QUICK REFERENCE (QR) VIDEO ACCESS

The images below are QR codes. Each code corresponds to a video from the *Goldman's Cecil Medicine 24* collection. For fast and easy video access, right from your mobile device, follow these instructions. The videos are also available on Expertconsult.com.

What You Need
- **A mobile device, such as a smartphone or tablet, equipped with a camera and Internet access**
- **A QR code reader application (If you do not already have a reader installed on your mobile device, look for free versions in your app store.)**

How It Works
- **Open the QR code reader application on your mobile device.**
- **Point the device's camera at the code and scan.**
- **Each code opens an individual video player for instant viewing—no log-on required.**

Confusion Assessment Method (CAM)
Chapter 26, Video 1 – Sharon K. Inouye

Stress Echocardiography
Chapter 55, Video 4 – Catherine M. Otto

Interlaminar Epidural Steroid Injection
Chapter 29, Video 1 – Ali Turabi

Dilated Cardiomyopathy
Chapter 55, Video 5 – Catherine M. Otto

Standard Echocardiographic Views
Chapter 55, Video 1 – Catherine M. Otto

A Moderate Pericardial Effusion (PE)
Chapter 55, Video 6 – Catherine M. Otto

Transthoracic Versus Transesophageal Echocardiography (TEE)
Chapter 55, Video 2 – Catherine M. Otto

Secundum Atrial Septal Defect
Chapter 69, Video 1 – Ariane J. Marelli

Contrast Echocardiography
Chapter 55, Video 3 – Catherine M. Otto

Perimembranous Ventricular Septal Defect
Chapter 69, Video 2 – Ariane J. Marelli

Coronary Stent Placement
Chapter 74, Video 1 – Paul S. Teirstein

VATS Wedge Resection
Chapter 101, Video 1 – Malcolm M. DeCamp

Guidewire Passage
Chapter 74, Video 2 – Paul S. Teirstein

Lung Recruitment in a Rat Lung
Chapter 105, Video 1 – Arthur S. Slutsky

Delivering the Stent
Chapter 74, Video 3 – Paul S. Teirstein

Renal Artery Stent
Chapter 127, Video 1 – Thomas D. DuBose, Jr., and Renato M. Santos

Inflating the Stent
Chapter 74, Video 4 – Paul S. Teirstein

Endoscopic View of Rectal Cancer
Chapter 199, Video 1 – Charles D. Blanke and Douglas O. Faigel

Final Result
Chapter 74, Video 5 – Paul S. Teirstein

Endoscopic Ultrasound
Chapter 199, Video 2 – Charles D. Blanke and Douglas O. Faigel

Superficial Femoral Artery (SFA) Stent Procedure
Chapter 79, Video 1 – Christopher J. White

Laparoscopic Roux-en-Y Gastric Bypass
Chapter 227, Video 1 – James M. Swain

Heart Transplant
Chapter 82, Video 1 – Y. Joseph Woo

Pituitary Surgery
Chapter 231, Video 1 – Ivan Ciric

Wheezing
Chapter 87, Video 1 – Jeffrey M. Drazen

Nasal Endoscopy
Chapter 259, Video 1 – Larry Borish

Skin Testing
Chapter 259, Video 2 – Larry Borish

Discectomy
Chapter 407, Video 7 – Jason H. Huang

Hip Arthroscopy Osteochondroplasty
Chapter 285, Video 1 – Bryan Kelly

Early Parkinson's Disease
Chapter 416, Video 1 – Anthony E. Lang

Cervical Provocation
Chapter 407, Video 1 – Richard L. Barbano

Freezing of Gait in Parkinson's Disease
Chapter 416, Video 2 – Anthony E. Lang

Spurling Maneuver
Chapter 407, Video 2 – Richard L. Barbano

Gunslinger Gait in Progressive Supranuclear Palsy (PSP)
Chapter 416, Video 3 – Anthony E. Lang

Cervical Distraction Test
Chapter 407, Video 3 – Richard L. Barbano

Supranuclear Gaze Palsy in PSP
Chapter 416, Video 4 – Anthony E. Lang

Straight Leg Raise
Chapter 407, Video 4 – Richard L. Barbano

Applause Sign in PSP
Chapter 416, Video 5 – Anthony E. Lang

Contralateral Straight Leg Raise
Chapter 407, Video 5 – Richard L. Barbano

Apraxia of Eyelid Opening (ALO) in PSP
Chapter 416, Video 6 – Anthony E. Lang

Seated Straight Leg Raise
Chapter 407, Video 6 – Richard L. Barbano

Cranial Dystonia in Multiple System Atrophy
Chapter 416, Video 7 – Anthony E. Lang

Anterocollis in Multiple System Atrophy
Chapter 416, Video 8 – Anthony E. Lang

Blepharospasm
Chapter 417, Video 4 – Anthony E. Lang

Stridor in Multiple System Atrophy
Chapter 416, Video 9 – Anthony E. Lang

Oromandibular Dystonia
Chapter 417, Video 5 – Anthony E. Lang

Alien Limb Phenomenon in Corticobasal Syndrome
Chapter 416, Video 10 – Anthony E. Lang

Cervical Dystonia
Chapter 417, Video 6 – Anthony E. Lang

Myoclonus in Corticobasal Syndrome
Chapter 416, Video 11 – Anthony E. Lang

Writer's Cramp
Chapter 417, Video 7 – Anthony E. Lang

Levodopa-Induced Dyskinesia in Parkinson's Disease
Chapter 416, Video 12 – Anthony E. Lang

Embouchure Dystonia
Chapter 417, Video 8 – Anthony E. Lang

Essential Tremor
Chapter 417, Video 1 – Anthony E. Lang

Sensory Trick in Cervical Dystonia
Chapter 417, Video 9 – Anthony E. Lang

Huntington's Disease
Chapter 417, Video 2 – Anthony E. Lang

Generalized Dystonia
Chapter 417, Video 10 – Anthony E. Lang

Hemiballism
Chapter 417, Video 3 – Anthony E. Lang

Tics
Chapter 417, Video 11 – Anthony E. Lang

Tardive Dyskinesia
Chapter 417, Video 12 – Anthony E. Lang

Bulbar Symptoms and Signs
Chapter 418, Video 2 – Pamela J. Shaw

Hemifacial Spasm
Chapter 417, Video 13 – Anthony E. Lang

Normal Swallowing
Chapter 418, Video 3 – Pamela J. Shaw

Limb Symptoms and Signs
Chapter 418, Video 1 – Pamela J. Shaw

Charcot-Marie-Tooth Disease (CMT) Exam and Walk
Chapter 428, Video 1 – Michael E. Shy

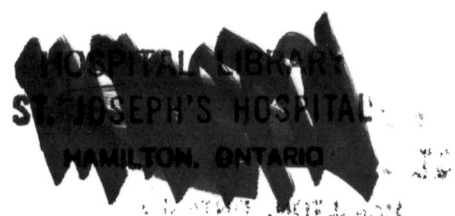

GOLDMAN'S
CECIL MEDICINE

GOLDMAN'S CECIL MEDICINE

24TH EDITION

LEE GOLDMAN, MD

Dean of the Faculties of Health Sciences and Medicine
Executive Vice President for Health and Biomedical Sciences
Harold and Margaret Hatch Professor of the University
Professor of Medicine and of Epidemiology
Columbia University
New York, New York

ANDREW I. SCHAFER, MD

Chairman, Department of Medicine
The E. Hugh Luckey Distinguished Professor of Medicine
Weill Cornell Medical College
Physician-in-Chief
New York-Presbyterian Hospital/Weill Cornell Medical Center
New York, New York

ELSEVIER
SAUNDERS

SAUNDERS

1600 John F. Kennedy Blvd.
Ste 1800
Philadelphia, PA 19103-2899

GOLDMAN'S CECIL MEDICINE, 24TH EDITION

ISBN: 978-1-4377-1604-7 (Single Volume)
978-1-4377-2788-3 (Two-Volume Set)
978-0-8089-2437-1 (International Edition)

Notices

Knowledge and best practice in this field are constantly changing. As new research and experience broaden our understanding, changes in research methods, professional practices, or medical treatment may become necessary.

Practitioners and researchers must always rely on their own experience and knowledge in evaluating and using any information, methods, compounds, or experiments described herein. In using such information or methods they should be mindful of their own safety and the safety of others, including parties for whom they have a professional responsibility.

With respect to any drug or pharmaceutical products identified, readers are advised to check the most current information provided (i) on procedures featured or (ii) by the manufacturer of each product to be administered, to verify the recommended dose or formula, the method and duration of administration, and contraindications. It is the responsibility of practitioners, relying on their own experience and knowledge of their patients, to make diagnoses, to determine dosages and the best treatment for each individual patient, and to take all appropriate safety precautions.

To the fullest extent of the law, neither the Publisher nor the authors, contributors, or editors, assume any liability for any injury and/or damage to persons or property as a matter of products liability, negligence or otherwise, or from any use or operation of any methods, products, instructions, or ideas contained in the material herein.

Library of Congress Cataloging-in-Publication Data

Goldman's Cecil medicine / [edited by] Lee Goldman, Andrew I. Schafer.—24th ed.
    p. ; cm.
  Cecil medicine
  Rev. ed. of: Cecil medicine. 23rd ed. c2008.
  Includes bibliographical references and index.
  ISBN 978-1-4377-1604-7 (single v. : alk. paper)—ISBN 978-1-4377-2788-3 (two v. set : alk. paper)—ISBN
978-0-8089-2437-1 (international ed. : alk. paper)—ISBN 978-1-4377-3665-6 (e-book)   1. Internal
medicine. I. Cecil, Russell L. (Russell La Fayette), 1881-1965. II. Goldman, Lee, MD. III. Schafer, Andrew I.
  IV. Cecil medicine. V. Title: Cecil medicine.
  [DNLM: 1. Medicine. WB 100]
  RC46.C423 2012
  616—dc23
                                            2011017824

Acquisitions Editor: Dolores Meloni
Developmental Editors: Catherine Carroll, Taylor Ball, Virginia Wilson
Publishing Services Manager: Patricia Tannian
Team Leader: Radhika Pallamparthy
Senior Project Manager: Linda Van Pelt
Project Manager: Anitha Sivaraj
Design Direction: Steven Stave
Marketing Manager: Helena Mutak

Printed in United States of America

Last digit is the print number: 9 8 7 6 5 4 3 2 1

ASSOCIATE EDITORS

PREFACE

The 24TH Edition of *Goldman's Cecil Medicine* symbolizes a time of extraordinary advances in medicine and in technological innovations for the dissemination of information. This textbook and its associated electronic products incorporate the latest medical knowledge in formats that are designed to appeal to learners who prefer to access information in a variety of ways.

The contents of *Cecil* have remained true to the tradition of a comprehensive textbook of medicine that carefully explains the *why* (the underlying normal physiology and pathophysiology of disease, now at the cellular and molecular as well as the organ level) and the *how* (now frequently based on Grade A evidence from randomized controlled trials). Descriptions of physiology and pathophysiology include the latest genetic advances in a practical format that strives to be useful to the nonexpert. Medicine has entered an era when the acuity of illness and the limited time available to evaluate a patient have diminished the ability of physicians to satisfy their intellectual curiosity. As a result, the acquisition of information, quite easily achieved in this era, is often confused with knowledge. We have attempted to counteract this tendency with a textbook that not only informs but also stimulates new questions and gives a glimpse of the future path to new knowledge. Grade A evidence is specifically highlighted in the text and referenced at the end of each chapter. In addition to the information provided in the textbook, the Cecil website supplies expanded content and functionality. In many cases, the full articles referenced in each chapter can be accessed from the Cecil website. The website is also continuously updated to incorporate subsequent Grade A information, other evidence, and new discoveries.

The sections for each organ system begin with a chapter that summarizes an approach to patients with key symptoms, signs, or laboratory abnormalities associated with dysfunction of that organ system. As summarized in Table 1-1, the text specifically provides clear, concise information regarding how a physician should approach more than 100 common symptoms, signs, and laboratory abnormalities, usually with a flow diagram, a table, or both for easy reference. In this way, *Cecil* remains a comprehensive text to guide diagnosis and therapy, not only for patients with suspected or known diseases but also for patients who may have undiagnosed abnormalities that require an initial evaluation.

Just as each edition brings new authors, it also reminds us of our gratitude to past editors and authors. Previous editors of *Cecil Medicine* include a short but remarkably distinguished group of leaders of American medicine: Russell Cecil, Paul Beeson, Walsh McDermott, James Wyngaarden, Lloyd H. Smith, Jr., Fred Plum, J. Claude Bennett, and Dennis Ausiello. As we welcome new associate editors—Wendy Levinson, Donald W. Landry, Anil Rustgi, and W. Michael Scheld—we also express our appreciation to Nicholas LaRusso and other associate editors from the previous editions on whose foundation we have built. Our returning associate editors—William P. Arend, James O. Armitage, David Clemmons, Jeffrey M. Drazen, and Robert C. Griggs—continue to make critical contributions to the selection of authors and the review and approval of all manuscripts. The editors, however, are fully responsible for the book as well as the integration among chapters.

The tradition of *Cecil Medicine* is that all chapters are written by distinguished experts in each field. We are also most grateful for the editorial assistance in New York of Theresa Considine and Silva Sergenian. These individuals and others in our offices have shown extraordinary dedication and equanimity in working with authors and editors to manage the unending flow of manuscripts, figures, and permissions. We also thank Faten Aberra, Reza Akari, Robert C. Brunham, Ivan Ciric, Seema Daulat, Gregory F. Erikson, Kevin Ghassemi, Jason H. Huang, Caron Jacobson, Lisa Kachnic, Bryan T. Kelly, Karen Krok, Heather Lehman, Keiron Leslie, Luis Marcos, Michael Overman, Eric Padron, Bianca Maria Piraccini, Don W. Powell, Katy Ralston, James M. Swain, Tania Thomas, Kirsten Tillisch, Ali Turabi, Mark Whiteford, and Y. Joseph Woo, who contributed to various chapters. At Elsevier, we are most indebted to Dolores Meloni and Linda McKinley, and also thank Cathy Carroll, Taylor Ball, Virginia Wilson, Linda Van Pelt, Suzanne Fannin, and Steve Stave, who have been critical to the planning and production process under the direction of Mary Gatsch. Many of the clinical photographs were supplied by Charles D. Forbes and William F. Jackson, authors of *Color Atlas and Text of Clinical Medicine*, Third Edition, published in 2003 by Elsevier Science Ltd. We thank them for graciously permitting us to include their pictures in our book. We have been exposed to remarkable physicians in our lifetimes and would like to acknowledge the mentorship and support of several of those who exemplify this paradigm—Robert H. Gifford, Lloyd H. Smith, Jr., Frank Gardner, and William Castle. Finally, we would like to thank the Goldman family—Jill, Jeff, Abigail, Mira, Daniel, and Robyn Goldman—and the Schafer family—Pauline, Eric, Pam, John, Evan, and Kate—for their understanding of the time and focus required to edit a book that attempts to sustain the tradition of our predecessors and to meet the needs of today's physician.

LEE GOLDMAN, MD
ANDREW I. SCHAFER, MD

CONTRIBUTORS

Charles S. Abrams, MD
Professor of Medicine, Associate Chief, Hematology-Oncology, Department of Medicine, University of Pennsylvania School of Medicine, Philadelphia, Pennsylvania
Thrombocytopenia

Frank J. Accurso, MD
Professor of Pediatrics, University of Colorado Denver School of Medicine, Denver, Colorado
Cystic Fibrosis

Nezam H. Afdhal, MD
Associate Professor of Medicine, Harvard Medical School; Chief of Hepatology, Beth Israel Deaconess Medical Center, Boston, Massachusetts
Diseases of the Gallbladder and Bile Ducts

Cem Akin, MD, PhD
Lecturer, Harvard Medical School; Department of Internal Medicine, Division of Rheumatology, Immunology and Allergy, Brigham and Women's Hospital, Boston, Massachusetts
Mastocytosis

Allen J. Aksamit, Jr., MD
Professor, Department of Neurology, Mayo Medical School; Consultant, Department of Neurology, Mayo Clinic, Rochester, Minnesota
Acute Viral Encephalitis; Poliomyelitis

Qais Al-Awqati, MB ChB
Robert F. Loeb Professor, Department of Medicine and Department of Physiology and Cellular Biophysics, Columbia University College of Physicians and Surgeons, New York, New York
Structure and Function of the Kidneys

Ban Mishu Allos, MD
Assistant Professor of Medicine and Preventive Medicine, Vanderbilt University School of Medicine, Nashville, Tennessee
Campylobacter *Infections*

David Altshuler, MD, PhD
Professor of Genetics and Medicine, Harvard Medical School; Department of Molecular Biology and Medicine, Massachusetts General Hospital, Boston, Massachusetts; Deputy Director and Chief Academic Officer, Broad Institute of MIT and Harvard, Cambridge, Massachusetts
The Inherited Basis of Common Diseases

Michael J. Aminoff, MD, DSc
Professor, Department of Neurology, University of California, San Francisco, School of Medicine, San Francisco, California
Approach to the Patient with Neurologic Disease

Jeffrey L. Anderson, MD, MACP
Professor, Department of Internal Medicine, University of Utah School of Medicine, Salt Lake City; Associate Chief of Cardiology, Intermountain Medical Center, Murray, Utah
ST Elevation Acute Myocardial Infarction and Complications of Myocardial Infarction

Karl E. Anderson, MD
Professor of Preventive Medicine and Community Health and Internal Medicine, University of Texas Medical Branch, Galveston, Texas
The Porphyrias

Larry J. Anderson, MD
Professor and Co-Director, Division of Pediatric Infectious Diseases, Emory University School of Medicine, Atlanta, Georgia
Coronaviruses

Karen H. Antman, MD
Provost, Boston University Medical Campus, and Dean, Boston University School of Medicine, Boston, Massachusetts
Primary and Metastatic Malignant Bone Lesions

Aśok C. Antony, MD
Professor of Medicine, Indiana University School of Medicine, Indianapolis, Indiana
Megaloblastic Anemias

Gerald B. Appel, MD
Professor of Clinical Medicine, Columbia University College of Physicians and Surgeons; Director of Clinical Nephrology, Department of Medicine, Columbia University Medical Center, New York, New York
Glomerular Disorders and Nephrotic Syndromes

Frederick R. Appelbaum, MD
Professor and Head, Division of Oncology, University of Washington School of Medicine; Director, Clinical Research Division, Fred Hutchinson Cancer Research Center, Seattle, Washington
The Acute Leukemias

William P. Arend, MD
Arend Endowed Chair in Rheumatogy and Distinguished Professor Emeritus, University of Colorado School of Medicine, Aurora, Colorado
Approach to the Patient with Rheumatic Disease

Paul Arguin, MD
Chief, Domestic Malaria Unit, Division of Parasitic Diseases, Centers for Disease Control and Prevention, Atlanta, Georgia
Approach to the Patient before and after Travel

James O. Armitage, MD
The Joe Shapiro Professor of Medicine, University of Nebraska College of Medicine, Section of Oncology and Hematology, University of Nebraska Medical Center, Omaha, Nebraska
Venomous Snake Bites; Approach to the Patient with Lymphadenopathy and Splenomegaly; Non-Hodgkin's Lymphomas

Cheryl A. Armstrong, MD
Professor and Chair, Department of Dermatology, University of Arkansas for Medical Sciences; Section Chief, Dermatology Section, Central Arkansas Veterans Healthcare System, Little Rock, Arkansas
Examination of the Skin and an Approach to Diagnosing Skin Diseases

M. Amin Arnaout, MD
Professor of Medicine, Harvard Medical School; Physician and Chief, Division of Nephrology, Department of Medicine, Massachusetts General Hospital, Boston, Massachusetts
Cystic Kidney Diseases

Robert Arnold, MD
Leo H. Criep Chair in Patient Care, Department of Medicine, Section of Palliative Care and Medical Ethics, University of Pittsburgh, Pittsburgh, Pennsylvania
Care of Dying Patients and Their Families

David Atkins, MD, MPH
Director, Quality Enhancement Research Initiative, Office of Research and Development, Department of Veterans Affairs, Washington, DC
The Periodic Health Examination

William L. Atkinson, MD, MPH
Medical Epidemiologist, National Center for Immunization and Respiratory Diseases, Centers for Disease Control and Prevention, Atlanta, Georgia
Immunization

Dennis Ausiello, MD
Jackson Professor of Clinical Medicine, Harvard Medical School; Physician-in-Chief, Massachusetts General Hospital, Boston, Massachusetts
Disorders of Sodium and Water Homeostasis

Bruce R. Bacon, MD
James F. King MD Endowed Chair in Gastroenterology, Professor of Internal Medicine, Division of Gastroenterology and Hepatology, Saint Louis University School of Medicine, St. Louis, Missouri
Inherited and Metabolic Disorders of the Liver; Iron Overload (Hemochromatosis)

Grover C. Bagby, MD
Professor, Department of Medicine, Department of Molecular and Medical Genetics, Oregon Health & Science University; Staff Physician, Hematology/Oncology, Portland Veterans Affairs Medical Center, Portland, Oregon
Aplastic Anemia and Related Bone Marrow Failure States

Barbara J. Bain, MB ChB
Professor in Diagnostic Haematology, Imperial College London; Consultant Haematologist, St Mary's Hospital, London, England
The Peripheral Blood Smear

Dean F. Bajorin, MD
Professor of Medicine, Department of Medicine, Weill Cornell Medical College; Attending Physician, Department of Medicine, Memorial Sloan-Kettering Cancer Center, New York, New York
Tumors of the Kidney, Bladder, Ureters, and Renal Pelvis

Mark Ballow, MD
Professor of Pediatrics, Chief, Division of Allergy and Clinical Immunology, University at Buffalo School of Medicine and Biomedical Sciences, Women & Children's Hospital of Buffalo, Buffalo, New York
Primary Immunodeficiency Diseases

Robert W. Baloh, MD
Professor of Neurology and Surgery (Head and Neck), David Geffen School of Medicine at UCLA, University of California, Los Angeles, California
Neuro-Ophthalmology; Smell and Taste; Hearing and Equilibrium

Jonathan Barasch, MD, PhD
Associate Professor of Medicine, Columbia University College of Physicians & Surgeons, New York, New York
Structure and Function of the Kidneys

Richard L. Barbano, MD, PhD
Professor of Neurology, University of Rochester; Chief of Neurology and Physical Medicine and Rehabilitation, Rochester General Hospital, Rochester, New York
Mechanical and Other Lesions of the Spine, Nerve Roots, and Spinal Cord; Videos

Murray G. Baron, MD
Professor of Radiology, Emory University School of Medicine, Atlanta, Georgia
Radiology of the Heart

Elizabeth Barrett-Connor, MD
Distinguished Professor and Chief, Division of Epidemiology, Department of Family and Preventive Medicine, University of California, San Diego, School of Medicine, La Jolla, California
Menopause

Michael J. Barry, MD
Professor of Medicine, Harvard Medical School; Medical Director, John D. Stoeckle Center for Primary Care Innovation, Massachusetts General Hospital, Boston, Massachusetts
Benign Prostatic Hyperplasia and Prostatitis

Bruce A. Barshop, MD, PhD
Professor, B. L. Maas Chair in Inherited Metabolic Disease, Department of Pediatrics, University of California, San Diego, School of Medicine, La Jolla, California
Homocystinuria and Hyperhomocysteinemia

John G. Bartlett, MD
Stanhope Bayne-Jones Professor of Medicine, Division of Infectious Diseases, Johns Hopkins University School of Medicine, Baltimore, Maryland
Bioterrorism

Mary Barton, MD, MPP
Scientific Director, U.S. Preventive Services Task Force, Center for Primary Care, Prevention and Clinical Partnerships, Agency for Healthcare Research and Quality, Rockville, Maryland
The Periodic Health Examination

Robert C. Basner, MD
Associate Professor of Clinical Medicine, Columbia University College of Physicians & Surgeons; Director, Cardiopulmonary Sleep and Ventilatory Disorders Center, Columbia University Medical Center, New York, New York
Obstructive Sleep Apnea

Stephen G. Baum, MD
Professor of Medicine and of Microbiology and Immunology, Albert Einstein College of Medicine; Senior Associate Dean for Students, Albert Einstein College of Medicine, Bronx, New York
Mycoplasma *Infections*

Daniel G. Bausch, MD, MPH&TM
Associate Professor, Department of Tropical Medicine and Section of Adult Infectious Diseases, Tulane University Health Sciences Center, New Orleans, Louisiana
Viral Hemorrhagic Fevers

Arnold S. Bayer, MD
Professor of Medicine, David Geffen School of Medicine at UCLA; Associate Chief, Adult Infectious Diseases, Senior Investigator, LA Biomedical Research Institute, Los Angeles, California
Infective Endocarditis

Hasan Bazari, MD
Associate Professor of Medicine, Harvard Medical School; Program Director, Internal Medicine Residency, Clinical Director, Nephrology Division, Massachusetts General Hospital, Boston, Massachusetts
Approach to the Patient with Renal Disease

John H. Beigel, MD
Medical Scientist, National Institute of Allergy and Infectious Diseases, National Institutes of Health, Bethesda, Maryland
Antiviral Therapy (Non-HIV)

George A. Beller, MD
Ruth C. Heede Professor of Cardiology, Division of Cardiovascular Medicine, Department of Medicine, University of Virginia Health System, Charlottesville, Virginia
Noninvasive Cardiac Imaging

Robert M. Bennett, MD
Professor of Medicine and Nursing, Oregon Health & Science University, Portland, Oregon
Fibromyalgia and Chronic Fatigue Syndrome

Joseph R. Berger, MD
Ruth L. Works Professor and Chairman, Department of Neurology, University of Kentucky, Lexington, Kentucky
Cytomegalovirus, Epstein-Barr Virus, and Other Slow Virus Infections of the Central Nervous System; Neurologic Complications of Human Immunodeficiency Virus Infection; Brain Abscess and Parameningeal Infections

Paul Berk, MD
Professor, Department of Medicine, Columbia University College of Physicians and Surgeons, New York, New York
Approach to the Patient with Jaundice or Abnormal Liver Tests

Nancy Berliner, MD
Professor of Medicine, Harvard Medical School; Chief, Division of Hematology, Department of Medicine, Brigham and Women's Hospital, Boston, Massachusetts
Leukocytosis and Leukopenia

James L. Bernat, MD
Louis and Ruth Frank Professor of Neuroscience, Professor of Neurology and Medicine, Dartmouth Medical School, Hanover, New Hampshire; Attending Neurologist, Dartmouth-Hitchcock Medical Center, Lebanon, New Hampshire
Coma, Vegetative State, and Brain Death

Philip J. Bierman, MD
Professor, Department of Internal Medicine, University of Nebraska Medical Center, Omaha, Nebraska
Non-Hodgkin's Lymphomas

Bruce R. Bistrian, MD, PhD, MPH
Professor of Medicine, Harvard Medical School; Chief, Clinical Nutrition, Beth Israel Deaconess Medical Center, Boston, Massachusetts
Nutritional Assessment

Joseph J. Biundo, MD
Clinical Professor of Medicine, Tulane Health Science Center, New Orleans, Louisiana
Bursitis, Tendinitis, and Other Periarticular Disorders and Sports Medicine

Charles D. Blanke, MD
Professor and Head, Medical Oncology, University of British Columbia; Vice President, Systemic Therapy, British Columbia Cancer Agency, Vancouver, British Columbia, Canada
Neoplasms of the Large and Small Intestine; Videos

Joel N. Blankson, MD, PhD
Associate Professor, Division of Infectious Diseases, Department of Medicine, Johns Hopkins University School of Medicine, Baltimore, Maryland
Immunopathogenesis of Human Immunodeficiency Virus Infection

Martin J. Blaser, MD
Frederick H. King Professor of Internal Medicine and Chair, Department of Medicine; Professor of Microbiology, New York University Langone Medical Center, New York, New York
Acid Peptic Disease

William A. Blattner, MD
Professor and Associate Director, Institute of Human Virology, University of Maryland School of Medicine, Baltimore, Maryland
Retroviruses Other Than Human Immunodeficiency Virus

Thomas P. Bleck, MD
Professor of Neurological Sciences, Neurosurgery, Medicine, and Anesthesiology and Assistant Dean, Rush Medical College; Associate Chief Medical Officer for Critical Care, Rush University Medical Center, Chicago, Illinois
Arboviruses Affecting the Central Nervous System

William E. Boden, MD
Clinical Chief, Division of Cardiovascular Medicine, Professor of Medicine and Preventive Medicine, University at Buffalo Schools of Medicine and Public Health; Medical Director, Cardiovascular Services, Kaleida Health, Chief of Cardiology, Buffalo General and Millard Fillmore Hospitals, Buffalo, New York
Angina Pectoris and Stable Ischemic Heart Disease

C. Richard Boland, MD
Chief, Division of Gastroenterology; Director, GI Cancer Research Laboratory, Baylor University Medical Center, Dallas, Texas
Cancer Genetics

Jean Bolognia, MD
Professor, Department of Dermatology, Yale University School of Medicine, New Haven, Connecticut
Infections, Hyper- and Hypopigmentation, Regional Dermatology, and Distinctive Lesions in Black Skin

Robert Bonomo, MD
Professor of Medicine, Pharmacology, and Molecular Biology and Microbiology, Case Western Reserve University School of Medicine; Director, VISN 10 GRECC, Louis Stokes Cleveland Veterans Affairs Medical Center, Cleveland, Ohio
Diseases Caused by Acinetobacter *and* Stenotrophomonas *Species*

Larry Borish, MD
Professor of Medicine, Asthma and Allergic Disease Center, University of Virginia, Charlottesville, Virginia
Allergic Rhinitis and Sinusitis; Videos

Patrick J. Bosque, MD
Associate Professor, Department of Neurology, University of Colorado Denver School of Medicine, Aurora, Colorado; Neurologist, Division of Neurology, Denver Health Medical Center, Denver, Colorado
Prion Diseases

Randall Brand, MD
Professor of Medicine and Academic Director, GI Division Shadyside; Director, GI Malignancy Early Detection, Diagnosis and Prevention, University of Pittsburgh Medical Center, Pittsburgh, Pennsylvania
Pancreatic Cancer

Itzhak Brook, MD, MSc
Professor, Department of Pediatrics and Medicine, Georgetown University, Washington, DC
Diseases Caused by Non–Spore-Forming Anaerobic Bacteria; Actinomycosis

Enrico Brunetti, MD
Assistant Professor of Infectious Diseases, University of Pavia; Attending Physician, Division of Infectious and Tropical Diseases, IRCCS San Matteo Hospital Foundation; Co-Director, WHO Collaborating Centre for Clinical Management of Cystic Echinococcosis, Pavia, Italy
Cestodes

David M. Buchner, MD, MPH
Professor, Department of Kinesiology and Community Health, University of Illinois at Urbana-Champaign, Champaign, Illinois
Physical Activity

Pierre A. Buffet, MD, PhD
Assistant Professor, Department of Parasitology, Pitié-Salpêtrière Hospital, Paris 6 University, Institut Pasteur, Paris, France
Leishmaniasis

H. Franklin Bunn, MD
Professor of Medicine, Harvard Medical School; Senior Physician, Brigham and Women's Hospital, Boston, Massachusetts
Approach to the Anemias

Peter A. Calabresi, MD
Professor of Neurology, Director, Johns Hopkins Multiple Sclerosis Center; Director, Division of Neuroimmunology and Neuroinfectious Diseases, Johns Hopkins University, Baltimore, Maryland
Multiple Sclerosis and Demyelinating Conditions of the Central Nervous System

David P. Calfee, MD, MSc
Associate Professor of Medicine and Public Health, Chief Hospital Epidemiologist, New York-Presbyterian Hospital/Weill Cornell Medical Center, New York, New York
Prevention and Control of Health Care–Associated Infections

Hugh Calkins, MD
Professor of Medicine, Director of Electrophysiology, Johns Hopkins Medical Institutions, Baltimore, Maryland
Principles of Electrophysiology

Douglas Cameron, MD, MBA
Emeritus Professor, Department of Ophthalmology, Mayo Medical School, Rochester, Minnesota
Diseases of the Visual System

Michael Camilleri, MD
Atherton and Winifred W. Bean Professor and Professor of Medicine and Physiology, Mayo Medical School; Consultant in Gastroenterology and Hepatology, Mayo Clinic, Rochester, Minnesota
Disorders of Gastrointestinal Motility

Grant W. Cannon, MD
Professor of Medicine, Division of Rheumatology, University of Utah School of Medicine; Associate Chief of Staff for Academic Affiliations, George E. Wahlen Veterans Affairs Medical Center, Salt Lake City, Utah
Immunosuppressing Drugs including Corticosteroids

Maria Domenica Cappellini, MD
Professor of Internal Medicine, Department of Internal Medicine, Università di Milano-Policlinico "Ca Granda" Foundation IRCCS, Milano, Italy
The Thalassemias

Blase A. Carabello, MD
Professor of Medicine, Baylor College of Medicine; Chief of Medicine, Michael E. DeBakey Veterans Affairs Medical Center, Houston, Texas
Valvular Heart Disease

Edgar M. Carvalho, MD, PhD
Professor of Clinical Medicine, Faculdade de Medicina da Bahia, Universidade Federal da Bahia, Salvador-BA, Brazil
Schistosomiasis (Bilharziasis)

Agustin Castellanos, MD
Professor of Medicine, Director, Clinical Electrophysiology, Division of Cardiovascular Medicine, University of Miami, Miller School of Medicine, Miami, Florida
Approach to Cardiac Arrest and Life-Threatening Arrhythmias

Naga P. Chalasani, MD
Professor of Medicine and Cellular and Integrative Physiology, Director, Division of Gastroenterology and Hepatology, Department of Medicine, Indiana University School of Medicine, Indianapolis, Indiana
Alcoholic and Nonalcoholic Steatohepatitis

Henry Chambers, MD
Professor of Medicine, University of California, San Francisco, School of Medicine; Chief, Division of Infectious Diseases, San Francisco General Hospital, San Francisco, California
Staphylococcal Infections

Mary Charlson, MD
William T. Foley Distinguished Professor of Medicine, Chief, Division of Epidemiology and Evaluative Sciences Research, Executive Director of Center for Integrative Medicine, Department of Medicine, Weill Cornell Medical College, New York, New York
Complementary and Alternative Medicine

William P. Cheshire, Jr., MD
Professor of Neurology, Director of Clinical Neurophysiology Laboratory, Mayo Clinic, Jacksonville, Florida
Autonomic Disorders and Their Management

Patrick F. Chinnery, MB BS
Director and Professor of Neurogenetics, Institute of Genetic Medicine, Newcastle University; Honorary Consultant Neurologist, Newcastle upon Tyne Hospitals NHS Trust, Newcastle upon Tyne, United Kingdom
Muscle Diseases

David C. Christiani, MD, MPH
Professor of Medicine, Harvard Medical School; Elkan Blout Professor of Environmental Genetics, Environmental Health, Harvard School of Public Health; Physician, Pulmonary and Critical Care Unit, Massachusetts General Hospital, Boston, Massachusetts
Physical and Chemical Injuries of the Lung

David R. Clemmons, MD
Kenan Professor of Medicine, University of North Carolina at Chapel Hill School of Medicine, Chapel Hill, North Carolina
Approach to the Patient with Endocrine Disease; Principles of Endocrinology

Jeffrey Cohen, MD
Chief, Laboratory of Infectious Diseases, National Institute of Allergy and Infectious Diseases, National Institutes of Health, Bethesda, Maryland
Varicella-Zoster Virus (Chickenpox, Shingles)

Myron S. Cohen, MD
J. Herbert Bate Distinguished Professor, Departments of Medicine, Microbiology and Public Health; Associate Vice Chancellor and Director, Institute of Global Health and Infectious Diseases, University of North Carolina at Chapel Hill School of Medicine, Chapel Hill, North Carolina
Approach to the Patient with a Sexually Transmitted Disease

Steven P. Cohen, MD
Associate Professor, Department of Anesthesiology, Johns Hopkins Medical Institutions, Baltimore, Maryland; Professor and Director of Pain Research, Department of Surgery, Walter Reed Army Medical Center, Washington, DC; Colonel, Medical Corps, U.S. Army Reserve
Pain

Steven L. Cohn, MD
Clinical Professor of Medicine, SUNY Downstate; Director, Medical Consultation Service, Kings County Hospital Center, Brooklyn, New York
Preoperative Evaluation

Robert Colebunders, MD, PhD
Professor, Department of Clinical Sciences, Institute of Tropical Medicine; Department of Epidemiology and Social Medicine, University of Antwerp, Antwerp, Belgium
Immune Reconstitution Inflammatory Syndrome in HIV/AIDS

Joseph M. Connors, MD
Clinical Professor, Division of Medical Oncology, Department of Medicine, University of British Columbia; Clinical Director, Centre for Lymphoid Cancer, British Columbia Cancer Agency, Vancouver, British Columbia, Canada
Hodgkin's Lymphoma

Deborah J. Cook, MD, MSc
Professor, Department of Medicine, Clinical Epidemiology, and Biostatistics, Academic Chair, Critical Care Medicine, McMaster University, Hamilton, Ontario, Canada
Approach to the Patient in a Critical Care Setting

C. Ralph Corey, MD
Gary Hock Distinguished Professor of Global Health, Director, Infectious Disease Research, Duke Clinical Research Institute; Director, Hubert/Yeargan Center for Global Health; Professor of Medicine and Pathology, Duke University Medical Center, Durham, North Carolina
Venomous Snake Bites

Kenneth H. Cowan, MD, PhD
Director, Eppley Cancer Center, University of Nebraska Medical Center; Director, Eppley Institute for Research in Cancer, University of Nebraska Medical Center, Omaha, Nebraska
Biology of Cancer

William A. Craig, MD
Professor Emeritus, Department of Medicine, University of Wisconsin School of Medicine and Public Health, Madison, Wisconsin
Antibacterial Chemotherapy

Simon L. Croft, PhD
Professor of Parasitology, Head, Faculty of Infectious and Tropical Diseases, London School of Hygiene and Tropical Medicine, London, England
Leishmaniasis

Mary K. Crow, MD
Joseph P. Routh Professor of Rheumatic Diseases in Medicine, Chief, Rheumatology Division, Department of Medicine, Weill Cornell Medical College; Physician-in-Chief and Chair, Rheumatology Division, Hospital for Special Surgery, New York, New York
Systemic Lupus Erythematosus

John A. Crump, MB ChB
Associate Professor of Medicine and Pathology, Division of Infectious Diseases and International Health, Duke University Medical Center; Director, Duke Tanzania Operations, Duke Global Health Institute, Duke University, Durham, North Carolina
Salmonella *Infections (including Typhoid Fever)*

Mark R. Cullen, MD
Professor of Medicine, Chief, Division of General Medical Disciplines, Stanford University School of Medicine, Stanford, California
Principles of Occupational and Environmental Medicine

Gary C. Curhan, MD, ScD
Associate Professor of Medicine, Harvard Medical School; Associate Professor of Epidemiology, Harvard School of Public Health; Physician, Renal Division and Channing Laboratory, Brigham and Women's Hospital, Boston, Massachusetts
Nephrolithiasis

Inger K. Damon, MD, PhD
Chief, Poxvirus and Rabies Branch, Centers for Disease Control and Prevention, Atlanta, Georgia
Smallpox, Monkeypox, and Other Poxvirus Infections

Troy E. Daniels, DDS, MSc
Professor, Department of Orofacial Sciences, University of California, San Francisco, School of Dentistry; Professor, Department of Pathology, University of California, San Francisco, School of Medicine, San Francisco, California
Diseases of the Mouth and Salivary Glands

Nancy Davidson, MD
Professor of Medicine and Pharmacology and Chemical Biology, University of Pittsburgh School of Medicine; Director, University of Pittsburgh Cancer Institute and UPMC Cancer Centers, Pittsburgh, Pennsylvania
Breast Cancer and Benign Breast Disorders

Lisa M. DeAngelis, MD
Professor of Neurology, Weill Cornell Medical College; Chair, Department of Neurology, Memorial Sloan-Kettering Cancer Center, New York, New York
Tumors of the Central Nervous System and Intracranial Hypertension and Hypotension

Malcolm M. DeCamp, MD
Fowler McCormick Professor of Surgery and Professor of Medicine, Northwestern University Feinberg School of Medicine; Chief, Division of Thoracic Surgery, Northwestern Memorial Hospital, Chicago, Illinois
Interventional and Surgical Approaches to Lung Disease; Video

Carlos Del Rio, MD
Hubert Professor and Chair, Hubert Department of Global Health, Rollins School of Public Health of Emory University; Professor of Medicine, Emory University School of Medicine, Atlanta, Georgia
Prevention of Human Immunodeficiency Virus Infection

George D. Demetri, MD
Associate Professor of Medicine, Harvard Medical School; Director, Ludwig Center at Dana-Farber Cancer Institute; Senior Vice President for Experimental Therapeutics, Dana-Farber Cancer Institute, Boston, Massachusetts
Sarcomas of Soft Tissue and Bone, and Other Neoplasms of Connective Tissues

Robert H. Demling, MD
Professor of Surgery, Harvard Medical School; Director of Education and Research, Department of Surgery, Brigham and Women's Hospital, Boston, Massachusetts
Medical Aspects of Trauma and Burn Care

Patricia A. Deuster, PhD, MPH
Professor and Scientific Director, Consortium for Health and Military Performance, Department of Military and Emergency Medicine, Uniformed Services University of the Health Sciences, Bethesda, Maryland
Rhabdomyolysis

Robert B. Diasio, MD
William J. and Charles H. Mayo Professor, Departments of Molecular Pharmacology and Experimental Therapeutics and Oncology, Mayo Medical School; Director, Mayo Clinic Cancer Center, Rochester, Minnesota
Principles of Drug Therapy

David J. Diemert, MD
Assistant Professor, Department of Microbiology, Immunology and Tropical Medicine, George Washington University; Director of Clinical Trials, Albert B. Sabin Vaccine Institute, Washington, DC
Intestinal Nematode Infections; Tissue Nematode Infections

Kathleen B. Digre, MD
Professor of Neurology and Ophthalmology, Adjunct Professor of Obstetrics and Gynecology, Director, Headache Clinic, University of Utah School of Medicine, Salt Lake City, Utah
Headaches and Other Head Pain

John M. Douglas, Jr., MD
Chief Medical Officer, National Center for HIV/AIDS, Viral Hepatitis, STD, and TB Prevention, Centers for Disease Control and Prevention, Atlanta, Georgia
Papillomavirus

Jeffrey M. Drazen, MD
Distinguished Parker B. Francis Professor of Medicine, Harvard Medical School; Senior Physician, Division of Pulmonary and Critical Care Medicine, Brigham and Women's Hospital; Editor-in-Chief, *New England Journal of Medicine,* Boston, Massachusetts
Asthma; Video

Stephen C. Dreskin, MD, PhD
Professor of Medicine and Immunology, Division of Allergy and Clinical Immunology, University of Colorado Denver School of Medicine, Aurora, Colorado
Urticaria and Angioedema

W. Lawrence Drew, MD, PhD
Professor, Laboratory Medicine and Medicine, University of California, San Francisco, School of Medicine, San Francisco, California
Cytomegalovirus

George L. Drusano, MD
Co-Director, Ordway Research Institute, Albany, New York
Antibacterial Chemotherapy

Thomas D. DuBose, Jr., MD
Tinsley R. Harrison Professor and Chair, Department of Internal Medicine, Wake Forest University School of Medicine, Winston-Salem, North Carolina
Vascular Disorders of the Kidney; Video

F. Daniel Duffy, MD
Steven Landgarten Professor in Medical Leadership, Dean, University of Oklahoma, School of Community Medicine, Tulsa, Oklahoma
Counseling for Behavior Change

Herbert L. DuPont, MD
H. Irving Schweppe, Jr., Chair of Internal Medicine and Vice Chairman, Department of Medicine, Baylor College of Medicine; Chief, Internal Medicine, St. Luke's Episcopal Hospital; Director, Center for Infectious Diseases, University of Texas–Houston School of Public Health, Houston, Texas
Approach to the Patient with Suspected Enteric Infection

Madeleine Duvic, MD
Professor of Dermatology and Medicine, Deputy Chairman, Department of Dermatology, The University of Texas M.D. Anderson Cancer Center, Houston, Texas
Urticaria, Drug Hypersensitivity Rashes, Nodules and Tumors, and Atrophic Diseases

Kathryn M. Edwards, MD
Sarah H. Sell Professor of Pediatrics, Vanderbilt University School of Medicine, Nashville, Tennessee
Parainfluenza Viral Disease

N. Lawrence Edwards, MD
Professor of Medicine, Vice Chairman, Department of Medicine, University of Florida College of Medicine; Chief, Section of Rheumatology, Veterans Administration Medical Center, Gainesville, Florida
Crystal Deposition Diseases

Lawrence H. Einhorn, MD
Distinguished Professor of Medicine, Lance Armstrong Foundation Professor of Oncology, Indiana University School of Medicine, Indianapolis, Indiana
Testicular Cancer

Ronald J. Elin, MD, PhD
A. J. Miller Professor and Chair, Department of Pathology and Laboratory Medicine, University of Louisville School of Medicine, Louisville, Kentucky
Reference Intervals and Laboratory Values

George M. Eliopoulos, MD
Professor of Medicine, Harvard Medical School; Division of Infectious Diseases, Beth Israel Deaconess Medical Center, Boston, Massachusetts
Principles of Anti-Infective Therapy

Perry Elliott, MBBS, MD
Reader in Inherited Cardiac Disease, The Heart Hospital, University College London, London, United Kingdom
Diseases of the Myocardium and Endocardium

Jerrold J. Ellner, MD
Professor of Medicine, Boston University; Chief, Section of Infectious Diseases, Boston Medical Center, Boston, Massachusetts
Tuberculosis

Louis J. Elsas II, MD
Professor and Chair, Department of Biochemistry and Molecular Biology, University of Miami; Professor, Department of Pediatrics, University of Miami, Miller School of Medicine, Miami, Florida
Approach to Inborn Errors of Metabolism

Dirk M. Elston, MD
Director, Department of Dermatology, Geisinger Medical Center, Danville, Pennsylvania
Arthropods and Leeches

Ezekiel J. Emanuel, MD, PhD
Chair, Department of Bioethics, The Clinical Center, National Institutes of Health, Bethesda, Maryland
Bioethics in the Practice of Medicine

Gregory F. Erickson, PhD
Professor Emeritus of Reproductive Medicine, Division of Reproductive Endocrinology, University of California, San Diego, School of Medicine, La Jolla, California
Ovaries and Development; Reproductive Endocrinology and Infertility

Armin Ernst, MD
Associate Professor of Medicine and Surgery, Harvard Medical School; Chief of Interventional Pulmonology, Beth Israel Deaconess Medical Center, Boston, Massachusetts
Interventional and Surgical Approaches to Lung Disease

Joel D. Ernst, MD
Professor, Departments of Medicine, Pathology, and Microbiology; Director, Division of Infectious Diseases, New York University School of Medicine, New York, New York
Leprosy (Hansen's Disease)

David S. Ettinger, MD
Alex Grass Professor of Oncology, Department of Oncology, The Sidney Kimmel Comprehensive Cancer Center at Johns Hopkins, Baltimore, Maryland
Lung Cancer and Other Pulmonary Neoplasms

Amelia Evoli, MD
Associate Professor, Department of Neuroscience, Catholic University, Rome, Italy
Disorders of Neuromuscular Transmission

Douglas O. Faigel, MD
Professor of Medicine, Mayo Medical School; Division of Gastroenterology and Hepatology, Mayo Clinic, Scottsdale, Arizona
Neoplasms of the Large and Small Intestine; Videos

Gary W. Falk, MD, MSc
Professor of Medicine, Division of Gastroenterology, University of Pennsylvania School of Medicine, Philadelphia, Pennsylvania
Diseases of the Esophagus

Murray J. Favus, MD
Professor of Medicine, Section of Endocrinology, Diabetes and Metabolism, University of Chicago Pritzker School of Medicine, Chicago, Illinois
Mineral and Bone Homeostasis

Gene Feder, MD
Professor of Primary Health Care, School of Social and Community Medicine, University of Bristol, Bristol, United Kingdom
Intimate Partner Violence

Stephan D. Fihn, MD, MPH
Professor, Medicine and Health Services, University of Washington School of Medicine; Director, Analytics and Business Intelligence, Department of Veterans Affairs, Seattle, Washington
Measuring Health and Health Care

Gary S. Firestein, MD
Professor of Medicine, Dean and Associate Vice Chancellor of Translational Medicine, University of California, San Diego, School of Medicine, La Jolla, California
Mechanisms of Inflammation and Tissue Repair

Neil Fishman, MD
Associate Professor of Medicine, University of Pennsylvania School of Medicine; Director, Department of Healthcare Epidemiology, Infection Prevention and Control; Director, Antimicrobial Stewardship Program, Hospital of the University of Pennsylvania, Philadelphia, Pennsylvania
Prevention and Control of Health Care–Associated Infections

Lee A. Fleisher, MD
Robert D. Dripps Professor and Chair of Anesthesiology, Professor of Medicine, University of Pennsylvania School of Medicine, Philadelphia, Pennsylvania
Overview of Anesthesia

Marsha D. Ford, MD
Adjunct Professor, Department of Emergency Medicine, University of North Carolina at Chapel Hill School of Medicine, Chapel Hill, North Carolina; Director, Carolinas Poison Center, Carolinas Medical Center, Charlotte, North Carolina
Acute Poisoning

Chris E. Forsmark, MD
Professor of Medicine, Chief, Division of Gastroenterology, Hepatology, and Nutrition, University of Florida College of Medicine, Gainesville, Florida
Pancreatitis

Vance G. Fowler, Jr., MD, MHS
Associate Professor, Department of Medicine, Division of Infectious Diseases, Duke University Medical Center, Durham, North Carolina
Infective Endocarditis

Jay W. Fox, PhD
Professor, Department of Microbiology, University of Virginia School of Medicine, Charlottesville, Virginia
Venoms and Poisons from Marine Organisms

Manuel A. Franco, MD, PhD
Director of Postgraduate Programs, School of Sciences, Pontificia Universidad Javeriana, Bogota, Colombia
Rotaviruses, Noroviruses, and Other Gastrointestinal Viruses

Martyn A. French, MD, MB ChB
Winthrop Professor in Clinical Immunology, School of Pathology and Laboratory Medicine, University of Western Australia; Consultant Clinical Immunologist, Royal Perth Hospital, Perth, Western Australia, Australia
Immune Reconstitution Inflammatory Syndrome in HIV/AIDS

Karen Freund, MD, MPH
Professor of Medicine, Director, Women's Health Interdisciplinary Research Center, Boston University School of Medicine; Professor of Epidemiology, Boston University School of Public Health, Boston, Massachusetts
Approach to Women's Health

Linda P. Fried, MD, MPH
Dean and DeLamar Professor of Public Health and of Medicine, Senior Vice President, Columbia University Medical Center; Professor of Epidemiology, Columbia University Mailman School of Public Health, New York, New York
Epidemiology of Aging: Implications of the Aging of Society

Cem Gabay, MD
Professor of Medicine, University of Geneva School of Medicine; Head, Division of Rheumatology, University Hospitals of Geneva, Geneva, Switzerland
Biologic Agents

Kenneth L. Gage, PhD
Chief, Flea-Borne Diseases Activity, Division of Vector-Borne Diseases, Centers for Disease Control and Prevention, Fort Collins, Colorado
Plague and Other Yersinia Infections

Robert F. Gagel, MD
Head, Division of Internal Medicine, Endocrine Neoplasia and Hormonal Disorders, The University of Texas M.D. Anderson Cancer Center, Houston, Texas
Endocrine Manifestations of Tumors: "Ectopic" Hormone Production

John N. Galgiani, MD
Professor of Medicine and Director, Valley Fever Center for Excellence, University of Arizona; Chief Medical Officer, Valley Fever Solutions Inc., Tucson, Arizona
Coccidioidomycosis

Patrick G. Gallagher, MD
Professor, Department of Pediatrics and Genetics, Yale University School of Medicine, New Haven, Connecticut
Hemolytic Anemias: Red Cell Membrane and Metabolic Defects

Eithan Galun, MD
Professor, Director, Goldyne Savad Institute of Gene Therapy, Hadassah Hebrew University Hospital, Jerusalem, Israel
Gene and Cell Therapy

Leonard Ganz, MD
Associate Professor of Medicine, University of Pittsburgh School of Medicine, UPMC-Shadyside, Pittsburgh, Pennsylvania
Electrocardiography

Guadalupe Garcia-Tsao, MD
Professor of Medicine, Section of Digestive Diseases, Yale University School of Medicine, New Haven, Connecticut; Chief, Digestive Diseases, VA-CT Healthcare System, West Haven, Connecticut
Cirrhosis and Its Sequelae

Jonathan D. Gates, MD, MBA
Assistant Professor of Surgery, Harvard Medical School; Director, Trauma Center and Vascular Surgeon, Brigham and Women's Hospital, Boston, Massachusetts
Medical Aspects of Trauma and Burn Care

William M. Geisler, MD, MPH
Associate Professor of Medicine and Epidemiology, University of Alabama at Birmingham School of Medicine, Birmingham, Alabama
Diseases Caused by Chlamydiae

Tony P. George, MD
Professor, Department of Psychiatry, Psychology and Medical Sciences, University of Toronto, Toronto, Ontario, Canada
Nicotine and Tobacco

Dale N. Gerding, MD
Professor, Department of Medicine, Loyola University Chicago Stritch School of Medicine, Maywood; Associate Chief of Staff for Research, Research Service, Hines Veterans Affairs Hospital, Hines, Illinois
Clostridial Infections

M. Eric Gershwin, MD
Distinguished Professor of Medicine, Chief, Division of Rheumatology, Allergy and Clinical Immunology, University of California, Davis, School of Medicine, Davis, California
Sjögren's Syndrome

Morie A. Gertz, MD
Professor and Chair, Department of Medicine, Mayo Medical School and Mayo Clinic, Rochester, Minnesota
Amyloidosis

Gordon D. Ginder, MD
Professor, Internal Medicine, Virginia Commonwealth University; Director, Massey Cancer Center, Virginia Commonwealth University, Richmond, Virginia
Microcytic and Hypochromic Anemias

Jeffrey Ginsberg, MD
Professor, Department of Medicine, McMaster University, Hamilton, Ontario, Canada
Peripheral Venous Disease

Geoffrey S. Ginsburg, MD, PhD
Professor of Medicine and Pathology, Duke University School of Medicine; Director, Center for Genomic Medicine, Institute for Genome Sciences and Policy; Director, Center for Personalized Medicine, Durham, North Carolina
Applications of Molecular Technologies to Clinical Medicine

Michael Glogauer, DDS, PhD
Associate Professor, Faculty of Dentistry, University of Toronto, Toronto, Ontario, Canada
Disorders of Phagocyte Function

John W. Gnann, Jr., MD
Professor of Medicine, Pediatrics, and Microbiology, University of Alabama at Birmingham School of Medicine and Birmingham Veterans Affairs Medical Center, Birmingham, Alabama
Mumps

Matthew R. Golden, MD, MPH
Associate Professor of Medicine, Director, PHSKC HIV/STD Program, University of Washington Center for AIDS and STD, Harborview Medical Center, Seattle, Washington
Neisseria Gonorrhoeae *Infections*

Lee Goldman, MD
Dean of the Faculties of Health Sciences and Medicine, Executive Vice President for Health and Biomedical Sciences, Harold and Margaret Hatch Professor of the University, Professor of Medicine and of Epidemiology, Columbia University, New York, New York
Approach to Medicine, the Patient, and the Medical Profession: Medicine as a Learned and Humane Profession; Approach to the Patient with Possible Cardiovascular Disease

Ellie J. Goldstein, MD
Clinical Professor of Medicine, David Geffen School of Medicine at UCLA, Los Angeles, California; Director, R.M. Alden Research Laboratory, Santa Monica, California
Diseases Caused by Non–Spore-Forming Anaerobic Bacteria

Lawrence T. Goodnough, MD
Professor of Pathology and Medicine, Stanford University School of Medicine; Director, Transfusion Service, Stanford University Medical Center, Stanford, California
Transfusion Medicine

Jörg J. Goronzy, MD, PhD
Professor of Medicine, Division of Immunology and Rheumatology, Stanford University School of Medicine, Stanford, California
The Innate and Adaptive Immune Systems

Eduardo Gotuzzo, MD
Principal Professor of Medicine, Universidad Peruana Cayetano Heredia; Director, Instituto de Medicina Tropical "Alexander von Humboldt," Lima, Peru
Cholera and Other Vibrio *Infections; Liver, Intestinal, and Lung Fluke Infections*

Deborah Grady, MD, MPH
Professor, Department of Medicine, University of California, San Francisco, School of Medicine; Associate Dean for Clinical and Translational Research, University of California, San Francisco, San Francisco, California
Menopause

Leslie C. Grammer, MD
Professor, Department of Medicine, Division of Allergy-Immunology, Northwestern University Feinberg School of Medicine, Chicago, Illinois
Drug Allergy

F. Anthony Greco, MD
Medical Director, Sarah Cannon Cancer Center, Nashville, Tennessee
Cancer of Unknown Primary Origin

Harry B. Greenberg, MD
Joseph D. Grant Professor of Medicine and Microbiology and Immunology; Senior Associate Dean of Research; Stanford University School of Medicine, Stanford, California
Rotaviruses, Noroviruses, and Other Gastrointestinal Viruses

Peter K. Gregersen, MD
Professor, Molecular Medicine, Director, Robert S. Boas Center for Genomics and Human Genetics, The Feinstein Institute for Medical Research, Hofstra University School of Medicine, Manhasset, New York
The Major Histocompatibility Complex

Robert C. Griggs, MD
Professor of Neurology, Medicine, Pediatrics, and Pathology and Laboratory Medicine, University of Rochester School of Medicine and Dentistry, Rochester, New York
Approach to the Patient with Neurologic Disease

Lisa M. Guay-Woodford, MD
Professor and Vice Chair, Department of Genetics; Pediatric Nephrologist, University of Alabama at Birmingham School of Medicine, Birmingham, Alabama
Hereditary Nephropathies and Developmental Abnormalities of the Urinary Tract

Richard L. Guerrant, MD
Thomas H. Hunter Professor of International Medicine, Infectious Diseases, and International Health, Director, Center for Global Health, University of Virginia School of Medicine, Charlottesville, Virginia
Escherichia Coli Enteric Infections; Cryptosporidiosis

Colleen Hadigan, MD, MPH
Staff Clinician, Laboratory of Immunoregulation, National Institute of Allergy and Infectious Diseases, National Institutes of Health, Bethesda, Maryland
Treatment of Human Immunodeficiency Virus Infection and Acquired Immunodeficiency Syndrome

John D. Hainsworth, MD
Chief Scientific Officer, Sarah Cannon Research Institute, Nashville, Tennessee
Cancer of Unknown Primary Origin

Anders Hamsten, MD, PhD
Professor of Cardiovascular Diseases, Department of Medicine, Center for Molecular Medicine, Karolinska University Hospital, Karolinska Institutet, Stockholm, Sweden
Atherosclerosis, Thrombosis, and Vascular Biology

Kenneth R. Hande, MD
Professor, Departments of Medicine and Pharmacology, Vanderbilt University School of Medicine, Nashville, Tennessee
Carcinoid Syndrome

H. Hunter Handsfield, MD
Clinical Professor of Medicine, Center for AIDS and STD, University
of Washington School of Medicine; Senior Research Leader, Battelle
Centers for Public Health Research and Evaluation, Seattle, Washington
Neisseria Gonorrhoeae Infections

Göran K. Hansson, MD, PhD
Professor, Center for Molecular Medicine, Department of Medicine,
Karolinska University Hospital, Karolinska Institutet, Stockholm, Sweden
Atherosclerosis, Thrombosis, and Vascular Biology

Rashidul Haque, MB, PhD
Senior Scientist and Head, Parasitology Laboratory, Laboratory Sciences
Division, International Centre for Diarrheal Disease Research, Bangladesh
(ICDDR,B), Dhaka, Bangladesh
Amebiasis

Raymond C. Harris, MD
Anne and Roscoe R. Robinson Professor of Medicine and Chief, Division of
Nephrology, Department of Medicine, Vanderbilt University School of
Medicine, Nashville, Tennessee
Diabetes and the Kidney

Stephen Crane Hauser, MD
Associate Professor of Medicine, Mayo Medical School; Consultant, Division
of Internal Medicine, Gastroenterology and Hepatology, Mayo Clinic,
Rochester, Minnesota
Vascular Diseases of the Gastrointestinal Tract

Frederick G. Hayden, MD
Richardson Professor of Clinical Virology, Professor of Medicine, University
of Virginia School of Medicine, Charlottesville, Virginia
Influenza

Letha Healey, MD
Staff Clinician, Critical Care Medicine Department, Clinical Center, National
Institutes of Health, Bethesda, Maryland
*Treatment of Human Immunodeficiency Virus Infection and Acquired
Immunodeficiency Syndrome*

Douglas C. Heimburger, MD, MS
Professor of Medicine, Associate Director for Education and Training,
Vanderbilt Institute for Global Health, Vanderbilt University School of
Medicine, Nashville, Tennessee
Nutrition's Interface with Health and Disease

Erik L. Hewlett, MD
Professor of Medicine and Pharmacology, Division of Infectious Diseases and
International Health, University of Virginia School of Medicine,
Charlottesville, Virginia
Whooping Cough and Other Bordetella *Infections*

David R. Hill, MD, DTM&H
Director, National Travel Health Network and Centre; Honorary Professor,
London School of Hygiene and Tropical Medicine, London, England
Giardiasis

Nicholas S. Hill, MD
Professor of Medicine, Tufts University School of Medicine; Chief, Division
of Pulmonary, Critical Care, and Sleep Medicine, Tufts Medical Center,
Boston, Massachusetts
Respiratory Monitoring in Critical Care

L. David Hillis, MD
Professor and Chair, Department of Medicine, University of Texas Health
Science Center at San Antonio, San Antonio, Texas
*Acute Coronary Syndrome: Unstable Angina and Non-ST Elevation Myocardial
Infarction*

Jack Hirsh, MD, DSc
Professor Emeritus, McMaster University, Hamilton, Ontario, Canada
Antithrombotic Therapy

V. Michael Holers, MD
Scoville Professor of Rheumatology, Department of Medicine, University of
Colorado Denver School of Medicine, Aurora, Colorado
Complement in Health and Disease

Steven M. Holland, MD
Chief, Laboratory of Clinical Infectious Diseases, National Institute
of Allergy and Infectious Diseases, National Institutes of Health,
Bethesda, Maryland
The Nontuberculous Mycobacteria

Steven Hollenberg, MD
Professor of Medicine, Robert Wood Johnson Medical School/UMDNJ;
Director, Coronary Care Unit, Cooper University Hospital, Camden,
New Jersey
Cardiogenic Shock

Edward W. Hook III, MD
Professor of Medicine, Epidemiology, and Microbiology, Director, Division
of Infectious Diseases, University of Alabama at Birmingham School of
Medicine, Birmingham, Alabama
Granuloma Inguinale (Donovanosis); Syphilis; Nonsyphilitic Treponematoses

Laurence Huang, MD
Professor of Medicine, University of California, San Francisco, School of
Medicine; Chief, HIV/AIDS Chest Clinic, San Francisco General
Hospital, San Francisco, California
*Pulmonary Manifestations of Human Immunodeficiency Virus and Acquired
Immunodeficiency Syndrome*

Leonard D. Hudson, MD
Professor of Medicine, Endowed Chair in Pulmonary Disease Research,
Division of Pulmonary and Critical Care Medicine, University of
Washington School of Medicine, Seattle, Washington
Acute Respiratory Failure; Mechanical Ventilation

Steven E. Hyman, MD
Provost, Harvard University, Cambridge, Massachusetts; Professor,
Department of Neurobiology, Harvard Medical School, Boston,
Massachusetts
Biology of Addiction

Michael Iannuzzi, MD, MBA
Edward C. Reifenstein Professor and Chair, Department of Medicine,
Upstate Medical University, Syracuse, New York
Sarcoidosis

Robert D. Inman, MD
Professor of Medicine and Immunology, University of Toronto; Director,
Arthritis Center of Excellence, Toronto Western Hospital, Toronto,
Ontario, Canada
The Spondyloarthropathies

Sharon K. Inouye, MD, MPH
Professor of Medicine, Harvard Medical School; Director, Aging Brain
Center, Milton and Shirley F. Levy Family Chair, Institute for Aging
Research, Hebrew SeniorLife; Faculty, Division of Gerontology, Beth Israel
Deaconess Medical Center, Boston, Massachusetts
*Neuropsychiatric Aspects of Aging; Delirium or Acute Mental Status Change in
the Older Patient; Video*

Karl L. Insogna, MD
Professor of Medicine, Section of Endocrinology, Department of Internal
Medicine, Director, Yale Bone Center, Yale University School of Medicine,
New Haven, Connecticut
The Parathyroid Glands, Hypercalcemia, and Hypocalcemia

Silvio E. Inzucchi, MD
Professor of Medicine, Clinical Director, Section of Endocrinology, Yale
University School of Medicine; Director, Yale Diabetes Center, Yale-New
Haven Hospital, New Haven, Connecticut
Type 1 Diabetes Mellitus; Type 2 Diabetes Mellitus

Eric M. Isselbacher, MD
Associate Professor of Medicine, Harvard Medical School; Associate Director, Heart Center and Co-Director, Thoracic Aortic Center, Massachusetts General Hospital, Boston, Massachusetts
Diseases of the Aorta

Ahmedin Jemal, DVM, PhD
Vice President, Surveillance Research, American Cancer Society, Inc., Atlanta, Georgia
The Epidemiology of Cancer

Joanna Jen, MD, PhD
Professor, Department of Neurology, David Geffen School of Medicine at UCLA, University of California, Los Angeles, California
Neuro-Ophthalmology; Smell and Taste; Hearing and Equilibrium

Dennis M. Jensen, MD
Professor of Medicine, David Geffen School of Medicine at UCLA, University of California, Los Angeles, CURE Digestive Diseases Research Center; Staff Physician, West Los Angeles Veterans Affairs Medical Center, Los Angeles, California
Gastrointestinal Hemorrhage and Occult Gastrointestinal Bleeding

Michael D. Jensen, MD
Professor of Medicine, Department of Endocrinology, Mayo Clinic, Rochester, Minnesota
Obesity

Robert T. Jensen, MD
Chief, Cell Biology Section, Digestive Diseases Branch, National Institute of Diabetes, Digestive and Kidney Diseases, National Institutes of Health, Bethesda, Maryland
Pancreatic Endocrine Tumors

Mariell Jessup, MD
Professor of Medicine, Department of Medicine, University of Pennsylvania School of Medicine; Medical Director, Penn Heart and Vascular Center, University of Pennsylvania Health System; Associate Chief, Clinical Affairs, Cardiovascular Division, University of Pennsylvania School of Medicine, Philadelphia, Pennsylvania
Cardiac Transplantation

Stuart Johnson, MD
Professor of Medicine, Loyola University Chicago Stritch School of Medicine, Maywood; Deputy Associate Chief of Staff for Research, Hines Veterans Affairs Hospital, Hines, Illinois
Clostridial Infections

Ralph F. Józefowicz, MD
Professor of Neurology and Medicine, Associate Chair for Education, Department of Neurology, University of Rochester School of Medicine and Dentistry, Rochester, New York
Approach to the Patient with Neurologic Disease

Stephen G. Kaler, MD
Molecular Medicine Program, Eunice Kennedy Shriver National Institute of Child Health and Human Development, Bethesda, Maryland
Wilson's Disease

Moses R. Kamya, MD, PhD
Professor of Medicine, Chair, Department of Medicine, School of Medicine, Makerere University College of Health Sciences, Kampala, Uganda
Malaria

Hagop Kantarjian, MD
Professor and Kelcie Margaret Kana Research Chair, Department of Leukemia, The University of Texas M. D. Anderson Cancer Center, Houston, Texas
The Chronic Leukemias

David R. Karp, MD, PhD
Professor and Chief, Rheumatic Diseases Division, The University of Texas Southwestern Medical Center at Dallas, Dallas, Texas
Complement in Health and Disease

Daniel L. Kastner, MD, PhD
NIH Distinguished Investigator, Scientific Director, Division of Intramural Research, National Human Genome Research Institute, National Institutes of Health, Bethesda, Maryland
The Systemic Autoinflammatory Diseases

David A. Katzka, MD
Professor of Medicine, Mayo Medical School, Rochester, Minnesota
Diseases of the Esophagus

Debra K. Katzman, MD
Professor of Pediatrics, Department of Pediatrics, University of Toronto; Head, Division of Adolescent Medicine, Senior Associate Scientist, Research Institute, The Hospital for Sick Children and University of Toronto, Toronto, Ontario, Canada
Adolescent Medicine

Carol A. Kauffman, MD
Professor, University of Michigan; Chief, Infectious Diseases Section, Veterans Affairs Ann Arbor Healthcare System, Ann Arbor, Michigan
Histoplasmosis; Blastomycosis; Paracoccidioidomycosis; Cryptococcosis; Sporotrichosis; Candidiasis

Kenneth Kaushansky, MD, MACP
Senior Vice President, Health Sciences, Dean, School of Medicine, Stony Brook University, Health Sciences Center, Stony Brook, New York
Hematopoiesis and Hematopoietic Growth Factors

Emmet B. Keeffe, MD
Professor of Medicine Emeritus, Division of Gastroenterology and Hepatology, Department of Medicine, Stanford University Medical Center, Stanford, California
Hepatic Failure and Liver Transplantation

Morton Kern, MD
Professor of Medicine, Associate Chief, Cardiology, University of California Irvine, Orange; Chief, Cardiology, Long Beach Veterans Administration Hospital, Long Beach, California
Catheterization and Angiography

Gerald T. Keusch, MD
Professor, International Health, Boston University School of Public Health; Associate Director, National Emerging Infectious Diseases Laboratory, Boston University, Boston, Massachusetts
Shigellosis

David H. Kim, MD
Associate Professor of Radiology, Section of Abdominal Imaging, University of Wisconsin School of Medicine and Public Health, Madison, Wisconsin
Diagnostic Imaging Procedures in Gastroenterology

Matthew Kim, MD
Instructor in Medicine, Harvard Medical School; Associate Physician, Division of Endocrinology, Diabetes and Hypertension, Brigham and Women's Hospital, Boston, Massachusetts
Thyroid

Louis V. Kirchhoff, MD, MPH
Professor, Departments of Internal Medicine (Infectious Diseases) and Epidemiology, University of Iowa; Staff Physician, Medical Service, Department of Veterans Affairs Medical Center, Iowa City, Iowa
Chagas' Disease

Michael J. Klag, MD, MPH
Dean, The Johns Hopkins Bloomberg School of Public Health, Baltimore, Maryland
Epidemiology of Cardiovascular Disease

Samuel Klein, MD
William H. Danforth Professor of Medicine and Nutritional Science, Director, Center for Human Nutrition, Washington University School of Medicine, St. Louis, Missouri
Protein-Energy Malnutrition

David S. Knopman, MD
Professor of Neurology and Consultant in Neurology, Mayo Clinic, Rochester, Minnesota
Regional Cerebral Dysfunction: Higher Mental Functions; Alzheimer's Disease and Other Dementias

Tamsin A. Knox, MD, MPH
Associate Professor of Medicine, Nutrition/Infection Unit, Tufts University School of Medicine, Boston, Massachusetts
Gastrointestinal Manifestations of HIV and AIDS

Albert I. Ko, MD
Associate Professor of Epidemiology and Medicine, Division Head, Epidemiology of Microbial Disease, Yale School of Public Health, New Haven, Connecticut; Collaborating Researcher, Oswaldo Cruz Foundation, Brazilian Ministry of Health, Salvador, Brazil
Leptospirosis

Rami S. Komrokji, MD
Associate Professor, Department of Oncologic Sciences, University of South Florida; Clinical Director, Department of Malignant Hematology, Associate Member, Moffitt Cancer Center and Research Institute, Tampa, Florida
Myelodysplastic Syndrome

Dimitrios P. Kontoyiannis, MD, ScD
Professor of Medicine and Deputy Chair, The University of Texas M.D. Anderson Cancer Center, Houston, Texas
Mucormycosis; Mycetoma

Barbara S. Koppel, MD
Professor of Clinical Neurology, New York Medical College, Valhalla, New York; Chief of Service, Metropolitan Hospital, New York, New York
Nutritional and Alcohol-Related Neurologic Disorders

Kevin Korenblat, MD
Associate Professor of Medicine, Washington University School of Medicine, St. Louis, Missouri
Approach to the Patient with Jaundice or Abnormal Liver Tests

Bruce R. Korf, MD, PhD
Professor and Wayne H. and Sara Crews Finley Chair in Medical Genetics, Department of Genetics; Director, Heflin Center for Genomic Sciences, University of Alabama at Birmingham, Birmingham, Alabama
Principles of Genetics

Neil J. Korman, MD, PhD
Professor, Department of Dermatology, Case Western Reserve University; Clinical Director, Murdough Family Center for Psoriasis, University Hospitals Case Medical Center, Cleveland, Ohio
Macular, Papular, Vesiculobullous, and Pustular Diseases

Joseph A. Kovacs, MD
Senior Investigator, Critical Care Medicine Department, National Institutes of Health, Bethesda, Maryland
Pneumocystis Pneumonia

Monica Kraft, MD
Professor of Medicine, Vice Chair for Research, Department of Medicine; Director, Duke Asthma, Allergy and Airway Center, Duke University Medical Center, Durham, North Carolina
Approach to the Patient with Respiratory Disease

Christopher M. Kramer, MD
Professor of Radiology and Medicine, Director, Cardiovascular Imaging Center, University of Virginia Health System, Charlottesville, Virginia
Noninvasive Cardiac Imaging

Donna M. Krasnewich, MD, PhD
Program Director, National Institute of General Medical Sciences, National Institutes of Health, Bethesda, Maryland
The Lysosomal Storage Diseases

Peter J. Krause, MD
Senior Research Scientist, Yale School of Public Health, Yale School of Medicine, New Haven, Connecticut
Babesiosis and Other Protozoan Diseases

Henry M. Kronenberg, MD
Professor of Medicine, Harvard Medical School; Chief, Endocrine Unit, Massachusetts General Hospital, Boston, Massachusetts
Polyglandular Disorders

Ernst J. Kuipers, MD, PhD
Professor of Medicine, Department of Gastroenterology and Hepatology, Department of Internal Medicine, Erasmus MC University Medical Center, Rotterdam, The Netherlands
Acid Peptic Disease

Paul Ladenson, MD
John Eager Howard Professor of Endocrinology; Professor of Medicine, Pathology, Oncology, Radiology and Radiological Sciences; Distinguished Service Professor, and Director, Division of Endocrinology and Metabolism, Johns Hopkins University School of Medicine, Baltimore, Maryland
Thyroid

Donald W. Landry, MD, PhD
Samuel Bard Professor of Medicine and Chair, Department of Medicine, Columbia University College of Physicians and Surgeons, New York, New York
Approach to the Patient with Renal Disease

Nancy E. Lane, MD
Professor of Medicine and Rheumatology, University of California, Davis, School of Medicine; Director, Aging Center, University of California at Davis Medical Center, Davis, California
Osteoarthritis

Anthony E. Lang, MD
Professor, Department of Medicine (Neurology), University of Toronto; Director, Movement Disorders Center, Toronto Western Hospital; Director, Division of Neurology, Jack Clark Chair for Parkinson's Disease Research, Toronto, Ontario, Canada
Parkinsonism; Other Movement Disorders; Videos

Richard A. Lange, MD, MBA
Professor and Executive Vice Chairman, Department of Medicine, University of Texas Health Science Center San Antonio, San Antonio, Texas
Acute Coronary Syndrome: Unstable Angina and Non-ST Elevation Myocardial Infarction

George V. Lawry, MD
Clinical Professor of Medicine, Chief, Division of Rheumatology, University of California Irvine, Orange, California
Approach to the Patient with Rheumatic Disease

Thomas H. Lee, MD, MSc
Professor of Medicine, Harvard Medical School; Network President, Partners Healthcare System, Boston, Massachusetts
Using Data for Clinical Decisions

William M. Lee, MD
Professor, Department of Internal Medicine, Division of Digestive and Liver Diseases, University of Texas Southwestern Medical Center, Dallas, Texas
Toxin- and Drug-Induced Liver Disease

James Leggett, MD
Associate Professor of Medicine, Oregon Health & Science University; Assistant Director of Medical Education, Providence Portland Medical Center, Portland, Oregon
Approach to Fever or Suspected Infection in the Normal Host

Adam Lerner, MD
Professor, Department of Medicine, Section of Hematology and Medical Oncology, Boston University School of Medicine, Boston, Massachusetts
Primary and Metastatic Malignant Bone Lesions

Stuart Levin, MD
The Ralph C. Brown, MD, Professor of Medicine and Chair, Department of Internal Medicine, Rush University Medical Center, Chicago, Illinois
Zoonoses

Stephanie M. Levine, MD
Professor of Medicine, Division of Pulmonary and Critical Care Diseases, University of Texas Health Science Center at San Antonio, San Antonio, Texas
Alveolar Filling Disorders

Gary R. Lichtenstein, MD
Professor of Medicine, Division of Gastroenterology, University of Pennsylvania School of Medicine; Director, Center for Inflammatory Bowel Diseases, Hospital of the University of Pennsylvania, Philadelphia, Pennsylvania
Inflammatory Bowel Disease

Henry W. Lim, MD, DSc
Chairman and C.S. Livingood Chair, Department of Dermatology, Henry Ford Hospital; Senior Vice President for Academic Affairs, Henry Ford Health System, Detroit, Michigan
Eczema, Photodermatoses, Papulosquamous (including Fungal) Diseases, and Figurate Erythemas

Aldo A. M. Lima, MD, PhD
Professor of Medicine and INCT-Biomedicine, Department of Physiology and Pharmacology, Federal University of Ceará, Fortaleza-Ceará, Brazil
Cryptosporidiosis; Schistosomiasis (Bilharziasis)

Andrew H. Limper, MD
Professor and Division Chair, Pulmonary and Critical Care Medicine, and Director, Thoracic Diseases Research Unit, Mayo Medical School; Consultant, Mayo Clinic, Rochester, Minnesota
Overview of Pneumonia

Geoffrey S. F. Ling, MD, PhD
Professor and Interim Chair, Department of Neurology, Uniformed Services University of the Health Sciences, Bethesda, Maryland; Director of Neuro Critical Care, Critical Care Medicine, Walter Reed Army Medical Center, Washington, DC
Traumatic Brain Injury and Spinal Cord Injury

Alan F. List, MD
Professor of Oncologic Sciences, University of South Florida; Executive Vice President and Physician-in-Chief, Moffitt Cancer Center; Senior Member, Malignant Hematology, Moffitt Cancer Center, Tampa, Florida
Myelodysplastic Syndrome

William C. Little, MD
McMichael Professor and Vice Chair, Department of Internal Medicine, Chief of Cardiology, Wake Forest University School of Medicine, Winston-Salem, North Carolina
Pericardial Diseases

Richard F. Loeser, MD
Professor of Internal Medicine, Section of Molecular Medicine, Wake Forest University School of Medicine, Winston-Salem, North Carolina
Connective Tissue Structure and Function

Bennett Lorber, MD
Thomas M. Durant Professor of Medicine, Professor of Microbiology and Immunology, Temple University School of Medicine, Philadelphia, Pennsylvania
Listeriosis

Donald E. Low, MD
Professor, Laboratory Medicine and Pathobiology, University of Toronto; Microbiologist-in-Chief, Mount Sinai Hospital/University Health Network; Medical Director, Public Health Laboratory–Toronto, Ontario Agency for Health Protection and Promotion, Toronto, Ontario, Canada
Nonpneumococcal Streptococcal Infections, Rheumatic Fever

Daniel R. Lucey, MD, MPH
Adjunct Professor of Microbiology and Immunology, Georgetown University Medical Center; Director, Center for Biologic Counterterrorism and Emerging Diseases, Washington Hospital Center, Washington, DC
Anthrax

James R. Lupski, MD, PhD
Cullen Professor and Vice Chair of Molecular and Human Genetics, Professor of Pediatrics, Baylor College of Medicine; Attending Medical Geneticist, Texas Children's Hospital, Ben Taub General Hospital, Houston, Texas
Gene, Genomic, and Chromosomal Disorders

Henry T. Lynch, MD
Chair, Preventive Medicine and Public Health, Professor of Medicine, Director, Creighton Hereditary Cancer Institute, Creighton University School of Medicine, Omaha, Nebraska
Cancer Genetics

Jeffrey M. Lyness, MD
Professor and Associate Chair for Education, Department of Psychiatry, University of Rochester School of Medicine and Dentistry; Medical Director for Continuing Medical Education, University of Rochester Medical Center, Rochester, New York
Psychiatric Disorders in Medical Practice

Bruce W. Lytle, MD
Chair, Heart and Vascular Institute, Department of Thoracic and Cardiovascular Surgery, The Cleveland Clinic, Cleveland, Ohio
Interventional and Surgical Treatment of Coronary Artery Disease

C. Ronald MacKenzie, MD
Associate Professor of Clinical Medicine, Department of Rheumatology, Hospital for Special Surgery and Weill Cornell Medical College, New York, New York
Surgical Treatment of Joint Disease

Harriet MacMillan, MD, MSc
Professor, Departments of Psychiatry and Behavioral Neurosciences, and Pediatrics, David R. (Dan) Offord Chair in Child Studies, Offord Centre for Child Studies, McMaster University, Hamilton, Ontario, Canada
Intimate Partner Violence

Robert D. Madoff, MD
Stanley M. Goldberg, MD, Professor of Surgery, Chief, Division of Colon and Rectal Surgery, University of Minnesota Medical School, Minneapolis, Minnesota
Diseases of the Rectum and Anus

Mark W. Mahowald, MD
Professor, Department of Neurology, University of Minnesota Medical School, Minneapolis, Minnesota
Disorders of Sleep

Atul Malhotra, MD
Associate Professor of Medicine, Harvard Medical School; Associate Physician, Brigham and Women's Hospital, Boston, Massachusetts
Disorders of Ventilatory Control

Lionel A. Mandell, MD
Professor of Medicine, Faculty of Health Sciences at McMaster University; Attending Physician, Department of Medicine, Henderson Division, Hamilton Health Sciences, Hamilton, Ontario, Canada
Streptococcus pneumoniae Infections

Peter Manu, MD
Professor of Medicine, Hofstra North Shore–LIJ School of Medicine at Hofstra University, Hempstead; Director of Medical Services, The Zucker Hillside Hospital, Glen Oaks, New York
Medical Consultation in Psychiatry

Marsha D. Marcus, PhD
Professor of Psychiatry and Psychology, University of Pittsburgh School of Medicine; Chief, Eating Disorders Program, Western Psychiatric Institute and Clinic, University of Pittsburgh Medical Center, Pittsburgh, Pennsylvania
Eating Disorders

Ariane J. Marelli, MD, MPH
Associate Professor, McGill University Health Center; Director, McGill Adult Unit for Congenital Heart Disease, McGill University, Montreal, Quebec, Canada
Congenital Heart Disease in Adults; Videos

Maurie Markman, MD
Vice President for Patient Oncology Services, National Director for Medical Oncology, Cancer Treatment Centers of America, Eastern Regional Medical Center, Philadelphia, Pennsylvania
Gynecologic Cancers

Andrew R. Marks, MD
Wu Professor and Chair, Department of Physiology and Cellular Biophysics and Director, Helen and Clyde Wu Center for Molecular Cardiology, Columbia University College of Physicians and Surgeons, New York, New York
Cardiac Function and Circulatory Control

Kieren A. Marr, MD
Professor of Medicine and Oncology, Director, Transplant and Oncology Infectious Disease Program, Johns Hopkins University School of Medicine, Johns Hopkins University, Baltimore, Maryland
Approach to Fever and Suspected Infection in the Compromised Host

Thomas J. Marrie, MD
Dean, Faculty of Medicine, Dalhousie University, Halifax, Nova Scotia, Canada
Legionella Infections

Paul Martin, MD
Professor of Medicine, Chief, Division of Hepatology, University of Miami, Miller School of Medicine, Miami, Florida
Approach to the Patient with Liver Disease

Joel B. Mason, MD
Professor of Medicine and Nutrition, Tufts University; Staff Physician, Tufts Medical Center; Director, Vitamins and Carcinogenesis Laboratory, U.S.D.A. Human Nutrition Research Center at Tufts University, Boston, Massachusetts
Vitamins, Trace Minerals, and Other Micronutrients

Barry M. Massie, MD
Professor of Medicine, University of California, San Francisco, School of Medicine; Chief, Cardiology Division, San Francisco VA Medical Center, San Francisco, California
Heart Failure: Pathophysiology and Diagnosis

Henry Masur, MD
Chief, Critical Care Medicine Department, Clinical Center, National Institutes of Health, Bethesda, Maryland
Treatment of Human Immunodeficiency Virus Infection and Acquired Immunodeficiency Syndrome

Eric L. Matteson, MD, MPH
Professor of Medicine, Division of Rheumatology and Division of Epidemiology, Mayo Medical School, Rochester, Minnesota
Infections of Bursae, Joints, and Bones

Toby Maurer, MD
Professor, Department of Dermatology, University of California, San Francisco, School of Medicine, San Francisco, California
Skin Manifestations in Patients with Human Immunodeficiency Virus Infection

Emeran A. Mayer, MD
Professor of Medicine, Physiology and Psychiatry; Director, Center for Neurobiology of Stress, Division of Digestive Diseases, David Geffen School of Medicine at UCLA, University of California, Los Angeles, California
Functional Gastrointestinal Disorders: Irritable Bowel Syndrome, Dyspepsia, and Functional Chest Pain of Presumed Esophageal Origin

Stephen A. McClave, MD
Professor of Medicine, Director of Clinical Nutrition, Division of Gastroenterology, Hepatology, and Nutrition, University of Louisville School of Medicine, Louisville, Kentucky
Enteral Nutrition

F. Dennis McCool, MD
Professor of Medicine, Alpert Medical School of Brown University, Providence, Rhode Island; Chief of Pulmonary Critical Care and Sleep Medicine, Memorial Hospital of Rhode Island, Pawtucket, Rhode Island
Diseases of the Diaphragm, Chest Wall, Pleura, and Mediastinum

Charles E. McCulloch, PhD
Professor and Head, Division of Biostatistics, Department of Epidemiology and Biostatistics, University of California, San Francisco, San Francisco, California
Statistical Interpretation of Data

Michael A. McGuigan, MDCM, MBA
Clinical Professor, Department of Emergency Medicine, State University of New York, Stony Brook; Medical Director, Long Island Regional Poison and Drug Information Center, Winthrop-University Hospital, Mineola, New York
Chronic Poisoning: Trace Metals and Others

John McHutchison, MD
Senior Vice President, Liver Disease Therapeutics, Gilead Sciences Inc., Foster City, California
Chronic Viral and Autoimmune Hepatitis

William McKenna, MD, DSc
Professor of Cardiology, Director, Institute of Cardiovascular Science, University College London, London, United Kingdom
Diseases of the Myocardium and Endocardium

Vallerie McLaughlin, MD
Professor of Medicine, Department of Internal Medicine, Division of Cardiovascular Medicine, and Director, Pulmonary Hypertension Program, University of Michigan, Ann Arbor, Michigan
Pulmonary Hypertension

John J. V. McMurray, MB, MD
Professor of Medical Cardiology, University of Glasgow; Honorary Consultant Cardiologist, Western Infirmary, Glasgow, Scotland, United Kingdom
Heart Failure: Management and Prognosis

Mary McNaughton-Collins, MD, MPH
Associate Professor of Medicine, Harvard Medical School, Boston, Massachusetts
Benign Prostatic Hyperplasia and Prostatitis

Kenneth McQuaid, MD
Professor of Clinical Medicine, University of California, San Francisco, School of Medicine; Chief, Gastroenterology Section, Veterans Affairs Medical Center, San Francisco, California
Approach to the Patient with Gastrointestinal Disease

Frederick W. Miller, MD, PhD
Chief, Environmental Autoimmunity Group, National Institute of Environmental Health Sciences, National Institutes of Health, Bethesda, Maryland
Polymyositis and Dermatomyositis

Kenneth L. Minaker, MD
Associate Professor of Medicine, Harvard Medical School; Chief, Geriatric Medicine Unit, Interim Chief, General Medicine Division, Massachusetts General Hospital, Boston, Massachusetts
Common Clinical Sequelae of Aging

Jonathan W. Mink, MD, PhD
Professor and Chief of Child Neurology, Departments of Neurology, Pediatrics, Brain and Cognitive Sciences, and Neurobiology and Anatomy, University of Rochester, Rochester, New York
Congenital, Developmental, and Neurocutaneous Disorders

Daniel R. Mishell, Jr., MD
Professor, Department of Obstetrics and Gynecology, University of Southern California, Keck School of Medicine, Los Angeles, California
Contraception

William E. Mitch, MD
Gordon Cain Chair in Nephrology and Director, Division of Nephrology, Department of Medicine, Baylor College of Medicine, Houston, Texas
Chronic Kidney Disease

Mark E. Molitch, MD
Professor of Medicine, Northwestern University Feinberg School of Medicine; Attending Physician, Northwestern Memorial Hospital, Chicago, Illinois
Neuroendocrinology and the Neuroendocrine System; Anterior Pituitary

Bruce A. Molitoris, MD
Professor of Medicine, Director of Nephrology, Director of the Indiana Center for Biological Microscopy, Indiana University School of Medicine, Indianapolis, Indiana
Acute Kidney Injury

José G. Montoya, MD
Associate Professor, Department of Medicine, Stanford University School of Medicine, Stanford, California; Director, Toxoplasma Serology Laboratory, Palo Alto Medical Foundation, Palo Alto, California
Toxoplasmosis

Fred Morady, MD
McKay Professor of Cardiovascular Diseases, Professor of Medicine, University of Michigan Health System, Ann Arbor, Michigan
Electrophysiologic Interventional Procedures and Surgery

Jeffrey A. Moscow, MD
Children's Miracle Network Professor, Chief, Hematology-Oncology, Department of Pediatrics, University of Kentucky, Lexington, Kentucky
Biology of Cancer

Andrew H. Murr, MD
Professor of Clinical Otolaryngology and Head and Neck Surgery, Roger Boles, MD, Endowed Chair in Otolaryngology Education and Vice Chair for Clinical Affairs, Department of Otolaryngology, University of California, San Francisco, School of Medicine; Chief of Service, San Francisco General Hospital, San Francisco, California
Approach to the Patient with Nose, Sinus, and Ear Disorders

Robert J. Myerburg, MD
Professor of Medicine and Physiology, Division of Cardiovascular Medicine, American Heart Association Chair in Cardiovascular Research, University of Miami, Miller School of Medicine, Miami, Florida
Approach to Cardiac Arrest and Life-Threatening Arrhythmias

Stanley Naguwa, MD
Clinical Professor, Division of Rheumatology, Allergy, Clinical Immunology, University of California, Davis, Davis, California
Sjögren's Syndrome

Stanley J. Naides, MD
Medical Director, Department of Immunology, Quest Diagnostics Nichols Institute, San Juan Capistrano, California
Arboviruses Causing Fever and Rash Syndromes

Theodore E. Nash, MD
Head, Gastrointestinal Parasites Section, Laboratory of Parasitic Diseases, National Institutes of Allergy and Infectious Diseases, National Institutes of Health, Bethesda, Maryland
Giardiasis

Avindra Nath, MD
Chief, Section of Infections of the Nervous System, National Institute of Neurological Diseases and Stroke, National Institutes of Health, Bethesda, Maryland
Cytomegalovirus, Epstein-Barr Virus, and Other Slow Virus Infections of the Central Nervous System; Neurologic Complications of Human Immunodeficiency Virus Infection; Meningitis: Bacterial, Viral, and Other; Brain Abscess and Parameningeal Infections

Eric G. Neilson, MD
Thomas Fearn Frist, Sr., Professor of Medicine and Cell Biology, Vanderbilt University School of Medicine, Vanderbilt University, Nashville, Tennessee
Tubulointerstitial Diseases

Lawrence S. Neinstein, MD
Professor of Pediatrics and Medicine, Keck School of Medicine; Executive Director, University Park Health Center, Chief, Division of College Health, Senior Associate Dean of Student Affairs, University of Southern California, Los Angeles, California
Adolescent Medicine

Thomas B. Newman, MD, MPH
Professor and Head, Division of Clinical Epidemiology, Departments of Epidemiology and Biostatistics and Pediatrics, University of California, San Francisco, School of Medicine, San Francisco, California
Statistical Interpretation of Data

William L. Nichols, MD
Associate Professor of Medicine and Laboratory Medicine, Hematology and Internal Medicine, Hematopathology and Laboratory Medicine, Mayo Medical School, Rochester, Minnesota
Von Willebrand Disease and Hemorrhagic Abnormalities of Platelet and Vascular Function

Lynnette K. Nieman, MD
Senior Investigator, Program on Reproductive and Adult Endocrinology, The Eunice Kennedy Shriver National Institute of Child Health and Human Development (NICHD), National Institutes of Health, Bethesda, Maryland
Adrenal Cortex

Dennis E. Niewoehner, MD
Professor, Department of Medicine, University of Minnesota Medical School; Chief, Pulmonary Section, Minneapolis Veterans Affairs Health Care System, Minneapolis, Minnesota
Chronic Obstructive Pulmonary Disease

S. Ragnar Norrby, MD, PhD
Director General, Swedish Institute for Infectious Disease Control, Solna, Sweden
Approach to the Patient with Urinary Tract Infection

David A. Norris, MD
Professor and Chair, Department of Dermatology, University of Colorado Denver School of Medicine, Aurora, Colorado
Structure and Function of the Skin

Susan O'Brien, MD
Professor of Medicine, Department of Leukemia, The University of Texas M.D. Anderson Cancer Center, Houston, Texas
The Chronic Leukemias

Francis G. O'Connor, MD, MPH
Associate Professor, Military and Emergency Medicine, Uniformed Services University, Bethesda, Maryland
Rhabdomyolysis

Patrick G. O'Connor, MD, MPH
Professor of Medicine, Yale University; Chief, General Internal Medicine, Yale University School of Medicine, Yale-New Haven Hospital, New Haven, Connecticut
Alcohol Abuse and Dependence

James R. O'Dell, MD
Professor and Chief of Rheumatology, Department of Internal Medicine, University of Nebraska Medical Center, Omaha, Nebraska
Rheumatoid Arthritis

Anne E. O'Donnell, MD
Professor of Medicine, Chief, Division of Pulmonary, Critical Care, and Sleep Medicine, Georgetown University Hospital, Washington, DC
Bronchiectasis, Atelectasis, Cysts, and Localized Lung Disorders

Jae K. Oh, MD
Professor, Internal Medicine, Co-Director, Echocardiography Laboratory, Division of Cardiovascular Diseases, Mayo Clinic, Rochester, Minnesota
Pericardial Diseases

Jeffrey E. Olgin, MD
Gallo-Chatterjee Distinguished Professor, Chief, Division of Cardiology, Co-Director of the Heart and Vascular Center, University of California, San Francisco, School of Medicine, San Francisco, California
Approach to the Patient with Suspected Arrhythmia

Jeffrey W. Olin, DO
Professor of Medicine, Director Vascular Medicine, Zena and Michael A. Wiener Cardiovascular Institute, Mount Sinai School of Medicine, New York, New York
Other Peripheral Arterial Diseases

Walter A. Orenstein, MD
Deputy Director for Immunization Programs, Vaccine Delivery, Global Health Program, Bill and Melinda Gates Foundation, Seattle, Washington
Immunization

Douglas R. Osmon, MD
Associate Professor of Medicine, Division of Infectious Diseases, Mayo Medical School, Rochester, Minnesota
Infections of Bursae, Joints, and Bones

Catherine M. Otto, MD
J. Ward Kennedy-Hamilton Endowed Chair of Medicine, Director, Training Programs in Cardiovascular Disease, University of Washington School of Medicine; Associate Director, Echocardiography, University of Washington Medical Center, Seattle, Washington
Echocardiography; Videos

Stephen A. Paget, MD
Professor of Medicine, Weill Cornell Medical College; Physician-in-Chief Emeritus, Hospital for Special Surgery, New York, New York
Polymyalgia Rheumatica and Temporal Arteritis

Mark Papania, MD, MPH
Medical Epidemiologist, Division of Viral Diseases, Centers for Disease Control and Prevention, Atlanta, Georgia
Measles

Peter G. Pappas, MD
Professor of Medicine, Division of Infectious Diseases, University of Alabama School of Medicine, Birmingham, Alabama
Dematiaceous Fungal Infections

Pankaj Jay Pasricha, MD
Professor of Medicine, Chief, Division of Gastroenterology and Hepatology, Stanford University School of Medicine, Stanford, California
Gastrointestinal Endoscopy

David L. Paterson, MD
Professor of Medicine, University of Queensland Centre for Clinical Research, Royal Brisbane and Women's Hospital Campus, Brisbane, Australia
Infections due to Other Members of the Enterobacteriaceae, including Management of Multidrug-Resistant Strains

Carlo Patrono, MD
Professor and Chair of Pharmacology, Catholic University School of Medicine, Rome, Italy
Prostaglandins, Aspirin, and Related Compounds

Jean-Michel Pawlotsky, MD, PhD
Professor of Medicine, University of Paris-Est; Director, National Reference Center for Viral Hepatitis B, C and Delta and Department of Virology, Henri Mondor University Hospital; Director, Department of Molecular Virology and Immunology, Institut Mondor de Recherche Biomédicale, Créteil, France
Acute Viral Hepatitis; Chronic Viral and Autoimmune Hepatitis

Richard D. Pearson, MD
Professor of Medicine and Pathology, Division of Infectious Diseases and International Health, University of Virginia School of Medicine, Charlottesville, Virginia
Antiparasitic Therapy

Eli N. Perencevich, MD, MSc
Professor of Internal Medicine, Department of Internal Medicine, University of Iowa, Carver College of Medicine; Core Investigator, Center for Research in the Implementation of Innovative Strategies in Practice, Iowa City Veterans Affairs Medical Center, Iowa City, Iowa
Enterococcal Infections

Trish M. Perl, MD, MSc
Professor, Department of Medicine, Pathology, and Epidemiology, Senior Health System Epidemiologist, Hospital Epidemiology and Infection Control, The Johns Hopkins Health System and University, Baltimore, Maryland
Enterococcal Infections

Michael C. Perry, MD, MSc
Professor of Medicine and Nellie B. Smith Chair of Oncology Emeritus, Departments of Hematology and Medical Oncology, University of Missouri, Ellis Fischel Cancer Center; Medical Director of Clinical Trials, Institute for Clinical and Translational Sciences, University of Missouri, Ellis Fischel Cancer Center, Columbia, Missouri
Approach to the Patient with Cancer

William A. Petri, Jr., MD, PhD
Professor of Medicine, Microbiology and Pathology, Wade Hampton Frost Professor of Epidemiology and Chief, Division of Infectious Diseases and International Health, University of Virginia, Charlottesville, Virginia
Relapsing Fever and Other Borrelia *Infections; African Sleeping Sickness; Amebiasis*

Marc A. Pfeffer, MD, PhD
Dzau Professor of Medicine, Harvard Medical School; Senior Physician, Cardiovascular Division, Brigham and Women's Hospital, Boston, Massachusetts
Heart Failure: Management and Prognosis

Perry J. Pickhardt, MD
Professor of Radiology and Chief, Gastrointestinal Imaging, University of Wisconsin School of Medicine and Public Health, Madison, Wisconsin
Diagnostic Imaging Procedures in Gastroenterology

Gerald B. Pier, PhD
Professor of Medicine (Microbiology and Molecular Genetics), Department of Medicine, Harvard Medical School; Microbiologist, Brigham and Women's Hospital, Boston, Massachusetts
Pseudomonas and Related Gram-Negative Bacillary Infections

David S. Pisetsky, MD, PhD
Professor of Medicine and Immunology, Duke University Medical Center; Chief of Rheumatology, Durham Veterans Affairs Medical Center, Durham, North Carolina
Laboratory Testing in the Rheumatic Diseases

Marshall R. Posner, MD
Professor of Medicine and of Gene and Cell Medicine, Director of Head and Neck Medical Oncology, and Director of Office of Cancer Clinical Trials, The Tisch Cancer Institute, Mount Sinai School of Medicine, New York, New York
Head and Neck Cancer

Charlene Prather, MD
Associate Professor of Internal Medicine, Saint Louis University School of Medicine, St. Louis, Missouri
Inflammatory and Anatomic Diseases of the Intestine, Peritoneum, Mesentery, and Omentum

Basil A. Pruitt, Jr., MD
Clinical Professor of Surgery and Dr. Ferdinand P. Herff Chair in Surgery, University of Texas Health Science Center at San Antonio; Consultant Surgeon, U. S. Army Institute of Surgical Research, Fort Sam Houston, San Antonio, Texas
Electric Injury

Reed E. Pyeritz, MD, PhD
Professor of Medicine and Genetics and Vice Chair for Academic Affairs, University of Pennsylvania School of Medicine, Philadelphia, Pennsylvania
Inherited Diseases of Connective Tissue

Thomas C. Quinn, MD, MSc
Professor of Medicine, Johns Hopkins University School of Medicine, Baltimore, Maryland; Associate Director for International Research, Division of Intramural Research, National Institute of Allergy and Infectious Diseases, National Institutes of Health, Bethesda, Maryland
Epidemiology of Human Immunodeficiency Virus Infection and Acquired Immunodeficiency Syndrome

Jai Radhakrishnan, MD, MSc
Associate Professor of Clinical Medicine, Department of Medicine, Division of Nephrology; Program Director, Nephrology Fellowship, Division of Nephrology, Columbia University Medical Center, New York, New York
Glomerular Disorders and Nephrotic Syndromes

Ganesh Raghu, MD
Professor of Medicine and Laboratory Medicine (Adjunct), Division of Pulmonary and Critical Care Medicine; Director, Interstitial Lung Disease, Sarcoid and Pulmonary Fibrosis Program; Medical Director, Lung Transplant Program, University of Washington, Seattle, Washington
Interstitial Lung Disease

Margaret V. Ragni, MD, MPH
Professor of Medicine and Clinical and Translational Science, Department of Medicine, Division of Hematology/Oncology, University of Pittsburgh School of Medicine; Director, Hemophilia Center of Western Pennsylvania, Pittsburgh, Pennsylvania
Hemorrhagic Disorders: Coagulation Factor Deficiencies

Srinivasa N. Raja, MD
Professor of Anesthesiology and Neurology; Director, Division of Pain Medicine, Johns Hopkins University School of Medicine, Baltimore, Maryland
Pain

S. Vincent Rajkumar, MD
Professor of Medicine and Chair, Myeloma Amyloidosis Dysproteinemia Group, Division of Hematology, Mayo Medical School and Mayo Clinic, Rochester, Minnesota
Plasma Cell Disorders

Didier Raoult, MD, PhD
Professor, Université de la Méditerranée, National Center for Scientific Research UMR 6236, Research and Development Institute 198, Université de la Méditerranée, Faculté de Médecine, Marseille, France
Bartonella Species Infections; Rickettsial Infections

Robert W. Rebar, MD
Volunteer Professor, Department of Obstetrics and Gynecology, Executive Director, American Society for Reproductive Medicine, University of Alabama at Birmingham School of Medicine, Birmingham, Alabama
Ovaries and Development; Reproductive Endocrinology and Infertility

Annette C. Reboli, MD
Professor of Medicine and Vice Dean, Cooper Medical School of Rowan University; Professor of Medicine, University of Medicine and Dentistry of New Jersey/Robert Wood Johnson Medical School, Department of Medicine, Division of Infectious Diseases, Cooper University Hospital, Camden, New Jersey
Erysipelothrix Infections

K. Rajender Reddy, MD
Professor of Medicine and of Medicine in Surgery, Director of Hepatology and Medical Director of Liver Transplantation, University of Pennsylvania School of Medicine, Philadelphia, Pennsylvania
Bacterial, Parasitic, Fungal, and Granulomatous Liver Diseases

Donald A. Redelmeier, MD, MSc
Professor of Medicine and of Health Policy Management and Evaluation, University of Toronto; Canada Research Chair, Sunnybrook Health Sciences Centre, Toronto, Ontario, Canada
Postoperative Care and Complications

Susan E. Reef, MD
Medical Epidemiologist, Global Immunization Division, Centers for Disease Control and Prevention, Atlanta, Georgia
Rubella (German Measles)

Neil M. Resnick, MD
Thomas Detre Professor of Medicine and Chief, Division of Gerontology and Geriatric Medicine; Director, University of Pittsburgh Institute on Aging, University of Pittsburgh, Pittsburgh, Pennsylvania
Incontinence

David B. Reuben, MD
Archstone Professor of Medicine; Director, Multicampus Program in Geriatric Medicine and Gerontology; Chief, Division of Geriatrics, David Geffen School of Medicine at UCLA, University of California, Los Angeles, California
Geriatric Assessment

Herbert Y. Reynolds, MD
Professor Emeritus, Department of Medicine, Penn State College of Medicine, Hershey, Pennsylvania; Adjunct Professor of Medicine, Uniformed Services University of the Health Sciences, F. Edward Hebert School of Medicine; Medical Officer, Division of Lung Diseases, National Heart, Lung, and Blood Institute, National Institutes of Health, Bethesda, Maryland
Respiratory Structure and Function: Mechanisms and Testing

Emanuel P. Rivers, MD, MPH
Clinical Professor and Senior Staff Attending, Departments of Emergency Medicine and Surgery (Critical Care), Wayne State University; Vice Chairman and Research Director, Department of Emergency Medicine, Henry Ford Hospital, Detroit, Michigan
Approach to the Patient with Shock

Robert A. Rizza, MD
Professor of Medicine, Department of Endocrinology, Mayo Clinic, Rochester, Minnesota
Hypoglycemia/Pancreatic Islet Cell Disorders

Lewis R. Roberts, MB ChB, PhD
Professor, Department of Medicine, Mayo Medical School; Consultant in Gastroenterology and Hepatology, Mayo Clinic, Rochester, Minnesota
Liver and Biliary Tract Tumors

Jean-Marc Rolain, PharmD, PhD
Professor, Université de la Méditerranée, National Center for Scientific Research UMR 6236, Research and Development Institute, Faculté de Médecine et de Pharmacie, Université de la Méditerranée, Marseille, France
Bartonella Species Infections

José R. Romero, MD
Professor of Pediatrics, University of Arkansas for Medical Sciences; Horace C. Cabe Professor of Pediatric Infectious Diseases, Arkansas Children's Hospital; Director, Pediatric Infectious Diseases Section; Director, Clinical Trials, Arkansas Children's Hospital Research Institute, Little Rock, Arkansas
Enteroviruses

G. David Roodman, MD, PhD
Professor of Medicine, University of Pittsburgh; Vice Chair for Research, University of Pittsburgh; Director, Center for Bone Biology, University of Pittsburgh Medical Center; University of Pittsburgh Cancer Institute, Pittsburgh, Pennsylvania
Paget's Disease of Bone

Clifford Rosen, MD
Professor, Department of Medicine, Tufts University School of Medicine, Boston, Massachusetts; Senior Scientist, Maine Medical Center Research Institute, Maine Medical Center, Portland, Maine
Osteoporosis

Karen Rosene-Montella, MD
Professor of Medicine and of Obstetrics and Gynecology, Vice Chair of Medicine for Quality and Outcomes, Alpert Medical School at Brown University; Senior Vice President, Women's Services and Clinical Integration, Lifespan; Chief of Medicine, Women and Infants Hospital, Providence, Rhode Island
Common Medical Problems in Pregnancy

Philip J. Rosenthal, MD
Professor, Department of Medicine, University of California, San Francisco, School of Medicine, San Francisco, California
Malaria

Marc E. Rothenberg, MD, PhD
Professor of Pediatrics, University of Cincinnati College of Medicine; Director, Division of Allergy and Immunology, Cincinnati Children's Hospital Medical Center, Cincinnati, Ohio
Eosinophilic Syndromes

Hope S. Rugo, MD
Clinical Professor of Medicine, Director, Breast Oncology Clinical Trials Program, University of California, San Francisco, Comprehensive Cancer Center, San Francisco, California
Paraneoplastic Syndromes and Other Non-Neoplastic Effects of Cancer

James A. Russell, MD
Professor, Department of Medicine, University of British Columbia; Principal Investigator, James Hogg Research Centre, Institute for Heart and Lung Health, St. Paul's Hospital, Vancouver, British Columbia, Canada
Shock Syndromes Related to Sepsis

Anil K. Rustgi, MD
T. Grier Miller Professor of Medicine and Genetics, Chief of Gastroenterology and American Cancer Society Research Professor, University of Pennsylvania School of Medicine, Philadelphia, Pennsylvania
Neoplasms of the Esophagus and Stomach

Robert A. Salata, MD
Professor and Vice Chair, Department of Medicine; Chief, Division of Infectious Diseases and HIV Medicine, Case Western Reserve University School of Medicine; Attending Physician and Consultant, University Hospitals Case Medical Center, Cleveland, Ohio
Brucellosis

Jane E. Salmon, MD
Professor, Department of Medicine, Weill Cornell Medical College; Collette Kean Research Chair, Divisions of Rheumatology and Research, Hospital for Special Surgery, New York, New York
Mechanisms of Immune-Mediated Tissue Injury

Renato M. Santos, MD
Assistant Professor of Internal Medicine; Associate Director, Cardiovascular Training Program, Wake Forest University School of Medicine, Winston-Salem, North Carolina
Vascular Disorders of the Kidney; Video

Michael N. Sawka, PhD
Chief, Thermal and Mountain Medicine Division, U.S. Army Research Institute of Environmental Medicine, Natick, Massachusetts
Disorders Due to Heat and Cold

Andrew I. Schafer, MD
Chairman, Department of Medicine; The E. Hugh Luckey Distinguished Professor of Medicine, Weill Cornell Medical College; Physician-in-Chief, New York-Presbyterian Hospital/Weill Cornell Medical Center, New York, New York
Approach to Medicine, the Patient, and the Medical Profession: Medicine as a Learned and Humane Profession; Approach to the Patient with Bleeding and Thrombosis; Hemorrhagic Disorders: DIC, Liver Failure, and Vitamin K Deficiency; Thrombotic Disorders: Hypercoagulable States

William Schaffner, MD
Professor and Chair, Department of Preventive Medicine; Professor of Medicine (Infectious Diseases), Vanderbilt University School of Medicine, Nashville, Tennessee
Tularemia and Other Francisella *Infections*

W. Michael Scheld, MD
Bayer-Gerald L. Mandell Professor of Infectious Diseases, Professor of Medicine, Clinical Professor of Neurosurgery, Director, Pfizer Initiative in International Health, Division of Infectious Diseases and International Health, Department of Medicine, University of Virginia Health System, Charlottesville, Virginia
Introduction to Microbial Disease: Host-Pathogen Interactions

Eileen Schneider, MD, MPH
Division of Tuberculosis Elimination, Centers for Disease Control and Prevention, Atlanta, Georgia
Coronaviruses

Thomas J. Schnitzer, MD, PhD
Professor, Physical Medicine, Rehabilitation, and Internal Medicine, Northwestern University Feinberg School of Medicine, Chicago, Illinois
Osteoarthritis

Robert T. Schooley, MD
Professor and Head, Division of Infectious Diseases, University of California, San Diego, School of Medicine, San Diego, California
Epstein-Barr Virus Infection

David L. Schriger, MD, MPH
Professor, Department of Emergency Medicine, David Geffen School of Medicine at UCLA, University of California, Los Angeles, California
Approach to the Patient with Abnormal Vital Signs

Steven A. Schroeder, MD
Distinguished Professor of Health and Healthcare, Department of Medicine, and Director, Smoking Cessation Leadership Center, University of California, San Francisco, San Francisco, California
Socioeconomic Issues in Medicine

Lynn M. Schuchter, MD
Professor of Medicine, Chief, Hematology/Oncology Division, University of Pennsylvania School of Medicine, Philadelphia, Pennsylvania
Melanoma and Nonmelanoma Skin Cancers

Sam Schulman, MD, PhD
Professor of Medicine, Department of Medicine, McMaster University, Hamilton, Ontario, Canada
Antithrombotic Therapy

Lawrence B. Schwartz, MD, PhD
Charles and Evelyn Thomas Professor of Medicine, Department of Internal Medicine, Medical College of Virginia, Virginia Commonwealth University, Richmond, Virginia
Systemic Anaphylaxis, Food Allergy, and Insect Sting Allergy

Robert S. Schwartz, MD
Distinguished Professor of Medicine, Tufts University School of Medicine, Boston, Massachusetts
Autoimmune and Intravascular Hemolytic Anemias

Carlos Seas, MD
Associate Professor of Medicine, Cayetano Heredia University; Attending Physician, Department of Tropical and Infectious Diseases, Cayetano Heredia National Hospital, Lima, Peru
Cholera and Other Vibrio *Infections*

Steven A. Seifert, MD
Professor, University of New Mexico School of Medicine; Medical Director, New Mexico Poison and Drug Information Center, Albuquerque, New Mexico
Venomous Snake Bites

Julian L. Seifter, MD
Associate Professor of Medicine, Harvard Medical School; Physician, Brigham and Women's Hospital, Boston, Massachusetts
Potassium Disorders; Acid-Base Disorders

Clay F. Semenkovich, MD
Herbert S. Gasser Professor and Chief, Division of Endocrinology, Metabolism and Lipid Research, Washington University School of Medicine, St. Louis, Missouri
Disorders of Lipid Metabolism

Carol E. Semrad, MD
Associate Professor of Medicine, Section of Gastroenterology, The University of Chicago Pritzker School of Medicine, Chicago, Illinois
Approach to the Patient with Diarrhea and Malabsorption

F. John Service, MD, PhD
Professor of Medicine, Mayo Clinic College of Medicine; Consultant in Endocrinology and Metabolism, Mayo Clinic, Rochester, Minnesota
Hypoglycemia/Pancreatic Islet Cell Disorders

George M. Shaw, MD, PhD
Professor, Division of Hematology/Oncology, Department of Medicine, University of Pennsylvania School of Medicine, Philadelphia, Pennsylvania
Biology of Human Immunodeficiency Viruses

Pamela J. Shaw, MB ChB, MD
Professor of Neurology, Academic Neurology Unit and Head of Neuroscience Department, University of Sheffield; Director, Sheffield Care and Research Centre for Motor Neuron Disorders, Sheffield, United Kingdom
Amyotrophic Lateral Sclerosis and Other Motor Neuron Diseases; Videos

Robert S. Sherwin, MD
CNH Long Professor of Medicine and Chief, Section of Endocrinology; Director, Yale Center for Clinical Investigation, Yale University School of Medicine, New Haven, Connecticut
Type 1 Diabetes Mellitus; Type 2 Diabetes Mellitus

Michael E. Shy, MD
Professor of Neurology and of Molecular Medicine and Genetics, Wayne State University School of Medicine, Detroit, Michigan
Peripheral Neuropathies; Video

Wilmer L. Sibbitt, Jr., MD
Professor of Internal Medicine, Rheumatology and Neurology, University of New Mexico Health Sciences Center, Albuquerque, New Mexico
Idiopathic Multifocal Fibrosclerosis

Ellen Sidransky, MD
Chief, Section of Molecular Neurogenetics, Medical Genetics Branch, National Human Genome Research Institute, National Institutes of Health, Bethesda, Maryland
The Lysosomal Storage Diseases

Robert F. Siliciano, MD, PhD
Professor of Medicine, Johns Hopkins University School of Medicine, Baltimore, Maryland
Immunopathogenesis of Human Immunodeficiency Virus Infection

Michael S. Simberkoff, MD
Professor of Medicine, New York University School of Medicine; Chief of Staff, Veterans Affairs New York Harbor Healthcare System, New York, New York
Haemophilus and Moraxella *Infections*

David L. Simel, MD, MHS
Professor and Vice Chair for Veterans Affairs, Department of Medicine, Duke University School of Medicine; Chief of Internal Medicine, Department of Medicine Service, Durham Veterans Affairs Medical Center, Durham, North Carolina
Approach to the Patient: History and Physical Examination

Karl Skorecki, MD
Annie Chutick Professor in Medicine (Nephrology) and Director, Rappaport Research Institute, Technion–Israel Institute of Technology; Director of Medical and Research Development, Rambam Health Care Campus, Haifa, Israel
Gene and Cell Therapy; Disorders of Sodium and Water Homeostasis

Arthur S. Slutsky, MD
Professor, Departments of Medicine, Surgery, and Biomedical Engineering, University of Toronto; Vice President of Research, St. Michael's Hospital, Toronto, Ontario, Canada
Acute Respiratory Failure; Mechanical Ventilation; Video

Eric J. Small, MD
Professor of Medicine and Urology, Chief, Division of Hematology and Oncology; Deputy Director and Director of Clinical Sciences, Helen Diller Family Comprehensive Cancer Center, University of California, San Francisco, California
Prostate Cancer

Gerald W. Smetana, MD
Associate Professor of Medicine, Harvard Medical School; Division of General Medicine and Primary Care, Beth Israel Deaconess Medical Center, Boston, Massachusetts
Principles of Medical Consultation

Frederick S. Southwick, MD
Professor of Medicine, Patient Quality Projects Manager, University of Florida and Shands Health System, Gainesville, Florida
Nocardiosis

Robert F. Spiera, MD
Associate Professor of Clinical Medicine, Weill Cornell Medical College; Director, Vasculitis and Scleroderma, The Hospital for Special Surgery, New York, New York
Polymyalgia Rheumatica and Temporal Arteritis

Stanley M. Spinola, MD
Professor and Chair, Department of Microbiology and Immunology; Professor of Medicine and of Pathology and Laboratory Medicine, Indiana University School of Medicine, Indianapolis, Indiana
Chancroid

Pawel Stankiewicz, MD, PhD
Associate Professor, Department of Molecular and Human Genetics, Baylor College of Medicine, Houston, Texas
Gene, Genomic, and Chromosomal Disorders

Paul Stark, MD
Professor of Clinical Radiology, University of California, San Diego, and Chief of Cardiothoracic Radiology, Radiology Service, Veterans Affairs San Diego Healthcare System, San Diego, California
Imaging in Pulmonary Disease

Lynne S. Steinbach, MD
Professor of Radiology and Orthopaedic Surgery, University of California, San Francisco, School of Medicine, San Francisco, California
Imaging Studies in the Rheumatic Diseases

Martin H. Steinberg, MD
Professor, Departments of Medicine, Pediatrics, and Pathology and Laboratory Medicine, Boston University School of Medicine; Director, Center of Excellence in Sickle Cell Disease, Boston Medical Center, Boston, Massachusetts
Sickle Cell Disease and Other Hemoglobinopathies

Theodore S. Steiner, MD
Associate Professor and Associate Head, Division of Infectious Diseases, University of British Columbia, Vancouver, British Columbia, Canada
Escherichia Coli Enteric Infections

David S. Stephens, MD
Stephen W. Schwarzmann Distinguished Professor of Medicine, Director, Division of Infectious Diseases, Department of Medicine, Emory University School of Medicine; Vice President for Research, Robert W. Woodruff Health Sciences Center, Emory University School of Medicine, Atlanta; Staff Physician, VA Medical Research Service (Atlanta), Decatur, Georgia
Neisseria Meningitidis Infections; Aspergillosis

David A. Stevens, MD
Professor, Department of Medicine, Stanford University, Stanford; Chief, Division of Infectious Diseases, Department of Medicine, Santa Clara Valley Medical Center, San Jose, California
Systemic Antifungal Agents; Aspergillosis

William G. Stevenson, MD
Professor of Medicine, Harvard Medical School; Director of Cardiac Electrophysiology, Brigham and Women's Hospital, Boston, Massachusetts
Ventricular Arrhythmias

Arthur E. Stillman, MD, PhD
William and Kay Casarella Professor, Department of Radiology, Emory University School of Medicine, Atlanta, Georgia
Radiology of the Heart

James K. Stoller, MD, MS
Jean Wall Bennett Professor of Medicine, Cleveland Clinic Lerner College of Medicine; Chair, Education Institute, Cleveland Clinic, Education Institute and Respiratory Institute, Cleveland Clinic, Cleveland, Ohio
Respiratory Monitoring in Critical Care

John H. Stone, MD, MPH
Associate Professor of Medicine, Harvard Medical School; Director, Clinical Rheumatology, Massachusetts General Hospital, Boston, Massachusetts
The Systemic Vasculitides

Edwin P. Su, MD
Assistant Professor, Clinical Orthopaedic Surgery, Weill Cornell Medical College; Assistant Attending, Department of Orthopaedic Surgery, Hospital for Special Surgery, New York, New York
Surgical Treatment of Joint Disease

Roland W. Sutter, MD, MPH&TM
Coordinator, Research and Product Development, Polio Eradication Department, World Health Organization, Geneva, Switzerland
Diphtheria and Other Corynebacteria Infections

Morton N. Swartz, MD
Professor of Medicine, Harvard Medical School; James Jackson Firm Chief of Medical Services, Massachusetts General Hospital, Boston, Massachusetts
Meningitis: Bacterial, Viral, and Other

Ronald S. Swerdloff, MD
Professor of Medicine, David Geffen School of Medicine at UCLA, Los Angeles; Chief, Division of Endocrinology and Metabolism, Harbor–UCLA Medical Center, Los Angeles Biomedical Research Institute, Torrance, California
The Testis and Male Sexual Function

Megan Sykes, MD
Michael J. Friedlander Professor of Medicine and Professor of Microbiology and Immunology and Surgical Sciences (in Surgery), Columbia University; Director, Columbia Center for Translational Immunology, Columbia University College of Physicians and Surgeons, New York, New York
Transplantation Immunology

Thomas A. Tami, MD
Medical Director, Group Health Associates; Director, Cincinnati Sinus Institute, Cincinnati, Ohio
Throat Disorders

Susan M. Tarlo, MB ChB
Professor, Department of Medicine and Dalla Lana School of Public Health, University of Toronto; Respiratory Physician, Toronto Western Hospital; Research Physician, Centre for Research Expertise in Occupational Disease, Gage Occupational and Environmental Health Unit, Toronto, Ontario, Canada
Occupational Lung Disease

Victoria M. Taylor, MD, MPH
Research Professor, Department of Health Services, University of Washington; Full Member, Cancer Prevention Program, Fred Hutchinson Cancer Research Center, Seattle, Washington
Cultural Context of Medicine

Ayalew Tefferi, MD
Professor of Medicine and Hematology, Mayo Medical School, Rochester, Minnesota
Polycythemias, Essential Thrombocythemia, and Primary Myelofibrosis

Paul S. Teirstein, MD
Visiting Professor of Medicine, Columbia University Medical Center, New York, New York; Chief of Cardiology and Director, Interventional Cardiology, Scripps Clinic, La Jolla, California
Interventional and Surgical Treatment of Coronary Artery Disease; Videos

Sam R. Telford III, ScD, MSc
Professor, Biomedical Sciences, Tufts University, North Grafton, Massachusetts
Babesiosis and Other Protozoan Diseases

Margaret Tempero, MD
Professor of Medicine, Division of Hematology and Oncology, University of California, San Francisco, School of Medicine; Leader, Pancreas Cancer Program, Director of Research Programs, Deputy Director, University of California, San Francisco, Helen Diller Family Comprehensive Cancer Center, San Francisco, California
Pancreatic Cancer

Michael J. Thun, MD, MSc
Vice President, Emeritus, Department of Epidemiology, American Cancer Society, Atlanta, Georgia
The Epidemiology of Cancer

Nina Tolkoff-Rubin, MD
Professor of Medicine, Harvard Medical School; Director of Dialysis and Renal Transplantation, Massachusetts General Hospital, Boston, Massachusetts
Treatment of Irreversible Renal Failure

Antonella Tosti, MD
Professor of Clinical Dermatology, Department of Dermatology and Cutaneous Surgery, University of Miami, Miller School of Medicine, Miami, Florida
Diseases of Hair and Nails

John J. Treanor, MD
Professor of Medicine and Chief, Infectious Diseases Division, University of Rochester Medical Center, Rochester, New York
Adenovirus Diseases

Ronald B. Turner, MD
Professor of Pediatrics, University of Virginia School of Medicine, Charlottesville, Virginia
The Common Cold

Arthur C. Upton, MD
Clinical Professor, Department of Environmental and Community Medicine, University of Medicine and Dentistry of New Jersey—Robert Wood Johnson Medical School, Piscataway, New Jersey; Professor Emeritus, Department of Environmental Medicine, New York University Medical School, New York, New York
Radiation Injury

Greet Van den Berghe, MD, PhD
Professor of Medicine, Katholieke Universiteit Leuven; Head, Department of Intensive Care Medicine, University Hospitals Leuven—Gasthuisberg, Leuven, Belgium
Parenteral Nutrition

John Varga, MD
John Hughes Professor of Medicine, Department of Medicine, Northwestern University Feinberg School of Medicine, Chicago, Illinois
Systemic Sclerosis (Scleroderma)

Adrian Vella, MD
Professor of Medicine, Division of Endocrinology and Metabolism, Mayo Clinic, Rochester, Minnesota
Hypoglycemia/Pancreatic Islet Cell Disorders

Joseph G. Verbalis, MD
Professor, Department of Medicine and Physiology, Georgetown University; Chief, Endocrinology and Metabolism, Georgetown University Hospital, Washington, DC
Posterior Pituitary

Ronald G. Victor, MD
Burns and Allen Professor of Medicine, David Geffen School of Medicine at UCLA, and Director, Hypertension Center; Co-Director, The Heart Institute, Cedars Sinai Medical Center, Los Angeles, California
Arterial Hypertension

Angela Vincent, MB ChB, MSc
Professor, Nuffield Department of Clinical Neurosciences, University of Oxford, Oxford, Oxon, United Kingdom
Disorders of Neuromuscular Transmission

Paul A. Volberding, MD
Professor and Vice Chair, Department of Medicine, University of California, San Francisco, School of Medicine; Co-Director, University of California, San Francisco–Gladstone Institute of Virology and Immunology Center for AIDS Research; Chief, Medical Service, San Francisco Veterans Affairs Medical Center, San Francisco, California
Hematology and Oncology in Patients with Human Immunodeficiency Virus Infection

Julie M. Vose, MD
Chief, Section of Hematology/Oncology, Professor of Medicine, University of Nebraska Medical Center, Omaha, Nebraska
Hematopoietic Stem Cell Transplantation

Robert M. Wachter, MD
Professor and Associate Chair, Department of Medicine, University of California, San Francisco, School of Medicine, San Francisco, California
Quality of Care and Patient Safety

Edward H. Wagner, MD, MPH
Professor of Public Health and Community Medicine, University of Washington and Director, MacColl Institute for Healthcare Innovation, Group Health Research Institute, Seattle, Washington
Comprehensive Chronic Disease Management

Edward E. Walsh, MD
Professor of Medicine, University of Rochester, Rochester, New York
Respiratory Syncytial Virus

Thomas J. Walsh, MD
Professor of Medicine, Division of Infectious Diseases, Weill Cornell Medical College, New York, New York
Aspergillosis

Christina Wang, MD
Professor of Medicine, David Geffen School of Medicine at UCLA; Program Director, General Clinical Research Center, Harbor–UCLA Medical Center, Los Angeles Biomedical Research Institute, Torrance, California
The Testis and Male Sexual Function

Christine Wanke, MD
Professor of Medicine and Public Health and Director, Division of Nutrition and Infection; Associate Chair, Department of Public Health, Tufts University School of Medicine, Boston, Massachusetts
Gastrointestinal Manifestions of HIV and AIDS

Stephen I. Wasserman, MD
Professor of Medicine, University of California, San Diego, School of Medicine, La Jolla, California
Approach to the Patient with Allergic or Immunologic Disease

Heiner Wedemeyer, MD
Professor, Department of Gastroenterology, Hepatology and Endocrinology, Hannover Medical School, Hannover, Germany
Acute Viral Hepatitis

Geoffrey A. Weinberg, MD
Professor of Pediatrics, University of Rochester School of Medicine and Dentistry; Director, Pediatric HIV Program, Golisano Children's Hospital at University of Rochester Medical Center, Rochester, New York
Parainfluenza Viral Disease

David A. Weinstein, MD, MMSc
Director, Glycogen Storage Disease Program, Division of Pediatric Endocrinology, University of Florida College of Medicine, Gainesville, Florida
Glycogen Storage Diseases

Robert S. Weinstein, MD
Professor of Medicine, University of Arkansas for Medical Sciences; Staff Physician, Department of Medicine, Central Arkansas Veterans Healthcare System, Little Rock, Arkansas
Osteomalacia and Rickets

Roger D. Weiss, MD
Professor of Psychiatry, Harvard Medical School, Boston, Massachusetts; Chief, Division of Alcohol and Drug Abuse, McLean Hospital, Belmont, Massachusetts
Drug Abuse and Dependence

Martin Weisse, MD
Professor, Department of Pediatrics, Uniformed Services University of the Health Sciences, Bethesda, Maryland; Colonel Army; Chief, Department of Pediatrics, Tripler Army Medical Center, Honolulu, Hawaii
Measles

Jeffrey I. Weitz, MD
Professor of Medicine and Biochemistry and Biomedical Sciences, McMaster University; Canada Research Chair in Thrombosis, Heart and Stroke Foundation of Ontario/J.F. Mustard Chair in Cardiovascular Research; Executive Director, Thrombosis and Atherosclerosis Research Institute, Hamilton, Ontario, Canada
Pulmonary Embolism

Samuel A. Wells, Jr., MD
Director, Thyroid Oncology Clinic, National Cancer Institute, Bethesda, Maryland
Medullary Thyroid Carcinoma and Calcitonin

Richard P. Wenzel, MD
Professor, Department of Medicine, Medical College of Virginia, Richmond, Virginia
Acute Bronchitis and Tracheitis

Victoria P. Werth, MD
Professor of Dermatology, University of Pennsylvania School of Medicine; Chief, Dermatology Section, Philadelphia Veterans Affairs Medical Center, Philadelphia, Pennsylvania
Principles of Therapy of Skin Diseases

Sterling G. West, MD
Professor of Medicine, Division of Rheumatology, University of Colorado Denver School of Medicine, Aurora, Colorado
Systemic Diseases in Which Arthritis Is a Feature

Cornelia M. Weyand, MD, PhD
Professor of Medicine, Division of Immunology and Rheumatology, Stanford University, Stanford, California
The Innate and Adaptive Immune Systems

A. Clinton White, Jr., MD
Paul R. Stalnaker, MD, Distinguished Professor and Director, Infectious Disease Division, Department of Internal Medicine, University of Texas Medical Branch, Galveston, Texas
Cestodes

Christopher J. White, MD
Professor and System Chairman for Cardiovascular Diseases, Ochsner Clinical School, University of Queensland, Ochsner Medical Institutions, New Orleans, Louisiana
Atherosclerotic Peripheral Arterial Disease; Video

Perrin C. White, MD
Professor, Department of Pediatrics, University of Texas Southwestern Medical Center; Chief, Department of Endocrinology, Children's Medical Center Dallas, Dallas, Texas
Disorders of Sexual Development

Richard J. Whitley, MD
Distinguished Professor of Pediatrics, Loeb Eminent Scholar Chair in Pediatrics, and Professor of Microbiology, Medicine and Neurosurgery, University of Alabama at Birmingham, Birmingham, Alabama
Herpes Simplex Virus Infections

Michael P. Whyte, MD
Professor of Medicine, Pediatrics, and Genetics, Division of Bone and Mineral Diseases, Washington University School of Medicine; Medical-Scientific Director, Center for Metabolic Bone Disease and Molecular Research, Shriners Hospital for Children, St. Louis, Missouri
Osteonecrosis, Osteosclerosis/Hyperostosis, and Other Disorders of Bone

Samuel Wiebe, MD, MSc
Professor and Head, Division of Neurology, Department of Clinical Neurosciences and Hotchkiss Brain Institute, University of Calgary, Calgary, Alberta, Canada
The Epilepsies

Jeanine P. Wiener-Kronish, MD
Henry Isaiah Dorr Professor of Research and Teaching in Anaesthetics, Harvard Medical School; Anesthetist-in-Chief, Department of Anesthesia, Critical Care and Pain Medicine, Massachusetts General Hospital, Boston, Massachusetts
Overview of Anesthesia

Jennifer E. Wildes, PhD
Assistant Professor of Psychiatry, University of Pittsburgh School of Medicine, Pittsburgh, Pennsylvania
Eating Disorders

Alexander Wilmer, MD, PhD
Professor of Medicine, Medical Intensive Care, Katholieke Universiteit Leuven, University Hospitals Leuven—Gasthuisberg, Belgium
Parenteral Nutrition

William Winkenwerder, Jr., MD, MBA
Chair, The Winkenwerder Company, Alexandria, Virginia
Disorders Due to Heat and Cold

Joseph I. Wolfsdorf, MB ChB
Professor of Pediatrics, Harvard Medical School; Clinical Director and Chair,
Division of Endocrinology, Children's Hospital Boston, Boston,
Massachusetts
Glycogen Storage Diseases

Gary P. Wormser, MD
Professor, Departments of Medicine and Pharmacology, New York Medical
College; Chief of Infectious Diseases and Vice Chair of Medicine, New
York Medical College; Chief of Infectious Diseases, Westchester Medical
Center, Valhalla, New York
Lyme Disease

John J. Wysolmerski, MD
Professor of Internal Medicine, Section of Endocrinology and Metabolism,
Department of Internal Medicine, Yale University School of Medicine,
New Haven, Connecticut
The Parathyroid Glands, Hypercalcemia, and Hypocalcemia

Myron Yanoff, MD
Professor and Chair, Department of Ophthalmology, Drexel University
College of Medicine; Adjunct Professor of Ophthalmology, University of
Pennsylvania School of Medicine, Philadelphia, Pennsylvania
Diseases of the Visual System

Neal S. Young, MD, MACP
Chief, Hematology Branch, National Heart, Lung, and Blood Institute;
Director, Center for Human Immunology, Autoimmunity, and
Inflammation, National Institutes of Health, Bethesda, Maryland
Parvovirus

William F. Young, Jr., MD, MSc
Tyson Family Clinical Endocrinology Professor in Honor of Vahab
Fatourechi, MD, and Professor of Medicine, Mayo Medical School;
Division of Endocrinology, Diabetes, Metabolism, and Nutrition, Mayo
Clinic, Rochester, Minnesota
Adrenal Medulla, Catecholamines, and Pheochromocytoma

Alan S. L. Yu, MB ChB
Solon E. Summerfield Professor of Medicine, Kansas University School of
Medicine; Director of the Kidney Institute and Division of Nephrology,
Kansas University Medical Center, Kansas City, Kansas
Disorders of Magnesium and Phosphorus

Mark L. Zeidel, MD
Herrman L. Blumgart Professor of Medicine, Department of Medicine,
Harvard Medical School; Physician-in-Chief and Chair, Department of
Medicine, Beth Israel Deaconess Medical Center, Boston, Massachusetts
Obstructive Uropathy

Peter Zimetbaum, MD
Associate Professor of Medicine, Harvard Medical School; Director, Clinical
Cardiology, Beth Israel Deaconess Medical Center, Boston, Massachusetts
Cardiac Arrhythmias with Supraventricular Origin

Justin A. Zivin, MD, PhD
Professor of Neurosciences, Department of Neurosciences, University
of California San Diego, La Jolla, California; Staff Neurologist,
San Diego Veterans Affairs Healthcare System, San Diego, California
*Approach to Cerebrovascular Diseases; Ischemic Cerebrovascular Disease;
Hemorrhagic Cerebrovascular Disease*

CONTENTS

SECTION XV: ONCOLOGY

SECTION XVI: METABOLIC DISEASES

SECTION XXIV: HIV AND THE ACQUIRED IMMUNODEFICIENCY SYNDROME

VIDEO CONTENTS

 This icon appears throughout the book to indicate chapters with accompanying video available on *Expertconsult.com*. For quick viewing, use your smartphone to scan the QR codes in the front of the book.

GOLDMAN'S
CECIL MEDICINE

SOCIAL AND ETHICAL ISSUES IN MEDICINE

1

APPROACH TO MEDICINE, THE PATIENT, AND THE MEDICAL PROFESSION: MEDICINE AS A LEARNED AND HUMANE PROFESSION

LEE GOLDMAN AND ANDREW I. SCHAFER

APPROACH TO MEDICINE

Medicine is a profession that incorporates science and the scientific method with the art of being a physician. The art of tending to the sick is as old as humanity itself. Even in modern times, the art of caring and comforting, guided by millennia of common sense as well as a more recent, systematic approach to medical ethics (Chapter 2), remains the cornerstone of medicine. Without these humanistic qualities, the application of the modern science of medicine is suboptimal, ineffective, or even detrimental.

The caregivers of ancient times and premodern cultures tried a variety of interventions to help the afflicted. Some of their potions contained what are now known to be active ingredients that form the basis for proven medications (Chapter 28). Others (Chapter 38) have persisted into the present era despite a lack of convincing evidence. Modern medicine should not dismiss the possibility that these unproven approaches may be helpful; instead, it should adopt a guiding principle that all interventions, whether traditional or newly developed, can be tested vigorously, with the expectation that any beneficial effects can be explored further to determine their scientific basis.

When compared with its long and generally distinguished history of caring and comforting, the scientific basis of medicine is remarkably recent. Other than an understanding of human anatomy and the later description, albeit widely contested at this time, of the normal physiology of the circulatory system, almost all of modern medicine is based on discoveries made within the past 150 years. Until the late 19th century, the paucity of medical knowledge was perhaps exemplified best by hospitals and hospital care. Although hospitals provided caring that all but well-to-do people might not be able to obtain elsewhere, there is little if any evidence that hospitals improved health outcomes. The term *hospitalism* referred not to expertise in hospital care but rather to the aggregate of iatrogenic afflictions that were induced by the hospital stay itself.

The essential humanistic qualities of caring and comforting can achieve full benefit only if they are coupled with an understanding of how medical science can and should be applied to patients with known or suspected diseases. Without this knowledge, comforting may be inappropriate or misleading, and caring may be ineffective or counterproductive if it inhibits a sick person from obtaining appropriate, scientific medical care. *Goldman's Cecil Textbook of Medicine* focuses on the discipline of *internal medicine,* from which neurology and dermatology, which are also covered in substantial detail in this text, are relatively recent evolutionary branches. The term *internal medicine,* which is often misunderstood by the lay public, was developed in 19th-century Germany. *Inneren medizin* was to be distinguished from clinical medicine because it emphasized the physiology and chemistry of disease, not just the patterns or progression of clinical manifestations. *Goldman's Cecil Textbook of Medicine* follows this tradition by showing how pathophysiologic abnormalities cause symptoms and signs and by emphasizing how therapies can modify the underlying pathophysiology and improve the patient's well-being.

Modern medicine has moved rapidly past organ physiology to an increasingly detailed understanding of cellular, subcellular, and genetic mechanisms. For example, the understanding of microbial pathogenesis and many inflammatory diseases (Chapter 264) is now guided by a detailed understanding of the human immune system and its response to foreign antigens (Chapters 44 to 48).

Health, disease, and an individual's interaction with the environment are also substantially determined by genetics. In addition to many conditions that may be determined by a single gene (Chapter 40), medical science increasingly understands the complex interactions that underlie multigenic traits (Chapter 41). In the not-so-distant future, the decoding of the human genome holds the promise that personalized health care can be targeted according to an individual's genetic profile, in terms of screening and presymptomatic disease management, as well as in terms of specific medications and their adjusted dosing schedules. Currently, knowledge of the structure and physical forms of proteins helps explain abnormalities as diverse as sickle cell anemia (Chapter 166) and prion-related diseases (Chapter 424). Proteomics, which is the normal and abnormal protein expression of genes, also holds extraordinary promise for developing drug targets for more specific and effective therapies.

Concurrent with these advances in fundamental human biology has been a dramatic shift in methods for evaluating the application of scientific advances to the individual patient and to populations. The randomized controlled trial, sometimes with thousands of patients at multiple institutions, has replaced anecdote as the preferred method for measuring the benefits and optimal uses of diagnostic and therapeutic interventions (Chapter 9). As studies progress from those that show biologic effect, to those that elucidate dosing schedules and toxicity, and finally to those that assess true clinical benefit, the metrics of measuring outcome has also improved from subjective impressions of physicians or patients to reliable and valid measures of morbidity, quality of life, functional status, and other patient-oriented outcomes (Chapter 10). These marked improvements in the scientific methodology of clinical investigation have expedited extraordinary changes in clinical practice, such as recanalization therapy for acute myocardial infarction (Chapter 73), and have shown that reliance on intermediate outcomes, such as a reduction in asymptomatic ventricular arrhythmias with certain drugs, may unexpectedly increase rather than decrease mortality. Just as physicians in the 21st century must understand advances in fundamental biology, similar understanding of the fundamentals of clinical study design as it applies to diagnostic and therapeutic interventions is needed. An understanding of human genetics will also help stratify and refine the approach to clinical trials by helping researchers select fewer patients with a more homogeneous disease pattern to study the efficacy of an intervention.

This explosion in medical knowledge has led to increasing specialization and subspecialization, defined initially by organ system and more recently by locus of principal activity (inpatient vs. outpatient), reliance on manual skills (proceduralist vs. nonproceduralist), or participation in research. Nevertheless, it is becoming increasingly clear that the same fundamental molecular and genetic mechanisms are broadly applicable across all organ systems and that the scientific methodologies of randomized trials and careful clinical observation span all aspects of medicine.

The advent of modern approaches to managing data now provides the rationale for the use of health information technology. Computerized health records, oftentimes shared with patients in a portable format, can avoid duplication of tests and assure that care is coordinated among the patient's various health care providers.

APPROACH TO THE PATIENT

Patients commonly have complaints (symptoms). These symptoms may or may not be accompanied by abnormalities on examination (signs) or on laboratory testing. Conversely, asymptomatic patients may have signs or laboratory abnormalities, and laboratory abnormalities can occur in the absence of symptoms or signs.

Symptoms and signs commonly define *syndromes,* which may be the common final pathway of a wide range of pathophysiologic alterations. The fundamental basis of internal medicine is that diagnosis should elucidate the pathophysiologic explanation for symptoms and signs so that therapy may improve the underlying abnormality, not just attempt to suppress the abnormal symptoms or signs.

When patients seek care from physicians, they may have manifestations or exacerbations of known conditions, or they may have symptoms and signs that suggest malfunction of a particular organ system. Sometimes the pattern of symptoms and signs is highly suggestive or even pathognomonic for a particular disease process. In these situations, in which the physician is focusing on a particular disease, *Goldman's Cecil Textbook of Medicine* provides scholarly yet practical approaches to the epidemiology, pathobiology, clinical manifestations, diagnosis, treatment, prevention, and prognosis of entities such as acute myocardial infarction (Chapter 73), chronic obstructive lung disease (Chapter 88), obstructive uropathy (Chapter 125), inflammatory bowel disease (Chapter 143), gallstones (Chapter 158), rheumatoid arthritis (Chapter 272), hypothyroidism (Chapter 233), tuberculosis (Chapter 332), and virtually any known medical condition in adults.

Many patients, however, have undiagnosed symptoms, signs, or laboratory abnormalities that cannot be immediately ascribed to a particular disease or cause. Whether the initial manifestation is chest pain (Chapter 50), diarrhea (Chapter 142), neck or back pain (Chapter 407), or a variety of more than 100 common symptoms, signs, or laboratory abnormalities, *Goldman's Cecil Textbook of Medicine* provides tables, figures, and entire chapters to guide the approach to diagnosis and therapy (see E-Table 1-1 or table on inside back cover). By virtue of this dual approach to known disease as well as to undiagnosed abnormalities, this textbook, similar to the modern practice of medicine, applies directly to patients regardless of their mode of manifestation or degree of previous evaluation.

The patient-physician interaction proceeds through many phases of clinical reasoning and decision making. The interaction begins with an elucidation of complaints or concerns, followed by inquiries or evaluations to address these concerns in increasingly precise ways. The process commonly requires a careful history or physical examination, ordering of diagnostic tests, integration of clinical findings with test results, understanding of the risks and benefits of the possible courses of action, and careful consultation with the patient and family to develop future plans. Physicians can increasingly call on a growing literature of evidence-based medicine to guide the process so that benefit is maximized while respecting individual variations in different patients. Throughout *Goldman's Cecil Textbook of Medicine,* the best current evidence is highlighted with specific grade A references that can be accessed directly in the electronic version.

The increasing availability of evidence from randomized trials to guide the approach to diagnosis and therapy should not be equated with "cookbook" medicine. Evidence and the guidelines that are derived from it emphasize proven approaches for patients with specific characteristics. Substantial clinical judgment is required to determine whether the evidence and guidelines apply to individual patients and to recognize the occasional exceptions. Even more judgment is required in the many situations in which evidence is absent or inconclusive. Evidence must also be tempered by patients' preferences, although it is a physician's responsibility to emphasize evidence when presenting alternative options to the patient. The adherence of a patient to a specific regimen is likely to be enhanced if the patient also understands the rationale and evidence behind the recommended option.

To care for a patient as an individual, the physician must understand the patient as a person. This fundamental precept of doctoring includes an understanding of the patient's social situation, family issues, financial concerns, and preferences for different types of care and outcomes, ranging from maximum prolongation of life to the relief of pain and suffering (Chapters 2 and 3). If the physician does not appreciate and address these issues, the science of medicine cannot be applied appropriately, and even the most knowledgeable physician will fail to achieve the desired outcomes.

Even as physicians become increasingly aware of new discoveries, patients can obtain their own information from a variety of sources, some of which are of questionable reliability. The increasing use of alternative and complementary therapies (Chapter 38) is an example of patients' frequent dissatisfaction with prescribed medical therapy. Physicians should keep an open mind regarding unproven options but must advise their patients carefully if such options may carry any degree of potential risk, including the risk that they may be relied on to substitute for proven approaches. It is crucial for the physician to have an open dialogue with the patient and family regarding the full range of options that either may consider.

The physician does not exist in a vacuum, but rather as part of a complicated and extensive system of medical care and public health. In premodern times and even today in some developing countries, basic hygiene, clean water, and adequate nutrition have been the most important ways to promote health and reduce disease. In developed countries, adoption of healthy lifestyles, including better diet (Chapter 220) and appropriate exercise (Chapter 15), is the cornerstone to reducing the epidemics of obesity (Chapter 227), coronary disease (Chapter 70), and diabetes (Chapter 237). Public health interventions to provide immunizations (Chapter 17) and to reduce injuries and the use of tobacco (Chapter 31), illicit drugs (Chapter 33), and excess alcohol (Chapter 32) can collectively produce more health benefits than nearly any other imaginable health intervention.

APPROACH TO THE MEDICAL PROFESSION

In a profession, practitioners put the welfare of clients or patients above their own welfare. Professionals have a duty that may be thought of as a contract with society. The American Board of Internal Medicine and the European Federation of Internal Medicine have jointly proposed that medical

TABLE 1-1 PROFESSIONAL RESPONSIBILITIES
Commitment to:
Professional competence
Honesty with patients
Patient confidentiality
Maintaining appropriate relations with patients
Improving the quality of care
Improving access to care
Just distribution of finite resources
Scientific knowledge
Maintaining trust by managing conflicts of interest
Professional responsibilities

From Brennan T, Blank L, Cohen J, et al. Medical professionalism in the new millennium: a physician charter. *Ann Intern Med.* 2002;1136:243-246.

professionalism should emphasize three fundamental principles: the primacy of patient welfare, patient autonomy, and social justice. As modern medicine brings a plethora of diagnostic and therapeutic options, the interactions of the physician with the patient and society become more complex and potentially fraught with ethical dilemmas (Chapter 2). To help provide a moral compass that is not only grounded in tradition but also adaptable to modern times, the primacy of patient welfare emphasizes the fundamental principle of a profession. The physician's altruism, which begets the patient's trust, must be impervious to the economic, bureaucratic, and political challenges that are faced by the physician and the patient (Chapter 5).

The principle of patient autonomy asserts that physicians make recommendations but patients make the final decisions. The physician is an expert advisor who must inform and empower the patient to base decisions on scientific data and how these data can and should be integrated with a patient's preferences.

The importance of social justice symbolizes that the patient-physician interaction does not exist in a vacuum. The physician has a responsibility to the individual patient and to broader society to promote access and to eliminate disparities in health and health care.

To promote these fundamental principles, a series of professional responsibilities has been suggested (Table 1-1). These specific responsibilities represent practical, daily traits that benefit the physician's own patients and society as a whole. Physicians who use these and other attributes to improve their patients' satisfaction with care are not only promoting professionalism but also reducing their own risk for liability and malpractice.

An interesting new aspect of professionalism is the increasing reliance on team approaches to medical care, as exemplified by physicians whose roles are defined by the location of their practice—historically in the intensive care unit or emergency department and more recently on the inpatient general hospital floor. Quality care requires coordination and effective communication across inpatient and outpatient sites among physicians who themselves now typically work defined hours. This transition from reliance on a single, always available physician to a team, ideally with a designated coordinator, places new challenges on physicians, the medical care system, and the medical profession.

The changing medical care environment is placing increasing emphasis on standards, outcomes, and accountability. As purchasers of insurance become more cognizant of value rather than just cost (Chapter 11), outcomes ranging from rates of screening mammography (Chapter 204) to mortality rates with coronary artery bypass graft surgery (Chapter 74) become metrics by which rational choices can be made. Clinical guidelines and critical pathways derived from randomized controlled trials and evidence-based medicine can potentially lead to more cost-effective care and better outcomes.

These major changes in many Western health care systems bring with them many major risks and concerns. If the concept of limited choice among physicians and health care providers is based on objective measures of quality and outcome, channeling of patients to better providers is one reasonable definition of better selection and enlightened competition. If the limiting of options is based overwhelmingly on cost rather than measures of quality, outcomes, and patient satisfaction, it is likely that the historic relationship between the patient and the truly professional physician will be fundamentally compromised.

Another risk is that the same genetic information that could lead to more effective, personalized medicine will be used against the very people whom it is supposed to benefit—by creating a stigma, raising health insurance costs, or even making someone uninsurable. The ethical approach to medicine

(Chapter 2), genetics, and genetic counseling (Chapter 39) provides means to protect against this adverse effect of scientific progress.

In this new environment, the physician often has a dual responsibility: to the health care system as an expert who helps create standards, measures of outcome, clinical guidelines, and mechanisms to ensure high-quality, cost-effective care and to individual patients who entrust their well-being to that physician to promote their best interests within the reasonable limits of the system. A health insurance system that emphasizes cost-effective care, that gives physicians and health care providers responsibility for the health of a population and the resources required to achieve these goals, that must exist in a competitive environment in which patients can choose alternatives if they are not satisfied with their care, and that places increasing emphasis on health education and prevention can have many positive effects. In this environment, however, physicians must beware of overt and subtle pressures that could entice them to underserve patients and abrogate their professional responsibilities by putting personal financial reward ahead of their patients' welfare. The physician's responsibility to represent the patient's best interests and avoid financial conflicts by doing too little in the newer systems of capitated care provides different specific challenges but an analogous moral dilemma to the historical American system in which the physician could be rewarded financially for doing too much.

In the current health care environment, all physicians and trainees must redouble their commitment to professionalism. At the same time, the challenge to the individual physician to retain and expand the scientific knowledge base and process the vast array of new information is daunting. In this spirit of a profession based on science and caring, *Goldman's Cecil Textbook of Medicine* seeks to be a comprehensive approach to modern internal medicine.

SUGGESTED READINGS

Ioannidis JP. Expectations, validity, and reality in omics. *J Clin Epidemiol.* 2010;63:945-949. *Perspectives on how modern biologic measurements and assays may individualize health care if appropriately validated.*

Mostaghimi A, Crotty BH. Professionalism in the digital age. *Ann Intern Med.* 2011;154:560-562. *Practical commentary.*

Qaseem A, Snow V, Gosfield A, et al. Pay for performance through the lens of medical professionalism. *Ann Intern Med.* 2010;152:366-369. *Explores how these two ideas can coexist successfully.*

Rogers W, Ballantyne A. Towards a practical definition of professional behavior. *J Med Ethics.* 2010;36:250-254. *Emphasizes the importance of responsibility; relationships with and respect for patients; probity and honesty; self awareness, and capacity for reflection.*

2

BIOETHICS IN THE PRACTICE OF MEDICINE

EZEKIEL J. EMANUEL

It commonly is argued that modern advances in medical technology, antibiotics, dialysis, transplantation, and intensive care units have created the bioethical dilemmas that confront physicians in the 21st century. In reality, however, concerns about ethical issues are as old as the practice of medicine itself. The Hippocratic Oath, composed sometime around 400 BC, attests to the need of ancient Greek physicians for advice on how to address the many bioethical dilemmas that they confronted. The Oath addresses issues of confidentiality, abortion, euthanasia, sexual relations between physician and patient, divided loyalties, and, at least implicitly, charity care and executions. Other Hippocratic works address issues such as termination of treatments to dying patients and telling the truth. Whether we agree with the advice dispensed or not, the important point is that many bioethical issues are not created by technology but are inherent in medical practice. Technology may make these issues more common and may change the context in which they arise, but there are underlying bioethical issues that seem timeless, inherent in the practice of medicine.

Many physicians have been educated that four main principles can be invoked to address bioethical dilemmas: autonomy, nonmaleficence, beneficence, and justice. Autonomy is the idea that people should have the right and freedom to choose, pursue, and revise their own life plans. Nonmaleficence is the idea that people should not be harmed or injured knowingly; this

principle is encapsulated in the frequently repeated phrase that a physician has an obligation to "first do no harm"—*primum non nocere.* This phrase is not found either in the Hippocratic Oath or in other Hippocratic writing; the only related, but not identical, Hippocratic phrase is "at least, do not harm." Whereas nonmaleficence is about avoiding harm, beneficence is about the positive actions that the physician should undertake to promote the well-being of his or her patients. In clinical practice, this obligation usually arises from the implicit and explicit commitments and promises surrounding the physician-patient relationship. Finally, there is the principle of justice as the fair distribution of benefits and burdens.

Although helpful in providing an initial framework, these principles have limited value because they are broad and open to diverse and conflicting interpretations. In addition, as is clear with the principle of justice, they frequently are underdeveloped. In any difficult case, the principles are likely to conflict. Conflicting ethical principles are precisely why there are bioethical dilemmas. The principles themselves do not offer guidance on how they should be balanced or specified to resolve the dilemma. These principles, which are focused on the individual physician-patient context, are not particularly helpful when the bioethical issues are institutional and systemic, such as allocating scarce vaccines or organs for transplantation or balancing the risks and benefits of mammograms for women younger than 50 years. Finally, these four principles are not comprehensive. Other fundamental ethical principles and values, such as communal solidarity, duties to future generations, trust, and professional integrity, are important in bioethics but not encapsulated except by deformation in these four principles.

There is no formula or small set of ethical principles that mechanically or magically gives answers to bioethical dilemmas. Instead, medical practitioners should follow an orderly analytic process. First, practitioners need to obtain the facts relevant to the situation. Second, they must delineate the basic bioethical issue. Third, it is important to identify all the crucial principles and values that relate to the case and how they might conflict. Fourth, because many ethical dilemmas have been analyzed previously and subjected frequently to empirical study, practitioners should examine the relevant literature, whether it is commentaries or studies in medical journals, legal cases, or books. With these analyses, the particular dilemma should be reexamined; this process might lead to reformulation of the issue and identification of new values or new understandings of existing values. Fifth, with this information, it is important to distinguish clearly unethical practices from a range of ethically permissible actions. Finally, it is important not only to come to some resolution of the case but also to state clearly the reasons behind the decisions, that is, the interpretation of the principles used and how values were balanced. Although unanimity and consensus may be desirable ideals, reasonable people frequently disagree about how to resolve ethical dilemmas without being unethical or malevolent.

A multitude of bioethical dilemmas arise in medical practice, including issues of genetics, reproductive choices, and termination of care. In clinical practice, the most common issues revolve around informed consent, termination of life-sustaining treatments, euthanasia and physician-assisted suicide, and conflicts of interest.

● PHYSICIAN-PATIENT RELATIONSHIP: INFORMED CONSENT

History

It commonly is thought that the requirement for informed consent is a relatively recent phenomenon. Suggestions about the need for a patient's informed consent can be found as far back as Plato, however. The first recorded legal case involving informed consent is the 1767 English case of *Slater v. Baker and Stapleton,* in which two surgeons refractured a patient's leg after it had healed improperly. The patient claimed they had not obtained consent. The court ruled:

> [I]t appears from the evidence of the surgeon that it was improper to disunite the callous without consent; this is the usage and law of surgeons: then it was ignorance and unskillfulness in that very particular, to do contrary to the rule of the profession, what no surgeon ought to have done.

Although there may be some skepticism about the extent of the information disclosed or the precise nature of the consent obtained, the notable fact is that an 18th-century court declared that obtaining prior consent of the patient is not only the usual practice but also the ethical and legal obligation of surgeons. Failure to obtain consent is incompetent and inexcusable. In contemporary times, the 1957 case of *Salgo v. Leland Stanford Junior University Board of Trustees* constitutes a landmark by stating that physicians have a positive legal obligation to disclose information about risks, benefits, and alternatives to patients; this decision popularized the term *informed consent*.

Definition and Justification

Informed consent is a person's autonomous authorization of a physician to undertake diagnostic or therapeutic interventions for himself or herself. In this view, the patient understands that he or she is taking responsibility for the decision while empowering someone else, the physician, to implement it. Not any agreement to a course of medical treatment qualifies as informed consent, however.

There are four fundamental requirements for valid informed consent: mental capacity, disclosure, understanding, and voluntariness. Informed consent assumes that people have the mental capacity to make decisions; disease, development, or medications can compromise patients' mental capacity to provide informed consent. Adults are presumed to have the legal competence to make medical decisions, and whether an adult is incompetent to make medical decisions is a legal determination. Practically, physicians usually decide whether patients are competent on the basis of whether patients can understand the information disclosed, appreciate its significance for their own situation, and use logical and consistent thought processes in decision making. Incompetence in medical decision making does not mean a person is incompetent in all types of decision making and vice versa. Crucial information relevant to the decision must be disclosed, usually by the physician, to the patient. The patient should understand the information and its implications for his or her interests and life goals. Finally, the patient must make a voluntary decision (i.e., one without coercion or manipulation by the physician). It is a mistake to view informed consent as an event, such as the signing of a form. Informed consent is viewed more accurately as a process that evolves during the course of diagnosis and treatment.

Typically, the patient's autonomy is the value invoked to justify informed consent. Other values, such as bodily integrity and beneficence, have also been cited, especially in early legal rulings.

Empirical Data

Fairly extensive research has been done on informed consent. In general, studies show that in clinical situations, physicians frequently do not communicate all relevant information for informed decision making. In a study of audiotapes from 1057 outpatient encounters, physicians mentioned alternatives in only 11.3% of cases, provided pros and cons of interventions in only 7.8% of situations, and assessed the patient's understanding of the information in only 1.5% of decisions. The more complex the medical decisions, the more likely it was that the elements of informed consent would be fulfilled. Importantly, data suggest that disclosure is better in research settings, both in the informed consent documents and in the discussions. For instance, in recorded interactions between researchers and prospective participants, the major elements of research, such as that the treatment was investigational and the risks and benefits, were disclosed in more than 80% of interactions. Greater disclosure in the research setting may be the consequence of requiring a written informed consent document. Some have suggested that for common medical interventions, such as elective surgery, standardized informed consent documents should include the risks and benefits as quantified in randomized controlled trials, as well as acceptable alternatives.

Patients frequently fail to recall crucial information disclosed, although they usually think they have sufficient information for decision making. Whether patients fail to recall key information because they are overwhelmed by the information or because they do not find much of it salient to their decision is unclear. The issue is what patients understand at the point of decision making, not what they recall later.

Studies aimed at improving informed consent in the clinical setting suggest that interactive media, such as videos, can improve understanding by patients. Conversely, data from the research setting suggest that interactive media do not improve participants' understanding, whereas more personal interaction, whether as an additional telephone call by a research nurse or as an additional face-to-face meeting, does enhance understanding.

One of the most important results of empirical research on informed consent is the gap between information and decision making. Many studies show that most patients want information, but far fewer prefer decision-making authority. One study showed that most patients wanted information, but only about one third desired decision-making authority, and patients' decision-making preferences were not correlated with their information-seeking preferences. Several investigators found that patients' preference for

TABLE 2-1	FUNDAMENTAL ELEMENTS FOR DISCLOSURE TO PATIENTS

Diagnosis and prognosis
Nature of proposed intervention
Reasonable alternative interventions
Risks associated with each alternative intervention
Benefits associated with each alternative intervention
Probable outcomes of each alternative intervention

decision-making authority increases with higher educational levels and declines with advancing age. Most important, the more serious the illness, the more likely patients are to prefer that physicians make the decisions. Several studies suggest that patients who have less of a desire to make their own decisions generally are more satisfied with how the decisions were made.

Practical Considerations

Implementing informed consent raises concerns about the extent of information to be disclosed and exceptions to the general requirement. A major area of ethical and legal disagreement has been what information to disclose and how to disclose it. As a practical matter, physicians should disclose at least six fundamental elements of information to patients: (1) diagnosis and prognosis; (2) nature of the proposed intervention; (3) alternative interventions, including no treatment; (4) risks associated with each alternative; (5) benefits of each alternative; and (6) likely outcomes of these alternatives (Table 2-1). Because risk is usually the key worry of physicians, it generally is recommended that physicians disclose (1) the nature of the risks, (2) their magnitude, (3) the probability that each risk will occur, and (4) when the consequence might occur. Some argue that minor risks need not be disclosed. In general, all serious risks, such as death, paralysis, stroke, or chronic pain, even if rare, should be disclosed, as should common risks.

The central problem is that the physician should provide this detailed information within reasonable time constraints and yet not overwhelm patients with complex information in technical language. The result has been various legal standards defining how much information should be disclosed. The *physician* or *customary* standard, adapted from malpractice law, states that the physician should disclose information "which a reasonable medical practitioner would make under the same or similar circumstances." Conversely, the *reasonable person* or *lay-oriented* standard states that physicians should disclose all information that a "reasonable person in the patient's circumstances would find material to" the medical decision. The physician standard is factual and can be determined empirically, but the patient-oriented standard, which is meant to engage physicians with patients, is hypothetical. Currently, each standard is used by about half the states.

There are exceptions to the requirements of informed consent. In emergency situations, consent can be assumed because patients' interests concentrate on survival and retaining maximal mental and physical functioning; as a result, reasonable persons would want treatment. In some circumstances, physicians may believe the process of informed consent could pose a serious psychological threat. In rare cases, the "therapeutic privilege" promoting a patient's well-being trumps autonomy, but physicians should be wary of invoking this exception too readily.

If patients are deemed incompetent, family members—beginning with spouse, children, parents, siblings, then more distant relatives—usually are selected as surrogates or proxies, although there may be concerns about conflicting interests or knowledge of the patient's wishes. In the relatively rare circumstance in which a patient formally designated a proxy, that person has decision-making authority.

The *substituted judgment* standard states that the proxy should choose what the patient would choose if he or she were competent. The *best interests* standard states that the proxy should choose what is best for the patient. Frequently, it is not clear how the patient would have decided because the situation was not discussed with the patient and he or she left no living will. Similarly, what is best for a patient is controversial because there are usually tradeoffs between quality of life and survival. These problems are exacerbated because a proxy's predictions about a patient's quality of life are poor; proxies tend to underestimate patients' functional status and satisfaction. Similarly, proxy predictions are inaccurate regarding life-sustaining preferences when the patient is mentally incapacitated; families tend to agree with patients less than 70% of the time in deciding whether to provide life-sustaining treatments if the patient became demented, when chance alone would generate agreement in 50% of the cases. Such confusion about how to decide for incapacitated patients can create conflicts among family members or between the family and medical providers. In such circumstances, an ethics consultation may be helpful.

TERMINATION OF MEDICAL INTERVENTIONS

History

Since the start of medicine, it has been viewed as ethical to withhold medical treatments from the terminally ill and "let nature take its course." Hippocrates argued that physicians should "refuse to treat those [patients] who are overmastered by their disease." In the 19th century, prominent American physicians advocated withholding of cathartic and emetic "treatments" from the terminally ill and using ether to ease pain at the end of life. In 1900, editors of *The Lancet* argued that physicians should intervene to ease the pain of death but did not have an obligation to prolong a clearly terminal life. The contemporary debate on terminating care began in 1976 with the *Quinlan* case, in which the New Jersey Supreme Court ruled that patients had a right to refuse life-sustaining interventions on the basis of a right of privacy and that the family could exercise the right for a patient in a persistent vegetative state.

Definition and Justification

It generally is agreed that all patients have a right to refuse medical interventions. Ethically, this right is based on the patient's autonomy and is implied by the doctrine of informed consent. Legally, state courts have cited the right to privacy, right to bodily integrity, or common law to justify the right to refuse medical treatment. In the 1990 *Cruzan* case and in the subsequent physician-assisted suicide cases, the U.S. Supreme Court affirmed that there is a "constitutionally protected right to refuse lifesaving hydration and nutrition." The Court stated that "[A] liberty interest [based on the 14th Amendment] in refusing unwanted medical treatment may be inferred from our prior decisions." All patients have a constitutional and an ethical right to refuse medical interventions. These rulings were the basis of the consistent state and federal court rulings to permit the husband to terminate artificial nutrition and hydration in the *Schiavo* case.

Empirical Data

Data show that termination of medical treatments is now the norm. More than 85% of Americans die without cardiopulmonary resuscitation, and more than 90% of decedents in intensive care units do not receive cardiopulmonary resuscitation. Of decedents in intensive care units, 90% die after the withholding or withdrawal of medical treatments, with an average of 2.6 interventions being withheld or withdrawn per decedent. Since the 1990s, the trend has been to stop medical interventions more frequently.

Despite extensive public support for use of advance care directives and the passage of the Patient Self-Determination Act mandating that health care institutions inform patients of their right to complete such documents, only about 47% of Americans have completed one. Data suggest that over 40% of patients required active decision-making about terminating medical treatments in their final days, yet 70% lack decision-making capacity, thereby emphasizing the importance of advance directives. Efforts to improve completion of advance care directives have generated mixed results. Unfortunately, even successful pilot efforts have not been adopted or easily scaled. A persistent problem has been that even when patients complete advance care directives, the documents frequently are not available, physicians do not know they exist, or they tend to be too general or vague to guide decisions. The widespread use of electronic health records should create the possibility that advance directives will be available whenever the patient presents to a health care provider.

Just as proxies are poor at predicting patients' wishes, data show that physicians are probably even worse at determining patients' preferences for life-sustaining treatments. In many cases, life-sustaining treatments are continued even when patients or their proxies desire them to be stopped; conversely, many physicians discontinue or never begin interventions unilaterally without the knowledge or consent of patients or their surrogate decision makers. These discrepancies emphasize the importance of engaging patients early in their care about treatment preferences.

Practical Considerations

There are many practical considerations in enacting this right (Table 2-2). First, patients have a right to refuse any and all medical interventions, from blood transfusions and antibiotics to respirators, artificial hydration, and

TABLE 2-2	PRACTICAL CONSIDERATIONS IN TERMINATION OF MEDICAL TREATMENTS
PRACTICAL QUESTION	**ANSWER**
Is there a legal right to refuse medical interventions?	Yes. The U.S. Supreme Court declared that competent people have a constitutionally protected right to refuse unwanted medical treatments based on the 14th Amendment.
What interventions can be legally and ethically terminated?	Any and all interventions (including respirators, antibiotics, intravenous or enteral nutrition, and hydration) can be legally and ethically terminated.
Is there a difference between withholding life-sustaining interventions and withdrawing them?	No. The consensus is that there is no important legal or ethical difference between withholding and withdrawing medical interventions. Stopping a treatment once begun is just as ethical as never having started it.
Whose view about terminating life-sustaining interventions prevails if there is a conflict between the patient and family?	The views of a competent adult patient prevail. It is the patient's body and life.
Who decides about terminating life-sustaining interventions if the patient is incompetent?	If the patient appointed a proxy or surrogate decision maker when competent, that person is legally empowered to make decisions about terminating care. If no proxy was appointed, there is a legally designated hierarchy, usually (1) spouse, (2) adult children, (3) parents, (4) siblings, and (5) available relatives.
Are advance care directives legally enforceable?	Yes. As a clear expression of the patient's wishes, they are a constitutionally protected method for patients to exercise their right to refuse medical treatments. In almost all states, clear and explicit oral statements are legally and ethically sufficient for decisions about withholding or withdrawing medical interventions.

nutrition. Although initiation of cardiopulmonary resuscitation was the focus of the early court cases, this issue is viewed best as addressing just one of the many medical interventions that can be stopped or withheld. The attempt to distinguish ordinary from extraordinary or heroic treatments has been unhelpful in determining which treatments may be stopped.

Second, there is no ethical or legal difference between withholding an intervention and withdrawing it. If a respirator or other treatment is started because physicians are uncertain whether a patient would have wanted it, they always can stop it later when information clarifies the patient's wishes. Although physicians and nurses might find stopping a treatment to be more difficult psychologically, withdrawal is ethically and legally permitted—and required—when it is consonant with the patient's wishes.

Third, competent patients have the exclusive right to decide about terminating their own care. If there is a conflict between a competent patient and his or her family, the patient's wishes are to be followed. It is the patient's right to refuse treatment, not the family's right. For incompetent patients, the situation is more complex; if the patients left clear indications of their wishes, whether as explicit oral statements or as written advance care directives, these wishes should be followed. Physicians should not be overly concerned about the precise form patients use to express their wishes; because patients have a constitutional right to refuse treatment, the real concern is whether the wishes are clear and relevant to the situation. If an incompetent patient did not leave explicit indications of his or her wishes or designate a proxy decision maker, the physician should identify a surrogate decision maker and rely on the decision maker's wishes while being cognizant of the potential problems noted.

Fourth, the right to refuse medical treatment does not translate into a right to demand any treatment, especially treatments that have no pathophysiologic rationale, have already failed, or are known to be harmful. Futility has become a justification to permit physicians unilaterally to withhold or withdraw treatments despite the family's requests for treatment. Some states, such as Texas, have enacted futility laws, which prescribe procedures by which

TABLE 2-3 DEFINITIONS OF ASSISTED SUICIDE AND EUTHANASIA

TERM	DEFINITION
Voluntary active euthanasia	Intentional administration of medications or other interventions to cause the patient's death with the patient's informed consent
Involuntary active euthanasia	Intentional administration of medications or other interventions to cause the patient's death when the patient was competent to consent but did not (e.g., the patient may not have been asked)
Nonvoluntary active euthanasia	Intentional administration of medications or other interventions to cause the patient's death when the patient was incompetent and was mentally incapable of consenting (e.g., the patient might have been in a coma)
Passive euthanasia	Withholding or withdrawal of life-sustaining medical treatments from a patient to let him or her die (termination of life-sustaining treatments)
Indirect euthanasia	Administration of narcotics or other medications to relieve pain with the incidental consequence of causing sufficient respiratory depression to result in the patient's death
Physician-assisted suicide	A physician provides medications or other interventions to a patient with the understanding that the patient can use them to commit suicide

physicians can invoke futility either to transfer a patient or to terminate interventions. However, the principle of futility is not easy to implement in medical practice. Initially, some commentators advocated that an intervention was futile when the probability of success was 1% or lower. Although this threshold seems to be based on empirical data, it is a covert value judgment. Because the declaration of futility is meant to justify unilateral determinations by physicians, it generally has been viewed as an inappropriate assertion that undermines physician-patient communication and violates the principle of shared decision making. Similar to the distinction between ordinary and extraordinary, futility is viewed increasingly as more obfuscating than clarifying, and it is being invoked much less often.

ASSISTED SUICIDE AND EUTHANASIA

History

Since Hippocrates, euthanasia and physician-assisted suicide have been controversial issues. In 1905, a bill was introduced into the Ohio legislature to legalize euthanasia; it was defeated. In the mid-1930s, similar bills were introduced and defeated in the British Parliament and the Nebraska legislature. As of 2010, physician-assisted suicide is legal in Oregon and Washington State, based on state-wide public referenda, and euthanasia and physician-assisted suicide are legal in the Netherlands, Belgium, Luxembourg, and Switzerland. Recently, the Montana Supreme Court did not recognize a constitutional right to physician-assisted suicide, but it ruled that the law permitting the termination of life-sustaining treatment protected physicians from prosecution if they helped hasten the death of a consenting, rational, terminally ill patient.

Definition and Justification

The terms *euthanasia* and *physician-assisted suicide* require careful definition (Table 2-3). So-called passive and indirect euthanasia are misnomers and are not instances of euthanasia, and both are deemed ethical and legal.

There are four arguments against permitting euthanasia and physician-assisted suicide. First, Kant and Mill thought that autonomy did not permit the voluntary ending of the conditions necessary for autonomy, and as a result, both philosophers were against voluntary enslavement and suicide. Consequently, the exercise of autonomy cannot include the ending of life because that would mean ending the possibility of exercising autonomy. Second, many dying patients may have pain and suffering because they are not receiving appropriate care, and it is possible that adequate care would relieve much pain and suffering (Chapter 3). Although a few patients still may experience uncontrolled pain and suffering despite optimal end-of-life care, it is unwise to use the condition of these few patients as a justification to permit euthanasia or physician-assisted suicide for any dying patient. Third, there is a clear distinction between intentional ending of a life and termination of life-sustaining treatments. The actual acts are different—injecting a life-ending medication, such as a muscle relaxant, or providing a prescription for one is not the same as removing or refraining from introducing an invasive medical intervention. Finally, adverse consequences of permitting euthanasia and physician-assisted suicide must be considered. There are disturbing reports of involuntary euthanasia in the Netherlands, and many worry about coercion of expensive or burdensome patients to accept euthanasia or physician-assisted suicide. Permitting euthanasia and physician-assisted suicide is likely to lead to further intrusions of lawyers, courts, and legislatures into the physician-patient relationship.

There are four parallel arguments for permitting euthanasia and physician-assisted suicide. First, it is argued that autonomy justifies euthanasia and physician-assisted suicide. To respect autonomy requires permitting individuals to decide when it is better to end their lives by euthanasia or physician-assisted suicide. Second, beneficence—furthering the well-being of individuals—supports permitting euthanasia and physician-assisted suicide. In some cases, living can create more pain and suffering than death; ending a painful life relieves more suffering and produces more good. Just the reassurance of having the option of euthanasia or physician-assisted suicide, even if people do not use it, can provide "psychological insurance" and be beneficial to people. Third, euthanasia and physician-assisted suicide are no different from termination of life-sustaining treatments that are recognized as ethically justified. In both cases, the patient consents to die; in both cases, the physician intends to end the patient's life and takes some action to end the patient's life; and in both cases, the final result is the same: the patient's death. With no difference in the patient's consent, the physician's intention, or the final result, there can be no difference in the ethical justification. Fourth, the supposed slippery slope that would result from permitting euthanasia and physician-assisted suicide is not likely. The idea that permitting euthanasia and physician-assisted suicide would undermine the physician-patient relationship or lead to forced euthanasia is completely speculative and not borne out by the available data.

In its 1997 decisions, the U.S. Supreme Court stated that there is no constitutional right to euthanasia and physician-assisted suicide but that there also is no constitutional prohibition against states legalizing these interventions. Consequently, the legalization of physician-assisted suicide in Oregon and Washington State was constitutional.

Empirical Data

Attitudes and practices related to euthanasia and physician-assisted suicide have been studied extensively. First, surveys indicate that about 60 to 70% of the American and British public support legalizing euthanasia and physician-assisted suicide for terminally ill patients who are suffering intractable pain. However, public support declines significantly for euthanasia and physician-assisted suicide in other circumstances. American and British physicians, however, are much less likely to support euthanasia and physician-assisted suicide, with oncologists, palliative care physicians, and geriatricians among the least supportive. Second, approximately 18 to 25% of American physicians have received requests for euthanasia or physician-assisted suicide; 43 to 63% of oncologists have received requests. Third, multiple studies indicate that less than 5% of American physicians have performed euthanasia or physician-assisted suicide. Among oncologists, 4% have performed euthanasia and 11% have performed physician-assisted suicide during their careers. Fourth, in many cases, the safeguards are violated. One study found that in 54% of euthanasia cases, it was the family who made the request; in 39% of euthanasia and 19% of physician-assisted suicide cases, the patient was depressed; in only half of the cases was the request repeated.

In the Netherlands and Belgium, where euthanasia and physician-assisted suicide are legal, less than 2% of all deaths are by these measures, with 0.4 to 1.8% of all deaths as the result of euthanasia without the patient's consent. In Oregon, about 0.2% of all deaths are by physician-assisted suicide.

Counterintuitively, data indicate that it is not pain that primarily motivates requests for euthanasia or physician-assisted suicide but rather psychological distress, especially depression and hopelessness. Interviews with physicians and with patients with amyotrophic lateral sclerosis, cancer, or infection with human immunodeficiency virus show that pain is not associated with interest in euthanasia or physician-assisted suicide; instead, depression and hopelessness are the strongest predictors of interest. Studies of patients in Australia and the Netherlands confirm the importance of depression in motivating requests for euthanasia. The desire to avoid dependence and loss of dignity are key motivations.

Finally, data from the Netherlands and the United States suggest that there are significant problems in performing euthanasia and physician-assisted suicide. Dutch researchers reported that physician-assisted suicide causes complications in 7% of cases, and in 15% of cases, the patients did not die, awoke from coma, or vomited up the medication. Ultimately, in nearly 20% of physician-assisted suicide cases, the physician ended up injecting the patient with life-ending medication, converting physician-assisted suicide to euthanasia. These data raise serious questions about how to address complications of physician-assisted suicide when euthanasia is illegal or unacceptable.

Practical Considerations

There is widespread agreement that if euthanasia and physician-assisted suicide are used, they should be considered only after all attempts at physical and psychological palliation have failed. A series of safeguards have been developed and embodied in the Oregon and the Dutch procedures, as follows: (1) the patient must be competent and must request euthanasia or physician-assisted suicide repeatedly and voluntarily; (2) the patient must have pain or other suffering that cannot be relieved by optimal palliative interventions; (3) there should be a waiting period to ensure that the patient's desire for euthanasia or physician-assisted suicide is stable and sincere; and (4) the physician should obtain a second opinion from an independent physician. Oregon and Washington State require patients to be terminally ill, whereas the Netherlands, Belgium, and Switzerland have no such requirement. Although there have been some prosecutions in the United States, there have been no convictions—except for Dr. Kevorkian—when physicians and others have participated in euthanasia and physician-assisted suicide.

● FINANCIAL CONFLICTS OF INTEREST

History

Worrying about how payment and fees affect medical decisions is not new. In 1899, a physician reported that more than 60% of surgeons in Chicago were willing to provide a 50% commission to physicians for referring cases. He subsequently argued that in some cases, this fee splitting led to unnecessary surgical procedures. A 1912 study by the American Medical Association confirmed that fee splitting was a common practice. Selling patent medicines and patenting surgical instruments were other forms of financial conflicts of interest thought to discredit physicians a century ago. In the 1990s, the ethics of capitation for physician services and pharmaceutical prescriptions and payments by pharmaceutical and biotechnology companies to clinical researchers raised the issue of financial conflicts of interest.

Definition and Justification

It commonly is argued that physicians have certain primary interests: (1) to promote the well-being of their patients, (2) to advance biomedical research, (3) to educate future physicians, and, more controversially, (4) to promote public health (Table 2-4). Physicians also have other, secondary interests, such as earning income, raising a family, and pursuing avocational interests. These secondary interests are not evil; typically, they are legitimate, even admirable. A conflict of interest occurs when one of these secondary interests compromises pursuit of a primary interest, especially the patient's well-being.

Conflicts of interest are problematic because they can or appear to compromise the integrity of physicians' judgment, compromising the patient's well-being or research integrity. Conflict of interest can induce a physician to do something—perform a procedure, fail to order a test, or distort data—that would not be in a patient's best interest. These conflicts can undermine the

trust of patients and the public, not only in an individual physician but also in the entire medical profession. The appearance of conflicts of interest can be damaging because it is difficult for patients and the public "to determine what motives have influenced a professional decision." The focus is on financial conflicts of interest, not because they are worse than other types of conflicts but because they are more pervasive and more easily identified and regulated compared with other conflicts. Since ancient times, the ethical norm on conflicts has been clear: the physician's primary obligation is to patients' well-being, and a physician's personal financial well-being should not compromise this duty.

Empirical Data

Financial conflicts are not rare. In Florida, it was estimated that nearly 40% of physicians were involved as owners of freestanding facilities to which they referred patients. Studies in the early 1990s consistently showed that self-referring physicians ordered more services, frequently charged more per service, and referred patients with less established indications. In one study, 4 to 4.5 times more imaging examinations were ordered by self-referring physicians than by physicians who referred patients to radiologists. Similarly, patients referred to joint-venture physical therapy facilities have an average of 16 visits compared with 11 at non–joint-venture facilities. Of great concern, licensed physical therapists at joint-venture facilities spent about 28 minutes per patient per visit compared with 48 minutes at non–joint-venture facilities. There are no comparable data on the influence of capitation on physicians' judgment.

Similarly, multiple studies have shown that interaction with pharmaceutical representatives can lead to prescribing of new drugs, nonrational prescribing, and decreased use of generic drugs by physicians. Industry funding for continuing medical education payment for travel to educational symposia increases prescribing of the sponsor's drug.

Regarding researcher conflicts of interest, the available data suggest that corporate funding does not compromise the design and methodology of clinical research; in fact, commercially funded research may be methodologically more rigorous than government- or foundation-supported research. Conversely, data suggest that financial interests do distort researchers' interpretation of data. The most important impact of financial interests, however, appears to be on dissemination of research studies. Growing evidence suggests the suppression or selective publication of data unfavorable to corporate sponsors but the repeated publication of favorable results.

Practical Considerations

First, financial conflicts of interest are inherent in any profession when the professional earns income from rendering a service. Second, conflicts come in many different forms, from legitimate payment for services rendered to investments in medical laboratories and facilities, drug company dinners and payment for attendance at meetings, payment for enrolling patients in clinical research trials, and consultation with companies.

Third, in considering how to manage conflicts, it is important to note that people are poor judges of their own potential conflicts. Individuals often cannot distinguish the various influences that guide their judgments, do not think of themselves as bad, and do not imagine that payment shapes their judgments. Physicians tend to be defensive about charges of conflicts of interest. In addition, conflicts tend to act insidiously, subtly changing practice patterns so that they then become what appear to be justifiable norms.

Fourth, rules—whether laws, regulations, or professional standards—to regulate conflicts of interest are based on two considerations: (1) the likelihood that payment or other secondary interests would create a conflict and (2) the magnitude of the potential harm if there is compromised judgment. Rules tend to be of three types: (1) disclosure of conflicts, (2) management of conflicts, and (3) outright prohibition. Federal law bans certain types of self-referral of physicians in the Medicare program. The American Medical Association and the Pharmaceutical Research and Manufacturers of America have established joint rules that permit physicians to accept gifts of minimal value but "refuse substantial gifts from drug companies, such as the costs of travel, lodging, or other personal expenses . . . for attending conferences or meetings."

Fifth, although there is much emphasis on disclosure of conflicts, which may be useful in publications, it is unclear whether this is a suitable safeguard in the clinical setting. Disclosure just may make patients worry more. Patients may have no context in which to place the disclosure or to evaluate the physician's clinical recommendation, and patients may have few

TABLE 2-4 PRIMARY INTERESTS OF PHYSICIANS
Promotion of the health and well-being of their patients
Advancement of biomedical knowledge through research
Education of future physicians and health care providers
Promotion of the public health

other options in selecting a physician or getting care, especially in an acute situation. Furthermore, self-disclosure often is incomplete, even when required.

Finally, some conflicts can be avoided by a physician's own action. Physicians can refuse to engage in personal investments in medical facilities or to accept gifts from pharmaceutical companies at relatively little personal cost. In other circumstances, the conflicts may be institutionalized, and minimizing them can occur only by changing the way organizations structure reimbursement incentives. Capitation encourages physicians to limit medical services, and its potentially adverse effects are likely to be managed by institutional rules rather than by personal decisions.

FUTURE DIRECTIONS

In the near future, as genetics moves from the research to the clinical setting, practicing physicians are likely to encounter issues surrounding genetic testing, counseling, and treatment. The use of genetic tests without the extensive counseling so common in research studies would alter the nature of the bioethical issues. Because these tests have serious implications for the patient and others, scrupulous attention to informed consent must occur. The bioethical issues raised by genetic tests for somatic cell changes, such as tests that occur commonly in cancer diagnosis and risk stratification, are no different from the issues raised with the use of any laboratory or radiographic test.

In some cases, ethics consultation services may be of assistance in resolving bioethical dilemmas, although current data suggest that consultation services are used mainly for problems that arise in individual cases and are not used for more institutional or policy problems.

SUGGESTED READINGS

Brezis M, Wiist WH. Vulnerability of health to market forces. *Med Care.* 2011;49:232-239. *Explores the tension between capitalism and the goals of social justice and public health.*
Education in Palliative and End-of-life Care. http://www.epec.net; 2010. Accessed March 27, 2011. *Frequently updated website.*
Okike K, Kocher MS, Wei EX, et al. Accuracy of conflict-of-interest disclosures reported by physicians. *N Engl J Med.* 2009;361:1466-1474. *Self-disclosure often is remarkably incomplete.*
Partnership for Caring. http://www.partnershipforcaring.org; 2010. Accessed March 27, 2011. *Frequently updated website.*

3

CARE OF DYING PATIENTS AND THEIR FAMILIES

ROBERT ARNOLD

By 2030, 20% of the U.S. population will be older than 65 years. Owing to successes in public health and medicine, many of these people will live the last years of their lives with chronic medical conditions such as cirrhosis, end-stage kidney disease, heart failure, and dementia. Even human immunodeficiency virus (HIV) and many cancers, once considered terminal, have turned into chronic diseases.

The burden associated with these illnesses is high. Patients report multiple physical and psychological symptoms that lower their quality of life. The economic pressures associated with medical care may adversely affect patients' socioeconomic status and cause family stress. In addition, these chronic illnesses are incurable and often will ultimately contribute to or result in death.

The discipline of palliative care was developed to decrease the burden associated with chronic illness. The recent National Consensus Project defines palliative care as follows:

The goal of palliative care is to prevent and relieve suffering and to support the best possible quality of life for patients and their families. Palliative care is operationalized through effective management of pain and other distressing symptoms, while incorporating psychosocial and spiritual care with consideration of family and patient needs, preferences, values, beliefs, and culture .... Palliative care affirms life by supporting the

patient and family's goals for the future, including their hopes for cure or life-prolongation, as well as their hopes for peace and dignity throughout the course of illness, the dying process, and death.

Four points deserve special emphasis. First, palliative care can be delivered at any time during the course of an illness and is often provided concomitantly with disease-focused, life-prolonging therapy. Waiting until a patient is dying to provide palliative care is a serious error. Prognostication is an inexact science. In addition, although most elderly patients with chronic incurable illnesses are in the last 10 years of their lives, they do not consider themselves to be dying. If palliative care is to have an impact on patients' lives, it should be provided earlier in a patient's illness, in tandem with other treatments.

Second, palliative care primarily focuses on the illness's burden rather than treating the illness itself. Because these burdens can be physical, psychological, spiritual, or social, good palliative care requires a multidisciplinary approach.

Third, palliative care takes the family unit as the central focus of care. Treatment plans must be developed for both the patient and the family.

Finally, palliative care recognizes that medical treatments are not uniformly successful and that patients die. At some point in a patient's illness, the treatments may cause more burden than benefit. Palliative care recognizes this reality and starts with a discussion of the patient's goals and the development of an individualized treatment plan.

Many people confuse palliative care with hospice—an understandable confusion because hospices epitomize the palliative care philosophy. The two, however, are different. In the United States, hospice provides palliative care, primarily at home, for patients who have a life expectancy of 6 months or less and who are willing to forgo life-prolonging treatments. However, the requirement that patients must have a life expectancy of less than 6 months limits hospice's availability because this degree of prognostication is difficult to achieve for many diseases. Moreover, doctors and patients often are unwilling to cease potentially life-prolonging treatments until very late in the disease course, and thus, most patients are not enrolled in hospice until a month before death.

Palliative care, both as a philosophy of care and as a subspecialty, now includes training of medical students and residents. Although every physician should have basic knowledge about palliative care, the creation of the new subspecialty of palliative medicine allows for a growing number of physicians capable of helping with difficult patient issues, educating other physicians, and expanding the knowledge base of palliative care.

PALLIATIVE CARE DOMAINS

Palliative care is a holistic discipline with physical, psychological, spiritual, existential, social, and ethical domains. When caring for patients with chronic life-limiting illness, good palliative care requires that the following questions be addressed:

Is the Patient Physically Comfortable?

Across many chronic conditions, patients have a large number of inadequately treated physical symptoms (Table 3-1). The reasons are multifactorial and range from inadequate physician education, to societal beliefs regarding the inevitability of suffering in chronic illness, to public concerns regarding opioids.

The first step to improve symptom management is a thorough assessment. Standardized instruments such as the Brief Pain Inventory (Fig. 3-1) measure both patients' symptoms and their effect on their lives. Use of standardized instruments assures that physicians will identify overlooked or underreported symptoms and, as a result, will enhance the satisfaction of both the patient and family.

The evidence for the treatment of end-stage symptoms continues to improve. Physicians now can use proven therapies to manage pain (Chapter 29), dyspnea (Chapters 50 and 83), and depression (Chapter 404). The use of nonsteroidal anti-inflammatory agents and opioids can result in effective pain management in more than 75% of patients with cancer. Advances such as intrathecal pumps and neurolytic blocks are helpful in the remaining 25%. Opioids are effective in patients with unrelieved dyspnea, and oxygen is helpful for short-term relief of hypoxemia. Depression can be treated effectively with medications and psychotherapy.

Is the Patient Psychologically Suffering?

Patients may be physically comfortable but still suffering. Psychological symptoms and syndromes such as depression, delirium, and anxiety are common in patients with life-limiting or chronic illnesses. It may be difficult

TABLE 3-1   APPROACHES TO THE MANAGEMENT OF PHYSICAL AND PSYCHOLOGICAL SYMPTOMS

SYMPTOM	ASSESSMENT	TREATMENT
Pain	How severe is the symptom (as assessed with the use of validated instruments) and how does it interfere with the patient's life? What is the etiology of the pain? Is the pain assumed to be neuropathic or somatic? What has the patient used in the past (calculate previous days' equal analgesic dose)?	Prescribe medications to be administered on a standing or regular basis if pain is frequent. For mild pain: use acetaminophen or a nonsteroidal anti-inflammatory agent (see Table 29-3 in Chapter 29). For moderate pain: titrate short-acting opioids (see Table 29-4 in Chapter 29). For severe pain: rapidly titrate short-acting opioids until pain is relieved or intolerable side effects develop; start long-acting opiates once pain is controlled. Rescue doses: prescribe immediate-release opioids—10% of the 24-hour total opiate every hour (orally) or every 30 minutes (parenterally) as needed. Concomitant analgesics (e.g., corticosteroids, anticonvulsants, tricyclic antidepressants, and bisphosphonates) should be used when applicable (particularly for neuropathic pain). Consider alternative medicine and interventional treatments for pain.
Constipation	Is the patient taking opioids? Does the patient have a fecal impaction?	Prescribe laxatives for all patients on opiates. If ineffective, add drugs from multiple classes (e.g., stimulant, osmotic laxatives, and enemas). Prescribe methylnaltrexone if still constipated.
Shortness of breath	Ask the patient to assess the severity of the shortness of breath. Does the symptom have reversible causes?	Prescribe oxygen to treat hypoxia-induced dyspnea, *but* not if the patient is not hypoxic. Opioids relieve breathlessness without measurable reductions in respiratory rate or oxygen saturation; effective doses are often lower than those used to treat pain. Aerosolized opiates do not work. Fans or cool air may work through a branch of the trigeminal nerve. Consider anxiolytics (e.g., low-dose benzodiazepines) and use reassurance, relaxation, distraction, and massage therapy.
Fatigue	Is the patient too tired to do activities of daily living? Is the fatigue secondary to depression? Is a disease process causing the symptom or is it secondary to reversible causes?	Provide cognitive education about conserving energy use. Treat underlying conditions appropriately.
Nausea	Which mechanism is causing the symptom (e.g., stimulation of the chemoreceptor trigger zone, gastric stimulation, delayed gastric emptying or "squashed stomach" syndrome, bowel obstruction, intracranial processes, or vestibular vertigo)? Is the patient constipated?	Prescribe an agent directed at the underlying cause (Chapter 134). If persistent, give antiemetic around the clock. Multiple agents directed at various receptors or mechanisms may be required.
Anorexia and cachexia	Is a disease process causing the symptom, or is it secondary to other symptoms (e.g., nausea and constipation) that can be treated? Is the patient troubled by the symptom or is the family worried about what not eating means?	A nutritionist may help find foods that are more appetizing (Chapter 220). Provide counseling about the prognostic implications of anorexia (Chapter 226).
Delirium	Is the confusion acute, over hours to days? Does consciousness wax and wane? Are there behavioral disturbances, marked by a reduced clarity in the patient's awareness of his environment, e.g., a problem of attention? Does the patient have disorganized thinking? Does the patient have an altered level of consciousness—either agitated or drowsy? Is there a reversible reason for the delirium? **D:** Drugs (opioids, anticholinergics, sedatives, benzodiazepines, steroids, chemotherapies and immunotherapies, some antibiotics) **E:** Eyes and ears (poor vision and hearing, isolation) **L:** Low-flow states (hypoxia, MI, CHF, COPD, shock) **I:** Infections **R:** Retention (urine/stool), Restraints **I:** Intracranial (CNS metastases, seizures, subdural, CVA, hypertensive encephalopathy) **U:** Underhydration, Undernutrition, Undersleep **M:** Metabolic disorders (sodium, glucose, thyroid, hepatic, deficiencies of vitamin B_{12}, folate, niacin, and thiamine) and toxic (lead, manganese, mercury, alcohol)	Identify underlying causes and manage symptoms (Chapter 27). Recommend behavioral therapies, including avoidance of excess stimulation, frequent reorientation, and reassurance. Ensure presence of family caregivers and explain delirium to them. Prescribe haloperidol, risperidone, or olanzapine.
Depression	Are you feeling down, depressed, or hopeless most of the time over the last 2 weeks? Do you find that little brings you pleasure or joy over the last 2 weeks? (Somatic symptoms are not reliable indicators of depression in this population.)	Recommend supportive psychotherapy, cognitive approaches, behavioral techniques, pharmacologic therapies (see Table 404-5 in Chapter 404), or a combination of these interventions; prescribe psychostimulants for rapid treatment of symptoms (within days) or selective serotonin reuptake inhibitors, which may require 3 to 4 weeks to take effect; tricyclic antidepressants are relatively contraindicated because of their side effects.
Anxiety (applicable also for family members)	Does the patient exhibit restlessness, agitation, insomnia, hyperventilation, tachycardia, or excessive worry? Is the patient depressed? Is there a spiritual or existential concern underlying the anxiety?	Recommend supportive counseling and consider prescribing benzodiazepines.
Spiritual distress	Are you at peace?	Inquire about spiritual support.

Modified from Morrison RS, Meier DE. Palliative care. *N Engl J Med.* 2004;350:2582-2590.

STUDY ID# _____   HOSPITAL ID# _____
DO NOT WRITE ABOVE THIS LINE
_____

Brief Pain Inventory (Short Form)

Date: _____/_____/_____   Time: _____

Name: _____   _____   _____
                   Last   First   Middle Initial

1.	Throughout our lives, most of us have had pain from time to time (such as minor headaches, sprains, and toothaches). Have you had pain other than these everyday kinds of pain today?

                    1. Yes   2. No

2.	On the diagram, shade in the areas where you feel pain. Put an X on the area that hurts the most.

Right   Left   Left   Right

3.	Please rate your pain by circling the one number that best describes your pain at its	worst	in the last 24 hours.

     0   1   2   3   4   5   6   7   8   9   10
     No   Pain as bad as
     pain   you can imagine

4.	Please rate your pain by circling the one number that best describes your pain at its	least	in the last 24 hours.

     0   1   2   3   4   5   6   7   8   9   10
     No   Pain as bad as
     pain   you can imagine

5.	Please rate your pain by circling the one number that best describes your pain on the	average.

     0   1   2   3   4   5   6   7   8   9   10
     No   Pain as bad as
     pain   you can imagine

6.	Please rate your pain by circling the one number that tells how much pain you have	right now.

     0   1   2   3   4   5   6   7   8   9   10
     No   Pain as bad as
     pain   you can imagine

FIGURE 3-1. Brief Pain Inventory (short form). (Copyright 1991. Charles S. Cleeland, PhD, Pain Research Group. All rights reserved.)

Continued

to determine whether increased morbidity and mortality are caused by the illness's physical effects or by the psychological effects of depression and anxiety on energy, appetite, or sleep. Screening questions focusing on mood (e.g., "Have you felt down, depressed, and hopeless most of the time for the last 2 weeks?") and anhedonism (e.g., "Have you found little brings you pleasure or joy in the last 2 weeks?") have been shown to help in diagnosing depression in this population.

For patients and families facing mortality, existential and spiritual concerns are common. Progressive illness often raises questions of love, legacy, loss, and meaning. A physician's role is not to answer these questions or to provide reassurance, but rather to understand the patient's concerns, how the patient is coping, and what resources might be of help. Spirituality often is a source of comfort, and physicians can screen regarding a patient's beliefs using a brief instrument such as the FICA spiritual assessment tool (Table 3-2). A single

7. What treatments or medications are you receiving for your pain?

_____

8. In the last 24 hours, how much relief have pain treatments or medications provided? Please circle the one percentage that most shows how much relief you have received.

0% No pain	10%	20%	30%	40%	50%	60%	70%	80%	90%	100% Complete relief

9. Circle one number that describes how, during the past 24 hours, pain has interfered with your:

A. General Activity

0 Does not interfere	1	2	3	4	5	6	7	8	9	10 Completely interferes

B. Mood

0 Does not interfere	1	2	3	4	5	6	7	8	9	10 Completely interferes

C. Walking Ability

0 Does not interfere	1	2	3	4	5	6	7	8	9	10 Completely interferes

D. Normal Work (includes both work outside the home and housework)

0 Does not interfere	1	2	3	4	5	6	7	8	9	10 Completely interferes

E. Relations with Other People

0 Does not interfere	1	2	3	4	5	6	7	8	9	10 Completely interferes

F. Sleep

0 Does not interfere	1	2	3	4	5	6	7	8	9	10 Completely interferes

G. Enjoyment of Life

0 Does not interfere	1	2	3	4	5	6	7	8	9	10 Completely interferes

FIGURE 3-1, cont'd.

screening question, such as "Are you at peace?," may identify patients who are in spiritual distress and facilitate referrals to hospital chaplains.

Is the Family Suffering?

Families are an important source of support for most patients. Families provide informal care-giving, often at the expense of their own physical, economic, and psychological health. Good palliative care requires an understanding of how the family is coping and a search for ways to provide family members with the social or clinical resources they need to improve their well-being. Comprehensive and individually targeted interventions can reduce caregivers' burdens, although the absolute benefits are relatively small.∎

Because patients in palliative care often die, the palliative care team must address bereavement. A letter of condolence or a follow-up phone call to the next of kin after a patient's death is respectful and offers the opportunity to clarify questions about the patient's care. Some family members suffer from complicated grief—a recently described syndrome associated with separation and traumatic distress, with symptoms persisting for more than 6 months. Primary care physicians, who have ongoing relationships with the loved one, and hospices, which provide bereavement services for a year after the patient's death, have the opportunity to assess whether the grief symptoms persist or worsen.

Is the Patient's Care Consistent with the Patient's Goals?

The sine qua non for palliative care is ensuring that the treatment plan is consistent with the patient's values. Most elderly, seriously ill patients are not focused on living as long as possible. Instead, they want to maintain a sense

TABLE 3-2 FICA SPIRITUAL ASSESSMENT TOOL

F—What is your **faith**/religion? Do you consider yourself a religious or spiritual person? What do you believe in that gives meaning/importance to life?

I—**Importance** and **influence** of faith. Is your faith/religion important to you? How do your beliefs influence how you take care of yourself? What are your most important hopes? What role do your beliefs play in regaining your health? What makes life most worth living for you? How might your disease affect this?

C—Are you part of a religious or spiritual **community**? Is this of support to you, and how? Is there a person you really love or is very important to you? How is your family handling your illness? What are their reactions/expectations?

A—How would you like me to **address** these issues in your health care? What might be left undone if you were to die today? Given the severity or chronicity of your illness, what is most important for you to achieve? Would you like me to talk to someone about religious/spiritual matters?

From Puchalski C, Romer A. Taking a spiritual history. *J Palliat Med.* 2000;3:129-137.

TABLE 3-3 CORE COMMUNICATION SKILLS

RECOMMENDED SKILL	EXAMPLE
A. IDENTIFYING CONCERNS AND RECOGNIZING CUES	
Elicit Concerns	
Open-ended questions	"Is there anything you wanted to talk to me about today?"
Active listening	Allowing patient to speak without interruption; allowing pauses to encourage patient to speak
Recognize Cues	
Informational concerns	Patient: "I'm not sure about the treatment options"
Emotional concerns	Patient: "I'm worried about that"
B. RESPONDING TO INFORMATIONAL CONCERNS	
"Ask-tell-ask"	Topic: communicating information about cancer stage
Ask	"Have any of the other doctors talked about what stage this cancer is?"
Tell	"That's right, this is a stage IV cancer, which is also called metastatic cancer…."
Ask	"Do you have questions about the staging?"
C. RESPONDING TO EMOTIONAL CONCERNS	
Nonverbal Empathy: S-O-L-E-R	
S	Face the patient **S**quarely
O	Adopt an **O**pen body posture
L	**L**ean toward the patient
E	Use **E**ye contact
R	Maintain a **R**elaxed body posture
Verbal Empathy: N-U-R-S-E	
N	**N**ame the emotion: "You seem worried"
U	**U**nderstand the emotion: "I see why you are concerned about this"
R	**R**espect the emotion: "You have shown a lot of strength"
S	**S**upport the patient: "I want you to know that I will still be your doctor whether you have chemotherapy or not"
E	**E**xplore the emotion: "Tell me more about what is worrying you"

From Back AL, Arnold RM, Tulsky JA. *Discussing Prognosis.* Alexandria, VA: American Society of Clinical Oncology; 2008.

of control, relieve their symptoms, improve their quality of life, avoid being a burden on their families, and have a closer relationship with their loved ones.

Ensuring that treatment is consistent with a patient's goals requires good communication skills (Table 3-3). The approaches to giving bad news, discussing goals of care, and talking about forgoing life-sustaining treatment have similar structures (Fig. 3-2). First, the patient needs to understand the basic facts about the diagnosis, possible treatments, and prognosis. The communication skill that helps physicians communicate information is *Ask-Tell-Ask*—exploring what the patient knows or wants to know, then explaining or answering questions, and then providing an opportunity for the patient to ask more. In the hospital, where discontinuity of care is common and misunderstandings frequent, it is important to determine what the patient knows before providing information so as to keep everyone well coordinated. When giving bad news, knowing what the patient knows allows the physician to anticipate the patient's reaction. Finally, information must be titrated based on the patient's preferences. Although most patients want to hear everything about their disease, a minority do not. There is no foolproof way to ascertain what any patient wants to know other than by asking.

When giving patients information, it is important to give small pieces of information, not use jargon, and check the patient's understanding. Giving information is like dosing a medication: one gives information, checks understanding, and then gives more information based on what the patient has heard.

After ensuring that the doctor and the patient have a shared understanding of the medical facts, the physician should engage in an open-ended conversation about the patient's goals as the disease progresses. This strategy requires that the patient be asked about both hopes and fears. One might ask: "What makes life worth living for you?" "If your time is limited, what are the things that are most important to achieve?" "What are your biggest fears or concerns?" "What would you consider to be a fate worse than death?" The clinician can use an understanding of these goals to make recommendations about which treatments to provide and which treatments would not be helpful. As a result, early palliative care can improve quality of life, mood, and even survival.[2]

Physicians find talking about prognosis particularly difficult for two reasons: first, it is hard to foretell the future accurately; and second, they fear this information will "take away patients' hope." Thus, they often avoid talking to patients about these issues unless specifically asked. Although some patients do not want to hear prognostic information, for many patients, this information helps them plan their lives. Given that one cannot guess how much information to provide, a physician can start these conversations by asking, "Are you the kind of person who wants to hear about what might happen in the future with your illness or would you rather take it day by day?" If the patient requests the latter, the physician can follow up by asking if there is someone else with whom he or she can talk about the prognosis. Second, before giving prognostic information, it is useful to inquire about the patient's concerns in order to provide information in the most useful manner. Finally, it is appropriate when discussing prognostic information to acknowledge uncertainty: "The course of this cancer can be quite unpredictable, and physicians don't have a crystal ball. I think you should be aware of the possibility that your health may deteriorate quickly, and you should plan accordingly. We probably are dealing with weeks to months, although some patients do better, and some do worse. Over time, the course may become clearer, and if you wish, I may be able to be a little more precise about what we are facing."

The physician must discuss these topics in an empathic way. Palliative care conversations are as much about emotions as facts. Talking about disease progression or death may elicit negative emotions such as anxiety, sadness, or frustration. These emotions decrease a patient's quality of life and interfere with the ability to hear factual information. Empathic responses strengthen the patient-physician relationship, increase the patient's satisfaction, and make the patient more likely to disclose other concerns. The first step is recognizing when the patient is expressing emotions. Once the physician recognizes the emotion being expressed, he or she can respond empathically.

It is also important for physicians to recognize their own emotional reactions to these conversations. The physician's emotional reactions color impressions of the patient's prognosis, thereby making it hard to listen to the patient, and may influence the physician to hedge bad news. The physician should become aware of her or his own emotional reactions to ensure that the conversation focuses on the patient rather than the health care provider's needs.

In addition to good communication skills, palliative care requires a basic knowledge of medical ethics and the law. For example, patients have the moral and legal right to refuse any treatment, even if refusal results in their death. There is no legal difference between withholding and withdrawing life-sustaining treatment. When confronted with areas of ambiguity, the physician should know how to obtain either a palliative care or ethics consultation.

Establishing Goals of Medical Care	Communicating Bad News	Withdrawing Treatment

Create the right setting: plan what to say, allow adequate time, and determine who else should be present at the meeting

Establish what the patient knows: clarify the situation and context in which the discussion about goals is occurring	Establish what the patient knows: clarify what the patient can comprehend, reschedule the talk if necessary	Establish and review the goals of care
Establish what the patient is hoping to accomplish: help distinguish between realistic and unrealistic goals	Establish how much the patient wants to know: recognize and support preferences; people handle information in different ways	Establish the context of the current discussion: discuss what has changed to precipitate the discussion
Suggest realistic goals: explore how goals can be achieved and work through unrealistic expectations	Share the information: avoid jargon, pause frequently, check for understanding, use silence; do not minimize the information	Discuss specific treatment in the context of the goals of care: talk about whether the treatment will meet the goals of care
		Discuss alternatives to the proposed treatment: talk about what will happen if the patient decides not to have the treatment

Respond empathetically to feelings: be prepared for strong emotions and allow time for response, listen, encourage description of feelings, allow silence

Make a plan and follow through: discuss which treatments will be undertaken to meet the goals, establish a concrete plan for follow-up, review and revise the plan periodically as needed	Follow-up: plan for next steps, discuss potential sources of support, share contact information, assess the patient's safety and support, repeat news of future visits	Plan for the end of treatment: document a plan for withdrawal of treatment and give it to the patient, the patient's family, and members of the health care team

FIGURE 3-2. A model for discussing different palliative care topics. Protocols for Communicating with Patients about Major Topics in Palliative Care. (Adapted from the EPEC Project: Education on Palliative and End-of-Life Care. Cited in Morrison, RS, Meier DE. Palliative care. *N Engl J Med.* 2004; 350:2582-2590; accessed January 4, 2010 from http://www.epec.net.)

During the past 10 years, there has been a societal push to encourage patients to designate health care proxies and to create advance care planning documents, typified by the use of living wills. These documents are meant to protect patients against unwanted treatments and to ensure that as they are dying, their wishes are followed. Unfortunately, there are few empirical data showing that these documents actually change practice. Still, discussions of the documents with health professionals and family members generally provoke important conversations about end-of-life care decisions and may help assuage the family in that they are respecting their loved one's wishes.

Is the Patient Going to Die in the Location of Choice?

Most patients say that they want to die at home. Unfortunately, most patients die in institutions—either hospitals or nursing homes. Good palliative care requires establishing a regular system of communication to minimize transitional errors. A social worker who knows about community resources is important in the development of a dispositional plan that respects the patient's goals.

Hospice programs are an important way to allow patients to die at home. In the United States, *hospice* refers to a specific, government-regulated form of end-of-life care, available under Medicare since 1982 but subsequently adopted by Medicaid and many other third-party insurers. Hospice care

typically is given at home, a nursing home, or specialized acute care unit. Care is provided by an interdisciplinary team, which usually includes a physician, nurse, social worker, chaplain, volunteers, bereavement coordinator, and home health aides, all of whom collaborate with the primary care physician, patient, and family. Bereavement services are offered to the family for a year after the death.

Hospices are paid on a per diem rate and are required to cover all the costs related to the patient's life-limiting illness. Because of this and the fact their focus is on comfort rather than life prolongation, many hospices will not cover expensive treatments such as inotropic agents in heart failure or chemotherapy in cancer, even if they have a palliative effect. This may be one of the reasons doctors are hesitant to refer patients until very late in a patient's course, and patients and families equate hospice with dying. Many hospices are experimenting with different service models in an attempt to enroll patients earlier in the course of their illness and increase access to their services.

1. Lorenz KA, Lynn J, Dy SM, et al. Evidence for improving palliative care at the end of life: a systematic review. *Ann Intern Med.* 2008;148:147-159.

2. Temel JS, Greer JA, Muzikansky A, et al. Early palliative care for patients with metastatic non-small-cell lung cancer. *N Engl J Med.* 2010;363:733-742.

SUGGESTED READINGS

End of Life/Palliative Education Resource Center. http://www.eperc.mcw.edu. Accessed March 27, 2011. *Peer-reviewed instructional and evaluation materials on end-of-life care, core resources for educators, and opportunities for training and funding.*

Kane RL. Finding the right level of posthospital care: "We didn't realize there was any other option for him." *JAMA.* 2011;305:284-293. *Review.*

Pallimed. A hospice and palliative medicine blog. http://www.pallimed.org. Accessed March 27, 2011. *Reviews recent scientific articles and promotes discussion of public policy. See also http://www.eperc.mcw.edu/ for short reviews of key topics.*

Silveira MJ, Kim SY, Langa KM. Advance directives and outcomes of surrogate decision making before death. *N Engl J Med.* 2010;362:1211-1218. *Advanced directives usually result in patients' receiving desired care.*

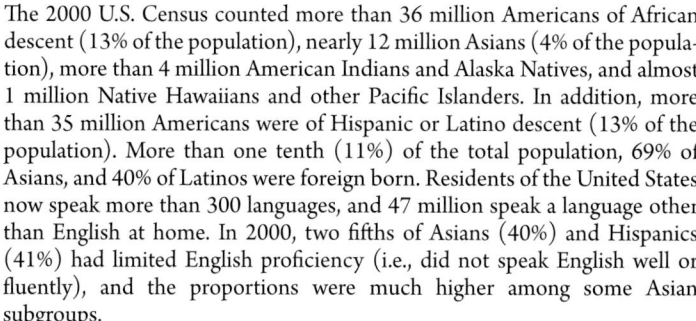

4

CULTURAL CONTEXT OF MEDICINE

VICTORIA M. TAYLOR

TABLE 4-1	HEALTH INSURANCE COVERAGE AMONG ADULTS AGED 18 YEARS AND OLDER BY RACE/ETHNICITY—CALIFORNIA
RACE/ETHNICITY	**CURRENTLY UNINSURED, % (95% CI)**
White	9.6 (9.0-10.3)
Black	13.0 (10.9-15.5)
American Indian/Alaska Native	18.9 (14.6-24.2)
Asian American	15.0 (13.5-16.7)
Chinese	12.3 (10.1-14.7)
Filipino	11.6 (8.4-15.7)
Korean	33.6 (28.6-39.1)
South Asian	11.9 (8.0-17.4)
Vietnamese	17.9 (13.8-22.8)
Latino	28.6 (27.1-30.1)
Foreign-born	36.1 (34.1-38.0)
U.S.-born	14.3 (12.6-16.1)
Mexican	28.7 (27.1-30.3)
Central American	33.2 (28.5-38.3)
Other Latino	21.3 (17.3-26.0)

CI = confidence interval.
From Holtby S, Zahnd E, Chia YJ, et al. *Health of California's Adults, Adolescents, and Children: Findings from CHIS 2005 and CHIS 2003.* Los Angeles: UCLA Center for Health Policy Research; 2008.

The 2000 U.S. Census counted more than 36 million Americans of African descent (13% of the population), nearly 12 million Asians (4% of the population), more than 4 million American Indians and Alaska Natives, and almost 1 million Native Hawaiians and other Pacific Islanders. In addition, more than 35 million Americans were of Hispanic or Latino descent (13% of the population). More than one tenth (11%) of the total population, 69% of Asians, and 40% of Latinos were foreign born. Residents of the United States now speak more than 300 languages, and 47 million speak a language other than English at home. In 2000, two fifths of Asians (40%) and Hispanics (41%) had limited English proficiency (i.e., did not speak English well or fluently), and the proportions were much higher among some Asian subgroups.

During the past two decades, a large body of literature has documented substantial disparities in health status, some based on socioeconomic status (Chapter 5), but many based on race, ethnicity, or other characteristics. For example, black men have a substantially higher age-adjusted prostate cancer incidence rate than do white men (240 per 100,000 versus 153 per 100,000). Mexican Americans and American Indians are more than twice as likely as non-Latino whites of a similar age to have diabetes. Compared with the general population, chronic hepatitis B infection is 25 to 75 times more common among Samoans and among immigrants from Cambodia, Laos, and Vietnam. Studies have documented high rates of suicidal behavior among gays and lesbians compared with heterosexuals. A major goal of Healthy People 2010 was to eliminate health differences among population subgroups for preventable and treatable conditions such as cancer, cardiovascular disease, diabetes, human immunodeficiency virus infection, and acquired immunodeficiency syndrome, among others.

Culture can be defined as a shared system of values, beliefs, and patterns of behavior, and it is not simply defined by race and ethnicity. Culture can also be shaped by factors such as country and region of origin, acculturation, language, religion, and sexual orientation. For instance, the black population of the northeastern United States includes individuals who moved from southern states decades ago as well as recent immigrants from Ethiopia. As the United States population becomes increasingly diverse and as pronounced differences in health status continue to be documented, consideration of the cultural context of medicine is becoming a national priority.

DISPARITIES IN HEALTH CARE ACCESS AND QUALITY

Components of health care access include the ability to get into the health care system as well as to obtain appropriate care once in the system. The availability of health care providers who meet an individual patient's needs is another key component of access to care. Quality care is based on scientific evidence (i.e., is effective), avoids injury to the patient (i.e., is safe), minimizes harmful delays (i.e., is timely), is responsive to the individual patient's needs (i.e., is patient centered), does not vary because of personal characteristics (i.e., is equitable), and avoids waste (i.e., is efficient) (Chapter 11).

Access and Communication

Racial and ethnic minority groups, particularly Latinos, are disproportionately represented among those with health care access problems. The proportions of Latinos who lack health insurance and have no regular source of medical care are more than twice the proportions among non-Latino whites (Table 4-1). Latinos are significantly more likely to report problems in obtaining health care for illness or injury, as well as referrals for specialist care, than are non-Latino whites, even after differences in education, income, and insurance coverage are taken into account. Black heterosexual women have significantly higher levels of health insurance coverage than do black lesbian or bisexual women.

Communication between patients and physicians is more of a problem among members of racial and ethnic minority groups than among whites. In one survey, 33% of Latinos, 27% of Asians, 23% of blacks, and 16% of whites reported one or more of the following problems with communication: the doctor did not listen to everything they said, they did not fully understand the doctor, or they had questions that they did not ask during the visit. In addition, Latinos who spoke Spanish as their primary language (43%) were more likely to have one or more communication problems than were those who spoke English as their primary language (26%).

Blacks (23%) and Latinos (26%) are far less likely than whites (82%) to have regular physicians of their own race and ethnicity. Research has shown that racial concordance between physicians and patients can improve the processes and outcomes of care. For instance, patients in race-concordant relationships with their physician rate his or her decision-making style as significantly more participatory and inclusive than do patients in race-discordant relationships. Furthermore, race-concordant office visits last significantly longer than do race-discordant visits.

Quality of Health Care

National surveys confirm population-level disparities in the quality of both preventive care and the management of chronic disease. American Indians/Alaska Natives and Latinos aged 50 years and older are far less likely to receive interval screening for colorectal cancer (Chapter 199) than are members of other racial/ethnic groups (Table 4-2). Compared with white diabetic adults, black and Latino adults with diabetes are more than 30% less likely to receive recommended preventive and screening services (Chapter 236) and are still less likely to receive them after adjustment for insurance coverage.

Racial and ethnic disparities exist in such specific clinical situations as the prescription of analgesia for pain control (blacks receive less pain medication than whites for extremity fractures), the surgical treatment of cancer (blacks are less likely than whites to receive potentially curative surgery for stage I or stage II non–small cell lung cancer), and the management of end-stage renal disease (blacks are less likely to be entered on the transplant list than are whites). Moreover, disparities in the quality of care are consistently found even when variations in such factors as insurance status, income, age, and comorbid conditions are taken into account.

Disparities in health care quality exist even in systems that are generally believed to provide equal access. For example, in Veterans Health Administration facilities, black patients who were ideal candidates to receive thrombolytic therapy (Chapter 73) on arrival were less likely to receive it than comparable white patients. Black patients were also significantly less likely to have coronary artery bypass graft surgery during their index hospitalization or within 90 days after a myocardial infarction even after adjustment for clinical characteristics and differences in patients' preferences. Similarly, of Medicare-managed care plans, black patients were less likely than white patients to receive diabetic retinal examination, post-infarction β-blockers, and post-hospitalization follow-up for mental illness after adjustment for clinical characteristics and for clustering within health plans.

CULTURAL COMPETENCE IN HEALTH CARE

Health disparities can be reduced or perhaps even eliminated by maintaining culturally competent health care systems. Cultural competence may be defined as a set of congruent attitudes, behaviors, and policies that come together both among professionals and within systems to enable effective work in cross-cultural situations (Fig. 4-1). Ongoing efforts to improve cultural competence in the U.S. health care system target organizational, structural, and clinical barriers. These initiatives aim to close gaps in health status, to decrease differences in the quality of care, to enhance patients' satisfaction, and to increase patients' trust.

Organizational Barriers and Interventions

Racial and ethnic minority physicians are more likely than their white colleagues to work in medically underserved communities. Moreover, they have a better understanding of barriers to health care (such as office hours that do not match community work patterns, bureaucratic intake processes that create fear of deportation among the undocumented, and long waiting times to get an appointment and, after arrival, to keep an appointment). Finally, minority physicians bring a nuanced awareness of the needs of diverse groups of patients and share it through the critical avenues of role modeling and teaching. However, only 6% of practicing physicians are black, Native American, or Latino, and only 15% of medical school applicants are from one of these groups.

Most (approximately two thirds) patients who receive care at federally funded community health centers in medically underserved areas are members of racial and ethnic minority groups. Further, the proportion of community health center patients who have limited English proficiency is 30% and has grown rapidly since 2000. The community health center model has proved effective not only in increasing access to care but also in improving continuity of care and health outcomes. For example, one study found that medically underserved communities with federally qualifying community health centers had 5.8 fewer preventable hospitalizations per 1000 population over 3 years than did similar communities without health centers. Consequently, ongoing efforts to increase the capacity of community health centers are likely to help reduce health disparities.

Structural Barriers and Interventions

The Department of Health and Human Services has created standards on culturally and linguistically appropriate interpreter services to guide

TABLE 4-2 COLORECTAL CANCER SCREENING LEVELS AMONG INDIVIDUALS AGED 50 YEARS AND OLDER BY RACE/ETHNICITY—UNITED STATES, 2006	
RACE/ETHNICITY	**FOBT LAST YEAR OR LOWER ENDOSCOPY LAST 10 YEARS % (95% CI)**
White	62.6 (62.1-63.0)
Black	59.0 (57.3-60.6)
American Indian/Alaska Native	48.4 (43.5-53.2)
Asian American/Pacific Islander	55.9 (51.0-60.7)
Latino	47.2 (44.5-49.9)

FOBT = fecal occult blood testing.
From Joseph DA, Rim SH, Seeff LC. Use of colorectal cancer tests—United States, 2002, 2004, and 2006. *MMWR Morb Mortal Wkly Rep.* 2008;57:253-258.

FIGURE 4-1. Analytic framework for evaluating the effectiveness of health care interventions to increase cultural competence. (From Anderson LM, Scrimshaw SC, Fullilove MT, et al, for the Task Force on Community Preventive Services. Culturally competent healthcare systems: a systemic review. *Am J Prev Med.* 2003;24[Suppl]:68-79).

providers. However, interpreter services often remain ad hoc, with family members and untrained nonclinical employees acting as interpreters. Use of ad hoc services has potentially negative clinical consequences, including breach of the patient's confidentiality and inaccurate communication. One major obstacle to the implementation of professional interpreter programs is a lack of reimbursement; Medicare and most private insurers do not pay for interpretation and related services (such as translation or telephone language lines), and only a few states currently pay for interpretation under Medicaid.

Accumulating evidence suggests that trained professional interpreters and bilingual providers can have a positive impact on the satisfaction of patients and quality of care among individuals with limited English proficiency. For example, in a health maintenance organization, the introduction of professional interpreter services for Portuguese- and Spanish-speaking patients increased their use of recommended preventive services, office visits, and number of prescriptions written and filled.

Assistance with "navigation" represents one promising model to enable racial and ethnic minority patients to move through the health system effectively and to be actively involved in decision making about their medical care. Navigator programs rely on personal guides to shepherd disadvantaged patients with chronic diseases into standard care. Guides help patients and their families navigate the treatment process, steering them around obstacles that may limit their access to quality care. For example, guides (who may be nurses, social workers, or volunteers who are familiar with the health care system) help patients choose doctors and assess treatment options. Currently, three major navigation programs (the National Cancer Institute, American Cancer Society, and Center for Medicare and Medicaid Services) are under way to address the needs of medically underserved cancer patients.

Community health workers are increasingly being used in attempts to close the gap in health care among various racial and ethnic minority populations. In general, community health workers live locally and share the language and culture of the population of patients served. Lay community health workers have several core functions; they provide cultural mediation between communities and the health care system, provide culturally appropriate and accessible health education and information, help people obtain the medical services they need, provide informal counseling and social support, and advocate for individuals within the health care system. The largest system formally to use the skills of community health workers is the Indian Health Service, which currently has about 1400 community health representatives who work with tribally managed or Indian Health Service programs in more than 550 American Indian/Alaska Native nations.

Evidence for the effectiveness of community health workers is provided by the breast and cervical cancer screening literature. For example, Vietnamese American women randomized to receive lay health worker group education are significantly more likely to obtain Papanicolaou tests than are women who do not.[1,2]

Clinical Barriers and Interventions

Patients who are members of racial and ethnic minority groups often have an understanding of health and disease (i.e., explanatory model) that differs from that of the general population. For example, many Vietnamese people believe that disease is caused by an imbalance of the humoral forces of yin and yang. When ill, they commonly use Chinese herbal medicine as well as indigenous folk practices known as Southern medicine in an effort to restore the balance of humoral forces. In addition, Vietnamese patients may think that Western medicine is too strong and will upset the internal balance. Consequently, a hypertensive patient, for example, may use Chinese herbal medicines (Chapter 38) instead of prescribed antihypertensive medication. Alternatively, the patient may take a lower dose of medication than prescribed by his or her physician.

Cultural competency training for health care providers generally includes some balance of cross-cultural knowledge and communication skills, taught while avoiding stereotypes. Examples include the effect of prejudice on gays and lesbians and how this prejudice shapes their interactions with the health care system, and common spiritual practices that might interfere with prescribed therapies (such as Ramadan fasting practices, when observed by diabetic Muslim patients). Communication skills that can be addressed in cultural competence training include approaches to eliciting patients' explanatory models and use of traditional treatments as well as methods for negotiating different styles of communication and levels of family participation in decision making. Overall, there is good evidence that cultural competency

training improves the attitudes and skills of health professionals as well as patient satisfaction, but less evidence that it improves clinical outcomes.[3]

Training in cultural diversity has recently become part of medical school curricula, often by "weaving" multiculturalism into the curriculum rather than teaching it as a separate course. Program components may include home visits that allow students to hear patients' stories of illness and treatment (and learn about patient-centered care) as well as discussions of clinical cases that allow students to explore issues related to health disparities, health care access, and unequal treatment.

● SUMMARY

The average life expectancy of Americans increased by more than 30 years between 1900 and 2000. However, some groups have not fully benefited from the medical and public health achievements of the last century. Although there are demonstrated correlations between racial and ethnic background and socioeconomic status (Chapter 5), poverty alone cannot explain all the gaps in health and health care that exist between minorities and whites. Although the disparities were first documented in blacks in the United States, a growing body of evidence indicates that Latinos and other racial/ethnic minority groups, as well as gays, lesbians, and bisexuals, also experience significant problems with health care access and quality, especially when their English is not proficient.

Efforts to improve cultural competence in health care, whether they are used alone or in conjunction with socioeconomic initiatives (Chapter 5), are likely to play a significant role in reducing health disparities across population subgroups. The dissemination of successful interventions through linkages with payers, policymakers, provider groups, community organizations, and the media will be critical.

Grade A

1. Mock J, McPhee SJ, Nguyen T, et al. Effective lay health worker outreach and media-based education for promoting cervical cancer screening among Vietnamese American women. *Am J Public Health.* 2007;97:1693-1700.
2. Taylor VM, Jackson JC, Yasui Y, et al. Evaluation of a cervical cancer control intervention using lay health workers for Vietnamese American women. *Am J Public Health.* 2010;100:1924-1929.
3. Sequist TD, Fitzmaurice GM, Marshall R, et al. Cultural competency training and performance reports to improve diabetes care for black patients: a cluster randomized, controlled trial. *Ann Intern Med.* 2010;152:40-46.

SUGGESTED READINGS

http://www.commonwealthfund.org/Publications/View-All.aspx?topic=Health+Care+Disparities *Website including key articles on health disparities.*
Walker R, St. Pierre-Hansen N, Cromarty H, et al. Measuring cross-cultural patient safety: identifying barriers and developing performance indicators. *Healthc Q.* 2010;13:64-71. *Review.*

5

SOCIOECONOMIC ISSUES IN MEDICINE

STEVEN A. SCHROEDER

All nations—rich and poor—struggle with how to improve the health of the public, obtain the most value from medical services, and restrain rising health care expenditures. Many developed countries also wrestle with the paradox that their citizens have never been so healthy or so unhappy with their medical care. Despite the reality that only 10% of premature deaths result from inadequate medical care, the bulk of professional and political attention focuses on how to obtain and pay for state-of-the-art medical care. By comparison, 40% of premature deaths stem from unhealthy behaviors—including smoking (about 44%; Chapter 31); excessive or unwise drinking (about 11%; Chapter 32), obesity and insufficient physical activity (about 15% but estimated to rise substantially in the years to come; Chapters 15 and 227), illicit drug use (about 2%; Chapter 33), and imprudent sexual behavior (about 3%; Chapter 293) (E-Fig. 5-1). Genetics (Chapter 39) account for an additional 30%; social factors—discussed next—account for 15%, and environmental factors (Chapter 18) account for 5%. Of the major behavioral causes of premature deaths (Fig. 5-1), tobacco use (Chapter 31) is by far the

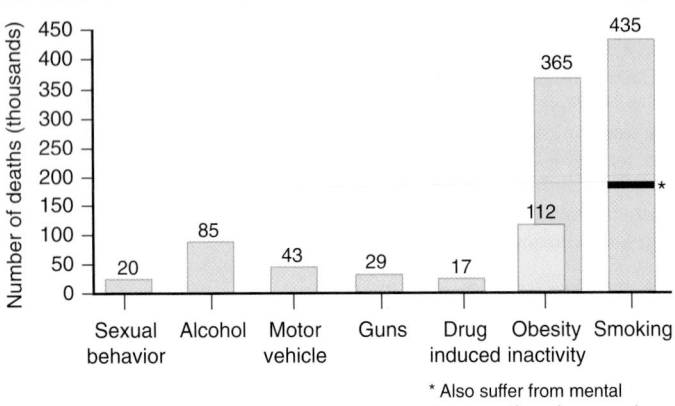

FIGURE 5-1. Number of U.S. deaths from behavioral causes. (Data from Mokdad AH, Marks JS, Stroup DF, Gerberding JL. Actual causes of death in the United States, 2000. *JAMA.* 2004;291:1238-1245; Mokdad AH, Marks JS, Stroup DF, Gerberding JL. Correction: actual causes of death in the United States, 2000. *JAMA.* 2005;293:293-294; Flegal KM, Graubard BI, Williamson DF, et al. Excess deaths associated with underweight, overweight, and obesity. *JAMA.* 2005;293:1861-1867. Adapted from Schroeder SA. Shattuck lecture: we can do better—improving the health of the American People. *N Engl J Med.* 2007;357: 1221-1228.)

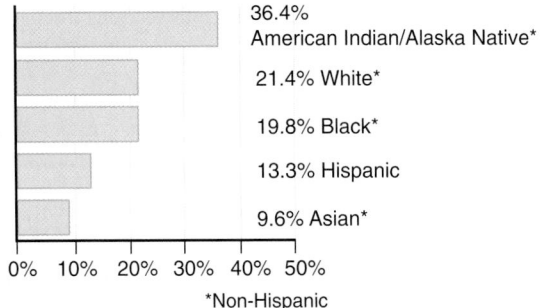

FIGURE 5-2. Prevalence of adult smoking by race/ethnicity, United States, 2007. (From Centers for Disease Control and Prevention. Cigarette smoking among adults—United States, 2007. *MMWR Morb Mortal Wkly Rep.* 2008;57:1221-1226.)

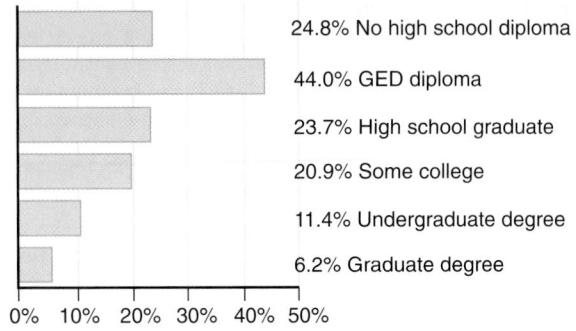

FIGURE 5-3. Age-adjusted prevalence of cigarette smoking in 2007, among persons 25 years of age or older, according to educational level. GED = General Education Development test. (From Centers for Disease Control and Prevention. Cigarette smoking among adults—United States, 2007. *MMWR Morb Mortal Wkly Rep.* 2008;57:1221-1226.)

isolation, and the anxiety derived from the feeling of having low status—is linked to poor health. This stress may trigger a variety of neuroendocrinologic responses that are useful for short-term adaptation and bring long-term adverse health consequences.

What can clinicians do with this knowledge? Clearly, it is difficult to write prescriptions for more income or for better schooling or neighborhoods or jobs, but physicians can encourage healthy behavior. At key times of transition, such as during discharge planning for hospitalized patients, clinicians should be attentive to social circumstances. For patients who are likely to be socially isolated, clinicians should encourage or arrange interactions with family, neighbors, religious organizations, or community agencies to improve the likelihood of optimal outcomes. In addition, physicians should seek to identify and to eliminate any aspects of racism in health care institutions. Finally, in their role as social advocates, physicians can promote such goals as safe neighborhoods, improved schools, and equitable taxation policies.

ECONOMIC ISSUES IN MEDICAL CARE

Medical care today is on a collision course. On the one hand, an ever-expanding science base continuously generates new technologies and drugs that promise a longer and healthier life. Add a public eager to obtain the latest breakthroughs touted in the media and over the Internet, plus a well-stocked medical industry eager to meet that demand, and it is easy to understand why expenditures continue to soar. On the other hand, payers for medical care—health insurance companies, government (federal, state, and local), and employers—increasingly bridle at medical care costs.

The United States continues to lead the world in health care expenditures (Fig. 5-4). In 2008, it spent about $2.4 trillion, amounting to 17% of its gross domestic product. It is projected that expenditures will continue to rise, exceeding 20% by 2014. Most policy analysts contend that this rate of increase in medical care expenditures is unsustainable, but the same has been said for many years. Few other countries have double-digit health care expenditures, and none comes close to 15% (see Fig. 5-4). A potent combination of supply and demand factors explains why the United States spends so much. On the supply side, it far exceeds other countries in the availability and use of expensive diagnostic technologies, such as magnetic resonance imaging and computed tomography (E-Fig. 5-2). For example, the United States has four times as many magnetic resonance imaging machines per capita as does Canada. Similar patterns exist for therapeutic technologies, whether coronary angioplasty, cancer chemotherapy, or joint prostheses. The differences are especially dramatic in older patients. For example, in the 65- to 69-year age group, the United States performed 1.95 more carotid endarterectomy procedures per capita than did Canada; but above the age of 80 years, the ratio was 8.7.

Other supply factors that drive high medical expenditures in the United States include a fee-for-service payment system that compensates physicians much more for using expensive technologies than when they do not; a medical professional work force that earns much higher incomes relative to the population than in other nations and that emphasizes specialist rather than generalist practice; accelerated development of new and costly medications that are directly marketed to consumers; much higher administrative costs; higher rates of fraud and abuse; and a high rate of defensive medicine in response to pervasive fears about medical malpractice suits. Supply factors that do not appear to be unique to the United States are the number of physicians or hospitals. Many other developed countries have a much larger

most important, although recent increases in obesity (Chapter 227) and physical inactivity (Chapter 15) are also alarming.

SOCIAL STATUS INFLUENCES HEALTH

Socioeconomic status, or class, is a composite of many different factors, including income, net wealth, education, occupation, and neighborhood. In general, people in lower classes are less healthy and die earlier than people at higher socioeconomic levels, a pattern that holds true in a stepwise fashion from the poorest to the richest. In the United States, the association between health and class is usually discussed in terms of racial and ethnic disparities; but in fact, race and class are independently associated with health status, and it can be argued that class is the more important factor. For example, U.S. racial disparities in adult smoking prevalence are relatively small among whites, blacks, and Hispanic Americans (Fig. 5-2), whereas there are huge differences among smoking rates by educational level (Fig. 5-3). U.S. physicians have reduced their smoking prevalence to a record low of only 1%.

In part, the relationship between class and health is mediated by the higher rates of unhealthy behaviors among the poor, such as the inverse relationship between educational attainment and cigarette smoking, but unhealthy behaviors do not fully explain the poor health of those in the lower socioeconomic classes. Even when behavior is held constant, people in lower socioeconomic classes are much more likely to die prematurely than are people of higher classes. Of interest is that first-generation immigrants appear to be more protected from the adverse health consequences of low socioeconomic status than are subsequent generations.

It is unclear which of the components of class—education, wealth (either absolute wealth or the extent of the gap between rich and poor), occupation, or neighborhood—makes the greatest impact on a person's health. Most likely, it is a combination of all of them. For example, the constant stress of a lower class existence—lack of control over one's life circumstances, social

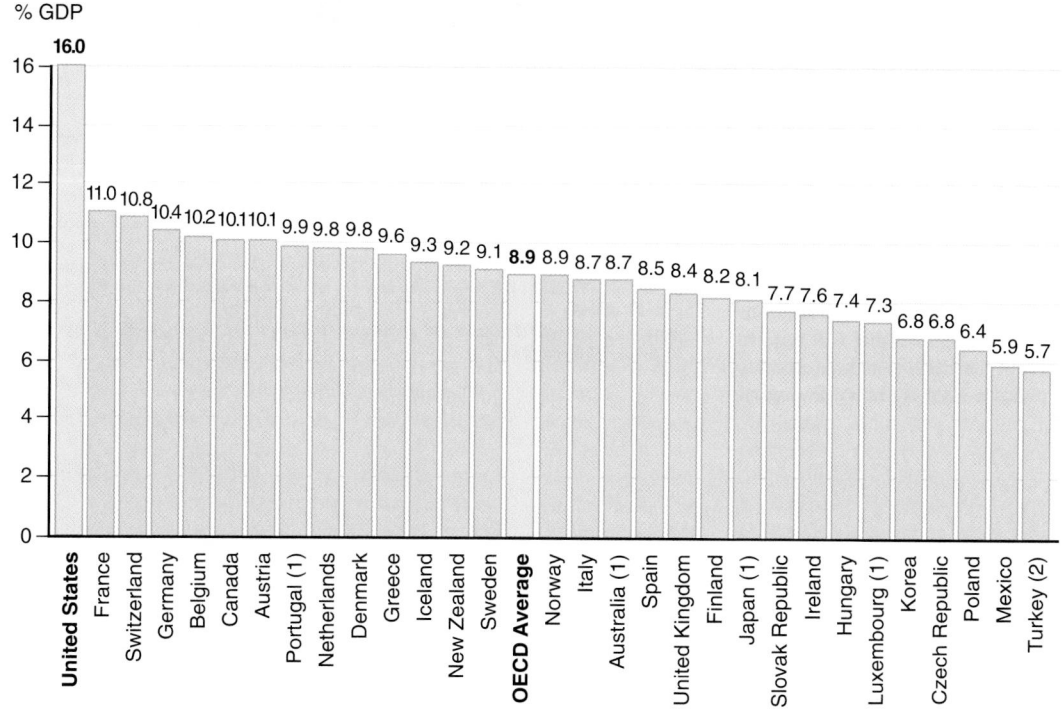

% GDP

FIGURE 5-4. Health expenditure as a share of gross domestic product (GDP), 2007. OECD = Organisation for Economic Co-operation and Development. (Data from Organisation for Economic Co-operation and Development Health, 2009.)

physician work force relative to their population, as well as a much higher ratio of primary care physicians to specialists. The number of hospitals and hospital beds, the frequency of hospitalizations, and the length of hospital stay are relatively low in the United States, although it does have a much greater proportion of intensive care beds. Finally, recent analyses suggest that a principal driver of high expenditures on health care in the United States is the much greater price charged per unit of service compared with other developed countries.

Demand factors also drive medical expenditures. The extent to which the media and the medical profession feature medical "breakthroughs" is extensive and one-sided. New promising treatments merit front-page stories and commercial advertisements, whereas subsequent disappointing results are buried or ignored. The cumulative result is to whet patients' appetite for more and to leave the impression that good health depends only on finding the right treatment. This same quest explains the popularity of alternative medicine, for which patients are willing to spend $34 billion annually out of their own pockets (Chapter 38).

It could be argued that rising expenditures for medical care are not a bad thing, as what could be more important than ensuring maximal health? There are several rebuttals to that argument. First, it is not clear that money spent on medical care brings appropriate value in the United States, given that its health statistics are worse than those of virtually every other developed country. Second, there are substantial regional differences in the supply and use of medical care, such as a two-fold difference in the supply of acute hospital beds in metropolitan regions (even with adjustment for demographic variables) and a four-fold difference in the risk of being hospitalized in an intensive care unit at the end of life. Similar regional differences exist for procedures such as transurethral prostatectomy, hysterectomy, and coronary artery bypass surgery. Yet there is no evidence that "more is better" on a regional basis. In fact, geographic areas with higher consumption of medical services have been shown to have worse outcomes for some conditions, such as acute myocardial infarction.

Money spent on medical care means less to spend on other important social priorities—schools, the environment, job creation, and competition with overseas manufacturers that spend less on health care. Furthermore, many businesses are reducing their health insurance contributions to employees and retirees, passing those costs along to the beneficiaries. Consequently, health insurance coverage has emerged as the most important issue in labor contract negotiations and strikes. In addition, rising health care expenditures are stressing public programs such as Medicare, Medicaid, the Veterans Administration health system, and municipal hospitals, with budget requests outstripping the tax base to pay for them. Medical debt is by far the most important cause of bankruptcy. Finally, as health care becomes less affordable

for businesses and government, the number of people without health insurance will continue to increase.

Since the mid-1970s, a variety of strategies to contain rising medical expenditures have yielded limited success. These attempts have tried to restrict the supply of costly medical technologies as well as the production of physicians, especially specialists; to promote health maintenance organizations that have incentives to spend less on medical care; to ration indirectly by limiting health insurance coverage; to institute prospective payment for hospital care; to use capitation payments or discounted fee schedules for physician reimbursement; to introduce gatekeeper mechanisms to reduce access to costly care; to put patients at more financial risk for their own medical care; to reform malpractice procedures; to reduce administrative costs; and to encourage less aggressive care at the end of life. The most recent suggestions—comparative effectiveness research to curtail unnecessary technology use, electronic medical records to avoid duplication of tests, and payment for performance—all hold the promise to improve quality, but their potential for substantial cost reduction is only theoretical at present. Fundamentally, all these strategies have failed because the political will to enforce them was missing. Americans—at least those with medical insurance—strongly resist limits on their choice of medical care, and the combined power of hospitals, medical professionals, and the pharmaceutical, medical device, and insurance industries overwhelms the meager forces pushing cost containment. Add to that the continuous production of new technologies and drugs plus the public's avidity for the latest innovations, and it is easy to see why medical costs are projected to keep rising. As a result, the costs of even modest health insurance plans are a challenge for most blue-collar and many middle-class families.

Payment for medical care varies by country. In the United States, health insurance coverage is an incomplete patchwork, consisting of government-sponsored programs for elderly people (Medicare), poor people (Medicaid), and veterans, plus employer-based coverage for workers and their families. Medicare covers acute care services in the hospital and in physicians' offices but has limited coverage for prescription drugs and long-term care. More than half of all Medicare subscribers also buy supplemental insurance. Medicaid covers more services than Medicare does, but Medicaid payments to physicians and hospitals are so low in many states that patients have restricted access to care. At any given time, more than 46 million Americans lack health insurance, and 70 million are without insurance at some point during the year. In addition, millions of immigrant workers are also uninsured. This large group must depend on charity care, often at community clinics and public hospitals, and it is well documented that lack of health insurance contributes to poor health, such as delayed diagnosis and undertreatment of asthma, diabetes, hypertension, and cancer.

The 2010 Patient Protection and Affordable Care Act (PPACA) contains insurance reform measures that took effect in 2010 and 2011, as well as coverage expansion that starts in 2014. About 32 million new people will be insured, about 50% privately and 50% in Medicaid. Revenue generating provisions are split about evenly between spending reductions and cost containment. In contrast to the passage of Medicare and Medicaid in 1965, the PPACA did not receive bipartisan support, and it is difficult to predict which of its components—if any—will survive.

Because medical care is both so valued and so expensive, physicians everywhere will inevitably become more involved in issues of medical economics. As cost-containment pressures force patients to assume more of their medical expenses, they will become more aware of costs and more demanding about the price and value of care. Informed clinical decision making will require that physicians have accurate information about the risks, benefits, and costs of medical care and better ways to communicate what is known and what is not.

SUGGESTED READINGS

Aaron HJ, Ginsburg PB. Is health care spending excessive? If so, what can we do about it? *Health Affairs.* 2009;28:1260-1276. *Analyzes the reasons the United States spends so much more on health care.*

Cubbin C, Vesely SK, Braveman PA, et al. Socioeconomic factors and health risk behaviors among adolescents. *Am J Health Behav.* 2011;35:28-39. *Shows the strong link in adolescents.*

Hajat A, Kaufman JS, Rose KM, et al. Long-term effects of wealth on mortality and self-rated health status. *Am J Epidemiol.* 2011;173:192-200. *Details the strong inverse relationship of wealth with poor health status and mortality.*

Marmot M, for the Commission on Social Determinants of Health. Achieving health equity: from root causes to fair outcomes. *Lancet.* 2007;370:1153-1163. *The quality of health and health services within and across countries corresponds with health outcomes.*

Schroeder SA. Shattuck lecture: we can do better—improving the health of the American People. *N Engl J Med.* 2007;357:1221-1228. *Reviews why, despite its high expenditures, the United States does so poorly in health outcomes.*

Seligman HK, Schillinger D. Hunger and socioeconomic disparities in chronic disease. *N Engl J Med.* 2010;363:6-9. *Perspective.*

PRINCIPLES OF EVALUATION AND MANAGEMENT

6

APPROACH TO THE PATIENT: HISTORY AND PHYSICAL EXAMINATION

DAVID L. SIMEL

OVERVIEW

Physicians may have multiple objectives with varying degrees of importance in their encounters with patients. These goals include but are not limited to the translation of symptoms and signs into diagnoses, assessment of stability or change in known conditions, provision of information and counseling for future prevention, and reaffirmation or alteration of therapeutic interventions.

The interaction between the patient and physician represents not only a scientific encounter but also a social ritual centered on locus of control and meeting each other's expectations. Patients may not be able to express their needs fully and may fear loss of control in determining their own medical fate. Conversely, physicians have expectations: a need to feel that they have not missed something important in addressing diagnostic challenges, a need to put limits on the time available for each interaction, and a need to maintain objectivity so that their evaluation and recommendations are not clouded by their emotional feelings about the patient. When the patient needs to establish the presence of health or the diagnosis for a symptom, a physician's expertise is expressed through the performance and interpretation of a rational clinical examination.

Physical Examination Begins with the History

It is almost impossible to consider the history as distinct from the physical examination because the clinical examination begins as soon as the physician sees or hears the patient. Cynics contend that physical diagnostic skills have diminished in importance because so many diagnoses are made during the history and then confirmed by a laboratory value or a radiograph. The problem may be lack of practice in detecting physical examination findings with proven accuracy. Even proponents of the clinical examination now demand proof of reasonable reproducibility and accuracy before they accept the value of specific components of the history and physical examination.

Quantitative Principles of the Clinical Examination

Data on the sensitivity, specificity, likelihood ratios (LRs), and observer variability of components of the clinical examination can be obtained by a literature search for evaluation of a disease-specific condition (e.g., melanoma) or a clinical finding (e.g., splenomegaly) (Table 6-1). For each component of the history and physical examination, there is an associated sensitivity (the percentage of patients with a disorder who have an abnormal finding), specificity (the percentage of patients without a disorder who have a normal finding), and measure of precision (the agreement beyond chance between two observers) (Chapter 9). Current research on the clinical examination uses LRs that inform clinicians how likely they are to observe a particular finding in a patient with a given condition as opposed to a patient without the condition. A patient with an abnormal glabellar tap has an LR of 4.5 for Parkinson's disease (Chapter 416), which means that the risk for parkinsonism increases 4.5-fold compared with a patient with the baseline risk. Similarly, a patient who insists that he or she does not have "shaking in the arms" has an LR of 0.25 for Parkinson's disease and is one fourth as likely (a reduced chance) to have the disease compared with the baseline risk. Evaluation of the precision of the examination uses the kappa (κ) statistic to describe the agreement beyond chance (0 = random agreement; +1 = perfect agreement).

MEDICAL HISTORY

The history begins by asking patients to describe, in their own words, the reason for seeking medical care (Table 6-2). Although patients may have many reasons for initiating a visit to the physician, they should be encouraged to select the one or two most important concerns they have. The physician should reassure the patient that he or she will not ignore other concerns but wants to understand what is most important to the patient.

History of the Present Illness

Open-ended questions facilitate descriptions of problems in the patient's own words. Subsequently, specific questions fill in gaps and help clarify important points. These questions should be asked in an order dictated by the story the patient tells and targeted to suit the individual problem. When the patient is acutely ill, the physician should limit the amount of time spent in open-ended discussion and move promptly to the most important features that allow quick evaluation and management. In general, the history of the problem under consideration includes the following:

- Description of onset and chronology
- Location of symptoms
- Character (quality) of symptoms
- Intensity
- Precipitating, aggravating, and relieving factors
- Inquiry into whether the problem or similar problems occurred before and, if so, whether a diagnosis was established at that time

It is often helpful to ask patients to express what they believe is the cause of the problem or what concerns them the most. This approach often uncovers other pertinent factors and helps establish that the physician is trying to meet the patient's needs.

Past Medical and Surgical History

An astute clinician recognizes that patients may not report all their prior problems because they may forget, may assume that previous events are unrelated to their current problem, or simply may not want to discuss past events. Open-ended statements such as "Tell me about other medical illnesses that we did not discuss" and "Tell me about any operations you had" prompt the patient to consider other items. The physician should ask the patient about unexplained surgical or traumatic scars.

A list of current medications includes prescriptions, over-the-counter medications, vitamins, and herbal preparations. Patients who do not recall the names of medications should bring all medication bottles to the next visit. Patients may not consider topical medications (e.g., skin preparations or eyedrops) as important, so they may need prompting.

Information about allergies (Chapter 262) is particularly important, but challenging, to collect. Patients may attribute adverse reactions or intolerances to allergies, but many supposed allergic reactions are not truly drug allergies. Less than 20% of patients who claim a penicillin allergy are allergic on skin testing. Eliciting the patient's actual response to medications facilitates a determination of whether the response was a true allergic reaction.

Social and Occupational History and Risk Factors

The social history not only reveals important information but also improves understanding of the patient's unique values, support systems, and social situation. The social history should be tailored to the individual patient and allow for physician-centered questioning and patient-centered expression of values and concerns.

Data that may influence risk factors for disease should be gathered, including a nonjudgmental assessment of substance abuse. The tobacco history should include the use of snuff, chewing tobacco, and cigar and cigarette smoking (Chapter 31). Alcohol use should be determined quantitatively and by the effect that it has had on the patient's life (Chapter 32). Past or present use of illicit substances, prescription pain medications or sedatives, and intravenous drugs should be assessed (Chapter 33). The sexual history should address sexual orientation as well as current and past sexual activity (including the number of partners). The employment history should include the current and past employment history, military experience, and any significant hobbies. Military veterans should be asked about their combat history, years of service, and areas of deployment.

The physician should also obtain information on socioeconomic status, insurance, the ability to afford or obtain medications, and past or current barriers to health care because of their impact on care of the patient (Chapter 5). Marital status and the living situation (i.e., whom the patient lives with, significant stressors for that patient) are important as risk factors for disease and to determine how best to care for the patient. A patient's culture (Chapter 4) and values should be known, including any prior advance directives or desire to overrule them (Chapter 3). The physician should explicitly elicit and record information regarding the next of kin; surrogate decision makers; emergency contacts; social support systems; and financial, emotional, and physical support available to the patient.

TABLE 6-1 MEDLINE SEARCH STRATEGY FOR IDENTIFYING QUANTITATIVE INFORMATION ON THE CLINICAL EXAMINATION USING THE OVID SEARCH SYSTEM*

1. exp physical examination/or physical exam$.mp
2. medical history taking.mp
3. professional competence.mp
4. (sensitivity and specificity).mp or (sensitivity and specificity).tw
5. (reproducibility of results or observer variation).mp
6. diagnostic tests, routine/
7. (decision support techniques or Bayes theorem).mp
8. 1 or 2 or 3 or 4 or 5 or 6 or 7
9. limit 8 to (Ovid full text available and human and English language)
10. exp melanoma
11. 9 and 10
12. exp splenomegaly
13. 9 and 12

*OVID Technologies, Inc. A condition and a physical finding are given as examples. Abbreviations or search term abbreviations are as follows: "exp" indicates that the topic is "exploded" to include all subheadings for the topic. The "$" is a wildcard designator, so "exam$" would include the words *examination, examining,* and *examiner.* "mp" searches for the word or phrase in the title, abstract, registry number word, or mesh subject heading. Step 9 limits the search to studies that involve humans only and where the full manuscript is available online and is written in English. If the search yields too few topics, the limitation of full text available can be removed and the search repeated. If too many results are obtained, some of the items from step 8 can be eliminated.

TABLE 6-3 REVIEW OF SYSTEMS*

FOCUS all questions on a specific time frame (e.g., within the past "month" or "now") and on items not already addressed during the clinical examination
Change in weight or appetite
Change in vision
Change in hearing
New or changing skin lesions
Chest discomfort or sensation of skipped beats
Shortness of breath, dyspnea on exertion
Abdominal discomfort, constipation, melena, hematochezia, diarrhea
Difficulty with urination
Change in menses
Joint or muscle discomfort not already mentioned
Problems with sleep
Difficulty with sexual function
Exposure to "street" drugs or medications not already mentioned
Depression (feeling "down, depressed, or hopeless"; loss of interest or pleasure in doing things)
A sensation of unsteadiness when walking, standing, or getting up from a chair

*Clinicians may start with this basic list and adapt the items to their specific patient population by considering factors such as age, gender, medications, and the problems identified during the examination. The process is facilitated by developing a routine personal approach to these questions, typically going through the systems from "head to toe."

TABLE 6-2 PATIENT'S MEDICAL HISTORY

Description of the patient
Age, gender, ethnic background, occupation
Chief reason for seeking medical care
State the purpose of the evaluation (usually in the patient's words)
Other physicians involved in the patient's care
Include the clinician that the patient identifies as his or her primary provider or the physician who referred the patient. Record contact information for all physicians who should receive information about the visit
History of the reason for seeking medical care
In chronologic fashion, determine the evolution of the indication for the visit and then each major symptom. It is best to address the patient's reason for seeking care first rather than what the physician ultimately believes is most important
Be careful to avoid "premature closure," in which a diagnosis is assumed before all the information is collected
Past medical and surgical history
List other illnesses and previous surgeries not related to the current problem
List all prescribed and over-the-counter medications with dose
Remember to ask about vitamin and herbal supplements
Allergies and adverse reactions
List allergic reactions to medications and food. Record the specific reaction (e.g., hives). Distinguish allergies from adverse reactions or intolerance to medication (e.g., dyspepsia from nonsteroidal anti-inflammatory agents)
Social and occupational history
Describe the patient's current family and a typical day for patient. The occupational history should focus on current and past employment as it might relate to the current problem. For veterans, inquire about their military history, including combat exposure, years of service, and areas of deployment
Risk factors
Include history of tobacco use, illegal drug use, and risk factors for sexually transmitted disease (including human immunodeficiency virus and hepatitis)
Family history
History of any diseases in first-degree relatives and a listing of family members with any conditions that could be risk factors for the patient (e.g., cardiovascular disease at a young age, malignancy, known genetic disorders, longevity)
Review of systems (see Table 6-3)

Family History

The family history is never diagnostic, but it allows risk stratification, which affects the pretest probability for an increasing number of disorders (e.g., heart disease, breast cancer, or Alzheimer's disease). For common diseases such as heart disease, additional inquiry into the age of onset in first-degree relatives and death attributed to the disease should be obtained (Chapter 51). When a patient reports that a first-degree relative had a myocardial infarction, the LR is 19 that the patient has a family history of myocardial infarction. Patients may lack appropriate information about the absence of disease, however, so a reported lack of a family history of myocardial infarction reduces the likelihood only by one third. In general, the specificity of the reported family history far exceeds its sensitivity; for example, only two thirds of patients with essential tremor (Chapter 417) report a family history, but 95% of such patients have first-degree relatives with tremor. The expansion of knowledge about genetic diseases (Chapter 39) requires clinicians not only to improve their skills in eliciting the family history but also to develop methods for confirming the information. For example, patients who report that a first-degree relative had carcinoma of the colon (LR 25), breast (LR 14), ovaries (LR 34), or prostate (LR 12) are usually providing accurate information.

Review of Systems

The review of systems, which is the structural assessment of each of the major organ systems, elicits symptoms or signs not covered, or overlooked, in the history of the present illness. In practice, the review of systems may be accomplished by direct questioning (Table 6-3) or by having the patient fill out a previsit questionnaire that constrains the answers to a specific time frame. When this review is directly obtained, physicians should not use open-ended questions but rather proceed with direct questions, such as "Has there been any recent change in your vision?" or "Have you recently had shortness of breath, wheezing, or coughing?" The relative value of these approaches has not been investigated fully, but restricting the symptoms to a narrower time frame prevents a complete retelling of the history. One estimate is that the review of systems yields a new important diagnosis about 10% of the time.

● PHYSICAL EXAMINATION

Chaperones

Surveys suggest that most patients of either sex and all ages report a lack of preference for a chaperone; it is not clear whether this response is their true feeling or a desire to give a "correct" response. Nevertheless, many adult women (29%) and adolescent girls (46%) do express a preference for a chaperone during a breast, pelvic, or rectal examination by a male physician (especially during their first examination). Examiners should offer patients the option of a chaperone, and a chaperone should be considered when the clinician and patient are of different genders. Many examiners prefer a chaperone to allay their own anxieties attributable to gender differences or to achieve a perceived need for protection should the patient become concerned during the procedure.

Vital Signs

Vital signs include the pulse rate, blood pressure, respiratory rate, body temperature, and the patient's quantitative assessment of pain. Marked abnormalities require a rapid, focused evaluation that may take precedence over the typical structural approach to the remainder of the evaluation (Chapter 7).

The pulse should be recorded as not just the rate but also the rhythm. Physicians may prefer to initiate the examination by holding the patient's hand while palpating the pulse. This nonthreatening initial contact with the patient allows the physician to determine whether the patient has a regular or irregular rhythm.

When the blood pressure is abnormal (Chapter 67), the measurement should be repeated, assuring that the cuff size is appropriate. Many adults require a large adult cuff; using a narrow cuff can alter systolic/diastolic blood pressure by −8 to +10/+2 to +8 mm Hg. The appearance of repetitive sounds (Korotkoff sounds, phase 1) constitutes systolic pressure. (Record the value rounded upward to the nearest 2 mm Hg.) After the cuff is inflated about 20 to 30 mm Hg above the palpated pressure, the Korotkoff sounds muffle and disappear as the pressure is released (phase 5). The level at which the sounds disappear is diastolic pressure.

Respirations should be assessed with the patient unaware that the rate is being observed. The examiner should decide whether patients have tachypnea (a rapid rate of breathing) or hypopnea (a slow or shallow rate of breathing). Tachypnea is not always associated with hyperventilation, which is defined by increased alveolar ventilation resulting in a lower arterial carbon dioxide level (Chapter 103). In the evaluation of patients suspected of having pneumonia, examiners agree on the presence of tachypnea only 63% of the time. The subjective sensation of dyspnea (Chapter 83) is caused by an increased work of breathing.

The body temperature of adults is measured with an oral electric thermometer. Rectal thermometers reliably record temperatures 0.4° C higher than oral thermometers. Tympanic thermometers may vary too much in comparison to oral thermometers (−1.2° to +1.6° C vs. the oral temperature) to be reliable in hospitalized patients.

As a vital sign measure, patients should self-rate any pain on a scale of 0 to 10 (no pain to worst pain ever) (Chapter 29). However, the validity, usefulness, and value of this approach as a screening tool for clinical diagnosis are uncertain.

Head and Neck
Face
The examiner can simplify the assessment by carefully judging for facial symmetry. Asymmetrical facial features should be noted and explained. Examples of asymmetry include skin lesions (Chapter 444), cranial nerve palsies (Chapter 403), parotid enlargement (Chapter 433), or the ptosis of Horner's syndrome (Chapter 432). A variety of disorders may cause symmetrical, abnormal facies; examples include acromegaly (Chapter 231), Cushing's syndrome (Chapter 234), and Parkinson's disease (Chapter 416).

Ears
Physicians may not recognize their patient's hearing impairment (Chapter 436). The inability to appreciate the whispered voice increases the likelihood of hearing loss (LR 6). Otoscopic evaluation of the tympanic membranes should reveal a translucent membrane and an obvious cone of light reflected where the eardrum meets the malleolus (see Fig. 434-6). Cerumen impaction is an easily treated cause of diminished hearing.

Nose
Patients frequently have nasal symptoms, such as a self-diagnosis of sinusitis (Chapter 434) or snoring (Chapter 412). The nares should be examined for the presence of polyps, which can be seen as obstructing, glistening mucosal masses. Transillumination performed in a dark room is useful for diagnosing sinusitis, especially when combined with visualization of a purulent discharge, a patient's report of a poor response to decongestants or antihistamines, a maxillary toothache, and the presence of discolored rhinorrhea (Chapter 434). These patients have an LR greater than 6 for rhinosinusitis.

Mouth
The quality of the patient's dentition directly affects nutrition. Generalist physicians can be confident that the patient requires dental care if periodontal disease or dental caries are detected (LR > 4). Premalignant oral lesions (e.g., leukoplakia [see Fig. 196-1], nodules, ulcerations) found by generalist physicians are usually verified by dentists (LR > 6.5) (Chapter 433). Patients who use smokeless tobacco products are at significantly increased risk for premalignant and malignant oral lesions (Chapter 31). Bimanual palpation of the cheeks and floor of the mouth facilitates identification of potentially malignant lesions (Chapter 433).

Eyes
The eye examination begins with simple visual inspection to look for symmetry in the lids, extraocular movements, pupil size and reaction, and the presence of redness (Chapters 431 and 432). Abnormalities in extraocular movements should be grouped into nonparalytic (usually chronic with onset in childhood) or paralytic causes (third, fourth, or sixth cranial nerve palsy). Pupillary abnormalities may be symmetrical or asymmetrical (anisocoria). Red eyes should be categorized by the pattern of ciliary injection, presence of pain, effect on vision, and papillary abnormalities. When the eye examination is approached systematically, the generalist physician can evaluate the likelihood of conjunctivitis, episcleritis or scleritis, iritis, and acute glaucoma.

Routine determination of visual acuity can help confirm or refute a patient's report of diminished vision but does not replace the need for formal ophthalmologic evaluation in patients with visual complaints (Chapter 431). Cataracts can be detected with direct ophthalmoscopy, but the generalist's proficiency in this evaluation is uncertain.

After identifying the optic disc by ophthalmoscopy, the examiner should note the border of the disc for clarity, color, and the size of the central cup in relation to the total diameter (usually less than half the diameter of the disc). A careful observer usually can see spontaneous venous pulsations that indicate normal intracranial pressure, but about 10% of patients with normal intracranial pressure will not have spontaneous pulsations. Abnormalities of the optic disc include optic atrophy (a white disc), papilledema (see Fig. 431-27) (blurry margins with a pink, hyperemic disc), and glaucoma (a large, pale cup with retinal vessels that dive underneath and that may be displaced toward the nasal side). The generalist's examination inadequately detects early glaucomatous changes, so high-risk patients should undergo routine ophthalmologic examination for glaucoma.

After inspecting the disc, the examiner should examine the upper and lower nasal quadrants for the appearance of vessels and the presence of any retinal hemorrhages (see Fig. 431-24) or lesions. Proceeding from the nasal quadrants to the temporal quadrants decreases the risk of papillary constriction from the bright light focused on the fovea. Dilating the pupils leads to an improved examination. Patients with diabetes (Chapter 236) should undergo routine examination by eye care experts because the sensitivity of a generalist's examination is not adequate to exclude diabetic retinopathy or monitor it over time.

Neck
Carotid Pulses
The carotid pulses should be palpated for contour and timing in relation to the cardiac impulse. Abnormalities in the carotid pulse contour reflect underlying cardiac abnormalities (e.g., aortic stenosis) but are generally appreciated only after detecting an abnormal cardiac impulse or murmur (Chapter 50).

Many physicians listen for bruits over the carotid arteries because asymptomatic carotid bruits are associated with an increased incidence of cerebrovascular and cardiac events in older patients (Chapters 413 and 414). In asymptomatic patients, the presence of a carotid bruit increases the likelihood of a 70 to 90% stenotic lesion (LR 4 to 10), but the absence of a bruit is of uncertain value. Unfortunately, clinical data do not provide adequate data for judging the importance of detecting bruits in asymptomatic patients.

Thyroid
The thyroid gland is felt best when standing behind the patient and using both hands to palpate the thyroid gland gently (Chapter 233). The palpatory examination is enhanced by asking the patient to swallow sips of water, which allows the thyroid to glide underneath the fingers. When viewed from the side, lateral prominence of the thyroid between the cricoid cartilage and the suprasternal notch indicates thyromegaly. The generalist physician should estimate the size of the thyroid gland as normal or enlarged; the impression of an enlarged thyroid gland by a generalist physician has an LR of almost 4, whereas assessment of normal size makes thyromegaly less likely (LR 0.4).

Lymphatic System
While palpating the thyroid, the examiner may also identify enlarged cervical lymph nodes (Chapter 171). Lymph nodes can also be palpated in the supraclavicular area, axilla, epitrochlear area, and inguinofemoral region. Simple lymph node enlargement confined to one region is common and does not usually represent an important underlying disorder. Unexpected gross lymph node enlargement in a single area or diffuse lymph node enlargement is more important. Patients with febrile illnesses, underlying malignancy, or inflammatory diseases should routinely undergo an examination of each of the aforementioned areas for lymph node enlargement.

Chest

Inspection of the patient's posture may reveal lateral curves in the back (scoliosis) or kyphosis that may be associated with loss of vertebral height from osteoporosis (Chapter 251). When patients have back pain, the spine and paravertebral muscles should be palpated for spasm and tenderness (Chapter 407). The patient may be placed through maneuvers to assess loss of mobility associated with ankylosing spondylitis (Chapter 273), but a history of loss of lateral mobility may be just as efficient in the early stages of spondylitis.

Lungs

Examination of the lungs begins with inspection for chest deformities. A barrel chest, thought to be typical of obstructive airways disease, is present only in severely affected patients (Chapters 83 and 88). The incremental value of palpation and percussion of the chest to supplement the history, auscultation, and eventual chest radiograph is unknown. Medical students show more consistency than pulmonary specialists do in recording auscultatory abnormalities. The presence or absence of adventitial sounds (wheezes, crackles, or rubs) has good interobserver reliability (κ 0.30 to 0.70). The best piece of information for increasing the likelihood of chronic obstructive pulmonary disease is a history of more than 40 pack years of smoking (LR 19). The presence of wheezing or downward displacement of the larynx to within 4 cm of the sternum (distance between the top of the thyroid cartilage and the suprasternal notch) increases the likelihood of obstructive pulmonary disease (LR of 4 for either). Auscultated wheezes are continuous sounds. Crackles (formerly called rales) are discontinuous lung sounds heard in conditions that create lung stiffening (heart failure, pulmonary fibrosis, and obstructive lung disease).

Heart

The patient should be examined in the sitting and lying positions (Chapter 50). Palpation of the apical impulse in the left lateral decubitus position helps detect a displaced apical impulse and can reveal a palpable S_3 gallop. When the apical impulse is lateral to the midclavicular line, radiographic cardiomegaly (LR 3.5) and an ejection fraction of less than 50% (LR 6) are more likely. Most examiners auscultate in sequence the aortic area, pulmonic area, left sternal border, and apex. First, listen to the heart sounds and concentrate on their timing, intensity, and splitting with respiration. The first and second heart sounds are heard best with the diaphragm, as are pericardial rubs. Gallops (S_3 and S_4) are heard best with the stethoscope bell. High-pitched versus low-pitched murmurs are detected by switching from the diaphragm to the bell (see Table 50-6). The location, timing, intensity, radiation patterns, and respiratory variation of murmurs should be noted. Special maneuvers during auscultation (e.g., Valsalva, auscultation during sudden squatting or standing) do not usually need to be performed if the results of routine precordial examination are entirely normal.

There is considerable concern about the reliability and accuracy of the cardiac examination. When performed on patients (as opposed to cardiac simulators), the reliability of perceiving an S_3 or S_4 is no better than chance, and agreement on the finding among examiners does not seem to improve with the examiner's experience. Nevertheless, the presence of an S_3 on any examination is useful for detecting left ventricular systolic dysfunction (LR > 4 for identifying patients with an ejection fraction <30%). The presence of a systolic thrill (palpable murmur, LR 12) or a holosystolic murmur increases the likelihood of moderate to severe aortic stenosis or mitral regurgitation. Quiet systolic murmurs (LR 0.08) are much less likely to herald important cardiac abnormalities. A loud, early diastolic murmur (LR 4) or a diastolic murmur associated with an S_3 suggests severe aortic regurgitation.

Breast

The most important determinants of the accuracy of the breast examination are the duration of the examination; the patient's position; careful evaluation of the breast boundaries; the pattern of the examination; and the position, movement, and pressure of the examiner's fingers (Chapter 204). Interobserver variability is substantial (κ about 0.3 to 0.6) because these aspects of the examination vary among physicians. To obtain the best sensitivity, the duration of the breast examination needs to be 5 to 10 minutes' total time, but few generalist physicians perform such a lengthy examination. Clinicians should recognize that the examination may make them (or their patient) feel uncomfortable—the presence of a chaperone may give the clinician the confidence to perform an intensive examination.

The patient should be examined with the pads of the fingers while she is supine, holding her hand first on her forehead (to flatten the lateral border of the breast) and then on her shoulder (to flatten the medial border). The examiner should make small circular motions with the fingers, moving up and down in parallel rows to span the entire breast-clavicle to the bra line. Cancerous breast lumps are difficult to distinguish from benign breast lumps on examination, but the presence of a fixed mass or a mass 2 cm in diameter has an LR of about 2 to 2.5 for cancer.

Abdomen

When patients have potential abdominal symptoms and the history suggests an acute problem, the examination should focus initially on identifying patients who may require surgical evaluation. Palpation and percussion of the abdomen of patients with no symptoms or risk factors for an abdominal disorder seldom reveal important abnormalities (Chapter 134) except for asymptomatic widening of the abdominal aorta in older patients (LR of 16 for detecting aneurysms >4 cm in diameter). However, palpation misses a substantial proportion of small to medium aneurysms (Chapter 78). After specific training in palpation techniques, general internists have good agreement on the presence or absence of an aortic aneurysm (κ = 0.53).

The presence of bowel sounds in patients with acute symptoms can be falsely reassuring because bowel sounds can be present despite an ileus and may be increased early in an obstruction. For patients without gastrointestinal symptoms or abnormalities on palpation, auscultation for bruits is important primarily to detect renal bruits in patients with hypertension (Chapters 67 and 127). The presence of an abdominal bruit in a hypertensive patient, if heard in systole and diastole, strongly suggests renovascular hypertension (LR $\approx$ 40).

Liver

Detection of liver disease depends mostly on the history and laboratory evaluations (Chapter 148). By the time that signs are present on physical examination, the patient usually has advanced liver disease. The first abnormalities on physical examination associated with liver disease are extrahepatic. The clinician should assess the patient for ascites, peripheral edema, jaundice, or splenomegaly as signs of liver disease. In patients with an enlarged liver, palpation should begin at the liver edge, but palpation of the edge below the costal margin increases the likelihood of hepatomegaly only slightly (LR 1.7). The upper border of the liver may be detected by percussion, and a span of less than 12 cm reduces the likelihood of hepatomegaly. In the absence of a known diagnosis (e.g., a hepatoma, which may cause a hepatic bruit), auscultation of the liver rarely is helpful.

Spleen

Examination for splenomegaly in patients without findings suggestive of a disorder associated with splenomegaly almost always reveals nothing (Chapter 171). Approximately 3% of healthy teenagers may have a palpable spleen. The examination for an enlarged spleen begins first with percussion in the left upper quadrant to detect dullness. Percussion is performed over the lowest left anterior axillary line during inspiration and expiration while the patient is supine. In the absence of dullness, the results of palpation do not establish or exclude splenomegaly, so a radiographic image (ultrasound or nuclear scintigraphy) is required. The presence of a palpable splenic edge in patients with dullness to percussion and clinical suspicion of splenomegaly confirms enlargement. Palpation can be performed by any of the following three approaches (κ about 0.2 to 0.4): palpating with the right hand while providing counterpressure with the left hand behind the spleen, palpating with one hand without counterpressure (with the patient in the right lateral decubitus position for both techniques), or placing the patient supine with the left fist under the left costovertebral angle while the examiner tries to hook the spleen with the hands.

Musculoskeletal System

The musculoskeletal examination in adult patients is almost always driven by symptoms (Chapters 264 and 271). Most patients have back pain at some point during their lives (Chapter 407). Back pain is second only to upper respiratory illness as a reason for seeking outpatient care. Most patients' musculoskeletal discomfort will be self limited. The patient's history helps assess the likelihood of an underlying systemic disease (age, history of systemic malignancy, unexplained weight loss, duration of pain, responsiveness to previous therapy, intravenous drug use, urinary infection, or fever). The most important physical examination findings for lumbar disc herniation in patients with sciatica all have excellent reliability, including ipsilateral straight leg raising causing pain, contralateral straight leg raising causing pain, and ankle or great toe dorsiflexion weakness (all with $\kappa > 0.6$).

The generalist physician should evaluate an adult patient with knee discomfort for torn menisci or ligaments. The best maneuver for demonstrating a tear in the anterior cruciate ligament is the anterior drawer or Lachman maneuver, in which the examiner detects the lack of a discrete end point as the tibia is pulled toward the examiner while the femur is stabilized. A variety of maneuvers that assess for pain, popping, or grinding along the joint line between the femur and tibia are used to evaluate for meniscal tears. As with many musculoskeletal disorders, no single finding has the accuracy of the orthopedist's examination, which factors in the history and a variety of clinical findings.

The shoulder examination is directed toward determining range of motion, maneuvers that cause discomfort, and assessment of functional disability. Hip osteoarthritis is detected by evidence of restriction of internal rotation and abduction of the affected hip. Generalist physicians often rely on radiographs to determine the need for referral to orthopedic physicians, but routine radiographs are not needed early in the course of shoulder or hip disorders. The degree of pain and disability experienced by the patient may prompt confirmation of the diagnosis and referral.

The hands and feet may show evidence of osteoarthritis (local or as part of a systemic process) (Chapter 270), rheumatoid arthritis (Chapter 272), gout (Chapter 281), or other connective tissue diseases. In addition to regional musculoskeletal disorders, such as carpal tunnel syndrome, a variety of medical and neurologic conditions should prompt routine examination of the distal ends of the extremities to prevent complications (e.g., diabetes [neuropathy or ulcers] or hereditary sensorimotor neuropathy [claw toe deformity]).

Skin

The skin should be examined under good lighting (Chapter 444). It is best to ask the patient to point out any spots on the skin of concern. Examiner agreement on some of the most important features of melanoma (asymmetry, haphazard color, border irregularity) is fair to moderate (Chapter 210). A lesion that is symmetrical, has regular borders, is only one color, is 6 mm or smaller, or has not enlarged in size is unlikely to represent a melanoma (LR 0.07). However, an increasing number of findings greatly enhances the likelihood of melanoma (LR 2.6 for two or more findings and LR 98 for the presence of all five findings) (Chapter 210).

Basal cell carcinoma and squamous cell carcinoma occur even more frequently than melanoma (Chapter 210). These lesions can be detected during routine examination by paying careful attention to sun-exposed areas of the nose, face, forearms, and hands.

Neurologic Examination

Full details of the neurologic examination are given in Chapter 403.

Psychiatric Evaluation

During the general examination, much of the psychiatric assessment (including cognition) is accomplished while eliciting the routine history and performing the review of systems (Chapter 404). Observation of the patient's mannerisms, affect, facial expression, and behavior may suggest underlying psychiatric disturbances. When a screening survey and review of systems are obtained by a questionnaire completed by the patient, the clinician should review the responses carefully to determine whether the patient exhibits symptoms of depression. Specific questioning for symptoms of depression is appropriate for all adult patients. Military veterans should be screened for post-traumatic stress disorder and possible prior traumatic brain injuries that may affect their behaviors. Delirium (Chapter 27) is common in both medical and surgical inpatients and is recognized by fluctuating mental status.

Genitalia and Rectum
Pelvic Examination

A complete examination includes a description of the external genitalia, appearance of the vagina and cervix as seen through a speculum, and bimanual palpation of the uterus and ovaries (Chapters 205 and 245). The precision of the pelvic examination is uncertain. In the emergency setting, there is poor agreement between resident physicians and emergency physicians on the presence of cervical motion tenderness, uterine tenderness, adnexal tenderness, and adnexal masses (κ about equal to 0.2 to 0.25)

(Chapter 293). Among gynecologists, assessment of uterine size by examination correlates reasonably well with measurement by pelvic ultrasound. Of asymptomatic women, 10 to 15% have some abnormality on examination, and 1.5% have abnormal ovaries. Screening for ovarian cancer is limited by the low sensitivity of the physical examination for detecting early-stage ovarian carcinoma (Chapter 205).

Male Genitalia

Examination of the male genitalia should begin with a description of whether the penis is circumcised and whether there are any visible skin lesions (e.g., ulcers or warts). Palpation should confirm the presence of bilateral testes in the scrotum. The epididymis and testes should be palpated for nodules. The low incidence of testicular carcinoma means than most nodules are benign (Chapter 206).

The prostate should be examined in all quadrants with attention focused on surface irregularities or differences in consistency throughout the prostate (Chapter 207). An estimate of prostate size may be confounded by the size of the examiner's fingers. It may be best to estimate the size of the prostate in centimeters of width and height.

Rectum

Patients can be examined while lying on their side, although this approach may place the examiner in an awkward stance (Chapters 134 and 147). The rectal examination in women can be performed as part of a bimanual examination, with the index finger in the vagina and the third finger in the rectum to permit palpation of the rectovaginal vault. Men may be asked to stand and lean over the examining table; alternatively, they may be examined while on their back with their hips and knees flexed. This latter maneuver is not used often, although it may facilitate examination of the prostate, which falls into the finger in this position.

The rectal examination begins with inspection of the perianal area for skin lesions. A well-lubricated, gloved finger is placed on the anus, and while applying gentle pressure, the examiner asks that the patient bear down as though having a bowel movement. This maneuver facilitates entry of the finger into the rectum. A normal rectal response includes tightening of the anal sphincter around the finger. The examiner should palpate circumferentially around the length of the fully inserted finger for masses. On withdrawing the gloved finger, the finger should be wiped on a stool guaiac card for fecal blood testing to assess for acute blood loss. As a screening test for colorectal carcinoma (Chapter 199), digital examination does not replace the need for testing stool samples collected by the patient (or using alternative screening strategies, such as flexible sigmoidoscopy or colonoscopy).

⬤ SUMMARIZING THE FINDINGS FOR THE PATIENT

The physician should summarize the pertinent positive and negative findings for the patient and be willing to express uncertainty to the patient, provided that it is accompanied by a plan of action (e.g., "I will reexamine you on your next visit"). The rationale for subsequent laboratory, imaging, or other tests should be explained. A plan should be established for providing further feedback and results to the patient, especially when there is a possibility that bad news may need to be delivered. Some physicians ask the patient if there is "anything else" to be covered. Patients who express additional new concerns at the end of the visit may have been fearful to address them earlier (e.g., "by the way, doctor, I'm getting a lot of chest pain"); when the problems seem non-urgent, it is acceptable to reassure the patient and offer the promise of evaluating them in a follow-up phone call or at the next visit.

⬤ FUTURE DIRECTIONS

The common assumption that physicians' diagnostic skills are deteriorating is not supported by evidence. There is considerable evidence that the scientific approach to understanding what is worthwhile and what is not worthwhile during the clinical examination identifies a core set of skills for clinical diagnosticians. Because good patient outcomes at good value are driven primarily by the quality of the information obtained during the clinical examination, continued application of scientific principles to the history and physical examination should improve diagnostic skills.

SUGGESTED READINGS

Boulware L, Marinopoulos S, Phillips K, et al. Systematic review: the value of the periodic health evaluation. *Ann Intern Med.* 2007;146:289-300. *A periodic health examination improves delivery of some recommended preventive services and may lessen patient worry.*

Society of General Internal Medicine. Website for Clinical Examination Research and Education Group. http://www.sgim.org/index.cfm?pageId=588. *Facilitates personal literature searches for topics on the clinical examination and a bibliography of the "Rational Clinical Examination Series" published in the Journal of the American Medical Association.*

APPROACH TO THE PATIENT WITH ABNORMAL VITAL SIGNS

DAVID L. SCHRIGER

Care of the patient is guided by integration of the chief complaint, history, vital signs, and physical examination findings (Chapter 6). Physicians should be keenly aware of a patient's vital signs but should seldom make them the centerpiece of the evaluation.

THE IMPORTANCE OF VITAL SIGNS

The importance of vital signs in medical care is a conundrum for proponents of an evidence-based approach to care of patients. No experienced physician would be willing to care for patients without them, yet a formal evaluation of the utility of vital signs for making specific diagnoses would conclude that they are not particularly useful because their likelihood ratios are too low to differentiate those who have a condition from those who do not (Chapter 6). For uncommon conditions, their predictive value is even worse. For example, the probability of tachycardia in a patient in thyroid storm is high, yet the probability of thyroid storm in a patient with isolated tachycardia is low. This application of Bayes' theorem (Chapter 9) demonstrates why there is no justification for ordering thyroid tests for every tachycardic patient and why attempts to say "When vital sign *x* is high [low], do *y*" fail. Each vital sign can be normal or abnormal in almost every acute condition (Table 7-1), and vital signs can be transiently abnormal in healthy individuals. An algorithmic approach to testing and treatment in response to abnormal vital signs would be too vague and too complex to be of use.

Predictive Value

How can it be that vital signs are poor predictors of diagnoses but central to the practice of medicine? First, although vital signs are insufficiently predictive to be of use in rigid algorithms, these algorithms are but one of several heuristics used by physicians to diagnose and to treat patients. Pattern recognition and the hypothetical-deductive model are heuristics that are based not on average tendencies of a single factor (e.g., hypotension is present in *x*% of cases of septic shock) or a small number of factors (hypotension and tachycardia are present in *y*% of cases of septic shock) but on the complex interaction of multiple factors (e.g., because this patient is an ill-appearing elderly man with an enlarged prostate and a history of urinary tract infections, is tachycardic and hypotensive, has clear lungs and an enlarged but nontender prostate, and has an oxygen saturation of 97%, he should be treated for urosepsis [Chapter 292] while awaiting results of urinalysis and urine culture).

Thus, vital signs can play an important function in medical decision making even though their likelihood ratios for specific complications are unimpressive. In one study, for example, the 16% of medical and surgical ward patients with abnormal vital signs had a 20-fold higher rate of transfer to a higher level of care, cardiac arrest, or death compared with patients with persistently normal vital signs.

Vital Signs as Symptoms

Abnormal vital signs are seldom the fundamental pathophysiologic problem. In shock (Chapter 106), hypotension and tachycardia are manifestations of pathophysiologic processes occurring at cellular and molecular levels. Given the circuitous links from clinical disease to fundamental pathophysiology to abnormal vital signs, it is not surprising that the relationships between the disease states and vital signs are not strong. Until new technologies enable direct measurement of primary pathologic processes, vital signs remain an important, albeit imperfect, proxy.

The five key vital signs are temperature, pulse, blood pressure, respiratory rate, and oxygen saturation (pulse oximetry). Pulse oximetry is included because it has become widely available in acute care settings, is noninvasive and relatively inexpensive, and provides information unique from the respiratory rate. Advocates have suggested that pain, smoking status, and weight be considered routine vital signs; although a case can be made for each, they are not considered here. Clinicians should never forget that the most important vital sign is what the patient looks like; general appearance is a sign that guides the intensity and urgency of the evaluation.

MEASURING VITAL SIGNS

Although obtaining vital signs is generally straightforward, the validity and reliability of measurement depend on proper technique and, for blood pressure and pulse oximetry, well-maintained equipment. Rectal and oral temperatures are generally accurate (Chapter 288), although oral temperatures can be falsely depressed in patients who breathe through their mouths. Axillary temperature is unreliable and should not be used. There is wide variability in the validity and reliability of measurements performed with tympanic membrane thermometers. A hypothermia thermometer is preferred in patients with suspected hypothermia, and core temperature should be measured with an esophageal, bladder, or rectal temperature sensor in patients with severe hypothermia or hyperthermia (Chapter 109).

Blood pressure must be measured with an appropriately sized cuff (Chapter 67). Automated blood pressure machines occasionally provide spurious results, and questionable values should be confirmed by manual auscultation and by checking other limbs. Pulse is best obtained by palpation because this technique provides the opportunity to assess regularity and contour; the pulse should be counted for sufficient time for an accurate rate to be obtained (at least 15 seconds). High heart rates on the readout of a cardiac monitor must be confirmed by palpation because these monitors can spuriously count large P waves, T waves, or pacemaker spikes as R waves, thereby reporting a heart rate double the actual rate. Orthostatic vital signs—the comparison of blood pressure and pulse in the supine, sitting, and standing positions—are advocated by some but have proved to be insensitive and nonspecific for hypovolemia.

Because the typical respiratory rate is between 12 and 20 breaths per minute and because there is considerable breath to breath variation, the respiratory rate should be assessed for at least 30 seconds and preferably 1 minute. Oxygen saturation is dependent on technology, so an understanding of the idiosyncrasies of the device being used is critical; valid measurements are unlikely unless there is good correlation of the machine's pulse reading and the patient's pulse. The probe should be placed on a part of the body that is warm and well perfused. Pulse oximeters compare the absorption of light at two wavelengths, so readings may be spuriously high under conditions that change the color of oxygenated or deoxygenated hemoglobin, including carbon monoxide poisoning (Chapter 94), methemoglobinemia (Chapter 164), and some of the less common hemoglobinopathies.

ROLE OF VITAL SIGNS IN MANAGEMENT OF THE PATIENT

Abnormal vital signs should be remeasured. Certain abnormalities require prompt evaluation (Table 7-2). Other vital sign abnormalities should be rechecked in the future unless they have been previously noted, in which case a work-up can be initiated, guided by the patient's past history and physical examination findings. It is critical that the physician always "treat the patient, not the vital signs."

TABLE 7-1	NORMAL AND PANIC RANGES FOR KEY VITAL SIGNS IN ADULTS*	
	NORMAL	**PANIC**
Temperature	36°-38° C (96.8°-100.4° F)	40° C (104° F)
Pulse	60-100 beats/min	<45 beats/min, >130 beats/min
Respirations	12-20 breaths/min	<10 breaths/min, >26 breaths/min
Oxygen saturation	95-100%	<90%
Systolic blood pressure	90-130 mm Hg	<80 mm Hg, >200 mm Hg
Diastolic blood pressure	60-90 mm Hg	<55 mm Hg, >120 mm Hg

*Normal values are for healthy adults. Values outside these ranges are common in patients who are ill or are anxious about their health care encounter. Panic values demand the health care provider's attention in any adult patient. These values are specific (rarely present in healthy patients) but not sensitive (most ill patients' vital signs will not include panic values). All vital signs must be interpreted in the context of the patient's presentation (see text).

TABLE 7-2   ABNORMALITIES REQUIRING RAPID EVALUATION IN THE ASYMPTOMATIC PATIENT

An irregularly irregular rapid pulse (if it is not known to be chronic) should trigger an evaluation of the patient's rhythm so that atrial fibrillation can be identified, evaluated, and treated (Chapter 64), thereby decreasing the patient's risk of stroke.

A heart rate above 130 beats/min warrants an electrocardiogram to determine the patient's rhythm and a consideration of the differential diagnosis of tachycardia (anemia and thyroid disease in particular).

A markedly elevated diastolic blood pressure (e.g., >115 mm Hg) should stimulate an evaluation for hypertensive urgencies (Chapter 67). Note that hypertension in the absence of signs of acute end-organ damage does not require acute treatment, which can reduce intracranial perfusion pressure and cause stroke. Patients with elevated blood pressure should be offered standard evaluation and treatment for chronic hypertension (Chapter 67).

Markedly low pulse or blood pressure in patients receiving cardioactive medications should lead to a confirmation that the patient is truly asymptomatic, an inquiry into the dosing of these medications, and a reconsideration of the regimen.

Markedly low pulse in elderly patients who are not receiving rate-controlling drugs should trigger an evaluation of the patient's cardiac conduction system.

Oxygen saturation below 93% in the absence of known pulmonary problems should prompt an evaluation of the patient's pulmonary status.

Patients without Systemic Complaints

In patients presenting for a routine evaluation or nonsystemic complaint (e.g., knee pain), an abnormal vital sign will seldom be the harbinger of acute illness. Most commonly, it will be a false reading or a transient finding due to random variation or anxiety that requires no evaluation or treatment and can be rechecked in the future. On occasion, it will be the only or most apparent manifestation of a chronic condition or risk factor. The measurement of an elevated blood pressure leading to a diagnosis of hypertension is the classic example of the value of vital signs in such patients.

Patients Who Complain of Systemic Illness but Do Not Appear to Be Ill

Vital signs serve two additional roles in symptomatic patients who do not appear particularly ill. First, abnormalities in vital signs provide information that may suggest or support a diagnosis. The presence of elevated temperature in a patient with productive cough, shortness of breath, and localized rales and egophony supports a diagnosis of infectious pneumonia. Vital signs may also play a role in defining therapy and triage. For example, guidelines for patients with community-acquired pneumonia (Chapter 97) formally incorporate vital signs.

The second role of vital signs in the stable symptomatic patient is to provide warning that the patient is sicker than he or she appears. For example, the presence of hypotension in a well-appearing patient thought to have pyelonephritis may be an indication of sepsis or hypovolemia. For vital signs to be of use, the physician must be aware of them and must incorporate them explicitly into a thought process that considers the dangerous diagnoses associated with the abnormal vital sign. The physician then must decide whether the likelihood of each potentially dangerous diagnosis is high enough to warrant specific evaluation. Unfortunately, no quick or easy rules differentiate spurious abnormalities that can be ignored from those that should trigger additional testing or treatment. What can be said is that the well-trained physician who is aware of abnormal vital signs and is willing to contemplate a change in treatment or disposition in response to them is less likely to make mistakes.

A few specific points bear mention. First, for most vital signs, "normal" is relative. Blood pressure must be interpreted in the context of the patient. For example, a blood pressure of 88/64 mm Hg may be reasonable for an otherwise healthy, young 50-kg woman but should cause concern in a 90-kg middle-aged man. Similarly, a blood pressure of 128/80 mm Hg would be fine in a 60-year-old man but worrisome in a 34-week pregnant woman. Second, because vital signs are insensitive measures of disease, normal vital signs should not dissuade the physician from pursuing potentially critical diagnoses. For example, young, well-conditioned adults may maintain normal vital signs well into the course of shock.

Use of Vital Signs in Patients Who Appear to Be Ill

For some patients, abnormal vital signs are expected on the basis of their appearance and their symptoms. For patients in extremis, care should proceed

according to established guidelines such as Advanced Cardiac Life Support (Chapter 63), Advanced Trauma Life Support, and algorithms for the treatment of shock (Chapters 107 and 108). For other ill-appearing patients, two processes must occur. In one, the physician, armed with knowledge of the differential diagnosis of each abnormal vital sign and the ability to take a thorough history and to perform an appropriate physical examination, narrows the list of potential diagnoses and decides which are of sufficient probability to warrant evaluation. Simultaneously, the physician considers the list of treatment options for all diagnoses associated with the abnormal vital sign and, before establishing a diagnosis, initiates those treatments for which the potential benefit of prompt administration exceeds potential harms. For example, antibiotics for febrile patients at risk for bacterial infection, hydrocortisone for hypotensive patients at risk for hypoadrenalism, and thiamine for hypothermic patients at risk for Wernicke's encephalopathy may improve outcome and are unlikely to cause harm even if the patient does not have the suspected condition. Although early presumptive treatment can be life-saving in selected patients, it should not be abused; physicians must avoid knee-jerk responses that can cause harm.

Differential Diagnosis and Treatment Options
Single Abnormal Vital Signs

Because vital signs can be abnormal in virtually any disease process, no differential diagnosis can be encyclopedic. The physician should focus initially on common diseases and diseases that require specific treatment. The thought process should begin with the chief complaint and history and then incorporate information about the vital signs and the remainder of the physical examination.

Multiple Abnormal Vital Signs

Patients who are acutely ill are likely to have several abnormal vital signs. Although certain patterns of abnormal vital signs predominate in specific conditions (e.g., hypotension, tachycardia, and hypothermia in profound sepsis), no pattern can be considered pathognomonic. The physician's goal is to work toward a diagnosis while simultaneously providing treatments whose benefits outweigh potential harms.

Fever is generally accompanied by tachycardia, with the general rule of thumb that the heart rate will increase by 10 beats per minute for every 1° C increase in temperature. The absence of tachycardia with fever is known as pulse-temperature dissociation and has been reported in typhoid fever (Chapter 316), legionnaires disease (Chapter 322), babesiosis (Chapter 361), Q fever (Chapter 335), infection with *Rickettsia* spp (Chapter 335), malaria (Chapter 353), leptospirosis (Chapter 331), pneumonia caused by *Chlamydia* spp (Chapter 326), and viral infections such as dengue fever (Chapter 390), yellow fever (Chapter 389), and viral hemorrhagic fevers (Chapter 389), although the predictive value of this finding is unknown.

Much can be learned by comparing the respiratory rate with pulse oximetry. Hyperventilation in the presence of high oxygen saturation suggests a central nervous system process or metabolic acidosis rather than a cardiopulmonary process. Low respiratory rates in the presence of low levels of oxygen saturation suggest central hypoventilation, which may respond to narcotic antagonists.

Hypertension and bradycardia in the obtunded or comatose patient are known as the Cushing reflex, a relatively late sign of elevated intracranial pressure. Physicians should strive to diagnose and treat this condition before the Cushing reflex develops.

Approach to Abnormalities of Specific Vital Signs
Elevated Temperature

Normal temperature is often cited as 37° C (98.6° F), but there is considerable diurnal variation and variation among individuals, so 38° C is the most commonly cited threshold for fever. Fever thought to be due to infection should be treated with antipyretics and appropriate antimicrobials (Chapter 288). The importance of early administration of antibiotics to potentially septic patients cannot be overstated (Chapters 108 and 288). Hyperthermia (temperature above 40° C) should be treated with cooling measures such as ice packs, cool misting in front of fans, cold gastric lavage, and, for medication-related syndromes, medications such as dantrolene (Chapter 109). Most hospital anesthesia departments will have a designated kit for the treatment of malignant hyperthermia (Chapters 440 and 442).

Low Temperature

The treatment of hypothermia is guided by its cause (Chapter 109). The body's temperature decreases when heat loss exceeds heat production. Every logically possible mechanism for this phenomenon has been observed. Decreased heat production can result from endocrine hypofunction (e.g., Addison's disease [Chapter 234], hypopituitarism [Chapter 231], hypothyroidism [Chapter 233]) and loss of the ability to shiver (e.g., drug-induced or neurologic paralysis or neuromuscular disorders). Malfunction of the hypothalamic regulatory system can be due to hypoglycemia (Chapter 236) and a variety of central nervous system disorders (Wernicke's encephalopathy [Chapter 425], stroke [Chapter 414], tumor [Chapter 195], and trauma [Chapter 406]). Resetting of the temperature set point can occur with sepsis. Increased heat loss can be due to exposure, behavioral and physical disorders that prevent the patient from sensing or responding to cold, skin disorders that decrease its ability to retain heat, and vasodilators (including ethanol). A careful history and physical examination should illuminate which of these possibilities is most likely.

Several considerations are worthy of emphasis. The spine of an obtunded hypothermic patient who is "found down" must be protected and evaluated because paralysis from a fall may have prevented the patient from seeking shelter and may have diminished the ability to produce heat. The physician should not forget to administer antibiotics to patients who may be septic (Chapter 108), thiamine to those who may have Wernicke's encephalopathy (Chapter 425), hydrocortisone to those who may be hypoadrenal (Chapter 234), and thyroid hormone to those who may have myxedema coma (Chapter 233). Severely hypothermic patients should be treated gently because any stimulation may trigger ventricular dysrhythmias (Chapter 109); even in the absence of pulses, cardiopulmonary resuscitation should be used only in patients with ventricular fibrillation or asystole.

Elevated Heart Rate

The rate, rhythm, and electrocardiogram differentiate sinus tachycardia from tachyarrhythmias (Chapters 62 to 65). Tachyarrhythmias can be instigated by conditions that may require specific treatment (e.g., sepsis [Chapter 108], electrolyte disorders [Chapters 118, 119, and 120], endocrine disorders [Chapter 233], and poisonings [Chapters 21 and 110]) before the arrhythmia is likely to resolve. For sinus tachycardia, treatment of the underlying cause is always paramount. Treatments may include antipyretics (for fever); anxiolytics; oral or intravenous fluids (for hypovolemia); nitrates, angiotensin-converting enzyme inhibitors, and diuretics (for heart failure and fluid overload [Chapter 59]); oxygen (for hypoxemia); α-blockers (for stimulant overdose); β-blockers (for acute coronary syndromes [Chapters 72 and 73] or thyroid storm [Chapter 233]); and anticoagulation (for pulmonary embolism [Chapter 98]). Tachycardia is often an appropriate response to a clinical condition and should not be treated routinely unless it is causing or is likely to cause secondary problems.

Low Pulse

Bradycardia can be physiologic (athletes and others with increased vagal tone), due to prescribed cardiac medications (e.g., β-blockers, calcium-channel blockers, digoxin), overdoses (e.g., cholinergics, negative inotropes), disease of the cardiac conducting system, electrolyte abnormalities (severe hyperkalemia), and inferior wall myocardial infarction (Chapters 64 and 73). Asymptomatic patients do not require immediate treatment. The goal of therapy is to produce a heart rate sufficient to perfuse the tissues and alleviate the symptoms (Chapter 63). Overdoses should be treated with specific antidotes (Chapter 110). Endocrine disorders should be treated with replacement therapy. In patients with acute coronary syndrome (Chapter 72), the goal is to restore perfusion and alleviate the ischemia. Patients with profound bradycardia or hypotension may require chronotropic drugs to increase perfusion even if they may increase myocardial oxygen demand. In normotensive patients with milder bradycardia, chronotropic agents should be used only if symptoms and ischemia cannot be resolved by other means. Atropine is the primary therapy for bradycardia; isoproterenol and cardiac pacing are reserved for those who do not respond (Chapter 63).

Elevated Blood Pressure

Elevated blood pressure does not require acute treatment in the absence of symptoms or signs of end-organ damage (Chapter 67). In patients whose blood pressure is markedly above their baseline, the history and physical examination should assess for the conditions that define "hypertensive emergency": evidence of encephalopathy, intracranial hemorrhage, ischemic stroke, heart failure, pulmonary edema, acute coronary syndrome, aortic dissection, renal failure, and preeclampsia. In the absence of these conditions, treatment should consist of restarting or adjusting the medications of patients with known hypertension and initiating a program of blood pressure checks and appropriate evaluation for those with no prior history of hypertension (Chapter 67).

The patient with a true hypertensive emergency should be treated with agents appropriate for the specific condition. Because rapid decreases in blood pressure can be as deleterious as the hypertensive state itself, intravenous agents with short half-lives, such as nitroprusside, labetalol, nitroglycerin, and esmolol, are preferred (Chapter 67).

Low Blood Pressure

Low blood pressure must be evaluated in the context of the patient's symptoms, general appearance, and physical examination findings. Treatment depends on context. The same blood pressure value may necessitate intravenous inotropic agents in one patient and no treatment in another.

In tachycardic hypotensive patients, the physician must rapidly integrate all available evidence to determine the patient's volume state, cardiac function, vascular capacitance, and primary etiology (Chapter 106). Not all patients with hypotension and tachycardia are in shock, and not all patients in shock will have hypotension and tachycardia. Patients in shock should be treated on the basis of the cause (Chapters 106 to 108).

Symptomatic hypotensive patients thought to be intravascularly volume depleted should receive intravenous fluid resuscitation with crystalloid or blood, depending on their hemoglobin level (Chapter 106). In patients with known heart disease, patients who are frail or elderly, and patients whose volume status is uncertain, small boluses of fluid (e.g., 250 mL of normal saline), each followed by reassessment, are preferred so that iatrogenic heart failure may be avoided. Inotropic support should be reserved for patients who do not respond to fluid resuscitation. High-output heart failure should be kept in mind in patients with possible thyroid storm or stimulant overdose.

Increased Respiratory Rate

Tachypnea is a normal response to hypoxemia (see later). Treatment of tachypnea in the absence of hypoxemia is directed at the underlying cause, which often is pain (Chapter 29). Anxiolytics (e.g., diazepam, 5 to 10 mg PO or IV; lorazepam, 1 to 2 mg PO, IM, or IV) or reassurance can calm patients with behavioral causes of hyperventilation. Breathing into a paper bag has been shown to be an ineffective treatment. Pulmonary embolism (Chapter 98) does not necessarily reduce the oxygen saturation or cause a low Po_2 and should always be considered in at-risk patients with unexplained tachypnea.

Decreased Respiratory Rate

Any perturbation of the respiratory center in the central nervous system can slow the respiratory drive (Chapter 86). Narcotics and other sedatives and neurologic conditions are common causes of a decreased respiratory rate. The primary treatment of apnea is mechanical ventilation (Chapter 105), but narcotic antagonists can be tried in patients with a history or physical examination findings (miosis, track marks, opiate patch) suggestive of narcotic use or abuse (Chapter 33). In nonapneic patients, mechanical ventilation is indicated for patients who are breathing too slowly to maintain an acceptable oxygen saturation and for patients who are retaining carbon dioxide in quantities sufficient to depress mental function. Patients who are unable to protect their airway should be intubated. Oxygen should be administered to all hypopneic patients who are hypoxemic (see earlier). Patients with chronic hypoventilation (Chapter 86) may have retained HCO_3^- to compensate for an elevated Pco_2 and so may depend on hypoxia to maintain respiratory drive; in these patients, overaggressive administration of oxygen can decrease the respiratory rate, increase the Pco_2, and increase obtundation (Chapter 104).

Decreased Oxygen Saturation

In hypopneic patients, initial efforts should try to increase the respiratory rate (see earlier) and tidal volume. Regardless of etiology, oxygen, in amounts adequate to restore adequate oxygen saturation ($Po_2 > 60$ mm Hg, oxygen saturation >90%), is the mainstay of therapy. When oxygen alone fails, noninvasive methods for improving ventilation or tracheal intubation are required (Chapter 104). Oxygen should increase the Po_2 in all patients except those who have severe right-to-left shunting (Chapter 69). Treatment of conditions that cause hypoxemia includes antibiotics (pneumonia), bronchodilators (asthma, chronic obstructive pulmonary disease), diuretics and vasodilators (pulmonary edema), anticoagulants (pulmonary embolism), hyperbaric oxygen (carbon monoxide poisoning), methylene blue (methemoglobinemia, sulfhemoglobinemia), and transfusion (anemia).

SUGGESTED READINGS

Glickman SW, Cairns CB, Otero RM, et al. Disease progression in hemodynamically stable patients presenting to the emergency department with sepsis. *Acad Emerg Med.* 2010;17:383-390. *About 25% of patients with sepsis and initially normal vital signs progress to shock within 72 hours.*

Lighthall GK, Markar S, Hsiung R. Abnormal vital signs are associated with an increased risk for critical events in US veteran inpatients. *Resuscitation.* 2009;80:1264-1269. *Emphasizes that abnormal vital signs carry a 20-fold increased risk for subsequent important deterioration among general medical and surgical patients.*

8

STATISTICAL INTERPRETATION OF DATA

THOMAS B. NEWMAN AND CHARLES E. MCCULLOCH

ROLE OF STATISTICS

Much of medicine is inherently probabilistic. Not everyone with hypercholesterolemia who is treated with a statin is prevented from having a myocardial infarction, and not everyone not treated does have one, but statins reduce the *probability* of a myocardial infarction in such patients. Because so much of medicine is based on probabilities, studies must be performed on *groups* of people to estimate these probabilities. Three component tasks of statistics are (1) selecting a sample of subjects for study, (2) describing the data from that sample, and (3) drawing inferences from that sample to a larger population of interest.

SAMPLING: SELECTING SUBJECTS FOR A STUDY

The goal of research is to produce generalizable knowledge, so that measurements made by researchers on samples of individuals will eventually help draw inferences to a larger group of people than was studied. The ability to draw such inferences depends on how the subjects for the study (the sample) were selected.

Sampling

The *intended sample* is the group of people who are eligible to be in the study based on meeting *inclusion criteria,* and not meeting *exclusion criteria.* For example, for a study of obesity, the intended sample (inclusion criteria) might be men and women 18 years or older who have a body mass index (BMI) of 30 kg/m^2 or higher. Exclusion criteria might include an inability to speak English or Spanish.

In some cases, the intended sample is a *simple random sample* of the target population, in which every member of the target population has an equal chance of being selected. Simple random samples are the easiest to handle statistically but are often impractical. An alternative is to take random samples of "clusters" (e.g., specific census tracts or geographic areas) and then attempt to study all of the subjects in each cluster.

Regardless of the method used to select the intended sample, the *actual sample* will almost always differ in important ways. Statistical methods address *only the effect of random variation on the inference from the intended sample to the target population.* Estimating the effects of differences between the intended sample and the actual sample depends on content knowledge about whether factors associated with being in the actual sample are related to those quantities.

DESCRIBING THE SAMPLE

Types of Variables

A key use of statistics is to describe sample data. Methods of description depend on the *type of variable. Categorical* variables consist of named characteristics, whereas *numerical* variables describe the data with numbers. Categorical variables can be further divided into *dichotomous* variables, which can take on only two possible values (e.g., alive/dead); *nominal*

variables, which can take on more than two values but have no intrinsic ordering (e.g., race); and *ordinal* variables, which have more than two values and an intrinsic ordering of the values (e.g., tumor stage). *Numerical* variables include *count* variables (e.g., the number of times a woman has been pregnant), *continuous* variables (those that have a wide range of possible values), and *time-to-event* variables (e.g., the time from initial treatment to recurrence of breast cancer).

Univariate Statistics for Continuous Variables: Mean, Median, and Standard Deviation

When describing data in a sample, it is a good idea to begin with *univariate* (one variable at a time) statistics. For continuous variables, univariate statistics typically measure *central tendency* and *variability.* The most common measures of central tendency are the *mean* (or average) and the *median* (i.e., the 50th percentile).

One of the most commonly used measures of variability is the *standard deviation* (SD). A useful property of the SD is that if the distribution of the variable is the familiar bell-shaped, or "normal," distribution, about 68% of the observations will be within 1 SD of the mean, and about 95% within 2 SD. Even when the distribution is not normal, these rules are often approximately true.

For variables that are not normally distributed, the mean and SD are not as useful for summarizing the data. In that case, the median may be a better measure of central tendency because it is not influenced by observations far below or far above the center. Similarly, the range and pairs of percentiles, such as the 25th and 75th percentiles, will provide a better description of the spread of the data than the SD.

Univariate Statistics for Categorical Variables: Proportions, Rates, and Ratios

For categorical variables, the main univariate statistic is the *proportion* of subjects with each value of the variable. Ordinal variables with many categories can be summarized by using proportions or by using medians and percentiles, as with continuous data that are not normally distributed.

It is worth distinguishing between *proportions, rates,* and *ratios* because these terms are often confused. *Proportions* are unitless, always between 0 and 1 inclusive, and express what fraction of the subjects have or develop a particular characteristic or outcome. Strictly speaking, *rates* have units of inverse time; they express the proportion of subjects in whom a particular characteristic or outcome develops over a specific time period. The term is frequently misused, however. For example, the term *false-positive rate* is widely used for the proportion of subjects without a disease who test positive, even though it is a proportion, not a rate. *Ratios* are the quotients of two numbers; they can range between zero and infinity. For example, the male-to-female ratio of people with a disease might be 3:1. As a rule, if a ratio can be expressed as a proportion instead (e.g., 75% male), it is more concise and easier to understand.

Incidence and Prevalence

Two terms commonly used (and misused) in medicine and public health are *incidence* and *prevalence. Incidence* describes the number of subjects who *contract* a disease *over time* divided by the population at risk. Incidence is usually expressed as a rate (e.g., 7 per 1000 per year), but it may sometimes be a proportion if the time variable is otherwise understood or clear, as in the lifetime incidence of breast cancer or the incidence of diabetes during pregnancy. *Prevalence* describes the number of subjects who *have* a disease at *one point in time* divided by the population at risk; it is always a proportion. At any point in time, the prevalence of disease depends on how many people contract it and how long it lasts: prevalence = incidence × duration.

Bivariate Statistics

Bivariate statistics summarize the relationship between two variables. In clinical research, it is often desirable to distinguish between *predictor* and *outcome* variables. Predictor variables include treatments received, demographic variables, and test results that are thought possibly to predict or cause the *outcome variable,* which is the disease or (generally bad) event or outcome that the test should predict or treatment prevent.

Dichotomous Predictor and Outcome Variables

A common and straightforward case is when both predictor and outcome variables are dichotomous and the results can thus be summarized in a 2 × 2 table. Bivariate statistics are also called *measures of association.*

Relative Risk

The *relative risk* or *risk ratio* (RR) is the ratio of the proportion of subjects in one group in whom the outcome develops divided by the proportion in the other group in whom it develops. For example, in the Women's Health Initiative (WHI) randomized trial, estrogen use was associated with an increased risk for stroke (RR = 1.37) and decreased risk for hip fracture (RR = 0.61).

Relative Risk Reduction

The *relative risk reduction* (RRR) is 1 − RR. In the aforementioned WHI example, estrogen had an RR of 0.61 for hip fracture, so the RRR would be 1 − 0.61 = 0.39, or 39%. The RRR is commonly expressed as a percentage.

Absolute Risk Reduction

The *risk difference* or *absolute risk reduction* (ARR) is the difference in risk between the groups, as defined earlier. In the WHI, the risk for hip fracture was 0.11% per year with estrogen and 0.17% per year with placebo, so the ARR = 0.06% per year, or 6 in 10,000 per year.

Number Needed to Treat

The *number needed to treat* (NNT) is 1/ARR. To see why this is the case, consider the WHI placebo group and imagine treating 10,000 patients for a year. All but 17 would not have had a hip fracture anyway because the fracture rate in the placebo group was 0.17% per year, and 11 subjects would sustain a fracture despite treatment because the fracture rate in the estrogen group was 0.11% per year. Thus, with treatment of 10,000 patients for a year, 17 − 11 = 6 fractures prevented, or 1 fracture prevented for each 1667 patients treated.

Risk Difference

When the treatment *increases* the risk for a bad outcome, the difference in risk between treated and untreated patients should still be calculated, but it is usually just called the risk difference rather than an ARR (because the "reduction" would be negative).

Odds Ratio

Another commonly used measure of association is the *odds ratio* (OR). The OR is the ratio of the *odds* of the outcome in the two groups, where the definition of the odds of an outcome is $p/(1 - p)$, with p being the probability of the outcome. From this definition it is apparent that when p is very small, $1 - p$ will be close to 1, so $p/(1 - p)$ will be close to p, and the OR will closely approximate the RR. When p is not small, however, the odds and probability will be quite different, and ORs and RRs will not be interchangeable.

Absolute versus Relative Measures

The choice of *absolute* versus *relative measures* of association depends on the use of the measure. RRs are more useful as summary measures of effect because they are more often generalizable across a wide variety of populations. RRs are also more helpful for understanding causality. However, absolute risks are more important for questions about clinical decision making because they relate directly to the tradeoffs between risks and benefits—specifically, the NNT, as well as the costs and side effects that need to be balanced against potential benefits. RRRs are often used in advertising because they are generally more impressive than ARRs. Unfortunately, the distinction between relative and absolute risks may not be appreciated by clinicians, thereby leading to higher estimates of the potential benefits of treatments when RRs or RRRs are used.

Risk Ratios versus Odds Ratios

The choice between RRs and ORs is easier: RRs are preferred because they are easier to understand. Because ORs that are not equal to 1 are always farther from 1 than the corresponding RR, they may falsely inflate the perceived importance of a factor. ORs are, however, typically used in two circumstances. First, in case-control studies (Chapter 10), in which subjects with and without the disease are sampled separately, the RR cannot be calculated directly. Second, in observational studies that use a type of multivariate analysis called *logistic regression* (see later), use of the OR is convenient because it is the parameter that is modeled in the analysis.

Dichotomous Predictor Variable, Continuous Outcome Variable

Many outcome variables are naturally continuous rather than dichotomous. For example, in a study of a new treatment of obesity, the outcome might be change in weight or BMI. Most measurements have units (e.g., kg, mm Hg), so differences between groups will have the same units and be meaningless without them. For measurements in unfamiliar units, such as a score on a new quality-of-life instrument, some benchmark is useful to help judge whether the difference in groups is large or small. What is typically done in that case is to express the difference in relation to the spread of values in the study, as measured by the SD. In this case, the *standardized mean difference* (SMD) is the difference between the two means divided by the SD of the measurement.

Continuous Predictor Variable

When predictor variables are continuous, the investigator can either group the values into two or more categories and calculate mean differences or SMDs between the groups as discussed earlier or use a *model* to summarize the degree to which changes in the predictor variable are associated with changes in the outcome variable. Perhaps the simplest model is to assume a linear relationship between the outcome and predictor. For example, one could assume that the relationship between systolic blood pressure (mm Hg) and salt intake (g/day) was linear over the range studied:

$$SBP_i = a + (b \times SALT_i) + \varepsilon_i$$

where SBP_i is the systolic blood pressure for study subject i, $SALT_i$ is that subject's salt intake, and ε_i is an error term that the model specifies must average out to zero across all of the subjects in the study. In this model, a is a constant, the *intercept,* and the strength of the relationship between the outcome and predictor can be summarized by the slope b, which has units equal to the units of SBP divided by the units of SALT, or mm Hg per gram of salt per day in this case.

It is important to keep in mind that use of a model to summarize a relationship between two variables may not be appropriate if the model does not fit. For example, if the effect of a 1-g/day change in salt intake differed in subjects ingesting low- and high-salt diets, the model would not fit and misleading conclusions could result.

When the outcome variable is dichotomous, the relationship with the continuous predictor variable is often modeled with a *logistic* model:

$$\Pr\{Y_i = 1\} = \frac{1}{1 + e^{-(a+bx_i)}}$$

where the outcome Y_i is coded 0 or 1 for study subject i, and x_i is that subject's value of the predictor variable. Once again, a is a constant, in this case related to the probability of the disease when the predictor is equal to zero, and b summarizes the strength of the association; in this case, it is the natural logarithm of the OR rather than the slope. The OR is the OR *per unit change* in the predictor variable. For example, in a study of lung cancer, an OR of 1.06 for pack years of smoking would indicate that the odds of lung cancer increase by 6% for each pack year increase in smoking.

Multivariable Statistics

In many cases, researchers are interested in the effects of multiple predictor variables on an outcome. Particularly in observational studies, it will be of interest to estimate the effects of each predictor variable *independent* of the effects of other variables. For example, in studying whether regular exercise decreases the risk for heart disease, investigators would try to take differences in race, sex, age, cigarette smoking, blood pressure, and cholesterol into account. Trying to stratify by all of these variables would require a massive data set and raise the issue of multiple testing (see expanded chapter at www.expertconsult.com). Instead, models are used because they enable the information about individual predictors to be summarized by using the full data set. These models are similar to those described earlier but include terms for the additional variables.

⬤ INFERRING POPULATION VALUES FROM A SAMPLE

The next step after describing the data is drawing inferences from a sample to the population. Statistics mainly quantify random error. Samples that were not randomly selected from populations may be unrepresentative because of *bias,* and statistics cannot help with this type of systematic (nonrandom) error.

Inferences from Sample Means: Standard Deviation versus Standard Error

The simplest case of inference from a sample to a population involves estimating a population mean from a sample. Intuitively, the larger the sample size,

N, the more likely that the sample mean will be close to the population mean. The more variability there is within the sample, the less accurate the estimate of the population mean is likely to be. To make inferences about a population mean from a sample mean, the *standard error of the mean* (SEM), which takes both of these factors into account, is as follows:

$$SEM = \frac{SD}{\sqrt{N}}$$

Confidence Intervals

The SEM has an interpretation pertaining to means that is parallel to the SD for individual observations. Just as about 95% of *observations* in a population are expected to be within ±1.96 SD of the mean, 95% of *sample means* are expected to be within 1.96 SEM of the population mean, thereby providing the 95% confidence interval (CI), which is the range of values for the population mean consistent with what was observed from the sample.

CIs can similarly be calculated for other quantities estimated from samples, including proportions, ORs, regression coefficients, and hazard ratios. In each case, they provide a range of values consistent with what was observed in the study in the target population.

Significance Testing and *P* Values

P values start with calculation of a *test statistic* that has a known distribution under the *null hypothesis,* which states that there is no association between variables. *P* values answer the question, "If the null hypothesis were true, what would be the probability of obtaining, by chance alone, a value of the test statistic this large or larger (suggesting an association between groups of this strength or stronger)?"

There are a number of common pitfalls in interpreting *P* values. The first is that because *P* values less than .05 are customarily described as being "statistically significant," results with *P* < .05 sometimes are described as "significant" when in fact the results may not be clinically significant (i.e., important) at all. This situation may arise when studies have a large sample size.

A second pitfall is concluding that no association exists simply because the *P* value is greater than .05. This problem is particularly likely if the sample size is small. It is then helpful to look at the 95% CI to see whether a clinically significant effect may have been missed.

Finally, a common misconception about *P* values is that they indicate the probability that the null hypothesis is true (e.g., that there is no association between variables). But calculation of *P* values is *based on the assumption* that the null hypothesis is true. The probability that an association is real depends not just on the probability of its occurrence under the null hypothesis but also on the probability of another basis for the association (see later)—an assessment that depends on information from outside the study, sometimes called the *prior probability.*

 Visit expertconsult.com for e-expanded chapter

SUGGESTED READINGS

Harvey BJ, Lang TA. Hypothesis testing, study power, and sample size. *Chest.* 2010;138:734-737. *Review.*
Walker E, Nowacki AS. Understanding equivalence and noninferiority testing. *J Gen Intern Med.* 2011;26:192-196. *Review.*

USING DATA FOR CLINICAL DECISIONS

THOMAS H. LEE

Key functions in the professional lives of all physicians are the collection and analysis of clinical data. Decisions must be made on the basis of these data, including which therapeutic strategy is most appropriate for the patient and whether further information should be gathered before the best strategy can be chosen. This decision-making process is a blend of science and art in which the physician must synthesize a variety of concerns, including the patient's most likely outcome with various management strategies, the patient's worst possible outcome, and the patient's preferences among these strategies.

Only rarely does the physician enjoy true certainty regarding any of these issues, so a natural inclination for physicians is to seek as much information as possible before making a decision. This approach ignores the dangers inherent in the collection of information. Some of these dangers are immediate, such as the risk of cerebrovascular accident associated with coronary angiography. Other dangers are delayed, such as the risk of a malignancy due to radiation exposure from diagnostic tests.

An additional concern is the cost of information gathering, including the direct costs of the tests themselves and the indirect costs that flow from decisions made on the basis of the test results. Substantial data demonstrate marked variation in use of tests among physicians located in different regions and even within the same group practice. Standards of medical professionalism endorse the need for physicians to exert their influence to minimize inefficiency, but this challenge grows increasingly complex as medical progress leads to proliferation of alternative testing strategies.

For the physician, there are three key questions in this sequence: Should I order a test to improve my assessment of diagnosis or prognosis? Which test is best? Which therapeutic strategy is most appropriate for this patient?

● SHOULD I ORDER A TEST?

The decision of whether to order a test depends on the physician's and the patient's willingness to pursue a management strategy with the current degree of uncertainty. This decision is influenced by several factors, including the patient's attitudes toward diagnostic and therapeutic interventions (e.g., a patient with claustrophobia might prefer an ultrasound to magnetic resonance imaging) and the information provided by the test itself. The personal tolerance of the patient and physician for uncertainty also frequently influences test-ordering approaches. A decision to watch and wait rather than to obtain a specific test also should be considered an information-gathering alternative because the information obtained while a patient is being observed often reduces uncertainty about the diagnosis and outcome. In other words, the "test of time" should be recognized as one of the most useful tests available when this tactic does not seem inappropriately risky.

Most tests do not provide a definitive answer about diagnosis or prognosis but instead reduce uncertainty. Accordingly, the impact of information from tests often is expressed as *probabilities* (Table 9-1). A probability of 1.0 implies that an event is certain to occur, whereas a probability of 0 implies that the event is impossible. When all the possible events for a patient are assigned probabilities, these estimates should sum to 1.0.

It is often useful to use *odds* to quantify uncertainty instead of probability. Odds of 1:2 suggest that the likelihood of an event is only half the likelihood that the event will not occur. The relationship between odds and probability is expressed in the following formula:

$$Odds = P/(1-P)$$

where *P* is the probability of an event.

TABLE 9-1	KEY DEFINITIONS*
Probability	A number between 0 and 1 that expresses an estimate of the likelihood of an event
Odds	The ratio of [the probability of an event] to [the probability of the event not occurring]
TEST PERFORMANCE CHARACTERISTICS	
Sensitivity	Percentage of patients with disease who have an abnormal test result
Specificity	Percentage of patients without disease who have a normal test result
Positive predictive value	Percentage of patients with an abnormal test result who have disease
Negative predictive value	Percentage of patients with a normal test result who do not have disease
BAYESIAN ANALYSIS	
Pretest (or prior) probability	The probability of a disease before the information is acquired
Post-test (or posterior) probability	The probability of a disease after new information is acquired
Pretest (or prior) odds	(Pretest probability of disease)/(1 − pretest probability of disease)
Likelihood ratio	(Probability of result in diseased persons)/ (probability of result in nondiseased persons)

Disease can mean a condition, such as coronary artery disease, or an outcome, such as postoperative cardiac complications.

Performance Characteristics

Sensitivity and *specificity* are key terms for the description of test performance. These parameters describe the test and are in theory true regardless of the population of patients to which the test is applied. Research studies that describe test performance often are based, however, on highly selected populations of patients; test performance may deteriorate when tests are applied in clinical practice. The result of a test for coronary artery disease, such as an electron beam computed tomography scan, rarely may be abnormal if it is evaluated in a low-risk population, such as high-school students. False-positive abnormal results secondary to coronary calcification in the absence of obstructive coronary disease are common when the test is performed in middle-aged and elderly people.

Although researchers are interested in the performance of tests, the true focus of medical decision making is the patient. Physicians are more interested in the implications of a test result on the probability that a patient has a specific disease or outcome, that is, the predictive values of abnormal or normal test results. These predictive values are extremely sensitive to the population from which they are derived (Table 9-2; see also Table 9-1). An abnormal lung scan result in an asymptomatic patient has a much lower positive predictive value than that same test result in a patient with dyspnea and a diminished oxygen saturation. Bayes' theorem (see later) provides a framework for analyzing the interaction between test results and a patient's pretest probability of a disease.

As useful as the performance characteristics may be, they are limited by the fact that few tests truly provide dichotomous (i.e., positive or negative) test results. Tests such as exercise tests have several parameters (e.g., ST segment deviation, exercise duration, hemodynamic response) that provide insight into the patient's condition, and the normal range for many blood tests (e.g., prostate-specific antigen) varies markedly according to the age of the tested population and one's willingness to "miss" patients with disease. Tests that require human interpretation (e.g., radiologic studies) are particularly subject to variability in the reported results.

Bayes' Theorem

The impact of a test result on a patient's probability of disease was first quantified by Bayes, an 18th-century English clergyman who developed a formula that describes the probability of disease in the presence of an abnormal test result. The classic presentation of Bayes' theorem is complex and difficult to use. A simpler form of this theorem is known as the *odds ratio* form, which describes the impact of a test result on the pretest odds (see Table 9-1) of a diagnosis or outcome for a specific patient.

To calculate the post-test odds of disease, the pretest odds are multiplied by the *likelihood ratio* (LR) for a specific test result. The mathematical presentation of this form of Bayes' theorem is as follows:

$$\text{Post-test odds} = (\text{Pretest odds}) \times (\text{LR})$$

The LR is the probability of a particular test result in patients with the disease divided by the probability of that same test result in patients without disease. In other words, the LR is the test result's sensitivity divided by the false-positive rate. A test of no value (e.g., flipping a coin and calling "heads" an abnormal result) would have an LR of 1.0 because half of patients with disease would have abnormal test results, as would half of patients without disease. This test would have no impact on a patient's odds of disease. The further an LR is above 1.0, the more that test result raises a patient's probability of disease. For LRs less than 1.0, the closer the LR is to 0, the more it lowers a patient's probability of disease.

When it is displayed graphically (Fig. 9-1), a test of no value (*dotted line*) does not change the pretest probability, whereas an abnormal or normal result from a useful test moves the probability up or down. For a patient with a high pretest probability of disease, an abnormal test result changes the patient's probability only slightly, but a normal test result leads to a marked reduction in the probability of disease. Similarly, for a patient with a low pretest probability of disease, a normal test result has little impact, but an abnormal test result markedly raises the probability of disease.

Consider how various exercise test results influence a patient's probability of coronary disease (see Table 9-2). For a patient whose clinical history, physical examination, and electrocardiographic findings suggest a 50% probability of disease, the pretest odds of disease are 1.0. LRs for various test results are developed by pooling data from published literature. The sensitivity of an exercise test with any amount of ST segment changes is the rate of such test results in patients with coronary disease, and the specificity is the percentage of patients without coronary disease who do *not* have this test result. The LR for no ST change is less than 1, whereas the LRs for patients with ST changes are greater than 1 (see Table 9-2). Therefore, when the LRs for various test results are multiplied by the pretest odds to calculate post-test odds, the odds decrease for patients without ST segment changes but increase for patients with 1 or 2 mm of ST segment change. Post-test odds can be converted to post-test probabilities according to the following formula:

$$\text{Probability} = \text{Odds}/(1 + \text{odds})$$

The calculations quantify how the absence of ST segment changes reduces a patient's probability of disease, whereas ST segment depression raises the probability of disease.

This form of Bayes' theorem is useful for showing how the post-test probability of disease is influenced by the patient's pretest probability of disease.

TABLE 9-2 EXAMPLE OF ODDS RATIO FORM OF BAYES' THEOREM

Question: What is the probability of coronary disease for a patient with a 50% pretest probability of coronary disease who undergoes an exercise test if that patient develops (a) no ST segment changes, (b) 1 mm of ST segment depression, or (c) 2 mm of ST segment depression?

Step 1. Calculate the pretest odds of disease:

$$P/(1-P) = 0.5/(1-0.5)$$
$$= 0.5/0.5$$
$$= 1$$

Step 2. Calculate the likelihood ratios for the various test results, using the formula LR = sensitivity/(1 − specificity). (Data from pooled literature.)

TEST RESULT	SENSITIVITY	SPECIFICITY	LIKELIHOOD RATIO
No ST segment changes	0.34	0.15	0.4
1-mm ST segment depression	0.66	0.85	4.4
2-mm ST segment depression	0.33	0.97	11

Step 3. Calculate the post-test odds of disease and convert those odds to post-test probabilities:

TEST RESULT	PRETEST ODDS	LIKELIHOOD RATIO	POST-TEST ODDS	POST-TEST PROBABILITY
No ST segment changes	1	0.4	0.4	0.29
1-mm ST segment depression	1	4.4	4.4	0.81
2-mm ST segment depression	1	11	11	0.92

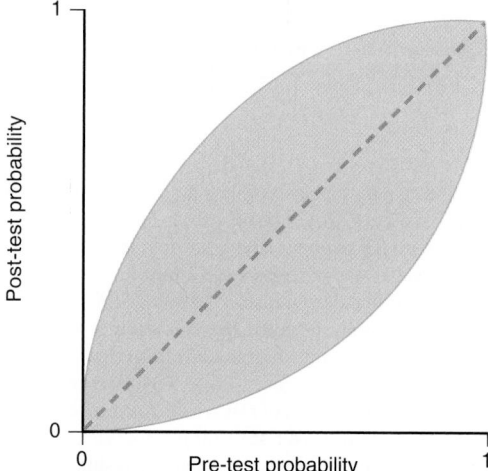

FIGURE 9-1. Impact of various test results on the patient's probability of disease. The x axis depicts a patient's probability of disease before a test. If the test is of no value, the post-test probability (*dotted line*) is no different from the pretest probability. An abnormal test result raises the post-test probability of disease, as depicted by the concave downward arc, whereas a normal test result lowers the probability.

TABLE 9-3 PRINCIPLES OF TEST ORDERING AND INTERPRETATION

The interpretation of test results depends on what is already known about the patient.

No test is perfect; clinicians should be familiar with their diagnostic performance (see Table 9-1) and never believe that a test "forces" them to pursue a specific management strategy.

Tests should be ordered if they may provide *additional* information beyond that already available.

Tests should be ordered if there is a reasonable chance that the data will influence the patient's care.

Two tests that provide similar information should not be ordered.

In choosing between two tests that provide similar data, use the test that has lower costs and/or causes less discomfort and inconvenience to the patient.

Clinicians should seek all of the information provided by a test, not just an abnormal or normal result.

The cost-effectiveness of strategies using noninvasive tests should be considered in a manner similar to that of therapeutic strategies.

FIGURE 9-2. Interpretation of test results in high-risk and low-risk patients. **A,** High-risk population (90% prevalence of disease). **B,** Low-risk population (5% prevalence of disease).

If a patient's clinical data suggest a *probability* of coronary disease of only 0.1, the *pretest odds* of disease would be only 0.11. For such a low-risk patient, an exercise test with no ST segment changes would lead to post-test probability of coronary disease of 4%, whereas 1- or 2-mm ST segment changes would lead to a post-test probability of disease of 33 or 55%.

Even if clinicians rarely perform the calculations that are described in Bayes' theorem, there are important lessons from this theorem that are relevant to principles of test ordering (Table 9-3). The most crucial of these lessons is that the interpretation of test results must incorporate information about the patient. An abnormal test result in a low-risk patient may not be a true indicator of disease. Similarly, a normal test result in a high-risk patient should not be taken as evidence that disease is not present.

Figure 9-2 provides an example of the post-test probabilities for positive and negative results for a test with a sensitivity of 85% and a specificity of 90% (e.g., radionuclide scintigraphy for diagnosis of coronary artery disease). In a high-risk population with a 90% prevalence of disease, the positive

predictive value of an abnormal result is 0.99 compared with 0.31 for the same test result obtained in a low-risk population with a 5% prevalence of disease. Similarly, the negative predictive value of a normal test result is greater in the low-risk population than in the high-risk population.

Multiple Testing

Clinicians frequently obtain more than one test aimed at addressing the same issue and at times are confronted with conflicting results. If these tests are truly independent (i.e., the tests do not have the same basis in pathophysiology), it may be appropriate to use the post-test probability obtained through performance of one test as the pretest probability for the analysis of the impact of the second test result.

If the tests are not independent, this strategy for interpretation of serial test results can be misleading. Suppose a patient with chronic obstructive pulmonary disease and a history vaguely suggestive of pulmonary embolism is found to have an abnormal lung ventilation-perfusion scan. Obtaining that same test result over and over would not raise that patient's probability of pulmonary embolism higher and higher. In this extreme case, the tests are identical; serial testing adds no information. More commonly, clinicians are faced with results from tests with related but not identical bases in pathophysiology, such as ventilation-perfusion scintigraphy and pulmonary angiography.

Regardless of whether tests are independent, the performance of multiple tests increases the likelihood that an abnormal test result will be obtained in a patient without disease. If a chemistry battery includes 20 tests and the normal range for each test has been developed to include 95% of healthy individuals, the chance that a healthy patient will have a normal result for any specific test is 0.95. However, the probability that all 20 tests will be normal is $(0.95)^{20}$, or 0.36. Most healthy people can be expected to have at least one abnormal result. Unless screening test profiles are used thoughtfully, false-positive results can subject patients to unnecessary tests and procedures.

Threshold Approach to Decision Making

Even if a test provides information, that information may not change management for an individual patient. Lumbar spine radiographs of a patient who is not willing to undergo surgery may reveal the severity of disease but expose the patient to needless radiation. Similarly, a test that merely confirms a diagnosis that already is recognized is a waste of resources (see Table 9-3).

Before ordering a test, clinicians should consider whether that test result could change the choice of management strategies. This approach is called the *threshold approach to medical decision making,* and it requires the physician to be able to estimate the threshold probability at which one strategy will be chosen over another. The management of a clinically stable patient with a high probability of coronary disease might not be changed by any of the post-test probabilities shown in Table 9-2. If that patient had no ST segment changes, the post-test probability of 0.29 still would be too high for a clinician to consider that patient free of disease. An abnormal test result that strengthened the diagnosis of coronary disease might not change management unless it suggested a greater severity of disease that might warrant another management strategy.

Testing for Peace of Mind

Physicians frequently order tests even when there is little chance that the outcomes will provide qualitatively new insights into a patient's diagnosis or prognosis or alter a patient's management. In such cases, the cited goal for testing may be to improve a patient's peace of mind. Although a decrease in uncertainty can improve quality of life for many patients, individuals with hypochondriasis and somatization disorders rarely obtain comfort from normal test results; instead, their complaints shift to a new organ system, and their demands focus on other tests. For such patients, management strategies using frequent visits and cognitive tactics are recommended.

⬤ WHICH TEST IS BEST?

If the clinician decided that more information is needed to reduce uncertainty, and if it appears possible that tests might lead to a change in management strategies, the question arises as to which test is most appropriate. Note that just because guideline-development committees have concluded that a specific test is "appropriate" in given clinical context, this does not mean that this test is the *most* appropriate option. Several factors influence the choice among diagnostic strategies, including patients' preferences, the costs and risks associated with the tests, and the diagnostic performance of alternative tests.

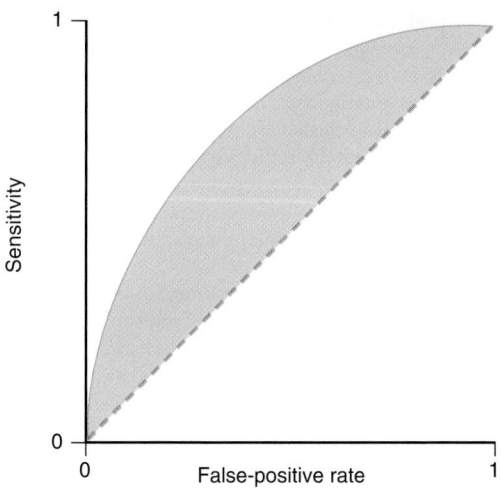

FIGURE 9-3. **Receiver operating characteristic curve.** The points on the curve reflect the sensitivity and false-positive (1 − specificity) rates of a test at various thresholds. As the threshold is changed to yield greater sensitivity for detecting the outcome of interest, the false-positive rate rises. The better the test, the closer the curve comes to the upper left corner. A test of no value (e.g., flipping a coin) would lead to a curve with the course of the *dotted line*. The area under the curve is used often to compare alternative testing strategies.

TABLE 9-4 STEPS IN PERFORMANCE OF DECISION ANALYSIS

Frame the question.
Create the decision tree.
   Identify the alternative strategies.
   List the possible outcomes for each of the alternative strategies.
   Describe the sequence of events as a series of decision nodes and chance nodes.
Choose a time horizon for the analysis.
Determine the probability for each chance outcome.
Assign a value to each outcome.
Calculate the expected utility for each strategy.
Perform sensitivity analysis.

Diagnostic performance of a test often is summarized in terms of sensitivity and specificity, but as shown in the example in Table 9-2, these parameters depend on which threshold (e.g., 1 vs. 2 mm of ST segment change) is used. A low threshold for calling a test result abnormal might lead to excellent sensitivity for detecting disease, but at the expense of a high false-positive rate. Conversely, a threshold that led to few false-positive results might cause a clinician to miss many cases of true disease.

The receiver operating characteristic (ROC) curve is a graphic form of describing this tradeoff and providing a method for comparing test performance (Fig. 9-3). Each point on the ROC curve describes the sensitivity and the false-positive rate for a different threshold for abnormality for a test. A test of no value would lead to an ROC curve with the course of the dotted line, whereas a misleading test would be described by a curve that was concave upward (not shown).

The more accurate the test, the closer its ROC curve comes to the upper left corner of the graph, which would indicate a test threshold that has excellent sensitivity and a low false-positive rate. The closer an ROC curve comes to the upper left corner, the greater the area under the curve. The area under ROC curves can be used to compare the information provided by two tests.

Even if one test is superior to another as shown by a greater area under its ROC curve, the question still remains as to what value of that test should be considered abnormal. The choice of threshold depends on the purpose of testing and on the consequences of a false-positive or false-negative diagnosis. If the goal is to screen the population for a disease that is potentially fatal and potentially curable, a threshold with excellent sensitivity is appropriate even if it leads to frequent false-positive results. In contrast, if a test is used to confirm a diagnosis that is likely to be treated with a high-risk invasive procedure, a threshold with high specificity is preferred. Only 1 mm of ST segment depression might be the appropriate threshold when exercise electrocardiography is used to evaluate the possibility of coronary disease in a patient with chest pain. If the question is whether to perform coronary angiography in a patient with stable angina in search of severe coronary disease that might benefit from revascularization, a threshold of 2 mm or more would be more appropriate.

● CHOOSING A STRATEGY

Physicians and patients ultimately must use clinical information to make decisions. These choices usually are made after consideration of a variety of factors, including information from the clinical evaluation, patients' preferences, and expected outcomes with various management strategies. Insight into the impact of these considerations can be improved through the performance of decision analysis (Table 9-4).

The first step in a decision analysis is to define the problem clearly; this step often requires writing out a statement of the issue so that it can be scrutinized for any ambiguity. After the problem is defined, the next step is to define the alternative strategies.

Consider the question of which test is most appropriate to screen patients for breast cancer: mammography with or without breast magnetic resonance imaging—a newer technology that is highly sensitive for detecting breast cancer but is more costly and less specific. The expected outcomes for these strategies depend on each test's sensitivity and specificity for detecting breast cancer, which is influenced in turn by other factors, such as the frequency with which the test is performed. Patients' outcomes also are influenced by their underlying risk for breast cancer and the likelihood that earlier detection of tumors reduces the risk for death.

Each of these variables must be known or estimated for calculations to be made of each strategy's predicted life expectancy and direct medical costs. These outcomes differ for patients according to age, medical history, family history, and presence or absence of genetic markers such as *BRCA* mutations. Optimal strategies for an elderly patient with a short life expectancy and low clinical risk of cancer are unlikely to be the same as for a younger patient with inherited mutations of the *BRCA1* or *BRCA2* gene, indicating a cumulative lifetime risk of breast cancer of 50 to 85% (Chapter 204).

The credibility of the decision analysis depends on the credibility of these estimates. Published reports often do not provide information on the outcomes of interest for specific subsets of patients, or there may not have been sufficient statistical power within subsets of patients for the findings to be statistically significant. Randomized trial data are relevant to the populations included in the trial; the extension of the findings to other genders, races, and age groups requires assumptions by individuals performing the analysis. For many issues, expert opinion must be used to derive a reasonable estimate of the outcome.

For many diseases, the potential outcomes are more complex than perfect health or death. With chronic diseases, patients may live many years in a condition somewhere between these two, and the goal of medical interventions may be to improve quality of life rather than to extend survival. The value of life in imperfect health must be reflected in decision analyses. These values by convention are expressed on a scale of 0 to 100, where 0 indicates the worst outcome and 100 indicates the best outcome.

Life-expectancy and quality-of-life estimates are combined in many decision analyses to calculate *quality-adjusted life years*. A strategy that leads to a 10-year life expectancy with such severe disability that utility of the state of health is only half that of perfect health would have a quality-adjusted life expectancy of 5 years. With such adjustments to life-expectancy data, the impact of interventions that improve quality of life but do not extend life can be compared with interventions that extend life but do not improve its quality or perhaps even worsen it.

After the value and the probability of the various outcomes have been estimated, the expected utility of each strategy can be calculated. In comparing the different strategies available at a decision node, the analysis generally selects the option with the highest expected utility. At chance nodes, the expected utility is the weighted average of the utility of the various possible branches.

After the analysis has been performed with the baseline assumptions, *sensitivity analyses* should be performed in which these assumptions are varied over a reasonable range. These analyses can reveal which assumptions have the most influence over the conclusions and identify threshold probabilities at which the conclusions would change. For example, the threshold at which breast magnetic resonance imaging should be added to mammography is likely to be influenced by the cost of the magnetic resonance imaging and the accuracy of the radiologists who interpret the images.

Cost-Benefit and Cost-Effectiveness Analyses

For clinicians and health care policymakers, the choices that must be addressed go beyond the choices within any single decision analysis. Because resources available for health care are limited, policymakers may have to choose among many competing "investments" in health. Although such decisions frequently are made on the basis of political considerations, cost-benefit and cost-effectiveness analyses can be informative in making the choices.

The methodology of these techniques is similar to that of decision analysis except that costs for the various possible outcomes and strategies also are calculated. *Discounting* is used to adjust the value of future benefits and costs because resources saved or spent currently are worth more than resources saved or expended in the future. In *cost-benefit* analyses, all benefits are expressed in terms of economic impact. Extensions in life expectancy are translated into dollars by estimating societal worth or economic productivity.

Because of the ethical discomfort associated with expressing health benefits in financial terms, *cost-effectiveness* analyses are used more commonly than cost-benefit analyses. In these analyses, the ratio of costs to health benefits is calculated; one frequently used method for evaluating a strategy is calculation of cost per quality-adjusted life year. These estimates can be used to compare strategies and to identify settings in which strategies that may be more expensive but more effective (e.g., coronary angiography) may "purchase" quality-adjusted life years at a lower cost than aggressive but less effective strategies (e.g., use of positron emission tomography scanning to diagnose coronary disease) (Table 9-5).

Cost-effectiveness analyses can provide important insights into the relative attractiveness of different management strategies and can help guide policymakers in decisions about which technologies to make available on a routine basis. No medical intervention can have an attractive cost-effectiveness if its effectiveness has not been proved. The cost-effectiveness of an intervention depends heavily on the population of patients in which it is applied. An

---

TABLE 9-5 ESTIMATED COST-EFFECTIVENESS OF COMMON HEALTH INTERVENTIONS

DISEASE CATEGORY	INTERVENTION VS. COMPARATOR IN TARGET POPULATION	COST PER QUALITY-ADJUSTED LIFE YEAR*
Circulatory	Coronary angiography vs. positron emission tomography (PET) in 55-year-old women with chest pain and risk factors that put them at intermediate pretest probability (25-75%) of coronary artery disease	Cost saving
	Angiography vs. exercise electrocardiography (ECG) in patients with no history of myocardial infarction presenting with mild chest pain (typical angina) who are able to undergo an exercise stress test	$47,000
	Exercise single-photon emission computed tomography (SPECT) vs. exercise ECG in patients with no history of myocardial infarction presenting with mild chest pain (typical angina) who are able to undergo an exercise stress test.	$52,000
	Angiography vs. exercise ECG in patients with no history of myocardial infarction presenting with mild chest pain (atypical angina) who are able to undergo an exercise stress test	$89,000
	In patients after a first stroke or transient ischemic attack, patients with heart disease receive transesophageal echocardiography and all others receive standard medical treatment vs. all receive standard medical treatment.	$240,000
	High-dose statin therapy vs. conventional-dose statin therapy in 60-year-old cohorts with acute coronary syndromes (ACS)	$14,000
	Prophylactic implantation of an implantable-cardioverter defibrillator (ICD) vs. control therapy in patients who are at risk for sudden death due to left ventricular systolic dysfunction—Sudden Cardiac Death in Heart Failure Trial (SCD HeFT) population (https://research.tufts-nemc.org/cear/search/detail.aspx?ArticleId=2005-01-01184&id=2005-01-01184-08C)	$77,000
	Cardiac resynchronization therapy (CRT-P) plus medical therapy vs. medical therapy in a 60-year-old patient with heart failure and cardiac dyssynchrony with moderate or severe symptoms (https://research.tufts-nemc.org/cear/search/detail.aspx?ArticleId=2007-01-02351&id=2007-01-02351-13C)	$9,900
Endocrine	Thyroid-stimulating hormone (TSH) screening vs. no TSH screening in women undergoing 5-year periodic health examinations, beginning at 35 years old	$13,000
	Annual diabetic retinopathy screening vs. no screening; diabetic patients receive routine medical care until they become blind in patients diagnosed with type 2 diabetes, aged 30 years or older, undergoing eye screening (https://research.tufts-nemc.org/cear/search/detail.aspx?ArticleId=2008-01-03569&id=2008-01-03569-01C)	Cost saving
	Intensive lifestyle intervention vs. usual care in 60-year-old cohort with impaired glucose tolerance	Cost saving
	Self-monitoring of blood glucose (SMBG) vs. no SMBG in patients with type 2 diabetes receiving insulin only (https://research.tufts-nemc.org/cear/search/detail.aspx?ArticleId=2006-01-02649&id=2006-01-02649-03C)	$9600
	Intensive glucose control, therapies designed to produce HbA1c (A1C) levels of 7.2% vs. conventional glucose control, therapies designed to produce HbA1c (A1C) levels of 10% in patients with new-onset type 2 diabetes at 60-65 years of age	$200,000
Digestive system	Endoscopic surveillance strategy vs. no therapy in man who has endoscopic biopsy-proven Barrett's esophagus—age 55 years	$150,000
	One-time colonoscopic screening for colorectal cancer at age 60-64 years old vs. no screening in men >40 years old	Cost saving
Infectious	One-time rapid HIV infection screening vs. no screening in U.S. communities with low to moderate HIV prevalence (0.05% to 1.0%) and annual incidence (0.0084% to 0.12%)	$35,000
	Treating patients with peginterferon alfa-2b plus ribavirin vs. no treatment in 55-year-old male naïve patients with genotypes 1, 2, and 3 chronic hepatitis C virus (HCV) infection	Cost saving
	Provision of influenza vaccine vs. no provision of service (no vaccine) in U.S. population age 50 years and older	$7,300
Injury	Driver air bag vs. no air bags in driving population (and passengers)	$36,000
	Dual air bag vs. driver air bag in driving population (and passengers)	$91,000
Obstetrics	Elective repeat cesarean section vs. vaginal birth (trial of labor) in 30-year-old patients who have had a previous low transverse cesarean delivery	$140,000
	Elective cesarean delivery vs. vaginal delivery in 25-year-old HIV-infected pregnant women with detectable HIV RNA	Cost saving
Oncology	Adjuvant chemotherapy plus trastuzumab vs. chemotherapy alone in patients with *HER2*-positive early breast cancer, from the U.S. health care system	$21,000
	MRI vs. mammography in women aged 40-49 years with *BRCA1* mutation	$16,000

*In 2008 U.S. dollars.
HIV = human immunodeficiency virus; RNA = ribonucleic acid; TSH = thyroid-stimulating hormone.
Center for the Evaluation of Value and Risk in Health. The Cost-Effectiveness Analysis Registry [Internet]. Boston: Institute for Clinical Research and Health Policy Studies, Tufts Medical Center. http://www.cearegistry.org 2009. Accessed Aug. 8, 2009.

inexpensive intervention would have a poor cost-effectiveness ratio if it were used in a low-risk population unlikely to benefit from it. In contrast, an expensive technology can have an attractive cost-effectiveness ratio if it is used in patients with a high probability of benefiting from it. Table 9-5 shows cost-effectiveness estimates from published literature for some common medical and nonmedical interventions. Such estimates should be used only with understanding of the population for which they are relevant.

SUGGESTED READINGS

Bonow RO. Should coronary calcium screening be used in cardiovascular prevention strategies? *N Engl J Med.* 2009;361:990-997. *Analysis of its potential value to improve risk stratification and management.*

CEA Registry. http://www.tufts-nemc.org/cearegistry; 2010. Accessed Nov. 11, 2010. *Through this website, the Harvard Center for Risk Analysis provides all published cost-effectiveness ratios, sorted by disease area and standardized according to 2008 dollars.*

Esserman L, Shieh Y, Thompson I. Rethinking screening for breast cancer and prostate cancer. *JAMA.* 2009;302:1685. *Assessment of the disappointing impact from breast and prostate cancer screening, with calls for new approaches.*

Kelly M, Morgan A, Ellis S, et al. Evidence based public health: a review of the experience of the National Institute of Health and Clinical Excellence (NICE) of developing public health guidance in England. *Soe Sci Med.* 2010;71:1056-1062. *Example of how data can guide health policy decisions.*

Wald NJ, Morris JK. Assessing risk factors as potential screening tests: A simple assessment tool. *Arch Intern Med.* 2011;171:286-291. *Shows when risk factors are and probably are not useful ways to screen for the probability of certain disease.*

10

MEASURING HEALTH AND HEALTH CARE

STEPHAN D. FIHN

The increasing emphasis on measuring and improving the quality of health care in the United States and elsewhere is based on several fundamental concerns. First, there is clear evidence that the health care system in the United States does not provide the highest quality of care possible. In one study, approximately 4600 randomly selected adults from 12 U.S. cities received recommended preventive, acute, or chronic care only slightly more than half the time. Second, substantial disparities in health care and outcomes persist, with women (Chapter 245), the poor (Chapter 5), and ethnic minorities (Chapter 4) typically faring less well than others. Third, there is growing concern that health care sometimes causes harm, as reflected by statistics indicating that 1 in 6.5 hospitalizations is complicated by a mistake in administering or prescribing medication, that 1 in 20 outpatient prescriptions is wrong, or that inpatient errors may cause as many as 44,000 to 98,000 deaths annually (Chapter 11). Fourth, health care is extraordinarily expensive, with an annual aggregate expenditure of more than $2 trillion (nearly $7500 per resident) that consumes nearly 17% of the U.S. gross domestic product (Chapter 5). If premiums for health insurance grow at the projected national rate of increase, the cost of family coverage will double from the 2008 average of $12,298 to $24,000 or even higher by 2020. Moreover, there is substantial evidence that the delivery system is inefficient and wasteful. Per capita expenditures for health care vary as much as 250% among communities of similar size, without any evidence that higher spending leads to better outcomes. In fact, observational data from Medicare suggest that there is actually an inverse relationship between the amount of overall health care spending at the state level and better quality.

Findings such as these have fueled demands from government, employers, and consumer groups for greater accountability and improved quality. In response, the information collected to measure health and health care has increased dramatically. Physicians and other health care providers are frequently confronted with these data in nearly every sphere of activity, including clinical care, education, and research. To interpret and apply this information correctly, health care providers should understand the basic principles of measuring the process and outcomes of health care.

● MEASUREMENT OF HEALTH CARE

The basic paradigm that guides assessment of quality includes three fundamental domains: structure, process, and outcome. *Structure* refers to the stable elements that make up the health care system, such as the physical plant, administrative organizations, and qualifications of the staff. Because structural characteristics, such as whether floors are clean or doctors are board certified, are often the easiest aspects of health care to observe and

measure, they were the main focus of early efforts to improve quality. Over time, however, it became clear that a clean environment and qualified providers are essential but insufficient to guarantee high quality unless the process of care is effective.

Process refers to how care is delivered, including medical interventions and interpersonal interactions. Thus it is important to know, for instance, whether the right physician has performed the right procedure on the right patient in the right way at the right time. Documenting these findings for the multitude of patients, however, can be expensive, difficult, and subjective because there may be a variety of acceptable approaches to a given clinical problem. Moreover, patients tend to be more concerned about achieving the best possible outcomes of care, such as curing disease, reducing symptoms, or improving function, than about how these outcomes are achieved.

Outcomes represent the presumptive results of care that is delivered. The concept of health outcomes encompasses a broad array of clinical indicators that include death, adverse clinical events, persistence or recurrence of disease, disability, discomfort, and pain. Outcomes from the patient's perspective include self-reported health, ability to function, burden imposed by disease, and satisfaction with care. In addition, there may be societal perspectives, such as cost-effectiveness and the cost-benefit ratio (Chapter 9). Judging care on the basis of outcomes is challenging because it may be difficult to measure outcomes reliably and because studies often fail to identify a relationship between high scores on process measures and better outcomes, such as lower in-hospital mortality. Indeed, recent studies of the quality of health care demonstrate that it is important to select measures that are adequately specified and provide a "tight" linkage between process and outcome.

● STANDARDS OF MEASUREMENT

Irrespective of what aspect of health care is being evaluated, the measures used should satisfy standards that help ensure the trustworthiness of the data generated. These standards include adequate specification, reliability, validity, responsiveness, and interpretability. A measure that is *adequately specified* has a well-defined numerator that explicitly describes patients who meet the relevant criteria (e.g., patients whose blood pressure is <140/90 mm Hg or who are followed up within 2 weeks), a well-defined denominator (e.g., patients with hypertension or those discharged with heart failure), and a clear description of patients who are excluded from the calculation (e.g., patients who are younger than 18 years, who have not had an appointment within 18 months, or for whom only comfort care is being provided).

A *reliable* measure yields consistent results when repeated under similar circumstances. Although random error can never be eliminated, one would expect, for example, that two reviewers examining the same medical records would classify the outcomes in the same fashion in all but a small minority of cases. The level of reliability can be compared with common diagnostic procedures in medicine, many of which demonstrate only moderate reliability. For example, common methods of echocardiographic determination of ejection fraction vary up to 24% (Chapter 55), the intraclass coefficient for exercise treadmill tests performed a day apart is only 0.70, and the interobserver correlation for ascertaining the presence of coronary stenosis by highly trained experts is approximately 0.75 (Chapter 57).

Validity refers to the accurate measurement of an intended effect or outcome. In the case of physiologic measures, such as diagnosis of coronary artery disease with electron beam computed tomography (Chapter 56), validity would be indicated by the likelihood of coronary stenoses demonstrated angiographically. In actuality, demonstrable coronary stenoses are present in only 55 to 84% of patients who have a positive result on electron beam computed tomography, which makes it a relatively invalid outcome measure. Validity for measures of subjective outcomes, such as pain, is typically documented through correlation with other related measures, such as the use of analgesic medications or limitation of activities.

Responsiveness reflects the sensitivity of a measure to clinically meaningful changes in status. Whereas a patient with worsening osteoarthritis might record no change on an instrument assessing activities such as bathing or dressing, this patient might exhibit declining scores on a measure that addresses more vigorous activities.

These principles of measurement apply to both quality improvement and research studies, although the standards used in research are generally more rigorous. Measures are typically developed initially for use in research studies and, when shown to possess acceptable performance, are applied to routine quality improvement activities.

Additional criteria should be applied to measures that are being considered for routine use in a clinical setting (Table 10-1), including whether a measure

TABLE 10-1	CRITERIA FOR EVALUATING SUITABILITY OF A CLINICAL PERFORMANCE MEASURE

1. Are the performance characteristics of the measure well established—i.e., valid and reliable?

   The measure appears to measure what is intended (face validity).

   The measure captures most meaningful aspects of care (content validity).

   The measure is reproducible over time and in multiple organizational settings (reliability).

2. Is the measure adequately specified?

   Numerator: definition of patients meeting measure (e.g., patients with blood pressure <140/90 mm Hg or followed up within 2 wk).

   Denominator: definition of patients qualifying for measure (e.g., patients with hypertension).

   Included populations.

   Excluded populations.

3. Is the measure likely to be useful in improving patient outcomes?

   Scientific basis for the measure is well established.

   The results of the measure are interpretable by individual(s) who are responsible for relevant activity.

   The measure is actionable—i.e., addresses an activity or function that is under the control of individual(s) who are responsible and that is amenable to change.

   Implementation of the measure is anticipated to promote the adoption of interventions that have the potential to improve patient outcomes substantially.

   The clinical burden of the condition(s) related to the measure in the affected population is sufficient to warrant measurement and corresponding intervention.

   Current levels of performance related to the measure within the health system indicate substantial opportunities of performance.

4. Can the measure feasibly be implemented?

   The data required for the measure are likely to be obtained with reasonable effort, at reasonable cost, and within a reasonable time frame.

   Data for the measure can be collected automatically when possible.

   The measure has undergone adequate field testing.

5. The measure is relevant to the strategic goals of the health care system.

is *interpretable, evidence based, actionable, feasible,* and *relevant.* An interpretable measure can be understood and applied in clinical settings. For example, although most physicians understand the clinical implications of a change in arterial pH from 7.42 to 7.30, they might not have the same appreciation of a 20-point change on a 100-point scale that measures physical function or satisfaction. Moreover, a measure should be closely related to an intervention that has the potential to improve outcomes that are linked to the burden of the condition in the population.

● TYPES OF MEASURES

Driven largely by efforts to compare the performance of providers and different health care systems, considerable effort has been expended to standardize measures at a national level. Examples include the Healthcare Effectiveness Data and Information Set (HEDIS), which is a set of standardized performance measures designed to assist purchasers and consumers in comparing the care and service provided by more than 90% of health plans in the United States. Another is ORYX, a set of national hospital quality measures collected by the Joint Commission on Accreditation of Healthcare Organizations (E-Table 10-1). Most of these are process measures, although some structural measures and intermediate outcome measures (see later) are included. The National Quality Forum (NQF), which is a quasi-public organization with more than 375 members from various sectors of the health care system, evaluates and issues endorsements for performance measures proposed by many different organizations.

Linkage between Process and Outcome Measures

Process measures are of greatest value when there is a close association, or tight linkage, between a process or action and an outcome. Numerous clinical trials, for example, have shown a substantial reduction in mortality when patients with hypercholesterolemia and ischemic heart disease are given a hydroxymethylglutaryl-coenzyme A reductase inhibitor (statin) to lower low-density lipoprotein cholesterol (LDL-C) levels (Chapter 213). Accordingly, the use of statins in appropriate patients is commonly used as an indicator of quality in many health care organizations. There are, however, limitations to using LDL-C measured at a single point in time; for instance, there may be a legitimate reason for LDL-C to be over the target range in as many as half of patients who would otherwise appear to have received

poor-quality care. Such reasons include having only recently started taking statins, and the dosage is still being titrated; having refused therapy; having a high LDL-C level despite maximal therapy; or having experienced an adverse effect of statins.

Intermediate and Combined Outcomes

Because many outcomes of interest, such as death or the occurrence of serious adverse events, may be relatively infrequent, *intermediate* or *surrogate outcomes* are sometimes measured instead of the true outcome of interest. Intermediate outcomes are often physiologic variables such as blood pressure, cholesterol level, or hemoglobin A_{1c} concentration. For example, the primary rationale for treating diabetes is to prevent complications such as blindness, amputation, or renal failure, and the efficacy of treatment should ultimately be determined by a reduction in risk for these complications. Though important in the pathophysiology of diabetes, a change in the measured hemoglobin A_{1c} level is meaningful as an outcome measure (particularly to the patient) only insofar as it reflects a reduction in risk afforded by treatment. As opposed to standard physiologic measures, other intermediate outcomes reflect subclinical disease; for example, microalbuminuria indicates subclinical renal disease in diabetes (Chapter 236). Intermediate outcomes are attractive because they are often familiar to clinicians and can readily be measured repeatedly in most or all patients, whereas the outcome of interest (e.g., amputation) is a relatively infrequent event in patients treated for diabetes. Using intermediate outcomes may be deceptive, however, particularly when the linkage to the true outcome of interest is loose. The presence of microalbuminuria in a patient with type 2 diabetes (Chapter 237), for instance, is associated with a 2½-fold increase in the relative odds of dying over a 6-year period when compared with diabetic patients who have no protein in their urine. This sizable increase in relative risk, however, translates into a relatively small increase in absolute risk for any individual in any given year. Thus, changes in quality as measured by rates of microalbuminuria would probably not be reflected in outcome measures such as the incidence of cardiovascular events or renal failure, except in extremely large populations. Moreover, it is possible for a treatment to have a salutary effect on a surrogate outcome but a deleterious effect overall. Such was the case for short-acting dihydropyridines such as nifedipine, which effectively lowered blood pressure in hypertensive patients but doubled the incidence of myocardial infarction.

Another strategy adopted when outcome events are infrequent is the use of combined end points. An example is the incidence of cardiovascular events, including stroke, myocardial infarction, unstable angina, and sudden cardiac death. This approach can improve the statistical power of a study, but it tends to exaggerate the perceived efficacy of a particular intervention and may obscure specific effects, such as when an intervention reduces the frequency of stroke more than it does myocardial infarction.

Patient-Oriented Measures

Although physiologic and standard clinical measures are important, the assessment of outcomes from the patient's perspective has increasingly been recognized as being of equal or even greater importance, especially when evaluating treatments intended to lessen symptoms or improve function rather than improve survival. Approaches that depend on a physician's perception of a patient's condition, such as the Canadian Cardiovascular Society Classification for cardiac symptoms (Chapter 50), are limited because physicians often tend to underestimate a patient's symptoms or disability, and such assessments are difficult to standardize. Self-reporting of health and function by patients themselves via standardized questionnaires overcomes these problems. The terminology used to describe the hundreds of questionnaires now available is evolving and, at times, confusing, but the resulting scales generally address various aspects of health-related quality of life, which is a complex, multidimensional concept. Facets or subscales of quality of life may include the severity of symptoms, pain, physical functioning, social functioning, general perceptions of health, overall burden of disease, emotional well-being, and coping, among others.

General measures of health status or health-related quality of life, such as the Short-Form 36 (SF-36), do not focus on a specific disease or condition but seek to assess overall health and functioning. General measures may, however, be insensitive to a specific yet clinically meaningful change in symptoms related to a particular condition. For this reason, more than 1000 *condition-specific measures* are now available. Whereas a patient's score on a questionnaire dealing with overall health might not change in response to successful treatment of a specific condition, such as gastroesophageal reflux, the score on a questionnaire specifically addressing symptoms of heartburn would register a substantial change.

In the past, measures of self-reported health were criticized as being "soft" and overly subjective. In fact, many general and condition-specific measures demonstrate reliability and validity that equal or exceed those of many physiologic or clinical measures commonly used in research or clinical settings. For example, among patients undergoing coronary artery bypass grafting (Chapter 74), a 10-point reduction in self-reported physical functioning (on a 100-point scale) increases the risk for death by the same magnitude that the presence of diabetes or chronic obstructive pulmonary disease does.

A shortcoming of nearly all outcome measures other than death is that it is difficult or impossible to use such measures to compare alternative treatments unless they are applied in precisely the same fashion. In the case of hypertension (Chapter 67), for example, different drugs might exhibit differential effects on the risk for stroke or heart failure and also on the risk for adverse events such as fatigue, hepatotoxicity, or renal insufficiency. *Utility measures,* which are derived from economic and decision theory, seek to provide a standard method of comparing such disparate outcomes. *Utility* is the value or preference that an individual places on a given state of health or condition. Utility is scored from 0 (generally equivalent to death) to 1.0 (ideal health). Multiplication of individual utilities for different health states by their probabilities of occurrence permits computation of the overall utility of a treatment or intervention and enables comparison with therapeutic alternatives through the technique of decision analysis. When combined with probabilities of survival, utility can be used to calculate quality-adjusted life years, yet another way of comparing outcomes of different treatment strategies (Chapter 9). Outside the research setting, however, utilities have not been widely used because they are difficult to elicit from patients.

Patients' experiences with health care are commonly measured by standardized questionnaires, such as the Consumer Assessment of Healthcare Providers and Systems (CAHPS) family of surveys, which were developed through a public-private partnership and include instruments used in both ambulatory and institutional settings. Like health-related quality of life, patient experience is a broad concept that can incorporate a number of different dimensions, including satisfaction with overall health care, systems of care, hospital care, outpatient care, specific types of treatments, individual health care providers, amenities, and other aspects. Because patients' perceptions of their care may not correlate highly with other aspects of the processes and outcomes of care, results must be interpreted in the context of these other measures.

Measures of Cost and Resource Use

Given the dramatically rising expense of health care, costs are frequently measured. Because of the complexity of the health care market, including contractual arrangements and complicated formulas for reimbursement, charges (prices) rarely represent the true underlying cost of services. Therefore, careful accounting methods are necessary to accurately ascertain cost. Because these methods can be laborious and expensive, *utilization* of health care services, such as average length of stay or number of days in intensive care units, is often measured as a proxy for cost. When actual costs are measured, the costs evaluated are generally those characterized as *direct,* or the actual fixed and variable expenses for labor, materials, and equipment necessary to provide a given clinical service. Because these costs are typically the responsibility of insurers and health systems, analyses that use direct costs assume their viewpoint. When more global perspectives are incorporated, including those of patients, it is also necessary to measure *indirect costs,* such as the loss of time and the inconvenience incurred by patients or the societal burdens of disability or loss of productivity. Naturally, indirect costs are even more difficult and expensive to measure than direct costs.

From a policy or decision-making perspective, information about cost is most useful when it permits comparisons of alternatives, such as different drugs to treat hypertension. *Cost-benefit* analysis attempts to summarize all costs of treatment and all potential benefits solely in monetary terms. This approach is controversial and is not frequently applied because it necessitates assigning dollar costs to outcomes such as death or disability. *Cost-effectiveness* analysis is performed more frequently because the results are expressed in more comprehensible clinical terms, such as cost per life saved or per quality-adjusted life year (using the utilities described earlier). When a new treatment is evaluated, it is desirable to calculate its *marginal cost-effectiveness,* which describes its costs and benefits in relation to an existing standard treatment.

SOURCES OF DATA FOR THE MEASUREMENT OF HEALTH AND HEALTH CARE

Under ideal circumstances, data for measuring health care are collected prospectively with techniques and instruments specifically designed for the patient population and the problem being assessed. In reality, the time and expense required to develop or identify measures and collect primary data are often too prohibitive to address many important questions. In these situations, it can be advantageous to use information collected for administrative or billing purposes that reflects the process of health care. Such secondary sources of data have increasingly been applied to a broad range of topics, including the use and outcomes of all types of health services.

Governmental Sources of Data

Historically, federal and state governments have collected data related to public health, such as the occurrence of communicable diseases or causes of death. With the expansion of publicly funded health programs such as Medicare and Medicaid, the rise in chronic illnesses as a major cause of morbidity and mortality, and the advent of programs to promote quality and consumer awareness through public reporting of performance data, governmental agencies now maintain a broad range of databases, many of which can be accessed via the Internet (E-Table 10-2). These databases make available vast amounts of information about the incidence and prevalence of various medical conditions, characteristics of patients and health care providers, types of health care services used, burdens and cost of illness, and other important health outcomes, such as adjusted mortality.

Clinical and Quality Data

Until the latter part of the 20th century, most statistics on health care delivery and on the health of groups of patients (with the exception of individual medical records) were maintained by governmental agencies. Today, there are hundreds of public and private entities that collect, process, analyze, or disseminate this information. The consolidation of health care delivery systems within markets and the wide use of electronic health records have led to the creation of very large and rich clinical databases that can be an excellent source for monitoring and improving the quality of care. These data sources can furnish clinical details about the severity and clinical course of illnesses not obtainable from administrative databases.

Another emerging source of data is quality measurement systems developed by peer review organizations, medical care organizations, health plans, professional organizations, consumer organizations, and bodies that perform accreditation. To a greater or lesser extent, all these groups have developed systems to measure and evaluate the performance of health care providers and systems. These data may be collected through the extraction of data from secondary sources, manual abstraction of physical or electronic medical records, or primary data collection by clinical or administrative personnel. Despite the relatively low expense, ready availability, and large size of secondary data sources, there are serious potential limitations to their use (Table 10-2).

DESIGN OF MEASUREMENT STUDIES

Data used to measure the structure, process, and outcomes of health care are obtained in a variety of ways. Investigators engaged in hypothesis-driven research often apply rigorous methods of measurement and research designs, whereas those evaluating the quality of care provided within and among health care organizations tend to rely on observational studies or secondary sources of data (i.e., data initially collected for a different purpose, such as clinical care or claims processing). However, progressive overlap in the methods used and the proliferation of computerized data sources have begun to blur the boundaries between certain types of research and quality improvement studies.

Experimental Studies

Evaluation of the effects of treatments on clinical outcomes should generally be performed in randomized, controlled trials in which the intervention is randomly assigned to ensure that patients who do (subjects) and do not (controls) receive it are as similar as possible. In double-blind studies, not only the patient but also the patient's physician and certain members of the investigative team are kept uninformed about the treatment assignment. Maintenance of blinding is more difficult in studies of interventions other than drugs, but even in studies of surgery or acupuncture, for example, control patients can undergo sham procedures. In studies evaluating more

TABLE 10-2 POTENTIAL LIMITATIONS OF SECONDARY DATA

FEATURE	POTENTIAL LIMITATIONS
Accuracy and precision of data	Basic information on patient characteristics, diagnoses, and procedures may be miscoded Data generally available only for people who use services or access the health care system during the period of interest Patients may be miscounted if they have multiple sites of residence or have undergone procedures in more than one system of care
Sample size	Large sample sizes may produce statistical significance without clinical or policy significance
Characterization of patients	Patients are incompletely characterized; key clinical data on processes and outcomes may be missing
Characterization of providers	Characteristics of providers may be missing, miscoded, or inconsistently recorded
Characterization of interventions	Services or procedures may be coded imprecisely or inaccurately
Ascertainment of outcomes	Outcomes of greatest relevance may not be captured (e.g., symptom relief, quality of life, out-of-hospital events, level of satisfaction)
Completeness of follow-up	Only data about discrete episodes of care may be coded; longitudinal follow-up requires data linkage, which may not be possible

Adapted from Huston P, Naylor CD. Health services research: reporting on studies using secondary data sources. *Can Med Assoc J.* 1996;155:1697-1702.

complex interventions, such as use of a team to manage diabetes or heart failure, blinding may be impractical. To help maintain equivalence in such cases, patients serving as controls may receive a less intensive intervention to help ensure that any observed difference in health outcome between the experimental and control groups is the result of genuine treatment effects rather than nonspecific effects of increased attention.

In trials of interventions that are applied directly to patients, such as medications or procedures, allocation of the experimental treatment is generally random by patient, and results are analyzed at the level of the patient. Conversely, in trials of interventions designed to improve how care is delivered, the unit of randomization and analysis may be the patient, the health care provider, or even the entire system of care, depending on the level at which the intervention is administered. In studying the clinical effects of an educational quality improvement program targeted toward physicians, for example, participating physicians should be randomized along with their patient panels, because the effects on patients within a panel would not be independent. Similarly, in a study of a new way to organize personnel within a practice to treat depression, entire practices might be the correct unit of randomization and analysis.

Although the randomized, controlled trial is the most rigorous method of assessing treatment effects, this approach has several shortcomings. To achieve equivalence between treatment and control groups with respect to key demographic and clinical characteristics, eligibility is often restricted to a narrow range of individuals who fulfill strict criteria. Although this approach enhances the internal validity of a trial's results, applicability of the results to groups of patients who would have been deemed ineligible for the trial (often elderly or chronically ill patients) remains uncertain. Moreover, to help ensure that patients fully comply with the treatment being tested, study personnel frequently provide substantially more support and assistance to participants than similar patients would receive in ordinary clinical settings. These differences often raise concerns about the *external validity* or generalizability of results. For this reason, tightly controlled randomized trials are often considered to establish the *efficacy* of an intervention—specifically, the potential benefit of an intervention under ideal conditions. To establish whether an intervention is successful in patients more typically seen in routine practice, investigators may conduct an *effectiveness trial,* also known as a *management* or *pragmatic trial.*

Other potential drawbacks of randomized trials are the long time required for planning and execution, the high expense, and the low statistical power to assess infrequent outcomes, especially for studies in which health care providers or systems of care are randomized. To compensate in part for these

drawbacks, *cluster randomized trials* are designed to permit randomization at the level of the provider or system, but they use sophisticated statistical techniques (e.g., multilevel or hierarchical regression) to perform analyses at the level of the patient so that statistical power is preserved. This approach is particularly well suited to effectiveness trials, which often involve testing of clinical strategies or programs. Other novel approaches are sequential methods, such as the *group sequential response* and *adaptive clinical trial* designs, which provide an opportunity to terminate a study, adjust the expected sample size, or modify the intervention as the trial progresses on the basis of interim analysis at predetermined points in time. These approaches, which are especially attractive when preliminary data are limited, can enhance efficiency by terminating positive or negative trials earlier than might be the case when using only initial sample size estimates.

Nonexperimental Designs

Although randomized trials remain the best approach to assess the efficacy of therapeutic interventions, other study designs, such as *observational* or *case-control* studies, are often used under certain circumstances. *Cohort* studies are a type of observational study in which one or more groups of patients are selected because they have or have not been exposed to a particular condition or intervention. Exposures can be broadly defined and can include the presence of a particular disease or condition (e.g., pneumonia or heart failure), receipt of a type of medication, provision of a certain medical service (e.g., surgical procedure) or set of services (e.g., care by a specialist physician or enrollment in a particular type of health plan), or exposure to a set of conditions (e.g., having health insurance). Cohort studies have numerous attractive features, including the ability to provide a direct estimate of the absolute risk for an outcome in exposed patients. The foremost liability of these approaches is that any observed difference in outcomes may be due to inherent differences between patients who do and do not receive the intervention because it is not randomly allocated. This dilemma can often be addressed by using statistical methods for *case mix adjustment* (described in the next section). In some circumstances, however, even extensive adjustment is inadequate, such as when there is *bias by indication.* This problem occurs in the study of a relationship between an exposure (e.g., a short-acting calcium-channel blocker) and an outcome (e.g., myocardial infarction) when one indication for the medication is treatment that is directly related to the outcome (i.e., angina pectoris). One solution to this problem is to eliminate patients for whom this bias is likely to be present. In the illustrative case, a heightened risk for myocardial infarction in patients taking short-acting calcium-channel blockers was initially demonstrated in a study restricted to persons with hypertension but no known cardiovascular disease.

In a *prospective cohort study,* participants are identified at the time of exposure and followed forward in time according to a predefined protocol and with standard measures. Prospective cohort studies often permit the enrollment of a broader cross section of patients than is possible in randomized trials and can be conducted under circumstances in which randomization is not feasible for ethical or logistic reasons. Like randomized trials, prospective cohort studies provide a means to ascertain that the exposure under study truly precedes the outcome of interest. Limitations of prospective cohort studies include the need to enroll large numbers of patients (especially when evaluating rare outcomes), the frequent loss of participants during follow-up, and the high expense, often related to the duration of follow-up.

In a *retrospective cohort study,* exposure is typically defined by using secondary data (e.g., an admitting diagnosis of acute myocardial infarction or a procedure code for spinal fusion on a hospital discharge abstract) at some point in the past, and patients are followed forward in time by using previously collected data for outcomes (e.g., death, reoperation, readmission). Formerly, retrospective cohort studies were limited in time and scope because they relied on the often tedious manual abstraction of medical charts. With the proliferation of secondary electronic data sources, this approach has become extremely popular and has several advantages—chiefly, the opportunity to study vast numbers of patients inexpensively, including those with relatively rare conditions. Standardized coding for many variables, such as diagnoses and procedures, helps reduce the variability introduced by human chart abstractors. Moreover, electronic records are far less apt to be unavailable or incomplete than paper records are. However, retrospective cohort studies are subject to a number of potentially serious flaws. Hypotheses are usually generated and studies designed well after the collection of data, which was generally done for a wholly different purpose. Thus, the reliability and validity of the data are often unknown and beyond the control of the investigator. This problem can lead to misclassification of both exposures and outcomes. For example, a diagnosis of pneumonia coded for billing purposes may not satisfy the rigorous criteria used in research. Although a patient's complete electronic record is rarely lost, missing data within records are common. Unlike with prospective studies, it may be difficult to be certain that an exposure preceded an outcome. For example, a patient might have had subclinical disease at the time of a given exposure, thereby leading to an erroneous impression of a temporal sequence when the disease was recognized clinically. Apart from methodologic limitations, the sheer volume of available data encourages investigators to conduct numerous analyses, often without prestated hypotheses. Multiple comparisons performed with very large sample sizes readily lead to erroneous conclusions that random associations are clinically meaningful because they are of marginal statistical significance.

Case-control studies differ from cohort studies in that the case and control groups are defined on the basis of whether subjects have experienced an outcome rather than on the basis of exposure. Data from existing records or gathered by interview (or both) are then used to ascertain the proportion of case and control patients who experienced the exposure of interest. As in cohort studies, exposures can be defined broadly, including a medication, a type of clinical event, or receipt of a service. Case-control studies are attractive in many settings because they require fewer patients than prospective studies do to achieve a similar level of statistical power. This attribute makes them especially useful for investigating uncommon outcomes. For example, pharmacoepidemiologists often use case-control studies to identify serious adverse effects of medications when the events are too rare to study with clinical trials or cohort studies. Case-control studies are nonetheless subject to a number of potential biases. As with cohort studies, the use of data from secondary sources can lead to misclassification of exposure or outcome. When exposure is determined by interview, differential recall by cases and controls can introduce bias. It may be even more difficult to be certain that an exposure truly occurred before the outcome than in retrospective cohort studies. Furthermore, the results of case-control studies do not yield estimates of absolute risk, as do randomized trials and cohort studies; they are expressed as the odds of an outcome in cases relative to controls. *Relative odds* only approximate the ratio of risk in cases to risk in controls.

Cross-sectional studies are performed when data on one or more groups of patients are collected at a single point in time. Although this approach is inexpensive and can provide estimates of the prevalence of a condition or outcome, it is highly subject to nearly all the biases mentioned and is the weakest method in terms of making inferences about whether a particular exposure directly causes a given outcome.

Case Mix Adjustment

Only in prospective, randomized trials is it possible to control which patients do and do not receive a specific treatment, and even then, it may not be possible to ensure the equivalence of all the characteristics that affect outcomes between subjects in the control and experimental groups. In all nonexperimental research designs, allocation of the experimental intervention is not random but is a function of a patient's personal and clinical characteristics and those of the system of care. Without consideration of such differences, it is impossible to differentiate the genuine effects of an intervention from bias related to allocation of the intervention to certain types of patients. Modern statistical techniques that can adjust for such differences are effective when many of the patient characteristics that exert an important influence on outcomes have been elucidated and relevant data are available. For example, the major factors that predict mortality after acute myocardial infarction include prolonged chest pain, tachycardia, hypotension, ST segment elevation on the admission electrocardiogram, poor left ventricular function, and initial laboratory measures that indicate a large infarct, such as a high troponin level. Thus, when comparing the outcomes of patients who are treated in different systems of care, it is essential to use multivariate statistical methods to adjust for these factors. Otherwise, differences observed between systems that are actually due to differing patient populations might erroneously be attributed to differences in quality of care. A related method is *propensity scoring*, which applies the results of modeling equations that predict how likely a person was to have received one intervention or the other based on personal and clinical characteristics. Even with sophisticated adjustments, however, studies of treatments that rely heavily on the judgment of physicians or the preference of patients are likely to have biases that cannot be addressed by statistical modeling and require randomized trials.

TABLE 10-3	EXPANDING AREAS OF STUDY FOR HEALTH CARE QUALITY AND OUTCOMES
GENERAL AREA OF STUDY	**EXAMPLE OF INTERVENTION OR OUTCOME EVALUATED**
Effectiveness of clinical programs	Disease management programs, specialized clinics, consultative services
Organization of care	Health maintenance organizations vs. private practice
Effects of different mechanisms of financing	Capitation vs. fee-for-service; different levels of pharmacy copayments
Outcomes of different types of providers	Generalists vs. specialists
Disparities among ethnic groups	Receipt of preventive services or sophisticated procedures
Patient safety	Occurrence of adverse drug effects or medical errors
Geographic variations in patterns of care	Use of expensive procedures

TRENDS IN OUTCOME MEASUREMENT

In recent years, the topics of studies evaluating the outcomes of health care interventions have expanded greatly. In addition to evaluating specific treatments, such as drugs or procedures, evaluations directly compare various types of clinical programs, systems of care, types of providers, mechanisms of financing, patient safety, disparities among ethnic groups, and geographic variations in patterns of care (Table 10-3). Recently, public attention has been focused on *comparative effectiveness,* which reflects the need to evaluate new and typically more expensive therapies in relation to older, well-established treatments, as opposed to the common practice of merely comparing them with placebo or clearly less effective regimens. Information from such trials is essential to identify the most cost-effective therapies.

It is safe to predict that studies on the processes and outcomes of health care will become even more ubiquitous with the expanding availability of electronic data, increasingly sophisticated statistical techniques, and growing public demand for accountability.

SUGGESTED READINGS

Fonarow GC, Peterson ED. Heart failure performance measures and outcomes: real or illusory gains. *JAMA.* 2009;302:792-794. *From 2002 to 2007, performance measures for heart failure improved 15 to 250%, but mortality, hospital readmissions, and costs remained constant.*

Nyweide DJ, Weeks WB, Gottlieb DJ, et al. Relationship of primary care physicians' patient caseload with measurement of quality and cost performance. *JAMA.* 2009;302:2444-2450. *Few primary care physicians have a sufficient number of patients to reliably detect a 10% relative difference on performance measures.*

Stulberg JJ, Delaney CP, Neuhauser DV, et al. Adherence to surgical care improvement project measures and the association with postoperative infections. *JAMA.* 2010;303:2479-2485. *Adherence was associated with fewer postoperative infections.*

11

QUALITY OF CARE AND PATIENT SAFETY

ROBERT M. WACHTER

During the past two decades, scores of studies have demonstrated that the quality and safety of modern health care leave much to be desired, despite the fact that most physicians are well trained and work very hard. Yet the evidence is undeniable, with clear documentation of stunning variations in patterns of care that are neither supported by evidence nor justified by outcomes, major gaps between evidence-based best practices and current practice, and staggering numbers of serious medical errors. The recognition of these quality and safety problems has catalyzed a major transformation in thinking and practice, with new technologies, regulations, training models, incentive systems, and more.

TABLE 11-1 THE INSTITUTE OF MEDICINE'S SIX QUALITY AIMS

Patient safety
Patient centeredness
Effectiveness
Efficiency
Timeliness
Equity

From Committee on Quality of Health Care in America, Institute of Medicine. *Crossing the Quality Chasm: A New Health System for the 21st Century.* Washington, DC: National Academy Press; 2001.

TABLE 11-2 COMPARISON OF THREE MEASURES OF CLINICAL QUALITY: THE DONABEDIAN TRIAD

MEASURE	SIMPLE DEFINITION	ADVANTAGES	DISADVANTAGES
Structure	How was care organized?	May be highly relevant in a complex health system	May fail to capture the quality of care by individual physicians
			Difficult to determine the "gold standard"
Process	What was done?	More easily measured and acted on than outcomes	A proxy for outcomes
			Not all may agree on "gold standard" processes
		May not require case-mix adjustment	May promote "cookbook" medicine, especially if physicians and health systems try to "game" their performance
		No time lag—can be measured when care is provided	
		May directly reflect quality (if carefully chosen)	
Outcomes	What happened to the patient?	What we really care about	May take years to occur
			May not reflect quality of care
			Requires case-mix and other adjustment to prevent "apples-to-oranges" comparisons

Modified from Donabedian A. The quality of care. How can it be assessed? *JAMA.* 1988;270:1743-1748; and Shojania KG, Showstack J, Wachter R. Assessing hospital quality: A review for clinicians. *Eff Clin Pract.* 2001;4:82-90.

To appreciate the problem and how to address it requires an understanding of quality measurement and improvement, the safety of patients, and value, which is the confluence of safety, quality, and cost.

QUALITY

Definition

Quality of care has been defined by the Institute of Medicine as "the degree to which health services for individuals and populations increase the likelihood of desired health outcomes and are consistent with current professional knowledge." It includes six aims for a quality health care system, emphasizing that quality involves more than the delivery of evidence-based care (Table 11-1). Nevertheless, evidence-based medicine (Chapter 9) provides much of the scientific underpinning for quality measurement and improvement. Previously, the lack of clinical evidence and the apprenticeship model of medical training promoted an idiosyncratic practice style by which a senior clinician or a marquee medical center determined the standard of care—a tradition now sometimes termed *eminence-based medicine.* Without discounting the value of experience and mature clinical judgment, the modern paradigm for determining optimal practice has changed, driven by the explosion in clinical research during the past 30 years; for example, the number of randomized clinical trials grew from 350 per year in 1970 to 18,000 per year in 2008. This research has helped define "best practices" in many areas of medicine, from preventive strategies for a healthy 62-year-old outpatient (Chapters 13 and 14) to the treatment of a patient with acute myocardial infarction and cardiogenic shock (Chapters 73 and 107).

Donabedian's triad, which divides quality measures into *structure* (how care is organized), *process* (what is done), and *outcomes* (what happens to the patient), represents the most popular construct for quality measurement. Each element of the triad has important advantages and disadvantages as a quality measure (Table 11-2). Most of the widely used quality measures are process measures for which clinical research has established a link between such processes and improved outcomes. An example is the rate at which aspirin or a β-blocker is given to survivors of a myocardial infarction before hospital discharge (Chapter 73). However, when processes are less relevant and the science of case-mix adjustment is suitably advanced (e.g., cardiac bypass surgery; Chapter 74), outcome measurement is often used. In other areas involving complex processes, structural measures are used as proxies for quality; examples here include the presence of intensivists to staff critical care units, a dedicated stroke service, and computerized physician order entry (CPOE) systems.

The Epidemiology of Quality-Related Problems

It is now well established that there are large and clinically indefensible variations in care from one city to another. Furthermore, U.S. practice adheres to the best evidence only slightly more than 50% of the time, even when adherence is known to correlate with ultimate clinical outcomes.

Levers for Change

For physicians, policymakers, administrators, and patients, evidence of major problems with quality has led to the recognition of structural problems that prevent the delivery of the highest quality of care. These problems include the lack of information regarding the performance of a provider or institution, the absence of incentives for quality improvement, the challenge for practicing physicians to stay abreast of modern evidence-based medicine, and the absence of an information technology support system for quality.

The first step in quality improvement is the creation of practice standards against which to measure quality. Scores of such measures have been promulgated by a variety of organizations, including payers (such as the Centers for Medicare and Medicaid Services), accreditors (such as the Joint Commission), and medical societies. These measures have identified many opportunities for improvement among individual physicians, practices, and hospitals.

Given the volume of new literature published each year, it is impossible for an individual physician to keep up with all the evidence-based advances in his or her field. *Practice guidelines,* such as those for the treatment of community-acquired pneumonia (Chapter 97) or the prophylaxis of deep venous thrombosis (Chapter 81), aim to synthesize evidence-based best practices into a set of summary recommendations. Although concerns about "cookbook medicine" linger, there is a growing consensus that best practices should be "hardwired" if possible. The major challenges are to update guidelines as new knowledge accumulates and to recognize the complexity of guidelines when patients have multiple, potentially overlapping illnesses. *Clinical pathways* are similar to guidelines but attempt to codify a series of steps, usually temporally (on day 1, do the following; on day 2, do the following; and so forth), making them more useful for stereotypical processes such as the postoperative management of patients after hip replacement.

Although professionalism (Chapter 1) should be a sufficient incentive for physicians to provide high-quality care, reaching this goal typically depends on the existence of a system organized to translate research into practice and to deliver the right care every time. Such a system requires significant investments (in educating physicians, hiring case managers or clinical pharmacists, building information systems, and developing guidelines). The historical payment system, which compensates physicians and hospitals equally whether quality is terrific or terrible, provides no incentive to make the requisite investments.

The Changing Environment for Quality

The recent recognition of major gaps in quality and of the need for systemic change to improve quality has led to a variety of initiatives to catalyze quality improvement. Virtually all involve several steps: defining reasonable quality measures (evidence-based measures; capturing appropriate structures, process, or outcomes), measuring the performance of providers or systems, and using these results to promote change. This final imperative creates the greatest degree of uncertainty and experimentation.

Although one might hope that simply giving a physician information about prior performance would generate meaningful improvement, this strategy yields only modest change at best. Increasingly, a more aggressive and transparent strategy, such as disseminating the results of quality measurement to key stakeholders, is being adopted. In some cases, simple transparency is the main strategy—the rationale being that providers will find the exposure of their gaps in quality to be sufficiently concerning or embarrassing to motivate improvement. Although there is little evidence that patients use such data to choose among physicians or hospitals, transparency itself has frequently resulted in impressive improvements in some publicly reported quality measures.

The newest strategy in the United States is to tie payments for service to quality performance (pay for performance, or P4P). A number of P4P programs are under way, and early results indicate that differential payment leads to modest gains beyond the improvements achieved by simple transparency. P4P also raises a host of concerns, including whether presently captured quality data are accurate, whether payments should go to the best performers or those with the greatest improvements, whether existing measures adequately measure quality in patients with complex diseases, and whether P4P will create undue focus on certain measurable practices, leading to relative inattention to other important processes that are not being compensated. A recent variation on the P4P theme is Medicare's "no pay for adverse events" program, in which hospital payments are withheld for certain "preventable" adverse events. As with P4P more generally, the jury is still out regarding the impact of such programs on quality and safety.

Quality Improvement Strategies

Whether the motivation is professionalism, embarrassment, or economics, the next question is how actually to improve the quality of care. There is no simple answer; successful institutions and physicians have used a variety of strategies. In general, most use a variation of a "plan, do, study, act" (PDSA) cycle, recognizing that quality improvement activities must be carefully planned and implemented, that their impact needs to be measured, and that the results of these activities are often imperfect and require retooling.

In addition to the PDSA cycle, several other types of activities are useful. For quality improvement practices that require predictable repetition, efforts to "hardwire" the practice or to use alternative providers who focus on the activity are often beneficial. For example, the best strategy to increase the rate of pneumococcal vaccination (Chapter 17) among hospitalized patients with pneumonia is to embed it in a standard order set, either paper based or computerized. Another example is that having a nurse remove patients' shoes before the physician's entry can increase rates of diabetic foot examinations in an outpatient practice (Chapter 236).

In some areas, though, quality improvement involves much more complex and interdependent activities. In these circumstances, bringing teams together to examine their practices and to participate in a PDSA cycle is the most likely path to success. For example, a group of cardiac surgeons in the northeastern United States participated in an experiment in which they observed one another's practices, agreed on best practices, and measured one another's outcomes; the result was a 24% reduction in mortality with cardiac surgery.

● PATIENT SAFETY

Epidemiology

The concept of "first, do no harm" began more than 2 millennia ago, and many hospitals host periodic forums (e.g., morbidity and mortality conferences) to discuss errors. Until recently, however, there has been little teaching about the nature of medical mistakes, investment in safety research, regulation of safety standards, or emphasis on safety improvements, despite the fact that an estimated 44,000 to 98,000 Americans die each year of medical mistakes— the equivalent of a jumbo jet crashing each day. Such deaths may be related to medication errors, gaps in the discharge process, communication problems in intensive care units, or retained sponges in surgical patients—in short, virtually every aspect of modern medical care. Moreover, detailed clinical and statistical evidence of suboptimal safety has been reinforced by several high-profile and disquieting errors, sometimes apparently related to inadequate

supervision and prolonged duty hours of trainees. These errors include the wrong patient getting a major procedure, the wrong limb being operated on, chemotherapy overdoses, mistaken mastectomies, and more.

Because patients may be harmed despite receiving perfect care (i.e., from an accepted complication of surgery or a side effect of medication), it is important to separate *adverse events* from *errors*. The patient safety literature commonly defines an error as "an act or omission that leads to an unanticipated, undesirable outcome or to substantial potential for such an outcome." Adverse events, in contrast, are injuries due to medical management rather than the patient's underlying illness. This distinction is crucial. For example, when a patient who was appropriately prescribed warfarin for chronic atrial fibrillation (Chapter 64) develops a gastrointestinal bleed despite a therapeutic international normalized ratio (INR), an adverse event, not a medical error, has occurred. Conversely, if the INR was supratherapeutic because the physician prescribed a new medication without checking for possible drug interactions, a medical error would have occurred.

The Modern Approach to Patient Safety

The historical approach to medical errors often has been to blame the provider who was most proximate: whoever performed the surgery, hung the intravenous medication, or mixed the chemotherapy. It is now recognized that this approach fails to appreciate that most errors are committed by hardworking, well-trained individuals, and such errors are unlikely to be prevented by admonishing people to be more careful or by shaming and suing them. Instead, the modern approach, known as *systems thinking*, holds that humans will inevitably err and that safety depends on creating systems that anticipate errors and either prevent or catch them before they cause harm. Such an approach has been the cornerstone of safety improvements in other high-risk industries for some time.

The "Swiss cheese" model of accidents, drawn from innumerable investigations of accidents in commercial aviation and the nuclear power industry, for example, emphasizes that single errors by one individual working in an otherwise safety-conscious system rarely cause harm. Instead, such errors must penetrate multiple incomplete layers of protection ("layers of Swiss cheese") to cause terrible harm. The lesson is to focus not on the futile goal of trying to perfect human behavior but rather on creating multiple overlapping layers of protection to decrease the probability that the holes in the Swiss cheese will ever align, allowing an error to slip through.

How to Improve Patient Safety

Drawing on these models, modern thinking emphasizes efforts to design and implement systems to prevent or catch errors. For example, errors in routine behaviors can best be prevented by building in redundancies and crosschecks in the form of checklists, read-backs, and other standardized safety procedures, such as counting sponges in the operating room, signing a surgical site before an operation, or asking patients their names before administering a medication. In recent years, the use of checklists for the placement of central lines and to prepare patients for surgery has resulted in remarkable reductions in morbidity and mortality. One way to decrease errors at the person-machine interface is by the use of "forcing functions," engineering solutions that decrease the probability of human error. The classic example outside of medicine is the modification of automobile braking systems to make it impossible to place a car in reverse when the driver's foot is off the brake. In health care, forcing functions include changing the gas nozzles and connectors so that anesthesiologists cannot mistakenly hook up the wrong gas, such as nitrogen instead of oxygen, and administer it to a patient. Given the ever-increasing complexity of modern medicine, building in such forcing functions in intravenous pumps, defibrillators, mechanical ventilators, and computerized order entry systems will be crucial to safety.

In addition to better systems, communication and teamwork must be improved. All commercial pilots must take "crew resource management" courses, in which they train for emergencies with other crew members, learn to flatten hierarchies that might stifle open communication, communicate clearly with standard language, and use checklists and other systemic approaches. Recent evidence supports that such interventions in medical care can lead to fewer errors and improved outcomes. The goal is a "culture of safety"—an environment in which teamwork, clear communication, and openness about errors, both with other health care professionals and with patients, is the norm. A tailored group of discharge services, emphasizing both process improvements and better collaboration among providers, can significantly reduce hospital readmissions,[1] and a multidisciplinary fall prevention program can reduce falls in hospitalized patients.[2]

Another key principle in ensuring the safety of patients is to learn from one's mistakes. Safe systems have a culture in which errors are openly discussed, often in morbidity and mortality conferences. To be most useful, these discussions should be interdisciplinary (involving doctors and other health professionals), identify when the errors occurred, and emphasize systems thinking and solutions; they should not be punitive. In addition to open discussions during conferences, safe organizations build in mechanisms to hear about errors from frontline staff, often through "incident reporting systems"; they also perform detailed "root cause" analyses of major errors or "sentinel events" in an effort to define all the layers of Swiss cheese that need improvement. The importance of open communication extends to patients as well. Disclosure of errors is now required by the Joint Commission. Patients and families value such openness, and preliminary evidence indicates that disclosure of errors might decrease the chance of a malpractice suit.

Finally, there is increasing appreciation of the importance of a well-trained, well-staffed, and well-rested work force for the delivery of safe care. Lower nurse-to-patient ratios, long work hours for residents, and lack of board certification are all linked to poor outcomes for patients. Safer systems cannot be created if the providers are overextended or poorly trained or supervised.

In the absence of comparative evidence, and in light of the high cost of interventions such as improved staffing, computerized order entry, and team-work training, even institutions committed to safety must often make difficult choices. Given the natural tendency to focus on practices that are measured, publicly reported, and compensated, institutions and physicians tend to focus first on areas that are subject to regulation or on initiatives with multiple potential benefits, such as computerization. Because improving culture is difficult to measure and to regulate, there is concern that it will not be as high a priority as it should be. Moreover, a safe culture depends on balancing the imperative to improve systems with the need to define and enforce accountability. The safety field is increasingly emphasizing more active enforcement of policies that address problems such as disruptive behavior by clinicians and failure to adhere to evidence-based safety practices.

VALUE: CONNECTING SAFETY AND QUALITY TO COST

Outside of health care, most purchasing decisions are based on perceived value: (quality + safety) ÷ cost. Health care decisions historically have not been made this way, in part because of the limited ability of patients and payers to make rational judgments about the quality and safety of a given provider or system, and in part because health care insurance insulates patients from the full cost of care. Much of the recent push to measure and to improve quality and safety should be seen as part of a broader effort to allow patients and payers to make rational judgments about value and to choose their providers on the basis of such judgments. Given the stakes, it is vital for physicians and other health care providers to participate in efforts to measure and improve the quality and safety of care and to do so while being mindful of the price tag.

1. Jack BW, Chetty VK, Anthony D, et al. A reengineered hospital discharge program to decrease rehospitalizations: a randomized trial. *Ann Intern Med.* 2009;150:178-187.
2. Dykes PC, Carroll DL, Hurley A, et al. Fall prevention in acute care hospitals: a randomized trial. *JAMA.* 2010;304:1912-1918.

SUGGESTED READINGS

Kachalia A, Kaufman SR, Boothman R, et al. Liability claims and costs before and after implementation of a medical error disclosure program. *Ann Intern Med.* 2010;153:213-221. *A before-after demonstrating lower liability costs after implementation of a program of disclosure and, where appropriate, settlement offers.*

Neily J, Mills PD, Young-Xu Y, et al. Association between implementation of a medical team training program and surgical mortality. *JAMA.* 2010;304:1693-1700. *A team training program was associated with an 18% reduction in surgical mortality.*

Wachter RM. Why diagnostic errors don't get any respect—and what can be done about them. *Health Aff (Millwood).* 2010;29:1605-1610. *Emphasizes potentially effective strategies to address diagnostic errors.*

12

COMPREHENSIVE CHRONIC DISEASE MANAGEMENT

EDWARD H. WAGNER

Although there is no clear definition of a chronic disease, the term generally refers to long-standing degenerative conditions of noninfectious origin. However, chronic infections, such as HIV or hepatitis C, and many mental and behavioral disorders also last for months, years, or a lifetime. Regardless of cause or pathophysiology, chronic conditions require ongoing attention and adjustments by patients and their loved ones and care by professionals. Patients with a wide variety of chronic health problems have similar needs to minimize morbidity and optimize quality of life (Table 12-1). Because these needs are shared across conditions, clinical management of these seemingly disparate illnesses requires similar practice capacities and functions. For example, the design and organization of care that leads to better outcomes are remarkably similar for diseases as clinically different as diabetes, depression, and HIV.

To live effectively with their health conditions and manage their treatments, patients must have access to the necessary information, skills, and encouragement. They must also receive evidence-based therapy and preventive care to improve disease control and reduce the risk of complications and exacerbations. The severity of most chronic conditions and the effectiveness of ongoing therapy wax and wane over time. As a consequence, regular monitoring and reassessment are required by patients and clinicians alike. When chronically ill patients experience periods of increased severity and risk, they benefit from an intensification of management and support. Care for the chronically ill generally involves multiple health professionals and care settings, for which transitions must be coordinated.

THE GOALS OF CHRONIC CARE MANAGEMENT

The goals of chronic care management are to meet the aforementioned needs of patients with chronic illness routinely and efficiently by delivering care in a system organized to do so. Chronic conditions, whether medical or psychiatric, present very different challenges for patients and their caregivers than do acute illnesses or injuries. Rarely cured and often changing in severity over time, chronic illness necessitates continuous monitoring and adjustments by patients (self-management) and caregivers alike.

The decisions made and behaviors undertaken by patients to deal with their illness, generally called *self-management*, influence the course and outcomes of most chronic diseases in major ways. Patients make decisions and take action in dealing with symptoms, coping with the social and emotional impacts of illness, monitoring their condition, taking medications, adjusting lifestyle, and interacting with the health care system. Most need training and ongoing support from their clinical providers to become competent managers of their health and their illness. The competence and confidence with which patients self-manage their illness have a major impact on outcome. For example, participants in diabetes or hypertension self-management training programs generally experience clinically significant reductions in hemoglobin A_{1c} or blood pressure levels without major changes in drug therapy.■ Self-management can be enhanced in patients of all socioeconomic

TABLE 12-1	COMMON NEEDS OF PATIENTS WITH CHRONIC ILLNESS

- Support and information that enables patients to be competent self-managers of their health and illness
- Effective clinical and behavioral treatment that keeps the disease under control and optimizes health status
- Effective preventive care to reduce the risk of complications and other morbidity
- Ongoing monitoring of the patient's condition to detect and respond to problems early in their course
- Intensification of management and support during high-risk periods
- Coordination of care to increase the efficiency and effectiveness of referrals and to prevent the mishaps that commonly occur during care transitions

groups by empowering, training, and supporting them. Modern self-management support is a collaborative rather than a didactic process that seeks concordance between providers' and patients' perspectives on the goals of treatment and the actions needed to reach those goals.

Whereas the primary goals of acute disease care are cure and recovery, cure is not an option for most chronic diseases, which are often characterized by slowly progressive deterioration, even with excellent care. Nevertheless, control of the metabolic or physiologic abnormalities or symptoms resulting from the underlying pathophysiologic processes (disease control) is now possible for many chronic conditions. Thus, a major goal for the management of many chronic illnesses is effective clinical treatment in accord with the best scientific evidence. Drugs, lifestyle modification, and other therapies attempt to minimize morbidity, limit further organ damage, reduce the risk of exacerbations and complications, and maintain quality of life and function. The metabolic or physiologic abnormalities or symptoms used to assess disease control often serve as clinical targets to guide therapy and as performance indicators to monitor the progress and quality of care for populations of patients (e.g., the percentage of diabetic patients with blood pressure <130/80 mm Hg). Disease control is best achieved through the systematic use of evidence-based treatment protocols that carefully step up or intensify treatment until clinical targets are reached.

Ongoing monitoring and assessment of chronically ill patients, including ensuring that they are not lost to follow-up, are essential to optimize therapy. Regular assessment of self-management activities reinforces their importance to the patient and to the overall management of the condition. Serious exacerbations and complications of common chronic illnesses are potentially preventable if identified early in their course and treated appropriately (e.g., recurrence of major depression, opportunistic infection in patients with HIV, lower extremity amputation among diabetic patients). The periodicity of assessments must change as the severity of illness waxes and wanes over time.

An increasingly important goal of effective chronic care management is to provide more intensive monitoring and management during periods of high risk, such as transitions from hospital to community or exacerbations. Clinical care or case management by nurses, pharmacists, or other nonphysician health professionals enables closer monitoring of patients, helps with medication adjustment, provides self-management support, and facilitates care coordination. Effective care management programs can reduce the likelihood of rehospitalization for chronically ill patients discharged from the hospital, reduce emergency room visits and hospitalizations among multiproblem ambulatory older adults, and improve disease control.

Chronically ill patients receive medical and supportive services from multiple providers with differing expertise in different settings. Without good coordination, many opportunities exist for errors, inefficiencies, and patient distress. Effective coordination of care can prevent or reduce hospital readmissions because of failures of post-discharge care, failed referrals, referrals without adequate information from the primary care provider, specialty visits without communication back to the primary care provider, duplicated testing, and so forth. Without assistance from their primary providers, patients or their loved ones must often assume responsibility for the onerous task of coordinating care.

● MATCHING PATIENT NEEDS AND CARE DELIVERY

Outpatients with diseases such as diabetes, hypertension, and major depression have been estimated to receive evidence-based interventions only about half the time, and less than half achieve optimal disease control. When individual practices are audited, omissions of evidence-based care appear almost randomly across different interventions and among patients within a practice, suggesting that these omissions are related to flaws in care systems rather than cognitive gaps.

The other goals of chronic care management are met even less often, because ambulatory care systems are largely organized to react to acute problems, not to address the ongoing needs of the chronically ill. The focus on making a diagnosis and initiating treatment for the problem at hand leaves little time for addressing less urgent needs such as medication adjustment, self-management support, and preventive care. Reimbursement systems that favor multiple short encounters aggravate the problem.

Lack of attention to patient self-management and inappropriate drug management by clinicians or patients are largely responsible for the poor control of chronic illness. Abundant evidence indicates that adherence to evidence-based treatment protocols substantially increases the proportion of patients reaching therapeutic targets and reduces the risk of morbidity and mortality. The protocols for most chronic conditions include recommendations to step up or intensify therapy when clinical targets are not reached. Failure to intensify treatment in patients who have not achieved therapeutic targets, called *clinical inertia*, has been found in a large percentage of patients with uncontrolled diabetes, hypertension, depression, and other chronic illnesses. Clinicians have an understandable reluctance to increase drug doses or add new drugs, but concerns about toxicity or patient nonadherence can be mitigated if practices have organized approaches to stepping up therapy and monitoring its impact.

Deficiencies in practice infrastructure and the professional environment compound the difficulties of meeting the needs of chronically ill patients. The majority of ambulatory practices in North America still has no electronic clinical record system, performance measurement program, or access to colleagues trained to provide self-management support or clinical care management. Primary care physicians are increasingly uninvolved or even unaware when their patients are hospitalized. Specialists' communications with and support of primary care practitioners have deteriorated because of complex provider network requirements. Efforts to improve the quality of chronic care must focus on improving the infrastructure and practice systems that busy clinicians require to meet the needs of their patients.

Interventions That Improve Care and Outcomes of Chronic Diseases

A wide array of interventions can improve the care and outcomes of major chronic diseases by changing the organization and functioning of the care delivery system, regardless of the specific condition. These changes fall into four general categories. *Patient-directed interventions* try to change patient knowledge, increase their involvement in care, and alter their behavior. *Provider-directed interventions* give providers feedback about the quality of their care and aim to change providers' knowledge and behavior through education and reminders. *Organizational changes* generally focus on the composition and functioning of the care team and the organization of office visits (e.g., group visits) and other encounters (e.g., telephone management). *Information technology (IT) interventions* include the use of computer reminders and other decision support programs, as well as the use of registries for population and patient management. Growing evidence suggests that the use of registries to measure performance, identify individuals needing care, and plan individual patient care may be the IT function that contributes the most to improving the care of the chronically ill.

Provider-directed interventions, especially educational programs, generally demonstrate weak effects. Conversely, interventions that change the composition or functioning of the practice team have the most salutary effects.[2,3] Across conditions, assigning patient care responsibilities to the nonphysician members of practice teams leads to the greatest improvements in disease control and other outcomes. Better informed patients have better outcomes when they receive care from more informed providers who are supported by a well-organized clinical team and appropriate IT.

The Chronic Care Model

The chronic care model identifies features of a health care system that encourage high-quality chronic disease care: self-management support, delivery system design, decision support, clinical information systems, health care organization, and community resources. Evidence-based changes in these six areas foster productive interactions between informed patients, who take an active part in their care, and providers with resources and expertise.[4]

This approach presumes that patients with one or more chronic illnesses have a primary care clinician who assumes responsibility for managing their care and coordinating the activities of other clinicians and institutions that provide advice and services. It posits that important patient outcomes, such as the prevention of morbidity, mortality, and avoidable emergency room visits and hospitalizations, can be affected by productive medical care.

Productive interactions are more likely to occur when patients actively participate in their care. To do so, patients need to be informed—that is, they must have the relevant information and skills to manage their illness. Patients also must be empowered to take an active role in their health care. More active patients are more likely to engage in relevant self-management behaviors and to use health care more effectively. A number of group and individual interventions increase the likelihood that patients have sufficient understanding of their illness and its treatment and the skills and confidence to be competent self-managers.

The other partner in productive interactions is the primary care clinician and the practice team. Before visits with chronically ill patients, practice teams should review accessible information to determine what services are needed, have clear assignments or standing orders for the delivery of those services, and include staff trained to perform them. Although all six elements of the chronic care model contribute to a delivery system that can effectively manage chronic illness, changes in two categories—delivery system design and self-management support—are essential to improve disease control and reduce morbidity and mortality.

Self-Management Support

Didactic patient education alone has been demonstrated to have little if any impact on patient behavior or disease control. To change their lifestyle, take medications as directed, deal with symptoms and stress, and address the other challenges of living with chronic illness, patients need to participate actively in their care, understand and agree with the clinician's assessment of the problems and recommendations, learn the skills needed to carry out the recommendations, develop goals and an action plan to guide behavior change, and review their progress regularly with the primary care team.

These needs can be met in either group or individual sessions that involve skill building, discussion, and negotiation related to recommendations, goals, barriers to reaching goals, and actions to overcome barriers. Although self-management courses facilitated by peer or professional leaders improve disease control in diabetes, hypertension, and other chronic diseases, their effects diminish after termination of the program. Sustained follow-up and reinforcement are essential.

Sustained self-management support is best accomplished by the primary care team in the context of ongoing chronic illness care. Although a physician's advice and encouragement are important, most primary care clinicians have neither the time nor the training to help patients set behavioral goals and develop action plans and then follow up by telephone or e-mail. Clinical staff such as nurses or medical assistants with good communication skills and additional training in counseling methods can and should perform these functions.

Delivery System Design
Team Care

The goal of delivery system design is to match the organization of care delivery to the needs of the chronically ill. Without the help of a team, it is unlikely that, in the course of a 15- to 20-minute visit, physicians can manage intercurrent problems, review and adjust treatment, provide recommended assessments and preventive care, discuss self-management goals and plans, and plan follow-up. Designing effective team care begins with a consideration of the various tasks required to meet the needs of the chronically ill and ensure adherence to guidelines. Some of these tasks, such as self-management counseling or medication reconciliation, are generic; others are disease specific. Key tasks are allocated to the most appropriate members of the practice team. The team's routine involvement in patient visits is facilitated by protocols and/or standing orders that guide independent action by nonclinician staff. Brief meetings, often termed *huddles*, before clinic sessions allow practice teams to review key data (often from registries) on scheduled patients to identify and plan the delivery of needed services. The goal is to maximize the productivity of every patient interaction.

Planned Interactions

Much of chronic care management involves predictable preventive care or disease management activities, which are often postponed when chronically ill patients initiate care for an acute problem. The availability of key patient data gives practice teams the opportunity to update chronic illness care even during visits for more urgent problems. Practice-initiated planned visits can focus on patients who are noncompliant with guidelines, have failed to reach treatment targets, or have been lost to follow-up. The practice tries to schedule longer visits that are structured to address these patients' needs. Another format for the delivery of planned care is the group visit, in which patients receive their primary medical care together as a group. Group sessions generally include the same check-in assessments that occur during an individual visit, followed by brief individual communications between the primary care provider and each patient, opportunities for private consultations, and an educational session with ample opportunity for peer-to-peer interaction. Approximately 30 to 50% of patients offered group visits attend them, and many prefer to receive much of their care in this setting.

Follow-up and Case Management

Follow-up tailored to a patient's needs and the clinical severity of the disease is a critical component of effective chronic care management. Traditionally, follow-up consists of periodic in-person physician visits whose frequency is limited by cost and convenience. Chronically ill individuals often experience periods when more intensive monitoring would be helpful, such as during exacerbations or intercurrent illnesses, following hospital discharge, or while medications are being changed. Ample evidence indicates that follow-up by telephone, e-mail, or telemedicine can be cost-effective and far more flexible than face-to-face return visits. Nonphysician team members, guided by protocols with clear referral criteria, can effectively manage electronic follow-up. Self-monitoring by patients is an important component of the follow-up plans for many chronic illnesses and is especially useful when patients use the results to adjust their therapy[5] as well as to inform their practice team. Collecting self-monitoring data for the sole purpose of bringing them to the doctor's office appears to be far less effective. A small number of chronically ill patients at high risk of hospitalization, nursing home placement, major complication, or death need even more intensive clinical case management services. Clinical case management appears to be effective for chronically ill patients discharged from the hospital; multiproblem, high-risk older patients in community practice; high-risk patients with type 2 diabetes and other diseases; and patients with major depression and other chronic psychiatric disorders.

Disease management programs have proliferated over the past decade. These generally involve nurse case managers who have limited if any involvement with the patients' physicians or their medical care. This disconnected case management system is relatively ineffective unless the case manager collaborates closely with the primary care clinician, influences the medication regimen directly or indirectly, and reviews his or her caseload regularly with the relevant medical specialist.

Decision Support

Efforts to educate health professionals have a very limited impact on clinical performance when compared with inserting information and alerts directly into the flow of decision making. Even the most carefully developed evidence-based guidelines will have no impact on practice if they are not integrated into clinical management through computer templates, alerts, protocols, standing orders, and other efforts to standardize practice.

Many chronically ill patients who are cared for by generalists benefit from the advice and involvement of medical specialists. Communication channels between generalists and specialists (Chapter 438) can be improved by creating systems whereby consultants respond to questions in real time by secure messaging within an electronic medical record system or by reviewing the caseloads of nurse care managers.

Involving patients in decision making improves patient satisfaction with their treatment, adherence with therapy, and even some health outcomes. To support their increasing role, a wide array of decision aids has been developed for patients.

Clinical Information Systems

Well-maintained registries that are either independent or incorporated in an electronic medical record enable practices to identify patients who need additional services, produce rapid summaries of key clinical data and services for future patient encounters, and measure clinical performance. Registries allow practices to both monitor and manage their chronically ill populations. For example, individuals overdue for important preventive interventions or who fail to keep appointments can be efficiently identified and contacted.

Electronic two-way communication between patients and providers is playing an increasing role in the management of chronic disease. Telehealth and web portals enable providers to obtain and respond to clinical data from patients, and they give patients an efficient mechanism for addressing their questions and concerns.

Community Resources

Programs and organizations in patients' local communities can most effectively meet many of their needs. Such needs include transportation, homemaker services, smoking cessation (Chapter 31), exercise (Chapter 15), weight control (Chapter 227), peer support, caregiver support and respite, self-management training, and financial counseling and assistance. For commonly needed services, practices should at least be able to provide information to advise patients on their best options.

● TRANSFORMING PRACTICE

Measures of disease control and other indicators of the quality of chronic care begin to improve only when practices have made system-wide changes in most of the elements of the chronic care model, such that the routine care of all their chronically ill patients has been affected. Practice routines and culture must change in ways that are initially foreign and uncomfortable for many practitioners. Team care means more meetings, new roles, and additional training for staff. To have useful registries and provide proactive care, busy practices must define their patient population and learn to manipulate software and data to get the information they need. Some of the changes may require additional financial investment. For all these reasons and more, improving chronic care management requires highly motivated physicians and practices that actively engage in continuous quality improvement. Practices must develop approaches that fit their patient population, resources, and practice style, and they must refine and adapt them using rapid cycle improvement methods.

Health Care Organization

Many practices caring for chronically ill individuals are parts of larger health care organizations that can either encourage and promote the improvement of chronic care or undermine and obstruct it. Helpful organizations promote continuous quality improvement, incorporate a trusted performance measurement system, and provide financial and/or nonfinancial incentives for high quality.

1. Chodosh J, Morton SC, Mojica W, et al. Meta-analysis: chronic disease self-management programs for older adults. *Ann Intern Med.* 2005;143:427-438.
2. Shojania KG, Ranji SR, McDonald KM, et al. Effects of quality improvement strategies for type 2 diabetes on glycemic control: a meta-regression analysis. *JAMA.* 2006;296:427-440.
3. Walsh JM, McDonald KM, Shojania KG, et al. Quality improvement strategies for hypertension management: a systematic review. *Med Care.* 2006;44:646-657.
4. Coleman K, Austin BT, Brach C, et al. Evidence on the chronic care model in the new millennium. *Health Aff (Millwood).* 2009;28:75-85.
5. Green BB, Cook AJ, Ralston JD, et al. Effectiveness of home blood pressure monitoring, web communication, and pharmacist care on hypertension control: a randomized controlled trial. *JAMA.* 2008;299:2857-2867.

SUGGESTED READINGS

Ahmed S, Gogovor A, Kosseim M, et al. Advancing the chronic care road map: a contemporary overview. *Healthc Q.* 2010;13:72-79. *Review.*

Hill MN, Miller NH, DeGeest S. American Society of Hypertension Writing Group. ASH position paper: Adherence and persistence with taking medication to control high blood pressure. *J Clin Hypertens.* 2010;12:757-764. *How to use the chronic care model to manage medications in hypertensive patients.*

Improving Chronic Care website. http://www.improvingchroniccare.org/index.php?p=Toolkit&s=244. *Advice for efficient and sustainable implementation of the chronic care model, with a downloadable copy and links to a variety of recommended tools.*

III

PREVENTIVE AND ENVIRONMENTAL ISSUES

13

COUNSELING FOR BEHAVIOR CHANGE

F. DANIEL DUFFY

Most office visits end with a brief conversation about diagnosis and a treatment recommendation, often including changes in long-standing behaviors. For clinicians, these conversations are routine, but for patients, these recommendations may challenge long-standing beliefs about well-being and begin repeated cycles of success and failure in replacing unhealthy habits with healthy ones. For patients with chronic illness, these habits typically include daily monitoring and medications for life.

Behavior change counseling is interpersonal therapy that changes mental models of health and internal motivational systems to reward healthy habits and extinguish unhealthy ones. The theory of behavior change counseling is grounded in cognitive behavior therapy, person-centered therapy, and social cognitive theory. Under experimental conditions and in practice, behavior change counseling delivered by trained counselors is efficacious in sustaining healthy diets, physical activity, abstinence from smoking, reduced alcohol consumption, safer sex, and daily self-care routines including adherence to medications.[1] The translation of behavior change counseling into a brief outpatient visit is challenging, owing to the long intervals between visits and the limited funding for counseling. Limited empirical evidence shows that brief office-based counseling using tailored patient-centered motivational methods and performed by trained clinicians successfully reduces smoking[2] and the hazardous use of alcohol.[3] Modest success can be achieved with brief office-based behavior change counseling for medication adherence, adopting safer sexual practices, making dietary change, and initiating physical activity.[4] The combination of direct counseling by the physician and a prepared office staff that supports patient self-care produces more effective outcomes. At a minimum, patient-centered motivational counseling improves the satisfaction of patients and physicians, forges therapeutic relationships, and influences modest changes in patients' health habits.

MODEL FOR OFFICE-BASED BEHAVIORAL CHANGE COUNSELING

Efficient behavior change counseling can be organized according to the transtheoretical model of change (Fig. 13-1), which cycles through five cognitive-experiential stages (*precontemplation, contemplation, determination, action,* and *maintenance*) and often through a sixth stage (*relapse*). Many patients recycle through the stages several times before establishing a new behavioral habit.

By identifying the stage of change, physicians can select efficient counseling strategies. For those who are not ready to change (precontemplation and contemplation), advice, education, and motivational counseling work best (Table 13-1). For those who are ready (determination and action), cognitive behavioral counseling based on self-determination theory works. For those who are already changing (maintenance and relapse), interventions based on social cognitive theory provides a good approach. An adaptation of the Counseling and Behavioral Interventions Work Group of the U.S. Preventive Services Task Force's "5 As" (assess, advise, agree, assist, and arrange) guides behavior change counseling in general health care settings.

Assess Risk for Unhealthy Behaviors

While taking a history of chronic illnesses (Chapter 6), physicians should ask about self-monitoring, adherence with medications, and self-care barriers and their solutions. In the personal and social history, physicians should ask about tobacco use, alcohol drinking, physical activity, diet, and sexual risks. In the family history, physicians uncover genetic and familial risks. Review of a patient's self-administered questionnaire by trained staff can help the physician obtain a health risk assessment efficiently.

Advise to Change Unhealthy Behaviors and Adopt Healthy Ones

There is strong evidence that direct, clear, nonjudgmental, and tailored advice delivered by a personal physician during a short office visit can help some patients stop smoking or reduce hazardous drinking.[4] Unfortunately, data also show that physicians rarely deliver information or advice about risky

behaviors, unless behavior change is the specific agenda for an encounter or treatment for a condition.

If the patient expresses interest and time permits, physicians should give personalized advice. If time is short, the physician should arrange a counseling conversation for the near future. How advice is given influences internal motivation and self-efficacy. For example, asking permission before giving advice and postponing the conversation if the patient declines demonstrate respect for patient autonomy and acknowledge that motivation to change is entirely an internal process.

If the patient agrees, the clinician begins not by giving information about behaviors and risk, but by asking the patient to share his or her values and beliefs about the unhealthy behavior. Asking "*What do you like most about … ?*" followed by, "*What concerns you about … ?*" changes the focus of behavior change counseling from a treatment to an understanding of patients' values and beliefs. The ensuing conversation should explore the patient's perceived advantages of continuing behaviors, thoughts about changing, and confidence in the ability to do so. The physician adds information to the conversation, often by asking probing questions. This technique creates an opportunity to empathize with patients' conflict and deliberately raise their conviction that changing is important for achieving valued personal goals and enhancing self-confidence in the ability to do so.

Based on the conversation, clinicians diagnose the patient's stage of change in order to agree on goals for progressing through the cycle of change. A diagnostic tool, the *Conviction-Confidence Ruler* (Fig. 13-2), helps assess internal motivation for change. The number patients select suggests their stage of change.

Patients who select a low (0 to 2) conviction and confidence number are in the precontemplation stage. If they select low conviction and confidence scores, express ambivalence or emotional distress about advice to change, and do not intend to change soon, they are in the contemplation stage.

Patients who select a midrange conviction and confidence score (3 to 7) and state their intention to change within the next month may be in the determination stage. When they select a high conviction (8 to 10) and moderate to high confidence number (5 to 9) or report already making attempts at change, they are in the action stage.

Maintenance-stage patients select high conviction and confidence numbers. They report successful experience with the healthy behavior and effective coping in response to situations in which the unhealthy behavior appears attractive or safe to do just once more. In the relapse stage, patients reported a period of success with a new behavior but then regressed. Feelings of low self-efficacy and unrealistic expectation for positive benefits from the old behavior win over their intention to maintain the change. Disappointed and discouraged, such patients select a low confidence number. If not demoralized, they select a high conviction number; otherwise their conviction number is also low, as they recycle back into resistant precontemplation.

Agree on Appropriate Goals for the Stage of Change

In this step, physicians elicit and clarify patients' self-determined goals, articulate their own goals, and find common ground or negotiate a compromise. The result is agreement on clear, realistic, and achievable goals appropriate for the patient's stage of change (Table 13-2). Unfortunately, such agreement on goals is infrequent after usual medical encounters. Few patients are in the determination or action stages, so using only action-based behavior change counseling is often ineffective and frustrating. Patients who are in the precontemplation or contemplation stages and not ready for a change goal can agree to learn more. Most patients are in maintenance or relapse stages, with experience with both success and failure; counseling that supports self-regulation is most effective and efficient in such situations.

Assist Patient in Developing a Self-Determined and Stage-Appropriate Plan

The assist step involves stage-specific counseling, which may require training to be effective. When physicians have insufficient time or training, they can refer patients to behavior change counseling professionals, either within the practice or elsewhere in the community.

Counseling patients in the precontemplation stage raises their personal conviction that change is necessary to achieve their life and health goals. This counseling elicits the patient's commitment to seek information from family members, friends, or people who have successfully made similar changes about the behavior and what changing might be like. This cognitive, attitudinal, and emotional exploration clarifies the internal conflict between current

TABLE 13-1 STAGES OF CHANGE CHARACTERISTICS

STAGE OF CHANGE	PATIENT RESPONSE	PATIENT COPING TASKS	CLINICIAN COUNSELING TASKS	COUNSELING RESOURCES
Precontemplation	Surprise Not thinking about changing Demoralized if had relapse	Learn about risks of behavior Develop self-awareness	Reflect Advise Inform	Information media Self-assessment logs or diary
Contemplation	Ambivalence Gives reasons for concern about behavior Gives rationalization for unconcern about behavior	Emotional disturbance Self-re-evaluation Raise conviction Raise confidence	Empathize with patient's ambivalence Avoid argument Develop discrepancy Roll with resistance	Conviction-Confidence Ruler Decisional balance Feedback logs Role models Referral for group training
Determination	I must change I can do it	Raise conviction Raise confidence Develop action plan Pick start date Go public	Support self-efficacy Negotiate action plan Anticipate problems Connect to social support	Menu of options Referral for formal counseling List of role models
Action	What will I do? Who or what might help? What problems might I have?	Take action steps to change Manage withdrawal from addiction	Manage cues to old behavior Alert to consequence of new behavior Add rewards Manage withdrawal	Written plan Menu of cues Menu of consequences Menu of rewards Referral for counseling
Maintenance	Satisfied with changed self Spontaneously tells about success and difficulties	Manage cues to old behavior Manage bad effects of the new behavior Seek and use social support Become a role model to others	Discuss signs and times of relapse danger Discuss the danger of "relapse thinking" Admire new lifestyle habits	Role-model for others Frequent social support Referral for maintenance counseling
Relapse	Tells about thinking old behavior was no longer a concern Loss of control Demoralization	Learn the antecedents of relapse Recognize "relapse thinking" Keep public Call for help	Reframe relapse to be a valuable lesson Evoke self-efficiency Move quickly back into action	Referral for formal relapse counseling Contact list of recovery role models Frequent follow-up

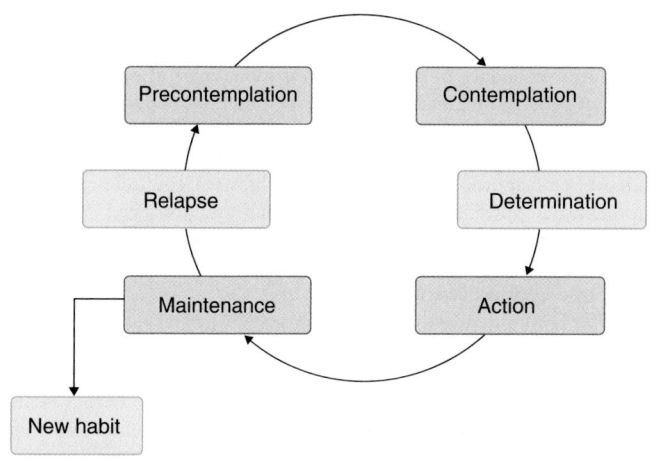

FIGURE 13-1. Cycle of change stages.

Conviction–Confidence Ruler

On a scale of 1–10, how *convinced* are you that it is important for you to change ... *(Name the behavior)* ... ?"

Not at all convinced	0 1 2 3 4 5 6 7 8 9 10	Totally convinced

On a scale of 1–10, how *confident* are you that you have the ability to change ... *(Name the behavior)* ... ?"

Not at all confident	0 1 2 3 4 5 6 7 8 9 10	Totally confident

FIGURE 13-2. Motivational counseling aid.

TABLE 13-2 SUGGESTED GOALS FOR EACH STAGE OF CHANGE

STAGE OF CHANGE	EXAMPLE GOALS FOR VITAL BEHAVIORS
Precontemplation	Learn about the risk of continuing unhealthy behavior
Contemplation	Re-evaluate one's life's goals in context of unhealthy behavior
Determination/action	Commit to a start/quit date and begin vital behaviors
Maintenance	Self-monitor behavior, success, and learning
Relapse recovery	Intensify social support and self-regulating behavior

behavior and life goals or moral values. Precontemplation is not influenced by professional argument or debate.

Motivational interviewing, which is best delivered during visits specifically scheduled for behavior change counseling, is effective for patients in contemplation, especially for those with addiction. Motivational interviewing helps patients explore and resolve their ambivalence about changing. Using open-ended questions such as *"What do you like about ... (the unhealthy behavior)... ?"* physicians inquire with genuine interest to reveal the patient's perceived advantages of the unhealthy habit or behavior. Turning to the healthy behavior, the physician asks with interest *"What concerns you about doing ... ?"* to clarify what patients believe the risks and the benefits of adopting vital behaviors might be. A *decisional balance table* (Table 13-3) can display patients' reasons for maintaining the current behavior compared with those for adopting the healthy one. Counselors should listen to patients' statements, repeating the exact words to elicit their self-motivating statements. By guiding patients in examining both sides of their ambivalence, resistance can be reduced and readiness to change can be assessed, without attempting premature change.

By helping patients "think out loud" about their conflicting reasons for change and their rationalizations for not changing, motivational interviewing amplifies the discomfort of ambivalence and motivates change. For example,

BEHAVIOR	REASONS NOT TO CHANGE	REASONS TO CHANGE
Unhealthy behavior	What do you like about it?	What are your concerns about it?
Healthy behavior	What are your concerns about it?	What do you like about it?

TABLE 13-3   DECISIONAL BALANCE

a conviction-confidence scale can clarify a patient's values and knowledge about the behavior, thereby allowing the counselor to ask, "*Why 4 and not lower?*" Asking questions like "*What would it take to raise your conviction level?*" helps patients to voice their values and beliefs and to understand their strengths and resources.

When patients express resistance to change, motivational interviewing recommends that counselors not argue but rather make empathic statements to demonstrate their understanding of the patient's painful ambivalence, beliefs, and feelings that rationalize a low conviction about the benefits of change. Using the conviction-confidence ruler, physicians can engage a patient's self-reflection by asking, "*What makes your commitment or confidence a "2" and not "0"?* If patients report a zero for commitment or confidence, the counselor might ask, "*Zero … that's as low as you can get….What would have to happen to make it a 1?*"

Determination/action counseling uses cognitive-behavioral methods to help patients develop a written plan to change lifestyle behaviors and to add self-monitoring and coping strategies to prevent relapse. The plan, which identifies the new behaviors patients will adopt to replace unhealthy ones, includes changing social situations that stimulate craving for the effects of the old behavior and using reminders and rewards for performing the new behavior. When the change requires an end to addictive behaviors, the plan must include treatments to manage withdrawal and craving. The plan asks partners and others who are making similar changes for support. The counseling helps patients anticipate challenges to sustaining the change and develop coping solutions for preventing and recovering from lapses. Plans work best when patients identify the people, resources, and coping strategies themselves. Exploring past experience with change may help identify strategies that were at least temporarily successful. Conversely, identifying what went wrong following a period of success clarifies how to cope with relapse situations.

Multidisciplinary teams of nurse educators, nutritionists, physical therapists, psychologists, and pharmacists can share education, counseling, and skills training. Referral is usually necessary for changing addictive behaviors and self-management of chronic illness.

The maintenance stage requires counseling in coping strategies to deal with the attraction or perceived safety of the unhealthy behavior, especially during the first months of change. Counseling aims at enhancing coping responses by self-monitoring of the positive effects of the healthy behavior, avoiding situations in which the unhealthy behavior becomes more attractive, and developing a strong social network that supports new coping responses.

Maintenance counseling conversations explore successes using questions like "*What has worked?*" and lapses using questions like "*Most people have difficulty; how has this change gone for you?*" It is useful to ask specifically about relapse thinking: "*Many people begin to think that after a while it's safe to … (return to the old habit) just one more time; how have you handled such thoughts?*" Regarding engaging social support, counselors might ask, "*Who or what has helped you sustain your new behavior?*" Planning for lapse recovery can be initiated by asking, "*Should you slip, what will you do, or who will you call?*"

If relapse occurs, counselors should remind patients that relapse, by definition, follows success, which proves that change is possible. Relapse must become a learning opportunity to revisit pre-relapse thinking and develop a new action plan.

Arrange Follow-up and Referral for Formal Counseling

At the conclusion of counseling, counselors ask patients to rehearse the plan verbally and state their confidence in being able to execute it. Confidence ratings less than 7 may be insufficient to undertake and sustain vital behaviors. Arranging for counseling at a future date aims to identify and resolve barriers until a patient's confidence level is at least 7, or to renegotiate a goal, with a confidence level of at least 7.

The arrange step involves scheduling future office visits within an appropriate interval for the stage of change. Longer counseling visits within a few months are appropriate for the precontemplation and contemplation stages.

In-person or telephone follow-up visits within a week or two are useful for counseling in the determination/action stage. For the maintenance stage, office follow-up counseling is as frequent as possible, usually monthly, and ideally combined with almost daily contact with other supporting persons or role models. When intensive counseling is necessary, counselors may arrange referral to patient education classes, behavioral counseling professionals, or self-help support groups to monitor the effectiveness of the referred behavior change counseling.

Grade A

1. Schedlbauer A, Davies P, Fahey T. Interventions to improve adherence to lipid lowering medication. *Cochrane Database Syst Rev.* 2010;3:CD004371.
2. McCambridge J, Slym RL, Strang J. Randomized controlled trial of motivational interviewing compared with drug information and advice for early intervention among young cannabis users. *Addiction.* 2008;103:1809-1818.
3. Solberg LI, Maciosek MV, Edwards NM. Primary care intervention to reduce alcohol misuse ranking its health impact and cost effectiveness. *Am J Prev Med.* 2008;34:143-152.
4. Goldstein MG, Whitlock EP, DePue E. Multiple behavioral risk factor interventions in primary care: summary of research evidence. *Am J Prev Med.* 2004;27:61-79.

SUGGESTED READINGS

Gardner B, Whittington C, McAteer J, et al. Using theory to synthesize evidence from behavior change interventions: the example of audit and feedback. *Soc Sci Med.* 2010;70:1618-1625. *Emphasizes the value of audit and feedback to change behavior.*

Novack DH, Clark WD, Saizow RB, et al, eds. doc.com—An interactive learning resource for healthcare communication. [Internet]: American Academy on Communication in Healthcare/ Drexel University College of Medicine; 2005. http://www.aachonline.org. Accessed Nov. 29, 2010.

14

THE PERIODIC HEALTH EXAMINATION

DAVID ATKINS AND MARY BARTON

Primary and secondary prevention is an essential part of primary care and the patient-centered medical home (Chapter 12). The appropriate services and their frequency vary with the age, gender, and individual risk factors of each patient. A periodic health examination focusing on prevention increases the delivery of appropriate screening and lifestyle counseling. The most comprehensive prevention recommendations are produced by the U.S. Preventive Services Task Force (USPSTF), an ongoing panel of experts supported by the federal Agency for Healthcare Research and Quality (*http://www.uspreventiveservicestaskforce.org*).

USPSTF recommendations are used by major primary care subspecialty groups, many health plans, and quality organizations. The USPSTF bases its recommendations on two factors: an estimate of the *net benefits* (benefits minus harms) of a service, and an assessment of the *certainty* of that estimate, based on the rigor of supporting studies. Grade A recommendations require high certainty of a substantial net benefit, most often from large, prospective, controlled studies that measure morbidity or mortality. USPSTF recommendations are thus more conservative than those of some subspecialty organizations that may give more weight to indirect evidence, such as earlier detection of disease, and less weight to potential harms of interventions. Clinicians can draw several general conclusions from an evidence-based approach to prevention: we should be selective in our use of screening tests and involve patients in decisions about specific services for which a small chance of benefit must be balanced against possible harm.

● HISTORY AND RISK ASSESSMENT

The history and risk assessment are important tools to identify individuals who may need additional screening tests or immunizations not generally recommended for their age group or who may benefit from specific counseling to address unhealthy behaviors. Formal health risk appraisals should be linked to a system to provide specific feedback and targeted interventions. Risk assessment should address the following:

- Use of tobacco, alcohol, and other drugs (especially injection drugs) (Chapters 31, 32, and 33)
- Diet (Chapter 220)
- Physical activity (Chapter 15)

- Sexual behavior that may increase the risk of sexually transmitted diseases or unintended pregnancy (Chapters 293, 392, and 395)
- Family history of cancer and heart disease
- Residence (community risk of infectious diseases)
- Presence of chronic diseases, such as diabetes, and of other cardiovascular risk factors (Chapter 51)

SCREENING FOR EARLY DISEASE OR ASYMPTOMATIC RISK FACTORS

Every year, new screening tests are introduced and marketed on the basis of their ability to detect unrecognized diseases or risk factors for disease. Other conditions need to be fulfilled for a screening test to be worthwhile for routine use, however (Table 14-1). Benefits of screening must be balanced against the potential harms, including false-positive results and the risks and costs of follow-up procedures or treatments. Even when tests have high specificity, the majority of positive results will be false-positives if the test is used to screen healthy populations for uncommon conditions such as cancer (Chapter 9). There is growing evidence that cancer screening can lead to "overdiagnosis"—detection of slow-growing cancers that would never have caused clinical symptoms in a patient's lifetime. Overdiagnosis subjects patients to the side effects of treatment with no benefits. A relatively small number of screening tests have been proved beneficial for the general population (Table 14-2), but additional tests are indicated for specific populations at risk (Table 14-3). Many commonly used tests are not recommended by the USPSTF (Table 14-4) because they provide little benefit or lack sufficient evidence to prove or disprove their value.

Depression

Depression is common and frequently undetected in primary care (Chapter 404). Simple screening instruments, including the following two questions— During the past 2 weeks, have you felt down, depressed, or hopeless? During the past 2 weeks, have you felt little interest or pleasure in doing things?— increase the detection of major depression. To improve outcomes, however, screening for depression must be linked to an organized system with staff support to ensure follow-up and treatment.[1]

High Blood Pressure, Abnormal Lipids, and Other Coronary Risk Factors

Blood pressure should be measured at least every 2 years (Chapter 67). The USPSTF recommends measuring total and high-density lipoprotein cholesterol, which can be done on fasting or nonfasting samples, beginning in middle age or earlier in the presence of other cardiovascular risk factors. The National Cholesterol Education Program guidelines recommend fasting lipoprotein analysis beginning at age 20 years (Chapter 213). Either strategy will detect the high-risk patients who need lipid-lowering therapy. Treatment decisions for elevated lipids and for blood pressure should be based on estimates of coronary heart disease risk (Chapter 51). Although factors such as C-reactive protein, homocysteine, and coronary calcification as assessed by computed tomography (CT) are associated with an increased risk of heart disease, the USPSTF found insufficient evidence to recommend their routine use.[2]

Abdominal Aortic Aneurysm

Between 5 and 9% of men older than 65 years have an abdominal aortic aneurysm (Chapter 78). The risk of aneurysm is higher in smokers and is substantially lower in women. The USPSTF recommends one-time screening with ultrasound examination in men aged 65 to 75 years who are current or former smokers, based on trials demonstrating as much as a 40% lower death rate from abdominal aortic aneurysm rupture in screened men.[3]

Colorectal Cancer

Screening can reduce both the incidence of and mortality from colorectal cancer. Options for screening men and women older than 50 years include an annual fecal occult blood test or fecal immunochemical test, flexible sigmoidoscopy every 5 to 10 years, or colonoscopy every 10 years (Chapter 199). Colonoscopy combines detection with the opportunity for biopsy and removal of lesions, so it is preferred in some guidelines. It carries higher costs and risks, however, and no single strategy has proved to be more effective or cost-effective than the alternatives.[4] In a randomized trial, a single flexible sigmoidoscopy screening between 55 and 64 years of age reduced the colorectal cancer incidence by 33% and the colorectal cancer mortality by 43% after 11 years of follow-up in people who were screened.[5] Evidence is not yet sufficient to support newer technologies such as CT colography or fecal tests for DNA markers of neoplasia. The USPSTF recommends stopping routine screening at age 75 years.

TABLE 14-2 PREVENTION RECOMMENDATIONS FOR THE GENERAL POPULATION: FROM THE U.S. PREVENTIVE SERVICES TASK FORCE AND OTHER SOURCES

SCREENING

Height, weight, and body mass index (BMI) calculation: periodically
Blood pressure: at least every 2 yr
Screen for problem drinking
Brief screen for depression*
Total blood cholesterol and HDL cholesterol: every 5 yr for men and women ≥20 yr with CHD risk factors and men ≥35 yr without CHD risk factors
Colorectal cancer screening: age ≥50 yr (see text for options)
Mammogram (± clinical breast examination): at least every 2 yr for women ≥50 yr; discuss with women 40–49
Papanicolaou (Pap) test: at least every 3 yr for sexually active women aged 21–65 yr
Chlamydia: sexually active women ≤24 yr and older women at risk
Bone mineral density test: women ≥65 yr and high-risk women <65 yr

COUNSELING

Substance use
    Tobacco cessation
    Reduction of risky or harmful alcohol use
Diet and exercise
    Limit saturated fat; maintain calorie balance; emphasize grains, fruits, and vegetables[‡]
    Regular physical activity[†]
Sexual behavior
    Unintended pregnancy: contraception
    STD prevention: avoid high-risk behavior, use condoms or female barrier with spermicide[†]
Injury prevention
    Lap and shoulder belts
    Motorcycle, bicycle, and ATV helmets[†]
    Smoke detector[†]
Dental health
    Regular visits to dental care provider[†]
    Floss, brush with fluoride toothpaste daily[†]

IMMUNIZATIONS

Pneumococcal vaccine (once, age ≥65 yr)
Influenza vaccine (annual, age ≥50 yr)
Tetanus-diphtheria (Td) boosters (every 10 yr)
Measles, mumps, rubella (MMR) vaccine (susceptible adults aged 19–49 yr)[§]
Varicella (2 doses, susceptible adults aged 30–49 yr)[§]
Human papillomavirus (HPV) vaccine (3 doses, women ≤26 yr)

CHEMOPREVENTION

Multivitamin with folic acid (women planning or capable of pregnancy)
Discuss benefits and harms of aspirin to prevent vascular disease in middle-aged adults and others at increased risk of vascular disease

*Depression screening is most effective where systems exist to improve its management.
[†]The ability of clinician counseling to influence this behavior is uncertain.
[‡]Diet counseling is most effective when it targets at-risk groups.
[§]Immunity can be verified by serologic testing, documented history of illness, or vaccination.
Other sources for Tables 14-2 and 14-3 include U.S. Department of Health and Human Services (diet, physical activity) and Centers for Disease Control and Prevention (injury prevention, immunizations, PPD).
ATV = all-terrain vehicle; CHD = coronary heart disease; HDL = high-density lipoprotein; STD = sexually transmitted disease.

TABLE 14-1 REQUIREMENTS OF AN EFFECTIVE SCREENING TEST

The disease being screened for is an important cause of morbidity and mortality
Screening can detect disease in an early, presymptomatic phase
Screening and treatment of patients with early disease or risk factors produce better health outcomes than does treatment of patients when they present with symptoms
Screening test is acceptable to patients and clinicians—safe, convenient, acceptable false-positive rate, acceptable costs
Benefits of early detection and treatment are sufficient to justify potential harms and costs of screening

TABLE 14-3   RECOMMENDED SCREENING AND INTERVENTIONS FOR HIGH-RISK POPULATIONS

POTENTIAL INTERVENTION	POPULATION
Ultrasound examination for abdominal aortic aneurysm	Current or former male smokers aged 65–75 yr
HIV test	High-risk sexual behavior or IV drug use; consider local epidemiology*
Syphilis (RPR/VDRL)	High-risk sexual behavior; consider local epidemiology*
Gonorrhea screen	High-risk sexual behavior; consider local epidemiology*
PPD	Specific immigrant groups, prisoners, HIV patients
Hepatitis B vaccine	Exposure to blood products; IV drug use; high-risk sexual behavior; travelers to high-risk areas
Hepatitis A vaccine	Persons living in or traveling to high-risk areas; institutionalized persons and workers in these institutions; those with certain chronic medical conditions
Meningococcal vaccine	First-year college students in dormitories; military recruits; those with asplenia; travelers to high-risk areas
Varicella vaccine	Adults born after 1980 without evidence of immunity
Breast cancer chemoprevention	Women at increased risk for breast cancer and with low risk of thromboembolic complications
Diabetes screen	Persons with elevated blood pressure

*Routine screening may be indicated in communities or settings where infection is prevalent.
HIV = human immunodeficiency virus; IV = intravenous; PPD = purified protein derivative; RPR = rapid plasma reagin; VDRL = Venereal Disease Research Laboratory.

TABLE 14-4   INTERVENTIONS NOT RECOMMENDED FOR ROUTINE USE IN ASYMPTOMATIC AVERAGE-RISK ADULTS*

Resting or exercise electrocardiography or helical CT for asymptomatic coronary disease
Ultrasound examination for asymptomatic carotid artery disease
Chest radiograph
Routine blood tests for anemia
Routine urine tests
Blood tests or ultrasound examination for ovarian cancer
Whole body CT
Brief tests of mental status
Vitamin supplements
Blood test for hepatitis C infection
Blood level of C-reactive protein to predict coronary risk
Prostate-specific antigen for prostate cancer

*These tests are not recommended for routine use because there is insufficient evidence that they improve clinical outcomes or because harms exceed benefits in the general population. Any of the tests may be appropriate for selected patients on the basis of clinical judgment, and some are under investigation for more widespread use.
CT = computed tomography.

Breast Cancer

In large trials, mammography screening (at intervals of 1 to 2 years, with or without clinical breast examination) reduces breast cancer mortality by 15 to 30% (Chapter 204). Most but not all trials suggest that the benefits of screening extend to women in their 40s, but the benefits are smaller and the risks of false-positive results are higher than in women aged 50 to 70 years.[6] No studies provide data on the benefits of screening women aged 75 and older. In a collaborative study, six independent models predicted that an average of 80% of the benefit of mammography could be achieved with biennial rather than annual mammography, whereas national mammography surveillance data indicate that false-positive results and other harms of screening would be reduced by about half if women were screened every other year instead of yearly. Although many cancers are discovered by patients, teaching women to perform breast self-examination increases the likelihood that a woman will undergo further evaluation for an unimportant finding, but it does not improve outcomes. Widespread screening for *BRCA1* or *BRCA2*, inherited mutations that increase the risk for breast cancer, is not recommended, but women with a suggestive family history (multiple first-degree relatives with breast or ovarian cancer) should be referred for genetic counseling.

Cervical Cancer

Papanicolaou (Pap) screening is highly effective in preventing invasive cervical cancer, but many low-risk women in the United States are screened more often than needed. The USPSTF and American College of Obstetrics and Gynecology endorse delaying screening until age 21, screening only every 2 to 3 years instead of annually in women with previous normal test results (Chapter 205), and offering low-risk women the option of discontinuing screening after 65 years of age. Screening is not indicated in women who have undergone a hysterectomy for benign disease. Liquid-based cytology specimens do not improve clinical outcomes significantly, but they allow testing for human papillomavirus (Chapters 205 and 381), which may help in managing borderline Pap smear results, such as atypical squamous cells. Primary screening for human papillomavirus, although sensitive for cervical neoplasia, is not recommended for routine use because it identifies many younger women with transient infection. Whether women who have received the human papillomavirus vaccine (Chapter 17) need less frequent screening is not yet known.

Prostate Cancer

Screening with prostate-specific antigen (PSA) can increase the detection of organ-confined prostate cancer, but two recent large trials provided conflicting results as to whether screening lowers morbidity or mortality from prostate cancer (Chapter 207). An American trial found no benefit of annual PSA testing, but it was hampered by a high rate of screening in the control group. A European study reported that men randomized to screening every 4 years had a 20% lower risk of dying from prostate cancer after 9 years; for each prostate cancer death prevented, 48 additional men were treated for prostate cancer and 1068 men had to undergo screening. Because of the significant morbidity associated with overdiagnosis and overtreatment, including incontinence and impotence, the USPSTF does not recommend routine PSA screening, but the American Cancer Society and some specialty groups recommend discussing PSA screening with men who have a life expectancy of at least 10 years.

Osteoporosis

Tests of bone mineral density can identify men and women with a high risk of fracture due to osteoporosis and who may benefit from medications proved to lower the risk of fracture (Chapter 251). The USPSTF recommends screening for osteoporosis in women older than 65 years or earlier in the presence of risk factors for osteoporosis. The most accurate predictor of risk of hip fracture is bone mineral density of the hip assessed with dual-energy x-ray absorptiometry. A tool developed by the World Health Organization (http://www.shef.ac.uk/FRAX/) incorporates bone mineral density and other risk factors, such as age and fracture history, to guide treatment decisions.

Thyroid Disease

Routine thyroid testing occasionally identifies patients with symptomatic but undiagnosed hypothyroidism (Chapter 233), but it more often detects subclinical hypothyroidism, a disorder marked by elevations in thyroid-stimulating hormone with normal levels of free thyroxine. Because the benefits of treating subclinical hypothyroidism remain uncertain, the USPSTF does not recommend routine thyroid testing in the absence of symptoms. Clinicians should be alert to subtle signs of thyroid disease and have a low threshold for testing patients in high-risk groups, including postpartum and postmenopausal women.

Diabetes

Routine screening for diabetes beginning at age 45 years is recommended by some groups, but the USPSTF recommends screening only in patients with elevated blood pressure (Chapter 237). Although tight glucose control can reduce the incidence of microvascular disease, the benefit of early presymptomatic detection on retinopathy, neuropathy, and nephropathy is likely to be small. The benefits of early detection of diabetes are much greater in persons with hypertension because more aggressive treatment of blood pressure in patients with diabetes has been shown to reduce cardiovascular events within 5 years.

HIV Infection

The USPSTF recommends screening for HIV infection in all pregnant women and in adolescents and adults at increased risk. In an effort to reduce the estimated 25% of infected patients who have not yet been diagnosed, however, the Centers for Disease Control and Prevention recommends that all adolescents and adults aged 13 to 64 years have at least one HIV test and annual tests if they are at high risk.

Sexually Transmitted Disease

Screening for chlamydia (Chapter 326) is recommended for all sexually active women ages 24 years and younger and for older women at risk. Nucleic acid amplification tests can be performed on cervical or urine specimens. Early detection can reduce pelvic inflammatory disease (Chapter 293), a risk factor for infertility and ectopic pregnancy. Similar benefits are likely from screening women for gonorrhea (Chapter 307), but the risk of gonorrhea infection is more concentrated in high-risk urban and southeastern rural populations.

Vision and Hearing

Undetected but correctable vision and hearing problems are common in older adults and can be discovered by asking about problems and performing simple tests of visual acuity and hearing. Regular visual acuity testing is recommended for older adults by many organizations, but a large trial did not find any lasting benefits of screening, despite detecting many correctable causes of vision problems.

● BEHAVIORAL INTERVENTIONS

Lifestyle factors contribute to a large proportion of preventable deaths in the United States. Brief interventions are effective for some behaviors such as smoking and problem drinking, but changing other behaviors usually requires more intensive approaches. The 5 *As* framework—ask, assess, advise, assist, and arrange—which was developed from smoking cessation research, provides a useful framework for counseling (Chapter 13).

Tobacco Use

Brief interventions can produce small but clinically important increases in quit rates among smokers. Effects increase with more intensive counseling and support, including the use of medication (Chapter 31).

Problem Drinking

A variety of screening instruments can detect patients with problems due to alcohol and those with risky patterns of alcohol consumption. Brief interventions can successfully reduce alcohol consumption in at-risk drinkers (Chapter 32).

Diet

Diet counseling can reduce the intake of saturated fat and increase the consumption of fruits and vegetables. Effects are most consistent with more intensive counseling (multiple sessions with trained counselors) and in higher risk patients, such as those with elevated lipid levels (Chapter 220).

Physical Activity

Moderate physical activity reduces the risk of obesity, diabetes, and coronary heart disease, among other benefits. Studies of counseling in the primary care setting, however, have reported inconsistent effects on long-term levels of physical activity (Chapter 15).

Injury Prevention

Motor vehicle injuries are the leading cause of years of potential life lost before age 65 years. In older persons, falls are a leading cause of unintentional injury and can be reduced with targeted interventions (Chapter 24).

● IMMUNIZATIONS

Recommendations regarding immunization (see Tables 14-2 and 14-3) are regularly updated by the Advisory Committee on Immunization Practices of the Centers for Disease Control and Prevention (*www.cdc.gov/vaccines*) (Chapter 17). Annual influenza immunization is effective in all adults but is most important in those older than 50 years and others at high risk because of chronic conditions or immunodeficiency. Pneumococcal immunization is recommended at least once at age 65 years or after for all adults and for younger adults with asplenia, chronic heart or lung disease, and other immune disorders. Revaccination is not generally recommended unless the initial immunization was before age 65 or the patient has immune-related risk factors. Two doses of varicella vaccine are recommended for all adults born in the United States after 1980 without other evidence of immunity, and one dose of zoster vaccine is recommended for all adults at age 60. Adults should be revaccinated once with the Tdap vaccine (tetanus, diphtheria, acellular pertussis) and every 10 years thereafter with Td, primarily to maintain levels of immunity against diphtheria.

● CHEMOPREVENTION

Aspirin, postmenopausal hormone replacement therapy, and breast cancer chemopreventive drugs carry both benefits and risks. Decisions need to consider the likely benefits (which increase with the underlying risk of the disease being prevented), the probability of harm, and the individual preferences of each patient.

Aspirin

In men and women without known vascular disease, aspirin reduces the combined risk of myocardial infarction, stroke, and other serious cardiovascular events by 12%, but it also increases the risk of serious gastrointestinal bleeding and hemorrhagic stroke and does not significantly reduce cardiovascular mortality.[7] Individuals and their physicians need to assess whether the benefits, which increase with the risk of vascular disease, outweigh the bleeding risks, which increase with age (Chapter 37).

Chemoprevention of Breast Cancer

Tamoxifen and raloxifene can reduce the incidence of invasive breast cancer by nearly 50% in women at increased risk, but both agents increase risk of thromboembolic events (including stroke) and worsen menopausal symptoms; tamoxifen also increases the risk of endometrial cancer (Chapter 204). The balance of benefits and harm is most favorable in women younger than 60 years who have an increased risk of breast cancer owing to family history.

Postmenopausal Hormone Therapy

Estrogen therapy reduces the risk of fracture, but it increases the risk of thromboembolism and gallbladder disease (Chapter 248). When given with progestin, postmenopausal estrogen modestly increases the risk of heart disease and stroke (primarily in women older than 60), breast cancer, and dementia.[8] Hormone replacement therapy is a reasonable option for women with persistent, troublesome menopausal symptoms, but it should not routinely be used for preventive purposes.

Vitamin Supplementation

The USPSTF does not recommend routine vitamin supplementation because multiple large trials have failed to demonstrate the benefits of vitamins A, C, and E or folic acid against heart disease or cancer. Several studies suggested that β-carotene may increase the risk of lung cancer in smokers, and a meta-analysis suggested that folic acid supplementation could increase cancer risk.

● FUTURE ISSUES

As the understanding of genetic factors that modify the risk of disease grows, clinicians may eventually be able to target screening, preventive treatments, or lifestyle interventions to those at greatest risk. The value of using currently available tests to screen average-risk individuals is limited by an incomplete understanding of the predictive value of specific genotypes in the general population, the uncertain effect of such information on clinical decisions, and concerns about the possible adverse effects of screening (e.g., anxiety or "labeling," false reassurance, discrimination).

With the current epidemic of obesity in the United States, and its attendant long-term health consequences, effective counseling tools and strategies may be more important in the coming decades than improved screening and early detection tools. Helping patients choose a healthier diet, increase their physical activity, and maintain a healthy weight is difficult, but the lessons of tobacco control over the past 30 years suggest that a combination of consistent clinical counseling and encouragement, complemented by public health messages and community strategies, can have an important health impact.

1. O'Connor EA, Whitlock EP, Beil TL, et al. Screening for depression in adult patients in primary care settings: a systematic evidence review. *Ann Intern Med.* 2009;151:793-803.

2. U.S. Preventive Services Task Force. Using nontraditional risk factors in coronary heart disease risk assessment: U.S. Preventive Services Task Force recommendation statement. *Ann Intern Med.* 2009;151:474-482.

3. Fleming C, Whitlock EP, Beil TL, et al. Screening for abdominal aortic aneurysm: a best-evidence systematic review. *Ann Intern Med.* 2005;142:203-211.

4. Whitlock EP, Lin JS, Liles E, et al. Screening for colorectal cancer: a targeted, updated systematic review for the U.S. Preventive Services Task Force. *Ann Intern Med.* 2008;149:638-658.

5. Atkin WS, Edwards R, Kralj-Hans I, et al. Once-only flexible sigmoidoscopy screening in prevention of colorectal cancer: a multicentre randomised controlled trial. *Lancet.* 2010;375:1624-1633.

6. Nelson HD, Tyne K, Naik A, et al. Screening for breast cancer: an update for the U.S. Preventive Services Task Force. *Ann Intern Med.* 2009;151:727-737.

7. Antithrombotic Trialists' Collaboration. Aspirin in the primary and secondary prevention of vascular disease: collaborative meta-analysis of individual participant data from randomized trials. *Lancet.* 2009;373:1849-1860.

8. Rossouw JE, Prentice RL, Manson JE, et al. Postmenopausal hormone therapy and risk of cardiovascular disease by age and years since menopause. *JAMA.* 2007;297:1465-1477.

SUGGESTED READINGS

Canadian Task Force on Preventive Health Care. http://www.canadiantaskforce.ca. *A Canadian counterpart to the USPSTF offers an independent perspective on preventive health interventions.*

National Guideline Clearinghouse. http://www.guidelines.gov. *Standardized descriptions of more than 1700 guidelines, with full text access to many of them. Guidelines can be searched by condition, intervention, or organization, and the site will construct a comparison of different guidelines on a given topic.*

U.S. Preventive Services Task Force. http://uspreventiveservicestaskforce.org. *This site includes all the recommendations and supporting reviews of the USPSTF.*

15

PHYSICAL ACTIVITY

DAVID M. BUCHNER

DEFINITIONS

Physical activity can be broadly defined as body movement that is produced by skeletal muscles and expends energy. When discussing the health benefits of activity, it is useful to divide body movements into two categories. *Baseline activity* refers to light-intensity activities of daily life, such as standing, walking slowly, and lifting lightweight objects. *Health-enhancing physical activity* is activity that when added to baseline activity produces important health benefits and generally involves the large muscle groups of the body and substantial energy expenditure. Herein, *physical activity* refers to health-enhancing physical activity. *Exercise* refers to the subset of physical activity that involves a structured program to improve physical fitness.

Regular physical activity improves *health-related physical fitness*—the physiologic components of fitness that influence risk of disease, functional limitations, disability, and premature mortality. These components include cardiorespiratory endurance (aerobic capacity); skeletal muscle strength, power, and endurance; body composition and bone strength; and balance, flexibility, and reaction time.

The primary attributes of physical activity are *type* (mode), *frequency, duration,* and *intensity.* Types of physical activity (e.g., walking, swimming, lifting, stretching) are grouped according to their main physiologic effects into well-known categories: *aerobic* (or "cardio"), *muscle strengthening, flexibility,* and *balance.* Intensity is the level of effort during activity. For aerobic activity, the *absolute intensity* is measured in metabolic equivalents (METs), with 1 MET being the resting metabolic rate—an oxygen consumption of roughly 3.5 mL/kg/minute. The *relative intensity,* which is the percentage of oxygen uptake (aerobic capacity) reserve required to perform an activity, ranges from 0 to 100%. In practice, the heart rate is used to monitor relative intensity because of the generally linear relationship between heart rate and percentage of oxygen uptake. The *volume* (or amount) of activity is the product of frequency, duration, and intensity. Volume can be measured as activity-related energy expenditure (e.g., kcal/week) or as MET-minutes per week (a sum of the MET intensity of all activities multiplied by the minutes each activity is performed).

EPIDEMIOLOGY

Levels of Physical Activity

Data on long-term trends in the level of physical activity among adults are limited. Even so, it is highly likely that Americans' level of physical activity has declined since the 1950s. Levels of activity around the home,

work-related activity, and transportation activity have apparently declined over the past 50 years. Trends in leisure-time physical activity are either stable or slightly improving.

In recent national surveys that track domestic, leisure-time, and transportation physical activity using questionnaires, about 45% of American adults are active at recommended levels. Using objective measurements (an accelerometer), however, less than 5% of adults meet the recommended levels of physical activity, suggesting that the lack of physical activity is a larger public health problem than previously realized.

Physical activity levels decline with age, and men report more activity than women. Higher levels of income and education are associated with greater physical activity. White Americans report higher levels of physical activity than other racial and ethnic groups do.

Preventive Health Benefits in Adults

There is strong evidence that regular moderate or vigorous physical activity (Table 15-1) reduces the risk for premature mortality and coronary artery disease (Chapter 51), stroke (Chapter 413), high blood pressure (Chapter 67), adverse lipid profile (Chapter 213), type 2 diabetes mellitus (Chapter 237), metabolic syndrome, osteoporosis (Chapter 251), colon cancer (Chapter 199), breast cancer (Chapter 204), and obesity (Chapter 227). Physical activity also reduces the risk for falls, cognitive impairment in older adults, age-related muscle loss, and depression (Chapters 24 and 404). There is moderate evidence that physical activity reduces the risk of hip fracture, lung cancer, endometrial cancer, and sleep disorders. Some evidence suggests that physical activity reduces the risk for anxiety disorders, osteoarthritis, and back pain. Observational studies consistently report that physical activity delays age-related functional limitations and loss of independence.

The benefits of physical activity are independent of other risk factors. For example, a sedentary obese smoker achieves health benefits from exercise, even if smoking and obesity persist.

Epidemiologic studies report that low levels of activity are associated with an increased risk for adverse health outcomes, including up to a 52% increase in overall mortality, a doubling of mortality from cardiovascular disease, and a 29% increase in mortality from cancer. When a healthy diet, regular activity, and abstinence from smoking are considered simultaneously, the effect of lifestyle is dramatic. For example, one study attributed 82% of coronary events in women to the lack of adherence to a healthy lifestyle.

The main determinant of the health benefits of physical activity is volume. Substantial health benefits begin to occur with a volume of 500 to 1000 MET-minutes/week. An adult can accumulate 500 MET-minutes by walking at 3.0 miles per hour (a 3.3-MET activity) on 5 days a week for 30 minutes (3.3 METs × 5 × 30 minutes = ≈500 MET-minutes). When measured by caloric expenditure, this volume of walking in a 75-kg (165-lb) adult expends an extra 430 kcal above the 190 kcal that would have been expended under resting conditions.

The dose-response relationship between volume and health benefits appears to be curvilinear, such that the marginal benefit of activity at lower

TABLE 15-1	EXAMPLES OF MODERATE-INTENSITY AND VIGOROUS-INTENSITY ACTIVITIES

MODERATE INTENSITY

Walking briskly (3 miles per hour or faster, but not race-walking)
Water aerobics
Bicycling slower than 10 miles per hour
Tennis (doubles)
Ballroom dancing
General gardening

VIGOROUS INTENSITY

Race-walking, jogging, or running
Swimming laps
Tennis (singles)
Bicycling 10 miles per hour or faster
Jumping rope
Heavy gardening (continuous digging or hoeing, with heart rate increases)
Hiking uphill or with a heavy backpack

From U.S. Department of Health and Human Services. *2008 Physical Activity Guidelines for Americans.* http://www.health.gov/paguidelines.

TABLE 15-2	RELATIVE RISK OF CARDIOVASCULAR DISEASE IN THE WOMEN'S HEALTH INITIATIVE OBSERVATIONAL STUDY (N = 73,743)

MEDIAN MET-MINUTES/WK	MULTIVARIATE ADJUSTED RELATIVE RISK OF CARDIOVASCULAR DISEASE
0	1.0
252	0.89
600	0.81
1050	0.78
1968	0.72

Data from Manson JE, Greenland P, LaCroix AZ, et al. Walking compared with vigorous exercise for the prevention of cardiovascular events in women. *N Engl J Med.* 2002;347:716-725.

levels is large, and the benefit decreases with higher activity levels. Data from the Women's Health Initiative Observational Study (Table 15-2) provide an example of the dose-response effect. Compared with the least active women, the risk for cardiovascular disease was 19% less in women who averaged 600 MET-minutes/week, yet just 28% less in women who averaged 1968 MET-minutes/week. Dose-response effects are also found in intervention studies. For example, a randomized trial of two doses of exercise (doses equivalent to jogging 12 and 20 miles/week) found that the lower volume of exercise significantly improved plasma lipoproteins, but the higher volume had greater beneficial effects.**1**

TREATMENT   Rx

Therapeutic Health Benefits in Adults

Clinical practice guidelines assign a substantial therapeutic role to physical activity in patients with coronary heart disease (Chapter 51), high blood pressure (Chapter 67), type 2 diabetes (Chapter 237), obesity (Chapter 227), osteoporosis (Chapter 251), osteoarthritis (Chapter 270), claudication (Chapter 79), and chronic obstructive pulmonary disease (Chapter 88). Physical activity also plays a role in the management of depression and anxiety disorders, elevated cholesterol levels, pain, heart failure, syncope, stroke, back pain, dementia, and constipation and in the prophylaxis of venous thromboembolism.

Physical activity effectively opposes age-related loss of fitness and functional limitations. Randomized controlled trials demonstrate that exercise by sedentary older adults improves health-related physical fitness (e.g., aerobic exercise improves aerobic capacity) and has beneficial effects on functional limitations, such as a slow gait speed. Generally, the benefits are most demonstrable in older adults with clinically significant functional limitations. Physical activity, especially balance training, prevents falls in older adults at increased risk for falling, such as those with impaired gait and balance.**3** It is probable that physical activity improves the ability to live independently, but evidence from randomized trials is incomplete.

Health Risks of Physical Activity

Physical activity and exercise have risks. Musculoskeletal injuries are by far the most common type of activity-related adverse event. The risk of injury depends on the type and volume of activity. Collision and contact sports have a much higher injury risk than noncontact activities such as walking, which is associated with about one musculoskeletal injury for every 1000 hours of walking for exercise. The weekly volume of activity is directly related to the risk of musculoskeletal injuries, but when following public health guidelines, which involves participating in about 500 to 1000 MET-minutes/week, the risk of injury is low. The risk of injury is directly related to the rate of increase in the dose of activity, with more rapid increases having higher risk. Previous musculoskeletal injuries and low fitness also increase the injury risk.

Overall, regular physical activity decreases the risk for sudden cardiac death and myocardial infarction; active adults have roughly a 70% lower risk of sudden death. However, relatively vigorous physical activity acutely increases the risk for these events in both active and inactive adults. About 5 to 10% of myocardial infarctions are associated with vigorous activity. Yet sudden death is a rare event during exercise, with published rates in the range of one death per year in 18,000 ostensibly healthy men and one death per 2.6 million workouts in fitness facilities.

Physical Activity Guidelines for Adults

For the first time, the U.S. Department of Health and Human Services has issued national physical activity guidelines: the *2008 Physical Activity Guidelines for Americans* (Table 15-3).

Recommended Amounts of Aerobic Activity for Prevention

To obtain substantial health benefits from physical activity, adults should do at least 150 minutes/week of moderate-intensity aerobic activity or 75

TABLE 15-3	KEY PHYSICAL ACTIVITY GUIDELINES FOR ADULTS

All adults should avoid inactivity. Some physical activity is better than none, and adults who participate in any amount of physical activity gain some health benefits.

For substantial health benefits, adults should do at least 150 min (2.5 hr)/wk of moderate-intensity aerobic activity or 75 min (1.25 hr)/wk of vigorous-intensity aerobic activity, or an equivalent combination of moderate- and vigorous-intensity aerobic activity.

Aerobic activity should be performed in episodes lasting at least 10 min and should be spread throughout the week.

For additional and more extensive health benefits, adults should increase their aerobic physical activity to 300 min (5 hr)/wk of moderate-intensity or 150 min (2.5 hr)/wk of vigorous-intensity aerobic physical activity, or an equivalent combination of moderate- and vigorous-intensity activity. Additional health benefits are gained by engaging in physical activity beyond this amount.

Adults should also do muscle-strengthening activities that are moderate or high intensity and involve all major muscle groups on 2 or more days/wk, as these activities provide additional health benefits.

From U.S. Department of Health and Human Services. *2008 Physical Activity Guidelines for Americans.* http://www.health.gov/paguidelines.

minutes/week of vigorous-intensity activity. Light-intensity activity is less than 3.0 METs, moderate-intensity activity is in the range of 3.0 to 5.9 METs, and vigorous-intensity activity is 6.0 METs or higher. There is insufficient evidence to determine whether the health benefits of 30 minutes of activity on 5 days a week differ from the health benefits of 50 minutes of activity on 3 days a week. Adults can also do an equivalent combination of both moderate- and vigorous-intensity activity, using the rule of thumb that one vigorous-intensity minute of activity counts the same as two moderate-intensity minutes.

Recommended Amounts of Muscle-Strengthening Activity for Prevention

Adults should perform activities that strengthen the major muscle groups of the body at least 2 days each week. The major muscle groups are the legs, hips, back, chest, abdomen, shoulders, and arms.

Flexibility Activity

Flexibility activities are an acceptable part of a physical activity regimen, but there is insufficient evidence that flexibility activities have any health benefits, even for preventing injuries. Flexibility training does increase flexibility, and it may facilitate the types of physical activity that do have health benefits. If so, flexibility training is more important for people with reduced flexibility, such as older adults with age- and disease-related changes in range of motion.

Balance Activity

Balance training is currently recommended only for adults at increased risk for falls, such as those older than 65 years with impaired gait or balance or frequent falls. Examples of balance exercises include sideways walking, backward walking, heel walking, and standing using a narrow base of support. Tai chi programs include exercises that improve balance. The optimal frequency, duration, and type of balance training are unknown. Preferably, adults at risk for falls should do balance training at least 3 days/week and follow an evidence-based program demonstrated to reduce the risk of falls.

Inactivity versus Sitting Time

Inactive adults engage in no activity that counts toward meeting the national guidelines. Doing some physical activity is clearly preferable to inactivity. A separate issue is whether more time spent sitting has an adverse effect on health, independent of a person's volume of moderate- to vigorous-intensity activity. It appears likely that spending more time in light-intensity baseline activity and less time sitting has an independent beneficial effect on health. Certainly, light-intensity activities expend calories and can be recommended as part of a plan to achieve and maintain a healthy weight. However, data are currently insufficient to issue guidelines on the amounts and patterns of sitting time that cause adverse health effects in adults.

Guidelines for Weight Management

The amount of activity required to maintain a healthy body weight varies widely among adults (Chapter 227). For some adults, the physical activity levels recommended in the guidelines will result in a stable, healthy body weight. Many adults, however, need higher levels of activity to achieve a healthy weight. These individuals should restrict their caloric intake and gradually increase their physical activity each week, to the point that is effective in achieving and maintaining a healthy body weight for them.

Additional Guidelines for Older Adults

In addition to balance training, the 2008 guidelines contain other recommendations specifically for older adults. Older adults who cannot do 150 minutes/week of moderate-intensity activity should be as active as their abilities and conditions allow. Progressive resistance strength training improves physical function in the elderly.[4] Older adults should determine their level of physical activity using relative intensity, not absolute intensity. This latter guideline seeks to avoid inappropriately high levels of effort in older adults with low fitness.

Recommending Physical Activity in Clinical Settings

Promoting physical activity in clinical settings involves essentially the same steps as the five As of smoking cessation: ask, advise, assess, assist, arrange. (1) Ask about the amount of physical activity a patient typically engages in each week by questionnaire or interview. (2) Advise all patients to participate in at least a moderate amount of physical activity each week. Advise patients who do not meet the recommendations to increase their physical activity gradually to a specified minimal level, and tailor the recommendations according to their medical conditions. (3) Assess the next step or steps a patient needs to take to become more active. (4) Assist the patient in taking these steps. (5) Arrange an appointment to follow up on efforts to increase activity.

Health care providers should ask and advise patients about physical activity regularly. One quality-of-care measure assesses whether asking and advising are done at least once a year in older adults. Some recommend that physical activity should be a "vital sign" that is assessed at every visit. Studies consistently report that adults (especially older adults) identify their health care providers as an important source of advice on physical activity.

The U.S. Preventive Services Task Force last reviewed the effectiveness of primary care–based counseling (i.e., assessing and assisting) in 2002. Counseling protocols vary among research studies; some have been effective, and some not. Overall, the task force concluded that the evidence was insufficient to recommend for or against counseling. In relatively healthy patients, a reasonable approach is to counsel selected patients who request information about physical activity, using a protocol that has been evaluated and shown to be effective. For example, a randomized trial demonstrated that an exercise prescription program increased physical activity and quality of life in women aged 40 to 76 over a 2-year period, although falls and injuries also increased.[5]

Exercise Prescription

For patients who want to exercise, a clinician can provide an exercise prescription. The prescription includes (1) the type, frequency, duration, and intensity of aerobic exercise; (2) the exercise movements (e.g., bench press), repetitions, and sets for resistance exercise; (3) other exercises such as stretching, balance exercises, warm-up, and cool-down; and (4) risk management strategies, such as increasing levels of activity gradually over time.

A prescription for vigorous-intensity aerobic exercise generally specifies a minimum frequency of at least 3 days/week, a minimum duration of 20 minutes, and an intensity of 70 to 85% of the maximal heart rate (HR_{max}). A prescription for moderate-intensity exercise would specify an intensity of 40 to 60% of oxygen uptake reserve (or 50 to 69% of HR_{max}) 3 or more days/week to reach an adequate volume. Training at the upper limits of vigorous intensity (85 to 89% of HR_{max}) is discouraged because of concern about injury and adherence. (Higher exercise intensities are commonly regarded as less pleasant.)

A prescription for resistance training generally specifies 8 to 10 separate exercises that train the major muscle groups, with at least one set of 8 to 12 repetitions of each exercise on 2 or 3 days/week. Some recommend that older adults do 10 to 15 repetitions in a set.

Lifestyle Prescription

A *lifestyle prescription* refers to approaches that integrate physical activity into daily life. For example, rather than walking specifically for exercise, a person walks to work or walks for pleasure as a recreational activity. Common ways to integrate physical activity into daily life are walking and biking for transportation and performing yard work and gardening.

Tailoring the Recommendation

Recommendations need to be tailored to individual abilities, individual preferences, medical conditions, and behavior techniques that improve adherence. Randomized trials show that home-based programs are superior to center-based programs in terms of long-term adherence.[6] Although center-based programs are preferred by some, in most cases they serve a short-term purpose, such as assisting adults to initiate regular exercise.

A target level of physical activity below that of preventive recommendations is appropriate for adults with very low fitness, a large burden of chronic disease (e.g., severe chronic obstructive lung disease), or major functional limitations. An assessment of the nature of the activity limitation and the individual's capabilities and preferences can determine the target activity level and other details of the activity recommendation. Often, promoting physical activity in such adults relies on health care and community resources designed for people with preexisting limitations, such as cardiac rehabilitation, pulmonary rehabilitation, and exercise classes for adults with arthritis.

Risk Management

Strategies to reduce injury include increasing physical activity gradually over time, selecting activities in which collision or contact with people or objects is unusual, increasing physical fitness, using appropriate gear and sports equipment (e.g., bike helmets), engaging in activities in safe environments, and following basic safety rules and policies. Popular activities such as walking, biking, swimming, and gardening have a low risk of injury. When increasing the level of physical activity, the guidelines recommend using relative intensity to determine the level of effort, starting with relatively moderate-intensity activity, then increasing the duration and frequency first and the intensity last. In general, adding 5 to 15 minutes of moderate-intensity activity per session, two to three times a week, to a person's usual activities carries a low risk of musculoskeletal injury and no known risk of sudden cardiac death.

There is no evidence of the protective value of a medical consultation in healthy people of any age who seek to increase their level of physical activity. The U.S. Preventive Services Task Force recommended against routine screening for coronary disease in adults at low risk for it and concluded that in adults at high risk for coronary disease, there is insufficient evidence to recommend for or against screening with resting electrocardiography, exercise treadmill test, or electron-beam computed tomography.

Coordination between Medical Care and Community

Many factors affecting physical activity levels are difficult to influence in medical care settings, such as the characteristics of the communal environment (e.g., parks and recreational facilities) and the social environment (e.g., crime and social support). Community-level interventions that address such characteristics are essential to promoting physical activity. Effective community-based interventions include school physical education, social support interventions, community-wide campaigns, enhancement of access to places where physical activity is possible, and interventions that involve community design, such as improving the connectivity of streets and the walkability of neighborhoods. Medical care and community efforts should be synergistic and mutually supportive. For example, health plans should be advocates for evidence-based community interventions. Community programs should serve as resources for evidence-based therapeutic activity for selected chronically ill adults, such as exercise classes designed to reduce the risk of falls.

1. Kraus WE, Houmard JA, Duscha BD, et al. Effects of the amount and intensity of exercise on plasma lipoproteins. *N Engl J Med.* 2002;347:1483-1492.
2. Pahor M, Blair SN, Espeland M, et al. Effects of a physical activity intervention on measures of physical performance: results of the lifestyle interventions and independence for elders pilot (LIFE-) study. *J Gerontol Series A.* 2006;61:1157-1165.
3. Gillespie LD, Robertson MC, Gillespie WJ, et al. Interventions for preventing falls in older people living in the community. *Cochrane Database Syst Rev.* 2009;2:CD007146.
4. Liu CJ, Latham NK. Progressive resistance strength training for improving physical function in older adults. *Cochrane Database Syst Rev.* 2009;3:CD002759.
5. Lawton BA, Rose SB, Elley CR, et al. Exercise on prescription for women age 40-74 recruited through primary care: two year randomized controlled trial. *Br J Sports Med.* 2009;43:120-123.
6. Ashworth NL, Chad KE, Harrison EL, et al. Home versus center based physical activity programs in older adults. *Cochrane Database Syst Rev.* 2005.1:CD004017.

SUGGESTED READINGS

Artinian NT, Fletcher GF, Mozaffarian D, et al. Interventions to promote physical activity and dietary lifestyle changes for cardiovascular risk factor reduction in adults: a scientific statement from the American Heart Association. *Circulation.* 2010;122:406-441. *Consensus guidelines.*

Katzmarzyk PT, Church TS, Craig CL, et al. Sitting times and mortality from all causes, cardiovascular disease, and cancer. *Med Sci Sports Exerc.* 2009;41:998-1005. *Showed a dose-response relationship between sitting time and all-cause mortality independent of the effect of moderate-to-vigorous physical activity.*

Physical Activity Guidelines Advisory Committee. Part G. Section 10. Adverse Events. In Physical Activity Guidelines Advisory Committee Report. www.health.gov/paguidelines. Accessed Dec. 4, 2010. *Reviews the determinants of activity-related adverse events and approaches to reduce injury risk.*

16

ADOLESCENT MEDICINE

DEBRA K. KATZMAN AND LAWRENCE S. NEINSTEIN

Adolescence, a period of transition between childhood and adulthood, is marked by critical biological, psychological, social, and cognitive changes. During this unique developmental period, patterns of behaviors and lifestyle choices are established that can influence current and future health, and unique medical and psychological problems can emerge. Adult-oriented health care providers play a pivotal role in engaging youth in their health and in providing health care to adolescents and young adults.

NORMAL PHYSICAL GROWTH AND DEVELOPMENT

Biologic growth and development in adolescents are signified by the onset of puberty (Chapter 243), which varies temporally among adolescents and explains why adolescents of the same chronologic age can vary greatly in physical appearance. Usually the first visible sign of puberty among females is thelarche, or the development of breast buds, which occurs on average at 10.5 years in white girls and 1 year earlier in African-American girls (Chapter 243).

Menarche occurs 2 to 4 years after the initial appearance of breast buds and pubic hair. The average age of menarche is 12.9 years for white girls and 12.2 years for African-American girls. Menstrual periods are not always regular during the first 2 years after menarche. At menarche, only 20% of cycles are ovulatory; it may take up to 4 years for 80% of cycles to be ovulatory. The average length for the completion of puberty in females is 4 years (range, 1.5 to 8.0 years).

Puberty begins about 2 years later in boys than in girls. The first physical sign of puberty in boys, testicular enlargement and thinning of the scrotum, occurs at 11.5 years. Adrenarche occurs 6 months later at an average age of 12.0 to 12.5 years (Chapter 242). Facial hair starts to grow about 3 years after pubic hair. The completion of puberty in males can take an average of 3 years (range, 2 to 5 years).

Pubertal weight gain accounts for about half of a person's ideal adult body weight. Peak weight gain follows the linear growth spurt by 3 to 6 months in adolescent girls and by about 3 months in adolescent boys. The average weight gain during puberty among adolescent females is 15 to 55 lb, or 7 to 25 kg (mean gain, 38.5 lb, or 17.5 kg). Overall, adolescent males gain 15 to 65 lb, or 7 to 30 kg, during puberty (mean gain, 52.2 lb or 23.7 kg).

Boys' body fat levels decrease during adolescence, dropping to 12% body fat by the end of puberty. On average, adolescent girls' lean body mass falls from 80 to 75%, whereas their average body fat levels increase from 16 to 27% by the end of adolescence. By the time adolescent girls are 16 years of age and adolescent boys are 18 years of age, they have accrued more than 90% of their adult skeletal mass. *Sexual maturity ratings* (SMRs), also known as Tanner staging, are used to describe the progression of secondary sexual characteristics that occur in adolescents, irrespective of chronologic age. SMR is based on the development of breasts and the appearance of pubic hair among girls (Fig. 16-1) and on testicular and penile development and the appearance of pubic hair among boys (Fig. 16-2). SMR 1 corresponds to the prepubertal stage; puberty has not begun, and no sexual development has occurred. SMR 2 to SMR 5 indicate the progression of puberty to adulthood. Once young people reach SMR 5, they have fully developed secondary sexual characteristics. Sexual maturation correlates with linear growth, changes in weight and body composition, and hormonal changes. Sexual maturation provides important assurance of the normal progression of puberty or identification of abnormal pubertal development.

NORMAL PSYCHOSOCIAL DEVELOPMENT

Adolescence is often divided into three psychosocial developmental phases: early adolescence (11 to 13 years), middle adolescence (14 to 16 years), and late adolescence (17 to 21 years). In early adolescence, adolescents begin to separate from their parents and establish an individual identity. As adolescents pull away from their parents in search of their own identity, their peer group takes on an important and special significance.

FIGURE 16-1. Female breast development. *Sexual maturity rating 1 (SMR 1)*: Preadolescent; no glandular tissue. Areola and papilla: Areola conforms to general chest line. *SMR 2*: Breast buds appear; areola is slightly widened and projects as small mound. *SMR 3*: Enlargement of the entire breast with protrusion of the papilla or of the nipple. Breast and areola enlarge with no separation of their contours. *SMR 4*: Enlargement of the breast and projection of areola and papilla as a secondary mound. *SMR 5*: Adult configuration of the breast with protrusion of the nipple; areola no longer projects separately from remainder of breast. (Redrawn from Daniel WA, Paulshock BZ. A physician's guide to sexual maturity rating. *Patient Care*. 1979;30:122. Original illustration by Paul Singh-Roy.)

At the beginning of adolescence, cognitive abilities are dominated by concrete thinking. Young adolescents lack abstract reasoning capabilities, problem-solving skills needed to overcome barriers to behavioral changes, and the ability to appreciate how their current behaviors can affect their future health status.

Middle adolescence is characterized by growth in emotional autonomy and increasing separation from family. The adolescents' peer groups play a powerful role, and adolescents are increasingly involved in partnering relationships that include dating, sexual experimentation, and adverse health behaviors such as smoking cigarettes, drinking alcohol, using street drugs, and being truant. Abstract reasoning skills emerge but often regress to concrete thinking when adolescents are faced with stressful situations. These adolescents begin to understand the relationship between health behaviors and future health status, but peer pressure makes it challenging to make health-related choices.

During late adolescence, young people become increasingly more economically and emotionally independent. Peer group values become less important, and young people spend more time in a relationship with one person. The late stage of adolescence is characterized by the development of a strong personal identity. Abstract reasoning skills expand, and older adolescents have problem-solving skills that help them overcome challenges to behavioral change.

VITAL STATISTICS

Although adolescents are generally perceived to be healthy, adolescent morbidity and mortality are the result of risky behaviors and social forces (Table 16-1). Adolescents increasingly engage in risky behaviors with each year of adolescence, especially between the ages of 11 and 16. Unintentional injury, homicide, and suicide are the leading causes of death in 15- to 24-year-olds and account for 71% of all adolescent and young adult deaths. About 75% of these causes of death and injury are preventable.

FIGURE 16-2. Male genital development. *SMR 1: Penis preadolescent. Testicular volume <4 mL. SMR 2: Penis slight or no enlargement. Beginning enlargement of testes; testicular volume 4 to 8 mL; scrotal skin reddened, thinner. SMR 3: Penis increased in length. Testicular volume 10 to 15 mL. Further enlargement of scrotum. SMR 4: Penis larger in breadth, glans penis develops. Testes and scrotum nearly adult; testicular volume 12-20 mL. SMR 5: Penis adult size; testicular volume greater than 25 mL.* **Female and male pubic hair development.** *Sexual maturity rating 1 (SMR 1): Prepubertal; no pubic hair. SMR 2: Small amount of scanty, long, slightly pigmented, along the base of the scrotum and phallus in the male and the medial border of the labia majora in females. SMR 3: Darker, coarser, starts to curl, small amount, extending laterally. SMR 4: Coarse, curly; resembles adult type but does not extend to the medial surface of the thighs. SMR 5: Abundant, adult-type pattern; hair extends onto the medial aspect of the thighs.* (Redrawn from Daniel WA, Palshock BZ. A physician's guide to sexual maturity rating. *Patient Care.* 1979;30:122. Original illustration by Paul Singh-Roy.)

TABLE 16-1	LEADING CAUSES OF DEATH IN U.S. ADOLESCENTS

CAUSE	PERCENTAGE OF DEATHS IN YOUTH AGED 15-24 YEARS
Unintentional injury	47
Homicide	16
Suicide	12
Malignancy	5
Heart disease	3
Congenital anomalies	1.3
Cerebrovascular disease	0.6
Human immunodeficiency virus	0.6
Influenza and pneumonia	0.5
Complicated pregnancy	0.5
All others	14

From U.S. Census Bureau, *2008 National Population Projections,* released August 2008.

Unintentional and Intentional Injuries

Unintentional injuries account for 44% of all injury deaths to children and adolescents. For every childhood death caused by injury, another 34 hospitalizations and 1000 emergency department visits occur. The major causes of unintentional injuries to adolescents are motor vehicle crashes, being struck by or against an object or person, cuts from sharp objects, and falls. Factors that contribute to adolescent injuries include socioeconomic factors (poor children are at greatest risk for injury), environmental factors (hazards such as all-terrain vehicles, backyard swimming pools, firearms, kerosene heaters, and gang activity), school environment, and developmental factors.

About 20% of all adolescents, especially adolescent girls in heterosexual relationships, report having experienced either psychological or physical violence from a dating partner. About 20 to 30% of students in grades 6 to 10 are involved in bullying, as a bully, victim, or bully-victim (those who are both aggressive to peers and victimized by peers). For younger adolescents, bullying can lead to a significantly higher risk of psychosomatic problems.

Homicide is the second leading cause of death in the 15- to 24-year-old population and the number one cause of death among African-American males 15 to 24 years of age. About 75% of homicides in older adolescents and young adults involve firearms.

Suicide (Chapter 404) is the third leading cause of death among adolescents and young adults 10 to 24 years of age. Native Americans and white youth 15 to 24 years of age have the highest suicides rates, whereas African-American youth 15 to 19 years of age and Asian youth 20 to 24 years of age have the lowest. The estimated ratio of attempted-to-completed suicides among adolescents ranges between 50:1 and 100:1. The most common methods used in suicide attempts are drugs or alcohol, whereas suffocation, hanging, or use of firearms is associated with completed suicides. Death rates caused by firearms are eight times higher in adolescent boys than in adolescent girls.

Prevention of Injuries

Clinicians should discuss the impact of alcohol and drugs on driving and stress the importance of routine use of seat belts when driving in a motor vehicle. Clinicians also should discuss safety during sports activities, such as use of bicycle helmets and sports-related protective gear.

Other Diseases

Excluding intentional and unintentional injuries, cancer is the leading cause of death in adolescents and is the leading cause of death by disease. Cancers with an increased incidence in adolescents include Hodgkin's disease (Chapter 192), germ cell tumors (Chapter 206), central nervous system tumors (Chapter 195), non-Hodgkin's lymphoma (Chapter 191), thyroid cancer (Chapter 233), malignant melanoma (Chapter 210), and acute lymphoblastic leukemia (Chapter 189). Human immunodeficiency virus (HIV) continues to be one of the ten leading causes of death among people 15 to 24 years of age.

● APPROACH TO THE ADOLESCENT PATIENT

When interviewing adolescent patients, the clinician should consider the adolescents' physical, cognitive, and psychosocial developmental stage, their growing autonomy and increasing role in taking responsibility for their own health and well-being, and their individual progression from childhood to adulthood. Chronologic age is not a guarantee that all adolescents will be at the same stage of physical, cognitive, and psychosocial development. The clinician should offer adolescent health care in a sensitive, flexible, and developmentally and culturally appropriate manner.

The clinician can meet with the adolescent alone at first to give the adolescent the message that she or he is the patient and the clinician is most eager to hear what the adolescent has to say. Conversely, the clinician can meet with the adolescent and her or his parents or guardians together for the initial part of the interview and then meet with the adolescent alone; this approach permits the clinician to develop an understanding of the reason for the visit from the perspective of the adolescent and his or her parents or guardians, and to communicate that input from both the adolescent and the parents or guardians is highly valued. This approach also provides an opportunity for the clinician to observe the interaction between the adolescent and parents or guardians. The final approach to the interview is to greet the adolescent and family, and request a meeting with the parents or guardians alone. This approach allows the parents or guardians to discuss concerns about the adolescent that they may not feel comfortable raising in the presence of the adolescent. Having this information may improve the focus of the visit. Using this approach, the encounter with the parents or guardians is then followed by the clinician meeting with the adolescent alone. With this interview structure, it is important that the adolescent be present from the time he or she meets with the clinician until the end of the visit, so that the adolescent does not perceive a breach of confidentiality.

Confidentiality

Issues of consent and confidentiality are central in the physician-adolescent interaction. Adolescents appreciate clinicians whom they trust and who can assure them of confidentiality. When guaranteed confidentiality, adolescents are more likely to seek necessary medical care, disclose sensitive information, and trust their clinician. Under these circumstances, most adolescents will involve their parents in their care. Parents appreciate education about the concept of confidentiality and recognize the importance of allowing the adolescent the opportunity to speak alone with their clinician. Confidentiality is also important for clinicians. To make an accurate diagnosis and provide treatment, the clinician must obtain all relevant information from the adolescent. If the adolescent fears that such information will not be kept confidential, she or he may not provide all the necessary factual information.

Confidentiality and defining the limits of confidentiality should be discussed with the adolescent and his or her parents or guardians at the beginning of the interview. The adolescent and family need to know that the clinician will intervene if he or she believes that the adolescent's actions may cause him or her, or another person, significant harm. Examples of situations in which the clinician would not maintain confidentiality when dealing with young people include disclosure of past or current sexual abuse, current suicidal intent, and disclosure of homicidal intent.

Those who work with young people must have a clear understanding of consent and confidentiality and should make sure that adolescents are aware of confidentiality policies and practices. The duty of confidentiality does not preclude encouraging and empowering adolescents to talk to their parents or guardians about important health care issues and include them in discussions of these issues. The legal definition of confidentiality varies, depending on geographic location. It is the clinician's responsibility to familiarize himself or herself with the legal issues of confidentiality (as they relate to the adolescent patient and his or her parents or guardians) in their locality.

Another goal of the interview is to build rapport with the adolescent and his or her parents or guardians. Clinicians can establish rapport with the adolescent at the start of the interview by creating an environment that is nonjudgmental, unintimidating, and supportive. The clinician's genuine interest in the adolescent is paramount. It is helpful to encourage the adolescent to talk about himself or herself—friends, hobbies, school. The clinician should listen carefully to the adolescent's statements and feelings. Sensitivity to and understanding of the adolescent's developmental stage and cultural background are important when interviewing an adolescent and interpreting answers accurately. The clinician should be respectful of the adolescent's growing need to be independent and desire to be treated as an individual person. Taking the time to build rapport is key to engaging the adolescent in a discussion of his or her personal health concerns with the clinician.

Preventive Health Care

Preventive health care for adolescents (Chapters 14 and 17) should promote physical and mental health and healthy physical, psychological, and social growth and development. Positive behaviors such as exercise (Chapter 15) and nutritious eating (Chapter 220) should be encouraged, and health risk behaviors such as unsafe driving, use of tobacco (Chapter 31), unsafe sexual behaviors, and excess alcohol (Chapter 32) should be discouraged. Because lifelong health habits are established during adolescence, it is an important time to invest in health promotion and preventive services.

Components of the Adolescent Care Health Visit
History

Open-ended, nonjudgmental, developmentally appropriate, and gender-neutral questions help put the adolescent at ease and produce informative answers (Chapter 14). In addition to a standard medical history, the assessment should include a psychosocial history from the adolescent, either through a screening questionnaire or during the interview with the adolescent alone. The HEEADSSS assessment, which is a valuable tool for obtaining a comprehensive psychosocial history, covers the following topics:
- **Home:** Family members, living arrangements, and relationships
- **Education/Employment:** Academic or vocational success and future plans
- **Eating:** Concerns about weight or body image or disordered eating attitudes and behaviors
- **Activities**: Recreational activities, dating, and relationships

- **Drugs:** Use of tobacco, alcohol, illicit drugs, anabolic steroids, and driving while intoxicated
- **Sexuality:** Sexual orientation, sexual activity, and sexual abuse
- **Suicide** (mental health): Feelings of sadness, loneliness, depression, or suicidal thoughts
- **Safety:** Risk of unintentional injury or violence, fighting, or weapon carrying

Physical Examination

In general, the adolescent physical examination should occur without a parent or guardian present. In some situations, the adolescent is asked whether he or she would prefer to have a parent in the room during the physical examination. A male clinician should request that a female health care provider be present during the physical examination of a female patient, especially during the breast and genital examination. In theory, a female clinician should request a male health care provider be present during the genital examination of a male patient.

Care should be taken to ensure the adolescent's privacy. Providing an examination gown that covers the trunk and genital area is important. Talking with the adolescent during the examination also tends to increase comfort; explaining the procedures and commenting on the results are helpful. A comprehensive physical examination (Chapter 14) should include measuring the adolescent's weight and height, calculating his or her body mass index, plotting these measurements on standardized growth charts, and determining the adolescent's SMR.

Young women who have HIV or who are immunosuppressed (e.g., those having chemotherapy, transplantation) should have a baseline Papanicolaou smear 3 years after their first sexual intercourse. Other indications for a pelvic examination in an adolescent include symptoms of vaginal or uterine infection, menstrual irregularities (e.g., amenorrhea, dysfunctional uterine bleeding, menorrhagia, and severe dysmenorrhea), undiagnosed abdominal and pelvic pain, tenderness, mass, trauma, sexual abuse, or assault. A careful sexual history, a review of symptoms, and urine or patient-obtained specimens may be an alternative to the pelvic examination.

Conclusion of the Health Visit

At the conclusion of the adolescent health visit, the clinician should review the findings with the adolescent and talk about what happens next. This discussion should not be rushed; the adolescent should have the opportunity to ask questions, get clarification, make comments, and respond to suggestions. The clinician should discuss with the adolescent what information will remain confidential. The clinician should then meet with the adolescent and the parents or guardians (if they have accompanied the adolescent to the health visit) to review the outcomes and discuss the nonconfidential issues.

Immunizations

Adolescents should be brought up-to-date on all recommended immunizations (Chapter 17).

⬤ REPRODUCTIVE HEALTH

Reproductive health care includes issues of adolescent sexual development, adolescent sexual behaviors, adolescent pregnancy, and contraception. In the United States, nearly 50% of high school boys and girls in grades 9 to 12 have had vaginal intercourse (50% of males, 46% of females) at least once. This number increases from 27% of females and 38% of males in grade 9 to about 65% of both boys and girls by their senior year. In addition, 4% of females and 10% of males in grades 9 to 12 started having sex before they were 13 years old, 14% of adolescents have had four or more sex partners during their lives, and 38% of sexually active high school students did not used a condom when they last had sexual intercourse. About 60% of adolescent girls who are 13 years of age or younger when they first had sexual intercourse report having involuntary intercourse. Adolescents are more likely to report engaging in oral than vaginal sex because they perceive oral sex as significantly less risky (fewer health, social, and emotional consequences) than vaginal sex, but adolescents who engage in oral sex also are more likely to engage in vaginal sex.

Every year about 800,000 pregnancies occur in females 15 to 19 years of age in the United States. About 50% of these pregnancies result in a live birth, about 35% end with an abortion, and about 15% end with a miscarriage or stillbirth. The birth rate for mothers 15 to 27 years of age decreased from 38.6 in 1991 to 22.1 in 2004 because of increased use of effective contraception and decreased sexual activity. Adolescent pregnancy is more common among black and Hispanic females as well as females from low-income families.

Positive outcomes of adolescent pregnancies are enhanced with good pre-natal care, adequate initial and follow-up prenatal visits, nutritional counsel-ing, assessment of psychosocial issues, and substance abuse counseling. Adolescents younger than 15 years are at increased risk for premature and low-birthweight infants; those older than 15 years who have adequate prena-tal care do not have increased adverse outcomes.

Contraception

The most commonly used contraceptive methods in adolescents are oral contraceptive pills (OCPs) and condoms, although new hormonal delivery systems such as transdermal patches, vaginal rings, and implants are conve-nient and effective (Chapter 246).

Sexually Transmitted Diseases

Every year, about 4 million adolescents in the United States acquire a sexu-ally transmitted disease (Chapter 293), representing 25% of the total cases of sexually transmitted disease diagnosed annually. *Chlamydia trachomatis,* which is the most commonly reported bacterial sexually transmitted disease, is reported annually in about 2.8% of female adolescents 15 to 19 years of age and 0.5% of male adolescents of the same age. The annual incidence of gonorrhea is about 0.6% for female adolescents 15 to 19 years of age and 0.4% for adolescent males of the same age. In adolescents, HIV (Chapter 395) is contracted primarily as a sexually transmitted disease, and adoles-cents and young adults 15 to 24 years of age represent 14% of all new HIV diagnoses in the United States. Human papillomavirus (Chapter 381), which is the most prevalent of all sexually transmitted diseases in 15- to 24-year-olds, has a prevalence of about 20% in adolescent girls 14 to 17 years of age.

Adolescents are at greater risk of acquiring sexually transmitted diseases because they are more likely to engage in unprotected sexual intercourse with concurrent partners who have multiple other partners. Adolescent girls may have persistent vaginal columnar epithelium that is more susceptible than squamous epithelium to *Neisseria gonorrhea, C. trachomatis,* and HPV, as well lower levels of immunoglobulin A in their cervical mucus. Treatment may be delayed owing to an inability to access confidential health care services, lack of health care coverage, poverty, and drug trafficking and use.

Chlamydial infections (Chapter 326), often asymptomatic or minimally symptomatic in women, usually present with a vaginal discharge in young adolescent girls. Otherwise, clinical presentations and treatments of sexually transmitted diseases (Chapter 293) in adolescents are similar to those in adults.

About 20% of adolescents given prescriptions for a sexually transmitted disease treatment fail to fill their prescriptions. Therefore, whenever avail-able, an observed single-dose therapy is recommended. In addition, expe-dited partner therapy (EPT), which is the treatment of sexual partners without requiring a prior clinical evaluation or prevention counseling, reduces the level of recurrent sexually transmitted diseases better than does standard management. Clinicians should consider the use of EPT for part-ners exposed within 60 days to heterosexual males and females with chla-mydia or gonorrhea infections when in-person evaluation and treatment are unlikely.

● ADOLESCENT EATING DISORDERS

Eating disorders (Chapter 226) commonly begin during adolescence. For adolescent-onset anorexia nervosa, bulimia nervosa, and other eating disor-ders, early recognition and aggressive treatment are critical to a successful outcome. The medical complications of eating disorders in adolescents include growth retardation, pubertal delay, low bone mineral density, and changes in brain structure and cognitive function. These complications, which occur early in the disease process, may not be completely reversible, thereby underscoring the need for early and aggressive treatment.

The goal of treatment is to restore physical health, normal eating-behavior patterns, and mental health and to reduce the impact of the eating disorder on the quality of life. Successful management strategies for adolescents with eating disorders include early restoration of a normal nutritional and physi-ologic state, involvement of the family in the treatment, and incorporation of an interdisciplinary team in the treatment. Adolescents should be treated at a facility where the health professionals understand eating disorders and have experience treating adolescents.

● SUBSTANCE ABUSE

Nearly half of adolescents try an illicit drug (Chapter 33) by the time they finish high school. About 75% of adolescents consume alcohol (Chapter 32) by the end of high school, and about half report having been drunk at least once in their life. Adolescents who begin using alcohol or drugs before 15 years of age are more than five times more likely to develop an addictive disorder later in life, compared with those who first use alcohol at 21 years of age. About 45% of adolescents use marijuana, and 20% of 12th graders are current smokers.

Adolescents start using drugs or alcohol primarily because of social pres-sures but report continuing them to feel good or cope with difficulties. Boys tend to initiate drug and alcohol use at younger ages than girls, but once girls begin to experiment, they are just as likely as boys to use drugs. Boys are more likely to consume marijuana, steroids, and smokeless tobacco, whereas girls are more likely to abuse amphetamines and methamphetamine.

Adolescents with poor self-esteem, low motivation, and poor academic achievement have a greater propensity for alcohol and drug abuse than those with positive self-esteem. Adolescents with a family member with a history of alcohol or other drug abuse are at greater risk. Adolescents are less likely to succumb to external pressures toward drug use if they have a strong sense of attachment to parents who clearly communicate their disapproval.

Signs and symptoms suggestive of substance abuse include changes in physical appearance, poor hygiene or dress, wearing long-sleeved shirts to hide scarring at injection sites, persistent cough or bronchitis, difficulty sleep-ing, sudden weight loss or weight gain, sudden changes in personality, aggres-sive behavior, irritability, nervousness, giddiness, changes in peer group, increased isolation from peers or family, depression, loss of interest in once favorite activities, decline in performance or attendance at school or work, forgetfulness, increased secretiveness, money or objects disappearing from the household, and prescription drugs that seem to be used up too quickly.

A validated screening tool for alcohol and substance abuse (Table 16-2) should be used in adolescents. Adolescents who answer "yes" to one of the six questions should receive advice on the adverse effects of substance abuse. Those who answer "yes" to two or more questions are at high risk and require further assessment or referral (Chapters 32 and 33). Urine drug testing has low sensitivity for detecting drug use, and there is no consensus about its role for screening adolescents.

Adolescent substance use can compromise psychological and social devel-opment, cause behavioral problems, and lead to a variety of high-risk behav-iors. Alcohol and drug use contributes to more than 40% of adolescent deaths from motor vehicle crashes, to suicide attempts, and to an increased risk for subsequent use and its related problems in adulthood.

Historically, substance abuse treatment has been based on abstinence. More recently, a harm-reduction approach has gained acceptance. Adoles-cents discontinue drug and alcohol use mainly because of concern about their negative effects, and community-based interventions can be effective.[1] To reduce alcohol abuse over time, individual interventions have a larger impact than family-based interventions.[2]

TABLE 16-2   CRAFFT SCREENING TOOL FOR DRUG AND ALCOHOL USE IN ADOLESCENTS

The adolescent is instructed, "Please answer these next questions honestly. Your answers will be kept confidential. During the past 12 months, did you..."
Drink any alcohol (more than a few sips)?
Smoke any marijuana or hashish?
Use anything else to get high?
If the adolescent answers "No" to the three opening questions, the provider only needs to ask the adolescent the first question—the CAR question. If the adolescent answers "Yes" to any one or more of the three opening questions, the provider asks all six CRAFFT questions.

   C—Have you ever ridden in a CAR driven by someone (including yourself) who was "high" or had been using alcohol or drugs?
   R—Do you ever use alcohol or drugs to RELAX, feel better about yourself, or fit in?
   A—Do you ever use alcohol/drugs while you are by yourself, ALONE?
   F—Do you ever FORGET things you did while using alcohol or drugs?
   F—Do your family or FRIENDS ever tell you that you should cut down on your drinking or drug use?
   T—Have you gotten into TROUBLE while you were using alcohol or drugs?
CRAFFT is a mnemonic acronym of first letters of key words in the six screening questions. The questions should be asked exactly as written.

CHRONIC ILLNESS AND TRANSITION

The prevalence of chronic diseases in adolescents has increased significantly because advances in medical technology and treatments have increased the survival of young people with childhood diseases formerly considered lethal. About 15% of adolescents in the United States live with a chronic illness. Chronic illness may affect the adolescent's development, or the adolescent's development may affect the illness. For example, cystic fibrosis (Chapter 89) may delay puberty and hinder normal peer development. Puberty can exacerbate diabetes mellitus (Chapter 236). Increased risk-taking by adolescents with diabetes, asthma, or chronic renal failure can hinder their compliance with their medication regimen.

Any chronic illness may limit age-appropriate activities and development. Adolescents with a chronic illness must have effective contraception and effective methods for preventing sexually transmitted diseases.

Adolescents in general, and those with special health care needs in particular, require a smooth, seamless, coordinated, and developmentally appropriate transition to the adult health care system. Barriers to a successful transition include a lack of adult physicians who can manage chronic childhood conditions (e.g., congenital heart disease; Chapter 69); patients, families, and pediatric subspecialists who are reluctant to terminate long-standing relationships; and patients and families who are poorly equipped to find their way in the adult health care system.

As adolescents move closer to the age of transfer, professionals should provide developmentally appropriate information and skills to support them and their families as they negotiate the adult health care system.

Adolescents benefit from an introductory visit with their adult-oriented care provider before leaving the pediatric health care system. This visit should give the adolescent a clearer idea about his or her new role as an adult patient, especially about expectations around decision making, giving consent, and the role of the family in his or her health care. The patient, family, and pediatric and adult health care systems should view the transition as a natural part of the developmental process of care for all adolescents.

1. Oesterle S, Hawkins JD, Fagan AA, et al. Testing the universality of the effects of the communities that care prevention system for preventing adolescent drug use and delinquency. *Prev Sci.* 2010; 11:411-423.
2. Tripodi SJ, Bender K, Litschge C, et al. Interventions for reducing adolescent alcohol abuse: a meta-analytic review. *Arch Pediatr Adolesc Med.* 2010;164:85-91.

SUGGESTED READINGS

Peter NG, Forke CM, Ginsburg KR, et al. Transition from pediatric to adult care: internists' perspectives. *Pediatrics.* 2009;123:417-423. *Emphasizes how internists should be better trained regarding childhood-onset conditions.*
http://www.cdc.gov/growthcharts. *Growth charts online.*
http://brightfutures.aap.org/web. Guidelines for prevention visits for children and adolescents. *A helpful resource.*
http://www.adolescenthealth.org. Position papers from the Society for Adolescent Medicine. *A catalog of useful reports.*

IMMUNIZATION

WALTER A. ORENSTEIN AND WILLIAM L. ATKINSON

Immunization is one of the most cost-effective means of preventing morbidity and mortality from infectious diseases. Routine immunization, particularly of children, has resulted in decreases of 90% or more in reported cases of measles, mumps, rubella, congenital rubella syndrome, poliomyelitis, tetanus, invasive *Haemophilus influenzae* and diphtheria. In many circumstances, immunization not only prevents morbidity and mortality but also, in the long run, reduces health care costs.

GENERAL CHARACTERISTICS OF IMMUNIZATIONS

Immunization protects against disease or the sequelae of disease through the administration of an immunobiologic—vaccines, toxoids, immune globulin preparations, and antitoxins. Protection induced by immunization can be active or passive.

Active Immunization

Administration of a vaccine or toxoid causes the body to produce an immune response against the infectious agent or its toxins. Vaccines consist of suspensions of live (usually attenuated) or inactivated microorganisms or fractions thereof. Toxoids are modified bacterial toxins that retain immunogenic properties but lack toxicity. Active immunization generally results in long-term immunity, although the onset of protection may be delayed because it takes time for the body to respond. With live attenuated vaccines, small quantities of living organisms multiply within the recipient until an immune response cuts off replication. In contrast, inactivated vaccines and toxoids contain large quantities of antigens. In most recipients, a single dose of a live vaccine generally induces an immune response that closely parallels natural infection and induces long-term immunity. Killed (inactivated) vaccines, in contrast, often require multiple doses.

Passive Immunization

Passive immunization with use of immune globulins or antitoxins delivers preformed antibodies to provide temporary immunity. Immune globulins obtained from human blood may contain antibodies to a variety of agents, depending on the pool of human plasma from which they are prepared. Specific immune globulins are made from the plasma of donors with high levels of antibodies to specific antigens, such as tetanus immune globulin. Most immune globulins must be injected intramuscularly, although an intravenous preparation is also available. Antitoxins are solutions of antibodies derived from animals immunized with specific antigens (e.g., diphtheria antitoxin). Passive immunization usually is indicated to protect individuals immediately before anticipated exposure or shortly after known or suspected exposure to an infectious agent (Table 17-1), when active immunization either is not possible or has not been adequate.

Route and Timing of Vaccination

Each immunobiologic has a preferred site and route of administration. In adults, vaccines containing adjuvants should be injected intramuscularly, preferably in the deltoid muscle. For most adults, intramuscular injections should be administered with a 1- to 1½-inch, 22- to 25-gauge needle. Use of the buttocks is discouraged except when large volumes are required because of the potential for damage to the sciatic nerve and because of diminished immune response to some vaccines, such as hepatitis B, probably because of injection into fat rather than into muscle. Subcutaneous vaccines also are usually administered in the triceps area. In general, inactivated vaccines and toxoids can be given at the same visit at different sites. Live and inactivated vaccines usually can be administered at the same time. For example, measles, mumps, and rubella (MMR) vaccine can be administered at the same time as inactivated poliovirus vaccine and live attenuated varicella vaccine. In general, injected and intranasally administered live vaccines not delivered on the same day should be separated by at least 4 weeks to avoid interference. Orally administered live vaccines, such as oral typhoid vaccine, can be administered at any interval before or after live injected or intranasal vaccines. Immune globulin may interfere with the replication of injected live vaccine viruses; ideally, most live vaccines should be administered at least 2 weeks before or 3 to 11 months after immune globulin. Immune globulin does not interfere with the response to yellow fever vaccine and is not believed to interfere with orally or intranasally administered live virus vaccines.

Adverse Reactions

No vaccine is completely safe or completely effective. Hypersensitivity to vaccine components, such as animal proteins, antibiotics, preservatives, and stabilizers, can lead to local and systemic reactions ranging from mild to severe. Minor reactions are common, but randomized trials caution that prophylactic antipyretic drugs at the time of vaccination reduce antibody reactions and should not be given routinely.◼ The egg protein contained in vaccines grown in chicken eggs (influenza and yellow fever vaccines) may cause reactions in persons severely allergic to eggs. In general, persons

TABLE 17-1 PASSIVE IMMUNIZATIONS FOR ADULTS

DISEASE	NAME OF MATERIAL	COMMENTS AND USE
Tetanus	Tetanus immune globulin, human	Management of tetanus-prone wounds in persons without adequate prior active immunization and treatment of tetanus
Cytomegalovirus	Cytomegalovirus immune globulin, intravenous	Prophylaxis for bone marrow and kidney transplant recipients
Diphtheria	Diphtheria antitoxin, equine	Treatment of established disease, high frequency of reactions to serum of nonhuman origin; in the United States, available only from CDC
Rabies	Rabies immune globulin, human	Postexposure prophylaxis of animal bites
Measles	Immune globulin, human	Prevention or modification of disease in contacts of cases, not for control of outbreaks
Hepatitis A	Immune globulin, human	Pre-exposure and postexposure prophylaxis for travelers and others who need protection before immunity can be achieved with hepatitis A vaccine
Hepatitis B	Hepatitis B immune globulin, human	Prophylaxis for needlestick or mucous membrane contact with HBsAg-positive persons, for sexual partners with acute hepatitis B or hepatitis B carriers, for infants born to mothers who are carriers of HBsAg, for infants whose mother or primary caregiver has acute hepatitis B
Varicella	Varicella-zoster immune globulin (VariZIG)	Persons with underlying disease and at risk for complications from chickenpox who have not had varicella or varicella vaccine and who are exposed to varicella; may be given after exposure to known susceptible adults, particularly if antibody negative. VariZIG is available under IND.
Vaccinia	Vaccinia immune globulin	Treatment of eczema vaccinatum, vaccinia necrosum, and severe inadvertent inoculations such as ocular vaccinia after vaccinia (smallpox) vaccination. Available only from the CDC.
Erythroblastosis fetalis	Rh immune globulin	Rh-negative women who give birth to Rh-positive infants or who abort
Hypogammaglobulinemia	Immune globulin, intravenous	Maintenance therapy
Idiopathic thrombocytopenic purpura	Immune globulin, intravenous	Therapy for acute episodes
Botulism	Bivalent A and B antitoxin, equine	Treatment of botulism; available through CDC
Snakebite	Antivenin, equine (North American coral snake antivenin)	Specific for North American coral snake, *Micrurus fulvius*
	Crotalidae, polyvalent	Effective for viper and pit viper bites, including rattlesnakes, copperheads, moccasins
Spider bite	Antivenin, equine	Specific for black widow spider, *Latrodectus mactans,* and other members of the genus

CDC = Centers for Disease Control and Prevention; HBsAg = hepatitis B surface antigen; IND = Investigational New Drug.

without anaphylactic-type allergies to eggs can be given these vaccines safely, but persons with anaphylactic reactions to eggs generally should not receive these vaccines except when it is absolutely necessary and then only under established protocols by physicians who are expert in such situations. Although measles and mumps vaccines are grown in chick embryo tissue culture, the risk of anaphylaxis even in persons with severe hypersensitivity to eggs is low, so they can be vaccinated without prior testing. Suspected adverse events temporally related to vaccinations should be reported to the Vaccine Adverse Events Reporting System (1-800-822-7967 or *www.vaers .hhs.gov*).

General Considerations

The major group that makes comprehensive, detailed recommendations regarding immunization of adults is the Advisory Committee on Immunization Practices of the Centers for Disease Control and Prevention (CDC), which publishes its information in *Morbidity and Mortality Weekly Report* (also available at *http://www.cdc.gov/vaccines/recs/schedules/adult-schedule. htm#print*). Immunizations for adults depend on age, lifestyle, occupation, and medical conditions. Two adult immunization schedules are available, one based on age group (Fig. 17-1 and E-Table 17-1) and one based on underlying risk (Fig. 17-2 and Table 17-2). All adults should have a primary series of tetanus and diphtheria toxoids with boosters of combined toxoids (Td) every 10 years. All adults should have a one-time dose of combined tetanus and diphtheria toxoids and acellular pertussis vaccine (Tdap) followed by Td every 10 years. Persons born in or after 1957 should have evidence of immunity to measles, mumps, and rubella (e.g., documentation of vaccination or presence of antibodies considered compatible with protection). Vaccination of susceptible adolescents and adults against varicella is desirable. Pneumococcal polysaccharide vaccine (PPSV23) is indicated for all adults 65 years and older and younger adults with certain medical conditions that place them at high risk of complications. Influenza vaccination also is recommended annually for all persons 6 months of age or older. Health care workers exposed to blood or blood products should receive hepatitis B vaccine. Health care workers likely to come in contact with persons transmitting measles, mumps, rubella, or varicella should be immune to those diseases.

Immunocompromise

Patients with conditions that compromise their immune systems generally should not receive live attenuated vaccines. Such patients include those with immunodeficiency diseases, leukemia, lymphoma, and generalized malignant disease and those who are immunosuppressed from therapy with corticosteroids, alkylating agents, antimetabolites, and radiation. An exception is infection with human immunodeficiency virus (HIV). Asymptomatic patients should receive MMR vaccine. MMR should be considered for symptomatic patients with HIV infection; however, severely immunocompromised persons should not be vaccinated. Varicella vaccination (2 doses, 3 months apart) may be considered in HIV-infected persons with CD4+ T-lymphocyte counts >200 cells/μL. Patients with leukemia in remission who have not been receiving any chemotherapy for at least 3 months may receive live virus vaccines. Short-course therapy (<2 weeks) with corticosteroids, alternate-day regimens with low to moderate doses of short-acting corticosteroids, and topical applications or tendon injections are not ordinarily contraindications to the administration of live vaccines.

Immunocompromised patients can receive inactivated vaccines and toxoids, although the efficacy of such preparations may be diminished. Patients with known HIV infection should receive pneumococcal vaccine and annual influenza vaccination.

Pregnancy

In general, live vaccines should not be given to pregnant women because of the theoretical concern that the vaccines could adversely affect the fetus. No significant adverse events attributable to vaccination of pregnant women with MMR or varicella have been documented; nevertheless, pregnant women should not receive MMR or varicella vaccine, and women who do receive these vaccines should wait 1 month before becoming pregnant. Poliomyelitis and yellow fever vaccines usually should not be given to pregnant women unless the risk of disease is substantial. Td vaccination is especially

Recommended Adult Immunization Schedule
UNITED STATES–2011

Note: These recommendations *must* be read with the footnotes that follow
containing number of doses, intervals between doses, and other important information.

Recommended adult immunization schedule, by vaccine and age group

Vaccine Age Group →	19–26 years	27–49 years	50–59 years	60–64 years	≥ 65 years
Influenza [1,*]	1 dose annually				
Tetanus, diphtheria, pertussis (Td/Tdap) [2,*]	Substitute 1-time dose of Tdap for Td booster; then boost with Td every 10 yrs				Td booster every 10 yrs
Varicella [3,*]	2 doses				
Human papillomavirus (HPV) [4,*]	3 doses (females)				
Zoster [5]				1 dose	
Measles, mumps, rubella (MMR) [6,*]	1 or 2 doses		1 dose		
Pneumococcal (polysaccharide) [7,8]	1 or 2 doses				1 dose
Meningococcal [9,*]	1 or more doses				
Hepatitis A [10,*]	2 doses				
Hepatitis B [11,*]	3 doses				

*Covered by the Vaccine Injury Compensation Program.

For all persons in this category who meet the age requirements and who lack evidence of immunity (e.g., lack documentation of vaccination or have no evidence of prior infection	Recommended if some other risk factor is present (e.g., based on medical, occupational, lifestyle, or other indications)

No recommendation

Report all clinically significant postvaccination reactions to the Vaccine Adverse Event Reporting System (VAERS). Reporting
   forms and instructions on filing a VAERS report are available at http://www.vaers.hhs.gov or by telephone, 800-822-7967.
Information on how to file a Vaccine Injury Compensation Program claim is available at htpp://www.hrsa.gov/vaccinecompensation
   or by telephone, 800-338-2382. Information about filing a claim for vaccine injury is available through the U.S. Court of Federal
   Claims, 717 Madison Place, N.W., Washington, D.C. 20005; telephone 202-357-6400.
Additional information about the vaccines in this schedule, extent of available data, and contraindications for vaccination are also
   available at http://www.cdc.gov/vaccines, or from the CDC-INFO Contact Center at 800-CDC-INFO (800-232-4636) in English or
   Spanish, 24 hours a day, 7 days a week.

FIGURE 17-1. Recommended adult immunization schedule, by vaccine and age group, United States, 2011. See E-Table 17-1 for footnotes. (From *http://www.cdc.gov/vaccines/recs/schedules/adult-schedule.htm#print.*)

indicated for pregnant women who are not appropriately vaccinated to prevent neonatal tetanus in their infants. Vaccination is done best after the first trimester to avoid attribution to a vaccine of an adverse outcome of pregnancy that was only coincidental. Most pregnant women should not receive TdaP. In such cases, however, TdaP should be administered postpartum. All pregnant women should be screened for hepatitis B surface antigen (HBsAg). Children born to mothers with active HBsAg infection should receive hepatitis B vaccine and hepatitis B immune globulin within 12 hours of birth. Women who will be pregnant during the influenza season should receive inactivated influenza vaccine. Pregnant women have been shown to be at particularly high risk of complications from influenza and are at high priority to receive this vaccine to protect them.

⬤ INDIVIDUAL IMMUNOBIOLOGICS

Hepatitis A

Two inactivated hepatitis A (Chapter 150) vaccines are available in the United States. Seroconversion rates after a single dose of either vaccine in persons older than 1 year exceed 95%. Antibody levels shown to be protective in animals develop in almost all persons.

Indications

The vaccine is indicated primarily for persons traveling to countries, generally the developing world, with high or intermediate endemicity for hepatitis A, but it is also recommended for other groups at high risk for infection or for development of severe hepatitis. In addition, vaccine is routinely recommended for children 12 to 23 months of age. Health care workers have not been shown to be at higher risk than the general population for hepatitis A and do not need routine immunization. Although food handlers are not at increased risk for hepatitis A compared with the general population, the consequences of infection or suspected infection in this group, which can lead to extensive public health investigations, may make vaccination cost-effective in some settings. Hepatitis A vaccine can be given to children 1 year of age or older to control outbreaks in communities with high rates of prior infection and be considered for communities with intermediate levels of prior infection (anti–hepatitis A seroprevalence of 10 to 25% by 5 years of age). Doses vary by age and product. All schedules call for a second dose at least 6 months after the first dose, with a permissible range for one of the products 18 months after the initial dose. Vaccines are not indicated for children younger than 1 year because adequate data on safety and efficacy are lacking.

Vaccines That Might Be Indicated for Adults Based on Medical and Other Indications

Vaccine Indication→	Pregnancy	Immuno-compromising conditions (excluding human immunodeficiency virus [HIV]) [3, 5, 6, 13]	HIV infection [3, 6, 12, 13] CD4+ T lymphocyte count <200 cells/μL	HIV infection [3, 6, 12, 13] CD4+ T lymphocyte count ≥200 cells/μL	Diabetes, heart disease, chronic lung disease, chronic alcoholism	Asplenia [12] (including elective splenectomy) and persistent complement component deficiencies	Chronic liver disease	Kidney failure, end-stage renal disease, receipt of hemodialysis	Healthcare personnel
Influenza [1,*]	1 dose TIV annually								1 dose TIV or LAIV annually
Tetanus, diphtheria, pertussis (Td/Tdap) [2,*]	Td	Substitute 1-time dose of Tdap for Td booster; then boost with Td every 10 yrs							
Varicella [3,*]	Contraindicated			2 doses					
Human papillomavirus (HPV) [4,*]		3 doses for females through age 26 yrs							
Zoster [5]	Contraindicated			1 dose					
Measles, mumps, rubella (MMR) [6,*]	Contraindicated			1 or 2 doses					
Pneumococcal (polysaccharide) [7,8]		1 or 2 doses							
Meningococcal [9,*]	1 or more doses								
Hepatitis A [10,*]	2 doses								
Hepatitis B [11,*]		3 doses							

*Covered by the Vaccine Injury Compensation Program.

☐ For all persons in this category who meet the age requirements and who lack evidence of immunity (e.g., lack documentation of vaccination or have no evidence of prior infection)

☐ Recommended if some other risk factor is present (e.g., on the basis of medical, occupational, lifestyle, or other indications)

☐ No recommendation

These schedules indicate the recommended age groups and medical indications for which administration of currently licensed vaccines is commonly indicated for adults ages 19 years and older, as of Febuary 4, 2011. For all vaccines being recommended on the adult immunization schedule, a vaccine series does not need to be restarted, regardless of the time that has elapsed between doses. Licensed combination vaccines may be used whenever any components of the combination are indicated and when the vaccine's other components are not contraindicated. For detailed recommendations on all vaccines, including those used primarily for travelers or that are issued during the year, consult the manufacturers' package inserts and the complete statement from the Advisory Committee on Immunization Practices (http://www.cdc.gov/vaccines/pubs/aclp-list.htm).

FIGURE 17-2. Recommended adult immunization schedule, by vaccine and medical and other indications, United States, 2011. See E-Table 17-1 for footnotes. (From *http://www.cdc.gov/vaccines/recs/schedules/adult-schedule.htm#print.*)

Side Effects

The most common side effect has been tenderness and soreness at the injection site. Although rare and more serious adverse events have been reported in temporal association with vaccination, a causal relationship has not been established.

Hepatitis B

Hepatitis B (Chapter 150) vaccine is the first vaccine that can prevent cancer (an estimated 800 persons per year in the United States die of hepatitis B–related liver cancer; many times more die in the developing world). It also can prevent acute and chronic complications of hepatitis B, including an estimated 4000 deaths annually from cirrhosis and 250 deaths annually from fulminant hepatic disease in the United States. Currently produced vaccines are derived from insertion of the gene for HBsAg into *Saccharomyces cerevisiae*. Hepatitis B vaccine, the first licensed vaccine made by use of recombinant techniques, produces adequate antibody responses in more than 90% of normal adults and more than 95% of normal infants, children, and adolescents when it is administered in a three-dose series. The dosage depends on the product, the age group, and the underlying clinical condition and can be determined by consulting the package insert. The duration of vaccine-conferred immunity is not known, although follow-up of vaccinees for more than 16 years indicates persistence of protection against clinically significant infections (i.e., detectable viremia and clinical disease). Booster doses are not currently recommended. Vaccine must be injected intramuscularly, preferably in the deltoid.

Indications

Hepatitis B vaccine is indicated for adults at high risk of infection (see Fig. 17-1 and E-Table 17-1). Because strategies targeting hepatitis B vaccine use only to high-risk populations have not had a significant impact on hepatitis B incidence, universal vaccination is recommended for infants and for all adolescents who have not been previously vaccinated. Universal screening for HBsAg is recommended for all pregnant women; administration of three doses of vaccine and one dose of hepatitis B immune globulin is recommended for infants of acutely or chronically infected mothers.

Side Effects

The major side effect is soreness at the injection site. Alopecia, which is usually reversible, has been reported rarely. Hepatitis B vaccine has not been shown to induce multiple sclerosis in controlled studies and has not been shown to exacerbate illness in patients with multiple sclerosis who are vaccinated.

Human Papillomavirus

Two human papillomavirus (HPV) vaccines are licensed. Both vaccines contain the L1 capsid protein of types 16 and 18, which account for about 70% of cases of cervical cancer. The quadrivalent vaccine also contains types 6 and 11, which are the most common causes of anogenital warts. Routine vaccination of 11- to 12-year-old girls is recommended in a three-dose schedule. The vaccine should be administered at 0, 1 to 2, and 6 months. Catch-up

Text continues on p. 71

TABLE 17-2 SELECTED IMMUNIZING AGENTS INDICATED FOR ADULTS*

DISEASE	IMMUNIZING AGENT	INDICATIONS	SCHEDULE	MAJOR CONTRAINDICATIONS AND PRECAUTIONS	COMMENTS
Anthrax	Anthrax vaccine, adsorbed, an inactivated vaccine	Pre-exposure prophylaxis of persons at high risk of exposure (e.g., military, certain laboratory workers) Consider with antibiotics for postexposure prophylaxis	0.5-mL dose IM at 0, 4, and 6 wk and 12 and 18 mo Manufacturer recommends booster annually thereafter If used after exposure, 3 doses at 0, 2, and 4 wk with antibiotics for at least 7-14 days after third dose	Severe allergic reaction to a vaccine component or after a prior dose Moderate or severe acute illness is a precaution to vaccination	Effectiveness against aerosol exposure inferred primarily from animal data Limited data on the benefits of postexposure use
Diphtheria	Tetanus and diphtheria toxoids combined	All adults	Two doses IM 4 wk apart, third dose 6-12 mo after second dose for primary series Booster every 10 yr No need to repeat if schedule is interrupted	History of neurologic reaction after a previous dose Severe allergic reaction to a vaccine component or after a prior dose Moderate or severe acute illness is a precaution	Tetanus and diphtheria toxoids combined with acellular pertussis vaccine (Tdap) preferred as one-time booster for all persons through 64 yr
Hepatitis A	Inactivated hepatitis A vaccine	Travelers to highly or intermediately endemic countries Men who have sex with men Illegal drug users (injection and noninjection) Persons who work with hepatitis A virus–infected primates or who do research with the virus Persons with chronic liver disease Recipients of clotting factors	Two doses at least 6 mo apart for persons aged ≥1 yr	Severe allergic reaction to a vaccine component or after a prior dose Moderate or severe acute illness is a precaution to vaccination	Recommended for all children Should be considered for outbreak control
Hepatitis B	Inactivated hepatitis B virus subunit vaccine containing HBsAg	Adolescents Health care and public safety workers potentially exposed to blood Clients and staff of institutions for the developmentally disabled Hemodialysis patients Men who have sex with men Users of illicit injectable drugs Recipients of clotting factors Household and sexual contacts of HBV carriers Inmates of long-term correctional facilities Heterosexuals treated for sexually transmitted diseases or with multiple sexual partners Travelers with close contact for ≥6 mo with populations with high prevalence of HBV carriage	Three doses IM at 0, 1, and 6 mo	Severe allergic reaction to a vaccine component or after a prior dose Moderate or severe acute illness is a precaution to vaccination	Pregnancy is not a contraindication Health care workers who have contact with patients or blood, sexual contacts of persons with chronic HBV infection, hemodialysis patients and other immunosuppressed persons, and recipients of clotting factor concentrates should be tested 1-2 mo after vaccination to determine serologic response
Human papilloma-virus	Inactivated L1 capsid proteins of types 6, 11, 16, and 18 (quadrivalent) and types 16 and 18 (bivalent)	Females at 11-12 yr; catch-up vaccination of females through 26 yr Males 9 through 26 yr for genital warts	Three 0.5-mL doses IM at 0, 1 to 2, and 6 mo	Severe allergic reaction to a vaccine component or to a prior dose Vaccine is not recommended for pregnant women	The vaccine will not protect against existing infections Because the types in the vaccine are not responsible for about 30% of infections associated with cervical cancer, screening for cancer should occur as for unvaccinated women
Influenza	Inactivated virus vaccine	All adults, with greatest priority for those ≥65 yr old, persons with underlying medical conditions, pregnant women, health care workers, and persons with close contact with children <5 years of age	Annual vaccination; see annual ACIP recommendation	Severe allergic reaction to an influenza vaccine component (including eggs) or after a prior dose Moderate or severe acute illness is a precaution to vaccination GBS within 6 wk of prior dose of influenza vaccine	Optimum timing for vaccination is October and November However, vaccination can occur in December and later, particularly for health care workers and persons at high risk for complications who were not vaccinated earlier Only one dose of influenza vaccine per season is recommended for adults

TABLE 17-2   SELECTED IMMUNIZING AGENTS INDICATED FOR ADULTS—cont'd

DISEASE	IMMUNIZING AGENT	INDICATIONS	SCHEDULE	MAJOR CONTRAINDICATIONS AND PRECAUTIONS	COMMENTS
Influenza (cont'd)	Live attenuated influenza virus	Persons 2 through 49 yr without underlying conditions that place them at high risk of complications from influenza	Annual vaccination; see annual ACIP statement Administered intranasally	Persons <2 yr or ≥50 yr Underlying disorders that place them at high risk of influenza complications History of GBS within 6 wk of prior dose of influenza vaccine Pregnant women Hypersensitivity to eggs or components of vaccine	Can be used for household contacts and health care workers caring for patients without severe immunocompromise
Japanese encephalitis	Inactivated Japanese encephalitis virus vaccine	Travelers to Asia spending at least 1 mo in endemic areas during transmission season	Two 0.5-mL doses IM on days 0 and 28 for persons 18 yr and older	Pregnancy	
Measles	Live virus vaccine	All adults born after 1956 without history of live vaccine on or after first birthday, physician-diagnosed measles, or detectable measles antibody Persons born before 1957 generally can be considered immune	One dose sufficient for most adults; 2 doses at least 1 mo apart indicated for persons entering college or medical facility employment, traveling abroad, or at risk of measles during outbreaks	Altered immunity (e.g., leukemia, lymphoma, generalized malignant disease, congenital immunodeficiency, immunosuppressive therapy) Immune globulin or other blood products within prior 3-11 mo, depending on dose of immune globulin or blood product received Untreated tuberculosis Anaphylactic hypersensitivity to neomycin or gelatin Pregnancy Thrombocytopenia	Persons with anaphylactic allergies to eggs may be vaccinated (see text) Vaccine should be administered to persons with asymptomatic HIV infection and should be considered for patients except those with severe immunocompromise
Meningococcal disease (2 vaccines)	1. Meningococcal conjugate vaccines containing polysaccharide of serogroups A, C, W135, and Y (age 2-55 yr) 2. Polysaccharide vaccine containing tetravalent A, C, W135, and Y (ages 56 yr and older)	All 11- to 18-year-old persons and all persons with persistent complement component deficiencies, anatomic or functional asplenia, persons who will travel to areas with hyperendemic or epidemic diseases; certain laboratory workers; may be useful during localized outbreaks	One dose with revaccination at age 16 yr of children who receive conjugate vaccine at 11-12 yr of age and every 5 yr for persons at high risk	1. Allergic reactions to a component of the vaccine including diphtheria toxoid and latex	Conjugate vaccine is preferred to polysaccharide alone for persons aged 2 through 55 yr
Mumps	Live virus vaccine	All adults born after 1956 without history of live vaccine on or after first birthday, physician-diagnosed mumps, or detectable mumps antibody Persons born before 1957 generally can be considered immune	One dose sufficient for most adults; 2 doses at least 1 mo apart indicated for persons entering college or medical facility employment, or traveling abroad	Altered immunity (e.g., leukemia, lymphoma, generalized malignant disease, congenital immunodeficiency, immunosuppressive therapy) Immune globulin or other blood products within prior 3-11 mo Anaphylactic hypersensitivity to neomycin or gelatin Pregnancy Thrombocytopenia if administered with measles vaccine	Although persons born after 1957 are generally immune, vaccine can be given to adults of all ages and may be particularly indicated for postpubertal males who are thought to be susceptible Persons with anaphylactic allergies to eggs may be vaccinated
Pertussis	Adult preparation of pertussis antigens combined with tetanus and diphtheria toxoids (Tdap)	All 11- to 12-year-olds Catch-up vaccination for all persons 13-64 yr of age Preferred interval of 5 yr from prior dose of Td but may be given at shorter intervals if risk of pertussis is high	One dose	Severe allergic reaction to a vaccine component or after a prior dose Moderate or severe acute illness is a precaution to vaccination	Two preparations are available, one licensed for 10- to 64-year-olds, one for 11- to 64-year-olds Administer one dose to persons 65 yr of age or older who have not previously received Td and who anticipate contact with infants younger than 1 yr of age

TABLE 17-2 SELECTED IMMUNIZING AGENTS INDICATED FOR ADULTS—cont'd

DISEASE	IMMUNIZING AGENT	INDICATIONS	SCHEDULE	MAJOR CONTRAINDICATIONS AND PRECAUTIONS	COMMENTS
Pneumococcal disease	23-Valent polysaccharide vaccine	Adults with cardiovascular disease, pulmonary disease (including asthma), diabetes mellitus, alcoholism, cirrhosis, cerebrospinal fluid leaks, splenic dysfunction or anatomic asplenia, Hodgkin's disease, lymphoma, multiple myeloma, chronic renal failure, nephrotic syndrome, immunosuppression, HIV infection, cigarette smokers 19 yr and older High-risk populations such as certain Native Americans and all adults ≥65 yr	One dose IM or SC; a second dose should be considered ≥5 yr later for adults at high risk of disease (e.g., asplenic patients) and those who lose antibody rapidly (e.g., nephrotic syndrome, renal failure, transplant recipients) Revaccinate adults who received a first dose when <65 yr who are now ≥65 yr and who received their vaccine at least 5 yr earlier	Severe allergic reaction to a vaccine component or after a prior dose Moderate or severe acute illness is a precaution to vaccination	Conjugate pneumococcal vaccine is not indicated for adults
Poliomyelitis	Inactivated poliovirus vaccine	Certain adults who are at greater risk of exposure to wild poliovirus than the general population, including travelers to countries where poliomyelitis is epidemic or endemic or specific populations with disease caused by wild poliovirus	For unvaccinated adults, two doses SC 4 wk apart and a third dose 6-12 mo after the second; if <4 wk available before protection is needed, a single dose of IPV For incompletely immunized adults, complete primary series that consists of three doses of IPV or prior OPV; no need to restart interrupted series A single dose of IPV can be given to adults who previously received a primary series but now are at high risk, such as travel to an endemic area	On theoretical grounds, pregnant women should not receive IPV, but if immediate protection is needed, IPV can be used Severe allergic reaction to a vaccine component or after a prior dose Moderate or severe acute illness is a precaution to vaccination	
Rabies	Inactivated vaccine, HDCV or PCEC	High-risk persons, including animal handlers, selected laboratory and field workers, and persons traveling for ≥1 mo to areas with high risk of rabies	Pre-exposure prophylaxis: three doses of 1 mL IM on days 0, 7, and 21 or 28	History of severe hypersensitivity reaction	Further doses needed after exposure
Rubella	Live virus vaccine	Adults, particularly women of childbearing age, who lack history of rubella vaccine and detectable rubella-specific antibodies in serum Males and females in institutions where rubella outbreaks may occur, such as hospitals, the military, and colleges Persons born before 1957, except women who can become pregnant, generally can be considered immune	One dose SC	Pregnancy, altered immunity (e.g., leukemia, lymphoma, generalized malignant disease, congenital immunodeficiency, immunosuppressive therapy) Immune globulin or other blood products within the 3-11 mo before vaccination Anaphylactic hypersensitivity to neomycin Administration of blood products should not contraindicate postpartum vaccination Thrombocytopenia if administered with measles vaccine	Women should be counseled to avoid pregnancy for 1 mo after vaccination

TABLE 17-2 SELECTED IMMUNIZING AGENTS INDICATED FOR ADULTS—cont'd

DISEASE	IMMUNIZING AGENT	INDICATIONS	SCHEDULE	MAJOR CONTRAINDICATIONS AND PRECAUTIONS	COMMENTS
Smallpox	Live vaccinia virus	Persons working with orthopox viruses Members of public health and health care response teams	One dose intracutaneously with a bifurcated needle Boosters every 10 yr and perhaps every 3 yr for persons working with virulent orthopox viruses	History or presence of eczema or other acute, chronic, or exfoliative skin condition Immunosuppression or pregnancy in patient or a close household or personal contact History of heart disease Breast-feeding Age <1 yr Allergy to a vaccine component No contraindications if exposed to smallpox	Some complications of vaccination are treatable with vaccinia immune globulin Vaccine is effective 3-4 days after exposure to variola and perhaps longer to prevent or to modify the illness Serious adverse events are rare but significant, including eczema vaccinatum, progressive vaccinia, myopericarditis, autoinoculation, and encephalitis Vaccinia is transmissible
Tetanus	Tetanus and diphtheria toxoids combined	All adults	Three doses IM needed for primary series: two doses 4 wk apart, third dose 6-12 mo after second dose Booster every 10 yr; no need to repeat if schedule is interrupted	History of neurologic or severe allergic reaction after a prior dose	Special recommendations for wound treatment (see text) Persons with GBS within the first 6 wk after immunization, particularly adults who received a prior primary series, probably should not be revaccinated in most circumstances Tetanus and diphtheria toxoids combined with acellular pertussis (Tdap) vaccine preferred for booster at age 11-12 yr One-time booster of Tdap for persons through 64 yr
Typhoid fever	Vi capsular polysaccharide vaccine Live attenuated Ty21a oral vaccine	Travelers to areas where the risk of prolonged exposure to contaminated food and water is high May be considered for family and intimate contacts of carriers and laboratory workers who work with *Salmonella typhi*	Vi polysaccharide vaccine: one dose IM 0.5 mL, boosters every 2 yr Oral vaccine: four doses on alternate days, repeat series every 5 yr if risk continues	Severe local or systemic reaction to a prior dose Ty21a vaccine should not be administered to persons with altered immunity or those receiving antimicrobial agents	Efficacy only 50-77% Food and water precautions essential
Varicella: chickenpox strain	Attenuated Oka strain of varicella virus	All persons without evidence of varicella immunity especially health care personnel, childbearing-age women, and persons with household or other contact with persons at high risk of complications of varicella (e.g., susceptible immunosuppressed persons)	Two 0.5-mL SC doses 4-8 wk apart for persons ≥13 yr A second dose is recommended for all persons who previously received one dose	Immunocompromise Pregnancy Allergy to vaccine components	Adults with a history of prior clinician-diagnosed or verified varicella can be considered immune Vaccine virus has rarely been transmitted to contacts from healthy vaccinees in whom rash developed Women who receive vaccine should not become pregnant for 1 mo
Varicella: zoster	Attenuated Oka strain of varicella virus, approximately 14 times more potent than varicella vaccine	Persons ≥60 years of age	One 0.65-mL dose SC	Immunocompromise Pregnancy Allergy to vaccine components	May be administered regardless of a prior history of shingles
Yellow fever	Live attenuated virus (17D strain)	Persons living or traveling in areas where yellow fever exists	One dose, booster every 10 yr	Immunocompromised persons History of anaphylactic allergies to eggs Pregnancy on theoretical grounds, although may be given if risk is high	Fever, jaundice, and multiple-organ system failure (viscerotropic disease) have been rarely reported in first-time recipients of 17D-derived yellow fever vaccinations Vaccinate only persons traveling to areas endemic to yellow fever

*See the text and package inserts for further details, particularly regarding indications, dosage, mode of administration, side effects, and adverse reactions and contraindications.

ACIP = Advisory Committee on Immunization Practices; GBS = Guillain-Barré syndrome; HBsAg = hepatitis B surface antigen; HBV = hepatitis B virus; HDCV = human diploid cell vaccine for rabies; HIV = human immunodeficiency virus; IM = intramuscularly; IPV = inactivated poliovirus vaccine; MMR = measles, mumps, and rubella vaccine; OPV = live trivalent oral poliovirus vaccine; PCEC = purified chick embryo cell culture rabies vaccine; SC = subcutaneously.

vaccination should be undertaken for females up through 26 years of age. Recipients of HPV vaccine should follow the same recommendations for Papanicolaou (Pap) smear screening as unvaccinated females. Persons with prior abnormal Pap smears or genital warts may be vaccinated to prevent persistent infection with types of HPV that are not in the vaccine. In 2009, the U.S. Food and Drug Administration (FDA) also licensed the quadrivalent vaccine for males, 9 through 26 years of age, for prevention of genital warts.

Side Effects

The most common reactions are local pain, swelling, and erythema, which may, in part, be explained by the aluminum-containing adjuvant rather than the L1 capsid protein. There is a slightly higher incidence of fever within 15 days of vaccination in vaccine recipients compared with placebo recipients.

Influenza

The two available influenza vaccines for seasonal influenza are the inactivated trivalent influenza vaccine (TIV) and the live attenuated influenza vaccine (LAIV). TIV, which contains split viruses of three major antigenic types, A (H3N2), A (H1N1), and B, is administered intramuscularly. LAIV, which consists of three cold-adapted, temperature-sensitive attenuated viruses, one for each of the expected circulating strains, is administered intranasally. LAIV is prepared by use of attenuated parent viruses that have been reassorted with circulating strains to contain six internal genes from the parent virus and genes for the surface hemagglutinin and neuraminidase of an A (H3N2), A (H1N1), or B strain. In 2009, a novel H1N1 virus emerged and caused a global pandemic. The 2009 H1N1 split virus vaccine is now the H1N1 component of the annual influenza vaccine.

Indications

Annual influenza (Chapter 372) vaccination with TIV is indicated for all adults but with a special emphasis on persons at high risk of complications from the disease: persons with chronic cardiopulmonary disorders, residents of nursing homes or other long-term care facilities, persons 50 years of age or older, patients with other chronic diseases (e.g., diabetes mellitus, kidney dysfunction, hemoglobinopathies, and immunosuppression) who have required regular medical follow-up or hospitalization in the prior year, adults and children who have any condition (e.g., cognitive dysfunction, spinal cord injuries, seizure disorders, or other neuromuscular disorders) that can compromise respiratory function or the handling of respiratory secretions or that can increase the risk for aspiration, and children receiving long-term aspirin therapy. Women who will be pregnant during the influenza season (usually late December through mid-March) also should be vaccinated. To reduce transmission of influenza to high-risk patients, health care workers and household contacts of high-risk patients should also be vaccinated annually, including contacts of children younger than 5 years of age. Annual vaccination is also recommended for all children 6 months through 18 years.

LAIV is licensed only for nonpregnant persons aged 2 through 49 years without underlying conditions that place them at high risk of complications from influenza. LAIV can be used for contacts of high-risk patients, if the contacts are of the appropriate age. LAIV, for theoretical concerns about live virus transmission, is not recommended for contacts of severely immunosuppressed patients such as patients with bone marrow transplants but can be given to contacts of persons with mild to moderate immunologic impairment.

The efficacy of TIV varies with the host's condition and the degree to which antigens in the vaccine match viruses in circulation the following season. Provided the match is good, the vaccine's efficacy is usually 70 to 90% in normal healthy young adults. Efficacy is substantially lower, often between 30 and 40%, in the institutionalized elderly; nevertheless, it seems to be 60 to 80% protective against pneumonia and death. LAIV has been found to be more than 85% effective in young children, even in a year when the circulating strain had antigenically drifted from the vaccine strain. Similar effects were seen in challenge studies in adults.

Ideally, seasonal vaccines should be administered as soon as they are available. If vaccine is available in December and January, vaccination should continue because it still can offer protection for many individuals. A review of influenza seasons from 1976-77 through 2008-09 documented that peak activity did not occur until January or later in more than 80% of those seasons and until February or later in more than 60%.

Side Effects

Persons with anaphylactic allergy to eggs generally should not be immunized. The most common side effect of TIV is soreness at the injection site. Fever, malaise, and myalgia may begin 6 to 12 hours after vaccination and persist for 1 to 2 days, although such reactions are most common in children exposed to vaccine for the first time. Severe allergic reactions are rare. If current influenza vaccines cause Guillain-Barré syndrome, it is likely to be rare, on the order of one case per 1 million doses. The most common adverse events after LAIV in adults are runny nose, headache, and sore throat.

Measles

Indications

Measles (Chapter 375) immunization is recommended for all persons born in or after 1957 who lack evidence of prior physician-diagnosed measles or laboratory evidence of immunity or appropriate vaccination. Before 1989, appropriate vaccination consisted of a single dose of live vaccine administered on or after the first birthday. Since then, a routine two-dose schedule has been recommended: the first dose, which is 93 to 98% effective, at 12 to 15 months of age, and the second dose at entry to primary school. All children from kindergarten through the 12th grade should have a second dose. Most adults are considered to have been appropriately vaccinated if they received one dose of vaccine administered on or after their first birthday. Some adults who are at increased risk of measles (health care workers with direct contact with patients, students in college, international travelers) should receive a second dose of vaccine, however, unless they have documentation of serologic evidence of immunity. Persons embarking on foreign travel ideally should have received two doses or have other evidence of measles immunity. Persons born before 1957 are usually immune as a result of natural infection and do not require vaccination, although vaccination is not contraindicated if they are believed to be susceptible.

During outbreaks of measles in institutions, all persons at risk who have not received two doses or who lack other evidence of measles immunity should be vaccinated. Measles vaccine is usually administered along with mumps and rubella vaccines as MMR to ensure immunity against all three diseases. Individuals already immune to one or more of the components may receive MMR without harm.

Measles vaccine is contraindicated for pregnant women on theoretical grounds, for persons with moderate to severe acute febrile illnesses, and for persons with altered immunocompetence, except those with HIV infection who are not severely immunocompromised. Patients with anaphylactic reactions to eggs can be vaccinated without prior skin testing.

Side Effects

In approximately 5 to 15% of susceptible recipients of measles vaccine, temperatures of 39.4° C or higher develop 5 to 12 days after vaccination and last 1 to 2 days. Transient rashes develop in about 5%. Thrombocytopenic purpura has been reported rarely after MMR. The overall rate of reactions after the second dose of a measles-containing vaccine is substantially lower than after the first dose. Encephalopathy or encephalitis after measles vaccination has been reported at a rate lower than the background or expected rate.

Meningococcal Vaccines

Three quadrivalent meningococcal polysaccharide vaccines against disease caused by serogroups A, C, Y, and W135 are available: meningococcal polysaccharide vaccine (MPSV4), which consists of 50 μg of polysaccharide of each of the four serogroups and is licensed for persons 2 years of age and older, and two meningococcal conjugate vaccines (MCV4). One conjugate consists of 4 μg of each polysaccharide covalently linked to 48 μg of diphtheria toxoid and licensed for persons 2 to 55 years of age. The other conjugate consists of polysaccharide linked to CRM_{197}. The four serogroups in each vaccine account for approximately two thirds of meningococcal disease in the United States and about 75% of the disease in persons 11 years of age or older (Chapter 306). Serogroup A and C polysaccharide vaccines have had 85 to 100% efficacy in epidemic settings, whereas polysaccharide vaccines for the other groups have documented good immunogenicity in adults. Meningococcal conjugate vaccine type C (MCV-C) has been associated with an estimated effectiveness of 88 to 98% in the year following vaccination in the United Kingdom, where it has been used widely. In addition, MCV-C has reduced colonization by 66% and decreased disease among unvaccinated persons by 67% in 1- to 17-year-olds and by 35% among those older than 25 years. In contrast to polysaccharide vaccines, conjugate vaccines induce immunologic memory, result in higher and more durable levels of high-avidity antibodies, and have been documented to induce herd immunity. The duration of immunity for both MPSV4 and MCV4 is thought to be about 5 years.

Indications

Routine vaccination with a single dose of MCV4 is recommended for all adolescents at 11 through 18 years of age who have not been previously vaccinated and for college freshmen who will live in dormitories. Vaccination is also recommended for very-high-risk persons, that is, those with persistent complement component deficiencies, persons with splenic dysfunction or without a spleen, microbiologists with frequent exposure to *Neisseria meningitidis* in culture, and persons who travel to or live in areas with hyperendemic or epidemic disease (e.g., the "meningitis belt" of sub-Saharan Africa, stretching from Mauritania to Ethiopia). MCV4 can be used for persons 2 to 10 years of age with high-risk conditions. It is not recommended routinely for this age group. For persons older than 55 years with an indication for vaccine, MPSV4 should be used. Meningococcal vaccination may be useful during localized epidemics of serogroups in the vaccine.

Re-vaccination is indicated at age 16 in children initially vaccinated between 11 and 12 years of age. For children initially vaccinated after age 12 years, re-vaccination recommendations are still being developed (*www.ccc. gov/vaccines*). For very high-risk persons, re-vaccination is recommended every 5 years.

Side Effects

The major side effects of MPSV4 are local reactions lasting 1 to 2 days. The incidence of local reactions and low-grade fever is slightly higher after MCV4 than with MPSV4. An excess risk of 1.25 cases of Guillain-Barré syndrome per million doses has been noted with the vaccination, although further studies have cast doubt on a causal association.

Mumps
Indications

Mumps (Chapter 377) vaccine is indicated for all persons, especially susceptible males, without evidence of immunity. For most adults, such evidence consists of a prior history of vaccination on or after the first birthday, physician-diagnosed mumps, or laboratory evidence of immunity. For adults at high risk, including health care workers, international travelers, and students at post–high school educational institutions, two doses of mumps vaccine constitute acceptable evidence of immunity. Most persons born before 1957 can be considered immune as a result of natural infection, although vaccination is not contraindicated if such persons are thought to be susceptible.

Side Effects

Adverse events after the Jeryl Lynn strain of mumps vaccine, the strain used in the United States, are uncommon—fever, parotitis, and allergic manifestations. Thrombocytopenic purpura has been reported rarely in persons administered MMR. Mumps vaccine is contraindicated for pregnant women on theoretical grounds, for persons with moderate to severe acute febrile illnesses, and for persons with altered immunocompetence. When combined with measles vaccine, it may be given to persons with asymptomatic HIV infection and considered for persons with symptomatic infection if they are not severely immunocompromised. Patients with anaphylactic reactions to eggs can be vaccinated without skin testing (see Measles earlier).

Pertussis Vaccine

In 2005, two vaccines were licensed for boosting immunity to pertussis. Both vaccines are combined with the adult preparation of tetanus and diphtheria toxoids and have a reduced content of pertussis antigens compared with the childhood pertussis-containing vaccines (Tdap). Boostrix (GlaxoSmith-Kline), which is licensed for adolescents and adults 10 through 64 years of age, contains three pertussis antigens—toxoid (PT), filamentous hemagglutinin (FHA), and pertactin (PRN). Adacel (Sanofi Pasteur, Inc.), which is licensed for 11- through 64-year-olds, contains five pertussis antigens, PT, FHA, PRN, and two fimbriae. Both vaccines, when administered to previously vaccinated adolescents and adults, induce serologic responses that are comparable to those induced during childhood vaccination with vaccines that have been proved effective. Adverse events, usually local reactions, are

similar with the adult preparation of tetanus and diphtheria toxoids (Td) alone. A single dose of Tdap is indicated for all adolescents at 11 to 12 years of age. Older adolescents should receive Tdap instead of Td if they have not received an adolescent Td booster. Tdap can be given at any interval. All adults younger than 65 years should receive a single dose of TdaP to replace a Td booster. Persons are 65 years and older who anticipate contact with an infant should receive a single dose of Tdap.

Pneumococcal Vaccine

Pneumococcal polysaccharide vaccine consists of purified polysaccharide capsular antigens from the 23 types of *Streptococcus pneumoniae* that are responsible for 85 to 90% of the bacteremic disease in the United States (Chapter 297). Most adults, including elderly patients and those with alcoholic cirrhosis and diabetes mellitus, have a two-fold or greater rise in type-specific antibodies within 2 to 3 weeks of vaccination. Although the serologic response is generally acceptable, estimates of vaccine efficacy in preventing disease vary widely. Efficacy may be lower in some patients, such as patients with alcoholic cirrhosis or Hodgkin's disease. There is good evidence that vaccination is approximately 60% effective against bacteremic pneumococcal disease, which accounts for an estimated 50,000 cases annually. Evidence regarding efficacy against pneumonia in high-risk populations is not clear, however.

Indications

The preponderance of information supports the use of pneumococcal vaccine in high-risk populations, including all persons older than 65 years. Two groups recently added to those recommended for vaccination include persons 19 years or older who smoke cigarettes or those who have asthma. Special efforts should target hospitalized patients. Approximately two thirds of patients who are admitted later with pneumococcal disease had been hospitalized for other reasons within the preceding 5 years.

Immunity may decrease 5 years or more after initial vaccination; a single booster dose should be considered at that time for adults at highest risk of disease, such as asplenic patients, and for adults who lose antibody rapidly, such as patients with nephrotic syndrome or renal failure. Persons older than 65 years who received a dose more than 5 years earlier when they were younger than 65 years should be revaccinated.

Side Effects

Local reactions are frequent. Less than 1% of vaccinees experience severe local reactions or systemic illness, such as fever and malaise. Severe events such as anaphylaxis are rare. Because of the rarity of severe reactions in revaccinated patients, persons with indications for vaccination but with unknown histories of prior vaccination should be vaccinated.

A pneumococcal conjugate vaccine in which the polysaccharides of 13 types are covalently linked to a protein carrier was licensed and recommended for universal use in children. This vaccine, which covers substantially fewer types than the 23-valent polysaccharide vaccine, is not approved for persons 9 years of age or older. Widespread vaccination of children in the United States has led to substantial reductions of invasive pneumococcal disease in adults, suggesting that children are the source for many adult infections. Trials of conjugate vaccines in adults are ongoing.

Poliomyelitis

The last documented cases of indigenously acquired poliomyelitis (Chapters 387 and 423) caused by wild polioviruses in the United States were reported in 1979. In 2000, an all inactivated poliovirus vaccine (IPV) schedule was recommended in the United States; this vaccine replaced the live attenuated oral poliovirus vaccine (OPV), which, although it had eliminated wild poliovirus in the United States, caused about eight cases per year on average among OPV recipients or their contacts. IPV is the only vaccine available in the United States. OPV is still the vaccine used in most countries around the world, however. Between 1988, when the goal was announced to eradicate wild poliovirus from the world, and 2010, cases of poliomyelitis worldwide decreased by an estimated 99%. Four countries (Nigeria, India, Pakistan, and Afghanistan) have never interrupted endemic transmission. However, because of spread from Nigeria and India, 16 countries were reinfected in 2010. Efforts to eradicate polio globally continue.

Indications

Routine vaccination of persons 18 years of age or older is not warranted given the small risk of exposure to wild virus in the United States. The major indication for adult vaccination is travel to areas where wild poliovirus is endemic or epidemic. Previously unvaccinated adults should receive IPV. Adult travelers who have histories of partial vaccination should complete a primary series of three doses with IPV. Adults who formerly received three doses of OPV or IPV should receive a single booster of IPV. A primary series of IPV consists of three doses. A fourth dose is administered to children at school entry.

Side Effects

No serious side effects of IPV have been reported.

Rabies
Indications

Rabies (Chapter 422) vaccine is indicated for pre-exposure prophylaxis of high-risk persons, including animal handlers, selected laboratory and field workers, and persons traveling for more than 1 month to areas where rabies is a constant threat. The pre-exposure regimen consists of three 1-mL intramuscular injections on days 0, 7, and 21 or 28 for all rabies vaccines. Postexposure treatment depends on prior exposure to vaccine (Chapter 422). Persons being treated for the first time should be given four doses at days 0, 3, 7, and 14. Human rabies immune globulin is also indicated for previously unvaccinated persons who are exposed.

Rubella
Indications

Rubella (Chapter 376) vaccine is indicated for susceptible adults born in 1957 or later and for susceptible women of any age who are considering becoming pregnant. Persons without a prior history of vaccination on or after the first birthday or laboratory evidence of immunity should be considered susceptible. A single dose of vaccine is 95% or more effective. Many persons receive two doses of rubella vaccine by the two-dose schedule of MMR.

Side Effects

Follow-up of susceptible pregnant women who received rubella vaccines within 3 months of the estimated date of conception has failed to reveal any evidence of defects compatible with congenital rubella syndrome in their offspring. Nevertheless, vaccine is contraindicated in pregnant women on theoretical grounds, and conception should be delayed for 1 month after rubella vaccination.

Adverse reactions occur only in susceptible persons. Arthralgia, usually of the small peripheral joints, develops in 40% of susceptible adults, and frank arthritis develops in 10 to 20%. Joint symptoms usually begin 1 to 3 weeks after vaccination and persist for 1 day to 3 weeks. Chronic recurrent or persistent joint symptoms have developed rarely after vaccination, but controlled studies have shown that the incidence of these events in vaccinees is similar to that in nonvaccinees. Other infrequent adverse events include transient peripheral neuritis and pain in the arms and legs. Thrombocytopenic purpura has been reported rarely when rubella vaccine is administered as MMR. Rubella vaccine is contraindicated for persons with moderate to severe acute illnesses and for persons with reduced immunocompetence. When given with measles vaccine, it may be administered to persons with asymptomatic HIV infection and considered for persons with symptomatic infection without severe immunocompromise. Rubella vaccine is grown in human diploid cells and can be administered without problems to persons with allergy to eggs.

Tetanus and Diphtheria

Tetanus (Chapter 304) toxoid is one of the most effective immunizations, with more than 95% protection after a primary series. A primary series consists of three doses. In persons aged 7 years or older, it should always be used in combination with diphtheria (Chapter 300) toxoid (Td), which is more than 85% effective in preventing disease. Combinations also including pertussis antigens (Tdap) are preferred to Td for routine immunization of adolescents. Doses need not be repeated if the schedule is interrupted. A booster dose of Td is recommended every 10 years. An easy way to remember is to schedule immunization at the middle of each decade (e.g., 25 years, 35 years).

Indications

After a wound, persons of unknown immunization status or persons who have received fewer than three doses of tetanus toxoid should receive a dose of Td regardless of the severity of the wound. Td also is indicated for persons who have previously received three or more doses if more than 10 years has elapsed since the last dose, in the case of clean and minor wounds, and if more than 5 years has elapsed for all other wounds. Persons who have never received a dose of TdaP should receive it in place of Td for wound management. Tetanus immune globulin should be administered simultaneously at a separate site to persons who have not received at least three doses of toxoid and who have wounds that are not clean and minor.

Side Effects

Most reactions to Td consist of local inflammation and low-grade fever. Guillain-Barré syndrome and brachial neuritis rarely have been associated with tetanus toxoid.

Varicella: Chickenpox

A live attenuated varicella vaccine (Oka strain) was licensed in 1995. A combination measles-mumps-rubella-varicella vaccine was licensed in 2005. One dose of the vaccine protects 70 to 90% of recipients against any disease and more than 95% of recipients against severe disease. Although some studies have suggested immunity may wane with increasing time since vaccination, others have not. Use of vaccine has been associated with dramatic decreases in the incidence of varicella. Breakthrough infections in persons who have previously seroconverted have been reported. Such breakthroughs are typically mild and average fewer than 50 lesions compared with several hundred lesions in unvaccinated persons with varicella. Breakthrough illnesses do not seem to increase in incidence or severity with increasing time since vaccination, a finding compatible with long-term protection after initial vaccination. Because of persistent transmission of varicella, a two-dose schedule is recommended for all persons.

Indications

Varicella vaccine is indicated routinely for all children without a contraindication. A two-dose schedule is recommended, generally at 12 to 15 months of age and 4 to 6 years of age. For persons who previously received a single dose, catch-up vaccination with a second dose is recommended, provided at least 3 months have elapsed since the first dose. Persons who received a second dose at least 28 days after the first dose do not need a third dose. Persons 13 years or older without evidence of immunity to varicella should receive two doses at least 4 weeks apart. Persons with a clinician-diagnosed or verified history of varicella disease can be considered immune and do not need vaccination. Although a negative or unknown history of disease is predictive of susceptibility in children, many adults with such histories are immune. Serologic screening of adults in some situations may be cost-effective, provided that identified susceptible adults are vaccinated. Serologic testing is not indicated after vaccination. The vaccine is contraindicated in the immunocompromised, persons with anaphylactic allergies to vaccine components, and pregnant women. Varicella vaccine is more temperature sensitive than other vaccines used in the United States. It must be stored frozen at −15° C or colder to retain potency, and it should be discarded if it is not used within 30 minutes of reconstitution.

Side Effects

The most common side effect is soreness at the injection site, which is reported in 25 to 35% of recipients 13 years or older. Varicella-like rashes at the injection site (median of two lesions) have been reported in 3% of recipients in this age group after the first dose and in 1% after the second dose. Nonlocalized rashes with a median of five lesions have been reported in 5.5% of recipients after the first dose and in 0.9% after the second dose. Although the vaccine virus can cause herpes zoster (shingles), the incidence is substantially lower than would be expected after natural varicella (Chapter 383). More severe events occurring in temporal relation to the vaccine have been reported rarely, although a causal relationship has not been established. Transmission of vaccine virus to a contact is extremely rare and appears to take place only with vaccinees in whom a varicella-like rash has developed.

Varicella: Zoster

Clinical trials of a varicella vaccine, approximately 14 times more potent than the varicella vaccine used routinely, among persons 60 years of age or older reported a 51% reduction in the incidence of zoster and a 67% decrease in postherpetic neuralgia. The efficacy against zoster declined with increasing age from 60 to 80 years or older, but there was evidence of continuing protection against postherpetic neuralgia. The vaccine requires special freezer storage.

Indications

Zoster vaccine is recommended as a single dose for persons 60 years of age or older. Persons with a prior history of zoster may be vaccinated. It is not necessary to elicit a history of varicella or to test for varicella immunity before administration of zoster vaccine. The vaccine is not recommended for immunocompromised persons or pregnant women.

Side Effects

The most common side effect attributed to the vaccine is local reactions.

● VACCINES INTENDED PRIMARILY FOR INTERNATIONAL TRAVELERS

Japanese Encephalitis Vaccine

Indications

Japanese encephalitis (Chapter 391) vaccine is indicated primarily for travelers to Asia who will spend a month or longer in endemic areas during the transmission season, especially if travel will include rural areas. In all instances, travelers should be advised to take personal precautions to reduce exposure to mosquito bites. An older vaccine was reported to be 80 to 91% effective in preventing clinical disease. The current whole virus inactivated vaccine (IXIARO, Intercell Biomedical) was licensed based on comparable immunogenicity. The primary series consists of two 0.5-mL doses given intramuscularly on days 0 and 28, with the second dose administered at least 1 week before travel (see Table 17-2). The duration of immunity is unknown. As of 2010, there were no recommendations for booster doses.

Side Effects

Headache and myalgia and local reactions (pain and tenderness) are common, occurring in more than 10% of vaccinees. However, the incidence rates of these events were similar to those in a comparison group, which received PBS and aluminum hydroxide.

Typhoid Vaccine

Indications

Two types of vaccines, a live attenuated Ty21a oral vaccine and a capsular polysaccharide vaccine (ViCPS), appear to be of comparable efficacy (50 to 77%). Typhoid (Chapter 316) vaccine is indicated primarily for travelers to areas where the risk of prolonged exposure to contaminated food and water is high. Because the vaccine is not always effective, food and water precautions are still essential. The vaccine also may be considered for family or other intimate contacts of typhoid carriers and laboratory workers who work with *Salmonella typhi*. For adults and children 6 years and older, either of the vaccines may be used. For Ty21a, one enteric-coated capsule is taken every other day for four doses. Alternatively, a single dose of the ViCPS vaccine may be given. The duration of protection with Ty21a is not known; repetition of the primary series is recommended every 5 years for persons at risk. Boosters are recommended every 2 years for the ViCPS vaccine if persons continue to be at risk. The ViCPS vaccine can be given to children as young as 2 years of age.

Side Effects

Adverse reactions are rare.

Yellow Fever Vaccine

Indications

Yellow fever (Chapter 389) occurs only in areas of South America and Africa. Vaccination with a single dose of the live attenuated 17D strain of virus confers protection to almost all recipients for at least 10 years. A booster dose is recommended every 10 years for persons at continued risk of exposure to yellow fever.

Side Effects

Side effects are uncommon. A rare syndrome of yellow fever vaccine, febrile multiple organ system failure or viscerotropic disease, has been reported, with high rates of mortality, primarily among older adults and persons who have undergone thymectomy or have severe thymic dysfunction being vaccinated for the first time. Yellow fever vaccine should be administered with caution and only after careful counseling to elderly patients who are going to spend time in yellow fever–endemic zones. Yellow fever vaccine should not be given to immunocompromised persons or persons with anaphylactic allergies to eggs. The vaccine is contraindicated in pregnant women on theoretical grounds, although if pregnant women must travel to a high-risk area, they may be vaccinated.

● VACCINES FOR POSSIBLE BIOTERRORISM AGENTS

Anthrax Vaccine

Anthrax vaccine adsorbed (AVA) is prepared from a cell-free filtrate of a nonencapsulated strain of anthrax and contains many cell products including protective antigen. Protective antigen is responsible for binding to cells, allowing transport of lethal factor and edema factor into host cells. A recombinant protective antigen (rPA) vaccine is in clinical trials.

Indications

Pre-exposure prophylaxis consists of five doses intramuscularly at 0 and 4 weeks and 6, 12, and 18 months followed by annual boosters. Protective efficacy of an earlier form of the vaccine against cutaneous anthrax was 92.5%. Animal models suggest efficacy against inhalation anthrax. Pre-exposure vaccination is recommended for persons engaged in work involving exposure to high concentrations of *Bacillus anthracis* or in activities with high potential for aerosol production. Vaccine may be given with antibiotics for postexposure prophylaxis (Chapters 20 and 302); the antibiotics should be continued for 7 to 14 days after the third dose of vaccine is given.

Side Effects

The most common adverse events are local reactions, including subcutaneous nodules, which are thought to be due to the deposition of the aluminum-containing adjuvant in subcutaneous tissue.

Smallpox Vaccine

Smallpox vaccine uses vaccinia virus, an orthopox virus that is distinct from variola and cowpox viruses and that provides cross-protection from smallpox. Smallpox vaccine is close to 100% effective when it is administered properly, with a bifurcated needle. Vaccination also prevents or modifies disease when it is administered within 3 to 4 days of exposure and perhaps even after greater delays. The skin usually does not need any special preparation. If alcohol is used for cleaning, the skin should be allowed to dry before vaccination to avoid inactivation of the vaccine. The needle is held perpendicular to the skin; 3 punctures for primary vaccination and 15 punctures for revaccination are made rapidly with enough vigor to ensure that a trace of blood appears within 15 to 20 seconds. With a primary take, the vaccination site should become reddened and pruritic by 3 or 4 days after vaccination; a large vesicle with a red areola forms and becomes pustular by 7 to 11 days. The lesion scabs by the third week. Fever is the most common adverse event. Other more serious complications include eczema vaccinatum, a local or disseminated vaccinia infection in persons with a history of eczema or other exfoliative dermatitis; vaccinia necrosum, which occurs in immunocompromised persons; autoinoculation, especially of the eye, which can cause keratitis and scarring; generalized vaccinia; myopericarditis; and encephalitis. The risk for death from vaccinia has been estimated to be approximately one case per 1 million primary vaccinations.

Indications

The vaccine is indicated for persons who work with orthopox viruses. To increase preparedness for a smallpox attack, vaccination is often recommended for persons who will serve on public health or health care response teams. The duration of immunity is unclear. Revaccination is recommended at least every 10 years for persons who continue to be at risk. Contraindications include history or presence of eczema, other chronic or exfoliative skin conditions, and immunosuppression or pregnancy in the patient or a close household or other contact. Persons who are younger than 1 year, are breast-feeding, or have allergies to vaccine components should not be vaccinated. Because of reports of postvaccination cardiac events, vaccination should be deferred in persons with ischemia or other severe heart diseases or at high risk for ischemic heart disease events (*www.cdc.gov/smallpox*). In the event of exposure to variola, there are no contraindications. Should variola be introduced into a community, vaccination would be indicated for all exposed persons and their close contacts to prevent further spread, and recommendations for more widespread vaccination would have to be evaluated on a case-by-case basis.

Other Agents

Other organisms or products that have been considered potential bioterrorism threats include plague (Chapter 320) and botulinum toxin (Chapter 304). Poisoning with botulinum toxin can be treated with a trivalent antitoxin, available from the Centers for Disease Control and Prevention (see *MMWR.* 2003;52:774; *www.cdc.gov/ncidod/srp/drugs/formulary.html*). An experimental pentavalent botulinum toxoid can be obtained from the Centers for Disease Control and Prevention for laboratory workers at high risk for exposure to toxin. Pre-exposure vaccination is not warranted or feasible for the general population.

🔴 OTHER VACCINES

A protein-conjugated vaccine for *Haemophilus influenzae* type b (Hib) may be considered for some adults at high risk for invasive Hib disease (e.g., asplenia, HIV infection).

1. Prymula R, Siegrist CA, Chlibek R, et al. Effect of prophylactic paracetamol administration at time of vaccination on febrile reactions and antibody responses in children: two open-label, randomized controlled trials. *Lancet.* 2009;374:1339-1350.

SUGGESTED READINGS

Advisory Committee on Immunization Practices. Recommended adult immunization schedule: United States, 2011. *Ann Intern Med.* 2011;154:168-173. *Consensus guidelines.*

Centers for Disease Control and Prevention. Recommendations of the Advisory Committee on Immunization Practices. *Comprehensive coverage on vaccine-preventable diseases, vaccines, indications, schedules, and adverse events. Published as available in the* Morbidity and Mortality Weekly Report *as "Recommendations and Reports" supplements and available at wwwnc.cdc.gov/vaccines/recs/acip/default .htm.*

Centers for Disease Control and Prevention. Traveler's Health. www.cdc.gov/travel/default.aspx. *A complete guide for the international traveler, including required and recommended vaccinations. Revised every 1 to 2 years.*

Centers for Disease Control and Prevention. Adult Immunization Schedule—United States, 2010. www.cdc.gov/vaccines/recs/schedules/adult-schedule.htm. *The schedule is divided in two parts: (1) vaccines recommended by age group and (2) vaccines recommended by underlying medical condition.*

National Center for Immunization and Respiratory Diseases (NCIRD) Centers for Disease Control and Prevention. *The CDC has established toll-free numbers for answering questions from the general public and physicians: 1-800-232-4636. Inquiries can be made to the CDC by e-mail: cdcinfo@cdc.gov or the CDC website at www.cdc.gov/vaccine.*

18

PRINCIPLES OF OCCUPATIONAL AND ENVIRONMENTAL MEDICINE

MARK R. CULLEN

In the first several decades after World War II, when many American workers came to enjoy coverage by health insurance—for everything but workplace injuries and illnesses—the myth grew that modern work was largely free of the risks of the industrial horrors of past eras. Starting in the 1970s, however, resurgence of societal and medical interest in these consequences of work found that diseases related to work were not truly extinct, just not well observed or studied. Occupational physicians, often cut off from mainstream medical practice, had difficulty changing the perception, and most practicing internists were largely oblivious. It is now recognized that a substantial burden of ill health and disability is due to work-associated physical, chemical, and biologic hazards. Another intriguing possibility, recognized by social epidemiologists, is that work may be injurious to health in ways beyond these tangible risks.

Although tens of thousands of toxic chemicals and other hazards can potentially cause or exacerbate a wide range of acute and chronic conditions, certain basic principles and clinical approaches apply broadly to general and specialty medical practice. This chapter outlines these basics, then briefly summarizes the most common occupational disorders seen by internists in developed countries, and finally reviews the effects of the environmental exposures most likely to be encountered.

🔴 PRINCIPLES OF OCCUPATIONAL AND ENVIRONMENTAL DISEASE

It is widely imagined that the major health effects of environmental and occupational exposures are unique disorders best recognized by their failure to fit easily into other diagnostic categories (e.g., arsenic poisoning). In reality, *the major consequences of chemical and physical exposures are, without further exploration of an environmental connection, indistinguishable in clinical presentations from disorders that make up the bulk of outpatient and inpatient medical practice:* rashes, abnormal liver function studies (Chapter 149), wheezing and irritative symptoms of the upper and lower respiratory tract (Chapter 87), various cancers (Chapter 183), peripheral neuropathies (Chapter 428), dysphoria (Chapter 404), and nonspecific cognitive dysfunction (Chapter 409). Although a handful of pathologically distinct disorders still occur, such as silicosis (Chapter 93) and lead poisoning (Chapter 21), when an environmental or workplace agent causes overt disease, physiologic and radiographic studies typically reveal manifestations completely consistent with common diagnoses such as asthma (Chapter 87), contact dermatitis (Chapter 446), fatty liver (Chapter 155), and lung cancer (Chapter 197).

The underlying cause may remain obscure unless the clinician adheres to a disciplined approach designed to investigate and exclude occupational or environmental causes whenever it is appropriate. The best approach is consistent use of the occupational and environmental history, a short series of questions that can be expanded on the basis of the replies (see later). The point is that the internist cannot "wait" to consider occupational or environmental issues until other diseases have been ruled out without running the risk of missing almost every occupational and environmental effect that he or she will encounter.

Whatever the pathway or time course, exposure dose is the major determinant of the risk for development of disease. As in pharmacology (Chapter 28), it is impossible to make any meaningful statement about cause and effect without appreciation of dose. Consider, for example, the difference in health effects among aspirin at 65 mg, 650 mg, and 6500 mg (Chapter 36). Over this two-order magnitude of change, the chemical goes from having one therapeutic target organ to having many and to being potentially lethal. It is no different with lead or organophosphate pesticides or solvents, except that there is rarely as simple a way to determine dose as in the drug situation, where pill bottles are labeled and drug prescriptions are recorded. This limitation is exacerbated because, unlike with drugs, the range of toxic exposures may vary far more widely. For example, water in a contaminated drinking well or poor indoor air in an office could have toxins at a level that is two, three, or even four orders of magnitude (i.e., 10,000 times) lower than the level that may have been evaluated in an epidemiologic study of workers or tested in animals. Fortunately, it is much easier to "range find" than one might presuppose (see later discussion of history), and eagerness for precision—often unattainable—should not interfere with obtaining the great amount of information that *can* be readily gleaned and is often sufficient to act on. The key point is that no attempt to apply clinical information in relation to work or environment can be useful without some effort to characterize exposure dose.

Environmental hazards may affect preferentially vulnerable populations—those with underlying disease, those at the extremes of life, those with atopy, and those with other serious health risks such as smoking or diabetes. Genetic differences may underlie some differences, but few relevant genes have been sufficiently characterized for use in practice. Clinical studies of a host of common occupational diseases have identified behavioral and constitutional cofactors; for example, smoking dramatically increases the risk of lung cancer in asbestos-exposed workers (Chapter 197). This interaction creates a double demand on the clinician—the presence of smoking or atopy in a young woman with cough does not preclude the possibility of an occupational cause of her asthma but rather actually increases the likelihood that such a consideration may be important.

The Occupational and Environmental History and Exposure Assessment

Key to determining whether work and other environmental exposures may be causing or contributing to adverse health is the history. The approach to obtaining this information and to the use of available resources to corroborate and complement it depends on the clinical context. In primary and much specialty medical care, where it is anticipated that a patient will be observed during a long period into the future, the most important step is to establish the hazards to which the patient may be exposed at work presently, the activities that may have resulted in past harmful exposures potentially relevant to future health (because of latency), and whether the present residential environment, including air and water and food sources, is thought to be contaminated by harmful materials. The recommended approach is to use a simple questionnaire, which can be self-administered or supervised by a medical extender (E-Fig. 18-1). These instruments can then be reviewed together by the patient and physician as time permits and updated over time. When jobs or materials are noted but the actual generic exposures are unknown, the patient and available reference sources can be enlisted to "translate" the history into specifics, such as which metals are being welded or what is actually contained in a cleaning agent or plastic. This information is obligatorily maintained and supplied on request by employers in most developed countries in the form of fact sheets termed *Material Safety Data Sheets*, many of which can be easily found online as well. In this way, the ongoing and former exposures, which may have an impact on health, can be noted and, where important, incorporated into routine preventive care or clinical surveillance for sequelae.

For patients with new clinical complaints or recently diagnosed conditions, the question of an environmental cause looms more urgently, so the approach must be more focused. If symptoms or signs of acute or subacute illness are suggested, the *timing* of recent or unusual environmental exposures in relation to the symptoms is key—more important than specific chemical detail. For example, if the patient develops shortness of breath shortly after the introduction of a new chemical or process at work or after a leak or spill, that fact should drive further questions, such as Did others get sick as well? For recurrent symptoms, such as cough or rash, cyclic changes are most often the strongest clue: Do symptoms get worse on workdays and improve on days off or holidays? For more insidious symptoms, such as weakness or numbness of the extremities or new-onset hepatic dysfunction, the appropriate question would be whether the onset of the abnormality has followed by weeks or months some demonstrable change in the work or home environment. Again, the coincidence of others similarly affected may be more valuable than detailed knowledge of the constituents of that environment. When such a temporal pattern is suggested, further efforts to establish what exposure has actually occurred are warranted, often with specialty consultation when it is available.

In the elucidation of evidently more chronic conditions, such as pulmonary fibrosis, chronic renal insufficiency, or a malignant neoplasm, an alternative approach is suggested because the exposure, if relevant, is usually remote. In this situation, a detailed query about current work or ambient environments is not likely to be helpful in differential diagnosis, although knowledge of a past exposure to an important hazard (such as silica, asbestos, or cadmium) might, on the basis of the knowledge of its effects, influence the sequence of the evaluation. However, it is generally more efficient to explore past exposures *after* the pathophysiologic disturbance has been characterized, focusing inquiry exclusively on factors known to cause or suspected of causing that disorder—as is easily found in suggested texts or literature searches.

In acute or chronic cases, information about *what* the exposure has been (generically) must be augmented by an estimation of exposure dose. A brief exposure to a fume containing a small percentage of lead will not, in general, cause acute lead poisoning (although hosts may differ in their responses), nor will trace contamination of a drinking well with benzene typically cause blood dyscrasias. The patient will rarely be able to supply detailed information about past or even current "dose" but often can provide valuable clues: Did the exposure continue during many years? Were fumes or fibers grossly visible in the air? Were respirators or other protective gear necessary or offered? Have episodes of unprotected exposure ever resulted in irritation or acute discomfort? A positive reply to any of these questions would suggest "high" exposure, where the reference point is the level at which the risk for development of a health effect becomes substantial. Conversely, if exposure has occurred in an otherwise typical office or around a home renovation, the levels of exposure are more likely "low." Nevertheless, such low-level exposure does not exclude a health effect, especially one caused by idiosyncratic mechanisms or occurring in hosts who are more "sensitive" to chemical exposures, a health characteristic found in 2 to 10% of the population. Although not to be condoned because of broader public health consequences, exposures in food and drinking water are uncommon causes of perceptible clinical problems. When concern about the exposure is high, information from

patients can be readily supplemented by information from employers (with the patient's consent!) and regulatory or health authorities or by consultation with specialists who should know the levels of most workplace hazards in the community. Finally, with an appropriate understanding of the limits of testing and awareness of "timing" issues in relation to exposure (as with measuring drug levels), an increasing number of hazardous chemicals can be biologically measured in blood or urine. Metals and some pesticides can be reliably tested now, and a broad array of organic chemicals should be amenable for testing in the near future. Random sampling for "unknowns" is rarely helpful and often leads to erroneous conclusions because trace chemicals are ubiquitous.

OCCUPATIONAL AND ENVIRONMENTAL HEALTH DISORDERS COMMON IN PRACTICE

Although almost any medical complaint or condition may have an occupational or environmental cause or contribution, certain conditions encountered in medical practice *commonly* do (Table 18-1). For these conditions, attention to the history is most important and most often rewarding.

Asthma

Men and women with preexisting airways disease tolerate irritants in the workplace poorly and may experience exacerbations in temporal relation to one or more exposures. More important, numerous antigens are extant in the workplace, from large proteins, such as latex and animal danders, to small molecules, such as isocyanates needed to set polyurethane. More than 250 agents have been well characterized, and many others are suspect. Virtually no profession or work is immune. Presentation is often nonspecific; timing of symptoms during or slightly staggered from exposure is the clue to diagnosis. The reward for early recognition of such causes is the likelihood that airway inflammation will abate when the noxious exposure is eliminated; otherwise lifelong, often generalized asthma is the rule (Chapter 87).

Chronic Interstitial and Parenchymal Lung Disorders

The rounded opacities of silicosis (Chapter 93) and coal workers' pneumoconiosis (Chapter 93) radiographically resemble sarcoid (Chapter 95); chronic beryllium disease (Chapter 93), a granulomatous disorder caused by sensitization to this widely used light metal, is clinically identical to sarcoid in almost all respects, but a reasonably specific test for blood and bronchoalveolar lavage fluid is now available to distinguish them. Asbestosis (Chapter 93) in every way is identical to idiopathic pulmonary fibrosis (Chapter 92) except that benign pleural changes often accompany asbestosis, which, unlike idiopathic pulmonary fibrosis, tends to run a far more indolent course and

TABLE 18-1	COMMON OCCUPATIONAL AND ENVIRONMENTAL HEALTH CONDITIONS IN GENERAL PRACTICE	
CONDITION	**EXPOSURE SETTINGS**	**COMMENT**
Asthma	Virtually any indoor or outdoor workplace	New-onset, recrudescent, or exacerbated asthma
Interstitial and parenchymal lung disorders	Dusts, metals, and organic materials	All parenchymal disorders have one or more environmental causes
Cancers of the respiratory tract	Asbestos, radon, silica, mineral oils, tars, and other carcinogens	Smokers are more likely to be affected
Sensorineural hearing loss	Noise, metals, and solvents	High-frequency loss, especially in younger workers
Musculoskeletal disorders of trunk and limbs	Heavy or stereotyped activities	Cold, vibration, and work stress contribute
Upper airway irritation	Dust and fumes	More common in smokers and atopic persons
Nonspecific building-related illness	Office work	Must exclude *specific* causes
Dermatitis, allergic or irritant	Repeated exposure to unprotected skin	Work and environmental exposures should be considered in every case
Multiple chemical sensitivities	Any	Complication of adverse environmental exposure

usually stops progressing when exposure ceases or within a few years thereafter. Hypersensitivity pneumonitis (Chapter 93) is rarely suspected outside of agricultural settings but is occurring far more often; the causes are likely to be microbial contaminants of work materials, but some chemicals, such as the isocyanates, may also be causal.

Cancers of the Respiratory Tract

Although most carcinomas of the lung and upper airway occur in smokers, occupational exposures to asbestos, silica, and the polyaromatic hydrocarbons in particulate air pollution, diesel exhaust, pitch, and asphalt contribute to the burden, as do radon and carcinogenic metals such as chromium and nickel found in most alloys (Chapter 197). Some organic materials, such as formaldehyde, are also likely culprits. Until there is an established strategy for secondary prevention, patients with these exposures should be observed expectantly; at a minimum, extraordinary efforts should be made to control smoking in these exposed individuals. Asbestos-exposed workers—smokers or otherwise—are additionally at risk for malignant mesothelioma (Chapters 99 and 197), but other than primary prevention, the only clinical implication is awareness for early diagnosis and compassionate care for this still largely incurable industrial disease.

Fatty Liver

With the widespread use of abdominal imaging, fatty liver has been recognized as more common than previously thought (Chapter 155). This disorder is common among individuals exposed regularly to organic solvents, a possibility that should be considered at the same time that infectious, metabolic, and pharmaceutical causes are considered. Once it is suspected, whether or not other factors are also present, exposure should be reduced. Improvement tends to be slow, but the risk of progression is likely to have been averted or at least diminished.

Sensorineural Hearing Loss

Aside from aging, noise is the most important cause of high-frequency sensorineural hearing loss, recognizable as early as in adolescence (Chapter 436). Hobbies such as shooting and loud music may combine with industrial and agricultural noise to accelerate hearing loss. Although it is the responsibility of employers to conduct routine audiograms and to control exposure, clinicians should test noise-exposed patients periodically and reinforce whatever control strategies may be in place at work. Exposure to metals such as lead and organic solvents may compound the risk further.

Musculoskeletal Disorders of the Upper Extremity and Trunk

The most common cause of work disability, including permanent disability, is injury to the back (Chapter 407) and wrist. Repetitive, heavy, awkward, and time-pressured activities are notorious contributors, as are cold and vibration. Although an anatomically localized lesion may be identified and specifically treated in a small fraction of cases, as in carpal tunnel syndrome (Chapter 428) or thoracic outlet obstruction, the most important modalities of care in most cases are early recognition and avoidance of further insult. Physical therapy and medications may hasten recovery but cannot prevent recurrences and even progression unless the causal work and avocational activities are modified.

Upper Airway Irritation

Virtually any smoke, fume, dust, or chemical has potential to irritate the upper respiratory tract (Chapter 93), causing acute or chronic symptoms indistinguishable from common allergic manifestations (Chapter 257) or upper respiratory infections (Chapter 96). Although the mucosae of the eyes, nose, sinuses, and throat tend to be forgiving, recurrent episodes are extremely nettlesome and cause substantial disability. Atopic patients and patients with frequent infections are often the most sensitive to these ubiquitous environmental insults, which must ultimately be addressed along with the symptoms themselves and secondary infections.

Dermatitis

Erythematous rashes are a common consequence of topical exposures to workplace, avocational, and household materials, including latex, plastics, and many foods (Chapter 446). Although the keys to recognition are timing and the anatomic relation to clothing, allergenic and irritating chemicals can find their way into unlikely places, such as the groin and belt lines. Specialty consultation and patch testing are warranted in intractable cases but should not supplant careful observation and history taking in most situations.

Sick Building Syndrome and Nonspecific Building-Related Illness

The effort to reduce the influx of "fresh" air into buildings to save heating and air-conditioning costs has resulted in upper airway and dermal irritation as well as vague central nervous system symptoms such as headache and fatigue, occurring shortly after beginning work and clearing minutes to hours after leaving the affected building. Many occupants are typically affected, especially those who spend the most time in one place. The cause is unknown, but recent evidence suggests that microbial materials may be the most common culprits. In every instance, a search for a specific allergen or irritant is worth undertaking (Chapter 257), but the most remedial sources are poor overall ventilation and dampness in which molds fester. When the cause is remedied, most building occupants typically experience symptomatic improvement. From a clinical perspective, the major consideration is whether any more serious problem, such as asthma, may have also developed.

Multiple Chemical Sensitivities

An environmental illness as transient as a single noxious inhalation or as persistent as a protracted course of nonspecific building-related illness can initiate a cycle of similar symptoms after exposures to odors or irritants at very low levels so that even everyday tasks such as shopping or driving become problematic. A patient typically complains of being "allergic" to everything, although there is no evidence for allergic mechanisms (Chapter 257); the cause of this vexing complication, most prevalent in women, is unknown and may involve psychological as well as physiologic factors. Despite the severity of complaints, which often include fatigue, muscle pain, stridor, chest tightness, and palpitations, laboratory test results are normal. Coexistent anxiety and depression often prompt psychiatric referral (Chapter 404), but the disorder has proved relatively refractory to all treatment modalities. Sympathetic support, environmental modification as needed to provide some symptomatic relief, and candor regarding the unknown nature of the disorder are appropriate; extensive clinical investigations often serve only to reinforce the patient's "sick" role and are best avoided. Despite all efforts, the most severely affected individuals will often seek the care of alternative practitioners (Chapter 38) with compelling if unproven theories and expensive, potentially harmful remedies.

● COMMON HAZARDOUS EXPOSURES IN THE WORKPLACE AND AMBIENT ENVIRONMENT

Tens of thousands of chemicals in the workplace, as well as important physical and biologic hazards, may be encountered in the general environment (Table 18-2). Several of these hazards are of major current concern in industrialized countries.

Metals

Exposures to lead and arsenic (Chapter 21), once commonplace in industry, are now generally controlled; concern remains highest for environmental settings, especially for children. There is now greater concern for mercury—entrained in large ocean fish worldwide—and manganese (Chapter 21), a potent neurotoxin in welding fumes and various alloys. For most metals—manganese being a notorious exception—blood or urine tests are available to quantify a patient's burden, but these tests must be mindful of timing, the form of metal, and possible "confounders," such as the largely benign form of arsenic excreted in urine for several days after even a single shellfish meal.

Organic Solvents

These petroleum derivatives remain ubiquitous in workplace and household products. All are irritating, potentially neurotoxic, and, to varying degrees, hepatotoxic (Chapter 110). A few, such as trichloroethylene and n-hexane, are more potent but no longer widely used. Benzene and the ethers of ethylene glycol are bone marrow toxins (Chapter 168).

Organohalides

Although these complex organic pesticides and industrial materials are no longer made and sold in developed countries, their remarkable biopersistence has resulted in entrainment into everyone's fat. Worse, the dread byproduct dioxin, once associated with herbicide manufacture, has now been recognized as a predictable consequence of combustion of any chlorine-containing materials. All are suspect carcinogens, although debate remains whether this effect is limited to soft tissue sarcomas (Chapter 209)—a relationship established for dioxin—or promotes cancers more globally.

19

TABLE 18-2 COMMON HAZARDS IN THE WORKPLACE AND AMBIENT ENVIRONMENT

HAZARD	HEALTH EFFECTS OF GREATEST CONCERN	COMMENTS
Metals	Neurotoxicity, cancer	Most can be measured in blood or urine to assess dose
Organic solvents	Respiratory and dermal irritation, neurotoxicity, hepatotoxicity	Benzene and a few others have unique effects
Organohalides (e.g., DDT, PCBs)	Cancer	Ubiquitous suspect carcinogens of high population concern
Herbicides and pesticides	Rare acute neurotoxicity, unknown long-term effects	Widespread hazards of high population concern
Electromagnetic radiation	Leukemia, glioblastoma	Ubiquitous exposures with unproven effects
Particulate matter	Acute and chronic atherosclerotic cardiovascular disease	Air pollution, workplace
Mold	Allergy	High population concern regarding putative chronic effects
Mineral dusts	Cancer	Old hazards still of high concern (e.g., asbestos, silica)

DDT = dichlorodiphenyltrichloroethane; PCBs = polychlorinated biphenyls.

Herbicides and Pesticides

The acute neurotoxicity and irritant properties of most herbicides and pesticides have been well studied (Chapter 110). These agents are generally well controlled, although both occupational and residential overexposures occasionally occur.

Electromagnetic Radiation

Electric wires, appliances, and, notoriously, cell phones emit low-frequency electromagnetic radiation at levels far below those that cause local thermal injuries (Chapter 19). These radiations are nonionizing, but there is some epidemiologic evidence of an increased risk of childhood leukemia with high-level exposure from household wiring and of excess brain tumors in adult workers with regular exposures. Moreover, recent reports from Europe suggest excess brain cancer in cell phone users. These data are difficult to interpret because study results differ according to how exposure is assessed; the only conclusion is that there is basis for concern and need for further study but not cause for widespread alarm or action other than precaution in the placement of new heavy power lines near schools and residences.

Particulate Matter

Evidence accumulated over the past decade points to the likelihood that ambient air pollution contributes measurably to the risk of cardiovascular disease. Focus has turned from the well-established respiratory irritants—the gases SO_2 and ozone—to the smallest particles, so-called $PM_{2.5}$. These particles are laden with polyaromatic hydrocarbons from diesel exhaust, coal burning, and industrial sources, which are proinflammatory. Unknown yet is whether this risk also accrues to more heavily exposed industrial workers, or those exposed to small particles of other composition, but it appears that controls on air quality have already resulted in reductions both of acute coronary events and overall mortality.

Mold

Molds are ubiquitous and long known for their unpleasant odors and potential for inducing allergic responses (Chapter 257), including asthma. Recently, concern has arisen over the potential for serious effects from various mycotoxins, long problems in veterinary medicine when domestic animals consume contaminated feed; however, a consensus panel concluded that there is no evidence of human risks beyond those well established from living or working in a moldy environment. Mold formation should be prevented wherever possible, especially in schools and offices, where molds contribute to problems with indoor air quality. Identification, with eradication of leaks and other sources of water accumulation, is key.

Mineral Dusts

Although asbestos has been largely abated, silica and human-made mineral fibers remain widely distributed in the environment. Silica (Chapter 93), present in virtually every form of "rock," is a potent cause of lung injury and cancer, so respiratory exposure should be carefully controlled in every setting. The evidence of serious risk from fibrous glass, mineral wool, and other human-made mineral fibers is less clear; probably only the finest fibers, such as slag wool, have cancer-causing potential, but many are potent dermal and upper respiratory irritants and should be well controlled for that reason alone.

SUMMARY

Occupational and environmental health problems remain prevalent, although their spectrum and nature have changed as rapidly as any in medicine and are likely to change even faster as technology, work, and knowledge continue to evolve. Physicians need not necessarily develop a large base of "facts"—themselves subject to revision frequently—but rather an approach that incorporates key elements and provides a foundation for efficient recognition and management of current and future clinical syndromes.

SUGGESTED READINGS

Schaafsma F, Schonstein E, Whelan KM, et al. Physical conditioning programs for improving work outcomes in workers with back pain. *Cochrane Database Syst Rev.* 2010;1:CD001822. *The effectiveness of physical conditioning programs when compared with usual care exercises in workers with back pain remains uncertain.*

Van Hee VC, Kaufman JD, Budinger GR, et al. Update in environmental and occupational medicine 2009. *Am J Respir Crit Care Med.* 2010;181:1174-1180. *Review.*

van Oostrom SH, Driessen MT, de Vet HC, et al. Workplace interventions for preventing work disability. *Cochrane Database Syst Rev.* 2009;2:CD006955. *Workplace interventions are effective to reduce sickness absence, not to improve health outcomes.*

RADIATION INJURY

ARTHUR C. UPTON

The term *radiation injury* denotes any abnormality of form or function caused by electromagnetic waves or accelerated atomic particles. The term is also often applied to the harmful effects of high-intensity ultrasound and electromagnetic fields. The different types of radiation differ markedly in their biologic effects, so each must be dealt with separately in considering the injuries it can cause.

IONIZING RADIATION INJURY

Ionizing radiation occurs as electromagnetic waves of extremely short wavelength (Fig. 19-1) and as accelerated atomic particles (e.g., electrons, protons, neutrons, α particles). The injuries they cause include mutagenic, carcinogenic, and teratogenic effects and various acute and chronic tissue reactions such as erythema, cataract of the lens, sterility, and depression of hematopoiesis.

EPIDEMIOLOGY

Precise data on the frequency of injuries caused by ionizing radiation are not available. Injuries attributable to excessive occupational exposure were prevalent among radiation workers in the era preceding modern safety standards but are seldom encountered in the United States today. The 1986 Chernobyl accident in Ukraine, however, caused radiation sickness in more than 200 emergency workers, injured 28 fatally, released enough radioactivity to require tens of thousands of inhabitants to be evacuated from the surrounding area, and resulted in a collective dose-equivalent commitment of 600,000 person-Sv for the population of the Northern Hemisphere. Less catastrophic but more numerous than reactor accidents are accidents involving medical and industrial γ-ray sources, which are occasionally serious enough to be fatal. Noteworthy in this context is the potential for terrorist attacks in which

FIGURE 19-1. The electromagnetic spectrum. (From Mettler FA, Upton AC. *Effects of Ionizing Radiation*, 3rd ed. Philadelphia: WB Saunders; 2008.)

TABLE 19-1 IONIZING RADIATION QUANTITIES AND DOSE UNITS

QUANTITY	DOSE UNIT*	DEFINITION
Radioactivity	Becquerel (Bq)	One disintegration per second
Absorbed dose	Gray (Gy)	Energy deposited in tissue (1 J/kg)
Equivalent dose	Sievert (Sv)	Absorbed dose weighted for the quality (potency) of radiation
Effective dose	Sievert (Sv)	Equivalent dose weighted for the sensitivity of exposed organs
Collective effective dose	Person-Sv	Effective dose applied to a population
Committed effective dose	Sievert (Sv)	Effective dose from a given intake of radioactivity to be received during a period extending into the future

*The units of measurement listed are those of the International System, which replaced earlier units such as the rad (1 rad = 0.01 Gy), the rem (1 rem = 0.01 Sv), and the curie (1 Ci = 3.7 × 10^10 Bq). Modified from Phillips TL. Radiation injury. In: Wyngaarden JB, Smith LH Jr, Bennett JC, eds. *Cecil Textbook of Medicine*, 19th ed. Philadelphia: WB Saunders; 1992:2351.

TABLE 19-2 AVERAGE AMOUNTS OF IONIZING RADIATION RECEIVED ANNUALLY FROM DIFFERENT SOURCES BY A U.S. RESIDENT

SOURCE	Dose* MSV	Dose* %
Natural		
Radon and thoron	2.28	37[†]
Cosmic	0.33	5
Terrestrial	0.21	3
Internal	0.29	5
Total natural	3.11	50
Artificial		
Computed tomography	1.47	24
X-ray diagnosis	0.33	5
Nuclear medicine	0.77	12
Interventional fluoroscopy	0.43	7
Consumer products	0.13	<0.3
Occupational	0.005	<0.3
Miscellaneous[‡]	<0.1	<0.3
Total artificial	3.138	50
Total natural and artificial	6.248	100

*Average effective dose.
†Average effective dose to bronchial epithelium.
‡Department of Energy, industrial, security, educational, research, and transportation facilities.
Modified from National Council on Radiation Protection and Measurements (NCRP). *Ionizing Radiation Exposure of the Population of the United States*. NCRP Report No. 160. Bethesda, MD: National Council on Radiation Protection and Measurements; 2009.

---

nuclear weapons, conventional explosives ("dirty bombs"), or other means may be used to disperse hazardous amounts of radioactivity.

Also of ongoing public health concern is the risk of cancer among the general population from exposure to ionizing radiation. Although no more than 3% of all cancers in the general population are thought to result from natural background ionizing irradiation, a substantially larger percentage of lung cancers are generally attributed to indoor radon. Another concern is the risk of heritable abnormalities resulting from the mutagenic and clastogenic effects of radiation, which have yet to be observed in humans but are well documented in other organisms.

Prenatal irradiation can also cause death, malformations, cataracts, mental retardation, impairment of growth, and behavioral disorders, depending on the dose and the developmental stage of the embryo at the time of exposure. Hence, special precautions are taken to avoid exposure of the embryo to irradiation.

PATHOBIOLOGY

The biologic effects of ionizing radiation result from damage to DNA and other vital molecules by locally deposited energy. Doses of ionizing radiation are therefore measured in terms of energy deposition (Table 19-1).

All humans are exposed continuously to natural background ionizing radiation from (1) cosmic rays; (2) radium and other radioactive elements in the earth's crust; (3) potassium 40, carbon 14, and other radionuclides normally present in human tissues; and (4) inhaled radon and its daughter elements (Table 19-2). In people residing at mile-high elevations, such as Denver, Colorado, the contribution from cosmic rays may be increased twofold; at jet aircraft altitudes, it may be increased more than 100-fold, exceeding 0.005 mSv/hour (1 Sv = 100 rem). Likewise, in regions where the earth's crust is rich in radium, the contribution from this radionuclide may be increased.

Among man-made sources of radiation, the largest is the use of x-rays and other radiographic procedures in medical diagnosis. Smaller amounts of radiation are also received from radioactive minerals in building materials, phosphate fertilizers, and crushed rock; radiation-emitting components of television sets, smoke detectors, and other consumer products; radioactive fallout from atomic weapons; and nuclear power.

Workers in various occupations are exposed to additional doses of ionizing radiation, depending on their job assignments and working conditions. The average annual effective dose received by monitored radiation workers in the United States is less than 1 mSv, and less than 1% of such workers approach the maximal permissible dose limit (50 mSv) in any given year.

Pathogenesis

Ionizing radiation, colliding randomly with atoms and molecules in its path, gives rise to ions and free radicals, which break chemical bonds, cause other molecular alterations, and can ultimately injure the absorbing cell and its neighbors. Any molecule can be altered, but DNA is the critical biologic target because of the limited redundancy of its genetic information. A dose of radiation large enough to kill the average dividing cell (2 Sv) causes hundreds of lesions in its DNA molecules. Most such lesions are reparable, but those produced by a densely ionizing radiation (e.g., proton or α particle) are generally less reparable than those produced by a sparsely ionizing radiation (e.g., x-ray or γ-ray).

Unrepaired or misrepaired damage to DNA may be expressed in the form of mutations, the frequency of which approximates 10^{-5} to 10^{-6} per locus per sievert. Because the mutation rate tends to increase in proportion to the dose, it is inferred that a single ionizing particle traversing a genetic target may suffice to cause a mutation. Radiation damage can also cause changes in chromosome number and structure, the yields of which are characterized

TABLE 19-3   SYMPTOMS, THERAPY, AND PROGNOSIS OF WHOLE BODY IONIZING RADIATION INJURY

	0-1 SV	1-2 SV	2-6 SV	6-10 SV	10-20 SV	>50 SV
Therapeutic needs	None	Observation	Specific treatment	Possible treatment	Palliative	Palliative
Vomiting	None	5-50%	>3 Gy, 100%	100%	100%	100%
Time to nausea, vomiting	—	3 hr	2 hr	1 hr	30 min	<30 min
Main locus of injury	None	Lymphocytes	Bone marrow	Bone marrow	Small bowel	Brain
Symptoms and signs	—	Moderate leukopenia, epilation	Leukopenia, hemorrhage, epilation	Leukopenia, hemorrhage, epilation	Diarrhea, fever, electrolyte imbalance	Ataxia, coma, convulsions
Critical period	—	—	4-6 wk	4-6 wk	5-14 days	1-4 hr
Therapy	Reassurance	Observation	Transfusion of granulocytes, platelets	Transfusion, antibiotics, bone marrow transplantation	Fluids and salts, possible bone marrow transplantation	Palliative
Prognosis	Excellent	Excellent	Guarded	Guarded	Poor	Hopeless
Lethality	0	0	0-80%	80-100%	100%	100%
Time of death	—	—	2 mo	1-2 mo	2 wk	1-2 days
Cause of death	—	—	Infection, hemorrhage	Hemorrhage, infection, pneumonitis	Enteritis, infection	Cerebral edema

Modified from Phillips TL. Radiation injury. In: Wyngaarden JB, Smith LH Jr, Bennett JC, eds. *Cecil Textbook of Medicine*, 19th ed. Philadelphia: WB Saunders; 1992:2354.

well enough so that their frequency in lymphocytes can serve as a biologic dosimeter.

Radiation damage to genes, chromosomes, and other vital organelles may kill cells, especially dividing cells, which are radiosensitive as a class. Measured in terms of proliferative capacity, the survival of dividing cells tends to decrease exponentially with increasing dose; rapid exposure to 1 to 2 Sv generally reduces the surviving population of such cells by about 50%. Except for lymphocytes and oocytes, which tend to die in interphase, most cells killed by irradiation die in mitosis.

Although the killing of cells is a stochastic process, too few cells are killed by a dose less than 0.5 Sv to cause clinically detectable injury in most organs, other than the testis and organs of the embryo. The killing of dividing progenitor cells, if sufficiently extensive, can interfere with the orderly replacement of senescent cells, especially in tissues such as the epidermis, bone marrow, and intestinal epithelium, which are normally characterized by high rates of cell turnover. The timing of the resulting atrophy varies, depending on the cell population dynamics within the tissue in question; in organs such as the liver and vascular endothelium, which are characterized by slow cell turnover, expression of the injury is delayed. Also, if the volume of tissue exposed is small or if the dose is accumulated slowly enough, the effects of irradiation may be counteracted in part by adaptive responses and by compensatory regenerative hyperplasia of surviving cells.

CLINICAL MANIFESTATIONS

Ionizing radiation injuries encompass a diversity of tissue reactions that vary markedly in their dose-response relationships, manifestations, timing, and prognosis. Except for mutagenic and carcinogenic effects, the reactions generally result from the killing of sizable numbers of cells in the exposed tissues and are not detectable unless the dose of radiation exceeds a substantial threshold. For this reason, the reactions are called *nonstochastic* (or *deterministic*) effects. In contrast, the mutagenic and carcinogenic effects of radiation are presumed to have no thresholds and are considered to be *stochastic* in nature. The existing data do not exclude the possibility, however, that the latter effects may have thresholds in the millisievert dose range, and the existence of adaptive responses to radiation (e.g., DNA repair processes) has been interpreted by some observers to support the hypothesis that the net effects of small doses may be beneficial (radiation hormesis).

Tissues in which cells proliferate rapidly are generally the first to exhibit radiation injury. In such tissues, mitotic inhibition and cytologic abnormalities may be detectable immediately after irradiation, whereas ulceration, fibrosis, and other degenerative changes may not appear until months or years later.

Skin

After rapid exposure to a dose of 6 Sv or more, erythema typically appears within 1 day, lasts a few hours, and is followed 2 to 4 weeks later by one or more waves of deeper and more prolonged erythema and epilation. Brief exposure to a dose greater than 10 to 20 Sv may cause transepithelial injury,

with moist desquamation, necrosis, and ulceration within 2 to 4 weeks. The ensuing fibrosis of the underlying dermis and vasculature may lead to atrophy and a second wave of ulceration months or years later.

Bone Marrow and Lymphoid Tissue

A dose of 2 to 3 Sv delivered rapidly to the whole body destroys enough lymphocytes to depress the lymphocyte count and immune response within hours. Such a dose also can damage enough hematopoietic cells to cause profound leukopenia and thrombocytopenia within 3 to 5 weeks. If the dose exceeds 5 Sv, fatal infection and hemorrhage are likely to result (Table 19-3).

Intestine

The killing of epithelial stem cells is sufficiently extensive after an acute dose of 10 Sv to cause rapid denudation of the overlying intestinal villi. If the area affected is large, death from a fatal dysentery-like syndrome may ensue within days.

Respiratory Tract

Rapid exposure of the lung to a dose of 6 to 10 Sv damages alveolar cells and the pulmonary vasculature sufficiently to result in acute pneumonitis within 1 to 3 months. If extensive, the process may lead to fatal respiratory failure within 6 months or pulmonary fibrosis and cor pulmonale months or years later.

Gonads

Spermatozoa are relatively radioresistant, but spermatogonia are highly radiosensitive; a dose of 0.15 Sv delivered rapidly to both testes causes oligospermia after a latent period of about 6 weeks, and a dose of 2 to 4 Sv may cause permanent sterility. Oocytes also are radiosensitive; a dose of 1.5 to 2 Sv delivered to both ovaries causes temporary sterility, and a larger dose causes permanent sterility, depending on the woman's age at the time of exposure.

Lens of the Eye

Acute exposure of the lens to more than 0.5 Sv may lead to a microscopic posterior polar opacity within months, and 2 to 3 Sv received in a single brief exposure or 5.5 to 14 Sv accumulated over months may result in a vision-impairing cataract.

Other Tissues and Organs

Other tissues and organs, except in the embryo, are relatively less radiosensitive. All tissues, however, are more radiosensitive when they are rapidly growing.

Whole Body Radiation Injury

Brief exposure of a major part of the body to more than 1 Sv may cause acute radiation syndrome, which is characterized by (1) an initial prodromal stage of malaise, anorexia, nausea, and vomiting; (2) an ensuing latent period; (3) a second (main) phase of illness; and (4) either recovery or death (see Table

19-3). The main phase of the illness usually takes one of four primary forms—hematologic, gastrointestinal, neurovascular, or pulmonary—depending on the size and anatomic distribution of the dose.

Localized or Regional Radiation Injury

In contrast to acute radiation syndrome, the manifestations of which are dramatic and relatively prompt, the reaction to localized irradiation in most tissues tends to evolve more slowly and does not produce symptoms or signs unless the volume of irradiated tissue or the dose is large. Injury produced by a radionuclide follows the anatomic distribution of the radionuclide and its emitted radiation, which may be influenced by the physicochemical state in which the radionuclide is encountered and its portal of entry into the body.

Heritable (Genetic) Effects of Radiation

Radiation-induced heritable mutations and chromosome abnormalities are well documented in other organisms but have yet to be observed in humans. Intensive study of more than 76,000 children of Japanese atomic bomb survivors has failed to detect definite evidence of heritable radiation effects in terms of untoward outcomes of pregnancy, neonatal death, malignant neoplasms, balanced chromosome rearrangements, sex chromosome aneuploidy, alterations in serum or erythrocyte protein phenotypes, changes in gender ratio, or disturbances in growth and development. On the basis of the existing evidence, it is inferred that a dose of at least 1 Sv is required to double the rate of heritable mutations in human germ cells and that, consequently, less than 1% of all genetically determined disease is attributable to natural background irradiation.

Carcinogenic Effects of Radiation

Many but not all types of benign and malignant growths are inducible by irradiation; however, these induced growths characteristically take years or decades to appear and possess no features distinguishing them from growths resulting from other causes. With few exceptions, such growths are detectable only after relatively large doses (>0.5 Sv) and vary in frequency based on the type of neoplasm and the age and gender of the exposed population. Because the existing data are insufficient to describe the dose-incidence relationship precisely or to define how long after irradiation the risk of cancer remains elevated in an exposed population, assessment of the risks of low-level irradiation must be based on models incorporating assumptions about these parameters (Table 19-4). Assessments depend heavily on findings in atomic bomb survivors, whose overall incidence of cancer can be inferred to increase as a linear nonthreshold function of their radiation dose. These estimates cannot be used to predict the risk of cancer attributable to a dose accumulated during weeks, months, or years, however, because experiments with laboratory animals have shown the carcinogenic potency of x-rays or γ-rays to decrease by a factor of 2 to 10 if the exposure is sufficiently prolonged. Furthermore, such estimates represent averages for a nominal population of males and females of all ages, whereas the estimates for breast cancer in women and for thyroid cancer in persons irradiated during childhood are substantially higher than those shown.

Effects on Lifespan

Mortality from cardiovascular, respiratory, and other non-neoplastic diseases as well as from various forms of cancer is increased in heavily irradiated populations. In lightly irradiated populations, however, these effects are not evident, and survival appears to be enhanced in some instances. This finding has prompted some to infer that the effects of small doses may be beneficial on balance (radiation hormesis), but this hypothesis is highly controversial and has yet to be validated.

Effects of Prenatal Irradiation

The embryo is especially vulnerable to death if it is exposed before implantation; it is susceptible to malformations and other developmental disturbances if it is exposed during subsequent stages of organogenesis, and it is sensitive throughout intrauterine life to the carcinogenic effects of radiation. Among the various disturbances in growth and development, the dose-dependent increase in the frequency of severe mental retardation and the dose-dependent decrease in IQ test scores in atomic bomb survivors who were irradiated between the 8th and 15th weeks and, to a lesser extent, the 16th and 25th weeks after conception are particularly noteworthy.

DIAGNOSIS

Any facility likely to encounter radiation injuries should be able to cope with these injuries and should have personnel on call who are trained and equipped appropriately to do so. At the outset, to evaluate the dose and determine whether the patient has been contaminated with radionuclides, the nature of the exposure and any measurements by film badges or other detectors should be reviewed in detail. If exposure to radionuclides is known or suspected, radioactivity measurements of the whole body, skin, other tissue, blood, urine, and body fluid may be indicated to identify the isotope and evaluate the dose. Malaise, anorexia, nausea, and vomiting suggest a total body dose larger than 1 Sv, as do signs of erythema, hemorrhage, or infection

---

TABLE 19-4 ESTIMATED LIFETIME RISK OF VARIOUS CANCERS ATTRIBUTABLE TO 0.1-SV RAPID IRRADIATION

TYPE OR SITE OF CANCER	Excess Cancer Deaths Per 100,000	
	No.	%*
Lung	205	3
Leukemia	86	14
Breast	73	2
Colon	61	3
Urinary bladder	25	5
Ovary	24	2
Stomach	22	4
Thyroid	8	16
Other	109	2
Total	613	3

*Percentage increase (rounded off) in the expected risk of death from cancer of that organ in a nonirradiated population.
Modified from National Research Council, National Academy of Sciences. *Health Risks from Exposure to Low Levels of Ionizing Radiation*. BEIR VII, phase 2. Washington, DC: National Academy Press; 2006.

TREATMENT

In managing radiation injury, good medical judgment and first aid are the priorities. Even a heavily irradiated patient should be evaluated for other types of injury, such as burns, mechanical trauma, and smoke inhalation. If radioactive contamination is known or suspected, rescue and medical personnel who handle the patient should wear gloves and other protective clothing and should take precautions to isolate all contaminated objects.

Apart from symptomatic treatment, management of the hematologic form of acute radiation syndrome is similar to that of pancytopenic leukemia, including reverse isolation, antibiotics to combat infection, granulocyte and platelet transfusions as needed, and intravenous fluids as required to combat dehydration and electrolyte loss (Chapter 189). Colony-stimulating factors and interleukin may be beneficial in patients exposed to 6 to 10 Sv. Bone marrow transplantation (Chapter 181) may be life-saving after a dose of 7 to 10 Sv if a suitably matched donor is available; therefore, specimens of marrow and peripheral blood should be obtained for tissue typing as early as possible.

For localized injuries, treatment depends on the anatomic location and severity. Dry and moist desquamation of the skin, which is the most common injury requiring treatment, is usually managed adequately by simple cleansing. Large or ulcerated lesions should be covered with lanolin and closed dressings that are changed regularly. Severe injuries may require resection of necrotic tissue and skin grafting.

In the event of radioactive contamination, steps should be taken to minimize the uptake and retention of the isotope. Contaminated areas should be rinsed; the mouth, nose, and bronchial tree should be lavaged; and the gastrointestinal tract should be purged, if necessary. Additional measures to inhibit the uptake and retention of specific radionuclides may be indicated. Radioactive iodine may be released during a radiation accident or nuclear detonation and can pose a significant risk of thyroid cancer, especially in children. Stable potassium iodide should be administered to potentially exposed persons (except those who are sensitive to iodine) to inhibit the uptake of radioactive iodine by the thyroid. Its protective effect persists for about 24 hours, and the optimal effect is achieved when potassium iodide is given before exposure or concurrently with exposure. The recommended dose varies, depending on the recipient's age, expected level of thyroid exposure to radioactivity, and pregnancy or lactation status; recommendations range from 130 mg for adults to 16 mg for neonates.

in the skin, conjunctivae, or mucous membranes. The extent of lymphopenia during the first 24 hours varies with the size of the total body dose. Although the granulocyte count may be elevated temporarily during the first 24 to 48 hours, the rapidity with which it and the platelet count fall in the ensuing 2 to 4 weeks also varies with the total body dose. Cytogenetic analysis of cultured lymphocytes for chromosome aberrations can be another useful index of exposure.

PREVENTION

Because the mutagenic and carcinogenic effects of ionizing radiation may have no thresholds, unnecessary exposure should be avoided, and any doses to radiation workers and patients should be kept as low as possible, with particular care taken not to exceed the relevant maximal permissible doses. Facilities using radiation or radiation sources should be designed and equipped appropriately and should provide specialized training and supervision for all workers who may be occupationally exposed. Because indoor radon and computed tomography account for the bulk of the public's exposure to ionizing radiation, measures to limit excessive doses from these sources are warranted.

PROGNOSIS

After a total body dose of 2 Sv or less, survival is probable with little or no treatment; in the 2- to 10-Sv range, appropriate treatment can afford a high rate of survival. If the injury is localized, the prognosis depends on the nature and severity of the reaction. Although recovery is the rule after minor, acute reactions, delayed reactions tend to be irreversible and progressive.

● NONIONIZING RADIATION INJURY
Ultraviolet Radiation

The ultraviolet (UV) radiation spectrum (see Fig. 19-1) is subdivided, for convenience, into three bands: UVA, or "black light," 315 to 400 nm; UVB, 280 to 315 nm; and UVC, which is germicidal, 200 to 280 nm. UV radiation does not penetrate deeply into human tissues, so the injuries it causes are confined chiefly to the skin and eyes.

EPIDEMIOLOGY

The largest source of UV radiation for the public is sunlight, which varies in intensity with latitude, elevation, and season. Important man-made sources include sun and tanning lamps, welding arcs, plasma torches, germicidal and black-light lamps, electric arc furnaces, hot-metal operations, mercury-vapor lamps, and some lasers. Low-intensity sources include fluorescent lamps and certain laboratory equipment.

Reactions of the skin to UV radiation, common among fair-skinned people, include sunburn, skin cancer (basal cell and squamous cell carcinoma and, to a lesser extent, melanoma), aging of the skin, solar elastosis, and solar keratosis. Injuries of the eye include photokeratitis, which may result from brief exposure to a high-intensity UV radiation source ("welder's flash") or more prolonged exposure to intense sunlight ("snow blindness"); cortical cataract; and pterygium.

PATHOBIOLOGY

The effects of UV radiation are primarily attributable to its absorption in DNA; pyrimidine dimers are produced and cause mutational changes in exposed cells. Sensitivity to UV radiation may be increased by DNA repair defects (as in xeroderma pigmentosum), by agents (e.g., caffeine) that inhibit repair enzymes, and by photosensitizing agents (e.g., psoralens, sulfonamides, tetracyclines, nalidixic acid, sulfonylureas, thiazides, phenothiazines, furocoumarins, and coal tar) that produce UV radiation–absorbing DNA photoproducts. The carcinogenic action of UV radiation is mediated through direct effects on the exposed cells and depression of local immunity.

CLINICAL MANIFESTATIONS

UVB in sunlight, although far less intense than UVA, plays a more important role in sunburn and skin carcinogenesis, but UVA also contributes to skin carcinogenesis, tanning, some photosensitivity reactions, and aging of the skin.

TREATMENT AND PREVENTION   Rx

Excessive exposure to sunlight or other sources of UV radiation should be avoided, especially in fair-skinned individuals. Protective clothing, UV radiation–screening lotions or creams, and UV radiation–blocking sunglasses should be used. To protect occupationally exposed workers, the American Conference of Governmental Industrial Hygienists has recommended 8-hour exposure limits for the unprotected eye that range from 3 mJ/cm^2 to 10^6 mJ/cm^2, depending on the wavelength of the radiation (note that 1 J/second = 1 W). The protective layer of ozone in the stratosphere is being depleted globally by chlorofluorocarbons and other air pollutants, and every 1% decrease in ozone is expected to increase the UV radiation reaching the earth by 1 to 2% and thus increase the rates of nonmelanotic skin cancer by 2 to 6%.

Visible Light

Visible light consists of electromagnetic waves varying in wavelength from 380 nm (violet) to 760 nm (red) (see Fig. 19-1).

PATHOBIOLOGY

Bright, continuously visible light normally elicits an aversion response to protect the eye against injury, so few sources of light other than a laser or the sun during a solar eclipse are large or bright enough to burn the retina under normal viewing conditions.

Photochemical reactions in the retina from sustained exposure to intensities exceeding 0.1 mW/cm^2, such as can result from fixing on a bright source of light, may suffice to produce photochemical blue-light injury. Brief exposure of the retina to intensities exceeding 10 W/cm^2, depending on image size, may cause a retinal burn.

CLINICAL MANIFESTATIONS

Too little illumination can cause eyestrain or seasonal affective disorder, whereas too bright a light can injure the retina (Chapter 431).

TREATMENT AND PREVENTION   Rx

Common sense usually suffices to prevent excessive exposure of the retina to light. However, in situations involving potential exposure to high-intensity sources, such as carbon arcs or lasers, appropriate training, proper design of equipment, and protective eye shields are important.

Infrared Radiation

Infrared radiation consists of electromagnetic waves ranging in wavelength from 7×10^{-5} m to 3×10^{-2} m. The injuries caused by infrared radiation are chiefly burns of the skin and cataracts of the lens of the eye.

EPIDEMIOLOGY

Potentially hazardous sources include furnaces, ovens, welding arcs, molten glass, molten metal, and heating lamps. The warning sensation of heat usually prompts aversion in time to prevent burning of the skin by infrared radiation; however, the lens of the eye is vulnerable because it lacks the ability to sense or dissipate heat.

CLINICAL MANIFESTATIONS

Glassblowers, blacksmiths, oven operators, and people working around heating and drying lamps are at increased risk of infrared radiation–induced cataracts (Chapter 431).

TREATMENT AND PREVENTION   Rx

Control of infrared radiation hazards requires appropriate shielding of its sources, training of potentially exposed persons, and use of protective clothing and goggles.

Microwave and Radio Frequency Radiation

Microwave and radio frequency radiation consists of electromagnetic waves ranging in frequency from about 3 kHz to 300 GHz.

EPIDEMIOLOGY

Sources of microwave and radio frequency radiation are used widely in radar, televisions, cellular phones, radios, other telecommunications systems, various industrial operations (e.g., heating, welding, and melting of metals; processing of wood and plastic; high-temperature plasma), household appliances (e.g., microwave ovens), and medical applications (e.g., diathermy and hyperthermia).

PATHOBIOLOGY

The biologic effects of microwave and radio frequency radiation are primarily thermal in nature, but there is growing evidence that some effects may be elicited through nonthermal mechanisms, such as DNA damage, as well. Because of the deep penetration of these types of radiation, the cutaneous burns they cause tend to involve dermal and subcutaneous tissues and to heal slowly.

CLINICAL MANIFESTATIONS

Isolated cases of skin burns, thermal injury to deeper tissues, and death from hyperthermia have been caused by industrial microwave and radio frequency radiation sources. Burns may also result from faulty or improperly used household microwave ovens and from the overexposure of patients with impaired cutaneous pain and temperature senses, which usually warn of impending injury. Other effects reported in the literature but not yet conclusively documented include cataract of the lens, impairment of fertility, developmental disturbances, neurobehavioral abnormalities, depression of immunity, and increased risk for certain cancers. Microwave and radio frequency radiation also can interfere with cardiac pacemakers (Chapter 66) and other medical devices.

TREATMENT AND PREVENTION

Microwave and radio frequency radiation sources must be designed and shielded properly, and potentially exposed persons, especially those with cardiac pacemakers or other sensitive devices, must be trained and supervised properly. In general, detectable heating of tissue requires microwave and radio frequency radiation power densities greater than 10 W/cm^2; avoidance of such exposure, as prescribed by existing federal standards, suffices to prevent such injuries. Further research is needed, however, to address the potential effects of long-term exposure, such as may result from repeated use of mobile phones, especially in children.

Extremely Low Frequency Electromagnetic Fields

Extremely low frequency electromagnetic fields range in frequency from 1 to 3000 Hz, including the 50- to 60-Hz fields associated with alternating currents in electric power distribution systems and appliances. Exposure to such fields is not known to be hazardous, but data suggesting that it may cause reproductive abnormalities and carcinogenic effects have aroused public health concern.

EPIDEMIOLOGY

The earth is surrounded by a naturally occurring electromagnetic field ranging from the low end of the extremely low frequency region to radio frequencies that exist briefly as a result of lightning discharges. Localized electromagnetic fields also are generated by electric power lines, transformers, motors, household appliances, video display tubes, and various medical devices, notably nuclear magnetic resonance imaging systems. These localized fields are generally stronger than naturally existing ones; electromagnetic field flux densities near common household appliances may range up to 270 mG, compared with the average value of 0.6 mG for the earth's magnetic field.

PATHOBIOLOGY

Evaluation of epidemiologic data is complicated by the lack of any known biologic basis for the effects of extremely low frequency electromagnetic fields on tissue, especially because the currents emanating from normal nerve and muscle activity are far stronger than the currents attributable to 1- to 10-mG external 60-Hz fields. Nevertheless, such fields have been reported to influence ion transport, melatonin secretion, and tumor promotion in some model systems.

CLINICAL MANIFESTATIONS

Exceptionally strong fields may affect electrically active tissues (nerves, neuromusculature, heart) and cardiac pacemakers and may raise body temperature. Conflicting epidemiologic studies have evaluated several possibilities:

that residential exposure of children to weaker electromagnetic fields may increase their risk of leukemia, that occupational exposure of male utility workers may increase their risk of brain cancer and leukemia, and that chronic exposure of pregnant women to video display tubes may increase their risk of miscarriage and of bearing children with birth defects. None of these links has been established.

TREATMENT AND PREVENTION

Persons with pacemakers should avoid electromagnetic fields stronger than 0.5 mT, which exist around transformers, accelerators, nuclear magnetic resonance imaging systems, and other electrical devices; areas containing such fields should be posted with warning signs. Exposure of workers should be limited in accordance with national guidelines.

Ultrasound

Although frequently classified with nonionizing radiation, ultrasound consists of mechanical vibrations at inaudibly high frequencies ($\geq$16 kHz) and is not a component of the electromagnetic spectrum.

EPIDEMIOLOGY

High-power, low-frequency ultrasound is used widely in science and industry for cleaning, degreasing, plastic welding, liquid extracting, atomizing, homogenizing, and emulsifying operations and in medicine for lithotripsy. Low-power, high-frequency ultrasound is used widely in analytic work and in medical diagnosis (e.g., ultrasonography).

PATHOBIOLOGY

The biologic effects of high-power ultrasound are similar in mechanism to those of mechanical vibration-localized heating, agitation, and fragmentation of tissues.

CLINICAL MANIFESTATIONS

Deleterious effects from prolonged exposure to high-power ultrasound include headache, malaise, tinnitus, vertigo, hypersensitivity to light and sound, and peripheral neuritis. Similar complaints may result from excessive exposure to high-frequency ultrasound through body contact with the source. However, adverse effects have not been shown to result from exposure to high-frequency ultrasound at the low power levels used in medical ultrasonography.

TREATMENT AND PREVENTION

Protection against ultrasound injury requires appropriate isolation and insulation of generating sources and proper training and ear protective devices for persons working around such sources. Yearly audiometric and neurologic examinations of workers are advisable.

SUGGESTED READINGS

American Conference of Governmental Industrial Hygienists. 2009 Threshold Limit Values and Biological Exposure Indices. Cincinnati, OH: American Conference of Governmental Industrial Hygienists; 2009. *An authoritative listing of maximal permissible occupational exposure limits for radiation of all types.*

Einstein AJ, Weiner SD, Bernheim A, et al. Multiple testing, cumulative radiation dose, and clinical indications for patients undergoing myocardial perfusion imaging. *JAMA.* 2010;304:2137-2144. *Multiple cardiac nuclear medicine tests result in substantial radiation exposure.*

Fazel R, Krumholz HM, Wang Y, et al. Exposure to low-dose ionizing radiation from medical imaging procedures. *N Engl J Med.* 2009;361:849-857. *Imaging procedures are an important source of exposure to ionizing radiation.*

International Commission on Non-Ionizing Radiation Protection. Exposure to high frequency electromagnetic fields, biological effects and health consequences (100 kHz-300 GHz). Oberschleissheim, Germany: International Commission on Non-Ionizing Radiation Protection; 2009. *Comprehensive overview of the sources, levels, and health effects of exposure to nonionizing, high-frequency electromagnetic radiation.*

20

BIOTERRORISM

JOHN G. BARTLETT

BIOLOGIC WEAPONS

DEFINITION

Weapons of mass destruction are classified as biologic, chemical, or nuclear. Biologic weapons are microbes or microbial products used for bioterrorism. The potential for mass destruction is evident from a report from the U.S. Office of Technology, which predicted that the release of 100 kg of anthrax spores upwind of Washington, DC, would cause 130,000 to 3 million deaths, matching the lethal potential of a hydrogen bomb. The Centers for Disease Control and Prevention (CDC) is responsible for orchestrating the public health response to a bioterrorism threat or attack in the United States, and the FBI is responsible for the criminal aspects. The CDC has reviewed and classified various potential bioweapons based on public health impact and the properties of such weapons in terms of health consequences, ease of delivery to large populations, potential for civil disruption, and sustainability by person-to-person transmission (Table 20-1). Those with the "best" potential (category A agents) include anthrax, smallpox, plague, botulism, tularemia, and selected viruses that cause viral hemorrhagic fever (Tables 20-1 and 20-2). Of these, the two agents that stand out are anthrax and smallpox.

Despite the enormous potential for mass destruction, the actual application of bioterrorism has been quite limited. During World War II there were major bioweapons programs in the United States, the Soviet Union, Japan, and Germany, but only Japan used its program in any well-established way. The Soviet Union had the largest bioweapons program, with approximately 50 facilities and 60,000 employees. In 1972 the Biologic and Toxin Weapons Convention, which was established to eliminate the threat of bioterrorism, was signed by 140 nations, including the United States and the Soviet Union. The subsequent destiny of the enormous volume of products (e.g., smallpox virus, botulinum toxin, anthrax spores) and most of the highly skilled

scientists in this area is largely unknown. Current estimates are that many nations continue to harbor bioweapons programs.

In addition to these large-scale national programs, there is the potential for individuals or dissident groups to use bioweapons. For example, in 1984 a religious cult in Oregon attempted to influence an election by contaminating restaurant salad bars with *Salmonella* to reduce voter turnout; the effort resulted in 751 cases of salmonellosis, but the election was not affected. Aum Shinrykio, a Japanese cult, was responsible for the release of sarin nerve gas, which killed 10 and injured 6000 in Tokyo.

More recently, there were 22 cases of anthrax in the United States during a 2-month period in 2001. Of the 22 cases, 20 were traced directly to six contaminated letters sent to different locations, all with the same molecular type of *Bacillus anthracis*. Some cases were cutaneous because the material in the letters was milled to a relatively large particle size that contaminated surfaces via gravity. By contrast, letters with anthrax that was milled to nearly the size of a single spore resulted in particles that were aerosolized and inhaled, causing inhalational anthrax. During this 2-month period, the CDC assigned 1000 personnel to deal with anthrax issues, prophylactic ciprofloxacin or doxycycline was delivered to 10,000 people who were exposed or possibly exposed, the New York City Health Department fielded more than 15,000 telephone calls, there were hundreds of false threats, and a hospital in Boston was closed for decontamination because of a white powder on the floor that turned out to be from a sugar donut. Ultimately, 11 cases of cutaneous anthrax and 11 of inhalational anthrax were diagnosed. Five of the 11 patients with inhalational anthrax died, despite good medical care. This experience clearly demonstrated the potential impact of a bioterrorism attack on a nation's citizenry.

The next important event was the decision to resume smallpox vaccinations in December 2002. The vaccine was mandatory for military personnel and voluntary for frontline medical personnel who were designated members of smallpox response teams. The concern was that smallpox is an ideal bioterrorism agent because vaccinations had been discontinued and the natural disease was considered to have been eradicated in 1977. The disease is contagious, highly lethal, and largely untreatable. Risk was difficult to assess, although the United States and Russia were the only countries known to have viable smallpox. The restarted vaccine program was hampered by the fact that few contemporary health care personnel knew how to deliver it and that the prior vaccine had been associated with severe complications. Despite these concerns, the experience with about 440,000 military personnel and 36,000

TABLE 20-1	CLASSIFICATION OF BIOTERRORISM AGENTS					
	Public Health Impact		**Dissemination***			
Agent	**Disease**	**Death**	**Delivery Potential**	**Person To Person**	**Public Perception**[†]	**Special Preparation**[‡]
Smallpox (A)	+	++	+	+++	+++	+++
Anthrax (A)	++	+++	+++	0	+++	+++
Plague (A)	++	+++	++	+	++	+++
Botulism (A)	++	+++	++	0	++	+++
Viral hemorrhagic fever (A)	++	+++	+	++	+++	++
Tularemia (A)	++	++	+	0	+	+++
Viral encephalitis (B)	++	+	+	0	++	++
Q fever (B)	+	+	++	0	+	++
Brucellosis (B)	+	+	++	0	+	++
Glanders (B)	++	+++	++	0	0	++
Melioidosis (B)	+	+	++	0	0	++
Psittacosis (B)	+	+	++	0	0	+
Ricin toxin (B)	++	++	++	0	0	++
Typhus (B)	+	+	++	0	0	+
Cholera (B)	+	+	++	+/−	+++	+
Shigellosis (B)	+	+	++	+	+	+

*Potential for rapid large-scale dissemination.
[†]Need for therapeutics, surveillance, laboratory demands.
[‡]Media reports with +++ include more than 45 titles in a survey of 233 newspapers and 70 TV and radio sources.
+++ = death in >50%; ++ = death in 21 to 49%; + = death in <20%.
A = greatest potential for bioterrorism; B = less likely or less important for bioterrorism.

TABLE 20-2 CLINICAL FEATURES OF CATEGORY A AGENTS

	ANTHRAX (INHALATIONAL)	SMALLPOX	PLAGUE (PNEUMONIA)	BOTULISM	VIRAL HEMORRHAGIC FEVER
Cases in U.S. per year	0-1	0	8-10	200-300	0
Clinical features	Flulike, then shock	Fever, then characteristic rash	Pneumonia, hemoptysis	Descending paralysis and involvement of cranial nerves	Hemorrhage and fever
Diagnosis	Blood culture, chest CT	BSL-4 laboratory for virus	Blood and sputum culture	Toxin assay of blood, GI specimens; EMG	BSL-4 laboratory for virus
Mortality	40-50%	30%	10-20%	60%	Variable
Treatment*	Cipro, doxy, or levo + 2nd agent,† 60-100 days	None	Gent/strep (cipro/doxy), 10 days	Antitoxin, ventilator	Ribavirin (some) 7 days
Prevention*	Cipro/doxy	Vaccine	Cipro/doxy	None	None
Infection control	Not transmitted Vaccine	Contact and airborne precautions	Masks	Not transmitted	Contact precautions

*Doses: cipro 400 mg IV q8-12h or 500-750 mg PO bid; levo 500-750 mg IV qd or 500 mg PO qd; doxy 100 mg PO or IV bid; gent 5 mg/kg/day IM or IV; strep 1 g IM bid; ribavirin 16 mg/kg/day IV × 4 days, then 8 mg/kg/day × 3 days or 1000-1200 mg/day PO × 7.
†Imipenem 500 mg IV q6h, rifampin 600 mg IV or PO qd, chloramphenicol 1 g IV q6h, clarithromycin 500 mg PO bid, vancomycin 1 g IV bid, or clindamycin 600 mg IV q8h.
BSL-4 = Biologic Safety Level 4; cipro = ciprofloxacin; CT = computed tomography; doxy = doxycycline; EMG = electromyography; gent = gentamicin; GI = gastrointestinal; levo = levofloxacin; strep = streptomycin; ( ) = alternative to preferred.

civilian medical professionals showed almost none of the previously described serious reactions, but about 50 cases of myocarditis or pericarditis were reported.

More recent planning for bioterrorism has been based on extensive reviews of the anthrax experience of 2001, the 9/11 experience, and two large national simulated bioterrorism attacks: TOPOFF, which was a simulated anthrax attack carried out in Denver in 2000, and Dark Winter, which was a simulated smallpox attack in 2001. The responses have included the Biomedical Advanced Research Development Authority (BARDA), the Project BioShield Act of 2004, and the Pandemic and All-Hazards Preparedness Act of 2006. These initiatives collectively provide extensive resources, organizational structure, and preemptive planning for bioterrorism, but many of these efforts share challenges that are common to pandemics such as influenza and natural disasters such as earthquakes, as well as to bioterrorism. A major concern is surge capacity—the ability of the health system to accommodate a large number of patients in terms of demands for emergency care, medical beds, medical personnel, medications, and equipment such as ventilators.

ANTHRAX
DEFINITION

Infection is caused by *B. anthracis* (Chapter 302). The three recognized forms reflect the portal of entry: inhalation, cutaneous exposure, and ingestion.

EPIDEMIOLOGY

The greatest concern for bioterrorism is the inhaled form of anthrax, which results from the inhalation of *B. anthracis* spores and causes a devastating disease with a mortality rate of about 50%, even with optimal management. The last naturally occurring case of inhalational anthrax in the United States was in 1976. The largest epidemic followed an accidental release of anthrax in Sverdlovsk, Russia, in 1979 and resulted in an estimated 80 to 250 cases. Cutaneous anthrax is the usual naturally occurring zoonotic form. An average of less than 1 case per year now occurs in the United States, with about 2000 naturally occurring cases in the world each year.

PATHOBIOLOGY

When inhalational anthrax is associated with bioterrorism, spores must be milled to less than 5 μm to permit both aerosolization and inhalation. The spores are taken up by alveolar macrophages and migrate to the mediastinal lymph nodes, where they revert to vegetative forms and produce toxins. The protective antigen combines with lethal toxin and edema toxin; these toxins are thought to account for the clinical features.

CLINICAL MANIFESTATIONS

The incubation period is usually 4 to 5 days, but the range is 2 to 43 days after exposure. Inhalational anthrax is a two-stage disease. The initial symptoms are nonspecific and flulike. Features that distinguish this stage from influenza are the lack of coryza and the anticipated exposure history. The second stage

is profound sepsis with chest pain, chest compression from large pleural effusions and mediastinal expansion, multiple organ failure, obtundation, cyanosis, hypotension, and death, which may occur within hours. Cutaneous anthrax is characterized by a vesicle that progresses to an eschar associated with substantial surrounding edema, often with regional adenopathy and systemic signs of infection.

DIAGNOSIS

The diagnosis is established by recovery of *B. anthracis* from blood or the infected site. Virtually all patients with inhalational anthrax have positive blood cultures, which frequently turn positive within 12 to 16 hours if cultures were obtained before therapy. Other highly characteristic features of the disease are a chest radiograph that shows a wide mediastinum and a computed tomography scan that shows hyperdense hilar and mediastinal lymph nodes, often with large pleural effusions. A highly characteristic feature of the disease is large, bloody pleural effusions. There may or may not be a pulmonary infiltrate.

TREATMENT Rx

The most important facets of treatment of inhalational anthrax are supportive care, drainage of pleural effusions, and rapid administration of antibiotics. The drugs approved by the Food and Drug Administration (FDA) for B. anthracis are intravenous penicillin, doxycycline, ciprofloxacin, and levofloxacin (see Table 20-2). In reality, a bioterrorism event involving inhaled anthrax would result in specific recommendations from the CDC. In 2001 the preferred agents were doxycycline or ciprofloxacin combined with a second agent such as penicillin, imipenem, rifampin, chloramphenicol, clarithromycin, vancomycin, or clindamycin, based on sensitivity tests of the epidemic strain. After clinical improvement, the intravenous administration may be changed to oral agents such as ciprofloxacin, levofloxacin, or doxycycline; the total recommended duration of treatment is 60 to 100 days, presumably owing to the persistence of spores. For cutaneous anthrax the recommended treatment is also ciprofloxacin or doxycycline for a total of 60 to 100 days, based on the assumption that a patient with cutaneous anthrax may have inhaled organisms as well.

PREVENTION

In the event of bioterrorism, prophylaxis appears to be critical because the disease is highly lethal, even with antibiotic treatment, and prophylaxis is highly effective. The recommendation for prophylaxis has been oral doxycycline or ciprofloxacin for 60 to 100 days, although more recent animal studies suggest that shorter courses are effective. In fact, anthrax did not develop in any exposed people who received even a single dose of these drugs before the onset of symptoms. An FDA-approved anthrax vaccine administered in six doses to wool sorters and other workers in high-risk occupations is very effective, but other anthrax vaccines appear to be effective with fewer administrations and result in fewer adverse reactions.

PROGNOSIS

Data from the Sverdlovsk outbreak in Russia suggest a mortality rate of 60 to 87%, despite appropriate antibiotics. In the 2001 epidemic in the United States, 5 of 11 patients (45%) with inhalational anthrax died, despite aggressive management. In the fatal cases, the interval between the onset of symptoms and death averaged 3 to 4 days. Survivors had long-term disability.

SMALLPOX

DEFINITION

Smallpox is a systemic infection caused by the virus *Variola major* or *Variola minor* (Chapter 380). The assumption is that any attempt at bioterrorism with smallpox would use *V. major*, which is associated with a substantially higher mortality rate. The virus is viewed as ideal for bioterrorism because it is easy to culture, survives well in aerosols, and is lethal in 30% of cases. Furthermore, most humans are now susceptible because immunization was stopped in the United States and most of the world by 1973.

EPIDEMIOLOGY

The global campaign to eradicate smallpox was initiated in 1966, and the last naturally occurring case was reported in 1977. In 1980 the World Health Organization (WHO) declared smallpox eradicated and recommended that all laboratories destroy their stocks of variola or transfer them to one of two WHO reference laboratories, one in Moscow and the other at the CDC in Atlanta. These remaining isolates were to be destroyed in 1999, but the WHO agreed to retain the supplies in an effort to develop an attenuated vaccine and antiviral drugs. The number of countries that have this virus other than Russia and the United States is not known.

Smallpox is spread from person to person in droplets from the oral pharynx. The greatest risk is to persons within 6 to 8 feet of an infected individual, and prior epidemics have consistently shown that most cases occur in household members and hospital contacts. The secondary attack rate in unvaccinated household members is 37 to 88%. Because the disease has been eradicated, any confirmed case of smallpox implies bioterrorism.

CLINICAL MANIFESTATIONS

The incubation period is usually 12 to 14 days. Initial symptoms are high fever, malaise, prostration, headache, and backache. These symptoms are severe, and most patients are bedridden. The rash usually appears on day 3 as a maculopapular eruption that subsequently evolves through the vesicular and then pustular stages; at 2 to 3 weeks it forms scabs that separate and leave a characteristic pitted scar. The rash begins on the face and forearms and then spreads to the trunk and legs. Pustules have a characteristic firm, round, deep-seated appearance and measure 7 to 10 mm in diameter. Lesions are more dense on the face and extremities, all are in the same stage, and the palms and soles may be involved. An important issue in terms of disease control is that transmission takes place during the rash phase and not during the early pre-rash period of illness.

DIAGNOSIS

Laboratory diagnosis requires fluid collected from a typical vesicular or pustular lesion, preferably by a vaccinated person with appropriate protection. Laboratory testing must be done in a maximum containment facility (Biologic Safety Level 4 [BSL-4] laboratory); tissue culture is used to recover the virus, and polymerase chain reaction and restriction fragment length polymorphism are used to characterize the viral strain. For the clinician, the major issue is the distinction of smallpox from chickenpox or other illnesses characterized by a vesicular rash (Table 20-3). With chickenpox (Chapter 383), the lesions are more superficial, have a centripetal distribution with greater involvement of the trunk and face, and are not all at the same stage of evolution. Patients are also less seriously ill.

Other conditions in the differential diagnosis for a vesicular or pustular rash include disseminated herpes zoster or herpes simplex (Chapter 382), drug eruptions (Chapter 448), erythema multiforme (Chapter 446), enteroviral infection (Chapter 387), secondary syphilis (Chapter 327), monkeypox (Chapter 380), molluscum contagiosum (Chapter 446), and generalized vaccinia. With a generalized maculopapular rash, the differential diagnosis includes measles (Chapter 375), rubella (Chapter 376), drug rash, erythema multiforme, and scarlet fever (Chapter 297).

TABLE 20-3   MAJOR AND MINOR CRITERIA FOR SMALLPOX AND PRIORITY FOR REPORTING TO CENTERS FOR DISEASE CONTROL AND PREVENTION

MAJOR CRITERIA

Fever (>38.3° C) 1-4 days before the onset of rash plus one of the following: headache, prostration, chills, vomiting, abdominal pain
Typical smallpox lesions: firm, round, deep-seated vesicles or pustules with evolution to umbilicated or confluent
Lesions at same stage of development

MINOR CRITERIA

Centrifugal distribution of rash (face and extremities)
First lesions on oral mucosa, palate, face, and arms
Patient appears toxic or moribund
Slow evolution of lesions—each stage lasts at least 1-2 days
Lesions on palms and soles

REPORTING PRIORITY

Report immediately: (1) febrile prodrome, (2) classic smallpox lesions, and (3) lesions in the same stage of development (all 3 present)
Urgent assessment: (1) febrile prodrome and one other major criterion *or* (2) febrile prodrome plus ≥4 minor criteria
Manage as clinically indicated: febrile prodrome and ≥4 minor criteria

---

TREATMENT   Rx

There is no therapy with established merit.

PREVENTION

Vaccination with vaccinia (cowpox) virus before exposure provides significant protection against smallpox. Persons in whom a vesicle or pustule develops or who have a pitted scar at a previous vaccination site have a "take" indicating an immune response. The duration of protection is not well known. Vaccination also provides some protection when given within 4 days after exposure because the immune response to vaccinia is faster than it is to smallpox. The major goal in the event of anticipated bioterrorism is to vaccinate persons with anticipated risks, such as military personnel or hospital-based smallpox response teams. In an outbreak, the highest priority would be first responders, household contacts, and others who have face-to-face contact with patients after the onset of fever.

Vaccination was associated with substantial risk when it was given routinely before 1973. The major currently recognized vaccine-associated complications (Chapter 17) include (1) postvaccinal encephalitis, which is probably an immune reaction; (2) progressive vaccinia, which is a progressive and rapidly lethal complication of disseminated vaccinia seen primarily in patients with defective cell-mediated immunity; (3) generalized vaccinia caused by dissemination of vaccinia; (4) accidental inoculation of other anatomic sites or other persons, usually bedmates; and (5) eczema vaccinatum in patients with a current or past history of eczema or atopic dermatitis. Complications that result from uncontrolled growth of vaccinia can be treated with vaccinia immune globulin. During the recent experience with smallpox vaccination in more than 500,000 U.S. military personnel and health care workers, the frequency of these adverse reactions was modest, and no deaths were recorded. However, another major complication—myoperi-carditis—was recognized; it was most common with primary vaccination, self-limited, and probably immune mediated.

PLAGUE

DEFINITION

Plague refers to infection by *Yersinia pestis* (Chapter 320).

EPIDEMIOLOGY

Approximately 10 cases of plague occur in the United States annually, but the pneumonic form of disease, which would be anticipated in the event of bioterrorism, is rare, with only about 7 cases in the past 50 years. Thus, any case of pneumonic plague, particularly if acquired in urban areas and outside endemic areas, should arouse suspicion of bioterrorism. An important clinical clue to the diagnosis is severe pneumonia associated with hemoptysis. It is known

TABLE 20-4 VIRAL HEMORRHAGIC FEVERS

AGENT	SOURCE	VECTOR	CLINICAL FEATURES	P-P TX	TREATMENT	MORTALITY (%)
Ebola	Africa	Not known	Fever, rash, DIC	Yes	Supportive	50-90
Marburg	Africa	Not known	Fever, rash	Yes	Supportive	20-70
Lassa fever	Africa	Rodent	Fever, conjunctivitis	Yes	Ribavirin	15-20
New World Arenaviridae	South America	Rodent	GI symptoms, conjunctivitis, adenopathy	Yes	Ribavirin	15-30
Rift Valley fever	Africa, Saudi Arabia	Mosquito	Fever, jaundice, photophobia	No	Ribavirin	<1
Yellow fever	Africa, Americas	Mosquito	Fever, jaundice, conjunctivitis	No	Supportive	20
Omsk hemorrhagic fever	Central Asia	Tick	Fever, cough, conjunctivitis, adenopathy	No	Supportive	1-10
Kyasanur	India	Tick	Biphasic encephalitis	No	Supportive	3-10

DIC = disseminated intravascular coagulation; GI = gastrointestinal; P-P Tx = person-to-person transmission.

that *Y. pestis* was produced in large quantities by Soviet scientists for bioterrorism before this program was abandoned in 1992. The WHO has estimated that a 50-kg release of *Y. pestis* over an urban area of 5 million people would result in 150,000 cases of plague pneumonia and 36,000 deaths.

CLINICAL MANIFESTATIONS

The incubation period is 1 to 6 days. The pneumonic form is associated with bloody sputum, fever, dyspnea, and frequent gastrointestinal symptoms, including nausea, vomiting, abdominal pain, and diarrhea. The course is rapidly progressive, with a sepsis syndrome at 2 to 6 days. Chest radiographs usually show consolidated infiltrates, and about 50% of patients have pleural effusions.

DIAGNOSIS

Y. pestis is a gram-negative coccobacillus that demonstrates bipolar staining and resembles a safety pin. Although the organism may be recognized by Gram stain of sputum, most laboratories require extended periods to identify it with standard methods. If this diagnosis is suspected, the laboratory should be warned so that one culture can be incubated at 28° C for rapid growth and a second at 37° C to permit identification of the capsular antigen. Rapid diagnostic tests are available in some state health departments, the CDC, and some military facilities. The differential diagnosis includes other severe forms of pneumonia or epidemic pneumonia, such as legionnaires' disease (Chapter 322), histoplasmosis (Chapter 340), anthrax (Chapter 302), tularemia (Chapter 319), and influenza (Chapter 372).

TREATMENT ℞

The preferred drugs are streptomycin or gentamicin; doxycycline and fluoroquinolones such as ciprofloxacin or levofloxacin are alternative agents. The duration of treatment is 10 days.

PREVENTION

Limited data define the efficiency of person-to-person transmission. Current recommendations are for contact and droplet precautions with the use of masks, gowns, gloves, and eye protection. Isolation may be discontinued after 48 hours of antibiotic treatment and clinical improvement. Prophylactic doxycycline or ciprofloxacin is recommended for 7 days for household members, health care workers, and other close contacts of patients. Prophylactic antibiotics are also advocated for other persons with a common-source exposure. As with anthrax, prophylaxis is virtually 100% effective, whereas treatment after the onset of symptoms is much less successful.

PROGNOSIS

The fatality rate of pneumonic plague approaches 100% without therapy. Mortality has been reduced to 5 to 14% with aminoglycoside treatment, but this experience is based largely on syndromes that are generally less severe than plague pneumonia.

● BOTULISM
See Chapter 304.

● TULAREMIA
See Chapter 319.

● VIRAL HEMORRHAGIC FEVER

DEFINITION

The hemorrhagic fever viruses (Chapter 389) include diverse organisms that cause a clinical illness characterized by fever and bleeding. These agents are grouped in four families: Filoviridae, Arenaviridae, Bunyaviridae, and Flaviviridae (Table 20-4). These viruses are attractive as bioweapons for several reasons: the minimal infecting dose may be as low as 10 virions, they can be distributed by aerosols, mortality rates are virus dependent but often high, they generate great fear, many are transmitted person to person, and no good treatment is available.

EPIDEMIOLOGY

The hemorrhagic fever viruses are not normally found in the United States, Europe, or Australia. They are transmitted by contact with infected animals or arthropod vectors, although the natural reservoir for Ebola and Marburg viruses is not known. Any case of viral hemorrhagic fever in a patient who has not been in an endemic area within the previous 22 days is presumed to represent bioterrorism.

CLINICAL MANIFESTATIONS

The onset of illness is generally nonspecific and consists of fever and myalgias. Additional symptoms are virus dependent (see Table 20-4) and include rash, encephalitis, pharyngitis, adenopathy, and gastrointestinal symptoms. The syndrome progresses to thrombocytopenia with petechiae, hematuria, hematemesis, hemoptysis, and melena. Disseminated intravascular coagulation with shock, delirium, convulsions, and coma may then develop.

DIAGNOSIS

Laboratory features include thrombocytopenia, as well as leukopenia, anemia, or hemoconcentration. All specimens from patients with suspected viral hemorrhagic fever should be referred to the CDC for testing in a BSL-4 laboratory. Personnel in the referring laboratory must be warned, and only designated technicians should be assigned to processing.

TREATMENT ℞

Ribavirin has activity in vitro against Lassa fever virus, New World arenaviruses, and bunyaviruses, but clinical experience is limited. It is assumed that a limited number of cases involving these viruses would permit the use of intravenous ribavirin, but a mass casualty setting would require oral administration. Treatment of other hemorrhagic fever viruses would largely be limited to supportive care.

PREVENTION

The major concern is nosocomial and household transmission by contact with blood and other body fluids. Patients should be kept in a single-occupant negative-pressure room, and health care personnel should use N95 respirators or powered air-purifying respirators, double gloves, impermeable gowns, goggles or face shields, and leg and shoe coverings. Nonessential staff and visitors should be excluded. Dedicated medical equipment such as stethoscopes and point-of-care analyzers should be available. Laboratory specimens should not be sent in pneumonic systems, contaminated objects should be cleaned with a 1 : 100 household bleach or similar disinfectant, and contaminated cloth items should be double-bagged and incinerated or autoclaved. Particular care must be exercised in managing corpses.

SUGGESTED READINGS

Friedlander AM, Little SF. Advances in the development of next-generation anthrax vaccines. *Vaccine.* 2009;27:D28-D32. *A short course of antibiotics prevents post-exposure disease in a macaque model.*

McFadden G. Killing a killer: what next for smallpox? *PloS Pathog.* 2010;6:e1000727. *A review of the current status of variola virus and smallpox vaccines and the debate on the destruction of smallpox.*

Merkel TJ, Perera PY, Kelly VK, et al. Development of a highly efficacious vaccinia-based dual vaccine against smallpox and anthrax, two important bioterror entities. *Proc Natl Acad Sci U S A.* 2010;107:18091-18096. *A single new vaccine appears to be efficacious against both agents.*

Wright JG, Quinn CP, Shadomy S, et al. Use of anthrax vaccine in the United States: recommendations of the Advisory Committee on Immunization Practices (ACIP), 2009. *MMWR Recomm Rep.* 2010;59:1-30. *Updated consensus guideline.*

21

CHRONIC POISONING: TRACE METALS AND OTHERS

MICHAEL A. MCGUIGAN

DEFINITION

The term *chronic poisoning* refers to toxicity that develops during repeated or continuous exposure to a substance over many months or years. A *trace metal,* which by definition is present in minute quantities, usually refers to metals that are essential to an organism's function; however, this chapter includes a number of metals that are not physiologically required and does not discuss acute poisoning (Chapter 110).

EPIDEMIOLOGY

The source of most of the substances discussed in this chapter is the environment—the home, the workplace, or the outdoors—and most exposures are unintentional. Because many of these metals are essential to normal physiologic functions, another source may be dietary supplements (Chapter 225). The most common site of absorption is the gastrointestinal tract.

The medical literature on chronic low-level exposure is uneven. Although the clinical toxicology of each metal is presented individually, most if not all exposures involve a number of different metals, and the clinical impact of metal-metal interactions is poorly understood.

Lead

EPIDEMIOLOGY

Lead poisoning was recognized more than 2000 years ago. Although lead poisoning is often considered primarily a problem among children of lower socioeconomic status living in dilapidated housing with peeling lead-based paint, lead poisoning also occurs in adults exposed through occupational or nonoccupational activities (Table 21-1). In the United States, approximately 95% of cases of blood lead levels 25 μg/dL or greater in adults are attributed to occupational exposure.

PATHOBIOLOGY

Inhaled fine particulates (<5 μm in diameter) of inorganic lead reach the alveoli and are readily absorbed; larger particles come in contact with airway mucus and are eventually swallowed. Only 20 to 30% of orally ingested lead is absorbed. Organic lead compounds can also be absorbed through the skin. Absorbed lead is distributed first to blood and soft tissue and then to bone, where more than 90% of total body lead is found. Factors contributing to bone demineralization (e.g., prolonged bedrest, pregnancy, menopause) promote the release of lead from bone. Lead is excreted primarily through

TABLE 21-1   COMMON SOURCES OF ADULT LEAD EXPOSURE

OCCUPATIONAL	NONOCCUPATIONAL

Manufacturing
    Manufacture of storage batteries
    Secondary smelting
    Manufacture of primary batteries
    Primary smelting
    Welding and cutting operations
	Shooting firearms
	Remodeling or renovation activities
	Hobbies (e.g., casting, ceramics, stained glass)
	Retained bullets or gunshot wounds
	Pica
	Contaminated food, liquid, or nontraditional medications

Construction
    Special trade contractors
    Painting, paperhanging, decorating
    Lead abatement workers	

Mining Mining of lead and zinc ores	
Wholesale trades Wholesale distribution of electrical apparatus and equipment, wiring supplies, and construction materials	
Retail trades Automobile repair shops	
Transportation, communication, electric, gas, and sanitary services	

TABLE 21-2   SUMMARY OF CLINICAL LEAD TOXICITY

BLOOD LEAD LEVEL (μG/DL)	EFFECTS
<10	Aminolevulinic acid dehydrase inhibition
15–30	Elevation of erythrocyte protoporphyrin
30–39	Mild elevations in blood pressure Altered testicular function
40–49	Increased coproporphyrins and urinary aminolevulinic acid Slowed peripheral nerve conduction
50–59	Reduced hemoglobin synthesis Neurologic symptoms
60–69	Reproductive effects in women
80–90	Anemia Encephalopathic symptoms Nephropathy
100	Encephalopathic signs

the kidneys at a rate of about 30 μg/day, which may increase to 200 μg/day with higher body burdens.

CLINICAL MANIFESTATIONS

Lead binds to sulfhydryl groups and adversely affects zinc- and calcium-dependent enzyme systems. This binding interferes with heme synthesis, DNA transcription, and calcium-dependent release of neurotransmitters and of protein kinase C, which regulate cell growth, learning, and memory. In addition, lead affects membrane integrity, steroid metabolism, and vitamin D synthesis in renal tubular cells, and it produces motor axon degeneration and segmental demyelination. The clinical manifestations of lead toxicity are roughly related to the blood lead level (Table 21-2).

Cardiovascular System

A cross-sectional study of 2165 women aged 40 to 59 years found that a change in blood lead levels from the lowest quartile (mean, 1.0 μg/dL; range, 0.5 to 1.6 μg/dL) to the highest quartile (mean, 6.3 μg/dL; range, 4.0 to 31.1 μg/dL) was associated with a significant increase in systolic (by 1.7 mm Hg) and diastolic (by 1.4 mm Hg) blood pressures. At blood lead levels between 10 and 40 μg/dL, lead increases systolic blood pressure by 1 to 2 mm Hg and diastolic pressure by 1.4 mm Hg for every doubling of the blood lead level. Workers with mean blood lead levels between 40 and 70 μg/dL have an increased risk of death from renal and hypertensive cardiovascular disease. The progression, mechanisms, and effects of therapeutic intervention are unclear in lead-associated hypertension.

Reproductive System

Workplace exposure to lead is associated with decreased fertility, spontaneous abortions, stillbirths, low birthweights, and increased infant mortality. At mean blood levels above 23 μg/dL, lead has a direct toxic effect on spermatogenesis, resulting in decreased sperm counts and abnormal sperm morphology and function.

Renal System

Lead accumulates in proximal tubule cells. Reported clinical findings include Fanconi's syndrome, increased urate excretion, chronic interstitial nephritis, and interference in the renin-aldosterone system. In a population with a mean blood lead level of 8.1 μg/dL, a 10 μg/dL increase in blood lead level was associated with a decrease in creatinine clearance of 10.4 mL/minute.

Nervous System

Chronic encephalopathy is more common than acute encephalopathy (Chapter 422). Early encephalopathic manifestations include changes in cognitive function and mood, early morning sleep disturbance, headache, irritability, lassitude, and loss of libido. Abnormalities in cognition or visual-motor function may be evident on psychometric testing. These findings may occur in workers with blood levels from 18 to 30 μg/dL but are more common in those with levels in the 40- to 60-μg/dL range. The decrease in neuropsychological performance may be comparable to that expected during aging of up to 20 years, although debate continues about the predictability of the effects of blood lead levels below 70 μg/dL. Many of these manifestations respond at least partially to a reduction in the blood lead level.

Lead affects peripheral nerve conduction. Lead-induced peripheral axonal neuropathy (Chapter 428) most commonly involves the motor nerves; it tends to be more severe in the upper extremities and on the dominant side. A subclinical decrease in ulnar nerve motor conduction velocity has been demonstrated at blood lead levels as low as 30 μg/dL. Lead poisoning also predisposes to the development of carpal tunnel and tarsal tunnel syndromes (Chapter 428).

Hematologic System

Lead affects the red cell membrane and interferes with enzymes involved in the synthesis of hemoglobin. The traditional findings in severe poisoning include a hypochromic microcytic anemia and basophilic stippling (Chapter 162).

DIAGNOSIS

The initial steps in the diagnosis of lead poisoning are to identify people involved in high-risk activities (see Table 21-1) and to determine the levels of lead in the venous (not capillary) blood. The diagnosis of lead poisoning should not rely on clinical symptoms and signs because these develop late and generally correlate poorly with blood lead levels. The blood lead level that triggers intervention is not well established for adults, and no national guidelines exist for managing adults with lead poisoning. It is in the best interest of the patient to follow the most conservative standards: a confirmed venous blood lead level of 40 μg/dL or greater should trigger intervention, including improved industrial hygiene, better dust control, and increased ventilation.

Mercury

DEFINITION

There are three chemical forms of mercury. Elemental or metallic mercury (Hg^0, quicksilver) is a silver liquid at room temperature. Inorganic mercury occurs in either a mercurous (Hg^+) or a mercuric (Hg^{++}) state. Organic mercurials are attached to short (ethyl or methyl) or long (alkyl or aryl) carbon chains. Each form of mercury can be found in a variety of occupations and products.

EPIDEMIOLOGY

The different chemical forms of mercury enter and are distributed throughout the body via different delivery systems. From a clinical perspective, the most

TREATMENT Rx

Treatment is designed to prevent further exposure, to reduce the blood lead level to an acceptable range, and to repair any existing damage. Removal of an individual from a lead environment is recommended if the blood lead level is 50 μg/dL or greater on three tests over 6 months or if a medical condition consistent with lead poisoning has been identified. Removal from the lead source is often associated with a gradual reduction in blood lead levels. Chelation therapy is generally recommended if symptoms or signs are present or if the blood lead level is above 60 μg/dL (Table 21-3).

Calcium disodium ethylenediaminetetraacetic acid ($CaNa_2EDTA$) is the first-line drug for treating asymptomatic adults with high blood lead levels. In the treatment of symptomatic lead poisoning (with or without encephalopathy), $CaNa_2EDTA$ is used in conjunction with dimercaprol (2,3-dimercaptopropanol or BAL). Larger doses of $CaNa_2EDTA$ (50 to 75 mg/kg/day) are used for more severely poisoned patients. A third chelator, succimer (meso-2,3-dimercapto-succinic acid, DMSA), is approved for the treatment of children with blood lead levels above 45 μg/dL; although succimer has not been approved by the Food and Drug Administration (FDA) for the treatment of adult lead poisoning, adults have been treated successfully with succimer, and it should be considered in place of $CaNa_2EDTA$ monotherapy. D-Penicillamine (3-mercapto-D-valine or penicillamine) is not recommended for the treatment of adult lead poisoning because of the high incidence of adverse drug reactions.

Chelation removes lead from the blood and soft tissues, but little is removed from bone. Redistribution of lead from deep stores after chelation may result in a rebound of blood lead levels and the redevelopment of clinical toxicity. For this reason, individuals should have their blood lead levels measured 2 weeks after the course of chelation has been completed. In general, the clinical response to chelation therapy is variable, and the data demonstrating improved outcomes are not robust. After chelation, if the blood lead level rises into the toxic range or symptoms recur, another course of chelation is indicated, with the same dose and duration used originally.

important target organ is the central nervous system, even though the kidney accumulates the most mercury regardless of the chemical type. Chronic poisoning with any of the chemical forms of mercury results in central nervous system toxicity. Ingestion of organic mercury is the most efficient way to get mercury into the brain, followed by the inhalation of elemental mercury vapor; ingestion of inorganic mercury is the least efficient.

PATHOBIOLOGY

Mercury produces toxicity by binding to sulfhydryl groups, thereby inhibiting enzyme systems and disrupting cell membrane integrity. Mercury also binds to amide, amine, carboxyl, and phosphoryl groups. Methyl mercury inhibits choline acetyltransferase, a critical enzyme in the formation of acetylcholine.

Elemental mercury is or has been used in dental amalgams, calibration instruments, electroplating, gold extraction, manometers, and thermometers. Elemental mercury pooled under carpets or floorboards in homes has resulted in clinical toxicity. Chronic parenteral injection of elemental mercury—no longer prescribed medically, but still rarely done by individuals—may produce neurotoxicity. However, ingested elemental mercury is poorly absorbed from the gastrointestinal tract and causes virtually no toxicity. Conversely, nearly 75% of inhaled elemental mercury vapor is absorbed through the lungs. Once it is absorbed, elemental mercury is distributed to the tissues and red blood cells, where it is oxidized to the mercuric form. Some elemental mercury crosses the blood-brain barrier, and oxidation within the central nervous system leads to an accumulation of divalent mercury in the brain because ionized mercury does not readily cross the blood-brain barrier.

Inorganic mercury may be a component of disinfectants, fireworks, preservatives, and photograph developing chemicals. Application of creams or ointments containing inorganic mercury to intact or damaged skin may result in systemic absorption of mercury. Inorganic mercury solutions are corrosive to the gastrointestinal tract, but up to 15% of ingested inorganic mercury is absorbed through the gastrointestinal mucosa. After absorption, the inorganic mercury salt is ionized and penetrates the blood-brain barrier poorly. However, absorbed divalent mercury can be reduced to the metallic form, which does cross the blood-brain barrier.

Organic mercurials are used as pesticides, preservatives, and disinfectants. Coal-fired power plants are a major source of mercury

TABLE 21-3 GENERAL GUIDELINES FOR CHELATION THERAPY

DRUG	ADULT DOSE	INDICATIONS	CONTRAINDICATIONS AND CAUTIONS
Dimercaprol, British antilewisite (BAL)	3–5 mg/kg (75 mg/m^2) IM every 4 hr for 2 days; then every 6 hr for 2 days; then every 12 hr for up to an additional 7 days	Lead: symptomatic poisoning	Administration is by deep intramuscular injections, which are painful Dimercaprol is often administered with CaNa$_2$EDTA The vehicle is peanut oil—do *not* use intravenously; use is contraindicated in those with peanut allergy
CaNa$_2$EDTA, edetate calcium disodium	20–30 mg/kg/day (1000–1500 mg/m^2/day) as a continuous infusion for 5 days	Lead: symptomatic poisoning or asymptomatic patients with high blood lead levels Manganese: symptomatic patients with blood, serum, or urine manganese levels above reference values	Do *not* use Na$_2$EDTA CaNa$_2$EDTA can be given IM in two or three divided doses High doses of CaNa$_2$EDTA increase zinc excretion and may be toxic to renal glomeruli and proximal tubules
Dimercaptopropanesulfonate (DMPS)	100 mg orally four times/day for 7 days; may repeat therapeutic course after 7 days without therapy if levels are still elevated	Arsenic: symptomatic patients with urine arsenic levels ≥50 µg/L; asymptomatic patients with urine arsenic levels >200 µg/L Manganese: symptomatic patients with blood, serum, or urine manganese levels above reference values Bismuth: symptomatic patients with bismuth blood levels >50 µg/L or urine levels >150 µg/L	
Deferoxamine	6 g as a continuous IV infusion given over 24 hr; may repeat if serum levels are still elevated	Aluminum: symptomatic patients with serum aluminum levels >100 µg/L	
Dimercaptosuccinic acid (DMSA), succimer	10 mg/kg (350 mg/m^2) orally every 8 hr for 5 days; then 10 mg/kg every 12 hr for 14 days	Lead: symptomatic poisoning or asymptomatic patients with high blood lead levels Mercury: symptomatic patients with mercury whole blood levels >10 µg/L or 24-hr urine levels ≥20 µg/L	Succimer has a sulfur-like odor

in the environment. Elemental and inorganic mercurials deposited in the environment are bioconverted into organic mercury compounds that are a recognized contaminant of the food chain, particularly in fish. Consumption of fish is the source of nearly all the methyl mercury in the general population. The FDA and the Environmental Protection Agency (EPA) recommend the avoidance of fish with the highest mercury concentrations—king mackerel, shark, swordfish, and tilefish from the Gulf of Mexico. Women of childbearing age and pregnant women should limit their consumption of medium-mercury fish: fresh tuna steak, canned white or albacore tuna, grouper, orange roughy, saltwater trout, bluefish, lobster, halibut, haddock, snapper, and crab. In addition, caution is urged regarding the consumption of fish from local lakes and ponds, which may be more polluted than commercial fish sources.

Organic mercury is highly lipid soluble, well absorbed through the gastrointestinal tract, and widely distributed throughout the body. Organic mercury compounds are metabolized in the body; longer chain mercury compounds are rapidly metabolized to inorganic mercury, whereas short-chain mercury compounds (e.g., methyl mercury) are slowly metabolized to inorganic mercury. Organic mercury readily crosses the blood-brain barrier, and oxidation within the central nervous system leads to the accumulation of mercuric ions in the brain.

CLINICAL MANIFESTATIONS

The chronic inhalation of elemental mercury vapor results in two syndromes. The first syndrome consists of neuropsychiatric manifestations, gingivostomatitis, and tremor. The tremor (Chapter 417) is evident at rest or with motion and may be aggravated with purposeful movement. The second syndrome is erythism, a neuropsychiatric constellation of findings that includes fatigue, insomnia, memory impairment, nervousness, irritability, shyness, social withdrawal, loss of confidence, timidity, and depression.

Chronic occupational exposure to inorganic mercury may cause subclinical psychomotor and neuromuscular abnormalities as well as long-term behavioral impairment. Neuropsychiatric abnormalities (inattention, memory, construction, and motor performance) appear to be dose related (Chapter 409).

Methyl mercury poisoning is cumulative and develops over several years. Based on epidemics of methyl mercury poisoning in Japan and Iraq in which large quantities of organic mercury were consumed, the initial symptoms are fatigue and perioral and extremity paresthesia, followed by difficulty with hand movements and disturbances of vision. The classic picture of methyl mercury poisoning is the gradual onset of ataxia, constricted visual fields, and dysarthria. Other findings are paresthesia, deafness, incoordination, loss of voluntary movement, and mental retardation. The full picture of toxicity is that of psychological, cerebellar, sensory, and motor abnormalities. However, moderate amounts of methyl mercury in the diet have not been linked to adverse effects in adults; most concern relates to potential toxic effects on the fetus and its developing central nervous system.

DIAGNOSIS

The diagnosis of mercury poisoning requires a history of exposure, compatible clinical findings, and elevated mercury levels in blood or urine.

The mean total mercury levels in whole blood and urine in the general population are 1 to 8 µg/L and 4 to 5 µg/L, respectively. Although elevated blood or urine mercury levels are consistent with clinical toxicity, clinical signs or symptoms are poorly correlated with blood or urine mercury levels because of substantial intraindividual and interindividual variation. For example, data in urban adults (mean age, 59 years) showed no significant association between blood mercury levels (mean, 2.1 µg/L; range, 0 to 16 µg/L) and neurobehavioral performance.

A 1 : 1 ratio of red blood cell to plasma mercury suggests inorganic mercury poisoning, whereas a ratio of 10 : 1 suggests organic mercury toxicity. Red blood cell and plasma mercury levels should be requested if the source and type of mercury exposure are unknown. Methyl mercury blood levels of 3 to 5 µg/dL may be found in patients with symptoms. Determination of a methyl mercury level is recommended if the exposure is to a contaminated environmental source.

Arsenic

DEFINITION

Arsenic is a naturally occurring omnipresent element that exists in three valence states: elemental or metallic arsenic (As^0), trivalent (arsenite, As^{3+}), and pentavalent (arsenate, As^{5+}). The trivalent form of arsenic (arsenite) is the most toxic and is responsible for the worldwide public health concern about chronic arsenic poisoning. Organic alkane arsenicals are of low toxicity, and elemental arsenic is virtually nontoxic.

TREATMENT   Rx

Asymptomatic patients with elevated urine mercury levels should have the analyses repeated after a 4-week period without fish consumption.

A patient with mercury poisoning should immediately be removed from the contaminated environment; the source of the mercury must then be identified and removed. Treatment is primarily symptomatic and supportive.

Chelation therapy (see Table 21-3) is used to increase the excretion of mercury, even though improved clinical outcomes have not been demonstrated; increased urinary excretion of mercury alone has become an accepted if empirical clinical goal. There is little agreement on the indications for the initiation or cessation of chelation therapy. The presence of clinical toxicity combined with elevated mercury levels is an accepted indication for chelation therapy, but its role in asymptomatic individuals with mercury levels above background values is controversial. A reasonable end point for chelation is the achievement of background levels of mercury in urine or blood (<20 µg/L or 10 µg/L, respectively). Fish eaters with elevated mercury levels should avoid eating any fish or shellfish for 1 month, after which mercury levels in blood or urine should be reanalyzed. If mercury levels have come down to reference values, low-mercury fish (shrimp, canned light tuna, salmon, pollock, catfish) can be reintroduced into the diet at a frequency of no more than two meals per week.

Succimer (see Table 21-3) is the chelator of choice because it can be given orally and has been effective in reducing brain levels of methyl mercury in animal studies. D-Penicillamine is less effective than succimer and has a higher adverse drug reaction rate. Dimercaprol is not recommended because of its potential to shift mercury from peripheral tissues into the brain. N-acetylcysteine has been proposed as a chelator of methyl mercury, and repeated oral administration may interrupt the enterohepatic recirculation of methyl mercury; however, use of the drug for this purpose has not undergone clinical trials and is not approved by the FDA.

EPIDEMIOLOGY

The major sources of human exposure to arsenic are the environment (mining, seafood, groundwater) and industry (pesticides, pigments, wood preservatives, glass or metal manufacturing, electronics, folk remedies). The arsenic content in the average North American adult diet is less than 1 µg/kg/day. Arsenic in seafood is primarily in the form of organic arsenicals, and the content is variable; freshwater fish may have up to 2 mg/kg, whereas lobster may have up to 22 mg/kg. The EPA drinking water standard is 10 µg/L.

PATHOBIOLOGY

Nearly 90% of ingested or inhaled arsenic is absorbed; little arsenic is absorbed through intact skin. Absorbed arsenic is widely distributed throughout the body, but no form of arsenic readily crosses the blood-brain barrier. Pentavalent arsenic and trivalent arsenic undergo oxidation-reduction reactions, converting one form to the other. Pentavalent arsenic is reduced by glutathione to the more toxic trivalent form. Methylation of trivalent arsenic produces the less toxic monomethylarsenate and dimethylarsenate metabolites, which are excreted in the urine. Organic arsenicals, such as those found in seafood, are essentially nontoxic; they are not metabolized to toxic forms of arsenic and are rapidly excreted in the urine, with an elimination half-life of 4 to 6 hours.

Arsenite (As^{3+}) binds to sulfhydryl groups, resulting in the inhibition of many enzyme systems (glycolysis, pyruvate dehydrogenase, Krebs cycle) and the decreased production of adenosine triphosphate. Arsenate (As^{5+}) replaces phosphate in microsomal enzyme systems, resulting in the uncoupling of oxidative phosphorylation and the decreased production of adenosine triphosphate. Pentavalent arsenate does not bind to sulfhydryl groups. Inorganic arsenic is a human carcinogen.

CLINICAL MANIFESTATIONS

Chronic poisoning develops after the ingestion or inhalation of arsenic over weeks to months, depending on the daily dose. Clinical manifestations develop gradually and are highly variable among exposed individuals. Typical initial manifestations include nonspecific complaints such as a metallic taste in the mouth, anorexia, weight loss, malaise, and weakness.

Skin lesions are some of the most common and earliest nonmalignant toxic effects. Typical dermal findings include melanosis (trunk and extremities), hyperpigmentation (tongue, oral mucosa, axilla), hyperkeratosis (palm,

sole), and brittle nails. Less common or late findings include alopecia and white transverse bands (Mees' lines) in the nails (Chapter 450).

Later findings involve the nervous system and carcinogenesis. Neurologic effects are both central and peripheral. Central effects include mild dementia (Chapter 409) and headache; cranial nerves are normal. Peripheral sensory and motor neuropathies (Chapter 428) develop in a stocking-and-glove distribution and cause muscle weakness, muscle atrophy, and ataxia.

Malignant neoplasms include Bowen's disease, basal cell carcinoma, and squamous cell carcinoma (Chapter 210). Lung cancer (Chapter 197) may result from the inhalation of dust containing high levels of arsenic. Arsenic in drinking water has been associated with leukemia, bladder cancer, renal cancer, hepatic cancer, and uterine cancer (Chapter 183). The cancer risk from arsenic in drinking water may be dose related. Studies of populations outside the United States show increases in cancer only when arsenic concentrations in drinking water measure more than several hundred micrograms per liter. Studies of U.S. populations exposed to average drinking water arsenic concentrations of about 190 µg/L have not demonstrated evidence of increased cancer.

Cardiovascular disease includes atherosclerosis, coronary artery disease, and hypertension. Blackfoot disease, peculiar to the southwestern coast of Taiwan, is a form of peripheral vascular disease that results in gangrene of the lower extremities. Other manifestations of exposure to arsenic in drinking water include chronic cough, type 2 diabetes, and reproductive abnormalities such as congenital malformations, miscarriages, and low birthweights.

DIAGNOSIS

The diagnosis of chronic arsenic poisoning depends on an appropriate history of exposure (including a source), compatible clinical manifestations, and documentation of an elevated body burden of arsenic. Principal sources of arsenic are environmental (contaminated water, air, soil) and occupational or industrial. Although seafood may be a source of organic arsenic, it is not associated with clinical toxicity.

Arsenic can be measured in the hair, blood, or urine. Hair analysis is a suboptimal method of determining chronic toxicity. Environmental arsenic is adsorbed to the external surface of the hair and is difficult to remove by washing. Arsenic levels vary within a single hair and among hairs, and there is significant interindividual variability in adsorption of arsenic to hair. Nonetheless, the normal arsenic hair levels are less than 1 µg/g dry weight, and arsenic levels in hair from people with chronic toxicity range from 1 to 5 µg/g or more.

Blood levels of arsenic reflect only very recent exposure and are not reliable indicators of chronic exposure to low levels of arsenic. For example, there is no correlation between blood arsenic levels and drinking water arsenic levels of 6 to 125 µg/L.

Normal urine arsenic levels are less than 50 µg/L or less than 25 µg/24 hours in the absence of seafood consumption. Among people aged 6 years and older in the United States, the 95th percentile for total urinary arsenic is 65.4 µg/L. Urine arsenic levels above 200 µg/L are abnormal. The average urine arsenic level among people with chronic toxicity is 207 µg of

TREATMENT   Rx

Treatment approaches can be stratified according to symptoms and urine levels of inorganic arsenic (Table 21-4). All patients who are symptomatic or who have urine inorganic arsenic levels of 50 µg/L or above should be removed from the source of the arsenic.

Dimercaptopropanesulfonate (DMPS) is the most widely studied chelating agent for chronic arsenic poisoning and is the drug of choice, although it is not approved by the FDA. DMPS forms a water-soluble complex with monomethyl arsenic that is excreted in the urine. In a randomized trial, DMPS therapy (100 mg orally four times/day on alternate weeks for 7 weeks) increased urine arsenic excretion and improved weakness, pigmentation, and lung disease, but it did not improve hematologic and blood chemistry abnormalities, neuropathy, hepatomegaly, keratosis, or skin histology.■ Chelation should continue until the urine arsenic level is below 50 µg/L. Succimer has not been successful in treating chronic arsenic toxicity, and dimercaprol is not recommended because the lipid-soluble dimercaprol-arsenic complex penetrates the blood-brain barrier. The effectiveness of selenium and vitamin E supplementation in ameliorating arsenic-induced skin changes is controversial.

TABLE 21-4 ARSENIC TREATMENT STRATIFICATION

INORGANIC ARSENIC LEVELS IN URINE (µG/L)	SYMPTOMATIC	ASYMPTOMATIC
<50	Supportive care	No treatment
50–200	Chelation*	Monitor 24-hr urine levels monthly
>200	Chelation*	Chelation*

*Using DMPS (see Table 21-3).

inorganic arsenic per gram of creatinine. Because urine analysis measures total arsenic, elevated levels should be speciated to determine the fractions of inorganic and organic arsenic. If this analysis is not possible, seafood should be eliminated from the patient's diet for 1 week, and the urine analysis repeated.

A nerve conduction study is not a reliable diagnostic tool for chronic arsenic toxicity. Among patients with elevated urine arsenic levels, the results of nerve conduction tests do not correlate well with the presence or absence of clinical neuropathy.

Cadmium

EPIDEMIOLOGY

Cadmium is found as a metal and in a number of industrial chemicals. Cadmium may enter the environment through contamination, fuel combustion, or fertilizer. The majority of cadmium is used occupationally in nickel-cadmium batteries and to protect polyvinyl chloride against heat and light. Cadmium is used as a pigment in coloring the red bags used for infectious hospital waste. When they are incinerated, these bags release cadmium into the environment, so medical waste incinerators are an important environmental source of cadmium. The largest source of most human exposure to cadmium is dietary, with an average daily intake of 10 to 30 µg. Cadmium exposure is doubled in people who smoke tobacco.

PATHOBIOLOGY

Approximately 25% of inhaled cadmium is absorbed. Although normally only 5% of ingested cadmium is absorbed, gastrointestinal absorption is increased in the presence of calcium or iron deficiency or high dietary fat. Cadmium concentrates in the liver and kidneys. Cadmium is poorly excreted from the body; the geometric mean terminal half-life for elimination in creatinine-adjusted urine is estimated to be 19 years. The kidney is the primary target organ in chronic toxicity.

CLINICAL MANIFESTATIONS

The clinical picture of chronic cadmium toxicity is one of irreversible renal toxicity (Chapter 124). Proximal tubule damage results in high urine concentrations of low-molecular-weight proteins, amino acids, glucose, phosphate, and calcium. Decreased glomerular filtration rate and nephrolithiasis may occur. Renal failure is common.

The renal pathophysiologic process may result in calcium deficiency, osteoporosis, osteomalacia, and bone fractures. Other clinical manifestations of chronic cadmium poisoning include male infertility, slowing of visual-motor functioning, and peripheral neuropathies.

The EPA and the International Agency for Research on Cancer have designated cadmium a probable human carcinogen. However, this designation is controversial, and chronic exposure to cadmium may not increase cancer rates. For example, residents of a cadmium-polluted village in England had no increase in cancer rates; a study of residents of a cadmium-polluted area in Belgium found no increase in prostate, kidney, or urinary tract cancers; a retrospective comparison of Japanese residents in high, low, and no cadmium-polluted areas found no differences in cancer mortality; and a study of copper-cadmium alloy workers found no increased risk of lung cancer.

DIAGNOSIS

A tentative diagnosis of chronic cadmium poisoning can be confirmed by measuring elevated urinary cadmium levels (>5 µg/L) and elevated urinary microprotein levels, particularly β_1-microglobulin.

TREATMENT   Rx

Treatment of the toxic effects of cadmium is symptomatic and supportive. There is no accepted way to reduce the body burden of cadmium. The use of CaNa$_2$EDTA or dimercaprol may increase nephrotoxicity. Succimer and N-acetylcysteine have achieved favorable results in animal studies, but neither has been adequately evaluated in human studies.

Manganese

DEFINITION

Manganese is an increasingly important toxin, both environmentally and occupationally. Manganese exists as a metal (metallic manganese, ferromanganese), as inorganic manganese (e.g., chloride or sulfate salts), or as organic manganese.

EPIDEMIOLOGY

Metallic manganese is used in steel production. Inorganic manganese (Mn^{2+}, Mn^{3+}, and Mn^{4+}) is most commonly found in industry and in the environment. Various inorganic manganese compounds are involved in the manufacture of animal feed, batteries, fertilizers, fireworks, fungicides, matches, and potassium permanganate. Organic manganese compounds are used as a fuel oil additive, as fungicides, and as a gasoline additive (methylcyclopentadienyl manganese tricarbonyl [MMT]). Neurotoxicity seen in methcathinone (street name "Cat") abusers has been attributed to manganese.

Manganese is an essential nutrient, acting as a cofactor in enzymatic reactions involving bone mineralization as well as protein and carbohydrate metabolism. As such, it is often a component of parenteral nutrition preparations, and chronic infusion can result in manganese toxicity. Substantial exposure to manganese occurs in people who work in welding, mining, and foundry occupations. People who work with gasoline or as automobile mechanics may be exposed to MMT.

PATHOBIOLOGY

Manganese is absorbed through the gastrointestinal and respiratory tracts and is distributed widely throughout the body. Manganese accumulates in the globus pallidus of the basal ganglia. Bile is the principal route of excretion. The elimination half-life is approximately 40 days, but it is longer for manganese in the central nervous system.

The primary target organ is the central nervous system. Despite the fact that manganese adversely affects enzymes, receptors, and transport systems, the exact mechanisms of toxicity are unclear. A characteristic finding in chronic manganese poisoning is the selective destruction of dopaminergic neurons. The pathophysiologic mechanism is uncertain, but one hypothesis is that Mn^{2+} causes oxidation, the production of free radicals or reactive oxygen species, or the depletion of antioxidants.

CLINICAL MANIFESTATIONS

People who work with manganese may develop a syndrome similar to but not identical with Parkinson's disease (Chapter 416). Findings include an extrapyramidal syndrome (masklike facies, tremor of the extremities at rest or on extension, bradykinesia, stooped posture, shuffling gait, propulsion abnormalities).

Several clinical characteristics may help distinguish between Parkinson's disease and manganese-induced parkinsonism. Manganese-poisoned patients have a "cock walk" and a propensity to fall backward when pushed. These patients often exhibit psychological disturbances early in the disease process. So-called manganese madness includes aggression, irritability, nervousness, and destructive behavior. Uncontrollable spasmodic crying or laughing, singing or dancing, or unfocused running around have been described.

DIAGNOSIS

The initial diagnosis of chronic manganese poisoning relies on a history of exposure and consistent clinical findings. In patients with significant central nervous system findings, T1-weighted magnetic resonance imaging that shows bilateral, symmetrical hyperdensities in the globus pallidus lends strong support to the diagnosis of chronic manganese poisoning.

Positron emission tomography may identify reduced striatal dopamine release.

Manganese levels in body fluids are helpful in establishing a diagnosis. Reference ranges have been established: blood, 40 to 140 μg/L; serum, 1.5 to 26.5 μg/L; and urine, 9.7 to 10.7 μg/L.

TREATMENT Rx

Treatment of chronic manganese toxicity starts with removing the source of the manganese and providing supportive care. The results of chelation with CaNa₂EDTA or DMPS (see Table 21-3) have been equivocal. Although levodopa responsiveness is a hallmark of Parkinson's disease, welders with manganese-induced parkinsonism treated with levodopa showed no improvement over placebo-treated control subjects.

Nickel

EPIDEMIOLOGY

Nickel is absorbed through the lungs, gastrointestinal tract, and skin. Water-soluble nickel compounds (e.g., nickel chloride or sulfate) are absorbed better than insoluble nickel is. Approximately 25% of the nickel in drinking water is absorbed. Nickel applied to the skin is absorbed into the skin but may not reach the circulation. The urine is the primary means of excretion of nickel from the body.

PATHOBIOLOGY

Nickel is used in a large number of metal alloys and in batteries, electroplating (e.g., table cutlery and some jewelry), coins, surgical staples, and some joint prostheses. Nickel is also present in drinking water; the EPA standard is 0.02 mg/kg/day.

Nickel appears to be an essential element in the body, but its physiologic role is unclear. Nickel crosses the cell membrane through calcium channels and competes with calcium for some receptors.

CLINICAL MANIFESTATIONS

Contact dermatitis (Chapter 446) is the most common manifestation of nickel toxicity. Exposure to consumer products containing nickel, particularly jewelry, causes sensitization and contact dermatitis in as many as 30% of people. Once sensitization has occurred, the severity of subsequent reactions is related to the dose of nickel.

Chronic occupational exposure to nickel dust and fumes has been associated with respiratory tract disease, including nasal, laryngeal, and lung cancers (Chapter 183). The EPA has identified nickel dust and nickel subsulfide as class A human carcinogens. Exposure to nickel in nonindustrial settings, such as ingestion of nickel in water or food or dermal contact, has not been associated with an increased risk of cancer.

DIAGNOSIS

Nickel levels in blood or urine are not useful in establishing either excessive exposure or risk of disease.

TREATMENT Rx

There is no specific treatment of nickel-induced dermal sensitivity.

OTHER TOXIC METALS
Aluminum

EPIDEMIOLOGY

Aluminum is the most abundant metal. It is widely available in consumer products such as food, water, cookware, food wraps, cans, antiperspirants, medications (especially antacids and phosphate binders), and dialysate fluids. North Americans consume 7 to 9 mg of aluminum in their diets each day. Industrial exposure to aluminum may result in significant toxicity.

PATHOBIOLOGY

Gastrointestinal tract absorption of aluminum ranges from 0.1 to 1%. Once it is absorbed, aluminum is bound to transferrin and distributed throughout the body, concentrating in bone and lung. The kidneys are the primary route of aluminum excretion, and a compromised ability to excrete aluminum is an important factor in the development of aluminum toxicity outside of the occupational setting. Rare individuals may accumulate significant amounts of aluminum from antiperspirants.

Aluminum blocks the incorporation of calcium into bones and inhibits osteoblastic and osteoclastic activity. In patients with renal failure, aluminum has been identified as a potential contributor to anemia, dialysis encephalopathy, and renal osteodystrophy.

CLINICAL MANIFESTATIONS

The central nervous system is a target organ for aluminum toxicity. The findings in dialysis encephalopathy (Chapters 132 and 133), which develops over months, include stuttering or stammering speech, directional disorientation, personality changes, myoclonus, motor apraxia, convulsions, and hallucinations. Industrial aluminum workers have developed cognitive defects, depression, incoordination, poor memory, and tremor. The relationship between aluminum exposure and Alzheimer's disease is controversial.

Chronic exposure to excessive aluminum may cause osteomalacia (Chapter 252), spontaneous fractures, and bone pain. Hypochromic, microcytic anemia (Chapter 162) that is unresponsive to iron therapy correlates with aluminum levels in the plasma or erythrocytes. Aluminum workers have an increased risk for the development of lung or bladder cancer (Chapter 203).

DIAGNOSIS

The background serum aluminum levels in normal individuals are less than 10 μg/L. Patients undergoing chronic dialysis may have serum aluminum levels up to 50 μg/L. Levels above 60 μg/L indicate increased absorption, serum levels above 100 μg/L are potentially toxic, and serum levels above 200 μg/L are usually associated with clinical symptoms and signs of toxicity.

TREATMENT Rx

Elevated serum aluminum levels can be brought down with extracorporeal clearance techniques, such as hemodialysis and hemofiltration. Deferoxamine (see Table 21-3) is indicated when serum aluminum levels exceed 100 μg/L. In hemodialysis patients, 2.5 mg/kg/week is as effective as the standard dose of deferoxamine (5 mg/kg/week) for treating aluminum overload.[2]

Beryllium

EPIDEMIOLOGY

Beryllium occurs naturally in rocks, coal, oil, soil, and volcanic dust. Commercially, beryllium is used in metal alloys for aerospace, aircraft, sports equipment (golf clubs, bicycle frames), and automotive manufacturing; in electronics and computers; in ceramics; and in defense weapons. Beryllium is naturally present in tobacco and may be inhaled during smoking.

PATHOBIOLOGY

Inhaled beryllium is cleared from the respiratory tract by mucociliary action and alveolar macrophages. Once it is absorbed, beryllium is distributed to the bones, liver, kidneys, lung parenchyma, and lymphatic system. The kidney is the primary route of beryllium excretion.

Repeated exposure to beryllium causes a cell-mediated immune response involving T lymphocytes and the release of T_H1 cytokines in genetically susceptible persons (Chapter 93). The cell-mediated response is persistent and results in the accumulation of immune effector cells (sensitized T lymphocytes, macrophages) that form granulomas and mononuclear cell infiltrations. A genetic predisposition to the development of chronic beryllium disease has been postulated. Dermal exposure to beryllium may cause irritative or atopic dermatitis as well as beryllium-containing foreign bodies and granulomas. The EPA considers beryllium to be a probable human carcinogen.

CLINICAL MANIFESTATIONS

Chronic beryllium disease is a progressive systemic hypersensitivity disease affecting the lungs and lymphatic system (Chapter 93). Clinical effects include progressive dyspnea, chest pain, weight loss, fatigue, anorexia, and fevers. Skin lesions, lymphadenopathy, and hepatosplenomegaly may occur. The pulmonary disease is progressive and may lead to respiratory failure within several years.

On pulmonary function testing, one third of patients have a predominantly obstructive pattern; one fourth have a predominantly restrictive pattern; one third have a reduced carbon monoxide diffusion capacity, with normal airflow and lung volumes; and some have a mix of obstruction and restriction (Chapter 85). A chest radiograph is normal early in the course, but later it shows diffuse bilateral infiltrates and hilar lymphadenopathy. Beryllium sensitivity is confirmed by the blood beryllium lymphocyte proliferation test. Tissue for histologic analysis from transbronchial or open lung biopsy may confirm the diagnosis.

TREATMENT Rx

Treatment involves removing the patient from exposure to beryllium, slowing or halting the progression of the disease with corticosteroids, and providing symptomatic and supportive care.

Bismuth

EPIDEMIOLOGY

Bismuth has been used in the treatment of gastrointestinal disorders such as ulcers, diarrhea, and *Helicobacter pylori* infection. Two forms of bismuth are toxic; lipid-soluble organic compounds (e.g., bismuth subgallate) are neurotoxic, and some water-soluble organic compounds (e.g., bismuth triglycollamate) are nephrotoxic.

PATHOBIOLOGY

Parenterally administered bismuth is distributed throughout the body but concentrates in the kidneys and liver. Elimination is through the kidneys, with a terminal elimination half-life of 3 to 10 weeks.

In the blood, bismuth binds to macroglobulins, immunoglobulins, lipoproteins, and haptoglobin. In the kidney, bismuth concentrates in the proximal tubule and causes necrosis. The mechanism of the neurologic effects is unclear.

CLINICAL MANIFESTATIONS

Chronic exposure to bismuth causes gastrointestinal, dermatologic, renal, and neurologic effects. Gastrointestinal effects include increased salivation, discoloration of the oral mucosa and gums, ulcerative stomatitis, nausea and vomiting, and diarrhea. Dermatologic effects are primarily a generalized rash after parenteral administration. Renal effects include nephritis, tubular necrosis, and renal failure.

The primary neurologic effect is an encephalopathy that develops in two distinct phases. The prodrome lasts up to several months and consists of asthenia, somnolence, depression, anxiety, and sometimes hallucinations. This prodrome is followed by the rapid onset (1 to 2 days) of encephalopathy characterized by confusion progressing to coma or dementia, dysarthria, disturbances of walking and standing, and tremor with myoclonic jerks. Chronic bismuth poisoning is associated with a distinctive electroencephalographic pattern: bilateral low-voltage diffuse beta frequencies that are maximal in the frontal and central regions and accentuated during hyperventilation.

The diagnosis of chronic bismuth toxicity is based on a history of exposure and a consistent clinical picture. Blood and urine levels of bismuth may be helpful. In chronic toxicity, the blood bismuth level is 50 to 1600 µg/L, and the urine level is 150 to 1250 µg/L. The median blood bismuth levels in patients with bismuth encephalopathy are in the range of 680 to 700 µg/L. In patients taking a bismuth product therapeutically, a blood bismuth level above 50 µg/L is a concern; a blood bismuth level above 100 µg/L is an indication to discontinue bismuth therapy.

TREATMENT Rx

Treatment of bismuth toxicity starts with stopping exposure to bismuth. DMPS administration (see Table 21-3) results in increased renal excretion of bismuth, but such therapy has not been shown to improve clinical outcomes.

Chromium

The most common forms of chromium in the environment are metallic chromium, trivalent chromium, and hexavalent chromium. Hexavalent chromium is the most toxic form. Trivalent chromium is essential for normal glucose tolerance; chromium picolinate is an alternative dietary supplement.

The trivalent and hexavalent chromiums are the most commonly used forms in industry. Chronic chromium toxicity is essentially an occupational disease related to tanning, metal alloys and electroplating (including surgical metals), photography, dyes, and cement.

Hexavalent chromium is absorbed primarily through the respiratory tract, with substantially smaller amounts absorbed through the gastrointestinal tract. The other valences are poorly absorbed. Hexavalent chromium is a skin and mucous membrane irritant. In dichromate compounds, hexavalent chromium binds to cellular and nuclear proteins and accumulates in red blood cells and platelets. Reduction of hexavalent to trivalent chromium creates intermediates that cause oxidative damage to DNA. Hexavalent chromium is a human carcinogen (lung cancer), but chromium and trivalent chromium are not classifiable. The EPA standard for chromium in drinking water is 100 µg/L.

Chronic occupational exposure to high levels of airborne hexavalent chromium has been associated with upper airway irritation (including nasal septum ulceration), bronchospasm, and an increased incidence of lung cancer. Repeated exposure to dichromate dust causes conjunctivitis and lacrimation. Dermal effects include irritation and chronic full-thickness ulcers. Chronic ingestion of high doses of chromium picolinate may cause renal impairment. The chronic drinking of water contaminated with hexavalent chromium may be associated with the development of stomach cancer. Reference levels of serum chromium are 0.05 to 0.16 µg/L. Treatment of chromium toxicity is symptomatic and supportive.

Cobalt

Cobalt is a naturally occurring element that exists as a metal, as a stable isotope, and as radioactive isotopes. The general public is rarely exposed to the radioactive isotopes (^{60}Co is used in radiation therapy). The metal is found in paints, enamels, and alloys used for household appliances, cutting tools, and joint replacements and surgical implants. Cobalt is a normal part of vitamin B$_{12}$. The average daily North American diet contains 5 to 40 µg of cobalt. Cobalt is absorbed through the gastrointestinal and respiratory tracts, distributed throughout the body, and excreted in the urine. Inhalation of cobalt is associated with obstructive and interstitial pulmonary disease. The interstitial pneumonitis is a fibrosing alveolitis, with leukocyte and multinucleated giant cell infiltration (Chapter 92). The process may be an immunoglobulin E–mediated response to cobalt reactivity. Chronic ingestion of or industrial exposure to cobalt produces a cardiomyopathy with pericardial effusions and biventricular heart failure (beer drinkers' cardiomyopathy of the 1960s). Cobalt levels are not useful in the diagnosis or management of chronic cobalt poisoning. The diagnosis is based on a history of exposure and compatible pulmonary findings. Medical evaluation should use standard methods for assessing pulmonary and cardiac function. Treatment consists of removing the patient from the source of cobalt and symptomatic and supportive care; both *N*-acetylcysteine and CaNa$_2$EDTA have been used, but there is no definitive clinical evidence of benefit.

Selenium

Selenium is used in the vulcanization of rubber, the manufacture of some red glass, the electronics and semiconductor industries, and some pharmaceutical products and dandruff shampoos. Selenium is absorbed through the gastrointestinal and respiratory tracts and accumulates primarily in the liver and kidneys. Selenium is cleared from the body in the urine and feces. The mechanism of toxicity is not clear, but one hypothesis is that selenium inhibits sulfhydryl enzymes, resulting in a reduction in intracellular oxidative reactions.

Chronic exposure to selenium compounds in animals results in hepatotoxicity and decreased growth. In humans, dermal effects include alopecia, abnormal nail formation, and discoloration and decay of the teeth. Chronic high-dose dietary selenium can cause neurologic effects such as paresthesia and paresis. Elevated selenium levels in body fluids have been associated with clinical toxicity. The diagnosis of selenium toxicity relies on identification of a source, compatible clinical findings, and elevated whole blood selenium levels. Whole blood selenium levels vary with dietary intake; people with a normal selenium intake (90 to 168 µg/day) have levels ranging from 0.143 to 0.211 µg/L. Treatment of chronic selenium toxicity consists of removing

FIGURE 21-1. Fifty-six-year-old woman (left) who has had discolored skin since age 14 years. At age 11 the patient was given nose drops of unknown composition for "allergies," and 3 years later her skin turned gray. She has argyria; a skin biopsy confirmed silver deposition. A person with normal-colored skin (right) is shown for comparison. (From Bouts BA. Images in clinical medicine: Argyria. *N Engl J Med.* 1999;340:1554).

the patient from the selenium source and providing symptomatic and supportive care. Chelating agents are not useful.

Silver

Silver is used widely in photography, electronics, electrical equipment, metal alloys, and antibacterial agents. Silver is ingested in water and foods. Silver toxicity develops after the ingestion of at least 25 g of silver over 6 months.

Silver is absorbed through the gastrointestinal tract, lungs, and skin. Ingested silver undergoes a significant hepatic first-pass effect. Silver has a high affinity for sulfhydryl groups and other proteins. Inorganic silver salts precipitate intracellularly and in turn are complexed with DNA, RNA, and other proteins; alternatively, ascorbic acid or catecholamines can reduce silver salts to the metallic form. Silver is not carcinogenic. Silver is eliminated primarily in the feces; little is excreted in the urine.

The dermal picture of chronic silver poisoning is argyria, an irreversible blue-gray pigmentation of the skin (Fig. 21-1). In the kidneys, silver is deposited in the basement membrane of the glomerulus; altered renal function would be expected but has not been documented clinically. Silver levels in body fluids have not been useful in establishing the diagnosis of chronic silver intoxication. Diagnosis is based on a history of exposure and a compatible clinical picture. Reference levels of serum silver are less than 0.5 µg/L. Treatment of chronic silver intoxication consists of removing the patient from the silver source and providing symptomatic and supportive care. Chelating agents are not useful.

Uranium

Uranium causes toxicity because of its chemical effects or its radiation effects (Chapter 19). Uranium compounds are used in photography and as dyes or fixatives; depleted uranium is used in military equipment. Uranium is poorly absorbed from all exposed sites. Two percent of the uranium in drinking water and food is absorbed into the body. Two thirds of the uranium in the body is in the bones, and about 15% is in the liver.

Uranium decays into radium and then into radon, a radioactive gas that seeps into building foundations in particular geographic areas. Although radon is a respiratory carcinogen (Chapter 197), uranium itself is not carcinogenic. The chemical toxicity of uranium affects the kidneys and lungs. Uranium is nephrotoxic but has not led to increased mortality from renal disease in uranium workers. The injury to the lungs involves nonmalignant damage to alveolar type II cells, but it does not increase mortality from respiratory disease in uranium workers. Treatment of uranium toxicity consists of removing the patient from the uranium source and providing symptomatic and supportive care. Chelators are not recommended.

Although alkalinization of the urine with sodium bicarbonate enhances removal of the uranium molecule from the body, no interventions reduce the effects of chronic uranium toxicity.

Zinc

Zinc is a common element found in air, soil, water, and food. It is widely used in metal alloys, cosmetics, and medications and as an alternative dietary supplement. The oral bioavailability of zinc is variable and depends on the formulation and amount ingested. After ingestion, zinc is concentrated in the liver before being distributed throughout the body. Muscle and bone contain 90% of the total body burden of zinc. High levels of zinc stimulate the synthesis of metallothionein in the liver and in the gastrointestinal mucosal cells. Zinc is eliminated from the body primarily through the gastrointestinal tract. Chronic ingestion of zinc in doses as low as 2 mg/kg/day may lead to microcytic anemia secondary to zinc-induced copper deficiency (a result of increased gastrointestinal mucosal cell metallothionein). Chronic ingestion of high doses of zinc causes nausea, vomiting, and abdominal cramping; variable increases in low-density lipoprotein levels and decreases in high-density lipoprotein levels; and impaired white blood cell function. Treatment of chronic zinc toxicity consists of removing the patient from the zinc source and providing symptomatic and supportive care. The use of chelating agents is not recommended.

1. Mazumder DNG, De KB, Santra A, et al. Randomized placebo-controlled trial of 2,3-dimercapto-1-propanesulfonate (DMPS) in therapy of chronic arsenicosis due to drinking arsenic-contaminated water. *J Toxicol Clin Toxicol.* 2001;39:665-674.
2. Kan WC, Chien CC, Wu CC, et al. Comparison of low-dose deferoxamine versus standard-dose deferoxamine for treatment of aluminium overload among haemodialysis patients. *Nephrol Dial Transplant.* 2010;25:1604-1608.

SUGGESTED READINGS

Argos M, Kalra T, Rathouz PJ, et al. Arsenic exposure from drinking water, and all-cause and chronic-disease mortalities in Bangladesh (HEALS): a prospective cohort study. *Lancet.* 2010;376:252-258. *Chronic arsenic exposure from drinking water is associated with about a 35 to 70% increase in all-cause mortality.*

Department of Health and Human Services, Public Health Service, Agency for Toxic Substances and Disease Registry: Toxicological Profiles. http://www.atsdr.cdc.gov/toxpro2.html. *The most comprehensive review of environmental toxins available; each profile includes a public health statement for consumers.*

Kosnett MJ. Chelation for heavy metals (arsenic, lead, and mercury): protective or perilous? *Clin Pharmacol Ther.* 2010;88:412-415. *Review of risks and benefits.*

Mozaffarian D, Shi P, Morris JS, et al. Mercury exposure and risk of cardiovascular disease in two U.S. cohorts. *N Engl J Med.* 2011;364:1116-1125. *Mercury exposure did not result in increased risk of cardiovascular disease.*

IV

AGING AND GERIATRIC MEDICINE

22

EPIDEMIOLOGY OF AGING: IMPLICATIONS OF THE AGING OF SOCIETY

LINDA P. FRIED

DEMOGRAPHIC REVOLUTION: TRANSITION TO AN AGING SOCIETY

There are now more than 39 million persons 65 years and older in the United States, or more than 12% of the population; in contrast, in 1900, there were 3 million persons 65 years and older, or just 4% of the population. By 2030, about 20% of the U.S. population will be older than 65. By 2050, the current population of older adults will more than double. These increases result from dramatic increases in life expectancy over the past century: in 1900, at birth, men could expect to live to 48 years, and women could expect to live to 51 years on average; by 2008, life expectancy had increased to 75 and 81 years, respectively. Substantial years are now lived after the age of 65 by a large proportion of the population.

With this significant demographic shift, older adults have become a large proportion of all persons with each of the major chronic diseases (Table 22-1). As a result of this burden of disease, people 65 years and older account for about 27% of U.S. health care expenditures, although they represent less than 13% of the U.S. population. Older adults make, on average, 11 outpatient visits per year. People age 75 years and older make almost twice as many emergency department visits as people of all younger ages combined.

HEALTH OF OLDER ADULTS

Changes in Health Status of Older Adults

By many measures, overall well-being is improving for the current generation of older adults compared with previous birth cohorts. In 2007, 39% of persons 65 years and older reported being in excellent or very good health. Educational status, a strong predictor of health behavior and health outcomes, is increasing. In 1950, 17.7% of persons 65 years and older had a high school diploma or higher, and 3.6% had a bachelor's degree or higher; by 2007, these percentages had increased to 74% and 19%. Physical disability, which is an adverse outcome of chronic diseases and aging, is reported by 37% of older adults; however, the remaining 63% are not disabled, and disability rates appear to have declined in the past 10 years.

In 1900, pneumonia and influenza, tuberculosis, diarrhea, and enteritis were the leading causes of death and accounted for 30% of all deaths in persons older than 65 years. Now, heart disease is the leading cause of death in persons 65 and older, followed by cancer, stroke, chronic lower respiratory diseases, Alzheimer's disease, diabetes mellitus, pneumonia, and influenza; the first three diseases accounted for nearly 60% of all deaths. Among persons 85 years and older, heart disease alone is responsible for about 35% of all deaths. Alzheimer's disease is the fourth leading cause of death in women 85 years and older, but it is a less common cause in men.

Death rates for people 65 years and older have declined substantially in the past three decades for heart disease, stroke, pneumonia, and influenza. The first two of these declines are due to a combination of improved medical care, risk factor reductions, and health-promoting changes in lifestyle. Conversely, mortality from chronic obstructive pulmonary disease and diabetes has increased dramatically.

Multiple Causes of Death in Older Adults

Mortality in older adults results from multiple contributing causes, even if one cause can be considered primary. One study of the predictors of 5-year mortality in older adults found that numerous types of health indices contribute: sociodemographic characteristics, health habits, cardiovascular risk factors, clinical and subclinical diseases, physical disability, and cognitive impairment (Table 22-2). After taking these risk factors and conditions into account, age itself becomes substantially less important as a predictor of mortality, up until the age of 85 years.

Disease Frequencies Rise with Increasing Age

The frequency of almost all chronic diseases increases with age, both before and after 65 years of age. For example, arthritis is reported by about 7% of adults aged 18 to 44 years, about 30% of adults aged 45 to 64 years, and about 50% of adults 65 years and older in 2007. The proportion of people who report very good or excellent health decreases with increasing age, from about 70% of persons aged 18 to 44, to about 55% of persons aged 45 to 64, to about 40% of persons 65 years and older. The prevalence of chronic diseases, especially for arthritis, diabetes, and hypertension, is higher in African Americans than in whites in the oldest age groups.

In addition to clinical diseases, subclinical disease is common in older adults. Among the 6000 men and women aged 65 years and older who participated in the Cardiovascular Health Study, 31% had evidence of clinical cardiovascular disease, whereas another 37% had subclinical disease by a variety of noninvasive measures. For example, brain infarct-like lesions, found on magnetic resonance imaging in 28% of Cardiovascular Health Study participants without a known history of stroke, are associated with falling, balance problems, and cognitive decline. Overall, subclinical cardiovascular disease is a stronger predictor of the older adults in whom clinical cardiovascular disease will develop than are other classic risk factors.

Onset of Geriatric Conditions

Health status in aging is a result of many factors, including the chronic diseases of aging and many other prevalent "geriatric" conditions that cannot be defined as classic "diseases" because they do not manifest in a single organ system or result from a single pathologic cause. Falls, which occur in one fourth of older adults, result in injuries, fractures, and high risk for disability and mortality (Chapter 24). Severe cognitive impairment, delirium (Chapters 26 and 27), and urinary incontinence (Chapter 25) have a substantial adverse impact on an older person, as does the sensory isolation resulting from hearing and visual impairment; all these conditions are frequent with aging. Frailty, occurring in 7% of community-dwelling older adults, is a geriatric syndrome that leads to heightened vulnerability to stressors and substantially increased risk for disability, falls, and mortality.

Why Geriatric Patients Are Different
Comorbid Conditions

Older patients differ from young or middle-aged adults who have the same disease in many ways. First, as a function of the high prevalences of many diseases, multimorbidity (or the co-occurrence of two or more diseases in the same individual) is common. Of people aged 65 years and older, 50% have two or more chronic diseases. The risk for becoming disabled or dependent increases with the number of diseases present, and some specific combinations of diseases synergistically increase the risk for disability. For example, arthritis and heart disease coexist in 18% of older adults; although the odds of developing disability are increased by 3-fold to 4-fold with either disease alone, the risk for disability increases 14-fold if both are present. Furthermore, one disease, such as cognitive impairment, may mask the symptoms of other important conditions, at least temporarily. Treatment of one disease may also affect another adversely, as in the use of aspirin to prevent stroke in individuals with a history of gastrointestinal bleeding.

Nonspecific Signs and Symptoms

Older adults differ also from younger adults in the greater likelihood that their diseases will have nonspecific symptoms and signs. For example, pneumonia and stroke may be associated with nonspecific changes in mentation as the primary presenting symptom. Similarly, the frequency of silent myocardial infarction increases with increasing age, as does the proportion of patients who manifest a myocardial infarction with a change in mental status, dizziness, or weakness rather than typical chest pain (Chapter 50). As a result, the diagnostic evaluation of geriatric patients must consider a wider spectrum of causes than would generally be considered in middle-aged adults.

Frailty

Another condition that is found primarily in older adults is frailty. Frailty, which is a state of decreased reserves and increased vulnerability to all kinds of stresses, from acute infection or injury to hospitalization, identifies individuals who likely will have a lower tolerance for any new medical or surgical condition. Frailty is thought to be a wasting syndrome with a characteristic clinical presentation, including weakness, poor exercise tolerance, slowed motor performance, low physical activity, and weight loss. Some estimates

TABLE 22-1 PREVALENCE OF SELECTED CONDITIONS REPORTED BY PERSONS 65 YEARS AND OLDER, UNITED STATES

	NUMBER OF PERSONS 65 YEARS AND OLDER WITH DISEASE (IN THOUSANDS)	PERCENTAGE OF PERSONS 65 YEARS AND OLDER REPORTING THE DISEASE	PERCENTAGE REPORTING THE DISEASE WHO ARE 65 YEARS AND OLDER, AMONG ALL INDIVIDUALS 18 YEARS AND OLDER REPORTING THE DISEASE, UNITED STATES
Hypertension*	19,442	54	37
Arthritis*	17,192	48	37
Disability†	13,467	37	41
Hearing impairment†	13,320	37	40
Heart disease*	11,239	31	45
Urinary incontinence†	9029[1]	25	N/A
Falls†	8379[1]	23	N/A
Malignant neoplasm*	7980	22	49
Obesity	7744	21	14
Influenza*	7744	22	N/A
Diabetes*	6748	19	39
Visual impairment†	5484	15	25
Alzheimer's disease*	4940[2]	13	96
Sinusitis*	4538	13	18
Ulcers*	4244	12	29
Stroke*	2985	8	55
Asthma*	2704	8	17
Frailty†	2528[3]	8	N/A
Emphysema*	1745	5	47
Kidney disease*	1359	4	41
Underweight	845	2	22
Liver disease*	526	2	20

*Clinical diseases.
†Geriatric conditions not associated with specific diseases.
Unless otherwise indicated, data provided by Pleis JR, Lucas JW. Summary health statistics for U.S. adults: National Health Interview Survey, 2007. National Center for Health Statistics. *Vital Health Stat.* 2009;10:240. [1]Lee PG, Cigolle C, Blaum C. The co-occurrence of chronic diseases and geriatric syndromes: the health and retirement study. *J Am Geriatr Soc.* 2009;57:511-516. [2]Hebert LE, Scherr PA, Bienias L, et al. Alzheimer's disease in the US population: prevalence estimates using the 2000 census. *Arch Neurol.* 2003;60:1119-1122. [3]Fried LP, Tangen CM, Walston J, et al. Frailty in older adults: evidence for a phenotype. *J Gerontol A Biol Sci Med Sci.* 2001;56:M146-M156.

indicate that the full syndrome is found in 7% of community-dwelling people aged 65 years and older and in 25% of community-dwelling people 85 years and older. Many institutionalized older adults are also frail. The syndrome of frailty is associated with a high risk for falls, need for hospitalization, poorer recovery after hospitalization, disability, and mortality. A core component of frailty is sarcopenia, or loss of muscle mass associated with aging, which occurs in 13 to 24% of persons aged 65 to 70 years and in 60% of persons 80 years and older. Energy dysregulation and abnormalities in multiple physiologic systems, including inflammation, immune function, hormonal status, and glucose metabolism, underlie the syndrome and decrease the ability to maintain homeostasis in the face of stress. Subclinical disease (e.g., atherosclerosis), end-stage chronic disease (e.g., heart failure, HIV/AIDS), or a combination of comorbid catabolic diseases may precipitate the clinically apparent syndrome. Evidence from randomized, controlled trials shows that resistance exercise, with (or without) nutritional supplements and home-based physical therapy, can increase lean body mass and strength in even the frailest older adults,[1,2] and that weight loss in obese, sedentary older adults has incremental benefit.[3]

Cognitive Impairment
Cognitive impairment, which increases in prevalence as people age (Fig. 22-1; Chapters 26 and 27), is a risk factor for a wide range of adverse outcomes, including falls, immobilization, dependency, institutionalization, and mortality. Cognitive impairment complicates the diagnosis of other medical conditions, necessitates targeted prevention of complications, compromises independence, and requires additional caregiving to ensure safety.

Physical Disability
A serious and common outcome of chronic diseases of aging is physical disability, defined as having difficulty or being dependent on others for the conduct of essential or personally meaningful activities of life from basic self-care (e.g., bathing or toileting) to tasks required to live independently (e.g., shopping, preparing meals, or paying bills) to a full range of activities considered to be productive or personally meaningful (Chapter 23). Among older adults, 37% report difficulty with tasks requiring mobility, and this difficulty with mobility predicts the future development of difficulty in instrumental activities of daily living (IADL; household management tasks) and activities of daily living (ADL; basic self-care tasks). In community-dwelling persons aged 65 years and older, difficulty with IADLs is reported by 20%, and difficulty with ADLs is reported by 11%; for both, the prevalence increases with age. People who have difficulty with IADLs and ADLs are at high risk of becoming dependent. Of persons older than 65 years, 3.5% reside in nursing homes, largely as a result of dependency in IADL or ADL (or both) secondary to severe disease. Generally, women live more years with disability, whereas men who become similarly disabled are more likely to die at a younger age. Although physical disability is primarily a result of chronic diseases and geriatric conditions, its onset and severity are modified by other factors, including treatments that control the underlying diseases, physical activity and rehabilitation, nutrition, smoking, and community-based services. Many intervention trials indicate that some disability can be prevented or its severity decreased.[4]

Relationships among Factors
Multimorbidity, frailty, and disability are recognized as distinct clinical entities (Fig. 22-2), although they are related in the same causal pathway. Multimorbidity may be a risk factor for frailty, and both are risk factors for disability. A vicious cycle may exist whereby inactivity resulting from disability precipitates or worsens frailty.

Thus, the health status of older adults includes a broader spectrum of issues than is found in middle-aged or younger patients, including prevalent chronic disease, recurrent disease, multimorbidity, and geriatric conditions, each of which can be an independent problem or interact with other problems

TABLE 22-2 PREDICTORS OF 5-YEAR AND LONG-TERM MORTALITY IN MEN AND WOMEN 65 YEARS AND OLDER IN THE CARDIOVASCULAR HEALTH STUDY*

RISK FACTOR CATEGORY	FIVE-YEAR MORTALITY PREDICTORS[†]	LONG-TERM MORTALITY PREDICTORS[‡]
Sociodemographic	Age (older) Gender (male) Income (<$50,000/yr)	Age (older) Gender (male) Race (black)
Anthropometric	Weight (lower)	Weight (lower)
Health habits	Physical activity (low) Smoking (pack years)	Physical activity (low) Smoking (pack years)
Cardiovascular risk factors	Brachial systolic blood pressure (elevated) Posterior tibial artery blood pressure (reduced) Diuretic use (in persons with severe CHF or liver disease) Fasting blood glucose (higher)	Fasting blood glucose (higher)
Serum measures	Albumin (lower) Creatinine (higher)	Albumin (lower) Creatinine (higher) IL-6 (greater) ApoE e4 allele
Clinically manifested disease	CHF	CHF Coronary heart disease
Subclinical disease, measured noninvasively	Forced vital capacity, mL (lower) Major ECG abnormality Ejection fraction abnormal Aortic stenosis (moderate to severe) Stenosis (maximal) of the internal carotid artery (greater)	Forced vital capacity, L (lower) Major ECG abnormality
Consequences of disease	Difficulty with instrumental activities of daily living (≥2) Cognitive impairment (greater) Poor self-assessed health	Difficulty with instrumental activities of daily living (≥2) DSST score (lower) Poor self-assessed health

ApoE = apolipoprotein E; CHF = congestive heart failure; DSST = Digit Symbol Substitution Test; ECG = electrocardiographic; IL-6, interleukin-6.
*Persons without cancer at the time of enrollment.
[†]Data from Fried LP, Kronmal RA, Newman AB, et al. Risk factors for 5-year mortality in older adults: the Cardiovascular Health Study. *JAMA.* 1998;279:585-592.
[†]Data from Newman AB, Sachs MC, Arnold AM, et al. Total and cause-specific mortality in the Cardiovascular Health Study. *J Gerontol.* 2009;64:1251-1261.

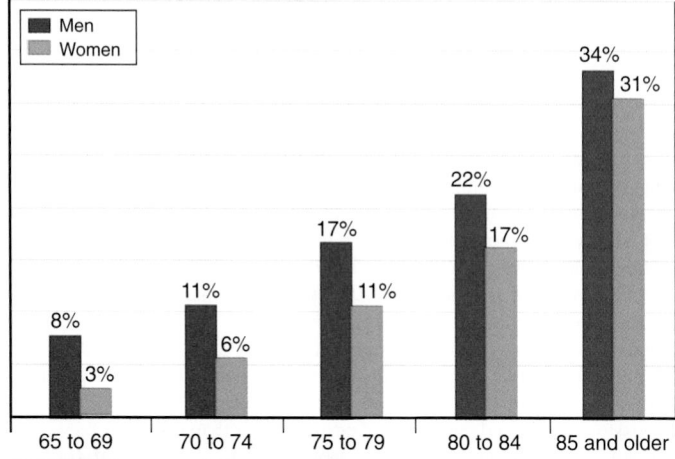

FIGURE 22-1. Percentage of persons 65 years or older with moderate or severe memory impairment (defined as ≤4 words recalled out of 20 on combined immediate and delayed recall tests). (Data from Lethbridge-Cejku M, Vickerie J. Summary health statistics for U.S. adults: National Health Interview Survey, 2003. National Center for Health Statistics. *Vital Health Stat.* 10;2005. Data also from Annual Estimates of the Population by Sex and Five-Year Age Groups for the United States April 1, 2000 to July 1, 2004 [NC-EST2004-01]. Source: Population Division, U.S. Census Bureau.)

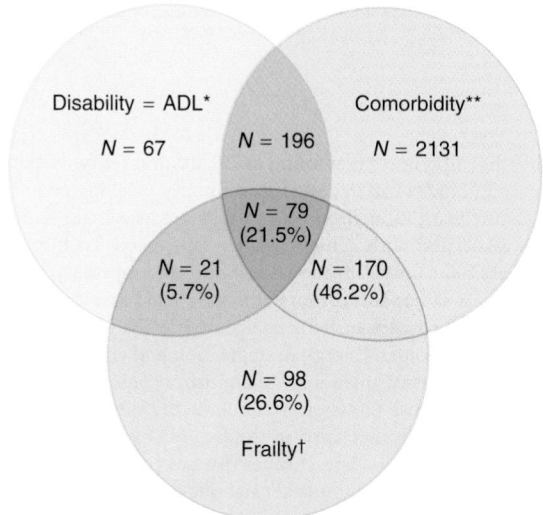

FIGURE 22-2. Overlap of frailty, disability, and comorbidity in community-dwelling older adults participating in the Cardiovascular Health Study. The total represented was 2762 subjects who had comorbidity, disability, or frailty, or any combination of these conditions. *N = 363 with a disability in activities of daily living (ADL); of these, 100 were frail. **N = 2576 with comorbidity, defined as two or more of the following nine diseases: myocardial infarction, angina, heart failure, claudication, arthritis, cancer, diabetes, hypertension, and chronic obstructive pulmonary disease. Of these, 249 were also frail. †N = 368 frail subjects. (Adapted from Fried LP, Tangen CM, Walston J, et al. Frailty in older adults: evidence for a phenotype. *J Gerontol A Biol Sci Med Sci.* 2001;56:M146-M156.)

to cause disability, dependency, or death. There is also, however, great heterogeneity in health status among older adults, with robust, independent individuals even in the oldest ages. Because of this heterogeneity, older patients may require primary, secondary, or tertiary preventive health care (Chapter 23) and an individualized titration of therapeutic and palliative care tailored to their individual health status, goals, and inherent risk. Overall, preventive health care is effective in older adults (Chapters 13 and 14), and attention to clinical practices and health habits—from immunization to physical activity—can prevent adverse outcomes into the oldest ages. Preventive measures should also be targeted to situations of acute stress (e.g., hospitalization or immobilization), when the risk of decline in function is high. Health status can change rapidly as people age, so clinical care, prevention, and services must evolve in concert with the health and function of the patient. Further, there is mounting evidence that social engagement, along with physical, cognitive, and social activity, can modify key health outcomes such as cognitive function and potentially frailty and disability.

1. Liu-Ambrose T, Nagamatsu LS, Graf P, et al. Resistance training and executive functions: a 12-month randomized controlled trial. *Arch Intern Med.* 2010;170:170-178.
2. Kemmler W, von Stengel S, Engelke K, et al. Exercise effects on bone mineral density, falls, coronary risk factors, and health care costs in older women: the randomized controlled senior fitness and prevention (SEFIP) Study. *Arch Intern Med.* 2010;170:179-185.
3. Santanasto AJ, Glynn NW, Newman MA, et al. Impact of weight loss on physical function with changes in strength, muscle mass, and muscle fat infiltration in overweight to moderately obese older adults: a randomized clinical trial. *J Obes.* 2011. [Epub ahead of print.]
4. The LIFE Study Investigators. Effects of a physical activity intervention on measures of physical performance: results of the Lifestyle Intervention and Independence for Elders Pilot (LIFE-P) Study. *J Gerontol A Biol Sci Med Sci.* 2006;61A:1157-1165.

SUGGESTED READINGS

Liu L. Social connections, diabetes mellitus, and risk of mortality among white and African-American adults aged 70 and older: an eight-year follow-up study. *Ann Epidemiol.* 2010;21:26-33. *In the elderly, the lack of social connections carries a risk similar to diabetes for predicting future mortality.*
Studenski S, Perera S, Patel K, et al. Gait speed and survival in older adults. *JAMA.* 2011;305:50-58. *Better gait speed is associated with better survival.*

GERIATRIC ASSESSMENT

DAVID B. REUBEN

Geriatric assessment is a broad term used to describe the evaluation of older patients, a process that recognizes the diverse medical and psychosocial conditions that influence the health status of older persons. In addition to the diseases that are common in the elderly population, these influences include social, psychological, and environmental factors. Geriatric assessment can range from brief screens by individual clinicians to an intensive interdisciplinary process that includes both evaluation and management.

Three fundamental concepts guide geriatric assessment and the resulting medical management. At the core of geriatric assessment is functional status, both as a dimension to be evaluated and as an outcome to be improved or maintained. A second overarching concept guiding geriatric assessment is prognosis, particularly life expectancy. Finally, geriatric assessment must be guided by the patient's goals.

FUNCTIONAL STATUS

Functional status can be viewed as a summary measure of the overall impact of health conditions in the context of an elderly person's environment and social support network. The underlying framework of functional status is a hierarchy of increasing complexity, beginning with specific physical movements (e.g., lifting, walking) that are integrated into higher level activities (e.g., fulfilling occupational and social roles). Impairment of functional status can be triggered by the onset of disease, deconditioning, changes in social support or environment, and advanced age.

Most commonly, older adults' functional status is assessed at two levels: activities of daily living (ADLs) and instrumental activities of daily living (IADLs). ADLs refer to self-care tasks such as bathing, dressing, toileting, maintaining continence, grooming, feeding, and transferring. Dependency in these tasks, which is present in up to 10% of older persons, usually requires full-time help at home or placement in a nursing home.

IADLs refer to tasks that are integral to maintaining an independent household, such as using the telephone, doing laundry, shopping for groceries, driving or using public transportation, preparing meals, taking medications, performing housework, and handling finances. Dependency in IADLs is more common, and almost 20% of persons aged 75 years or older are impaired in at least one task. With the progressive loss of multiple IADL functions, older persons find it more difficult to remain in their homes. Accordingly, many social services (e.g., meals-on-wheels, homemaker services, transportation services) are available to compensate for these deficiencies. A move to an assisted living facility can provide most IADL functions, but many facilities do not routinely provide assistance with ADLs except at an additional cost. In the United States, the costs of assisted living facilities are not covered by Medicare.

At a higher level of function, advanced activities of daily living (AADLs) refer to the ability to fulfill societal, community, and family roles, as well as participate in recreational or occupational tasks. These advanced activities vary considerably from individual to individual but may be valuable in monitoring functional status before the development of disability.

The choice of functional assessment tool depends on the characteristics of the population being assessed. For example, nursing home residents are almost always completely dependent in IADLs, so the focus should be on assessing ADLs and other basic dimensions of health. Hospitalized older persons should be assessed with regard to their prehospitalization functional status to provide insight into what may be achievable, as well as their functional status at the time of discharge to identify any existing gap and facilitate plans to close it.

Functional status is usually measured by self-report or proxy report. However, physical and occupational therapists often add objective information using structured clinical examinations or assessments. In addition, dimensions such as mobility and balance that contribute to function can be assessed by objective measures (described later).

Functional status should be assessed periodically: at the time of an initial visit, after a major illness, and at the time of social milestones, such as the illness of a spouse or a change in living or working situation. Changes in functional status should always prompt further diagnostic evaluation and intervention unless the change is expected and reflects a trajectory that is consistent with the patient's wishes. Measurement of functional status can be valuable in monitoring response to treatment (especially of chronic diseases) and can provide prognostic information that is useful in planning short- and long-term care.

PROGNOSIS

Life expectancy affects both the assessment process and the management decisions based on that assessment. For some older patients, comorbidities can worsen prognosis, such that screening tests (e.g., mammography) and treatments (e.g., for hypertension) with demonstrated effectiveness would not be beneficial within the expected survival period.

Clinicians can estimate remaining years of life by age, gender, and race using life tables (Table 23-1). These tables, however, do not consider clinical characteristics or functional status, which can lead to wide variations in how long an individual patient will live.

PATIENT GOALS

As people age, their current and future health may become a prominent factor in determining and achieving their life goals. Among very old patients, goals may be limited to achieving a functional or health state (e.g., being able to walk independently), controlling symptoms (e.g., pain, dyspnea), maintaining their living situation (e.g., remaining at home), or short-term survival (e.g., living long enough to reach a personal milestone, such as an upcoming holiday). Sometimes the goals of patients and physicians differ. For example, a patient may want a cure, whereas the physician believes that only symptom management is possible. Conversely, the physician may believe that a better outcome is possible, but the patient declines to pursue the recommended path (e.g., hip replacement to restore mobility).

COMPONENTS OF GERIATRIC ASSESSMENT

Geriatric assessment begins with a medical evaluation. Some aspects (described later) that are rarely abnormal in younger adults (e.g., mobility, cognition) may cause substantial morbidity in older persons. In addition, some clusters of abnormal findings, such as muscle wasting, poor hygiene, bruises, pressure sores, and contractures, should raise the suspicion of elder mistreatment, neglect, or abuse. In such cases, patients should be questioned and examined without family members or caregivers present. Patients should then be queried whether anyone has threatened or hurt them, whether they have been receiving enough care, and whether anyone has taken their things. Answers to these questions may provide confirmatory information and prompt a report to adult protective services.

Nonmedical assessments are also important because they can identify problems that should be addressed and may be key to achieving the patient's goals. In addition to an assessment of functional status, older persons' environmental, financial, and nonfinancial support should be assessed. In some situations, particularly when older persons become acutely ill or experience caregiver stress or loss of a loved one, assessment of spiritual needs, with appropriate referral, may be valuable.

TABLE 23-1	LIFE EXPECTANCY (IN YEARS) FOR OLDER PERSONS BY AGE, RACE, AND SEX			
	White		Black	
AGE	MALE	FEMALE	MALE	FEMALE
65	17.2	20	15.2	18.6
70	13.7	16.2	12.4	15.3
75	10.7	12.8	9.9	12.2
80	8.1	9.7	8.0	9.6
85	6.0	7.1	6.3	7.5
90	4.3	5.1	4.9	5.7
95	3.1	3.6	3.8	4.3
100	2.2	2.5	2.9	3.2

Advance Directives

Clinicians should discuss older patients' preferences for specific treatments while they still have the cognitive capacity to make these decisions. Patients should be asked to identify a spokesperson to make medical decisions for them if they cannot speak for themselves. This information should be conveyed through a durable power of attorney for health care, which also allows patients to specify treatments they do not want. Many states have allowed the use of Physician Orders for Life-Sustaining Treatment, a specific advance directive that documents a patient's end-of-life treatment preferences and serves as an order sheet. The standardized form is signed by both the physician and the patient and must be honored in all settings of care.

Medical Assessment

The medical assessment includes vision; hearing; cognition; mood and affect; falls, mobility, and balance; medication review; nutrition; and urinary incontinence. Numerous screening instruments have been developed that assess many of these dimensions. Other important medical components of geriatric assessment include a review of the patient's medications and a determination of whether preventive services are up-to-date.

Vision

Each of the four major eye diseases—cataract, age-related macular degeneration, diabetic retinopathy, and glaucoma (Chapter 431)—increases in prevalence with age. Moreover, presbyopia is virtually universal, and the vast majority of older persons require eyeglasses. Visual impairment has been associated with increased risk of falls, functional and cognitive decline, immobility, and depression. Corrective lenses or other treatments may restore vision or prevent further decline of visual function.

A single question can be used to screen for visual impairment: Do you have difficulty driving, watching television or reading, or doing any of your daily activities because of your eyesight, even while wearing glasses?

The Snellen eye chart is the standard method of screening for visual acuity. The patient is asked to stand 20 feet from the chart and read letters. Inability to read letters on or below the 20/40 line with their best-corrected vision (using glasses) indicates the need for further evaluation.

Hearing

Hearing loss (Chapter 436), which affects 30% of community-dwelling older adults older than 65 years and 75% of residents living in nursing home settings, is associated with reduced cognitive, social, emotional, and physical functioning. When hearing loss is detected, amplification by hearing aids or assistive listening devices can improve quality of life and functional status.

To assess hearing, the physician can administer the whisper voice test, which involves whispering three different random words in each ear at distances of 6, 12, and 24 inches from the patient's ear and then asking the patient to repeat the words. Patients who fail the screen—that is, are unable to repeat half the whispered words correctly—should be referred to an audiologist for further evaluation. Alternatively, the Hearing Handicap Inventory for the Elderly, a 10-item self-report instrument, has been used widely.

A more accurate screening tool for hearing impairment is the Welch Allyn AudioScope. This handheld otoscope has a built-in audiometer that can be set at different levels of intensity. A pretone at 60 dB is delivered to the patient, and then four tones of 500, 1000, 2000, and 4000 Hz at 40 dB are presented. The inability to hear either the 1000- or 2000-Hz frequency in both ears or both the 1000- and 2000-Hz frequencies in one ear indicates a positive screen and identifies the need for formal audiometric testing.

Cognitive Assessment

The incidence of dementia (Chapters 26 and 409) increases with age, especially among those older than 85 years. Early detection of memory problems can lead to the identification of treatable conditions that contribute to cognitive impairment and the development of a proactive management plan with the patient's full participation.

The most commonly used screen is the Mini-Mental State Examination (MMSE), a 30-item interviewer-administered assessment of several dimensions of cognitive function (see Table 26-4). However, the MMSE is too long for most practitioners to incorporate routinely into their clinical practices, and the instrument must be purchased for use. Several shorter screens have also been validated, including recall of three items at 1 minute and the Mini-Cog test (see Table 26-5), which combines three-item recall and the clock-drawing test.

Another component of cognitive assessment is decision-making capacity. In cognitively intact older persons, capacity is assumed. However, among those with cognitive impairment, decision making must be determined before many treatments are initiated. As a rule, capacity is specific to the decision the patient is being asked to make. Ask the following questions to determine a patient's decision-making capacity:
- Can the patient make and express personal preferences at all?
- Can the patient comprehend the risks and benefits?
- Does the patient comprehend the implications?
- Can the patient give reasons for the alternative selected?
- Are supporting reasons rational?

If the answer to all these questions is yes, the patient is competent to make the decision at hand. If not, then a surrogate (the durable power of attorney for health care, if the patient has identified one) should make the decision. If a durable power of attorney for health care has not been identified, the decision can be made by a family member, friend, or caregiver who knows the patient well. The order of surrogates is determined by state law. If no one is available, the health care provider should make the decision based on the patient's known value system or what the health care provider believes to be in the best interest of the patient.

Mood and Affect

Although major depression (Chapter 404) is no more common among the elderly than among the younger population, minor depression and other affective disorders are common and cause considerable morbidity. Moreover, depression may present atypically, and it may be masked in patients with cognitive impairment or other neurologic disorders such as Parkinson's disease (Chapter 416).

A two-item version of the Patient Health Questionnaire (PHQ-9) can effectively screen for depression symptoms. The screener asks the patient: Over the past 2 weeks, how often have you been bothered by any of the following problems?
- Little interest or pleasure in doing things.
- Feeling down, depressed, or hopeless.

Responses are scored as follows: 0 = not at all, 1 = several days, 2 = more than half the days, 3 = nearly every day. Persons who score a total of 3 points or higher on the two-item screen have a 75% probability of having a depressive disorder. More detailed information can be gathered using instruments such as the Geriatric Depression Scale.

Falls, Mobility, and Balance

Approximately one third of community-dwelling persons older than 65 and half of those older than 80 fall each year. Ten percent of these falls result in a serious injury. Patients who have fallen or have gait or balance problems are at higher risk of another fall. Performing a falls assessment (measuring orthostatic blood pressure; assessing vision; reviewing medications; and testing balance, gait, and lower extremity strength) and treating risk factors for falling can reduce falls by 30 to 40%.

All older patients should be asked at least annually if they have fallen, and frail older persons should be asked about falls at every visit. In addition, asking about fear of falling can identify patients at risk of future falls.

Patients who have fallen or have a fear of falling should have their balance and gait assessed by direct observation of their ability to perform specific tasks. Tests of balance include the ability to maintain a side-by-side, semitandem, and full-tandem stance for 10 seconds; resistance to a nudge; and stability during a 360-degree turn. Quadriceps strength can be assessed by observing an older person rising from a hard armless chair without using his or her hands.

In addition, direct qualitative and quantitative observation of gait to determine stability is a quick and important component of assessment. Qualitative aspects include evaluation of hesitancy; sway; step length, height, symmetry, and continuity; and path deviation. Gait speed is also a helpful marker for recurrent falls. Patients who take more than 13 seconds to walk 10 meters are more likely to have recurrent falls.

The timed "up-and-go" test combines some features of strength and gait. It is a timed test of the patient's ability to rise from a standard armchair, walk 3 meters (10 feet), turn, walk back, and sit down again. Patients who take longer than 20 seconds to complete the test should receive further evaluation.

Medication Review

Older persons often see several different health care providers who prescribe multiple medications that increase the risk for drug-drug interactions and adverse drug events. At a minimum, the clinician should review the patient's updated and accurate medication list at each visit. A good method of detecting potential problems is to have patients bring in all their medications (prescription and nonprescription) in their bottles. Entering a patient's medication list into commercially available computer drug interaction programs can help prevent adverse events.

Nutrition

Malnutrition in older adults includes obesity (Chapter 227), undernutrition (Chapter 221), and specific vitamin deficiencies (Chapter 225). Obesity in older adults is defined as a body mass index (BMI) of 30 kg/m^2 or greater. High BMI is associated with poorer function and more comorbidities, such as type 2 diabetes mellitus (Chapters 236 and 237), osteoarthritis (Chapter 270), hyperlipidemia (Chapter 213), coronary artery disease (Chapter 51), and sleep apnea (Chapter 100).

At the initial visit, patients should be weighed and asked about weight loss in the previous 12 months. They should be weighed at all follow-up visits. BMI should be calculated on the initial visit and periodically thereafter (e.g., yearly or when a change in weight suggests the need to recalculate). Serum markers, including serum albumin, prealbumin, and cholesterol levels, are nonspecific indicators of nutritional status and can be affected by inflammatory states, physiologic stress, and trauma.

Weight loss of 4% or more over 12 months predicts increased mortality and should prompt an evaluation of medical (e.g., malignancy, gastrointestinal disorders, hyperthyroidism, diabetes), psychiatric (e.g., depression, dementia), dental, and social or functional (e.g., poverty, inability to shop or prepare meals) causes.

Urinary Incontinence

Approximately one third of community-dwelling older adult women have some degree of urinary incontinence (Chapter 25), and 75% of older men have abnormal urinary tract symptoms. Complications of incontinence include skin irritation, pressure ulcers, urinary tract infections, sleep disruption, and falls. Identification of urinary incontinence is important because effective behavioral and pharmacologic treatments are available.

A simple screen for urinary incontinence asks the following question: Have you had urinary incontinence (do you "lose" your urine) to the extent that it is bothersome and you would like to know how it can be treated? This may be valuable in determining which patients want further evaluation and therapy. Patients who answer yes should be asked how much urine is leaked, how much it interferes with daily life, and when the leakage occurs. Further evaluation and treatment depend on whether the incontinence is overflow incontinence, urge incontinence, or stress incontinence (see Table 25-3).

● PREVENTIVE SERVICES

Preventive services include lifestyle advice, screening tests to detect asymptomatic disease, and vaccinations. Recommended adult immunization schedules include annual influenza vaccination, one-time pneumonia vaccination, one-time pneumococcal vaccination, one-time herpes zoster vaccination (even if the patient reports a past episode of herpes zoster), and tetanus toxoid vaccination every 10 years (Chapter 17).

To help the clinician decide what is appropriate for a specific patient, the U.S. Preventive Services Task Force has created an interactive website (*http://epss.ahrq.gov/ePSS/search.jsp*) with recommendations based on the patient's age, gender, tobacco use, and current sexual activity (Chapter 14). For younger elderly persons, recommendations include screening for blood pressure, diabetes, hyperlipidemia, obesity, alcohol misuse, colorectal cancer, and osteoporosis, as well as breast cancer in women, with appropriate counseling and treatment if these disorders are detected. Aspirin may be recommended to prevent cardiovascular disease in this population. Other recommendations depend on patient-specific risk factors.

With increasing age, fewer preventive services are recommended because of limited life expectancy and greater comorbidities. Accordingly, some preventive measures (e.g., aspirin to prevent cardiovascular disease) and cancer screenings are not recommended in the very elderly. When the evidence base for preventive services is sparse, decisions should be individualized, based on the patient's personal values, goals, and preferences.

● NONMEDICAL ASSESSMENTS

Environmental Assessment

Assessing a patient's environment includes evaluating three components: the person's ability to access community services (e.g., getting to the bank and stores if the patient cannot drive), the safety of the physical environment, and the appropriateness of the living situation for the person's functional ability and cognitive status. A brief screen for safety of the physical environment can be accomplished by using a checklist that is in the public domain (*http://www.cdc.gov/ncipc/pub-res/toolkit/Falls_ToolKit/DesktopPDF/English/booklet_Eng_desktop.pdf*). For home-bound older patients, a home safety evaluation by a home health agency is more appropriate.

Social Support Assessment

When older persons become frail, the adequacy of their social support network may be the determining factor in whether they can remain at home or need institutionalization. A brief screen of social support includes taking a social history, including asking who would be available to help if the patient becomes ill. For patients with functional impairment, the clinician should ascertain who can help the patient perform ADLs or IADLs. Early identification of problems with social support can help avoid crisis situations if the patient has a sudden medical or functional decline. Caregivers should be screened periodically for symptoms of depression or caregiver burnout and referred for counseling or support groups if necessary.

Financial Assessment

Although clinicians do not have the training or expertise to explore financial resources in detail, knowing the patient's insurance status may be helpful. For example, patients with Medicaid coverage may qualify for additional medical or social support benefits. Some may be eligible for other state or local benefits, depending on their income. Others may have long-term care insurance or veterans' benefits that can help pay for caregivers, obviating the need for institutionalization.

● A STRATEGIC APPROACH TO GERIATRIC ASSESSMENT FOR THE PRACTICING CLINICIAN

Although assembling an interdisciplinary assessment team is beyond the capability of most practitioners, even small group practices can use teamwork and simple practice design to perform geriatric assessments efficiently and comprehensively. These assessments can lead to local implementation of or referral to comprehensive care models that can improve the outcomes of elderly individuals with a variety of chronic conditions.[1][2] Because of time constraints, screening is increasingly delegated to staff and to patients and their families using standing orders, forms, and questionnaires (Table 23-2). For example, previsit questionnaires can be used to gather information about past medical and surgical history; medications and allergies; social history, including available social support resources, preventive services, ability to perform functional tasks, and need for assistance; home safety; and advance directives. In addition, the previsit questionnaire can include specific questions that assess vision, hearing, falls, urinary incontinence, and depressive symptoms. A reasonable approach is to assess these issues annually beginning at age 75 years. Persons who are younger than 75 but have multiple comorbidities should also be screened and reassessed annually. In addition, some elements of geriatrics assessment (assessing ADLs and IADLs; gait, balance, and falls; mood and affect; and cognition) should be performed after major illnesses, especially those requiring hospitalization.

TABLE 23-2	APPROACHES TO ASSESSING FUNCTION IN ELDERLY INDIVIDUALS				
	Previsit Questionnaire			**Office Staff Administered**	
ASPECT BEING ASSESSED	LENGTH OF SCREEN*	INSTRUMENTS	LENGTH OF SCREEN*	INSTRUMENTS	
Functional status	D	Activities of daily living Instrumental activities of daily living			
Advance directives	B	Specific question about advance directives			
MEDICAL ASSESSMENT					
Visual impairment	B	Single-item question	B	Snellen eye chart (see Table 431-1)	
Hearing impairment	B	Hearing Handicap Inventory for the Elderly	B (if needed)	Whisper test Audioscope	
Cognitive problems			B	Mini-cog 3-item recall (see Table 26-5)	
Mind, affective problems	D	Geriatric depression scale (see Table 26-3)	B		
Falls, mobility, balance	B	Simple questions	B	Timed up-and-go test	
Medication review			D	Inspection of medication bottles	
Malnutrition	D	Single question	B	Weight	
Urinary incontinence	B	Single question	B	International Consultation on Incontinence Modular Questionnaire -UI short form if single question is positive	
Preventive services	D	Specific questions			
OTHER DIMENSIONS					
Environment	D	Home safety checklist			
Social support	B	Single question			
Financial status			B	Insurance status	

*B = brief screen (e.g., <2 min); D = detailed evaluation (usually ≥5 min).

1. Boult C, Green AF, Boult LB, et al. Successful models of comprehensive care for older adults with chronic conditions: evidence for the Institute of Medicine's "Retooling for an Aging America" report. *J Am Geriatr Soc.* 2009;57:2328-2337.
2. Wenger NS, Roth CP, Shekelle PG, et al. A practice-based intervention to improve primary care for falls, urinary incontinence, and dementia. *J Am Geriatr Soc.* 2009;57:547-555.

SUGGESTED READINGS

Berry SD, Ngo L, Samelson EJ, et al. Competing risk of death: an important consideration in studies of older adults. *J Am Geriatr Soc.* 2010;58:783-787. *Emphasizes that the elderly receive less benefit from an intervention because of other adverse prognostic factors.*

Formiga F, Ferrer A, Chivite D, et al. Predictors of long-term survival in nonagenarians: the NonaSantfeliu study. *Age Ageing.* 2011;40:111-116. *Better cognitive status and lesser comorbidity are the best predictors of 5-year survival in nonagenarians.*

Reuben DB. Medical care for the final years of life: "When you're 83, it's not going to be 20 years." *JAMA.* 2009;302:2686-2694. *A practical approach to functionally impaired elderly patients.*

24

COMMON CLINICAL SEQUELAE OF AGING

KENNETH L. MINAKER

EPIDEMIOLOGY

Increased longevity throughout the world is influencing medical care dramatically as more and more older individuals survive with more complex medical conditions. Although some elderly individuals present classically with single-system disease, others have presentations and responses to treatments that are different from those in younger patients. This variation in presentation and behavior of illnesses, which is due to the combined effect of aging and comorbid disease, must be understood if elderly patients are to receive successful care.

PATHOBIOLOGY

Age-associated changes in health and disease are the result of (1) variations in the underlying physiologic changes that occur with age; (2) the presence of other diseases and medical conditions that have developed over time; (3) genetic predispositions for certain diseases; (4) lifestyle factors, including health-seeking behavior, diet, exercise, and exposure to medications and toxins; and (5) the variability intrinsic to diseases and medical conditions in general. Although no single hypothesis fully explains the process of aging at this time (Chapter 22), two major approaches have emerged (Table 24-1). The first concerns programmed causes, which are dominated by genetic theories. The second concerns stochastic causes, so-called process-of-living theories, in which genetic or environmental influences limit viability.

Spectrum of Changes Produced by Aging Processes

Perhaps the most important observation regarding normal aging is how much does not change. Most hormone levels, liver enzyme activities, electrolyte levels, body temperature, and basal glucose concentration remain constant throughout the lifespan. Long-term studies have indicated that there is no age-related anemia (Chapter 161), although the hematocrit declines slightly in men presumably because of the age-related decline in testosterone.

The passage of time results in changes that are not due to aging per se but rather may be considered "dose-time" related. For example, prolonged exposure results in the emergence of abnormalities and illnesses, such as skin cancer due to cumulative actinic injury (Chapter 210). Much of the lifetime exposure to sun is received before the age of 20 years, yet the resulting cancers follow decades later. Another example is polycystic kidney disease, which is an inheritable condition that does not appear until well into adulthood (Chapter 129); the passage of time allows the "full expression" of the genetic phenotype, but aging itself is not the key factor.

Some conditions become less likely with advancing age because of changes in the immune system. Immune disorders such as systemic lupus erythematosus (Chapter 274) and multiple sclerosis (Chapter 419) rarely appear in late life, presumably because changes in the immune system lead to less aggressive autoimmune activity. Similarly, although many cancers are more common in elderly people, many of the most aggressive tumors occur at a young age, suggesting that immune tolerance develops with advancing age.

TABLE 24-1 PATHOBIOLOGY OF AGING

THEORY	DEFINITION	CAUSE: GENETIC (G) OR ENVIRONMENTAL (E)	
PROGRAMMED THEORIES			
Programmed senescence	Aging results from gene interference with the ability of the cells to reproduce	Master clock, cancer protection	G
Hormonal	Biologic clock alters hormone secretion, resulting in tissue changes	Decrease in levels of insulin-like growth factor-I and the hormones estrogen, testosterone, DHEA, and melatonin	G
Immunologic	T-cell function declines, increasing the chances for development of infections and cancer	Alteration in the cytokines that are responsible for communication between immune cells	G
Telomere shortening	Shortening of telomeres in somatic cells lessens the ability of cells to divide	Cells cannot divide	G, E
STOCHASTIC THEORIES			
Metabolic rate	The higher the basal metabolic rate (the rate at which the body, at rest, uses energy), the shorter the lifespan	Energy demands to maintain basal metabolism	G
Glycation	Glycation (browning) causes proteins to be joined, resulting in rigidity and decreased function	Elevated glucose	G, E
Somatic mutation	Mutations in genes occur with aging, eventually causing cells to stop functioning	Errors in the transmission of genetic messages over time	G
Wear and tear	Parts of cells wear out over time	Accumulated debris mechanically disrupts cell function	E
Oxygen free radicals	Tissue damage is caused by free radicals, such as superoxide or hydroxyl radicals; this is a specific form of the wear-and-tear theory	Oxygen free radicals are unstable chemical compounds that can oxidize cell components such as DNA and proteins	E

DHEA = dehydroepiandrosterone.

Physiologic aging modulates the ways in which illnesses cause signs and symptoms. The elderly individual with hyperthyroidism often presents not with the systemic findings of agitation, irritability, hyperactivity, hyperphagia, and increased bowel movements but rather with apathy, anorexia, and atrial fibrillation (Chapter 233). The underlying pathophysiologic process may be no different, but age-related changes in physiology alter the body's sensitivity to dysfunction and influence the clinical presentation.

The most important physiologic change of aging is the predisposition to more generalized clinical syndromes and more severe disease. The lung function of a healthy 70-year-old is about 50% that of a 30-year-old (Chapters 83 and 85). Renal function commonly declines by 50% or more by the age of 70 years (Chapter 117). The resultant lack of physiologic reserve capacity does not affect day-to-day function but can affect the ability to recover from an extreme illness that exhausts the body's reserve capacity.

Geriatric syndromes emerge from these age-related changes. Many systems that maintain our upright posture are compromised by age, leading to increased postural sway. An older individual is much more likely to fall after a slip or a push. The consequences of that fall are more serious because of the age-related loss of bone mass (Chapter 251), resulting in fall-related fractures and spinal cord injuries.

Some physiologic changes imitate illness when they may be a normal part of aging. Diabetes mellitus may "appear" and "disappear" in elderly people (Chapters 236 and 237). The ability of insulin to stimulate glucose uptake declines with age and usually is manifested as postprandial hyperglycemia, but with normal fasting insulin and glucose levels. Under stress situations, older individuals can appear to be diabetic, but when the stressful situation is relieved, they no longer have chemical evidence of diabetes. Nevertheless, this loss of physiologic reserve understandably contributes to the increasing prevalence of diabetes with advancing age.

The age-related changes that make elderly people more vulnerable in daily life are often subtle. Older individuals are more likely to develop hypothermia or hyperthermia (Chapter 109) during extreme environmental exposure because of neurologic and thermoregulatory changes. The loss of brain stem neurotransmitters in older persons not only may cause a senile gait pattern but also predisposes to genetically determined conditions such as Parkinson's disease (Chapter 416). Decreases in the function of the frontal lobe inhibitory center predispose to urgency of urination.

Some age-related changes cause specific medical sequelae. Menopause (Chapter 248) is a normal aging process that produces symptoms and predisposes to future bone loss, urogenital atrophy, and atherosclerosis. Senile cataracts are caused by post-translational modifications in lens proteins combined with the inability of the lens to dispose of breakdown products associated with these processes; as a result, the lens becomes stiffer, thicker, and more opaque with age (Chapter 431).

EFFECTS OF AGING ON SPECIFIC ORGANS AND SYSTEMS

Cardiovascular System

Aging and Its Clinical Sequelae

Many important physiologic changes occur in the aging heart and help explain common age-associated cardiac disorders. Perhaps the most important physiologic change is the delay in left ventricular filling, which declines 50% between the ages of 20 and 80 years. Cardiac filling becomes more dependent on active filling late in diastole during atrial contraction (Chapter 52). This phenomenon commonly is related to thickening and stiffening of the left ventricular wall. Under normal conditions, systolic function remains unchanged, but the thickened ventricle will not produce normal output when volumes are low or be able to avoid elevated filling pressures and the resulting pulmonary congestion when volume is high. As a result, brain natriuretic peptide levels increase with age as myocardial sensors detect greater pressures in the heart.

The resting heart rate slows slightly with advancing age, and maximal and submaximal exercise-induced heart rates show an age-related decline. The loss of sinus node pacemaker cells—up to 90% at 80 years—contributes to these changes. There also are changes in central and baroreflex-mediated heart rate control (Chapter 62). Heart valves thicken and stiffen, particularly in the mitral and aortic locations (Chapter 75). The functional significance of heart valve stiffening is minimal, but 25% of older individuals have flow murmurs (Chapter 50). The aorta dilates and its walls thicken as medial walls calcify; with this loss of elasticity, there is a secondary increase in systolic blood pressure (Chapter 67). The arteriosclerosis that is due to intimal disease further causes arterial walls to thicken, calcify, and lose their elasticity, thereby predisposing aging vessels to occlude or rupture (Chapter 70).

In most industrialized countries, there is a progressive increase in blood pressure with advancing age (Chapter 67). In general, systolic blood pressure increases after the age of 30 years, continues to rise until the mid-70s, then tends to fall slightly through the 80s and 90s. Diastolic blood pressure tends to parallel the usual increase in body weight that peaks in the early 50s in men and the early 60s in women; diastolic pressures subsequently fall slightly in older age. These changes in blood pressure are not universal, suggesting varied genetic and environmental causes, such as stress, sodium and potassium intake, and obesity.

Age-Related Cardiovascular Syndromes

Although atherosclerosis is the most important cause of symptomatic cardiac disease in elderly people, age-associated vascular stiffness predisposes to left ventricular stiffness, impaired diastolic filling, and the clinical syndrome of diastolic heart failure (Chapter 58). The most common arrhythmia in older individuals is atrial fibrillation (Chapter 64), which may occur in one third of older individuals undergoing surgery and may affect 4% of community-dwelling elderly individuals. Although thyroid disease, coronary artery disease, valvular heart disease, and intrinsic conduction system disease are common causes, atrial fibrillation in elderly people is often "lone" atrial fibrillation without a detectable underlying illness.

The combination of sensitivity to filling volumes and impaired heart rate response to stress may explain the increasingly prevalent syndrome of postural hypotension that is present in 20% of older individuals (Chapter 62). Postural hypotension is also common in elderly individuals after large meals; during infections severe enough to depress salt and water intake; and during volume-depleting stresses, such as diarrhea, diuretic therapy, and bowel preparation for colonoscopy. Stiffening of vessels in which baroreceptors reside also reduces the ability to modulate blood pressure with advancing age.

Perhaps the most important principle in the approach to cardiovascular signs and symptoms with advancing age is to recognize the narrowed homeostatic capacity of elderly people. Volume status must be managed carefully, attention should be paid to standing as opposed to sitting blood pressure in patients predisposed to postural hypotension, side effects of medications must be anticipated and monitored, and cardiovascular instability must be expected during almost any major illness that an older person may experience.

Respiratory System

The most characteristic change in the chest wall with advancing age is stiffening (Chapter 85). Cartilages thicken and calcify, and spinal ligaments and joints become stiffer. The primary internal change in the lungs is the loss of the elastic recoil. The result is a modest expansion of the chest wall with the appearance of a mild barrel chest. Although resting lung mechanics do not appear to change in any major way, maximal breathing capacity declines by approximately 40%. At the alveolar level, the capacity to exchange oxygen and carbon monoxide decreases by approximately 50% between the ages of 30 and 65 years, in part as a result of ventilation-perfusion mismatching (Chapter 85). Although these changes are not noticeable at rest, individuals experience fatigue or shortness of breath when the respiratory system is under stress (e.g., during exercise or major illness). Pulmonary reflexes such as coughing and ciliary function decrease, predisposing elderly individuals to the pooling of secretions.

These changes do not produce substantial abnormalities in resting oxygen saturation, but they produce a steady decline in arterial Po_2. The arterial Po_2 of many individuals older than 80 years is about 70 to 75 mm Hg. As with other age-related physiologic findings, these changes do not interfere with function under resting conditions but dramatically affect survival during severe respiratory illness.

Age-Related Respiratory Syndromes

The major clinical impact of normal physiologic aging in the lungs is an earlier appearance of shortness of breath as a warning signal of underlying disease. Myocardial infarction and heart failure can present primarily with shortness of breath, mainly owing to age-related mechanical changes, an inability to clear blood from the lungs, and a decline in resting pulmonary function to near the threshold for clinical hypoxia. Aspiration pneumonia increases with age in association with impaired swallowing, reflux, and reduced clearance of lung secretions.

Gastrointestinal System

A broad series of changes occur in gastroenterologic tissues, but the redundancy of overall gastrointestinal function usually prevents clinical symptoms. Age-related changes in the mouth include slower production of dentine, shrinkage of the root pulp, and decreasing bone density of the jaw. Taste and smell decline progressively with advancing age, with rising thresholds for tasting salt, sweetness, and certain proteins (Chapter 435). The overall net effect is that food may taste more bitter, and more sugar is required before something tastes sweet. Salivary gland function normally does not change with age (Chapter 433). The loss of bone and tongue musculature makes the tongue appear to be enlarged.

The esophagus appears to function relatively normally. The strength of muscle contraction declines, however, and peristaltic waves slow with advancing age. There is also a tendency for the lower esophageal sphincter to become lax (Chapter 140). These changes predispose to aspiration.

The gastric mucosa secretes less acid with advancing age. Although these changes do not appear to affect digestion in most individuals, associated conditions, such as atrophic gastritis, may further decrease the absorption of nutrients to the point of producing illness. Most studies suggest that delayed gastric emptying is a feature of aging, leading to a sense of early satiety, which can impair subsequent food ingestion (Chapter 138).

Liver weight declines by one third between the ages of 30 and 90 years, primarily because of the loss of hepatocytes. The result is a decreased ability to process medications such as benzodiazepines, which require two steps for metabolism, and vitamin K–blocking agents. Doses of drugs often must be adjusted, and their blood levels should be monitored when possible.

Aging is associated with a significant reduction in small intestinal surface area with the consequence of reduced absorption of some dietary components, such as calcium. Colonic function declines with advancing age. Motility up to the rectosigmoid area, measured by passage of markers, does not appear to decline with advancing age (Chapter 138). Distal to this point, however, evacuation is characteristically slower with advancing age. Stool frequency tends to decline, and hardness of stools appears to increase with advancing age. Diverticula are present in approximately 50% of people older than 80 years and are likely to be related to reduced dietary fiber and the resulting greater intracolonic pressure (Chapter 144).

Age-Related Gastroenterologic Syndromes

The most important age-related symptom is constipation (Chapter 138), which may affect 60% of individuals in late life. Obstipation can present atypically with confusion, nausea, and vomiting or as obscure fever resulting from stercoral ulcerations. Perhaps the most common abnormality related to declining hepatic function is increased sensitivity to medications that require hepatic metabolism.

Renal and Urinary Excretory System

Overall kidney size declines by approximately one third, and blood flow through the kidney declines by about 1% per year. Beginning in the late 30s, cortical nephrons appear to drop out and sclerose at a much higher rate than medullary nephrons, creating a hyperfiltration syndrome that limits maximal concentrating capacity (Chapter 117). Resulting functional changes include decreased ability to excrete a salt load, declining glomerular filtration rate, delayed ability to regain sodium and potassium balance during deprivation states, and difficulty in conserving water under situations of dehydration. Excretion of water loads is not strikingly impaired with age, but modest and perhaps clinically significant reductions in acid secretion have been shown in older individuals.

The bladder tends to become more irritable with advancing age and may generate less power during contraction. Because of the delay in sodium excretion and orthostatic changes, nocturia is common; older individuals appear to produce more urine at night than during the day. The most important bladder change may be the slight increase in residual bladder urine volume. Atrophy of vaginal and urethral tissues due to postmenopausal estrogen deprivation predisposes women to urinary tract infections (Chapter 248).

Age-Related Renal and Urinary Tract Syndromes

The age-related increases in asymptomatic bacteriuria and urinary tract infections are almost certainly due to increased residual bladder volume and loss of protective factors in the normal anatomic structures. As the prostate gland grows with advancing age, benign prostatic hypertrophy causes urinary retention in men (Chapter 131). Urinary incontinence (Chapter 25) is more prevalent in women. The kidney is more susceptible to the effects of medications, particularly nonsteroidal anti-inflammatory drugs, which can result in sodium and fluid retention and subsequent hypertension. In elderly individuals, a slight acidemia results from impaired acid excretion and may contribute to the development of osteoporosis.

Dehydration or volume depletion, which is increasingly prevalent with advancing age, often accompanies acute infections and increases the morbidity and mortality of pneumonia or urinary tract infections. Dehydration is the most common fluid and electrolyte disorder in the frail elderly patient because of decreased fluid intake and increased fluid losses. Vomiting and diarrhea are the most common causes of isotonic dehydration. Fever associated with delirium is the leading cause of hypertonic dehydration. Hypotonic dehydration is seen most commonly with overuse of diuretics. Signs and symptoms of dehydration are notoriously vague or absent. Orthostatic tachycardia and hypotension are important clinical findings, and an acute decline in weight may be documented. Perhaps the most useful clinical parameter is a history of having missed one or more meals. A day's food contains about 1 liter of water, which may become a major water source for older individuals with impaired thirst. Laboratory tests should measure the electrolytes, osmolality, creatinine, and blood urea nitrogen; a blood urea nitrogen–to-creatinine ratio greater than or equal to 25 is suggestive of dehydration.

Anticipation and prevention of dehydration are crucial. Adequate food intake should be maintained. The total water ingested per day in persons over age 70 years ideally should be 3.7 liters for men and 2.7 liters for women. At a minimum, 30 mL of daily fluid intake per kilogram of body weight is recommended. In patients suffering from an acute medical event, it is important to review any long-term medications, particularly diuretics, that may have contributed to dehydration and to define the ethically appropriate approach to future episodes. In terminally ill patients, death from dehydration becomes a natural event in which symptom-focused care relieves discomfort from dry mucous membranes (Chapter 3).

Endocrine System

Growth hormone levels fall with advancing age, with initial loss of nocturnal growth hormone spikes (Chapter 231). These declines contribute to the decreased muscle strength, thinning of bones and skin, and increased central fat associated with aging. It is currently unclear whether replacement of growth factors can induce a permanent reversal of muscle, bone, and skin changes with advancing age.

The production rates and clearance rates of thyroxine, triiodothyronine, and calcitonin appear to be constant with advancing age despite the increased prevalence of thyroid disease in late life (Chapter 233). There is an increase in parathyroid hormone levels, particularly in women, with advancing age, perhaps in compensation for the age-related decline of the kidney's ability to maintain normal levels of phosphorus and calcium in the blood (Chapter 253).

The adrenal glands maintain their ability to secrete cortisone with advancing age (Chapter 234). Dehydroepiandrosterone declines 85 to 90% by the age of 70 years, however, perhaps contributing to impaired immune or cardiovascular function. Renin and aldosterone secretion rates decline progressively with advancing age and do not contribute to the increased rates of hypertension with advancing age.

The insulin content of the elderly pancreas is increased, but the release of insulin in response to stimulation may be blunted with advancing age (Chapters 236 and 237). There is also a concomitant decline in insulin clearance with advancing age, with the net result that plasma insulin levels in response to glucose appear to be relatively preserved. Insulin resistance may increase with advancing age, but glucagon secretion appears to be well preserved.

The ovaries show dramatic declines in estrogen and progesterone as fibrosis and scarring occur. Menopause occurs at an average age of 51 years, with subsequent hot flashes, accelerated bone loss, and atrophy of estrogen-sensitive tissues (Chapter 248). Levels of testosterone decrease in some men beginning around 50 years, but declines do not appear to affect the potency of semen. Sexual function is relatively well preserved, albeit with an increase in the refractory period, increase in the time to arousal, and a loss of tissue turgor (Chapter 242).

Age-Related Endocrine Syndromes

The most important age-related endocrine syndrome occurring with advancing age is menopause (Chapter 248). Most other endocrine changes with age may enhance the prevalence of common disorders seen with aging, especially diabetes.

Immune System

Normal aging produces an obvious decrease in the size of the thymus gland between puberty and 50 or 60 years of age, at which time the gland becomes difficult to identify anatomically. This decrease in size is accompanied by a corresponding drop in thymosin levels, which are related directly to the number of functional T cells found in older adults. T cells also appear to be less active in responding to the presence of foreign proteins, and they tend to reproduce more slowly than those in younger adults. Functional studies of immune responsiveness suggest that although antibody responses are produced by older individuals, they tend to be less robust and less long lasting than in younger individuals (Chapters 44 and 257).

Clinical Syndromes of Aging

There are increased morbidity and mortality associated with influenza and pneumonia with advancing age and reactivation of infections such as tuberculosis and herpes zoster. The decline in immune function also may make it

less likely that older adults will develop autoimmune diseases, such as systemic lupus erythematosus.

Vaccine therapy, which is recommended for the prevention of herpes zoster (Chapters 17 and 383), reduces zoster-related adverse effects on functional status and quality of life.[1] It is even more critical to maintain annual immunization against influenza (Chapter 17). Pneumovax and tetanus vaccination are also important in elderly people (Chapter 17).

Hematopoietic System

The pluripotent stem cell and the erythroid and myeloid progenitor cells show no age-related reduction, indicating that there is minimal or no change in basal hematopoiesis during aging (Chapter 159). The aging hematopoietic system is less able to respond to increased demands, however, as evidenced by a slower recovery from anemia and less of a rise of hemoglobin during hypoxia. The older marrow also appears to respond less well to erythropoietin.

Neutrophils from elderly individuals show less prekilling activity and lower levels of lysozyme (Chapter 172), with a significant reduction in signal transduction and less release of inositol 1,4,5-trisphosphate and diacylglycerol during stimulation. During nutritional deprivation, there appears to be impairment in the reserve capacity to kill phagocytosed bacteria, a change that may contribute to the high prevalence of serious bacterial infections among nutritionally compromised elderly patients.

Age-Related Hematopoietic Syndromes

There are no specific syndromes of impaired hematopoiesis, aside from the clinical observation that during a comparable illness stress, hematologic abnormalities are more likely in elderly patients.

Musculoskeletal System

Bone mass and density decrease with age after reaching maximum in the 20s. In women, this loss may be about 1% per year until menopause, when it can increase to 2 to 3% per year (Chapters 248 and 251). By 5 to 10 years after menopause, bone loss returns to a rate of loss of 1% per year, but it may accelerate again in the late 80s. Because men have more bone mass than women do and lose bone mass at a similar rate of about 1% per year, the clinical effects in men are not seen until advanced age.

Tendons and ligaments become less elastic with advancing age, contributing to a higher incidence of rupture, especially of the Achilles tendon, in older individuals. Cartilage and ligaments of the ribs and spine are more likely to become calcified and less elastic.

Muscles reach their ultimate size and strength in the 20s and 30s. By 70 years of age, muscle mass declines by approximately 25% for men and women unless it is offset by exercise. By the age of 80 years, muscle size and strength in most sedentary adults decrease by 30 to 40% from the mid-30s peak. Muscle mass in late life depends on exercise earlier in life to reach a higher early mass and exercise late in life to stimulate muscle preservation.

Age-Related Musculoskeletal Syndromes

The most important age-related clinical syndrome associated with advancing age is osteoporosis (Chapter 251). Sarcopenia, or diminished muscle mass, is a clear predisposing factor for falls, which is the leading cause of accidental death at home in older individuals. Bone and muscle mass respond well to gravitational stress and resistance exercises, respectively, even in the oldest age ranges.

Falls are a major age-related syndrome involving neural, musculoskeletal, and cardiovascular systems. Most falls in older adults are due to a combination of several factors rather than a single event. Internal contributors to falls include sensory impairment from poor eyesight, hearing loss, and balance disturbances; diseases of the brain, including motor and sensory disorders, cognitive impairment that produces poor judgment or apraxia, and depression; cardiovascular, respiratory, and metabolic diseases; and musculoskeletal conditions, such as lower limb weakness, poor grip strength, osteoporosis, rheumatoid arthritis, osteoarthritis, and foot disorders. External causes of falls include medications. The risk of falling increases in patients who receive four or more prescription medications; drugs specifically shown to increase the risk of falling include hypnotics, muscle relaxants, antihypertensives, diuretics, and antidepressants. Environmental problems increase the risk of falls. Inside the home, risks include stairs (coming down is more hazardous than climbing up, as the first and last steps often have no railing or an unusable one); loose objects, such as furniture, cords, and rugs; poor lighting, particularly in areas with dark and light variability; poorly fitting shoes; surfaces with glare or patterning; and lack of bathroom safety equipment. Outdoor risks include uneven pavements and surface roads made slippery from ice, water, or fallen leaves.

For a person who has fallen, the evaluation should include a detailed history of the circumstances surrounding the fall, medications, medical problems, and mobility; an examination of vision, gait, balance, and lower extremity joint function; an examination of neurologic function, including muscle strength; and an examination of the cardiovascular system. The investigations for falls and syncope (Chapters 50 and 62) are similar. Tests are needed only if the history and physical examination do not reveal the cause of falling or if they point to a particular abnormality that requires laboratory evaluation. These tests may include the following:

- Blood tests to exclude anemia, infection, and metabolic problems such as diabetes and thyroid disease
- Electrocardiogram to evaluate heart disease
- 24-Hour electrocardiogram recording or loop monitor to evaluate arrhythmias (Chapter 62)
- Echocardiogram for patients with significant heart murmurs (Chapter 55)
- Drug levels to determine whether a patient is being undertreated or overtreated with a particular drug
- If focal neurologic signs or symptoms are present, a computed tomographic scan of the brain
- If suggestive symptoms are present, a radiograph of the neck or spine to look for spinal stenosis (Chapter 407)

The risk of falls can be reduced by exercise interventions in community-dwelling elderly persons **2** and by multifactorial interventions in elderly persons in nursing facilities and hospitals. **3**

Prevention of Fractures

The prevention of fractures has three components. First, persons with lower bone densities are more likely to fracture a bone, given the same amount of trauma, than are persons with higher bone densities. Women should be assessed for osteoporosis and treated accordingly (Chapter 251). Osteoporosis often is underdiagnosed in men, and men with fractures or repeated falls should be evaluated for possible osteoporosis; however, screening strategies for elderly men have not been defined.

Fractures can be prevented if falls can be prevented. Older people who have recurrent falls should have regular exercise and balance training after their risk factors for falling are fully addressed. The optimal type, duration, and intensity of exercise are unclear, but balance training for 10 weeks or more has the best-proven benefit. Exercise must be sustained for continued benefit. Vitamin D improves muscle strength but may not reduce falls.

When someone falls, the damage may be reduced by the intrinsic padding of fat or by devices such as mechanical hip protectors. Randomized controlled trials of hip protectors to reduce fractures in nursing home patients and in ambulatory older individuals have shown mixed results in the United States. Compliance with these cumbersome devices is only 25 to 70%.

Nervous System

Brain size decreases with advancing age; after the age of 60 years, its size declines by 5 to 10%. The decrease in size is caused primarily by a decrease in the cerebral cortex. Novel adjustments to cell loss include the formation of new connections between remaining neurons. Aging is associated with a progressive decline in the synthesis of neurotransmitters and a decline in their corresponding receptors. A major functional change is slower reaction times, which may be the result of a slower nerve conduction or trans-synaptic speed.

The farsightedness of aging is caused by the diminished ability of the lens to focus on nearby objects because of its thickening and stiffening (Chapter 431). There is reduced ability to distinguish colors, particularly blue, because of yellowing of the lens. Overall transmission of light through the lens may decline by 50 to 65% between the ages of 25 and 60 years; as a result, individuals require more ambient light. Older individuals experience more glare because light scatters through the thickened lens. Older individuals also notice more floaters as the vitreous jelly becomes slightly more liquefied and mobile with advancing age. Tear production is decreased, leading to a sense of grittiness in the older eye. Overall visual acuity tends to decrease with age; by age 65 years, 40% of men and 60% of women have a visual acuity of 20/70 or worse.

Approximately 25% of individuals older than 65 years experience hearing loss with age (Chapter 436), with men affected more than women. The degeneration of neural transmission from the ear to the brain results in difficulty in identifying a voice or understanding a spoken message when there is background noise. Presbycusis results in high-frequency sound loss and more difficulty in distinguishing high-pitched consonants and voices compared with lower-pitched vowels and sounds.

Sleep patterns change with advancing age (Chapter 412). Functionally, older adults are more wakeful during the night and spend much more time in bed. The pattern of sleep characteristically changes from the fairly regular stepwise patterns of childhood and young adulthood to a more fragmented pattern, with frequent awakenings in late life.

Defined changes in brain function also occur with age, even in persons who do not meet standardized criteria for cognitive impairment. For example, the older brain does less well with divided attentional tasks, and it processes more slowly.

Age-Related Neurologic Syndromes

Age-associated memory dysfunction is common (Chapters 26 and 409), and delirium (Chapter 27) may occur, especially during illnesses. Prevention of delirium is possible with a proactive consultation intervention, which can reduce the incidence of hospital delirium by about 40 to 50%.

Sleep-disordered breathing associated with sleep apnea appears to rise in prevalence with advancing age (Chapter 100). Anatomic changes, such as tissue laxity and diseases of the nose and sinuses, may contribute to sleep-disordered breathing. Sleep apnea may have a neurologic basis either in the sleep cycling center, leading to central sleep apnea, or in neurologic control of pharyngeal tissues.

Integumentary System

Thinning of the subcutaneous tissue begins in most people in their mid-40s, independent of the degree of sun exposure or protection from injury. The epidermis and dermis adhere less tightly, making the skin feel looser and increasing its tendency to blister and to be subject to friction burns or pressure ulceration (Chapter 443). This phenomenon also leads to senile purpura (Fig. 24-1) that results from tears in small venules when the skin is bumped or abraded (Chapter 448).

Environmental exposures, including ultraviolet sunlight, wind, and smoking, help promote the development of wrinkles by damaging the subcutaneous tissues and the epidermis, especially the elastin fibers. The process of photo injury (Chapter 446) leads to slow repair, particularly of tissues of the distal forearm and lower leg. Ultraviolet light exposure also predisposes to the development of skin cancers, the most common of which is basal cell cancer, but squamous cell cancer and melanoma are also age dependent (Chapter 210). Approximately two thirds of aging individuals experience at least one skin problem, and about 40% have two underlying skin disorders.

The most profound consequence of environmental exposure and age-related changes is that wound repair rates are significantly prolonged. In individuals older than 65 years, healing takes about 50% longer compared with individuals in their 30s; complete skin healing can take 5.5 weeks instead of 3.5 weeks.

Rates of epithelial cell regeneration decrease by about 50% from maturity to 70 years of age. A similar pattern is seen in hair, which grows more slowly.

FIGURE 24-1. Senile purpura is a common and benign condition that results from impaired collagen production and capillary fragility in elderly people. In the absence of other signs of disease, no investigation is necessary. (From Forbes CD, Jackson WF. *Color Atlas and Text of Clinical Medicine,* 3rd ed. London: Mosby; 2003.)

With advancing age, graying is variable but universal because the number of melanocytes within hair bulbs declines with age (Chapter 450). Changes in skin cell size and shape cause irregular patterning and may predispose to water-induced or environment-induced cracking.

Age-Related Integumentary Syndromes

Specific illnesses affecting the skin include basal cell cancer and rosacea (Chapters 446 to 449). Aging skin syndromes also include xerosis, thermoregulatory changes, skin thinning, and hair loss. The primary therapy for xerosis is the external application of treatments to protect and moisturize the skin (Chapter 445).

Diminished sweating poses a threat during times of high ambient and environmental temperatures or in the context of fever (Chapters 109 and 289). The absence of sweating lessens heat loss by conduction and evaporation, and it diminishes the urge to move to a more protected environment. Because few elderly individuals experience thirst, dehydration may occur quickly in these settings. Environmental protection from temperature extremes is crucial (Chapter 109).

Pressure sores are necrotic areas of muscle, subcutaneous fat, and skin as a result of compression and subsequent ischemia (Fig. 24-2). Pressure sores usually occur between underlying bone and a hard surface or a soft surface during a prolonged time. Among elderly patients in acute care hospitals, the incidence rate is 8%, and the prevalence rate is 16%. Rates are even higher in patients who are in intensive care units or who have hip fractures.

A standard mattress can generate pressures as high as 150 mm Hg, well above the 30- to 35-mm Hg continuous-pressure threshold needed to cause pressure sores. In addition to pressure injury, shear injury is important. Shear injury, which occurs when local blood vessels are stretched and separated from underlying perforating vessels, is more likely when the patient is in a sloped position or is rubbing constantly against underlying surfaces. Burning injury also can result from friction of the superficial skin layers. A complicating feature of all pressure ulcers is moisture, which leads to softening of the skin, sticking to underlying surfaces, and easy access for infection.

Individuals at higher risk include those who are immobile; those who are incontinent of bowel or bladder; and those who have compromised circulation due to hypotension, dehydration, or vascular disease. Neurologic disease, particularly peripheral neuropathy that impairs sensation, can predispose to pressure ulcers, as can any neurologic condition that causes spasticity, contractures, or poor mobility.

Preventive strategies encourage safe positioning, regular turning, and avoidance of direct pressure. Judicious use of pressure-reducing beds may lower the incidence of pressure ulcers after hip fractures. Deep foam mattresses and air suspension beds are even more effective.

When pressure sores appear, they should be photographed to establish a baseline. Nutrition should be improved, all pressure on the wound should be removed, and active vigilance should be focused to prevent additional pressure ulcers. Débridement of necrotic tissue should be considered; wet-to-dry dressings and surgical or chemical débridement are often used. Infections may require topical or systemic antibiotics. Semiocclusive and occlusive dressings also can be helpful. Most pressure ulcers heal within 6 months, but operative repair is sometimes necessary.

Clinical Pharmacology

Of all prescription medications (Chapter 28), about 30% are taken by elderly people, even though they compose only 14% of the population. Nonprescription medications are disproportionately consumed by older individuals and are increasingly implicated in drug-drug interactions.

The gastrointestinal absorption of medications generally does not change with advancing age, despite the theoretical possibility that medications requiring acidification in the stomach may be absorbed less well because of the higher frequency of atrophic gastritis and reduced gastric acid. Drug distribution changes significantly with advancing age because medications distribute to fat or muscle. As muscle mass declines with advancing age, fat increases as a proportion of total body weight. As a result, older individuals are more sensitive to the effects of water-soluble drugs (heart) and have prolonged effects from lipophilic drugs (brain).

The decline in renal function with normal aging reduces the clearance of many drugs, especially digoxin, aminoglycosides, and cimetidine. Hepatic metabolism also may decline with age. Oxidative reactions, so-called phase 1 reactions, become impaired with normal aging, whereas phase 2 reactions (conjugation and glucuronidization) are relatively spared. A clinical example is that diazepam, which requires phase 1 and phase 2 metabolism, has a prolonged half-life with advancing age, but oxazepam, which requires only phase 2 reactions to be metabolized, does not.

The overall impact of these pharmacokinetic changes is that the half-life, which is proportional to the volume of distribution divided by drug clearance, increases for many lipophilic drugs. Poorly nourished or frail elderly persons may have a low serum albumin level. The normal age-related decline in the serum albumin level is clinically insignificant. When the albumin level is less than 3 g/dL, however, drug levels have to be interpreted on the basis of their binding to albumin; albumin levels this low are associated with an increased risk of in-hospital death and longer lengths of hospital stay.

Independent of pharmacokinetic issues, elderly people are more sensitive to many medications. The brain appears to be increasingly sensitive to many compounds, including opiates, benzodiazepines, and neuroleptics. As a result, lower doses cause effects equivalent to those seen with higher doses in younger individuals. Warfarin, which acts primarily on the liver, will maintain therapeutic anticoagulation profiles at lower doses in elderly patients because the aging liver is increasingly sensitive to blockage of vitamin K–dependent systems.

Elderly people are at higher risk for nonadherence to prescribed regimens. Factors influencing nonadherence include the number of medications and their cost, inadequate education of the patient, unacceptable side effects, and complexity of the medical regimen. Individuals who take more than three prescription drugs have lower adherence. Below three medications per day, elderly individuals in general have high adherence rates. Unfortunately, no intervention has reliably improved adherence rates in elderly people.

Perhaps the most important phenomenon in multiple-drug regimens in older individuals is the progressive accumulation of anticholinergic effects, including dry mouth, constipation, poor vision, urinary retention, balance disorders, and cognitive difficulties. Anticholinergic drugs include neuroleptics, antispasmodics, antianxiety agents, antihistamines, and medications used for urinary incontinence.

An Integrated Approach

Because elderly people commonly have many medical conditions, some of which are age-related and others exacerbated by age-related conditions, a multidisciplinary approach is often useful. For example, integrated and home-based geriatric care management improve quality of care and reduce acute care utilization among high-risk community-dwelling elderly people. Collaborative care interventions are more effective for depression in older people than usual care and are also of high value. Similarly, geriatric intervention improved functional abilities and mental well-being of vulnerable older people. Physicians should become aware of such community resources that can benefit these patients.

FIGURE 24-2. Severe sacral pressure sore, one of the serious but preventable complications of immobility. (From Forbes CD, Jackson WF. *Color Atlas and Text of Clinical Medicine*, 3rd ed. London: Mosby; 2003.)

1. Schmader KE, Johnson GR, Saddier P, et al. Effect of a zoster vaccine on herpes zoster-related interference with functional status and health-related quality-of-life measures in older adults. *J Am Geriatr Soc.* 2010;58:1634-1641.
2. Gillespie LD, Robertson MC, Gillespie WJ, et al. Interventions for preventing falls in older people living in the community. *Cochrane Database Syst Rev.* 2009;2:CD007146.

3. Cameron ID, Murray GR, Gillespie LD, et al. Interventions for preventing falls in older people in nursing care facilities and hospitals. *Cochrane Database Syst Rev.* 2010;1:CD005465.
4. Melis RJ, van Eijken MI, Teerenstra S, et al. A randomized study of a multidisciplinary program to intervene on geriatric syndromes in vulnerable older people who live at home (Dutch EASYcare Study). *J Gerontol A Biol Sci Med Sci.* 2008;63:283-290.
5. Chang-Quan H, Bi-Rong D, Zhen-Chan L, et al. Collaborative care interventions for depression in the elderly: a systematic review of randomized controlled trials. *J Investig Med.* 2009;57:446-455.

SUGGESTED READINGS

Basaria S, Coviello AD, Travison TG, et al. Adverse events associated with testosterone administration. *N Engl J Med.* 2010;363:109-122. *Testosterone gel in elderly men with low testosterone levels improved strength but increased adverse cardiac events almost 5-fold.*
Delbaere K, Close JC, Heim J, et al. A multifactorial approach to understanding fall risk in older people. *J Am Geriatr Soc.* 2010;58:1679-1685. *Balance-related impairments are the critical predictors.*
Ko FC. The clinical care of frail, older adults. *Clin Geriatr Med.* 2011;27:89-100. *Review of biology and treatment.*
Steinman MA, Hanlon JT. Managing medications in clinically complex elders: "There's got to be a happy medium." *JAMA.* 2010;304:1592-1601. *Review.*

25

INCONTINENCE

NEIL M. RESNICK

DEFINITION

Urinary incontinence is the involuntary leakage of urine sufficient to be a health or social problem.

EPIDEMIOLOGY

More than twice as common in women as in men, the prevalence of incontinence increases with age. But at no age does it affect the majority of individuals—even over age 85 years. Incontinence afflicts 15 to 30% of older adults living at home, one third of those in acute care settings, and half of those in nursing homes. It predisposes to perineal rashes, pressure ulcers, urinary tract infections, urosepsis, falls, and fractures, and it is associated with embarrassment, stigmatization, isolation, depression, anxiety, sexual dysfunction, and risk of institutionalization. Its cost in the United States exceeds $26 billion annually.

Despite these considerations, geriatric incontinence remains largely neglected, by patients and physicians alike. This is unfortunate because its increased prevalence with age relates more to age-associated diseases and functional impairments than to age itself. Most importantly, incontinence is usually treatable and often curable at all ages, even in frail elderly people, although the approach in older patients must be broader than that employed in younger patients.

PATHOBIOLOGY

At any age, continence depends not only on the integrity of lower urinary tract function but also on the presence of adequate mentation, mobility, motivation, and manual dexterity. Although incontinence in younger patients is rarely associated with deficits in these domains, such deficits occur commonly in older patients in whom they can cause or exacerbate incontinence or influence therapeutic approaches.

With age, bladder capacity does not change, but bladder sensation and contractility decrease. At the cellular level, detrusor smooth muscle develops a "dense band pattern" characterized by dense sarcolemmal bands with depleted caveolae. This depletion may mediate the age-related decline in bladder contractility. In addition, an incomplete dysjunction pattern characterized by scattered protrusion junctions develops and may underlie the high prevalence of involuntary bladder contractions (detrusor overactivity) in older adults of both sexes. Urethral length and sphincter strength decrease in women, whereas the prostate enlarges in most men and causes measurable obstruction in about half. The postvoid residual volume (PVR) in the bladder also increases but normally to less than 100 mL. In addition, elderly people often excrete most of their fluid intake at night, even in the absence of venous insufficiency, renal disease, heart failure, or prostatism. Coupled with an age-associated increase in sleep disorders, most older adults have one or two episodes of nocturia per night.

None of these changes causes incontinence, but all predispose to it. This predisposition, combined with the increased likelihood that an older person will encounter an additional pathologic, physiologic, or pharmacologic insult, explains the increased prevalence of incontinence with age. The implications are equally important. The onset or exacerbation of incontinence in an older person is likely to be due to precipitants that are outside the lower urinary tract and that are amenable to medical intervention. Furthermore, treatment of the precipitants alone may be sufficient to restore continence, even if there is coexisting urinary tract dysfunction. For example, a flare of hip arthritis in a woman with age-related detrusor overactivity may decrease mobility sufficiently to convert her urinary urgency into incontinence. Treatment of the arthritis, rather than the involuntary detrusor contractions, will not only restore continence but also lessen pain and improve mobility. Because of their frequency, reversibility, and association with morbidity beyond incontinence, the transient precipitant causes should be addressed first.

Causes of Transient Incontinence

Incontinence is transient in up to one third of community-dwelling elderly people and in up to half of acutely hospitalized patients. Although most transient causes are outside the lower urinary tract (Table 25-1), three points warrant emphasis. First, the risk of transient incontinence is increased if, in addition to physiologic changes of the lower urinary tract, there also are pathologic changes. Anticholinergic agents are more likely to cause overflow incontinence in individuals with a weak or obstructed bladder, whereas excess urine output is more likely to cause urge incontinence in people with detrusor overactivity or impaired mobility. Second, these transient causes may persist if left untreated and should not be dismissed merely because incontinence is long-standing. Third, identification of the most common cause is of little value because causes vary among individuals, and geriatric incontinence is rarely due to just one cause.

Causes of Established Incontinence Related to the Lower Urinary Tract

Detrusor overactivity, which also is called involuntary bladder contraction or *overactive bladder*, generally causes *urge incontinence* and is the most common type of lower urinary tract dysfunction in incontinent elderly people, accounting for about two thirds of cases. Histologically, detrusor overactivity is associated with the complete dysjunction pattern, with widening of the intercellular space, reduction of normal (intermediate) muscle cell junctions, and emergence of novel protrusion junctions and ultraclose abutments that connect cells together in chains. These connections may mediate a change in cell coupling from a mechanical to an electrical mechanism that results in involuntary bladder contraction. Other potential causes include ischemia, abnormalities in suburothelial myofibroblasts, and changes in central nervous system structural and functional control mechanisms.

At any age, detrusor overactivity is usually idiopathic, but it can be associated with a variety of other causes that may affect prognosis and management. Such conditions include an upper motor neuron lesion (Chapters 407 and 418), urethral obstruction, stress incontinence, bladder calculus, and bladder carcinoma (Chapter 203).

Detrusor overactivity exists as two subsets in elderly people: one in which contractile function is preserved and one in which it is impaired. The latter condition, termed *detrusor hyperactivity with impaired contractility*, has several implications. First, because the bladder is weak, these patients commonly develop urinary retention, which is also seen in patients with outlet obstruction and detrusor underactivity. Second, even in the absence of retention, detrusor hyperactivity with impaired contractility mimics other lower urinary tract causes of incontinence. For instance, if the involuntary detrusor contraction occurs coincident with a stress maneuver and if the weak contraction is not detected, detrusor hyperactivity with impaired contractility will be misdiagnosed as stress incontinence. Alternatively, because detrusor hyperactivity with impaired contractility may be associated with urinary urgency, frequency, weak flow rate, elevated residual urine, and bladder trabeculation, in men it may mimic prostatic obstruction. Third, anticholinergic therapy of detrusor hyperactivity with impaired contractility may result in urinary retention owing to bladder weakness, thereby requiring alternative therapeutic approaches.

Stress incontinence, which is the second most common cause of incontinence in older women and the dominant cause in middle-aged women, usually reflects urethral hypermobility plus some degree of sphincter

TABLE 25-1 CAUSES OF TRANSIENT INCONTINENCE: DIAPERS MNEMONIC

Delirium	Result of underlying illness or medication; incontinence is secondary and abates once the cause of delirium is corrected
Infection—*symptomatic* UTI	Acute, symptomatic UTI causes incontinence, but the far more common asymptomatic bacteriuria does not
Atrophic urethritis/vaginitis	Characterized by vaginal erosions, telangiectasia, petechiae, and friability; may cause or contribute to incontinence. Although oral estrogen may worsen incontinence, a 3- to 12-month course of topical estrogen can be useful

Pharmaceuticals	*Drug type:*	*Potential effects on continence:*
	Sedative-hypnotics (e.g., long-acting benzodiazepines; alcohol)	Sedation, delirium, decreased mobility
	Anticholinergics (dicyclomine, disopyramide, sedating antihistamines, antipsychotics, tricyclic antidepressants, anti-Parkinson's, antidepressants)(*not* SSRIs)	Urinary retention, overflow incontinence, delirium, impaction; the antipsychotics also decrease mobility
	Opiates	Urinary retention, stool impaction, sedation, delirium
	α-Adrenergic antagonists	Relax sphincter; may induce stress incontinence in women
	α-Adrenergic agonists	Urinary retention in men (tighten sphincter, prostate)
	Calcium channel blockers, especially the dihydropyridines	Urinary retention; nocturnal diuresis due to fluid retention
	"Loop" diuretics (thiazide-like agents only rarely cause it)	Polyuria, frequency, urgency
	NSAIDs	Nocturnal diuresis due to fluid retention
	Thiazolidinediones	Nocturnal diuresis due to fluid retention
	Dopamine receptor agonists (e.g., ropinirole, pramipexole)	Nocturnal diuresis due to fluid retention
	Angiotensin-converting enzyme inhibitors	Drug-induced cough leads to stress incontinence in women
	Vincristine	Urinary retention due to neuropathy

Excess urine output	From large intake, diuretic agents (theophylline, caffeinated beverages, alcohol), and metabolic disorders (hyperglycemia, hypercalcemia); nocturnal incontinence may result from mobilization of peripheral edema (CHF, venous insufficiency)
Restricted mobility	Often results from overlooked, correctable conditions such as arthritis, pain, foot problems, postprandial hypotension
Stool impaction	May cause both fecal and urinary incontinence that remit with disimpaction

CHF = congestive heart failure; NSAIDs = nonsteroidal anti-inflammatory drugs; SSRI = selective serotonin reuptake inhibitor; UTI = urinary tract infection.
Adapted from Resnick NM, Tadic SD, Yalla SV. Geriatric incontinence and voiding dysfunction. In: Wein AJ, Novick AC, Partin AW, et al, eds. *Campbell-Walsh Urology*, 10th ed. St. Louis: Elsevier; 2010.

weakness. Stress incontinence is rare in men but can result from sphincter damage following radical but not transurethral prostatectomy.

Urethral obstruction is the second most common cause of established incontinence in older men, although most obstructed men are not incontinent. When obstruction is associated with incontinence, it usually presents as urge incontinence owing to the associated detrusor overactivity; overflow incontinence is uncommon. Outlet obstruction is rare in women but may result from a bladder neck suspension or from urethral kinking associated with a large cystocele.

Detrusor underactivity is usually idiopathic. When it causes incontinence, it is associated with overflow incontinence (<10% of incontinence).

Damage to lower urinary tract innervation can cause several types of dysfunction. A brain lesion may cause detrusor overactivity. A spinal cord lesion (Chapters 195 and 407) above the sacral level can cause both detrusor overactivity and detrusor-sphincter dyssynergia, a condition in which the sphincter contracts rather than relaxes during detrusor contraction; the result can be severe outlet obstruction and hydronephrosis. A spinal cord lesion below the sacral level can cause detrusor underactivity, sphincter weakness, or both. Peripheral and autonomic nerve damage can cause still additional problems. Because *neurogenic bladder* is such a nonspecific term, it is preferable to refer to the dysfunction that it causes.

Causes of Incontinence Unrelated to the Lower Urinary Tract (Functional Incontinence)

"Functional" incontinence, which is often cited as a distinct type of geriatric incontinence and attributed to deficits of cognition and mobility, implies that urinary tract function is normal. However, normal urinary tract function is the exception, even in continent elderly people, and is rarely observed in incontinent elderly people. Incontinence is not inevitable, even with dementia or immobility. Among the most severely demented institutionalized residents, nearly 20% are continent; among those who can transfer from a bed to a chair, nearly half are continent. Functionally impaired individuals also are the most likely to suffer from factors that cause transient incontinence, and a diagnosis of functional incontinence may result in failure to detect these reversible causes. Finally, if functionally impaired individuals also have urethral obstruction or stress incontinence, they may benefit from targeted therapy. Nonetheless, functional impairment often contributes to incontinence, and addressing its causes and those of transient incontinence may ameliorate incontinence sufficiently to obviate the need for further investigation.

CLINICAL MANIFESTATIONS

The manifestations of transient incontinence depend on the underlying condition. For established incontinence, detrusor overactivity usually manifests as *urge incontinence*, characterized by leakage that follows the abrupt onset or intensification of a desire to void, leakage of a moderate to large amount, urinary frequency (>8 voids/day), nocturia, and nocturnal incontinence. However, some patients with detrusor overactivity may present without the urge component. *Stress incontinence* causes leakage that coincides with both the onset and cessation of a cough or other cause of increased abdominal pressure; nocturnal leakage is rare. Some patients report both types of incontinence, or *mixed incontinence*, but it is useful to determine which component is the most bothersome. Occasionally, patients present with incontinence that is more difficult to characterize clinically without further testing.

DIAGNOSIS

In addition to a targeted clinical evaluation (Table 25-2), a bladder diary can provide diagnostic clues and guide therapy (Fig. 25-1). For example, incontinence occurring only between 8 AM and noon may be caused by a morning loop diuretic. Incontinence that occurs at night in a demented man with heart failure, but not during a 4-hour nap in his wheelchair, is likely due to nocturnal diuresis associated with his heart failure and not to dementia, impaired mobility, or prostatic obstruction. A woman with volume-dependent stress incontinence may leak only on the way to void after a full night's sleep, when her bladder contains more than 400 mL—more than it ever does during her continent waking hours.

Because urinary retention is difficult to detect by examination and can affect diagnosis and therapy, the PVR volume should be determined routinely, except possibly in middle-aged women with a classic presentation of stress incontinence. Urodynamic testing is generally unnecessary unless diagnostic certainty is required, such as before surgical repair or if there is evidence of a serious underlying cause of the incontinence, such as a brain or spinal cord lesion, carcinoma of the bladder or prostate, hydronephrosis, or bladder calculus. Urodynamic evaluation comprises a battery of tests designed to assess the lower urinary tract during the filling and voiding phases of micturition. The selection among tests depends on the clinical setting and question to be answered; for instance, measuring detrusor pressure and urine flow during voiding can determine whether urethral obstruction is present, whereas monitoring bladder and urethral pressures during the filling phase and with coughing may be helpful for patients with an atypical presentation of mixed incontinence.

TABLE 25-2 CLINICAL EVALUATION OF THE INCONTINENT PATIENT

HISTORY

Type (urge, stress, overflow, or mixed)
Incontinence frequency, severity, duration
Pattern (diurnal, nocturnal, or both; also, e.g., after taking medications)
Associated symptoms (straining to void, incomplete emptying, dysuria, hematuria, suprapubic/perineal discomfort)
Alteration in bowel habit/sexual function (because of proximity to the bladder and shared innervation)
Other relevant factors (cancer, acute illness, neurologic disease, pelvic or lower urinary tract surgery/radiation therapy)
Medications, including nonprescription agents (see Table 25-1)
Brief assessment of cognitive and physical function

PHYSICAL EXAMINATION

Identify other relevant medical conditions (e.g., congestive heart failure, peripheral edema)
If stress incontinence suspected, determine whether leakage *coincides* with the onset *and* cessation of a single, forceful cough
Palpate for bladder distention after voiding
Pelvic examination to detect atrophic vaginitis, pelvic muscle laxity, pelvic mass
Rectal examination (skin irritation, resting tone and voluntary control of anal sphincter, prostate nodule; fecal impaction (*note:* prostate size correlates poorly with presence of urethral obstruction)
Neurologic examination (mental status and elemental examination, including sacral reflexes and perineal sensation)

INITIAL INVESTIGATION

Bladder diary (see Fig. 25-1)
Metabolic survey (electrolytes, calcium, glucose, and urea nitrogen as appropriate)
Measure postvoid residual (PVR) volume, by portable ultrasound if available
Urinalysis to detect sterile hematuria or infection; culture if new-onset or worsening incontinence
Renal ultrasound to detect hydronephrosis in men whose PVR urine exceeds about 200 mL
Urine cytology for patients with hematuria, pain, or unexplained new-onset or worsening incontinence
Uroflowmetry for men in whom urethral obstruction is suspected
Cystoscopy for patients with hematuria, suspicion of lower urinary tract pathology (e.g., bladder fistula, stone, or tumor; urethral diverticulum), or need for lower urinary tract surgery

Adapted from Resnick NM, Yalla SV. Management of urinary incontinence in the elderly. *N Engl J Med.* 1985;313:800-805.

Date	Time	Volume Voided (mL)	Are You Wet or Dry?	Approximate Volume of Incontinence	Comments
4/5	3:40 pm	240	Wet	Slight	
	6:05 pm	210	Dry		
	8:15 pm	150	Dry		Running water
	10:20 pm	150	Wet	15 mL	Bowel movement
	10:30 pm	30	Dry		
4/6	3:15 am	270	Wet	Slight	
	6:05 am	300	Wet	Slight	
	7:40 am	200	Dry		
	9:50 am	?	Dry		
	11:20 am	200	Dry		
	12:50 pm	180	Dry		
	1:40 pm	240	Dry		
	3:35 pm	160	Dry		
	6:00 pm	170	Dry		
	8:20 pm	215	Wet	Slight	Running water
	10:25 pm	130	Dry		

FIGURE 25-1. Sample bladder diary. Bladder diary of an incontinent 75-year-old man. Urodynamic evaluation excluded urethral obstruction and confirmed a diagnosis of detrusor hyperactivity with impaired contractility (detrusor hyperactivity with impaired contractility). Note the 24-hour urine output of nearly 3 liters due to the belief that drinking 10 glasses of fluid per day was "good for my health." (He did not mention this until queried about the voiding record.) Given the typical voided volume of 150 to 250 mL and a measured postvoid residual of 150 mL, excess fluid intake was overwhelming his usual bladder capacity of 400 mL (150 + 250 mL). Although involuntary bladder contractions were present, the easily reversible volume component of the problem, combined with the risk of precipitating urinary retention with an anticholinergic agent, prompted treatment with volume restriction alone. After daily urinary output dropped to 1500 mL, frequency abated, and incontinence resolved. (Adapted from DuBeau CE, Resnick NM. Evaluation of the causes and severity of geriatric incontinence: a critical appraisal. *Urol Clin North Am.* 1991;18:243-256.)

TREATMENT Rx

Optimal therapy requires a multifactorial approach (Table 25-3), including treatment of transient causes, underlying medical conditions, functional impairments, and the urinary tract abnormality itself. Although pads and diapers have a role, they remain an adjunct to more specific therapy.

Behavioral Therapy

Behavioral therapy includes education, self-monitoring with a bladder diary, adjustment of fluid intake, weight loss for overweight women with stress incontinence,[1] use of aids (e.g., a bedside urinal), and various types of bladder retraining and urethral sphincter exercises (e.g., progressively increasing voiding intervals, strategies to cope with urgency, and pelvic muscle exercises).[1-3] The efficacy of behavioral therapy is equivalent to pharmacotherapy for urge incontinence and is superior to drugs for stress incontinence.[2,3] Moreover, combining behavioral and pharmacologic therapy may prove more beneficial than either treatment alone, especially for urge incontinence, because neither therapy generally abolishes involuntary bladder contractions. For institutionalized patients who are cognitively impaired but can state their name and are partly mobile, regular daytime reminders to void ("prompted voiding")

have proved effective for daytime incontinence; pads and diapers are appropriate for the others.[4]

Pharmacotherapy

Currently approved drugs have generally proved ineffective for stress incontinence and overflow incontinence, but several bladder relaxants are available for urge incontinence (see Table 25-3). Each has proved superior to placebo in well-conducted trials, and most have also proved effective in trials targeting older patients.[2,3] All have antimuscarinic properties, such as dry mouth, constipation, visual blurring, and occasional confusion. Yet each is well tolerated even in cognitively impaired elderly patients when prescribed properly, although cognitive status should be monitored. These drugs also can be well tolerated in patients taking cholinesterase inhibitors. The choice among drugs often hinges on other considerations. For instance, immediate-release oxybutynin has the quickest onset of action, making it an inexpensive and effective choice for patients who need excellent control at predictable times. The other drugs, although more expensive, can be used less often and can be better tolerated for daily use.

Regardless of the agent selected, the key is to begin with a low dose and increase it slowly, realizing that the full benefit is generally not apparent for

TABLE 25-3 STEPWISE APPROACH TO TREATMENT OF URINARY INCONTINENCE*

CONDITION	CLINICAL TYPE OF INCONTINENCE†	TREATMENT
Detrusor overactivity with normal contractility	Urge	1. Bladder retraining or prompted voiding regimens 2. ± Bladder relaxant medication if needed and not contraindicated (see drug list below) 3. Indwelling catheterization alone is often unhelpful because detrusor spasms often increase, leading to leakage around the catheter 4. In selected cases, induce urinary retention pharmacologically and add intermittent or indwelling catheterization‡
Detrusor hyperactivity with impaired contractility	Urge§	1. If bladder empties adequately, behavioral methods (as above) ± bladder relaxant medication (low doses; especially feasible if sphincter incompetence coexists) 2. If residual urine >150 mL, augmented voiding techniques¶ or intermittent catheterization (± bladder relaxant medication). If neither feasible, undergarment or indwelling catheter‡ 3. In selected cases, induce urinary retention pharmacologically and add intermittent or indwelling catheterization‡
Stress incontinence	Stress	1. Conservative methods (weight loss if obese; treatment of cough or atrophic vaginitis; physical maneuvers to prevent leakage [e.g., tighten pelvic muscles before cough, cross legs]; occasionally, use of tampon or pessary is helpful) 2. If leakage threshold ≥150 mL identified, adjust fluid excretion and voiding intervals appropriately 3. Pelvic muscle exercises ± biofeedback/weighted intravaginal cones; must continue indefinitely 4. Surgery (sling, artificial sphincter, periurethral bulking injections)
Urethral obstruction	Urge/overflow‖	1. Conservative methods (including adjustment of fluid excretion, bladder retraining/prompted voiding) if hydronephrosis, recurrent symptomatic UTI, and hematuria have been excluded 2. α-Adrenergic antagonist 3. Also consider adding a bladder relaxant if detrusor overactivity coexists, PVR is small, and surgery not desired/feasible; *monitor PVR!* 4. Finasteride, if not contraindicated and the patient either prefers it or is not a surgical candidate 5. Surgery (incision, prostatectomy) is an effective alternative before or after these steps
Underactive detrusor	Overflow	1. Decompress for at least several days (the larger the PVR, the longer should be the decompression [up to a month]) and then perform a voiding trial 2. Exclude urethral obstruction if this has not already been done 3. If cannot void or PVR remains large, try augmented voiding techniques¶ ± α-adrenergic antagonist, but only if some voiding possible; bethanechol *rarely* useful 4. If fails, or voiding is not possible, intermittent or indwelling catheterization‡

*These treatments should be initiated only after adequate toilet access has been ensured, contributing conditions have been treated (e.g., atrophic vaginitis, UTI, fecal impaction, heart failure), fluid management has been optimized, and unnecessary or exacerbating medications have been addressed. For additional details, see text.
†*Urge:* leakage in the absence of stress maneuvers and urinary retention, usually preceded by *abrupt* onset or intensification of the need to void; *stress:* leakage that coincides *instantaneously* with stress maneuvers, in the absence of urinary retention or detrusor contraction; *overflow:* frequent leakage of small amounts associated with urinary retention.
‡UTI prophylaxis can be used for recurrent symptomatic UTIs, but only if catheter is not indwelling.
§May also mimic stress or overflow incontinence.
‖Also can cause postvoid "dribbling" alone, which is treated conservatively (e.g., by sitting to void and allowing more time, "double voiding," and in men by gently "milking" the urethra after voiding).
¶Augmented voiding techniques include Credé (application of suprapubic pressure) and Valsalva (straining) maneuvers, and double voiding. They should be performed only *after* voiding has begun.
Anticholinergic bladder relaxant agents for urge incontinence:
Oxybutynin IR, 7.5-20 mg daily (2.5-5 mg tid-qid); oxybutynin XL, 5-30 mg once daily; oxybutynin patch twice weekly; oxybutynin 10% gel (1 g topically per day)
Tolterodine, 2 mg twice daily; tolterodine LA, 4 mg once daily
Darifenacin, 7.5-15 mg once daily
Solifenacin, 5-10 mg once daily
Trospium, 20 mg daily to twice daily; XL now available
Fesoterodine, 4-8 mg once daily
PVR = postvoid residual; UTI = urinary tract infection.
Adapted and updated in 2011 from Resnick NM. Voiding dysfunction and urinary incontinence. In: Beck JC, ed. *Geriatric Review Syllabus.* New York: American Geriatrics Society, 1991:141-154.

about 2 months and that side effects may offset the benefit. With such titration, urge incontinence can be controlled in about one third of patients and substantially improved in another one third.

Surgical Procedures

Surgery for stress incontinence has proved effective for women of all ages, including elderly women, and is relatively durable. Periurethral bulking injections can help frail women or those with mild stress incontinence, but it does not generally restore continence. However, urethral sling and midurethral tape suspension procedures can cure most women for at least 5 years.**5** For women with more complex stress incontinence and for men with stress incontinence more than a year after radical prostatectomy, an artificial sphincter has proved effective and relatively durable. Experience with the "male sling" is still limited.

Surgical interventions for urge incontinence, including neuromodulation, tibial nerve stimulation, and injections of botulinum toxin are successful in selected situations. However, they have not been studied adequately in elderly people, and the limited preliminary data suggest that older patients may not fare as well as younger ones.

PREVENTION

There are scant data regarding the prevention of incontinence, but one randomized trial of an educational and behavioral modification program for women older than 55 years found that it reduced the risk of incontinence for a year.**6** A secondary analysis of the Diabetes Prevention Program found that, at the end of 3 years, an intensive lifestyle intervention was associated with reduced risk of self-reported incontinence, with most of the benefit explained by weight loss and a reduced risk of stress incontinence.**7**

PROGNOSIS

Limited data suggest that incontinence progresses in about one third of patients and remits in about 10 to 15%, although it is unclear how much of the remission reflects intervention or improvement in functional or medical status.

1. Subak LL, Wing R, West DS, et al. Weight loss to treat urinary incontinence in overweight and obese women. *N Engl J Med.* 2009;360:481-490.
2. Shamliyan TA, Kane RL, Wyman J, et al. Systematic review: randomized, controlled trials of nonsurgical treatments for urinary incontinence in women. *Ann Intern Med.* 2008;148:459-473.
3. Hartmann KE, McPheeters ML, Biller DH, et al. Treatment of overactive bladder in women. Evidence Report/Technology Assessment No. 187. AHRQ Publication No. 09-E017. Rockville, MD: Agency for Healthcare Research and Quality, 2009.
4. DuBeau CE, Kuchel GA, Johnson T, et al. Incontinence in the frail elderly. *Neurourol Urodyn.* 2010;29:165-179.
5. Albo ME, Richter HE, Brubaker L, et al. Burch colposuspension versus fascial sling to reduce urinary stress incontinence. *N Engl J Med.* 2007;356:2143-2155.
6. Diokno AC, Sampselle CM, Herzog AR. Prevention of urinary incontinence by behavioral modification program: a randomized controlled trial among older women in the community. *J Urol.* 2004;171:1165-1171.
7. Brown JS, Wing RA, Barrett-Connor E, et al. Lifestyle intervention is associated with lower prevalence of urinary incontinence. *Diabetes Care.* 2006;29:385-390.

SUGGESTED READINGS

Goode PS, Burgio KL, Richter HE, et al. Incontinence in older women. *JAMA*. 2010;303:2172-2181. *Evidence-based review*.

Guzzo TJ, Drach GW. Major urologic problems in geriatrics: assessment and management. *Med Clin North Am*. 2011;95:253-264. *Review*.

26

NEUROPSYCHIATRIC ASPECTS OF AGING

SHARON K. INOUYE

DEFINITION

The process of aging produces important physiologic changes in the central nervous system (Table 26-1), including neuroanatomic, neurotransmitter, and neurophysiologic changes. These processes result in age-related symptoms and manifestations (Table 26-2) for many older persons. These physiologic changes develop at dramatically variable rates among older persons, however, and the decline may be modified by factors such as diet, exercise, environment, lifestyle, genetic predisposition, disability, disease, and side effects of drugs. These changes can result in the common age-related symptoms of benign senescence, slowed reaction time, postural hypotension, vertigo or giddiness, presbyopia, presbycusis, stiffened gait, and sleep difficulties. In the absence of disease, these physiologic changes usually result in relatively modest symptoms and little restriction in activities of daily living. These changes decrease physiologic reserve, however, and increase the susceptibility to challenges posed by disease-related, pharmacologic, and environmental stressors.

EPIDEMIOLOGY

Neuropsychiatric disorders, the leading cause of disability in older persons, account for nearly 50% of functional incapacity. Severe neuropsychiatric conditions have been estimated to occur in 15 to 25% of older adults worldwide. These conditions are due to diseases that increase with age but are not part of the normal aging process. Alzheimer's disease and related dementias occur in approximately 10% of adults aged 65 years and older and in 40% of those older than 85 years (Chapter 409). Delirium occurs in 5 to 10% of all persons older than 65 years and in up to 80% of older persons during hospitalizations for acute illnesses (Chapter 27). Severe depression (Chapter 404) occurs in approximately 5% of older adults, with 15% having significant depressive symptoms. Anxiety disorders occur in 10% of older adults. Older individuals are also subject to substantial morbidity and functional disability from cerebrovascular disease (Chapters 413 through 415), Parkinson's disease (Chapter 416), peripheral neuropathies (Chapter 428), degenerative myelopathies (Chapters 407 and 430), spinal stenosis and disc disease (Chapter 407), seizure disorders (Chapter 410), sleep apnea (Chapter 100),

visual disturbances (Chapter 431), falls (Chapter 24), incontinence (Chapter 25), and impotence (Chapter 242).

DIAGNOSIS

To diagnose these conditions, physicians must understand and perform a mental status examination and an assessment of functional capacity and know the uses and side effects of psychoactive drugs in geriatric patients.

Mental Status Examination

In addition to a detailed neurologic examination, evaluation of neuropsychiatric disturbances in older persons requires a careful mental status examination, including an assessment of mood, affect, and cognition. Brief screening tests are available to evaluate these domains and to assist in the detection of potential problems requiring further evaluation and treatment. For depression screening, scores of 6 or more on the 15-item short-form Geriatric Depression Scale (Table 26-3) indicate substantial depressive symptoms requiring further evaluation. Alternative depression screening instruments include the Center for Epidemiologic Studies Depression Scale (CES-D). For cognitively impaired patients, observer-rated depression scales, such as the Hamilton Depression Scale or Cornell Scale, are recommended.

TABLE 26-2	NEUROPSYCHIATRIC MANIFESTATIONS OF AGE-RELATED PHYSIOLOGIC CHANGES
SYSTEM	**MANIFESTATION**
Cognition	Forgetfulness
	Processing speed declines throughout adult life
	Neuropsychological declines: selective attention, verbal fluency, retrieval, complex visual perception, logical analysis
Reflexes	Stretch reflexes lose sensitivity
	Decreased or absent ankle reflexes
	Decreased autonomic and righting reflexes, postural instability
Sensory	Presbycusis (high-frequency hearing loss), tinnitus
	Deterioration of vestibular system, vertigo
	Presbyopia (decreased lens elasticity)
	Slowed pupil reactivity, decreased upgaze
	Olfactory system deterioration
	Decreased vibratory sensation
Gait and balance	Gait stiffer, slowed, forward flexed
	Increased body sway and mild unsteadiness
Sleep	Decreased sleep efficiency, fatigue
	Increased awakenings, insomnia
	Decrease in sleep stages 3 and 4
	Sleep duration more variable, more naps

TABLE 26-1	AGE-RELATED PHYSIOLOGIC CHANGES IN THE CENTRAL NERVOUS SYSTEM

Neuroanatomic changes
  Brain atrophy
  Decreased neuron counts
  Increased neuritic plaques
  Increased lipofuscin and melanin

Neurotransmitter changes
  Decline in cholinergic transmission
  Decreased dopaminergic synthesis
  Decreased catecholamine synthesis

Neurophysiologic changes
  Decreased cerebral blood flow
  Electrophysiologic changes (slowing of alpha rhythm, increased latencies in evoked responses)

TABLE 26-3	GERIATRIC DEPRESSION SCALE—SHORT FORM
1. Are you basically satisfied with your life?	yes/**NO**
2. Have you dropped many of your activities and interests?	**YES**/no
3. Do you feel that your life is empty?	**YES**/no
4. Do you often get bored?	**YES**/no
5. Are you in good spirits most of the time?	yes/**NO**
6. Are you afraid that something bad is going to happen to you?	**YES**/no
7. Do you feel happy most of the time?	yes/**NO**
8. Do you feel helpless?	**YES**/no
9. Do you prefer to stay home rather than going out and doing new things?	**YES**/no
10. Do you feel you have more problems with memory than most?	**YES**/no
11. Do you think it is wonderful to be alive now?	yes/**NO**
12. Do you feel pretty worthless the way you are now?	**YES**/no
13. Do you feel full of energy?	yes/**NO**
14. Do you feel that your situation is hopeless?	**YES**/no
15. Do you think that most people are better off than you are?	**YES**/no

Scoring: Answers indicating depression are highlighted; six or more highlighted answers indicate depressive symptoms.
Modified from Yesavage J, Brink T, Rowe T, et al. Development and validation of a geriatric depression screening scale: a preliminary report. *J Psychiatr Res*. 1983;17:37-49.

FIGURE 26-1. Montreal Cognitive Assessment (MOCA).

TABLE 26-4 MINI-COG TEST

1. Instruct the patient to listen carefully to and remember 3 unrelated words and then to repeat the words: BANANA, SUNRISE, CHAIR.
2. Instruct the patient to draw the face of a clock, either on a blank sheet of paper or on a sheet with a large circle already drawn on the page. After the patient puts the numbers on the clock face, ask him or her to draw the hands of the clock to read a specific time, such as 11:10. These instructions can be repeated, but no additional instructions should be given. Allow up to 3 minutes to complete the clock drawing.
3. Ask the patient to repeat the 3 previously presented words.
4. Give 1 point for each correct word and 2 points for a correctly drawn clock. Scores <3 suggest cognitive impairment.

Adapted from Borson S, Scanlan J, Watanabe J, et al. Improving identification of cognitive impairment in primary care. *Int J Geriatr Psychiatry.* 2006; 21:349-355. Reprinted by permission of the copyright holder (S. Borson).

Early cognitive deficits can easily be missed during conversation because intellectual impairment can be masked with intact social skills. Given the high frequency of cognitive impairment, formal cognitive screening is recommended for all older persons. Ideally, cognitive testing should evaluate at least the general domains of attention, orientation, language, memory, visuospatial ability, and conceptualization. To exclude delirium, attention should be assessed first by asking the patient to perform a task, such as repeating five digits or reciting the months backward; the remainder of cognitive testing would not be useful in an inattentive patient. For further cognitive testing, many brief, practical screening instruments are available. Historically, the most widely used instrument has been the Mini-Mental State Examination, a 19-item, 30-point scale that can be completed in 10 minutes. This copyrighted instrument now requires a per-use fee if the official version is used. A useful, brief alternative instrument is the Mini-Cog test, which can be completed in 2 to 4 minutes (Table 26-4); scores <3 suggest cognitive impairment. More detailed testing can be conducted with the Montreal Cognitive Assessment (Figure 26-1), which requires 10 to 15 minutes; scores less than 26 indicate cognitive impairment. Questions to evaluate judgment and problem-solving ability in hypothetical situations, such as in a fire or when driving, can provide crucial insight into the patient's ability to function safely and independently.

Functional Assessment

Functional impairment, defined as difficulty in performing daily activities, is common among elderly persons. Although it is not routinely evaluated in the standard medical assessment, determination of the patient's degree of functional incapacity based on medical and neuropsychiatric conditions is crucial to understanding the burden of disease and its impact on the individual's daily life. The important relationship between functional status and health in older persons is reflected by the finding that functional measures are stronger predictors of mortality after hospitalization than are admitting diagnoses. Functional measures strongly predict other important hospital outcomes in the elderly, such as length of stay, functional status at discharge, future care

needs, caregiver burden, risk for institutionalization, and long-term prognosis. Functional independence is critical if patients are to remain living independently in the community, and functional decline represents a leading risk factor for nursing home placement.

The functional assessment should include an assessment of the patient's ability to perform basic self-care activities of daily living and instrumental activities of daily living, the higher level activities needed for independent living. Activities of daily living include basic self-care skills such as feeding, grooming, bathing, dressing, toileting, transferring, and walking. Instrumental activities of daily living are more complex tasks, including shopping, preparing meals, managing finances, housekeeping, using the telephone, taking medications, and driving or using public transportation. The functional assessment is conducted with the patient or the family, and the questions ascertain whether the patient can perform these activities independently. Other related domains that should be assessed include vision, hearing, continence, nutritional status, safety, falls, living situation, social support, and socioeconomic status.

The onset of acute cognitive or functional decline is often the first and sometimes the only sign of serious acute illness in older persons, and it warrants immediate medical attention. Similarly, the onset or worsening of related conditions, such as delirium, falls, incontinence, depression, frailty, or failure to thrive, heralds the need for prompt medical evaluation.

TREATMENT   Rx

Psychoactive Effects of Drugs in Older Patients
Adverse Drug Events in the Elderly

Iatrogenic complications occur in 29 to 38% of older hospitalized patients, with a three- to five-fold increased risk in older compared with younger patients. Adverse drug events, the most common type of iatrogenic complication, account for 20 to 40% of all complications. The elderly are particularly vulnerable to adverse drug reactions because of multiple-drug regimens, multiple chronic diseases, relative renal and hepatic insufficiency, decreased physiologic reserve, and altered drug metabolism with aging. Inappropriate drug use has been reported in about 40% of hospitalized older patients, with more than one quarter of these patients having absolute contraindications to the drug and the others being given a drug that was unnecessary. Because 50% of adverse drug events occur in patients receiving inappropriate drugs, the potential for reducing these adverse events is substantial.

Drugs with Psychoactive Effects

Nearly every class of drug has the potential to cause mental status changes in a vulnerable patient, but specific drugs are commonly implicated (Table 26-5) and should be used with caution in older patients. Many cases of delirium or cognitive decline in older patients may be preventable through avoidance, substitution, or dose reduction of these psychoactive drugs. Long-acting benzodiazepines (e.g., flurazepam, diazepam) are particularly problematic medications for the elderly and should be avoided whenever possible. If nonpharmacologic approaches to the management of insomnia are unsuccessful, short-term use of an intermediate-acting benzodiazepine without active metabolites (e.g., lorazepam 0.5 mg, half-life of 10 to 15 hours) is recommended. Drugs with anticholinergic effects (e.g., antihistamines, antidepressants, neuroleptics, antispasmodics) produce a panoply of poorly tolerated side effects in older patients, including delirium, postural hypotension, urinary retention, constipation, and dry mouth. Of the narcotics, meperidine causes

TABLE 26-5 DRUGS WITH PSYCHOACTIVE EFFECTS

Sedative-hypnotics
  Benzodiazepines (especially flurazepam, diazepam)
  Barbiturates
  Sleeping medications (chloral hydrate)

Narcotics (especially meperidine)

Anticholinergics
  Antihistamines (diphenhydramine, hydroxyzine)
  Antispasmodics (belladonna, Lomotil)
  Heterocyclic antidepressants (amitriptyline, imipramine, doxepin)
  Neuroleptics (chlorpromazine, haloperidol, thioridazine)
  Antiparkinson drugs (benztropine, trihexyphenidyl)
  Atropine, scopolamine

Cardiac drugs
  Digitalis glycosides
  Antiarrhythmics (quinidine, procainamide, lidocaine)
  Antihypertensives (β-blockers, methyldopa)

Gastrointestinal drugs
  H_2-antagonists (cimetidine, ranitidine, famotidine, nizatidine)
  Proton pump inhibitors (esomeprazole, lansoprazole, omeprazole, pantoprozole)
  Metoclopramide (Reglan)

Miscellaneous drugs
  Nonsteroidal anti-inflammatory drugs
  Corticosteroids
  Anticonvulsants
  Levodopa
  Lithium

Over-the-counter drugs
  Cold and sinus preparations (antihistamines, pseudoephedrine)
  Sleep aids (diphenhydramine, alcohol-containing elixirs)
  Stay Awake (caffeine)
  Nausea, gastrointestinal relief (Donnagel, meclizine, H_2-antagonists, loperamide)

TABLE 26-6 GUIDELINES FOR DRUG THERAPY IN THE ELDERLY

GENERAL PRINCIPLES

Remember that the elderly are highly sensitive to the psychoactive effects of all drugs.
Know the pharmacology of the drugs you prescribe. Know a few drugs well.

RECOMMENDED APPROACH

Use nonpharmacologic approaches whenever possible.
Avoid *routine* use of "as needed" drugs for sleep, anxiety, pain.
Choose the drug with the least toxic potential.
Substitute less toxic alternatives whenever possible (antacid or sucralfate for an H_2-blocker or proton pump inhibitors, metamucil or kaopectate for imodium, or Lomotil, scheduled acetaminophen regimen for pain management).
Reduce the dosage.
"Start low and go slow."
  Start with 25-50% of the standard dose of psychoactive drugs in the elderly.
  Titrate the drug slowly.
  Set realistic end points: titrate to improvement, not elimination of symptoms.
Keep the regimen simple.
Regularly reassess the medication list. Have the patient bring in all bottles and review what is being taken.
Re-evaluate long-time drug use because the patient is changing.
Review over-the-counter medication use.

---

delirium more frequently than other agents because of an active metabolite, normeperidine. Cardiac drugs, such as digitalis and antiarrhythmic agents, have prolonged half-lives, narrowed therapeutic windows, and decreased protein binding in older patients. The clinician should be aware that toxicity with these agents (e.g., digoxin) can occur even at therapeutic drug levels. The H_2-receptor antagonists (e.g., cimetidine, ranitidine, famotidine, nizatidine) are among the most common causes of drug-induced delirium in the elderly because of their frequent use; clinicians should strongly consider the use of less toxic alternatives (e.g., sucralfate, antacids) or dosage reductions for older patients, especially when the medication is being used for prophylaxis rather than treatment of active disease. Proton pump inhibitors have been associated with delirium in case reports; however, the overall rate of this adverse effect has not been systematically determined. The Beers list, which is updated regularly, includes drugs that are potentially inappropriate for the elderly and drugs associated with high rates of adverse events in the elderly, including mental status changes and falls.

Psychoactive drugs account for nearly 50% of preventable adverse drug events, often in patients who have been prescribed three or more psychoactive drugs, frequently at inappropriately high doses in the elderly. Delirium and cognitive impairment are the most frequent adverse outcomes of psychoactive drugs. The use of any psychoactive drug is associated with a 4-fold increased risk of delirium or cognitive decline, but the outcomes of these conditions depend on the type or class of drug administered and the total number of drugs received. Sedative-hypnotic drugs are associated with a 3- to 12-fold increased risk for delirium or cognitive decline, narcotics are associated with a 2- to 3-fold increased risk, and anticholinergic drugs are associated with a 5- to 12-fold increased risk. Each drug carries its own individual risk for adverse outcomes, and when multiple drugs are used, the overall risk is compounded by the heightened potential for drug-drug interactions. If more than three drugs are added in a 24-hour period, the risk of delirium increases 4-fold. Similarly, the risk of cognitive decline increases directly with the number of drugs prescribed, from a 3-fold increased risk with two or three drugs to a 14-fold increased risk with six or more drugs.

Principles of Drug Therapy in the Elderly

Physicians always should consider whether nonpharmacologic approaches (Chapter 38) may be used as alternatives to medications in older persons. Relaxation techniques, massage, and music are highly effective for the treatment of insomnia and anxiety; localized pain can often be managed effectively with local measures such as injection, heat, ultrasound, and transcutaneous electrical stimulation.

When drug therapy is required in the elderly, physicians should choose the drug with the least toxic potential and emphasize drugs that have been well tested in older populations (Table 26-6). It is often wise to start with 25 to 50% of the standard adult dosage for any psychoactive drug and increase the dose slowly. Drug regimens should be kept simple, with the fewest drugs and the fewest number of pills possible. Most important, the medication list should be reassessed frequently. Systematic interventions involving geriatricians, clinical pharmacists, and computer-based systems can significantly reduce the frequency of adverse drug reactions in older persons.

Even long-standing medications should be reevaluated because the patient is changing with age and illness. Long-term use does not justify continued use. The physician should review with the patient all prescribed and over-the-counter medications on a regular basis, preferably by having the patient bring in all medication bottles and indicate how each is being taken. Patients frequently underestimate the toxic potential of over-the-counter medications and herbal remedies, and they may be using a variety of such agents that could potentiate the side effects or directly counteract the desired effects of prescription medications (Chapter 28). For example, high-risk over-the-counter medications for older persons include nonsteroidal anti-inflammatory agents, H_2-blockers, and antihistamines. In addition, herbal remedies such as gingko biloba may interact with warfarin to cause bleeding; others (such as kava kava and Chinese herbal preparations) are associated with the risk of hepatotoxicity.

FUTURE DIRECTIONS

Screening methods for cognitive and functional decline should be used for high-risk older persons. An important goal for the future is to incorporate these screening and interventional measures into the routine care of all older persons in physicians' offices, clinics, hospitals, nursing homes, and other settings.

Grade A

1. Schnipper JL, Hamann C, Ndumele CD, et al. Effect of an electronic medication reconciliation application and process redesign on potential adverse drug events: a cluster-randomized trial. *Arch Intern Med.* 2009;169:771-780.

SUGGESTED READINGS

Kåreholt I, Lennartsson C, Gatz M, et al. Baseline leisure time activity and cognition more than two decades later. *Int J Geriatr Psychiatry.* 2011;26:65-74. *Various forms of engagement in mid-life can protect cognition later in life.*

Ting C, Rajji TK, Ismail Z, et al. Differentiating the cognitive profile of schizophrenia from that of Alzheimer disease and depression in late life. *PLoS One.* 2010;5:e10151. *Guidance for making these important diagnostic distinctions.*

27

DELIRIUM OR ACUTE MENTAL STATUS CHANGE IN THE OLDER PATIENT

SHARON K. INOUYE

Mental status change, one of the most common presenting symptoms in acutely ill elders, is estimated to account for 30% of emergency evaluations among older patients. Mental status often serves as a barometer of the underlying health of an elderly patient and is commonly the only symptom of serious underlying disease. A broad range of medical, neurologic, and psychiatric conditions can lead to mental status changes (Chapters 404 and 409). A systematic approach aids in the evaluation of suspected mental status change in an older patient (Fig. 27-1).

The first step in evaluating suspected altered mental status in an older patient is to obtain a detailed history from a reliable informant to establish the patient's baseline level of cognitive function and the clinical course of any cognitive changes. Chronic changes (those occurring over months to years) most likely represent an underlying dementing illness and should be evaluated accordingly (Chapter 409). Acute changes (those occurring over days to weeks)—even if superimposed on an underlying dementia—should be evaluated by a detailed cognitive assessment to determine whether delirium is present. If features of delirium (e.g., inattention, disorganized thinking, altered level of consciousness, fluctuating symptoms) are not present, further evaluation for depression, acute nonorganic psychotic disorders, or other psychiatric conditions is indicated.

 DELIRIUM

Delirium, a clinical syndrome characterized as an acute disorder of attention and cognitive function, is the most frequent complication of hospitalization for elders and is a potentially devastating problem. Delirium is often unrecognized despite sensitive methods for its detection, and its complications may be preventable.

DEFINITION

The definition of and diagnostic criteria for delirium are evolving. The fourth edition of the *Diagnostic and Statistical Manual of Mental Disorders* (text revision) has been used widely (Table 27-1), but the criteria in this manual were based on expert consensus, and their diagnostic sensitivity and specificity have not been determined. The Confusion Assessment Method (CAM) provides a simple, operationalized diagnostic algorithm. In studies of more than 1000 subjects, it had a sensitivity of 94%, a specificity of 89%, and a high interrater reliability.

EPIDEMIOLOGY

In persons older than 65 years, the prevalence of delirium at hospital admission is 13 to 60%. Delirium develops in 6 to 56% of patients during hospitalization. Higher rates are found when frequent surveillance is performed in older, surgical, and intensive care populations. Delirium occurs in 15 to 74% of postoperative patients, 60 to 80% of patients in medical intensive care units, up to 60% of nursing home patients, and at least 80% of patients at the end of life.

The hospital mortality rates for delirium are 25 to 33%—as high as those associated with acute myocardial infarction and sepsis. The problem of delirium in hospitalized elderly patients has assumed particular prominence because patients aged 65 years and older currently account for more than 50% of all inpatient days of hospital care. Based on U.S. vital health statistics, delirium complicates hospital stays for at least 20% of the 12.5 million older persons hospitalized each year and increases hospital costs by more than $2500 per patient, amounting to more than $6.9 billion (2004 U.S. dollars) of Medicare expenditures yearly. Substantial additional costs are incurred after hospital discharge because of the increased need for rehabilitation services, nursing home placement, home care, and rehospitalization. Health care costs associated with delirium range from $38 billion to $152 billion per year. These extrapolations highlight the extensive economic and health policy implications of delirium.

TABLE 27-1   DIAGNOSTIC CRITERIA FOR DELIRIUM

DSM-IV TR DIAGNOSTIC CRITERIA

A. Disturbance of consciousness (i.e., reduced clarity of awareness of the environment) with reduced ability to focus, sustain, or shift attention
B. A change in cognition (e.g., memory deficit, disorientation, language disturbance) or the development of a perceptual disturbance that is not better accounted for by a preexisting, established, or evolving dementia
C. The disturbance develops over a short period (usually hours to days) and tends to fluctuate during the course of the day
D. Evidence from the history, physical examination, or laboratory findings indicates that the disturbance is caused by the direct physiologic consequences of a general medical condition

CAM DIAGNOSTIC ALGORITHM*

Feature 1. Acute onset and fluctuating course. This information is usually obtained from a family member or nurse and is shown by positive responses to the following questions: Is there evidence of an acute change in mental status from the patient's baseline? Did the (abnormal) behavior fluctuate during the day—that is, tend to come and go or increase and decrease in severity?
Feature 2. Inattention. This feature is shown by a positive response to the following question: Did the patient have difficulty focusing attention—for example, was he or she easily distracted or did he or she have difficulty keeping track of what was being said?
Feature 3. Disorganized thinking. This feature is shown by a positive response to the following question: Was the patient's thinking disorganized or incoherent, such as rambling or irrelevant conversation, unclear or illogical flow of ideas, or unpredictable switching from subject to subject?
Feature 4. Altered level of consciousness. This feature is shown by any answer other than "alert" to the following question: Overall, how would you rate this patient's level of consciousness: alert (normal), vigilant (hyperalert), lethargic (drowsy, easily aroused), stupor (difficult to arouse), or coma (unable to arouse)?

*The diagnosis of delirium requires the presence of features 1 and 2 and either 3 or 4.
CAM = Confusion Assessment Method, from Inouye SK, van Dyck CH, Alessi CA, et al: Clarifying confusion: The Confusion Assessment Method. A new method for detection of delirium. *Ann Intern Med.* 1990;113:941-948. Training manual available at http://elderlife.med.yale.edu/pdf/The Confusion Assessment Method.pdf; DSM-IV = American Psychiatric Association. *Diagnostic and Statistical Manual of Mental Disorders*, 4th ed., text revision. Washington, DC: American Psychiatric Association; 2000.

PATHOBIOLOGY

Similar to other common geriatric syndromes (Chapter 24), delirium usually has multiple causes. A search for the innumerable potential underlying contributors requires clinical astuteness and a thorough medical evaluation, especially because many of these factors are treatable but may result in substantial morbidity and mortality if left untreated. The process is made more challenging by the frequently nonspecific, atypical, or muted features of the underlying illness in older persons. Delirium is commonly the only initial sign of an underlying life-threatening illness such as pneumonia (Chapter 97), urosepsis (Chapter 292), or myocardial infarction (Chapter 73) in the older population.

The development of delirium usually involves a complex interrelationship between a vulnerable patient with pertinent predisposing factors and exposure to noxious insults or precipitating factors. Delirium may develop in vulnerable patients, such as cognitively impaired or severely ill patients, after a relatively benign insult, such as a single dose of sleeping medication. Conversely, in patients who are not vulnerable, delirium may develop only after exposure to multiple noxious insults. Previous studies have shown that the effects of these risk factors may be cumulative. Recognition of this multifactorial causation is important to the clinician because the removal or treatment of one factor in isolation usually is not sufficient to resolve the delirium. The full spectrum of vulnerability and precipitating factors should be addressed.

Predisposing factors, or factors that increase vulnerability, include preexisting cognitive impairment or dementia, severe underlying illness, high levels of comorbidity, functional impairment, advanced age, chronic renal insufficiency, dehydration, malnutrition, and vision or hearing impairment. Dementia is an important and consistent risk factor for delirium; demented patients have a twofold to fivefold increased risk for delirium. Of delirious patients, 30 to 50% have underlying dementia. Delirious patients commonly have evidence of underlying chronic brain disease, particularly conditions associated with cognitive impairment such as Alzheimer's disease, Parkinson's disease, or cerebrovascular disease.

Medications, the most common remediable cause of delirium, contribute to delirium in 40% of cases (Chapter 26). Insufficiency or failure of any major

FIGURE 27-1. Algorithm for the evaluation of suspected mental status change in older patients. PRN = as needed; TFTs = thyroid function tests.

organ system, particularly renal or hepatic failure, can precipitate delirium. Hypoxemia and hypercarbia have been associated with delirium. Clinicians must be attuned to occult respiratory failure, which in the elderly often lacks the usual signs and symptoms of dyspnea and tachypnea and can be missed by the measurement of oxygen saturation alone. Acute myocardial infarction or heart failure can manifest as delirium in an elderly patient without the usual symptoms of chest pain or dyspnea. Occult infection is a particularly notable cause of delirium. Older patients frequently fail to mount the febrile or leukocytotic response to infection, and clinicians must assess them carefully for signs of pneumonia, urinary tract infection, endocarditis, abdominal abscess, or infected joints. A variety of metabolic disorders may contribute to delirium, including hypernatremia and hyponatremia, hypercalcemia, acid-base disorders, hypoglycemia and hyperglycemia, and thyroid or adrenal disorders. Immobilization and immobilizing devices (e.g., indwelling bladder catheters, physical restraints, bed alarms) are important factors in precipitating delirium. Dehydration and volume depletion and nutritional decline during hospitalization (e.g., weight loss, fall in serum albumin concentration) are well-documented factors contributing to delirium. Drug and alcohol withdrawal are important and often unsuspected causes of delirium in the elderly. Environmental factors, such as unfamiliar surroundings, sleep deprivation, deranged schedule, frequent room changes, sensory overload, and sensory deprivation, may aggravate delirium in the hospital. Psychosocial factors, such as depression, psychological stress, pain, and lack of social supports, also may precipitate delirium.

The basic pathogenesis of delirium is unclear. Most investigators agree that delirium seems to be a functional rather than a structural lesion. Electroencephalographic studies show global functional derangements in patients with delirium, characterized by generalized slowing of cortical background activity with the appearance of delta and theta activity. Neuroimaging studies coupled with cognitive testing demonstrate a generalized disruption in higher cortical function, with dysfunction in the prefrontal cortex, frontal and temporoparietal cortex, fusiform cortex, lingual gyri, subcortical structures, thalamus, and basal ganglia. The leading hypotheses for the pathogenesis of delirium focus on the roles of neurotransmission and inflammation. The most widely postulated mechanism for delirium is the failure of cholinergic transmission. Evidence supporting this hypothesis includes the frequent association of anticholinergic drugs with delirium, the reversal of delirium with procholinergic drugs such as physostigmine, the increased levels of serum anticholinergic activity in some delirious patients, and the benefit of cholinesterase inhibitors in some cases of delirium. Other neurotransmitter systems, such as dopamine, serotonin, tryptophan, norepinephrine, and γ-aminobutyric acid, may also play a role in delirium, but the evidence is less well developed. In some circumstances, such as infection or cancer, delirium may be mediated through cytokines, such as interleukin-2 and tumor necrosis factor. Although delirium has long been considered a transient syndrome, several of these basic mechanisms may not be completely reversible, particularly those resulting in hypoxic damage. Acute stress with high levels of cortisol may also contribute to delirium. The dose and duration of the noxious insult, along with the degree of vulnerability of the patient, also may exert great influence on the ultimate reversibility of the delirium.

CLINICAL MANIFESTATIONS

The cardinal features of delirium include acute onset and inattention. Establishing the acuteness of onset requires accurate knowledge of the patient's baseline cognitive function. Patients with delirium are inattentive; that is, they have difficulty focusing, maintaining, and shifting attention. They appear easily distracted and have difficulty maintaining conversation and following commands. Objectively, patients may have difficulty with simple repetitive tasks, digit spans, and recitation of months backward. Other key features include disorganized thought processes, which are usually a manifestation of underlying cognitive or perceptual disturbances; altered level of consciousness, which typically consists of lethargy with reduced awareness of the environment; and fluctuation of cognitive symptoms. Although not cardinal elements, other features that frequently occur during delirium include disorientation, cognitive deficits, psychomotor agitation or retardation, perceptual disturbances such as hallucinations and illusions, paranoid delusions, and sleep-wake cycle reversal.

DIAGNOSIS

The cornerstone of the evaluation of delirium is a comprehensive history and physical examination (Table 27-2). The first step is to establish the diagnosis

---

TABLE 27-2 EVALUATION OF DELIRIUM IN ELDERLY PATIENTS

Perform cognitive testing and determine baseline cognitive functioning: establish the diagnosis of delirium

Obtain a comprehensive history and perform a physical examination, including a careful neurologic examination for focal deficits and a search for occult infection

Review the patient's medication list: discontinue or minimize all psychoactive medications; check the side effects of all medications

Perform a laboratory evaluation (tailored to the individual): complete blood count, electrolytes, blood urea nitrogen, creatinine, glucose, calcium, phosphate, liver enzymes, oxygen saturation

Search for occult infection: physical examination, urinalysis, chest radiography, selected cultures (as indicated)

When no obvious cause is revealed after these steps, further targeted evaluation is considered in selected patients, as follows:
  Laboratory tests: magnesium, thyroid function, vitamin B$_{12}$ level, drug levels, toxicology screen, ammonia level
  Arterial blood gas analysis: indicated in patients with dyspnea, tachypnea, any acute pulmonary process, or history of significant respiratory disease
  Electrocardiography: indicated in patients with chest or abdominal discomfort, shortness of breath, or cardiac history
  Cerebrospinal fluid examination: indicated when meningitis or encephalitis is suspected
  Brain imaging: indicated in patients with new focal neurologic signs or with a history or signs of head trauma
  Electroencephalography: useful in diagnosing occult seizure disorder and in differentiating delirium from nonorganic psychiatric disorders

---

of delirium through cognitive assessment and to determine whether the present condition represents an acute change from the patient's baseline cognitive function. Because cognitive impairment may not be apparent during conversation, brief cognitive screening tests, such as the Mini-Cog Test (Chapter 26) and the Confusion Assessment Method, should be used. Attention should be assessed further with other simple tests, such as a forward digit span (inattention is indicated by an inability to repeat five digits forward) or recitation of the months backward. A delirium assessment for nonverbal (e.g., intubated) patients, called the CAM-ICU, has been developed. The history, which should be obtained from a reliable informant, is targeted to establish the patient's baseline cognitive function and the time course of any mental status change and to obtain clues about potential precipitating factors, such as recent medication changes, intercurrent infection, or medical illness. Physical examination should include a detailed neurologic examination for focal deficits and a careful search for signs of occult infection or an acute abdominal process.

Review of the patient's medication list, including over-the-counter medications, is crucial, and the use of medications with psychoactive effects should be discontinued or minimized whenever possible. In the elderly, these medications may cause psychoactive effects even at doses and measured drug levels within the "therapeutic range." Consideration should also be given to the possibility that withdrawal from alcohol or other medications is a contributor to delirium.

Laboratory Findings

Laboratory evaluation must be tailored to the individual situation (see Table 27-2). In patients with preexisting cardiac or respiratory diseases or related symptoms, electrocardiography or arterial blood gas determination may be indicated. The need for cerebrospinal fluid examination is controversial except when it is clearly indicated, such as in a febrile delirious patient. Brain imaging should be reserved for patients with new focal neurologic signs, those with a history or signs of head trauma, and those without another identifiable cause of the delirium. Electroencephalography, with a false-negative rate of 17% and a false-positive rate of 22% for distinguishing delirious from nondelirious patients, has a limited role and is most useful for detecting an occult seizure disorder and differentiating delirium from psychiatric disorders.

Differential Diagnosis

A crucial difficulty is distinguishing a long-standing confusional state (dementia) from delirium alone or delirium superimposed on dementia (see Fig. 27-1). These two conditions are differentiated by the acute onset of

TABLE 27-3　DELIRIUM RISK FACTORS AND POTENTIAL INTERVENTIONS

RISK FACTOR	INTERVENTION
Cognitive impairment	Reality orientation program (reorienting techniques, communication) Therapeutic activities program
Sleep deprivation	Noise reduction strategies Scheduling of nighttime medications, procedures, and nursing activities to allow uninterrupted period of sleep
Immobilization	Early mobilization (e.g., ambulation or bedside exercises) Minimal use of immobilizing equipment (e.g., bladder catheters)
Psychoactive medications	Restricted use of "as needed" sleep and psychoactive medications (e.g., sedative-hypnotics, narcotics, anticholinergic medications) Nonpharmacologic protocols for management of sleep and anxiety
Vision impairment	Provision of vision aids (e.g., magnifiers, special lighting) Provision of adaptive equipment (e.g., illuminated phone dials, large-print books)
Hearing impairment	Provision of amplifying devices Repair of hearing aids
Dehydration	Early recognition and volume repletion

symptoms in delirium (dementia is much more insidious) and the impaired attention and altered level of consciousness associated with delirium. The differential diagnosis also includes depression and nonorganic psychotic disorders. Although paranoia, hallucinations, and affective changes can occur with delirium, the key features of acute onset, inattention, altered level of consciousness, and global cognitive impairment assist in the recognition of delirium. At times, the differential diagnosis can be difficult, particularly with an uncooperative patient or when an accurate history is unavailable. Because of the potentially life-threatening nature of delirium, it is prudent to manage the patient as if he or she has delirium and to search for and treat underlying precipitants (e.g., intercurrent illness, metabolic derangement, drug toxicity) until further information can be obtained.

TREATMENT　Rx

Prevention

The most effective strategy to reduce delirium and its associated complications is primary prevention before delirium occurs. Preventive strategies should address important risk factors and target moderate- to high-risk patients at baseline (Table 27-3). Randomized trials have shown that a geriatrics consultation or a multidisciplinary intervention aimed at the risk factors for delirium can reduce the incidence of delirium by 40%. To date, no drug treatments, including cholinesterase inhibitors, have been effective in preventing delirium.[1] On a larger scale, preventive efforts require systemwide changes to educate physicians and nurses and thus improve their recognition of delirium and heighten their awareness of its clinical implications, to provide incentives to change practice patterns that lead to delirium (e.g., immobilization, sleep medications, bladder catheters, physical restraints), and to create systems that enhance high-quality geriatric care (e.g., geriatric expertise, case management, clinical pathways, quality monitoring).

Medical Therapy

In general, nonpharmacologic approaches should be used in all delirious patients, and these are usually successful in managing symptoms. Pharmacologic approaches should be reserved for patients whose symptoms may result in the interruption of needed medical therapies (e.g., intubation, intravenous lines) or may endanger the safety of the patient or other persons. No drug is ideal for the treatment of delirium, however; any drug can cloud the patient's mental status further and obscure efforts to monitor the course of the mental status change. The drug should be given at the lowest dose and for the shortest time possible. Neuroleptics are the preferred agents. Haloperidol, the most widely used agent, causes less orthostatic hypotension and fewer anticholinergic side effects than thioridazine and is available in parenteral form; however, it has a higher rate of extrapyramidal side effects and acute dystonias. Second-generation antipsychotics have not proved superior to haloperidol.[2] If parenteral administration is required, intravenous use results in a rapid onset of

action, short duration of effect, and risk of hypotension and torsades de pointes; intramuscular use has a more optimal duration of action and is preferred. The recommended starting dose is 0.25 to 0.5 mg of haloperidol orally or intramuscularly, repeated every 30 minutes after the vital signs have been rechecked, until sedation has been achieved. The end point should be an awake but manageable patient. The average elderly patient who has not been treated previously with neuroleptics should require a total loading dose of no more than 3 to 5 mg of haloperidol. Subsequently, a maintenance dose consisting of half the loading dose should be administered in divided doses during the next 24 hours, with doses tapered over the next few days as the agitation resolves.

Benzodiazepines are not recommended as the first-line treatment of delirium because of their tendency to cause oversedation and exacerbate the confusional state. They remain the drugs of choice, however, for the treatment of withdrawal syndromes from alcohol and sedative drugs (Chapters 32 and 33).

Nonpharmacologic Management

Multicomponent geriatric interventions may be effective in improving quality of life without increasing health care costs.[3] Nonpharmacologic management techniques recommended for every delirious patient include encouraging the presence of family members, using "sitters" as orienting influences, and transferring a disruptive patient to a private room or closer to the nurse's station for increased supervision. Interpersonal contact and communication, including verbal reorientation strategies, simple instructions and explanations, and frequent eye contact, are vital. Patients should be involved in their own care and allowed to participate in decision making as much as possible. Eyeglasses and hearing aids may reduce sensory deficits. Mobility, self-care, and independence should be encouraged, and physical restraints and bed alarms should be avoided, if possible, because of their tendency to increase agitation, their lack of efficacy, and their potential to cause injury. Attention must be focused on minimizing the disruptive influences of the hospital environment. Clocks and calendars should be provided to assist with orientation. Room and staff changes should be kept to a minimum. A quiet environment with low-level lighting is optimal for delirious patients. Perhaps the most important intervention is to schedule the checking of vital signs, the administration of medications, and the performance of procedures to allow the patient's uninterrupted sleep at night. Nonpharmacologic approaches to relaxation, including music, relaxation tapes, and massage, can be highly effective in managing agitation.

End-of-Life Care

Delirium occurs in at least 80% of patients at the end of life and is considered part of the dying process by many hospice care providers (Chapter 3). Establishing the goals for care in advance with the patient and family is critical to guide appropriate management. For example, some patients may prioritize the preservation of alertness and the ability to communicate with loved ones as long as possible; others may prioritize comfort above all else. Physicians must be aware that even in terminal patients, many causes of delirium are potentially reversible with simple interventions such as adjusting medications, providing oxygen, or treating dehydration; however, aggressive diagnostic evaluation is usually inappropriate in this population. Nonpharmacologic measures to treat agitation and delirium should be instituted in all patients (including massage, music, and relaxation therapies). Haloperidol remains the first-line therapy for delirium in terminally ill patients. If more sedation is indicated, a short-acting benzodiazepine such as lorazepam (starting dose, 0.5 to 1.0 mg PO, IM, or SL), which is easily titrated, is recommended in this setting. Because sedation may result in decreased interaction and communication, increased confusion, and respiratory depression, this choice should be made in conjunction with the family.

PROGNOSIS

Delirium is an important independent determinant of prolonged hospital stay, increased mortality, higher health care costs, increased rates of institutional placement, and functional and cognitive decline—even after controlling for age, gender, dementia, illness severity, and baseline functional status. Delirium was previously considered a reversible, transient condition, but more recent studies on the duration and persistence of symptoms document that delirium may be much more persistent than previously believed. Delirium typically lasts for 30 days or more, and only 20% of patients have complete resolution of all symptoms at 6-month follow-up. Delirium seems to have greater deleterious effects in patients with underlying cognitive impairment. The long-term detrimental effects are most likely related to the duration, severity, and underlying cause of the delirium and the vulnerability of the patient.

FUTURE DIRECTIONS

Because delirium is common, frequently iatrogenic, and linked to processes of care, it is considered to be a marker of the quality of care and patient safety in the hospital setting. Strategies to prevent delirium are a priority. It is hoped that future research will elucidate the pathophysiologic mechanisms of delirium by the use of neuroimaging modalities, neuropsychological testing, and genetic and laboratory markers; clarify the contribution of delirium to irreversible cognitive impairment; and improve the evidence-based management of delirium.

1. Overshott R, Karim S, Burns A. Cholinesterase inhibitors for delirium. Cochrane Database Syst Rev 2008, Issue 1, Art. No. CD005317.

2. Campbell N, Boustani MA, Ayub A, et al. Pharmacological management of delirium in hospitalized adults: a systemic evidence review. *J Gen Intern Med.* 2009;24:848-853.

3. Pitkala KS, Laurila JV, Strandberg TE, et al. Multicomponent geriatric intervention for elderly inpatients with delirium: effects on costs and health-related quality of life. *J Gerontol Med Sci.* 2008;63:56-61.

SUGGESTED READINGS

Clegg A, Young JB. Which medications to avoid in people at risk of delirium: a systematic review. *Age Ageing.* 2011;40:23-29. *Benzodiazepines, opioids, dihydropyridines, and antihistamine H₁ antagonists carry the highest risks.*

Witlox J, Eurelings LS, de Jonghe JF, et al. Delirium in elderly patients and the risk of postdischarge mortality, institutionalization, and dementia: a meta-analysis. *JAMA.* 2010;304:443-451. *In-hospital delirium correlates with a 2-fold increase in mortality, a 2.4-fold increase in institutionalization, and a 13-fold increase in subsequent dementia.*

Wong CL, Holroyd-Leduc J, Simel DL, et al. Does this patient have delirium?: value of bedside instruments. *JAMA.* 2010;304:779-786. *Review suggesting that the Confusion Assessment Method, which takes 5 minutes to administer, is the preferred diagnostic instrument.*

V

CLINICAL PHARMACOLOGY

28

PRINCIPLES OF DRUG THERAPY

ROBERT B. DIASIO

Under different conditions, a drug may produce diverse effects ranging from no effect to a desirable effect to an undesirable toxic effect. Physicians must learn how to individualize the drug dosage under different conditions to ensure effective and safe therapy. This necessitates understanding the pharmacokinetics—the movement of a drug over time through the body—and the pharmacodynamics—the relationship between drug concentration and drug effect (Fig. 28-1). This chapter reviews the basic concepts of pharmacokinetics and pharmacodynamics, followed by guidelines on how to use this information to optimize therapeutic applications. Drug interactions and adverse drug responses are briefly discussed, with advice on how both can be recognized and minimized in clinical practice.

● PHARMACOKINETIC PRINCIPLES

Administration

The most efficient and straightforward means of administering a drug into the systemic circulation is by intravenous injection of the drug as a bolus. With this route, the full amount of a drug is delivered to the systemic circulation almost immediately. The same dose also may be administered as an intravenous infusion over a longer period, resulting in a decrease in the peak plasma concentration and an accompanying increase in the time the drug is present in the circulation. Many other routes of administration can be used, including sublingual, oral, transdermal, rectal, inhalational, subcutaneous, and intramuscular; each of these routes carries not only a potential delay in the time it takes the drug to enter the circulation but also the possibility that a large fraction of it will never reach the circulation.

Absorption

Absorption refers to the transfer of a drug from the site of administration to the systemic circulation. Many drugs cross a membrane barrier by passive diffusion and enter the systemic circulation. Because passive diffusion in this setting depends on the concentration of the solute at the membrane surface, the rate of drug absorption is affected by the concentration of free drug at the absorbing surface. Factors that influence the availability of free drug thus affect drug absorption from the administration site; this effect can be exploited to design medications that release a drug slowly into the circulation by prolonging drug absorption. With certain sustained-released oral preparations, the rate of dissolution of the drug in the gastrointestinal tract determines the rate at which the drug is absorbed (e.g., timed-release antihistamines). Similarly, a prolonged drug effect can be obtained by the use of transdermal medications (e.g., nitroglycerin) or intramuscular depot preparations (e.g., benzathine penicillin G).

First-Pass Effect

Some drugs that are administered orally are absorbed relatively well into the portal circulation but are metabolized by the liver before they reach the systemic circulation. Because of this "first-pass" or "presystemic" effect, the oral route may be less suitable than other routes of administration for such drugs. A good example is nitroglycerin, which is well absorbed but efficiently metabolized during the first pass through the liver. The same drug can achieve adequate systemic levels when it is given sublingually or transdermally.

Bioavailability

The extent of absorption of a drug into the systemic circulation may be incomplete. The bioavailability of a particular drug is the fraction (F) of the total drug dose that ultimately reaches the systemic circulation from the site of administration. This fraction is calculated by dividing the amount of the drug dose that reaches the circulation from the administration site by the amount of the drug dose that would enter the systemic circulation after direct intravenous injection into the circulation (essentially the total dose). Bioavailability, or F, can range from 0, in which no drug reaches the systemic circulation, to 1.0, in which essentially all the drug is absorbed. The bioavailability of a drug may vary in different formulations because the overall absorption differs. This variability has become a concern with the increasing use of generic preparations.

Distribution

After delivery of a drug into the systemic circulation either directly by intravenous injection or after absorption, the drug is transported throughout the body, initially to the well-perfused tissues and later to areas that are less perfused. The distribution phase can be assessed best by plotting the drug's plasma concentration on a log scale versus time on a linear scale (Fig. 28-2). For an intravenously administered drug, when absorption is not a factor, the initial phase—from immediately after administration through the rapid fall in concentration—represents the distribution phase, during which a drug rapidly disappears from the circulation and enters the tissues. This is followed by the elimination phase (see later), when drug in the plasma is in equilibrium with drug in the tissues. During this latter phase, the drug's plasma concentration is thought to be related to drug effect.

Volume of Distribution

The volume of distribution (VD) relates the amount of drug in the body to the concentration of drug in the plasma. It is calculated by dividing the dose that ultimately gets into the systemic circulation by the plasma concentration at time zero (C_{p0}):

$$VD = dose/C_{p0} \tag{1}$$

The C_{p0} can be calculated by extrapolating the elimination phase back to time zero (see Fig. 28-2). The VD is best considered the "apparent VD" because it represents the apparent volume needed to contain the entire amount of the drug, assuming it is distributed throughout the body at the same concentration as in the plasma. Table 28-1 lists pharmacokinetic data for commonly used drugs from several drug classes, showing the wide variation in VD. Digoxin, for example, has a large VD (>5 L), whereas glimepiride has a relatively small VD (0.18 L). As discussed later, VD is a useful pharmacokinetic tool for calculating the loading dose and appreciating how various changes can affect a drug's half-life.

Elimination

Drugs are removed from the body by two major mechanisms: hepatic elimination, in which drugs are metabolized in the liver and excreted through the biliary tract; and renal elimination, in which drugs are removed from the circulation by either glomerular filtration or tubular secretion. For most drugs, the rates of hepatic and renal elimination are proportional to the plasma concentration of the drug. This relationship is often described as a "first-order" process. Two measurements, clearance and half-life, are used to evaluate elimination.

Clearance

The efficiency of elimination can be assessed by quantifying how fast the drug is cleared from the circulation. Drug clearance is a measure of the volume of plasma cleared of drug per unit of time. It is similar to the clinical measurement used to assess renal function—creatinine clearance, which is the volume of plasma from which creatinine is removed per minute. Total drug clearance (Cl_{tot}) is the rate of elimination by all processes (El_{tot}) divided by the plasma concentration of the drug (C_p):

$$Cl_{tot} = El_{tot}/C_p \tag{2}$$

Drugs may be cleared by several organs, but as noted earlier, renal clearance and hepatic clearance are the two major mechanisms. Total drug clearance (Cl_{tot}) can best be described as the sum of clearances by each organ. For most drugs, this is essentially the sum of renal clearance and hepatic clearance:

$$Cl_{tot} = Cl_{Ren} + Cl_{Hep} \tag{3}$$

Table 28-1 shows the wide variation in clearance values among commonly used medications; some drugs (e.g., phenobarbital) have relatively low clearances (<5 mL/minute), and other drugs (e.g., aspirin) have relatively high clearances (>500 mL/minute). Tobramycin is cleared almost entirely by the kidneys, whereas aspirin, carbamazepine, and phenytoin are cleared less than 5% by the kidneys.

Drug clearance is affected by several factors, including blood flow through the organ of clearance, protein binding to the drug, and activity of the clearance processes in the organs of elimination (e.g., glomerular filtration rate and tubular secretion in the kidney, enzyme activity in the liver). Drug clearance

FIGURE 28-1. Schematic of a drug's movement through the body, from the site of administration to production of a drug effect. The relationship between pharmacokinetics and pharmacodynamics is shown.

FIGURE 28-2. Representative drug concentration versus time plot used in pharmacokinetic studies. Concentration of drug is plotted with a logarithmic scale on the ordinate, and time is plotted with a linear scale on the abscissa. The resultant curve has two phases: the distribution phase, which is the initial portion of the plotted line when the concentration of drug decreases rapidly; and the later elimination phase, during which there is an exponential disappearance of drug from the plasma over time. The dotted line extrapolated from the elimination phase back to time zero is used to calculate plasma concentration at time zero (C_{p0}). During the elimination phase, the half-life ($t_{1/2}$) can be calculated as the time it takes to decrease the concentration by half (shown here as the time needed to decrease from concentration C_a to $\frac{1}{2} C_a$).

is not affected by the distribution of drug throughout the body (VD) because clearance mechanisms act only on drug in the circulation.

Half-life

The amount of time needed to eliminate a drug from the body depends on the clearance and the VD. The first-order elimination constant (K_e) represents the proportion of the apparent VD that is cleared of drug per unit of time during the drug's exponential disappearance from the plasma over time (elimination phase):

$$K_e = Cl/VD \qquad (4)$$

The value of this constant for a particular drug can be determined by plotting drug concentration versus time on a log-linear plot (see Fig. 28-2) and measuring the slope of the straight line obtained during the exponential (elimination) phase.

The time needed to eliminate the drug is best described by its half-life ($t_{1/2}$), which is the time required during the elimination phase (see Fig. 28-2) for the plasma concentration of the drug to be decreased by half. Mathematically, the half-life is equal to the natural logarithm of 2 (representing a reduction of drug concentration to half) divided by K_e. Substituting for K_e from

Equation 4 and calculating the natural logarithm of 2, the half-life can be represented by the following equation:

$$t_{1/2} = 0.693 \, VD/Cl \qquad (5)$$

From this equation, one can predict that at a given clearance, as the VD increases, the half-life increases. Similarly, at a given VD, as the clearance increases, the half-life decreases. Clinically, many disease states (see later) can affect VD and clearance. Because disease affects VD and clearance differently, the half-life may increase, decrease, or not change much at all. Therefore, the half-life by itself is not a good indicator of the extent of abnormality in elimination.

The half-life is useful to predict how long it takes for a drug to be eliminated from the body. For any drug that has a first-order elimination, one would expect that by the end of the first half-life, the drug would be reduced to 50%; by the end of the second half-life, to 25%; by the end of the third half-life, to 12.5%; by the end of the fourth half-life, to 6.25%; and by the end of the fifth half-life, to 3.125%. In general, a drug can be considered essentially eliminated after three to five half-lives, when less than 10% of the effective concentration remains. Table 28-1 shows the wide variation in half-life for several commonly used drugs.

⬤ APPLYING PHARMACOKINETIC PRINCIPLES
Using a Loading Dose

To attain a desired therapeutic concentration rapidly, a loading dose is often used. In determining the amount of drug to be given, the physician must consider the "volume" within the body into which the drug will be distributed. This volume is best described by the apparent VD. The loading dose can be calculated by multiplying the desired concentration by the VD:

$$\text{Loading dose} = \text{desired concentration} \times \text{VD} \qquad (6)$$

Rapid administration of the entire loading dose may produce an initially high peak concentration that results in toxicity. This problem can be avoided either by administering the loading dose as a divided dose or by varying the rate of access to the circulation, such as by administering the drug as an infusion (with an intravenous drug) or by taking advantage of the slower access to the circulation from various other routes (e.g., oral dosing). This approach is illustrated by phenytoin (see Table 28-1), which may need to be administered with a loading dose to achieve a therapeutic level (10 to 20 mg/L) rapidly. Because the VD for phenytoin is approximately 0.6 L/kg, the loading dose calculated from Equation 6 is 420 mg/L to attain a minimally therapeutic level of 10 mg/L in a 70-kg adult. However, administration of 420 mg of phenytoin by intravenous bolus carries the risk of cardiac arrest and death. By taking advantage of the reduced bioavailability (F = 0.8) and slow absorption of oral phenytoin, the loading dose can be administered safely as an oral dose of 500 mg.

The equation for the loading dose can also be used to calculate the dose needed to "boost" an inadequate blood level of drug to a desired therapeutic range. If therapeutic monitoring shows that the phenytoin level is 5 mg/L and the desired level is 15 mg/L, it is necessary to multiply the difference needed to achieve the desired concentration (10 mg/L) by the VD

TABLE 28-1 PHARMACOKINETIC PARAMETERS FOR SOME COMMONLY USED DRUGS

DRUG	VD (L/KG)	PROTEIN BINDING (%)	TOTAL CLEARANCE (ML/MIN)	% OF TOTAL CLEARANCE AS RENAL CLEARANCE	HALF-LIFE (HR)	THERAPEUTIC RANGE (MG/L)
Amoxicillin	0.47	17-18		86	1.2	2-8
Aspirin (acetylsalicylic acid)	0.14-0.18	80-90	575-725	<2	0.2-0.3	20-250
Carbamazepine	1.2	75-90	50-125	1-3	12-17	4-12
Digoxin	5-7.3	20-30	75	50-70	34-44	0.5-2
Glimepiride	0.18	>99.5	0.62 ± 0.26	<0.5	3.4 ± 2.0	
Lidocaine	3	60-80	700	<10	1.5-2	1-5
Lithium carbonate	0.7-1	0	20-40	95-99	20-270	0.4-1.4*
Penicillin G	0.5-0.7	45-68	—	20	0.4-0.9	Variable
Phenobarbital	0.6-0.7	20-45	4	25	2-6 days	<10-40*
Phenytoin	0.4-0.8	88-93	—	<5	7-26	10-20
Procainamide	2.2	14-23	470-600	40-70	2.5-4.7	4-8
Theophylline	0.3-0.7	60	36-50	<10	4-16	5-20
Tobramycin	0.25-0.30	<10	70	>95	2-4	0.5-2 (TR) 4-8 (PK)
Vancomycin	0.4-1	52-60	65	85	4-6	5-10 (TR) 25-35 (PK)

*Therapeutic range varies according to the indication for the drug. For example, lithium carbonate in the range of 0.4-1.3 mg/L is appropriate for affective schizophrenia disorder; a range of 1.0-1.4 mg/L is appropriate for mania. Phenobarbital concentration below 10 mg/mL is appropriate for anticonvulsant therapy; 40 mg/L is appropriate as a hypnotic.
PK = peak value; TR = trough value; VD = volume of distribution.

(0.6 L/kg) to determine the dose (in milligrams per kilogram) necessary to achieve this drug level after distribution. In a 70-kg individual, 0.6 mg/kg is multiplied by 70 kg to obtain the calculated loading dose (420 mg) that can be administered safely. A 500-mg oral dose with a bioavailability of less than 1 (e.g., F = 0.8) would deliver to the systemic circulation the approximate amount needed and avoid the risks associated with rapid intravenous administration.

Determining Drug Accumulation

Continuing to administer a drug, either as a prolonged infusion or as repeated doses, results in accumulation until a steady state occurs. Steady state is the point at which the amount of drug being administered equals the amount being eliminated so that the plasma and tissue levels remain constant. The elimination half-life determines not only the time course of drug elimination but also the time course of drug accumulation. This "mirror image" pattern of drug accumulation and elimination is illustrated in Figure 28-3. As with drug elimination, three to five half-lives determine the time it takes to reach steady state during drug accumulation. Whereas drugs with short half-lives accumulate rapidly, drugs with long half-lives require a longer time to accumulate, with a potential delay in achieving therapeutic levels. For drugs with long half-lives, a loading dose may be needed to obtain rapid drug accumulation and a more rapid therapeutic effect.

With each change in drug dose or rate of infusion, a change in steady state occurs. Although it is not obvious for drugs with short half-lives, the effects of dose adjustments for drugs with longer half-lives are delayed, and the time varies directly with the drug's half-life.

Using a Maintenance Dose

After steady state is reached in three to five half-lives with either a continuous infusion or intermittent doses, the rate of drug administered equals the rate of drug eliminated. For an intravenous drug, the administration rate is the infusion rate (I); for a drug administered by another route (e.g., orally), the administration rate is the dose per unit of time (D/t). Equation 7 shows that the rate of elimination (total) equals $Cl_{tot} \times C_p$. With an intravenously administered drug, because the infusion rate equals the elimination rate at steady state, it follows that

$$I = Cl_{tot} \times C_p \tag{7}$$

Similarly, with an orally administered drug, the dose administered per unit of time equals the elimination rate at steady state, with the result that

$$D/t = Cl_{tot} \times C_p \tag{8}$$

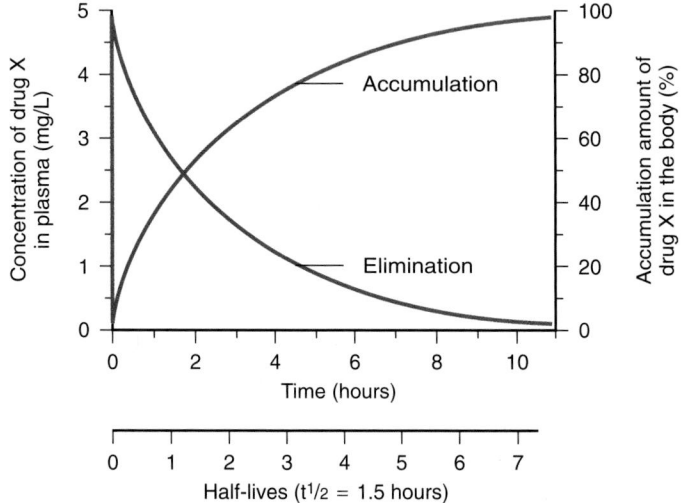

FIGURE 28-3. Representative plot of the "mirror image" relationship between the elimination of drug (after drug is discontinued) and the accumulation of drug (during infusion). The plot shows the concentration on the left *y*-axis and time on the upper *x*-axis. The lower *x*-axis shows the time in half-lives, and the *y*-axis on the right shows the percentage of drug in the body. After three to five half-lives, elimination is essentially complete, and accumulation is essentially at a steady state.

These equations show the direct relationship between the dose and the resultant plasma concentration at steady state. This relationship is independent of the distribution of the drug. By use of these equations, it is possible to determine the infusion rate or the interval and dose needed to achieve and maintain a specified drug concentration in the plasma.

When a drug is administered intermittently, it approaches steady-state concentration over time, with a pattern similar to that observed with continuous infusion (Fig. 28-4). With intermittent drug administration, such as with an oral dose, the drug concentration fluctuates; the magnitude of fluctuation between the peak and trough concentrations depends on the interval of administration, drug half-life, absorption characteristics, and site of administration. The effect of a change in the interval of administration for an oral drug is shown in Figure 28-4. As the intervals decrease below the half-life, the fluctuation decreases and approaches the curve produced by an intravenous infusion. Orally administered drugs may reach the blood stream more

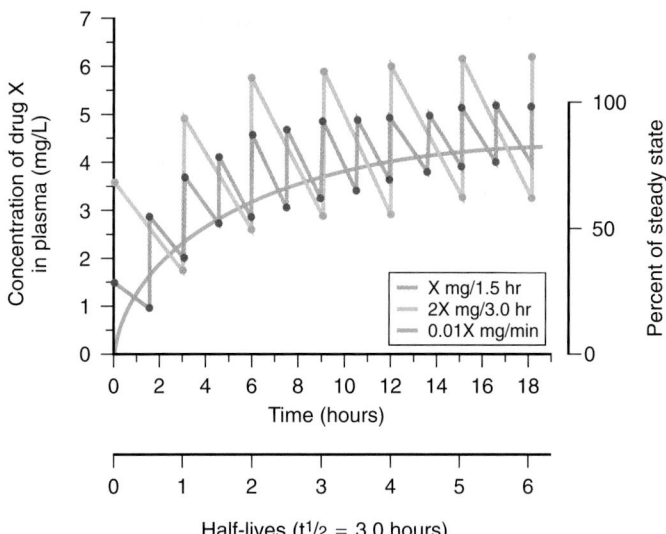

FIGURE 28-4. Accumulation of drug over time, approaching a steady state. Time is depicted in hours (upper *x*-axis) and half-lives (lower *x*-axis, showing that steady state is reached in three to five half-lives). The green line depicts the pattern produced by an infusion of a hypothetical drug at a dose of 0.01X. The orange line shows the pattern resulting from oral administration of a 2X dose every 3 hours, and the blue line represents the pattern produced by oral administration of dose X every 1.5 hours.

rapidly, attaining a higher peak concentration with one formulation, whereas the same drug administered as a timed-release formulation is absorbed more slowly, with a lower peak concentration but lasting longer in the plasma. Finally, the same drug administered by different routes may have different plasma profiles not only because of differing absorption characteristics but also because of other effects, such as first-pass metabolism.

Decreasing the Drug Level

At times, it may be necessary to decrease the plasma drug level while maintaining therapy (e.g., when signs of toxicity become apparent or a potentially dangerously high concentration of drug is noted; see later). The most effective and rapid response is to discontinue the drug; the length of time for which the drug is discontinued is determined by the estimated half-life of the drug in the specific patient. After discontinuation of the drug for a time based on its half-life, the total clearance (Cl_{tot}) of the drug can be used to determine what infusion rate (I, Equation 7) or dose and interval (D/t, Equation 8) must be used to achieve the new desired concentration (C_p).

Effect of Dose Increases on Elimination Kinetics

Although the previously discussed pharmacokinetic principles can be a guide to the dose of most drugs, not all drugs behave the same when the dose is increased. The elimination of most drugs follows first-order or linear kinetics; the amount of drug eliminated is directly proportional to the concentration of drug in the plasma (Fig. 28-5A). A few drugs have a different pattern of elimination. Three of the most commonly used drugs that exhibit this different pharmacokinetic pattern are ethanol, phenytoin, and salicylate. These drugs have dose-dependent, nonlinear saturation kinetics. As the dose of drug increases and the concentration of drug in the plasma rises, the relative amount of drug being eliminated falls (i.e., the clearance decreases) until the rate of drug metabolism is at its maximum. At this point, drug elimination is said to be zero order, and the drug concentration in plasma starts to increase much more (no longer linearly) with each subsequent increase in dose (Fig. 28-5B).

● MONITORING DRUG CONCENTRATION AS A GUIDE TO THERAPY

Although published pharmacokinetic data (usually population averages) such as those in Table 28-1 are useful to determine initial drug dosing, modification of the dose may be needed in an individual patient. For some drugs (e.g., certain antihypertensives or anticoagulants), the therapeutic effects (e.g., blood pressure or coagulation) can be quantified easily over a range of concentrations, permitting adequate drug adjustment. For many other drugs (e.g., some antiarrhythmics or antiseizure medications), therapeutic effects

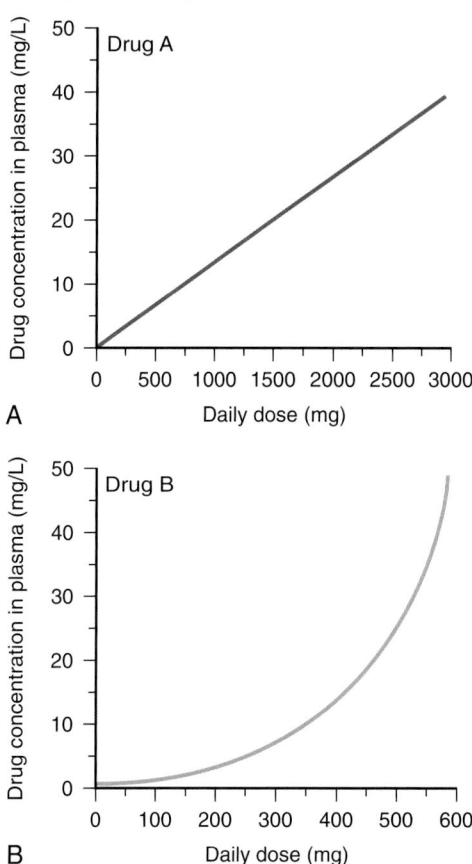

FIGURE 28-5. Effect of increasing the dose of a drug on its serum concentration. **A,** Drug A follows first-order or linear kinetics. **B,** Drug B follows zero-order or nonlinear (or saturable) kinetics.

over a range of concentrations are not readily detectable. With these drugs, the plasma concentration may provide further guidance in optimizing therapy if the plasma concentration of the drug is a reflection of its concentration at the site of action and the drug effects are reversible. A third, much smaller group of drugs produces irreversible effects (e.g., aspirin inhibition of platelet aggregation). With these drugs, plasma drug concentration does not correlate with drug effect, and drug monitoring is not useful.

To use drug concentration as a guide to therapy, it is necessary to establish a range of concentrations from minimally to maximally efficacious with tolerable toxicity. This range of concentrations, or the *therapeutic window,* is usually determined from a dose-response curve generated from a population of patients who have been examined closely for therapeutic and toxic effects (Fig. 28-6). This graph also may be used to determine the *therapeutic index,* a useful measure of drug toxicity calculated by dividing the 50% value from the toxicity curve by the 50% value from the efficacy curve. Because these curves are generated from population data, the values may not be applicable to all individuals.

Table 28-1, in addition to providing useful pharmacokinetic data, lists therapeutic ranges of several common drugs for which measuring the concentration and knowing the therapeutic range may be useful in clinical management. Many of these drugs are used to treat serious or life-threatening diseases. In these cases, it is essential to avoid inadequate doses because a therapeutic effect is needed. Excessive doses must also be avoided because of the risk of toxicity with drugs that have a small therapeutic index. In contrast, it is not necessary to assay levels of drugs used to treat noncritical diseases (when inadequate treatment is not a serious problem) or for which the therapeutic index is large (when relative overtreatment is not likely to produce toxicity).

Problems with Interpreting Drug Concentration

The time of blood collection, perhaps more than any other factor, contributes to the misinterpretation of drug levels. As can be seen in Figure 28-2, if sampling is performed too early, while the drug is still in the distribution phase, the drug level may be high and not reflect drug concentration at the site of action. It is therefore important to sample after the distribution phase.

For many drugs administered intermittently, a trough level, obtained immediately before the next dose is administered, is most useful for making decisions about dose adjustments (see Table 28-1). For drugs administered by infusion or intermittently at short intervals (see Fig. 28-4), the best time to draw blood is during steady state.

Protein binding is another major factor that contributes to the misinterpretation of drug levels. Free drug (not bound to protein and able to equilibrate with tissues and to interact with the site of action) is the critical drug concentration when therapeutic decisions are being made. Many drugs are tightly bound to plasma protein, however. Table 28-1 shows that many commonly used drugs, such as aspirin, carbamazepine, phenytoin, and glimepiride, have protein binding of more than 75%. Because many of the commonly used drug assays determine total drug concentration (which includes protein-bound drug and free drug), assessment of the "true" free drug concentration may be inaccurate, particularly if the fraction of drug bound to protein varies. In addition, the drug's binding may be decreased by disease or by other drugs, leading to increased unbound drug levels that alter

the interpretation of the measured drug concentrations. Kidney and liver disease can change the binding of certain drugs (e.g., phenytoin) to protein because of a decrease in protein (e.g., decreased albumin, as in nephrotic syndrome or liver disease) or as a result of competition for protein binding by endogenously produced substances (e.g., uremia in kidney disease, hyperbilirubinemia in liver disease). Similarly, other drugs may compete for binding to protein. A major problem secondary to these changes in protein binding is that free drug is not typically measured in many of the common drug assays used by clinical laboratories. Last, changes in drug binding to protein can affect the pharmacokinetics of the drug, the main effect being on the VD, which increases as protein binding decreases.

The usefulness of a drug assay is also limited by physiologic changes that may alter the response at a particular drug concentration. An example of this pharmacodynamic change is the response produced by a certain level of digoxin in the presence of altered electrolyte concentrations (e.g., potassium, calcium, magnesium). Tolerance, a reduced response to a given concentration of drug with continued use, is another pharmacodynamic change that may alter how a drug concentration is interpreted. Tolerance is commonly observed with the continued use of narcotics (e.g., in terminal cancer patients); initially, adequate pain control is noted at a given drug concentration, but after long-term administration, the same drug concentration is no longer associated with pain relief.

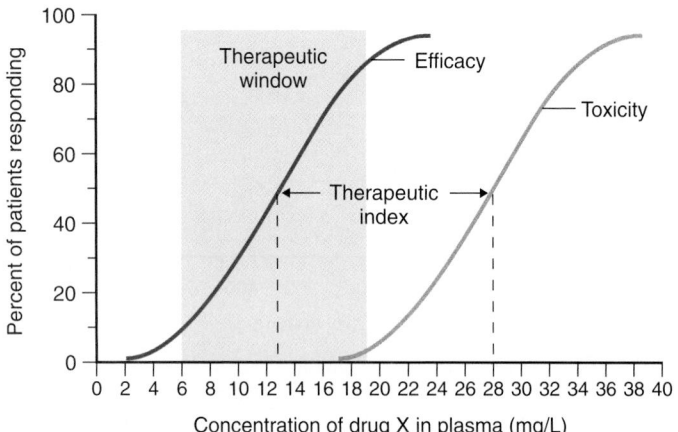

FIGURE 28-6. Pattern produced in a dose-response population study in which both effect and toxicity are measured. The therapeutic window is shown as the range of therapeutically effective concentrations, which includes most of the efficacy curve and less than 10% of the toxicity curve. The therapeutic index is calculated by dividing the 50% value on the toxicity curve by the 50% value on the efficacy curve.

● ADJUSTING DRUG DOSE WITH DISEASE
Kidney Disease

The major questions to be answered when determining whether a drug dosage needs to be adjusted in the setting of kidney disease are the following: Is the drug primarily excreted through the kidneys? Are increased drug levels likely to be associated with toxicity? If the answer to both is yes, it is likely that with decreased renal clearance, a drug will accumulate and become toxic. With renal failure, it is necessary to adjust the dosing regimen of such drugs, particularly for a drug with a long half-life and a small therapeutic index (e.g., digoxin).

To obtain the desired concentration over time in the presence of decreased clearance, adjustments can be made by decreasing the dose while maintaining the dose interval (DD), maintaining the dose but increasing the interval between doses (II), or a combination of both (DD and II). Table 28-2 shows how these three different methods are used to adjust the dosages of several common drugs to account for renal dysfunction (see Table 28-1 for their pharmacokinetic properties with normal renal function). With these

TABLE 28-2   ADJUSTMENT OF DRUG DOSAGE IN RENAL FAILURE

DRUG	TYPE OF ELIMINATION	Half-Life (hr) NORMAL	Half-Life (hr) END-STAGE RENAL DISEASE	METHOD*	GFR >50 ML/MIN	GFR 10-50 ML/MIN	GFR <10 ML/MIN	REMOVED BY DIALYSIS†
Amikacin	Renal	2-3	30	DD II	60-90% 12 hr	30-70% 12-18 hr	20-30% 24 hr	Yes
Aspirin	Hepatic (renal)	2-19	Unchanged	II	4 hr	4-6 hr	Avoid	Yes
Carbamazepine	Hepatic (renal)	35	?	DD	Unchanged	Unchanged	75%	No
Digoxin	Renal (nonrenal 15-40%)	36-44	80-120	DD II	Unchanged 24 hr	25-75% 36 hr	10-25% 48 hr	No
Lidocaine	Hepatic (renal <20%)	1.2-2.2	1.3-3	DD	Unchanged	Unchanged	Unchanged	No
Lithium carbonate	Renal	14-28	Prolonged	DD	Unchanged	50-75%	25-50%	Yes
Penicillin G	Renal (hepatic)	0.5	6-20	DD II	Unchanged 6-8 hr	75% 8-12 hr	25-50% 12-16 hr	Yes
Phenobarbital	Hepatic (renal 30%)	60-150	117-160	II	Unchanged	Unchanged	12-16 hr	Yes
Phenytoin	Hepatic (renal)	24	8	DD	Unchanged	Unchanged	Unchanged	No
Procainamide	Renal (hepatic 7-24%)	2.5-4.9	5.3-5.9	II	4 hr	6-12 hr	8-24 hr	Yes
Theophylline	Hepatic	3-12	?	DD	Unchanged	Unchanged	Unchanged	Yes
Tobramycin	Renal	2.5	56	DD II	60-90% 8-12 hr	30-70% 12 hr	20-30% 24 hr	Yes
Vancomycin	Renal	6-8	200-250	II	24-72 hr	72-240 hr	240 hr	No

*DD (alone) = decrease dose (maintain same interval); II (alone) = increase interval between doses (maintain dose); DD and II (together) = combination of both approaches.
†Dialysis refers to hemodialysis.
GFR = glomerular filtration rate.

adjustments, it may be possible to achieve an average concentration similar to that obtained with normal renal function; however, there may be concomitant marked changes in the magnitude of peak and trough values. In choosing the type of drug adjustment, the physician should consider not only the therapeutic index of the drug but also (1) whether an effective concentration must be achieved quickly and maintained within a narrow range (i.e., maintaining an average drug concentration and avoiding trough levels at which the drug is ineffective) and (2) whether toxicity is associated with elevated (i.e., peak) drug concentrations.

Renal drug clearance correlates with creatinine clearance (whether the drug uses glomerular filtration or tubular secretion); therefore, any adjustment of drug dose in kidney disease can use the creatinine clearance to calculate the dose needed because renal drug clearance is proportional to creatinine clearance. The creatinine clearance (Cl_{Cr}), which is used as an estimate of glomerular filtration rate, may be calculated directly from the serum creatinine concentration by the following equation:

$$Cl_{cr} = [(140 - age) \times weight\ (kg)] / [72 \times serum\ creatinine\ (mg/dL)] \quad (9)$$

The calculated creatinine clearance should be multiplied by 0.85 for females. (*Note:* This calculation applies only when the serum creatinine concentration is less than 5 mg/dL and renal function is not rapidly changing.)

Using Clearance for Dose Adjustment

The dose of a drug used in renal insufficiency ($dose_{D-RI}$) is proportional to the dose used with normal renal function ($dose_D$) in the same ratio as clearance of the drug in renal insufficiency (Cl_{D-RI}) to clearance with normal renal function (Cl_D). By rearranging, $dose_{D-RI}$ is defined as:

$$Dose_{D-RI} = dose_D \times [Cl_{D-RI} / Cl_D] \quad (10)$$

One can estimate the Cl_{D-RI} by multiplying Cl_D by the ratio of the creatinine clearance in renal insufficiency (Cl_{Cr-RI}) over Cl_{Cr} with normal renal function:

$$Cl_{D-RI} = Cl_D \times [Cl_{Cr-RI} / Cl_{Cr}] \quad (11)$$

As shown in Equation 3, total clearance is the sum of clearance by renal and nonrenal (typically hepatic) mechanisms. Any nonrenal clearance is assumed to remain normal, and only the renal clearance is adjusted, with total clearance being reduced only to the extent that renal clearance is reduced. The dose may be calculated from the total (adjusted) clearance and the desired plasma concentration by either Equation 7 or Equation 8. The calculated dose is only an initial guide to the dose needed, however. By monitoring the drug response or the plasma drug concentration at various times after initial dosing, further dose adjustments can be made as necessary. From a practical perspective, most clinical dose adjustments in the presence of renal dysfunction can be guided by published tables based on changes in glomerular filtration rate (see Table 28-2) and the effectiveness of dialysis in removing the drug. Computerized decision support systems are particularly effective in guiding medication dosing for inpatients with renal insufficiency.

Loading Dose in Renal Insufficiency

For drugs typically administered with a loading dose in patients with normal renal function, the same approach can be used in those with renal insufficiency to ensure that the desired concentration is achieved rapidly. For drugs typically administered without a loading dose, the presence of a prolonged half-life resulting from renal insufficiency may delay drug accumulation to steady state. In this setting, a loading dose (equal to the amount needed to reach steady state with normal renal function) is required.

Additional Considerations in Renal Insufficiency

Because of individual differences among patients, the approaches outlined earlier should be considered only initial approximations to prevent ineffective (too low) or toxic (too high) doses. For maintenance therapy, it is desirable to monitor blood levels to guide dosing.

If a metabolite of the drug is responsible for its effect or toxicity and the metabolite accumulates in the setting of renal failure, the drug level alone may not provide sufficient guidance for planning therapy. For example, the major metabolite of procainamide is N-acetylprocainamide, which has a toxicity similar to that of the parent drug but only modest antiarrhythmic activity. In the setting of renal failure, N-acetylprocainamide may accumulate dramatically because it is more dependent on renal elimination. Measurement of procainamide levels alone does not accurately assess either the levels needed for antiarrhythmic effect or the risk of toxicity.

Liver Disease

Although many drugs are biotransformed in the liver, it is not possible to make any general recommendations for drug dose adjustments in liver disease. In contrast to renal disease, no useful laboratory test is available on which to base dose adjustments. It has been suggested that if the liver's capacity to produce protein (reflected by albumin concentration and prothrombin time) is reduced significantly, the clearance of drugs metabolized by the cytochrome P-450 enzymes is probably reduced as well.

One special situation that can develop with chronic liver disease and may require dose adjustment is the portacaval shunt. This condition produces not only a potential hemodynamic alteration, leading to decreased hepatic blood flow and accompanying decreased clearance, but also a possible bypassing of the first-pass effect, resulting in higher concentrations of drug reaching the systemic circulation. Drugs with a large hepatic extraction that are typically administered orally (e.g., propranolol) may appear in the systemic circulation at higher, potentially toxic concentrations.

Hemodynamic Diseases

Decreased cardiac output and hypotensive conditions lead to decreased perfusion of the organs, including those responsible for eliminating drugs. As noted earlier with regard to primary kidney disease, the dose can be adjusted for decreased renal perfusion by the use of creatinine clearance. The effect of decreased hepatic blood flow on pharmacokinetics is more difficult to assess. For drugs that have a high hepatic extraction (e.g., lidocaine), decreased hepatic blood flow suggests a need for dose reduction.

Altered hemodynamics also may affect the distribution of selected drugs. Drugs that have a relatively large VD (e.g., lidocaine, procainamide, quinidine) may be affected by conditions leading to hypotension, such as shock, resulting in a decrease in the apparent VD. With a reduced VD, the loading dose of a drug should be reduced to avoid potentially toxic drug levels.

In general, in the setting of severely compromised hemodynamics, it is advisable to be conservative, avoiding potentially toxic loading and maintenance doses of drugs. Drug levels and the clinical status should be monitored closely, and drug doses should be adjusted as necessary.

APPROACH TO DRUG OVERDOSE

The pharmacokinetic principles discussed earlier can be used to determine the best approach to drug removal in the setting of a drug overdose, particularly if hemodialysis or hemoperfusion is contemplated. The major goal is to increase the overall clearance of the drug, removing a substantial fraction of the total body load of drug. Examination of the VD and clearance values can provide some guidance. For drugs with a large VD (e.g., digoxin; see Table 28-1), only a small amount can be removed because clearance affects only the amount of drug present in the plasma, and a large portion of the drug is outside the plasma compartment. Similarly, for drugs with high clearance values, hemoperfusion may increase the overall clearance only minimally and is not indicated. Table 28-2 provides data for determining whether hemodialysis is likely to be useful to remove several commonly prescribed drugs.

USING DRUGS IN THE ELDERLY

Administering drugs to the elderly is perhaps the most challenging area of adult therapeutics because of several factors: the increasing likelihood of multiple illnesses, often with multisystemic involvement; the need for these patients to take multiple drugs (often prescribed by different physicians); and the increasing probability of altered pharmacokinetics and pharmacodynamics. These factors together contribute to a significantly increased frequency of drug interactions and adverse drug responses in this group of patients.

Pharmacokinetic Changes with Age

These changes can be secondary to the general physiologic effects of aging, such as alteration in body composition, or to specific changes in pharmacokinetically important organs (e.g., kidneys, liver). The distribution of drugs tends to change dramatically with age, mainly because of changes in body composition. Most typical is the increase in total body fat, with the accompanying decrease in lean body mass and total body water. The concentration of plasma proteins may also change; in particular, albumin decreases as the liver ages. Changes in drug distribution are manifested as a change in the apparent VD. For water-soluble drugs that are not bound to plasma proteins, the apparent VD is reduced; in contrast, for lipid-soluble drugs, the VD is increased. Minimal changes in metabolism accompany aging, but these alone cannot account for altered pharmacokinetics.

Excretion can be altered in the elderly, and the clearance of many drugs is decreased. Cardiac output and blood flow to the kidneys and liver also may be decreased. Glomerular filtration rate may be reduced by 50%. Hepatic elimination of drugs is less affected, except for drugs with a high hepatic clearance (e.g., lidocaine). The elimination half-life of many drugs is increased with aging as a consequence of a larger apparent VD and a decreased hepatic or renal clearance (see Equation 5).

Pharmacodynamic Changes with Age

These changes are a result of changes in the responsiveness of the target organ. They require the use of smaller drug doses in the elderly, even if the pharmacokinetics are unchanged. This affects many drugs commonly used in the elderly; for example, antianxiety drugs and drugs from the sedative-hypnotic class may produce increased central nervous system depression in the elderly at concentrations that are well tolerated in younger adults. Similarly, anticoagulants (e.g., warfarin) may produce hemorrhage in the elderly at concentrations that are well tolerated in younger adults.

General Recommendations for Drug Use in the Elderly

- Clearance of drugs eliminated by the kidneys may be reduced by 50%.
- Drugs eliminated primarily by the liver typically do not require dose adjustments for age, except for drugs with high hepatic clearances, which may be affected by the age-related decrease in hepatic blood flow.
- Because of the potential for increased target organ sensitivity in the elderly, only the lowest effective dose should be used.
- Frequent reviews of the patient's drug history should be conducted, including both prescription and over-the-counter medications, keeping in mind the increased potential risk for drug interactions and adverse drug responses.

⬤ INTERACTIONS BETWEEN DRUGS

Because patients are typically treated with multiple agents, even for a single disease, the possibilities for drug interactions are great. Most clinically important drug interactions typically involve a drug with a low therapeutic index (e.g., warfarin) and an easily detectable pharmacologic effect (e.g., bleeding), such that a small increase in the amount of drug produces a significant effect (toxicity).

It is difficult to accurately assess the prevalence of drug interactions in either the inpatient or the ambulatory setting, particularly because no formal and comprehensive surveillance mechanism is available. The risk for drug interactions seems to be increasing, particularly for critically ill, hospitalized patients, who are frequently taking more than 10 medications.

There are basically two types of drug interaction: (1) pharmacokinetic drug interactions, caused by a change in the amount of drug or active metabolite at the site of action; and (2) pharmacodynamic drug interactions (without a change in pharmacokinetics), caused by a change in drug effect.

Pharmacokinetic Drug Interactions
Less Drug at the Site of Action
Decreased Absorption

The gastrointestinal lumen is perhaps the best example of an area where drug interactions can result in decreased drug absorption. Some commonly used drugs can illustrate this type of interaction. For many drugs, a physicochemical interaction prevents the drug from being absorbed. Drugs such as colestipol and cholestyramine (resins used to lower cholesterol and bind bile acids) can also bind other drugs present in the gastrointestinal lumen, including digoxin and warfarin. Because of the potential for many other drugs to be bound, it is generally recommended that other drugs not be administered within 2 hours of colestipol or cholestyramine. Another type of interaction occurs when metal ions (e.g., aluminum, calcium, and magnesium in antacids and iron in supplements to treat iron deficiency) form insoluble complexes with tetracyclines, which can act as chelating agents. Other commonly used medications that decrease absorption include kaolin-pectin suspensions to treat diarrhea. These medications can significantly inhibit the absorption of coadministered drugs (e.g., digoxin).

Drugs that are particularly susceptible to pH changes may have decreased absorption when they are administered with other drugs that either affect gastric acidity or alter the extent of exposure to low pH. Protein pump inhibitors or H_2-receptor antagonists may elevate gastric pH, which can inhibit the dissolution and subsequent absorption of drugs that are weak bases (e.g., ketoconazole). Medications that delay gastric emptying (e.g., belladonna

alkaloids) can increase the degradation of a coadministered acid-labile drug (e.g., levodopa), resulting in decreased absorption.

Altered Distribution

Drugs that use the same active transport process to reach their site of action can compete at the level of transport, resulting in lower levels of drug reaching that site. The classic example of this type of interaction is the coadministration of guanidinium-type antihypertensives with tricyclic antidepressants, phenothiazines, and certain sympathomimetic amines (e.g., ephedrine), which block the effects of the antihypertensive drug.

Increased Metabolism

Many drugs (e.g., phenobarbital, phenytoin, ethanol, glutethimide, griseofulvin, rifampin) and toxic compounds (e.g., cigarette smoke, certain chlorinated hydrocarbons) can increase the hepatic metabolism of other drugs (e.g., corticosteroids, cyclophosphamide, cyclosporine, certain β-adrenergic blockers, theophylline, warfarin) by inducing the activity of the cytochrome P-450 mixed function oxidase (CYP) system.

More Drug at the Site of Action
Increased Absorption

Any drug that increases the rate of gastric emptying (e.g., metoclopramide) can potentially increase the absorption of acid-unstable drugs. Also, drugs that decrease intestinal motility (e.g., anticholinergics) may increase the absorption of drugs that are relatively poorly absorbed (e.g., digoxin tablets) by increasing the drug's contact time with the absorbing surface.

Altered Distribution

Drugs bound to protein are limited in their distribution (particularly to the site of action) and are not available for metabolism or excretion. Drugs can compete with each other for binding to plasma proteins, resulting in drug interactions. Sulfonamides can displace barbiturates bound to serum albumin, leading to increased levels of free barbiturates and possible toxicity.

Decreased Metabolism

One of the most impressive drug interactions is produced when one drug inhibits the metabolism of another, leading to the second drug's accumulation and a significant risk of toxicity. This type of interaction results when 6-mercaptopurine, an antileukemic drug with a low therapeutic index, is used with allopurinol, often administered to control hyperuricemia. The interaction may result in potentially life-threatening toxicity.

Some drugs can inhibit the metabolism of many other drugs. For example, cimetidine can inhibit the metabolism of diazepam, imipramine, lidocaine, propranolol, quinidine, theophylline, and warfarin. Amiodarone inhibits the metabolism of calcium-channel blockers, phenytoin, quinidine, and warfarin. Of particular importance with amiodarone is its half-life of 1 to 2 months; it continues to inhibit drug metabolism for several months after it has been discontinued.

Other drugs are notable because their metabolism is inhibited by a variety of different drugs. The metabolism of the commonly used anticoagulant warfarin is inhibited not only by cimetidine and amiodarone but also by many other drugs, including alcohol, allopurinol, disulfiram, metronidazole, phenylbutazone, sulfinpyrazone, and trimethoprim-sulfamethoxazole. Similarly, the metabolism of phenytoin is inhibited by chloramphenicol, clofibrate, dicumarol, disulfiram, isoniazid (slow acetylators), phenylbutazone, and valproic acid.

Although most of these examples involve enzymes that metabolize the drug in the liver, drug-metabolizing enzymes outside the liver also may be affected by certain drugs. The best-known example is monoamine oxidase, which can be affected by nonspecific monoamine oxidase inhibitors, resulting in the accumulation of catecholamines at multiple sites after their release in response to the eating of tyramine-containing foods such as aged cheese, aged or cured meats, and any spoiled meat, poultry, or fish.

Decreased Excretion

Drugs can compete for the active transporters present in the kidney. Most of these interactions involve the acid transporters. The best-known interaction is probenecid's inhibition of penicillin transport, leading to decreased penicillin clearance and thus higher plasma levels, an interaction that was used in the past to maximize penicillin therapy. A similar inhibitory effect on the renal excretion of methotrexate can be produced by salicylates, phenylbutazone, and probenecid. The active transport of basic drugs (e.g., procainamide) can also be inhibited by other drugs (e.g., cimetidine, amiodarone).

Pharmacodynamic Drug Interactions

With pharmacodynamic interactions, drugs interact at the level of the receptor (target) or may produce additive effects by acting at separate sites on cells. An example of the first is the interaction of propranolol and epinephrine, which blocks β-adrenergic receptors; as a result, the α-adrenergic effects of epinephrine are unopposed. This undesirable interaction can result in severe hypertension.

Many examples exist of the additive effects of drugs. Aspirin, which can produce increased bleeding time by acting on platelets, can interact with warfarin, which affects clotting. The result is an increased risk of hemorrhage. Similarly, cardiac drugs, such as β-adrenergic blockers and calcium-channel blockers, have additive negative inotropic effects when they are coadministered, resulting in an increased risk of cardiac failure.

DIAGNOSIS AND PREVENTION OF DRUG INTERACTIONS

For a drug interaction to be recognized, the index of suspicion must be high whenever multiple drugs are used together. Because of the ever-increasing list of known and suspected drug interactions, it is impossible for a clinician to remember all or even many of the possible interactions.

Several clinical settings should raise concern about the possibility of drug interactions:

- The use of any drug with a low therapeutic index (Table 28-3) should be suspect.
- As the number of drugs being used concurrently increases, there is a disproportionately greater risk of drug interactions, particularly with more than 10 drugs.
- Critically ill patients who have multisystemic disease with compromised renal, hepatic, cardiac, or pulmonary function have an increased risk of drug interactions. This risk may be higher for patients with acquired immunodeficiency syndrome, who have an immunocompromised state and take a large number of drugs.
- Patients with various behavioral and psychiatric disorders (e.g., drug abusers taking a large number of prescription drugs as well as illicit drugs and alcohol) are at risk for drug interactions.

Another type of drug interaction that is becoming increasingly important is that between components of food (e.g., grapefruit juice) or natural products (e.g., herbs) and drugs. By inhibiting the intestinal cytochrome P-450 3A4 enzyme system, grapefruit juice can raise levels of drugs metabolized by this pathway (e.g., saquinavir, cyclosporine, verapamil) and result in toxicity or adverse drug effects.

Several steps can be taken to prevent drug interactions:

- When taking the medical history, it is important to document all drugs the patient is taking (and has recently taken), including prescription, over-the-counter, and other addictive drugs.
- It is desirable to minimize the number of drugs being taken by frequently reviewing the patient's drug list to ensure that each drug continues to be needed.
- There should be a high degree of suspicion when medications with a low therapeutic index known to have a high risk of drug interactions (see Table 28-3) are used.
- High-risk clinical settings, such as occur with critically ill patients, should raise the suspicion of adverse drug interactions.
- Adverse drug interactions should be considered in the differential diagnosis whenever any change occurs in a patient's course.

TABLE 28-3	DRUGS WITH LOW THERAPEUTIC INDICES AT HIGH RISK FOR ADVERSE DRUG RESPONSES AND DRUG INTERACTIONS

Anticoagulants

Antiarrhythmics

Anticonvulsants

Digoxin

Lithium carbonate

Oral hypoglycemics

Theophylline

ADVERSE REACTIONS TO DRUGS

An adverse drug response (ADR) is an undesired effect produced by a drug at standard doses, which typically necessitates reducing or stopping the suspected agent and may require treatment of the noxious effect produced. Further harm may occur with continued or future therapy with the drug.

EPIDEMIOLOGY

The financial impact of ADRs is estimated to be more than $100 billion per year. The actual incidence of ADRs is difficult to quantify because many cases are either not recognized or not reported. Several large studies have shown that the incidence may approach 20% for outpatients (even higher for patients taking more than 15 drugs) and 2 to 7% for inpatients. The incidence of ADRs increases exponentially with more than four drugs. Meta-analyses of several prospective studies suggest that ADRs are now the third leading cause of death in hospitalized patients. It is clear from more recent surveys that a relatively small group of drugs (see Table 28-3) continues to be implicated in most of the reported ADRs. Current trends suggest that the incidence of ADRs is likely to increase as a result of more prescribed and over-the-counter medications being used.

ETIOLOGY

Most ADRs are caused by an exaggerated (but predictable) pharmacologic effect of the drug or by a toxic or immunologic effect of the drug or a metabolite (not typically expected).

Predictable Toxic Responses to Drugs

Exaggerated drug responses that cause adverse drug effects may be due to any condition that causes altered pharmacokinetics or pharmacodynamics (discussed earlier). There has been increasing interest in the discipline of pharmacogenomics, which explores the role of genetic factors in altered pharmacokinetics or pharmacodynamics and the resultant increased susceptibility to ADRs. There is now ample evidence that molecular changes in the genes coding for drug-metabolizing enzymes can account for the variability in pharmacokinetics and drug effects observed in population studies. There are now many examples of the role of pharmacogenomics in altered drug response and effect. Three of the best-studied examples are genetic polymorphisms associated with debrisoquine-sparteine, N-acetylation, and mephenytoin. Each is associated with autosomal recessive inheritance, and together they are responsible for the metabolism of approximately 40 drugs (Table 28-4). Individuals with autosomal recessive genes are typically "poor metabolizers," with potentially altered pharmacokinetics that result in elevated plasma drug concentrations and can lead to toxicity. Recent studies have focused on genomic alterations associated with the variability in response to some commonly used drugs. Thus, the variability of response to warfarin (Chapter 37) is now understood to be due to single nucleotide polymorphisms in the cytochrome P-450 2C9 (CYP2C9) and vitamin K epoxide reductase (VKOR) genes. These single nucleotide polymorphisms have a significant effect on warfarin dose requirements. Similarly, polymorphisms in transporter genes can have profound effects on the pharmacokinetics of statins (Chapter 213). A common genetic variant of the organic anion-transporting polypeptide 1B1 can reduce the hepatic uptake of many statins, increasing the risk of statin-induced myopathy. Also, it is now appreciated that genetically impaired adenosine triphosphate–binding cassette G2 transporter efflux activity can result in an increase in systemic exposure to various statins. Of particular importance to therapeutics is that the effects of these genetic polymorphisms differ, depending on the specific statin used. This provides a rational basis for an individualized approach to the use of lipid-lowering therapeutic agents.

A particularly impressive example occurs with certain cancer chemotherapy agents that have a relatively narrow therapeutic window and the potential to produce severe cytotoxicity (e.g., deficiency in dihydropyrimidine dehydrogenase activity can result in life-threatening toxicity after the administration of 5-fluorouracil). These defects typically are not recognized until the patient is given the drug. They are often described as "pharmacogenetic" syndromes.

Other genetic alterations do not affect metabolism specifically and do not produce a range of quantitative changes. These defects can produce "qualitative" defects and are often associated with structural defects. The classic example is glucose-6-phosphate dehydrogenase. Individuals who are deficient in this enzyme cannot tolerate the oxidative stress produced by some

TABLE 28-4 GENETIC POLYMORPHISMS OF DRUG-METABOLIZING ENZYMES

TYPE	PRIMARY DRUG EXAMPLES	OTHER DRUGS THAT ARE SUBSTRATES	INCIDENCE OF "POOR METABOLIZERS" IN WHITES (%)	ENZYME INVOLVED
Debrisoquine-sparteine polymorphism	Amitriptyline, codeine, tamoxifen	Antidepressants, antiarrhythmics, β-adrenergic receptor–blocking drugs, codeine, dextromethorphan, neuroleptics	5-10	Cytochrome P-450 IID6 (CYP2D6)
Mephenytoin polymorphism	Mephenytoin	Mephobarbital, hexobarbital, diazepam, omeprazole	4 (Japanese, Chinese, 15-20)	Cytochrome P-450 IIC (CYP2C)
N-acetylation polymorphism	Isoniazid, sulfadiazine	Hydralazine, phenelzine, procainamide, dapsone, sulfamethazine, sulfapyridine, aminoglutethimide, aminosalicylic acid, sulfasalazine	40-70 (Japanese, 10-20)	N-acetyltransferase (NAT2)
Methyl conjugation polymorphism	Catecholamines	L-Dopa, methyldopa	25-30	Catechol-O methyltransferase (COMT)

drugs, leading to hemolysis (Chapter 164). Drugs that can produce this clinical picture include aspirin, nitrofurantoin, primaquine, probenecid, quinidine, quinine, sulfonamides, sulfones, and vitamin K. Another similar defect is deficiency of methemoglobin reductase, which results in an inability to maintain iron in hemoglobin in the ferrous state, causing methemoglobinemia (Chapter 161) after exposure to oxidizing drugs such as nitrites, sulfonamides, and sulfones.

Unpredictable Toxic Responses to Drugs

Other toxic or immunologic ADRs are not predictable and are not obviously due to an increase in drug concentration (pharmacokinetic) or drug effect (pharmacodynamic). Unpredictable toxic responses include direct reactions between a drug and a specific organ (e.g., platinum-containing drugs, such as cisplatin, can produce direct toxicity in the kidney and the eighth cranial nerve). With other drugs, metabolism to an active intermediate must occur first. With a standard dose of acetaminophen, no untoward effects occur because the relatively small amount of reactive metabolite formed by oxidative metabolism is detoxified rapidly by reduced glutathione. In the presence of an overdose, the glutathione is depleted, and the remaining reactive metabolite can damage the liver. Understanding the mechanism of this toxicity has provided a rationale for treating acetaminophen overdose. Sulfhydryl-containing compounds (e.g., N-acetylcysteine), which can complex with the reactive metabolite, can be administered to reduce the amount of free toxic metabolite present, protecting the liver.

Immunologic reactions to drugs are generally not produced by the drug alone. Similar to other low-molecular-weight compounds (<1000 D), they are typically not antigenic themselves. When a drug or reactive metabolite combines with a protein to form a drug-protein complex, it can become antigenic, capable of eliciting an immune response.

Perhaps the most impressive form of drug allergy is anaphylaxis, which is due to an immunoglobulin E–mediated hypersensitivity. Many drugs from different classes have been shown to produce this type of drug allergy. The best-known example is the anaphylactic response produced by penicillin, which can occur after its administration by any route. Skin testing with penicillin G, penicilloic acid, or penicilloyl polylysine can identify patients at risk and should be performed in those with a suspected penicillin allergy who need treatment with penicillin. If the skin test result is positive, the patient must undergo desensitization before receiving penicillin. If the skin test result is negative, penicillin can be administered with caution.

DIAGNOSIS OF ADVERSE DRUG RESPONSES

Although many of the well-known adverse drug effects are due to a relatively small group of drugs, every drug has the potential to cause an ADR. A physician should always consider the possibility of an ADR in the differential diagnosis even if none has been reported previously for the particular drug. In earlier editions of this book, we provided a table listing many diverse clinical presentations associated with ADRs. The reader is now referred to the numerous websites providing more complete and up-to-date information on ADRs than can be detailed here. For example, www.prosoftedc.com/aers/aers.php allows one to monitor drug safety with unlimited access to

up-to-date information from the Food and Drug Administration's Adverse Event Reporting System (AERS).

In many instances, it is readily apparent that a specific drug has produced an ADR, such as the appearance of a rash in an otherwise healthy patient who was recently prescribed a single drug (e.g., penicillin). In other cases, the effect produced by the drug may be difficult to discern from other disease states. In still other cases, the adverse effect may mimic the illness being treated (e.g., development of an arrhythmia in a patient being treated with an antiarrhythmic drug).

From a public health perspective, it is highly desirable to have a mechanism available to detect, catalog, and track the incidence and severity of ADRs not only for drugs at various stages of development but also for drugs that were approved earlier. The Food and Drug Administration tracks adverse drug events through a voluntary reporting program, MedWatch. Health care professionals are encouraged to report any adverse events or product problems on a one-page form that can be sent by mail, fax, or electronically to the Food and Drug Administration. Although various methods for surveying ADRs have been proposed, ultimately, the cooperation of alert clinicians and health care professionals must be encouraged.

SUGGESTED READINGS

De Gregori M, Allegri M, De Gregori S, et al. How and why to screen for CYP2D6 interindividual variability in patients under pharmacological treatments. *Curr Drug Metab.* 2010;11:276-282. *The polymorphisms of CYP2D6 significantly affect the pharmacokinetics of about 50% of the drugs in clinical use, which are CYP2D6 substrates.*

Evans BJ. Establishing clinical utility of pharmacogenetic tests in the post-FDAAA era. *Clin Pharmacol Ther.* 2010;88:749-751. *The FDA Amendments Act, when fully implemented, will offer new sources of evidence and new regulatory mechanisms during the postmarket phase of drug life.*

Guest EJ, Rowland-Yeo K, Rostami-Hodjegan A, et al. Assessment of algorithms for predicting drug-drug interactions via inhibition mechanisms: comparison of dynamic and static models. *Br J Clin Pharmacol.* 2011;71:72-87. *Assessment of methods to predict drug-drug interactions and their clinical relevance.*

Kamali F, Wynne H. Pharmacogenetics of warfarin. *Annu Rev Med.* 2010;61:63-75. *Reviews the role of various genetic factors in warfarin therapeutics.*

Kennedy DA, Seely D. Clinically based evidence of drug-herb interactions: a systematic review. *Expert Opin Drug Saf.* 2010;9:79-124. *Overview of clinically important interactions that can result from coexposure to commonly used herbal medicines and prescription drugs.*

Kunac DL, Tatley MV. Detecting medication errors in the New Zealand pharmacovigilance database: a retrospective analysis. *Drug Saf.* 2011;34:59-71. *The most commonly involved medications were antibacterials for systemic use and anti-inflammatory agents, with gastrointestinal and respiratory system disorders the most common adverse events reported.*

Moyer TP, O'Kane DJ, Baudhuin LM, et al. Warfarin sensitivity genotyping: a review of the literature and summary of patient experience. *Mayo Clin Proc.* 2009;84:1079-1094. *Up-to-date review of warfarin use from a pharmacogenomic perspective.*

Pai MP. Estimating the glomerular filtration rate in obese adult patients for drug dosing. *Adv Chronic Kidney Dis.* 2010;17:53-62. *Explores current approaches and controversies for estimating of GFR and creatinine clearance among obese patients in clinical practice.*

Seden K, Dickinson L, Khoo S, et al. Grapefruit-drug interactions. *Drugs.* 2010;70:2373-2407. *Review of its interactions with calcium channel blockers, immunosuppressants, antihistamines, and other drugs.*

Steinman MA, Hanlon JT. Managing medications in clinically complex elders: "there's got to be a happy medium." *JAMA.* 2010;304:1592-1601. *Systematic approach to addressing the medication regimen in the context of the clinical reality, social situation, and goals of care.*

Wang L, McLeod HL, Weinshilboum RM. Genomics and drug response. *N Engl J Med.* 2011;364:1144-1153. *Review.*

Woodcock J. Assessing the clinical utility of diagnostics used in drug therapy. *Clin Pharmacol Ther.* 2010;88:765-773. *Examination of the clinical utility and challenges of diagnostics in drug therapy.*

29

PAIN

STEVEN P. COHEN AND SRINIVASA N. RAJA

Pain is ubiquitous in life, usually serving as a warning sign of impending or actual injury to the organism. As such, pain is older than humans, dating back to our most primitive ancestors. Pain is also a vital diagnostic clue for physicians. Physicians should be intimately familiar with pain because it is the most common symptom for which patients seek medical attention. According to the U.S. government's annual report on Americans' health, one in four adults suffered a day-long bout of pain within the past 30 days, and 10% suffer from pain every day. Among the various types of pain, back pain is the most common, followed by headaches and arthralgias. Spinal pain is the leading cause of disability in industrialized nations, with the economic costs exceeding $100 billion annually in the United States by some estimates. Special populations at particular risk for chronic pain include elderly people and individuals with physical and psychological morbidities. Several conditions characterized by chronic pain, such as irritable bowel syndrome, interstitial cystitis, fibromyalgia, and complex regional pain syndrome, are more prevalent in females than males.

DEFINITION

The International Association for the Study of Pain defines pain as "an unpleasant sensory and emotional experience associated with actual or potential tissue damage, or described in terms of such damage." This definition recognizes that pain may be experienced in some circumstances in the absence of ongoing tissue damage, such as phantom pain after a healed amputation. One implication of this construct is the assumption that pain is always subjective; hence, a patient's report of pain should always be accepted at face value in the absence of evidence to the contrary.

PATHOBIOLOGY

Classification of Pain States

Multiple classifications have been used to describe pain states based on duration, anatomic source, or etiology. *Acute pain* usually results from injury or inflammation, has survival value, and may play a role in the healing process by promoting behaviors that minimize reinjury. In contrast, *chronic pain* is

perhaps best construed as a "disease" that serves no useful purpose. Although there is no clear threshold at which acute pain transitions to a chronic state, it is generally accepted that pain persisting beyond the expected healing period is pathologic. In most cases, this period is between 3 and 6 months. The intensity of pain can be classified as mild (1 to 3), moderate (4 to 5), or severe (≥6 on a 0 to 10 numerical rating scale).

Somatic and Visceral Pains

Pain can originate from somatic or visceral structures. *Somatic pain* is well localized and generally results from injury or disease of the skin, musculoskeletal structures, and joints. *Visceral pain* arises from internal organ dysfunction and can result from inflammation, ischemia, occlusion of flow resulting in capsular or organ distension (e.g., renal stones, bowel obstruction, cholecystitis) or from functional pathology (e.g., irritable bowel syndrome). In contrast to somatic pain, visceral pain is usually diffuse and poorly localized, is often referred to somatic regions (e.g., myocardial ischemia radiating into the arm), and tends to be associated with exaggerated autonomic reflexes and greater emotional features.

Neuropathic, Nociceptive, and Mixed Pain

Pain can be etiologically classified as neuropathic, nociceptive, or mixed (Table 29-1). *Neuropathic pain* has been defined as pain resulting from disease or injury to the peripheral or central nervous somatosensory system. Common neuropathic pain states include postherpetic neuralgia, diabetic neuropathy, and radicular pain. *Nociceptive pain* usually results from an injury or disease affecting somatic structures such as skin, muscle, tendons and ligaments, bone, and joints. Pain associated with cancer can result from the tumor itself or can be a consequence of therapy (e.g., surgery, chemotherapy, and radiation therapy). In light of the often multiple different etiologies, advanced cancer pain is a typical example of a mixed pain state.

Dysfunctional Pain

There is a group of pain syndromes that have been characterized by amplification of pain signaling in the absence of either inflammation or injury (as in nociceptive pain) or damage to the nervous system (as in neuropathic pain). These conditions include pain states such as fibromyalgia, irritable bowel syndrome, and interstitial cystitis. The precise pathophysiologic mechanisms of pain in these disorders are unclear, although they share some features of neuropathic pain. Other chronic pain states, such as primary erythromelalgia and paroxysmal extreme pain disorder, are perhaps best described as hereditary channelopathies associated with mutations of the voltage-gated sodium channel Nav1.7. These mutations lead to increased excitability of nociceptive

TABLE 29-1 CLASSIFICATION AND PREVALENCE OF COMMON PAIN CONDITIONS

| Neuropathic | | Nociceptive | | |
PERIPHERAL	CENTRAL*	SOMATIC	VISCERAL	MIXED
Peripheral neuropathy (1-3%)	Central post-stroke pain (8%)	Arthritis (25-40% in people >40 years)	Endometriosis (10% in women of reproductive age)	Headache (15% for migraine, 20-30% for tension-type)
Postherpetic neuralgia (annual incidence 0.1-0.2%)	Spinal cord injury (30-50%)	Myofascial pain (5-10%)	Irritable bowel syndrome (5-15%)	Cancer§ (lifetime prevalence 30-40%)
Chronic postsurgical pain (2-10% after surgery)	Multiple sclerosis (25%)	Fibromyalgia† (2-4%)	Interstitial cystitis (0.2-1% of women)	Low back pain‖ (point prevalence 10-30%)
Phantom limb pain (30-60% of patients with major limb amputation)	Parkinson's disease (10%)	Connective tissue disorders (0.2-0.5%)	Ulcers/gastritis/esophagitis (3-9%)	Neck pain‖ (annual incidence 20-30%)
Trigeminal neuralgia (0.01%)	Seizure disorder (1-3%)	Burn pain‡ (annual incidence of burns requiring hospitalization 0.01%)	Cholecystitis/appendicitis	Ischemic pain§
Radiculopathy/spinal stenosis (3-10%)				
Complex regional pain syndrome (0.03%, 3-20% after orthopedic surgery)				
Nerve entrapment syndromes (e.g., carpal tunnel, thoracic outlet, meralgia paresthetica; 2-4%)				

*Prevalence rates represent proportion of patients with condition who develop pain.
†Some cases may represent a variant of central pain.
‡Third-degree burns often associated with neuropathic pain.
§Neuropathic pain occurs in 20-50% of cases and may occur secondary to tumor invasion, surgery, chemotherapy, and radiation treatment.
‖Neuropathic pain may accompany nociceptive pain in 10-35% of cases.
§Typically nociceptive, but long-standing pain may result in ischemic neuropathy.

afferent fibers and ongoing activity in sensory neurons, resulting in spontaneous pain.

Pain Mechanisms

Pain results from activation of specialized peripheral receptors (*nociceptors*) by a noxious event (stimulus). These stimuli fall into one of three categories: *mechanical* (e.g., pressure, tumor growth, incision), *thermal* (e.g., hot or cold), or *chemical* (e.g., ischemia or infection). The stimulus is then converted into an electrical nerve signal (*transduction*), which is conveyed along the axons of thinly myelinated (A-delta) or unmyelinated (C) nerve fibers through specific pathways (*transmission*). *Modulation* refers to the attenuation of pain signals through intrinsic inhibitory activity within the peripheral and the central nervous systems before being perceived as an unpleasant sensation (*perception*). *Pathologic pain* is the result of injury- or disease-induced changes in the peripheral or central nervous system leading to alterations in the pain signaling process. One important example of pathologic pain from injury to the nervous system is *peripheral sensitization*. This form of pain is characterized by the development of spontaneous ectopic activity in injured nerves and dorsal root ganglion cells, as well as enhanced sensitivity to mechanical, thermal, or chemical stimuli. Recent studies have shown an important role for cytokines, such as tumor necrosis factor-α (TNF-α) and interleukins, released by macrophages and other inflammatory cells, in the peripheral sensitization process.

The prolonged and repeated activation of nociceptive afferent fibers produces *central sensitization*, a state of increased sensitivity of central pain signaling neurons. Activation of *N*-methyl-D-aspartate (NMDA) receptors by glutamate is thought to be an important mechanism for central sensitization. Recent studies indicate that in addition to functional changes in neurons, microglia and astrocytes may also play an important role in the central sensitization process. Other central neuroplastic changes that may contribute to neuropathic pain states include deafferentation hyperactivity that may occur after spinal cord or avulsion injuries, loss of large fiber afferent inhibition, reorganization of central connections of primary afferent fibers, and excitatory descending modulatory mechanisms. Central and, to a lesser extent, peripheral sensitization are considered to be the prime culprits responsible for pain induced by innocuous stimuli (*allodynia*), and increased pain to normally noxious stimuli (*hyperalgesia*), that are commonly observed in neuropathic pain states.

DIAGNOSIS

History

Similar to the work-up of any symptom, the evaluation of pain begins with a thorough history. One of the primary tenets of pain assessment is that subjective complaints should always be taken seriously. There is currently no diagnostic test that can measure pain or even ascertain its existence. The most promising techniques involve functional brain imaging that reflects cerebral metabolism. Presently, these techniques are research tools that have helped us understand that the brains of chronic pain patients undergo morphologic alterations such as a diminution in gray matter in the areas involved in pain perception. A comprehensive history should include the anatomic region of pain, its quality, exacerbating and relieving factors, temporal aspects, associated symptoms and signs (e.g., numbness or weakness), interference with activities of daily living, and response to current and prior treatments. The temporal aspects of pain can provide valuable clues to etiology and help guide treatment. Most cases of acute pain develop subsequent to a specific inciting event (e.g., surgery, trauma), whereas chronic pain conditions are usually more insidious in onset. Because acute pain tends to be self-limited and the relationship to a precipitant event is more tangible, it may be better tolerated and associated with fewer psychological sequelae.

The severity of pain can be measured through a variety of different rating scales. Some of the more common instruments include categorical scales, verbal and numerical rating scales (0 to 10), and the visual analogue scale, in which a 10-cm line is anchored on each side by two points designated as "no pain" and "worst possible pain." Because there are subtle differences between different types of scales, repeat assessments and response to therapy are ideally gauged using the same instrument. For young children and mentally incapacitated patients, the use of age-appropriate substitute scales or facial expressions has been validated.

Recent guidelines from experts across multiple specialties and sectors have concluded that pain scores represent only one component of pain management. Other important aspects of treatment include assessments of functional capacity (e.g., Oswestry disability index for back pain), psychological

TABLE 29-2	CATEGORIZATION OF NEUROPATHIC AND NOCICEPTIVE PAIN	
CLINICAL CHARACTERISTIC	**NEUROPATHIC PAIN**	**NOCICEPTIVE PAIN**
Etiology	Nerve injury or peripheral/central sensitization	Tissue or potential tissue damage
Descriptors	Lancinating, shooting, electrical-like, stabbing	Throbbing, aching, pressure-like
Sensory deficits	Frequent (e.g., numbness, tingling, pricking)	Infrequent and, if present, in nondermatomal or non-nerve distribution
Motor deficits	Neurologic weakness may be present if motor nerve affected	May have pain-induced weakness
Hypersensitivity	Pain frequently evoked with nonpainful (allodynia) or painful (exaggerated response) stimuli	Uncommon except for hypersensitivity in the immediate area of an acute injury
Character	Distal radiation common	Distal radiation less common; proximal radiation frequent
Paroxysms	Exacerbations common and unpredictable	Exacerbations less common and associated with activity
Autonomic signs	Color changes, temperature changes, swelling, and/or sudomotor (sweating) activity occur in one third to one half of patients	Autonomic signs uncommon in chronic nociceptive pain

and emotional functioning (e.g., SF-36), satisfaction ratings, adverse treatment effects, and disposition (i.e., work status). It is therefore imperative that realistic goals are established, and individually tailored treatment regimens are developed to achieve these ends.

Distinguishing between neuropathic and nociceptive pain can have important treatment implications (Table 29-2). Neuropathic pain is characterized by positive and negative symptoms. Negative symptoms, such as a loss of sensation, are usually the result of axon and neuron loss, whereas the positive symptoms reflect abnormal excitability of the nervous system. Numbness, tingling, and other symptoms suggestive of sensory dysfunction are strongly indicative of neuropathic pain, especially when they occur in a dermatomal or solitary nerve distribution. Descriptors such as "burning," "shooting," and "electrical" are more apt to be associated with neuropathic pain, whereas adjectives such as "squeezing," "throbbing," and "aching" tend to be strongly identified with nociceptive pain states such as acute inflammatory pain or arthralgias. Other positive symptoms observed in neuropathic pain states include pain evoked by normally innocuous stimuli (allodynia) and an exaggerated or prolonged pain to noxious stimuli (hyperalgesia or hyperpathia). Although neuropathic pain tends to be more intermittent than nociceptive pain, mechanical spinal pain is classically exacerbated by movement. As alluded to earlier, some conditions such as cancer may be characterized by aspects of both nociceptive and neuropathic pain.

The proper evaluation of the patient in pain includes a psychosocial history. Between one half and two thirds of chronic pain patients exhibit varying degrees of major psychopathology, with depression being the most common comorbidity, followed by anxiety disorders, somatoform disorders, and substance abuse. Many of these coexisting psychological conditions have been associated with poor treatment prognosis. People seeking chronic pain care may also be more likely to carry a concomitant axis II diagnosis (i.e., personality disorder). Patients with axis II diagnoses are more likely to be designated as "difficult patients," which can act as an additional barrier to effective treatment. Potential social factors that can negatively affect treatment should be identified, including low job satisfaction, secondary gain, and ongoing litigation. A focused psychosocial history that includes prior psychiatric diagnoses, suicidal ideation, work history, legal history, and substance abuse, is therefore essential in the formulation of a treatment plan.

Physical Examination

Examination of the patient in pain should encompass all bodily systems because pain is a frequent manifestation of systemic disease. A physical examination finding by itself is almost never pathognomonic but usually functions to confirm suspicions garnered from the history and to select patients for imaging studies or invasive diagnostic testing. Unlike acute pain, *chronic pain is usually not associated with increased vital signs or facial grimacing.* Thorough neurologic and musculoskeletal examinations are particularly useful in evaluating pain. Sensory symptoms can precede other neurologic findings by months or weeks. The most common forms of neuropathy are associated with sensory deficits in a glove-stocking distribution, but other patterns occur as well (Chapter 428). Numbness in the distribution of a nerve root or single nerve strongly suggests neuropathic pain, but nondermatomal sensory changes can accompany nociceptive pain (e.g., fibromyalgia or arthritis) as well. Allodynia and hyperalgesia are hallmarks of neuropathic pain. Postural and gait abnormalities may be either causative factors for rheumatologic conditions (e.g., bursitis) or consequences of the underlying condition.

A careful evaluation of passive and active range of motion is useful because generalized and regional pain complaints are often accompanied by decreases in range of motion. Distinctions should be drawn between pain-induced and neurologic weakness, with the latter often occurring in conjunction with muscle atrophy or asymmetry in reflexes. Sometimes, reflex assessment is the only way to distinguish between a true neurologic condition and non-organic etiologies; hence, deep tendon reflexes are a useful component of the pain exam.

Diagnostic Tests

Imaging has largely supplanted history and physical examination as the gold standard for diagnosing pathology, but is not without drawbacks. There is a poor correlation between findings on magnetic resonance imaging (MRI) and the intensity of spinal pain, with greater than 50% of asymptomatic individuals having abnormalities on lumbar, thoracic, and cervical films. Previous studies found that neither radiographs nor MRI studies affect treatment outcomes and are unlikely to affect decision making[1]; in fact, redundant imaging can lead to unnecessary procedures. Absolute indications for MRI in patients with back pain are (1) serious or progressive neurologic deficits, (2) new-onset bowel and bladder dysfunction, (3) suspected metastatic disease, or (4) when referring patients for procedural interventions. The presence of "red flags" suggestive of more serious pathology (e.g., extremes of age, trauma history, immunosuppressed state, persistent fever, infection, or history of intravenous drug abuse) should also alert the practitioner to seek further evaluation. Electromyography and nerve conduction studies (Chapter 428) can be used to diagnose injury to large nerve fibers. However, because these studies are associated with significant false-negative and false-positive rates and are not sensitive in detecting impairment of small fiber (nociceptive afferent fibers) function, a normal neurophysiologic study does not rule out neuropathic pain. For small fiber neuropathies, a skin biopsy demonstrating decreased density of epidermal nerve fibers is a sensitive test.

For nonspinal pain conditions, MRI is ideal for detecting inflammation and soft tissue pathology, whereas computed tomography (CT) scanning is indicated for disease processes associated with bone destruction or ossification. The main advantages of ultrasound are that it is safe, is inexpensive, does not utilize ionizing radiation, and is relatively cheap.

TREATMENT Rx

The goals of treatment should include elucidating the cause of pain and alleviating suffering. Consequently, the goal of pain treatment should not be limited to pain reduction but should encompass improving functional status, mood, and social interactions (i.e., quality of life). Chronic pain may result from diverse etiologies, including physical trauma, disease, infection, and therapies such as radiation, chemotherapy, and surgery. It has been argued that treatment should be mechanism based rather than etiology based, but at the present time, simple clinical tools to correlate symptoms and signs with mechanisms are lacking. Hence, treatment is primarily etiology based, or symptomatic. The future development and validation of diagnostic methods to identify mechanisms (e.g., intravenous infusion tests) may help develop novel target-specific pharmacologic agents.

Pain is a complex perceptual experience affected by a multitude of factors that include not only activation of nociceptors but also emotions (e.g., fear, anxiety), memory and cognition, social and cultural context, and expectations. Thus, it is not surprising that despite a paucity of studies evaluating a multidisciplinary approach to pain management, a strong consensus exists that this approach is beneficial.

Pharmacologic Therapies

Antipyretic Analgesics

Today, aspirin (Chapter 36) is the most widely used analgesic in the world. Along with its pharmacologic cousins, nonsteroidal anti-inflammatory drugs (NSAIDs) and the antipyretic drugs acetaminophen and phenacetin, this group forms the backbone of pharmacologic pain treatment. Antipyretic analgesics exert their antinociceptive effects by the inhibition of cyclooxygenase, the rate-limiting enzyme in the production of prostaglandins, which are lipid-based compounds that sensitize nociceptors and regulate inflammation. There are several pharmacologic distinctions between NSAIDs and their counterparts, phenazone and acetaminophen. Whereas NSAIDs act both centrally and peripherally, making them effective topical agents for nociceptive inflammatory conditions, the primary site of enzyme inhibition for acetaminophen is in the central nervous system. Acetaminophen is also a weaker analgesic than NSAIDs and is largely devoid of anti-inflammatory effects.

The main drawback of nonopioid antipyretic analgesics is their ceiling effect, which can render them ineffective as stand-alone agents for severe pain. For cancer pain, the World Health Organization treatment paradigm advocates adding opioids to an analgesic regimen uncontrolled by NSAIDs, not replacing them. NSAIDs may act synergistically with opioids and have proven opioid-sparing effects. It is well acknowledged that aspirin, NSAIDs, and acetaminophen are more effective in treating nociceptive than neuropathic pain, although a significant proportion of neuropathic pain sufferers regularly take NSAIDs.

The second major concern about nonopioid antipyretic agents is side effects. For NSAIDs, these include bleeding, gastrointestinal ulceration, renal toxicity, and an increased risk of cardiovascular events. Although the use of cyclooxygenase-2 selective inhibitors like celecoxib and rofecoxib may attenuate the risk of bleeding and ulcers, the risk of renal failure and cardiovascular events from these drugs remains a significant cause of morbidity and mortality. These risks are significantly increased in elderly patients and with polypharmacy. In view of its more favorable safety profile, acetaminophen is often considered a first-line therapy ahead of NSAIDs, even for pain conditions associated with inflammation.

Adjuvant Analgesics

Multiple evidence-based guidelines for the treatment of chronic pain states, particularly neuropathic pain, have been recently published. In general, these suggest that antidepressants and anticonvulsants should be the two first-line classes of medications for chronic neuropathic pain. Depending on the particular drug and condition, these medications have been demonstrated to provide significant pain relief above and beyond that observed with placebo in 20 to 40% of ideal pharmacologic candidates (i.e., number needed to treat is between 2.5 and 5 in randomized trials). Whereas opioids have shown similar efficacy for neuropathic pain, anticonvulsants and antidepressants carry a lower risk of serious adverse events (e.g., addiction) and long-term tolerance, rendering them preferable to opioids for long-standing noncancer pain (Table 29-3). In terms of efficacy, tricyclic antidepressants (TCAs) are superior to serotonin-norepinephrine reuptake inhibitors, which in turn are more effective than serotonin-specific reuptake inhibitors. Among the various TCAs, amitriptyline is the most studied but is probably comparable in efficacy to its metabolite nortriptyline and its cousin imipramine. However, the latter two drugs' more favorable side effect profiles (e.g., less sedation and anticholinergic activity) make them the preferred choices for neuropathic pain. In patients who cannot tolerate TCAs, serotonin-norepinephrine reuptake inhibitors such as duloxetine can be beneficial. In addition to neuropathic pain, antidepressants have also been shown to be effective in headache prophylaxis, chest pain, abdominal and pelvic pain, fibromyalgia, arthritis, and spinal pain.

Anticonvulsants are probably effective for neuropathic pain by virtue of their membrane-stabilizing-properties. Although anticonvulsant drugs may be slightly more effective than antidepressants for prototypical "lancinating-type" neuropathic pain, antidepressants may be more versatile in that they have proven benefit in myriad other pain conditions. Owing to their high efficacy and favorable side-effect profiles, gabapentin and its pharmacologic relative pregabalin are first-line agents for most forms of neuropathic pain. In addition to independent pain-relieving properties, these drugs may act synergistically with opioids, provide anxiolysis, and exhibit preemptive analgesic effects when administered before surgery.

When gabapentinoid drugs are ineffective or intolerable, alternative anticonvulsants that act through different cellular mechanisms such as lamotrigine and oxcarbazepine may be employed. For trigeminal neuralgia, carbamazepine remains the treatment of choice, although adverse effects, such as the risk of agranulocytosis, limit its utility for other conditions. Other classes of adjuvants that may be effective in certain contexts include topical creams (e.g., NSAIDs, capsaicin, lidocaine), N-methyl-D-aspartate antagonists (e.g., dextromethorphan), skeletal muscle relaxants (e.g., baclofen, cyclobenzaprine), cannabinoids, and antiarrhythmics (mexiletine). Topical lidocaine patches have been shown to reduce the pain and allodynia in patients with postherpetic neuralgia, and anecdotal evidence has suggested lidocaine may be useful in the treatment of certain types of back pain. Recently, a

TABLE 29-3   ADJUVANT ANALGESIC DRUGS FOR CHRONIC PAIN

DRUG	DOSAGE	INDICATIONS	ADVERSE EFFECTS	COMMENTS
TRICYCLIC ANTIDEPRESSANTS				
Amitriptyline, imipramine, desipramine, nortriptyline	10-150 mg/day	Peripheral neuropathy, postherpetic neuralgia, other types of peripheral neuropathic pain, central pain, facial pain, fibromyalgia, headache prophylaxis, irritable bowel syndrome, and chronic low back pain with or without radiculopathy	Sedation, dry mouth, confusion, weight gain, constipation, urinary retention, ataxia, cardiac conduction delay (QTc prolongation)	First-line agents for neuropathic pain and headache prophylaxis Secondary amine drugs (e.g., nortriptyline) have fewer side effects than tertiary amines (e.g., amitriptyline) Contraindicated in glaucoma
SEROTONIN-NOREPINEPHRINE REUPTAKE INHIBITORS				
Venlafaxine	75-225 mg/day	Peripheral neuropathy, headache prophylaxis	Sedation, dry mouth, constipation, ataxia, hypertension, hyperhidrosis	Dose adjustment in patients with renal dysfunction
Duloxetine	60-120 mg/day	Peripheral neuropathy, fibromyalgia, chronic back pain	Sedation, dry mouth, constipation, hyperhidrosis	U.S. Food and Drug Administration (FDA) approved for fibromyalgia and diabetic neuropathy Contraindicated in glaucoma
ANTICONVULSANTS				
Gabapentin	600-3600 mg/day	Peripheral neuropathy, postherpetic neuralgia, other types of peripheral neuropathic pain, central pain, pelvic pain, headache prophylaxis, radiculopathy, chronic postsurgical pain	Sedation, weight gain, dry mouth, ataxia, edema	First-line agent for neuropathic pain FDA approved for postherpetic neuralgia Effective preemptively for postoperative pain
Pregabalin	150-600 mg/day	Peripheral neuropathy, postherpetic neuralgia, central pain, fibromyalgia	Sedation, weight gain, dry mouth, ataxia, edema	First-line agent for neuropathic pain FDA approved for diabetic neuropathy, postherpetic neuralgia, fibromyalgia Effective preemptively for postoperative pain Same mechanism of action as gabapentin
Carbamazepine	200-1600 mg/day	Facial neuralgias, diabetic neuropathy	Sedation, ataxia, diplopia, hyponatremia, agranulocytosis, diarrhea, aplastic anemia, hepatotoxicity, Stevens-Johnson syndrome	First-line agent and FDA approved for trigeminal and glossopharyngeal neuralgia Contraindicated in patients with porphyria and atrioventricular conduction block
Topiramate	50-400 mg/day	Headache prophylaxis, chronic low back pain with or without radiculopathy	Sedation, ataxia, diplopia, weight loss, diarrhea, metabolic acidosis, kidney stones	First-line agent and FDA approved for migraine prophylaxis Often used as appetite suppressant
CORTICOSTEROIDS (SYSTEMIC)				
Prednisone	5-60 mg/day	Inflammatory arthritis, other inflammatory pain conditions (e.g., inflammatory bowel disease), traumatic nerve injury, complex regional pain syndrome	Myriad psychiatric, gastrointestinal, neurologic, and cardiac side effects; immunosuppression, weakness, edema, weight gain, elevated glucose, poor wound healing, others	Stronger evidence supports local (i.e., injection) administration More effective for acute pain Strong anti-inflammatory effects
MISCELLANEOUS				
Muscle relaxants	Variable depending on drug	Skeletal muscle spasm, acute spinal pain, temporomandibular disorder Baclofen effective for spasticity, dystonia, and trigeminal neuralgia	Sedation, ataxia, blurred vision, confusion, asthenia, xerostomia and other gastrointestinal effects, palpitations	First-line agents for acute back pain and skeletal muscle spasm
Lidocaine patch	1-3 patches every 12 hr	Postherpetic neuropathy, peripheral neuropathy, other types of neuropathic and possibly myofascial pain associated with allodynia	Minimal systemic side effects when applied appropriately	Second-line agent and FDA approved for postherpetic neuralgia
Capsaicin cream	0.025% applied 3 or 4 times per day	Postherpetic neuralgia, peripheral neuropathy and other types of neuropathic pain, chronic postsurgical pain, arthritis and other musculoskeletal conditions	Burning on application Minimal systemic side effects when applied appropriately	FDA approved for arthritis Second-line agent for postherpetic neuralgia and third-line agent for peripheral neuropathy Single application 8% patch providing up to 3 months of pain relief was recently approved for postherpetic neuralgia
Cannabinoids	Variable depending on drug and delivery route	Strongest evidence is for multiple sclerosis May be effective for peripheral neuropathy and other types of neuropathic pain spasticity	Myriad psychiatric, neurologic, and cardiac effects; xerostomia, abdominal pain, and other gastrointestinal effects	Fourth-line agent with narrow therapeutic index Modest analgesic effect comparable to codeine

high-concentration (8%) topical patch of capsaicin (the pungent chemical in chili pepper) has been approved for the treatment of postherpetic neuralgia. A single 1-hour application of the capsaicin patch can result in attenuation of pain for up to 12 weeks. Topical NSAIDs (e.g., diclofenac) have been shown to be effective in the short term for the treatment of osteoarthritis and other rheumatologic disorders and have been touted as having fewer adverse effects than systemic NSAIDs.

Opioid Analgesics

Opioid analgesics, such as morphine, oxycodone, hydromorphone, and methadone, are the cornerstone of treatment for cancer pain (Table 29-4). Several randomized studies have also demonstrated their usefulness in non-cancer pain conditions such as chronic osteoarthritis and neuropathic pain states.[2] Maximizing the therapeutic effects of opioid analgesics requires careful attention to balancing the beneficial effects with the undesirable adverse effects. Understanding the clinical pharmacology of opioids, including their relative potency, duration of action, oral bioavailability, and pharmacokinetics, is essential for rational use (see Table 29-4). Their use for chronic pain management is limited primarily by their myriad side effects that include nausea, vomiting, constipation, sedation, itch, respiratory depression, and endocrine deficiency leading to sexual dysfunction and accelerated osteoporosis. Attentive treatment to opioid-induced side effects can facilitate dose titration, maximize analgesia, and minimize adverse effects. Aggressive management with stool softeners and agents that enhance bowel motility such as docusate, lactulose, and senna, can minimize constipation. Whereas most opioids are devoid of end-organ toxicity, an exception is meperidine. A metabolite, normeperidine, can accumulate after several days of treatment, causing myoclonus and anxiety; at higher concentrations, confusion, delirium, and seizures can ensue. Opioids that are predominantly renally eliminated, such as morphine, should be used with caution in patients with renal dysfunction. Two metabolites of morphine, morphine-6-glucuronide, which contains analgesic properties, and morphine-3-glucuronide, which may amplify pain in certain contexts, can accumulate in patients with renal dysfunction and are largely responsible for the adverse effects of morphine. Alternate drugs in such patients are fentanyl and methadone.

For treatment of acute pain (e.g., postoperative pain) or an acute exacerbation of chronic pain in hospitalized patients (e.g., sickle cell crisis), patient-controlled analgesia (PCA) provides a convenient means of administering opioids. Intravenous morphine, fentanyl, or hydromorphone is commonly administered using an infusion device designed to prevent overdose. With or without a basal infusion (which can be used to replace a sustained-release opioid in a patient who is NPO), the bolus dose, lockout time interval between doses, and the maximal dose per hour can be programmed in and adjusted based on clinical circumstances. PCA devices are safe and allow patients to control their pain management with less dependence on health care providers. Studies comparing PCA with conventional administration of opioids have generally found PCAs to be associated with better pain relief and higher satisfaction rates, albeit with larger amounts of medication consumed.

The long-term use of opioids can be associated with tolerance and physical dependence. Cross-tolerance among opioids is not complete, and a strategy that is often used when tolerance to an opioid is suspected is rotation to an alternate opioid drug. Although addiction (Chapter 33) to opioids when used

TABLE 29-4 FORMULATIONS, DOSAGES, AND PHARMACOLOGIC INFORMATION ON COMMONLY PRESCRIBED OPIOIDS

DRUG	EQUIANALGESIC DOSAGE (ORAL UNLESS SPECIFIED)	READILY AVAILABLE ROUTES OF ADMINISTRATION	DURATION OF ACTION	COMMENTS
Morphine	30 mg	IV, IM, PO, PR; SR formulation	3-6 hr for short-acting, 8-12 hr for SR	Reference standard for all opioids Renally excreted active metabolite
Oxycodone	20 mg	PO, PR; SR formulation	3-6 hr for short-acting, 8-12 hr for SR	Widely available in combination form with nonopioid analgesics; SR form popular among recreational users
Hydromorphone	3-6 mg	PO, PR, IV, IM	3-6 hr	Higher PO/IV conversion ratio than other opioids
Hydrocodone	30-60 mg	PO	3-6 hr	Wide variation in morphine equivalent dose Most commonly prescribed opioid in U.S. Typically used in combination form with nonopioid analgesic Formulations containing <15 mg hydrocodone are schedule III in U.S.
Methadone	2-20 mg	PO, PR, IV	6-12 hr for pain	Morphine: methadone conversion varies according to dose and length of opioid use, ranging from 2 : 1 to >20 : 1 in patients on very high doses Any physician with a schedule II DEA license may prescribe for pain May take 5-7 days to reach steady state due to extended half-life (i.e., accumulation) Electrocardiogram monitoring recommended with higher doses Other properties such as NMDA receptor antagonism and reuptake inhibition of serotonin and norepinephrine may slow the development of tolerance and increase efficacy for neuropathic pain
Fentanyl	12.5 µg/hr (TD) 800-1000 µg (TM) 200-400 µg (B)	TD, TM, B	72 hr for TD; 1 hr-2 hr for TM and B	TD, TM, and B formulations may be useful in patients with poor bowel function TD: wide variation in conversion ratios Delivery system may be associated with fewer gastrointestinal side effects TM and B: delivery systems associated with more rapid (10-min) onset than immediate-release oral opioids. U.S. Food and Drug Administration (FDA) approved for breakthrough cancer pain in opioid-tolerant patients
Codeine	200 mg	PO, PR	3-6 hr	Often used in combination with nonopioid analgesics Efficacy and side effects may be affected by rate of metabolism to morphine Popular as cough suppressant
Propoxyphene	200 mg	PO, PR	3-6 hr	Wide variation in morphine equivalent dose Often used in combination form with nonopioid analgesic Toxic metabolite may accumulate with excessive use, especially in elderly patients Weak antagonist at NMDA receptor
Meperidine	300 mg	PO, PR, IV	2-4 hr	Toxic metabolite may accumulate with excessive use, especially in patients with renal insufficiency Associated with tachycardia and hypertension May cause more "euphoria" than other opioids
Buprenorphine	0.4 mg SL	SL, PR, IV, TD	6-8 hr	Partial opioid agonist that may precipitate withdrawal in opioid-dependent patients Lower abuse potential, and fewer psychomimetic effects, than pure agonists Not readily reversed by naloxone Schedule III drug in U.S. Primary use of SL preparation is to treat addiction

B = buccal; IV = intravenous; NMDA = N-methyl-D-aspartate; PO = oral; PR = rectal; SL = sublingual; SR = sustained release; TD = transdermal; TM = transmucosal.

for the treatment of chronic pain is reported to be relatively uncommon, guidelines for responsible prescribing of opioids have been published as a monograph by the Federation of State Medical Boards. The critical suggested steps in the management of chronic pain patients with opioids include appropriate patient evaluation, creating and maintaining clear and detailed documentation, creating a function-based treatment plan with well-defined patient goals that include an exit strategy, obtaining a written patient-physician agreement that includes informed consent and patient education, periodic review that focuses on progress toward functional goals, and making specialist referrals when managing difficult patients. Diversion of opioids and the increasing abuse of prescription opioids, particularly in teenagers and young adults, is another growing societal concern (Chapter 33).

Tramadol and tapentadol comprise part of a new class of analgesic drugs that have a dual mechanism of action. Tramadol is a weak agonist and inhibits the reuptake of norepinephrine and serotonin. Along with the usual side effects associated with opioids, seizures have been reported with tramadol, and adverse drug interactions can occur in patients taking warfarin sodium (Coumadin) and selective serotonin reuptake inhibitors (SSRIs). Tapentadol also has a dual mode of action as a μ–opioid agonist and a norepinephrine reuptake inhibitor. Nausea, dizziness, constipation, and sedation are reported side effects of this drug. Tramadol is presently approved for moderate to moderately severe pain, whereas tapentadol, which is currently a schedule II drug in the United States, is approved for moderate to severe acute pain.

Butorphanol, nalbuphine, and pentazocine are opioid agonist-antagonist drugs that can antagonize the actions of μ–opioid agonists and can cause psychotomimetic effects owing to their actions on the κ-opioid receptor. These drugs should be used with caution, particularly in patients receiving other μ–opioid agonists. Buprenorphine, a partial agonist at the μ–opioid receptor and an antagonist at other opioid receptors, is available as a sublingual pill that is approved for the treatment of opioid addiction. A transdermal formulation is approved in Europe for the treatment of chronic pain.

Combination Therapies

Most clinical trials have studied the effects of individual drugs in specific chronic pain states. However, no one drug is universally effective, and often the drug only provides partial pain relief. In clinical practice, two or more drugs are often used in combination to achieve an additive beneficial effect or to decrease the adverse effects associated with the use of a single drug. The rational use of polypharmacy should include drugs that act at different sites in the pain signaling process or modulate different neurotransmitter systems, or both (Fig. 29-1). Although results are conflicting, a preponderance of recent randomized trials suggest that combination therapy with opioids and either anticonvulsants or antidepressants may be more effective than using either drug class as a stand-alone treatment.[3] Similarly, combining two adjuvant medication classes (e.g., gabapentin and nortriptyline) was recently shown to be more efficacious than giving either drug alone for neuropathic pain,[4] and combination treatment with pregabalin and celecoxib was found to be superior to monotherapy in a mixed population of patients with chronic low back pain.[5] Additional studies are needed to help develop guidelines for rational polypharmacy based on pain pathophysiology, mechanisms of action, and genetic medicine.

Psychological Treatment

The relationship between pain and psychopathology is complex. The lifetime prevalence rate of coexisting psychiatric illness in chronic pain patients ranges from 50% to upward of 80%. Between 30% and 60% of chronic pain sufferers experience symptoms of depression, making it the most common comorbidity. For anxiety disorders and substance abuse, the coprevalence rates are about 30% and 10 to 15%, respectively.

Viewed from a different perspective, the relationship is even more striking. More than 60% of patients with major depression and more than half of all patients with anxiety and substance abuse disorders experience moderate to severe chronic pain. Although it is widely acknowledged that disease states and injuries that result in chronic pain can predispose patients to depression, anxiety, and even self-destructive behavior, what is less commonly appreciated is the effect preexisting psychiatric conditions have on pain perception. There is a plethora of literature demonstrating that coexisting psychopathology is a strong predictor for the development of chronic pain after an acute, traumatic event (e.g., back pain episode, surgery, motor vehicle crash).

It is necessary to screen all pain patients for psychological conditions that can adversely affect treatment (Table 29-5). Not only major psychiatric conditions such as depression and generalized anxiety but also maladaptive behaviors and secondary diagnoses such as somatization disorder and poor coping skills can negatively influence treatment. Psychological screening is mandated for pain patients being considered for neuromodulation (e.g., spinal cord stimulation), and many spine surgeons will defer surgery until major psychiatric issues are adequately addressed.

Relaxation techniques such as biofeedback, self-hypnosis, and guided imagery have proved effective in a wide array of acute and chronic pain conditions but may be especially useful in those with high levels of anxiety. Cognitive behavioral therapy is a highly structured form of psychotherapy predicated

FIGURE 29-1. Rational choice of combination therapies for pain should be based on the mechanisms of drug actions. Combining drugs with disparate actions can have additive or synergistic analgesic effects and minimize adverse effects. NMDA = *N*-methyl-D-aspartate; PAG = periaqueductal gray; RVM = rostral ventromedial medulla.

TABLE 29-5 PSYCHOSOCIAL FACTORS ASSOCIATED WITH CHRONIC PAIN

Multiple pain complaints

Poor job satisfaction/low pay

Inadequate coping skills

Fear-avoidance behavior

Manual labor/physically stressful job

Obesity

Somatization

Smoking

Low baseline activity levels

Ongoing litigation

Low education level

Greater baseline disability

Anxiety

Depressed mood

Emotional distress

on the replacement of negative thought patterns and behaviors with more positive, constructive ones. These therapies may enhance the modulation of afferent pain signals. Ideal candidates include educated, motivated patients in whom distorted thinking (e.g., "catastrophization") and counterproductive behaviors serve to amplify pain behavior. In patients with personality disorders and ingrained maladaptive behaviors, long-term psychotherapy may be necessary.

Interventional Therapies: Nerve Blocks, Neuromodulation, and Neurosurgery
Nerve Blocks

Nerve blocks and injections may be done for therapeutic, diagnostic, and sometimes prognostic purposes (i.e., to select candidates for surgery or radio frequency denervation). Mechanistically, injections performed with local anesthetic may work by releasing entrapped nerves, enhancing blood flow, and interrupting processes involved in central sensitization (i.e., "breaking the cycle of pain"). Additional benefits of adding corticosteroid to local anesthetic include blocking the inflammatory cascade, suppressing ectopic discharges from injured nerves, and inhibiting the synthesis of prostaglandins, some of which serve to sensitize nociceptors.

Nerve blocks are almost never a panacea for noncancer pain, but in appropriate candidates, blocks may provide intermediate-term pain relief, facilitate rehabilitative therapy, and improve quality of life for several weeks to months. Translating this relief into long-term improvement inevitably necessitates addressing the underlying etiologies and predisposing factors, which often entails physical therapy, psychotherapy, and rehabilitation. Injections that can afford benefit in well-selected individuals include trigger point injections with local anesthetic for myofascial pain and nerve blocks with corticosteroid for entrapment syndromes (e.g., carpal tunnel syndrome, occipital neuralgia). Among spinal injections, the strongest evidence is for epidural steroid injections in patients with radicular pain of less than 6 months' duration. Neurolytic procedures, such as celiac plexus neurolysis with alcohol or phenol, have been shown to provide significant pain relief lasting several months in patients with pain associated with cancer of the pancreas, liver, and gastrointestinal tract.

Spinal Cord Stimulation

Spinal cord stimulation is an effective, minimally invasive neuromodulatory technique for managing a variety of chronic pain states refractory to more conservative measures. It was developed based on the gate-control theory, which postulates that activation of peripheral sensory A-fibers can attenuate pain signaling by slower-conducting pain C-fibers. Common indications include failed back surgery syndrome, complex regional pain syndromes, and outside of the United States, ischemic pain.

Surgery

Surgical interventions are often advocated in chronic pain patients who have failed more conservative measures, but surgery is fraught with the same limitations as nerve blocks. A traumatic neuroma is an inexorable consequence of cutting or burning a nerve, formed as a result of unregulated and disorganized nerve regeneration. Neuromas have been shown to fire ectopic pain signals and are often quite painful. Hence, neurolytic procedures are rarely successful in the long-term treatment of neuropathic pain. Part of the challenge in deciding when operative therapy is indicated revolves around the difficulty involved in establishing a causative relationship between the targeted pathology and pain. Roughly 10% of women of reproductive age have endometriosis, but many patients with endometriosis have minimal symptoms, and pelvic pain is a frequent occurrence in young females with no detectable pathology. With respect to inguinal hernia repair and spinal decompression, the incidence of chronic postsurgical pain is inversely correlated with the size of the bowel and disc herniation, respectively. This illustrates that in many of these individuals, the targeted pathology may not have been the primary cause of symptoms. On a similar note, scar tissue is a predictable sequela of surgical treatment, but lysis of adhesions is only infrequently associated with long-term symptom palliation because of the high recurrence rate and absence of any means to correlate the presence of adhesions with pain. Not surprisingly, surgery done solely to remove a painful body part (e.g., hysterectomy, orchiectomy) rarely results in long-term benefit.

Back Pain

Back pain is the leading cause of disability in people younger than 45 years in the industrialized world and thus deserves separate mention when discussing interventional therapies. In patients who present with serious spinal pathology (primarily infection, tumor, and trauma), decompression, stabilization, and fusion can be highly beneficial, but outcomes are strongly dependent on the primary pathology and patient. Decompression procedures done for spinal stenosis or radiculopathy are also effective for short-term relief, but the benefits diminish with time.[6,7] With respect to fusion or disc replacement done for axial pain associated with common degenerative changes, less than 40% of patients can expect a highly functional outcome.

Physical Treatments

The use of "physical" therapies to provide pain relief and enhance function forms a cornerstone in the multimodal approach to the patient with pain. Physical therapists evaluate, educate, and provide minimally invasive and noninvasive procedural interventions to patients to help prevent and alleviate the pain and dysfunction associated with physical and mental maladies. These interventions include both addressing causative mechanisms of pain (e.g., core strengthening, correcting gait and postural abnormalities) and providing treatments (e.g., ultrasound, hot and cold packs, joint manipulation).

Exercise has been used for decades as a treatment for chronic pain and as a means to prevent injury. Exercise may work through a variety of mechanisms, including enhancing blood flow, releasing endorphins, exerting anti-inflammatory effects, activating descending inhibitory pathways, and improving sleep and mood. Whereas the largest body of research has been conducted in patients with spinal pain, benefits have also been demonstrated in those with fibromyalgia, headaches, arthritis, neuropathic pain, and cancer.

Complementary and Alternative Therapies

Physicians are referring patients for complementary and alternative medical (CAM) treatments with increasing frequency, with utilization rates exceeding one third for certain conditions. CAM therapies have been used to treat myriad pain conditions, including cancer and noncancer pain and both neuropathic and nociceptive conditions (Chapter 38). Some of the most popular and studied CAM modalities are acupuncture, chiropractic, yoga, and dietary supplements, all of which have been shown in clinical trials to reduce pain and improve functional capacity in certain contexts. However, the effect size tends to be modest for these treatments, and there is little evidence to support the superiority of any one "proven" modality over another.

Pain Management in Older Persons

Older adults often have varied and multiple pain conditions that exist with other comorbidities. Pharmacologic management of pain in this population can be challenging because of the potential for drug-drug and drug-disease interactions. The potential for drug-related adverse effects is the basis for the popular recommendation of "start low and go slow" in the titration of analgesic drugs. The potential interaction between anticoagulants, such as warfarin and aspirin, and NSAIDs can result in an increased risk for bleeding. Age-related decrease in hepatic blood flow and decreased first-pass effect can result in higher bioavailability of opioids, such as morphine. Significant interactions between analgesic drugs metabolized hepatically by CYP2D6, such as codeine, hydrocodone, oxycodone, tramadol, and antidepressants, may result in decreased metabolism and increased toxicity. Several drugs used for the management of chronic pain and their active metabolites, such as duloxetine, gabapentin, pregabalin, oxycodone, and tramadol, are primarily renally eliminated. Their dose should be adjusted accordingly. An updated guideline for the pharmacologic management of persistent pain in older persons based on a synthesis of the best available evidence has been recently published.

FUTURE DRUGS AND PREVENTION OF PAIN

Much research is being done to develop new routes of drug administration, abuse-deterrent opioids, and novel nonopioid drug treatments, which can optimize outcomes and reduce risks and side effects for pharmacotherapy. Two other areas ripe for investigation are the development of drugs that exploit the unique genetic makeup of pain patients, and refining selection criteria for various therapies. The conceptual appeal of these and other endeavors is that treatment tailored to individuals is likely to result in greater benefit and less risk than the "shotgun" approach to pain treatment that is too often used.

Regenerative therapies, which seek to facilitate the body's ability to repair, replace, restore and regenerate diseased or damaged tissue, is another frontier in pain medicine. These treatments are currently in preliminary stages of development but may someday be used to treat central, joint, and spinal pain.

Finally, identifying patients at high risk of developing pain and employing strategies to either prevent pain or minimize the disease burden represent other areas that have been henceforth underinvestigated. In patients at high risk for chronic postsurgical pain (e.g., young patients with preexisting pain and psychological comorbidities), these measures might include the use of preemptive analgesics, such as NSAIDs and anticonvulsants, and employment of surgical techniques associated with less trauma. For patients with musculoskeletal complaints, this might entail educational initiatives, extensive rehabilitation, fall-reduction classes, and increased reimbursement for walking aids and wheelchairs.

1. Modic MT, Obuchowski NA, Ross JS, et al. Acute low back pain and radiculopathy: MR imaging findings and their prognostic role and effect on outcome. *Radiology.* 2005;237:597-604.
2. Noble M, Treadwell JR, Tregear SJ, et al. Long-term opioid management for chronic noncancer pain. *Cochrane Database Syst Rev.* 2010;1:CD006605.
3. Gilron I, Bailey JM, Tu D, et al. Morphine, gabapentin, or their combination for neuropathic pain. *N Engl J Med.* 2005;352:1324-1334.
4. Gilron I, Bailey JM, Tu D, et al. Nortriptyline and gabapentin, alone and in combination for neuropathic pain: a double-blind, randomised controlled crossover trial. *Lancet.* 2009;374:1252-1261.
5. Romano CL, Romano D, Bonora C, et al. Pregabalin, celecoxib, and their combination for treatment of chronic low-back pain. *J Orthop Traumatol.* 2009;10:185-191.
6. Weinstein JN, Tosteson TD, Lurie JD, et al. Surgical vs nonoperative treatment for lumbar disk herniation. The Spine Patient Outcomes Research Trial (SPORT): a randomized trial. *JAMA.* 2006;296:2441-2450.
7. Weinstein JN, Tosteson TD, Lurie JD, et al, for the SPORT Investigators. Surgical versus nonsurgical therapy for lumbar spinal stenosis. *N Engl J Med.* 2008;358:794-810.

SUGGESTED READINGS

American Geriatrics Society Panel on the Pharmacological Management of Persistent Pain in Older Persons. Pharmacological management of persistent pain in older persons. *J Am Geriatr Soc.* 2009;57:1331-1346. *Updated guidelines developed and written by a multidisciplinary panel of the American Geriatrics Society.*

Chou R, Fanciullo GJ, Fine PG, et al, for the American Pain Society–American Academy of Pain Medicine Opioids Guidelines Panel. Clinical guidelines for the use of chronic opioid therapy in chronic noncancer pain. *J Pain.* 2009;10:113-130. *Practical guidelines on opioid use for noncancer pain by a multidisciplinary panel.*

Dunn KM, Saunders KW, Rutter CM, et al. Opioid prescriptions for chronic pain and overdose: a cohort study. *Ann Intern Med.* 2010;152:85-92. *Emphasizes the need for close supervision because higher doses of opioids increase the risk of overdose.*

Dworkin RH, O'Connor AB, Audette J, et al. Recommendations for the pharmacological management of neuropathic pain: an overview and literature update. *Mayo Clin Proc.* 2010;85(suppl):S3-S14. *A review providing an evidence-based recommendation for the pharmacological treatment of neuropathic pain.*

Morlion B. Pharmacotherapy of low back pain: targeting nociceptive and neuropathic pain components. *Curr Med Res Opin.* 2011;27:11-33. *The combination of pregabalin or antidepressants to target the neuropathic component of pain with opioids or nonsteroidal agents to target nociceptive pain may be preferable to either alone.*

30

BIOLOGY OF ADDICTION

STEVEN E. HYMAN

DEFINITION

Drug addiction is defined as compulsive substance use despite serious negative consequences. Harmful drug use and addiction are significant contributors to medical morbidity and mortality both directly as a result of the toxic effects of abused drugs and indirectly through accidents, violence, nonsterile needle use, and other health hazards. By far the greatest contributors to illness and death are the widely used legal drugs, tobacco (Chapter 31) and alcohol (Chapter 32), although illegal addictive drugs and abused prescription drugs (Chapter 33) also exact a significant toll. In addition, addiction creates enormous burdens on society by impairing the function of the addicted person in multiple life roles, disrupting families and neighborhoods, and motivating crime.

Compulsive use, the cardinal feature of addiction, means that the affected person cannot control substance use for a significant period of time, despite powerful reasons to do so such as drug-related health problems, drug-associated arrest, or the threat of losing one's job or spouse. In the clinic, addiction can be remarkably frustrating to treat: drug seeking and administration are apparently voluntary behaviors that an otherwise sentient person seems unwilling to control. Even after significant efforts have been exerted to get an addicted patient into drug treatment, relapse is common, even long after the last withdrawal symptom has cleared. Relapses are often precipitated by stress or by reminders of drug use ("cues") that may range from familiar drug use contexts (such as smoking after a meal), to interactions with drug-using friends, to the smell of marijuana or tobacco smoke, to bodily feelings previously associated with drug-seeking (interoceptive cues). Cellular and molecular studies of drug action, animal models of drug use, and noninvasive human neuroimaging studies are providing significant insights into the neurobiology underlying compulsive drug taking and its persistence. Other important frontiers of research include the human genetics of addiction risk and more recently, the neurobiology of what have been called "behavioral addictions," such as compulsive gambling.

Drug users may repeatedly take drugs in order to gain pleasure or escape from negative feelings, including the aversive feelings that may occur when drugs wear off. As a result of repeated drug administration over time, drug receptors and their downstream signaling pathways (Table 30-1) are excessively stimulated and may thus undergo homeostatic adaptations. These adaptations can produce tolerance (the need for increasing drug doses to achieve desired affects) or dependence (revealed by withdrawal symptoms between drug doses or with drug cessation). Both tolerance and dependence can contribute to ongoing drug use and to dosage increases; however, neither tolerance nor dependence explains compulsive use. First, tolerance and dependence occur not only with repeated use of many addictive drugs (e.g., heroin), but also with many nonaddictive drugs (e.g., bronchodilators, nitrates, selective serotonin reuptake inhibitor [SSRI] antidepressants). Second, some highly addictive drugs such as cocaine may produce little dependence and withdrawal in some individuals who nonetheless exhibit compulsive use. Finally, if dependence and withdrawal were necessary factors in addiction, the phenomenon of late, post-detoxification relapse would not be the major clinical problem that it is. Although these forms of homeostatic adaptation play a role in addiction, as will be described, other types of plasticity within the nervous system are more significant.

The term *dependence* was selected to signify *addiction* within the *Diagnostic and Statistical Manual of Mental Disorders* of the American Psychiatric Association (DSM-IV) presumably because the term *addiction* was thought to be stigmatizing. This choice unfortunately has contributed to the confusion of physiologic dependence (the type of adaptation described previously) with addiction by physicians and patients alike. This confusion creates unnecessary obstacles to the treatment of many conditions, including cancer pain, anxiety disorders, and depression.

RISK FACTORS FOR ADDICTION

Only a minority of individuals who use drugs go on to become addicted. The best-established risk factors for addiction are male sex and family history. Across countries and cultures, males have a greater risk for both heavy drug use and addiction with risk ratios in the range of 1.4 : 1 to 2 : 1. In recent years, however, the sex ratios have narrowed in many countries, especially for tobacco use and alcohol.

Genes play the preponderant role in familial risk as evidenced by twin and adoption studies. Twin studies consistently show higher rates of concordance for heavy drug use and addiction within monozygotic twin pairs than within dizygotic twin pairs. Adoption studies that have been performed in several Scandinavian countries and in the United States have focused mostly on alcoholism. These studies demonstrate that individuals adopted early in life

TABLE 30-1	PROPERTIES OF ADDICTIVE DRUGS		
DRUG	**NEUROTRANSMITTER**	**DRUG TARGET**	**EFFECT AFTER BINDING**
Opiates (morphine, heroin, oxycodone)	Endorphins	μ and δ opioid (agonist)	Activate G_i/G_o Activate K^+ channels
Psychostimulants (cocaine, amphetamines)	Dopamine (DA)	Dopamine transporter (DAT)* (antagonist)	Increase synaptic DA; stimulate presynaptic and postsynaptic DA receptors
Nicotine	Acetylcholine	Nicotinic acetylcholine receptors (nAChRs) (agonist)	Stimulate cation channel (may desensitize)
Alcohol	γ-Aminobutyric acid (GABA) Glutamate	$GABA_A$ receptor (agonist) N-methyl-D-aspartate (NMDA) receptor (antagonist)	Activate Cl^- channel Inhibit Ca^{2+} entry
Marijuana (Δ^9-tetrahydrocannabinol)	Anandamide	Cannabinoid CB_1 (agonist)	Activate G_i/G_o
Phencyclidine, ketamine		NMDA receptor channel (antagonist)	Inhibit Ca^{2+} entry

*The psychostimulants also interact with the norepinephrine and serotonin transporters, but under normal conditions, it is the DAT that is critical for rewarding and addictive properties. Unlike cocaine, amphetamines enter dopamine through the DAT and interact with a second target, the vesicular monoamine transporter (VMAT), to release DA into the cytoplasm and thence, through the DAT, to release it into the synapse.
Adapted from Hyman SE, Malenka RC, Nestler EJ. Neural mechanisms of addiction: the role of reward-related learning and memory. *Annu Rev Neurosci.* 2006;29:565-598.

tend to resemble their biologic rather than their adoptive parents with respect to patterns of alcohol use.

Although genes clearly play a significant role in vulnerability to addiction, few of the specific genetic variants that confer risk have been identified with certainty. Like all common neuropsychiatric disorders, addiction risk is highly genetically complex; there is evidence from linkage and association studies for contributions by a large number of genetic variants of relatively small effect. Large genome-wide association studies and other applications of modern genomic methods are continuing. However, the task of gene identification is also complicated by the challenges of phenotype definition. There are no objective medical tests with which to make the diagnosis, and there may be independent genetic and nongenetic risk factors for different stages of substance use disorders such as drug experimentation, addiction, and treatment responsiveness. Moreover, twin and family studies suggest that there may be both shared and unshared genetic risk factors underlying different drug preferences. As in other genetically complex disorders, it is hoped that with the identification of multiple risk-conferring variants, systems biology approaches can be brought to bear that will identify biochemical pathways involved in pathogenesis and suggest potential treatment targets.

REWARD CIRCUITRY: THE NEURAL SUBSTRATE OF ADDICTION

The survival and perpetuation of species require that animals, including humans, learn to predict threats and also learn the circumstances under which they can obtain food, water, shelter, and opportunities for mating. Neural circuits that have been highly conserved in evolution underlie these survival functions. A "fear circuit" centered on the amygdala regulates responses to threats, and a "reward circuit" centered on dopamine-releasing neurons that project from the ventral tegmental area (VTA) of the midbrain to the nucleus accumbens (NAc), prefrontal cortex, and other forebrain structures (Fig. 30-1) controls the pursuit of positive survival goals or "rewards." A simple operational definition of reward is a stimulus that elicits approach and consummatory behaviors.

Based on lesioning and physiologic studies in animals and more recently imaging in humans, the NAc (see Fig. 30-1), especially its outer region, called the *shell*, has been shown to play a necessary role in assigning motivational properties (desire, incentive salience) on rewards and to the stimuli that predict them. Thus, for example, in rat and mouse models, an intact NAc is required if the animal is to learn to work (e.g., lever pressing) to obtain natural rewards, such as palatable foods, or to learn how to self-administer drugs such as cocaine. Once an animal learns how to obtain a reward, and the relevant behaviors become ingrained, reward seeking no longer depends on the NAc and is supported by the dorsal striatum (called the *caudate* and *putamen* in humans), the brain structure that underlies well-learned behaviors and habits.

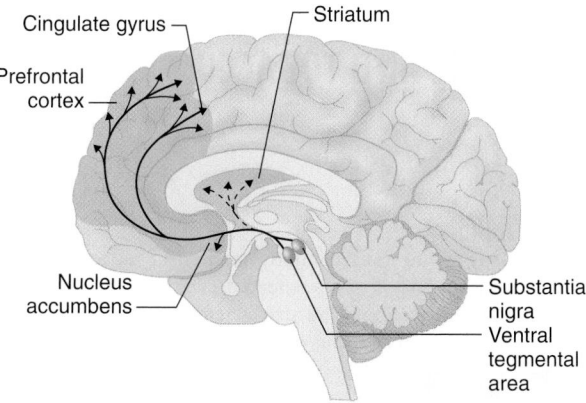

FIGURE 30-1. Brain reward circuits. The major dopaminergic projections to the forebrain that underlie brain reward are shown superimposed on a diagram of the human brain: projections from the ventral tegmental area to the nucleus accumbens, amygdala (not shown), hippocampus (not shown), and prefrontal cerebral cortex. Also shown are projections from the substantia nigra to the dorsal striatum (caudate and putamen and related structures) that play a role in habit formation and other deeply ingrained motor behaviors, including cue-dependent drug-seeking and self-administration. (From Hyman SE, Malenka RC, Nestler EJ. Neural mechanisms of addiction: the role of reward-related learning and memory. *Annu Rev Neurosci.* 2006;29:565-598.)

Under natural conditions, speed and efficiency in gaining food, water, and shelter improve the probability of survival. Thus, a critical role of reward circuitry is to facilitate the rapid learning of cues that predict the proximity of reward and of the behaviors that maximize the chances of successfully obtaining it. Once learned, predictive cues automatically activate cognitive, physiologic, and behavioral responses aimed at obtaining the predicted reward. In the laboratory, the simplest example of reward-related learning is classic (or pavlovian) conditioning in which a neutral stimulus, such as the sound of a bell, is reliably paired with a natural reward (an unconditioned stimulus) such as food. The sound of the bell quickly becomes a learned (conditioned) stimulus that henceforth activates physiologic and behavioral preparedness to obtain and consume the food.

The neurotransmitter dopamine, released from VTA neurons in the NAc, plays the key (albeit not the only) role in binding rewards and reward-associated cues to adaptive reward-seeking responses. In animals, implanted electrodes can record firing of dopamine neurons; microdialysis catheters and electrochemical methods can be used to detect dopamine that has been released from presynaptic neurons. In humans, positron emission tomography (PET) permits indirect measures of dopamine release by observing the displacement of a positron-emitting D_2 dopamine receptor ligand previously bound to receptors following a stimulus or pharmacologic challenge. Using such methods in multiple paradigms, it has been well established that natural rewards cause firing of VTA neurons and dopamine release in the NAc and other forebrain regions. When dopamine action is blocked, whether by lesioning dopamine neurons, blocking post-synaptic dopamine receptors, or inhibiting dopamine synthesis, rewards no longer motivate the behaviors necessary to obtain them.

New insights into the role of dopamine have emerged from studies of patients with Parkinson's disease (PD). PD results from the death of midbrain dopamine neurons; however, neurons within the substantia nigra (SN), which project to the caudate and putamen, are more severely affected than neurons within the VTA. Patients are generally treated with L-DOPA, a dopamine precursor, but as the disease progresses, other drugs may be needed, including selective D_2 dopamine receptor agonists. Relevant to this discussion is that a minority of patients treated with D_2 dopamine receptor agonists develop new risky, goal-directed behaviors such as compulsive gambling or compulsive shopping. These behaviors generally cease when the drug is withdrawn. It is thought that dopamine receptor agonists produce therapeutic effects on motor behavior in the more fully denervated caudate and putamen but combine with endogenous dopamine from preserved VTA neurons to overstimulate the NAc and other components of reward circuitry. These observations not only underscore the role of dopamine in motivation and reward seeking, but also suggest that what have been called *behavioral addictions* such as compulsive gambling share neural substrates with drug addiction.

Electrophysiologic recordings from nonhuman primates and functional magnetic resonance imaging (fMRI) studies in humans have converged on new views of how dopamine acts. Contrary to earlier ideas, dopamine does not appear to function as a neural representation of pleasure; rather, it serves as a learning signal in diverse forebrain circuits that are involved in responding to rewards. Dopaminergically innervated circuits underlie such functions as connecting reward-related stimuli to desire (NAc), learning and automatizing new motor behaviors (caudate and putamen), response selection, and relative valuation of experiences (orbital prefrontal cortex). Other neurotransmitters, perhaps endogenous opioid peptides, may be involved in hedonic responses (i.e., signaling pleasure). In this regard, it is noteworthy that nicotine, which is highly addictive—and causes dopamine release—does not produce significant euphoria of the sort produced by cocaine or heroin.

Much evidence suggests that the precise pattern of dopamine neuron firing, and the resulting synaptic release of dopamine in forebrain circuits, act to shape behavior so as to maximize future reward. In a basal state, dopamine neurons have a slow tonic pattern of firing. When a reward is encountered that is new, unexpected, or greater than expected, there is a phasic burst of firing of dopamine neurons causing a transient increase in synaptic dopamine. When a reward is predicted from known cues and is exactly as expected, there is no change from the tonic pattern of firing, that is, no additional dopamine release. When a predicted reward is omitted or less than expected, dopamine neurons pause their firing to levels below their tonic rate. Phasic increases in synaptic dopamine signify that the world is better than expected, facilitate learning of new predictive information, and bind the newly learned predictive cues to action.

PROPERTIES OF ADDICTIVE DRUGS

Addictive drugs are chemically diverse and interact with different molecular targets in the nervous system (see Table 30-1). They also exhibit significant differences from each other in many of their physiologic and behavioral effects. For example, cocaine and amphetamines are stimulants; they increase arousal, may cause anxiety, and at lower doses enhance cognitive performance. Alcohol is a depressant, is anxiolytic at low doses, and degrades cognitive performance. Heroin and other opiates are analgesic and cause drowsiness, constipation, and pupillary constriction. The shared behavioral effect of all addictive drugs is the liability, in vulnerable individuals, of causing compulsive use. The shared pharmacologic property that is required to cause addiction is the ability to increase levels of synaptic dopamine in the forebrain. For example, cocaine blocks the dopamine uptake transporter (DAT) that normally clears dopamine from synapses. Amphetamines cause reverse transport of dopamine into synapses through the DAT. Opiates, nicotine, alcohol, and cannabinoids cause dopamine release, acting by different initial mechanisms to release VTA neurons from resting inhibitory control.

Natural rewards, such as food or sexual opportunities, regulate the firing of dopamine neurons through highly processed sensory information, both external and interoceptive. Addictive drugs short-circuit this kind of information processing by acting directly on receptors and cells that regulate VTA dopamine neurons. Acting by such direct pharmacologic mechanisms, addictive drugs may produce greater quantities of synaptic dopamine over longer times than natural rewards. In addition, addictive drugs provide a grossly pathologic learning signal by occluding pauses in dopamine neuron firing even when drug use proves less pleasurable than expected or even aversive. For example, when the inhalation of a smoker causes painful coughing, it might seem that the brain would signal an experience that is worse than expected with a resulting decrement in VTA neuron firing rate. Because, however, nicotine causes dopamine release pharmacologically, independent of the smoker's actual experience, forebrain circuits, unavailable to conscious introspection, still receive a positive message that reinforces nicotine seeking and nicotine use. In short, addictive drugs, by virtue of their effects on dopamine, always signal "better than expected."

DRUG-INDUCED NEURAL PLASTICITY RELEVANT TO ADDICTION

In recent years, much neurobiologic research on addiction has focused on compulsive aspects of drug use, the ability of specific cues to activate drug seeking and craving, and the long persistence of stress and cue-dependent relapse risk. As described previously, compulsive drug use and the power of drug-associated cues reflect the usurpation of brain reward circuitry by drugs that directly cause dopamine release. The persistence of addiction reflects long-term changes in neurons, synapses, and circuits. Research over more than a decade has identified long-term changes in gene expression resulting from use of addictive drugs; recently, some long-lived alterations in gene expression have been attributed to drug-induced epigenetic mechanisms such as modification of chromatin.

Long-term changes in gene expression may render the addicted person susceptible to stress and may also create persistent changes in hedonic state and mood regulation that may motivate drug taking. By themselves, however, changes in gene expression do not explain the ability of exquisitely specific cues to activate drug seeking or, if seeking is impeded, intense subjective drug craving. The ability of specific cues to activate drug seeking and wanting is based on long-term associative memories consolidated under the influence of dopamine. Long-term memory formation represents perhaps the most persistent changes in brain function that may occur in adult life. The neural substrates of memory likely include alterations in synaptic weights, such as long-term potentiation (LTP) or long-term depression (LTD), and physical remodeling of dendritic spines.

The centrality of associative learning mechanisms for addiction was first recognized from clinical observation: much drug taking, and most notably late relapses, follows exposure to cues previously associated with drug use. Cues that can reinitiate drug use include environmental stimuli (e.g., persons with whom drugs have been used, drug paraphernalia) and bodily feelings. Because addictive drugs reliably increase synaptic dopamine as a result of their direct pharmacologic actions—indeed, they produce an excessive and grossly distorted dopamine signal—the brain receives a powerful impetus to connect the circumstances in which the drugs have been used with the motivation to take drugs again. Even if the drug is no longer pleasurable, the

release of dopamine continues to reinforce drug wanting and seeking. Moreover, the reliability and quantity of dopamine release give drugs a marked advantage over natural rewards and other learned goals, including prosocial goals.

In the laboratory, it has been possible to study the effects of drug cues on neural circuits, physiology, and subjective responding in addicted human subjects. For example, drug-associated cues have been shown to elicit drug urges and physiologic responses (such as sympathetic activation), as well as activation of reward circuits in addicted human subjects. Using PET, cocaine-related cues have been shown to elicit dopamine release in the dorsal striatum in addicted subjects.

Investigations at the cellular and molecular levels have begun to identify the physiologic and molecular changes that underlie the effects of addictive drugs on reward-related memory processes. Among psychotropic drugs that have been examined, only those drugs that can cause addiction produce LTP in brain reward circuits including the VTA. Addictive drugs also activate transcription factors such as the cyclic adenosine monophosphate response element binding protein (CREB) and to alter the composition of activator protein 1 (AP-1) complexes in brain reward circuits. Dopamine and cocaine have been shown to regulate many genes downstream of CREB, AP-1, and other transcription factors. It has proved challenging, however, to determine which drug-regulated proteins are causally involved in addiction, as opposed to other processes such as physiologic dependence and withdrawal, or have no critical role at all. Part of the challenge is that while rodent models, including transgenic mouse models, have provided many insights into drug action and behavior, it is difficult to model human compulsion in animals, that is, to model a free-living and independent person who loses control over drug use while experiencing the negative consequences of that use. That said, a great body of detail is beginning to emerge about the neural processes that produce addiction.

SUGGESTED READINGS

Dagher A, Robbins TW. Personality, addiction, dopamine: insights from Parkinson's disease. *Neuron.* 2009;61:502-510. *Administration of dopamine agonists to patients with Parkinson's disease provides compelling new insight into the role of dopamine in addiction and into the biology of behavioral addictions.*

Haberstick BC, Zeiger JS, Corley RP, et al. Common and drug-specific genetic influences on subjective effects to alcohol, tobacco and marijuana use. *Addiction.* 2011;106:215-224. *Review.*

Hyman SE, Malenka RC, Nestler EJ. Neural mechanisms of addiction: the role of reward-related learning and memory. *Annu Rev Neurosci.* 2006;29:565-598. *Reviews behavioral and neurobiologic evidence that addictive drugs usurp normal systems underlying reward-related memory.*

Khokhar JY, Ferguson CS, Zhu AZ, et al. Pharmacogenetics of drug dependence: role of gene variations in susceptibility and treatment. *Annu Rev Pharmacol Toxicol.* 2010;50:39-61. *Reviews the genetic risk factors for drug addiction.*

Koob G. A role for brain stress systems in addiction. *Neuron.* 2008;59:11-14. *Reviews the role of stress and especially of corticotrophin releasing hormone in addictive disorders.*

31

NICOTINE AND TOBACCO

TONY P. GEORGE

DEFINITIONS

Cigarette smoking is the most common method of tobacco use (>90%), although other forms, including pipe tobacco, cigars, and smokeless tobacco, are common as well. Nicotine is the active ingredient that functions to reinforce tobacco addiction in all forms of tobacco.

EPIDEMIOLOGY

Cigarette smoking is the most preventable cause of morbidity and mortality in the Western world. In the United States, approximately 20% of the population uses tobacco, compared with 47% in 1965. Since the release of the surgeon general's report in 1965, smoking prevalence has been substantially reduced, but this reduction appears to have slowed in recent years, likely because the remaining smokers are refractory to tobacco treatment. Approximately 450,000 people die each year in the United States as a result of smoking-attributable medical illnesses such as lung cancer, chronic obstructive pulmonary disease, cardiovascular disease, and stroke; the economic and health care costs of tobacco use exceed $400 billion annually. The use of smokeless tobacco (e.g., chewing tobacco) has increased, contributing to higher rates of oral pathologies such as precancerous oral lesions and cancers of the mouth and nasopharynx. Moreover, the health risks of environmental tobacco smoke have become increasingly clear, prompting widespread tobacco bans in public settings.

Worldwide, it is estimated that approximately 1.1 billion people use tobacco on a regular basis, including approximately 65 million in the United States. Tobacco smoking is increasing rapidly throughout the developing world, and it is estimated that cigarette smoking will cause about 450 million deaths worldwide in the next 50 years. Smoking begins at a younger age in new smokers, the rates of smoking in women are increasing, and more smokers are of a lower socioeconomic status. Reducing smoking prevalence by 50% would prevent 20 million to 30 million premature deaths in the first quarter of this century and 150 million in the second quarter.

For most smokers, quitting is the single most important thing they can do to improve their health. A recent prospective cohort study in Norway suggests that even with sustained reductions (>50%) in daily smoking consumption, there is little if any reduction in cardiovascular disease and lung or other smoking-related cancer risk, further substantiating the merits of quitting versus only reducing smoking.

PATHOBIOLOGY

Nicotine is the primary reinforcer in tobacco smoke, but more than 4000 components contribute to the sensory (non-nicotinic) aspects of cigarette smoking. The primary site of action of nicotine is the $\alpha_4\beta_2$ nicotinic acetylcholine receptor, and the endogenous neurotransmitter acting on this receptor is acetylcholine. Nicotinic acetylcholine receptors in the central nervous system are pentameric ion channel complexes comprising two α and three β subunits; the eight α subunits are designated α_2 through α_9, and the three β subunits are designated β_2 through β_4. This produces considerable diversity in subunit combinations, which may explain in part the region-specific and functional selectivity of nicotine's effects in the central nervous system. Activation of nicotinic acetylcholine receptors leads to Na^+/Ca^{2+} ion channel fluxes and neuronal membrane depolarization. The receptors are located presynaptically on several neurotransmitter-secreting neuron types in the central nervous system, including mesolimbic dopaminergic (DA) neurons that project from the ventral tegmental area to the nucleus accumbens. Activation of the nicotinic acetylcholine receptors on mesolimbic DA neurons leads to dopamine secretion in the nucleus accumbens.

At low concentrations of nicotine, $\alpha_4\beta_2$ nicotinic acetylcholine receptor stimulation of afferent GABAergic projections onto mesoaccumbal DA neurons predominates, leading to reduced mesolimbic DA neuron firing and dopamine release. At higher nicotine concentrations, $\alpha_4\beta_2$ nicotinic acetylcholine receptors desensitize, and activation of α_7 nicotinic acetylcholine receptors on glutamatergic projections predominates, leading to increased mesolimbic DA neuron firing and release. Within milliseconds of activation by nicotine, nicotinic acetylcholine receptors desensitize; after overnight abstinence, they resensitize. This may explain why most smokers report that the first cigarette in the morning is the most satisfying. Interestingly, recent positron emission tomography neuroimaging studies have shown that two to three puffs on a cigarette saturate the nicotinic acetylcholine receptors in the brain reward system, suggesting that although binding to these central receptors is an important first step in the effects of nicotine, it does not fully explain continued smoking behaviors.

CLINICAL MANIFESTATIONS

Although there is a subset of cigarette smokers who do not smoke every day, most smokers are daily users and have some degree of physiologic dependence on nicotine. Smokers typically describe a "rush" and feelings of alertness, relaxation, and satisfaction when smoking, and it is well known that nicotine has both stimulating and anxiolytic effects, depending on the basal level of arousal. Airway stimulation is an important aspect of smoking behavior, and additives such as menthol enhance the experience by increasing the taste and reducing the harshness of smoked tobacco.

Interestingly, the positive effects of cigarette smoking (e.g., taste, satisfaction) appear to be mediated by non-nicotine components of tobacco such as tar. Besides positive reinforcement, withdrawal, and craving, there are several secondary effects of nicotine and tobacco use that may contribute to both the maintenance of smoking and smoking relapse, including mood modulation (e.g., reduction of negative affect), stress reduction, and weight control. In

addition, conditioned cues can elicit the urge to smoke even after prolonged periods of abstinence. Specific effects might be particularly relevant to smokers wishing to lose weight and those with psychiatric disorders (mood modulation, cognitive enhancement, stress reduction). These secondary effects may present additional targets for pharmacologic intervention in certain subgroups of smokers (e.g., schizophrenic, depressed, or weight-concerned smokers).

DIAGNOSIS

Nicotine dependence is established clinically by historical documentation of daily smoking (typically 10 to 40 cigarettes/day) for several weeks, evidence of tolerance (e.g., lack of adverse effects of nicotine, such as nausea), and the presence of symptoms of nicotine withdrawal upon smoking cessation. These withdrawal symptoms, which peak within 12 to 24 hours of cessation, include dysphoria, anxiety, irritability, decreased heart rate, insomnia (waking in the middle of the night), increased appetite, and craving for cigarettes. In addition, most dependent smokers state that they smoke their first cigarette of the day within 5 minutes of awakening. Timeline follow-back procedures and smoking diaries have been used successfully to monitor smoking consumption over time. Scales such as the Fagerstrom Test for Nicotine Dependence allow an assessment of the level of nicotine dependence, with a score of 4 or greater (on a scale of 0 to 10) consistent with physiologic dependence. Nicotine craving and withdrawal can be reliably monitored with validated scales such as the Tiffany Questionnaire for Smoking Urges and the Minnesota Nicotine Withdrawal Scale. These scales have excellent test-retest reliability and internal consistency in smokers with schizophrenia when compared with nonpsychiatric control smokers, suggesting that they can be used in psychiatric populations.

TREATMENT   Rx

Psychosocial Treatments

Behavioral therapies (Table 31-1) are based on the theory that learning processes operate in the development, maintenance, and cessation of smoking. Behavioral treatments for smoking can facilitate the motivation to quit, emphasize the social and contextual aspects of smoking, and enhance overall success at smoking cessation. In most reviews, 6-month quit rates with behavioral therapies are 20 to 25%, and behavioral therapy typically increases quit rates up to twofold over standard medical advice. The primary goals of behavioral therapies in the treatment of tobacco dependence are to provide smokers with the necessary skills to help them quit smoking and avoid smoking in high-risk situations.

Brief Interventions

Brief interventions can increase the rate of smoking cessation and are strongly endorsed in the latest Department of Health and Human Services Guidelines on Tobacco Dependence Treatment. It is recommended that physicians use the five As with all patients: ask patients if they smoke, advise patients to quit, assess patients' level of motivation to quit, assist with attempts to quit, and arrange follow-up contacts. Providing self-help material is a form of brief intervention used to increase the motivation to quit and impart smoking cessation skills. Several recent studies have documented that minimal behavioral interventions such as community support groups, telephone counseling, and computer-generated tailored self-help materials can augment smoking cessation rates in controlled settings.

Motivational Interventions

The goal of motivational interviewing interventions is to elicit change by addressing ambivalence, increasing the patient's intrinsic motivation for change, and creating an atmosphere of acceptance in which patients take responsibility for making change happen. Brief motivational interventions have been developed for smoking cessation, and there is some evidence of increased smoking cessation using such techniques.

Cognitive-Behavioral Therapies

In cognitive-behavioral therapy, patients learn to identify situations in which they are likely to smoke and then plan to cope with these situations using behavioral (e.g., substitution of behavior) and cognitive (e.g., challenging thoughts) techniques. Some degree of efficacy has been observed in smokers using both individual and group counseling formats.

Relapse-Prevention (Coping Skills) Therapies

A large number of smokers relapse within 6 months of quitting. Focusing on relapse-prevention skills, including recognizing high-risk situations and coping with lapses, can be included in initial smoking cessation treatment or after a quit attempt.

Pharmacologic Treatments

Three classes of smoking cessation pharmacotherapies—nicotine replacement therapies (NRTs), sustained-release bupropion, and varenicline (Table 31-2)—have been approved by the Food and Drug Administration (FDA). Other off-label and novel medications are also discussed in this section.

Nicotine Replacement Therapies

The goal of NRT is to alleviate tobacco withdrawal, which allows smokers to focus on habit and conditioning factors when attempting cessation. After smoking cessation, NRT is gradually reduced so that minimal withdrawal occurs. NRTs rely on systemic venous absorption and thus do not produce the rapid high levels of arterial nicotine achieved when cigarette smoke is inhaled. Thus, individuals are unlikely to become addicted to NRTs. NRTs should be discontinued if the person restarts smoking, although safety concerns regarding smoking while using a nicotine patch appear to be less serious than previously thought. All commercially available forms of NRT are effective and increase quit rates by approximately 1.5- to 2.5-fold compared with placebo.[1] The transdermal patch, gum, and lozenge are sold over the counter (OTC); the nasal spray and inhaler require a prescription.

Nicotine Gum

Nicotine ingested orally is extensively metabolized on the first pass through the liver. Nicotine polacrilex gum avoids this problem through buccal absorption. Nicotine gum, which was approved as an OTC medication in the United States in 1996, contains 2 or 4 mg of nicotine that is released from a resin by chewing. Nicotine gum should be administered by scheduled dosing (e.g., 1 piece of 2-mg gum/hour). The original recommended duration of treatment was 3 months, but many experts believe longer treatment is more effective. Nicotine absorption peaks 30 minutes after beginning to chew the gum. Venous nicotine levels from 2- and 4-mg gum are about one third and two thirds, respectively, of the steady-state nicotine levels (i.e., between cigarettes) achieved with cigarette smoking. Nicotine delivered by cigarettes is absorbed directly into the pulmonary arterial circulation. Thus, arterial levels from smoking are 5 to 10 times higher than those from the 2- and 4-mg gums. Absorption of nicotine in the buccal mucosa is decreased by an acidic environment, so patients should not drink beverages (e.g., coffee, soda, juice) immediately before, during, or after nicotine gum use.

Several placebo-controlled trials established the safety and efficacy of nicotine gum for smoking cessation.[1] There appears to be some evidence to support the use of higher doses of nicotine gum (4-mg pieces) in more highly dependent cigarette smokers (≥25 cigarettes/day), which supports the idea of matching the nicotine gum dose to the smoker's dependence level. Side effects from nicotine gum are rare and include those of mechanical origin (e.g., difficulty chewing, sore jaw) or local pharmacologic origin (e.g., burning in mouth, throat irritation). Tolerance to most side effects develops over the first week, and education about proper use of the gum (e.g., not chewing too vigorously) decreases side effects.

Nicotine Lozenges

Lozenges that deliver nicotine (2- and 4-mg preparations) by buccal absorption were approved for OTC use in the United States in 2002. Lozenges offer additional nicotine replacement options for smokers and allow greater absorption of nicotine compared with nicotine gum. Mild throat and mouth irritation were reported in preliminary trials. Nicotine lozenges have shown their superiority to placebo lozenges, with a significant reduction in nicotine craving and withdrawal.[1] Furthermore, higher doses of lozenges may be more efficacious in more highly dependent smokers, suggesting that similar to nicotine gum, lozenge dose can be matched to dependence level. Interestingly, the combination of nicotine lozenge with nicotine patch may lead to the highest long-term quit rates compared with nicotine replacement monotherapies and bupropion.[2]

TABLE 31-1	BEHAVIORAL TREATMENTS FOR TOBACCO DEPENDENCE	
TREATMENT	**MECHANISM OF ACTION**	**EFFECTIVENESS RATING***
Brief interventions	Increase motivation to quit and impart cessation skills (e.g., community support, telephone counseling)	2
Cognitive-behavioral and relapse-prevention therapies	Use behavioral strategies to manage triggers; use cognitive coping strategies to target maladaptive thoughts and prevent relapse	1
Motivational interviewing	Promote patient's self-motivational statements to gain greater awareness of the problems related to smoking and increase intention to stop smoking	2

*1 = strong evidence to support efficacy; 2= moderate evidence to support efficacy; 3= little evidence to support efficacy.

TABLE 31-2	PHARMACOLOGIC TREATMENTS FOR TOBACCO DEPENDENCE	
TREATMENT	**MECHANISM OF ACTION**	**EFFECTIVENESS RATING***
NICOTINE REPLACEMENT THERAPIES†		
Gum (OTC)	Slow nicotine absorption gradually reduces nicotine craving and withdrawal	1
TNP (OTC)	Slow nicotine absorption gradually reduces nicotine craving and withdrawal	1
Lozenge (OTC)	Slow nicotine absorption gradually reduces nicotine craving and withdrawal	1
Vapor inhaler (prescription)	Fast nicotine absorption leads to stimulation of nicotinic acetylcholine receptors, which rapidly reduces nicotine craving and withdrawal	1
Nasal spray (prescription)	Fast nicotine absorption leads to stimulation of nicotinic acetylcholine receptors, which reduces craving and withdrawal	1
NON-NICOTINE PHARMACOTHERAPIES		
Bupropion SR†	Blocks re-uptake of dopamine and norepinephrine; high-affinity, noncompetitive nicotinic acetylcholine receptor antagonism reduces nicotine reinforcement, withdrawal, and craving	1
Varenicline†	Acts as partial agonist of $\alpha_4\beta_2$ nicotinic acetylcholine receptors	1
Nortriptyline	Blocks re-uptake of norepinephrine and serotonin; probably reduces withdrawal symptoms and comorbid depressive symptoms; side effects limit utility	1-2
Clonidine	α_2-Adrenoreceptor agonist reduces nicotine withdrawal symptoms	2
Mecamylamine	Noncompetitive, high-affinity nicotinic acetylcholine receptor antagonist combined with TNP reduces nicotine reinforcement, craving, and withdrawal	2
Naltrexone	Endogenous μ-opioid peptide receptor antagonist reduces nicotine craving and withdrawal in combination with TNP; may reduce alcohol use and obviate cessation-induced weight gain	3
Monoamine oxidase inhibitors	Increased monoamine levels can reduce nicotine reinforcement, withdrawal, and craving; might be helpful for smokers with comorbid mood disorders	2
Rimonabant	Endocannabinoid receptor (CB₁) antagonist; has shown efficacy in smoking cessation trials and may be particularly useful in weight-concerned smokers	2
Nicotine vaccine	Limited evidence of efficacy for smoking cessation in early human trials; may have utility in relapse prevention	2

*1 = strong evidence to support efficacy; 2 = moderate evidence to support efficacy; 3 = little evidence to support efficacy.
†Approved by the Food and Drug Administration.
OTC = over the counter; SR = sustained release; TNP = transdermal nicotine patch.

Transdermal Nicotine Patch

The four transdermal nicotine patch (TNP) formulations take advantage of the ready absorption of nicotine through the skin. Three of the patches are for 24-hour use, and one is for 16-hour use. Starting doses are 21 or 22 mg/24-hour patch and 15 mg/16-hour patch. Patches are applied daily each morning. Nicotine administered by the patches is absorbed slowly, so that on the first day, venous nicotine levels peak 6 to 10 hours after application of the patch. Thereafter, nicotine levels remain fairly steady, with a decline from peak to trough of 25 to 40% with 24-hour patches. Nicotine levels obtained with the use of patches are typically half those obtained by smoking. After 4 to 6 weeks on a high-dose patch (21 or 22 mg/24 hours or 15 mg/16 hours), smokers are tapered to a medium dose (14 mg/24 hours or 10 mg/16 hours) and then, after another 2 to 4 weeks, to the lowest dose (7 mg/24 hours or 5 mg/16 hours). Most studies suggest that abrupt cessation of the use of patches causes no significant withdrawal. The recommended treatment is usually 6 to 12 weeks, but a 24-week course may be up to 50% more effective than an 8-week course.[3]

The overall efficacy of the TNP for smoking cessation has been well documented.[1] The effects are independent of patch type, treatment duration, tapering procedures, and behavioral therapy format or intensity, although it should be noted that behavioral treatment enhances outcomes compared with TNP alone. Severe adverse events have not been associated with nicotine patches. The most common minor side effects are skin reactions (50%), insomnia and increased or vivid dreams (15% with 24-hour patches), and nausea (5 to 10%). Tolerance to these side effects usually develops within a week. Rotation of patch sites decreases skin irritation. Insomnia reported in the first week after smoking cessation appears to be due to nicotine withdrawal rather than the nicotine patch itself. A 24-hour patch can be removed before bedtime to determine whether the insomnia is due to the nicotine patch. Without treatment, insomnia usually abates after 4 to 7 days. There appears to be little risk of dependence associated with patch use; only 2% of patch users continue to use it for an extended period after a cessation trial.

Nicotine Nasal Spray

Nicotine nasal spray is a nicotine solution in a nasal spray bottle similar to those used for saline sprays. This NRT was approved for the treatment of nicotine dependence in the United States in 1996. Nasal spray delivers droplets that average about 1 mg nicotine per administration, and the patient administers the spray (10 mg/mL) to each nostril every 4 to 6 hours. This formulation produces a more rapid rise in nicotine levels than does nicotine gum; the nicotine levels produced by nicotine spray fall between those produced by nicotine gum and by cigarettes. Peak nicotine levels occur within 10 minutes, and venous nicotine levels are about two thirds of between-cigarette levels. Smokers can use the nasal spray as needed up to 30 times/day for 12 weeks. Randomized, double-blind, placebo-controlled trials of nasal spray versus placebo spray have established the safety and efficacy of nasal spray for smoking cessation.[1] These trials employed treatment for 3 to 6 months, and nicotine nasal spray led to a doubling of quit rates during active use. Differences were reduced or absent with extended follow-up, suggesting the need to continue using this agent. However, such long-term studies have not been published. Major side effects from nicotine nasal spray are nasal and throat irritation, rhinitis, sneezing, coughing, and watering eyes. Nicotine nasal spray may have some risk of dependence; prolonged use occurs in about 10% of smokers using the nasal spray, so follow-up is recommended.

Nicotine Inhaler

Cartridges (plugs) of nicotine (containing about 1 mg of nicotine each) are placed inside hollow cigarette-like plastic rods. The cartridges produce a nicotine vapor when warm air is passed through them. Absorption from a nicotine inhaler is primarily buccal rather than respiratory. More recent versions of inhalers produce a more rapid rise in venous nicotine levels compared with nicotine gum but a less rapid rise compared with nicotine nasal spray, with nicotine blood levels of about one third that of between-cigarette levels. Smokers are instructed to puff continually on the inhaler (0.013 mg/puff) during the day, and the recommended dosing is 6 to 16 cartridges daily. The inhaler is used as needed for about 12 weeks. No serious medical side effects have been reported with nicotine inhalers. Fifty percent of subjects report throat irritation or coughing. Randomized, double-blind, placebo-controlled trials have demonstrated the superiority of the nicotine inhaler to placebo inhalers for smoking cessation.[1] Results revealed a two- to threefold increase in quit rates (17 to 26%) at trial end point compared with placebo inhalers, and smaller differences at follow-up periods of 1 year or longer. These data support the short-term efficacy of inhalers in cigarette smokers, but longer-term trials are needed. There is also some modest concern about the risk of abuse, based on long-term use of the product in less than 10% of smokers.

Sustained-Release Bupropion

Bupropion, a phenylaminoketone atypical antidepressant agent, in the sustained-release (SR) formulation (Zyban), is a non-nicotine first-line pharmacologic treatment for nicotine-dependent smokers who want to quit. The mechanism of action in the treatment of nicotine dependence likely involves dopamine and norepinephrine reuptake blockade, as well as antagonism of high-affinity nicotinic acetylcholine receptors. The exact mechanism by which bupropion exerts antismoking effects is unclear. The goals of bupropion therapy are smoking cessation, reduction of nicotine craving and withdrawal symptoms, and prevention of cessation-induced weight gain.

The target dose of this agent in nicotine-dependent patients is 300 mg daily (150 mg twice a day). It is typically started 7 days before the target quit date (TQD) at 150 mg daily, then increased to 150 mg twice a day after 3 to 4 days. Unlike NRTs, there is no absolute requirement that smokers completely cease smoking by the TQD, although many smokers report a significant reduction in the urge to smoke and cravings, which facilitates cessation at the TQD when drug levels reach steady-state plasma levels. Some smokers gradually reduce their cigarette smoking over several weeks before quitting completely.

A pivotal multicenter study established the efficacy and safety of bupropion SR for the treatment of nicotine dependence, which led to its FDA approval in 1998. In a 7-week double-blind, placebo-controlled multicenter trial, four doses of bupropion SR (0, 100, 150, and 300 mg/day in twice-a-day dosing), in combination with weekly individual cessation counseling, were prescribed to 615 cigarette smokers using at least 15 cigarettes/day. At 1-year follow-up, cessation rates were 12.4%, 19.6%, 22.9%, and 23.1%, respectively. Bupropion SR treatment dose-dependently reduced weight gain associated with smoking cessation and significantly reduced nicotine withdrawal symptoms at doses of 150 and 300 mg/day.

Subsequently, the efficacy of combined bupropion SR and TNP was studied in a double-blind, placebo-controlled, randomized multicenter trial. A total of 893 cigarette smokers, using at least 15 cigarettes/day, were randomized to one of four experimental groups: (1) placebo bupropion + placebo patch; (2) placebo bupropion + TNP; (3) bupropion (300 mg/day) + placebo patch; or (4) bupropion + TNP. Cessation rates at the 1-year follow-up assessment were 15.6%, 16.4%, 30.3%, and 35.5% respectively. The bupropion groups did significantly better than the placebo and TNP alone groups, but the combination of bupropion and TNP was not significantly better than bupropion alone. Weight suppression after cessation was most robust in the combination therapy group.

Finally, a randomized, controlled trial demonstrated the efficacy of bupropion SR in relapse prevention after smoking cessation.[4] In individuals who had quit smoking with 7 weeks of bupropion (300 mg/day) treatment, bupropion SR versus placebo for 12 months delayed smoking relapse and resulted in weight gain.

Common side effects reported with bupropion administration in cigarette smokers are headache, nausea and vomiting, dry mouth, insomnia, and activation, most of which occur during the first week of treatment. The main contraindication for the use of bupropion is a past history of seizures of any cause. The rates of de novo seizures are low with this agent (<0.5%) at doses of 300 mg/day or less, but they have been observed when daily dosing exceeds 450 mg/day.

Varenicline

Varenicline tartrate (Chantix in the United States; Champix in Europe and Canada), a partial $\alpha_4\beta_2$ nicotinic acetylcholine receptor agonist, was approved as a first-line smoking cessation agent in the United States in 2006 and in Canada and Europe in 2007. The initial phase II trials of varenicline established its safety and efficacy in comparison to placebo and suggested an optimal dose of 2 mg/day.[5] Two independent but identical 12-week phase III trials comparing varenicline (2 mg/day) to bupropion SR (300 mg/day) were then conducted.[6,7] The quit rates for both studies were similar for continuous abstinence over the last 4 weeks (weeks 9 to 12) of the study. For study 1, the quit rates were as follows: varenicline, 43.9%; bupropion SR, 29.8%; and placebo, 17.6%.[6] For study 2, they were varenicline, 44.0%; bupropion SR, 29.5%; and placebo, 17.7%.[7] Quit rates were significantly higher for participants taking varenicline compared with bupropion SR, and both drugs resulted in significantly higher quit rates than placebo. Continuous abstinence over the follow-up period (weeks 9 to 52) was lower, but participants taking varenicline continued to show a higher rate of abstinence than those taking bupropion and placebo. Varenicline is also more effective in smoking relapse prevention compared with placebo.[8]

Varenicline reduces tobacco cravings and smoking satisfaction and is generally well tolerated. The most common adverse events reported in the initial studies were nausea and insomnia. Since the drug's approval, however, concerns have arisen over treatment-emergent neuropsychiatric events, including agitation, suicidal and homicidal ideation, mania, and psychosis. Thus, close monitoring of smokers, especially those with a history of psychiatric illness, is strongly advised when prescribing this agent.

Off-Label Medications

Other medications (see Table 31-2) have demonstrated some efficacy for tobacco treatment but are not approved for this indication and should be considered second-line treatments.

Novel Medications on the Horizon: Cannabinoid Antagonists and Nicotine Vaccines

Two novel pharmacologic strategies not yet approved in the United States may offer some additional strategies for smoking cessation and smoking relapse prevention. The cannabinoid receptor (CB_1) antagonist rimonabant demonstrated promising results in clinical trials in the United States and Europe; at the 20 mg/day dose, it doubled the chance of quitting compared with placebo. Most notably, it potently suppresses smoking cessation–related weight gain. Side effects, which include nausea, vomiting, and tremors, are dose dependent. Unfortunately, rimonabant was not approved for smoking cessation by the FDA and was recently withdrawn as a pharmacologic treatment for obesity by the European Medications Agency owing to safety concerns related to the emergence of clinical depression. Trials with other CB_1 antagonists are in progress.

Nicotine vaccines are being developed by a number of companies. They appear to be well tolerated and enhance smoking cessation rates. Higher abstinence rates are observed as a function of higher serum antibody titers. The nicotine vaccine also shows promise for the prevention of smoking initiation or relapse and will likely be tested for these indications. Side effects include soreness at the injection site and hypersensitivity reactions to vaccine components.

PREVENTION

Tobacco dependence remains one of the leading preventable causes of morbidity and mortality in the Western world. Although smoking cessation therapies are among the most cost-effective and proven therapies in medicine, most health care providers do not identify tobacco use in their patients. The U.S. Public Health Service recently published updated clinical practice guidelines for nicotine dependence that provide standards for the treatment of tobacco dependence. In addition, effective tobacco policies such as state taxes and prevention efforts targeted at reducing the initiation of tobacco use by youths and adults are critical elements in the overall strategy to reduce the burden of tobacco-related disease and related social and health care costs.

PROGNOSIS

The prognosis for tobacco smokers who quit is excellent in terms of years of life and quality of life gained. Bans on smoking in public places can reduce local rates of acute myocardial infarction by about 17%.

Although medications and behavioral treatments have documented efficacy in treating tobacco dependence, these therapies must be used in combination to achieve the best overall results and ensure adequate skill acquisition and treatment adherence. Novel treatment and prevention interventions, such as the nicotine vaccine and the employment of personalized medicine—matching the right medications to smokers with preferential responses using pharmacogenetic approaches—are generating considerable excitement in the tobacco treatment field and may be available within the next decade. Further, given the high rates of tobacco use and dependence in psychiatric populations and the lower rates of quitting in this subset of smokers compared with the general population, the specific adaptation of tobacco treatments to mentally ill smokers will be of paramount importance in improving prognosis and outcome in these hard-to-treat smokers. Additional future challenges include developing safer and more effective smoking cessation therapies and making these therapies available to all smokers who wish to quit.

Grade A

1. Silagy C, Lancaster T, Stead L, et al. Nicotine replacement therapies for smoking cessation. *Cochrane Database Syst Rev.* 2004;3:CD000146.
2. Piper ME, Smith SS, Schlam TR, et al. A randomized placebo-controlled clinical trial of 5 smoking cessation pharmacotherapies. *Arch Gen Psychiatry.* 2009;66:1253-1262.
3. Schnoll RA, Patterson F, Wileyto EP, et al. Effectiveness of extended-duration transdermal nicotine therapy: a randomized trial. *Ann Intern Med.* 2010;152:144-151.
4. Hays JT, Hurt RD, Rigotti NA, et al. Sustained-release bupropion for pharmacologic relapse-prevention after smoking cessation: a randomized, controlled trial. *Ann Intern Med.* 2001;135:423-433.
5. Oncken C, Gonzales D, Nides M, et al. Efficacy and safety of the novel selective nicotinic acetylcholine receptor partial agonist, varenicline, for smoking cessation. *Arch Intern Med.* 2006;166:1571-1577.
6. Gonzales D, Rennard SI, Nides M, et al. Varenicline, an alpha$_4$ beta$_2$ nicotinic acetylcholine receptor partial agonist, vs. sustained release bupropion and placebo for smoking cessation. *JAMA.* 2006;296:47-55.
7. Jorenby DE, Hays JT, Rigotti NA, et al. Efficacy of varenicline, an alpha$_4$ beta$_2$ nicotinic acetylcholine receptor partial agonist, vs. placebo or sustained release bupropion for smoking cessation. *JAMA.* 2006;296:56-63.
8. Tonstad S, Tonnesen P, Hajek P, et al. Effect of maintenance therapy with varenicline on smoking cessation. *JAMA.* 2006;296:64-71.

SUGGESTED READINGS

Hamer M, Stamatakis E, Kivimaki M, et al. Objectively measured secondhand smoke exposure and risk of cardiovascular disease: what is the mediating role of inflammatory and hemostatic factors? *J Am Coll Cardiol.* 2010;56:18-23. *Secondhand smoke elevates the CRP level, which accounts for about 50% of its effect on increasing the risk of cardiovascular disease.*

Piano MR, Benowitz NL, Fitzgerald GA, et al. Impact of smokeless tobacco products on cardiovascular disease: implications for policy, prevention, and treatment: a policy statement from the American Heart Association. *Circulation.* 2010;122:1520-1544. *Policy statement emphasizing their risks.*

Strand BH, Mishra G, Kuh D, et al. Smoking history and physical performance in midlife: results from the British 1946 birth cohort. *J Gerontol A Biol Sci Med Sci.* 2010;66:142-149. *Lifetime cigarette pack years are strongly related to poorer midlife physical performance.*

32

ALCOHOL ABUSE AND DEPENDENCE

PATRICK G. O'CONNOR

DEFINITION

A variety of terms have been used to describe the spectrum of medical, psychological, behavioral, and social problems associated with excessive consumption of alcohol (*alcohol problems*). *Alcoholism* is perhaps the most widely used term to describe patients with alcohol problems. In an attempt to define *alcoholism* more precisely, a panel of 23 experts convened by the National Council on Alcoholism and Drug Dependence and the American Society of Addiction Medicine developed a definition of alcoholism that included "a primary chronic disease with genetic, psychosocial and environmental factors . . . often progressive and fatal . . . characterized by impaired control over drinking, preoccupation with the drug alcohol, use of alcohol despite future consequences, and distortions of thinking, most notably denial." Because the term *alcoholism* is so broad, it also can be imprecise in defining the entire spectrum of alcohol problems.

Abstainers are individuals who consume no alcohol. *Moderate drinking* is defined by the National Institute on Alcohol Abuse and Alcoholism as the average number of drinks consumed daily that places an adult at low risk for alcohol problems. There is some epidemiologic evidence to suggest that moderate drinking may have some health benefits by reducing the risk of cardiovascular disease (Chapter 51). The scope of alcohol consumption that imparts this benefit may be low, however (e.g., less than one drink per day).

At-risk drinking is a level of alcohol consumption that imparts health risks (Table 32-1). This category of drinking behavior has been identified on the

TABLE 32-1   TERMS AND CRITERIA FOR PATTERNS OF ALCOHOL USE

AT-RISK DRINKING

Men: >14/week or >4 drinks/day
Women: >7/week or >3 drinks/day

ALCOHOL ABUSE

Maladaptive pattern of alcohol use leading to clinically significant impairment or distress, manifested within a 12-month period by one or more of the following:
    Failure to fulfill role obligations at work, school, or home
    Recurrent use in hazardous situations
    Legal problems related to alcohol
    Continued use despite alcohol-related social or interpersonal problems
Symptoms have never met criteria for alcohol dependence

ALCOHOL DEPENDENCE

Maladaptive pattern of alcohol use leading to clinically significant impairment or distress, manifested within a 12-month period by three or more of the following:
    Tolerance (either increasing amounts used or diminished effects with the same amount)
    Withdrawal (withdrawal symptoms or use to relieve or avoid symptoms)
    Use of larger amounts for a longer period than intended
    Persistent desire or unsuccessful attempts to cut down or control use
    Great deal of time spent obtaining, using, or recovering from use
    Important social relationships, occupations, or recreational activities given up or reduced
    Use despite knowledge of alcohol-related physical or psychological problems

basis of epidemiologic evidence that certain threshold levels of alcohol consumption are associated with increased risk of specific health problems. At-risk drinking is defined differently for men younger than 65 years than for women of all ages because of generally lower body weights and lower rates of metabolism of alcohol in women; the definition in men older than 65 years is the same as in women because of the age-related increased risk of alcohol problems, in part due to changes in alcohol metabolism in older individuals. *Binge drinking* or *heavy drinking* is the episodic consumption of large amounts of alcohol, usually five or more drinks per occasion for men and four or more drinks per occasion for women. One standard drink contains 12 g of pure alcohol, an amount equivalent to that contained in 5 ounces of wine, 12 ounces of beer, or 1.5 ounces of 80-proof spirits. *Problem drinking* refers to a level of alcohol consumption that causes any problems for the patient (medical, psychiatric, behavioral, or social—*alcohol problems*).

Alcohol abuse and *alcohol dependence*, which are alcohol use disorders defined in the *Diagnostic and Statistical Manual of Mental Disorders,* 4th edition, require the presence of specific social or clinical phenomena (see Table 32-1). *Alcohol abuse* includes criteria that indicate social dysfunction or use in high-risk situations (e.g., driving). *Alcohol dependence* includes social consequences along with criteria related to physiologic aspects of dependence (e.g., tolerance, loss of control) and use despite physical or psychological problems. The distinction between *alcohol abuse* and *alcohol dependence* is important given the general need for more intensive treatment services for patients who are alcohol dependent.

EPIDEMIOLOGY

In national surveys, 64% of American adults reported that they use alcoholic beverages (liquor, wine, or beer), whereas 36% reported that they were abstinent. Among individuals who use alcohol, many experience problems because of their drinking. It has been estimated that more than $100 billion is spent by American society each year to treat alcohol use disorders and to recover the costs of alcohol-related economic losses. Excessive alcohol consumption ranks as the third leading preventable cause of death in the United States after cigarette smoking and obesity. More than 100,000 deaths per year in the United States are attributed to alcohol use disorders.

Population-based epidemiologic studies have shown that alcohol use disorders are among the most prevalent medical, behavioral, or psychiatric disorders in the general population. An epidemiologic survey of the general population in the United States documented a prevalence of alcohol abuse and dependence estimated to be between 7.4 and 9.7%. The lifetime prevalence of abuse and dependence is estimated to be even higher. Despite higher thresholds and tolerance, men are at least twice as likely as women to meet criteria for alcohol abuse and dependence by standard diagnostic survey techniques. Although sociodemographic features, such as young age, low income, and low education level, have been associated with an increased risk for problem drinking, alcohol use disorders are prevalent throughout all sociodemographic groups, and all individuals should be screened carefully. The "skid row" stereotype of the alcohol-dependent patient is much more the exception than the rule.

The prevalence of alcohol use disorders is higher in most health care settings than it is in the general population because alcohol problems often result in treatment-seeking behaviors. The prevalence of problem drinking in general outpatient and inpatient medical settings has been estimated between 15 and 40%. These data strongly support the need for physicians to screen all patients for alcohol use disorders.

PATHOBIOLOGY

Beverage alcohol contains ethanol, which acts as a sedative-hypnotic drug. Alcohol is absorbed rapidly into the blood stream from the stomach and intestinal tract. Because women have lower levels of gastric alcohol dehydrogenase, the enzyme primarily responsible for metabolizing alcohol, they experience higher blood alcohol concentrations than do men who consume similar amounts of ethanol per kilogram of body weight. The absorption of alcohol can be affected by other factors, including the presence of food in the stomach and the rate of alcohol consumption. By means of metabolism in the liver, alcohol is converted to acetaldehyde and acetate (Fig. 32-1). Metabolism is proportional to an individual's body weight, but a variety of other factors can affect how alcohol is metabolized. A genetic variation in a significant proportion of the Asian population alters the structure of an aldehyde hydrogenase isoenzyme, resulting in the development of an alcohol flush reaction, which includes facial flushing, hot sensations, tachycardia, and hypotension.

FIGURE 32-1. Ethanol metabolism. Alcohol dehydrogenase predominates at low to moderate ethanol doses. The microsomal ethanol-oxidizing system is induced at high ethanol levels of chronic exposure and by certain drugs. Aldehyde dehydrogenase inhibition (genetic or drug induced) leads to acetaldehyde accumulation.

In the brain, alcohol seems to affect a variety of receptors, including γ-aminobutyric acid (GABA), N-methyl-D-aspartate, and opioid receptors. Glycinuric and serotoninergic receptors also are thought to be involved in the interaction between alcohol and the brain. The phenomena of reinforcement and cellular adaptation are thought, at least in part, to influence alcohol-dependent behaviors. Alcohol is known to be reinforcing because withdrawal from ethanol and ingestion of ethanol itself are known to promote further alcohol consumption. After chronic exposure to alcohol, some brain neurons seem to adapt to this exposure by adjusting their response to normal stimuli. This adaptation is thought to be responsible for the phenomenon of tolerance, whereby increasing amounts of alcohol are needed over time to achieve desired effects. Although much has been learned about the variety of effects alcohol can have on various brain receptors, no single receptor site has been identified. A variety of neuropsychological disorders are seen in association with chronic ethanol use, including impaired short-term memory, cognitive dysfunction, and perceptual difficulties.

Although the brain is the primary target of alcohol's actions, a variety of other tissues have a major role in how alcohol affects the human body. Direct liver toxicity may be among the most important consequences of acute and chronic alcohol use (Chapter 155). A variety of histologic abnormalities ranging from inflammation to scarring and cirrhosis have been described. The pathophysiologic mechanism of these effects is thought to include the direct release of toxins and the formation of free radicals, which can interact negatively with liver proteins, lipids, and DNA. Alcohol also has substantial negative effects on the heart and cardiovascular system. Direct toxicity to myocardial cells frequently results in heart failure (Chapter 58), and chronic heavy alcohol consumption is considered to be a major contributor to hypertension (Chapter 67). Other organ systems that experience significant direct toxicity from alcohol include the gastrointestinal tract (esophagus, stomach), immune system (bone marrow, immune cell function), and endocrine system (pancreas, gonads).

CLINICAL MANIFESTATIONS

Alcohol has a variety of specific acute and chronic effects. The acute effects seen most commonly are alcohol intoxication and alcohol withdrawal. Chronic clinical effects of alcohol include almost every organ system.

Acute Effects
Alcohol Intoxication
After entering the blood stream, alcohol rapidly passes through the blood-brain barrier. The clinical manifestations of alcohol intoxication are related directly to the blood level of alcohol. Because of tolerance, individuals chronically exposed to alcohol generally experience less severe effects at a given blood alcohol level than do individuals who are not chronically exposed to alcohol.

The symptoms of mild alcohol intoxication in nontolerant individuals typically occur at blood alcohol levels of 20 to 100 mg/dL and include euphoria, mild muscle incoordination, and mild cognitive impairment. At higher blood alcohol levels (100 to 200 mg/dL), more substantial neurologic dysfunction occurs, including more severe mental impairment, ataxia, and prolonged reaction time. Individuals with blood alcohol levels in these ranges can be obviously intoxicated with slurred speech and lack of coordination.

These effects progress as the blood alcohol level rises to higher levels, to the point at which stupor, coma, and death can occur at levels equal to or greater than 300 to 400 mg/dL, especially in individuals who are nontolerant to the effects of alcohol. The usual cause of death in individuals with very high blood levels of alcohol is respiratory depression and hypotension.

Alcohol Withdrawal Syndrome

Alcohol withdrawal can occur when individuals decrease their alcohol use or stop using alcohol altogether. The severity of symptoms can vary greatly. Many individuals experience alcohol withdrawal without seeking medical attention, whereas others require hospitalization for severe illness. Because ethanol is a central nervous system depressant, the body's natural response to withdrawal of the substance is a hyperexcitable neurologic state. This state is thought to be the result of adaptive neurologic mechanisms being unrestrained by alcohol, with an ensuing release of a variety of neurohumoral substances, including norepinephrine. In addition, chronic exposure to alcohol results in a decrease in the number of GABA receptors and impairs their function.

The clinical manifestations of alcohol withdrawal include hyperactivity resulting in tachycardia and diaphoresis. Patients also experience tremulousness, anxiety, and insomnia. More severe alcohol withdrawal can result in nausea and vomiting, which can exacerbate metabolic disturbances. Perceptual abnormalities, including visual and auditory hallucinations and psychomotor agitation, are common manifestations of more moderate to severe alcohol withdrawal. Grand mal seizures commonly occur during alcohol withdrawal, although they do not generally require treatment beyond the acute withdrawal phase.

The time course of the alcohol withdrawal syndrome can vary within an individual and by symptom complex, and the overall duration of symptoms can be a few to several days (Fig. 32-2). Tremor is typically among the earliest symptoms and can occur within 8 hours of the last drink. Symptoms of tremulousness and motor hyperactivity typically peak within 24 to 48 hours. Although mild tremor typically involves the hands, more severe tremors can involve the entire body and greatly impair a variety of basic motor functions. Perceptual abnormalities typically begin within 24 to 36 hours after the last drink and resolve within a few days. When withdrawal seizures occur, they are typically generalized tonic-clonic seizures and most often occur within 12 to 24 hours after reduction of alcohol intake. Seizures can occur, however, at later time periods as well.

The most severe manifestation of the alcohol withdrawal syndrome is delirium tremens. This symptom complex includes disorientation, confusion, hallucination, diaphoresis, fever, and tachycardia. Delirium tremens typically begins after 2 to 4 days of abstinence, and the most severe form can result in death.

Chronic Effects

Acute manifestations, including intoxication and withdrawal, are generally stereotypical in their appearance and time course, but chronic manifestations tend to be more varied. Many patients with alcohol dependence may be without evidence of any chronic medical manifestations for many years. As time goes on, however, the likelihood that one or more of these manifestations will occur increases considerably. All major organ systems can be affected, but the primary organ systems involved are the nervous system, cardiovascular system, liver, gastrointestinal system, pancreas, hematopoietic

system, and endocrine system (Table 32-2). Patients who drink are at risk for a variety of malignant neoplasms, such as head and neck, esophageal, and liver cancers (Chapters 196, 198, and 202). Excessive alcohol use often causes significant psychiatric and social morbidity that can be more common and more severe than the direct medical effects, especially earlier in the course of problem drinking.

Nervous System

In addition to the acute neurologic manifestations of intoxication and withdrawal, alcohol has major chronic neurologic effects. About 10 million Americans have identifiable nervous system impairment from chronic alcohol use. Individual predisposition to these disorders is highly variable and is related to genetics, environment, sociodemographic features, and gender; the relative contribution of these factors is unclear.

In the central nervous system, the major effect is cognitive impairment. Patients may present with mild to moderate short-term or long-term memory problems or may have severe dementia resembling Alzheimer's disease (Chapter 409). The degree to which the direct toxic effect of alcohol is responsible for these problems or the impact of alcohol-related nutritional deficiencies is uncertain (Chapter 425). The deficiency of vitamins such as thiamine may play a major role in promoting alcoholic dementia and severe cognitive dysfunction, as is seen in Korsakoff's syndrome. Alcohol also causes a polyneuropathy that can present with paresthesias, numbness, weakness, and chronic pain (Chapters 425 and 428). As with the central nervous system, peripheral nervous system effects are thought to be caused by a combination of the direct toxicity of alcohol and nutritional deficiencies. A small proportion (<1%) of patients with alcohol dependence may develop midline cerebellar degeneration, which presents as an unsteady gait.

Cardiovascular System

The most common cardiovascular complications of chronic alcohol consumption are cardiomyopathy, hypertension, and supraventricular arrhythmias. Alcoholic cardiomyopathy can present clinically in a manner similar to

TABLE 32-2	ALCOHOL-RELATED COMPLICATIONS
SYSTEM/REALM OF PROBLEM	**COMPLICATIONS**
Nervous system	Intoxication
	Withdrawal
	Cognitive impairment
	Cerebellar degeneration
	Peripheral neuropathy
Cardiovascular system	Cardiac arrhythmias
	Chronic cardiomyopathy
	Hypertension
Liver	Fatty liver
	Alcoholic hepatitis
	Cirrhosis
Gastrointestinal tract	
Esophagus	Chronic inflammation
	Malignant neoplasms
	Mallory-Weiss tears
	Esophageal varices
Stomach	Gastritis
	Peptic ulcer disease
Pancreas	Acute pancreatitis
	Chronic pancreatitis
Other medical problems	Cancers: mouth, oropharynx, esophagus
	Hepatoma
	Pneumonia
	Tuberculosis
Psychiatric	Depression
	Anxiety
	Suicide
Behavioral and psychosocial	Injuries
	Violence
	Crime
	Child or partner abuse
	Tobacco, other drug abuse
	Unemployment
	Legal problems

FIGURE 32-2. Time course of alcohol withdrawal.

other causes of heart failure (Chapter 58). It is the most common cause of nonischemic cardiomyopathy in Western countries, accounting for about 45% of cases. Like these other causes, alcoholic cardiomyopathy also responds to conventional treatments of heart failure (Chapter 59). Abstinence from alcohol can result in significant improvement in cardiomyopathy in some patients. Increasing levels of alcohol consumption also are associated with increasing levels of systolic and diastolic hypertension (Chapter 67).

The most common arrhythmias associated with chronic alcohol use include atrial fibrillation and supraventricular tachycardia; these are seen commonly in the setting of acute intoxication and withdrawal (Chapter 64). The prevalence of alcohol-induced arrhythmias is unclear. Alcoholic cardiomyopathy also is associated with arrhythmias, in particular, ventricular arrhythmias (Chapter 65).

Liver

Alcohol abuse is the major cause of morbidity and mortality from liver disease in the United States. It has been estimated that there are more than 2 million people with known alcoholic liver disease in the United States. Factors that predispose to early liver disease include the quantity and duration of alcohol exposure, female gender, and malnutrition. The range of clinical manifestations includes acute fatty liver, alcoholic hepatitis, and cirrhosis (Chapter 156). Fatty liver associated with alcohol ingestion can be asymptomatic or associated with nonspecific abdominal discomfort; it generally improves with abstinence from alcohol. Alcoholic hepatitis can present as an asymptomatic condition identified through abnormalities in liver enzymes or as an acute episode with abdominal pain, nausea, vomiting, and fever. Patients with alcoholic hepatitis have particularly high levels of aspartate aminotransferase in the blood and elevated levels of γ-glutamyltransferase. Alcoholic hepatitis typically improves with abstinence from alcohol.

Alcohol-related cirrhosis is a major cause of death in the United States (Chapter 157). Although patients are often asymptomatic, patients with more advanced cirrhosis may present with a variety of symptoms and signs, including jaundice, ascites, and coagulopathy. Cirrhosis also is associated with gastrointestinal bleeding from esophageal varices (Chapter 140). Although there is some controversy about the use of liver transplantation to treat patients with alcoholic cirrhosis, many believe that patients in established recovery are good candidates for liver transplantation (Chapter 157).

Gastrointestinal Disease

Chronic alcohol use is associated with a variety of esophageal problems, including esophageal varices, Mallory-Weiss tears, and squamous cell carcinoma of the esophagus. The risk of squamous cell carcinoma is increased further in patients who smoke tobacco and drink alcohol. Patients with these problems can present with difficulty swallowing, chest pain, gastrointestinal blood loss, and weight loss. Acute alcoholic gastritis typically presents with abdominal discomfort, nausea, and vomiting (Chapter 137).

Pancreas

The risk of pancreatitis in individuals with alcohol dependence is approximately four times that in the general population. Quantity and duration of alcohol exposure and a history of pancreatitis are predictive of future episodes. Acute alcoholic pancreatitis, which may present with severe abdominal pain, nausea, vomiting, fever, and hypotension, can be life-threatening (Chapter 146). Individuals who have recurrent acute pancreatitis may develop chronic pancreatitis, which typically presents with chronic abdominal pain, malabsorption, weight loss, and malnutrition.

Hematopoietic System

The anemia that commonly is seen in patients with chronic alcohol problems can be multifactorial (e.g., blood loss, nutrient deficiency, secondary to liver disease and hypersplenism). Studies of selected inpatients with alcohol dependence showed the prevalence of anemia to range from about 10 to 60%. Gastrointestinal blood loss due to Mallory-Weiss tears (Chapter 137), alcoholic gastritis (Chapter 134), or esophageal varices (Chapters 137 and 156) may be a key factor, and many patients develop subsequent iron deficiency. Dietary folate deficiency can be associated with megaloblastic anemias (Chapter 167). Alcohol also has a direct toxic effect on the bone marrow, which can lead to sideroblastic anemia that resolves after abstinence. Alcohol can suppress megakaryocyte production and cause thrombocytopenia, which may manifest as petechiae or bleeding (Chapter 175); the

thrombocytopenia is particularly sensitive to abstinence, with platelet counts usually rebounding or returning to normal within 5 to 7 days after cessation of alcohol intake. Alcohol also appears to interfere directly with platelet function. Alcohol-related immune dysfunction, as evidenced by decreased production and function of white blood cells and derangement in humoral and cell-mediated immunity, partly explains why alcohol-dependent individuals are at higher risk for infectious diseases, such as pneumonia and tuberculosis.

Malignant Neoplasms

Alcohol intake has been associated with upper digestive, respiratory, and liver malignant neoplasms. Alcohol use is associated with squamous cell carcinomas of the esophagus (Chapter 198) and of the head and neck (Chapter 196). The co-occurrence of alcohol and tobacco abuse seems to be synergistic. Either heavy alcohol use or smoking individually increases the rate of oropharyngeal cancer by about six or seven times that of the general population, whereas the rate for people with both risk factors is about 40 times that of the general population. Patients with alcohol-induced liver disease who also have a history of hepatitis B or C are at particularly increased risk for hepatocellular carcinoma (Chapter 202).

Chronic alcohol use also has been associated with malignant neoplasms of the breast (Chapter 204), prostate (Chapter 207), pancreas (Chapter 200), cervix (Chapter 205), lung (Chapter 197), and colon (Chapter 199). Women who have more than one or two alcoholic drinks per day may increase their breast cancer risk 1.5-fold or more. Hormonal mechanisms and direct carcinogenic effects of alcohol have been postulated as causes of this association. The association of cervical cancer with alcohol dependence may be due to alcohol-associated high-risk sexual behaviors that are thought to increase the risk of cervical cancer.

Other Medical Issues

Gout has been associated with alcohol abuse, and flares can occur at lower serum urate levels than in nonalcoholic patients (Chapter 281). Alcoholic ketoacidosis (Chapter 120), which usually follows an alcoholic binge, presents as nausea, vomiting, abdominal pain, and volume depletion. Typically, ketoacidosis is seen with low or normal glucose readings. Mild or nonspecific abnormalities in thyroid function, especially in patients with underlying liver disease, may reflect abnormalities in the clearance of thyroid-stimulating hormone or the impact of elevated circulating estrogens. Infertility and menstrual irregularities have been associated with chronic alcohol consumption, presumably due to alcohol-induced hypothalamic-pituitary dysfunction, gonadal toxicity, and impaired hepatic metabolism of circulating hormones. Hypogonadism is highly prevalent in male alcoholics with cirrhosis. Alcohol dependence also is associated with higher rates of dental and periodontal disease (Chapter 433) and with a variety of dermatologic problems, including spider angiomas and, in patients with poor hygiene, skin infestations. Both at-risk drinking and alcohol dependence have been shown to be associated with an increased risk of hospital-acquired infections, sepsis, and mortality, especially in intensive care patients.

Psychiatric Issues

Psychiatric symptoms and illnesses are exceedingly common among individuals with alcohol problems. The prevalence of anxiety disorders is about 40%, and the prevalence of affective disorders is about 30%. Antisocial personality disorder is also more common in individuals with alcohol problems than in the general population. These psychiatric problems are more prevalent during periods of heavy drinking and withdrawal. All patients with alcohol use disorders require careful screening for psychiatric illnesses. Effective treatment of underlying psychiatric disorders may result in improved drinking behaviors.

Other Behavioral and Psychosocial Issues

Alcohol commonly is the underlying cause of domestic abuse, injuries, trauma, motor vehicle crashes, and burns. Patients presenting with injuries should be questioned carefully about their alcohol use. Tobacco (Chapter 31) and other drug abuse (Chapter 33) is more prevalent in people with alcohol problems than in the general population.

DIAGNOSIS

Data from the history, physical examination, and laboratory generally are needed to provide a complete picture of the extent of alcohol problems in affected patients (Table 32-3).

TABLE 32-3   DIAGNOSIS OF ALCOHOL PROBLEMS

HISTORY

Step 1: Ask all patients about current and past use.
    Do you drink alcohol (ever or currently)?
    Do you have a family history of alcohol problems?
Step 2: Obtain detailed history regarding quantity and frequency of alcohol use.
    What types of alcohol do you consume?
    How often do you drink?
    How much do you usually drink?
    Do you ever drink more, and if so, how much?
Step 3: Standardized questionnaire
    CAGE questions:
    Have you ever felt that you should *c*ut down on your drinking?
    Have people *a*nnoyed you by criticizing your drinking?
    Have you ever felt bad or *g*uilty about drinking?
    Have you ever taken a drink first thing in the morning (*e*ye opener) to steady your
        nerves or get rid of a hangover?
Step 4: Assess specific areas in suspected or known problem drinkers.
    Criteria for alcohol abuse and dependence
    Evidence of medical and psychiatric problems
    Evidence of behavioral or social problems
    Use of other substances
        Tobacco
        Mood-altering prescription drugs
        Illicit drugs (e.g., heroin, cocaine)
    Prior alcohol or substance abuse treatment

PHYSICAL EXAMINATION

Thorough and complete examination important in all patients
Focus attention to system with identified problems
In all patients, carefully examine
    Central and peripheral nervous systems
    Cardiovascular system
    Liver
    Gastrointestinal tract

LABORATORY STUDIES (IN SELECTED PATIENTS)

Liver enzymes
Coagulation studies
Complete blood count
Carbohydrate-deficient transferrin

Discussing the Diagnosis with Patients

In discussing alcohol problems, it is crucial that physicians be sensitive to the stigma and shame that may be felt by patients with alcohol problems and by their families. Alcohol-related diagnoses or problems should be discussed in a nonjudgmental manner, which forges a partnership and indicates commitment to helping with whatever problems the patients might have. Setting the stage for the discussion should include educating patients about the various levels of alcohol problems (e.g., at-risk drinking, alcohol abuse, alcohol dependence) so that patients have an understanding of the spectrum of alcohol problems. Many patients may have a skewed view of what qualifies as problem drinking and may believe that only individuals with severe alcohol problems are truly problem drinkers. The history, physical examination, and laboratory studies should be provided as "proof" that a problem may or does exist.

History

A four-step approach to the alcohol history includes comprehensive questions about alcohol use and a thorough evaluation for alcohol-related problems.

Step 1: Ask All Patients about Current and Past Alcohol Use

A single question—Do you currently or have you ever used alcohol?—can identify quickly patients who are not lifetime abstainers and require further screening. Patients who answer yes to this question should proceed through the subsequent three steps. Patients who answer no can be classified as lifetime abstainers from alcohol and require no further questioning unless their answer changes over time. It is crucial to ask about current and past alcohol use because many patients who meet lifetime criteria for alcohol dependence but who are currently in recovery answer no to the question about current use; unless it is specifically asked about, important past use information may be missed.

Step 2: Obtain Detailed History Regarding Quantity and Frequency of Alcohol Use

A question to be asked routinely is, What type or types of alcoholic drinks (beer, wine, spirits) do you consume? Many patients do not consider the use of beer or wine "drinking." Quantity should be determined for typical use—How much do you usually drink on a typical drinking day?—and for range of use—Do you ever drink more than your usual amount, and if so, how much? This second question can be particularly important for identifying binge drinking. Quantity questions offer easy identification of at-risk drinking. Asking about the frequency of alcohol consumption—How often do you drink?—helps distinguish daily from nondaily alcohol users. Binge drinkers who drink only on weekends tend to have significant alcohol problems yet not be daily drinkers. A major goal of step 2 is to acquire a complete characterization of current alcohol use behaviors and the pattern of quantity and frequency of alcohol use during the patient's lifetime.

Step 3: Use Standardized Screening Instruments

Many standardized questionnaires have been developed to detect alcohol abuse and dependence. The two questionnaires that have been evaluated most extensively in medical settings are the CAGE (Cut down, Annoyed, Guilty, and Eye opener) questionnaire (see Table 32-3) and the Alcohol Use Disorder Identification Test (AUDIT). The CAGE questionnaire includes four questions and is scored by giving 1 point for each positive response. Given that the word *ever* is used in the CAGE questions, by definition this instrument is designed to detect lifetime alcohol problems and does not distinguish between lifetime problems and current problems. To screen for alcohol abuse and dependence, the CAGE has a sensitivity of 43 to 94% and a specificity of 70 to 97% when a cutoff score of 2 is used to indicate a "positive" result.

The AUDIT's ten questions cover the quantity and frequency of alcohol use, drinking behaviors, adverse psychological symptoms, and alcohol-related problems. It was developed by the World Health Organization to identify hazardous (e.g., at-risk) drinking and harmful (e.g., alcohol use that results in physical or psychological harm) drinking. In contrast to the CAGE questionnaire, the AUDIT focuses on recent (current to past year) drinking behaviors. Each question is scored 0 to 4 (range for total score is 0 to 40), and a total score of 8 is considered to be a positive result.

Step 4: Assess Specific Areas in Suspected or Known Problem Drinkers

Questions asked in step 4 are based on the results of the questions asked in steps 2 and 3 to obtain more detailed information in patients with potential alcohol problems. Even patients who do not screen positive on the CAGE questionnaire may warrant detailed questioning about alcohol abuse and dependence (see Table 32-1), especially if they are drinking at or above at-risk levels or there is other evidence of possible alcohol problems. A detailed review for evidence of alcohol-related medical and psychiatric problems should occur, and the need for further medical and psychiatric evaluation should be determined. The physician should look for evidence of behavioral and social problems commonly associated with alcohol use and screen for family and occupational dysfunction and other problems, such as domestic violence. Patients should be asked about their use of tobacco, mood-altering prescription medications, and illicit drugs such as heroine and cocaine.

Finally, many patients with alcohol problems have prior treatment episodes that should be detailed. The inquiry should include questions not only about formal alcohol treatment (including number of episodes, duration of treatment, and inpatient versus outpatient treatment) but also about more informal treatments, such as attendance at self-help groups like Alcoholics Anonymous (AA). For patients who require a referral for treatment, knowledge of prior treatment experience is a crucial determinant of future referral recommendations.

The National Institute on Alcohol Abuse and Alcoholism has published *Helping Patients Who Drink Too Much: A Clinician's Guide*, which provides a similar approach to screening and evaluating patients for alcohol-related problems and includes an appendix of useful supporting materials.

Physical Examination

Patients with potential alcohol use disorders require a detailed physical examination to complement the history. In addition, attention should be focused on detecting common alcohol-related problems, including the nervous system, cardiovascular system, liver, and gastrointestinal system (see Table 32-2).

Laboratory Findings

A variety of laboratory tests have been proposed to aid screening for alcoholic abuse and dependence. Aminotransferase levels, red blood cells, mean corpuscular volume, and carbohydrate-deficient transferrin, alone or in combination, are not as effective as screening questionnaires, such as the CAGE and the AUDIT.

Laboratory tests do have a role in diagnosis and assessment of patients with potential alcohol problems. Routine laboratory testing including liver enzymes (Chapter 149), bilirubin, complete blood count, and prothrombin time should be obtained in all patients with alcohol problems on a regular basis so that an appropriate and complete picture of the effects of alcohol on the individual can be obtained.

PROGNOSIS

Alcohol abuse and dependence are chronic disorders that are characterized by exacerbations and remissions. The prognosis is better for patients who seek treatment and receive it in a systematic way (Table 32-6), but it can be poor for patients with advanced liver disease and continued alcohol use. In addition, the use of combinations of medications (e.g., naltrexone plus acamprosate) is under investigation.

PREVENTION AND TREATMENT

The relationship of change in alcohol use with prevention of subsequent problems has been well established. Treatment of alcohol use disorders should be based on the severity of potential or actual alcohol problems and tailored to meet the needs of individual patients. Separate advice and management approaches are suggested for nondependent at-risk or problem drinkers compared with individuals who are alcohol dependent (Table 32-4).

Treatment of At-Risk Drinkers

Evidence confirms that generalist physicians, in a cost-effective manner, can help patients reduce their alcohol intake and prevent subsequent alcohol-related problems by using brief (5 to 20 minutes), focused counseling techniques (brief interventions) that are well suited for primary care and other medical settings. The brief counseling strategy includes four main components: motivational techniques, feedback about the problems with alcohol use, discussion of the adverse effects of alcohol, and setting recommended drinking limits. Motivational techniques are designed to motivate patients to change their alcohol use behavior by identifying potential or actual problems with which their alcohol use is associated. Feedback about these problems can

TABLE 32-4   ADVICE FOR PATIENTS WITH ALCOHOL PROBLEMS

State your medical concern:
Be specific about your patient's drinking patterns and related health risks.
Ask: How do you feel about your drinking?

Agree on a plan of action:
Ask: Are you ready to try to cut down or abstain?
Talk with patients who are ready to make a change in their drinking about a specific plan of action.

For patients who are not alcohol dependent:
Advise the patient to cut down if drinking is at or above at-risk drinking amounts (see Table 32-1) and there is no evidence of alcohol dependence.
Ask the patient to set a specific drinking goal: Are you ready to set a drinking goal? Some patients choose to abstain for a period of time or for good; others prefer to limit the amount they drink. What do you think will work best for you?
Provide patient education materials and tell the patient: It helps to think about your reasons for wanting to cut down and examine what situations trigger unhealthy drinking patterns. These materials will give you some useful tips on how to maintain your drinking goal.

For patients with evidence of alcohol dependence:
Advise to abstain if:
    Evidence of alcohol dependence
    History of repeated failed attempts to cut down
    Pregnant or trying to conceive
    Contraindicated medical condition or medication
Refer for additional diagnostic evaluation or treatment.
Procedures for patient in making referral decisions:
    Involve your patient in making referral decisions.
    Discuss available alcohol treatment services.
    Schedule a referral appointment while the patient is in the office.

make it clear to the patient that the problems exist. For at-risk and problem drinkers who do not meet criteria for alcohol dependence, setting recommended drinking limits below at-risk levels (e.g., less than one drink per day for women and less than two drinks per day for men) is a realistic and suitable goal. Epidemiologic evidence suggests that drinking below these levels is less likely to be associated with problems. Several randomized clinical trials confirm that patients who receive brief interventions significantly decrease their alcohol intake, often to "safe" levels, and can decrease health care use as well.

Treatment of Alcohol Dependence

Patients who meet criteria for alcohol dependence typically require more intensive services than do patients who meet criteria for at-risk drinking. Most patients can be managed in outpatient treatment settings, whereas patients with more severe alcohol dependence or comorbid problems initially may require inpatient management, specific counseling programs, and pharmacologic therapy. Before entering a formal program to maintain remission, many patients first require medical management of alcohol withdrawal. Professional organizations have published practice guidelines that provide useful recommendations for how to select among treatment options for patients with alcohol dependence.

Management of Alcohol Withdrawal

Many patients may not present for medical management of alcohol withdrawal and deal with it on their own. However, a substantial subset do present for alcohol withdrawal treatment. Patients with mild to moderate withdrawal generally can be managed safely as outpatients with close follow-up. Patients with moderate to severe withdrawal, as manifested by hypertension, tremor, and any mental status changes, especially patients with significant comorbid medical or psychiatric illnesses, generally are treated best as inpatients. Patients who have a history of severe withdrawal in the past (e.g., delirium tremens) or who have a history of alcohol withdrawal seizures also generally should be managed as inpatients. The three major goals of medical management of alcohol withdrawal are to minimize the severity of withdrawal-related symptoms; to prevent specific withdrawal-related complications, such as seizures and delirium tremens; and to provide referral to relapse prevention treatment.

A wide variety of medications have been evaluated for their effectiveness in managing the alcohol withdrawal syndrome (Table 32-5). Longer-acting benzodiazepines are preferred because they provide a smoother withdrawal. Shorter-acting benzodiazepines, such as oxazepam, may be indicated in individuals with severe liver disease. The most common approach is to administer a standing dose of a benzodiazepine, with additional medication being given "as needed" on the basis of withdrawal symptoms. The specific benzodiazepine and dose often depend on the experience of the prescribing physician and the characteristics of the patient, including the severity of withdrawal (higher doses are used if withdrawal is more severe), the presence of liver disease (patients with severe liver disease should receive lower doses or shorter-acting medications), and the response to prior doses of medication (higher doses are given if symptom control is inadequate; lower doses are given if adverse effects, such as oversedation, have occurred). In general, the amount of medication per dosing period is decreased gradually as the withdrawal syndrome abates. An individualized "symptom-triggered" dosing approach, in which benzodiazepines are administered on a dose-by-dose basis as guided by withdrawal symptoms, is safe and effective in certain patients and can reduce the total doses of benzodiazepines needed to treat withdrawal. β-Blockers (atenolol and propranolol), α-agonists (clonidine), and antiepileptics (carbamazepine) improve signs and symptoms of alcohol withdrawal but are viewed best as adjunctive medications to be used in addition to benzodiazepines.

Prevention of Relapse
Counseling Strategies Used by Alcohol Treatment Programs

Three commonly used psychotherapeutic techniques are motivational enhancement therapy, 12-step facilitation, and cognitive-behavioral coping skills. Two of these techniques are designed to give patients specific tools to help them avoid relapse to alcohol use. In motivational enhancement therapy, patients identify reasons for staying away from alcohol. The 12-step facilitation therapy uses the principles of AA to help patients focus their attention on abstinence. In cognitive-behavioral coping skills therapy, the patient identifies triggers to alcohol use and develops strategies to help deal with the triggers when they are present.

Project MATCH (Matching Alcohol Treatments to Client Heterogenicity) showed equivalence among three counseling approaches (cognitive-behavioral coping skills therapy, motivational enhancement therapy, or 12-step facilitation therapy) to treat alcohol dependence. At 1-year follow-up, most enrolled patients either remained abstinent or significantly decreased their alcohol use.

Self-Help Groups

Self-help groups such as AA and Rational Recovery are an important source of support and treatment for many patients with alcohol dependence. AA has

TABLE 32-5   MEDICATIONS FOR THE TREATMENT OF ALCOHOL DEPENDENCE*

MEDICATION	DOSE AND ROUTE	FREQUENCY	EFFECTS	MAJOR COMMON ADVERSE EFFECTS
ALCOHOL WITHDRAWAL				
Benzodiazepines[†]				
Chlordiazepoxide*	25-100 mg, PO/IV/IM[‡]	Every 4-6 hr	Decreased severity of withdrawal; stabilization of vital signs; prevention of seizures and delirium tremens	Confusion, oversedation, respiratory depression
Diazepam[†]	5-10 mg, PO/IV/IM[‡]	Every 6-8 hr		
Oxazepam[†]	15-30 mg, PO[‡]	Every 6-8 hr		
Lorazepam[†]	1-4 mg, PO/IV/IM[‡]	Every 4-8 hr		
β-Blockers				
Atenolol	25-50 mg, PO	Once a day	Improvement in vital signs	Bradycardia, hypotension
Propranolol	10-40 mg, PO	Every 6-8 hr	Reduction in craving	
α-Agonists				
Clonidine	0.1-0.2 mg, PO	Every 6 hr	Decreased withdrawal symptoms	Hypotension, fatigue
Antiepileptics				
Carbamazepine	200 mg, PO	Every 6-8 hr	Decreased severity of withdrawal; prevention of seizures	Dizziness, fatigue, red blood cell abnormalities
PREVENTION OF RELAPSE				
Disulfiram[†]	125-500 mg, PO	Daily	Decreased alcohol use among those who relapse	Disulfiram-alcohol reaction, rash, drowsiness, peripheral neuropathy
Naltrexone[†]	50 mg, PO 380 mg, IM	Daily Every 4 wk	Increased abstinence, decreased drinking days	Nausea, abdominal pain, myalgias-arthralgias
Acamprosate[†]	666 mg, PO	Three times a day	Increased abstinence	Diarrhea

*Most commonly used medications listed.
[†]Currently approved by U.S. Food and Drug Administration for the indication noted.
[‡]Dose and routes given for standard fixed-dose regimens, which include dose tapers over time.

TABLE 32-6   OVERVIEW OF TREATMENT APPROACH FOR PATIENTS WITH ALCOHOL PROBLEMS

Evaluate all patients
For patterns of problem alcohol use (Table 32-1)
For alcohol-related complications, if indicated (Table 32-2)
With use of data collected from history, physical examination, and laboratory testing (Table 32-3)

For at-risk and nondependent problem drinkers
Advise to decrease alcohol use to below at-risk levels (Table 32-4)
Advise patients who cannot decrease use to below at-risk levels to abstain

For patients who are alcohol dependent
Assess for need for withdrawal management medications (Table 32-5)
Refer to an alcohol treatment program
Consider medication to prevent relapse (Table 32-5)

---

the advantage of being widely available throughout the United States and is free of charge. The overall approach to treatment is based on the 12 steps for maintaining abstinence and dealing with the various effects of alcohol. AA meetings can be either "open" to anybody in the community or "closed" for active members only. The meetings vary in format, size, location, and demographic makeup. In counseling patients about attending AA, it is important for physicians to make them aware that variations in the nature of specific meetings, especially location and demographics of participants, require patients to be willing to attend more than one meeting site on a trial basis so that they find a comfortable setting.

Research of the effectiveness of AA has been limited, and there are no large controlled studies. Indirect evidence suggests, however, a significant improvement in alcohol use behaviors.

Pharmacotherapy to Prevent Relapse to Alcohol Use

The addition of medication to enhance the effectiveness of counseling therapies has been the subject of research for the past 40 years. As the neurobiology of alcohol use disorders has become more clearly understood, the potential to develop medications that may promote abstinence or decreased alcohol use has grown. Three medications—disulfiram, naltrexone, and acamprosate—are approved for the treatment of alcohol dependence in the United States[1] (see Table 32-5).

Disulfiram

Disulfiram is designed to prevent alcohol use by causing a severe adverse reaction when patients use alcohol. The disulfiram reaction, which includes flushing, nausea, vomiting, and diarrhea, is mediated by the inhibition of alcohol dehydrogenase and the resulting increase in serum levels of acetaldehyde and acetate after ingestion of alcohol. Disulfiram also affects monoamine metabolism, and the alcohol-disulfiram reaction may be related to changes in central monoamine functioning. Although disulfiram offers little benefit to most patients, it is effective in reducing alcohol intake in highly motivated patients who are supervised in an alcohol treatment program.

Naltrexone

Naltrexone is thought to decrease alcohol use by diminishing the euphorigenic effects of alcohol and by decreasing craving in alcohol-dependent patients. Randomized, placebo-controlled trials generally have shown that alcohol-dependent patients who receive naltrexone (50 mg/day) are more likely to decrease their alcohol use or remain abstinent compared with patients who receive placebo,[2] and the effects persist after discontinuation of treatment, although one randomized trial did not show benefit in male veterans with severe alcohol dependence. Although most studies of naltrexone were performed in a specialty alcohol treatment setting and observed subjects for only 10 to 12 weeks, one study demonstrated that naltrexone can be effective in primary care settings in patients who were observed for up to 34 weeks.[3] Side effects of naltrexone are infrequent, most notably self-limited nausea in about 10% of patients. Dose-related hepatotoxicity has been reported in patients treated for obesity with high-dose naltrexone (300 mg/day). Mild liver enzyme abnormalities are not a contraindication to naltrexone, but patients should be followed with repeated liver enzyme studies. Patients with acute hepatitis or liver failure should not use naltrexone. In addition to the oral naltrexone, a newer long-acting injectable form of naltrexone was approved by the U.S. Food and Drug Administration (FDA) in 2006.[4] Injectable naltrexone is typically administered at a dose of 380 mg intramuscularly every 4 weeks. Before beginning naltrexone, it is important to be sure that the patient is not opioid dependent in order to avoid a potentially severe opioid withdrawal reaction. Complete opioid abstinence for at least 7 to 10 days is recommended. Adverse reactions seen most commonly in patients who receive injectable naltrexone include injection site reactions (e.g., induration, itching) and symptoms such as nausea and headache, which are generally self-limited.

Acamprosate

Approved by the FDA in 2004, acamprosate (calcium acetylhomotaurinate) has been identified as an effective agent for treatment of alcohol dependence. The precise mechanism of action of acamprosate is uncertain, but it may be related to its effects on neuroexcitatory amino acids and the inhibitory GABA system. In a randomized, placebo-controlled clinical trial, subjects who received acamprosate were more likely to remain abstinent compared with subjects who received placebo.**5** Side effects are minimal and typically include diarrhea. Like naltrexone, acamprosate is given as an adjunctive therapy to psychological treatments for alcohol dependence.

Other Pharmacologic Approaches to Prevent Relapse

There has been much interest in evaluation of the effectiveness of combinations of drug therapies to treat alcohol dependence. One study of 160 patients suggested that the combination of naltrexone and acamprosate was more effective than either medication alone. A larger federally funded study that enrolled 1383 subjects, Project COMBINE, examined naltrexone and acamprosate alone and in combination with two different psychological therapies to see which combination of pharmacologic and behavioral therapies is most effective.**6** The behavioral therapies were medical management, which was designed to approximate counseling that can be provided in primary care and other medical settings, and combined behavioral intervention, which incorporated counseling techniques that are provided in alcohol treatment specialty settings. Results from this study demonstrated that patients receiving medical management with naltrexone, combined behavioral intervention, or both fared best, lending further support to the idea that alcohol-dependent patients can be effectively treated in primary care and other medical settings. Interestingly, acamprosate was not shown to be effective in this study.

Topiramate, a fructopyranose derivative, has been shown to be an effective treatment of alcohol dependence in randomized clinical trials at a dose of up to 300 mg/day.**7** Other medications that have shown promise include ondansetron, bromocriptine, and sodium valproate. Other drugs have shown possible benefits in patients with concurrent depression (e.g., fluoxetine) or anxiety (e.g., buspirone) or no effect (e.g., lithium).

FUTURE DIRECTIONS

To date, most studies have focused on shorter-term outcomes, from a few months to a year. It is important to understand more clearly what happens to these patients over time, especially the need for "booster sessions" to sustain improvements provided by brief interventions. Newer pharmacologic therapies may help many patients.

Grade A

1. Laaksonen E, Koski-Jannes A, Salaspuro M, et al. A randomized, multicentre, open-label, comparative trial of disulfiram, naltrexone and acamprosate in the treatment of alcohol dependence. *Alcohol Alcohol.* 2008;43:53-61.
2. Rösner S, Hackl-Herrwerth A, Leucht S, et al. Opioid antagonists for alcohol dependence. *Cochrane Database Syst Rev.* 2010;12:CD001867.
3. O'Malley SS, Rounsaville BJ, Farren C, et al. Initial and maintenance naltrexone treatment for alcohol dependence using primary care vs specialty care: a nested sequence of 3 randomized trials. *Arch Intern Med.* 2003;163:1695-1704.
4. Garbutt JC, Kranzler HR, O'Malley SS, et al, for the Vivitrex Study Group. Efficacy and tolerability of long-acting injectable naltrexone for alcohol dependence: a randomized controlled trial. *JAMA.* 2005;293:1617-1625.
5. Rösner S, Hackl-Herrwerth A, Leucht S, et al. Acamprosate for alcohol dependence. *Cochrane Database Syst Rev.* 2010;9:CD004332.
6. Anton RF, O'Malley SS, Ciraulo, DA, et al, for the COMBINE Study Research Group. Combined pharmacotherapies and behavioral interventions for alcohol dependence. The COMBINE study: a randomized controlled trial. *JAMA.* 2006;295:2003-2017.
7. Flórez G, Saiz PA, Garcia-Portilla P, et al. Topiramate for the treatment of alcohol dependence: comparison with naltrexone. *Eur Addict Res.* 2011;17:29-36.

SUGGESTED READINGS

Amato L, Minozzi S, Vecchi S, et al. Benzodiazepines for alcohol withdrawal. *Cochrane Database Syst Rev.* 2010;3:CD005063. *Benzodiazepines protect against alcohol withdrawal symptoms, especially seizure.*

Johnson BA. Medication treatment of different types of alcoholism. *Am J Psychiatry.* 2010;6:630-639. *Review.*

Minozzi S, Amato L, Vecchi S, et al. Anticonvulsants for alcohol withdrawal. *Cochrane Database Syst Rev.* 2010;3:CD005064. *Anticonvulsants have no obvious benefit for treating alcohol withdrawal.*

Saitz R. Alcohol screening and brief intervention in primary care: absence of evidence for efficacy in people with dependence or very heavy drinking. *Drug Alcohol Rev.* 2010;29:631-640. *These interventions are disappointingly ineffective.*

Schuckit MA. Alcohol-use disorders. *Lancet.* 2009;373:492-501. *Review of diagnosis and treatment, emphasizing importance of clinicians routinely screening for alcohol disorders.*

Zarkin GA, Bray JW, Aldridge A, et al. The effect of alcohol treatment on social costs of alcohol dependence: results from the COMBINE study. *Med Care.* 2010;48:396-401. *Combined pharmacotherapies and behavioral intervention are a cost-savings strategy for patients who are alcohol dependent.*

33

DRUG ABUSE AND DEPENDENCE

ROGER D. WEISS

DEFINITION

The terms *drug abuse* and *drug dependence* refer to a clinical syndrome characterized by the following statement from the fourth edition of the American Psychiatric Association's *Diagnostic and Statistical Manual of Mental Disorders*: "The essential feature of dependence is a cluster of cognitive, behavioral, and physiological symptoms indicating that the individual continues substance use despite significant substance-related problems." There is no single pathognomonic symptom that is diagnostic of drug dependence. Rather, the syndrome of drug dependence as described in the text above is a series of seven symptoms, of which the individual needs to meet three in the same 12-month period to warrant a diagnosis of dependence (Table 33-1). Several points are important to keep in mind when considering the diagnosis of drug dependence.

The criteria for the diagnosis are the same regardless of the substance used. Thus, the criteria for opioid dependence are the same as those for nicotine dependence and cocaine dependence, although different drugs are more likely to produce symptoms.

The diagnostic term *drug dependence* should only be used with people whose drug use is problematic; tolerance and physical dependence are neither necessary nor sufficient for a diagnosis of drug dependence. If someone is using legitimately prescribed medications as intended (e.g., opioids for chronic pain or benzodiazepines for panic disorder), and those medications are helping the person to function better, that person will not meet criteria for drug dependence, even if the person is tolerant to the medication and is physically dependent.

Finally, the 5th edition of the American Psychiatric Association's *Diagnostic and Statistical Manual of Mental Disorders* may no longer distinguish between abuse and dependence, using the term *substance abuse disorder* instead. However, that decision has not yet been finalized.

EPIDEMIOLOGY

Use of illicit drugs and nonmedical use of prescribed drugs is quite common. In 2009, approximately 22 million Americans reported using an illicit drug in

TABLE 33-1 DIAGNOSTIC CRITERIA FOR DRUG DEPENDENCE AND DRUG ABUSE

"A maladaptive pattern of substance use, leading to clinically significant impairment or distress."

DEPENDENCE (≥3 IN 12-MONTH PERIOD)

1. Tolerance
2. Withdrawal
3. The substance is often taken in larger amounts for a longer period than intended
4. Unsuccessful efforts or a persistent desire to cut down or to control substance use
5. A great deal of time is spent in activities necessary to obtain the substance or to recover from its effects
6. Important social, occupational, or recreational activities given up or reduced because of substance use
7. Continued substance use despite knowledge of having had persistent or recurrent physical or psychological problems that are likely to be caused or exacerbated by the substance

ABUSE (≥1 IN A 12-MONTH PERIOD)

1. Recurrent substance use resulting in failure to fulfill major role obligations at work, school, or home
2. Recurrent substance use in situations in which it is physically hazardous
3. Recurrent substance-related legal problems
4. Continued substance use despite having persistent or recurrent social or interpersonal problems caused or exacerbated by the effects of the substance

and

Never met criteria for dependence

From American Psychiatric Association. *Diagnostic and Statistical Manual of Mental Disorders*, 4th ed. Washington DC: American Psychiatric Association; 1994.

the previous month, representing approximately 9% of the population: when asked about their substance use in the past month, 17 million people reported using marijuana, 7 million reported using potentially psychoactive prescription drugs nonmedically, 2 million people used cocaine, and 1 million people used hallucinogens; in fact, 10% of youths aged 12 to 17 years reported using an illicit drug in the past month. Drug abuse produces substantial medical morbidity and mortality as well as tremendous social and economic costs.

PATHOBIOLOGY

Drug abuse and dependence are complex disorders involving the interaction between the pharmacology of a specific drug, an individual's genetic makeup, psychological strengths and weaknesses, environmental circumstances, and societal influences such as physical and perceived drug availability, legal status and cost of the drug, religious and cultural mores, and presence of alternative rewarding activities. Thus, one can conceptualize the etiology of drug abuse by employing the public health model frequently cited when studying infectious disease, that is, as an interaction among the host (i.e., the potential drug user), the agent (a specific drug in this case, as opposed to an infectious microorganism), and the environment (the person's family life, peer group, and the social, cultural, and religious attitudes toward use of that substance).

The Host

A host factor that is well known to heighten vulnerability to drug abuse problems is a positive family history of a substance use disorder, which has been shown to increase the likelihood of development of both alcohol and drug dependence. Twin studies and adoption studies have shown that both genetic and environmental factors contribute to this vulnerability, although the precise nature by which this occurs is still unknown and a subject of active research. One area of great research interest relates to whether people can be vulnerable to drug dependence in general (e.g., as a result of a risk-taking temperament or poor decision making) or whether they are at high risk to abuse particular substances (perhaps because of a highly reinforcing response to a specific drug).

Psychiatric illness and personality disorders have been shown to influence the likelihood of developing drug abuse problems. For example, the presence of conduct disorder in childhood and adolescence and antisocial personality disorder in adulthood have both been shown to predispose to subsequent drug abuse problems. Psychiatric disorders such as mood disorders are frequently found in people with drug abuse problems. However, it is important to note that the presence of these two disorders in the same person does not necessarily imply causation, even if one of the disorders manifests first.

In addition to the risk factors mentioned previously, certain individual protective factors may reduce the likelihood of an addictive disorder. Individuals who have positive familial relationships, success in academic activities, and meaningful religious affiliation have a lower likelihood of developing drug abuse problems. The fact that many people have a mixture of risk and protective factors speaks to the complex etiologic nature of drug abuse problems.

The Agent

Most drugs of abuse are inherently reinforcing; animals typically will self-administer most of the commonly abused drugs. Not all drugs are equally reinforcing in general, however, and there is a great deal of individual variation in drug preference. Some people like the stimulating effects of drugs such as cocaine and amphetamine, whereas others experience that level of stimulation as extremely uncomfortable. Some people like the relaxation induced by drugs such as marijuana and sedative-hypnotics, whereas others feel deadened and overly slowed down by these drugs. Although some people gravitate toward particular drugs of abuse because of their specific pharmacologic properties, other will use a variety of drugs indiscriminately, based on level of availability; some of these people are primarily seeking to alter their current emotional state, regardless of the direction in which it is changed. The reinforcing properties of many drugs of abuse appear to be mediated through dopaminergic pathways, although other neurotransmitters, including γ-aminobutyric acid (GABA), serotonin, and norepinephrine are also involved in mediating drug-induced reinforcement.

The Environment

The third critical factor in the development, maintenance, and (perhaps) cessation of drug abuse is the environment in which the use occurs. Drug use does not occur in a vacuum. Rather, many societal factors, including legal status, availability, price, perception of dangerousness, social desirability, peer group, and religious beliefs influence behavior relating to substance use. Drug availability is known to be a substantial influence on likelihood of substance use. For example, alcohol consumption has been shown to increase when the hours during which alcohol can be sold are extended. The restriction of alcohol availability by restricting hours of sale or by increasing its cost through taxation, in turn, reduces consumption. Illicit drugs are, of course, by definition less available than alcohol or tobacco. A major factor that influences use of these agents is the potential user's perception of the drug's safety, social cachet (or lack thereof), likelihood of incurring legal consequences, and peer group behavior. Treatment research has shown that environmental influences can have a powerful effect on drug use: studies have shown, for example, that offering an alternative positive reward (e.g., a voucher that can be exchanged for desired goods and services such as movie tickets or clothes) in response to abstaining from drugs may help drug-dependent individuals overcome their severe craving and reduce their substance use. In fact, this type of treatment approach, based on the use of motivational incentives for abstinence, has been shown to be one of the most powerful treatment interventions available for the treatment of drug dependence. The responsiveness of drug-dependent individuals to environmental contingencies demonstrates the importance of appreciating the complexity of the interaction among the individual, the drug, and the environment in the determination of drug use.

CLINICAL MANIFESTATIONS

Medical Complications Related to Drug Abuse and Dependence

Drug abuse is associated with significant medical morbidity and sometimes with mortality. Medical complications related to drug abuse are often directly related to the pharmacology of the abused agent, for example, the vasoconstrictor properties of cocaine; drug-specific complications are described later in the sections focusing on particular drugs of abuse.

In addition to these drug-specific sequelae, however, many medical complications incurred by drug-dependent patients occur not as a result of the particular drug being abused. Rather, serious complications may occur as a result of three factors that cut across many of the drugs of abuse: (1) paraphernalia, particularly unsterile needles; (2) adulterants; and (3) lifestyle issues.

Paraphernalia

Some of the most serious medical problems that occur in individuals with drug abuse and dependence occur as a result of the route of administration rather than from the actual drug being used. The use of unsterile needles, particularly if shared with other drug users, can lead to a variety of localized and systemic infections, some of which can be life-threatening. Skin infections and cellulitis are relatively common among injection drug users. Systemic infections related to needle use are often quite serious; individuals who inject drugs may develop infective endocarditis (Chapter 76). Other relatively common infections among injection drug users include hepatitis B, hepatitis C, and HIV infection.

Adulterants

Drugs that are purchased and sold illicitly are often adulterated or "cut" with other similar-looking products, with the intention of increasing the dealer's profit margin. For example, other white powdery substances are typically added to cocaine and heroin during the dealing process, to dilute their purity. Some of these adulterants can, in turn, cause medical problems. At times, these complications occur because of the combined toxicity of the adulterant and the route of administration. Thus, for example, a patient may have a granuloma in the lung or liver as a result of talc use; talc is commonly added to street heroin and can also cause difficulties in users who crush talc-containing pharmaceutical tablets (e.g., opioids) and then inject them. Other common adulterants in street drugs include quinine (frequently used with heroin) and lidocaine (often added to cocaine), but such toxic materials as strychnine and ground glass have been found in samples of street drugs, leading to serious medical sequelae.

Lifestyle Issues

Many drug-dependent patients expose themselves to multiple risks due to intoxication, participating in dangerous illegal activities, and associating with potentially violent people. As a result, these individuals experience a high rate of traumatic injuries and are at greater risk of being victims of assault, homicide, or suicide. Suicide is far more common among people with substance abuse problems than among the general population; this may be related to a combination of the effects of acute intoxication, the high prevalence of depression among drug-dependent patients, and the higher rate of antisocial personality disorder in this population, which is associated with a propensity toward impulsiveness, risk taking, and violence. Although it is well known that intoxication can lead to motor vehicle crashes, intoxication can also serve as a risk factor for becoming a victim of someone else's vehicle; one study reported that one third of pedestrians who are killed by motor vehicles have alcohol in their blood, perhaps a reflection of the combination of risk taking, poor judgment, and impaired motor coordination that can occur during periods of intoxication.

TREATMENT Rx

General Treatment Principles

Drug abuse and dependence represent a relatively heterogeneous group of disorders, based on type of drug or drugs used, frequency and amount of use, severity of medical, behavioral, and social consequences, presence and severity of comorbid medical and psychiatric illness, and motivation to change. Treatment thus requires a careful medical and psychiatric assessment, including a detailed substance use history and laboratory testing. It is often helpful to enlist the help of a family member or significant other (with the patient's permission) in obtaining historical information. Intoxication and withdrawal syndromes need to be treated acutely; longer-term treatment involves helping the patient to reduce or (ideally) abstain from substances of abuse and thus improve overall functioning.

Among the common drugs of abuse, medications with approval by the U.S. Food and Drug Administration (FDA) are only available for opioids. However, researchers are actively studying a number of compounds for the treatment of other drugs of abuse, particularly stimulants and marijuana. Behavioral treatments are critically important in the treatment of substance use disorders. A number of behavioral treatments have a substantial evidence base supporting their efficacy; these include cognitive-behavioral therapy, motivational enhancement therapy, contingency management (also referred to as *motivational incentive*) therapy, 12-step facilitation therapy, and behavioral couples therapy. In addition to professional treatment, peer support groups such as the 12-step-oriented Alcoholics or Narcotics Anonymous and non-12-step groups such as SMART Recovery can be extremely helpful in facilitating recovery from drug abuse problems.

MAJOR DRUGS OF ABUSE

Opioids

For centuries, opioids have been a core part of the medical pharmacopoeia, primarily because of their capacity to treat pain, but also because of their antitussive and antidiarrheal properties. Unfortunately, opioids are also powerful euphoriants and thus have substantial abuse liability. Although opium itself has been used for centuries, the isolation of morphine and codeine from opium in the 19th century, along with the introduction of the hypodermic needle, led to the increased prevalence of intravenous opioid use. Ironically, heroin was introduced near the end of the 19th century as a treatment for morphine addiction.

Opioids can be divided into four categories: (1) natural opium alkaloids, including opium, morphine, and codeine; (2) semisynthetic derivatives of morphine, including heroin and oxycodone; (3) synthetic opioids that are not derived from morphine, including methadone and meperidine; and (4) opioid-containing preparations such as elixir of terpin hydrate.

EPIDEMIOLOGY

Opioid dependence represents a significant public health problem and accounts for more admissions for substance use disorder treatment than any substance other than alcohol. In the past decade, there has been a shift in the epidemiology of opioid abuse, however, with a reduction in heroin use and an increase in the abuse of opioid analgesic drugs; the latter has occurred as a result of either misuse of prescription opioids or illicit use of these agents. Approximately 600,000 people reported using heroin in 2009, with 180,000 trying the drug for the first time. During the same year, over 12 million people either misused prescription opioids or used them illicitly, with 2 million doing so for the first time; opioids are currently the most commonly misused prescription drugs. Most people who use opioid analgesics in this way report that they obtained them from a friend or relative. It is thus likely that a portion of these people might, for example, have used a relative's opioid for the

treatment of a temporary painful condition such as a migraine headache. However, the number of people seeking treatment for dependence on opioid analgesics has increased dramatically in the past decade.

PATHOBIOLOGY

Opioids are readily absorbed when taken orally, intranasally, or by smoking or injection. Heroin, which is almost immediately converted to morphine in the liver, is most commonly injected but may be smoked or used intranasally.

Opioids work by binding to specific opioid receptors and then exerting their activity. Three major subtypes of opioid receptors have been identified and well described for many years. Most of the commonly abused opioids bind as agonists to the μ-receptor and typically produce the effects most commonly associated with opioids: miosis, respiratory depression, analgesia, euphoria, and drowsiness. Opioids that bind to the κ-receptor, unlike μ-receptor agonists, often produce dysphoria rather than euphoria. The other two receptors, δ- and N/OFQ-receptors, do not appear to play a known significant role in opioid dependence.

Opioid analgesics are ordinarily taken by the oral route, but they may be altered to be used through a different route of administration. This is particularly common with the extended release preparations, which may be altered by chewing the pill (facilitating a rapid release of the opioid medication) or by crushing the pill, dissolving it in water, and then injecting it or using it intranasally.

CLINICAL MANIFESTATIONS

The initial response to the administration of heroin, particularly when used intravenously, is a "rush," often described as orgasmic, lasting 30 to 60 seconds. This sensation is generally followed by a profound sense of relaxation that is sometimes referred to as being "wrapped in warm cotton." During this period, the user generally feels drowsy and may be seen to be "nodding," with mental clouding and a sense of tranquility. A reduction in respiratory rate occurs, along with miosis, reduced contractility of smooth muscle, and reduced secretions in the stomach, pancreas, and biliary tract. Thus, constipation and urinary hesitancy may occur. Itching is commonly seen during opioid intoxication. Many people experience nausea and vomiting in their initial use of opioids, although tolerance tends to develop to this effect over time. Tolerance also occurs to some other effects rather quickly, particularly the analgesic, respiratory depressant, and euphoriant properties of opioids. In contrast, relatively little tolerance occurs to constipation or to pupillary constriction. It is important to be aware, then, that miosis is a manifestation of opioid use, but it is not diagnostic of opiate overuse or intoxication.

Physical Dependence

Physical dependence on opioids leads to a characteristic withdrawal syndrome, the key signs of which include elevated heart rate and blood pressure, mydriasis, abdominal cramps, sweating, gooseflesh, rhinorrhea, lacrimation, and gastrointestinal distress, particularly diarrhea, nausea, and vomiting. Insomnia is common, particularly difficulty falling asleep; this is often the most long-lasting complaint among people who experience opioid withdrawal. Yawning, muscle twitches, and difficulty with body temperature regulation are also commonly seen. The severity of withdrawal can be highly variable, depending on the dose of opioids taken, the length of time that they have been taken, and individual factors. For short-acting opioids such as heroin and hydrocodone, the earliest stages of withdrawal typically occur approximately 6 to 12 hours after the last use. Peak symptoms tend to occur 48 to 72 hours after the last dose, and most clinical symptoms usually resolve within 7 to 10 days. For longer-acting opioids such as methadone, each of these time periods associated with withdrawal from short-acting opioids should be approximately doubled or tripled.

Other Medical Complications

The most common serious medical complications that occur from opioid use are typically related to factors other than the opioids themselves, particularly needle use and adulterants; these were discussed previously. Common medical problems among those dependent on heroin include hepatitis B, hepatitis C, infective endocarditis, talc granulomatosis, HIV infection, cellulitis, and abscesses, all typically related to needle use.

An important noninfectious complication that has been reported with opioid abuse is alteration of the cardiac conduction system, with a prolongation of the QT interval; this can lead to potentially serious arrhythmias, including torsades de pointes. This complication has been particularly noted with the long-acting opioid L-α-acetylmethadol (LAAM) and with methadone.

Chronic pain is commonly seen among opioid-dependent individuals, not just those who have received opioids for the treatment of pain. Pain can occur in opioid-dependent individuals for numerous reasons. In addition to the possibility that a chronic painful condition led to the use of opioids in the first place, those dependent on opioids are more likely to experience accidents, violence, and other forms of physical trauma that could produce chronic pain. There is also some evidence that chronic opioid use may lead to hyperalgesia, although there is some controversy regarding this issue. As with all substance use disorders, psychiatric illnesses (particularly mood disorders) are more common in opioid-dependent patients than in the general population. Moreover, it is important to note that the use of multiple drugs is extremely common in patients with opioid dependence, particularly among those using heroin. Indeed, the use of more than one drug is typically the rule rather than the exception in most substance use disorders.

TREATMENT   Rx

Opioid Withdrawal

Opioid detoxification can be accomplished by switching patients from their current drug of abuse (e.g., heroin, hydrocodone) to methadone or buprenorphine and then tapering that medication. Although the details of accomplishing this vary, one method commonly used in hospital settings is to administer methadone 10 mg orally whenever a patient experiences objective signs of opioid withdrawal (e.g., mydriasis, tachycardia, hypertension, and sweating). This process can be repeated every 2 to 4 hours for 24 hours after the initial dose; the total amount of methadone given in that 24-hour period is the "stabilization dose," which should not ordinarily exceed 40 mg. The stabilization dose is then reduced by 5 mg a day until the detoxification is completed.

Buprenorphine can also be used successfully for opioid detoxification[1]: patients who demonstrate objective signs of opioid withdrawal (often measured with a standardized withdrawal severity scale) can be stabilized on buprenorphine over a 1- to 2-day period; the subsequent taper from buprenorphine may occur either right away or after a period of stabilization on buprenorphine. The dose of buprenorphine will depend on whether the medication will be used for a brief, several-day detoxification or for longer-term stabilization or maintenance treatment.

Longer-Term Opioid Dependence Treatment

There are three effective medications that are approved by the FDA for the treatment of opioid dependence: methadone (a full opioid agonist), buprenorphine (a partial agonist), and naltrexone (an opioid antagonist). Methadone has been used successfully for both detoxification from opioids and maintenance treatment for many years.[2] Unlike buprenorphine and naltrexone, which can be prescribed by physicians in their offices (although physicians wishing to prescribe buprenorphine for the treatment of opioid dependence must receive specialized training and certification to do so), methadone is available for the treatment of opioid dependence only in specially licensed treatment programs. Methadone is a long-acting μ-receptor agonist with a slow onset of peak effects (typically approximately 2 to 6 hours) and a slow offset of action, allowing for once-a-day administration. Methadone reduces opioid craving and induces cross-tolerance, thus blocking or attenuating the effects of other opioid use. Although the therapeutic dose of methadone for a particular individual may vary, doses of 60 mg or higher have typically been shown to be more effective than lower doses; there is some evidence that even higher doses (e.g., 80 mg a day or more) may be more effective than 60 mg. Methadone treatment has been shown to reduce opioid use, increase employment, decrease criminal behavior, and reduce the rate of development of HIV infection.

When a patient enrolled in a methadone treatment program experiences pain (e.g., postoperatively) requiring opioid analgesia, the patient should continue to receive the baseline methadone maintenance treatment dose for the addiction and should receive a different opioid for treatment of the pain (Chapter 29); before administering methadone, it is a good idea to confirm the methadone dose with the patient's treatment program whenever possible. The fact that the patient is receiving methadone every day does not obviate the need for opioid analgesia, however. In fact, many patients receiving methadone treatment for opioid dependence will require a dose of opioids that is relatively high as a result of cross-tolerance to other opioid drugs.

The Drug Addiction Act of 2000 revolutionized the treatment of opioid dependence by enabling the approval of the partial opioid agonist buprenorphine for the treatment of opioid dependence and allowing treatment with buprenorphine to be administered in physicians' offices rather than only in specialized opioid treatment programs. To prescribe buprenorphine, physicians must apply to the Substance Abuse and Mental Health Services Administration (SAMHSA) for a waiver that allows them to prescribe buprenorphine,

after taking an 8-hour training course on buprenorphine. At the time of this writing, physicians may treat up to 100 patients with buprenorphine in their office practice. Buprenorphine, a partial μ-agonist and κ-antagonist, has a more favorable safety profile than methadone because of its partial agonist properties. Respiratory depression, which can be induced by full agonists, and which is responsible for some overdose deaths, is far less likely to occur with buprenorphine because its partial agonist properties cause a plateau of opioid effects as the dose increases. Buprenorphine is administered sublingually for the treatment of opioid dependence either as buprenorphine alone (sometimes referred to as the "mono" product) or (more commonly, in the United States) as a combination product of buprenorphine and naloxone; the naloxone is added to discourage users from dissolving the tablet and injecting the medication because the naloxone in the combination product will precipitate withdrawal when injected. Buprenorphine has been shown to be effective for both opioid detoxification and for maintenance treatment. A randomized trial has shown that extended treatment with buprenorphine-naloxone for 12 weeks improved outcome compared with short-term detoxification in opioid-addicted youth (aged 15 to 21 years).[3] Typical doses of 12 to 16 mg of sublingual buprenorphine per day appear to be as effective as methadone in doses up to approximately 60 mg a day. However, individuals who require much higher doses of methadone may respond better to that agent than to buprenorphine.[4]

Naltrexone, a pure opioid antagonist, blocks the effects (including euphoria) of opioids. As a result, individuals taking naltrexone should have a reduced desire to use opioids because the latter drug will have no desired effect. When used orally (50 mg/day) or in its long-acting form (380 mg intravenously every 4 weeks), naltrexone is highly effective at suppressing illicit opioid use. However, naltrexone suffers from very low acceptability; few patients are interested in being treated with naltrexone. Moreover, among those who initially accept this treatment, the dropout rate is extremely high. Nevertheless, naltrexone can be a useful medication for patients who are willing (either as the result of external pressure or for internal motivation) to use it.

Methadone, buprenorphine, and naltrexone are not designed to be delivered alone but should be given along with counseling to be effective. It has been well demonstrated that the administration of methadone in the absence of counseling is an inadequate treatment approach; less is known about the optimal combination of buprenorphine and counseling. One study demonstrated that counseling delivered within a medical office setting can be quite effective in conjunction with buprenorphine treatment, suggesting that general physicians who are trained to use buprenorphine can effectively treat at least a portion of patients with opioid dependence in their offices with a combination of buprenorphine and counseling.

Central Nervous System Stimulants: Cocaine and Amphetamines

The two most important central nervous system stimulants, cocaine and amphetamine (including methamphetamine), are derived from different sources; the former is extracted from coca leaves, whereas the latter is a synthetic compound. However, both induce similar psychoactive activity when taken illicitly and can produce similar adverse consequences. Amphetamine has been used over the years to treat obesity and to combat fatigue and depression. Cocaine is still used as a topical anesthetic for otolaryngologic surgery. Ironically, its vasoconstrictor action, which is responsible for many of the cocaine-related medical complications described later, can be valuable for surgeons because of the resultant reduction of blood flow in the operating field. Although cocaine was not extracted from the coca leaf until the 19th century, coca leaves have been chewed for more than 1500 years for medicinal and religious purposes, as well as to combat work-related fatigue. Sigmund Freud was one of the foremost advocates of cocaine, both extolling its psychoactive properties and discovering its ability to relieve pain, thus eventually leading to its discovery as the first local anesthetic. Cocaine was seen in the late 19th century as a "cure-all" and was included in numerous patent medicines as well as in Coca-Cola. The Harrison Narcotic Act of 1914 restricted the use of cocaine, and the drug was not widely used until the late 1970s, when there was a resurgence in cocaine use in the United States.

Like cocaine, amphetamine was synthesized for the first time in the late 19th century. It was used for clinical purposes for the first time in the 1920s. Reports of amphetamine abuse first occurred in the 1930s, with intermittent epidemics since that time. In recent years, methamphetamine abuse has been particularly prevalent and worrisome in the United States, with particularly high concentration of its use in the Midwestern and Western states, including Hawaii.

Cocaine can be used either intranasally, by intravenous injection, or by smoking. Cocaine hydrochloride, which is the form of the drug used in medical therapeutics, is a water-soluble compound that can be used intranasally ("snorted") or injected. Adding an alkaline compound such as baking soda to an aqueous solution of cocaine hydrochloride produces a rocklike compound known as *crack,* which can be smoked. Smoking cocaine produces the most rapid onset of intoxication (6 to 10 seconds) and the shortest period of drug effect (10 to 15 minutes). Methamphetamine can also be used in multiple ways—either orally, by smoking, or intravenously. Methamphetamine effects last much longer than those produced by cocaine; psychiatric symptoms such as paranoia that typically last only a matter of hours in cocaine users may persist for days to weeks after methamphetamine use and occasionally may result in a chronic psychotic state.

EPIDEMIOLOGY

Approximately 37 million Americans have used cocaine during their lifetime. In 2009, just under 5 million people used cocaine; 1.6 million people, or 0.7% of the population, reported using cocaine in the past month. Of these past-month cocaine users, 30% (492,000) used crack, an increase from 2008. There were 600,000 new users in 2009, a number that has been in decline since 2002. Cocaine had the third highest rate of drug abuse or dependence in 2009 and was the second most common drug associated with a recent treatment episode; cocaine use is also associated with 28% of emergency room visits associated with drug abuse.

Other stimulant use is less common; approximately 22 million Americans have used stimulants nonmedically during their lifetime, with 12.8 million lifetime methamphetamine users. Methamphetamine use in the past month was reported by 500,000 people in the United States in 2009, a number comparable to the number of past-month crack cocaine users.

PATHOBIOLOGY

Both cocaine and amphetamine increase the accumulation and activity of specific neurotransmitters in the synaptic cleft, including dopamine, norepinephrine, and serotonin. Cocaine is believed to exert this effect by binding to the dopamine transporter. Increased dopaminergic activity, particularly in the nucleus accumbens, is thought to be responsible for the reinforcing effects of cocaine. Amphetamines appear to increase the level of dopamine in the synaptic cleft primarily by stimulating presynaptic dopamine release as opposed to reuptake blockade.

CLINICAL MANIFESTATIONS

Both cocaine and amphetamines reliably produce euphoria, wakefulness, a sense of initiative, increased self-confidence (sometimes to the point of grandiosity), and in some instances, sexual stimulation. With higher doses, users may feel "wired," a syndrome characterized by anxiety, irritability, and perhaps paranoia. Withdrawal from either of these agents leads to opposite effects from those of intoxication: increased appetite, hypersomnia, and depression, which can occasionally be serious. Medical complications related to cocaine use are related to a combination of cocaine's stimulant activity (increased heart rate and blood pressure) and its vasoconstrictor properties. Local complications that result from the drug's vasoconstrictor activity include ulcerations of the nasal mucosa, perforation of the nasal septum, and decreased pulmonary diffusion capacity. Systemic complications include myocardial infarction, intracranial hemorrhage, grand mal seizures (as a result of intoxication, not withdrawal), and ventricular tachyarrhythmias, which may be responsible for sudden death. Physicians seeing a patient in an emergency room for an unexplained seizure should consider drug abuse as a potential cause (not only cocaine, but also phencyclidine and meperidine intoxication may lead to seizures, as can sedative-hypnotic or alcohol withdrawal). A serum or urine toxicology screen may thus be an important diagnostic tool in such a situation.

TREATMENT Rx

The treatment of central nervous system stimulant abuse and dependence primarily consists of behavioral therapies, including individual and group therapy, and self-help groups. Specific forms of treatment, such as cognitive-behavioral therapy, individual drug counseling using a 12-step-oriented disease model, and a behavioral treatment in which patients are reinforced for positive outcomes (e.g., drug-free urine screens), have been found to be successful. A great deal of research has been conducted in search of an effective pharmacotherapeutic treatment for stimulant dependence, but there is as yet no medication that has consistently been found to be effective enough to warrant approval by the FDA for this purpose.

Sedative-Hypnotic and Anxiolytic Drugs

Benzodiazepines and other sedative-hypnotic and anxiolytic medications such as barbiturates and zolpidem are frequently prescribed for the treatment of anxiety and sleep difficulties. Although different classifications of these drugs have very different chemical structures, they are grouped together according to their therapeutic applications. Most of these drugs act at the γ-aminobutyric acid type A (GABA$_A$) receptor and can cause physical dependence and both dispositional and pharmacodynamic tolerance. According to epidemiologic studies, approximately 9 million people, or 3.6% of the population aged 12 years and over, have used a sedative-hypnotic drug nonmedically.

Because the benzodiazepines are far and away the most commonly prescribed sedative-hypnotics, they are also the most widely abused. There are two major patterns of benzodiazepine abuse. Many people who ultimately abuse these medications have initially received a legitimate benzodiazepine prescription for the treatment of anxiety or insomnia. However, a combination of tolerance and decreased effectiveness of the agent over time may lead some people to increase their dose on their own. In such circumstances, attempts by the physician to taper the person off of the medication can be very difficult.

A second pattern of benzodiazepine abuse occurs among individuals who are using other drugs of abuse, most commonly opioids or stimulants. For example, many individuals who are dependent on heroin or other opioids may use benzodiazepines as a means of either enhancing the opioid effect or buffering symptoms of opioid withdrawal. Such individuals typically use relatively large doses of benzodiazepines intermittently, and therefore many of these patients do not develop physical dependence on benzodiazepines, unlike the first category of patients described previously, for whom physical dependence is common.

TREATMENT Rx

The treatment of people who are abusing benzodiazepines depends to some extent on the pattern of abuse. For individuals who have an anxiety disorder and have been misusing a legitimately prescribed medication, a common approach would be to taper the benzodiazepine and to institute a different type of treatment, such as an antidepressant along with cognitive-behavioral therapy. Tapering a benzodiazepine that a person has been taking for an extended period of time (sometimes many years) often requires a slow process, with careful monitoring of withdrawal symptoms (anxiety, agitation, insomnia, tachycardia, palpitations). Because benzodiazepine withdrawal, like alcohol withdrawal, can precipitate a seizure, gradual withdrawal is preferred. Most patients tolerate a benzodiazepine dose reduction initially with relatively little difficulty. However, as with most drug withdrawal regimens, people experience their greatest difficulty toward the end of the taper. One reason for this is that the percent dose reduction at the low end of a taper regimen continues to increase over time; a reduction from 2 mg to 1.5 mg of clonazepam, for instance, is a 25% reduction, whereas the same half-milligram dose reduction from 1 mg to 0.5 mg represents a 50% drop.

For patients who are abusing benzodiazepines as part of a pattern of multiple substance use, medical detoxification from the benzodiazepine itself will often not be necessary; for this population, psychosocial approaches that advocate abstinence from all substances of abuse, in conjunction with appropriate pharmacotherapy as needed (e.g., in the case of opioid dependence), is the preferred approach. It is important to note, however, that some deaths have been reported in France and elsewhere as a result of combinations of buprenorphine and benzodiazepines, usually used parenterally. Thus, physicians who are treating patients who are abusing both opioids and benzodiazepines need to be mindful of this issue when considering the use of buprenorphine.

Marijuana

Marijuana, which refers to the dried leaves and flowers of the plant *Cannabis sativa,* has been used for its psychoactive and medicinal properties for centuries. The major psychoactive substance in marijuana is δ-9-tetrahydrocannabinol (THC); the concentration of THC has increased from 1 to 3% in 1970 to nearly 8% in 2005; more potent varieties such as sinsemilla may contain nearly twice as much THC.

EPIDEMIOLOGY

Marijuana is the most commonly used illicit drug worldwide; it is estimated that approximately 160 million people have used marijuana. More than 16 million Americans state that they have used marijuana in the past month, with 104 million people in the United States having used marijuana during their lifetime.

PATHOBIOLOGY

Marijuana and other cannabinoids such as hashish (dried cannabis resin) exert their effects by binding to the cannabinoid receptors, of which two are currently known. Binding to the CB1 receptor, which is located primarily in the brain, appears to be responsible for the psychoactive effects of THC, whereas the CB2 receptor may be associated with immune system responses.

CLINICAL MANIFESTATIONS

When marijuana is smoked, its psychoactive effects occur almost immediately, with peak intensity approximately 30 minutes later; effects tend to disappear within 3 hours. Oral administration of marijuana leads to a delayed onset of action, but the effects of the drug persist for a longer period of time. Because THC is highly soluble in lipids, it can be stored in fat depots of regular users for several weeks, sometimes longer, with resultant positive urine tests for THC. Physiologic effects of marijuana intoxication include increased heart rate and conjunctival injection. Psychological effects include a sense of euphoria and well-being, friendliness, increased appetite, a distorted sense of time, impaired short-term memory, and sometimes a feeling of having achieved special insights. Cannabis has the capacity to cause tolerance in regular users, and some regular heavy users experience withdrawal symptoms on cessation of use, including irritability, difficulty sleeping, and anxiety.

TREATMENT Rx

The most common acute adverse event that occurs in marijuana smokers is a sense of acute panic, most common in inexperienced smokers, when the user's level of intoxication is greater than expected and the individual feels out of control. This can be best managed with reassurance that the effects will go away as the drug wears off. Recent evidence has shown that cannabis use, particularly during adolescence, may increase the likelihood of development of a psychotic disorder such as schizophrenia later in life.

Compared with alcohol, opioids, and stimulants, it is relatively uncommon for people to seek treatment of cannabis dependence itself. However, that situation has gradually changed in recent years, and an increasing number of people have sought treatment because of difficulty stopping marijuana use. There are no medications approved by the FDA for the treatment of cannabis dependence. Psychosocial approaches similar to the treatment of other substance use disorders are currently the treatment of choice.

Hallucinogens

Hallucinogens are a group of plant-based and synthetic drugs that lead to (primarily visual) perceptual alterations such as illusions and hallucinations, along with an alteration in the experience of external stimuli; ordinary events can appear quite profound to people while they are under the influence of these agents. The most common hallucinogens are lysergic acid diethylamide (LSD), mescaline, and psilocybin. Methylene dioxymethamphetamine (MDMA), also known as *ecstasy*, has both mild stimulant and potentially hallucinogenic properties and is thus sometimes categorized with the hallucinogens and sometimes as a stimulant.

EPIDEMIOLOGY

Approximately 1.3 million people in the United States report having used a hallucinogen in the previous month; approximately 37 million people have used these drugs during their lifetime. LSD is the most commonly used hallucinogen, with 24 million lifetime users in the United States; approximately 60% of that number have used MDMA.

PATHOBIOLOGY

LSD is thought to exert its action through serotonin agonist activity, particularly at the 5-HT$_{2A}$ receptor. Other neurotransmitters may be involved in hallucinogenic activity as well. Hallucinogens can produce tolerance in a matter of days, but they do not produce physical dependence.

CLINICAL MANIFESTATIONS

In addition to their effects on perception and behavior, hallucinogens can produce sympathomimetic effects such as tachycardia, increased blood pressure and body temperature, and pupillary dilatation. Hyperreflexia and muscle weakness can also be seen. The most commonly seen medical consequence of hallucinogen use is hyperthermia, which can occur most commonly in users of MDMA.

The most common acute psychological adverse event, similar to marijuana, is a feeling of panic over the sense of loss of control that a person may

feel as a result of intoxication; as is the case with marijuana, this is most likely to occur in inexperienced users. Some hallucinogen users will develop psychotic symptoms that fail to remit after the drug has worn off. Some hallucinogen use can also lead to longer-term perceptual difficulties. When these occur, a spontaneous return of very brief hallucinogen-induced symptoms long after the drug has worn off is known as a *flashback*. People who have perceptual difficulties that are much more pervasive may be said to have *hallucinogen persisting perception disorder*, which can at times be quite disabling.

TREATMENT Rx

Symptomatic treatment is focused on the specific adverse medical and psychiatric sequelae described previously. If a psychotic episode that occurs after use of a hallucinogen persisted over time, it would be treated like any other psychotic disorder. There is no specific treatment for abuse of or dependence on hallucinogens per se, and it is very uncommon for people to seek treatment specifically because they want to stop using hallucinogens.

Phencyclidine

Phencyclidine (PCP) was originally developed as a human general anesthetic, but its use for that purpose was stopped in the 1960s because it frequently led to psychosis and hallucinations in the postoperative period. Approximately 120,000 individuals report that they used PCP during 2009, which represents more than a 40% decline from 5 years previous to that. Low doses of PCP can lead to symptoms that resemble alcohol intoxication, with slurred speech, ataxia, and a subjective feeling sometimes described as "feeling dead." PCP intoxication typically is accompanied by increased muscle tone, hyperreflexia, nystagmus, and ataxia.

When taken in high doses, PCP can have serious medical and psychiatric consequences. High-dose users may experience psychosis, catatonia, and extremely violent behavior. Medical sequelae of PCP intoxication can include muscle rigidity, seizures, hyperthermia, coma, and occasionally death.

Anabolic-Androgenic Steroids

Anabolic-androgenic steroids differ from other drugs described in this chapter because the motivation for use is typically related to the drug's physical rather than behavioral effects. Anabolic-androgenic steroids such as testosterone and its synthetic analogues have traditionally been used primarily to enhance strength and thus athletic performance, although in recent years, an increasing number of people have used these drugs primarily in an attempt to improve their physical appearance. Anabolic-androgenic steroids can have a legitimate medical purpose; they have most commonly been used to treat testosterone deficiency in men and more recently have been used to treat wasting syndromes in patients with AIDS.

Abuse of anabolic-androgenic steroids can cause a number of medical and psychiatric problems, including hypertension, elevated low-density lipoprotein cholesterol, cardiomyopathy, hepatotoxicity, acne, feminization (gynecomastia and reduced testicular size) in men, and masculinization (hirsutism, reduction in breast tissue, deeper voice) in women. Behavioral effects include aggressiveness (sometimes leading to violence) and an increased prevalence of mood disorders. There is no specific treatment to help people abusing anabolic steroids to stop. Rather, behavioral treatment approaches that are commonly used to treat other substance use disorders should be employed with this population.

● CONCLUSION AND FUTURE DIRECTIONS

The ever-changing epidemiology of drug abuse means that the next decade will likely present new challenges as new drugs of abuse become increasingly popular. Recent research has focused on developing and testing effective pharmacologic and behavioral treatments for drug abuse and dependence. Screening for these disorders in general medical practice and combining office-based interventions with referrals to specialty drug abuse treatment as indicated can lead to successful outcomes for many of these patients.

1. Gowing L, Ali R, White JM. Buprenorphine for the management of opioid withdrawal. *Cochrane Database Syst Rev.* 2009;3:CD002025.
2. Mattick RP, Breen C, Kimber J, et al. Methadone maintenance therapy versus no opioid replacement therapy for opioid dependence. *Cochrane Database Syst Rev.* 2009;3:CD002209.
3. Woody GE, Poole SA, Subramaniam GA, et al. Extended vs. short-term buprenorphine-naloxone for treatment of opioid-addicted youth: a randomized trial. *JAMA.* 2008;300:2003-2011.

4. Mattick RP, Kimber J, Breen C, et al. Buprenorphine maintenance versus placebo or methadone maintenance for opioid dependence. *Cochrane Database Syst Rev.* 2008;2:CD002207.

SUGGESTED READINGS

Benotsch EG, Koester S, Luckman D, et al. Non-medical use of prescription drugs and sexual risk behavior in young adults. *Addict Behav.* 2011;36:152-155. *Young adults who use prescription medication recreationally also use marijuana, ecstasy, cocaine, methamphetamine, and poppers and tend to engage in risky sexual behaviors.*

Haber PS, Demirkol A, Lange K, et al. Management of injecting drug users admitted to hospital. *Lancet.* 2009;374:1284-1293. *Review.*

Ling W, Casadonte P, Bigelow G, et al. Buprenorphine implants for treatment of opioid dependence: a randomized controlled trial. *JAMA.* 2010;304:1576-1583. *Buprenorphine implants (4 implants of 80 mg each) reduce opioid use, with about twice as many patients (40% vs. 20%) drug free for 16 weeks.*

Meader N. A comparison of methadone, buprenorphine and alpha(2) adrenergic agonists for opioid detoxification: a mixed treatment comparison meta-analysis. *Drug Alcohol Depend.* 2010;108:110-114. *Buprenorphine and methadone appear to be the most effective detoxification treatments.*

Oviedo-Joekes E, Brissette S, Marsh DC, et al. Diacetylmorphine versus methadone for the treatment of opioid addiction. *N Engl J Med.* 2009;361:777-786. *In a randomized trial, diacetylmorphine treatment resulted in a 40% greater decrease in the rate of illicit-drug use or other illegal activity as compared with methadone.*

Strang J, Metrebian N, Lintzeris N, et al. Supervised injectable heroin or injectable methadone versus optimised oral methadone as treatment for chronic heroin addicts in England after persistent failure in orthodox treatment (RIOTT): a randomised trial. *Lancet.* 2010;375:1885-1895. *Injectable heroin is more effective than oral methadone for lowering street heroin use.*

34

IMMUNOSUPPRESSING DRUGS INCLUDING CORTICOSTEROIDS

GRANT W. CANNON

IMMUNOSUPPRESSIVE DRUGS

The immune response is an essential host defense mechanism to control and fight infection. The ability to suppress immune reactions is a critical component in autoimmune disease treatment and transplantation management. During autoimmune diseases, the basic immune physiology is altered, and one or more components of this process do not function properly. Current challenges related to the selection, dosing, monitoring, and development of immunosuppressive drugs involve identifying the component of the immune system to be altered by the immunosuppressive therapy while maintaining a competent immune response to fight infection and perform other important immunoregulatory functions. After organ transplantation, most patients have an immune response to reject the implanted organ. Thus, immunosuppression during transplantation management involves the suppression of normal immune reactions rather than a pathologic process, as in the treatment of autoimmune disease. Suppression of natural host immune responses inevitably affects the ability of these protective mechanisms to fight infection. The general principles for selecting immunosuppressive therapy in transplantation patients involve specific monitoring for organ rejection and the selection of immunosuppressive therapy proportionate to the degree of rejection or to maintain tolerance of the implanted organ. Selection of the most effective therapy requires an individualized treatment program. These decisions require an understanding of the underlying pathophysiologic process, prognosis, and potential adverse events associated with the agents selected.

This chapter describes the mechanism of action—including the components of the immune response affected by the therapy—indications, and adverse events associated with commonly used immunosuppressive agents in autoimmune diseases and transplantation. Although each of these agents is discussed individually, these drugs are frequently used in combination to take advantage of their complementary effects. An understanding of the principles and adverse events associated with immunosuppressive therapy is important for all physicians as the use of these drugs becomes more widespread; however, the initiation and management of immunosuppressive therapy, particularly in patients with organ transplants and severe autoimmune diseases, should generally be limited to specialists with specific training in its use.

Corticosteroids

Historically, the initial enthusiasm related to the marked clinical benefit of corticosteroids in the treatment of rheumatoid arthritis was dampened by the significant adverse effects that developed after prolonged use. As opposed to allergic and idiosyncratic reactions to medications, the majority of adverse effects related to corticosteroid therapy are a direct consequence of the physiologic effects of the drug. This observation sparked a determined effort to understand the mechanisms of action of corticosteroids at physiologic levels and therapeutic doses. The objectives of these investigations have been to modify the naturally occurring hormones to exploit their clinical benefits while avoiding the associated adverse effects.

Mechanism of Action

Corticosteroids affect multiple physiologic functions at the molecular, cellular, and organ levels. The final result of corticosteroid treatment represents the composite effects of the drug on these multiple functions, which vary with the particular agent, dose, route, and duration of treatment (Table 34-1).

Molecular Action

Genomic Effects

Corticosteroids are lipophilic and rapidly cross cell membranes into the cytosol, where they bind to the glucocorticoid receptor. The complex of glucocorticoid and its receptor then enters the nucleus and affects gene transcription by binding to glucocorticoid response elements. The complex may either stimulate or suppress gene transcription and subsequent protein production. This mechanism may have an impact on the function of 1% of all genes and suppresses the production of cytokines and other important inflammatory proteins. In addition to binding to glucocorticoid response elements, the glucocorticoid–glucocorticoid receptor complex suppresses signal transduction pathways such as transcription factor activator protein-1, nuclear factor-κB, and nuclear factor of activator of T cells. Corticosteroids may also affect post-transcription and post-translation steps of protein synthesis. The anti-inflammatory actions of corticosteroids may be related to

TABLE 34-1	MECHANISM OF ACTION OF IMMUNOSUPPRESSIVE AGENTS

CORTICOSTEROIDS

Binding to cytosol glucocorticoid receptor results in suppression of pro-inflammatory cytokines (genomic effects)
Inhibition of arachidonic acid release and binding to surface receptor (nongenomic effects)
Results of corticosteroid actions:
    Leukocyte numbers
        Increase in circulating neutrophils
        Decrease in circulating lymphocytes, monocytes, eosinophils, and basophils
    Leukocyte function
        Decreased trafficking of neutrophils
        Decrease in leukocytes' cellular immune functions and immunoglobulin production
    Cytokines
        Decrease in pro-inflammatory cytokines: IL-1, IL-2, IL-6, and tumor necrosis factor-α
        Increase in anti-inflammatory cytokines: IL-4, IL-10, and IL-13
    Decreased production of prostaglandins and leukotrienes

PURINE PATHWAY INHIBITORS

Azathioprine: inhibition of DNA synthesis and purine synthesis
Mycophenolate mofetil: inhibition of purine synthesis

PYRIMIDINE PATHWAY INHIBITORS

Leflunomide: inhibition of pyrimidine synthesis by inhibiting dihydroorotate dehydrogenase

IMMUNOPHILIN-BINDING AGENTS

Calcineurin inhibition
    Cyclosporine: binds with cyclophilin to inhibit calcineurin, resulting in decreased T-cell activation
    Tacrolimus: binds with FKBP12 to inhibit calcineurin, resulting in decreased T-cell activation
Mammalian target of rapamycin (mTOR) inhibition
    Sirolimus: binds to FKBP12 to inhibit mTOR, resulting in decreased T-cell activation

ALKYLATING AGENTS

Cyclophosphamide: alkylation of nucleic acids with cytotoxic action

FKBP12 = 12-kD FK-binding protein; IL = interleukin.

their action on the nuclear factor-κB and activator protein-1 pathways; the adverse events produced are related more to the activation or suppression of gene transcription.

Nongenomic Effects

The genomic effects of corticosteroids require the diffusion of the drug into the cell, binding to the receptor, entry into the nucleus, and alteration of transcription. The ultimate effect on protein synthesis is not immediate, and it generally takes at least 30 minutes before any response is seen. The observation that some actions of corticosteroids are seen immediately has directed a search for nongenomic effects of these drugs. The glucocorticoid–glucocorticoid receptor complex can inhibit arachidonic acid release. In addition to the cytosol glucocorticoid receptor, a membrane-bound receptor may be present that mediates nongenomic functions.

Systemic Effects

Impact on Leukocytes

Corticosteroids affect the activation, production, circulation, function, and survival of leukocytes. Whereas these impacts appear to be modulated principally by the genomic effects of corticosteroids on cytokines, corticosteroids act on adhesion molecules and other mechanisms as well. The effects are on neutrophils, monocytes, macrophages, lymphocytes, eosinophils, and basophils. With corticosteroid therapy, neutrophils increase in the peripheral circulation, primarily because of demargination; in contrast, there is a decrease in monocytes, lymphocytes, eosinophils, and basophils. Although the number of circulating neutrophils may increase, trafficking appears to be impaired. The impact on T cells is more pronounced than the effects on B cells, with the induction of apoptosis particularly in immature and activated T cells. Although the function of B cells and neutrophils is not affected as strongly as that of T cells, prolonged use of high-dose corticosteroids can lead to suppression of antibody production.

Changes in Inflammatory Mediators

Corticosteroids result in a decrease in multiple pro-inflammatory cytokines and interleukins (ILs), including IL-1, IL-2, IL-6, and tumor necrosis factor-α, at the same time that there is an increase in anti-inflammatory cytokines such as IL-4, IL-10, and IL-13. Corticosteroids have been associated with a reduction in the production of prostaglandins, leukotrienes, and other arachidonic acid metabolites, probably related to the reduced production of cyclooxygenase 2 and phospholipase A_2–related pro-inflammatory compounds (Chapter 36).

TREATMENT

Specific Issues with Corticosteroid Therapy

Multiple corticosteroid compounds and preparations are available (Table 34-2). These compounds have differences in potency, half-life, and sodium-retaining properties. In many conditions, the local administration of corticosteroids provides clinical benefit without the systemic toxicity associated with oral therapy. Local therapies include topical, ophthalmic, inhaled, and local injection, such as soft tissue and intra-articular injections. Although the potential for adverse events is generally reduced with local therapy, local toxicities as well as systemic effects can develop if large doses of topical corticosteroids are used.

Whereas most conditions can be treated with local or oral corticosteroids, intravenous administration can provide pulse doses if desired. Intravenous therapy can also be used when the patient cannot take oral medication or the absorption of oral agents is impaired. Pulse therapy generally consists of high-dose intravenous treatment that is often administered as divided doses over 3 to 5 days. High-dose pulse therapy has been advocated in acute organ transplantation rejection, severe systemic lupus erythematosus (SLE), aggressive vasculitis, and other acute and severe autoimmune disorders. The use of high-dose corticosteroid pulse therapy has been associated with the development of sudden cardiac arrhythmias and sudden death. However, many of these patients had serious concurrent diseases that could have been partly responsible for electrolyte abnormalities and other associated morbidities contributing to these complications. Because of this possible association, close monitoring of patients receiving high-dose corticosteroid pulse therapy is warranted.

Indications

Corticosteroids are employed in a wide range of autoimmune disorders and transplantation procedures. A listing of each indication for which corticosteroids have been used and proved effective is beyond the scope of this chapter, but indications range from multiple rheumatologic disorders and

many other inflammatory conditions to transplantation. For example, the demonstration that inflammation plays a significant role in reactive airway disease has dramatically increased the use of systemic and inhaled corticosteroids in asthma and chronic obstructive pulmonary disorders. The challenge is to determine the appropriate dose, route, and duration of therapy. For severe autoimmune disorders, high doses of corticosteroids are indicated. In many cases, oral prednisone, 60 to 80 mg/day as single or divided doses, can be employed. If patients cannot take oral medication or higher doses of corticosteroids are indicated, they can be administered intravenously. Comparative data on the most appropriate doses and routes of administration are generally not available. Clinical judgment and empirical literature form the basis of these treatment regimens.

Adverse Effects

With most medications, adverse events are the result of allergic and idiosyncratic reactions. The adverse events associated with corticosteroids, however, are generally caused by the drug's physiologic action. Investigations are ongoing to determine whether separate mechanisms might account for the therapeutic benefits of corticosteroids, whereas other pathways are involved in the adverse events related to these drugs. Currently available forms of corticosteroids do not allow the separation of adverse events from therapeutic effects. For example, the increase in infection associated with corticosteroids is a result of the drug's impact on leukocyte function and antibody production; it is not an allergic reaction. The prevalence and severity of these adverse effects increase in proportion to the dose and duration of therapy. The key to reducing adverse events is to use the lowest dose needed for the shortest possible duration. Data also suggest that intermittent and every-other-day dosing may be associated with less toxicity than daily or divided daily doses.

Despite these limitations, corticosteroids are the only viable treatment option in many conditions, and efforts must be made to prevent, detect the development of, and monitor these adverse events. In most situations, education of the patient coupled with vigilant surveillance can detect these adverse events and often reduce their serious impact.

The following discussion is not a comprehensive list of all reported adverse events associated with corticosteroids. Infection, osteoporosis, metabolic abnormalities, and cardiovascular effects are highlighted because specific interventions can have an impact on these problems through proper education of the patient, monitoring, or prophylactic therapy.

Infection

Infections are increased in patients taking corticosteroids, particularly bacterial, fungal, and mycobacterial infections. These opportunistic infections are seen much less frequently in healthy individuals with normal immune function. The increased incidence and general severity of these infections are complicated by the anti-inflammatory actions of corticosteroids, which can mask many of the cardinal signs of infection such as fever, inflammation, and local discomfort. Patients taking corticosteroids should be alerted to the possibility of these "subclinical" infections, and the provider must be vigilant in investigating signs and symptoms that might be less concerning in patients not taking corticosteroids. Management of infections in patients receiving corticosteroids requires close monitoring. Appropriate diagnostic procedures, antimicrobial therapy, and supportive measures are key to the successful management of infections in immunocompromised hosts. Patients with adrenal suppression may require "stress doses" of corticosteroids during the initial treatment. However, when a reduction in corticosteroid dose is possible, this may help restore the host immune response to the infection, particularly with chronic infections.

Preventive measures to reduce infections include proper immunizations. For example, in a patient being evaluated for future transplantation, immunizations should be given before the immunosuppressive therapy, if possible. In many cases, however, a delay of immunosuppressive therapy is not possible to allow immunizations to be updated. In patients receiving chronic immunosuppressive therapy, routine immunizations should be offered when the disease is stable. Prophylactic antibiotics are generally not recommended to prevent infections in patients receiving corticosteroid therapy. However, two notable exceptions are the use of antituberculosis therapy in purified protein derivative (PPD)–positive patients and trimethoprim-sulfamethoxazole therapy in patients receiving high-dose corticosteroid therapy for *Pneumocystis jirovecii* (previously *Pneumocystis carinii*) prophylaxis.

TABLE 34-2 GLUCOCORTICOID PREPARATIONS

	ANTI-INFLAMMATORY POTENCY	EQUIVALENT DOSE (MG)	SODIUM-RETAINING POTENCY	PLASMA HALF-LIFE (MIN)	BIOLOGIC HALF-LIFE (HR)
Hydrocortisone	1	20	2+	90	8-12
Cortisone	0.8	25	2+	30	8-12
Prednisone	4	5	1+	60	12-36
Prednisolone	4	5	1+	200	12-36
Methylprednisolone	5	4	0	180	12-36
Triamcinolone	5	4	0	300	12-36
Betamethasone	20-30	0.6	0	100-300	36-54
Dexamethasone	20-30	0.75	0	100-300	36-54

From Garber EK, Targoff C, Paulus HE. Glucocorticoid preparations. In: Paulus HE, Furst DE, Droomgoole SH, eds. *Drugs for Rheumatic Diseases.* New York: Churchill Livingstone; 1987:446.

Osteoporosis

Bone loss associated with corticosteroids affects multiple sites and has a greater impact on trabecular bone than cortical bone. Common sites of involvement are the spine and femur; associated fracture rates may be as high as 20%, depending on the dose and duration of therapy. On initiation of long-term corticosteroid therapy, all patients should be evaluated for osteoporosis prophylactic therapy (Chapter 251). Unless it is contraindicated, patients should be receiving adequate calcium and vitamin D through diet or supplements. In many patients, bisphosphonates provide significant protection. Postmenopausal women may be evaluated for potential estrogen replacement therapy, which may be helpful if the benefits of therapy with corticosteroids outweigh the risks for cardiovascular disease and malignancy. If osteoporosis develops in a patient receiving corticosteroids, efforts should be made to discontinue therapy or reduce the dose. Agents used for the treatment of osteoporosis should also be administered (Chapter 251). Effective therapies include bisphosphonates and anabolic agents such as parathyroid hormone preparations. These agents are generally used in association with calcium and vitamin D supplementation. An algorithm for the prevention and treatment of glucocorticoid-induced osteoporosis is provided in Figure 34-1.

Metabolic Effects

The metabolic effects of corticosteroids may influence glucose metabolism, with results ranging from mild glucose intolerance to frank diabetes. Patients beginning corticosteroid therapy should be monitored for glucose intolerance and treated if significant hyperglycemia develops. The management of patients with existing diabetes is particularly challenging during corticosteroid therapy; they require close monitoring and adjustments to their diabetes management programs.

Exogenous corticosteroids suppress the hypothalamic-pituitary-adrenal (HPA) axis (Chapters 230 and 234). The likelihood of adrenal suppression increases with the dose and duration of therapy. HPA axis suppression should be considered in patients receiving doses of 20 mg/day or more for 3 weeks or longer, although suppression can occur with lower doses. Formal evaluations can be performed to test the integrity of the HPA axis, but in most cases, a scheduled tapering of corticosteroid dose over several weeks allows the return of HPA axis function without signs of adrenal insufficiency. The ideal rate for the tapering of corticosteroids has not been evaluated by clinical trials. The rate of reduction in corticosteroid dose is often limited more by the relapse of disease activity than by the development of adrenal insufficiency. In general, a rapid reduction in dose (about 10 mg prednisone-equivalent/day), as tolerated by the patient's clinical disease, can be undertaken until a dose reflecting the normal physiologic production of cortisol is achieved. After this point, reductions of 1 to 2.5 mg/day every 1 to 2 weeks are generally well tolerated and can be accomplished by decreasing the dose of alternate-day treatment over 6 to 8 weeks. However, with an acute medical illness, patients who received corticosteroid doses in the past sufficient to cause HPA suppression should receive stress doses of steroids for up to 1 year after steroid treatment. Other metabolic complications of corticosteroid treatment include weight gain with truncal obesity; electrolyte abnormalities, including hypokalemia; and fluid retention.

Cardiovascular Effects

Corticosteroids may induce or exacerbate cardiovascular risk factors, including hypertension, hyperlipidemia, and diabetes. Multiple mechanisms have been proposed for these effects, but the end result is that patients taking corticosteroids have an increased prevalence of atherosclerotic diseases and their associated complications. This problem is complicated by the recent observation that many patients with inflammatory conditions, including rheumatoid arthritis and SLE, may have an increased risk for cardiovascular disease above that predicted by traditional risk factors. These observations emphasize the need to monitor corticosteroid-treated patients closely for cardiovascular risk factors (Chapter 51) and to treat detected abnormalities aggressively.

Other Adverse Effects

Many other adverse events have been reported with corticosteroid therapy and are listed in Table 34-3. Osteonecrosis (avascular necrosis) is common during corticosteroid therapy and often involves the femoral head. Peptic ulcer disease is increased independent of concurrent nonsteroidal anti-inflammatory therapy. Cataracts and a variety of dermatologic abnormalities are more common. Muscle weakness or steroid myopathy, alteration of mood and behavior, and psychosis may develop. This broad spectrum of clinical complications requires the prescriber of corticosteroids to be aware of and alert to the development of these adverse events.

Purine Inhibition

Purines are critical components of nucleic acids and are particularly important in proliferating cells as part of cell growth and division. The inhibition of purines by competitive inhibitors (azathioprine and 6-mercaptopurine) and the blocking of critical enzymes (mycophenolate mofetil) in the purine pathway are effective methods of immunosuppression.

Azathioprine and 6-Mercaptopurine
Mechanism of Action

Azathioprine is an inactive compound that is metabolized to the active compound 6-mercaptopurine (6-MP). The exact mechanisms of action of 6-MP and its metabolites have not been fully established. At high doses, 6-MP may be incorporated into RNA and DNA, resulting in a cytotoxic effect; however, this effect is probably not the drug's major action at the usual doses employed. Most likely through the feedback inhibition of de novo purine synthesis, 6-MP and its metabolites may reduce cell proliferation and thus produce immunosuppression. Genetically controlled differences in the activity of enzymes involved in the metabolism of 6-MP have been identified. The enzyme thiopurine S-methyltransferase is responsible for the metabolism of 6-MP to the metabolite methyl-6-MP. A rare homozygous (0.3%) and heterozygous (10%) defect in thiopurine S-methyltransferase is associated with increased toxicity, with severe hematologic toxicity in homozygous patients.

The drug is eventually metabolized by xanthine oxidase. Because xanthine oxidase is inhibited by allopurinol, the concurrent use of allopurinol and azathioprine or 6-MP can result in a significant reduction in the metabolism of the active compounds and a significant increase in drug toxicity. For this reason, the combination of allopurinol and azathioprine should be avoided.

Indications

Azathioprine is approved by the Food and Drug Administration (FDA) for the prevention of renal transplant rejection and for the treatment of rheumatoid arthritis. Clinical trials and reports suggest that azathioprine also has efficacy in other types of organ transplantation and autoimmune diseases. Azathioprine has been particularly effective as an adjunct to corticosteroid

TABLE 34-3 MAJOR ADVERSE EVENTS ASSOCIATED WITH IMMUNOSUPPRESSIVE THERAPIES*

CORTICOSTEROIDS

Serious and opportunistic infections
Osteoporosis
Metabolic disorders: hyperglycemia, adrenal suppression, hyperlipidemia, electrolyte abnormalities, fluid retention, hypertension, truncal obesity
Cardiovascular
Miscellaneous: osteonecrosis, peptic ulcer disease, cataracts, dermatologic abnormalities, steroid myopathy, psychosis, growth retardation, altered mood and behavior

AZATHIOPRINE

Serious and opportunistic infections
Hematologic abnormalities: leukopenia, thrombocytopenia, anemia
Gastrointestinal: nausea, vomiting, rare hepatitis
Reproductive: pregnancy class D
Miscellaneous: pancreatitis, interstitial pneumonitis, rashes

MYCOPHENOLATE MOFETIL

Serious and opportunistic infections
Leukopenia
Gastrointestinal: diarrhea, nausea, dyspepsia, elevated transaminases
Reproductive: pregnancy class C

CYCLOSPORINE

Serious and opportunistic infections
Renal disease and hypertension
Potential for increased malignant neoplasms
Reproductive: pregnancy class C
Miscellaneous: hirsutism, gingival hyperplasia, hyperuricemia, electrolyte abnormalities

TACROLIMUS

Serious and opportunistic infections
Renal disease and hypertension (perhaps lower than with cyclosporine)
Potential for increased malignant neoplasms
Post-transplantation diabetes mellitus
Neurotoxicity: tremor, headaches, motor function abnormalities, mental status alteration, sensory changes
Reproductive: pregnancy class C
Miscellaneous: hirsutism, gingival hyperplasia, myocardial hypertrophy

SIROLIMUS

Serious and opportunistic infections
Renal disease and hypertension
Potential for increased malignant neoplasms
Reproductive: pregnancy class C
Miscellaneous: hyperlipidemia, pneumonitis, interstitial lung disease

CYCLOPHOSPHAMIDE

Serious and opportunistic infections
Increased incidence of malignant neoplasms
Hematologic toxicity: leukopenia, thrombocytopenia, anemia
Reproductive: pregnancy class D, premature ovarian failure, oligospermia, fetal abnormalities
Urologic: hemorrhagic cystitis, bladder cancer
Miscellaneous: nausea, vomiting, diarrhea, pulmonary fibrosis

*This list highlights the most serious and common adverse events but does not include all reported adverse events with these agents.

therapy, allowing a reduction in corticosteroid dose and avoiding the associated adverse events.

Adverse Effects

Serious infection has been reported during treatment with azathioprine, similar to that seen with other immunosuppressive drugs. Opportunistic infections are a particular concern. Hematologic abnormalities include leukopenia, thrombocytopenia, and anemia. A complete blood count (CBC) is recommended on a regular basis, with greater frequency at the initiation of therapy. Current guidelines recommend a CBC weekly during the first month of azathioprine therapy, every 2 weeks during the second and third months, and monthly thereafter. Genotyping of the enzyme thiopurine S-methyltransferase may identify subjects at the highest risk for hematologic toxicity, but it does not substitute for monitoring of the CBC. Gastrointestinal toxicity is usually minor, but patients may have significant symptomatic

complaints of nausea, vomiting, diarrhea, and epigastric pain; these are often self limited and reversible. Severe hepatic toxicity has been rarely reported, leading to a recommendation for regular monitoring of serum transaminases, alkaline phosphatase, and bilirubin, particularly during the first 6 months of therapy. Rare complications of azathioprine treatment include fever, arthralgia, rash, pancreatitis, and interstitial pneumonitis.

Azathioprine use in pregnancy is classified as category D and has been associated with fetal abnormalities in animals. The use of azathioprine should be avoided, if possible, in pregnant women and nursing mothers, although patients with organ transplants and autoimmune disease have had successful pregnancies while receiving azathioprine.

The association between azathioprine treatment and the development of malignant neoplasms is controversial. In most clinical situations, azathioprine is used in conditions and in combination or temporal sequence with other drugs that are associated with the development of malignancies. For example, patients with systemic vasculitis or SLE may initially be treated with cyclophosphamide and then with azathioprine. An increase in malignant neoplasms in this population could be related to azathioprine treatment, but the prior cyclophosphamide therapy may be a greater risk factor. In addition, patients with solid organ transplantation, another circumstance in which azathioprine is frequently used, appear to have a higher rate of malignant neoplasms unrelated to the use of immunosuppressive drugs. Extensive efforts to identify an independent increased risk for malignant neoplasms with azathioprine have not produced consistent results. These results suggest that the risk for malignant transformation with azathioprine is very low, if it exists at all.

Azathioprine is an important and effective therapy in organ transplantation and autoimmune disease. It is often used in combination with other agents and as a corticosteroid-sparing drug. Surveillance for infection and monitoring for hematologic toxicity are important. Concurrent treatment with allopurinol should be avoided to prevent serious toxicity from an interaction of the two drugs.

Mycophenolate Mofetil

Mechanism of Action

Mycophenolate mofetil is a prodrug that is converted in vivo to the active compound mycophenolic acid. Mycophenolic acid acts through inhibition of the enzyme inosine monophosphate dehydrogenase, resulting in an increase in 6-thionosinic acid, which is normally metabolized by this enzyme. The accumulation of 6-thionosinic acid acts via a negative feedback loop to suppress the de novo synthesis of purines and associated DNA production. Although it is not a cytotoxic agent, the actions of mycophenolic acid are most pronounced on proliferating cells, such as lymphocytes, reducing cell division and associated functions of these critical cells in the immune response.

Indications

Mycophenolate mofetil is approved by the FDA for the prevention of allograft rejection in renal, hepatic, and cardiac transplantation. In addition to these approved indications, mycophenolate mofetil has been evaluated in SLE; its principal use is in patients with lupus nephritis, although the drug has been used for other manifestations. Current studies are seeking to determine whether this agent can replace cytotoxic agents, such as cyclophosphamide, in the treatment of SLE, particularly as initial and maintenance therapy for lupus nephritis. Limited use has been reported in other autoimmune diseases such as rheumatoid arthritis, vasculitis, and polymyositis.

Adverse Effects and Monitoring

Common adverse events with mycophenolate mofetil include hematologic and gastrointestinal complications. Leukopenia is reported in 20 to 35% of patients receiving this drug for organ transplantation; however, severe neutropenia is seen in only 2 to 3% of subjects. Patients receiving mycophenolate mofetil have a higher susceptibility to infections, including opportunistic infections, similar to that seen with other immunosuppressive agents. Diarrhea, nausea, and dyspepsia are frequent. Abnormalities of liver enzymes are commonly noted and appear to be dose dependent. Rare complications include pulmonary fibrosis and malignant neoplasms. Mycophenolate mofetil is classified as category C by the FDA for use in pregnant women. Although the agent should be avoided in patients who are pregnant or not practicing adequate contraception, this drug appears to have less impact on the reproductive system than does cyclophosphamide. Patients with SLE who are concerned about cyclophosphamide's potential

FIGURE 34-1. Algorithm for the prevention of steroid-induced osteoporosis on initiation of glucocorticoid (GC) therapy. FRAX = World Health Organization Fracture Assessment Tool. (Modified from American College of Rheumatology 2010 recommendations for the prevention and treatment of glucocorticoid-induced osteoporosis. *Arthritis Rheum.* 2010;62:1515-1526.)

severe impact on reproductive organs may elect to use mycophenolate mofetil instead.

Monitoring of patients receiving mycophenolate mofetil should include a monthly CBC and hepatic enzyme activities. Monitoring for gastrointestinal and infectious complications should be conducted during regular clinical follow-up.

Mycophenolate mofetil is an important and effective agent in the management of transplant patients. Ongoing studies are evaluating the role of this drug in other autoimmune diseases. It is hoped that mycophenolate mofetil can provide effective therapy for rheumatic and autoimmune disorders with less toxicity than that associated with currently available agents. It has particular potential for use in lupus nephritis.

Immunophilin-Binding Agents

The development of immunophilin inhibitors has significantly advanced organ transplantation. Each of these drugs—cyclosporine, tacrolimus (also known as FK506), and sirolimus (also known as rapamycin)—has significant immunosuppressive activity on T-cell–mediated functions. Although the mechanism of action for each drug differs, they all bind to a cytosolic protein. This binding results in a decrease in T-cell cytokine production and T-cell proliferation. These separate sites of action allow these agents to be used in combination in transplantation management. In addition, because of these differences in action and binding, each drug has a unique adverse event profile.

Cyclosporine

Mechanism of Action

Cyclosporine acts by binding to the cytosolic protein cyclophilin to form a cyclosporine-cyclophilin complex. The cyclosporine-cyclophilin complex inhibits the enzyme calcineurin, which is involved in multiple T-cell functions and is of particular importance in enhancing the transcription of genes for pro-inflammatory cytokines. The use of cyclosporine inhibits the production of IL-2, resulting in a decrease in T-cell activation. Cyclosporine also inhibits the production of other cytokines, including IL-3, IL-4, granulocyte-macrophage colony-simulating factor, tumor necrosis factor-α, and interferon-γ. The overall impact of these actions is to reduce immune function and inflammation.

Indications

The use of cyclosporine and other calcineurin inhibitors has revolutionized treatment after solid organ transplantation. The specific FDA-approved indications include renal, liver, and heart transplantation. Most often the drug is used in conjunction with other immunosuppressive agents, including corticosteroids and azathioprine. The critical clinical challenge is to balance the potent immunosuppressive effects of the drug against its adverse effects, with particular attention to the avoidance of infectious complications and monitoring for hypertension and renal toxicity. Because of these critical issues, prescription of this drug is limited to physicians experienced in the use of immunosuppressive agents.

Oral cyclosporine is also approved for the treatment of rheumatoid arthritis as a disease-modifying antirheumatic drug (DMARD), either alone or in combination with methotrexate. Although it is effective in the treatment of rheumatoid arthritis and other rheumatic diseases, cyclosporine does not have substantially greater efficacy than the other DMARDs. Cyclosporine is also approved for the treatment of psoriasis. Because of its significant adverse event profile, cyclosporine is generally reserved for patients with autoimmune diseases who have failed therapy with more traditional and less toxic agents.

Topical cyclosporine is effective and is approved to increase tear production, presumed to be suppressed secondary to inflammation, in patients with keratoconjunctivitis sicca syndrome. Topical treatment is associated with a much lower frequency of adverse drug events than is systemic cyclosporine therapy.

Adverse Effects

Close monitoring is required during cyclosporine therapy. Blood levels can be measured, which is useful to ensure that the drug remains within the therapeutic range and below levels associated with increased toxicity. Because many potential drug and food interactions can either raise or lower cyclosporine levels, such as increased levels seen with the ingestion of grapefruit and grapefruit juice, patients should be constantly monitored, and blood levels should be obtained when indicated. These evaluations should ensure that when medical therapy is added, changed, or deleted, these adjustments do not have an impact on the effects of the cyclosporine.

Infection

Patients receiving cyclosporine and other calcineurin inhibitors have an increased risk of developing infections. Opportunistic infections associated with impaired cell-mediated immunity are particularly increased in these patients.

Renal Disease and Hypertension

Renal disease and hypertension are common adverse events during cyclosporine therapy and increase in prevalence with increased doses and duration of therapy. Close monitoring of blood pressure and serum creatinine concentration is critical during treatment with cyclosporine. In many cases, these conditions are reversible if they are detected early and appropriate dose adjustments are implemented. In many patients, a mild increase in serum creatinine concentration may be tolerated if the level remains stable. Although renal abnormalities and hypertension are commonly identified during treatment with cyclosporine, most patients can continue taking the drug if adjustments in dose or other interventions are implemented to avoid these complications.

Malignant Neoplasia

Malignant neoplasms, particularly lymphomas, are more common in patients receiving solid organ transplants and immunosuppressive therapy. However, the exact cause of these malignant neoplasms has not been determined. In vitro mutagenesis assays with cyclosporine have been negative. In vivo animal studies have yielded equivocal results, with some data suggesting a possible increased rate of malignant neoplasms in rats and mice.

Reproductive Issues

Cyclosporine is a pregnancy class C drug. Data in animals have demonstrated toxicity to both the embryo and the fetus. Patients should practice effective contraception while receiving this drug. Data from pregnant transplant patients are difficult to interpret because cyclosporine is generally not the only medical therapy being given to these women, and the impact of the disease associated with organ transplantation may be difficult to separate from the impact of therapy. Despite these limitations, normal pregnancies and early childhood development have been reported in many women receiving cyclosporine and their children. Premature birth and low birthweight are more common among women receiving cyclosporine. Therefore, although the use of cyclosporine during pregnancy and breast-feeding should be avoided if possible, in patients who become pregnant, an assessment can determine whether the immunosuppressive therapy should be continued. In some cases, the risk of organ rejection with the discontinuation of cyclosporine therapy may exceed the risk of exposure to the fetus during pregnancy.

Other Adverse Effects

Cyclosporine has also been associated with the development of hirsutism, gingival hyperplasia, hyperuricemia, and electrolyte abnormalities.

Tacrolimus
Mechanism of Action

Whereas cyclosporine binds to cyclophilin, tacrolimus binds to a different protein, the 12-kD FK-binding protein (FKBP12). The binding of FKBP12 and tacrolimus forms a complex that inhibits calcineurin in a fashion similar to cyclosporine. Through this mechanism, tacrolimus has similar inhibitory effects on T-cell function and cytokine production.

Indications

Tacrolimus is approved for the prophylactic treatment of organ rejection after kidney and liver transplantation. Its efficacy and safety in rheumatoid arthritis are limited but encouraging. Experience with this agent is less extensive than that with cyclosporine.

Adverse Effects

The major adverse events associated with tacrolimus are similar to those associated with cyclosporine and include increased susceptibility to infection, renal disease, and hypertension. An increase in malignant neoplasia is also reported, with a pattern similar to that in patients receiving cyclosporine.

In addition to the adverse events similar to those reported with other calcineurin inhibitors, some specific complications have been reported with tacrolimus, including the development of post-transplantation diabetes mellitus. This was seen in 20% of subjects in phase III clinical trials of tacrolimus, with the onset generally occurring within the first 3 months of therapy. In many patients, post-transplantation diabetes mellitus resolves after the drug is discontinued. Neurotoxicity has been reported, including tremor, headache, motor function abnormalities, mental status alterations, and sensory changes. Myocardial hypertrophy has also been reported. Tacrolimus, like cyclosporine, is pregnancy class C; patients receiving this drug should practice effective contraception.

Sirolimus
Mechanism of Action

Sirolimus (or rapamycin) in not a calcineurin inhibitor, but it has many actions and mechanisms similar to that class of drug. The mechanism of action of sirolimus involves binding to FKBP12, the binding protein for tacrolimus, but the effect of this binding is different. Instead of acting on calcineurin, the sirolimus-FKBP12 complex binds to another protein, the mammalian target of rapamycin (mTOR), which is a key regulatory kinase. The inhibition of mTOR results in significant immunosuppression by decreasing T-cell proliferation and the progression from G_1 phase to S phase in the cell cycle. Because sirolimus works through a different mechanism of action from cyclosporine, the two drugs have been studied in combination. In renal transplantation patients, these two agents in combination have a greater immunosuppressive effect than that of cyclosporine alone.

Indications

Sirolimus is approved for the prophylaxis of organ rejection in renal transplantation patients older than 12 years, in combination with cyclosporine and corticosteroids. Data on the use of sirolimus in other populations, including subjects with autoimmune diseases, are limited and are generally derived from animal models.

Adverse Effects

The adverse event profile of sirolimus in terms of infections and malignant neoplasms is similar to that of the calcineurin inhibitors. Renal disease in patients taking cyclosporine and sirolimus in combination has been reported more frequently than in those receiving cyclosporine alone. Adverse reactions specific for sirolimus include hyperlipidemia, interstitial lung disease, and the syndrome of calcineurin-induced hemolytic-uremic syndrome, thrombotic thrombocytopenic purpura, and thrombotic microangiopathy.

Alkylating Agents

Alkylating agents are an important component of immunosuppressive therapy in autoimmune diseases. The use of these agents is limited by their toxicity, particularly the potential for the development of malignant neoplasia, reproductive toxicity, and an increased incidence of infection. Patients considered candidates for alkylating therapy should be fully informed of the potential risks and benefits of these drugs and should concur with the decision to use them. Regular monitoring of the CBC and urinalysis is important in patients receiving these drugs.

Cyclophosphamide

Cyclophosphamide has been used primarily as a cytotoxic drug for the treatment of malignant neoplasms; it is currently approved for this indication as well as for biopsy-proven minimal change nephrotic disease in children. Several severe autoimmune diseases are also responsive to cyclophosphamide, which is often given in conjunction with initial high-dose corticosteroid therapy. Because of the significant toxicities associated with these drugs, a benefit-to-risk assessment and discussion should be undertaken with each patient for whom cyclophosphamide is being considered. In most cases, the diseases warranting cyclophosphamide therapy are life-threatening conditions with a poor prognosis, justifying the use of such a toxic agent.

Mechanism of Action

Cyclophosphamide is an inactive compound that can be administered either orally or intravenously. It is metabolized to the active drug by the cytochrome P-450 mixed-function oxidase system. This process produces the active compounds phosphoramide mustard and the toxic metabolite acrolein. The cytotoxic effect of this drug results from the alkylation of various cellular constituents, especially nucleic acids. Changes in immune function with cyclophosphamide include depletion of lymphoid tissues, with decreases in both B and T cells, suppression of cellular immune function, and decreased antibody production.

Indications

The use of cyclophosphamide in the treatment of rheumatic diseases is most common and well studied in lupus nephritis and severe systemic vasculitis. Controlled clinical trials have demonstrated improved outcomes in these conditions, with reduced progression to end-stage renal disease in patients with SLE and improved survival in those with systemic vasculitides such as Wegener's granulomatosis. The evaluation of cyclophosphamide in patients with SLE has demonstrated the benefit of intermittent, usually monthly, intravenous pulse therapy as a method to avoid some of the most severe toxic side effects while maintaining therapeutic efficacy. However, pulse intravenous cyclophosphamide is not as effective as continuous oral cyclophosphamide in all conditions, particularly Wegener's granulomatosis. Patients with other conditions, such as polyarteritis nodosa, Takayasu's arteritis, and Churg-Strauss syndrome, reportedly benefit from cyclophosphamide therapy; however, the low prevalence of these diseases has prohibited the conduct of controlled clinical trials to prove its efficacy. Cyclophosphamide is also effective in the treatment of rheumatoid arthritis, but it is generally not used in this condition because of its toxicity and the availability of other effective agents. Although the advent of cyclophosphamide has been a tremendous advance in the treatment of these life-threatening diseases, the use of less toxic medications with similar clinical efficacy is currently under investigation.

Adverse Effects

Before the initiation of cyclophosphamide therapy, a frank discussion with the patient about potential serious and even life-threatening adverse events should be undertaken and documented.

MALIGNANT NEOPLASIA. Malignant neoplasms may develop in patients receiving cyclophosphamide for the treatment of both malignant and nonmalignant diseases. The risk of malignant change appears to increase with the duration and dose of cyclophosphamide. The most common malignant neoplasms are bladder, myeloproliferative, and lymphoproliferative disorders. The use of intravenous pulse cyclophosphamide may reduce but not eliminate the risk of bladder cancer. These malignant neoplasms may develop years after discontinuation of the drug.

REPRODUCTIVE ISSUES. Cyclophosphamide can be teratogenic, affect female reproduction, and reduce male fertility. Cyclophosphamide is pregnancy category D and should not be used in pregnant women unless life-threatening disease is present that warrants this treatment. Although successful pregnancies have been reported in patients receiving cyclophosphamide during pregnancy, fetal abnormalities are well documented secondary to chromosome damage. The use of cyclophosphamide in premenopausal women can induce premature ovarian failure. The use of gonadotropin-releasing hormone analogues during intravenous pulse cyclophosphamide therapy may reduce but not eliminate the risk of premature ovarian failure in patients with SLE. In males, a temporary or permanent decrease in sperm count may occur with cyclophosphamide. Because the recovery of fertility after cyclophosphamide therapy is variable, sperm banking should be considered before treatment is begun.

OTHER ADVERSE EFFECTS. As with other immunosuppressive agents, infections are more frequent and potentially more serious in patients receiving cyclophosphamide. Opportunistic infections are more likely to be seen in these subjects. Hematologic abnormalities can involve all cell lines. The CBC should be monitored regularly, and cyclophosphamide should be discontinued or the dose reduced when cytopenias develop. Cyclophosphamide treatment may be complicated by hemorrhagic cystitis and bladder cancer, which are probably related to the toxic metabolite acrolein. Efforts to reduce the potential for hemorrhagic cystitis and malignant bladder neoplasms include the use of intravenous pulse therapy, hydration, frequent voiding, and treatment with agents containing sulfhydryl groups to scavenge acrolein. Regular urinalysis for blood is indicated to monitor for bladder toxicity. Patients may develop severe nausea, vomiting, and diarrhea with cyclophosphamide therapy.

Chlorambucil

Chlorambucil has not been evaluated as extensively as cyclophosphamide, but this agent appears to have similar properties and a similar adverse event profile. Like cyclophosphamide, chlorambucil is associated with the development of malignant neoplasms and should be avoided during pregnancy.

Miscellaneous Agents

Although principally prescribed for other indications, methotrexate and leflunomide have been evaluated and used for their potential immunosuppressive effects. Leflunomide blocks the enzyme dihydroorotate dehydrogenase, resulting in the inhibition of pyrimidine synthesis and a reduction in T-cell activation. Methotrexate has multiple mechanisms of action, but its major effect in autoimmune diseases is mediated by inhibition of the enzyme aminoimidazole-4-carboxamide ribonucleotide transformylase. This inhibition affects purine synthesis, increasing the intracellular concentration of aminoimidazole-4-carboxamide ribonucleotide, which stimulates the release of adenosine, a potent anti-inflammatory compound. Methotrexate has principally been advocated for its corticosteroid-sparing effects. Both methotrexate and leflunomide are effective DMARDs in the treatment of rheumatoid arthritis.

SUGGESTED READINGS

Grossman JM, Gordon R, Ranganath VK, et al. American College of Rheumatology 2010 recommendations for the prevention and treatment of glucocorticoid-induced osteoporosis. *Arthritis Care Res.* 2010;62:1515-1526. *Consensus guidelines.*

Kuypers DR. Immunotherapy in elderly transplant recipients: a guide to clinically significant drug interactions. *Drugs Aging.* 2009;26:715-737. *A detailed review of medications that interact with immunosuppressive medications.*

Lui JC, Baron J. Effects of glucocorticoids on the growth plate. *Endocr Dev.* 2011;20:187-193. *Glucocorticoids inhibit chondrocyte proliferation, hypertrophy, and cartilage matrix synthesis, but after their discontinuation, the growth plate grows more rapidly than normal for age.*

35

BIOLOGIC AGENTS

CEM GABAY

Biologic agents are a new class of therapeutic agents that target different mediators involved in the pathogenesis of human diseases. The development of these therapies has markedly improved the management of many diseases. In addition, their use has greatly increased our understanding of the pathophysiology of these diseases. One of the most compelling examples is the efficacy of tumor necrosis factor (TNF)-α inhibitors in rheumatoid arthritis and inflammatory bowel disease.

Classification systems for the different biologic therapies have been established (Table 35-1). The pharmaceutical company usually provides the prefix of the name, and the suffix defines whether this is a monoclonal antibody (mab), a soluble receptor (cept), or a kinase inhibitor (inib). Monoclonal antibodies, by far the largest group of biologic agents today, also include in their names the type of target (immune system, cancer, cardiovascular system, bone), as well as their origin (chimeric, humanized, human). Rather than providing an exhaustive review of all tested approaches, this chapter reviews the currently approved treatments.

TUMOR NECROSIS FACTOR-α INHIBITORS

The cytokine TNF-α binds to two different receptors, TNF-R55 and TNF-R75, and exerts important functions in the control of host responses against infection. However, uncontrolled TNF-α production may lead to chronic inflammation and subsequent tissue damage.

Types of TNF Inhibitors

Different agents have been developed to inhibit the biologic activity of TNF-α, including monoclonal antibodies and soluble receptors. Monoclonal antibodies include infliximab (Remicade), adalimumab (Humira), and golimumab (Simponi). Infliximab is a chimeric antibody, whereas the other two are fully human antibodies. Certolizumab-pegol (Cimzia) is a pegylated humanized anti–TNF-α antibody Fab' fragment. Etanercept (Enbrel) is a fusion protein that contains the extracellular portion of TNF-R75 coupled to the Fc domain of human immunoglobulin (Ig) G1. All these agents bind to TNF-α and block its biologic activity. Etanercept also binds to lymphotoxin-α (previously termed TNF-β). Infliximab has been shown to exert cytotoxic effects on macrophages and T lymphocytes expressing TNF-α on their surface.

Indications

TNF-α antagonists are approved for the treatment of rheumatoid arthritis (Chapter 272). They exert marked anti-inflammatory effects and prevent the progression of structural joint damage. TNF-α inhibitors are efficacious in

TABLE 35-1	NOMENCLATURE OF MONOCLONAL ANTIBODIES

Nomenclature for monoclonal antibodies (mAbs) are composed of a prefix, a subsystem A, a subsystem B, and a suffix.

The common stem for all mAbs is –*mab*, placed as a suffix.

Substems B and A preceding –*mab* represent source identifiers of the antibody, as follows:

TARGET (MOLECULE, CELL, ORGAN)	SUBSTEM A
Immunomodulating	-*l(i)*-
Cardiovascular	-*c(i)*-
Bone	-*o(s)*-
Interleukin	-*k(i)*-
Tumor	-*t(u)*-
SOURCE	**SUBSTEM B**
Human	-*u*-
Humanized	-*zu*-
Chimeric	-*xi*-
Rat	-*a*-
EXAMPLE	**INDICATES**
Ri*tu*ximab	Tumor, chimeric
Deno*su*mab	Bone, human
Tras*tuzu*mab	Tumor, humanized
Beva*ci*zumab	Cardiovascular, humanized

From the International Nonproprietary Names (INN) Program of the World Health Organization, 2009: www.who.int/medicines/services/inn/Generalpoliciesformonoclonalantibodies2009.pdf.

early rheumatoid arthritis and in long-standing disease refractory to conventional disease-modifying antirheumatic drugs (DMARDs) such as methotrexate. TNF-α inhibitors are also approved for the treatment of ankylosing spondylitis refractory to nonsteroidal anti-inflammatory drugs (NSAIDs) and psoriatic arthritis refractory to DMARDs (Chapter 273). Anti–TNF-α antibodies, but not etanercept, have proven efficacy in severe Crohn's disease (Chapter 143) by reducing the disease activity score, inducing closure of draining fistulas, and allowing a decrease in the dose of chronic glucocorticoid medication. Infliximab is approved for the treatment of ulcerative colitis refractory to conventional therapy. Infliximab, adalimumab, and etanercept are also approved for the treatment of chronic plaque psoriasis (Chapter 446) refractory to phototherapy or systemic therapy.

Adverse Effects

TNF-α inhibitors can cause allergic reactions. Postmarketing data have shown that TNF-α inhibitors are associated with an increased risk of infections, including all types of bacterial and opportunistic infections. In particular, the use of TNF-α inhibitors has been associated with an increased risk of reactivation of latent tuberculosis. The results of cohort studies do not support an increased risk of cancer. Rare cases of demyelinating disorders, lupus-like manifestations, and cytopenia have also been reported.

INTERLEUKIN-1 INHIBITORS

Interleukin (IL)-1 (both IL-1α and IL-1β) binds to IL-1 receptors (type I IL-1R and IL-1R accessory protein) to induce a vast array of inflammatory signals. IL-1 receptor antagonist (IL-1Ra) competitively inhibits the interaction of IL-1 with its receptors.

Types of IL-1 Inhibitors

Anakinra (Kineret), recombinant human IL-1Ra, was the first IL-1 inhibitor used in clinical trials. Rilonacept (Arcalyst) is a fusion protein including the IL-1 binding motifs of IL-1 receptors coupled to the Fc domain of human IgG1. Canakinumab (Ilaris) is a fully human monoclonal antibody against IL-1β.

Indications

Anakinra is approved for the treatment of rheumatoid arthritis refractory to conventional DMARDs, but it has relatively modest efficacy. Anakinra, canakinumab, and rilonacept exert marked anti-inflammatory effects in hereditary systemic autoinflammatory diseases (Chapter 269) characterized by enhanced IL-1β production, leading to their approval for this indication. Anakinra is effective in some patients with systemic inflammatory diseases, including systemic-onset juvenile idiopathic arthritis, adult-onset Still's disease, and other autoinflammatory conditions. Clinical trials have reported encouraging results in crystal-induced arthritis such as gout and chondrocalcinosis. Promising results have also been reported from the use

of anakinra in type 2 diabetes mellitus and smoldering/indolent multiple myeloma.

Adverse Effects

Anakinra is frequently associated with injection site reactions. A modest increase in serious infections has been reported with anakinra. The combination of anakinra and etanercept (and probably other TNF-α antagonists as well) increases the risk of infections and is not recommended.

INTERLEUKIN-6 INHIBITORS

IL-6 is a pro-inflammatory cytokine that binds to a heterodimeric receptor, including IL-6Rα and gp130. Tocilizumab (Actemra) is a humanized monoclonal antibody against IL-6Rα that inhibits its interaction with IL-6.

Indications

Tocilizumab is approved for the treatment of rheumatoid arthritis refractory to conventional DMARDs and TNF-α antagonists.■ In clinical trials, tocilizumab prevented the progression of radiographic damage. Tocilizumab is also effective in controlling the inflammatory manifestations of systemic-onset juvenile idiopathic arthritis. Clinical trials are in progress in other inflammatory rheumatic diseases.

Adverse Effects

Tocilizumab has been associated with an increased risk of serious infections. A transient increase in transaminase levels has been reported. Hypercholesterolemia and cytopenia may appear in some patients.

ANTIBODY AGAINST INTERLEUKIN-12 AND INTERLEUKIN-23

IL-12 and IL-23 are heterodimeric cytokines, including a common p40 subunit and a specific subunit—p35 for IL-12, and p19 for IL-23. IL-23 participates in the differentiation of T$_H$17 cells that produce IL-17. Recent experimental findings indicate that IL-23 and IL-17 are critical for the development of autoimmune pathologies. Ustekinumab (Stelara) is a human monoclonal antibody against p40 that targets both IL-12 and IL-23 and blocks their biologic activities.

Indications

Ustekinumab is approved for the treatment of psoriasis in patients who have had prior exposure to phototherapy or other systemic therapies. In clinical trials, ustekinumab was associated with the successful treatment of Crohn's disease. In addition, ustekinumab was effective in patients with psoriatic arthritis refractory to conventional DMARDs. Anti–IL-17 antibodies are also in clinical trials for the treatment of psoriasis and rheumatoid arthritis.

Adverse Effects

Ustekinumab has been well tolerated in clinical trials.

INHIBITORS OF ANGIOGENESIS

Vascular endothelial growth factor (VEGF) is a family of growth factors involved in vasculogenesis and angiogenesis. VEGF-A binds to the tyrosine kinase receptors VEGFR1 and VEGFR2. VEGF has been implicated in tumor growth and metastasis, in diabetic retinopathy, and in age-related macular retinopathy.

Types of Angiogenesis Inhibitors

Bevacizumab (Avastin) is a humanized monoclonal antibody against VEGF that acts as an angiogenesis inhibitor. VEGF Trap is a fusion protein containing extracellular immunoglobulin motifs of VEGFR1 and VEGFR2 coupled to human IgG1. Sunitinib (Sutent) and sorafenib (Nexavar) are two orally available tyrosine kinase inhibitors that block not only VEGFR2 but also platelet-derived growth factor receptor β, C-kit, and Flt3 receptor.

Indications

Bevacizumab is approved for the treatment of glioblastoma (Chapter 195) and also for some patients with non–small cell lung cancer (Chapter 197) and metastatic colorectal cancer (Chapter 199). The absence of clear benefit on survival in patients with metastatic breast cancer led to the removal of the indication by the FDA. Bevacizumab is still approved in Europe in combination with placitaxel for this indication. Intraocular injections of ranibizumab (Lucentis), an antibody fragment derived from bevacizumab, are effective in maintaining vision in the vast majority of patients with wet macular degeneration (Chapter 431) and are approved for this indication.

Sunitinib is approved for the treatment of metastatic renal cell carcinoma (Chapter 203) and gastrointestinal stromal tumor refractory to imatinib (Chapter 209). Sorafenib is approved for advanced renal cell carcinoma and some cases of hepatocarcinoma (Chapter 202).

Adverse Effects

Bevacizumab has been associated with a heightened risk of bleeding and gastrointestinal tract perforation. Delayed wound healing and hypertension have also been reported. Sunitinib and sorafenib are generally well tolerated. Reported adverse events include hypertension, fatigue, asthenia, diarrhea, and some abnormal laboratory tests, including lipase, amylase, leukocytes, and platelets.

⬤ INHIBITORS OF TUMOR GROWTH FACTORS

Epidermal growth factor receptor (EGFR), a member of the ErbB-1 (HER-1) family of receptors, is a cell surface receptor for EGF and transforming growth factor-α. Binding of EGFR tyrosine kinase activity leads to increased gene transcription, cell proliferation, and inhibition of apoptosis. Human epithelial growth factor receptor (HER)-2 (also known as ErbB-2) is a receptor with tyrosine kinase activity that is expressed at high levels in 20 to 30% of breast cancers and other types of cancers and may cause uncontrolled tumor cell proliferation.

Types of Tumor Growth Factor Inhibitors

Two types of strategies target the EGFR pathway: monoclonal antibodies to the extracellular domain of EGFR, and orally available tyrosine kinase inhibitors. Cetuximab (Erbitux) is a chimeric monoclonal IgG1 anti-EGFR antibody that inhibits EGFR signaling and may also induce tumor cell death by antibody-dependent cellular cytotoxicity. Panitumumab (Vectibix) is a fully human monoclonal IgG2 antibody directed against EGFR. Erlotinib (Tarceva) and gefitinib (Iressa) are the two most commonly studied EGFR tyrosine kinase inhibitors.

Trastuzumab (Herceptin) is a humanized monoclonal IgG1 antibody that binds to the extracellular domain of HER-2. Lapatinib (Tykerb) is a small molecule with inhibitory activity on EGFR and HER-2 tyrosine kinases.

Indications

Cetuximab is an approved second- and third-line treatment for colorectal cancer and squamous cell carcinoma of the head and neck.**2** Positive results were also reported in clinical trials of cetuximab as first- or second-line treatment in patients with non–small cell lung cancer. Panitumumab is approved for the treatment of metastatic colorectal cancer. Erlotinib is approved for the treatment of metastatic non–small cell lung carcinoma and advanced pancreatic cancer, and gefitinib is approved for the treatment of advanced non–small cell lung carcinoma. Trastuzumab and lapatinib are approved for the treatment of metastatic breast cancer expressing HER-2.

Adverse Effects

Cetuximab is sometimes associated with severe allergic reactions during infusion. Acne-like skin rash is commonly reported. Erlotinib and gefitinib are associated with acne-like rash and mild gastrointestinal symptoms. Cardiotoxicity is a major problem in patients treated with trastuzumab. Approximately 10% of patients are unable to tolerate this drug because of preexisting heart problems. The risk of cardiomyopathy is increased when combined with anthracycline (which itself is associated with cardiac toxicity). Lapatinib is generally well tolerated, but some cases of hepatotoxicity have been reported.

⬤ OTHER TYROSINE KINASE INHIBITORS

Imatinib mesylate (Gleevec, Glivec) works by binding to the adenosine triphosphate (ATP) binding site of Bcr-abl, resulting in competitive inhibition of its enzymatic activity. Imatinib also inhibits the tyrosine kinase activity of C-kit and platelet-derived growth factor receptor.

Indications

Imatinib represents a major advance over conventional treatments for chronic myelogenous leukemia (Chapter 190), with more than 90% of patients obtaining a complete hematologic response and 70 to 80% achieving a complete cytogenetic response. Resistance to imatinib is often a result of point mutations causing a conformation change in Bcr-abl, which impairs imatinib binding. Dasatinib (Sprycel) and nilotinib (Tasigna), two other tyrosine kinase inhibitors, are approved for the treatment of chronic myelogenous leukemia that is not responsive or is intolerant to imatinib, and dasatinib can provide more rapid and possibly durable responses than does imatinib.**3**

Imatinib is also approved for the treatment of patients with C-kit–positive advanced gastrointestinal stromal tumor (Chapter 209). Early clinical trials also showed imatinib's potential beneficial effects in systemic mastocytosis, hypereosinophilic syndrome, and dermatofibrosarcoma protuberans. Imatinib is in clinical trials for systemic sclerosis.

Adverse Effects

Imatinib has been associated with cytopenia, edema, nausea, and rash, as well as rare cases of congestive heart failure. Cytopenia and congestive heart failure are also reported with dasatinib, and cytopenia can occur with nilotinib. The latter drug also carries a potential risk of severe cardiac arrhythmias.

⬤ BIOLOGIC AGENTS TARGETING T LYMPHOCYTES

T cells play a central role in immune responses and are thus important targets for therapies against graft rejection and autoimmune diseases.

Types of Agents Modulating T-Cell Activity

The agents targeting T cells include antibodies against T cells, soluble receptors inhibiting costimulation signals, and antibodies blocking T-cell migration. Therapies targeting CD3 were developed more than 30 years ago with a mouse monoclonal IgG2 antibody called OKT3. These antibodies were used in the treatment of kidney transplant rejection but were associated with limiting side effects due to the occurrence of a "cytokine release syndrome." A series of non-Fc binding humanized anti-CD3 monoclonal antibodies was developed to overcome this problem, along with the development of antimurine immunoglobulin antibodies.

Abatacept (Orencia) is a fusion protein containing the extracellular portion of cytotoxic T-lymphocyte antigen-4 coupled to the Fc portion of human IgG1; it inhibits costimulatory signals between CD28 and CD80/86. Alefacept (Amevive) is a recombinant fully human fusion protein in which the extracellular domain of CD2 has been linked to the Fc portion of IgG1; it inhibits costimulatory signals between CD2 and LFA-3.

Natalizumab (Tysabri), a humanized monoclonal antibody against α_4-integrin, inhibits the migration of T cells by blocking the interaction between α_4-integrin and adhesion molecules expressed on endothelial cells.

Indications

Different monoclonal anti-CD3 antibodies are used in clinical trials for the prevention of transplant rejection (Chapter 48), as well as for the treatment of acute graft-versus-host disease and type 1 diabetes mellitus.

Abatacept is approved for the treatment of rheumatoid arthritis refractory to conventional DMARDs and TNF-α inhibitors. Positive results have been reported in psoriasis and psoriatic arthritis. Alefacept is approved for the treatment of chronic plaque psoriasis. Natalizumab is approved for the treatment of patients with highly active remitting-relapsing multiple sclerosis on monotherapy (Chapter 419) and for severe Crohn's disease.

Adverse Effects

Abatacept is generally well tolerated, but serious infections may occur. Lymphopenia may occur with alefacept, and infections, malignancies, and hepatotoxicity have been reported in clinical trials. Natalizumab can be associated with allergic reactions and hepatotoxicity. Some cases of multifocal progressive leukoencephalopathy (Chapter 378), a fatal neurologic complication of JC virus reactivation in immunosuppressed individuals, have been reported, thus limiting the use of natalizumab.

⬤ BIOLOGIC AGENTS TARGETING B LYMPHOCYTES

The B-cell lineage plays a critical role in immune responses through the production of immunoglobulins, the presentation of antigen to T cells, and the production of cytokines. Therapies targeting B cells are used in B-cell lymphoma and autoimmune diseases.

Mode of Action

B cells can be targeted either by the use of monoclonal antibodies depleting B cells or by the inhibition of cytokines essential for their maturation and survival, such as B-cell activating factor of the TNF family (BAFF) and a proliferation-inducing ligand (APRIL). Rituximab (Rituxan, MabThera), ofatumumab (Arzerra), and ocrelizumab are B-cell–depleting monoclonal antibodies binding to CD20. Belimumab is a fully human monoclonal antibody against BAFF. Atacicept is a fusion protein containing the extracellular domain of TACI (BAFF and APRIL receptor), which inhibits BAFF and APRIL biologic activities.

Indications

Rituximab is approved for the treatment of non-Hodgkin's B-cell lymphoma (Chapter 191). More recently, rituximab has also been approved for rheumatoid arthritis patients with an inadequate response to TNF-α inhibitors. Ofatumumab is approved for the treatment of chronic lymphocytic leukemia (Chapter 190). Ocrelizumab is currently in clinical trials in multiple sclerosis and systemic lupus erythematosus. Epratuzumab, a humanized monoclonal anti-CD22 B-cell–depleting antibody, is in clinical trials for non-Hodgkin's B-cell lymphoma and systemic lupus erythematosus.

The administration of belimumab in patients with systemic lupus erythematosus has led to positive results regarding the number of flares and disease activity. Atacicept is in clinical trials for rheumatoid arthritis and systemic lupus erythematosus.

Adverse Effects

Rituximab is associated with an allergic reaction during infusions, a systemic reaction due to tumoral B-cell lysis, and an increased risk of infections. Rare cases of multifocal progressive leukoencephalopathy have been reported. Hypogammaglobulinemia may occur, particularly after several series of infusions.

CONCLUSIONS

The use of biologic agents has led to major advances in the management of many severe diseases refractory to conventional therapies. These agents have also provided a unique way to confirm the role of basic mechanisms in human diseases. New developments in this field will take different directions, including the refinement of existing strategies (using more selective inhibitors or human rather than chimeric antibodies), the extension to indications other than those for which the agents were primarily designed, and the selection of novel targets.

1. Singh JA, Beg S, Lopez-Olivo MA. Tocilizumab for rheumatoid arthritis. *Cochrane Database Syst Rev.* 2010;7:CD008331.
2. Liu L, Cao Y, Tan A, et al. Cetuximab-based therapy versus non-cetuximab therapy for advanced cancer: a meta-analysis of 17 randomized controlled trials. *Cancer Chemother Pharmacol.* 2010;65: 849-861.
3. Kantarjian H, Shah NP, Hochhaus A, et al. Dasatinib versus imatinib in newly diagnosed chronic-phase chronic myeloid leukemia. *N Engl J Med.* 2010;362:2260-2270.

SUGGESTED READINGS

Devine EB, Alfonso-Christancho R, Sullivan SD. Effectiveness of biologic therapies for rheumatoid arthritis: an indirect comparisons approach. *Pharmacotherapy.* 2011;31:39-51. *All approved biologic agents are significantly better than placebo, with the TNFα inhibitor certolizumab perhaps the most efficacious.*
Gabay C, Lamacchia C, Palmer G. IL-1 pathways in inflammation and human diseases. *Nat Rev Rheumatol.* 2010;6:232-241. *Describes some basic findings on IL-1 biology and their implications for the use of IL-1 inhibitors in the management of different inflammatory diseases.*
Graudal N, Jürgens G. Similar effects of disease-modifying antirheumatic drugs, glucocorticoids, and biologic agents on radiographic progression in rheumatoid arthritis: meta-analysis of 70 randomized placebo-controlled or drug-controlled studies, including 112 comparisons. *Arthritis Rheum.* 2010;62:2852-2863. *All agents were beneficial, thereby suggesting that biologic agents should be reserved for patients resistant to DMARD therapy.*
Grothey A, Galanis E. Targeting angiogenesis: progress with anti-VEGF treatment with large molecules. *Nat Rev Clin Oncol.* 2009;6:507-518. *Discusses the rationale for using antiangiogenic compounds in the treatment of cancer, with a focus on antibodies that target the VEGF system.*

36

PROSTANOIDS, ASPIRIN, AND RELATED COMPOUNDS

CARLO PATRONO

Arachidonic acid, or 5,8,11,14-eicosatetraenoic acid, is a 20-carbon polyunsaturated fatty acid esterified in the phospholipid domain of cell membranes. In response to chemical, physical, and hormonal stimuli, arachidonic acid is released from the glycerol backbone sn-2 position by the action of various phospholipases A_2, and can be subjected to rapid enzymatic conversion to a series of oxygenated derivatives collectively called *eicosanoids*. The enzymes catalyzing various structural modifications of free arachidonic acid include prostaglandin H synthases (commonly known as *cyclooxygenases* [COX]), *lipoxygenases*, and *cytochrome P-450 isozymes*. The resulting eicosanoids include prostanoids (prostaglandins and thromboxane A_2), leukotrienes, lipoxins, and epoxylins. Esterified arachidonic acid can also be subjected to in situ peroxidation, catalyzed by oxygen radicals, to form a series of corresponding isomers called *isoeicosanoids*.

Eicosanoids are not stored but are produced in response to diverse stimuli, with a pattern that reflects the cell-specific distribution of arachidonic acid–metabolizing enzymes and downstream isomerases and synthases. Eicosanoids are not circulating hormones but rather ubiquitous autacoids that modulate the intensity and duration of many important cellular responses in an autocrine (acting on the same cells that produced them) or paracrine (acting on nearby cells) fashion.

BIOSYNTHESIS AND ACTION OF PROSTANOIDS

Prostanoids include prostaglandins D_2, E_2, $F_{2\alpha}$, and I_2 (prostacyclin) and thromboxane A_2. They are formed through the sequential actions of phospholipase A_2 to release arachidonic acid from membrane phospholipids, prostaglandin H synthase to catalyze the cyclooxygenation of arachidonic acid to form the unstable intermediate prostaglandin G_2 and its reduction to prostaglandin H_2, and specific isomerases and synthases to catalyze the conversion of prostaglandin H_2 to different prostanoids (Fig. 36-1). Once formed, prostanoids interact with specific G protein–coupled receptors to evoke a variety of cellular responses, depending on the site of their biosynthesis (see Fig. 36-1).

Two prostaglandin H synthases have been identified: prostaglandin H synthase-1 is expressed constitutively in all cells; prostaglandin H synthase-2 is constitutively expressed in some cells (e.g., neurons and renal cells) and is induced in other cell types in response to cytokines (e.g., in monocytes), tumor promoters (e.g., in intestinal epithelial cells), growth factors (e.g., in bone marrow–derived stem cells), and laminar shear stress (e.g., in endothelial cells). Because nonsteroidal anti-inflammatory drugs (NSAIDs) target the COX activity of these enzymes, they have become known colloquially as COX-1 and COX-2. Both enzymes are homodimers that convert arachidonic acid, two O_2 molecules, and two electrons from one or more unknown reductants to prostaglandin H_2. COX-1 and COX-2 are found predominantly in the same cellular organelles, at the luminal surface of the endoplasmic reticulum and nuclear envelope of cells. Only one monomer of a dimer catalyzes arachidonic acid oxygenation at any given time. The cross-talk between monomers serves as a way for COX-2 to exhibit selectivity toward arachidonic acid, even when it is a minor component of the available fatty acid pool, and to sustain a "late phase" of prostanoid production. In contrast, COX-1 may efficiently oxygenate arachidonic acid in the early phase of prostanoid production, when this substrate represents a large fraction of free fatty acids, but may be inhibited by other competing fatty acids in the late phase.

Phenotypical analyses of COX-1-deficient and COX-2-deficient mice, as well as studies with isoform-selective inhibitors, suggest that there are processes in which each isozyme is uniquely involved (e.g., platelet aggregation for COX-1, ovulation and neonatal development for COX-2) and others in which both isozymes function coordinately (e.g., inflammation and its resolution, gastrointestinal ulceration and healing, and carcinogenesis). A way in which the two biosynthetic pathways may be dissociated metabolically is by a preferential coupling of the COX isozymes to various upstream phospholipases and downstream synthases, conditioning preferential formation of a particular prostanoid by a given cell type (e.g., COX-2-dependent prostacyclin by vascular endothelial cells).

Moreover, COX-2 oxygenation may play a unique role in a novel signaling pathway dependent on agonist-induced release of endocannabinoids. Among the products of COX-2 oxygenation of endocannabinoids are glyceryl prostaglandins, some of which (e.g., glyceryl prostaglandin E_2 and glyceryl prostaglandin I_2) exhibit interesting biologic activities in inflammatory, neurologic, and vascular systems.

MEASUREMENTS OF THE PROSTAGLANDIN H SYNTHASE PATHWAY

Prostanoids are formed in vivo at a relatively low rate (e.g., 0.1 ng/kg per minute for both prostacyclin and thromboxane A_2) and are metabolized extensively by lung and liver enzymes to form chemically stable, but biologically inactive, derivatives that are excreted primarily through the kidney. Given the chemical instability and extremely low concentrations (1 to 2 pg/

FIGURE 36-1. **Production and actions of prostaglandins and thromboxane.** Arachidonic acid, a 20-carbon fatty acid containing four double bonds, is liberated from the *sn*2 position in membrane phospholipids by phospholipase A$_2$, which is activated by diverse stimuli. Arachidonic acid is converted by prostaglandin H synthases, which have both cyclooxygenase (COX) and hydroperoxidase (HOX) activity, to the unstable intermediate prostaglandin H$_2$. The synthases are colloquially termed *cyclooxygenases* and exist in two forms, cyclooxygenase-1 and cyclooxygenase-2. Prostaglandin H$_2$ is converted by tissue-specific isomerases to multiple prostanoids. These bioactive lipids activate specific cell membrane receptors of the superfamily of G protein–coupled receptors. Some of the tissues in which individual prostanoids exert prominent effects are indicated. IP denotes prostacyclin receptor, TP thromboxane receptor, DP prostaglandin D$_2$ receptor, EP prostaglandin E$_2$ receptor, and FP prostaglandin F$_{2\alpha}$ receptor.

mL) of prostanoids in the systemic circulation, assessment of their production in humans is largely based on measurements of stable urinary metabolites (e.g., 11-dehydro-thromboxane B$_2$, a major enzymatic derivative of thromboxane A$_2$, and 2,3-dinor-6-keto-PGF$_{1\alpha}$, a major enzymatic derivative of prostacyclin). These analytical measurements have established that thromboxane metabolite excretion is primarily derived from platelet thromboxane biosynthesis and largely reflects the rate of platelet activation in vivo. Similarly, prostacyclin metabolite excretion largely reflects the rate of vascular prostacyclin biosynthesis in vivo. Thromboxane biosynthesis is persistently enhanced in association with the major cardiovascular risk factors (e.g., diabetes mellitus). Both thromboxane and prostacyclin biosynthesis are episodically increased in patients with acute coronary syndromes, perhaps reflecting a homeostatic response to accelerated platelet-vascular interactions.

Studies of the human pharmacology of COX inhibitors have largely relied on the development of whole blood assays of platelet COX-1 (based on serum thromboxane B$_2$ measurements) and monocyte COX-2 (based on lipopolysaccharide-induced prostaglandin E$_2$ production) activities. These assays have been useful in characterizing the variable potency of NSAIDs in inhibiting COX-1 and COX-2 in vitro (a measure of isozyme selectivity) and in determining ex vivo the dose- and time-dependence of their inhibitory effects in health and disease.

● CLINICAL PHARMACOLOGY OF PROSTAGLANDIN H SYNTHASE INHIBITION

Most traditional NSAIDs inhibit COX-1 and COX-2 with similar potency (Fig. 36-2). Some traditional NSAIDs (e.g., nimesulide and diclofenac) and a class of COX-2 inhibitors called coxibs (e.g., celecoxib and etoricoxib) are more potent in inhibiting COX-2 than COX-1 (see Fig. 36-2). These drugs fall into three general categories based on their mechanism of action. One category of inhibitors includes freely reversible competitive inhibitors, such as ibuprofen and mefenamic acid. Binding of these inhibitors to the COX sites of both monomers comprising a dimer is required for inhibition of COX-2 oxygenation of the substrate. A second group of inhibitors, including flurbiprofen, meclofenamate, diclofenac, and indomethacin, comprises time-dependent, noncovalent inhibitors. These NSAIDs are allosteric inhibitors that bind to one monomer of COX to inhibit its activity. Aspirin is unique to a third group of inhibitors that cause a time-dependent, covalent inhibition. Binding of aspirin to COX-1 or COX-2 leads to irreversible acetylation of a highly conserved serine residue (Ser-529 and Ser-516 in human COX-1 and

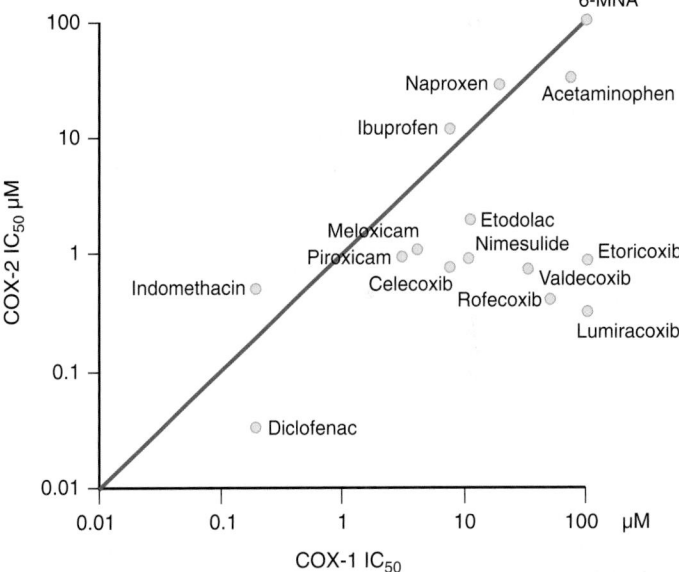

FIGURE 36-2. **COX-2 selectivity as a continuous variable.** Concentrations of various COX-2 inhibitors to inhibit the activity of platelet COX-1 and monocyte COX-2 by 50% (IC$_{50}$) are plotted on the abscissa and ordinate scales, respectively. The *solid line* describes equipotent inhibition of both COX-1 and COX-2. Symbols to the left of this line denote greater inhibition of COX-1 than COX-2. Symbols to the right of this line indicate progressively greater inhibition of COX-2 than COX-1, that is, increasing degrees of COX-2 selectivity. Aspirin is not shown in the figure because the long-term incubation required for monocyte COX-2 expression in human whole blood affects the chemical stability of the drug and underestimates its inhibitory potency. 6-MNA denotes 6-methoxy-2-naphthylacetic acid, the active metabolite of nabumetone.

COX-2, respectively). Aspirin acetylates only one monomer of a COX-1 dimer to cause complete loss of COX activity. Aspirin also maximally acetylates one monomer of human COX-2. The acetylated monomer of aspirin-treated COX-2 forms 15-hydroperoxyeicosatetraenoic acid from arachidonic acid, whereas the nonacetylated partner monomer forms mainly prostaglandin H$_2$ but only at 15 to 20% of the rate of native COX-2. Thus, the effect of

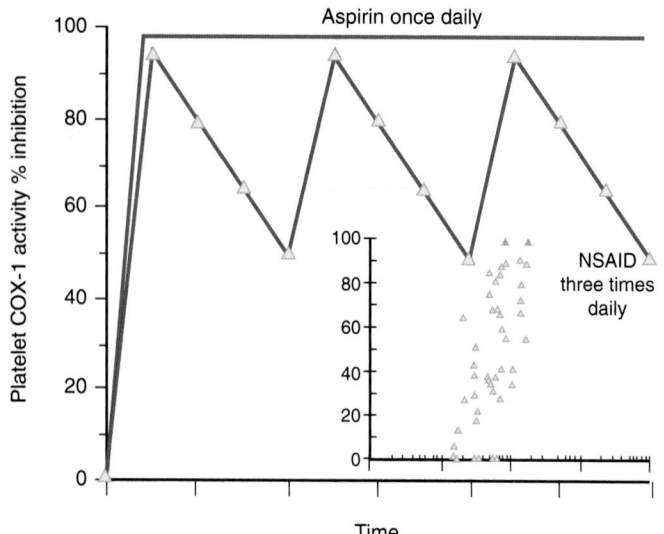

FIGURE 36-3. Time-dependent inhibition of platelet COX-1 activity by aspirin and a traditional nonsteroidal anti-inflammatory drug (NSAID). The average time course of inhibition of serum TXB_2, an ex vivo index of platelet COX-1 activity, is depicted over 24 hours following the administration of low-dose aspirin once daily and a traditional NSAID with short half-life given every 8 hours. The *inset* depicts the interindividual variability in the relationship between NSAID plasma levels plotted on the abscissa log scale and the corresponding level of inhibition of platelet COX-1 plotted on the ordinate.

TABLE 36-1	VASCULAR DISORDERS FOR WHICH ASPIRIN HAS BEEN SHOWN TO BE EFFECTIVE AND THE LOWEST EFFECTIVE DOSE	
DISORDER	**LOWEST EFFECTIVE DAILY DOSE (MG)**	
TIA and ischemic stroke*	50	
Men at high cardiovascular risk	75	
Essential hypertension	75	
Chronic stable angina	75	
Unstable angina or NSTEMI*	75	
Severe carotid artery stenosis*	75	
Polycythemia vera	100	
Acute ischemic stroke*	160	
Acute STEMI	162	

*Higher doses were tested and not found to confer any greater risk reduction.
NSTEMI = non–ST elevation myocardial infarction; STEMI = ST elevation myocardial infarction; TIA = transient ischemic attack.

aspirin on COX-2 is an incomplete allosteric inhibition compared with that seen with COX-1.

Traditional NSAIDs typically inhibit platelet COX-1 and monocyte COX-2 by 50 to 90%, depending on dose; this effect is usually transient, depending on dose and half-life (Fig. 36-3). Coxibs inhibit monocyte COX-2 to the same extent as other NSAIDs, while substantially sparing platelet (and presumably other cells) COX-1 in most patients exposed to therapeutic doses. In contrast, aspirin achieves virtually complete (i.e., >97%) and persistent (i.e., ≥ 24 hour) inactivation of platelet COX-1 by virtue of its irreversible mechanism of action and inability of anucleate platelets to resynthesize the enzyme. Aspirin is equally potent in acetylating COX-1 and COX-2 in vitro. However, its unique mechanism of action and unusual pharmacokinetic features (20-minute half-life; presystemic encounter with the platelet target in the portal blood before first-pass liver metabolism) allow selective, cumulative inhibition of platelet COX-1 at low doses while substantially sparing vascular COX-2. The effect of aspirin on COX-1-dependent TXA_2 production is saturable at daily doses as low as 30 to 50 mg; in contrast, its inhibitory effect on COX-2-dependent prostaglandin I_2 biosynthesis is dose dependent up to daily doses of 650 to 1300 mg.

The relationships among inhibition of COX isozyme activity, reduced prostanoid formation, and changes in prostanoid-dependent cell function in vivo are not necessarily linear. The strikingly nonlinear relationship between inactivation of platelet COX-1 and inhibition of thromboxane-dependent platelet activation in vivo has important clinical implications for the cardiovascular effects of low-dose aspirin versus traditional NSAIDs (see later). In addition, interindividual variability in drug plasma levels as well as in the corresponding level of COX isozyme inhibition contributes to substantial unpredictability of the individual clinical response to COX inhibitors (E-Fig. 36-1).

Low-Dose Aspirin as an Antithrombotic and Anti-cancer Agent

The efficacy and safety of aspirin as an antithrombotic agent have been evaluated in several populations, ranging from apparently healthy persons at low risk of vascular complications (so-called primary prevention) to high-risk patients presenting with or surviving an acute myocardial infarction or an acute ischemic stroke (so-called secondary prevention). The clinical efficacy of aspirin was demonstrated at doses ranging from 50 to 162 mg given once daily (Table 36-1), consistent with the irreversible nature of its mechanism of action. Furthermore, higher doses (e.g., 300 to 325 mg) were not found to confer additional benefits, consistent with saturability of platelet COX-1 acetylation at low doses.**1**

In the six primary prevention trials among 95,000 low-risk individuals, aspirin allocation yielded a 12% relative risk reduction in serious vascular events (myocardial infarction, stroke, or vascular death).**2** This protective effect was mainly due to a reduction in nonfatal myocardial infarction. The net effect on stroke was not significant, reflecting a small reduction in presumed ischemic stroke and counterbalancing effects on hemorrhagic stroke and other (probably ischemic) stroke. There was no significant reduction in vascular mortality. Aspirin increased gastrointestinal (or other extracranial) bleeds by approximately 50%.**2**

In 16 secondary prevention trials in 17,000 high-risk patients with prior myocardial infarction, or prior stroke or transient cerebral ischemia, aspirin allocation yielded 19% fewer serious vascular events, with similar proportional reductions in coronary events (20% relative risk reduction) and ischemic stroke (22% relative risk reduction) but a nonsignificant increase in hemorrhagic stroke.**2** The absolute benefit of aspirin was about 25 times larger in secondary than in primary prevention (15 vs. 0.6 fewer vascular events per 1000 per year). In both primary and secondary prevention trials, the proportional reductions in serious vascular events appeared similar for men and women and for older and younger people. The risks of serious vascular events and of major extracranial bleeds were predicted by the same independent risk factors (age, male gender, diabetes mellitus, current smoking, blood pressure, and body mass index), so those with high risk of vascular complications also had a high risk of bleeding.

For secondary prevention of cardiovascular disease, the net benefits of adding aspirin to other preventive measures (e.g., statins) substantially exceed the bleeding hazards, irrespective of age and gender. In addition, aspirin, 75 mg daily or more for at least several years, reduces the incidence and mortality of colorectal cancer.**3**

Traditional Nonsteroidal Anti-inflammatory Drugs and Coxibs

NSAIDs constitute a chemically heterogeneous group of compounds that provide symptomatic relief of pain and inflammation associated with a variety of human disorders, including the rheumatic diseases. Their shared therapeutic actions (i.e., analgesic, anti-inflammatory, and antipyretic) are usually accompanied by mechanism-based adverse effects on gastrointestinal, cardiovascular, and renal functions. Prostanoids reproduce the main signs and symptoms of the inflammatory response and cause hyperalgesia and fever. Because of the redundancy of mediators of these responses, it is not surprising that NSAIDs only exert a moderate anti-inflammatory effect, are effective only against pain of low to moderate intensity and reduce fever, but do not interfere with the physiologic control of body temperature. The analgesic, anti-inflammatory, and antipyretic actions of traditional NSAIDs are largely reproduced by coxibs, a class of selective inhibitors of COX-2.

COX-2 selectivity is a continuous variable (see Fig. 36-2). Thus, one can pragmatically characterize three levels of COX-2 selectivity in terms of the probability of sparing COX-1 at therapeutic plasma levels: low (e.g., acetaminophen), intermediate (e.g., celecoxib, nimesulide, and diclofenac), and high (e.g., rofecoxib, etoricoxib, and lumiracoxib).

NSAIDs can modify the pharmacokinetics or pharmacodynamics of other drugs given concurrently, resulting in clinically important drug interactions. A pharmacodynamic interaction may occur between most NSAIDs and several classes of antihypertensive drugs. Reduced production of vasodilator prostacyclin and natriuretic prostaglandin E_2, as a consequence of renal

COX-2 inhibition, results in vasoconstriction and sodium and water retention that in turn tend to elevate blood pressure, regardless of the mechanism of action of antihypertensive drugs. This pharmacodynamic interaction has been described with most traditional NSAIDs (including acetaminophen) and coxibs, but not with low-dose aspirin.

Some NSAIDs favoring COX-1 over COX-2 inhibition, such as ibuprofen and naproxen, may interfere with the antiplatelet effect of low-dose aspirin by competing with acetylsalicylic acid for a common docking site (arginine-120) within the COX-1 channel. Drugs favoring COX-2 versus COX-1 inhibition, such as acetaminophen and diclofenac, do not interfere with the pharmacodynamic effect of low-dose aspirin, similarly to celecoxib and rofecoxib.

Upper gastrointestinal complications (bleeds, perforations, and obstructions) occur in 1 to 2% of NSAID-treated patients (Chapter 141). The mortality rate associated with hospitalization due to major gastrointestinal events is 5 to 6% in recent studies. Mortality rates associated with upper or lower gastrointestinal complications due to NSAIDs are similar. The major risk factors for upper gastrointestinal bleeding are represented by age and a prior history of gastrointestinal disorders (E-Fig. 36-1). Male gender, cigarette smoking, and heavy alcohol intake increase this risk by less than twofold, as do oral glucocorticoids. Oral anticoagulants, thienopyridines, and low-dose aspirin increase the risk of NSAID-induced bleeding complications by two- to three-fold. The excess of these complications due to traditional NSAIDs has been estimated to range between 3 and 30 events per 1000 patients treated per year depending on the absence or presence of risk factors (E-Fig. 36-1).

Highly selective COX-2 inhibitors are associated with a statistically significant 50 to 66% relative risk reduction in ulcer complications compared with naproxen or ibuprofen.**4** However, no such agent is available on the U.S. market.

A meta-analysis of tabular data from 138 randomized trials of five different coxibs in approximately 145,000 patients has revealed that, in placebo comparisons, allocation to a coxib was associated with a 42% increased incidence of vascular events with no statistically significant heterogeneity among the different coxibs.**5** This excess risk of vascular events was derived primarily from a two-fold increased risk of myocardial infarction. Overall, there was no significant difference in the incidence of vascular events between a coxib and any traditional NSAID, but there was evidence of significant heterogeneity between naproxen and the other traditional NSAIDs (largely represented by ibuprofen and diclofenac).**5**

Current evidence suggests that the risk of myocardial infarction depends on the extent of COX-2 inhibition and not on the variable COX-2 selectivity of the inhibitor. This risk appears to be modulated by concomitant high-grade and persistent inhibition of platelet COX-1 activity, as suggested by the neutral cardiovascular phenotype associated with a high-dose regimen of naproxen. However, in patients at high cardiovascular risk, whose platelet COX-1 is completely and persistently inactivated by low-dose aspirin, the administration of any COX-2 inhibitor (including naproxen) is likely to produce detrimental cardiovascular consequences.

Given the nonlinear relationship between inhibition of platelet COX-1 activity and inhibition of platelet activation in vivo, it is perhaps not surprising that the cardiovascular safety profiles of coxibs and some traditional NSAIDs appear similar because they both fail to inhibit platelet activation adequately irrespective of their COX-2 selectivity. Early appearance, dose dependence, and slow dissipation of risk are important features of COX-2-related cardiotoxicity.

Grade
Ⓐ

1. CURRENT-OASIS 7 Investigators, Mehta SR, Bassand JP, et al. Dose comparisons of clopidogrel and aspirin in acute coronary syndromes. *N Engl J Med.* 2010;363:930-942.
2. Baigent C, Blackwell L, Collins R, et al, for the Antithrombotic Trialists' (ATT) Collaboration. Aspirin in the primary and secondary prevention of vascular disease: collaborative meta-analysis of individual participant data from randomised trials. *Lancet.* 2009;373:1849-1860.
3. Rothwell PM, Wilson M, Elwin CE, et al. Long-term effect of aspirin on colorectal cancer incidence and mortality: 20-year follow-up of five randomised trials. *Lancet.* 2010;376:1741-1750.
4. Schnitzer TJ, Burmester GR, Mysler E, et al, for the TARGET Study Group. Comparison of lumiracoxib with naproxen and ibuprofen in the Therapeutic Arthritis Research and Gastrointestinal Event Trial (TARGET), reduction in ulcer complications: randomised controlled trial. *Lancet.* 2004;364:665-674.
5. Kearney PM, Baigent C, Godwin J, et al. Do selective cyclooxygenase-2 inhibitors and traditional non-steroidal anti-inflammatory drugs increase the risk of atherothrombosis? Meta-analysis of randomized trials. *BMJ.* 2006;332:1302-1308.

SUGGESTED READINGS

Patrono C, Baigent C. Low-dose aspirin, coxibs, and other NSAIDs: a clinical mosaic emerges. *Mol Interv.* 2009;9:31-39. *This review discusses the mechanisms underlying the cardiovascular effects of low-dose aspirin, traditional NSAIDs, and coxibs.*

Patrono C, Rocca B. The future of antiplatelet therapy in cardiovascular disease. *Annu Rev Med.* 2010;61:49-61. *This review discusses different mechanisms of platelet inhibition with emphasis on the pharmacokinetic and pharmacodynamic determinants of clinical efficacy and safety of antiplatelet drugs.*

Stavrakis S, Stoner JA, Azar M, et al. Low-dose aspirin for primary prevention of cardiovascular events in patients with diabetes: a meta-analysis. *Am J Med Sci.* 2011;341:1-9. *Argues against low-dose aspirin for primary prevention of cardiovascular events in patients with diabetes.*

Sung JJ, Lau JY, Ching JY, et al. Continuation of low-dose aspirin therapy in peptic ulcer bleeding: a randomized trial. *Ann Intern Med.* 2010;152:1-9. *In a small randomized trial, low-dose aspirin therapy increased the risk of recurrent bleeding from 5.4 to 10.3%, but reduced mortality by 11.6%.*

ANTITHROMBOTIC THERAPY

SAM SCHULMAN AND JACK HIRSH

Antithrombotic therapy suppresses the natural hemostatic mechanisms (Chapter 174) and is effective for preventing and treating venous, cardiac, and arterial thromboembolism. A variety of medications are now available that interfere with different steps in coagulation and platelet activation, sometimes with synergistic effects. In recent years, randomized clinical trials have produced a substantial body of evidence-based literature to guide the use of antithrombotic therapy for a wide range of clinical conditions.

PHARMACOLOGIC AGENTS

Vitamin K Antagonists

For more than 60 years, vitamin K antagonists have been the only oral anticoagulants available for clinical use. Now, with the development of novel oral agents that target single coagulation enzymes (see later), the situation is changing. Coumarins are vitamin K antagonists, of which warfarin is the most widely used. Coumarins inhibit a vitamin K reductase that catalyzes the reduction of 2,3-epoxide (vitamin K epoxide), thereby leading to the depletion of vitamin KH_2, which is required for the production of functionally active (γ-carboxylated) coagulation proteins (factors II [prothrombin], VII, IX, and X) and anticoagulant proteins (protein C and protein S) (Chapter 178). Vitamin K_1 in food sources can reverse these effects of coumarins because it is reduced to vitamin KH_2 by a warfarin-insensitive vitamin K reductase (Fig. 37-1).

Warfarin is rapidly and almost completely absorbed from the gastrointestinal tract. It has a half-life of about 40 hours, a delayed onset of action (2 to 7 days, depending on dose), and a residual anticoagulant effect for up to 5 days after treatment is discontinued. The dose-response relationship of warfarin varies widely among individuals and is influenced by many factors, including age, body weight, liver disease, dietary vitamin K_1, genetic factors, concomitant drug use, compliance of the patient, and inappropriate dosage adjustments.**1** Of these factors, inappropriate dosage adjustment and improved compliance through patient education are the most readily correctable.

The effect of warfarin must be monitored closely to prevent overdosing or underdosing. Laboratory monitoring is performed by measuring the prothrombin time and is reported as an international normalized ratio (INR). During initiation of warfarin therapy, the INR reflects primarily the depression of factor VII, which has a half-life of only 6 hours. There is evidence that the reliability of warfarin monitoring is improved by having the dosage controlled by an anticoagulation management service and by using computer-assisted algorithms. The convenience of monitoring is increased with a portable point-of-care instrument. Pharmacogenetic-guided dosing of warfarin has been evaluated in four randomized trials without producing evidence that the rate of major hemorrhage or thromboembolic complications is reduced, and the current cost is $100 to $200 per patient.

Indications for Warfarin

Warfarin is effective in the primary and secondary prevention of systemic embolism in patients with atrial fibrillation (Chapter 64); in the prevention of systemic arterial embolism in patients with valvular heart disease

FIGURE 37-1. Warfarin inhibits vitamin K epoxide reductase and leads to the intracellular depletion (in the hepatocyte) of vitamin KH_2. Vitamin KH_2 is required for the conversion (by γ-carboxylation) of functionally inactive to active coagulation proteins. The anticoagulant effect of warfarin can be reversed by vitamin K_1 in food because it is reduced to vitamin KH_2 by a warfarin-insensitive vitamin K reductase.

TABLE 37-1	RECOMMENDED MANAGEMENT OF ELEVATED INR WITH OR WITHOUT BLEEDING IN PATIENTS TREATED WITH WARFARIN			
INR	**BLEEDING**	**WARFARIN**	**VITAMIN K_1**	**FFP/PCC/rFVIIa**
<5.0	Negligible	Hold 1 dose or reduce dose	No	No
5.0-9.9	Negligible	Hold 1-2 doses	1-2.5 mg PO*	No
≥10	Negligible	Hold	2.5-5 mg PO	No
Any	Serious or life-threatening	Hold	10 mg IV⁺ and repeat PRN	Yes

*Only for patients at increased risk of bleeding.[26]
⁺Intravenous (IV) infusion should be given slowly.
FFP = fresh-frozen plasma; INR = International Normalized Ratio; PCC = prothrombin complex concentrate; PO = orally; PRN = as needed; rFVIIa, recombinant factor VIIa.

Warfarin-induced skin necrosis occurs in 1 in 5000 patients, more frequently in women, and affects mainly breasts, buttocks, and thighs. An imbalance between moderately reduced procoagulant factors and severely depressed natural inhibitors may cause this hypercoagulable state in patients with congenital deficiency of protein C or protein S (Chapter 179), dietary deficiency of vitamin K, cancer, or heparin-induced thrombocytopenia with premature start of vitamin K antagonists (Chapter 175).

Reversing the Effect of Warfarin

The anticoagulant effect of warfarin can be reversed in one of three ways: by discontinuation of therapy, with the expectation that the INR will return to baseline in about 5 days; by administration of vitamin K_1, with the expectation that the anticoagulant effect will be reduced in 6 hours and reversed in 24 hours; and by infusion of fresh-frozen plasma (FFP), prothrombin complex concentrate (PCC), or recombinant coagulation factor VIIa (rFVIIa), which produce immediate reversal (Table 37-1).

Heparin and Low-Molecular-Weight Heparins
Heparin

Heparin binds to antithrombin (AT), thereby increasing the rate at which AT inactivates thrombin, activated factor X (factor Xa), and other coagulation enzymes. Heparin accelerates the inactivation of thrombin by AT by providing a template to which both the enzyme and the inhibitor bind to form a ternary complex (Fig. 37-2). In contrast, the inactivation of factor Xa by the AT-heparin complex does not require ternary complex formation and is achieved by binding of the heparin-bound AT to factor Xa. Heparin binds to a number of plasma, platelet, and endothelial cell–derived proteins that compete with AT for heparin binding. Binding of heparin to plasma proteins contributes to the variability of its anticoagulant response, whereas binding to hepatic macrophages is responsible for its dose-dependent clearance. Both properties contribute to the unpredictable anticoagulant effect of heparin and the need for laboratory monitoring.

Heparin is effective for the prevention and treatment of venous thromboembolism,[3-5] for the early treatment of patients with unstable angina and acute myocardial infarction,[6,7] for patients who have cardiac surgery under cardiopulmonary bypass,[8] for patients undergoing vascular surgery,[9] and during and after coronary angioplasty and coronary stent placement.[8]

The anticoagulant effects of heparin are usually monitored by the activated partial thromboplastin time (aPTT). A therapeutic effect is achieved when the aPTT ratio is equivalent to a heparin level of 0.3 to 0.7 anti–factor Xa units, which for many reagents is an aPTT ratio of 1.5 to 2.5.[4] The risk of bleeding complications is increased with increasing heparin dosage, which in turn is related to the anticoagulant response. However, other clinical factors, such as recent surgery, trauma, and invasive procedures, are also important as predictors of bleeding during heparin treatment.

For the treatment of venous thromboembolism, heparin is given in doses of 80 U/kg followed by 18 U/kg per hour by continuous infusion; the dose is adjusted according to the aPTT result at 6 hours by use of a validated nomogram. Lower doses (70 U/kg or 5000 U followed by 15 U/kg/h or 1000 U/hour) of heparin are used in patients with acute myocardial ischemia, who also receive aspirin and platelet glycoprotein IIb/IIIa complex (GPIIb-IIIa) antagonists or thrombolytic therapy.

The main complications of heparin are bleeding and heparin-induced thrombocytopenia. Less common complications are heparin-induced

The anticoagulant effect of warfarin (bioprosthetic and mechanical heart valves [Chapter 75]); in the primary and secondary prevention of venous thromboembolism (Chapters 81 and 98); in the prevention of acute myocardial infarction in high-risk patients (Chapters 72 and 73); and in the prevention of stroke (Chapter 414), recurrent infarction, and death in patients with acute myocardial infarction (Chapter 73).[2] A target INR of 2.5 (range, 2.0 to 3.0) is recommended for almost all indications. Exceptions are mechanical prosthetic heart valve in the mitral position or caged-ball or caged-disk valve in the aortic position or any mechanical aortic valve in combination with atrial fibrillation, anterior myocardial infarction, left atrial enlargement, or low ejection fraction, when an INR of 3.0 (range, 2.5 to 3.5) is recommended.

Dosing and Monitoring

If a rapid anticoagulant effect is required, heparin and warfarin should be started at the same time and overlapped for at least 5 days. Warfarin is started with the estimated maintenance dose of about 5 mg/day, with the first INR measurement after 2 to 3 days, and patients usually reach an INR of 2.0 in 4 or 5 days. If there is no increase of the INR after two or three doses, the daily dose should be progressively increased until an INR response is observed. In patients with a low risk of bleeding, warfarin may be started at a dose of 10 mg and then adjusted according to daily INR results. Heparin treatment is discontinued when the INR has been in the therapeutic range for 2 days. The INR is then performed two or three times weekly for 1 to 2 weeks and then weekly up to a maximal interval of 4 weeks, depending on the stability of INR results, and more frequently when a new drug is added to the treatment.

Adjustments to the dose when the INR drifts out of the therapeutic range should be gradual and based on the weekly dose (e.g., a 10 to 20% change in weekly dose). Patients should be encouraged to keep a log of their dose and their INR response.

Adverse Effects

Warfarin-related bleeding is increased by the level of the INR. The risk of bleeding is also increased with concomitant aspirin use, in persons older than 65 years, in those with a history of stroke or gastrointestinal bleeding, and in those with serious comorbid conditions. Elderly patients are more sensitive to warfarin, requiring lower doses to reach the therapeutic range, and have an increased tendency to bleed, including intracranially, even when their INR is in the therapeutic range (Chapter 23).

osteoporosis and hyperkalemia. Heparin-related bleeding is dose related, and the risk is increased in patients who undergo an invasive procedure and if heparin is used in combination with a platelet GPIIb-IIIa antagonist or a thrombolytic agent.

If heparin-induced thrombocytopenia (Chapter 175) is suspected on clinical grounds and anticoagulant treatment is indicated, heparin should be stopped and replaced with a thrombin inhibitor, either hirudin (lepirudin) or argatroban. Warfarin should not be used alone to treat acute heparin-induced thrombocytopenia because it can aggravate the thrombotic process, but it is safe in combination with a thrombin inhibitor after the platelet count has risen above 100×10^9/L.

Low-Molecular-Weight Heparins
LMWHs are fragments produced by either chemical or enzymatic depolymerization of heparin. LMWHs are approximately one third the size of

Heparin and LMWH (MW > 5400)

LMWH (MW < 5400)

☐ = high-affinity pentasaccharide

FIGURE 37-2. Only one third of high-affinity pentasaccharide-containing heparin molecules and one fifth of pentasaccharide-containing low-molecular-weight heparin (LMWH) molecules activate antithrombin (AT). Virtually all of the high-affinity heparin molecules are large enough to bridge between AT and factor IIa (thrombin). In contrast, only 25 to 50% of LMWH molecules have a molecular weight (MW) of 5400 or more, and although these smaller molecules inactivate factor Xa, they do not inactivate factor IIa. Although heparin has equal anti–factor IIa and anti–factor Xa activities, LMWH has reduced anti–factor IIa activity.

heparin (Table 37-2). Depolymerization of heparin changes the anticoagulant profile. As a result, LMWHs have less protein and cellular binding and, as a consequence, have a more predictable dose response, better bioavailability, and a longer plasma half-life than regular heparin. LMWHs can therefore be administered subcutaneously once daily without laboratory monitoring.

Compared with heparin, which has a ratio of anti–factor Xa to anti–factor IIa activity of approximately 1:1, the various commercial LMWHs have ratios of anti–factor Xa to anti–factor IIa varying between 4:1 and 2:1, depending on their molecular size distribution. LMWHs are cleared principally by the renal route. LMWHs are associated with a lower incidence of heparin-induced thrombocytopenia and heparin-induced osteoporosis than is heparin.

LMWHs are effective in the prevention and treatment of venous thromboembolism (VTE) (Chapter 81),**3-5** in the treatment of patients with unstable angina and non–ST elevation myocardial infarction (Chapters 72 and 73),**7** and as an adjunct to fibrinolytic therapy in patients with acute ST elevation myocardial infarction (Chapter 73).**6**

Pentasaccharides
On the basis of knowledge of the AT-binding sequence on heparin, a pentasaccharide, fondaparinux, with high affinity for AT has been synthesized. The structure of fondaparinux has been modified to increase its affinity to AT. Fondaparinux inactivates factor Xa through an AT-mediated mechanism. Because it is too short to bridge AT to thrombin, fondaparinux has no activity against thrombin.

After subcutaneous injection, fondaparinux is rapidly and completely absorbed and exhibits a bioavailability of 100%. The volume of distribution is similar to the blood volume. The drug is mainly excreted unchanged in the urine, with a terminal half-life of 17 hours in young volunteers and 21 hours in elderly volunteers.**4**

Fondaparinux circulates extensively bound to AT with minimal binding to other plasma proteins. Limited experimental and clinical studies suggest that fondaparinux has a lower risk of heparin-induced thrombocytopenia than that of heparin or LMWH as well as a lower risk of bone loss and of local skin reactions.

Fondaparinux is effective in the prevention and treatment of VTE**3,5** and is also effective in the treatment of acute coronary syndromes.**6,7**

New Anticoagulants
The limitations of established anticoagulants have prompted the development of a variety of new anticoagulant agents that target various specific steps in the coagulation mechanism.

Direct Thrombin Inhibitors
Direct thrombin inhibitors act independently of AT to inactivate both free thrombin and thrombin bound to fibrin. The direct thrombin inhibitors include hirudin, synthetic hirudin fragments (hirugen, lepirudin, and

TABLE 37-2 ANTICOAGULANT PROFILES, MOLECULAR WEIGHTS, PLASMA HALF-LIVES, AND RECOMMENDED DOSES OF COMMERCIAL LOW-MOLECULAR-WEIGHT HEPARINS

AGENT	ANTI-X_a/ANTI-II_a RATIO	MOLECULAR WEIGHT	PLASMA HALF-LIFE (MIN)	Recommended Dose (International Anti-Xa Units)		
				GENERAL SURGERY PROPHYLAXIS	ORTHOPEDIC SURGERY PROPHYLAXIS	ACUTE TREATMENT
Enoxaparin	2.7:1	4500	129-180	4000 U SC daily	4000 U SC daily or 3000 U SC bid	7000 U SC bid*† or 10,500 U SC daily*
Dalteparin	2:1	5000	119-139	2500 U SC daily	2500 U SC bid or 5000 U SC daily	8400 U SC bid*† or 14,000 U SC daily*
Nadroparin	3.2:1	4500	132-162	2850 U SC daily	2700 U SC daily,* 4000 U SC daily* from day 4	13,300 U SC daily*
Tinzaparin (Innohep)	1.9:1	4500	111	3500 U SC daily	3500 U SC daily* or 4500 U SC daily*	12,250 U daily*
Ardeparin	2:1	6000	200		50 U/kg SC bid	
Danaparoid‡	20:1	6500	1100	750 U SC daily	750 U SC bid	2500 U IV, then 4 hr each of 400 U/hr and 300 U/hr, then 200 U/hr; or 2000 U SC bid

*Weight-adjusted dose; stated dose for 70-kg patient.
†The higher daily dose is for acute coronary syndromes; the lower dose is for deep vein thrombosis.
‡Danaparoid sodium is a heparinoid.
IV = intravenously; SC = subcutaneously.

bivalirudin [Hirulog]), and low-molecular-weight inhibitors that react with the active site of thrombin (dabigatran and argatroban).[10]

Bivalirudin is approved for use in coronary angioplasty (Chapter 73),[11] and both argatroban and lepirudin are approved in patients with heparin-induced thrombocytopenia (Chapter 175). Data comparing argatroban with hirudin in heparin-induced thrombocytopenia are too limited for conclusions to be drawn about their relative efficacy and safety. Argatroban is metabolized in the liver and can be used in patients with renal failure, whereas the other direct thrombin inhibitors depend on elimination through renal excretion, and they may be used in patients with liver disease.

Dabigatran etexilate is metabolized by ubiquitous esterases to dabigatran, a reversible, active-site thrombin inhibitor. The bioavailability after oral administration is 6%; the half-life is 12 to 17 hours with substantial prolongation in case of renal failure, owing to predominant elimination through the kidneys. Dabigatran etexilate has been approved in Europe and several other countries for prophylaxis against VTE after hip or knee arthroplasty (first dose, 110 mg; then 220 mg once daily; for patients over 70 years of age or with creatinine clearance, 30 to 50 mL/minute, first dose 75 mg and then 150 mg daily). The effect is similar to that of enoxaparin (40 mg subcutaneously daily).[12] Dabigatran (150 mg twice daily) is more effective than warfarin for stroke prophylaxis in atrial fibrillation, whereas a lower dose (110 mg twice daily) is equally effective with lower risk for major bleeding. Both doses resulted in fewer intracranial hemorrhages than warfarin.[13] Dabigatran has been approved for this use in the United States and Canada. In the treatment of VTE, dabigatran (150 mg twice daily) has comparable effect to warfarin and is at least as safe regarding bleeding.[14]

Direct Factor Xa Inhibitors

A number of orally available low-molecular-weight active site-directed factor Xa inhibitors have been designed and are in various stages of clinical development (rivaroxaban, apixaban, betrixaban, edoxaban). Unlike heparins and pentasaccharides, direct inhibitors inactivate factor Xa without the need for AT as a cofactor.[10]

Rivaroxaban, an oxazolidinone derivative, has a bioavailability of 80%, reaches maximal plasma concentration 1 to 4 hours after oral administration, and has a half-life of 5 to 9 hours in young volunteers and 11 to 13 hours in elderly volunteers. Elimination occurs to one third each through the hepatofecal route, intact through the kidneys, and as a metabolite through the kidneys. Rivaroxaban (10 mg daily for 30-39 days) is more effective than enoxaparin in patients undergoing hip or knee arthroplasty but with a trend to more bleeding.[15]

Apixaban has also a high bioavailability, mixed pathway elimination, and a half-life of 12 hours. Given for prophylaxis against VTE after knee arthroplasty, apixaban (2.5 mg twice daily) has similar or better efficacy than LMWH and similar or lower risk of bleeding.[16,17]

Platelet-Active Drugs

The platelet-active drugs inhibit different steps in either platelet activation (aspirin, ticlopidine, clopidogrel, prasugrel, cilostazol, and dipyridamole) or platelet recruitment (GPIIb-IIIa antagonists abciximab, tirofiban, and eptifibatide) (Fig. 37-3).[10,18]

Aspirin and Other Cyclooxygenase Inhibitors
Mechanism of Action and Pharmacology

Aspirin permanently inactivates cyclooxygenase isoenzymes (COX-1 and COX-2) that catalyze the conversion of arachidonic acid to prostaglandin H_2, a precursor of a variety of eicosanoids including thromboxane A_2 in platelets and prostacyclin (prostaglandin I_2) in vascular endothelial cells.

Aspirin is rapidly absorbed in the stomach and upper intestine, attaining peak plasma levels about 30 minutes after ingestion; it has a half-life of about 15 minutes. Inhibition of platelet function is evident by 1 hour with uncoated aspirin but can be delayed after administration of enteric-coated aspirin. Therefore, if only enteric-coated tablets are available when a rapid effect is required, the tablets should be chewed.

Aspirin potentiates the antithrombotic effects of warfarin (in high-risk subjects), dipyridamole (in those with ischemic stroke), clopidogrel (in those with coronary stents or acute myocardial ischemia), and heparin (in the prevention of recurrent miscarriages in pregnant women with antiphospholipid antibody syndrome and in patients with acute coronary ischemia). Aspirin produces a small increase in major bleeding and a very small increase in the risk of cerebral hemorrhage. It also potentiates bleeding when it is added to another antithrombotic agent.

FIGURE 37-3. Sites of action of platelet inhibitors. ADP = adenosine diphosphate; GPIIb-IIIa = glycoprotein IIb/IIIa complex; TXA_2 = thromboxane A_2.

Aspirin causes gastrointestinal side effects that are dose dependent. Aspirin is contraindicated in individuals with active peptic ulcer disease or aspirin-induced asthma or if gastrointestinal side effects are severe.

Clinical Uses

Based on the results of a meta-analysis, there is evidence that aspirin reduces vascular death by approximately 15% and nonfatal vascular events by about 30% in patients with cardiovascular disease (Table 37-3).[18] These effects are achieved in patients with silent myocardial ischemia or stable angina, unstable angina, non–ST elevation myocardial infarction, ST elevation myocardial infarction, and ischemic cerebrovascular disease.[6-8,19] Aspirin is also effective in patients after coronary angioplasty or coronary artery bypass surgery[8] and in preventing symptomatic coronary events in asymptomatic men and women older than 50 years.[8,18] Aspirin has a favorable risk-to-benefit ratio for secondary prevention in patients with overt vascular disease, but the risk-to-benefit ratio is marginal when aspirin is used as primary prevention in asymptomatic individuals, even individuals with type 2 diabetes.[20] Aspirin is less effective than oral anticoagulants in the prevention of recurrent stroke in atrial fibrillation[21] and less effective than LMWH or warfarin in preventing venous thromboembolism.[3]

Phosphodiesterase Inhibitors

Dipyridamole and cilostazol are phosphodiesterase inhibitors, which elevate platelet cyclic adenosine and guanine monophosphate (cAMP and cGMP) levels. They block platelet reactivity and also inhibit vasoconstriction. The most common side effect is headache.

Dipyridamole is a pyrimidopyrimidine derivative with a terminal half-life of 10 hours and elimination primarily by biliary excretion. Favorable results were obtained with a modified-release preparation in patients with prior stroke or transient ischemic attack, in whom the risk of stroke was reduced by 16% with dipyridamole alone and by 37% with aspirin and dipyridamole in combination, compared with placebo.[18,19]

In a meta-analysis, cilostazol (100 mg twice daily) was shown to improve maximal and pain-free walking distance in patients with intermittent claudication.[22] Cilostazol is contraindicated in patients with congestive heart failure, owing to reports of fatal events with similar drugs.

Thienopyridines

Ticlopidine, clopidogrel, and prasugrel are thienopyridines that inhibit adenosine diphosphate–induced platelet aggregation through the action of their active metabolites at the $P2Y_{12}$ receptor level. The drugs are administered orally, but their onset of action is delayed until their active metabolites are formed. Similarly, recovery of platelet function is delayed until the circulating affected platelets are replaced by newly formed, unaffected platelets.

Based on a better safety profile and equal efficacy, clopidogrel has replaced ticlopidine. Clopidogrel is rapidly absorbed and metabolized, producing inhibition of platelet aggregation as soon as 90 minutes after an oral loading dosing of 300 mg. With repeated daily administration of low doses (75 mg), there is cumulative inhibition of platelet function with a return to normal 7 days after the last dose of clopidogrel.

Clopidogrel is more effective than aspirin in patients who have experienced a recent stroke or recent myocardial infarction and in patients presenting with symptomatic peripheral arterial disease.[6,9,19] The additional benefit over aspirin is modest and similar to that observed with ticlopidine (about 10% relative risk reduction). The combination of clopidogrel and aspirin is also more effective than aspirin alone in patients with unstable angina and non–ST elevation myocardial infarction (20% risk reduction)[7] and in patients with atrial fibrillation,[23] but at a cost of a modest increase in bleeding. The combination of clopidogrel and aspirin is also more effective than

---

TABLE 37-3 SUMMARY OF GRADE A RECOMMENDATIONS FOR ANTITHROMBOTIC THERAPY

Grade 1A indicates that experts are certain that benefits do or do not outweigh risks, burdens, and costs. Grade 2A indicates that they are less certain, resulting in a weaker recommendation.

PREVENTION OF VENOUS THROMBOEMBOLISM (Chapters 81 and 98)[3]

General Recommendations

Every general hospital should develop a formal, active strategy to prevent venous thromboembolism, such as computer decision support systems (grade 1A).
Patients at high risk for or with active bleeding: mechanical methods—elastic stockings or intermittent pneumatic compression (grade 1A)

General Surgery

Moderate-risk general surgery: LMWH, low-dose unfractionated heparin or fondaparinux (grade 1A)
Higher-risk general surgery: LMWH, low-dose unfractionated heparin or fondaparinux; for major procedures until discharge from hospital (grade 1A)
Major gynecologic surgery for benign disease: LMWH, or low-dose unfractionated heparin every 12 hours (grade 1A)
Extensive gynecologic surgery for malignant disease: low-dose unfractionated heparin every 8 hours, higher doses of LMWH, or intermittent pneumatic compression as long as patient is not ambulating (grade 1A)

Major Orthopedic Surgery

Elective total hip replacement surgery: subcutaneous LMWH, started either 12 hours before or 12-24 hours after surgery or 4-6 hours after surgery at half dose; fondaparinux, started 6-24 hours after surgery; or adjusted-dose warfarin (INR target of 2.5; range, 2.0 to 3.0), started preoperatively or immediately after surgery (grade 1A)
Elective total knee replacement surgery: LMWH, fondaparinux, or adjusted-dose warfarin (grade 1A)
Hip fracture surgery: fondaparinux (grade 1A)
Anticoagulant prophylaxis should be continued for at least 10 days (grade 1A). Extended prophylaxis should be given for up to 35 days with LMWH after total hip replacement and with fondaparinux after hip fracture surgery (grade 1A). Routine duplex ultrasonography screening at the time of hospital discharge or during outpatient follow-up is not recommended in asymptomatic patients after total hip replacement or total knee replacement (grade 1A).
Isolated distal lower-extremity injuries: routine thromboprophylaxis is not recommended (grade 2A)

Neurosurgery, Burns, Trauma, and Acute Spinal Cord Injury

Neurosurgery: intermittent pneumatic compression (grade 1A) or LMWH started after surgery (grade 2A)
Trauma or burn patients: all burn patients with at least one risk factor for VTE and all patients with major trauma or acute spinal cord injury should receive thromboprophylaxis, if it is not contraindicated (grade 1A). LMWH is started as soon as it is considered safe (grade 1A).

Medical Conditions

Acutely ill medical patients, confined to bed and with at least one additional risk factor for VTE: low-dose unfractionated heparin, LMWH or fondaparinux (grade 1A)

Critical Care

Most patients should, after appropriate assessment of the risk for VTE, receive thromboprophylaxis: if medically ill or postoperative—with unfractionated heparin or LMWH; with major trauma or orthopedic surgery—with LMWH (grade 1A).

TREATMENT OF VENOUS THROMBOEMBOLIC DISEASE
(Chapters 81 and 98)[5]

Acute Treatment

Acute treatment: LMWH, or unfractionated heparin IV, adjusted dose SC or fixed dose SC, or fondaparinux (grade 1A)
Start treatment with vitamin K antagonists on the first day (grade 1A).
Patients with DVT: early ambulation when feasible (grade 1A)

Long-Term Anticoagulation

Patients with VTE and cancer: treat with LMWH for the first 3-6 months (grade 1A).
Patients with a first episode of VTE and reversible or time-limited risk factors: treat with vitamin K antagonists for 3 months (grade 1A).
Patients with a first episode of unprovoked VTE: treat for at least 3 months and extend long-term if risk factors for bleeding are absent and good anticoagulation monitoring is achievable (grade 1A).
After two or more episodes: treat long-term (grade 1A).
Adjust the dose of vitamin K antagonist to maintain a target INR of 2.5 with a range of 2.0 to 3.0 for all treatment durations (grade 1A). In patients with a strong preference for less frequent INR testing after the first 3 months, continue with INR range 1.5 to 1.9 (grade 1A).
Prescribe an elastic compression stocking with an ankle pressure of 30 to 40 mm Hg for 2 years after a proximal DVT (grade 1A).
Women treated with warfarin after VTE and who become pregnant: substitute with unfractionated heparin or LMWH (grade 1A).
Women using warfarin or unfractionated heparin and who wish to breast-feed: continue the medication (grade 1A).

ATRIAL FIBRILLATION (Chapter 64)[21]

Patients with Previous Ischemic Stroke, TIA, Systemic Embolism, or at Least One Other Risk Factor for Stroke

Standard approach: warfarin anticoagulation (INR of 2.5; range, 2.0 to 3.0) (grade 1A)
Warfarin contraindicated or declined by patient: aspirin, 75 to 325 mg daily
Aspirin plus low-, fixed-dose warfarin should not be used.

VALVULAR AND STRUCTURAL HEART DISEASE (Chapter 75)[27]

Mitral Valve Disease

Rheumatic mitral valve disease with atrial fibrillation, previous systemic embolism, or left atrial thrombus: warfarin anticoagulation (INR of 2.5; range, 2.0 to 3.0) (grade 1A)
Mitral valve prolapse with documented but unexplained TIA: long-term aspirin, 50 to 162 mg daily (grade 1A)

Mechanical Heart Valves

Warfarin anticoagulation (grade 1A)

Patent Foramen Ovale

Patent foramen ovale and stroke: platelet-active drug

ACUTE ST SEGMENT ELEVATION MYOCARDIAL INFARCTION AND CORONARY THROMBOLYSIS (Chapter 73)[6,7]

All patients with acute myocardial infarction should receive aspirin (160 to 325 mg), chewed and swallowed, at initial evaluation by health care personnel (grade 1A).
Maintenance dose of 75 to 162 mg daily should be continued indefinitely (grade 1A).
All patients should also receive clopidogrel, 300 mg for patients less than 75 years old and 75 mg for older patients without reperfusion therapy, followed by 75 mg daily for up to 28 days (grade 1A).
All patients should also receive anticoagulation (grade 1A), with fondaparinux for patients with no reperfusion therapy (first dose 2.5 mg IV, then SC daily for up to 9 days) (grade 1A), or with enoxaparin for patients with fibrinolytic therapy and preserved renal function (grade 2A).
Anticoagulation should be extended for at least 3 months, using warfarin (INR 2.0 to 3.0), for patients with large anterior myocardial infarction, significant heart failure, intracardiac thrombus, or atrial fibrillation (grade 2A).
Patients with ischemic symptoms characteristic of myocardial infarction of less than 12 hours' duration and persistent ST segment elevation should be rapidly evaluated for reperfusion therapy with primary percutaneous coronary intervention or thrombolysis (grade 1A).
Thrombolytic therapy should be given before arrival to the hospital, when feasible (grade A), and otherwise ideally within 30 minutes from arrival (grade 1A).
Choice of fibrinolytic agent for patients with symptom duration <12 hours: streptokinase, anistreplase, reteplase, tenecteplase, or alteplase (grade 1A).
Choice of fibrinolytic agent for patients with symptom duration <6 hours: alteplase and tenecteplase are superior to streptokinase (grade 1A).

TABLE 37-3 SUMMARY OF GRADE A RECOMMENDATIONS FOR ANTITHROMBOTIC THERAPY—cont'd

NON–ST SEGMENT ELEVATION ACUTE CORONARY SYNDROMES AND PERCUTANEOUS CORONARY INTERVENTIONS (Chapters 72 and 74)[7,8]

Platelet-Active Drugs

Aspirin, non–enteric-coated, at an initial dose of 162 to 325 mg to chew and swallow as soon as possible after the clinical impression of unstable angina is formed (grade 1A). Aspirin by mouth, 75 to 100 mg, should be continued indefinitely (grade 1A).

In cases of aspirin allergy or intolerance: clopidogrel at a bolus dose of 300 mg orally and then 75 mg indefinitely (grade 1A).

Patients at a moderate to high risk for an ischemic event and planned for early invasive strategy: "upstream" clopidogrel (300-mg bolus orally, followed by 75 mg daily) or a GPIIb-IIIa antagonist IV (eptifibatide or tirofiban) (grade 1A) or both (grade 2A).

Clopidogrel should be continued, in addition to aspirin, for 12 months (grade 1A).

Anticoagulants

Unfractionated heparin, LMWH, bivalirudin or fondaparinux (grade 1A). For patients with early conservative strategy: fondaparinux (grade 1A)

CHRONIC CORONARY ARTERY DISEASE (Chapter 71)[8]

Primary Prevention

Moderate or high risk for a coronary event: aspirin, 75 to 100 mg daily (grade 2A)

Very high risk with easily monitored INR: warfarin targeted at INR of approximately 1.5 (grade 2A)

CORONARY ARTERY BYPASS GRAFTS (Chapter 74)[8]

Aspirin, 75 to 100 mg (75 to 162 mg for internal mammary bypass grafting) indefinitely (grade 1A), starting after surgery (grade 2A)

Discontinue clopidogrel 5 days before the operation (grade 2A).

ANTITHROMBOTIC THERAPY IN PATIENTS UNDERGOING PERCUTANEOUS CORONARY INTERVENTION (Chapters 72 and 74)[8]

Platelet-Active Drugs

Aspirin, 162 to 325 mg, should be administered before PCI (grade 1A).

Aspirin, 75 to 100 mg daily, should be used for secondary prevention of cardiovascular events (grade 1A).

Thienopyridines

Clopidogrel should be combined with aspirin for 12 months after bare metal stent placement (grade 1A) and for at least 12 months after drug-eluting stent (grade 1A).

Platelet Glycoprotein IIb/IIIa Antagonists

Abciximab (0.25 mg/kg bolus and 12-hour infusion at 10 μg/min) or eptifibatide (two bolus doses of 180 μg/kg 10 minutes apart) should be considered in all patients undergoing percutaneous coronary intervention, particularly patients with refractory unstable angina or with other high-risk features (grade 1A).

ANTITHROMBOTIC THERAPY IN PERIPHERAL ARTERIAL OCCLUSIVE DISEASE (Chapter 79)[9]

Patients should be treated indefinitely with a platelet-active agent (grade 1A).

Moderate to severe disabling intermittent claudication, not responding to exercise and not candidate for invasive procedures: cilostazol (grade 1A)

Patients with carotid endarterectomy should be treated preoperatively and continued indefinitely with aspirin, 75 to 100 mg daily (grade 1A).

Adding warfarin to aspirin for peripheral arterial disease is not more effective but increases life-threatening bleeding.[28]

Peripheral Vascular Reconstructive Surgery

Patients having infrainguinal bypass operations: aspirin, 75 to 100 mg/day, begun preoperatively (grade 1A)

Intraoperative Anticoagulation Therapy

Patients undergoing major vascular reconstructive operations should be systemically anticoagulated with heparin at the time of application of cross-clamps (grade 1A).

ANTITHROMBOTIC AND THROMBOLYTIC THERAPY FOR ISCHEMIC STROKE (Chapter 414)[19]

Acute ischemic stroke treatment within 3 hours of onset of symptoms:

Thrombolytic therapy: in eligible patients, IV t-PA in a dose of 0.9 mg/kg (maximum of 90 mg), with 10% of the total dose given as an initial bolus and the remainder infused during 60 minutes (grade 1A).

Streptokinase is not recommended (grade 1A).

Acute ischemic stroke patients not receiving thrombolysis:

Aspirin, 150 to 325 mg/day, started early (grade 1A)

DVT or Pulmonary Embolism Prophylaxis

For acute stroke patients with restricted mobility: low-dose subcutaneous heparin or LMWH, provided there are no contraindications to anticoagulation (grade 1A)

Stroke Prevention

Noncardioembolic cerebral ischemic events (stroke or TIA; atherothrombotic, lacunar, or cryptogenic): platelet-active drugs (grade 1A); preferably the combination of aspirin and extended-release dipyridamole (25/200 mg bid) (grade 1A) or otherwise aspirin, 50 to 100 mg/day or clopidogrel (75 mg daily) are acceptable options for initial therapy.

Patients with recent acute coronary syndrome: clopidogrel plus aspirin (75 to 100 mg daily) (grade 1A)

Stroke and aortic atherosclerotic lesions: platelet-active drugs

Cardioembolic ischemic events: long-term warfarin (target INR of 2.5; range, 2.0 to 3.0) for atrial fibrillation (grade 1A)

Carotid endarterectomy: aspirin, 50 to 100 mg/day, before carotid endarterectomy and continued long-term after the procedure

---

aPTT = activated partial thromboplastin time; DVT = deep vein thrombosis; ECG = electrocardiogram; FFP = fresh-frozen plasma; INR = International Normalized Ratio; IV = intravenous; LMWH = low-molecular-weight heparin; PCC = prothrombin complex concentrate; PCI = percutaneous coronary intervention; rFVIIa = recombinant factor VIIa; SC = subcutaneously; TIA = transient ischemic attack; t-PA = tissue plasminogen activator; VTE = venous thromboembolism.

---

aspirin alone in patients who have percutaneous coronary intervention procedures. Clopidogrel appears to be as well tolerated as aspirin.[18]

Prasugrel is more potent and has a more rapid onset of action than clopidogrel.[10] Given as a bolus dose of 60 mg, followed by 10 mg daily, when compared with clopidogrel, prasugrel reduces the absolute risk of cardiovascular death or nonfatal myocardial infarction or stroke by 2.2%, which is partly offset by an absolute increase of serious bleeding of 0.5%.[24]

Ticagrelor, an oral direct and reversible P2Y$_{12}$ receptor inhibitor, provides a faster response than the thienopyridines.[10] In a randomized trial in patients with acute coronary syndromes, ticagrelor was more effective than clopidogrel, providing an absolute risk reduction for cardiovascular death, myocardial infarction, or stroke of 1.9% without any significant increase of major bleeding.[25]

Integrin α$_{IIb}$β$_3$ (GPIIb-IIIa) Receptor Antagonists

The final common pathway of platelet aggregation is mediated by the binding of fibrinogen to the functionally active integrin α$_{IIb}$β$_3$ (GPIIb-IIIa) on the platelet surface. Inhibitors of this process include monoclonal antibodies, synthetic peptides containing Arg-Gly-Asp (RGD) or Lys-Gly-Asp (KGD), and peptidomimetic and nonpeptide RGD mimetics. These compounds are administered intravenously and inhibit platelet function by competing with fibrinogen (and von Willebrand factor) for occupancy on the platelet integrin receptor.[18] Abciximab (ReoPro), a mouse-human chimeric 7E3 Fab antibody, inhibits platelet aggregation in a concentration-dependent manner. Platelet function is impaired rapidly after an intravenous bolus of abciximab and gradually recovers over 24 to 48 hours. Tirofiban (MK-383, Aggrastat) is a nonpeptide derivative of tyrosine. It has a plasma half-life of 1.6 hours, and its effect on hemostasis is reversed within 4 hours of stopping treatment. Eptifibatide (Integrilin) is a synthetic disulfide-linked cyclic heptapeptide. It has a rapid onset and offset of action, and its effect on platelet function is reduced by more than 50% after 4 hours.

All three GPIIb-IIIa receptor antagonists are effective intravenous agents in patients undergoing percutaneous coronary interventions[8] (Chapter 74), and tirofiban and eptifibatide are effective in patients with unstable angina or non–ST elevation myocardial infarction.[7] The GPIIb-IIIa receptor antagonists are administered in combination with heparin and aspirin. Orally active nonpeptide GPIIb-IIIa inhibitors have been developed for long-term use, but the results of clinical trials have been disappointing.

Fibrinolytic Agents

Fibrinolytic agents convert plasminogen to the enzyme plasmin, which then degrades fibrin to soluble fragments, thereby lysing the thrombus. Of the available fibrinolytic agents, streptokinase and urokinase are not fibrin specific; in contrast, recombinant tissue-type plasminogen activator (rt-PA, alteplase) and the rt-PA variant tenecteplase are relatively fibrin specific (Chapter 73).

Streptokinase is an indirect fibrinolytic agent. It binds to plasminogen, converting it into a plasmin-like molecule that in turn converts plasminogen to plasmin. Streptokinase has a number of disadvantages. It is antigenic, rendering its repeated use problematic, and allergenic, producing chills, fever, and rigors in some patients and, in rare instances, anaphylaxis. Anistreplase (APSAC) is an acylated complex of streptokinase and Lys-plasminogen. Compared with streptokinase, it is more fibrin specific, has a longer plasma half-life, and is inactive until it is selectively activated by deacylation on the fibrin surface. Its side-effect profile, antigenicity, and efficacy are similar to those of streptokinase.

Urokinase is a naturally occurring plasminogen activator that differs from streptokinase in that it directly activates plasminogen and is not antigenic. Urokinase was used extensively to treat peripheral vascular occlusions, but production problems have curtailed its availability.

In its natural state, tissue plasminogen activator is produced by vascular endothelium; rt-PA (alteplase) is produced by recombinant DNA technology. Alteplase is not antigenic or allergenic, and it has greater fibrin specificity than does streptokinase. It has a short half-life of about 3.5 minutes and therefore is given as a continuous intravenous infusion.

Truncated forms of rt-PA have been developed; the first was reteplase (r-PA), a single-chain deletion mutant that lacks certain domains. As a result, its half-life is about twice that of rt-PA, permitting double-bolus therapy 30 minutes apart. r-PA has lower affinity for fibrin than does rt-PA, but fibrinogen depletion with r-PA is less than that with streptokinase. No antigenicity has been reported with this compound.

Tenecteplase (TNK-tPA) is a mutant tissue plasminogen activator with amino acid substitution at three sites. Compared with rt-PA, it has a longer half-life, allowing single-bolus administration, increased fibrin specificity, and increased resistance to inhibition by plasminogen activator inhibitor 1.

Grade A

1. Ansell J, Hirsh J, Hylek E, et al. Pharmacology and management of the vitamin K antagonists. *Chest.* 2008;133:160S-198S.
2. Schulman S. Care of patients receiving long-term anticoagulant therapy. *N Engl J Med.* 2003; 349:675-683.
3. Geerts WH, Bergqvist D, Pineo GF, et al. Prevention of venous thromboembolism: American College of Chest Physicians Evidence-Based Clinical Practice Guidelines, 8th ed. *Chest.* 2008;133:381S-453S.
4. Hirsh J, Bauer KA, Donati MB, et al. Parenteral anticoagulants: American College of Chest Physicians Evidence-Based Clinical Practice Guidelines. 8th ed. *Chest.* 2008;133:141S-159S.
5. Kearon C, Kahn SR, Agnelli G, et al. Antithrombotic therapy for venous thromboembolic disease: American College of Chest Physicians Evidence-Based Clinical Practice Guidelines, 8th ed. *Chest.* 2008;133:454S-545S.
6. Goodman SG, Menon V, Cannon CP, et al. Acute ST-segment elevation myocardial infarction: American College of Chest Physicians Evidence-Based Clinical Practice Guidelines. 8th ed. *Chest.* 2008;133:708S-775S.
7. Harrington RA, Becker RC, Cannon CP, et al. Antithrombotic therapy for non-ST-segment elevation acute coronary syndromes: American College of Chest Physicians Evidence-Based Clinical Practice Guidelines. 8th ed. *Chest.* 2008;133:670S-707S.
8. Becker RC, Meade TW, Berger PB, et al. The primary and secondary prevention of coronary artery disease: American College of Chest Physicians Evidence-Based Clinical Practice Guidelines. 8th ed. *Chest.* 2008;133:776S-814S.
9. Sobel M, Verhaeghe R. Antithrombotic therapy for peripheral artery occlusive disease: American College of Chest Physicians Evidence-Based Clinical Practice Guidelines. 8th ed. *Chest.* 2008;133:815S-843S.
10. Weitz JI, Hirsh J, Samama MM. New antithrombotic drugs: American College of Chest Physicians Evidence-Based Clinical Practice Guidelines. 8th ed. *Chest.* 2008;133:234S-256S.
11. Stone GW, Witzenbichler B, Guagliumi G, et al. Bivalirudin during primary PCI in acute myocardial infarction. *N Engl J Med.* 2008;358:2218-2230.
12. Wolowacz SE, Roskell NS, Plumb JM, et al. Efficacy and safety of dabigatran etexilate for the prevention of venous thromboembolism following total hip or knee arthroplasty: a meta-analysis. *Thromb Haemost.* 2009;101:77-85.
13. Connolly SJ, Ezekowitz MD, Yusuf S, et al. Dabigatran versus warfarin in patients with atrial fibrillation. *N Engl J Med.* 2009;361:1139-1151.
14. Schulman S, Kearon C, Kakkar AK, et al. Dabigatran versus warfarin in the treatment of acute venous thromboembolism. *N Engl J Med.* 2009;361:2342-2352.
15. Eriksson BI, Kakkar AK, Turpie AG, et al. Oral rivaroxaban for the prevention of symptomatic venous thromboembolism after elective hip and knee replacement. *J Bone Joint Surg Br.* 2009;91:636-644.
16. Lassen MR, Raskob GE, Gallus A, et al. Apixaban or enoxaparin for thromboprophylaxis after knee replacement. *N Engl J Med.* 2009;361:594-604.
17. Lassen MR, Raskob GE, Gallus A, et al. Apixaban versus enoxaparin for thromboprophylaxis after knee replacement (ADVANCE-2): a randomized double-blind trial. *Lancet.* 2010;375:807-815.
18. Patrono C, Baigent C, Hirsh J, et al. Antiplatelet drugs: American College of Chest Physicians Evidence-Based Clinical Practice Guidelines. 8th ed. *Chest.* 2008;133:199S-233S.
19. Albers GW, Amarenco P, Easton JD, et al. Antithrombotic and thrombolytic therapy for ischemic stroke: American College of Chest Physicians Evidence-Based Clinical Practice Guidelines. 8th ed. *Chest.* 2008;133:630S-669S.
20. De Berardis G, Sacco M, Strippoli GF, et al. Aspirin for primary prevention of cardiovascular events in people with diabetes: meta-analysis of randomised controlled trials. *BMJ.* 2009;339:b4531.
21. Singer DE, Albers GW, Dalen JE, et al. Antithrombotic therapy in atrial fibrillation. *Chest.* 2008;133:546S-592S.
22. Robless P, Mikhailidis DP, Stansby GP. Cilostazol for peripheral arterial disease. *Cochrane Database Syst Rev.* 2008;1:CD003748.
23. Connolly SJ, Pogue J, Hart RG, et al. Effect of clopidogrel added to aspirin in patients with atrial fibrillation. *N Engl J Med.* 2009;360:2066-2078.
24. Wiviott SD, Braunwald E, McCabe CH, et al. Prasugrel versus clopidogrel in patients with acute coronary syndromes. *N Engl J Med.* 2007;357:2001-2015.
25. Wallentin L, Becker RC, Budaj A, et al. Ticagrelor versus clopidogrel in patients with acute coronary syndromes. *N Engl J Med.* 2009;361:1045-1057.
26. Crowther MA, Ageno W, Garcia D, et al. Oral vitamin K versus placebo to correct excessive anticoagulation in patients receiving warfarin: a randomized trial. *Ann Intern Med.* 2009;150:293-300.
27. Salem DN, O'Gara PT, Madias C, et al. Valvular and structural heart disease: American College of Chest Physicians Evidence-Based Clinical Practice Guidelines. 8th ed. *Chest.* 2008;133:593S-629S.
28. Anand S, Yusuf S, Xie C, et al. Oral anticoagulant and antiplatelet therapy and peripheral arterial disease. *N Engl J Med.* 2007;357:217-227.

SUGGESTED READINGS

Baigent C, Blackwell L, Collins R, et al. Aspirin in the primary and secondary prevention of vascular disease: collaborative meta-analysis of individual participant data from randomised trials. *Lancet.* 2009;373:1849-1860. *The net benefit of aspirin is more convincing in secondary than in primary prevention of vascular disease.*

Gurbel PA, Tantry US. Combination antithrombotic therapies. *Circulation.* 2010;121:569-583. *Review.*

Krishnaswamy A, Lincoff AM, Cannon CP. Bleeding complications of unfractionated heparin. *Expert Opin Drug Saf.* 2011;10:77-84. *Practical approaches to dosing and monitoring.*

Matchar DB, Jacobson A, Dolor R, et al. Effect of home testing of international normalized ratio on clinical events. *N Engl Med.* 2010;363:1608-1620. *In a randomized trial, weekly INR self-testing was not effective for delaying the time until first stroke, major bleed, or death compared with monthly high-quality standard testing.*

38

COMPLEMENTARY AND ALTERNATIVE MEDICINE

MARY CHARLSON

COMPLEMENTARY AND INTEGRATIVE INTERVENTIONS

Despite tremendous strides by modern medicine in understanding the mechanisms of disease and improving treatments, many patients faced with illness find that conventional therapies do not completely alleviate their suffering. As a result, many patients, particularly those who have experienced life-threatening illnesses, turn to alternative or complementary therapies that they believe will make them feel better.

Most complementary therapies are provided in community settings, not in health institutions. In 2007 a nationally representative sample showed that almost 40% of adults and 11% of children in the United States had used complementary or alternative medical (CAM) therapies in the prior year. CAM modalities include biologically based therapies, body-based practices, mind-body therapies, energy medicine, and whole medical systems; the proportion of U.S. adults using these CAM modalities in 2007 is shown in Table 38-1. Of note, adults had more visits with CAM practitioners, including acupuncturists, massage therapists, and herbalists, than they had with primary care physicians. Most people who use CAM modalities do not disclose this to their physicians because they are concerned that their physicians may not understand or support the use of such approaches.

The use of CAM modalities is particularly high in cancer patients. Eighty percent of patients who are undergoing treatment for cancer use one or more CAM modalities, and about half tell their oncologists. The use of CAM modalities does not stop when treatment is over; in fact, patients may seek such modalities even more aggressively after treatment is completed, much to the surprise of their physicians. When oncologists tell patients that their treatment is over and that they have an excellent prognosis or that the critical time frame for recurrence has passed, they expect the patients to be enormously relieved. All too often, patients experience distress when told that they can go back to their usual lives, asking, "What life?" The growing field

TABLE 38-1 USE OF COMPLEMENTARY OR ALTERNATIVE MEDICINE BY U.S. ADULTS IN 2007

MODALITY	% OF ADULTS WHO USED IT
BIOLOGICALLY BASED THERAPIES	
Herbal or natural products	17.7
Dietary supplements	N/A
Diet-based therapy	3.5
BODY-BASED PRACTICES	
Chiropractic or osteopathic manipulation	8.6
Massage	8.3
Movement therapies*	1.5
MIND-BODY THERAPIES	
Biofeedback	0.2
Hypnosis	0.2
Meditation	9.4
Guided imagery	2.2
Progressive relaxation	2.9
Deep breathing	12.7
Yoga	6.1
Tai chi	1.0
Qi gong	0.3
ENERGY MEDICINE†	
Reiki, biofield, and other therapies	0.5
WHOLE MEDICAL SYSTEMS	
Naturopathy	0.3
Homeopathy	1.8
Ayurveda	0.1
Traditional Chinese medicine (acupuncture)	1.4
Traditional healers	0.4

*Pilates, Trager, Feldenkrais, and Alexander.
†Energy medicine is based on the theory that there are energy fields surrounding and penetrating the human body. Energy therapies are intended to manipulate these energy fields.

TABLE 38-2 QUESTIONS PHYSICIANS CAN ASK TO EXPLORE PATIENTS' BELIEFS

What do you think this illness does?
What worries you with this illness?
Why did you think you got this illness?
How do you think it should be treated?
Who do you ask for advice about illness?

of survivorship medicine recognizes that patients who have had cancer may face ongoing physical, psychological, and spiritual challenges.

Most often, patients who are feeling distressed are referred to support groups. Surprisingly, support groups were not shown to improve quality of life in breast cancer survivors in randomized trials. Cognitive-behavioral therapy may also be recommended for patients who experience anxiety after treatment for cancer. Randomized trials have shown that cognitive-behavioral therapy may be effective in improving mood in cancer patients. More and more, cancer survivors reach for complementary or integrative approaches to healing and health to address their psychological, physical, and spiritual needs.

Integrative health is a broad framework that encompasses complex biologic, psychological, cultural, and social pathways to health and disease. *Complementary medicine* encompasses adjunctive approaches to conventional medicine for preventing or treating illness or distress. These alternative approaches are embraced in many different communities and cultures.

THE IMPORTANCE OF PATIENT BELIEFS, EXPECTATIONS, AND CULTURES

Beliefs about illness and health and about the risks and benefits of treatment are deeply rooted at a cultural and social network level. Americans rely on family and social networks for advice about how to handle most illnesses and see physicians for only 10 to 20% of illness episodes. Social networks in many communities help determine many individuals' beliefs and expectations with regard to health and the use of different treatment modalities. Emerging data suggest that apart from determining expectations about disease and treatment, social networks can have a profound impact on health and affect. A recent analysis of the Framingham data showed that obesity spreads through social networks. The chance of becoming obese increased by 171% if a friend became obese or 40% if a sibling became obese. Obesity was not higher in neighbors, suggesting that the findings were not due to environmental confounding. Instead, obesity appears to be propagated through social networks. A similar analysis of the Framingham data suggested that happiness is also spread through social networks. Such social network influences are rarely considered in modern medicine, except in approaches to HIV and drug addiction.

Physicians are often not aware that their patients have beliefs about the cause of their illness (i.e., their explanatory model). As a result, it is common for patient-doctor discussions to involve major discrepancies in understanding, expectations, and goals. For example, Hmong parents in Minnesota who placed heated cups on their children's skin to relieve chest congestion (a traditional practice) were mistakenly reported for child abuse because the cups caused erythematous patches. Puerto Rican women who reported having visions during religious ceremonies (as was expected) were incorrectly diagnosed as having schizophrenia. Understanding and addressing patients' beliefs is critical to overcoming otherwise hidden barriers to adopting effective treatments and preventing unintended consequences. Questions that can be employed to elucidate patients' beliefs are shown in Table 38-2. Explanatory models of illness are deeply rooted in culture and embedded in indigenous medical systems and healing practices.

INDIGENOUS MEDICAL SYSTEMS AND TRADITIONAL HEALING PRACTICES

Having evolved over thousands of years, most indigenous medical systems frame health as balance or harmony and illness as imbalance. To treat illness, indigenous systems seek to restore balance using a combination of foods, herbs, physical manipulation, movement, prayer, and social interventions. Each has its own methods of diagnosis, using the patient's symptoms and often his or her family or social situation.

For Native Americans, health means staying strong in spirit, mind, and body and staying in harmony with oneself, one's community, and the earth. Efforts to restore health focus on healing the spirit of the person who is ill and healing the community and the environment. Ceremonies and rituals such as the sweat lodge as well as herbal remedies may be used. Ayurvedic (ancient Indian) medicine focuses on achieving a balance of three elements—vata (air), pita (bile), and kapha (phlegm)—through the use of foods, herbs, yoga, meditation, and massage. Traditional Chinese medicine draws on ancient theory to achieve a balance of yin and yang (opposites) and the five elements (water, wood, fire, earth, and metal) through acupuncture, herbs, foods, and massage. The life force or energy, called *Qi*, is believed to flow through meridians; acupuncture, tai chi, and qi gong are all thought to balance the flow of energy. Tibetan medicine combines elements from Ayurvedic, Greek, and Chinese medical systems with the Buddhist philosophy that all illness and suffering come from the mind; it emphasizes guided meditation as central to harmony and healing. African traditional medicine frames illness as a physical or mental problem caused by a disruption of a person's own balance or his or her social relationships. Diagnosis involves identifying the spiritual cause of the illness; treatments are designed to restore spiritual and social balance and may involve herbals, prayers to ancestors, and family interventions, as well as rituals and ceremonies. Obviously, these descriptions are too short to do justice to any of these traditions, but they emphasize that each of these indigenous medical systems has specific theories about the cause of, susceptibility to, and treatment for certain conditions and specific strategies for diagnosis. These traditional systems are currently being used to treat millions of people worldwide. In Asia and Africa, the World Health Organization estimates that 80% of people currently depend primarily on traditional medicine.

There is limited research about the effectiveness of indigenous medical systems as a whole because these systems are deeply intertwined with culture. Most Western research has taken one element or tool from a traditional system and tested its use to treat a specific condition or disease. For example, acupuncture has been shown to reduce nausea and vomiting induced by chemotherapy. Iyengar yoga improves function and reduces pain in patients with chronic back pain. Tai chi reduces pain and improves function among patients with osteoarthritis of the knee. Our knowledge is limited about the effectiveness of specific practices across diverse communities; specifically, we do not know whether responses to therapies differ between populations that have used "alternative" approaches for many years as part of their healing traditions and those that have only recently begun to incorporate them.

● TRADITIONAL VERSUS MODERN MEDICINE: THE MIND AND THE BODY

In traditional medical systems, the mind and spirit were not viewed as separate from the body; the health of the mind and spirit was viewed as central to physical health. Many traditional systems held that physical illness is caused by disturbances of the mind or spirit. As a result, many interventions were designed to improve the health of the mind and spirit.

In the Indo-Tibetan Buddhist tradition, healing focuses on building the discipline of attention through healing visualization, recitation, and deep breathing. The Tibetans developed a comprehensive system of self-healing and learning called the *gradual path*, which deals with the causes of suffering and the approaches to end suffering. Self-healing is taught through meditation guided by a mentor. Recently, guided meditation in this tradition has been shown to improve quality of life in breast cancer survivors.

African traditional medicine focuses on the spiritual causes of illness and then on the physical manifestations. The traditional healer understands the beliefs and normative values of the community and interprets what the patient has done wrong to cause the illness. The intervention may involve prayer, dancing, singing, drumming, ritual, or community ceremonies. Recently, traditional healers have developed rituals for the rehabilitation of children who were abducted and forced to become soldiers. Reconciliation with their dead ancestors and with those who died is a central part of the ritual. These rituals were adapted from those used for centuries to peacefully reintegrate returning warriors into the community.

Native American healing focuses on restoring health and harmony with the community and with nature. Illness is believed to stem from spiritual imbalances. Purifying and cleansing the body and spirit through sweat lodge ceremonies is an important healing tradition. Other rituals may include the whole community and involve drumming, singing, chanting, and prayers. Sweat lodge rituals have improved the success of interventions designed to change addictive behaviors.

For the most part, Western medicine does not have equivalent approaches. The focus of Western medicine has been medical and surgical treatments for the physical body. Most interventions target the individual patient. Community-based rituals or interventions for improving health are still largely the province of religious institutions. The difference between modern medicine and indigenous systems grew out of the mind-body dichotomy. Introduced by Descartes in the West, the philosophy that the mind and the body are separate and distinct provided the foundation for modern medicine. The physical body became the focus of Western medicine, while the mind and the spirit were exclusively the domain of the church.

● THE MIND-BODY CONNECTION

For some time it has been clear that psychosocial states such as stress, social isolation, and depression alter the risk of developing chronic illness and increase the risk of adverse outcomes. For example, depression increases the risk of developing heart disease. Depressive symptoms also increase the risk of morbidity and mortality among patients who have heart disease. Lack of emotional support increases mortality in patients who have had a myocardial infarction. Sudden emotional stress can precipitate heart failure in patients without coronary artery disease.

Psychosocial stress may be caused by a discrete life event such as the death of a family member, chronic situations related to social role or work, or small day-to-day hassles. The impact of a given event depends on how the individual perceives it: is the event a threat, and if so, how severe? An individual's interpretation of events as physical or psychological threats is based on his or her own experience and that of the individual's social network. Once an event is perceived as a potential threat, an individual may experience negative emotions, such as anger or anxiety. Such emotions activate emotional memory and trigger reaction patterns learned in response to prior stresses, initiating the neuroendocrine stress response. People react to stress with their own patterned behavioral responses, and most resultant behaviors tend to increase the negative impact of stress (e.g., eating unhealthy food, gaining weight, smoking, living a sedentary life, not taking medications). The impact of negative psychosocial states on health has been clear for several decades; however, we have recently gained a greater understanding of the potential mechanisms.

How Does Psychosocial Stress Impact Health?

The repeated triggering of the stress cascade can adversely affect multiple aspects of health and adaptation. There is emerging evidence that psychosocial stress is one of the most salient, potentially modifiable mechanisms linking illness and health.

Allostatic Load

An approach has been defined to measure the cumulative toll exacted by adverse behavioral, psychological, social, physiologic, and environmental stressors. Stress causes specific neural and endocrine responses, with sympathetic activation resulting in the release of catecholamines from the adrenal medulla and cortisol from the adrenal cortex. The acute stress response is designed to protect against threats to survival. However, chronic stress, especially psychosocial stress, can have a negative impact on health. Chronic stress interferes with biologic regulatory processes central to homeostasis. Chronic stress disrupts the hypothalamic-pituitary-adrenal (HPA) axis, resulting in abnormal circadian cortisol rhythms, with elevated and flattened diurnal cortisol levels and elevated overnight urinary cortisol. Stress also disrupts the autonomic balance, resulting in an increase in sympathetic versus parasympathetic function and elevated levels of urinary catecholamines. There are multiple biologic markers of the stress response that indicate cumulative stress-related wear and tear, which is called *allostatic load*. The potential adverse consequences of allostatic load were evaluated in the MacArthur Studies of Successful Aging, which followed 736 healthy men and women between 70 and 79 years of age. Among patients without cardiovascular disease at baseline, patients with a higher allostatic load had a higher mortality and greater functional decline that those with a lower allostatic load. Of note, older men with more social network ties and greater social integration had lower allostatic load scores. Therefore, individuals under chronic stress had greater neuroendocrine and cardiovascular responses and subsequent adverse health outcomes.

Stress Reactivity

Efforts to measure sympathetic-parasympathetic balance have focused on measures of stress reactivity, including heart rate variability and blood pressure. Studies measuring cardiovascular reactivity in the context of daily life have yielded valuable insights. For example, day-to-day social interactions may be associated with changes in cardiovascular reactivity; the changes depend on the relationships involved. Negative social relationships may cause activation of the sympathetic nervous system, leading to increased cardiovascular reactivity. People who have increased reactivity to stress have a larger, longer-lasting increase in negative affect. In contrast, during positive social interaction with one's partner, blood pressure levels are lower than during interactions with other people.

In some studies, the health impact of heightened cardiovascular reactivity depended on socioeconomic status. Thus, social context and social support may alter stress reactivity. Increased cardiovascular reactivity to stressors may predict cardiovascular disease.

Chronic work stress has significant health consequences. The Whitehall study showed that workers with higher chronic work-related stress had a higher incidence of coronary heart disease and higher death rates from heart disease. Higher work stress was associated with four components of the metabolic syndrome (higher fasting glucose, higher triglycerides, greater waist circumference, and lower high-density lipoprotein cholesterol), as well as worse health behaviors (lower physical activity, poor diet) and the development of obesity.

Importantly, higher work stress was also associated with lower heart rate variability. Lower heart rate variability indicates lower vagal tone—that is, reduced parasympathetic and increased sympathetic activity. Lower heart rate variability predicts increased all-cause mortality and increased risk of coronary heart disease. There is a correlation between heart rate variability (the high-frequency component reflecting vagal activity) and emotion-specific changes in blood flow in the medial prefrontal cortex.

The Cholinergic Inflammatory Pathway

The vagus nerve, which controls parasympathetic tone and heart rate variability, also mediates the release of pro- and anti-inflammatory cytokines. Through the vagus nerve, the nervous system has the ability to sense and suppress inflammation through the cholinergic anti-inflammatory pathway. Stimulation of the vagus nerve leads to the release of acetylcholine, which in turn inhibits the inflammatory response by inhibiting the release of pro-inflammatory cytokines (interleukin-6 and tumor necrosis factor). When pro-inflammatory cytokines are released to defend against pathogens, the release is a rapid and localized reflex; however, if pro-inflammatory cytokines are released over a prolonged period, they can create a systemic humoral response, leading to or exacerbating diseases such as rheumatoid arthritis, inflammatory bowel disease, and atherosclerosis.

Stress and the Brain

A large body of literature highlights the effects of chronic stress on the structure and function of the hippocampus and amygdala. The hippocampus is important for both contextual and declarative memory. Severe stress and elevated steroid levels impair memory reversibly and may affect the reliability of contextual memories, which are important in evaluating a potential threat. High levels of stress hormones also impair declarative memory reversibly. Chronic stress can cause a reduction in the size of the hippocampus (which provides negative feedback to the HPA axis). However, there is some evidence of plasticity at least in the dentate gyrus in the hippocampus: in primates, new cells are increased by exercise and enriched environments. A study showed that older patients who are socially disengaged experience cognitive decline, leading to speculation that social engagement may buffer against stress-related damage to the hippocampus.

The amygdala and the prefrontal cortex are also involved in the affective and attentional response to stress. The amygdala is important to threat recognition and fear, as well as emotional learning. Chronic stress causes increases in the amygdala (which provides positive feedback to the HPA axis). The prefrontal cortex likely exerts a major inhibitory influence on the amygdala. Chronic stress interferes with the prefrontal cortex and results in decreased working memory and impaired problem solving. It has been shown that among medical students experiencing the same examination stress, those with higher perceived stress levels also had more impairment in attentional control compared with those whose perceived stress levels were lower. Importantly, after 1 month of vacation, the impairment in prefrontal cortex function was reversible. Thus, stress results in both reversible and irreversible changes in the hippocampus, amygdala, and prefrontal cortex that are involved in multiple aspects of cognition, attention, and emotion.

Stress and Telomere Length

Chronic stress is also associated with telomere length, a marker of cellular age. When telomeres shorten sufficiently, the cell becomes senescent. An important study evaluated mothers of healthy children versus mothers of chronically ill children; the hypothesis was that mothers of ill children would have greater perceived stress than mothers of healthy children and thus shorter telomeres. Instead, the investigators found no difference in telomere length, telomerase activity, or oxidative stress. However, in both groups of mothers, telomere length was correlated with perceived stress; specifically, the higher the mother's perceived stress, the shorter her telomeres were. High-stress mothers had the equivalent of 1 decade of aging in telomere length in contrast to the low-stress mothers. Because the study was cross-sectional, it could not establish whether the correlation represented causation.

Thus, if the stress response, which is designed to protect against acute events, becomes a chronic response, it can have an adverse impact on cellular aging and multiple aspects of regulatory systems, including the HPA axis, parasympathetic-sympathetic tone, the vagus nerve, and the central nervous system.

How Do Integrative Interventions Reduce the Impact of Stress?

Reducing the impact of stress is likely a key mechanism through which many integrative interventions work. It is important to realize that it is not the actual magnitude of the stressor that has the adverse health impact; it is the individual's perception of the stressor. Thus, in two mothers with chronically ill children, telomeres are shortened in the mother with high perceived stress but not in the mother with a low level of perceived stress. Medical students with high levels of perceived stress about an upcoming examination have attentional shifts and impairment in prefrontal cortex function, whereas those with low perceived stress do not.

Integrative interventions are almost uniformly designed to increase confidence in one's own control and in one's ability to self-regulate emotion and mood. Many of these interventions focus on the individual's being present in the moment and achieving nonjudgmental awareness. They are also designed, using different theories, to create greater harmony between the mind and the body.

Cognitive neuroscience has begun to understand meditation as a discipline of attention; stress reduction is achieved through learning. This model is consistent with the view of traditional medical systems that use meditation, prayer, guided imagery, recitation, singing, drumming, and chanting to build present awareness, attention, and harmony. Yoga, tai chi, and qi gong are examples of practices that involve movement and meditation.

Studies of clinically stressed populations indicate that interventions aimed at reducing stress by promoting the cognitive regulation of attention and affective behavior yield enhancements in neuroendocrine and immune function and clinically significant improvements in quality of life. A few small studies have reported changes in heart rate variability in response to an intervention. Transcendental meditation[1] and biofeedback can increase heart rate variability in cardiac patients; acupuncture may also increase heart rate variability. It has been suggested that interventions designed to increase heart rate variability should target patients whose conditions are associated with high levels of pro-inflammatory cytokines, such as inflammatory bowel disease or rheumatoid arthritis. Meditation may also improve blood pressure and insulin resistance.[1] With regard to brain plasticity and telomere shortening, studies have only begun to evaluate interventions' potential to effect changes.

⬤ WHY DO PATIENTS SEEK INTEGRATIVE INTERVENTIONS?

First, patients want to play an active role in their recovery and return to health—that is, self-healing. Self-healing is a concept that may seem strange to physicians, yet we know that self-healing (i.e., regeneration) allows repair to occur after injury.

Patient empowerment and active engagement are major determinants of health outcomes. An overwhelming body of literature has shown that confidence in one's ability to do something—that is, self-efficacy—is a powerful predictor of success. More and more studies have shown the importance of whether patients believe they can influence their own health outcomes. People who think they can influence their own outcomes (those with an internal locus of control) fare better than those who believe that what they do does not matter (those with an external locus of control). Of note, it has been known for more than 20 years that locus of control can predict health outcomes and behaviors. Ten-year-olds who believed they could influence events by their own actions had a reduced risk of obesity and psychological distress than those with a greater external locus of control.

Self-efficacy can be enhanced; that is, patients can learn strategies to increase confidence in their ability to cope with illness and thereby improve their health outcomes, at least over the short term.[2] A self-management course, including action planning, modeling of behaviors, problem solving, and a decision-making model, may increase self-efficacy and reduce hospitalizations. Many disease management courses cite this model but miss the critical ingredients of improving self-efficacy, decision making, and problem solving, focusing instead on specific things the patient should monitor and report to the nurse or doctor, potentially undermining self-efficacy and reinforcing the external locus of control.

To date, only a few complementary approaches have achieved widespread use in medical centers. Among commonly used complementary and alternative medical therapies, acupuncture is beneficial for tension-type headache[3]; can improve nausea, vomiting, and other symptoms in cancer patients[4]; can lower blood pressure by about 5.4/2.0 mm Hg during treatment but not after it is stopped[5]; has some benefit for chronic lower back pain,[6] but has small and probably not clinically relevant benefits for peripheral joint osteoarthritis.[7] Tai Chi may be an effective treatment for fibromyalgia.[8] By comparison, Echinacea is not effective for the common cold,[9] hypnotherapy is not effective for smoking cessations,[10] and glucosamine and chondroitin are not beneficial for osteoarthritis of the hip or knee.[11]

1. Paul-Labrador M, Pol D, Dwyer JH, et al. Effects of a randomized controlled trial of transcendental meditation on components of the metabolic syndrome in subjects with coronary heart disease. *Arch Intern Med.* 2006;166:1218-1224.

2. Foster G, Taylor SJ, Eldridge SE, et al. Self-management education programmes by lay leaders for people with chronic conditions. *Cochrane Database Syst Rev.* 2007;4:CD005108.

3. Linde K, Allais G, Brinkhaus B, et al. Acupuncture for tension-type headache. *Cochrane Database Syst Rev.* 2009;1:CD007587.

4. Capodice JL. Acupuncture in the oncology setting: clinical trial update. *Curr Treat Options Oncol.* 2010;11:87-94.

5. Flachskampf FA, Gallasch J, Gefeller OY, et al: Randomized trial of acupuncture to lower blood pressure. *Circulation.* 2007;115:3121-3129.

6. Berman BM, Langevin HH, Witt CM, et al. Acupuncture for chronic low back pain. *N Engl J Med.* 2010;363:454-461.

7. Manheimer E, Cheng K, Linde K, et al. Acupuncture for peripheral joint osteoarthritis. *Cochrane Database Syst Rev.* 2010;1:CD001977.

8. Wang C, Schmid CH, Rones R, et al. A randomized trial of tai chi for fibromyalgia. *N Engl J Med.* 2010;363:743-754.

9. Barrett B, Brown R, Rakel D, et al. Echinacea for treating the common cold: a randomized trial. *Ann Intern Med.* 2010;153:769-777.

10. Barnes J, Dong CY, McRobbie H, et al. Hypnotherapy for smoking cessation. *Cochrane Database Syst Rev.* 2010;10:CD001008.

11. Wandel S, Jüni P, Tendal B, et al. Effects of glucosamine, chondroitin, or placebo in patients with osteoarthritis of hip or knee: network meta-analysis. *BMJ.* 2010;341:c4675.

SUGGESTED READINGS

Kennedy DA, Seely D. Clinically based evidence of drug-herb interactions: a systemic review. *Expert Opin Drug Saf.* 2010;9:79-124. *Review.*

Liston C, McEwen BS, Casey BJ. Psychosocial stress reversibly disrupts prefrontal processing and attentional control. *Proc Natl Acad Sci U S A.* 2009;106:912-917. *Documents the effect of stress on mental function.*

VI
GENETICS

39

PRINCIPLES OF GENETICS

BRUCE R. KORF

The elucidation of the structure and function of the genome is one of the great scientific triumphs of the 20th century. The relevance of inheritance to health and disease probably has been recognized throughout history, but it is only during the last century that the rules governing inheritance and the mechanisms whereby genetic information is stored and used have come to light. The application of this knowledge to medical practice so far has focused on relatively rare monogenic and chromosomal disorders. Major contributions have been made in these areas in the form of approaches to genetic counseling, genetic testing, prenatal diagnosis, newborn screening, carrier screening, and, to a limited extent, treatment. As important as these contributions are, however, their impact has been limited by the rarity of these disorders. Powerful tools resulting from the Human Genome Project are changing this situation (Chapter 42). Genetic factors that contribute to common and rare disorders are being identified, leading to new approaches to diagnosis, prevention, and treatment. Genetics and genomics are increasingly occupying center stage in medical practice, guiding treatment decisions and preventive strategies. This chapter reviews the paradigm whereby genetics is being integrated into the routine practice of medicine.

● GENETIC CONTRIBUTION TO DISEASE

It may be argued that no disorder is either completely determined genetically or completely determined by nongenetic factors. Even monogenic conditions, such as phenylketonuria, are modified by the environment, in this case by dietary intake of phenylalanine. Genetically determined host factors are known to modify susceptibility to infection or other environmental agents. Even individuals who are victims of trauma may find themselves at risk in part because of genetic traits that affect behavior or ability to perceive or escape from danger.

Multifactorial Inheritance

Complex traits that are important for both health and disease are the result of an interaction of multiple genes with one another and with the environment (Fig. 39-1). In some cases, individual genes or environmental factors contribute overwhelmingly to the cause of a disorder, as with a genetic condition, such as neurofibromatosis or Marfan syndrome, or an acquired disorder, such as bacterial infection or trauma. Other times, there may be interplay among many factors, making it difficult to dissect out the specific genes or environmental exposures.

From a medical perspective, it is helpful to divide the genetic contribution to disease into three categories: high-penetrance monogenic or chromosomal disorders, monogenic versions of common disorders, and complex, multifactorial disorders. Each of these has an impact on medical practice in distinctive ways.

High-Penetrance Monogenic or Chromosomal Disorders

High-penetrance monogenic or chromosomal disorders are the disorders that most clinicians think of as "genetic conditions." They include rare but familiar single-gene disorders, such as neurofibromatosis, Marfan syndrome, and cystic fibrosis, and chromosomal abnormalities, such as trisomy 21 (Down syndrome). Several thousand distinct human genetic disorders have been described and cataloged in *Mendelian Inheritance in Man* (available at www.ncbi.nlm.nih.gov/Omim/). These include mendelian dominant or recessive disorders, sex-linked disorders, and conditions that are due to mutations within the 16.6-kilobase mitochondrial genome. They also include major chromosomal aneuploidy syndromes and syndromes associated with duplication or deletion of small regions of the genome that result in either reproducible syndromes, such as Williams syndrome (deletion of contiguous loci from a region of chromosome 7), or nonspecific mental retardation.

Role of the Nonspecialist

Because of the rarity of many of these conditions, most practitioners have limited experience with a given disorder and are likely to need to refer the patient to an appropriate specialist for assistance with diagnosis and management. Nevertheless, the nonspecialist has many distinct roles in the care of these patients. These roles begin with the recognition of the fact that the patient may have a disorder and arrangement for appropriate diagnostic evaluation. Many genetic disorders produce obvious signs or symptoms that at least prompt referral even if they are not immediately suggestive of a diagnosis. Others can be more subtle, with nevertheless significant consequences if the diagnosis is missed. An example is Marfan syndrome (Chapter 268). The physician needs to be alert to the physical characteristics of patients with Marfan syndrome because life-threatening aortic dissection can be avoided with appropriate monitoring and treatment. Table 39-1 lists examples of some adult-onset monogenic conditions with which the internist should be familiar.

Treatment of Patients with Genetic Disorders

The treatment of patients with genetic disorders may require the assistance of a specialist, but the nonspecialist is likely to be the first contact when an affected individual is ill. The primary care physician needs to be familiar with the disorder and major potential complications. For example, the patient with neurofibromatosis who experiences chronic back pain may be presenting with a malignant peripheral nerve sheath tumor, requiring more aggressive evaluation than would be typical for an unaffected individual with back pain. Formation of a good working relationship between the specialist and nonspecialist is crucial to ensure effective care.

The nonspecialist also has an important role in supporting the patient and helping to explain the difficult choices that may be offered for management. This includes providing support for patients who have disorders that cannot be treated and for the emotional impact that accompanies knowledge that a disorder may be transmitted to one's offspring or shared with other relatives. Most patients have little understanding of the mechanisms of genetics and genetic disease. Although the responsibility to explain these issues may reside with specialists and counselors, the primary care provider has an important supportive role.

Advances in Genetics

Many of the disorders in this group have been known for a long time, but more recent advances in genetics have had a substantial impact on approaches to diagnosis and management. Genetic testing has been refined with the advent of molecular diagnostic tests that detect mutations within individual genes. Even rare disorders may be amenable to diagnostic testing; a database of testing laboratories can be found on the Internet (available at www.genetests.org). Whole-genome scanning for small deletions or duplications is revealing mutations in patients with disorders such autism, for which standard chromosomal analysis had previously been unrevealing. Population screening for carrier status of some disorders now is offered routinely. Some tests are targeted to particular ethnic groups, such as Ashkenazi Jews (Tay-Sachs disease, Canavan disease, cystic fibrosis, Gaucher's disease) or individuals of African, Mediterranean, or Asian ancestry (hemoglobinopathies) (Table 39-2). Pan-ethnic screening is now being made available for cystic fibrosis, although risks differ in different ethnic groups. Newborn screening is being expanded beyond inborn errors of metabolism such as phenylketonuria and galactosemia, with the advent of tandem mass spectrometry and the availability of a standardized panel of tests. Finally, treatment of some monogenic disorders is becoming feasible. Life expectancy for patients with cystic fibrosis has been increasing gradually with better treatments for chronic lung disease; dietary therapy is available for many inborn errors of metabolism; novel therapies that use either pharmaceuticals or gene or enzyme replacement strategies are in use or being tested for many conditions. The principles of management of genetic disorders are evolving rapidly so that care of patients increasingly requires active partnership of specialists and primary care providers. Moreover, individuals with congenital disorders such as Down syndrome are routinely surviving to adulthood and require primary care providers who are familiar with their special needs.

Monogenic Versions of Common Disorders

Not all monogenic disorders produce obscure phenotypes, and not all common disorders are due to complex multifactorial causes. Some common disorders occur in some families as single-gene traits (Table 39-3). This is usually true for only a proportion of affected individuals, but in some cases it is a significant proportion and represents an important group of patients to be recognized.

Breast Cancer

An example is breast cancer (Chapter 204). About 10% of cases of this common form of cancer can be attributed to mutation in one of two genes, *BRCA1* or *BRCA2*. Women who inherit a mutation in one of these genes face a high risk of eventually developing breast or ovarian cancer—more than 80% by age 70 years for breast cancer. Women at risk because of mutation do not look different from women with sporadic breast cancer but can be distinguished by many features, including family history of breast or ovarian cancer in multiple relatives, early age at onset of cancer, and multifocality of the cancer (e.g., bilateral breast cancer or breast and ovarian cancer).

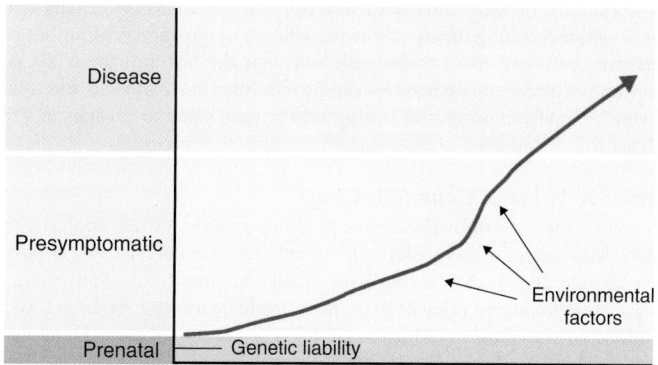

FIGURE 39-1. Multifactorial etiology of disease. An individual is born with a genetic liability but remains in a presymptomatic state for some time until additional events occur, including exposure to environmental factors, that result in crossing a threshold that is identified as *disease*. In instances of high-penetrance monogenic disorders, the genetic liability may be overwhelming. In other instances, genetic factors may contribute only slightly to disease risk.

Colon Cancer and Other Common Disorders

Another example from cancer genetics is colon cancer (Chapter 199). Two syndromes, familial adenomatous polyposis and hereditary nonpolyposis colon cancer, are autosomal dominantly inherited and convey a high risk of colon cancer. Other noncancer examples are hemochromatosis (Chapter 219), in which cirrhosis, cardiomyopathy, diabetes, joint disease, and other problems ensue from excessive iron absorption; 10% of whites carry an allele that predisposes to this recessive disorder. Mutations in the factor V gene or the prothrombin gene occur commonly and predispose to deep venous thrombosis (Chapter 179). Rarer examples include inherited forms of cardiomyopathy, hypertension, and familial hypercholesterolemia.

Management

The physician may be called on to address these disorders in many ways. There is a compelling reason to make an early diagnosis of hemochromatosis because the complications can be prevented, but not reversed, by phlebotomy and subsequent monitoring of iron stores. Individuals at risk of colon cancer can be offered surveillance with colonoscopy or surgical resection of the colon to reduce the risk of cancer. Individuals at risk of breast and ovarian cancer likewise can be offered surveillance, chemoprevention, or surgery. The benefits of knowledge of genetic risks are less clear in some instances. Carriers of the factor V Leiden mutation would not be treated with anticoagulation until after an event of thrombosis, and the treatment may not be different for a carrier versus a noncarrier. In some cases, however, knowledge of carrier status might help ensure prompt diagnosis or avoid situations of high risk.

TABLE 39-2	MAJOR RECESSIVE DISORDERS FOR WHICH CARRIER SCREENING COMMONLY IS OFFERED IN THE UNITED STATES	
DISORDER	**MAJOR AT-RISK POPULATION**	**CARRIER FREQUENCY**
Cystic fibrosis	White	1:25
	Ashkenazi Jewish	1:29
Sickle cell anemia	African American	1:10
β-Thalassemia	Mediterranean	1:30
α-Thalassemia	Southeast Asian, Chinese	1:30
Tay-Sachs disease	Ashkenazi Jewish	1:30
	French Canadian	1:30
Canavan's disease	Ashkenazi Jewish	1:40
Familial dysautonomia	Ashkenazi Jewish	1:30

TABLE 39-1	HIGH-PENETRANCE SINGLE-GENE DISORDERS THAT MAY PRESENT IN ADULTHOOD, WITH SOME MAJOR MEDICAL IMPLICATIONS*	
DISORDER	**INHERITANCE**	**MAJOR MEDICAL IMPLICATIONS**
CARDIOVASCULAR		
Marfan syndrome	AD	Risk of aortic dissection; lens dislocation
Long QT syndrome	AD, AR	Arrhythmia, sudden death
RENAL		
Adult polycystic kidney disease	AD	Renal failure
PULMONARY		
α₁-Antitrypsin deficiency	AR	Emphysema, cirrhosis
NEUROLOGIC		
NF1	AD	Benign and malignant nerve sheath tumors, gliomas
NF2	AD	Schwannomas (especially vestibular), meningiomas
Von Hippel-Lindau	AD	Hemangioblastoma of cerebellum, brain stem, eye; pheochromocytoma; renal cell carcinoma
Huntington disease	AD	Movement disorder, psychiatric disorder, dementia
HEMATOLOGIC		
Globin disorders	AR	Stroke, iron overload
ENDOCRINE		
MEN syndromes	AD	Tumors of thyroid and parathyroid, pheochromocytoma

*See Table 39-3 for examples of lower penetrance disorders.
AD = autosomal dominant; AR = autosomal recessive; MEN = multiple endocrine neoplasia; NF = neurofibromatosis.

TABLE 39-3	SINGLE-GENE DISORDERS WITH INCOMPLETE PENETRANCE THAT MAY ACCOUNT FOR INHERITED FORMS OF SELECTED COMMON DISORDERS	
DISORDER	**INHERITANCE: GENES**	**MAJOR MEDICAL IMPLICATIONS**
Hemochromatosis	AR: *HFE*	Cirrhosis, cardiomyopathy, diabetes mellitus
Thrombophilia	AD, AR: multiple genes	Deep venous thrombosis
Breast and ovarian cancers	AD: *BRCA1, BRCA2*	Breast and ovarian cancers
Familial adenomatous polyposis	AD: *APC*	Multiple colonic polyps, colon cancer
Hereditary nonpolyposis colorectal cancer	AD: DNA mismatch repair genes	Colorectal cancer, endometrial cancer
Maturity-onset diabetes of the young	AD: multiple genes	Diabetes mellitus
Cardiomyopathy	AD: genes involved in cardiac contractile apparatus	Arrhythmia, heart failure

AD = autosomal dominant; AR = autosomal recessive.

Genetic Testing

As with other medical tests, the physician should carefully consider risks, benefits, and clinical utility in deciding to use a genetic test. Some distinct ethical and legal risks may apply to some genetic tests. These may include anxiety, stigmatization, guilt, and possibly discrimination for insurance or employment. Some of these risks may be addressed by legislation to maintain privacy of genetic information, such as the Genetic Information Nondiscrimination Act, but the risks of anxiety, guilt, and stigmatization cannot be legislated away. To some extent, further research may improve the basis for surveillance or lead to effective treatments. For now, many of these disorders present a double-edged sword of potentially useful knowledge and potentially harmful information.

Role of the Physician

The role of the physician in dealing with monogenic disorders includes recognition of individuals at risk and participation in formulation of a care plan. Individuals at risk cannot be identified by physical appearance and usually are not evident from medical history or physical examination findings. The most valuable screening tool is the family history. Directed questioning about a family history of major monogenic disorders, especially breast, ovarian, and colon cancer, as well as hypercholesterolemia, hypertension, deep venous thrombosis, cirrhosis, and diabetes, can identify the occasional patient with mendelian segregation of these common disorders. Even if the information is of uncertain reliability, eliciting a family history can prompt referral for further evaluation, documentation of the family history, and consideration for genetic testing. The physician's job is not simply to identify individuals at risk; some people believe they are at high risk even in the absence of well-documented risk factors. Addressing these misconceptions can bring peace of mind and usually does not require genetic testing.

Complex, Multifactorial Disorders

Understanding the genetics of common disorders is one of the great challenges of modern medicine, with the promise of major returns in terms of prevention, diagnosis, and treatment. The etiology of these disorders is complex in that they result from an interaction of multiple genes with one another and with environmental factors. The specific genes that are relevant may be different from one person to the next. Identification of these genes is difficult given this heterogeneity and the relatively small impact that any particular gene may have in a particular person.

Population Studies

Dissection of the genetic contribution to common disease cannot be accomplished by the standard genetic approaches involving study of rare variants or family-based linkage studies. Most recent efforts have focused on study of large groups of patients, comparing the prevalence of particular genetic markers in case patients and control subjects. The availability of markers has been boosted by the identification of single-nucleotide polymorphisms (SNPs) (Chapter 42). These are differences in single DNA bases between individuals that occur every several hundred bases. Some of these account for common genetic differences between people, including differences that may contribute to disease. The catalog of SNPs currently includes several million variants; it has been found that the genome has evolved as blocks of clusters of genes, making it possible to use only a limited number of SNPs within a given region to determine whether there is a gene in that region that is associated with a disease. Since completion of the HapMap Project, there has been a dramatic increase in the number of SNPs found to be associated with common disorders. As genetic risk factors for common disorders come to light, it is likely that there will be advances in risk assessment, disease stratification, and developing new approaches to treatment.

Genetic Risk Assessment

The goal of genetic risk assessment is the identification of individuals at risk of disease before the onset of signs or symptoms. In principle, the genetic factors could be identified at birth, or any time in life, by testing a DNA sample. Individuals found to be at risk might be offered treatment in advance of onset of the disease to avoid complications or might be advised to modify their lifestyle to avoid exposure to environmental factors that might increase their risk of disease. Several companies have begun to offer "personalized genomic testing." Tests are usually accessed through an Internet site without intervention of a health professional and involve analysis of hundreds of thousands of SNPs in a clinical laboratory. Results are provided through a secure Internet site, sometimes with an option for genetic counseling.

Although the concept of genomic risk assessment would appear to be an attractive paradigm, many questions may be raised about its practicality and implementation. First, predictive testing is useful only insofar as it guides further management. This is likely to be a moving target because ability to test for risk can be developed more quickly than ability to modify that risk. The utility of interventions may be valued differently by different people. This already has been the case for testing of disorders such as breast cancer. Some women at risk choose not to know their *BRCA* status because the options, including surveillance or prophylactic surgery, are unacceptable to them. If there were a low-cost, safe, and effective treatment that would neutralize any risk the decision to test would be simple, but short of that, there are reasonable arguments on both sides of the issue of whether to test. For many disorders, it will take a long time to show the efficacy of any intervention because there may be a period of many years between the test and the onset of a disorder. Unless surrogate markers can be identified and followed, the task of proving a benefit to predictive testing may require years to decades in some instances.

Predictive Value of Genetic Testing

A second issue surrounds the degree to which genetic testing would be predictive. Most genetic tests are likely to involve detection of relatively common polymorphic alleles that account for small increments of relative risk of disease. The predictive value of these tests would be modest, perhaps too low to induce an individual to modify behavior or to take medication. Here, again, much depends on the efficacy of any intervention that can be offered. There may be some disorders for which testing would have substantial predictive value and clinical utility and others for which testing would not be justified.

Social and Ethical Issues

A third concern relates to social and ethical issues. Will people use test results as an excuse to pursue self-destructive behaviors, having received what may be false reassurance of "immunity"? Will genetic testing further exacerbate the divide between individuals who can afford to pay for their care and those who cannot? Will people misinterpret results of testing in terms of a simplistic notion of genetic determinism, erroneously believing that their futures have been written, leaving them no recourse but to meet their fate? The rapid pace of technologic change is going to challenge the ability of the social and legal systems to keep pace.

Service Models

Finally, there are questions of the ideal context in which to offer such testing. The personal genomics companies provide their services directly to the consumer in most cases. This creates the obvious risk for incorrect interpretation of results by the patient, although it is not clear that the health care work force is otherwise prepared to deal with the challenges of interpretation of genome-wide studies. The challenges will only increase if whole-genome sequencing at modest cost (e.g., <$1,000) becomes available, as is widely anticipated.

Disease Stratification

A second application of genomics in medical practice entails stratification of disease. Even if genetic testing is not used to predict individuals at risk, it may well be used to determine the most appropriate treatment for a clinically diagnosed disorder. Most common disorders, such as hypertension and diabetes, are symptom complexes that probably result from a variety of causes. The particular combination of causes may differ in different individuals and may respond to different types of treatments. Choice of antihypertensive drug may come to depend on genetic testing to determine the specific cause of hypertension in a patient. There are already examples of genotypes that predict response to drugs, for example, in lung cancer. It is possible that genetic tests eventually will accompany many if not most treatment decisions.

Effects and Identification of Drugs

Aside from helping to choose the most efficacious drug, genetic testing may play a role in avoidance of side effects and in appropriate dosing. Many drugs are known to be associated with rare side effects, some of which are sufficiently severe as to lead the drug to be withdrawn from use. Some of these side effects may occur only in individuals who are susceptible on the basis of having a particular allele at a polymorphic locus. An example is the

TABLE 39-4	GENES IN WHICH COMMON POLYMORPHISMS AFFECT RATES OF DRUG METABOLISM OR ACTION
GENE	**MEDICATIONS (EXAMPLES)**
CYP2C9	Phenytoin, warfarin
CYP2D6	Debrisoquin, β-blockers, antidepressants
VKORC1	Warfarin
UGT1A1	Irinotecan
Thiopurine methyltransferase	Mercaptopurine, azathioprine
N-acetyltransferase	Isoniazid, hydralazine
CYP2C19	Clopidogrel

multidisciplinary workshop. *Genet Med.* 2009;11:559-567. *Report of a workshop on issues related to personal genomic testing.*

Limdi NA, Veenstra DL. Expectations, validity, and reality in pharmacogenetics. *J Clin Epidemiol.* 2009;63:960-969. *Review of the use of pharmacogenetics in medicine.*

Rotimi CN, Jorde LB. Ancestry and disease in the age of genetic medicine. *N Engl J Med.* 2010;363:1551-1558. *Review.*

40

GENE, GENOMIC, AND CHROMOSOMAL DISORDERS

PAWEŁ STANKIEWICZ AND JAMES R. LUPSKI

association of polymorphisms in certain sodium or potassium channel genes with risk of arrhythmia on exposure to specific drugs.

Absorption and metabolism of drugs are largely under genetic control. Several polymorphisms are known to lead to particularly rapid or slow metabolism, accounting for individuals who experience dose-related side effects or lack of efficacy at standard dosages (Table 39-4). Detection of these polymorphisms would allow customization of drug dosage to an individual's pattern of metabolism, increasing the likelihood of efficacy without a prolonged period of trial-and-error dosing. There has been a major interest in applying this paradigm to warfarin dosing, although questions remain about the cost-effectiveness and practicality of genetic testing in routine use of this drug.

The greatest gift of genetics and genomics to medicine may be in the ability to identify new drug targets and develop new approaches to treatment. Identification of genes that contribute to common disorders is revealing the cellular mechanisms that lead to disease. This knowledge offers the opportunity to develop new pharmaceutical agents that would target the physiologic mechanisms more precisely, leading to drugs that work better and cause fewer side effects. New approaches to gene replacement or insertion of genes into cells as localized drug delivery systems also may be developed. The treatment of common disorders likely would entail the use of approaches developed as a result of genomics even in cases in which genetic testing is not used to predict individuals who are at risk.

CONCLUSION

The Human Genome Project began after most practicing physicians completed their medical training, and few are familiar with the methods and approaches of medical genetics and genomics. Nevertheless, physicians will be using the products of the genome project increasingly in their day-to-day practice during the coming years. Whether they are providing care for a patient with a rare genetic disorder or for a patient with a common condition not usually regarded as genetic, management choices increasingly will be informed by tests and treatments that in some way are based on information from the genome sequence.

The essence of the encounter between a physician and a patient can be distilled to two questions: Why this person? Why this time? A person who seeks medical care is doing so as the product of human evolution, having an ancestry associated with certain genetic vulnerabilities, because of inheritance of certain familial risk factors, because of exposure to some environmental factors, because of a particular physiologic process gone awry, because of behavioral traits that lead the person to seek medical care, because of prompting by family or friends to go to the doctor, because society makes medical services available, and because the person can afford to seek care. Genetics cannot answer all of these questions, but it is providing the key to addressing many of the biologic questions that underlie the medical mysteries that have puzzled humankind for generations.

SUGGESTED READINGS

Ginsburg GS, Willard HF. Genomic and personalized medicine: foundations and applications. *Transl Res.* 2009;154:277-278. *Overview of the role genetics and genomics increasingly will play in medical practice.*

Guttmacher AE, McGuire AL, Ponder B, et al. Personalized genomic information: preparing for the future of genetic medicine. *Nat Rev Gen.* 2010; 11:161-165. *Four experts with different insights into the field of genomic medicine.*

Khoury MJ, McBride CM, Schully SD, et al. The Scientific Foundation for personal genomics: recommendations from a National Institutes of Health-Centers for Disease Control and Prevention

THE HUMAN GENOME

Unprecedented technologic advances in molecular biology during the past two decades have enabled the determination of the entire DNA (deoxyribonucleic acid) sequence content of the human genome (Human Genome Project, HGP; *www.ornl.gov/sci/techresources/Human_Genome/home.shtml*) and establishment of a reference haploid genome. To date, a few other personal diploid human genomes have been sequenced, and the enormous amount of available DNA sequence data has expanded our view of the genetic bases of disease.

Human genomic DNA is packaged within the nucleus in 23 chromosome pairs, 22 autosomes, and two sex chromosomes, XX in females and XY in males. The diploid genome (2n) in each cell consists of two identical haploid copies of about 3×10^9 base pairs (bp), thus equaling in total 6 billion nucleotides. Most of the human genome consists of repetitive elements: tandem repeats (e.g., satellite sequences in centromeres), telomeric repeats, microsatellites, minisatellites, and short and long interspersed retrotransposable elements (e.g., *Alu* elements and LINE elements, respectively) (Table 40-1). These elements form heterochromatin; however, their functional role remains largely unknown. The unique DNA sequences constituting euchromatin compose the minority of our genome and include 20,000 to 25,000 genes, 700 micro-RNA genes, pseudogenes, gene fragments, nongenic sequences, and regulatory elements. Although protein coding sequences occupy only about 2% of the human genome, it has been demonstrated recently that the majority of our DNA may be transcribed into RNA.

Approximately 4 to 5% of the human genome, including both repetitive and unique sequences, is present in two or more copies in the haploid genome. DNA fragments larger than 1 kb in size and of DNA sequence identity greater than 90% have been termed *low-copy repeats* (LCRs) or segmental duplications (SDs). Most LCRs have arisen during primate speciation. A subset of LCRs with DNA sequence identity greater than 95 to 97% and longer than 10 kb can lead to local genome instability during both meiotic (constitutional) and mitotic (somatic) cell divisions, resulting in genomic rearrangements.

GENE

The concept of a gene can be traced back to 1865 when Gregor Mendel observed the inheritance of phenotypic traits in the garden pea, *Pisum sativum*. Mendel noted that two *factors*, which we now know to be corresponding DNA loci (alleles) located on homologous chromosomes, separate from each other during meiosis and segregate to two different gametes. This phenomenon of independent segregation is now known as *Mendel's First Law*. *Mendel's Second Law* described the independent segregation of two different (nonallelic) loci during gamete formation. The *inheritance factors* or *units of heredity* encoding the genetic information were later defined as *genes*. We now define *gene* as a fragment of DNA that carries the information used to transcribe it into a functional RNA (ribonucleic acid).

The DNA double helix is composed of four nucleotides: two purine bases, adenine (A) and guanine (G), and two pyrimidine bases, thymine (T) and cytosine (C), all connected to deoxyribose sugars and linked by phosphodiester bonds at the 5′ and 3′ carbons of the sugar (in RNA, thymine is replaced by uracil, U). Three consecutive nucleotides (triplet codon) of the coding DNA encode an amino acid. There are 64 possible different codons (4^3 combinations) but only 20 amino acids; therefore, the genetic code has been termed *degenerate*. Most of the genes in our genome comprise several coding

TABLE 40-1. STRUCTURE OF THE HUMAN GENOME

CHROMATIN FEATURE	SEQUENCE TYPE	HUMAN GENOME (HAPLOID)		SIZE (% OF 3 MILLION BASE PAIRS)*	
Euchromatin	Protein coding	20,000-25,000 genes		~2	
	Noncoding	RNA genes			
		Regulatory elements			
		Pseudogenes	}	~38	
		Gene fragments			
		Conserved sequences			
Heterochromatin	Repetitive			~60	
		Tandem: Satellite DNA, minisatellites, microsatellites		~14	
		Interspersed (transposons):		~45	
		Retro-transposons			~8
		LTR			
		Non-LTR			
		SINE (*Alu*)			~13
		LINE			~21
		DNA transposons			~3

*Estimated.
LTR = Long-terminal repeat.

regions or exons that are separated by noncoding introns. The entire gene (exons and introns) is transcribed into messenger RNA (mRNA) by RNA polymerase II starting from its 5′ end and continuing beyond the polyA recognition signal at the 3′ end. Typically, mRNA begins with a cap and terminates with a polyadenylated (polyA) tail at the 3′ end. In the subsequent process of splicing, the intervening noncoding introns are deleted, and the spliced, mature mRNA is translated into a polypeptide. The polypeptides start at the 5′ end (NH₂) with a methionine encoded by the AUG triplet. At the 3′ end (COOH), the polypeptides are terminated by one of three termination codons: UAA, UAG, or UGA (Fig. 40-1).

Micro-RNAs are single-stranded, 21- to 24-bp RNA molecules encoded by their own genes or introns of other genes but not translated into protein (i.e., they are noncoding RNAs). Micro-RNAs are thought to regulate (usually downregulate) gene expression of more than half of all human protein-coding genes. The phenotypic consequences of micro-RNAs are mainly unknown; they are believed to prevent the development of cancer and other diseases.

⬤ GENETIC VARIATION

In addition to the HGP, the International HapMap (*http://hapmap.ncbi.nlm.nih.gov*), Human Genome Diversity (*www.stanford.edu/group/morrinst/hgdp.html*), ENCODE (*www.genome.gov/10005107*), and ongoing personal genome sequencing projects have revealed the tremendous and underappreciated extent of variation in our genome. Genetic variation

consists of two major types: (1) nucleotide sequence changes, or single nucleotide variation (SNV), and (2) genome structural changes, or copy-number variation (CNV) (Fig. 40-2).

Single Nucleotide Variation

A genetic polymorphism is defined as a heterozygous DNA variation present in greater than 1% of the population. Genome-wide nucleotide variation has been uncovered in the early phase of DNA sequencing analyses, which showed that human genomes differ mainly by single nucleotide changes. These differences have been termed *single nucleotide polymorphisms* (SNPs) and defined as a nucleotide change at a given position generated by substitution (usually there are two alleles per SNP). Only a minority of SNPs map to exons; however, SNPs located outside of the protein-coding regions can still exert phenotypic effects, such as by modifying gene regulatory elements or transcription factor binding sites, generating splicing mutations, or affecting noncoding RNAs. Any two humans differ on average by about 3.5 million SNVs or SNPs, about 0.1% of the 3.0×10^9 reference haploid genome (phase 3 of the International HapMap project).

A set of consecutive SNPs (or other markers) is defined as a *haplotype*. A nonrandom association of markers in a population not interrupted by meiotic recombination (*crossing-over*) is described as *linkage disequilibrium*. (Note that linkage disequilibrium exemplifies the exception to Mendel's Second Law.)

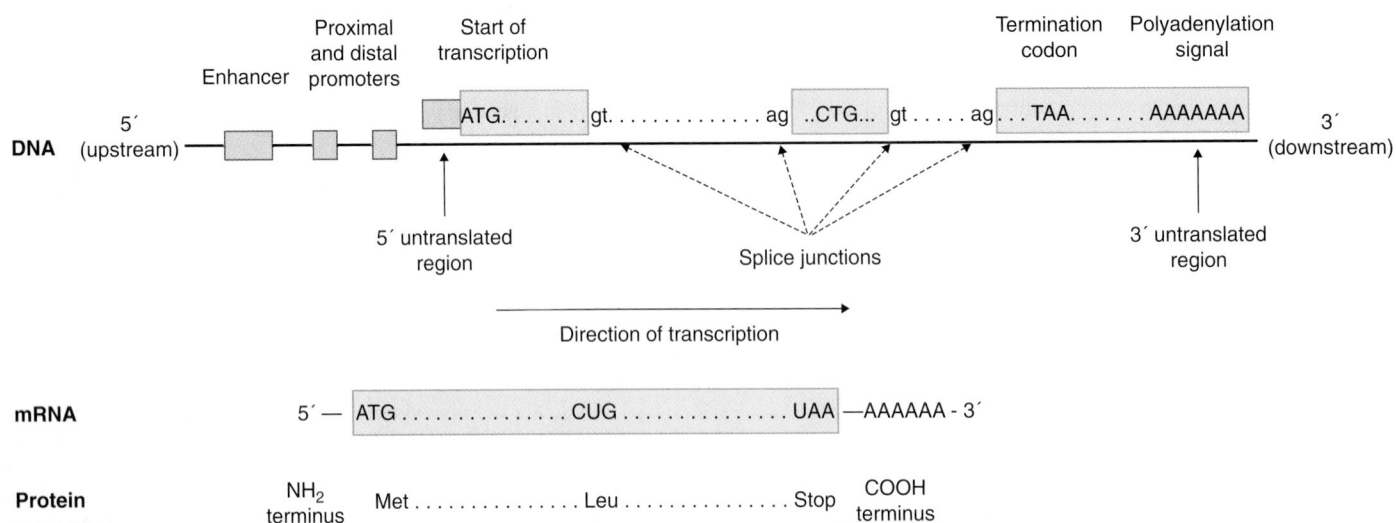

FIGURE 40-1. Gene structure. Schematic representation of the general structure of a typical human gene. Three exons are depicted as *orange open rectangles*. Note that the transcription usually starts with an ATG triplet encoding methionine. The 5′ (upstream) portion of a gene corresponds to the NH₂ terminus, and the 3′ (downstream) segment encodes the COOH terminus of the polypeptide. Enhancers and promoters are shown as *blue rectangles*.

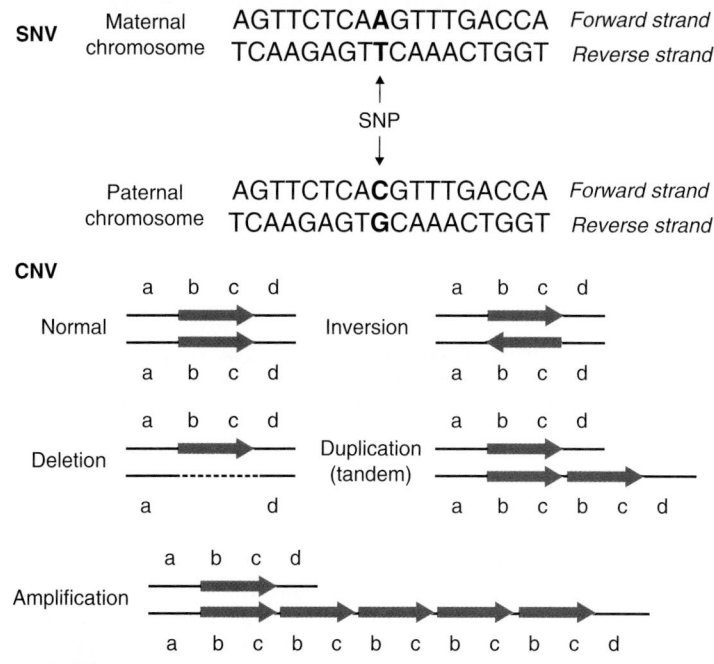

FIGURE 40-2. **Genetic variation.** *Top,* Heterozygous single nucleotide polymorphism (SNP, or single nucleotide variation SNV) representing the most common transition C→T is shown. *Bottom,* Structural genomic changes: a balanced inversion and the unbalanced copy-number variations (CNVs), deletion, duplication, and amplification are shown with *black arrows* on two homologous chromosomes (*black lines*). The *dashed line* represents a deleted fragment of one chromosome.

Tandem Repeats

Variable number of tandem repeats (VNTRs), or *minisatellites*, and short tandem repeats (STRs) such as unstable dinucleotides, trinucleotides, and tetranucleotides, $(GT)_n$, $(CAA)_n$, or $(GATA)_n$, referred to as *microsatellites*, are highly variable. Both minisatellites and microsatellites have been successfully used in linkage and association studies that enable the mapping of traits and the identification of genes and loci responsible for both mendelian disorders and complex traits. These highly polymorphic sequence repeats are extremely variable in the copy number of their repeating subunits; this property enables the use of a number of such markers to derive a unique pattern of marker genotypes for each human individual. Thus, such markers have been useful for identity testing and DNA forensics.

Repetitive Elements

The other group of polymorphic elements in the human genome is represented by retrotransposons, long and short interspersed nuclear elements (LINEs and SINEs) (see Table 40-1). The most common *Alu* and L1 elements introduce recombinogenic genomic instability and insertional mutagenic activity; their positions within an individual human personal diploid genome can vary tremendously.

Copy-Number Variation

A more recently characterized group of major polymorphic genetic variation in the human genome is represented by structural changes. In this postgenomic era, high-resolution genome-wide analysis of human genome sequences has revealed higher-order architectural features, with a potential to cause genomic instability and extensive submicroscopic structural variations. These structural variations consist of unbalanced CNVs, including deletions, duplications, triplications, insertions, and translocations, that differ from the normal diploid state, as well as balanced rearrangements, such as genomic inversions. Both CNVs and SNVs have been shown to play a major role in human genetic diversity, evolution, and susceptibility to diseases. Surprisingly, it has been found that any two human genomes contain more base pair differences due to CNVs than SNVs.

Recent analyses have revealed over 38,000 CNVs (greater than 100 bp) that occupy more than 29% of the reference human genome. A validated subset of these CNVs overlaps 13% of the Reference Sequence (*www.ncbi.nlm.nih.gov/projects/RefSeq/RSG*) genes and 12% of the Online Mendelian Inheritance in Man (OMIM) (*www.ncbi.nlm.nih.gov/sites/*

entrez?db=omim) genes and was predicted by conceptual translation to alter the structure of 12.5% gene transcripts and 5.5% mRNAs. Despite all these recent achievements, the total number, position, size, gene content, and population distribution of CNVs remain obscure because we still do not have accurate and reliable molecular methods to study smaller CNVs on a genome-wide scale in different populations, particularly when copy-number changes are greater than 4 or 5.

CNVs have been shown to be responsible for mendelian diseases, nonmendelian traits such as complex diseases, and common traits (including neurobehavioral traits) or to represent benign polymorphic variation. CNVs can lead to an abnormal phenotype by disrupting the gene structure or changing the copy number of dosage-sensitive genes. However, long-range effects of CNVs involving nongenic sequences, leaving a gene intact, have been also demonstrated. Furthermore, evidence suggests that a combination of two or more CNVs at the same or different loci may be responsible for phenotypic variation. The genome-wide scale of phenotypic effects exerted by CNVs (genomic load) are unknown and await further studies.

Any two individuals differ by about 1000 CNVs ranging in size from about 500 bp to 1 Mb. An updated summary of CNVs can be found in the Toronto Database of Genomic Variants (*http://projects.tcag.ca/variation*). Many clinically relevant CNVs can be found in the Database of Chromosomal Imbalance and Phenotype in Humans using Ensembl Resources (DECIPHER) (*https://decipher.sanger.ac.uk/information*).

CHROMOSOMES

The recombined haploid (1n) human genome formed during meiosis is stored as chromosomes in female and male gametes. They merge at conception, and this diploid genome instructs the development of a zygote; the diploid human genome is subsequently transmitted to the mitotically dividing daughter cells. Human chromosomes can be distinguished from each other in a light microscope by differences in size and characteristic banding patterns after specific chemical staining (e.g., G-banding with Giemsa) when the chromosomes are arrested in a condensed phase (metaphase) of mitotic divisions.

Each human metaphase chromosome is composed of two chromatids that form short (p) and long (q) arms connected by a centromere built with α-satellite DNA. Based on the relative position of the centromere along the chromosome, chromosomes have been described as metacentric (similarly sized p and q arms), submetacentric (q arm significantly longer than p), and acrocentric (chromosomes 13, 14, 15, 21, and 22, with centromeres located close to the end of a chromosome) (Fig. 40-3).

Telomeres consist of repetitive DNA sequences (thousands of copies of TTAGGG repeats) located at the ends of both chromosome arms that are stabilized by a reverse transcriptase enzyme, telomerase, which adds TTAGGG sequence to the 3′ end of DNA strands. In contrast to germline and cancer cells, human somatic cells lacking telomerase gradually lose the telomeric sequences. As a result, cells reach the limit of their replicative capacity and fall into senescence.

Chromosomal Aberrations
Numerical Aberrations

Microscopically visible chromosomal aberrations have been divided into numerical and structural aberrations and are found in 1 in about 160 live births. The numerical aberrations are usually lethal. Polyploidies (multiplication of a haploid set of 23 chromosomes), such as triploidies (3n), 69,XXX, 69,XXY, and 69,XYY, and tetraploidies (4n), 92,XXYY or 92,XXXX, are caused by abnormal egg fertilization by two sperms or by a failure in zygote division, respectively.

The most commonly detected viable chromosomal aneuploidies, trisomies and monosomies, involve chromosomes X, Y, 21, 18, and 13 and arise as a result of meiotic nondisjunctions. Sex chromosome aneuploidies are more common and are found in 1 in 440 newborns. Monosomy X (45,X cell line) in female patients with Turner's syndrome is identified in every 4000 female newborns. However, this birth rate represents only 1% of all fetuses with 45,X because more than 99% are spontaneously aborted (this is similar to the most frequent fetal aneuploidy, trisomy 16, that results in 100% miscarriages). In most cases, the 45,X cell line is found as a mosaic along with another cell line that has either a normal karyotype or a structural rearrangement of the X chromosome (e.g., deletion of the short arm, ring chromosome, or isochromosome of the long or short arms). One in every 1000 males has a 47,XXY chromosome complement that is responsible for Klinefelter's syndrome.

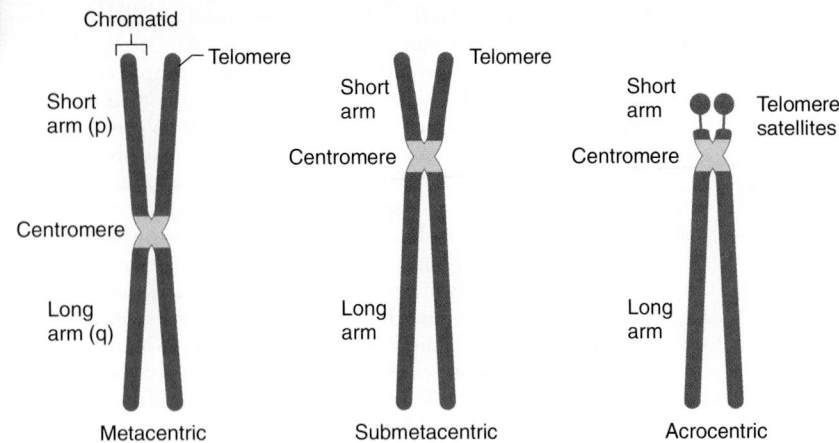

FIGURE 40-3. Types of metaphase chromosomes. Metacentric, submetacentric, and acrocentric chromosomes are composed of two arms connected by a centromere. Each chromosome arm consists of two chromatids.

In contrast to gonosomes, monosomies of all autosomes are lethal. The only trisomies compatible with life are found in patients with Down syndrome (trisomy 21 in every 670 newborns), Edwards' syndrome (trisomy 18 in 1 in 5000 newborns), and Patau's syndrome (trisomy 13 in every 10,000 newborns).

Incomplete supernumerary chromosomes are termed *marker chromosomes.* They usually originate from acrocentric autosomes (~ 50% from chromosome 15) and are found in every 4000 newborns. The severity of the abnormal phenotype in carriers of marker chromosomes varies among different chromosomes and is estimated as 28% in de novo cases.

Structural Aberrations

Chromosomal deletions and duplications have been categorized as microscopically visible or submicroscopic, terminal or interstitial, recurrent or nonrecurrent. The most frequent are recurrent common-sized rearrangements flanked by directly oriented LCRs or SDs that mediate nonallelic homologous recombination (NAHR). For example, an about 3 Mb microdeletion in chromosome 22q11.2 occurs in patients with DiGeorge velocardiofacial syndrome and is found in 1:4000 newborns. The 1.4-Mb Charcot-Marie-Tooth disease type 1A (CMT1A) duplication causes greater than half of all adult-onset inherited Charcot-Marie-Tooth neuropathy, and de novo events account for up to 90% of sporadic cases. The phenotypic consequences of deletion/duplication CNVs depend on whether the CNVs harbor a dosage-sensitive (e.g., haploinsufficient for deletion) gene.

Balanced reciprocal translocations result from an exchange of the DNA material between two chromosomes and are found in 1 in about 600 individuals. During meiosis, the translocation chromosomes form a pachytene tetrad structure and, depending on the segregation type (alternate or adjacent, symmetric or asymmetric), either balanced or unbalanced products are transmitted to progeny. The unbalanced products often lead to either spontaneous abortions or births of clinically affected children. Recently, it has been shown by high-resolution genome analyses that up to 40% of apparently balanced translocations found in subjects with abnormal phenotypes are associated with additional imbalances at or near the translocation breakpoint or somewhere else in the genome.

Translocations involving short arms (or centromeres) of acrocentric chromosomes are described as robertsonian translocations. Balanced robertsonian translocations (45-chromosome complement) are present in 1 in 900 newborns; thus, these are the most common chromosome rearrangements in humans. The most frequent robertsonian translocation, t(13;14), is found in 1 in 1300 individuals. The carriers of balanced robertsonian translocations have a significantly increased risk for an unbalanced karyotype in progeny (e.g., trisomy 21 or trisomy 13) or uniparental disomy for chromosomes 14 and 15 that are known to contain imprinted genes.

Constitutional nonrobertsonian chromosomal translocations are nonrecurrent, with the exception of five recurrent translocations: t(11;22) (q11.2;q23.3) and t(8;22)(q24.13;q11.21), that use AT-rich cruciforms, and translocations t(4;8)(p16;p23), t(8;12)(p23.1p13.31), and t(4;11) (p16;p15.2) that are mediated by LCR gene clusters.

When a fragment of one chromosome is translocated into another chromosome's arm, the aberration is termed an *insertion* or *insertional translocation.* Insertional translocations have been recently shown by high-resolution human genome analyses to occur more than 100 times more frequently than recognized previously. The carrier of a balanced insertion has up to a 50% chance of an unbalanced offspring.

An inversion is defined when a chromosome fragment is reversed end to end. Inversions harboring the centromere are termed *pericentric,* and those with breakpoints mapping in the same chromosome arm are termed *paracentric.* Usually, only the products of pericentric inversions (unbalanced terminal deletion of one chromosome arm accompanied by a terminal duplication of the second arm) are found in a progeny. The acentric or dicentric products of paracentric inversions are unstable and thus not transmitted.

Other, less common structural chromosomal abnormalities include ring chromosomes, isochromosomes, complex chromosome rearrangements, and heterochromatin variants. Rings arise when two broken ends of the same chromosome fuse. Usually, chromosome material telomeric to the breakpoints is lost and leads to an abnormal phenotype. Rings are commonly unstable mitotically and often form double ring structures. Isochromosomes arise when one part of the chromosome is duplicated and separated from the other. Isochromosomes can be monocentric (breakpoint in the centromere) or dicentric and thus unstable, unless one of the centromeres becomes inactivated (pseudoisodicentric). Chromosome aberrations with more than two breakpoints on two or more chromosomes are termed *complex chromosome rearrangements* and often result in an unbalanced product of meiotic division.

Mosaicism and Chimeras

The presence of two or more cell lines with different chromosome complements in one individual is termed *mosaicism* when they originate from the same zygote or *chimeras* when the cells originate from different zygotes. Chromosomal mosaicism is a common phenomenon, observed in about 50% of embryos at the eight-cell stage and in up to 75% of blastocysts. Somatic chromosomal mosaicism is found, for example, in patients with hypomelanosis of Ito and Pallister-Killian syndrome (tetrasomy 12p).

⬤ MUTATION

Mutation is defined as a change in nucleotide sequence due to errors of DNA replication, recombination, or repair or to radiation, chemical mutagens, viruses, or transposons. Gene mutations can be inherited from a parent (hereditary, germline, or constitutional) and thus present in every cell. Alternatively, mutations can be acquired in some tissues at some time either during an individual's development or at any time throughout a person's life (somatic) (Fig. 40-4). Recent whole genome sequencing of lung cancer tissue suggests one new point mutation for every pack of cigarettes smoked. Point mutations, usually involving only one or a few nucleotides, have been divided into substitutions, insertions, and deletions. Mutations mapping in protein-coding sequences and changing the protein structure have been termed *nonsynonymous,* whereas those that do not lead to protein change are known as *synonymous* or silent mutations. The latter mutations can still have functional consequences (e.g., by generating a cryptic splice site, an exon splice enhancer, or affecting the regulatory elements).

Based on the functional consequences, mutations have been divided into loss-of-function and gain-of-function mutations. The former, also known as *hypomorphic* (partial loss) or *amorphic* or *null* (complete *loss*), affect the dosage-sensitive or haploinsufficient genes, in which a decreased amount of protein is not sufficient for normal function. Gain-of-function mutations

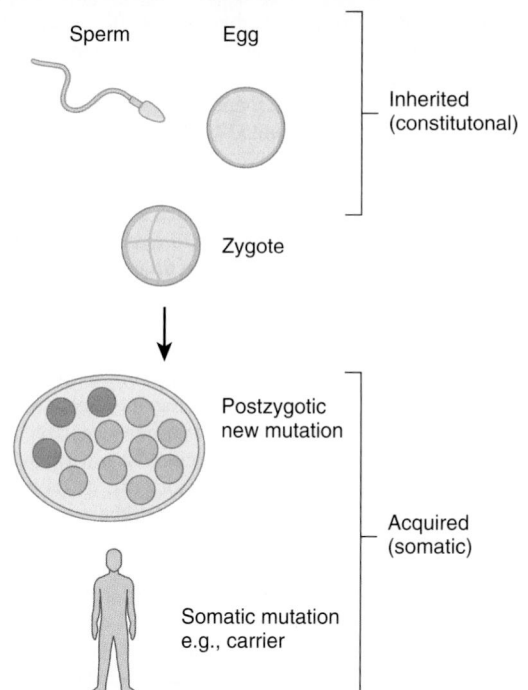

FIGURE 40-4. Mutation. Constitutional mutations are inherited from one of the parents. They can be present in the somatic cells of a parent (carrier) or can arise during gametogenesis (de novo). Mutations that occur postzygotically (acquired, somatic) are usually found in a mosaic state.

increase or add a new function for the protein (*neomorphic*), and dominant negative mutations are translated into a protein that interacts antagonistically with the normal product from the other allele (*antimorphic*).

The situation in which one allele is mutated and the second is normal (wild-type) is referred to as *heterozygous*. A combination of the same two mutations in each of the alleles of the same locus (e.g., in consanguineous families) is defined as *homozygous* mutations, or compound heterozygotes when the two mutant alleles are distinct. Two mutant alleles at different loci are described as *double heterozygote*. When one of the autosomal alleles is absent (e.g., because of a deletion CNV and for most of the X chromosome genes in males), the locus is referred to as *hemizygous*.

Different mutations in one gene can manifest with the same or distinct phenotypes, phenomena called *allelic heterogeneity* or *allelic affinity*, respectively. By contrast, the same abnormal clinical phenotype can be caused by mutations in different genes (genetic or locus heterogeneity).

Single Nucleotide Variation

Nonsynonymous mutations can lead to a single amino acid change (*missense*), modify the downstream protein structure (*frameshift*), introduce a stop codon (*premature termination codon [PTC]*) that truncates the protein prematurely (*nonsense*), or abolish the specific site at which splicing of an intron takes place during the processing of precursor mRNA into mature mRNA (*splice site*). The PTC-mutated mRNAs are inactivated and removed from cells by a surveillance mechanism called *nonsense mediated decay* that is initiated by a premature termination codon in any exon, except the last and a 50- to 55-bp portion of the second to last (i.e., penultimate) exon that usually escape nonsense mediated decay.

Transition mutations refer to changes from pyrimidine to pyrimidine (e.g., C to T) or purine to purine (e.g., A to G), and are more frequent than exchanges from purine to pyrimidine (e.g., A to C) or pyrimidine to purine (e.g., T to G), that is, transversions. The most common C-to-T transition (about ten-fold relative to other bases) occurs in the methylated CpG dinucleotide because methylated C is subject to deamination and becomes T.

Mutations that are unstable have been termed *dynamic*. Pathogenic dynamic expansion of trinucleotide, tetranucleotide, and pentanucleotide repeat sequences can be located in coding (e.g., CAG triplet in Huntington's disease) or noncoding regions such as introns (e.g., GAA in Friedreich's ataxia) or untranslated regions, either 5′ (e.g., CGG in fragile X syndrome, OMIM 300624) or 3′ (e.g., CTG in myotonic dystrophy). The mutations convey phenotypes that can be inherited as autosomal dominant (e.g., myotonic

dystrophy), autosomal recessive (e.g., Friedreich's ataxia), or X-linked (e.g., fragile X syndrome) traits due to gain- or loss-of-function mutations. For each of the dynamic mutation diseases, there is a specific repeat number limit, above which the disease is manifested. The number of repeats below that threshold but greater than in normals is referred to as a *premutation*. However, in some "disease genes," premutations are also associated with a milder, nonspecific phenotype (e.g., ovarian failure in females and late-onset neurologic disorders in males with premutations in the fragile X *FMR1* gene). The number of repeats tends to expand in the next generations, a phenomenon called *anticipation*; this typically occurs in a sex-specific manner.

Copy-Number Variation

It has now become apparent that the Watson-Crick DNA base pair changes are not the only mutational mechanism responsible for mendelian monogenic diseases and complex traits. Higher-order genomic architectural features can lead to a regional instability and susceptibility to DNA rearrangements or CNVs, which can be a frequent cause of diseases in humans. Such conditions due to structural genome changes or CNV have been referred to as *genomic disorders*.

A major mechanism by which rearrangements convey phenotypes is gene dosage due to a variation in gene copy number. CNVs can lead to deletion, duplication, or disruption of the dosage-sensitive gene, generate gene fusions, exert position effects, or unmask mutations in the coding region or other functional SNPs in the second allele, as when a deletion CNV results in a hemizygous state.

Different calculations have shown that the de novo locus-specific mutation rates for genomic rearrangements are between 10^{-4} and 10^{-5}, at least 1000 to 10,000 fold more frequent than de novo point mutations. Thus, new mutation CNV can contribute significantly to sporadic disease.

Many genomic disorders occur sporadically and are often caused by de novo rearrangements. Recurrent rearrangements (deletions, duplications, or inversions) are caused by NAHR between LCR that are located less than 5 to 10 Mb from each other and have greater than 97% DNA sequence identity. The fixed position of these LCRs and SDs in the human genome result in recurrent rearrangements having a common size for a given region. NAHR between directly oriented LCRs leads to deletions or reciprocal duplications of the genomic region located between them, and NAHR between the oppositely oriented LCRs results in an inversion of the intervening genomic segment. Interestingly, the strand exchanges for NAHR sites are not scattered throughout the entire length of homology within LCRs, but instead cluster in recombination hot spots.

Most nonrecurrent CNVs appear to occur by nonhomologous recombination mechanisms, and one often observes microhomology at the breakpoints. One prominent mechanism, particularly for complex (e.g., deletion/normal/duplication) rearrangements is the microhomology-mediated break-induced replication mechanism. The remainder of nonrecurrent different-sized rearrangements likely result from a nonhomologous end-joining recombination mechanism.

Microduplication and Microdeletion Syndromes

Some of the microduplication and microdeletion syndromes are caused by a copy-number change of the dosage-sensitive or haploinsufficient gene. Among the best characterized genomic disorders are common autosomal dominant peripheral neuropathies, CMT1A and hereditary neuropathy with liability (HNPP) to pressure palsies, that in more than 99% of cases are caused by duplication and deletion CNV, respectively, of an about 1.4-Mb genomic interval within 17p12 harboring a dosage-sensitive myelin gene *PMP22*. This genomic segment is flanked by two about 24-kb and about 98.7% identical LCRs, called the *proximal CMT1A-REP* and the *distal CMT1A-REP*, which serve as substrates for NAHR. Another example of common predominantly monogenic reciprocal microdeletion and microduplication syndromes include Potocki-Lupski syndrome due to dup(17)(p11.2p11.2), reciprocal to del(17)(p11.2p11.2) found in patients with Smith-Magenis syndrome. When two or more dosage-sensitive genes that are usually functionally unrelated are involved, these are referred to as *contiguous gene deletion* or *duplication syndromes*, for example, Potocki-Shaffer syndrome resulting from deletion del(11)(p11.2p11.2).

LCR-mediated recurrent microdeletion and microduplication syndromes usually have similar prevalence in different populations; however, for a few genomic disorders, significant differences in incidences in different world populations have been observed, likely demonstrating that variation of genomic architecture is a significant factor for disease susceptibility (e.g.,

17q21.31 microdeletion syndrome, Sotos' syndrome, 5q35). Examples of well-known and characterized microdeletion syndromes include Williams-Beuren syndrome (7q11.23), Prader-Willi and Angelman syndromes (15q11.2q12), DiGeorge velocardiofacial syndrome (22q11.2), microdeletion 17q21.31 syndrome, and Sotos' syndrome. For all these microdeletions, the reciprocal microduplications predicted by the NAHR model have been reported with phenotypes typically being milder. Recent studies revealed that some fraction of patients with autism and of patients with schizophrenia have deletion or duplication CNV involving specific loci (e.g., 1q21.1, 15q13.3, and 16p11.2); for 16p11.2, deletion CNV is more frequently associated with an autism phenotype, whereas duplication CNV can cause schizophrenia.

⬤ PATTERNS OF INHERITANCE

Mendelian Inheritance

Most characterized disease-associated mutations in humans can be assigned to a single gene (monogenic) or locus and segregate as a mendelian trait in an autosomal dominant, autosomal recessive, or X-linked fashion.

Autosomal dominant mutation is present in only one allele and thus is transmitted in meiosis to 50% of the gametes and is expected to manifest in half the offspring unless the trait is incompletely penetrant (e.g., in Marfan syndrome), represents variable expressivity (e.g., in cystic fibrosis), is age dependent (e.g., in Huntington disease), or lethal (e.g., alveolar capillary dysplasia). In pedigree analysis, autosomal dominant inheritance is revealed as a vertical transmission of the trait.

In an autosomal recessive trait, the affected individuals carry two mutant alleles at a specific locus that are either the same (usually in consanguineous families) or different. In general, both mutations are inherited from unaffected carrier parents (note that occasionally heterozygous carriers of the mutated allele may manifest a mild phenotype or have an increased susceptibility to complex or multifactorial traits). Theoretically, affected probands represent 25% of the progeny; two thirds of the unaffected siblings carry one mutated allele, and the remaining one fourth of all progeny (one third of unaffected) have two wild-type alleles. In pedigree analysis, autosomal recessive inheritance is observed as horizontal transmission of the trait.

In X-linked (both dominant and recessive) diseases, no male-to-male transmission is observed, and all daughters of affected fathers are obligate carriers of the mutated allele. X-linked dominant diseases are more rare than X-linked recessive disorders and present both in males and in females. Usually, there are twice as many affected females as males; however, if the disease is lethal in males, only females are affected (e.g., Rett's syndrome). Because of X-inactivation, the phenotype in females is milder than in males. In an X-linked recessive trait, only males are affected; in female carriers, the X chromosome harboring a mutated recessive allele is preferentially inactivated by nonrandom X-inactivation. However, females with an incomplete or skewed X inactivation, females with only one X chromosome (Turner's syndrome), or females carrying a balanced translocation between the X chromosome and an autosome (X material on the derivative chromosomes is not inactivated) can manifest the X-linked recessive disease.

Nonmendelian Inheritance

The occurrence of sporadic cases of the disease can be explained by a classic mendelian inheritance, such as de novo autosomal dominant, autosomal recessive, or X-linked mutation; however, one has to consider other possibilities, including nonmendelian inheritance—genomic imprinting, uniparental disomy, mosaicism, mitochondrial DNA mutations, and digenic or triallelic inheritance.

Some genes acquire different activity status (usually methylation) after passage through spermatogenesis compared with oogenesis. As a result, a gene can be silenced (imprinted), depending on the parent of origin. This parent-of-origin effect is observed for the *UBE3A* gene on chromosome 15q12 that is imprinted during spermatogenesis, and only the maternal copy is active. When the active maternal copy of *UBE3A* is mutated, deleted, or inactivated in a different way, the offspring is affected with Angelman's syndrome.

Sporadically, a chromosome pair may not be inherited from both parents. This distortion from biparental inheritance, termed *uniparental disomy* (UPD), may have clinical consequences when the uniparental chromosomes contain an autosomal recessive mutation or an imprinted gene. When both homologues are inherited from one parent, it is referred as *heterodisomy*. In isodisomy, both homologues in an offspring originate from only one of the parental homologues. The most common mechanism for UPD is trisomy

rescue, in which an early postzygotic embryo is trisomic, as a result of chromosome nondisjunction in meiosis I, and the extra chromosome is then lost during further development to restore disomy. Because this is a random event, in one third of cases, the disomic chromosomes remaining after trisomy to disomy rescue will represent UPD. Consequently, UPD is associated with advanced maternal age.

In some diseases, pathogenic mutations have been found in single alleles of two different genes with the other alleles at each given locus being normal. This double heterozygous phenomenon of two interacting genes has been reported, for example, for *ROM1* and *RDS* in retinitis pigmentosa and *GJB6* and *GJB2* in deafness.

In some patients, three abnormal alleles in two different genes have been identified. The phenomenon of triallelic (or oligogenic) inheritance has been observed, for example, in Bardet-Biedl syndrome, familial hypercholesterolemia, and cortisone reductase deficiency. Monogenic chromosomal microduplication syndromes (e.g., CMT1A) can also be categorized as triallelic given the presence of three alleles at a given locus owing to duplication CNV.

Another distortion from mendelian inheritance can be caused by mosaicism. Two or more cell lines can be present either in the gonads only (germline mosaicism) or in somatic cells. Mosaicism should be suspected when healthy parents have two or more children with a dominant disease. Mosaicism can be particularly relevant when mutational processes involve DNA replication errors and occur mitotically (e.g., point mutation and microhomology-mediated break-induced replication).

Very rarely, a disease trait is transmitted to daughters and sons only from mothers. In such cases, one should consider a mitochondrial disease. Mitochondrial DNA (mtDNA) is present in multiple copies in the cell cytoplasm and is transmitted to progeny only through the oocytes. Initial clinical signs and symptoms typically originate from the most energy-dependent tissues (e.g., eyes, brain, skeletal muscle, and heart), and the phenotypic expression among family members varies and depends mainly on the proportion of mtDNA in the cytoplasm that carries the mutation, that is, heteroplasmy.

⬤ ASSAYING GENETIC VARIATION

Chromosome aberrations larger than about 5 Mb can be detected by light microscopy after specific staining that reveals characteristic banding patterns (e.g., G-banded karyotype analysis). Submicroscopic rearrangements, such as microdeletions or microduplications (30 kb to 5 Mb), have been analyzed for the past two decades using molecular cytogenetic techniques such as fluorescence in situ hybridization. In these routine clinical cytogenetic techniques, usually a subpopulation of peripheral blood phytohemagglutinin-stimulated T lymphocytes is analyzed. Rearrangements of similar size (i.e., 30 kb to 5 Mb in size) can be analyzed also using pulsed-field gel electrophoresis. However, both these technologies are limited to the analysis of specific genomic regions, that is, locus-specific testing.

The recent development of array-based comparative genomic hybridization (array CGH) has enabled screening of the entire human genome for imbalances, with the level of genome resolution depending only on the number, size, and distance between the arrayed interrogating probes. These genome-wide imaging techniques are analogous to digital photography wherein the resolution observed is dependent on the pixels used. Initial clinical array CGH used large genomic clones, BACs and PACs (bacterial or P1 artificial chromosomes), as interrogating probes. Recently, they have been replaced by oligonucleotides, of which millions can be synthesized on one glass slide. Oligonucleotide probes are also used on SNP arrays that, in contrast to microarray-based CGH, enable association studies or detection of uniparental disomies.

For detection of genomic imbalances, an alternative quantitative polymerase chain reaction–based technique, multiplex ligation-dependent probe amplification (MLPA) has been developed. MLPA is an inexpensive, simple, rapid, and sensitive tool to detect dosage alterations in selected genomic regions.

Most recently, several next-generation sequencing (NGS) technologies have been developed that enable massively parallel DNA sequencing reactions simultaneously and thus whole genome sequencing, or sequencing of the entire genome of an individual, to enable the determination of a Personal Genome Sequence (Fig. 40-5). In NGS, DNA sequencing uses chemistries other than the traditional Sanger dideoxy chain termination method. NGS methods generate far larger quantities of data at less expense; however, the individual raw sequence reads that are generated from individual amplified DNA template sequences have shorter read lengths and lower quality. Nevertheless, massive redundant sequencing of a personal diploid human genome (e.g., 30-fold coverage with respect to the haploid human reference genome sequence) can provide a robust and accurate Personal Genome Sequence.

CONCLUSION

Mutations in humans are caused by SNVs and CNVs. New mutations can contribute to sporadic disease. The total genomic load can be important to a clinical phenotype. Individual genetic variation is extensive. It is a sobering thought that for more than 90% of the annotated genes in the reference human genome, a function remains to be elucidated for the potential clinical consequences of mutations. Furthermore, 98% of the human genome is non-coding, and the functional consequences of variation within it cannot be assisted using the genetic code.

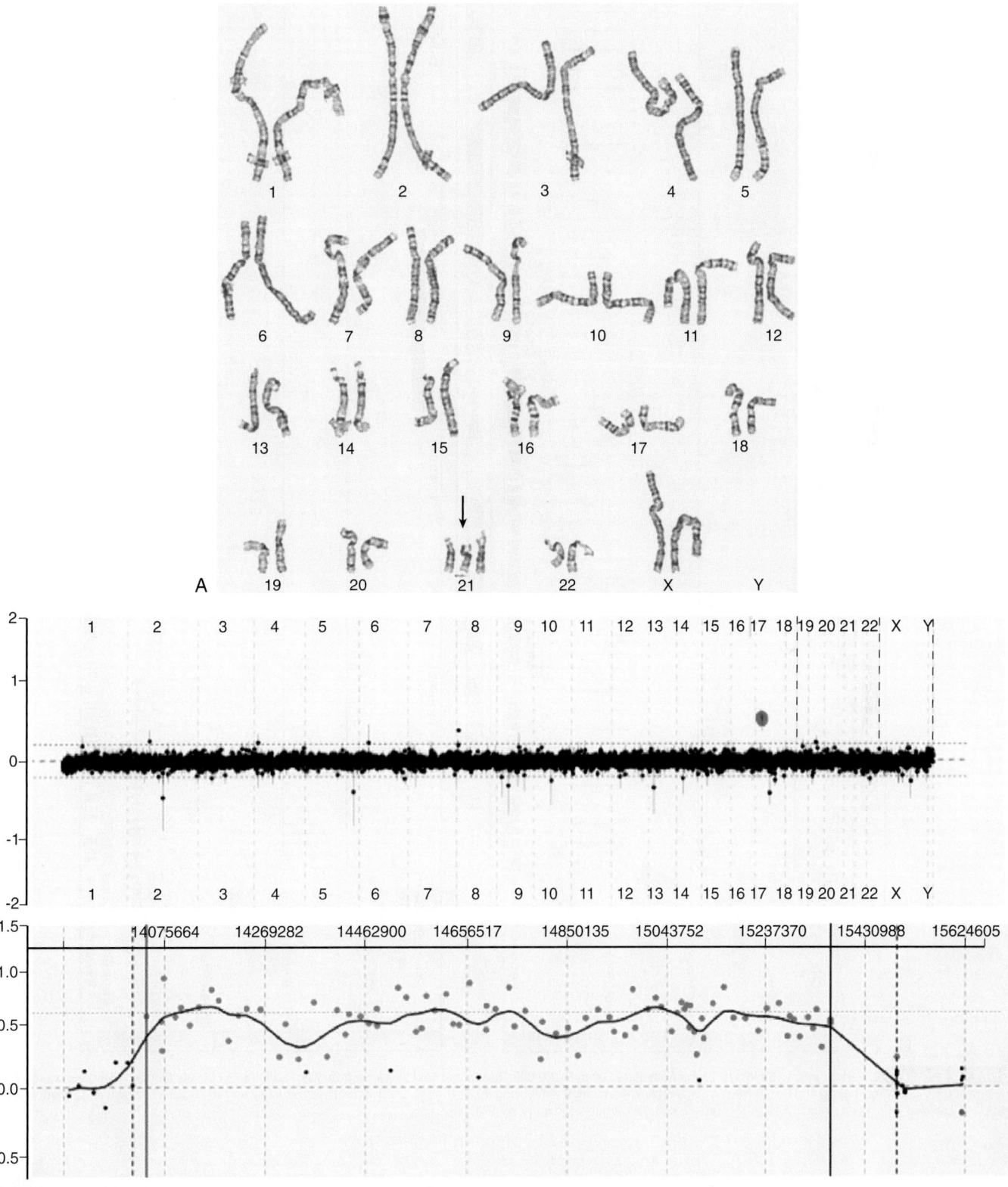

FIGURE 40-5. Assaying copy-number variation (CNV). **A,** G-banded metaphase chromosomes (karyogram) in a female (two X chromosomes) with trisomy 21 (Down syndrome). **B,** The genome-wide (*upper*) and region-specific (*bottom*) plots of the oligonucleotide-based array comparative genomic hybridization (array CGH) showing a 1.4-Mb CMT1A duplication (*green*) on chromosome 17p12. Oligonucleotides presented with *green color* and displaced upward, indicating a gain of chromosome material in the patient versus the reference DNA.

Continued

C

FIGURE 40-5, cont'd. C, Heterozygous CNV loss (*black bar* from 55,124,00 to 55,207,000) (*upper*) and gain (*black bar* from 73,071,000 to 73,114,000) (*bottom*) identified using oligonucleotide array CGH (Agilent Technology and Roche-NimbleGen) and next-generation sequencing (NGS) 454 Life Sciences (Roche). Low-copy repeats (LCRs) are shown at the bottom as *orange, dark yellow*, and *gray* bars representing >99%, >98%, and 90-98% DNA sequence identity, respectively.

SUGGESTED READINGS

Conrad DF, Pinto D, Redon R, et al. Origins and functional impact of copy number variation in the human genome. *Nature*. 2010;464:704-712. *Describes the most updated set of CNVs greater than 443 base pairs detected using tiling oligonucleotide microarrays with 42 million probes.*

Dietz HC. New therapeutic approaches to Mendelian disorders. *N Engl J Med*. 2010;363:852-863. *Review.*

Lupski JR, Reid JG, Gonzaga-Jauregui C, et al. Complete genome sequencing reveals *SH3TC2* mutations causing CMT1 neuropathy. *N Engl J Med*. 2010;362:1181-1191. *First use of personal whole genome sequencing to identify the genetic basis of disease in a single patient.*

Sheehan NA, Meng S, Didelez V. Mendelian randomization: a tool for assessing causality in observational epidemiology. *Methods Mol Biol*. 2011;713:153-166. *Methods for determining independent importance of a genetic variant based on epidemiologic data.*

Stankiewicz P, Lupski JR. Structural variation in the human genome and its role in disease. *Annu Rev Med*. 2010;61:437-455. *Reviews the role of CNV in disease.*

41

THE INHERITED BASIS OF COMMON DISEASES

DAVID ALTSHULER

A central question in medicine is to understand why some people get sick and others do not. We seek these answers for multiple reasons: to provide explanations to our patients, to improve our ability to predict disease risk, and most importantly, to understand pathophysiology as a foundation for designing rational approaches to prevention and therapy. In some cases, a single environmental exposure is found to play a major role in disease (e.g., smoking and lung cancer, or human immunodeficiency virus infection [HIV] and acquired immunodeficiency syndrome [AIDS]). In others, such as Huntington's disease or cystic fibrosis, mutation of a single gene is necessary and can be sufficient to cause illness. Such singular answers are the exception; in most cases, disease is attributable neither to a single environmental factor nor to mutation of a single gene. Rather, most cases of disease result from the combined action of inborn and somatically acquired alterations in gene sequence, environmental and behavioral exposures, and bad luck. Such disorders, which make up most of the morbidity and mortality in the population, are termed *complex traits*.

Human genetics is a unique tool for generating new hypotheses about the root causes of disease, based on genome-wide searches in the human population that are unlimited by prior assumptions about underlying pathophysiologic processes. Because the sequence of the human genome and much of its common variation is now known, and given emerging tools and methods to directly determine genome sequences of individuals, we are entering an era in which medicine can be informed by knowledge of the specific genes and variants that contribute to risk for common human diseases.

HERITABILITY: INHERITED VARIATION IN DISEASE RISK

Susceptibility to disease varies within and across human populations. Studies of *familial aggregation* can determine the extent to which inheritance contributes to these patterns. These studies are simple in concept and ask whether members of the same family display more similar rates of disease than do individuals chosen at random from the population. Of course, familial clustering can reflect not only shared genes but also shared environment. The contribution of shared genotype can be dissected further by comparing rates of disease within families as a function of the extent of genetic relatedness. The cleanest such design involves the comparison of disease concordance among dizygotic and monozygotic twin pairs. For common diseases such as types 1 and 2 diabetes mellitus, obesity, hypertension, coronary artery disease, autoimmune diseases, common cancers, schizophrenia, and bipolar disease, twin studies have documented that rates of concordance are significantly higher in monozygotic than in dizygotic twin pairs. For many other traits of clinical interest (e.g., most drug responses), formal tests of heritability have not yet been performed, and the role of inheritance in these characteristics is less well documented.

Data about familial aggregation allow the calculation of *heritability,* or the fraction of interindividual variability in disease risk attributable to additive genetic influences. The remaining variability among individuals is due to all other contributions: environmental influences on disease, nonadditive (*epistatic*) genetic effects (e.g., gene-gene interactions or gene-environment interactions), error in the measurement of relatedness or disease, and random chance. For most clinically important traits (diseases and risk factors), empirical estimates of heritability range from 20 to 80% (see Online Mendelian Inheritance in Man, available at *www.ncbi.nlm.nih.gov:80/entrez/query.fcgi?db=OMIM,* for comprehensive information).

When interpreting estimates of heritability, it is important to consider two crucial factors: the effect of measurement errors and the environmental context. *Measurement errors* can decrease the estimate of the heritability of a trait. A single measurement of blood pressure is much less heritable than a composite score based on serial measures of blood pressure over time. That is, day-to-day variability and imprecision in clinical measures can obscure an underlying biologic susceptibility that is entrained by inheritance. For the patient and physician, this means that although the blood pressure on a given day may not be particularly heritable, the blood pressure over time (which is presumably the relevant risk factor for vascular disease) is heritable to a much greater extent.

Second, estimates of heritability must be interpreted in the context of the environment in which the study was performed. In the case in which environmental triggers of disease are relatively constant across a study population, inherited factors may explain much of the variation in rates of disease. In contrast, in the case in which exposure to environmental causes of disease is highly varied across the study population, nongenetic factors may outweigh the contribution of inborn susceptibility. For example, the rate and diversity of smoking behavior will have a major impact on how much of the variability in rates of lung cancer (in any given study or patient cohort) may be explained by inheritance. If nobody smoked (or everyone smoked), little of the variation in lung cancer risk would be due to smoking behavior; if, in contrast, half the population smoked multiple packs a day, and the other half not at all, this behavior would no doubt dominate over inborn susceptibility.

For these reasons, heritability is not a fixed characteristic of a given disease, but an assessment of a given population, set of measurements, and the extent to which variability in genetic and environmental exposure explains disease risk. This sheds light on what is sometimes thought to be a contradiction between rates of disease being highly heritable (in a given population) and yet varying dramatically across populations separated by time, geography, or socioeconomic status. In broad comparisons across groups, environmental exposure and methods of clinical ascertainment can vary substantially and contribute to secular changes in patterns of disease. Conversely, within a group exposed to a relatively uniform environment and studied in a standardized manner, genetic susceptibility may play a major role in determining individual risk.

HETEROZYGOSITY: INHERITED VARIATION IN GENOME SEQUENCE

Heritability expresses the patterns of inherited variation in rates of disease; *heterozygosity* expresses the rate of inherited variation in genome sequences (Table 41-1). Heterozygosity is defined as the proportion of sites on the chromosome at which two randomly chosen copies differ in DNA sequence. Because cells are *diploid* (carry two copies of the genome sequence) and because these two copies were selected in a semirandom manner from the population, heterozygosity is equivalent to the fraction of base pairs that vary between the two copies each of us inherited from our mother and our father. That is, heterozygosity is the rate of genetic variation in the individual.

Single-nucleotide polymorphisms (SNPs) are sites at which a single letter in the DNA code has been swapped for a single alternate letter. Such variants are observed at approximately 1 in 1000 positions in the human genome sequence. In the protein coding regions of genes, rates of genetic variation are lower—less than 1 in every 2000 bases; the rate of variation that substantially alters the sequence of the encoded protein is lower still (see Table 41-1). These rates can be understood in light of darwinian selection against changes that alter the amino acid sequence of encoded proteins.

Genomes also contain larger scale variation: insertions and deletions of nucleotides, alteration in the number of copies of particular genes and sequences, and larger-scale alterations such as inversions and translocations. Both SNPs and larger-scale alterations can influence gene function and contribute to disease.

TABLE 41-1 CHARACTERISTICS OF HUMAN GENOME SEQUENCE VARIATION

Length of the human genome sequence (base pairs)	3,000,000,000
Number of human genes (estimated)	20,000
Fraction of base pairs that differ between the genome sequence of a human and a chimpanzee	1.3% (1 in 80)
Fraction of base pairs that vary between the genome sequence of any two humans	0.1% (1 in 1000)
Fraction of coding region base pairs that vary in a manner that substantially alters the sequence of the encoded protein	0.2% (1 in 5000)
Number of sequence variants present in each individual as heterozygous sites	3,000,000
Number of amino acid–altering variants present in each individual as heterozygous sites	12,000
Number of sequence variants in any given human population with frequency of >1%	10,000,000
Number of amino acid polymorphisms present in the human genome with a population frequency of >1%	75,000
Fraction of all human heterozygosity attributable to variants with a frequency of >1%	98%

The genetic variation in each of us is due largely to common variants. Empirically, more than 98% of the heterozygous sites in each individual display frequency of greater than 1% in the worldwide human population. Because most human heterozygosity is due to common variants, a database containing all common (>1% frequency) sequence variants in the human population can be constructed by sequencing the genomes of only hundreds of individuals, and yet would capture most of the genetic variation in any individual.

Built on the foundation of the human genome project, a catalogue of common DNA variants has been created by a series of public-private projects, including the SNP Consortium, International HapMap, and 1000 Genomes Projects. At the time of this writing, the public database contains more than 17 million human genetic variants (*www.ncbi.nlm.nih.gov:80/SNP/index.html*). Not all these entries represent common variants (some are rare), and some may represent technical false-positive findings. Nonetheless, the existing collection represents most of the common variants in each individual and has fueled efforts to systematically measure genetic variants for their contribution to disease.

The major role of common variation in human sequence diversity is explained by the unique demographic history of the human population. Despite the global distribution of the current human population, it is now clear that all people on the planet are the descendants of a single population that lived in Africa only 10,000 to 40,000 years ago. The ancestral population was small (with an effective size of perhaps 10,000 individuals), lived a hunter-gatherer existence at low population densities (relative to other humans and later domesticated animals), and had evolved in Africa over millions of years. Most human genetic variation arose in this phase of human history, before the more recent migrations, expansions, and invention of technologies (e.g., farming) that resulted in widespread population of the globe. Most common human genetic variation predates the Diaspora and is shared by all populations on earth.

A second factor is the slow rate of change in human DNA. Mutation and recombination occur at very low rates: on the order of 10^{-8} per base pair per generation. And yet, any pair of human genes traces a lineage back to a shared ancestor who lived on the order of 10^3 to 10^4 generations ago (if a generation is 20 years, then 10^4 generations is 200,000 years). In other words, considering the typical nucleotide in two unrelated humans, it is more likely that they trace back to a shared ancestor without any mutation having occurred than it is that a mutation has arisen in the intervening time. This explains why 99.9% of base pairs are identical when any two copies of the human genome are compared.

Another aspect of human variation is explained by these simple mathematical and population genetic relationships: the extent of human DNA sequence diversity attributable to rare and common variants. Each of us inherits from our parents some 3 million common polymorphisms (classically defined as those with frequency of >1%). We inherit common variants that are shared by apparently unrelated individuals but do not reach a frequency of 1% or

higher. Finally, we inherit thousands of variants that are unique to each individual and their closest relatives. The question of how these different classes of variants influence disease is of central interest and importance to medical genetics.

The shared ancestry of human populations explains another aspect of human genetic variation: the correlations among nearby variants known as *linkage disequilibrium*, or *haplotypes*. Empirically, individuals who carry a particular variant at one site in the genome are observed to be more likely than chance to carry a particular set of variants at nearby positions along the chromosome. That is, not all combinations of nearby variants are observed in the population, but rather only a small subset of the possible combinations. These correlations reflect the fact discussed earlier that most variants in our genomes arose once in human history (typically long ago) and did so on an arbitrary but unique copy carried by some individual in the population. The ancestral copy of the genome on which the mutation occurred can be recognized in the current population as a stretch of particular alleles (known as a *haplotype*) that track together in the population. That is, although most variations in our genome arose before written human history, the DNA sequence in each of us carries a record of the evolution and demographic history of the human population.

These ancestral haplotypes, passed down from shared prehistoric ancestors in Africa, can be recognized in the current human population. The haplotype structure of the human genome offers a practical tool in association studies of human disease because it is not necessary to measure directly each nucleotide in order to capture much of the information. Such haplotype-based methods are the foundation for genome-wide association studies, discussed later.

THE SEARCH FOR GENES UNDERLYING MONOGENIC DISEASES

The *genetic architecture* of a disease refers to the number and magnitude of genetic risk factors that exist in each patient and in the population and their frequencies and interactions. Diseases can be due to a single gene (*monogenic*) in each family or to multiple genes (*polygenic*). It is easiest to identify genetic risk factors when only a single gene is involved and this gene has a large impact on disease in that family. In cases in which a single gene is necessary and sufficient to cause disease, the condition is termed a *mendelian* disorder because the disease tracks perfectly with a mutation (in the family) that obeys Mendel's simple laws of inheritance.

Some single-gene disorders are caused by the same gene in all affected families; for example, cystic fibrosis is always caused by mutations in *CFTR*. Although many individuals with cystic fibrosis carry the same founder mutation (δ-508), others carry any pair of a wide variety of different mutations in *CFTR*. The existence of many different mutations at a given disease gene is known as *allelic heterogeneity*.

A mendelian disorder can be due to a single genetic lesion in any given family, but in different families can be due to mutations in a variety of genes. This phenomenon, termed *locus heterogeneity*, is illustrated by retinitis pigmentosa. Although mutation in a single gene is typically necessary and sufficient to cause retinitis pigmentosa, there are dozens of different genes in which retinitis pigmentosa mutations have been found (Online Mendelian Inheritance in Man #268000). In each family, however, only one such gene is mutated to cause disease.

Most single-gene disorders are rare (present in <1% of the population) and are manifested early in life. Many are severe and cause death before reproduction in the absence of modern medical care. The fact that most monogenic disorders are severe in childhood and rare in the population is probably not a coincidence, but reflects the impact of *natural selection*. The deleterious effect of these mutations results in a decrease in reproductive fitness (in individuals unlucky enough to inherit them), and the mutations and the disease are therefore unlikely to drift to high frequency in the population.

There are exceptions to this general idea: cases in which the mutation causing a severe monogenic disease (such as *HbS*, the cause of sickle cell anemia) is common in the population at large. Such cases appear to be the result of a different kind of selection, known as *balancing selection*—situations in which a gene mutation is beneficial in one circumstance (a genotype or environment) but deleterious in another. Heterozygous carriers for *HbS* are relatively protected against malaria, and this benefit balances the deleterious effect of sickle cell disease in homozygotes.

Starting in the 1980s, the advent of genome-wide linkage analysis led to rapid success at identifying the specific genetic mutations that cause mendelian disorders, with hundreds of genes identified for clinically important conditions (for comprehensive information, see *www.ncbi.nlm.nih.gov:80/entrez/query.fcgi?db=OMIM*). Progress was sparked by the development of a suite of powerful research techniques—*family-based linkage analysis* followed by *positional cloning*—in which a genome-wide search is undertaken for the causal gene, which is first localized to a chromosomal region. (The initial idea of genetic linkage mapping traces to Sturtevant in fruit flies in 1913 but did not become practical in humans until the 1980s.)

Once the search has been focused by the discovery of linkage between a chromosomal region and a disease, that chromosomal neighborhood is scoured for the genetic culprit, which is recognized based on the observation of mutations that alter the protein coding sequence, and are enriched in cases of disease compared with unaffected relatives and population-based controls. The power of these approaches prompted and was fuelled by the Human Genome Project, which provided the foundation of information on DNA structure, sequence, and genetic variation required to undertake such searches.

GENETIC INVESTIGATION OF COMMON DISEASES

Similar to mendelian disorders, most common diseases are influenced by inheritance. In contrast to mendelian disorders, however, the genetic contribution to common diseases appears to be due to the action of many genes rather than a single gene in each family. Empirical evidence in favor of this model comes from efforts to use the same approach (positional cloning) for complex traits that was applied successfully to monogenic disorders.

In the 1990s, the tools of family-based linkage analysis were applied to nearly all common disorders. Much of this work was done in isolated founder populations (such as Finland and Iceland) with the goal of simplifying the genetic architecture and accessing extended pedigrees. Excepting a few notable successes, however, these studies revealed few strong signals that localized the genes responsible for disease. In most of the hundreds of such studies that have been published, there are many weak statistical signals (few if any are statistically significant given the large number of hypotheses tested) and little agreement between different studies of the same disease.

In view of the well-understood statistical power of family-based linkage methods (based on their extensive use for monogenic disorders) and their relatively limited success despite extensive efforts in common diseases, it was concluded by most investigators that rare variants in single genes do not explain a large fraction of the risk for common diseases. If a single gene contained rare mutations of large effect that explained 20% or more of the inherited risk for type 2 diabetes, hypertension, or schizophrenia, it is likely that its location would long since have been found based on linkage analysis.

A next potential shortcut to understanding the genetic determinants of common diseases is to identify and study rare, early-onset forms of diseases that clearly demonstrate mendelian patterns of inheritance. Because these families display patterns of inheritance consistent with a major gene of large effect, the powerful tools of positional cloning can be and have been used successfully to identify the genes responsible. Important examples include the role of *BRCA1* and *BRCA2* in early-onset breast cancer, maturity-onset diabetes of the young as a form of type 2 diabetes, many monogenic disorders of blood pressure and electrolyte regulation, early-onset Alzheimer's disease, and many others.

These successes provide diagnostic information for families burdened with severe, early-onset forms of disease and insight into the underlying pathways responsible for disease. For example, more than 20 genes have been identified that, when mutated, cause rare mendelian disorders of blood pressure and electrolyte regulation. So far, every one of these genes is active in the kidney, and most are involved in the renin-angiotensin-aldosterone pathway. This result is a compelling demonstration of the central importance of the kidney in human blood pressure regulation and has suggested new therapeutic targets of substantial promise.

It was hoped that the genes found to be responsible for early-onset, monogenic forms of common diseases would contribute to the more common forms of disease in the population. In this scenario, severe mutations might cause early-onset forms, and more prevalent but subtle alterations in the same genes might contribute to common forms of disease. A comprehensive test of this hypothesis awaited tools from the human genome project and improved methods of genetic epidemiologic analysis.

ASSOCIATION STUDIES: FROM CANDIDATE GENES TO GENOME-WIDE ASSOCIATION STUDIES

Genome-wide association studies (GWAS) are simple in concept. A genetic variant is identified, its frequency is measured in individuals with the disease of interest, and it is compared with well-matched controls (drawn from the population at large or unaffected family members). This process can be repeated for as many genetic variants as exist—up to and including a genome-wide collection. Appropriate analyses need be performed to rule out alternative explanations for an association to disease, such as mismatching of cases and controls, or technical artifacts. Because the null distribution is well described (under the hypothesis of no association between genotype and phenotype), it is possible to calibrate such analyses and to identify reproducible associations from out of the large sea of benign polymorphisms.

Genetic association studies were pioneered in the context of the *HLA* locus on chromosome 6. The *HLA* was discovered based on its role in transplantation tolerance and is characterized by diverse allelic variation that can be measured based on interactions of antibodies and antigens. By measuring these protein-based (immunologic) readouts of the underlying genetic variation, *HLA* alleles were found to be a major determinant of susceptibility to infectious and autoimmune diseases. Starting in the 1960s, empirical data on human population genetics and genetic association studies were developed in the context of the *HLA*.

By the 1980s, tools of molecular biology made it possible to directly measure DNA variation (rather than using protein or phenotype measurements as surrogates for the underlying genetic variation), ushering in the modern era of human genetic research. In this pregenomic era, it was only practical to measure one or a small number of genetic variations in each study, limiting association studies to incomplete assessments of individual "candidate" genes selected based on biologic criteria.

The study of candidate genes led to a modest number of robust and reproducible associations, such as the contribution of Apo-ε4 to Alzheimer's disease; factor V Leiden to deep venous thrombosis; a 32-base deletion in the chemokine receptor CCR5 to HIV infection; common variants in the insulin gene to type 1 diabetes; SNPs in the peroxisome proliferator-activated receptor γ (PPAR-γ) and the β-cell potassium channel Kir6.2 to the risk for type 2 diabetes.

By early in the 2000s, comprehensive surveys of published genetic association studies showed that valid associations were few and far between, with many initial claims of association proving irreproducible, likely representing false-positive claims. One such analysis estimated that, in the pre-GWAS era, only 10 to 20 bona fide associations had been documented of common genetic variants with common diseases.

A major reason for the state of this literature was the intrinsically low likelihood of finding a gene and variant contributing to any given disease. Each genome contains millions of genetic variants, and presumably only a small fraction of these influence disease. This is often described as a problem of "multiple hypothesis testing," with the investigative community searching for associations between multiple genes, multiple variants in each gene, and multiple diseases. An alternative (bayesian) statistical framework frames this issue based on low prior probabilities of association. Regardless, it is conceptually clear that much more stringent statistical thresholds (than the traditional $P < .05$) are required for declaring association of genetic variants and disease.

As in linkage analysis for mendelian traits, a key to success in association studies was the advent of genome-wide search, unbiased by prior hypotheses about biologic mechanisms. With the sequencing of the human genome, development of large-scale SNP databases, and tools for genotyping up to 1M SNPs per individual, by 2005 it became practical to perform GWAS to identify genomic loci harboring allelic variation. With a recognition that any given variant had a very low likelihood of truly being associated with disease, much more stringent statistical thresholds were deployed (typically requiring a P value of 10^{-7} or lower to declare "genome-wide significance").

Age-related macular degeneration (AMD) provided an early success of GWAS. AMD is a typical common, polygenic disease (Chapter 431); siblings of affected patients are perhaps three to six times as likely as unrelated individuals to become afflicted, and yet family-based linkage analysis revealed only modestly significant (and modestly reproducible) linkage results. The pathophysiologic defects that underlie AMD were largely unknown until it was found that a common coding polymorphism in the gene for complement factor H is a major risk factor for AMD. The variant (*Y402H*) has a high population frequency (approximately 35% in European populations) and increases risk by 2.5- to 3-fold in heterozygotes and by 5- to 7-fold in homozygotes. Multiple other complement factors have since been found to harbor common genetic variation that influences the risk for AMD in a highly reproducible manner, providing unambiguous information about the primary role of complement in this common disease.

Since 2005, GWAS has been used to identify literally hundreds of novel genetic variants that show reproducible associations to a large variety of common human diseases. The field evolved a set of criteria and standards that largely eliminated the previous difficulties with irreproducible claims of association, making association studies a reliable method to identify genomic loci related to human diseases. The National Human Genome Research Institute of the National Institutes of Health maintains a catalogue of GWAS findings (www.genome.gov/26525384) that, at the time of this writing, included 904 such associations for 165 traits. This represents rapid progress compared with the two dozen or so such findings known at the start of the decade.

The results of GWAS support a number of conclusions about the role of common genetic variants in common disease. First, most diseases investigated by GWAS have yielded novel findings, suggesting that the approach has general utility. Second, only a small fraction of these findings were previously known, indicating that new clues can be obtained by genetic mapping of common diseases. Third, most of the associations demonstrate extremely modest odds ratios (on the order of 1.1-fold to 1.5-fold), indicating that natural selection has purged alleles of large effect from the pool of common variants. Fourth, most of the associated SNPs lie in noncoding regions, suggesting that they act through effects on gene regulation rather than directly altering protein-coding sequences. Fifth, only a modest fraction of the estimated heritability of each disease has yet been explained, indicating a role for other common variants of more modest effect, rare variants, genetic interactions, or other (as yet unanticipated) influences.

Because GWAS are genome-wide (not limited to "candidate" genes), they provide a test of the hypothesis that prior investigations had identified sets of genes relevant to each disease (relevant, that is, through the lens of genetic variation and inheritance). In the case of autoimmune diseases, many (perhaps half) of the 100 or more findings from GWAS lie near a gene previously known to play a role in the immune system. Similarly, a substantial fraction of the genetic variants found to influence lipid levels lie near genes that were previously known to play a role in lipid biology (because they were known already either through rare mutations that contribute to mendelian forms of hyperlipidemia or through biologic investigations). These findings confirm that the basic pathophysiologic mechanisms already known can be "validated" through the lens of inherited risk factors and encourage investigation of the new findings offered by GWAS.

In contrast, for some diseases, most of the genetic variants found are novel and do not lie near genes previously studied. One such case is type 2 diabetes, for which 35 independent genomic loci have been found to influence risk for disease, and yet only a handful were previously implicated by other methods. This may indicate and illuminate gaps in our previous knowledge of the pathophysiology of type 2 diabetes.

Although tantalizing, the results of GWAS have raised many more questions than they have answered. These discoveries implicate particular genomic regions, but to date in only a few cases have the causal genes been proved. This is challenging in large part because so many of these common variants are noncoding, and it remains difficult to connect noncoding variation to the genes thereby regulated. To the extent that truly novel genes are identified, much work is needed to discover their biologic and physiologic functions. Finally, GWAS findings explain only a modest fraction of the estimated heritability of most diseases, leaving open the question of which genes, and which types of variants and genetic effects, explain the remainder.

FROM COMMON VARIANTS TO INDIVIDUAL GENOMES

Although much of human genetic variation is due to common DNA variants (such as those tested through GWAS), each of us also inherits many thousands of variants that arose more recently and that tend to be lower in frequency and more population specific. To the extent that such variants have very large effects on phenotype, they may have been previously identified based on family-based linkage studies of mendelian disorders. However, there almost certainly exists a large universe of lower-frequency variations that are too rare to have been captured by the first generation of GWAS and that have effects too modest to have been recognized and identified in family-based linkage analyses.

The study of such lower-frequency and rare variants is now becoming practical owing to advances in technology for DNA sequencing. With dramatic drops in price and increases in throughput, it is increasingly practical to sequence individual genomes in the context of medical research (and, in the future, clinical practice). Such an approach will provide a much more complete assessment of genetic variation than was previously obtainable and will incorporate common as well as rare variants.

The first task will be to develop methods to interpret the millions of variants in each genome. Variants of high frequency have already been well studied by GWAS, and each is increasingly annotated with information about disease association. For variants that are lower in frequency, but still observed in a substantial number of unrelated individuals, the basic association methodology can be applied. That is, the frequencies of each specific variant can be measured in affected cases and in unaffected controls and compared with an appropriately constructed null distribution and statistical threshold. Moreover, the availability of a much more complete database of DNA variation (as is being created by the 1000 Genomes Project) will lead to a second generation of GWAS that is more complete for lower-frequency variation.

Many DNA variants will be unique to individuals (and their close relatives), however, and will require different approaches. If the analysis includes a large pedigree, with multiple affected and unaffected relatives, it may be possible to perform the association analysis in single families. More typically, however, it will be necessary to analyze large sets of samples, measure the rate of different (individually rare) variants in each gene, and compare these rates between cases and controls.

In the distant future, we may learn to "read" genome sequences and predict the effect of a variant never before observed. For the foreseeable future, however, interpretation will require statistical analysis of genomes, documenting that variation in particular genes is robustly and reproducibly associated with each particular disease.

IMPLICATIONS AND FUTURE DIRECTIONS

Inherited factors contribute substantially to common as well as rare diseases. Mendelian disorders are typically caused by rare mutations in the protein-coding regions of genes. Common variants, investigated through GWAS, have typically modest effects and often act through noncoding effects on gene regulation. Each of us carries a deep reservoir of less common variation that will soon be tested for a role in disease using methods of next-generation DNA sequencing. It seems reasonable to expect that an integrative analysis of this information will result in a defined list of genes and variants in those genes (both common and rare) that contribute to each human disease.

Success identifying genes and mutations will only prove of value if it leads to improved prediction, diagnosis, understanding, and treatment. Prediction and personalized medicine require a foundation of evidence that demonstrates clinical benefit. This will involve incorporating DNA variation in epidemiologically valid cohorts and testing particular approaches to genetic prediction in clinical trials. The fact that some genetic tests may prove predictive in no way means that routine genome sequencing will be useful to patients, and much work will be needed to offer the public and physicians guidance in interpreting such data.

Biologic understanding requires bedside-to-bench research, in which genes found as mutated in patients are studied in the laboratory. It will be necessary to place these new genes into known (and as yet unrecognized) biologic pathways and to understand how dysfunction and dysregulation lead to disease. In some cases, such as the role of complement in AMD (see earlier), initial answers may come quickly; in others, in which the relevant pathobiology is as yet unknown, the information to be gleaned from following these clues is unpredictable. Presumably, in the fullness of time, the genetic insights gleaned from patients will lead to a new generation of therapies that more directly target the underlying root causes of risk in the population. What is most certain is that genetic and genomic information is accumulating at a staggering rate and holds both much potential and much challenge for the future of medicine.

SUGGESTED READINGS

Altshuler D, Daly MJ, Lander ES. Genetic mapping in human disease. *Science.* 2008;322:881-888. *A review of genetic mapping of human disease.*

Lifton RP. Individual genomes on the horizon. *N Engl J Med.* 2010;362:1235-1236. *A commentary previewing the use of individualized genome sequences in clinical medicine.*

Manolio TA. Genomewide association studies and assessment of the risk of disease. *N Engl J Med.* 2010;363:166-176. *Review.*

Fark YJ, Claus R, Weichenhan D, et al. Genome-wide epigenetic modifications in cancer. *Prog Drug Res.* 2011;67:25-49. *Review.*

42

APPLICATION OF MOLECULAR TECHNOLOGIES TO CLINICAL MEDICINE

GEOFFREY S. GINSBURG

MOLECULAR TECHNOLOGIES ALONG THE CONTINUUM FROM HEALTH TO DISEASE

Along the continuum from health to disease (as shown in Fig. 42-1), there are now several important points in clinical decision making for which molecular technologies are being applied to health care (Table 42-1). Using DNA-based approaches, risk estimates for developing some diseases can now be quantified during health and possibly even at birth. Molecular signatures from technology platforms that measure the expressed genome (RNA, proteins, metabolites) now allow interventions at the level of the individual by defining physiologic states in response to our environment that predict future clinical outcomes. These methods can also provide more precise ways to screen for and to detect disease at its earliest molecular manifestations. Similarly, they are the basis for a new molecular classification of disease and diagnosis that foretells prognosis. The selection of certain drugs now may be guided by a patient's underlying genetic makeup as well as the molecular makeup of the disease. Given that a disease's evolution from baseline risk often occurs over many years, molecular profiling over time defines a novel form of health care that focuses on disease prevention and proactive management rather that the current paradigm of acute intervention and crisis management.

GENES, GENOMES, DISEASE, AND TREATMENT

A key question in medicine is to what extent genetic variation influences the likelihood of disease onset, affects the natural history of disease in combination with the environment, or provides clues relevant to the management of disease. And it is not just the human genome that is relevant to an individual's state of health—the genomes of thousands of microorganisms are relevant to human phenotypes, and insights from their genomes are providing new approaches for the diagnosis, study, and treatment of disease (see Microbiome).

Variation in the Human Genome

It is now estimated that any two randomly selected individuals have sequences that are 99.5% identical, or that an individual genome would be heterozygous

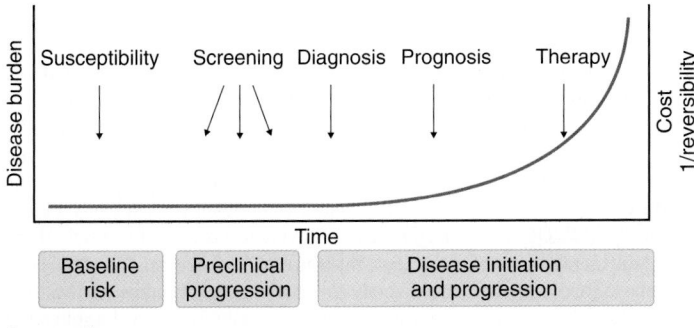

FIGURE 42-1. Use of molecular technologies across the continuum from health to disease. Various molecular technologies may be used to complement the traditional approach to evaluating at the time points indicated. SNP = single nucleotide polymorphism. (Adapted from Snyderman R. The role of genomics in enabling prospective health care. In: Willard H, Ginsburg G, eds. *Genomic and Personalized Medicine.* Burlington, Mass: Elsevier; 2009:378-385.)

at approximately 15 to 25 million positions. Most of the differences involve a single base in the DNA code, referred to as single nucleotide polymorphisms (SNPs). The remaining variation consists of insertions or deletions of short sequence stretches, and copy-number variation (CNV) in the number of repeated elements at a particular locus in the genome. These types of variation can influence disease, and this must be accounted for in any attempt to understand the contribution of genetics to human health.

Genome-wide Association Studies

The "common allele, common disease" hypothesis has been explored with notable success in a number of conditions, using large cohorts of well-phenotyped patients and high-throughput methods to genotype up to 1 million variants in the genome. Genome-wide association studies (GWAS) report the statistical association of one or more variants in a narrow genomic region with the presence or absence of the clinical condition. The reported SNPs define risk factors for that condition, at least in the populations under study, and can provide novel insights into the biology of the disease. As of December 2010, more than 3500 SNPs have been reported to be associated with more than 50 phenotypes in published studies (www.genome.gov/gwastudies/). It should be stressed that in most instances, *causality* of the reported SNP and the increased risk has not been proved; it may be that the actual causal variant is not the SNP itself but is a currently undetected variant that lies in linkage disequilibrium with the SNP. In most instances, the functional impact of the associated SNP is obscure, and it will require integrated genomic and functional studies to elucidate the precise basis for the roles of genome variation in disease.

Medical Resequencing

Resequencing specific genes in a cohort of affected individuals with disease is an alternative or complementary approach to GWAS to uncover rare variants responsible for the disease in question. It may indeed be that these more rare variants are responsible for most genetic risk, but there are insufficient data to draw conclusions. Most efforts have focused on one or several genes that are believed to be strong candidates for the phenotype under study. Using this approach, rare variants in relevant candidate genes have been detected at a statistically significant higher frequency in the genomes of patients with common clinical conditions. These early successes suggest a strategy of resequencing relevant genes in individuals at the extremes of the population distribution for measurable traits.

Somatic Mutations

It has been of interest to use medical resequencing to search for somatic mutations in tumor tissue in order to identify genes potentially relevant to cancer progression. The Cancer Genome Atlas (http://cancergenome.nih.gov/index.asp), started in 2006, has begun to explore systematically the entire spectrum of genomic changes in human cancers and has already published its first results for glioblastoma. The genes implicated in these studies tend to be different from those identified as inherited risk factors in previous genetic studies and provide novel insights into the biology of human cancer and suggest candidates for exploring mechanisms of tumorigenesis or metastasis or for developing therapeutic approaches.

Copy-Number Variation

There has been an unanticipated prevalence of structural variants in the genome that collectively account for more variation in genome sequence than do SNPs. The most common types of structural variations are CNVs. A dedicated effort is under way to catalogue CNVs in the human genome and to associate these with clinical phenotypes. Although most CNVs are inherited, some occur de novo or even in somatic cells; in these cases, an individual will have different repeat lengths from either of his or her parents. CNVs can contribute to human diseases in at least two ways:

1. *Pathogenic* CNVs are certain genomic imbalances that appear to cause neurodevelopmental diseases directly. Pathogenic CNVs are usually de novo in nature and have associated specific genomic imbalances with as many as 50 genetic syndromes (*www.sanger.ac.uk/PostGenomics/decipher/*).
2. *Benign* CNVs have been identified in healthy individuals and may have more subtle consequences on human health.

Epigenetics and the Epigenome

Epigenetic changes, in DNA methylation or in histone modification over time, in the genome may result in aberrant gene expression and human

TABLE 42-1 APPLICATION OF MOLECULAR DIAGNOSTICS ALONG THE CONTINUUM FROM HEALTH TO DISEASE: EXAMPLES

TIME POINT IN CLINICAL DECISION MAKING	Cancer		Cardiovascular Disease	
	Test	*Indication*	*Test*	*Indication*
Risk/susceptibility	*BRCA1, BRCA2* *HNPCC* *TP53, PTEN*	Breast Colon Sarcomas	*KIF6, 9p21* Familion 5-gene profile	CAD LQTS
Screening	HPV genotypes	Cervical	Corus CAD	CAD
Diagnosis	Pathwork Tissue of Origin	Cancer of unknown primary	Corus CAD	CAD
Prognosis	Oncotype DX (21-gene assay) MammaPrint (70-gene assay) HER2/neu, ER, PR	Breast	TnI, BNP, CRP	ACS
Pharmacogenomics	HER2/neu *UGT1A1* *KRAS* *EGFR* AmpliChip; DMET *CYP2D6/* *CYP2C19*	Herceptin Irinotecan Cetuximab Erlotinib, gefitinib Various (see Table 42-2)	*KIF6, SLCO1B1* AmpliChip; DMET *CYP2D6/CYP2C19* *VKORC1*	Statins Various (see Table 42-2) Warfarin
Monitoring	CTCs	Tumor recurrence or progression	AlloMap gene profile	Transplant rejection

ACS = acute coronary syndromes; BNP = brain natriuretic peptide; CAD = coronary artery disease; CRP = C-reactive protein; CTCs = circulating tumor cells; ER = estrogen receptor; HPV = human papillomavirus; LQTS = long QT syndrome; PR = progesterone receptor; TnI = troponin I.

disease in response to environmental influences. It has become clear during the past two decades that epigenetic changes (methylation) play a crucial role in carcinogenesis. Similar research is emerging on DNA methylation in other diseases, especially autoimmune and cardiovascular disorders. For example, aberrantly hypomethylated DNA in circulation in systemic lupus erythematosus (SLE) (Chapter 274) might induce an immune response because of its similarity to unmethylated microbial DNAs. Further contributions of defective methylation to SLE pathogenesis could be due to the transcription of endogenous retroviruses or the increase in the expression of certain genes related to autoreactivity. In cardiovascular disease, global DNA hypomethylation and coexisting hyperhomocystinemia have been observed. Taken together, these data reinforce the notion that methylation profiles can be highly valuable to study the pathogenesis of a variety of conditions. The National Institutes of Health have initiated the Human Epigenome Project, whose goal is to indentify, catalogue, and interpret widespread DNA methylation patterns of all human genes in all major tissues; this effort has now been expanded internationally.

Microbiome
The genome sequences of thousands of microorganisms have been determined and are being used to provide rapid diagnostic tests in clinical settings; to predict antibiotic or antifungal efficacy; to identify the source of airborne, water, or soil contaminants; to monitor hospital or community environments; and to understand better the contribution of microbial ecosystems and various environmental exposures to diverse human phenotypes. For example, the human colon contains more than 400 bacterial species comprising some 10^{13} to 10^{14} microorganisms. The gastrointestinal tract (as well as other body cavities and the skin) provides a unique environment for microorganisms, the microbiome, whose impact on human health and disease is just being explored. The genomes of the microbiota are significantly different from the human genome and have the capacity to alter the metabolic profile of different individuals or different populations, with clinically meaningful effects on drug metabolism, toxicity, and efficacy. The applications to microbiomes of approaches in genomics are revolutionizing clinical diagnostics, for example, to identify unknown viral infections or to diagnose antibiotic resistance in infections such as methicillin-resistant *Staphylococcus aureus* (MRSA). A number of diseases have been associated with large-scale imbalances in the gut microbiome, including inflammatory bowel disease, antibiotic-resistant diarrhea, and obesity.

Personal Genomics
The delivery of information from individual genomes is a fast-moving area of technology development that is spawning a social and information revolution

among consumers. Dramatic improvements in sequencing technology have reduced the cost and time of resequencing projects to approach the long awaited personal "$1000 genome." What remains unsettled for now is what degree of genome surveillance will be most useful, either for research or for clinical practice. The push for incorporation of genome information into clinical practice may come as much or more from consumers as from professionals. Several companies offer genome-wide SNP profiles to the public, some with associated risk estimates for relevant clinical conditions. There is a clear and important research agenda that needs to be developed in concert with these technologic breakthroughs that allows health providers and the public to understand the information and, more importantly, to believe that it is accurate, informative, and actionable. With the vast amount of information contained in the human genome sequence, it will be critically important that the proper reading, interpretation, and communication of the information are carried out. This may be a "disruptive technology" in health care delivery, providing health and disease risk information to consumers without physician intervention and guidance. Patients are already bringing reports from these analyses to their health providers and requesting guidance. What are providers, armed with a paucity of genomic training, telling them?

Pharmacogenetics
DNA variation that is associated with response to drugs is referred to as *pharmacogenetics*, and there are now numerous examples of molecularly guided therapies that use DNA assays (E-Table 42-1). To assist clinicians in the practice of pharmacogenetics across a broad number of medications, the first microarray-based gene chip, approved both in the United States and European Union, was released in 2003 as the AmpliChip CYP450. The product was designed to identify key genetic polymorphisms in two CYP450 enzymes, *CYP2D6* and *CYP2C19*, cumulatively responsible for much of the first-pass metabolism of many currently prescribed drugs. The regulatory agencies cleared this test based solely on analytic performance and validity information, but indicated that its utility specifically for clinical application needed to be proved. Thus, clinicians remain unclear about the impact of these tests on clinical decision-making guidelines.

Perhaps the best example of a pharmacogenetic association for which the clinical relevance is clear features management of treatment with warfarin. The oral anticoagulant warfarin (Chapter 37) is prescribed for the long-term treatment and prevention of thromboembolic events, with more than 31 million prescriptions annually in the United States alone. However, because of the drug's narrow therapeutic index, a variety of complications are associated with its treatment, even after dose adjustment according to age, gender, weight, disease state, diet, and concomitant medications. Investigation of pharmacokinetic and pharmacodynamic drug properties indicated the additive involvement of two genes in determination of warfarin maintenance dose. One of these genes encodes CYP2C9, which is responsible for most of the metabolic clearance (~80%) of the more pharmacologically potent S-enantiomer of warfarin. Both *CYP2C9*2* and **3* cause a reduction in S-warfarin clearance, with ten-fold variation seen from the genotype linked with the highest (*CYP2C9*1/*1*) to lowest (*CYP2C9*3/*3*) activity. It is estimated that *CYP2C9* variants account for 10 to 20% of the total variation in warfarin dose, with additional genetic and environmental factors playing larger roles in dose determination. The second gene is the vitamin K epoxide reductase complex protein 1 (*VKORC1*), targeted by warfarin. Consideration of *VKORC1* genotype, together with *CYP2C9* genotype and factors such as age and body size, is estimated to account for 35 to 60% of the variability in warfarin dosing requirements. Although further studies are under way, the clinical pharmacology advisory panel to the U.S. Food and Drug Administration (FDA) acknowledged the importance and potential for genotyping of *CYP2C9* and *VKORC1* during the early phase of warfarin therapy, and the drug label was amended accordingly in August 2007; however, the Center for Medicare and Medicaid Services announced in 2009 that it would not reimburse for testing until there was more evidence of a clinical benefit.

THE EXPRESSED GENOME

Gene Expression

Information from (RNA, protein, or metabolite) expression informs three areas relevant to clinical decision making:

- Disease diagnosis and classification
- Disease prognosis
- Pharmacogenomics

Disease Diagnosis and Classification

Whole-genome RNA expression data can be used to identify subtypes of cancer not previously recognized by traditional methods of analysis (Table 42-2). Among many examples, patterns of RNA expression have identified subclasses of tumors that define the acute leukemias or Burkitt's lymphoma from diffuse large B-cell lymphomas (DLBCL). Breast cancer profiling has defined four different gene expression subtypes; these molecularly defined subtypes have important prognostic relevance. Outside of cancer, complementary DNA microarray technology has proved useful for classifying a broad range of diseases, such as rheumatoid arthritis, Crohn's disease, schizophrenia, and multiple sclerosis, and for differentiating between ischemic and nonischemic cardiomyopathy.

Disease Prognosis

The first prognostic application of gene expression signatures described two molecularly distinct forms of DLBCL previously not appreciated using traditional histopathology techniques: germinal center B-like DLBCL and activated B-like DLBCL. Their clinical significance is that patients with germinal center B-like DLBCL have significantly better overall survival when treated with standard chemotherapy. Similarly, microarray studies of breast cancer have proved more powerful than traditional methods for predicting a patient's outcome, such as tumor size, lymph node status, and estrogen receptor status; for example, a 70-gene expression signature was found to be a strong predictor of metastasis, outperforming all currently used clinical predictors.

In 2009, oncologists used RNA expression signatures (Oncotype DX) for risk stratification and prognosis in more than 40,000 breast cancer patients and had cumulatively ordered more than 135,000. A prospective cooperative group clinical trial in Europe (MINDACT) aims to measure the effectiveness of a gene expression predictor of breast cancer prognosis in guiding adjuvant chemotherapy when compared with predictions based solely on the traditional clinical parameters for prognoses. A current study sponsored by the National Cancer Institute aims to use the Oncotype DX test from Genomic Health, Inc., to identify low-risk breast cancer patients unlikely to benefit from chemotherapy. For lung cancer, a similar opportunity now exists to refine prognosis and redirect treatment in early-stage disease and a clinical trial has been developed that uses this signature to randomize patients to surgical treatment with or without adjuvant chemotherapy.

Pharmacogenomics

The use of complex molecular information from the genome (as opposed to DNA variation) is often referred to as *pharmacogenomics*. (As described earlier, *pharmacogenetics* refers to individual responses to drugs as a function of DNA variation.) The expressed genome has provided several important

TABLE 42-2 PERIPHERAL BLOOD GENE EXPRESSION SIGNATURES TO CLASSIFY DISEASE STATES

	TARGET CELL	RESULTS	CHAPTER
Autoimmune	Whole blood RNA	A 41-gene signature differentiates **infliximab** responders from nonresponders.	35
	Whole blood RNA	A 29-gene signature best differentiates active from inactive **systemic lupus erythematosus.**	274
Inflammatory	Peripheral monocytes	A 53-gene signature distinguishes between patients with active **multiple sclerosis** and healthy controls.	419
	Peripheral monocytes	A 136-gene signature distinguishes active **multiple sclerosis** patients on TNF-α therapy from treatment-naïve patients.	419
	Whole blood RNA	A 10-gene-based composite score for diagnosing **atopy** and **asthma** performs better than the total IgE count, with a sensitivity and specificity of 96% and 92%, respectively.	257
Neoplasm	CD27⁺ and CD19⁺ B cells; CD4⁺ T cells	A 2984-gene signature can distinguish subtypes of **diffuse large B-cell lymphoma**.	191
	Bone marrow mononuclear cell RNA	A 50-gene signature is highly correlated with **AML-ALL distinction** and is used to develop a classification scheme.	189
	CD34⁺ blast cells RNA	A 2856-gene signature allows **classification of AML** into 16 distinct groups.	189
Transplant	CD4⁺ and CD8⁺ T-cell RNA	A 17-gene signature identifies donor samples **likely to cause GVHD** with 80% accuracy.	181
	Whole blood RNA	A 91-gene signature distinguishes between **transplant rejection** (grade 3A) and controls (grade 0).	48
Environmental Exposure	Whole blood RNA	A 216-gene profile differentiates **oxidative damage** from active oxidative damage in active and passive smokers.	31
	Whole blood RNA	A 62-gene profile correlates with severity of **arsenic poisoning.**	21
	Whole blood RNA	A 25-gene signature identifies **exposure to ionizing radiation** with overall accuracy of 90%.	19
Cardiovascular Disease	Platelet RNA	A 54-gene signature classifies **STEMI and stable CAD**. Moreover, MRP8/14 predicts risk for a future cardiovascular event.	71, 73
	Whole blood RNA	A 160-gene signature correlates with extent of **coronary stenosis** and is associated with atherosclerotic vascular disease.	70
	Whole blood RNA	A 14-gene signature confirmed by PCR is associated with the **presence and extent of CAD.**	71

ALL = acute lymphoblastic leukemia; AML = acute myelogenous leukemia; CAD = coronary artery disease; GVHD = graft-versus-host disease; IgE = immunoglobulin E; PCR = polymerase chain reaction; STEMI = ST elevation myocardial infarction; TNF = tumor necrosis factor.
Adapted from Aziz H, Zaas A, Ginsburg G. Peripheral blood gene expression profiling for cardiovascular disease assessment. *Genomic Med.* 2007;1:105-112.

TABLE 42-3 MOLECULAR MARKER INFORMED CANCER THERAPIES (TARGETED THERAPEUTICS)

BIOMARKER	DRUG	CANCER TYPE	DRUG EFFECT	FDA DRUG LABELING RECOMMENDED OR REQUIRED
Estrogen receptor	Tamoxifen	Breast	Response	Yes
HER2/neu	Trastuzumab	Breast	Response	Yes
EGFR	Cetuximab	Colorectal	Response	Yes
Kras	Cetuximab	Colorectal	Response	Yes
EGFR	Panitumumab	Colorectal	Response	Yes
Kras	Panitumumab	Colorectal	Response	Yes
DPYD	5-FU	Breast/colorectal	Response	No
EGFR	Erlotinib	Lung	Response	No
EGFR	Gefitinib	Lung	Response	No
BCR-ABL	Imatinib	CML	Response	Yes
C-KIT	Imatinib	CML/ALL	Response	Yes

5-FU, 5-fluorouracil; ALL = acute lymphocytic leukemia; CML = chronic myelogenous leukemia; DPD = dihydropyrimidine dehydrogenase; EGFR = epidermal growth factor receptor.
Adapted from Freedman A, Sansbury L, Figg W, et al. Cancer pharmacogenomics and pharmacoepidemiology: setting a research agenda to accelerate translation. *J Natl Cancer Inst.* 2010;102:1698-1705.

examples of novel biomarkers that can be used to guide therapy selection. An iconic form of pharmacogenomics is "targeted therapy," of which there are now several examples in clinical practice (E-Table 42-1 and Table 42-3). Trastuzumab therapy (a monoclonal antibody specifically targeting *HER2/neu*-overexpressing breast tumors) is an example of a protein therapeutic for which an obligatory biomarker assay and diagnostic test have been developed to identify the patients most likely to benefit from this drug. Trastuzumab is marketed solely for the subset of patients (~10%) who overexpress *HER2/neu* (Chapter 204). Given the low prevalence of marker-positive breast cancers, it has been suggested that if it were not for the use of the diagnostic marker the drug would not have been successfully developed. In cardiovascular medicine, a targeted approach to acute coronary syndromes has been practiced for more than a decade with the use of cardiac troponin I (cTnI) measurements to dictate the beneficial use of glycoprotein IIb/IIIa inhibitors.

Recently, a series of gene expression signatures have been developed to predict the activation state of various oncogenic signaling pathways, thereby portending the advent of personalized cancer treatment based on a tumor's gene expression pattern. When evaluated in several large collections of human cancers, these gene expression signatures identify patterns of pathway deregulation in tumors and clinically relevant associations with disease outcomes, including prognosis. Linking pathway deregulation with sensitivity to therapeutics that target components of the pathway provides an opportunity to make use of these "oncogenic signatures" to guide the use of target therapeutics.

Proteomics

Proteomics is the large-scale study of proteins. The *proteome* often refers to the full complement of proteins and their various derivatives (e.g., splice variants or post-translational modification). In the context of health and disease, proteomics seeks to define the full set of proteins associated with a particular physiologic state. The capabilities and direction of proteomics is evolving in terms of both protein identification and differential expression between two physiologic states (such as health and a specific disease). Quantitative proteomics, in which global differences in protein abundances are measured, continues to be a priority area for biomarker discovery and molecular medicine. This area has been dominated by stable isotope approaches, but recent label-free quantitative methods have been developed that rely on the measured intensity of a peptide ion and compares this to its intensity in other samples. Label-free methods have the advantage of higher throughput and fewer sample manipulation steps. Multiple-reaction monitoring of specific peptides within biofluids allows quantitation of absolute abundance of proteins in clinical samples. Although this technology is relatively immature in its applications to human health and disease compared with RNA and metabolic profiling, it is anticipated that these methods, combined with the development of mass spectroscopy (MS) technology, will advance proteomics to more routine use in

disease classification and diagnosis, prognosis, and pharmacogenomics within the next several years.

Metabolic Profiling

A metabolic profile is very similar to some of the traditional targeted profiles, such as a lipid profile, although it is more comprehensive. Metabolomics measures changes in the metabolic or chemical milieu that are downstream of genomic and proteomic alterations. It is estimated that humans contain approximately 5000 discrete small molecule metabolites, and the identification of metabolic fingerprints for specific diseases may have particular practical utility for the development of therapies because metabolic changes immediately suggest enzymatic drug targets. Similar to genomics and proteomics, metabolomics may be useful in disease diagnosis, prognosis, and drug development. In particular, metabolomics will likely be a valuable tool in assessing drug toxicity. Targeted MS-based metabolic profiling has also been increasingly applied to studies of human diseases and conditions. These tools are being applied to diverse areas, such as diabetes, obesity, cardiovascular disease, cancer, and mental disorders.

● ASSEMBLING MOLECULAR INFORMATION FOR CLINICAL DECISION MAKING

Despite the potential for molecular information to transform health care, past experience indicates that new molecular interventions, like any new medical intervention, will remain substantially underused for many years unless a robust infrastructure is established for supporting their appropriate use. Moreover, molecular interventions may face even greater barriers to clinical adoption compared with more traditional medical interventions, owing to such factors as limited clinician familiarity with molecular technologies, the volume and complexity of the underlying data that may need to be considered, and financial coverage of additional testing in an already financially challenged health care system.

Of the many strategies that have been evaluated for promoting evidence-based care, one strategy has been found to be particularly effective: clinical decision support (CDS), which entails providing clinicians, patients, and other health care stakeholders with pertinent knowledge or person-specific information, intelligently filtered or presented at appropriate times, to enhance health and health care. Clinician-directed CDS interventions evaluated in randomized controlled trials have significantly improved patient care, provided that the CDS was delivered automatically as a part of clinician workflow, offered at the time and location of decision making, recommended a specific course of action, and used a computer to generate the recommendations.

Extended to molecular medicine, CDS supports its consistent and evidence-based application in health care. For example, when initiating warfarin therapy using an electronic prescribing system, a clinician could be provided with recommendations on dosing and monitoring that account for the patient's *CYP2C9* and *VKORC1* genotypes. As another example, to

TABLE 42-4 CLINICAL DECISION SUPPORT REQUIREMENTS TO APPLY MOLECULAR TECHNOLOGIES TO CLINICAL MEDICINE

NEED	AVAILABLE RESOURCES
Centrally managed repositories of medical knowledge	Authoritative knowledge on how molecular interventions should be used in clinical practice (e.g., U.S. Preventive Services Task Force, U.S. Evaluation of Genomic Applications in Practice and Prevention initiative) Repositories of structured experimental genomic and molecular data (e.g., PharmGKB for pharmacogenetic and pharmacogenomic experimental data and curated knowledge; NCBI dbGaP for data from studies evaluating the interaction between genotypes and phenotypes; and NCBI GEO for gene expression data) Large-scale efforts at managing medical information in health systems (Intermountain Healthcare, Partners HealthCare)
Standardized representation of molecular and patient data	Standardized information terminologies for both molecular and traditional patient data (e.g., HL7 data standards, including HL7 Clinical Genomics data standards and emerging HL7 virtual medical record standard; openEHR Archetypes; SNOMED CT; LOINC; BSML; MAGE-ML; National Cancer Institute/caBIG Common Data Elements)
Standard approaches for locating and retrieving patient and molecular data	Approaches for locating and retrieving patient data across systems (e.g., HL7 Retrieve, Locate, and Update Service draft standard and corresponding OMG technical specification) Regional and national initiatives for secure health data exchange (e.g., U.K. National Health Service Connecting for Health, U.S. Nationwide Health Information Network prototypes, caBIG, Indiana Health Information Exchange)
Sharing and coordination of information	Initiatives to share medical knowledge (e.g., Morningside Initiative, U.S. Federal CDS Collaboratory) Efforts to specify functional requirements of EHR systems (e.g., HL7 EHR System Functional Model standard) Coordinated use of available health information technology standards (e.g., U.S. Health Information Technology Standards Panel, Integrating the Healthcare Enterprise)

BSML = Bioinformatic Sequence Markup Language; caBIG = cancer Biomedical Informatics Grid; dbGaP = database of Genotype and Phenotype; EHR = electronic health record; GEO = Gene Expression Omnibus; LOINC = Logical Observation Identifiers Names and Codes; MAGE-ML = microarray and gene expression markup language; NCBI = National Center for Biotechnology Information; PharmGKB = Pharmacogenomics and Pharmacogenetics Knowledge Base; SNOMED CT = Systematized Nomenclature of Medicine, Clinical Terms.
Adapted from Kawamoto K, Lobach D, Willard H, Ginsburg G. National clinical decision support infrastructure to enable the widespread and consistent application of genetics and genomics in healthcare. PMCID: PMC2666673 2009;9:17.

support a clinician in his or her treatment of a patient with breast cancer, an electronic health record (EHR) system could consider the gene expression profile of the patient's cancer biopsy and provide an individually tailored prediction of how the patient is likely to respond to various therapeutic options. Critical to the vision of molecular medicine supported by information technologies will be a national CDS infrastructure (Table 42-4) that enables authoritative, centrally curated knowledge of molecular information that can be consistently leveraged in clinical practices across the nation. The true application of molecular technologies will require robust CDS systems that (1) access molecular and other patient data located within the EHR, (2) evaluate and integrate this information in relation to rule sets, and (3) deliver the information in a fashion that allows real-time actionable recommendations for the individual patient.

SUGGESTED READINGS

Chadwick R. Personal genomes: no bad news? *Bioethics*. 2011;25:62-65. *Thoughtful review of whole genome sequencing's potential effects on people and their lives.*
Ginsburg GS, Willard HF, eds. *Genomic and Personalized Medicine*. 2nd ed. Philadelphia: Elsevier; 2011. *A comprehensive work on the discovery, translational, clinical, and policy research and evidence to guide molecular information and technologies from bench to bedside.*

43

CELL AND GENE THERAPY

KARL SKORECKI AND EITHAN GALUN

CELL THERAPY

Cell therapy refers to the provision of living cells to patients for the prevention or treatment of human disease. The best established and most widely practiced form of cell therapy is the administration of blood and blood products in transfusion medicine. Other emerging applications of cell therapy involve the use of cells as vehicles for the delivery of genes or gene products, as discussed in the section on gene therapy.

In regenerative medicine, cells from various sources are administered to augment, repair, or replace tissues or organs damaged by disease, injury, or congenital anomaly. In this regard, solid organ transplantation can be considered a form of cell therapy. Like blood and blood product transfusion (Chapter 180), solid organ transplantation provides fully differentiated,

functioning replacement cells of the transplanted organ (Chapter 48). One of the most important practical limitations of solid organ transplantation is the shortage of available organs relative to the growing demand. In certain forms of irreversible organ system failure, such as neurodegenerative disease, organ transplantation is not a therapeutic option. For these reasons, the development of safe and effective cell therapies is progressing rapidly.

Stem Cells of Human Origin

Stem cells possess two defining properties: (1) the capacity for self-renewal, and (2) the capacity to differentiate into cell types with specialized cellular functions. This may occur at the individual stem cell level through the process of asymmetrical cell division (Fig. 43-1) or at the cell population level wherein a subset of cells differentiate and the remaining stem cells remain dormant or replicate themselves as stem cells. After asymmetrical cell division, non–stem cell derivatives may either generate a pool of organ system–restricted, transit-amplifying cells with enhanced proliferative capacity or differentiate by epigenetic and gene expression profile changes until reaching the terminally differentiated state. This framework was developed after the discovery of bone marrow cells that were capable of reconstituting the adult hematopoietic system. These hematopoietic stem cells constitute the basis for hematopoietic stem cell transplantation, the only form of stem cell therapy currently well established in clinical practice (Chapter 181). Besides these two cardinal properties of self-renewal and differentiation capacity, stem cells can also be classified according to three additional attributes. These are replicative capacity (limited versus unlimited), the scope or potency of differentiation (e.g., pluripotent, multipotent, oligopotent, unipotent), and their place in the life history of the organism (developmental or postdevelopmental). Thus, more recent terminology has broadened use of the term *stem cells* to cover a wider array of cell types that contribute to organ development or have the capacity to repopulate tissues and organ systems. The term *stem cell*, together with the formulations noted previously, has also recently been extrapolated to describe certain cellular subpopulations that may be principally responsible for the growth of malignant tumors. However, because cancer stem cells (Chapter 185) have no role in tissue regeneration, they are not considered further in this chapter.

Embryonic and Induced Pluripotent Stem Cells

The fertilized egg, or zygote, develops first into a blastocyst, then an embryo, and then a fetus. The blastocyst is evident on day 5 after fertilization and consists of 200 to 250 cells, 30 to 34 of which consist of the inner cell mass, or epiblast. The remaining cells are the outer cell mass (Fig. 43-2). After the entire blastocyst attaches to the lining of the uterus, embryonic and extraembryonic development begins. At the blastocyst stage, each cell in the inner cell mass has the capacity to differentiate into derivatives of all three germline layers (ectoderm, mesoderm, and endoderm). In normal development, these cells do not persist beyond the blastocyst stage. Unused preimplantation

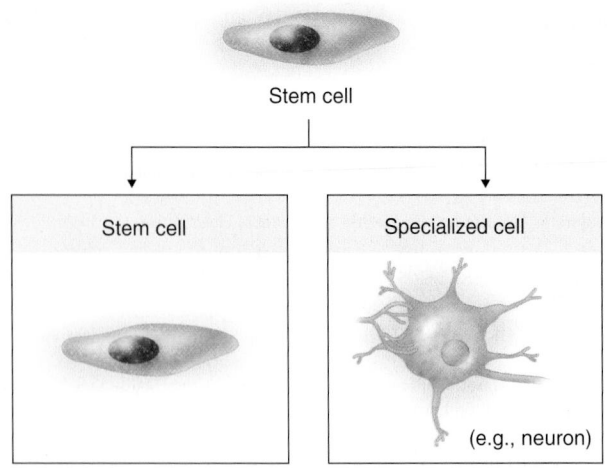

Stem cell

Stem cell   Specialized cell

(e.g., neuron)

FIGURE 43-1. **Asymmetrical cell division.** Although this first characteristic was considered a *required characteristic* for stem cells based on their original description in the adult hematopoietic system, not all cell types currently named as stem cells necessarily display this property. For instance, human embryonic stem cells divide by symmetrical cell division.

blastocysts generated for in vitro fertilization can be used to generate human embryonic stem cells (hESCs) from the microdissected inner cell mass. Under appropriate culture conditions, these hESCs exhibit unlimited self-renewal in cell culture in the undifferentiated state without undergoing replicative senescence (i.e., losing the ability to divide). This occurs by virtue of the expression of high levels of the telomerase enzyme, which protects against senescence-associated attrition of the telomeric ends of linear chromosomes during repeated rounds of cell division. Under appropriate cell culture conditions, hESCs are pluripotent; they can differentiate into any of the known cell types of the body.

A major goal of embryonic stem cell research is to direct the differentiation process to enable enrichment to homogeneity of a replacement cell type by adding growth factors that activate cell signaling pathways used in normal embryonic development. This approach has yielded partial enrichment of cells with properties similar to those of authentic fetal pancreatic β cells, vascular endothelial cells, and cardiomyocytes, as well as more mature cells with properties similar to those of bone, connective tissue, and retinal, neuronal, and hepatic cells.

More recently, methods have been developed to reprogram differentiated adult somatic cells into a state of pluripotency, thereby generating induced pluripotent stem cells (iPSCs; Fig. 43-3). The methods to achieve this were enabled by identifying the various cell signaling and gene regulatory pathways that confer pluripotency on hESCs—including the transcription factors Nanog, Oct-4, and Sox-2. The availability of iPSCs from a given patient in need of replacement cells potentially avoids problems of immune rejection because the iPSCs will be recognized as autologous or self rather than allogeneic in origin. In addition, the use of iPSCs appears to invoke fewer ethical concerns, as outlined later. iPSCs derived from patients with certain genetic diseases also provide a unique experimental platform for studying the cellular and molecular pathways that go awry during the development of the affected cell types and tissues.

During the later stages of prenatal human development, cells of fetal origin often show enhanced proliferative capacity as well as the ability to differentiate into more than one type of mature or specialized cell. Thus, these cells have also been used as sources of cell therapy in regenerative medicine and can also be considered stem or progenitor cells—but with more restricted replicative capacity and differentiation potential than is the case for hESCs and iPSCs. To date, the only fetal-derived stem cells that have been used with documented success in human clinical applications are the dopaminergic cells derived from the developing fetal nervous system for the treatment of Parkinson's disease (Chapter 416).

Translating hESCs and iPSCs into a therapeutic platform has the potential for the development of teratomas and malignant tumors from residual undifferentiated cells, following administration of what appears to be a homogeneous population of fully differentiated replacement cells. Progress to clinical trials requires definitive clarification of this concern.

Adult (Postnatal) Stem Cells

After birth, many tissues are thought to contain a subpopulation of cells with the capacity for extended self-renewal, combined with the ability to differentiate into more mature cell types with specialized functions. Adult stem cells generate an intermediate state characterized by enhanced proliferation (transit-amplifying cells or progenitor cells), before reaching full terminal differentiation (Fig. 43-4).

Adult stem cells, thought to represent less than 0.01% of the total number of cells, are located in specialized supportive niche compartments at various sites within the hematopoietic system and elsewhere, and respond to cues in their local microenvironment. As a result of the success of hematopoietic stem cell transplantation in the treatment of bone marrow failure or in conjunction with myeloablative therapy in malignancy, scientists have been motivated to find adult stem cells in other organs and other organ systems. Adult tissues and organ systems reported to contain stem cells include bone marrow (hematopoietic and mesenchymal compartments) and peripheral blood, the central nervous system, blood vessel endothelium, dental pulp, epithelia of the skin, adipose tissue, digestive system, cornea, retina, testis, and liver. Controversy exists regarding the existence of adult stem cells in the kidney, pancreas, and heart. Whether adult stem cells represent remnants of developmental stem cells that persist into adulthood for purposes of organ maintenance and repair or represent a distinct cell type dedicated for this latter purpose is not clear.

Given their low percentage, dispersed tissue distribution, and markers that are not fully defined, isolation of adult stem cells for therapeutic use has been technically challenging, with the greatest successes to date reported for mesenchymal stem cells. Mesenchymal stem cells represent a type of multipotential adult progenitor cell found in the bone marrow niche that supports hematopoiesis. Mesenchymal stem cells have also been isolated from adipose tissue, blood, umbilical cord, and muscle. Although mesenchymal and other multipotential adult progenitor cells have been shown in some experimental animal models to differentiate into a wide variety of cell types representing all three germ layers, they do not possess the capacity to develop into every cell type, as do hESCs and iPSCs.

There is some evidence that beyond the therapeutic value to hematopoietic reconstitution, bone marrow transplantation may also make some contribution to restoration of organ system function after certain forms of solid organ transplantation. Although adult stem cells are classically thought to be committed to a narrow spectrum of differentiation within the organ system, some studies have suggested the possibility that certain adult stem cells may display unexpected degrees of plasticity. *Plasticity* refers to the ability of differentiated cells to undergo transdifferentiation into mature cell derivatives of another germline origin. Such plasticity would allow bone marrow-derived hematopoietic or mesenchymal stem cells to transdifferentiate into cardiac, vascular endothelial, connective tissue, neuronal, or other cells that show promise in clinical trials of regenerative medicine.

Like iPSCs, postnatal or adult stem cells have the potential to circumvent two of the obstacles in developmental stem cell therapy: ethical concerns regarding the use of cells of developmental origin, and alloimmunologic rejection. Adult stem cells may have the additional advantage of being less prone to teratoma and tumor development. hESCs and their derivatives generally emanate from a source not related to the potential recipient and can therefore be considered an allogeneic graft. Research studies have confirmed the immunogenicity of hESCs despite their very early developmental origin. Adult stem cells and iPSCs of autologous origin should not elicit an alloimmunologic response and therefore offer a potential solution. On the other hand, when the underlying disease is an active autoimmune destructive process (e.g., type 1 diabetes mellitus), it can be expected that replacement cells of autologous origin might also be targets of the immune-mediated pathophysiologic process.

Specific Disease Applications in Cell Therapy

Except for hematopoietic stem cell and solid organ transplantation, experimental cell therapies have been implemented in a limited number of patient trials.

Neurodegenerative Disease and Neuronal Injury

Parkinson's disease (Chapter 416) involves loss of melanin-containing dopaminergic neurons within the substantia nigra pars compacta of the midbrain, coupled with accompanying depletion of striatal dopamine. This cellular loss is responsible for the major motor features of the disease. Although

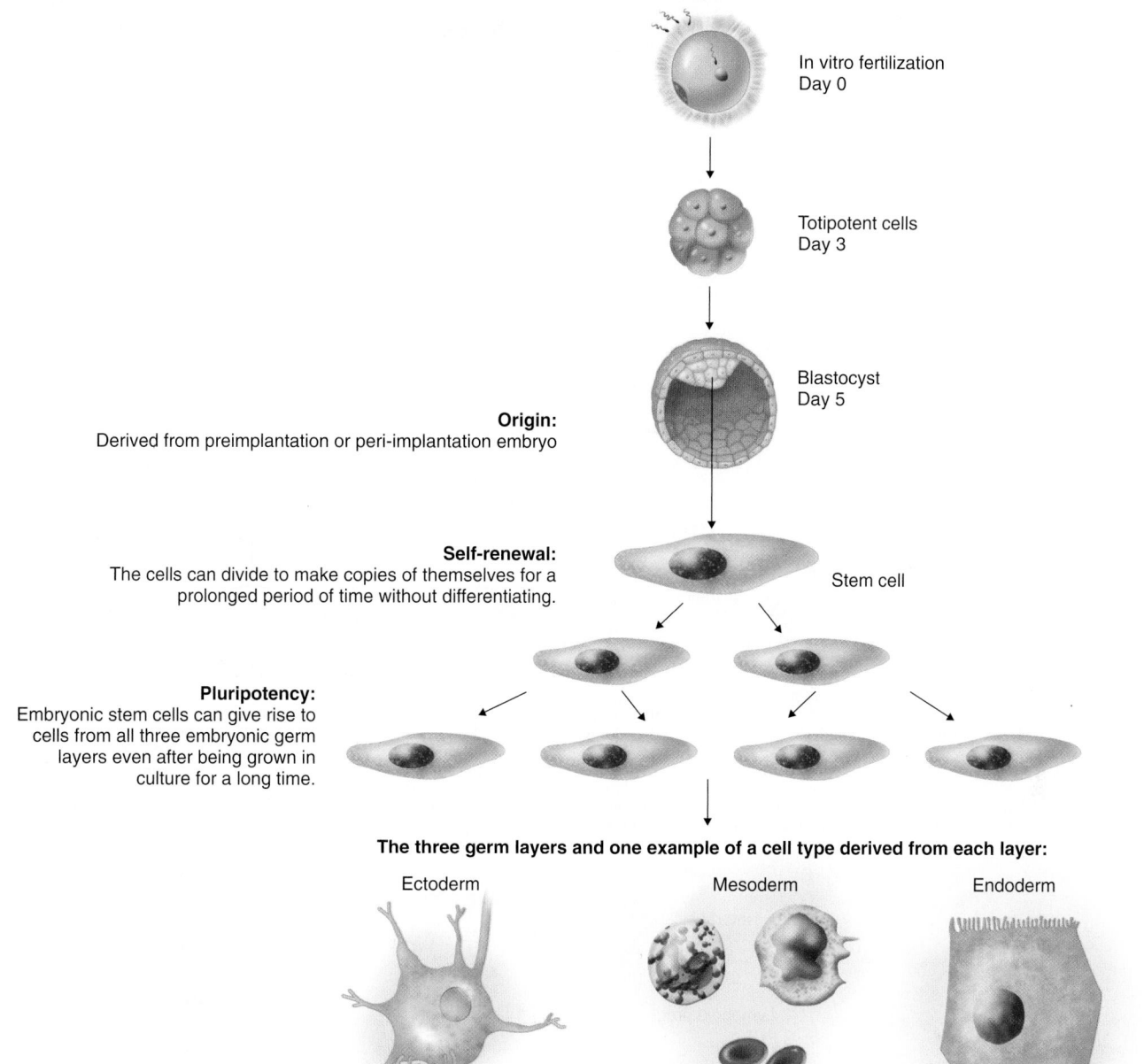

In vitro fertilization
Day 0

Totipotent cells
Day 3

Blastocyst
Day 5

Origin:
Derived from preimplantation or peri-implantation embryo

Stem cell

Self-renewal:
The cells can divide to make copies of themselves for a
prolonged period of time without differentiating.

Pluripotency:
Embryonic stem cells can give rise to
cells from all three embryonic germ
layers even after being grown in
culture for a long time.

The three germ layers and one example of a cell type derived from each layer:

Ectoderm

Mesoderm

Endoderm

Neuron

Blood cells

Liver cell

Ectoderm gives rise to:
brain, spinal cord, nerve cells,
hair, skin, teeth, sensory cells
of eyes, ears, nose, and
mouth, and pigment cells.

Mesoderm gives rise to:
muscles, blood, blood
vessels, connective
tissues, and the heart.

Endoderm gives rise to:
the gut (pancreas,
stomach, liver, etc.), lungs,
bladder, and germ cells
(egg or sperm).

FIGURE 43-2. Embryonic stem cells. *Totipotency* refers to the capacity to differentiate into all cell types in an organism, including extraembryonic tissues, placenta, and umbilical cord, a property confined to the fertilized egg itself, including the cells derived from the first few cell divisions after fertilization. *Pluripotency* refers to the capacity to differentiate into all the specialized cell types derived from the three germ layers (ectoderm, mesoderm, endoderm) of the developing embryo and is a hallmark feature of embryonic stem and germ cells.

pharmacologic dopaminergic replacement therapy is effective in the early stages of illness, prolonged treatment with pharmacologic agents alone is associated with refractoriness and complications and fails to halt the underlying neurodegeneration. In the search for more definitive therapy, early reports of cell replacement suggested significant improvement in motor function after intrastriatal implantation of mesencephalic tissue, obtained from aborted human fetuses aged 6 to 9 weeks after conception. Long-term immunosuppressive treatment is essential to allow transplanted dopaminergic neurons to develop into their full functional potential despite the notion of an immunologic sanctuary within the brain. Clinical assessment standards have provided evidence of long-lived graft survival and clinical benefit after therapy with cells of fetal origin that has now lasted up to 10 years or longer

in some patients. Further progress is limited by lack of sufficient source tissue to treat a large number of affected patients, prohibitive variability in functional outcome, reports of serious dyskinesias in a subset of treated patients, and ethical considerations.

Investigations of stem cell–based approaches for the treatment of other neurodegenerative diseases, including Alzheimer's disease, Batten's disease, amyotrophic lateral sclerosis, stroke, and brain and spinal cord injury, are now moving between experimental animal model studies to planning of clinical trials. Recent reports have shown a major clinical benefit in animal models on directed differentiation and transplantation of hESCs toward a retinal pigment epithelium. Human studies with these cells may be soon initiated for patients suffering from age-related macular degeneration.

Adult cell

iPS cell reprogramming factors

iPS cells

Mesoderm
(Middle layer)

Endoderm
(Internal layer)

Ectoderm
(External layer)

Cardiac muscle

Skeletal muscle cells

Tubule cell of the kidney

Red blood cells

Smooth muscle (in gut)

Lung cell (alveolar cell)

Thyroid cell

Pancreatic cell

Skin cells of epidermis

Neuron cell

Pigment cell

FIGURE 43-3. Induced pluripotent stem (iPS) cells. Introduction of three growth factors and a chemical agent that modifies gene expression is sufficient to restore pluripotency to adult somatic cells. (Adapted from http://www.sigmaaldrich.com/life-science/stem-cell-biology/ipsc.html.)

Bone

Natural killer (NK) cell

T lymphocytes

Neutrophil

Basophil

Lymphoid progenitor cell

B lymphocyte

Eosinophil

Monocyte/ macrophage

Hematopoietic stem cell

Multipotent stem cell

Myeloid progenitor cell

Red blood cells

Platelets

Bone matrix

Stromal cell

Blood vessel

Stromal stem cell

Osteoclast

Adipocyte

Bone (or cartilage)

Osteoblast

Lining cell

Osteocyte

Pre-osteoblast

Skeletal muscle stem cell?

Hepatocyte muscle stem cell?

Hematopoietic supportive stroma

Marrow adipocyte

Hematopoietic stem cell

FIGURE 43-4. Adult stem cells. Adult stem cells can be multipotent and have the capacity to differentiate into a limited number of different cell types, often restricted to a given tissue or organ system, as in the case of adult hematopoietic or epidermal stem cells. Two stem cell types have been isolated from adult bone marrow—the hematopoietic stem cell and the mesenchymal stem cell. Adult mesenchymal stem cells of bone marrow origin, although their range of differentiation has been shown to be broader than that of any other adult stem cell type, do not reach pluripotency. It is thought that in some organ systems, such as the gastrointestinal epithelium, a unipotent pool of progenitors exists for repopulating a rapid population turnover of only one type of cell—although it is difficult to be certain whether such progenitors can be distinguished from the overall population of fully differentiated cells in tissues with high cellular turnover.

Muscular Dystrophies and Other Disorders of the Musculoskeletal System

In the major genetic forms of muscular dystrophy (Chapter 429), a range of approaches have been developed that aim to correct the genetic defect, restore functional expression of the missing gene product (e.g., dystrophin), and thereby slow disease progression. Implantation of myoblast muscle precursor cells might enable the improved repopulation of degenerating dystrophic muscles in these disease states. Although initial success in harvesting myoblasts was reported, clinical benefit did not ensue because of an inflammatory response that destroys most injected myoblasts. Furthermore, failure of myoblasts to migrate meaningful distances from the injection site renders implantation by direct needle injection impractical in acute muscular dystrophy disorders.

Protocols have been devised for the development of mixed biomechanical substitutes for bone, tendon, cartilage, and other connective tissues that incorporate or produce relevant surrounding matrix. For these forms of cell therapy, connective tissue scaffold can be produced in vitro and then repopulated with endogenous recipient cells in the patient, thus potentially preempting immune rejection and other problems related to the presence of cells of allogeneic origin.

Heart Disease

In heart failure (Chapters 58 and 59), limitations of clinical therapy have motivated the search for cell-based therapies to restore or augment myocardial contractile function or reestablish functional cardiomyocytes in damaged cardiac regions.

Autologous skeletal myoblasts have been shown in clinical trials to grow in scarred cardiac tissue after direct intracardiac injection. However, histologic or functional evidence of electrical or mechanical coupling has not been demonstrated. Currently, most experimental work selects a specific preparation of bone marrow and peripheral stem cells and progenitors. In some cases, the apparent differentiation of bone marrow cells into cardiac myocyte phenotypes has been subsequently refuted. In cell culture, hESCs are easily induced into a cardiomyocyte phenotype, including the following features: rhythmic contraction, gene and protein expression markers for cardiomyocyte differentiation, electrical coupling through gap junctions, responsiveness to chronotropic and inotropic agents, and electromechanical coupling with heterotypic cardiomyocytes derived from other sources. Cardiomyocytes of human embryonic stem cell origin have been shown to serve as a biologic pacemaker after conduction system ablation in experimental animals. They have also been shown to enhance cardiac contractility after myocardial infarction induced by coronary ligation in experimental animals. For the treatment of refractory cardiac rhythm disturbances, a combination of cell and gene therapy involves the stable expression of potassium conductance or other ion channels in skin fibroblasts derived from patients suffering from refractory rhythm disturbances, followed by their implantation into electrically unstable regions of the heart by guided endomyocardial injection. A major experimental effort in the use of bone marrow–derived cells through intracoronary administration aims to improve left ventricular function after acute myocardial infarction. Clinical experience with more than 1000 patients who received stem cell therapy indicates a favorable safety profile with a modest improvement in cardiac function and structural remodeling in the setting of acute myocardial infarction or chronic heart failure. Direct intracardiac muscle administration was more frequently associated with lesser degrees of improvement and sometimes with arrhythmias.

Diabetes Mellitus

Successful pancreatic transplantation and improved glucocorticoid-free protocols for transplantation of islets of Langerhans have been shown not only to restore glucose control in patients with diabetes mellitus but also to prevent or even reverse some of the disease's complications (Chapters 236 and 237). However, whole organ or islet-based transplantation approaches are limited both by immunologic rejection and by limitation of an available source of transplantable tissues. This has motivated the search for cell types that can replace (type 1 diabetes mellitus) or augment (type 2 diabetes mellitus) deficient β-cell function. Although no clinical applications have been reported, significant progress has been made with cells of human origin tested in cell culture and in animal models. Strategies that have been pursued include the developmental reprogramming of hepatic cells along the endocrine pancreatic lineage differentiation to provide these cells with the appropriate machinery for glucose-mediated insulin release. Protocols have also been established for differentiation of hESCs to either a precursor or mature β-cell phenotype. Because the pathogenesis of type 1 diabetes mellitus involves autoimmune destruction of pancreatic islet cells, the β cells derived from autologous sources, such as the patient's own iPSCs, might also become a target for autoimmune destructive processes unless preemptive measures are taken. In addition, because glucose monitoring and insulin delivery systems are constantly improving, any cell therapy–based approach must provide a clear advantage over existing therapeutic modalities while meeting the most rigorous standards of patient safety.

Stem Cell–Derived Platforms in Gene and Drug Discovery

In addition to the generation of cells for regenerative applications, the ability to grow a wide variety of different specialized cell types of human origin in culture provides unparalleled opportunities for gene and drug discovery and testing. For example, the ability to grow human cardiomyocytes in culture provides a preclinical human cellular-based experimental platform for screening newly developed drugs in terms of their potential to cause QT-interval prolongation and hence the risk for arrhythmia in the clinical setting. Other examples include the creation of an experimental tissue microenvironment of human origin for studying the stromal response to tumor growth and testing anticancer drugs that target tumorigenic responses such as angiogenesis. By combining technologies such as RNA interference (RNAi) with human stem cell growth and technology (E-Fig. 43-1), it will also be possible to uncover the role of certain gene products in the biochemical pathways and cellular responses in gene therapy.

Societal, Ethical, and Legal Considerations in Stem Cell Research and Therapy

Societal, ethical, and legal concerns about defining the concept of personhood status before birth have emerged among countries and political or religious constituencies in the field of stem cell research and therapy. Although there is a broad consensus that full personhood sanctity and associated rights should be accorded to each individual from at least the moment of birth, similar consensus does not apply to the status of an individual before birth. Various guidelines for research have been developed worldwide based on milestones in embryonic development. Bioethicists and legislators are often concerned about the possibility that research scientists and clinicians will move beyond allowable activities into prohibited domains. Previous concerns about therapeutic cloning, in which the first step is oocyte somatic nuclear transfer, or replacement of the haploid nucleus of a harvested oocyte with the diploid nucleus derived from the somatic cell of a potential cell therapy recipient were based mostly on the fear of a slippery slope to reproductive cloning. However, the successful generation of human iPSCs has for the most part supplanted the incentive for oocyte somatic nuclear transfer. Continued civil discourse and strict regulatory guidelines to ensure patient safety in clinical trials will remain key in resolving the bioethical dilemmas and societal concerns raised by stem cell and related emerging biomedical technologies.

⬤ GENE THERAPY

The use of genes as therapeutic platforms emerged during the mid-20th century, and in the 1990s, the first regulated registered studies were performed in the United States. Since then, more than 10,000 patients have been treated in more than 1000 studies in 15 countries across all continents with various modalities of gene therapy for a variety of diseases. About 50 studies have been performed for tracking gene delivery and more than 1000 for therapeutic assessment. One hundred studies involved monogenic diseases, and 1000 involved cancer patients, which is also the most common disease category for gene therapy studies worldwide. Two gene therapy agents are currently available on the market. Fomivirsen (Vitravene) is used for the treatment of cytomegalovirus retinitis (Chapter 384) in patients with acquired immunodeficiency syndrome (AIDS). The *p53* tumor suppressor coding sequence in an adenovirus vector is used for the treatment of head and neck cancer patients and is registered only in China. Most patients who participated in the first gene therapy clinical trials were administered marker or reporter genes rather than actual therapeutic genes. Of the thousands treated, two deaths have been attributed directly to gene therapy. The mortality statistics attributed to gene therapy are very low when compared with those associated with chemotherapy and transplantation, two therapeutic modalities frequently used today in clinical practice for disease targets of gene therapy.

Genetic Material

The therapeutic payload in most cases, the core of every gene therapy drug, is composed of an expression cassette. Essential clinical objectives of gene therapy are based on controlling gene expression through regulation of a tissue-specific promoter for expression. Although a few systems have been developed in the experimental setting, none has yet received approval for clinical use by the U.S. Food and Drug Administration or any other regulatory authority, other than the expression of *p53* in head and neck tumors by regulatory authorities in China.

Gene Therapy Delivery Methods

Gene therapy agents are often composed of two elements: the genetic material and the delivery system. The latter is usually the more complex and limiting component, and it is important to select the most efficient delivery method for any genetic therapy. Unfortunately, many gene therapy delivery methods are associated with potential adverse effects, thus necessitating tailoring of therapy to specific clinical considerations. The most commonly used delivery systems have used retrovirus- and adenovirus-based approaches. Virus-based approaches take advantage of the fact that viruses have been designed through evolution to serve as genetic material delivery systems. However, for each specific virus-based gene therapy vector, there have been major disadvantages that should be balanced against potential therapeutic benefits. Nonviral methods have also been used in many studies. The most commonly used nonviral delivery methods involve the use of naked/plasmid DNA and liposome-mediated delivery. In cancer gene therapy, the immune response to the delivery vehicle carrying the anticancer genetic material can be used to advantage by serving as an adjuvant. However, the system for delivery of a gene to be expressed for a prolonged period to replace or supplement a missing gene product in monogenic disease states should preferably be ignored by the immune system.

Naked/Plasmid DNA

In theory, the most straightforward approach to gene therapy would be the introduction of genetic material, such as an antisense molecule, short interfering RNA (siRNA), or an expression cassette, directly into the targeted cellular compartment (i.e., DNA into the nucleus or RNA into the cytoplasm). However, in clinical practice, this turns out not to be efficient. Systemic administration of naked DNA into the blood stream generally results in loss of the delivered genetic material, nonspecific interactions with serum proteins, and active degradation mediated by the innate immune system (e.g., tissue macrophages). Direct administration or application to target organs or tissues may circumvent some of these problems, but certain barriers must also be overcome. When the payload is a DNA expression cassette, it will need to interact with the cellular membrane and penetrate it, escape the endosomal compartment and cytosolic degradation by nucleases, and traverse the nuclear pores to reach the nucleus of the cell. This is a long process that is prone to failure unless supported by additional means that allow the DNA to pass the cellular barriers. Electroporation is an approach that has been applied to well-circumscribed body compartments or masses, such as muscle, skin, and tumors. Patients treated with electroporation have experienced tissue damage and associated pain. Additional methods have also been developed for the administration of naked DNA, including the different types of gene guns used for DNA vaccination and ultrasound energy for the transduction of endothelial cells, which could be used for cardiovascular applications and against tumor angiogenesis.

Naked DNA has also been formulated as part of DNA vaccination approaches to the treatment of cancer and immune and infectious diseases. Although preclinical studies have been promising, successful extrapolation to the clinic has not yet been achieved.

Nonviral Vectors

Nonviral vectors have been designed to overcome the cell membrane barrier and, in some cases, intracytoplasmic compartmentalization of the administered genetic material. These nonviral vectors are efficient at enhancing membrane penetration in vitro; however, their efficiency in vivo is significantly reduced. There are additional advantages to nonviral delivery systems: they are inexpensive and can carry large DNA molecules, and their structure can be modified to comply with specific needs, such as conjugation to short peptides for targeting. After systemic and, in some cases, local administration, these nonviral vectors stimulate the innate immune response by serving as adjuvants. They interact with serum proteins as well as cells that were not meant to be targeted, and with extracellular matrix. Once the DNA reaches the nucleus, it is subject to silencing. After cell division, expression is significantly reduced. Currently, nonviral vectors are used in specific selected cases. Local and systemic delivery of nonviral delivery systems could induce reciprocal immune effects with an undesirable inflammatory clinical response.

Adenovirus as a Viral Vector

Adenovirus is a nonenveloped DNA virus with the capacity to carry a large genetic payload. Adenoviruses, as well as adenovectors (the virally based vector), transduce nondividing cells, a property that is important for gene therapy for many cell types, such as hepatocytes (<0.1% of hepatocytes are replicating in humans at any given time). These vectors have been modified to prevent their replication in healthy tissues. Replication-defective (RD) adenovectors are used for short-term expression. Additional modifications of the viral genome and the cellular system supporting production of the viral particles have enabled deletion of all the viral coding sequences, thereby converting it into a "gutted" vector (helper-dependent [HD] adenovector). It is possible to clone the therapeutic genes into the RD adenovirus and generate recombinant adenovectors in a relatively short time. An additional advantage of adenovectors is that the relatively simple production system enables the generation of a very high titer. High viral titers are essential when administration is parenteral or when production of a large amount of a given protein is needed, such as in disease states in which secretion of a protein is impaired and each cell needs to encode its own normal protein. The HD adenovectors, which do not harbor virus-encoded genes, are able to support the transgene expression for months and possibly for more than a year. RD adenovector-transduced cells express viral proteins and induce an immune response. They are thus used in clinical cases in which the therapeutic gene needs to be expressed at high levels for a short period. High-titer systemic administration of adenovectors could be associated with severe adverse effects, such as disseminated intravascular coagulopathy (Chapter 178).

Retroviral Vectors

Retroviral vectors are an RNA group of viruses that harbor two RNA genomic copies in each viral particle, which is composed of a capsid and surrounded by an envelope. For gene therapy applications, two groups of viruses have been modified for clinical assessment and use: the oncoretroviruses and the lentiviruses. Vectors generated from both groups have already entered clinical testing.

Gammaretroviral Vectors

Gammaretroviral vectors are derived from different gammaretroviruses, including the murine leukemia virus and the Moloney murine leukemia virus. RD viruses are produced in special packaging cells that supply all the essential components in *trans* for viral replication and structural proteins. The viral gene therapy vector is composed of (1) a genome without any encoded viral sequences that is responsible for the production of viral proteins; (2) the therapeutic genetic payload and the structural components; and (3) the capsid and envelope. These viral vectors can carry transgenic payloads up to 8 kilobases (kb) in length. Retroviral vectors are capable of transducing only dividing cells. If the DNA reaches the nucleus, integration of the viral genome into the host cell chromosome can occur and lead to stable, long-term transgene expression. At its peak, a multiplicity of infection (MOI) integration occurs at numerous sites. Therefore, if long-term correction of a genetic disorder is required, the target cells must first be induced to replicate. The integration is a random event, with preference within an approximately 5-kb nucleotide window around the transcription initiation site. Thus, there is concern that interference with normal cell function could occur, including the activation of oncogenes or the disruption of tumor suppressor genes. Such events have occurred and have led to the development of malignant transformation both in animal models (rodents and primates) and in humans. There is evidence that "young" cells of the hematopoietic system and hepatocytes are more susceptible to malignant transformation than are terminally differentiated cells. On the other hand, the selectivity for dividing cells is advantageous if one aims to deliver a toxin gene to a growing tumor surrounded by quiescent normal parenchyma. The production of retroviral vectors is less efficient than that of adenovectors. As a result, the application of retroviruses is, in most cases, not by systemic administration but by ex vivo or direct injection into normal or tumor tissue.

Lentiviral Vectors

This group of viruses has been developed more recently for gene therapy applications. Human immunodeficiency virus (HIV) and the feline, simian, and equine immunodeficiency virus (FIV, SIV, and EIV, respectively) lentivirus family members were converted to become lentivectors for gene therapy. These vectors are deprived of the structural and most nonstructural and accessory genomic sequences that are supplied in *trans* in the packaging cell line for vector production. In addition, the envelope glycoprotein is of nonlentivirus origin, and for safety measures, the origin of replication is inactivated to generate a self-inactivating vector. All these genomic manipulations have been introduced to improve the safety of the lentivector and to enable a large cloning capacity of up to 8 kb. The lentivectors have been applied in only a few gene therapy studies, mainly for the treatment of AIDS patients. However, additional studies using lentivirus-based delivery systems are under way in patients with hemoglobinopathies, Parkinson's disease, X-linked adrenoleukodystrophy, and other genetic and degenerative diseases, with promising results. The long-term risk of using retroviral vectors, including gammaretroviral and lentiviral vectors, is not known. The possible development of clonal dominance, transformation, and cancer in the case of retroviral stem cell transduction is judiciously monitored in all appropriately registered studies.

Adenovirus-Associated Virus

Adenovirus-associated virus (AAV) is a single-strand DNA, nonenveloped, nonpathogenic human parvovirus. Viral vectors were derived from several serotypes, which exhibit different tissue and cell tropism. The capacity of AAV vectors is smaller, which is a limitation for certain AAV vector gene therapy approaches. The capacity for high titers (10^{12} transducing units per milliliter) of AAV serotypes enables systemic injections with reasonable MOI in targeted cells and tissues. Additional advantages of AAV vectors are that they transduce nondividing cells and do not integrate into the target cell genome. The innate immune system detects the AAV and responds to it, and antibodies generated against the viral capsid after a single injection attenuate the effect of a second administration of AAV vector. Long-term expression is detected with the use of AAV vectors. Phase I to III clinical studies have assessed the AAV vector for genetic, viral, inflammatory, degenerative, and malignant diseases. A study with AAV coagulation factor IX showed short-term efficacy owing to the development of an immune attack against the transduced hepatocytes. Studies both in Europe and the United States have shown a long-term benefit for patients with Leber's congenital amaurosis treated by subretinal administration of AAV to express retinal pigment epithelium-specific 65-kD protein (RPE65). Success was also reported in Parkinson's disease. Furthermore, more than 2 years of follow-up showed no significant side effects.

Special Virus-Derived Vectors

In addition to the adenoviral, retroviral, and AAV vectors, numerous, more specialized virus-based vectors with interesting properties and clinical objectives have been developed during the past 10 years.

Herpes simplex virus type 1 (HSV-1) is a DNA virus that can be manipulated to become RD and accommodate a large amount of foreign DNA for gene delivery. Expression of the transgene payload is transient. The HSV-1 amplicon has been used in numerous clinical trials of gene therapy for neurologic diseases.

Virus-like particles (VLPs) were recently developed for vaccination or gene therapy. VLPs of human papillomavirus were recently used as empty particles for vaccination against cervical cancer with significant success. Viruses of the same group, including SV40, which is also a DNA virus, are used for the generation of VLPs to carry gene therapy payloads. One advantage of SV40 is the low immune response against the virus. Again, similar barriers will slow the development of these vehicles, such as limitation of titers and production capacity.

Recombinant vaccinia virus (rVV) was initially developed for the expression of proteins in transduced tissues. Clinical studies in this avenue have encountered limited success. However, recent development of rVV for the treatment of malignant diseases through the expression of antigens might yield clinical benefit.

Oncolytic Viruses

Oncolytic viruses replicate in tumor cells and induce a cytopathic effect or kill tumor cells through other means, such as induction of apoptosis. The major obstacle facing the current development of antitumor drugs is not their potency, but rather their low selectivity for tumor cells. High therapeutic selectivity is essential to enable a safe therapeutic window. Virotherapy has such properties, but these viruses are still waiting to be proved clinically effective. Tumor-targeted oncolytic viruses are composed of two groups. Genetically engineered viruses are designed to replicate in tumor cells preferentially. This group includes adenoviruses that can replicate only in the presence of a nonfunctioning tumor suppressor gene, such as *p53* or *Rb*. The latter viruses will selectively replicate in tumor cells and induce their killing. The engineered HSV-1 and rVV viruses can also be included in this group. The second group consists of inherently antitumor-selective viruses found to possess antitumor effects through specific protein expression (reovirus) or viruses that activate the innate or adaptive immune response against the tumor, such as the Newcastle disease virus, measles virus strains, Sindbis virus, poliovirus, and vesicular stomatitis virus. The rationale for the use of reovirus in a virotherapeutic approach against cancer is based on the observation that reovirus infection activates host protein kinases to shut down protein production, an essential protection against the infection. Activated Ras signaling is known to interfere with protein kinase activation and with its signaling after reovirus infection. This allows the reovirus to continue to replicate in tumor cells and spare normal tissues. Such replication induces a specific cytopathic effect in malignant cells. Genetically engineered viruses and inherently antitumor-selective viruses have been tested in early clinical trials and are awaiting studies to determine their effectiveness in specific types of cancer. Virotherapy, in combination with standard chemotherapy, has the potential to further increase the antitumor activity of oncolytic virotherapy in a synergistic manner.

Diseases Treated by Gene Therapy
Inherited Immunodeficiency

More than 30 patients reported to date worldwide have undergone treatment with different retroviral vectors for inherited immunodeficiencies (Chapter 258). Patients with one of the following three diseases are included in this group: two types of severe combined immunodeficiency (SCID), both of which are characterized by dysregulation of lymphocyte development, and X-linked chronic granulomatous disease (X-CGD), an inherited immune deficiency with absent phagocyte reduced nicotinamide adenine diphosphate (NADPH) oxidase activity caused by mutations in the *gp91* (*phox*) gene. Individuals with adenosine deaminase (ADA) SCID suffer from premature death of T, B, and natural killer (NK) cells as a result of the accumulation of purine metabolites; patients with this condition have been treated with vectors expressing the *ADA* gene. In the first patients with ADA SCID, transduced T cells expressing transgenic *ADA* have been shown to persist for longer than 10 years; however, the therapeutic effect of gene therapy resulted in incomplete correction of the metabolic defect. More recently, an improved gene transfer protocol of bone marrow CD34-positive cells, combined with low-dose busulfan, resulted in multilineage, stable engraftment of transduced progenitors at substantial levels, restoration of immune function, correction of the *ADA* metabolic defect, and proven clinical benefit. Overall, no adverse effect or toxicity has been observed in patients treated with *ADA* gene transfer in mature lymphocytes or hematopoietic progenitors.

The X-linked type (X-SCID group), in which there is defective cytokine-dependent survival signaling in T and NK cells, was shown to be corrected by introduction of the wild-type sequence of the common γ-C chain, which is an essential component of five cytokine receptors. In one clinical study, hematologic malignancies developed in four patients. One of the four died of this complication. A group of ten patients treated with a different viral transduction protocol were successfully treated, with one reported malignancy in up to 8 years of follow-up. Two adult X-CGD patients who suffered recurrent bacterial infections have been treated with CD34-positive cells transduced with a gammaretroviral vector expressing *gp91 phox*, with significant clinical improvement in the short term. However, in both of these patients, there was an expansion of gene-transduced cells caused by the transcriptional activation of growth-promoting genes leading to myelodysplasia and gradual loss of efficacy.

In summary, of the close to 30 patients worldwide treated with gene therapy for immunodeficiency disorders, significant clinical improvement has been observed in many. However, severe and even life-endangering adverse consequences have been encountered with certain viral vectors and protocols. Additional clinical information from long-term observation and new clinical studies will be important for a clearer assessment of clinical benefit.

Hematologic Disorders

Additional inherited diseases treated in recent years with gene therapy have included mostly hematologic conditions in which a low amount of a secreted protein could reverse the clinical phenotype, and partial success has been achieved in various inherited bleeding disorders. However, the response has not usually been sustained or has been accompanied by adverse reactions, such as increases in hepatic enzymes in the case of hepatic artery administration.

Cardiovascular and Pulmonary Conditions

The most common cardiovascular-related syndromes are related to atherosclerotic arterial occlusive disease. To overcome arterial occlusions, especially when conventional treatments fail to improve blood supply to the ischemic organs, therapeutic angiogenesis has been advocated as a therapeutic option. Transfer of genes encoding angiogenic growth factors (vascular endothelial growth factor and fibroblast growth factor), delivered by nonviral and viral vectors, has been tested in phase II and III studies in patients with coronary and peripheral arterial disease.

Cystic Fibrosis

Experimental protocols for gene therapy for cystic fibrosis (CF) (Chapter 89) have been implemented since 1990. The cystic fibrosis transmembrane conductance regulator (CFTR) protein is mutated in patients with CF. Transducing the epithelium of the nasal and bronchial tree is potentially feasible through nonsystemic approaches. Nonviral gene therapy methods that deliver a copy of the *CFTR* gene to the airway of CF patients have been developed. Several placebo-controlled clinical trials of liposome-mediated *CFTR* gene transfer to the nasal epithelium have confirmed its safety and demonstrated variable degrees of functional correction.**1** In addition, several clinical studies have assessed the potential of retrovectors, adenovectors, and AAV vectors for gene therapy for CF.**2,3** With both nonviral and viral delivery systems, there were only mild side effects. However, the long-term clinical benefit has been marginal. Improved vectors are being assessed in preclinical studies.

Cancer

Gene therapy approaches to treatment of cancer have been based on perturbation of pathways in the tumorigenesis process (Chapter 185), which has led to diverse anticancer gene therapy approaches.

Tumor-Specific Expression of Anticancer Proteins

Certain promoters are activated in many types of tumors (e.g., human telomerase or survivin), whereas others are activated in specific types of tumors (probasin in prostate cancer, ceruloplasmin in ovarian cancer, HER2 in breast cancer, carcinoembryonic antigen in colon cancer). Targeting of tumor-specific promoters constitutes a rational basis for anticancer therapeutics, which may fall into different categories, including cellular proteins that are involved in apoptosis or antiproliferation, or both (e.g., p53, Fas, p202, E1A, and BAX). Their expression induces tumor-specific killing. The most clinically advanced gene therapy drug against cancer is the RD adenovector expressing the human *p53* gene. This therapy (Gendicine) is approved in China for the treatment of patients with head and neck squamous cell carcinoma by direct administration into the tumor bed. According to the results emanating from China**4** and clinical phase III studies in the United States, this treatment has therapeutic benefits. Additionally, the use of suicide genes is one of the most promising approaches for cancer gene therapy.

DNA Vaccines

Human clinical trials using DNA vaccines against cancer (as well as infectious diseases) have been conducted in the past several years. Although these studies have consistently demonstrated the safety of such DNA vaccines, the resultant immunologic responses have not been encouraging, including lack of or low antibody response detected in most cases and somewhat weak cellular response in some trials. Disappointing results were also reported with the use of DNA vaccines against HIV and other infectious agents. However, new methods are currently being assessed for DNA vaccination, such as electroporation and new generations of gene guns. Tumor gene knockdown has been used in many different clinical studies. This approach involves the use of antisense oligonucleotides (ASOs) to target genes involved in cancer progression. ASOs inhibit translation through a mechanism that involves the formation of an mRNA-ASO duplex, which leads to RNase-H-mediated cleavage of the target mRNA. The disappointing lack of clinical efficacy for some first-generation ASOs indicates that challenges remain to be confronted and overcome.

RNA Interference

RNA interference regulates gene expression by a highly precise mechanism of sequence-directed gene silencing at the stage of translation by degrading specific messenger RNAs or by blocking its translation into protein. Research into the use of RNAi for therapeutic applications has gained considerable momentum. It has been suggested that many of the novel disease-associated targets that have been identified are amenable to conventional small molecule drug blockade and can potentially be targeted with RNAi. In the coming years, the concept of RNAi will be actively translated into a therapeutic option, with numerous phase I and II trials currently being conducted. Local and systemic approaches of delivery are under development.

Gene Therapy Ethics and Regulation

There are major differences in the ethical issues pertaining to somatic as opposed to germline gene therapy. In most countries, germline gene therapy, because of its potential effect on future generations, is appropriately outlawed. Our limited understanding of the complex interactions that have shaped human evolution, together with societal and cultural considerations, precludes the possibility of conceiving of responsible programs for germline genetic modifications in humans, as well as germline gene therapy approaches. However, somatic gene therapy is encouraged and performed worldwide under strict regulatory authority with remarkable congruency of guidelines in different countries and global constituencies. The concept that gene therapies constitute novel biologic drugs provides an appropriate framework for regulatory oversight.

Future Directions

In recent years, the genetic payload/transgene and delivery systems have experienced significant improvements. Rapid advances in understanding the molecular underpinnings of pathogenetic processes have facilitated translation to novel biologically based therapeutics, including gene therapy approaches. The major developments in recent years have been in the design of new types of transgenes. The discovery of RNAi (see E-Fig. 43-1) and the biogenesis and potential role of siRNA, including their apparent efficiency in the knockdown of gene expression, suggests that these developments will revolutionize gene therapy in the coming years. Viral infections still pose a major threat to humanity. Because viruses are developing resistance to the current available therapies, there is an ongoing battle between the viruses and our ability to develop novel strategies to fight them. In vitro and in vivo experiments demonstrate the effectiveness of RNAi in inhibiting many viruses that cause severe health and economic problems, including respiratory syncytial, hepatitis C, and influenza viruses.

The tragic occurrence of tumors in patients after retroviral vector-based treatment of X-SCID has motivated researchers to direct the integration of transgenes to specific human genomic sites. It is hoped that assessment of these transgene insertion navigation tools will reduce the random occurrence of insertional mutagenic events. In addition to the development of novel transgenes, there is progress with viral and nonviral vectors. The AAV vector has experienced significant improvement as a delivery system in recent years because of its capacity for targeting with different capsid serotypes and more efficient production, and this has resulted in high-level AAV transgene expression early after transduction. The lentivectors are safer now than in earlier generations and will be the subject of newly planned clinical trials.

1. Lee T, Southern KW. Topical cystic fibrosis transmembrane conductance regulator gene replacement for cystic fibrosis-related lung disease. *Cochrane Database Syst Rev.* 2007;18:CD005599.
2. Moss RB, Milla C, Colombo J, et al. Repeated aerosolized AAV-CFTR for treatment of cystic fibrosis: a randomized placebo-controlled phase 2B trial. *Hum Gene Ther.* 2007;18:726-732.
3. Moss RB, Rodman D, Spencer LT, et al. Repeated adeno-associated virus serotype 2 aerosol-mediated cystic fibrosis transmembrane regulator gene transfer to the lungs of patients with cystic fibrosis: a multicenter, double-blind, placebo-controlled trial. *Chest.* 2004;125:509-521.
4. Zhang SW, Xiao SW, Liu CQ. Recombinant adenovirus-p53 gene therapy combined with radiotherapy for head and neck squamous-cell carcinoma. *Zhonghua Zhong Liu Za Zhi.* 2005;27:426-428.

SUGGESTED READINGS

Aiuti A, Cattaneo F, Galimberti S, et al. Gene therapy for immunodeficiency due to adenosine deaminase deficiency. *N Engl J Med.* 2009;360:447-458. *Gene therapy, combined with reduced-intensity conditioning, can be a safe and effective treatment for SCID in patients with ADA deficiency.*

Castanotto D, Rossi JJ. The promises and pitfalls of RNA-interference-based therapeutics. *Nature.* 2009;457:426-433. *The ability of short RNA sequences to modulate gene expression has provided a powerful tool with which to study gene function and is set to revolutionize the treatment of disease.*

Daley GQ. Stem cells: roadmap to the clinic. *J Clin Invest.* 2010;120:8-10. *Introduces a series of articles providing a balanced and realistic perspective on some of the major advances that might lead to clinical applications of stem cells in regenerative medicine.*

Davies JC, Alton EW. Gene therapy for cystic fibrosis. *Proc Am Thorac Soc.* 2010;7:408-414. *Review.*

Hyun I. The bioethics of stem cell research and therapy. *J Clin Invest.* 2010;120:71-75. *Consideration of the bioethics of human stem cell research taking into account recent scientific developments.*

Katz MG, Swain JD, Tomasulo CE, et al. Current strategies for myocardial gene delivery. *J Mol Cell Cardiol.* 2011;50:766-776. *Review.*

Kitchen SG, Zack JA. Stem cell-based approaches to treating HIV infection. *Curr Opin HIV AIDS.* 2011;6:68-73. *Review of recent trials.*

Maguire AM, High KA, Auricchio A, et al. Age-dependent effects of RPE65 gene therapy for Leber's congenital amaurosis: a phase 1 dose-escalation trial. *Lancet.* 2009;374:1597-1605. *Gene therapy has the potential to reverse disease or prevent further deterioration of vision in patients with otherwise incurable inherited retinal degeneration.*

Parmacek MS, Epstein JA. Cardiomyocyte renewal. *N Engl J Med.* 2009;361:86-88. *Thoughtful review indicating that progress toward regenerative therapy for heart disease should be based on a sound formulation of cardiac cell and developmental biology.*

VII

PRINCIPLES OF IMMUNOLOGY AND INFLAMMATION

44

THE INNATE AND ADAPTIVE IMMUNE SYSTEMS

JÖRG J. GORONZY AND CORNELIA M. WEYAND

GENERAL PRINCIPLES OF THE IMMUNE SYSTEM

The immune system has evolved as a complex network of molecules, cells, and organs to defend against pathogenic microorganisms and noninfectious foreign substances. Beyond its role in host protection, it regulates tissue homeostasis and tissue repair. Cells of the immune system identify and remove injured, dead, and malignant cells. Immune system cells derive from hematopoietic stem cells in the bone marrow, circulate in the blood and lymph, form complex microstructures in specialized lymphoid organs, and infiltrate virtually every tissue. These cells express characteristic profiles of surface molecules, also referred to as *cluster of differentiation* (CD) molecules, with which they sense soluble or cell-bound ligands in their microenvironment. Molecular structure, ligands, and main functions of more than 300 molecules have been defined; a selected list is given in E-Table 44-1. The anatomic organization of immune system cells in lymphoid organs and their ability to circulate throughout the body and to migrate between blood and lymphoid tissues are crucial components of host defense. On activation, these cells transcribe and release cytokines, small soluble proteins that communicate between cells within the immune system or between immune system cells and cells in other tissues (Table 44-1).

Innate and Adaptive Immunity

Principally, host protection is accomplished by two types of immunity: innate and adaptive. The *innate immune system* is present in all vertebrates and is widely conserved among species. It provides the first line of defense and functions through immediate responses that use preformed proteins and pre-existing cells. *Innate immunity,* broadly defined, includes physical barriers, such as epithelial layers, and chemical impediments, such as antimicrobial substances at these surfaces. Using a narrower definition, the innate immune system mediates nonspecific protection through a diverse set of cells, including monocytes, macrophages, dendritic cells, natural killer (NK) cells, eosinophils, basophils, neutrophils, and mast cells. A variety of chemical mediators, such as members of the complement system, acute phase reactants, and cytokines, contribute to inflammatory responses that develop to prevent tissue invasion by pathogens. The need for immediacy is irreconcilable with selectivity and adaptivity. Response patterns of the innate immune system are broad, and collateral tissue damage is often unavoidable. Despite the lack of specificity, innate immunity is highly effective; microbial invasion is frequently controlled, and pathogens are often eliminated. The pathogenicity of microorganisms is largely related to their ability to resist and overcome the first line of defense mounted by the innate immune system.

If invading microorganisms succeed in escaping the host's nonspecific defense mechanisms, a second line of defense, *adaptive immunity,* secures host survival. Adaptive immune responses depend on innate immunity for supplementation and augmentation and to provide crucial information about the nature of the attacker. The term *adaptive* relates to the ability of the system to adapt to the microbial challenge; it is also called *acquired* or *specific immunity.* The adaptive immune system has unique attributes, such as specificity, diversity, memory, specialization, tolerance, and homeostasis.

Immune specificity relies on two major cell types: B lymphocytes and T lymphocytes. These cells possess receptors that specifically recognize antigenic determinants and that distinguish subtle differences. To contend with the gamut of possible antigens, the adaptive immune system requires an enormous spectrum of specific receptors. An extremely high degree of discriminatory specificity is achieved by clonal distribution of the recognition structures; each individual T cell and B cell expresses a unique receptor.

The diversity of the adaptive immune system is not inherited; it is acquired somatically and is called the *lymphocyte repertoire.* The frequency of T or B cells in the naïve repertoire specific for a particular antigenic determinant is less than 1 in 10^5 and is therefore extremely low. On recognition of an antigen, the adaptive immune system reacts with clonal expansion of these infrequent antigen-responsive cells to build up a line of defense. Proliferating antigen-specific cells acquire new properties, including effector functions and the ability to function as memory cells. Specificity and memory are prerequisites for heightened reactivity to recurrent or persistent infections and also provide the basis for vaccination. Another example of the adaptive power of the specific immune system lies in specialized responses to different classes of microbes (e.g., parasites vs. viral infections). Specialization is a consequence of differentiation during the evolution of the immune response; it results in selection of the most appropriate effector pathway for a particular microbial challenge.

Molding the responding lymphocyte population to the antigenic profile of the invading pathogen inevitably involves the risk of generating cells that respond to self-antigens. To prevent injury to the host, the adaptive immune system discriminates between self and nonself. Nonreactivity to self is actively acquired and is maintained by several mechanisms, collectively called *self-tolerance.* Distinguishing self and nonself is individualized for each host and requires the selection of an individual set of nonself-reactive receptors. Consequently, the outcome of self/nonself discrimination is not transferred from generation to generation and is devoid of evolutionary pressure. In contrast, innate immunity relies on genetically programmed recognition structures and receptors that have been evolutionarily selected to recognize pathogens but not self.

Together with the capability of generating tremendous diversity and specificity, the adaptive immune system has a built-in ability to self-limit responses and to regain homeostasis. This mechanism is crucial in preventing excessive immune responses and in providing space for emerging lymphocytes that are required for a new specific immune response.

Leukocyte Migration and Homing

Mobility of the cellular constituents is fundamental to innate and adaptive immunity. To home to the site of tissue injury or to enter lymphoid organs, cells use a multistep process of adherence and activation. Initially, leukocytes roll on activated endothelial cells, activate chemokine receptors, increase adhesiveness, and eventually migrate through the endothelial layer across a chemokine gradient. The selectin family of proteins mediates the first steps of leukocyte migration. Selectins have a lectin domain and bind to carbohydrate ligands. L-selectin is present on virtually all leukocytes; P-selectin and E-selectin are expressed on activated endothelial cells, and P-selectin is also stored in platelets. Selectins capture floating leukocytes and initiate their attachment and rolling on activated endothelial cells. To transform attachment and rolling into firm adhesion, the concerted action of chemokines, chemokine receptors, and integrins is necessary. Integrins are heterodimers formed of many different α chains and β chains; different α/β combinations are expressed on different cell subsets. Only after activation can integrins interact with ligands on endothelial cells. Activation involves modification of the cytoplasmic domain of the β chain, which leads to a structural change of the extracellular domains. This process is termed *inside-out signaling.* The last step of homing is transendothelial migration. Here, the firmly attached leukocytes migrate through the endothelial cell monolayer and the basement membrane.

INNATE IMMUNE SYSTEM

Principles of Innate Immune System Activation

Activation by Pattern Recognition Receptors

The strategy of the innate immune system is to focus on the recognition of a few highly conserved structures that are preserved in large groups of microorganisms shared by entire classes of pathogens and essential for their survival and pathogenicity. The system uses a few hundred receptor structures to identify microbial invaders. This set of receptors is insufficient to cover the entire spectrum of antigens expressed on infectious agents. Structures recognized by pattern recognition receptors (PRRs) are collectively referred to as *pathogen-associated molecular patterns* (PAMPs). Examples of PAMPs are bacterial lipopolysaccharides, peptidoglycans, mannans, bacterial DNA, double-stranded RNA, and glucans.

PAMP-binding receptor families share structural characteristics, such as leucine-rich repeated domains, calcium-dependent lectin domains, and scavenger-receptor protein domains. They can be secreted to act as opsonins; the best-characterized receptor of this class is the mannose-binding lectin that binds to microbial carbohydrates and activates the lectin pathway of complement activation. Another functional class of PRRs is expressed on the

TABLE 44-1 CYTOKINES AND CYTOKINE FUNCTION

CYTOKINES	MAJOR PRODUCER CELLS	PRINCIPAL ACTION
HEMATOPOIETIN FAMILY		
IL-2	T cells	Proliferation of T cells, B cells, and NK cells
IL-3	T cells	Early hematopoiesis
IL-4	T cells, mast cells	B-cell activation, IgE switch, inhibition of T_H1 cells
IL-5	T cells, mast cells	Eosinophil growth and differentiation
IL-6	Macrophages, endothelial cells	T-cell and B-cell growth and differentiation, induction of acute phase proteins
IL-7	Bone marrow, thymic epithelium	Growth of pre-B cells and pre-T cells
IL-9	T cells	Stimulation of mast cells and T_H2 cells
IL-11	Stromal fibroblasts	Hematopoiesis
IL-13	T cells	B-cell growth and differentiation, inhibition of T_H1 cells and macrophages
G-CSF	Fibroblasts and monocytes	Neutrophil development and differentiation
IL-15	Non-T cells	Growth of T cells and NK cells
GM-CSF	Macrophages, T cells	Growth and differentiation of myelomonocytic lineage cells
INTERFERON FAMILY		
IFN-α	Leukocytes	Antiviral; increases MHC class I expression
IFN-β	Fibroblasts	Antiviral; increases MHC class I expression
IFN-γ	T cells, NK cells	Macrophage activation; increases expression of MHC molecules, Ig class switching, inhibition of T_H2 cells
TNF FAMILY		
TNF-α	Macrophages, NK cells, T cells	Induction of pro-inflammatory cytokines, endothelial cell activation, apoptosis
TNF-β (LT-α)	T cells, B cells	Cell death, endothelial activation, lymphoid organ development
LT-β	T cells, B cells	Cell death, lymphoid organ development
OTHERS		
TGF-β	Monocytes, T cells	Anti-inflammatory; inhibits cell growth, induces IgA secretion
IL-1α, IL-1β	Macrophages, endothelial cells	Acute phase response, fever, macrophage activation, costimulation
IL-10	T cells, macrophages	Suppression of macrophage functions
IL-12	Macrophages, dendritic cells	NK cell activation, T_H1 cell differentiation
IL-16	T cells, mast cells, eosinophils	Chemoattractant for CD4 T cells, monocytes, and eosinophils
IL-17	CD4 memory cells	Cytokine production by epithelia, endothelia, and fibroblasts
IL-18	Macrophages	IFN-γ production by T cells and NK cells
IL-23	Macrophages, dendritic cells	T_H17 cell differentiation

CD = cluster of differentiation; G-CSF = granulocyte colony-stimulating factor; GM-CSF = granulocyte-macrophage colony-stimulating factor; IFN = interferon; Ig = immunoglobulin; IL = interleukin; LT = lymphotoxin; MHC = major histocompatibility complex; NK = natural killer; TGF = transforming growth factor; T_H = helper T lymphocyte; TNF = tumor necrosis factor.

surface of phagocytes and facilitates endocytosis. The macrophage mannose receptor and the macrophage scavenger receptor are the best-known examples. These receptors are essential for the clearance of microbes from the circulation. A third class of PRRs controls cell activation (Fig. 44-1); the most important members are toll-like receptors (TLRs). TLRs are expressed on either the cell membrane or the endosome to sense extra- or intracellular pathogens. They function by regulating the activity of nuclear factor-κB (NF-κB) and interferon signaling pathways and control the expression of many inflammatory cytokines and cell surface molecules. Prominent members of the TLR family are TLR4, which, in conjunction with other cell surface molecules, binds bacterial lipopolysaccharides; TLR2, which recognizes bacterial peptidoglycans and lipoproteins; and TLR9, which binds to bacterial DNA motifs.

PRRs used by the innate immune system are fundamentally different from the antigen-specific receptors generated in the adaptive immune system. The receptors of the innate immune system are encoded in the germline and are under evolutionary pressure. They are shared by many different cells, including macrophages and dendritic cells, and are not clonally distributed (i.e., different cell types display identical specificity). Finally, PRRs do not recognize self, so they do not carry the risk for autoimmune injury, although exceptions to this rule (e.g., recognition of heat shock proteins) have been described.

Regulation by Major Histocompatibility Complex Class I–Recognizing Receptors

Several cells of the innate immune system require reversal of inhibition to enter the activation cycle. Loss of inhibitory signals in constitutively activated cells is particularly important for NK cells. NK cells are poised to attack, but they are held in check by inhibitory receptors that recognize major histocompatibility complex (MHC) class I or MHC class I–like molecules. The observation that NK cells kill target cells lacking MHC class I molecules led to the

missing-self hypothesis. The principle that immune cells are kept in check by recognizing self-determinants is appreciated now as fundamental in the immune system.

Provision of negative signals is closely linked to the recognition of MHC class I molecules. Currently, three types of MHC class I–recognizing receptors are known. C-type lectin receptors (CD159) recognizing human leukocyte antigen E (HLA-E) and killer immunoglobulin-like receptors (CD158) specific for HLA-C and, to a lesser extent, HLA-A and HLA-B are expressed predominantly on NK cells. Immunoglobulin-like transcript receptors (CD85) are more widely expressed. Immunoglobulin-like transcript receptor 2 is expressed on NK cells, B cells, monocytes, dendritic cells, and macrophages. Immunoglobulin-like transcript receptors 3 and 4 are encountered on monocytes, dendritic cells, and macrophages. By screening cell surfaces for the expression of MHC class I molecules, the innate immune system collects information about the intactness of tissues, emphasizing the crucial role of MHC class I molecules as markers of tissue integrity. Recognition of MHC class I molecules provides a negative signal that suppresses cell activity. However, all receptor families also include stimulatory isoforms that mediate an activating signal. The balance between these opposing signals is finely tuned, ultimately determining whether innate immunity is initiated.

Activation by Fc Receptors

Most cells of the innate immune system possess immunoglobulin crystallizable fragment (Fc) receptors (FcRs) and can bind antibodies attached to antigens (see Fig. 44-1). FcRs specifically interact with the constant region (Fc portion) of immunoglobulins. Each member of the FcR family displays specificity for one or a few immunoglobulin isotypes. The isotype of the antibody determines which cell type is activated in a given response. Triggering of most FcRs transmits activating signals; however, inhibitory FcRs do exist. Phagocytic cells, such as neutrophils and macrophages, are equipped with FcγRs that are activated by immunoglobulin G (IgG) antibodies,

FIGURE 44-1. Activation pathways in the innate immune system. Cells of the innate immune system recognize microorganisms and tissue damage caused by either infection or malignancy. Dendritic cells and monocytes/macrophages use a multitude of receptors to sense constituents of pathogens—often bacterial molecules common to many classes of microorganisms—and respond to cytokines and endogenous stimulators released from injured cells. Binding of complement factors can also trigger cell activation. Self-recognition of major histocompatibility complex (MHC) class I molecules by natural killer (NK) cells can deliver positive or negative signals. Lack of MHC class I molecules on the target cell surface activates NK cells to kill the target. IFN = interferon; IL = interleukin; TNF = tumor necrosis factor.

particularly IgG1. Ligation of an FcγR triggers phagocytosis of the antigen, activation of respiratory burst, and induction of cytotoxicity. On NK cells, FcγRs initiate antibody-dependent cell-mediated cytotoxicity. In this process, the cytolytic machinery of NK cells is triggered by the binding of IgG1-coated or IgG3-coated target cells. FcRs on mast cells, basophils, and activated eosinophils are specific for IgE. In contrast to other FcRs, they bind monomeric antibody molecules with extremely high affinity. Cross-linking of the constitutively cell surface–bound IgE induces cell activation and the release of cytoplasmic granules.

Activation by Cytokines
Generally, cells of the innate immune system are exquisitely sensitive to the action of cytokines. Cytokines are soluble, low-molecular-weight glycoproteins that derive from many tissue sources. They are chemical messengers that convey information between cells, regulate the differentiation of effector cells, and modulate immune responses. Important examples of cytokine-mediated signals in the innate immune system are interferon-γ (IFN-γ), produced by NK cells, which is the most potent activator of macrophages; interleukin-6 (IL-6), which induces acute phase reactants; IL-12, IL-23, and IL-27, derived from macrophages and dendritic cells, which coordinate the development of adaptive immune responses; IL-15, which regulates the activity and proliferation of NK cells; and type I IFN secreted at the time of injury, which activates NK cells and dendritic cells (see Fig. 44-1).

Cellular Elements of the Innate Immune System
Monocytes and Macrophages
Monocytes circulate in the peripheral blood with a half-life of 1 to 3 days. Macrophages arise from monocytes that have migrated out of the circulation and have proliferated and differentiated in tissue. Tissue macrophages are common in lymphoid organs, but they are also present in connective tissues, such as the perivascular space, and in the lining of serous cavities (pleura and peritoneum). Specialized macrophages include alveolar macrophages in the lung, Kupffer cells in the liver, osteoblasts in bone, microglia in the central nervous system, and type A synoviocytes in the synovial membrane. Macrophages are activated through the triggering of PRRs or FcRs, and they respond

vigorously to IFN-γ (see Fig. 44-1). They secrete myriad products, including hydrolytic enzymes, reactive oxygen species, cytokines (tumor necrosis factor-α [TNF-α], IL-1, IL-6, IL-10, IL-12, IL-15, and IL-18), and chemokines. They phagocytose and expose the engulfed microorganism to a wide range of toxic intracellular molecules, including reactive oxygen species, nitric oxide, antimicrobial cationic proteins and peptides, and lysosomal enzymes. In addition to attacking microbial organisms, macrophages remove dying and dead host cells. They recognize molecules expressed on apoptotic cells and eliminate them without initiating an inflammatory response. Finally, they play a crucial role in the recruitment of adaptive immune responses. After capturing antigen, they function as antigen-presenting cells for T lymphocytes. In this function, however, they are less important than dendritic cells.

Dendritic Cells/Langerhans Cells
Dendritic cells represent the major cell type linking the innate and adaptive immune systems. Their primary function is the presentation of antigens to T cells. They are the only cell type that can activate naïve T cells and initiate adaptive immune responses. Two major lineages of dendritic cells exist: myeloid and plasmacytoid dendritic cells. When positioned in the skin, myeloid dendritic cells are referred to as *Langerhans cells*. They constantly endocytose and digest extracellular molecules but usually do not display these molecules at a sufficient density to activate T cells. On receiving a stimulatory signal, they convert into highly efficient antigen-presenting cells. Activation signals can derive from PAMPs or from host cells that react to injury and secrete mediators such as TNF-α or heat shock proteins (see Fig. 44-1). Activation causes dendritic cells to change their expression profile of chemokine receptors and to migrate from the local tissue to lymph nodes. In parallel, they begin expressing accessory molecules on their cell surface, a prerequisite for T-cell activation, and to secrete cytokines (e.g., IFN-α by plasmacytoid dendritic cells, or IL-12 and IL-23 by myeloid dendritic cells) that orchestrate T-cell differentiation. When they arrive in the T-cell zone of the lymph node, they display MHC–peptide complexes with peptides derived from endocytosed and digested antigens. With high surface expression of MHC and accessory molecules, dendritic cells optimize the process of antigen presentation and T-cell priming (Fig. 44-2).

FIGURE 44-2. Interface between the innate and adaptive immune systems. Dendritic cells (DCs) reside in the tissue, where they recognize and ingest antigens. If they also receive an activating signal (e.g., by binding pathogen-associated molecular patterns or cytokines), they enter lymph vessels and travel to regional lymph nodes. In parallel, they mature into efficient antigen-presenting cells that express high levels of cell surface major histocompatibility complex (MHC) and costimulatory molecules. In the T-cell zones, DCs present the antigen engulfed in the peripheral tissue to prime naïve T cells. By capturing and transporting antigens and priming naïve T cells, DCs integrate responses of the innate and adaptive immune systems. HEV = high endothelial venules.

Natural Killer Cells

NK cells provide the first line of defense against viral infections and other intracellular pathogens while adaptive responses are generated. NK cells are sensitized by cytokines released from macrophages and dendritic cells. They function by secreting cytokines, mainly IFN-γ, which activate macrophages and other cells. They also are poised to kill virus-infected cells. NK cells induce apoptosis of the target cells by injecting pore-forming enzymes and granzymes. One of the interesting features of NK biology is the activation of these lymphocytes when MHC class I molecules on target cells are lost (see Fig. 44-1). NK cells are important in tumor surveillance because they are able to kill MHC class I–deficient tumor cells that are no longer susceptible to adaptive immune responses.

Neutrophils, Eosinophils, and Basophils
Neutrophils

Neutrophils are the most abundant circulating white blood cells. They are recruited rapidly to inflammatory sites and are capable of phagocytosing and digesting microbes. Activation of neutrophils and phagocytosis is facilitated through the triggering of FcRs or complement receptors. During phagocytosis, the pathogen is first surrounded by the phagocyte membrane, and then internalized in membrane-bound vesicles known as *phagosomes*. Phagosomes fuse with lysosomes, which contain enzymes, proteins, and peptides that inactivate and digest microbes. Beyond their phagocytic capability, neutrophils produce a variety of toxic products. The release of toxic products is known as the *respiratory burst* because it is accompanied by an increase in oxygen consumption. During the respiratory burst, oxygen radicals are generated by lysosomal reduced nicotinamide adenine dinucleotide phosphate (NADPH) oxidases. Neutrophils are short-lived cells, dying soon after they have been activated. Secretion of their granule products, in particular enzymes (myeloperoxidase, elastase, collagenase, and lysozyme), causes direct cellular injury and damages macromolecules at inflamed sites.

Eosinophils

In contrast to macrophages and neutrophils, eosinophils (Chapter 173) are only weakly phagocytic. They are potent cytotoxic effector cells against parasites. Their major effector mechanism is the secretion of various cationic proteins (major basic protein, eosinophil cationic protein, and eosinophil-derived neurotoxin). These proteins are released into the extracellular space,

where they directly destroy the invading microorganism, but they can also damage host tissue.

Basophils

Basophils and tissue mast cells are important reservoirs of inflammatory mediators such as histamines, prostaglandins, leukotrienes, and selected cytokines. Basophils and tissue mast cells have high-affinity receptors for monomeric IgE. They play a role in atopic allergies, in which allergens bind immunoglobulin (IgE) and cross-link FcεRs. Their function in normal immune responses is incompletely understood.

Soluble Factors in Innate Defenses

Effector functions of the cells of the innate immune system are enhanced by many circulating proteins. A particularly important contribution derives from the complement system, a group of plasma enzymes and regulatory proteins that are converted from inactive pro-enzymes to active enzymes in a controlled and systematic cascade, which is crucial in linking microbial recognition to cellular effector function (Chapter 47). Mannose-binding lectin circulates in the plasma, functioning as an opsonin, and is involved in activation of the complement pathway. C-reactive protein, an acute phase protein, participates in opsonization by binding to bacterial phospholipids. Finally, the innate immune system could not work without the cytokines that regulate the recruitment and activation of leukocytes (see Table 44-1). Cells of the innate immune system are not only the principal producers of such cytokines but also their targets.

● ADAPTIVE IMMUNE SYSTEM

Principles of Adaptive Immune System Activation: Recognition of Antigen
Structure of Antigen-Specific Receptors

The innate immune system recognizes structural patterns that are common in the microbial world, whereas the adaptive immune system is designed to respond to the entire continuum of antigens. This goal is achieved through two principal types of antigen recognition receptors: antibodies and T-cell receptors (TCRs). Antibodies are expressed as cell surface receptors on B cells or are secreted. They recognize conformational structures formed by the tertiary configuration of proteins. In contrast, α/β TCRs fit specifically to epitopes formed by a small linear peptide embedded into MHC molecules on the surface of antigen-presenting cells.

Antibodies consist of two identical heavy chains and two identical light chains, which are covalently linked by disulfide bonds. The amino (N)-terminal domain of each chain is variable and represents the recognition structure that interacts with the antigen. Each antibody has two binding arms of identical specificity. The carboxy (C)-terminal ends of the heavy and light chains form the constant region, which defines the subclass of the antibody (κ or λ for light chains; IgM, IgA, IgD, IgE, or IgG for heavy chains). Additional subclasses can be distinguished for IgG and IgA. The constant region of antibodies includes the Fc region. Fc regions can polymerize (IgA) or pentamerize in the presence of a J (joining) chain (IgM). Fc regions are also the ligand for the FcRs on cells of the innate immune system.

TCRs are dimers of α chains and β chains or of γ chains and δ chains, each of which contains three complementary-determining binding sites in the N-terminal domain. These complementary-determining sites define the specificity. α/β TCRs exclusively recognize peptide fragments in the context of MHC molecules. γ/δ TCRs are more variable and can recognize certain glycolipid antigens in the context of MHC-like molecules or even unprocessed antigens, functioning similar to antibodies. The repertoires of antibodies and TCRs are extremely diverse and have been estimated in the human to account for 10^8 to 10^9 unique (of 10^{15} possible) combinations. This enormous diversity cannot be genetically encoded; it must be acquired. Its foundation consists of fewer than 400 genes that are recombined and modified. Immunoglobulin heavy chains are formed from four gene segments encoded on chromosome 14—the variable, diversity, joining, and constant region gene segments. Also, TCR β chains and δ chains are assembled by the recombination of variable, diversity, joining, and constant region segments of TCR genes. Immunoglobulin light chains and TCR α chains and γ chains lack the diversity segment and are composed of three gene segments. During antibody or TCR rearrangement, gene segments are cut out by nucleases and spliced together at the DNA level to form linear coding units for each receptor gene. Through the combination of several different mechanisms, an enormous diversity of receptors is generated. First, the genome contains multiple forms of gene segments; each receptor or antibody uses a different combination of these gene segments. Second, the splicing process is imprecise, introducing nucleotide variations at the variable-diversity, diversity-joining, and variable-joining junctions. These inaccuracies lead to frame shifts and result in completely different amino acid sequences. Finally, random nucleotides can be inserted at the junctional region by an enzyme, deoxyribonucleotidyl transferase.

Once generated, TCR sequences remain unchanged. This rule does not apply to immunoglobulins, which can undergo editing. Immunoglobulin editing includes replacement of an entire variable region (receptor editing); class switching during immune responses, in which the variable-diversity-joining unit combines with different constant region genes (isotype switching); or somatic hypermutation, in which the antigen contact areas of the antibody undergo mutations during an immune response to improve the affinity (affinity maturation).

Antigen Processing

T cells do not recognize native antigens but rather peptide fragments that are displayed in the context of MHC class I and class II molecules. The two classes of MHC molecules are used as restriction elements by two different subsets of T cells. CD4+ T cells recognize antigen peptides embedded into MHC class II molecules, whereas CD8+ T cells are directed against peptides complexed with MHC class I molecules. Generally, MHC class II molecules are expressed only on specialized antigen-presenting cells, such as dendritic cells, monocytes, macrophages, and B cells. Peptides bound to MHC class II molecules derive from extracellular antigens that are captured and internalized into endosomes to be digested by proteinases, notably cathepsin. Occasionally, intracellular proteins or membrane proteins are also funneled into this pathway. MHC class II molecules are assembled in the endoplasmic reticulum in association with a protein called the *invariant chain* (Fig. 44-3).

The molecules are transported to the endosome, where the invariant chain is removed from the peptide-binding cleft, making the cleft accessible to peptides derived from extracellular proteins. MHC class II molecules, stabilized by peptides of 10 to 30 amino acids, are displayed on the cell surface, where they can be recognized by CD4+ T cells.

MHC class I–associated peptides are produced in the cytosol by the proteosome, a large cytoplasmic multiprotein enzyme complex (see Fig. 44-3). Specialized transporter proteins, called *transporter in antigen processing* (TAP), facilitate translocation from the cytosol to the endoplasmic reticulum. There, the peptides bind to newly formed MHC class I molecules and are transported to the cell surface, where they are recognized by antigen-specific CD8+ T cells.

The nature of the antigen-processing pathway determines the sequence of events in immune responses. Extracellular antigens, in general, enter the endosomal pool and associate with MHC class II molecules to stimulate CD4+ T cells. Cytosolic antigens, including antigens from intracellular infectious agents, are degraded and displayed in the context of MHC class I molecules to initiate CD8+ T-cell responses.

Cellular Elements of the Adaptive Immune System
T Cells
T-Cell Development

T precursor cells are derived from hematopoietic stem cells seeded into the thymus, where all the subsequent stages of T-cell maturation occur (Fig. 44-4). Pre-T cells express two enzymes, recombinase and terminal

FIGURE 44-3. Pathways of antigen processing and delivery to major histocompatibility complex (MHC) molecules. Cytosolic proteins are broken down by the proteosome to generate peptide fragments, which are transported into the endoplasmic reticulum by specialized peptide transporters (TAP). After peptides are bound to MHC class I molecules, MHC-peptide complexes are released from the endoplasmic reticulum and travel to the cell surface, where they are ligands for CD8+ T-cell receptors (TCRs). Extracellular foreign antigens are taken into intracellular vesicles, called *endosomes*. As the pH in the endosomes gradually decreases, proteases are activated that digest antigens into peptide fragments. After fusing with vesicles that contain MHC class II molecules, antigenic peptides are placed in the antigen-binding groove. Loaded MHC class II–peptide complexes are transported to the cell surface, where they are recognized by the TCRs of CD4+ T cells.

FIGURE 44-4. Maturation of T cells in the thymus. Precursors committed to the T-cell lineage arrive in the thymus and begin to rearrange their T-cell receptor (TCR) genes. Immature T cells with receptors binding to self–major histocompatibility complex (MHC) on cortical epithelial cells receive signals for survival (positive selection). At the corticomedullary junction, surviving T cells probe self-antigens presented by dendritic cells and macrophages. T cells reacting strongly to self-antigens are deleted by apoptosis (negative selection). T cells released into the periphery are tolerant toward self and recognize foreign antigens in the context of self-MHC.

deoxynucleotidyl transferase, enabling them to recombine TCR genes. The β chain of the TCR is rearranged first and is expressed together with a pre-TCR α chain. Signals from the immature TCR complex inhibit rearrangement of the second β-chain allele and induce T-cell proliferation and expression of the CD4 and CD8 molecules. Subsequently, the TCR α chain is recombined. From here, the T cell undergoes many differentiation and selection steps modulated by the thymic microenvironment. Early stages of thymocytes reside in the thymic cortex, where they mostly interact with epithelial cells. They then migrate toward the medulla, encountering dendritic cells and macrophages at the corticomedullary junction. Thymic stromal cells regulate T-cell proliferation by secreting lymphopoietic growth factors, such as IL-7. Interactions of the TCR with MHC molecules expressed on epithelial cells and on dendritic cells or macrophages determine the fate of the thymocyte. Low-avidity recognition of peptide-MHC complexes on thymic epithelial cells by the TCR results in positive selection. This recognition event rescues cells from apoptotic cell death and ensures that only T cells with functional receptors survive. Thymocytes that express a receptor not fitting any MHC antigen complex die by neglect. High-affinity interaction between the TCR and peptide-MHC complex induces apoptotic death of the recognizing T cell. This process of negative selection eliminates T cells with specificity for self-antigens and is responsible for central tolerance to many autoantigens. It has been estimated that approximately 1% of thymocytes survive the stringent selection process. While undergoing selection, T cells continue to differentiate, with orderly expression of cell surface molecules. Thymocytes expressing CD4 and CD8 molecules develop into single-positive CD4$^+$ helper T cells that have been selected on MHC class II complexes or CD8$^+$ cytotoxic T cells that are restricted to MHC class I complexes.

T-Cell Stimulation and Accessory Molecules

T-cell activation is initiated when TCR complexes recognize antigenic peptides in the context of the appropriate MHC molecule on the surface of an antigen-presenting cell. Antigen recognition by T cells results in proliferation and differentiation and triggers various effector functions. Stimulation of the TCR is not sufficient and needs to be complemented by the interaction of accessory molecules on the T cell and their ligands on the antigen-presenting cell. A spectrum of accessory molecules is known (see E-Table 44-1). The coreceptors CD4 and CD8 interact with MHC class II and class I molecules and support activation signals through the TCR. Adhesion molecules (integrins) stabilize the interactions between T cells and antigen-presenting cells. Finally, specialized costimulatory molecules provide a second signal in addition to the TCR signal. In the absence of such a second signal, T cells undergo apoptosis or are rendered nonresponsive and anergic.

The best-known and best-studied costimulatory molecule expressed on T cells is the CD28 molecule, which binds to the CD80/CD86 ligands expressed on activated antigen-presenting cells. CD28-mediated signals are mandatory for the expression of many activation markers on the responding T cell and, in particular, for the secretion of IL-2.

Signals from the TCR result in the activation of many genes and entry of the T cell into the cell cycle. The signals are transmitted by a cascade of cytoplasmic events. Cross-linking of the TCR and associated CD3 molecules results in the recruitment and activation of phosphotyrosine kinases and the phosphorylation of molecular constituents of the TCR and various adapter molecules; signals mediated through the TCR activate several biochemical pathways, which collectively lead to the activation of transcription factors that regulate gene expression.

Three major variables determine the outcome of TCR stimulation: the duration and affinity of the TCR-antigen interaction, the maturation stage of the responding T cell, and the nature of the antigen-presenting cell. Antigen-presenting cells are gatekeepers in the initiation of T-cell responses. They can upregulate the expression of accessory molecules that provide costimulatory signals. MHC-peptide complexes are particularly dense on dendritic cells, enabling them to activate naïve T cells. In contrast, memory and effector cells have a lower threshold for activation and can react to antigens presented on peripheral tissue cells.

T-Cell Differentiation and Effector Functions

T-cell activation induces T-cell proliferation, with the goal of clonally selecting and expanding antigen-specific T cells. The extent of clonal proliferation is impressive. Antigen-specific CD8$^+$ T cells expand by a factor of 50,000; CD4$^+$ T cells expand slightly less. During the phase of rapid growth, T cells differentiate from naïve T cells that are essentially devoid of effector functions into effector T cells. The transition into effector cells is associated with

a fundamental shift in functional profiles. First, effector T cells have a lower activation threshold; they do not require costimulation and can scan tissues that lack professional antigen-presenting cells. Second, they switch the expression of chemokine receptors and adhesion molecules to gain access to peripheral tissues. Finally, they gain effector functions. The principal effector function of CD8$^+$ T cells is to lyse antigen-bearing target cells. CD4$^+$ T cells produce many cytokines and express cell surface molecules that are important in the activation of phagocytes and other lymphocytes. CD8$^+$ T cells are committed to differentiating into cytotoxic T cells as they emerge from the thymus; the spectrum of options for CD4$^+$ T cells is larger. Different subsets of CD4$^+$ effector T cells can be distinguished based on the preferential production of certain cytokines (see Table 44-1). T$_H$1 T cells produce predominantly IFN-γ and TNF-α and are involved in cell-mediated immunity, such as delayed-type hypersensitivity reactions. T$_H$2 T cells preferentially produce IL-4, IL-5, and IL-13, cytokines that regulate B-cell responses and the activation of eosinophils. T$_H$17 T cells producing IL-17 and IL-22 induce an intense inflammatory response to eliminate difficult to clear pathogens. Follicular T helper cells home to lymphoid follicles, where they express CD40 ligand (CD154) and secrete IL-21 and other cytokines to provide B-cell help. The decision as to which differentiation pathway to take is made during the early stages of T-cell activation and depends on many factors, including the cytokines produced by cells of the innate immune system in the microenvironment, the nature of costimulatory signals, and the avidity of the TCR–MHC antigen interaction. Lineage development is generally correlated with the expression of specific transcription factors (T-bet for T$_H$1 cells, GATA3 for T$_H$2 cells, or RORγt for T$_H$17 cells). Lineage commitment is not absolute and is not terminal, and transition between different effector types is possible.

Cytotoxic T-cell effector functions are also triggered by antigen recognition by the TCR. On recognizing the appropriate MHC class I–peptide complex, CD8$^+$ T cells induce apoptosis in target cells. The T cell polarizes toward the area of antigen contact; specialized lytic granules are clustered in the contact area. A pore-forming protein, perforin, is released from the lytic granules and inserted into the target cell membrane. Proteases (granzymes) are injected into the target cells to initiate the apoptotic process by activating enzyme cascades. Mechanisms deployed by CD8$^+$ T cells are essentially identical to those of NK cells. CD4$^+$ T cells can also induce apoptosis, but by a different mechanism from CD8$^+$ T cells. Upon activation, they express cell surface molecules such as Fas ligand (CD178) and TRAIL, which initiate the apoptotic cascade selectively in cells expressing the respective ligands Fas (CD95) or the death receptors DR4 and DR5.

Regulatory T Cells

Depending on their cytokine profile, CD4$^+$ T cells have the ability to cross-regulate each other, influence T-cell differentiation, and suppress T-cell effector activity. Classic examples of T cells with regulatory activity cells generated during the normal immune response are IL-10– and transforming growth factor-β (TGF-β)–producing cells. In addition, specialized subsets of regulatory T (Treg) cells are characterized by expression of the transcription factor forkhead box P3 (Foxp3). Naturally occurring Foxp3$^+$ Treg cells are generated during T-cell development in the thymus and recognize self-antigens. Foxp3$^+$ Treg cells can also arise from conventional CD4$^+$ T cells in the periphery. Phenotypically and functionally, natural and inducible Treg cells are indistinguishable; their development and function depend on Foxp3, and they are able to suppress T-cell expansion and constitutively express several cell surface markers. However, none of these markers is specific for Treg, as activated T cells can also express them. Treg cells are important in peripheral tolerance, controlling the expansion of autoreactive T cells, and they also play a role in immune responses to pathogens by virtue of their ability to suppress T-cell effector function. Despite extensive studies in various models, the mechanism by which Treg cells functions in vivo remains poorly understood.

T-Cell Homeostasis

Effective immunity depends on the ability of the immune system to generate large numbers of antigen-specific T cells rapidly, yet the space in the T-cell compartment is limited. To avoid competition for space and resources and to prevent perturbation of T-cell diversity by lifelong exposure to antigens, the adaptive immune system employs several counterbalancing mechanisms. In the later stages of the activation process, a strong negative signal derives from interaction of the T-cell molecule cytotoxic T-lymphocyte antigen (CTLA)-4 (CD152) with CD80/CD86 on antigen-presenting cells. In addition, T cells undergo activation-induced cell death. Activated CD4$^+$ T cells begin to secrete Fas ligand and acquire sensitivity to Fas-mediated death, inducing apoptotic suicide and fratricide in neighboring T cells. These mechanisms impose constraints in the early stages of the T-cell antigen response. Other mechanisms control the rapid decline of expanded antigen-specific T cells when elimination of the antigen has been achieved. Removal of the driving antigen causes a deprivation of cytokines and costimulatory molecules, and growth factor–deprived T cells die from apoptosis. It has been estimated that only 5% of the antigen-expanded population survives after antigen clearance.

B Lymphocytes

B-Cell Development

B cells are generated in the bone marrow. Supported by a specialized microenvironment of nonlymphoid stromal cells, lymphoid stem cells differentiate into distinctive B-lineage cells. Driven by chemokines (stromal cell–derived factor 1) and cytokines (IL-7), precursor B cells enter a process of tightly controlled sequential rearrangements of heavy chain and light chain immunoglobulin genes. On pre-B cells, the membrane μ chain is associated with a surrogate light chain to form a pre-B-cell receptor (BCR). Signals provided through this receptor induce proliferation of a progeny that subsequently rearranges different light chain gene segments.

It is estimated that only 10% of B cells generated in the bone marrow reach the circulating pool. Losses are mostly due to negative selection and clonal deletion of immature B cells that express receptors directed against selfantigens. Cross-linking of surface IgM by multivalent self-antigens causes immature B cells to die. Such self-reactive B cells can be rescued from death by replacing the light chain with a newly rearranged light chain that is no longer self-reactive (receptor editing). On maturation, B cells begin to express surface IgD. B cells positive for IgD and IgM are exported from the bone marrow and seed peripheral lymphoid tissues (Fig. 44-5).

B-Cell Stimulation

Mature B cells are activated by soluble and cell-bound antigens to develop into antibody-secreting effector cells. B cells respond to a large variety of antigens, including proteins, polysaccharides, and lipids. Binding of antigen to cell surface IgM molecules induces BCR clustering. In addition to the antigen-binding immunoglobulin, the BCR comprises two proteins, Ig-α and Ig-β. The Ig-α/Ig-β heterodimer functions to transduce a signal and initiates the intracellular signaling cascade. The composition of the BCR, with a ligand-binding and a signal-transducing unit, and the signaling events that lead to gene induction are similar to those of the TCR. BCR triggering can be enhanced by coreceptors. The coreceptor complex is composed of CD81, CD19, and CD21; CD21 binds to complement fragments on opsonized antigens.

Naïve B cells require accessory signals in addition to triggering of the immunoglobulin receptor. They receive second signals either from helper T cells or from microbial components. Microbial constituents, such as bacterial polysaccharides, can induce antibody production in the absence of helper T cells (thymus-independent antigens). In the case of protein antigens (thymus-dependent antigens), the initial BCR stimulation prepares the cell for subsequent interaction with helper T cells. These activated B cells start to enter the cell cycle; upregulate cell surface molecules, such as CD80 and CD86, that provide costimulatory signals to T cells; and upregulate certain cytokine receptors. These B cells are prepared to activate helper T cells and to respond to cytokines secreted by those T cells, but they cannot differentiate into antibody-producing cells in the absence of T-cell help.

B-Cell Differentiation

Differentiation of antigen-activated B cells depends on interaction with helper T cells. B cells use their antigen receptor not only to recognize antigens but also to internalize them. After processing endocytosed antigens, MHC class II–peptide complexes appear on the cell surface, where antigen-specific CD4$^+$ T cells detect them. Also, B cells express costimulatory molecules and provide optimal conditions for T-cell activation. On activation, CD4$^+$ T cells express CD154 on their surface and are able to stimulate the CD40 molecule on their B-cell partner. CD40-CD154 interaction is essential for subsequent B-cell proliferation and differentiation. Cytokines secreted by the helper T cells act in concert with CD154 to amplify B-cell differentiation and to determine the antibody type by controlling isotype switching. Isotypes greatly influence the versatility of antibodies as effector molecules, and cytokines drive isotype switching by stimulating the transcriptional activation of heavy chain constant region genes. T-cell–dependent B-cell differentiation and maturation take place in germinal centers, specialized structures in secondary lymphoid tissues (see Fig. 44-5). There, the variable regions of B cells are altered by somatic hypermutation, leading to the production of large amounts of high-affinity antibodies. Subsequently, B cells that possess immunoglobulin receptors with high affinity for antigens in the germinal center are selected for survival (affinity maturation).

Lymphocytes and Lymphoid Tissue

The initiation of adaptive immune responses depends on rare antigenspecific T cells and B cells meeting antigen-presenting cells and their relevant antigen. The recognition of a specific antigen in the tissue by uncommon T

FIGURE 44-5. B-cell development and differentiation. The early stages of B-cell development occur in the bone marrow, with cells progressing through a developmental program determined by the rearrangement and expression of immunoglobulin (Ig) genes. Immature B cells with receptors for multivalent self-antigens die in the bone marrow. Surviving B cells coexpress IgD and IgM surface receptors. They are seeded into peripheral lymphoid organs, where they home to selected locations and receive signals to survive and become longer-lived naïve B cells. Antigen-binding B cells and antigen-presenting B cells that receive help from antigen-specific T cells are activated through membrane-bound and secreted molecules. Activated B cells migrate into the follicles, leading to the formation of germinal centers. B cells in germinal centers undergo somatic hypermutation of immunoglobulin genes; cells with high affinity for antigens presented on the surface of follicular dendritic cells are selected to differentiate into either memory B cells or plasma cells.

cells has a low probability, and it is unlikely that sufficient numbers of antigen-presenting cells and lymphocytes can be brought together to provide crucial momentum. The immune system uses specialized lymphoid microstructures to bring antigens to the site of lymphocyte traffic and accumulation. Secondary lymphoid organs include the spleen for blood-borne antigens, the lymph nodes for antigens encountered in peripheral tissues, and the mucosa-associated, bronchial-associated, and gut-associated lymphoid tissues, where antigens from epithelial surfaces are collected. Lymphocytes circulate through secondary lymphoid organs, constantly searching for their antigen. Their homing to secondary lymphoid organs is facilitated by specialized microvessels, called *high endothelial venules*. Secondary lymphoid tissues have developed several strategies to sequester the relevant antigen. Antigens in peripheral tissue are encountered first by dendritic cells that, after activation, are mobilized to transport antigens into the local lymph nodes by the draining lymph. These antigen-bearing dendritic cells enter the lymph nodes through the afferent lymphatic vessel and settle in the T-cell–rich zones to present processed antigens to T cells. The net result of this process is an accumulation and concentration of the antigen in an environment that can be readily screened by infrequent antigen-specific T cells (see Fig. 44-2).

B cells are segregated from T cells in the lymph nodes and are localized in follicles. If B cells find their cooperating T cells, they enter germinal centers. Germinal centers contain a network of follicular dendritic cells that capture particulate antigen or immune complexes on the cell surface. This unprocessed antigen is taken up by antigen-specific B cells, processed and presented, and recognized by antigen-specific T cells. These T cells provide cytokines and cell-cell contact signals to support the germinal center reaction, a process that includes somatic hypermutation, affinity selection, and isotype switching (see Fig. 44-5). Germinal centers are essential for generating antibody-secreting plasma cells and memory B cells.

Lymphoid organ development is highly dependent on environmental cues. The symbiotic relationship between the host immune system and microorganisms is best exemplified in the gastrointestinal tract. Development of gut-associated lymphoid tissue is absolutely dependent on bacterial colonization. Increasing evidence suggests that host-symbiont interactions regulate adaptive immune functions throughout life. Disturbances in the bacterial microbiota and failure to maintain intestinal homeostasis are important in diverse diseases, including inflammatory bowel disease (Chapter 143) and HIV-associated immune defects.

Memory

An important consequence of adaptive immunity is the generation of immunologic memory, the basis for long-lived protection after a primary infection. Memory induction by vaccination is one of the landmark successes in medicine. Immunologic memory is defined as the ability to respond more rapidly and effectively to pathogens that have been encountered previously. The bases of immunologic memory are qualitative and quantitative changes in antigen-specific T cells and B cells. As a direct result of clonal expansion and selection in antigen-driven responses, the frequencies of antigen-specific memory B cells and memory T cells are increased 10-fold to 1000-fold compared with the naïve repertoires. The mechanisms through which memory T cells and B cells escape clonal downsizing in the terminal stages of the primary immune response are not clear. The enrichment of antigen-specific B cells and T cells enhances the sensitivity of the system to renewed challenges and provides a head start of 4 to 10 cell divisions. In addition to increased frequencies, memory T cells and B cells are functionally different from their naïve counterparts. Memory cells are long-lived and survive in the presence of certain cytokines without the need for continuous antigenic stimulation, guaranteeing immunologic memory for the life expectancy of the individual cell. Memory B cells produce predominantly IgG and IgA antibodies with evidence of somatic hypermutation and high affinity for the antigen. Cell surface expression of high-affinity antibodies allows more efficient antigen uptake, which enhances the crucial interaction with T cells. High affinity also gives memory B cells a competitive advantage over naïve B cells in antigen binding, leading to progressive affinity maturation of somatically mutated antibody molecules.

Because the TCR does not undergo isotype switching or affinity maturation, memory T cells are more difficult to distinguish from naïve or effector T cells. In contrast to effector cells, memory T cells lack activation markers and need antigen stimulation to resume effector functions. In contrast to naïve T cells, memory T cells have a lower activation threshold and are less dependent on costimulatory signals. In essence, their requirements for

antigen stimulation are fewer, and their clonal size is larger, permitting fast, efficient responses to secondary antigen encounters. Also, memory T cells resume effector functions without having to undergo cell divisions.

Immunologic Tolerance and Autoimmunity

Unresponsiveness to self is a fundamental property of the immune system and is a condition, sine qua non, to maintain tissue integrity of the host. Self/nonself distinction is relatively straightforward for the innate immune system, in which receptors to nonself molecules are genetically encoded and evolutionarily selected. Self/nonself discrimination is much more complex for the adaptive immune system, in which antigen-specific receptors are generated randomly and the entire spectrum of antigens can be recognized. The adaptive immune system must acquire the ability to distinguish between self and nonself. Several different mechanisms are used, collectively called *tolerance*. Tolerance is antigen specific; its induction requires the recognition of antigen by lymphocytes in a defined setting. Failure of self-tolerance results in immune responses against self-antigens. Such reactions are called *autoimmunity* and may give rise to chronic inflammatory autoimmune disease.

Central and peripheral tolerance mechanisms can be distinguished. In central tolerance, self-reactive lymphocytes are deleted during development. This process of negative selection is particularly important for T cells. During thymic development, T cells that recognize antigen with high affinity, in particular antigens that are constitutively expressed on antigen-presenting cells, are deleted. Central tolerance for B cells follows the same principles. Recognition of antigen by developing B cells in the bone marrow induces apoptosis. Negative selection is particularly important for B cells that recognize multivalent antigens because they do not depend on T-cell help and cannot be controlled peripherally.

Not all self-reactive T cells are centrally purged from the repertoire; certain antigens are not encountered at sufficient densities in the thymus. Also, all T cells have some degree of self-reactivity, which is necessary for positive selection in the thymus and for peripheral survival. Mechanisms of peripheral T-cell tolerance include anergy, peripheral deletion, clonal ignorance, and suppression of immune responses by regulatory T cells. T-cell anergy is transient and is actively maintained. It is induced if CD4+ T cells recognize antigens without receiving costimulatory signals. In general, costimulatory molecules are restricted to antigen-presenting cells, and their expression is activation dependent. Antigen recognition on immature or resting antigen-presenting cells or on any cell other than peripheral antigen-presenting cells results in anergy. Tissue-residing immature dendritic cells need to be activated by cytokines or recognition of PAMPs to stimulate and not to anergize T cells. Peripheral deletion is induced as a consequence of hyperstimulation. Hyperstimulation of T cells (e.g., by high doses of antigen and high concentrations of IL-2) preferentially activates pro-apoptotic pathways and causes elimination of the responding T-cell specificity. This mechanism may be responsible for the elimination of T cells specific for plentiful peripheral self-antigens and for foreign antigens abundantly present during infection. Whereas induction of anergy and activation-induced cell death are active consequences of antigen recognition, the third tolerance mechanism, clonal ignorance, is less well understood. Clonal ignorance is defined as the presence of self-reactive lymphocytes that fail to recognize or to respond to peripheral antigens. These cells remain responsive to antigenic challenge if given in the right setting. An example of clonal ignorance is nonresponsiveness to sequestered antigens that are not accessible to the immune system. Other mechanisms must exist, however, because clonal ignorance has also been shown for accessible antigens. Treg cells play a pivotal role in maintaining peripheral tolerance. During an immune response, T cells can acquire the ability to produce regulatory cytokines, such as TGF-β, IL-10, or IL-4, that dampen or suppress immune responses. A dedicated subset of Treg cells, Foxp3 CD4+ T cells, has been identified and characterized. Harnessing the frequencies and function of these cells may offer a promising approach to restoring peripheral tolerance in treating autoimmune diseases or facilitating transplantation tolerance; their elimination or functional suppression may potentiate cancer immunotherapy.

Peripheral tolerance of B cells is maintained through the absence of T-cell help. B cells require signals from T cells to differentiate into effector cells. B lymphocytes that recognize self-antigens in the periphery in the absence of T-cell help are rendered anergic or are unable to enter lymphoid follicles, where they could receive T-cell help, effectively excluding them from immune responses.

Generation and maintenance of self-tolerance can fail, in which case autoimmune responses are generated. Overall, chronic inflammatory diseases induced by tolerance failure occur in about 5% of the general population. Given the complexity of regulation, it is surprising that autoimmune diseases are not more frequent. It is thought that most autoimmune diseases result from dysfunction of the adaptive immune system. Many models of autoimmunity rely on the hypothesis that peripheral anergy is broken. Aberrant expression of costimulatory molecules on nonprofessional antigen-presenting cells or inappropriate activation of tissue-residing dendritic cells sets the stage for the induction of "forbidden" T-cell responses. Also, autoreactive B cells that recognize self-antigen complexed with foreign antigen may engulf this complex and receive help from T cells specific for the foreign antigen. Autoimmunity also may emerge if antigen ignorance is broken. This could happen if tissue barriers break down and antigens that are usually sequestered from the immune system, such as antigens from the central nervous system or the eye, become accessible. Tolerance mechanisms of anergy or clonal ignorance can also fail if a foreign antigen is sufficiently different from a self-antigen to initiate an immune response but sufficiently similar for activated T cells to elicit T-cell and B-cell effector functions (molecular mimicry).

SUGGESTED READINGS

Bonilla FA, Oettgen HC. Adaptive immunity. *J Allergy Clin Immunol.* 2010;125:S33-S40. *Concise review of the current understanding of the mechanisms of adaptive immunity.*

Delano MJ, Thayer T, Gabrilovich S, et al. Sepsis induces early alterations in innate immunity that impact mortality to secondary infection. *J Immunol.* 2011;186:195-202. *Sepsis impairs innate immunity and increases susceptibility to secondary infections.*

Iwasaki A, Medzhitov R. Regulation of adaptive immunity by the innate immune system. *Science.* 2010;327:291-295. *Review of mechanisms by which pathogen-specific innate immune recognition activates antigen-specific adaptive immune responses.*

Littman DR, Rudensky AY. Th17 and regulatory T cells in mediating and restraining inflammation. *Cell.* 2010;140:845-858. *Discussion of how immune balance is achieved by interactions of different T-lymphocyte classes with pro- or anti-inflammatory activities in the context of genetic and environmental factors.*

Von Boehmer H, Melchers F. Checkpoints in lymphocyte development and autoimmune disease. *Nat Immunol.* 2010;11:14-20. *Discussion of how failures at B-cell and T-cell developmental checkpoints result in autoimmunity.*

45

THE MAJOR HISTOCOMPATIBILITY COMPLEX

PETER K. GREGERSEN

HUMAN LEUKOCYTE ANTIGENS

The major histocompatibility complex (MHC) occupies a unique position in the nexus of clinical medicine, immunology, and genetics. Hundreds of diseases and clinical phenotypes have been associated with genes located within the MHC. The most important of these genes encode the human leukocyte antigens (HLAs), a family of cell surface proteins that are essential for normal immune function. HLA genes display a remarkably high degree of genetic variation among individuals in the population, and this variability is largely responsible for individual differences in immune responsiveness. These effects on immune responsiveness are in turn related to individual differences in susceptibility to a variety of autoimmune, inflammatory, and infectious disorders. Thus, the structural variability of the HLA molecules themselves underlies most but not all of the HLA disease associations reported over the past 3 decades.

Structure of HLA Molecules

Discovery of the x-ray crystallographic structure of an HLA molecule had a major impact on understanding the molecular basis of immune recognition by T cells. A ribbon diagram of the structure of an HLA class I molecule is shown in Figure 45-1. The "business end" of the molecule contains a peptide-binding cleft formed by the two membrane distal domains (α_1 and α_2) of the HLA class I heavy chain, as seen in the side view in Figure 45-1A. A view from the top of this cleft is shown in Figure 45-1B, which can be thought of as the "T-cell view" of the HLA molecule. It illustrates that the base of the peptide-binding cleft is formed by β-pleated sheets, with two α-helical structures forming the sides of the cleft. It is now known that the T-cell receptor physically interacts with both the HLA molecule and the peptide bound within the cleft to form a "trimolecular complex" (E-Fig. 45-1). Thus, it is not surprising that structural differences in HLA molecules, particularly in amino acids surrounding the peptide-binding cleft, have a major role in many immunologically mediated diseases.

Properties of HLA Class I and Class II Isoforms

There are two major isoforms of HLA molecules, termed *class I* and *class II*. Both isoforms are anchored in the cell membrane and contain a peptide-binding cleft similar to that shown in Figure 45-1. However, their specific structural and functional features differ, as summarized in Table 45-1 (E-Fig. 45-2). In the case of class I molecules, a highly variable α chain (45 kD) forms a noncovalent heterodimer with an invariant β_2-microglobulin (12 kD) and is anchored to the cell by a single transmembrane segment on the α chain. In contrast, HLA class II molecules are formed by α chain (32 kD) and β chain (28 kD) heterodimers, and in many cases both chains exhibit structural variability among individuals. HLA class I molecules are expressed on nearly all nucleated cells. HLA class II molecules are found on more restricted cell populations, including B cells, monocytes, macrophages, dendritic cells, and other "professional" antigen-presenting cells such as Langerhans cells in the skin. Certain subsets of T cells also express class II molecules. In addition, HLA class II molecules are expressed on thymic epithelium, where they are involved in thymic selection of the T-cell receptor repertoire (see later). The size of the peptides bound to HLA class I molecules is

FIGURE 45-1. Two views of an HLA class I molecule. **A,** Ribbon diagram showing the x-ray crystallographic structure of an HLA class I molecule (side view). The β-strand structures are indicated by *thick green arrows* (oriented in an amino to carboxy direction), whereas connecting loops are indicated as *thin lines*. The α-helices are shown flanking a peptide-binding cleft at the top (membrane distal portion) of the molecule. The base (membrane proximal portion) of the molecule is formed by the noncovalent association between the α_3 domain of the class I α chain and β_2-microglobulin (β_2m). **B,** View from the top of the molecule emphasizing that the base of the peptide-binding cleft consists of β-pleated sheets flanked by α-helical structures. C = C terminal; N = N terminal. (Adapted from Bjorkman PJ, Saper MA, Samraoi B, et al. Structure of the class I histocompatibility antigen HLA-A2. *Nature.* 1987;329:506-512.)

circumscribed to 8 or 9 amino acids in length, whereas the peptides presented by HLA class II molecules are longer and more variable in size, with lengths usually ranging from 10 to 20 amino acids. HLA class I molecules generally present peptides for recognition by CD8$^+$ T cells, such as in cytotoxic CD8$^+$ T-cell responses against virally infected tissues. In contrast, HLA class II molecules are primarily involved in presenting antigenic peptides to CD4$^+$ T cells.

TABLE 45-1	COMPARISON OF STRUCTURAL AND FUNCTIONAL FEATURES OF HLA CLASS I AND CLASS II ISOTYPES	
FEATURE	**HLA CLASS I**	**HLA CLASS II**
Chain structure of heterodimer	45-kD α chain 12-kD β$_2$-microglobulin	34-kD α chain 28-kD β chain
Tissue distribution	All nucleated cells	Antigen-presenting cells (monocytes, B cells, dendritic cells, Langerhans cells), thymic epithelium, and some T cells; inducible on other cell types by interferon-γ
Size of bound peptides	8-9 amino acids	10-20 amino acids
Source peptides	Cytosolic	Endosomal
Functions	Presentation of antigenic peptides to CD8$^+$ T cells; ligands for natural killer cell receptors	Presentation of antigenic peptides to CD4$^+$ T cells

Sources of the peptide antigens presented by class I and class II molecules are quite distinct. In the case of class I molecules, the bound peptides are derived from cytosol and are loaded onto the class I molecules during their synthesis in the endoplasmic reticulum. Thus, either host or virally derived peptides may be present in the peptide cleft, and a peptide is required for proper folding and surface expression of class I molecules. In contrast, HLA class II molecules present peptides that are present in endosomes, and peptide loading onto class II molecules occurs in endocytic vesicles. These peptides are derived from sources exogenous to the cell, such as soluble proteins, particles, cell debris, or whole organisms. In the case of B cells, surface immunoglobulin can facilitate the internalization of highly specific antigens, whereas in macrophages and other antigen-presenting cells, endocytosis and phagocytosis mediate less specific cellular internalization of antigens. Mycobacteria and intracellular parasites such as *Leishmania* replicate inside vesicular compartments of the cell; therefore, peptides from these agents are generally presented on class II molecules.

Organization of HLA Molecules
Genetic Map of HLA Genes

The MHC is contained within a 3.6 million–base pair region located at chromosome 6p21 and encodes more than 200 different genes, approximately 40% of which appear to have some role in immune function. Figure 45-2 shows a simplified map of the major HLA loci. The HLA class I and class II regions are separated by a gene-dense region often referred to as the *central MHC*. This central region encodes a number of genes of immunologic importance, including several complement components and tumor necrosis factor-α and -β, to name only a few. The class I heavy chains for HLA-A, HLA-B, and HLA-C are encoded on the telomeric side of the MHC, along with a number of other class I–like molecules, as shown in Figure 45-2. The HLA class II region is considerably more complicated, with multiple α and

FIGURE 45-2. Map of the human major histocompatibility complex (MHC) spanning approximately 3.5 million base pairs on the short arm of chromosome 6. The HLA class I and class II molecules are encoded in distinct regions of the MHC. The HLA class II region contains three subregions: DR, DQ, and DP. Each of these subregions contains a variable number of α- and β-chain genes. HLA class II loci with known functional protein products are labeled in bold. In the case of DR, different numbers of DRB genes are present in different haplotypes, some of which are nonfunctional pseudogenes (ψ). A summary of the most common of these is shown in the *box*. The DQ and DP subregions each contain one pair of functional α- and β-chain genes. The HLA class I region contains the three "classic" class I genes—HLA-A, HLA-B, and HLA-C—as well as other related "nonclassic" class I molecules such as MICA, MICB, HLA-E, and HLA-G. The gene for familial hemochromatosis (HFE) is found just telomeric to the HLA class I region, about 3 million base pairs distant from HLA-A. The "central" MHC also contains a number of genes related to immune function, including the complement components (C4A, C4B, C2, and factor B), as well as tumor necrosis factor (TNF)-α and -β. Not shown in the figure are more than 100 additional genes, many of which are located in the central MHC. A complete listing of MHC-encoded genes can be found in Horton R, Wilming L, Rand V, et al. Gene map of the extended human MHC. *Nat Rev Genet.* 2004;5:889-899.

β chains encoded for each of the major HLA class II isotypes: HLA-DR, HLA-DQ, and HLA-DP. Of these, HLA-DR exhibits additional complexity, in that a different gene organization of β chains is seen, depending on the particular DR haplotype.

HLA Typing Nomenclature and Patterns of Allelic Sequence Variation

In addition to the organizational complexity of the HLA region, the nomenclature for HLA typing of different alleles at each locus presents some challenges for the nonexpert. In the past decade, hundreds of HLA alleles have been sequenced, and each HLA allelic variant is defined by its locus and sequence. For example, B*2701 indicates allele 2701 at the HLA-B locus, and DRB1*0401 indicates allele 0401 at the DRB1 locus. This nomenclature is, in principle, quite straightforward. However, there are many different alleles at each of these loci; for example, more than 100 alleles have been identified at the HLA-B locus, and similar allelic diversity is seen at HLA-A and HLA-C, as well as in many of the HLA class II loci. The sequence relationships between alleles are both complex and informative for understanding HLA associations with disease, and the nomenclature reflects this to some degree. It is therefore worth understanding the origins of these naming conventions.

The current HLA nomenclature contains traces of the early history of HLA typing. A serologic approach was initially used for HLA typing. HLA protein variation is highly immunogenic between individuals; therefore, typing alloantisera can be derived either from multiply transfused individuals (who make an antibody response to HLA molecules on the donor white cells) or from multiparous women (who commonly form antibodies to the paternal HLA antigens expressed by the fetus). Thus, by screening large numbers of individuals, panels of alloantisera were developed as the first HLA typing reagents. These original HLA typing sera did not distinguish all the variation at a particular locus, and it is now apparent that serologic typing actually detects rather large groups of structurally related alleles. For example, the serologically defined allele HLA-DR4 contains well over 30 different alleles at the DRB1 locus, although only a few of these alleles are common in the population. Table 45-2 summarizes the major allelic groups at the DRB1 locus and shows the relationship between the original serologic typing and the various groups of alleles defined at the sequence level. For some allelic groups, such as HLA-DR3, there is little sequence diversity within the group, depending on the population; thus, almost all white Europeans carry just one type of DR3 allele, DRB1*0301. As a result, the term *DR3* is often used in conversation to refer to the DRB1*0301 allele and is reasonably precise when talking about a white population. In contrast, *DR4* could refer to any one of several different alleles (see Table 45-2).

In addition to having large numbers of alleles at each locus, the frequency distribution of these alleles is highly variable in human populations. As shown in Table 45-2, five DRB1 alleles predominate in the northern European white population (shown in bold), with frequencies ranging from 10 to 30%. This frequency distribution would be quite different in a different population group, even among white subgroups, such as a comparison of northern and southern European populations. The population differences emphasize the importance of matching controls to cases by ethnic origin when comparing allele frequencies between them.

HLA Associations with Disease: The Concept of Disease Susceptibility

Table 45-3 provides a representative sample of some well-established HLA associations with human disease. The overwhelming majority of these studies were conducted with a case-control design in which the frequency of alleles was compared in subjects with appropriately matched controls. Matching of controls is a critical part of the study design because HLA alleles can differ greatly between different populations; as a result, many early reports in the literature turned out to be false positives. Nevertheless, hundreds of diseases and medically relevant phenotypes have confirmed associations with HLA alleles.

As shown in Table 45-3, the strength of many of these disease associations is rather modest, with an estimated relative risk of 10 or less. Therefore, HLA alleles confer a state of susceptibility, or risk, for disease. Because the HLA risk alleles are usually quite common in the population, and the diseases are relatively uncommon, many individuals who carry these risk alleles do not contract the disease. Conversely, a substantial number of individuals with the disease do not carry the known HLA risk-conferring alleles. Thus, in a practical sense, HLA typing alone is not very useful in a clinical setting for most diagnostic purposes. Even for a disease such as ankylosing spondylitis (Chapter 273), where the relative risk approaches 100, the disease develops in only a fraction of the HLA-B27 carriers in the population because the carrier frequency of HLA-B27 in a white population is approximately 8%. When confronting a patient with typical symptoms of ankylosing spondylitis, testing for B27 can be confirmatory; however, it is not diagnostic by itself because the prevalence of ankylosing spondylitis is very low (≈0.12%) in the population. The recently described association of B57 with adverse reactions to abacavir is one of the first examples in which HLA testing may be directly useful in a clinical setting. Knowledge of this association has now been shown to reduce the incidence of drug reactions in treated populations.

This pattern of association, in which HLA alleles confer a state of risk or susceptibility to disease, implies that other factors must be involved for a disease to actually manifest. In general, these other factors can include other genes, environmental factors, and nongenetic factors such as stochastic or "epigenetic" events that may occur at any time during development. Somatic rearrangements of T-cell and B-cell receptor genes are one example of such a stochastic process. These factors explain why concordance rates for many autoimmune disorders in monozygotic twins are only in the 30% range, even though these diseases all exhibit significant genetic associations with particular HLA alleles and have a strong genetic component. The genetic predisposition conferred by the MHC is only part of the overall genetic contribution to most autoimmune disorders, and the MHC component varies in importance, depending on the particular disease.

Linkage Disequilibrium

An understanding of the concept of linkage disequilibrium is critical to the proper interpretation of HLA associations or, indeed, any genetic associations with human diseases. The term *linkage disequilibrium* is used to describe the fact that alleles at adjacent loci are often found together on the same chromosomal segment, or haplotype, more frequently than would be predicted by chance. This phenomenon occurs throughout the genome, and the MHC is no exception. Indeed, because of the high degree of allelic diversity at HLA loci, the pattern of linkage disequilibrium between HLA alleles can be quite complicated and, like the alleles themselves, often varies among different population groups. For example, in most white populations, the DRB1*0301 allele is almost always found on the same haplotype with the DQB1*0201 allele at the DQB1 locus. (Note that the DQB1 locus is situated several hundred thousand base pairs away from the DRB1 locus; see Fig. 45-2.) Likewise, DR4 alleles (at DRB1) are often found to be in linkage

| TABLE 45-2 | SUMMARY OF MAJOR ALLELIC GROUPS AT THE DRB1 LOCUS AND THEIR RELATIONSHIP TO COMMON DRB1 ALLELES DEFINED AT THE SEQUENCE LEVEL |

Allelic Groups (Serologic Typing)		EXAMPLES OF COMMON ALLELES (NORTHERN EUROPEAN WHITE INDIVIDUALS) DEFINED BY SEQUENCE*
MAJOR GROUPS	**SEROLOGIC "SPLITS"**	
DR1		DRB1***0101**, 0102, 0103
DR2	DR15	DRB1***1501**, 1502
	DR16	DRB1*1601
DR3		DRB1***0301**
DR4		DRB1***0401**, 0402, 0403, 0404, 0405, 0406, 0407, 0408
DR5	DR11	DRB1*1101, 1102, 1103, 1104
	DR12	DRB1*1201
DR6	DR13	DRB1*1301, 1302, 1303
	DR14	DRB1*1401
DR7		DRB1***0701**
DR8		DRB1*0801, 0802, 0803, 0804, 0806
DR9		DRB1*0901
DR10		DRB1*1001

*Alleles in bold are found in at least 10% of individuals in the population.
From Williams F, Meenagh A, Single R, et al. High resolution HLA-DRB1 identification of a Caucasian population. *Hum Immunol.* 2004;65:66-77.

TABLE 45-3 SELECTED HLA ASSOCIATIONS WITH HUMAN DISEASES

DISEASE	MAJOR HLA ASSOCIATION (ALLELIC GROUP OR HAPLOTYPE)	EFFECT/APPROXIMATE RELATIVE RISK/RELATIVE HAZARD
AUTOIMMUNE DISEASES		
Type 1 diabetes	DR3-DQ2 DR4-DQ3	10
Multiple sclerosis	DR2-DQ1	3-5
Celiac disease	DR3-DQ2 DR4-DQ3	30
Rheumatoid arthritis	DR1, DR4	2-5
Systemic lupus erythematosus	DR2, DR3, DR8	2-10
Ankylosing spondylitis	B27	100
Psoriasis	Cw6	10
INFECTIOUS DISEASES		
Progression to AIDS	B35	2-3
Severe malaria	B53	0.5 (protective)
Transient vs persistent hepatitis C infection	DR11-DQ3	5-10
OTHER		
Hemochromatosis	A3	10
Adverse drug reaction (allopurinol)	B58	>100
Cervical cancer	DR11-DQ3	2-3

AIDS = acquired immunodeficiency syndrome; HFE = hereditary hemochromatosis gene.

disequilibrium with DQB1*0302. These two haplotypes are both associated with type 1 diabetes (see Table 45-3).

Occasionally, linkage disequilibrium can extend to very long chromosomal segments. For example, a common haplotype in northern European white populations extends to several million base pairs and contains the HLA alleles A*0101-B*0801-DRB1*0301-DQB1*0201, often referred to as the *A1-B8-DR3* or *8.1 haplotype*. This particular haplotype accounts for about a third of all DR3 haplotypes in a U.S. white population and is of particular interest because it is associated with a variety of diseases, some of which are listed in Table 45-4. Because haplotypes such as these are inherited as a unit, it can be difficult to determine which specific genes on the haplotype are actually responsible for the disease association in a population.

There are a number of possible explanations for linkage disequilibrium. In part, it reflects the fact that meiotic recombination in the genome is discontinuous, and some loci have very low recombination rates between them—such as between the DRB1 and DQB1 loci. In addition, population migrations can introduce haplotypes into new population groups and thereby generate common "founder" haplotypes. Finally, some haplotypes may be kept intact because of selection. For example, it may be that the combination of genes found on the A1-B8-DR3 haplotype confers a survival advantage. Whatever the underlying reason, it is important to keep in mind that any HLA association may reflect the presence of linkage disequilibrium with another allele at another locus on the same haplotype.

HLA Associations with Autoimmune and Infectious Diseases

The majority of autoimmune disorders exhibit some association with HLA class II alleles, although because of linkage disequilibrium, it is not always clear which locus is actually responsible for the association. In the case of type 1 diabetes, the bulk of evidence suggests that alleles at the HLA-DQ locus play a predominant role by virtue of specific amino acid substitutions that are present on multiple different DQB1 alleles; aspartic acid at amino acid position 57 of the DQβ chain is thought to be of particular importance. Rheumatoid arthritis is another autoimmune disorder in which the molecular basis of HLA class II associations has been partially worked out. In this case, a series of DRB1 alleles, including DRB1*0101, *0401, *0404, *0405, all share a common amino acid sequence (Q-K or R-R-A-A) at positions 70 to 74 of the DRβ1 chain, located on the rim of the peptide-binding cleft (see

TABLE 45-4 DISEASES AND PHENOTYPES ASSOCIATED WITH THE A1-B8-DR3 (8.1) HAPLOTYPE

IgA deficiency
Common variable immunodeficiency
Myasthenia gravis
Dermatitis herpetiformis
Rheumatoid arthritis (central portion of the 8.1 haplotype only)
Rapid loss of CD4+ T cells in HIV infection
Low antibody response to hepatitis B immunization
Increases (tumor necrosis factor) or decreases (interleukin-5) in cytokine production in vitro

Fig. 45-1). This sequence is known as the *shared epitope* and provides an appealing unifying explanation for the complex patterns of HLA-DR associations with rheumatoid arthritis. However, for both type 1 diabetes and rheumatoid arthritis, there are exceptions to these observations, and certain combinations of HLA alleles can confer very high degrees of risk. For most of the HLA-associated diseases, the exact molecular basis of the association has not been definitively established, and in some cases, even the causative locus is uncertain (see Table 45-3). For ankylosing spondylitis, it appears that most allelic variants of HLA-B27 are associated with disease. Recent genetic data provide support for the C*0601 allele being causative for psoriasis. However, in the case of systemic lupus erythematosus and multiple sclerosis, the relative importance of DRB1 versus DQB1 alleles is not clear.

For infectious diseases, such as the role of HLA-B35 in the progression of acquired immunodeficiency syndrome (AIDS), there is evidence that particular amino acid residues on the HLA-B molecule are especially important. The amino acids that distinguish risk alleles (B*3502, B*3503) from nonrisk alleles (B*3501) alter the structure of a "pocket" within the peptide-binding cleft on the various HLA-B35 proteins and therefore can affect the kinds of human immunodeficiency virus (HIV) antigenic peptides that are bound by these alleles. Other HLA-B alleles, such as B27 and B58, protect against progression of HIV, apparently by similar mechanisms. Aside from HLA-B associations with HIV outcome, specific structural explanations have not yet been defined for most HLA associations with infectious diseases.

Mechanisms Explaining HLA Associations with Disease

It is fair to say that the mechanisms underlying HLA disease associations are still not fully explained for any disorder, and the mechanisms clearly differ for different diseases. However, there are two general categories of mechanisms that are likely to be important. First, a pattern of immune responsiveness, or lack of immune responsiveness, can be related to the ability of an individual's HLA molecules to bind and present antigenic peptides (either foreign or self) to T cells. This mechanism is often referred to as *determinant selection*, which means that HLA molecules are involved in selecting which antigenic determinants are selected for presentation to responding T cells. As mentioned earlier, this probably underlies the contrasting HLA-B allelic associations with AIDS progression.

An alternative mechanism invokes the role of HLA molecules in regulating thymic selection of the mature T-cell repertoire. During thymic development, thymocytes either survive or die of apoptosis, depending in large part on their ability to recognize "self" HLA molecules (and associated "self" peptides) on thymic epithelium or on other antigen-presenting cells in the thymus. This recognition is mediated through the α/β T-cell receptor. Thus, the structural repertoire of T-cell receptors in the mature circulating T-cell population is shaped by the structural variation of the selecting HLA molecules. This may lead to "holes" in the T-cell repertoire or, alternatively, enrichment for particular T-cell specificities. In this view, the presence of particular sets of potentially responding T cells provides a risk factor for response, or lack of response, to autoantigens or foreign antigens. It implies the need for an environmental trigger to actually cause this risk to manifest as overt clinical disease.

In addition to these two basic models, it has been proposed that HLA molecules can themselves serve as a source of antigenic peptides and may predispose to disease by means of molecular mimicry or other more complex mechanisms. However, none of these proposed mechanisms has been definitively proved for any disorder.

HLA Associations with Disease May Reflect Linkage Disequilibrium with Non-HLA Genes

In most cases, HLA associations such as those listed in Table 45-3 probably reflect the mechanistic involvement of the HLA molecules themselves in the disease or phenotype under study. However, the MHC is one of the most gene-dense segments in the human genome, and other genes in the region may in fact be responsible for the observed disease association. A good example of this is hemochromatosis (Chapter 219). Early studies showed that certain HLA class I alleles, such as HLA-A3, were highly associated with this disorder. However, it is now clear that the causative gene, *HFE*, is actually more than 3 million base pairs distant from the HLA-A locus (see Fig. 45-2). The HLA-A3 association is observed because the *HFE* C282Y allele (causative for hemochromatosis) is frequently found on the same haplotype as HLA-A3 in many white populations.

Some of the associations with the A1-B8-DR3 haplotype almost certainly reflect linkage disequilibrium with genes other than HLA class I and class II genes (see Table 45-3). Although the HLA genes may contribute to some of these disorders, it is likely that other genes on the 8.1 haplotype also contribute to risk. The central portion of the MHC in particular (see Fig. 45-2) is very dense with many genes of uncertain function, as well as genes for important inflammatory cytokines such as tumor necrosis factor and complement components C2 and C4. Indeed, the combination of several different genes may well explain why this haplotype is associated with so many different immunologic disorders.

HLA Typing and Bone Marrow Transplantation

As the term *histocompatibility* implies, the ability of the MHC to control graft rejection in experimental animals led to the realization that HLA matching is important for transplant survival. For solid organ transplantation, treatment with immunosuppressive agents often prevents the rejection of HLA-mismatched transplants. However, for bone marrow transplantation (Chapter 181), careful matching of the major HLA class I and class II loci is important for a successful outcome, regardless of whether the donor is related or unrelated to the recipient. Because of the extensive sequence diversity of HLA alleles, very large numbers of unrelated donors are required to ensure a reasonable probability of a match for any given recipient who does not have a living related donor. This has led to the development of international bone marrow donor registries that now contain more than 10 million potential donors who have been screened for HLA type. If transplantation is performed in the presence of a significant mismatch at either class I or class II loci, T cells from the recipient may recognize the donor HLA molecules or their bound peptides as foreign and initiate an immune response, leading to graft rejection. Interestingly, even when HLA molecules are completely matched, T cells still occasionally initiate rejection because of individual differences in "minor" histocompatibility antigens that are not encoded within the MHC but are processed and presented as antigenic peptides that appear foreign to the host.

HLA Class I: Alternative Forms and Functions

The HLA class I region of the MHC contains a number of genes that encode so-called nonclassic class I genes, including HLA-E, HLA-G, MICA, and MICB (see Fig. 45-2). These molecules do not present peptides to α/β T cells but rather interact with a variety of other ligands that are generally found on natural killer cells and some other types of T cells. In addition, certain allelic subsets of the "classic" class I molecules (e.g., HLA-A, -B, and -C) can interact with some of these other ligands. Among these ligands, the killer cell immunoglobulin-like receptor (KIR) family displays a large degree of genetic variation in both gene structure and gene number and has been associated with human disease. For example, certain combinations of HLA class I alleles and KIR alleles have been associated with risk for rheumatoid vasculitis as well as outcome of HIV infection. These genetic relationships are complex, and this aspect of HLA class I function in disease has been relatively understudied.

HLA and Clinical Medicine

The identification of risk genes within the MHC may hold the key to understanding a large number of immunologically related disorders. However, we are far from identifying all of these genes, and in the few cases in which the actual risk alleles are known with confidence, their mechanism of action is not clear. Moreover, most HLA-associated disorders are complex, and additional genetic or environmental factors (or both) are likely to be involved, most of which have not yet been identified. Therefore, in most cases, HLA typing alone has limited diagnostic utility. HLA typing may be diagnostically important in the future if used in combination with other biomarkers, and HLA typing remains critical to successful bone marrow transplantation. Thus, it is likely that future advances in immunology and genetics will lead to greater clinical use of genetic typing of HLA genes, as well as other genes, within the MHC.

SUGGESTED READINGS

Claas FH. Clinical relevance of circulating donor-specific HLA antibodies. *Curr Opin Organ Transplant.* 2010;15:462-466. *Which HLA antibodies are the direct cause of graft failure remains uncertain.*

Howell WM, Carter V, Clark B. The HLA system: immunobiology, HLA typing, antibody screening and crossmatching techniques. *J Clin Pathol.* 2010;63:387-390. *Overview of biology and methodologies.*

Shiina T, Hosomichi K, Inoko H, et al. The HLA genomic loci map: expression, interaction, diversity and disease. *J Hum Genet.* 2009;54:15-39. *A detailed review of the genetics and disease associations within the HLA region.*

Zachary AA, Eng HS. Desensitization: achieving immune détente. *Tissue Antigens.* 2011;77:3-8. *Desensitization can increase the rate of transplantation among sensitized patients.*

46

MECHANISMS OF IMMUNE-MEDIATED TISSUE INJURY

JANE E. SALMON

THE ADAPTIVE IMMUNE RESPONSE

Definition

The adaptive immune response is a crucial component of host defense against infection. Its distinguishing and unique feature is the ability to recognize pathogens specifically, based on clonal selection of lymphocytes bearing antigen-specific receptors. Antigens unassociated with infectious agents also may elicit adaptive immune responses. Many clinically important diseases are characterized by normal immune responses directed against an inappropriate antigen, typically in the absence of infection. Immune responses directed at noninfectious antigens occur in allergy, in which the antigen is an innocuous foreign substance, and in autoimmunity, in which the response is to a self-antigen.

Effector mechanisms that eliminate pathogens in adaptive immune responses are essentially identical to those of innate immunity. The specific antigen recognition feature of the adaptive immune response seems to have been appended to the preexisting innate defense system. As a result, the inflammatory cells and molecules of the innate immune system are essential for the effector functions of B and T lymphocytes. In addition to initiating protective responses, they mediate tissue injury in allergy, hypersensitivity, and autoimmunity.

Effector Mechanisms

Effector actions of antibodies depend on recruiting cells and molecules of the innate immune system. Antibodies are adapters that bind antigens to nonspecific inflammatory cells and direct their destructive effector responses. Antibodies also activate the complement system, which enhances opsonization of antigens, recruits phagocytic cells, and amplifies (or "complements") antibody-triggered damage. The isotype or class of antibodies produced determines which effector mechanisms are engaged.

Cell-bound receptors for immunoglobulin (Ig) constitute the link between humoral and cellular aspects of the immune cascade and play an integral part in the process by which foreign and endogenous opsonized material is identified and destroyed. These cell-based binding sites for antibodies, termed *Fc receptors,* interact with the constant region (Fc portion) of the immunoglobulin heavy chain of a particular antibody class regardless of its antigen specificity. Accessory cells that lack intrinsic specificity, such as neutrophils, macrophages, and mast cells, are recruited to participate in inflammatory responses through the interaction of their Fc receptors with antigen-specific antibodies. Distinct receptors for different immunoglobulin isotypes are expressed on different effector cells.

Receptors for IgG (FcγRs) are a diverse group of receptors expressed as hematopoietic cell surface molecules on phagocytes (macrophages, monocytes, neutrophils), platelets, mast cells, eosinophils, and natural killer (NK) cells. FcγRs often are expressed as stimulatory and inhibitory pairs. Triggering of stimulatory FcγRs initiates a series of events, including phagocytosis; antibody-dependent, cell-mediated cytotoxicity; secretion of granules; and release of inflammatory mediators, such as cytokines, reactive oxidants, and proteases. Extensive structural diversity among FcγR family members leads to differences in binding capacity, signal transduction pathways, and cell type–specific expression patterns. This diversity allows IgG complexes to activate a broad program of cell functions relevant to inflammation, host defense, and autoimmunity. Phagocyte activation is triggered by stimulatory FcγRs, facilitating the recognition, uptake, and destruction of antibody-coated targets, whereas multivalent IgG binding to FcγRs on platelets leads to platelet aggregation and thrombosis, and binding to FcγRs on NK cells mediates cytotoxicity of antibody-coated targets.

IgE binds to high-affinity FcεRs on mast cells, basophils, and activated eosinophils. In contrast to FcγRs, which are low affinity and bind to multivalent IgG rather than circulating individual IgG molecules, FcεRs can bind monomeric IgE. A single mast cell may be armed with IgE molecules specific for different antigens, all bound to surface FcεRs. Mast cells, localized beneath the mucosa of the gastrointestinal and respiratory tracts and the dermis of the skin, await exposure to multivalent antigens, which cross-link surface IgE bound to FcεRs and cause release of histamine-containing granules and generation of cytokines and other inflammatory mediators. IgE-mediated activation of eosinophils, cells normally present in the connective tissue of underlying respiratory, urogenital, and gut epithelium, leads to the release of highly toxic granule proteins, free radicals, and chemical mediators such as prostaglandins, cytokines, and chemokines. These amplify local inflammatory responses by activating endothelial cells and recruiting and activating more eosinophils and leukocytes. Prepackaged granules and high-affinity FcεRs that bind to free monomeric IgE enable an immediate response to pathogens or allergens at the first site of entry, a location where FcεR-bearing cells reside.

Inhibitory FcγRs, which modulate activation thresholds and terminate stimulating signals, are key elements in the regulation of effector function. Given that inhibitory and stimulatory Fc receptors are often coexpressed on the same cells, the effector response to a specific stimulus in a particular cell represents the balance between stimulatory and inhibitory signals. Inhibitory

FcγRs can dampen responses triggered by FcεRs on mast cells and FcγR-mediated inflammation at sites of immune complex deposition.

Effector activities targeted by IgG and IgM also may be mediated by components of the complement system (Chapter 49). Antigen-bound multimeric immunoglobulin can initiate activation of the classical pathway of complement, causing enhanced phagocytosis of antigen-antibody complexes, increased local vascular permeability, and recruitment and activation of inflammatory cells. The target of injury is specified by the antibody, and the extent of damage is determined by the synergistic activities of immunoglobulin and complement.

Antigen-specific effector T cells also may initiate tissue injury. On exposure to an appropriate antigen, memory T cells are stimulated to release cytokines and chemokines that activate local endothelial cells and recruit and activate macrophages and other inflammatory cells. The effector cells directed by T-cell–derived cytokines, or cytolytic T cells themselves, mediate tissue damage. T_H1 cells produce interferon-γ (IFN-γ) and activate macrophages to cause injury, whereas T_H2 cells produce interleukin-4 (IL-4), IL-5, and eotaxin (an eosinophil-specific chemokine) and trigger inflammatory responses in which eosinophils predominate.

⬤ HYPERSENSITIVITY REACTIONS

In predisposed individuals, innocuous environmental antigens may stimulate an adaptive immune response, immunologic memory, and, on subsequent exposure to the antigen, inflammation. These "overreactions" of the immune system to harmless environmental antigens (allergens), called *hypersensitivity* or *allergic reactions,* produce tissue injury and can cause serious disease. Hypersensitivity reactions are grouped into four types according to the effector mechanisms by which they are produced (Table 46-1). The effectors for types I, II, and III hypersensitivity reactions are antibody molecules, whereas type IV reactions are mediated by antigen-specific effector T cells.

Autoimmune disease is characterized by the presence of antibodies and T cells specific for self-antigens expressed on target tissues. The mechanisms of antigen recognition and effector function that lead to tissue damage in autoimmune disease are similar to the mechanisms elicited in response to pathogens and environmental antigens. These mechanisms resemble certain hypersensitivity reactions and may be classified accordingly (Table 46-2). Autoimmune disease caused by antibodies directed against cell surface or extracellular matrix antigens corresponds to type II hypersensitivity reactions; disease caused by formation of soluble immune complexes that subsequently are deposited in tissue corresponds to type III hypersensitivity; and disease caused by effector T cells corresponds to type IV hypersensitivity. Typically, several of these pathogenic mechanisms are operative in autoimmune disease. However, IgE responses are not associated with damage in autoimmunity.

Type I Hypersensitivity Reactions

Type I hypersensitivity reactions (Fig. 46-1) are triggered by the interaction of antigen with antigen-specific IgE bound to FcεRs on mast cells, which causes mast cell activation. Proteolytic enzymes and toxic mediators, such as histamine, are released immediately from preformed granules, and chemokines, cytokines, and leukotrienes are synthesized after activation. Together, these mediators increase vascular permeability, break down tissue matrix proteins, promote eosinophil production and activation (IL-3, IL-5, and granulocyte-macrophage colony-stimulating factor [GM-CSF]), and cause influx of effector leukocytes (tumor necrosis factor-α [TNF-α], platelet-activating factor, and macrophage inflammatory protein [MIP-1]), constriction of smooth muscle, stimulation of mucus secretion, and amplification of T_H2 cell responses (IL-4 and IL-13). Eosinophils and basophils, activated through cell surface FcεRs, rapidly release highly toxic granular proteins (major basic protein, eosinophil peroxidase, and collagenase) and, over a longer period, produce cytokines (IL-3, IL-5, and GM-CSF), chemokines (IL-8), prostaglandins, and leukotrienes that activate epithelial cells, leukocytes, and eosinophils to augment local inflammation and tissue damage.

FcεR-bearing effectors act in a coordinated fashion. The immediate allergic inflammatory reaction initiated by mast cell products is followed by a late-phase response that involves recruitment and activation of eosinophils, basophils, and T_H2 lymphocytes. The manifestations of IgE-mediated reactions depend on the site of mast cell activation. Mast cells reside in vascular and epithelial tissue throughout the body. In a sensitized host (an individual with IgE responses to antigens), re-exposure to antigen leads to type I hypersensitivity responses only in the mast cells exposed to the antigen. Inhalation of antigens produces bronchoconstriction and increased mucus secretion

TABLE 46-1 FOUR MAJOR TYPES OF IMMUNOLOGICALLY MEDIATED HYPERSENSITIVITY REACTIONS*

IMMUNOLOGIC SPECIFICITY	TYPE I (IgE ANTIBODY)	TYPE II (IgG ANTIBODY)	TYPE III (IgG ANTIBODY)	Type IV (T Cells)			
				T$_H$1 CELLS	T$_H$2 CELLS	T$_H$17 CELLS	T CELLS
Antigen	Soluble antigen allergen	Cell- or matrix-associated antigen	Soluble antigen	Soluble antigen	Soluble antigen	Soluble antigen	Cell-associated antigen
Effector mechanism	FcεRI- or FcγRIII-dependent mast cell activation, with release of mediators/cytokines	FcγR$^+$ cells (phagocytes, NK cells), complement	FcγR$^+$ cells, complement	Macrophage activation	Eosinophil activation	Macrophage activation Neutrophil activation	Direct cytotoxicity
Examples	Systemic anaphylaxis, asthma, allergic rhinitis, urticaria, angioedema	Certain drug reactions and reactions to incompatible blood transfusions	Arthus reaction and other immune complex–mediated reactions (e.g., serum sickness, subacute bacterial endocarditis)	Contact dermatitis, tuberculin reaction	Chronic allergic inflammation (e.g., chronic asthma, chronic allergic rhinitis)	Contact dermatitis, atopic dermatitis, asthma, rheumatoid arthritis	Contact dermatitis (e.g., poison ivy), reactions to certain virus-infected cells, some instances of graft rejection

*Hypersensitivity reactions were classified into four types by Coombs and Gell (1963) and modified by Janeway and colleagues (2001).
FcγR = Fc receptor for immunoglobulin G; FcεR = Fc receptor for immunoglobulin E; NK = natural killer.
(From Coombs RRA, Gell PGH: Classification of allergic reactions responsible for clinical hypersensitivity and disease. In Gell PGH, Coombs RA [eds]: *Clinical Aspects of Immunology.* Oxford, UK: Blackwell; 1963; and Janeway C, Travers P, Walport M, Shlomchick M: *Immunobiology: The Immune System in Health and Disease.* 5th ed. New York: Garland Publishing; 2001.)

TABLE 46-2 CLASSIFICATION OF AUTOIMMUNE DISEASES ACCORDING TO MECHANISM OF TISSUE INJURY

HYPERSENSITIVITY REACTION	AUTOIMMUNE DISEASE	AUTOANTIGEN
TYPE II		
Antibody against cell-surface antigens	Autoimmune hemolytic anemia	Rh blood group antigens, I antigen
	Autoimmune thrombocytopenic purpura	Platelet integrin glycoprotein IIb:IIIa
Antibody against receptors	Graves' disease	Thyroid-stimulating hormone receptor (agonistic antibodies)
	Myasthenia gravis	Acetylcholine receptor (antagonistic antibodies)
Antibody against matrix antigens	Goodpasture's syndrome	Basement membrane collagen (α$_3$-chain of type IV collagen)
	Pemphigus vulgaris	Epidermal cadherin (desmoglein)
TYPE III		
Immune complex diseases	Mixed essential cryoglobulinemia	Rheumatoid factor IgG complexes (with or without hepatitis C antigens)
	Systemic lupus erythematosus	DNA, histones, ribosomes, binuclear proteins
TYPE IV		
T-cell-mediated diseases	Insulin-dependent diabetes mellitus	Pancreatic B-cell antigen
	Rheumatoid arthritis	Unknown synovial joint antigen
	Multiple sclerosis	Myelin basic protein, proteolipid protein

FIGURE 46-1. Type I hypersensitivity. Type I responses are mediated by immunoglobulin E (IgE), which induces mast cell activation. Cross-linking of the Fc receptor for IgE (FcεR) on mast cells, triggered by the interaction of multivalent antigen with antigen-specific IgE bound to FcεR, causes the release of preformed granules containing histamine and proteases. Cytokines, chemokines, and lipid mediators are synthesized after cell activation. IL = interleukin; TNF = tumor necrosis factor.

(asthma and allergic rhinitis); ingestion of antigens causes increased peristalsis and secretion (diarrhea and vomiting); and the presence of subcutaneous antigens initiates increased vascular permeability and swelling (urticaria and angioedema). Blood-borne antigens cause systemic mast cell activation, increased capillary permeability, hypotension, tissue swelling, and smooth muscle contraction—the characteristics of systemic anaphylaxis.

Type II Hypersensitivity Reactions

Type II hypersensitivity reactions (Fig. 46-2) are caused by chemical modification of cell surface or matrix-associated antigens that generates "foreign" epitopes to which the immune system is not tolerant. B cells respond to this antigenic challenge by producing IgG, which binds to these modified cells and renders them susceptible to destruction through complement activation, phagocytosis, and antibody-dependent cytotoxicity.

This phenomenon is seen clinically when drugs interact with blood constituents and alter their cellular antigens. Hemolytic anemia caused by immune-mediated destruction of erythrocytes (Chapter 163) and thrombocytopenia caused by destruction of platelets (Chapter 175), both type II hypersensitivity reactions, are adverse effects of certain drugs. Chemically reactive drug molecules bind covalently to the surface of red cells or platelets creating new epitopes that in a small subset of individuals are recognized as foreign antigens by the immune system and stimulate production of IgM and IgG antibodies reactive with the conjugate of drug and cell surface protein. Penicillin-specific IgG binds to penicillin-modified proteins on red blood cells and triggers activation of the complement cascade. Activation of complement components C1 through C3 results in covalent binding of C3b to the red cell membrane and renders circulating red cells susceptible to phagocytosis by FcγR and complement receptor–bearing macrophages in the spleen or liver. Activation of complement components C1 through C9 and formation of the membrane attack complex cause intravascular lysis of red cells. The factors that predispose only some people to drug-induced type II hypersensitivity reactions are unknown. Penicillin, quinidine, and methyldopa have been associated with hemolytic anemia and thrombocytopenia through this mechanism. Another example is heparin-induced

FIGURE 46-2. Type II hypersensitivity. Type II responses are mediated by immunoglobulin G (IgG) directed against cell surface or matrix antigens, which initiates effector responses through the Fc receptor for IgG (FcγR) and complement. The relative contributions of these pathways vary with the IgG subclass and the nature of the antigen. Only FcγR-mediated phagocytosis by macrophages (MΦ) is depicted in this figure. Activation of complement components would result in binding of C3b to the red blood cell membrane, rendering red blood cells susceptible to phagocytosis and leading to formation of the membrane attack complex and cell lysis.

FIGURE 46-3. Type III hypersensitivity. Type III responses are mediated by immunoglobulin G (IgG) directed against soluble antigens. Localized deposition of immune complexes activates mast cells, monocytes, neutrophils, and platelets bearing the Fc receptor for IgG (FcγR), and initiates the complement cascade, all effectors of tissue damage. Generation of complement components C3a and C5a recruits and stimulates inflammatory cells and amplifies effector functions. PMN = polymorphonuclear leukocyte (also called *neutrophil*).

thrombocytopenia or thrombosis, a severe, life-threatening complication that occurs in 1 to 3% of patients exposed to heparin (Chapter 175). Interactions among heparin, human platelet factor 4, antibodies to the human platelet factor 4–heparin complex, platelet FcγRIIA, and splenic FcγRs (which remove opsonized platelets) are involved in the pathogenesis of this disease.

Autoantibodies directed at antigens on the cell surface or extracellular matrix cause tissue damage by mechanisms similar to type II hypersensitivity reactions. IgG or IgM antibodies against erythrocytes lead to cell destruction in autoimmune hemolytic anemia because opsonized cells (coated with IgG or IgM and complement) are removed from the circulation by phagocytes in the liver and spleen or are lysed by formation of the membrane attack complex. Platelet destruction in autoimmune thrombocytopenic purpura occurs through a similar process. Because nucleated cells express membrane-bound complement regulatory proteins, they are less sensitive to lysis through the membrane attack complex, but when coated with antibody, they become targets for phagocytosis or antibody-dependent cytotoxicity. This mechanism is responsible for autoimmune and alloimmune neutropenia (Chapter 170).

IgM and IgG antibodies recognizing antigens within tissue or binding to extracellular antigens cause local inflammatory damage through FcγR and complement mechanisms. Pemphigus vulgaris (Chapter 447) is a serious blistering disease that results from a loss of adhesion between keratinocytes caused by autoantibodies against the extracellular portions of desmoglein 3, an intercellular adhesion structure of epidermal keratinocytes. Another example of a type II hypersensitivity reaction is Goodpasture's disease (Chapter 123), in which antibodies against the α_3-chain of type IV collagen (the collagen in basement membranes) are deposited in glomerular and lung basement membrane. Tissue-bound autoantibodies activate monocytes, neutrophils, and basophils through FcγRs, initiating release of proteases, reactive oxidants, cytokines, and prostaglandins. Local activation of complement, particularly C5a, recruits and activates inflammatory cells and amplifies tissue injury. Neighboring cells are lysed by assembly of the membrane attack complex or by FcγR-initiated, antibody-dependent cytotoxicity.

Autoantibodies against cell surface receptors produce disease by stimulating or blocking receptor function. In myasthenia gravis (Chapter 430), autoantibodies against the acetylcholine receptors on skeletal muscle cells bind the receptor and induce its internalization and degradation in lysosomes, reducing the efficiency of neuromuscular transmission and causing progressive muscle weakness. In contrast, Graves' disease (Chapter 233) is characterized by autoantibodies that act as agonists. Autoantibodies to thyroid-stimulating hormone receptors bind the receptor, mimicking the natural ligand, inducing thyroid hormone overproduction, disrupting feedback regulation, and causing hyperthyroidism.

Type III Hypersensitivity Reactions

Type III hypersensitivity reactions (Fig. 46-3) are caused by tissue deposition of small soluble immune complexes that contain antigens and high-affinity IgG antibodies directed at these antigens. Localized deposition of immune complexes activates FcγR-bearing mast cells and phagocytes and initiates the complement cascade, all effectors of tissue damage.

Immune complexes are generated in all antibody responses. The formation and the fate of immune complexes depend on the biophysical and immunologic properties of the antigen and the antibody. These properties include the size, net charge, and valence of the antigen; the class and subclass of the antibody; the affinity of the antibody-antigen interaction; the net charge and concentration of antibody; the molar ratio of available antigen and antibody; and the ability of the immune complex to interact with the proteins of the complement system. The lattice size of the immune complex is influenced strongly by the physical size and valence of the antigen, the association constant of antibody for that antigen, the molar ratio of antigen and antibody, and the absolute concentrations of the reactants. Larger aggregates fix complement more efficiently, present a broader multivalent array of ligands for complement and FcγRs to bind, and are taken up more readily by mononuclear phagocytes in the liver and spleen and thereby removed from the circulation. Smaller immune complexes, which form in antigen excess—as occurs early in an immune response—circulate in the blood and are deposited in blood vessels, where they initiate inflammatory reactions and tissue damage through interactions with FcγRs and complement receptors.

Serum sickness is a systemic type III hypersensitivity reaction, historically described in patients injected with therapeutic horse antiserum for the treatment of bacterial infections. In general, serum sickness occurs after the injection of large quantities of a soluble antigen. Clinical features include chills, fever, rash, urticaria, arthritis, and glomerulonephritis. Disease manifestations become evident 7 to 10 days after exposure to the antigen, when antibodies are generated against the foreign protein and form immune complexes with these circulating antigens. Immune complexes are deposited in blood vessels, where they activate phagocytes and complement, producing widespread tissue injury and clinical symptoms. The effects are transient, however, and resolve after the antigen is cleared.

A syndrome similar to serum sickness occurs in chronic infections in which pathogens persist in the face of continued immune response. In subacute bacterial endocarditis (Chapter 76), antibody production continues but fails to eliminate the infecting microbes. As the pathogens multiply, generating new antigens, immune complexes form in the circulation and are deposited in small blood vessels, where they lead to inflammatory damage of skin, kidney, and nerve. Hepatitis B virus infection (Chapters 150 and 151) may be associated with immune complex deposition early in its course,

FIGURE 46-4. **Type IV hypersensitivity.** Type IV responses are mediated by T cells through three different pathways. In the first, type 1 helper T (T_H1) cells recognize soluble antigens (Ag) and release interferon-γ (IFN-γ) to activate effector cells, in this case macrophages (MΦ), and cause tissue injury. In T_H2-mediated responses, eosinophils predominate. T_H2 cells produce cytokines to recruit and activate eosinophils, leading to their degranulation and tissue injury lymphocytes (CTLs). In the third pathway, damage is caused directly by cytolytic T cells. IL = interleukin.

during a period of antigen excess, because antibody production in response to hepatitis B surface antigen is as yet relatively insufficient; some anicteric patients may present with acute arthritis. Mixed essential cryoglobulinemia, which may be associated with hepatitis C viral infection, is an immune complex–mediated vasculitis in which deposition of complexes containing IgG, IgM, and hepatitis C antigens causes inflammation in peripheral nerves, kidneys, and skin. Serum sickness also can develop in transplant recipients who are treated with mouse monoclonal antibodies specific for human T cells to prevent rejection, and in patients with myocardial infarction who are treated with the bacterial enzyme streptokinase to effect thrombolysis.

Systemic lupus erythematosus (Chapter 274), the prototypical immune complex–mediated autoimmune disease, is characterized by circulating IgG directed against common cellular constituents, typically DNA and DNA-binding proteins. Small immune complexes are deposited in skin, joints, and glomeruli and initiate local tissue damage.

Type IV Hypersensitivity Reactions

Type IV hypersensitivity reactions (Fig. 46-4), also known as *delayed-type hypersensitivity reactions,* are mediated by antigen-specific effector T cells. They are distinguished from other hypersensitivity reactions by the lag time from exposure to the antigen until the response is evident (1 to 3 days). Antigen is taken up, processed, and presented by macrophages or dendritic cells. Type 1 helper T (T_H1) effector cells that recognize the specific antigen (these are scarce and take time to arrive) are stimulated to release chemokines, which recruit macrophages to the site and release cytokines that mediate tissue injury. IFN-γ activates macrophages and enhances their release of inflammatory mediators, whereas TNF-α and TNF-β activate endothelial cells, enhance vascular permeability, and damage local tissue. The prototypical type IV hypersensitivity reaction is the tuberculin test, but similar reactions can occur after contact with sensitizing antigens (e.g., poison ivy, certain metals) and lead to epidermal reactions characterized by erythema, cellular infiltration, and vesicles. CD8$^+$ T cells also may mediate damage by direct toxicity.

In contrast to T_H1-mediated hypersensitivity reactions, in which the effectors are macrophages, eosinophils predominate in T_H2-mediated responses.

T_H2 effector T cells are associated with tissue damage in chronic asthma (Chapter 87). T_H2 cells produce cytokines to recruit and activate eosinophils (IL-5 and eotaxin), leading to degranulation, further tissue injury, and chronic, irreversible airway damage.

T_H17 cells, members of the helper T-cell lineage, produce IL-17 family cytokines that regulate innate effectors and orchestrate local inflammation by inducing release of proinflammatory cytokines and chemokines, recruiting neutrophils, and enhancing T_H2 cytokine production to amplify allergic and autoimmune responses. T_H17 cells have been implicated in contact dermatitis, atopic dermatitis, asthma, and rheumatoid arthritis.

In some autoimmune diseases, effector T cells specifically recognize self-antigens to cause tissue damage, either by direct cytotoxicity or by inflammatory responses mediated by activated macrophages. In type 1 insulin-dependent diabetes mellitus, T cells mediate destruction of B cells of the pancreatic islets. IFN-γ–producing T cells specific for myelin basic proteins have been implicated in multiple sclerosis. Rheumatoid arthritis is another autoimmune disease caused, at least in part, by activated T_H1 cells.

SUGGESTED READINGS

Khosroshahi A, Stone JH. Treatment approaches to IgG4-related systemic disease. *Curr Opin Rheumatol.* 2011;23:67-71. *Review of this systemic fibroinflammatory condition.*

Klareskog L, Gregersen PK, Huizinga TW. Prevention of autoimmune rheumatic disease: state of the art and future perspectives. *Ann Rheum Dis.* 2010;69:2062-2066. *Review of suspected inciting antigens.*

Mauri C. Regulation of immunity and autoimmunity by B cells. *Curr Opin Immunol.* 2010;22:761-767. *Review.*

47

MECHANISMS OF INFLAMMATION AND TISSUE REPAIR

GARY S. FIRESTEIN

THE INFLAMMATORY RESPONSE

Host defense mechanisms have evolved to recognize pathogens rapidly, render them harmless, and repair the damaged tissue. This complex and highly regulated sequence of events can also be triggered by environmental stimuli such as noxious mechanical and chemical agents. Under normal circumstances, tightly controlled responses protect against further injury and clear damaged tissue. In disease states, however, pathologic inflammation can lead to marked destruction of the extracellular matrix (ECM) and organ dysfunction.

Initiation of the Inflammatory Response

When normal tissue encounters a pathogen, resident cells are stimulated by engagement of pattern recognition receptors that activate an ancient arm of host defense known as *innate immunity*. In contrast to *adaptive immunity*, which provides exquisite antigen specificity, innate immune responses recognize common motifs on pathogens (Chapter 44). Additional cytoplasmic receptors can sense "danger" signals from a toxic environment or cellular stress, such as urate or adenosine triphosphate (ATP). Innate mechanisms are designed for rapid responses (minutes to hours) compared with the more leisurely adaptive system that can take days to weeks to develop. In addition to orchestrating early events that are critical to host defense, cells of the innate system like dendritic cells orchestrate the subsequent adaptive cascade through the generation of chemokines that organize lymphoid tissue and presentation of antigens to lymphocytes. Innate immunity provides intergenerational continuity in that the receptors are encoded in the germline and are passed unchanged to progeny to protect the species. In contrast, each individual must generate his or her own adaptive immune system through complex somatic mutations and gene rearrangements. This provides defense tailored for each member of the species; its complexity and beauty permit specificity but also provide opportunities for error such as responses against self-antigens in autoimmunity.

Pattern Recognition Receptors and Innate Immunity

The toll-like receptor (TLR) family of proteins, which bind molecular structures on microbial pathogens that normally are not found in mammalian cells, are critical members of the innate immune system. Some are expressed on the cell surface, such as TLR2, which is activated primarily by bacterial peptidoglycan and lipoproteins, and TLR4, which is activated by lipopolysaccharide (LPS, or endotoxin). Others are expressed mainly on the inner leaflet of cytoplasmic vesicles, like TLR9, which is activated by unmethylated bacterial sequences that are enriched for CpG motifs, or TLR3 and TLR7, which are important for antiviral defense because they bind double-stranded and single-stranded viral RNA, respectively. In addition to exogenous molecules, some endogenous structures can bind to TLRs, including heat shock proteins and oxidized low-density lipoproteins (oxLDLs). The latter might be especially important in the pathogenesis of atherosclerosis, where LDL activates TLR4 within vascular plaques. Local endothelial cell– and macrophage-derived chemotactic factors can then recruit activated T cells into the atheroma.

Signaling by TLR2 and TLR4 progresses through adaptor proteins and often converges on a kinase known as MyD88, which orchestrates several downstream cascades. By directing the phosphorylation of IκB kinase-β (IKKβ), MyD88 activates nuclear factor-κB (NF-κB), a master switch for inflammatory genes. Translocation of NF-κB to the cell nucleus stimulates the production of cytokines (e.g., interleukin-6 [IL-6], IL-8, and tumor necrosis factor [TNF]), the machinery for prostaglandin release (e.g., cyclooxygenase 2 [COX2]), and genes that regulate the ECM (e.g., metalloproteinases). This rapid response is normally transient, although it can persist in pathogenic states. MyD88-independent pathways that stimulate innate immunity also exist. For instance, TLR3 stimulation by RNA viruses uses a separate pathway involving IKKβ and interferon regulating factor-3 (IRF-3). IRF-3, in combination with several other transcription factors, induces the expression of genes such as interferon-β (IFN-β) to establish an antiviral state.

These genes primarily offer protection against pathogens by initiating key defense mechanisms. However, these same pathways can create a hazardous milieu that is toxic to normal cells through the production of oxygen radicals, nitric oxide, and other reactive intermediaries. These molecules can damage DNA and harm bystander cells, or even lead to neoplasia (E-Table 47-1). For instance, long-standing inflammation in the colon, as in ulcerative colitis, is associated with adenocarcinoma. Increased COX2 expression as a result of NF-κB translocation is another mechanism that contributes to the development of tumors at inflammatory sites. An unanticipated finding is that NF-κB itself can also directly augment carcinogenesis by serving as a survival signal for damaged cells that would normally be deleted by apoptosis.

The TLR signal transduction mechanisms, initiated by broad categories of nonmammalian structures, integrate the environmental stimuli and generate a broadly antipathogenic response. Fine-tuning of host defenses against unique pathogen structures to provide long-lived immunity requires the slower, more precise adaptive immune system. Although it is more cumbersome and primitive, innate immunity provides signals that activate adaptive responses. For instance, TLRs can stimulate dendritic cells (Chapter 44), which have internalized and processed antigen, to migrate from peripheral tissues to central lymphoid organs. The dendritic cells can also produce cytokines and, after maturation, present antigens to T cells in the context of class II major histocompatibility molecules and surface costimulatory proteins. The activated T cells can then migrate to the tissue to enhance and amplify the host response. T cells also provide help to B cells, thereby stimulating antibody production and activating other components of innate immunity (e.g., the complement system).

The Inflammasome and Innate Immune Responses

Receptors that can recognize "danger" signals and potential pathogens are present in the cell cytoplasm. The inflammasome is among the best characterized systems and includes the 22-family-member human Nod-like receptor (NLR) family of cytoplasmic proteins. The activated NLR proteins recruit additional proteins to form a complex with caspase-1 and adaptor molecule apoptosis-associated specklike protein (ASC). Activation of caspase-1 is one of the critical functions of inflammasomes, with resultant cleavage and activation of IL-1, IL-18, and IL-33.

Disorders of the inflammasome can lead to autoinflammatory diseases. The prototypic syndromes known as familial cold autoinflammatory disease, Muckle-Wells disease, and neonatal-onset multisystem inflammatory disease (NOMID) are due to nonconserved mutations in the NLR gene that encodes cryopyrin (also known as NALP3). These three rare diseases are characterized by abnormal inflammasome activation with aberrant release of processed IL-1β. The clinical manifestations, including fever, rash, hearing impairment, and arthritis, depend on the specific amino acid substitution as well as other less well-defined genetic influences. The critical role of IL-1 has been proved by studies using treatment with IL-1 inhibitors, which prevent flares and, in some cases, appear to reverse end-organ disease. The inflammasome also appears to play a key role in other more common diseases, such as gout, in which urate crystals can activate the inflammasome. IL-1 inhibitors also appear to be effective in some patients, although long-term controlled studies are needed.

Immune Complexes and Complement

The complement system (Chapter 49) is another ancient defense mechanism that links innate immunity and the humoral arm of adaptive immunity. Both the classical complement pathway, activated by immunoglobulin G (IgG)– and IgM-containing immune complexes, and the alternative pathway, activated by bacterial products, converge at the third component of complement, C3, with proteolytic release of fragments that amplify the inflammatory response and mediate tissue injury. The anaphylotoxins C3a and C5a directly increase vascular permeability and contraction of smooth muscle. C3a and C3a desArg also induce TNF and IL-1β production by peripheral blood mononuclear cells. C5a induces mast cell release of histamine, thereby indirectly mediating increased vascular permeability. C5a also activates leukocytes and enhances their chemotaxis, adhesion, and degranulation, with release of proteases and toxic metabolites. C5b attaches to the surface of cells and microorganisms and is the first component in the assembly of the C5b-9 membrane attack complex.

Individuals with abnormalities of the early complement components, especially C1q, C2, and C4, usually have a minimally increased incidence of infection but demonstrate an enhanced risk of developing autoimmune diseases such as systemic lupus erythematosus (SLE) (Chapter 274). The mechanism of increased disease susceptibility is probably related to inefficient clearance of immune complexes. Enhanced activation and consumption of complement proteins can also occur in SLE accompanied by low plasma C3 and C4 levels, especially in association with disease exacerbations. C3 or C5 deficiency causes increased susceptibility to bacterial infections, whereas defects in the late components that form the membrane attack complex result in an increased incidence of *Neisseria* sp bacteremia.

Environmental Stress and Tissue Damage

Tissue injury due to direct trauma or noxious stimulus also initiates an inflammatory response and is associated with microvascular damage, extravasation of leukocytes through vascular walls, and leakage of plasma and proteins into the tissue. As noted previously, the inflammasome acts as a sensor that can initiate this program in some cases. In other cases, such as ischemia, acid-sensitive ion channels on the cell surface can detect the environmental stress due to a decrease in tissue pH. Thrombus formation at the site of vascular damage begins the inflammatory cascade through the release of vasoactive amines (e.g., serotonin), release of lysosomal proteases, and formation of eicosanoid products. The platelets can also later regulate healing with release of growth factors such as platelet-derived growth factor (PDGF) and transforming growth factor-β (TGF-β).

Second Wave of the Inflammatory Response

Activation of innate immunity quickly leads to the robust influx of inflammatory cells. Resident cells, such as vascular endothelial cells, mast cells, dendritic cells, and interstitial fibroblasts, respond by releasing soluble mediators, including eicosanoids and pro-inflammatory cytokines (E-Table 47-2). These mediators amplify the inflammatory response and recruit additional leukocytes. Locally stimulated cells, along with the newly arrived inflammatory cells, release toxic reactive intermediates of nitrogen and oxygen as well as a myriad of proteases, principally matrix metalloproteinases (MMPs), serine proteases, and cysteine proteases. These molecules are designed to help destroy infectious agents and remove damaged cells, thus clearing the injured site for tissue repair. Prolonged stimulation of acute inflammatory mechanisms can cause severe tissue destruction. However, in most situations, the normal physiologic response is an exquisitely coordinated program that uses proteolytic enzymes to remodel the ECM and promote a supportive environment for wound healing rather than tissue damage.

Cellular Response

Inflammatory cell infiltration at the site of initial tissue damage typically progresses in an orderly fashion. The process begins with release of chemokines and soluble mediators from resident cells, including interstitial fibroblasts, mast cells, and vascular endothelial cells. Signaling from these events alters the local adhesion molecule profile and creates a chemotactic gradient that recruits cells from the blood stream. Mast cells, in particular, act as sentinels and can degranulate within seconds to release vasoactive amines. In most acute responses, polymorphonuclear leukocytes (PMNs) are the first inflammatory cells to extravasate from the circulation and arrive at the site of injury, followed later by mononuclear cells under the influence of separate signals.

Most tissue fibroblasts and vascular endothelial cells are quiescent before migration of PMNs into the tissue. However, these resident cells can be triggered to proliferate and migrate toward the site of injury as well as to synthesize cytokines, proteases, and ECM components. Growth factors are released, such as basic fibroblast growth factor (bFGF) and vascular endothelial growth factor (VEGF), stimulating new blood vessel formation. Together with granulocyte-macrophage colony-stimulating factor (GM-CSF), these locally released growth factors contribute to cellular proliferation and amplification of the inflammatory response and also induce maturation of dendritic cells that process antigens. In addition, fibroblasts and endothelial cells secrete new ECM proteins, MMPs, and other ECM-digesting enzymes. The balance of protease and ECM production varies as tissue is remodeled during the course of inflammation. Initially, the response favors proteolytic activity to clear damaged infrastructure. This is followed by a shift to increased production of new ECM to allow tissue repair and wound healing.

Increased vascular permeability, caused by disruption of endothelial cell tight junctions, allows blood-borne proteins such as fibrinogen, fibronectin, and vitronectin to extravasate into the perivascular ECM. Interaction with preexisting ECM allows the assembly of new ligands for a subset of adhesion molecules (e.g., integrins $\alpha5\beta1$ and $\alpha v\beta3$). This increased vascular permeability and change in the profiles of adhesion molecules and ligands, in conjunction with release of chemoattractant molecules, lead to the recruitment of leukocytes to sites of inflammation. Some of the chemokines involved are IL-8 (for neutrophils), macrophage chemoattractant protein-1 (MCP-1) for monocytes, RANTES (regulated on activation, T-cell expressed and secreted) for monocytes and eosinophils, and IL-16 (for CD4$^+$ T cells). In addition, chemokines recruit specific subsets of cells by binding to chemokine receptors.

The precise combination of chemokines and vascular adhesion molecules present in an inflammatory lesion determines the specificity of time and event for the recruitment of subsets of inflammatory cells. Ligation of integrins on leukocytes also prolongs cell survival once they have moved into the tissue, by preventing apoptosis. The central role of certain specific adhesion molecule-ligand pairs has been confirmed in human diseases. For instance, $\alpha4\beta1$ plays a key role in the recruitment of lymphocytes to the central nervous system in multiple sclerosis, and blocking this interaction suppresses disease activity (Chapter 419). Eosinophils also use the same adhesion receptors to migrate into the lung in allergen-induced asthma (Chapter 87).

Increased expression of intracellular adhesion molecule 1 (ICAM-1) and vascular cell adhesion molecule 1 (VCAM-1), as well as increased chemokine expression, is also evident in other cell types, such as the airway epithelium after allergen challenge in asthma. Rapid and transient influx of neutrophils occurs in allergic airway disease, along with activation of the local T cells and mast cells. These neutrophils produce lipid mediators, reactive oxygen intermediates, and proteases such as elastase, which may contribute to airflow obstruction, epithelial damage, and remodeling. Neutrophil elastase, together with chemokines released by both recruited and allergen-activated T cells and mast cells, serves to recruit eosinophils.

Soluble Mediators
Pro-inflammatory Cytokines
Pro-inflammatory cytokines, often derived from macrophages and fibroblasts, are mediators that activate the immune system. The pro-inflammatory members of the IL-1 family (IL-α, IL-1β, IL-18, and IL-33) and TNF have pleiotropic activities and can enhance adhesion molecule expression on endothelial cells, induce proliferation of endogenous cells, and stimulate antigen presentation. IL-1 and TNF also increase expression of matrix-degrading enzymes, such as collagenase and stromelysin. In addition, they stimulate synthesis of other inflammatory mediators such as prostaglandin E$_2$ (PGE$_2$) from fibroblasts. Inhibitors of TNF are effective therapeutic agents in inflammatory diseases such as psoriasis, rheumatoid arthritis, and inflammatory bowel disease, and IL-1 inhibitors are beneficial in genetic diseases such as Muckle-Wells syndrome and familial cold autoinflammatory syndrome.

IL-1 and TNF comprise only a small fraction of the acute cytokine response. Many other factors also participate, including IL-6 and its related

cytokines (IL-11, osteopontin, and leukemia inhibitory factor), which can both induce acute phase reactants and bias an immune response toward a helper T type 1 (T$_H$1) or T$_H$2 phenotype (Chapter 46). GM-CSF can regulate dendritic cell maturation, increase expression of human leukocyte antigen (HLA-DR) on these cells, and enhance antigen presentation. The T$_H$1 lymphokine IFN-γ, although often considered part of the secondary wave that ensues after T-cell activation, can also induce expression of HLA-DR, increase expression of endothelial cell adhesion molecules, and inhibit collagen production. IL-1, IL-6, and IL-23 coordinate differentiation toward Th17 cells, a phenotype that is thought to play a major role in inflammation and autoimmunity owing to the production of IL-17 family members (IL-17A through F). Of these, IL-17A and perhaps IL-17F are especially important because they can synergize with IL-1 and TNF. The growth factor TGF-β biases cells toward the regulatory T cell (Treg) phenotype, which can suppress antigen-specific responses of other T cells (see later).

Cytokines play a key role in the establishment and perpetuation of inflammatory diseases. In rheumatoid arthritis (Chapter 272), autocrine and paracrine cytokine networks play a critical role in the perpetuation of inflammation. Effects of IL-1 and TNF are often central to continued synovitis, and there is increasing evidence that IL-15 participates by enhancing TNF production. IL-17A contributes to synoviocyte activation, and IL-18 can trigger T-cell differentiation toward a T$_H$1 phenotype. Factors such as MCP-1 recruit and activate macrophages into atheromas containing oxLDLs and foam cells. In allergic asthma (Chapter 87), IL-13 is emerging as a central inflammatory cytokine. IL-13 functions through binding to cell surface IL-4 receptors, and IL-4R–deficient mice are relatively resistant to the development of asthma. An IL-23 inhibitor, ustekinemab, has shown dramatic efficacy in psoriasis, indicating a major role for this pathway in inflammatory skin disease.

Eicosanoids
In addition to cytokines and immune complexes, local inflammatory responses lead to the release of eicosanoids, which are lipid-derived molecules. Because lipids are present in the cell membrane, they are readily available substrates for the synthesis of mediators. These molecules are functional immediately adjacent to sites of synthesis, and their half-lives range from seconds to minutes. Eicosanoids are not stored but are produced de novo from membrane lipids when cell activation by mechanical trauma, cytokines, growth factors, or other stimuli leads to release of arachidonic acid. Cytosolic phospholipase A$_2$ (cPLA$_2$) is the key enzyme in eicosanoid production. Cell-specific and agonist-dependent events coordinate the translocation of cPLA$_2$ to the nuclear envelope, endoplasmic reticulum, and Golgi apparatus, where interaction with cyclooxygenase (COX) (in the case of prostaglandin synthesis) or 5-lipoxygenase (in the case of leukotriene synthesis) can occur.

Prostaglandins
Prostanoids are produced when arachidonic acid is released from the plasma membrane of injured cells by phospholipases and metabolized by cyclooxygenases and specific isomerases (Chapter 36). These molecules act both at peripheral sensory neurons and at central sites within the spinal cord and brain to evoke pain and hyperalgesia. Their production is increased in most acute inflammatory conditions, including arthritis and inflammatory bowel disease. In response to exogenous and endogenous pyrogens, PGE$_2$ derived from COX2 mediates a central febrile response. In addition, prostaglandins synergize with bradykinin and histamine to enhance vascular permeability and edema. The levels of prostaglandins are usually very low in normal tissues and increase rapidly with acute inflammation, well before leukocyte recruitment. COX2 induction with inflammatory stimuli most likely accounts for the high levels of prostanoids in chronic inflammation.

COX2 also plays a key role in platelet-endothelial cell interactions by increasing the production of prostacyclin (PGI$_2$) in endothelial cells (Chapter 36). Increased risk of myocardial infarction associated with the use of selective COX2 inhibitors might be related to unopposed production of thromboxane A$_2$ by COX1 in platelets. Prostacyclin production also protects against atherosclerosis in female mice, and COX2 blockade abrogates this beneficial effect. Thus, COX inhibitors can potentially increase thrombotic events.

Leukotrienes
In addition to prostaglandins, a distinct set of enzymes direct arachidonic acid metabolites toward the synthesis of leukotrienes (Chapter 87). Their relative importance depends on the specific target organ of an inflammatory response. For instance, leukotriene receptor antagonists have demonstrated

efficacy in asthma, whereas similar approaches have been less impressive in rheumatoid arthritis. Unlike prostaglandins, leukotrienes are primarily produced by inflammatory cells such as neutrophils, macrophages, and mast cells. 5-Lipoxygenase is the key enzyme in this cascade, transforming released arachidonic acid to the epoxide leukotriene A_4 (LTA_4) in concert with 5-lipoxygenase-activating protein (FLAP). LTA_4 can be hydrolyzed by cytosolic LTA_4 hydrolase to LTB_4, a potent neutrophil chemoattractant and stimulator of leukocyte adhesion to endothelial cells. LTA_4 can also conjugate with glutathione to form LTC_4 by LTC_4 synthase at the nuclear envelope. LTC_4 migrates out of the cell, using transporters such as the multidrug resistance–associated protein, and can be metabolized extracellularly to LTD_4 and LTE_4. These three cysteinyl leukotrienes comprise the "slow-reacting substance of anaphylaxis" for their slow and sustained smooth muscle–contracting abilities. They promote plasma leakage from postcapillary venules, upregulation of expression of cell surface adhesion molecules, and bronchoconstriction.

Histamine

Histamine is a vasoactive amine produced by basophils and mast cells that markedly increases capillary leakage. In basophils, histamine is released in response to bacterial formylmethionyl-leucyl-phenylalanine (f-MLP) sequences, complement fragments C3a and C5a, and IgE. The resultant edema can be readily observed clinically in urticaria (Chapters 260 and 448) and allergic rhinitis (Chapter 259). Despite the production of histamine in asthma and in acute synovitis, histamine blockers have minimal therapeutic effect in these conditions. The stimulus for release of histamine from mast cell granules is the same as in basophils, except for the absence of f-MLP receptors in this cell type. Histamine can also synergize with locally produced LTB_4 and LTC_4. In addition, histamine enhances leukocyte rolling and firm adhesion, and induces gaps in the endothelial cell lining, enhancing leukocyte extravasation.

Kinins

Kinins induce vasodilation, edema, and smooth muscle contraction, as well as pain and hyperalgesia, through stimulation of C fibers. They are formed from high- and low-molecular-weight kininogens by the action of serine protease kallikreins in plasma and peripheral tissues. The primary products of kininogen digestion are bradykinin and lysyl-bradykinin. These products have high affinity for the B2 receptor, which is widely expressed and is responsible for the most common effects of kinins. The peptides desArg-BK and Lys-desArg-BK are generated by carboxypeptidases and bind the kinin B1 receptor subtype, which is not expressed in normal tissues but is rapidly upregulated by TLR ligands and cytokines. The kinin B2 receptor is internalized rapidly and desensitized, whereas the B1 receptor remains highly responsive. Kinin actions are associated with the secondary production of other mediators of inflammation, including nitric oxide, mast cell–derived products, and the pro-inflammatory cytokines IL-6 and IL-8. In addition, kinins can increase IL-1 production through initial stimulation of TNF and can increase prostanoid production through activation of phospholipase A_2 and release of arachidonic acid.

Mechanisms of Tissue Damage in Inflammation
Reactive Oxygen and Nitrogen

Macrophages, neutrophils, and other phagocytic cells can generate large amounts of toxic reactive oxygen intermediates (ROIs) and reactive nitrogen intermediates (RNIs) that can directly kill pathogens. ROIs and RNIs also serve as critical signal transduction molecules that regulate expression of inflammatory genes.

These molecules can have deleterious effects on normal tissue by damaging DNA, oxidizing membrane lipids, and nitrosylating proteins. Release of reactive intermediates can be initiated by microbial products such as LPS and lipoproteins, by cytokines such as IFN-γ and IL-8, and by engagement of Fc receptors by IgG. These events cause translocation of several cytosolic proteins, including Rac2 and Rho-family guanosine triphosphatase (GTPase) to the membrane-bound complex carrying cytochrome c, with subsequent activation of reduced nicotinamide adenine dinucleotide phosphate (NADPH) oxidase. The reaction catalyzed by NADPH oxidase leads to superoxide production, which, in turn, increases hydrogen peroxide, hydroxyl radicals and anions, hypochlorous acid, and chloramines.

In some cases, ROIs can contribute directly to the initiation of chronic disease. Lipid oxidation produces aldehydes that substitute lysine residues in apolipoprotein B-100. This altered moiety either binds to TLR2 to induce

cytokine production or is internalized by macrophages, leading to the production of foam cells and fatty streaks, the primary lesions of atherosclerosis (Chapter 70). Subsequently, altered epitopes in damaged host proteins can be presented to T cells to initiate an adaptive immune response that amplifies the inflammatory vascular lesion.

Nitric oxide synthases (NOS) convert L-arginine and molecular oxygen to L-citrulline and nitric oxide (NO). There are three known isoforms of NOS: neuronal NOS (ncNOS or NOS1) and endothelial cell NOS (ecNOS or NOS3) are both constitutively expressed, whereas macrophage NOS (macNOS, iNOS, or NOS2) is induced by inflammatory cytokines such as TNF-α and IFN-γ, as well as by products of viruses, bacteria, protozoa, and fungi and by low oxygen tension and low environmental pH.

Together with prostaglandins, the production of NO by NOS2 and ROIs by NADPH oxidase is a key mechanism by which macrophages paradoxically impair T-cell proliferation. This might control inflammatory processes or delete autoreactive T cells and partially accounts for the immunosuppression observed in certain infections and malignancies.

Proteases

Production of enzymes that degrade the ECM represents a key mechanism of tissue turnover in inflammation. Reconfiguring of the matrix remodels damaged tissue, releases matrix-bound growth factors and cytokines, prepares the tissue for the ingrowth of new blood vessels, and alters the local milieu to permit adherence and retention of newly recruited cells.

The MMPs are a family of more than 20 extracellular endopeptidases that participate in degradation and remodeling of the ECM matrix (Table 47-1). They are produced as pro-enzymes and require limited proteolysis or partial denaturation to expose the catalytic site. Their name is derived from their dependence on metal ions (zinc/metzincin superfamily) for activity and from their potent ability to degrade structural ECM proteins. MMPs can also cleave cell surface molecules and other pericellular nonmatrix proteins, thereby regulating cell behavior. For instance, MMPs can alter cell growth by digesting matrix proteins associated with growth factors. FGF and TGF-β

TABLE 47-1 COMMON MATRIX METALLOPROTEINASES (MMPS) AND THEIR SUBSTRATES

MMP FAMILY	MATRIX SUBSTRATES	OTHER SUBSTRATES
Collagenases	Collagen I, II, III, VII, and X Aggrecan	Pro-MMP-1, -2, -8, -9, and -13 Pro-TNF-α
Entactin	α_1-Proteinase inhibitors Gelatin Tenascin	
Gelatinases	Aggrecan Denatured collagen Elastin Fibronectin Laminin Vitronectin	Pro-MMP-1, -2, and -13 Pro-TNF-α Pro-IL-1β Latent TGF-β
Matrilysins	Proteoglycans Denatured collagens Entactin Fibrin, fibrinogen Fibronectin Gelatin Laminin Tenascin Vitronectin	Pro-MMP-2 and -7 Pro-TNF-α Membrane-bound Fas ligand (FasL) Plasminogen β4 Integrins
Stromelysins	Proteoglycans Aggrecan Collagen III, IV, V, IX, X, and XI Entactin Fibrin, fibrinogen Fibronectin Gelatin Laminin Tenascin Vitronectin	Pro-MMP-1, -3, -7, -8, -9, -10, and -13 Pro-TNF-α Pro-IL-1β Plasminogen α_1-Proteinase inhibitors

IL = interleukin; MMP = matrix metalloproteinase; TGF = transforming growth factor; TNF = tumor necrosis factor.

have high affinities for matrix molecules that serve as depots for storage of these cytokines in their activation state. Matrix proteolysis releases some growth factors and can make them available to cell surface receptors. In addition, MMPs can directly cleave and activate growth factors. MMPs affect cell migration by altering cell-matrix or cell-cell receptor sites. For instance, the adhesion molecule β4 integrin is cleaved by MMP-7. MMP-3 and MMP-7 digest E-cadherin and not only disrupt endothelial cell junctions but also stimulate cell migration.

Degradation of the ECM is usually initiated by collagenases, which cleave native collagen. Denatured collagen is then recognized and further degraded by gelatinases and stromelysins. Unlike the collagenases, stromelysins demonstrate broad substrate specificity and act on many ECM proteins, such as proteoglycan, fibronectin, laminin, and many cartilage proteins. Stromelysins can also amplify the remodeling process by activating collagenase through limited proteolysis. MMP gene expression can be induced by many pro-inflammatory cytokines, including TNF, IL-1, IL-17, and IL-18, through MAP kinase signal transduction pathways.

Several other classes of proteases remodel the matrix, including serine proteases and cysteine proteases. High levels of active serine proteases, such as trypsin, chymotrypsin, and elastase, are released by infiltrating PMNs at sites of inflammation and can directly digest the ECM or activate the pro-enzyme forms of secreted MMPs. The ADAM (a disintegrin and metalloproteinase) family can cleave the extracellular domain of cytokine receptors. These ECM proteases include two members of the aggrecanase family. One of the aggrecanases (aggrecanase 2, or ADAMTS5) has been implicated in osteoarthritis because mice deficient in this enzyme have decreased cartilage destruction in models of osteoarthritis.

Tissue Repair and Resolution of Inflammation

Inflammation is a normal physiologic response, but it can cause serious host injury if it is allowed to persist. Hence, additional mechanisms are required to reestablish homeostasis once this response is initiated. Suppression of acute inflammation by removal or deactivation of mediators and effector cells permits the host to repair damaged tissues through elaboration of appropriate growth factors and cytokines (Fig. 47-1). As in the initial generation of an inflammatory response, components of resolution include a cellular response (apoptosis and necrosis), formation of soluble mediators (such as anti-inflammatory cytokines and antioxidants), and production of direct effectors (such as protease inhibitors).

Deletion of Inflammatory Cells

Cells can be removed from an inflammatory site by several mechanisms. First, the influx of cells can be decreased by suppressing chemotactic factor production and vascular adhesion molecule expression. Second, cells, especially lymphocytes, can be released from the tissue and return to the circulation through lymphatics. Third, stressed cells can undergo necrosis with the release of their contents into the local environment. Perhaps the most critical mechanism for clearing cells from an inflammatory site is programmed cell death, or apoptosis.

Apoptosis is a highly regulated process in eukaryotic cells that leads to cell death and marks the surface membrane for rapid removal by phagocytes. This clearance process does not elicit an inflammatory response, in contrast to cell death by necrosis. PMN phagocytes have a very short half-life in the tissue, and the persistence or release of their contents into the microenvironment after death can be deleterious. In some pathologic conditions, such as leukocytoclastic vasculitis (Chapter 278), abundant neutrophil apoptosis is readily apparent on histopathologic examination; in fact, it is one of the pathologic criteria for this diagnosis. Other cells, including T lymphocytes, undergo postactivation apoptosis to prevent their overwhelming of host responses. Defective apoptosis or even persistence of apoptotic cells that escape clearance may contribute to chronic inflammatory and autoimmune diseases. For instance, loss of tolerance to self-antigens might participate in autoimmune responses in SLE.

Commitment of a cell to apoptosis can be initiated by a number of factors, including the ROIs in the cellular microenvironment as well as signaling through several death receptor pathways (e.g., FasL/Fas and TNF-related apoptosis-inducing ligand [TRAIL]). The former can damage DNA, which is a common byproduct of the genotoxic environment created by inflammation. If DNA damage is excessive, repair by tightly regulated mismatch repair mechanisms is terminated, and programmed cell death begins. The burden of mutations induced by ROIs or RNIs in chronic inflammation can potentially accumulate over time and eventually lead to amino acid substitutions in key regulatory proteins. Ultimately, as has been observed in ulcerative colitis, neoplastic disease can ensue.

Removal of apoptotic bodies, or the remnants of packaged apoptotic cells, is rapid and can be accomplished by macrophages, fibroblasts, epithelial and endothelial cells, muscle cells, and dendritic cells. The surface receptors used in recognition and engulfment of apoptotic cells include integrins (e.g., αvβ3), lectins, scavenger receptors, adenosine triphosphate (ATP)-binding cassette transporter 1, LPS receptor, CD14, and complement receptors CR3 and CR4. However, some of these membrane molecules can be used in both pro-inflammatory and apoptotic pathways, the divergence of which may be based on differing ligands and accessory molecules. Apoptotic cells display a series of membrane-associated molecular patterns that interact with receptors on phagocytes. The details of interactions between apoptotic cells and phagocytes are only partially understood. A general feature of apoptotic cells is loss of phospholipid asymmetry, with external presentation of phosphatidylserine. Externalized phosphatidylserine may be sufficient to trigger phagocytosis, but other apoptotic cell surface structures exist.

Although some inflammatory and immune cells are being deleted, other cell lineages expand during the resolution phase. Mesenchymal cells, especially fibroblasts, proliferate and produce new matrix that can contract to form

FIGURE 47-1. Anti-inflammatory mechanisms that resolve inflammation and lead to repair of the extracellular matrix. IL = interleukin; SERPINs = serine protease inhibitors; TGF = transforming growth factor; TIMPs = tissue inhibitor of metalloproteinases; TNF = tumor necrosis factor.

a fibrotic scar. Locally produced growth factors such as PDGF and TGF-β induce DNA synthesis of these stromal cells. In addition, mesenchymal stem cells that either reside in the tissue or migrate from the peripheral blood can differentiate into the appropriate organ-specific lineage. The pluripotential cells, in the presence of the appropriate milieu, can become adipocytes, chondrocytes, bone cells, or other terminally differentiated stromal cells.

Soluble Mediators
Anti-inflammatory Cytokines

A variety of anti-inflammatory cytokines are released by resident and infiltrating cells. TGF-β and IL-10 are examples that are produced by macrophages, interstitial fibroblasts, or T cells. Some T-cell cytokines, including IL-4, IL-10, and IL-13, suppress the expression of MMP by cells stimulated by IL-1 or TNF. In addition to increasing fibroblast proliferation, TGF-β suppresses collagenase production, increases collagen deposition, and decreases MMP activity by inducing production of the tissue inhibitors of metalloproteinases (TIMPs). The repair phase is abnormal in diseases in which tissue fibrosis represents a major pathologic manifestation. For example, scleroderma (Chapter 275) is marked by diffuse fibrosis and is accompanied by high levels of TGF-β and increased production of ECM.

Cytokine decoy receptors can also downregulate the inflammatory response. Receptors can also be shed from the cell surface after proteolytic cleavage and can absorb cytokines, thereby preventing them from ligating functional receptors on cell membranes. These cytokine inhibitors can be released as a coordinated attempt to prevent unregulated inflammation, as in septic shock (Chapter 108), in which endotoxin induces production of soluble receptors after initial massive production of TNF and IL-1. Other types of cytokine-binding proteins are also produced as counter-regulatory mechanisms, including IL-18-binding protein (IL-18BP), which is an Ig superfamily-related receptor that captures IL-18. In bone remodeling (Chapter 251), interactions of receptor activator of NF-κB (RANK) with RANK ligand are required for osteoclast-mediated resorption. The competitive antagonist osteoprotegerin is a member of the TNF receptor family that binds to RANK ligand and inhibits osteoclast activation.

The need for tight control of the pro-inflammatory cytokine IL-1 is demonstrated by the existence of two separate mechanisms. An IL-1 decoy receptor, known as the type II IL-1R, has both cell membrane and soluble forms that neutralize IL-1 activity. In addition, a natural IL-1 antagonist, IL-1Ra, can bind to functional IL-1 receptors and compete with IL-1α or IL-1β. However, IL-1Ra does not transduce a signal to the cell and blocks the biologic functions of ambient IL-1. The balance of IL-1 and IL-1Ra production depends on many influences. For instance, monocytes produce more IL-1, whereas mature macrophages produce IL-1Ra.

Prostanoids and Cyclooxygenase

COX2 induced by pro-inflammatory mediators appears early and can contribute to inflammatory responses. However, COX2 expression late in the process has led to speculation that it also functions in the resolution of inflammation. This regulation might occur through formation of the cyclopentenone prostaglandins (CyPG). The prostanoids can serve as ligands for peroxisome proliferator-activated receptors (PPARs) (Chapter 213). There are three main classes of PPAR receptors—PPARα, PPARβ/δ, and PPARγ—all of which bind to DNA as heterodimers in association with the retinoid X receptor. Activation of PPARγ by CyPG is associated with the suppression of activator protein 1 (AP-1) and signal transducer and activator of transcription (STAT) transcriptional pathways in macrophages. A variety of natural and synthetic PPAR agonists have demonstrated efficacy in models of ischemia-reperfusion injury, arthritis, and inflammatory airway disease.

Inhibitors of Direct Effectors
Antioxidants

Antioxidant enzymes that can inactivate the toxic intermediates and protect normal tissues include catalase and superoxide dismutase. Catalase is a peroxisomal enzyme that catalyzes the conversion of hydrogen peroxide to water and oxygen. Superoxide dismutases (SOD) catalyze the dismutation of superoxide to hydrogen peroxide, which is then removed by catalase or glutathione peroxidase. Glutathione peroxidases and glutathione reductase are additional mechanisms for maintaining redox balance and removal of toxic metabolites. Insufficient production of intracellular antioxidants such as glutathione can suppress lymphocyte responses and could account for defective T-cell receptor signaling and blunted immunity in T cells derived from rheumatoid arthritis synovium (Chapter 272).

Interactions of free radicals with surrounding molecules can generate secondary radical species in a self-propagating chain reaction. Chain-breaking antioxidants are small molecules that can receive or donate an electron and thereby form a stable byproduct with a radical. These antioxidant molecules are categorized as either aqueous phase (vitamin C, albumin, reduced glutathione) or lipid phase (vitamin E, ubiquinol-10, carotenoids, and flavonoids). In addition, transition metal-binding proteins (ceruloplasmin, ferritin, transferrin, and lactoferrin) can serve as antioxidants by sequestering cationic iron and copper and thereby inhibiting the propagation of hydroxyl radicals.

Protease Inhibitors

Protease inhibitors regulate the function of endogenous proteases and reduce the likelihood of collateral damage to tissues. These proteins form two functional classes, active site inhibitors and α2-macroglobulin (α2M). The latter class of protease inhibitors acts by covalently linking the protease to the α2M chain and thereby blocking access to substrates. α2M binds to all classes of proteases and, after forming a covalent bond, conveys them to cells through receptor-mediated endocytosis with subsequent enzymatic inactivation. The family of inhibitors of serine proteases (SERPINs) are the most abundant members of the former class of protease inhibitors and play a major role in regulation of blood clot resolution and inflammation, as indicated by many of their names: antithrombin III, plasminogen activator inhibitors 1 and 2, α2-antiplasmin, α1-antitrypsin, and kallistatin.

The tissue inhibitor of metalloproteinases (TIMP) family blocks the function of most MMPs. The TIMPs bind to activated MMPs and irreversibly block their catalytic sites. Examples of disease states with an unfavorable balance between TIMPs and MMPs include loss of cartilage in arthritis and regulation of tumor metastasis. TIMP-MMP imbalance in destructive forms of arthritis appears be caused by the limited production capacity for protease inhibitors, which is overwhelmed by the prodigious expression of MMPs. Whereas IL-1 and TNF-α induce MMPs, IL-6, TGF-β, and several other growth factors suppress production of MMPs and increase levels TIMPs. Therefore, the cytokine profile has a pivotal influence on the status of remodeling. When pro-inflammatory cytokines predominate, the balance favors matrix destruction; in the presence of pro-inflammatory cytokine inhibitors and growth factors, matrix protein production increases, and MMPs are inhibited by TIMPs.

SUGGESTED READINGS

Davis DM. Mechanisms and functions for the duration of intercellular contacts made by lymphocytes. *Nat Rev Immunol.* 2009;9:543-555. *Detailed discussion of structure and function relationships in key adhesion molecules as they relate to cell-cell communication.*

Karin M. The IκB kinase: a bridge between inflammation and cancer. *Cell Res.* 2008;18:334-342. *Discusses mechanisms that link inflammation and cancer, with an emphasis on NF-κB.*

Lee SB, Kaluri R. Mechanistic connection between inflammation and fibrosis. *Kidney Int.* 2010;78:S22-S26. *Review.*

Martinon F, Mayor A, Tschopp J. The inflammasomes: guardians of the body. *Annu Rev Immunol.* 2009;27:229-265. *Review of how the inflammasome regulates innate immunity and host defense.*

Wang J, Hori K, Ding J, et al. Toll-like receptors expressed by dermal fibroblasts contribute to hypertrophic scarring. *J Cell Physiol.* 2011;226:1265-1273. *Rationale for manipulating these receptors to ameliorate scarring.*

48

TRANSPLANTATION IMMUNOLOGY

MEGAN SYKES

DEFINITION

Clinical transplantation encompasses the transplantation of organs and islets of Langerhans, in which it is necessary to overcome the host-versus-graft (HVG) immune response to avoid rejection, as well as hematopoietic cell transplantation (HCT; Chapter 181), in which not only the HVG but also the graft-versus-host (GVH) immune response must be contended with. Because preparations of marrow or mobilized peripheral blood stem cells contain mature T cells, their administration to conditioned, and consequently immunoincompetent, recipients is associated with the risk of GVH disease. Organs transplanted include the cornea, kidney, liver, heart, lung,

TABLE 48-1 LYMPHOCYTES INVOLVED IN GRAFT REJECTION

CELL TYPE	ANTIGENS RECOGNIZED	FUNCTION	ROLE IN TRANSPLANTATION
CD4$^+$ T cells	Allogeneic MHC class II ($\pm$ peptide) Self–MHC class II + donor peptide	1. Assistance (cytokines and costimulation) in CD8$^+$ T-cell activation, expansion, and CTL differentiation; B-cell Ig class switching, expansion, and effector differentiation 2. Cytotoxicity 3. Regulatory function	Organ allografts Cellular allografts Xenografts GVHD
CD8$^+$ T cells	Allogeneic MHC class I ($\pm$ peptide) Self–MHC class I + donor peptide	1. Cytotoxicity 2. Cytokine production 3. Regulatory function	Organ allografts Cellular allografts Xenografts GVHD
NK cells	MHC class I (activates or inhibits NK cell function) Other activating ligands	1. Cytotoxicity 2. Cytokine production	? Organ allografts Cellular allografts Xenografts
B cells	MHC class I and II Blood group antigens Xenogeneic carbohydrates	1. Antibody-mediated rejection (hyperacute, acute humoral, and chronic rejection)	Organ allografts Cellular allografts Xenografts

CTL = cytotoxic T lymphocyte; GVHD = graft-versus-host disease; Ig = immunoglobulin; MHC = major histocompatibility complex; NK = natural killer.

small intestine, and pancreas, and even the hand and face. The list of transplanted allogeneic cells is likely to expand in the future to include other cell types such as hepatocytes, myoblasts, and stem cell–derived replacement cells. Transplants originating from a member of the same species are referred to as *allotransplants.* However, many believe that transplants from other species, termed *xenografts,* represent a promising solution to the severely inadequate supply of allogeneic organs and tissues, and such grafts may be used in the future.

● ANTIGENS IN TRANSPLANTATION

The major antigens recognized during graft rejection and the cell types targeting them are summarized in Table 48-1.

Major Histocompatibility Antigens

The major histocompatibility complex (MHC; Chapter 45)—consisting of human leukocyte antigens (HLAs) in humans—presents the strongest immunologic obstacle to all types of allografts. Because of its uniquely extensive polymorphism, truly MHC-identical, unrelated donors are difficult to find in an outbred species such as humans. The strong immunogenicity of allogeneic MHC molecules relates to the manner in which T cells are selected in the thymus; developing thymocytes do not survive unless they can weakly recognize a self-MHC/peptide complex on a thymic stromal cell. This process is termed *positive selection*. However, because thymocytes whose receptors have high affinity for self-MHC complexes are deleted, strongly autoreactive T cells rarely make it into the peripheral T-cell pool. Allogeneic antigens are not part of this *negative selection* process. The net result of these two selection steps is that the human T-cell "repertoire" is strongly biased to have cross-reactivity to allogeneic MHC molecules, providing a barrier to organ and hematopoietic cell transplantation. In the case of organ transplantation, in which long-term pharmacotherapy with powerful immunosuppressive drugs is used in an effort to prevent graft rejection, this can translate into improved results with matched organs in some situations. However, for unrelated, cadaveric donor transplantation, the benefits of HLA matching may be counterbalanced by the disadvantages associated with prolonged graft ischemia when attempts are made to transport organs to the most closely matched recipient. For HCT, the risks of GVH disease and marrow graft failure are so greatly amplified in the presence of extensive HLA mismatches that such transplants are generally avoided; if a sufficiently matched, related donor cannot be found, a search is conducted through large registries containing millions of volunteer unrelated donors.

Minor Histocompatibility Antigens

Minor histocompatibility antigens are peptides derived from polymorphic peptides presented by an MHC molecule. Even genotypically HLA-identical siblings have different minor histocompatibility antigens. These are sufficient to induce graft rejection if immunosuppressive pharmacotherapy is not used. In the case of HCT, significant GVH disease frequently (about 30 to 50% of the time) complicates transplantation between HLA-identical siblings, even with the use of pharmacologic immunoprophylaxis.

Other Antigens

The major blood group (ABO) antigens can be the target of a dramatic "hyperacute" rejection process that occurs when mismatched vascularized grafts are transplanted. Recognition of blood group antigens on the endothelial surface of the graft vessels by recipient "natural" antibodies (antibodies without known sensitization to the antigens) activates the complement and coagulation cascades, resulting in rapid graft thrombosis and ischemia. A similar outcome can occur after transplantation to an individual with preformed antidonor HLA antibodies resulting from presensitization by prior transplantation, transfusion, or pregnancy. Antibodies against other polymorphic antigens, such as MHC class I–related chain A, have been associated with graft rejection. Until recently, successful transplantation was not possible in the presence of a positive antidonor crossmatch. However, considerable success has now been achieved in the transplantation of ABO-mismatched kidneys, livers, and hearts (the last in the neonatal period only) and in the transplantation of kidneys to highly presensitized patients. In the case of kidney and liver transplantation, initial removal of the antibody and sometimes depletion of B cells, as well as the infusion of intravenous immunoglobulin, have led to success. ABO-mismatched neonatal heart transplantation has been successful because the transplant is performed before the recipient has developed high levels of anti–blood group antigen antibodies, and the B cells seem to be rendered tolerant to the donor blood group antigen by the grafting process. Recognition of blood group antigens can also be of significance in HCT, in which ABO barriers are routinely crossed in both directions. This can cause hemolysis of recipient erythrocytes if the mismatch is in the GVH direction, but this complication can be avoided by washing the cellular product before infusion. Mismatches in the HVG direction can cause more persistent problems due to ongoing destruction of donor erythropoietic cells, resulting in pure red cell aplasia. More often, however, donor erythropoiesis is established, and antidonor isohemagglutinins disappear from the circulation.

A and B blood group antigens are caused by the presence or absence of specific glycosylation enzymes in different individuals. Likewise, an antigenic specificity of the utmost importance in xenotransplantation is a carbohydrate epitope, Galα1-3Galα1-4GlcNAc (αGal), which is produced by a specific galactosyl transferase. Humans and Old World monkeys lack a functional αGal transferase and produce high levels of natural antibodies against the ubiquitous αGal epitope. Because animals of interest as xenograft sources (e.g., pigs) express αGal at high levels on their vascular endothelium, transplantation of vascularized organs from pigs results in hyperacute rejection unless something is done to absorb the antibodies or inactivate complement. The recent development of αGal-knockout pigs is therefore an important milestone, and encouraging results have been obtained in initial studies of pig-to-primate transplantation.

In another type of transplant reaction, recognition as foreign results not from the presence of an antigen but, paradoxically, from the absence of a self-MHC molecule. Natural killer (NK) cells express a series of surface inhibitory and activating receptors that determine, collectively, whether the NK cell does or does not kill a potential target cell. The ligands for the inhibitory receptors are MHC class I molecules, and the receptors recognize specific groups of alleles. An NK cell may kill an allogeneic target that lacks a self-MHC inhibitory ligand. In animal models, this phenomenon results in rapid bone marrow rejection when the donor marrow cells are not given in excess numbers or when a fraction of them is destroyed by an incompletely suppressed T-cell response. A similar phenomenon has not been clearly demonstrated in clinical HCT. The possibility that NK cells play a role in organ allograft rejection has long been an area of controversy. NK cells may be of particular importance in xenotransplantation, where they appear early in infiltrates of organ xenografts undergoing acute vascular rejection. NK cells clearly play a strong role in the rejection of xenogeneic bone marrow, an observation that is relevant in one approach to inducing tolerance (see the later discussion).

● MECHANISMS OF REJECTION AND GRAFT-VERSUS-HOST DISEASE

Cellular Mediators

Many different cell types participate in rejection responses, and there is considerable redundancy. T cells are key players in most forms of rejection, with the exception of rejection that can be induced by antibodies in the absence of T-cell help. These include hyperacute and acute vascular rejection processes that may be induced by natural antibodies, as described earlier, or by antibodies that are present due to presensitization. The possible role of NK cells has already been discussed.

Direct and Indirect Allorecognition

T-cell responses are induced by antigen-presenting cells (APCs) that present alloantigens. There are two forms of alloantigen recognition—direct and indirect (Fig. 48-1). Direct allorecognition denotes recognition of donor antigens on donor APCs provided by the graft. The extraordinarily high frequency of T cells with alloreactivity is caused by direct recognition of allogeneic MHC. Indirect recognition is the recognition of donor antigens that are picked up and presented on recipient MHC molecules on recipient APCs. The indirect response is more similar to "normal" T-cell responses, in which professional APCs present peptide antigens to T cells that are present at relatively low frequency in the naïve repertoire.

Direct alloreactivity is particularly important in the early post-transplantation period, when APCs within the transplanted organ are still present; many of these cells migrate to the lymphoid tissues, where they initiate the alloresponse. However, the APC supply that comes with the donor graft is not renewable; therefore, if the direct response is not maintained by the recognition of donor antigens on endothelial cells or other cells in the graft, it recedes in importance. The indirect response, in contrast, can be maintained by the constantly renewed pool of recipient APCs. The indirect response is of particular importance in inducing antibody responses.

Effector Mechanisms of Rejection

T cells can promote graft rejection through several effector mechanisms. One is the antibody-dependent processes that have already been discussed, which can be induced by CD4$^+$ helper T cells that promote the differentiation and immunoglobulin (Ig) class switching of B cells that recognize other specificities on the same alloantigens. T cells provide cognate help to B cells when they recognize complexes of self-MHC with donor MHC-derived peptide antigens (produced by B cells whose surface Ig receptors recognize and pick up the donor MHC antigen). If antidonor antibody is not present before transplantation but is induced afterward, the response can lead to the pathologic picture of acute humoral rejection. Antibodies may also participate in a slower, poorly understood process of chronic rejection, which, in the case of kidney and heart transplantation, is characterized by unique vascular lesions with intimal thickening and loss of the vessel space and, in the case of lung transplantation, by obliterative bronchiolitis. The mechanisms underlying these chronic rejection lesions are not well understood, and several different immune processes may in fact lead to similar lesions.

Another major effector pathway leading to graft rejection involves cytotoxic T lymphocytes (CTLs), which are predominantly members of the CD8$^+$ T-cell subset but also include CD4$^+$ T cells. Several effector mechanisms lead to the killing of target cells by CTLs; these include the granzyme/perforin-mediated pathway and the pathways involving Fas/Fas ligand (FasL) and other members of the tumor necrosis factor (TNF) receptor family and their ligands (Chapter 46). Because CD8$^+$ cells recognize MHC class I molecules, which are widely expressed, it is not difficult to envision graft destruction by CD8$^+$ CTLs. CD8$^+$ CTLs may be activated via an APC that is initially stimulated through contact with an alloreactive CD4$^+$ cell. This is one form of CD4 "help" for CD8$^+$ cells. In addition, CD8$^+$ cells may be dependent on cytokines such as interleukin-2 (IL-2) from CD4$^+$ cells for their expansion and cytotoxic differentiation. However, there are also many examples of CD8$^+$ cell-mediated rejection that is independent of "help" from CD4$^+$ cells. MHC class II, which is recognized by CD4$^+$ T cells, is less widely expressed on graft tissues than is MHC class I, although it may be induced on endothelial cells and graft parenchymal cells in the presence of inflammatory cytokines such as interferon-γ (IFN-γ).

In addition to cytotoxic mechanisms resulting from direct allorecognition, CD4$^+$ and CD8$^+$ T cells with indirect specificity seem to be capable of causing graft destruction under some circumstances. Cytokines such as IFN-γ have been implicated in some instances, but the pathways of indirect graft destruction are not well understood. A CD8$^+$ cell-mediated form of skin graft rejection dependent on donor antigens cross-presented on recipient MHC molecules (a form of indirect allorecognition for CD8$^+$ cells) has been described in an animal model. This form of graft rejection may be directed at antigen presented on the endothelial cells of recipient vessels that revascularize the graft. This mechanism would not apply to primarily vascularized organ allografts.

The Role of T-Cell Trafficking

All the rejection processes described require trafficking of T cells into the graft. This process is made possible after the initial activation of naïve T cells in the lymphoid tissues. Naïve T cells can migrate into lymph nodes because of their expression of the CCR7 chemokine receptor and the adhesion molecule L-selectin. These T cells are activated by migratory graft APCs that also enter the lymph nodes. T-cell activation is associated with the loss of CCR7 and L-selectin expression and the acquisition of a new set of chemokine receptors and adhesion molecules that allow rolling and adhesion on the graft endothelium and entry into the graft parenchyma (Chapter 46). Inflammation in the graft, such as that induced by ischemia-reperfusion injury and the transplantation procedure itself, as well as that induced by initially responding T cells, is associated with the upregulation of chemokines and adhesion ligands that promote the entry of lymphocytes into the graft. Nevertheless, well-healed grafts can be slowly rejected by adoptively transferred memory T cells, demonstrating that acute graft injury and inflammation are not essential for rejection in the presence of an established memory T-cell response. Rejection of hematopoietic cell grafts may involve many of the same mechanisms involved in solid organ rejection, although less work has been done in this area.

Mechanisms of Graft-versus-Host Disease

Initiation of GVH disease (Chapter 181) requires that donor T cells recognize host alloantigens. The disease attacks a variety of recipient epithelial

Direct Allorecognition

Indirect Allorecognition

FIGURE 48-1. Direct and indirect allorecognition. Direct allorecognition involves the recognition by a T-cell receptor of major histocompatibility complex (MHC) molecules (with or without a peptide) on a donor antigen-presenting cell (APC). Indirect allorecognition involves recognition by the T-cell receptor of a donor peptide presented on a recipient APC that has picked up and processed donor antigens.

TABLE 48-2 EXPERIMENTAL STRATEGIES TO PREVENT GRAFT-VERSUS-HOST DISEASE

STRATEGY	ADVANTAGES	LIMITATIONS
Donor T-cell T_H2 polarization (e.g., conditioning with ATG and TLI, in vitro stimulation with cytokine exposure)	May preserve GVL	May limit GVL; T_H2 can contribute to acute and chronic GVHD
Tolerance induction of donor T cells (e.g., costimulatory blockade, regulatory cells)	Some strategies may selectively tolerize GVH-reactive T cells (e.g., in vitro antigen exposure with costimulatory blockade)	Global immunosuppression may limit GVL and anti-infectious immunity; tolerance (i.e., GVH protection) may be incomplete
Donor T-cell depletion plus NK-cell infusion with class I mismatched transplantation	NK cells do not cause GVHD but may mediate antitumor effects; donor NK cells may eliminate host APCs that trigger GVHD	May require very large numbers of donor NK cells; antitumor effect may not apply to all tumors; requires appropriate MHC disparity and expression of polymorphic NK cell receptors; insufficient T-cell immunity to infection
Donor T-cell depletion followed by delayed DLI	Preserves high level of GVL due to GVH reactivity; GVHD does not occur if host inflammation from conditioning has subsided and initial HCT was devoid of donor T cells	Antitumor effect delayed until time of DLI; most applicable for indolent lymphohematopoietic tumors; GVHD more difficult to control in humans than in animal models
Depletion of donor T cells recognizing host alloantigens by in vitro activation/depletion (i.e., "allodepletion")	Preserves anti-infectious immunity and tumor antigen-specific responses	Loss of GVH reactivity limits GVL; highly efficient allodepletion methods not yet available; residual T cells may cause GVHD
Donor T-cell depletion with infusion of expanded infection-specific T cells (e.g., CMV or EBV-specific)	Reduced GVHD potential while protecting against significant infectious organisms	Lack of GVL effect; lack of broad anti-infectious immunity; expense and inefficiency of in vitro T-cell expansion; loss of survival/homing potential of cultured T cells
Donor T-cell depletion with infusion of expanded tumor antigen-specific T cells	GVL without GVHD	Lack of anti-infectious immunity; expense and inefficiency of in vitro expansion of tumor-specific T cells; loss of survival/homing potential of cultured T cells
Insertion of suicide gene (e.g., thymidine kinase) into donor T cells	Drugs targeting inserted gene (e.g., gancyclovir) kill donor T cells to treat GVHD after GVL initiated	Expense and inefficiency of in vitro transduction of T cells; loss of function/survival/homing potential of cultured T cells; risk of GVHD if transduction incomplete; curtailment of GVL when donor T cells killed in vivo
Block T-cell trafficking to epithelial GVHD target tissues (e.g., blockade of adhesion molecules or chemokines, sphingosine 1 phosphate agonists)	Permits lymphohematopoietic GVH reactions to occur, with associated GVL effects	Redundancy of trafficking pathways in inflammatory environment may limit efficacy; tumors outside of lymphohematopoietic system not targeted
Block injury/promote repair in epithelial target tissues (e.g., keratinocyte growth factor)	Permits lymphohematopoietic GVH reactions to occur, with associated GVL effects	Efficacy may be limited

APC = antigen-presenting cell; ATG = antithymocyte globulin; CMV = cytomegalovirus; DLI = donor lymphocyte infusion; EBV = Epstein-Barr virus; GVH = graft versus host; GVHD = graft-versus-host disease; GVL = graft-versus-leukemia effects; HCT = hematopoietic cell transplantation; MHC = major histocompatibility complex; NK = natural killer; T_H2 = helper T lymphocytes type 2; TLI = total lymphoid irradiation.

tissues, including the skin, intestine, and liver. Animal models have demonstrated clear roles for both CD4$^+$ and CD8$^+$ cells in initiating GVH disease, and each subset can do so independently of the other. The mechanisms of GVH disease include activation of alloreactive donor T cells by recipient APCs, leading to the differentiation of effector cells with direct cytotoxic activity and cytokine production in response to host antigens. A prominent role is played by TNF-α, whose production is induced in part by the translocation of bacteria across the intestinal wall, promoting activation of the innate immune system via toll-like receptors (Chapter 44). An intensely proinflammatory environment is produced by the combination of conditioning-induced tissue injury and disruption of mucosal barriers, bacterial activation of the innate immune system, and the GVH alloresponse. It is now appreciated that the inflamed microenvironment in target tissues plays an important role in promoting the trafficking of GVH-reactive T cells into these tissues.

● STRATEGIES TO PREVENT GRAFT-VERSUS-HOST DISEASE

In view of the critical role of donor T cells in inducing GVH disease (Chapter 181), an obvious strategy to prevent this complication is to remove mature T cells from the marrow graft. In both animal models and clinical studies, this approach has been effective in preventing GVH disease; however, it has several disadvantages. One is that adult humans, particularly those who have undergone prior chemotherapy and radiotherapy, have little remaining thymic tissue and therefore demonstrate sluggish T-cell recovery, leading to serious opportunistic infections.

The second disadvantage applies to the most common indication for allogeneic HCT—the treatment of hematologic malignancies (Chapter 181). In this setting, T-cell depletion is often associated with an increased relapse rate due to the loss of a graft-versus-tumor effect, which is in large part mediated by GVH alloreactivity. Separation of GVH disease from graft-versus-tumor

effects is a major goal of research in HCT, and some promising strategies are being explored (Table 48-2). These include the control of T-cell trafficking so that the GVH alloresponse is confined to the lymphohematopoietic tissues where the tumor resides, as well as host conditioning with total lymphoid irradiation in combination with antithymocyte globulin in an attempt to enrich NKT cells, which may inhibit GVH disease without impeding graft-versus-tumor effects.

The third disadvantage of donor T-cell depletion in HCT is that it increases the rate of engraftment failure. GVH alloreactivity and a "veto" effect of donor T cells help overcome host resistance to donor engraftment. A "veto" cell, which may be a T cell or an NK cell, kills a CTL that recognizes it. Although this phenomenon has been well established in animal models, its mechanisms have not been clearly determined, and its potential role in humans is uncertain. NK-cell recognition in the GVH direction, resulting from the absence in the recipient of an MHC class I ligand (E-Fig. 48-1) that can trigger a donor NK-cell inhibitory receptor (KIR), may promote donor marrow engraftment and antitumor effects in the setting of T-cell–depleted, HLA-mismatched HCT.

Clinically, pharmacologic immunosuppressive prophylaxis is usually used for at least 6 months after HCT to minimize the complication of GVH disease. Additionally, HLA-matched or closely matched donors are chosen whenever possible, because GVH disease increases in frequency and severity as more HLA barriers are transgressed. These measures are insufficient, however, and GVH disease remains a major complication of HCT. Therefore, many of the new strategies being explored in organ transplantation and other fields are also being examined for the prevention of GVH disease in experimental models. It should be borne in mind, however, that donor T cells' tolerance to recipient alloantigens (see the later discussion) might not be entirely beneficial in the setting of HCT for the treatment of malignant disease, because the loss of GVH alloreactivity is likely to come with a loss of antitumor effects.

STRATEGIES TO PREVENT ALLOGRAFT REJECTION

Nonspecific Immunosuppression

Immunosuppressive drugs are the mainstay of clinical organ transplantation, and improvements in these drugs have allowed the transplantation of hearts, lungs, pancreatic islets, and livers. The mechanisms of action of these agents are discussed in Chapter 34. However, it is noteworthy that despite these improvements and their enormous impact on early graft survival, these agents have been less effective in attenuating late graft loss. Because chronic immunologic rejection processes and the side effects of immunosuppressive drugs themselves are responsible for much of this late graft loss, better immunosuppressive agents and the induction of immune tolerance (see the later discussion) are major research goals.

Costimulatory Blockade

As our understanding of immune responses has increased, efforts to improve allograft survival have focused on numerous biologic agents, including antibodies and small molecules that target receptors of the immune system, as well as cell-based therapies. Because of the central role played by T cells in the immune response, considerable attention has been paid to blockers of T-cell costimulation. When a naïve T cell recognizes antigen through its unique T-cell receptor, additional costimulatory signals are required to allow full activation, expansion, and differentiation to occur. These signals are often provided by APCs in the form of ligands (e.g., B7-1, B7-2) for costimulatory receptors (e.g., CD28) on the T cell. Cross-talk between the T cell and the APC (e.g., due to CD40 activation by CD154 upregulation on the activated T cell) further amplifies the costimulatory activity of the APC, allowing it to effectively activate other T cells as well. The CD154 (T cell)–CD40 (B cell) interaction also promotes Ig class switching and the functioning of B cells as APCs. Blockade of these processes (e.g., by CTLA4Ig and anti-CD154 monoclonal antibodies) has led to marked prolongation of allograft survival in stringent rodent and large-animal models. Robust, systemic tolerance to donor antigens has been achieved in rodents receiving bone marrow transplants with costimulatory blockade and little or no additional conditioning. Some of these agents have been or are currently being evaluated in clinical trials of transplantation and autoimmune diseases. Anti-CD154 antibodies have been associated with thromboembolic complications, however, and their evaluation in transplantation trials is currently on hold. Numerous additional costimulatory and inhibitory pathways that affect T-cell responses have been described, and these are all potential targets for further manipulation of the alloresponse.

Immune Tolerance

Immune tolerance denotes a state in which the immune system is specifically unreactive to the donor graft (or recipient, in the case of GVH reactivity), while remaining normally responsive to other antigens. Tolerance is distinct from the state produced by nonspecific immunosuppressive agents, which increases the risk of infection and malignancy. Numerous approaches to tolerance induction have been described in rodent models, largely owing to the strong tolerogenicity of primarily vascularized heart, liver, and kidney grafts in these animals. Because such grafts are less tolerogenic in humans, none of these strategies has been applied clinically to date. Therefore, tolerance strategies that are appropriate for clinical evaluation must first be tested in stringent models, including relatively nontolerogenic grafts such as MHC-mismatched skin in rodents and vascularized organ graft models in large animals. In most of the models, only a superficial understanding of the mechanisms leading to tolerance has been achieved.

The three major mechanisms of T-cell tolerance are deletion, anergy, and suppression (often referred to as *regulation*). *Deletion* denotes the destruction of T cells with receptors that recognize donor antigens; it can be achieved during T-cell development in the thymus, for example, by the induction of mixed chimerism in T-cell–depleted hosts. Deletion can also be applied to mature T cells in the periphery, for example, by transplantation of a tolerogenic organ or marrow graft in combination with blockade of costimulatory molecules. *Anergy* denotes the inability of T cells to respond fully to antigens they recognize, and it can be induced by antigen presentation without costimulation. *Suppression* has attracted considerable interest since the discovery that constitutively CD25$^+$ T cells of the CD4$^+$ subset have suppressive activity that is dependent on expression of the transcription factor forkhead box protein 3 (Foxp3). These and other types of suppressive T cells (e.g., NKT cells) have been implicated in rodent transplantation tolerance models and

in the prevention of autoimmunity. However, it seems likely that large numbers of regulatory cells recognizing the relevant antigens would be needed to apply this type of cellular therapy clinically, and the ultimate practicality of the approach remains to be determined. Nevertheless, an improved understanding of this type of immune regulation may lead to effective strategies for activating or expanding regulatory T cells in vivo, thereby favoring the suppressive immune response over destructive alloimmunity.

These developments in animal models and in the understanding of immune mechanisms have encouraged efforts to achieve immune tolerance in the setting of clinical transplantation. Every transplantation center has anecdotal cases of patients who have removed themselves from chronic immunosuppression without experiencing graft rejection. However, for every such patient, there are dozens more who have experienced rejection episodes with dose reductions or discontinuation of immunosuppressive drugs. Although trials of minimization and slow withdrawal of nonspecific immunosuppressive therapy are under way in organ transplant recipients, a major limitation is the absence of good predictors of success. It remains to be seen whether recently identified molecular "tolerance signatures" will provide markers with sufficient predictive value to allow such withdrawal to be undertaken safely.

One approach developed in animal models has been successfully applied to the induction of immune tolerance in a small group of patients receiving renal allografts. This approach involves bone marrow transplantation after nonmyeloablative conditioning, which is much less toxic than standard HCT conditioning. It was shown to be effective in the most stringent rodent and large-animal models before being evaluated clinically. Initial success using combined kidney and bone marrow transplantation in patients with renal failure due to multiple myeloma led to pilot studies in patients with renal failure without malignant disease, with encouraging preliminary results. This approach and others that have emerged from ongoing investigations provide hope that, in the future, transplant recipients might not need chronic immunosuppressive therapy, with its attendant complications and its limited ability to control chronic rejection. Because autoimmune diseases are major contributors to end-stage renal disease, diabetes, and other types of organ failure, the potential of tolerance strategies to reverse autoimmunity while inducing allograft tolerance is a source of hope for those patients as well. All these approaches must be undertaken with the caution, however, because successful regimens could lead to immune tolerance to active infectious organisms as well.

SUGGESTED READINGS

Gooley TA, Chien JW, Pergam SA, et al. Reduced mortality after allogeneic hematopoietic-cell transplantation. *N Engl J Med.* 2010;363:2091-2101. *Mortality from allogeneic hematopoietic stem cell transplantation decreased from 63% in 1993-1997 to 47% in 2003-2007, but the risk of relapse or progression of the underlying disease did not change.*

Locascio SA, Morokata T, Chittenden M, et al. Mixed chimerism, lymphocyte recovery, and evidence for early donor-specific unresponsiveness in patients receiving combined kidney and bone marrow transplantation to induce tolerance. *Transplantation.* 2010;90:1607-1615. *Potential role of chimerism to induce tolerance.*

Sánchez-Fueyo A, Strom TB. Immunologic basis of graft rejection and tolerance following transplantation of liver or other solid organs. *Gastroenterology.* 2011;140:51-64. *Review.*

Sarwal MM. Deconvoluting the "omics" for organ transplantation. *Curr Opin Organ Transplant.* 2009;14:544-551. *An overview of the role of genomics, proteomics, and the like in transplantation medicine.*

Sykes M. Hematopoietic cell transplantation for tolerance induction: animal models to clinical trials. *Transplantation.* 2009;87:309-316. *A review of animal studies and recent clinical studies of tolerance induction using hematopoietic cell transplantation.*

49

COMPLEMENT IN HEALTH AND DISEASE

DAVID R. KARP AND V. MICHAEL HOLERS

The complement system consists of more than 30 serum and membrane proteins that participate in both host defense and a wide variety of pathologic states. This system serves many protective functions ascribed to the innate immune system (Chapter 44). It helps to maintain blood sterility by depositing the membrane attack complex (MAC) in bacterial cell walls and lysing them. It also participates in the opsonization of pathogens for phagocytic removal. The peptide *anaphylatoxins* produced during complement activation promote inflammatory responses with microbicidal effects. The deposition of complement on immune complexes helps to keep them soluble and remove them from the circulation.

There also is increasing evidence that complement can shape the adaptive immune response (Chapter 44). Antigens decorated by complement proteins are taken up by B cells and other antigen-presenting cells, resulting in T-cell activation. Complement activation is needed for optimal antibody production by B cells. Lastly, humans and experimental animals that are deficient in early complement components are often predisposed to autoimmune diseases, particularly systemic lupus erythematosus (SLE) (Chapter 274). This observation suggests that complement is required in some way to identify soluble self-antigens and eliminate self-reactive B cells.

Complement is activated immediately on exposure to immune complexes, but it lacks the immunologic memory of T or B cells with clonotypic receptors that discriminate between self and non-self. Activated complement can be deposited on host and pathogenic surfaces. This potentially dangerous situation is controlled by a series of genetically, structurally, and functionally similar proteins termed the *regulators of complement activation* (RCA). These proteins provide species-specific downregulation of complement activation on host tissues.

Inappropriate complement action occurs when the nondiscriminating activating proteins function in excess of the regulatory proteins that limit damage on self-tissues. This can be seen in almost any inflammatory disease. Some conditions are obvious, such as autoimmune hemolytic anemia, lupus nephritis, and immune complex vasculitis. In other diseases, the role of complement may be contributory but is less clear. These include myocardial infarction, stroke, cardiopulmonary bypass, and hemodialysis. Table 49-1 lists conditions in which complement activation is associated with pathology rather than protection.

In each of these conditions, inhibition of complement activation potentially would limit tissue damage. Many strategies have been developed to discover inhibitors that can work at various sites in the complement activation cascades for use as possible therapeutic agents in human diseases. These potential complement inhibitors include small molecules designed similarly to traditional drugs and newer biologic agents, particularly antibodies that inhibit complement activation.

Although the complement system plays important roles in infection and inflammatory responses, it also has many deleterious effects that must be controlled in conditions ranging from immune complex injury to reproduction. The critical feature of complement-mediated pathology is the alternative pathway amplification loop. As shown in Figure 49-1, failure to control this response results in the generation of potent inflammatory signals and the recruitment of tissue-damaging neutrophils, monocytes, and mast cells. Because more than half of the proteins associated with the complement system are dedicated to the control of activation or effector functions, it is

clear that discrimination between "self" and "non-self" must occur even in the innate immune system.

Knowledge of how complement is activated and how it can be controlled offers new opportunities for the development of therapeutic agents for human diseases. Recently, anti-C5 monoclonal antibody therapy has been approved for treatment of paroxysmal nocturnal hemoglobinuria (Chapter 163), and it is anticipated that within the next few years, many additional complement-targeted drugs will be approved for clinical use. The diseases most likely to be improved by complement inhibition are autoimmune and inflammatory injuries to retina and the kidney.

ACTIVATION OF COMPLEMENT

As an essential component of the innate immune system, complement is endowed with redundant yet carefully controlled activation pathways. The molecular events that occur during activation not only are responsible for the pathology of complement-associated disease states but also offer opportunities for the rational design of inhibitors. For simplicity, it is convenient to think of the different parts of the complement activation pathways as involving *recognition, convertase/amplification,* and *effector* mechanisms.

Classical Pathway

Although traditionally thought of as activated only by immune complexes containing immunoglobulin M (IgM) or IgG, the classical pathway has been shown to be activated by targets other than immune complexes (Fig. 49-2). Notably, apoptotic cells bind C1q and activate the C1 proteases. C1 also is

TABLE 49-1	PATHOLOGIC CONDITIONS PRIMARILY ASSOCIATED WITH COMPLEMENT ACTIVATION
Allotransplantation	Macular degeneration
Alzheimer's disease	Meconium pneumonitis
ARDS	Multiple sclerosis
Arthus reaction	Multisystem organ failure
Asthma	Myasthenia gravis
Bullous pemphigoid	Post–cardiopulmonary bypass
Burns	Psoriasis
Crohn's disease	Recurrent spontaneous abortion
Glomerulonephritis (many causes)	Rheumatoid arthritis
Hemodialysis	Septic shock
Hemolytic anemia	Stroke
Hereditary angioedema	Systemic lupus erythematosus
Immune complex vasculitis	Traumatic brain injury
Ischemia-reperfusion injury	Xenotransplantation

ARDS = adult respiratory distress syndrome.

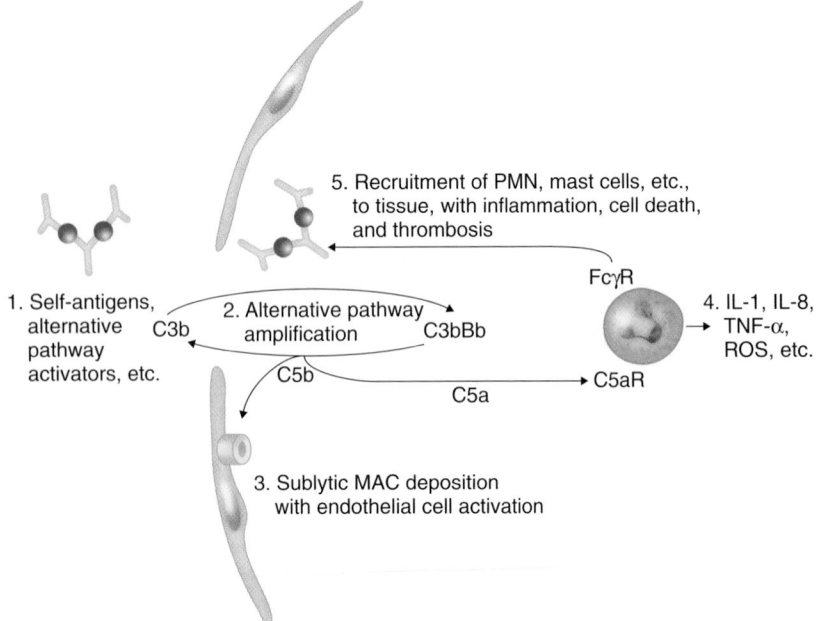

FIGURE 49-1. Pathogenic effect of complement. **1,** Complement is activated by immune complexes or the exposure of surfaces that lack regulatory proteins. **2,** In the absence of effective regulation, the alternative pathway activation loop produces large amounts of both C5a and C5b. **3,** C5b initiates the deposition of sublytic amounts of the membrane attack complex (MAC), leading to cellular activation and proliferation. **4,** C5a is a potent chemoattractant and activator of polymorphonuclear neutrophils (PMN), mast cells, and other leukocytes, resulting in production of inflammatory cytokines and chemokines. **5,** Leukocytes also express Fc receptors (e.g., FcγR) that interact with immunoglobulin G bound to damaged tissue, further amplifying the generation of inflammatory mediators and activating coagulation pathways. IL = interleukin; ROS = reactive oxygen species; TNF-α = tumor necrosis factor-α.

FIGURE 49-2. Schematic representation of the activation of the classical pathway and generation of its C3 convertase. Included are naturally occurring regulators (inhibitors) of this pathway. Ag-Ab = antigen-antibody complex; C1-INH = C1 inhibitor; C4bp = C4-binding protein; CR = complement receptor; CRP = C-reactive protein; DAF = decay-accelerating factor; MCP = membrane cofactor protein; oxLDL = oxidized low-density lipoprotein; SAP = serum amyloid protein.

FIGURE 49-3. Schematic representation of the activation of the lectin pathway and generation in concert with the classical pathway of a C3 convertase. Included are naturally occurring regulators (inhibitors) of this pathway. CR = complement receptor; C4bp = C4-binding protein; DAF = decay-accelerating factor; IgG = immunoglobulin G; MASP = MBL-associated serine protease; MBL = mannose-binding lectin; MCP = membrane cofactor protein.

activated by the accumulated Aβ protein found in the neuritic plaques of patients with Alzheimer's disease. C-reactive protein (CRP) and serum amyloid protein bind to chromatin and other ribonucleoprotein complexes released from apoptotic cells. The CRP–nuclear antigen complexes bind and activate C1. C1q and the classical pathway appear to play a role in the opsonization and removal of nuclear materials that frequently contain autoantigens. The few patients with hereditary C1q deficiency all eventually develop SLE. The addition of CRP and enzymatically modified low-density lipoprotein to human serum causes the activation of complement, as determined by the almost quantitative conversion of C3 to C3b. Finally, deposits of CRP and activated C1 have been shown in infarcted human myocardium. Together, these observations suggest that activation through the antibody-independent classical pathway is important in protective immune responses and in pathogenic inflammatory reactions.

Regulation of the classical pathway activation occurs at several levels. First is the serine protease inhibitor (serpin), C1-inhibitor (C1-INH). C1-INH blocks the activity of many proteases, including factor XIIa, kallikrein, and factor XIa of the clotting system and C1r and C1s in the complement system. The importance of C1-INH is seen in hereditary angioedema (Chapter 260). In this instance, the heterozygous deficiency of C1-INH allows uncontrolled proteolysis of C2 and C4 after minor trauma. A vasoactive peptide is released from C2 and leads to painless (but occasionally life-threatening) soft tissue swelling. Treatment of acute attacks of hereditary angioedema includes purified C1-INH and antifibrinolytic drugs such as ε-aminocaproic acid.

Classical pathway activation also is regulated by RCA proteins. These proteins form the basis for the ability of the complement system to discriminate self from nonself targets. They are discussed in depth later in this chapter. The RCA proteins C4-binding protein (C4-bp) and complement receptor 1 (CR1) provide classical pathway regulation.

Lectin Pathway

The most recently described complement recognition and activation pathway is the lectin pathway (Fig. 49-3). The protein mannose-binding lectin (MBL) is a member of the collectin family that includes pulmonary surfactants A and D. MBL has a structure similar to C1q, in that it consists of several subunits, each having a globular recognition domain and a collagen-like portion that interacts with serine proteases. In the case of MBL, the globular domain is a lectin that binds to repeating carbohydrates (mannose and N-acetylglucosamine) on the surface of pathogens. Many microorganisms are recognized by MBL, including gram-positive and gram-negative bacteria, mycobacteria, fungi, parasites, and viruses, including human immunodeficiency virus 1 (HIV-1). In general, mammalian glycoproteins and glycolipids are not recognized by MBL. One notable exception is agalactosyl IgG. The levels of this modified immunoglobulin are increased in inflammatory conditions such as rheumatoid arthritis, raising the possibility that excessive activation of the lectin pathway is clinically relevant.

Three serine proteases, MASP-1, MASP-2, and MASP-3, associate with MBL, presumably through the collagen-like domain. Although not formally proved, this is analogous to the association of C1r and C1s with C1q. Activation of MASP-1 and MASP-2 results in cleavage of C2 and C4, with the subsequent formation of the classical pathway C3 convertase (C4b2a).

Variation in the structural and regulatory portions of the MBL gene leads to wide individual differences in serum levels. Low levels of MBL have been associated with recurrent infections in children and adults and have been shown to be a minor risk factor for the development of SLE. More striking is

FIGURE 49-4. Schematic representation of the activation of the alternative pathway and generation of its C3 convertase. Included are naturally occurring regulators (inhibitors) of this pathway. C3Nef = C3-nephritic factor; CR = complement receptor; DAF = decay-accelerating factor; IgA = immunoglobulin A; MCP = membrane cofactor protein.

the association of low levels of MBL with infection in SLE. In a study of Danish lupus patients, heterozygous MBL deficiency was associated with a fourfold increase in the risk of bacterial pneumonia, and homozygous deficiency with a more than 100-fold increase.

Alternative Pathway

The alternative pathway is much less stringent in its recognition requirements. It takes advantage of the fact that C3 undergoes spontaneous low-grade activation in the fluid phase (Fig. 49-4). This allows the covalent attachment of C3 to the polysaccharides of fungi and bacteria and to other appropriately charged targets, such as endotoxin and virally infected cells. Other alternative pathway activators include IgA immune complexes and biomaterials, such as cardiopulmonary bypass and hemodialysis membranes.

During spontaneous activation, called *tickover*, C3 acquires a C3b-like conformation and binds factor B, which is cleaved by the serine protease factor D to form the alternative pathway C3 convertase C3bBb. This complex has a short half-life. It is stabilized by properdin (factor P) during physiologic complement activation. This convertase cleaves more C3, which leads to additional C3bBb production. In fact, the C3b can also come from either the classical or alternative pathway. Thus, the activation of complement from any of the three pathways is greatly amplified. The alternative pathway C3 convertase is negatively regulated by the RCA proteins factor H, decay-accelerating factor (DAF), and CR1.

The central role of the alternative pathway as an essential amplifier of complement activation is borne out in its association with a number of clinicopathologic states. For example, membranoproliferative glomerulonephritis type II (Chapter 123) is associated with excessive C3 deposition in the kidney due either to the presence of autoantibodies (C3 nephritic factor) that stabilize the alternative C3 convertase or to genetic deficiencies in the complement regulatory proteins factor H and factor I. Likewise, the atypical form of hemolytic-uremic syndrome (i.e., not associated with shiga-like toxin) (Chapter 175) is found in families that harbor heterozygous mutations in factor H or I or have activating mutations in factor B or C3. Strong genetic associations have linked age-related macular degeneration (Chapter 431) to functional mutations in factor H as well as factor B and C3. Finally, rodent models of many of the complement-associated diseases listed in Table 49-1 are ameliorated when the alternative pathway is genetically disrupted.

C3 and C5 Convertases

The three activation pathways converge at C3. C3 (and C4) contains a reactive glutamic acid residue buried within the three-dimensional structure of the protein. Normally the γ-carboxy group of the reactive glutamic acid in C3 (and C4) is linked to a nearby cysteine in an "internal thioester." On activation, the thioester is exposed to the surface of the protein, where it can react with amino or hydroxyl groups. Most of the thioesters are hydrolyzed by water to form inactive C3 or C4. Some of the thioesters form amide or ester bonds to proteins or carbohydrates, covalently attaching C3b (and C4b) to target surfaces. This enables cells bearing CR1 to bind these targets and opsonize them, representing one of the effector mechanisms of complement.

The covalently bound C3b associates with C4b2a (classical or lectin pathway) or with C3bBb (alternative pathway) to form a convertase for C5. C3b is part of the alternative-pathway C3 convertase, and its product generates an amplification loop that can deposit thousands of C3b molecules on a target, regardless of the initial activation step.

Regulators of Complement Activation

The major function of the protein regulators of complement activation (RCA) (E-Fig. 49-1) as a group is to limit the production of C3b by either the classical or the alternative C3 convertases. Because the addition of C3b to a C3 convertase makes it a C5 convertase, regulation of the two enzyme complexes is linked. Modulation of their activity on host cells limits tissue destruction and the production of inflammatory mediators.

There are six RCA proteins that control the C3/C5 convertases, listed in Table 49-2. The genes for all of these proteins are found in a cluster on human chromosome 1.q32. Structurally, they are composed of repeating subunits termed *short consensus repeats* (SCRs), sometimes referred to as *complement control protein* modules. Each SCR has about 60 amino acids with four invariant cysteine residues. The pairing of the disulfides leads to a four- to five-β pleated sheet structure, causing the SCRs to appear like beads on a string.

Although the SCRs are structurally related, the individual RCA proteins may recognize different parts of the C3 molecule. They do so using specific combinations of SCRs. The RCA proteins function to control complement activation by two processes. First is *decay acceleration*. This refers to the process whereby the RCA protein binds to C3b or C4b in the convertase and dissociates the other members of the complex, rendering it enzymatically inactive. The second effect is *cofactor* activity. Some of the RCA proteins facilitate the recognition of C3b or C4b by a serum protease, factor I. Cleavage of C3b or C4b by factor I renders the convertase irreversibly inactive.

Despite their relatedness, the RCA proteins exhibit differences in their overall structure, distribution, and function (see Table 49-2). All of the RCA

proteins except MCP and CR2 have decay acceleration activity; it is the only function of DAF. This glycosyl phosphatidylinositol-linked protein is widely expressed and causes the removal of C2a or Bb from the C3 and C5 convertases. DAF lacks the cofactor activity seen with the other RCA proteins (except CR2). Factor H and C4bp are serum proteins. MCP and DAF are ubiquitously expressed membrane proteins. CR1 and CR2 are membrane proteins expressed primarily on hematopoietic cells.

RCA proteins have been linked to several disease states. DAF is missing from the abnormal erythrocytes of patients with paroxysmal nocturnal hemoglobinuria (Chapter 163). Although the hemolysis of these cells is ultimately due to the fact that the cells also lack CD59 (see later discussion), the DAF deficiency promotes complement activation on these cells. The association between genetic factor H deficiency and type II membranoproliferative glomerulonephritis and familial hemolytic-uremic syndrome has been mentioned. Lastly, low levels of CR1 and/or CR2 have been seen in patients with SLE. CR1 has cofactor and decay activity, and its major role is in the removal of immune complexes from the circulation. CR2 is necessary for optimal B-cell regulation, including the downmodulation of autoreactive B cells.

Membrane Attack Complex

The cleavage of C5 by either convertase generates C5a, the most potent of the complement anaphylatoxins, and C5b. C5b associates with C6 and C7 to create a lipophilic trimer as part of the MAC (E-Fig. 49-2). On the surface of a target cell, fewer than 1% of the C5b67 trimers that are formed insert into the lipid bilayer and serve as binding sites for C8. This attracts C9 to the membrane, and C9 has the capacity to self-polymerize. A total of 12 to 18 C9 molecules form a ring structure, completing the MAC. In its complete form, the MAC appears like a doughnut with a 10-nm pore running through the center. This pore can allow water and ions to enter the cells, ultimately leading to cell lysis. A MAC with only one or two C9 molecules also can cause lysis, however, suggesting that the MAC disrupts the lipid integrity in its general vicinity, rather than creating holes in the membrane.

The MAC itself appears to be largely redundant in terms of protection against infection. It appears to be essential only for efficient elimination of *Neisseria* species. Individuals who are homozygous deficient for C6, C7, or C8 are at risk for meningococcal and gonococcal infection (Chapters 306 and 307). C9 deficiency is the most common immunodeficiency in Japan, with a heterozygote frequency of 3 to 5%, which notably is not associated with an increased risk of *Neisseria* infection. Absence of an efficient MAC is not deleterious to the population in general and may have some selective advantage.

Extensive complement activation during an inflammatory response can result in sufficient MAC deposition to cause host cell lysis. Most nucleated cells have mechanisms to resist the osmotic changes caused by the MAC, however, and they may "disassemble" the MAC as it is formed. Rather, the nonlethal effects of sublytic MAC deposition are more likely to contribute to pathology. In most cells, this occurs through a general activation of multiple cell signaling pathways. Calcium enters the cell, activating protein kinases and phospholipase C, and upregulates the production of cyclic adenosine monophosphate (cAMP). G proteins and their associated factors are concentrated at the cell membrane, perhaps localized to C9 directly. The mitogen-activated protein kinase pathways (extracellular signal-regulated kinase [ERK], c-Jun N-terminal kinase [JNK], and p38) are activated, resulting in the induction of transcription factors such as c-jun and c-fos, cell proliferation, and inhibition of apoptosis.

The response to MAC deposition depends on the cell type (E-Table 49-1). In phagocytic cells, such as polymorphonuclear neutrophils or macrophages, sublytic MAC activation leads to the production of reactive oxygen species (e.g., superoxide, hydrogen peroxide), as well as prostaglandins and leukotrienes. Platelets undergo the exposure of phosphatidylserine on their outer membrane, facilitating formation of blood coagulation enzyme complexes with a potentially procoagulant effect. On endothelial cells, MAC deposition induces the synthesis of interleukin-1α (IL-1α), which leads to further autocrine and paracrine endothelial cell activation; stimulates a procoagulant state by altering the phospholipid composition of the endothelial membrane, inducing the synthesis of tissue factor and upregulating the synthesis of plasminogen activator inhibitor; induces the expression of adhesion molecules, including intercellular adhesion molecule 1 (ICAM-1) and E-selectin; and stimulates endothelial cells to proliferate through growth factor production. Despite the fact that cell death does not occur, deposition of the sublytic levels of MAC leads to a potentially more dangerous situation, with increased inflammation, coagulation, and cellular proliferation.

TABLE 49-2	DISTRIBUTION AND FUNCTION OF REGULATORS OF COMPLEMENT ACTIVATION (RCA) PROTEINS	
RCA PROTEIN	**DISTRIBUTION**	**FUNCTION**
C4-binding protein	Serum	Cofactor for C4b; decay of classical C3/C5 convertases
Factor H	Serum	Cofactor for C3b; decay of alternative C3/C5 convertases
Decay-accelerating factor	Widely distributed on most cell types	Decay of classical and alternative C3/C5 convertases
Membrane cofactor protein	Widely distributed on most cell types	Cofactor for C3b and C4b (not RBCs)
Complement receptor 1	Most blood cells; mast cells	Cofactor for C3b and C4b; decay of C3/C5 convertases; receptor for C3b/C4b
Complement receptor 2	B cells; follicular dendritic cells	Receptor for C3b fragments; regulation of B cells

RBCs = red blood cells.

Regulation of MAC formation is important clinically and has become an area of therapeutic research. Two fluid-phase proteins, clusterin and S-protein (vitronectin), bind the C5b-7 complex and prevent its association with the lipid membrane. C8 and usually two to four C9 molecules bind to this soluble complex, termed *sC5b-9*, which is lytically inactive. CD59 is a membrane-bound inhibitor of MAC formation. This small glycoprotein is attached to the cell membrane through a glycosyl phosphatidylinositol tail. It binds tightly to C5b-8, preventing the binding and polymerization of C9. CD59 shows strong species restriction, being most effective in the inhibition of MAC formation by the same or closely related species. The expression of CD59 is defective in patients with paroxysmal nocturnal hemoglobinuria, owing to the failure to synthesize the glycosyl phosphatidylinositol tail on this and many other cell surface proteins, including DAF. The clinical features of paroxysmal nocturnal hemoglobinuria are protean. The hemolysis is believed to be caused by low-grade complement activation on red blood cells due to the lack of DAF; without CD59, MAC formation then proceeds and allows hemolysis (Chapter 163).

Anaphylatoxins

In addition to the MAC, the other major source of pathologic damage resulting from complement activation comes from the action of the anaphylatoxins. These are the peptides C3a, C4a, and C5a, which are cleaved from their respective proteins during activation. They were named by Friedberger in 1910 to describe toxic effects after the transfer of complement-activated serum into laboratory animals. They are 77 (C3a and C4a) or 74 (C5a) amino acids long and contain a carboxy (C)-terminal arginine. The structures of C3a and C5a have been determined by x-ray crystallography and nuclear magnetic resonance; they exhibit a compact amino (N)-terminal region that is held together by conserved disulfide bonds. This part of the molecule contains cationic amino acids that are believed to interact with the anaphylatoxin receptors. The C-terminal regions of the anaphylatoxins are extended sequences. Only the last five amino acids are required for activity. In plasma, the C-terminal arginine is removed rapidly by carboxypeptidase N from anaphylatoxins not bound to their receptors. Depending on the response studied, this removal totally inactivates the anaphylatoxin or reduces its potency by 1000-fold.

The C5a receptor (C5aR [CD88]) was the first anaphylatoxin receptor to be characterized. It is a seven-transmembrane-spanning protein that couples ligand binding to G-protein signaling. Expressed on myeloid cells, particularly neutrophils and eosinophils, it mediates the potent chemoattractant property of C5a for both of these cell types. Signaling through CD88 leads to rapid secretion of all granule contents. These include proteases, peroxidases, and lactoferrin from neutrophils, and peroxidase, major basic protein, and eosinophil cationic protein from eosinophils. C5a also induces the release of cytokines, such as tumor necrosis factor (TNF), IL-1, IL-6, and IL-8, and adhesion molecules, promoting the inflammatory response. The C5aR also has been found on numerous other tissues (E-Table 49-2). These include hepatocytes, bronchial and alveolar epithelium, vascular endothelium, renal mesangial and tubular epithelial cells, and brain neuronal cells. The function of C5a in these tissues is not clear. In vitro experiments have shown that these cells are activated by exposure to the anaphylatoxins, leading to production of cytokines, chemokines, and prostaglandins, and to cell proliferation.

The C3a receptor is also a seven-transmembrane-domain protein. It is expressed on almost all myeloid cells, including mast cells, where it mediates the release of allergic mediators. The C3aR also has been detected on many tissues, including in the brain.

The anaphylatoxins have many biologic effects. In general, they cause smooth muscle contraction and recruitment of granulocytes, monocytes, and mast cells. In theory, they can contribute to the pathophysiology of any inflammatory condition. C3a and C5a have been shown to play a role in diseases such as adult respiratory distress syndrome, multisystem organ failure, septic shock, myocardial ischemia-reperfusion injury, asthma, rheumatoid arthritis, SLE, and inflammatory bowel disease. The anaphylatoxin peptides also are responsible for the "postpump" syndrome seen in patients undergoing cardiopulmonary bypass or hemodialysis. Exposure of blood to dialysis or perfusion membranes leads to complement activation. Within minutes of starting bypass, there is a sharp increase in the levels of C3a and C5a in the extracorporeal circuit being returned to the patient. This increase can be associated with respiratory distress, pulmonary hypertension, and pulmonary edema. It has been shown that the length of time that patients stay on the ventilator after bypass surgery depends on the level of C3a generated during reperfusion.

C3a and C5a have been implicated in the initiation and prolongation of adult respiratory distress syndrome (Chapter 104) and multisystem organ failure (Chapter 106). After severe trauma (Chapter 112), levels of C3a have been measured that suggest activation of the entire circulating C3 pool. This activation leads to bronchoconstriction, increased vascular permeability, and vascular plugging with leukocytes. The activation of white blood cells continues the cycle of tissue damage with further complement activation. Continued elevation of C3a in shock or adult respiratory distress syndrome is a poor prognostic sign. C3a also appears to play a major role in the pathogenesis of asthma (Chapter 87).

● COMPLEMENT INHIBITORS

Given the many disease states in which complement is one of the central mediators of pathology, it is no surprise that several complement inhibitors are in preclinical or clinical development for treatment of human diseases. These inhibitors take several different forms. Some are variations of physiologic inhibitors, whereas others are the products of molecular biologic searches for novel compounds.

It is important to consider where in the complement pathway to design an inhibitor to act. Inhibition of the activation pathways limits the production of biologically active peptides. All three pathways need to be inhibited, however, for this approach to be effective. Inhibiting the activation of C3 not only prevents the generation of the C3a anaphylatoxin but also may leave the patient susceptible to infection by limiting the deposition of C3b on targets as an opsonin. Inhibition of C3b deposition also theoretically would decrease the patient's ability to clear immune complexes, resulting in renal, pulmonary, and vascular damage. It also might promote the development of antibodies to self-antigens.

Inhibition of the C5 convertases is an attractive goal because it would prevent the generation of the C5a anaphylatoxin and the MAC. This strategy would inhibit complement activation from any cause without the potentially immunosuppressive effects of limiting C3b deposition. Inhibitors based on this concept are the farthest along in clinical treatment.

Other concerns about complement inhibition include whether it is short-term or long-term and whether it is systemic or localized. Long-term inhibition of complement, particularly at early steps, is likely to predispose the patient to infection. Short-term (hours to days) inhibition at any step is unlikely to cause problems. Given that inflammation is usually a local phenomenon, there are several mechanisms being tested to target complement inhibitors to these sites. In this way, higher levels of inhibition can be achieved where needed with lower doses of inhibitor.

Natural Complement Inhibitors

Naturally occurring compounds that control complement activation include products or extracts of plants, fungi, insects, venoms, and cell lines. The mechanism of complement inhibition by some of these natural products is known and is of clinical and experimental importance. Cobra venom factor isolated from *Naja naja* is a 144,000-D glycoprotein that forms an alternative pathway convertase in association with Bb; this leads to massive activation of complement that causes pulmonary microvascular injury in experimental animals. Perhaps the most widely used natural inhibitor of complement activation is heparin. It decreases activation of the classical and the alternative pathways. In clinical practice, the anticomplementary effect of heparin has been used to prevent complement activation during cardiopulmonary bypass. Measurement of complement activation products such as C3a or soluble C5b-9 after bypass showed decreases of 35 to 70% for adult and pediatric patients when heparin-coated extracorporeal circuits (e.g., Duraflo II) were used. Although numerous studies have looked at the decrease in complement activation by heparin-coated bypass circuits, there have been few attempts to correlate this with clinical outcome.

Anti-C5

The complement inhibitor that has achieved the widest attention as a therapeutic agent is a monoclonal antibody to C5. The advantage to this strategy is that it prevents the generation of C5a, the most potent of the anaphylatoxins, and of the MAC. The generation of C3b and C4b opsonins still would occur, allowing proper clearance of pathogens and immune complexes even if C5 conversion were inhibited chronically. Because there is evidence that activation of early complement components is important for the maintenance of tolerance to self-antigens, inhibition of C5 activation may be less worrisome than inhibition of C3 activation. Lastly, there appears to be little detrimental effect of genetic C5 deficiency. The only consequence of C5 deficiency in humans seems to be an increased risk of *Neisseria* infection.

The anti-C5 monoclonal antibody eculizumab has been approved for use in patients with paroxysmal nocturnal hemoglobinuria to block intravascular hemolysis and stabilize hemoglobin levels.[1] Several groups have also reported the favorable use of an anti-C5 monoclonal antibody in animal model systems of arthritis and lupus nephritis.

Soluble CR1

Soluble CR1 (sCR1) was the first rationally designed complement inhibitor to undergo extensive testing. The idea behind the use of this RCA protein was that it had multiple mechanisms of action. It has two separate binding sites for C3b and one for C4b. It not only serves as a cofactor for the enzymatic degradation of C3b and C4b but also can dissociate the classical (C3b4b) and the alternative (C3b2) C5 convertases. It is produced by recombinant methodology in animal cells. A modified version, produced in a manner that decorates the protein with the carbohydrate sialyl Lewis[x], the ligand for P-selectin and E-selectin, targets sCR1 directly to activated (inflamed) endothelium. Another modified form of sCR1 targets the protein to the lipid membrane of cells. This technique has been shown to be experimentally effective in situations in which sCR1 can be delivered locally, such as intra-articular injections or the perfusion of donor organs before transplantation.

Soluble CR1 blocks activation of complement in many experimental animal models of disease, including myocardial ischemia-reperfusion injury, intestinal ischemia, and middle cerebral artery ligation in rodents. In each case, the administration of sCR1 was associated with decreased tissue injury, less neutrophil accumulation, and lower concentrations of inflammatory mediators such as leukotriene B$_4$. In allograft transplantation, the donor organ undergoes significant ischemia-reperfusion injury. Animal models of allogeneic renal and lung transplantation have shown that sCR1 prolongs graft survival, which may prevent early rejection episodes. In pig-to-primate cardiac xenotransplantation, sCR1 prolonged graft survival remarkably. In one study of human lung transplantation, patients were randomly assigned to receive or not receive a single infusion of 10 mg/kg of sCR1 before restoration of blood flow in the graft. Complement activation was suppressed for 2 days after surgery. There were trends for all patients toward decreased time on the ventilator and in the intensive care unit that did not reach statistical significance. For patients who had been receiving cardiopulmonary bypass during surgery (and may have had more complement activation), however, there was a 56% decrease in time spent on the ventilator postoperatively if they were treated with sCR1.

sCR1 has also been found to have salutary effects in animal models of autoimmune disease, including collagen-induced arthritis, experimental autoimmune neuritis, a model for Guillain-Barré syndrome, and models of myasthenia gravis, multiple sclerosis, and glomerulonephritis.

Transgenic Animals

Xenotransplantation offers a solution to the chronic lack of solid organs for transplantation. The most studied donor animal is the pig because swine have many desirable experimental and practical characteristics, such as size and ease of production. Although immunosuppression and other strategies may be able to overcome cellular immune barriers, the most pressing current problem facing xenotransplantation is hyperacute rejection. This is the immediate (within minutes) cessation of graft function owing to natural IgM antibodies that react with the vascular endothelium of the xenograft. The target of these antibodies is mainly the carbohydrate moiety galactose-(α1,3)-galactose present on the graft. These antibodies quickly activate complement, leading to intravascular coagulation, tissue edema, hemorrhage,

and endothelial activation. Prevention of hyperacute rejection would require reducing the levels of antibodies or of their antigens, inhibiting complement activation, or a combination of all three. Because complement regulatory proteins display species specificity, the approach to limit complement activation in xenografts has been to make transgenic pigs that express one or more membrane proteins of human origin. In one study, kidneys from the triple-transgenic pigs were transplanted into bilaterally nephrectomized baboons. No immunosuppression or pretreatment of the recipients was given. Under these circumstances, the function of a nontransgenic pig kidney ceases within 3 minutes, and the graft rapidly becomes nonviable. The function of transgenic kidneys was maintained with good urine output for 3 to 5 days in the six baboons that received these grafts.

C3a and C5a Receptor Antagonists

The profound biologic effects of the anaphylatoxins and the many conditions in which C3a and C5a are believed to play a pathologic role make the development of specific inhibitors of these proteins attractive. Because the active portion of the anaphylatoxins is contained in the C-terminal part of the protein, it is possible that small-molecule antagonists could be developed that are orally available, easy to synthesize, and inexpensive. These are all advantages over the use of biologics such as monoclonal antibodies or recombinant RCA proteins. To date, several synthetic C5a antagonists have been described. C5a inhibitors are in early human clinical trials. Finally, a potent small-molecule inhibitor of C3a has been found to be active in vitro as an inhibitor of C3a-mediated cellular activation, chemotaxis, and smooth muscle contraction.

Anti–Factor B

Inactivation of the factor B gene in mice prevents a number of autoimmune or inflammatory diseases. Presumably, this represents the necessity for an intact alternative pathway to amplify subclinical complement activation. Inhibition of the alternative pathway activation loop is an attractive target for therapy because it would allow for protective immunity against pathogens through the classical pathway. The efficacy of this approach has been demonstrated using a monoclonal antibody to factor B that inhibits its function. This antibody blocks activation of the alternative pathway in the serum of a number of species, including mice, rats, nonhuman primates, and humans. In a mouse model of complement-mediated pregnancy loss, administration of the anti–factor B antibody resulted in a 50% decrease in fetal death. In models of asthma and renal ischemia-reperfusion injury, this antibody ameliorated disease. This strategy could have wide applicability in a number of disease states.

1. Hillmen P, Young NS, Schubert J, et al. The complement inhibitor eculizumab in paroxysmal nocturnal hemoglobinuria. *N Engl J Med.* 2006;355:1233-1243.

SUGGESTED READINGS

Dunkelberger JR, Song WC. Complement and its role in innate and adaptive immune responses. *Cell Res.* 2010;20:34-50. *Review.*

Lynch AM, Gibbs RS, Murphy JR, et al. Early elevations of the complement activation fragment C3a and adverse pregnancy outcomes. *Obstet Gynecol.* 2011;117:75-83. *Elevated C3a as early as the first trimester of pregnancy is an independent predictor of adverse pregnancy outcomes.*

Ram S, Lewis LA, Rice PA. Infections of people with complement deficiencies and patients who have undergone splenectomy. *Clin Microbiol Rev.* 2010;23:740-780. *Practical review.*

Rutkowski MJ, Sughrue ME, Kane AJ, et al. Cancer and the complement cascade. *Mol Cancer Res.* 2010;8:1453-1465. *Complement proteins can promote carcinogenesis by a variety of mechanisms via dysregulation of mitogenic signaling pathways.*

VIII

CARDIOVASCULAR DISEASE

50

APPROACH TO THE PATIENT WITH POSSIBLE CARDIOVASCULAR DISEASE

LEE GOLDMAN

Patients with cardiovascular disease may present with a wide range of symptoms and signs, each of which may be caused by noncardiovascular conditions. Conversely, patients with substantial cardiovascular disease may be asymptomatic. Because cardiovascular disease is a leading cause of death in the United States and other developed countries, it is crucial that patients be evaluated carefully to detect early cardiovascular disease, that symptoms or signs of cardiovascular disease be evaluated in detail, and that appropriate therapy be instituted. Improvements in diagnosis, therapy, and prevention have contributed to a 70% or so decline in age-adjusted cardiovascular death rates in the United States since the 1960s. However, the absolute number of deaths from cardiovascular disease in the United States has not declined proportionately because of the increase in the population older than 40 years as well as the aging of the population in general.

In evaluating a patient with known or suspected heart disease, the physician must determine quickly whether a potentially life-threatening condition exists. In these situations, the evaluation must focus on the specific issue at hand and be accompanied by the rapid performance of appropriately directed additional tests. Examples of potentially life-threatening conditions include acute myocardial infarction (Chapter 73), unstable angina (Chapter 72), suspected aortic dissection (Chapter 78), pulmonary edema (Chapter 59), and pulmonary embolism (Chapter 98).

⬤ USING THE HISTORY TO DETECT CARDIOVASCULAR SYMPTOMS

Patients may complain spontaneously of a variety of cardiovascular symptoms (Table 50-1), but sometimes these symptoms are elicited only by obtaining a careful, complete medical history. In patients with known or suspected cardiovascular disease, questions about cardiovascular symptoms are key components of the history of present illness; in other patients, these issues are a fundamental part of the review of systems.

Chest Pain

Chest discomfort or pain is the cardinal manifestation of myocardial ischemia resulting from coronary artery disease or any condition that causes myocardial ischemia by an imbalance of myocardial oxygen demand compared with myocardial oxygen supply (Chapter 71). New, acute, often ongoing pain may indicate an acute myocardial infarction, unstable angina, or aortic dissection; a pulmonary cause, such as acute pulmonary embolism or pleural irritation; a musculoskeletal condition of the chest wall, thorax, or shoulder; or a gastrointestinal abnormality, such as esophageal reflux or spasm, peptic ulcer disease, or cholecystitis (Table 50-2). The chest discomfort of myocardial infarction commonly occurs without an immediate or obvious precipitating clinical cause and builds in intensity for at least several minutes; the sensation can range from annoying discomfort to severe pain (Chapter 73). Although a variety of adjectives may be used by patients to describe the sensation, physicians must be suspicious of any discomfort, especially if it radiates to the neck, shoulder, or arms. The probability of an acute myocardial infarction can be estimated by integrating information from the history, physical examination, and electrocardiogram (Fig. 50-1).

The chest discomfort of unstable angina is clinically indistinguishable from that of myocardial infarction except that the former may be precipitated more clearly by activity and may be more rapidly responsive to antianginal therapy (Chapter 72). Aortic dissection (Chapter 78) classically presents with the sudden onset of severe pain in the chest and radiating to the back; the location of the pain often provides clues to the location of the dissection. Ascending aortic dissections commonly present with chest discomfort radiating to the back, whereas dissections of the descending aorta commonly present with back pain radiating to the abdomen. The presence of back pain or a history of hypertension or other predisposing factors, such as Marfan syndrome, should prompt a careful assessment of peripheral pulses to determine whether the great vessels are affected by the dissection and of the chest radiograph to evaluate the size of the aorta. If this initial evaluation is suggestive, further testing with transesophageal echocardiography, computed tomography (CT), or magnetic resonance imaging (MRI) is indicated. The pain of pericarditis (Chapter 77) may simulate that of an acute myocardial infarction, may be primarily pleuritic, or may be continuous; a key physical finding is a pericardial rub. The pain of pulmonary embolism (Chapter 98) is commonly pleuritic in nature and is associated with dyspnea; hemoptysis also may be present. Pulmonary hypertension (Chapter 68) of any cause may be associated with chest discomfort with exertion; it commonly is associated with severe dyspnea and often is associated with cyanosis.

Recurrent, episodic chest discomfort may be noted with angina pectoris and with many cardiac and noncardiac causes (Chapter 71). A variety of stress tests (Table 50-3) can be used to provoke reversible myocardial ischemia in susceptible individuals and to help determine whether ischemia is the pathophysiologic explanation for the chest discomfort (Chapter 71).

Dyspnea

Dyspnea, which is an uncomfortable awareness of breathing, is commonly due to cardiovascular or pulmonary disease. A systematic approach (see Fig. 83-3 in Chapter 83) with selected tests nearly always reveals the cause. Acute dyspnea can be caused by myocardial ischemia, heart failure, severe hypertension, pericardial tamponade, pulmonary embolism, pneumothorax, upper airway obstruction, acute bronchitis or pneumonia, or some drug overdoses (e.g., salicylates). Subacute or chronic dyspnea is also a common presenting or accompanying symptom in patients with pulmonary disease (Chapter 83). Dyspnea also can be caused by severe anemia (Chapter 161) and can be confused with the fatigue that often is noted in patients with systemic and neurologic diseases (Chapters 264 and 403).

In heart failure, dyspnea typically is noted as a hunger for air and a need or an urge to breathe. The feeling that breathing requires increased work or effort is more typical of airway obstruction or neuromuscular disease. A feeling of chest tightness or constriction during breathing is typical of bronchoconstriction, which is commonly caused by obstructive airway disease (Chapters 87 and 88) but also may be seen in pulmonary edema. A feeling of heavy breathing, a feeling of rapid breathing, or a need to breathe more is classically associated with deconditioning.

In cardiovascular conditions, chronic dyspnea usually is caused by increases in pulmonary venous pressure as a result of left ventricular failure (Chapters 58 and 59) or valvular heart disease (Chapter 75). Orthopnea, which is an exacerbation of dyspnea when the patient is recumbent, is due to increased work of breathing because of either increased venous return to the pulmonary vasculature or loss of gravitational assistance in diaphragmatic effort. Paroxysmal nocturnal dyspnea is severe dyspnea that awakens a patient at night and forces the assumption of a sitting or standing position to achieve gravitational redistribution of fluid.

Palpitations

Palpitations (Chapter 62) describe a subjective sensation of an irregular or abnormal heartbeat. Palpitations may be caused by any arrhythmia (Chapters 64 and 65) with or without important underlying structural heart disease. Palpitations should be defined in terms of the duration and frequency of the episodes; the precipitating and related factors; and any associated symptoms of chest pain, dyspnea, lightheadedness, or syncope. It is crucial to use the history to determine whether the palpitations are caused by an irregular or a regular heartbeat. The feeling associated with a premature atrial or ventricular contraction, often described as a "skipped beat" or a "flip-flopping of the heart," must be distinguished from the irregularly irregular rhythm of atrial fibrillation and the rapid but regular rhythm of supraventricular tachycardia. Associated symptoms of chest pain, dyspnea, lightheadedness, dizziness, or diaphoresis suggest an important effect on cardiac output and mandate further evaluation. In general, evaluation begins with ambulatory electrocardiography (ECG) (Table 50-4), which is indicated in patients who have palpitations in the presence of structural heart disease or substantial accompanying symptoms. Depending on the series, 9 to 43% of patients have important underlying heart disease. In such patients, more detailed evaluation is warranted (see Fig. 62-1).

Lightheadedness or *syncope* (Chapter 62) can be caused by any condition that decreases cardiac output (e.g., bradyarrhythmia, tachyarrhythmia, obstruction of the left ventricular or right ventricular inflow or outflow, cardiac tamponade, aortic dissection, or severe pump failure), by

TABLE 50-1 CARDINAL SYMPTOMS OF CARDIOVASCULAR DISEASE

Chest pain or discomfort
Dyspnea, orthopnea, paroxysmal nocturnal dyspnea, wheezing
Palpitations, dizziness, syncope
Cough, hemoptysis
Fatigue, weakness
Pain in extremities with exertion (claudication)

reflex-mediated vasomotor instability (e.g., vasovagal, situational, or carotid sinus syncope), or by orthostatic hypotension (see Table 62-1 in Chapter 62). Neurologic diseases (e.g., migraine headaches, transient ischemic attacks, or seizures) also can cause transient loss of consciousness. The history, physical examination, and ECG are often diagnostic of the cause of syncope (see Table 62-2 in Chapter 62). Syncope caused by a cardiac arrhythmia usually occurs with little warning. Syncope with exertion or just after conclusion of exertion is typical of aortic stenosis and hypertrophic obstructive cardiomyopathy. In many patients, additional testing is required to document central nervous system disease, the cause of reduced cardiac output, or carotid sinus

TABLE 50-2 CAUSES OF CHEST PAIN

CONDITION	LOCATION	QUALITY	DURATION	AGGRAVATING OR RELIEVING FACTORS	ASSOCIATED SYMPTOMS OR SIGNS
CARDIOVASCULAR CAUSES					
Angina	Retrosternal region; radiates to or occasionally isolated to neck, jaw, epigastrium, shoulder, or arms (left common)	Pressure, burning, squeezing, heaviness, indigestion	<2-10 min	Precipitated by exercise, cold weather, or emotional stress; relieved by rest or nitroglycerin; atypical (Prinzmetal's) angina may be unrelated to activity, often early morning	S_3 or murmur of papillary muscle dysfunction during pain
Rest or unstable angina	Same as angina	Same as angina but may be more severe	Usually <20 min	Same as angina, with decreasing tolerance for exertion or at rest	Similar to stable angina but may be pronounced; transient heart failure can occur
Myocardial infarction	Substernal and may radiate like angina	Heaviness, pressure, burning, constriction	≥30 min but variable	Unrelieved by rest or nitroglycerin	Shortness of breath, sweating, weakness, nausea, vomiting
Pericarditis	Usually begins over sternum or toward cardiac apex and may radiate to neck or left shoulder; often more localized than the pain of myocardial ischemia	Sharp, stabbing, knifelike	Lasts many hours to days; may wax and wane	Aggravated by deep breathing, rotating chest, or supine position; relieved by sitting up and leaning forward	Pericardial friction rub
Aortic dissection	Anterior chest; may radiate to back	Excruciating, tearing, knifelike	Sudden onset, unrelenting	Usually occurs in setting of hypertension or predisposition, such as Marfan syndrome	Murmur of aortic insufficiency, pulse or blood pressure asymmetry; neurologic deficit
Pulmonary embolism (chest pain often not present)	Substernal or over region of pulmonary infarction	Pleuritic (with pulmonary infarction) or angina-like	Sudden onset; minutes to <1 hr	May be aggravated by breathing	Dyspnea, tachypnea, tachycardia; hypotension, signs of acute right ventricular failure, and pulmonary hypertension with large emboli; rales, pleural rub, hemoptysis with pulmonary infarction
Pulmonary hypertension	Substernal	Pressure; oppressive	Similar to angina	Aggravated by effort	Pain usually associated with dyspnea; signs of pulmonary hypertension
NONCARDIAC CAUSES					
Pneumonia with pleurisy	Localized over involved area	Pleuritic, localized	Brief or prolonged	Painful breathing	Dyspnea, cough, fever, dull to percussion, bronchial breath sounds, rales, occasional pleural rub
Spontaneous pneumothorax	Unilateral	Sharp, well localized	Sudden onset, lasts many hours	Painful breathing	Dyspnea; hyperresonance and decreased breath and voice sounds over involved lung
Musculoskeletal disorders	Variable	Aching	Short or long duration	Aggravated by movement; history of muscle exertion or injury	Tender to pressure or movement
Herpes zoster	Dermatomal in distribution	Burning, itching	Prolonged	None	Vesicular rash appears in area of discomfort
Esophageal reflux	Substernal, epigastric	Burning, visceral discomfort	10-60 min	Aggravated by large meal, postprandial recumbency; relief with antacid	Water brash
Peptic ulcer	Epigastric, substernal	Visceral burning, aching	Prolonged	Relief with food, antacid	
Gallbladder disease	Epigastric, right upper quadrant	Visceral	Prolonged	May be unprovoked or follow meals	Right upper quadrant tenderness may be present
Anxiety states	Often localized over precordium	Variable; location often moves from place to place	Varies; often fleeting	Situational	Sighing respirations, often chest wall tenderness

Modified from Andreoli TE, Carpenter CCJ, Griggs RC, et al. Evaluation of the patient with cardiovascular disease. In: *Cecil Essentials of Medicine*, 6th ed. Philadelphia: WB Saunders; 2004:34-35.

FIGURE 50-1. Flow diagram to estimate the risk for acute myocardial infarction in emergency departments in patients with acute chest pain. For each clinical subset, the numerator is the number of patients with the set of presenting characteristics who had a myocardial infarction; the denominator is the total number of patients presenting with that characteristic or set of characteristics. CHF = congestive heart failure; DVT = deep vein thrombosis. (Modified from Pearson SD, Goldman L, Garcia TB, et al. Physician response to a prediction rule for the triage of emergency department patients with chest pain. *J Gen Intern Med.* 1994;9:241-247.)

TABLE 50-3 COMMON EXERCISE TEST PROTOCOLS*

PROTOCOL	STAGE	DURATION (min)	GRADE (%)	RATE (mph)	METABOLIC EQUIVALENTS AT COMPLETION	FUNCTIONAL CLASS
Modified Bruce protocol[†]	1	3	0	1.7	2.5	III
	2	3	10	1.7	5	II
	3	3	12	2.5	7	I
	4	3	14	3.4	10	I
	5	3	16	4.2	13	I
Naughton protocol[‡]	0	2	0	2	2	III
	1	2	3.5	2	3	III
	2	2	7	2	4	III
	3	2	10.5	2	5	II
	4	2	14	2	6	II
	5	2	17.5	2	7	I

*Ramp protocols in which the workload is gradually increased on the basis of the patient's estimated functional capacity to achieve maximal effort in approximately 10 minutes are also useful.
[†]Commonly used in ambulatory patients.
[‡]Commonly used in patients with recent myocardial infarction, unstable angina, or other conditions that are expected to limit exercise.
Modified from Braunwald E, Goldman L, eds. *Primary Cardiology*, 2nd ed. Philadelphia: WB Saunders; 2003.

TABLE 50-4 AMERICAN HEART ASSOCIATION/AMERICAN COLLEGE OF CARDIOLOGY GUIDELINES FOR USE OF DIAGNOSTIC TESTS IN PATIENTS WITH PALPITATIONS*

AMBULATORY ELECTROCARDIOGRAPHY

Class I	Palpitations, syncope, dizziness
Class II	Shortness of breath, chest pain, or fatigue (not otherwise explained, episodic, and strongly suggestive of an arrhythmia as the cause because of a relation of the symptom with palpitation)
Class III	Symptoms not reasonably expected to be due to arrhythmia

ELECTROPHYSIOLOGIC STUDY

Class I	Patients with palpitations who have a pulse rate documented by medical personnel as inappropriately rapid and in whom electrocardiographic recordings fail to document the cause of the palpitations Patients with palpitations preceding a syncopal episode
Class II	Patients with clinically significant palpitations, suspected to be of cardiac origin, in whom symptoms are sporadic and cannot be documented; studies are performed to determine the mechanisms of arrhythmias, to direct or provide therapy or to assess prognosis
Class III	Patients with palpitations documented to be due to extracardiac causes (e.g., hyperthyroidism)

ECHOCARDIOGRAPHY

Class I	Arrhythmias with evidence of heart disease Family history of genetic disorder associated with arrhythmias
Class II	Arrhythmias commonly associated with, but without evidence of, heart disease Atrial fibrillation or flutter
Class III	Palpitations without evidence of arrhythmias Minor arrhythmias without evidence of heart disease

*Class I, general agreement the test is useful and indicated; class II, frequently used, but there is a divergence of opinion with respect to its utility; class III, general agreement the test is not useful.
From Braunwald E, Goldman L, eds. *Primary Cardiology*, 2nd ed. Philadelphia: WB Saunders; 2003:132.

TABLE 50-5 A COMPARISON OF THREE METHODS OF ASSESSING CARDIOVASCULAR DISABILITY

CLASS	NEW YORK HEART ASSOCIATION FUNCTIONAL CLASSIFICATION	CANADIAN CARDIOVASCULAR SOCIETY FUNCTIONAL CLASSIFICATION	SPECIFIC ACTIVITY SCALE
I	Patients with cardiac disease but without resulting limitations of physical activity Ordinary physical activity does not cause undue fatigue, palpitation, dyspnea, or anginal pain.	Ordinary physical activity, such as walking and climbing stairs, does not cause angina. Angina with strenuous or rapid or prolonged exertion at work or recreation	Patients can perform to completion any activity requiring ≥7 metabolic equivalents, e.g., can carry 24 lb up 8 steps; carry objects that weigh 80 lb; do outdoor work (shovel snow, spade soil); do recreational activities (skiing, basketball, squash, handball, jog or walk 5 mph)
II	Patients with cardiac disease resulting in slight limitation of physical activity They are comfortable at rest. Ordinary physical activity results in fatigue, palpitations, dyspnea, or anginal pain.	Slight limitation of ordinary activity Walking or climbing stairs rapidly, walking uphill, walking or stair climbing after meals, in cold, in wind, or when under emotional stress, or only during the few hours after awakening Walking >2 blocks on the level and climbing >1 flight of ordinary stairs at a normal pace and in normal conditions	Patient can perform to completion any activity requiring ≥5 metabolic equivalents but cannot and does not perform to completion activities requiring ≥7 metabolic equivalents, e.g., have sexual intercourse without stopping, garden, rake, weed, roller skate, dance foxtrot, walk at 4 mph on level ground
III	Patients with cardiac disease resulting in marked limitation of physical activity They are comfortable at rest. Less than ordinary physical activity causes fatigue, palpitations, dyspnea, or anginal pain.	Marked limitation of ordinary physical activity Walking 1 or 2 blocks on the level and climbing >1 flight in normal conditions	Patient can perform to completion any activity requiring ≥2 metabolic equivalents but cannot and does not perform to completion any activities requiring ≥5 metabolic equivalents, e.g., shower without stopping, strip and make bed, clean windows, walk 2.5 mph, bowl, play golf, dress without stopping
IV	Patients with cardiac disease resulting in inability to carry on any physical activity without discomfort Symptoms of cardiac insufficiency or of the anginal syndrome may be present even at rest. If any physical activity is undertaken, discomfort is increased.	Inability to carry on any physical activity without discomfort—anginal syndrome may be present at rest	Patient cannot or does not perform to completion activities requiring ≥2 metabolic equivalents; cannot carry out activities listed above (Specific Activity Scale, class III)

From Goldman L, Hashimoto B, Cook EF, et al. Comparative reproducibility and validity of systems for assessing cardiovascular functional class: advantages of a new specific activity scale. *Circulation.* 1981;64:1227-1234. Reproduced by permission of the American Heart Association.

syncope. When the history, physical examination, and ECG do not provide helpful diagnostic information that points toward a specific cause of syncope, it is imperative that patients with heart disease or an abnormal ECG be tested with continuous ambulatory ECG monitoring to diagnose a possible arrhythmia (see Fig. 62-1 in Chapter 62); in selected patients, formal electrophysiologic testing may be indicated (Chapter 62). In patients with no evident heart disease, tilt testing (Chapter 62) can help detect reflex-mediated vasomotor instability.

Other Symptoms

Nonproductive *cough* (Chapter 83), especially a persistent cough (see Fig. 83-1 in Chapter 83), can be an early manifestation of elevated pulmonary venous pressure and otherwise unsuspected heart failure. *Fatigue* and *weakness* are common accompaniments of advanced cardiac disease and reflect an inability to perform normal activities. A variety of approaches have been used to classify the severity of cardiac limitations, ranging from class I (little or no limitation) to class IV (severe limitation) (Table 50-5). *Hemoptysis*

(Chapter 83) is a classic presenting finding in patients with pulmonary embolism, but it is also common in patients with mitral stenosis, pulmonary edema, pulmonary infections, and malignant neoplasms (see Table 83-5 in Chapter 83). *Claudication,* which is pain in the extremities with exertion, should alert the physician to possible peripheral arterial disease (Chapters 79 and 80).

Complete Medical History

The complete medical history should include a thorough review of systems, family history, social history, and past medical history (Chapter 14). The review of systems may reveal other symptoms that suggest a systemic disease as the cause of any cardiovascular problems. The family history should focus on premature atherosclerosis or evidence of familial abnormalities, such as may be found with various causes of the long QT syndrome (Chapter 65) or hypertrophic cardiomyopathy (Chapter 60).

The social history should include specific questioning about cigarette smoking, alcohol intake, and use of illicit drugs. The past medical history may reveal prior conditions or medications that suggest systemic diseases, ranging from chronic obstructive pulmonary disease, which may explain a complaint of dyspnea, to hemochromatosis, which may be a cause of restrictive cardiomyopathy. A careful history to inquire about recent dental work or other procedures is crucial if bacterial endocarditis is part of the differential diagnosis.

● PHYSICAL EXAMINATION FOR DETECTION OF SIGNS OF CARDIOVASCULAR DISEASE

The cardiovascular physical examination, which is a subset of the complete physical examination, provides important clues to the diagnosis of asymptomatic and symptomatic cardiac disease and may reveal cardiovascular manifestations of noncardiovascular diseases. The cardiovascular physical examination begins with careful measurement of the pulse and blood pressure (Chapter 7). If aortic dissection (Chapter 78) is a consideration, blood pressure should be measured in both arms and, preferably, in at least one leg. When coarctation of the aorta is suspected (Chapter 69), blood pressure must be measured in at least one leg and in the arms. Discrepancies in blood pressure between the two arms also can be caused by atherosclerotic disease of the great vessels. Pulsus paradoxus, which is more than the usual 10 mm Hg drop in systolic blood pressure during inspiration, is typical of pericardial tamponade (Chapter 77).

General Appearance

The respiratory rate may be increased in patients with heart failure. Patients with pulmonary edema are usually markedly tachypneic and may have labored breathing. Patients with advanced heart failure may have Cheyne-Stokes respirations.

Systemic diseases, such as hyperthyroidism (Chapter 233), hypothyroidism (Chapter 233), rheumatoid arthritis (Chapter 272), scleroderma (Chapter 275), and hemochromatosis (Chapter 219), may be suspected from the patient's general appearance. Marfan syndrome (Chapter 268), Turner's syndrome (Chapter 243), Down syndrome (Chapter 40), and a variety of congenital anomalies also may be readily apparent.

Ophthalmologic Examination

Examination of the fundi may show diabetic (see Fig. 431-24 in Chapter 431) or hypertensive retinopathy (see Fig. 67-11 in Chapter 67) or Roth's spots (see Fig. 431-28 in Chapter 431) typical of infectious endocarditis. Beading of the retinal arteries is typical of severe hypercholesterolemia. Osteogenesis imperfecta, which is associated with blue sclerae, also is associated with aortic dilation and mitral valve prolapse. Retinal artery occlusion (see Fig. 431-29 in Chapter 431) may be caused by an embolus from clot in the left atrium or left ventricle, a left atrial myxoma, or atherosclerotic debris from the great vessels. Hyperthyroidism may present with exophthalmos and typical stare (see Fig. 431-6 in Chapter 431), whereas myotonic dystrophy, which is associated with atrioventricular block and arrhythmia, often is associated with ptosis and an expressionless face (see Fig. 429-2 in Chapter 429).

Jugular Veins

The external jugular veins help in assessment of mean right atrial pressure, which normally varies between 5 and 10 cm H₂O; the height (in centimeters) of the central venous pressure is measured by adding 5 cm to the height of the observed jugular venous distention above the sternal angle

FIGURE 50-2. Jugular venous distention is defined by engorgement of the internal jugular vein more than 5 cm above the sternal angle at 45 degrees. The central venous pressure is the observed venous distention above the sternal angle plus 5 cm. (From American Academy of Family Physicians Online. http://www.aafp.org/afp/20000301/1319.html. Accessed June 9, 2010.)

FIGURE 50-3. Typical distention of the internal jugular vein. (From http://courses.cvcc.vccs.edu/WisemanD/jugular_vein_distention.htm.)

of Louis (Fig. 50-2). The normal jugular venous pulse, best seen in the internal jugular vein (and not seen in the external jugular vein unless insufficiency of the jugular venous valves is present), includes an *a* wave, caused by right atrial contraction; a *c* wave, reflecting carotid artery pulsation; an *x* descent; a *v* wave, which corresponds to isovolumetric right ventricular contraction and is more marked in the presence of tricuspid insufficiency; and a *y* descent, which occurs as the tricuspid valve opens and ventricular filling begins (Fig. 50-3). Abnormalities of the jugular venous pressure (Fig. 50-4) and arterial pulse are useful in detecting conditions such as heart failure, pericardial disease, tricuspid valve disease, and pulmonary hypertension (Table 50-6).

Carotid Pulse

The carotid pulse should be examined in terms of its volume and contour. The carotid pulse (Fig. 50-5) may be increased in frequency and may be more intense than normal in patients with a higher stroke volume secondary to aortic regurgitation, arteriovenous fistula, hyperthyroidism, fever, or anemia. In aortic regurgitation or arteriovenous fistula, the pulse may have a bisferious quality. The carotid upstroke is delayed in patients with valvular aortic stenosis (Chapter 75) and has a normal contour but diminished amplitude in any cause of reduced stroke volume.

Cardiac Inspection and Palpation

Inspection of the precordium may reveal the hyperinflation of obstructive lung disease or unilateral asymmetry of the left side of the chest because of right ventricular hypertrophy before puberty. Palpation may be performed with the patient either supine or in the left lateral decubitus position; the latter position moves the left ventricular apex closer to the chest wall and increases the ability to palpate the point of maximal impulse and other phenomena. Low-frequency phenomena, such as systolic heaves or lifts from the left ventricle (at the cardiac apex) or right ventricle (parasternal in the third or fourth intercostal space), are felt best with the heel of the palm. With the patient in the left lateral decubitus position, this technique also may allow palpation of an S_3 gallop in cases of advanced heart failure or an S_4 gallop in cases of poor left ventricular distensibility during diastole. The left ventricular apex is more diffuse and sometimes may be frankly dyskinetic in patients with advanced heart disease. The distal palm is best for feeling thrills, which are the tactile equivalent of cardiac murmurs. By definition, a thrill denotes a murmur of grade 4/6 or louder. Higher-frequency events may be felt best with the fingertips; examples include the opening snap of mitral stenosis or the loud pulmonic second sound of pulmonary hypertension.

Auscultation

The first heart sound (Fig. 50-6), which is largely produced by closure of the mitral and—to a lesser extent—the tricuspid valves, may be louder in patients with mitral valve stenosis and intact valve leaflet movement and less audible in patients with poor closure due to mitral regurgitation (Chapter 75). The second heart sound is caused primarily by closure of the aortic valve, but closure of the pulmonic valve is also commonly audible. In normal individuals, the louder aortic closure sound occurs first, followed by pulmonic closure. With expiration, the two sounds are virtually superimposed. With inspiration, by comparison, the increased stroke volume of the right ventricle commonly leads to a discernible splitting of the second sound. This splitting may be fixed in patients with an atrial septal defect (Chapter 69) or a right bundle

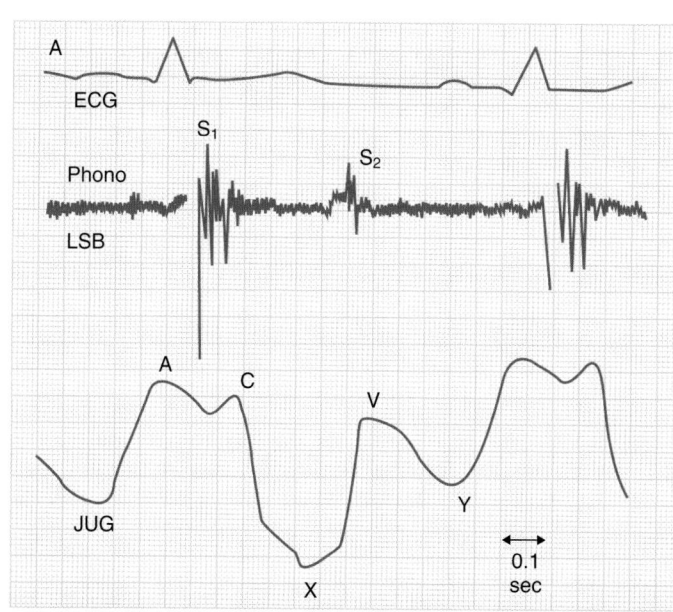

FIGURE 50-4. Normal jugular venous pulse. ECG = electrocardiogram; JUG = jugular vein; LSB = left sternal border; phono = phonocardiogram; S_1 = first heart sound; S_2 = second heart sound.

TABLE 50-6	**ABNORMALITIES OF VENOUS PRESSURE AND PULSE AND THEIR CLINICAL SIGNIFICANCE**
Positive hepatojugular reflux	Suspect heart failure, particularly left ventricular systolic dysfunction (echocardiography recommended)
Elevated systemic venous pressure without obvious x or y descent, quiet precordium, and pulsus paradoxus	Suspect cardiac tamponade (echocardiography recommended)
Elevated systemic venous pressure with sharp y descent, Kussmaul's sign, and quiet precordium	Suspect constrictive pericarditis (cardiac catheterization and MRI or CT recommended)
Elevated systemic venous pressure with a sharp brief y descent, Kussmaul's sign, and evidence of pulmonary hypertension and tricuspid regurgitation	Suspect restrictive cardiomyopathy (cardiac catheterization and MRI or CT recommended)
A prominent a wave with or without elevation of mean systemic venous pressure	Exclude tricuspid stenosis, right ventricular hypertrophy due to pulmonary stenosis, and pulmonary hypertension (echo-Doppler study recommended)
A prominent v wave with a sharp y descent	Suspect tricuspid regurgitation (echo-Doppler or cardiac catheterization to determine etiology)

CT = computed tomography; MRI = magnetic resonance imaging.
From Braunwald E, ed. *Heart Disease: A Textbook of Cardiovascular Medicine,* 5th ed. Philadelphia: WB Saunders; 1997.

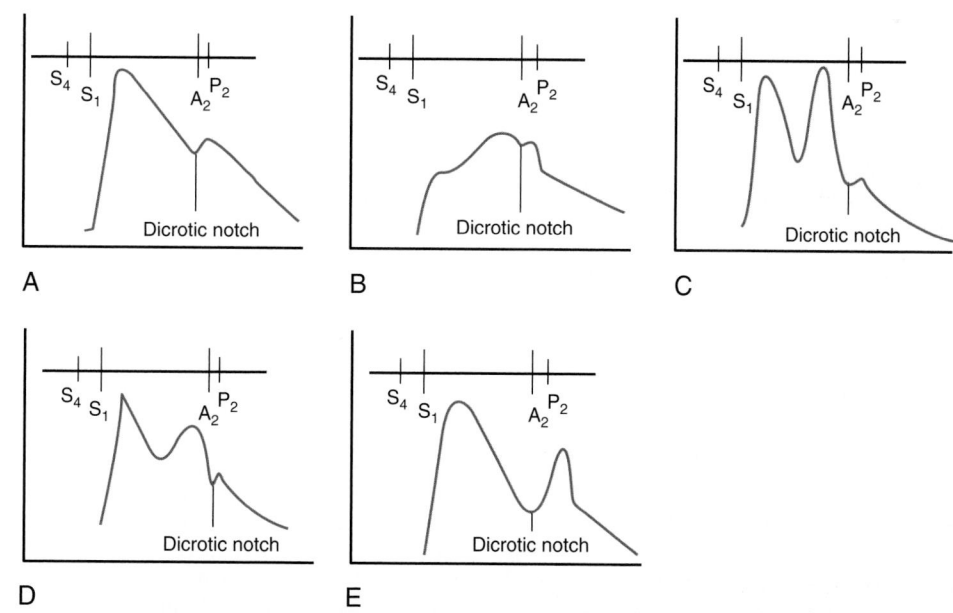

FIGURE 50-5. Schematic diagrams of the configurational changes in the carotid pulse and their differential diagnosis. Heart sounds also are illustrated. **A,** Normal. **B,** Anacrotic pulse with slow initial upstroke. The peak is close to the second heart sound. These features suggest fixed left ventricular outflow obstruction, such as valvular aortic stenosis. **C,** Pulsus bisferiens, with percussion and tidal waves occurring during systole. This type of carotid pulse contour is observed most frequently in patients with hemodynamically significant aortic regurgitation or combined aortic stenosis and regurgitation with dominant regurgitation. It rarely is observed in patients with mitral valve prolapse or in normal individuals. **D,** Pulsus bisferiens in hypertrophic obstructive cardiomyopathy. This finding rarely is appreciated at the bedside by palpation. **E,** Dicrotic pulse results from an accentuated dicrotic wave and tends to occur in sepsis, severe heart failure, hypovolemic shock, and cardiac tamponade and after aortic valve replacement. A_2 = aortic component of the second heart sound; P_2 = pulmonary component of the second heart sound); S_1 = first heart sound; S_4 = atrial sounds. (From Chatterjee K. Bedside evaluation of the heart: the physical examination. In: Chatterjee K, Chetlin MD, Karliner J, et al, eds. *Cardiology: An Illustrated Text/Reference.* Philadelphia: JB Lippincott; 1991:3.11-3.51.)

A S_4 Atrial or presystolic gallop (S_4)

B M_1 T_1 Split first heart sound

C   EC   Aortic or pulmonary systolic ejection click (EC)

D A_2 P_2 Split second heart sound

E   OS   Opening snap of mitral stenosis (OS)

F S_3 Third heart sound (S_3)

G S_1 SC S_2 Midsystolic click (SC)

FIGURE 50-6. **Timing of the different heart sounds and added sounds.** (Modified from Wood P. *Diseases of the Heart and Circulation*, 3rd ed. Philadelphia: JB Lippincott; 1968.)

branch block. The split may be paradoxical in patients with left bundle branch block or other causes of delayed left ventricular emptying. The aortic component of the second sound is increased in intensity in the presence of systemic hypertension and decreased in intensity in patients with aortic stenosis. The pulmonic second sound is increased in the presence of pulmonary hypertension.

Early systolic ejection sounds are related to forceful opening of the aortic or pulmonic valve. These sounds are common in congenital aortic stenosis, with a mobile valve; in hypertension, with forceful opening of the aortic valve; and in healthy young individuals, especially when cardiac output is increased. Midsystolic or late systolic clicks are caused most commonly by mitral valve prolapse (Chapter 75). Clicks are relatively high-frequency sounds that are heard best with the diaphragm of the stethoscope.

An S_3 corresponds to rapid ventricular filling during early diastole. It may occur in normal children and young adults, especially if stroke volume is increased. After about 40 years of age, however, an S_3 should be considered abnormal; it is caused by conditions that increase the volume of ventricular filling during early diastole (e.g., mitral regurgitation) or that increase pressure in early diastole (e.g., advanced heart failure). A left ventricular S_3 gallop is heard best at the apex, whereas the right ventricular S_3 gallop is heard best at the fourth intercostal space at the left parasternal border; both are heard best with the bell of the stethoscope. An S_4 is heard rarely in young individuals but is common in adults older than 40 or 50 years because of

reduced ventricular compliance during atrial contraction; it is a nearly ubiquitous finding in patients with hypertension, heart failure, or ischemic heart disease.

The opening snap of mitral and, less commonly, tricuspid stenosis (Chapter 75) occurs at the beginning of mechanical diastole, before the onset of the rapid phase of ventricular filling. An opening snap is high pitched and is heard best with the diaphragm; this differential frequency should help distinguish an opening snap from an S_3 on physical examination. An opening snap commonly can be distinguished from a loud pulmonic component of the second heart sound by the differential location (mitral opening snap at the apex, tricuspid opening snap at the left third or fourth intercostal space, pulmonic second sound at the left second intercostal space) and by the longer interval between S_2 and the opening snap.

Heart murmurs may be classified as systolic, diastolic, or continuous (Table 50-7). Murmurs are graded by intensity on a scale of 1 to 6. Grade 1 is faint and appreciated only by careful auscultation; grade 2, readily audible; grade 3, moderately loud; grade 4, loud and associated with a palpable thrill; grade 5, loud and audible with the stethoscope only partially placed on the chest; and grade 6, loud enough to be heard without the stethoscope on the chest. Systolic ejection murmurs usually peak in early to mid systole when left ventricular ejection is maximal; examples include fixed valvular, supravalvular, or infravalvular aortic stenosis and pulmonic stenosis. The murmur of hypertrophic obstructive cardiomyopathy has a similar ejection quality, although its peak may be later in systole when dynamic obstruction is maximal (Chapter 60). Pansystolic murmurs are characteristic of mitral or tricuspid regurgitation or with a left-to-right shunt from conditions such as a ventricular septal defect (left ventricle to right ventricle). A late systolic murmur is characteristic of mitral valve prolapse (Chapter 75) or ischemic papillary muscle dysfunction. Ejection quality murmurs also may be heard in patients with normal valves but increased flow, such as occurs with marked anemia, fever, or bradycardia secondary to congenital complete heart block; they also may be heard across a valve that is downstream from increased flow because of an intracardiac shunt. Maneuvers such as inspiration, expiration, standing, squatting, and hand gripping can be especially useful in the differential diagnosis of a murmur; however, echocardiography commonly is required to make a definitive diagnosis of cause and severity (Table 50-8).

High-frequency, early diastolic murmurs are typical of aortic regurgitation and pulmonic regurgitation from a variety of causes. The murmurs of mitral and tricuspid stenosis begin in early to mid-diastole and tend to diminish in intensity later in diastole in the absence of effective atrial contraction, but they tend to increase in intensity in later diastole if effective atrial contraction is present.

Continuous murmurs may be caused by any abnormality that is associated with a pressure gradient in systole and diastole. Examples include a patent ductus arteriosus, ruptured sinus of Valsalva aneurysm, arteriovenous fistula (of the coronary artery, pulmonary artery, or thoracic artery), and a mammary soufflé. In some situations, murmurs of two coexistent conditions (e.g., aortic stenosis and regurgitation; atrial septal defect with a large shunt and resulting flow murmurs of relative mitral and pulmonic stenosis) may mimic a continuous murmur.

Abdomen

The most common cause of hepatomegaly in patients with heart disease is hepatic engorgement from elevated right-sided pressures associated with right ventricular failure of any cause. Hepatojugular reflux is elicited by pressing on the liver and showing an increase in the jugular venous pressure; it indicates advanced right ventricular failure or obstruction to right ventricular filling. Evaluation of the abdomen also may reveal an enlarged liver caused by a systemic disease, such as hemochromatosis (Chapter 219) or sarcoidosis (Chapter 95), which also may affect the heart. In more severe cases, splenomegaly and ascites also may be noted. Large, palpable, polycystic kidneys (Chapter 129) commonly are associated with hypertension. A systolic bruit suggestive of renal artery stenosis (Chapter 127) or an enlarged abdominal aorta (Chapter 78) is a clue of atherosclerosis.

Extremities

Extremities should be evaluated for peripheral pulses, edema, cyanosis, and clubbing. Diminished peripheral pulses suggest peripheral arterial disease (Chapters 79 and 80). Delayed pulses in the legs are consistent with coarctation of the aorta and are seen after aortic dissection.

TABLE 50-7 SOME COMMON CAUSES OF HEART MURMURS*

	USUAL LOCATION	COMMON ASSOCIATED FINDINGS
SYSTOLIC		
Holosystolic		
Mitral regurgitation	Apex → axilla	↑ with handgrip; S_3 if marked mitral regurgitation; left ventricular dilation common
Tricuspid regurgitation	LLSB	↑ with inspiration; right ventricular dilation common
Ventricular septal defect	LLSB → RLSB	Often with thrill
Early–mid systolic		
Aortic valvular stenosis	RUSB	
Fixed supravalvular or subvalvular	RUSB	Ejection click if mobile valve; soft or absent A_2 if valve immobile; later peak associated with more severe stenosis
Dynamic infravalvular	LLSB → apex + axilla	Hypertrophic obstructive cardiomyopathy; murmur louder if left ventricular volume lower or contractility increased, softer if left ventricular volume increased†; can be later in systole if obstruction delayed
Pulmonic valvular stenosis	LUSB	↑ with inspiration
Infravalvular (infundibular)	LUSB	↑ with inspiration
Supravalvular	LUSB	↑ with inspiration
"Flow murmurs"	LUSB	Anemia, fever, increased flow of any cause‡
Mid–late systolic		
Mitral valve prolapse	LLSB or apex → axilla	Preceded by click; murmur lengthens with maneuvers that decrease left ventricular volume†
Papillary muscle dysfunction	Apex → axilla	Ischemic heart disease
DIASTOLIC		
Early diastolic		
Aortic regurgitation	RUSB, LUSB	High-pitched, blowing quality; endocarditis, diseases of the aorta, associated aortic valvular stenosis; signs of low peripheral vascular resistance
Pulmonic valve regurgitation	LUSB	Pulmonary hypertension as a causative factor
Mid–late diastolic		
Mitral stenosis, tricuspid stenosis	Apex, LLSB	Low pitched; in rheumatic heart disease, opening snap commonly precedes murmur; can be due to increased flow across normal valve‡
Atrial myxomas	Apex (L), LLSB (R)	"Tumor plop"
Continuous		
Venous hum	Over jugular or hepatic vein or breast	Disappears with compression of vein or pressure of stethoscope
Patent ductus arteriosus	LUSB	
Arteriovenous fistula		
Coronary	LUSB	
Pulmonary, bronchial, chest wall	Over fistula	
Ruptured sinus of Valsalva aneurysm	RUSB	Sudden onset

*See also Chapters 69 and 75.

†Left ventricular volume is decreased by standing or during prolonged, forced expiration against a closed glottis (Valsalva maneuver); it is increased by squatting or by elevation of the legs; contractility is increased by adrenergic stimulation or in the beat after an extrasystolic beat.

‡Including a left-to-right shunt through an atrial septal defect for tricuspid or pulmonic flow murmurs, and a ventricular septal defect for pulmonic or mitral flow murmurs.

LLSB = left lower sternal border (4th intercostal space); LUSB = left upper sternal border (2nd-3rd intercostal spaces); RLSB = right lower sternal border (4th intercostal space); RUSB = right upper sternal border (2nd-3rd intercostal spaces).

Edema (Fig. 50-7) is a cardinal manifestation of right-sided heart failure. When it is caused by heart failure, pericardial disease, or pulmonary hypertension, the edema is usually symmetrical and progresses upward from the ankles; each of these causes of cardiac edema commonly is associated with jugular venous distention and often with hepatic congestion. Unilateral edema suggests thrombophlebitis or proximal venous or lymphatic obstruction (Fig. 50-8). Edema in the absence of evidence of right-sided or left-sided heart failure suggests renal disease, hypoalbuminemia, myxedema, or other noncardiac causes. Among unselected patients with bilateral edema, about 40% have an underlying cardiac disease, about 40% have an elevated pulmonary blood pressure, about 20% have bilateral venous disease, about 20% have renal disease, and about 25% have idiopathic edema.

Cyanosis (Fig. 50-9) is a bluish discoloration caused by reduced hemoglobin exceeding about 5 g/dL in the capillary bed. Central cyanosis is seen in patients with poor oxygen saturation resulting from a reduced inspired oxygen concentration or inability to oxygenate the blood in the lungs (e.g., as a result of advanced pulmonary disease, pulmonary edema, pulmonary arteriovenous fistula, or right-to-left shunting); it also may be seen in patients with marked erythrocytosis. Methemoglobinemia (Chapter 161) also can present with cyanosis. Peripheral cyanosis may be caused by reduced blood flow to the extremities secondary to vasoconstriction, heart failure, or shock.

Clubbing (Fig. 50-10), which is loss of the normal concave configuration of the nail as it emerges from the distal phalanx, is seen in patients with pulmonary abnormalities such as lung cancer (Chapter 197) and in patients with cyanotic congenital heart disease (Chapter 69).

Examination of the Skin

Examination of the skin may reveal bronze pigmentation typical of hemochromatosis (Chapter 219); jaundice (see Fig. 149-2 in Chapter 149) characteristic of severe right-sided heart failure or hemochromatosis; or capillary hemangioma typical of Osler-Weber-Rendu disease (see Fig. 176-1 in Chapter 176), which also is associated with pulmonary arteriovenous fistulas and cyanosis. Infectious endocarditis may be associated with Osler's nodes (see Fig. 76-2 in Chapter 76), Janeway's lesions, or splinter hemorrhages (Fig. 50-11) (Chapter 76). Xanthomas (Fig. 50-12) are subcutaneous deposits of cholesterol seen on the extensor surfaces of the extremities or on the palms and digital creases; they are found in patients with severe hypercholesterolemia.

Laboratory Studies

All patients with known or suspected cardiac disease should have an ECG and chest radiograph. The ECG (Chapter 54) helps identify rate, rhythm,

TABLE 50-8 SENSITIVITY AND SPECIFICITY OF BEDSIDE MANEUVERS IN THE IDENTIFICATION OF SYSTOLIC MURMURS

MANEUVER	RESPONSE	MURMUR	SENSITIVITY (%)	SPECIFICITY (%)
Inspiration	↑	RS	100	88
Expiration	↓	RS	100	88
Valsalva maneuver	↑	HC	65	96
Squat to stand	↑	HC	95	84
Stand to squat	↓	HC	95	85
Leg elevation	↓	HC	85	91
Handgrip	↓	HC	85	75
Handgrip	↑	MR and VSD	68	92
Transient arterial occlusion	↑	MR and VSD	78	100

HC = hypertrophic cardiomyopathy; MR = mitral regurgitation; RS = right sided; VSD = ventricular septal defect.
Modified with permission from Lembo NJ, Dell'Italia IJ, Crawford MH, et al. Bedside diagnosis of systolic murmurs. *N Engl J Med.* 1988;318:1572-1578. Copyright 1988 Massachusetts Medical Society. All rights reserved.

FIGURE 50-7. Pitting edema in a patient with cardiac failure. A depression ("pit") remains in the edema for some minutes after firm fingertip pressure is applied. (From Forbes CD, Jackson WD. *Color Atlas and Text of Clinical Medicine*, 3rd ed. London: Mosby; 2003.)

Unilateral or bilateral?

— Unilateral —

R/O DVT

Yes → Anticoagulation

No → Pain?

Yes → Fever or increased WBC?

Yes → Cellulitis or other infection? → Antibiotic treatment

No → Characteristic physical signs of popliteal cyst or gastrocnemius rupture
- Yes → Initiate symptomatic therapy
- No → Consider MRI

No → Postphlebitic syndrome?

Yes → Continue anticoagulation

No → R/O malignancy Detailed history Pelvic exam Rectal exam

— Bilateral —

Detailed history Physical exam

Urine dipstick

− → Obvious findings of CHF?

Yes → Initiate appropriate therapy → Pursue further diagnostic work-up as appropriate

No → Creatinine Electrolytes Albumin Cholesterol Prothrombin time Liver enzymes TSH Chest x-ray Cardiac echo
- Renal disease
- Occult CHF
- Cirrhosis
- Hypo-thyroidism
- Other or idiopathic

Follow-up abnormalities
Initiate appropriate therapy

+ → R/O concurrent cardiac and hepatic disease → Consider renal biopsy → Initiate appropriate therapy

FIGURE 50-8. Diagnostic approach to patients with edema. CHF = congestive heart failure; DVT = deep venous thrombosis; MRI = magnetic resonance imaging; R/O = rule out; TSH = thyroid-stimulating hormone; WBC = white blood cell count. (From Chertow G. Approach to the patient with edema. In: Braunwald E, Goldman L, eds. *Primary Cardiology*, 2nd ed. Philadelphia: WB Saunders; 2003.)

FIGURE 50-9. Arterial embolism causing acute ischemia and cyanosis of the leg. Initial pallor of the leg and foot was followed by cyanosis. (From Forbes CD, Jackson WD. *Color Atlas and Text of Clinical Medicine*, 3rd ed. London: Mosby; 2003.)

FIGURE 50-10. Severe finger clubbing in a patient with cyanotic congenital heart disease. (From Forbes CD, Jackson WD. *Color Atlas and Text of Clinical Medicine*, 3rd ed. London: Mosby; 2003.)

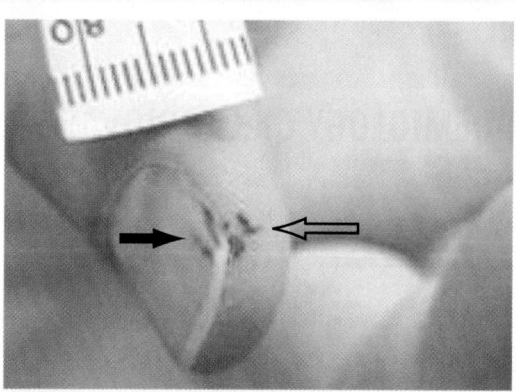

FIGURE 50-11. Splinter hemorrhage (*solid arrow*) and Janeway's lesions (*open arrow*). These findings should stimulate a work-up for endocarditis. (From American Academy of Family Physicians Online. http://www.aafp.org/afp/20040315/1417.html. Accessed June 9, 2010.)

FIGURE 50-12 Eruptive xanthomas of the extensor surfaces of the lower extremities. This patient had marked hypertriglyceridemia. (From Massengale WT, Nesbitt LT Jr. Xanthomas. In: Bolognia JL, Jorizzo JL, Rapini RP, eds. *Dermatology*. Philadelphia: Mosby; 2003:1449.)

conduction abnormalities, and possible myocardial ischemia. The chest radiograph (Chapter 53) yields important information on chamber enlargement, pulmonary vasculature, and the great vessels.

Blood testing in patients with known or suspected cardiac disease should be targeted to the conditions in question. In general, a complete blood cell count, thyroid indices, and lipid levels are part of the standard evaluation. Point-of-care biomarker measurements in the emergency department can decrease unnecessary admissions and reduce median length-of-stay.

Echocardiography (Chapter 55) is the most useful test to analyze valvular and ventricular function. By use of Doppler flow methods, stenotic and regurgitant lesions can be quantified. Hand-held ultrasonography performed by generalists can improve the assessment of left ventricular function, cardiomegaly, and pericardial effusion. Transesophageal echocardiography is the preferred method to evaluate possible aortic dissection and to identify clot in the cardiac chambers. Radionuclide studies (Chapter 56) can measure left ventricular function, assess myocardial ischemia, and determine whether ischemic myocardium is viable. CT can detect coronary calcium, which is a risk factor for symptomatic coronary disease (Chapter 56). In the setting of acute chest pain, multislice CT is effective in diagnosing coronary disease, but it currently cannot adequately determine the physiologic significance.▪

Stress testing by exercise or pharmacologic stress is useful to precipitate myocardial ischemia that may be detected by ECG abnormalities, perfusion abnormalities on radionuclide studies, or transient wall motion abnormalities on echocardiography. These tests are often crucial in diagnosis of possible myocardial ischemia (Chapter 71) and in establishment of prognosis in patients with known ischemic heart disease.

Cardiac catheterization (Chapter 57) can measure precise gradients across stenotic cardiac valves, judge the severity of intracardiac shunts, and determine intracardiac pressures. Coronary angiography provides a definitive diagnosis of coronary disease and is a necessary prelude to coronary revascularization with a percutaneous coronary intervention (Chapter 74) or coronary artery bypass graft surgery (Chapter 74).

Continuous ambulatory ECG monitoring can help diagnose arrhythmias. A variety of newer technologies allow longer-term monitoring in patients with important but infrequently occurring symptoms (Chapter 62). Formal invasive electrophysiologic testing can be useful in the diagnosis of ventricular or supraventricular wide-complex tachycardia, and it is crucial for guiding a wide array of new invasive electrophysiologic therapies (Chapter 66).

● SUMMARY

The history, physical examination, and laboratory evaluation should help the physician establish the cause of any cardiovascular problem; identify and quantify any anatomic abnormalities; determine the physiologic status of the valves, myocardium, and conduction system; determine functional capacity; estimate prognosis; and provide primary or secondary prevention. Key preventive strategies, including diet modification, recognition and treatment of hyperlipidemia, cessation of cigarette smoking, and adequate physical exercise, should be part of the approach to every patient, with or without heart disease.

Grade **A** ○

1. Goodacre SW, Bradburn M, Cross E, et al. The randomised Assessment of Treatment using Panel Assay of Cardiac Markers (RATPAC) trial: a randomised controlled trial of point-of-care cardiac markers in the emergency department. *Heart.* 2011;97:190-196.

SUGGESTED READINGS

Amsterdam EA, Kirk JD, Bluemke DA, et al. Testing of low-risk patients presenting to the emergency department with chest pain: a scientific statement from the American Heart Association. *Circulation.* 2010;122:175-1776. *Guidelines.*

Brown AF, Cullen L, Than M. Future developments in chest pain diagnosis and management. *Med Clin North Am.* 2010;94:375-400. *Review.*

Martin LD, Howell EE, Ziegelstein RC, et al. Hand-carried ultrasound performed by hospitalists: does it improve the cardiac physical examination? *Am J Med.* 2009;122:35-41. *It improves the accuracy of the assessment of left ventricular dysfunction, cardiomegaly, and pericardial effusion.*

51

EPIDEMIOLOGY OF CARDIOVASCULAR DISEASE

MICHAEL J. KLAG

DEFINITION OF CARDIOVASCULAR DISEASES

Cardiovascular diseases, which encompass congenital malformations (Chapter 69) and acquired diseases of the circulatory system, include coronary heart disease (Chapters 70 to 74), arrhythmias (Chapters 62 to 65), valvular heart disease (Chapter 75), cardiomyopathy (Chapter 60), pericardial disease (Chapter 77), heart failure (Chapter 59), stroke (Chapter 413), peripheral arterial disease (Chapter 79), aortic diseases (Chapter 78), venous diseases (Chapter 81), and pulmonary vascular diseases (Chapter 68). However, because of their incidence and prevalence, their impact on survival and quality of life, and their shared pathogenesis (Chapter 70), this chapter mainly focuses on the epidemiology of coronary heart disease, stroke, and heart failure.

BURDEN OF CARDIOVASCULAR DISEASE

Impact in the United States

The age-adjusted mortality rate for cardiovascular disease has decreased substantially in the past few decades, with a 69% decline for coronary heart disease and a 76% decline for stroke in 2006 compared with 1950 (Fig. 51-1). This decline is considered to be about equally attributable to reductions in major risk factors and to evidence-based medical therapies.

Despite this decline in the cardiovascular disease mortality rate, heart disease (about 620,000 out of about 2.4 million deaths total) and stroke (about 135,000 deaths) are still the first and third leading causes of deaths in the United States. Because of a growing and aging population, the total number of cardiovascular disease deaths has decreased only modestly, by about 16% since 1979. Cardiovascular disease, including congenital defects, still accounts for more than one of every three deaths in the United States.

An estimated 17.6 million American adults currently have coronary heart disease, about 6.4 million have had a stroke, and 5.8 million have heart failure. The prevalence of peripheral arterial disease is estimated to be 8 million, and about 2.2 million people are estimated to have atrial fibrillation.

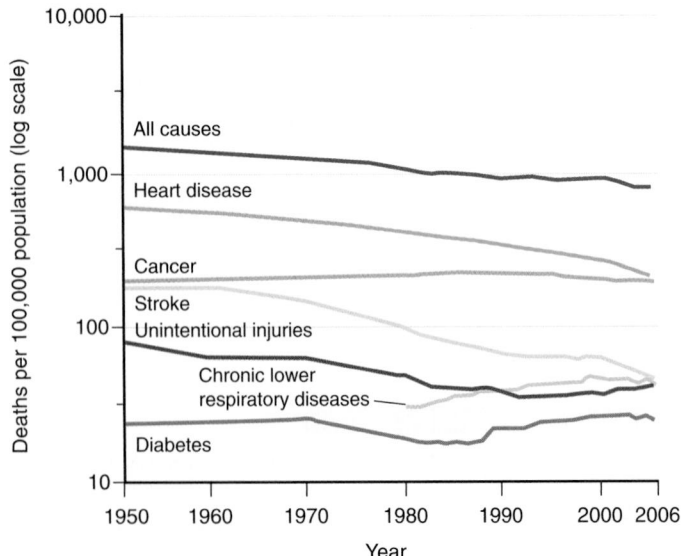

FIGURE 51-1. Age-adjusted death rates for selected leading causes of death: United States, 1958-2006. (From CDC/NCHS, Health United States, 2009. Figure 18. Data from the National Vital Statistics System.)

The annual estimated incidence in the United States is 785,000 for coronary heart disease, 610,000 for stroke, and 670,000 for heart failure. Importantly, heart disease and stroke are the 3rd and 12th leading chronic conditions that limit activity, and stroke is the leading cause of serious long-term disability.

Hospitalization rates for myocardial infarction and stroke have been relatively steady in the United States over the past few decades. However, diagnostic measures have improved substantially during this time period, likely leading to hospitalization of milder cases. Improved survival of patients with severe disease, who are at greater risk for recurrence, may also have contributed to this constant hospitalization rate. In contrast, hospitalization rates for heart failure and atrial fibrillation have substantially increased (two- to three-fold) in the past few decades.

In 2010, cardiovascular diseases are projected to cost $324 billion in health care expenditures (direct costs) and $189 billion in lost productivity (indirect costs). Direct and indirect costs are estimated to be $96 billion and $81 billion for coronary heart disease, $48 billion and $26 billion for stroke, and $35 billion and $4 billion for heart failure, respectively.

Worldwide Impact

Coronary heart disease and stroke are the leading causes of death in both economically developed and developing countries. Each year, more than 17 million people die from cardiovascular disease worldwide. Currently, 80% of deaths due to coronary heart disease or stroke take place in developing countries. Cardiovascular disease occurs at a younger age in developing countries than in developed countries, thereby resulting in serious loss of productivity. For example, 50% of cardiovascular disease deaths in India occur before 70 years of age, whereas only about 25% of cardiovascular disease deaths in developed countries occur before age 70 years. Traditional risk factors play an important role in the excess risk for cardiovascular disease in developing countries, thereby emphasizing the urgent need to develop cost-effective programs to control these risk factors in settings with limited resources.

PRIMARY AND SECONDARY PREVENTION

Primary prevention is defined as preventing cardiovascular disease among persons without clinically apparent cardiovascular disease. *Secondary prevention* denotes preventing the recurrence of cardiovascular disease among those who already have it. Preventive interventions are largely the same for primary and secondary intervention, except that the targeted levels of low-density lipoprotein cholesterol (LDL-C) are lower when cardiovascular disease is present (Chapter 213), and some medications, such as aspirin, are recommended for every patient with coronary heart disease.[1] Cardiovascular disease is also an indication for influenza vaccination.

The absolute risk of a future cardiovascular disease event is substantially higher in persons who already have cardiovascular disease. Because the reduction in absolute risk is greater for secondary than primary prevention, secondary prevention is more cost-effective than primary prevention. Nevertheless, the control of blood pressure (Chapter 67) and the use of statins (Chapter 213) can markedly lower the risk of cardiovascular disease in apparently healthy individuals, with low rates of adverse effects.[2]

RISK FACTORS FOR CARDIOVASCULAR DISEASE

Atherosclerotic disease in the arteries of the heart and brain is the most common cause of clinically apparent coronary heart disease and stroke. Heart failure most commonly occurs as a result of coronary heart disease or hypertension, although valvular heart disease (Chapter 75) and cardiomyopathy (Chapter 60) also can lead to heart failure.

Risk factors for cardiovascular disease can be categorized as traditional (i.e., those identified in the Framingham Heart Study) or novel (Table 51-1). Risk factors can also be grouped as modifiable or nonmodifiable.

Individual Risk Factors

Age

Older age is one of the strongest risk factors for coronary heart disease, stroke, and heart failure. An age over 45 years in men and 55 years in women is considered a risk factor for coronary heart disease, and every 10 years of older age imparts a risk of coronary heart disease equivalent to the presence of hypertension or diabetes. In general, traditional risk factors are more strongly associated with the risk of cardiovascular disease at younger compared with older ages.

TABLE 51-1   RISK FACTORS FOR CORONARY HEART DISEASE AND/OR STROKE

	TRADITIONAL (OR ESTABLISHED)*	NOVEL (OR LESS ESTABLISHED)
Modifiable	Hypertension Diabetes Dyslipidemia† Smoking Obesity Physical inactivity Kidney dysfunction/damage Left ventricular hypertrophy Alcohol Atrial fibrillation‡	Socioeconomic status Psychological factors Inflammatory markers Infection Homocysteine Thrombotic factors Natriuretic peptide Troponin†
Nonmodifiable	Age Gender Ethnicity Family history	Genetic polymorphism Coronary artery calcification†

*Factors incorporated in multiple risk scoring systems or dealt with in clinical guidelines and potentially affecting clinical decisions for cardiovascular disease prevention.
†Risk factor mainly for coronary heart disease.
‡Risk factor mainly for stroke.

Gender

Before age 60, men have a 1.5- to 2-fold higher risk of coronary heart disease and stroke than do women. After 60 years of age, however, the risk of coronary heart disease and stroke in women increases at a faster rate than men, and the risk becomes equivalent in both sexes at 80 years of age. This gender difference at younger ages is thought to be primarily due to differences in levels of estrogen and other endogenous sex hormones. Clinical trials of hormone replacement therapy in postmenopausal women, however, have not reduced the risk of cardiovascular disease.[3]

Race and Ethnicity

The incidence and prevalence of cardiovascular disease vary substantially across ethnic groups. For example, the incidence of stroke and heart failure in the United States is 1.5- to 2-fold higher in blacks compared with whites, whereas the incidence of coronary heart disease is relatively comparable between these groups. Asians are less prone to developing coronary heart disease than whites or blacks. These differences in the incidence of cardiovascular disease among ethnic groups are largely attributable to differences in risk factor profiles. Numerous studies demonstrate that migrants assume the cardiovascular disease risk of their new environment within two generations. Thus, lifestyle and other environmental factors appear to be more important than ethnicity in influencing the risk of cardiovascular disease. There are also ethnic differences in awareness of traditional modifiable risk factors. Individual ancestry, as estimated by genetic markers, may provide better information for differentiating the genetic and environmental contributions to ethnic differences.

Hypertension

Hypertension (Chapter 67), defined as systolic/diastolic blood pressure of 140/90 mm Hg or higher, is the most prevalent modifiable risk factor for coronary heart disease, stroke, and heart failure. Hypertension affects one third of U.S. adults. Systolic pressure is a stronger risk predictor than diastolic blood pressure, and each 20-mm Hg increase in systolic blood pressure is associated with two-fold increased risk of coronary heart disease in middle-aged populations. Numerous studies have demonstrated that blood pressure control by antihypertensive drug therapy decreases cardiovascular disease risk when used in either primary or secondary prevention.[4] Adoption of a diet that is rich in potassium, magnesium, calcium, protein, and fiber can reduce blood pressure to a degree equivalent to using one antihypertensive medication, and substituting additional protein or unsaturated fats leads to additional improvement in blood pressure and the lipid profile.[5]

Diabetes Mellitus

Diabetes mellitus (Chapters 236 and 237), which is defined as fasting plasma glucose of 126 mg/dL or higher, a nonfasting plasma glucose or a plasma glucose 2 hours after an oral glucose tolerance test of 200 mg/dL or higher, or a hemoglobin A_{1c} level of 6.5% or higher, is associated with a two-fold increased risk for cardiovascular disease. Diabetes is often considered as equivalent to a history of coronary heart disease in terms of predicting the risk for coronary heart disease events. Intensive glucose control among diabetic patients has been associated with a reduction in the incidence or progression of microvascular disease, such as retinopathy or nephropathy, but not necessarily with that of macrovascular disease.[6] By comparison, aggressive blood pressure reduction in persons with diabetes prevents both microvascular and macrovascular disease.[7]

Dyslipidemia

Elevated LDL-C is a strong risk factor, particularly for coronary heart disease (Chapter 213). Each 1-mg/dL increase in the LDL-C level is associated with approximately a 1% higher risk of coronary heart disease. Decreased HDL-C levels and elevated triglyceride levels are also associated with the risk of coronary heart disease. Current clinical guidelines for treatment of hyperlipidemia (Chapter 213) are based mainly on LDL-C levels, but the nonfasting non-HDL cholesterol level (total cholesterol minus HDL-C) and the HDL cholesterol level are sufficient to estimate the risk of coronary heart disease.

The effectiveness of statins to reduce coronary heart disease risk is established in both primary and secondary prevention.[8] In contrast, drugs that specifically increase HDL-C and reduce triglycerides have not demonstrated consistent benefits for reducing cardiovascular events.[9,10]

Serum total cholesterol and triglyceride levels are inversely associated with the risk of hemorrhagic stroke in many, but not all, studies. Persons with the highest blood pressures and lowest serum cholesterol levels are at the greatest risk. Several studies have reported neutral or weak associations of dyslipidemia with ischemic stroke. Nevertheless, statin treatment reduces the incidence of stroke.[8]

Smoking

Current smokers have an approximately two-fold higher risk of cardiovascular disease compared with former and never smokers. Second-hand smoke is also associated with a 30% or greater increase in the risk of coronary heart disease. Bans on smoking in public places have been associated with a 20% reduction in incident coronary heart disease.

In patients with coronary heart disease, the risk for recurrent coronary heart disease events is substantially reduced by smoking cessation, and the risk in former smokers returns to the level of nonsmokers within 3 years. Smoking cessation is associated with increased risk of incident diabetes, in part due to weight gain. Thus, body weight and glucose metabolism should be carefully monitored among persons who attempt to quit smoking.

Obesity

Obesity (Chapter 227) is closely associated with hypertension, dyslipidemia, and diabetes. Even accounting for these traditional cardiovascular risk factors, obesity may be an independent predictor of coronary heart disease, stroke, and heart failure. Each 5-kg/m² higher body mass index (BMI) is associated with 40% increased risk for cardiovascular mortality in middle-aged populations. Among individuals with morbid obesity (BMI ≥ 35 kg/m²), weight reduction through bariatric surgery may reduce the risk of coronary heart disease by more than 50%.

Among patients with established coronary heart disease or heart failure, higher adiposity is paradoxically associated with better prognosis, probably because of weight loss in persons with severe illness, especially heart failure, who also experience high mortality. In addition, persons with severe heart disease who are very obese probably die earlier than persons who weigh less. Thus, prevalent patients with heart disease and obesity likely have less severe disease, thereby imparting a survival advantage.

Physical Inactivity

Physical inactivity and sedentary lifestyle (Chapter 15) are associated with increased risk for cardiovascular disease. Exercise is an important adjunct to diet for achieving and maintaining weight loss, and exercise improves lipid and glucose metabolism and decreases blood pressure. In patients who have survived an acute myocardial infarction, exercise-based cardiac rehabilitation is associated with reduction of mortality but not of recurrent myocardial infarction.[11]

Kidney Dysfunction or Damage

Chronic kidney disease (Chapter 132), defined as a persistently reduced glomerular filtration rate of less than 60 mL/minute/1.73 m^2 or kidney damage, usually detected by albuminuria, raises the risk of incident cardiovascular disease. Cardiovascular mortality increases exponentially with lower glomerular filtration rate and increases linearly on a log-log scale at higher levels of albuminuria. Cardiovascular mortality is two-fold higher at a glomerular filtration rate of 30 to 45 mL/minute/1.73 m^2 or albuminuria of more than 100 mg/day, compared with normal levels of about 90 mL/minute/1.73 m^2 and about 5 mg/day, respectively, independently of each other and of traditional risk factors.

Left Ventricular Hypertrophy

Left ventricular hypertrophy usually represents target-organ damage from hypertension, although multiple factors play a role in its development. The regression of left ventricular hypertrophy by antihypertensive treatment may be associated with more favorable outcomes.

Socioeconomic Status

Most of the evidence for the link between socioeconomic status, an individual's social position relative to other members of a society, and cardiovascular disease comes from economically developed countries. In general, low socioeconomic status is associated with increased risk of cardiovascular disease. The mechanism for this association is multifactorial, perhaps mediated through in utero and childhood exposures and lack of educational opportunities that result in deleterious health behaviors and risk factor patterns (Chapter 4). In addition, a reduced accessibility to health care (Chapter 5) and greater exposure to residential and occupational harmful exposures almost certainly play a role. For example, neighborhood characteristics, such as accessibility to healthy food and walkability, are associated with higher prevalence of obesity, and air pollution predicts incident coronary heart disease.

Psychological Factors

Acute and chronic stress, in daily life or due to a natural disaster, is associated with an increased risk for cardiovascular disease. Acute or chronic stress may raise blood pressure, alter glucose or lipid metabolism, and increased blood viscosity.

Inflammation

Higher levels of inflammatory markers are associated with a higher risk of cardiovascular disease, consistent with the concept that atherosclerosis is an inflammatory process (Chapter 70). C-reactive protein, which is the most studied inflammatory marker, is undoubtedly associated with the future risk for cardiovascular disease, although this association is considerably attenuated by the adjustment for conventional risk factors. Genotypes associated with elevated levels of C-reactive protein are not associated with the risk of coronary heart disease, suggesting that C-reactive protein itself is not a cause of cardiovascular disease. Nevertheless, the C-reactive protein can be used for risk stratification beyond traditional risk factors.

Infection

Infection with microorganisms such as *Chlamydophila pneumoniae* (Chapter 326), *Helicobacter pylori* (Chapter 141), cytomegalovirus (Chapter 384), hepatitis A virus (Chapter 150), and influenza virus (Chapter 372) has been reported to be associated with the risk of coronary heart disease. However, antibiotic treatment of these pathogens has not reduced risk.[12] In contrast, vaccination for influenza virus may help prevent recurrent coronary heart disease and is currently recommended for secondary prevention.

Homocysteine

Blood homocysteine levels are associated with the risk of cardiovascular disease, but reducing blood homocysteine levels using folic acid alone or in combination with other B vitamins is not effective for either primary or secondary prevention.[13]

Alcohol

A J-shaped association between alcohol consumption (Chapter 32) and the risk of incident coronary heart disease has been noted in both primary and secondary prevention settings, with the lowest risk at light (<3 drinks per week) to moderate (3 to 7 [for female] or 14 [for male] per week) alcohol consumption. Alcohol use, however, is also associated with injuries and other harmful outcomes, including hypertension and atrial fibrillation. Thus, persons who do not drink should not be encouraged to initiate regular alcohol consumption.

Family History

Premature coronary heart disease in a first-degree relative (male relative <55 years and female <65 years or <60 years in both genders) is associated with increased risk of coronary heart disease. Family history of premature coronary heart disease likely integrates genetic predisposition to cardiovascular disease or cardiovascular risk factors, lifestyle preferences, and environmental factors.

Genetic Factors

Numerous single nucleotide polymorphisms have been associated with cardiovascular disease risk factors or the incidence of cardiovascular disease. Nevertheless, current genetic risk scoring using 101 single nucleotide polymorphisms has not yet improved the prediction of incident cardiovascular disease after accounting for traditional risk factors. However, single nucleotide polymorphisms have been associated with differing response to specific antihypertensive and antiplatelet drugs.

Thrombotic and Fibrinolytic Factors

Various thrombotic and fibrinolytic factors, such as fibrinogen and plasminogen activator inhibitor, have been associated with incident cardiovascular disease. Whether such information improves the prediction of prognosis over prediction based on traditional risk factors alone and, if so, whether such factors provide targets for prevention, are not yet clear.

Risk Prediction

Although clinical interventions to prevent cardiovascular disease usually target individual risk factors, methods to predict the risk of cardiovascular disease use information on multiple risk factors, including age, gender, smoking, hypertension, diabetes, and lipids. Of these, the Framingham Risk Score is most commonly used in the United States. Some clinical guidelines use an individual's probability of coronary heart disease within 10 years to make clinical decisions about treatment with statins and aspirin. Although the original Framingham Risk Score estimated coronary heart disease risk, a new score predicting global cardiovascular disease risk (coronary heart disease, stroke, heart failure, and peripheral artery disease) has recently been published (Tables 51-2 and 51-3).

New Aspects of Traditional Risk Factors

Global risk prediction and the management of traditional risk factors in clinical practice are generally based on the most recent assessments of risk factors or the average of multiple measurements over a short period of time. However, change over time or the duration of an abnormal risk factor level may be associated with future risk independent of baseline values. The association of traditional risk factors with cardiovascular disease risk is generally graded and continuous, such that higher levels of the risk factors impart greater risk; as a result, cutoffs to define elevated levels of risk factors are somewhat arbitrary. In general, the definition of normal is becoming stricter with increasing recognition that "borderline" levels of risk factors are associated with cardiovascular risk, that the greatest population burden may be in persons with lower elevations of risk because they are much more numerous than persons with very high levels of risk, and because interventions are becoming safer and more effective. For example, diabetes is now defined as a fasting glucose level of 126 mg/dL rather than 140 mg/dL.

● NEW BIOMARKERS OF SUBCLINICAL DAMAGE OR DISEASE

New biomarkers of subclinical cardiovascular disease include the coronary artery calcium score (Chapter 56), troponin level, and natriuretic peptide levels. Because these biomarkers are related to ongoing pathophysiologic processes, it is not surprising that they may be better predictors of future events than are traditional risk factors.

TABLE 51-2 POINTS OF FRAMINGHAM RISK SCORE FOR CARDIOVASCULAR DISEASE PREDICTION ACCORDING TO TRADITIONAL RISK FACTORS

POINTS	AGE (YR)	HDL-C (MG/DL)	TOTAL CHOLESTEROL (MG/DL)	SBP NOT TREATED	SBP TREATED	SMOKER	DIABETES
WOMEN							
−3					<120		
−2		60+					
−1		50-59			<120		
0	30-34	45-49	<160	120-129		No	No
1		35-44	160-199	130-139			
2	35-39	<35		140-149	120-129		
3			200-239		130-139	Yes	
4	40-44		240-279	150-159			Yes
5	45-49		280+	160+	140-149		
6					150-159		
7	50-54				160+		
8	55-59						
9	60-64						
10	65-69						
11	70-74						
12	75+						
MEN							
−2		60+		<120			
−1		50-59					
0	30-34	45-49	<160	120-129	<120	No	No
1		35-44	160-199	130-139			
2	35-39	<35	200-239	140-159	120-129		
3			240-279	160+	130-139		Yes
4			280+		140-159	Yes	
5	40-44				160+		
6	45-49						
7							
8	50-54						
9							
10	55-59						
11	60-64						
12	65-69						
13							
14	70-74						
15	75+						

HDL-C = high-density lipoprotein cholesterol; SBP = systolic blood pressure.

TABLE 51-3 CARDIOVASCULAR RISK ACCORDING TO TOTAL POINTS OF FRAMINGHAM RISK SCORE

Women		Men	
POINTS	10-YEAR RISK, %	POINTS	10-YEAR RISK, %
		≤−3	<1
≤−2	<1	−2	1.1
−1	1.0	−1	1.4
0	1.2	0	1.6
1	1.5	1	1.9
2	1.7	2	2.3
3	2	3	2.8
4	2.4	4	3.3
5	2.8	5	3.9
6	3.3	6	4.7
7	3.9	7	5.6
8	4.5	8	6.7
9	5.3	9	7.9
10	6.3	10	9.4
11	7.3	11	11.2
12	8.6	12	13.2
13	10.0	13	15.6
14	11.7	14	18.4
15	13.7	15	21.6
16	15.9	16	25.3
17	18.5	17	29.4
18	21.5	18+	>30
19	24.8	—	—
20	28.5	—	—
21+	>30	—	—

Grade A

1. Smith SC Jr, Allen J, Blair SN, et al. AHA/ACC guidelines for secondary prevention for patients with coronary and other atherosclerotic vascular disease: 2006 Update. Endorsed by the National Heart, Lung, and Blood Institute. *Circulation.* 2006;113:2363-2372.
2. Ridker PM, Danielson E, Fonseca FA, et al. Rosuvastatin to prevent vascular events in men and women with elevated C-reactive protein. *N Engl J Med.* 2008;359:2195-2207.
3. Sare GM, Gray LJ, Bath PMW. Association between hormone replacement therapy and subsequent arterial and venous vascular events: a meta-analysis. *Eur Heart J.* 2008;29:2031-2041.
4. Turnbull F. Effects of different blood-pressure-lowering regimens on major cardiovascular events: results of prospectively-designed overviews of randomised trials. *Lancet.* 2003;362:1527-1535.
5. Appel LJ, Giles TD, Black HR, and American Society of Hypertension Writing Group. ASH position paper: dietary approaches to lower blood pressure. *J Am Soc Hypertens.* 2009;5:321-331.
6. Ray KK, Seshasai SRK, Wijesuriya S, et al. Effect of intensive control of glucose on cardiovascular outcomes and death in patients with diabetes mellitus: a meta-analysis of randomised controlled trials. *Lancet.* 2009;373:1765-1772.
7. UK Prospective Diabetes Study Group. Tight blood pressure control and risk of macrovascular and microvascular complications in type 2 diabetes: UKPDS 38. *BMJ.* 1998;317:703-713.
8. Baigent C, Keech A, Kearney PM, et al. Efficacy and safety of cholesterol-lowering treatment: prospective meta-analysis of data from 90,056 participants in 14 randomized trials of statins. *Lancet.* 2005;366:1267-1278.
9. The ACCORD Study Group. Effects of combination lipid therapy in type 2 diabetes mellitus. *N Engl J Med.* 2010;362:1563-1574.
10. Barter PJ, Caulfield M, Eriksson M, et al, for the ILLUMINATE Investigators. Effects of torcetrapib in patients at high risk for coronary events. *N Engl J Med.* 2007;357:2109-2122.
11. Lavie CJ, Thomas RJ, Squires RW, et al. Exercise training and cardiac rehabilitation in primary and secondary prevention of coronary heart disease. *Mayo Clin Proc.* 2009;84:373-383.
12. Andraws R, Berger JS, Brown DL. Effects of antibiotic therapy on outcomes of patients with coronary artery disease: a meta-analysis of randomized controlled trials. *JAMA* 2005;293:2641-2647.
13. Clarke R, Halsey J, Lewington S, et al. Effects of lowering homocysteine levels with B vitamins on cardiovascular disease, cancer, and cause-specific mortality: meta-analysis of 8 randomized trials involving 37,485 individuals. *Arch Intern Med.* 2010;170:1622-1631.

SUGGESTED READINGS

Bui AL, Horwich TB, Fonarow GC. Epidemiology and risk profile of heart failure. *Nat Rev Cardiol.* 2011;8:30-41. *Review.*
Greenland P, Alpert JS, Beller GA, et al. 2010 ACCF/AHA guideline for assessment of cardiovascular risk in asymptomatic adults: executive summary: a report of the American College of Cardiology Foundation/American Heart Association Task Force on practice guidelines. *Circulation.* 2010;122:2748-2764. *Guidelines.*

Lloyd-Jones D, Adams RJ, Brown TM, et al. Heart disease and stroke statistics—2010 update: a report from the American Heart Association. *Circulation.* 2010;121:e46-e215. *Updated U.S. statistics.*
Wijeysundera HC, Machado M, Farahati F, et al. Association of temporal trends in risk factors and treatment uptake with coronary heart disease mortality, 1994-2005. *JAMA.* 2010;303:1841-1847. *The decline in CHD mortality in 1994 and 2005 in Ontario, Canada, was about equally attributable to reductions in risk factors and to improvements in treatment.*

52

CARDIAC FUNCTION AND CIRCULATORY CONTROL

ANDREW R. MARKS

The heart has the daunting task of pumping sufficient amounts of blood to meet both its own metabolic demands and those of the other organs. Uniquely among all the organs, the heart's failure to perform its task for even a few minutes causes death. The heart continuously fulfills this physiologic role with a variety of electrical, contractile, and structural functions that control the flow of blood to the organs.

STRUCTURE OF THE HEART

Cardiac Development
In humans, the formation of a linear heart tube from the primary cardiac crescent occurs between days 21 and 23 of gestation. Looping of the heart tube and trabecular formation of the ventricle occurs at 26 days of gestation (E-Fig. 52-1). At 6 weeks, the embryonic interventricular communication closes, followed by thickening and remodeling of the ventricular walls in the first trimester. By the end of week 7, heart development is essentially finished, although the heart continues to enlarge throughout gestation.

Electrical Cells
The heart is a muscular pump controlled by regular electrical discharges from specialized muscle cells in the conduction system (Chapter 61). The molecular basis for the electrical activity of the heart is the activation of specific ion-conducting channels (Fig. 52-1). Coordinated activation and inactivation of cardiac ion channels regulate the membrane potential of the cardiac cells, thereby resulting in a rapid sequence of depolarization followed by repolarization. This electrical activity, which is manifested on the body surface as the electrocardiogram (ECG), is known as the action potential, and it is responsible for activating the contraction of the cardiac muscle. At a typical heart rate of 70 beats per minute, the heart beats about 100,000 times per day, or 37 million beats a year, corresponding to 3 billion beats over a lifespan of 80 years. Failure to propagate the signal throughout the heart (e.g., heart block), or abnormal rhythms (arrhythmias) that are either too slow (bradycardia) or too fast (tachycardia), can result in death (Chapter 63).

Ion Channels
Sodium, potassium, and calcium channels determine the electrical activity of the heart by opening and closing in a highly choreographed pattern that determines the action potential of the heart. The electrical regulation of the heart, which is reflected in the relative concentrations of ions inside and outside the heart muscle cells, determines the five phases of the action potential. The action potential is initiated when the opening of sodium channels results in a rapid influx of sodium (phase 0) down its concentration gradient (~145 mmol outside the heart muscle cell, ~10 mmol inside). After a brief early repolarization owing to activation of potassium channels (phase 1), the rapid sodium influx depolarizes the cell, thereby activating calcium channels that allow calcium influx (phase 2) down its concentration gradient (~3 mmol outside, ~100 nmol inside). This calcium influx triggers excitation-contraction coupling that results in pumping by the heart. Potassium channels then open and cause repolarization (phase 3) as potassium fluxes out of the cell down its concentration gradient (~4 mmol outside, ~135 mmol inside). The membrane potential returns to the resting level of about −90 mV (phase 4).

Conduction System
Specialized pacemaker cells in the sinoatrial (SA) node (Fig. 52-2) have slightly higher (less negative) resting potentials and gradually depolarize

FIGURE 52-1. Cardiac action potential and ion channels. Myocardial contraction begins when sodium channels open and positively charged sodium ions flow into the cell and cause membrane depolarization (phase 0). During phases 1, 2, and 3, calcium ions flow into the cell through L-type calcium channels, while potassium flows out of the cell through voltage-gated potassium channels. These three phases correspond to the myocardial contraction, which corresponds to the QRS complex on the surface electrocardiogram (ECG). The sodium-potassium adenosine triphosphatase (NKA) helps return the system to its resting state.

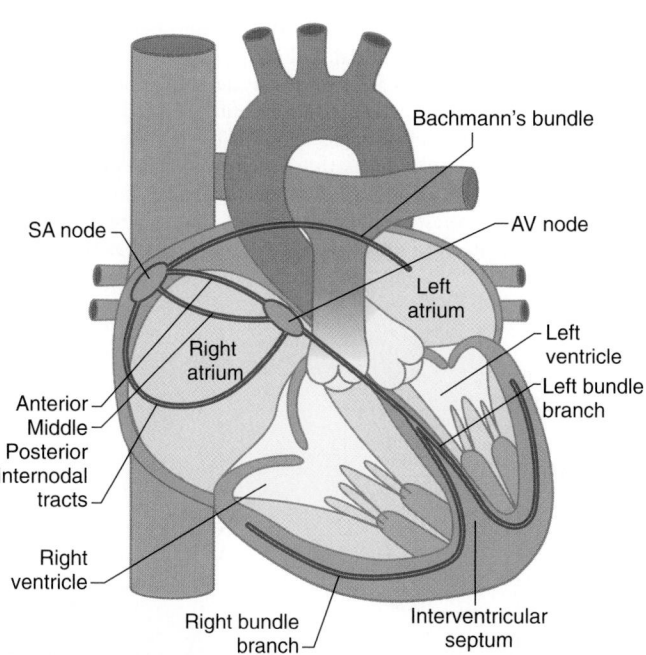

FIGURE 52-2. Cardiac anatomy. Cardiac anatomy comprises electrical and structural components. The electrical impulse that directs cardiac contraction originates in the sinoatrial (SA) node and is rapidly conducted through the atria by specialized conduction tracts. The impulses merge at the atrioventricular (AV) node where, after a brief pause, they are rapidly conducted into the ventricles through the bundle of His, which is composed of specialized Purkinje cells. Blood moves from the atria into the ventricles through the tricuspid and mitral valves during diastole. During systole, blood from the ventricles is pumped into the pulmonary artery and aorta through the pulmonic and aortic valves.

the depolarizing signal enters the bundle of His, where conduction is rapid. The bundle of His divides into the right and left bundle branches, which conduct the depolarizing signals into the ventricles and account for the QRS complex on the ECG. Repolarization is represented by the ST segment and the T and U waves of the ECG.

Contractile Cells

Heart muscle is composed of millions of individual cells, which are known as *cardiomyocytes* and which contain an elaborate machinery required for coordinated contraction that pumps blood. Each cardiomyocyte is connected to its neighbors through specialized junctions that enable them to work as a single contractile unit.

Ultrastructure

The basic unit of the contractile system is the sarcomere, which is defined anatomically as the distance between two Z lines that anchor thin filaments composed of actin, tropomyosin, and troponin. Thin filaments slide past thick filaments (composed of myosin and titin) in a calcium-dependent manner to shorten the sarcomere length. The contractile proteins are surrounded by a calcium-filled membrane called the *sarcoplasmic reticulum*. The sarcoplasmic reticulum forms specialized associations with the transverse tubules, which are invaginations of the plasma membrane and contain voltage-gated calcium channels. When the muscle is activated by depolarization of its membrane, this electrical signal travels deep into the muscle through the transverse tubules. Inside the muscle, the electrical depolarizing signal activates the voltage-gated channels, which open to allow a small amount of calcium to enter the muscle cells. This influx of calcium in turn activates the type 2 ryanodine receptor (RyR2)–calcium release channels on the sarcoplasmic reticulum. The RyR channels open and release enough calcium from the sarcoplasmic reticulum to raise the calcium concentration in the myoplasm about ten-fold. As a result, calcium binds to troponin C in the thin filaments and causes a conformational change that enables crossbridging between actin and myosin, thereby leading to sliding of the filaments, shortening of the sarcomere, and muscle contraction. Hydrolysis of adenosine triphosphate (ATP) provides the energy required for the generation of force by the actin-myosin interaction. The conversion of electrical energy (depolarization of the cell membrane) to mechanical energy is known as excitation-contraction coupling. Relaxation of the heart muscle occurs when calcium is pumped back into the sarcoplasmic reticulum through the sarcoendoplasmic reticulum ATPase. Contractile force can be enhanced during stress by activation of the β-adrenergic pathway, which increases both the amount of calcium released and the rate of calcium uptake in the sarcoplasmic reticulum (E-Fig. 52-3).

during phase 5 owing to the activity of the potassium and calcium channels and the hyperpolarization-activated cyclic nucleotide gated (HCN) channels that are responsible for a small inward (depolarizing) current. In the normal heart, pacemaker cells are the first cells to depolarize, and they trigger the subsequent depolarization of the cells in specialized conducting fibers that propagate the electrical signal throughout the heart muscle in a highly regular and integrated fashion. Electrical activation (depolarization) spreading through the atria to the atrioventricular (AV) node is reflected as the P wave on the ECG (Chapter 54). The slowing of conduction in the AV node accounts for the PR interval on the ECG. After passing through the AV node,

Although the heart is a muscular pump, 60 to 70% of its cells are cardiac fibroblasts, not muscle cells. These fibroblasts provide critical components of the extracellular matrix that determine the structure of the heart.

● ANATOMY OF THE HEART

The primary pumping chamber of the heart is the thick-walled left ventricle, which is composed of billions of cardiomyocytes connected end to end through gap junctions. The right ventricle is a thinner-walled chamber, divided from the left ventricle by the *interventricular septum*. Above the ventricles are the right and left atria, which are thin-walled chambers that receive low-pressure venous blood; they are separated from the ventricles by the *tricuspid valve* on the right side and the *mitral valve* on the left side. These valves are attached to *papillary muscles* that emerge from the ventricular walls through *chordae tendineae*. The pressure gradient between the ventricles and the atria opens the AV valves. The papillary muscles help establish the positions of the valve leaflets and prevent regurgitant flow during contraction. The *aortic and pulmonary valves* separate the left and right ventricles from their arterial connections and enable blood flow out of the ventricles.

Coronary Blood Flow

The coronary arteries receive blood from the aorta, directly above the aortic valve, and travel through the epicardium that surrounds the heart to supply blood to the heart muscle (see Fig. 57-3 in Chapter 57). The diastolic blood pressure in the ascending aorta just above the aortic valve determines most of the flow of blood into the normal (nonstenosed) coronary arteries while the heart is relaxed. During systole, coronary flow is determined by the left ventricular intracavitary pressure, which equals the pressure within the inner myocardial wall, where coronary arteries are compressed during systole. Coronary blood flows to the epicardium during both systole and diastole but flows to the endocardium predominantly during diastole.

Metabolic Regulation of the Cardiovascular System

Cardiac muscle requires constant coronary perfusion to supply oxygen and other metabolites. Increased energy consumption owing to enhanced contractility necessitated by increased pressures or higher heart rates (e.g., during exercise) can be met only by increased coronary blood flow. Signals that augment coronary blood flow (by up to six-fold) include nitric oxide, adenosine, bradykinins, prostaglandins, and carbon dioxide. The breakdown of ATP is the source of adenosine, whereas nitric oxide is produced by the action of nitric oxide synthases that metabolize the amino acid L-arginine. Autoregulatory mechanisms, including constriction in response to increased luminal pressures and dilation in response to reduced pressure, also play a role in determining coronary artery blood flow. Other metabolic factors that cause vasoconstriction include endothelin peptides, serotonin, 5-hydroxytryptamine, thromboxane, angiotensin II, and β_1-adrenergic stimulation.

Sympathetic and parasympathetic pathways of the autonomic nervous system and the renin-angiotensin system exert potent regulatory effects on cardiovascular function. The sympathetic nervous system plays the key role in the response to stress (e.g., the fight-or-flight response) by increasing heart rate and myocardial contractility and decreasing vascular tone. Regulation of cardiovascular function by the sympathetic nervous system is mediated by norepinephrine that is released at the nerve endings and by epinephrine from the adrenal gland. β-Adrenergic signaling is mediated by epinephrine, which increases the heart rate and vasodilates the central arterial bed, thereby resulting in reduced afterload, which in turn helps augment cardiac output.

● PHYSIOLOGY OF THE HEART AND CIRCULATORY CONTROL

Cardiac Energetics

The major immediate source of energy in the heart is the oxidation of fatty acids and glucose. When oxygen supply is limited, glucose metabolism is favored because it generates more ATP per oxygen consumed. The heart has virtually no ability to conduct anaerobic metabolism (i.e., glycolysis) and therefore is dependent on oxygen for its function. For example, heart function deteriorates immediately under conditions of hypoxia, ischemia, and carbon monoxide poisoning.

Basal metabolism, total mechanical work performed by the heart, contractility, and heart rate determine the oxygen and energy consumption of the heart. During excitation-contraction coupling, two key steps require energy consumption (ATP hydrolysis): release of the myosin head–actin interaction, and reuptake of calcium into the sarcoplasmic reticulum.

The mechanical work of the heart is determined by the total *pressure-volume area* (E-Fig. 52-4), which is related to the number of actin-myosin cross-bridges formed during the contraction. It is the sum of the external work performed by the heart in pumping blood from the ventricle to the aorta (represented by the area inside the pressure-volume loop) plus energy stored in the myocardium at the end of contraction. Enhanced contractility requires increased oxygen consumption because an increased amount of calcium released from the sarcoplasmic reticulum requires increased ATP and oxygen consumption to pump the released calcium back into the sarcoplasmic reticulum through the sarcoplasmic reticular ATPase. Based on these principles, increasing the heart rate requires increased oxygen consumption. If the heart rate increases from 70 to 140 beats per minute during exercise or stress, oxygen consumption increases almost two-fold over the basal value.

Contractility and Relaxation

The Cardiac Cycle

In resting humans, the heart beats approximately once per second. With each beat, the heart cycles through a series of four hemodynamic events represented by changes in pressures and volumes (Fig. 52-3) as well as electrical activity as represented by the ECG. When the heart muscle is relaxed at end diastole, the ventricular pressure is at its resting level (*end-diastolic pressure*) and the ventricular volumes are at their maximal value (*end-diastolic volume*). Aortic pressure declines as the blood ejected into the aorta during the previous ventricular contraction flows to the peripheral circulation. Atrial contraction provides a final boost to ventricular volume immediately before ventricular systole. Ventricular contraction increases the pressure in the ventricle; when this pressure exceeds the pressure in the atrium, the mitral valve closes. However, because ventricular pressure remains less than aortic pressure, the aortic valve remains closed, and no blood enters or leaves the ventricle during this first phase of the cardiac cycle, the *isovolumic contraction* phase. During systole, ventricular pressure eventually exceeds aortic pressure, at which time the aortic valve opens, blood is ejected into the aorta, and ventricular volume decreases during the *ejection* phase of the cycle. At the end of systole when contraction is maximum, ejection ends, and the ventricular volumes are at their lowest (*end-systolic volume*). The volume of the ejected blood, which is termed the *stroke volume* (SV), is defined as the difference between the end-diastolic and end-systolic volumes. The ejection fraction

FIGURE 52-3. Wiggers's diagram. Changes in aortic, left ventricular, and left atrial pressures represented graphically as a function of time, with the corresponding electrocardiogram signal for each. LVP = left ventricular pressure.

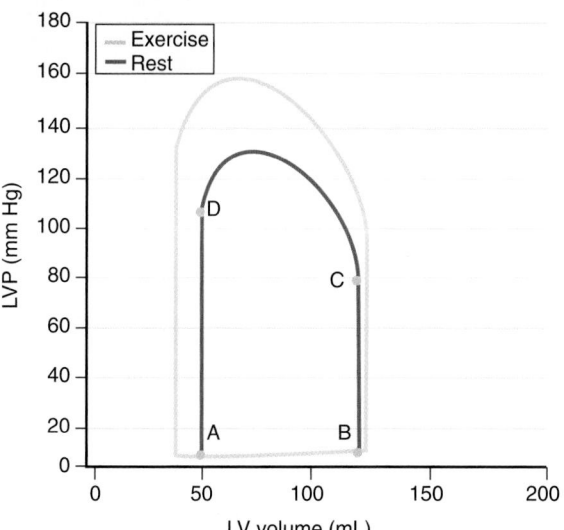

FIGURE 52-4. Pressure-volume loop. The left ventricle (LV) begins to fill when pressure in the chamber falls below that of the left atrium, and the mitral valve opens (point A). Pressure in the ventricle slowly rises as the muscle fibers are stretched by the increasing volume. When the myocardium contracts (point B), pressure in the left ventricle rises, causing the mitral valve to close and trapping the blood inside the chamber (isovolumic contraction). When the pressure in the left ventricle is higher than in the aorta, the aortic valve opens (point C), and blood is ejected out of the left ventricle. As the left ventricle stops contracting, pressure in the aorta becomes higher than that in the left ventricle, and the aortic valve closes (point D). During this period of isovolumic relaxation, the ventricle rapidly relaxes until it starts filling again. During exercise, the release of norepinephrine from sympathetic nerve terminals leads to enhanced myocardial contractility. As a result, the left ventricle generates higher pressures and ejects a greater volume of blood during each beat. LVP = left ventricular pressure.

TABLE 52-1	RANGE OF NORMAL RESTING HEMODYNAMIC VALUES

PRESSURE

Central venous (mean): 0-5 mm Hg
Right atrial (mean): 0-5 mm Hg
Right ventricular (systolic/diastolic): 20-30/0-5 mm Hg
Pulmonary artery (systolic/diastolic): 20-30/8-12 mm Hg
Left atrial (mean): 8-12 mm Hg
Left ventricular (systolic/diastolic): 100-150/8-12 mm Hg
Aortic (systolic/diastolic): 100-150/70-90 mm Hg

VOLUME-RELATED MEASURES

Right ventricular end-diastolic volume: 70-100 mL
Left ventricular end-diastolic volume: 70-100 mL
Stroke volume: 40-70 mL
Cardiac index: 2.5-4 L/min/m^2
Ejection fraction: 55-70%

ARTERIAL RESISTANCE

Systemic vascular resistance: 10-20 mm Hg · min/L
Pulmonary vascular resistance: 0.5-1.5 mm Hg · min/L

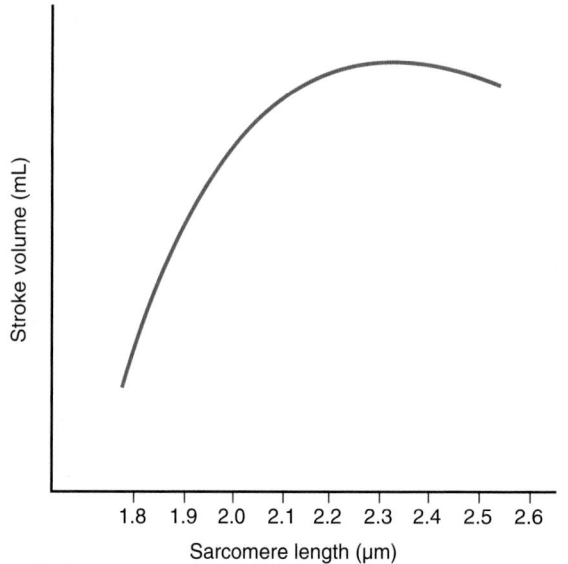

FIGURE 52-5. Starling's law. Cardiac output, represented as stroke volume (end-systolic volume minus end-diastolic volume), as a function of initial sarcomere stretch. The greater the initial stretch on the fibers during diastole, referred to as *preload*, the more force is generated during systole.

(EF), defined as the percentage of end-diastolic volume (EDV) ejected during a contraction (EF = 100 × SV/EDV), is an index of heart function. The next phase in the cycle occurs when the heart muscle relaxes, ventricular pressures are less than the aorta pressure, and the aortic valve closes. During this *isovolumic relaxation* phase, ventricular volumes remain constant because, once again, both the mitral and aortic valves are closed. When ventricular pressures fall below atrial pressures, the mitral and tricuspid valves open, and blood flows from the atria into the ventricles during the *filling* phase.

These four phases of the cardiac cycle can be represented by a *pressure-volume diagram* (Fig. 52-4), which plots the instantaneous ventricular pressure versus volume to calculate the *pressure-volume loop*. Similar effects occur on the left and right sides of the heart, but with higher pressures on the left side (Table 52-1).

Pressure-Volume Relationships

The volume of a ventricular chamber correlates with length of its muscles and sarcomeres. In the left ventricle, with its circular cross section, Laplace's law defines the relationship among pressure in the chamber (P), muscle tension (T, force/unit cross-sectional area of the muscle), chamber wall thickness (h), and the internal radius of the chamber (R): $P \approx 2 \cdot T \cdot h/R$. Both calcium and the length of the heart muscle determine force (Fig. 52-5). Each muscle is composed of a linear array of sarcomere bundles. Maximal force is achieved at a sarcomere length of about 2.2 to 2.3 mm, which results in the optimal overlap of thick and thin filaments. When the sarcomere length is less than 2.0 mm, the ends of the thin filaments contact each other, thereby resulting in a reduction in force. Conversely, when sarcomeres are stretched beyond 2.3 mm, force decreases owing to reduced overlap between myosin heads and actin.

Force-length relationships, which are determined by measuring the force developed at different muscle lengths while preventing the muscle from shortening (isometric contractions), characterize the systolic and diastolic contractile properties of cardiac muscle. With increasing muscle length, end-systolic force increases to a greater degree than does end-diastolic force. The difference in force at end diastole versus end systole increases as muscle length increases as a result of the greater developed force of the stretched muscle. This relationship of force to length is referred to as the Frank-Starling law of the heart.

Work of the Heart

Cardiovascular performance is reflected in the arterial blood pressure and cardiac output (mean arterial blood flow), which in turn are dependent on four factors: preload, afterload, ventricular contractility, and heart rate.

Preload, which refers to the degree to which sarcomeres are stretched just before systole, is defined as the end-diastolic pressure or volume. The Frank-Starling law of the heart dictates that ventricular pressure and output vary with preload, so a decrease in preload decreases end-diastolic volume and pressure, peak pressure, and stroke volume. Conversely, increased preload increases ventricular pressure and output, subject to the limits to which preload pressures can be increased. Left ventricular end-diastolic pressures of 20 to 25 mm Hg and greater cause exudation of fluid into the alveoli and pulmonary edema (Chapter 58).

Afterload refers to the stress that the ventricle must overcome to eject blood. Peak arterial pressure reflects the peak stress imposed on cardiomyocytes according to Laplace's law (described previously as $P \approx 2 \cdot T \cdot h/R$). As long as there is no left ventricular outflow obstruction, arterial pressure reflects myocyte afterload, as does *total peripheral resistance* (TPR), which corresponds to the tone of the resistance vessels. TPR is the ratio between the mean pressure decrease across the arterial system (mean arterial pressure [MAP] minus mean central venous pressure [CVP]) and cardiac output (CO): TPR = (MAP − CVP)/CO. When TPR is increased, the pressure-volume relationship shifts such that peak pressure is increased whereas stroke volume and ejection fraction are decreased.

Contractility of cardiac muscle (*myocardial contractility*) or a ventricle (*ventricular contractility*) is the intrinsic ability to generate force independent of preload or afterload. When contractility is increased, the pressure-volume relationship shifts so that pressure, stroke volume, and ejection fraction are increased at constant preload volume and arterial resistance.

Cardiac output is measured in liters per minute and is equal to the amount of blood ejected at each heartbeat (stroke volume in liters per beat) multiplied by the number of beats per minute. As a result, *heart rate* is a powerful determinant of cardiac performance. Cardiac output and mean arterial pressure can be related to preload, afterload, contractility, and heart rate through the Frank-Starling curves, which plot end-diastolic pressure versus cardiac output or mean arterial pressure, to yield an overall picture of left ventricular function.

● CARDIOVASCULAR RESPONSES TO STRESSORS

Exercise
Exercise requires dramatic increases in cardiac function combined with remodeling of the peripheral circulation to meet the enhanced metabolic demands of critical organs and redirect blood flow to those organs. Indeed, the oxygen consumption during exercise can increase as much as 18-fold. About one third of the requirement for increased oxygen consumption is met by improved extraction of oxygen from the blood in the muscles (reducing venous saturation from about 75% to about 25%) and the remainder by increasing cardiac output as much as 6-fold. Increased cardiac function is achieved largely through sympathetic stimulation and reduction in vagal tone, which combine to increase the heart rate, contractility, ejection fraction, filling rates, and systolic blood pressure and to decrease aortic impedance. In young healthy individuals, heart rate can increase from a baseline of 60 to 70 beats per minute at rest to as much as 170 to 200 beats per minute with exercise. To increase rather than decrease cardiac output at these high heart rates, which can limit ventricular filling and stroke volume, contractility must also increase, through a phenomenon known as the positive force frequency relationship or Bowditch phenomenon. Along with increased cardiac contractility, arterial vasodilation in the aorta and other major arteries reduces the resistance to cardiac outflow. Both enhanced cardiac contractility and arterial vasodilation are triggered by the same sympathetic nervous system signals. With increased cardiac outflow, venous return also must increase, so preload can be maintained as well as possible to enhance cardiac function by the Frank-Starling mechanism.

Heart Failure
Heart failure can be defined as the inability of the heart to provide sufficient blood flow to meet the metabolic demands of the organs (Chapter 58). Heart failure can be due to systolic dysfunction with volume overload, most often as the consequence of ischemic heart disease (myocardial infarction) or as the end-stage consequence of hypertension. Systolic heart failure is characterized by increases in the size of the various cardiac chambers (rightward shift of the end-diastolic pressure-volume relationship). In another form of heart failure, known as *diastolic heart failure*, the heart is not necessarily increased in size, and systolic function is preserved.

Aging
Prolongation of contraction and relaxation times, which are common abnormalities in older individuals, may be related to cardiac hypertrophy as a consequence of the high prevalence of hypertension with advancing age (Chapter 67). A progressive "stiffening" of the large arteries with advancing age increases resistance, although the mechanism underlying this change is not understood. The heart rate and contractile responses to sympathetic signals are reduced and lead to a diminished ability to respond to conditions of acute overload, such as increased blood pressure or an acute myocardial infarction.

 Visit expertconsult.com for e-expanded chapter

SUGGESTED READINGS

Burkhoff D, Dickstein ML, Ferber P. The Heart Simulator. http://www.columbia.edu/itc/hs/medical/heartsim. Accessed Sept. 22, 2010. *A useful web-based learning tool for cardiac physiology.*

Gandhi MS, Kamalov G, Shahbaz AU, et al. Cellular and molecular pathways to myocardial necrosis and replacement fibrosis. *Heart Fail Rev.* 2011;16:23-34. *Review.*

Rawlins J, Carre F, Kervio G, et al. Ethnic differences in physiological cardiac adaptation to intense physical exercise in highly trained female athletes. *Circulation.* 2010;121:1078-1085. *Addresses the question of "what is normal" cardiac physiology.*

RADIOLOGY OF THE HEART

MURRAY G. BARON

53

The heart casts a homogeneous shadow on the chest film. No internal detail can be seen within its contours because the radiodensities of blood, myocardium, and other cardiac tissues are so similar that one cannot be distinguished from the others. Only two borders of the heart, where it contacts the radiolucent, air-containing lung, can be discerned in any one projection. Changes in the size or shape (or both) of the chambers of the heart and the great vessels usually alter the shape of the cardiac silhouette. However, because the heart is a three-dimensional structure, multiple views are required for complete radiographic evaluation. With the advent of echocardiography, the need for this "cardiac series" has disappeared. However, a remarkable amount of information regarding the heart is contained on standard frontal and lateral chest films, which remain a useful tool for detecting disease, evaluating the severity of known disease, documenting the progress of disease, and assessing the efficacy of treatment.

● RADIOLOGIC ANATOMY
Except for the more complex cardiac anomalies, which are rare, especially in adults, the positions and spatial relationships of the cardiac chambers and the great vessels are the same from one patient to the next and are not significantly affected by disease. On a frontal chest film, the right cardiac border is composed of a straight vertical upper half formed by the superior vena cava and a gently convex lower half representing the lateral wall of the right atrium (Fig. 53-1). The break in the contour of this border of the heart indicates the

FIGURE 53-1. Normal radiographic anatomy, magnetic resonance images. **A,** Coronal section at the level of the aortic valve. The right border of the cardiac silhouette is formed by the superior vena cava (S) and the right atrium (RA). The *arrow* indicates the caval-atrial junction. The lower portion of the left cardiac border is formed by the left ventricle (LV). A = ascending aorta; P = main pulmonary artery. **B,** Coronal section at the level of the left atrium. The upper portion of the left cardiac border is formed by the aorta (A), main pulmonary artery (P), and left atrial appendage (LAA), see *arrow.* I = inferior vena cava; LA = left atrium; T = trachea. **C,** Sagittal section near the midline. The right ventricle (RV) forms the anterior surface of the heart, which abuts the sternum. The pulmonary artery (P) extends upward and posteriorly from the ventricle. The posterior border of the heart is formed by the left atrium (LA) and left ventricle (LV). The aorta (A) is behind the heart.

caval-atrial junction. Some patients are able to inhale deeply enough to uncover a small, straight segment of the inferior vena cava between the diaphragm and the right atrium.

Abnormalities of the caval segment are usually due to dilation of the ascending aorta. A localized bulge in its midportion usually indicates post-stenotic dilation secondary to aortic valve stenosis, whereas aortic insufficiency is commonly associated with a more generalized dilation of the aorta. A bulge in the region of the caval-atrial junction may be due to an aneurysm of either the right coronary artery or the noncoronary sinus of Valsalva or to a markedly enlarged left atrium. Dilation of either atrium tends to extend the cardiac silhouette to the right, whereas dilation of either ventricle enlarges the silhouette to the left.

The left cardiac border is composed of four distinct segments. The uppermost bulge represents the aortic knob, the most distal portion of the aortic arch where it turns downward to become the descending aorta. The prominence below the knob is formed by the main pulmonary artery and the subvalvular portion of the outflow tract of the right ventricle. The lowermost third of this border represents the anterolateral wall of the left ventricle. Between this bulge and that of the pulmonary artery is a short, flat, or slightly concave segment where the left atrial appendage reaches the border of the heart.

Aneurysms of the descending thoracic aorta commonly involve its most proximal portion in the region of the ligamentum arteriosum and appear as a dilated aortic knob. Prominence of the pulmonary artery segment is common in younger individuals, but after the age of 35 to 40 years, such dilation is almost always an indicator of pulmonary arterial hypertension.

In the lateral view (see Fig. 53-1C), the anterior border of the cardiac silhouette is formed by the body and the outflow tract of the right ventricle. The heart lies in the anterior portion of the chest, and the right ventricle abuts the lower third of the sternum. Both the outflow tract and the pulmonary artery slope posteriorly. Air-containing lung interposed between this portion of the heart and the anterior chest wall forms the "retrosternal clear space." The posterior border of the heart extends from the level of the pulmonary carina to the diaphragm. Its upper half is formed by the back of the left atrium, and the lower half represents the posterior wall of the left ventricle. The shadow of the inferior vena cava is usually seen in the lateral projection extending obliquely upward and anteriorly from the diaphragm to enter the posterior aspect of the right atrium. The lowermost contour of the normal left ventricle curves anteriorly and crosses the inferior vena cava about 2 cm above the left side of the diaphragm.

Alterations in the contour of the heart usually reflect dilation or hypertrophy of the chambers, or both. Many times the pattern of these changes, together with the appearance of the pulmonary vasculature, points to a specific underlying cardiac abnormality. Chest films are most sensitive for detecting chamber dilation. Cardiac hypertrophy is more difficult to recognize because the thickened myocardium tends to encroach on the ventricular lumen more than extending outward and enlarging the cardiac silhouette. With severe hypertrophy, as in hypertrophic cardiomyopathy, the heart enlarges to the left and the apex becomes blunted, but this appearance is not pathognomonic.

HEART SIZE

A normal-sized heart does not guarantee the absence of cardiac disease. Angina, for example, no matter how severe, does not affect heart size until the left ventricle decompensates. Similarly, patients with restrictive cardiomyopathy may be in severe heart failure with a normal-appearing heart. Conversely, an enlarged heart always indicates the presence of cardiac or pericardial disease. Therefore, accurate evaluation of heart size is important.

Heart size, in the absence of disease, is directly related to the habitus of the patient. The cardiothoracic ratio, which compares the transverse diameter of the heart with the width of the chest, gives a readily obtainable, rough estimate of heart size. This ratio is measured by dropping a vertical line through the heart and summing the greatest distance to the right and left cardiac borders (Fig. 53-2) to give the transverse cardiac diameter. The transverse thoracic diameter, the greatest width of the chest, is measured from the inner surfaces of the ribs. Dividing the cardiac diameter by the chest diameter gives the cardiothoracic ratio. A value of less than 0.6 can be considered within the limits of normal. Setting this value at 0.5, as is often done, produces too many false-positive results.

In most cases, exact measurement of the cardiac silhouette is not necessary, and a reasonably experienced observer can achieve an acceptable degree of accuracy by visual estimation. With either method, several cautions must be

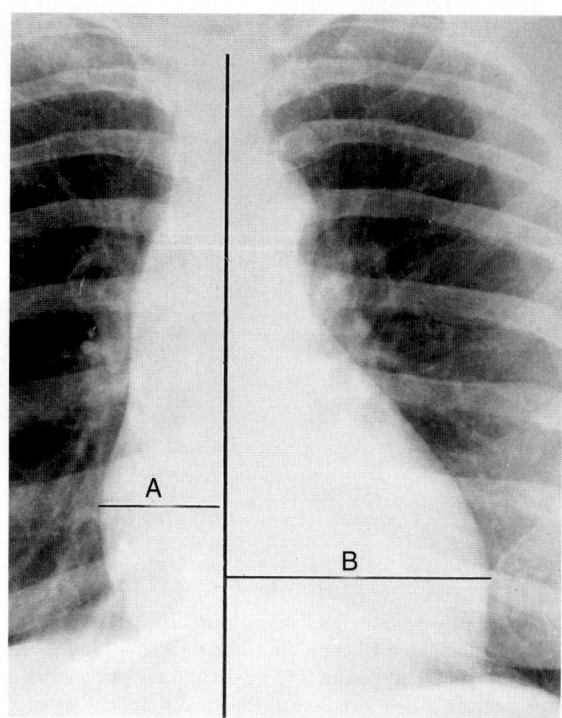

FIGURE 53-2. Measurement of the transverse cardiac diameter. Severe aortic stenosis with a 95-mm systolic gradient across the valve is present. The heart, though considerably hypertrophied, is normal in size and configuration. A *vertical line* is drawn through the heart. The greatest distances to the right cardiac border (A) and to the left cardiac border (B) are then measured. Transverse cardiac diameter = A + B.

observed. The single greatest effect on apparent cardiac size is the degree of inspiration. The volume of the heart is essentially constant throughout the cardiac cycle. As the diaphragm moves up with expiration, the vertical diameter of the heart is shortened, and its transverse diameter increases. Because heart size is estimated primarily from its width, the heart appears larger on expiratory films. The degree of inspiration can be determined from the relationship of the diaphragm to the ribs. On a properly positioned frontal chest film, a reasonable degree of inspiration is indicated if the diaphragm is lowered to at least the level of the posterior portion of the ninth rib.

When the anteroposterior diameter of the chest is small, the heart may be compressed between the sternum and the spine so that it splays to one or both sides. For this reason, the heart often appears enlarged in patients with the straight back syndrome or with a pectus excavatum deformity of the sternum. An epicardial fat pad (actually it is extrapleural fat outside the pericardium) can occur in one or both cardiophrenic angles and make the heart appear larger than it actually is. The fat pad can be recognized because the cardiophrenic angle appears obtuse or the cardiac apex is indistinct. In addition, the slightly greater density of the heart can usually be distinguished from the more radiolucent image of the fat.

A change in size of the cardiac silhouette can also occur between systole and diastole. This point is important because chest films are exposed at random with reference to the cardiac cycle, so a change in heart size between two examinations may be solely due to the timing of filming. In most cases, the difference in the transverse cardiac diameter between systole and diastole is small, no more than several millimeters. However, in younger patients, especially the more athletic with a slow heart rate and a large stroke volume, phasic change in the normal cardiac diameter can be as large as 2 cm.

CHAMBER ENLARGEMENT

Left Atrium

Dilation of the left atrium alone, in the absence of a left-to-right shunt, is most often due to disease of the mitral valve, although it can also result simply from atrial fibrillation. The two "popular" radiologic signs of left atrial enlargement—a double contour within the right cardiac border and elevation of the left main bronchus—are accurate when present, but they are insensitive and seen in only about half the cases of mitral valve disease. To produce a discernible margin within the cardiac silhouette in the frontal projection, the thickness of the heart must increase sharply at some point. This increase in thickness occurs in mitral disease when the left atrium enlarges and

FIGURE 53-3. Left atrial enlargement in mitral valve disease. **A,** Patient 1: The enlarged left atrium is causing the central portion of the cardiac silhouette to be abnormally dense. The right border of the atrium is seen within the right side of the cardiac silhouette. The left main bronchus *(black arrows)* is elevated. The region of the left atrial appendage *(white arrow)* is slightly concave because this structure was resected at a previous mitral commissurotomy. **B,** Patient 2: The enlarged left atrial appendage bulges from the left side of the heart *(white arrow)*, whereas the body of the atrium *(arrowheads)* extends beyond the right atrium to form a part of the right heart border. No double density is seen within the heart, and the left main bronchus *(black arrows)* is not elevated.

protrudes posteriorly from the back of the heart. The right border of the left atrium is then silhouetted where it abuts the right lung, and its contour is seen within the cardiac silhouette (Fig. 53-3A). This pattern is not apparent with lesser degrees of left atrial enlargement. Conversely, when the right atrium also enlarges, as is common in long-standing mitral valve disease, it forms a continuous curve on the posterior cardiac border with the enlarged left atrium. Thus, the double contour is not seen with mild left atrial enlargement or in severe cases of mitral valve disease. Furthermore, because the radiologic technique used for chest films is chosen to provide optimal images of the lungs, the enlarged heart is underexposed and the double contour may be hidden within its opaque silhouette. For the same reason, the position of the left main bronchus often cannot be clearly visualized through the mediastinal shadow.

A more sensitive sign of left atrial enlargement in the frontal projection is dilation of the left atrial appendage. The appendage extends anteriorly from the atrium along the left side of the heart, below the level of the pulmonary artery (see Fig. 53-1B). It forms the part of the left heart border between the pulmonary artery segment and the left ventricular segment. Normally, the border of the appendage is flat or slightly concave. Any convexity is abnormal and usually indicates left atrial enlargement.

Left Ventricle

The shape of the dilated left ventricle depends to a large extent on the underlying cause. When it is due to insufficiency of the aortic or mitral valve, the ventricle elongates and its apex is displaced downward, to the left, and posteriorly (Fig. 53-4). When the dilation is due to coronary artery disease or primary myocardial disease, the ventricle tends to assume a more globular shape. In the lateral view, the downward extension of the enlarged left ventricle covers more of the vena cava shadow than normal, and the crossing point of their posterior borders occurs nearer to the diaphragm than normal. Unfortunately, the usefulness of this sign is limited because of the distortion produced by even slight rotation of the patient from the true lateral position.

Enlargement of the left ventricle produces a smoothly curved dilation of the lower portion of the cardiac silhouette. A localized bulge in this contour most often represents a ventricular aneurysm (Fig. 53-5). Dilation of the left ventricle is usually associated with elevated left ventricular end-diastolic pressure. The latter increases resistance to left atrial emptying and can result in dilation of the atrium. Therefore, left atrial enlargement in the presence of a large left ventricle does not necessarily indicate the presence of mitral valve disease.

Right Atrium

Enlargement of only the right chambers of the heart is seen in severe pulmonary hypertension without coexisting left heart failure, in bacterial endocarditis of the tricuspid or pulmonic valve (or both), and in carcinoid syndrome. Dilation of the right atrium causes an accentuation and outward bowing of the curvature on the lower half of the right cardiac contour in the frontal view. With greater degrees of dilation, the cardiac silhouette enlarges to the right (Fig. 53-6).

FIGURE 53-4. Left ventricular dilation, aortic insufficiency. The apex of the heart is displaced downward and to the left. The ascending aorta *(arrow)* is diffusely dilated. The pulmonary vasculature is normal.

Right Ventricle

The right ventricle is the most difficult of the four cardiac chambers to evaluate on chest films. Except for a small area in the subpulmonic region, the chamber is not border-forming in the frontal projection. Even moderate right ventricular enlargement may produce no abnormality in this view other than some prominence of the main pulmonary artery. As right ventricular size increases, the transverse diameter of the heart enlarges to the left, and the cardiac apex becomes blunted and elevated (see Fig. 53-6). Enlargement of either or both ventricles displaces the apex of the heart to the left. It is not often possible to distinguish between biventricular enlargement and dilation of one or the other ventricle.

As the right ventricle enlarges, its area of contact with the sternum increases and tends to obliterate the retrosternal clear space in the lateral view. This sign is nonspecific inasmuch as it also depends on the shape of the chest and the size of the left ventricle, as well as the size of the right ventricle.

CALCIFICATION

Most calcifications involving the heart occur in cardiac structures as a result of inflammatory or necrotic processes (or both) or degenerative disease. Because the calcific deposits have greater radiodensity than cardiac tissues, they can often be seen within the cardiac silhouette.

The aortic and mitral valves abut each other, both inserting on the central fibrous tendon of the heart. On a frontal chest film, the two valves lie next to each other in the midportion of the cardiac silhouette, to the left of the spine (Fig. 53-7A), the aortic valve being slightly higher. It is often difficult to determine which valve is calcified in this view. They can be separated by fluoroscopy because the aortic valve tends to move in a vertical direction as the heart beats, whereas the motion of the mitral valve approximates the horizontal. This distinction can also be made accurately from the lateral chest film. If a line is drawn from the left main bronchus, seen as a dark circular shadow over the lower end of the trachea, to the anterior costophrenic angle, the mitral valve lies below the line and the aortic valve above it (Fig. 53-7B).

In the United States, calcification of only the aortic valve is most likely to represent degenerative disease of the cusps (a process in older patients akin to coronary artery calcification) or deterioration of a congenitally bicuspid valve (Chapter 75). In developing countries, calcification of the aortic or mitral valves, or both, is usually a late sequela of rheumatic fever. Calcification of the mitral annulus, which is seen in patients older than 70 years and is about four times more frequent in women than in men, is only rarely of clinical significance. The pattern of calcification is characteristic and should not be confused with that of the mitral valve. Calcium is deposited mainly between the base of the posterior mitral leaflet and the posterior wall of the left ventricle. It is seen as a broad, curvilinear band of calcium in a C shape, open superiorly and to the right on the frontal film and anteriorly on the lateral. In severe cases, the calcific deposits may also extend across the base of the anterior mitral leaflet and then form an O encircling the mitral orifice.

Calcification of the myocardium almost always indicates a previous transmural infarction and, frequently, a ventricular aneurysm. The calcified scar appears as a fine, curvilinear density, most commonly on the anterolateral

FIGURE 53-5. Left ventricular aneurysm. A bulge on the lower portion of the left cardiac border, formed by the anterolateral wall of the left ventricle, represents a ventricular aneurysm. The patient had suffered a myocardial infarction 1 year previously. The left atrial appendage segment *(arrow)* is normal. A transvenous pacemaker has been inserted through the right subclavian vein. The electrode tip is situated in the apex of the right ventricle.

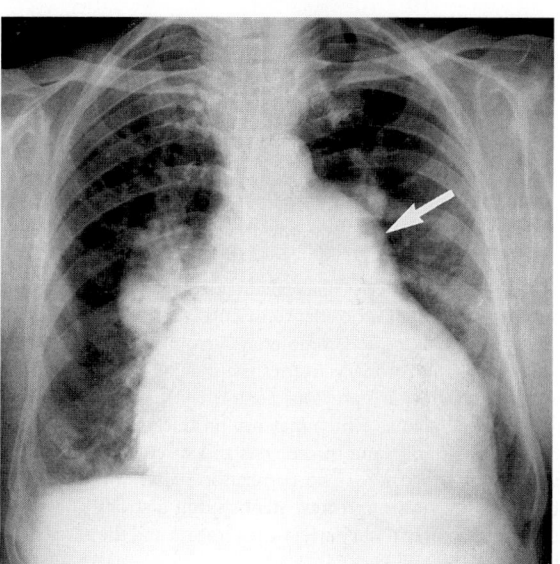

FIGURE 53-6. Right ventricular enlargement seen in a patient with resistive pulmonary hypertension secondary to an atrial septal defect. The main pulmonary artery *(arrow)* and the right pulmonary artery are markedly dilated. The left pulmonary artery was also dilated but is hidden by the heart in this view. The sudden "cutoff" of the vascular shadows just beyond the hila is characteristic of resistive pulmonary hypertension. Enlargement of the right ventricle is elevating the cardiac apex and displacing it to the left. Accentuation of the curvature of the lower right cardiac border and enlargement of the cardiac silhouette to the right are caused by dilation of the right atrium.

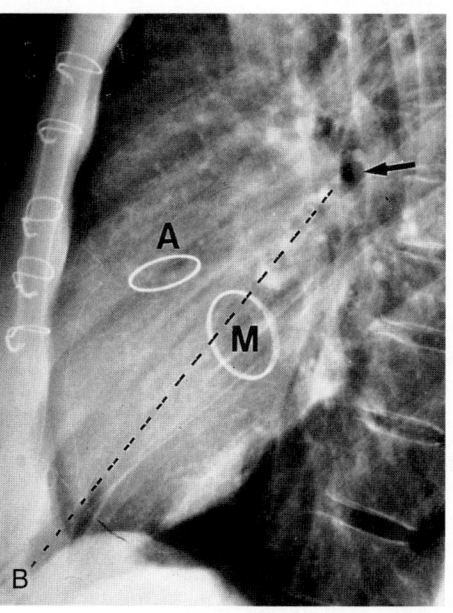

FIGURE 53-7. Location of the mitral and aortic valves. Both the mitral (M) and aortic (A) valves have been replaced by porcine heterografts. The circular stents indicate the location and tilt of each valve. **A,** Frontal projection. The two valves are normally in contact with each other, and it is difficult to separate them in the frontal projection. Furthermore, on a routinely exposed film, calcific deposits are not easily seen because of the overlapping shadows of the descending aorta *(arrows)* and the spine. **B,** Lateral projection. The valves can be differentiated on the lateral view by drawing a line from the left main bronchus *(arrow)* to the anterior costophrenic sulcus. The aortic valve lies above this line and the mitral valve below it.

FIGURE 53-8. Calcified myocardial infarctions. **A,** Patient 1: frontal projection of an anterolateral left ventricular aneurysm. The fine calcific line outlines an anterolateral aneurysm of the left ventricle. The calcific deposit is much finer than that seen with pericardial calcification. The patient had suffered a myocardial infarction several years earlier. **B,** Patient 2: lateral projection of a septal infarction. The curvilinear calcific deposit is within the scarred lower portion of the ventricular septum. The infarction extended posteriorly along the base of the heart to involve the diaphragmatic wall of the left ventricle (arrow).

aspect of the heart, best seen on the frontal view (Fig. 53-8A), or in the lower portion of the interventricular septum, best seen on the lateral projection (see Fig. 53-8B). Calcification of the pericardium is usually coarser and tends to occur in clumps. Often, pericardial calcium is distributed primarily over the interventricular sulcus and the atrioventricular grooves, but when extensive, the deposits may coalesce and completely surround the heart (Fig. 53-9).

Calcification of the coronary arteries is a specific sign of complicated atheromatous plaques in which previous hemorrhage has occurred. Not uncommonly, this type of plaque, which may not produce significant narrowing of the vessel, is the site of acute thrombosis and vascular occlusion leading to myocardial infarction. There is no correlation between the sites of calcium deposition and the sites of greatest stenosis, but a strong correlation exists between the extent of coronary artery calcification and the extent of coronary arterial sclerosis.

Calcification of the coronary arteries is difficult to visualize on chest films because the deposits are thin and their shadows are blurred by the motion of the heart. Ultrafast computed tomography (CT) scanning using either electron beam or helical CT is very sensitive and accurate for detecting and quantifying the extent of coronary arterial calcification (Chapter 56). However, the data accumulated to date have not clearly shown a correlation between the volume of coronary calcification and the clinical status of the patient. Although high calcium scores indicate extensive atherosclerosis, acute events, such as myocardial infarction or sudden death, can occur in patients with little or no calcification of their coronary arteries.

⬤ PERICARDIAL EFFUSION

The pericardium completely invests the heart, except for a small area on its posterior surface between the entrances of the pulmonary veins and the superior and inferior venae cavae. When fluid accumulates in the pericardium, the sac distends smoothly to enlarge the cardiac silhouette and give it a flask-shaped appearance. A similar shape can occur with a dilated, failing heart.

The two conditions are readily differentiated by the appearance of the pulmonary hila on a frontal chest film. The pericardial sac extends onto the great vessels and up to or slightly above the level of the bifurcation of the main pulmonary artery (Fig. 53-10). As the sac distends with fluid, it tends to overlap and obscure the hilar vessels. Conversely, when the heart fails, the vessels become congested and appear more prominent than normal (Fig. 53-11).

Posterior displacement of the epicardial fat line is a second reliable sign of pericardial effusion (Chapter 77). In adults, fat is often insinuated between the myocardium and the visceral pericardium (the epicardium) and is sometimes seen on the lateral projection as a curvilinear, radiolucent shadow paralleling the anterior aspect of the heart. The anterior surface of the parietal pericardium borders the retrosternal mediastinal fat. The soft tissue density between these two fat lines therefore represents the

FIGURE 53-9. Calcific pericarditis. **A,** Frontal projection. A large, thick, calcific plaque (arrow) lies just below the level of the left upper lobe bronchus. More caudad, the calcific deposits become confluent and cover the diaphragmatic surface of the heart. **B,** The dense calcific peel around the cardiac apex and the diaphragmatic aspect of the heart is better seen. Linear calcific deposits (arrows) lie within the atrioventricular sulcus. **C,** Nonenhanced computed tomography shows the irregular, thick, calcific peel almost encircling the heart.

pericardium, the epicardium, and the fluid between them. When normal, this stripe is no more than 2 to 4 mm thick. As fluid accumulates in the pericardial sac, the epicardial fat line is displaced posteriorly and the pericardial stripe widens (Fig. 53-12).

⬤ PULMONARY VASCULATURE

Almost all of the linear shadows in the lung represent large and medium-sized pulmonary arteries and veins. The terminal branches of the vessels are too small to be visualized as individual structures. The same is true of the interstitial tissues that support the alveoli and form the primary and secondary interlobular septa. However, summation of the minimal densities cast by these structures gives the pulmonary fields an overall grayish cast. The large vessels are seen because their soft tissue density is contrasted against the surrounding air-containing alveoli.

The caliber of the pulmonary vessels reflects the volume of blood flowing through the lungs. When this volume is diminished because of a right-to-left shunt, venous blood bypasses the pulmonary vessels, and, as a result, these vessels are smaller in caliber and the lungs appear abnormally radiolucent. Increased size and prominence of the pulmonary vessels, both central and peripheral, usually indicate an increase in pulmonary blood flow secondary to a left-to-right shunt (Fig. 53-13A). The vessels in the lower as well as the upper lung fields are dilated. Although pulmonary arteries and veins also become abnormally prominent in patients with heart failure, the vessels are not usually sharply outlined, and additional signs of pulmonary venous hypertension or interstitial edema are present (Chapter 58).

The vessels to the lower lobes carry about 60 to 70% of the pulmonary blood flow and are normally of greater caliber than the vessels to the upper lobes. As pulmonary venous pressure increases, the lower lobe vessels become constricted, so more blood is distributed to the upper lobes, which makes their vessels more prominent. This redistribution of the pulmonary vasculature is a reliable sign of pulmonary venous hypertension (see Fig. 53-13B),

although it is often difficult to recognize unless quite marked. With a sufficient further increase in venous pressure, pulmonary edema develops.

Pulmonary Edema

Normally, extravascular circulation of fluid in the lungs from the capillaries through the interstitium and back to the blood stream by way of the lymphatics is constant. When pulmonary venous pressure increases, more and more fluid leaks from the capillary bed, the capacity of the lymphatics to remove the fluid is exceeded, and the interstitium becomes waterlogged. Because the interlobular septa in the outer portions of the lung bases are oriented parallel to the x-ray beam on an erect film, when thickened, they are seen as parallel, short horizontal lines extending to the pleural surfaces (Kerley B lines). Kerley A lines also represent thickened interlobular septa, but they are longer and are seen in the upper lung fields. These lines are within the depth of the lung and do not usually reach the pleural surface. Most of the other septa, even when thickened, are too fine to be identified as individual structures. However, the summation pattern creates random "noise" on the film that obscures the shadows of the pulmonary vessels (Fig. 53-14). A ground-glass appearance of the lung fields without identifiable vascular markings within them is characteristic of interstitial pulmonary edema (Chapter 58). The patient is generally severely tachypneic at this stage, but rales may not be

FIGURE 53-10. Superior pericardial reflection with effusion after a tap. During pericardiocentesis, some of the fluid withdrawn was replaced with air. The normal pericardium is now outlined between the intrapericardial air and the air in the lungs and is seen as a thin linear shadow along the outer border of the cardiac silhouette. The film is made in the erect position, and the air has risen to the highest point of the pericardial cavity *(arrows),* above the level of the pulmonary hila and almost reaching the aortic arch.

FIGURE 53-12. Pericardial effusion with posterior displacement of the epicardial fat line. The *two lines of arrows* point to the substernal fat and the subepicardial fat layers. **A,** Normal. The fine line of soft tissue density between the fat layers represents the epicardium, the pericardium, and the fluid between them. **B,** Same patient with a pericardial effusion. The epicardial fat line is displaced posteriorly, and the pericardial stripe is abnormally wide.

FIGURE 53-11. Hilum overlay sign. **A,** Pericardial effusion. The heart is diffusely enlarged. Its silhouette extends outward and is obscuring the hilar shadows in each lung. **B,** Dilated cardiomyopathy. The heart is diffusely enlarged. The failing left ventricle has caused congestion of the hilar vessels, and they are more prominent than normal.

present. Interstitial edema also causes thickening of the bronchial walls and peribronchial connective tissue, best seen when they are projected on end. This "peribronchial cuffing" is best visualized in the superior portion of the pulmonary hila, where the anterior segmental bronchus of the upper lobes is viewed on end. When the interstitium can no longer accommodate the excess fluid, it spills into the alveoli (Fig. 53-15). At this point, as air bubbles through the fluid, the typical auscultatory findings of pulmonary edema appear.

Pulmonary Arterial Hypertension

Resistive pulmonary hypertension can result from a left-to-right intracardiac shunt, mitral valve disease, or extracardiac disease, such as repeated episodes of pulmonary embolization (Chapter 98). The central pulmonary arteries become grossly dilated. Instead of gradually tapering as they bifurcate, a sudden, sharp change in the caliber of the vessels is noted. The size and number of the smaller arterial branches decrease, and they take on the appearance of a "pruned tree" (see Fig. 53-6). With severe pulmonary hypertension,

the right heart chambers may dilate. The radiographic appearance of pulmonary hypertension is relatively specific but not sensitive, and clinically significant pulmonary hypertension can be present with a normal-appearing pulmonary vascular bed.

The Cardiac Veins

Almost all coronary blood returns to the heart through the coronary sinus. The orifice of the coronary sinus is in the base of the right atrium just above the entrance of the inferior vena cava and behind the tricuspid valve. Three major cardiac veins drain through the coronary sinus. The great cardiac vein runs upward in the anterior portion of the interventricular sulcus to the atrioventricular sulcus, where it turns to the right (Fig. 53-16) and is joined by the posterior vein of the left ventricle. The drainage area of the latter vein roughly corresponds to the distribution of the circumflex coronary artery. These combined veins continue in the atrioventricular sulcus around the back of the heart as the coronary sinus, which empties into the right atrium. The third vein, the middle cardiac vein, courses in the posterior portion of the interventricular sulcus together with the posterior descending branch of the right coronary artery and joins the coronary sinus near its entrance into the right atrium.

Although percutaneous ventricular pacing initially was limited to the right ventricle, an electrode can now be safely placed percutaneously into a cardiac vein. If a venous catheter in the right atrium curves anteriorly in the lateral view, it extends into the right ventricle. However, if it curves posteriorly, it almost certainly enters the coronary sinus. In the frontal projection, the courses of a catheter in the coronary sinus and a catheter in the right ventricle are almost identical, although one is located on the back of the heart and the

FIGURE 53-13. Pulmonary vasculature. **A,** Atrial septal defect, left-to-right shunt. All pulmonary vessels, to the lower lobes as well as to the upper lobes, are dilated, which is indicative of increased blood flow. **B,** Mitral stenosis, pulmonary venous hypertension with redistribution of the pulmonary vasculature. The lower lobe vessels are constricted and the upper vessels, which now carry more blood, are of greater caliber.

FIGURE 53-15. Alveolar pulmonary edema, acute myocardial infarction. Patchy areas of consolidation can be seen in the perihilar regions of both lungs. Dilation of the heart after a massive myocardial infarction may not be seen for the first 24 to 48 hours.

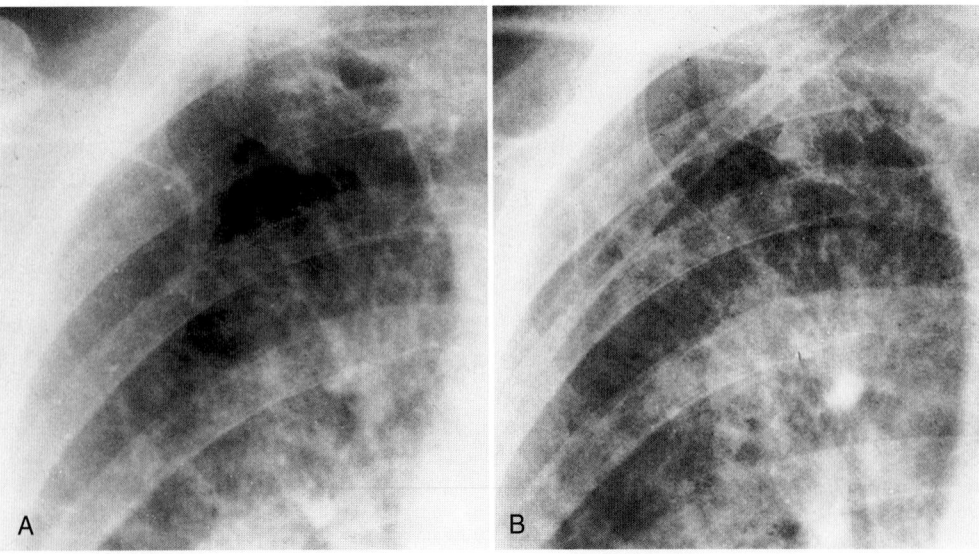

FIGURE 53-14. Interstitial pulmonary edema. **A,** Close-up of the right upper lobe; portable film of a patient with an acute myocardial infarction. The pulmonary vessels are well outlined. **B,** Two days later, the patient became tachypneic. No abnormal auscultatory findings were present in the lungs. Radiographically, the lung fields are noisy, with numerous random shadows obscuring the outline of the pulmonary vessels. The appearance and the time sequence of the changes are characteristic of interstitial pulmonary edema.

other is more anterior in the right ventricular cavity. Because the coronary sinus courses directly above the attachment of the posterior leaflet of the mitral valve (Fig. 53-17), it can be used for the percutaneous placement of a device to constrict the mitral orifice, thereby producing the same effect as a surgical mitral annuloplasty (Chapter 75).

FIGURE 53-16. Biventricular pacemaker, frontal view. The left ventricular lead extends retrograde through the coronary sinus into the great cardiac vein (GV), running in the anterior interventricular sulcus. The section of the coronary sinus between the *arrowheads* is the portion adjacent to the insertion of the posterior mitral leaflet. RA = right atrial lead; RV = right ventricular lead.

THE HEART AND PORTABLE FILMS

Not uncommonly, cardiac patients are too ill to be transported, so their studies must be performed with portable equipment at the bedside. The resulting images are less sharp and have less contrast, and the degree of magnification of the intrathoracic structures can vary considerably. Portable images can also vary from one to the next because the positioning of the patient and the film and the distance between the patient and the x-ray tube are all dependent, in practice, on visual estimation of the technologist. Despite these differences, the same principles of interpretation also apply to portable images, with a few important caveats:

1. The size of the heart, especially relative to the width of the chest, is magnified on a portable image, so the cardiothoracic ratio is not particularly useful. Furthermore, small changes in cardiac size from one portable film to the next have little significance because of the likelihood of variations in technique. Conversely, if the heart appears smaller on a portable than on an erect film, the decrease in size is almost certainly real.

2. If the technologist tilts the x-ray tube even slightly toward the patient's head, the heart will appear even larger and will be projected over the hilar vessels, thereby mimicking the "hilum overlay" sign of a pericardial effusion. Thus, this sign is not useful with portable images.

3. Free pleural fluid collects in the dependent portions of the pleural space, at first in the costophrenic sulci. With fixed equipment in which the x-ray beam is horizontal, the lateral costophrenic sulci are usually obliterated by the fluid, and the upper level of the fluid can be seen. When the patient is supine or slightly tilted, the fluid flows out of the costophrenic sulci and layers along the posterior chest wall. The x-ray beam, although still at right angles to the patient, is no longer horizontal, so the fluid, now viewed en face, appears as an ill-defined haze.

4. Portable films are frequently used to confirm the position of various inserted devices. Without any sense of depth, however, all that is really known is that the object is "projected over" the region of interest; it could actually be some distance away.

SUGGESTED READINGS

Kasznia-Brown J. Cardiac disease on chest x-ray: a pictorial view. *Br J Hosp Med (Lond).* 2010;71:182-184. *Practical clinical pearls.*

Miller RR, Ely EW. Radiographic measures of intravascular volume status: the role of vascular pedicle width. *Curr Opin Crit Care.* 2006;12:255-262. *Assessment of the value of radiographic markers of volume status.*

FIGURE 53-17. Left subclavian biventricular pacemaker. Frontal (A) and lateral (B) images. The right ventricular lead (RV) is seen in the lateral view to curve anteriorly through the tricuspid valve. Its tip is in the apex of the right ventricle. The left ventricular lead curves posteriorly in the atrium and enters the coronary sinus (CS), continuing to the posterior vein of the left ventricle (PV). Note how the right ventricular lead and coronary sinus are superimposed in the frontal projection (RA) right atrial lead.

54

ELECTROCARDIOGRAPHY

LEONARD GANZ

Electrocardiography, which has changed surprisingly little since it was initially introduced by Einthoven in the early 1900s, allows recording of myocardial activation from several vantage points on the body's surface, thereby permitting analysis of electrical activation in different myocardial regions. Surface electrocardiography may be supplemented with intracardiac recordings, which are particularly helpful in the diagnosis and management of cardiac arrhythmias (Chapter 62).

● NORMAL FUNCTION AND ELECTROCARDIOGRAM

Normal Cardiac Activation

Electrical activation of the heart depends on the spread of a depolarizing wave front from pacemaker cells through cardiac muscle, as well as specialized conducting tissues (Fig. 54-1). Under normal circumstances, cells in the sinoatrial (SA) nodal complex in the high lateral aspect of the right atrium have the highest spontaneous depolarization rate and are therefore the dominant cardiac pacemaker (Chapter 61). This electrical wave front spreads throughout the right and left atria; specialized conducting tracts called *Bachmann's* bundle speed the depolarizing wave front to the left atrium. Electrical atrial activation triggers atrial muscular contraction, which pumps blood through the tricuspid and mitral valves into the right and left ventricles. Normally, the atrioventricular (AV) node, where conduction delay is physiologic, serves as the only electrical connection linking the atria and ventricles; the AV valve rings are insulated. The depolarizing wave front exits the AV node into the bundle of His, a specialized conducting tissue capable of rapid conduction. The bundle of His bifurcates into right and left bundle branches; the left bundle branch divides into the left anterior and left posterior fascicles. The bundle branches, as well as their more distal ramifications of specialized conducting tissue, are called the *Purkinje system*. From these specialized conducting tissues, the depolarizing wave front enters into and then moves through ventricular muscle. As in the atria, ventricular electrical activation begets muscular contraction, which pumps blood through the semilunar valves into the pulmonary and systemic circulations. After electrical activation, or depolarization, a period of electrical recovery, or repolarization, is necessary before repeated activation.

At the cellular level, a complex orchestration of ion channels opening and closing determines the membrane potential throughout this process. The flow of ions into and out of the myocardial cells inscribes an action potential, which reflects depolarization and repolarization, as well as spontaneous depolarization of pacemaker cells (Chapter 61).

The Electrocardiographic Waves

Labeled alphabetically, beginning with the P wave, the basic waves of the electrocardiogram (ECG) correspond to these electrical events (Fig. 54-2). The P wave represents atrial muscular depolarization; in severe hyperkalemia, atrial electrical activation may be unaccompanied by atrial muscular activation, and no P wave is inscribed. The QRS complex represents ventricular muscular depolarization; because of the disparity between ventricular and atrial muscle mass, the QRS complex is typically much larger in voltage amplitude than the P wave is. Recorded from multiple vantage points, the QRS complex harbors tremendous information about the structure and function of ventricular tissue. Under normal circumstances, the PR interval, which is the segment from the onset of the P wave to the onset of the QRS complex, represents the delay between atrial and ventricular depolarization. The ST segment and T wave (and occasionally the U wave) reflect ventricular repolarization, a process of electrical recovery that must take place before the ventricle can be depolarized again. Atrial muscle also requires repolarization before the next depolarizing wave front. Because ventricular mass far exceeds atrial muscular mass, the low-amplitude atrial repolarization wave is buried underneath the QRS complex and is rarely manifested on the ECG.

Electrocardiography Standards

A standard ECG is recorded on paper with 1-mm ("small" boxes) as well as 5-mm ("big" boxes) gridlines. Voltage amplitude is measured on the vertical axis (typically 10 mm equaling 1 mV) and time on the horizontal axis. Because the usual ECG recording speed is 25 mm per second, each 1-mm gridline ("small" box) represents 0.04 second (40 msec), and each 5-mm gridline ("big" box) equals 0.2 second (200 msec). These parameters are the usual calibration or standardization. Necessary for proper interpretation, the standardization parameters are typically printed on the ECG.

A standard ECG is recorded over a 10-second period, although a rhythm or monitor strip can be recorded for substantially longer if necessary. Multiple leads are typically recorded simultaneously from the top to the bottom of the page. The usual groupings of leads include I, II, and III; aVR, aVL, and aVF; V_1, V_2, and V_3; and V_4, V_5, and V_6 (see later). Each group of leads is recorded for 2.5 seconds. A single lead (or multilead) rhythm strip is recorded below for the entire 10 seconds. Thus, as the ECG is scanned from left to right, one sees 10 seconds of cardiac activity, with each complex recorded simultaneously in multiple leads.

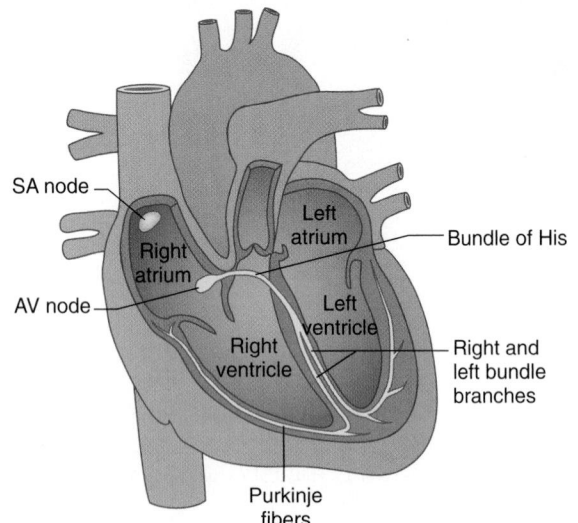

FIGURE 54-1. Cardiac conduction system. The normal conducting system consists of pacemaker cells in the sinoatrial (SA) nodal complex, specialized intra-atrial conducting tracts (including Bachmann's bundle), the atrioventricular (AV) node, the His-Purkinje system, and working atrial and ventricular myocardium.

FIGURE 54-2. Inscription of a normal electrocardiogram (ECG). Sinoatrial nodal depolarization is not visible on the surface ECG; the P wave corresponds to atrial mechanical contraction. The PR interval denotes conduction through the atrial muscle, atrioventricular node, and His-Purkinje system. The QRS complex reflects ventricular muscle depolarization. The ST segment and T wave correspond to ventricular repolarization. Atrial repolarization also occurs, but the signal is of low amplitude and buried underneath the QRS complex. Note the gridlines. On the horizontal axis, each 1-mm line ("small" box) denotes 0.04 second (40 msec); a "big" box denotes 0.2 second (200 msec). On the vertical axis, 1 mm ("small" box) corresponds to 0.1 mV; 10 mm (two "big" boxes) therefore denotes 1 mV.

TABLE 54-1 NORMAL ELECTROCARDIOGRAPHIC INTERVALS	
Heart rate	50-100 beats per minute
P wave duration	<0.12 sec (120 msec)
PR interval	0.09 (90 msec) to 0.20 sec (200 msec)
QRS duration	0.075 (75 msec) to 0.11 sec (110 msec)
QTc	0.45 sec (450 msec) males, 0.46 sec (460 msec) females
QRS axis	−30 to + 90 degrees

Normal Intervals

Each of the various ECG waves and intervals has normal ranges, defined from large numbers of electrocardiographic recordings in (presumably) healthy subjects (Table 54-1; see Fig. 54-2).

The RR interval (or PP interval), which is the measurement from R wave to R wave (or P wave to P wave), allows calculation of the heart rate. Because there are 60,000 msec in a minute, the heart rate (HR) in beats per minute can be easily calculated from the RR or PP interval in milliseconds:

$$HR = \frac{60,000}{RR}$$

Although traditionally the normal resting heart rate has been defined as 60 to 100 beats per minute, a range of 50 to 90 at rest may actually be more reflective of normal physiology. When the heart rate is grossly irregular, as in atrial fibrillation (Chapter 64), the RR interval can be averaged over a number of cardiac cycles to estimate the heart rate. Because a standard ECG records 10 seconds in time, the heart rate (beats per minute) will equal the number of QRS complexes recorded on a standard ECG multiplied by 6.

P Wave Duration

The P wave duration, from the beginning to the end of a P wave, is typically less than 0.12 second (120 msec, three small boxes) in length. A broader P wave reflects an intra-atrial or interatrial conduction delay, or both. Abnormalities in P wave amplitude, morphology, and axis may reflect atrial enlargement.

PR Interval

The PR interval, which is measured from the onset of the P wave to the onset of the QRS complex, is normally between 0.09 and 0.2 second (90 to 200 msec). One-to-one AV conduction with a PR interval greater than 0.2 second has traditionally been called first-degree AV block, but *delayed AV conduction* may be a more appropriate term. Conduction through the atrial tissue, the AV node, and the His-Purkinje system contributes to the PR interval. When the PR interval is prolonged, delay is usually present in the AV node, although other sites of delay are possible. Prolongation of the PR interval is associated with an increased risk of atrial fibrillation, need for a pacemaker, and higher overall mortality. A short PR interval may reflect ventricular preexcitation (Wolff-Parkinson-White syndrome), a junctional rhythm, or other conditions.

QRS Complex

The QRS complex, which reflects ventricular muscular electrical activation, carries important information in patients with coronary artery disease, cardiomyopathy, metabolic abnormalities, and other conditions. Capital letters (Q, R, S) denote large-amplitude deflections (≥5 mm or 0.5 mV), whereas lowercase letters (q, r, s) signify low-amplitude deflections (<5 mm or 0.5 mV). Q, q, S, and s waves are negative excursions from the isoelectric baseline, whereas R and r waves are positive deflections. Q and q waves are initial negative deflections, and S and s waves are negative deflections that follow a positive deflection (R or r wave); a QS complex is an entirely negative deflection. An R′ or r′ wave refers to a second positive deflection after an S (or s) wave. The duration of the QRS complex reflects the time required for ventricular depolarization. Ventricular activation usually requires at least 0.075 second (75 msec, nearly two small boxes). There is some debate regarding the upper limit of the normal range for QRS duration; a recent consensus document specified 0.11 second (110 msec, nearly three small boxes). If the QRS duration is prolonged, an intraventricular or interventricular conduction delay (IVCD), or both, is present. Particular patterns of IVCD have been termed *bundle branch block* (see later).

QT Interval

The QT interval, which reflects ventricular repolarization, is measured from the onset of the QRS complex to the end of the T wave. Accurate assessment of the repolarization interval is important inasmuch as patients with prolonged repolarization, either congenital or acquired, may be at risk for torsades de pointes ventricular tachycardia (Chapter 65). The QT interval must be corrected to allow comparison of this interval at differing heart rates. Bazett's formula defines a corrected QT interval (QTc):

$$QTc = \frac{QT}{\sqrt{RR}}$$

Bazett's formula works reasonably well at heart rates in the normal range but overcorrects at high rates and undercorrects at low rates. Although more complex regression formulas have been developed to correct the QT interval at different heart rates, none has achieved widespread clinical use. Irregular rhythms (notably atrial fibrillation) complicate calculation of the QTc. Calculating multiple QTc intervals and then taking the average is reasonable; alternatively, the QTc after the longest RR interval can be considered the "worst-case scenario" of the repolarization interval.

The presence of a U wave complicates measurement of the QT (and therefore QTc) interval because it is not always clear where the T wave ends and whether the U wave should be included in a QTU interval. If the isoelectric baseline is reached between the T and U waves, the U wave is not generally included in the QT interval. If the T wave "merges" into the U wave without reaching the isoelectric baseline, the U wave is included in the QT (or QTU) interval. Short QTc intervals are unusual. The QTc in a given patient may vary somewhat over the course of the day and tends to be slightly longer in young and middle-aged women than in men. The upper limit of a normal QTc is somewhat debatable, but a cutoff of 0.45 second (450 msec) in men and 0.46 second (460 msec) in women was proposed recently in a consensus document. The QT interval is quite sensitive to drug effects, as well as to electrolyte and metabolic derangements.

Electrocardiographic Leads

Recording a single ECG lead allows calculation of the heart rate and, frequently, accurate diagnosis of the heart rhythm. When the ECG is recorded from multiple skin leads simultaneously, the direction (or vector) of activation as the electrical wave front moves through the heart can be inferred. Although a number of different lead systems are possible (and some are actually used in research settings), standard electrocardiography uses 12 leads from 12 vantage points, recorded with 10 electrodes, 6 on the chest wall and 4 on the limbs. In reality, only three limb leads are actually used to generate recordings; the right leg lead serves as an electrical ground. The limb leads, called the *frontal plane leads,* generate bipolar and augmented unipolar lead recordings. The chest or precordial electrodes record unipolar recordings. Bipolar leads record the potential difference between two skin electrodes. In unipolar recordings, the lead of interest, the exploring electrode, is compared with a reference electrode. By convention, a positive deflection is recorded if the electrical wave front is moving toward the positive electrode in a bipolar pair or toward the exploring electrode in a unipolar lead.

The bipolar limb leads measure potential differences between electrodes on pairs of limb electrodes. Lead I compares the right arm (negative) and left arm (positive), lead II the right arm (negative) and left leg (positive), and lead III the left arm (negative) and left leg (positive) (Fig. 54-3). Because the direction of both atrial and ventricular depolarization is away from the right arm and toward the left arm, a positive P wave and QRS complex are generally recorded in lead I. Similarly, the P wave and QRS complexes are positive in leads II and III in normal SA to AV conduction because atrial and ventricular activation proceeds in a craniocaudal direction. The bipolar limb leads closely resemble Einthoven's original string galvanometer recordings.

Leads aVR, aVL, and aVF are augmented unipolar leads in which the potential in each limb is compared with a reference electrode. For lead aVR, the potential of the right arm is compared with a reference composed of the left arm and left leg electrodes. Lead aVL compares the left arm potential with a reference combining the right arm and left leg; aVF compares the left leg with a right and left arm reference. Because atrial and ventricular activation normally moves from right to left and in a craniocaudal direction, the P wave and QRS complex are negative in lead aVR but positive in lead aVF. In lead aVL, P waves and QRS complexes are generally upright, although an rS complex may be recorded, particularly in young patients.

The precordial electrodes are positioned at specific points on the chest wall (Fig. 54-4A). These unipolar leads compare electrical potential between the

Lead I

Lead II

Lead III

Lead aVR

Lead aVL

Lead aVF

FIGURE 54-3. Normal cardiac activation as manifested in the limb leads. Under normal circumstances, P waves and QRS complex are typically upright in leads I, II, III, and aVF and inverted in aVR. In lead aVL, P waves are usually upright, although QRS complexes may be either upright or inverted. The right leg electrode serves to ground the system.

A   B

V₁ V₂ V₃ V₄ V₅ V₆

FIGURE 54-4. Precordial leads. **A,** Positioning of the precordial leads on the chest wall. **B,** Normal cardiac activation as manifested in the precordial leads. Note the small r wave and deep S wave in lead V₁, the transition at around V₃ or V₄, and the "septal" q wave and large R wave in lead V₆.

A   B

FIGURE 54-5. Axis of electrical activation. **A,** Vectors for the limb leads (LL) in the frontal plane. **B,** Hexaxial reference for determining the frontal plane axis. Note that the vectors for leads I, II, and III are in the same direction as in **A,** but now, like the augmented limb leads, these standard limb lead vectors have been moved so that they emanate from the center of the figure. LA = left atrium; RA = right atrium.

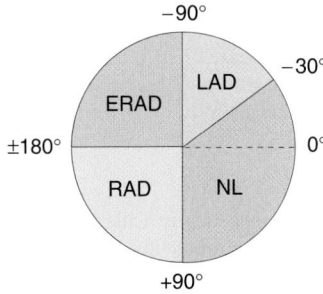

FIGURE 54-6. Chart of frontal plane axes. Normal (NL) = −30 to +90 degrees; left axis deviation (LAD) = −30 to −90 degrees (moderate, −30 to −45 degrees; marked, −45 to −90 degrees); right axis deviation (RAD) = +90 to +180 degrees (moderate, +90 to +120 degrees; marked, +120 to +180 degrees); extreme right axis deviation (ERAD) = −90 to ±180 degrees. Mild RAD is considered normal in children, adolescents, and young adults.

chest electrode and a reference electrode called the *Wilson central terminal.* The Wilson central terminal combines the right arm, left arm, and left leg potentials through 5000-Ω resistors. The six precordial leads define atrial and ventricular activation with respect to a somewhat transverse plane through the chest wall (see Fig. 54-4B). In this plane, atrial activation moves from right to left. Initial ventricular activation involving the septum is directed from left to right; left ventricular depolarization, which dominates right ventricular depolarization because of the differential in myocardial mass, then moves apically and laterally. In lead V₁, to the right of the sternum, the P wave is biphasic (reflecting right and then left atrial activation). Initial ventricular activation of the septum inscribes an r wave, whereas subsequent activation away from lead V₁ records a dominant S wave. In lead V₆, the P wave is positive. Initial septal depolarization inscribes a tiny "septal" q wave (usually ≤0.02 second), and subsequent ventricular depolarization records a dominant R wave.

Right-sided chest leads should be recorded when right ventricular abnormalities are suspected. RV₃, the mirror image of lead V₃, is routinely recorded in pediatric patients because of the possibility of congenital heart disease. In adults, ST elevation in lead RV₃ is quite specific for acute right ventricular infarction in those being evaluated for an acute inferior wall myocardial infarction.

Axis

An axis of electrical activation can be defined in the frontal plane axis by combining the bipolar and augmented unipolar limb leads (Fig. 54-5A). By convention, the axis parallel to lead I, toward the left arm, is called 0 degrees. A frontal plane axis between −30 and +90 degrees is normal; other axes are abnormal (Fig. 54-6). Right axis deviation is a normal variant in children and

adolescents. The frontal plane axis can be estimated by identifying the limb lead in which the QRS complex is most nearly isoelectric (similar positive and negative deflections); the axis is perpendicular to this lead (see Fig. 54-5B). Because two lines pointing 180 degrees apart can be drawn perpendicular to any given line, examination of the other limb leads defines the direction in which the axis points. If the QRS complex is positive in any given limb lead, the axis will be oriented toward that limb lead, not away from it. Alternatively, the axis is in the normal range if the QRS complexes are primarily positive in both leads I and II.

An axis per se is not defined in the precordial leads. Rather, because the typical progression from leads V_1 to V_6 is from a predominantly negative to a positive QRS complex, the transition point is usually defined as the point at which the amplitude of the R wave begins to exceed the amplitude of the S wave.

APPROACH TO INTERPRETING THE ELECTROCARDIOGRAM

A stepwise approach to interpreting the ECG ensures that no features of the tracing will be overlooked (Table 54-2).

Normal Electrocardiogram

Figure 54-7 is an example of a normal ECG. Sinus rhythm occurs at about 78 beats per minute, with minor variations in the RR intervals (sinus arrhythmia). The PR interval, QRS duration, and QTc are all normal. The QRS complex is most nearly isoelectric in lead aVL, so the QRS axis will be perpendicular to lead aVL. Because aVL points to −30 degrees, the QRS axis must be approximately −120 or +60 degrees. Because the QRS complex is positive in leads I and II (large R waves), the QRS axis is approximately +60 degrees. The transition in the precordial leads is between leads V_3 and V_4. The P wave is biphasic in lead V_1 and then positive in the other precordial leads. "Septal" q waves, reflecting not lateral infarction but rather normal early septal depolarization, are present in leads V_5 and V_6. Tiny q waves, a normal variant, are seen in the inferior leads.

Abnormal Electrocardiogram

Electrocardiography in patients with coronary artery disease is reviewed in Chapters 71 to 73 and arrhythmias in Chapters 61 to 66.

Conduction Abnormalities and Axis Deviation

Abnormalities of the specialized conduction system (i.e., His-Purkinje system) reflect slow or absent conduction in a particular structure, but fascicular blocks do not prolong QRS duration beyond 120 msec (Table 54-3). An IVCD is generally defined as a QRS duration of more than 0.11 second (110 msec). When the QRS has a duration of at least 0.12 second (120 msec), it often has the configuration of a specific bundle branch block (Fig. 54-8).

Chamber Hypertrophy

A number of criteria for defining left ventricular hypertrophy (LVH; Fig. 54-9) and right ventricular hypertrophy (RVH) have been proposed. All of the LVH criteria suffer from poor sensitivity (ranging from 30 to 50%), although the specificity is good (85 to 95%). The Cornell voltage criterion, developed with an echocardiographic standard for LVH, simply adds the S wave amplitude in V_3 and the R wave amplitude in aVL; a total greater than

TABLE 54-2	STEPWISE APPROACH TO INTERPRETING THE ELECTROCARDIOGRAM

Estimate the heart rate
Define the heart rhythm (regular vs. irregular; relationship of P waves to QRS complexes)
Measure intervals (PR, QRS duration, QT)
Calculate/estimate QTc
Estimate QRS axis
Examine P wave morphology, duration, and axis
Examine QRS progression and transition in precordial leads
Examine QRS complexes in regional groupings (septal leads [V_1,V_2], anterior leads [V_2, V_3, V_4], lateral leads [I, aVL, V_5, V_6], inferior and posterior leads [II, III, aVF, V_1, V_2])
Examine ST segments in regional groupings
Examine T waves in regional groupings

TABLE 54-3	FASCICULAR AND BUNDLE BRANCH BLOCKS			
	QRS DURATION	**AXIS**	**QRS MORPHOLOGY**	**ST SEGMENTS AND T WAVES**
LAFB	<0.12 sec (120 msec)	−45 to −90 degrees	Delayed transition across the precordium qR aVL	Normal
LPFB	<0.12 sec (120 msec)	+90 to +180 degrees	Delayed transition across the precordium rS in I, aVL qR in III, aVF	Normal
RBBB	≥0.12 sec (120 msec)	Normal	rsr′, rsR′, rSR′ in V_1 (and usually V_2); wide S in V_6 and I	Discordant in V_1 and V_2
RBBB with LAFB	≥0.12 sec (120 msec)	−45 to 90 degrees	rsr′, rsR′, rSR′ in V_1 (and usually V_2); wide S in V_6 and I	Discordant in V_1 and V_2
RBBB with LPFB	≥0.12 sec (120 msec)	+ 90 to +180 degrees	rsr′, rsR′, rSR′ in V_1 (and usually V_2); wide S in V_6 and I	Discordant in V_1 and V_2
LBBB	≥0.12 sec (120 msec)	Variable	rS or QS in V_1 (S wide and notched); wide notched R without q in V_5, V_6, and I Wide notched R with or without small q in aVL	Discordant in V_1 to V_6

LAD = left axis deviation; LAFB = left anterior fascicular block; LBBB = left bundle branch block; LPFB = left posterior fascicular block; RBBB = right bundle branch block.

FIGURE 54-7. Normal electrocardiogram. The heart rate is approximately 78 beats per minute, with minor irregularity. Sinus arrhythmia is present. The axis is approximately +60 degrees. The PR, QRS, and QT intervals are approximately 140, 90, and 360 msec, respectively. P wave morphology, duration, and axis are normal. The transition is between leads V_3 and V_4. No abnormal Q waves are present. ST segments are isoelectric, and T waves are concordant with QRS complexes.

FIGURE 54-8. Fascicular and bundle branch blocks. **A,** Left anterior fascicular block (LAFB). Left axis deviation is present; the axis is approximately −60 degrees. The QRS duration is normal, and there is a delay in R wave progression across the precordial leads (late transition). Small q waves are present in leads I and aVL and small r waves in leads II, III, and aVF. **B,** Right bundle branch block (RBBB). The QRS is widened, with an rsR′ pattern in lead V₁ and a wide terminal S wave in lead V₆. ST segments are downsloping, and T waves are discordant with the QRS complex in the right precordial leads. The axis is normal, and signs of normal septal activation (q waves in lead V₆) are present. **C,** RBBB and LAFB. In addition to features diagnostic of RBBB, an axis of −60 degrees is present.

D

FIGURE 54-8, cont'd. **D,** Left bundle branch block (LBBB). The QRS is widened, with a broad, notched complex in leads I, aVL, and the left precordial leads. Small r waves and broad, deep S waves are present in the right precordial leads. With LBBB, the axis is usually normal or deviated to the left. ST segments and T waves are discordant with the QRS complex throughout the precordium.

FIGURE 54-9. Left ventricular hypertrophy. Note the striking S wave amplitude in the right precordial leads and R wave amplitude in the left precordial leads. Repolarization abnormalities are present in the left precordial leads, as well as the limb leads. The S wave amplitude in V_3 (2.4 mV) plus the R wave amplitude in aVL (1.0 mV) total 3.4 mV, easily satisfying the Cornell voltage criteria in this 76-year-old hypertensive man. Sinus bradycardia (50 beats per minute) is present as well.

2.0 mV in women and 2.8 mV in men implies LVH. In many clinical settings, the Cornell criterion has replaced the more complicated Romhilt-Estes criteria, which assign points for QRS amplitude, repolarization abnormalities ("strain" pattern), left axis deviation, and other electrocardiographic features. RVH is much less common than LVH. Electrocardiographic criteria for diagnosing RVH have even lower sensitivity (10 to 20%) than for LVH, although the specificity is similar. The Sokolow-Lyon criterion for RVH adds the R wave amplitude in lead V_1 to the S wave amplitude in lead V_5 or V_6; a sum of 1.05 mV or greater implies RVH.

Low QRS Voltage

Low QRS voltage is defined as limb lead voltage less than 5 mm (0.5 mV) in all leads or precordial voltage less than 10 mm (1 mV) in all leads. The differential diagnosis is broad (Table 54-4), and no underlying explanation is defined in many cases.

Repolarization Abnormalities

Abnormalities of the ST segment or T waves, or both, are extremely common (Table 54-5). Electrolyte and other metabolic abnormalities, drug effects (particularly digoxin and antiarrhythmic drugs), and secondary effects caused by LVH or bundle branch block are all commonly encountered. Early repolarization, a relatively common pattern of ST segment elevation previously thought to be benign, occurs more commonly in patients with

TABLE 54-4 CAUSES OF LOW QRS VOLTAGE
Normal variant
Pericardial effusion
Myocardial infarction
Cardiomyopathy
Hypothyroidism
Obesity
Sarcoidosis
Amyloidosis
Chronic obstructive pulmonary disease
Anasarca

idiopathic ventricular fibrillation than in controls and has also been associated with an increased risk of cardiac mortality.

Pitfalls of Automated Computerized Electrocardiographic Readings

Automatic interpretations of ECG tracings are generally quite accurate for calculating heart rates, axes, and intervals. Interpretation of the significance of repolarization abnormalities may be less accurate, and diagnosis of rhythms

TABLE 54-5 CAUSES OF REPOLARIZATION ABNORMALITIES

Athlete's heart
Early repolarization (normal variant)
Myocardial ischemia/injury
Pericarditis
Electrolyte abnormalities
Left ventricular hypertrophy
Intraventricular conduction delay/bundle branch block
Drug effects (digitalis, antiarrhythmic drugs, etc.)
Long QT syndrome
Stroke/neurologic catastrophe

is the striking weakness of these programs. Thus, over-reading of the computerized interpretation by the physician and comparison with previous tracings, when available, remain mandatory.

SUGGESTED READINGS

Cheng S, Keyes MJ, Larson MG, et al. Long-term outcomes in individuals with prolonged PR interval or first-degree atrioventricular block. *JAMA.* 2009;301:2571-2585. *Prolongation of the PR interval increases the risk of atrial fibrillation, need of a pacemaker, and overall mortality by 10 to 20%.*

Steinvil A, Chundadze T, Zeltser D, et al. Mandatory electrocardiographic screening of athletes to reduce their risk for sudden death: proven fact or wishful thinking? *J Am Coll Cardiol.* 2011;57:1291-1296. *Mandatory ECG does not change risk of sudden death.*

Tikkanen JT, Anttonen O, Junttila MJ, et al. Long-term outcome associated with early repolarization on electrocardiography. *N Engl J Med.* 2009;361:2529-2537. *In Finnish men and women with mean follow-up of 30 ± 11 years, an early repolarization pattern in the inferior leads was associated with a significantly increased risk of cardiac death.*

55

ECHOCARDIOGRAPHY

CATHERINE M. OTTO

Echocardiography is the clinical standard for evaluating cardiac function in patients with known or suspected heart disease. This chapter reviews the basic principles of echocardiography, echocardiographic approaches, quantitative measurements, and clinical indications. The specific use of echocardiography and additional images is shown in other chapters on individual types of cardiovascular diseases.

ECHOCARDIOGRAPHIC IMAGING

Principles

Echocardiography is based on the use of a piezoelectric crystal that converts electrical to mechanical energy, and vice versa, allowing both transmission and reception of an ultrasound signal. The frequency of ultrasound waves used for diagnostic imaging ranges from 2 to 10 MHz, with lower frequencies having greater tissue penetration and higher frequencies providing better image resolution. Each transducer consists of a complex array of piezoelectric crystals arranged to provide images in a fanlike two-dimensional image, with the narrow top of this sector scan indicating the origin of the ultrasound signal. Transducers also include an acoustic lens that determines the focal depth, height, and width of the ultrasound beam.

Images are generated based on the reflection of ultrasound from acoustic interfaces: for example, the boundary between the blood in the left ventricle and the myocardium. The time delay between transmission and reception is used to determine the depth of origin of the ultrasound reflection. The depths of the reflected signals from multiple ultrasound beams are combined to generate a two-dimensional image. The speed of signal analysis allows acquisition of two-dimensional ultrasound images at frame rates of 30 to 60 per second. Ultrasound is strongly attenuated by bone and air, so echocardiography relies on acoustic "windows" where, for example, ultrasound can penetrate to the heart while avoiding the ribs and lungs. With transthoracic imaging, the patient is positioned to bring the cardiac structures close to the chest wall, usually in a left lateral decubitus position, and the transducer is placed on the chest, using gel to provide acoustic coupling between the transducer and skin. Standard acoustic windows are parasternal, apical, subcostal, and suprasternal notch.

Standard Image Planes

From the parasternal window, the image plane is adjusted manually by an experienced physician or sonographer to provide long and short axis views. Standard cardiac imaging planes are aligned relative to the axis of the heart, with the long axis defined as the plane that intersects the cardiac apex and the middle of the aortic valve. Short axis views are perpendicular to this long axis, with standard image planes at the cardiac base (aortic valve level), mitral valve, and midventricular levels. From the apical window, the transducer is rotated to provide three views oriented 60 degrees from each other, producing a four-chamber, a two-chamber, and a long axis view (Fig. 55-1).

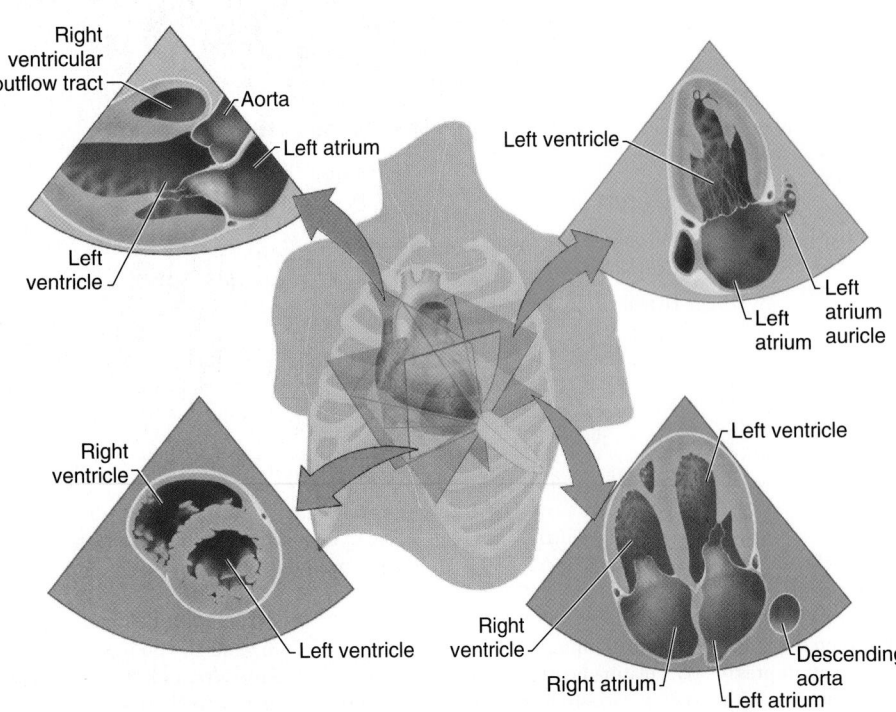

FIGURE 55-1. The four basic image planes used in transthoracic echocardiography. A parasternal transducer position or "window" is used to obtain long and short axis views. The long axis view *(purple outline)* extends from the left ventricular apex through the aortic valve plane. The short axis view is perpendicular to the long axis view, resulting in a circular view of the left ventricle *(red outline)*. The transducer is placed at the ventricular apex to obtain the two-chamber *(blue outline)* and four-chamber *(green outline)* views, each of which is about a 60-degree rotation from the long axis view and perpendicular to the short axis view. The four-chamber view includes both ventricles and both atria. The two-chamber view includes the left ventricle and left atrium; sometimes the atrial appendage is visualized. (From Otto CM. *Textbook of Clinical Echocardiography,* 4th ed. Philadelphia: Elsevier Saunders; 2009:32, Fig. 2-1.)

Measurements

Echocardiography provides accurate cardiac dimensions from two-dimensional or two-dimensional-guided linear depth (M-mode) recordings. The measurements typically provided include left ventricular (LV) end-diastolic and end-systolic internal dimensions, LV wall thickness, left atrial anterior-posterior diameter, and aortic sinus dimension. LV ejection fraction (EF) is determined by visual estimation or, more accurately, by tracing the endocardial borders at end diastole and end systole in two orthogonal views. End-diastolic and end-systolic ventricular volumes (EDV and ESV, respectively) are calculated using validated formulas, and the EF is determined as follows:

$$EF = (EDV - ESV)/EDV$$

Limitations

Echocardiography is a very accurate, widely available, and widely used imaging approach. However, the quality of images can be suboptimal because of poor tissue penetration (e.g., excessive adipose tissue, position of the lungs relative to the heart), although images are nondiagnostic in fewer than 5% of patients with current instrumentation. Reflections are stronger when the interface is perpendicular to the ultrasound beam, so structures that are parallel to the beam may not be visible, an artifact called *echo dropout*. This potential limitation may be avoided by the use of appropriate imaging planes and the integration of data from multiple transducer positions. Ultrasound artifacts, such as beam width, shadowing, and reverberations, may be misinterpreted by inexperienced observers.

⬤ DOPPLER ECHOCARDIOGRAPHY

Principles

Ultrasound energy that is backscattered from moving red blood cells is shifted to a higher frequency when the blood is moving toward the transducer and a lower frequency when it is moving away. The magnitude of this Doppler shift corresponds to the velocity of blood flow.

Modalities

Pulsed Doppler allows measurement of flow velocity at a specific intracardiac site with the advantages of high spatial and temporal resolution. However, spatial localization is based on intermittent sampling at a time interval corresponding to the depth of interest. The sampling frequency, which is depth dependent, limits the maximum detectable velocity because of a phenomenon called *signal aliasing*. Normal intracardiac flow velocities are about 1 m/second, which can usually be recorded with pulsed Doppler.

Continuous-wave Doppler allows measurement of high velocities along the entire length of the ultrasound beam, but the origin of the high-velocity signal must be inferred from the two-dimensional images. With stenotic and regurgitant valves, blood flow velocities may be as high as 5 to 6 m/second, requiring the use of the continuous-wave Doppler mode. Both pulsed and continuous-wave Doppler velocities are displayed as a graph of velocity versus time, with the density of the spectral display corresponding to signal strength.

Color flow Doppler imaging is a modification of pulsed Doppler in which the flow velocity is displayed across a two-dimensional image using a color scale to indicate direction and velocity. The advantage is a visually appealing display of intracardiac flow patterns. Disadvantages are low temporal resolution (frame rates of 10 to 30 per second) and poor velocity resolution due to signal aliasing.

Tissue Doppler uses the Doppler principle to record the velocity of motion of the myocardial wall. Tissue Doppler recordings of the myocardium adjacent to the mitral annulus are used to evaluate diastolic ventricular function.

Measurements

A standard echocardiographic study includes pulsed Doppler measurement of antegrade flow velocities (transmitral and transaortic) and evaluation for valve regurgitation using continuous-wave and color Doppler modalities. Other Doppler measurements depend on the specific clinical indication.

Quantitative measurements using Doppler data are derived from two basic concepts: volume flow rate and the pressure-velocity relationship. Stroke volume (in cubic centimeters) can be calculated as the volume of a cylinder, where the base is the spatial cross-sectional area (CSA, in square centimeters) of flow, determined as the area of a circle from a two-dimensional diameter measurement. The height of the cylinder is the distance the average blood cell travels in one cardiac cycle, which is the velocity time integral (VTI, in centimeters) of flow. Therefore,

$$SV\,(cm^3) = CSA\,(cm^2) \times VTI\,(cm)$$

This approach has been validated for measurement of transaortic, transmitral, and transpulmonic flow. Measurement of volume flow rate at two different intracardiac sites allows quantitation of intracardiac shunts and valvular regurgitation.

The relationship between the pressure gradient (ΔP) across a narrowing and the velocity (v) of blood flow is described by the simplified Bernoulli equation:

$$\Delta P = 4v^2$$

This equation allows calculation of maximum and mean gradients across stenotic valves, estimation of pulmonary systolic pressure, and detailed evaluation of intracardiac hemodynamics with regurgitant valves.

⬤ ECHOCARDIOGRAPHIC APPROACHES

Several echocardiographic modalities are in clinical use. If it is unclear which modality is optimum in a specific clinical setting, consultation with the echocardiographer is appropriate.

Transthoracic echocardiography (TTE) is the standard clinical approach in most patients with suspected or known cardiac disease. Advantages are that it is noninvasive, has no known adverse effects, and provides detailed data on cardiac anatomy and physiology. Limitations include poor image quality in some patients, limited visualization of structures distant from the transducer (e.g., atrial septum, left atrial appendage), and the inability to visualize structures immediately distal to prosthetic heart valves (acoustic shadowing).

Transesophageal echocardiography (TEE) offers superior image quality because of a shorter distance between the transducer and the heart, the absence of interposed bone or lung, and the use of a higher-frequency transducer. TEE usually is well tolerated, but intubation of the esophagus entails some risk, and most clinicians do this procedure with the patient under conscious sedation. TEE is much more sensitive than TTE for detection of left atrial thrombus (95% vs. 50%), valvular vegetations (99% vs. 60%), and prosthetic mitral valve regurgitation (Fig. 55-2).

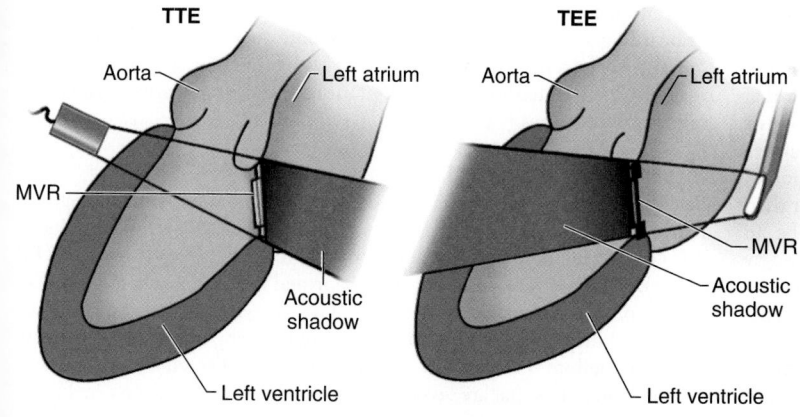

FIGURE 55-2. The problem of acoustic shadowing from a prosthetic mitral valve replacement (MVR). On the left, with transthoracic echocardiography (TTE), the acoustic shadow distal to the prosthetic valve obscures the left atrium, limiting assessment of valve regurgitation by Doppler techniques. On the right, with transesophageal echocardiography (TEE), the left atrium now can be evaluated for valvular regurgitation. However, the acoustic shadow now obscures the left ventricle. (From Otto CM. *Textbook of Clinical Echocardiography,* 4th ed. Philadelphia: Elsevier Saunders; 2009:117, Fig. 5-9.)

A   B

Handheld echocardiography refers to the use of smaller, less expensive ultrasound systems that can be carried by the physician, who can perform quick, limited examinations in the office or at the bedside. These laptop-sized echocardiography units range from the very simple, with only two-dimensional imaging and limited controls, to systems with high-quality imaging and all Doppler modalities. Handheld echocardiography does not replace a complete imaging study but can serve as an adjunct to the physical examination, particularly in the acute care setting, such as to distinguish ventricular dilation from a pericardial effusion or to estimate ventricular systolic performance.

Contrast echocardiography may be performed using intravenous injection of agitated saline to opacify the right-sided heart chambers. These microbubbles are relatively large and do not pass through pulmonary capillaries. Therefore, appearance of contrast in the left side of the heart within one or two beats after right heart opacification is consistent with an intracardiac shunt. Although most atrial-level shunts are predominantly left-to-right shunts, a small amount of right-to-left shunting occurs, which is the basis of this approach.

Contrast echocardiography also may be performed with commercially available microbubbles in the range of 1 to 5 µm. Because these microbubbles are smaller than the pulmonary capillaries, right heart opacification is followed by left heart opacification, which can enhance the evaluation of systolic function when image quality is suboptimal, especially during stress echocardiography (Fig. 55-3).

Three-dimensional echocardiography is increasingly available and is useful in some clinical settings, particularly for the evaluation of complex structural heart disease and for transcatheter interventions (Fig. 55-4).

Stress echocardiography is a standard approach for evaluating patients with known or suspected coronary artery disease; it has a sensitivity (85 to 95%) and a specificity (80 to 90%) similar to those of radionuclide stress imaging (Chapters 56 and 71). Myocardial infarction results in thinning and akinesis of the affected wall. However, in the absence of infarction, resting myocardial function is normal, even when severe epicardial coronary disease is present. The increased myocardial demand associated with exercise or pharmacologic stress leads to myocardial ischemia, which results in a regional wall motion abnormality, often before the onset of chest pain or electrocardiographic changes (Fig. 55-5).

In patients who can exercise, standard views of the left ventricle are recorded at baseline and immediately after maximal treadmill or bicycle exercise. If endocardial definition is suboptimal, left-sided contrast is used. The rest and exercise images are compared in a side-by-side cine loop format. Myocardial ischemia is present if resting wall motion is normal but hypokinesis or akinesis is seen after exercise. The pattern of regional wall motion accurately identifies the area of myocardium at risk and is reasonably reliable for identification of the affected coronary artery. With three-vessel coronary disease, rather than a regional wall motion abnormality, the only clue on imaging may be an absence of the expected decrease in chamber size at peak exercise, caused by diffuse ischemia. Interpretation of an exercise echocardiogram includes exercise duration, hemodynamic response, symptoms, and electrocardiographic changes, in addition to the echocardiographic images (see Fig. 55-5).

In patients who are unable to exercise, stress testing is performed using a graded intravenous infusion of dobutamine, beginning at 5 to 10 µg/kg/

minute and increasing every 3 minutes to a maximum dose of 40 µg/kg/minute. If needed, atropine is used to achieve 85% of the maximum predicted heart rate. In addition to evaluation for myocardial ischemia, dobutamine stress echocardiography can assess myocardial viability in areas of stunning or hibernation, based on an improvement in endocardial motion from baseline to low-dose dobutamine, with subsequent worsening of function at higher doses—the "biphasic" response.

Intracardiac echocardiography (ICE) is performed using an ultrasound probe on a catheter that is inserted into the right side of the heart through the femoral vein. ICE is used in the cardiac catheterization laboratory to guide percutaneous closure of a patent foramen ovale (PFO) and other procedures. In the electrophysiology laboratory, ICE helps guide catheter positioning and identify complications.

● CARDIAC FUNCTION MEASUREMENTS

In addition to qualitative descriptions of cardiac anatomy and physiology, echocardiography provides precise and accurate quantitation of cardiac function, including ventricular systolic and diastolic function, an estimate of the severity of valve stenosis and regurgitation, and a noninvasive estimate of pulmonary pressures.

Systolic Ventricular Function

Overall LV systolic function is graded by visual estimation, with an approximate correspondence to EF as follows: normal (EF > 55%), mildly reduced (EF, 40 to 55%), moderately reduced (EF, 20 to 40%), severely reduced (EF < 20%). More precise quantitation is performed when clinically indicated by calculation of a biplane ejection fraction. Cardiac output calculations are not routine but may be helpful for noninvasive monitoring of therapy in patients with heart failure. Because EF measurements are affected by preload and afterload, measures that are less dependent on loading conditions, including

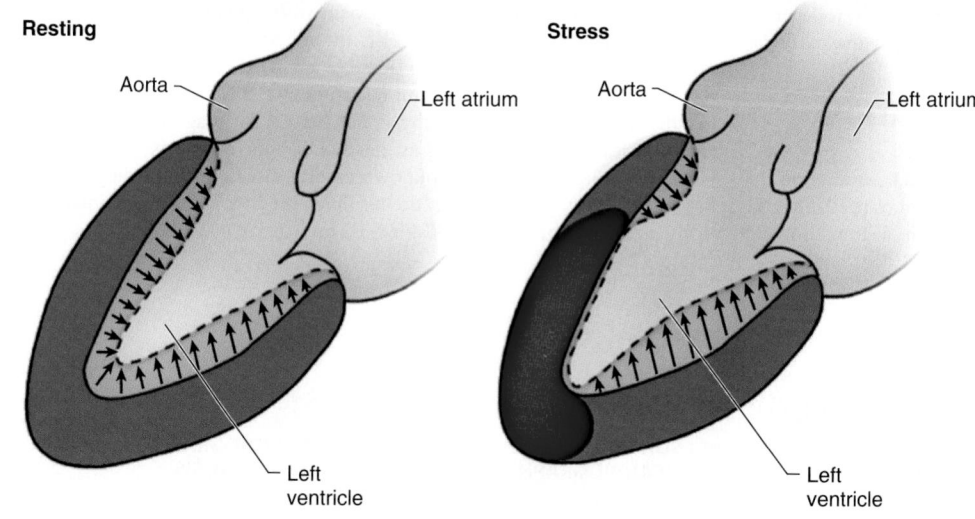

Resting

Aorta — — Left atrium

— Left ventricle

Stress

Aorta — — Left atrium

— Left ventricle

FIGURE 55-5. The concept of stress echocardiography in a patient with 70% stenosis in the proximal third of the left anterior descending (LAD) coronary artery. At rest *(left)*, endocardial motion and wall thickening are normal. After stress *(right)*, either exercise or pharmacologic, the middle and apical segments of the anterior wall become ischemic, showing reduced endocardial wall motion and wall thickening. If the LAD extends around the apex, the apical segment of the posterior wall also will be affected, as shown here. The normal segment of the posterior wall shows compensatory hyperkinesis. (From Otto CM. *Textbook of Clinical Echocardiography,* 4th ed. Philadelphia: Elsevier Saunders; 2009:191, Fig. 8-9.)

the end-systolic dimension or volume, are generally preferred for clinical decision making in situations such as the timing of surgery for chronic valvular regurgitation.

Diastolic Ventricular Function

Evaluation of diastolic ventricular function is challenging because the patterns of ventricular filling are affected by preload, heart rate, and coexisting valvular regurgitation in addition to the diastolic properties of the ventricle. However, echocardiography can classify diastolic function based on the combination of LV inflow, pulmonary vein flow, tissue Doppler velocities, and the isovolumic relaxation time. An estimate of LV filling pressure (e.g., LV end-diastolic pressure) also can be inferred using these approaches.

Valvular Stenosis

Echocardiography is the clinical standard for evaluation of aortic valvular heart disease (see Fig. 75-1). Cardiac catheterization can be reserved for cases in which echocardiography is nondiagnostic, clinical data are discrepant with echocardiographic findings, or coronary anatomy needs to be assessed (Chapter 75).

In patients with aortic stenosis, the most direct measure of stenosis severity is the antegrade velocity across the valve, indicating mild (<3 m/second), moderate (3 to 4 m/second), or severe (>4 m/second) valve obstruction. The maximum and mean transaortic pressure gradients also can be calculated using the Bernoulli equation. Accurate evaluation depends on a careful examination by an experienced echocardiographer.

Aortic valve area (AVA) is calculated using the continuity equation, based on the concept that volume flow rates proximal to and within the narrowed orifice are equal:

$$\text{AVA} \times \text{VTI}_{AS} = \text{CSA}_{LVOT} \times \text{VTI}_{LVOT}$$

or

$$\text{AVA} = (\text{CSA}_{LVOT} \times \text{VTI}_{LVOT})/\text{VTI}_{AS}$$

where LVOT = left ventricular outflow tract, VTI = velocity time integral, CSA = cross-sectional area, and AS = aortic stenosis (Fig. 55-6). It is especially important to calculate the AVA when LV systolic dysfunction accompanies aortic valve disease. In some patients, dobutamine stress echocardiography is helpful in distinguishing ventricular dysfunction caused by severe aortic stenosis from primary myocardial disease with concurrent moderate stenosis.

The evaluation of mitral stenosis (see Fig. 75-3) includes measurement of the mean transmitral gradient from the velocity curve and calculation of the valve area, both from two-dimensional planimetry of a short-axis image of the orifice and from the deceleration slope of the Doppler curve (pressure half-time method).

Valvular Regurgitation

The current approach to evaluating valvular regurgitation is based on the proximal geometry of the regurgitant jet, with measurement of the narrowest jet width (vena contracta; see Fig. 75-5). When further quantitation is

CW:2MHz APX AV

m/s

←V$_{max}$

$\Delta P = 4v^2$

8.0

FIGURE 55-6. In a patient with aortic stenosis, the aortic jet velocity is recorded with continuous wave Doppler from the window that yields the highest velocity signal. Maximum velocity (V$_{max}$) is used to calculate the maximum systolic gradient. The Doppler curve is traced, as shown, to calculate the mean systolic gradient, using the Bernoulli equation, by which the pressure gradient (ΔP) equals four times the square of the velocity.

needed, regurgitant volume (RV), regurgitant fraction (RF), and regurgitant orifice area (ROA) are calculated. Although color flow visualization of the flow disturbance may be helpful for detection of regurgitation and for understanding the mechanism of valve dysfunction, this approach should no longer be used to evaluate severity.

For aortic regurgitation, a narrow vena contracta (<3 mm) indicates mild regurgitation, whereas a wide vena contracta (>6 mm) indicates severe regurgitation. Additional evaluation of the severity of aortic regurgitation is based on the presence of holodiastolic flow reversal in the abdominal aorta and the density and slope of the continuous wave Doppler velocity curve. The approach to evaluating mitral regurgitation (see Fig. 75-5) is similar, beginning with measurement of the vena contracta. In addition to calculation based on transmitral versus transaortic volume flow rates, the proximal acceleration of flow into the regurgitant orifice allows evaluation with central regurgitant jets. Color flow shows a proximal isovelocity surface area (PISA).

Pulmonary Pressures

Estimation of pulmonary artery systolic pressure (PAP) is a standard component of a complete examination. The systolic pressure difference between the right ventricle and right atrium is calculated from the peak velocity in the tricuspid regurgitant (V$_{TR}$) jet, using the Bernoulli equation. Then, the right atrial pressure (RAP) is estimated from the size and appearance of the inferior vena cava. Because right ventricular and pulmonary artery systolic pressures are equal (in the absence of pulmonic stenosis),

$$\text{PAP} = 4(\text{V}_{TR})^2 + \text{RAP}$$

A small amount of tricuspid regurgitation is present in most patients, so pulmonary pressures can be estimated with this approach in more than 90%

of patients. Because this approach measures only pulmonary systolic pressure, not pulmonary vascular resistance, invasive evaluation may still be needed in some clinical situations (Chapter 68).

THE ECHOCARDIOGRAPHIC EXAMINATION

Clinical Indications

Echocardiography is an effective approach to the initial evaluation of many cardiac signs and symptoms (Table 55-1). Even when transesophageal imaging might be helpful, most clinicians begin with a transthoracic examination; exceptions are for the patient with a possible acute aortic dissection (Chapter 78), in whom TEE should be performed as quickly as possible, and in the evaluation of possible left atrial thrombosis before cardioversion without anticoagulation (Chapter 64). It is important to remember that resting echocardiography is not helpful for diagnosis of coronary artery disease; stress imaging is needed if this diagnosis is suspected (Chapter 71). In patients with known cardiac disease, echocardiography is used to evaluate severity, assess the results of medical and surgical interventions, and guide procedures (Table 55-2).

TABLE 55-1 COMMON SYMPTOMS AND SIGNS EVALUATED BY ECHOCARDIOGRAPHY

REASON FOR ECHOCARDIOGRAPHY	POSSIBLE ECHOCARDIOGRAPHIC FINDINGS OR DIAGNOSIS	REASON FOR ECHOCARDIOGRAPHY	POSSIBLE ECHOCARDIOGRAPHIC FINDINGS OR DIAGNOSIS

Chest pain	Coronary artery disease
	  Acute myocardial infarction on resting echocardiography
	  Stress echocardiography needed to detect coronary disease
	Aortic dissection
	Pericarditis
	Valvular aortic stenosis
	Hypertrophic cardiomyopathy
		Cardiac murmur
		  Systolic
		
		  Diastolic
			Flow murmur (no valve abnormality)
			Aortic stenosis—valvular or subaortic
			Hypertrophic cardiomyopathy
			Mitral regurgitation
			Ventricular septal defect
			Pulmonic stenosis
			Tricuspid regurgitation
			Mitral stenosis
			Aortic regurgitation
			Pulmonic regurgitation
			Tricuspid stenosis

Heart failure	Left ventricular systolic dysfunction (global or segmental) Valvular heart disease Left ventricular diastolic dysfunction Pericardial disease Right ventricular dysfunction	Cardiomegaly on chest radiography	Pericardial effusion Dilated cardiomyopathy Specific chamber enlargement (e.g., left ventricle in chronic aortic regurgitation)
Palpitations	Left ventricular systolic dysfunction Mitral valve disease Congenital heart disease (e.g., ASD, Ebstein's anomaly) Pericarditis No structural cardiac disease	Systemic embolic event	Left ventricular systolic function and segmental wall motion abnormalities (aneurysms) Left ventricular thrombus Aortic valve disease Mitral valve disease Left atrial thrombus (TTE has low sensitivity, TEE required) Atrial septal defect or patent foramen ovale

ASD = atrial septal defect; TEE = transesophageal echocardiography; TTE = transthoracic echocardiography.
From Otto CM. *Textbook of Clinical Echocardiography,* 4th ed. Philadelphia: Elsevier Saunders; 2009:114-115, Tables 5-1 and 5-2.

TABLE 55-2 INDICATIONS FOR ECHOCARDIOGRAPHY BY KNOWN DIAGNOSIS

CLINICAL DIAGNOSIS	KEY ECHOCARDIOGRAPHIC FINDINGS	LIMITATIONS OF ECHOCARDIOGRAPHY	ALTERNATIVE APPROACHES
VALVULAR HEART DISEASE (CHAPTER 75)			
Valve stenosis	Etiology of stenosis, valve anatomy Transvalvular ΔP, valve area Chamber enlargement and hypertrophy LV and RV systolic function Associated valvular regurgitation	Possible underestimation of the severity of stenosis Possible coexisting coronary artery disease	Cardiac catheterization; MRI
Valve regurgitation	Mechanism and etiology of regurgitation Severity of regurgitation Chamber enlargement LV and RV systolic function PA pressure estimate	TEE may be needed to evaluate mitral regurgitant severity and valve anatomy (especially before MV repair)	Cardiac catheterization; MRI
Prosthetic valve function	Evidence for stenosis Detection of regurgitation Chamber enlargement Ventricular function PA pressure estimate	Imaging of prosthetic valves is limited by shadowing and reverberations TEE is needed for suspected prosthetic MR due to "masking" of the LA on TTE	Cardiac catheterization
Endocarditis (Chapter 76)	Detection of vegetations (TTE sensitivity 70-85%) Presence and degree of valve dysfunction Chamber enlargement and function Detection of abscess Possible prognostic implications	TEE more sensitive for detection of vegetations (>90%) A definite diagnosis of endocarditis also depends on bacteriologic criteria TEE more sensitive for detecting an abscess	Blood cultures and clinical findings also are diagnostic criteria for endocarditis

TABLE 55-2 INDICATIONS FOR ECHOCARDIOGRAPHY BY KNOWN DIAGNOSIS—cont'd

CLINICAL DIAGNOSIS	KEY ECHOCARDIOGRAPHIC FINDINGS	LIMITATIONS OF ECHOCARDIOGRAPHY	ALTERNATIVE APPROACHES
CORONARY ARTERY DISEASE			
Acute myocardial infarction (Chapters 72 and 73)	Segmental wall motion abnormality reflects "myocardium at risk" Global LV function (EF) Complications: Acute MR vs. VSD Pericarditis LV thrombus, aneurysm RV infarct	Coronary artery anatomy itself is not directly visualized	Coronary angiography Radionuclide LV angiography Cardiac catheterization
Angina (Chapter 71)	Global and segmental LV systolic function Exclude other causes of angina (e.g., AS, HOCM)	Resting wall motion may be normal despite significant CAD Stress echocardiography is needed to induce ischemia and wall motion abnormality	Coronary angiography Stress thallium ETT
Pre-revascularization/ post-revascularization	Assess wall thickening and endocardial motion at baseline Improvement in segmental function after procedure	Dobutamine stress and/or contrast echocardiography is needed to detect viable but nonfunctioning myocardium	MRI PET Thallium ETT Contrast echocardiography
End-stage ischemic disease	Overall LV systolic function (EF) PA pressures Associated MR LV thrombus RV systolic function	—	Coronary angiography Radionuclide EF
CARDIOMYOPATHY (CHAPTERS 58-60)			
Dilated	Chamber dilation (all four) LV and RV systolic function (qualitative and EF) Coexisting atrioventricular valve regurgitation PA systolic pressure LV thrombus	Indirect measures of LVEDP Accurate EF may be difficult if image quality is poor	Radionuclide EF LV and RV angiography
Restrictive	LV wall thickness LV systolic function LV diastolic function PA systolic pressure	Must be distinguished from constrictive pericarditis	Cardiac catheterization with direct, simultaneous RV and LV pressure measurement after volume loading
Hypertrophic	Pattern and extent of LV hypertrophy Dynamic LVOT obstruction (imaging and Doppler) Coexisting MR Diastolic LV dysfunction	—	—
Hypertension (Chapter 67)	LV wall thickness and chamber dimensions LV mass LV systolic function Aortic root dilation	—	—
PERICARDIAL DISEASE (CHAPTER 77)			
	Pericardial thickening Detection, size, and location of PE 2D signs of tamponade physiology Doppler signs of tamponade physiology	Diagnosis of tamponade is a hemodynamic and clinical diagnosis Constrictive pericarditis is a difficult diagnosis Not all patients with pericarditis have an effusion	Intracardiac pressure measurements for tamponade or constriction MRI or CT to detect pericardial thickening
DISEASES OF THE AORTA (CHAPTER 78)			
Aortic root dilation	Etiology of aortic dilation Accurate aortic root diameter measurements Anatomy of sinuses of Valsalva (especially Marfan syndrome) Associated aortic regurgitation	—	CT, MRI, aortography
Aortic dissection	2D images of ascending aorta, aortic arch, descending thoracic and proximal abdominal aorta Imaging of dissection "flap" Associated aortic regurgitation Ventricular function	TEE more sensitive (97%) and more specific (100%) Cannot assess distal vascular beds	Aortography CT MRI TEE
CARDIAC MASSES (CHAPTER 60)			
LV thrombus	High sensitivity and specificity for diagnosis of LV thrombus Suspect with apical wall motion abnormality or diffuse LV systolic dysfunction	Technical artifacts can be misleading 5-MHz or higher frequency transducer and angulated apical views needed TEE is needed to detect LA thrombus reliably	LV thrombus may not be recognized on radionuclide or contrast angiography
LA thrombus	Low sensitivity for detection of LA thrombus, although specificity is high Suspect with LA enlargement, MV disease	—	TEE

TABLE 55-2 INDICATIONS FOR ECHOCARDIOGRAPHY BY KNOWN DIAGNOSIS—cont'd

CLINICAL DIAGNOSIS	KEY ECHOCARDIOGRAPHIC FINDINGS	LIMITATIONS OF ECHOCARDIOGRAPHY	ALTERNATIVE APPROACHES
Cardiac tumors	Size, location, and physiologic consequences of tumor mass	Extracardiac involvement is not well seen Cannot distinguish benign from malignant tumor or tumor from thrombus	TEE CT MRI (with cardiac gating) Intracardiac echocardiography
PULMONARY HYPERTENSION (CHAPTER 68)			
	Estimate of PA pressure Evidence of left-sided heart disease to account for increased PA pressures RV size and systolic function (cor pulmonale) Associated TR	Indirect PA pressure measurement Cannot determine pulmonary vascular resistance accurately	Cardiac catheterization
CONGENITAL HEART DISEASE (CHAPTER 69)			
	Detection and assessment of anatomic abnormalities Quantitation of physiologic abnormalities Chamber enlargement Ventricular function	No direct intracardiac pressure measurements Complicated anatomy may be difficult to evaluate if image quality is poor (TEE is helpful)	MRI with 3D reconstruction Cardiac catheterization TEE

2D = two-dimensional; 3D = three-dimensional; AS = aortic stenosis; CAD = coronary artery disease; CT = computed tomography; EF = ejection fraction; ETT = exercise treadmill test; HCM = hypertrophic cardiomyopathy; LA = left atrial; LV = left ventricular; LVEDP = left ventricular end-diastolic pressure; LVOT = left ventricular outflow tract; MR = mitral regurgitation; MRI = magnetic resonance imaging; MV = mitral valve; ΔP = pressure gradient; PA = pulmonary artery; PE = pericardial effusion; PET = positron emission tomography; RV = right ventricular; TEE = transesophageal echocardiography; TR = tricuspid regurgitation; TTE = transthoracic echocardiography; VSD = ventricular septal defect.
From Otto CM. *Textbook of Clinical Echocardiography*, 4th ed. Philadelphia: Elsevier Saunders; 2009:475-478.

Normal Findings

Trace to mild regurgitation is considered "physiologic" and is seen with 70 to 80% of mitral valves, 80 to 90% of tricuspid valves, and 70 to 80% of pulmonic valves in normal individuals. The prevalence of aortic regurgitation increases with age, but it is found in only 5% of young normal adults; the presence of aortic regurgitation raises the possibility of subtle aortic valve or root abnormalities.

A PFO (Chapter 69) is present in 25 to 35% of normal individuals and may be identified by color Doppler or by contrast echocardiography. Use of the Valsalva maneuver enhances identification of a PFO because the slight elevation in right atrial pressure may lead to a brief right-to-left shunt. The significance of a PFO in patients without clinical events is unclear. Other common anatomic variants seen on echocardiography include aberrant chords (or "webs") in the left ventricle; small, linear, mobile echoes associated with the valves (Lambl's excrescences); and normal ridges in the left and right atrium.

Unexpected abnormal findings also may be found on studies requested for other indications. A bicuspid aortic valve is present in 1 to 2% of the population; most of these patients are asymptomatic until late in life, so many cases are diagnosed "incidentally" by echocardiography. Aortic valve sclerosis, which is a frequent unexpected echocardiographic diagnosis, is a marker of cardiovascular disease and an increased risk of myocardial infarction even if valve function is normal.

INTEGRATING THE ECHOCARDIOGRAPHIC AND CLINICAL FINDINGS

The echocardiographic request should indicate the specific reason for the study and any relevant symptoms or signs. The echocardiographic examination then can be tailored to answer the clinical question. The echocardiographic results should be interpreted in conjunction with other clinical data. If the echocardiographic data seem discrepant with the clinical data, the requesting physician should review the images with the echocardiographer to identify areas of uncertainty and to determine the next best diagnostic step.

SUGGESTED READINGS

Melamed R, Sprenkle MD, Ulstad VK, et al. Assessment of left ventricular function by intensivists using hand-held echocardiography. *Chest.* 2009;135:1416-1420. *A small bedside diagnostic ultrasound imaging system can allow intensivists, after a short training period, to estimate left ventricular systolic function.*

Mitiku TY, Heidenreich PA. A small pericardial effusion is a marker of increased mortality. *Am Heart J.* 2011;161:152-157. *Even a small asymptomatic pericardial effusion is associated with a 17% increased mortality after adjustment for other clinical factors.*

Pepi M, Evangelista A, Nihoyannopoulos P, et al. Recommendations for echocardiography use in the diagnosis and management of cardiac sources of embolism: European Association of Echocardiography (EAE) (a registered branch of the ESC). *Eur J Echocardiogr.* 2010;11:461-476. *Consensus guidelines.*

56

NONINVASIVE CARDIAC IMAGING

CHRISTOPHER M. KRAMER AND GEORGE A. BELLER

NUCLEAR CARDIOLOGY

The techniques of nuclear cardiology permit the noninvasive imaging of myocardial perfusion under stress and resting conditions and of resting regional and global function by use of radionuclide imaging agents and gamma or positron cameras with associated computer processing. All these techniques are based on acquiring images of radioactivity emanating from tracers localized in heart muscle or in the blood pools of the left and right ventricles. Myocardial perfusion imaging is the most commonly performed nuclear cardiology technique, most often in conjunction with either exercise or pharmacologic stress intended to produce flow heterogeneity between relatively hypoperfused and normally perfused myocardial regions. Radionuclide angiography, in which technetium-99m (^{99m}Tc)-labeled red blood cells or other ^{99m}Tc-labeled agents are injected intravenously, is used for measurement of left ventricular ejection fraction and assessment of regional wall motion, especially to monitor changes in global left ventricular function in patients undergoing chemotherapy with cardiac toxic drugs. Positron emission tomography (PET) can assess regional myocardial metabolism to estimate myocardial viability, most often with fluorine-18–labeled 2-deoxyglucose (FDG), as well as myocardial perfusion by use of rubidium-82 (^{82}Rb). Hybrid cameras with computed tomography (CT) permit multimodality imaging of coronary anatomy and physiologic perturbations in flow or myocardial function.

Myocardial Perfusion Imaging
Imaging Agents

For the assessment of myocardial perfusion, ^{99m}Tc-labeled perfusion agents, which provide higher-quality images more quickly, are used more commonly than thallium-201 (^{201}Tl) for exercise or pharmacologic stress perfusion imaging to evaluate patients with suspected or known coronary heart disease (CHD). Of the various ^{99m}Tc-labeled agents, ^{99m}Tc-sestamibi and ^{99m}Tc-tetrofosmin are the most common. These ^{99m}Tc agents permit simultaneous assessment of regional and global left ventricular function and volumes with gated single-photon emission computed tomography (SPECT) technology.

Some laboratories use dual-isotope rest ^{201}Tl/stress ^{99m}Tc-sestamibi imaging, in which patients undergo ^{201}Tl imaging at rest and then, immediately

FIGURE 56-1. Short-axis images showing a moderately large, reversible defect of the apex, anterior wall, and septum. This defect is consistent with disease of the proximal left anterior descending coronary artery.

afterward, undergo ^{99m}Tc-sestamibi imaging during stress. Reversibility is identified by comparing the perfusion pattern on the stress ^{99m}Tc-sestamibi images with the pattern on the baseline resting ^{201}Tl images. The major advantage of this technique is the marked decrease in total imaging time, but the disadvantage is a substantially higher radiation dose. In patients with a low to intermediate pretest probability of CHD, a normal stress myocardial perfusion study obviates the need for a resting study, reducing both cost and radiation.

Detection of Coronary Heart Disease

The major indications for stress and rest myocardial perfusion imaging are to diagnose CHD, to assess prognosis, and to detect myocardial viability. Exercise or pharmacologic stress myocardial perfusion imaging in patients with chest pain yields a sensitivity for detecting CHD in the 85 to 90% range (Fig. 56-1). The specificity for excluding CHD is in the 85% range for ^{99m}Tc-sestamibi SPECT imaging and increases to 90% with gated SPECT. Exercise or pharmacologic stress SPECT perfusion imaging have sensitivities and specificities that are superior to those of exercise electrocardiogram (ECG) testing alone. The specificity of gated SPECT for detecting CHD with use of one of the ^{99m}Tc-labeled perfusion agents is 20 to 30% higher than that of ^{201}Tl SPECT in women.

Radionuclide stress perfusion imaging is of particular value compared with exercise ECG testing alone in (1) patients with resting ECG abnormalities, such as those seen with left ventricular hypertrophy, digitalis effect, Wolff-Parkinson-White syndrome, and intraventricular conduction abnormalities; and (2) patients who fail to achieve more than 85% of maximal predicted heart rate. Approximately 40% of patients with a low to intermediate pretest likelihood of CHD who manifest 1.0 mm or more of horizontal or downsloping ST segment depression have no evidence of CHD (false-positive findings). The addition of stress perfusion imaging can assist in differentiating true-positive from false-positive ST depression. Detection of proximal left anterior descending stenoses and proximal multivessel CHD is enhanced by identifying regional systolic thickening or wall motion abnormalities on the gated SPECT images compared with assessment based on perfusion alone. If possible, drugs such as long-acting nitrates, β-blockers, and rate-lowering calcium blockers should be discontinued for 24 hours before exercise stress testing that is performed to diagnose or to exclude CHD as the cause of chest pain.

Pharmacologic Stress Imaging

In patients who are unable to exercise to adequate heart rates and workloads on exercise stress testing protocols, pharmacologic stress testing with use of vasodilators (e.g., dipyridamole), adenosine, regadenoson, or inotropic agents (e.g., dobutamine) is an alternative to exercise for detecting physiologically significant coronary artery stenoses. Sensitivity and specificity for CHD detection are comparable for dipyridamole and adenosine. The addition of limited exercise to dipyridamole or adenosine imaging can prevent the vasodilator-induced hypotension, improve the ECG detection of ischemia, and enhance image quality by increasing the heart-to-liver ratio of tracer uptake. Dobutamine stress is preferred in patients who have bronchospasm or a history of asthma or who have consumed caffeine, which is an adenosine receptor antagonist, within 12 hours before testing. Patients who experience side effects such as hypotension and chest pain during dipyridamole or adenosine infusion should be treated with intravenous aminophylline, an adenosine antagonist that immediately reverses these side effects. Regadenoson has fewer side effects than adenosine. PET myocardial perfusion imaging, which is performed only with vasodilator stress, has a higher specificity and better ability to detect multivessel disease than SPECT.

Assessment of Prognosis

The extent of hypoperfusion on post-stress SPECT perfusion images provides important incremental prognostic information when added to clinical characteristics, the resting left ventricular ejection fraction, exercise ECG stress test variables, and even coronary artery anatomy. Nondiabetic patients with chest pain and a normal myocardial perfusion scan at peak exercise or under vasodilator stress have a subsequent cardiac death or infarction rate of less than 1% per year and are generally appropriate candidates for medical therapy (Chapter 71) or require further diagnostic evaluation for a noncardiac cause of chest pain (Chapters 50 and 139). Conversely, patients with high-risk imaging results may benefit from early referral for invasive strategies, including coronary revascularization (Chapter 74), even if symptoms are mild. Patients who show inducible ischemia involving more than 20% of the left ventricular myocardium may have a better outcome with coronary revascularization compared with medical therapy.

Transient ischemic left ventricular cavity dilation, by which the left ventricular cavity appears more dilated on stress images compared with rest images, is a particularly high-risk finding on SPECT. This finding occurs when subendocardial ischemia after stress causes a decrease in tracer uptake in the subendocardium, thereby yielding what appears to be a larger left ventricular cavity than was observed on the resting images.

Patients with abnormal pharmacologic stress studies have a worse prognosis than patients with comparable defect patterns seen on exercise scans, perhaps because their inability to exercise is also a prognostic factor. Assessment of regional left ventricular function on post-stress gated SPECT images enhances the detection of three-vessel CHD. Exercise or pharmacologic stress perfusion imaging also provides useful prognostic information for pre-discharge risk stratification in clinically low- to intermediate-risk patients who have experienced an uncomplicated myocardial infarction or unstable angina. Demonstration of defects remote from the zone of infarction (which indicate underlying multivessel disease), evidence for residual ischemia within the infarct zone, or both identify patients with an increased risk of reinfarction and subsequent cardiac death.

Exercise or pharmacologic stress perfusion imaging is superior to exercise ECG testing alone for detection of coronary restenosis in patients presenting with recurrence of symptoms after a percutaneous coronary intervention (Chapter 74). Stress perfusion imaging also has proved useful for identifying high-risk asymptomatic patients who have undergone previous coronary artery bypass graft surgery (Chapter 74) and patients who have intermediate or nonevaluable stenoses on coronary angiography.

Determination of Myocardial Viability with Single-Photon Emission Computed Tomography or Positron Emission Tomography

SPECT perfusion imaging is performed in the resting state to identify residual myocardial viability in zones corresponding to severe regional wall motion abnormalities in patients with CHD and depressed left ventricular function. When severe left ventricular dysfunction is caused by "hibernation" (a state of chronic reduced contractility because of substantial ischemia), and not by irreversible myocardial necrosis, areas of resting hypoperfusion that are viable and contributing to hibernation show initial defects on early images but no or less severe defects on 3-hour delayed images. If uptake ultimately exceeds 50 or 60% of peak uptake in these regions, there is a high probability (65 to 75%) that regional myocardial function will improve after successful revascularization, compared with only a 10 to 20% probability for myocardial zones showing less than 50% of peak uptake on resting images.

Regional myocardial metabolism can be assessed noninvasively by PET with FDG and a flow tracer such as [^{13}N]ammonia or ^{82}Rb. FDG is a glucose analogue that is taken up initially in myocardial cells and is trapped by conversion to FDG-6-phosphate. FDG is cell membrane impermeable and remains within viable cells at high concentrations for more than 40 to 60 minutes. Increased FDG activity on clinical PET images in areas of diminished regional blood flow, as determined by [¹³N]ammonia imaging, is characteristic of myocardial viability. These areas of blood flow/FDG mismatch usually show improved regional function after coronary revascularization. Regions of the heart that show both diminished perfusion and FDG uptake (a "match" pattern) represent predominantly nonviable myocardium, with only a 10 to 15% probability of showing improved systolic function after revascularization. Patients who have an ischemic cardiomyopathy with poor viability on either resting SPECT or PET have a worse outcome after coronary revascularization compared with patients with predominantly viable myocardium.

Imaging of Ventricular Function

Global and segmental left and right ventricular function can be evaluated accurately by gated cardiac blood pool imaging to provide a radionuclide angiogram or ventriculogram. The equilibrium radionuclide angiographic approach is performed after thorough mixing of ⁹⁹ᵐTc-labeled blood cells within the intravascular compartment. Because ⁹⁹ᵐTc remains within the blood pool, serial imaging studies can be acquired during several hours. Acquisition of the images is synchronized with the QRS complex on the ECG through a multigated approach by which each cardiac cycle is divided into multiple frames. A uniform diminution of left ventricular systolic function without segmental wall motion abnormalities suggests nonischemic dilated cardiomyopathy (Chapter 60), whereas depressed global left ventricular function associated with segmental wall motion abnormalities suggests ischemic heart disease.

● CARDIAC COMPUTED TOMOGRAPHY

For CT, imaging with high spatial and temporal resolution and ECG gating during a breath-hold yields snapshots of the heart reconstructed from the same phase of the cardiac cycle. Multidetector computed tomography (MDCT), which has almost entirely replaced electron beam CT, can capture a three-dimensional image of the heart in one to two heartbeats on the latest generation scanners as well as provide coronary artery calcium scoring without the use of contrast and with only 1 to 3 millisievert (mSv) of radiation. MDCT coronary arteriography requires 60 to 100 mL of iodinated contrast and average radiation doses less than 5 mSv. However, without careful planning of the imaging approach, radiation doses on the order of 10 to 25 mSv have been reported on 64-detector scanners. β-Blockade is often used to achieve a heart rate of less than 60 beats per minute to optimize imaging, and irregular rhythms such as atrial fibrillation may diminish image quality.

Coronary Artery Calcium Scoring

Coronary calcium is an indicator of the burden of atherosclerotic plaque, and very high levels confer an increased risk of future cardiac events (Fig. 56-2). Calcium scores are generally calculated as an Agatston score, which corresponds to each coronary lesion's calcium area multiplied by the maximal CT attenuation value of that lesion, and then summed for the entire coronary tree. Calcium scores are age, gender, and race dependent and must be normalized by these factors. In a large prospective, population-based study, the

coronary calcium score predicted coronary events independently of either standard risk factors or C-reactive protein and was a better predictor than the Framingham risk score. Calcium scores above 300 were associated with an increased risk of myocardial infarction and cardiac death at every risk level. The utility of calcium scoring is highest in intermediate-risk patients on the basis of Framingham risk data, and there is no evidence that a calcium score in otherwise low- or high-risk groups would change risk factor management. Importantly, there is no correlation between coronary calcium and the physiologic or anatomic significance of a stenosis. Consensus guidelines suggest that stress testing may be indicated in patients with high calcium scores (>300 to 400).

Computed Tomographic Coronary Angiography

MDCT is an excellent technique to diagnose anomalous coronary arterial anatomy in adults (Fig. 56-3). For detection of coronary artery disease, 64-detector scanners have consistently demonstrated sensitivities on a per-segment basis in the 95% range, specificities of 85 to 98%, positive-predictive values of 64 to 91%, and negative-predictive values of 99%. Thus, the technique appears to be an excellent way to exclude significant coronary artery disease (Fig. 56-4). Initial studies with 256- and 320-detector row scanners are even more promising. A limitation of the technique, however, is its lower specificity in heavily calcified vessels, which are more common in elderly patients. MDCT tends to overestimate the percentage of stenosis when compared with intravascular ultrasound. The accuracy for detecting stenoses in bypass grafts is quite high, although evaluation of native vessel coronary artery disease is limited in postbypass patients owing to extensive calcification and smaller size vessels. Stents less than 3 mm in diameter cannot be

FIGURE 56-3. Contrast-enhanced computed tomographic angiogram in a young patient with chest pain and an anomalous right coronary artery (RCA). The RCA originates with a slit-like origin from the left coronary cusp (arrow) and passes anteriorly between the aorta and right ventricular outflow tract. The left main coronary artery originates normally from the left cusp.

FIGURE 56-2. Non–contrast-enhanced computed tomography axial slices through the heart at two locations for coronary calcium scoring as risk assessment in an asymptomatic patient. On the left, the slice includes the left anterior descending artery with extensive calcification in its proximal portion (arrow). On the right, the slice includes the right coronary artery with proximal spotty calcification (arrow). This patient's calcium score was 457, putting him in a higher risk group regardless of his Framingham risk score.

FIGURE 56-4. Contrast-enhanced computed tomographic coronary angiogram obtained on a dual source 64-detector scanner in a patient with atypical chest pain. The left anterior descending (LAD) artery has a nonobstructive lesion *(arrow)* containing both noncalcified (soft) plaque, which appears dark, and a focal area of calcification. The right coronary artery (RCA) and left circumflex coronary artery (LCx) are normal.

adequately evaluated by MDCT, although accuracy in larger stents is improving with the use of advanced postprocessing techniques.

MDCT coronary angiography is not recommended as a routine screening test, but it can be useful in selected situations, such as in low- or low-intermediate-risk patients who present to emergency departments with chest pain but without ECG changes or elevations of cardiac biomarkers (Chapter 50). The high negative-predictive value of MDCT often can exclude important CHD and avoid the need for other testing in this patient group. MDCT also may be useful in patients with equivocal or nondiagnostic stress testing or new-onset heart failure. The extent and severity of coronary disease found at CT coronary angiography correlate with subsequent all-cause mortality in a similar fashion to catheter-based coronary angiography.

Other Cardiac Applications

The same data acquired by MDCT for coronary artery imaging can be reformatted and used for functional cardiac imaging, including measurement of left ventricular volumes, ejection fraction, wall thickness, and global and segmental wall motion. In acute and chronic myocardial infarction, contrast-enhanced MDCT can demonstrate late enhancement in a manner similar to cardiovascular magnetic resonance imaging (CMR), albeit with a lower signal and contrast-to-noise ratio. MDCT also can complement echocardiography to evaluate cardiac anatomy in patients with congenital heart disease, especially in patients with contraindications to CMR. MDCT can evaluate pericardial thickness and calcification in patients with suspected constrictive pericarditis (see Fig. 77-10 in Chapter 77) and can evaluate native and prosthetic valvular structures and cardiac masses when imaging with other modalities is inadequate.

Cardiac CT is often used to image the left atrium and pulmonary venous anatomy for preprocedural planning for pulmonary vein ablations for atrial fibrillation (Chapter 66). Cardiac venous anatomy may be imaged to aid in the implantation of left ventricular pacemakers in the cardiac venous system for biventricular pacing for heart failure (Chapters 59 and 66).

● CARDIOVASCULAR MAGNETIC RESONANCE IMAGING

Indications, Contraindications, and Pulse Sequences

CMR is a tremendously versatile and flexible imaging modality. CMR is typically performed on 1.5-Tesla (T) scanners, although problems with ECG gating and off-resonance effects previously encountered at higher field strength (3 T) have largely been overcome. Advantages of CMR include the lack of ionizing radiation, the variety of tissues that can be characterized, and the ability to image the heart in any arbitrary plane. Images typically are obtained using ECG gating and breath-hold techniques.

In addition to general restrictions regarding magnetic resonance (e.g., certain intracranial aneurysm clips, transcutaneous electrical nerve stimulation units, intra-auricular implants), patients with cardiac pacemakers and

implantable cardioverter-defibrillators generally should *not* undergo CMR because of concern regarding reprogramming of the device, direct stimulation of the heart during gradient switching, or localized heating in the lead system. Newer pacemaker systems and defibrillator models may not be susceptible, but even in these cases, careful precautions must be taken, including close monitoring and device testing and reprogramming after the procedure. CMR is safe for all prosthetic heart valves, although image distortions immediately around the prosthesis will obscure nearby pathology. CMR is safe for patients with intracoronary stents, including at 3 T. Gadolinium-based contrast agents are now contraindicated in patients with a glomerular filtration rate of less than $30 \text{ mL/minute}/1.83 \text{ m}^2$, owing to the recently identified complication of nephrogenic systemic fibrosis (Chapter 275) in a small subset of patients with severe chronic kidney disease, especially those on dialysis.

A comprehensive CMR study includes evaluation of cardiac structure, function, tissue characteristics, perfusion, and scarring or fibrosis. The components of the examination are tailored to the particular diagnostic question at hand.

Specific Clinical Applications
Coronary Disease

For detection of myocardial ischemia, gadolinium perfusion imaging during vasodilator stress with adenosine or regadenoson shows defects, generally in the subendocardium, that persist for at least 5 heartbeats during the first pass of contrast. Imaging is often repeated at rest after approximately 10 minutes to be sure any defect seen with stress was not either artifactual or due to an infarct (the latter is excluded in combination with late gadolinium enhancement). Head-to-head comparisons of vasodilator stress perfusion CMR and dobutamine stress CMR suggest a higher sensitivity for contrast-enhanced perfusion imaging and higher specificity for dobutamine wall motion imaging. MDCT has superior spatial resolution and accuracy compared with CMR for imaging of the coronary arteries. However, CMR coronary imaging is ideal for the diagnosis of anomalous coronary arteries.

CMR with late gadolinium enhancement is the gold standard technique for assessment of myocardial scar owing to myocardial infarction, with a better accuracy than nuclear imaging approaches, especially for smaller non–Q wave infarctions (Fig. 56-5). In acute myocardial infarction, CMR techniques assess the myocardium at risk and estimate the amount of salvaged myocardium owing to reperfusion. Areas of low signal in the subendocardial core of the infarction represent regions of microvascular obstruction with severe capillary destruction and are a marker of subsequent adverse left ventricular remodeling and poorer outcome.

Cardiomyopathies

CMR is increasingly used to identify the underlying etiology of cardiomyopathies and is the best test to diagnose arrhythmogenic right ventricular

FIGURE 56-5. Late gadolinium-enhanced four-chamber long-axis image in a patient with a scar *(arrow)* from a prior anterior myocardial infarction.

FIGURE 56-7. Gadolinium-enhanced image in a 22-year-old man shows patchy subepicardial enhancement *(arrows)*, characteristic of acute myocarditis.

FIGURE 56-6. Magnetic resonance image in a 27-year-old woman with arrhythmogenic right ventricular cardiomyopathy demonstrates regional right ventricular (RV) systolic dysfunction, which is the hallmark of the disease. The *arrow* points to a region of RV dyskinesis at end systole, and the RV appears like an accordion at end systole.

FIGURE 56-8. Late gadolinium-enhanced magnetic resonance image in a 47-year-old man with heart failure, heart block, and hilar lymphadenopathy shows patchy late gadolinium enhancement in a noncoronary distribution, including subepicardial anterior wall enhancement *(upper arrow)* and near transmural apical enhancement *(lower arrow)* consistent with myocardial sarcoidosis.

dysplasia (Fig. 56-6), which is associated with an increased risk of sudden death (Chapters 60 and 65). Arrhythmogenic right ventricular cardiomyopathy is characterized by regional or global right ventricular dilation and dysfunction. Late gadolinium enhancement may be seen but can be difficult to identify in the thin-walled right ventricle in this disease. Fat is a nonspecific finding.

In patients who present in acute heart failure or with chest pain, elevated troponins, but a negative coronary arteriogram, CMR is ideally suited to identify myocarditis (Chapter 60) noninvasively (Fig. 56-7), with changes most often in the basal lateral wall pattern seen as chronic midwall enhancement, which is a poor prognostic marker in the setting of dilated cardiomyopathy. CMR is more sensitive than echocardiography to measure regional wall thickness and left ventricular outflow tract gradients in patients with hypertrophic cardiomyopathy (Chapter 60). Cardiac amyloidosis (Chapters 60 and 194) can be seen as diffuse subendocardial enhancement, patchy enhancement, or simply difficulty in nulling normal myocardium. Patchy fibrosis is readily identified in cardiac sarcoidosis (Chapters 60 and 95) (Fig.

56-8) and may be more sensitive than endomyocardial biopsy. In iron overload conditions such as thalassemia (Chapter 165), multi-echo T1-weighted imaging of T2* can identify the extent of iron overload. Rarer causes of cardiomyopathy, such as ventricular noncompaction, Chagas' disease (Chapters 60 and 355), and takotsubo cardiomyopathy (Chapter 60), also have characteristic CMR findings. CMR is highly accurate for the noninvasive quantitative assessment of left and right ventricular volumes and ejection fraction but is rarely needed clinically for this purpose unless adequate echocardiography (Chapter 55) cannot be obtained.

Aortic Dissection, Pericardial Disease, and Masses
CMR is an excellent test to detect aortic dissection (see Fig. 78-5 in Chapter 78) or intraluminal aortic hematoma (see Fig. 78-6 in Chapter 78) in patients who are stable enough for it and have no contraindications. CMR is also an excellent test for the evaluation of chronic pericardial disease (Fig. 56-9) because it accurately identifies pericardial thickness as well as adherence of the pericardium to the epicardium in constrictive pericarditis. Real-time

FIGURE 56-9. Magnetic resonance image of a 35-year-old man with dyspnea many years after mantle radiation for Hodgkin's lymphoma shows a thickened pericardium *(arrows)* circumferentially around the left and right ventricles.

FIGURE 56-10. Diastolic magnetic resonance image of a large left atrial myxoma *(arrow)* showing that it is attached to the atrial septum and is prolapsing across the mitral valve.

FIGURE 56-11. Three-dimensional contrast-enhanced magnetic resonance angiogram in a patient with an aortic coarctation *(arrow)*.

SUGGESTED READINGS

Flotats A, Knuuti J, Gutberlet M, et al. Hybrid cardiac imaging: SPECT/CT and PET/CT. A joint position statement by the European Association of Nuclear Medicine (EANM), the European Society of Cardiac Radiology (ESCR) and the European Council of Nuclear Cardiology (ECNC). *Eur J Nucl Med Mol Imaging.* 2011;38:201-212. *Consensus guidelines.*

Harrington RA, Bates ER, Bridges CR, et al. ACCF/ACR/AHA/NASCI/SAIP/SCAI/SCCT 2010 expert consensus document on coronary computed tomographic angiography: a report of the American College of Cardiology Foundation Task Force on Expert Consensus Documents. *Circulation.* 2010;121:2509-2543. *Consensus guidelines.*

Hundley WG, Bluemke DA, Finn JP, et al. ACCF/ACR/AHA/NASCI/SCMR 2010 expert consensus document on cardiovascular magnetic resonance: a report on the American College of Cardiology Foundation Task Force on Expert Consensus Documents. *Circulation.* 2010;121:2462-2508. *Consensus guidelines.*

Pennell DJ. Cardiovascular magnetic resonance. *Circulation.* 2010;121:692-705. *A comprehensive review.*

imaging can demonstrate ventricular interdependence, a hallmark of this disease.

CMR is also an ideal tool to diagnose intracardiac (Fig. 56-10) and extracardiac masses such as myxomas, thrombus, and tumors, owing to its high spatial resolution and ability to perform tissue characterization.

Congenital Heart Disease

CMR is useful for the assessment of both simple and complex congenital heart disease (Chapter 69). Although atrial septal defects and ventricular septal defects in adults are generally well appreciated by echocardiography, phase velocity CMR readily quantifies blood flow through the major blood vessels, thereby facilitating accurate assessment of the ratio of pulmonary to systemic blood flow. CMR is particularly valuable for assessing abnormalities of the great vessels, such as aortic coarctation (Fig. 56-11), extracardiac anatomy, or anomalous pulmonary venous drainage, and in patients with complex congenital heart disease who have undergone prior corrective or palliative shunt surgery, such as in tetralogy of Fallot. CMR is uniquely able to measure right ventricular volumes accurately, an often important determination in this setting.

57

CATHETERIZATION AND ANGIOGRAPHY

MORTON KERN

Cardiac catheterization is insertion and passage of small plastic tubes (catheters) into arteries and veins to the heart to obtain radiographic images of coronary arteries and cardiac chambers (angiography and ventriculography) and to measure pressures in the heart (hemodynamics). Coronary angiography defines the site, severity, and morphology of atherosclerotic lesions, and it identifies collateral blood supply beyond occluded vessel segments. Cardiac catheterization is used not only to diagnose coronary artery, valvular (Chapter 75), and myocardial diseases (Chapter 60), but also to perform therapeutic (interventional) procedures to relieve obstructing arterial stenoses (Chapter 74), open narrowed valves, or close intracardiac defects (Chapter 69) through catheter-based, minimally invasive percutaneous techniques. These same diagnostic and therapeutic techniques are also used in the peripheral arterial circulation in a modified fashion to address carotid, renal, and peripheral vascular disease (Chapter 80), aortic aneurysms (Chapter 78), and vascular shunts (Table 57-1).

● INDICATIONS AND CONTRAINDICATIONS FOR CARDIAC CATHETERIZATION

The indications to perform cardiac catheterization include the need to diagnose atherosclerotic coronary artery disease, abnormalities of cardiac muscle

TABLE 57-1 PROCEDURES THAT MAY ACCOMPANY CORONARY ANGIOGRAPHY

PROCEDURE	COMMENTS
Central venous access: femoral, internal jugular, subclavian	Uses IV access for emergency medications or fluids, temporary pacemaker; pacemaker not mandatory for most coronary angiography
Hemodynamic assessment, left heart pressures, aorta, and left ventricle	Routine for all studies
Right and left heart combined pressures	Not routine for coronary artery disease but mandatory for valvular heart disease and routine for heart failure, right ventricular dysfunction, pericardial disease, cardiomyopathy, intracardiac shunts, congenital abnormalities
Left ventriculography	Routine for all studies; may be excluded with high-risk patients and those with left main coronary or aortic stenosis, severe congestive heart failure, or renal failure
Internal mammary selective angiography	Routine for coronary bypass conduit
Pharmacologic studies: Complication of coronary spasm, use of ergonovine or acetylcholine conducted in specialized centers Use of vasodilators	Conducted routinely for coronary angiography with nitroglycerin and commonly nitric oxide used for pulmonary hypertension
Aortography	Routine for aortic insufficiency, aortic dissection, and aneurysm and may be performed with or without aortic stenosis; routine to locate bypass graft conduits not visualized by selective angiography
Cardiac pacing electrophysiologic studies	Arrhythmia evaluation routine
Interventional and special techniques	Percutaneous coronary angioplasty including balloon stenting, Rotablator, and coronary atherectomy Intracoronary pressure flow assessment of lesion severity routine Balloon catheter valvuloplasty, myocardial biopsy, atrial septal defect or patent foramen ovale defect closure, transseptal or direct left ventricular function to assess valvular heart disease and invasive interventional electrophysiologic catheter ablation
Vascular closure devices	Routinely available for patients prone to femoral artery access bleeding

From Kern MJ, ed. *The Cardiac Catheterization Handbook*, 5th ed. St. Louis: Mosby; 2010.

TABLE 57-2 INDICATIONS AND CONTRAINDICATIONS FOR CARDIAC CATHETERIZATION

INDICATIONS

1. Identification of the extent and severity of coronary artery disease and evaluation of left ventricular function
2. Assessment of the severity of valvular or myocardial disorders such as aortic stenosis and/or insufficiency, mitral stenosis and/or insufficiency, and various cardiomyopathies to determine the need for surgical correction
3. Collection of data to confirm and complement noninvasive studies
4. Determination of the presence of coronary artery disease in patients with confusing clinical presentations or chest pain of uncertain origin

ABSOLUTE CONTRAINDICATIONS

1. Inadequate facilities
2. Patient refusal

RELATIVE CONTRAINDICATIONS

1. Severe uncontrolled hypertension
2. Ventricular arrhythmias
3. Recent acute stroke
4. Severe anemia
5. Active gastrointestinal bleeding
6. Allergy to radiographic contrast
7. Acute renal failure
8. Uncompensated congestive failure (patient cannot lie flat)
9. Unexplained febrile illness and/or untreated active infection
10. Electrolyte abnormalities (e.g., hypokalemia)
11. Severe coagulopathy
12. Pregnancy
13. Uncontrolled arrhythmias, hypertension
14. Uncooperative patient or patient refusal

function, valvular abnormalities, and congenital heart disease (Table 57-2). Contraindications to cardiac catheterization are few. Absolute contraindications involve only inadequate facilities or equipment for catheterization. Relative contraindications depend on the urgency of the procedure and conditions.

TECHNIQUE OF CATHETERIZATION

After the procedure and its indications, risks, and benefits are explained to the patient, the patient is placed on the cardiac catheterization table and centered under the C-arm of the radiographic gantry (E-Fig. 57-1). After sterile preparation and draping, local anesthetic is administered over the vascular access site (most commonly the femoral but, alternatively, the radial artery). The artery is punctured, and a vascular sheath is inserted, through which the angiographic catheter is advanced over a soft spring-tipped 0.035-inch guidewire that permits safe, atraumatic passage of the catheter to the heart. The specially shaped catheters are seated and connected to a manifold to measure pressure and inject radiographic contrast media.

Coronary arteriography records the images from multiple angles by rotating the C-arm. The images are displayed and preserved on digital imaging systems.

After coronary angiography, the catheter is exchanged for a ventriculography catheter that is inserted into the left ventricle. After left ventricular (LV) pressure is measured, radiographic contrast media (approximately 35 to 45 mL) is injected under high pressure (1000 psi) to assess LV wall motion, chamber size, presence of mitral valve regurgitation, and the shape of the aortic root. The LV ejection fraction (normal is 50 to 70%), a measure of the heart function, is computed as a percentage of the diastolic volume ejected.

After the diagnostic angiograms are completed, the need for coronary revascularization (Chapter 74) is assessed. If suitable symptomatic coronary artery obstructions are present, percutaneous coronary intervention (PCI) may be performed at the same time, if discussed and consented to in advance. Alternatively, the patient may be referred for later PCI or for coronary artery bypass graft (CABG) surgery.

At the conclusion of the catheterization procedure, the catheters are removed. For the femoral artery, hemostasis is achieved either by manual compression, which requires the patient to remain stationary in bed for 4 hours, or by use of a vascular closure device while the patient remains in bed for 1 to 2 hours. For the radial approach, the arterial sheath is removed with the simple application of a specialized compression wrist band; the patient can ambulate immediately.

COMPLICATIONS OF CARDIAC CATHETERIZATION

For the diagnostic cardiac catheterization, risks are less than 0.2% for death, less than 0.5% for myocardial infarction, less than 0.07% for stroke, less than 0.5% for serious arrhythmia, and less than 1% for major vascular complications, including thrombosis and bleeding requiring transfusion or pseudoaneurysm (Table 57-3). Vascular complications occur more frequently with the femoral artery approach than with the radial artery approach; the brachial artery approach, which is used only when neither femoral nor radial access is possible, has the highest rate of vascular complications, and the radial artery has the lowest.

Patients are not routinely anticoagulated for a diagnostic catheterization, and special preparations must be made for patients who are receiving anticoagulants, patients who have diabetes or renal insufficiency, and patients who may have a potential allergy to radiographic contrast media. For the anticoagulated patient, provisions to withhold warfarin or heparin must be made

TABLE 57-3 COMPLICATIONS OF CARDIAC CATHETERIZATION

MAJOR COMPLICATIONS

1. Death
2. Cerebrovascular accident
3. Myocardial infarction, shock
4. Ventricular tachycardia/fibrillation

RARE BUT SERIOUS COMPLICATIONS

1. Aortic dissection
2. Cardiac perforation
3. Tamponade
4. Congestive heart failure
5. Contrast reaction/anaphylaxis
6. Nephrotoxicity
7. Arrhythmias, including heart block, asystole, supraventricular tachyarrhythmias
8. Hemorrhage, including local or retroperitoneal
9. Infection
10. Protamine reaction
11. Vascular complications, including thrombosis, embolus, vascular injury, pseudoaneurysm

FIGURE 57-1. Normal left ventricular (LV) and aortic (Ao) pressures measured with high-fidelity pressure transducers.

to reduce the potential for femoral puncture site bleeding complications (e.g., retroperitoneal hematoma or pseudoaneurysm). For example, a patient taking warfarin after an aortic valve replacement would have the warfarin withheld for about 3 days before the catheterization, the international normalized ratio would be monitored, and the patient might be administered bridging heparin to the time of the procedure; warfarin would be restarted after the procedure.

For elective catheterizations in patients with insulin-dependent diabetes, half of the usual morning dose of insulin generally is given the morning of the procedure to provide reasonable diabetic coverage and to avoid hypoglycemia. Metformin should be withheld before study. Medications for hypertension and other medical conditions are continued up to and including the morning of the procedure.

Contrast-induced nephropathy, which generally becomes clinically apparent 2 to 3 days after the catheterization, is uncommon. Patients with diabetes or renal insufficiency and patients who are dehydrated from any cause are at a three- to five-fold increased risk for contrast-induced renal failure. For patients with renal insufficiency and those at high risk for contrast-induced renal failure because of diabetes or dehydration, hydration and treatment with *N*-acetylcysteine (Mucomyst, 600 mg evening and morning of procedure) are used routinely in most catheterization laboratories in an attempt to reduce the risk for contrast-induced renal failure.

Contrast media reactions are rare, with an overall incidence of 5% or less, but potentially serious. Adverse reactions occur in 10 to 12% of patients with a history of allergy and in 15% of patients with reported reaction on a previous contrast radiographic examination. There are three types of contrast allergies: cutaneous and mucosal manifestations, smooth muscle and minor anaphylactoid responses, and cardiovascular and major anaphylactoid responses involving laryngeal or pulmonary edema. Pretreatment with corticosteroids is helpful in reducing all types of reactions except urticaria. Patients reporting previous allergic reactions to contrast media should be premedicated with prednisone (60 mg orally the evening before and morning of the procedure) and diphenhydramine (25 to 50 mg orally the morning of the procedure). Patients with known prior anaphylactoid reactions should be pretreated with steroids in the same dose as above. Routine treatment with a histamine-2 blocker (e.g., cimetidine) does not appear to have any benefit.

Hypotension during and after cardiac catheterization may occur from a vasovagal response, bleeding (often occult), myocardial ischemia or infarction, or cardiac tamponade. Vasovagal hypotension is treated with volume and atropine (0.5 to 1.0 mg intravenously). Hypotension due to cardiac tamponade, which may occur during or after PCI, requires reversal of anticoagulation and urgent pericardiocentesis (Chapter 77).

Pulmonary congestion may develop in patients with marginal LV function or critical valvular heart disease. Congestion compromising respiratory and hemodynamic function is an emergency treated with oxygen, diuretics,

nitroglycerin, inotropic agents, and intraaortic balloon pumping as indicated (Chapter 107).

Chest pain during coronary angiography is unusual, but myocardial ischemia with pain and ST segment changes may occur during PCI (Chapter 74). Treatment with nitroglycerin, heparin, and antiplatelet medications usually controls myocardial ischemia before revascularization (Chapter 72). Minor arrhythmias (e.g., atrial or ventricular premature beats, brief episodes of supraventricular tachycardia) are common and usually resolve without treatment. Ventricular tachycardia or fibrillation is a rare occurrence but requires prompt defibrillation (Chapter 63).

HEMODYNAMIC DATA OBTAINED DURING CARDIAC CATHETERIZATION

Hemodynamic data are the pressure and flow measurements generated by the heart and recorded during the catheterization procedure. A pressure wave is created by cardiac muscular contraction and is transmitted from the cardiac chamber through the arterial circuit (Fig. 57-1). The pressure waves are measured using the fluid-filled catheters with a pressure transducer, which converts the mechanical pressure to an electrical signal that is displayed on a video monitor.

Simultaneous pressure measurements across the heart valves are used to diagnose valve function. Hemodynamic data also include sampling multiple blood oxygen saturations throughout the right and left sides of the heart for intracardiac shunt identification. Cardiac output is commonly measured by a thermodilution technique. Hemodynamic data permit calculation of vascular and pulmonary resistances and cardiac valve areas (see Table 52-1 in Chapter 52). Complete hemodynamic data requiring right and left heart catheterization are indicated to evaluate dyspnea of any cause; to confirm echocardiographic findings when data are not concordant with clinical or other testing results; and to determine the status of valvular heart disease, cardiomyopathy, and constrictive or restrictive coronary physiology.

Complications of right heart catheterization are rare. The most common problem is transient arrhythmia resulting from mechanical stimulation by the catheter as it passes through the right ventricular outflow tract. In patients with left bundle branch block, a temporary pacemaker may be needed if right bundle branch block occurs during right-sided heart catheterization.

Examples of Hemodynamics for Valvular Heart Disease

The severity of a valvular stenosis is based on the pressure gradient and flow across the valve. In patients with suspected aortic stenosis, a transvalvular pressure gradient should be obtained whenever there is conflicting clinical or echocardiographic data. The pressure recordings most commonly used to assess the aortic valve gradients are the left ventricle and the femoral artery through a side arm of the femoral artery sheath (Fig. 57-2). The normal aortic valve area is 2.5 to 3.5 cm^2 in adults. Severe aortic valve stenosis is associated with valve areas smaller than 1.0 cm^2.

In patients with mitral stenosis, the valve gradient usually is measured using the LV and pulmonary capillary wedge pressures (Fig. 57-3). The most accurate method to compute the mitral stenosis gradient uses the left atrial

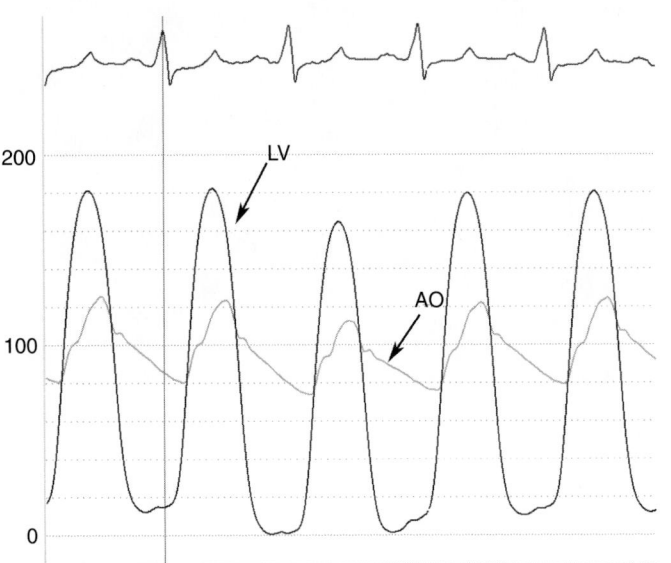

FIGURE 57-2. Hemodynamics of aortic stenosis. Left ventricular (LV) and aortic (AO) pressures are measured simultaneously. Aortic pressure is measured from a central position.

FIGURE 57-3. Examples of the hemodynamic findings in aortic and mitral stenosis. *Left panel,* Simultaneous recording of aortic (AO) and left ventricular (LV) pressure shows a 50-mm Hg systolic pressure gradient. *Right panel,* There is a 15-mm Hg diastolic gradient between the pulmonary capillary wedge pressure (PCW) and the LV pressure. The a wave in the PCW tracing is larger than the v wave, indicating increased resistance to LV filling in this patient. ECG = electrocardiogram.

(obtained by transseptal puncture) and LV pressures. The normal mitral valve area is 4 to 6 cm^2. Valve areas smaller than 1.0 to 1.2 cm^2 are considered severe mitral stenosis.

In patients with mitral regurgitation, the hemodynamics often show a characteristic large v wave on the pulmonary capillary wedge (PCW) tracing (Fig. 57-4). The grading of mitral regurgitation is on a semiquantitative 1 to 4 severity scale based on the amount of contrast seen passing backward from the left ventricle through the incompetent mitral valve into the left atrium. Grade 1 angiographic mitral regurgitation demonstrates a brief puff of contrast filling the left atrium and emptying immediately; grade 2 shows contrast filling the left atrium on 3 beats with moderate density; grade 3 shows contrast filling immediately and moderate density persisting for 2 to 3 beats; and grade 4 shows contrast filling the entire left atrium, often including the appendage, with a density equal to that of the left ventricle for several beats after injection.

CORONARY ANGIOGRAPHY

Coronary angiography visualizes the epicardial arteries, branches, collaterals, and anomalies to diagnose and treat in patients with coronary artery disease (Fig. 57-5). In anticipation of PCI, the angiogram documents not only the presence and location of stenoses but also proximity to major and minor side branches, luminal abnormalities (e.g., thrombi), areas of calcification, and collateral supply, which will influence the decision and techniques used for revascularization. For the two-dimensional radiographic images to depict the three-dimensional coronary tree, multiple angulations of the radiographic imaging system are required.

Assessment of Coronary Stenoses

The degree of a stenosis is most often reported as the estimated percentage diameter luminal reduction of the most severely narrowed segment compared with the adjacent angiographically normal vessel segment, seen in the worst radiographic projection (Fig. 57-6). Because the operator uses visual estimations, an exact evaluation is impossible with less than 20% variation between readings of two or more experienced angiographers. The severity of a stenosis alone should not always be assumed to be associated with abnormal physiology (flow) and ischemia. Moreover, coronary artery disease is a diffuse process, so minimal luminal irregularities on angiography may represent significant, albeit nonobstructive, coronary artery disease at the time of angiography. The precise physiologic impact or morphologic detail of stenosis can be made with specialized catheters and sensor-tipped guidewires. For example, intermediately severe lesions (40 to 70% narrowed) without prior evidence of ischemia can be assessed using a pressure sensor guidewire to measure the translesional pressure during maximal blood flow (e.g., hyperemia induced by adenosine). This pressure measurement, which is called the *fractional flow reserve* (FFR), represents the percentage of normal flow across the stenosis. FFR values higher than 0.80 are considered nonischemic and do not require revascularization. Conversely, if the FFR is lower than 0.80, PCI may be undertaken. The lesion's length, true diameter, eccentricity, and degree of calcium involvement can be determined by intravascular ultrasound catheter-based imaging (IVUS); such information can help guide subsequent PCI (Fig. 57-7).

Coronary Artery Anomalies

Coronary artery anomalies may be present in patients with chest pain syndromes or in young individuals who have survived sudden death. The

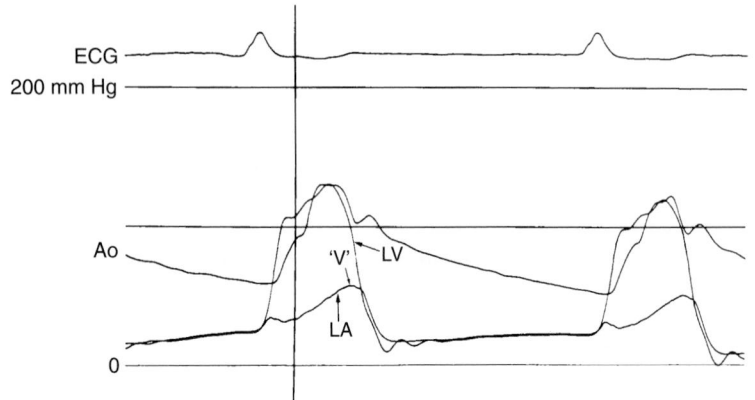

FIGURE 57-4. Hemodynamic tracings in a patient with mitral regurgitation characterized by giant v wave ('V') in the left atrial pressure (LA). This v wave corresponds to marked increase in flow and volume into the left atrium. Ao = aortic pressure; LV = left ventricular pressure.

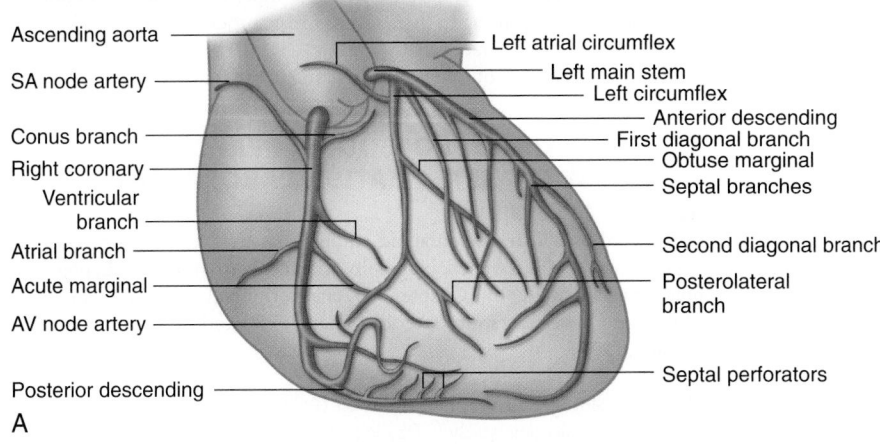

Ascending aorta
SA node artery
Conus branch
Right coronary
Ventricular branch
Atrial branch
Acute marginal
AV node artery
Posterior descending

Left atrial circumflex
Left main stem
Left circumflex
Anterior descending
First diagonal branch
Obtuse marginal
Septal branches
Second diagonal branch
Posterolateral branch
Septal perforators

A

SA node artery
Conus branch
Right coronary
Ventricular branch
Acute marginal
AV node artery

Ascending aorta
Left atrial circumflex
Left main stem
Left anterior descending
First diagonal branch
Left circumflex
Obtuse marginal branch
Posterolateral branch
Second diagonal branch
Septal branches
Distal right coronary

B

Posterior descending

FIGURE 57-5. Coronary vessels. The right anterior oblique (**A**) and left anterior oblique (**B**) views are shown. The major arteries are the left main, left anterior descending, circumflex, and right coronary arteries. AV = atrioventricular; SA = sinoatrial. (Modified from Yang SS, Bentivoglio LG, Maranhao V, et al, eds. *From Cardiac Catheterization Data to Hemodynamic Parameters.* Philadelphia: Oxford University Press; 1988.)

FIGURE 57-6. Example of a significant stenosis in the right coronary artery.

FIGURE 57-7. Angiographic monitor display of intravascular ultrasound (IVUS) image of coronary artery during percutaneous coronary intervention. Precise dimensions of the artery and lumen are provided.

angiographic appearance of coronary anomalies is not always straightforward, and computed tomographic angiography (Chapter 56) has become the diagnostic modality best suited to delineate the origin and course of the anomaly (Fig. 57-8).

At the time of coronary angiography, the misdiagnosis of an unsuspected anomalous origin of a coronary artery is a potential problem. Because the natural history of a patient with an anomalous origin of a coronary artery may depend on the anatomic pathway of the anomalous vessel, it is important to define accurately the origin and course of the vessel. Even experienced angiographers have difficulty delineating the true course of the anomalous vessel.

The most critical coronary anomaly is when the left main coronary artery arises from the right cusp and traverses a course between the aorta and pulmonary artery. The artery's initial course through the aortic wall creates a narrow oval opening; with aortic stretch during exercise, coronary blood flow is limited.

Ventriculography

The left ventriculogram, an integral part of nearly every coronary angiographic study, provides information on the motion of the walls of the heart (Fig. 57-9), LV volumes during systole and diastole, the LV ejection fraction, the rate of ejection, the quality of contractility, the presence of hypertrophic myopathy, and valvular regurgitation. The normal pattern of LV contraction is a coordinated, uniform, almost concentric inward motion of all points along the ventricular inner surface during systole. Uncoordinated contractions are named according to their severity (e.g., moderate or severe hypokinesis, akinesis, and aneurysm-dyskinesis). Focal abnormal wall motion indicates the presence of ischemia, infarction, or aneurysm.

● ADDITIONAL PROCEDURES PERFORMED IN THE CATHETERIZATION LABORATORY

Noncardiac Angiography

Other cardiovascular angiographic studies that may accompany coronary angiography and left ventriculography include aortography (Chapter 78), pulmonary angiography (Chapter 98), and peripheral vascular angiography of iliac and lower extremity arteries (Chapters 80 and 81) or renal arteries (Chapter 127).

Electrophysiologic Studies and Ablation Techniques

An electrophysiologic study (EPS) is an invasive procedure that involves the placement of multipolar catheter electrodes at various intracardiac sites (Chapter 62). The general purposes of an EPS are to characterize the electrophysiologic properties of the conduction system, induce and analyze the mechanism of arrhythmias, and evaluate the effects of therapeutic interventions. Electrode catheters are routinely placed in the right atrium, across the tricuspid valve annulus in the area of the atrioventricular node and His bundle, the right ventricle, the coronary sinus, and sometimes the left ventricle. EPS is routinely used in the clinical management of patients who have supraventricular and ventricular arrhythmias (Chapters 64 and 65).

Transseptal Heart Catheterization

Transseptal access using a long catheter with a needle to puncture the thin atrial septal membrane at the fossa ovalis permits placement of a catheter into the left atrium and then the LV. It is an established technique used to acquire precise, high-quality hemodynamic data for patients with aortic stenosis, mitral valve disease (both stenosis and regurgitation), and hypertrophic cardiomyopathy (outflow tract obstructive gradient) and to provide access for valvuloplasty techniques (Chapter 75). The risks of transseptal catheterization, which include punctures of the aortic root, the coronary sinus, or the posterior free wall of the atrium, are potentially lethal problems.

Endomyocardial Biopsy

Endomyocardial biopsy procedures use venous access from the internal jugular vein or femoral vein to insert a flexible metal bioptome to obtain four to six 1-mm^3 pieces of right ventricular myocardium. There are two definitive indications for endomyocardial biopsy: monitoring for cardiac transplant rejection (Chapter 82) and detection of anthracycline cardiotoxicity (Chapter 60). Other indications in selected patients include diagnosis of cardiomyopathy and myocarditis and differentiation between restrictive and constrictive cardiomyopathies.

Other Procedures

Pericardiocentesis (Chapter 77) and PCI (Chapter 74) are performed in the catheterization laboratory for specific indications. Other procedures include balloon valvuloplasty for stenotic heart valves (Chapter 75) and closure of an atrial septal defect or patent foramen ovale (Chapter 69), which is confirmed by typical oxygen saturations detected at catheterization. Percutaneous implantation of prosthetic heart valves is a newer procedure that may become routine for many laboratories in the future.

FIGURE 57-8. Frame from a computed tomographic angiographic study showing the origin of the left main coronary artery arising from the right sinus of Valsalva and coursing anteriorly between the aorta and pulmonary artery.

FIGURE 57-9. Example of left ventriculography. The ventricular contour is seen in diastole (*left panel*) and in systole (*right panel*).

SUGGESTED READINGS

Kern MJ, Samady H. Current concepts of integrated coronary physiology in the cath lab. *J Am Coll Cardiol.* 2010;55:173-185. *How to use coronary pressure and flow measurements to achieve optimal outcomes.*

Patel MR, Peterson ED, Dai D, et al. Low diagnostic yield of elective coronary angiography. *N Engl J Med.* 2010;362:886-895. *Among patients who do not have known coronary disease but undergo elective coronary angiography for suspected coronary disease, only about one third have obstructive coronary disease.*

58

HEART FAILURE: PATHOPHYSIOLOGY AND DIAGNOSIS

BARRY M. MASSIE

HEART FAILURE

DEFINITION

Heart failure is a heterogeneous syndrome in which abnormalities of cardiac function are responsible for the inability of the heart to pump blood at an output sufficient to meet the requirements of metabolizing tissues or the ability to do so only at abnormally elevated diastolic pressures or volumes. The heart failure syndrome is characterized by signs and symptoms of intravascular and interstitial volume overload (shortness of breath, rales, elevated jugular venous pressure, and edema) or manifestations of inadequate tissue perfusion (impaired exercise tolerance, fatigue, signs of hypoperfusion, renal dysfunction), or both. Heart failure may occur as a result of (1) impaired myocardial contractility (systolic dysfunction, commonly characterized as reduced left ventricular [LV] ejection fraction [EF]); (2) increased ventricular stiffness or impaired myocardial relaxation in the absence of systolic dysfunction (diastolic dysfunction, which is commonly associated with a relatively normal LVEF and is often termed *heart failure with preserved EF*); (3) a variety of other cardiac abnormalities, including obstructive or regurgitant valvular disease, intracardiac shunting, or disorders of heart rate or rhythm; or (4) states in which the heart is unable to compensate for increased peripheral blood flow or metabolic requirements. In adults, LV involvement is almost always present even if the manifestations are primarily those of right ventricular (RV) dysfunction (fluid retention without dyspnea or rales). Heart failure may result from an acute insult to cardiac function, such as a large myocardial infarction (MI), or, more commonly, from a chronic process. The focus in this chapter is on the syndrome of *chronic* heart failure, including its presentation in an acutely decompensated state. The most common causes of de novo acute heart failure, such as MI (Chapter 73), valvular disease (Chapter 75), myocarditis (Chapter 60), and cardiogenic shock (Chapter 107), are discussed elsewhere.

Both the incidence and the prevalence of heart failure are growing, as is the resulting burden of deaths and hospitalizations. Although these trends primarily reflect the strong association between heart failure and advancing age, they also are influenced by the rising prevalence of precursors such as hypertension, diabetes, dyslipidemia, and obesity in industrialized societies and the improved long-term survival of patients with ischemic and other forms of heart disease. The annual incidence of heart failure rises from less than 1 per 1000 patient years among those younger than 45 years, to 10 per 1000 patient years for those older than 65 years, to 30 per 1000 patient years (3%) for those older than 85 years. Prevalence figures follow a similar exponential pattern, increasing from 0.1% before 50 to 55 years of age to almost 10% after age 80 years. About 20% of U.S. adults will develop heart failure in their lifetimes. Overall in the United States, the estimated prevalence of heart failure is 5.8 million patients, with an annual incidence of 670,000 new cases per year. Heart failure results in 1.1 million hospital discharges and causes or contributes to 280,000 deaths per year. Although the relative incidence and prevalence of heart failure are lower in women than men, women constitute at least half of the cases because of their longer life expectancy. Any condition that causes myocardial necrosis or produces chronic pressure or volume overload can induce myocardial dysfunction and heart failure. In developed countries, the causes of heart failure have changed greatly over several decades. Valvular heart disease, with the exception of calcific aortic stenosis, has declined markedly, whereas coronary heart disease has become the predominant cause in men and women, being responsible for 60 to 75% of cases. Hypertension, although less frequently the primary cause of heart failure than in the past, continues to be a major factor in 75%, including most of the patients with coronary disease.

Prevention of Heart Failure

Treatment of hypertension, with a focus on the systolic pressure, reduces the incidence of heart failure by 50%. This intervention remains effective even in patients older than 75 years (Chapter 67). Any intervention that reduces the risk of a first or recurrent MI (Chapter 51) will also reduce the incidence of heart failure. In patients with reduced LVEF, angiotensin-converting enzyme (ACE) inhibitors, aldosterone blockers, and β-blockers prevent or delay progressive LV dysfunction and dilation and the onset or worsening of heart failure. Well-timed intervention for progressive valvular disease affords another opportunity to prevent eventual heart failure (Chapter 75).

Stages of Heart Failure

The recognition that most patients who develop heart failure have underlying risk factors or predisposing clinical conditions that precede its development, usually by many years, has led to a greater emphasis on early detection and treatment of predisposing factors, on the staging of heart failure (Fig. 58-1), and on early intervention. *Stage A* heart failure includes patients who are at risk for development of heart failure but do not as yet have either symptoms or apparent structural abnormalities of the heart; this includes patients with hypertension, atherosclerotic disease, diabetes, obesity, or the

At Risk for Heart Failure

Stage A At high risk for HF but without structural heart disease or symptoms of HF	**Stage B** Structural heart disease but without signs or symptoms of HF
e.g., Patients with: • hypertension • atherosclerotic disease • diabetes • obesity • metabolic syndrome or Patients • using cardiotoxins • with FHx CM	e.g., Patients with: • previous MI • LV remodeling including LVH and low EF • asymptomatic valvular disease

Heart Failure

Stage C Structural heart disease with prior or current signs or symptoms of HF
e.g., Patients with: • known structural heart disease and • shortness of breath and fatigue, reduced exercise tolerance

Structural heart disease →

Development of symptoms of HF →

Therapy See Figure 59–1

FIGURE 58-1. Stages of heart failure. EF = ejection fraction; FHx CM = family history of cardiomyopathy; HF = heart failure; LV = left ventricle; LVH = left ventricular hypertrophy; MI = myocardial infarction. (Modified from Hunt SA. ACC/AHA 2005 guideline update for the diagnosis and management of chronic heart failure in the adult: a report of the American College of Cardiology/American Heart Association Task Force on Practice Guidelines [Writing Committee to Update the 2001 Guidelines for the Evaluation and Management of Heart Failure]. *J Am Coll Cardiol.* 2005;46:e1-e82.)

metabolic syndrome and individuals with ongoing excessive alcohol intake, use of cardiotoxic drugs, a familial history of cardiomyopathy, or a known genetic abnormality associated with cardiomyopathy (Chapter 60). *Stage B* encompasses asymptomatic patients who have demonstrable structural abnormalities that predispose to heart failure, such as prior MI, LV hypertrophy diagnosed by electrocardiography or echocardiography, reduced LVEF or LV dilation, or asymptomatic but hemodynamically significant valvular heart disease. *Stage C* heart failure includes patients who have exhibited symptoms or signs of heart failure. These patients may have improved to the point of being relatively asymptomatic, but they still are classified as stage C and usually continue to receive treatment with agents that are known to improve their natural history, such as β-blockers and inhibitors of the renin-angiotensin-aldosterone system.

PATHOBIOLOGY

Differing Mechanisms of Heart Failure

Heart failure is a syndrome that may result from many cardiac and systemic disorders (Table 58-1). Some of these disorders, at least initially, do not involve the heart, and the term *heart failure* may be confusing. Even in high-output states, however, the patient may present with the classic findings of exertional dyspnea and edema (*high-output heart failure*) that resolve if the underlying disorder is eliminated. If they persist, these conditions may impair myocardial performance secondarily as a result of chronic volume overload or direct deleterious effects on the myocardium. Other conditions, including mechanical abnormalities, disorders of rate and rhythm, and pulmonary abnormalities, do not primarily affect myocardial function but are frequent causes of heart failure.

Abnormalities of Cardiac Function

Systolic Function

In the normal left ventricle, stroke volume increases over a wide range of end-diastolic volumes (the Frank-Starling effect). If contractility (or the inotropic state of the myocardium) is enhanced, such as during exercise or catecholamine stimulation, this increase is correspondingly greater (Table 58-2). In the failing heart with depressed contractility, there is relatively little increment in systolic function with further increases in LV volume, and the ventricular function curve is shifted downward and flattened (Chapter 52). In the clinical setting, systolic dysfunction is characterized by depressed stroke volume despite elevated ventricular filling pressures. The resulting symptoms are those of pulmonary or systemic congestion, activity intolerance, and organ dysfunction.

Assessment of systolic function clinically is more problematic. The most useful measure is the LVEF (stroke volume/end-diastolic volume, usually expressed as a percentage), which reflects a single point on the ventricular function curve. The EF is *load dependent*, however, meaning that alterations in afterload (see later discussion) can affect it independently of contractility. In addition, mitral regurgitation, which facilitates ejection into the low-pressure left atrium, may lead to an overestimation of systolic function by the EF. Nonetheless, with the exceptions indicated earlier, when the EF is normal (>50 to 55% in most laboratories), systolic function is usually adequate. LVEFs that are mildly (40 to 50%), moderately (30 to 40%), or severely (<30%) depressed are associated with reduced survival and, in the severe range, with reduced functional reserve, if not overt symptoms of heart failure. Cardiac output, in contrast, is a poor measure of systolic function because it can be affected markedly by heart rate, systemic vascular resistance, and the degree of LV dilation.

Diastolic Function

Diastole is the portion of the cardiac cycle between aortic valve closure and mitral valve closure. Diastole consists of three phases: (1) active relaxation, (2) the conduit phase, and (3) atrial contraction. If relaxation is delayed or if the myocardium is abnormally stiff (e.g., an excessively steep relationship between change in pressure and change in volume [$\Delta P/\Delta V$]), passive filling may be impaired and atrial pressures are abnormally elevated. In this setting of a noncompliant ventricle (compliance is the inverse of stiffness—the change in volume for a given change in pressure), atrial contraction is responsible for a disproportionately large amount of diastolic filling.

The importance of abnormalities of diastolic function in the pathogenesis of heart failure is increasingly appreciated. Because relaxation is energy dependent, it frequently is impaired in the presence of ischemia or hypoxemia. Recurring myocardial ischemia, myocardial hypertrophy, and aging all are associated with interstitial fibrosis and impaired diastolic function.

TABLE 58-1　PATHOGENESIS OF HEART FAILURE

IMPAIRED SYSTOLIC (CONTRACTILE) FUNCTION

Ischemic damage or dysfunction
  Myocardial infarction
  Persistent or intermittent myocardial ischemia
  Hypoperfusion (shock)
Chronic pressure overloading
  Hypertension
  Obstructive valvular disease
Chronic volume overload
  Regurgitant valvular disease
  Intracardiac left-to-right shunting
  Extracardiac shunting
Nonischemic dilated cardiomyopathy
  Familial/genetic disorders
  Toxic/drug-induced damage
  Immunologically mediated necrosis
  Infectious agents
  Metabolic disorders
  Infiltrative processes
  Idiopathic conditions

IMPAIRED DIASTOLIC FUNCTION (RESTRICTED FILLING, INCREASED STIFFNESS)

Pathologic myocardial hypertrophy
  Primary (hypertrophic cardiomyopathies)
  Secondary (hypertension)
Aging
Ischemic fibrosis
Restrictive cardiomyopathy
  Infiltrative disorders (amyloidosis, sarcoidosis)
  Storage diseases (hemochromatosis, genetic abnormalities)
Endomyocardial disorders

MECHANICAL ABNORMALITIES

Intracardiac
  Obstructive valvular disease
  Regurgitant valvular disease
  Intracardiac shunts
  Other congenital abnormalities
Extracardiac
  Obstructive (coarctation, supravalvular aortic stenosis)
  Left-to-right shunting (patent ductus arteriosus)

DISORDERS OF RATE AND RHYTHM

Bradyarrhythmias (sinus node dysfunction, conduction abnormalities)
Tachyarrhythmias (ineffective rhythms, chronic tachycardia)

PULMONARY HEART DISEASE

Cor pulmonale
Pulmonary vascular disorders

HIGH-OUTPUT STATES

Metabolic disorders
  Thyrotoxicosis
  Nutritional disorders (beriberi)
Excessive blood flow requirements
  Chronic anemia
  Systemic arteriovenous shunting

TABLE 58-2　MAJOR DETERMINANTS OF CARDIAC PERFORMANCE

Ventricular systolic function (contractility)
Ventricular diastolic function
Relaxation
Stiffness
Ventricular preload
Ventricular afterload
Cardiac rate and conduction
Myocardial blood flow

Ventricular Preload

In the intact heart, preload is best characterized by the end-diastolic volume or pressure, which are indirect indicators of end-diastolic fiber length (Chapter 52). The performance of the normal left ventricle is highly preload dependent, but the failing heart operates at high preloads and on the flat part of the LV function curve (see Fig. 52-3 in Chapter 52). In contrast to the normal ventricle, an increase in preload does not improve systolic function but worsens pulmonary congestion further. Preload reduction by diuresis or by reduction of venous return with venodilating agents generally has a beneficial effect on symptoms of heart failure.

Ventricular Afterload

LV afterload frequently is equated with arterial pressure or systemic vascular resistance, but a more accurate measurement of afterload is systolic wall stress (Chapter 52), defined as follows:

$$\text{Systolic wall stress} = (\text{Pressure} \times \text{radius of left ventricle}) \div \\ (2 \times \text{thickness of left ventricle})$$

At any given arterial pressure, afterload is increased with a dilated, thin-walled ventricle and decreased with a smaller or thicker ventricle. Increased afterload has an effect similar to that of depressed contractility, so afterload reduction can improve cardiac performance.

Heart Rate and Rhythm

Heart rate affects cardiac performance by two mechanisms. First, increasing the heart rate enhances the inotropic state by upregulating cytosolic calcium concentrations. Second, heart rate is an important determinant of cardiac output and is the primary mechanism by which cardiac output is matched to demand in situations such as exercise. Because stroke volume is relatively fixed in the failing heart, heart rate becomes a major determinant of cardiac output. Chronic tachycardia impairs ventricular performance, however, and cardiac function can decline rapidly with sustained tachyarrhythmias (as seen in atrial fibrillation, atrial flutter, chronic atrial tachycardia, and even inappropriate sinus tachycardia).

Optimal cardiac performance depends on a well-coordinated sequence of contraction. Normal atrioventricular conduction times (0.16 to 0.20 second) enhance the contribution of atrial contraction to LV filling, which is particularly important in the noncompliant ventricle. Patients with heart failure frequently have intraventricular conduction abnormalities, which result in dyssynchronous contractions, such that the septum and parts of the anterior wall begin contracting only after systole has ended in other regions. Cardiac resynchronization therapy can prevent the onset of heart failure in patients with significant ventricular dyssynchrony, usually manifest electrically as a left bundle branch block.

Myocardial Blood Flow and Oxygen Requirements

In the normal heart, myocardial blood flow is closely coupled to oxygen requirements, and it is not ordinarily considered a determinant of cardiac performance. However, myocardial ischemia is associated with a rapid decline in contractile function that may persist long beyond the episode (myocardial stunning). Chronically inadequate blood flow may lead to a reduction in contractility, which reestablishes the balance between oxygen delivery and demands (hibernation). Low arterial diastolic pressures may interfere with the autoregulatory reserve of the coronary circulation, which is limited at diastolic pressures of less than 60 mm Hg. Endothelial dysfunction, which is common in patients with heart failure, also may limit blood flow. At the same time, tachycardia, increased afterload, and substantial LV hypertrophy increase myocardial oxygen requirements. Inadequate myocardial blood flow plays an important role in the pathogenesis of cardiac dysfunction, sometimes even in patients without obstructive coronary disease.

Genetic Causes of Dilated Cardiomyopathy

Although much less is known about the genetics of dilated cardiomyopathy than that of hypertrophic cardiomyopathy (Chapter 60), several forms of familial cardiomyopathy have been recognized, most of which are inherited in an autosomal dominant pattern. Mutations of genes encoding for nuclear membrane proteins (emerin, lamin) or for contractile or cytoskeletal proteins (desmin, a cardiac myosin, vinculin) have been identified. Cardiomyopathy also is associated with muscular dystrophies (Duchenne's, Becker's, and limb-girdle dystrophies; Chapter 429) and other forms of myopathy. As research

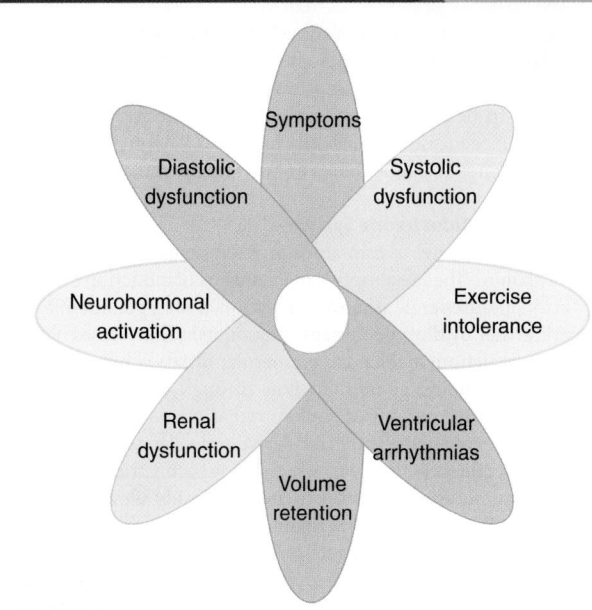

FIGURE 58-2. Pathophysiology of heart failure, illustrated by Venn diagram.

TABLE 58-3	NEUROHORMONES THAT MAY BE INCREASED IN CHRONIC HEART FAILURE
Norepinephrine	Natriuretic peptides
Epinephrine	Endothelin
Plasma renin activity	Endorphins
Angiotensin II	Calcitonin gene–related peptide
Aldosterone	Growth hormone
Prostaglandins	Cortisol
Vasopressin	Proinflammatory cytokines
Neuropeptide Y	Neurokinin A
Vasoactive intestinal peptides	Substance P

in this area burgeons, it is estimated that genetic abnormalities may be involved in 20 to 30% of cases of idiopathic dilated cardiomyopathy.

Heart Failure Syndrome

Chronic heart failure is a multifaceted syndrome with diverse presentations (Fig. 58-2). The initial manifestations of hemodynamic dysfunction are a reduction in stroke volume and a rise in ventricular filling pressures, perhaps in the basal state but consistently under conditions of increased systemic demand for blood flow. These changes have downstream effects on cardiovascular reflexes and systemic organ perfusion and function, which in turn stimulate a variety of interdependent compensatory responses involving the cardiovascular system, neurohormonal systems, and alterations in renal physiology. It is this constellation of responses that leads to the characteristic pathophysiology of the heart failure syndrome. Recognition of the role of neurohormonal activation in heart failure has grown with the increasing understanding of its pathophysiology and with evidence that blockade of some of these responses can have a profound effect on the natural history of the disease (Table 58-3). The number of hormonal systems that are known to be activated in heart failure continues to grow.

Neurohormonal Responses
Sympathetic Nervous System

Initial activation of the sympathetic nervous system probably results from reduced pulse pressures, which activate arterial baroreceptors, and renal hypoperfusion. Evidence for its activation comes from elevated levels of circulating norepinephrine, direct sympathetic nerve recordings showing increased activity, and increased release of norepinephrine by several organs, including the heart. As cardiac function deteriorates, responsivity to norepinephrine diminishes, as evidenced by baroreceptor desensitization and downregulation of cardiac adrenergic receptors and signal transduction. This desensitization may further stimulate sympathetic responses.

The adaptive role of norepinephrine is to stimulate heart rate and myocardial contractility and to produce vasoconstriction. These actions reverse the depression of cardiac output and blood pressure. Increased levels of plasma norepinephrine are associated with a worse prognosis, although it is unclear whether this is a cause-and-effect relationship. There is also convincing, albeit circumstantial, evidence that norepinephrine has adverse effects on the myocardium. In this regard, β-adrenoceptor blockade, which once was considered dangerous in heart failure because it would interfere with important compensatory mechanisms, consistently improves LV function and prognosis. The roles of other catecholamines in heart failure remain undefined.

Renin-Angiotensin-Aldosterone System

Elements of the renin-angiotensin-aldosterone system are activated relatively early in heart failure. The presumptive mechanisms of induction include renal hypoperfusion, β-adrenergic system stimulation, and hyponatremia. All may be activated further by diuretic therapy. Angiotensin II increases blood pressure by vasoconstriction; it enhances glomerular filtration by increasing renal pressure and maintaining glomerular flow through its intrarenal hemodynamic effects. Aldosterone causes sodium retention, which restores normal cardiac output by enhancing intravascular volume. These adaptations have deleterious consequences, however. Excessive vasoconstriction can depress LV function, and sodium retention increases already elevated ventricular filling pressures. There also is experimental evidence indicating that angiotensin II may have pathologic effects on the myocardium and may induce vascular hypertrophy, whereas aldosterone induces myocardial fibrosis. The striking success of ACE inhibitors and aldosterone blockers in improving the natural history of heart failure suggests that the adverse effects of renin-angiotensin-aldosterone activation may outweigh the benefit in patients with or at risk of heart failure.

Other Neurohormonal Systems

Levels of several natriuretic peptides are elevated consistently in heart failure, and they may counterbalance the vasoconstricting and sodium-retaining actions of the renin-angiotensin-aldosterone and sympathetic nervous systems. However, the renal responses to these natriuretic hormones are often downregulated in patients with heart failure, so they do not have the same natriuretic effects in patients with chronic heart failure that they manifest in normal individuals. Elevated circulating and tissue levels of vasodilating prostaglandins may improve glomerular hemodynamics, and inhibitors of prostaglandin synthesis (including aspirin and other nonsteroidal anti-inflammatory agents) interfere with the hemodynamic and renal actions of ACE inhibitors.

Endothelin and arginine vasopressin are elevated in many patients with heart failure, and interference with their actions may promote vasodilation and aquaresis. Arginine vasopressin induces vasoconstriction through a vascular (V-1) receptor and reduces free water clearance through a renal tubular (V-2) receptor. Endothelin causes prolonged vasoconstriction, reductions in glomerular filtration, and pulmonary arteriolar constriction. Although endothelin is a theoretically attractive target for therapy, clinical trials with endothelin antagonists have been negative or even shown harm, thereby indicating that interdiction of neurohormonal activation is not uniformly beneficial.

Cytokine Activation

Circulating levels of many proinflammatory cytokines, including tumor necrosis factor-α (TNF-α), interleukin-1β, and interleukin-6, are elevated in patients with relatively severe heart failure and may be involved in the syndrome of cardiac cachexia. These cytokines also may induce contractile dysfunction, myocardial fibrosis, and myocyte necrosis, perhaps by mediating some of the deleterious responses to catecholamines and angiotensin II. Nonetheless, trials using antagonists of TNF-α have not shown clinical benefit.

Altered Renal Physiology

In most patients with chronic heart failure, the kidneys are anatomically and structurally normal. Reduced blood pressure, diminished stroke volume, and reduced renal perfusion pressure and flow are sensed as reduced blood volume by the high-pressure baroreceptors and the juxtaglomerular apparatus, which maintain cardiovascular homeostasis. In chronic heart failure, these receptors become desensitized, generating reduced afferent responses. The low-pressure intracardiac pressure and volume receptors also are desensitized. Thirst and fluid intake may be increased as a result of activation of the cerebral thirst center. Although heart failure usually is associated with a normal or increased blood volume, it paradoxically is characterized by activation of the same homeostatic responses as those that act in hemorrhage and shock; the result is abnormal retention of sodium and water. In advanced heart failure, which is usually characterized by low cardiac output or

hypotension (or coexisting renal vascular disease), the glomerular filtration rate may become so severely reduced that sodium and fluid retention becomes refractory to diuretic therapy.

Left Ventricular Remodeling and Progression of Heart Failure

After an initial insult precipitates heart failure, progressive alterations occur in myocardial structure and function owing to continuing damage by the underlying process and responses to hemodynamic stresses and neurohormonal activation. The left ventricle progressively dilates and changes from the normal ellipsoid shape to a more spherical geometry. This "remodeling" is accompanied by changes in the cardiac interstitium that lead to altered orientation of the myofibrils and progressive fibrosis. The result is more discoordinate and less effective contraction. Inhibitors of the renin-angiotensin-aldosterone system and β-blockers slow, halt, or reverse this remodeling process, preventing LV dilation, geometric distortion, and deterioration in contractile function.

CLINICAL MANIFESTATIONS

Heart failure may manifest acutely in a de novo manner, chronically, or as recurring exacerbations of chronic heart failure.

Acute Decompensation of Heart Failure

Most episodes of acute worsening of heart failure occur in patients with previously recognized symptoms of chronic heart failure. Patients with such decompensations usually present with shortness of breath, generally after a period of fluid retention or signs of congestion, as manifested by worsening edema and some degree of worsening dyspnea (Fig. 58-3).

Occasionally, the initial presentation may be more acute, with rapid progression to resting dyspnea or pulmonary edema, or both. The acute presentation is often associated with severe hypertension and is particularly characteristic of patients who have diastolic dysfunction and whose stiff left ventricle tolerates fluid retention poorly. In patients without a preceding history of heart failure, other precipitating factors, such as acute MI (Chapter 73), tachyarrhythmias (Chapters 64 and 65), previously unrecognized or new valvular abnormalities (Chapter 75), toxic damage (including alcohol excess), or acute myocarditis (Chapter 60), should be considered. Rapid diagnosis by noninvasive testing and early cardiac catheterization is essential. In patients whom myocarditis is suspected, particularly when the clinical presentation suggests giant cell myocarditis, early endomyocardial biopsy is recommended. Treatment is cause specific and may include early coronary revascularization, valve repair or replacement, or supportive care (e.g., inotropic support, intra-aortic balloon pumping, ventricular assist devices). If the condition does not improve, cardiac transplantation (Chapter 82) may be the best option for appropriate candidates.

Chronic Heart Failure
Left-Sided and Right-Sided Heart Failure

Most adult patients with heart failure have abnormalities of the left ventricle as the underlying cause. Nonetheless, the clinical presentation may be

FIGURE 58-3. Number of days from onset of worsening of selected symptoms of heart failure to admission to hospital: cumulative percentage of patients. (Reprinted with permission from Schiff GD, Fung S, Speroff T, et al. Decompensated heart failure: symptoms, patterns of onset, and contributing factors. *Am J Med.* 2003;114:625-630.)

variable, sometimes suggesting predominantly or even exclusively RV dysfunction. The manifestations of LV dysfunction are related to elevated filling (diastolic) pressures, which are transmitted backward to the left atrium and pulmonary veins, or inadequate cardiac output. The former results in dyspnea (sometimes at rest but usually with activity) and, when severe, pulmonary edema (classically associated with rales and possibly pleural effusions). The cardiac output may be insufficient to support peripheral organ function, causing exertional muscle fatigue, impaired renal function and salt excretion, or depressed mentation.

Right-sided heart failure results from either chronic RV pressure overload (e.g., pulmonary hypertension resulting from cor pulmonale, pulmonary vascular disease or pulmonary embolism) or intrinsic dysfunction of the right ventricle or its valves. However, the most common cause of RV pressure overload is left-sided heart dysfunction, which results in pulmonary hypertension. If the symptoms and signs of left-sided heart failure are absent or difficult to elicit, the physician inappropriately may seek a primarily right-sided pathology. The primary manifestations of right-sided failure are related to chronically elevated right atrial and systemic venous pressures: jugular venous distention, peripheral edema, ascites, hepatic and bowel edema, and varied gastrointestinal complaints. These patients are especially vulnerable to renal dysfunction because elevated venous pressures may cause renal medullary ischemia and depress renal function.

Heart Failure with Preserved Ejection Fraction

Myocardial mechanisms that lead to the syndrome of heart failure can be differentiated into conditions that depress LV systolic function and conditions that occur despite normal or relatively preserved contractility. Although it is arbitrary, an LVEF threshold of 45 to 50% often is used for this distinction

Until the widespread use of noninvasive assessments of LV function, heart failure with preserved EF was considered unusual in the absence of valvular abnormalities or other specific and uncommon causes. It is now recognized that at least 40-50% of patients with heart failure have relatively normal EFs. In the ongoing Cardiovascular Health Study, a population-based study of more than 5000 patients aged 65 years and older, more than 70% of the patients developing heart failure had normal or only mildly impaired EFs. As the population ages and as interventional and pharmacologic approaches reduce infarct sizes and prevent LV remodeling, it is likely that heart failure with preserved EF will become increasingly common.

Although there are many potential causes of heart failure with preserved EF, most patients have current hypertension or a history of treated hypertension; the resulting LV hypertrophy and fibrosis are probably responsible for increased chamber stiffness. Ischemic heart disease also may contribute to heart failure with preserved systolic function, probably by virtue of subendocardial fibrosis or as a result of acute, intermittent ischemic dysfunction. Diabetes mellitus is often present, especially in women. Age itself is a crucial predisposing factor because it causes loss of myocytes (apoptosis), increased fibrosis with shifts to more rigid forms of collagen, and loss of vascular compliance.

The mortality rate of patients with heart failure with preserved systolic function is somewhat lower than the rate for those with low EFs but still is high, often owing to the significant comorbid conditions that are common in these older-aged individuals. Hospitalization and rehospitalization rates for these patients are comparable to those for patients with reduced EFs. Unfortunately, clinical trials have yet to identify any therapeutic interventions that improve the outcomes of the patients with heart failure with preserved systolic function.

Although patients who have heart failure with preserved systolic function are often considered to have *diastolic dysfunction*, other explanations for this presentation must be considered, some of which are reversible or warrant specific therapy (Table 58-4). The first two questions to consider are whether the patient's symptoms are caused by heart failure of any type and whether important valvular abnormalities are present. LVEF measurements may be inaccurate, particularly if their technical quality is suboptimal. Regurgitant valve disease may lead to a dissociation between the LVEF and underlying myocardial dysfunction because afterload may be low in this setting. There also are many conditions in which LV function is impaired transiently, but subsequently measured EFs may be normal. Intermittent ischemia, presenting as episodic heart failure (*flash pulmonary edema*), is the most important of these conditions because revascularization may be indicated. Severe hypertension with subsequent control and transient tachyarrhythmias also may have temporary effects on EF. Some patients

---

TABLE 58-4	CAUSES OF (AND ALTERNATIVE EXPLANATIONS FOR) HEART FAILURE WITH PRESERVED LEFT VENTRICULAR EJECTION FRACTION (>45-50%)

Inaccurate diagnosis of heart failure (e.g., pulmonary disease, obesity)

Inaccurate measurements of ejection fraction

Systolic function overestimated by ejection fraction (e.g., mitral regurgitation)

Episodic, unrecognized systolic dysfunction

Intermittent ischemia

Arrhythmia

Severe hypertension

Alcohol abuse

Diastolic dysfunction

Abnormalities of myocardial relaxation
  Ischemia
  Hypertrophy

Abnormalities of myocardial compliance
  Hypertrophy
  Aging
  Fibrosis
  Diabetes
  Infiltrative disease (amyloidosis, sarcoidosis)
  Storage disease (hemochromatosis)
  Endomyocardial disease (endomyocardial fibrosis, radiation, anthracyclines)

Pericardial disease (constriction, tamponade)

TABLE 58-5	FACTORS THAT MAY PRECIPITATE ACUTE DECOMPENSATION OF CHRONIC HEART FAILURE

Discontinuation of therapy (patient noncompliance or physician initiated)

Initiation of medications that worsen heart failure (calcium antagonists, β-blockers, nonsteroidal anti-inflammatory drugs, antiarrhythmic agents)

Iatrogenic volume overload (transfusion, fluid administration)

Dietary indiscretion

Alcohol consumption

Increased activity

Pregnancy

Exposure to high altitude

Arrhythmias

Myocardial ischemia or infarction

Worsening hypertension

Worsening mitral or tricuspid regurgitation

Fever or infection

Anemia

---

with alcoholic cardiomyopathy exhibit rapid recovery in EF when they cease drinking.

The remaining patients most likely have diastolic dysfunction as the underlying disorder. The noninvasive measurement of diastolic function remains problematic. The most commonly used test, Doppler echocardiography, is neither sensitive nor specific for diastolic dysfunction. Particularly in elderly patients, Doppler mitral valve filling patterns show impaired early diastolic filling in most subjects, whether or not they have evidence of heart failure. Diastolic dysfunction is basically a diagnosis of exclusion based on accompanying conditions and circumstantial evidence.

Factors Precipitating Acute Decompensation of Chronic Heart Failure

Many patients with chronic heart failure maintain a stable course, and then abruptly present with acutely or subacutely worsening symptoms. Although this decompensation may reflect unrecognized gradual progression of the underlying disorder, many precipitating events must be considered and, if present, addressed (Table 58-5). An important focus is on changes in medications (by patient or physician), diet, or activity. Superimposed new or altered cardiovascular conditions, such as arrhythmias, ischemic events, hypertension, or valvular abnormalities, should be considered. Systemic processes, such as fever, infection, declining renal function, or anemia, also can cause cardiac decompensation.

DIAGNOSIS

The diagnosis of heart failure is straightforward when a patient presents with classic symptoms and accompanying physical findings. In patients with chronic heart failure, however, the diagnosis is often delayed or missed entirely because no single sign or symptom is diagnostic.

CLINICAL EVALUATION

The most frequent symptoms, dyspnea and fatigue, are not specific for heart failure, especially in older individuals, but their presence always should lead to a more complete evaluation. The more specific symptoms of orthopnea, paroxysmal nocturnal dyspnea, and severe edema are much less common. Although the physical examination may be helpful, characteristic physical findings may be absent. The chest radiograph (Chapter 53), on which many physicians rely, adds relatively little to the clinical evaluation except when pulmonary edema is present (see Fig. 53-15 in Chapter 53).

The key to making the timely diagnosis of chronic heart failure is to maintain a high degree of suspicion, particularly in high-risk patients with coronary artery disease, chronic hypertension, diabetes, a history of heavy alcohol use, or advanced age. If such patients present with any of the symptoms or physical findings suggestive of heart failure, additional testing (see later discussion) should be undertaken, typically beginning with echocardiography (Chapter 55).

The common symptoms of heart failure are well known but are frequently absent and variably specific for this condition. The symptoms generally reflect, but may be dissociated from, the hemodynamic derangements of elevated left-sided and right-sided pressures and impaired cardiac output or cardiac output reserve.

Dyspnea

Dyspnea (Chapter 83), or perceived shortness of breath, is the most common symptom of heart failure. In most patients, dyspnea is present only with activity or exertion. The underlying mechanisms are multifactorial. The most important is pulmonary congestion with increased interstitial or intra-alveolar fluid, which activates juxtacapillary J receptors, stimulating a rapid and shallow pattern of breathing. Increased lung stiffness may enhance the work of breathing, leading to a perception of dyspnea. Central regulation of respiration may be disturbed in those with more severe heart failure, resulting in disordered sleep patterns and sleep apnea. Cheyne-Stokes respiration, or periodic breathing, is common in advanced heart failure, is usually associated with low-output states, and may be perceived by the patient (and the patient's family) as either severe dyspnea or transient cessation of breathing. Hypoxia, which is uncommon in heart failure unless there is accompanying pulmonary disease, suggests the presence of pulmonary edema. Dyspnea is a relatively sensitive symptom of heart failure when patients maintain or attempt a moderate level of activity. However, in patients who are inactive, dyspnea may not be prominent, and the diagnosis of heart failure is often delayed or overlooked. In addition, dyspnea may become less prominent with the onset of RV failure and tricuspid regurgitation, which may lead to lower pulmonary venous pressures. Dyspnea, moreover, is also a common symptom of patients with pulmonary disease (Chapter 83), obesity, or anemia and of sedentary individuals.

Orthopnea and Paroxysmal Nocturnal Dyspnea

Orthopnea is dyspnea that is positional, occurring in the recumbent or semi-recumbent position. It occurs as a result of the increase in venous return from the extremities and splanchnic circulation to the central circulation with changes in posture, with resultant increases in pulmonary venous pressures and pulmonary capillary hydrostatic pressure. Nocturnal cough may be a manifestation of this process and is an under-recognized symptom of heart failure. Orthopnea is a relatively specific symptom of heart failure, although it may occur in patients with pulmonary disease who breathe more effectively in an upright posture and in individuals with significant abdominal obesity or ascites. Most patients with mild or moderate heart failure do not experience orthopnea if they are treated adequately.

Paroxysmal nocturnal dyspnea is an attack of acute, severe shortness of breath that awakens the patient from sleep, usually 1 to 3 hours after the patient retires. Symptoms usually resolve over 10 to 30 minutes after the patient arises, often gasping for fresh air from an open window. Paroxysmal nocturnal dyspnea results from increased venous return and mobilization of interstitial fluid from the extremities and elsewhere, with accumulation of alveolar edema. Paroxysmal nocturnal dyspnea almost always represents heart failure, but it is a relatively uncommon finding.

Acute Pulmonary Edema

Pulmonary edema results from transudation of fluid into the alveolar spaces due to acute rises in capillary hydrostatic pressures caused by an acute depression of cardiac function or an acute rise in intravascular volume. The initial symptoms may be cough or progressive dyspnea. Because alveolar edema may precipitate bronchospasm, wheezing is common. If the edema is not treated, the patient may begin coughing up pink (or blood-tinged), frothy fluid and become cyanotic and acidotic.

Exercise Intolerance

Activity or exercise intolerance is, together with dyspnea, the most characteristic symptom of chronic heart failure. Intuitively, it might be assumed that exercise would be limited by shortness of breath because of rising pulmonary venous pressures and pulmonary congestion. Although this mechanism may contribute, it is only one of many operating. Blood flow to exercising muscles is impaired as a result of reduced cardiac output reserve and impaired peripheral vasodilation; oxygen delivery is limited, and early fatigue ensues. Heart failure is associated with additional abnormalities of skeletal muscle itself, including biochemical changes and alterations in fiber types, which increase muscle fatigue and impair muscle function. Finally, heart failure may affect adversely respiratory muscle function and ventilatory control.

Fatigue

Fatigue is a common, if nonspecific, complaint of patients with heart failure. Perhaps the most common origin of this complaint is muscle fatigue. Fatigue also may be a nonspecific response to the systemic manifestations of heart failure, such as chronic increases in catecholamines and circulating levels of cytokines, sleep disorders, and anxiety.

Edema and Fluid Retention (Ascites, Pleural Effusion, Pericardial Effusion)

Elevated right atrial pressures increase the capillary hydrostatic pressures in the systemic circulation, with resultant transudation. The location of edema fluid is determined by position (e.g., dependent) and by the accompanying pathology. Most commonly, edema accumulates in the extremities and resolves at night, when the legs are not dependent. Edema may occur only in the feet and ankles, but if it is more severe, it may accumulate in the thighs, scrotum, and abdominal wall. Edema is more likely and more severe in patients with accompanying venous disease, in those who have had veins harvested for coronary bypass surgery, and in patients taking calcium channel blockers, which themselves cause edema. Fluid retention associated with thiazolidinediones (Chapter 237) and nonsteroidal anti-inflammatory drugs may precipitate heart failure or mimic it.

Fluid also may accumulate in the peritoneal cavity and in the pleural or pericardial spaces. Ascites occurs as a result of elevated pressures in the hepatic, portal, and systemic veins draining the peritoneum. Ascites is unusual in heart failure and almost always is associated with peripheral edema. Most commonly, there is severe tricuspid regurgitation, with potential damage to the liver. Otherwise, significant primary liver disease should be suspected as an exacerbating factor or cause of ascites. Pleural effusions are fairly common in chronic heart failure, especially when they are accompanied by left-sided and right-sided manifestations. The effusions result from an increase in transudation of fluid into the pleural space and from impaired lymphatic drainage caused by elevated systemic venous pressures. Pericardial effusions are far less frequent but may occur.

Abdominal and Gastrointestinal Symptoms

Passive congestion of the liver may lead to right upper quadrant pain and tenderness and mild jaundice. Usually only mild elevations of transaminase levels and modest increases in bilirubin levels are observed. With severe, acute rises in central venous pressures, especially if associated with systemic hypotension, a severe congestive and ischemic hepatopathy may occur, with striking elevations in liver function markers and hypoglycemia. Recovery is usually rapid and complete if the hemodynamic abnormalities are corrected.

Bowel wall edema may lead to early satiety (a common symptom in heart failure), nausea, diffuse abdominal discomfort, malabsorption, and a rare form of protein-losing enteropathy. The potential role of heart failure in producing these nonspecific gastrointestinal symptoms is often overlooked, leading to extensive diagnostic testing or unnecessary discontinuation of medications.

Sleep Disorders and Central Nervous System Manifestations

Periods of nocturnal oxygen desaturation to less than 80 to 85% are relatively common in patients with heart failure; they coincide with episodes of apnea (Chapter 100) and often are preceded or followed by episodes of hyperventilation. These are similar to, and may represent truncated forms of, Cheyne-Stokes respiration. These episodes reflect altered central nervous system ventilatory control and have been associated with diminished heart rate variability. Supplemental oxygen appears to reverse some of the ventilatory disorders, and the apneic spells respond to nasal positive-pressure ventilation. In some patients, these interventions have a striking beneficial effect on fatigue and other symptoms of heart failure.

Aside from the common complaint of fatigue, which originates in part in the central nervous system, brain function is not affected in most patients with heart failure. In advanced heart failure, cerebral hypoperfusion can cause impairment of memory, irritability, limited attention span, and altered mentation.

Cardiac Cachexia

In chronic, severe heart failure, unintentional chronic weight loss may occur, leading to a syndrome of cardiac cachexia. The mechanisms underlying this syndrome are unclear, but it may result from many factors, including increased levels of pro-inflammatory cytokines (e.g., TNF), elevated metabolic rates, loss of appetite, and malabsorption. Cardiac cachexia carries a poor prognosis.

PHYSICAL EXAMINATION

The physical findings associated with heart failure generally reflect elevated ventricular filling pressures and, to a lesser extent, reduced cardiac output. In chronic heart failure, many of these findings are absent, often obscuring the correct diagnosis.

Appearance and Vital Signs

Compensated patients may be comfortable, but patients with more severe symptoms are often restless, dyspneic, and pale or diaphoretic. Although the heart rate is usually at the high end of the normal range or higher (>80 beats per minute), it may be lower in patients with chronic, stable heart failure. Premature beats and arrhythmias are common. Pulsus alternans (alternating amplitude of successive beats) is a sign of advanced heart failure (or of a large pericardial effusion). The blood pressure may be normal or high, but in advanced low-output heart failure, it is usually on the low end of normal or lower.

Jugular Veins and Neck Examination

Examination of the jugular veins is one of the most useful aspects of the evaluation of patients with heart failure. The jugular venous pressure should be quantified in centimeters of water (normal = 8 cm H_2O) (see Figs. 50-2 and 50-3 in Chapter 50), estimating the level of pulsations above the sternal angle (and arbitrarily adding 5 cm H_2O in any posture). The presence of abdominal-jugular reflux should be assessed by putting pressure on the right upper quadrant of the abdomen for 30 seconds and avoiding an induced Valsalva maneuver; a positive finding is a rise in the jugular pressure of at least 1 cm. Either an elevated jugular venous pressure or an abnormal abdominal-jugular reflux has been reported in 80% of patients with advanced heart failure. No other simple sign is nearly as sensitive.

An additional important finding in the neck is evidence of tricuspid regurgitation—a large "cv" wave, usually associated with a high jugular venous pressure. This finding is confirmed by hepatic pulsations, which can be detected during the abdominal-jugular reflux determination. The carotid pulses should be evaluated for evidence of aortic stenosis, and thyroid abnormalities should be sought.

Pulmonary Examination

Although dyspnea is the most common symptom of patients with heart failure, the pulmonary examination is usually unremarkable. Rales, representing alveolar fluid, are a hallmark of heart failure; when they are present in patients without accompanying pulmonary disease, they are highly specific for the diagnosis. In chronic heart failure, they are often absent, however, even in patients known to have pulmonary capillary wedge pressures greater than 20 mm Hg (normal, <12 mm Hg). LV failure cannot be excluded by the absence of rales. Pleural effusions, which tend to lateralize on the right side because of the greater surface area of the lungs, are not uncommon, but large effusions are relatively rare in chronic heart failure.

Cardiac Examination

The cardiac examination is a crucial part of the evaluation of the patient with heart failure, but it is more useful for identification of associated cardiac abnormalities than for assessment of the severity of the heart failure (Chapter 50). Assessment of the point of maximal impulse may provide information concerning the size of the heart (enlarged if displaced below the fifth intercostal space or lateral to the midclavicular line) and its function (if sustained beyond one third of systole or palpable over two interspaces). Additional precordial pulsations may indicate an LV aneurysm. A parasternal lift is valuable evidence of pulmonary hypertension.

The first heart sound (S_1) may be diminished in amplitude when LV function is poor, and the pulmonic component of the second heart sound (P_2) may be accentuated when pulmonary hypertension is present. An apical third heart sound (S_3) is a strong indicator of significant LV systolic dysfunction, but it is present only in a minority of patients with low EFs and elevated LV filling pressures. A fourth heart sound (S_4) is not a specific indicator of heart failure, but it is usually present in patients with diastolic dysfunction. An S_3 at the lower left or right sternal border or below the xiphoid indicates RV dysfunction. Murmurs may indicate the presence of significant valvular disease as the cause of heart failure, but mitral and tricuspid regurgitation also are common secondary manifestations of severe ventricular dilation and dysfunction.

Examination of the Abdomen and Extremities

The size, pulsatility, and tenderness of the liver should be evaluated as evidence of passive congestion and tricuspid regurgitation. Ascites and edema should be sought and quantified.

Characterization: Essential and Contingent Tests

Essential Tests

Chest Radiography

Although the standard posteroanterior and lateral chest radiographs provide limited information about chamber size, the presence of overall cardiomegaly (a cardiothoracic ratio of >0.50, especially if >0.60) is a strong indicator of heart failure or another cause of cardiomegaly (especially valvular insufficiency) (see Fig. 53-4 in Chapter 53). However, almost 50% of patients with heart failure do not have this high a cardiothoracic ratio.

Most patients with acute heart failure, but only a minority of those with chronic heart failure, have clear evidence of pulmonary venous hypertension (upper lobe redistribution, enlarged pulmonary veins), interstitial edema (haziness of the central vascular shadows or increased central interstitial lung markings), or pulmonary edema (perihilar or patchy peripheral infiltrates). The absence of these findings reflects the subjectivity of interpretation and the increased capacity of the lymphatics to remove interstitial and alveolar fluid in chronic heart failure. This absence of radiographic findings is consistent with the absence of rales in most patients with chronic heart failure despite markedly elevated pulmonary venous pressures. Pleural effusions are important adjunctive evidence of heart failure. Characteristically, these are more common and larger on the right than on the left side, reflecting the greater pleural surface area of the right lung.

Electrocardiography

The major importance of the electrocardiogram is to evaluate cardiac rhythm, identify prior MI, and detect evidence of LV hypertrophy (Chapter 54). Prior MI suggests that the cause is ischemic cardiomyopathy with systolic dysfunction. LV hypertrophy is a nonspecific finding but may point toward LV diastolic dysfunction if the EF is not depressed.

Echocardiography

Noninvasive cardiac imaging is a crucial part of the diagnosis and evaluation of heart failure. The most useful procedure is transthoracic echocardiography (Chapter 55), which provides a quantitative assessment of LV function; in the presence of appropriate symptoms and signs, it can confirm the presence of heart failure resulting from systolic dysfunction or indicate whether the patient has heart failure with preserved systolic function. The echocardiogram also provides a wealth of additional valuable information, including assessment of LV and RV size and regional wall motion (as an indicator of prior MI), evaluation of the heart valves, and diagnosis of LV hypertrophy. Particularly valuable are quantitative measurements of pulmonary artery and central venous pressures. The echocardiogram generally has replaced the chest radiograph in the diagnostic assessment of heart failure, and it can provide useful hemodynamic measurements without cardiac catheterization.

Measurements of Natriuretic Peptides

Serum levels of natriuretic peptides can be measured quickly and accurately, including point-of-care testing at the bedside. B-type natriuretic peptide (BNP) and amino (N)-terminal pro-BNP are relatively sensitive and specific markers for clinically confirmed heart failure These peptides have been found to be useful adjuncts in the diagnosis of patients presenting in the acute care setting with possible heart failure, particularly when the diagnosis remains uncertain.[1] However, levels of both BNP and N-terminal pro-BNP increase with age in the absence of clinical heart failure, especially in women, probably reflecting increased ventricular stiffness associated with aging and hypertension. BNP levels may also be increased slightly in patients with chronic obstructive pulmonary disease, in whom elevations may reflect diastolic dysfunction or RV dysfunction but nonetheless may lead to a false-positive clinical diagnosis of heart failure. Elevated natriuretic peptide measurements are associated with a worse prognosis and may be helpful in assessing the response to therapy. Randomized clinical trials that have assessed the clinical value of serial measurements in guiding therapy suggest a reduction in all-cause mortality compared with usual clinical practice.[2]

Contingent Tests

After the diagnosis of heart failure is made, the goal of additional testing is to identify potentially correctable or specifically treatable causes and to obtain further information that is necessary for future management.

Laboratory Testing

An extensive battery of laboratory tests is not required for most patients with heart failure. Routine testing should include a complete blood cell count (to detect anemia and systemic diseases with hematologic manifestations); measurement of renal function and electrolytes, including magnesium (to exclude renal failure and to provide a baseline for subsequent therapy); liver function tests (to exclude accompanying liver pathology and provide a baseline); and blood glucose and lipid testing (to diagnose diabetes and dyslipidemia, both of which should be managed aggressively in patients with heart failure).

A few additional tests may be indicated. Thyrotoxicosis, and to a lesser extent hypothyroidism, may cause heart failure and may be difficult to diagnose clinically, especially in older patients (Chapter 233). Many guidelines recommend thyroid function tests for all patients, or at least all elderly patients and those with atrial fibrillation. Hemochromatosis (Chapter 219) is a potentially treatable cause of heart failure; particularly if there is accompanying diabetes or hepatic disease, measurement of serum ferritin levels is indicated. Sarcoidosis (Chapter 95) is another potentially treatable cause, although it would be unusual not to have evidence of accompanying lung disease. Amyloidosis (Chapter 194) should be considered in patients with other manifestations, but treatment of the cardiac manifestations is rarely successful except with heart transplantation.

Assessment of Left Ventricular Function

Although heart failure is a syndrome with many pathogenic mechanisms, the most common are LV systolic dysfunction and LV diastolic dysfunction. In some patients, it is almost impossible to distinguish between these two forms of heart failure by clinical evaluation because both may present with the same symptoms and with only subtle differences on physical examination. However, it is important to distinguish between these two entities because they may require different diagnostic evaluations and different therapeutic approaches (Chapter 59). The most useful and practical test is the echocardiogram (Chapter 55); alternative approaches include radionuclide measurements of LVEF (Chapter 56) and left ventriculography if cardiac catheterization (Chapter 57) is being performed. All these tests allow the detection of significant systolic dysfunction; diastolic dysfunction sometimes can be documented (Chapter 55) but often is identified primarily as a process of exclusion in patients with preserved systolic function. Randomized trials have found no benefit, in terms of days alive and out of hospital or in a number of other relevant end points, among patients who were

monitored with pulmonary artery catheterization compared with those who were not.[3]

DIAGNOSTIC EVALUATION

Assessment for Coronary Artery Disease

Coronary artery disease is the most common cause of heart failure in industrialized societies, particularly in men. Often it is known that a patient has coronary disease based on a prior history of MI or positive results on an angiogram or noninvasive test, but in some patients, MI can be silent. There are two reasons to identify the coexistence of heart failure and coronary disease: first, to treat symptoms that may be caused by ischemia and, second, to improve prognosis (Chapters 71, 72, and 73). A prudent approach is to divide patients with heart failure into three groups: (1) those with clinical evidence of ongoing ischemia (active angina or a possible ischemic equivalent), (2) those who have had a prior MI but do not currently have angina, and (3) those who may or may not have underlying coronary disease. The first group of patients may be evaluated most expeditiously by coronary angiography because they stand to benefit in terms of symptoms and probably have more extensive ischemia. In the second group are patients with heart failure and prior MI who by other criteria (age, absence of other major comorbid conditions) are good candidates for coronary revascularization; they generally should undergo noninvasive stress testing in conjunction with nuclear myocardial perfusion imaging or echocardiography to assess regional function and myocardial viability (Chapter 71). CT angiography is a useful screening test to evaluate coronary anatomy (Chapter 56), but it provides little physiologic information. These procedures identify individuals with extensive ischemic but viable myocardium, whose prognosis and symptoms also may be improved with revascularization. The third group, patients without either angina or prior MI, are much less likely to benefit from an evaluation for asymptomatic coronary disease.

Myocardial Biopsy

There is no rationale for routine myocardial biopsy in patients with heart failure, even in the subgroup without apparent coronary disease. Few entities that might be detected are amenable to specific therapy, and those that are (hemochromatosis, sarcoidosis) usually can be detected by their other manifestations or other procedures. A possible exception is acute fulminant myocarditis (Chapter 60), particularly eosinophilic and giant cell myocarditis, which may respond to immunosuppressive therapy. Another exception is in the patient being evaluated for cardiac transplantation (Chapter 82) because the presence of some entities may preclude this procedure.

Assessment of Exercise Capacity

Quantitative assessment of exercise capacity provides additional insight into prognosis beyond the clinical evaluation and measurements of cardiac function, particularly when a detailed history of activity tolerance cannot be obtained. Exercise testing with measurements of peak oxygen uptake by respiratory gas exchange has become a routine part of the evaluation for transplantation (Chapter 82) because it provides an indication of need for early intervention and an additional method for follow-up. In most patients, testing is not necessary, however. Emphasis should be placed on eliciting each patient's maximum tolerated activity and the minimum activity associated with symptoms; both can be monitored from visit to visit as a guide to management.

Assessment of Arrhythmias

Ventricular arrhythmias are extremely common in patients with chronic heart failure, with 50 to 80% of patients exhibiting nonsustained ventricular tachycardia during 24-hour monitoring. Because approximately 50% of cardiac deaths in these patients are sudden, these arrhythmias have been viewed with concern. In multivariate analyses, asymptomatic ventricular arrhythmias carry little independent prognostic significance when the severity of symptoms, EF, and presence of concurrent coronary disease are taken into account. Arrhythmias are no more predictive of sudden death than of total mortality. Ventricular arrhythmias associated with syncope or hemodynamic compromise must be taken seriously and require further evaluation and treatment (Chapter 65). Selected patients with advanced heart failure will benefit from implantable cardioverter defibrillators (Chapters 59 and 66).

Differential Diagnosis

Although it is not difficult to make the definitive diagnosis of heart failure in a patient who presents with the classic symptoms and signs, several alternative diagnoses need to be considered in less clear-cut situations, such as in the patient with normal LV function and less definitive clinical evidence. The most common alternative diagnosis is pulmonary disease, for which pulmonary function testing is usually helpful (Chapter 85). If LV systolic function is normal, it may be difficult to make a conclusive determination of the relative role of diastolic heart failure compared with other concomitant conditions, such as severe obesity, chronic anemia, or other systemic illnesses; in some patients, a therapeutic trial of treatment for heart failure (Chapter 59) may be diagnostic.

Follow-Up Testing

After the diagnosis of heart failure is confirmed and the initial evaluation is complete, there is little need for further testing beyond the laboratory tests necessary to monitor therapy (primarily renal function and electrolytes). If the status of ventricular function is known, there are few indications for retesting. Exceptions are monitoring for transplantation and important changes in clinical status, such as marked deterioration in a patient previously known to have preserved LV function or the occurrence of new murmurs in conjunction with declining status.

1. Lam LL, Cameron PA, Schneider HG, et al. Meta-analysis: effect of B-type natriuretic peptide testing on clinical outcomes in patients with acute dyspnea in the emergency setting. *Ann Intern Med.* 2010;153:728-735.
2. Porapakkham P, Zimmet H, Billah B, et al. B-type natriuretic peptide-guided heart failure therapy: a meta-analysis. *Arch Intern Med.* 2010;170:507-514.
3. The ESCAPE Investigators. Evaluation study of congestive heart failure and pulmonary artery catheterization effectiveness. The ESCAPE trial. *JAMA.* 2005;294:1625-1633.

SUGGESTED READINGS

Al-Mohammad A, Mant J. The diagnosis and management of chronic heart failure: review following the publication of the NICE guidelines. *Heart.* 2011;97:411-416. *Review.*
Heart Failure Society of America. 2010 Comprehensive guideline: executive summary. *J Cardiac Failure.* 2010;16:475-539. *Consensus guidelines.*
Hunt SA. Focused update incorporated into the ACC/AHA 2005 guidelines for the diagnosis and management of heart failure in adults. *Circulation.* 2009;119:e391-479. *Consensus guideline update.*
McMurray JJ. Clinical practice: systolic heart failure. *N Engl J Med* 2010;362:228-238. *Practical overview.*

59

HEART FAILURE: MANAGEMENT AND PROGNOSIS

JOHN J. V. MCMURRAY AND MARC A. PFEFFER

EVALUATION AND MANAGEMENT OF HEART FAILURE

Heart failure is an overarching term for a syndrome (i.e., a constellation of signs and symptoms) that encompasses a vast spectrum of cardiovascular disorders and is associated with a greatly heightened risk for death and nonfatal adverse cardiovascular events (Chapter 58). Treatment is initially directed toward prevention of cardiac injury (e.g., due to hypertension or myocardial infarction) or toward limiting structural progression if cardiac damage has already occurred (e.g., left ventricular remodeling with declining left ventricular ejection fraction) and delaying the development of symptomatic heart failure. Once symptoms develop, treatments are also directed at improving functional status as well as prognosis.

Approximately one in five adults will develop heart failure. In the United States, 5.8 million people have heart failure, and U.S. hospitals annually admit 1.1 million patients with a primary diagnosis of heart failure. The estimated cost of heart failure in the United States is about $39 billion per year. Randomized controlled clinical trials (RCTs) supply the framework for quantifying what different therapeutic approaches can offer. Even when they are definitive, RCTs only generate data about average risks and benefits of the

tested therapeutic option in a selected cohort. Because an individual patient's responses can only be implied from the overall estimated group responses, RCTs cannot definitively direct the approach of every patient or answer the myriad questions that confront the practitioner regarding the specific circumstances of the patient. Another major limitation of RCTs is the relatively narrow time frame of observation, generally only months to several years, compared with epidemiologic experiences during decades. Despite these limitations, RCTs are the premier tool of evidence-based medicine, and the field of heart failure has fortunately been the focus of relatively high-quality RCTs that have provided robust evidence to improve clinical care and prognosis (Table 59-1). Indeed, the implementation of evidence from RCTs into clinical practice has resulted in impressive temporal improvements in survival after discharge from a first hospital admission for heart failure. Moreover, the age at which symptomatic heart failure first becomes evident has increased. Despite these tangible advances, heart failure continues to be a leading cause of morbidity and mortality in elderly people.

STAGES OF HEART FAILURE

The American Heart Association/American College of Cardiology Guidelines for the Evaluation and Management of Chronic Heart Failure in the Adult use a staging classification to underscore the evolution and progression of heart failure severity (Fig. 59-1). This classification emphasizes the use of different strategies and therapeutic options across the full spectrum of the syndrome, from prevention of heart failure to palliation of patients with end-stage disease.

Stage A: Individuals at Risk for Development of Heart Failure

Stage A designates patients at risk for development of heart failure based on concomitant cardiovascular diseases such as hypertension, coronary artery disease, and diabetes mellitus. Also included in stage A are individuals with prior exposure to cardiotoxic agents such as doxorubicin (Chapter 182) and those with a family history of a cardiomyopathy (Chapter 60). Although these predisposing factors do not by themselves technically constitute the syndrome of heart failure, the guidelines stress the importance of identifying individuals with modifiable factors because this represents an important opportunity to reduce the reservoir of patients at risk.

Population-based preventive approaches can reduce the incidence of heart failure. For example, public health programs targeting the eradication of the insect vector for *Trypanosoma cruzi* (Chapter 355) have reduced the incidence of Chagas' cardiomyopathy (Chapter 60) in endemic regions of South and Central America.

Other population-based approaches to reduce the incidence of heart failure require specific screening efforts to identify individuals with modifiable risk factors. The most important, although unfortunately nonmodifiable, risk factor for the development of heart failure is advanced age; the incidence of heart failure rises sharply per decade after the age of 45 years (Chapter 58). For each decade of age after 45 years, the incidence of heart failure doubles, and heart failure is the leading hospital diagnosis for patients older than 65 years in the United States.

Hypertension

Of the modifiable factors, hypertension (Chapter 67) undoubtedly contributes the greatest population-attributable risk for heart failure. In other words, even though the increased risk of heart failure in an individual with hypertension is modest, the high prevalence of hypertension in the general population means that at a population level, hypertension is the major cause of heart failure.

The contribution of hypertension to the risk of heart failure was a consistent finding from all major cardiovascular epidemiologic studies, and the earliest RCTs of antihypertensive therapy showed unambiguous reductions in the risk of heart failure. Of the components of blood pressure, elevated systolic pressure has a greater influence on the incidence of heart failure than does diastolic pressure. In fact, aging is associated with a progressive rise in systolic blood pressure and fall in diastolic pressure as the compliance of the arterial tree diminishes (Chapter 67). In community-based studies, isolated systolic hypertension and elevated pulse pressure have been the most predictive blood pressure measurements for development of heart failure. In the Systolic Hypertension in the Elderly Program, antihypertensive treatment with chlorthalidone followed by atenolol reduced the incidence of new heart failure by about 50%, a treatment effect size recently exceeded (relative risk reduction, 64%) with indapamide followed by perindopril in the Hypertension in Very Elderly Trial, probably the last placebo-controlled

TABLE 59-1 CONTROLLED TRIALS* IN SYMPTOMATIC HEART FAILURE WITH REDUCED SYSTOLIC FUNCTION

TRIAL, TREATMENT, AND YEAR PUBLISHED	N	SEVERITY OF HEART FAILURE	ESTIMATED FIRST-YEAR PLACEBO/CONTROL GROUP MORTALITY	BACKGROUND TREATMENT[+]	TREATMENT ADDED	TRIAL DURATION (YR)	PRIMARY END POINT	RELATIVE RISK REDUCTION (%)[‡]	Events Prevented Per 1000 Patients Treated[§‖]		
									DEATH	HF HOSP.	DEATH OR HF HOSP.
ACE INHIBITORS											
CONSENSUS, 1987[5]	253	End stage	52	Spironolactone	Enalapril, 20 mg bid	0.54[+]	Death	40	146	—	—
SOLVD-T, 1991[6]	2569	Mild-severe	15.7	—	Enalapril, 20 mg bid	3.5	Death	16	45	96	108
β-BLOCKERS											
CIBIS-2, 1999[a]	2647	Moderate-severe	13.2	ACE-I	Bisoprolol, 10 mg qd	1.3[+]	Death	34	55	56	—
MERIT-HF, 1999[b]	3991	Mild-severe	11.0	ACE-I	Metoprolol CR/XL, 200 mg qd	1.0[+]	Death	34	36	46	63
COPERNICUS, 2001[10]	2289	Severe	19.7	ACE-I	Carvedilol, 25 mg bid	0.87[+]	Death	35	55	65	81
SENIORS, 2005[c]	2128	Mild-severe	10.4	ACE-I + spironolactone	Nebivolol, 10 mg qd	1.75	Death or CV hosp.	14	23	0	—
ANGIOTENSIN RECEPTOR BLOCKERS											
Val-HeFT, 2001[8]	5010	Mild-severe	~8.0	ACE-I	Valsartan, 160 mg bid	1.9	CV death or morbidity	13	0	35	33[§]
CHARM-Alternative, 2003[7]	2028	Mild-severe	12.6	BB	Candesartan, 32 mg qd	2.8	CV death or HF hosp.	23	30	31	60
CHARM-Added, 2003[9]	2548	Moderate-severe	10.6	ACE-I + BB	Candesartan, 32 mg qd	3.4	CV death or HF hosp.	15	28	47	39
ALDOSTERONE BLOCKADE											
RALES, 1999[11]	1663	Severe	~25	ACE-I	Spironolactone, 25-50 mg qd	2.0[+]	Death	30	113	95	—
EMPHASIS-HF, 2011[13]	2737	Mild	8.1	ACE-I + BB	Eplerenone, 50 mg qd	1.75	Death or HF hosp.	37	30	64	66
HYDRALAZINE-ISDN											
V-HeFT-1, 1986[d]	459	Mild-severe	26.4	—	Hydralazine, 75 mg tid-qid ISDN, 40 mg qid	2.3	Death	34	52	0	—
A-HeFT, 2004[15]	1050	Moderate-severe	~9.0	ACE-I + BB + spironolactone	Hydralazine, 75 mg tid ISDN, 40 mg tid	0.83[+]	Composite	—	40	80	—

	n	Severity		Background therapy	Test treatment		Primary end point				
DIGITALIS GLYCOSIDES											
DIG, 1997[14]	6800	Mild-severe	~11.0	ACE-I	Digoxin	3.1	Death	0	0	79	73
SHIFT, 2010	6558	Mild-severe	~7.5	ACE-I + BB + spironolactone	Ivabradine 7.5 mg bid	1.9	CV death or HF hosp.	18	14	47	—
CRT											
COMPANION, 2004[20]	925	Moderate-severe	19.0	ACE-I + BB + spironolactone	CRT	1.35‡	Death or any hospital admission	19	38	—	87
CARE-HF, 2005[21]	813	Moderate-severe	12.6	ACE-I + BB + spironolactone	CRT	2.45	Death or CV hospital admission	37	97	151	184
CRT-D											
COMPANION, 2004[20]	903	Moderate-severe	19.0	ACE-I + BB + spironolactone	CRT-ICD	1.35‡	Death or any hospital admission	20	74	—	114
MADIT-CRT, 2009[23]	1820	Mild	~3.0%	ACE-I + BB + spironolactone + ICD	CRT-ICD	2.4‡	Death or HF event**	34	5	—	—
RAFT, 2010[22]	1798	Mild-moderate	~6.5	ACE-I + BB + spironolactone + ICD	CRT-ICD	3.3	Death or HF hosp.	25	53	66	70
IMPLANTABLE CARDIOVERTER-DEFIBRILLATOR											
SCD-HeFT, 2005[19]	1676	Mild-severe	~7.0	ACE-I + BB	ICD	3.8	Death	23	—	—	—
VENTRICULAR ASSIST DEVICE											
REMATCH, 2001[e]	129	End stage	75	ACE-I + spironolactone	LVAD	1.8	Death	48	282	—	—
EXERCISE TRAINING											
HF-ACTION, 2009[17]	2231	Mild-severe	~6.0	ACE-I + BB + spironolactone	Exercise training	2.5	Death or any hosp.	7	6	—	—

*Excluding active-controlled trials.

†In more than one third of patients, ACE-I + BB means that ACE inhibitors were used in almost all patients and BB in the majority; most patients were also taking diuretics, and many digoxin (except in DIG). Spironolactone was used at baseline in 5% Val-HeFT, 8% MERIT-HF, 17% CHARM-Added, 19% SCD-HeFT, 20% COPERNICUS, and 24% CHARM-Alternative.

‡Relative risk reduction in primary end point.

§Stopped early for benefit.

||Individual trials may not have been designed or powered to evaluate effect of treatment on these outcomes.

¶Primary end point that also included treatment of heart failure with intravenous drugs for 4 hours or more without admission and resuscitated cardiac arrest (both added small numbers).

aThe Cardiac Insufficiency Bisoprolol Study II (CIBIS-II): a randomised trial. Lancet. 1999;353:9-13.

bEffect of metoprolol CR/XL in chronic heart failure: metoprolol CR/XL Randomised Intervention Trial in Congestive Heart Failure (MERIT-HF). Lancet. 1999;353:2001-2007.

bCohn JN, Archibald DG, Ziesche S, et al. Effect of vasodilator therapy on mortality in chronic congestive heart failure: results of a Veterans Administration Cooperative Study. N Engl J Med. 1986;314:1547-1552.

cFlather MD, Shibata MC, Coats AJ, et al. Randomized trial to determine the effect of nebivolol on mortality and cardiovascular hospital admission in elderly patients with heart failure (SENIORS). Eur Heart J. 2005;26:215-225.

dRose EA, Gelijns AC, Moskowitz AJ, et al. Long-term mechanical left ventricular assistance for end-stage heart failure. N Engl J Med. 2001;345:1435-1443.

ACE-I = ACE inhibitor; BB = β-blocker; CRT = cardiac resynchronization therapy (biventricular pacing); CRT-D = CRT device that also defibrillates; CV = cardiovascular; HF hosp. = patients with at least one hospital admission for worsening heart failure—some patients had multiple admissions; ICD = implantable cardioverter-defibrillator; ISDN = isosorbide dinitrate; LVAD = left ventricular assist device.

Modified from McMurray JJ, Pfeffer MA. Heart failure. Lancet. 2005;365:1877-1889.

Trials

Therapy	Stage A	Stage B	Stage C	Stage D
Antihypertensives	VA Study I and II SHEP HOT ALLHAT			
Statins	HPS WOSCOPS ASCOT-LLA AFCAPS-Texcaps	HPS 4S CARE		
β-Blockers		BHAT Norwegian β-blocker trial CAPRICORN	CIBIS II MERIT HF COPERNICUS COMET SENIORS	
ACE inhibitors	HOPE EUROPA (PEACE)	SAVE SOLVD-P AIRE TRACE	SOLVD-T CONSENSUS	
Angiotensin II receptor blockers (ARBs)		VALIANT	CHARM alternative CHARM added Val-HeFT	
Hydralazine/nitrates			V-HeFT I and II A-HeFT	
Digoxin			DIG	
Aldosterone antagonists		EPHESUS ————→ RALES ——→		
Implantable cardioverter-defibrillator (ICD)		MADIT II	SCD-HeFT ——→	
Cardiac resynchronization therapy (CRT)			COMPANION CARE HF MADIT-CRT	
Left ventricle assist device (LVAD)				REMATCH

Stage A	Stage B	Stage C	Stage D
High risk for HF without structural heart disease or symptoms of HF	**Structural heart disease but without signs or symptoms of HF**	**Structural heart disease with prior or current symptoms of HF**	**Refractory HF requiring specialized interventions**
Patients with • Hypertension • Artherosclerotic disease • Diabetes • Obesity • Metabolic syndrome or Patients using • Cardiotoxins with family history of cardiomyopathy (FHx CM)	Patients with • Previous MI • LV remodeling including LVH and low EF • Asymptomatic valvular disease	Patients with • Known structural heart disease • Shortness of breath and fatigue, reduced exercise tolerance	Patients with marked symptoms at rest despite maximal medical therapy (e.g., those who are recurrently hospitalized or cannot be safely discharged from the hospital without specialized interventions)

THERAPY	THERAPY	THERAPY	THERAPY
Goals • Treat hypertension • Encourage smoking cessation • Treat lipid disorders • Encourage regular exercise • Discourage alcohol intake, illicit drug use • Control metabolic syndrome **Drugs** • ACEI or ARB as appropriate patients for vascular or diabetes	**Goals** • Treat hypertension • Encourage smoking cessation • Treat lipid disorders • Encourage regular exercise • Discourage alcohol intake, illicit drug use • Control metabolic syndrome **Drugs** • ACEI or ARB as appropriate patients for vascular or diabetes • β-Blockers in appropriate patients **Devices in selected patients** • Implantable defibrillators	**Goals** • Treat hypertension • Encourage smoking cessation • Treat lipid disorders • Encourage regular exercise • Discourage alcohol intake, illicit drug use • Control metabolic syndrome • Dietary salt restriction **Drugs for routine use** • Diuretics for fluid retention • ACEI • β-Blockers in appropriate patients **Drugs in selected patients** • Aldosterone antagonist • ARBs • Digitalis • Hydralazine/nitrates **Devices in selected patients** • Biventricular pacing • Implantable defibrillators	**Goals** • Appropriate measures under stages A, B, C • Decision re: appropriate level of care **Options** • Compassionate end-of-life care/hospice • Extraordinary measures • Heart transplantation • Chronic inotropes • Permanent mechanical support • Experimental surgery or drugs

antihypertensive trial. In general, the actual extent of blood pressure lowering achieved, not the agent used, is the most important factor in reducing overall rates of major cardiovascular events. However, the greatest reduction in risk of heart failure seems to be seen when initial therapy is based on a diuretic and angiotensin-converting enzyme (ACE) inhibitor. By comparison, treatment with α-blockers increases the risk of heart failure compared with other antihypertensive drugs. Most important, it is estimated that effective treatment of hypertension (Chapter 67) will substantially reduce the age-adjusted incidence of heart failure by approximately 60% in women and 50% in men.

Other Risk Factors

Treatment of atherosclerotic risk factors, such as hypercholesterolemia (Chapter 213), and promotion of measures that encourage healthier lifestyles, such as smoking cessation (Chapter 31), weight control (Chapter 227), and aerobic exercise (Chapter 15), should also reduce the number of individuals who progress from stage A to stage B (structural heart disease but without symptoms of heart failure). ACE inhibitors protect against the development of heart failure in patients with diabetes mellitus or with evidence of atherosclerosis. Although obesity is correlated with hypertension, lipid abnormalities, and glucose intolerance, an elevated body mass index is also an independent risk factor for the development of heart failure.

Stage B: Asymptomatic Structural or Functional Heart Disease

Stage B identifies asymptomatic (class I; Chapter 58) patients who have a structural or functional cardiac disorder (e.g., left ventricular hypertrophy, enlargement, or dysfunction and valvar abnormalities) but do not have the signs and symptoms, such as dyspnea and fatigue, of the heart failure syndrome. In addition to history, physical examination, and electrocardiography (Chapter 54), more extensive screening with echocardiography (Chapter 55) or other imaging modalities (Chapter 56) is often required to detect patients with asymptomatic cardiac structural abnormalities.

A patient who has an acute myocardial infarction not complicated by early heart failure is an obvious example of someone who transitions from stage A to stage B. Rapid pharmacologic or mechanical coronary reperfusion is one of the immediate goals of therapy, with the aim of limiting the extent of myocardial injury and reducing the risk for death and future development of heart failure (Chapters 72 and 73). Survivors of the acute phase of myocardial infarction, a well-studied stage B cohort, are at particularly high risk for the future development of heart failure, with an overall annual incidence of 2% per year—but higher in patients who are older, have a lower left ventricular ejection fraction (LVEF), do not routinely perform at least moderate exercise, or have concomitant hypertension or diabetes mellitus. For example, a clinically stable asymptomatic patient who has recovered from a myocardial infarction but who is older than 60 years with an LVEF of less than 50% and a history of diabetes and hypertension has an estimated 30% 5-year likelihood of experiencing death or heart failure; without diabetes or hypertension, the 5-year estimated rate becomes 12%. By comparison, a younger myocardial infarction survivor who has an LVEF over 50% and does not have hypertension or diabetes would be anticipated to have a 5-year rate for heart failure or death of only 3%. Data also suggest that an assessment of right ventricular function provides further independent incremental prediction for the risk of developing heart failure. With the continued improvements in care of patients with acute myocardial infarction (Chapters 72 and 73) and the use of implantable cardioverter-defibrillators (ICDs) after myocardial infarction in patients with reduced LVEF, this pool of stage B patients, who represent a reservoir for new-onset heart failure, has been expanding.

The impaired left ventricle, often due to a prior myocardial infarction, can undergo progressive chamber enlargement. This process, also termed *left ventricular remodeling*, describes the time-dependent and often insidious structural alterations of the impaired left ventricle, whereby the relationship of the left ventricular cavity volume increases out of proportion to mass, so the overall ventricular geometry becomes more distorted, usually more spherical. This distortion of left ventricular geometry often leads to mitral regurgitation. These structural changes produce regional and global increases in myocardial wall stress, which can promote further remodeling and contribute to the progressive deterioration of cardiac function and structure often associated with the later stages of symptomatic heart failure.

TREATMENT   Rx

ACE Inhibitors and Angiotensin Receptor Blockers

Mechanistic studies confirm that ACE inhibitors inhibit progressive left ventricular enlargement by reducing wall stress during the entire cardiac cycle as well as by more direct inhibition of the intracellular signaling pathways involved in myocardial hypertrophy and interstitial fibrosis. This attenuation of ventricular remodeling by ACE inhibitors reduces the development of symptomatic heart failure and death in stage B asymptomatic patients with left ventricular dysfunction by about 20%.[1,2] In addition, deaths, often sudden and unexpected, attributed to cardiovascular causes, are reduced in stage B patients by ACE inhibitor therapy.

Several ACE inhibitors are effective as prophylactic therapy for high-risk stage B patients (see Fig. 59-1), and the target dose of each agent is established (Table 59-2). The angiotensin receptor blocker (ARB) valsartan (Table 59-3) is as effective as captopril in reducing risk for cardiovascular death and other nonfatal cardiovascular outcomes,[3] thereby providing an alternative pharmacologic class of agents. Importantly, in patients with left ventricular dysfunction or acute heart failure in the context of a myocardial infarction, the combination of an ACE inhibitor and ARB is not better than either alone, so combination therapy is not recommended in this setting.

β-Blockers

β-Adrenergic receptor blockers (β-blockers) have long been known to reduce death and recurrent myocardial infarction when they are administered during the acute phase of myocardial infarction in patients without pulmonary congestion (Chapter 73). However, carvedilol (Table 59-4) also improves survival, reduces subsequent nonfatal myocardial infarctions, and has a favorable trend for reduced hospitalizations for heart failure in patients with a recent myocardial infarction and reduced LVEF (≤40%) when it is added to an ACE inhibitor.[4] For stage B patients whose left ventricular dysfunction does not have an ischemic etiology, the evidence for β-blockers is less firm.

Treatment of Arrhythmias

Functional as well as structural problems may lead to the development of heart failure. For example, a persistently rapid ventricular rate in patients with atrial fibrillation can cause a rate-related (tachycardia-induced) cardiomyopathy (Chapter 64). Adequate pharmacologic control of the ventricular rate or interventions to restore sinus rhythm or to ablate re-entry pathways (Chapter 66) may reduce the risk for heart failure.

Other Therapies

Any treatments that control hypertension or reduce the risk of myocardial infarction will benefit stage B patients. Examples include statins, antiplatelet agents, and smoking cessation.

FIGURE 59-1. Stages of heart failure (HF). 4S = Scandinavian Simvastatin Survival Study; AFCAPS-Texcaps = Air Force/Texas Coronary Atherosclerosis Prevention Study; A-HeFT = African American Heart Failure Trial; AIRE = Acute Infarction Ramipril Efficacy study; ALLHAT = Antihypertensive and Lipid Lowering to Prevent Heart Attack Trial; ASCOT-LLA = Anglo-Scandinavian Cardiac Outcomes Trial—Lipid Lowering Arm; BHAT = The Beta-Blocker Heart Attack Trial; CAPRICORN = Carvedilol Post-Infarct Survival Control in LV Dysfunction; CARE HF = Cardiac Resynchronization in Heart Failure; CHARM added = Candesartan in Heart Failure—Added Trial; CHARM alternative = Candesartan in Heart Failure—Alternative Trial; CIBIS II = Cardiac Insufficiency Bisoprolol Study II; COMET = Carvedilol or Metoprolol European Trial; COMPANION = Comparison of Medical Therapy, Pacing, and Defibrillation in Heart Failure; CONSENSUS = Cooperative North Scandinavian Enalapril Survival Study; COPERNICUS = Carvedilol Prospective Randomized Cumulative Survival Trial; DIG = Digitalis Investigation Group; EPHESUS = Eplerenone Post-Acute Myocardial Infarction Heart Failure Efficacy and Survival Study; EUROPA = European Trial on Reduction of Cardiac Events with Perindopril in Stable Coronary Artery Disease; HOPE = Heart Outcomes Prevention Evaluation; HOT = Hypertension Optimal Treatment; HPS = Heart Protection Study; MADIT II = Multicenter Automatic Defibrillator Implantation Trial II; MERIT-HF = Metoprolol CR/XL Randomized Intervention Trial in Congestive Heart Failure; PEACE = Prevention of Events with ACE inhibition; RALES = Randomised Aldactone Evaluation Study; REMATCH = Randomized Evaluation of Mechanical Assistance for the Treatment of Congestive Heart Failure; SAVE = Survival and Ventricular Enlargement trial; SCD-HeFT = Sudden Cardiac Death in Heart Failure Trial; SHEP = Systolic Hypertension in the Elderly Program; SOLVD-P = Studies of Left Ventricular Dysfunction-Prevention; SOLVD-T = Studies of Left Ventricular Dysfunction-Treatment; TRACE = Trandolapril Cardiac Evaluation; VALIANT = Valsartan in Acute Myocardial Infarction Trial; VHeFT = Vasodilator-Heart Failure Trials; WOSCOPS = West of Scotland Coronary Prevention Study.

TABLE 59-2 PRACTICAL GUIDANCE ON THE USE OF ANGIOTENSIN-CONVERTING ENZYME INHIBITORS IN PATIENTS WITH HEART FAILURE DUE TO LEFT VENTRICULAR SYSTOLIC DYSFUNCTION

WHY?

Two major randomized trials (CONSENSUS I and SOLVD-T) and a meta-analysis of smaller trials have conclusively shown that angiotensin-converting enzyme (ACE) inhibitors increase survival, reduce hospital admissions, and improve NYHA class and quality of life in patients with *all* grades of symptomatic heart failure. Other major randomized trials in patients with systolic dysfunction after acute myocardial infarction (SAVE, AIRE, TRACE) have shown that ACE inhibitors increase survival. In patients with heart failure (ATLAS), the composite end point of death or hospital admission was reduced by higher doses of ACE inhibitor compared with lower doses. ACE inhibitors have also been shown to delay or to prevent the development of symptomatic heart failure in patients with *asymptomatic* left ventricular systolic dysfunction.

IN WHOM AND WHEN?

Indications:
  Potentially *all* patients with heart failure and a low ejection fraction
  First-line treatment (along with β-blockers) in patients with NYHA class II-IV heart failure; start as early as possible in course of disease. ACE inhibitors are also of benefit in patients with asymptomatic left ventricular systolic dysfunction (NYHA class I).
Contraindications:
  History of angioedema
  Known bilateral renal artery stenosis
Cautions/seek specialist advice:
  Significant hyperkalemia (K$^+$ > 5.0 mmol/L)
  Significant renal dysfunction (creatinine >221 μmol/L or >2.5 mg/dL)
  Symptomatic or severe asymptomatic hypotension (systolic blood pressure <90 mm Hg)
Drug interactions to look out for:
  K$^+$ supplements/K$^+$-sparing diuretics, e.g., amiloride and triamterene (beware combination preparations with furosemide)
  Aldosterone antagonists (spironolactone, eplerenone), angiotensin receptor blockers, NSAIDs*
  "Low-salt" substitutes with a high K$^+$ content

WHERE?

In the community for most patients
Exceptions—see *Cautions/seek specialist advice*

WHICH ACE INHIBITOR AND WHAT DOSE?

	Starting Dose	Target Dose
Captopril	6.25 mg thrice daily	50 mg thrice daily
Enalapril	2.5 mg twice daily	10-20 mg twice daily
Lisinopril	2.5-5.0 mg once daily	20-35 mg once daily
Ramipril	2.5 mg once daily	5 mg twice daily or 10 mg once daily
Trandolapril	0.5 mg once daily	4 mg once daily

HOW TO USE?

Start with a low dose (see above).
Double dose at not less than 2-week intervals.
Aim for target dose (see above) or, failing that, the highest tolerated dose.
Remember: some ACE inhibitor is better than no ACE inhibitor.
Monitor blood pressure and blood chemistry (urea/blood urea nitrogen, creatinine, K$^+$).
Check blood chemistry 1-2 weeks after initiation and 1-2 weeks after final dose titration.
When to stop up-titration, reduce dose, stop treatment—see Problem Solving.
A specialist heart failure nurse may assist with education of the patient, follow-up (in person or by telephone), biochemical monitoring, and dose up-titration.

ADVICE TO PATIENT

Explain expected benefits (see Why?).
Treatment is given to improve symptoms, to prevent worsening of heart failure leading to hospital admission, and to increase survival.
Symptoms improve within a few weeks to a few months of starting treatment.
Advise patients to report principal adverse effects, (i.e., dizziness/symptomatic hypotension, cough)—see Problem Solving.
Advise patients to avoid NSAIDs* not prescribed by a physician (self-purchased over-the-counter) and salt substitutes high in K$^+$—see Problem Solving.

PROBLEM SOLVING

Asymptomatic low blood pressure
  Does not usually require any change in therapy
Symptomatic hypotension
  If dizziness, lightheadedness, or confusion and a low blood pressure, reconsider need for nitrates, calcium-channel blockers,† and other vasodilators.
  If no signs or symptoms of congestion, consider reducing diuretic dose.
  If these measures do not solve problem, seek specialist advice.
Cough
  Cough is common in patients with heart failure, many of whom have smoking-related lung disease.
  Cough is also a symptom of pulmonary edema, which should be excluded when a new or worsening cough develops.
  ACE inhibitor–induced cough rarely requires treatment discontinuation.
  When a troublesome cough does develop (e.g., one stopping the patient from sleeping) and can be proved to be due to ACE inhibition (i.e., recurs after ACE inhibitor withdrawal and rechallenge), substitution of an angiotensin receptor blocker can be considered (see Table 59-3).
Worsening renal function
  Some rise in urea (blood urea nitrogen), creatinine, and potassium is to be expected after initiation of an ACE inhibitor; if an increase is small and asymptomatic, no action is necessary.
  An increase in creatinine of up to 50% above baseline, or ≤266 μmol/L (3 mg/dL), whichever is the smaller, is acceptable.
  An increase in potassium to ≤5.5 mmol/L is acceptable.
  If urea, creatinine, or potassium does rise excessively, consider stopping concomitant nephrotoxic drugs (e.g., NSAIDs*) and other potassium supplements or retaining agents (triamterene, amiloride, spironolactone-eplerenone‡) and, if no signs of congestion, reducing the dose of diuretic.
  If greater rises in creatinine or potassium than those outlined above persist despite adjustment of concomitant medications, the dose of the ACE inhibitor should be halved and blood chemistry rechecked within 1-2 weeks; if there is still an unsatisfactory response, specialist advice should be sought.
  If potassium rises to >5.5 mmol/L or creatinine increases by >100% or to above 310 μmol/L (3.5 mg/dL), the ACE inhibitor should be stopped and specialist advice sought.
  Blood chemistry should be monitored frequently and serially until potassium and creatinine have plateaued.

Note: It is very rarely necessary to stop an ACE inhibitor, and clinical deterioration is likely if treatment is withdrawn. Ideally, specialist advice should be sought before treatment discontinuation.
*Avoid nonsteroidal anti-inflammatory drugs (NSAIDs) unless essential.
†Calcium-channel blockers should be discontinued unless absolutely essential (e.g., for angina or hypertension).
‡The safety and efficacy of an ACE inhibitor used with an angiotensin receptor blocker and spironolactone (as well as β-blocker) are uncertain, and the use of all three inhibitors of the renin-angiotensin-aldosterone system together is not recommended.
Modified from McMurray J, Cohen-Solal A, Dietz R, et al. Practical recommendations for the use of ACE inhibitors, β-blockers, aldosterone antagonists and angiotensin receptor blockers in heart failure: putting guidelines into practice. *Eur J Heart Fail.* 2005;7:710-721.

Stages C and D: Symptomatic Heart Failure

The development of symptoms and signs of the heart failure syndrome defines the transition from patients in the asymptomatic "at-risk" stages (A and B) to those who fulfill the clinical diagnosis of symptomatic heart failure (Chapter 58). This transition to the symptomatic phase underscores the progressive nature of heart failure and heralds a marked decline in prognosis. In one study, for example, the 2-year mortality rate was 27% in symptomatic patients compared with 10% in asymptomatic patients despite similarly reduced LVEFs and comorbidities.

TABLE 59-3 PRACTICAL GUIDANCE ON THE USE OF ANGIOTENSIN RECEPTOR BLOCKERS IN PATIENTS WITH HEART FAILURE DUE TO LEFT VENTRICULAR SYSTOLIC DYSFUNCTION

WHY?

Added to standard therapy, including an angiotensin-converting enzyme (ACE) inhibitor, in patients with all grades of symptomatic heart failure, the angiotensin receptor blockers (ARBs) valsartan and candesartan have been shown, in two major randomized trials (Val-HeFT and CHARM), to reduce heart failure hospital admissions, to improve NYHA class, and to maintain quality of life. The two CHARM low-left ventricular ejection fraction trials (CHARM-Alternative and CHARM-Added) also showed that candesartan reduced all-cause mortality. In patients previously intolerant of an ACE inhibitor, candesartan has been shown to reduce the risk of the composite outcome of cardiovascular death or heart failure hospitalization, to reduce the risk of heart failure hospital admission, and to improve NYHA class. These findings in heart failure are supported by another randomized trial in patients with left ventricular systolic dysfunction, heart failure, or both complicating acute myocardial infarction (VALIANT) in which valsartan was as effective as the ACE inhibitor captopril in reducing mortality and cardiovascular morbidity.

IN WHOM AND WHEN?

Indications:
    Potentially *all* patients with heart failure
    First-line treatment (along with β-blockers) in patients with NYHA class II-IV heart failure intolerant of an ACE inhibitor
    Second-line treatment (after optimization of ACE inhibitor and β-blocker*) in patients with NYHA class II-IV heart failure
Contraindications:
    Known bilateral renal artery stenosis
Cautions/seek specialist advice:
    Significant hyperkalemia (K^+ > 5.0 mmol/L)
    Significant renal dysfunction (creatinine, >221 μmol/L or >2.5 mg/dL)
    Symptomatic or severe asymptomatic hypotension (systolic blood pressure < 90 mm Hg)
Drug interactions to look out for:
    K^+ supplements/K^+-sparing diuretics, e.g., amiloride and triamterene (beware combination preparations with furosemide)
    Aldosterone antagonists (spironolactone, eplerenone), ACE inhibitors, NSAIDs†
    "Low-salt" substitutes with a high K^+ content

WHERE?

In the community for most patients
Exceptions—see *Cautions/seek specialist advice*

WHICH ARB AND WHAT DOSE?

	Starting Dose	Target Dose
Candesartan	4 or 8 mg once daily	32 mg once daily
Valsartan	40 mg twice daily	160 mg twice daily
Losartan	50 mg once daily	150 mg daily

HOW TO USE?

Start with a low dose (see above).
Double dose at not less than 2-week intervals.
Aim for target dose (see above) or, failing that, the highest tolerated dose.
Remember: some ARB is better than no ARB.
Monitor blood pressure and blood chemistry (urea/blood urea nitrogen, creatinine, K^+).
Check blood chemistry 1-2 weeks after initiation and 1-2 weeks after final dose titration.
When to stop up-titration, reduce dose, stop treatment—see Problem Solving.
A specialist heart failure nurse may assist with education of the patient, follow-up (in person or by telephone), biochemical monitoring, and dose up-titration.

ADVICE TO PATIENT

Explain expected benefits (see Why?).
Treatment is given to improve symptoms, to prevent worsening of heart failure leading to hospital admission, and to increase survival.
Symptoms improve within a few weeks to a few months of starting treatment.
Advise patients to report principal adverse effect (i.e., report dizziness/symptomatic hypotension)—see Problem Solving.
Advise patients to avoid NSAIDs† not prescribed by a physician (self-purchased over-the-counter) and salt substitutes high in K^+—see Problem Solving.

PROBLEM SOLVING

Asymptomatic low blood pressure
    Does not usually require any change in therapy
Symptomatic hypotension
    If dizziness, lightheadedness, or confusion and a low blood pressure, reconsider need for nitrates, calcium-channel blockers,‡ and other vasodilators.
    If no signs or symptoms of congestion, consider reducing diuretic dose.
    If these measures do not solve problem, seek specialist advice.
Worsening renal function
    Some rise in urea (blood urea nitrogen), creatinine, and potassium is to be expected after initiation of an ARB; if the increase is small and asymptomatic, no action is necessary.
    An increase in creatinine of up to 50% above baseline, or ≤266 μmol/L (3 mg/dL), whichever is the smaller, is acceptable.
    An increase in potassium to ≤5.5 mmol/L is acceptable.
    If urea, creatinine, or potassium does rise excessively, consider stopping concomitant nephrotoxic drugs (e.g., NSAIDs†) and potassium supplements or retaining agents (triamterene, amiloride, spironolactone-eplerenone*) and, if no signs of congestion, reducing the dose of diuretic.
    If greater rises in creatinine or potassium than those outlined above persist despite adjustment of concomitant medications, the dose of the ARB should be halved and blood chemistry rechecked within 1-2 weeks; if there is still an unsatisfactory response, specialist advice should be sought.
    If potassium rises to >5.5 mmol/L or creatinine increases by >100% or to above 310 μmol/L (3.5 mg/dL), the ARB should be stopped and specialist advice sought.
    Blood chemistry should be monitored frequently and serially until potassium and creatinine have plateaued.

Note: It is very rarely necessary to stop an ARB, and clinical deterioration is likely if treatment is withdrawn. Ideally, specialist advice should be sought before treatment discontinuation.

*The safety and efficacy of an ARB used with an ACE inhibitor and spironolactone (as well as a β-blocker) are uncertain, and the use of all three inhibitors of the renin-angiotensin-aldosterone system together is not recommended.

†Avoid nonsteroidal anti-inflammatory drugs (NSAIDs) unless essential.

‡Calcium-channel blockers should be discontinued unless absolutely essential (e.g., for angina or hypertension).

Modified from McMurray J, Cohen-Solal A, Dietz R, et al. Practical recommendations for the use of ACE inhibitors, β-blockers, aldosterone antagonists and angiotensin receptor blockers in heart failure: putting guidelines into practice. *Eur J Heart Fail.* 2005;7:710-721.

TREATMENT   (Rx)

The goals of treatment for patients with stage C and stage D heart failure are relief of symptoms, avoidance of hospital admission, and prevention of premature death. In general, the preventive measures that are of value during stages A and B should be sustained in patients with stages C and D heart failure.

Heart Failure with Reduced Left Ventricular Ejection Fraction

Pharmacologic Treatment

Drugs are the mainstay of the treatment of patients with symptomatic heart failure on the basis of the cumulative experiences from RCTs (see Table 59-1), particularly for patients with reduced LVEF. However, devices and surgery have an important and increasing role in patients with advanced symptomatic heart failure (stages C and D; see Fig. 59-1). Exercise clearly improves well-being and clinical outcomes (see Table 59-1), but the evidence base for other lifestyle interventions is less robust. The organization and delivery of care can also have a substantial impact on outcomes.

Diuretics

Mechanism of Action. Diuretics act by blocking sodium reabsorption at specific sites in the renal tubule, thereby enhancing urinary excretion of sodium and water.

Clinical Benefits. Although not proven to improve mortality and morbidity in large trials, diuretics are required in nearly all patients with symptomatic heart failure (stages C and D) to relieve dyspnea and the signs of sodium and water retention ("congestion"), that is, peripheral and pulmonary edema. No other treatment relieves symptoms and the signs of sodium and water overload as rapidly and effectively. Once a patient needs a diuretic, treatment is usually necessary for the rest of the patient's life, although the dose and type of diuretic may vary.

TABLE 59-4 PRACTICAL GUIDANCE ON THE USE OF β-BLOCKERS IN PATIENTS WITH HEART FAILURE DUE TO LEFT VENTRICULAR SYSTOLIC DYSFUNCTION

WHY?

Several major randomized controlled trials (i.e., USCP, CIBIS II, MERIT-HF, COPERNICUS) have shown, conclusively, that certain β-blockers increase survival, reduce hospital admissions, and improve NYHA class and quality of life when added to standard therapy (diuretics, digoxin, and angiotensin-converting enzyme [ACE] inhibitors) in patients with *stable* mild and moderate heart failure and in some patients with severe heart failure. In the SENIORS trial, which differed substantially in design from the aforementioned studies (older patients, some patients with preserved left ventricular systolic function, longer follow-up), nebivolol appeared to have a smaller treatment effect, although direct comparison is difficult. One other trial (BEST) did not show a reduction in all-cause mortality but did report a reduction in cardiovascular mortality and is otherwise broadly consistent with the aforementioned studies. The COMET trial showed that carvedilol was substantially more effective than a low dose of short-acting metoprolol tartrate* (long-acting metoprolol succinate was used in MERIT-HF).

IN WHOM AND WHEN?

Indications:
  Potentially *all* patients with *stable* mild and moderate heart failure; patients with severe heart failure should be referred for specialist advice
  First-line treatment (along with ACE inhibitors) in patients with *stable* NYHA class II-III heart failure; start as early as possible in course of disease
Contraindications:
  Asthma
  Second- or third-degree atrioventricular block
Cautions/seek specialist advice:
  Severe (NYHA class IV) heart failure
  Current or recent (<4 wk) exacerbation of heart failure (e.g., hospital admission with worsening heart failure, heart block, or heart rate <60/min)
  Persisting signs of congestion, hypotension/low blood pressure (systolic <90 mm Hg), raised jugular venous pressure, ascites, marked peripheral edema
Drug interactions to look out for:
  Verapamil, diltiazem (should be discontinued)[†]
  Digoxin, amiodarone

WHERE?

In the community in stable patients (NYHA class IV/severe heart failure patients should be referred for specialist advice)
Not in unstable patients hospitalized with worsening heart failure
Other exceptions—see *Cautions/seek specialist advice*

WHICH β-BLOCKER AND WHAT DOSE?

	Starting Dose	Target Dose
Bisoprolol	1.25 mg once daily	10 mg once daily
Carvedilol	3.125 mg twice daily	25-50 mg twice daily
Metoprolol CR/XL	12.5-25 mg once daily	200 mg once daily*
Nebivolol	1.25 mg once daily	10 mg once daily

HOW TO USE?

Start with a low dose (see above).
Double dose at not less than 2-week intervals.
Aim for target dose (see above) or, failing that, the highest tolerated dose.
Remember: some β-blocker is better than no β-blocker.
Monitor heart rate, blood pressure, and clinical status (symptoms, signs—especially signs of congestion, body weight).
Check blood chemistry 1-2 weeks after initiation and 1-2 weeks after final dose titration.
When to stop up-titration, reduce dose, stop treatment—see Problem Solving.
A specialist heart failure nurse may assist with education of the patient, follow-up (in person or by telephone), and dose up-titration.

ADVICE TO PATIENT

Explain expected benefits (see Why?).
Treatment is given to improve symptoms, to prevent worsening of heart failure leading to hospital admission, and to increase survival.
Symptomatic improvement may develop slowly after starting treatment, taking 3-6 months or longer.
Temporary symptomatic deterioration may occur during initiation or up-titration phase; in the long term, β-blockers improve well-being.
Advise patient to report deterioration (see Problem Solving) and that deterioration (tiredness, fatigue, breathlessness) can usually be easily managed by adjustment of other medication; patients should be advised not to stop β-blocker therapy without consulting the physician.
To detect and to treat deterioration early, patients should be encouraged to weigh themselves daily (after waking, before dressing, after voiding, before eating) and to increase their diuretic dose should their weight increase, persistently (>2 days), by >1.5-2.0 kg.[‡]

PROBLEM SOLVING

Worsening symptoms or signs (e.g., increasing dyspnea, fatigue, edema, weight gain)
  If increasing congestion, increase dose of diuretic or halve dose of β-blocker (if increasing diuretic does not work).
  If marked fatigue (or bradycardia—see below), halve dose of β-blocker (rarely necessary); review patient in 1-2 weeks; if not improved, seek specialist advice.
  If serious deterioration, halve dose of β-blocker or stop this treatment (rarely necessary); seek specialist advice.
Low heart rate
  If <50 beats/min and worsening symptoms, halve dose of β-blocker or, if severe deterioration, stop β-blocker (rarely necessary).
  Review need for other heart rate–slowing drugs (e.g., digoxin, amiodarone, diltiazem, or verapamil[†]).
  Arrange electrocardiogram to exclude heart block.
  Seek specialist advice.
Asymptomatic low blood pressure
  Does not usually require any change in therapy
Symptomatic hypotension
  If dizziness, lightheadedness, or confusion and a low blood pressure, reconsider need for nitrates, calcium-channel blockers,† and other vasodilators.
  If no signs or symptoms of congestion, consider reducing diuretic dose or ACE inhibitor.
  If these measures do not solve problem, seek specialist advice.

Note: β-Blockers should not be stopped suddenly unless absolutely necessary (there is a risk for a "rebound" increase in myocardial ischemia or infarction and arrhythmias). Ideally, specialist advice should be sought before treatment discontinuation.

*Metoprolol tartrate should not be used in preference to an evidence-based β-blocker in heart failure.

†Calcium-channel blockers should be discontinued unless absolutely necessary, and diltiazem and verapamil are generally contraindicated in heart failure.

‡This is generally good advice for all patients with heart failure.

Modified from McMurray J, Cohen-Solal A, Dietz R, et al. Practical recommendations for the use of ACE inhibitors, β-blockers, aldosterone antagonists and angiotensin receptor blockers in heart failure: putting guidelines into practice. *Eur J Heart Fail.* 2005;7:710-721.

Practical Use. The key principle is to prescribe the minimum dose of diuretic needed to maintain an edema-free state ("dry weight"). Excessive use can lead to electrolyte imbalances, such as hyponatremia, hypokalemia (and risk of digitalis toxicity), hyperuricemia (and risk of gout), and uremia. The risk of renal dysfunction is increased by concomitant use of nonsteroidal anti-inflammatory drugs (NSAIDs). Diuretic-induced hypovolemia may also cause symptomatic hypotension and prerenal azotemia. Restriction of dietary sodium intake may help reduce but does not eliminate the requirement for diuretics. Diuretic dosing should be flexible, with temporary increases for evidence of fluid retention (e.g., increasing symptoms, weight gain, edema) and decreases for evidence of hypovolemia (e.g., as a consequence of increased electrolyte loss due to gastroenteritis, decreased fluid intake, or both).

In some patients with milder symptoms of heart failure and preserved renal function (stage C), a thiazide diuretic such as chlorthalidone may suffice. In more advanced heart failure (stage D) or in patients with concomitant renal dysfunction, a loop diuretic such as furosemide is often needed. Loop diuretics cause a rapid onset of an intense but relatively short-lived diuresis compared with the longer-lasting but gentler effect of a thiazide diuretic. The timing of administration of a loop diuretic, which need not be taken first thing every morning, can be adjusted according to the patient's social activities. The dose may be postponed or even temporarily omitted if the patient has to travel or has another activity that might be compromised by the prompt action of the diuretic. In severe heart failure (stage D), the effects of long-term administration of a loop diuretic may be diminished by increased sodium reabsorption at the distal tubule. This problem can be offset by use of the combination of a loop diuretic and a thiazide or thiazide-like diuretic (e.g., hydrochlorothiazide or metolazone), which act in synergy with a loop diuretic by blocking sodium reabsorption in different segments of the nephron. This combination requires more frequent monitoring of electrolytes and renal function for diuretic-induced hyponatremia, abnormalities of the serum potassium level, and prerenal azotemia.

A period of intravenous loop diuretic, given either as bolus injections or by continuous infusion, may be required in patients who become resistant to the action of oral diuretics. Why this resistance develops is uncertain, but factors thought to be important include impaired absorption of oral diuretics due to gut edema, hypotension, reduced renal blood flow, and adaptive changes in the nephron.

In patients with advanced heart failure (stage D), an aldosterone antagonist, such as spironolactone, which increases excretion of sodium but not of potassium, usually should be added. Patients receiving a combination of diuretics require careful monitoring of blood chemistry and clinical status. The use of an aldosterone antagonist (or, rarely, a potassium-sparing diuretic) along with an ACE inhibitor or ARB (treatment with all three is not recommended) requires particular care and surveillance for hyperkalemia.

Although they are highly effective in relieving symptoms and signs, diuretics alone are not sufficient for treatment of heart failure. In cases of severe resistant volume overload, mechanical removal of fluid by ultrafiltration may be considered. The addition of other treatments will better maintain clinical stability, slow structural progression, and reduce the risk of hospital admission and premature death.

ACE Inhibitors

Mechanism of Action. These drugs act by inhibiting the enzyme that converts the inactive decapeptide angiotensin I to the active octapeptide angiotensin II (and that also breaks down bradykinin). In patients with heart failure, excessive angiotensin II is thought to exert myriad harmful actions mediated through stimulation of the angiotensin II type 1 receptor subtype (AT_1R), including vasoconstriction (which increases ventricular afterload), excessive growth of myocytes and the extracellular matrix (contributing to maladaptive left ventricular remodeling), activation of the sympathetic nervous system, prothrombotic actions, and augmentation of the release of arginine vasopressin and the retention of sodium (both directly and through stimulation of aldosterone secretion).

ACE inhibitors also reduce the breakdown of bradykinin (as ACE is identical to kininase II), and the resultant accumulation of bradykinin is directly or indirectly responsible for two of the specific adverse effects of ACE inhibitors, cough and angioedema. Bradykinin may, however, also have beneficial effects (vasodilation, inhibition of adverse cardiovascular remodeling, and antithrombotic actions), although the importance of these bradykinin-mediated actions to the clinical benefits of ACE inhibition is uncertain.

Clinical Benefits. Clinical trials have shown that treatment with an ACE inhibitor, when it is used alone or added to diuretics and digoxin, decreases left ventricular size, improves systolic function, reduces symptoms and hospital admissions, and prolongs survival (see Table 59-1).[5,6] These agents also reduce the risk for development of myocardial infarction, diabetes, and atrial fibrillation. Consequently, treatment with an ACE inhibitor is recommended for all patients with systolic dysfunction, irrespective of symptoms or etiology. ACE inhibitors are not a substitute for a diuretic but mitigate diuretic-induced hypokalemia.

Practical Use. ACE inhibitors should be introduced as early as possible in a patient's treatment. The only contraindications are current symptomatic

hypotension and bilateral renal artery stenosis (Chapter 127); the latter is often associated with a prompt and marked increase in serum levels of blood urea nitrogen and creatinine when renal perfusion is reduced precipitously by inhibiting the production and actions of angiotensin. Treatment should be started in a low dose (see Table 59-2), with the dose gradually increased toward a target dose proven of benefit in a clinical trial. The patient should be evaluated for symptomatic hypotension, uremia, and hyperkalemia after each dose increment; these adverse effects are uncommon and can usually be resolved by reduction in the dose of diuretic (if the patient is edema free) or concomitant hypotensive or nephrotoxic medications (e.g., nitrates, calcium-channel blockers, or NSAIDs). A dry, nonproductive cough occurs in approximately 15% of patients treated with an ACE inhibitor, and if it is troublesome, substitution of an ARB is recommended. In the rare cases of angioedema (Chapter 260), the ACE inhibitor should be stopped and not used again; an ARB can be cautiously substituted.

Angiotensin Receptor Blockers

Mechanism of Action. Instead of inhibiting the production of angiotensin II through ACE, ARBs block the binding of angiotensin II to the AT_1R. This pharmacologically distinct mechanism of action may be important because angiotensin II is also believed to be produced by other enzymes, such as chymase. ARBs do not inhibit kininase II or the breakdown of bradykinin, so they do not cause cough and cause less angioedema than do ACE inhibitors.

Clinical Benefits. When they are used as the sole agent in heart failure, ARBs produce benefits similar to those of ACE inhibitors and can be substituted for them in patients who have cough or angioedema with ACE inhibitors.[7,8] When they are used in clinically effective doses, other adverse effects such as hypotension, renal dysfunction, and hyperkalemia are encountered as frequently as with an ACE inhibitor. As with an ACE inhibitor, the specific agents, dosing regimens, and target doses that were of demonstrable benefit in clinical trials are recommended (see Table 59-1).

In the broader population of patients with symptomatic (stage C or stage D, functional class II to class IV) heart failure that can be treated with an ACE inhibitor, an ARB *in combination with* an ACE inhibitor (and β-blocker) further improves LVEF, relieves symptoms, reduces the risk of hospital admission for worsening heart failure, and can also reduce the risk for cardiovascular death (see Table 59-3).[8,9] Consequently, the addition of an ARB to both an ACE inhibitor and a β-blocker may be considered in any patient with persisting symptoms (stages C and D). There is, however, also strong evidence that addition of an aldosterone antagonist to an ACE inhibitor is of benefit in patients with advanced (classes III to IV) heart failure (see later), but the efficacy and safety of the four-drug combination of an ACE inhibitor, β-blocker, ARB, and aldosterone antagonist are uncertain. Consequently, either an ARB or an aldosterone antagonist, but not both, should be added to an ACE inhibitor and a β-blocker in such patients.

The approach to initiation, titration, and monitoring of an ARB is similar to that of an ACE inhibitor (see Table 59-3). The adverse effects, with the exception of cough and angioedema, are similar. Use of multiple inhibitors of the renin-angiotensin-aldosterone system requires even more diligent monitoring, especially in patients at higher risk for uremia, hypotension, or hyperkalemia (i.e., patients 75 years of age and older or with a systolic blood pressure below 100 mm Hg, diabetes, or renal impairment) because combined treatment with an ACE inhibitor and an ARB significantly increases the risks of worsening renal function, hyperkalemia, and symptomatic hypotension.

As with ACE inhibitors, β-blockers, and aldosterone antagonists, treatment with ARBs should be indefinite unless there is intolerance.

β-Blockers

Mechanism of Action. Heart failure is characterized by excessive activation of the sympathetic nervous system, which causes vasoconstriction and sodium retention, thereby increasing cardiac preload and afterload and often inducing myocardial ischemia or arrhythmias. In addition, norepinephrine can cause hypertrophy of myocytes and augment their apoptosis. β-Blockers counteract many of these harmful effects of the hyperactivity of the sympathetic nervous system.

Clinical Benefits. The long-term addition of a β-blocker to an ACE inhibitor (and diuretic and digoxin) further improves left ventricular function and symptoms, reduces hospital admissions, and strikingly improves survival.[10] Consequently, a β-blocker is recommended for all patients with symptomatic systolic dysfunction, irrespective of etiology and severity, and the combination of a β-blocker with an ACE inhibitor is now the cornerstone of the treatment of symptomatic heart failure (see Fig. 59-1).

Practical Use. The major contraindications to use of a β-blocker in heart failure are asthma (although it is important to note that the dyspnea caused by pulmonary congestion can be confused with reactive airway disease) and second- or third-degree atrioventricular block. Initiation of treatment during an episode of acute decompensated heart failure should also generally be avoided. In addition, caution is advised in patients with a heart rate below 60 beats per minute or a systolic blood pressure below 90 mm Hg. It is recommended that a β-blocker shown to produce benefits in a randomized trial be used (see Table 59-1).

Like ACE inhibitors, β-blockers should be introduced as early as possible in a patient's treatment, started in a low dose (see Table 59-4), and increased gradually toward a target dose used in a clinical trial (the "start low–go slow" approach). The patient should be checked for symptomatic hypotension and excessive bradycardia after each dose increment, but both of these side effects are uncommon, and hypotension can often be resolved by reduction in the dose of other nonessential blood pressure–lowering medications (e.g., nitrates and calcium-channel blockers). Bradycardia is more likely in patients who are also taking digoxin or amiodarone, and the simultaneous use of these agents should be reviewed if excessive bradycardia occurs. On occasion, symptomatic worsening and fluid retention (e.g., weight gain or edema) may occur after initiation of a β-blocker or during dose up-titration; these side effects usually can be resolved by a temporary increase in the diuretic dose without necessitating discontinuation of the β-blocker.

Treatment with a β-blocker should be given for life, although the dose may need to be decreased (or, rarely, treatment discontinued) during episodes of acute decompensation if the patient shows signs of circulatory underperfusion or refractory congestion.

Aldosterone Antagonists

Mechanism of Action. Aldosterone, which is the second effector hormone in the renin-angiotensin-aldosterone cascade, has detrimental vascular, renal, autonomic, and cardiac actions when it is produced in excess in patients with heart failure. Excessive aldosterone promotes sodium retention and hypokalemia, and it is believed to contribute to myocardial fibrosis, all of which predispose to arrhythmias. Aldosterone antagonists block these undesirable actions and act as potassium-sparing diuretics.

Clinical Benefits. The aldosterone antagonist spironolactone (Table 59-5) improves symptoms, reduces hospital admissions, and increases survival when it is added to an ACE inhibitor (and diuretics and digoxin) in patients with a

reduced LVEF and severely symptomatic heart failure.[11] Eplerenone, another aldosterone antagonist, reduces mortality and morbidity when it is added to both an ACE inhibitor and β-blocker in patients with a reduced LVEF and heart failure or diabetes after a recent myocardial infarction (see Table 59-5)[12] and when added to an ACE inhibitor/ARB and β-blockers in class II heart failure.[13] Consequently, an aldosterone antagonist should be considered in patients who remain in severe heart failure (class III or IV) despite treatment with a diuretic, ACE inhibitor (or ARB), and β-blocker. When begun, it should be given indefinitely. The combination of an ACE inhibitor, an ARB, and an aldosterone antagonist has not been adequately evaluated and is not recommended.

Treatment with an aldosterone antagonist should be initiated with a low dose (see Table 59-5) with careful monitoring of serum electrolytes and renal function. Hyperkalemia and uremia are the adverse effects of greatest concern (as with ACE inhibitors and ARBs), and an aldosterone antagonist should not be given to patients with a serum potassium concentration of more than 5.0 mmol/L, serum creatinine concentration above 2.5 mg/dL (>221 μmol/L) or other evidence of markedly impaired renal function. The importance of selection of patients and dose is underscored by reports of a worrisome incidence of serious hyperkalemia in community practice settings. Spironolactone can have antiandrogenic effects, especially painful gynecomastia, in men; because eplerenone has less of an action on the androgen receptor, it is a reasonable substitute in patients who experience this adverse effect.

Digoxin

Mechanism of Action. Digitalis glycosides inhibit the cell membrane Na^+,K^+-ATPase pump, thereby increasing intracellular calcium and myocardial contractility. In addition, digoxin is thought to enhance parasympathetic and reduce sympathetic nervous activity as well as to inhibit renin release.

TABLE 59-5 PRACTICAL GUIDANCE ON THE USE OF SPIRONOLACTONE IN PATIENTS WITH HEART FAILURE DUE TO LEFT VENTRICULAR SYSTOLIC DYSFUNCTION

WHY?

The RALES study showed that low-dose spironolactone increased survival, reduced hospital admissions, and improved NYHA class when added to standard therapy (diuretic, digoxin, angiotensin-converting enzyme [ACE] inhibitor, and, in a minority of cases, β-blocker) in patients with severe (NYHA class III or IV) heart failure. In patients with left ventricular systolic dysfunction and heart failure (or diabetes) complicating *acute* myocardial infarction (EPHESUS) and in patients with NYHA class II symptoms on an ACE inhibitor/ARB and β-blocker (EMPHASIS-HF), another aldosterone antagonist, eplerenone, increased survival and reduced hospital admissions for cardiac causes.

IN WHOM AND WHEN?

Indications:
Potentially all patients with symptomatic heart failure (class II-IV NYHA)
Second-line therapy (after ACE inhibitors and β-blockers*) in patients with NYHA class II-IV heart failure
Cautions/seek specialist advice:
Significant hyperkalemia (K^+ > 5.0 mmol/L)[†]
Significant renal dysfunction (creatinine > 221 μmol/L or 2.5 mg/dL)[†]
Drug interactions to look out for:
K^+ supplements/K^+-sparing diuretics (e.g., amiloride and triamterene; beware combination preparations with furosemide)
ACE inhibitors, angiotensin receptor blockers, NSAIDs[‡]
"Low-salt" substitutes with a high K^+ content

WHERE?

In the community or in the hospital
Exceptions—see *Cautions/seek specialist advice*

WHICH DOSE?[†]

	Starting Dose	Target Dose
Spironolactone	25 mg once daily or on alternate days	25-50 mg once daily
Eplerenone	25 mg once daily	50 mg once daily

HOW TO USE?

Start with a low dose (see above).
Check blood chemistry at 1, 4, 8, and 12 weeks; 6, 9, and 12 months; every 6 months thereafter.
If K^+ rises above 5.5 mmol/L or creatinine rises to ≥221 μmol/L (2.5 mg/dL), reduce dose to 25 mg on alternate days and monitor blood chemistry closely.
If K^+ rises to ≥6.0 mmol/L or creatinine to ≥310 μmol/L (3.5 mg/dL), stop spironolactone immediately and seek specialist advice.
A specialist heart failure nurse may assist with education of the patient, follow-up (in person or by telephone), biochemical monitoring, and dose up-titration.

ADVICE TO PATIENT

Explain expected benefits (see Why?).
Treatment is given to improve symptoms, to prevent worsening of heart failure leading to hospital admission, and to increase survival.
Symptom improvement occurs within a few weeks to a few months of starting treatment.
Avoid NSAIDs[‡] not prescribed by a physician (self-purchased over-the-counter) and salt substitutes high in K^+.
If diarrhea or vomiting occurs, patients should stop spironolactone and contact the physician.

PROBLEM SOLVING

Worsening renal function/hyperkalemia
  See How to Use?
Major concern is hyperkalemia (>6.0 mmol/L); although this was uncommon in RALES, it has been seen more commonly in clinical practice.
  Conversely, a high-normal potassium level may be desirable in patients with heart failure, especially if they are taking digoxin.
  It is important to avoid other K^+-retaining drugs (e.g., K^+-sparing diuretics such as amiloride and triamterene) and nephrotoxic agents (e.g., NSAIDs[‡]).
  The risk for hyperkalemia and renal dysfunction when an aldosterone antagonist is given to patients already taking an ACE inhibitor and angiotensin receptor blocker is higher than when an aldosterone antagonist is added to just an ACE inhibitor or angiotensin receptor blocker given singly; close and careful monitoring is mandatory.*
Some "low-salt" substitutes have a high K^+ content.
Male patients treated with spironolactone may develop breast discomfort or gynecomastia (these problems are significantly less common with eplerenone).

---

*The safety and efficacy of spironolactone used with an ACE inhibitor *and* an angiotensin receptor blocker (as well as a β-blocker) are uncertain, and the use of all three inhibitors of the renin-angiotensin-aldosterone system together is not recommended.

[†]It is extremely important to adhere to these cautions and doses in light of recent evidence of serious hyperkalemia with spironolactone in usual clinical practice in Ontario.

[‡]Avoid nonsteroidal anti-inflammatory drugs (NSAIDs) unless essential.

Modified from McMurray J, Cohen-Solal A, Dietz R, et al. Practical recommendations for the use of ACE inhibitors, β-blockers, aldosterone antagonists and angiotensin receptor blockers in heart failure: putting guidelines into practice. *Eur J Heart Fail.* 2005;7:710-721.

Clinical Benefits. Only one large RCT has examined the effects of starting (as opposed to withdrawing) digoxin on mortality and morbidity in patients with heart failure in sinus rhythm. In that trial, digoxin did not reduce mortality but did decrease the risk for admission to hospital for worsening heart failure when it was added to a diuretic and an ACE inhibitor.[14] In patients in sinus rhythm, addition of digoxin is recommended only for those whose heart failure remains symptomatic despite standard three-drug treatment with a diuretic, ACE inhibitor, and β-blocker plus an ARB or aldosterone antagonist. In patients with atrial fibrillation, digoxin may be used at an earlier stage if a β-blocker fails to control the ventricular rate (ideally less than 70 beats per minute at rest and less than 100 beats per minute during exercise; Chapter 64). Digoxin can also be used to control the ventricular rate when β-blocker treatment is being initiated or up-titrated.

If the effect of digoxin is needed urgently, loading with 10 to 15 µg/kg *lean* body weight, given in three divided doses 6 hours apart, may be used. The maintenance dose should be one third of the loading dose. Smaller maintenance doses (e.g., one fourth of the loading dose and not more than 62.5 µg/day) should be used in elderly patients and in patients with reduced renal function as well as in patients with a low body mass. Monitoring of the serum digoxin concentration is recommended because of the narrow therapeutic window. A steady state is reached 7 to 10 days after treatment is started; blood should be collected at least 6 hours (and ideally 8 to 24 hours) after the last dose. The currently recommended therapeutic range is 0.5 to 1.0 ng/mL.

Digoxin can cause anorexia, nausea, arrhythmias, confusion, and visual disturbances, especially if the serum concentration is above 2.0 ng/mL. Hypokalemia increases susceptibility to the adverse effects. The dose of digoxin should be reduced in elderly patients and patients with renal dysfunction. Certain drugs increase serum digoxin concentration, including amiodarone.

Hydralazine and Isosorbide Dinitrate

Mechanism of Action. Hydralazine is a powerful direct-acting arterial vasodilator. Its mechanism of action is not understood, although it may inhibit enzymatic production of superoxide, which neutralizes nitric oxide and may induce nitrate tolerance. Nitrates dilate both veins and arteries, thereby reducing preload and afterload by stimulating the nitric oxide pathway and increasing cyclic guanosine monophosphate in vascular smooth muscle. Neither drug on its own nor any other direct-acting vasodilator has been demonstrated to be beneficial in heart failure.

Clinical Benefits. Although this combination has been known for some time to improve systolic function and probably to reduce death in classes II to IV heart failure compared with placebo, head-to-head comparison showed that an ACE inhibitor is superior for improving survival. Nevertheless, on the basis of subgroup analyses suggesting that African Americans responded better to hydralazine and isosorbide dinitrate, a subsequent RCT showed that the addition of hydralazine and isosorbide dinitrate in African Americans, most of whom were receiving an ACE inhibitor and β-blocker and many of whom were taking spironolactone, further reduced mortality and hospital admissions for heart failure and improved quality of life.[15]

A fixed combination of 37.5 mg of hydralazine and 20 mg of isosorbide dinitrate was used in the trial; one tablet was given and if tolerated, a second was given 12 hours later. One tablet was then prescribed three times daily for 3 to 5 days, at which point the dose was increased to the target maintenance of two tablets three times daily, that is, a daily dose of 225 mg hydralazine and 120 mg isosorbide dinitrate. Because of the limited inclusion criteria of this RCT, however, it is uncertain whether this combination of vasodilators is an effective addition in other populations of patients.

Practical Use. Other than for African Americans, the main indication for hydralazine and isosorbide dinitrate is in patients with intolerance to an ACE inhibitor and an ARB. Hydralazine and isosorbide dinitrate should be used as additional treatment in African Americans and considered for other patients who remain symptomatic with other proven therapies. The main dose-limiting adverse effects are headache and dizziness. A rare adverse effect of higher doses of hydralazine, especially in slow acetylators, is a systemic lupus erythematosus–like syndrome (Chapter 274).

Omega-3 Polyunsaturated Fatty Acids (n-3 PUFA)

A trial of 1 g of n-3 PUFA (850 to 852 mg eicosapentaenoic acid and docosahexaenoic acid as ethyl esters in the average ratio of 1:1.2) per day led to a small reduction in cardiovascular morbidity and mortality in patients with heart failure. However, in light of negative trials in post-MI patients and for the prevention of AF, the role of these agents remains uncertain.

Other Pharmacologic Issues

Ivabradine, a specific inhibitor of the sinus node (at 7.5 mg twice daily), reduces mean heart rate from 75 to 64 beats per minute and reduced subsequent hospital admission in patients with chronic heart failure by about 25%. However, this agent has not reduced mortality, and the risks of symptomatic bradycardia and other side effects offset much of its benefits. Some therapies that are of proven value for cardiovascular conditions that underlie or are associated with heart failure are of uncertain benefit (antiplatelet treatment, Chapter 37) or do not improve outcomes (statins, Chapter 213) in patients

with persistent, symptomatic heart failure. Warfarin is indicated in patients with atrial fibrillation, provided there is no contraindication to its use (Chapter 64). Warfarin may also be used in patients with evidence of intracardiac thrombus (e.g., detected during echocardiographic examination) or systemic thromboembolism. The many interactions of warfarin with other drugs, including some statins and amiodarone (Chapter 37), must always be considered when warfarin or another drug in a patient taking warfarin is initiated. Heparin prophylaxis (Chapter 37) against deep venous thrombosis is indicated when patients with heart failure are bed bound, such as during hospital admission.

Vaccination against influenza and pneumococcal infection is advised (Chapter 17) in all patients with heart failure because infection can lead to clinical deterioration.

The aforementioned treatments are the only pharmacologic therapies shown to be of benefit in patients with heart failure and a reduced LVEF. Other treatments have been tested in randomized trials and shown to have a neutral (e.g., amlodipine) or uncertain (e.g., bosentan and etanercept) effect on mortality and morbidity or to increase mortality (e.g., milrinone, flosequinan, vesnarinone, and moxonidine).

Drugs to Use with Caution in Heart Failure

Patients with heart failure, especially if it is severe, often have renal and hepatic dysfunction, so any drug excreted predominantly by the kidneys or metabolized by the liver may accumulate (Chapter 28). Similarly, because of their extensive comorbidity, patients with heart failure are inevitably treated with multiple drugs, thereby increasing the risk of drug interactions.

Drugs that should be avoided, if possible, in heart failure include thiazolidinediones (because of the risk of fluid retention), most antiarrhythmic drugs (including dronedarone, although amiodarone and dofetilide may be used), most calcium-channel blockers (with the exception of amlodipine), corticosteroids, NSAIDs, cyclooxygenase 2 inhibitors, many antipsychotics (e.g., clozapine), and antihistamines. Metformin (because of the risk of lactic acidosis) should be used with caution. Some salt substitutes contain substantial amounts of potassium and must be used cautiously. Other dietary constituents (e.g., grapefruit and cranberry juice) and supplements such as St. John's wort can interact with drugs taken by patients with heart failure, especially warfarin and digoxin.

Organization of Care

Several studies have shown that organized, nurse-led, multidisciplinary care can improve outcomes in patients with heart failure, particularly by reducing recurrent hospital admissions. The most successful approach seems to involve education of the patients, their families, and caregivers about heart failure and its treatment (including flexible diuretic dosing and reinforcing the importance of adherence), recognizing (and acting on) early deterioration (dyspnea, sudden weight gain, edema), and optimizing proven pharmacologic treatments.[16] A home-based rather than clinic-based approach may be best, although trials are needed to compare these types of interventions directly. Even telephone follow-up is of value. New technology enabling noninvasive home telemonitoring of physiologic measures (e.g., heart rate and rhythm, blood pressure, temperature, respiratory rate, weight, and estimated body water content) and implanted devices, which collect similar data and may be interrogated remotely, are also being tested as aids to monitoring and management. Despite the usefulness of B-type natriuretic peptide (BNP) in the diagnosis of heart failure and as a prognostic measure, treatment guided by BNP levels has not been shown in randomized trials to be any better than standard, evidence-based care.

Education

Education of the patient, family, and caregivers is invaluable (Table 59-6). Self-detection of early signs and symptoms of deterioration provides for earlier intervention. Counseling on the proper use of therapies, with an emphasis on adherence, is critical.

Useful patient-oriented material is available from several reliable sources the Heart Failure Society of America (*www.abouthf.org/education_modules.htm*), American Heart Association (*www.americanheart.org/presenter.jhtml?identifier=1486*), National Heart, Lung, and Blood Institute (*www.nhlbi.nih.gov/health/dci/Diseases/Hf/HF_WhatIs.html*), the Heart Failure Association of the European Society of Cardiology (*www.heartfailurematters.org/EN/Pages/index.aspx*), and other organizations.

Medication Use Counseling. When appropriate, a patient should be taught how to adjust the dose of diuretic within individualized limits. The dose should be increased (or a supplementary diuretic added) if there is evidence of fluid retention (symptoms of congestion) and decreased if there is evidence of hypovolemia (e.g., increased thirst associated with weight loss or postural dizziness, especially during hot weather or an illness causing decreased fluid intake or sodium and water loss). If hypovolemia is more marked, the doses of other medications also will have to be reduced.

The expected effects, beneficial and adverse, of other drugs should also be explained in detail (e.g., possible association of cough with ACE inhibitor). It is useful to inform patients that improvement with many drugs is gradual and may become fully apparent only after several weeks or even months of

TABLE 59-6 TOPICS THAT SHOULD BE DISCUSSED WITH A PATIENT WITH HEART FAILURE AND WITH HIS OR HER FAMILY AND CAREGIVERS

General advice
  Explain what heart failure is and why symptoms occur
    Causes of heart failure
    How to recognize symptoms
    What to do if symptoms occur
    Self-weighing (to identify fluid retention)
  Rationale for treatments
  Importance of adhering to pharmacologic and nonpharmacologic (e.g., dietary) treatments
  Smoking advice
  Prognosis
Drug counseling
  Rationale (i.e., benefits of individual drugs)
  Dose and time of administration
  Potential adverse effects (and what, if any, action to take)
  What to do in case of missed or skipped doses
  Self-management (e.g., flexible diuretic dosing)
Rest and exercise
  Rest
  Exercise and activities related to work
  Daily physical activity
  Sexual activity
  Rehabilitation
Vaccinations and immunizations
Travel
Driving
Dietary and social habits
  Control sodium intake when necessary (e.g., some patients with severe heart failure)
  Avoid excessive fluids in severe heart failure
  Avoid excessive alcohol intake

Modified from Swedberg K, Cleland J, Dargie H, et al, for the Task Force for the Diagnosis and Treatment of Chronic Heart Failure of the European Society of Cardiology. Guidelines for the diagnosis and treatment of chronic heart failure: executive summary (update 2005). *Eur Heart J.* 2005;26:1115-1140.

treatment. It is also important to explain the need for gradual titration with ACE inhibitors, ARBs, and β-blocking drugs to a desired dose level, which again may take weeks or even months to achieve. Patients should be advised not to use NSAIDs without consultation and to be cautious about using herbal or other nonproprietary preparations (Chapter 38).

Adherence. Education and counseling of the patient, caregiver, and family promote adherence, which is associated with better outcomes. Drug adherence can also be helped by certain pharmacy aids, such as dose allocation (dosette) boxes.

Exercise. Tailored, structured, supervised aerobic exercise is safe and improves functional capacity and quality of life in patients with heart failure (see Table 59-1).**17** An appropriate exercise prescription may also reduce hospitalizations and mortality in patients with heart failure.

Diet, Nutrition, Alcohol. Most guidelines advocate avoidance of foods containing relatively high salt content in the belief that doing so may reduce the need for diuretic therapy. This recommendation is based on clinical experience, which suggests that excess sodium intake can be a precipitant of clinical decompensation. Some salt substitutes have a high potassium content, which can lead to hyperkalemia.

Restriction of fluid intake is indicated only during episodes of decompensation associated with peripheral edema or hyponatremia. In these situations, daily intake should be restricted to 1.5 to 2.0 L to help facilitate reduction in extracellular fluid volume and to avoid hyponatremia.

Reducing excessive weight will reduce the work of the heart and may lower blood pressure (Chapter 67). Conversely, malnutrition is common in severe heart failure, and the development of cardiac cachexia is an ominous sign. Reduced food intake is sometimes caused by nausea (e.g., related to digoxin use or hepatosplenic congestion) or abdominal bloating (e.g., due to ascites). In these cases, small frequent meals and high-protein and high-calorie liquids may be helpful. In severe decompensated heart failure, eating may be difficult because of dyspnea.

Moderate alcohol intake is not thought to be harmful in heart failure, although excessive intake can cause cardiomyopathy and atrial arrhythmias in susceptible individuals. In patients with suspected alcoholic cardiomyopathy, abstinence from alcohol may improve cardiac function.

Smoking. Smoking causes peripheral vasoconstriction, which is detrimental in heart failure. Nicotine replacement therapy (Chapter 31) is believed to be safe in heart failure. The safety of bupropion in heart failure is uncertain, especially as it is known to increase blood pressure.

Sexual Activity. Sexual activity need not be restricted in patients with compensated heart failure, although dyspnea may be limiting. In men with erectile dysfunction (Chapter 242), treatment with a cyclic guanine monophosphate phosphodiesterase type 5 inhibitor can be useful, but these drugs must not be taken within 24 hours of prior nitrate use, and nitrates must not be restarted for at least 24 hours afterward.

Driving. Patients with heart failure can continue to drive, provided their condition does not induce undue dyspnea, fatigue, or other incapacitating symptoms. Patients with recent syncope, cardiac surgery, percutaneous coronary intervention, or device placement may be restricted from driving, at least temporarily, according to local regulations. Patients holding an occupational or commercial license may also be subject to additional restrictions.

Traveling. Short flights are unlikely to cause problems for a patient with compensated heart failure. Cabin pressure is generally maintained to provide an oxygen level no lower than equivalent to 6000 feet above sea level, which should be well tolerated in patients without severe pulmonary disease or pulmonary hypertension. Longer journeys may cause limb edema and dehydration, thereby predisposing to venous thrombosis. Adjustment of the dose of diuretics and other treatments should be discussed with the patient wishing to travel to a warm climate or a country where the risk of gastroenteritis is high. It is also advisable for heart failure patients to carry a list of medications and contact information for their health care provider.

Comorbidity

Comorbid conditions, which are common and important in patients with heart failure, may be due to the underlying cardiovascular disease that caused or contributed to heart failure (e.g., hypertension, coronary artery disease, diabetes mellitus), may arise as a complication of heart failure (e.g., arrhythmias), or can result from an adverse effect of treatment given for heart failure (e.g., gout). The exact causes of other comorbidities in heart failure, such as diabetes (Chapters 236 and 237), depression (Chapter 404), sleep apnea (Chapter 100), renal dysfunction (Chapter 132), and anemia (Chapter 161), are complex and uncertain. These and other comorbid conditions, such as chronic obstructive pulmonary disease and asthma, are important because they are a major determinant of prognosis and may limit the use of certain treatments for heart failure (e.g., renal dysfunction limiting use of ACE inhibitors or asthma limiting β-blockers) and because treatment of comorbidities may affect the stability of heart failure (e.g., NSAIDs needed for rheumatic conditions can cause salt and water retention and renal dysfunction). Both prevention (e.g., diabetes mellitus) and treatment (e.g., anemia) of comorbidities are being evaluated as a potential new therapeutic goal in heart failure.

Angina. β-Blockers are of benefit in both angina (Chapter 71) and heart failure. Ivabradine, which is an inhibitor of the I_f current in the sinus node, reduces heart rate, is an effective antianginal agent at 2.5 to 7.5 mg twice daily, and is safe in patients with left ventricular systolic dysfunction. Nitrates relieve angina but on their own are not of proven value in chronic heart failure. Calcium-channel blockers should generally be avoided in heart failure because they have a negative inotropic action and cause peripheral edema; only amlodipine has been shown to have no adverse effect on survival. Trimetazidine, ranolazine, and nicorandil are antianginal drugs that are available in certain countries; their safety in patients with heart failure is uncertain. Percutaneous and surgical (Chapter 74) revascularization is also of value in relieving angina in selected patients with heart failure (see below).

Atrial Fibrillation. Atrial fibrillation (Chapter 64) may be the cause of or a consequence of heart failure in a patient presenting with atrial fibrillation and a rapid ventricular rate, and the distinction can be difficult, especially because prolonged atrial fibrillation may lead to a rate-related cardiomyopathy. Thyrotoxicosis (Chapter 233) and mitral valve disease (Chapter 75), especially stenosis, must be excluded. Alcohol abuse should also be considered. β-Blockers and digoxin are given to control the ventricular rate. The patient should be supervised closely after the initiation of these treatments because underlying sinus node dysfunction may raise the risk of bradycardia. Unless the patient presents emergently with symptoms or signs of heart failure, myocardial ischemia, or hypertension, there is little or no evidence to support a strategy of restoring sinus rhythm rather than controlling the ventricular rate in most patients with heart failure (Chapter 64).**18** Atrioventricular node ablation and pacing may be required to control ventricular rate (Chapter 66). The use of catheter ablation to cure atrial fibrillation in patients with heart failure is promising but is not currently recommended routinely (Chapter 66). There is a strong indication for thromboembolism prophylaxis with warfarin in patients with heart failure and atrial fibrillation (Chapter 64).

Asthma and Reversible Airways Obstruction. Asthma is a contraindication for use of a β-blocker, but most patients with chronic obstructive pulmonary disease (Chapter 88) can tolerate a β-blocker. Pulmonary congestion can mimic chronic obstructive pulmonary disease. Systemic administration of a corticosteroid to treat reversible airways obstruction may cause sodium and water retention and exacerbate heart failure, whereas inhalation therapy is better tolerated.

Diabetes Mellitus. Diabetes mellitus is discussed in detail elsewhere (Chapters 236 and 237). The prevalence and incidence of diabetes mellitus are high in heart failure, and the risk for development of type 2 diabetes may be reduced by ACE inhibitors and ARBs. β-Blocker treatment is not contraindicated and is of benefit in patients with diabetes and heart failure. Thiazolidinediones cause sodium and water retention, may lead to decompensation, and are not recommended in patients with or at risk of heart failure. Metformin may cause lactic acidosis and is not recommended in patients with severe heart failure.

Abnormal Thyroid Function. Both thyrotoxicosis and hypothyroidism can cause heart failure (and thyrotoxicosis can cause atrial fibrillation, which may precipitate heart failure). Amiodarone can also induce both hypothyroidism and hyperthyroidism, the latter being particularly difficult to diagnose. The risk of thyroid dysfunction may be less with the related antiarrhythmic agent dronedarone, but dronedarone increases mortality in severe heart failure and should be avoided in patients with stage C or D heart failure or recently decompensated heart failure.

Gout. Hyperuricemia and gout (Chapter 281) are common in heart failure and can be caused or aggravated by diuretic treatment. Allopurinol may prevent gout, and acute attacks are better treated with colchicine, oral steroids, or intra-articular steroids rather than by an NSAID.

Renal Dysfunction. Most patients with heart failure have a reduced glomerular filtration rate. ACE inhibitors, ARBs, and aldosterone antagonists often cause a further small reduction in glomerular filtration rate and rise in serum blood urea nitrogen and creatinine levels, which, if limited, should not lead to discontinuation of treatment. Marked increases in blood urea nitrogen and creatinine, however, should prompt consideration of underlying renal artery stenosis (Chapter 127). Renal dysfunction may also be caused by sodium and water depletion, leading to relative hypovolemia (e.g., due to excessive diuresis, diarrhea, and vomiting) or hypotension. Nephrotoxic agents such as NSAIDs are also a common cause of renal dysfunction in heart failure.

Prostatic Obstruction. For prostatic disease (Chapter 131), a 5α-reductase inhibitor may be preferable to an α-adrenoceptor antagonist, which can cause hypotension and salt and water retention. Prostatic obstruction should also be considered in male patients with deteriorating renal function.

Anemia. A normocytic, normochromic anemia (Chapter 161) is also common in heart failure, in part because of the high prevalence of renal dysfunction. Malnutrition and blood loss may also contribute. Intravenous iron treatment with 200 mg of ferric carboxymaltose improves quality of life and reduces symptoms in patients with class II or III heart failure and iron deficiency without adverse effects.[19]

Depression. Depression (Chapter 404) is common in patients with heart failure, perhaps partly owing to disturbance of the hypothalamic-pituitary axis and other neurochemical pathways but also as a result of social isolation and the adjustment to chronic disease. Depression is associated with worse functional status, reduced adherence to treatment, and poor clinical outcomes. Both psychosocial interventions and pharmacologic treatment are helpful. Selective serotonin reuptake inhibitors are believed to be the best tolerated pharmacologic agents, whereas tricyclic antidepressants should be avoided because of their anticholinergic actions and potential to cause arrhythmias.

Cancer. Many anticancer drugs, particularly anthracyclines, cyclophosphamide, and trastuzumab (Herceptin), can cause myocardial damage and heart failure, as can mediastinal radiotherapy. Pericardial constriction can be a result of previous radiotherapy, and malignant pericardial involvement can cause effusion and tamponade (Chapter 77).

Devices and Surgery
Implantable Cardioverter-Defibrillators
About half of patients with heart failure die suddenly, mainly as the result of a ventricular arrhythmia. The relative risk of sudden death, as opposed to death from progressive heart failure, is greatest in patients with milder heart failure. In patients with more advanced heart failure, progressive pump failure deaths are relatively more common. Antiarrhythmic drugs have not been shown to improve survival in heart failure, but ICDs (Chapter 66) reduce the risk of death in selected patients after myocardial infarction (Chapter 73) and improve survival in patients with class II or III heart failure and systolic dysfunction who were otherwise treated with optimal medical therapy.[20,21] All patients with class II or class III heart failure, irrespective of etiology, and an LVEF of 35% or less should be considered for an ICD provided they have no other conditions greatly limiting life expectancy (i.e., have an anticipated survival of at least a year) or quality of life.

Cardiac Resynchronization Therapy
About 30% of patients with heart failure have substantial prolongation of the QRS duration on the surface electrocardiogram, which is a marker of abnormal electrical activation of the left ventricle causing dyssynchronous contraction, less efficient ventricular emptying, and, often, mitral regurgitation. Atrioventricular coupling may also be abnormal, as reflected by a prolonged PR interval, as may interventricular synchrony. Cardiac resynchronization therapy (CRT) with atrial-biventricular or multisite pacing optimizes atrioventricular timing and improves synchronization of cardiac contraction. In selected patients with marked systolic dysfunction (LVEF ≤ 35%), severe symptoms (functional class III or IV), and a wide QRS (120 milliseconds or more, usually manifest with left bundle branch block morphology), CRT improves

pump function, reduces mitral regurgitation, relieves symptoms, and significantly prolongs exercise capacity. CRT reduces the composite of death or hospital admission in such patients (see Table 59-1) by more than 35%,[21] and in one trial, it also reduced the risk of death from any cause by 36%.[21] Many other outcome measures, including quality of life, were also improved. The combination of CRT plus an ICD also reduces all-cause mortality by 25% in patients with an LVEF <30%, a QRS >120 milliseconds, and functional class II or III heart failure.[22] In patients with New York Heart Association (NYHA) class I and II symptoms, an LVEF of 30% or less, and a QRS duration of 130 milliseconds or more, CRT (plus an ICD) improved ventricular function and reduced the risk of worsening heart failure, compared with an ICD alone (see Table 59-1); these effects were most pronounced in individuals with a QRS 150 milliseconds or more. CRT did not reduce the risk of death in this population with a relatively low mortality.[23]

The current debate focuses on whether additional patients will benefit from CRT. CRT appears to be beneficial in patients in sinus rhythm, class I or II symptoms, LVEF of 30% or less, a left bundle branch block morphology, and a QRS duration of at least 130 milliseconds. The combination of a CRT plus an ICD improves ventricular function and reduces the risk of worsening heart failure compared with an ICD alone (see Table 59-1), especially in patients with a QRS ≥150 milliseconds.[23] CRT has not been shown to help patients with echocardiographic dyssynchrony but a narrow QRS (<120 milliseconds).

Whether patients with right bundle branch block and atrial fibrillation are helped by CRT is still uncertain. There is no consensus yet about whether (or in whom) CRT alone or a CRT with implantable cardioverter-defibrillator capabilities should be used.

Surgery
With the exception of cardiac transplantation and ventricular assist devices, there are no generally accepted criteria for surgical intervention. Use of operative procedures is variable among centers and greatly dependent on local experience and expertise. Expert imaging and detailed hemodynamic and functional assessments are usually required when any patient with heart failure is considered for surgery, and close liaison between the relevant experts in these fields is essential. The collective expertise in surgical centers is often used to make highly individualized decisions about whether to operate and what procedures will be attempted. "Established" operative treatments for patients with heart failure include coronary artery bypass grafting, surgery for mitral valve incompetence, left ventricular remodeling surgery (including aneurysmectomy), implantation of ventricular assist devices, and heart transplantation. "Experimental" approaches include ventricular constraint devices and intramyocardial cell transplantation.

A recent trial showed no benefit (in symptoms or rates of death or hospitalization for cardiac causes) of surgical ventricular reconstruction. Cardiomyoplasty and partial left ventriculectomy are other recently developed operations for heart failure now thought to be without benefit.

Percutaneous Coronary Intervention or Coronary Artery Bypass Grafting. Percutaneous coronary intervention or coronary artery bypass grafting (Chapter 74), as appropriate, is indicated for relief of angina. The extent of ischemia and residual myocardial viability can be determined by noninvasive assessments such as dobutamine echocardiography (Chapter 55), magnetic resonance imaging (Chapter 56), and positron emission tomographic scanning (Chapter 56) in patients with impaired LVEF. In patients with coronary artery disease and an ejection fraction ≤35%, coronary artery bypass surgery plus optimal medical therapy can significantly reduce cardiovascular mortality but not overall mortality compared with optimal medical therapy alone.[24] As a result, the role of surgery in such patients should be individualized.

Cardiac Transplantation. Cardiac transplantation (Chapter 82) remains the most accepted surgical intervention in end-stage heart failure. Selection criteria usually focus on patients with refractory heart failure, that is, those with severe symptoms and functional limitations (peak oxygen consumption of less than 10 mL/kg/min), as well as a particularly worrisome clinical course and prognosis attributed to their cardiac condition. These patients are often dependent on intravenous inotropic agents and mechanical support.

Left Ventricular Assist Devices. Given the scarcity of organ donors, left ventricular assist devices are used as a "bridge to transplantation" or even as a permanent, definitive, procedure ("destination therapy") for some patients with advanced heart failure. A pulsatile volume-displacement left ventricular assist device can provide a short but significant prolongation of survival in patients who have end-stage heart failure and are ineligible for transplantation (see Table 59-1), but the rates of bleeding, infective and thrombotic complications, and mechanical dysfunction necessitating repeat surgery were high with this older device. In patients with end-stage heart failure ineligible for transplantation, a new continuous-flow device is significantly better than this older device in terms of 2-year survival without repeat device surgery or disabling stroke (46% versus 11%).[25]

A recent trial showed no benefit (in symptoms or rates of death or hospitalization for cardiac causes) of surgical ventricular reconstruction. Cardiomyoplasty and partial left ventriculectomy are other recently developed operations for heart failure now thought to be without benefit.

Heart Failure with Preserved Left Ventricular Ejection Fraction (Diastolic Dysfunction)

Although all patients with symptomatic heart failure share a constellation of signs and symptoms, impaired physical capacity, and reduced quality of life, some have a preserved LVEF (generally above 40 or 50%) and many are thought to have diastolic dysfunction (Chapter 58). Diastolic heart failure often has a cause different from that of systolic heart failure and a better survival rate (Chapters 52, 58, and 60), but sometimes it is an early manifestation of what will evolve into heart failure with a reduced LVEF. The distinction is important, however, because most of the RCTs that generated the evidence for treatment of heart failure included only patients with reduced LVEFs (see Table 59-1). Treatment of the underlying cardiovascular and other disorders that contribute to symptomatic stage C and stage D of heart failure with preserved LVEF, such as hypertension, myocardial ischemia, and diabetes, is critical and is as for stages A and B (see earlier). In patients with atrial fibrillation, control of the ventricular rate with a β-blocker or a rate-limiting calcium-channel blocker (or restoration of sinus rhythm) is particularly important (Chapter 64). Diuretics are used empirically to treat sodium and water retention, according to the same principles as in heart failure with reduced LVEF. In one trial of patients with an LVEF higher than 40% (mean, 54%), treatment with the ARB candesartan decreased the risk of hospital admission for heart failure but did not improve survival or the composite outcome of cardiovascular death or hospital admission for worsening heart failure. In a more recent study of patients with an LVEF of 45% or higher (mean, 60%), the ARB irbesartan had no beneficial effect, raising the possibility that the benefit of candesartan in the earlier trial was largely in patients with borderline systolic dysfunction (i.e., LVEF of 40-50%).[26] Smaller studies in patients in sinus rhythm have shown that the calcium-channel blocker verapamil or the nonselective β-adrenergic blocker propranolol can improve symptoms and exercise capacity in patients with heart failure and preserved LVEF, possibly by reducing heart rate and thereby increasing the duration of diastolic left ventricular filling as well as by directly enhancing myocardial relaxation. There are, however, no current RCTs in which these drugs decisively reduced mortality or morbidity in patients with heart failure and preserved LVEF, so treatment currently is aimed to relieve symptoms.

Heart Failure Due to Valvular Heart Disease

Heart failure also can arise as a result of regurgitant and stenotic valve disease (Chapter 75). It can sometimes be difficult to determine whether mitral regurgitation is primary or secondary in a patient with heart failure and left ventricular dilation, although a prior history of known valve disease or rheumatic fever may suggest a primary valve problem. The objective of treatment of primary valve disease is the prevention of heart failure by surgical repair or replacement of the diseased valve or valves (Chapter 75). The development of overt heart failure is an ominous sign, sometimes requiring emergent valve replacement (e.g., aortic stenosis) but sometimes indicating that valve replacement may not be possible (e.g., because of severe pulmonary hypertension).

Aortic Stenosis

Evaluation of the aortic valve (Chapter 75) can be difficult in patients with poor left ventricular systolic function. Such patients may have insufficient cardiac output to generate a high gradient across even a severely stenotic valve. Conversely, a calcified and degenerate but nonstenotic aortic valve may appear stenosed simply because it does not open normally in patients with very low cardiac output. A calculated valve area provides a better assessment of the severity of aortic stenosis in these patients. Stress echocardiography (Chapter 55) may help assess the potential for ventricular recovery after relief of aortic stenosis. Consideration should be given as to whether concomitant myocardial ischemia from coronary artery disease may also be contributing to a reversible depression of systolic function. Transcatheter valve replacement is a promising new technique for patients who have aortic stenosis but are at very high risk for open valve replacement.

Mitral Regurgitation

Mitral regurgitation can be a primary cause or a secondary manifestation in a patient with heart failure and left ventricular dilation (Chapter 75). Surgery sometimes will result in clinical improvement, but some patients with advanced left ventricular dysfunction will not achieve substantial benefit (e.g., mitral valve surgery in a patient with long-standing severe mitral regurgitation). Valve repair or annuloplasty may, however, be beneficial in carefully selected patients with secondary mitral regurgitation caused by or exacerbated by left ventricular dilation. Valve repair is generally preferable to valve replacement.

Heart Failure Due to Nonischemic Dilated Cardiomyopathy

Patients with heart failure and normal coronary arteries should be evaluated for possible reversible causes. Untreated hypertension is now an unusual cause of dilated cardiomyopathy in the United States, but hypertension was once a leading cause in the United States and remains a major consideration in many parts of the world. Infiltrative cardiomyopathies (e.g.,

hemochromatosis, amyloid, sarcoid) and arteritides sometimes have specific recommended therapies (Chapters 60, 95, 194, and 219). Chagas' disease (Chapter 355) must be considered in patients from endemic areas. Alcohol and other toxins (e.g., chemotherapeutic agents) are other recognized causes of dilated cardiomyopathy. Dilated cardiomyopathy can also develop in the peripartum period. Most cases of nonischemic dilated cardiomyopathy are usually labeled idiopathic (i.e., no specific etiology can be determined), although many may have a genetic origin, especially if there is a positive family history. Irrespective of etiology, patients with nonischemic dilated cardiomyopathy should be treated in the same way as patients whose dilated, poorly contracting left ventricle is a result of coronary artery disease.

Heart Failure Due to Hypertrophic Cardiomyopathy

Heart failure can arise in patients with hypertrophic cardiomyopathy because of predominant diastolic dysfunction, associated mitral incompetence, or the development of systolic dysfunction. The management of hypertrophic cardiomyopathy and its complications is often very different from the management of dilated cardiomyopathy (Chapter 60), thereby underscoring the value of echocardiography in the evaluation of the patient with heart failure.

Acute Decompensated Heart Failure and Pulmonary Edema

Patients presenting with acute heart failure include those who develop heart failure de novo as a consequence of another cardiac event, usually a myocardial infarction, and those who present for the first time with decompensation of previously asymptomatic and often unrecognized cardiac dysfunction (patients previously in stage B, a transition with profound prognostic implications). However, because of frequent recurrences, most episodes of acute decompensation occur in patients with established, chronic heart failure that has worsened as a result of the unavoidable natural progression of the syndrome, with an intercurrent cardiac (e.g., arrhythmia) or noncardiac (e.g., pneumonia) event, or as a consequence of an avoidable reason, such as nonadherence with treatment or use of an agent that can alter renal function. Although it is not always identified, searching for a reversible precipitant is an important aspect of the initial therapy plan (Table 59-7).

Most patients with acute heart failure require admission to the hospital, especially if pulmonary edema is present. In contrast to chronic heart failure, data from RCTs generally are not available to guide effective therapy for patients with acute decompensated heart failure. The principal goals of management of this heterogeneous group of patients are to relieve symptoms, the most important of which is extreme dyspnea, and to maintain or restore vital organ perfusion. An intravenous bolus or infusion of a loop diuretic (e.g., furosemide, 50 to 100 mg intravenous bolus twice daily, or 10 mg per hour continuous intravenous infusion, titrated according to the symptom response,[27] the reduction in edema, and renal function) and, in hypoxemic patients, oxygen are the key first-line treatments. An intravenous opiate may also be given to relieve anxiety and distress. Noninvasive ventilation using a tight-fitting mask to provide positive-pressure ventilation reduces respiratory distress and metabolic disturbances more rapidly than does standard oxygen therapy but has not reduced short-term mortality.[28] Intravenous infusion of a nitrate (e.g., continuous intravenous infusion of 20 to 200 µg/mm of nitroglycerin, titrated according to the symptomatic response and hemodynamic measurements, particularly arterial blood pressure) is also valuable in patients with a systolic blood pressure of 100 mm Hg or higher (Fig. 59-2). Intravenous nesiritide (human BNP as a 2.0 µg/kg intravenous bolus followed by a continuous intravenous infusion of 0.01 to 0.03 µg/kg/mm titrated according to the symptomatic response and hemodynamic measurements, particularly arterial blood pressure) can reduce the pulmonary capillary wedge pressure more promptly than intravenous nitroglycerin, but the effect of this short-term

TABLE 59-7	SOME COMMON PRECIPITATING CAUSES OF HEART FAILURE

Myocardial ischemia or infarction
Atrial fibrillation or other supraventricular tachycardias
Uncontrolled hypertension
Valvular disease
Ventricular tachycardia
Pulmonary embolism
Pericardial disease
Sepsis
Anemia
Nutritional and medical noncompliance
Adverse drug effects
Hyperthyroidism or hypothyroidism

From Kimmelstiel CD, DeNofrio D, Konstam MA. Heart failure. In: Wachter RM, Goldman L, Hollander H, eds. *Hospital Medicine*, 2nd ed. Philadelphia: Lippincott Williams & Wilkins; 2005:360.

Acute Pulmonary Edema

↓

Exclude/treat arrhythmia[1]
+/or acute mechanical problem[2]
+/or acute coronary syndrome

↓

IV diuretic (e.g., 50 mg furosemide[3])
High flow oxygen[4]
IV opiate + antiemetic (e.g., 4-8 mg
morphine + 10 mg metoclopramide[5])

— Hypotension/shock — Persisting hypoxemia —

Consider IV inotrope, e.g., dobutamine[6]/invasive hemodynamic monitoring/mechanical support[7]

Assess response[8]

Consider CPAP[9]/ invasive ventilation

— Unsatisfactory — Satisfactory —

Consider IV vasodilator (e.g., NTG,[10] SNP, nesiritide)

Continue

[1] Causal arrhythmia (e.g., ventricular tachycardia). It can be difficult to determine whether atrial fibrillation is a primary cause of acute pulmonary edema or secondary to it. An ECG is an essential investigation.

[2] Acute mechanical problems include ventricular septal rupture and mitral valve papillary muscle rupture. Mechanical support (e.g., an intra-aortic balloon pump) and urgent surgery should be considered. An echocardiogram should be performed as soon as possible, especially in a patient without a prior diagnosis of heart failure/other relevant heart disease (e.g., prior myocardial infarction or valve disease).

[3] Dose of diuretic depends on prior diuretic use and renal function—a lower dose may suffice if preserved renal function and no prior diuretic use.

[4] Oxygen causes an increase in systemic vascular resistance and a reduction in heart rate and cardiac output and should only be administered to patients with hypoxemia.

[5] Consider if patient agitated/distressed/in pain; may cause respiratory depression and dose should be reduced in very elderly.

[6] An intravenous infusion of dobutamine may be started at a dose of 2.5 µg/kg/min, doubling every 15 minutes according to response and tolerability (dose titration usually limited by excessive tachycardia, arrhythmias, or ischemia). A dose above 20 µg/kg/min is rarely needed.

[7] E.g., an intra-aortic balloon pump

[8] Improvement in symptoms and peripheral perfusion and adequate urine output—patient should be monitored closely, and usually a response will occur within 30 minutes. Bladder catheterization may help in monitoring urine output.

[9] Continuous positive airways pressure (CPAP) is valuable in severe pulmonary edema, especially if associated with hypoxemia. Endotracheal intubation and invasive mechanical ventilation should be considered in patients with persisting hypoxemia and physical ventilatory exhaustion.

[10] An intravenous infusion of nitroglycerin (NTG) should be started at a dose of 10 µg/min and doubled every 10 minutes according to response and tolerability (usually dose up-titration is limited by hypotension). A dose of more than 100 µg/min is rarely needed.

FIGURE 59-2. Approach to the patient with acute pulmonary edema. ECG = electrocardiogram.

therapy on other clinical outcomes is controversial. In volume-overloaded patients with severe heart failure unresponsive to diuretics, ultrafiltration is an option at specialized centers.

In patients with marked hypotension or other evidence of organ hypoperfusion, an inotropic agent such as dobutamine (continuous intravenous infusion of 2.5 to 25 µg/kg/mm, titrated according to hemodynamic and heart rate response and induction of arrhythmias or myocardial ischemia) or a phosphodiesterase inhibitor (e.g., milrinone) should be considered, although neither treatment has ever been shown to reduce in-hospital deaths. In some countries, the calcium sensitizer levosimendan is also available for use in these patients. In general, potent inotropic agents should be used in a cardiac-monitored setting at the lowest clinically effective dose and for the shortest duration possible (Chapter 107). Although there are limited data supporting a benefit, low-dose dopamine (intravenous infusion of 2.5 µg/kg/mm) may be administered in an attempt to improve renal function. Patients with severe hyponatremia may benefit from the arginine vasopressin antagonist tolvaptan (15 to 60 mg orally once daily).

In more critically ill patients, mechanical support (e.g., with an intra-aortic balloon pump) may also be considered (Chapter 107). The aim of treatment is to support the patient's circulation and vital organ function until either the patient's heart recovers or a definitive operative procedure can be performed (e.g., transplantation or permanent implantation of a ventricular-assist device).

In patients admitted to the hospital, discharge planning and subsequent management to reduce the risk of readmission are important. Ideally, an effective oral diuretic regimen should have been identified, and fluid-volume and biochemical stability should have been achieved. This optimization of volume status and development of a stable oral regimen before discharge is thought to reduce the risk of early readmission. Treatment with an ACE inhibitor, β-blocker, and ARB or aldosterone antagonist, as appropriate, should also be started and titrated in the stabilized patient before discharge. Outpatient follow-up should be arranged to ensure that any of those treatments that have not been started before discharge are initiated after discharge and that the dose of each drug is increased, as tolerated, to the appropriate target.

Outpatient Follow-Up

The key to successful follow-up is the careful tracking of clinical symptoms and the patient's weight, which often involves interviewing not only the patient but also family members, who may be more aware of changes in status than the patient (see Organization of Care, earlier). Continuity of care and seamless transitions from the inpatient to the outpatient setting are crucial aspects of optimal management. Patients with advanced heart failure and patients requiring frequent hospitalization require special handling. Programs that provide telephone-based tracking of daily weights and symptoms can detect deterioration in time to intervene before the need for hospitalization. Although these programs may be costly, several evaluations have found them to be cost-effective. Because the management of these patients requires considerable experience and expertise, specialized heart failure programs and clinics have been developed and may provide additional benefit compared with traditional care.

PROGNOSIS

The prognosis of patients with heart failure is poor despite advances in therapy. Of patients who survive the acute onset of heart failure, only 35% of men and 50% of women are alive after 5 years. Although it is difficult to predict prognosis in individual patients, patients with symptoms at rest (class IV) have a 30 to 50% annual mortality rate, patients who are symptomatic with mild activity (class III) have mortality rates of 10 to 20% annually, and patients with symptoms only with moderate activity (class II) have a 5 to 10% annual mortality rate. Mortality rates are higher in older patients, men, and patients with a reduced LVEF or underlying coronary heart disease.

⬤ END-OF-LIFE CONSIDERATIONS

Although predicting the trajectory of illness in patients with advanced heart failure is notoriously difficult, it is often apparent when a patient has progressed to end-stage heart failure, commonly associated with concomitant renal failure. In these circumstances, the expertise of the palliative care team may be especially helpful (Chapter 3). Useful websites providing information on palliative care relevant to heart failure are available (*www.goldstandardsframework.nhs.uk/* and *www.palliativecarescotland.org.uk/assets/files/AR%2031%20March%202009.pdf*). Medications such as parenteral opiates (with an antiemetic) and benzodiazepines may be particularly helpful in relieving dyspnea, anxiety, and pain that arises from ascites, hepatic congestion, lower limb edema, and pressure points. At this stage in the patient's illness, it may be appropriate to discuss withdrawal of conventional treatment, deactivation of an ICD to avoid undesired and unpleasant electrical discharges, and a do-not-resuscitate order if the patient and others involved in the patient's care agree that "comfort care" is appropriate. Hospice care may be chosen by some at this point.

⬤ FUTURE DIRECTIONS

The discovery of primitive pluripotent stem cells that have the potential to differentiate into contractile tissue has generated considerable optimism about their transplantation into patients with impaired systolic function. Stimulation of the small population of resident stem cells in adult myocardium may also be possible.

1. Pfeffer MA, Braunwald E, Moyé LA, et al. Effect of captopril on mortality and morbidity in patients with left ventricular dysfunction after myocardial infarction: results of the survival and ventricular enlargement trial. The SAVE Investigators. *N Engl J Med.* 1992;327:669-677.
2. The SOLVD Investigators. Effect of enalapril on mortality and the development of heart failure in asymptomatic patients with reduced left ventricular ejection fractions. *N Engl J Med.* 1992;327:685-691.
3. Pfeffer MA, McMurray JJ, Velazquez EJ, et al. Valsartan, captopril, or both in myocardial infarction complicated by heart failure, left ventricular dysfunction, or both. *N Engl J Med.* 2003;349:1893-1906.
4. Dargie HJ. Effect of carvedilol on outcome after myocardial infarction in patients with left-ventricular dysfunction: the CAPRICORN randomised trial. *Lancet.* 2001;357:1385-1390.
5. The CONSENSUS Trial Study Group. Effects of enalapril on mortality in severe congestive heart failure: results of the Cooperative North Scandinavian Enalapril Survival Study (CONSENSUS). *N Engl J Med.* 1987;316:1429-1435.
6. The SOLVD Investigators. Effect of enalapril on survival in patients with reduced left ventricular ejection fractions and congestive heart failure. *N Engl J Med.* 1991;325:293-302.
7. Granger CB, McMurray JJ, Yusuf S, et al. Effects of candesartan in patients with chronic heart failure and reduced left-ventricular systolic function intolerant to angiotensin-converting-enzyme inhibitors: the CHARM-Alternative trial. *Lancet* 2003;362:772-776.
8. Cohn JN, Tognoni G: A randomized trial of the angiotensin-receptor blocker valsartan in chronic heart failure. *N Engl J Med.* 2001;345:1667-1675.
9. McMurray JJ, Östergren J, Swedberg K, et al. Effects of candesartan in patients with chronic heart failure and reduced left-ventricular systolic function taking angiotensin-converting-enzyme inhibitors: the CHARM-Added trial. *Lancet.* 2003;362:767-771.
10. Packer M, Coats AJ, Fowler MB, et al. Effect of carvedilol on survival in severe chronic heart failure. *N Engl J Med.* 2001;344:1651-1658.
11. Pitt B, Zannad F, Remme WJ, et al. The effect of spironolactone on morbidity and mortality in patients with severe heart failure: randomized Aldactone Evaluation Study Investigators. *N Engl J Med.* 1999;341:709-717.
12. Pitt B, Remme W, Zannad F, et al. Eplerenone, a selective aldosterone blocker, in patients with left ventricular dysfunction after myocardial infarction. *N Engl J Med.* 2003;348:1309-1321.
13. Zannad F, McMurray JJ, Krum H, et al. Eplerenone in patients with systolic heart failure and mild symptoms. *N Engl J Med.* 2011;364:11-21.
14. The Digitalis Investigation Group. The effects of digoxin on mortality and morbidity in patients with heart failure. *N Engl J Med.* 1997;336:525-533.
15. Taylor AL, Ziesche S, Yancy C, et al. Combination of isosorbide dinitrate and hydralazine in blacks with heart failure. *N Engl J Med.* 2004;351:2049-2057.
16. Sochalski J, Jaarsma T, Krumholz HM, et al. What works in chronic care management: the case of heart failure. *Health Aff (Millwood).* 2009;28:179-189.
17. O'Connor CM, Whellan DJ, Lee KL, et al. HF-ACTION Investigators. Efficacy and safety of exercise training in patients with chronic heart failure: HF-ACTION randomized controlled trial. *JAMA.* 2009;301:1439-1450.
18. Roy D, Talajic M, Nattel S, et al. Atrial Fibrillation and Congestive Heart Failure Investigators. Rhythm control versus rate control for atrial fibrillation and heart failure. *N Engl J Med.* 2008;358:2667-2677.
19. Anker SD, Comin Colet J, Filippatos G, et al. Ferric carboxymaltose in patients with heart failure and iron deficiency. *N Engl J Med.* 2009;361:2436-2448.
20. Bardy GH, Lee KL, Mark DB, et al. Amiodarone or an implantable cardioverter-defibrillator for congestive heart failure. *N Engl J Med.* 2005;352:225-237.
21. Cleland JG, Daubert JC, Erdmann E, et al. The effect of cardiac resynchronization on morbidity and mortality in heart failure. *N Engl J Med.* 2005;352:1539-1549.
22. Tang AS, Wells GA, Talajic M, et al. Cardiac-resynchronization therapy for mild-to-moderate heart failure. *N Engl J Med.* 2010;363:2385-2395.
23. Moss AJ, Hall WJ, Cannom DS, et al. Cardiac-resynchronization therapy for the prevention of heart-failure events. *N Engl J Med.* 2009;361:1329-1338.
24. Velazquez EJ, Lee KL, Deja MA, et al, for the STICH Investigators. Coronary-artery bypass surgery in patients with left ventricular dysfunction. *N Engl J Med.* 2011;364:1607-1616.
25. Slaughter MS, Rogers JG, Milano CA, et al. Advanced heart failure treated with continuous-flow left ventricular assist device. *N Engl J Med.* 2009;361:2241-2251.
26. Massie BM, Carson PE, McMurray JJ, et al. I-PRESERVE Investigators. Irbesartan in patients with heart failure and preserved ejection fraction. *N Engl J Med.* 2008;359:2456-2467.
27. Felker GM, Lee KL, Bull DA, et al. Diuretic strategies in patients with acute decompensated heart failure. *N Engl J Med.* 2011;364:797-805.
28. Weng CL, Zhao YT, Liu Qh, et al. Meta-analysis: noninvasive ventilation in acute cardiogenic pulmonary edema. *Ann Intern Med.* 2010;152:590-600.

SUGGESTED READINGS

Joynt KE, Orav EJ, Jha AK. The association between hospital volume and processes, outcomes, and costs of care for congestive heart failure. *Ann Intern Med.* 2011;154:94-102. *Experience is associated with better outcomes but a higher cost.*

McMurray JJV. Systolic heart failure. *N Engl J Med.* 2010;362:32-42. *Concise review.*

Weintraub NL, Collins SP, Pang PS, et al. Acute heart failure syndromes: emergency department presentation, treatment, and disposition: current approaches and future aims: a scientific statement from the American Heart Association. *Circulation.* 2010;122:1975-1996. *Guidelines.*

60

DISEASES OF THE MYOCARDIUM AND ENDOCARDIUM

WILLIAM McKENNA AND PERRY ELLIOTT

⬤ MYOCARDIAL DISEASE

A substantial minority of cases of heart failure result from familial (genetic) or nonfamilial (acquired) disorders, which can be confined to the heart or be multisystem disorders. The term *cardiomyopathy* refers to myocardial disorders in which the heart muscle is structurally and functionally abnormal in the absence of coronary artery disease (Chapter 73), hypertension (Chapter 67), valvular disease (Chapter 75), or congenital heart disease (Chapter 69) sufficient to cause the observed myocardial abnormality. Cardiomyopathies are classified according to ventricular morphology and pathophysiology into four major types: dilated cardiomyopathy, hypertrophic cardiomyopathy, restrictive cardiomyopathy, and arrhythmogenic right ventricular cardiomyopathy (ARVC) (Table 60-1; Fig. 60-1). Diseases that do not fit into these groups (such as endocardial fibroelastosis and left ventricular noncompaction) are termed *unclassified cardiomyopathies.* Mixed phenotypes can exist; for example, patients with hypertrophic and dilated cardiomyopathies frequently have a restrictive left ventricular physiology or develop ventricular dilation.

Hypertrophic Cardiomyopathy

DEFINITION AND EPIDEMIOLOGY

Hypertrophic cardiomyopathy is defined as unexplained left ventricular hypertrophy in the absence of abnormal loading conditions (valve disease, hypertension, congenital heart defects) sufficient to explain the degree of hypertrophy. The disease occurs in all racial groups, with a prevalence of between 0.2 and 0.5%.

PATHOBIOLOGY

Hypertrophic cardiomyopathy is usually familial with autosomal dominant inheritance. Mutations in sarcomeric contractile protein genes (Table 60-2) account for approximately 50 to 60% of cases. More than 400 different

TABLE 60-1 PROFILES OF MYOCARDIAL DISEASE

	HYPERTROPHIC	DILATED	RESTRICTIVE	ARVC
Causes	Genetic (see Table 60-2)	Myocarditis (see Table 60-4) Metabolic/endocrine Genetic (see Table 60-2)	Infiltrative or storage diseases (see Table 60-8) Endomyocardial (e.g., Löffler's, carcinoid) Genetic (see Table 60-2)	Genetic (see Table 60-2)
Ejection fraction	Increased	Reduced	25-50%	Normal until end stage 30% regional LV disease
Left ventricular	Usually decreased	Increased	Normal	Normal until end stage
End-diastolic dimension				Right ventricle dilated
Left ventricular wall thickness	Increased	Normal	Normal or mildly increased	Normal
Atrial size	Increased	Increased	Increased; may be massive	Left atrium normal; right dilated in severe disease
Valvular disease	Mitral regurgitation (SAM)	Mitral (functional); tricuspid regurgitation in late stages	Mitral and tricuspid regurgitation, rarely severe	Tricuspid regurgitation in severe disease
Common symptoms	Dyspnea; chest pain, syncope Late: orthopnea, PND	Dyspnea, fatigue Late: orthopnea, PND	Dyspnea Late: orthopnea, PND, right heart failure	Palpitations, syncope Late: right heart failure
Arrhythmia	Atrial fibrillation, ventricular tachycardia; conduction block in PRKAG2, mitochondrial; Fabry's disease	Ventricular tachyarrhythmias; heart block in Chagas' disease, giant cell myocarditis, laminopathies	Atrial fibrillation; conduction block in sarcoid, amyloidosis, desminopathy	Ventricular ectopy and tachycardia

ARVC = arrhythmogenic right ventricular cardiomyopathy; LV = left ventricular; SAM = systolic anterior motion of mitral valve; PND = paroxysmal nocturnal dyspnea.

FIGURE 60-1. Initial approach to classification of cardiomyopathy. The evaluation of symptoms or signs consistent with heart failure first includes confirmation that they can be attributed to a cardiac cause. Although this conclusion is often apparent from routine physical examination and electrocardiography, echocardiography serves to confirm cardiac disease and provides clues to the presence of other cardiac diseases, such as focal abnormalities, suggesting primary valve disease or congenital heart disease. Having excluded these conditions, cardiomyopathy is generally considered to be dilated, restrictive, or hypertrophic, as shown in Table 60-1. Patients with apparently normal cardiac structure and contraction are occasionally found to demonstrate abnormal intracardiac flow patterns consistent with diastolic dysfunction but should also be evaluated carefully for other causes of their symptoms. Most patients with so-called diastolic dysfunction also demonstrate at least borderline criteria for left ventricular hypertrophy, frequently in the setting of chronic hypertension and diabetes. A moderately decreased ejection fraction without marked dilation or a pattern of restrictive cardiomyopathy is sometimes referred to as *minimally dilated cardiomyopathy*, which may represent either a distinct entity or a transition between acute and chronic disease.

mutations have been identified, with marked variation in disease penetrance and clinical expression. A similar clinical phenotype is seen in association with other uncommon genetic disorders, including Noonan's syndrome (Chapter 69), Friedreich's ataxia (Chapter 429), neurofibromatosis (Chapter 426), hereditary spherocytosis (Chapter 164), respiratory chain disorders, glycogen storage diseases (Chapter 214), and lysosomal storage disorders (Chapter 215) (see Table 60-2).

PATHOLOGY

In the common form of autosomal dominant hypertrophic cardiomyopathy, myocardial hypertrophy usually affects the interventricular septum more than other regions of the left ventricle. Other patterns, including concentric, mid-ventricular (sometimes associated with a left ventricular apical diverticulum), and apical also occur. Coexistent right ventricular hypertrophy is

TABLE 60-2 GENETIC CAUSES OF CARDIOMYOPATHY

GENE	SYMBOL	INHERITANCE	PHENOTYPES	FREQUENCY
SARCOMERIC PROTEINS				
Cardiac β-myosin heavy chain	MYH7	AD	Variable: moderate to severe prognosis; HCM; LVNC; DCM; Laing distal myopathy	HCM 30-40%; DCM 4-6%
Cardiac troponin T	TNNT2	AD	HCM: possible high incidence of sudden death; DCM	HCM 5%; DCM 3%
Cardiac troponin I	TNNI3	HCM, AD; DCM, AR	Can present with restrictive physiology/cardiomyopathy; HCM; DCM	HCM 5%, DCM <1%
Cardiac troponin C	TNNC	AD	DCM	<1%
Cardiac myosin binding protein C	MYBPC3	AD	Late onset of the disease described; cases of children with a severe hypertrophy also reported; DCM	HCM 30-40%; DCM (?)
Cardiac α-myosin heavy chain	MYH6	AD	DCM, HCM	DCM (?) 2-3%; HCM <1%
Titin	TTN	AD	DCM, HCM	DCM (?); HCM rare
Cardiac actin	ACTC	DCM and HCM AD	DCM, LVNC, HCM	DCM <1%; HCM ≈1%
Essential myosin light chain	MYL3	AD	HCM	(?)
Regulatory myosin light chain	MYL2	AD	HCM	≈1%
α-Tropomyosin	TPM1	AD	HCM, DCM	HCM ≈1-2%; DCM <1%
Z-DISC PROTEINS				
Cypher/ZASP	LDB3		LVNC	
Metavinculin	VCL	AD	DCM, HCM	DCM <1-1%; HCM rare
LIM binding domain 3	LDB3	AD	DCM, HCM	DCM <1-1%; HCM rare
Titin-cap or telethonin	TCAP	AD	DCM, HCM	DCM <1-1%; HCM <1%
Myozenin 2	MYOZ2	AD	HCM	<1%
Muscle LIM protein	CSRP3	AD	DCM, HCM	DCM <1%; HCM rare
CYTOSKELETAL PROTEINS				
Desmin	DES	AD	DCM	<1-1%
α- and β-dystroglycans	DAG1	NA	DCM	NA
α-, β-, γ-, and δ-sarcoglycans	SGCA, SGCB, SGCG, SGCD	SGCD AD	DCM	SGCD <1%
Caveolin-3	CAV3	AD	DCM, HCM	HCM rare
Lamin A/C	LMNA	DCM, AD; EMD2, AD; EMD3, AR; LGMD1B, AD	LVNC, DCM, DCM in Emery-Dreifuss muscular dystrophy types 2 and 3 (EMD2 and EMD3), DCM in limb girdle muscular dystrophy (LGMD) 1B	DCM 4-8%
Syntrophin	SNT	NA	DCM	NA
Dystrobrevin	DTN	NA	DCM	NA
Dystrophin	DMD	XL	DCM in Duchenne muscular dystrophy (DMD), Becker muscular dystrophy (BMD)	(?)
DESMOSOMAL PROTEINS				
Plakoglobin	JUP	Naxos disease, AR	ARVC, ARVC in Naxos disease	Rare
Desmoplakin	DSP	Carvajal syndrome, AR; ARVC, AD	ARVC, DCM in Carvajal syndrome	ARVC 6-16%
Desmoglein 2	DSG2	AD	ARVC	12-40%
Desmocollin 2	DSC2	AD	ARVC	Rare
Plakophilin-2	PKP2	AD, AR	ARVC	AD 11-43%, AR rare
SARCOPLASMIC RETICULUM				
Phospholamban	PLN	AD	DCM, HCM	DCM (?); HCM rare
METABOLIC PROTEINS				
Protein kinase, AMP-activated, γ₂ noncatalytic subunit	PRKAG2	AD	HCM in Wolff-Parkinson-White syndrome	NA
α-Galactosidase A	GLA	XL	HCM in Anderson-Fabry disease	NA
Lysosomal-associated membrane protein 2	LAMP2	XL	HCM in Danon disease	NA
OTHERS				
Hereditary hemochromatosis	HFE	AR	DCM and RCM in hereditary hemochromatosis	NA
Hereditary amyloidosis	TTR	AD	HCM and RCM in hereditary amyloidosis	NA
RAS-MAPK pathway genes	PTPN11/RAF1/SOS1/KRAS/HRAS/BRAF/MEK1-2	AD	HCM in Noonan syndrome and LEOPARD syndrome	NA
Frataxin	FRDA	AR	HCM in Friedreich ataxia	NA

AD = autosomal dominant; AR = autosomal recessive; ARVC = arrhythmogenic right ventricular cardiomyopathy; DCM = dilated cardiomyopathy; HCM = hypertrophic cardiomyopathy; NA = not available; RCM = restrictive cardiomyopathy; XL = X-linked.

present in up to 17% of cases. The papillary muscles are often displaced anteriorly, thereby contributing to systolic anterior motion of the anterior mitral valve leaflet in 25% of patients and of the posterior leaflets in 10% of cases in the resting state. Often, the mitral valve is structurally abnormal, with elongation of the anterior leaflet and occasional direct insertion of the papillary muscle into the anterior leaflet. The histologic hallmark of hypertrophic cardiomyopathy is a triad of myocyte hypertrophy, myocyte disarray, and interstitial fibrosis. Myocyte disarray refers to architectural disorganization of the myocardium, with adjacent myocytes aligned obliquely or perpendicular to each other in association with increased interstitial collagen. The myofibrillar architecture within the myocyte is also disorganized. Although myocyte disarray occurs in aortic stenosis, long-standing hypertension, and some forms of congenital heart disease, the presence of extensive disarray (more than 10% of ventricular septal myocytes) is thought to be a highly specific marker for hypertrophic cardiomyopathy. Small intramural coronary arteries are often dysplastic and narrowed owing to wall thickening by smooth muscle cell hyperplasia.

PATHOPHYSIOLOGY

Abnormal ventricular geometry, wall thickening, myocyte hypertrophy, myocyte and myofibrillar disarray, and myocardial fibrosis all contribute to impairment of left ventricular diastolic function. The net result is elevation of left ventricular end-diastolic pressures, symptoms of heart failure, and reduced exercise tolerance. Global measures of left ventricular systolic function are often normal, but regional myocardial dysfunction and progressive systolic impairment are relatively common.

Approximately 25% of patients have left ventricular outflow tract obstruction at rest caused by contact between the anterior leaflet of the mitral valve and the interventricular septum during ventricular systole. Many patients without outflow obstruction at rest develop it during physiologic and pharmacologic interventions that reduce left ventricular end-diastolic volume or increase left ventricular contractility (e.g., amyl nitrate inhalation, Valsalva maneuver, and administration of intravenous inotropic agents).

CLINICAL MANIFESTATIONS

Most patients are asymptomatic or have only mild or intermittent symptoms. Symptomatic progression is usually slow, age related, and associated with a gradual deterioration in left ventricular function over decades. Fewer than 5% of patients may have rapid, symptomatic deterioration. Symptoms can develop at any age, even many years after the appearance of electrocardiographic (ECG) or echocardiographic manifestations of left ventricular hypertrophy. Occasionally, sudden death may be the initial presentation. However, most individuals with hypertrophic cardiomyopathy have few if any symptoms, and the diagnosis is often made as a result of family screening or the incidental detection of a heart murmur or an abnormal ECG.

Approximately 20 to 30% of adults develop chest pain (Chapters 50 and 71), which may occur on exertion, at rest, or nocturnally. Postprandial angina associated with mild exertion is typical. Mild to moderate dyspnea on exertion is relatively common, and some patients develop paroxysmal nocturnal dyspnea that may be caused by transient myocardial ischemia or arrhythmia. Approximately 20% of patients experience syncope (Chapters 50 and 62), and a similar proportion complain of presyncope. Palpitations (Chapter 62) are frequent and are usually attributable to supraventricular or ventricular ectopy or to forceful cardiac contraction. Sustained palpitations are usually caused by supraventricular tachyarrhythmias, but initial presentation with a symptomatic arrhythmia is uncommon. Patients with distal or apical hypertrophy have fewer symptoms, better exercise capacity, no arrhythmias, and good prognosis. Occasionally, however, patients with distal or apical hypertrophy may have severe refractory chest pain or may present with troublesome supraventricular arrhythmias.

DIAGNOSIS

A three- to four-generation family history, which should be obtained in all patients with a new diagnosis of cardiomyopathy, helps to determine the probability of familial disease and its mode of inheritance. The initial diagnostic evaluation includes a family history focusing on premature cardiac disease or death, a comprehensive medical history focusing on cardiovascular symptoms, a careful physical examination, a 12-lead ECG, and a two-dimensional echocardiogram.

The general evaluation may provide diagnostic clues in patients whose hypertrophic cardiomyopathy is associated with syndromes or metabolic disorders. For example, Noonan's syndrome (Chapter 69) is characterized by short stature, developmental delay, cutaneous abnormalities (café au lait spots), hypertelorism, ptosis, low-set posteriorly rotated ears, and a webbed neck. These features are shared with the less common LEOPARD syndrome. Angiokeratomas, anhidrosis, Raynaud's-like symptoms with neuropathy, cornea verticillata, retinal vascular dilation, tinnitus, diarrhea, and proteinuria are typical features of Fabry's disease (Chapter 215).

Clinical examination of the cardiovascular system is often normal. In the presence of left ventricular outflow tract obstruction, the arterial pulse has a rapid upstroke and downstroke (sometimes with a bisferiens character), the apex beat is sustained or double (reflecting a palpable atrial impulse followed by left ventricular contraction), and auscultation will demonstrate a systolic ejection murmur that is heard loudest at the left sternal edge and that radiates to the right upper sternal edge and apex (Chapter 50). Most patients with left ventricular outflow tract obstruction also have the murmur of mitral regurgitation, which results from failure of the mitral valve leaflets to coapt owing to the systolic anterior motion of the mitral valve. Physiologic and pharmacologic maneuvers that decrease afterload or venous return (e.g., standing, Valsalva maneuver, inhalation of amyl nitrite) or increase contractility (e.g., a post-extrasystole beat) will increase the intensity of the murmur, whereas interventions that increase afterload and venous return (e.g., squatting or handgrip) will reduce it (see Table 50-2 in Chapter 50). In contrast, physical signs in most patients who do not have left ventricular outflow tract obstruction are subtle and are limited to features that reflect the hyperdynamic contraction (rapid upstroke pulse) and poorly compliant right (prominent a wave in jugular venous pressure) and left (S_4 gallop, double-apex beat) ventricles (Chapter 50).

Diagnostic Testing

More than 90% of patients have abnormal ECG findings, but no changes are disease specific. The most common abnormalities are increased QRS voltage consistent with left ventricular hypertrophy, left axis deviation (15 to 20%), abnormal Q waves (25 to 30%, most commonly in inferolateral leads), and ST segment or T wave changes (>50%). An isolated increase in the QRS voltage without ST segment changes or T wave inversion is rare in hypertrophic cardiomyopathy. The presence of predominantly distal or apical thickening is associated with giant negative T wave inversion on the ECG tracing.

Two-dimensional echocardiography (Chapter 55) is the mainstay of diagnostic imaging, but magnetic resonance imaging (Chapter 56) and computed tomography (Chapter 56) provide alternatives if the echocardiogram is of poor quality. In most patients, the hypertrophy is asymmetrical and involves the anterior and posterior intraventricular septum (Fig. 60-2). The hypertrophy, however, may be more generalized and involve the free wall of the left ventricle, or it may be localized and confined to areas other than the septum, such as the lateral or posterior wall of the left ventricle. The echocardiogram can measure left ventricular outflow tract obstruction, both at rest and after provocative maneuvers. Patients with an outflow tract gradient of 30 mm Hg or more typically have systolic anterior motion of the mitral valve, with contact of either the anterior or (less commonly) the posterior mitral leaflet with the intraventricular septum during systole, in association with a posteriorly directed jet of mitral regurgitation, the severity of which is proportionate to the severity of the obstruction. Most patients with hypertrophic cardiomyopathy have left atrial enlargement as well as echocardiographic evidence of diastolic dysfunction.

When available, cardiopulmonary exercise testing with metabolic gas exchange measurements provides an accurate and reproducible assessment of exercise capacity, which can be followed serially. Cardiac catheterization is rarely required for diagnosis or management, but it may be indicated when measurement of intracardiac pressures is required to guide therapeutic decisions (e.g., in patients with severe mitral regurgitation) and for the exclusion of coexistent coronary artery disease in patients with chest pain.

Diagnostic Criteria

A wall thickness of more than 2 standard deviations above the mean, corrected for age, gender, and height, is generally accepted as diagnostic. In adults, this value is typically 1.5 cm or greater in men and 1.3 cm or greater in women. In the presence of other causes of left ventricular hypertrophy such as long-standing systemic hypertension or aortic stenosis, the diagnosis of hypertrophic cardiomyopathy may be problematic. However, secondary hypertrophy from other causes rarely exceeds 1.8 cm. Hypertrophy in the

FIGURE 60-2. Hypertrophic obstructive cardiomyopathy. **A,** The two-dimensional long-axis parasternal view shows the chambers of the heart. The left ventricle posterior wall (LVPW) is thickened, and the most striking abnormality is the hypertrophy of the interventricular septum (IVS). Another characteristic feature is a Venturi effect: as blood leaves the left ventricle (LV), it sucks the anterior leaflet of the mitral valve forward, a phenomenon called *systolic anterior motion* (SAM). **B,** This phenomenon is more clearly shown in the parasternal long-axis M-mode echocardiogram. The massive thickening of the septum is also obvious in the M-mode image (IVS). AO = aorta; LA = left atrium; RV = right ventricle. (From Forbes CD, Jackson WF. *Color Atlas and Text of Clinical Medicine,* 3rd ed. London: Mosby; 2003.)

TABLE 60-3 DIAGNOSTIC CRITERIA FOR HYPERTROPHIC CARDIOMYOPATHY IN FIRST-DEGREE RELATIVES OF AFFECTED PATIENTS*

MAJOR CRITERIA	MINOR CRITERIA
ECHOCARDIOGRAPHY	
Left ventricular wall thickness ≥13 mm in the anterior septum or posterior wall or ≥15 mm in the posterior septum or free wall	Left ventricular wall thickness of 12 mm in the anterior septum or posterior wall or of 14 mm in the posterior septum or free wall
Severe SAM of the mitral valve (septal-leaflet contact)	Moderate SAM of the mitral valve (no mitral leaflet-septal contact)
	Redundant mitral valve leaflets
ELECTROCARDIOGRAPHY	
Left ventricular hypertrophy with repolarization changes (Romhilt and Estes)	Complete bundle branch block or (minor) interventricular conduction defects (in left ventricular leads)
T wave inversion in leads I and aVL (≥3 mm with QRS-T wave axis difference ≥30 degrees), V_3-V_6 (≥3 mm) or II and III and aVF (≥5 mm)	Minor repolarization changes in left ventricular leads
	Deep S wave in lead V_2 (>25 mm)
Abnormal Q waves (>40 msec or >25% R wave) in at least two leads from II, III, aVF (in absence of left anterior hemiblock), and V_1-V_4; or I, aVL, V_5-V_6	Unexplained chest pain, dyspnea, or syncope

*The diagnosis of hypertrophic cardiomyopathy in first-degree relatives of patients with the disease is based on the presence of one major criterion or two minor echocardiographic criteria or one minor echocardiographic and two minor electrocardiographic criteria.
aVF = augmented voltage unipolar left foot lead; aVL = augmented voltage unipolar left arm lead; SAM = systolic anterior motion.
Adapted from McKenna WJ, Spirito P, Desnos M, et al. Experience in clinical genetics in hypertrophic cardiomyopathy. *Heart.* 1997;77:130-132.

highly trained athlete is usually less than 1.6 cm in males and 1.4 cm in females, and typically occurs in association with an increased left ventricular end-diastolic dimension and stroke volume. An ECG tracing showing Q waves or inferolateral repolarization changes in an athlete favors the diagnosis of hypertrophic cardiomyopathy.

Given the 50% probability of disease in a first-degree relative of a patient with hypertrophic cardiomyopathy, modified diagnostic criteria (Table 60-3) consider the high probability that their otherwise unexplained ECG and echocardiographic findings reflect incomplete disease expression, with the corresponding risks for complications and for passing the gene to their children.

TREATMENT   Rx

Clinical management is based mainly on symptoms (Fig. 60-3). Exceptions include specific therapies for lysosomal storage diseases, such as Pompe's (Chapter 214) and Fabry's disease (Chapter 215), and for Friedreich's ataxia (Chapter 429). The treatment of the remaining patients with hypertrophic cardiomyopathy focuses on the counseling of family members, the management of symptoms, and the prevention of disease-related complications.

Family Evaluation

All patients with hypertrophic cardiomyopathy should be counseled on the implications of the diagnosis for their families. Careful pedigree analysis can reassure relatives who are not at risk for inheriting the disease. For those who are at risk, current guidelines recommend screening with a 12-lead ECG and echocardiogram at intervals of 12 to 18 months, usually starting at the age of 12 years (unless there is a "malignant" family history of premature sudden death, the child is symptomatic or a competitive athlete, or there is a clinical suspicion of left ventricular hypertrophy) until full growth and maturation are achieved (usually by the age of 18 to 21 years). Thereafter, if there are no signs of disease expression, screening approximately every 5 years is advised because the onset of left ventricular hypertrophy may be delayed until well into adulthood in some families. Modified diagnostic criteria (see Table 60-3) consider the high probability that otherwise unexplained ECG and echocardiographic findings in first-degree relatives reflect incomplete disease expression.

When available, genetic testing can identify a disease-causing mutation in an index case and thereby provide presymptomatic diagnosis of family members. Whenever genetic testing is considered, individuals should be informed about the purpose of the test, the most probable mode of inheritance, and the potential hazards and limitations of genetic testing.

Symptom Management
Medical Therapy

Therapeutic options in patients *without* left ventricular outflow gradients are limited predominantly to pharmacologic therapy. β-Blockade may improve chest pain and dyspnea. The dose (starting at a dose equivalent to propranolol, 120 mg/day) should be titrated to achieve a target heart rate of 50 to 70 beats per minute at rest and 130 to 140 beats per minute at peak exercise. Calcium antagonists such as verapamil (starting at a dose of 120 mg/day) and diltiazem (starting at a dose of 180 mg/day) are useful alternatives, particularly in patients with refractory chest pain, but high doses (e.g., verapamil >480 mg/day, diltiazem >360 mg/day) may be required. In patients with paroxysmal nocturnal dyspnea and no evidence of ventricular outflow obstruction, a transient mechanism such as myocardial ischemia or arrhythmia may be the cause, although investigations usually fail to identify the precise cause. Such patients, as well as those with chronically raised pulmonary pressures, may require diuretics (e.g., furosemide, 20 to 40 mg orally as needed, followed by 20 mg/day if required). The dose and duration of diuretic therapy should be minimized because injudicious use of these drugs can be dangerous, particularly in patients with severe diastolic impairment or labile obstruction.

In patients with symptoms caused by left ventricular outflow tract obstruction, the main aim of treatment is to reduce the outflow tract gradient. Options include negative inotropic drugs, surgery, atrioventricular sequential pacing, and percutaneous alcohol ablation of the interventricular septum. Approximately 60 to 70% of patients improve with β-blockers, although high doses (equivalent to propranolol at 480 mg/day) are frequently required, and side effects are often limiting. When β-blockade alone is ineffective, disopyramide, titrated to the maximal tolerated dose (usually between 400 and 600 mg/day), may be effective in up to two thirds of patients, but side effects related to the anticholinergic effects (e.g., dry eyes and mouth) limit its use. Disopyramide should be given concomitantly with a small to medium dose of a β-blocker (e.g., propranolol, 120 to 240 mg/day), which will slow the heart rate and also blunt rapid atrioventricular nodal conduction should supraventricular arrhythmias develop. In patients who have left ventricular outflow tract obstruction and are taking a β-blocker and disopyramide, other antiarrhythmic drugs that alter repolarization (e.g., sotalol or amiodarone) must be avoided because of the potential proarrhythmic effect. In patients with outflow tract gradients, verapamil can be effective, but caution is required in patients with severe obstruction or elevated pulmonary pressures.

Interventional Therapy

Surgery should be considered for significant outflow obstruction (gradient >50 mm Hg) in patients who have symptoms refractory to medical therapy. The most commonly performed surgical procedure, ventricular septal myectomy, either abolishes or substantially reduces the gradient in 95% of cases, reduces mitral regurgitation, and improves exercise capacity and symptoms. Surgery should be performed in an experienced center, where mortality rates should be less than 1% for isolated myomectomy. The main complications (atrioventricular block, ventricular septal defects) are rare. In some patients, concomitant mitral valve repair or replacement may be required.

In experienced centers, the selective injection of alcohol into a septal perforator branch of the left anterior descending coronary artery to create a localized septal scar yields outcomes similar to surgery. The main nonfatal complication is atrioventricular block requiring a pacemaker in 5 to 20% of patients.

Dual-chamber pacing using a short-programmed atrial ventricular delay to produce maximal pre-excitation while maintaining effective atrial transport can reduce the outflow gradient by 30 to 50% but provides little objective improvement in exercise capacity in most patients.

Supraventricular Arrhythmia

Atrial fibrillation in hypertrophic cardiomyopathy is associated with a high risk for systemic embolization, so anticoagulation (international normalized ratio in the range of 2.0 to 3.0) should be considered in all patients with sustained or paroxysmal atrial fibrillation (Chapter 64). Treatment with low-dose amiodarone, 1000 to 1400 mg/week, is effective in maintaining sinus rhythm and in controlling the ventricular response during breakthrough episodes. The addition of a low-dose β-blocker, verapamil, or diltiazem may be required for rate control. Serious side effects on low-dose amiodarone are uncommon. β-blockers, particularly those with class III action (e.g., sotalol), are less effective alternatives. In general, the principles of managing atrial fibrillation in patients with hypertrophic cardiomyopathy are similar to those in other conditions (Chapter 64), with the provision that the threshold to use anticoagulation should be low because of the significant embolic risk.

Prevention of Sudden Death

The overall risk for sudden death in children and adults with hypertrophic cardiomyopathy is approximately 1% per year, but a minority of individuals have a much greater risk for ventricular arrhythmia and sudden death. The most powerful predictor of sudden cardiac death in hypertrophic cardiomyopathy is a history of previous cardiac arrest. In patients without such a history, the most useful markers of risk are a family history of premature (<40 years of age) sudden cardiac death; unexplained syncope (unrelated to neurocardiogenic mechanisms); a flat or hypotensive blood pressure response to upright exercise; nonsustained ventricular tachycardia on ambulatory electrocardiographic monitoring or during exercise; and severe left ventricular hypertrophy on echocardiography (defined as a maximal left ventricular wall thickness of 30 mm or more). Patients with two or more of these markers have an annual mortality rate of 3 to 6% and should receive an implantable cardioverter-defibrillator (ICD) (Chapter 66). All patients with hypertrophic cardiomyopathy should be advised to avoid competitive sports and intense physical exertion. Patients without any risk factors do not warrant an ICD. For patients with one risk factor, decisions regarding an ICD should be individualized based on the patient's age and severity of disease.

FIGURE 60-3. Approach to the management of hypertrophic cardiomyopathy (HCM). ICD = implantable cardioverter-defibrillator. (Adapted from Maron BJ, McKenna WJ, Danielson GK, et al. American College of Cardiology/European Society of Cardiology clinical expert consensus document on hypertrophic cardiomyopathy. *J Am Coll Cardiol.* 2003;42:1687-1713.)

PROGNOSIS

Most patients with hypertrophic cardiomyopathy follow a stable and benign course with a low risk for adverse events and a survival similar to that of age- and gender-matched normal populations, but many experience progressive symptoms caused by atrial arrhythmia and gradual deterioration in left ventricular systolic and diastolic function. About 1% of affected individuals die suddenly each year. The annual incidence of stroke varies from 0.56 to 0.8%/year, rising to 1.9% in patients older than 60 years, and 23% of strokes are fatal. The development of severe systolic heart failure is associated with a poor prognosis, with an overall mortality rate of up to 11% per year. The incidence of infective endocarditis is 1.4 per 1000 person-years overall but 3.8 per 1000 person-years in patients with obstruction.

Myocarditis

DEFINITION AND EPIDEMIOLOGY

Myocarditis, which is an inflammatory process involving the myocardium, can be caused by infections, immune-mediated damage, or toxins (Table 60-4). The incidence and prevalence of myocarditis are difficult to estimate because the clinical presentation varies from asymptomatic ECG abnormalities to hemodynamic collapse and sudden death. Population estimates of the prevalence of myocarditis range from 1 in 100,000 to 1 in 10,000, whereas postmortem studies report myocarditis in up to 12% of young victims of sudden cardiac death.

Worldwide, the most common infective myocarditis is Chagas' disease, caused by *Trypanosoma cruzi,* a protozoan organism endemic in rural areas of South and Central America (Chapter 355). In the Western world, viral myocarditis is the most common cause of inflammatory heart disease. Human immunodeficiency virus (HIV) infection (Chapter 392) is associated with lymphocytic monocarditis and is a strong predictor of poor prognosis. Smallpox vaccination (Chapter 17) causes myopericarditis, with a reported incidence of 7.8 cases per 100,000 vaccine administrations. Other rare myocarditises include giant cell myocarditis, myocarditis complicating autoimmune disorders such as systemic lupus erythematosus (Chapter 274), and cocaine abuse (Chapter 33).

PATHOBIOLOGY

Myocarditis is defined histologically by the presence of myocyte injury, with degeneration or necrosis, and an inflammatory infiltrate not due to ischemia. Four patterns are recognized: *active myocarditis,* with myocyte degeneration or necrosis and definite cellular infiltrate with or without fibrosis; *borderline myocarditis,* with a definite cellular infiltrate without evidence of myocardial cellular injury; *persistent myocarditis,* with continued active myocarditis on repeat biopsy; and *resolving or resolved myocarditis,* characterized by a diminished or absent infiltrate with evidence of connective tissue healing on repeat biopsy. Despite their widespread use, these criteria have low specificity and sensitivity, with a diagnostic yield as low as 10 to 20% in some series. Therefore, newer virology techniques used in conjunction with conventional light microscopy include nested polymerase chain reaction (PCR) or reverse transcription PCR on RNA and DNA extracted from endomyocardial biopsy specimens, as well as immunohistochemical staining for subtypes of infiltrating lymphocytes and abnormal expression of cellular adhesion molecules on interstitial or endothelial cells.

Viral Myocarditis

Most data on the pathology of viral myocarditis come from murine models. Initially, there is direct invasion of the myocardium by cardiotropic viruses, which enter the cardiomyocyte through receptor-mediated endocytosis. The viral genome, which translated intracellularly to produce viral protein or is incorporated into the host cell genome, may contribute to myocyte dysfunction by cleaving dystrophin. In the second phase, activation of the host immune system, including recruitment of natural killer cells and macrophages, increases the expression of proinflammatory cytokines such as interleukin-1 and tumor necrosis factor. Activation of CD4$^+$ T lymphocytes promotes clonal expansion of B lymphocytes, thereby resulting in further myocardial cell damage, inflammation, and the production of circulating anti-heart antibodies directed against contractile, structural, and mitochondrial proteins. This autoimmune response may result in long-term ventricular remodeling owing to direct effects on myocardial structural components or alterations in the extracellular matrix.

TABLE 60-4 CAUSES OF MYOCARDITIS

INFECTION

Viral

Coxsackievirus, human immunodeficiency virus, echovirus, adenovirus, influenza, measles, mumps, parvovirus, poliovirus, rubella, varicella-zoster virus, herpes simplex virus, cytomegalovirus, hepatitis C virus, rabies virus, respiratory syncytial virus, vaccine virus, dengue virus, yellow fever virus

Protozoal

Trypanosoma cruzi, Toxoplasma gondii

Bacterial

Brucella, Corynebacterium diphtheriae, Salmonella, Haemophilus influenzae, Mycoplasma pneumoniae, Neisseria meningitidis (meningococcus), *Streptococcus pneumoniae, Staphylococcus, Mycobacterium, Neisseria gonorrhoeae* (gonococcus), *Vibrio cholerae*

Spirochetal

Treponema pallidum, Borrelia, Leptospira

Fungal

Aspergillus, Candida, Cryptococcus, Actinomyces, Blastomyces, Histoplasma, Coccidioides

Rickettsial

Coxiella burnetii, Rickettsia rickettsii, Rickettsia tsutsugamushi

Parasitic

Trichinella spiralis, Echinococcus granulosus, Taenia solium

IMMUNE-MEDIATED DISORDERS

Alloantigens

Heart transplant rejection

Autoantigens

Churg-Strauss syndrome, celiac disease, Whipple's disease, giant cell myocarditis, Kawasaki disease, systemic lupus erythematosus, systemic sclerosis, sarcoidosis, scleroderma, polymyositis, thrombocytopenic purpura

Allergens (Drugs)

Penicillin, sulfonamides, tetracycline, methyldopa, streptomycin, tricyclic antidepressants, thiazide diuretics, dobutamine, indomethacin

TOXIC CAUSES

Drugs

Anthracyclines, catecholamines, amphetamines, cocaine, cyclophosphamide, 5-fluorouracil, Herceptin, interferon, interleukin-2

Physical Agents

Electric shock, radiation, hyperpyrexia

Heavy Metals

Copper, iron, lead

Others

Arsenic, snake bite, scorpion bite, wasp and spider stings, phosphorus, carbon monoxide

GENETIC DISORDERS

Inherited cardiomyopathies with immune-mediated pathogenesis (dilated and right ventricular cardiomyopathy)

CLINICAL MANIFESTATIONS

Some patients report prodromal symptoms of viremia, including fever, myalgia, coryzal symptoms, or gastroenteritis, but many individuals with myocarditis are asymptomatic and manifest only transient ECG abnormalities such as nonspecific ST segment and T wave abnormalities, pathologic Q waves, and low QRS voltages. Less common ECG presentations include acute myocardial infarction (Chapter 73), atrioventricular block (Chapter 64), and ventricular arrhythmias (Chapter 65). Patients with impairment of left ventricular function may present with symptoms and signs of fulminant cardiogenic shock (Chapter 107) with acute cardiovascular collapse. In some cases, sudden cardiac death is the first presentation.

DIAGNOSIS

The diagnosis of myocarditis requires a high index of suspicion because it may mimic other common conditions. On echocardiography, evidence of impaired left ventricular systolic performance, often without significant left ventricular dilatation, is typical. Regional wall motion abnormalities are common, and left (or right) ventricular thrombus may be present. Evidence of left ventricular diastolic impairment and pericardial effusions is common. Cardiac magnetic resonance imaging can detect myocardial inflammation and myocyte injury, with pericellular and cellular edema.

Routine blood tests such as full blood count and erythrocyte sedimentation rate are usually unhelpful, but serum markers of myocardial injury such as troponin T and I may be elevated. Creatine kinase and its cardiac isoform CK-MB are less sensitive and specific than troponin and are not useful as screening tests. Increased levels of autoantibodies against myocardial proteins (such as myosin and the adenine nucleotide translocator protein) correlate with progressive worsening of ventricular function.

Cardiac catheterization with right ventricular endomyocardial biopsy remains the gold standard diagnostic test for myocarditis. However, it is generally reserved for patients with heart failure refractory to standard management, features suggestive of systemic disease (e.g., connective tissue disease [Chapter 268], amyloidosis [Chapter 193], hemochromatosis [Chapter 219], sarcoidosis [Chapter 95]), or suspicion of giant cell myocarditis because of new-onset heart failure associated with tachyarrhythmias or conduction disease.

Specific Causes

Viral myocarditis may be suspected from the clinical picture of recent febrile illness, often with prominent myalgias, followed by angina-like chest pain, dyspnea, or arrhythmias. Elevated troponin levels support the diagnosis, and increasing viral titers (to coxsackievirus, echovirus, adenovirus, or influenza virus) confirm recent infection. Clinical cardiomyopathy occurs in 10 to 40% of patients infected with HIV, owing to the HIV itself or to coinfection with cytomegalovirus.

Giant cell myocarditis, which accounts for 10 to 20% of biopsy-positive cases of myocarditis, presents with the rapid onset of chest pain, fever, and hemodynamic compromise, often with ventricular tachycardia or atrioventricular block. When ventricular tachyarrhythmias are a major feature of myocarditis, particularly in a young person, endomyocardial biopsy is generally recommended to determine whether giant cell myocarditis is present, even though the diagnosis is statistically unlikely.

Toxoplasmosis (Chapter 357) *myocarditis,* owing to intermittent rupture of cysts in the myocardium, can cause atypical chest pain, arrhythmias, pericarditis, and symptomatic heart failure. Diagnosis is made from antibody titers. Lyme carditis (Chapter 329) classically presents with conduction system abnormalities resulting from infection with *Borrelia burgdorferi,* which is diagnosed serologically.

Immune-mediated myocarditis can be associated with polymyositis (Chapter 277) or systemic lupus erythematosus (Chapter 274), although pericarditis and coronary artery vasculitis are more common. Hypersensitivity reactions, especially to drugs (Chapter 262), can cause myocarditis that is often associated with peripheral eosinophilia and can be confirmed by endomyocardial biopsy.

TREATMENT ⟨Rx⟩

The first-line treatment of myocarditis is supportive with afterload reduction and diuresis (Chapter 59). Patients with fulminant acute myocarditis may require inotropic support, mechanical assist devices, or extracorporeal membrane oxygenation (Chapter 107). Following initial stabilization, patients with symptoms and signs of heart failure should receive angiotensin-converting enzyme inhibitors, diuretics, β-blockers, and anticoagulants in accordance with standard guidelines (Chapter 59). Patients with intractable and deteriorating heart failure may require cardiac transplantation (Chapter 82).

The role of immunosuppression is uncertain. In one randomized, placebo-controlled trial of 111 adults with biopsy-proven myocarditis, there was no difference in mortality or improvement in left ventricular function in patients treated with prednisolone plus either cyclosporine or azathioprine.[1] Conversely, in a randomized trial of patients who had major histocompatibility complex expression on endomyocardial biopsy samples and who were randomized to prednisolone (1 mg/kg/day tapering to a maintenance dose of 0.2 mg/kg/day for a total of 90 days) and azathioprine (1 mg/kg/day for a total of 100 days) versus placebo, left ventricular ejection fraction improved in the immunosuppressed group, but no difference was observed in mortality or rates of transplantation or rehospitalization over a 2-year follow-up period.[2] At present, immunosuppression is generally reserved for patients with giant cell myocarditis, in whom there is some benefit,[3] although the optimal regimen is yet to be determined. Intravenous immunoglobulin therapy is not helpful.[4]

PROGNOSIS

Patients with acute myocarditis with mild heart failure or symptoms suggestive of myocardial ischemia or infarction typically improve within weeks without sequelae. An acute presentation of myocarditis with advanced heart failure (ejection fraction <35%) may resolve but can lead to chronic left ventricular dysfunction (dilated cardiomyopathy) or progress to death or cardiac transplantation. Patients who present with acute fulminant myocarditis, however, have an excellent prognosis, with survival rates of more than 90%. Giant cell myocarditis is usually fatal without heart transplantation.

Dilated Cardiomyopathy

DEFINITION AND EPIDEMIOLOGY

Dilated cardiomyopathy is a heart muscle disorder defined by dilation and impaired systolic function of the left or both ventricles, in the absence of coronary artery disease, valvular abnormalities, or pericardial disease. In adults, prevalence estimates range from 14 to 36 per 100,000. In children, dilated cardiomyopathy is the most common cardiomyopathy, accounting for up to 58% of cases. Overall, males and females are approximately equally affected, except for dilated cardiomyopathy associated with neuromuscular disorders or inborn errors of metabolism, for which there is male predominance, because some of these conditions have an X-linked inheritance.

PATHOBIOLOGY

A number of conditions are associated with dilated cardiomyopathy, including neuromuscular disorders, inborn errors of metabolism, and malformation syndromes. In most patients, no identifiable cause is found, and the disease is termed *idiopathic dilated cardiomyopathy.*

Genetic Dilated Cardiomyopathy

Between 20 and 50% of individuals with dilated cardiomyopathy have evidence of familial disease (see Table 60-2). Autosomal dominant inheritance, which accounts for 68% of familial cases, has two major forms: isolated dilated cardiomyopathy and dilated cardiomyopathy associated with conduction system disease. The latter patients may also have an associated skeletal myopathy. Genes implicated in isolated dilated cardiomyopathy include cytoskeletal and sarcomeric protein genes. Mutations in the lamin A/C gene, which encodes a nuclear envelope protein, cause atrial arrhythmia and progressive atrioventricular conduction disease, which precede the development of dilated cardiomyopathy by several years.

X-linked inheritance accounts for between 2 and 5% of familial cases of dilated cardiomyopathy Neuromuscular disorders account for 26% of cases, 90% of which are Duchenne, Becker's, and Emery-Driefuss muscular dystrophies (Chapter 429). Isolated X-linked dilated cardiomyopathy, also caused by mutations in the dystrophin gene, is characterized by raised serum creatine kinase muscle isoforms but does not result in clinical signs or symptoms of skeletal muscular dystrophy.

Acquired Dilated Cardiomyopathy

Common acquired causes of dilated cardiomyopathy include infectious myocarditis, chemotherapy (Chapter 182), radiotherapy (Chapter 19), alcohol (Chapter 32), cocaine (Chapter 33), nutritional deficiencies (Chapter 222), iron overload (Chapter 219), inflammatory and autoimmune disorders (Chapters 274 and 278), endocrinopathies (Chapter 233), and pregnancy (Chapter 247). Tachycardia-mediated cardiomyopathy (tachycardiomyopathy) is rare and usually reverses once the tachycardia is controlled.

CLINICAL MANIFESTATIONS

The symptoms and signs associated with dilated cardiomyopathy depend on the age of the patient and the degree of left ventricular dysfunction. Although the first presentation may be with sudden death or a thromboembolic event, most patients present with symptoms of high pulmonary venous pressure or low cardiac output (Chapter 58), which can be acute, sometimes precipitated by intercurrent illness or arrhythmia, or chronic. Increasingly, dilated cardiomyopathy is diagnosed incidentally in asymptomatic individuals during family screening.

Adults initially present with reduced exercise tolerance and dyspnea on exertion. With worsening left ventricular function, patients may develop dyspnea at rest, orthopnea, paroxysmal nocturnal dyspnea, peripheral edema, and ascites. Symptoms related to mesenteric ischemia, such as abdominal pain after meals, nausea, vomiting, and anorexia, may dominate, especially in children. Arrhythmia symptoms, such as palpitations, presyncope, and syncope, can occur at any age.

In advanced disease, features of low cardiac output include sinus tachycardia, weak peripheral pulses, and hypotension. The jugular venous pressure may be elevated, and the apical impulse is displaced. Peripheral edema, hepatomegaly, and ascites are common in patients with heart failure. Auscultation of the chest typically reveals basal crackles. Auscultation of the heart may reveal the presence of a third (and sometimes also a fourth) heart sound. In patients with functional mitral regurgitation, a pansystolic murmur may be heard at the apex and radiate to the axilla, but frequently no murmurs are heard, even in the presence of mitral incompetence, especially if cardiac output is very low.

DIAGNOSIS

The ECG may be normal but more typically shows sinus tachycardia, non-specific ST segment and T wave changes (most commonly in the inferior and lateral leads), atrial enlargement, and voltage criteria for ventricular hypertrophy. Atrioventricular block raises the possibility of mutations in the lamin A/C gene. Supraventricular and ventricular arrhythmias are common. The chest radiograph is usually abnormal, with an increased cardiothoracic ratio (greater than 0.5) reflecting left ventricular and left atrial dilation. Patients with pulmonary edema have increased pulmonary vascular markings and pleural effusion.

On echocardiography, the presence of ventricular end-diastolic dimensions greater than 2 standard deviations above body surface area–corrected means (or greater than 112% of predicted dimension) and fractional shortening less than 25% are sufficient to make the diagnosis. Other common features include functional mitral and tricuspid regurgitation and abnormalities of diastolic left ventricular function. Cardiac magnetic resonance imaging may show areas of myocardial fibrosis.

Other recommended tests (Table 60-5) include a complete blood count and tests of renal, thyroid, and hepatic function. Levels of serum creatine kinase should be measured in all patients with dilated cardiomyopathy because this may provide important clues to the etiology. Other cardiac biomarkers, such as troponin I and troponin T, can be elevated. Plasma B-type natriuretic peptide levels predict survival, hospitalization rates, and listing for

cardiac transplantation. Symptom-limited exercise testing, combined with respiratory gas analysis, is a useful technique to assess functional limitation and disease progression in patients with stable dilated cardiomyopathy.

Cardiac catheterization is rarely needed except perhaps to exclude severe coronary artery disease or to provide more precise information about possible valvular heart disease. Endomyocardial biopsy may be diagnostic for myocarditis and for some metabolic or mitochondrial disorders but is rarely advised. Hemodynamic assessment of left ventricular end-diastolic and pulmonary artery pressures may be necessary before transplantation.

TREATMENT   Rx

Supportive therapy includes sodium and fluid restriction, avoidance of alcohol and other toxins, and use of established heart failure medications (Chapter 59). Although older recommendations emphasized rest and avoidance of exercise, this advice should be limited to patients with myocarditis or peripartum cardiomyopathy; for other patients, a submaximal exercise regimen is desirable to sustain mobility, to avoid deconditioning, and to maintain physical and psychological health. Patients with atrial fibrillation or with echocardiographic evidence of a left atrial or left ventricular mural thrombosis should be anticoagulated to an international normalized ratio of 2.0 to 3.0. An ICD is preferred over medication for ventricular arrhythmias,[5] and some patients require management for advanced heart failure (Chapter 59) with biventricular pacing, inotropic medications, ventricular assist devices, and cardiac transplantation (Chapter 82).

Family Screening

Familial evaluation of first-degree relatives by history and physical examination and with 12-lead ECG and two-dimensional echocardiographic studies is warranted at the time of diagnosis and serially thereafter. Precise algorithms to guide the interval of evaluation remain to be determined; because disease progression is usually slow, evaluation about every 5 years until age 50 years appears appropriate. The detection of early disease in a family member offers an opportunity to initiate treatment, usually with an angiotensin-converting enzyme inhibitor or β-blocker, but the efficacy of such therapy remains to be proved.

PROGNOSIS

The prognosis of idiopathic and genetically determined dilated cardiomyopathy is related to the severity of disease at the time of presentation and the response to treatment. Most patients improve with treatment, but 5-year survival is less than 50% in patients who present with severe disease (e.g., ejection fraction <25%, left ventricular end-diastolic dimension >65 mm, peak oxygen consumption <12 mL/kg/minute).

Specific Causes of Dilated Cardiomyopathy

Alcoholic Cardiomyopathy

In the United States, excess alcohol consumption (Chapter 32) contributes to more than 10% of cases of heart failure. Alcohol and its metabolite, acetaldehyde, are cardiotoxins. Myocardial depression is initially reversible but, if alcohol consumption is sustained, can lead to myocyte vacuolization, mitochondrial abnormalities, and myocardial fibrosis. Even in chronic stages, however, the heart failure represents a sum of both reversible and irreversible myocardial dysfunction. The amount of alcohol necessary to produce symptomatic cardiomyopathy in susceptible individuals is not known but has been estimated to be six drinks (~4 oz of pure ethanol) a day for 5 to 10 years. Frequent binging without heavy daily consumption may also be sufficient. Alcoholic cardiomyopathy can develop in patients without social evidence of an alcohol problem. Abstinence leads to improvement in at least 50% of patients with severe symptoms, some of whom normalize their left ventricular ejection fractions. Patients with other causes of heart failure also should limit alcohol consumption.

Chemotherapy

Anthracycline (doxorubicin, daunorubicin, epirubicin) cardiotoxicity (Chapter 182) causes characteristic histologic changes on endomyocardial biopsy with overt heart failure in 5 to 10% of patients who receive doses greater than or equal to 450 mg/m^2 of body surface area. Patients who have received anthracyclines in the prepubertal period without apparent cardiotoxicity may develop cardiac failure in young adulthood. The risk is higher in patients who have lower baseline ejection fractions, concomitant radiation therapy, or higher doses of anthracycline. *Cyclophosphamide* and

---

TABLE 60-5	LABORATORY EVALUATION OF CARDIOMYOPATHY

CLINICAL EVALUATION

History and physical examination to identify cardiac and noncardiac disorders*
Assessment of ability to perform routine and desired activities*
Assessment of volume status*

LABORATORY EVALUATION

Electrocardiogram*
Chest radiograph*
Two-dimensional and Doppler echocardiogram*
Chemistry
   Serum sodium,* potassium,* glucose, creatinine,* blood urea nitrogen,* calcium,*
      magnesium*
   Albumin,* total protein,* liver function tests,* serum iron, ferritin
   Urinalysis
   Creatine kinase
   Thyroid-stimulating hormone*
Hematology
   Hemoglobin/hematocrit*
   White blood cell count with differential,* including eosinophils
   Erythrocyte sedimentation rate

INITIAL EVALUATION IN SELECTED PATIENTS ONLY

Titers for suspected infection
   Acute viral (coxsackievirus, echovirus, influenza virus)
   Human immunodeficiency virus, Epstein-Barr virus
   Lyme disease, toxoplasmosis
   Chagas' disease
Catheterization with coronary angiography in patients with angina who are
   candidates for intervention*
Serologic studies for active rheumatologic disease
Endomyocardial biopsy

*Level I recommendations from Hunt SA, Abraham WT, Chin MH, et al. ACC/AHA 2005 Guideline Update for the Diagnosis and Management of Chronic Heart Failure in the Adult. *Circulation.* 2005;112:e154-e235.

ifosfamide can cause acute severe heart failure and malignant ventricular arrhythmias. Some *tyrosine kinase inhibitors* (e.g., sunitinib) cause a reduction in systolic function, especially in the presence of coronary artery disease, but there is good response to withdrawal and conventional medical therapy (Chapter 190). *5-Fluorouracil* can cause coronary artery spasm and depressed left ventricular contractility. Up to 11% of patients who receive *trastuzumab* (Chapter 204), a recombinant monoclonal antibody that binds to human epidermal growth factor type 2, develop dilated cardiomyopathy, which is reversible after withdrawal and conventional drug treatment. The risk for cardiotoxicity increases with previous anthracycline and radiation treatment. *Interferon-α* may be associated with hypotension and arrhythmias in up to 10% of patients, and *interleukin-2* rarely has been associated with cardiotoxicity.

Metabolic and Endocrine Disease

Excess catecholamines, as in *pheochromocytoma* (Chapter 235), may injure the heart by compromising the coronary microcirculation or by direct toxic effects on myocytes. *Cocaine* (Chapter 33) increases synaptic concentrations of catecholamines by inhibiting reuptake at nerve terminals; the result may be an acute coronary syndrome or chronic cardiomyopathy.

Thiamine deficiency from poor nutrition or alcoholism (Chapter 225) can cause beriberi heart disease, with vasodilation and high cardiac output followed by low output. *Calcium deficiency* resulting from hypoparathyroidism, gastrointestinal abnormalities, or chelation directly compromises myocardial contractility.

Hypophosphatemia (Chapter 121), which may occur in alcoholism, during recovery from malnutrition, and in hyperalimentation, also reduces myocardial contractility. Patients with *magnesium depletion* owing to impaired absorption or increased renal excretion (Chapter 121) also may present with left ventricular dysfunction.

Hypothyroidism (Chapter 233) depresses contractility and conduction and may cause pericardial effusions, whereas *hyperthyroidism* increases cardiac output, can worsen underlying heart failure, and may rarely be the sole cause of heart failure.

The presenting sign of *diabetes* (Chapter 236) can be cardiomyopathy, especially with diastolic dysfunction, independent of epicardial coronary atherosclerosis, for which it is a major risk factor.

Obesity (Chapter 227) can cause cardiomyopathy with increased ventricular mass and decreased contractility, which improve after weight loss, or it can aggravate underlying heart failure from other causes.

Peripartum Cardiomyopathy

Peripartum cardiomyopathy appears in the last month of pregnancy or in the first 5 months after delivery in the absence of preexisting cardiac disease (Chapter 247). The incidence is between 1 in 3000 and 1 in 15,000 deliveries, with increased risk in older mothers or in the setting of twins, malnutrition, tocolytic therapy, toxemia, or hypertension. Lymphocytic myocarditis, found in 30 to 50% of biopsy specimens, suggests an immune component, perhaps cross-reactivity between uterine and cardiac myocyte proteins or an enhanced susceptibility to viral myocarditis. More recently, it has been suggested that enhanced oxidative stress triggers activation of cathepsin D, a ubiquitous lysosomal enzyme, which cleaves serum prolactin in its antiangiogenic and proapoptotic 16-kD form. The latter appears to promote endothelial inflammation and impair cardiomyocyte metabolism and contraction. Presentation is usually with orthopnea and dyspnea on minimal exertion, most often within the first weeks after delivery when the excess volume of pregnancy would normally be mobilized. Preexisting cardiac disease must be excluded. Diuretics facilitate postpartum diuresis, and angiotensin-converting enzyme inhibitors improve symptoms (Chapter 59). In a small randomized trial, oral bromocriptine (2.5 mg twice daily for 2 weeks, then daily for 6 weeks) significantly improved recovery of left ventricular function and may reduce deaths.[6] The prognosis is improvement to normal or near-normal ejection fraction during the next 6 months in more than 50% of patients. About 4% require heart transplantation, and about 9% die suddenly or from complications of heart transplantation.

Overlap with Restrictive Cardiomyopathy

Diseases causing primarily restrictive cardiomyopathies can occasionally overlap to cause a picture consistent with dilated cardiomyopathy. For example, *hemochromatosis* (Chapter 219) and *sarcoidosis* (Chapter 95) should be considered when evaluating any patient with a cardiomyopathy, although these conditions are more often considered with the restrictive diseases.

Amyloidosis (Chapter 194) is less commonly confused with dilated than with hypertrophic cardiomyopathy but should be considered in a patient with a thick-walled ventricle with moderately depressed contractile function.

Arrhythmogenic Right Ventricular Cardiomyopathy

DEFINITION AND EPIDEMIOLOGY

ARVC (Chapter 65) is a genetically determined heart muscle disorder characterized histologically by loss of cardiomyocytes with replacement by fibrous or fibrofatty tissue in the right ventricular myocardium; clinically by ventricular arrhythmias, heart failure, and sudden death; and histologically by cardiomyocyte loss and replacement. It is associated with arrhythmia, heart failure, and premature sudden death. The disease is seen in patients of European, African, and Asian descent, with an estimated prevalence between 1 in 1000 and 1 in 5000 adults.

PATHOBIOLOGY

ARVC is inherited as an autosomal dominant disease, with incomplete penetrance, although recessive forms with cutaneous manifestations are recognized (see Table 60-2). Most cases are caused by heterozygous mutations in genes encoding components of the desmosome and adherens junction of cardiomyocytes. The most common occur in plakophilin-2, desmocollin-2, desmoplakin, and desmoglein-2. Homozygous mutations in plakoglobin are responsible for the rare autosomal recessive form, Naxos disease. Recently, a mutation in the transmembrane cytoplasmic protein 43 (TNEM43) has been described. Two other nondesmosomal genes, the cardiac ryanodine receptor and transforming growth factor-β3 (TGF-β3), have been linked with ARVC but are probably not important in most patients.

Pathology

The main pathologic feature is progressive loss of right ventricular myocardium, which is replaced by adipose and fibrous tissue. These changes begin in the inflow, outflow, and apical regions of the right ventricle. Aneurysm formation in these areas is typical. Progressive myocardial involvement may lead to global right ventricular dilation. Severe right ventricular disease is often associated with fibrofatty substitution of the left ventricular myocardium, with the posterolateral wall preferentially affected.

Mutations in desmosomal protein genes may increase the susceptibility of the myocardium to the damaging effects of mechanical stress, thereby predisposing to cardiomyocyte detachment, death, and eventual replacement with fibrofatty tissue. The acute phase of myocardial injury may be accompanied by inflammation. The predilection for the right ventricle has been explained by its thin wall and greater distensibility. As desmosomal proteins interact with many other proteins, including components of the cellular cytoskeleton and intermediate filaments, it is possible that ventricular dysfunction occurs as the result of reduced cytoskeletal integrity and impaired force transduction. Some desmosomal proteins, in particular plakoglobin, are also important signaling molecules that regulate the transcription of many other genes. Finally, a reduction in the number and size of gap junctions may result in a electrical coupling defect, thereby increasing the propensity to arrhythmia without significant morphologic changes.

CLINICAL MANIFESTATIONS

By convention, the natural history of ARVC is divided into four phases, but it is not inevitable that patients will progress through all phases. In the early phase, patients are usually asymptomatic, but resuscitated cardiac arrest and sudden death may be the initial manifestations, particularly in adolescents and young adults. The overt arrhythmic phase usually begins in adolescents and young adults, when patients note palpitations or syncope. Symptomatic sustained arrhythmias are usually accompanied by morphologic and functional abnormalities of the right ventricle. The third phase, characterized by diffuse right ventricular disease, occurs in the middle and later decades; patients may present with right-sided heart failure despite relatively preserved left ventricular function. In the advanced stage, left ventricular involvement and biventricular heart failure are seen.

DIAGNOSIS

Clinical evaluation includes inquiry for symptoms of arrhythmia (syncope, presyncope, sustained palpitation); a family history of premature cardiac symptoms or sudden death; 12-lead, 24-hour, and maximal exercise ECG testing; and two-dimensional echocardiography with specific right ventricular views. Contrast echocardiography may be required to obtain better endocardial definition of the right ventricular myocardium and apex of the left ventricle. Magnetic resonance imaging may provide accurate assessment of ventricular volumes as well as noninvasive characterization of fibrous tissue and fat.

Ventricular arrhythmias with a left bundle branch block morphology, consistent with a right ventricular origin, are characteristic. However, the ECG and arrhythmic manifestations are not specific to ARVC and overlap with many other disease states, so standard criteria are recommended for diagnosis (Table 60-6). Because these criteria are highly specific but lack sensitivity for detecting early disease, more sensitive criteria are recommended for first-degree relatives of known cases (Table 60-7). The diagnosis of ARVC in a proband also raises the possibility of mutation analysis in the family to identify those at risk and in need of serial evaluation as well as those who need no specific follow-up.

Differential Diagnosis

The differential diagnosis includes other inherited cardiomyopathies, the inherited arrhythmia syndromes (long QT syndrome, Brugada's syndrome, and catecholaminergic polymorphic ventricular tachycardia; Chapter 65), and causes of right ventricular dilation such as intracardiac or extracardiac shunts (Chapter 69). The differentiation from so-called benign right ventricular outflow tract tachycardia may be problematic, although in the latter the 12-lead ECG and right ventricular imaging studies are typically normal, and no familial disease is present. Some patients with desmosomal protein

---

TABLE 60-6 REVISED TASK FORCE CRITERIA FOR ARRHYTHMOGENIC RIGHT VENTRICULAR CARDIOMYOPATHY IN PROBANDS*

Criteria	
MAJOR	**MINOR**
I. GLOBAL OR REGIONAL DYSFUNCTION AND STRUCTURAL ALTERATIONS*	
By two-dimensional echo:	**By two-dimensional echo:**
• Regional RV akinesia, dyskinesia, or aneurysm	• Regional RV akinesia or dyskinesia
• *and* 1 of the following (end diastole):	• *and* 1 of the following (end diastole):
PLAX RVOT ≥32 mm (corrected for body size [PLAX/BSA] ≥19 mm/m²)	PLAX RVOT ≥29 to <32 mm (corrected for body size [PLAX/BSA] ≥16 to <19 mm/m²)
PSAX RVOT ≥36 mm (corrected for body size [PLAX/BSA] ≥21 mm/m²)	PSAX RVOT ≥32 to <36 mm (corrected for body size [PSAX/BSA] ≥18 to <21 mm/m²)
or fractional area change ≤33%	*or* fractional area change >33% to ≤40%
By MRI:	**By MRI:**
• Regional RV akinesia or dyskinesia or dyssynchronous RV contraction	• Regional RV akinesia or dyskinesia or dyssynchronous RV contraction
• *and* 1 of the following:	• *and* 1 of the following:
RV end-diastolic volume indexed to BSA ≥110 mL/m² (male) or ≥100 mL/m² (female)	RV end-diastolic volume indexed to BSA ≥100 to <110 mL/m² (male) or ≥90 to <100 mL/m² (female)
or RV ejection fraction ≤40%	*or* RV ejection fraction >40% to ≤45%
By RV angiography:	
• Regional RV akinesia, dyskinesia, or aneurysm	
II. TISSUE CHARACTERIZATION OF WALL	
• Residual myocytes <60% by morphometric analysis (or <50% if estimated), with fibrous replacement of the RV free wall myocardium in ≥1 sample, with or without fatty replacement of tissue on endomyocardial biopsy	• Residual myocytes 60% to 75% by morphometric analysis (or 50% to 65% if estimated), with fibrous replacement of the RV free wall myocardium in ≥1 sample, with or without fatty replacement of tissue on endomyocardial biopsy
III. REPOLARIZATION ABNORMALITIES	
• Inverted T waves in right precordial leads (V₁,V₂, and V₃) or beyond in individuals >14 years of age (in the absence of complete right bundle-branch block QRS ≥120 msec)	• Inverted T waves in leads V₁ and V₂ in individuals >14 years of age (in the absence of complete right bundle branch block) or in V₄, V₅, or V₆ • Inverted T waves in leads V₁, V₂, V₃, and V₄ in individuals >14 years
IV. DEPOLARIZATION/CONDUCTION ABNORMALITIES	
• Epsilon wave (reproducible low-amplitude signals between end of QRS complex to onset of the T wave) in the right precordial leads (V₁ to V₃)	• Late potentials by SAECG in ≥1 of 3 parameters in the absence of a QRS duration ≥110 msec on the standard ECG • Filtered QRS duration (fQRS) ≥114 msec • Duration of terminal QRS <40 µV (low-amplitude signal duration) ≥38 msec • Root-mean-square voltage of terminal 40 msec ≤20 µV • Terminal activation duration of QRS ≥55 msec measured to the end of the QRS, including R′, in V₁, V₂, or V₃, in the absence of complete right bundle-branch block
V. ARRHYTHMIAS	
• Nonsustained or sustained ventricular tachycardia of left bundle branch morphology with superior axis (negative or indeterminate QRS in leads II, III, and aVF and positive in lead aVL)	• Nonsustained or sustained ventricular tachycardia of RV outflow configuration, left bundle branch block morphology with inferior axis (positive QRS in leads II, III, and aVF and negative in lead aVL) or of unknown axis • >500 ventricular extrasystoles per 24 hours (Holter)
VI. FAMILY HISTORY	
• ARVC confirmed in a first-degree relative who meets current Task Force criteria • ARVC confirmed pathologically at autopsy or surgery in a first-degree relative • Identification of a pathogenic mutation† categorized as associated or probably associated with ARVC in the patient under evaluation	• History of ARVC in a first-degree relative in whom it is not possible or practical to determine whether the family member meets current Task Force criteria • Premature sudden death (<35 years of age) due to suspected ARVC in a first-degree relative

*Hypokinesis is not included in this or subsequent definitions of right ventricular (RV) regional wall motion abnormalities for the proposed modified criteria.
†A pathogenic mutation is a DNA alteration associated with ARVC that alters or is expected to alter the encoded protein, is unobserved or rare in a large non-ARVC control population, and either alters or is predicted to alter the structure or function of the protein or has demonstrated linkage to the disease phenotype in a conclusive pedigree.
ARVC = arrhythmogenic right ventricular cardiomyopathy; aVF = augmented voltage unipolar left foot lead; aVL = augmented voltage unipolar left arm lead; BSA = body surface area; PLAX = parasternal long-axis view; PSAX = parasternal short-axis view; RVOT = right ventricular outflow tract.
Diagnostic terminology for original criteria: this diagnosis is fulfilled by the presence of 2 major, 1 major plus 2 minor, or 4 minor criteria from different groups.
Diagnostic terminology for revised criteria: definite diagnosis: 2 major, 1 major and 2 minor, or 4 minor criteria from different categories; borderline: 1 major and 1 minor or 3 minor criteria from different categories; possible: 1 major or 2 minor criteria from different categories.
From Marcus FI, McKenna WJ, Sherrill D, et al. Diagnosis of arrhythmogenic right ventricular cardiomyopathy/dysplasia: proposed modification of the task force criteria. *Circulation.* 2010;121:1533-1541.

TABLE 60-7 ARRHYTHMOGENIC RIGHT VENTRICULAR CARDIOMYOPATHY: CRITERIA FOR DIAGNOSIS OF FIRST-DEGREE RELATIVES WHO DO NOT FULFILL CRITERIA AS PROBANDS*

ARVC in a first-degree relative plus one of the following:	
ECG	T wave inversion in right precordial leads (V_2 and V_3)
Signal-averaged ECG	Late potentials seen on signal-averaged ECG
Arrhythmia	Left bundle branch block–type ventricular tachycardia on ECG, Holter monitoring, or during exercise testing; >200 extrasystoles over a 24-hour period
Structural or functional abnormality of the right ventricle	Mild global right ventricular dilation or reduction in ejection fraction with normal left ventricle; mild segmental dilation of the right ventricle; regional right ventricular hypokinesia

*Any one criterion is adequate for the diagnosis.
ARVC = arrhythmogenic right ventricular cardiomyopathy; ECG = electrocardiogram.
From Hamid MS, Norman M, Quraishi A, et al: Prospective evaluation of relatives for familial arrhythmogenic right ventricular cardiomyopathy reveals a need to broaden diagnostic criteria. *J Am Coll Cardiol* 2002;40:1445-1450.

TABLE 60-8 CAUSES OF RESTRICTIVE CARDIOMYOPATHIES

INFILTRATIVE DISORDERS

Amyloidosis
Sarcoidosis

STORAGE DISORDERS

Hemochromatosis
Fabry's disease
Glycogen storage diseases

FIBROTIC DISORDERS

Radiation
Scleroderma
Drugs (e.g., doxorubicin, serotonin, ergotamine)

METABOLIC DISORDERS

Carnitine deficiency
Defects in fatty acid metabolism

ENDOMYOCARDIAL DISORDERS

Endomyocardial fibrosis
Hypereosinophilic syndrome (Löffler's endocarditis)

MISCELLANEOUS CAUSES

Carcinoid syndrome

gene mutations demonstrate left ventricular involvement early in the disease may have a predominant left ventricular dilated cardiomyopathy phenotype.

TREATMENT

Rx

Pharmacologic treatment is the first-line therapy for patients with well-tolerated, non–life-threatening ventricular arrhythmias, such as frequent ventricular extrasystoles. Treatment of patients with symptomatic ventricular arrhythmias is with an ICD, with supplemental sotalol (160 to 240 mg/day) or even amiodarone (maintenance dose of 200 mg/day). Catheter ablation (Chapter 66) is indicated in patients with drug-refractory incessant ventricular arrhythmia or frequent recurrences of ventricular tachycardia after implantation of an ICD, although recurrence is common.

Retrospective analyses of clinical and pathologic series have identified a number of possible predictors of adverse outcome in probands, including an early age of onset of symptoms; competitive sporting activity; a malignant family background; severe right ventricular dilation; left ventricular involvement; syncope; episodes of complex ventricular arrhythmias or VT; and increased QRS dispersion on 12-lead ECG. ICD implantation is recommended for the prevention of sudden cardiac death in patients with documented sustained ventricular tachycardia or ventricular fibrillation and a reasonable expectation of survival with a good functional status for longer than 1 year. ICD implantation may also be appropriate in patients with extensive disease, including those with left ventricular involvement, or undiagnosed syncope when ventricular tachycardia or ventricular fibrillation has not been excluded as the cause.

Standard heart failure therapy, including diuretics, angiotensin-converting enzyme inhibitors, and β-blockers is indicated in patients in whom ARVC has progressed to severe heart failure or biventricular systolic dysfunction (Chapter 59). Anticoagulation should be considered in the presence of atrial fibrillation (Chapter 64), marked ventricular dilation, or ventricular aneurysms. In patients in whom heart failure is refractory, cardiac transplantation (Chapter 82) should be considered.

PROGNOSIS

Most data on prognosis in ARVC are derived from small, high-risk populations. By the age of 40 years, event-free survival is 50 to 60% in patients with Naxos disease and some autosomal dominant forms. In patients who have syncope or sustained ventricular arrhythmias and are treated with an ICD, freedom from appropriate shock therapy is about 75% at 48 months after implantation, with 96% of patients alive. Risk factors for sudden cardiac death include severe right ventricular disease, left ventricular involvement, and a history of unexplained syncope.

Restrictive Cardiomyopathy

DEFINITION AND EPIDEMIOLOGY

The incidence and prevalence of restrictive cardiomyopathy in adults are unknown. Restrictive cardiomyopathies (Table 60-8) are characterized by stiffness, impaired filling, elevated left ventricular diastolic pressures, and reduced diastolic volume of the left or right ventricle despite normal or near-normal systolic function and wall thickness. Primary forms are uncommon, whereas secondary forms, in which the heart is affected as a part of a multisystem disorder, usually present at the advanced stage of an infiltrative disease (e.g., amyloidosis or sarcoidosis) or a systemic storage disease (e.g., hemochromatosis). Idiopathic restrictive cardiomyopathy affects both male and female patients and may manifest in children and young adults.

PATHOBIOLOGY

Approximately 30% of patients with idiopathic restrictive cardiomyopathy have familial disease. Mutations in the gene encoding desmin (an intermediate filament) cause restrictive cardiomyopathy associated with skeletal myopathy and cardiac conduction system abnormalities. Mutations in the cardiac sarcomere protein genes also cause restrictive cardiomyopathy.

The macroscopic features of restrictive cardiomyopathy include biatrial dilation and small ventricular cavities. In many hearts, there is thrombus in the atrial appendages and patchy endocardial fibrosis. The histologic features of idiopathic restrictive cardiomyopathy are typically nonspecific with patchy interstitial fibrosis, but myocyte disarray is not uncommon in patients with pure restrictive cardiomyopathy. Amyloidosis, hemochromatosis, and sarcoidosis are among the systemic diseases that cause restrictive cardiomyopathy (see later).

CLINICAL MANIFESTATIONS

Most patients present with symptoms and signs of heart failure and arrhythmia. Common symptoms include dyspnea on exertion, recurrent respiratory tract infections, general fatigue, and weakness. Symptoms may progress rapidly to dyspnea at rest, orthopnea, and paroxysmal nocturnal dyspnea. Many patients complain of chest pain and palpitation. Syncope is a presenting symptom in 10% of children. Rarely, sudden death is the initial manifestation of the disease.

Physical examination typically reveals an elevated jugular venous pressure, which has a prominent y descent and fails to fall (or rises) during inspiration (Kussmaul's sign). On cardiac auscultation, the pulmonary component of the second heart sound may be loud if pulmonary vascular resistance is high. A third heart sound and occasionally a fourth heart sound commonly produce a gallop rhythm. Peripheral edema, ascites, and hepatomegaly are common.

DIAGNOSIS

The most frequent ECG abnormalities include p-mitrale and p-pulmonale, nonspecific ST segment and T wave abnormalities, ST segment depression, and T wave inversion, usually in the inferolateral leads. Voltage criteria for left and right ventricular hypertrophy may be present, although patients with amyloidosis have low-voltage QRS complexes. Conduction abnormalities include intraventricular conduction delay and abnormal Q waves.

FIGURE 60-4. **Idiopathic restrictive cardiomyopathy.** Right ventricular (RV) and left ventricular (LV) pressure electrocardiographic (ECG) tracings in a patient with idiopathic restrictive cardiomyopathy. A dip-and-plateau pattern is seen in both ventricles, and diastolic filling pressures are elevated. The plateaus occur at different pressures, approximately 16 mm Hg for the RV tracing compared with 20 mm Hg for the LV tracing. The diagnosis of restrictive disease was confirmed by thoracotomy. (Redrawn from Benofti JR, Grossman W, Cohn PF. The clinical profile of restrictive cardiomyopathy. *Circulation.* 1980;61:1206.)

On cardiac imaging, both atria are markedly dilated and can dwarf the size of the ventricles in patients with normal global systolic function and a non-hypertrophied, nondilated left ventricle. Pulsed-wave Doppler velocities typically show increased early diastolic filling velocity, decreased atrial filling velocity, an increased ratio of early diastolic filling to atrial filling, decreased E wave deceleration time, and decreased isovolumic relaxation time. Pulmonary vein and hepatic vein pulsed-wave Doppler velocities demonstrate higher diastolic than systolic velocities, increased atrial reversal velocities, and an atrial reversal duration greater than mitral atrial filling duration. Tissue Doppler imaging usually shows reduced diastolic annular velocities and an increased ratio of early diastolic tissue Doppler annular velocity to mitral early diastolic filling velocity, reflecting elevated left ventricular end-diastolic pressures.

The characteristic hemodynamic feature on cardiac catheterization is a deep and rapid early decline in ventricular pressure at the onset of diastole, with a rapid rise to a plateau in early diastole ("dip-and-plateau" or "square root sign") (Fig. 60-4). Left ventricular end-diastolic, left atrial, and pulmonary capillary wedge pressures are markedly elevated, usually 5 mm Hg or more above right atrial and right ventricular end-diastolic pressures. Volume loading and exercise accentuate the difference between left-sided and right-sided pressures.

The diagnostic evaluation aims to exclude potentially reversible conditions. In such cases, the cardiac manifestations may provide the clues, but definitive diagnosis relies on the demonstration of disease-specific features, such as amyloid protein in amyloidosis (Chapter 194), noncaseating granulomas in sarcoidosis (Chapter 95), abnormal iron studies in hemochromatosis (Chapter 219), or reduced α-galactosidase A levels in Fabry's disease (Chapter 215). Endomyocardial biopsy is rarely required to make these diagnoses.

TREATMENT   **Rx**

Diuretics are the main therapy for heart failure symptoms (Chapter 59), but they must be carefully administered so as not to reduce left ventricular filling pressures to the point of hypotension. Angiotensin-converting enzyme inhibitors and β-blockers are commonly recommended despite few data on their benefit. In patients with secondary restrictive cardiomyopathies, specific treatment of the underlying systemic disease is often appropriate (see later). Referral for transplant assessment should be considered early because pulmonary hypertension may develop and necessitate heart and lung transplantation.

PROGNOSIS

In adults with restrictive cardiomyopathy, the clinical course is usually slow and protracted. Survival from the time of diagnosis is often 10 years or more, except for amyloidosis, which progresses much more rapidly. Symptoms of heart failure are generally progressive and respond poorly to treatments for heart failure.

Specific Clinical Syndromes

SARCOIDOSIS

The frequency of myocardial involvement in patients with sarcoidosis (Chapter 95) is difficult to determine because it is frequently subclinical and patchy in nature. Postmortem studies suggest that the heart is involved in at least 25% of patients, but clinical cardiac involvement occurs in fewer than 10% of patients. Clinical manifestations of sarcoid include heart failure, conduction abnormalities, atrial and ventricular arrhythmias, pericardial effusion, valvular dysfunction, and, rarely, sudden cardiac death. Right heart failure secondary to pulmonary hypertension may occur in patients with extensive fibrotic lung disease. Myocardial infiltration by sarcoid granulomas results in restrictive or dilated cardiomyopathy. The most common site is in the lateral wall of the left ventricle. Papillary muscle involvement is responsible for the most common valvulopathy, mitral regurgitation. Granuloma formation in the basal interventricular septum may cause conduction abnormalities. Ventricular arrhythmias are also frequent. Biopsy of extracardiac sites is usually adequate for the diagnosis, but a gallium scan often demonstrates cardiac inflammation. A myocardial biopsy may show granulomas but, because of the focal distribution of the lesions, may be nondiagnostic. Corticosteroid therapy may improve arrhythmias, but heart failure may worsen despite such therapy. An ICD is generally indicated for ventricular arrhythmias.

AMYLOIDOSIS

EPIDEMIOLOGY AND PATHOBIOLOGY

Amyloidosis can result in deposition of amyloid protein in the atria, ventricles, coronary vessels, conduction system, and valves. The degree of cardiac involvement varies among subtypes. Hematologic disorders (Chapter 193) associated with excessive light chain (AL) immunoglobulin production are the most common cause of cardiac amyloid. Familial forms caused by the accumulation of mutant proteins (transthyretin or A-apolipoprotein) (Chapter 194) have variable cardiac involvement. Secondary amyloidosis, due to deposition of serum amyloid A protein in chronic inflammatory diseases, rarely affects the heart. In senile systemic amyloidosis, cardiomyopathy is by caused deposition of normal wild-type transthyretin; this disease nearly always affects elderly persons (>70 years), with a clinical course that is considerably slower than other types of amyloid.

DIAGNOSIS

The ECG tracing in most forms of cardiac amyloid characteristically shows decreased voltage despite increased wall thickness on echocardiography. Characteristic two-dimensional echocardiographic findings in advanced cardiac amyloidosis are biventricular hypertrophy, thickened valves and interatrial septum, dilated atria, and a small pericardial effusion. The myocardium has a hyperreflective granular texture (Fig. 60-5), best seen on digital image

FIGURE 60-5. **Amyloidosis.** An apical four-chamber echocardiographic image demonstrates biventricular hypertrophy in a patient with biopsy-proved amyloidosis. RA = right atrium; RV = right ventricle. (From Levine RA. Echocardiographic assessment of the cardiomyopathies. In: Weyman AE, ed. *Principles and Practice of Echocardiography,* 2nd ed. Philadelphia: Lea & Febiger; 1994:810.)

analysis. Echo Doppler in advanced disease demonstrates a restrictive left ventricular filling pattern. Cardiac magnetic resonance imaging may show subendocardial late gadolinium enhancement with abnormal gadolinium kinetics. Nuclear scans with ^{123}I-labeled serum amyloid P component are highly specific.

A definitive diagnosis of amyloidosis requires a tissue biopsy, which can be obtained from other sites. For example, fine-needle aspiration of abdominal fat is positive for amyloid deposits in more than 70% of patients with AL amyloidosis. If negative, endomyocardial biopsy has a very high sensitivity.

TREATMENT AND PROGNOSIS   Rx

Specific therapies to impede precursor protein production and fibril formation should be implemented whenever possible (Chapter 194). Diuretics, often in high doses (e.g., furosemide 40 to 80 mg daily), are the mainstay of the palliative heart failure regimen. Angiotensin-enzyme converting or angiotensin II inhibitors should be used very cautiously because they are often poorly tolerated and of unproven efficacy in cardiac amyloid. Aldosterone inhibitors might be helpful in advanced cases. Patients may be hypersensitive to digoxin because of enhanced drug binding with amyloid fibrils. Patients with atrial fibrillation in AL amyloidosis should receive anticoagulation with warfarin (Chapter 37) because of a very high rate of thromboembolism. Cardiac transplantation remains controversial, but heart transplantation (Chapter 82) with high-dose chemotherapy and with stem cell transplantation (Chapter 181) has been used in patients with AL amyloidosis.

Patients with amyloidosis with heart failure have a median survival time of less than 1 year and a 5-year survival rate of less than 5%. Most deaths occur suddenly. Patients with familial amyloidosis have a slower course than do patients with a monoclonal gammopathy.

HEREDITARY HEMOCHROMATOSIS

Hereditary hemochromatosis (Chapter 219) is an autosomal recessive disorder caused by excessive iron deposition in various organs, including the liver, spleen, pancreas, endocrine glands, and heart. In whites, its prevalence is between 1 in 200 and 1 in 500, with an even higher prevalence in the Irish population. The most common form is caused by mutations in the *HFE* gene, with two missense mutations accounting for most cases (C282Y and H63D).

Most patients with classical disease present between the ages of 40 and 60 years with hyperpigmentation, diabetes mellitus, and hepatomegaly. Up to 35% of patients with hemochromatosis experience heart failure, and 36% develop arrhythmias. Restrictive physiologic features dominate early in the disease, followed by ventricular dilation. The diagnosis is generally made from the clinical picture, an elevated serum iron level, and a high transferrin saturation. Genetic testing is helpful, and the diagnosis can be confirmed by endomyocardial biopsy. Phlebotomy and iron chelation therapy with deferoxamine (Chapter 219) may improve cardiac function before cell injury becomes irreversible. Standard heart failure treatment (Chapter 59) is generally recommended. Death from hemochromatosis results more often from cirrhosis and liver carcinoma than from cardiac disease.

Unclassified Cardiomyopathies
LEFT VENTRICULAR NONCOMPACTION

Failure of the trabecular or spongiform layer of the myocardium to compact may occur with congenital heart disease, including atrial and ventricular septal defects and coarctation of the aorta (Chapter 69), and with the rare X-linked multisystem disorder, Barth's syndrome. With recent improvements in imaging technology, it has also been recognized in patients with hypertrophic and dilated cardiomyopathy. The prevalence of localized areas of noncompaction is unknown, but clinically significant isolated left ventricular noncompaction in the absence of other cardiac abnormalities is uncommon.

Areas of noncompacted myocardium may be best delineated from normal myocardium by the demonstration of flow within the myocardium by Doppler or contrast echocardiography. When extensive areas are involved, systolic performance may be impaired, and there is a risk of ventricular arrhythmias and systemic emboli. Treatment, when necessary, is for associated heart failure (Chapter 59), arrhythmias (Chapters 64 and 65), and the risk of emboli (Chapter 59). Natural history and prognosis are not well established.

TAKOTSUBO CARDIOMYOPATHY

Takotsubo cardiomyopathy is a syndrome of transient apical left ventricular dysfunction that mimics myocardial infarction (Chapter 73). Postulated mechanisms include coronary artery spasm, myocarditis, and dynamic mid-cavity obstruction.

The clinical syndrome classically includes chest pain, ST segment elevation, and raised cardiac biomarkers in association with emotional or physical stress. Coronary arteriography reveals normal epicardial vessels. Conservative treatment with rehydration and removal of the determinants of stress usually results in rapid resolution within hours of the symptoms, ECG changes, and wall motion abnormalities.

DISEASES OF THE ENDOCARDIUM

Endocardial fibrosis, fibroelastosis, and thrombosis are subclassified into endomyocardial diseases with hypereosinophilia (hypereosinophilic syndromes) and endomyocardial disease without hypereosinophilia (e.g., endomyocardial fibrosis) (see Table 60-8).

Hypereosinophilic Syndrome

Hypereosinophilic syndromes are a rare and heterogeneous group of disorders defined as persistent blood eosinophilia ($>1.5 \times 10^9$/L) for more than 6 consecutive months, associated with evidence of eosinophil-induced organ damage in the absence of causes of hypereosinophilia, such as allergic, parasitic, and malignant disorders (Chapter 173). Pathogenic mechanisms include stem cell mutations that lead to expression of PDGFRA-containing fusion genes, mainly the *FIP1L1-PDGFRA* fusion gene, with constitutive tyrosine kinase activity and sustained overproduction of interleukin-5 by activated T-cell subsets. Clinically, hypereosinophilic syndrome can be classified into chronic eosinophilic leukemia, lymphocytic hypereosinophilic syndrome, myeloproliferative hypereosinophilic syndrome, and idiopathic hypereosinophilic syndrome. The term *organ-restricted eosinophilic disease*, such as eosinophilic gastroenteritis, dermatitis, or pneumonia, is used when a specific organ or tissue is the exclusive target of eosinophilic infiltration and damage. The term *Löffler's fibroplastic endocarditis* with eosinophilia has been used to describe cardiac damage caused by direct toxicity of circulating eosinophils in patients with persistent hypereosinophilia, but its use is now discouraged.

CLINICAL MANIFESTATIONS AND DIAGNOSIS

Hypereosinophilic syndrome is a rare disorder that tends to occur in patients 20 to 50 years of age, but all age groups are affected. Cardiac involvement generally evolves in three phases: an early necrotic stage that involves the endomyocardium, which is usually asymptomatic but can present as acute heart failure; a thrombotic stage, in which thrombi develop on the ventricular endocardium, sometimes causing peripheral emboli; and the final fibrotic stage, endomyocardial fibrosis, which causes restrictive cardiomyopathy and damage to atrioventricular valves. Chest pain, cough, dyspnea or orthopnea, and edema of the lower extremities are typical symptoms. Some patients may develop arrhythmias.

The characteristic two-dimensional echocardiographic findings include endocardial thickening, apical obliteration of one or both ventricles by an echogenic material, hyperdynamic contraction of the spared ventricular walls with bilateral atrial enlargement, and a restrictive pattern on echo Doppler.

TREATMENT   Rx

Patients with the F/P fusion gene chromosomal rearrangement should be treated with the tyrosine kinase inhibitor, imatinib (100 mg daily for 1 week, increasing by 100 mg each week to 400 mg as guided by toxicity and hematologic response); the duration of therapy is still under investigation. Because some patients develop severe congestive heart failure within days after initiation of therapy, pretreatment with corticosteroids is recommended by some authorities. For patients without the F/P fusion gene, corticosteroids (median maximal daily dose of prednisone 40 mg, range 5 to 625 mg; duration 2 months to 20 years; median maintenance dose of 10 mg daily, range 1 to 40 mg/day) are the most common first-line therapy. Steroid-sparing and second-line drugs include hydroxyurea (median maximal daily dose of 1000 mg, range 500 to 2000 mg, adjusted to response), interferon-α (median maximal dose of 14 million units per week, range 3 to 40 million units per week, adjusted to response), and imatinib (as above).

Tropical Endomyocardial Fibrosis

Tropical endomyocardial fibrosis is probably the most common type of restrictive cardiomyopathy worldwide. The disease occurs predominantly within the tropics and affects mostly children and adolescents, usually from low socioeconomic backgrounds. Its cause is unknown, but potential contributors include infection, autoimmunity, genetic predisposition, ethnicity, diet, climate, and poverty.

Severe hypereosinophilia is found in some patients early in the initial stage of the illness, which is characterized by febrile illness, pancarditis, facial and periorbital swelling, pruritus, urticaria, and neurologic symptoms. This phase is followed by ventricular thrombosis that affects the apices and the subvalvular apparatus and then evolves to endocardial fibrosis. The final stage is characterized by restrictive physiology, atrioventricular valve regurgitation, and marked atrial dilation. Death results from complications of chronic heart failure but can occur suddenly owing to thromboembolism or arrhythmia.

Atrial fibrillation is common at presentation. In advanced disease, the ECG shows low-voltage QRS complexes, nonspecific ST-T wave changes, and conduction abnormalities. Echocardiography demonstrates apical obliteration, reduction of ventricular cavity size, and tethering or retraction of mitral or tricuspid leaflets, or both. There is no specific laboratory test, and hypereosinophilia is present only early in the disease.

There is no specific treatment for endomyocardial fibrosis. Medical treatment is used to control the heart failure (Chapter 59) and arrhythmias (Chapters 64 and 65). Surgical endocardial resection, combined with valve repair or replacement, has an early postoperative mortality between 15 and 30%. The overall prognosis is poor, with a 44% mortality rate at 1 year, increasing to nearly 90% at 3 years.

Carcinoid Syndrome

EPIDEMIOLOGY AND PATHOBIOLOGY

Carcinoid tumors are rare (1 in 100,000) neuroendocrine malignancies originating mostly from enterochromaffin cells in the gastrointestinal tract (Chapter 240). Carcinoid syndrome, with flushing, diarrhea, and bronchospasm, occurs after tumor cells metastasize to the liver and the vasoactive substances produced by the tumors enters the systemic circulation through the hepatic vein. Carcinoid heart disease occurs in up to 70% of cases of carcinoid syndrome.

The typical cardiac lesion is the carcinoid plaque, which is composed of smooth muscle cells, myofibroblasts, and elastic tissue that forms a fibrous layer on the endocardial surface of the right ventricle and atrium, the valve leaflets, and the subvalvular apparatus, including the chordae and papillary muscles. The tricuspid valve plaques tend to develop on the ventricular side of the leaflets, where they adhere to the mural endocardium and cause valvular regurgitation. On the pulmonary valve, the predominant lesion is stenosis. In patients with a patent foramen ovale, left-sided valvular involvement can occur. Occasional patients may have concomitant myocardial metastases and pericardial effusions from direct tumor invasion.

The most common presentation is dyspnea with signs and symptoms of right-sided heart failure. The ECG and radiograph are nonspecific. Echocardiography shows thickening of the tricuspid valve, the subvalvular apparatus, and the pulmonary valve. In severe disease, the tricuspid leaflets are retracted and fixed, with loss of normal coaptation. Similar findings can be seen on cardiac magnetic resonance imaging.

TREATMENT AND PROGNOSIS   Rx

Treatment of the underlying carcinoid with a somatostatin analogue can improve systemic symptoms (Chapter 240). Valve replacement now has an operative mortality of less than 10% (Chapter 240). Without treatment, patients with carcinoid heart disease have a mean life expectancy of 1.6 years. In one series, cardiac surgery for valve disease was associated with about a 50% risk reduction.

Nonbacterial Thrombotic (Marantic) Endocarditis

EPIDEMIOLOGY AND PATHOBIOLOGY

Platelet-fiber masses that are adherent to the mitral or aortic valves are seen in about 20% of patients with malignant tumors, especially mucin-producing adenocarcinomas, melanomas, leukemias, and lymphomas. The lesions are sterile, commonly verruciform, and without accompanying inflammation.

CLINICAL MANIFESTATIONS AND DIAGNOSIS

Nonbacterial thrombotic endocarditis is virtually always asymptomatic but occasionally is a source of systemic emboli. Because of the small size of many of the emboli, the first presentation is often with cerebral symptoms. Larger lesions are detectable by echocardiography, but even transesophageal echocardiography is not sufficiently sensitive to identify lesions that may be found at autopsy and that may have been the source of systemic emboli.

TREATMENT   Rx

No treatment has been proved efficacious. However, systemic anticoagulation similar to that used in patients with tumor-associated deep vein thrombosis is often tried (Chapters 81 and 187).

CARDIAC TUMORS

Myocardial Tumors

Most primary cardiac tumors (Table 60-9) are benign. However, all tumors that extend from other tissues into the heart are malignant, as are metastatic lesions.

EPIDEMIOLOGY AND PATHOBIOLOGY

Primary tumors of the heart are unusual, with a prevalence of 1 in 2000 to 1 in 4000 in autopsy series. Nearly all these primary tumors are benign myxomas, although fibromas, lipomas, and fibroelastomas also occur. Rhabdomyomas are seen in children, especially with tuberous sclerosis (Chapter 426). The rare primary malignant tumors include sarcomas, especially angiosarcomas (see Table 60-9). Rarely, a primary mesothelioma or lymphoma may originate in the heart.

Up to 20% of advanced cancers may involve the pericardium, epicardium, or cardiac chambers either by direct extension of the primary tumor or by metastatic disease. Direct extension occurs principally from cancers of the lung, breast, esophagus, and mediastinum. Extension through the inferior vena cava to the right atrium and even to the right ventricle occurs with cancers of the kidney, adrenal gland, and liver. Metastatic spread is most common with melanomas or lymphomas.

TABLE 60-9   CARDIAC TUMORS

PRIMARY
Benign
Myxoma
Lipoma
Fibroma
Rhabdomyoma
Fibroelastoma
Malignant
Sarcoma
Mesothelioma
Lymphoma
SECONDARY
Direct Extension
Lung cancer
Breast cancer
Mediastinal tumors
Metastatic Tumors
Malignant melanoma
Leukemia
Lymphoma
Venous Extension
Renal cell cancer
Adrenal cancer
Liver cancer

Pericardial Tumors

CLINICAL MANIFESTATIONS

Pericardial tumors almost always result from direct extension of tumors, principally lung and breast, which produce a pericardial effusion that can progress to cardiac tamponade (Chapter 77). Patients typically are asymptomatic or minimally symptomatic in terms of the cardiac involvement until the effusion is very large, although they often may be very ill owing to progressive tumor elsewhere.

DIAGNOSIS

The diagnosis is often suspected in a patient with advanced malignant disease based on evidence of heart failure, hypertension, or arrhythmia and is confirmed by echocardiography. The differentiation between pericardial involvement by tumor and postradiation pericarditis depends on pericardiocentesis, often guided by echocardiography, and cytologic examination.

TREATMENT   Rx

Cardiac tamponade must be treated with urgent pericardiocentesis, preferably under echocardiographic or radiologic guidance (Chapter 77). Although such a procedure can be life-saving and provide short-term to immediate-term palliation, control of the effusion often requires prolonged drainage, administration of intrapericardial chemotherapeutic agents, or limited or full pericardiectomy (Chapter 77). Some patients with pericardial tumors may respond to aggressive systemic chemotherapy, but recurrent accumulation of fluid is sufficiently likely that creation of a pericardial window should be considered before hospital discharge.

PROGNOSIS

In many cases, a tumor that is causing pericarditis has extended or will eventually extend through the pericardial space and into the myocardium, so no therapy is likely to be successful. The prognosis is very poor, except in unusual cases in which the tumor responds dramatically to systemic therapy.

Intracavitary Tumors
MYXOMA

DEFINITION AND EPIDEMIOLOGY

A *myxoma* is a benign polypoid neoplasm that originates from endocardial cells and is attached to the interatrial septum, usually protruding into the left atrium but occasionally into the right atrium and rarely into the ventricles. Myxomas are more common in women, especially between the ages of 30 and 60 years, than in men. These tumors can be familial and are rarely associated with other systemic abnormalities.

CLINICAL MANIFESTATIONS

Myxomas are slow growing and usually do not produce symptoms or signs until they enlarge. The typical presentation is with a tumor embolus, whereby usually small portions of the myxoma break loose and cause a single embolism or a shower of emboli. However, a large embolism from a myxoma can be of sufficient size to obstruct a medium-sized artery. Some patients have systemic symptoms, including fever, malaise, and arthralgias, as part of a clinical syndrome that may be confused with bacterial endocarditis (Chapter 76) or a collagen vascular disease. Large myxomas can prolapse into the mitral valve orifice during diastole, or they may obstruct blood flow from the left atrium to the left ventricle and mimic rheumatic mitral stenosis.

DIAGNOSIS

A myxoma large enough to obstruct the mitral orifice can produce an audible "tumor plop" when the myxoma prolapses and obstructs blood flow during diastole, at the same time that the opening snap of mitral stenosis would typically be heard. If obstruction is incomplete, the tumor plop may be followed by a diastolic rumble. As obstruction becomes more severe, cardiac output may fall precipitously. Echocardiography (Chapter 53) is usually definitive; transesophageal echocardiography provides a higher sensitivity than does transthoracic echocardiography, and magnetic resonance imaging can be helpful.

TREATMENT   Rx

Surgical removal is generally curative, although myxomas can be multiple or recur in about 5% of cases. Follow-up postoperative echocardiography is generally recommended. However, the optimal frequency and duration for follow-up screening are uncertain.

OTHER PRIMARY INTRACAVITARY TUMORS

Papillary fibroelastomas are rare, typically frondlike tumors that may arise from a cardiac valve, often the mitral valve, and are generally detected incidentally by echocardiography. However, like myxomas, they can manifest with systemic or even coronary emboli. Surgical excision is usually successful.

Angiosarcomas, which are more frequent in men than in women, typically involve the pericardium and right atrium. They cause obstruction with clinical signs and symptoms of right-sided heart failure. These sarcomas are generally not amenable to therapy.

EXTENSION OF TUMOR INTO THE CARDIAC CAVITIES

Direct extension of tumor up the inferior vena cava into the right atrium can be seen with renal cell carcinomas and less commonly with liver and adrenal cancers. In some cases, tumor extension is accompanied by adherent clot, and either the tumor or the clot may cause obstruction or pulmonary emboli (Chapter 98). No treatments are generally successful, and the prognosis is grim.

Intramyocardial Tumors

Benign tumors in the myocardium include lipomas, fibromas, and rhabdomyomas. Primary malignant tumors include sarcomas, lymphomas, and mesotheliomas. Metastatic tumors include melanomas, lymphomas, and leukemias. The tumors may be clinically silent, or they may produce arrhythmias or even impinge on coronary arteries, thereby causing ischemic syndromes. Large tumors may protrude into the cardiac chamber and cause obstruction. Therapies are not successful, except for occasional patients whose metastatic tumors may respond to systemic chemotherapy or whose primary tumors have been cured by heart transplantation.

Grade **A**

1. Mason JW, O'Connell JB, Herskowitz A, et al. A clinical trial of immunosuppressive therapy for myocarditis: the Myocarditis Treatment Trial Investigators. *N Engl J Med*. 1995;333:269-275.
2. Wojnicz R, Nowalany-Kozielska E, Wojciechowska C, et al. Randomized, placebo-controlled study for immunosuppressive treatment of inflammatory dilated cardiomyopathy: two-year follow-up results. *Circulation* 2001;104:39-45.
3. Cooper LT Jr, Hare JM, Tazelaar HD, et al. Usefulness of immunosuppression for giant cell myocarditis. *Am J Cardiol*. 2008;102:1535-1539.
4. Robinson J, Hartling L, Vandermeer B, et al. Intravenous immunoglobulin for presumed viral myocarditis in children and adults. *Cochrane Database Syst Rev*. 2005;25:CD004370.
5. Kadish A, Dyer A, Daubert JP, et al. Prophylactic defibrillator implantation in patients with non-ischemic dilated cardiomyopathy. *N Engl J Med*. 2004;350:2151-2158.
6. Sliwa K, Blauwet L, Tibazarwa K, et al. Evaluation of bromocriptine in the treatment of acute severe peripartum cardiomyopathy: a proof-of-concept pilot study. *Circulation*. 2010;121:1465-1473.

SUGGESTED READINGS

Basso C, Corrado D, Marcus FI, et al. Arrhythmogenic right ventricular cardiomyopathy. *Lancet*. 2009;373:1289-1300. *Review of the genetics, pathology, and clinical manifestations of ARVC.*
Blauwet LA, Cooper LT. Myocarditis. *Prog Cardiovasc Dis*. 2010;52:274-288. *Review.*
Cardinale D, Colombo A, Lamantia G, et al. Anthracycline-induced cardiomyopathy: clinical relevance and response to pharmacologic therapy. *J Am Coll Cardiol*. 2010;55:213-220. *Prompt treatment can reduce the risk of major cardiac events.*
Gujja P, Rosing DR, Tripodi DJ, et al. Iron overload cardiomyopathy: better understanding of an increasing disorder. *J Am Coll Cardiol*. 2010;56:1001-1012. *Review.*
Jeffries JL, Towbin JA. Dilated cardiomyopathy. *Lancet*. 2010;375:752-762. *Review.*
Seward JB, Casaclang-Verzosa G. Infiltrative cardiovascular diseases. *J Am Coll Cardiol*. 2010;55:1769-1779. *Review.*
Sorajja P, Nishimura RA, Gersh BJ, et al. Outcome of mildly symptomatic or asymptomatic obstructive hypertrophic cardiomyopathy: a long-term follow-up study. *J Am Coll Cardiol*. 2009;5:234-241. *Patients with obstructive HCM and with mild or no symptoms are at a very small increased risk for mortality unless they have very elevated resting gradients.*
van Spaendonck-Zwarts KY, van Tintelen JP, van Veldhuisen DJ, et al. Peripartum cardiomyopathy as a part of familial dilated cardiomyopathy. *Circulation*. 2010;121:2169-2175. *Some cases of peripartum cardiomyopathy represent the first presentation of a familial dilated cardiomyopathy.*

61

PRINCIPLES OF ELECTROPHYSIOLOGY

HUGH CALKINS

The function of the human heart requires rhythmic beatings occurring on the average 70 times a minute, 24 hours a day, for 80 or more years. The close to 3 billion contractions of the cardiac musculature that must occur without fail are coordinated by an intricate network of specialized electrically active cells that are integrated with the myocytes that comprise the predominant mass of the heart. Any loss of electrical activity, even for a few seconds, results in syncope (Chapters 50 and 62); loss of electrical activity for a few minutes may end in death.

CARDIAC ELECTROPHYSIOLOGY

Ion channels are integral membrane-spanning proteins, which allow the rapid movement of specific ions, most importantly Na^+, K^+, Cl^-, and Ca^{2+}, across the cell membrane at rates of 10^8 ions per second (E-Fig. 61-1). The opening and closing of the channels occur through a process of gating, whereby changes in the voltage, ligand, or receptor associated with the channel lead to alterations in the conformation of the proteins that activate or inactivate the channel pore. Voltage gating is the predominant method of regulating ion channels in the heart and is found in sodium and various potassium channels. Ligand-gated ion channels use ligands such as neurotransmitters, ions such as intracellular calcium, and metabolic products such as adenosine triphosphate (ATP) to activate a variety of channels, including those for potassium. Receptor-gated channels use changes in the physical environment, such as stretch, to activate channels, including those for chloride, which regulate intracellular volume.

The coordinated activity of numerous ion channels contributes to the creation of the cardiac action potential (Fig. 61-1). There are five phases to the cardiac action potential. At rest, the transmembrane potential of the cell exists close to −90 mV (the inside of the cell is positive with respect to the outside). With depolarization of the cell either from depolarization of adjacent cells or from an external change in voltage, sodium channels change from a closed to an open state and rapidly move sodium ions down a gradient into the interior of the cell, creating the sodium current I_{Na} and the rapid upstroke of phase 0 of the action potential. At the peak of depolarization, approximately +40 mV, the sodium current is inactivated, and the transient outward current I_{to} is activated with the opening of various voltage-gated potassium channels, resulting in the rapid decrease in voltage and phase 1 of the action potential. The plateau of the action potential, phase 2, follows and is an amalgamation of multiple currents representing inward and outward movement of ions. Contributors to this phase include the rapid component of the delayed rectifier potassium current I_{Kr}, the slow component of the delayed rectifier potassium current I_{Ks}, the L-type calcium channel, and the Na^+-Ca^{2+} exchanger. As the outward potassium currents increase and the calcium current decreases at the end of phase 2, the action potential progresses to phase 3, the phase of rapid repolarization. The inward rectifier potassium current I_{K1} contributes significantly to this final phase of repolarization and brings the action potential to its resting membrane potential. During phase 4, the heart is in diastole, with most cells at −85 to −90 mV. Specialized cells located in the sinoatrial and atrioventricular nodes repolarize to approximately −60 mV and contain currents that contribute to spontaneous depolarization during phase 4. These pacemaker cells contain the inward activation, or funny, current I_f activated by hyperpolarization and carried by sodium, and the background sodium current I_{Na-B}. The calcium currents $I_{Ca,L}$ and $I_{Ca,T}$, the sodium-potassium pump $I_{Na,K}$, and the sodium calcium exchanger $I_{Na,Ca}$ additionally may contribute to diastolic depolarization.

Variations in the duration and shape of the cardiac action potential depend on its location in the heart (Fig. 61-2). Likewise, alterations of ion channel expression and activity in disease states contribute to prolongation of the action potential. The atrial action potential has a typical duration of 100 to 200 msec, whereas the ventricular action potential typically lasts 250 to 300 msec. Different layers of the ventricle exhibit marked changes in the action potential. Epicardial cells have a prominent phase 1 compared with endocardial cells, in which phase 1 is blunted. The phase 2 plateau is decreased in epicardial cells, leading to less activation of the delayed rectifier currents

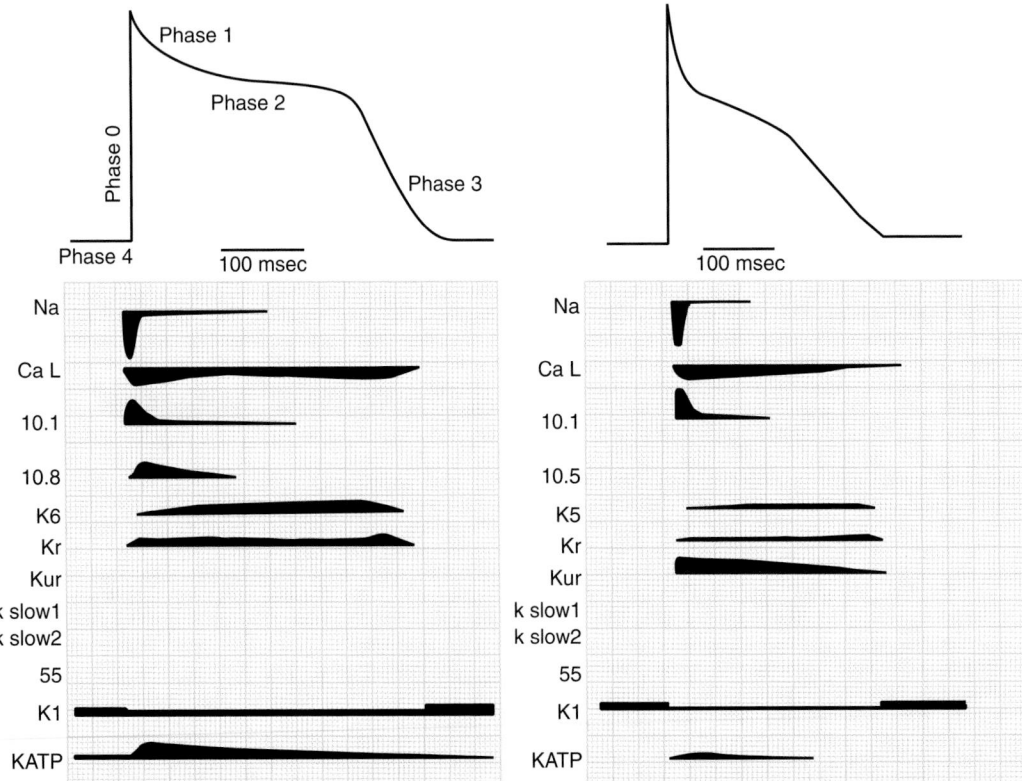

FIGURE 61-1. The cardiac action potential waveforms and underlying ionic currents in adult human and ventricular (*left*) and atrial (*right*) myocytes. The time- and voltage-dependent properties of the voltage-gated inward Na^+ (Nav) and Ca^{2+} (Cav) currents expressed in human atrial and ventricular myocytes are similar. In contrast, multiple types of K^+ currents, particularly Kv currents, contribute to atrial and ventricular action potential repolarization. The properties of the various Kv currents are distinct, and, in contrast to the inward currents, there are multiple Kv currents expressed in individual myocytes throughout the myocardium. (From Kass R. Molecular physiology of cardiac repolarization. *Physiol Rev.* 2005;85:1207.)

Sinus Rhythm with Preexcitation

A

Re-entrant Tachycardia

B

FIGURE 61-2. Accessory pathway in sinus rhythm and in ortho-dromic re-entrant tachycardia. (From Bassam CT. A molecular basis for Wolff-Parkinson-White syndrome. *N Engl J Med.* 2001;344:1861. Copyright © 2001 Massachusetts Medical Society. All rights reserved.)

and a prolonged action potential in epicardial cells. M cells found in the mid-myocardium have the longest action potential duration and may contribute to the U wave seen on the surface electrocardiogram (ECG). The J (Osborne) wave seen on the ECG in cases of hypothermia (see Fig. 109-2 in Chapter 109) may be due to the increased prominence of I_{to} in the epicardial cells. Prolongation of the action potential is seen in cardiac hypertrophy or failure. At the molecular level, downregulation of the transient outward current I_{to} plays a prominent role in these disease states.

In a normal heart, the source of initial depolarizations occurs in the pacemaker cells of the sinus node (E-Fig. 61-2). The sinoatrial (SA) node is found at the lateral border of the superior vena cava and right atrial junction in the sulcus terminalis. It is an ovoid structure measuring up to 2 cm long by 0.5 cm wide. The sinus node artery, branching from either the right coronary artery (55 to 60%) or the left coronary artery (40 to 45%), runs through the middle of the sinus node. Pacemaker cells, seen as spider-shaped and spindle-shaped cells in the node, spontaneously depolarize during diastole. The wave of depolarization spreads through the sinus node and into the surrounding myocardium. The sympathetic and parasympathetic nervous systems affect the sinus rate. Adrenergic stimulation increases the rate by increasing $I_{Ca,L}$ and I_f activity. Cholinergic stimulation decreases the rate by decreasing $I_{Ca,L}$ and I_f activity. Stretch mediators found in the node and coupled to chloride channels also may increase the atrial rate with increasing atrial pressure. The SA node is the predominant pacemaker in the heart owing to its rapid rates of depolarization and overdrive suppression of secondary pacemakers.

Depolarization occurs through the atria to the atrioventricular (AV) node and from the right atrium to the left atrium. Three intra-atrial pathways—anterior, middle, and posterior—connect the right and left atria. Three intra-nodal pathways—superior, middle, and inferior tracts—also may connect the SA node to the AV node, although various investigators have disputed their presence. The P wave on the ECG is formed by atrial depolarization. The AV node is found at the apex of the triangle of Koch, formed by the tendon of Todaro on one side and the tricuspid annulus on the other, on the right side of the heart and anterior to the os of the coronary sinus. The arterial supply of the AV node arises from the right coronary artery in 85 to 90% of cases. The AV node itself is complex and can be divided into three general regions, with further subdivisions possible. A transitional zone contains multiple atrial inputs that extend to the compact AV node, which penetrates the central fibrous body and becomes the bundle of His. The compact AV node ranges from 5 to 7 mm by 2 to 5 mm in size. At least two distinct populations of AV node cells, rod-shaped and ovoid, have been described. These cells spontaneously depolarize because of a strong I_f current. Most ovoid cells lack I_{Na} and I_{to}, leading to slower depolarization. Conduction is relatively slow through the AV node compared with atrial and ventricular tissue, in part because of the decreased density of gap junction proteins, such as connexin 43, which is 33 times less prevalent in the AV node compared with ventricular cells. This reduction in gap junctions and intercalated discs leads to slower depolarization of neighboring cells. On the surface ECG, most of the PR interval depends on this slow AV node conduction.

The bundle of His arises from the compact AV node as it enters the central fibrous body. Conduction through the His bundle is rapid, on the order of

35 to 55 msec to the ventricles, owing to the presence of rapidly acting sodium channels. The arterial supply of the bundle of His originates from the left anterior descending artery in 90% of cases, with 10% emanating from the right coronary artery. The right and left bundle branches originate from the bundle of His. The left bundle branch further subdivides into the left anterior fascicle and left posterior fascicle before supplying the ventricular endocardium with Purkinje fibers. The right bundle branch trifurcates distally into a network that supplies the anterolateral papillary muscle, the low right septum, and the parietal band. Activation of the His-Purkinje system can be seen as the later portion of the PR interval on the surface ECG.

Ventricular activation occurs first from the left to right septum, followed by the synchronized depolarization of both ventricles from apex to base and endocardium to epicardium. The rapid activation of myocardial cells is due in part to the strong presence of the gap junction protein connexin 43. Knockout mice homozygous for connexin 43 deletions die with conotruncus malformations early in life, whereas mice heterozygous for connexin 43 deletion (Cx43+/−) have significant decreases in ventricular conduction in otherwise normal ventricles. Ventricular depolarization can be seen as the QRS complex on the surface ECG and is followed by repolarization seen as the ST, T, and U waves.

Normally the only connection between the atria and the ventricles is through the AV node and His bundle because the fibrous rings surrounding the tricuspid valve and mitral valve are electrically insulating. In a small percentage of the population (0.15 to 0.25%), anomalous myocardial bypass tracts join atrium to ventricle (Kent bundle) or, less frequently, atrium to AV node (James fiber), atrium to His bundle (Brechenmacher fiber), or AV node or His to Purkinje fiber or ventricle (Mahaim fiber). The classic AV bypass tract involved in the Wolff-Parkinson-White syndrome is composed of fibers containing I_{Na} and conducts rapidly in a nondecremental manner similar to that seen in the atria, His-Purkinje, or ventricular tissue (Fig. 61-2). A missense mutation in the γ2 regulatory subunit of adenosine monophosphate (AMP)-activated protein kinase gene *PRKAG2* can cause the Wolff-Parkinson-White syndrome, with a possible effect of interfering with muscle fiber regression during embryogenesis. The surface ECG often shows a δ wave (see Fig. 64-19 in Chapter 64), the hallmark of ventricular preexcitation, preceding the QRS complex.

The heart is innervated by the sympathetic and the parasympathetic nervous systems, with their influence on ion channels manifested as changes in the heart rate, refractoriness, and contractility. Sympathetic stimulation causes the release of norepinephrine at the postganglionic nerve terminal, leading to β₁-adrenergic and β₂-adrenergic receptor activation, followed by G protein–mediated adenylyl cyclase production, which increases production of cyclic AMP (cAMP), which leads to the activation of protein kinase A, ultimately resulting in the phosphorylation of ion channels, which alter their gating and function. Parasympathetic activity leads to release of acetylcholine at the nerve terminal, which stimulates muscarinic cholinergic receptors, followed by direct G protein–mediated activation of channels, or indirect G protein–mediated secondary messenger activation using cAMP. Multiple membrane currents are influenced by sympathetic or parasympathetic activity. The L-type calcium channel current $I_{Ca,L}$ is increased four times with β-adrenergic stimulation, leading to increased conduction of the SA and AV nodes. β-Adrenergic stimulation also leads to a cAMP-mediated change in the activation of I_f, with the result being increased activity of cardiac pacemaker cells and higher heart rates. Parasympathetic stimulation leads to activation of the acetylcholine-activated potassium current I_{KACh}, which results in decreased pacemaker activity and slowing of conduction over the AV node. Purinergic receptors are a third family of G protein–coupled receptors that are activated by adenosine. Exposure to adenosine leads to activation of I_{KACh} and inhibition of $I_{Ca,L}$, resulting in slowing of the pacemaker activity for SA and AV nodes and conduction delay through the AV node.

Mechanisms of Cardiac Tachyarrhythmias

A cardiac arrhythmia is an abnormality in the timing or sequence of cardiac depolarization. There are two predominant types of cardiac arrhythmias: (1) tachyarrhythmia—an abnormally rapid cardiac rhythm (heart rate >100 beats per minute) and (2) bradyarrhythmia—a slow cardiac rhythm (heart rate <60 beats per minute) (Chapters 62, 64, and 65). The mechanism of cardiac tachyarrhythmias can be grouped into two general categories, abnormalities of impulse formation and re-entry (E-Fig. 61-3). Abnormalities of impulse formation can be subdivided further into abnormal automaticity and triggered activity. In the normal heart, the sinus node is the predominant pacemaker, with secondary pacemakers located in the atria, AV node, and His-Purkinje system, which function in the event that normal initiation or propagation is affected by disease or drugs. Automaticity is the ability to initiate spontaneous impulses. Under normal circumstances, there is a hierarchical sequence in the rate of firing of the heart cells that have the capacity for automaticity. Normally, spontaneous firing is fastest in the sinus node (70 to 80 beats per minute under resting conditions), and the sinus node is the predominant pacemaker. The AV node and His bundle fire at 50 to 60 beats per minute, and the Purkinje fibers fire at 30 to 40 beats per minute. The lower pacemaker may take over the pacemaking function of the heart if the faster pacemaker fails or slows. Variations in autonomic tone may have a major effect on normal automaticity. In general, activation of the sympathetic nervous system increases automaticity, whereas activation of the parasympathetic nervous system decreases automaticity. Under pathologic conditions that depolarize cells, myocardial cells outside the specialized conduction system also may acquire automaticity, a phenomenon termed *abnormal automaticity*.

Triggered activity is an uncommon mechanism of cardiac arrhythmias. Triggered activity occurs when a preceding depolarization does not repolarize completely before depolarizing again. *Early afterdepolarizations* (EADs) occur during phase 2 and phase 3 of the action potential. The basis for EADs appears to involve the L-type calcium channel. EADs are facilitated by increased repolarization times, as seen in either congenital or acquired long QT syndromes. With drugs that prolong the QT interval, such as erythromycin, quinidine, sotalol, and procainamide, the block of potassium channels involved in repolarization leads to prolongation of the action potential. The ultimate effect of EADs may be in initiating polymorphic ventricular tachycardia or torsades de pointes (Chapter 65). *Delayed afterdepolarizations* (DADs) arise during phase 4 of the action potential, when the cell membrane is completely repolarized. Transient inward currents, which are not normally present, may be initiated by the action of elevated intracellular calcium on the sodium-calcium exchanger or by release of calcium from the sarcoplasmic reticulum, and they may form the basis for DADs. Rapid heart rates, increased extracellular calcium, and adrenergic stimulation all may contribute to DADs. DADs are thought to form the basis of arrhythmias resulting from digitalis, idiopathic ventricular tachyarrhythmias, and idioventricular rhythms, and they may be reduced by drugs that block the uptake of calcium by the sarcoplasmic reticulum. Multifocal atrial tachycardia is another example of an arrhythmia that results from DAD-mediated triggered activity. The third type of automaticity, *depolarization-induced automaticity*, has been reproduced in cardiac tissues but may not lead to clinically relevant arrhythmias. Depolarization-induced automaticity arises from the constant application of current to muscle, a process that leads to spontaneous firing of the muscle.

Re-entry is the most common mechanism of cardiac arrhythmias. Re-entry generally occurs in the setting of abnormalities in impulse conduction. The abnormalities in impulse conduction may result from an anomalous electrical connection in the heart (i.e., an accessory pathway) or from poor impulse propagation. The basis for poor propagation of the depolarizing wave front in the heart may be attributed to pathology, drugs, or hormonal modulation of the conduction system. Fibrosis or calcification of the AV node, His bundle, or right and left bundle branches may lead to AV block or right and

left bundle-branch blocks. AV nodal block may be a result of high vagal tone, as seen during sleep or in a well-conditioned athlete, or may be due to agents that act on the AV node, such as digitalis, β-adrenergic blockers, or calcium-channel blockers. Slowing of conduction in the atrium and ventricles also may be affected directly by hyperkalemia or ischemia.

The basis for poor propagation of the depolarizing wave front in the heart usually results from pathologic changes in patients with structural heart disease, including coronary artery disease, left ventricular hypertrophy, and heart failure. Fibrotic changes in the heart, with increases in collagen and intracellular matrix as seen in hypertrophy or infarction, can lead to areas of slow conduction and provide portals for re-entry. Changes in the gap junction proteins have been noted in hypertrophy with increases of connexin 43. These changes typically result from advanced age or the presence of structural heart disease, such as a prior myocardial infarction or a cardiomyopathy. In ischemia, the action potential is abbreviated owing to activation of I_{KACh}; in hypertrophy and failure, action potential prolongation from loss of I_{to} is found. Other influences on remodeling include catecholamines, free radicals, angiotensin-converting enzyme, angiotensin II, aldosterone, cytokines, and nitric oxide. Re-entry occurs when there is continuation of a propagating wave front, which reactivates areas of the heart that previously have depolarized and are not refractory. The refractory period, which is the time interval in which the cells are unable to depolarize after a second stimulus, often persists until the transmembrane voltage is +60mV at the activation threshold of I_{Na}.

Three types of re-entry have been described: circus movement re-entry, reflection, and phase 2 re-entry. The simplest model of circus movement tachycardia, the ring model, requires the presence of unidirectional block, in which the wave front can travel only in one direction, and a long enough circuit, in which recovery from refractoriness occurs before the approach of the leading edge of depolarization (Fig. 61-3). The length of the circuit must be equal to or greater than the wavelength (conduction velocity × refractory period) of the tachycardia. Three criteria for circus movement tachycardia include the presence of unidirectional block, the presence of a distinct path of recurrent propagation, and the fact that disrupting the circuit at any point along the path terminates the tachycardia. AV reciprocating tachycardia is an example of a re-entrant tachycardia (see Fig. 64-20 in Chapter 64). During sinus rhythm, the cardiac impulse activates the ventricle through the AV node and the accessory pathway. The tachycardia is initiated when a premature atrial impulse blocks the accessory pathway and conducts down the AV node (owing to differences in refractoriness). The impulse then returns to the atria by conduction through the accessory pathway, resulting in a re-entrant or circus movement tachycardia. Atrial fibrillation is the most common type of arrhythmia that results from re-entry. In contrast to arrhythmias with an accessory pathway in which there is only a single fixed re-entrant circuit, however, atrial fibrillation results from the presence of many functional re-entrant wavelets that propagate throughout the atria simultaneously. It has been estimated that at least three re-entrant wavelets must coexist for atrial fibrillation to be sustained. *Re-entry resulting from reflection* occurs when an

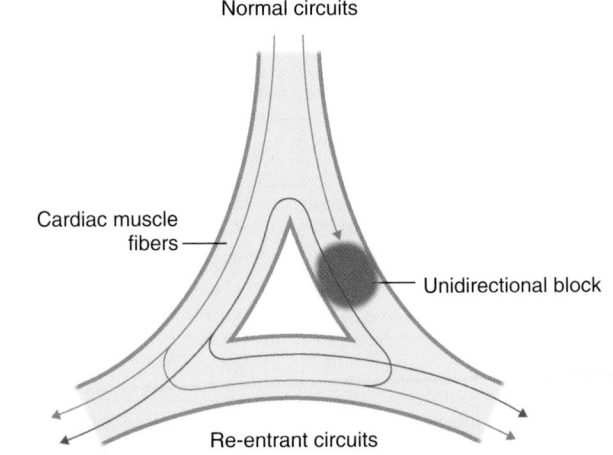

Normal circuits

Cardiac muscle fibers

Unidirectional block

Re-entrant circuits

FIGURE 61-3. Unidirectional block as a result of abnormal repolarization, conduction, or intracellular calcium homeostasis. *Red arrows* show normal conduction, and *blue arrows* show re-entry through previously refractory tissue. (From Keating MT, Sanguinetti MC. Molecular and cellular mechanisms of cardiac arrhythmias. *Cell.* 2001;104:569.)

impulse proceeds back and forth over a functionally unexcitable pathway, depolarizing proximal tissue on each return cycle. *Phase 2 re-entry* occurs when an action potential dome during phase 2 is propagated from normal myocytes to myocytes lacking the dome, followed by local reexcitation, extrasystolic beats, and circus movement re-entry. Phase 2 re-entry notably is found in Brugada's syndrome (Chapter 65). Brugada's syndrome is the result of a sodium channel mutation in the α-subunit SCN5A. The hallmark of Brugada's syndrome is ST segment elevation and a right bundle branch pattern in V_1 to V_3 on the ECG. The ECG abnormalities can be explained by the loss of a phase 2 action potential dome in the epicardium but not in the endocardium owing to a failure of I_{Na} to reach a more positive voltage before phase 1. Endocardium-to-epicardium phase 2 re-entry occurs, leading to the ventricular tachycardia or ventricular fibrillation that is seen in Brugada's syndrome.

Multiple intrinsic and extrinsic factors can affect the initiation and propagation of cardiac arrhythmias (E-Fig. 61-4). At the molecular level, multiple mutations contribute to the inherited long QT syndrome and to idiopathic ventricular fibrillation (Brugada's syndrome). Twelve different subtypes of long QT syndrome have been described, and the genetic mutations of each have been identified. Genetic testing now can find a mutation in approximately two thirds of patients with long QT syndrome. The three most common types are LQT1 and LQT2, which account for approximately 90% of genotyped cases, and LQT3, which accounts for an additional 5% to 8% of cases. The mutations in long QT syndrome affect the sodium channel and potassium channels involved in repolarization with either gain of function for the sodium channel or loss of function for the potassium channels, resulting in a prolonged phase 2. The most common subtype, LQT1, is a disorder of the potassium channel α-subunit KVLQT1 responsible in part for I_{Ks}. LQT2 is due to mutations in HERG, a component of I_{Kr}. LQT3 affects the sodium channel SCN5A at a site leading to incomplete inactivation, and a continuing inward current Brugada's syndrome has been shown to be due to mutations in SCN5A, causing faster inactivation of the sodium channel. Familial polymorphic ventricular tachycardia has been linked to mutations in the cardiac ryanodine receptor (*RyR2*) gene of the cardiac sarcoplasmic reticulum, mutations that may lead to changes in calcium-induced activation.

Mechanism of Bradyarrhythmias

Cardiac bradyarrhythmias may result from either abnormalities in impulse formation or abnormalities in impulse conduction. Sinus bradycardia is the most common type of bradyarrhythmia. Sinus bradycardia results from a decreased rate of firing of the sinus node, which may be physiologic and result from increased parasympathetic tone (i.e., during sleep) or pathologic and result from a fibrosis of the sinus node, such as occurs with aging. Bradyrrhythmias also occur when abnormalities of conduction interrupt the normal sequence of cardiac depolarization. Depending on the site of block, subsidiary pacemakers begin to fire, creating an "escape" rhythm. Conduction block usually is due to fibrosis or calcification of the AV node, His bundle, or right and left bundle branches. Conduction block also may result from increased parasympathetic tone, however, as seen during sleep or in a well-conditioned athlete, or may be due to agents that act on the AV node, such as digitalis, β-adrenergic blockers, or calcium channel blockers.

SUGGESTED READINGS

Boyett MR. 'And the beat goes on.' The cardiac conduction system: the wiring system of the heart. *Exp Physiol.* 2009;94:1035-1049. *Detailed overview.*

Park DS, Fishman GI. The cardiac conduction system. *Circulation.* 2011;123:904-915. *Review.*

Trayanova NA. Whole-heart modeling: application to cardiac electrophysiology and electromechanics. *Circ Res.* 2011;108:113-128. *Review.*

62

APPROACH TO THE PATIENT WITH SUSPECTED ARRHYTHMIA

JEFFREY E. OLGIN

CLINICAL MANIFESTATIONS

Patients with suspected arrhythmias can present in a variety of ways. Typical symptoms include palpitations, syncope, and presyncope (dizziness). On occasion, arrhythmias can manifest more subtly as exercise intolerance, lethargy, and vague complaints of malaise or without any symptoms at all. Conversely, arrhythmias occasionally manifest as aborted sudden cardiac death (cardiac arrest) (Chapter 63). The specific differential diagnosis, prognosis, and treatment of these symptoms are determined by the severity of the symptom (i.e., whether it results in syncope) and whether the patient has underlying structural heart disease. In general, the likelihood of a life-threatening arrhythmia, such as ventricular tachycardia or ventricular fibrillation, in a patient with symptoms of palpitations or syncope is significantly greater in a patient who has structural heart disease. Therefore, the determination of whether structural heart disease is present is a key step in the diagnosis and prognosis of patients with suspected arrhythmias.

Palpitations

Palpitations, defined as an awareness of an irregular or rapid heartbeat, are most commonly due to ectopic beats—namely, premature atrial contractions (PACs; Chapter 64) and premature ventricular contractions (PVCs; Chapter 65)—or to tachyarrhythmias. A careful history can often distinguish benign palpitations from those that need further evaluation. It can be useful to have the patient tap out with a finger what the palpitations feel like. An irregularly irregular pattern suggests atrial fibrillation, whereas a more regular, rapid pattern suggests a sustained tachycardia. A reliable symptom suggesting that palpitations are caused by a tachyarrhythmia, particularly a supraventricular tachycardia, is the sensation of a regular, rapid-pounding sensation in the neck. Conversely, most patients who complain of symptoms from PACs or PVCs are often more aware of the post-extrasystolic pause or the accentuated output of the post-extrasystolic beat than of the actual premature beat itself. The majority of patients who have symptoms suggestive of premature beats but not of sustained tachycardia do not require further evaluation if they have no other symptoms and no evidence of structural heart disease—that is, an otherwise normal cardiac history, physical examination, and electrocardiogram (ECG) (see Table 50-4 in Chapter 50). If, however, the symptoms are not due to a single occasional extrasystole or are accompanied by presyncope or syncope, further evaluation is required (Fig. 62-1). Antiarrhythmic therapy is usually not necessary to treat PACs or PVCs unless the symptoms are frequent or severe. β-Blockers (e.g., metoprolol 25 mg/day or atenolol 25 mg/day) are first-line therapy in highly symptomatic patients with documented PACs or PVCs.

Palpitations are the most common presentation of tachyarrhythmias. The majority of tachyarrhythmias in patients without structural heart disease are due to supraventricular tachycardias (Chapter 64) that resolve spontaneously within several seconds. When the tachyarrhythmia is more prolonged, it often resolves with simple interventions. Patients themselves can cough several times, perform the Valsalva maneuver, exhale forcefully against a closed glottis for several seconds, or even rub gently on their eyeballs. A physician can use carotid sinus massage (Chapter 64), performed by pressing and rubbing the carotid pulse just below the angle of the mandible for 5 to 15 seconds. This maneuver should be avoided in elderly patients and in patients with a history of cerebrovascular accident, known carotid artery stenosis, or carotid bruit on auscultation. In patients with structural heart disease, palpitations may signify ventricular tachycardia (Chapter 65), particularly if they occur with syncope or presyncope. Rarely do bradyarrhythmias manifest as palpitations.

Presyncope and Syncope

Syncope, defined as a sudden loss of consciousness, and presyncope, or light-headedness, are caused by global impairment of blood flow to the brain

Evaluation of Patients with Palpitations, Dizziness, and/or Syncope

FIGURE 62-1. Algorithm for evaluating patients with symptoms of palpitation, dizziness, or syncope. ARVD = arrhythmogenic right ventricular dysplasia; AV = atrioventricular; CAD = coronary artery disease; ECG = electrocardiogram; echo = echocardiogram; EP = electrophysiology; ICD = implantable cardioverter-defibrillator; LQTS = long QT syndrome; SCD = sudden cardiac death; SVT = supraventricular tachycardia; WPW = Wolff-Parkinson-White syndrome.

(Table 62-1). Syncope can be a manifestation of tachyarrhythmias, bradyarrhythmias, or neurocardiogenic syncope, or it can be unrelated to any arrhythmia. A careful history and physical examination are necessary to exclude other cardiac causes (e.g., acute ischemia, aortic stenosis) or neurologic causes. Important historical features that suggest an arrhythmic cause are an association with palpitations and the lack of any neurologic deficits preceding or following the event. Important differential diagnoses include conditions other than lightheadedness that may be termed dizziness by the patient. Vertigo (Chapter 436), a sense of imbalance or of the "room spinning," and ataxia (Chapter 417) can usually be distinguished by the history and physical examination. The possibility of seizures (Chapter 410) must also be evaluated; syncope from an arrhythmia or neurocardiogenic syncope occasionally results in seizure-like activity, and seizures can sometimes be confused with syncope. The most important distinguishing feature is that postictal symptoms, a key feature of seizure disorders, are absent when syncope is the result of an arrhythmia. Patients with syncope from an arrhythmia usually awaken without any neurologic residual, unless the patient experienced a cardiac arrest with prolonged hypoxia and required resuscitation.

Because most spells of episodic loss of consciousness occur outside medical observation, the history is the most critical part of the evaluation (Table 62-2). Each syncopal episode should be reviewed in detail, with special attention to symptoms preceding the episode, events during unconsciousness, and the symptoms and time course of regaining orientation after consciousness is restored. Information from a witness can be essential to the evaluation.

The patient's presymptomatic activity and positioning, as well as symptoms when the syncopal episode began, are important clues to diagnosis. Seizures or cardiac arrhythmias can occur in any body position, but recumbent patients rarely develop neurocardiogenic (vasovagal) syncope and never have orthostatic hypotension. Prodromal lightheadedness, dizziness (but uncommonly vertigo), bilateral tinnitus, nausea, diffuse weakness, and dimming of vision are symptoms of cerebral hypoperfusion and support the diagnosis of syncope, which may be from a cardiac, orthostatic, or neurocardiogenic cause. Loss of consciousness so rapid that a prodrome is absent may occur with seizures and with some cardiac arrhythmias such as asystole, which typically causes loss of consciousness within 4 to 8 seconds in the

TABLE 62-1   CAUSES OF SYNCOPE AND THEIR PREVALENCE

NEUROCARDIOGENIC CAUSES

Vasovagal (8–41% of patients)
Situational (1–8% of patients)
    Micturition
    Defecation
    Swallow
    Cough
Carotid sinus syncope (0.4% of patients)
Neuralgias
Psychiatric disorders
Medications, exercise

ORTHOSTATIC HYPOTENSION (4–10% OF PATIENTS)

DECREASED CARDIAC OUTPUT

Obstruction to flow (1–8% of patients)
    Obstruction to left ventricular outflow or inflow: aortic stenosis, hypertrophic obstructive cardiomyopathy, mitral stenosis, myxoma
    Obstruction to right ventricular outflow or inflow: pulmonic stenosis, pulmonary embolism, pulmonary hypertension, myxoma
Other heart disease
    Pump failure, myocardial infarction, coronary artery disease, coronary spasm, tamponade, aortic dissection

ARRHYTHMIAS (4–38% OF PATIENTS)

Bradyarrhythmias: sinus node disease, second- and third-degree atrioventricular block, pacemaker malfunction, drug-induced bradyarrhythmias
Tachyarrhythmias: ventricular tachycardia, torsades de pointes (e.g., associated with congenital long QT syndrome or acquired QT prolongation), supraventricular tachycardia

NEUROLOGIC AND PSYCHIATRIC DISEASES (3–32% OF PATIENTS)

Migraine
Transient ischemic attacks

UNKNOWN (13–41% OF PATIENTS)

Adapted from Kapoor W. Approach to the patient with syncope. In: Braunwald E, Goldman L, eds. *Primary Cardiology*, 2nd ed. Philadelphia: Saunders; 2003.

TABLE 62-2 CLINICAL FEATURES SUGGESTING SPECIFIC CAUSES

SYMPTOM OR FINDING	DIAGNOSTIC CONSIDERATION
After sudden unexpected pain, fear, or unpleasant sight, sound, or smell	Vasovagal
Prolonged motionless standing	Vasovagal
Well-trained athlete after exertion (without heart disease)	Vasovagal
During or immediately after micturition, cough, swallowing, or defecation	Situational syncope
Syncope with throat or facial pain (glossopharyngeal or trigeminal neuralgia)	Neurocardiogenic syncope with neuralgia
With head rotation, pressure on the carotid sinus (as in tumors, shaving, tight collars)	Carotid sinus syncope
Immediately on standing	Orthostatic hypotension
Medication that may lead to long QT syndrome, orthostasis, or bradycardia	Drug induced
Associated with headaches	Migraine, seizures
Associated with vertigo, dysarthria, diplopia	Transient ischemic attack, subclavian steal, basilar migraine
With arm exercise	Subclavian steal
Confusion after a spell or loss of consciousness for >5 min	Seizure
Differences in blood pressure or pulse in the two arms	Subclavian steal or aortic dissection
Syncope and murmur with changing position (from sitting to lying, bending, turning over in bed)	Atrial myxoma or thrombus
Syncope with exertion	Aortic stenosis, pulmonary hypertension, mitral stenosis, obstructive hypertrophic cardiomyopathy, coronary artery disease
Family history of sudden death	Long QT syndrome, Brugada's syndrome
Brief loss of consciousness, no prodrome, with heart disease	Arrhythmias
Frequent syncope, somatic complaints, no heart disease	Psychiatric illness

From Kapoor WN. Syncope. *N Engl J Med.* 2000;343:1856-1862.

upright position but usually requires 12 to 15 seconds in the recumbent position. Palpitations during the prodrome suggest a tachyarrhythmia. The activity of the patient immediately before the onset of symptoms may also provide clues. Syncope associated with the cessation of exertion or with anxiety or pain suggests neurocardiogenic syncope, whereas symptoms during exertion suggest an arrhythmia. Syncope associated with a change in posture suggests orthostatic causes, whereas symptoms while straining at urination suggests situational neurocardiogenic syncope.

A witness's description of the events during the episode of unconsciousness is very helpful. Although body stiffening and limb jerking occur with generalized seizures, similar movements can result from cerebral hypoperfusion, especially if perfusion is not restored rapidly. Such muscle jerking is often multifocal and can be synchronous or asynchronous. In contrast to epileptic seizures, which generally produce tonic-clonic activity for at least 1 to 2 minutes, muscle jerking in syncope rarely persists for longer than 30 seconds. If an arrhythmia continues or the patient is physically maintained upright, tonic stiffening of the body followed by jerking movements of the limbs can occur. Occasionally, motor movements identical to a tonic-clonic seizure occur, and a mistaken diagnosis of epilepsy can be made. Urinary incontinence during the spell is frequently used to support or refute a diagnosis of epilepsy; however, fainting with a full bladder can result in incontinence, whereas seizures with an empty bladder will not. Tongue biting favors seizures.

The time frame over which consciousness and orientation are regained is perhaps the most important clue in differentiating seizures from syncope. Recovery of orientation after neurocardiogenic syncope occurs within seconds of regaining consciousness. Recovery of orientation after self-reversible arrhythmia-associated syncope is usually proportional to the duration of the unconsciousness and is usually rapid (0 to 10 seconds). Life-threatening arrhythmias (e.g., prolonged asystole or ventricular fibrillation) usually do not resolve without resuscitation, and the confusion after regaining consciousness may be permanent owing to ischemic brain injury (Chapter 63). By comparison, the period of confusion after seizures, often accompanied by agitation, continues for 2 to 20 minutes after recovery of consciousness.

DIAGNOSIS

Arrhythmias are generally categorized as bradyarrhythmias (slow heart rates), tachyarrhythmias (fast heart rates), or premature beats (single extrasystoles from the atrium or the ventricle—PACs [see Fig. 64-12 in Chapter 64] or PVCs [see Fig. 65-3 in Chapter 65], respectively) (see Table 62-1). Although not a primary arrhythmia, neurocardiogenic syncope is a related diagnostic and management issue because its symptoms are frequently similar to those of arrhythmias and because neurocardiogenic syncope secondarily results in bradycardia (see later).

Bradyarrhythmias

Bradyarrhythmias (Chapter 64) can be due to dysfunction in the sinoatrial node, atrioventricular (AV) node, or His-Purkinje system (below the AV node). Sinus bradycardia manifests as a slow atrial (sinus) rate and can occur at rest or as an inappropriately slow rate during exercise (chronotropic incompetence). Sinus arrest can be intermittent, when transient loss of sinus activity (loss of the P wave on the ECG) causes brief sinus pauses, or persistent, with prolonged loss of atrial activation. The sinus rate and even the presence of sinus pauses are influenced by autonomic tone. Therefore, healthy individuals—particularly younger patients and well-trained athletes (with high vagal tone)— have occasional sinus slowing, often during sleep. A sinus pause of more than 3 seconds is considered pathologic when it is associated with symptoms. Sinus bradycardia and sinus arrest can also be the result of medications, typically β-blockers and calcium-channel blockers. When not "physiologic" or due to medications, sinus bradycardia and sinus arrest are the result of intrinsic conduction system disease. Sinus bradycardia, especially if it is intermittent, can also signify disease of the right coronary artery.

Bradyarrhythmias from AV nodal disease result from the failure of impulse conduction from the atrium to the ventricle. Like the sinus node, the AV node is dramatically affected by autonomic tone. Mobitz type I second-degree AV block (Wenckebach block; see Fig. 64-8 in Chapter 64) can be seen during periods of high vagal tone and is not necessarily pathologic; for example, it does not progress to complete heart block and is not associated with a widened QRS. Many drugs, such as β-blockers and calcium-channel blockers, commonly cause first-degree AV block and should be considered a potential cause of any degree of AV block. Mobitz type II block (see Fig. 64-9 in Chapter 64) signifies that the level of AV block is below the AV node in the His-Purkinje system, which is not sensitive to autonomic tone; the resulting QRS is widened, and there is a high likelihood of progression to complete heart block (third-degree AV block; see Figs. 64-10 and 64-11 in Chapter 64). Intermittent complete heart block, which can result in drop attacks or Stokes-Adams attacks, is usually preceded by abnormal baseline findings on the ECG, such as a bundle branch block or second-degree AV block. The treatment of choice for symptomatic bradyarrhythmias or those likely to progress to complete heart block is implantation of a permanent pacemaker (Chapter 66).

Tachyarrhythmias

Tachyarrhythmias can arise from the atrium or AV node (supraventricular tachycardia) or from the ventricle (ventricular tachycardia). Supraventricular tachyarrhythmias that may be associated with palpitations, presyncope, or syncope include atrial tachycardia (see Fig. 64-18 in Chapter 64), AV nodal re-entrant tachycardia (see Fig. 64-19 in Chapter 64), AV junctional tachycardia (see Fig. 64-20 in Chapter 64), atrial flutter (see Fig. 64-23 in Chapter 64), and atrial fibrillation (see Fig. 64-24 in Chapter 64), sometimes in association with accessory conduction pathways that facilitate the re-entry needed to sustain the arrhythmia. Ventricular tachyarrhythmias include the various forms of ventricular tachycardia (see Fig. 65-3 in Chapter 65). Treatment is guided by the specific tachyarrhythmia and its underlying cause (see Table 62-3 and Tables 64-6 and 64-7 in Chapters 62 and 64, respectively) (Chapters 63 through 66).

Neurocardiogenic Syncope and Related Syndromes

Neurocardiogenic syncope is the sudden onset of lightheadedness or loss of consciousness as a result of autonomic reflexes and is more common in

TABLE 62-3   ARRHYTHMIC CAUSES OF PALPITATIONS AND SYNCOPE

ETIOLOGY	SPECIFIC ARRHYTHMIA	Symptoms			TREATMENT	COMMENTS
		PALPITATIONS	DIZZINESS	SYNCOPE		
BRADYARRHYTHMIAS						
Sinus node dysfunction	Sinus bradycardia	No	Occasional	Rare	Pacemaker (if symptoms)	Can be seen in association with neurocardiogenic syncope
	Sinus arrest	Occasional	Yes	Occasional	Pacemaker	Pause >3 sec
	Sick sinus syndrome	Occasional	Yes	Occasional	Pacemaker	
AV nodal disease	First-degree AV block	No	No	No	None	
	Type I second-degree AV block	Occasional	No	No	None	Can be seen in association with neurocardiogenic syncope
	Type II second-degree AV block	Occasional	Rare	No	Pacemaker if severe	Can progress to complete heart block
	Third-degree AV block	Yes	Yes	Yes	Pacemaker	
Tachy-brady syndrome		Yes	Yes	Occasional	Treat tachycardia if possible Pacemaker	Can also be manifestation of sick sinus syndrome
TACHYARRHYTHMIAS						
SVT	Atrial tachycardia	Yes	Occasional	Rare	Ablation β-Blockers (e.g., metoprolol, atenolol)* Calcium-channel blockers (e.g., diltiazem)*	
	Atrial flutter	Yes	Occasional	Rare	Ablation Antiarrhythmic drugs (e.g., amiodarone)* Cardioversion (acute episode)	Often difficult to control rate
	Atrial fibrillation	Yes	Occasional	Rare	Ventricular rate control Warfarin Antiarrhythmic drugs (e.g., amiodarone)* Cardioversion (acute episode) Ablation	
	AV nodal re-entrant tachycardia	Yes	Yes	Rare	Ablation β-Blockers (e.g., metoprolol, atenolol)* Calcium-channel blockers (e.g., diltiazem)*	
	AV re-entrant tachycardia (WPW)	Yes	Yes	Rare	Ablation Antiarrhythmic drugs*	
VT	Idiopathic (RV outflow tract, fascicular)	Yes	Yes	Occasional	Ablation	Absence of structural heart disease Low risk of sudden death
	VT secondary to CAD, cardiomyopathy	Yes	Yes	Yes	ICD Amiodarone (400 mg qd)* Ablation	Increased incidence of sudden death
	Bundle branch re-entry	Yes	Yes	Yes	Ablation	Usually in the setting of LV dysfunction and baseline intraventricular conduction delay
	Genetic syndromes (e.g., long QT syndrome, Brugada's, arrhythmic right ventricular dysplasia)	Occasional	Yes	Yes	ICD	Not always a clear family history Increased incidence of sudden death
Ectopy	PACs	Occasional	No	No	None β-Blockers (e.g., atenolol, metoprolol) if symptomatic*	
	PVCs	Occasional	No	No	None β-Blockers (e.g., atenolol, metoprolol) if symptomatic*	Benign in absence of structural heart disease
NEUROCARDIOGENIC SYNCOPE		No	Yes	Yes	Behavioral (hydration, avoid triggers, abort episodes) Midodrine (10 mg tid)	

*See Table 64-7 in Chapter 64 for drug doses.

AV = atrioventricular; CAD = coronary artery disease; ICD = implantable cardioverter-defibrillator; LV = left ventricle; PACs = premature atrial contractions; PVCs = premature ventricular contractions; RV = right ventricle; SVT = supraventricular tachycardia; VT = ventricular tachycardia; WPW = Wolff-Parkinson-White syndrome.

younger patients (teenage to third decade of life). It is sometimes called a vasovagal episode, a common faint, or situational syncope if it is clearly induced by a particular activity (e.g., micturition syncope). In this form of neurocardiogenic syncope, heightened parasympathetic output, either due to direct stimulation (e.g., micturition, defecation, abdominal pain or other gastrointestinal conditions) or as a reflex in response to sympathetic stimulation (e.g., seeing blood, abrupt cessation of exercise), results in arterial dilation (called the vasodilatory response) and an inhibition of sinus and AV node activity (the cardioinhibitory response). The result is a transient decrease in blood pressure, often manifested as lightheadedness or syncope. Because they are associated with parasympathetic (vagal) output, episodes are frequently accompanied by nausea, diaphoresis, and salivation.

Treatment of this form of syncope can be challenging. The most effective therapies are behavioral (avoidance of triggers), wearing of compression stockings, and maintenance of adequate hydration and salt intake. Lying down with the feet elevated and performing isometric hand exercises may abort an acute episode. Medical therapy, including β-blockers (pindolol 5 to 15 mg twice daily), mineralocorticoids (fludrocortisone 0.1 mg/day), paroxetine (10 to 20 mg/day), and midodrine (an α-adrenergic agonist and vasoconstrictor; 2.5 to 5 mg three times daily), has shown some efficacy in reducing recurrence rates, although the efficacy of β-blockers for reducing syncopal episodes has been inconsistent. Even though bradycardia is a dominant feature of neurocardiogenic syncope, a pacemaker is not effective for the prevention of episodes because most patients also have a major vasodilatory component.

Rarely, situational syncope is associated with swallowing or coughing. Swallowing can trigger brain stem reflexes that lead to vagally induced bradyarrhythmias, with resultant syncope. This phenomenon may or may not be associated with severe pain in the tonsillar pillar, which may radiate to the ear (i.e., glossopharyngeal neuralgia; Chapter 405). The pain can usually be prevented by carbamazepine (400 to 1000 mg/day orally); in refractory cases, 300 mg/day of phenytoin can be added. Cough-related syncope can occur with severe, repeated coughing, which may increase thoracic pressure and result in increased vagal tone or a transient reduction in outflow from the intracranial veins, followed by a transient increase in intracranial pressure and impaired blood flow.

A related cause of syncope is carotid body hypersensitivity, in which vagal tone is increased by direct stimulation of the carotid body. This condition is frequently seen in older patients (particularly men older than 60 years), in whom episodes are associated with mechanical stimulation of the neck (e.g., turning the head, shaving, wearing a tight collar or necktie). Use of β-blockers, calcium-channel blockers, and digitalis can exacerbate or predispose to this condition. This form of syncope is diagnosed by documenting pauses longer than 3 seconds in response to carotid sinus massage and is curable with a pacemaker because carotid body stimulation does not cause significant vasodilation.

Postural or orthostatic hypotension can result in recurrent syncope. The history confirms that the patient is in the upright posture during spells, that the prodromal symptoms are those of cerebral hypoperfusion, and that the symptoms are relieved with recumbency. The diagnosis is supported by detecting a decrease of 30 mm Hg or greater in systolic blood pressure or a decrease of 10 mm Hg or greater in diastolic blood pressure between recumbent and upright postures. The many causes include drugs, polyneuropathies (Chapter 428), and neurodegenerative disorders (Chapter 416).

Cerebrovascular syncope results from cerebral hypoperfusion due to vascular phenomena, as opposed to generalized hypotension caused by arrhythmias or neurocardiogenic reflexes. Loss of consciousness can be a component of a basilar artery transient ischemic attack, but other brain stem symptoms nearly always precede or accompany the unconsciousness. Vertigo is most frequent, but diplopia or visual field disturbances, hemifacial or perioral numbness, and dysarthria or ataxia are also common. Recovery of consciousness may require 30 to 60 minutes. Although the diagnosis is suggested by the history and clinical presentation, imaging studies can be useful to confirm the diagnosis. Carotid Doppler studies may show various degrees of stenosis, especially in older patients. However, unconsciousness requires bihemispheric dysfunction; thus, unilateral carotid stenosis alone does not cause syncope. Transcranial Doppler studies or magnetic resonance angiography of the basilar artery is indicated only if brain stem ischemic symptoms are present in addition to loss of consciousness; false-positive tests are common, especially with increasing age. These patients, who are at risk for basilar artery stroke, should be treated with aspirin and should be considered for other treatments (e.g., surgery, stent placement) appropriate for their symptoms and anatomy (Chapter 414).

Other syndromes that can cause syncope include subclavian artery stenosis, which may result in retrograde blood flow from the vertebral artery to one arm, with resultant brain stem hypoperfusion (i.e., subclavian steal syndrome). Asymmetry in upper extremity systolic blood pressure, typically averaging 45 mm Hg, is nearly always present. Brain stem symptoms are similar to those in basilar transient ischemic attacks, including loss of consciousness, but a subsequent stroke from subclavian steal is rare. Repair of the stenosis is the treatment of choice. Syncope may also occur in up to 10% of patients with basilar artery migraine (Chapter 405). It can have a postural (orthostatic) manifestation or be associated with other basilar artery symptoms.

Neuropsychiatric syncope is a diagnosis of exclusion but is suggested by young age, frequent spells, multiple symptoms (e.g., dizziness, vertigo, lightheadedness, numbness), and duplication of the patient's symptoms by hyperventilation with the mouth open for 2 to 3 minutes. Whereas syncope and seizures occur with the eyes open, often with gaze deviation, psychogenic events frequently begin with eye closing.

Seizures (Chapter 410) can cause loss of consciousness and occasionally present clinically as syncope. However, seizures usually have a characteristic presentation and include a postictal phase, whereas most patients experiencing a syncopal episode quickly regain consciousness, except when cerebral perfusion is so compromised as to cause a secondary seizure or persistent anoxia and brain damage.

Diagnostic Tests
Electrocardiography
The baseline ECG is critical in the evaluation of a patient with palpitations or syncope. The presence of ventricular preexcitation, as manifested by a short PR interval and a delta wave (see Fig. 64-21 in Chapter 64), establishes the likely diagnosis of Wolff-Parkinson-White syndrome in a patient with palpitations and AV reciprocating tachycardia (Chapter 64); it can also be used to determine the location of the responsible accessory pathway. The baseline ECG provides useful predictive information about the likelihood of conduction system abnormalities being responsible for bradyarrhythmias (e.g., sinus bradycardia suggests sinus node dysfunction, a prolonged PR interval suggests AV nodal disease, and a widened QRS suggests disease below the AV node). The ECG is also useful in diagnosing prior myocardial infarction (i.e., pathologic Q waves), which raises the likelihood of ventricular tachycardia as a potential cause of syncope or palpitations. Abnormalities such as a prolonged QT interval in a patient with syncope and a family history of syncope or sudden death suggest one of the congenital long QT syndromes (Chapter 65). An incomplete right bundle branch block with coved ST segment elevation in ECG lead V_1 or V_2 in a patient with syncope or palpitations suggests Brugada's syndrome, whereas an epsilon wave, incomplete right bundle branch block, and inverted T waves in V_1 are suggestive of right ventricular dysplasia (Chapter 65). All these syndromes carry an increased risk of recurrent syncope and sudden death if untreated (Chapters 63 through 65).

Performing an ECG during an episode of palpitations is extremely useful in making a definitive diagnosis. For narrow–QRS complex tachycardias, the specific supraventricular tachycardia can often be surmised from the 12-lead ECG obtained during symptoms (Fig. 62-2). Moreover, for wide–QRS complex tachycardias, the 12-lead ECG is useful in distinguishing a supraventricular tachycardia (with aberrancy) from a ventricular tachycardia (Fig. 62-3). The presence of fusion beats or AV dissociation during a wide–QRS complex tachycardia leads to the diagnosis of ventricular tachycardia. For ventricular tachycardias, the morphology of the QRS complex is useful in determining the location of the ventricular tachycardia focus and in identifying idiopathic ventricular tachycardia (right ventricular outflow tract or fascicular), which has a much more benign course than ventricular tachycardia in the setting of coronary disease (Chapter 65).

The effect of carotid sinus massage, vagal maneuvers, or adenosine (given as a rapid intravenous bolus of 6 mg and repeated at a dose of 12 mg if the initial dose is ineffective) is also useful in narrowing the differential diagnosis of a tachycardia. These maneuvers slow conduction through the AV node. Therefore, tachycardias that terminate with either maneuver are likely to involve the AV node as a critical component of the re-entrant circuit (AV nodal re-entrant tachycardia or AV re-entrant tachycardia). If the maneuver induces AV block but does not terminate the arrhythmia, likely causes are atrial fibrillation, atrial flutter, and atrial tachycardias (or occasionally ventricular tachycardia if the QRS is wide). On rare occasions, atrial tachycardias and some idiopathic ventricular tachycardias terminate in response to

FIGURE 62-2. ECG algorithm for diagnosis of narrow-complex tachycardias. AVNRT = atrioventricular nodal reciprocating tachycardia; AVRT = atrioventricular reciprocating tachycardia; MAT = multifocal atrial tachycardia; PJRT = permanent form of junctional reciprocating tachycardia. (From Blomstrom-Lundqvist C, Scheinman MM, Aliot EM, et al. ACC/AHA/ESC guidelines for the management of patients with supraventricular arrhythmias—executive summary. *Circulation.* 2003;108:1871-1909.)

adenosine. Important clues to the specific mechanism can be obtained at the onset or termination of tachycardia, so obtaining a continuous 12-lead ECG during carotid sinus massage or the administration of adenosine is useful.

During bradycardias, the ECG is useful in determining the level of the conduction system (sinus node, AV node, or His bundle) responsible for the bradycardia. Sinus bradycardia is diagnosed when a slow (<50/minute at rest) atrial rate (P wave) conducts to the ventricle. Sinus arrest or sinus pauses (see Fig. 64-6 in Chapter 64) are diagnosed by absent or dropped P waves. First-degree AV block (see Fig. 64-7 in Chapter 64) is defined as a prolonged PR interval (>200 msec), and second-degree AV block is defined by P waves that occasionally do not conduct to the ventricle (P wave without an ensuing QRS); Mobitz type I second-degree AV block (also known as Wenckebach block; see Fig. 64-8 in Chapter 64) is characterized by progressive lengthening of the PR interval until one P wave does not conduct to the ventricle. This form of AV block is often seen in younger patients, is usually benign, and rarely progresses to complete AV (third-degree) block. Mobitz type II second-degree AV block (see Fig. 64-9 in Chapter 64), which is characterized by the sudden, unexpected loss of conduction of a P wave to the ventricle (dropped QRS), signifies disease of the His-Purkinje system and often progresses to complete heart block. Complete heart block or third-degree AV block (see Figs. 64-10 and 64-11 in Chapter 64) is diagnosed by the dissociation of P waves from QRS complexes, with an atrial rate faster than the ventricular rate.

Ambulatory Monitoring

For intermittent symptoms such as palpitations, dizziness, or syncope, it is often difficult to obtain a 12-lead ECG while the symptoms are occurring. Therefore, ambulatory monitoring, which allows ECG monitoring over long periods, is a vital diagnostic tool. There are currently three types of ambulatory monitors: Holter monitors, which continuously record the ECG for 24 to 48 hours; event recorders, which are wearable loop recorders that record only during specific events (when the patient activates the recorder because of symptoms or the recorder detects a heart rate above or below a specified threshold) and can be worn for 1 month or more; and implantable loop recorders, which function similarly to event recorders but can be used for up to 14 months. More recently, home telemetry units have been developed, allowing patients to undergo prolonged continuous remote monitoring by wireless or Internet connections. The choice of ambulatory monitoring method is largely determined by the frequency of the symptoms and the likelihood of capturing an episode during a given monitoring period.

Ambulatory monitoring is diagnostic only if abnormalities occur during symptoms or if the patient has typical symptoms without any concurrent abnormalities. A "normal" monitoring record is nondiagnostic if the patient does not have symptoms during the period.

Holter Monitors

Holter monitors use either a tape (in older devices) or digital media (in newer devices) to record a 3-, 5-, or 12-lead surface ECG continuously for 24 to 48 hours. Processing, printing, and analysis of the recordings are performed offline with commercial systems. In addition to recording the rhythm, analyses of heart rate variability and ST segment changes and accurate counts of PACs and PVCs can be automated. Some systems allow extrapolation to produce a "virtual" 12-lead recording at any time during the monitoring period. Holter monitoring is useful for detecting symptoms that are frequent (multiple times daily) and for diagnosing sinus node dysfunction (sinus node arrest, sick sinus syndrome) or intermittent AV block. It can also be useful to assess the adequacy of control of the ventricular rate in a patient with atrial fibrillation.

Event Monitors

Event monitors, also known as loop recorders, are designed to record intermittent episodes during long periods (weeks to months) and are thus useful for patients with less frequent symptoms. The system records the ECG into a loop buffer that is continuously updated and overwritten. The duration of memory varies from a few seconds to a few minutes and is usually programmable. When activated, the information is "locked" into memory and continues to record forward for a preprogrammed amount of time. Newer systems allow both patient-activated (when symptoms occur) and event-triggered (when the heart rate is above or below a preset threshold) recording. Some recorders have algorithms to detect and record atrial fibrillation automatically, regardless of the heart rate. After episodes have been recorded, the patient transmits the recording over the telephone to centralized receivers. Some event monitors require leads similar to Holter monitors, whereas others are worn on the wrist or are put into small credit card–sized devices that are placed on the chest during symptoms. The latter type is useful only in patients whose symptoms last for several minutes and who do not have syncope.

IMPLANTABLE LOOP RECORDERS. Implantable loop recorders are small devices with integrated leads that are implanted in a small subcutaneous pocket during a simple surgery, usually performed in the electrophysiology

FIGURE 62-3. ECG algorithm for diagnosis of wide-complex tachycardias. A = atrial; AP = accessory pathway; AT = atrial tachycardia; AV = atrioventricular; AVRT = atrioventricular reciprocating tachycardia; BBB = bundle branch block; LBBB = left bundle branch block; RBBB = right bundle branch block; SR = sinus rhythm; SVT = supraventricular tachycardia; V = ventricular; VT = ventricular tachycardia. (From Blomstrom-Lundqvist C, Scheinman MM, Aliot EM, et al. ACC/AHA/ESC guidelines for the management of patients with supraventricular arrhythmias—executive summary. *Circulation.* 2003;108:1871-1909.)

laboratory. They function similarly to event recorders in terms of recording ECGs. Patients can activate the device with a small transmitter, or the device can be autotriggered on the basis of preprogrammed heart rates. The device can be interrogated by a computer, similar to the way pacemakers are interrogated to program the device's parameters and to retrieve ECGs that have been recorded. In patients with recurrent, difficult-to-diagnose syncope, an implantable loop recorder is better than the combination of tilt testing, an external loop recorder, and electrophysiologic testing.

Tilt Table Testing

Tilt table testing is used to confirm the diagnosis of neurocardiogenic syncope. The test involves continuous heart rate and blood pressure monitoring during head-up tilting. After baseline measurements in the supine position, the patient is tilted head-up at 60 to 80 degrees for 60 minutes. Some laboratories use isoproterenol or nitroglycerin as additional provocation. A positive result is a sudden and precipitous fall in blood pressure and heart rate, with concurrent reproducibility of symptoms (syncope). Because there is an appreciable false-positive rate, the test is best used as a confirmatory test in patients with a history suggestive of neurocardiogenic syncope or in patients with syncope in whom structural heart disease and other causes of syncope have been excluded.

Electrophysiologic Studies

Electrophysiologic studies involve the placement of several transvenous catheters in the heart to make temporary measurements of intracardiac electrograms and to perform pacing. Electrophysiologic studies are useful to identify the precise mechanism of tachyarrhythmias and are a necessary prelude to curative ablation (Chapter 66). Most arrhythmias, especially those with re-entrant mechanisms, can be readily induced during electrophysiologic studies. In addition, the existence and characteristics of accessory AV pathways (i.e., those responsible for Wolff-Parkinson-White syndrome or other re-entrant tachyarrhythmias) can be readily assessed by an electrophysiologic study. In patients with previous myocardial infarction, electrophysiologic studies are useful in determining the existence of a substrate for ventricular arrhythmias (Chapter 65), which may be treated with ablation or implantable defibrillators (Chapter 66). Electrophysiologic studies are also useful to determine the integrity of the conduction system and the precise mechanism of bradyarrhythmias that may be causing syncope. Therefore, electrophysiologic studies are indicated in patients with documented or suspected tachyarrhythmias as a prelude to curative ablation; in patients with a previous myocardial infarction and syncope, presyncope, or palpitations to exclude ventricular tachycardia; and in patients with severe or prolonged symptoms and no apparent diagnosis by history or ambulatory monitoring, especially in the setting of an abnormal ECG.

Other Tests

Echocardiography

Echocardiography (Chapter 55) can be useful to ensure that a patient does not have underlying structural heart disease, which can be an important prognostic factor in patients with ventricular tachycardia or syncope. Echocardiography should be performed in patients who present with syncope that is not obviously neurocardiogenic to ensure that there is no valvular or myocardial cause.

Exercise Testing

Exercise testing (Chapter 50) can be useful to assess arrhythmias, particularly in patients whose symptoms are exercise related. Exercise testing can also be useful in the evaluation of patients with bradyarrhythmias to diagnose chronotropic incompetence, and it can differentiate AV block due to autonomic tone (improves with exercise) from intrinsic conduction disease (generally worsens with an increasing rate).

Neurologic Testing

Routine electroencephalography (Chapter 403) is not helpful because a single study may be normal, even in epileptic patients. Structural brain diseases rarely cause episodic loss of consciousness, and routine brain imaging studies are indicated only in patients with focal neurologic findings. Carotid Doppler (Chapter 414) studies can document stenosis, but unconsciousness requires bihemispheric dysfunction. Transcranial Doppler or magnetic resonance angiography of the basilar artery is indicated only in patients with symptoms suggestive of brain stem ischemia.

TREATMENT   Rx

Treatment of syncope depends on the underlying cause. Proximate to the syncopal episode, hospital admission (e.g., observation in a chest pain unit or its equivalent) is recommended when the cause of syncope is unclear, especially in elderly patients, otherwise fragile or worrisome patients, or those suspected of having a cardiac or cerebrovascular cause, or if the syncope resulted in significant injury. Patients at highest risk have a systolic blood pressure below 90 mm Hg, a history of myocardial infarction or heart failure, a complaint of shortness of breath, an abnormal initial ECG, or a hematocrit less than 30%.

Until the cause of the syncope is determined and treated, patients should be instructed to avoid situations that may cause injury as a result of the syncope, especially if there is no prodrome and episodes are frequent. Careful consideration should be given to driving restrictions, which may be mandatory depending on local laws, and restrictions on dangerous work-related activity (e.g., for pilots, heavy machine operators, bus drivers) until definitive therapy is given.

In patients with a cardiac cause of syncope, targeted treatments include valve replacement for aortic stenosis (Chapter 75); medications for hypertrophic cardiomyopathy (Chapter 60); cardioversion, a pacemaker, an implantable cardioverter-defibrillator, ablation, or medications for tachyarrhythmias (Table 62-3; Chapters 63 through 65); and fluid repletion for orthostatic hypotension.

In patients with neurocardiogenic syncope, behavioral guidance should encourage an increased intake of fluid and salt, as well as the avoidance of situations that precipitate symptoms. Patients should also be taught how to tense their arms and legs and grip their hands during prodromal symptoms to increase peripheral resistance and systemic blood pressure. If neurocardiogenic syncope recurs despite education and lifestyle changes, fludrocortisone (0.1 mg/day, starting dose) can expand intravascular volume but has not been proved to prevent syncope. Midodrine (usually 10 mg three times daily), an α₁-receptor agonist and vasoconstrictor, has shown potential benefit, but other α-agonists have not. Paroxetine (20 mg/day), a selective serotonin re-uptake inhibitor, reduced recurrent neurocardiogenic syncope in one trial of very symptomatic patients but otherwise has been disappointing. In randomized trials, β-blockers have not been useful. Pacemakers do not reduce recurrent neurocardiogenic syncope, but they are very effective in patients with cardioinhibitory syncope as a result of severe bradycardia.

PROGNOSIS

One syncopal event predicts a substantial risk for recurrent syncope. Although syncope itself does not appear to increase the risk of death, patients with cardiac or cerebrovascular causes have higher mortality rates than patients with definable noncardiac causes or those without a definable cause. Among patients who come to an emergency department, the overall death rate of about 7.5% at 1 year reflects patients' underlying abnormalities.

1. Krahn AD, Klein GJ, Yee R, et al. Randomized assessment of syncope trial: conventional diagnostic testing versus a prolonged monitoring strategy. *Circulation.* 2001;104:46-54.
2. van Dijk N, Quartieri F, Blanc JJ, et al. Effectiveness of physical counterpressure maneuvers in preventing vasovagal syncope: the Physical Counterpressure Manoeuvres Trial (PC-Trial). *J Am Coll Cardiol.* 2006;48:1652-1657.
3. Moya A, Sutton R, Ammirati F, et al. Guidelines for the diagnosis and management of syncope (version 2009): the Task Force for the Diagnosis and Management of Syncope of the European Society of Cardiology (ESC). *Eur Heart J.* 2009;30:2631-2671.
4. Connelly SJ, Sheldon R, Thorpe KE, et al. Pacemaker therapy for prevention of syncope in patients with recurrent severe vasovagal syncope: Second Vasovagal Pacemaker Study (VPS II): a randomized trial. *JAMA.* 2003;289:2224-2229.

SUGGESTED READINGS

Duncan GW, Tan MP, Newton JL, et al. Vasovagal syncope in the older person: differences in presentation between older and younger patients. *Age Ageing.* 2010;39:465-470. *Older patients were more likely to fall and less likely to report palpitations or to lose consciousness totally.*

Thavendiranathan P, Bagai A, Khoo C, et al. Does this patient with palpitations have a cardiac arrhythmia? *JAMA.* 2009;302:2135-2143. *Review.*

Zimetbaum P, Goldman A. Ambulatory arrhythmia monitoring: choosing the right device. *Circulation.* 2010;122:1629-1636. *Review emphasizing the role of loop recorders and post-event recorders.*

63

APPROACH TO CARDIAC ARREST AND LIFE-THREATENING ARRHYTHMIAS

ROBERT J. MYERBURG AND AGUSTIN CASTELLANOS

Cardiac arrest is characterized by an abrupt loss of consciousness because of absence of blood flow owing to loss of cardiac pumping action. If not treated promptly, it will lead to central nervous system injury or death within minutes. Cardiac arrest is often forewarned by a change in cardiovascular status, as indicated by the appearance or worsening of symptoms related to transient arrhythmias, such as palpitations, lightheadedness, or near-syncope or syncope (Chapter 62). Other forewarnings may include new or worsening chest pain, dyspnea, or weakness. These warning symptoms, however, are limited by their sensitivity and predictive power in individual patients. Moreover, cardiac arrest may occur unexpectedly as a first cardiac event in an apparently healthy individual, in a patient with known previous cardiac disease, or as the final event in any fatal disease.

The most common electrical mechanisms of cardiac arrest are the ventricular tachyarrhythmias (Chapter 65)—ventricular fibrillation (VF) or pulseless ventricular tachycardia (VT). In a substantial minority of cardiac arrests, severe bradyarrhythmia, asystole, or pulseless electrical activity is the first rhythm abnormality noted. The latter may be the primary mechanism of the cardiac arrest or a result of deterioration of VT/VF. Pulseless electrical activity or asystole may also be seen after termination of VT/VF by electrical cardioversion. Pulseless electrical activity is defined as secondary when it occurs in the setting of predisposing factors, such as hypoxia or other metabolic disorders, and primary when it is the initial rhythm noted in patients with predisposing cardiac disorders. The probability of survival after intervention is far better for ventricular tachyarrhythmias than for bradyarrhythmic or asystolic mechanisms. The interval between cardiac arrest and the initiation of resuscitation and cardioversion is the major determinant of survival.

● PREDISPOSING WIDE–QRS COMPLEX TACHYCARDIAS

Sustained tachycardias with wide QRS complexes should be considered of ventricular origin and potentially high risk until determined otherwise. Most wide-QRS tachycardias are initially approached as a medical urgency or emergency, whereas most narrow-QRS tachycardias of supraventricular origin are approached with less urgency (Chapters 64 and 65).

Management of Sustained Ventricular Tachycardia

Sustained VT occurs most commonly in the presence of structural heart disease and must be interpreted as a forewarning of fatal arrhythmia in that setting. It is characterized by QRS complexes that are usually longer than 0.12

Monomorphic Nonsustained Ventricular Tachycardia

A

Polymorphic Nonsustained Ventricular Tachycardia

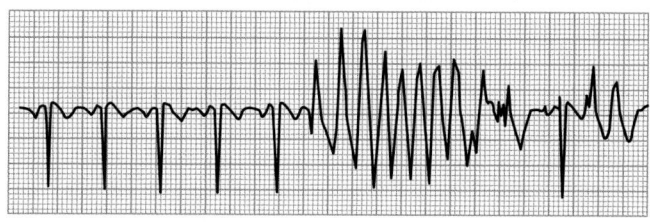

B

FIGURE 63-1. Nonsustained ventricular tachycardia. Monomorphic patterns (**A**) are characterized by a slower and more stable electrical pattern than polymorphic patterns (**B**). Both have long-term prognostic implications in patients with advanced structural heart disease, but monomorphic patterns tend to be more stable over the short term.

second, with a mean vector that is markedly different from the QRS vector of normally conducted impulses. The rate of most VTs is between 140 and 200 impulses per minute, but rates may be slower or faster. VT may be electrically stable (such as monomorphic VT patterns at relatively slow rates; Fig. 63-1A) or unstable (such as polymorphic VTs or monomorphic VTs at rates exceeding 190 to 200 per minute; see Fig. 63-1B) (Chapter 65). Slower monomorphic VT may be better tolerated, whereas rapid VT is often associated with hemodynamic instability. In the latter circumstance, VT must be managed as a life-threatening or imminently fatal event, analogous to a VT/VF cardiac arrest (see later) that is usually treated with electrical cardioversion as initial therapy. Long-term management strategies, often involving consideration of implantable cardioverter-defibrillator therapy, are based on consideration of the likelihood of recurrent tachycardias and the extent of underlying disease (Chapter 65). Some well-tolerated, slow monomorphic VTs, especially in the absence of structural heart disease, may be more benign and treated with less urgency, usually with antiarrhythmic drugs or β-adrenergic blocking agents (see Table 64-5 in Chapter 64).

Distinguishing Supraventricular from Ventricular Tachycardias

It is important to distinguish between supraventricular tachycardia (SVT) (Chapter 64) and VT for both risk prediction and therapy. Although it is generally assumed that narrow-QRS tachycardias are supraventricular in origin, VT occasionally has a narrow QRS complex on a one- or two-lead rhythm strip, thereby mimicking SVT. Whenever possible, the diagnosis of tachycardia should be based on a 12-lead electrocardiogram (ECG). However, a standard ECG will not always suffice because patients with intraventricular conduction abnormalities (such as a left or right bundle branch block) will have wide-complex tachycardias during SVTs, usually with a QRS vector similar to that seen in normal sinus rhythm. In addition, when an SVT is very rapid, a functional bundle branch block may generate a widened QRS duration and shift the axis transiently. In both these examples, the wide QRS may mimic VT, and it may be necessary to perform an electrophysiologic study to determine the diagnosis (Chapter 62).

When wide-complex SVT is suspected clinically, transient vagal stimulation by carotid sinus massage or an atrioventricular nodal blocking agent, such as intravenous adenosine (see Table 64-5 in Chapter 64), may be useful for slowing the rate or terminating an SVT. Intravenous calcium-blocking agents generally should not be used for the diagnosis or treatment of wide-QRS tachycardias, especially in the presence of structural heart disease, because of their myocardial depressant effects. The exception is when it is known with certainty that the tachycardia is an SVT in a patient with normal or near-normal left ventricular function.

SVTs can result in a risk for generating life-threatening ventricular arrhythmias in two circumstances. One is in patients with high-grade coronary artery stenoses, in whom rapid heart rates can cause myocardial ischemia because

of the dependence of coronary blood flow on the diastolic interval; the arrhythmia should be treated urgently, usually by electrical direct current (DC) cardioversion (Chapter 66), unless specific medical therapy is available and controls the rate promptly (Chapter 64). The second is in patients with Wolff-Parkinson-White syndrome, who may have ventricular rates greater than 300 beats per minute during atrial fibrillation when the accessory pathway has a short refractory period (see Fig. 64-19 in Chapter 64). This arrhythmia, which can cause hypotensive VT or VF, requires prompt therapy (Chapter 64).

● GENERAL MANAGEMENT OF CARDIAC ARREST

Basic life-support (BLS) and advanced cardiac life support (ACLS) strategies for initial and definitive responses to cardiac arrest have improved survival in victims of cardiac arrest. The principles of BLS and ACLS apply to both in-hospital and out-of-hospital cardiac arrest, but their applications and outcomes depend on the setting. In the hospital, the probability of survival is determined by the specific patient category (acute syndromes better than end-stage diseases), the mechanism of cardiac arrest (better for tachyarrhythmias than for bradyarrhythmias, asystole, or pulseless electrical activity), and the hospital site (better in intensive care units or other monitored settings than on an unmonitored general care unit). In many acute care settings, including patients with acute coronary syndromes (Chapters 72 and 73), outcomes can be excellent. For other in-hospital settings and most out-of-hospital settings, the absolute number and proportion of survivors remain low, except in unique out-of-hospital settings that can provide an extraordinarily rapid response time to victims in VF or VT. When immediate defibrillation in highly protected environments is available, such as monitored intensive care units and electrophysiology laboratories, where response times of less than 60 seconds are the norm, the survival rate after VF is greater than 90% in the absence of pathophysiologic conditions that favor persistence of the potentially fatal arrhythmia.

Once 2 to 3 minutes have elapsed from the onset of cardiac arrest to attempted defibrillation, the survival probability falls below 50% in most in-hospital and out-of-hospital circumstances. Survival rates continue to fall rapidly thereafter, decreasing to 25% or less by 4 to 6 minutes and less than 10% by 10 minutes. Although immediate defibrillation is the preferred method within the first few minutes after the onset of cardiac arrest, a brief period of cardiopulmonary resuscitation (CPR) to provide oxygenation of the victim improves survivability when the time to defibrillation exceeds 4 to 5 minutes.

Basic Life Support

The activities included within BLS encompass the initial responses for diagnostic evaluation, followed by a seamless flow into establishing ventilation and perfusion through the techniques of CPR or the newly proposed concept of cardiocerebral resuscitation (see later). The first action is to confirm that the collapse is the result of a cardiac arrest. After an initial evaluation for response to voice or tactile stimulation, observation for respiratory movements and skin color, and simultaneous palpation of major arteries for the presence of a pulse, the determination that a life-threatening incident is in progress should immediately prompt a call to an emergency medical rescue system (911).

The absence of respiratory efforts, or the presence of only gasping agonal respirations in conjunction with an absent pulse, is diagnostic of cardiac arrest. Although the absence of a carotid or femoral pulse is a primary diagnostic criterion for the health care professional, palpation for a pulse is no longer recommended for lay responders. The absence of respiratory efforts or severe stridor with *persistence of a pulse* suggests a primary respiratory arrest that may lead to cardiac arrest in a short time; skin color may be pale or intensely cyanotic. In the latter circumstance, initial efforts should include oropharyngeal exploration in search of a foreign body and the Heimlich maneuver, which entails wrapping the arms around the victim from the back and delivering a sharp thrust to the upper part of the abdomen with a closed fist, particularly in a setting in which aspiration is likely (e.g., collapse in a restaurant).

Once a pulseless cardiac arrest is established, a blow to the chest (precordial thump) may be attempted by a properly trained rescuer as part of an initial response when monitoring and a defibrillator are not immediately available. A precordial thump should not be used in an unmonitored patient with a perceptible rapid tachycardia or without complete loss of consciousness because of concern about converting organized electrical activity into VF. The technique involves one or two blows delivered firmly to the junction of the middle and lower thirds of the sternum from a height of 8 to 10 inches, but the effort should be abandoned if a spontaneous pulse does not immediately occur or if the patient begins to breathe.

The precordial thump should be followed immediately by the initiation of CPR so as to maintain viability of the central nervous system, heart, and other vital organs until a definitive intervention can be carried out. CPR can be performed by professional and paraprofessional personnel, by experienced emergency medical technicians, and by trained laypersons. Time is the key element for success, and there should be minimal delay between the diagnosis and preparatory efforts in the initial response and institution of CPR. If only one witness is present, the only activity that should precede BLS is telephone contact (911) of emergency personnel.

Clearing the airway, which is a critical step in preparing for successful resuscitation, includes tilting the head backward and lifting the chin, in addition to exploring the airway for foreign bodies—including dentures—and removing them. The Heimlich maneuver should be performed if there is reason to suspect a foreign body lodged in the oropharynx, as suggested by severe respiratory stridor rather than by slow agonal respirations or apnea. When the person at the scene has insufficient physical strength to perform the maneuver, mechanical dislodgement of a foreign body can sometimes be achieved by abdominal thrusts with the unconscious patient in a supine position. If there is suspicion that respiratory arrest precipitated the cardiac arrest, particularly in the presence of a mechanical airway obstruction, a second precordial thump should be delivered after the airway has been cleared.

With the head properly placed and the oropharynx clear, mouth-to-mouth respiration can be initiated, but bystander compression-only CPR is as good as, if not better than, compression plus mouth-to-mouth respiration.[1] A variety of devices are available for establishing ventilation, including plastic oropharyngeal airways, esophageal obturators for establishing ventilation, a masked Ambu bag, and endotracheal tubes. Intubation is the preferred procedure, but time should not be sacrificed, even in the in-hospital setting, while awaiting an endotracheal tube or a person trained to insert it quickly and properly. Temporary support with Ambu bag ventilation is the usual method in the hospital until endotracheal intubation can be accomplished; in the out-of-hospital setting, mouth-to-mouth resuscitation is performed while awaiting emergency rescue personnel. The lungs should be inflated twice in succession after every 30 chest compressions.

The third element of BLS, circulation, is intended to maintain blood flow until definitive steps can be taken. The rationale is based on the hypothesis that chest compression maintains an externally driven pump function by sequential emptying and filling of its chambers, with competent valves favoring the forward direction of flow. The palm of one hand is placed over the lower part of the sternum while the heel of the other rests on the dorsum of the lower hand. The sternum is then depressed with the resuscitator's arms straight at the elbows to provide a less tiring and more forceful fulcrum at the junction of the shoulders and back. With this technique, sufficient force is applied to depress the sternum about 4 to 5 cm, with abrupt relaxation. The cycle is carried out at a rate of about 100 compressions per minute. In the 2005 modification of guidelines for emergency cardiac care, the integration of respiratory and compression actions was changed to a compression-ventilation ratio of 30:2 for single responders to victims from infancy (excluding newborns) through adulthood, and two responders for adults.

For two-rescuer CPR for infants and children, the former compression-ventilation ratio of 15:2 was retained. Another recently suggested modification, which is intended to encourage more bystander CPR by untrained or remotely trained bystanders who lack confidence, is the "hands-only" (cardiac-only, compression-only) technique, which uses 200 successive compressions without interruption. This variation, which may be more effective than compression-ventilation sequences, also allays concerns about bystander mouth-to-mouth ventilation of unknown victims in the absence of mechanical airway devices.

Automated External Defibrillators—Intermediate Life Support

Because time to defibrillation is the major determinant of survival, despite any temporizing benefit of BLS, and because ACLS strategies are generally implemented by in-hospital personnel or out-of-hospital emergency medical rescue system responders, an intermediate strategy has emerged that is based on the availability of automated external defibrillators (AEDs) for use by nonconventional first responders. Referred to as public access defibrillation or lay first-responder systems, the strategy relies on devices that prompt the user to deliver a defibrillation shock when deemed appropriate by a computerized rhythm detection system in the device. The operators can be trained police officers, security guards, airline personnel, or trained (or even untrained) lay responders (Table 63-1). A number of studies have suggested improved survival rates when such strategies are deployed in public sites, but an initial study of a home deployment strategy was disappointing.[2] Further study is warranted because most out-of-hospital cardiac arrests occur at home. AED programs are not a replacement for ACLS (see later), but rather an intermediate supplement to the BLS-ACLS sequence that is intended to attempt earlier defibrillation while awaiting the arrival of ACLS-trained emergency rescue personnel.

Advanced Cardiac Life Support

ACLS methods, other than those directly related to control of tachyarrhythmias, have led to the generation of comprehensive protocols to guide responders over a broad expanse of clinical circumstances and mechanisms of cardiac arrest ranging from transient clinical events to end-stage multisystem disease. The general goals of ACLS are to restore a hemodynamically effective cardiac rhythm, optimize ventilation, and maintain and support the restored circulation. During ACLS, the patient's cardiac rhythm is promptly cardioverted or defibrillated as the first priority, if appropriate equipment is immediately available. If cardiac arrest has lasted for 4 to 5 minutes before the availability of a defibrillator, a short period of closed-chest cardiac compression immediately before defibrillation increases the probability of survival.[3] Additional survival benefit has not been observed for delays greater than 10 minutes.

After the initial attempt to restore a hemodynamically effective rhythm, the patient is intubated and oxygenated, if needed, and the heart is paced if a bradyarrhythmia or asystole occurs. An intravenous line is established to deliver medications. After intubation, the goal of ventilation is to reverse hypoxemia and not merely to achieve a high alveolar Po_2. When available, oxygen rather than room air should be used to ventilate the patient, and arterial O_2 saturation should be monitored, when possible. In the out-of-hospital setting, a face mask or an Ambu bag by means of an endotracheal tube is generally used.

TABLE 63-1	AUTOMATED EXTERNAL DEFIBRILLATOR STRATEGIES FOR RAPID RESPONSE TO CARDIAC ARRESTS CAUSED BY VENTRICULAR FIBRILLATION			
DEPLOYMENT	**EXAMPLES**	**RESCUERS**	**ADVANTAGES**	**LIMITATIONS**
Emergency vehicles	Police cars Fire engines Ambulances	Trained emergency personnel	Experienced users Broad deployment Objectivity	Deployment time Arrival delays Community variations
Public access sites	Public buildings Stadiums, malls Airports Airliners	Security personnel Designated rescuers Random laypersons	Population density Shorter delays Lay and emergency personnel access	Low event rates Inexperienced users Panic and confusion
Multifamily dwellings	Apartments Condominiums Hotels	Security personnel Designated rescuers Family members	Familiar locations Defined personnel Shorter delays	Infrequent use Low event rates Geographic factors
Single-family dwellings	Private homes Apartments Neighborhood "Heart Watch"	Family members	Immediate access Familiar setting	Acceptance Victim may be alone One-time user; panic

FIGURE 63-2. General algorithm for advanced cardiac life support (ACLS) response to ventricular fibrillation (VF) or pulseless ventricular tachycardia (VT). For more detail, see the ACLS guidelines in Suggested Readings. *Note:* In a 2008 advisory, 200 compression-only sequences were suggested as an alternative to standard CPR cycles between shocks, and this approach is under consideration for future guidelines. CPR = cardiopulmonary resuscitation; ECG = electrocardiogram.

intervals with defibrillator shocks in between, but high-dose epinephrine does not appear to provide added benefit. Vasopressin, 40 U given IV once, is an equally good alternative to epinephrine,[4] but the combination does not appear to be better than either one alone.[5]

This algorithm is based on the 2005 update. In a 2008 advisory, use of 200 compression-only sequences was suggested as an alternative to standard CPR cycles between shocks.

Pharmacotherapy for Resistant Arrhythmias

For a patient who continues in VF or pulseless VT despite multiple attempts at DC cardioversion after epinephrine, or who has recurrent episodes of VF or VT after cardioversion, electrical stability may be achieved by administering intravenous antiarrhythmic agents while continuing resuscitative efforts (see Fig. 63-2). Amiodarone (150 mg IV over a 10-minute period, followed by 1 mg/minute for up to 6 hours and 0.5 mg/minute thereafter) is the initial treatment of choice.[6] Additional bolus dosing, to a maximum of 500 mg, can be tried if the initial bolus is unsuccessful. Amiodarone need not be given as a routine to individuals who respond to initial defibrillation with a persistently stable rhythm, but it is preferred for those who have recurrent episodes of VT or VF after initial defibrillation and oxygenation.

If there is sufficient clinical evidence that the cardiac arrest was heralded by the onset of an acute coronary syndrome, lidocaine (1.0- to 1.5-mg/kg bolus given IV, with the dose repeated in 2 minutes) may be used instead of amiodarone, or if amiodarone has failed. When acute or intermittent ischemia is not thought to be the mechanism, intravenous amiodarone is the preferred initial drug, but lidocaine may be tried if amiodarone fails. Intravenous procainamide (loading infusion of 100 mg/5 minutes to a total dose of 500 to 800 mg, followed by a continuous infusion at 2 to 5 mg/minute) is now rarely used but may be tried in those with persisting, hemodynamically unstable arrhythmias.

In patients with acute hyperkalemia as the triggering event for resistant VF, hypocalcemia, or arrest potentially caused by excess doses of calcium-blocking drugs, 10% calcium gluconate (5 to 20 mL infused at a rate of 2 to 4 mL/minute) may be helpful. Otherwise, calcium should not be used routinely during resuscitation, even though ionized Ca^{2+} levels may be low during resuscitation from cardiac arrest.

Some resistant forms of polymorphic VT (*torsades de pointes*), rapid monomorphic VT, ventricular flutter (rate > 260/minute), or resistant VF respond to $MgSO_4$ (1 to 2 g IV given over a 1- to 2-minute period) or to β-blocker therapy (propranolol, 1-mg boluses IV to a total dose of up to 15 to 20 mg; or metoprolol, 5 mg IV, up to 20 mg). $MgSO_4$ is specifically indicated for polymorphic VTs due to inherited or acquired (drug-induced) long QT patterns (Chapter 65). This VT pattern also occurs with marked hypokalemia, so 20 mEq/hour of intravenous potassium chloride should be included in the treatment of patients who have a serum K^+ of less than 3 mEq/L and whose polymorphic VT is resistant to other therapies. However, hypokalemia also may follow the acid-base and electrolyte shifts associated with prolonged arrests and should not be considered a primary cause of the cardiac arrest in that circumstance.

● MANAGEMENT OF TACHYARRHYTHMIC CARDIAC ARRESTS

Direct Current Cardioversion

When VF or a rapid VT is identified on a monitor or by telemetry, defibrillation should be performed immediately (Fig. 63-2). When a reversible cause, such as an acute ischemic syndrome or electrolyte disturbance, is the mechanism, normal rhythm can be successfully restored in up to 90% of VF victims weighing up to 90 kg with a DC monophasic shock of up to 360 J, or a with a biphasic shock of up to 200 J, delivered within 2 to 3 minutes. Failure of the initial shock to restore an effective rhythm is a poor prognostic sign. Although some algorithms suggest a succession of monophasic shock energies from 200 to 360 J, or biphasic waveforms from 100 to 200 Joules, during a sequence of attempts to defibrillate, there is little to be gained from beginning with energies less than 300 J monophasic or less than 150 J biphasic during a cardiac arrest response.

After a single shock at 300 or 360 J of monophasic energy, or 150 or 200 J biphasic, the patient should be checked for restoration of a spontaneous pulse; CPR should be continued for five cycles if a pulse remains absent. Subsequently, a second shock should be delivered, followed by epinephrine, 1 mg intravenously (IV). If a pulse is still absent, CPR is repeated for five cycles before the next shock. Epinephrine may be repeated at 3- to 5-minute

● MANAGEMENT OF CARDIAC ARREST CAUSED BY ASYSTOLE, BRADYARRHYTHMIAS, OR PULSELESS ELECTRICAL ACTIVITY

The approach to a patient with bradyarrhythmic or asystolic arrest or with pulseless electrical activity differs from the approach to patients with tachyarrhythmic events (VT/VF). Once this form of cardiac arrest is recognized, efforts should focus on first establishing control of the patient's cardiorespiratory status (i.e., continue CPR, intubate, and establish intravenous access), then reconfirming the rhythm (in two leads if possible), and finally taking actions that favor the emergence of a stable spontaneous rhythm or attempt to pace the heart. Possible reversible causes, particularly for bradyarrhythmia and asystole, should be considered and excluded (or treated) promptly (Fig. 63-3), including hypovolemia, hypoxia, cardiac tamponade, tension pneumothorax, preexisting acidosis, drug overdose, hypothermia, and hyperkalemia. Epinephrine (1.0 mg IV every 3 to 5 minutes) and atropine (1.0 to 2.0 mg IV) or isoproterenol (up to 15 to 20 µg/minute IV), which are commonly used in an attempt to elicit spontaneous electrical activity or increase the rate of a bradycardia, have only limited success. In the absence of an intravenous line, epinephrine (1 mg, i.e., 10 mL of a 1 : 10,000 solution) may be given by the intracardiac route, but there is danger of coronary or myocardial laceration. Sodium bicarbonate, 1 mEq/kg, may be tried for known or

FIGURE 63-3. General algorithm for advanced cardiac life support response to brady-cardic or asystolic cardiac arrest or pulseless electrical activity. For more detail, see Suggested Readings. CHF = congestive heart failure; CPR = cardiopulmonary resuscitation; MI = myocardial infarction.

1. Hüpfl M, Selig HF, Nagele P. Chest-compression-only versus standard cardiopulmonary resuscitation: a meta-analysis. *Lancet.* 2010;376:1552-1557.
2. Bardy GH, Lee KL, Mark DB, et al. Home use of automated external defibrillators for sudden cardiac arrest. *N Engl J Med.* 2008;358:1793-1804.
3. Wik L, Hansen TB, Fylling F, et al. Delaying defibrillation to give basic cardiopulmonary resuscitation to patients with out-of-hospital ventricular fibrillation: a randomized trial. *JAMA.* 2003;289:1389-1395.
4. Aung K, Htay T. Vasopressin for cardiac arrest: a systematic review and meta-analysis. *Arch Intern Med.* 2005;165:17-24.
5. Gueugniaud PY, David JS, Chanzy E, et al. Vasopressin and epinephrine vs. epinephrine alone in cardiopulmonary resuscitation. *N Engl J Med.* 2008;359:21-30.
6. Dorian P, Cass D, Schwartz B, et al. Amiodarone as compared with lidocaine for shock-resistant ventricular fibrillation. *N Engl J Med.* 2002;346:884-890.
7. Arrich J, Holzer M, Herkner H, et al. Hypothermia for neuroprotection in adults after cardiopulmonary resuscitation. *Cochrane Database Syst Rev.* 2009;4:CD004128.
8. Connolly SJ, Hallstrom AP, Cappato R, et al. Meta-analysis of the implantable cardioverter defibrillator secondary prevention trials. AVID, CASH and CIDS studies. Antiarrhythmics vs Implantable Defibrillator study. Cardiac Arrest Study Hamburg. Canadian Implantable Defibrillator study. *Eur Heart J.* 2000;21:2071-2078.

SUGGESTED READINGS

Brooks SC, Bigham BL, Morrison LJ. Mechanical versus manual chest compressions for cardiac arrest. *Cochrane Database Syst Rev.* 2011;1:CD007260. *Review finding no benefit from mechanical devices.*
Field JM, Hazinski MF, Sayre MR, et al. Executive summary: 2010 American Heart Association Guidelines for Cardiopulmonary Resuscitation and Emergency Cardiovascular Care. *Circulation.* 2010;122:S640-S656. *Review.*
Kong MH, Fonarow GC, Peterson ED, et al. Systematic review of the incidence of sudden cardiac death in the United States. *J Am Coll Cardiol.* 2011;57:794-801. *Review.*
Maron BJ, Estes NA 3rd. Commotio cordis. *N Engl J Med.* 2010;362:917-927. *Review.*
Nichol G, Aufderheide TP, Eigel B, et al. Regional systems of care for out-of-hospital cardiac arrest: a policy statement from the American Heart Association. *Circulation.* 2010;121:709-729. *Advocates national implementation of systems known to be effective.*
Stub D, Bernard S, Duffy SJ, et al. Post cardiac arrest syndrome: a review of therapeutic strategies. *Circulation.* 2011;123:1428-1435. *Review.*

strongly suspected preexisting hyperkalemia or bicarbonate-responsive acidosis.

External pacing systems (Chapter 66) should be used for out-of-hospital bradycardic or asystolic arrest, although its influence on outcome is not well documented. In the hospital setting, external pacing is generally used during the initial response to a bradycardic or asystolic arrest, but it should be superseded by transvenous pacing if the arrest is prolonged, if continuous pacing is needed, or if the external device fails to pace. Unfortunately, an *asystolic* patient continues to have a very poor prognosis despite available techniques.

ADJUNCTIVE THERAPEUTIC ACTIONS

During or after therapy targeted to restoration of an electrically stable cardiac rhythm, the patient's general metabolic state should be addressed by improving oxygenation and reversing acidosis. Intravenous sodium bicarbonate (1 mEq/kg), with up to 50% of this dose repeated every 10 to 15 minutes during the course of CPR, is recommended for patients with known or suspected preexisting bicarbonate-responsive causes of acidosis, for certain drug overdoses (Chapter 110), and after prolonged and unsuccessful attempts at resuscitation. Caution must be exercised, however, because excessive quantities of sodium bicarbonate can be deleterious by causing alkalosis, hypernatremia, and hyperosmolality. When possible, arterial pH, Po_2, and Pco_2 should be monitored during the resuscitation. In addition, moderate therapeutic hypothermia (32° to 34° C) is now recommended for post–cardiac arrest improvement of cerebral function and of survival[7] as part of the concept of "cardiocerebral resuscitation."

LONG-TERM MANAGEMENT

Survivors of a cardiac arrest that is not due to transient factors remain at high risk for recurrent cardiac arrest and sudden cardiac death. An implantable defibrillator improves outcomes in survivors of cardiac arrest.[8]

64

CARDIAC ARRHYTHMIAS WITH SUPRAVENTRICULAR ORIGIN

PETER ZIMETBAUM

Supraventricular arrhythmias are divided into bradyarrhythmias and tachyarrhythmias. Any rhythm that originates above where the His bundle bifurcates into the right and left bundle branches is considered to be supraventricular in origin.

ANATOMY AND NORMAL ELECTROPHYSIOLOGY

The normal cardiac impulse begins in the sinus node complex, which is located at the junction of the right atrium and the superior vena cava. It then travels through the right atrium and primarily activates the left atrium through the coronary sinus. The time it takes to activate the atria is represented by the P wave on the electrocardiogram (ECG). After depolarizing the atria, the impulse enters the atrioventricular (AV) node, which is located in the inferior septal region of the right atrium, where a delay occurs. This delay allows time for the atria to contract and fill the ventricles. In most individuals, the impulse travels through the AV node over a uniform functional pathway or route. Some people have two or more functional pathways called dual AV nodal pathways (fast and slow pathways). The delay in the AV node represents most of the isoelectric portion of the PR interval on the ECG (E-Fig. 64-1). The usual duration of atrial activation including delay in the AV node is up to 140 msec and can be measured directly as the atrial-His interval. The impulse then travels into the specialized infranodal conducting system, i.e., through the His bundle, then right and left bundle branches, and into the Purkinje network. The Purkinje network extends or fans out throughout the ventricular endocardium. Impulses conduct rapidly through the Purkinje network, thereby allowing nearly simultaneous activation of the ventricles. A small portion of the isoelectric segment of the PR interval represents infranodal conduction. This infranodal conduction through the His-Purkinje system can also be measured directly (His-ventricle interval) and should take between 40 and 60 msec. Once out of the Purkinje network, the impulse proceeds relatively slowly from the endocardial to epicardial surface of the ventricles. The QRS complex on ECG represents depolarization of the bundle branches and ventricular myocardium. Patients who have ventricular preexcitation activate the ventricles through an alternative route to the normal ventricular conduction system. These patients have bypass tracts or accessory pathways over which the ventricular myocardium can be activated directly rather than traveling over the AV node and His-Purkinje network. These pathways, which develop as a failure of the normal fibrous separation of the atria and ventricles, are located in proximity to the tricuspid and mitral valves. Direct activation of the ventricular myocardium without the usual delay in the AV node results in a slurred upstroke of the QRS complex called a delta (δ) wave (E-Fig. 64-2).

The normal heart rate is generated by tissues or pacemaker cells with intrinsic automaticity. The sinus node cells produce the greatest rate (60 to 100 beats/minute) of automaticity and suppress other potentially automatic (AV junctional, 40 to 55 beats/minute; His-Purkinje cells, 15 to 40 beats/minute) tissues with slower rates of depolarization. The sinus node and AV node are heavily influenced by the parasympathetic (vagal) and sympathetic (adrenergic) nervous system. At rest, the parasympathetic system controls sinus node automaticity. With exertion or emotional or physical stress, a withdrawal of parasympathetic tone and an increase in heart rate, which is then perpetuated by sympathetic tone, further increase heart rate. Sinus arrhythmia refers to the normal variation in heart rate with inspiration and expiration. With inspiration, a withdrawal of vagal tone increases heart rate; by comparison, expiration is associated with a drop in heart rate (Fig. 64-1). During sleep, a dominance of vagal tone slows heart rate.

⬤ BRADYARRHYTHMIAS

Bradyarrhythmias may be caused by sinus node, AV node, or His-Purkinje dysfunction (Table 64-1).

Sinus Bradycardia and Sinus Node Dysfunction

Sinus bradycardia (Fig. 64-2) is generally defined as a sinus rate of less than 60 beats per minute. It should be noted, however, that sinus rates as low as 45 to 50 beats per minute, particularly at rest, can be physiologically normal. Sinus node dysfunction encompasses a group of disorders including sinus bradycardia, sinoatrial (SA) exit block, sinus arrest (pause of >2 to 3 seconds) during sinus rhythm, chronotropic incompetence, and tachycardia-bradycardia (tachy-brady) syndrome. Sinus node dysfunction in combination with symptoms such as fatigue, dizziness, near or complete syncope

(Chapters 50 and 62), or worsening of heart failure (Chapter 58) is called sick sinus syndrome. The tachy-brady syndrome is often identified by a prolonged delay in sinus node recovery following the termination of atrial fibrillation (AF) (Fig. 64-3). SA exit block refers to the electrophysiologic phenomenon of sinus node firing with delay or block of the impulse as it travels from the sinus node to the surrounding atrial tissue (Fig. 64-4). SA exit block can be first degree, second degree (type 1 or 2), and third degree. First-degree SA block is difficult to diagnose from the surface ECG. Second-degree SA exit block type 1 is manifest by progressive PP shortening preceding the sinus pause. The PP interval following the pause must be greater than twice the PP interval that preceded the pause. Second-degree SA exit block type 2 is characterized by a pause equaling an exact multiple of the sinus rate (i.e., constant PP interval before and after the pause). High-degree SA exit block refers to the absence of multiple P waves with a pause still corresponding to an absolute multiple of the underlying PP intervals, and third-degree AV block results in a complete absence of sinus P waves.

Chronotropic incompetence refers to the inability to increase the sinus rate appropriately in response to exercise or other physiologic demand. In most patients, chronotropic incompetence is manifest by a maximal heart rate of less than 100 beats per minute.

TABLE 64-1 BRADYCARDIAS
SINUS NODE DYSFUNCTION
Sinus bradycardia < 45 beats/min
Sinoatrial exit block
First-degree
Second-degree
Third-degree
Sinus arrest
Bradycardia-tachycardia syndrome
ATRIOVENTRICULAR BLOCK
First-degree
Second-degree
Mobitz type I (Wenckebach phenomenon)
Mobitz type II
Higher degree (e.g., 2:1, 3:1)
Third-degree
Atrioventricular node
His-Purkinje system

FIGURE 64-1. Sinus arrhythmia. Note the variation in sinus rates, which fluctuate with normal variations in autonomic tone.

FIGURE 64-2. Sinus bradycardia. Progressive sinus bradycardia—in this case related to heightened vagal tone while sleeping.

FIGURE 64-3. Electrocardiographic evidence of tachy-brady syndrome. Atrial fibrillation with a tachycardic ventricular response followed by conversion to sinus bradycardia.

FIGURE 64-4. Sinoatrial block. Sinoatrial exit block, probably type 2, is characterized by a pause equaling an exact multiple of the sinus rate.

FIGURE 64-5. First-degree atrioventricular (AV) block. Note the prolonged (>200 msec) AV conduction.

FIGURE 64-6. Mobitz I block. Progressive PR prolongation from 320 to 615 msec, followed by a blocked P wave. The subsequent conducted PR interval is less than the PR interval before the dropped P wave.

FIGURE 64-7. Two-to-one conduction in the atrioventricular (AV) node and below the AV node. **A,** Two-to-one conduction, with the conducted beats demonstrating a prolonged PR interval (>300 msec) and a narrow QRS, indicating Mobitz I block in the AV node. **B,** Normal-duration conducted PR interval and a wide QRS duration favoring Mobitz II block into an infranodal site of block.

Atrioventricular Conduction Disturbances

AV conduction disturbances refer to abnormal conduction in the AV node or in the His-Purkinje system (HPS) below the AV node. Electrical transmission through the AV conduction system is primarily limited by the AV node, which conducts in a decremental fashion to prevent excessively rapid conduction to the ventricles. The normal AV node rarely conducts faster than 200 beats per minute and slows with aging. The AV node is heavily influenced by autonomic tone and may conduct more than 200 beats per minute in the presence of heightened sympathetic and withdrawal of parasympathetic tone. Conduction through the HPS system is faster and nondecremental.

The AV blocks are classified as first, second, high, and third degree. First-degree AV block is a misnomer because nothing is actually blocked—rather, there is delay, usually in the AV node, manifest by a prolonged PR interval (Fig. 64-5). Second-degree AV block is divided into Mobitz type I (Wenckebach) or Mobitz type II. Mobitz type I is defined by progressive PR prolongation with eventual block after a P wave (Fig. 64-6). The initial PR prolongation is longest, the subsequent RR intervals shorten, and the PR interval following the blocked P wave is shorter than the last conducted PR interval before the blocked P wave. Mobitz type I usually occurs in the AV node. Mobitz type II, which is characterized by the abrupt failure of conduction after a P wave without preceding PR prolongation, usually represents conduction disease below the AV node. In patients with 2 : 1 block (two P waves for every QRS), it can be difficult to determine whether the block is Mobitz I in the AV node or Mobitz II below the AV node. Clues to conduction disease in the AV node include a prolonged PR interval (i.e., more than 300 msec) and a narrow QRS duration. Clues to conduction disease below the node include a normal PR interval but with bundle branch block (Fig. 64-7).

High-degree or advanced AV block, which is a form of second-degree block with multiple or successive nonconducted P waves, or both (Fig. 64-8), frequently recurs or persists. Third-degree block (or complete heart block) refers to a rhythm in which the atrial and ventricular activity occur independently, and the atrial rate usually exceeds the ventricular rate. Third-degree heart block can be seen with sinus rhythm or any atrial tachyarrhythmia with a regular escape rhythm in the AV junction or below (Fig. 64-9). Sometimes there is no escape rhythm, and heart block results in asystole. Complete heart block, particularly when it is acute and accompanied by an escape rhythm, can be associated with marked QT prolongation, which signifies a risk of torsades de pointes (Chapter 65). For this reason, patients who undergo AV node ablation have their pacemakers set at 80 beats per minute for at least 6

weeks after the procedure to prevent QT prolongation and torsades de pointes. Eventually, the pacing rate can be reduced to more physiologic levels without the ongoing risk of ventricular arrhythmia. Complete heart block and other types of severe bradyarrhythmia may present with syncope if there is a prolonged pause before an escape rhythm develops. More often, these rhythms present with fatigue and dyspnea. The blood pressure is often elevated owing to peripheral vasoconstriction, and there may be renal insufficiency secondary to reduced cardiac output.

The term AV dissociation refers to any rhythm in which the atria and ventricles beat independently of one another. If the atrial rate is faster than the ventricular rate, it is called complete heart block or third-degree AV block. AV dissociation with an atrial rate slower than the subsidiary pacemaker is usually seen with junctional or ventricular tachycardias.

CLINICAL MANIFESTATIONS

Sinus bradycardia and various degrees of AV nodal blocks can occur asymptomatically during sleep in healthy individuals. Asymptomatic first- and second-degree AV block, particularly when partially or completely reversed by exercise, is usually benign. Persistent second-degree and third-degree AV nodal block is abnormal and is often associated with dizziness, fatigue, exertional dyspnea, worsening of heart failure, near-syncope, or syncope. Third-degree AV block with a good junctional escape mechanism that accelerates during exercise, as often noted in patients with congenital AV block, may remain asymptomatic. Patients with congenital heart block may not appreciate their potential for a more active lifestyle because of the lack of a reference point but often feel much better when an appropriate heart rate acceleration can be achieved after pacemaker therapy.

DIAGNOSIS

Bradycardias are typically diagnosed by the ECG. In symptomatic patients with symptoms suggestive of bradyarrhythmia, 24-hour Holter monitoring or prolonged loop monitoring usually can make the diagnosis, but some patients may require formal electrophysiologic testing (Chapter 62). Any bradycardias, including sinus node dysfunction (Table 64-2) and AV nodal block (Table 64-3), can be caused at least in part by vagal influences, such as vasovagal episodes, vomiting, abdominal surgery, and upper and lower gastrointestinal invasive procedures. Syncope, sometimes caused by the bradycardia and sometimes by vasodepression with hypotension, may result (Chapters 50 and 62). Medications, infiltrative diseases, fibrocalcific degeneration, and a variety of other causes must be considered.

TREATMENT   Rx

The treatment of sinus node dysfunction and AV blocks consists of first removing any medications that may precipitate dysfunction (see Table 64-2). Although some patients will recover normal conduction, the susceptibility to medications usually indicates an underlying conduction abnormality that may worsen over time.

Asymptomatic sinus node dysfunction requires no therapy. Asymptomatic atrioventricular nodal block can also be managed without intervention unless the QT interval is markedly prolonged, in which case a pacemaker should be considered. For symptomatic sinus node dysfunction and second- and third-degree AV block, acute management includes intravenous atropine (1 mg) or isoproterenol (usually 1 to 2 μ/minute infusion) to increase the heart rate. Temporary cardiac pacing (Chapter 66) may be required. If sinus node dysfunction or AV block is due to transient abnormalities, such as drug-induced or acute ischemic syndromes, temporary pacing is usually sufficient; however, when infra-His or intra-His block is suspected (e.g., exercise-induced AV block or asymptomatic Mobitz type II block) and the site can be documented with His bundle recording, permanent pacing (see Tables 66-1 and 66-2 in Chapter 66) is the only effective chronic therapy, and consensus recommendations for pacemaker implantation should guide its use. For all forms of persistent symptomatic sinus node dysfunction or second- or third-degree AV block, permanent pacing is the therapy of choice (Chapter 66).

FIGURE 64-8. **High-degree atrioventricular block.** Periods of complete heart block with three nonconducted P waves (the first of which is buried in the first QRS complex) followed by two P waves, the second of which is conducted to the ventricle with a long PR interval. The subsequent three P waves are once again nonconducted, with the last P wave buried in the last QRS complex.

FIGURE 64-9. **Complete heart block** with the atrial beats *(black arrows)* dissociated from the ventricular beats *(red arrows)*. Note the ST elevation in leads III and aVF indicating acute inferior myocardial infarction as the cause of complete heart block.

TABLE 64-2	CAUSES OF SINUS NODE DYSFUNCTION

INTRINSIC

Hypothyroidism
Fibrocalcific degeneration
Increased vagal tone, especially in sleep apnea
Congenital mutations
Scleroderma
Amyloidosis
Chagas' disease

EXTRINSIC

Trauma, including cardiac surgery
Drugs
    Calcium-channel blockers
    β-Blockers
    Digoxin
    Antiarrhythmic medications (amiodarone, dronedarone, sotalol, flecainide, propafenone)
    Lithium

FIGURE 64-10. **Atrial premature beat.** Sinus rhythm with an atrial premature beat as the third complex in the rhythm strip. The P wave is buried in the preceding T wave.

FIGURE 64-11. **Junctional premature beat.** The premature beat is narrow but slightly different in morphology compared with the surrounding sinus beats. This premature beat is from the atrioventricular junction or slightly more distal in the fascicles. The inverted P wave following the QRS represents retrograde activation of the atria.

TABLE 64-3	CAUSES OF ATRIOVENTRICULAR BLOCK

All causes of sinus node dysfunction and
    Lyme disease
    Bacterial endocarditis with abscess formation
    Cardiac sarcoidosis with granuloma
    Inferior myocardial infarction
    Anterior myocardial infarction (less common and often associated with cardiogenic shock)
    Congenital mutations (possibly associated with maternal lupus erythematosus and transmission of anti-Ro and La antibodies)

Corrected transposition of the great vessels

Chagas' disease

Some neurologic conditions (especially myotonic dystrophy)

Drugs as in Table 64-2

FIGURE 64-12. **Ectopic atrial rhythm.** The inverted P waves in leads II, III, and aVF indicate a nonsinus P wave originating in the low right atrium.

Supraventricular Rhythms with a Normal Rate

Atrial premature beats (APBs) can arise from the right or left atrium or the pulmonary veins. The P wave, which differs from the P wave of sinus rhythm unless the APB originates near the sinus node, always precedes the QRS complex (Fig. 64-10). If the P wave is blocked, however, it is not followed by a QRS complex. A blocked premature atrial contraction may be confused with second-degree AV block, unless its prematurity is recognized, or with sinus node dysfunction, if it is inconspicuous. Altered appearance of the ST-T segment is often a clue to the presence of a P wave. A premature QRS complex with the morphology of the underlying sinus rhythm in the absence of a premature P wave represents an AV junctional beat (Fig. 64-11).

An ectopic atrial rhythm refers to a nonsinus atrial rhythm from a single focus with a single P wave morphology (Fig. 64-12). Wandering atrial pacemaker refers to an ectopic atrial rhythm with at least three distinct P wave morphologies at rates between 50 and 100 beats per minute (Fig. 64-13).

FIGURE 64-13. **Wandering atrial pacemaker.** Rhythm with three distinct P wave morphologies.

CLINICAL MANIFESTATIONS

APBs are most often asymptomatic but can occasionally be experienced as palpitations (Chapter 62). Similarly, ectopic atrial rhythms, including a wandering atrial pacemaker, are virtually always asymptomatic. Rarely, ectopic atrial rhythm can be very slow and associated with symptoms of fatigue.

DIAGNOSIS

The diagnosis of atrial premature beats, ectopic atrial rhythms, and wandering atrial pacemakers are all made by ECG or on an ambulatory Holter monitor or loop event recorder (Chapter 62).

TREATMENT   Rx

Premature atrial contractions do not generally require treatment unless they are associated with significant symptoms. Treatment consists primarily of β-blockers (e.g., atenolol, 25 to 100 mg daily) or calcium-channel blockers (e.g., long-acting diltiazem, 180 to 300 mg daily). Ectopic atrial rhythms and wandering atrial pacemakers are rarely symptomatic and are not treated with medications. Rarely, a slow ectopic rhythm associated with fatigue can be treated with atrial pacing at a rate faster than the ectopic atrial rhythm.

Supraventricular Tachyarrhythmias

The supraventricular tachycardias (SVTs) are defined as arrhythmias with three or more beats at a rate of greater than 100 beats per minute (Table 64-4). The beats, which can be regular or irregular, are usually narrow complex but can be wide complex when associated with bundle branch block

TABLE 64-4   SUPRAVENTRICULAR TACHYCARDIAS

	R-R REGULARITY	P WAVE MORPHOLOGY
ATRIAL TACHYCARDIAS		
Sinus tachycardia	Regular	Positive in II, III, aVF; negative in aVR
Sinus node re-entry	Regular	Positive in II, III, aVF; negative in aVR
Atrial tachycardia, unifocal	Regular	P different from sinus
Atrial tachycardia, multifocal	Irregular	Three or more different P wave morphologies
Atrial flutter, common, counterclockwise	Regular; irregular if variable AV block	Sawtooth flutter waves; regular waveform; negative in II, III, aVF, positive in V₁, negative in V₆
Clockwise		Positive in II, III, aVF; negative in V₁; positive in V₆
Atrial flutter, uncommon	Regular; irregular if variable AV block	Pattern different than common atrial flutter (counterclockwise or clockwise)
Atrial fibrillation	Irregularly irregular	Irregular fibrillation waves
AV JUNCTIONAL TACHYCARDIAS		
AV re-entry (using accessory pathways)		
Orthodromic	Regular	Retrograde P in ST-T wave
Antidromic	Regular preexcited	Retrograde P, short RP
Slow conducting	Regular	Retrograde P at end of T wave or later (long RP)
Atriofascicular (antidromic)	Regular preexcited	Retrograde P, short RP
AV nodal re-entry		
Common (slow-fast)	Regular	Retrograde P obscured by QRS or alters the end of QRS (short RP)
Uncommon (fast-slow)	Regular	Retrograde P at end of T wave or later (long RP)
Others (slow-slow)	Regular	PR-RP approximately equal
Nonparoxysmal junctional tachycardia*	Regular, slow rate	AV dissociation
Automatic junctional tachycardia*	Regular	AV dissociation

*Site of origin usually infranodal.
AV = atrioventricular.

(aberration) or conduction over an accessory pathway. Atrial dilation, acute myocardial infarction, pulmonary embolism, acute or chronic inflammatory states, or scars from prior surgery involving atrial myocardium or pericardium are among the causes of atrial tachyarrhythmias.

Sinus Tachycardia

Sinus tachycardia (Fig. 64-14) is an arrhythmia that is almost always a physiologic response to an emotional or physical stress such as anxiety, exercise, anemia, hypotension, hypoxemia, fever, thyrotoxicosis, or heart failure. It is characterized by a gradual increase and decrease in heart rate and rarely exceeds 180 beats per minute. In rare cases, it may be a nonphysiologic condition called inappropriate sinus tachycardia, which is characterized by sinus tachycardia that develops in response to minimal stress and that continues beyond the time when the normal response would have slowed. This disorder is difficult to manage but is sometimes responsive to β-blockade.

Sinus node re-entry is a rare form of SVT caused by re-entry in the sinus node. As opposed to physiologic ST, it begins abruptly, is often triggered by a premature atrial beat, and ends abruptly. The P wave morphology is identical to sinus rhythm, and β-blockers are the treatment of choice if required for symptoms.

Atrial Tachycardia

The term atrial tachycardia refers to a group of SVTs that originate from focal anatomic locations in the atria and propagate in a centrifugal pattern (Fig. 64-15). These locations include the pulmonary veins, crista terminalis in the right atrium, tricuspid or mitral annulus, coronary sinus, or regions of scar tissue from previous cardiac surgery. Atrial tachycardias, which are usually regular rhythms that rarely exceed 200 beats per minute, may present in young age but more often develop later in life. Atrial tachycardias can be re-entrant, triggered, or automatic in mechanism. Some forms of atrial tachycardia are incessant and can predispose to a tachycardia-related cardiomyopathy (Chapter 60). Other forms of atrial tachycardia are paroxysmal and may remit spontaneously without treatment. When persistent, atrial tachycardias can be managed with medications (calcium-channel or β-blockers or other antiarrhythmic drugs). Electrical mapping and ablation (Chapter 66) of atrial

FIGURE 64-14. Sinus tachycardia at 120 beats/min.

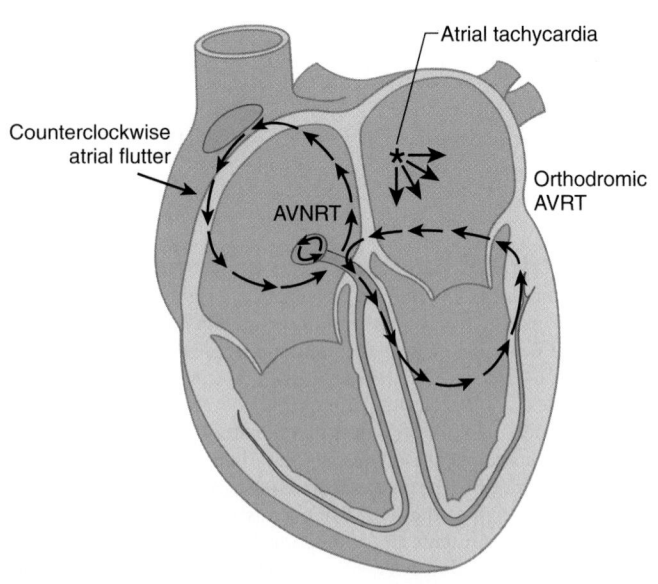

FIGURE 64-15. Diagram of the site and mechanism of common forms of supraventricular tachycardia. AVNRT = atrioventricular nodal re-entrant tachycardia; AVRT = atrioventricular re-entrant tachycardia.

tachycardia are highly effective and are increasingly offered as first-line therapy. Multifocal atrial tachycardia (Fig. 64-16), which is a unique form of atrial tachycardia characterized by three or more P wave morphologies, is distinguished from wandering atrial pacemaker when the rate is 100 beats per minute or more rather than less than 100 beats per minute. It is an irregular rhythm and occurs almost exclusively in patients with advanced pulmonary disease.

Atrioventricular Nodal Re-entrant Tachycardia

Atrioventricular nodal re-entrant tachycardia (AVNRT), which is a common form of SVT in all age groups, presents most often in young adulthood and frequently occurs after a change in position. It is more common in women than men and may develop or be exacerbated by pregnancy or certain phases of the menstrual cycle. Patients with AVNRT have two functional AV nodal pathways (dual pathways). Typically, an atrial premature beat blocks in one pathway (fast pathway) and conducts slowly over the other pathway (slow pathway). If this beat conducts back up the fast pathway and then re-enters the slow pathway, AV nodal re-entry occurs (Fig. 64-17). This re-entrant circuit is confined to the AV node, and the result is that both the atria and ventricles are activated nearly simultaneously. P waves may not be visible on the ECG because they are buried in the QRS complex. When P waves are present, they usually are seen just after the QRS and have a negative or superior axis (negative in leads II, III, and aVF; short RP tachycardia) (see Fig. 64-15). Atypical AVNRT is rare and occurs with conduction down the fast pathway and up the slow pathway, with a long interval between the preceding R wave and subsequent negative P wave (e.g., long RP tachycardia).

Junctional Tachycardia

Junctional tachycardia refers to a focal (non-re-entrant) tachycardia originating in the AV junction (Fig. 64-18). A number of different forms of junctional tachycardia have differing clinical patterns. Nonparoxysmal junctional

tachycardia is a benign arrhythmia that rarely exceeds 120 beats per minute and typically exhibits a "warm-up" and "cool-down" pattern. A more rapid paroxysmal form of junctional tachycardia occurs in young adults and is often associated with exercise. Congenital junctional ectopic tachycardia, which occurs in the pediatric population, is associated with very rapid rates and a risk of tachycardia-related cardiomyopathy.

Accessory Pathway Tachycardias

Tachycardias associated with an accessory pathway or bypass tract are called atrioventricular re-entrant tachycardia (AVRT). These tachycardias most often conduct down the normal AV conducting system and back up the accessory pathway (orthodromic AVRT) (see Fig. 64-15). Antidromic tachycardia is rare and represents conduction down the accessory pathway and back up the normal conducting system or less commonly, a second accessory pathway. Wolff-Parkinson-White syndrome is defined by the presence of delta waves or preexcitation on the ECG in sinus rhythm (Fig. 64-19), often with a

FIGURE 64-18. Junctional tachycardia. A tachycardia without evident P waves. The negative deflections at the end of leads II, III, and aVF represent retrograde P waves. This rhythm is impossible to distinguish from atrioventricular nodal re-entrant tachycardia on the surface electrocardiogram.

FIGURE 64-16. Multifocal atrial tachycardia. An atrial tachycardia with three different P wave morphologies.

FIGURE 64-17. Electrocardiograms demonstrating different rhythms in the same patient. **A,** Atrioventricular nodal re-entrant tachycardia, with *arrows* indicating retrograde P waves (negative in lead II, positive in V₁). **B,** Same patient in sinus rhythm. The absence of a negative deflection at the end of the QRS in lead II and positive deflection in V₁ confirms that those findings in panel **A** were retrograde P waves.

Atrial Fibrillation with Preexcitation

Sinus Rhythm with Preexcitation

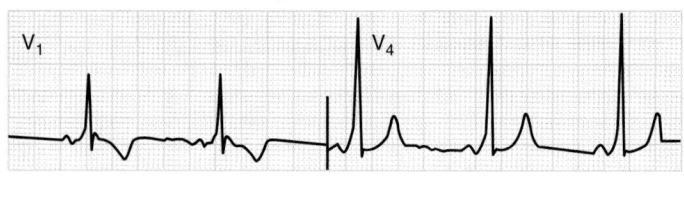

FIGURE 64-19. Two panels of the same patient with ventricular preexcitation. The rhythm on the left is fast, broad, and irregular, indicating atrial fibrillation with conduction over an accessory pathway. The rhythm on the right is sinus with conduction over an accessory pathway.

history of AVRT, but many patients with ventricular preexcitation never get AVRT. Up to 40% of patients with accessory pathways have AF. Because accessory pathway tissue, unlike the AV node, is usually nondecremental, a rapidly conducting accessory pathway may allow AF to conduct to the ventricles at excessive rates and precipitate ventricular fibrillation. Drugs like digoxin, which accelerate accessory pathway conduction, should be avoided in these patients.

The ECG during orthodromic AVRT can have a narrow complex, but a wide QRS complex will be seen if there is aberration from a bundle branch block, especially at more rapid rates. The retrograde P wave is negative in leads I and aVL if it conducts over a left lateral accessory pathway and negative in leads II, III, and aVF if it conducts over a septal or postural septal accessory pathway (Fig. 64-20). The P wave occurs later (after the preceding R wave) compared with AVNRT because in AVRT, the impulse must conduct beyond the AV node and into the ventricle before returning to the atria over an accessory pathway. In antidromic AVRT, the QRS complex is wide with a slurred upstroke and resembles that seen with ventricular tachycardia as opposed to a bundle branch block. Antidromic conduction with AF is often fast, broad, and irregular (see Fig. 64-19).

Atrial Flutter

Atrial flutter is an arrhythmia with an atrial rate of approximately 300 beats per minute and a ventricular response of 150 (2:1), 100 (3:1), or slower multiples. Typical atrial flutter is a macro-re-entrant circuit that circulates in the right atrium in a clockwise or counterclockwise loop (Fig. 64-21). The inferior portion of typical flutter uses the narrow region between the inferior vena cava and tricuspid annulus as a critical isthmus of conduction. Typical atrial flutter almost always occurs in patients with underlying cardiovascular or pulmonary disease. It can also develop in patients who receive anti-arrhythmic drugs (e.g., sodium-channel blocking drugs) for AF. Atypical atrial flutter refers to macro-re-entrant atrial circuits that do not use this critical cavotricuspid isthmus of tissue. These atypical forms of atrial flutter often occur in the left atrium after mitral valve surgery or catheter ablation of AF. Typical atrial flutter can be recognized by a "sawtooth" P wave morphology, which is predominantly negative in leads II, III, and aVF and positive in V$_1$ (counterclockwise atrial flutter) or positive in leads II, III, and aVF and negative in V$_1$ (clockwise atrial flutter).

Atrial Fibrillation

AF is identified by the absence of P waves and the presence of an irregularly irregular ventricular rate. Coarse AF, which describes the presence of residual atrial activity on the ECG, is generally best seen in lead V$_1$ with the absence of P wave–like activity in other leads (Fig. 64-22). AF can be present with a regular ventricular rate when there is concomitant AV dissociation (e.g., complete heart block or ventricular tachycardia).

AF, which is the most common arrhythmia in clinical practice, afflicts over two million Americans. The likelihood of developing AF increases with aging, with an anticipated three-fold increase in prevalence as the U.S. population ages in the next 20 years. AF is almost always a recurrent disorder with the possible exception of AF that develops in association with hyperthyroidism (Chapter 233) and surgery (Chapter 441). AF can be paroxysmal (terminates spontaneously) or persistent (persists for at least 7 days or until cardioverted). Paroxysmal AF can occur as self-remitting arrhythmia for decades or can progress to permanent AF. Patients with persistent AF generally progress to permanent AF unless sinus rhythm is restored with cardioversion.

In addition to its association with aging, AF frequently occurs in association with hypertension (Chapter 67) or other comorbid conditions such as

FIGURE 64-20. Atrioventricular re-entrant tachycardia. Negative P waves are seen in leads II, III, and aVF indicative of retrograde conduction to the atria over a septal accessory pathway.

FIGURE 64-21. Two examples of atrial flutter. A, Typical counterclockwise right atrial flutter with classic sawtooth flutter waves seen in leads II, III, and aVF. B, Clockwise right atrial flutter.

FIGURE 64-22. Coarse atrial fibrillation. The wavy baseline is suggestive of atrial activity and can be misinterpreted as P waves or flutter waves. The irregularity of the QRS complexes indicates that this is atrial fibrillation.

diabetes mellitus, thyrotoxicosis, heart failure, coronary artery disease, valvular heart disease, or lung disease such as chronic obstructive pulmonary disease or obstructive sleep apnea. About 20% of patients have no associated comorbidity and have what may be termed *lone AF*. Some patients develop AF after binges of alcohol use ("holiday heart") or after parasympathetic surges such as after vigorous exercise or a large meal (vagally induced AF). Excessive caffeine intake is an often cited but very rare cause of AF. AF requires a trigger in the form of atrial premature depolarizations, which often originate in the pulmonary veins and which, in the susceptible individual, result in AF. The susceptibility to AF may relate to changes in the electrical function of the left atrium. Prolonged periods of AF can lead to electrical and structural remodeling of the atria and promote the further perpetuation of AF ("AF begets AF").

AF results in the loss of the atrial contribution to ventricular filling. This so-called loss of atrial kick is generally well tolerated in normal individuals, in whom only about 15% of ventricular filling is the result of atrial contraction. In patients who have stiff, noncompliant ventricles (e.g., patients with aortic stenosis, hypertrophic or restrictive cardiomyopathy, or long-standing hypertension), however, up to 40% of ventricular filling may be related to atrial contraction, so stroke volume may fall noticeably in such patients.

The primary morbidity associated with AF is thromboembolism. Thromboembolism in patients with nonvalvular AF typically results from thrombus formation in and dislodgement from the left atrial appendage. The risk of thromboembolism is unrelated to the pattern of AF (paroxysmal or persistent) but is increased in the first 3 to 4 weeks after cardioversion, when the gradual return of atrial mechanical function can result in a particularly high risk of thromboembolism. The risk of thromboembolism in AF increases with age, diabetes mellitus, hypertension, previous embolic episodes, and heart failure. The lowest incidence (<1% annually) is in patients younger than 65 years with lone AF.

CLINICAL MANIFESTATIONS

SVTs can produce symptoms specifically related to the rhythm itself, including fatigue, palpitations (Chapter 62), dizziness, shortness of breath, chest discomfort, presyncope, and syncope. These symptoms are mostly related to the rapidity of the ventricular response and are most prevalent at the onset of the arrhythmia. In contrast to other forms of SVT, asymptomatic episodes of AF are common in patients who also have symptomatic AF.

Incessant SVT and uncontrolled ventricular rates can cause tachycardia-related cardiomyopathy, which is reversible with control of these arrhythmias. In some situations, however, the clinical presentation may be dominated by the underlying condition that precipitates the arrhythmia, such as fever, physical stress, hypovolemia, heart failure (Chapter 58), hypoxia, sympathomimetic or parasympatholytic medications, thyrotoxicosis (Chapter 233), and pheochromocytoma (Chapter 235).

Re-entrant tachycardias begin and end abruptly, whether without treatment or when terminated with vagal maneuvers or intravenous medications. An accessory pathway with ventricular preexcitation can be undiagnosed into adulthood, when it can mimic myocardial infarction or right ventricular hypertrophy on the electrocardiogram.

DIAGNOSIS

The key to diagnosis is the 12-lead ECG if the symptoms are very frequent. A Holter monitor is useful if the arrhythmia is likely to be detected by 24 to 48 hours of monitoring, whereas a continuous loop event recorder, which can be worn for up to a month and activated by the patient for symptoms, is preferred if the arrhythmia is less frequent (Chapter 62). Another alternative is a device that records data continuously and transmits to a central station, capturing both symptomatic and asymptomatic arrhythmias over a period of up to a month.

On physical examination, patients with a blocked atrial beat or AVNRT may have large (cannon) "a" waves detected in their jugular veins (see Fig. 50-4 in Chapter 50). Carotid sinus massage, which has a vagal effect on the AV node, can terminate SVTs that depend on the AV node as part of the circuit (AVNRT and AVRT). Carotid sinus massage also can occasionally terminate atrial tachycardia but more often will slow the pulse by reducing the number of atrial inputs conducted through the AV node. Similarly, carotid sinus massage will slow but not terminate atrial flutter and AF.

Electrophysiologic testing (Chapter 66) is the definitive way to distinguish SVT from VT (see Table 65-2 in Chapter 65). The SVT can often be initiated by paced premature beats, after which the mechanism and location of the arrhythmia can be determined.

TREATMENT   Rx

Acute Therapy
Sinus, Atrial, Atrioventricular Nodal Re-entrant, and Junctional Tachycardias

Sinus tachycardia rarely should be treated directly. Instead, treatment should focus on identifying and treating any precipitating underlying conditions, especially heart failure, pulmonary disease, fever, and thyroid disease. Multifocal atrial tachycardia is relatively unresponsive to medical therapy, is very difficult to ablate, and is best treated by management of the underlying pulmonary disorder. Nondihydropyridine calcium-channel blocking drugs (diltiazem, verapamil; Table 64-5) are most often used if a therapy is absolutely required.

Sustained or repeated episodes of nonsustained SVT, however, generally require effective therapy. If rapid control is desired (e.g., in patients with myocardial ischemia or hypotension), cardioversion is the best solution (Chapter 66). Atrial tachycardias, including atrial flutter or AF, may also convert spontaneously or convert after treatment of an underlying cause, such as hypoxia or heart failure, or after cessation of precipitating medications.

An acute episode of either AVNRT or junctional tachycardia can often be terminated with vagal maneuvers, such as carotid massage. In most atrial tachycardias, adenosine or vagal stimulation (or both) produces enough AV block to unmask the atrial origin of the tachycardia. However, some atrial tachycardias and most episodes of AVNRT terminate after administration of adenosine. Intravenous β-blockers or calcium-channel blockers (see Table 64-5) can be used for the same purpose. For sustained control of the ventricular rate during atrial tachycardia, intravenous esmolol and diltiazem are effective.

Accessory Pathway Tachycardia

The acute management of SVTs that use an accessory pathway (AVRT) depends on the mechanism of the rhythm. If the tachycardia uses the AV node as one limb of the circuit, it may terminate with vagal maneuvers such as carotid sinus massage. If the tachycardia uses an accessory pathway as the antegrade limb (antidromic AVRT), it is important to avoid measures that may accelerate the conduction properties of the accessory pathway. For example, digoxin and epinephrine will increase conduction over the accessory pathway and potentially accelerate the tachycardia. Patients may have an adrenergic response to a drop in blood pressure induced by the vasodilating properties of β-blockers and calcium-channel blockers, particularly when AF conducts over an accessory pathway. As a result of these potential complications, adenosine (see Table 64-5) is the drug of choice for the acute termination of antidromic AVRT, but a true antiarrhythmic drug, such as intravenous amiodarone, or cardioversion should be considered for antidromically conducted AF. In orthodromic AVRT, in which the AV node is the antegrade limb of the tachycardia, β-blockers or calcium-channel blockers can be used as well as adenosine.

Atrial Flutter

It can be very difficult to control the rate of acute atrial flutter, which generally must be treated by restoring sinus rhythm. Intravenous ibutilide is approximately 60% effective for converting atrial flutter to sinus rhythm. Direct current electrical cardioversion, which is highly (>95%) effective for restoring sinus rhythm, should not be performed unless the episode of atrial flutter is believed to be less than 48 hours in duration, or transesophageal echocardiogram has excluded clot in the left atrial appendage, or until the risk of stroke has been minimized by achieving a therapeutic international normalized ration (INR) of 2 to 3 for the prior 4 weeks.

Atrial Fibrillation

For acute AF without hypotension, rate control is crucial and can be accomplished with esmolol, metoprolol, verapamil, or diltiazem (see Table 64-5); digoxin is usually a third-line agent (Fig. 64-23). All patients with new-onset AF should receive anticoagulation acutely with heparin (Chapter 37). The decision of whether to restore and maintain sinus rhythm or allow recurrences or progression to permanent AF is a fundamental component of AF management. Trials of a strategy of rate control compared with a

TABLE 64-5 ANTIARRHYTHMIC DRUGS: DOSES AND SIDE EFFECTS

ANTIARRHYTHMIC DRUG AND COMMON USE	DOSE/METABOLISM	SIDE EFFECTS AND REQUIRED MONITORING	SELECTED DRUG INTERACTIONS
Quinidine	Hepatic CYP 3A4 (70%), renal (30%) Dose: sulfate—600 mg tid, gluconate—324 to 648 mg q8h Dose reduced for renal failure	Thrombocytopenia Cinchonism Pruritus, rash QT prolongation/torsades de pointes	↑ Digoxin and amiodarone concentrations Quinidine inhibits CYP 2D6 and may increase drugs metabolized by this enzyme, e.g., ↑ effect of tricyclic antidepressants, haloperidol, some β-blockers, fluoxetine, narcotics Quinidine metabolism inhibited by cimetidine Quinidine metabolism increased by phenobarbital, phenytoin, and rifampicin
Procainamide	Mostly hepatic—rapid acetylators produce more NAPA; NAPA renally cleared PO dose: 50 mg/kg/24 hr IV dose: 1 g over 25 min, then 20-60 µg/kg/min infusion Reduce dose for renal dysfunction or low cardiac output	Rash, fever, arthralgias, drug-induced lupus, particularly in slow acetylators Agranulocytosis QT prolongation/torsades de pointes	Procainamide clearance reduced by trimethoprim, cimetidine, and ranitidine
Disopyramide	Renal, hepatic (CYP 3A4) Dose: 100-400 mg q8-12h; max dose, 800 mg/24 hr Reduce dose for renal or hepatic dysfunction	Anticholinergic (contraindicated for narrow-angle glaucoma): dry mouth, urinary retention, constipation, blurry vision QT prolongation/torsades de pointes	None
Propafenone	Hepatic: 150-300 mg q8h or sustained release 225-425 mg bid	Metallic taste, dizziness, SIADH Atrial flutter, ventricular tachycardia	May decrease the metabolism of warfarin Increase digoxin levels
Flecainide	Renal, hepatic CYP 2D6 50-100 mg bid; max dose, 300-400 mg/day	Dizziness, headache, visual blurring Atrial flutter, ventricular tachycardia	May increase digoxin levels Flecainide levels increased by amiodarone, haloperidol, quinidine, cimetidine, and fluoxetine
β-Blockers (selected)	Hepatic, renal Only renal (atenolol, nadolol) IV esmolol: 250-500 µg over 1 min, then 50-300 µg/kg/min over 4 min Acebutolol, 200-600 mg bid; atenolol, 25-100 mg qd; carvedilol, 3.125-50 mg bid; metoprolol, 25-150 mg bid; nadolol, 20-120 mg qd; nebivolol, 5-40 mg qd; propranolol, 10-120 mg bid	Fatigue, depression, bronchospasm, impotence	Minimal, except for carvedilol and metoprolol, whose levels may be increased by amiodarone, propafenone, quinidine, fluoxetine, haloperidol, paroxetine, and cimetidine
Sotalol	Renal: 80-120 mg bid Max dose, 240 mg bid	Bronchospasm QT prolongation/torsades de pointes	No significant interactions
Dofetilide	Renal, hepatic CYP 3A4 CrCl > 60 (500 µg bid), CrCl 40-60 (250 µg bid), CrCl 20-39 (125 µg bid)	QT prolongation and torsades de pointes Three days of in-hospital monitoring is required during drug initiation	Contraindicated with verapamil, ketoconazole, cimetidine, megestrol, prochlorperazine, and trimethoprim Hydrochlorothiazide increases dofetilide levels Must discontinue amiodarone at least 3 mo before dofetilide initiation
Ibutilide	Hepatic CYP 3A4 1 mg IV over 10 min, repeat after 10 min if necessary	Nausea QT prolongation and torsades de pointes Must monitor for 4 hr after drug initiation	None
Amiodarone	Hepatic half-life 50 days PO load 10 g over 7-10 days, then 400 mg for 3 wk, then 200 mg/day for atrial fibrillation Maintenance dose of 400 mg/day for VT Dose reduce load for bradycardia or QT prolongation IV: 150-300 mg bolus, then 1 mg/min infusion for 6 hr, followed by 0.5 mg/min thereafter	Pulmonary (acute hypersensitivity pneumonitis, chronic interstitial infiltrates), hepatitis Thyroid (hypo- or hyperthyroidism) Photosensitivity, blue-gray discoloration with chronic high dose, nausea, ataxia, tremor, alopecia Avoid if identified thyroid nodule LFTs two to three times a year, TFTs twice yearly, PFTs and CXR at initiation and CXR yearly thereafter. QT prolongation expected; reduce dose if exceeds 500 msec	Inhibits CYP 450 enzymes—increases concentrations of warfarin, digoxin, cyclosporine, alprazolam, carbamazepine, HMG-CoA inhibitors, phenytoin, and quinidine
Dronedarone	Hepatic CYP 3A4 half-life 30 hr PO 400 mg bid Improved absorption with food	Reduces the secretion of creatinine without a reduction in GFR Hepatic failure Avoid in heart failure	Increases digoxin levels (dose reduce digoxin by half) May increase myositis with simvastatin Avoid grapefruit
Calcium-channel blocker (nondihydropyridine)	Hepatic Inhibit CYP 3A4 IV diltiazem, 20 mg bolus over 2 min, then 5-15 mg per hour maintenance infusion Verapamil long-acting 120-480 mg qd Diltiazem long-acting 180-300 mg qd	Constipation, rash, peripheral edema	Inhibits CYP 3A4—will increase levels of alprazolam, carbamazepine, dihydropyridine, cyclosporine, HMG-CoA inhibitors. Verapamil (but not diltiazem) increases digoxin levels

TABLE 64-5 ANTIARRHYTHMIC DRUGS: DOSES AND SIDE EFFECTS—cont'd

ANTIARRHYTHMIC DRUG AND COMMON USE	DOSE/METABOLISM	SIDE EFFECTS AND REQUIRED MONITORING	SELECTED DRUG INTERACTIONS
Adenosine	Erythrocyte, endothelial cell 6-mg IV push, followed if necessary by 12 mg after 1-2 min	Nausea, headache, flushing, chest pain, bronchospasm (contraindicated if asthma)	Methylxanthines compete for adenosine receptors with adenosine Dipyridamole decreases the metabolism of adenosine
Digoxin	Renal, hepatic, gastrointestinal, 0.125-375 mg/day	Anorexia, nausea, fatigue, confusion, altered vision with green-yellow halos	Levels of or sensitivity to digoxin increased by hypokalemia, quinidine, verapamil, amiodarone, propafenone, renal failure, hypoxia, decreased muscle mass Levels of or sensitivity to digoxin decreased by malabsorption, hyperkalemia, hypocalcemia

CXR = chest x-ray; CYP = cytochrome P-450; GFR = glomerular filtration rate; HMG-CoA = 3-hydroxy-3-methylglutaryl coenzyme A; IV = intravenous administration; LFT = liver function test; NAPA = N-acetyl procainamide; PFT = pulmonary function test; PO = oral administration; SIADH = syndrome of inappropriate diuretic hormone; TFT = thyroid function test; VT = ventricular tachycardia.

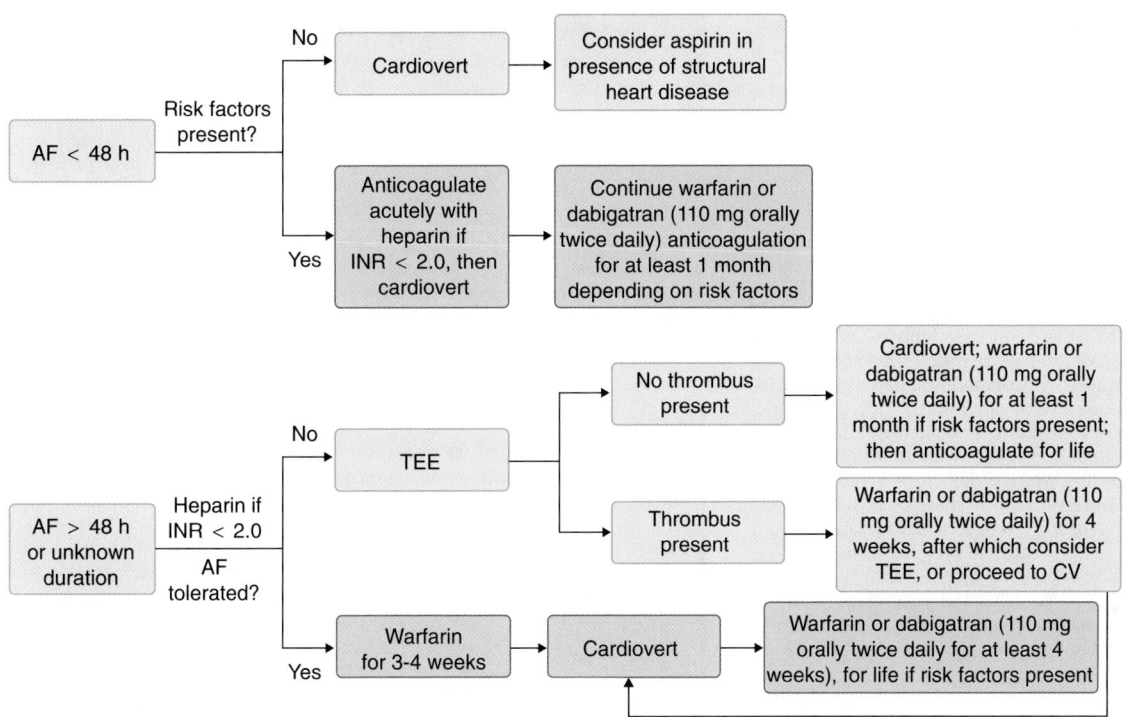

FIGURE 64-23. Management of recent-onset atrial fibrillation (AF). CV = Cardioversion; INR = International Normalized Ratio; TEE = Transesophageal echocardiography.

strategy of rhythm control with antiarrhythmic drugs have demonstrated no difference in total or arrhythmic mortality associated with these two approaches,[1-3] even in patients with a reduced ejection fraction.[4] Because a significant component of the adverse events experienced in the rhythm control arms of these studies was due to stroke in un-anticoagulated patients and toxicity from antiarrhythmic drugs, advances in antiarrhythmic and anti-coagulant medications as well as the advent of reliable ablative therapies for AF may necessitate a reevaluation of this question.

If a strategy of rate control is chosen, it is important to confirm a heart rate of 80 to 110 beats per minute at rest and less than 140 beats per minute with exercise, preferably by monitoring the heart rate during exercise on an exercise treadmill test or with an ambulatory monitor. More strict rate control is not beneficial.[5] Failure to confirm rate control can result in the development of tachycardia-induced cardiomyopathy. First-line therapy for rate control includes β-blockers or calcium-channel blockers; digoxin can also be used but is generally less effective. Patients commonly require a combination of mediations to achieve goal heart rates.

If a strategy of rhythm control is chosen, many patients will first require cardioversion, either pharmacologic or electrical (Chapter 66). The risk of clot formation must be mitigated before cardioversion in all patients with AF of more than 48 hours' duration. The first step generally is to perform transesophageal echocardiography (TEE) (Chapter 55). If TEE shows no evidence of a left atrial clot, cardioversion can be undertaken without systemic anticoagulation; if the patient has risk factors for stroke in association arrith AF, however, most clinicians administer anticoagulation during the cardioversion and for the subsequent 4 weeks. If the TEE shows evidence of clot, 4 consecutive weeks of anticoagulation with an INR of at least 2 is required, and anticoagulation must be maintained for at least 3 to 4 weeks after cardioversion. Electrical cardioversion, which should be performed with a minimum of 200 joules, is successful in more than 90% of cases. Pharmacologic cardioversion can be

performed with intravenous drugs such as ibutilide, which is more successful for atrial flutter (60% efficacy) than AF (50%). Oral medications can also be used as a "pill in the pocket" strategy. Patients can take a single dose of propafenone (600 mg) or flecainide (300 mg) with a conversion rate for recent-onset AF (<48 hours' duration) of approximately 50% without the need for a screening TEE. Oral amiodarone (typically loaded with 10 g over the first week, followed by 400 to 600 mg a day for the next 3 weeks) can also be used for cardioversion and is successful in approximately 50% of patients with both recent and more prolonged AF.

Long-Term Management
AVNRT, AVRT, Atrial Tachycardias, and Atrial Flutter
Chronic therapy for AVNRT is guided by the frequency and severity of symptoms. Many patients are able to live with this rhythm with infrequent recurrences, which terminate spontaneously or with adenosine. If chronic therapy is required, β-blockers or calcium-channel blockers and less commonly digoxin are used. Ablation of AVNRT (Chapter 66) is highly effective and should be considered before using sodium- or potassium-channel blocking drugs.

Most patients with symptomatic AVRT are treated with catheter ablation (Chapter 66). Ablation of an accessory pathway located near the AV node or His bundle carries a 1% risk of complete heart block, whereas ablation of accessory pathways on the left side of the heart and distant from the AV node and His bundle region is not associated with a risk of heart block but carries a small risk of stroke. At present, it is not standard of care to ablate accessory pathways in patients without symptomatic arrhythmias.

The long-term management of atrial tachycardia depends on symptoms. If the rhythm is highly symptomatic, it is generally managed with a β-blocker or calcium-channel blocker. If these medications are unsuccessful or not tolerated, ablation is frequently recommended, but antiarrhythmic medications are an alternative.

In patients with atrial flutter, ventricular rate control is possible by achieving AV nodal block with β-blockers, calcium-channel blockers, and digitalis. However, radio frequency ablation, which is curative, is now the preferred choice for most patients with atrial flutter (Chapter 66), especially recurrent atrial flutter. Because atrial flutter carries a 3% per year risk of thromboembolism, patients with atrial flutter should also receive long-term anticoagulation similar to what is recommended for AF (see later). If atrial flutter is successful, the risk of recurrence is very small, and long-term anticoagulation is not necessary.

Atrial Fibrillation

Therapies for the chronic maintenance of sinus rhythm in patients with AF include pharmacologic and procedural approaches. The procedural approaches include catheter-based ablation inside the left atrium with the goal of electrically isolating the pulmonary veins from the left atrium. Similarly, a minimally invasive surgical approach can electrically isolate the pulmonary veins from the external surface of the heart with the additional resection of the left atrial appendage. Both these procedures have become standard options for AF, especially in patients who have recurrent AF despite at least one antiarrhythmic drug.[6,7] The catheter approach carries a small risk of cardiac perforation, including pericardial tamponade and atrioesophageal fistula formation, and a 1% risk of stroke. There is also a small risk of pulmonary vein stenosis, which has been reduced by newer technologies. The surgical approach carries a higher risk of cardiac bleeding, particularly during the resection of the left atrial appendage, and is associated with a significantly longer recovery time than the percutaneous approach. However, there should be no stroke risk associated with the surgical procedure because it is performed completely from the epicardial surface of the heart. In addition, the exclusion of the left atrial appendage may prove protective in regard to future thromboembolic risk.[8] Both procedures appear to be equally effective, with approximately 60 to 70% of patients experiencing a significant reduction or absence of AF following either procedure. It is typical to offer a second procedure to patients who have recurrent AF following a first catheter-based procedure. Finally, a more extensive surgical operation, called the maze procedure, requires a full thoracotomy and is most often performed concomitantly as part of open coronary artery bypass surgery or an open valve operation. In this procedure, electrical lines of block are created in the left atrium to interrupt the perpetuation of AF, the pulmonary veins are isolated, and the left atrial appendage is resected. Success rates for this procedure, which should be reserved for refractory, symptomatic AF, exceed 80%. However, none of these procedures has yet been demonstrated to reduce the risk of stroke risk, so anticoagulation should be maintained for 6 months after the procedure in patients without clinical risk factors for stroke and chronically in patients with risk factors. Catheter-based procedures directed at excluding the left atrial appendage from the systemic blood stream may become options in patients who have a high risk of stroke and who cannot tolerate systemic anticoagulation owing to an excessive risk of bleeding.

The pharmacologic options for the treatment of AF work by blocking sodium, potassium, or a combination of cardiac channels. Blockade of these channels results in slowing of cardiac conduction (sodium channels) and prolongation in cardiac repolarization (potassium channels) as well as additional effects from modulation of the autonomic nervous system. The choice of antiarrhythmic drug is based on the patient's underlying clinical condition (Table 64-6).

Amiodarone is the most widely used medication for AF with an efficacy of 60 to 70% at 1 year. It is associated with a number of drug interactions, most notably with warfarin and digoxin. Its associated risk of thyroid, liver, and lung toxicities, related in part to the iodine moieties on this compound, necessitate careful follow-up. For prevention of recurrent AF, oral amiodarone is significantly more effective than propafenone and sotalol, which are the recommended alternatives. Another alternative is 400 mg twice daily of dronedarone, which is related to amiodarone but has no iodine and a 24-hour half-life, significantly reduced cardiovascular hospitalizations by 16% and death from 3.9% to 2.7% at 21 months in patients with AF.[9] Dronedarone is currently thought to be safe, however, only in patients with an ejection fraction greater than 35% and no evidence of advanced heart failure.

Quinidine, procainamide, and disopyramide are predominantly sodium-channel blocking drugs that also block potassium channels at slow heart rates. Each of these drugs is moderately successful in AF, with about 50% of treated patients in sinus rhythm at 1 year, but each also has idiosyncratic noncardiovascular toxicities that can significantly limit their utility (see Table 64-5). Propafenone and flecainide are also sodium-channel blockers that are widely used for the maintenance of sinus rhythm. These drugs are moderately effective, with a 50% rate of sinus rhythm at 1 year, and are generally well tolerated but must be avoided in patients with structural heart disease, particularly with a history of prior myocardial infarction and impaired left ventricular function, because of a risk for drug-induced ventricular arrhythmia. Dofetilide is a potassium-channel blocking medication that is moderately effective for suppressing AF but carries a dose-dependent risk of QT prolongation and torsades de pointes.

TABLE 64-6	SELECTION OF ANTIARRHYTHMIC DRUGS
PATIENT CHARACTERISTICS	**ANTIARRHYTHMIC DRUG CHOICES**
No structural heart disease	*First line:* flecainide, propafenone, dronedarone, sotalol *Second line:* amiodarone, dofetilide
Depressed left ventricular ejection fraction with heart failure	*First line:* amiodarone, dofetilide *Avoid:* dronedarone, flecainide, propafenone
Coronary artery disease without congestive heart failure	*First line:* sotalol, dronedarone, dofetilide, amiodarone *Avoid:* flecainide, propafenone
Hypertrophic cardiomyopathy	*First line:* amiodarone, sotalol, dronedarone *Second line:* disopyramide

TABLE 64-7	CURRENT RECOMMENDATIONS FOR THROMBOEMBOLIC PROPHYLAXIS FOR PATIENTS WITH ATRIAL FIBRILLATION BASED ON RISK FACTORS FOR STROKE
No risk	Aspirin (81 to 325 mg/day) or nothing
One moderate risk factor (age ≥ 75 yr, hypertension, heart failure, left ventricular ejection fraction ≤ 35%, diabetes mellitus)	Warfarin (INR 2-3) or dabigatran (110 mg orally twice daily) preferred in patients age ≥ 65 yr with heart failure or age 65-74 yr with diabetes or coronary disease; otherwise aspirin (81 or 325 mg)
At least two moderate risk factors or one high risk factor (prior stroke or transient ischemic attack, mitral stenosis, prosthetic valve)	Warfarin (INR 2-3, or 2.5-3.5 with prosthetic valve) or dabigatran (110 mg orally twice daily)

Anticoagulation

The presence or absence of associated conditions help determine which patients with AF require chronic anticoagulation with warfarin or other systematic coagulants (Table 64-7). Long-term anticoagulation therapy with warfarin or dabigatran is generally recommended in all patients who have persistent or paroxysmal AF, who are older than 65 years, and who have no contraindications to anticoagulation.[10] Warfarin alone is superior to aspirin[11] or the combination of clopidogrel and aspirin, with meta-analysis showing that adjusted-dose warfarin and antiplatelet agents reduce stroke by approximately 60% and 20%, respectively.[12] Although there is some protective effect at an INR as low as 1.8, the target INR for chronic anticoagulation with warfarin should be 2 to 3 to avoid INRs less than 1.8. For patients who do not require or cannot tolerate warfarin, aspirin is a reasonable alternative. Clopidogrel (75 mg/day), in addition to aspirin, reduces the risk of major vascular events from 7.6% per year to 6.8% per year compared with aspirin alone, but increases the risk of major bleeding from 1.3% per year to 2% per year.[13] Dabigatran at 110 mg twice daily is as effective as warfarin but causes less bleeding.[14] Newer alternatives include direct thrombin inhibitors and factor Xa inhibitors. For example, in a randomized study of patients unable to tolerate warfarin, the factor Xa inhibitor apixaban (5 mg daily) reduced stroke and systemic embolism without major increases in bleeding.[15] These new classes of anticoagulants do not require monitoring with blood tests and do not interact with food or medications. Aspirin may be better than no treatment for patients who cannot tolerate warfarin. The addition of aspirin to moderate-intensity warfarin in anticoagulation (INR 2 to 3) can decrease vascular events and is recommended in high-risk patients.[16]

Grade **A**

1. Hohnloser SH, Kuck K-H, Lilienthal J. Rhythm or rate control in atrial fibrillation. Pharmacological Intervention in Atrial Fibrillation (PIAF): a randomized trial. *Lancet.* 2000;356:1789-1794.
2. Wyse DG, Waldo AL, DiMarco JP, et al. A comparison of rate control and rhythm control in patients with atrial fibrillation. *N Engl J Med.* 2002;347:1825-1833.
3. Van Gelder IC, Hagens VE, Bosker HA, et al. A comparison of rate control and rhythm control in patients with recurrent persistent atrial fibrillation. *N Engl J Med.* 2002;347:1834-1840.
4. Roy D, Talajic M, Nattel S, et al. Rhythm control versus rate control for atrial fibrillation and heart failure. *N Engl J Med.* 2008;358:2667-2677.
5. Van Gelder I, Groenveld H, Crijns H. Lenient versus strict rate control in patients with atrial fibrillation. *N Engl J Med.* 2010;362:1363-1373.
6. Wilber DJ, Pappone C, Neuzil P, et al. Comparison of antiarrhythmic drug therapy and radiofrequency catheter ablation in patients with paroxysmal atrial fibrillation: a randomized controlled trial. *JAMA.* 2010;303:333-340.
7. Terasawa T, Balk EM, Chung M, et al. Systematic review: comparative effectiveness of radiofrequency catheter ablation for atrial fibrillation. *Ann Intern Med.* 2009;151:191-202.

8. Holmes DR, Reddy VY, Turi ZG, et al. Percutaneous closure of the left atrial appendage versus warfarin therapy for prevention of stroke in patients with atrial fibrillation: a randomized non-inferiority trial. *Lancet.* 2009;374:534-542.
9. Hohnloser SH, Crijns HJ, van Eickels M, et al. Effect of dronedarone on cardiovascular events in atrial fibrillation. *N Engl J Med.* 2009;360:668-678.
10. Perez-Gomez F, Alegria E, Berjon J, et al. Comparative effects of antiplatelet, anticoagulant, or combined therapy in patients with valvular and nonvalvular atrial fibrillation: a randomized multicenter study. *J Am Coll Cardiol.* 2004;44:1557-1566.
11. Mant J, Richard FD, Fletcher K, et al. Warfarin versus aspirin for stroke prevention in an elderly community population with atrial fibrillation (the Birmingham atrial fibrillation treatment of the aged study, BAFTA). *Lancet.* 2007;370:493-503.
12. Hart RG, Pearce LA, Aguilar MI, et al. Meta-analysis: antithrombotic therapy to prevent stroke in patients who have nonvalvular atrial fibrillation. *Ann Intern Med.* 2007;146:857-867.
13. Connolly SJ, Pogue J, Hart RG, et al, for the ACTIVE Investigators. Effect of clopidogrel added to aspirin in patients with atrial fibrillation. *N Engl J Med.* 2009;360:2066-2078.
14. Connolly SJ, Ezekowitz MD, Yusuf S, et al. Dabigatran versus warfarin in patients with atrial fibrillation. *N Engl J Med.* 2009;361:1139-1151.
15. Connolly SJ, Eikelboom J, Joyner C, et al. Apixaban in patients with atrial fibrillation. *N Engl J Med.* 2011;364:806-817.
16. Taylor FC, Cohen H, Ebrahim S. Systematic review of long term anticoagulation or antiplatelet treatment in patients with non-rheumatic atrial fibrillation. *BMJ.* 2001;322:321-326.

SUGGESTED READINGS

Dobrev D, Nattel S. New antiarrhythmic drugs for treatment of atrial fibrillation. *Lancet.* 2010;375:1212-1223. *Review.*
Wann LS, Curtis AB, January CT, et al. 2011 ACCF/AHA/HRS focused update on the management of patients with atrial fibrillation (updating the 2006 guideline). A report of the American College of Cardiology Foundation/American Heart Association Task Force on Practice Guidelines. *Circulation.* 2011;123:104-123. *Consensus guidelines.*
Zimetbaum P, Goldman A. Ambulatory arrhythmia monitoring: choosing the right device. *Circulation.* 2010;122:1629-1636. *Comprehensive review.*

65

VENTRICULAR ARRHYTHMIAS

WILLIAM G. STEVENSON

Ventricular arrhythmias originate below the atrioventricular (AV) node in the ventricular myocardium or His-Purkinje system. These include premature ventricular beats, ventricular couplets, nonsustained and sustained ventricular tachycardias (VTs), and ventricular fibrillation (VF). These arrhythmias occur in all forms of heart disease and can be the initial presentation of disease. Sustained arrhythmias are an important cause of sudden death. Arrhythmias associated with genetic abnormalities of cardiac ion channels can cause sudden death despite the absence of identifiable structural heart disease. Ventricular arrhythmias that occur in the absence of structural heart disease or a defined ion channel abnormality are referred to as *idiopathic* and are usually benign. Evaluation and management are guided by the risk of arrhythmic death, which is determined by the presenting symptoms, type of arrhythmia, and associated underlying heart disease.

EPIDEMIOLOGY

Premature ventricular contractions (PVCs) are encountered on a standard electrocardiogram (ECG) in fewer than 1% of subjects younger than 20 years of age. The prevalence increases with age to greater than 2% of patients older than 50 years. Premature ventricular beats can be a sign of increased sympathetic tone, myocardial ischemia, hypoxia, and electrolyte abnormalities, particularly hypokalemia (Table 65-1), or underlying heart disease.

Sustained ventricular arrhythmias are usually caused by underlying structural heart disease, and the prevalence of arrhythmias increases with the severity of the heart disease. Ventricular arrhythmias are responsible for most of the 150,000 to 350,000 sudden deaths (Chapter 63) that occur annually in the United States and account for approximately 13% of all mortality. VF due to acute myocardial ischemia (Chapter 73) in the setting of coronary artery disease is the most common cause. The annual incidence of out-of-hospital VF is approximately 8 per 100,000. A 24-hour ECG recording will show premature ventricular beats and nonsustained VT in more than half of patients with advanced heart failure (Chapter 59). In the heart failure population, sustained VT or VF develops at a rate of approximately 2% per year or less when the left ventricular ejection fraction is above about 30%, but the rate doubles for patients with worse ventricular function.

TABLE 65-1 POTENTIAL FACTORS AGGRAVATING VENTRICULAR ARRHYTHMIAS

Elevated sympathetic tone
  Acute illness
  Central nervous system injury
  Hypovolemia
  Exertion/emotion
Fever
Myocardial ischemia/infarction
Tachycardia
  Atrial fibrillation
  Sinus tachycardia
Bradycardia
Electrolyte abnormalities
  Hypokalemia, hypomagnesemia, hypocalcemia
Hypoxia
Hyperthyroidism
Sleep apnea
Toxins
  Amphetamines, caffeine, ephedrine, pseudoephedrine
  QT prolonging drugs/toxins (see Table 65-3)
  Digitalis glycosides

PATHOBIOLOGY

Ventricular arrhythmia can be caused by automaticity or re-entry. Purkinje fibers have the capability for spontaneous automaticity that emerges normally at rates slower than 50 beats per minute. Abnormal automaticity occurs in partially depolarized ventricular or Purkinje myocytes. Triggered automaticity results from afterdepolarizations, which may be early or delayed in relation to the completion of ventricular repolarization. Delayed afterdepolarizations, which are membrane depolarizations that follow the completion of repolarization (i.e., usually after the completion of the T wave on the ECG), can occur when intracellular calcium overload increases the activity of the sodium-calcium exchanger, thereby producing a depolarizing inward flux of sodium. This mechanism is implicated in the ventricular arrhythmias seen in digitalis toxicity, familial catecholaminergic polymorphic VT, and some idiopathic right ventricular outflow tract arrhythmias. Rapid pacing and β-adrenergic stimulation promote delayed afterdepolarizations, so these arrhythmias are often exercise induced. Early afterdepolarizations occur before the completion of repolarization, that is, before the end of the T wave on the ECG, because a prolonged time to repolarization allows recovery of ion channels before the end of repolarization. Early afterdepolarizations are involved in the genesis of polymorphic VT associated with QT prolongation in the long QT syndromes and possibly during myocardial ischemia.

Re-entry in regions of myocardial scar is the most common cause of sustained VT associated with structural heart disease. The scar contains areas of fibrous tissue as well as surviving myocyte bundles that can create channels for propagation through the scar. Separation of myocyte bundles by fibrous tissue and uncoupling of adjacent bundles leads to slow conduction through these regions, thereby promoting re-entry (Fig. 65-1).

Re-entry can also occur in the absence of a fixed structural abnormality in the tissue. Spiral wave re-entry is one such formation that can be provoked in normal tissue by electrical stimulation (Fig. 65-2). The core of the spiral wave may wander through the tissue, thereby changing the ventricular activation sequence and producing polymorphic VT (see later). Alternatively, the spiral wave may anchor on anatomic discontinuities to produce a consistent beat-to-beat ventricular activation. Spiral waves that encounter refractory tissue can break into daughter waves and disorganize to VF.

CLINICAL MANIFESTATIONS AND DIAGNOSES

Ventricular arrhythmias can be asymptomatic and be detected by an irregular pulse, on a routine ECG, on routine monitoring in the hospital, or on an exercise test. Ventricular arrhythmias also can present symptomatically as palpitations (Chapters 50 and 62), dizziness, exercise intolerance, syncope (Chapters 50 and 62), or sudden cardiac arrest (Chapter 63). The diagnosis should be confirmed with an ECG. Individuals often have substantial hour-to-hour and day-to-day variation in the frequency of ventricular arrhythmias, so ambulatory monitoring is useful to record the cardiac rhythm at the time of symptoms (Chapter 62) if the arrhythmia is not present on the resting ECG. Exercise testing should be considered in patients with exercise-induced symptoms.

FIGURE 65-1. Initiation of scar-related re-entry. At the *top* are cardiac electrograms recorded by an implanted cardioverter-defibrillator. The *top tracing* is an atrial electrogram. The *bottom tracing* is the electrogram recorded from the lead in the right ventricular apex. Three beats of sinus rhythm are followed by a premature beat, which initiates ventricular tachycardia. The schematics below the tracings illustrate a potential mechanism of initiation of scar-related re-entry. In each panel, a cross section through the myocardium includes a region of scar *(white and gray regions)* that contains surviving myocyte bundles. A dense region of fibrosis *(solid gray region)* causes conduction block that creates a channel for conduction along the right-hand side of the fibrosis region. **A,** During sinus rhythm, wave fronts *(yellow arrows)* enter the channel from both sides and collide within the channel, thereby preventing re-entry. **B,** A premature beat *(star)* produces a wave front that reaches the superior end of the channel and finds it refractory, where it blocks *(dashed white line)*. The wave front that reaches the lower end of the channel enters the channel. **C,** Conduction through the channel is slow, allowing time for the initial region of block to recover. The wave front emerges from the exit of this channel, where it produces the first beat of ventricular tachycardia. **D,** The complete re-entry circuit.

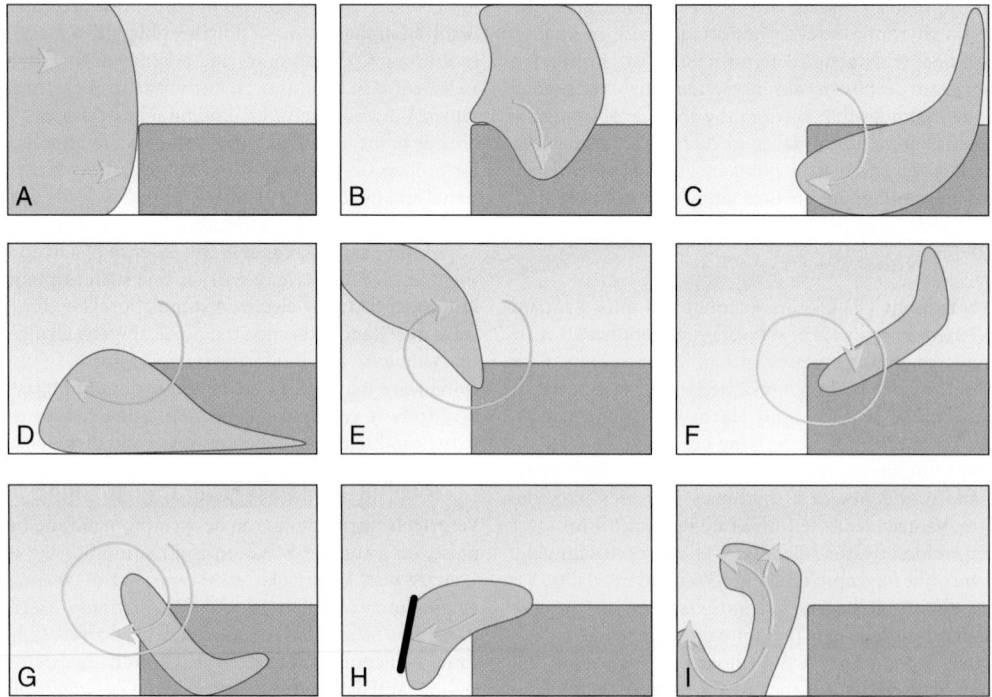

FIGURE 65-2. Spiral wave re-entry. The area of *blue* represents an excitation wave of depolarization. **A,** A wave front propagates from left to right and encounters a region of incompletely recovered tissue *(dark red region)*. **B,** The wave front propagates along the margin of refractory tissue until it reaches recovered tissue and propagates inferiorly (C). **D** to **G,** The wave front continues re-entering and establishing a circuit that continues to spiral through the tissue *(yellow arrow)*. **H,** The spiral wave encounters a region of block *(black line)*, which splits the wave front (I). Multiple potential wave fronts can be generated, thereby leading to fibrillation.

A

B

C

FIGURE 65-3. Ventricular arrhythmias. **A,** Multifocal premature ventricular beats. **B,** Nonsustained monomorphic ventricular tachycardia. Note dissociated P waves indicated by *arrows.* **C,** Sustained monomorphic ventricular tachycardia. Dissociated P waves are indicated by *arrows.*

⬤ TYPES OF VENTRICULAR ARRHYTHMIAS

A single beat is referred to as a *premature ventricular beat* (Fig. 65-3). Two consecutive beats are *ventricular couplets.* Three or more consecutive beats at a rate faster than 100 beats per minute are *VT* (see Fig. 65-3B and C). Three or more consecutive beats at slower rates are designated *idioventricular rhythms.* VT that terminates spontaneously within 30 seconds is *nonsustained* (see Fig. 65-3B), whereas *sustained VT* persists longer than 30 seconds.

The QRS morphology of the arrhythmia is determined by the sequence of ventricular activation. Conduction through the ventricular myocardium is slower than activation of the ventricles over the Purkinje system, so the QRS complex will be wide, typically more than 0.12 second. When VT is caused by repetitive activation from the same source, the QRS complexes are the same from beat to beat, and VT is monomorphic (see Fig. 65-3B and C). A continually changing activation sequence produces polymorphic VT with a changing QRS morphology (Fig. 65-4A). VF has continuous irregular activation with no discrete QRS complexes (see Fig. 65-4D). Although underlying structural heart disease is usually present, these arrhythmias do not require a fixed structural substrate.

The QRS morphology of an individual beat is determined largely by the site of initial ventricular activation. Arrhythmias that originate from the right ventricle or septum result in late activation of much of the left ventricle, thereby producing a prominent S wave in V₁, referred to as a *left bundle branch block–like configuration* (Fig. 65-5). Arrhythmias that originate from the free wall of the left ventricle have a prominent positive deflection in V₁, thereby producing a right bundle branch block–like morphology (Fig. 65-6). The axis of the QRS is also useful. A frontal plane axis that is directed inferiorly, as indicated by dominant R waves in leads II, III, and aVF, suggests initial activation of the cranial portion of the ventricle, whereas a frontal plane axis that is directed superiorly (dominant S waves in II, III, and aVF) suggests initial activation at the inferior wall.

Very rapid monomorphic VT has a sinusoidal appearance, also called *ventricular flutter,* because it is not possible to distinguish the QRS complex from the T wave (see Fig. 65-4B). Relatively slow sinusoidal VTs have a wide QRS indicative of slowed ventricular conduction (see Fig. 65-4C). Hyperkalemia, toxicity from excessive effects of drugs that block sodium channels (e.g., flecainide, propafenone, or tricyclic antidepressants), and severe global myocardial ischemia are causes.

⬤ PREMATURE VENTRICULAR CONTRACTIONS AND NONSUSTAINED VENTRICULAR TACHYCARDIA

PVCs can be due to automaticity or re-entry. PVCs that have the same QRS morphology, which indicates that they have the same origin, are unifocal

PVCs (see Fig. 65-5). PVCs from more than one focus give rise to PVCs with different QRS morphologies and are known as *multifocal premature ventricular beats* (see Fig. 65-3A).

During myocardial ischemia or in association with other heart disease, PVCs can be a harbinger of sustained VT or VF. When encountered during acute illness or as a new finding, the possibility of myocardial ischemia and other aggravating factors (Table 65-1) should be considered, and evaluation for underlying heart disease is warranted.

Three or more consecutive ventricular beats that occur at a rate faster than 100 beats per minute and that terminate spontaneously are nonsustained VT (see Fig. 65-3B). In patients with heart disease, nonsustained VT is associated with more severe disease and increased mortality. However, suppression of nonsustained VT with antiarrhythmic drugs does not improve survival. In ambulatory patients, nonsustained VT is usually monomorphic, with rates of less than 200 beats per minute and a duration of less than 8 beats. Nonsustained VT that is rapid, polymorphic, or with a first beat that occurs before the peak of the T wave ("short coupled") (see Fig. 65-4A) is uncommon and should prompt careful evaluation for causes of sustained VT and diseases associated with a high risk of sudden death (Table 65-3).

Idiopathic PVCs and nonsustained VT occur in the absence of structural or genetic heart disease. Most frequently, these PVCs originate from the right ventricular outflow tract and have a left bundle branch block configuration, with an inferiorly directed frontal plane axis (see Fig. 65-5). Less common sites of origin are the aortic and mitral valve annuli, the left ventricular papillary muscles, and the Purkinje system.

Once the diagnosis is established, further evaluation assesses the possible presence and severity of underlying heart disease. A family history of sudden death should prompt evaluation for genetic syndromes associated with sudden death, including cardiomyopathy (Chapter 60), long QT syndrome (see later), and arrhythmogenic right ventricular cardiomyopathy (Chapter 60). Any abnormality on the 12-lead ECG warrants further evaluation. Repolarization abnormalities are seen in a number of genetically determined syndromes associated with sudden death, including the long QT syndrome, Brugada's syndrome, arrhythmogenic right ventricular cardiomyopathy, and hypertrophic cardiomyopathy (Chapter 60). An echocardiogram (Chapter 55) is often warranted to assess ventricular function, wall motion abnormalities, and valvular heart disease. Cardiac magnetic resonance imaging is also useful for this purpose and for the detection of ventricular scarring that is the substrate for sustained VT. Exercise stress testing should be performed in patients who have exertional symptoms and for those who are at risk for coronary artery disease.

A

B

C

D

FIGURE 65-4. **A,** Polymorphic ventricular tachycardia associated with QT prolongation. Sinus rhythm, with a couplet of premature ventricular contractions, is followed by a sinus beat, and then by a polymorphic ventricular tachycardia. The QT interval of the sinus beats is markedly prolonged, exceeding 0.56 second. **B,** Rapid sinusoidal ventricular tachycardia with a rate approximating 250 beats/minute. **C,** Sinusoidal ventricular tachycardia owing to hyperkalemia. The rate is slower than 150 beats/minute, but the QRS duration exceeds 200 msec, thereby creating the sinusoidal appearance. **D,** Ventricular fibrillation.

FIGURE 65-5. **Twelve-lead electrocardiogram with simultaneous two-lead rhythm strip (V₂ and V₅) showing premature ventricular beats that originated from the right ventricular outflow tract.** Sinus rhythm and frequent premature ventricular beats are present. The premature ventricular contractions all have the same morphology, best appreciated in the bottom two continuous leads, with a left bundle branch block–like configuration in V₁ consistent with an origin in the right ventricle or septum. The frontal plane axis is directed inferiorly, indicating initial depolarization from the cranial aspect of the ventricle.

FIGURE 65-6. Sustained monomorphic ventricular tachycardia (VT) originating from an inferior left ventricular infarct region. VT has a right bundle branch block–like configuration in V$_1$, consistent with an origin in the left ventricle. The frontal plane axis is directed superiorly, consistent with initial depolarization of the inferior wall of the left ventricle.

TABLE 65-2 DISTINGUISHING VENTRICULAR TACHYCARDIA FROM SUPRAVENTRICULAR TACHYCARDIA WITH ABERRANT CONDUCTION

VENTRICULAR TACHYCARDIA	SUPRAVENTRICULAR TACHYCARDIA
AV dissociation	Same QRS morphology as preexisting
AVR: initial R > S or initial r or q > 40 msec	bundle branch block in sinus
V$_1$ to V$_6$: absence of rs	rhythm
V$_1$ to V$_6$: onset of R to S > 100 msec in any lead	V$_1$: rsR′
V$_6$: QS or QR	

TREATMENT Rx

Idiopathic Ventricular Tachycardia

For idiopathic PVCs and nonsustained VT in the absence of underlying heart disease, no specific therapy is needed unless the patient has significant symptoms or evidence that ectopy is depressing ventricular function. Reassurance that the arrhythmia is benign is often sufficient to allow the patient to cope with the symptoms, which will often wax and wane in frequency over years. Avoiding stimulants, such as caffeine, is helpful in some patients. If symptoms require treatment, β-adrenergic blockers and nondihydropyridine calcium-channel blockers (verapamil and diltiazem) are sometimes helpful (see Table 64-7 in Chapter 64). Suppression with more potent antiarrhythmic drugs can be effective but warrants careful consideration of the risks. Catheter ablation can be considered, particularly if unifocal PVCs are causing significant symptoms or contributing to depressed ventricular function, but the potential benefit must be carefully weighed against the procedure risks (Chapter 66).

For PVCs and nonsustained VT that have an impact on quality of life or are extremely frequent such that they may be contributing to ventricular dysfunction, chronic therapy with β-adrenergic blockers (Table 64-7) should be considered. Amiodarone and catheter ablation may be considered if β-adrenergic blockers are ineffective (see later).

Acute Coronary Syndromes

During and early after acute myocardial infarction (MI) (Chapter 73), PVCs and nonsustained VT are common and can be an early manifestation of ischemia and a harbinger of subsequent VF. Treatment with β-adrenergic blockers and correction of hypokalemia and hypomagnesemia reduce the risk of VF. Routine administration of the antiarrhythmic drug lidocaine does not reduce mortality.

Following recovery from acute MI, frequent PVCs (typically more than 10 PVCs per hour), repetitive PVCs with couplets, and nonsustained VT are markers for depressed ventricular function and increased mortality, but suppression of the arrhythmias with antiarrhythmic drug therapy does not improve survival and is

not recommended. For survivors of an acute MI, an implantable cardioverter-defibrillator (ICD) reduces mortality in certain high-risk groups: patients who have survived more than 40 days after the acute MI and have a left ventricular ejection fraction of 30% or less or who have an ejection fraction of less than 0.35% and have symptomatic heart failure (functional class II or III); and patients more than 5 days after MI who have a reduced left ventricular ejection fraction, nonsustained VT, and inducible sustained VT or VF on electrophysiologic testing.[1] ICDs do not reduce mortality when routinely implanted soon after MI or in patients after recent coronary artery revascularization surgery.[2]

Depressed Ventricular Function and Heart Failure

Premature ventricular beats and nonsustained VT are common in patients with depressed ventricular function and heart failure, in whom they are markers for disease severity and increased mortality. Suppression of PVCs with antiarrhythmic drug therapy does not improve survival and is not routinely warranted. For example, in patients with prior MI and a depressed left ventricular ejection fraction, chronic antiarrhythmic drug therapy with the sodium-channel blocking antiarrhythmic drugs flecainide or moricizine increases mortality despite suppression of ventricular ectopy, apparently because of their proarrhythmic and negative inotropic effects. Therefore, antiarrhythmic drugs whose major action is blockade of the cardiac sodium channel (flecainide, propafenone, mexiletine, quinidine, disopyramide) are avoided in patients with structural heart disease. Therapy with dofetilide (see Table 64-7 in Chapter 64), which blocks the repolarizing current IKr, does not improve survival. In patients with heart failure and depressed left ventricular function, amiodarone suppresses ventricular ectopy and reduces sudden death but does not appear to improve survival,[3,4] whereas insertion of an ICD reduces the mortality rate by 20%, from 36% to 29%, over 5 years.[4]

Other Cardiac Disease

Ventricular ectopy is associated with increased mortality in patients with *hypertrophic cardiomyopathy* (Chapter 60) or with *congenital heart disease* (Chapter 69) associated with right or left ventricular dysfunction. In these patients, management is similar to what is recommended in patients with ventricular dysfunction. Pharmacologic suppression of the arrhythmia does not improve mortality, and ICDs are warranted for high-risk patients.

Premature Ventricular Contraction–Induced Ventricular Dysfunction

Very frequent ventricular ectopy can depress ventricular function, probably by a mechanism similar to that by which any chronic tachycardia causes tachycardia-induced cardiomyopathy. PVCs rarely contribute to depressed ventricular function unless they account for more than 10% of beats. The PVCs that cause ventricular depression typically are unifocal, most commonly originating from the left ventricular papillary muscles or outflow tract regions. The distinction between PVC-induced ventricular dysfunction compared with a cardiomyopathy that causes ventricular dysfunction independent of the ventricular arrhythmia is difficult and often can be made only retrospectively by observing an improvement in ventricular function after the arrhythmia is suppressed with amiodarone or catheter ablation.

FIGURE 65-7. Images from a patient with an area of scar in the anterior left ventricular wall. **A,** Echocardiography shows a region of akinesis *(arrow).* **B,** Cardiac magnetic resonance imaging shows the same area of akinesis *(arrow).* **C,** Magnetic resonance imaging after administration of gadolinium contrast shows a region of delayed enhancement *(arrow)* consistent with scar.

IDIOVENTRICULAR RHYTHMS

Three or more ventricular beats at a rate slower than 100 beats/minute is an *idioventricular rhythm.* Automaticity is the likely mechanism. Idioventricular rhythms are common during acute MI (Chapter 73), when atropine therapy is occasionally indicated, and are seen as an escape rhythm during bradycardias. This rhythm is more common in patients with cardiomyopathies or sleep apnea, and it also can be idiopathic, often emerging when the sinus rate slows during sleep. Therapy targets any underlying cause and correction of bradycardia (Chapter 64).

SUSTAINED MONOMORPHIC VENTRICULAR TACHYCARDIA

CLINICAL MANIFESTATIONS

Sustained monomorphic VT presents as a wide QRS tachycardia. Presentations include palpitations, dyspnea, lightheadedness, syncope (Chapters 50 and 62), cardiac arrest, and sudden death (Chapter 63). During cardiac arrest, VT often deteriorates to VF, which may be the initial cardiac rhythm recorded. Structural heart disease with ventricular scarring that allows re-entry is the most common cause. Scars can be due to prior MI (Chapter 73), cardiomyopathies (Chapter 60), sarcoidosis (Chapter 95), and prior ventricular surgery, such as repair of tetralogy of Fallot (Chapter 69). Less commonly, VT is related to re-entry or automaticity in a diseased Purkinje system. Idiopathic VT occurs in the absence of structural heart disease. Management is determined by the underlying heart disease and the frequency and severity of symptoms.

DIAGNOSIS

All patients with monomorphic VT must be evaluated for possible underlying heart disease. When left ventricular function is depressed or there is evidence of structural myocardial disease, scar-related re-entry is the most likely diagnosis. Scars are suggested by pathologic Q waves on the ECG (see Fig. 73-1 in Chapter 73), segmental left or right ventricular wall motion abnormalities on echocardiogram (Fig. 65-7) or nuclear imaging, and areas of delayed gadolinium enhancement during magnetic resonance imaging (see Fig. 65-7). Patients who present with sustained VT associated with coronary artery disease typically have had large MIs and may present years after the acute infarct with a remodeled ventricle and markedly depressed left ventricular function.

TREATMENT AND PROGNOSIS　Rx

Initial management is according to advanced cardiac life support (ACLS) guidelines (Chapters 7 and 63). Following restoration of sinus rhythm, hospitalization and evaluation to define underlying heart disease are required. Sustained monomorphic VT must be distinguished from supraventricular tachycardia with aberrancy (Chapter 64) to guide further therapy. The presence of AV dissociation is the most reliable maker for VT (see Fig. 65-3C), but P waves can be difficult to define, and 1:1 conduction from ventricle to atrium occurs in some VTs, so a 1:1 relationship of P waves to the QRS does not exclude the diagnosis of VT. A number of QRS morphologic criteria for distinguishing VT from supraventricular tachycardia with aberrancy (Table 65-2)

have been described but are less reliable in patients with severe heart disease. The presence of underlying structural heart disease, particularly a history of prior MI, favors a diagnosis of VT rather than supraventricular tachycardia with aberrancy. An electrophysiologic study (Chapter 62) is sometimes required for definitive diagnosis.

Following restoration of sinus rhythm, assessment of cardiac biomarkers for evidence of MI (Chapter 72) is appropriate, but acute MI is rarely a cause of sustained monomorphic VT, and elevations in troponin or CK-MB are more likely to indicate MI that is secondary to hypotension and ischemia from the VT. Even when there is evidence of acute MI, a preexisting scar from previous MI should be suspected as the cause of the VT. Scar-related re-entry is not dependent on recurrent acute myocardial ischemia, so coronary revascularization cannot be anticipated to prevent recurrent VT, even when it may be appropriate for other indications (Chapter 74).

Scars provide a durable substrate for sustained VT, and up to 70% of patients have a recurrence of the arrhythmia within 2 years. Most patients with sustained monomorphic VT have depressed ventricular function, which is a risk factor for sudden death. ICDs reduce annual mortality from 12.3% to 8.8% and reduce arrhythmic deaths by 50% in patients with hemodynamically significant sustained VT or a history of cardiac arrest compared with pharmacologic therapy,**5** and they are usually warranted in such patients, provided that there is a reasonable expectation of survival with acceptable functional status for the next year after recovery from the VT episode. Chronic amiodarone therapy may be considered for patients who are not candidates for or who decline ICD placement.**3** Patients with frequent symptomatic VT require antiarrhythmic drug therapy or catheter ablation**5,6** to reduce recurrences.

Following ICD implantation, patients remain at risk for heart failure, recurrent ischemic events, and recurrent VT, with a 5-year mortality rate that exceeds 30%. Attention to therapies with survival benefit, including β-adrenergic blocking agents, angiotensin-converting enzyme inhibitors, and statins (Chapter 73) is critical.

Nonischemic Dilated Cardiomyopathy

Sustained monomorphic VT associated with cardiomyopathy is usually due to areas of ventricular scar. The etiology of scar is often unclear, but progressive fibrosis is a potential cause. On magnetic resonance imaging, scars are detectable as areas of delayed gadolinium enhancement and are more often intramural or subepicardial in location compared with those in patients with prior MI. Scars that cause VT are often located adjacent to a valve annulus and can occur in either ventricle. Any cardiomyopathic process can cause scars and VT, but cardiac sarcoidosis (Chapters 60 and 95) and Chagas' disease (Chapter 355) are particularly associated with monomorphic VT. An ICD is usually warranted.**7** Antiarrhythmic drugs and catheter ablation are used to control recurrent episodes in patients with an ICD.

Arrhythmogenic Right Ventricular Cardiomyopathy

Arrhythmogenic right ventricular cardiomyopathy (ARVC) (Chapter 60) is a rare genetic disorder with an estimated prevalence of 1 in 5000. Patients typically present between the second and fifth decades with palpitations, syncope, or cardiac arrest owing to sustained monomorphic VT, although polymorphic VT can also occur. Most cases are due to genetic mutations involving desmosomal proteins, including plakoglobin, plakophilin-2, desmin, desmocollin, and desmoglein-2. Inheritance is usually autosomal dominant with variable penetrance. Fibrosis and fibrofatty replacement of right ventricular myocardium, and less often the left ventricle, provide the substrate for reentrant VT that usually has a left bundle branch block–like configuration, consistent with a right ventricular origin.

The sinus rhythm ECG suggests the disease in more than 90% of patients, most often showing T wave inversions in V_1 to V_3 (Fig. 65-8C). Delayed activation of the right ventricle may cause a widened QRS (≥110 msec) in the right precordial leads and a prolonged S wave upstroke in those leads. Cardiac imaging may show right ventricular enlargement or areas of abnormal motion, or reveal areas of scar on magnetic resonance imaging with gadolinium. Distinction from idiopathic right ventricular outflow tract VT can be difficult.

A

B

C

FIGURE 65-8. Sinus rhythm electrocardiogram findings in three genetic sudden death syndromes. **A,** QT prolongation during sinus rhythm in a patient with long QT syndrome. **B,** ST elevation in V_1 and V_2 in a patient with Brugada's syndrome. **C,** T wave inversion in V_1-V_3 in a patient with arrhythmogenic right ventricular dysplasia.

Left ventricular function is usually preserved, heart failure is rare, and survival to advanced age can be anticipated provided that VT can be controlled. An ICD is routinely recommended. When VT is exercise induced, it may respond to β-adrenergic blockers and prohibition of exercise. Sotalol, amiodarone, and catheter ablation have been used to reduce recurrences.

Tetralogy of Fallot
Ventricular tachycardia occurs in approximately 3 to 14% of patients late after repair of tetralogy of Fallot (Chapter 69) and contribute to a 2% per decade risk of sudden death. Factors associated with VT risk include age more than 5 years at repair, high-grade ventricular ectopy, inducible VT on an electrophysiologic study, abnormal right ventricular hemodynamics, and sinus rhythm QRS duration of more than 180 msec. An ICD is usually warranted for patients who have a spontaneous episode of VT, but criteria for a prophylactic ICD in other patients has not been established.

Bundle Branch Re-entry Ventricular Tachycardia
Re-entry through the Purkinje system occurs in approximately 5% of patients with monomorphic VT in the presence of structural heart disease. The re-entry circuit typically revolves retrograde up the left bundle and anterograde down the right bundle, thereby producing VT that has a left bundle branch block configuration. Catheter ablation of the right bundle branch abolishes this VT. Other scar-related VTs are often present and may require additional therapy.

IDIOPATHIC MONOMORPHIC VENTRICULAR TACHYCARDIA
CLINICAL MANIFESTATIONS AND DIAGNOSIS
Idiopathic VT in patients without structural heart disease usually presents with palpitations, lightheadedness, and occasionally syncope, often provoked by sympathetic stimulation during exercise or emotional upset. The QRS morphology of the arrhythmia suggests the diagnosis (see later). The sinus rhythm ECG is normal. Cardiac imaging shows normal ventricular function and no evidence of ventricular scar. Occasionally, a patient with structural heart disease is found to have concomitant idiopathic VT, unrelated to the structural disease. Sudden death is rare.

TREATMENT Rx

Treatment is required for symptoms or when frequent or incessant arrhythmias depress ventricular function. β-Adrenergic blockers are first-line therapy. Nondihydropyridine calcium-channel blockers (diltiazem and verapamil) are sometimes effective. Catheter ablation is warranted for severe symptoms or when β-blockers or calcium-channel blockers are not effective or not desired. Efficacy and risks of catheter ablation vary with the specific site of origin of the VT, being most favorable for arrhythmias originating in the right ventricular outflow tract.

Outflow tract VTs originate from a focus, usually with features consistent with triggered automaticity. The arrhythmia may present with sustained VT, nonsustained VT or PVCs, often provoked by exercise or emotional upset. Repeated bursts of nonsustained VT, which may occur incessantly, are known as repetitive monomorphic VT and can cause tachycardia-induced cardiomyopathy with depressed ventricular function that recovers after suppression of the arrhythmia.

Origin in the right ventricular outflow tract, which is the most common site of origin, gives rise to VT that has a left bundle branch block configuration in V_1 and an axis that is directed inferiorly, with tall R waves in leads II, III, and aVF (see Fig. 65-5). The arrhythmia can also arise in the left ventricular outflow tract or in sleeves of myocardium that extend along the aortic root. Left ventricular origin should be suspected when lead V_1 or V_2 has prominent R waves. Although the typical outflow tract QRS morphology favors idiopathic VT, cardiomyopathies can also cause PVCs or VT from this region; in such cases, management is the same as for arrhythmias in patients with structural heart disease (see earlier).

Left ventricular intrafascicular verapamil-sensitive VT arrhythmia presents with sustained VT that has a right bundle branch block–like configuration. It is often exercise induced and occurs more often in men than women. The mechanism is re-entry in or near the septal ramifications of the left ventricular Purkinje system. VT can be terminated by intravenous administration of verapamil, although chronic therapy with oral verapamil is not always effective. Catheter ablation is recommended if β-adrenergic blockers or calcium-channel blockers are ineffective or not desired.

TABLE 65-3 POLYMORPHIC VENTRICULAR TACHYCARDIA

ETIOLOGY	MECHANISM/CAUSES	CLINICAL FEATURES
Acute myocardial infarction/ischemia	Re-entry through the ischemic border zone	VT degenerating to VF, greatest risk during the first hour of infarction Common cause of sudden death
Ventricular hypertrophy, cardiomyopathy, heart failure, myocarditis	Multiple factors likely contribute (ion channel remodeling, abnormal calcium handling, ischemia)	Sudden death
Idiopathic VF		PVCs from the Purkinje system or RVOT initiating VF
Idiopathic VT with acquired QT prolongation	Early afterdepolarizations Bradycardia Hypokalemia, hypomagnesemia, hypocalcemia Antiarrhythmic drugs: disopyramide, dofetilide, ibutilide, procainamide, quinidine, sotalol, amiodarone (rare) Psychotropic drugs: haloperidol, droperidol, phenothiazines, pimozide, mesoridazine, tricyclic antidepressants Antibiotics: chloroquine, erythromycin, pentamidine, halofantrine, sparfloxacin, trimethoprim-sulfamethoxazole Other drugs: arsenic, methadone, others	Torsades de pointes causing syncope or cardiac arrest
GENETIC SUDDEN DEATH SYNDROMES		

Congenital long QT syndrome
  LQTS-1
  LQTS-2
  LQTS-3
	Abnormal gene and ion current
	  $KCNQ1$ Iks
	  $KCNQ2$ Ikr
	  $SCN5A$ Ina
		Sudden death or syncope due to torsades de pointes
		Events during swimming, exertion
		Events with emotional or auditory stimuli
		Events at rest and sleep

Short QT syndrome	Mutations affecting IKr, IKs, IK1	QTc < 320 msec
Brugada's syndrome	$SCN5A$ mutations affecting INa account for approximately 25% of cases	J-point elevation in leads V_1-V_3 Events at night, during fever
Catecholaminergic polymorphic VT	Mutations affecting the ryanodine receptor or calsequestrin	Events during exertion or emotional upset

LQTS = long QT syndrome; PVC = premature ventricular contraction; RVOT = right ventricular outflow tract; VF = ventricular fibrillation; VT = ventricular tachycardia.

● POLYMORPHIC VENTRICULAR TACHYCARDIA

Sustained polymorphic VT (see Fig. 65-4A) can be seen with any form of structural heart disease. However, unlike sustained monomorphic VT, polymorphic VT does not always indicate a structural abnormality or focus of automaticity. Re-entry with multiple or moving wave fronts, spiral wave re-entry (see Fig. 65-2), and multiple automatic foci are potential mechanisms. Sustained polymorphic VT usually degenerates rapidly into VF. Causes include acute MI or ischemia, ventricular hypertrophy, and a number of gene mutations that affect cardiac ion channels (Table 65-3).

Acute Myocardial Infarction and Ischemia

Acute MI or ischemia is a common cause of polymorphic VT and always should be considered immediately. Approximately 10% of patients with acute MI develop VT that degenerates to VF, related to re-entry through the infarct border zone. The risk is greatest in the first hour of acute MI. Following resuscitation (Chapter 63), management is as for acute MI (Chapter 73). β-Adrenergic blockers, intravenous amiodarone, and correction of hypokalemia and hypomagnesemia are warranted. Repeated episodes of polymorphic VT suggest ongoing myocardial ischemia and warrant assessment of whether coronary reperfusion has been re-established. Episodes that occur within the first 48 hours of acute MI do not necessarily confer a long-term risk, and long-term therapy usually is not required after recovery from the MI.

Acquired Long QT Syndrome

QT prolongation is associated with polymorphic VT that often has a characteristic waxing and waning QRS amplitude (see Fig. 65-4A) and is called *torsades de pointes* (twisting about the points). The VT often has a characteristic initiation sequence of PVCs that induces a pause, followed by a sinus beat that has a longer QT interval and interruption of the T wave by the PVC that is the first beat of the polymorphic VT. This characteristic initiation is called *pause dependent*. Causes of QT prolongation include electrolyte abnormalities, chronic bradycardia, and a large number of medications that block repolarizing potassium currents, notably the antiarrhythmic drugs sotalol, dofetilide, and ibutilide, but also a number of other medications used for noncardiac diseases, including erythromycin, pentamidine, haloperidol, phenothiazines, and methadone (see Table 65-3). Individual susceptibility may be related to genetic polymorphisms or mutations that influence repolarization.

Patients present with near-syncope, syncope, or cardiac arrest. Sustained episodes degenerate to VF requiring defibrillation. PVCs and nonsustained VT often precede episodes of sustained VT. Prevention of further episodes can usually be achieved by administration of 1 to 2 g of MgSO₄ intravenously. If bradycardia is present, the heart rate should be increased sufficiently to suppress PVCs, often to 100 beats per minute, with temporary pacing or administration of isoproterenol (starting at 1 μg/minute and titrating to the desired heart rate, up to 10 μg/minute). Rapid pacing in addition to MgSO₄ (1 to 2 g) administration is sometimes required. Potential contributing factors should be corrected, including removal of all medications that prolong the QT interval and correction of electrolyte abnormalities. Drug interactions that elevate levels of the offending agent are an important cause. Patients who experience a polymorphic VT induced by QT prolongation should be considered to have a susceptibility to the arrhythmia, and medications known to prolong the QT interval are contraindicated.

Congenital Long QT Syndrome

The congenital long QT syndrome (LQTS) is caused by mutations that interfere with ventricular repolarization, prolong the QT interval, and predispose to polymorphic VT. The syndrome is rare, with a prevalence of approximately 1 in 7000. The most frequently encountered mutations, LQTS-1 and -2 (see Table 65-3), cause abnormalities of potassium channels, but mutations affecting the sodium channel (LQTS-3) and calcium channels have also been described.

Patients present with syncope or cardiac arrest, often in childhood. In LQTS-1, episodes tend to occur during exertion, particularly swimming. In LQTS-2, sudden auditory stimuli or emotional upset predispose to events. Asymptomatic patients may be discovered in the course of family screening or on a routine ECG. Penetrance is variable, such that the QT interval is usually, but not always, prolonged to more than 0.44 second (see Fig. 65-8A). LQTS-1 responds well to chronic therapy with β-adrenergic blockers (e.g., nadolol, 0.5 to 3.5 mg/kg daily). ICDs are recommended for patients with arrhythmias despite β-adrenergic blocker therapy or other high-risk disease features, including a (QTc > 0.5 second). Family members of the proband should be screened with an ECG. The type of LQTS identified by genetic testing can help guide management decisions and family screening, but the clinical utility of genotype-phenotype correlations are still being defined. All mutations have not been identified, and failure to identify a known mutation does not exclude the syndrome.

Brugada's Syndrome and Other Repolarization Syndromes

Brugada's syndrome is a rare familial syndrome characterized on the ECG by more than 0.2 mV of ST segment elevation with a coved ST segment and negative T wave in more than one anterior precordial lead (V_1 to V_3) (see Fig. 65-8B) and clinically by episodes of polymorphic VT that present as syncope or cardiac arrest in the absence of structural heart disease. Cardiac arrest may occur during sleep or be provoked by febrile illness. Males are more commonly affected than females. Mutations involving cardiac sodium channels are identified in approximately 25% of cases. Distinction from patients with similar ST elevation owing to left ventricular hypertrophy, pericarditis (Chapter 77), myocardial ischemia or MI (Chapter 72), hyperkalemia (Chapter 119), hypothermia (Chapter 109), right bundle branch block (see Fig. 54-8B in Chapter 54), and ARVC is often difficult. Furthermore, the characteristic ST segment elevation can wax and wane over time. Administration of sodium-channel blocking drugs, such as flecainide, causes further ST elevation in affected individuals. An ICD is recommended. Quinidine has been used successfully to suppress frequent VT.

The short QT syndrome is a very rare familial disorder characterized by a short QTc interval (<0.32) and susceptibility to polymorphic VT and sudden death due to mutations involving cardiac potassium channels. Rare patients with idiopathic polymorphic VT and VF associated with ST elevation in inferior and lateral ECG leads have been reported. This type of ECG pattern, known as *early repolarization,* can also be a normal variant.

Catecholaminergic Polymorphic Ventricular Tachycardia

This rare familial syndrome causes exercise-induced PVCs, a characteristic VT with alternating QRS morphologies termed *bidirectional tachycardia,* polymorphic VT, and VF. Mutations involving the cardiac ryanodine receptor and calsequestrin are identified causes. Patients usually present during childhood with exercise- or emotion-induced palpitations, syncope, or cardiac arrest. β-Adrenergic blockers (e.g., nadolol, 1 to 2 mg/kg/day, or propranolol, 2.5 to 3.5 mg/kg/day) and an implantable defibrillator are recommended. Verapamil (240 to 480 mg daily), or flecainide (50 to 100 mg twice daily), or surgical left cardiac sympathetic denervation reduces or prevents recurrent VT in some patients.

● VENTRICULAR FIBRILLATION

VF is characterized by disordered electrical ventricular activation without identifiable QRS complexes (see Fig. 65-4C). Spiral wave re-entry (see Fig. 65-2) and multiple circulating re-entry wave fronts are possible mechanisms. Sustained polymorphic or monomorphic VT that degenerates to VF is a common cause of out-of-hospital cardiac arrest. Treatment follows ACLS guidelines (Chapters 7 and 63), with defibrillation to restore sinus rhythm. If resuscitation is successful, further evaluation is performed to identify and treat underlying heart disease and potential causes of the arrhythmia, including the possibility that VF was initiated by monomorphic or polymorphic VT. If a transient reversible cause, such as acute MI, is not identified, therapy to reduce the risk of sudden death is often warranted. An ICD is often warranted provided the patient has reasonable expectation for survival over the following year with acceptable functional capacity. Chronic amiodarone therapy may be considered for individuals who are not ICD candidates.**3**

● INCESSANT VENTRICULAR TACHYCARDIA AND ELECTRICAL STORM

VT is incessant when it continues to recur shortly after electrical, pharmacologic, or spontaneous conversion to sinus rhythm. "VT storm" or "electrical storm" refers to three or more separate episodes of VT within 24 hours. Slow incessant VT is sometimes asymptomatic, but it can cause heart failure or tachycardia-induced cardiomyopathy. More commonly, these presentations are life-threatening and require emergent therapy. Measures to reduce sympathetic tone, including β-adrenergic blockade, sedation, and general anesthesia, have been used effectively. Intravenous administration of amiodarone can be effective. Urgent catheter ablation can be life-saving. Rare patients with idiopathic VF due to rapid polymorphic VT from the Purkinje system

or outflow tract in the absence of heart disease benefit from catheter ablation of the initiating focus.

● VENTRICULAR ARRHYTHMIAS IN PATIENTS WITH IMPLANTABLE DEFIBRILLATORS

ICDs effectively terminate VT when it occurs and markedly reduce the risk of death from arrhythmias. ICDs do not, however, prevent the arrhythmia. ICDs can be programmed to provide antitachycardia pacing in an attempt to terminate VT by rapid pacing (Fig. 65-9B), which is painless and often asymptomatic. If antitachycardia pacing fails or is not a programmed treatment for rapid VT or VF, an ICD shock is administered. Interrogation of the ICD, which commonly can be performed remotely and communicated by the Internet, allows assessment of any arrhythmias detected by the ICD and of therapies delivered (Fig. 65-9).

Despite effective termination of VT by the ICD, the occurrence of VT predicts an increased risk of mortality and heart failure. VT episodes can be evidence of deteriorating heart failure or myocardial ischemia. Evaluation for progression of heart disease and optimization of medical therapy are warranted.

ICD shocks are painful, reduce quality of life, and can cause post-traumatic stress syndrome. Patients with recurrent episodes of symptomatic VT warrant therapy to prevent episodes. Amiodarone is more effective than β-adrenergic blockers or sotalol.**5** Changes in antiarrhythmic drug therapy can alter the VT rate and the energy required for defibrillation, thereby necessitating programming changes in the ICD algorithms for detection and therapy. Catheter ablation reduces episodes of VT in more than 70% of patients with monomorphic VT.**6**

● ANTIARRHYTHMIC DRUGS FOR VENTRICULAR ARRHYTHMIAS

Use of antiarrhythmic drugs (see Table 64-5 in Chapter 64 for dosing) is based on consideration of the risks and potential benefit for individual patients. Many drugs have the potential to induce "proarrhythmia," thereby increasing the frequency of the arrhythmia or causing a new arrhythmia, such as torsades de pointes for QT interval–prolonging drugs.

β-Adrenergic Blockers

Many ventricular arrhythmias are sensitive to sympathetic stimulation, and β-adrenergic stimulation also diminishes the electrophysiologic effects of many antiarrhythmic drugs. The safety of β-blocking agents makes them the first choice of therapy for most ventricular arrhythmias. They are particularly effective for exercise-induced arrhythmias and idiopathic arrhythmias. Bradyarrhythmias are the major cardiac toxicity.

Calcium-Channel Blockers

The nondihydropyridine calcium-channel blockers diltiazem and verapamil can be effective for ventricular arrhythmias and for some idiopathic ventricular arrhythmias.

Sodium-Channel Blockers

Antiarrhythmic drugs with prominent sodium-channel blocking effects can suppress ventricular arrhythmias. Mexiletine, quinidine, disopyramide, flecainide, and propafenone are available for chronic oral therapy. Quinidine, disopyramide, and procainamide also have potassium-channel blocking effects that prolong the QT interval. These agents have potential proarrhythmic effects and, with the possible exception of quinidine, also have negative inotropic effects that may contribute to the increased mortality observed in patients with prior MI. Long-term therapy is generally avoided in patients with structural heart disease but may be used to reduce symptomatic arrhythmias in some patients with ICDs. Lidocaine and procainamide can be used for acute intravenous therapy.

Potassium-Channel Blockers

Sotalol and dofetilide block the delayed rectifier potassium channel IKr, thereby prolonging the QT interval. Sotalol also has nonselective β-adrenergic blocking activity. Sotalol has been shown to reduce ICD shocks, but it is less effective than amiodarone for this purpose.**5** Proarrhythmia with torsades de pointes occurs in 3% of patients. These drugs are excreted by the kidney, so dose adjustment is required according to renal function. These drugs must be avoided in patients with other risk factors for torsades de pointes, including QT prolongation and hypokalemia.

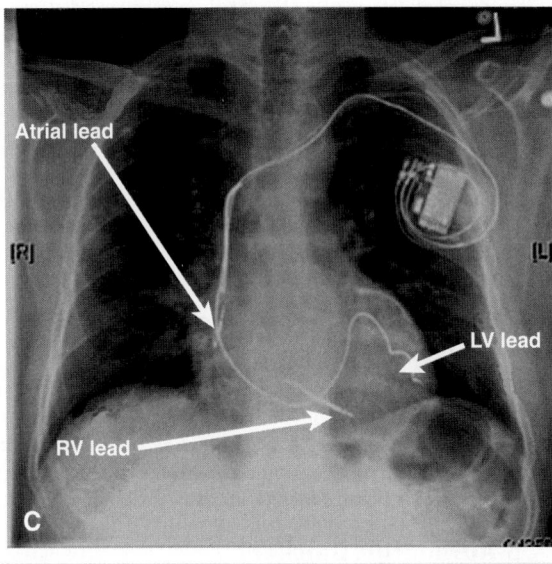

FIGURE 65-9. Implantable cardioverter-defibrillator (ICD). **A,** An electrocardiogram (ECG) tracing of sustained monomorphic ventricular tachycardia (VT) terminated by a shock from an ICD. **B,** Two-lead ECG tracing showing sustained monomorphic VT that is detected by the implanted ICD. A burst of rapid pacing terminates VT. The ICD then provides atrioventricular (A-V) pacing to prevent bradyarrhythmia. **C,** Anterior-posterior radiograph showing an ICD that incorporates a lead to the right atrium, right ventricular (RV) apex, and through the coronary sinus to an epicardial vein over the lateral left ventricle (LV). The pulse generator is evident in the left infraclavicular region.

Amiodarone and Dronedarone

Amiodarone, which blocks multiple cardiac ionic currents and has sympatholytic activity, suppresses a variety of ventricular arrhythmias. It is administered intravenously for life-threatening arrhythmias. During chronic oral therapy, electrophysiologic effects develop over several days, depending on dosing. It is more effective than sotalol in reducing ICD shocks and is the preferred drug in patients who are not candidates for an ICD.**3,5** Bradyarrhythmia is the major cardiac adverse effect. Ventricular proarrhythmia can occur, but torsades de pointes is uncommon. Noncardiac toxicities contribute to drug discontinuation in approximately one third of patients during long-term therapy. Pneumonitis or pulmonary fibrosis occurs in approximately 1% of patients. Photosensitivity is common, and neuropathy and ocular toxicity can occur. Systematic monitoring is recommended during chronic therapy: assessment for thyroid and liver toxicity with thyroid-stimulating hormone and aminotransferase levels every 6 months, and lung toxicity with a chest radiograph and determination of lung diffusing capacity annually. In a randomized study, dronedarone, which is related to amiodarone but without iodine in it, resulted in a 2.13-fold increase in mortality in patients with heart failure.**8**

1. Goldenberg I, Gillespie J, Moss AJ, et al. Long-term benefit of primary prevention with an implantable cardioverter-defibrillator: an extended 8-year follow-up study of the Multicenter Automatic Defibrillator Implantation Trial II. *Circulation.* 2010;122:1265-1271.
2. Steinbeck G, Andresen D, Seidl K, et al. Defibrillator implantation early after myocardial infarction. *N Engl J Med.* 2009;361:1427-1436.
3. Piccini JP, Berger JS, O'Connor CM. Amiodarone for the prevention of sudden cardiac death: a meta-analysis of randomized controlled trials. *Eur Heart J.* 2009;30:1245-1253.
4. Bardy GH, Lee KL, Mark DB, et al. Amiodarone or an implantable cardioverter-defibrillator for congestive heart failure. *N Engl J Med.* 2005;352:225-237.
5. Connolly SJ, Dorian P, Roberts RS, et al. Comparison of beta-blockers, amiodarone plus beta-blockers, or sotalol for prevention of shocks from implantable cardioverter defibrillators. The OPTIC Study: a randomized trial. *JAMA.* 2006;295:165-171.
6. Kuck KH, Schaumann A, Eckardt L, et al. Catheter ablation of stable ventricular tachycardia before defibrillator implantation in patients with coronary heart disease (VTACH): a multicentre randomized controlled trial. *Lancet.* 2010;375:4-6.
7. Kadish A, Dyer A, Daubert JP, et al. Prophylactic defibrillator implantation in patients with non-ischemic dilated cardiomyopathy. *N Engl J Med.* 2004;350:2151-2158.
8. Kober L, Torp-Pedersen C, McMurray JJ, et al. Increased mortality after dronedarone therapy for severe heart failure. *N Engl J Med.* 2008;358:2678-2687.

SUGGESTED READINGS

Aliot EM, Stevenson WG, Almendral-Garrote JM, et al. EHRA/HRS Expert consensus on catheter ablation of ventricular arrhythmias. *Heart Rhythm.* 2009;6:886-933. *Consensus statement on outcomes and risks.*

Heist EK, Ruskin JN. Drug-induced arrhythmia. *Circulation.* 2010;122:1426-1435. *Review.*

Jacobson JT, Weiner JB. Management of ventricular tachycardia in patients with structural heart disease. *Cardiovasc Ther.* 2010;28:225-263. *Review.*

Manuchehry A, Agusala K, Montevecchi M, et al. Ventricular tachyarrhythmias in patients receiving an implantable cardioverter-defibrillator for primary versus secondary prophylaxis indications. *Pacing Clin Electrophysiol.* 2011. [Epub ahead of print.] *Monomorphic VT is the most common cause of appropriate ICD therapy regardless of implant indication thereby suggesting it is the most common trigger of SCD.*

Probst V, Veltmann C, Eckardt L, et al. Long-term prognosis of patients diagnosed with Brugada syndrome: results from the FINGER Brugada Syndrome Registry. *Circulation.* 2010;121:635-643. *The rate of cardiac events at 32-month follow-up was 7.7% in patients with aborted SCD, 1.9% in patients with syncope, and 0.5% in patients with no symptoms.*

Vest RN 3rd, Gold MR. Risk stratification of ventricular arrhythmias in patients with systolic heart failure. *Curr Opin Cardiol.* 2010;25:268-275. *Emphasizes that symptomatic heart failure is the most powerful predictor of sudden cardiac death from ventricular arrhythmias.*

ELECTROPHYSIOLOGIC INTERVENTIONAL PROCEDURES AND SURGERY

FRED MORADY

PACEMAKERS

Pacemaker Generators and Leads

Pacemaker batteries, which are lithium iodide cells that typically have a lifespan of 7 to 8 years, now often weigh less than 30 g. They are usually implanted subcutaneously in the infraclavicular area (Fig. 66-1). The programmability of many different variables has become standard, as has the ability of the pacemaker to provide diagnostic and telemetric data.

Pacemaker leads are generally bipolar, with the distal electrode serving as the cathode. Unipolar leads are less commonly used because of the potential for pacing chest wall muscles and for inhibition of pacing by skeletal muscle myopotentials. The leads are inserted into the heart either percutaneously through a subclavian vein or by cutdown into a cephalic vein. Atrial leads are usually positioned in the right atrial appendage, and ventricular leads are placed in the right ventricular apex. Fixation to the myocardium is achieved either passively with tines or actively with a screw mechanism. Newer lead

FIGURE 66-1. Site of implantation of a permanent pacemaker or automatic implantable cardioverter-defibrillator. The pacemaker is usually implanted in the left pectoral region, but it may be placed elsewhere if necessary. (From Forbes CD, Jackson WF. *Color Atlas and Text of Clinical Medicine*, 3rd ed. London: Mosby; 2003.)

and electrode designs, such as high-impedance leads and carbon-tipped electrodes, have resulted in lower acute and chronic pacing thresholds.

Pacing Modes

The mode of pacing is described in shorthand fashion by a three- to five-letter code. The first letter designates the chamber being paced (A for atrium, V for ventricle, D for dual chamber); the second letter designates the chamber in which the depolarizations are sensed by the pacemaker (A, V, D, or O for no sensing); the third letter designates whether the pacemaker functions in an inhibited (I) or tracking mode (T), in both modes (D), or asynchronously (O); and the fourth letter indicates whether the pacemaker is capable of rate modulation independent of atrial activity. An additional fifth letter may be used to designate the capability for antitachycardia pacing (P), delivery of shocks (S), or both (D). The most commonly used pacing modes are VVI (pacing and sensing within the ventricle in inhibited fashion), VVIR (VVI plus rate responsiveness), and DDD (pacing and sensing of the atrium and ventricle in both inhibited and tracking fashion).

The most appropriate pacing mode must always be determined on an individual basis, the goal being to meet the patient's physiologic needs with the simplest system possible. For example, in a patient with chronic atrial fibrillation who has symptomatic pauses but not chronotropic incompetence, a VVI pacemaker is sufficient. However, if the patient also has chronotropic incompetence, a VVIR pacemaker is necessary to restore a normal rate response to exercise. In a patient with a high-degree atrioventricular (AV) block and normal sinus node function, DDD pacing is optimal. However, if a patient with a high-degree AV block also has sinus node dysfunction, the ideal pacing mode is DDDR.

In patients who have paroxysmal atrial fibrillation and a high-degree AV block, no single pacing mode is optimal. DDD pacing is ideal when the patient is in sinus rhythm, but during atrial fibrillation, DDD pacing may result in tracking of the atrium at the upper rate limit of the pacemaker. Conversely, VVIR pacing, which is ideal during atrial fibrillation, will not provide AV synchrony during periods of sinus rhythm. The development of mode-switching pacemakers has solved this dilemma. Mode-switching pacemakers are capable of pacing in the DDD mode during sinus rhythm and automatically switching to rate-responsive ventricular pacing during atrial fibrillation or other supraventricular arrhythmias (Fig. 66-2).

The choice between ventricular (VVIR) and atrial (AAIR) or dual-chamber (DDDR) pacing remains controversial. Although a randomized trial of 225 patients with sinus node dysfunction reported a significant reduction in cardiovascular death at 8 years with AAIR versus VVIR pacing,[1] studies of nearly 5000 patients have shown no survival differences when patients were randomized to DDDR or VVIR pacing. Dual-chamber pacing, like atrial pacing, reduces the incidence of atrial fibrillation and appears to result in slightly better quality of life.[2] In these randomized trials, 5 to 25% of patients who initially received VVIR pacemakers "crossed over" to DDDR pacing because of physician-diagnosed pacemaker syndrome (see Complications of Pacemakers).

Several studies have demonstrated that the ventricular dyssynchrony induced by right ventricular pacing may have deleterious effects on ventricular function and functional capacity and may also predispose to the development of atrial fibrillation. Therefore, pacemakers should always be programmed to minimize the amount of ventricular pacing.

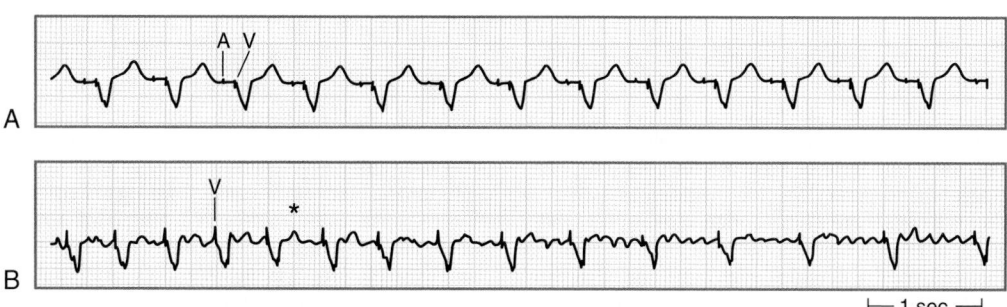

FIGURE 66-2. Rhythm strips from a Holter monitor in a patient with complete atrioventricular block, sinus bradycardia, paroxysmal atrial fibrillation, and a rate-responsive dual-chamber pacemaker with mode-switching capability. **A,** When the patient is in sinus rhythm, the pacemaker functions in a DDDR mode, with synchronized atrial and ventricular pacing at 105 beats per minute while the patient is walking. **B,** At the onset of an episode of atrial fibrillation, there is tracking of the atrium that results in ventricular pacing at 140 beats per minute, which is the upper rate limit of the pacemaker. Within 2 seconds *(asterisk),* the mode-switch feature results in VVIR pacing, and the ventricular pacing rate gradually falls to 70 beats per minute, which is the lowest rate limit of the pacemaker. A = atrial stimulus; V = ventricular stimulus.

TABLE 66-1 CLASS I INDICATIONS* FOR IMPLANTATION OF A PERMANENT PACEMAKER

SINUS NODE DYSFUNCTION

1. Symptomatic sinus bradycardia
2. Symptomatic chronotropic incompetence
3. Symptomatic sinus bradycardia resulting from required drug therapy

ATRIOVENTRICULAR (AV) BLOCK

1. Third-degree and advanced second-degree AV block associated with symptomatic bradycardia
2. Third-degree and advanced second-degree AV block in an awake patient with asystole of >3 seconds or an escape rate of <40 beats per minute or with an infranodal escape rhythm
3. Atrial fibrillation with a pause of ≥5 seconds
4. Third-degree and advanced second-degree AV block due to postoperative AV block that is not expected to resolve
5. Third-degree and advanced second-degree AV block with neuromuscular diseases such as myotonic muscular dystrophy, Kearns-Sayre syndrome, and Erb dystrophy
6. Asymptomatic third-degree AV block if cardiomegaly or left ventricular dysfunction is present, or if the block is below the AV node

CHRONIC BIFASCICULAR BLOCK

1. Advanced second-degree or intermittent third-degree AV block
2. Type II second-degree AV block
3. Alternating bundle branch block

AFTER ACUTE PHASE OF MYOCARDIAL INFARCTION

1. Second-degree infranodal AV block with alternating bundle branch block
2. Third-degree infranodal AV block
3. Transient advanced second-degree or third-degree infranodal AV block and associated bundle branch block
4. Persistent symptomatic second-degree or third-degree AV block

CAROTID SINUS SYNDROME

1. Recurrent syncope caused by spontaneous carotid sinus stimulation or carotid sinus pressure that induces asystole of >3 seconds in duration

*Class I indications are conditions for which a pacemaker is indicated.
Adapted from Epstein AE, DiMarco JP, Ellenbogen KA, et al. ACC/AHA/HRS 2008 guidelines for device-based therapy of cardiac rhythm abnormalities: executive summary. *J Am Coll Cardiol.* 2008;51:2085-2105.

TABLE 66-2 CLASS IIA INDICATIONS* FOR IMPLANTATION OF A PERMANENT PACEMAKER

SINUS NODE DYSFUNCTION

1. Heart rate of <40 beats per minute when a clear association between symptoms consistent with bradycardia and the actual presence of bradycardia has not been demonstrated
2. Syncope of unclear etiology when sinus node dysfunction is demonstrated by electrophysiologic testing

ATRIOVENTRICULAR (AV) BLOCK

1. Persistent third-degree AV block with an escape rate of >40 beats per minute in an asymptomatic adult without cardiomegaly
2. Asymptomatic second-degree infranodal AV block
3. First-degree or second-degree AV block associated with symptoms similar to pacemaker syndrome
4. Asymptomatic type II second-degree AV block with a narrow QRS

CHRONIC BIFASCICULAR BLOCK

1. Syncope, when other potential causes of syncope have been excluded
2. An HV interval of ≥100 msec
3. Pathologic pacing-induced infranodal AV block during electrophysiologic testing

CAROTID SINUS SYNDROME

1. Syncope without clear provocative events and with asystole of >3 seconds during carotid sinus pressure

*Class IIA indications are conditions for which a pacemaker is reasonable.
Adapted from Epstein AE, DiMarco JP, Ellenbogen KA, et al. ACC/AHA/HRS 2008 guidelines for device-based therapy of cardiac rhythm abnormalities: executive summary. *J Am Coll Cardiol.* 2008;51:2085-2105.

Indications for a Permanent Pacemaker

In general, pacemakers are implanted either to alleviate symptoms caused by bradycardia or to prevent severe symptoms in patients in whom symptomatic bradycardia is likely to develop (Tables 66-1 and 66-2). The most common bradycardia-induced symptoms are dizziness or lightheadedness, syncope or near-syncope (Chapters 50 and 62), exercise intolerance, and symptoms of heart failure. Because these symptoms are nonspecific, documentation of an association between symptoms and bradycardia should be obtained before pacemaker implantation. If the bradycardia is persistent, such as in a patient with a complete AV block, a simple electrocardiogram may be sufficient to document the need for a pacemaker. If the bradycardia is intermittent, other diagnostic testing, such as 24-hour ambulatory monitoring, a continuous loop recorder, an implantable event monitor, or an electrophysiology test (Chapter 62), may be needed to document a relationship between symptoms and bradycardia.

After a symptomatic bradycardia has been documented, a correctable cause for the bradycardia should be excluded before a pacemaker is implanted. Correctable causes of symptomatic bradycardia include hypothyroidism, an overdose with drugs such as digitalis, electrolyte disturbances, and several categories of medications, most commonly β-adrenergic blocking agents (administered either orally or in the form of eyedrops for glaucoma), calcium-channel blocking agents, and antiarrhythmic medications (Chapter 64). At times, a pacemaker is necessary to allow continued treatment with a medication that is responsible for the bradycardia, such as in a patient in whom symptomatic sinus bradycardia develops after initiation of therapy with a β-adrenergic blocking agent for paroxysmal atrial fibrillation associated with a rapid ventricular response.

Complications of Pacemakers

Complications related to the implantation procedure occur in less than 2% of patients and include pneumothorax, perforation of the atrium or ventricle,

lead dislodgement, infection, and erosion of the pacemaker pocket. Thrombosis of the subclavian vein occurs in 10 to 20% of patients and is more likely in the presence of multiple leads; it rarely causes symptoms.

Pacemaker-mediated tachycardia is a possible complication of DDD pacing when the atrial lead senses retrograde depolarizations because of ventriculoatrial conduction. The resulting tachycardia often has a rate equal to the upper rate limit of the pacemaker. Pacemaker-mediated tachycardia can be eliminated by various reprogramming maneuvers, such as lengthening of the postventriculoatrial refractory period. Patients with dual-chamber pacemakers for sinus node disease are at risk for future atrial fibrillation. In a randomized study, minimizing dual-chamber ventricular pacing reduced the risk of atrial fibrillation by 40%.[3]

The pacemaker syndrome consists of symptoms of weakness, lightheadedness, exercise intolerance, or palpitations caused by the absence of AV synchrony during ventricular pacing. It is treated by restoring AV synchrony with DDD pacing or, if AV conduction is intact, with AAI pacing. During long-term follow-up after pacemaker implantation, potential problems include failure to pace, failure to capture, and changes in the pacing rate. These problems may be a manifestation of suboptimal programming, fracture of a lead or a break in the insulation, generator malfunction, or battery depletion.

Temporary Pacemakers

Temporary pacemaker leads are generally inserted percutaneously into an internal jugular or subclavian vein or by cutdown into a brachial vein and then positioned under fluoroscopic guidance in the right ventricular apex and attached to an external generator. Temporary pacing is used to stabilize patients awaiting permanent pacemaker implantation, to correct a transient symptomatic bradycardia caused by drug toxicity or a metabolic defect, or to suppress torsades de pointes by maintaining a rate of 85 to 100 beats per minute until the causative factor has been eliminated. Temporary pacing may also be used in prophylactic fashion in patients at risk for symptomatic bradycardia during a surgical procedure or high-degree AV block in the setting of an acute myocardial infarction. The most common complication of temporary pacemakers is infection; this risk is minimized by limiting the use of a pacemaker lead to 48 hours. In emergency situations, ventricular pacing can be instituted immediately by transcutaneous pacing with electrode pads applied to the chest wall.

TRANSTHORACIC CARDIOVERSION AND DEFIBRILLATION

Mechanism of Action

Direct current defibrillators store an electrical charge and discharge it across two paddle electrodes in a damped, sinusoidal waveform. The shock terminates arrhythmias caused by re-entry by simultaneously depolarizing large portions of the atria or ventricles, thereby causing the re-entry circuits to extinguish (Chapters 61, 64, and 65).

A nonsynchronized shock that is delivered coincident with the T wave during supraventricular tachycardia (SVT) or ventricular tachycardia (VT) may precipitate ventricular fibrillation (VF). *Cardioversion* refers to the termination of SVT or VT by delivery of a shock in synchrony with the QRS complex. When shocks are delivered to terminate VF, synchronization to the QRS complex is not necessary, and this process is referred to as *defibrillation.*

Technique

Whenever cardioversion or defibrillation is performed on an elective basis, the patient should be in a fasting state. Intravenous access to a peripheral vein should be established, and oxygen, suction, and equipment needed for airway management should be readily available. Transthoracic shocks are painful, and drugs commonly used for anesthesia or amnesia include short-acting barbiturates such as methohexital or a short-acting amnestic agent such as midazolam. In the anteroapical configuration, one electrode is positioned to the right of the sternum at the level of the second intercostal space, and the second electrode is positioned at the midaxillary line, lateral to the apical impulse. In the anteroposterior configuration, an electrode is placed to the left of the sternum at the fourth intercostal space, and the second electrode is positioned posteriorly, to the left of the spine, at the same level as the anterior electrode. These two-electrode configurations result in similar success rates of cardioversion and defibrillation.

Important variables affecting the success of cardioversion or defibrillation are the shock waveform and shock strength. Defibrillators that deliver biphasic shocks are now clinically available and have a significantly higher success rate than conventional defibrillators. Other technique-dependent variables that maximize delivery of energy to the heart include firm paddle pressure, delivery of the shock during expiration, and repetitive shocks. Patient-related variables that may decrease the probability of successful cardioversion and defibrillation include metabolic disturbances, long arrhythmia duration, some antiarrhythmic drugs such as amiodarone, and body weight in excess of 80 kg.

Because cardioversion of atrial fibrillation (Chapter 64) may be complicated by thromboembolism, anticoagulation with warfarin is generally necessary for 3 weeks before cardioversion and for 1 month after cardioversion whenever atrial fibrillation has been present for 48 hours or longer. The 3-week period of anticoagulation before cardioversion can be eliminated if no atrial thrombi are seen on a transesophageal echocardiogram, but anticoagulation for 1 month after cardioversion is still necessary to prevent thrombus formation secondary to transient, postconversion atrial stunning.

Indications

The most common arrhythmias treated by cardioversion and defibrillation are VF, VT, atrial fibrillation, and atrial flutter (Chapters 63, 64, and 65). Treatment of VF is always an emergency, and a 200-J shock should be delivered as quickly as possible, followed by one or more 360-J shocks if necessary. Depending on the patient's hemodynamic status, cardioversion of VT may be performed electively or on an emergency basis; if elective, an initial shock strength of 50 J is appropriate, followed by higher energy levels if additional shocks are needed. An initial energy level of 50 J is appropriate for cardioversion of atrial flutter. In atrial fibrillation, in which cardioversion is generally performed on an elective basis, an initial shock of 100 to 200 J is appropriate, depending on the patient's body weight. Shocks of 300 to 360 J are then used if necessary. If atrial fibrillation must be treated on an urgent basis, for example, in a patient with Wolff-Parkinson-White syndrome who has a very rapid ventricular rate and hemodynamic compromise, an initial shock of 200 J should be followed by 360-J shocks, as needed. Because the defibrillation energy requirement is a probability function and not a discrete value, subsequent shocks may be effective for cardioversion and defibrillation even when the first 360-J shock is ineffective.

Complications

Asynchronous shocks may precipitate VF. Rarely, VF may occur even when shocks are synchronized to the QRS complex. The risk for post-shock ventricular arrhythmias is increased in the presence of a supratherapeutic plasma concentration of digitalis, so cardioversion in patients with digitalis toxicity should be avoided.

Transient ST segment elevation may occur after cardioversion and is usually of no clinical consequence. Mild myocardial necrosis may occasionally occur if a total energy exceeding 425 J is delivered in a short period. Another rare complication of cardioversion is pulmonary edema, which may be due to transient left ventricular dysfunction.

Post-shock bradycardia or asystole may occur because of vagal discharge or an underlying sick sinus syndrome. At times, atropine or emergency transcutaneous pacing may be necessary. In patients who have a pacemaker or implantable cardioverter-defibrillator (ICD), the shocking electrodes should be positioned as far away from the generator as possible, and the generator and pacing threshold should be checked afterward.

IMPLANTABLE CARDIOVERTER-DEFIBRILLATORS

ICD Pulse Generators and Leads

ICDs now weigh as little as 60 g, are multiprogrammable, have improved detection algorithms, are capable of antitachycardia and antibradycardia (including dual-chamber) pacing, can deliver biphasic shocks at strengths of less than 1 to 42 J, and provide a record of the electrograms recorded during arrhythmic episodes. With the development of pulse generators small enough to implant in the infraclavicular area and endocardial leads that are inserted transvenously, the implantation procedure has been greatly simplified and is now very similar to that for permanent pacemakers.

ICDs that deliver shocks to terminate atrial fibrillation, as well as VT and VF, are clinically available. Biventricular ICDs are available for patients who need an ICD and have advanced (class III or IV) heart failure and a bundle branch block.

A single lead that contains a pacing-sensing electrode and two defibrillating coils can be used. If adequate defibrillation is not achieved with a single-lead configuration, a subcutaneous patch electrode or subcutaneous array can be added. In another commonly used configuration, the pulse generator itself functions as an electrode, and a lead that has a pacing-sensing electrode at its tip and a distal defibrillating coil electrode is positioned at the right ventricular apex. Multiple other combinations of a chest wall patch electrode and defibrillating electrodes in the right ventricular apex, superior vena cava, or coronary sinus can also be used. When a biventricular ICD is implanted, a lead is inserted into a branch of the coronary sinus for left ventricular pacing.

Indications

ICDs have become first-line therapy in patients who have survived an episode of VF not associated with acute myocardial infarction or who have had an episode of hemodynamically significant, sustained VT (Chapter 65).[4] ICDs are also implanted in individuals at high risk for cardiac arrest, including patients with idiopathic, dilated cardiomyopathy and unexplained syncope or patients with coronary artery disease (CAD), an ejection fraction of less than 35%, spontaneous episodes of nonsustained VT, and inducible sustained VT in the electrophysiology laboratory (Chapter 65).[5] Based on the results of large-scale clinical trials, the indications for implantation of an ICD include patients with a previous myocardial infarction and an ejection fraction of 30% or less, as well as patients with dilated cardiomyopathy (ischemic or nonischemic), an ejection fraction of 35% or less, and class II or III heart failure.[6-8]

Programming of ICDs

Testing is performed at the time of implantation to determine the energy requirement for defibrillation. A safety margin of at least 10 J should be present; for example, if the maximum output of the pulse generator is 32 J, successful defibrillation should be achieved with shocks of 22 J or less in strength. If the patient has had episodes of VT, antitachycardia pacing can be evaluated and programmed as needed to terminate the VT. Appropriate programming of the device is performed during predischarge testing.

With ICDs that are tiered-therapy devices, as many as two VT zones and one VF zone are available to provide individualized therapy for ventricular arrhythmias that have different rates. The rate threshold and various sequences of antitachycardia pacing and low- or high-energy shocks can be programmed for each of the two VT zones. The VF zone is a high-rate zone in which high-energy shocks are delivered. Optimal programming is important for many reasons, including minimizing patient discomfort, reducing the chance of

FIGURE 66-3. Examples of stored electrograms obtained several hours after three different patients had experienced a flurry of shocks from an implantable cardioverter-defibrillator and showing the rhythm recorded by the device immediately before a shock was delivered. **A,** In this patient, the stored electrogram demonstrates ventricular tachycardia at a rate of 300 beats per minute, thus indicating that the shock was appropriate. He was treated with amiodarone to reduce the frequency of episodes of ventricular tachycardia. **B,** This patient received shocks because of paroxysmal supraventricular tachycardia at a rate of 206 beats per minute, which exceeded the programmed rate cutoff of 170 beats per minute. He underwent radio frequency ablation of the paroxysmal supraventricular tachycardia and received no further inappropriate shocks. **C,** The stored electrograms in this patient indicate that the patient received inappropriate shocks that were triggered by atrial fibrillation at a rate of 180 beats per minute. The rate cutoff of the device in this patient was 150 beats per minute. This patient was treated with a β-blocker to keep the ventricular rate less than 150 beats per minute during atrial fibrillation.

syncope with an arrhythmia episode, maximizing the battery life of the pulse generator, and preventing inappropriate shocks.

Complications

Complications related to the implantation procedure include pneumothorax, myocardial perforation, and infection, all of which should have an incidence of less than 1%. Complications associated with the subcutaneous or submuscular pocket into which the device is placed include hematoma formation and erosion of the pocket. The endocardial leads that are used in the ICD system occasionally become dislodged shortly after implantation, thus necessitating a second procedure to reposition the leads. Other lead complications include fracture or breakdown of the insulation, either of which may result in failure to defibrillate. Fracture of a lead may also result in an artifact that mimics VF and triggers inappropriate shocks.

Patients who have an ICD do not require evaluation every time that they experience a device discharge. However, urgent evaluation is necessary if the patient experiences flurries of discharges. Analysis of stored electrograms often reveals the underlying problem (Fig. 66-3). The frequent shocks may be appropriate shocks triggered by flurries of VT or VF; if a correctable cause such as a metabolic defect or proarrhythmic drug cannot be identified, antiarrhythmic drug therapy or catheter ablation, or both, should be used to eliminate these arrhythmia flurries. Flurries of shocks may be triggered by atrial fibrillation with a rapid ventricular response, in which case aggressive management of the atrial fibrillation is indicated. In addition, flurries of shocks may be a manifestation of a lead fracture, in which case lead replacement is necessary.

● RADIO FREQUENCY CATHETER ABLATION

Tissue Effects of Radio Frequency Energy

Radio frequency ablation is a percutaneous catheter technique that can permanently eliminate a variety of SVTs and VTs that previously required either chronic pharmacologic treatment for suppression or surgery for cure. Radio frequency energy is delivered through an electrode catheter whose tip is in contact with tissue that is critical to maintenance of the tachycardia. The radio frequency energy results in resistive heating of the tissue and irreversible tissue destruction when the tissue temperature exceeds 50° C. Depending on the type of catheter and the power settings, the lesions that are created are up to 7 to 8 mm in diameter and up to 6 to 8 mm deep. Chronic lesions demonstrate coagulation necrosis and are well demarcated.

Procedural Aspects

Diagnostic electrophysiologic testing (Chapter 62) and radio frequency ablation are often performed during the same procedure, sometimes on an outpatient basis, such as in patients with paroxysmal SVT. Various pacing techniques or infusions of isoproterenol (or both) are used to induce the patient's arrhythmia and allow the specific mechanism of the tachycardia to

be determined. Depending on the type of tachycardia, the sites in the heart targeted for ablation are determined by the results of mapping or as guided by specific anatomic landmarks. Radio frequency energy is delivered, typically in applications of 1 minute, at a power setting sufficient to result in adequate tissue heating of 60° to 70° C.

Radio Frequency Ablation of Supraventricular Arrhythmias

AV nodal re-entrant tachycardia (Chapter 64), the most common type of paroxysmal SVT, is eliminated by radio frequency ablation of the "slow" limb of the re-entry circuit. Target sites for ablation are located in the posteroseptal aspect of the right atrium, near the ostium of the coronary sinus. In experienced hands, slow-pathway ablation has a success rate of 98% and is associated with a less than 1% risk of high-degree AV block.

Cryoablation, which is an alternative to radio frequency ablation, is associated with a lower risk for AV block but a lower long-term success rate. Cryoablation is useful in patients at higher risk for AV block, such as small children.

Left-sided accessory pathways are ablated by using either a retrograde aortic or a transseptal approach, and those that are right sided or septal are ablated with a venous approach. Detailed mapping of the accessory pathway is essential for identification of an appropriate ablation site, and the ablation catheter is positioned on either the atrial or the ventricular aspect of the mitral or tricuspid annulus. The success rate of accessory pathway ablation is 90 to 98%, and the complication rate is 2 to 3%. A fatal complication occurs in less than 0.1% of patients. The most common nonfatal but serious complications are cardiac tamponade as a result of mechanical perforation of the heart by an electrode catheter and high-degree AV block in patients with a septal accessory pathway. Cryoablation is associated with a lower risk for AV block and is useful for ablation of accessory pathways located near the AV node.

Detailed mapping is also needed to identify sites for ablation of atrial tachycardias. Most atrial tachycardias arise in the right atrium and are mapped by using a venous approach, but left atrial tachycardias are mapped via a transseptal approach. Assuming that the atrial tachycardia is arising only at one site, the success rate of ablation is approximately 90%, and complications are rare.

Type I atrial flutter (Chapter 64) arises in the right atrium and can be eliminated by radio frequency ablation directed at a critical isthmus in the low right atrium, between the tricuspid annulus and the inferior vena cava. The success rate of this type of ablation is greater than 90%, and the risk for a serious complication is less than 1%.

Catheter ablation aimed at the elimination of atrial fibrillation is useful in patients with symptomatic, drug-refractory atrial fibrillation.**9** The 1-year efficacy of catheter ablation appears to be in the range of 75 to 85% for paroxysmal atrial fibrillation and 65 to 75% for chronic atrial fibrillation. The most serious complications are myocardial perforation, thromboembolism, and atrioesophageal fistula, with an overall risk of 1 to 2%. Pulmonary vein stenosis is a potentially serious complication that can be avoided by not delivering radio frequency energy applications within the tubular portion of the pulmonary veins.

In patients with refractory atrial fibrillation (Chapter 64) associated with an uncontrolled ventricular rate, radio frequency ablation of the AV node can improve symptoms, functional capacity, and left ventricular function. In AV node ablation, a third-degree AV block is intentionally induced; the success rate is 100%, and all patients require a permanent pacemaker.

Inappropriate sinus tachycardia can also be managed with radio frequency ablation, but this approach should be recommended only as a last resort. The sinus node, located in the high lateral portion of the right atrium, is targeted for ablation. The success rate is 80%, and 10% of patients require a pacemaker because of an inadequate atrial escape rate.

Because of a very favorable risk-benefit ratio, radio frequency ablation is appropriate first-line therapy for any patient with paroxysmal SVT, Wolff-Parkinson-White syndrome, or type I atrial flutter that is symptomatic enough to warrant therapy (Chapter 64). For atrial flutter other than type I and inappropriate sinus tachycardia, an ablation procedure is appropriate only in patients with severe symptoms who are refractory to medication.

Ablation techniques and new technologies for ablation of atrial fibrillation are still evolving, and their long-term efficacy is not yet established. After 1 year, rates of recurrent atrial fibrillation have been reduced by catheter ablation, but rates of stroke and mortality have not.[10]

Radio Frequency Ablation of Ventricular Tachycardia

Radio frequency ablation has been used as first-line treatment of idiopathic VT. The most common type of idiopathic VT arises in the outflow tract of the right ventricle and has a left bundle branch block configuration and superior axis. Another type of idiopathic VT has a right bundle branch block configuration and a superior axis and arises in the inferoapical aspect of the left ventricle (Chapter 65). The success rate of radio frequency ablation of these types of VT has been 85 to 100%, and complications have been rare.

In patients with CAD, VT usually arises in diseased tissue adjacent to an area of previous infarction in the left ventricle. Because the disease process is diffuse instead of focal and because VT may originate at multiple sites, radio frequency ablation of VT is not usually curative in patients with CAD. More often, radio frequency ablation is used as adjunctive therapy with an ICD or with antiarrhythmic drug therapy. In the setting of CAD, the success rate of radio frequency ablation of VT has been 65 to 95%, with serious complications occurring in approximately 5% of patients.

● ARRHYTHMIA SURGERY

Wolff-Parkinson-White Syndrome

At present, surgical ablation of an accessory pathway may be indicated for the rare patient with Wolff-Parkinson-White syndrome who has potentially dangerous arrhythmias and in whom catheter ablation is unsuccessful. When performed by an experienced surgeon, the success rate of surgical ablation of an accessory pathway approaches 100%, and the risk for a serious complication is low. Intraoperative mapping is necessary to establish the location of the accessory pathway, which then can be ablated either cryosurgically using an epicardial approach or by direct dissection using an endocardial approach.

Ventricular Tachycardia in Patients with Coronary Artery Disease

The substrate for monomorphic VT in patients with CAD usually lies within visually apparent scar tissue surrounding an area of previous myocardial infarction (Chapter 65). Subendocardial resection has been successful in eliminating VT when performed either on a visual basis, with resection or cryoablation of all visually apparent scar tissue, or on a map-guided basis, with resection or cryoablation limited to the areas found to be participating in generation of the VT. At centers experienced in this type of surgery, the success rate of subendocardial resection has been 85 to 90%, and the operative mortality rate has been in the range of 5 to 10%. Although subendocardial resection has the potential advantage of preventing recurrences of VT, the relatively high operative mortality rate and the widespread availability of ICDs have discouraged its use.

Atrial Fibrillation

In the maze procedure, a series of incisions or linear lesions or both (created by cryoablation or radio frequency ablation) are made in specific regions of the left and right atria to subdivide the atria into parts too small to sustain atrial fibrillation. The operative mortality rate associated with the maze

procedure is less than 2%, and more than 90% of patients have had no recurrences of atrial fibrillation during long-term follow-up. However, because it requires extensive surgery, the maze procedure is performed by only a small number of surgeons.

A variety of simpler operative procedures for atrial fibrillation have been developed, some of which can be performed with minimally invasive surgery. The long-term efficacy of these simpler "mini-maze" procedures is lower than that of the maze procedure, but because of their ease and low risk, their use has become widespread, mostly as an adjunct to valve or coronary bypass surgery.

1. Connelly SJ, Kerr CR, Gent M, et al. Effects of physiological pacing versus ventricular pacing on the risk of stroke and death due to cardiovascular causes. *N Engl J Med.* 2000;342:1385-1391.
2. Lamas GA, Lee KL, Sweeney MO, et al. Ventricular pacing or dual-chamber pacing for sinus-node dysfunction. *N Engl J Med.* 2002;346:1854-1862.
3. Sweeney MO, Bank AJ, Nsah E, et al. Minimizing ventricular pacing to reduce atrial fibrillation in sinus-node disease. *N Engl J Med.* 2007;357:1000-1008.
4. The Antiarrhythmics versus Implantable Defibrillators (AVID) Investigators. A comparison of antiarrhythmic-drug therapy with implantable defibrillators in patients resuscitated from near-fatal ventricular arrhythmias. *N Engl J Med.* 1997;337:1576-1583.
5. Buxton AE, Lee KL, Fisher JD, et al. A randomized study of the prevention of sudden death in patients with coronary artery disease. Multicenter Unsustained Tachycardia Trial Investigators. *N Engl J Med.* 1999;341:1882-1890.
6. Goldenberg I, Gillespie J, Moss AJ, et al. Long-term benefit of primary prevention with an implantable defibrillator: an extended 8-year follow-up study of the Multicenter Automatic Defibrillator Implantation Trial II. *Circulation.* 2010;122:1265-1271.
7. Bardy GH, Lee KL, Mark DB, et al. Amiodarone or an implantable cardioverter-defibrillator for congestive heart failure. *N Engl J Med.* 2005;352:225-237.
8. Bristow MR, Saxon LA, Boehmer J, et al. Cardiac-resynchronization therapy with or without an implantable defibrillator in advanced chronic heart failure. *N Engl J Med.* 2004;350:2140-2150.
9. Jaïs P, Cauchemez B, Macle L, et al. Catheter ablation versus antiarrhythmic drugs for atrial fibrillation: the A4 study. *Circulation.* 2008;118:2498-2505.
10. Wilber DJ, Pappone C, Neuzil P, et al. Comparison of antiarrhythmic drug therapy and radiofrequency catheter ablation in patients with paroxysmal atrial fibrillation: a randomized controlled trial. *JAMA.* 2010;303:333-340.

SUGGESTED READINGS

Bardy GH, Smith WM, Hood MA, et al. An entirely subcutaneous implantable cardioverter-defibrillator. *N Eng J Med.* 2010;363:36-44. *In a non-randomized study, an entirely subcutaneous ICD detected and treated tachyarrhythmias.*
Weerasooriya R, Khairy P, Litalien J, et al. Catheter ablation for atrial fibrillation: are results maintained at 5 years of follow-up? *J Am Coll Cardiol.* 2011;57:160-166. *Arrhythmia-free survival rates after a single ablation were 40%, 37%, and 29% at 1, 2, and 5 years.*

67

ARTERIAL HYPERTENSION

RONALD G. VICTOR

DEFINITION

Hypertension has been defined as a usual blood pressure of 140/90 mm Hg or higher (Table 67-1), blood pressure levels for which the benefits of drug treatment have been shown in randomized controlled trials. This conservative definition has been called into question by epidemiologic data showing continuous positive relationships between the risk for death from coronary artery disease (CAD) and stroke with systolic or diastolic blood pressure values as low as 115/75 mm Hg (Fig. 67-1). Thus, an artificial dichotomy between "hypertension" and "normotension" may delay medical treatment until vascular health has been irreversibly compromised by elevated blood pressure values previously considered normal. For certain high-risk patients, such as those with CAD, the recommended medical treatment threshold recently has been lowered to 130/80 mm Hg.

EPIDEMIOLOGY

Affecting one fourth of the adult population (70 million people in the United States and 1 billion people worldwide), arterial hypertension is the leading cause of death in the world and the most common cause for an outpatient visit to a physician; it is the most easily recognized treatable risk factor for

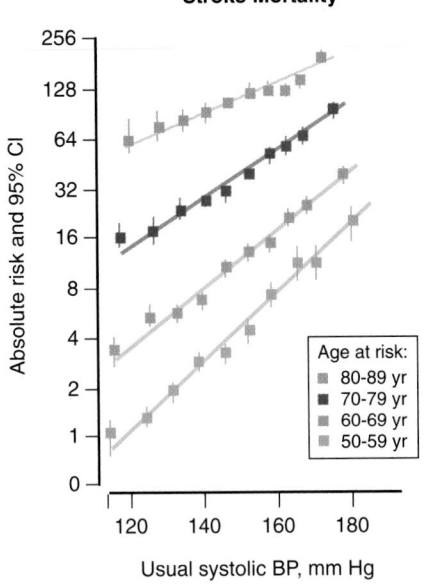

FIGURE 67-1. Absolute risk of coronary artery disease and stroke mortality by usual systolic blood pressure (BP) levels. (From Lewington S, Clarke R, Qizilbash N, et al, for the Prospective Studies Collaboration. Age-specific relevance of usual blood pressure to vascular mortality: a meta-analysis of individual data for one million adults in 61 prospective studies. *Lancet.* 2002;360:1903-1913.)

TABLE 67-1	STAGING OF OFFICE BLOOD PRESSURE*	
BLOOD PRESSURE STAGE	**SYSTOLIC BLOOD PRESSURE (mm Hg)**	**DIASTOLIC BLOOD PRESSURE (mm Hg)**
Normal	<120	<80
Prehypertension	120-139	80-89
Stage 1 hypertension	140-159	90-99
Stage 2 hypertension	≥160	≥100

*Calculation of seated blood pressure is based on the mean of two or more readings on two separate office visits.
From Chobanian A, Bakris G, Black H, et al. The Seventh Report of the Joint National Committee on the Prevention, Evaluation, and Treatment of High Blood Pressure: the JNC 7 report. *JAMA.* 2003;289:2560-2572.

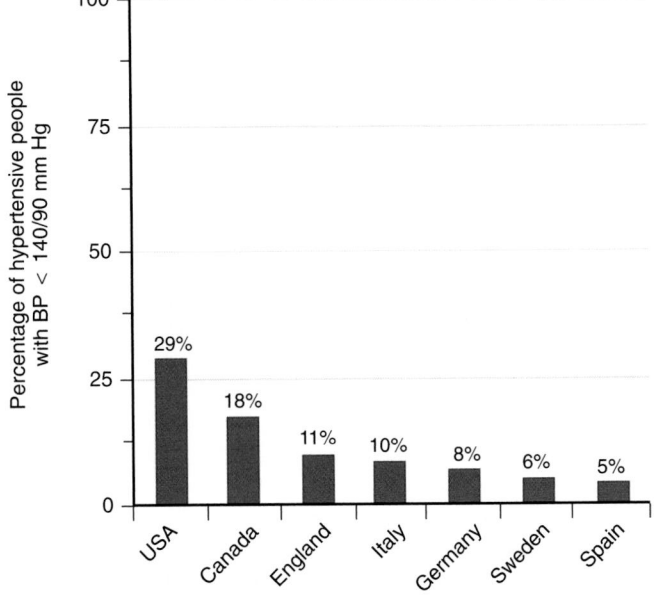

FIGURE 67-2. Hypertension control rates in North America and Europe. (From Wolf-Maier K, Cooper RS, Kramer H, et al. Hypertension treatment and control in five European countries, Canada, and the United States. *Hypertension.* 2004;43:10-17.)

stroke (Chapters 413, 414, and 415), myocardial infarction (Chapters 72 and 73), heart failure (Chapters 58 and 59), peripheral vascular disease (Chapter 79), aortic dissection (Chapter 78), atrial fibrillation (Chapter 64), and end-stage kidney disease (Chapter 132). Because of increasing rates of obesity and aging of the population, hypertension is projected to affect 1.5 billion persons, one third of the world's population, by the year 2025. Presently, about 54% of strokes and 47% of ischemic heart disease worldwide is attributable to high blood pressure. Half of this disease burden is in people who meet the definition of hypertension, and the remainder is in people with lesser degrees of high blood pressure (*prehypertension*).

The asymptomatic nature of most cases of hypertension and the inherent variability in blood pressure can delay diagnosis and treatment. Most cases of hypertension are multifactorial. Blood pressure control typically requires empirical treatment with several classes of prescription medication. Pill burden, prescription drug costs, medication side effects, and insufficient time for patient education contribute to nonadherence to medications. Physicians can be too slow to initiate and intensify blood pressure medication. Lifestyle modification (particularly diet and exercise) can lower blood pressure somewhat, but the reduction rarely is enough to eliminate the need for medication. For all these reasons, blood pressure is controlled to a value below 140/90 mm Hg in less than one third of affected individuals, even in higher-income countries with the most advanced systems of health care (Fig. 67-2). Effective management requires continuity of care by a knowledgeable physician and continued active involvement by an educated patient.

Aging and Pulse Pressure

Patients often ask: Is systolic or diastolic blood pressure more important? Both are (Fig. 67-3). In industrialized societies, systolic pressure rises progressively with age; if individuals live long enough, almost all (>90%) will develop hypertension. This age-dependent rise in blood pressure is not an essential part of human biology. In less developed countries where

consumption of calories and salt is low, blood pressures remain low and do not rise with age. In developed countries, diastolic pressure rises until the age of 50 years and decreases thereafter, producing a progressive rise in pulse pressure (systolic pressure minus diastolic pressure) (Fig. 67-4).

Different hemodynamic faults underlie hypertension in younger and older persons. Patients who develop hypertension before the age of 50 years typically have *combined systolic and diastolic hypertension*: systolic pressure above 140 mm Hg *and* diastolic pressure above 90 mm Hg. The main hemodynamic fault is vasoconstriction at the level of the resistance arterioles. In contrast, most patients who develop hypertension after the age of 50 years have *isolated systolic hypertension*: systolic pressure above 140 mm Hg but diastolic pressure below 90 mm Hg (often below 80 mm Hg). In isolated systolic hypertension, the primary hemodynamic fault is decreased distensibility of the large conduit arteries. Collagen replaces elastin in the elastic lamina of the aorta, a process that is accelerated by both aging and hypertension. When pulse wave velocity increases sufficiently, the rapid return of the arterial pulse wave from the periphery augments central systolic (rather than diastolic) pressure. The augmented systolic load on the left ventricle increases myocardial oxygen demands, whereas the rapid diastolic runoff compromises myocardial perfusion. As the population ages, most uncontrolled hypertension occurs in older patients with isolated systolic hypertension.

Gender and Race/Ethnicity

Before the age of 50 years, hypertension is less common in women than men, suggesting a protective effect of estrogen. After menopause, hypertension is more common in women than men.

One in three African American individuals has hypertension, compared with one in four or five white and Mexican American individuals. In African Americans, hypertension also starts at a younger age, is more severe, and causes more target organ damage, leading to premature disability and death. In the Bogalusa Heart Study, African American children already had higher blood pressures than white children by grade school. However, hypertension is more prevalent in the white populations of several European countries (e.g., Finland, Germany, Spain) than in African Americans and is rare among Africans living in Africa (Fig. 67-5). These international data emphasize the importance of environmental factors.

PATHOBIOLOGY

In 90 to 95% of hypertensive patients, a single reversible cause of the elevated blood pressure cannot be identified, hence the term *primary hypertension*. However, in most patients with primary hypertension, readily identifiable behaviors—habitually excessive consumption of calories, salt, or alcohol—contribute to the elevated blood pressure. In the remaining 5 to 10%, a more discrete mechanism can be identified, and the condition is termed *secondary or identifiable hypertension*. At the organ-system level, hypertension results from a gain in function of pathways that promote vasoconstriction and renal sodium retention or a loss in function of pathways that promote vasodilation and renal sodium excretion. Neural, hormonal, renal, and vascular mechanisms are involved. There is increasing evidence that neurohormonal activation contributes to the early pathogenesis by compromising vascular function (e.g., endothelium-dependent vasodilation) and structure (e.g., inward remodeling) that precede hypertension.

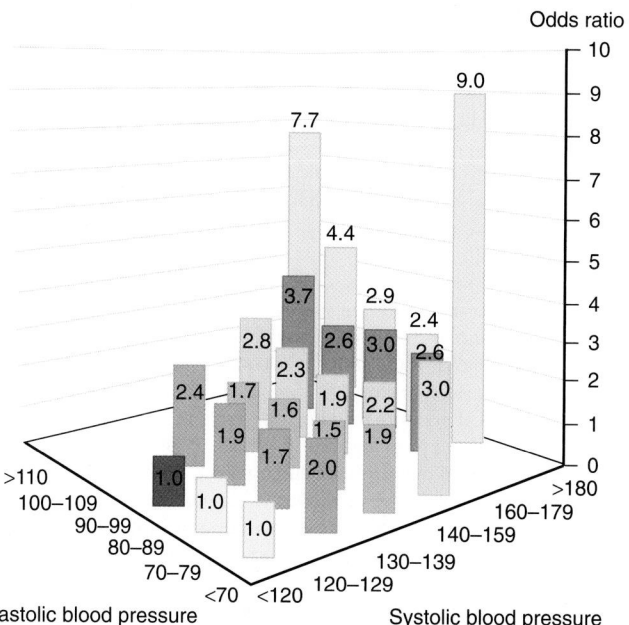

FIGURE 67-3. Joint influences of systolic blood pressure and diastolic blood pressure on the risk (odds ratio) of a cardiovascular event. (Modified from Franklin SS, Lopez VA, Wong ND, et al. Single versus combined blood pressure component and risk for cardiovascular disease: the Framingham Heart Study. *Circulation.* 2009;119:243-250.)

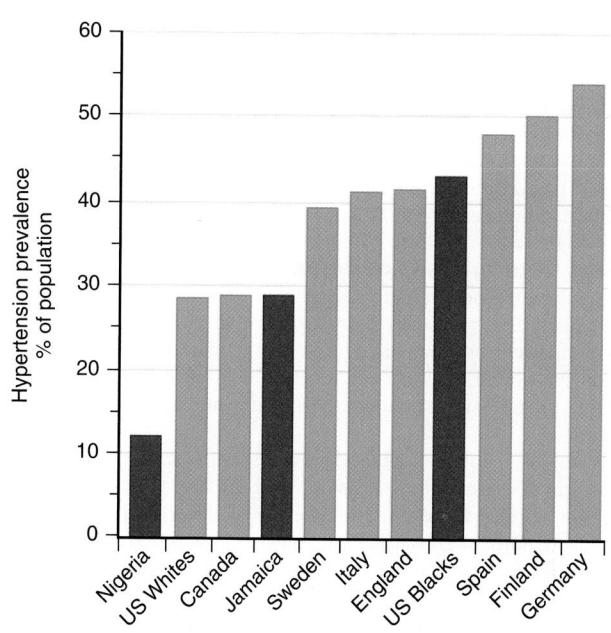

FIGURE 67-5. Geographic variation in hypertension prevalence in populations of African and European ancestries. (From Cooper RS, Wolf-Maier K, Luke A, et al. An international comparative study of blood pressure in populations of European vs. African descent. *BMC Med.* 2005;3:1-8.)

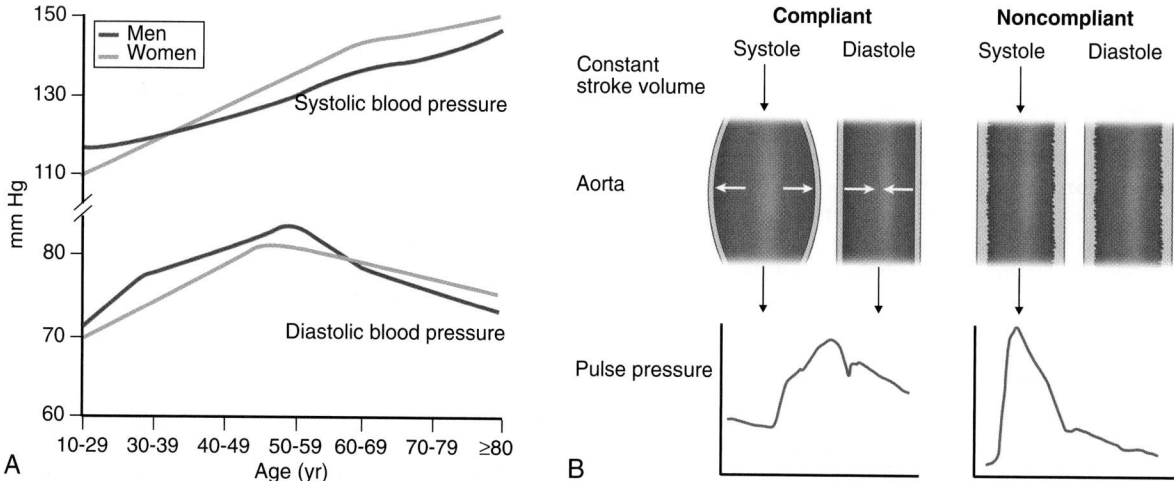

FIGURE 67-4. Aging and pulse pressure. **A,** Age-dependent changes in systolic and diastolic blood pressure in the United States. **B,** Schematic diagram showing the relation between aortic compliance and pulse pressure. (**A,** From Burt V, Whelton P, Rocella EJ, et al. Prevalence of hypertension in the U.S. adult population: results from the Third National Health and Nutrition Examination Survey, 1988-1991. *Hypertension.* 1995;25:305-313; **B,** Courtesy of Dr. Stanley Franklin, University of California at Irvine.)

Behavioral Determinants of Human Blood Pressure Variation

The most important behavioral determinants of blood pressure are related to dietary consumption of calories and salt. Across populations, the prevalence of hypertension increases linearly with average body mass index. With the unrelenting obesity epidemic in both developed and developing societies, increasing attention is being paid to the *metabolic syndrome* (Chapter 237) that often accompanies hypertension. The metabolic syndrome refers to the frequent clustering of elevated blood pressure with abdominal ("male pattern") adiposity, insulin resistance with glucose intolerance, and a dyslipidemic pattern consisting typically of elevated plasma triglyceride and low high-density lipoprotein cholesterol levels. In the Framingham Heart Study, obesity has been estimated to account for as much as 60% of the new cases of hypertension. The underlying mechanisms by which weight gain leads to hypertension are incompletely understood, but there is mounting evidence for an expanded plasma volume plus sympathetic overactivity. The sympathetic overactivity is thought to be a compensatory attempt to burn fat but at the expense of peripheral vasoconstriction, renal salt and water retention, and hypertension. In some obese individuals, sleep apnea (Chapter 100) is an important cause of hypertension. Repeated arterial desaturation sensitizes the carotid body chemoreceptors, causing sustained sympathetic overactivity even during waking hours.

Dietary sodium intake is another key behavioral determinant of human hypertension. In the INTERSALT study of 52 locations around the world, the risk for development of hypertension during three decades of adult life was linearly and tightly related to dietary sodium intake. Interindividual variability in blood pressure responses to dietary sodium loading and sodium restriction indicates an important genetic underpinning.

Genetic Determinants of Human Blood Pressure Variation

Concordance of blood pressures is greater within families than in unrelated individuals, greater between monozygotic twins than between dizygotic twins, and greater between biologic siblings than between adoptive siblings living in the same household. As much as 70% of the familial aggregation of blood pressure is attributed to shared genes rather than to shared environment.

The complex regulation of blood pressure has thwarted the genetic dissection of primary human hypertension, with the first positive genome-wide association studies suggesting multiple risk alleles, each having very small effects. Mutations in 20 salt-handling genes cause ultra-rare syndromes of severe, early-onset hypotension (salt-wasting syndromes) or hypertension (all inherited as mendelian traits). The clinical relevance of these mutations to common primary hypertension has been limited, although recent data indicate that heterozygous mutations in genes underlying the pediatric salt-wasting syndromes (Bartter's and Gitelman's) are present in 1 to 2% of the general adult population and confer resistance against primary hypertension.

CLINICAL MANIFESTATIONS

Hypertension has been called the silent killer, an asymptomatic chronic disorder that silently damages the blood vessels, heart, brain, and kidneys if it is undetected and untreated. Although headaches (Chapter 405) are common in patients with mild to moderate hypertension, episodes of headaches do not correlate with fluctuations in blood pressure. Rather, they correlate with a person's awareness of his or her diagnosis.

DIAGNOSIS

Initial Evaluation for Hypertension

The initial evaluation for hypertension should accomplish three goals: (1) stage the blood pressure, (2) assess the patient's overall cardiovascular risk, and (3) detect clues of secondary hypertension that require further evaluation.

Goal 1: Accurate Assessment of Blood Pressure
Office Blood Pressure

Traditionally, blood pressure has been staged as normal, prehypertension, or hypertension based on the average of two or more readings taken at two or more office visits (see Table 67-1). The blood pressure should be measured at least twice after 5 minutes of rest with the patient seated, the back supported, and the arm bare and at heart level. A large adult-sized cuff should be used to measure blood pressure in overweight adults because the standard-sized cuff will cause falsely elevated readings. Tobacco and caffeine should be avoided for at least 30 minutes. Blood pressure should be measured in both arms, to exclude coarctation of the aorta, and after 5 minutes of standing, to exclude a significant postural fall, particularly in older persons and persons with diabetes or other conditions (e.g., Parkinson's disease) that predispose to autonomic insufficiency.

Home and Ambulatory Blood Pressure Monitoring

A person's blood pressure varies so much throughout a 24-hour period that it is impossible to characterize it accurately except by repeated measurements under various conditions. Out-of-office readings are the only way to obtain a clear picture of a person's usual blood pressure for accurate diagnosis and management. These readings are more predictive of cardiovascular events than office readings and overcome many of the pitfalls of office measurement, including physician errors and "white coat" reactions. Home blood pressure monitoring also improves medication adherence by actively involving patients in their own medical care.

New recommendations include the following: (1) home blood pressure monitoring should become a routine part of the clinical management of patients with known or suspected hypertension the same way that home blood glucose monitoring is essential to the management of patients with diabetes; (2) two (or three) readings should be taken in the morning and at night for 1 week, with a total of at least 12 readings being averaged before making clinical decisions; and (3) the target treatment goal is an average home blood pressure of less than 135/85 mm Hg for most patients and less than 130/80 mm Hg for high-risk patients, such as those with CAD, heart failure, diabetes, or chronic kidney disease.

A validated electronic oscillometric monitor with an arm cuff should be chosen from the dabl Educational Web site (*www.dableducational.org*). Each patient's monitor should be checked in the physician's office for its accuracy and appropriate cuff size. Patients must be taught correct measurement techniques and to avoid reporting bias. Wrist monitors are inaccurate and thus not recommended. The oscillometric method may not work well in patients with atrial fibrillation or frequent extrasystoles, for whom manual sphygmomanometry is required. Rare patients become obsessed about taking their blood pressure and need to stop.

Ambulatory blood pressure monitoring (Table 67-2) provides automated measurements of blood pressure during a 24-hour period while patients are engaged in their usual activities, including sleep (Fig. 67-6). Ambulatory blood pressure measurement is superior to standard office measurement in predicting fatal and nonfatal myocardial infarction and stroke. Recommended normal values are an average daytime blood pressure below 135/85 mm Hg, nighttime blood pressure below 120/70 mm Hg, and 24-hour blood pressure below 130/80 mm Hg. Some experts have recommended a lower cutoff value of 130/80 mm Hg as a more stringent definition of normal daytime blood pressure.

About 20% of patients with elevated office blood pressures have normal home or ambulatory blood pressures. If the daytime blood pressure is below 135/85 mm Hg (or preferably below 130/80 mm Hg) and there is no target organ damage despite consistently elevated office readings, the patient has

TABLE 67-2	RECOMMENDED INDICATIONS FOR AMBULATORY BLOOD PRESSURE MONITORING

Suspected "white coat hypertension" (high office blood pressure readings in patients with otherwise low total cardiovascular risk)*

Considerable variability of clinic blood pressure readings

Marked discrepancy between home and office blood pressure readings (e.g., suspected masked hypertension)

Suspected nocturnal hypertension

Suspected resistance to drug treatment

Suspected orthostatic hypotension or autonomic failure, particularly in elderly or diabetic patients

Elevated office blood pressure in pregnant women or suspected preeclampsia

*Medicare currently reimburses for ambulatory monitoring only to confirm the diagnosis of white coat hypertension that is suspected on the basis of three normal home readings in patients with no evidence of target organ damage despite repeatedly elevated office blood pressure readings (ICD 796.2).
Modified from Mancia G, DeBacker G, Dominickak A, et al. 2007 Guidelines for the management of arterial hypertension of the European Society of Hypertension (ESH) and the European Society of Cardiology (ESC). *Eur Heart J.* 2007;23:1462-1536.

"office-only" or "white coat" hypertension, caused by a transient adrenergic response to the measurement of blood pressure in the physician's office. The cardiovascular risk is intermediate to that in persons with consistently normal blood pressure and those with consistently high blood pressure. Many patients do not have pure white coat hypertension but rather white coat aggravation, a white coat reaction superimposed on a milder level of out-of-office hypertension that nevertheless needs treatment. For example, up to 30% of treated patients who have persistently elevated office blood pressure readings will be shown by ambulatory monitoring to have adequate or even excessive control of their hypertension, thereby eliminating overtreatment (see Fig. 67-6). In other patients, office readings underestimate ambulatory blood pressures, presumably because of sympathetic overactivity (e.g., owing to job stress, home stress, or tobacco smoke) that dissipates when the patient comes to the office. Such "masked hypertension," present in up to 10% of patients, increases cardiovascular risk.

Ambulatory monitoring is the only way to detect hypertension during sleep. Blood pressure normally dips during sleep and increases sharply when a person awakens and becomes active (see Fig. 67-6). Nocturnal hypertension increases the aggregate blood pressure burden on the cardiovascular system and is a stronger predictor of cardiovascular outcomes than daytime ambulatory blood pressure or office measurements. Nocturnal hypertension is particularly common in patients with chronic kidney disease (Chapter 132), presumably because of their sustained sympathetic overactivity, which does not shut down during sleep, and centralization of blood volume with nocturnal recumbence.

Goal 2: Cardiovascular Risk Stratification

Although cardiovascular risk increases with increasing blood pressure, it also increases if the patient has hypertensive target organ damage or additional cardiovascular risk factors. More than 75% of hypertensive patients meet current U.S. criteria for initiation of lipid-lowering medication (low-density lipoprotein cholesterol more than 130 mm Hg), and 25% have diabetes. Thus, the minimal laboratory testing required for the initial evaluation of hypertension is determination of blood electrolyte, fasting glucose, and serum creatinine levels (with calculated glomerular filtration rate [GFR]), a fasting lipid panel, hematocrit, spot urinalysis (including urine albumin-to-creatinine ratio), and a resting 12-lead electrocardiogram (ECG).

The gradient of increasing levels of blood pressure with cardiovascular risk steepens as additional risk factors are added (Fig. 67-7). As the overall risks multiply, blood pressure control becomes more important. Current U.S. guidelines recommended a usual blood pressure of 140/90 mm Hg as the threshold for initiating antihypertensive medication in most patients, with a lower threshold of 130/80 mm Hg for high-risk patients with diabetes or chronic kidney disease. Based on more recent data, the operational definition of high-risk patients has been expanded to include most patients with established CAD, carotid artery disease, peripheral artery disease, abdominal aortic aneurysm, heart failure, or high risk for CAD (10-year Framingham risk score of >10%) (Table 67-3). Because cardiovascular risk increases so

steeply with age (see Fig. 67-1), most hypertensive men older than 55 years and most hypertensive women older than 65 years will have a Framingham risk score higher than 10% (*http://hp2010.nhlbihin.net/atpiii/calculator.asp*).

Goal 3: Identification and Treatment of Secondary (Identifiable) Causes of Hypertension

The third goal of the initial evaluation is to screen for identifiable causes of hypertension (Table 67-4), in the hope of finding a cure. A thorough search for secondary causes, which is not cost-effective in most patients with hypertension, becomes critically important in two circumstances: (1) when there is a compelling finding on the initial evaluation and (2) when the hypertensive process is so severe that it either is refractory to intensive multiple-drug therapy or requires hospitalization.

Renal Parenchymal Hypertension

Chronic kidney disease (Chapter 132) is the most common cause of secondary hypertension. Hypertension is present in more than 85% of patients with

TABLE 67-3	RECOMMENDED (TARGET) BLOOD PRESSURE VALUES*

BP < 150/80 mm Hg
  Very elderly persons (80+ years of age)
BP < 140/90 mm Hg
  Uncomplicated hypertension
BP < 130/80 mm Hg
  Diabetes mellitus
  Chronic kidney disease
    GFR <60 mL/min/1.73 m^2
    Urine albumin-to-creatinine ratio ≥30 mg/g (consider <120/80 mm Hg if >1 g of proteinuria per day)
  Other patients at high risk for coronary artery disease (primary prevention)
  Coronary artery disease risk equivalents
  Carotid artery disease
  Peripheral arterial disease
  Abdominal aortic aneurysm
  10-year Framingham risk score > 10% (most men over age 55, most women over age 65)
  Established coronary artery disease: stable or unstable (secondary prevention)
  Secondary prevention of stroke or TIA
  Heart failure or left ventricular systolic dysfunction (consider BP < 120/80 mm Hg)

*Values are for office readings; target values for home or daytime ambulatory monitoring are generally set 5 mm Hg lower.
BP = blood pressure; GFR = glomerular filtration rate; TIA = transient ischemic attack.
Adapted from Rosendorff C, Black HR, Cannon CP, et al. Treatment of hypertension in the prevention and management of ischemic heart disease: a scientific statement from the American Heart Association Council for High Blood Pressure Research and the Councils on Clinical Cardiology and Epidemiology and Prevention. *Circulation.* 2007;115:2761-2788.

FIGURE 67-6. The 24-hour ambulatory blood pressure (BP) monitor tracings of two different patients. **A,** Optimal blood pressure in a healthy 37-year-old woman. Note the normal variability in blood pressure, the nocturnal dip in blood pressure during sleep, and the sharp increase in blood pressure on awakening. **B,** Pronounced white coat effect in an 80-year-old woman referred for evaluation of medically refractory hypertension. Documentation of the white coat effect prevented overtreatment of the patient's isolated systolic hypertension. (**A,** Courtesy of Ronald G. Victor, MD, Hypertension Division, Department of Internal Medicine, University of Texas Southwestern Medical Center, Dallas, Texas; **B,** Courtesy of Wanpen Vongpatanasin, MD, Hypertension Division, Department of Internal Medicine, University of Texas Southwestern Medical Center, Dallas, Texas.)

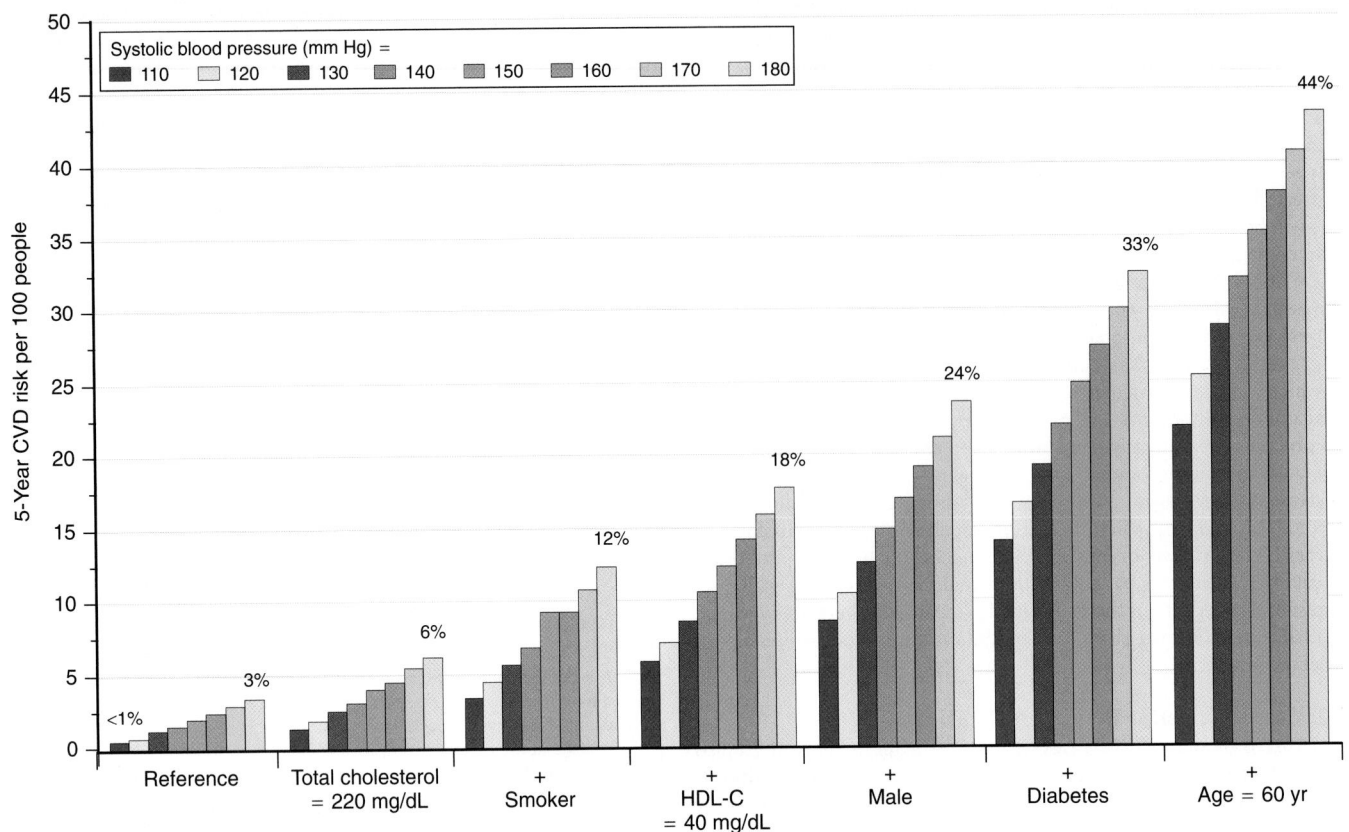

FIGURE 67-7. Absolute risk of cardiovascular disease (CVD) during 5 years in patients by systolic blood pressure at specified levels of other risk factors. The reference category is a nondiabetic, nonsmoking woman aged 50 years with a total cholesterol value of 190 mg/dL and a high-density lipoprotein cholesterol (HDL-C) value of 60 mg/dL. Risks are given for systolic pressures of 110, 120, 130, 140, 150, 160, 170, and 180 mm Hg. In the other categories, additional risk factors are added consecutively. (From Jackson R, Lawes CMM, Benett DA, et al. Treatment with drugs to lower blood pressure and blood cholesterol based on an individual's absolute cardiovascular risk. *Lancet.* 2005;365:434-441.)

TABLE 67-4   GUIDE TO EVALUATION OF IDENTIFIABLE CAUSES OF HYPERTENSION

SUSPECTED DIAGNOSIS	CLINICAL CLUES	DIAGNOSTIC TESTING
Chronic kidney disease	Estimated GFR <60 mL/min/1.73 m² Urine albumin-to-creatinine ratio ≥30 mg/g	Renal sonography
Renovascular disease	New elevation in serum creatinine, marked elevation in serum creatinine with ACEI or ARB, drug-resistant hypertension, flash pulmonary edema, abdominal or flank bruit	Renal sonography (atrophic kidney), CT or MR angiography, invasive angiography
Coarctation of the aorta	Arm pulses > leg pulses, arm BP > leg BP, chest bruits, rib notching on chest radiography	MR angiography, TEE, invasive angiography
Primary aldosteronism	Hypokalemia, drug-resistant hypertension	Plasma renin and aldosterone, 24-hour urine aldosterone and potassium after oral salt loading, adrenal vein sampling
Cushing's syndrome	Truncal obesity, wide and blanching purple striae, muscle weakness	1 mg dexamethasone-suppression test, urinary cortisol after dexamethasone, adrenal CT
Pheochromocytoma	Paroxysms of hypertension, palpitations, perspiration, and pallor; diabetes	Plasma metanephrines, 24-hour urinary metanephrines and catecholamines, abdominal CT or MR imaging
Obstructive sleep apnea	Loud snoring, large neck, obesity, somnolence	Polysonography

ACEI = angiotensin-converting enzyme inhibitor; ARB = angiotensin receptor blocker; BP = blood pressure; CT = computed tomography; GFR = glomerular filtration rate; MR, magnetic resonance; TEE = transesophageal echocardiography.

chronic kidney disease and is a major factor causing their increased cardiovascular morbidity and mortality. The mechanisms causing the hypertension include an expanded plasma volume and peripheral vasoconstriction; the peripheral vasoconstriction is caused by both activation of vasoconstrictor pathways (renin-angiotensin and sympathetic nervous systems) and inhibition of vasodilator pathways (nitric oxide).

Measurement of serum creatinine alone is an inadequate screening test for renal insufficiency. A spot urine specimen should be obtained to screen for microalbuminuria, which is defined as a urine albumin-to-urine creatinine ratio of 30 to 300 mg/g (equivalent to excretion of 30 to 300 mg of albumin per 24 hours); higher levels of albuminuria indicate more advanced kidney disease. Using the spot urine specimen, creatinine clearance should be

calculated (*www.nephron.com*; *www.newtech.kidney.org*) (Chapter 116) to screen for an estimated GFR below 60 mL/min/1.73 m².

In patients with mild (stage 2: GFR of 60 to 90 mL/min/1.73 m²) or moderate (stage 3: GFR of 30 to 60 mL/min/1.73 m²) proteinuric chronic kidney disease, stringent blood pressure control is imperative both to slow the progression to end-stage renal disease and to reduce the excessive cardiovascular risk. In patients with severe chronic kidney disease, hypertension often becomes difficult to treat and may require either (1) intensive medical treatment with loop diuretics, potent vasodilators (e.g., minoxidil), high-dose β-adrenergic blockers, and central sympatholytics; or (2) initiation of chronic hemodialysis as the only effective way to reduce plasma volume. In chronic hemodialysis patients, the challenge is to control interdialytic hypertension without exacerbating dialysis-induced hypotension. The annual mortality rate in the hemodialysis population is 25%; half of this excessive mortality is caused by cardiovascular events that are related, at least in part, to hypertension.

Renovascular Hypertension

PATHOBIOLOGY AND CLINICAL MANIFESTATIONS

The two main causes of renal artery stenosis (Chapter 127) are atherosclerosis (85% of cases), typically in older persons with other clinical manifestations of systemic atherosclerosis, and fibromuscular dysplasia (15% of cases), typically in young women who are otherwise healthy. Although renal artery stenosis and hypertension frequently coexist, the presence of a renal artery stenosis does not prove that the patient's hypertension is renovascular in origin or that revascularization will improve renal perfusion and blood pressure.

Unilateral renal artery stenosis can lead to underperfusion of the juxtaglomerular cells, thereby causing renin-dependent hypertension even though the contralateral kidney is able to maintain normal blood volume. In contrast, bilateral renal artery stenosis (or unilateral stenosis with a solitary kidney) constitutes a potentially reversible cause of progressive renal failure and volume-dependent hypertension. The following clinical clues increase the suspicion of renovascular hypertension: any hospitalization for urgent or emergent hypertension; recurrent "flash" pulmonary edema; recent worsening of long-standing, previously well-controlled hypertension; severe hypertension in a young adult or after the age of 50 years; precipitous and progressive worsening of renal function in response to angiotensin-converting enzyme (ACE) inhibition or angiotensin II receptor blockade; unilateral small kidney by any radiographic study; extensive peripheral arteriosclerosis; and a flank bruit.

DIAGNOSIS

Contrast-enhanced computed tomography (CT) and magnetic resonance angiography are the preferred screening tests for renal artery stenosis, but gadolinium-enhanced magnetic resonance imaging (MRI) is contraindicated in patients with advanced chronic kidney disease to avoid potentially fatal gadolinium-induced nephrogenic systemic fibrosis (Chapter 275). Fibromuscular dysplasia classically causes a "string of beads" lesion in the midportion of a renal artery (Fig. 67-8A), whereas atherosclerotic renal artery lesions are proximal and discrete (see Fig. 67-8B). Invasive renal angiography is the "gold standard" for confirming the diagnosis of renal artery stenosis.

TREATMENT ℞

Balloon angioplasty is the treatment of choice for fibromuscular dysplasia, with overall favorable outcomes. In contrast, medical management of hypertension and the associated atherosclerotic risk factors is first-line treatment for atherosclerotic renal artery stenosis. Truly drug-resistant hypertension and a progressive decline in renal function (ischemic nephropathy) currently are the only two firm indications for balloon angioplasty. Most atherosclerotic renal artery lesions do not cause hypertension or progressive renal failure, and most patients will not benefit from revascularization (balloon angioplasty or stenting), which carries substantial risks of serious complications.[1] About 15% of patients undergoing cardiac catheterization will have a renal artery lesion when coronary angiography is followed by routine ("drive-by") renal angiography, but evidence does not support this diagnostic practice or therapy based on it.

Mineralocorticoid-Induced Hypertension Due to Primary Aldosteronism

PATHOBIOLOGY

The most common causes of primary aldosteronism (Chapter 234) are a unilateral aldosterone-producing adenoma and bilateral adrenal hyperplasia. Because aldosterone is the principal ligand for the mineralocorticoid receptor in the distal nephron, excessive aldosterone production causes excessive renal Na^+-K^+ exchange, often resulting in hypokalemia.

CLINICAL MANIFESTATIONS AND DIAGNOSIS

The diagnosis should always be suspected when hypertension is accompanied by either unprovoked hypokalemia (serum potassium concentration below 3.5 mmol/L in the absence of diuretic therapy) or a tendency to develop excessive hypokalemia during diuretic therapy (serum potassium concentration below 3.0 mmol/L). However, more than one third of patients do not have hypokalemia on initial presentation, and the diagnosis should also be considered in any patient with resistant hypertension.

Screening for hyperaldosteronism should be restricted to the small fraction of hypertensive patients with hypokalemia or severe drug-resistant hypertension. If such patients have a positive screening test—a high serum aldosterone level and a suppressed plasma renin activity level— and want to consider laparoscopic adrenalectomy, the patient should be referred to an experienced center for further evaluation: salt-loading to test for nonsuppressible aldosteronism and, if present, adrenal vein sampling to test for lateralization.

Fibromuscular Dysplasia

Atherosclerosis

FIGURE 67-8. Computed tomographic angiogram with three-dimensional reconstruction. **A,** The classic "string of beads" lesion of fibromuscular dysplasia (bilateral in this patient). **B,** A severe proximal atherosclerotic stenosis of the right renal artery and mild stenosis of the left renal artery. (Images courtesy of Bart Domatch, MD, Radiology Department, University of Texas Southwestern Medical Center, Dallas, Texas.)

TREATMENT

CT has too many false-positive and false-negative results to be used as a noninvasive alternative to invasive adrenal vein sampling. Laparoscopic adrenalectomy and mineralocorticoid receptor blockade with eplerenone (50 to 100 mg per day) constitute highly effective therapeutic options that target the disease-causing mechanism with a favorable risk-to-benefit ratio.

Mendelian Forms of Mineralocorticoid-Induced Hypertension

Almost all the rare mendelian forms of hypertension are mineralocorticoid induced and involve excessive activation of the epithelial Na^+ channel (ENaC), the final common pathway for reabsorption of sodium from the distal nephron (Fig. 67-9). Thus, salt-dependent hypertension can be caused both by gain-of-function mutations of ENaC or the mineralocorticoid receptor and by increased production or decreased clearance of mineralocorticoid receptor ligands, which are aldosterone, deoxycorticosterone, and cortisol.

Pheochromocytomas and Paragangliomas

Pheochromocytomas are rare catecholamine-producing tumors of the adrenal chromaffin cells, whereas paragangliomas are even rarer tumors of the extra-adrenal chromaffin cells (Chapter 235). The diagnosis should be suspected when hypertension is drug resistant or paroxysmal, particularly when accompanied by paroxysms of headache, palpitations, pallor, or diaphoresis. In some patients, pheochromocytoma is misdiagnosed as panic disorder. A family history of early-onset hypertension may suggest pheochromocytoma as part of the multiple endocrine neoplasia syndromes (Chapter 239). An increasing number of pheochromocytomas are being detected incidentally on abdominal imaging studies for nonadrenal indications. If the diagnosis is missed, outpouring of catecholamines from the tumor can cause unsuspected hypertensive crisis during unrelated surgical procedures, in which case mortality rates exceed 80%.

Other Neurogenic Causes

Other causes of neurogenic hypertension that can be confused with pheochromocytoma include sympathomimetic agents (cocaine, methamphetamine; Chapter 33), baroreflex failure, and obstructive sleep apnea (Chapter 100). A history of surgery and radiation therapy for head and neck tumors (Chapter 196) raises suspicion of baroreceptor damage. Snoring and somnolence suggest sleep apnea, but continuous positive airway pressure to treat the sleep apnea rarely improves blood pressure substantially (Chapter 100).

Other Causes of Secondary Hypertension

Coarctation of the aorta typically occurs just distal to the origin of the left subclavian artery, so the blood pressure is lower in the legs than in the arms (opposite of the normal situation) (see Fig. 69-7 in Chapter 69). The clue is that the pulses are weaker in the lower than in the upper extremities, indicating the need to measure blood pressure in the legs as well as in both arms. Intercostal collaterals can produce bruits on examination and rib notching on the chest radiograph. Coarctations can be cured with surgery or angioplasty.

Hyperthyroidism tends to cause systolic hypertension with a wide pulse pressure, whereas hypothyroidism tends to cause mainly diastolic hypertension. Treatment is for the underlying disease. Hyperparathyroidism (Chapter 253) also has been associated with hypertension. Cyclosporine and tacrolimus are important causes of secondary hypertension in transplant recipients, apparently by inhibition of calcineurin, the calcium-dependent phosphatase that is expressed not only in lymphoid tissue but also in neural, vascular, and renal tissue. In the absence of outcomes data, nondihydropyridine calcium-channel blockers (CCBs) have become the drugs of first choice, but they increase cyclosporine blood levels. Combination therapy with diuretics, CCBs, and central sympatholytics often is required.

PREVENTION AND TREATMENT OF HYPERTENSION

At the population level, the primary prevention of hypertension requires large-scale societal changes, including further efforts to influence the food industry to reduce salt in processed foods, efforts to increase exercise, and the availability of fresh fruits and vegetables. Once a person's blood pressure rises to prehypertension levels, lifestyle modifications alone are almost never enough to return blood pressure to normal, and recidivism is almost universal.

Although short-term pharmacologic therapy with a low-dose angiotensin receptor blocker (ARB) has been advocated to prevent conversion from prehypertension to full-blown hypertension, blood pressure quickly rises again once the ARB is discontinued.[2] Thus, lifelong prescription medication is the cornerstone of effective therapy for primary hypertension, with lifestyle modification serving as an adjunct but not as an alternative. The objective is to reduce the blood pressure and associated metabolic abnormalities sufficiently to reduce the risk for cardiovascular events and end-stage renal disease without compromising the patient's quality of life.

FIGURE 67-9. Mendelian forms of hypertension that cause mineralocorticoid-induced hypertension. AME = apparent mineralocorticoid excess; Ang = angiotensin; BP = blood pressure; GRA = glucocorticoid-remediable aldosteronism; 17αHD and 11βHD = 17α- and 11β-hydroxylase deficiency; 11β-HSD2 = 11β-hydroxysteroid dehydrogenase type 2; DOC = deoxycorticosterone; ENaC = epithelial Na^+ channel; HEP = hypertension exacerbated by pregnancy; MR = mineralocorticoid receptor; NCCT = sodium-chloride cotransporter; PHA2 = pseudohypoaldosteronism type 2; ROMK = rectifying outer medullary K^+ channel; WNK = with no lysine kinases. See text for explanation. (Modified from Lifton RP, Gharavi AG, Geller DS. Molecular mechanisms of human hypertension. *Cell.* 2001;104:545-556.)

Randomized trials have proved beyond any doubt that antihypertensive drug therapy reduces cardiovascular risk, with benefits that are proportional to the reduction in blood pressure achieved.[3] However, in practice, most treated patients do not achieve the same low risk levels of truly normotensive persons because their blood pressures remain higher than optimal owing to the threshold levels of guidelines, the hesitation of practicing physicians to start and intensify drug treatment, the costs of medications, and nonadherence despite the generally declining costs of medications as they become generic.

Multidrug regimens with two, three, or even more medications of different drug classes are almost always required to achieve currently recommended blood pressure goals, particularly for high-risk patients. Low-dose drug combinations exert synergistic effects on blood pressure while minimizing dose-dependent side effects. For most patients with hypertension, lipid-lowering therapy and antiplatelet therapy are indicated as part of a comprehensive cardiovascular risk-reduction strategy (Chapter 51).

Lifestyle Modification

Every antihypertensive regimen should include lifestyle modification. The Seventh Report of the Joint National Committee on Prevention, Detection, Evaluation, and Treatment of High Blood Pressure (JNC 7) recommended a trial of lifestyle modification alone for an unspecified time (6 to 12 months in prior guidelines) before antihypertensive medication is prescribed, even for high-risk patients. This is wishful thinking and may be a cause of therapeutic inertia. More recent data, however, support greater urgency in achieving pharmacologic control of high blood pressure to reduce cardiovascular risk, at least in patients with multiple risk factors. In sufficiently motivated individuals, lifestyle modification can decrease medication requirements, have a favorable impact on associated cardiovascular risk factors, and emphasize the active role patients can play in controlling their blood pressure.

Moderate dietary sodium reduction (Chapter 220) reduces renal potassium wasting during diuretic therapy and lowers blood pressure by 2/2 mm Hg on average. Most dietary sodium comes from processed foods rather than from the salt shaker. Without draconian measures, daily salt consumption can be reduced from 10 to 6 g by teaching patients to read food labels (6 g of NaCl = 2.4 g of sodium = 100 mmol of sodium). The Dietary Approaches to Stop Hypertension (DASH) study showed that individuals with prehypertension or stage 1 hypertension can lower their blood pressures, at least over the short term, by as much as 11/6 mm Hg even without restricting calorie or sodium intake if they adhere to a diet rich in fresh fruits and vegetables (for high potassium content) and low-fat dairy products.[4] This diet (*www.nhlbi.nih.gov/health/public/heart/hbp/dash/*) is strongly recommended because the blood pressure–lowering effects can approach the magnitude of drug monotherapy, can be enhanced by an additional 2/1 mm Hg by dietary sodium restriction, and are seen in all ethnic groups, especially African Americans.

Smokers should be counseled to quit because tobacco (Chapter 31) is such a potent risk factor for coronary heart disease, stroke, and progression of hypertensive nephrosclerosis to end-stage renal disease. Because blood pressure increases transiently by 10 to 15 mm Hg after each cigarette, smokers of more than 20 cigarettes per day often have higher blood pressures out of the office than in the smoke-free medical office. Blood pressure increases similarly with the first morning cup of coffee, but the pressor response to caffeine usually (but not always) habituates throughout the day. Thus, caffeine consumption need not be eliminated.

Moderate alcohol (Chapter 32) consumption (one or two drinks per day) does not increase the risk for hypertension in Western populations; but in Japanese populations, hypertension is more common in men who are moderate drinkers than in men who cannot drink because of a loss-of-function mutation in the alcohol dehydrogenase gene. In all populations, heavy drinking (three or more standard-sized drinks per day) and especially binge drinking activate the sympathetic nervous system the next day during withdrawal and are associated with an increased incidence and severity of hypertension, which is reversible if alcohol consumption decreases.

After a bout of aerobic exercise (Chapter 15), a small reduction in blood pressure can persist for several hours. Relaxation techniques (e.g., meditation, biofeedback, breathing exercises) can decrease blood pressure transiently but generally produce little if any demonstrable effect on ambulatory blood pressure (Chapter 38). However, in some individuals in whom overwhelming home or job strain or anger is a major determinant of high blood pressure, cognitive behavior therapy and anxiolytics (Chapter 404) may be beneficial. Patients often associate hypertension directly with life stress, but stress management alone rarely is sufficient to control their hypertension.

Pharmacologic Therapy

More than 100 antihypertensive medications are marketed (Table 67-5). Lowering blood pressure with medication reduces but does not eliminate cardiorenal risks.

Classes of Oral Antihypertensive Drugs

The various classes of oral antihypertensive drugs have different mechanisms of actions, which explain the therapeutic principles of their use as well as their major contraindications and side effects (Table 67-6).

Diuretics

Mechanism of Action. With initiation of diuretic therapy, contraction of blood volume causes the initial fall in blood pressure. With continued therapy, blood volume is partially restored, and vasodilator mechanisms (e.g., opening of adenosine triphosphate [ATP]-sensitive K^+ channels) sustain the antihypertensive action. Loop diuretics block Na^+-K^+-$2Cl^-$ transport in the thick ascending loop of Henle, where a large portion of the filtered sodium is reabsorbed. Thiazide diuretics and the indoline derivative indapamide block Na^+-Cl^- cotransporter in the distal convoluted tubule, where a smaller portion of the filtered sodium is reabsorbed. Spironolactone and eplerenone prevent aldosterone from activating the mineralocorticoid receptor, thereby inhibiting the downstream activation of ENaC, whereas triamterene and amiloride block ENaC directly; because less sodium is presented to the Na^+,K^+-ATPase on the vascular side of the collecting duct cells, less potassium is excreted in the urine.

Therapeutic Principles. Diuretics are the oldest, least expensive, and still among the most effective antihypertensive medications. In the Antihypertensive and Lipid-Lowering Treatment to Prevent Heart Attack Trial (ALLHAT), the thiazide-type diuretic chlorthalidone was at least as effective as (and in some instances more effective than) newer and more expensive agents (the ACE inhibitor lisinopril or the dihydropyridine CCB amlodipine) in lowering blood pressure and preventing the attendant cardiovascular complications in all subgroups of patients.[5] Combined with other classes of antihypertensive medications, diuretics exert a synergistic effect on blood pressure. The most common cause of apparently drug-resistant hypertension is the failure to include a diuretic in the therapeutic regimen or to dose it correctly.

Because of their long half-lives, thiazides are more effective than short-acting loop diuretics for most patients with hypertension. Chlorthalidone, the thiazide-type diuretic used in the ALLHAT and many other trials, is more potent and has a much longer duration of action than hydrochlorothiazide, which for decades has replaced chlorthalidone as the main thiazide-type diuretic in clinical practice. Low-dose hydrochlorothiazide (12.5 mg/day), often in fixed-dose combination with an ACE inhibitor or ARB, is recommended for mild uncomplicated hypertension, whereas chlorthalidone (typically 25 mg/day, which has a potency equivalent to about 40 mg of hydrochlorothiazide [HCTZ]) is recommended for more severe or more difficult hypertension.

When the GFR falls below 50 mL/min/1.73 m^2, standard doses of hydrochlorothiazide become ineffective, although chlorthalidone or much higher doses of HCTZ can be effective. Loop diuretics are the diuretics of choice for treating hypertension in patients with chronic kidney disease or heart failure. Because the duration of action of furosemide is less than 6 hours, torsemide is a better choice owing to its longer half-life. The addition of chlorthalidone to a loop diuretic can sometimes restore blood pressure responsiveness in patients with resistant hypertension due to volume expansion in the setting of advanced chronic kidney disease.

Thiazides can aggravate glucose intolerance (especially when used in combination with a β-blocker), cause hypokalemia and hyponatremia (especially in older persons), precipitate gout, elevate serum lipids, and rarely cause severe photosensitive dermatitis. They are more likely than any other antihypertensive drugs to cause erectile dysfunction.

With its more favorable side-effect profile, eplerenone (50-100 mg/day) has replaced spironolactone as the drug of choice for primary aldosteronism. Low-dose eplerenone (12.5 to 50 mg/day) and low-dose spironolactone (6.25 to 50 mg/day) have been understudied and underused in primary hypertension. Both drugs are powerful antihypertensives and avoid hypokalemia. Either drug can be remarkably effective as add-on therapy for otherwise drug-resistant hypertension. Hyperkalemia must be avoided when using these agents in patients with kidney disease.

Angiotensin-Converting Enzyme Inhibitors and Angiotensin Receptor Blockers

Mechanism of Action. The renin-angiotensin-aldosterone system is one of the most important targets for antihypertensive drugs. The interaction of angiotensin II with G protein–coupled receptors, termed AT_1 receptors, accelerates numerous cellular processes that contribute not only to hypertension but also to its end-organ damage. The ACE inhibitors block the conversion of angiotensin I to angiotensin II, initially leading to a dramatic fall in plasma angiotensin II levels; with continued treatment, however, plasma angiotensin II levels return to normal (the phenomenon of "ACE escape") because ACE inhibitors do not block alternative pathways that generate angiotensin II. The sustained antihypertensive action of ACE inhibitors is explained in part by their ability to block the metabolism of bradykinin, a potent endothelium-dependent vasodilator. These agents slow the deterioration of renal function in patients with chronic kidney disease by causing greater dilation of the efferent renal arteriole, thereby reducing intraglomerular pressure.

By comparison, ARBs lower blood pressure specifically by blocking the interaction of angiotensin II on the AT_1 receptors. Thus, ARBs do not increase bradykinin, which has been implicated in both the therapeutic benefits and the side effects of ACE inhibitors (i.e., cough, angioedema).

Therapeutic Principles. Because of their favorable side-effect profiles and putative ancillary benefits on vascular health, ACE inhibitors and ARBs have gained popularity for the general treatment of hypertension. As monotherapy,

TABLE 67-5 ORAL ANTIHYPERTENSIVE AGENTS

DRUG	DOSE RANGE, TOTAL, MG/DAY (DOSES PER DAY)	USUAL STARTING DOSE, MG/DAY (DOSES PER DAY)	DRUG	DOSE RANGE, TOTAL, MG/DAY (DOSES PER DAY)	USUAL STARTING DOSE, MG/DAY (DOSES PER DAY)
DIURETICS			Moexipril	7.5-30 (1)	7.5 (1)
Thiazide Diuretics			Perindopril	4-16 (1)	4 (1)
Chlorthalidone	6.25-50 (1)	12.5 (1)	Quinapril	5-80 (1-2)	40 (2)
HCTZ	6.25-50 (1)	12.5 (1)	Ramipril	2.5-20 (1)	2.5 (1)
Indapamide	1.25-5 (1)	1.25 (1)	Trandolapril	1-8 (1)	2 (1)
Metolazone	2.5-5 (1)	2.5 (1)	**ANGIOTENSIN RECEPTOR BLOCKERS**		
Loop Diuretics			Candesartan	8-32 (1)	16 (1)
Bumetanide	0.5-2 (2)	1 (2)	Eprosartan	400-800 (1-2)	400 (1)
Ethacrynic acid	25-100 (2)	25 (2)	Irbesartan	150-300 (1)	150 (1)
Furosemide	20-160 (2)	20 (2)	Losartan	25-100 (2)	50 (1)
Torsemide	2.5-20 (1-2)	5 (2)	Olmesartan	5-40 (1)	20 (1)
Potassium Sparing			Telmisartan	20-80 (1)	40 (1)
Amiloride	5-20 (1)	10 (2)	Valsartan	80-320 (1-2)	160 (2)
Eplerenone	25-100 (1-2)	25 (1)	**DIRECT RENIN INHIBITOR**		
Spironolactone	6.25-400 (1-2)	6.25 (1)	Aliskiren	150-300 (1)	150 (1)
Triamterene	25-100 (1)	37.5 (1)	**α-BLOCKERS**		
β-BLOCKERS			Doxazosin	1-16 (1)	1 (1)
Acebutolol	200-800 (2)	200 (2)	Prazosin	1-40 (2-3)	1 (2)
Atenolol	25-100 (1)	25 (1)	Terazosin	1-20 (1)	1 (1)
Betaxolol	5-20 (1)	5 (1)	Phenoxybenzamine for pheochromocytoma	20-120 (2)	20 (2)
Bisoprolol	2.5-20 (1)	2.5 (1)	**CENTRAL SYMPATHOLYTICS**		
Carteolol	2.5-10 (1)	2.5 (1)	Clonidine	0.2-1.2 (2-3)	0.2 (2)
Metoprolol	50-450 (2)	50 (2)	Clonidine patch	0.1-0.6 (weekly)	0.1 (weekly)
Metoprolol XL	50-200 (1-2)	50 (1)	Guanabenz	2-32 (2)	2 (2)
Nadolol	20-320 (1)	40 (1)	Guanfacine	1-3 (1) (qhs)	1 (1)
Penbutolol	10-80 (1)	10 (1)	Methyldopa	250-1000 (2)	250 (2)
Pindolol	10-60 (2)	10 (1)	Reserpine	0.05-0.25 (1)	0.05 (1)
Propranolol	40-180 (2)	40 (2)	**DIRECT VASODILATORS**		
Propranolol LA	60-180 (1-2)	60 (1)	Hydralazine	10-200 (2)	20 (2)
Timolol	20-60 (2)	20 (2)	Minoxidil	2.5-100 (1)	2.5 (1)
α-/β-BLOCKERS/VASODILATING β-BLOCKERS			**FIXED-DOSE COMBINATIONS**		
Carvedilol	6.25-50 (2)	6.25 (2)	Aliskiren/HCTZ	150/12.5-300/25 (1)	150/12.5 (1)
Carvedilol CR	20-80 (1)	20 (1)	Amiloride/HCTZ	5/50 (1)	5/50 (1)
Labetalol	200-2400 (2)	200 (2)	Amlodipine/benazepril	2.5-5/10-20 (1)	2.5/10 (1)
Nebivolol	5-40 (1)	5 (1)	Amlodipine/olmesartan	5/20-10/40 (1)	5/20 (1)
CALCIUM-CHANNEL BLOCKERS			Amlodipine/telmisartan	5/20-10/80 (1)	5/20 (1)
Dihydropyridines			Amlodipine/valsartan	5/160-10/320 (1)	5/160 (1)
Amlodipine	2.5-10 (1)	2.5 (1)	Atenolol/chlorthalidone	50-100/25 (1)	50/25 (1)
Felodipine	2.5-20 (1-2)	2.5 (2)	Benazepril/HCTZ	5-20/6.25-25 (1)	20/6.25 (1)
Isradipine CR	2.5-20 (2)	2.5 (2)	Bisoprolol/HCTZ	2.5-10/6.25 (1)	2.5/6.25 (1)
Nicardipine SR	30-120 (2)	30 (2)	Candesartan/HCTZ	16-32/12.5-25 (1)	16/12.5 (1)
Nifedipine XL	30-120 (1)	30 (1)	Enalapril/HCTZ	5-10/25 (1-2)	5/25 (1)
Nisoldipine	10-40 (1-2)	10 (2)	Eprosartan/HCTZ	600/12.5-25 (1)	600/12.5 (1)
Nondihydropyridines			Fosinopril/HCTZ	10-20/12.5 (1)	10/12.5 (1)
Diltiazem CD	120-540 (1)	180 (1)	Irbesartan/HCTZ	150-300/12.5-25 (1)	150/12.5 (1)
Verapamil HS	120-480 (1)	180 (1)	Losartan/HCTZ	50-100/12.5-25 (1)	50/12.5 (1)
ANGIOTENSIN-CONVERTING ENZYME INHIBITORS			Olmesartan/HCTZ	20-40/12.5 (1)	20/12.5 (1)
Benazepril	10-80 (1-2)	20 (1)	Spironolactone/HCTZ	25/25 ($^1/_2$-1)	25/25 (1/2)
Captopril	25-150 (2)	25 (2)	Telmisartan/HCTZ	40-80/12.5-25 (1)	40/12.5 (1)
Enalapril	2.5-40 (2)	5 (2)	Trandolapril/verapamil	2-4/180-240 (1)	2/180 (1)
Fosinopril	10-80 (1-2)	20 (2)	Triamterene/HCTZ	37.5/25 ($^1/_2$-1)	37.5/25 (1/2)
Lisinopril	5-80 (1-2)	40 (2)	Valsartan/HCTZ	80-160/12.5-25 (1)	160/12.5 (1)

HCTZ = hydrochlorothiazide.

TABLE 67-6 MAJOR CONTRAINDICATIONS AND SIDE EFFECTS OF ANTIHYPERTENSIVE DRUGS

DRUG CLASS	MAJOR CONTRAINDICATIONS	SIDE EFFECTS
Diuretics		
Thiazides	Gout	Insulin resistance, new-onset type 2 diabetes
		Hypokalemia, hyponatremia
		Hypertriglyceridemia
		Hyperuricemia, precipitation of gout
		Erectile dysfunction (more than other drug classes)
		Potentiate nondepolarizing muscle relaxants
		Photosensitivity dermatitis
Loop diuretics	Hepatic coma	Interstitial nephritis
		Hypokalemia
		Potentiate succinylcholine
		Potentiate aminoglycoside ototoxicity
Potassium-sparing diuretics	Serum potassium concentration > 5.5 mEq/L GFR < 30 mg/mL/1.73 m^2	Hyperkalemia
ACEIs	Pregnancy	Cough
	Bilateral renal artery stenosis	Hyperkalemia
	Hyperkalemia	Angioedema
		Leukopenia
		Fetal toxicity
		Cholestatic jaundice (rare fulminant hepatic necrosis if the drug is not discontinued)
Dihydropyridine CCBs	As monotherapy in chronic kidney disease with proteinuria	Headaches
		Flushing
		Ankle edema
		CHF
		Gingival hyperplasia
		Esophageal reflux
Nondihydropyridine CCBs	Heart block	Bradycardia, AV block (especially with verapamil)
	Systolic heart failure	Constipation (often severe with verapamil)
		Worsening of systolic function, CHF
		Gingival edema or hypertrophy
		Increase cyclosporine blood levels
		Esophageal reflux
ARBs, DRI	Pregnancy	Hyperkalemia
	Bilateral renal artery stenosis	Angioedema (very rare)
	Hyperkalemia	Fetal toxicity
β-Adrenergic blockers	Heart block	New-onset type 2 diabetes (especially in combination with a thiazide)
	Asthma	Heart block, acute decompensated CHF
	Depression	Bronchospasm
	Cocaine and methamphetamine abuse	Depression, nightmares, fatigue
		Cold extremities, claudication (β_2 effect)
		Stevens-Johnson syndrome
		Agranulocytosis
α-Adrenergic blockers	Orthostatic hypotension	Orthostatic hypotension
	Systolic heart failure	Drug tolerance (in the absence of diuretic therapy)
	Left ventricular dysfunction	Ankle edema
		CHF
		First-dose effect (acute hypotension)
		Potentiate hypotension with PDE-5 inhibitors (e.g., sildenafil)
Central sympatholytics	Orthostatic hypotension	Depression, dry mouth, lethargy
		Erectile dysfunction (dose dependent)
		Rebound hypertension with clonidine withdrawal
		Coombs' test–positive hemolytic anemia and elevated liver enzymes with α-methyldopa
Direct vasodilators	Orthostatic hypotension	Reflex tachycardia
		Fluid retention
		Hirsutism, pericardial effusion with minoxidil
		Lupus with hydralazine

ACE = angiotensin-converting enzyme; ARBs = angiotensin receptor blockers; AV = atrioventricular; CCBs = calcium-channel blockers; CHF = congestive heart failure; DRI = direct renin inhibitor; GFR = glomerular filtration rate; NSAIDs = nonsteroidal anti-inflammatory drugs; PDE-5 = phosphodiesterase-5.

they generally are less potent than diuretics or CCBs, particularly in African Americans, but they amplify the effects of these other drug classes when they are used in combination. An ACE inhibitor or an ARB is considered the basis for antihypertensive drug therapy in mild or moderate chronic kidney disease (Chapter 116) because they rarely precipitate hyperkalemia or acute renal failure and appear to provide renoprotection. Serum creatinine and potassium concentrations must be monitored in all patients receiving an ACE inhibitor or ARB. In patients with chronic kidney disease, initiation of an ACE inhibitor or ARB often causes small and transient increases in serum creatinine concentration that do not necessitate discontinuation. ACE inhibitors and ARBs can precipitate acute renal failure in patients with bilateral renal artery stenosis

(Chapter 127) or hypovolemia. After correction of hypovolemia, the ACE inhibitor or ARB usually can be restarted safely at a lower dose.

The most common side effect of ACE inhibitors is a dry cough. Patients may complain not of a cough but rather of having to clear the throat or loss of voice later in the day. These symptoms occur in 3 to 39% of patients, resolve in a few days after the drug is discontinued, and can be eliminated by switching the patient to an ARB. The incidence is higher in African Americans than in whites and is highest in Asians.

The ARBs are less effective than dihydropyridine CCBs in controlling hypertension but are increasingly popular because they have a more favorable side-effect profile than ACE inhibitors. Their efficacy is enhanced by addition of low-dose HCTZ or a dihydropyridine CCB. An increasing number of fixed-dose combinations are available (see Table 67-5). Losartan, the prototype, differs from the other ARBs in two ways: a shorter duration of action, requiring twice-daily dosing if it is used as monotherapy; and a uricosuric effect, which may be beneficial in patients with hyperuricemia. Newer ARBs vary in potency and duration of action. The putative special metabolic benefit of telmisartan, which shares structural homology with the insulin sensitizer pioglitazone, remains unproved.

Direct Renin Inhibitors

Aliskiren is the first in a new class of orally effective, nonpeptide, low-molecular-weight renin inhibitors. Direct renin inhibitors block the renin-angiotensin-aldosterone system at its origin without increasing bradykinin. By eliminating the reactive rise in plasma renin activity seen with ACE inhibitors and ARBs, direct renin inhibition may prevent more hypertensive complications, particularly renal complications. Short-term studies in patients with mild or moderate hypertension suggest that once-daily low-dose (150 mg) or high-dose (300 mg) aliskiren is equivalent to an ARB in terms of both blood pressure–lowering effect and favorable side-effect profile. The contraindications are the same. Randomized trials of cardiovascular outcomes compared with other drugs are pending.

Calcium-Channel Blockers

Mechanism of Action. The CCBs are antiarrhythmic, antianginal, and antihypertensive because they block the opening of voltage-gated (L-type) Ca^{2+} channels in cardiac myocytes and vascular smooth muscle cells. The resultant decrease in the cytosolic Ca^{2+} signal decreases heart rate and ventricular contractility and relaxes vascular smooth muscle. Blood pressure lowering is related mainly to peripheral arterial vasodilation, with the rank order of potency being dihydropyridines > diltiazem >> verapamil. In contrast, for negative chronotropic and inotropic effects, the rank order of potency is verapamil >> diltiazem > dihydropyridines.

Therapeutic Principles. *Short-acting dihydropyridines should not be used to treat hypertension.* By triggering an abrupt fall in blood pressure with reflex sympathetic activation, these rapidly acting arterial vasodilators can precipitate myocardial ischemia, infarction, stroke, and death. By comparison, the safety and efficacy of long-acting dihydropyridine CCBs was confirmed by ALLHAT and the VALUE (Valsartan Antihypertensive Long-term Use Evaluation) trial.[6] For most hypertensive patients, these are among the most potent, best tolerated, and safest antihypertensive medications available, but there are some caveats. For comparable degrees of blood pressure lowering, dihydropyridine CCBs exert protection against myocardial infarction and stroke equivalent to that of diuretics, but their use is associated with a greater risk for heart failure. For patients with renal insufficiency and proteinuria, dihydropyridine CCB-based therapy is less renoprotective than ARB- or ACE inhibitor–based therapy. However, in most patients with renal disease, multiple classes of medications, including dihydropyridines, are required to achieve blood pressure goals. Thus, dihydropyridine CCBs should not be used as first-line therapy for hypertension in patients with proteinuria, but they may be used as adjunctive therapy once the dose of the ACE inhibitor or ARB has been maximized in combination with an appropriate diuretic.

Verapamil is a weak antihypertensive and of limited utility because of dose-dependent constipation. Diltiazem is intermediate in potency between verapamil and the dihydropyridines; it is usually well tolerated. Verapamil and diltiazem can cause heart block, especially in older patients and in patients taking digoxin.

Adrenergic Receptor Blockers and Central Sympatholytics

Sympathetic drive to the sinus node increases heart rate and cardiac output through β-adrenergic receptors, whereas sympathetic drive to the peripheral vasculature causes neurogenic vasoconstriction through α-adrenergic receptors. Sustained activation of the sympathetic nervous system is thought to contribute to chronic hypertension by vascular remodeling, renin release, and attenuation of renal sodium excretion by an action on the distal tubules.

β-Adrenergic Blockers

Mechanism of Action. Interaction of epinephrine or norepinephrine with $β_1$-adrenoreceptors in the heart causes G protein–linked activation of adenylate cyclase, resulting in positive chronotropic and inotropic effects. Interaction of catecholamines with $β_2$-adrenoreceptors relaxes bronchiolar and arteriolar smooth muscle. With the initiation of β-blocker therapy, blood pressure at first is little affected because the fall in cardiac output is offset by a compensatory increase in peripheral resistance. Over time, blood pressure falls progressively as the peripheral vasculature relaxes. Thus, the antihypertensive effect of β-blockade involves decreases in cardiac output ($β_1$-receptors), renin release ($β_1$-receptors), and norepinephrine release (prejunctional $β_2$-receptors).

The prototype β-blocker, propranolol, nonselectively blocks both $β_1$- and $β_2$-receptors. Other standard β-blockers (metoprolol, atenolol, acebutolol, and bisoprolol) are *relatively* cardioselective. In low doses, they exert a greater inhibitory effect on $β_1$- than on $β_2$-receptors, but selectivity is lost at high doses. In contrast, combined α- and β-blockers (labetalol, carvedilol, nebivolol)

cause vasodilation by blocking $α_1$-adrenoreceptors on vascular smooth muscle and possibly by increasing the bioavailability of nitric oxide.

Therapeutic Principles. Although standard β-blockers are first-line medical therapy for ischemic heart disease (Chapters 72 and 73) and heart failure (Chapter 59), they are no longer first-line or even second-line agents for uncomplicated hypertension. They predispose to diabetes, particularly when combined with a thiazide, and offer less stroke protection than other antihypertensive drugs.[7] In addition to being rather weak antihypertensives, they are less effective than other agents in lowering central aortic blood pressure because bradycardia allows more time for wave reflection and thus central pressure augmentation. β-blockers can cause fatigue, limit exercise tolerance, and worsen depression.

Compared with standard β-blockers, combined α-/β-blockers are better antihypertensives. They lower blood pressure more and have a more favorable metabolic profile. Generic carvedilol is now widely affordable ($10 for a 90-day supply), but its patent has expired, and no outcomes trials have been performed. Labetalol, which rarely causes severe hepatotoxicity, should be reserved for hypertensive urgencies, perioperative management, or very difficult hypertension. All β-blockers can precipitate heart block, and they can aggravate preexisting asthma.

α-Adrenergic Blockers

Mechanism of Action. By blocking the interaction of norepinephrine on vascular α-adrenergic receptors, these drugs cause peripheral vasodilation, thereby lowering blood pressure. By increasing skeletal muscle blood flow, they increase insulin sensitivity. By dilating urethral smooth muscle, they improve symptoms of prostatism. Prazosin, doxazosin, terazosin, and intravenous phentolamine selectively block $α_1$-adrenoreceptors; phenoxybenzamine blocks both $α_1$- and $α_2$-receptors.

Therapeutic Principles. Phenoxybenzamine remains the drug of choice for preoperative management of pheochromocytoma (Chapter 235); after α-blockade is achieved, a β-blocker should be added to block an otherwise excessive reflex tachycardia. The selective $α_1$-blockers are not first-line agents and should not be used as monotherapy because their propensity to cause fluid retention can lead to tachyphylaxis and unmask or exacerbate heart failure. However, when they are prescribed as part of a combination regimen that includes a diuretic, they are effective fourth- or fifth-line therapy for difficult hypertension and are particularly useful in older men with prostatism. Although marketed specifically for prostatism and not as an antihypertensive agent, the selective $α_{1A}$-blocker tamsulosin lowers blood pressure in some men.

Central Sympatholytics

Mechanism of Action. Stimulation of postsynaptic $α_2$-adrenergic receptors and imidazoline receptors in the central nervous system lowers central sympathetic outflow, whereas stimulation of presynaptic $α_2$-receptors causes feedback inhibition of norepinephrine release from peripheral sympathetic nerve terminals. The combined effect is reduced sympathetic drive to the heart and peripheral circulation, thereby leading to decreased heart rate, cardiac output, and peripheral vascular resistance.

Therapeutic Principles. The central sympatholytics are best reserved for short-term oral treatment of severe uncontrolled hypertension. They are potent antihypertensive agents that may be needed as fourth- or fifth-line therapy for very difficult hypertension, but their troublesome central nervous system side effects often reduce quality of life. To avoid rebound hypertension between doses, short-acting clonidine must be given every 6 to 8 hours or, whenever possible, discontinued using a gradual tapering schedule. Rebound hypertension is less of a problem with longer-acting preparations (guanfacine, clonidine patch). α-Methyldopa remains the drug of choice for chronic hypertension in pregnancy (Chapter 247).

Direct Vasodilators

Mechanism of Action. Minoxidil and hydralazine are potent hyperpolarizing arterial vasodilators that work by opening vascular ATP-sensitive K^+ channels.

Therapeutic Principles. By causing selective and rapid arterial dilation, both drugs cause profound reflex sympathetic activation and tachycardia as well as ankle edema. For this reason, hydralazine has largely been replaced by the longer-acting dihydropyridine CCBs. However, hydralazine remains the treatment of choice for acute severe hypertension in pregnancy (Chapter 247). A combination of hydralazine plus nitroglycerin now is recommended for the treatment of heart failure specifically in African Americans, in whom hypertensive heart disease is the most common cause of heart failure (Chapter 58). Severe hypertension accompanying advanced chronic kidney disease (Chapter 132) is the main indication for minoxidil, which must be combined with a β-blocker to prevent excessive reflex tachycardia and with a loop diuretic to prevent excessive fluid retention. Institution of hemodialysis is usually a more effective means of controlling hypertension.

Antihypertensive Drug Interactions

By inhibiting the kidney's ability to excrete sodium, nonsteroidal anti-inflammatory drugs (including aspirin in daily doses above 81 mg), can negate the antihypertensive action of diuretics and renin-angiotensin system inhibitors, but they do not interfere with CCBs. However, even a single glass of grapefruit juice increases the bioavailability of dihydropyridine CCBs by inhibiting the intestinal cytochrome P-450 3A4 system, which is responsible for the first-pass metabolism of many oral medications. Acetaminophen per se does not appear to cause salt retention, but in Great Britain, and not in the United States, each acetaminophen tablet contains 1000 mg of sodium. A high-fat meal will impair aliskiren absorption. Verapamil and diltiazem will increase blood levels of cyclosporine and digoxin.

Which Drugs for Which Patients?

Choosing the best drugs to treat hypertension in a given patient is based primarily on effective lowering of blood pressure and prevention of hypertensive complications with minimal side effects (see Table 67-6) and cost. A secondary consideration is concomitant treatment of comorbid cardiovascular diseases (e.g., angina, heart failure). According to a strict evidence-based approach, a "compelling indication" is defined as a comorbid condition for which the use of a specific antihypertensive drug has been shown to improve disease outcomes in a randomized controlled trial (Table 67-7).

Choice of Therapy for the Patient with "Uncomplicated" Primary Hypertension

To date, a few DNA sequence variations have been proposed to identify individual patients whose blood pressure is particularly sensitive to a specific drug class. However, pharmacogenetic research has yet to affect the clinical treatment of hypertension.

In the absence of such ideal scientific information, the now outdated 2003 JNC 7 guidelines recommended a thiazide-type diuretic as cost-effective first-line therapy for most patients with hypertension. They also recommended initiation of therapy with two drugs (one being a thiazide) for stage 2 hypertension. In contrast, the European Society of Hypertension–European Society of Cardiology makes no specific drug class recommendation, arguing that the most effective drugs are those that the patient will tolerate and take. The revised guidelines of the British Hypertension Society previously advocated initiation of therapy with an ACE inhibitor or ARB ("A" drug) for young white patients (<55 years), who often have high-renin hypertension, but a CCB or diuretic ("C" or "D" drug) for older and black patients, who often have low-renin hypertension.

In contrast, there is growing evidence and consensus about the overriding importance of lowering blood pressure with combinations of drugs with different mechanisms of action (see Table 67-5), rather than belaboring the choice of the single best initial agent, to reach currently recommended blood pressure treatment targets (see Table 67-3). For example, tight control (goal systolic pressure of <130 mm Hg) of systolic blood pressure in nondiabetic patients is significantly more effective than usual control (goal systolic pressure of <140 mm Hg) in reducing subsequent left ventricular hypertrophy by electrocardiography, and it can reduce important cardiovascular events by 50%.[8] Systolic blood pressure targets are achieved in only 50 to 60% of hypertensive patients, even when they receive an average of three drugs in the idealized setting of a randomized trial.

Low-dose combination drug therapy is not only the best way to control blood pressure but also the best way to minimize side effects because the dose-response relationship for blood pressure is rather flat, occurring at the lower end of the dose range for most medications, whereas many of the side effects are steeply dose dependent. Synergistic combinations achieve blood pressure control at lower doses.

The question is: Which drug combinations are best?

Dual therapy with an ACE inhibitor plus amlodipine (the longest-acting, best studied, and now generic dihydropyridine CCB) was found in recent trials to offer more cardiovascular protection, particularly against stroke, than dual therapy with either a β-blocker plus a thiazide[9] or an ACE inhibitor plus thiazide.[10] Other recent data indicate that ACE inhibitors or ARBs offer similar cardiovascular protection[11] and thus are interchangeable, except for higher cost of ARBs and almost no cough. All the ACE inhibitors and ARBs are available as fixed-dose combinations with a low dose of hydrochlorothiazide (see Table 67-5). Lotrel is the prototype ACE inhibitor–amlodipine fixed-dose combination, and several new (branded) ARB-CCB combinations recently have been marketed (see Table 67-5).

Amlodipine and other dihydropyridine CCBs cause dose-dependent ankle edema because they preferentially dilate arteries rather than veins, thereby elevating hydrostatic pressure; the resulting ankle edema often can be relieved by the addition of an ACE inhibitor, ARB, or aliskiren, which dilate the veins as well as the arteries. Standard β-blockers are no longer recommended to treat uncomplicated hypertension. In contrast, generic carvedilol is being used increasingly as third- or fourth-line therapy. Central sympatholytic agents should be reserved as fifth-line therapy for patients with difficult hypertension.

Despite much compelling basic research on ancillary (pleiotropic) benefits of ACE inhibitors or ARBs to block multiple adverse effects of angiotensin II, in clinical trials most of the cardiovascular benefit derived from these and all

TABLE 67-7 "COMPELLING" INDICATIONS AND PUBLISHED EVIDENCE

COMPELLING INDICATION	DRUG CLASS (RELEVANT CLINICAL TRIALS*)
Systolic heart failure	ACEI (CONSENSUS, SAVE) ARB (Val-HeFT, CHARM) β-Blocker (MERIT-HFCOMET) Aldosterone antagonist (RALES)
Recent MI	β-Blockers (ISIS)
Reduced left ventricular function after MI	ACEI (SAVE, TRACE) Aldosterone antagonist (EPHESUS) β-Blocker (CAPRICORN)
Type 1 diabetes	ACEI (CCSG)
Type 2 diabetes	ACEI (MICRO-HOPE)
Type 2 diabetic nephropathy	ARB (IDNT, RENAAL, IRMA-2, MOSES, ONTARGET)
Nondiabetic chronic kidney disease	ACEI (REIN, AIPRI, AASK, ONTARGET)
CV disease	ACEI (HOPE, EUROPA) ARB (ONTARGET)
Prior stroke or TIA	ACEI + thiazide (PROGRESS)
Isolated systolic hypertension in older persons	DHP-CCB (Syst-Eur, Syst-China, STOP-2) Thiazide (SHEP) ACEI (STOP-2) ARB (SCOPE, second-line)
Hypertension in the very elderly	ACEI + thiazide (HYVET)
Left ventricular hypertrophy by electrocardiography	ARB plus thiazide (LIFE)

*CONSENSUS, Cooperative North Scandinavian Enalapril Survival Study (N Engl J Med. 1987;316:1429-1435); SAVE, Survival and Ventricular Enlargement study (N Engl J Med. 1992;327:669-677); Val-HeFT, Valsartan Heart Failure Trial (N Engl J Med. 2001;345:1667-1675); CHARM, Candesartan in Heart Failure: Assessment of Reduction in Morbidity and Mortality (Lancet. 2003;362:759-766); MERIT-HF, Metoprolol Randomized Intervention Trial in Congestive Heart Failure (JAMA. 2000;283:1295-1302); COMET, comparison of carvedilol and metoprolol on clinical outcomes in patients with chronic heart failure in the Carvedilol Or Metoprolol European Trial (Lancet. 2003;362:7-13); RALES, Randomized Aldactone Evaluation Study (N Engl J Med. 1999;341:709-717); ISIS, International Study of Infarct Survival (Lancet. 1986;2:57-66); TRACE, Trandolapril Cardiac Evaluation (N Engl J Med. 1995;333:1670-1676); EPHESUS, Eplerenone Post-Myocardial Infarction Heart Failure Efficacy and Survival Study (N Engl J Med. 2003;348:1309-1321); CAPRICORN, effect of carvedilol on outcome after myocardial infarction in patients with left-ventricular dysfunction (Lancet. 2001;357:1385-1390); CCSG, Captopril Cooperative Study Group (N Engl J Med. 1993;323:1456-1462); MICRO-HOPE, Microalbuminuria, Cardiovascular and Renal Outcomes substudy of the Heart Outcomes Prevention Evaluation (Lancet. 2000;355:253-259); IDNT, Irbesartan Diabetic Nephropathy Trial (N Engl J Med. 2001;345:841-860); RENAAL, Reduction of Endpoints in NIDDM with the Angiotensin II Antagonist Losartan (N Engl J Med. 2001;345:861-869); IRMA-2, Irbesartan Microalbuminuria study 2 (N Engl J Med. 2001;345:870-878); REIN, Ramipril Evaluation in Nephropathy trial (Lancet. 1998;352:1252-1256); AIPRI, ACE Inhibition in Progressive Renal Insufficiency (Kidney Int. 1997;63[Suppl]:S63-S67); AASK, African American Study of Kidney Disease and Hypertension (JAMA. 2002;288:2421-2431); ONTARGET, Ongoing Telmisartan Alone and in combination with Ramipril Global Endpoint Trial (N Engl J Med. 2008;358:1547-1559; Lancet. 2008;372:547-553); HOPE, Heart Outcomes Prevention Evaluation (N Engl J Med. 2000;342:145-153); EUROPA, European Reduction of Cardiac Events with Perindopril in Stable Coronary Artery Disease (Lancet. 2003;362:782-788); PROGRESS, Perindopril Protection Against Recurrent Stroke Study (Lancet. 2001;358:1033-1041); Syst-Eur, Systolic Hypertension in Europe trial (Lancet. 1997;360:757-764); Syst-China, Systolic Hypertension in China trial (J Hypertens. 1998;16:1823-1829); STOP-2, Swedish Trial in Old Patients with Hypertension 2 (Lancet. 1999;354:1751-1756); SHEP, Systolic Hypertension in the Elderly Program (JAMA. 1991;265:3255-3264); SCOPE, Study on Cognition and Prognosis in the Elderly (J Hypertens. 2003;21:875-886); HYVET, Hypertension in the Very Elderly Trial (N Engl J Med. 2008;358:1887-1898); LIFE, Losartan Intervention for Endpoint Reduction (Lancet. 2002;359:995-1003).
ACE = angiotensin-converting enzyme; ACEI = angiotensin-converting enzyme inhibitor; ARB = angiotensin receptor blocker; CHF = congestive heart failure; CV = cardiovascular; DHP-CCB = dihydropyridine calcium-channel blocker; MI = myocardial infarction; TIA = transient ischemic attack.
Modified and updated from Elliott WJ. Compelling Indications for Antihypertensive Drugs. ASH Clinical Hypertension Review Course. New York: American Society of Hypertension; 2005:333-351.

other classes of antihypertensive agents comes directly from lowering blood pressure (Fig. 67-10). Dual therapy with an ACE inhibitor and ARB provides no more cardiovascular protection than either alone and is associated with more hypotension and renal failure.[11]

Along with antihypertensive medication and lifestyle modification, additional cardiovascular risk reduction with low-dose aspirin (81 mg) (Chapter 37) and lipid-lowering medication (Chapter 213) should be strongly considered as an integral part of cardiovascular risk reduction. In treated hypertensive

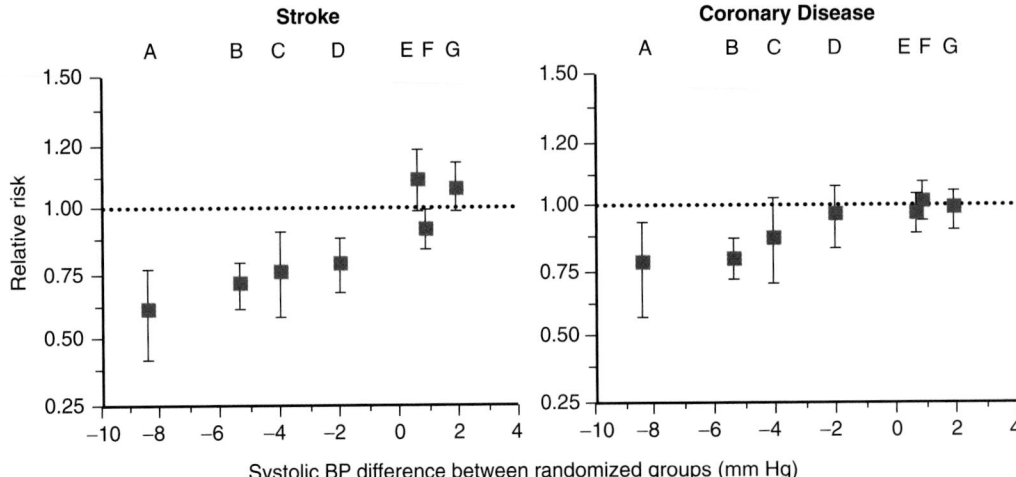

FIGURE 67-10. Meta regression analysis of randomized controlled intervention trials. (12 trials, N = 94,338 patients with hypertension, coronary artery disease, or diabetic nephropathy who were assigned to treatment with amlodipine or an angiotensin receptor blocker.) Systolic blood pressure (BP) differences were obtained by subtracting the mean change in the amlodipine or ARB group from the corresponding mean change in the reference group. Regardless of drug class, most of the protection against stroke and myocardial infarction was related to lowering of systolic BP. (From Wang J-G, Li Y, Franklin SS, et al. Prevention of stroke and myocardial infarction by amlodipine and angiotensin receptor blockers: a quantitative review. *Hypertension.* 2007;50:181-188.)

patients, low-dose aspirin reduces the risk for myocardial infarction by 36% without increasing the risk for intracerebral hemorrhage. In patients with moderate hypertension, additional cardiovascular risk factors, and an average low-density lipoprotein cholesterol level of 130 mg/dL, the addition of 10 mg of atorvastatin to the antihypertensive regimen results in a 36% reduction in fatal and nonfatal myocardial infarction and a 27% reduction in fatal and nonfatal stroke.**12** Thus, statin therapy should be used in such patients with the goal of reducing the low-density lipoprotein cholesterol level to below 100 mg/dL or even lower (Chapter 213).

Hypertension in Minority Populations

Mexican Americans have the lowest rate of control of hypertension of all U.S. race/ethnic groups but also have the highest risk for diabetes. Thus, antihypertensive regimens should be tailored to avoid causing more new cases of diabetes. In African Americans, hypertension not only is more prevalent than in the general population but also starts at a younger age, is less well controlled, and causes disproportionate and premature disability and death. African Americans commonly have lower plasma renin levels and have less response to monotherapy with an ACE inhibitor, ARB, or β-blocker than do white hypertensive patients. In one randomized trial, African American participants in the ALLHAT had a 40% higher risk for fatal stroke when taking an ACE inhibitor than when taking a diuretic, probably because blood pressure remained higher on the ACE inhibitor. However, when high doses of an ACE inhibitor or ARB are used in combination with a diuretic, antihypertensive efficacy is amplified, and racial/ethnic differences disappear. ACE inhibitors or ARBs can help achieve excellent control of hypertension in African American patients when used as part of an appropriate multidrug regimen.

Hypertensive Nephrosclerosis: A Misnomer?

Second only to diabetes, hypertension is thought to be the next most common cause of end-stage renal disease (ESRD; Chapter 132). Because African Americans are at increased risk for both hypertension and chronic kidney disease, most cases of nondiabetic kidney disease in African Americans have been attributed to *hypertensive nephrosclerosis*—small shrunken kidneys caused by chronic glomerular ischemia owing to severe constriction of the afferent renal arteriole. However, most cases of presumed hypertensive nephrosclerosis are due primarily to a West African ancestral gene locus on chromosome 21 (ApoL1), which both confers resistance against trypanosomiasis and is a powerful risk factor for non-diabetic chronic kidney disease. This risk allele, which is present in 30% of African Americans, may explain why intensive lowering of blood pressure failed to prevent ESRD in the African American Study of Kidney Disease trial.**13**

Mild to moderate nondiabetic chronic kidney disease has been considered a compelling indication for ACE inhibitors, but the renal benefit of an ACE inhibitor–based regimen in nondiabetic chronic kidney disease has been confined to short-term trials and was not demonstrated during long-term follow-up.**13** A recommended multidrug regimen for hypertension in patients with stage II or stage III chronic kidney disease is a loop diuretic (for effective control of obligatory sodium retention), a low-dose ACE inhibitor or ARB (to reduce intraglomerular hypertension), and a central sympatholytic (to reduce sympathetic overactivity from a pressor reflex arising in the failing kidneys). If proteinuria is present, the blood pressure should be lowered gradually to 130/80 mm Hg, if possible, without causing a progressive rise in serum creatinine levels. The ACE inhibitor and loop diuretic will need to be held

temporarily if the rise in serum creatinine concentration exceeds 30% of the baseline value or the serum potassium concentration increases to more than 5.6 mmol/L; they often can be restarted at lower doses once the acute deterioration in renal function has resolved.

Hypertension in Patients with Diabetes

Compared with its 25% prevalence in the general adult population, hypertension is present in 75% of diabetic patients and is a major factor contributing to an excessive risk for myocardial infarction, stroke, heart failure, microvascular complications, and diabetic nephropathy progressing to ESRD (Chapter 237). Compared with less intensive treatment, more intensive reduction of blood pressure has been proved to reduce stroke and microvascular end points dramatically in patients with diabetes. To reduce these risks, blood pressures should be lowered to 130/80 mm Hg, a goal that typically requires three to five drugs.**14** On the basis of data from randomized trials, type 1 diabetes (Chapter 236) with renal insufficiency is a compelling indication for ACE inhibitor–based antihypertensive therapy, whereas type 2 diabetes (Chapter 237) with renal insufficiency is now considered to be a compelling indication for ARB-based antihypertensive therapy because similar data do not exist for ACE inhibitor–based regimens in type 2 diabetic patients (see Table 67-7). However, an ACE inhibitor or ARB alone rarely achieves the stringent blood pressure goals; a loop diuretic is usually needed to shrink the expanded plasma volume, and a dihydropyridine CCB is usually needed for antihypertensive synergy. To optimize renal protection, the CCB should not be started until antihypertensive therapy has been initiated with an ACE inhibitor or ARB. A β-blocker should be added if the patient has coronary disease, which is prevalent in diabetes or heart failure. The α- and β-blocker carvedilol has a better metabolic profile than the pure β-blockers.

Systolic Hypertension in Older Persons

In older persons with isolated systolic hypertension, lowering systolic pressure from above 160 to below 150 mm Hg has been shown to reduce the risk for stroke by 30%, myocardial infarction by 23%, and overall cardiovascular mortality by 18%; it also reduces heart failure admissions and slows the progression of dementia. Even hypertensive patients older than 80 years have benefited from treatment with an ACE inhibitor and thiazide regimen (perindopril plus indapamide) compared with placebo.**15**

However, because of slower drug metabolism and reduced postural autonomic reflexes in older persons, it is important to start with low doses of antihypertensive medication and titrate slowly. If orthostatic hypotension is present, medication should be titrated to standing blood pressure. The same triple combination therapy for systolic and diastolic hypertension should be used for isolated systolic hypertension: an ACE inhibitor (or ARB), a dihydropyridine CCB, and thiazide. In some older patients, even low-dose thiazides cause unacceptable degrees of hyponatremia. β-blockers should be restricted to patients with coronary disease or heart failure and should be used with caution because they are more likely to precipitate heart block, to impair exercise tolerance, and to cause depression.

Blood Pressure Lowering for Secondary Prevention of Stroke

Most neurologists recommend minimal or no blood pressure reduction during an acute ischemic stroke unless the patient is a candidate for thrombolytic therapy (Chapters 414 and 415). Once the patient's condition has stabilized, however, lowering blood pressure by 12/5 mm Hg with a combination of the thiazide diuretic indapamide plus the ACE inhibitor perindopril reduces the risk for recurrent stroke by 43%.[16]

Hypertension in Patients with Ischemic Heart Disease

In patients with stable coronary disease, 130/80 mm Hg is an appropriate threshold for starting an antihypertensive regimen. Blood pressure should be lowered slowly, and caution is advised in lowering diastolic blood pressure below 60 mm Hg to avoid the potential risk for subendocardial ischemia. To lower myocardial oxygen demands in patients with coronary disease, the antihypertensive regimen should reduce blood pressure without causing reflex tachycardia. Thus, a β-blocker is often prescribed in conjunction with a dihydropyridine CCB. β-Blockers are indicated for hypertensive patients who have sustained a myocardial infarction (Chapters 72 and 73) and for most patients with chronic heart failure (Chapter 59), and they are typically first-line therapy in patients with angina (Chapter 71). ACE inhibitors are indicated for almost all patients with left ventricular systolic dysfunction (Chapters 59 and 60) and may be considered for post–myocardial infarction patients even in the absence of ventricular dysfunction (Chapters 72 and 73). In patients with very high cardiovascular risk profiles but without known left ventricular dysfunction, the ACE inhibitor ramipril (10 mg/day) reduces cardiovascular events, an effect that may or may not be beyond what can be explained by blood pressure reduction alone. In normotensive patients with stable coronary artery disease, data are conflicting as to whether the addition of an ACE inhibitor reduces the risk for subsequent cardiovascular events.

The CCBs, including amlodipine, and the α-blockers have a greater propensity than other antihypertensive drugs to precipitate heart failure and should be avoided in hypertensive patients with known heart failure and those with asymptomatic left ventricular systolic dysfunction. Optimal control of hypertension is perhaps the best way to prevent diastolic heart failure.

Hypertension Associated with Oral Contraceptives and Estrogen Replacement

Oral contraceptives, particularly current low-dose estrogen preparations, cause a small increase in blood pressure in most women but rarely cause a large increase into the hypertensive range. The mechanism is unknown, but women older than 35 years and those who smoke or are overweight appear to be at increased risk. Drospirenone, a progestin with structural homology to spironolactone, is claimed to have neutral or beneficial effects on blood pressure from mineralocorticoid reception antagonism. If hypertension develops, oral contraceptive therapy should be discontinued in favor of other methods of contraception. Oral estrogen replacement therapy after menopause appears to cause a small increase in blood pressure, whereas transdermal estrogen (which bypasses first-pass hepatic metabolism) appears to cause a small decrease in blood pressure.

Hypertension in Pregnancy

Hypertension, the most common nonobstetric complication of pregnancy, is present in about 10% of all pregnancies (Chapter 247). About one third is caused by chronic hypertension, defined as an increase in blood pressure to 140/90 mm Hg or more after the 20th week of gestation, accompanied by proteinuria (>300 mg/24 hours) and pathologic edema. Preeclampsia sometimes also is accompanied by seizures (eclampsia) and the multisystem HELLP syndrome (Chapters 153 and 247) of hemolysis, elevated liver enzymes, and low platelets. Preeclampsia is the most common cause of maternal mortality and perinatal mortality. Given the current trend of childbearing in women older than 35 years, the prevalence of chronic hypertension in pregnancy is rising. In the absence of randomized trials, α-methyldopa remains the drug of choice for chronic hypertension in pregnancy, and hydralazine (plus bedrest) for preeclampsia. In preeclampsia, magnesium sulfate is predictably effective in preventing seizures but, despite being a vasodilator, has inconsistent effects on blood pressure.

Resistant Hypertension

One in five hypertensive patients has drug-resistant hypertension, in which blood pressure remains above goal values despite concurrent treatment with three antihypertensive drugs of different classes. Most such patients actually have *pseudoresistance* from (1) improper blood pressure measurement technique, (2) white coat reactions, (3) medication nonadherence, (4) ingestion of pressor substances (e.g., nonsteroidal anti-inflammatory drugs, excessive alcohol, psychiatric drugs), or (5) an inadequate blood pressure regimen. Common correctable issues are clonidine rebound (especially with as-needed dosing), inadequate diuretic therapy, inappropriate use of a loop diuretic in a patient with normal renal function, infrequent dosing with a short-acting loop diuretic (e.g., once-a-day furosemide), and low-dose thiazide in a patient with impaired renal function. Significant impairment in renal function can be present with serum creatinine concentrations in the range of 1.2 to 1.4 mg/dL or even lower, particularly in older patients with little muscle mass. GFR should be estimated by standard equations (Chapter 116), and urinary albumin-to-creatinine ratio from a spot urine specimen should be obtained.

Truly drug-resistant patients should be screened for secondary hypertension, especially unrecognized chronic kidney disease, obstructive sleep apnea, and primary aldosteronism. In the absence of an identifiable cause for the

hypertension, a mineralocorticoid receptor antagonist and an α-/β-blocker are recommended as highly effective fourth- and fifth-line therapy. Low-dose eplerenone or spironolactone can be remarkably effective for resistant hypertension—even when serum aldosterone is within the normal range. An implantable carotid baroreceptor pacemaker and radio frequency ablation of the renal nerves are potentially useful device-based treatments currently undergoing evaluation for drug-resistant hypertension.

Acute Severe Hypertension

Twenty-five percent of all emergency department patients present with an elevated blood pressure (Chapter 7). *Hypertensive emergencies* are acute, often severe, elevations in blood pressure, accompanied by rapidly progressive target organ dysfunction, such as myocardial or cerebral ischemia or infarction, pulmonary edema, or renal failure. *Hypertensive urgencies* are severe elevations in blood pressure without severe symptoms and without evidence of acute or progressive target organ dysfunction. The key distinction depends on the state of the patient and the assessment of target organ damage, not just the absolute level of blood pressure.

The full-blown clinical picture of a hypertensive emergency is a critically ill patient who presents with a blood pressure above 220/140 mm Hg, headaches, confusion, blurred vision, nausea and vomiting, seizures, pulmonary edema, oliguria, and grade 3 or grade 4 hypertensive retinopathy (Fig. 67-11). Hypertensive emergencies require immediate intensive care unit (ICU) admission for intravenous therapy and continuous blood pressure monitoring. Hypertensive emergencies often can be managed with oral medications and appropriate outpatient follow-up in 24 to 72 hours. The most common hypertensive cardiac emergencies include acute aortic dissection (Chapter 78), hypertension after cardiac surgery (Chapter 74), acute myocardial infarction (Chapter 73), and unstable angina (Chapter 72). Other hypertensive emergencies include cocaine-induced sympathetic crisis, eclampsia (Chapter 247), head trauma (Chapter 406), severe body burns (Chapter 112), postoperative bleeding from vascular suture lines, and epistaxis that cannot be controlled with anterior and posterior nasal packing. Neurologic emergencies—acute ischemic stroke, hemorrhagic stroke, subarachnoid hemorrhage, and hypertensive encephalopathy—can be difficult to distinguish from one another (Chapters 413 to 415). Hypertensive encephalopathy (Chapter 415) is characterized by severe hypertensive retinopathy (retinal hemorrhages and exudates, with or without papilledema) and a posterior leukoencephalopathy (affecting mainly the white matter of the parieto-occipital regions) seen on cerebral MRI or CT. A new focal neurologic deficit suggests a stroke in

FIGURE 67-11. Hypertensive retinopathy is traditionally divided into four grades. **A,** Grade 1 shows early and minor changes in a young patient. Increased tortuosity of a retinal vessel and increased reflectiveness (silver wiring) of a retinal artery are seen at 1 o'clock in this view. Otherwise, the fundus is completely normal. **B,** Grade 2 also shows increased tortuosity and silver wiring (*arrowheads*). In addition, there is "nipping" of the venules at arteriovenous crossings. **C,** Grade 3 shows the same changes as grade 2 plus flame-shaped retinal hemorrhages and soft "cotton-wool" exudates. **D,** In grade 4, there is swelling of the optic disc (papilledema), retinal edema is present, and hard exudates may collect around the fovea, producing a typical "macular star." (From Forbes CD, Jackson WF. *Color Atlas and Text of Clinical Medicine,* 3rd ed. London: Mosby; 2003.)

evolution, which demands a much more conservative approach to the elevated blood pressure (Chapter 414).

In most other hypertensive emergencies, the goal of parenteral therapy is to achieve a controlled and gradual lowering of blood pressure. A good rule of thumb is to lower the initially elevated arterial pressure by 10% in the first hour and by an additional 15% during the next 3 to 12 hours to a blood pressure of no less than 160/110 mm Hg. Blood pressure can be reduced further during the next 48 hours. Exceptions to this rule are aortic dissection (Chapter 78) and postoperative bleeding from vascular suture lines, two situations that demand much more rapid normalization of blood pressure. In most other cases, unnecessarily rapid correction of the elevated blood pressure to completely normal values places the patient at high risk for worsening cerebral, cardiac, and renal ischemia. In chronic hypertension, cerebral autoregulation is reset to higher than normal blood pressures. This compensatory adjustment prevents tissue overperfusion (increased intracranial pressure) at very high blood pressures, but it also predisposes to tissue underperfusion (cerebral ischemia) when an elevated blood pressure is lowered too quickly (Chapter 414). In patients with coronary disease, overly rapid or excessive reduction in diastolic blood pressure in the ICU can precipitate an acute myocardial ischemia or infarction.

Intravenous Drugs for Hypertensive Emergencies. Among parenteral agents for hypertensive emergencies (Table 67-8), no definitive comparisons of efficacy and safety exist. Sodium nitroprusside, which is a nitric oxide donor that causes both venous and arterial dilation, has been the most widely used agent for hypertensive emergencies because it can be titrated rapidly to control blood pressure. Disadvantages are reflex tachycardia, rebound hypertension after discontinuation, and thiocyanate toxicity in patients with renal insufficiency. Intravenous nitroglycerin, another nitric oxide donor, is a potent coronary vasodilator and therefore the drug of choice for hypertension in the setting of acute coronary syndromes, when it typically is combined with intravenous β-blockade (metoprolol) to reduce the double product (systolic blood pressure times heart rate) and thus myocardial oxygen demands. Nitroglycerin also is a potent venodilator that lowers preload in patients with hypertension in the setting of exacerbated heart failure. However, nitroprusside may be necessary if pulmonary edema results from severe hypertension (increased afterload). Compared with nitroprusside, the fall in blood pressure is less predictable with nitroglycerin. Intravenous labetalol is an effective treatment of hypertensive crisis, particularly in the setting of myocardial ischemia with preserved ventricular function. Nicardipine is a parenteral dihydropyridine CCB that is used most often in the postoperative cardiac surgery patient. Clevidipine, a new dihydropyridine CCB with an ultrafast onset and offset of action of 1 minute, is a pure arterial vasodilator that does not depress cardiac output and appears safe for patients with heart failure. Fenoldopam mesylate is a selective dopamine-1 receptor agonist that causes both systemic and renal vasodilation as well as increased glomerular filtration, natriuresis, and diuresis; it is a good choice for hypertensive emergencies in the setting of acute renal failure. Hydralazine (intravenous or intramuscular) is recommended only for hypertension during pregnancy because of the marked reflex tachycardia it precipitates.

After the blood pressure has been brought under acute control, oral labetalol and dihydropyridine CCBs are particularly useful agents in weaning patients from parenteral therapy so they can be transferred from the ICU. A few doses of intravenous furosemide are often needed to overcome drug resistance due to secondary volume expansion resulting from parenteral vasodilator therapy.

Secondary hypertension should be suspected in patients admitted to the ICU with hypertensive crisis. Normal 24-hour urinary catecholamine values or normal plasma normetanephrine and metanephrine values collected when the blood pressure is the highest (first 24 hours in ICU) effectively rule out pheochromocytoma (Chapter 235). Bilateral renal artery stenosis (Chapter 127) and other secondary causes should be excluded after the patient has been transferred out of the ICU but before discharge from the hospital.

Oral Medications for Hypertensive Urgencies. Most patients who present to the emergency department with hypertensive urgencies either are not adhering to their medical regimen or are being treated with an inadequate regimen. To expedite medication changes, outpatient follow-up should be arranged within 72 hours. Uncontrolled severe chronic hypertension may not require acute treatment in the emergency department if the patient clearly has adequate outpatient follow-up. Otherwise, for management of the patient during the short interim period, labetalol is effective in a dose of 200 to 300 mg, which can be repeated in 2 to 3 hours and then prescribed in twice-daily dosing. If a β-blocker is contraindicated, clonidine is effective in an initial dose of 0.1 or 0.2 mg followed by additional hourly doses of 0.1 mg. Captopril, a short-acting ACE inhibitor, lowers blood pressure within 15 to 30 minutes of oral dosing. A small test dose of 6.25 mg should be used to avoid an excessive fall in blood pressure in hypovolemic patients; then, the full oral dose is 25 mg, which can be repeated in 1 to 2 hours and prescribed as 25 to 75 mg twice daily.

Incidental Blood Pressure Elevation in the Emergency Department

Blood pressures above 160/110 mm Hg are a common incidental finding among patients who present to emergency departments and other acute care settings for urgent medical or surgical care of symptoms that are unrelated to blood pressure (e.g., musculoskeletal pain, orthopedic injury). The elevated blood pressure more often is the first indication of chronic hypertension than a simple physiologic stress reaction, so there is an important opportunity to initiate primary care referral for formal evaluation of possible chronic hypertension. Home or ambulatory blood pressure monitoring is indicated to determine whether the patient's blood pressure normalizes completely once the acute illness has resolved.

PROGNOSIS

An important prognostic factor in hypertension is electrocardiographic or echocardiographic left ventricular hypertrophy (LVH), with the latter already present in as many as 30% of patients with newly diagnosed hypertension and

TABLE 67-8   PARENTERAL AGENTS FOR MANAGEMENT OF HYPERTENSIVE EMERGENCIES

AGENT	DOSE	ONSET OF ACTION	PRECAUTIONS
PARENTERAL VASODILATORS			
Sodium nitroprusside	0.25-10 µg/kg/min IV infusion	Immediate	Thiocyanate toxicity, rebound hypertension
Nitroglycerin	5-100 µg/min IV infusion	2-5 min	Headache, tachycardia, tolerance
Nicardipine	5-15 mg/hr IV infusion	5-10 min	Protracted hypotension after prolonged use
Clevidipine	1-2 mg as rapid IV infusion, rapidly increase dose to 16 mg	2-4 min	Minimal
Fenoldopam mesylate	0.1-0.3 µg/kg/min IV infusion	1-5 min	Headache, tachycardia, increased intraocular pressure
Hydralazine	5-10 mg as IV bolus or 10-40 mg IM; repeat q4-6h	10 min IV; 20 min IM	Unpredictable and excessive falls in pressure; reflex tachycardia, angina exacerbation
Enalaprilat	0.625-1.25 mg q6h IV bolus	15-60 min	Unpredictable and excessive falls in pressure; acute renal failure (in bilateral renal stenosis)
PARENTERAL ADRENERGIC INHIBITORS			
Labetalol	20-80 mg as slow IV injection q10min, or 0.5-2 mg/min IV as infusion hypotension	5-10 min	Bronchospasm, heart block, orthostatic hypotension
Metoprolol	5 mg IV q10min × 3 doses	5-10 min	Bronchospasm, heart block, heart failure, exacerbation of cocaine-induced MI
Esmolol	500 µg/kg IV during 3 min, then 25-100 mg/kg/min as IV infusion	1-5 min	Bronchospasm, heart block, heart failure
Phentolamine	5-10 mg IV bolus q5-15min	1-2 min	Tachycardia, orthostatic hypotension

90% of patients with severe hypertension. LVH is associated with an increased risk for heart failure, stroke, and kidney failure. All drugs that lower blood pressure will reduce left ventricular mass, but the reduction averages only 12% or less and is less with β-blockers. With regression of LVH, the associated risks are reduced but not eliminated.

Because of their relatively short duration (typically <5 years), randomized trials may underestimate the lifetime protection against disability and death afforded by several decades of antihypertensive therapy in clinical practice. In the Framingham Heart Study, treatment of hypertension for 20 years in middle-aged adults reduced total cardiovascular mortality by 60%, which is considerably greater than the results of most randomized controlled trials despite the less intense treatment guidelines when therapy was initiated in the 1950s to 1970s. Further benefits may be seen with lower blood pressure treatment thresholds and goals than those presently endorsed, along with better control of associated cardiovascular risk factors.

1. The ASTRAL Investigators. Revascularization versus medical therapy for renal-artery stenosis. *N Engl J Med.* 2009;361:1953-1962.
2. Julius S, Nesbitt SD, Egan BM, et al. Feasibility of treating prehypertension with an angiotensin-receptor blocker. *N Engl J Med.* 2006;354:1685-1697.
3. Law MR, Morris JK, Wald NJ. Use of blood pressure lowering drugs in the prevention of cardiovascular disease: meta-analysis of 147 randomized trials in the context of expectations from prospective epidemiological studies. *BMJ.* 2009;338:1665-1684.
4. Elmer PJ, Obarzanek E, Vollmer WM, et al. Effects of comprehensive lifestyle modification on diet, weight, physical fitness, and blood pressure control: 18-month results of a randomized trial. *Ann Intern Med.* 2006;144:485-495.
5. The ALLHAT Officers and Coordinators for the ALLHAT Collaborative Research Group. The major outcomes in high-risk hypertensive patients randomized to angiotensin-converting enzyme inhibitor or calcium channel blocker vs. diuretic: the Antihypertensive and Lipid-Lowering Treatment to Prevent Heart Attack Trial (ALLHAT). *JAMA.* 2002;288:2981-2997.
6. Julius S, Kjeldsen SE, Weber M, et al. Outcomes in hypertensive patients at high cardiovascular risk treated with regimens based on valsartan or amlodipine: the VALUE randomised trial. *Lancet.* 2004;363:2022-2031.
7. Lindholm LH, Carlberg B, Samuelsson O. Should beta blockers remain first choice in the treatment of primary hypertension? A meta-analysis. *Lancet.* 2005;366:1545-1553.
8. Verdecchia P, Staessen JA, Angeli F, et al. Usual versus tight control of systolic blood pressure in non-diabetic patients with hypertension (Cardio-Sis): an open-label randomized trial. *Lancet.* 2009;374:525-533.
9. Dahlof B, Sever PS, Poulter NR, et al. Prevention of cardiovascular events with antihypertensive regimen of amlodipine adding perindopril as required versus atenolol adding bendroflumethiazide as required, in the Anglo-Scandinavian Cardiac Outcomes Trial—Blood Pressure Lowering Arm (ASCOT-BPLA): a multicentre randomised controlled trial. *Lancet.* 2005;366:895-906.
10. Jamerson K, Weber MA, Bakris GL, et al. Benazepril plus amlodipine or hydrochlorothiazide for hypertension in high-risk patients. *N Engl J Med.* 2008;359:2417-2428.
11. The ONTARGET Investigators. Telmisartan, ramipril, or both in patients at high risk for vascular events. *N Engl J Med.* 2008;358:1547-1559.
12. Sever PS, Dahlof B, Poulter NR, et al. Prevention of coronary and stroke events with atorvastatin in hypertension patients who have average or lower-than-average cholesterol concentrations, in the Anglo-Scandinavian Cardiac Outcomes Trial—Lipid Lowering Arm (ASCOT-LLA): a multicentre randomized controlled trial. *Lancet.* 2003;361:1149-1158.
13. Appel LJ, Wright JT, Greene T, et al. Long-term effects of renin-angiotensin system-blocking therapy and a low blood pressure goal on progression of hypertensive chronic kidney disease in African Americans. *Arch Intern Med.* 2008;168:832-839.
14. The ACCORD Study Group. Effects of intensive blood-pressure control in type 2 diabetes mellitus. *N Engl J Med.* 2010;362:1575-1585.
15. Beckett NS, Peters R, Fletcher AE, et al. Treatment of hypertension in patients 80 years of age or older. *N Engl J Med.* 2008;358:1887-1898.
16. PROGRESS Collaborative Group. Randomised trial of a perindopril-based blood-pressure-lowering regimen among 6,105 individuals with previous stroke or transient ischaemic attack. *Lancet.* 2001;358:1033-1041.

SUGGESTED READINGS

Appel LJ, Frohlich ED, Hall JE, et al. The importance of population-wide sodium reduction as a means to prevent cardiovascular disease and stroke: a call to action from the American Heart Association. *Circulation.* 2011;123:1138-1143. *Recommendation for primordial prevention of hypertension by population-wide reduction in the sodium content of processed food.*
Drazner MH. The progression of hypertensive heart disease. *Circulation.* 2011;123:327-334. *Review.*
Rothwell PM, Howard SC, Dolan E, et al. Prognostic significance of visit-to-visit variability, maximum systolic blood pressure, and episodic hypertension. *Lancet.* 2010;375:895-905. *High visit-to-visit variability in systolic blood pressure is associated with an increased risk of stroke.*

PULMONARY HYPERTENSION

VALLERIE MCLAUGHLIN

DEFINITION

The normal pulmonary vasculature is a low-pressure system, with less than one tenth the resistance to flow observed in the systemic vasculature. Pulmonary hypertension refers to the hemodynamic state in which the pressure in the pulmonary artery is elevated above a mean of 25 mm Hg. A specific type of pulmonary hypertension, pulmonary arterial hypertension, also requires that the left heart filling pressure (pulmonary capillary wedge pressure, left ventricular end-diastolic pressure, or left atrial pressure) be 15 mm Hg or less. The syndrome of pulmonary arterial hypertension results when blood flow through the pulmonary circulation is restricted, thereby leading to pathologic increases in pulmonary vascular resistance and, ultimately, to right ventricular failure. Pulmonary hypertension may also be a consequence of many other chronic diseases, including left heart failure (Chapter 58), a variety of parenchymal lung diseases, and thromboembolic disease (Chapter 98) (Table 68-1).

EPIDEMIOLOGY

Normal pulmonary blood pressure is 20/10 (mean 15) mm Hg at rest at sea level, rising to 30/13 (mean 20) mm Hg with mild exercise. Pressures rise with altitude, and at an altitude of about 15,000 feet, normal resting pulmonary artery pressures are about 38/14 (mean 20) mm Hg. Pulmonary arterial systolic pressure rises gradually with age, and each 10-mm Hg increase is associated with a 2.7-fold greater risk for mortality.

Idiopathic pulmonary arterial hypertension, formerly called primary pulmonary hypertension, is the prototype of group 1 pulmonary arterial hypertension. This disease affects women more than men in a 2:1 ratio. It may present at any age, with a mean age of onset of 37 years. The prevalence of pulmonary arterial hypertension is between 15 and 26 per million persons. Heritable pulmonary arterial hypertension occurs in a familial context, most often (70%) owing to a mutation in the bone morphogenic protein receptor type 2. Less commonly, mutations in activin receptor–like kinase type 1, or endoglin, have been identified in patients with pulmonary arterial hypertension, predominately with coexistent hereditary hemorrhagic telangiectasia (Chapter 176). Drug- and toxin-induced pulmonary arterial hypertension has been most clearly linked to anorexigens, including aminorex, fenfluramine, and dexfenfluramine. Although these agents are no longer used, observational studies suggest that amphetamines, methamphetamines, and L-tryptophan are likely related to the development of pulmonary arterial hypertension.

One of the most common types of group 1 pulmonary arterial hypertension occurs in the setting of connective tissue diseases. For example, the prevalence of pulmonary arterial hypertension in patients with scleroderma (Chapter 275) is in the range of 7 to 12%. It is less common in systemic lupus erythematosus (Chapter 274), rheumatoid arthritis (Chapter 272), and other systemic vasculitides (Chapter 278). Pulmonary arterial hypertension is a rare but well established complication of human immunodeficiency virus (HIV) infection, with a prevalence of 0.5%. Prospective hemodynamic studies show that 2 to 6% of patients with portal hypertension (Chapter 148) develop pulmonary arterial hypertension, although the reason for the association is not clear.

A significant proportion of patients with untreated systemic-to-pulmonary shunts, commonly owing to congenital heart disease (Chapter 69), develop pulmonary arterial hypertension. Persistent exposure of the pulmonary vasculature to increased blood flow and pressure leads to an elevated pulmonary vascular resistance. In some cases, Eisenmenger's syndrome (Chapter 69), with a reversal of flow across the defect, results in right-to-left shunting. Pulmonary veno-occlusive (Chapter 98) disease and pulmonary capillary hemangiomatosis are rare disorders that directly affect the pulmonary vasculature. The presentation of each is often similar to pulmonary arterial hypertension, but the prognosis is particularly poor.

Pulmonary hypertension owing to left heart disease probably represents the most frequent cause of pulmonary hypertension seen in practice (group 2 patients). Left-sided ventricular (Chapter 58) or valvular disease

TABLE 68-1   UPDATED CLINICAL CLASSIFICATION OF PULMONARY HYPERTENSION

GROUP 1

Pulmonary arterial hypertension (PAH)
  Idiopathic PAH
  Heritable
    BMPR2
    ALK1, endoglin (with or without hereditary hemorrhagic telangiectasia)
    Unknown
  Drug and toxin induced
  Associated with
    Connective tissue diseases
    HIV infection
    Portal hypertension
    Congenital heart diseases
    Schistosomiasis
    Chronic hemolytic anemia
Persistent pulmonary hypertension of the newborn
Pulmonary veno-occlusive disease with left to right shunts and/or pulmonary capillary hemangiomatosis

GROUP 2

Pulmonary hypertension owing to left heart disease
  Systolic dysfunction
  Diastolic dysfunction
  Valvular disease

GROUP 3

Pulmonary hypertension owing to lung diseases and/or hypoxia
  Chronic obstructive pulmonary disease
  Interstitial lung disease
Other pulmonary diseases with mixed restrictive and obstructive pattern
  Sleep-disordered breathing
  Alveolar hypoventilation disorders
  Chronic exposure to high altitude
  Developmental abnormalities

GROUP 4

Chronic thromboembolic pulmonary hypertension

GROUP 5

Pulmonary hypertension with unclear multifactorial mechanisms
  Hematologic disorders: myeloproliferative disorders, splenectomy
  Systemic disorders: sarcoidosis, pulmonary Langerhans cell histiocytosis: lymphangioleiomyomatosis, neurofibromatosis, vasculitis
  Metabolic disorders: glycogen storage disease, Gaucher's disease, thyroid disorders
  Others: tumoral obstruction, fibrosing mediastinitis, chronic renal failure on dialysis

ALK1 = activin receptor-like kinase type 1; BMPR2 = bone morphogenetic protein receptor type 2; HIV = human immunodeficiency virus.
Reprinted from Simonneau G, Robbins IM, Beghetti M, et al. Updated clinical classification of pulmonary hypertension. *J Am Coll Cardiol.* 2009;54:S43-S54.

(Chapter 75) may increase left atrial pressure, which then is transmitted back to the pulmonary vasculature. Often, the transpulmonary gradient and pulmonary vascular resistance are normal. In such cases, optimal treatment of the left heart disease results in reduction of the left heart filling pressures and, consequently, a reduction in the pulmonary artery pressures. On occasion, patients with left heart disease have an elevation of pulmonary artery pressure greater than expected based on the elevation of left heart filling pressures, with a transpulmonary gradient of more than 12 mm Hg and a pulmonary vascular resistance of more than 3 Wood units (Wood units = [pulmonary artery pressure minus mean pulmonary capillary wedge pressure] divided by cardiac output). This difference may be due to an increase in pulmonary artery vasomotor tone or pulmonary vascular remodeling in the setting of persistently elevated left heart filling pressures.

Group 3 patients have pulmonary hypertension owing to lung diseases or hypoxia. Any disorder that results in hypoxemia (e.g., chronic obstructive lung disease [Chapter 88], interstitial lung disease [Chapter 92], sleep-disordered breathing [Chapter 100]) may result in pulmonary hypertension, although the pressure elevation tends to be modest, with a mean pulmonary artery pressure of 25 to 35 mm Hg. Echocardiography-based observations have suggested that up to 80% of patients with chronic obstructive lung disease and idiopathic pulmonary fibrosis have elevated pulmonary artery pressures. In patients who have more advanced parenchymal lung disease and undergo evaluation for lung volume reduction surgery or lung transplantation, 40 to 50% have pulmonary hypertension at the time of right heart catheterization. Most often, the elevations in pulmonary artery pressures are modest, but a small proportion of patients have more substantial elevations.

Group 4 patients have chronic thromboembolic pulmonary hypertension (Chapter 98), which must be differentiated from the other groups because the treatment is quite different. Approximately 4% of patients who have suffered an acute pulmonary embolism progress to develop chronic thromboembolic pulmonary hypertension. Approximately half of those ultimately diagnosed with chronic thromboembolic pulmonary hypertension do not have a known history of an acute pulmonary embolism. Patients with a significant clot burden can be candidates for a pulmonary thromboendarterectomy, which is a potentially curative procedure for this disorder.

Group 5 pulmonary arterial hypertension consists of several forms for which the etiology is unclear or multifactorial. Among these conditions are a number of hematologic, systemic, and metabolic disorders.

PATHOBIOLOGY

The pathobiology of pulmonary arterial hypertension is complex and incompletely elucidated (Fig. 68-1). The pulmonary arterial hypertension phenotype is characterized by endothelial dysfunction, a decreased ratio of apoptosis to proliferation in pulmonary artery smooth muscle cells, and a thickened, disordered adventitia in which adventitial metalloproteases are excessively activated. The evolution of pulmonary vascular disease frequently originates with the interaction of a predisposing state and one or more inciting stimuli, a concept referred to as the "multiple-hit hypothesis."

In group 1 pulmonary arterial hypertension, patients have a panvasculopathy predominantly affecting the small pulmonary arterioles. It is characterized by a variety of arterial abnormalities, including intimal hyperplasia, medial hypertrophy, adventitial proliferation, thrombosis in situ, varying degrees of inflammation, and plexiform lesions. An individual patient may manifest all or some of these lesions, and the distribution of the lesions may be diffuse or focal.

The genetic defect best characterized in heritable pulmonary arterial hypertension is that of the bone morphogenetic protein receptor type 2, a member of the transforming growth factor-β signaling family. This defect accounts for 70% of heritable pulmonary arterial hypertension cases, although it has also been detected in 11 to 40% of patients with apparently idiopathic pulmonary arterial hypertension and no family history. Characteristics of this gene include incomplete penetrance (20%) and genetic anticipation. Less commonly, mutations in activin receptor–like kinase type 1, or endoglin, have been identified, usually in families with coexistent hereditary hemorrhagic telangiectasia.

The imbalance in the production or metabolism of vasoactive mediators in the pulmonary vasculature includes a reduction in prostacyclin and nitric oxide, which have vasodilator and antiproliferative properties, and an increase in thromboxane and endothelin, which are vasoconstrictors as well as mitogens. The reduction in nitric oxide synthase in pulmonary arterial hypertension diminishes nitric oxide and, subsequently, cyclic guanosine monophosphate production. Endothelin-1 is a potent vasoconstrictor and smooth muscle mitogen that may contribute to the development of pulmonary arterial hypertension. Prostacyclin synthase is reduced in pulmonary arterial hypertension, resulting in an inadequate production of prostacyclin I_2, which is a vasodilator with potent antiproliferative effects. Other aberrations include those of the voltage-dependent potassium channels and serotonin pathways. Disorders of inflammatory and coagulation pathways have also been described.

Chronic changes in the pulmonary vasculature also occur as a result of other types of pulmonary hypertension. Chronic elevation of left heart filling pressures causes a backward transmission of pressure to the pulmonary venous system and triggers vasoconstriction in the pulmonary arterial bed. Histologically, the veins thicken abnormally, and a neointima is formed. As secondary features, medial hypertrophy and thickening of the neointima on the arterial side of the pulmonary circulation occur. These changes can be reversed with therapies that result in chronic reduction of left heart filling pressures.

In parenchymal lung disease, changes in the distal pulmonary arterial vessels are related to hypoxia. Hypoxia induces muscularization of the distal

FIGURE 68-1. Potential mechanisms involved in the development of pulmonary arterial hypertension (PAH). Ang = angiopoietin; AVD = apoptotic volume decrease; BMP = bone morphogenetic protein; BMPR = bone morphogenetic protein receptor; CaM = calmodulin; CREB = cAMP-response element binding protein; DAG = diacylglycerol; E_m = membrane potential; EGF = epidermal growth factor; EGFR = epidermal growth factor receptor; ET = endothelin; GAP = GTPase-activating protein; GPCR = G protein–coupled receptor; HHV = human herpesvirus; HT = hydroxytryptamine (serotonin); HTT = hydroxytryptamine (serotonin) transporter; IP_3 = inositol 1,4,5-trisphosphate; Kv = voltage-gated K⁺; MAPK = mitogen-activated protein kinase; MLC = myosin light chain; MLCK = myosin light chain kinase; NA(D)PH = nicotinamide adenine dinucleotide phosphate; NO = nitric oxide; PASMC = pulmonary artery smooth muscle cell; PDGF = platelet-derived growth factor; PGI_2 = prostacyclin; PKC = protein kinase C; PLC = phospholipase C; ROC = receptor-operated Ca^{2+} channels; ROS = reactive oxygen species; RTK = receptor tyrosine kinase; SR = sarcoplasmic reticulum; SRF = serum response factor; TCF = T-cell factor; TIE = endothelial-specific tyrosine kinase; VDCC = voltage-dependent calcium channel. (Modified from Morrell NW, Adnot S, Archer SL, et al. Cellular and molecular basis of pulmonary hypertension. *J Am Coll Cardiol.* 2009;54:S20-S31.)

vessels and medial hypertrophy of the more proximal vessels. Neither neo-intima formation nor the development of plexiform lesions is observed.

The pathology of chronic thromboembolic pulmonary hypertension is often distinct from idiopathic pulmonary arterial hypertension. The lesions are frequently more variable, with some arterial pathways that appear relatively unaffected and others that show recanalized vascular thromboses. However, the involvement of distal microvessels, particularly when thromboses have occurred in subsegmental arteries, can resemble idiopathic pulmonary arterial hypertension with the formation of plexiform lesions.

Pathophysiology

The normal pulmonary vasculature bed has a remarkable capacity to dilate and recruit unused vasculature to accommodate increases in pulmonary blood flow. In pulmonary hypertension, the pulmonary artery pressure and pulmonary vascular resistance are increased at rest and further increase with exertion. In response to this increased afterload, the normally very thin right ventricle hypertrophies and eventually dilates. Early on in the process, the right ventricle may be capable of maintaining normal cardiac output at rest, although it may fail to augment cardiac output with exercise, thereby leading to exertional dyspnea. As the disease progresses, the right ventricular dysfunction may progress to the point that resting cardiac output is impaired.

Right ventricular function is a major determinant of functional capacity and prognosis in pulmonary arterial hypertension. Although the left ventricle is not affected by pulmonary vascular disease itself, progressive right ventricular dilation can impair left ventricular filling and lead to mildly increased left heart filling pressure. The pathophysiology of pulmonary hypertension related to left heart and lung disease is further complicated by those underlying disorders.

The two most frequent mechanisms of death are progressive right ventricular failure and sudden death. Right ventricular failure, as evidence by elevated jugular venous pressure, lower extremity edema, and occasionally ascites, may also be accompanied by evidence of poor forward flow owing to inadequate filling of the left ventricle. Hypotension, hypoperfusion, and renal insufficiency may result. Other potential causes of death include pneumonia, sepsis, and pulmonary embolism.

CLINICAL MANIFESTATIONS

History

Dyspnea, which is the most common symptom of pulmonary hypertension, initially may be attributed to underlying disorders such as heart failure or obstructive lung disease, but the dyspnea of pulmonary hypertension typically is insidious in progression and reproducible. Dyspnea is classified by the

World Health Organization (WHO) system, which is similar to the New York Heart Association classification system for angina and heart failure (see Table 50-5 in Chapter 50), and may progress to dyspnea at rest.

Other common symptoms of pulmonary hypertension include fatigue, lightheadedness, chest pain (Chapter 50), and palpitations (Chapters 50 and 62). Syncope (Chapter 62), which is an ominous finding, is often exertional in nature; it signifies the inability of the right ventricle to augment cardiac output as needed for physical activity. Symptoms of right heart failure, including edema and ascites, signify advanced disease.

Patients often have symptoms associated with their underlying disease, which typically is far advanced by the time pulmonary arterial hypertension develops. For example, patients with pulmonary hypertension associated with left heart disease often have paroxysmal nocturnal dyspnea and orthopnea. Patients with pulmonary hypertension related to hypoxic lung disease may have cough, sputum production, or wheezing.

Physical Examination

Distention of jugular veins (see Fig. 50-3 in Chapter 50) may signify right ventricular failure, and prominent v ways (see Fig. 50-4 in Chapter 50) may be a result of tricuspid regurgitation. The amplitude of the carotid upstroke may give some insight into the cardiac output. The classic physical examination finding in pulmonary hypertension is a loud pulmonic component to the second heart sound, which reflects high pulmonary pressures that increase the force of the pulmonic valve closure. Palpation of the sternum often reveals a parasternal lift as the hypertrophied, pressure-overloaded right ventricle obliterates the retrosternal air space. A right ventricular fourth heart sound reflects diastolic filling of the hypertrophied, noncompliant right ventricle, akin to the left-sided fourth heart sound in a patient with systemic hypertension and left ventricular hypertrophy. The murmur of tricuspid regurgitation, which is holosystolic, located at the left lower sternal border, and augments with inspiration, is common in patients with moderate to severe pulmonary hypertension. Other findings on auscultation may include an early systolic click and the murmur of pulmonic regurgitation. A right ventricular third heart sound often signifies advanced disease and right heart failure. Other signs consistent with right ventricular failure include hepatomegaly, peripheral edema (see Fig. 50-7 in Chapter 50), ascites, hypotension, diminished pulse pressure, and cool extremities.

Other physical examination findings may give some insight into the etiology of the pulmonary hypertension. For example, central cyanosis and clubbing may suggest an intracardiac shunt and Eisenmenger's physiology. Sclerodactyly, telangiectasias (see Fig. 275-3 in Chapter 275), arthritis, Raynaud's phenomenon (see Fig. 80-5 in Chapter 80), and skin rashes may increase the suspicion of an underlying connective tissue disease. Splenomegaly, spider angioma, palmar erythema (see Fig. 148-2 in Chapter 148), icterus (see Fig. 148-1 in Chapter 148), and caput medusa may suggest portal hypertension as an etiology. Signs of left heart disease, such as pulmonary congestion, a left-sided third heart sound, or findings of mitral or aortic valve disease on auscultation may signify pulmonary hypertension as a result of left heart disease. Fine rales, accessory muscle use, wheezing, protracted expiration, and productive cough may denote group 3 pulmonary hypertension as a result of hypoxic lung disease. Pulmonary vascular bruits suggest chronic thromboembolic pulmonary hypertension.

DIAGNOSIS

Initial assessments include an electrocardiogram (ECG) and chest radiograph. The ECG may show right axis deviation, right ventricular enlargement, right atrial enlargement, and ST and T wave changes across the anterior precordium that reflect right ventricular strain (Fig. 68-2). The chest radiograph may demonstrate enlarged proximal pulmonary arteries (see Fig. 53-6 in Chapter 53) with peripheral tapering or pruning of the pulmonary vasculature (Fig. 68-3A). The lateral may reveal the reduction in retrosternal air space as a result of right ventricular enlargement (see Fig. 68-3B).

If, based on the history, physical examination, ECG, and chest radiograph, there is a reasonable suspicion for pulmonary hypertension, a series of diagnostic evaluations should follow (Fig. 68-4), usually beginning with an echocardiogram, and with further testing guided by the patient subtype (Table 68-2). The echocardiogram gives insight not only into the presence of pulmonary hypertension but also into the presence of common disorders of the left heart that may result in pulmonary hypertension. Two-dimensional echocardiographic findings reflective of elevated pulmonary artery pressures include right atrial enlargement, right ventricular enlargement, flattening of the intraventricular septum, and an underfilled left ventricle (Fig. 68-5). The right ventricular systolic pressure may be estimated based on the velocity of the tricuspid regurgitant jet using the modified Bernoulli equation (Chapter 55) (Fig. 68-6), although a reliable estimate of right ventricular systolic pressure is not always obtainable, and this measurement is prone to error, particularly in patients with parenchymal lung disease, The echocardiogram is also useful to assess for left heart causes of pulmonary hypertension, such

25 mm/sec   10mm/mV   150 Hz 7.1.1   12SL 233   CID: I   EID:6 EDT: II:46 06-JUN-2007 ORDER:

FIGURE 68-2. Electrocardiogram demonstrating sinus rhythm, right axis deviation, and right ventricular hypertrophy with a strain pattern.

FIGURE 68-3. Posterior-anterior **(A)** and Lateral **(B)** chest radiographs demonstrating enlarged proximal pulmonary arteries and right ventricular enlargement.

FIGURE 68-4. **Diagnostic approach to pulmonary arterial hypertension (PH).** Because the suspicion of PH may arise in various ways, the sequence of tests may vary. However, the diagnosis of PH requires that certain data support a specific diagnosis. In addition, the diagnosis of idiopathic pulmonary arterial hypertension (IPAH) is one of excluding all other reasonable possibilities. *Pivotal tests* are those that are essential to establishing a diagnosis of any type of PH by either identification of criteria of associated disease or exclusion of diagnoses other than IPAH. All pivotal tests are required for a definitive diagnosis and baseline characterization. An abnormality of one assessment (such as obstructive pulmonary disease on pulmonary function tests [PFTs]) does not preclude that another abnormality (chronic thromboembolic disease on VQ scan and pulmonary angiogram) is contributing or predominant. *Contingent tests* are recommended to elucidate or confirm results of the pivotal tests and need only be performed in the appropriate clinical context. The *combination* of pivotal and appropriate contingent tests contributes to assessment of the differential diagnoses in the right-hand column. It should be recognized that definitive diagnosis may require additional specific evaluations not necessarily included in this general guideline. 6MWT = 6-minute walk test; ABGs = arterial blood gases; ANA = antinuclear antibody serology; CHD = congenital heart disease; CPET = cardiopulmonary exercise test; CT = computed tomography; CTD = connective tissue disease; CXR = chest X-ray; ECG = electrocardiogram; HIV = human immunodeficiency virus screening; Htn = hypertension; LFTs = liver function tests; PE = pulmonary embolism; RA = rheumatoid arthritis; RAE = right atrial enlargement; RH cath = right heart cath; RVSP = right ventricular systolic pressure; RVE = right ventricular enlargement; RVSP = right ventricular systolic pressure; SLE = systemic lupus erythematosus; TEE = transesophageal echocardiography; VHD = valvular heart disease; VQ scan = lung ventilation-perfusion scintigram. (From McLaughlin VV, Archer SL, Badesch DB, et al. ACCF/AHA 2009 expert consensus document on pulmonary hypertension: a report of the American College of Cardiology Foundation Task Force on Expert Consensus Documents and the American Heart Association developed in collaboration with the American College of Chest Physicians; American Thoracic Society, Inc.; and the Pulmonary Hypertension Association. *J Am Coll Cardiol.* 2009;53:1573-1619.)

TABLE 68-2 APPROACH TO SPECIFIC PATIENT SUBGROUPS

	FURTHER ASSESSMENT	RATIONALE
BMPR2 mutation	Echocardiogram yearly; RHC if echocardiogram demonstrates evidence of PAH (high right ventricular systolic pressure or right heart chamber enlargement)	Early detection of PAH; 20% chance of developing PAH
First-degree relative of patient with BMPR2 mutation or within pedigree of two or more patients with a diagnosis of PAH	Genetic counseling and recommendation for BMPR2 genotyping; proceed as above if positive	Autosomal dominant transmission
Systemic sclerosis	Echocardiogram yearly; RHC if echocardiogram demonstrates evidence of PAH (high right ventricular systolic pressure or right heart chamber enlargement)	About 8% (by RHC): 27% (by echo screening) prevalence of PAH in systemic sclerosis
HIV infection	Echocardiogram if symptoms or signs suggestive of PAH; RHC if echo demonstrates evidence of PAH (high right ventricular systolic pressure or right heart chamber enlargement)	0.5% prevalence of PAH
Portal hypertension	Echocardiogram if OLT considered; RHC if echocardiogram demonstrates evidence of PAH (high right ventricular systolic pressure or right heart chamber enlargement)	4% prevalence of PAH in candidates for OLT; PAH is predictive of poor OLT outcome
Prior appetite suppressant use (fenfluramine)	Echocardiogram only if symptomatic	Incidence of PAH is approximately 0.005% if agent used >3 mo
Congenital heart disease with shunt	Echocardiogram and RHC at time of diagnosis; consider repair of defect if significant left-to-right shunt present	High probability of PAH developing in unrepaired shunt (Eisenmenger's syndrome)
Recent acute pulmonary embolism	Ventilation-perfusion (V/Q) scintigraphy 3 mo after event if symptomatic; pulmonary angiogram if positive	3% risk of chronic thromboembolic PH; negative V/Q scan excludes chronic thromboembolism
Sickle cell disease	Echocardiogram yearly; RHC if echocardiogram demonstrates evidence of PAH (high right ventricular systolic pressure or right heart chamber enlargement)	Increased mortality if PH present, early detection of PH, 30% develop PH, about 10% develop PAH

BMPR2 = bone morphogenic protein receptor 2; HIV = human immunodeficiency virus; OLT = orthotopic liver transplantation; PAH = pulmonary arterial hypertension; RHC = right heart catheterization.
From McLaughlin VV, Archer SL, Badesch DB, et al. ACCF/AHA 2009 expert consensus document on pulmonary hypertension: a report of the American College of Cardiology Foundation Task Force on Expert Consensus Documents and the American Heart Association developed in collaboration with the American College of Chest Physicians; American Thoracic Society, Inc.; and the Pulmonary Hypertension Association. *J Am Coll Cardiol.* 2009;53:1573-1619.

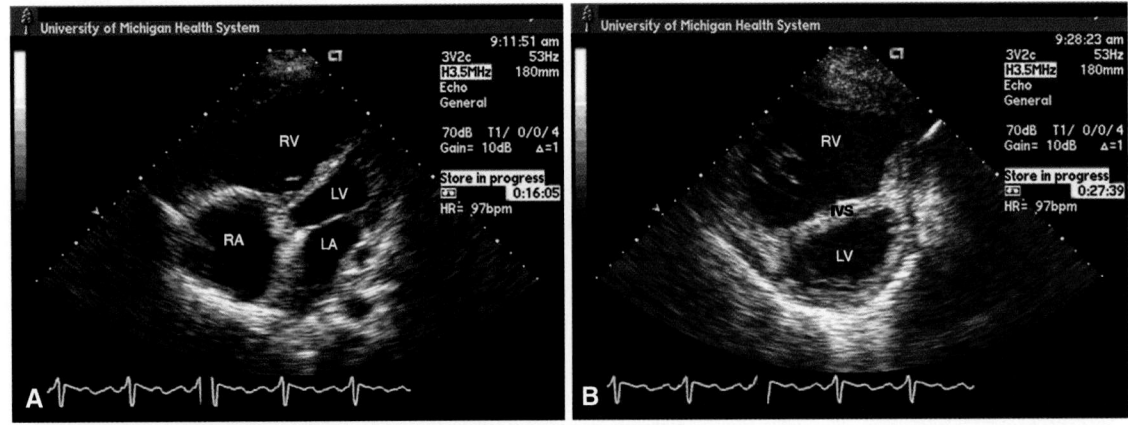

FIGURE 68-5. Echocardiographic images of the heart. **A,** Four-chamber view. Right atrial (RA) enlargement, right ventricular (RV) enlargement. The left atrium (LA) and left ventricle (LV) are small and underfilled. **B,** Short axis view. RV enlargement is present. Flattening of the intraventricular septum (IVS) results from pressure and volume overload of the RV.

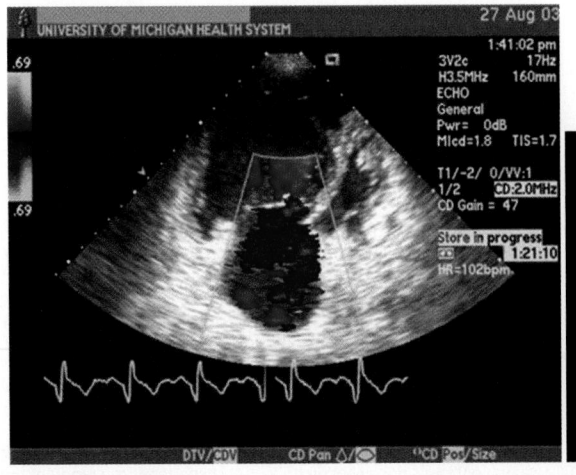

Modified Bernoulli's Equation:
$$4 \times (V)^2 + RAP = RVSP \ (PASP)$$

FIGURE 68-6. Calculation of estimated pulmonary artery pressure based on the velocity of the tricuspid regurgitant jet. RAP = right atrial pressure; RVSP = right ventricular systolic pressure; PASP = pulmonary artery systolic pressure; V = tricuspid jet velocity (m/sec).

as systolic dysfunction, diastolic dysfunction, and valvular heart disease. Occasionally, a previously unknown congenital heart defect is discovered during this evaluation. In approximately 25% of patients, a previously trivial patent foramen ovale may shunt blood from the right atrium to the left atrium, owing to the high pulmonary vascular resistance, and thereby worsen systemic oxygenation.

In a patient with unexplained dyspnea and evidence of pulmonary hypertension on echocardiogram, chronic thromboembolic pulmonary hypertension must be excluded. The study of choice for this assessment is the ventilation-perfusion scan (see Fig. 98-4 in Chapter 98), which often shows multiple perfusion defects that are not matched on ventilation. Although spiral computed tomography (CT) is excellent for the assessment of acute pulmonary embolus, it sometimes fails to detect surgically accessible chronic thromboembolic disease. If either of these studies is abnormal, further evaluation with a pulmonary angiogram may be required to determine whether chronic thrombolic disease is the diagnosis and, if so, whether it is surgically accessible.

Pulmonary function tests in patients with pulmonary arterial hypertension may show mild restrictive disease and a mildly reduced diffusing capacity for carbon monoxide. Patients with the scleroderma spectrum of diseases tend to have more substantial reductions in the diffusing capacity for carbon monoxide, which may even precede the development of pulmonary hypertension. Pulmonary function tests may disclose evidence of obstructive or restrictive lung disease; further evaluation with chest CT may be necessary. Overnight oximetry is useful to screen for obstructive sleep apnea (Chapter 100). If indicated, formal polysomnography may be required.

Recommended serologic testing, given the known associations, includes an antinuclear antibody test and HIV serology, in addition to liver function tests to assess for chronic liver disease. A study of functional capacity, most commonly the 6-minute walk test, is useful to assess the severity of disease, to determine the potential need for oxygen, and to establish a baseline against which to assess subsequent changes in exercise capacity as a result of medical interventions.

If pulmonary arterial hypertension is suspected based on the noninvasive evaluation, the diagnosis must be confirmed with a right heart catheterization that measures right atrial pressure, right ventricular pressure, pulmonary artery (systolic, diastolic, and mean) pressures, pulmonary arterial wedge pressure (reflective of left ventricular end-diastolic pressure or left atrial pressure), cardiac output and index, heart rate, systemic blood pressure, and oxygen saturations in the superior vena cava, inferior vena cava, pulmonary artery, and a systemic artery. From this information, pulmonary vascular resistance and systemic vascular resistance may be calculated, right ventricular performance can be assured, and an intracardiac or intrapulmonary shunt can be confirmed or excluded.

In patients with left heart or parenchymal lung disease, however, optimal management of the underlying condition is often undertaken before considering right heart catheterization. Patients with suspected chronic thromboembolic disease often undergo both right heart catheterization and pulmonary angiography (Chapter 98) to assess surgical candidacy and operative risk.

Measurement of the wedge pressure, a surrogate for left atrial pressure in the absence of pulmonary vein obstruction, is useful to exclude pulmonary hypertension caused by left heart disease or, in rare cases, pulmonary veno-occlusive disease. If an optimal wedge pressure tracing cannot be obtained, or if there is any question about the accuracy of the wedge pressure tracing, a left ventricular end-diastolic pressure should be obtained.

Acute vasodilator testing is often performed at the time of the initial right heart catheterization, not only for its prognostic implications but also to identify patients who might be candidates for therapy with calcium-channel blockers. Although the data regarding vasodilator testing and treatment with calcium-channel blockers are largely restricted to patients with idiopathic pulmonary arterial hypertension, vasodilator testing is often performed in patients with other types of pulmonary arterial hypertension. However, acute vasodilator testing is not indicated and may be harmful in patients with significantly elevated left heart filling pressures because pulmonary edema may ensue.

The three agents most commonly used for acute vasodilator testing in the cardiac catheterization laboratory are inhaled nitric oxide, intravenous epoprostenol, and intravenous adenosine. A positive response to an acute vasodilator is a decrease in mean pulmonary artery pressure by at least 10 mm Hg, to a mean pulmonary artery pressure of less than 40 mm Hg, without a decrease in cardiac output. If a patient meets these criteria, it is reasonable to administer a trial of oral calcium-channel blockers.

TREATMENT Rx

General Measures

Important goals of therapy in patients with pulmonary arterial hypertension include alleviation of symptoms, particularly dyspnea; improvement of functional capacity, which is often measured by the 6-minute walk test; and improvement of hemodynamics by lowering pulmonary artery pressure and increasing cardiac output. Another important goal of therapy is to reverse, or at least prevent, disease progression, often measured in clinical trials as hospitalization, escalation of therapy, and lung transplantation.

Patients are encouraged to engage in low-level graded aerobic exercise, such as walking, as tolerated. Patients are advised to avoid heavy physical exertion or isometric exercise because this may provoke exertional syncope. Exposure to high altitudes may contribute to hypoxic pulmonary vasoconstriction and may not be well tolerated. A sodium-restricted diet (<2400 mg/day) is advised and is particularly important to manage volume status in patients with right ventricular failure. Routine immunizations, such as those against influenza and pneumococcal pneumonia, are advised. Because hypoxia is a potent pulmonary vasoconstrictor, supplemental oxygen is recommended to maintain saturations above 90% at rest, with exertion, and during sleep. In patients with intracardiac shunting and Eisenmenger's physiology (Chapter 69), this goal may not be possible.

Patients with pulmonary arterial hypertension are advised against pregnancy because the hemodynamic fluctuations of pregnancy, labor, delivery, and the postpartum period are potentially life-threatening, with a 30 to 50% mortality rate in some series. Current guidelines recommend that pregnancy be avoided or terminated early in women with pulmonary arterial hypertension. Women of childbearing potential should be counseled on contraception options at the time of diagnosis.

For patients with idiopathic, heritable, anorexigen-induced, and connective tissue disease–associated pulmonary arterial hypertension (group 1 pulmonary arterial hypertension), clinical trial data can guide effective therapy (Fig. 68-7). For all other types of pulmonary hypertension, the safety and efficacy of pulmonary arterial hypertension–specific therapies have not been demonstrated, so treatment should instead be targeted at the underlying disease.

Treatment of the Underlying Conditions

The initial treatment should be directed at any underlying or associated conditions, especially lung disease, that also directly affect exercise tolerance and systemic diseases that have effective therapies. After these disorders have been optimally treated, specific therapy of the pulmonary arterial hypertension itself should be considered.

Background Therapy

In three uncontrolled observational series in patients with primarily idiopathic pulmonary arterial hypertension, warfarin coagulation improved survival. Consensus recommendations advocate the use of warfarin titrated to an INR of 1.5 to 2.5 in patients with idiopathic pulmonary arterial hypertension. Although no data are available to guide recommendations in patients with other types of pulmonary arterial hypertension, warfarin is generally recommended in patients with advanced disease and severe right heart failure, in the absence of contraindications. Diuretics (e.g., furosemide, initiated at 20 mg and titrated as needed) are indicated to manage right ventricular volume overload; in some patients, intravenous diuretics may be necessary. Serum electrolytes and renal function must be closely monitored. Digoxin, 0.125 to 0.25 mg/day, is sometimes used in patients with right ventricular failure and a low cardiac output and in patients with atrial arrhythmias, despite the paucity of data; if the patient experiences any evidence of digoxin toxicity, the drug should be discontinued because of the unfavorable risk-to-benefit ratio.

Vasodilator Therapy
Calcium-Channel Blockers

Approximately 7% of adult patients with idiopathic pulmonary arterial hypertension have a favorable response to acute vasodilator testing and excellent prognosis with calcium-channel blockers. Long-acting nifedipine, diltiazem, and amlodipine are the most commonly used calcium-channel blockers. Because of its potential negative inotropic effects, verapamil should be avoided. Patients must be followed closely for both the safety and efficacy of this therapy. If a patient who meets the definition of an acute response does not improve to WHO class I or II on calcium-channel blocker therapy, the patient should not be considered a chronic responder; alternative or additional pulmonary arterial hypertension specific therapy should be instituted.

Targeted Therapies

In clinical trials, intravenous epoprostenol improves functional class, exercise endurance, hemodynamics, and survival in patients with idiopathic pulmonary arterial hypertension,[1] and it also improves exercise tolerance and hemodynamics in patients with pulmonary arterial hypertension related to

FIGURE 68-7. Pulmonary hypertension treatment algorithm. CCB = calcium-channel blocker; ERA = endothelin receptor antagonist; IV = intravenous; PDE-5I = phosphodiesterase type 5 inhibitor; SC = subcutaneous. (From McLaughlin VV, Archer SL, Badesch DB, et al. ACCF/AHA 2009 expert consensus document on pulmonary hypertension: a report of the American College of Cardiology Foundation Task Force on Expert Consensus Documents and the American Heart Association developed in collaboration with the American College of Chest Physicians; American Thoracic Society, Inc.; and the Pulmonary Hypertension Association. *J Am Coll Cardiol.* 2009; 53:1573-1619.)

the scleroderma spectrum of diseases.[2] Uncontrolled studies have also reported favorable effects with intravenous epoprostenol in patients with numerous forms of associated pulmonary arterial hypertension. Observational series suggest a long-term survival benefit with intravenous epoprostenol compared with historical controls. Epoprostenol must be delivered by continuous intravenous infusion, commonly initiated in the hospital at a dose of 2 ng/kg/minute, with the dose titrated up based on symptoms of pulmonary arterial hypertension and side effects of the therapy. Each patient must learn the techniques of sterile preparation of the medication, operation of the ambulatory infusion pump, and care of the central venous catheter. Although dosing must be highly individualized, maintenance doses in the range of 25 to 40 ng/kg/minute are typically needed for patients on monotherapy. Common side effects include headache, jaw pain, flushing, nausea, diarrhea, skin rash, and musculoskeletal pain. Infections and infusion interruption can be life-threatening.

Subcutaneous treprostinil can provide a modest but statistically significant improvement in exercise tolerance.[3] The main limitation of this therapy is pain and erythema at the site of the subcutaneous infusion, a complication that occurs in 85% of patients. Other prostanoid-type side effects, including headache, diarrhea, rash, and nausea, also occur. Subcutaneous treprostinil is often started in the home, with the dose titrated up based on symptoms of pulmonary arterial hypertension and drug side effects. Treprostinil is less potent than epoprostenol, and higher doses are required to achieve the desired efficacy. Inhaled treprostinil four times daily[4] and inhaled iloprost six to nine times daily[5] also are effective for improving exercise capacity. However, cough is an additional side effect with this method of administration.

The endothelin receptor antagonist bosentan (initiated orally at 62.5 mg twice daily and titrated up to 125 mg twice daily after 1 month) improves hemodynamics and exercise capacity and the clinical course of pulmonary arterial hypertension.[6,7] Ambrisentan (administered orally at doses of either 5 mg or 10 mg once daily) has similar benefits.[8] Liver enzymes must be monitored on a monthly basis; the dose should be reduced if liver enzymes rise to greater than three to five times the upper limits of normal and discontinued if they rise to five times the upper limit of normal. Other side effects include lower extremity edema, headache, and nasal congestion.

The chronic administration of inhaled nitric oxide is cumbersome and not clinically useful. However, the phosphodiesterase type 5 antagonists sildenafil and tadalafil are effective and useful for pulmonary arterial hypertension.[9,10] Sildenafil is approved at a dose of 20 mg three times daily and tadalafil at a dose of 40 mg once daily. The most common side effects of the phosphodiesterase inhibitors are headache, flushing, dyspepsia, and epistaxis.

Given the availability of therapies that target different pathologic processes, combination therapy is an attractive theoretical option in pulmonary arterial hypertension. Emerging data support the incremental benefit of combining more than one targeted therapy[4,11-12] under careful observation, usually in a specialized center.

Invasive Therapies

Despite advances in medical therapies for pulmonary arterial hypertension, many patients experience progressive functional decline, largely related to worsening right heart failure. In carefully selected patients, atrial septostomy may improve symptoms. Atrial septostomy creates a right-to-left interatrial shunt, thereby decreasing right heart filling pressures and improving right heart function and left heart filling. Although the right-to-left shunting decreases systemic arterial oxygen saturation, it is anticipated that the improvement in cardiac output will result in overall augmentation in systemic oxygen delivery. Contraindications to performing atrial septostomy include severe right ventricular failure on cardiorespiratory support, mean right atrial pressure of more than 20 mm Hg, pulmonary vascular resistance index of more than 55 U/m^2, resting oxygen saturation of less than 90% on room air, and left ventricular end-diastolic pressure of more than 18 mm Hg. Because of the high morbidity and mortality associated with this procedure, it should be performed only by experienced operators in specialized centers.

Bilateral lung (Chapter 101) or heart-lung transplantation (Chapter 82) is the final option for selected patients with pulmonary arterial hypertension when medical therapy fails. The 1-, 3-, 5-, and 10-year survival rates are 66%, 57%, 47%, and 27%, respectively, in patients with idiopathic pulmonary arterial hypertension who undergo transplantation. Transplantation as a potential therapeutic option should be discussed with selected patients at the time of diagnosis, although timing of referral is challenging. Patients who are otherwise good transplant candidates should be referred when they have an unacceptable response to medical therapies.

Assessing Response to Therapy

Given the complexity of the disease, the variable response to therapy, and the goal of optimizing and individualizing care, patients with pulmonary arterial hypertension must be followed closely. The usual recommendation is every 3 to 6 months in stable patients and every 1 to 3 months in patients with worsening or unstable symptoms or signs.

PROGNOSIS

Several clinical factors are correlated with prognosis (Table 68-3). The natural history of idiopathic pulmonary arterial hypertension is a median survival of 2.8 years with 1-, 3-, and 5-year survival rates of 68%, 48%, and 34%, respectively. Patients with pulmonary arterial hypertension related to the scleroderma spectrum of diseases tend to have a poorer prognosis than those with idiopathic pulmonary arterial hypertension, whereas patients with pulmonary arterial hypertension related to congenital heart disease tend to have a better prognosis, perhaps because they have better right ventricular function. Observational series suggest survival benefits for modern treatments, including epoprostenol, treprostinil, bosentan, and ambrisentan, but data are limited. Nevertheless, studies have demonstrated the 1-year survival on current medical therapy to be in the 85 to 88% range.

The natural history of patients with groups 2 and 3 pulmonary hypertension are influenced by their left heart and lung disease. In most cases, the presence of pulmonary hypertension in addition to the underlying disease portends a poor prognosis.

TABLE 68-3 PULMONARY ARTERIAL HYPERTENSION: DETERMINANTS OF PROGNOSIS*

DETERMINANTS OF RISK	LOWER RISK (GOOD PROGNOSIS)	HIGHER RISK (POOR PROGNOSIS)
Clinical evidence of RV failure	No	Yes
Progression of symptoms	Gradual	Rapid
WHO class†	II, III	IV
6-MW test‡	Longer (>400 m)	Shorter (<300 m)
CPET	Peak Vo_2 > 10.4 mL/kg/min	Peak Vo_2 < 10.4 mL/kg/min
Echocardiography	Minimal RV dysfunction	Pericardial effusion, significant RV enlargement or dysfunction, right atrial enlargement
Hemodynamics	RAP < 10 mm Hg, CI > 2.5 L/min/m^2	RAP > 20 mm Hg, CI < 2.0 L/min/m^2
BNP§	Minimally elevated	Significantly elevated

*Most data available pertain to idiopathic pulmonary arterial hypertension. Few data are available for other forms of PAH. One should not rely on any single factor to make risk predictions.
†WHO class is the functional classification for PAH and is a modification of the New York Heart Association functional class.
‡6-MW test is also influenced by age, gender, and height.
§Because there are currently limited data regarding the influence of BNP on prognosis, and many factors including renal function, weight, age, and gender may influence BNP, absolute numbers are not given for this variable.
6-MW = 6-minute walk; BNP = brain natriuretic peptide; CI = cardiac index; CPET = cardiopulmonary exercise testing; peak Vo_2 = average peak oxygen uptake during exercise; RAP = right atrial pressure; RV = right ventricle; WHO = World Health Organization.
From McLaughlin VV, Archer SL, Badesch DB, et al. ACCF/AHA 2009 expert consensus document on pulmonary hypertension: a report of the American College of Cardiology Foundation Task Force on Expert Consensus Documents and the American Heart Association developed in collaboration with the American College of Chest Physicians; American Thoracic Society, Inc.; and the Pulmonary Hypertension Association. *J Am Coll Cardiol.* 2009;53:1573-1619.

1. Barst RJ, Rubin LJ, Long WA, et al. A comparison of continuous intravenous epoprostenol (prostacyclin) with conventional therapy for primary pulmonary hypertension. *N Engl J Med.* 1996;334:296-301.
2. Badesch DB, Tapson VF, McGoon MD, et al. Continuous intravenous epoprostenol for pulmonary hypertension due to the scleroderma spectrum of disease: a randomized, controlled trial. *Ann Intern Med.* 2000;132:425-434.
3. Simonneau G, Barst RJ, Galiè N, et al. Continuous subcutaneous infusion of treprostinil, a prostacyclin analogue, in patients with pulmonary arterial hypertension. *Am J Respir Crit Care Med.* 2002;165:800-804.
4. McLaughlin VV, Benza RL, Rubin LJ, et al. Addition of inhaled treprostinil to oral therapy for pulmonary arterial hypertension: a randomized controlled clinical trial. *J Am Coll Cardiol.* 2010; 55:1915-1922.
5. Olschewski H, Simonneau G, Galiè N, et al. Inhaled iloprost for severe pulmonary hypertension. *N Engl J Med.* 2002;347:322-329.
6. Channick RN, Simonneau G, Sitbon O, et al. Effects of the dual endothelin-receptor antagonist bosentan in patients with pulmonary hypertension: a randomised placebo-controlled study. *Lancet.* 2001;358:1119-1123.
7. Rubin LJ, Badesch DB, Barst RJ, et al. Bosentan therapy for pulmonary arterial hypertension. *N Engl J Med.* 2002;346:896-903.
8. Galiè N, Olschewski H, Oudiz R, et al. Ambrisentan for the treatment of pulmonary arterial hypertension: results of the ambrisentan in pulmonary arterial hypertension, randomized, double-blind, placebo-controlled, multicenter, efficacy (ARIES) study 1 and 2. *Circulation.* 2008;117:3010-3019.
9. Galiè N, Ghofrani HA, Torbicki A, et al. Sildenafil citrate therapy for pulmonary arterial hypertension. *N Engl J Med.* 2005;353:2148-2157.
10. Galiè N, Brundage BH, Ghofrani HA, et al. Tadalafil therapy for pulmonary arterial hypertension. *Circulation.* 2009;119:2894-2903.
11. McLaughlin VV, Oudiz RJ, Adaani F, et al. Randomized study of adding inhaled iloprost to existing bosentan in pulmonary arterial hypertension. *Am J Respir Crit Care Med.* 2006;174:1257-1263.
12. Simonneau G, Rubin LJ, Galiè N, et al. Addition of sildenafil to long-term intravenous epoprostenol therapy in pulmonary arterial hypertension: a randomized trial. *Ann Intern Med.* 2008;149:521-530.

SUGGESTED READINGS

Humbert M, Sitbon O, Chaouat A, et al. Survival in patients with idiopathic, familial, and anorexigen-associated pulmonary arterial hypertension in the modern management era. *Circulation.* 2010;122:156-163. *Estimated survivals are 86% at 1 year, 70% at 2 years, and 55% at 3 years.*
Kaw R, Pasupuleti V, Deshpande A, et al. Pulmonary hypertension: an important predictor of outcomes in patients undergoing non-cardiac surgery. *Respir Med.* 2011;105:619-624. *Mean pulmonary arterial pressure is an independent predictor of post-operative morbidity.*

McLaughlin VV, Archer SL, Badesch DB, et al. ACCF/AHA 2009 expert consensus document on pulmonary hypertension: a report of the American College of Cardiology Foundation Task Force on Expert Consensus Documents and the American Heart Association developed in collaboration with the American College of Chest Physicians; American Thoracic Society, Inc.; and the Pulmonary Hypertension Association. *J Am Coll Cardiol.* 2009;53:1573-1619. *Expert consensus document.*
Nef HM, Möllmann H, Hamm C, et al. Pulmonary hypertension: updated classification and management of pulmonary hypertension. *Heart.* 2010;96:552-559. *Review.*

69

CONGENITAL HEART DISEASE IN ADULTS

ARIANE J. MARELLI

The convergence of major progress in medicine, pediatrics, and cardiovascular surgery has resulted in the survival of an increasingly large number of adult patients with congenital heart disease. Adult physicians are becoming increasingly responsible for these patients, commonly in concert with a cardiologist and a tertiary care facility.

DEFINITIONS

Patients can be divided into three categories according to the surgical status: unoperated, surgically palliated, or physiologically repaired. Congenital heart lesions can be classified as *acyanotic* or *cyanotic. Cyanosis* refers to a blue discoloration of the mucous membranes resulting from an increased amount of reduced hemoglobin. Central cyanosis occurs when the circulation is mixed because of a right-to-left shunt.

A *native lesion* refers to an anatomic lesion present at birth. Acquired lesions, naturally occurring or as a result of surgery, are superimposed on the native anatomy. *Palliative* interventions are performed in patients with cyanotic lesions and are defined as operations that either increase or decrease pulmonary blood flow while allowing a mixed circulation and cyanosis to persist (Table 69-1). *Physiologic* repair applies to procedures that provide total or nearly total anatomic and physiologic separation of the pulmonary and systemic circulations in complex cyanotic lesions and result in patients who are acyanotic.

Eisenmenger's complex refers to flow reversal across a ventricular septal defect (VSD) when pulmonary vascular resistance exceeds systemic levels. *Eisenmenger's physiology* designates the physiologic response in a broader category of shunt lesions in which a right-to-left shunt occurs in response to an elevation in pulmonary vascular resistance. *Eisenmenger's syndrome* is a term applied to common clinical features shared by patients with Eisenmenger's physiology.

Each congenital lesion can influence the course of another. For example, the physiologic consequences of a VSD are different if it occurs in isolation or in combination with pulmonary stenosis. A *simple lesion* is defined as either a shunt lesion or an obstructive lesion of the right or left heart occurring in isolation. A *complex lesion* is a combination of two or more abnormalities.

EPIDEMIOLOGY

Genetic Determinants

In 90% of patients, congenital heart disease is attributable to multifactorial inheritance; only 5 to 10% of malformations are due to primary genetic factors, either chromosomal or related to a single mutant gene. The most common defect observed in patients with chromosomal aberrations is a VSD, which occurs in 90% of patients with trisomy 13 and trisomy 18. Defects of the endocardial cushions and the ventricular septum are found in 50% of patients with Down syndrome (trisomy 21). The most frequently observed defects in patients with Turner's syndrome (45,X) are aortic coarctation, aortic stenosis, and atrial septal defect (ASD). About 15% of patients with tetralogy of Fallot have a deletion on chromosome 22q11; prevalence is higher in those with a right aortic arch. Abnormalities involving the chromosomal band 22q11 can also result in a group of syndromes, the most common of which is DiGeorge syndrome. The shared phenotypic features are designated CATCH-22 syndromes, that is, a combination of *c*ardiac defects, *a*bnormal facies, *t*hymic hypoplasia, *c*left palate, and *h*ypocalcemia. The

TABLE 69-1	PALLIATIVE SURGICAL SHUNTS FOR CONGENITAL HEART LESIONS
PALLIATIVE SHUNT	**ANASTOMOSIS**
SYSTEMIC ARTERIAL TO PULMONARY ARTERY SHUNTS	
Classic Blalock-Taussig	Subclavian artery to PA
Modified Blalock-Taussig	Subclavian artery to PA (prosthetic graft)
Potts anastomosis	Descending aorta to left PA
Waterston shunt	Ascending aorta to right PA
SYSTEMIC VENOUS TO PULMONARY ARTERY SHUNTS	
Classic Glenn	SVC to right PA
Bidirectional Glenn	SVC to right and left PA
Bilateral Glenn	Right and left SVC to right and left PA

PA = pulmonary artery; SVC = superior vena cava.
From Marelli A, Mullen M. Palliative surgical shunts for congenital heart lesions. *Clin Paediatr.* 1996;4:189.

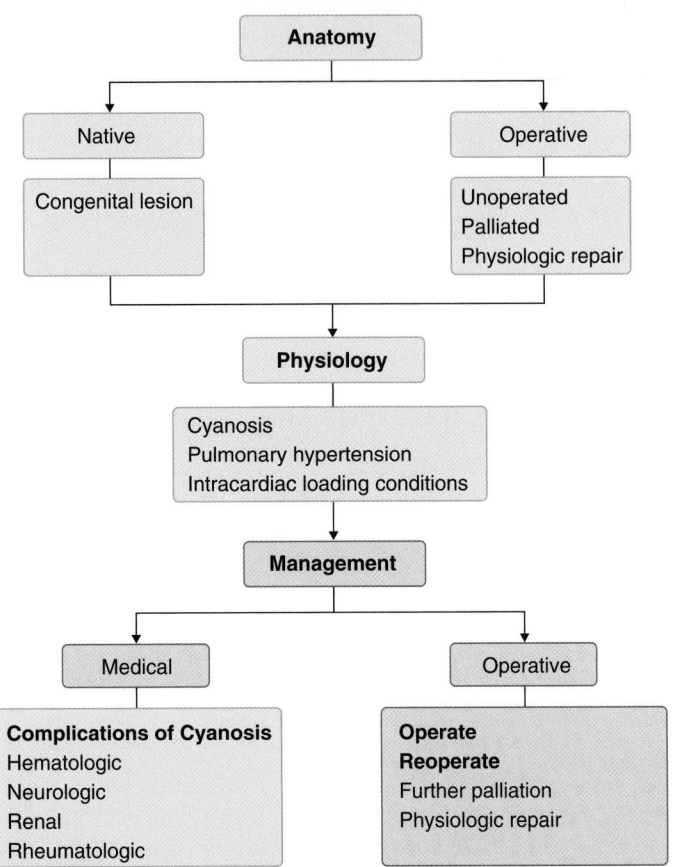

FIGURE 69-1. The goals of complete clinical assessment in congenital heart disease are to define the anatomy and physiology to determine appropriate management.

recurrence risk for families with a child who carries a congenital cardiac malformation due to a chromosomal anomaly is related to the recurrence risk of the chromosomal anomaly itself.

Typically, single mutant genes are also associated with syndromes of cardiovascular malformations, although not every patient with the syndrome has the characteristic cardiac anomaly. Examples include osteogenesis imperfecta (autosomal recessive), associated with aortic valve disease; Jervell and Lange-Nielsen syndrome (autosomal recessive) and Romano-Ward syndrome (autosomal dominant), associated with a prolonged QT interval and sudden death; and Holt-Oram syndrome (autosomal dominant), in which an ASD occurs with a range of other skeletal anomalies. Osler-Weber-Rendu telangiectasias are associated with pulmonary arteriovenous fistulas. Williams syndrome occurs with supravalvular aortic stenosis in most cases. Noonan's syndrome is associated with pulmonary stenosis, ASD, and hypertrophic cardiomyopathy. Although autosomal dominant inheritance has been implicated for both, most cases are sporadic. Deletion at chromosome 7q11.23 has been identified in patients with Williams syndrome, and a gene defect has been mapped to 12q22-qter in patients with Noonan's syndrome.

The risk for recurrence when the mother carries a sporadically occurring congenital lesion varies from 2.5 to 18%, depending on the lesion. Obstructive lesions of the left ventricular outflow tract have the highest recurrence rates in offspring. When the father carries the lesion, 1.5 to 3% of the offspring are affected. When a sibling has a congenital cardiac anomaly, the risk for recurrence in another sibling varies from 1 to 3%.

Incidence and Prevalence

Cardiac malformations occur at a rate of 8 per 1000 live births, or 32,000 infants with new diagnoses yearly in the United States. The prevalence of congenital heart disease has increased in the general population, with the steepest rise observed in adults with severe or complex lesions. An estimated 20% die in the first year of life—a substantial decrease from the late 1960s. An overall prevalence of 4 per 1000 adults has been documented. The median age of patients with severe lesions has increased from childhood to late adolescence. Currently, more than 1 million patients are thought to be alive in the United States with congenital heart disease.

Bicuspid aortic valve occurs in about 2% of the general population, is the most common congenital cardiac anomaly encountered in adult populations, and accounts for up to half of surgical cases of aortic stenosis in adults (Chapter 75). ASDs constitute 30 to 40% of cases of congenital heart disease in adults, with ostium secundum ASD accounting for 7% of all congenital lesions. A solitary VSD represents 15 to 20% of all congenital lesions and is the most common congenital cardiac lesion observed in children; its high spontaneous closure rates explain the lesser prevalence in adults. Patent ductus arteriosus (PDA) accounts for 5 to 10% of all congenital cardiac lesions in infants with a normal birthweight. Pulmonary stenosis and coarctation of the aorta represent 3 to 10% of all congenital lesions.

Tetralogy of Fallot is the most common cyanotic congenital anomaly observed in adults. Together with complete transposition of the great arteries, these lesions account for 5 to 12% of congenital heart disease in infants. More complex lesions such as tricuspid atresia, univentricular heart,

congenitally corrected transposition of the great arteries, Ebstein's anomaly, and double-outlet right ventricle account for 2.5% or less of all congenital heart disease.

CLINICAL MANIFESTATIONS

Congenital heart disease is a lifelong condition during which the patient and the lesion evolve concurrently. A patient may have been monitored for many years because of an erroneous diagnosis made in infancy or childhood when diagnostic techniques were more limited. The differential diagnosis of native and surgical anatomy in the adult with an unknown diagnosis depends on whether the patient is cyanotic or acyanotic. On completion of the evaluation, the following questions should be answered (Fig. 69-1): What is the native anatomy? Has this patient undergone surgery for the condition? What is the physiology? What can and should be done for this patient both medically and surgically, and importantly, who should do it?

If the patient has not undergone surgery, the question is, Why not? If the patient is palliated, has the degree of cyanosis progressed as evidenced by a drop in systemic saturation or a rise in hemoglobin? If the patient has undergone a physiologic repair, what procedure was performed? Are residual lesions present, and have new lesions developed as a consequence of surgery? The patient's physiology is determined by the presence or absence of cyanosis, pulmonary hypertension, adequate filling of the cardiac chambers, and any resulting medical complications.

A clinical assessment, 12-lead electrocardiogram (ECG), chest radiograph, and baseline oxygen saturation should be part of every initial assessment. Two-dimensional transthoracic echocardiography (Chapter 55) and Doppler and color flow imaging are used to establish the diagnosis and to monitor the evolution of documented hemodynamic complications. Transesophageal echocardiographic examination is particularly useful in adults and is increasingly important during interventional catheter-guided therapy and surgery. Magnetic resonance imaging (Chapter 56) and computed tomography (Chapter 56) are useful adjuncts. Cardiac catheterization for congenital heart disease has shifted from pure diagnosis to include intervention. Coronary arteriography is recommended for adults older than 40 years in whom surgical intervention is contemplated.

Pulmonary Hypertension and Its Complications

Pulmonary hypertension secondary to structural disease of the heart or circulation can occur with or without an increase in pulmonary vascular resistance. Pulmonary vascular obstructive disease occurs when pulmonary vascular resistance rises and becomes fixed and irreversible. In the most common congenital anomalies, pulmonary hypertension is a result of increased pulmonary blood flow because of a native left-to-right shunt. Examples include ASD, a moderately sized VSD, PDA, and a variety of complex lesions. The rate at which pulmonary hypertension progresses to become pulmonary vascular obstructive disease varies from one lesion to another and depends at least in part on the source of pulmonary blood flow. Pulmonary hypertension typically develops in patients with an ASD after the fourth decade; Eisenmenger's syndrome is a late complication seen in only 5 to 10% of cases. In contrast, in patients with a large VSD or persistent PDA, progressive elevation in pulmonary vascular resistance occurs rapidly because the pulmonary vascular bed is exposed not only to the excess volume of the left-to-right shunt but also to systemic arterial pressures. As a result, Eisenmenger's complex develops in approximately 10% of patients with a large VSD during the first decade. Surgical pulmonary artery banding is a palliative measure aimed at decreasing pulmonary blood flow and protecting the pulmonary vascular bed against the development of early pulmonary vascular obstructive disease.

If forward flow from the right side of the heart is insufficient, native collaterals or surgical shunts provide an alternative source of pulmonary blood flow (see Table 69-1). With large surgical shunts, however, direct exposure of the pulmonary vascular bed to the high pressures of the systemic circulation causes pulmonary vascular obstructive disease. As a result, systemic to pulmonary arterial shunts are currently less favored in neonates and infants, in whom systemic venous to pulmonary arterial shunts are now preferred.

The term *Eisenmenger's syndrome* should be reserved for patients in whom pulmonary vascular obstructive disease is present and pulmonary vascular resistance is fixed and irreversible. These findings, in combination with the absence of left-to-right shunting, render the patient inoperable.

The clinical manifestations of Eisenmenger's syndrome include dyspnea on exertion, syncope, chest pain, congestive heart failure, and symptoms related to erythrocytosis and hyperviscosity. On physical examination, central cyanosis and digital clubbing are hallmark findings. Systemic oxygen saturations typically vary between 75 and 85%. The pulse pressure narrows as the cardiac output falls. Examination of jugular venous pressure can reveal a dominant a wave reflecting a noncompliant right ventricle until tricuspid insufficiency is severe enough to generate a large v wave. A prominent right ventricular impulse is felt in the left parasternal border in end expiration or in the subcostal area in end inspiration. A palpable pulmonary artery is commonly felt. The pulmonary component of the second heart sound is increased and can be felt in most cases. Pulmonary ejection sounds are common when the pulmonary artery is dilated with a structurally normal valve. Right atrial gallop is heard more frequently when the a wave is dominant. A murmur of tricuspid insufficiency is common, but the inspiratory increase in the murmur (Carvallo's sign) disappears when right ventricular failure occurs. In diastole, a pulmonary insufficiency murmur is often heard. The 12-lead ECG shows evidence of right atrial enlargement, right ventricular hypertrophy, and right axis deviation. Chest radiographic findings include a dilated pulmonary artery segment, cardiac enlargement, and diminished pulmonary vascular markings. Echocardiography confirms the right-sided pressure overload and pulmonary artery enlargement as well as the tricuspid and pulmonary insufficiency. Cardiac catheterization is indicated if doubt exists about the potential reversibility of the elevated pulmonary vascular resistance in a patient who might otherwise benefit from surgery.

Cyanosis occurs when persistent venous to arterial mixing results in hypoxemia. Adaptive mechanisms to increase oxygen delivery include an increase in oxygen content, a rightward shift in the oxyhemoglobin dissociation curve, a higher hematocrit, and an increase in cardiac output. When cyanosis is not relieved, chronic hypoxemia and erythrocytosis result in hematologic, neurologic, renal, and rheumatic complications.

Hematologic complications of chronic hypoxemia include erythrocytosis, iron deficiency, and bleeding diathesis. Hemoglobin and hematocrit levels, as well as red blood cell indices, should be checked regularly and correlated with systemic oxygen saturation levels. Symptoms of hyperviscosity include headaches, faintness, dizziness, fatigue, altered mentation, visual disturbances, paresthesias, tinnitus, and myalgia. Symptoms are classified as mild to moderate when they interfere with only some activities, or they can be marked to severe and interfere with most or all activities. Patients with compensated erythrocytosis establish an equilibrium hematocrit at higher levels in an iron-replete state with minimal symptoms. Patients with decompensated erythrocytosis manifest unstable, rising hematocrit levels and experience severe hyperviscosity symptoms.

Hemostatic abnormalities can occur in up to 20% of cyanotic patients with erythrocytosis. Bleeding is usually mild and superficial and leads to easy bruising, skin petechiae, or mucosal bleeding, but epistaxis, hemoptysis, or even life-threatening postoperative bleeding can occur. A variety of clotting factor deficiencies and qualitative and quantitative platelet disorders have been described.

Neurologic complications, including cerebral hemorrhage, can be caused by hemostatic defects and are most often seen after inappropriate use of anticoagulant therapy. Patients with right-to-left shunts may be at risk for paradoxical cerebral emboli. Focal brain injury may provide a nidus for brain abscess if bacteremia supervenes. Attention should be paid to the use of air filters in peripheral intravenous lines to avoid paradoxical emboli through a right-to-left shunt.

Prophylactic phlebotomy has no place in the prevention of cerebral arterial thrombosis. Indications for phlebotomy are the occurrence of symptomatic hyperviscosity in an iron-repleted patient and prevention of excessive bleeding perioperatively.

Pulmonary complications include massive pulmonary hemorrhage and in situ arterial thrombosis. A rapid clinical deterioration associated with progressive hypoxemia often marks the terminal stage of disease. No clear benefits are observed with the use of anticoagulants (systemic or intrapulmonary) because of the risk for prolonged bleeding due to the underlying coagulopathy. The chronic disease process and high mortality prohibit pulmonary endarterectomy.

Renal dysfunction can be manifested as proteinuria, hyperuricemia, or renal failure. Focal interstitial fibrosis, tubular atrophy, and hyalinization of afferent and efferent arterioles can be seen on renal biopsy. Increased blood viscosity and arteriolar vasoconstriction can lead to renal hypoperfusion with progressive glomerulosclerosis. Hyperuricemia is commonly seen in patients with cyanotic congenital heart disease and is thought to be due mainly to the decreased reabsorption of uric acid rather than overproduction from erythrocytosis. Asymptomatic hyperuricemia need not be treated because lowering of uric acid levels has not been shown to prevent renal disease or gout.

Rheumatologic complications include gout and hypertrophic osteoarthropathy, which is thought to be responsible for the arthralgias affecting up to one third of patients with cyanotic congenital heart disease. In patients with right-to-left shunting, megakaryocytes released from the bone marrow bypass the lung and are entrapped in systemic arterioles and capillaries, where they release platelet-derived growth factor, which promotes local cell proliferation. Digital clubbing and new osseous formation with periostitis occur and cause the symptoms of arthralgia. Symptomatic hyperuricemia and gouty arthritis can be treated as necessary with colchicine, probenecid, or allopurinol; nonsteroidal anti-inflammatory drugs are best avoided, given the baseline hemostatic anomalies in these patients.

TREATMENT ℞

In patients with Eisenmenger's syndrome, bosentan (62.5 mg twice daily for 4 weeks, then 125 mg twice daily) improves hemodynamics and exercise capacity for at least 40 weeks.■ Chronic oxygen therapy is unlikely to benefit hypoxemia secondary to right-to-left shunting in the setting of a fixed pulmonary vascular resistance. Chronic oxygen therapy results in mucosal dehydration with an increased incidence of epistaxis and is therefore not recommended.

In the iron-replete state, moderate to severe hyperviscosity symptoms typically occur when hematocrit levels exceed 65%. If no evidence of dehydration is present, removal of 500 mL of blood during a 30- to 45-minute period should be followed by quantitative volume replacement with normal saline or dextran (Fig. 69-2). The procedure may be repeated every 24 hours until symptomatic improvement occurs.

Treatment of spontaneous bleeding is dictated by its severity and the abnormal hemostatic parameters (Fig. 69-3). For severe bleeding, platelet transfusions, fresh-frozen plasma, vitamin K, cryoprecipitate, and desmopressin have been used. Reduction in erythrocyte mass also improves hemostasis, so cyanotic patients undergoing surgery should have prophylactic phlebotomy if the hematocrit is greater than 65%.

Iron deficiency is common in cyanotic adult patients because of excessive bleeding or phlebotomy. In contrast to normocytic erythrocytosis, which is rarely symptomatic at hematocrit levels less than 65%, iron deficiency may manifest with hyperviscosity symptoms at hematocrit levels well below 65%. The treatment of choice is not phlebotomy but oral iron repletion until a rise in hematocrit is detected, typically within 1 week.

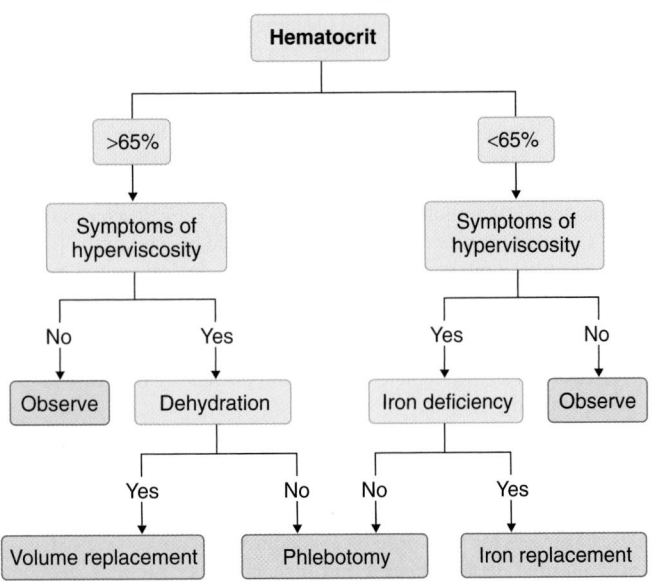

FIGURE 69-2. Treatment algorithm for erythrocytosis of cyanotic congenital heart disease.

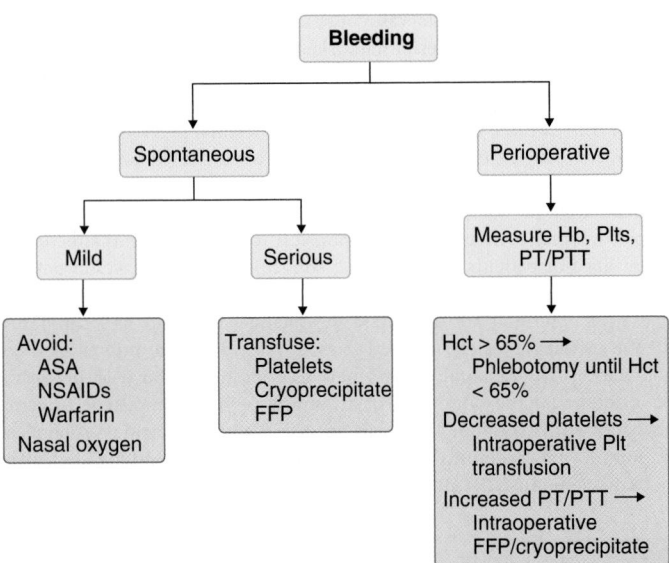

FIGURE 69-3. Treatment algorithm for bleeding diathesis of cyanotic congenital heart disease. ASA = acetylsalicylic acid; FFP = fresh-frozen plasma; Hb = hemoglobin; Hct = hematocrit; NSAIDs = nonsteroidal anti-inflammatory drugs; Plts = platelets; PT = prothrombin time; PTT = partial thromboplastin time.

● SIMPLE LESIONS
Isolated Shunt Lesions

Hemodynamic complications of significant shunts relate to volume overload and chamber dilation of the primary chamber receiving the excess left-to-right shunt and to secondary complications of valvular dysfunction and damage to the pulmonary vascular bed. The size and duration of the shunt determine the clinical course and therefore the indications for closure. The degree of shunting is a function of both the size of the communication and, depending on its location, biventricular compliance or pulmonary and systemic vascular resistance. Clinically apparent hemodynamic sequelae of shunts are typically apparent or can be expected to occur when pulmonary to systemic flow ratios exceed 1.5:1.

Shunt size can be inferred and measured with cardiac ultrasonography. Secondary enlargement of the cardiac chambers receiving excess shunt flow in diastole occurs as the shunt size becomes hemodynamically significant; in addition, the pulmonary artery becomes enlarged as pulmonary pressure rises. When tricuspid insufficiency occurs primarily from right ventricular dilation or secondary to pulmonary hypertension, the regurgitant jet can be used to estimate the pulmonary pressure as another indicator of shunt significance. When the pulmonary to systemic flow $(\dot{Q}_p:\dot{Q}_s)$ exceeds 2:1, the volume of blood in both circulations can be estimated by comparing the stroke volume at the pulmonary and aortic valves. Shunt detection and quantification can also be obtained by a first-pass radionuclide study. As a bolus of radioactive substance is injected into the systemic circulation, the rise and fall of radionuclide activity can be measured in the lungs. When a shunt is significant, the rate of persistent activity in the lungs over time can be used to calculate the shunt fraction. For both echocardiographic and radionuclide quantification of shunt size, sources of error are multiple. The most predictable results are obtained only in experienced laboratories. Uncertainty about the physiologic significance of a borderline shunt can be minimized by integrating serial determinations from multiple clinical and relevant diagnostic sources rather than basing management decisions on a single calculated shunt value.

Atrial Septal Defect

Classification of ASDs is based on anatomic location. Most commonly, an ostium secundum ASD occurs in the central portion of the interatrial septum as a result of an enlarged foramen ovale or excessive resorption of the septum primum. The combination of a secundum ASD and acquired mitral stenosis is known as *Lutembacher's syndrome,* the pathophysiology of which is determined by the relative severity of each. Abnormal development of the embryologic endocardial cushions results in a variety of atrioventricular canal defects, the most common of which consists of a defect in the lower part of the atrial septum in the ostium primum location, typically accompanied by a cleft mitral valve and mitral regurgitation. The sinus venosus defect, which accounts for 2 to 3% of all interatrial communications, is located superiorly at the junction of the superior vena cava and right atrium and is generally associated with anomalous drainage of the right-sided pulmonary veins into the superior vena cava or right atrium. Less commonly, interatrial communications can be seen at the site of the coronary sinus, typically associated with an anomalous left superior vena cava.

The pathophysiology is determined by the effects of the shunt on the heart and pulmonary circulation. Right atrial and right ventricular dilation occurs as shunt size increases with pulmonary to systemic flow ratios greater than 1.5:1. Superimposed systemic hypertension and coronary artery disease modify left ventricular compliance and favor left-to-right shunting. Mitral valve disease can occur in up to 15% of patients older than 50 years. Right-sided heart failure, atrial fibrillation, or atrial flutter can occur as a result of chronic right-sided volume overload and progressive ventricular and atrial dilation. Stroke can result from paradoxical emboli, atrial arrhythmias, or both. A rise in pulmonary pressure occurs because of the increased pulmonary blood flow. Pulmonary hypertension is unusual before 20 years of age but is seen in 50% of patients older than 40 years. The overall incidence of pulmonary vascular obstructive disease is 15 to 20% in patients with ASD. Eisenmenger's disease with reverse shunting, a late and rare complication of isolated secundum ASD, is reported in 5 to 10% of patients.

▶ DIAGNOSIS ◀

Although most patients are minimally symptomatic in the first three decades, more than 70% become impaired by the fifth decade. Initial symptoms include exercise intolerance, dyspnea on exertion, and fatigue caused most commonly by right-sided heart failure and pulmonary hypertension. Palpitations, syncope, and stroke can occur with the development of atrial arrhythmias.

On physical examination, most adults have a normal general physical appearance. When Holt-Oram syndrome is present, the thumb may have a third phalanx or may be rudimentary or absent. With an uncomplicated nonrestrictive communication between both atria, the a and v waves are equal in amplitude. Precordial palpation typically discloses a normal left ventricular impulse unless mitral valve disease occurs. Characteristically, if the shunt is significant, a right ventricular impulse can be felt in the left parasternal area in end expiration or in the subxiphoid area in end inspiration. A dilated pulmonary artery can sometimes be felt in the second left intercostal space. On auscultation, the hallmark of an ASD is the wide and fixed splitting of the second heart sound. Pulmonary valve closure, as reflected by P_2, is delayed because of right ventricular overload and the increased capacitance of the pulmonary vascular bed. The A_2-P_2 interval is fixed because the increase in venous return elevates the right atrial pressure during inspiration, thereby decreasing the degree of left-to-right shunting and offsetting the usual phasic respiratory changes. In addition, compliance of the pulmonary circulation is reduced from the high flow, thus making the vascular compartment less susceptible to any further increase in blood flow. A soft midsystolic murmur generated by the increased flow across the pulmonary valve is usually heard in the second left interspace. In the presence of a high left-to-right shunt volume, increased flow across the tricuspid valve is heard as a mid-diastolic murmur at the lower left sternal border. With advanced right-sided heart failure, evidence of systemic venous congestion is present.

The ECG characteristically shows an incomplete right bundle branch block pattern (Fig. 69-4). Right axis deviation and atrial abnormalities, including a prolonged PR interval, atrial fibrillation, and flutter, are also seen. Typically, the chest radiograph shows pulmonary vascular plethora with increased markings in both lung fields consistent with increased pulmonary blood flow (see Fig. 53-13 in Chapter 53). The main pulmonary artery and both its branches are dilated. Right atrial and right ventricular dilation can be seen. Cardiac ultrasonography is diagnostic and provides important prognostic information (Fig. 69-5). Ostium primum and secundum ASDs are easily identifiable with transthoracic imaging, but a sinus venosus ASD can be missed unless it is specifically sought. For more accurate visualization of the superior interatrial septum and localization of the pulmonary veins, transesophageal echocardiography is useful. With Doppler study, pulmonary artery pressures can be quantified, and the $\dot{Q}:\dot{Q}$ can be measured.

TREATMENT Rx

Closure of an ASD either percutaneously or surgically is indicated in the presence of right heart enlargement, with or without symptoms. Centrally located defects measuring up to 3.5 cm can be occluded by transcatheter techniques in a cardiac catheterization laboratory. Advantages of this approach include the avoidance of sternotomy and cardiopulmonary bypass. Uncomplicated secundum ASDs may be closed surgically in children and adults with minimal operative mortality, although surgical closure is usually reserved for patients in whom concomitant repair of associated valvular anomalies is required, anomalous pulmonary veins are present, or device closure is not technically feasible.

In patients older than 40 years with symptoms and significant shunts, closure improves functional status and survival.[2] In the presence of a significant shunt, closure of an ASD before 25 years of age without evidence of pulmonary hypertension results in a long-term outcome that is similar to that of age- and sex-matched controls. Advanced age (60 years) is not a contraindication to ASD closure in the presence of a significant shunt because a significant number of patients will show evidence of symptomatic improvement. Preoperative pulmonary artery pressure and the presence or absence of pulmonary vascular disease are important predictors of successful interventional outcome.

FIGURE 69-4. Electrocardiographic hallmark in atrial septal defect. Right precordial leads V_1 and V_2 illustrate two variants of an incomplete right bundle branch block pattern, the rSrT pattern (**A**) and the rsR' pattern (**B**).

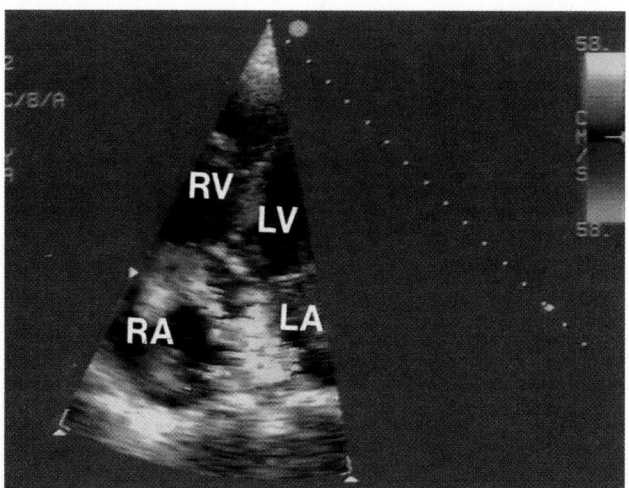

FIGURE 69-5. Color flow Doppler apical four-chamber view showing blood flow from the left atrium (LA) to the right atrium (RA) through a moderately sized atrial septal defect. LV = left ventricle; RV = right ventricle. (From Forbes CD, Jackson WF. *Color Atlas and Text of Clinical Medicine,* 3rd ed. London: Mosby; 2003.)

Patent Foramen Ovale

Integrity of the fetal circulation depends on the patency of the foramen ovale. In most cases, the fall in pulmonary vascular resistance at birth induces the foramen to become sealed. Necropsy studies have revealed that the foramen ovale remains patent beyond the first year of life in about 30% of individuals, and clinical studies have demonstrated that the prevalence of patent foramen ovale is three times greater in patients with cryptogenic stroke (Chapter 414), particularly before the age of 55 years, because of right-to-left shunting and paradoxical embolization of material from the venous circulation. Cardiac investigation of the patient with cryptogenic stroke includes transesophageal echocardiography with agitated saline injection to visualize the presence of a right-to-left shunt (Chapter 55). Patent foramen ovale most likely to result in future paradoxical embolization is found in patients younger than 55 years with a prior cryptogenic stroke, in association with a hypermobile septum with aneurysm formation, and when a significant amount of right-to-left shunting is present at rest without provocative maneuvers. Some data suggest that a patent foramen ovale also may be associated with migraine headaches.

TREATMENT Rx

Currently there are no data to support closure of a patent foramen ovale for primary stroke prevention in a patient in whom it is fortuitously diagnosed on routine echocardiography. Ongoing randomized trials are addressing the benefit of closure versus medical therapy after a stroke; in the meantime, warfarin to an international normalized ratio of 2.0 to 3.0 is usually recommended over aspirin for secondary stroke prevention. Primary closure of a patent foramen ovale is indicated when a patient has contraindications to medical therapy, if medical therapy has failed, or in the presence of a hypercoagulable state not treatable by medical therapy. Device closure in experienced centers is usually preferred to surgical closure, although surgical closure is performed if the patient undergoes cardiac surgery for other reasons. Device closure appears to be associated with a low incidence of yearly recurrence rates. Despite the potential link with migraine headaches, closure of a patent foramen ovale does not result in symptomatic improvement.[3]

Ventricular Septal Defect

For anatomic classification of VSDs, the interventricular septum can be divided into four regions. Defects of the membranous septum, or infracristal VSDs, are located in a small translucent area beneath the aortic valve and account for up to 80% of VSDs. These VSDs typically show a variable degree of extension into the inlet or outlet septum, hence their designation as perimembranous. Infundibular defects or supracristal outlet VSDs occur in the conal septum above the crista supraventricularis and below the pulmonary valve. Inlet defects are identified at the crux of the heart between the tricuspid and mitral valves and are usually associated with other anomalies of the atrioventricular canal. Defects of the trabecular or muscular septum can be multiple and occur distal to the septal attachment of the tricuspid valve and toward the apex.

The pathophysiology and clinical course of VSDs depend on the size of the defect, the status of the pulmonary vascular bed, and the effects of shunt size on intracardiac hemodynamics. Unlike ASDs, a VSD may decrease in size with time. Approximately half of all native VSDs are small, and more than half of them close spontaneously; moderate or even large VSDs may also close in 10% or less of cases. The highest closure rates are observed in the first decade of life; spontaneous closure in adult life is unusual.

Patients who have a small defect with trivial or mild shunts are defined as those with a $\dot{Q}:\dot{Q}$ of less than 1.5 and normal pulmonary artery pressure and vascular resistance. Patients with moderate defects have a $\dot{Q}:\dot{Q}$ ratio of greater than 1.2 and elevated pulmonary artery pressure but not elevated pulmonary vascular resistance. Patients with a large and severe defect have an elevated $\dot{Q}:\dot{Q}$ ratio with high pulmonary pressure and elevated pulmonary vascular resistance. Eisenmenger's complex develops in about 10% of patients with VSDs, usually when there is no resistance to flow at the level of the defect, which can be as large as the aorta. When a systolic pressure gradient is present between the ventricles, the physiologic severity may be trivial or mild but can also be moderate or severe.

Minimal or mild defects usually cause no significant hemodynamic or physiologic abnormality. A moderate or severe defect causes left atrial and ventricular dilation consistent with the degree of left-to-right shunting. Shunting across the ventricular septum occurs predominantly during systole when left ventricular pressure exceeds that on the right; diastolic filling abnormalities occur in the left atrium. With moderate or severe defects, the right side of the heart becomes affected as a function of the rise in pulmonary pressure and pulmonary blood flow.

DIAGNOSIS

An adult with a VSD most commonly has a small restrictive lesion that either was small at birth or has undergone some degree of spontaneous closure. A second group of patients consists of those with large, nonrestrictive VSDs that have not been operated on; these patients have had Eisenmenger's complex for most of their lives. Patients with a moderately sized defect are typically symptomatic as children and are therefore more likely to have repair at a young age.

Patients with a trivial or mild shunt across a small, restrictive VSD are usually asymptomatic. Physical examination discloses no evidence of systemic or pulmonary venous congestion, and jugular venous pressure is normal. A thrill may be palpable at the left sternal border. Auscultation reveals normal S_1 and S_2 without gallops. A grade 4 or louder, widely radiating, high-frequency, pansystolic murmur is heard maximally in the third or fourth intercostal space and reflects the high-pressure gradient between the left and right ventricles throughout systole. The striking contrast between a loud murmur and an otherwise normal cardiac examination is an important diagnostic clue. The ECG and chest radiograph are also normal in patients with small VSDs.

At the other end of the spectrum are patients with Eisenmenger's complex (see earlier). Between these two extremes are patients with a moderate defect, whose pathology reflects a combination of pulmonary hypertension and left-sided volume overload resulting from a significant left-to-right shunt. In adults, shortness of breath on exertion can be the result of both pulmonary venous congestion and elevated pulmonary pressure. On physical examination, a diffuse palpable left ventricular impulse occurs with a variable degree of right ventricular hypertrophy and an accentuated second heart sound. A systolic murmur persists as long as pulmonary vascular resistance is below systemic resistance. The ECG commonly shows left atrial enlargement and left ventricular hypertrophy. The chest radiograph shows shunt vascularity with an enlarged left atrium and ventricle. The degree of pulmonary hypertension determines the size of the pulmonary artery trunk.

Echocardiography can identify the defect and determine the significance of the shunt by assessing left atrial and ventricular size, pulmonary artery pressure, and the presence or absence of right ventricular hypertrophy. Cardiac catheterization is reserved for those in whom surgery is considered. Adults with a small defect of no physiologic significance need not be studied invasively. Those with Eisenmenger's complex have severe pulmonary vascular disease and are not surgical candidates. Patients who have a moderately sized shunt that appears hemodynamically significant and in whom pulmo-

nary pressures are elevated are most likely to benefit from direct measurements of pulmonary vascular resistance and reactivity.

TREATMENT

Patients with Eisenmenger's complex have pulmonary vascular resistance that is prohibitive to surgery. For this group of patients, management centers on the medical complications of cyanosis (see earlier). In a few patients with small defects, complications can relate to progressive tricuspid insufficiency caused by septal aneurysm formation or to acquired aortic insufficiency when an aortic cusp becomes engaged in the high-velocity jet flow generated by the defect. The intermediate group of patients with a defect of moderate physiologic significance should have surgical closure unless it is contraindicated by high pulmonary vascular resistance.

Late results after operative closure of isolated VSDs include residual patency in up to 20% of patients, only about 5% of whom need a reoperation. Rhythm disturbances after surgical closure of VSDs include tachyarrhythmias and conduction disturbances. Right bundle branch block occurs in one third to two thirds of patients, whereas first-degree atrioventricular block and complete heart block occur in less than 10%. Sudden cardiac death after surgical repair of VSD occurs in 2% of patients.

Patent Ductus Arteriosus

The ductus arteriosus connects the descending aorta to the main pulmonary trunk near the origin of the left subclavian artery (Fig. 69-6). Normal postnatal closure results in fibrosis and degenerative changes in the ductal lumen, leaving in its place the residual ligamentum arteriosum, which rarely can become part of an abnormal vascular ring. When the duct persists, significant calcification of the aortic ductal end is observed.

The physiologic consequences of a PDA are determined by its size and length as well as by the ratio of pressure and resistance of the pulmonary and aortic circulations on either end of the duct. If systolic and diastolic pressure in the aorta exceeds that in the pulmonary artery, aortic blood flows continuously down a pressure gradient into the pulmonary artery and then returns to the left atrium. The left atrium and subsequently the left ventricle dilate, whereas the right side of the heart becomes progressively affected as pulmonary hypertension develops.

A small PDA has continuous flow throughout the entire cardiac cycle without left-sided heart dilation, pulmonary hypertension, or symptoms. Patients with a small PDA, although protected from hemodynamic complications of a significant left-to-right shunt, remain at risk for infectious endarteritis, which usually develops on the pulmonary side of the duct and occurs at a rate of about 0.45% per year after the second decade. Because endarteritis accounts for up to one third of the total mortality in patients with PDA, ductal closure should be considered even when the PDA is small.

FIGURE 69-6. Anatomy of a patent ductus arteriosus. Note the relationships among the position of the ductus, left subclavian artery, and pulmonary artery bifurcation. Ao = aorta; BCA = brachiocephalic; CCA = common carotid artery; LPA = left pulmonary artery; PDA = patent ductus arteriosus; PT = pulmonary trunk; RPA = right pulmonary artery; SCA = subclavian artery. (From Perloff JK, ed. Clinical Recognition of Congenital Heart Disease, 4th ed. Philadelphia: WB Saunders; 1994:510.)

A PDA is of moderate or large size but still restrictive when a left-to-right shunt occurs throughout systole and diastole is of variable duration. Left atrial or ventricular dilation and pulmonary hypertension will vary with the quantity of left-to-right shunting as well as with the secondary effects on the pulmonary vascular bed. Symptoms generally increase by the second and third decades and include dyspnea, palpitations, and exercise intolerance. As heart failure, pulmonary hypertension, or endarteritis develops, mortality rises to 3 to 4% per year by the fourth decade, and two thirds of patients die by 60 years of age. Eisenmenger's physiology with systemic or suprasystemic pulmonary pressure and a right-to-left shunt develops in 5% of patients with an isolated PDA.

DIAGNOSIS

In patients with Eisenmenger's physiology, a right-to-left shunt from the pulmonary artery to the descending aorta results in decreased oxygen saturation in the lower extremities compared with the upper extremities. This difference in cyanosis and clubbing is most prominent in the toes; the left arm is variably affected through the left subclavian artery, and the right arm is typically spared. With a large left-to-right shunt, the pulse pressure widens as diastolic flow into the pulmonary artery lowers systemic diastolic pressure. The arterial pulse becomes bounding as a result of increased stroke volume. Precordial palpation discloses variable left and right ventricular impulses as determined by the relative degree of left-sided volume overload and pulmonary hypertension. In the presence of a continuous aortopulmonary gradient, the classic "machinery" murmur of a PDA can be heard at the first or second left intercostal space below the left clavicle. As the pulmonary pressure rises, the diastolic component of the murmur becomes progressively shorter. With the development of Eisenmenger's physiology and equalization of aortic and pulmonary pressure, the entire murmur may disappear, and the clinical findings are dominated by pulmonary hypertension.

In adult patients with a significant left-to-right shunt, the ECG shows a bifid P wave in at least one limb lead consistent with left atrial enlargement and a variable degree of left ventricular hypertrophy. The PR interval is prolonged in about 20% of patients. In older patients, the chest radiograph shows calcification at the location of the PDA. Characteristically, the ascending aorta and pulmonary artery are dilated, and the left-sided chambers are enlarged. Echocardiography may not directly visualize the PDA but can accurately identify it by a Doppler signal that often parallels the length of the murmur. Left-sided heart dilation and pulmonary hypertension can be quantified and monitored. Cardiac catheterization to assess pulmonary vascular resistance is commonly indicated before closure.

TREATMENT (Rx)

After ligation of a PDA in infancy or early childhood, cardiac function is commonly normal, and no special follow-up is required. If pulmonary artery pressure and pulmonary vascular resistance are substantially elevated, preoperative evaluation should assess the degree of reversibility. With Eisenmenger's disease, closure is contraindicated. Closure of a PDA either percutaneously or surgically is indicated in the presence of left heart enlargement or if prior endarteritis has occurred. Reported operative mortality rates vary from less than 1 to 8%, depending on the presence of calcification and the degree of pulmonary hypertension. Transcatheter or coil occlusion is an accepted procedure in adults. Residual shunt rates vary from 0.5 to 8%, depending on the device used. Small residual defects that are detected by echocardiography but are not associated with an audible murmur or hemodynamic findings do not appear to carry a significant risk for endarteritis.

Aortopulmonary Window

An aortopulmonary window is typically a large defect across the adjacent segments of both great vessels above their respective valves and below the pulmonary artery bifurcation. The pathophysiology is similar to that of a PDA. The shunt is usually large, so pulmonary vascular resistance rises rapidly and abolishes the aortopulmonary gradient in diastole. The murmur is usually best heard at the third left intercostal space. With a right-to-left shunt, differential cyanosis never occurs because the shunt is proximal to the brachiocephalic vessels. Differentiation of an aortopulmonary window from a PDA can usually be confirmed with echocardiography; the left-to-right shunt is seen in the main pulmonary artery in the aortopulmonary window compared with the left pulmonary artery bifurcation in PDA. Cardiac cath-eterization confirms the diagnosis and hemodynamics. Surgical repair is necessary unless pulmonary vascular obstructive disease precludes closure.

Pulmonary Arteriovenous Fistulas

Pulmonary arteriovenous fistulas can occur as isolated congenital disorders or as part of generalized hereditary hemorrhagic telangiectasia (Osler-Weber-Rendu syndrome). These fistulas typically occur in the lower lobes or the right middle lobe and can be small or large, single or multiple. The arterial supply usually comes from a dilated, tortuous branch of the pulmonary artery.

The most common finding is that of abnormal opacity on a chest radiograph in a patient with buccal ruby patches or in an otherwise healthy adult who has mild cyanosis. Shunting between deoxygenated pulmonary arterial blood and the oxygenated pulmonary venous blood results in a physiologic right-to-left shunt. The degree of shunting is typically small and not significant enough to result in dilation of the left atrium and ventricle. Heart failure is unusual. Hemoptysis can result if a fistula ruptures into a bronchus. In patients with hereditary hemorrhagic telangiectasia, angiomas occur on the lips and mouth as well as in the gastrointestinal tract and on pleural, liver, and vaginal surfaces. Epistaxis is most common, but cerebrovascular accidents can also occur. Patients with hereditary hemorrhagic telangiectasia can have symptoms that resemble those of a transient ischemic attack even in the absence of right-to-left shunting. On physical examination, cyanosis and clubbing can be notable or barely detectable. Auscultation can disclose soft systolic or continuous noncardiac murmurs on the chest wall adjacent to the fistula. The murmur typically increases with inspiration. The ECG is usually normal. The chest radiograph shows one or more densities, typically in the lower lobes or in the right middle lobe. An echocardiogram can confirm the presence of the fistula by showing early opacification of the left atrium in the absence of any other intracardiac communication when saline is injected into a peripheral vein. The absence of a hemodynamically significant shunt can be confirmed by documenting normal cardiac chamber size.

If the hypoxemia is progressive or if a neurologic complication is documented to have occurred because of paradoxical emboli, fistula closure should be considered. Options include percutaneous catheter techniques if the fistula is small and accessible or a pulmonary wedge resection or lobectomy if the fistula is large. Multiple or recurrent fistulas create a major therapeutic challenge.

Isolated Obstructive Lesions of the Right and Left Ventricular Outflow Tract

Complications of obstructive lesions of the outflow tract relate to the secondary effects of exposure to pressure overload in the chamber proximal to the obstruction. The inability to increase systemic or pulmonary blood flow in the face of a fixed obstruction can cause exercise intolerance, inadequate myocardial perfusion, ventricular arrhythmias, and sudden death.

RIGHT VENTRICULAR OUTFLOW TRACT OBSTRUCTION

Obstruction of the right ventricular outflow tract can occur at the level of the pulmonary valve (see later), above it in the main pulmonary artery or its branches, or below it in the right ventricle itself. Supravalvular and branch pulmonary artery stenoses are important and common complications in patients with tetralogy of Fallot (see later). Residual supravalvar pulmonary stenosis is sometimes seen after palliative pulmonary artery banding to decrease pulmonary blood flow in patients with large left-to-right shunts. Congenital branch pulmonary artery stenosis can occur in isolation or with valvar pulmonary stenosis, shunt lesions, or a variety of syndromes. Patients with Noonan's syndrome have a characteristic phenotypic facial appearance, short stature, and webbed neck; cardiac lesions may include a dysplastic pulmonary valve, left ventricular hypertrophic cardiomyopathy, and peripheral pulmonary artery stenosis. Supravalvular pulmonary stenosis can be seen with supravalvular aortic stenosis in Williams (elfin facies) syndrome.

Pulmonary atresia refers to an absent, imperforate, or closed pulmonary valve, which typically occurs in conjunction with other malformations. Pulmonary atresia with a nonrestrictive VSD is a complex cyanotic malformation that is discussed later.

Primary infundibular stenosis with an intact ventricular septum can result from a fibrous band just below the infundibulum. In a double-chambered right ventricle, obstruction is caused by anomalous muscle bundles that divide the right ventricle into a high-pressure chamber below the hypertrophied muscle bundles and a low-pressure chamber above the bundles and below the valve. The clinical features vary according to the presence or absence of other lesions, such as pulmonary valvular stenosis or VSD.

VALVULAR PULMONARY STENOSIS

Isolated congenital valvular pulmonary stenosis (Chapter 75) is a common lesion due to a bicuspid valve in 20% of cases, a dysplastic valve caused by myxomatous changes and severe thickening in 10% of cases, and an abnormal trileaflet valve in most of the remaining cases. Fusion of the leaflets results in a variable degree of thickening and calcification in older patients.

The 25-year survival of patients with valvular pulmonary stenosis is greater than 95% but is worse in those with severe stenosis and peak systolic gradients greater than 80 mm Hg. For patients with mild (<50 mm Hg gradients) and moderate (50 to 80 mm Hg gradients) pulmonary stenosis, bacterial endocarditis, complex ventricular arrhythmias, and progression of the stenosis are uncommon.

DIAGNOSIS

A patient with moderate or even severe pulmonary stenosis may be asymptomatic. With severe stenosis, exercise intolerance can be associated with presyncope and ventricular arrhythmias. Progressive right-sided heart failure is the most common cause of death. On physical examination of patients with significant pulmonary stenosis, jugular venous pressure has a dominant a wave, reflecting a noncompliant right ventricle. Palpation discloses a sustained parasternal lift of right ventricular hypertrophy. An expiratory systolic ejection click is characteristic if the leaflets are still mobile. In moderate or severe stenosis, a grade 3 or louder systolic murmur can be heard and felt in the second left interspace. The length of the murmur increases as it peaks progressively later in systole with an increasing degree of obstruction. If right-sided heart failure occurs, tricuspid insufficiency and systemic venous congestion develop. The ECG can show right axis deviation and tall, peaked right atrial P waves in lead II. With more than mild stenosis, the R wave exceeds the S wave in lead V_1. On chest radiography, the main pulmonary artery can be dilated even if the stenosis is mild. Characteristically, the left pulmonary artery is more dilated than the right because of the leftward direction of the high-velocity jet. A variable degree of right ventricular hypertrophy is manifested as right-sided chamber enlargement. Echocardiography can establish the diagnosis and determine the severity by Doppler ultrasound examination. Patients with valvar pulmonary stenosis do not require cardiac catheterization. The mean gradient at echocardiography correlates well with the gradient measured at cardiac catheterization and should be used for therapeutic decisions because peak instantaneous Doppler gradients tend to overestimate the severity of disease.

TREATMENT Rx

Depending on symptoms, percutaneous balloon valvotomy should be considered for patients with isolated valvar pulmonary stenosis and mean Doppler gradients of 30 mm Hg or greater unless there is moderate or severe pulmonary regurgitation. In the presence of a doming valve, pulmonary angioplasty is the procedure of choice for adults, who achieve persistently good results at 10-year follow-up. For patients with hypoplastic pulmonary arteries or subvalvular stenosis (double-chambered right ventricle), surgical resection of right ventricular muscle bands can be performed.

LEFT VENTRICULAR OUTFLOW TRACT OBSTRUCTION

Stenosis of the left ventricular outflow tract can occur at, below, or above the aortic valve. Discrete subaortic stenosis, most commonly caused by a fibromuscular ring just below the valve, accounts for 15 to 20% of all cases of congenital obstruction of the left ventricular outflow tract. Concomitant aortic insufficiency occurs in 50% of cases. Supravalvular aortic stenosis results from thickened media and intima above the aortic sinuses; early coronary atherosclerosis or even ostial coronary obstruction can occur.

CONGENITAL VALVULAR AORTIC STENOSIS

The normal aortic valve has three cusps and commissures. A unicuspid aortic valve accounts for most cases of severe aortic stenosis in infants (Chapter 75). A bicuspid aortic valve, which is the most common congenital cardiac malformation, functions normally at birth but often becomes gradually obstructed as calcific and fibrous changes occur; prolapse of one or both cusps can cause aortic insufficiency.

The pathophysiology of aortic stenosis depends not only on its severity but also on the age at diagnosis. When a bicuspid aortic valve becomes stenotic in adulthood because of degenerative changes, criteria for diagnosis and intervention parallel those for other forms of acquired aortic stenosis (Chapter 75). The estimated overall 25-year survival rate for patients with

congenital valvular aortic stenosis diagnosed in childhood is 85%. Children with initial peak cardiac catheterization gradients of less than 50 mm Hg have long-term survival rates of higher than 90%, as opposed to survival rates of 80% in those with gradients of 50 mm Hg or greater.

DIAGNOSIS

Symptoms include angina, exertional dyspnea, presyncope, and syncope and may progress to heart failure. The auscultatory hallmark of a bicuspid aortic valve is an audible systolic ejection click that is typically of a higher pitch than the first heart sound and is best heard not at the cardiac base but at the apex. The sound is caused by sudden movement of the stenotic valve as it moves superiorly in systole and is followed by the typical aortic stenosis murmur (Chapter 75). When significant calcification of the valve results in reduced mobility, the ejection sound is no longer heard. The diagnosis is easily confirmed by two-dimensional echocardiography, with which the number and orientation of aortic cusps can readily be identified.

TREATMENT Rx

Conservative management is generally indicated for mild stenosis with a peak gradient of less than 25 mm Hg, but close supervision is required because 20% of these patients require an intervention during long-term follow-up. Unlimited athletic participation is allowed only for asymptomatic patients with peak gradients of less than 20 to 25 mm Hg, a normal ECG, and a normal exercise test. For children who are symptomatic or have gradients greater than 30 mm Hg but do not have significant aortic insufficiency, transcatheter aortic valvotomy is preferred. Aortic valvuloplasty can be considered in young adults, but calcification limits its success, and valve replacement is usually required (Chapter 75). For adults, treatment decisions are similar to those for aortic stenosis from other causes. For patients with subvalvular aortic stenosis, surgical intervention is indicated in the presence of peak gradients above 50 mm Hg, symptoms, or progressive aortic insufficiency.

COARCTATION OF THE AORTA

Aortic coarctation typically occurs just distal to the left subclavian artery at the site of the aortic ductal attachment or its residual ligamentum arteriosum. Less commonly, the coarctation ridge lies proximal to the left subclavian. A bicuspid aortic valve is the most common coexisting anomaly, but VSDs and PDAs are also seen. Pseudocoarctation refers to buckling or kinking of the aortic arch without the presence of a significant gradient.

The most common complications of aortic coarctation are systemic hypertension (Chapter 67) and secondary left ventricular hypertrophy with heart failure. Systemic hypertension is caused by decreased vascular compliance in the proximal aorta and activation of the renin-angiotensin system in response to renal artery hypoperfusion below the obstruction. Left ventricular hypertrophy occurs in response to chronic pressure overload. Congestive heart failure occurs most commonly in infants and then after 40 years of age. The high pressure proximal to the obstruction stimulates the growth of collateral vessels from the internal mammary, scapular, and superior intercostal arteries to the intercostals of the descending aorta. Collateral circulation increases with age and contributes to perfusion of the lower extremities and the spinal cord. This mechanism, although adaptive in a patient who has not undergone surgery, accounts for significant morbidity during surgery when the motor impairment results from inadequate protection of spinal perfusion. Aneurysms occur most notably in the ascending aorta and in the circle of Willis. Premature coronary disease is thought to be related to the resulting hypertension. Complications, including bacterial endarteritis at the coarctation site or, more commonly, endocarditis at the site of a bicuspid aortic valve, cerebrovascular complications, myocardial infarction, heart failure, and aortic dissection, occur in 2 to 6% of patients, more frequently in those with advancing age who have not undergone surgery.

DIAGNOSIS

Young adults may be asymptomatic with incidental systemic hypertension and decreased lower extremity pulses. Coarctation should always be considered in adolescents and young adult men with unexplained upper extremity hypertension. The pressure differential can cause epistaxis, headaches, leg fatigue, or claudication. Older patients have angina, symptoms of heart failure, and vascular complications.

On physical examination, the lower half of the body is typically slightly less developed than the upper half. The hips are narrow and the legs are short, in contrast to broad shoulders and long arms. Blood pressure measurements

FIGURE 69-7. Chest radiograph of a patient with coarctation of the aorta. The radiographic *3* formed by the dilated subclavian artery above and the dilated aorta below (*short arrow*) is shown. Note the notching, best seen at the level of the seventh and eighth ribs (*long arrows*). The dilated ascending aortic segment can also be seen.

should be obtained in each arm and one leg; an abnormal measurement is an increase of less than 10 mm Hg in popliteal systolic blood pressure compared with arm systolic blood pressure. The diastolic pressure should be the same in the upper and lower extremities. A pressure differential of more than 30 mm Hg between the right and the left arms is consistent with compromised flow in the left subclavian artery. Right brachial palpation characteristically reveals a strong or even bounding pulse compared with a slowly rising or absent femoral, popliteal, or pedal pulse. Examination of the eyegrounds can reveal tortuous or corkscrew retinal arteries. Precordial palpation is consistent with left ventricular pressure overload. On auscultation, a systolic ejection sound reflecting the presence of a bicuspid aortic valve should be sought. The coarctation itself generates a systolic murmur heard posteriorly, in the midthoracic region, the length of which correlates with the severity of the coarctation. Over the anterior of the chest, systolic murmurs reflecting increased collateral flow can be heard in the infraclavicular areas and the sternal edge or in the axillae.

In adult coarctation, the most common finding on the ECG is left ventricular hypertrophy. Chest radiographic findings are diagnostic. Location of the coarctation segment between the dilated left subclavian artery above and the leftward convexity of the descending aorta below results in the "3 sign" (Fig. 69-7). Bilateral rib notching as a result of dilation of the posterior intercostal arteries is seen on the posterior of the third to eighth ribs when the coarctation is below the left subclavian. Unilateral rib notching sparing the left ribs is observed when the coarctation occurs proximal to the left subclavian artery. Transthoracic echocardiography documents the gradient in the descending aorta and determines the presence of left ventricular hypertrophy. Magnetic resonance imaging (Chapter 56) is the best modality for visualizing the anatomy of the descending aorta. Cardiac catheterization should measure pressures and assess collaterals when surgery is contemplated.

TREATMENT **Rx**

Intervention is recommended in patients who have gradients of 20 mm Hg or more on cardiac catheterization (Chapter 57) or who have evidence of significant collateral flow on imaging studies. The choice between catheter interventional and surgical intervention, which should be made in conjunction with a specialist, depends on the associated anomalies and the anatomy of the coarctation segment. Fifty percent of patients repaired when they are older than 40 years have residual hypertension, whereas those who have undergone surgery between the ages of 1 and 5 years have a less than 10% prevalence of hypertension on long-term follow-up. Balloon angioplasty is the treatment of choice for focal recoarctation in patients who have previously been operated on. The incidence of incomplete relief and restenosis is decreased in adults by endovascular stent placement. Focal complications include aortic aneurysms and, rarely, aortic rupture.

Anomalies of the Sinuses of Valsalva and Coronary Arteries
SINUS OF VALSALVA ANEURYSMS
At the base of the aortic root, the aortic valve cusps are attached to the aortic wall, above which three small pouches, or sinuses, are seated. The right coronary artery originates from one sinus and the left main coronary artery from a second; the third is called the *noncoronary sinus.* A weakness in the wall of the sinus can result in aneurysm formation with or without rupture. In more than 90% of cases, the aneurysm involves the right or noncoronary cusp. Rupture typically occurs into the right side of the heart at the right atrial or ventricular level with a resulting large left-to-right shunt driven by the high aortic pressure.

A previously asymptomatic young man typically has chest pain and rapidly progressing shortness of breath sometimes after physical strain. The physical examination is consistent with significant heart failure. Even if the communication is between the aorta and the right side of the heart, biventricular failure is not unusual. The classic murmur is loud and continuous, often with a thrill. A murmur of aortic insufficiency secondary to damage to the adjacent aortic valve may be superimposed. The chest radiograph shows volume overload of both ventricles with evidence of shunt vascularity and pulmonary venous congestion. The echocardiogram is diagnostic. Cardiac catheterization can verify the integrity of the coronary artery adjacent to the ruptured aneurysm.

Even though symptoms may abate as the heart dilates, progressive cardiac decompensation typically results in death within 1 year of the rupture. A ruptured sinus of Valsalva aneurysm therefore requires urgent surgical repair.

CORONARY ARTERY FISTULAS
Fistulas arise from the right or left coronary arteries and in 90% of cases drain into the right ventricle, the right atrium, or the pulmonary artery in order of decreasing frequency. Typically, young patients are asymptomatic, but supraventricular arrhythmias are seen with progressive dilation of the intracardiac chambers. Angina can occur as the fistula creates a coronary steal by diverting blood away from the myocardium. Heart failure is seen with large fistulas. A continuous murmur heard in a young, otherwise normal acyanotic, asymptomatic patient should suggest the diagnosis. Most fistulas are associated with a small shunt, and hence the murmur is often less than grade 3 and is heard in the precordial area. Unless the shunt is large, the ECG is normal, as is the chest radiograph. The echocardiogram, especially the transesophageal echocardiogram, is diagnostic. Percutaneous transcatheter closure with coil embolization is preferred, but surgical ligation is also an alternative.

ANOMALOUS ORIGIN OF THE CORONARY ARTERIES
The left main coronary artery normally arises from the left sinus of Valsalva and courses leftward, posterior to the right ventricular outflow tract. The right coronary artery arises from the right sinus of Valsalva and courses rightward to the right ventricle. Isolated ectopic or anomalous origins of the coronary arteries (see Fig. 57-8 in Chapter 57) are seen in 0.6 to 1.5% of patients undergoing coronary angiography.

The most common anomaly is ectopic origin of the left circumflex artery from the right sinus of Valsalva, followed by anomalous origin of the right coronary artery from the left sinus and anomalous origin of the left main coronary artery from the right sinus. If the anomalous coronary artery does not course between the pulmonary artery and aorta, the prognosis is favorable. Risks of ischemia, myocardial infarction, and death are greatest when the left main coronary artery courses between both great vessels.

Coronary arteries can also originate from the pulmonary trunk. If both the right and left arteries originate from the pulmonary trunk, death usually occurs in the neonatal period. If only the left anterior descending coronary artery originates from the pulmonary trunk, the rate of survival to adulthood is approximately 10%, depending on the development of collateral retrograde flow to the anomalous artery from a normal coronary artery. This collateral flow may cause a continuous murmur along the left sternal border, congestive heart failure from the large shunt, and a coronary steal syndrome as blood is diverted away from the normal artery.

A single coronary ostium can provide a single coronary artery that branches into right and left coronary arteries, the left then giving rise to the circumflex and the anterior descending arteries. The ostium can originate from the right or left aortic sinus. The coronary circulation is functionally normal unless one of the branches passes between the aorta and the pulmonary artery.

Diagnostic procedures include angiography, magnetic resonance imaging, and transesophageal echocardiography. For an anomalous coronary artery that originates from the pulmonary artery, surgical reimplantation into the aorta is preferred. For an anomalous artery that courses between the pulmonary artery and aorta, a bypass graft to the distal vessel is preferred.

● SPECIFIC COMPLEX LESIONS
Tetralogy of Fallot

Tetralogy of Fallot, the most common cyanotic malformation, is characterized by superior and anterior displacement of the subpulmonary infundibular septum, which causes the tetrad of pulmonary stenosis, VSD, aortic override, and right ventricular hypertrophy. The VSD is perimembranous in 80% of cases. Additional cardiac anomalies include a right-sided aortic arch in up to 25% of patients. An anomalous left anterior descending artery originating from the right coronary cusp and crossing over the right ventricular outflow tract is seen in 10% of cases. Other associated anomalies include ASD, left superior vena cava, defects of the atrioventricular canal, and aortic insufficiency. With pulmonary atresia, pulmonary blood flow occurs through aortic to pulmonary collaterals. Life expectancy is limited unless staged reconstructive surgery is performed.

The physiology in unrepaired tetralogy of Fallot is determined by the severity and location of the pulmonic outflow obstruction and by the interaction of pulmonary and systemic vascular resistance across a nonrestrictive VSD. Because the pulmonary stenosis results in a relatively fixed pulmonary resistance, a drop in systemic vascular resistance as occurs with exercise is associated with increased right-to-left shunting and increasing cyanosis. A child who squats after running is attempting to reverse the process by increasing systemic vascular resistance by crouching with bent knees. Native pulmonary blood flow is typically insufficient. Unless a PDA has remained open, a cyanotic adult will typically have undergone a palliative procedure to increase pulmonary blood flow.

Examination of unrepaired patients reveals central cyanosis and clubbing. The right ventricular impulse is prominent. The second heart sound is single and represents the aortic closure sound with an absent or inconspicuous P_2. Typically, little or no systolic murmur is heard across the pulmonary valve because the more severe the obstruction, the more right-to-left shunting occurs and the less blood flows across a diminutive right ventricular outflow tract. A diastolic murmur of aortic insufficiency is often heard in adults. In the presence of a palliative systemic arterial to pulmonary artery shunt, the high-pressure gradient generates a loud continuous murmur. In a patient who has not undergone surgery, progressive infundibular stenosis and cyanosis occur. Before the advent of palliative surgery, mortality rates were 50% in the first few years of life, and survival past the third decade was unusual.

Complete surgical repair consists of patch closure of the VSD and relief of the right ventricular outflow tract obstruction. Adequate pulmonary blood flow is ensured by reconstruction of the distal pulmonary artery bed. Previous palliative shunts are usually taken down. Complete repair in childhood yields a 90 to 95% 10-year survival rate with good functional results, and 30-year survival rates may be as high as 85%. Total correction with low mortality and a favorable long-term follow-up is possible even in adulthood.

After repair, residual pulmonary stenosis, proximal or distal, with a right ventricular pressure greater than 50% of systemic occurs in up to 25% of patients. Some degree of pulmonary insufficiency is common, particularly if a patch has been inserted at the level of the pulmonary valve or if a pulmonary valvotomy has been performed. Residual VSDs can be found in up to 20% of patients. Patients may be asymptomatic or may have symptoms related to long-term complications after surgical repair. Symptoms can reflect residual right ventricular pressure or volume overload or arrhythmias at rest or with exercise. Angina can occur in a young patient if surgical repair has damaged an anomalous left anterior descending artery as it courses across the right ventricular outflow tract. In acyanotic adults, clubbing commonly regresses. A right ventricular impulse is often felt as a result of residual pulmonary insufficiency or stenosis. Typically, no functioning pulmonary valve is present, and hence the second heart sound is still single. A systolic murmur can represent residual pulmonary stenosis, residual VSD, or tricuspid insufficiency. A diastolic murmur can reflect aortic or pulmonary insufficiency. Ventricular arrhythmias are common after repair, with an incidence of sudden death as high as 5%.

The ECG in unrepaired tetralogy of Fallot shows right axis deviation, right atrial enlargement, and dominant right ventricular forces over the precordial leads. The most common finding after repair is complete right bundle branch block, which is seen in 80 to 90% of patients. The chest radiograph typically

FIGURE 69-8. Chest radiograph of an adult after tetralogy of Fallot repair. A right aortic arch with rightward indentation of the trachea *(long arrow)* can be seen. The right ventricular apex remains upturned *(short arrow)*. Note the sternal wires consistent with intracardiac repair, clarifying the fullness of the pulmonary artery segment often seen after extensive enlargement of the right ventricular outflow tract.

shows an upturned apex with a concave pulmonary artery segment giving the classic appearance of a boot-shaped heart. Figure 69-8 demonstrates the findings in an adult after repair. The apex is persistently upturned, although the pulmonary artery segment is no longer concave. Echocardiography can confirm the diagnosis and document intracardiac complications in repaired and unrepaired patients. Shunt patency can be determined by Doppler examination. Magnetic resonance imaging can accurately document stenosis in the distal pulmonary artery bed. Cardiac catheterization is reserved for patients in whom operative or reoperative treatment is contemplated or in whom the integrity of the coronary circulation needs to be verified.

Patients with a change in exercise tolerance, angina, or evidence of heart failure and those with symptomatic arrhythmias or syncope should be referred for complete evaluation. Surgical reintervention is generally considered when right ventricular pressure is more than two thirds as high as systemic pressure because of residual right ventricular outflow tract obstruction, free pulmonary regurgitation occurs with right ventricular dysfunction or sustained arrhythmias, or a residual VSD causes a significant shunt.

Complete Transposition of the Great Arteries

Complete transposition of the great arteries is the second most common cyanotic lesion, and surgically corrected adults are increasingly common. In simple transposition of the great arteries, the atria and ventricles are in their normal positions, but the aorta arises from the right ventricle, and the pulmonary artery arises from the left ventricle. When the aorta is anterior and rightward with respect to the pulmonary artery, as is most common, D-transposition is present. The native anatomy has the pulmonary and systemic circulations in parallel, with deoxygenated blood recirculating between the right side of the heart and the systemic circulation, whereas oxygenated blood recirculates from the left side of the heart to the lungs. The condition is incompatible with life unless a VSD, PDA, or ASD is present or an ASD is created; a hemodynamically significant VSD is present in 15% of cases. Subpulmonary obstruction of the left ventricular outflow tract occurs in 10 to 25% of cases.

The Senning or Mustard atrial baffle repairs, which were the first corrective procedures, redirect oxygenated blood from the left atrium to the right ventricle so that it may be ejected into the aorta while deoxygenated blood detours the right atrium and heads for the left ventricle and into the pulmonary artery. Although this operation results in acyanotic physiology, the right ventricle assumes a permanent position under the aorta and pumps against systemic pressures, a lifelong task for which it was not designed. When the subpulmonary obstruction is significant, the Rastelli procedure reroutes blood at the ventricular level by tunneling the left ventricle to the aorta inside the heart through a VSD. A conduit is then inserted outside the heart between the left ventricle and aorta. More recently, the arterial switch operation transects the aorta and pulmonary artery above their respective valves and switches them to become realigned with their physiologic outflow tracts and appropriate ventricles. The proximal coronary arteries are translocated from the sinuses of the native aorta to the neoaorta (native pulmonary artery). In this operation, each ventricle reassumes the role that it was embryologically destined to fulfill.

If an adult patient is cyanotic and has a native intracardiac shunt or a palliative shunt, referral to an appropriate facility should be undertaken to explore the possibility of intracardiac repair. At present, adults with transposition of the great arteries most commonly have undergone an atrial baffle repair, with an expected 15-year survival rate of 75% and a 20-year survival rate of 70%. For patients with an atrial baffle procedure, symptoms include exercise intolerance, palpitations caused by bradyarrhythmias or atrial flutter, and right ventricular failure. The patient is typically acyanotic unless a baffle leak exists. The clinical findings are determined by the presence or absence of systemic right ventricular failure. On auscultation, the second heart sound is classically single. The ECG reveals sinus bradycardia, but nodal rhythms and heart block occur as the patient ages. The chest radiograph shows a variable degree of right ventricular enlargement. Echocardiography can be used to confirm the diagnosis and to explore related abnormalities. Cardiac catheterization is performed when an operation or reoperation is contemplated. Reoperation is performed in approximately 20% of patients for baffle-related complications, progressive left ventricular outflow tract stenosis, or severe tricuspid regurgitation.

Congenitally Corrected Transposition of the Great Arteries

In congenitally corrected transposition of the great arteries, the great arteries are transposed, the ventricles are inverted, but the atria remain in their normal position. The systemic circulation (left atrium, morphologic right ventricle, and aorta) and pulmonary circulation (right atrium, morphologic left ventricle, and pulmonary artery) are in series. The patient is therefore acyanotic unless an intracardiac shunt is also present. The right ventricle is aligned with the aorta and performs lifelong systemic work, which accounts in part for its eventual failure. Associated lesions include a VSD, pulmonary stenosis, and Ebstein's malformation of the left-sided tricuspid valve. Complete heart block develops at a rate of 2% per year. Patients with congenitally corrected transposition of the great arteries and no other associated defects can remain free of symptoms until the sixth decade, at which time significant atrioventricular valve regurgitation, failure of the right (systemic) ventricle, supraventricular arrhythmias, and heart block occur.

Right-Sided Ebstein's Anomaly

The septal and posterior cusps of the tricuspid valve are largely derived from the right ventricle as it liberates a layer of muscle that skirts away from the cavity to become valve tissue. When this process occurs abnormally, the posterior and septal cusps of the tricuspid valve remain tethered to the muscle and adhere to the right ventricular surface—hence the diagnostic hallmark of Ebstein's anomaly, apical displacement of the septal tricuspid leaflet.

In right-sided Ebstein's anomaly of the tricuspid valve, the right side of the heart consists of three anatomic components: the right atrium proper, the true right ventricle, and the atrialized portion of the right ventricle between the two. The displaced septal and posterior tricuspid leaflets lie between the atrialized right ventricle and the true right ventricle. In mild Ebstein's anomaly, the degree of tricuspid leaflet tethering is only mild, the anterior leaflet retains mobility, and the size of the true right ventricle is only mildly reduced. Severe Ebstein's anomaly is associated with severe tethering of the tricuspid leaflet tissue and a diminutive, hypocontractile true right ventricle. Functionally, the valve is regurgitant because it is unable to appose its three leaflets during ventricular contraction. Valvular regurgitation and asynchronous, abnormal right ventricular function cause the dilation and right-sided heart failure observed in the more severe forms of the lesion. The wide spectrum of severity of the anomaly is based on the degree of tricuspid leaflet tethering and the relative proportion of atrialized and true right ventricle. The most common associated cardiac defect, a secundum ASD or patent foramen ovale, is reported in more than 50% of patients. On physical examination, a clicking "sail sound" is heard as the second component of S_1 when tricuspid valve closure becomes loud and delayed.

The 12-lead ECG typically shows highly peaked P waves with a wide, often bizarre-looking QRS complex. Preexcitation occurs in 20% of patients; supraventricular tachyarrhythmias, atrial fibrillation, and atrial flutter occur in 30

to 40% of patients and constitute the most common findings in adolescents and adults with right-sided Ebstein's anomaly.

When patients of all ages are taken together, the predicted mortality is approximately 50% by the fourth or fifth decade. Complications include atrial arrhythmias due to severe right atrial enlargement and cyanosis caused by a right-to-left atrial shunt as tricuspid insufficiency increases and the right ventricle fails. Atrial arrhythmias, cyanosis, and the presence of an intra-atrial communication also increase the risk for stroke.

Intervention is considered when functional status or cyanosis worsens, significant atrial arrhythmias are documented, or a cerebrovascular accident occurs. Surgical options include replacement or repair of the tricuspid valve and closure of the ASD. The feasibility of tricuspid valvuloplasty depends on the size and mobility of the anterior tricuspid leaflet, which is used to construct a unicuspid right-sided valve.

Atrioventricular Canal Defect

Embryologic septation of the atrioventricular canal results in closure of the inferior portion of the interatrial septum and the superior portion of the interventricular septum. Septation is achieved with the growth of endocardial cushions, which also contribute to development of the mitral and tricuspid valves. Hence, the nomenclature *atrioventricular canal defect* or *endocardial cushion defect* is used to designate this group of anomalies.

A partial atrioventricular canal defect refers to an ostium primum ASD with a cleft mitral valve. The anomaly is manifested as a hemodynamic combination of an ASD with a variable degree of mitral regurgitation. The 12-lead ECG shows the typical findings of left axis deviation with a Q wave in leads I and aVL and a prolonged PR interval. The echocardiogram shows a defect in the inferior portion of the interatrial septum and a cleft mitral valve.

A complete atrioventricular canal defect is an uncommon defect consisting of a primum ASD, an inlet VSD that usually extends to the membranous interventricular septum, and a common atrioventricular valve. Adults who have not been operated on usually have Eisenmenger's syndrome unless concomitant pulmonary stenosis has protected the pulmonary vascular bed or the VSD has undergone spontaneous closure, in which case the physiologic consequences are similar to those of a partial atrioventricular canal.

Surgical repair of an atrioventricular defect consists of closing the interatrial or interventricular communication with reconstruction of the common atrioventricular valve or closure of the cleft in the mitral valve. An adult who has undergone repair may have significant residual regurgitation of the mitral or tricuspid valve. Even after surgery, acquired subaortic obstruction can occur in the long left ventricular outflow tract, which has a classic gooseneck deformity on cardiac angiography.

Univentricular Heart and Tricuspid Atresia

The terms *single ventricle, common ventricle,* and *univentricular heart* have been used interchangeably to describe the double-inlet ventricle, in which one ventricular chamber receives flow from both the tricuspid and mitral valves. In 75 to 90% of cases, the single ventricle is a morphologic left ventricle. Obstruction of one of the great arteries is common, and life expectancy is short without an operation. The patients most likely to survive to adulthood palliated or, rarely, without surgery have a single ventricle of the left morphologic type, with pulmonary stenosis protecting the pulmonary vascular bed.

In tricuspid atresia, no orifice is found between the right atrium and right ventricle, and an underdeveloped or hypoplastic right ventricle is present. The morphologic left ventricle is consistently normally developed and therefore becomes the single functional ventricle. Typically, blood flows into the right atrium, then through an obligatory ASD and to the left atrium, where it then proceeds to the left ventricle. Variable features include a VSD, the abnormal position of the great arteries, and the relative degree of pulmonary stenosis, all of which are used to classify tricuspid atresia. Without surgery, 50% of patients die in the first 6 months and 90% in the first decade.

Adult patients rarely have not been operated on. They may be acyanotic after the Fontan operation; if cyanotic and palliated, the patient may benefit from further palliation or may be eligible for the Fontan operation. With the Glenn shunt or the Fontan operation, a direct anastomosis is created between the systemic venous and pulmonary circulations. Venous blood flows passively from the systemic veins to the pulmonary circulation and returns oxygenated to a left-sided atrium and into the single functional ventricle, which then pumps oxygenated blood into the systemic circulation. The Glenn anastomosis diverts part of the systemic venous return to the lungs, whereas the Fontan procedure makes the patient acyanotic by diverting the entire systemic venous circulation to the pulmonary vascular bed. For optimal results, a successful Fontan operation requires low pulmonary vascular resistance, preserved single ventricular function, and unobstructed anastomosis between the systemic veins and the pulmonary arteries. At 5-year follow-up, 80% or more of Fontan survivors are in New York Heart Association functional class I or II, with successful pregnancy reported in a small number of patients. When patients of all ages are considered together, 10-year survival rates vary from 60 to 70%. Late deaths are due to reoperation, arrhythmia, ventricular failure, and protein-losing enteropathy.

Vascular Malformations
AORTIC ARCH ANOMALIES
Vascular Rings and Other Arch Anomalies
One of the most frequent developmental errors of the aortic arch is an aberrant right subclavian artery originating distal to the left subclavian and coursing rightward behind the esophagus at the level of the third thoracic vertebrae. Although the finding is frequent, symptoms are uncommon. When symptoms occur, the term *dysphagia lusoria* has been used in reference to swallowing difficulties that result from esophageal compression. Abnormal development of the brachial arches and dorsal aorta can result in a variety of anomalies that lead to the formation of vascular rings around the trachea and esophagus. The outcome is often benign, but symptoms of respiratory compromise or dysphagia warrant surgery. When the left pulmonary artery arises from the right and passes leftward between the trachea and esophagus, a pulmonary artery sling occurs. Symptoms of tracheal compression warrant correction.

A right aortic arch occurs when the aortic arch courses toward the right instead of the left. Mirror-image branching is the most common anatomic variant. In most cases, this anomaly coexists with other congenital lesions, notably tetralogy of Fallot.

ANOMALOUS VENOUS CONNECTIONS
Anomalies of Systemic Venous Return
A persistent left superior vena cava can be fortuitously diagnosed on chest radiography or on echocardiography. Its clinical relevance depends on development of the coronary sinus. If the coronary sinus is normally formed, typically the left superior vena cava drains into the right atrium through the coronary sinus. If the coronary sinus is not normally developed, the persistent left superior vena cava drains into the left atrium, and cyanosis results from the obligatory right-to-left shunt. The latter commonly occurs with an ASD or a complex cardiac anomaly.

Venous return above the renal veins can be abnormal with inferior vena cava interruption and azygos or hemiazygos continuation. In the former, inferior vena cava flow above the renal veins continues into the azygos vein, which courses normally up the right of the spine to empty into the junction between the superior vena cava and right atrium. In a less common anatomic arrangement, the caval flow empties into a hemiazygos vein, which empties into a persistent left superior vena cava. The finding rarely occurs in isolation but can be seen in patients with associated simple or complex malformations.

Anomalies of Pulmonary Venous Return
In partial anomalous pulmonary venous return, one or more, but not all four, pulmonary veins are not connected to the left atrium. The most common pattern has the right pulmonary veins connected to the superior vena cava, usually with a sinus venosus ASD. Anomalous connection of the right pulmonary veins to the inferior vena cava results in a chest radiographic shadow that resembles a Turkish sword, hence the designation *scimitar syndrome*. Associated anomalies include hypoplasia of the right lung, anomalies of the bronchial system, hypoplasia of the right pulmonary artery, and dextroposition of the heart. Partial anomalous pulmonary venous return results in a left-to-right shunt physiology similar to that of an ASD.

In total anomalous pulmonary venous return, all the pulmonary veins connect abnormally to either the right atrium or one of the systemic veins above or below the diaphragm. Concurrent obstruction of the pulmonary veins is present when drainage occurs below the diaphragm and variable when drainage occurs above it. An ASD is essential to sustain life. One third of cases occur with major complex cardiac malformations.

In cor triatriatum, the pulmonary veins drain into an accessory chamber that is usually connected to the left atrium through an opening of variable size. The hemodynamic consequences are determined by the size of this opening and are similar to those of mitral stenosis. If symptoms of pulmonary venous hypertension occur, surgical treatment is indicated.

CARDIAC MALPOSITIONS
The normal heart is left sided and hence the designation *levocardia*. Cardiac malpositions are defined in terms of the intrathoracic position of the heart in relation to the position of the viscera (visceral situs), which are usually concordant with the position of the atria. That is, when the liver is on the right and the stomach is on the left, the atrium receiving systemic venous blood (right atrium) is right sided and the atrium receiving pulmonary venous blood (left atrium) is left sided. Asplenia and polysplenia syndromes are associated with a variety of complex cardiovascular malformations.

Dextrocardia and Mesocardia
In dextrocardia, the heart is on the right side of the thorax with or without situs inversus. When the heart is right sided with inverted atria, the stomach is right sided, and the liver is left sided, the combination is dextrocardia with situs inversus. In this arrangement, also called *mirror-image dextrocardia*, the ventricles are inverted, but so are the viscera and therefore the atria. The heart usually functions normally, and the diagnosis is often fortuitous. The heart sounds are louder on the right side of the chest, and the liver is palpable on the left. The chest radiograph shows a right-sided cardiac apex with a lower left hemidiaphragm and a right-sided stomach bubble. The ECG shows an inverted P and T wave in lead I with a negative QRS deflection and a reverse pattern between aVR and aVL. A mirror-image progression is seen from V_1 to a right-sided V_6 lead. An echocardiogram should be performed to ensure that intracardiac anatomy is normal.

When dextrocardia with situs solitus occurs, the ventricles are inverted but not the viscera and therefore not the atria. Associated severe cardiac malformations are typical.

In mesocardia, the heart is centrally located in the chest with normal atrial and visceral anatomy. The apex is central or rightward displaced on the chest radiograph. Typically, no associated cardiac malformations are present.

SPECIALIZED ISSUES
Endocarditis Prophylaxis
Prolonged survival of patients with complex congenital heart disease has resulted in a population at increased risk for infective endocarditis (Chapter 76). Adults with congenital heart disease should be informed about the risks of endocarditis. Any unexplained fever requires blood cultures to be drawn before antibiotics are initiated. Thorough transthoracic and transesophageal echocardiograms should be performed to assess the presence of vegetations. If infection of prosthetic material is suspected, early consultation with a specialist who has access to a congenital heart surgeon should be initiated because of the potential for rapid deterioration.

Antibiotic prophylaxis before dental procedures that involve manipulation of the gingiva, periapical regions of the teeth, or mucosal tissue is indicated in patients with previous infective endocarditis; unrepaired cyanotic lesions; palliative shunts or conduits; prosthetic valves or prosthetic materials used for valve repair; repaired congenital heart disease with prosthetic material or transcatheter device within 6 months of intervention; and repaired congenital heart disease with residual lesions at or adjacent to the site of a prosthetic patch or device (Chapter 76). It is also reasonable to consider prophylaxis against endocarditis before vaginal delivery at the time of membrane rupture in such patients. Prophylaxis is not indicated for nondental procedures in the absence of active infection.

Exercise
The goal of exercise evaluation is to assess the functional results of therapeutic interventions and to provide guidelines for exercise prescriptions. Patients with residual hemodynamic lesions or unrepaired congenital cardiac anomalies should be evaluated on an annual basis with a physical examination, an ECG, and a cardiac ultrasonographic examination if indicated. Pertinent additional tests may include Holter monitoring and exercise testing. Attention should be directed to the detection of pulmonary hypertension, arrhythmias, myocardial dysfunction, and symptoms such as exercise-induced dizziness, syncope, dyspnea, or chest pain.

A series of exercise guidelines have been proposed for major groups of congenital heart defects (Table 69-2). Patients beyond 6 months after repair of a single shunt lesion without pulmonary hypertension, arrhythmias, or evidence of myocardial dysfunction can participate in all sports. With

TABLE 69-2 EXERCISE RECOMMENDATIONS IN ADULTS WITH CONGENITAL HEART DISEASE

CONDITION	UNRESTRICTED	LOW-MODERATE INTENSITY*	PROHIBITED
ASD†	No PHT; no arrhythmia; normal ventricular function	PA pressure >40 mm Hg *with* normal ETT; no arrhythmia	Eisenmenger's
VSD†	Small; no PHT; no arrhythmia; normal ventricular function	Moderate VSD	Eisenmenger's
PDA†	Small; no PHT; no arrhythmia; normal ventricular function	PA pressure >40 mm Hg *with* normal ETT; no arrhythmia	Eisenmenger's
Coarctation‡	Gradient ≤20 mm Hg arm to leg; normal BP at rest and exercise	Gradient ≥20 mm Hg arm to leg *with* normal BP and normal ETT	Gradient ≥50 mm Hg arm to leg *or* aortic aneurysm
PS	Gradient <50 mm Hg; no arrhythmia; normal ventricular function	Gradient ≥50 mm Hg	Gradient ≥70 mm Hg *or* ventricular arrhythmia
AS	Gradient ≤20 mm Hg; normal ECG; normal ETT; asymptomatic	Gradient >20 mm Hg *with* normal ECG, normal ETT; asymptomatic	Gradient ≥50 mm Hg *or* ventricular arrhythmia
TOF after repair	Normal RV pressure; no shunt; no arrhythmia	Increased RV pressure *or* moderate PR *or* SVT	RV pressure ≥65% systemic *or* ventricular arrhythmia on ETT *or* severe PR
Mustard or Senning		No cardiomegaly, arrhythmia, or syncope; normal ETT	Cardiomegaly *or* arrhythmia at rest or exercise
c-TGA unoperated	No cardiomegaly; mild TR; no arrhythmia; normal ETT	Moderate RV dysfunction, moderate TR; no arrhythmia	Severe TR *or* uncontrolled arrhythmia
Ebstein's	Mild Ebstein's; no arrhythmia; operated with mild TR	Moderate TR *with* no arrhythmia	Severe Ebstein's *or* uncontrolled arrhythmia
Fontan		Normal O₂ saturation *with* near-normal ETT and ventricular function	Moderate-severe MR or TR *or* uncontrolled arrhythmia

*Based on peak dynamic and static components of exercise during competition for individual sports (see credit line).
†Unoperated or 6 months after surgery.
‡Unoperated or 1 year after surgery.
AS = aortic stenosis; ASD = atrial septal defect; BP = blood pressure; c-TGA = corrected transposition of the great arteries; ECG = electrocardiogram; ETT = exercise tolerance test; MR = mitral regurgitation; PA = pulmonary artery; PDA = patent ductus arteriosus; PHT = pulmonary hypertension; PR = pulmonary regurgitation; PS = pulmonary stenosis; RV = right ventricle; SVT = supraventricular tachyarrhythmia; TOF = tetralogy of Fallot; TR = tricuspid regurgitation; VSD = ventricular septal defect.
Based on guidelines recommended in Graham TP, Bricker TJ, James FW, et al. 26th Bethesda conference: recommendations for determining eligibility for competition in athletes with cardiovascular abnormalities. Task Force 1: Congenital heart disease. *J Am Coll Cardiol.* 1994;24:867. Reprinted with permission of the American College of Cardiology.

residual shunts, if the peak pulmonary artery pressure is less than 40 mm Hg in the absence of ventricular dysfunction or significant arrhythmias, patients can enjoy a free range of activity. Patients with elevated pulmonary vascular resistance are at risk of sudden death during intense exercise; although most self-limit their activity, participation in competitive sports is contraindicated. Patients with aortic and pulmonary stenosis should be counseled as recommended earlier, according to gradient severity. For patients with uncomplicated aortic coarctation, athletic participation is permitted if the arm-leg blood pressure gradient is 20 mm Hg or less at rest and the peak systolic blood pressure during exercise is normal. For patients after tetralogy of Fallot repair, repair of transposition of the great arteries, and the Fontan operation, exercise recommendations vary according to residual ventricular function and the presence or absence of arrhythmias.

1. Gatzoulis MA, Beghetti M, Galiè N, et al. Longer-term bosentan therapy improves functional capacity in Eisenmenger syndrome: results of the BREATHE-5 open-label extension study. *Int J Cardiol.* 2008;127:27-32.
2. Attie F, Rosas M, Granados N, et al. Surgical treatment for secundum atrial septal defects in patients >40 years old: a randomized clinical trial. *J Am Coll Cardiol.* 2001;38:2035-2042.
3. Dowson A, Mullen MJ, Peatfield R, et al. Migraine intervention with STARFlex Technology (MIST) trial: a prospective, multicenter, double-blind, sham-controlled trial to evaluate the effectiveness of patent foramen ovale closure with STARFlex septal repair implant to resolve refractory migraine headache. *Circulation.* 2008;117:1397-1404.

SUGGESTED READINGS

Penny DJ, Vick GW 3rd. Ventricular septal defect. *Lancet.* 2011;377:1103-1112. *Review.*
Silversides CK, Marelli A, Beauchesne L, et al. Canadian Cardiovascular Society 2009 Consensus Conference on the Management of Adults with Congenital Heart Disease: executive summary. *Can J Cardiol.* 2010;26:143-150. *Practical guidelines.*
Thaler DE, Kent DM. Rethinking trial strategies for stroke and patent foramen ovale. *Curr Opin Neurol.* 2010;23:73-78. *Review of potential risks and benefits.*
Warnes CA, Williams RG, Bashore TM, et al. ACC/AHA 2008 Guidelines for the Management of Adults with Congenital Heart Disease: a report of the American College of Cardiology/American Heart Association Task Force on Practice Guidelines (writing committee to develop guidelines on the management of adults with congenital heart disease). *Circulation.* 2008;118:e714-833. *Consensus guidelines.*

70

ATHEROSCLEROSIS, THROMBOSIS, AND VASCULAR BIOLOGY

GÖRAN K. HANSSON AND ANDERS HAMSTEN

Atherosclerosis is the underlying cause of most cases of myocardial infarction, ischemic stroke, and peripheral arterial disease. It is also a major cause of chronic heart failure and vascular dementia. Atherosclerosis, which is a chronic inflammatory response to the accumulation of lipid in the artery wall, initially is typically characterized by clinically silent intimal plaques in arteries for years and even decades. Fissuring or erosion of atherosclerotic plaques triggers the formation of a thrombus that accumulates over seconds to minutes to cause acute ischemia of the end organ. This ischemia, in turn, results in the dramatic clinical manifestations. It is estimated that approximately 90% of cases of myocardial infarction (Chapter 73), 60% of strokes (Chapter 414), most cases of heart failure (Chapter 58), and up to one third of all cases of dementia (Chapter 409) are due to atherosclerosis.

RISK FACTORS FOR ATHEROSCLEROSIS

The major risk factors that promote the development of atherosclerosis are an elevated low-density lipoprotein (LDL) cholesterol level, a low high-density lipoprotein (HDL) level (Chapter 213), cigarette smoking, type 2 diabetes (Chapter 237), hypertension (Chapter 67), and a family history of coronary heart disease, ischemic stroke, or peripheral arterial disease. Other conditions thought to increase the risk of atherosclerotic disease include abdominal obesity, hypertriglyceridemia, high plasma levels of lipoprotein (a) [Lp(a)], hyperfibrinogenemia, the inflammatory marker C-reactive protein (CRP), and physical inactivity. Other emerging risk factors, including uric acid, psychosocial stress, encompassing external stressors (e.g., job stress, life events, and financial problems), and reactions to stress (e.g., depression [Chapter 404], anxiety, psychosocial distress, and sleep disturbances [Chapter 100]), also appear to contribute. Elevation of plasma total homocysteine is also associated with increased cardiovascular risk, but it is possible that chronic renal dysfunction accounts for at least some of the vascular pathology seen in hyperhomocysteinemia.

An atherogenic lipoprotein phenotype has been defined as the presence of a predominance of small, dense LDL particles, hypertriglyceridemia, and low plasma HDL cholesterol concentration. This lipoprotein phenotype, which is strongly linked to obesity, insulin resistance, hypertension, and abnormalities in postprandial lipoprotein metabolism, is similar to the so-called metabolic syndrome, in that both are associated with a cluster of atherogenic and thrombotic risk factors—raised plasma levels of fibrinogen, plasminogen activator inhibitor-1 (PAI-1), and coagulation factor VII, as well as platelet hyperactivity.

FORMATION OF ATHEROSCLEROTIC LESIONS

Atherosclerosis is thought to be initiated when apolipoprotein B (apoB100)-containing lipoproteins, predominantly LDL, accumulate in the vascular intima, the innermost layer of the artery (Fig. 70-1). Small dense LDL particles are particularly prone to accumulate in the intima, where they associate with proteoglycans of the extracellular matrix. Lipoprotein lipase produced locally in the artery can bridge LDL to the extracellular matrix, and phospholipase and sphingomyelinase actions may contribute to the entrapment of LDL. Once trapped in the artery wall, LDL particles can be attacked by enzymes such as myeloperoxidase and NADPH oxidases; they may also be modified by nonenzymatic oxidation. During oxidative modification of LDL, certain biologically active oxidized phospholipid species are released and activate endothelial cells and macrophages. Such activation leads to production of chemokines and expression of leukocyte adhesion molecules that together instigate recruitment of monocytes and T cells to the intima. Local growth factors induce recruited monocytes to develop into macrophages.

In the intima, macrophages take up oxidized LDL through their scavenger receptors, start to accumulate cholesterol, and are gradually transformed into cholesterol-laden foam cells. Some macrophages in the intima produce proinflammatory mediators, including tumor necrosis factor (TNF), interleukin-1 (IL-1), proinflammatory eicosanoids, radical oxygen and nitrogen species, and prothrombotic factors.

T cells that are stimulated to enter the intima may recognize antigens presented by macrophages. These antigens include components of LDL, other endogenous proteins, and possibly microbial antigens. Activated intimal T cells produce T$_H$1-type cytokines, such as interferon-γ, TNF, and lymphotoxin, all of which are strongly proatherogenic. With the entry and activation of T cells and macrophages, the accumulation of lipid in the intima leads to the chronic inflammatory disease process of atherosclerosis.

Although adaptive immunity is believed to exert a net proatherogenic effect, antiatherogenic immune responses against LDL involve activation of regulatory T cells, secretion of the anti-inflammatory cytokines IL-10 and transforming growth factor-β, and production of anti-LDL antibodies. In addition to T cells and macrophages, atheroma formation is also stimulated by dendritic cells that take up and present antigen and by mast cells that secrete enzymes and bioactive mediators.

Triglyceride-rich lipoprotein remnant particles, which have adverse effects on endothelial function, penetrate into the subendothelial space of normal intima and atherosclerotic plaques, where they are retained. The LDL-like Lp(a) lipoprotein particle exerts both proatherogenic and prothrombotic actions.

Conversely, antiatherogenic HDL particles counteract the formation of atherosclerotic lesions. These particles mediate cholesterol efflux from cells by acting as acceptors of cholesterol delivered from specific transport proteins termed adenosine triphosphate–binding cassette (ABC) A1 and G1. In addition, HDL particles carry anti-inflammatory and antioxidant proteins.

GROWTH, DEATH, AND THE PROGRESSION OF DISEASE

Early atherosclerotic lesions grow by the accumulation of cholesterol; infiltration of inflammatory cells; the activation, proliferation, and death of such cells; and the gradual development of a core that contains cellular debris and lipids. As a tissue response to this process, smooth muscle cells form a

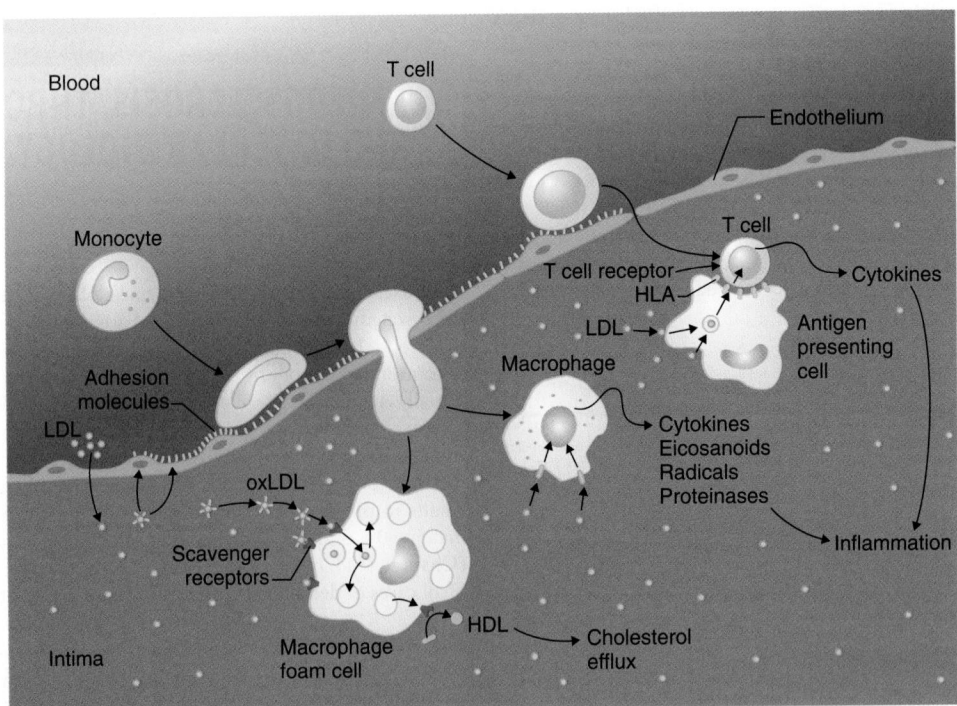

FIGURE 70-1. Formation of atherosclerotic plaques. Low-density lipoproteins (LDL) transit from the blood stream to the arterial intima and accumulate under the endothelial cell layer. LDL particles undergo oxidative modification in the intima (denoted by spikes on LDL particles), thereby leading to their binding to scavenger receptors and uptake by macrophages, which accumulate cholesterol and develop into foam cells. Cholesterol efflux to high-density lipoprotein (HDL) counteracts the tendency to foam cell formation. Molecules released from oxidatively modified LDL activate endothelial cells to express leukocyte adhesion molecules that promote binding of monocytes and T cells to the surface of the artery. Chemokines stimulate monocytes and T cells to migrate into the intima, where the monocytes differentiate into macrophages. Although many macrophages develop into foam cells, some are activated, thereby leading to release of proinflammatory cytokines, eicosanoids, radicals, and proteases. T cells entering through similar mechanisms as monocytes can recognize local antigens, such as LDL components, which are presented to them by antigen-presenting cells (dendritic cells and macrophages) that express HLA molecules. T cells whose receptors can recognize local antigens are activated, thereby leading to release of a host of cytokines that can activate macrophages and enhance vascular inflammation. (Modified from Hansson GK. Inflammation, atherosclerosis, and coronary artery disease. *N Engl J Med.* 2005;352:1685-1695.)

subendothelial cap structure dominated by collagen fibers that are produced by these cells. The collagen cap mechanically stabilizes the plaque and creates a barrier between the hemostatic components of the blood and the thrombogenic material of the plaque. Until the plaque is far advanced, compensatory enlargement ("remodeling") of the arterial wall prevents it from significantly protruding into the arterial lumen. However, after the plaque enlarges to a sufficient size, the lumen narrows as the plaque grows, and the artery remodels inward, often accompanied by exaggerated or paradoxical vasoconstriction.

PLAQUE ACTIVATION, THROMBOSIS, AND INFARCTION

The atherosclerotic process typically is silent for months, years, and even decades, and it may never result in clinical manifestations. However, if and when the plaque's surface is damaged, thrombotic occlusion of the artery may ensue. Surface continuity may be damaged by fissuring (so-called plaque rupture, observed in 60 to 80% of cases of acute coronary syndrome) or surface erosion (present in 20 to 40% of cases with coronary thrombosis, especially women and young victims of sudden coronary death). Fissures and erosions stimulate atherothrombosis by exposing thrombogenic material inside the plaque, such as phospholipids, tissue factor, and matrix molecules, to platelets and coagulation factors (Fig. 70-2). Platelet aggregates formed on exposed surfaces are stabilized by a fibrin network. Tissue factor, expressed in vascular smooth muscle cells and macrophages of the atherosclerotic plaque, is the primary cellular initiator of the blood coagulation cascade that leads to fibrin formation. Atherothrombi expand rapidly and can fill the lumen within minutes, thereby leading to ischemia and infarction.

The cause of plaque rupture remains unclear. Clinical studies have associated ischemic atherothrombotic events such as myocardial infarction (Chapter 73) and stroke (Chapter 414) with infections and stressful events. Histopathologic analysis shows increased inflammation with infiltration of macrophages, activated T cells, dendritic cells, and mast cells, as well as reduced thickness of the fibrous cap and increased neovascularity at sites of plaque rupture and thrombosis. Ruptured plaques also tend to have a large necrotic lipid core. In contrast, plaques underlying erosions do not have a large lipid core and show less inflammation compared with ruptured plaques.

Several members of the matrix metalloproteinase and cysteine proteinase families are found at sites of plaque rupture and have been implicated in plaque rupture, but their effects on the composition and size of lesions are complex. Apoptosis of inflammatory cells and smooth muscle cells, which are contained in the plaque and are likely to contribute to plaque rupture, may be initiated by activation of the death receptor group of the TNF receptor superfamily. Apoptotic macrophages release tissue factor, and a reduced number of smooth muscle cells leads to matrix depletion and destabilizes the plaque. In addition, activated T cells inhibit matrix synthesis by production of interferon-γ, a cytokine that inhibits collagen fiber formation as well as proliferation of smooth muscle cells.

Although a range of factors contribute to atherothrombosis, the precise sequence of events is not yet known. Similarly, the precise role of the activation of coagulation pathways and platelets, combined with the inhibition of fibrinolysis, remains to be defined. Importantly, plaque rupture frequently occurs without clinical manifestations, possibly reflecting variation in the thrombotic response depending on the thrombogenicity of exposed plaque constituents, local hemorrheology, shear-induced platelet activation, systemic clotting activity, fibrinolytic function, and the sensitivity of the end organ to ischemia.

PRINCIPLES OF ANTIATHEROSCLEROTIC THERAPY

Current treatment of atherosclerosis aims at controlling risk factors and maintaining perfusion in affected arteries. However, progress in understanding the pathogenesis of atherosclerosis is expected to result in more direct approaches. To date, firmly established interventions include smoking cessation, dietary and pharmacologic reduction of LDL cholesterol (Chapter 213), and management of blood pressure (Chapter 67). Available data also strongly support intervention directed toward hyperglycemia (Chapter 237), low HDL cholesterol levels (Chapter 213), hypertriglyceridemia (Chapter 213), obesity (Chapter 227), and physical inactivity (Chapter 15). Statins clearly reduce atherosclerotic lesions and inhibit their progression.[1][2] Statins also can prevent nitroglycerin-induced endothelial dysfunction and nitrate tolerance.[3] Aspirin and other inhibitors of platelet aggregation, β-adrenergic receptor blockers, and angiotensin-converting enzyme inhibitors[4] or angiotensin II antagonists are also part of the routine secondary prevention of coronary heart disease (Chapter 71). Inhibitors of platelet aggregation are widely used for secondary prevention of atherosclerotic cardiovascular disease. Aspirin inhibits formation of proaggregatory prostaglandins, whereas other inhibitors of platelet aggregation modulate

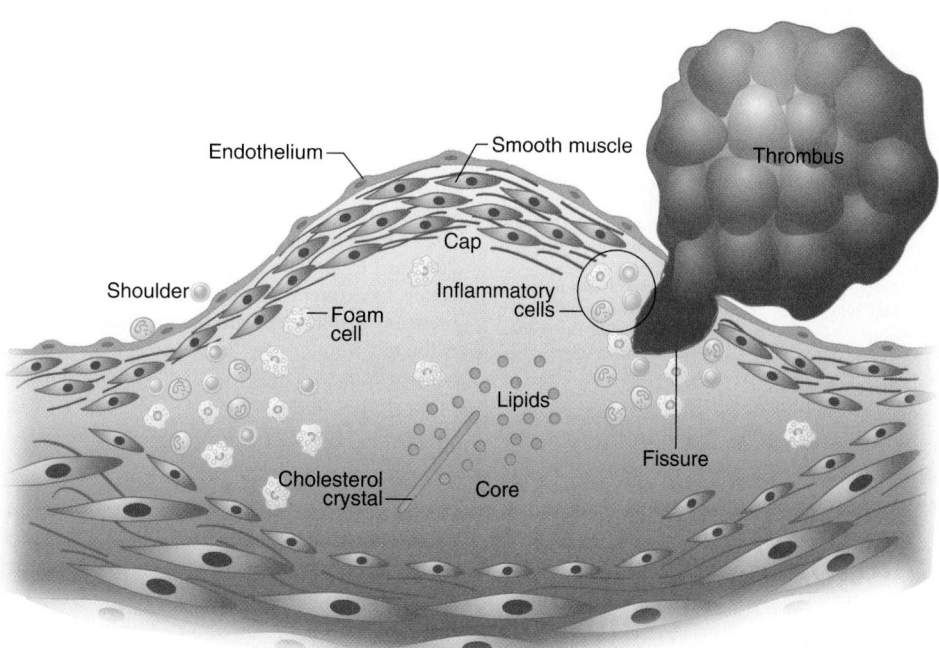

FIGURE 70-2. **Plaque rupture and atherothrombosis.** The advanced atherosclerotic plaque has a central core with lipids, especially cholesterol, live and dead cells, necrotic material from dead foam cells, and calcium salts. The plaque is overlaid by a fibrous cap that consists of smooth muscle cells and collagen (produced by the muscle cells) and covered by an intact layer of endothelial cells. Inflammatory cells (macrophages, T cells, mast cells, dendritic cells, and occasional B cells) are interspersed with these components and are particularly abundant in the shoulder regions of plaques, where fissures (also called ruptures) may expose thrombogenic core material (e.g., lipids, collagen, tissue factor) to blood components. This event triggers platelet aggregation and humoral coagulation, thereby leading to thrombus formation at the site of fissuring. Thrombi may expand locally to obstruct blood flow or they may detach to cause embolization. (Modified from Hansson GK. Inflammation, atherosclerosis, and coronary artery disease. *N Engl J Med.* 2005;352:1685-1695.)

expression of platelet adhesion molecules. Nitroglycerin and similar compounds that mimic the action of endogenous nitric oxide remain the most important vasodilators used in secondary prevention (Chapter 71). In one preliminary trial, eicosapentaenoic acid reduced coronary events for 4 to 6 years after treatment.[5]

FUTURE DIRECTIONS

Novel therapeutic opportunities that are currently being considered include new targets for lipid-lowering treatment, use of new immunosuppressing and anti-inflammatory compounds, and vaccination with disease-related antigens. Investigational agents targeting atherogenic lipoproteins include inhibitors of squalene synthase, microsomal triglyceride transfer protein, proprotein convertase subtilisin kexin type 9 (PCSK9), and antisense oligonucleotides to apoB. Compounds targeting HDL include liver X receptor (LXR) agonists, inhibitors of endothelial lipase, and apoA-I mimetic peptides. Statins (Chapter 213) have an array of beneficial actions that are independent of LDL cholesterol reduction, including attenuation of inflammation and inhibition of antigen presentation. Besides their beneficial effects on lipid and blood glucose levels, peroxisome proliferator-activated receptor (PPAR) agonists (Chapter 237) exhibit direct antiatherosclerotic effects in experimental studies.

Members of the TNF superfamily of proinflammatory proteins, eicosanoids, and cell surface proteins promoting antigen-specific T-cell activation are particularly promising targets of anti-inflammatory therapy, whereas stimulation of anti-inflammatory signaling pathways represents a different potential antiatherosclerotic therapy. Inhibition of secreted and lipoprotein-associated phospholipase A_2 is already being examined in clinical trials. Similarly, vaccination against immunogenic epitopes in the protein and lipid moieties of LDL may induce anti-inflammatory regulatory immunity and reduce LDL uptake in cells of the atherosclerotic lesion.

1. Corti R, Fuster V, Fayad ZA. Effects of aggressive versus conventional lipid-lowering therapy by simvastatin on human atherosclerotic lesions: a prospective, randomized, double-blind trial with high-resolution magnetic resonance imaging. *J Am Coll Cardiol.* 2005;46:106-112.
2. Crouse JR 3rd, Raichlen JS, Riley WA, et al. Effect of rosuvastatin on progression of carotid intima-media thickness in low-risk individuals with subclinical atherosclerosis: the METEOR trial. *JAMA.* 2007;297:1344-1353.
3. Liuni A, Luca MC, Di Stolfo G, et al. Coadministration of atorvastatin prevents nitroglycerin-induced endothelial dysfunction and nitrate tolerance in healthy humans. *J Am Coll Cardiol.* 2011;57:93-98.
4. Dagenais GR, Pogue J, Fox K, et al. Angiotensin-converting-enzyme inhibitors in stable vascular disease without left ventricular systolic dysfunction or heart failure: a combined analysis of three trials. *Lancet.* 2006;368:581-588.
5. Yokoyama M, Origasa H, Matsuzaki M, et al. Effects of eicosapentaenoic acid on major coronary events in hypercholesterolaemic patients (JELIS): a randomised open-label, blinded endpoint analysis. *Lancet.* 2007;369:1090-1098.

SUGGESTED READINGS

Alsheikh-Ali AA, Kitsios GD, Balk EM, et al. The vulnerable atherosclerotic plaque: scope of the literature. *Ann Intern Med.* 2010;153:387-395. *Review.*

Bäck M, Ketelhuth DF, Agewall S. Matrix metalloproteinases in atherothrombosis. *Prog Cardiovasc Dis.* 2010;52:410-428. *Proteolytic enzymes may play a key role in plaque rupture and myocardial infarction.*

Khera AV, Cuchel M, de la Llera-Moya M, et al. Cholesterol efflux capacity, high-density lipoprotein function, and atherosclerosis. *N Engl J Med.* 2011;364:127-135. *Cholesterol efflux capacity is negatively associated with carotid intima-media thickness and the likelihood of angiographic coronary artery disease.*

71

ANGINA PECTORIS AND STABLE ISCHEMIC HEART DISEASE

WILLIAM E. BODEN

DEFINITION

Ischemic heart disease is most commonly caused by obstruction or stenosis of one or more of the coronary arteries by atheromatous plaque (Chapter 70). Obstruction can result in myocardial ischemia and infarction (Chapters 72 and 73) with associated symptoms of angina, ischemia, myocardial remodeling, heart failure (Chapter 58), arrhythmic complications (Chapters 63, 64, 65), and ultimately death.

Angina pectoris is generally a consequence of a supply-demand imbalance between an activity that increases cardiac workload or "demand," thereby resulting in an increase in heart rate, blood pressure, or both, and the inability of the narrowed epicardial coronary arteries (Chapter 57) to augment antegrade flow or "supply" in response to this increase in demand. Such an imbalance classically results in chest discomfort (Chapter 50) of varying intensity and duration. Angina pectoris is generally defined as a discomfort in the chest or adjacent areas caused by myocardial ischemia. Often, angina is described incorrectly as "chest pain." The term *angina*, however, derives from a neologism of two Latin words, "angor animi," which literally translates into "fear of life being extinguished ('from the breast')," according to Heberden's original description in 1768. Had Heberden been trying to convey the term for chest pain, he would more likely have used the Latin term *dolor pectoris*.

Grading of Angina Pectoris

The Canadian Cardiovascular Society (CCS) angina grading scale is a widely used four-point ordinal scale that classifies angina pectoris from mild (class I: angina occurring only during strenuous or prolonged physical activity) to severe (class IV: inability to perform any activity without angina, or angina at rest) and includes the full spectrum of angina from chronic stable to unstable (see Table 50-5 in Chapter 50). Operationally, the CCS angina scale permits clinicians to categorize patients as mild or stable (generally CCS classes I and II) versus severe or unstable (typically CCS classes III and IV). Other grading systems include a specific activity scale, which is based on the metabolic cost of specific activities, and an anginal score, which integrates the clinical features and tempo of angina with electrocardiographic (ECG) changes and offers independent prognostic information beyond that provided by age, gender, ventricular function, and coronary anatomy.

EPIDEMIOLOGY

It is currently estimated that 17,600,000 adults in the United States have heart disease, 10,200,000 of whom have angina pectoris and 8,500,000 of whom have had acute myocardial infarction (MI). Approximately 785,000 Americans will experience a new ischemic heart disease event annually, and about 470,000 will have a recurrent event. In 2006, ischemic heart disease accounted for 52% of all deaths caused by cardiovascular disease and was the single most frequent cause of death in American men and women, resulting in more than one in every six deaths. The economic burden of ischemic heart disease in the United States in 2010 has been estimated at $177.1 billion. Despite the sustained decline in age-specific case-fatality rates from coronary artery disease over the past several decades, ischemic heart disease is now the leading cause of death worldwide, and it is expected that this rate of rise will continue to accelerate over the coming decade as a consequence of the epidemic rise in obesity (Chapter 227), type 2 diabetes (Chapter 237), and the metabolic syndrome, which may give rise to an increasing risk of developing premature coronary artery disease in younger generations. The World Health Organization has projected that, over the next decade, the global number of deaths from coronary artery disease will increase by 46% from 7.6 million in 2005 to 11.1 million in 2020. An estimated 8 million patients come to emergency departments annually for chest pain, and approximately 1.5 million of them are hospitalized with the acute coronary syndrome (ACS; Chapter 72). Although women may have typical angina less frequently than men, more women than men in the United States die annually of ischemic heart disease or its complications, and, overall, ischemic heart disease is the most common cause of death in women.

PATHOBIOLOGY

Angina is the most frequent clinical expression of myocardial ischemia. Ischemia, which rapidly develops when a mismatch arises between myocardial oxygen needs and myocardial oxygen supply, can manifest clinically in many different ways besides angina, from no symptoms (e.g., silent ischemia) to unstable angina, MI, or sudden cardiac death. It may remain stable for many years in selected patients or may be rapidly progressive with an abrupt change in frequency and tempo over days to weeks. Conversely, atherosclerosis, which is the most common cause of myocardial ischemia, may evolve for years without any manifestations of ischemia.

In contrast to the inherent pathogenetic complexity mediated by differing mechanisms associated with abrupt plaque rupture, fissuring, or erosion in patients with ACS (Chapters 70 and 72), the pathogenesis of chronic stable angina is, by comparison, seemingly less complicated and heterogeneous because it fundamentally involves a myocardial supply-demand mismatch. In most patients with stable ischemic heart disease, the process of atherosclerosis involves a fundamentally different histopathology (small lipid core with a thick or very thick fibrous cap and a low proclivity to rupture) compared with ACS or unstable angina, in which the principal histopathologic picture is that of a large lipid core subtended by a thinned, inflamed cap, which harbors the high-risk or vulnerable plaque with a high proclivity for rupture (Chapter 70).

Two major pathogenetic mechanisms may result in myocardial ischemia and angina in the chronic setting: so-called demand angina, which is caused by an increase in myocardial oxygen requirements and workload, and supply angina, which is caused by diminished oxygen delivery to myocardial tissue. Demand angina is a consequence of the increased myocardial oxygen (O_2) requirements that occur with increased physical activity, emotion, or stress. In a patient with chronic, restricted O_2 delivery owing to atherosclerotic narrowing of a coronary artery, this increased demand may precipitate angina. Other extracardiac precipitants of angina include the excessive metabolic demands imposed by fever, thyrotoxicosis (Chapter 233), severe anemia (Chapter 161) from blood loss, tachycardia from any cause (Chapters 62, 63, 64), and hypoglycemia (Chapter 238).

By contrast, supply angina may occur in patients with either unstable angina (Chapter 72) or chronic stable angina by transient reductions in myocardial O_2 delivery as a consequence of coronary vasoconstriction with resulting dynamic coronary stenosis. In the presence of coronary luminal narrowing due to atherosclerosis, superimposed platelet thrombi and leukocytes may elaborate vasoconstrictor substances, such as serotonin and thromboxane A_2, whereas endothelial damage in diseased coronary arteries may decrease production of vasodilator substances such as nitric oxide and adenosine. The result is an abnormal vasoconstrictor response to exercise and other stimuli, such as exogenously administered adenosine or the paradoxical vasoconstrictor response to the typical flow-mediated reactive hyperemia associated with brachial artery compression. In some clinical settings, patients who have normal coronary arteries or non–flow-limiting stenoses may exhibit dynamic obstruction alone, which can cause myocardial ischemia and result in angina at rest (Prinzmetal's [variant] angina). Conversely, in patients with severe fixed obstruction to coronary blood flow, only a minor increase in dynamic obstruction can reduce blood flow below a critical level and cause myocardial ischemia.

The pathophysiologic basis for angina and ischemia in patients with stable ischemic heart disease has important implications for the selection of anti-ischemic agents. The greater the contribution from increased myocardial O_2 requirements to the imbalance between supply and demand, the greater the likelihood that agents such as β-blockers or heart rate–lowering calcium antagonists will provide clinical benefit, whereas nitrates and calcium antagonists with more potent vasodilatory properties (particularly the dihydropyridines) will be more beneficial to alleviate angina and ischemia mediated by coronary vasoconstriction.

Although the most common cause of ischemic heart disease is atherosclerotic narrowing of the epicardial coronary arteries resulting in flow-limiting obstruction to blood flow, obstructive coronary artery disease may also have nonatherosclerotic causes, such as congenital abnormalities of the coronary arteries (Chapter 69), vasospasm, myocardial bridging, coronary arteritis in association with systemic vasculitides (Chapter 278), and radiation-induced coronary disease (Chapter 19). Myocardial ischemia and angina pectoris may also occur in the absence of obstructive coronary artery disease, as in the case of aortic valve disease (Chapter 75), hypertrophic cardiomyopathy (Chapter 60), and idiopathic dilated cardiomyopathy. Moreover, ischemic heart disease may coexist with these other forms of heart disease.

CLINICAL MANIFESTATIONS

History

It is important to recognize that there are many causes of chest pain (see Table 50-2 in Chapter 50), that angina-like chest pain may not represent ischemic heart disease (Table 71-1), that ischemic heart disease causes symptoms other than anginal pain (Table 71-2), and that nonatherosclerotic coronary artery abnormalities may cause ischemic chest pain (Table 71-3).

Angina pectoris has four cardinal clinical features: the character of the discomfort, its site and distribution, its provocation, and its duration. The character of anginal discomfort is typically described as a pressure sensation that conveys a feeling of strangling and anxiety (Chapter 50). Other adjectives frequently used to describe this discomfort include heavy,

TABLE 71-1	PROBABILITY (%) OF CORONARY ARTERY DISEASE BY AGE, GENDER, AND SYMPTOMS			
GENDER	AGE (yr)	DEFINITE ANGINA	ATYPICAL ANGINA	NONCARDIAC CHEST PAIN
Men	30-39	83	46	3
	40-49	88	57	12
	50-59	94	71	18
	60-69	95	78	31
	≥70	97	94	63
Women	30-39	—	20	4
	40-49	56	31	4
	50-59	68	30	6
	60-69	81	48	10
	≥70	96	56	—

From Chaitman BR, Bourassa MG, Davis K, et al. Angiographic prevalence of high-risk coronary artery disease in patient subsets (CASS). *Circulation*. 1981;64:360-367.

TABLE 71-2	NON–CHEST PAIN SYMPTOMS OF CHRONIC ISCHEMIC HEART DISEASE

DYSPNEA

Dyspnea on exertion
Dyspnea at rest
Paroxysmal nocturnal dyspnea
Temporal change of increasing exertional dyspnea with declining effort tolerance

NON–CHEST LOCATIONS OF DISCOMFORT (EITHER EXERTIONAL OR AT REST)

Neck or mandibular discomfort or pain
Throat tightness
Shoulder discomfort
Upper arm or forearm discomfort (more often left-sided)
Interscapular or infrascapular discomfort

MID-EPIGASTRIC OR ABDOMINAL

Mid-epigastric burning, often postprandially
Sharp abdominal pain (atypical, but more common in women)
Right-upper quadrant discomfort (may mimic gallbladder disease or pancreatitis)
Nausea and/or vomiting (often associated with increased vagal tone secondary to inferior myocardial ischemia or infarction)

DIAPHORESIS

EXCESSIVE FATIGUE AND WEAKNESS

Often a discernible prodrome of increasing fatigue with declining effort tolerance

DIZZINESS AND SYNCOPE

Uncommon, unless precipitated or exacerbated by alterations in heart rate or rhythm (e.g., bradyarrhythmia, tachyarrhythmia, heart block), blood pressure (e.g., hypotension), or cardiac output (e.g., decreased cerebral perfusion)

squeezing, constricting, viselike, suffocating, and, at times, crushing. In some patients, the quality of the sensation is more vague and atypical (often in women and elderly patients), and these patients may describe the discomfort as a burning sensation in the mid-epigastrium or as an uncomfortable, numb sensation. Anginal equivalents (i.e., symptoms of myocardial ischemia other than angina), such as dyspnea, fatigue, lightheadedness or dizziness, and gastric eructations, may likewise be described.

The site and distribution of anginal discomfort are predominantly midsternal or retrosternal but can be precordial. Radiation is common, usually to the left neck and shoulder and down the ulnar surface of the left arm; the right arm and the outer surfaces of both arms may also be involved. Discomfort that radiates to the jaw may be confused with dental pain. Epigastric discomfort alone or in association with chest pressure may occur. Provocation of angina is classically caused by physical exertion or activity, emotional stress, exposure to the cold, sexual intercourse, or eating a large meal. Angina that occurs at rest or nocturnally often heralds a change in the pattern from stable to unstable and may indicate that there is an incipient plaque rupture leading

TABLE 71-3	NONATHEROSCLEROTIC CAUSES OF ISCHEMIC CHEST PAIN

PRIMARY CARDIAC CAUSE

Coronary artery abnormalities
   Coronary spasm
   Coronary arteritis
   Coronary dissection
   Coronary artery anomalies
   Radiation-induced coronary disease
Myocardial bridging
Aortic stenosis
Hypertrophic cardiomyopathy
Dilated cardiomyopathy
Tachycardia

PRIMARY NONCARDIAC CAUSE

Anemia
Sickle cell disease
Hypoxemia
Carbon monoxide poisoning
Hyperviscosity (e.g., polycythemia)
Hyperthyroidism
Pheochromocytoma

to ACS. Vasospastic (or Prinzmetal's) angina may occur spontaneously at rest or nocturnally without provocation.

The typical duration of an episode of angina pectoris is brief. An episode usually begins gradually and reaches its maximal intensity over a period of minutes before abating. It is unusual for angina pectoris to peak and trough in less than a minute, and it is common that patients with exertional angina usually prefer to rest, sit, or stop walking during episodes that may be precipitated by the offending activity. Chest discomfort that persists for more than 15 to 20 minutes, especially at rest or nocturnally, is likely to represent ACS or MI. By contrast, features that suggest a noncardiac etiology of angina pectoris include pleuritic pain, pain reproduced by movement or palpation of the chest wall or arms, sharp or constant pain lasting for many hours, pain or discomfort that a patient can localize to the chest wall with the tip of one finger, or very brief episodes of pain lasting seconds (Chapter 50). Typical angina pectoris is generally relieved within minutes by rest or the use of sublingual, oral, or cutaneous nitroglycerin. The response to sublingual nitroglycerin is often a helpful diagnostic tool, although it should be emphasized that some noncardiac pain (e.g., esophageal spasm) may also respond to nitroglycerin.

Although chest discomfort is usually the predominant symptom in chronic (stable) angina, unstable angina, Prinzmetal's (variant) angina, microvascular angina, and acute MI, chest discomfort is absent, atypical, or not prominent in some patients. Patients with chronic ischemic heart disease may complain predominantly or exclusively of dyspnea, diminishing exercise tolerance or weakness. Others will first present with an abnormal exercise test result or other evidence of myocardial ischemia without any symptoms. Some patients will present with cardiac arrhythmias or even sudden cardiac death.

Physical Examination

Many patients with stable ischemic heart disease present with normal physical findings, but a diligent physical examination may reveal findings that represent either the consequences of myocardial ischemia or evidence of risk factors for coronary artery disease. Inspection of the eyes may reveal a corneal arcus, and examination of the skin may show xanthomas (see Fig. 50-12 in Chapter 50). Retinal arteriolar changes are common in patients with coronary artery disease who have hypertension or diabetes mellitus (see Figs. 431-26 and 431-24 in Chapter 431).

The cardiac examination is generally of limited benefit in evaluating patients with chest pain or establishing a diagnosis of ischemic heart disease. During an episode of chest discomfort, myocardial ischemia may produce either a third or fourth heart sound.

Myocardial ischemia also can cause a transient holosystolic or mid-late systolic apical murmur owing to reversible papillary muscle dysfunction that results in mitral regurgitation. These murmurs are more prevalent in patients with extensive coronary artery disease, especially with inferior or inferoposterior ischemia owing to right coronary artery disease. It is important to distinguish such a murmur from the murmur of aortic stenosis or obstructive

hypertrophic cardiomyopathy (see Tables 50-7 and 50-8 in Chapter 50). A displaced left ventricular (LV) apical impulse, particularly if dyskinetic, is a sign of significant LV systolic dysfunction.

If patients have coexisting heart failure, an elevated jugular venous pressure, pulmonary rales, and peripheral edema may be present (Chapter 58). The physical examination may reveal other implicating or contributing conditions, such as thyroid enlargement (Chapter 233) or severe anemia (Chapter 161).

DIAGNOSIS AND EVALUATION

In addition to a careful history and physical examination, assessment of patients with stable ischemic heart disease includes the 12-lead ECG, measurement of biochemical and inflammatory markers, and noninvasive diagnostic testing. The first goal is to assess the patient's probability of ischemia so that an appropriate evaluation can expedite effective therapy (Fig. 71-1).

Resting Electrocardiogram

Although there may be focal, diagnostic findings of ST segment depression and T wave inversions (Fig. 71-2) on the resting ECG in chronic ischemic heart disease, even patients with extensive anatomic coronary artery disease may have a normal tracing at rest. In addition to myocardial ischemia, other conditions that can produce ST-T wave abnormalities include LV hypertrophy and dilation due to long-standing hypertension and valvular heart disease (e.g., aortic stenosis, hypertrophic cardiomyopathy), electrolyte abnormalities, neurogenic effects, and antiarrhythmic drugs. The presence of new ST-T wave abnormalities on the resting ECG, however, can be helpful in the diagnosis of coronary artery disease and may correlate with the severity of the underlying heart disease.

In addition to focal ST-T wave abnormalities, the ECG may reveal various conduction disturbances, most frequently left bundle branch block and left anterior fascicular block (Chapter 54). The finding of abnormal Q waves is relatively specific for the presence of previous MI but may not help to determine when such an event occurred. Arrhythmias, especially ventricular premature beats (Chapter 65), may be present on the ECG but have a low sensitivity and specificity for coronary artery disease.

During a spontaneous episode of angina pectoris or during exertion or stress, the ECG becomes abnormal in 50% or more of patients with normal resting ECGs. The most common abnormality observed is focal ST segment depression, usually in one or more ECG lead groups, which signifies the presence of subendocardial ischemia. On occasion, transient, but diminutive, ST segment elevation and normalization of previous resting ST-T wave depression or inversion (pseudonormalization) may develop during chronic angina and ischemia, although ST segment elevation is far more commonly observed in ACS patients with plaque rupture.

Laboratory Testing

In patients with new-onset or worsening symptoms, a troponin level can distinguish MI and ACS from stable ischemic heart disease (Chapters 72 and 73). An elevated plasma concentration of brain natriuretic peptide does not help diagnose stable ischemic heart disease but is suggestive of heart failure (Chapter 58) and is associated with a higher risk of future cardiovascular events. High-sensitivity C-reactive protein, an acute phase reactant of inflammation, has a strong and consistent relationship to the risk of future cardiovascular events, and an elevated level may warrant more aggressive diagnostic evaluation and therapy.

All patients with chronic angina should have biochemical evaluation of total cholesterol, low-density lipoprotein (LDL) cholesterol, high-density lipoprotein (HDL) cholesterol, triglyceride, serum creatinine (estimated glomerular filtration), and fasting blood glucose levels (Table 71-4). Other biochemical markers that are not routinely recommended but are associated with higher risk of future cardiovascular events include lipoprotein (a), apoprotein B, small dense LDL cholesterol, and lipoprotein-associated phospholipase A_2 (Lp-PLA$_2$). Homocysteine levels correlate with the risk of developing coronary heart disease, but randomized trials have failed to demonstrate a reduction of clinical events when elevated homocysteine levels are reduced; as a result, screening for an elevated homocysteine level is not recommended.

Noninvasive Testing

Noninvasive stress testing with a standard ECG treadmill or bicycle exercise, radionuclide imaging (Chapter 56), stress echocardiography (Chapter 55), or newer diagnostic modalities such as cardiac magnetic resonance (CMR;

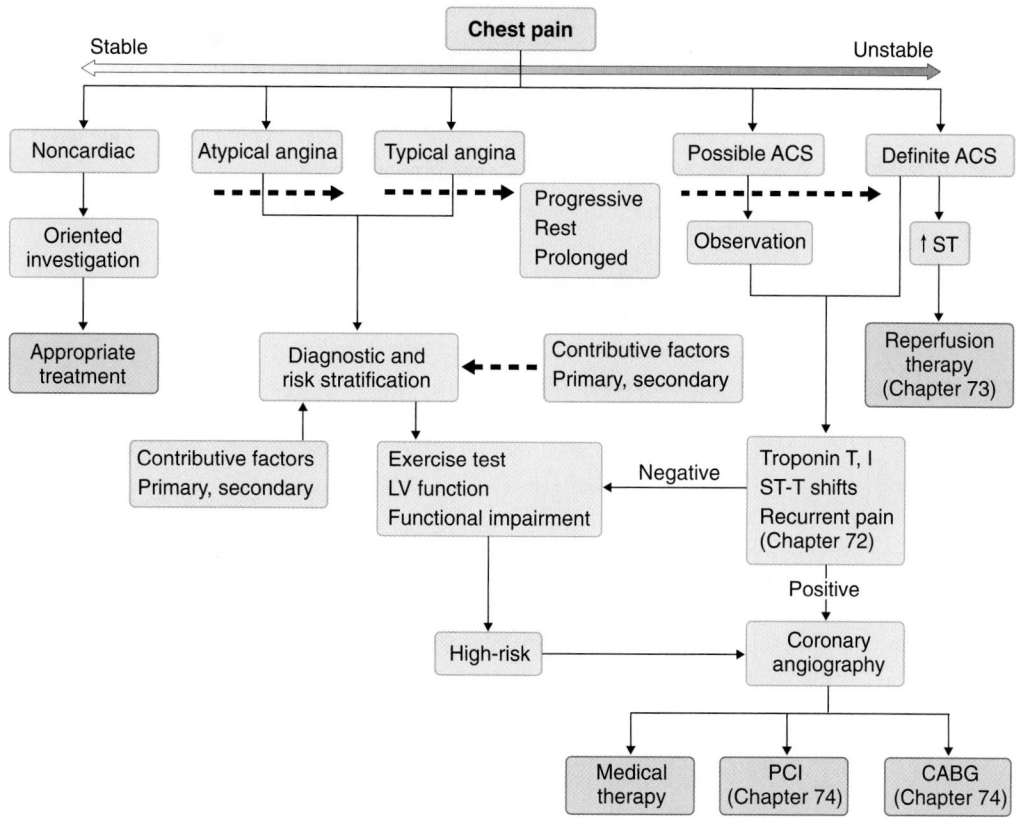

FIGURE 71-1. Evaluation of chest pain. ACS = acute coronary syndrome; CABG = coronary artery bypass graft; LV = left ventricular; PCI = percutaneous coronary intervention. (Adapted from Théroux P. Angina pectoris. In: Goldman L, Ausiello DA, eds. *Cecil Textbook of Medicine,* 23rd ed. Philadelphia: Saunders Elsevier; 2008.)

FIGURE 71-2. Ischemic ST segment shifts and repolarization changes on electrocardiogram (ECG).

TABLE 71-4 BLOOD TESTS TO OBTAIN ROUTINELY (OR SELECTIVELY*) IN PATIENTS WITH CHRONIC STABLE ISCHEMIC HEART DISEASE

LIPID LEVELS

Low-density lipoprotein (LDL) and high-density lipoprotein (HDL) cholesterol
Triglyceride level
*LDL electrophoresis (especially apoprotein B and small dense LDL)
*Lipoprotein (a)
*Lipoprotein-associated phospholipase (Lp-PLA2)

METABOLIC EVALUATION

Fasting plasma glucose
Serum creatinine
Thyroxine level
*Hemoglobin A_{1c} in patients with known or suspected diabetes

MARKERS OF INFLAMMATION OR CARDIAC FUNCTION

*High-sensitivity C-reactive protein (hs-CRP)
*Brain natriuretic peptide (BNP)

PROTHROMBOTIC ASSESSMENT

Plasma fibrinogen
Platelet count
*Factor V Leiden
*D-dimer
*Plasminogen activator inhibitor (PAI) type 1

TO ASSESS OTHER POTENTIAL CARDIAC RISK FACTORS

*Serum homocysteine

Chapter 56) or positron-emission tomography (PET; Chapter 56) (Fig. 71-3) is a useful and clinically important approach to establishing the diagnosis and prognosis in patients with stable ischemic heart disease. The predictive accuracy of these tests is defined not only by their sensitivity and specificity but also by the prevalence of disease (or pretest probability) in the population under study. Noninvasive testing should be performed only if the incremental information is likely to alter the planned management strategy. Thus, the value of noninvasive stress testing is greatest when the pretest likelihood is intermediate because the test result is likely to have the greatest effect on the post-test probability of coronary artery disease and, hence, on clinical decision making.

Each noninvasive test has a sensitivity and specificity (Table 71-5), which, when combined with a patient's pretest probability (see Table 71-1), can yield a post-test probability for coronary artery disease (Fig. 71-4). The choice among tests depends on the patient's characteristics (Table 71-6).

Exercise Electrocardiography

An exercise ECG is the preferred test in patients who have suspected angina pectoris and are considered to have a moderate probability of coronary artery disease if the resting ECG is normal (i.e., ST segments are not obscured by structural heart disease or medication), provided that subjects are capable of achieving an adequate workload. Interpretation of the exercise ECG should include the exercise capacity achieved (duration and metabolic equivalents of the external workload; see Table 50-3 in Chapter 50), the magnitude and extent of ST segment deviation, and clinical and hemodynamic responses to exercise.

The exercise test protocol is usually adjusted to a patient's tolerance, aiming for 6 to 12 minutes of exercise time (i.e., Bruce protocol stages II to

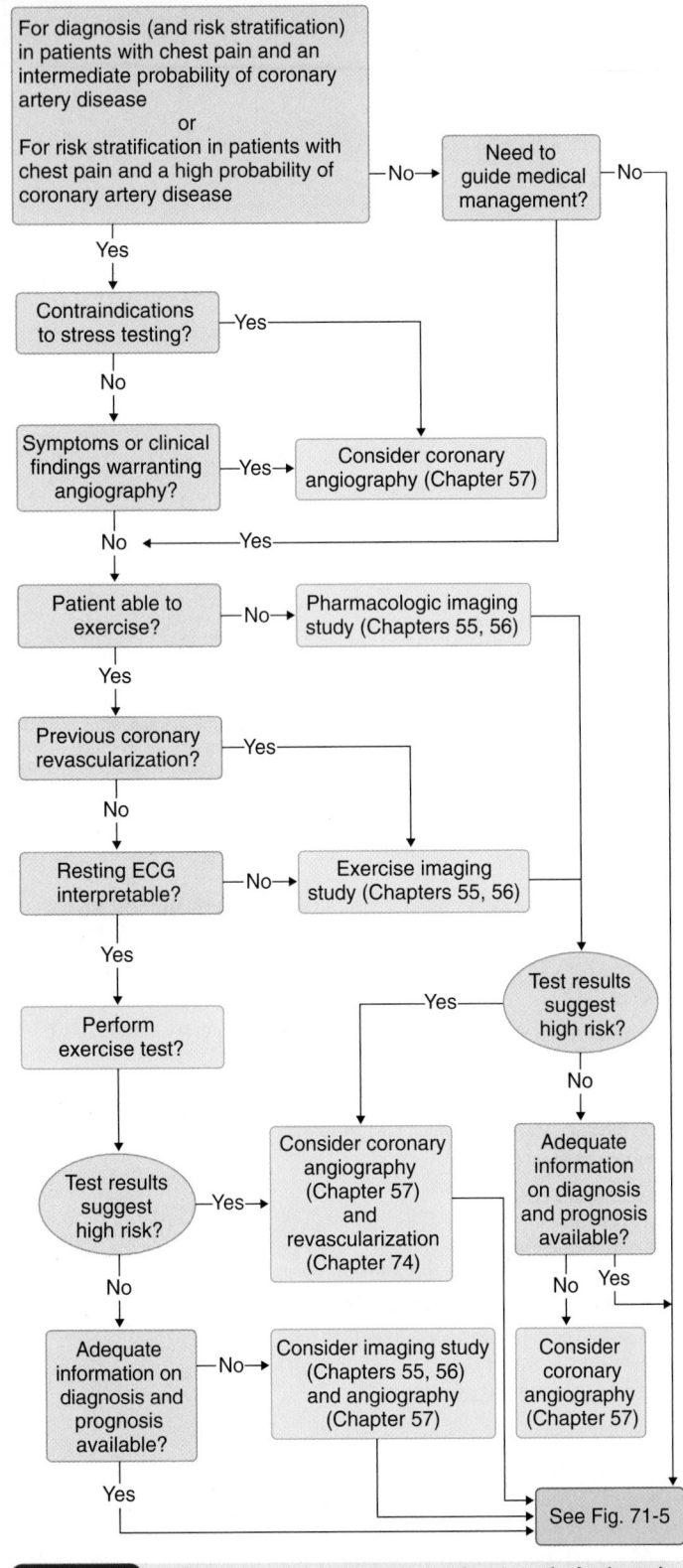

FIGURE 71-3. Approach to the use of stress testing and angiography for the evaluation of chronic stable angina. ECG = electrocardiogram. (Modified from American College of Cardiology/American Heart Association Task Force on Practice Guidelines. *Management of Patients with Chronic Stable Angina. ACC/AHA/ACP-ASIM Pocket Guidelines.* Philadelphia: Elsevier Science; 2000.)

TABLE 71-5   APPROXIMATE SENSITIVITY AND SPECIFICITY OF COMMON TESTS TO DIAGNOSE CORONARY ARTERY DISEASE

	SENSITIVITY	SPECIFICITY
EXERCISE ELECTROCARDIOGRAPHY		
>1 mm ST depression	0.70	0.75
>2 mm ST depression	0.33	0.97
>3 mm ST depression	0.20	0.99
PERFUSION SCINTIGRAPHY		
Exercise SPECT	0.88	0.72
Pharmacologic SPECT	0.90	0.82
ECHOCARDIOGRAPHY		
Exercise	0.85	0.81
Pharmacologic stress	0.81	0.79
PET	0.95	0.95

PET = positron emission tomography; SPECT = single-photon emission computed tomography. From Gibbons RJ, Abrams J, Chatterjee K, et al. ACC/AHA 2002 guideline update for the management of patients with chronic stable angina—summary article: a report of the American College of Cardiology/American Heart Association Task Force on Practice Guidelines (Committee on Management of Patients with Chronic Stable Angina). *Circulation.* 2003;107:149-158.

TABLE 71-6   SUGGESTED NONINVASIVE TESTS IN DIFFERENT TYPES OF PATIENTS WITH STABLE ANGINA

Exertional angina, mixed angina, walk-through angina, postprandial angina with or without prior myocardial infarction	
Normal resting ECG	Treadmill exercise ECG test
Abnormal, uninterpretable resting ECG	Exercise myocardial perfusion scintigraphy (^{201}Tl, ^{99m}Tc-sestamibi) or exercise echocardiography
Unsuitable for exercise	Dipyridamole, adenosine, or regadenoson myocardial perfusion scintigraphy, dobutamine stress echocardiography
Atypical chest pain with normal or borderline abnormal resting ECG or with nondiagnostic stress ECG, particularly in women	Exercise myocardial perfusion scintigraphy, exercise echocardiography
Vasospastic angina	ECG during chest pain, ST segment ambulatory ECG, exercise test
Dilated ischemic cardiomyopathy with typical angina or for assessment of hibernating or stunned myocardium	Regional and global ejection fraction by radionuclide ventriculography or two-dimensional echocardiography, radionuclide myocardial perfusion scintigraphy; in selected patients, flow and metabolic studies with positron emission tomography
Syndrome X	Treadmill exercise stress ECG, coronary blood flow by positron emission tomography, Doppler probe
Known severe aortic stenosis or severe hypertrophic cardiomyopathy with stable angina	Exercise stress tests contraindicated; dipyridamole, adenosine, or regadenoson myocardial perfusion scintigraphy in selected patients; coronary angiography preferred
Mild aortic valvar disease or hypertrophic cardiomyopathy with typical exertional angina	"Prudent" treadmill myocardial perfusion scintigraphy, dipyridamole or adenosine or regadenoson myocardial perfusion scintigraphy

ECG = 12-lead electrocardiogram. Modified from Braunwald E, Goldman L, eds. *Primary Care Cardiology,* 2nd ed. Philadelphia: WB Saunders; 2003.

IV) to achieve maximal oxygen consumption and to elicit objective evidence of inducible ischemia, if present. Exercise stress testing is generally very safe, with death or MI occurring in less than one case per 2500 tests, when such provocative testing is avoided in patients with severe aortic stenosis, severe hypertension, or uncontrolled heart failure. Other contraindications are acute MI, symptomatic arrhythmias, acute pulmonary embolism, and suspected acute aortic dissection. Relative contraindications are hypertension greater than 200 mm Hg systolic or 110 mm Hg diastolic, hypertrophic cardiomyopathy, and high-degree atrioventricular block.

FIGURE 71-4. Approximate probabilities of coronary artery disease in different patient groups. **A,** Approximate probability of coronary artery disease before and after noninvasive testing in a patient with typical angina pectoris. These percentages demonstrate how the sequential use of an electrocardiogram (ECG) and an exercise thallium test may affect the probability of coronary artery disease in a patient with typical angina pectoris. **B,** Approximate probability of coronary artery disease before and after noninvasive testing in a patient with atypical angina symptoms. **C,** Approximate probability of coronary artery disease before and after noninvasive testing in an asymptomatic subject in the coronary artery disease age range. (Redrawn from Branch WB Jr, ed. *Office Practice of Medicine,* 3rd ed. Philadelphia: WB Saunders; 1994:45.)

Concomitant antianginal therapy (notably the use of β-blockers) reduces the sensitivity of exercise testing as a screening tool. If the purpose of the exercise test is to diagnose ischemia, it should be performed, whenever possible, before initiating β-blockers, or 2 to 3 days after their discontinuation.

Nuclear Cardiology Imaging

Stress myocardial perfusion imaging (Chapter 56) using single-photon emission computed tomography (SPECT) with simultaneous electrocardiographic testing (see Fig. 56-1 in Chapter 56) is particularly helpful in the diagnosis of coronary artery disease in patients with abnormal resting ECGs and among those in whom ST segment responses cannot be interpreted accurately, such as patients with repolarization abnormalities caused by LV hypertrophy, those with left bundle branch block, and those receiving digitalis. Its sensitivity and specificity are superior to exercise

electrocardiography alone in detecting coronary artery disease, especially multivessel disease, in identifying regional perfusion defects that may localize to and correlate with diseased vessels, and in delineating the magnitude and extent of ischemic and infarcted myocardium. Treadmill testing is preferred for patients who are capable of performing such physical activity because of the additional diagnostic and prognostic information achieved with graded exercise. In the 40 to 50% of patients who are unable to exercise adequately, however, pharmacologic vasodilator stress with dipyridamole, adenosine, or regadenoson may be the preferred approach to noninvasive testing.

Stress Echocardiography

Stress two-dimensional echocardiography using exercise or pharmacologic stress can detect regional ischemia by identifying new wall motion abnormalities (see Fig. 55-5 in Chapter 55). Additional clinical information regarding associated structural heart disease, chamber dimensions, and valve function can be readily obtained. Exercise echocardiography can detect the presence of coronary artery disease with a similar accuracy as achieved with stress myocardial perfusion imaging and is useful for localizing and quantifying ischemic myocardial segments. Pharmacologic stress is usually performed with dobutamine in patients who are unable to exercise and in those unable to achieve adequate heart rates with exercise.

Ambulatory Ischemic Monitoring

Patients with symptomatic myocardial ischemia have episodes of silent ischemia that occur with the activities of daily living and are detectable on ambulatory monitoring but go unrecognized clinically because of the absence of angina or anginal equivalents. Although such "silent myocardial ischemia" may be detected during 24-hour ambulatory ECG recordings and may provide a quantitative estimate of the frequency and duration of ischemic episodes, its sensitivity for detecting coronary artery disease is much less reliable than that of exercise ECG.

Stress Cardiac Magnetic Resonance Imaging

Pharmacologic stress perfusion with CMR imaging is becoming increasingly available in many centers and may provide additional diagnostic capability in detecting the presence of structural heart disease, in addition to suspected coronary artery disease. CMR with gadolinium enhancement is the most accurate way to diagnose a scar from a prior MI (see Fig. 56-7 in Chapter 56).

Chest Roentgenography

Unless there is no history of prior MI, heart failure, or structural heart disease, the chest radiograph (Chapter 53) is usually normal in patients with chronic angina or stable ischemic heart disease. If an enlarged cardiac silhouette is present, it is generally indicative of a previous MI with LV dilation and cardiac remodeling. Other causes of cardiomegaly include long-standing hypertension, concomitant valvular heart disease, pericardial effusion, or nonischemic cardiomyopathy.

Cardiac Computed Tomographic Angiography

Cardiac computed tomographic angiography (CCTA; Chapter 56) is a highly sensitive method to detect coronary calcification (see Fig. 56-2 in Chapter 56), which is strongly associated with coronary atherosclerosis and can also provide noninvasive angiography of the proximal coronary arteries. Although coronary calcification is a highly sensitive (approximately 90%) finding in patients with coronary artery disease, the specificity for identifying patients with obstructive coronary artery disease is much lower (approximately 50%). Because of the potential unnecessary testing from false-positive results, CCTA is currently not recommended as a routine screening approach for suspected obstructive coronary artery disease in individuals at low risk (<10% 10-year estimated risk of coronary events). CCTA can be coupled with PET imaging in a hybrid PET and computed tomography scanner, which can provide a quantitative assessment of coronary anatomy along with regional myocardial blood flow and cardiac metabolism.

Diagnostic Coronary Angiography

Despite the continued evolution of noninvasive diagnostic testing, invasive coronary angiography (Chapter 57) remains the gold standard for anatomic definition of coronary artery disease. Among patients with the clinical diagnosis of stable ischemic heart disease referred for coronary angiography, a 70% or more luminal diameter narrowing is found in one (about 25%), two (about 25%), or all three (about 25%) epicardial coronary arteries, in about 75% of cases; another 5 to 10% of patients have obstruction of the left main

TABLE 71-7   CORONARY ANGIOGRAPHY FOR DIAGNOSIS AND RISK STRATIFICATION IN PATIENTS WITH CHRONIC ANGINA AND STABLE ISCHEMIC HEART DISEASE

FOR INITIAL DIAGNOSTIC INDICATION

Recommended on the basis of evidence or general consensus
Patients with suspected angina and evidence of intermediate-high risk, moderate-severe ischemia on noninvasive testing, or a changing angina pattern who have survived sudden cardiac death or serious ventricular arrhythmia

Weight of evidence or opinion is in favor
Uncertain diagnosis after noninvasive testing, and the benefit of a more certain diagnosis outweighs the risk and cost of coronary angiography
Inability to undergo noninvasive testing because of disability, illness, or morbid obesity
Occupational requirement for a definitive diagnosis
Suspected nonatherosclerotic cause of myocardial ischemia
Suspicion of a coronary spasm
High pretest probability of left main or three-vessel disease
Recurrent hospitalization for chest pain in the absence of definitive diagnosis
Overriding desire for a definitive diagnosis and a greater than low probability of CAD

Not recommended
Significant comorbidity in patients in whom the risk of coronary arteriography outweighs the benefit of the procedure
Overriding personal desire for a definitive diagnosis and a low probability of CAD

FOR INITIAL RISK STRATIFICATION OR TREATMENT INDICATION

Recommended on the basis of evidence or general consensus
With disabling (CCS class III and class IV) chronic stable angina despite medical therapy
With high-risk criteria on noninvasive testing regardless of anginal severity
Patients with angina who have survived sudden cardiac death or serious ventricular arrhythmia
Angina and symptoms and signs of congestive heart failure
Clinical characteristics that indicate a high likelihood of severe CAD

Weight of evidence or opinion is in favor
Significant left ventricular dysfunction (EF < 45%), CCS class I or class II angina, and demonstrable ischemia but less than high-risk criteria on noninvasive testing
High-risk criteria suggesting ischemia on noninvasive testing
Inadequate prognostic information after noninvasive testing
Clinical characteristics that indicate a high likelihood of severe CAD
CCS class I or class II angina, preserved left ventricular function (EF > 45%), and less than high-risk criteria on noninvasive testing
CCS class III or class IV angina that improves to class I or class II with medical therapy
CCS class I or class II angina but intolerance (unacceptable side effects) to adequate medical therapy

Not recommended
CCS class I or class II angina in patients who respond to medical therapy and who have no evidence of ischemia on noninvasive testing
Patients who prefer to avoid revascularization after adequate explanation

CAD = coronary artery disease; CCS = Canadian Cardiovascular Society; CHD = coronary heart disease; EF = ejection fraction.
Modified from Gibbons RJ, Abrams J, Chatterjee K, et al. ACC/AHA 2002 guideline update for the management of patients with chronic stable angina—summary article: a report of the American College of Cardiology/American Heart Association Task Force on Practice Guidelines (Committee on Management of Patients with Chronic Stable Angina). *Circulation.* 2003;107:149-158.

coronary artery; and the remaining 15 to 20% have no flow-limiting coronary obstructions. These data emphasize the persisting role of coronary angiography for diagnostic purposes (Table 71-7), but angiography is also helpful for risk stratification in patients with clear-cut angina and ischemic heart disease. In patients with less severe coronary stenoses (i.e., 50 to 70% on angiography), coronary intravascular ultrasonography (see Fig. 57-7 in Chapter 57) can substantially enhance the quantification of obstruction and vulnerability of the coronary atheroma to future instability. A pressure wire positioned proximal and distal to a coronary stenosis can measure the severity of the stenosis and determine whether functionally significant flow reduction may be ameliorated by myocardial revascularization.

Differential Diagnosis of Angina

Many common noncardiac disorders may present with clinical features that can be confused with angina pectoris (see Table 50-2 in Chapter 50). In some instances, symptoms may be indistinguishable from ischemic heart disease. For example, many patients with angina have coexisting esophageal disorders (Chapter 140), and both angina and esophageal discomfort may be relieved by nitroglycerin (Chapter 50). A distinguishing feature from angina is that esophageal discomfort is often relieved by antacids, proton pump inhibitors, or food.

Costochondritis can mimic angina but can typically be distinguished by the presence of well-localized pain on palpation. However, pressure, if applied too firmly to the anterior chest wall during examination of a patient with suspected angina pectoris, may elicit symptoms of discomfort even in normal subjects. Cervical radiculopathy may cause pain radiating to the shoulders, neck, or upper arms and can be confused with angina. However, this condition typically causes a constant ache that is often exacerbated by neck movement or rotation and may be accompanied by a focal sensory deficit or radiculopathy.

Pulmonary hypertension (Chapter 68) can cause exertional chest discomfort that may share many of the characteristics of angina pectoris. It is believed that right ventricular ischemia during physical exertion may cause this discomfort along with associated symptoms of exertional dyspnea, dizziness, and syncope. Findings on physical examination typically include a parasternal lift, a loud (and sometimes palpable) pulmonary component of the second heart sound, and findings of right ventricular hypertrophy on ECG.

Chest pain may also be an important presenting clinical feature of pulmonary embolism (Chapter 98). Physical findings typically include tachycardia and tachypnea, an accentuated pulmonic component of the second heart sound, and occasionally a right-sided S_4 gallop. Pleuritic discomfort suggests pulmonary infarction, whereas a history of pain exacerbated by inspiration or deep breathing, along with a pleural friction rub, usually helps distinguish it from angina pectoris.

Acute pericarditis (Chapter 77) may be confused with the discomfort of angina pectoris, but pericarditis tends to cause chest pain that is generally sharp, is not relieved by rest or nitroglycerin, is exacerbated by movement or deep breathing, and is associated with a pericardial friction rub that may be evanescent. Aortic dissection (Chapter 78), which may present with acute, severe chest pain, may be confused with an acute MI but generally not with angina.

Risk Stratification

Clinical and noninvasive criteria can be used in a complementary fashion to refine the estimate of risk for the individual patient with stable ischemic heart disease (Table 71-8). Clinical characteristics that include age, male sex, diabetes mellitus, previous MI, and the presence of symptoms typical of angina are predictive of the presence of coronary artery disease. Heart failure and LV dysfunction (generally defined by an ejection fraction < 50%), the severity and extent of angina, and associated symptoms such as dyspnea are also important predictors of outcome in patients with stable ischemic heart disease.

The simple classification of disease into single-, double-, or triple-vessel or left main coronary artery disease remains the most widely used approach (Table 71-9). Additional prognostic information is provided by the severity and extent of coronary luminal narrowing and its location. For example, high-grade lesions of the left main coronary artery or its equivalent, as defined by severe proximal left anterior descending and proximal left circumflex coronary artery disease, are particularly life-threatening. The SYNTAX trial has permitted the identification of subsets of coronary artery disease patients into three tertiles of low-, moderate-, and high-risk anatomic findings, based on multiple lesional characteristics (see Tables 71-8 and 71-9). It should be kept in mind, however, that the plaque causing the most severe chronic stenosis is not necessarily the one that will subsequently rupture to cause acute coronary syndrome or acute MI.

TREATMENT   Rx

Comprehensive management of angina and stable ischemic heart disease (Fig. 71-5) entails multiple therapeutic approaches to the identification and treatment of associated diseases that can precipitate or worsen angina and ischemia (Table 71-10): cardiac risk factor identification and intervention; application of pharmacologic and nonpharmacologic interventions for secondary prevention; pharmacologic and symptomatic management of angina and ischemia; and myocardial revascularization with percutaneous coronary intervention (PCI) or coronary artery bypass graft (CABG) surgery, when indicated (Table 71-11). A multidimensional management approach integrates all of these considerations, often simultaneously, in each patient. Among pharmacotherapies, three drug classes are classified as being "disease modifying" in that they have been demonstrated to reduce mortality and morbidity in patients with stable ischemic heart disease and preserved LV function: aspirin,

TABLE 71-8 USING THE RESULTS OF NONINVASIVE RISK STRATIFICATION TO GUIDE CLINICAL DECISION MAKING

HIGH RISK (>3% ANNUAL MORTALITY RATE)

Severe resting left ventricular dysfunction (LVEF < 35%)
High-risk treadmill score (≤ −11)*
Severe exercise left ventricular dysfunction (exercise LVEF < 35%)
Stress-induced large perfusion defect (particularly if anterior)
Stress-induced multiple perfusion defects of moderate size
Large, fixed perfusion defect with left ventricular dilation or increased lung uptake (^{201}Tl)
Stress-induced moderate perfusion defect with left ventricular dilation or increased lung uptake (^{201}Tl)
Echocardiographic wall motion abnormality (involving more than two segments) developing at low dose of dobutamine or at a low heart rate (<120 beats/min)
Stress echocardiographic evidence of extensive ischemia

INTERMEDIATE RISK (1-3% ANNUAL MORTALITY RATE)

Mild to moderate resting left ventricular dysfunction (LVEF = 35-49%)
Intermediate-risk treadmill score (−11 < score < 5)*
Stress-induced moderate perfusion defect without left ventricular dilation or increased lung intake (^{201}Tl)
Limited stress echocardiographic ischemia with a wall motion abnormality only at higher doses of dobutamine involving two segments or less

LOW RISK (<1% ANNUAL MORTALITY RATE)

Low-risk treadmill score (≥ 5)*
Normal or small myocardial perfusion defect at rest or with stress†
Normal stress echocardiographic wall motion or no change of limited resting wall motion abnormalities during stress†

*Score = (duration of exercise in minutes) − (5 × mm of ST segment depression) − (4 × angina score), where 0 = no angina, 1 = nonlimiting angina, and 2 = angina that causes discontinuation of the test.
†Although the published data are limited, patients with these findings will probably not be at low risk in the presence of either a high-risk treadmill score or severe resting left ventricular dysfunction (LVEF < 35%).
LVEF = left ventricular ejection fraction.
From Gibbons RJ, Abrams J, Chatterjee K, et al. ACC/AHA 2002 guideline update for the management of patients with chronic stable angina—summary article: a report of the American College of Cardiology/American Heart Association Task Force on practice guidelines (Committee on the Management of Patients with Chronic Stable Angina). *J Am Coll Cardiol.* 2003;41:159-168.

TABLE 71-9 CORONARY ARTERY DISEASE PROGNOSTIC INDEX

EXTENT OF CORONARY ARTERY DISEASE	5-YEAR MORTALITY RATE (%)*
1-vessel disease, 75%	7
>1-vessel disease, 50-74%	7
1-vessel disease, ≥95%	9
2-vessel disease	12
2-vessel disease, both ≥95%	14
1-vessel disease, ≥95% proximal LAD	17
2-vessel disease, ≥95% LAD	17
2-vessel disease, ≥95% proximal LAD	21
3-vessel disease	21
3-vessel disease, ≥95% in at least 1	27
3-vessel disease, 75% proximal LAD	33
3-vessel disease, ≥95% proximal LAD	41

*Assuming medical treatment only.
LAD = left anterior descending coronary artery.
From Califf RM, Armstrong PW, Carver JR, et al. Task Force 5: stratification of patients into high, medium and low risk subgroups for purposes of risk factor management. *J Am Coll Cardiol.* 1996;27:1007-1019.

angiotensin-converting enzyme (ACE) inhibition, and effective lipid lowering. Other therapies such as nitrates, β-blockers, calcium antagonists, and ranolazine have been shown to improve angina, exercise performance, and reduce ischemia, but have not been proved to reduce mortality in patients with stable ischemic heart disease.

Disease-Modifying Therapies

Careful attention to lifestyle and the management of coronary risk factors is essential (Fig. 71-6). Such secondary prevention strategies can reduce the risk of progressive coronary disease, morbidity, and mortality.

Drugs That Alter Lipid Metabolism

Each 1% increase in the LDL cholesterol level results in a 2 to 3% increase in risk for coronary events (Chapter 51). Large, randomized clinical trials in patients with ischemic heart disease have shown a consistent and significant reduction in mortality and cardiac events with statin therapy (Chapter 213). Patients with stable angina should routinely be treated with statins to a target of less than 70 mg/dL [1] using any of a variety of specific statin drugs (see Table 213-5 in Chapter 213).

Gemfibrozil, a fibrate at 1200 mg daily, can reduce fatal and nonfatal MI in men who have coronary heart disease and normal levels of LDL cholesterol but who also have low levels of HDL cholesterol and elevated triglycerides, [2] but fibrates have not been shown to reduce overall mortality despite about a 10% reduction in major cardiovascular events. [3] Other cholesterol-lowering agents such as ezetimibe or bile acid sequestrants can be used instead of statins in those who are intolerant or can be added to high-dose statins in those in whom the LDL goal has not been achieved, but there are no studies to indicate whether these agents reduce cardiac events or mortality.

Each 1-mg/dL decline in HDL cholesterol is associated with a 2 to 3% increase in the risk of MI and death from cardiac causes. Nicotinic acid raises HDL cholesterol by about 25 to 30% on an average at doses of 1 to 2 g/day, but its use has been limited by side effects, notably flushing. Nicotinic acid reduces carotid artery intimal media thickness, a surrogate for atherosclerotic progression, but clinical outcomes data are lacking. Cholesteryl ester transfer protein inhibitors may be quite effective in raising HDL levels but have had no benefit in clinical trials to date.

Angiotensin-Converting Enzyme Inhibitors

ACE inhibitor administration (see Table 67-5 in Chapter 67) reduces cardiac events, cardiovascular mortality, and all-cause mortality in patients with risk factors for or with previously diagnosed coronary artery disease, [1][4] including high-risk patients with vascular disease or diabetes and patients with stable coronary artery disease and no clinical evidence of heart failure. By contrast, ACE inhibitors do not appear to prevent future cardiac events in post-MI patients with preserved LV function. Whether angiotensin receptor blockers have similar benefits in patients with chronic angina and stable ischemic heart disease is not yet known.

Antiplatelet Agents and Anticoagulants

Aspirin reduces the risk of adverse cardiovascular events by 33% in patients with stable angina. The reduction in vascular events is comparable for doses of 75 to 150 mg daily and 160 to 325 mg daily, but daily doses of less than 75 mg have less benefit. [5] Therefore, in the absence of contraindications, aspirin, 75 to 325 mg once daily, should be administered routinely in all patients with angina and stable ischemic heart disease.

Clopidogrel (Chapter 37), which is the most widely used thienopyridine in the treatment of patients with coronary artery disease, is of proven benefit when combined with aspirin to reduce the composite end point of death, MI, or stroke in patients after an acute coronary event. The standard regimen is an initial loading dose of 300 to 600 mg orally, followed by a maintenance dose of 75 mg daily. In patients with angina and stable ischemic heart disease, however, adding clopidogrel to low-dose (75 to 162 mg/day) aspirin does not reduce the primary composite end point of MI, stroke, or death from cardiovascular causes, [6] so clopidogrel should be reserved for patients who cannot tolerate aspirin or who have had an acute coronary event (Chapter 72) or a stent implantation (Chapter 74). Prasugrel is a new thienopyridine that is approved in patients with ACS and in those who undergo PCI with stent placement, but it has not yet been studied in the medical management of patients with chronic angina and stable coronary artery disease.

Warfarin is generally as effective as aspirin for preventing coronary events in patients with angina and is preferred over aspirin for patients with concomitant atrial fibrillation (Chapter 66), but it is associated with a higher risk of bleeding. Combination therapy with warfarin plus aspirin is superior to aspirin alone if the international normalized ratio is maintained above 2.0, but the benefit of the combination must be weighed against a 1 per 100 patient years risk of bleeding. [7] Anticoagulants are more commonly used in Europe than in America.

Therapeutic Agents to Reduce Angina and Ischemia

The goal of antianginal therapy is to reduce symptoms of cardiac ischemia and to improve quality of life. β-Blockers, which prevent the binding of catecholamines to the β-adrenergic receptor, lower heart rate and myocardial contractility, thereby reducing myocardial workload, myocardial oxygen demand, and ischemia and anginal symptoms. β-Blockers raise the ischemic threshold and delay or prevent the onset of angina with exercise. β-Blockers also reduce the rate of secondary cardiac events and sudden cardiac death in post-MI patients, but there have been no placebo-controlled outcome trials in angina patients. All β-blockers appear to be equally effective in patients with chronic stable angina (Table 71-12). The β-blocker dose should be titrated to a target resting heart rate of 50 to 60 beats per minute as tolerated by the patient.

Calcium-channel blockers (Table 71-13) reduce afterload owing to their peripheral vasodilatory effects and thus lower myocardial workload and myocardial oxygen demand. Calcium-channel blockers also reduce coronary vascular resistance and inhibit coronary vasospasm by preventing coronary arterial smooth muscle contraction. This favorable reduction in myocardial oxygen demand, coupled with an increase in myocardial oxygen supply, results in a reduction in angina and ischemia. Nondihydropyridine calcium-channel blockers, such as verapamil and diltiazem, also reduce heart rate.

Conversely, dihydropyridine calcium channel antagonists, such as amlodipine, have greater effect on vascular smooth muscle, are better peripheral and coronary vasodilators, and hence may have advantages for use in the hypertensive patient with angina. In randomized clinical trials, calcium-channel blockers and β-blockers are generally equally effective in relieving angina, improving time to onset of angina, and improving time to ischemic ST depression during exercise. Because calcium-channel blockers have not been shown to reduce death or MI in patients with stable or previously unstable ischemic heart disease, these agents are usually used in patients who cannot tolerate β-blockers or who require additional pharmacotherapy to control their symptoms. When used with β-blockers, care must be taken not to cause symptomatic bradycardia with verapamil and diltiazem. When used alone, diltiazem is

FIGURE 71-5. Algorithm for the treatment of stable angina. AS = aortic stenosis; CABG = coronary artery bypass graft; CAD = coronary artery disease; MI = myocardial infarction; NTG = nitroglycerin; PTCA = percutaneous transluminal coronary angioplasty. (Modified from American College of Cardiology/American Heart Association Task Force on Practice Guidelines. *Management of Patients with Chronic Stable Angina. ACC/AHA/ACP-ASIM Pocket Guidelines.* Philadelphia: Elsevier Science; 2000.)

TABLE 71-10 TREATMENT OF PATIENTS WITH STABLE ANGINA

GENERAL MEASURES

Rule out and control aggravating conditions
    Associated noncardiac diseases
    Associated cardiac disease
    Use of drugs aggravating angina
Smoking cessation
Dietary counseling for body weight and lipid control
Exercise prescription
Treat to targets
    Hypertension
    Blood lipids
    Diabetes

PHARMACOLOGIC THERAPY: RECOMMENDATIONS FOR PHARMACOTHERAPY TO PREVENT MI AND DEATH AND TO REDUCE SYMPTOMS

Recommended on the basis of evidence or general consensus
Aspirin in the absence of contraindications
β-Blockers as initial therapy in the absence of contraindications in patients with prior MI or without prior MI
Angiotensin-converting enzyme inhibitor in all patients with CAD who also have diabetes or left ventricular systolic dysfunction
Low-density lipoprotein-lowering therapy in patients with documented or suspected CAD and LDL cholesterol greater than 130 mg/dL, with a target LDL of less than 100 mg/dL
Sublingual nitroglycerin or nitroglycerin spray for the immediate relief of angina
Calcium-channel antagonists or long-acting nitrates as initial therapy for reduction of symptoms when β-blockers are contraindicated
Calcium-channel antagonists or long-acting nitrates in combination with β-blockers when initial treatment with β-blockers is not successful
Calcium-channel antagonists and long-acting nitrates as a substitute for β-blockers if initial treatment with β-blockers leads to unacceptable side effects

Weight of evidence or opinion is in favor
Clopidogrel when aspirin is contraindicated
Long-acting nondihydropyridine calcium-channel antagonists instead of β-blockers as initial therapy
In patients with documented or suspected CAD and LDL cholesterol level of 100 to 129 mg/dL, several therapeutic options are available (Level of Evidence: B)
Lifestyle and/or drug therapies to lower LDL to less than 100 mg/dL
Weight reduction and increased physical activity in persons with the metabolic syndrome
Institution of treatment of other lipid or nonlipid risk factors; consider use of nicotinic acid or fibric acid for elevated triglycerides or low HDL cholesterol
Angiotensin-converting enzyme inhibitor in patients with CAD or other vascular disease

Usefulness unclear
Low-intensity anticoagulation with warfarin in addition to aspirin

Not recommended
Dipyridamole
Chelation therapy

CAD = coronary artery disease; HDL = high-density lipoprotein; LDL = low-density lipoprotein; MI = myocardial infarction.
From Gibbons RJ, Abrams J, Chatterjee K, et al. ACC/AHA 2002 guideline update for the management of patients with chronic stable angina—summary article: a report of the American College of Cardiology/American Heart Association Task Force on practice guidelines (Committee on the Management of Patients with Chronic Stable Angina). *J Am Coll Cardiol.* 2003;41:159-168.

TABLE 71-11 CURRENT RECOMMENDATIONS FOR MYOCARDIAL REVASCULARIZATION IN PATIENTS WITH CHRONIC STABLE ANGINA

CABG SURGERY VERSUS MEDICAL THERAPY

Among patients with medically refractory angina pectoris, CABG surgery is indicated for symptom improvement.

Among patients with medically stable angina pectoris, CABG surgery is indicated to prolong life in left main coronary artery disease or three-vessel disease (regardless of left ventricular function) and, possibly, to help symptoms.

CABG surgery may be indicated for prolongation of life if the proximal left anterior descending coronary artery is involved (regardless of the number of diseased vessels).

CABG surgery may reduce the composite end point of death, myocardial infarction, or stroke in diabetic patients with extensive multivessel (two- to three-vessel) coronary artery disease compared with medical therapy.

PCI VERSUS MEDICAL THERAPY

For the initial management of patients with stable ischemic heart disease, PCI does not reduce the risk of death, myocardial infarction, or other major cardiovascular events when added to optimal medical therapy.

Among patients with medically refractory angina pectoris, PCI is indicated for symptom improvement.

PCI may be indicated in the presence of severe myocardial ischemia, regardless of symptoms. PCI does not appear to improve survival compared with medical treatment among patients with one- or two-vessel disease.

In the absence of symptoms or myocardial ischemia, PCI is not indicated (merely for the presence of an anatomic stenosis).

PCI VERSUS CABG SURGERY

For single-vessel disease, PCI and CABG surgery provide excellent symptom relief, but repeated revascularization procedures are required more frequently after PCI. Intracoronary stenting is preferred to regular PCI, but direct comparison with CABG surgery is limited.

For treated diabetic patients with two- or three-vessel disease, CABG surgery is the treatment of choice.

For nondiabetic patients, multivessel PCI and CABG surgery are acceptable alternatives. The choice of PCI or CABG surgery for initial treatment depends primarily on local expertise and the patient's and physician's preferences.

In general, PCI is preferred for patients at low risk and CABG surgery for patients at high risk.

CABG = coronary artery bypass graft; PCI = percutaneous coronary intervention.

---

or tachyphylaxis, an 8- to 12-hour nitrate-free interval daily is recommended. Nitroglycerin and nitrates can cause vasodilation-induced headache, a decrease in blood pressure, and, more rarely, severe hypotension with bradycardia due to activation of the vagal Bezold-Jarisch reflex. Because the vasodilation by nitroglycerin is markedly exaggerated and prolonged in the presence of the phosphodiesterase inhibitors sildenafil (Viagra), vardenafil (Levitra), and tadalafil (Cialis), these agents and nitrates should not be used concurrently.

Ranolazine (initiated at a dose of 500 mg twice daily and titrated up to a maximal dose of 1000 mg twice daily) is the newest U.S. Food and Drug Administration–approved antianginal agent and the first new drug class for angina since calcium-channel blockers were introduced clinically 30 years ago. Ranolazine acts by reducing intracellular calcium overload in ischemic myocytes by inhibiting late inward sodium current entry. The net effect of reduced late inward sodium current is a reduction in LV wall tension and myocardial oxygen demand, thereby reducing angina and ischemia. Ranolazine increases exercise tolerance in patients with stable angina, reduces episodes of recurrent ischemia, and provides additional antianginal benefit in patients who are already on intensive antianginal therapy with β-blockers and calcium-channel blockers. In patients with ACS, ranolazine also reduces hemoglobin A_{1c} concentrations in diabetic patients, and it is associated with a reduction in arrhythmic events, in particular, episodes of ventricular tachycardia and atrial fibrillation.[8] Although ranolazine can minimally prolong the QT interval (on average, 6 to 8 msec), it has not been shown to increase the risk of torsades de pointes. Its precise role in the management of stable angina remains to be determined.

Nonpharmacologic Treatment

Enhanced external counterpulsation (EECP) is an alternative treatment for patients with refractory angina. EECP is generally administered as 35 sequential treatments (1 hour daily; 5 days/week) over 7 weeks. EECP does not reduce ischemia on myocardial perfusion imaging, and the mechanisms underlying

---

often preferred because the dihydropyridine calcium-channel blockers can increase the heart rate.

Nitrates (Table 71-14) continue to be widely prescribed for antianginal treatment and are effective when administered sublingually, orally, or topically. They act as vasodilators by entering vascular smooth muscle, where they are metabolized to nitric oxide, which relaxes vascular smooth muscle, including in coronary arteries. These effects reduce angina by improving coronary blood flow. Nitrates also lower preload owing to their venodilator effects, with a resulting reduction in LV end-diastolic pressure and wall tension, which, in turn, lowers subendocardial oxygen demand. When used in patients with stable angina, nitrates improve exercise tolerance, time to onset of angina, and ST segment depression during treadmill exercise testing. Long-acting nitrates, which are frequently combined with β-blockers and calcium-channel blockers, have additive antianginal and anti-ischemic effects in patients with stable ischemic heart disease. Sublingual nitroglycerin or oral spray can terminate an angina attack and can be used as prophylaxis to prevent exertional angina. Long-acting nitrates administered orally or transdermally are used to prevent angina and to improve exercise tolerance. For avoidance of nitrate tolerance

FIGURE 71-6. Approach to lifestyle interventions and pharmacotherapy. ACE = angiotensin-converting enzyme; ARB = angiotensin receptor blocker; HbA$_{1c}$ = hemoglobin A$_{1c}$; LVEF = left ventricular ejection fraction; MI = myocardial infarction; Rx = prescribe.

its effects are poorly understood. Possible mechanisms include durable hemodynamic changes that reduce myocardial O$_2$ demand, improvement in myocardial perfusion by diastolic augmentation of retrograde coronary flow, and improved endothelial function. Although EECP increased the time to ST segment depression during exercise testing, reduced angina, and improved health-related quality of life for at least 1 year in one randomized, double-blind study of patients with chronic stable angina, its role in the treatment of angina remains unclear.[9]

Myocardial Revascularization

Coronary revascularization with either PCI or CABG (Chapter 74) can prolong life, reduce major cardiovascular events, and improve health status, quality of life, and functional capacity in selected patients with chronic, stable ischemic heart disease.

Comparisons of PCI with Optimal Medical Therapy

Randomized clinical trials comparing PCI with medical therapy in patients with stable coronary heart disease are few in number, and many recruited patients predominantly with single-vessel disease and were completed before the routine use of coronary stenting and contemporary aggressive preventive medical therapy. In general, these studies showed benefits of PCI in terms of symptoms[10] but not in terms of subsequent MI or death.[11] In the most recent trial of modern PCI (the Clinical Outcomes Utilizing Revascularization and Aggressive druG Evaluation [COURAGE] trial), including stents, versus aggressive medical therapy, there were no significant differences in the composite primary outcome of all-cause mortality or

nonfatal MI or in stroke or hospitalization for ACS between the two strategies during a 2.5- to 7.0-year (median, 4.6-year) follow-up period.[12] PCI improved symptoms for 2 years, especially in patients with more severe angina, but differences were no longer present at 36 months, at which time both PCI and intensive medical therapy led to better symptom control than was noted at baseline. Because PCI as an initial management strategy in patients with stable coronary artery disease does not reduce death, MI, or other major cardiovascular events when added to optimal medical therapy, the importance of preventive pharmacotherapy and lifestyle modification for secondary prevention of major cardiovascular events in patients with stable CHD must be paramount.

Comparisons of CABG with Medical Therapy

Randomized trials comparing CABG with medical therapy indicate that a greater severity of ischemia, a greater extent of disease, and the presence of LV dysfunction favor a greater magnitude of benefit of CABG over medical therapy on survival. CABG prolongs survival in patients with significant left main coronary artery disease irrespective of symptoms, in patients with multivessel coronary artery disease and impaired LV function (ejection fraction < 50%), and in patients with three-vessel coronary artery disease that includes the proximal left anterior descending coronary artery. Patients with extensive multivessel coronary artery disease appear to benefit more from CABG surgery, particularly if they also have diabetes, whereas PCI is most appropriate for patients with one- or two-vessel coronary artery disease. Of note is that these randomized trials found little difference in mortality between CABG surgery and medical therapy at 1 year, but the benefits of CABG surgery over medical therapy steadily emerged over the next 3 to 5 years. Thereafter, the benefits of CABG surgery diminished, perhaps as a result of late occlusion of saphenous vein grafts, progression of disease in the nonbypassed native coronary arteries, and increasing rates of CABG surgery in the medical group among those with high-risk anatomy and severe symptoms ("crossovers"). It is important to emphasize that very few patients in these early trials received arterial grafts (which would likely improve the long-term results of CABG surgery), aspirin to prevent graft occlusion, lipid-lowering drugs to mitigate late graft disease progression, or inhibitors of the renin-angiotensin-aldosterone system. With improvements in operative techniques, more common use of antiplatelet-agents, more intensive use of disease-modifying therapies, and more aggressive risk factor management over the past decade, the benefits of modern-day CABG surgery compared with contemporary medical therapy may have changed.

Comparisons of PCI with CABG Surgery for Multivessel Coronary Artery Disease

Of the randomized outcomes trials that have compared PCI with CABG in patients with multivessel coronary artery disease, most excluded patients with significant left main coronary artery disease and were conducted in an era before the advent of stents and other advances in PCI technology, including newer adjunctive medical therapies that are increasingly in widespread clinical use. The Bypass Angioplasty Revascularization Investigation (BARI) trial found no overall difference in survival or MI rates between percutaneous balloon angioplasty and CABG surgery at 10 years, but CABG provided a significantly better survival advantage in patients with diabetes.[13] CABG also was associated with a greater initial improvement in angina and with a diminished frequency of repeat revascularization procedures compared with balloon angioplasty. A significant survival advantage was observed in patients with previously treated diabetes who underwent CABG rather than angioplasty.

More recently, the BARI-2D trial of 2368 diabetic patients with coronary artery disease who were randomized to prompt revascularization with PCI or CABG versus delayed or no revascularization with optimal medical therapy found no significant difference for the primary end point of total mortality.[14] Thus, the BARI-2D results replicate the principal finding of the COURAGE trial[10]—namely, that an initial strategy of PCI provides no incremental clinical benefit over intensive medical therapy and lifestyle intervention alone, and that an "optimal medical therapy first" instead of a "PCI first" strategy seems justifiable in many diabetic patients with coronary disease.

In a randomized trial of CABG or PCI patients with three-vessel or left main coronary artery disease, rates of major adverse cardiac or cerebrovascular events (i.e., death from any cause, stroke, MI, or repeat revascularization) at 12 months were significantly higher in the PCI group (18% vs. 12% for CABG), in large part because of an increased rate of repeat revascularization (14% vs. 6%).[15] At 12 months, the rates of death and MI were similar between the two groups, although stroke was significantly more likely to occur with CABG (2.2% vs. 0.6% with PCI). Thus, based on these 1-year findings, CABG still is generally considered the preferred option for patients with three-vessel or left main coronary artery disease.

In summary, among those who remain symptomatic despite intensive treatment, or who have substantial ischemia or extensive coronary artery disease, revascularization with either PCI or CABG is appropriate, depending on the anatomic complexity of disease (see Table 71-11; Chapter 73). CABG surgery appears to be preferable to PCI in symptomatic patients with three-vessel or

TABLE 71-12 CLINICAL USE OF β-BLOCKERS

COMPOUND BY RECEPTOR ACTIVITY	INTRINSIC SYMPATHOMIMETIC ACTIVITY*	MEMBRANE STABILITY EFFECT	HALF-LIFE (hr)	EXCRETION	USE
β₁ AND β₂					
Propranolol	−	++	1-6	Hepatic	20-80 mg bid-tid
Propranolol long-acting	−	++	8-11	Hepatic	80-360 mg/day
Nadolol	−	−	40-80	Renal	40-80 mg/day
Pindolol	+	+	3-4	Renal	2.5-7.5 mg tid
Sotalol	−	−	7-18	Renal	40-160 mg bid
Timolol	−	−	4-5	Hepatic-renal	10-15 mg bid
β₁ SELECTIVE					
Acebutolol	+	+	3-4	Hepatic	200-600 mg bid
Atenolol	−	−	6-9	Renal	50-200 mg/day
Bisoprolol	−	−	9-12	50% renal	5-20 mg/day
Metoprolol	−	−	3-7	Hepatic	50-200 mg bid
Metoprolol long-acting	−	−	14-25	Hepatic	100-400 mg
Esmolol	−	−	4.5 min	Esterases in red cells	Bolus 500 μg/kg 50-300 μg/kg/min IV
β₁, β₂, α₂					
Labetalol	+	−	6	Hepatic	200-600 mg bid
Carvedilol	−	+	6-10	Hepatic	2.5-25 mg bid

*Presence commonly associated with maintenance of or increase in heart rate; absence associated with decrease in heart rate.
From Théroux P. Angina pectoris. In: Goldman L, Ausiello DA, eds. *Cecil Textbook of Medicine*, 23rd ed. Philadelphia: Saunders Elsevier; 2008.

TABLE 71-13 PROPERTIES OF CALCIUM-CHANNEL BLOCKING DRUGS IN CLINICAL USE

DRUGS	USUAL DOSE	ELIMINATION HALF-LIFE (HR)	Hemodynamic Effect HR	Hemodynamic Effect PVR	SIDE EFFECTS
DIHYDROPYRIDINES					
Nifedipine PA*	10-40 mg bid	10	↑↑	↓↓↓	Hypotension, dizziness, flushing, edema, constipation
Nifedipine XL*	30-120 mg/day	24	↑	↓↓	
Amlodipine	2.5-10 mg/day	30-50	=	↓↓↓	Headache, edema
Felodipine	2.5-10 mg/day	11-16	↑	↓↓↓	Headache, dizziness
Isradipine	2.5-10 mg bid	8	=	↓↓↓	Headache, fatigue
Nicardipine	20-40 mg tid	2-4	↑	↓↓↓	
Nicardipine SR*	30-60 mg bid	8-10	↑	↓↓	Headache, dizziness, flushing, edema
Nisoldipine	10-40 mg/day	7-12	=	↓↓↓	As for nifedipine
Nitrendipine	20 mg/day or bid	5-12	↑	↓↓↓	As for nifedipine
OTHERS					
Bepridil	200-400 mg/day	24-40	↓	↓	Arrhythmias, dizziness, nausea
Diltiazem	30-90 mg tid	4-6	↓	↓	Hypotension, dizziness, bradycardia, edema
Diltiazem CD*	120-540 mg/day	—	↓	↓	
Verapamil	80-160 mg tid	3-8	↓	↓↓	
Verapamil SR*	120-480 mg/day	—	↓	↓↓	Hypotension, heart failure, edema, bradycardia

*PA, XL, SR, CD: long acting.
HR = heart rate; PVR = peripheral vascular resistance.
From Théroux P. Angina pectoris. In: Goldman L, Ausiello DA, eds. *Cecil Textbook of Medicine*, 23rd ed. Philadelphia: Saunders Elsevier; 2008.

TABLE 71-14 CLINICAL USE OF NITROGLYCERIN AND NITRATES

	DOSE	DURATION OF ACTION	INDICATION
NITROGLYCERIN			
Sublingual or buccal spray	0.15-1.5 mg	Relief of angina	Before or at onset of pain
Ointment	7.5-40 mg	8-12 hr	Prophylaxis of angina
Transdermal	0.2-0.8 mg/hr	8-16 hr	Prophylaxis of angina
Intravenous	5-400 µg/hr	Ongoing; increasing doses as needed	Recurrent chest pain, systemic hypertension, left-sided heart failure
ISOSORBIDE DINITRATE			
Oral	5-40 mg tid	6-8 hr	Prophylaxis of angina
ISOSORBIDE-5-MONONITRATE			
Oral	20 mg bid	8-12 hr	Prophylaxis of angina
Oral, slow release	30-240 mg/day	12-20 hr	Prophylaxis of angina

From Théroux P. Angina pectoris. In: Goldman L, Ausiello DA, eds. *Cecil Textbook of Medicine*, 23rd ed. Philadelphia: Saunders Elsevier; 2008.

left main coronary artery disease and in diabetic patients with stable ischemic heart disease. PCI provides equivalent survival outcomes, but repeat procedures are more often needed, and symptomatic outcomes are generally not as good as after CABG.[16] Whether newer stent technologies will alter these findings remains unclear.

Other Anginal Syndromes

Variant Angina or Prinzmetal's Angina

The diagnosis of variant or Prinzmetal's angina is based on the documentation of transient ST segment elevation during an episode of chest pain in the absence of a severe, fixed coronary stenosis. Prinzmetal's variant angina typically is caused by an occlusive spasm superimposed on a nonsevere coronary artery stenosis. In some patients, however, no underlying stenoses are seen, or the underlying stenosis may be severe. Associated Raynaud's phenomenon and migraine headache have been described in some patients, suggesting that the syndrome may be part of a more generalized vasospastic disorder.

The chest pain occurs predominantly at rest, although approximately one third of patients may also experience pain during exercise. There is a predilection for the pain to wake the patient in the early morning hours when sympathetic activity is increasing. The syndrome is often cyclical, with periods of exacerbation with repetitive episodes of chest pain that may persist only for seconds or be more prolonged and severe, alternating with periods with few or no symptoms. The pain is typically relieved by nitroglycerin. The ST segment elevation accompanying the pain signifies transmural ischemia owing to total abrupt occlusion of a nonsignificant stenosis in the absence of adequate collateral circulation. The subsequent rapid reperfusion may explain the high prevalence of severe life-threatening arrhythmias.

Coronary angiography, with a provocative test for spasm such as injection of acetylcholine into the affected coronary artery, usually precipitates the syndrome. Such testing is useful to establish the diagnosis and to assess the response to therapy, especially in patients with normal or nearly normal coronary angiograms, in whom the diagnosis is otherwise unclear. Dihydropyridine calcium-channel blockers (e.g., amlodipine, 5 to 10 mg orally per day) are preferred in patients with Prinzmetal's angina.

Microvascular Angina with Normal Coronary Angiography

Angina can occur despite normal coronary arteries, even after an acetylcholine challenge. More detailed testing may reveal increased coronary resistance and an inability to increase coronary resistance and increase coronary flow in response to stimuli such as exercise, adenosine, dipyridamole, and atrial pacing.

Symptoms occur most frequently at rest and often in relation to emotional stress. Periods of exacerbation commonly alternate with symptom-free periods. The syndrome is more frequent in women, and some patients have an altered perception of pain or hypersensitivity to certain stimuli.

The diagnosis requires objective documentation of ischemia based on ST-T segment changes, a metabolic abnormality, a transient regional perfusion defect or new wall motion abnormality on echocardiography, or endothelial dysfunction that limits blood flow reserve. Abnormal endothelium-dependent vasoreactivity can be associated with regional myocardial perfusion defects on SPECT and PET imaging.

β-blockers may be useful, particularly when a relative tachycardia, hypertension, or decreased heart rate variability on Holter monitoring is present. Nitroglycerin can relieve symptoms in approximately 50% of patients, and long-acting nitrates or calcium antagonists are sometimes helpful.

The prognosis in general is favorable and not different from that of a general age-matched population in the absence of coronary artery disease. However, some studies have indicated that an ischemic response to exercise is associated with increased mortality.

Silent Myocardial Ischemia

Up to 20% of patients with ischemic heart disease may not present with angina. Such patients are often described as having silent myocardial ischemia. Some patients are totally asymptomatic despite obstructive coronary artery disease, which may be severe. Others have silent ischemia after a prior documented MI. The third and most common form occurs in patients who may also exhibit the usual forms of chronic stable angina, unstable angina, and Prinzmetal's angina. When monitored, these patients, who typically have silent ischemia episodes in addition to symptomatic ischemia, are sometimes referred to as having *mixed angina*. This mixed angina is estimated to be present in approximately one third of all treated patients with angina, although an even higher prevalence has been reported in diabetic patients. In these patients, about 85% of ambulant ischemic episodes occur without chest pain, and 66% of angina episodes are not accompanied by ST segment depression, suggesting that overt angina pectoris is merely the "tip of the ischemic iceberg." Pharmacologic agents that reduce or abolish episodes of symptomatic ischemia also reduce or abolish episodes of silent ischemia.

PROGNOSIS WITH OPTIMAL MANAGEMENT

Modern treatments have improved the prognosis of patients with stable ischemic heart disease to an annual mortality rate of 1 to 3% and a 1 to 2% rate of major ischemic events. The 1-year rate of cardiovascular death is now 1.9% (95% confidence interval [CI], 1.7 to 2.1), with a 2.9% (95% CI, 2.6 to 3.2) rate of all-cause mortality, and a 4.5% (95% CI, 4.2 to 4.8) rate of the combined outcome of cardiovascular death, MI, or stroke.

Recurrent angina is a common subsequent complaint in many patients with stable ischemic heart disease—even those who were initially treated successfully with PCI. About 30% of patients continue to experience angina one or more times per week, with associated greater physical limitation and worse quality of life, and almost 80% of patients who underwent initially successful PCI for chronic angina still take one or more antianginal agents at 1 year.

Selection of optimal treatment requires a full understanding of the potential risks and benefits of each treatment approach. In patients with stable symptoms who have not had an adequate trial of medical therapy (e.g., 8 to 12 weeks of multifaceted medical therapy and lifestyle intervention), such an initial approach of aggressive medical therapy is recommended. For patients whose angina or quality of life is not adequately controlled with optimal medical therapy, revascularization with either PCI or CABG surgery should be considered. Although the results of randomized trials must be individualized for specific patients, a multidisciplinary approach to clinical decision making can ensure that all therapeutic options are fully and transparently discussed so that patients are offered the most appropriate evidence-based treatment recommendations.

1. Cannon CP, Braunwald E, McCabe CH, et al. Intensive versus moderate lipid lowering with statins after acute coronary syndromes. *N Engl J Med.* 2004;350:1495-1504.
2. Tenkanen L, Mänttäri M, Kovanen PT, et al. Gemfibrozil in the treatment of dyslipidemia: an 18-year mortality follow-up of the Helsinki Heart Study. *Arch Intern Med.* 2006;166:743-748.
3. Jun M, Foote C, Lv J, et al. Effects of fibrates on cardiovascular outcomes: a systematic review and meta-analysis. *Lancet.* 2010;375:1875-1884.
4. Dagenais GR, Pogue J, Fox K, et al. Angiotensin-converting enzyme inhibitors in stable vascular disease without left ventricular systolic dysfunction or heart failure: a combined analysis of three trials. *Lancet.* 2006;368:581-588.
5. Lièvre M, Cucherat M. Aspirin in the secondary prevention of cardiovascular disease: an update of the APTC meta-analysis. *Fundam Clin Pharmacol.* 2010;24:385-391.
6. Bhatt DC, Fox KA, Hacke W, et al. Clopidogrel and aspirin versus aspirin alone for the prevention of atherothrombotic events. *N Engl J Med.* 2006;354:1706-1717.
7. Anand SS, Yusuf S. Oral anticoagulants in patients with coronary artery disease. *J Am Coll Cardiol.* 2003;41:62S-69S.
8. Morrow DA, Scirica BM, Karwatowska-Prokupczok E, et al. Effects of ranolazine on recurrent cardiovascular events in patients with non-ST-segment elevation acute coronary syndromes: the MERLIN TIMI-36 randomized trial. *JAMA.* 2007;297:1775-1784.
9. McKenna C, McDaid C, Suekarran S, et al. Enhanced external counterpulsation for the treatment of stable angina and heart failure: a systematic review and economic analysis. *Health Technol Assess.* 2009;13:1-90.
10. Weintraub WS, Spertus JA, Kolm P, et al. Effect of PCI on quality of life in patients with stable coronary disease. *N Engl J Med.* 2008;359:677-687.
11. Trikalinos TA, Alsheikh-Ali AA, Tatsioni A, et al. Percutaneous coronary interventions for non-acute coronary artery disease: a quantitative 20-year synopsis and a network meta-analysis. *Lancet.* 2009;373:911-918.
12. Boden WE, O'Rourke RA, Teo KK, et al. Optimal medical therapy with or without PCI for stable coronary disease. *N Engl J Med.* 2007;356:1503-1516.
13. BARI Investigators. The final 10-year follow-up results from the BARI randomized trial. *J Am Coll Cardiol.* 2007;49:1600-1606.
14. Frye R, August P, Brooks M, et al. BARI 2D: a randomized clinical trial of treatment strategies for type 2 diabetes and coronary artery disease. *N Engl J Med.* 2009;360:2503-2515.
15. Serruys PW, Morice MC, Kappetein AP, et al. Percutaneous coronary intervention versus coronary artery bypass grafting for severe coronary artery disease. *N Engl J Med.* 2009;360:961-972.
16. Hlatky MA, Boothroyd DB, Bravata DM, et al. Coronary artery bypass surgery compared with percutaneous coronary interventions for multivessel disease: a collaborative analysis of individual patient data from 10 randomised trials. *Lancet.* 2009;373:1190-1197.

SUGGESTED READINGS

Patel MR, Peterson ED, Dai D, et al. Low diagnostic yield of elective coronary angiography. *N Engl J Med.* 2010;362:886-895. *Only about one third of patients had significant coronary disease.*

Pfister ME, Zellweger MJ, Gersh BJ. Management of stable coronary artery disease. *Lancet.* 2010;375:763-772. *Review.*

Wijeysundera HC, Nallamothu BK, Krumholz HM, et al. Meta-analysis: effects of percutaneous coronary intervention versus medical therapy on angina relief. *Ann Intern Med.* 2010;152:370-379. *In a meta-analysis, PCI was associated with better relief of angina than was medical therapy, although the benefit is attenuated in contemporary studies with better use of evidence-based medical therapies.*

72

ACUTE CORONARY SYNDROME: UNSTABLE ANGINA AND NON–ST ELEVATION MYOCARDIAL INFARCTION

RICHARD A. LANGE AND L. DAVID HILLIS

DEFINITION

The term *acute coronary syndrome* (ACS) is used to describe the continuum of myocardial ischemia (unstable angina pectoris) or infarction (with or without concomitant ST segment elevation). The patient with *unstable angina* has cardiac chest pain that is new, worsening (i.e., more severe, prolonged, or frequent than previous episodes of angina), or occurring at rest, *without* serologic evidence of myocyte necrosis (i.e., no elevation of serum concentrations of troponin or the MB isoenzyme of creatine kinase [CK-MB]). The patient with cardiac chest pain *with* serologic evidence of myonecrosis and without ST segment elevation is said to have a *non–ST segment elevation myocardial*

infarction (MI). Because unstable angina and non–ST segment elevation MI are characterized by the absence of ST segment elevation, they are collectively termed *non–ST segment elevation ACS*, or NSTE-ACS (Fig. 72-1). The patient with acute-onset cardiac chest pain, serologic evidence of myonecrosis, and persistent (>20 minutes) ST segment elevation is said to have an *ST segment elevation MI* (Chapter 73).

EPIDEMIOLOGY

More than 1.4 million individuals in the United States are hospitalized annually with ACS, of whom approximately two thirds have NSTE-ACS. More than half of those with NSTE-ACS are older than 65 years, and almost half are women. NSTE-ACS is more common in individuals with one or more risk factors for atherosclerosis (Chapter 51), peripheral vascular disease, or a chronic inflammatory disorder, such as rheumatoid arthritis, psoriasis, or infection.

Most subjects with ACS have so-called *primary* ACS, which is precipitated by rupture of a coronary arterial atherosclerotic plaque, with subsequent platelet aggregation and thrombus formation, leading, in turn, to compromised blood flow in the involved artery. An occasional individual has so-called *secondary* ACS, which is caused by a transient or sustained marked imbalance between myocardial oxygen supply and demand. Substantial reductions in oxygen supply, for example, can be caused by severe systemic arterial hypotension, anemia, or hypoxemia; dramatic increases in oxygen demand can be caused by fever, tachycardia, severe systemic arterial hypertension, or thyrotoxicosis. In the subject thought to have secondary ACS, therapy should be directed at correcting the underlying cause.

PATHOBIOLOGY

The precipitating event in almost all subjects with NSTE-ACS is atherosclerotic coronary arterial plaque rupture or erosion, with subsequent platelet aggregation and thrombus formation, leading to subtotal occlusion of the involved artery. In an occasional patient with extensive collateral blood supply to the region of myocardium that is perfused by an occluded artery, total thrombotic occlusion of the artery leads to NSTE-ACS rather than to ST segment elevation MI.

Rarely, intense vasospasm of a segment of an epicardial coronary artery, due to focal endothelial dysfunction (i.e., Prinzmetal's angina) or drug ingestion (caused, for example, by cocaine, chemotherapeutic agents, or one of the serotonin receptor agonist "triptans"), causes a transient or sustained compromise of coronary arterial blood flow, with resultant NSTE-ACS. Spontaneous coronary arterial dissection, which occurs most often in peripartum women and patients with vasculitis, may result in NSTE-ACS.

Plaque Rupture

Atherosclerotic coronary arterial plaque rupture (Chapter 70) or erosion is the initiating event in most patients with NSTE-ACS. Several factors may play a role in the deterioration of the protective fibrous cap that separates the atheroma in the vessel wall from the coronary arterial lumen. Local and systemic inflammation, mechanical features, and anatomic changes contribute to the transformation of a stable atherosclerotic plaque to a so-called "vulnerable" plaque, the rupture of which triggers platelet adherence, activation, and aggregation, with subsequent thrombus formation.

The deposition of oxidized low-density lipoprotein (LDL) in the coronary arterial wall stimulates an inflammatory response, which results in the accumulation of macrophages and T lymphocytes at the plaque border. These inflammatory cells secrete cytokines (e.g., interferon-γ), which inhibit collagen synthesis and deposition, as well as enzymes (e.g., matrix metalloproteinases and cathepsins), which promote collagen and elastin degradation, thereby rendering the overlying fibrous cap vulnerable to rupture.

Systemic inflammation may play a role in plaque rupture as evidenced by the predisposition of individuals with chronic gingivitis, rheumatoid arthritis, and chronic or acute infection to develop ACS. Angiographic and angioscopic studies of the coronary arteries of ACS patients often demonstrate plaque ulceration and thrombosis at more than one site, thereby suggesting that a systemic and diffuse inflammatory process is present.

The mechanical characteristics and location of coronary arterial plaques appear to influence their stability. For example, thin fibrous caps are more likely to erode or rupture than are thick ones. Sites of low shear stress, such as vessel bifurcations, have reduced production of endothelial vasodilator substances (i.e., nitric oxide and prostacyclin), accelerated accumulation of lipids and inflammatory cells, increased degradation of the extracellular matrix, and thinning of the fibrous cap, all of which contribute to plaque instability.

Non–ST segment elevation ACS

Acute ST segment elevation myocardial infarction

ECG

No ST elevation

ST elevation

Cardiac Biomarker

Neg   ↑↑

↑↑

DX

USA   NSTEMI

STEMI

FIGURE 72-1. Acute coronary syndrome (ACS). Symptomatic, morphologic, electrocardiographic (ECG), and serologic findings in patients with various kinds of ACS. Subjects with ACS usually complain of chest pain. If the involved coronary artery is totally occluded by fresh thrombus (shown on the *right*), the patient's ECG reveals ST segment elevation; cardiac biomarkers subsequently are elevated; and he or she is diagnosed with an ST segment elevation myocardial infarction (STEMI). If the involved coronary artery is partially occluded by fresh thrombus (shown on the *left*), the patient's ECG does not show ST segment elevation. If cardiac biomarkers are not elevated, he or she is diagnosed with unstable angina (USA). If cardiac biomarkers are elevated, the patient is diagnosed with a non–ST segment elevation MI (NSTEMI). Dx = diagnosis.

Detailed histologic examination of evolving atherosclerotic plaques reveals a rich neovascularization that is the result of angiogenic peptides, such as fibroblast growth factors, vascular endothelial growth factor, placental growth factor, oncostatin M, and hypoxia-inducible factor, which are secreted by smooth muscle cells, inflammatory cells, and platelets. This neovascularization contributes to the growth of atheroma and to leukocyte trafficking, plaque hemorrhage, and destabilization.

Thrombus Formation

Platelets play a pivotal role in the pathobiology of ACS. Following erosion or rupture of a "vulnerable" plaque, circulating platelets *adhere* to the exposed subendothelial proteins, after which they are *activated*. With activation, the platelets change shape from discoid to stellate, thereby increasing the surface area on which thrombin formation can occur. The platelets then release the contents of their intracellular granules (i.e., thromboxane, serotonin, adenosine diphosphate, von Willebrand factor, fibrinogen) into the immediate environment and promote focal vasoconstriction of the adjacent arterial segment and activation of nearby platelets. Platelets also augment their number of surface glycoprotein IIb/IIIa receptors and the affinity of these receptors to bind circulating fibrinogen. The result is platelet *aggregation*, which occurs as fibrinogen binds to the glycoprotein IIb/IIIa receptors of adjacent platelets, thereby creating a "platelet plug."

Simultaneously with formation of the platelet plug, activation of the coagulation system with the generation of thrombin is a powerful stimulator of platelet activation and aggregation. In addition, thrombin converts fibrinogen to fibrin, which is incorporated into the thrombus. Subtotal coronary arterial occlusion by this platelet-rich thrombus compromises blood flow in the involved artery, thereby resulting in an imbalance of oxygen supply and demand of the myocytes perfused by the artery. Distal embolization of platelet-rich thrombi from the site of a ruptured plaque contributes to the compromise in blood flow. If the supply-demand imbalance is transient, the involved myocytes become ischemic but do not die because the ischemia is of insufficient duration to cause necrosis. The patient typically complains of cardiac chest pain at rest, but serologic evidence of myonecrosis, as evidenced by elevated serum concentrations of troponin or CK-MB, is absent; a diagnosis of *unstable angina* is made. In contrast, if the supply-demand imbalance is sustained, ischemic myocytes begin to die, and infarction occurs. The patient typically complains of cardiac chest pain at rest, and serologic evidence of myonecrosis confirms the diagnosis of *non–ST segment elevation MI.*

CLINICAL MANIFESTATIONS

Symptoms

The patient with NSTE-ACS typically complains of retrosternal pressure, squeezing, or heaviness that may be intermittent and recurrent or persistent (Chapter 50). If the episodes are intermittent and recurrent, the duration of each episode may range from only a few minutes to several hours. The chest pain may radiate to the left arm, neck, or jaw, and it may be accompanied by diaphoresis, nausea, abdominal pain, dyspnea, or syncope.

Atypical presentations of NSTE-ACS are not uncommon and may include aching or vague chest discomfort, epigastric pain, acute-onset indigestion, unexplained fatigue, or dyspnea. Such atypical complaints are often observed in younger (25 to 40 years of age) and older (>75 years of age) patients, women, and patients with diabetes mellitus, chronic renal insufficiency, or dementia.

Women with NSTE-ACS are more likely to have diabetes mellitus, hypertension, hyperlipidemia, and heart failure and to be older than men. They are less likely to be smokers or to have had a previous MI or coronary revascularization.

Physical Examination

The patient with NSTE-ACS often has a normal physical examination. On occasion, evidence of left ventricular dysfunction (Chapter 58), such as basilar rales or a ventricular gallop, hypotension, or peripheral hypoperfusion, may accompany an episode of NSTE-ACS or appear shortly thereafter. An important goal of the physical examination is to exclude noncardiac causes of the subject's symptoms (i.e., costochondritis, pneumothorax, pulmonary embolism, pneumonia) and nonischemic cardiac disorders (i.e., aortic dissection, pericarditis, severe systemic arterial hypertension) that can cause chest pain, other symptoms, or an elevation of cardiac biomarkers (Chapter 50). Accordingly, differences in blood pressure between the upper and lower limbs, decreased lung sounds, friction rubs, and pain on sternal palpation suggest a diagnosis other than NSTE-ACS. Other findings on physical examination—such as an elevated blood pressure, pallor, or increased sweating or tremor—point toward precipitating conditions, such as uncontrolled hypertension (Chapter 67), anemia (Chapter 161), or thyrotoxicosis (Chapter 233), respectively.

DIAGNOSIS

The patient with suspected ACS should be evaluated promptly because an expedient and accurate diagnosis permits the timely initiation of appropriate therapy, which can reduce the rate of complications. The initial assessment should be directed at determining whether the subject's symptoms are likely caused by myocardial ischemia, MI, or some other disorder. The likelihood of ACS can be estimated from the history, physical examination, and electrocardiogram (ECG) (Table 72-1).

In the acute setting, the presence or absence of traditional risk factors for atherosclerosis is far less important for determining the presence or absence of ACS than are the patient's symptoms, ECG findings, and serologic evidence of myonecrosis. As a result, these long-term risk factors are not the key factors that should be used to determine whether an individual should be evaluated, hospitalized, or treated for ACS.

HIGH LIKELIHOOD

Any of the following features:

Chest or left arm pain as the main symptom, similar in nature to previously noted angina

Known coronary artery disease

Evidence on physical exam of transient mitral regurgitation murmur, hypotension, diaphoresis, or pulmonary edema

New or transient ST segment deviation (≥1 mm) or T wave inversion in multiple precordial leads

Elevated serum troponin or CK-MB concentration

INTERMEDIATE LIKELIHOOD

Absence of high-likelihood features and any of the following:

Chest or left arm discomfort as main symptom

Age > 70 yr

Male gender

Diabetes mellitus

Extracardiac vascular disease

Q waves, ST segment depression (0.5-1 mm), or T wave inversion (>1 mm) in leads with dominant R waves

Normal cardiac troponin or CK-MB

LOW LIKELIHOOD

Absence of high- or intermediate-likelihood features, but may have:

Probable ischemic symptoms in the absence of any of the intermediate likelihood characteristics

Recent cocaine use

Chest discomfort reproduced by palpation

T wave flattening or inversion < 1 mm in leads with dominant R waves

Normal electrocardiogram

Normal serum troponin or CK-MB concentration

Modified from Anderson JL, Adams CD, Antman EM, et al. ACC/AHA 2007 Guidelines for the management of patients with unstable angina/non-ST-elevation myocardial infarction. *Circulation.* 2007;116:e148-e304.

Conditions that increase the likelihood that the symptomatic patient is experiencing myocardial ischemia or MI include older age, male gender, diabetes mellitus, extracardiac vascular disease, and chest pain radiating to the left arm, neck, or jaw as the presenting symptom. Myocardial ischemia is highly likely if anginal symptoms are accompanied by ECG abnormalities (i.e., ST segment depression or elevation ≥1 mm in magnitude or T wave inversion in multiple precordial leads), elevated serum concentration of troponin or CK-MB, or evidence of left ventricular dysfunction.

In a patient with known coronary artery disease, typical symptoms are likely to be caused by myocardial ischemia or MI rather than by another condition, particularly if the patient confirms that his or her symptoms are similar to previous anginal episodes. Conversely, a young individual who has a normal ECG and no risk factors for atherosclerosis is unlikely to be having ACS even when complaining of chest pain with features consistent with ischemia or infarction.

It is important to inquire about the use of cocaine and methamphetamines in the patient with suspected ACS, especially patients who are less than 40 years of age or have few traditional risk factors for atherosclerosis. These drugs can increase myocardial oxygen demand and concomitantly decrease oxygen supply by causing vasospasm and thrombosis. A urine toxicologic analysis should be considered when substance abuse is suspected as a cause of or contributor to ACS.

Electrocardiogram

An ECG should be obtained and examined promptly in the patient with suspected ACS. An ECG obtained during a symptomatic episode is particularly valuable. If the patient has persistent (>20 minutes) ST segment elevation, prompt reperfusion therapy should be initiated (Chapter 73). Transient ST segment abnormalities that develop during a symptomatic episode at rest and resolve when the patient is asymptomatic strongly suggest NSTE-ACS. ST segment depression (or transient ST segment elevation) and T wave abnormalities occur in up to 50% of NSTE-ACS patients.

A completely normal ECG does not exclude the possibility of NSTE-ACS; in fact, about 5% of patients who are discharged from the emergency department and ultimately diagnosed with ACS have a normal ECG. Ischemia or infarction in the territory of the left circumflex coronary artery often escapes detection with a standard 12-lead ECG, but it may be detected with right-sided leads (V_{4R} and V_{3R}) or posterior leads (V_7 to V_9). In the patient whose initial ECG is normal, subsequent ECGs should be obtained in the first 24 hours and during symptomatic episodes, and they should be compared with previous tracings to identify new ST segment or T wave abnormalities. Deep (>2 mm), symmetrical T wave inversion in the anterior chest leads is often associated with a hemodynamically significant stenosis of the left main or proximal left anterior descending coronary artery.

More than half of all episodes of myocardial ischemia are asymptomatic. On-line continuous computer-assisted 12-lead ST segment monitoring is a valuable diagnostic tool for detecting such episodes. Continuous ST segment monitoring also adds independent prognostic information to the resting ECG, serum cardiac enzymes, and other variables.

Serum Biomarkers

Troponin (Chapter 73) is detectable in the blood with conventional assays within 3 to 4 hours of the onset of myonecrosis, but in some individuals, its detection may be delayed for up to 8 hours. As a result, single negative assessment of serum troponin is insufficient to exclude MI in a patient with recent symptoms. To demonstrate or to exclude myonecrosis, repetitive blood sampling and troponin measurements should be performed 6 to 12 hours after the initial evaluation of the patient and following any additional episodes of chest pain. High sensitivity troponin assays can detect extremely small amounts of troponin in the blood, thereby improving the early (i.e., within 2 hours of symptom onset) diagnosis of MI. Troponin levels can be measured in the hospital's central chemistry laboratory or with point-of-care instruments at the patient's bedside using desktop devices or handheld bedside rapid qualitative assays. The advantage of point-of-care systems for avoiding delays must be weighed against their higher costs and the need for stringent quality control. In addition, point-of-care assays are qualitative or semiquantitative and observer dependent, whereas the central laboratory provides more accurate quantitative information concerning biomarker concentrations.

Up to one third of ACS patients whose serum CK-MB concentrations are normal have detectable serum concentrations of troponin T and I, indicating that myonecrosis has occurred and establishing the diagnosis of NSTE-MI. Current recommendations call for the use of the serum troponin concentration for acute risk stratification at the time of the patient's arrival to hospital.

Noninvasive Testing

The patient considered to have a low likelihood for ACS (based on the history, physical examination, ECG, and serum biomarkers) should undergo timely stress testing (Chapter 50), which does not absolutely establish or exclude the presence of coronary artery disease but has a high enough predictive value to guide acute decision making. Alternatively, multidetector computed tomographic (CT) coronary angiography has a high (>98%) negative predictive value to exclude coronary artery disease when performed and interpreted at centers experienced in its use. Conversely, the patient who is believed to be at intermediate or high risk for ACS and who continues to have typical ischemic chest pain with ECG abnormalities or elevated cardiac biomarkers should not undergo urgent diagnostic stress testing or CT coronary angiography; when such patients become symptom free with medical therapy and otherwise do not have indications for coronary angiography (see later), stress testing, often with myocardial perfusion imaging, should be performed before hospital discharge.

An echocardiogram may be helpful in the patient with chest pain if the ECG is nondiagnostic (i.e., minimal ST segment or T wave abnormalities). If left ventricular hypokinesis or akinesis is observed during an episode of chest pain and then improves when symptoms resolve, myocardial ischemia is likely. In the patient with T wave inversion in the anterior leads of uncertain etiology, hypokinesis of the left ventricular anterior wall suggests that the observed T wave abnormality is due to a severe stenosis of the left anterior descending coronary artery. Because echocardiography can help evaluate and identify alternative causes for the patient's chest pain, such as myocarditis (Chapter 60), aortic dissection (Chapter 78), or pulmonary embolism (Chapter 98), it is recommended in patients whose diagnosis is uncertain.

Coronary Angiography

Coronary angiography (Chapter 57) should be performed in patients who are thought to be at high risk for a cardiac ischemic event (death, MI, or recurrent ischemia) in the ensuing days, weeks, and months (see later); have spontaneous or inducible myocardial ischemia despite appropriate medical therapy; or have a confusing or difficult clinical presentation and a subsequent inconclusive noninvasive evaluation. The results of angiography help determine whether revascularization is appropriate and, if so, whether it should be attempted surgically (through coronary artery bypass grafting [CABG]) or percutaneously (through percutaneous coronary intervention [PCI]) (Chapter 74).

In patients with NSTE-ACS, coronary angiography demonstrates more than 50% luminal diameter narrowing of the left main coronary artery in about 15% of patients, of all three major epicardial coronary arteries in about 30 to 35% of patients, of two of the three epicardial arteries in about 20 to 30% of patients, and of one major epicardial artery in 20 to 30% of patients. About 15% of patients have no coronary arterial narrowing of hemodynamic significance. Women with NSTE-ACS are likely to have less extensive coronary artery disease than men, and patients with non–ST segment elevation MI on average have more extensive disease than those with unstable angina.

The coronary arterial lesion responsible for NSTE-ACS (the so-called culprit lesion) typically is asymmetrical or eccentric, with scalloped or overhanging edges and a narrow base or neck. These angiographic features reflect underlying plaque disruption and thrombus formation. Although obvious thrombus is visible angiographically in only one third of patients with NSTE-ACS, coronary angioscopy shows plaque rupture with overlying thrombus in most.

If the patient had previous coronary angiography, the culprit lesion usually can be seen to have progressed substantially. Interestingly, the lesion that is the nidus for ACS often is not severely stenotic when assessed on the previous angiogram; in fact, two thirds of culprit lesions previously had less than 50% luminal diameter narrowing (and, therefore, would not have been considered appropriate for surgical or percutaneous revascularization).

During the months after a NSTE-ACS, the culprit coronary arterial lesion is more likely to progress and to precipitate another ACS than are other lesions in the same patient. Lesions with irregular borders, overhanging edges, or obvious thrombus at angiography are more likely to precipitate another ACS in the ensuing months when compared with those that do not display these morphologic characteristics.

Risk Assessment and Triage

The initial evaluation of the patient with possible or suspected ACS should focus on an assessment of his or her risk of acutely sustaining a cardiac ischemic event (death, MI, or recurrent ischemia). Patients may be admitted immediately to a coronary intensive care unit or to an intermediate care unit, watched carefully in a monitored chest pain evaluation unit, or discharged home based on their risk of an MI (Fig. 72-2; see Fig. 50-1 in Chapter 50). Patients considered to be at low risk for a cardiac ischemic event should be discharged home, with further evaluation performed as an outpatient. Conversely, patients not at low risk should be hospitalized for further evaluation and treatment.

After the initial triage decision is made, urgent therapeutic interventions are based on the risk of adverse events in the coming hours, days, weeks, and months—estimated by using either the Thrombolysis in Myocardial Infarction (TIMI) or Global Registry of Acute Coronary Events (GRACE) risk algorithm—balanced against the risk of a bleeding complication from intensive medical therapy (Table 72-2) or an adverse event from an invasive cardiac procedure. Based on this initial assessment, the patient's therapy can be tailored, thereby reducing the likelihood of adverse events.

Although serum markers of myonecrosis comprise only one of the TIMI or GRACE risk variables, the presence of this variable alone appears to identify the patient as being "high risk." However, although elevated serum markers indicate myonecrosis, they provide no insight into its cause: in some subjects, myonecrosis occurs with disease entities other than coronary artery disease (e.g., pulmonary embolism, decompensated heart failure, severe hypertension or tachycardia, anemia, sepsis). Thus, when evaluating the patient with possible ACS, the presence of elevated serum markers should be assessed in conjunction with other variables.

Increasing age is associated with a higher incidence of both ACS-related cardiac ischemic events and complications from intensive medical therapy

TABLE 72-2   RISK VARIABLES FOR ISCHEMIC EVENTS AND BLEEDING COMPLICATIONS

1. RISK VARIABLES PREDICTIVE OF DEATH, MYOCARDIAL INFARCTION, OR RECURRENT ISCHEMIA

A. Thrombolysis in Myocardial Infarction (TIMI) Score*

Age > 65 yrs
Three or more risk factors for atherosclerosis
Known coronary artery disease (previous coronary arteriography or myocardial infarction)
Two or more episodes of anginal chest pain in the 24 hr before hospitalization
Use of aspirin in the 7 days before hospitalization
ST segment deviation ≥ 0.5 mV
Elevated serum concentrations of troponin or CK-MB

B. Global Registry of Acute Coronary Events (GRACE)†

Age
Heart failure class
Heart rate
Systolic blood pressure
ST segment deviation
Cardiac arrest during presentation
Serum creatinine concentration
Elevated serum markers of myonecrosis

2. RISK FACTORS FOR BLEEDING COMPLICATIONS WITH INTENSIVE THERAPY‡

Female gender
Older age
Renal insufficiency
Low body weight
Tachycardia
Systolic arterial pressure (high or low)
Anemia
Diabetes mellitus

*Individuals with three or more of these variables are considered to be "high risk," whereas those with 0, 1, or 2 are considered to be "low risk." (From Diez JG, Cohen M. Balancing myocardial ischemic and bleeding risks in patients with non-ST-segment elevation myocardial infarction. *Am J Cardiol.* 2009;103:1396-1402.)

†Each variable is assigned a numerical score based on its specific value, and the eight scores are summed to yield a total score, which is applied to a reference nomogram to determine the patient's risk. The GRACE application tool is available online at www.outcomes-umassmed.org/grace. (From Brieger D, Fox KA, Fitzgerald G, et al. Predicting freedom from clinical events in non-ST-elevation acute coronary syndromes: the Global Registry of Acute Coronary Events. *Heart.* 2009;95:888-894.)

‡The patient's bleeding risk can be estimated with the tool available at www.crusadebleedingscore.org. (From Subherwal S, Bach RG, Chen AY, et al. Baseline risk of major bleeding in non-ST-segment-elevation myocardial infarction: the CRUSADE [Can Rapid risk stratification of Unstable angina patients Suppress ADverse outcomes with Early implementation of the ACC/AHA Guidelines] Bleeding Score. *Circulation.* 2009;119:1873-1882.)

and invasive cardiac procedures. Even though elderly people are at increased risk of such treatment-related complications, they nonetheless derive a greater absolute and relative benefit from such intensive therapy when compared with younger individuals. Apart from this initial risk assessment, the ACS patient's general medical and cognitive status, anticipated life expectancy, risk of treatment-related complications, and, most importantly, personal preferences should be evaluated and considered.

Once the risk status of the ACS patient is established, management is initiated and tailored to the patient's risk of sustaining a subsequent ischemic cardiac event or a treatment-related complication (Table 72-3). For example, the patient considered to be at low risk of a subsequent ischemic event does not benefit from intensive antithrombotic therapy or routine coronary angiography and revascularization.[1] Conversely, in patients considered to be at high risk of sustaining an ischemic event, optimal therapy—including coronary angiography and revascularization (if appropriate)—results in a substantial 20 to 40% decrease in the risk of recurrent ischemia and MI and an approximately 10% reduction in mortality.[2,3] In short, the magnitude of benefit of intensive therapy correlates with the patient's level of risk.

Differential Diagnoses

Several cardiac and noncardiac conditions, some of which are potentially life-threatening, may mimic NSTE-ACS. The patient with a pulmonary

FIGURE 72-2. Initial triage for patients with symptoms suggestive of an acute coronary syndrome (ACS). ECG = electrocardiogram; LV = left ventricular. (Modified from Anderson JL, Adams CD, Antman EM, et al. ACC/AHA 2007 guidelines for the management of patients with unstable angina and non-ST-segment elevation myocardial infarction. A report of the American College of Cardiology/American Heart Association Task Force on Practice Guidelines. *Circulation.* 2007;116:e148-e304.)

embolism (Chapter 98) often complains of dyspnea and chest pain and may have ECG abnormalities and elevated serum concentrations of troponin and CK-MB. Aortic dissection (Chapter 78) should be considered and excluded because the therapies for NSTE-ACS are contraindicated in patients with this condition. Stroke (Chapter 414) and subarachnoid hemorrhage (Chapter 415) may be accompanied by ECG abnormalities, segmental wall motion abnormalities, and elevated serum biomarker concentrations. Underlying chronic cardiac conditions, such as valvular heart disease (i.e., aortic stenosis, aortic regurgitation) and hypertrophic cardiomyopathy (Chapter 60), may be associated with symptoms similar to those of NSTE-ACS, elevated serum biomarker concentrations, and ECG abnormalities. Myocarditis (Chapter 60), pericarditis (Chapter 77), and myopericarditis often cause chest pain that resembles angina, ECG abnormalities, and elevated serum biomarker concentrations. A flu-like or upper respiratory tract infection often precedes or accompanies these conditions. Patients with "stress cardiomyopathy" (takotsubo syndrome) typically have chest pain, ST segment abnormalities and deeply inverted T waves, and mildly elevated serum biomarker concentrations (Chapter 60).

PREVENTION AND TREATMENT   Rx

The goals of treatment of the patient with NSTE-ACS are to prevent recurrent ischemia by correcting the imbalance between myocardial oxygen supply and demand; to prevent thrombus propagation; and to stabilize the "vulnerable" plaque. Antianginal medications, such as nitroglycerin, β-adrenergic blockers, and calcium-channel blockers, favorably affect myocardial oxygen supply and demand, thereby preventing recurrent ischemia. Antiplatelet and antithrombotic agents retard thrombus propagation, and statins promote plaque stabilization. Once the risk status of the ACS patient is established, treatment is initiated (see Table 72-3).

Every NSTE-ACS patient, regardless of the level of risk, should promptly receive antianginal medications, antiplatelet therapy (aspirin and clopidogrel), and a statin, unless contraindicated. A "low-risk" patient should also receive unfractionated heparin but not more intensive antiplatelet or anticoagulant therapy because anticoagulation beyond aspirin, clopidogrel, and heparin increases the risk of bleeding without further reducing the risk of an ischemic cardiac event. Routine coronary angiography and revascularization are not beneficial and should be reserved for the patient with recurrent ischemia despite intensive medical therapy.

TABLE 72-3 MANAGEMENT STRATEGIES FOR PATIENTS WITH ACUTE CORONARY SYNDROME

THERAPY	INITIATION	DURATION	DOSE, ROUTE, AND DURATION	BENEFIT VS. PLACEBO (REDUCED INCIDENCE OF …)
LOW-RISK PATIENT				
Antianginal				
β-Blocker*	Immediately	Hospitalization ± indefinitely	Metoprolol, 5 mg IV boluses (three given 2 to 5 minutes apart) then 50 mg orally twice daily titrated up to 100 mg twice daily or atenolol, 5-10 mg IV bolus then 100 mg orally daily	Recurrent ischemia
Nitroglycerin	Immediately	Hospitalization ± indefinitely	0.3 to 0.6 mg sublingually or 5 to 10 μg/min IV initially and increased by 10 μg/min every 5 min	Not studied
Diltiazem or verapamil*	Immediately	Hospitalization ± indefinitely	30 to 90 mg orally four times daily or up to 360 mg of long-acting preparation orally daily	MI, recurrent ischemia
Lipid Lowering				
Statin	Before hospital discharge	Indefinitely	Atorvastatin, up to 80 mg orally daily	Recurrent ischemia
Antiplatelet				
Aspirin	Immediately	Indefinitely	162-325 mg orally initial dose then 81 mg orally daily	Death, MI
Clopidogrel	Immediately	1-12 mo	300 mg orally initial dose then 75 mg orally daily	MI, recurrent ischemia
Anticoagulant				
Unfractionated heparin	Immediately	2 to 5 days	60 U/kg IV bolus then 12 U/kg IV adjusted to achieve an aPTT of 50 to 70 sec	Death or MI (combined)
HIGH-RISK PATIENT				
Antianginal				
β-Blocker*	Immediately	Hospitalization ± indefinitely	Metoprolol, 5 mg IV boluses (three given 2 to 5 minutes apart) then 50 mg orally twice daily titrated up to 100 mg twice daily or atenolol, 5-10 mg IV bolus then 100 mg orally daily	Death, MI, recurrent ischemia
Nitroglycerin	Immediately	Hospitalization ± indefinitely	0.3 to 0.6 mg sublingually or 5 to 10 μg/min IV initially and increased by 10 μg/min every 5 min	Not studied
Diltiazem or verapamil*	Immediately	Hospitalization ± indefinitely	30 to 90 mg orally four times daily or up to 360 mg of long-acting preparation orally daily	MI, recurrent ischemia
Lipid Lowering				
Statin	Before hospital discharge	Indefinitely	Atorvastatin, up to 80 mg orally daily	Recurrent ischemia
Antiplatelet				
Aspirin	Immediately	Indefinitely	162-325 mg orally initial dose then 81 mg orally	Death, MI
Clopidogrel	Immediately	≥12 mo	300 mg orally initial dose then 75 mg orally daily	MI, recurrent ischemia
Glycoprotein IIb/IIIa inhibitor (eptifibatide, tirofiban, or abciximab)	At time of PCI	12-24 hr post-PCI	Abciximab, 0.25 mg/kg IV bolus then 0.125 μg/kg/min IV (max 10 μg/min) for 12 hr or eptifibatide, 180 μg/kg IV bolus then 2.0 μg/kg/min IV for 18-24 hr or tirofiban, 0.4 μg/kg/min IV for 30 min then 0.1 μg/kg/min IV for 12 to 24 hr	MI
Anticoagulants				
Unfractionated heparin or	Immediately	2 to 5 days; discontinue after successful PCI	60 U/kg IV bolus then 12 U/kg IV adjusted to achieve an aPTT of 50 to 70 sec	Death or MI (combined)
Enoxaparin or	Immediately	Duration of hospitalization (up to 8 days); discontinue after successful PCI	1 mg/kg subcutaneously twice daily	MI, recurrent ischemia[†]
Bivalirudin	Immediately	Up to 72 hr; discontinue 4 hr after PCI	0.1 mg/kg IV bolus then 1.75 mg/kg/hr IV	Bleeding[‡]
Invasive Management				
Coronary angiography followed by revascularization (if appropriate)	Up to 36-80 hr after hospitalization; within 24 hr in "very high risk" patients			MI, recurrent ischemia

*Avoid in the patient with decompensated heart failure, hypotension, or hemodynamic instability.
†As compared with unfractionated heparin.
‡As monotherapy compared with heparin and glycoprotein IIb/IIIa inhibitor combination.
aPTT = activated partial thromboplastin time; IV = intravenous; MI = myocardial infarction; PCI = percutaneous coronary intervention.
Modified from Lange RA, Hillis LD. Optimal management of acute coronary syndromes. *N Engl J Med.* 2009;260:2237-2240.

Conversely, the high-risk patient should receive antianginal medications, antiplatelet therapy (aspirin and clopidogrel), a statin, a more intensive anticoagulant therapy, and coronary angiography followed by revascularization (if indicated). In the patient whose coronary anatomy is suitable, revascularization reduces the incidence of ischemia and recurrent MI, and in certain patients (see later), it improves survival.

Antianginal Therapy

Nitroglycerin

Nitroglycerin (Chapter 71), which is a venodilator at low doses and an arteriolar dilator at higher doses, may prevent recurrent ischemia in patients with unstable angina, but no studies of sufficient statistical power have determined whether it reduces the risk of MI in this patient population. In patients who complain of recurrent symptoms, nitroglycerin should be given sublingually or by buccal spray (0.3 to 0.6 mg). Patients with ongoing or recurrent chest pain should receive intravenous nitroglycerin (5 to 10 µg/minute using nonabsorbable tubing), with escalation of the dose in increments of 10 µg/minute until symptoms resolve or adverse effects develop. Nitroglycerin's most common adverse effects are headache, nausea, dizziness, hypotension, and reflex tachycardia.

Nitrate tolerance can be avoided by providing the patient with a "nitrate-free" period (i.e., a brief cessation of drug administration). Nitroglycerin should not be given to the patient who has received a phosphodiesterase-5 inhibitor (i.e., sildenafil, tadalafil, or vardenafil) within the previous 24 to 48 hours, as severe hypotension may ensue.

β-Adrenergic Blockers

β-Adrenergic blockers diminish symptoms and the risk of MI in patients who are not already taking a β-blocker at the time of hospital admission. In the normotensive patient without ongoing chest pain or tachycardia, metoprolol should be initiated at 50 mg orally every 6 to 8 hours, with the dose increased (to 100 mg twice daily) as necessary to control heart rate, blood pressure, and symptoms. In high-risk patients and in patients with tachycardia or elevated systemic arterial pressure, metoprolol should be administered intravenously (3 boluses of 5 mg each given 5 minutes apart) initially, after which an oral dose should be initiated. A reasonable target heart rate is 50 to 60 beats per minute at rest.

β-Blockers should not be administered to patients with decompensated heart failure, hypotension, hemodynamic instability, or advanced atrioventricular block. Because most patients with chronic obstructive pulmonary disease or peripheral vascular disease tolerate β-blockers without difficulty, these conditions should not preclude their use.

Calcium-Channel Blockers

Calcium-channel blockers, which cause coronary and systemic arterial vasodilation, increase coronary arterial blood flow and lower systemic arterial pressure. The nondihydropyridine calcium-channel blockers, diltiazem and verapamil, slow heart rate and are recommended for the patient with a contraindication to a β-adrenergic blocker or persistent or recurrent symptoms despite treatment with nitroglycerin or a β-blocker. Oral diltiazem (30 to 90 mg four times daily of the short-acting preparation or up to 360 mg once daily of the long-acting preparation) is the preferred agent because studies have shown that it reduces the incidence of myocardial ischemia and recurrent MI in patients with NSTE-ACS.[4] Diltiazem is contraindicated in patients with left ventricular dysfunction or pulmonary vascular congestion. Caution should be exercised when combining a β-blocker with diltiazem because the two drugs may act synergistically to depress left ventricular systolic function as well as sinus and atrioventricular nodal conduction. Short-acting nifedipine should not be administered to the patient with ACS unless the patient is already receiving a β-blocker because it may increase the risk of death. The risks and benefits of long-acting dihydropyridines in patients with NSTE-ACS are undefined.

Antiplatelet Agents

In patients with NSTE-ACS, *aspirin* (Chapter 36), 75 to 1300 mg daily, reduces the risk of death or MI by roughly 50%.[5] Because high-dose aspirin increases the risk of gastrointestinal bleeding but is no more efficacious than low-dose aspirin, the patient should be treated with 75 to 162 mg daily, unless contraindicated (i.e., the patient has an aspirin allergy or active bleeding). Once initiated, aspirin therapy should be continued indefinitely.

Clopidogrel (Chapter 37) is a thienopyridine that blocks the P2Y$_{12}$ adenosine diphosphate (ADP) receptor, thereby diminishing ADP-mediated platelet activation. Its antiplatelet activity is synergistic with aspirin because the two agents inhibit different platelet-activating pathways. Clopidogrel is a prodrug that must be metabolized by the cytochrome P-450 system to the active form. Polymorphisms in the cytochrome P-450 isoform CYP2C19, present in 15 to 20% of individuals, slow metabolism of the prodrug to the active form, thereby reducing the magnitude of platelet inhibition.

In patients with NSTE-ACS, the addition of clopidogrel to aspirin reduces the composite end point of cardiovascular death, nonfatal MI, or stroke by 20% (2.1% reduction in absolute risk) compared with treatment with aspirin

alone.[6] The benefit of an aspirin-clopidogrel combination is seen as early as 24 hours after drug initiation and persists for the 12 months of the study; an increase in minor bleeding is observed in those receiving both agents.

Dual antiplatelet therapy (aspirin and clopidogrel) should be administered routinely to the ACS patient, unless contraindicated. The patient who is allergic to or intolerant of aspirin should receive clopidogrel alone. Because maximal platelet inhibition occurs 3 to 5 days after clopidogrel is initiated unless a large dose is given initially, the patient should receive a loading dose of 300 to 600 mg, then 75 mg daily for at least 1 year.

Clopidogrel treatment increases the risk of bleeding in the patient undergoing CABG. Clopidogrel should not be initiated in likely candidates for CABG; if already begun, it should be discontinued 5 days before the planned surgery. Drugs that are potent inhibitors of the CYP2C19 enzyme should not be administered with clopidogrel because they affect the metabolism to its active form and reduce its antiplatelet effects. Such drugs include omeprazole, esomeprazole, cimetidine, fluconazole, ketoconazole, voriconazole, etravirine, felbamate, fluoxetine, and fluvoxamine. For clopidogrel-treated patients who need antacid therapy, treatment with ranitidine or pantoprazole is recommended.

Prasugrel (Chapter 37) is another thienopyridine with a greater antiplatelet effect and a more rapid onset of action than clopidogrel. In patients with ACS who are referred for PCI, prasugrel in combination with aspirin reduces ischemic events (i.e., a combination of cardiovascular death, nonfatal MI, and stroke) by 20% compared with concomitant clopidogrel and aspirin (2.2% absolute risk reduction) therapy.[7] However, this benefit is obtained at a 0.5% increased risk of life-threatening bleeding and a 0.3% increased risk of fatal bleeding. At present, prasugrel is approved for use in the ACS patient who is referred for PCI. In combination with aspirin, it is administered as a 60 mg oral loading dose followed by a 10 mg daily maintenance dose. Because prasugrel-associated bleeding complications are highest in patients with a previous stroke or transient ischemic attack, age older than 75 years, or a body weight of less than 60 kg, its use should be avoided in the patient with any of these features.

Glycoprotein IIb/IIIa inhibitors (Chapter 37) block platelet aggregation in response to all potential agonists and are the most potent antiplatelet agents available. Three glycoprotein IIb/IIIa inhibitors, each of which must be administered parenterally, are available: abciximab is the Fab fragment of a monoclonal antibody to the receptor; eptifibatide is a peptide; and tirofiban is a peptidomimetic molecule.

Glycoprotein IIb/IIIa inhibitors reduce the incidence of recurrent ischemic events in patients with NSTE-ACS who undergo PCI, but not in patients who are managed with medical therapy alone. If a glycoprotein IIb/IIIa inhibitor is administered, it should be initiated at the time of angiography because previously published studies have shown that its routine administration beforehand carries an increased bleeding risk and no improvement in outcomes.[8] The glycoprotein IIb/IIIa inhibitor infusion (see Table 72-3) typically is continued for 12 to 24 hours following PCI.

Anticoagulants

Anticoagulant therapy should be administered to all patients with ACS unless a contraindication, such as active bleeding, is present. For the patient in whom a noninvasive, ischemia-guided management strategy is selected, treatment with unfractionated heparin, low-molecular-weight heparin (LMWH), or fondaparinux is appropriate, with fondaparinux recommended for the patient at increased risk of bleeding. For the patient in whom an invasive management strategy is selected, unfractionated heparin and LMWH are the agents of choice. Bivalirudin may be preferred in the individual undergoing PCI, but it should not be used in the initial management of the patient with ACS.

Heparin

Unfractionated heparin (Chapter 37) exerts its anticoagulant effect by accelerating the action of circulating antithrombin and prevents thrombus propagation but does not lyse existing thrombi. In the patient with NSTE-ACS, the addition of heparin to aspirin reduces the rate of in-hospital ischemic events (i.e., death or MI) by 33%.[9]

Unfractionated heparin should be initiated with an intravenous bolus of 60 U/kg, followed by a continuous infusion of approximately 12 U/kg/hour (maximum, 1000 U/hour), adjusted to maintain the activated partial thromboplastin time (aPTT) at 1.5 to 2.5 times control (i.e., 50 to 70 seconds) or a heparin concentration at 0.3 to 0.7 U/mL (by anti–factor Xa determinations). The infusion should be continued for 48 hours or until revascularization is performed, whichever occurs sooner. Frequent monitoring of the aPTT or heparin concentration is necessary because the anticoagulant response to a standard dose of unfractionated heparin varies widely among individuals; even when a weight-based nomogram (see Table 81-4 in Chapter 81) is followed, the aPTT is outside the therapeutic range more than one third of the time.

Mild thrombocytopenia occurs in 10 to 20% of patients treated with unfractionated heparin. In 1 to 5% of patients, a more severe form of thrombocytopenia develops. This antibody-mediated response usually occurs 4 to 14 days after the initiation of treatment, although it may become manifest far more quickly in the subject who received heparin within the preceding 6 months. Such antibody-mediated thrombocytopenia is associated with thromboembolic sequelae in 30 to 80% of subjects.

Low-Molecular-Weight Heparin

LMWHs (Chapter 37), which are fragments of unfractionated heparin, exert a more predictable anticoagulant effect, have a longer half-life, and are less likely to cause thrombocytopenia compared with unfractionated heparin. Because they provide predictable and sustained anticoagulation with once- or twice-daily subcutaneous administration, monitoring of their anticoagulant effect is not required.

LMWH is superior to unfractionated heparin in preventing MI or death during hospitalization in patients with NSTE-ACS who have elevated serum cardiac biomarkers as well as in those considered to be at high risk for recurrent ischemia (i.e., the subject with three or more TIMI risk factors).[10] In the low-risk subject, unfractionated heparin and LMWH have similar efficacy.[10] In the patient who is likely to undergo CABG surgery during the hospitalization, unfractionated heparin is preferred over LMWH because its anticoagulant effects can be more readily reversed with protamine.

Two LMWHs are approved for the treatment of the patient with NSTE-ACS, enoxaparin and dalteparin. The dose of enoxaparin is 1 mg/kg subcutaneously twice daily, and the dose of dalteparin is 120 IU/kg (maximum, 10,000 IU) subcutaneously twice daily. Therapy should be continued for the duration of the hospitalization, up to 8 days, or until revascularization is performed (whichever occurs first). In obese (>120 kg), thin (<60 kg), or renally impaired (creatinine clearance < 30 mL/minute) patients, the LMWH dose should be adjusted to achieve an anti–factor Xa concentration of 0.5 to 1.5 IU/mL 4 to 6 hours after drug administration.

LMWH should be avoided in the patient with a history of heparin-induced thrombocytopenia. In the patient with renal failure, treatment with LMWH has been associated with the development of hyperkalemia.

Fondaparinux

Fondaparinux (Chapter 37), which is a selective factor Xa inhibitor, does not require dose adjustment and monitoring. Fondaparinux does not cause thrombocytopenia. Fondaparinux is as effective as enoxaparin in preventing ischemic cardiac events but with 50% fewer major bleeding episodes (from 4.1% to 2.2%).[11] An increased incidence of catheter-related thrombosis has been reported following fondaparinux treatment, so it is not recommended for the patient who is likely to undergo coronary angiography. Thus, fondaparinux is a desirable anticoagulant for the patient with ACS who is managed with a noninvasive approach, especially if he or she is at higher risk of a bleeding complication with anticoagulant therapy, but not for other patients.

For the patient with ACS, fondaparinux is administered as a 2.5-mg subcutaneous injection once daily for up to 5 days or until hospital discharge. Its use is contraindicated in patients with severe renal impairment and in those who weigh 50 kg or less, and it should not be used as the sole anticoagulant during a PCI.

Bivalirudin

Bivalirudin, a direct thrombin inhibitor, is currently recommended as an alternative anticoagulant for patients undergoing PCI. It has not been tested in the patient with ACS who is managed with an ischemia-guided strategy. Hence, the administration of bivalirudin in a setting other than the cardiac catheterization laboratory is not recommended. In the patient undergoing PCI, bivalirudin (0.75 mg/kg intravenous bolus followed by an infusion of 1.75 mg/kg/hr for up to 4 hours after the PCI) is as effective as combination heparin and glycoprotein IIb/IIIa inhibitor therapy in preventing ischemic events, but it causes fewer major bleeding episodes.[12] Bivalirudin is the anticoagulant of choice for the patient with ACS who has heparin-induced thrombocytopenia.

Statins

Prompt initiation of statin therapy is recommended in all patients with NSTE-ACS to promote plaque stabilization and to restore endothelial function. Moreover, when statin therapy is initiated during the patient's hospitalization (rather than at hospital discharge), long-term medical compliance is substantially improved. In the absence of contraindications, high-dose atorvastatin (80 mg daily) should be given orally to the patient with NSTE-ACS, regardless of the baseline serum LDL cholesterol concentration; a lower dose is not as effective in reducing ischemic events.[13]

Recurrent or Refractory Unstable Angina

In most patients hospitalized with NSTE-ACS, symptoms do not recur after the institution of appropriate antianginal therapy. The occasional patient with continued or recurrent chest pain despite optimal medical therapy is at high risk for an MI. For the patient with refractory myocardial ischemia or hemodynamic instability despite optimal medical therapy, intraaortic balloon counterpulsation can reduce the ischemic episodes until revascularization can be performed. Intra-aortic balloon function is synchronized with the patient's ECG so that it inflates during diastole and deflates during systole, thereby augmenting coronary arterial blood flow and reducing myocardial oxygen demand by decreasing afterload. Intra-aortic balloon counterpulsation causes lower limb ischemia in approximately 3% of patients in whom the device is placed, but this complication usually resolves with its removal.

Coronary Revascularization

Coronary revascularization is performed to relieve angina that is persistent or recurrent despite optimal medical therapy, to prevent recurrent ischemia or MI in patients at high risk for a subsequent ischemic event, and to improve survival in patients with suitable anatomy.

Coronary revascularization is successful in relieving symptoms in 90% of the patients with angina refractory to medical therapy. Whether coronary bypass surgery or PCI is the more appropriate method of revascularization is determined by the location and severity of coronary arterial stenoses and the presence of comorbid medical conditions that may affect the performance or safety of the revascularization procedure.

The patient who has been rendered symptom free with optimal medical therapy should undergo an assessment to determine whether he or she is at high risk or relatively low risk of sustaining a cardiac ischemic event (death, MI, or recurrent ischemia) in the ensuing days, weeks, and months and a bleeding complication from intensive medical therapy or an invasive cardiac procedure. Patients who are at low risk of having an ischemic event (those with a normal serum troponin concentration, age less than 75 years, and zero, one, or two TIMI risk variables) should be evaluated noninvasively for inducible ischemia before hospital discharge. If the patient has spontaneous or provocable ischemia, coronary angiography and, if appropriate, revascularization should be performed.

The ACS patient with a detectable serum troponin concentration, age more than 75 years, or three or more TIMI risk variables is considered to be high risk and should be referred for routine coronary angiography and revascularization (if appropriate) during the hospitalization because this management strategy reduces the incidence of subsequent ischemic cardiac events.[3,14] In most subjects, early (within 24 hours of hospitalization) invasive therapy is no better at preventing death, MI, or stroke than somewhat delayed (median, 50 hours) invasive management, although it is associated with a modest decrease in the occurrence of recurrent ischemia.[2] In contrast, in the one third of subjects considered to be very high risk (GRACE risk score of >140, corresponding to an incidence of in-hospital death or MI of >20%), an early invasive management strategy is superior to a delayed strategy in reducing the incidence of death, MI, or stroke.[2]

The patient with clinical features or noninvasive test results suggestive of severe coronary artery disease (i.e., left ventricular dysfunction, hemodynamic instability, life-threatening ventricular arrhythmias, or extensive inducible ischemia) should be referred for coronary angiography to determine whether left main or three-vessel coronary arterial disease is present because patients with these coronary anatomic findings derive a survival benefit with coronary revascularization compared with medical therapy (Chapter 74).

Complications

Patients with NSTE-ACS can develop recurrent ischemic events or any of the complications associated with ST segment elevation MI, including arrhythmias, heart failure, and mechanical complications (Chapter 73). However, the acute complications other than recurrent ischemia occur less often in subjects with NSTE-ACS because the amount of myocardial damage usually is less.

Because intensive medical therapy in conjunction with invasive management can lead to life-threatening bleeding complications, the patient's risk of such should be assessed before these therapies are instituted. Female gender, older age, renal insufficiency, low body weight, tachycardia, systolic arterial pressure, hematocrit, and diabetes mellitus predict an increased risk of major bleeding, often due to excessive dosing of antiplatelet or anticoagulant agents. The bleeding risk can be estimated with the tool available at *www.crusadebleedingscore.org*.

Integrated Approach to Treatment

Although the treatment of the subject with NSTE-ACS should be individualized, taking into account the specific features of the disease and the particular circumstances of the patient, algorithms nonetheless provide a useful framework (Fig. 72-3).

NSTE-ACS is an acute episode related to one active culprit lesion, but the patient often has diffuse atherosclerosis. Smoking cessation (Chapter 31), cholesterol lowering (Chapter 213), control of blood pressure (Chapter 67), and diabetes mellitus (Chapters 236 and 237) are important long-term prevention strategies. Maintaining compliance long-term with medical therapy appears to reduce the risk of a future ischemic event by up to 80%.

PROGNOSIS

Because the number of ECG leads demonstrating ST segment depression and the magnitude of such depression are indicative of the extent and severity of myocardial ischemia and MI, it is not surprising that ST segment depression correlates with the patient's prognosis. Compared with subjects without

FIGURE 72-3. Approach to the patient with acute coronary syndrome (ACS). Low-risk patients have age < 75 years, no elevation in serum troponin concentration, and two or fewer Thrombolysis in Myocardial Infarction (TIMI) risk variables. Intermediate- or high-risk patients are those with age > 75 years, elevated serum troponin concentration, or three or more TIMI risk variables. The Global Registry of Acute Coronary Events (GRACE) score is available at *www.outcomes-umassmed.org/grace.* GP = glycoprotein; LMWH = low-molecular-weight heparin; NSTE = non–ST segment elevation.

ST segment depression, the patient with NSTE-ACS who has ST segment depression of 1 mm or greater in two or more leads is almost four times as likely to die within 1 year, and the patient with ST segment depression of 2 mm or greater in magnitude is almost six times as likely to die within 1 year. If ST segment depression of 2 mm or greater is present in more than one region of the ECG, the mortality is increased ten-fold. Even the 20% of patients with ACS who have only 0.5 to 1 mm of ST segment depression have an adverse prognosis. Patients with ST segment depression also have a higher risk for subsequent cardiac events compared with patients with only T wave inversion (>1 mm).

The magnitude of the serum troponin concentration predicts short-term (30 days) and long-term (1 year) risks of recurrent MI and death, independent of ECG abnormalities or markers of inflammatory activity. C-reactive protein measured with a highly sensitive assay, which is a widely used marker of inflammation, has no role in the diagnosis of ACS but is predictive of long-term (6 months) mortality among patients with troponin-negative NSTE-ACS. Elevated levels of natriuretic peptides (B-type natriuretic peptide [BNP] or its N-terminal prohormone [NT-proBNP]) are associated with a three- to five-fold increased mortality in patients with NSTE-ACS, although they have limited value for diagnosis, initial risk stratification, and selection of an initial management strategy. Natriuretic peptide concentrations measured a few days after the onset of symptoms have better predictive value than those measured at the time of hospitalization. In patients with NSTE-ACS, a simultaneous assessment of troponin, hsCRP, and BNP is superior to a single biomarker assessment at predicting short-term (in-hospital and 30-day) outcome.

During the past two decades, the prognosis of patients with ACS has improved dramatically with the introduction of more effective medical therapy and revascularization techniques. In contrast to individuals with ST segment elevation MI, in whom most events occur before or shortly after presentation to the hospital, patients with NSTE-ACS continue to have these events during the ensuing days, weeks, and months. Although in-hospital mortality is higher in patients with ST segment elevation MI than among those with NSTE-ACS (7 vs. 5%, respectively), the mortality rates at 6 months are similar for the two conditions (12 vs. 13%, respectively). During long-term follow-up of patients hospitalized with ACS, rates of death are actually higher in those with NSTE-ACS than in those with ST segment elevation MI, with a two-fold difference after 4 years. As a result, treatment strategies for NSTE-ACS should address the issues related to both the acute event and longer-term treatment.

1. Morrow DA, Cannon CP, Rifai N, et al. Ability of minor elevations of troponins I and T to predict benefit from an early invasive strategy in patients with non-ST elevation myocardial infarction: results from a randomized trial. *JAMA.* 2001;286:2405-2412.
2. Mehta SR, Granger CB, Boden WE, et al. Early versus delayed invasive intervention in acute coronary syndromes. *N Engl J Med.* 2009;360:2165-2175.
3. O'Donoghue M, Boden WE, Braunwald E, et al. Early invasive vs conservative treatment strategies in women and men with unstable angina and non-ST-segment elevation myocardial infarction: a meta-analysis. *JAMA.* 2008;300:71-80.
4. Gibson RS, Boden WE, Theroux P, et al. Diltiazem and reinfarction in patients with non-Q-wave myocardial infarction: results of a double-blind, randomized, multicenter trial. *N Engl J Med.* 1986;315:423-429.
5. Collaborative meta-analysis of randomised trials of antiplatelet therapy for prevention of death, myocardial infarction, and stroke in high risk patients. *BMJ.* 2002;324:71-86.
6. Yusuf S, Mehta SR, Zhao F, et al. Early and late effects of clopidogrel in patients with acute coronary syndromes. *Circulation.* 2003;107:966-972.
7. Wiviott SD, Braunwald E, McCabe CH, et al. Prasugrel versus clopidogrel in patients with acute coronary syndromes. *N Engl J Med.* 2007;357:2001-2015.
8. Giugliano RP, White JA, Bode C, et al. Early versus delayed, provisional eptifibatide in acute coronary syndromes. *N Engl J Med.* 2009;360:2176-2190.
9. Eikelboom JW, Anand SS, Malmberg K, et al. Unfractionated heparin and low-molecular-weight heparin in acute coronary syndrome without ST elevation: a meta-analysis. *Lancet.* 2000;355: 1936-1942.
10. Antman EM, Cohen M, Bernink PJ, et al. The TIMI risk score for unstable angina/non-ST elevation MI: a method for prognostication and therapeutic decision making. *JAMA.* 2000;284:835-842.

11. Yusuf S, Mehta SR, Chrolavicius S, et al. Comparison of fondaparinux and enoxaparin in acute coronary syndromes. *N Engl J Med.* 2006;354:1464-1476.
12. Stone GW, McLaurin BT, Cox DA, et al. Bivalirudin for patients with acute coronary syndromes. *N Engl J Med.* 2006;355:2203-2216.
13. Cannon CP, Braunwald E, McCabe CH, et al. Intensive versus moderate lipid lowering with statins after acute coronary syndromes. *N Engl J Med.* 2004;350:1495-1504.
14. Cannon CP, Weintraub WS, Demopoulos LA, et al. Comparison of early invasive and conservative strategies in patients with unstable coronary syndromes treated with the glycoprotein IIb/IIIa inhibitor tirofiban. *N Engl J Med.* 2001;344:1879-1887.

SUGGESTED READINGS

Anderson JL, Adams CD, Antman EM, et al. ACC/AHA 2007 guidelines for the management of patients with unstable angina/non ST-elevation myocardial infarction: a report of the American College of Cardiology/American Heart Association Task Force on Practice Guidelines (Writing Committee to Revise the 2002 Guidelines for the Management of Patients With Unstable Angina/Non ST-Elevation Myocardial Infarction): developed in collaboration with the American College of Emergency Physicians, the Society for Cardiovascular Angiography and Interventions, and the Society of Thoracic Surgeons: endorsed by the American Association of Cardiovascular and Pulmonary Rehabilitation and the Society for Academic Emergency Medicine. *Circulation.* 2007;116:e148-304. *Comprehensive guidelines.*

Chew DP, Anderson FA, Avezum A, et al. Six month survival benefits associated with clinical guideline recommendations in acute coronary syndromes. *Heart.* 2010;96:1201-1206. *PCI, CABG, statins, and clopidogrel were the major contributors to better outcomes with guideline-driven care.*

Hillis LD, Lange RA. Optimal management of acute coronary syndromes. *N Engl J Med.* 2009;360:2237-2240. *Review.*

Stone GW, Maehara A, Lansky A, et al. A prospective natural-history study of coronary atherosclerosis. *N Engl J Med.* 2011;364:226-235. *Coronary lesions responsible for ACS are often initially angiographically mild (~30% stenosis) with a thin-cap fibroatheroma, large plaque burden, small luminal area, or some combination of these.*

73

ST SEGMENT ELEVATION ACUTE MYOCARDIAL INFARCTION AND COMPLICATIONS OF MYOCARDIAL INFARCTION

JEFFREY L. ANDERSON

DEFINITION

Conceptually, myocardial infarction (MI) is myocardial necrosis caused by ischemia. Practically, MI can be diagnosed and evaluated by clinical, electrocardiographic, biochemical, radiologic, and pathologic methods. Technologic advances in detecting much smaller amounts of myocardial necrosis than previously possible (e.g., by troponin determinations) have required a redefinition of MI. Given these developments, the term *MI* now should be qualified with regard to size, precipitating circumstance, and timing. This chapter focuses on acute MI associated with ST segment elevation on the electrocardiogram (ECG). This category of acute MI is characterized by profound ("transmural") acute myocardial ischemia affecting relatively large areas of myocardium. The underlying cause essentially always is *complete* interruption of regional myocardial blood flow (resulting from coronary occlusion, usually atherothrombotic) (Chapter 70). This clinical syndrome should be distinguished from non–ST segment elevation MI, in which the blockage of coronary flow is incomplete and for which different acute therapies are appropriate (Chapter 72).

EPIDEMIOLOGY

Cardiovascular disease is responsible for almost one half of all deaths in the United States and other developed countries and for one fourth of deaths in the developing world (Chapter 51). By 2020, cardiovascular disease will cause one of every three deaths worldwide. Cardiovascular disease causes almost 1 million deaths in the United States each year; it accounts for 37% of all deaths and contributes to 58% of deaths. Annually, an estimated 1.2 million U.S. residents suffer a fatal or nonfatal acute MI. Coronary heart disease, the leading cause of cardiovascular death, underlies or is a contributing cause of 650,000 deaths annually. Half of coronary heart disease deaths (250,000/year) are directly related to acute MI, and at least half of these acute MI–related deaths occur within 1 hour of onset of symptoms and before patients reach a hospital emergency department.

More than 5 million people visit emergency departments in the United States each year for evaluation of chest pain and related symptoms, and almost 1.5 million are hospitalized for an acute coronary syndrome (Chapter 50). The presence of ST segment elevation or new left bundle branch block (LBBB) on the ECG distinguishes patients with acute MI who require consideration of immediate recanalization therapy from other patients with an acute coronary syndrome (non–ST segment elevation MI/unstable angina; Chapter 72). Changing demographics, lifestyles, and medical therapies have led to a decrease in the ratio of ST segment elevation MI to non–ST segment elevation acute coronary syndromes over the past 10 to 15 years, so ST segment elevation MI now accounts for about 30% of all MIs. However, ST segment elevation MI is associated with greater in-hospital (but not posthospital) mortality than non–ST segment elevation MI, and it remains an important contributor to total population mortality.

PATHOBIOLOGY

Erosion, fissuring, or rupture of vulnerable atherosclerotic plaques has been determined to be the initiating mechanism of coronary thrombotic occlusion, thereby precipitating intraplaque hemorrhage, coronary spasm, and occlusive luminal thrombosis (Chapter 70). Plaque rupture most frequently occurs in lipid-laden plaques with an endothelial cap weakened by internal collagenase (metalloproteinase) activity derived primarily from macrophages. These macrophages are recruited to the plaque from blood monocytes responding to inflammatory mediators and adhesion molecules.

With plaque rupture, elements of the blood stream are exposed to the highly thrombogenic plaque core and matrix containing lipid, tissue factor, and collagen. Platelets adhere, become activated, and aggregate; vasoconstrictive and thrombogenic mediators are secreted; vasospasm occurs; thrombin is generated and fibrin formed; and a partially or totally occlusive platelet- and fibrin-rich thrombus is generated. When coronary flow is occluded, electrocardiographic ST segment elevation occurs (ST segment elevation acute MI). Partial occlusion, occlusion in the presence of collateral circulation, and distal coronary embolization result in unstable angina or non–ST segment elevation MI (Chapter 72). Ischemia from impaired myocardial perfusion causes myocardial cell injury or death, ventricular dysfunction, and cardiac arrhythmias.

Although most MIs are caused by atherosclerosis, occasional patients can develop complete coronary occlusions owing to coronary emboli, in situ thrombosis, vasculitis, primary vasospasm, infiltrative or degenerative diseases, diseases of the aorta, congenital anomalies of a coronary artery, or trauma (Table 73-1). In a canine model of coronary occlusion and recanalization, myocardial cell death begins within 15 minutes of occlusion and proceeds rapidly in a wave front from endocardium to epicardium. Partial myocardial salvage can be achieved by releasing the occlusion within 3 to 6 hours; the degree of salvage is inversely proportional to the duration of ischemia and occurs in a reverse wave front from epicardium to endocardium. The extent of myocardial necrosis can also be altered by modification of metabolic demands and collateral blood supply. The temporal dynamic of infarction in human disease, although more complex, is generally similar.

CLINICAL MANIFESTATIONS

Traditionally, the diagnosis of acute MI has rested on the triad of ischemic-type chest discomfort, ECG abnormalities, and elevated serum cardiac markers. Acute MI was considered present when at least two of the three were present. With their increasing sensitivity and specificity, serum cardiac markers (e.g., troponin I [TnI] or troponin T [TnT]) have assumed a dominant role in confirming the diagnosis of acute MI in patients with suggestive clinical or ECG features.

History

Ischemic-type chest discomfort is the most prominent clinical symptom in most patients with acute MI (see Table 50-1 in Chapter 50). The discomfort is characterized by its quality, location, duration, radiation, and precipitating and relieving factors. The discomfort associated with acute MI is qualitatively similar to that of angina pectoris but more severe. It often is perceived as heavy, pressing, crushing, squeezing, bandlike, viselike, strangling, constricting, aching, or burning; it rarely is perceived as sharp pain and generally not as stabbing pain (Chapters 50 and 71).

The primary location of typical ischemic pain is most consistently retrosternal, but it also can present left parasternally, left precordially, or across the anterior chest (Chapter 50). Occasionally, discomfort is

TABLE 73-1 CONDITIONS OTHER THAN CORONARY ATHEROSCLEROSIS THAT CAN CAUSE ACUTE MYOCARDIAL INFARCTION

Coronary emboli	Causes include aortic or mitral valve lesions, left atrial or ventricular thrombi, prosthetic valves, fat emboli, intracardiac neoplasms, infective endocarditis, and paradoxical emboli
Thrombotic coronary artery disease	Can occur with oral contraceptive use, sickle cell anemia and other hemoglobinopathies, polycythemia vera, thrombocytosis, thrombotic thrombocytopenic purpura, disseminated intravascular coagulation, antithrombin III deficiency and other hypercoagulable states, macroglobulinemia and other hyperviscosity states, multiple myeloma, leukemia, malaria, and fibrinolytic system shutdown secondary to impaired plasminogen activation or excessive inhibition
Coronary vasculitis	Seen with Takayasu's disease, Kawasaki disease, polyarteritis nodosa, lupus erythematosus, scleroderma, rheumatoid arthritis, and immune-mediated vascular degeneration in cardiac allografts
Coronary vasospasm	Can be associated with variant angina, nitrate withdrawal, cocaine or amphetamine abuse, and angina with "normal" coronary arteries
Infiltrative and degenerative coronary vascular disease	Can result from amyloidosis, connective tissue disorders (e.g., pseudoxanthoma elasticum), lipid storage disorders and mucopolysaccharidoses, homocystinuria, diabetes mellitus, collagen vascular disease, muscular dystrophies, and Friedreich's ataxia
Coronary ostial occlusion	Associated with aortic dissection, luetic aortitis, aortic stenosis, and ankylosing spondylitis syndromes
Congenital coronary anomalies	Including Bland-White-Garland syndrome of anomalous origin of the left coronary artery from the pulmonary artery, left coronary artery origin from the anterior sinus of Valsalva, coronary arteriovenous fistula or aneurysms, and myocardial bridging with secondary vascular degeneration
Trauma	Associated with and responsible for coronary dissection, laceration, or thrombosis (with endothelial cell secondary to trauma such as angioplasty) and with radiation and cardiac contusion
Augmented myocardial oxygen requirements exceeding oxygen delivery	Encountered with aortic stenosis, aortic insufficiency, hypertension with severe left ventricular hypertrophy, pheochromocytoma, thyrotoxicosis, methemoglobinemia, carbon monoxide poisoning, shock, and hyperviscosity syndromes

predominantly perceived in the anterior neck, jaw, arms, or epigastrium. It generally is somewhat diffuse; highly localized pain (finger point) is rarely angina or acute MI. The most characteristic pattern of radiation is to the left arm, but the right arm or both arms can be involved. The shoulders, neck, jaw, teeth, epigastrium, and interscapular areas also are sites of radiation. Discomfort above the jaws or below the umbilicus is not typical of acute MI. Associated symptoms often include nausea, vomiting, diaphoresis, weakness, dyspnea, restlessness, and apprehension.

The discomfort of acute MI is more severe and lasts longer (typically 20 minutes to several hours) than angina, and it is not reliably relieved by rest or nitroglycerin. The onset of acute MI usually is unrelated to exercise or other apparent precipitating factors. Nevertheless, acute MI begins during physical or emotional stress and within a few hours of arising more frequently than explained by chance.

It is estimated that at least 20% of acute MIs are painless ("silent") or atypical (unrecognized). Elderly patients and patients with diabetes are particularly prone to painless or atypical MI, which occurs in as many as one third to one half of such patients. Because the prognosis is worse in elderly patients and in those patients with diabetes, diagnostic vigilance is required. In these patients, acute MI can present as sudden dyspnea (which can progress to pulmonary edema), weakness, lightheadedness, nausea, and vomiting. Confusional states, sudden loss of consciousness, a new rhythm disorder, and an unexplained fall in blood pressure are other uncommon presentations. The differential diagnosis of ischemic chest discomfort also should include gastrointestinal disorders (e.g., reflux esophagitis; Chapter 140), musculoskeletal pain (e.g., costochondritis), anxiety or panic attacks, pleurisy or pulmonary embolism (Chapter 98), and acute aortic dissection (see Table 50-2 in Chapter 50 and Chapter 78).

Physical Examination

No physical findings are diagnostic or pathognomonic of acute MI. The physical examination can be entirely normal or may reveal only nonspecific abnormalities. An S_4 gallop frequently is found if carefully sought. Blood pressure often is initially elevated, but it may be normal or low. Signs of sympathetic hyperactivity (tachycardia, hypertension, or both) often accompany anterior wall MI, whereas parasympathetic hyperactivity (bradycardia, hypotension, or both) is more common with inferior wall MI.

The examination is best focused on an overall assessment of cardiac function. Adequacy of vital signs and peripheral perfusion should be noted. Signs of cardiac failure, both left and right sided (e.g., S_3 gallop, pulmonary congestion, elevated neck veins) should be sought, and observation for arrhythmias and mechanical complications (e.g., new murmurs) is essential. If hypoperfusion is present, determination of its primary cause (e.g., hypovolemia, right heart failure, left heart failure) is critical to management.

DIAGNOSIS

Electrocardiogram

In patients with a possible acute MI, an ECG must be obtained immediately. Although the initial ECG is neither perfectly specific nor perfectly sensitive in all patients who develop acute ST segment elevation myocardial infarction (STEMI), it plays a critical role in initial stratification, triage, and management (Chapter 50). In an appropriate clinical setting, a pattern of regional ECG ST segment elevation suggests coronary occlusion causing marked myocardial ischemia; hospital admission is indicated with triage to the coronary care unit (CCU). An emergency recanalization strategy (primary angioplasty or fibrinolysis) should be used unless it is contraindicated. Other ECG patterns (ST segment depression, T wave inversion, nonspecific changes, normal ECG) in association with ischemic chest discomfort are consistent with a non–ST segment elevation acute coronary syndrome (non–ST segment elevation MI or unstable angina) and are treated with different triage and initial management strategies (Chapter 72).

Electrocardiographic Evolution

Serial ECG tracings improve the sensitivity and specificity of the ECG for the diagnosis of acute MI and assist in assessing the outcomes of therapy. When typical ST segment elevation persists for hours and is followed within hours to days by T wave inversions and Q waves, the diagnosis of acute MI can be made with virtual certainty. The ECG changes in ST segment elevation acute MI evolve through three overlapping phases: (1) hyperacute or early acute, (2) evolved acute, and (3) chronic (stabilized).

Early Acute Phase

This earliest phase begins within minutes, persists, and evolves over hours. T waves increase in amplitude and widen over the area of injury (hyperacute pattern). ST segments evolve from concave to a straightened to a convex upward pattern (acute pattern). When prominent, the acute injury pattern of blended ST-T waves can take on a tombstone appearance (Figs. 73-1 and 73-2). ST segment depressions that occur in leads opposite those with ST segment elevation are known as *reciprocal changes* and are associated with larger areas of injury and a worse prognosis but also with greater benefits from recanalization therapy.

Other causes of ST segment elevation must be considered and excluded. These conditions include pericarditis (Chapter 77), left ventricular (LV) hypertrophy with J point elevation, and normal variant early repolarization (Chapter 54). Pericarditis (or perimyocarditis) is of particular concern because it can mimic acute MI clinically, but fibrinolytic therapy is *not* indicated and can be hazardous.

FIGURE 73-1. Electrocardiographic tracing shows an acute anterolateral myocardial infarction. Note ST segment elevation in leads I, L, and V$_1$ to V$_6$ with Q waves in V$_1$ to V$_4$.

FIGURE 73-2. Electrocardiographic tracing shows an acute inferoposterior myocardial infarction.

Evolved Acute Phase

During the second phase, ST segment elevation begins to regress, T waves in leads with ST segment elevation become inverted, and pathologic Q or QS waves become fully developed (>0.03-second duration or depth >30% of R wave amplitude, or both).

Chronic Phase

Resolution of ST segment elevation is quite variable. It is usually complete within 2 weeks of inferior MI, but it can be delayed further after anterior MI. Persistent ST segment elevation, often seen with a large anterior MI, is indicative of a large area of akinesis, dyskinesis, or ventricular aneurysm. Symmetrical T wave inversions can resolve over weeks to months or can persist for an indefinite period; hence, the age of an MI in the presence of T wave inversions is often termed *indeterminate*. Q waves usually do not resolve after anterior MI but often disappear after inferior wall MI.

Early recanalization therapy accelerates the time course of ECG changes so that, on coronary recanalization, the pattern can evolve from acute to chronic over minutes to hours instead of days to weeks. ST segments recede rapidly, T wave inversions and losses of R wave occur earlier, and Q waves may not develop or progress and occasionally may regress. Indeed, failure of ST segment elevation to resolve by more than 50 to 70% within 1 to 2 hours suggests failure of fibrinolysis and should prompt urgent angiography for "rescue angioplasty."

True Posterior Myocardial Infarction and Left Circumflex Myocardial Infarction Patterns

"True posterior" MI presents a mirror-image pattern of ECG injury in leads V$_1$ to V$_2$ to V$_4$ (Fig. 73-2). Anatomically, the location of injury of "true posterior MI" by magnetic resonance imaging actually involves portions of the *lateral* left ventricular wall and is typically caused by occlusion of a nondominant left circumflex artery. The acute phase is characterized by ST segment depression, rather than ST segment elevation. The evolved and chronic phases show increased R wave amplitude and widening instead of Q waves. Recognition of a true posterior acute MI pattern is challenging but important because the diagnosis should lead to an immediate recanalization strategy. Extending the ECG to measure left posterior leads V$_7$ to V$_9$ increases sensitivity for detecting acute left circumflex–related injury patterns (i.e., ST segment elevation) with excellent specificity (Chapter 54). Other causes of prominent upright anteroseptal forces include right ventricular (RV) hypertrophy, ventricular preexcitation variants (Wolff-Parkinson-White syndrome; Chapter 64), and normal variants with early R wave progression. New appearance of these changes or the association with an acute or evolving inferior MI usually allows the diagnosis to be made.

Right Ventricular Infarction

Proximal occlusion of the right coronary artery before the acute marginal branch can cause RV as well as acute inferior MI in about 30% of cases. Because the prognosis and treatment of acute inferior MI differ in the presence of RV infarction, it is important to make this diagnosis. The diagnosis is assisted by obtaining right precordial ECG leads, which are routinely indicated for inferior acute MI (Chapter 54). Acute ST segment elevation of at least 1 mm (0.1 mV) in one or more of leads V$_{4R}$ to V$_{6R}$ is both sensitive and specific (>90%) for identifying acute RV injury, and Q or QS waves effectively identify RV infarction.

Diagnosis in the Presence of Bundle Branch Block

The presence of LBBB often obscures ST segment analysis in patients with suspected acute MI. The presence of a new (or presumed new) LBBB in association with clinical (and laboratory) findings suggesting acute MI is associated with high mortality; patients with new-onset LBBB benefit substantially from recanalization therapy and should undergo triage and treatment in the same way as patients with ST segment elevation MI. Certain ECG patterns, although relatively insensitive, suggest acute MI if present in

TABLE 73-2 CONDITIONS THAT CAN MIMIC ST SEGMENT ELEVATION MYOCARDIAL INFARCTION

Early repolarization with non-coronary chest pain
Myocarditis
Pericarditis
Takotsubo cardiomyopathy

the setting of LBBB: Q waves in two of leads I, aVL, V_5, V_6; R wave regression from V_1 to V_4; ST segment elevation of 1 mm or more in leads with a positive QRS complex; ST segment depression of 1 mm or more in leads V_1, V_2, or V_3; and ST segment elevation of 5 mm or more associated with a negative QRS complex. The presence of right bundle branch block (RBBB) usually does not mask typical ST-T wave or Q wave changes, except for rare cases of isolated true posterior acute MI, characterized by tall right precordial R waves and ST segment depressions.

Differential Diagnosis

Although ST-segment elevation MI is often an easy diagnosis to make based on the presentation and test results (see later), other considerations include acute pericarditis (Chapter 77), acute myocarditis (Chapter 60), stress-induced takotsubo syndrome (Chapter 60), and early repolarization (Table 73-2). All but early repolarization can be associated with abnormal biomarkers, but none is associated with a coronary occlusion. Early coronary angiography is advised when any of these conditions is suggested or when MI may be related to a cause other than atherosclerosis (see Table 73-1).

Serum Cardiac Markers

Ideal markers are not normally present in serum, become rapidly and markedly elevated during acute MI, and are not released from other injured tissues (see Table 73-2). The increasing sensitivity and specificity of serum cardiac markers, which are macromolecules (proteins) released from myocytes undergoing necrosis, have made them the "gold standard" for detection of myocardial necrosis. However, because of the 1- to 12-hour delay after the onset of symptoms before markers become detectable or diagnostic, and given laboratory delays even when markers are positive, the decision to proceed with an urgent recanalization strategy (primary angioplasty or fibrinolysis) must be based on the patient's clinical history and initial ECG (Chapter 50).

Troponins I and T

Troponins have replaced other markers because they are more specific in the setting of injuries to skeletal muscle or other organs and also are more sensitive in the setting of minimal myocardial injury. Cardiac-derived TnI (cTnI) and TnT (cTnT), proteins of the sarcomere, are not normally present in the blood with standard sensitivity assays and have amino acid sequences distinct from their skeletal muscle isoforms. With even small acute MIs, troponins increase to 20-fold or more above the lower limits of the assay, and elevations persist for several days.

The troponins generally are first detectable 2 to 4 hours after the onset of acute MI, are maximally sensitive at 8 to 12 hours, peak at 10 to 24 hours, and persist for 5 to 14 days. Their long persistence has allowed them to replace other markers for the diagnosis of acute MI in patients presenting late (>1 to 2 days) after symptoms. However, this persistence can obscure the diagnosis of an early recurrent MI, for which more rapidly cleared markers (i.e., CK-MB) are more useful. Clinically, cTnI and cTnT appear to be of approximately equivalent utility, except renal failure is more likely to be associated with false-positive elevations of cTnT than of cTnI.

Ultrasensitive troponin assays increase assay sensitivity and enable even earlier diagnosis. However, because troponins also may be present in low concentration in a number of nonischemic cardiovascular conditions, specificity for MI remains an issue.

Other Laboratory Tests

On admission, routine assessment of complete blood count and platelet count, standard blood chemistry studies, a lipid panel, and coagulation tests (prothrombin time, partial thromboplastin time) are useful. Results assist in assessing comorbid conditions and prognosis and in guiding therapy. Hematologic tests provide a useful baseline before initiation of antiplatelet, antithrombin, and fibrinolytic therapy or coronary angiography or angioplasty.

Myocardial injury precipitates polymorphonuclear leukocytosis, commonly resulting in an elevation of white blood cell count of up to 12,000 to 15,000/μL, which appears within a few hours and peaks at 2 to 4 days. The metabolic panel provides a useful check on electrolytes, glucose, and renal function. On hospital admission or the next morning, a fasting lipid panel is recommended to assist in decision making for inpatient lipid lowering (e.g., statin therapy if low-density lipoprotein is greater than 70 mg/dL (Chapter 213). Unless carbon dioxide retention is suspected, finger oximetry is adequate to titrate oxygen therapy. The C-reactive protein level increases with acute MI, but its incremental prognostic value in the acute setting is unknown. B-type natriuretic peptide, which increases with ventricular wall stress and relative circulatory fluid overload, may provide useful incremental prognostic information in the setting of acute MI.

Imaging

A chest radiograph is the only imaging test *routinely* obtained on admission for acute MI. Although the chest radiograph is often normal, findings of pulmonary venous congestion, cardiomegaly, or widened mediastinum can contribute importantly to diagnosis and management decisions. For example, a history of severe, "tearing" chest and back pain in association with a widened mediastinum should raise the question of a dissecting aortic aneurysm (Chapter 78). In such cases, fibrinolytic therapy must be withheld pending more definitive diagnostic imaging of the aorta. Other noninvasive imaging (e.g., echocardiography [Chapter 55], cardiac nuclear scanning [Chapter 56], and other testing) is performed for evaluation of specific clinical issues, including suspected complications of acute MI. Coronary angiography (Chapter 57) is performed urgently as part of an interventional strategy for acute MI or later for risk stratification in higher-risk patients who are managed medically.

Echocardiography

Two-dimensional transthoracic echocardiography with color-flow Doppler imaging is the most generally useful noninvasive test obtained on admission or early in the hospital course (Chapter 55). Echocardiography efficiently assesses global and regional cardiac function and enables the clinician to evaluate suspected complications of acute MI. The sensitivity and specificity of echocardiography for regional wall motion assessment are high (>90%), although the age of the abnormality (new versus old) must be distinguished clinically or by ECG. Echocardiography is helpful in determining the cause of circulatory failure with hypotension (relative hypovolemia, LV failure, RV failure, or mechanical complication of acute MI). Echocardiography also can assist in differentiating pericarditis and perimyocarditis from acute MI. Doppler echocardiography is indicated to evaluate a new murmur and other suspected mechanical complications of acute MI (papillary muscle dysfunction or rupture, acute ventricular septal defect, LV free wall rupture with tamponade or pseudoaneurysm). Later in the course of acute MI, echocardiography may be used to assess the degree of recovery of stunned myocardium after recanalization therapy, the degree of residual cardiac dysfunction and indications for angiotensin-converting enzyme (ACE) inhibitors and other therapies for heart failure, and the presence of LV aneurysm and mural thrombus (requiring oral anticoagulants).

Radionuclide, Magnetic Resonance, and Other Imaging Studies

Radionuclide techniques generally are too time consuming and cumbersome for routine use in the acute setting. More commonly, they are used in risk stratification before or after hospital discharge to augment exercise or pharmacologic stress testing (Chapter 56). Thallium-201 and, increasingly, technetium-99m sestamibi (alone or together—dual isotope imaging) remain the most frequently used "cold spot" tracers to assess myocardial perfusion and viability, as well as infarct size, although additional tracers are becoming available. Infarct-avid tracers to identify, locate, and size recent myocardial necrosis are available but are rarely required for ST segment elevation MI. Computed tomography (Chapter 56) and magnetic resonance imaging (Chapter 56) can be useful to evaluate patients with a suspected dissecting aortic aneurysm and, together with positron emission tomography, for research purposes and in selected clinical applications such as for assessment of myocardial viability (infarct sizing). When the issue of a non-atherosclerotic cause of myocardial necrosis is raised (e.g., perimyocarditis simulating acute MI), contemporary multislice (e.g., 64-slice) coronary computed tomography (Chapter 56) can assess coronary artery disease qualitatively and semiquantitatively, and it can also distinguish other causes of chest pain syndromes (Chapters 50 and 56).

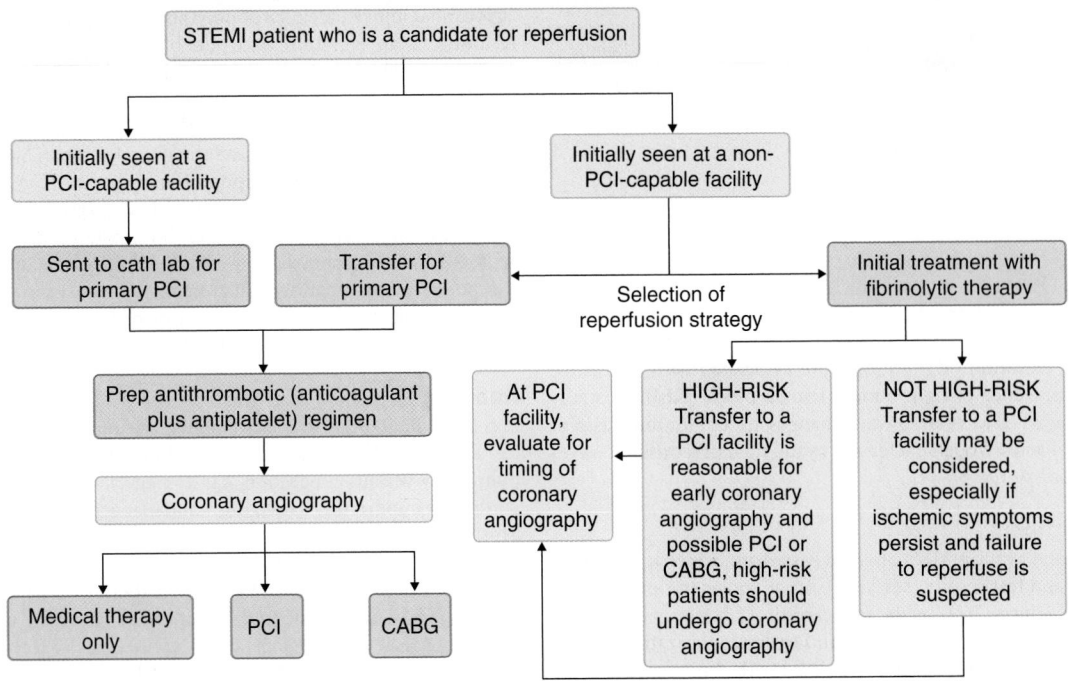

FIGURE 73-3. Evidence-based approach to percutaneous coronary intervention (PCI) and coronary artery bypass grafting (CABG) after ST segment elevation myocardial infarction (STEMI). (Adapted from Kushner FG, Hand M, Smith SC Jr, et al. 2009 Focused updates: ACC/AHA guidelines for the management of patients with ST-elevation myocardial infarction and the ACC/AHA/SCAI guidelines on percutaneous coronary intervention. *J Am Coll Cardiol.* 2009;54:2205-2241.)

TREATMENT   Rx

Assessment and Management

Prehospital Phase

More than one half of deaths related to acute MI occur within 1 hour of onset of symptoms and before the patient reaches a hospital emergency department. Most of these deaths are caused by ischemia-related ventricular fibrillation (VF) and can be reversed by defibrillation (Chapters 63 and 66). Rapid defibrillation allows resuscitation in 60% of patients when treatment is delivered by a bystander using an on-site automatic external defibrillator or by a first-responding medical rescuer (Chapter 63). Moreover, the first hour represents the best opportunity for myocardial salvage with recanalization therapy. Thus, the three goals of prehospital care are as follows: (1) to recognize symptoms promptly and seek medical attention; (2) to deploy an emergency medical system team capable of cardiac monitoring, defibrillation and resuscitation, and emergency medical therapy (e.g., nitroglycerin, lidocaine, atropine); and (3) to transport the patient expeditiously to a medical care facility staffed with personnel capable of providing expert coronary care, including recanalization therapy (primary angioplasty or fibrinolysis).

The greatest time lag to recanalization therapy is the patient's delay in calling for help. Public education efforts have yielded mixed results, and innovative approaches are needed. The feasibility of initiating fibrinolytic therapy by highly trained ambulance personnel in coordinated ambulance and emergency department systems has been shown. More recently, data indicate that high-dose prehospital tirofiban (25 µg/kg bolus, then 0.15 µg/kg/minute for 18 hours) can improve intermediate outcomes in patients with acute ST elevation MI who undergo percutaneous coronary intervention and is equivalent to abciximab.**1** In coordinated systems and when transportation delays are substantial, initiation of fibrinolytic or other antithrombotic therapy in the field may be considered, thereby shortening the time to recanalization.

Hospital Phases

Emergency Department

The goals of emergency department care are to identify patients with acute myocardial ischemia rapidly, to stratify them into acute ST segment elevation MI as compared with other acute coronary syndromes (see Fig. 72-1 in Chapter 72 and Fig. 73-1), to initiate a recanalization strategy and other appropriate medical care in qualifying patients with acute ST segment elevation MI, and to prioritize by triage rapidly to inpatient care (CCU, step-down unit, observation unit) or outpatient care (patients without suspected ischemia) (see Fig. 72-2 in Chapter 72).

The evaluation of patients with chest pain and other suspected acute coronary syndromes begins with a 12-lead ECG even as the physician is beginning a focused history, including contraindications to fibrinolysis, and a targeted physical examination. Continuous ECG monitoring should be started, an intravenous line should be established, and admission blood tests should be drawn (including cardiac markers such as cTnI or cTnT). As rapidly as possible, the patient should be stratified as having a probable ST segment elevation acute MI, a non–ST segment elevation acute MI, probable or possible unstable angina, or likely noncardiac chest pain.

In patients with ST segment elevation acute MI by clinical and ECG criteria, a recanalization strategy must be selected: alternative choices are primary percutaneous coronary intervention (primary PCI; the patient is transferred directly to the cardiac catheterization laboratory with a goal of door-to-balloon time of less than 90 minutes) or fibrinolysis (begun immediately in the emergency department with a goal of door-to-needle time of less than 30 minutes) (Fig. 73-3).

Aspirin (162 to 325 mg) should be given to all patients unless it is contraindicated (see Fig. 73-3). A loading dose of a thienopyridine (e.g., clopidogrel, 600 mg, or prasugrel, 60 mg) also is recommended for STEMI patients for whom PCI is planned. In addition, it is reasonable to start treatment with a glycoprotein IIb/IIIa (GPIIb-IIIa) receptor antagonist (abciximab, 0.25 mg/kg IV bolus, then 0.125 µg/kg/minute [maximum, 10 µg/minute] for up to 12 hours), tirofiban (25 µg/kg IV bolus, then 0.15 µg/kg/minute for 12 to 18 hours; reduce infusion rate by 50% for estimated creatinine clearance less than 30 mL/minute) or eptifibatide (180 µg/kg IV bolus, second bolus after 10 minutes, then 2.0 µg/kg/minute for up to 18 hours; reduce infusion by 50% for estimated creatinine clearance less than 50 mL/minute) at the time of primary PCI for STEMI in selected patients, such as those with a large burden of thrombus or those who have not received adequate thienopyridine loading. It is uncertain whether there is any incremental usefulness of starting GPIIb-IIIa receptor antagonists "upstream," before arrival in the catheterization laboratory.

Intravenous heparin (initial bolus 60 IU/kg, maximum, 4000 IU, then 12 IU/kg/hour, maximum 1000 IU/hour, for patients >70 kg, adjusted to maintain activated partial thromboplastin time 1.5 to 2 times the control value) or low-molecular-weight heparin (LMWH; e.g., enoxaparin, 30 mg intravenous bolus, then 1 mg/kg subcutaneously twice daily, for patients <75 years old without renal insufficiency) or bivalirudin (for those undergoing a primary PCI strategy—0.75 mg/kg bolus, then 1.75 mg/kg/hour infusion) is appropriate in most patients. In STEMI patients who are undergoing PCI who are at higher risk for bleeding, evidence supports using bivalirudin anticoagulation with a thienopyridine but without a GPIIb-IIIa receptor antagonist.**2**

Patients with chest pain should be given sublingual nitroglycerin (0.4 mg every 5 minutes for up to three doses), after which an assessment should be made of the need for intravenous nitroglycerin. Persistent ischemic pain may be treated with titrated intravenous doses of morphine (i.e., 2 to 4 mg intravenously [IV], repeated every 5 to 15 minutes to relieve pain). Initiation of β-blocker therapy is usually indicated, especially in patients with hypertension, tachycardia, and ongoing pain; however, decompensated heart failure is a contraindication to the acute initiation of β-blocker therapy, particularly by the intravenous route. Oxygen should be used in doses sufficient to avoid hypoxemia (e.g., initially at 2 to 4 L/minute by nasal cannula; fingertip oximetry may be used to monitor effect). The ideal systolic blood pressure is 100 to 140 mm Hg. Excessive hypertension usually responds to titrated nitroglycerin, β-blocker therapy, and morphine (also given for pain). Relative hypotension could require discontinuation of these medications, fluid administration, or other measures as appropriate to the hemodynamic subset (Table 73-3). Atropine (0.5 to 1.5 mg IV) should be available to treat symptomatic bradycardia and hypotension related to excessive vagotonia. Direct transfer to the catheterization laboratory or fibrinolysis followed by transfer to the CCU should occur as expeditiously as possible.

Early Hospital Phase: Coronary Care

Coronary care for early hospital management of acute MI has reduced in-hospital mortality by more than 50%. The goals of CCU care include (1) continuous ECG monitoring and antiarrhythmic therapy for serious arrhythmias (i.e., rapid defibrillation of VF), (2) initiation or continuation of a coronary recanalization strategy to achieve myocardial reperfusion, (3) initiation or continuation of other acute medical therapies, (4) hemodynamic monitoring and appropriate medical interventions for different hemodynamic subsets of patients, and (5) diagnosis and treatment of mechanical and physiologic complications of acute MI. General care and comfort measures also are instituted. A sample of CCU admission orders is given in Table 73-4.

General care measures include attention to activity, diet, and bowels, education, reassurance, and sedation. Bedrest is encouraged for the first 12 hours. In the absence of complications, dangling, bed to chair, and self-care activities can begin within 24 hours. When stabilization has occurred, usually within 1 to 3 days, patients may be transferred to a step-down unit where progressive reambulation occurs. The risk for emesis and aspiration or the anticipation of angiography or other procedures usually dictates nothing by mouth or clear liquids for the first 4 to 12 hours. Thereafter, a heart-healthy diet in small portions is recommended. In patients at high risk for bleeding gastric stress ulcers, a proton pump inhibitor or an H$_2$-antagonist is recommended for prophylaxis in patients receiving antithrombotic therapy. Many patients benefit from an analgesic (e.g., morphine sulfate, in 2- to 4-mg increments) to relieve ongoing pain and an anxiolytic or sedative during the CCU phase. A benzodiazepine is frequently selected. Sedatives should not be substituted for education and reassurance from concerned caregivers to relieve emotional distress and improve behavior; routine use of anxiolytics is neither necessary nor recommended. Constipation often occurs with bedrest and narcotics; stool softeners and a bedside commode are advised.

The ECG should be monitored continuously in the CCU (and usually in the step-down unit) to detect serious arrhythmias and to guide therapy. Measures to limit infarct size (i.e., coronary recanalization) and to optimize hemodynamics also stabilize the heart electrically. Routine antiarrhythmic prophylaxis (e.g., with lidocaine or amiodarone) is not indicated, but specific arrhythmias require treatment (see later text).

Hemodynamic evaluation is helpful in assessing prognosis and in guiding therapy (see Table 73-3). Clinical and noninvasive evaluation of vital signs is adequate for normotensive patients without pulmonary congestion. Patients with pulmonary venous congestion alone can usually be managed conservatively. Invasive monitoring is appropriate when the cause of circulatory failure is uncertain and when titration of intravenous therapies depends on hemodynamic measurements (e.g., pulmonary capillary wedge pressure and cardiac output). Similarly, an arterial line is not necessary in all patients and may be associated with local bleeding after fibrinolysis or potent antiplatelet and antithrombin therapy. Arterial catheters are appropriate and useful in clinically unstable, hypotensive patients who do not respond to intravenous fluids to replete or expand intravascular volume (see the later discussion of complications).

Later Hospital Phase

Transfer from the CCU to the step-down unit usually occurs within 1 to 3 days, when the cardiac rhythm and hemodynamics are stable. The duration of this late phase of hospital care is usually an additional 2 to 3 days in uncomplicated cases. Activity levels should be increased progressively under continuous ECG monitoring. Medical therapy should progress from parenteral and short-acting agents to oral medications appropriate and convenient for long-term outpatient use.

Risk stratification and functional evaluations are critical to assess prognosis and to guide therapy as the time for discharge approaches. Functional evaluation also can be extended to the early period after hospital discharge. Education must be provided about diet, activity, smoking, and other risk factors (e.g., lipids, hypertension, diabetes).

Specific Therapeutic Measures
Recanalization Therapy

Early reperfusion of ischemic, infarcting myocardium represents the most important conceptual and practical advance for ST segment elevation acute MI and is the primary therapeutic goal. Coronary recanalization is accomplished by using primary PCI with angioplasty and, commonly, stenting or with fibrinolytic (thrombolytic) therapy. With broad application of recanalization therapy, 30-day mortality rates from ST segment elevation acute MI have progressively declined over the past 3 decades (from 20 to 30% to 5 to 10%). Each community should develop and follow a multidisciplinary STEMI system of care that provides consistently optimal STEMI care within the resources available.

Fibrinolytic Therapy

Various fibrinolytic agents (Table 73-5) are useful in patients with ST segment elevation or new or presumed-new LBBB who present for treatment within 12 hours of the onset of symptoms and who have no contraindications to the use of these agents (Table 73-6). Compared with no recanalization therapy, older fibrinolytics such as streptokinase reduced mortality by 18% (from 11.5 to 9.8%) at 5 weeks. Patients with anterior ST segment elevation benefit more (37 lives saved per 1000) than those with inferior ST segment elevation only (8 lives saved per 1000), and younger patients benefit more than elderly (>75 years) patients. No benefit or a slight adverse effect is seen in patients presenting with normal ECGs or ST depression alone. Benefit is time dependent; it declines from about 40 lives or more saved per 1000 within the first hour, to 20 to 30 lives saved per 1000 for hours 2 to 12, to a nonsignificant 7 lives saved per 1000 for hours 13 to 24. An accelerated regimen of tissue plasminogen activator (t-PA plus intravenous heparin) further reduces mortality at 30 days (by 14%, from 7.3 to 6.3%), compared with streptokinase because the patency rate of the infarct-related artery at 90 minutes is higher with t-PA (81%) than with streptokinase (53 to 60%). Longer-acting variants of t-PA, given by single-bolus (tenecteplase) or double-bolus (reteplase) injections are now in widespread clinical use because they are more convenient to give, but they have not improved survival further.

The major risk of fibrinolytic therapy is bleeding. Intracerebral hemorrhage is the most serious and frequently fatal complication; its incidence rate is 0.5 to 1% with currently approved regimens. Older age (>70 to 75 years), female gender, hypertension, and higher relative doses of t-PA and heparin increase

TABLE 73-3 HEMODYNAMIC SUBSETS OF ACUTE MYOCARDIAL INFARCTION

	BLOOD PRESSURE (RELATIVE)	TYPICAL PHYSICAL FINDINGS	CARDIAC INDEX (L/min/m²)	PA WEDGE PRESSURE (mm Hg)	SUGGESTED INTERVENTIONS
Normal	Normal	±S$_4$	>2.5	≤12	None required
Hyperdynamic	Normal or high	Anxious	>3	<12	Control pain, anxiety; β-blocker; treat SBP to <140 mm Hg
Hypovolemia	Low	Dry	≤2.7	≤9	Add fluids to maintain normal pressure; can develop pulmonary edema if hypotension caused by unrecognized LV failure
Mild LV failure	Low to high	Rales, ±S$_3$	2-2.5	>15	Diuresis; nitrates, ACE inhibitor; consider low-dose β-blocker
Severe LV failure	Low to normal	Above +S$_3$, ± ↑ JVP, ± edema	<2	>20	Diuresis; nitrates; low-dose ACE inhibitor; avoid β-blockers; consider inotropes, urgent revascularization
Cardiogenic shock	Very low	Above + cool, clammy; ↓ mental or renal function	≤1.5	>25	Avoid hypotensive agents; place intra-aortic balloon pump; urgent revascularization if possible
RV infarct	Very low	↑ JVP with clear lungs	<2.5	≤12	Give IV fluids; avoid nitrates and hypotensive agents; dobutamine if refractory to fluids

↑ = increased; ↓ = decreased; ACE = angiotensin-converting enzyme; IV = intravenous; JVP = jugular venous pressure; LV = left ventricle; PA = pulmonary artery; RV = right ventricle; SBP = systolic blood pressure.

Adapted from Forrester JS, Diamond G, Chatterjee K, et al. Medical therapy of acute myocardial infarction by application of hemodynamic subsets (second of two parts). *N Engl J Med.* 1976;295:1404-1413.

TABLE 73-4 SAMPLE ADMISSION ORDERS FOR ST SEGMENT ELEVATION ACUTE MYOCARDIAL INFARCTION

Diagnosis:	Acute ST segment elevation myocardial infarction
Admit:	Coronary care unit with telemetry
Condition:	Serious
Vital signs:	q½h until stable, then q1-4h and PRN; pulse oximetry × 24 hr; notify if heart rate <50 or >100; respiratory rate <8 or >20; SBP <90 or >150 mm Hg; O₂ saturation <90%
Activity:	Bedrest × 12 hr with bedside commode; thereafter, light activity if stable
Diet:	NPO except for sips of water until pain free and stable; then 2 g sodium, heart-healthy diet as tolerated, unless on call for catheterization (or other test requiring NPO)
Laboratory tests:*	Troponin I or T and CK/CK-MB q8h × 3; comprehensive blood chemistry, magnesium, CBC with platelets; PT/INR, aPTT; BNP; lipid profile (fasting in morning); portable CXR
IV therapy:	D₅W or NS to keep vein open (increase fluids for relative hypovolemia); second IV if IV medication given
Recanalization therapy:*	Emergency primary coronary angioplasty, or fibrinolysis (if appropriate) 1. Primary angioplasty (preferred if available within 90 min) 2. Tenecteplase, alteplase, reteplase, or streptokinase (see Table 73-5 for doses)
Medications:	1. Nasal O₂ at 2 L/min × 6 hr, then by order (titrate to keep O₂ saturation >90%) 2. Aspirin 162-325 mg chewed on admission, then 81-162 mg PO daily 3. IV heparin, 60 U/kg bolus (maximum, 4000 U) and 12 U/kg/hr (maximum, 1000 U/hr), titrate to target aPTT 1.5-2.0 × control (about 50-70 sec), OR enoxaparin (preferred with fibrinolytic), 30 mg IV, then 1 mg/kg SC q12h (maximum SC doses, 100 mg on day 1; reduce to 0.75 mg/kg for age ≥75, increase interval to q24h for CrCl <30 mL/min), OR bivalirudin (with primary PCI), 0.75 mg/kg IV bolus, then 1.75 mg/kg/hr (delay 30 min if heparin given) 4. Metoprolol, 12.5 PO q6h, incremented to 25-50 mg q6h as tolerated (hold for SBP < 100 mm Hg, pulse < 50 beats/min, asthma, heart failure); may consider IV metoprolol if immediate effect required (tachyarrhythmia, severe hypertension, unrelieved pain) in the absence of heart failure 5. Consider IV nitroglycerin drip × 24-48 hr (titrated to SBP 100-140 mm Hg) 6. Morphine sulfate, 2-4 mg IV and increment at 5-15 min PRN for unrelieved pain 7. Stool softener 8. Anxiolytic or hypnotic if needed 9. ACE inhibitor for hypertension, anterior acute MI, or LV dysfunction, in low oral dose (e.g., captopril, 6.25 mg q8h), begun within 24 hours or when stable (SBP > 100 mm Hg) and adjusted upward 10. Lipid-lowering therapy (i.e., statin) regardless of LDL: target LDL at least <100 mg/dL (<70 mg/dL reasonable); clopidogrel, 300-600 mg PO, then 75 mg PO daily, or prasugrel 60 mg PO, then 10 mg PO daily (with PCI strategy), begun immediately after PCI (if CABG not planned) 11. Specific treatments for hemodynamic subgroups (see Table 73-3)

*If not ordered in the emergency department.

ACE = angiotensin-converting enzyme; aPTT = activated partial thromboplastin time; BNP = brain natriuretic peptide; CABG = coronary artery bypass graft surgery; CBC = complete blood count; CK = creatine kinase; CrCI = creatinine clearance; CXR = chest radiograph; D₅W = 5% dextrose in water; GP = glycoprotein; INR = International Normalized Ratio; IV = intravenous; LDL = low-density lipoprotein; LV = left ventricle; MI = myocardial infarction; NPO = nothing by mouth; NS = normal saline; PCI = percutaneous coronary intervention; PO = orally; PRN = as needed; PT = prothrombin time; daily = once daily; SBP = systolic blood pressure; SC = subcutaneous.

Adapted from Kushner FG, Hand M, Smith SC Jr, et al. 2009 Focused updates: ACC/AHA guidelines for the management of patients with ST-elevation myocardial infarction and the ACC/AHA/SCAI guidelines on percutaneous coronary intervention. *Circulation.* 2009;120:2271-306.

TABLE 73-5 CHARACTERISTICS OF INTRAVENOUS FIBRINOLYTIC AGENTS APPROVED BY THE FOOD AND DRUG ADMINISTRATION

	STREPTOKINASE (SK)	ALTEPLASE (T-PA)	RETEPLASE (R-PA)	TENECTEPLASE (TNK-T-PA)
Dose	1.5 MU in 30-60 min	100 mg in 90 min*	10 U + 10 U, 30 min apart	30-50 mg[†] over 5 sec
Circulating half-life (min)	≅20	≅4	≅18	≅20
Antigenic	Yes	No	No	No
Allergic reactions	Yes	No	No	No
Systemic fibrinogen depletion	Severe	Mild to moderate	Moderate	Minimal
Intracerebral hemorrhage	≅0.4%	≅0.7%	≅0.8%	≅0.7%
Patency (TIMI-2/3) rate, 90 min[‡]	≅51%	≅73-84%	≅83%	≅77-88%
Lives saved per 100 treated	≅3[§]	≅4[¶]	≅4	≅4
Cost per dose (approximate U.S. dollars)	300	1800	2200	2200

*Accelerated t-PA given as follows: 15-mg bolus, then 0.75 mg/kg over 30 min (maximum, 50 mg), then 0.50 mg/kg over 60 min (maximum, 35 mg).

[†]TNK-t-PA is dosed by weight (supplied in 5-mg/mL vials): <60 kg = 6 mL; 61-70 kg = 7 mL; 71-80 kg = 8 mL; 81-90 kg = 9 mL; >90 kg = 10 mL.

[‡]TIMI = Thrombolysis in Myocardial Infarction. Data from Granger CB, Califf RM, Topol EJ. Thrombolytic therapy for acute myocardial infarction: a review. *Drugs.* 1992;44:293-325; and Bode C, Smalling RW, Berg G, et al. Randomized comparison of coronary thrombolysis achieved with double-bolus reteplase (recombinant plasminogen activator) and front-loaded, accelerated alteplase (recombinant tissue plasminogen activator) in patients with acute myocardial infarction: the RAPID[II] Investigators. *Circulation.* 1996;94:891-898.

[§]Patients with ST segment elevation or bundle branch block, treated <6 hr.

[¶]Based on the finding from the GUSTO trial that t-PA saves one more additional life per 100 treated than does SK. Data from The GUSTO Investigators. An international randomized trial comparing four thrombolytic strategies for acute myocardial infarction. *N Engl J Med.* 1993;329:673-682; and Simes RJ, Topol EJ, Holmes DR Jr, et al. Link between the angiographic substudy and mortality outcomes in a large randomized trial of myocardial reperfusion: importance of early and complete infarct artery reperfusion. GUSTO-I Investigators. *Circulation.* 1995;91:1923-1928.

TABLE 73-6 INDICATIONS AND CONTRAINDICATIONS TO FIBRINOLYTIC THERAPY

INDICATIONS

Ischemic-type chest discomfort or equivalent for 30 min-12 hr with new or presumed new ST segment elevation in two contiguous leads of ≥2 mm (≥0.2 mV) in leads V_1, V_2, or V_3 or ≥1 mm in other leads

New or presumed-new left bundle branch block with symptoms consistent with myocardial infarction

Absence of contraindications

CONTRAINDICATIONS, ABSOLUTE

Active bleeding or bleeding diathesis (menses excluded)

Prior hemorrhagic stroke, ischemic stroke within 3 months, except acute ischemic stroke within 3-4.5 hours

Intracranial or spinal cord neoplasm or arteriovenous malformation

Suspected or known aortic dissection

Closed head or facial trauma within 3 months

CONTRAINDICATIONS, RELATIVE

Severe, uncontrolled hypertension by history or on presentation (>180/110 mm Hg)

Anticoagulation with therapeutic or elevated international normalized ratio (>2-3)

Old ischemic stroke (>3 mo ago); intracerebral disease other than above

Recent (<3 wk) major trauma/surgery or prolonged (>10 min) cardiopulmonary resuscitation or internal bleeding

Active peptic ulcer

Recent noncompressible vascular punctures

Pregnancy

For streptokinase/anistreplase: prior exposure (especially if >5 days ago) or allergic reaction

Adapted from Kushner FG, Hand M, Smith SC Jr, et al. 2009 Focused updates: ACC/AHA guidelines for the management of patients with ST-elevation myocardial infarction and the ACC/AHA/SCAI guidelines on percutaneous coronary intervention. *Circulation.* 2009;120:2271-2306.

TABLE 73-7 INDICATIONS FOR PRIMARY ANGIOPLASTY AND COMPARISON WITH FIBRINOLYTIC THERAPY

INDICATIONS

Alternative recanalization strategy for ST segment elevation or LBBB acute MI within 12 hr of symptom onset (or >12 hr if symptoms persist)

Cardiogenic shock developing within 36 hr of ST segment elevation/Q wave acute MI or LBBB acute MI in patients <75 yr old who can be revascularized within 18 hr of shock onset

Recommended only at centers performing >200 PCI/yr with backup cardiac surgery and for operators performing >75 PCI/yr

ADVANTAGES OF PRIMARY PCI

Higher initial recanalization rates

Reduced risk of intracerebral hemorrhage

Less residual stenosis; less recurrent ischemia or infarction

Usefulness when fibrinolysis contraindicated

Improvement in outcomes with cardiogenic shock

DISADVANTAGES OF PRIMARY PCI (COMPARED WITH FIBRINOLYTIC THERAPY)

Access, advantages restricted to high-volume centers, operators

Longer average time to treatment

Greater dependence on operators for results

Higher system complexity, costs

LBBB = left bundle branch block; MI = myocardial infarction; PCI = percutaneous coronary intervention (includes balloon angioplasty, stenting).

---

the risk for intracranial hemorrhage. The risk-to-benefit ratio should be assessed in each patient when fibrinolysis is considered and specific regimens are selected.

For failed fibrinolysis, rescue PCI is more effective than repeat fibrinolysis.[3] After fibrinolysis, regardless of its apparent success, the best strategy is to transfer all STEMI patients with high-risk features rapidly to a hospital with PCI facilities to undergo angiography, rather than to transfer only selected patients in whom fibrinolysis failed or recurrent ischemia developed.[4,5] This early transfer and angiography strategy at a median of 3 hours after fibrinolysis reduces the risk for recurrent ischemia, reinfarction, heart failure, cardiogenic shock or death by 36%.

Primary Percutaneous Coronary Intervention

Prompt PCI is the preferred recanalization strategy (Table 73-7).[6,7] PCI achieves mechanical recanalization by inflation of a catheter-based balloon centered within the thrombotic occlusion. Percutaneous transluminal coronary angioplasty (PTCA) is generally augmented by placing a stent at the site of occlusion as a scaffold to enlarge the lumen and to retain optimal postangioplasty expansion. Preference is often given to drug-eluting stents (e.g., sirolimus, paclitaxel), which markedly reduce the rates of restenosis but can increase the risk of late thrombosis (Chapter 74). Factors favoring a bare metal stent include inability to maintain at least 1 year of dual antiplatelet therapy because of an increased risk for bleeding, need for concomitant anticoagulation, risk for poor adherence or anticipated need for surgery requiring interruption of thienopyridine.

The relative benefits of primary PTCA or PCI over fibrinolysis are confirmed by a meta-analysis that found a significantly lower mortality rate (4.4 versus 6.5%; odds ratio, 0.66) and lower rates of nonfatal reinfarction (2.9 versus 5.3%; odds ratio, 0.53) and intracerebral hemorrhage with primary PTCA compared with fibrinolysis. PCI yields better outcomes than fibrinolysis across all age groups when it is performed within 1 to 2 hours of presentation to a health care facility.

Currently, a primary PCI strategy begins with initiation of a thienopyridine in the emergency department, together with aspirin and an anticoagulant (e.g., heparin or bivalirudin), followed by rapid application of coronary angioplasty with stenting. Augmented antiplatelet therapy with a GPIIb-IIIa inhibitor may be added in selected patients, generally at the time of catheterization. The addition of a reduced dose of a plasminogen activator to GPIIb-IIIa therapy in the field or emergency department may further improve outcomes only in selected patients who undergo early PCI, but this approach is generally not recommended.[8] Facilitated PCI, whereby patients at hospitals without PCI capabilities are given adjusted doses of fibrinolytic or GPIIb-IIIa inhibitors, or both, and then are transferred to other hospitals for emergent (i.e., within 1 to

2 hours) PCI, overall appears to be no better than rapid transfer for primary PCI within 1 to 2 hours.[8,9]

Operator and institutional experience is an issue more important to outcomes with primary PCI than fibrinolysis and has been incorporated into current recommendations (see Table 73-7). Primary PCI is feasible in community hospitals without surgical capability, but concerns about timing and safety remain. Current guidelines allow that primary PCI "might be considered" in hospitals without on-site cardiac surgery, provided (1) there is a proven plan for rapid and safe transport to a nearby hospital with cardiac surgery capability and availability, and (2) the PCI is done by a skilled operator (≥75 PCIs/year) in a hospital with adequate experience (≥36 primary PCIs/year).

Mechanical reperfusion, primarily with stenting and a GPIIb-IIIa receptor antagonist, for patients presenting more than 12 hours but less than 48 hours after the onset of symptoms, also can reduce infarct size and perhaps adverse events.[10] Extending PCI to ST segment elevation MI beyond 12 hours deserves further testing in larger studies.

An additional important indication is cardiogenic shock occurring within 36 hours of the onset of acute MI and treated within 18 hours of the onset of shock (Chapter 107). However, benefit was not established for patients older than 75 years, and benefit was greater with earlier PCI.

Increasing positive experience with PCI of the left main coronary artery with stents, especially drug-eluting stents, suggests that it may be an alternative to coronary artery bypass grafting (CABG) in patients with an amenable anatomy, a low risk of PCI procedural complications, and an increased risk of adverse surgical outcomes.

Mechanical thrombus aspiration at the time of angiography may improve outcomes of patients with STEMI undergoing primary PCI.[11] To reduce the risk for contrast-induced nephropathy, an isosmolar or a low-molecular-weight contrast medium together with preprocedure hydration is recommended in patients undergoing angiography.

Selecting a Recanalization Regimen

Whether to use PCI or fibrinolytic therapy depends on local resources and experience as well as on patient factors. Outcomes appear to be determined both by timing and by institutional and operator experience. In general, in experienced facilities (≥200 PCIs/center; surgical capability; ≥75 PCIs/operator annually; frequent primary PCI, e.g., ≥36/year/center; ≥4/operator/year) that are able to mobilize and treat patients quickly (<90 minutes to balloon inflation), primary PCI is considered the preferred strategy, with stenting preferred over balloon PTCA. PCI is particularly preferred for patients at higher risk for mortality (including shock), for later presentations (>3 hours), and for patients with greater risk of intracerebral hemorrhage (age >70 years, female gender, therapy with hypertensive agents). Ancillary antithrombotic therapy with primary PCI includes aspirin, unfractionated heparin or LMWH or bivalirudin, and a GPIIb-IIIa inhibitor (preferably initiated on admission before catheterization). Clopidogrel is begun directly after PCI and is continued after discharge.

For other situations, fibrinolytic therapy becomes the recommended recanalization strategy. If time since the onset of symptoms is within 3 hours and the difference between expected time to PCI and fibrinolytic administration is more than 1 hour, fibrinolysis is often the preferred strategy. Fibrinolysis also is preferred in centers without sufficient PCI experience or capability. In hospitals with long ambulance transport times (>60 to 90 minutes), a strategy for initiating prehospital fibrinolysis may be considered. Very early or prehospital fibrinolysis followed by a routine emergent (i.e., within 1 to 2 hours) invasive strategy on hospital arrival, that is, "pharmacoinvasive therapy," although an appealing concept, appears to cause a *higher* rate of in-hospital mortality, cardiac ischemic events, and strokes compared with primary PCI alone or by a more delayed invasive approach after fibrinolysis in stabilized patients,[4,5,12] and its use cannot be recommended as a primary recanalization strategy. Whether fibrinolysis before PCI will be beneficial in selected subgroups with MI, such as patients seen within the first hour of symptoms and with an expected delay to PCI of 2 hours or more, deserves further testing. Currently, however, efforts should be made to provide primary PCI to a larger percentage of patients with acute MI.

The selection of a specific fibrinolytic regimen is based on the risk of complications of the acute MI, the risk of intracerebral hemorrhage, and a consideration of economic constraints. Using these factors, longer-acting variants of t-PA (i.e., tenecteplase and reteplase) have become dominant in the United States and other affluent medical markets; in other countries, less costly streptokinase is still widely used. A nonimmunogenic fibrinolytic agent is preferred for patients with a history of prior streptokinase use. Streptokinase is associated with a lower risk for intracerebral hemorrhage than other regimens if excessive heparin is avoided. Tenecteplase combined with enoxaparin was more effective than tenecteplase with standard heparin or with a GPIIb-IIIa inhibitor (abciximab) and heparin in one but not another trial. Reteplase with abciximab showed no mortality advantage when combined (in half-dose) with abciximab than with heparin alone; ischemic events decreased, but intracerebral hemorrhage increased, especially in elderly patients. Over the past decade, the application of recanalization therapy has remained relatively constant in the United States and other Western countries at 70 to 75% of "eligible" patients with acute MI. Primary PCI use has increased substantially over time, although fibrinolytic therapy continues to be more commonly applied, particularly in developing countries.

Ancillary and Other Therapies
Antiplatelet Therapy
Aspirin

Platelets form a critical component of coronary thrombi. Aspirin inhibits platelet aggregation by irreversibly blocking cyclooxygenase 1 activity by selective acetylation of serine at position 530. Cyclooxygenase 1 catalyzes the conversion of arachidonic acid to thromboxane-A_2, a potent platelet aggregator (Chapter 36).

Aspirin has been extensively tested to prevent coronary heart disease (Chapter 37). Aspirin trials in ST segment elevation acute MI have been more limited but positive. The most important trial of aspirin in ST segment elevation acute MI randomized more than 17,000 patients with "suspected acute MI" (representing mostly, but not entirely, ST segment elevation acute MI) to aspirin or control and to intravenous streptokinase or control. At 5 weeks, the relative risk for vascular death was reduced 21% by aspirin alone, 25% by streptokinase alone, and 40% by aspirin in combination with streptokinase. Since that time, aspirin has been included as standard therapy in most treatment regimens for ST segment elevation acute MI.

Current guidelines strongly recommend aspirin (class I indication) on admission in a dose of 162 to 325 mg, preferably chewed. Aspirin administration is continued throughout hospitalization and then indefinitely in a maintenance dose of 75 to 162 mg/day on an outpatient basis (enteric-coated forms are popular).

Adenosine Diphosphate Receptor Antagonists

The thienopyridine clopidogrel exerts potent antiplatelet effects by blocking the platelet membrane adenosine diphosphate receptor (Chapter 37). For patients allergic to aspirin, clopidogrel has become the alternative of choice for short- and long-term therapy of ST segment elevation acute MI. A single loading dose is given, usually 300 mg with fibrinolytic therapy but 600 mg with PCI. The maintenance dose is 75 mg/day.

In patients who can take aspirin, the addition of clopidogrel (300 mg followed by 75 mg/day) to aspirin and fibrinolytic therapy in patients 75 years or younger reduces predischarge occlusion rates of infarct-related arteries (by 41%) and reduces ischemic complications at 30 days (by 20%) without increasing rates of intracerebral hemorrhage.[13] When given without a loading dose but also without an upper age restriction, clopidogrel reduces 15-day ischemic complications by 9% and death from any cause by 7%.[14] Hence, clopidogrel appears to represent a beneficial initial adjunctive therapy in patients with STEMI who are treated with fibrinolytic agents. However, clopidogrel increases the risk for bleeding with CABG, so it is commonly initiated only after coronary angiography has been performed and early surgery has been excluded as a therapeutic choice; if CABG is planned, clopidogrel should be withheld for 5 to 7 days unless the urgency of surgery outweighs the risk of excessive bleeding.

Prasugrel, a new and more potent thienopyridine, may reduce ischemic events at the cost of a small increase in bleeding compared with clopidogrel after PCI in patients with acute STEMI.[15] Prasugrel is contraindicated in patients with a prior history of stroke or transient ischemia attack and should be used with caution (or in reduced doses) in older (≥75 years) and smaller (<60 kg) patients.

Clopidogrel added to aspirin on admission for patients with non–ST segment elevation acute MI or unstable angina (Chapter 72) or after a PCI reduces vascular events (by 22%) at 3 to 12 months compared with aspirin alone. Extrapolation of these findings led to the recommendations that clopidogrel be used for 3 to 12 months as an alternative antiplatelet agent in patients with ST segment elevation acute MI when aspirin is contraindicated and that it be considered routinely (in addition to aspirin) in patients after primary PCI.

Glycoprotein IIB/IIIA Inhibitors

Inhibitors of the platelet membrane GPIIb-IIIa receptor, a fibrinogen receptor, have been shown to benefit high-risk patients with non–ST segment elevation acute coronary syndrome (Chapters 37 and 72) on admission or after PCI. The benefit in STEMI is smaller when routine stenting is used and when GPIIb-IIIa therapy is administered only in the catheterization laboratory. Earlier ("upstream") glycoprotein inhibition before hospital admission or in the emergency department (precatheterization) is effective in improving coronary patency by the time of emergency angiography, but incremental benefit on clinical outcomes has not been established. If early CABG is a possibility after angiography, a shorter-acting inhibitor (eptifibatide, tirofiban) may impart a lower perioperative risk for bleeding than abciximab.

Antithrombin Therapy
Low-Molecular-Weight Heparins

Compared with unfractionated heparins, LMWHs have enhanced inhibitory activity for factor Xa (Chapter 37). They also have more reliable bioavailability and longer durations of action, thus permitting subcutaneous administration once or twice daily in fixed (weight-adjusted) doses. Evidence suggests that in patients with ST segment elevation acute MI who are treated with fibrinolytic therapy, LMWH can improve angiographic outcomes and can reduce reinfarction rates by 25% and mortality by about 10% compared with unfractionated heparin.[16] Enoxaparin may thus be preferred over unfractionated heparin as an antithrombotic agent for ST segment elevation acute MI in most patients treated with a fibrinolysis strategy. When used as ancillary therapy with a fibrinolytic agent, enoxaparin may be given to patients younger than 75 years who do not have renal insufficiency as a 30-mg intravenous bolus, followed by 1 mg/kg subcutaneously twice daily until hospital discharge, and to those 75 years and older as 0.75 mg/kg subcutaneously twice daily without a bolus.

Unfractionated Heparin

Unfractionated heparin can be used in patients undergoing primary PCI and in those receiving fibrin-specific lytic agents (i.e., alteplase, reteplase, or tenecteplase; see Fig. 73-3 and Table 73-4). It also can be used with intravenous streptokinase or anistreplase for patients at high risk for systemic emboli (e.g., large or anterior acute MI with LV thrombus, atrial fibrillation [AF]). Excessive bleeding when heparin is used in combination with antithrombotic regimens has led to reductions in heparin doses, with improved safety. When given with a fibrinolytic agent, intravenous heparin is begun concurrently and is given for 48 hours. Currently recommended doses include a 60 U/kg bolus (maximum, 4000 U), followed initially by a 12 U/kg/hour infusion (maximum, 1000 U/hour), with adjustment after 3 hours based on activated partial thromboplastin time (target of 50 to 70 seconds, 1.5 to 2 times control). Experimental regimens including a GPIIb-IIIa inhibitor and a fibrinolytic agent have used even lower heparin doses. During primary PCI, high-dose heparin is used (activated clotting time, 300 to 350 seconds). Given together with a GPIIb-IIIa inhibitor during PCI, the dose of heparin is adjusted to a lower activated clotting time range (150 to 300 seconds).

Factor Xa Inhibitors

Selective factor Xa inhibitors (e.g., fondaparinux, 2.5 mg subcutaneously once daily for up to 8 days during index hospitalization) reduce the end point of death or reinfarction at 30 days by 18 to 23% independent of heparin use in patients who receive fibrinolysis or no recanalization therapy but have no benefit in patients who have undergone PCI.[18] These results suggest that fondaparinux may be a preferred alternative to unfractionated heparin or no heparin (e.g., in patients who present later, in patients treated with streptokinase) in patients with STEMI who are not undergoing a primary PCI strategy.

Direct Antithrombins

Bivalirudin, a synthetic hirudin analogue with direct antithrombin activity (Chapter 37), compares favorably with heparin and a glycoprotein IIb/IIIa inhibitor for ST segment elevation acute MI managed by primary PCI, with better survival rates at 1 year.[18] However, an increased risk of ischemic events and stent thrombosis occurs in bivalirudin patients who do not receive upstream therapy with a 600-mg loading dose of clopidogrel. As a result, bivalirudin, together with early administration of clopidogrel, has become a

FIGURE 73-4. Algorithm to aid in selection of implantable cardioverter-defibrillator (ICD) in patients with ST segment elevation myocardial infarction (STEMI) and diminished ejection fraction (EF). The appropriate management path is selected based on left ventricular EF measured at least 1 month after STEMI. All patients, whether an ICD is implanted or not, should receive medical therapy. EPS = electrophysiologic studies; LOE = level of evidence; NSVT = nonsustained ventricular tachycardia; VF = ventricular fibrillation; VT = ventricular tachycardia. (Adapted from Antman EM, Anbe DT, Armstrong PW, et al. 2004 Update: ACC/AHA guidelines for the management of patients with ST-elevation myocardial infarction—executive summary. A Report of the American College of Cardiology/American Heart Association Task Force on Practice Guidelines. *Circulation.* 2004;110:588-536.)

widely used antithrombotic regimen in primary PCI for ST segment elevation acute MI.

Other Pharmacologic Therapies

Nitrates

Nitroglycerin and other organic nitrates (isosorbide dinitrate and isosorbide mononitrate) induce vascular smooth muscle relaxation by generating vascular endothelial nitric oxide. The resulting vasodilation of veins and peripheral and coronary arteries can beneficially reduce excessive cardiac preload and afterload, increase coronary caliber in responsive areas of stenosis, reverse distal small coronary arterial vasoconstriction, improve coronary collateral flow to ischemic myocardium, and inhibit platelet aggregation in acute MI (Chapter 71). The results are improved oxygen delivery and reduced oxygen consumption. Potential clinical benefits include relief of ischemia, limitation of infarct size, prevention of dilative remodeling, control of hypertension (afterload), and relief of congestion (preload).

In the era before reperfusion, nitrates appeared to confer a mortality benefit in acute MI. In the context of fibrinolytic therapy and aspirin, however, mortality benefits are modest, with a relative survival benefit of about 4 lives saved per 1000 patients treated. Nitroglycerin is definitely recommended for the first 24 to 48 hours for patients with acute MI and pulmonary congestion, large anterior MI, persistent ischemia, or hypertension. For other patients without contraindications, nitrates are possibly useful.

When nitrates are clearly indicated early in acute MI, intravenous nitroglycerin is preferred. Intravenous nitroglycerin may begin with a bolus injection of 12.5 to 25 μg followed by an infusion of 10 to 20 μg/minute. The infusion rate is increased by 5 to 10 μg every 5 to 10 minutes up to about 200 μg/minute during hemodynamic monitoring until clinical symptoms are controlled or blood pressure targets are reached (blood pressure decreased by 10% in normotensive patients or by 30% in hypertensive patients but not less than 80 mm Hg mean or 90 mm Hg systolic).

β-Blockers

β-Adrenoceptor blockers reduce heart rate, blood pressure, and myocardial contractility, and they stabilize the heart electrically. These actions provide clinical benefit to most patients with acute MI by limiting myocardial oxygen consumption, relieving ischemia, reducing infarct size, and preventing serious arrhythmias.

In the era before fibrinolysis, a meta-analysis of 28 randomized trials involving 27,500 patients found a modest early benefit on mortality (14% odds reduction), cardiac arrest (16% reduction), and nonfatal reinfarction (19% reduction). In patients with acute MI who are receiving fibrinolytic therapy, immediate (intravenous then oral) metoprolol reduces recurrent ischemic events and reinfarction compared with deferred oral therapy. Further experience has shown that moderate to severe heart failure should preclude the early use of intravenous β-blockers, but not predischarge and outpatient oral therapy initiated in small doses and carefully adjusted once stability is achieved.

Early (first-day) initiation of oral β-blockade is generally recommended for patients with acute MI who have ongoing or recurrent ischemic pain or

tachyarrhythmias if they do not have heart failure or other contraindications (asthma, hypotension, severe bradycardia), regardless of concomitant fibrinolysis or PCI. Intravenous initiation (e.g., metoprolol, 5 mg over 2 minutes to a total of 15 mg over 10 to 15 minutes, or atenolol, 2.5 to 5 mg over 2 minutes to a total of 10 mg over 10 to 15 minutes) is reasonable in the absence of contraindications if an indication for immediate therapy is present, such as a tachyarrhythmia or hypertension. However, the routine, short-term initiation of intravenous β-blockade should be avoided because it is not associated with benefit and, indeed, causes a small excess of early death from cardiogenic shock, primarily in patients with preexisting heart failure.[14] All patients without contraindications or intolerance to β-blocker therapy should receive oral doses, titrated to tolerance or goal (e.g., metoprolol, 25 to 100 mg twice daily; atenolol, 50 to 100 mg/day; or carvedilol, 6.25 to 25 mg twice daily). β-Blocker therapy should begin promptly, in the absence of heart failure and if not otherwise contraindicated, and should be continued during the in-hospital convalescent phase of STEMI and beyond.

Renin-Angiotensin-Aldosterone System Inhibitors

The renin-angiotensin-aldosterone system is activated in acute MI and heart failure. Use of an ACE inhibitor has been shown to improve remodeling after acute MI (especially after large anterior MI). ACE inhibitors also have demonstrated efficacy in heart failure, wherein they prevent disease progression, hospitalization, and death (Chapter 59). A meta-analysis of three major trials and 11 smaller ones involving more than 100,000 patients showed an overall mortality reduction of 6.5%, representing about 5 lives saved per 1000 patients treated. Benefit is concentrated and greater in higher-risk patients with large or anterior MI and with LV dysfunction or heart failure, although patients with lesser degrees of LV dysfunction and only moderate cardiovascular risk can also benefit in the long term.

Oral *ACE inhibitor therapy* should begin within the first 24 hours in patients with anterior infarction, pulmonary congestion, or low ejection fraction (<0.40) in the absence of hypotension (systolic pressure <100 mm Hg or >30 mm Hg less than usual baseline) or known contraindications. An *angiotensin receptor blocker* (ARB) should be given to otherwise qualifying patients who are intolerant of ACE inhibitors. An ACE inhibitor or an ARB also should be considered for other patients with STEMI, especially those with a relative indication (e.g., hypertension, diabetes, or mild renal insufficiency), with the expectation of a smaller but worthwhile benefit. All patients without contraindications or intolerance to initial ACE inhibitor or ARB therapy also should receive these drugs during the in-hospital convalescent phase. ACE inhibitor therapy should begin with low oral doses and should be progressively adjusted to full dose as tolerated. For example, the short-acting agent captopril may be started in a dose of 6.25 mg or less and adjusted over 1 to 2 days to 50 mg twice daily. Before discharge, a transition may be made in graded dose schedules to longer-acting agents such as ramipril (2.5 mg titrated to 10 mg/day), lisinopril (2.5 to 5 mg titrated to 10 mg/day), or enalapril (2.5 mg, titrated to up to 20 mg twice daily). In patients who cannot tolerate ACE inhibitors (e.g., because of cough), graded doses of an ARB may be substituted (e.g., valsartan, 80 to 160 mg twice daily, or losartan, 50 to 100 mg/day).

Selective *aldosterone receptor blockade* with eplerenone (25 to 50 mg/day) reduces total and cardiovascular mortality (including sudden death) as well as cardiovascular hospitalizations in post-MI patients who have an ejection fraction of 0.40 or less and heart failure or diabetes and who are already receiving other optimal therapies, including ACE inhibitors.[19] Spironolactone also benefits patients with advanced heart failure, including those in whom it is caused by a remote MI. Hence, aldosterone receptor blockade should be added to other standard therapies during convalescence in patients with these characteristics. Hyperkalemia, which is the most common side effect, requires monitoring (Chapter 59).

Antiarrhythmic Agents

Antiarrhythmic therapy is reserved for treatment of, or short-term prevention after, symptomatic or life-threatening ventricular arrhythmias, together with other appropriate measures (cardioversion, treatment of ischemia and metabolic disturbances). An implantable cardioverter-defibrillator (ICD) is indicated in patients with VF or hemodynamically significant sustained ventricular tachycardia (VT) occurring more than 2 days after STEMI or in patients with inducible VT or VF at electrophysiologic study and a depressed ejection fraction (≤0.40) at least 1 month after STEMI (Chapter 65). An ICD also may be considered for patients with severe LV dysfunction (ejection fraction ≤0.30) at least 1 month after STEMI and 3 months after CABG without spontaneous or induced VT or VF.[20] These differences reflect an apparent time dependence, in which the benefit of an ICD appears to be delayed until the early post-MI and post-revascularization periods (Chapter 66). By comparison, early ICD implantation is not beneficial in a broader group of patients because its usefulness in preventing similar deaths is offset by the high rate of nonsudden deaths.[21]

Inotropes

Digitalis and intravenous inotropes can increase oxygen demand, provoke serious arrhythmias, and extend infarction. Current recommendations support the use of digoxin in selected patients recovering from acute MI who develop supraventricular tachyarrhythmias (e.g., AF) or heart failure refractory to ACE inhibitors and diuretics. Intravenous inotropes (e.g., dobutamine, dopamine, milrinone, and norepinephrine) are reserved for temporary support of patients with hypotension and circulatory failure that is unresponsive to volume replacement (Chapters 59 and 107). Other treatment measures for these patients (e.g., intra-aortic balloon pump, early revascularization) are discussed herein.

Lipid-Lowering Therapy

Lipid lowering, particularly with hydroxymethylglutaryl–coenzyme A reductase inhibitors (statins), reduces event rates in patients with coronary disease, and a more aggressive approach appears to provide superior benefits (Chapter 213).[22] A fasting lipid profile should be obtained on admission, so a statin can be started promptly in the hospital with a low-density lipoprotein cholesterol goal of less than 70 mg/dL.

Other Medical Therapies

Calcium channel blockers, although anti-ischemic, also are negatively inotropic and have not been shown to reduce mortality after ST segment elevation acute MI. With certain agents and in specific groups of patients, harm has been suggested. For example, short-acting nifedipine has been reported to cause reflex sympathetic activation, tachycardia, hypotension, and increased mortality. Verapamil or diltiazem (heart rate–slowing drugs) may be given to patients in whom β-blockers are ineffective or contraindicated for control of rapid ventricular response with AF or relief of ongoing ischemia *in the absence of heart failure, LV dysfunction, or atrioventricular (AV) block.*

Magnesium is of no benefit in patients with acute MI who are treated with fibrinolysis. Supplementation is recommended if the magnesium level is lower than normal or in patients with torsades de pointes–type VT associated with a prolonged QT interval.

Glucose-insulin-potassium affords no benefit on mortality, cardiac arrest, or cardiogenic shock when this combination is added to usual care in patients with acute STEMI. However, *glucose control,* using an insulin-based regimen to achieve and maintain glucose levels less than 180 mg/dL while avoiding hypoglycemia, is recommended in the acute phase of STEMI. After the acute phase, individualized treatment is indicated using agents or combinations of agents that best achieve glycemic control and are well tolerated (Chapters 236 and 237).

Management of Complications
Recurrent Chest Pain

When chest pain recurs after acute MI, the diagnostic possibilities include post-infarction ischemia, pericarditis, infarct extension, and infarct expansion. Characterization of the pain, physical examination, ECG, echocardiography, and cardiac marker determinations assist in the differential diagnosis. CK-MB often discriminates reinfarction better than cTnI or cTnT.

Post-infarction angina developing spontaneously during hospitalization for acute MI despite medical therapy usually merits coronary angiography. β-blockers (IV, then orally) and nitroglycerin (IV, then orally or topically) are recommended medical therapies. Pain with recurrent ST segment elevation or recurrent elevation of cardiac markers may be treated with (re)administration of t-PA or, possibly, a GPIIb-IIIa inhibitor, together with nitroglycerin, β-blockade, and heparin. Streptokinase, which induces neutralizing antibodies, generally should not be readministered after the first few days. If facilities for angiography, PCI, and surgery are available, an invasive approach is recommended to relieve discomfort occurring hours to days after an acute MI that is associated with objective signs of ischemia. Radionuclide perfusion stress testing can be helpful in patients with discomfort that is transient or of uncertain ischemic origin. For lesions with questionable degrees of stenosis at angiography, coronary pressure (fractional flow reserve) or Doppler velocimetry can determine whether PCI is warranted.

Infarct expansion implies circumferential slippage with thinning of the infarcted myocardium. Infarct expansion can be associated with chest pain but without recurrent elevation of cardiac markers. Expansive remodeling can lead to an LV aneurysm. The risk for remodeling is reduced with early recanalization therapy and administration of ACE inhibitors.

Acute pericarditis most commonly manifests on days 2 to 4 in association with large, "transmural" infarctions causing pericardial inflammation. Occasionally, hemorrhagic effusion with tamponade develops; thus, excessive anticoagulation should be avoided. Pericarditis developing later (2 to 10 weeks) after acute MI could represent Dressler's syndrome, which is believed to be immune mediated. The incidence of this post-MI syndrome has decreased dramatically in the modern reperfusion era. Pericardial pain is treated with aspirin (preferred, especially in the acute setting) or other nonsteroidal agents (e.g., indomethacin); patients with severe symptoms could require corticosteroids.

Rhythm Disturbances
Ventricular Arrhythmias

Acute MI is associated with a proarrhythmic environment that includes heterogeneous myocardial ischemia, heightened adrenergic tone, intracellular electrolyte disturbance, lipolysis and free fatty acid production, and oxygen free radical production on recanalization. Arrhythmias thus are common early during acute MI. Micro-re-entry is likely the most common electrophysiologic mechanism of early-phase arrhythmias, although enhanced automaticity and triggered activity also are observed in experimental models.

Primary VF, the most serious MI-related arrhythmia, contributes importantly to mortality within the first 24 hours. It occurs with an incidence of 3 to 5% during the first 4 hours and then declines rapidly over 24 to 48 hours. Polymorphic VT and, less commonly, monomorphic VT are associated life-threatening arrhythmias that can occur in this setting. Clinical features (including warning arrhythmias) are not adequately specific or sensitive to identify patients at risk for sustained ventricular tachyarrhythmias, so all patients should be continuously monitored. Prophylactic lidocaine, which reduces primary VF but does not decrease (and may increase) mortality, is not recommended. Primary VF is associated with a higher rate of in-hospital mortality, but long-term prognosis is unaffected in survivors.

Accelerated idioventricular rhythm (60 to 100 beats per minute) frequently occurs within the first 12 hours and is generally benign (i.e., is not a risk factor for VF). Indeed, accelerated idioventricular rhythm frequently heralds recanalization after fibrinolytic therapy. Antiarrhythmic therapy is not indicated except for sustained, hemodynamically compromising accelerated idioventricular rhythm.

Late VF, which is defined as VF developing more than 48 hours after the onset of acute MI, often occurs in patients with larger MIs or heart failure, portends a worse prognosis for survival, and is an indication for aggressive measures (e.g., consideration of an ICD). Monomorphic VT resulting from re-entry in the context of a recent or old MI also can appear late after MI, and patients may require long-term therapy (e.g., an ICD).

Electrical cardioversion is required for VF and sustained polymorphic VT (unsynchronized shock) and for sustained monomorphic VT that causes hemodynamic compromise (synchronized shock) (Chapters 65 and 66). Brief intravenous sedation is given to conscious, "stable" patients. For slower, stable VT and nonsustained VT requiring therapy, intravenous amiodarone or intravenous lidocaine is commonly recommended. After episodes of VT or VF, infusions of antiarrhythmic drugs may be given for 6 to 24 hours; the ongoing risk for arrhythmia then is reassessed. Electrolyte and acid-base imbalance and hypoxia should be corrected. β-Blockade is useful in patients with frequent polymorphic VT associated with adrenergic activation ("electrical storm"). Additional, aggressive measures should be considered to reduce cardiac ischemia (e.g., emergency PCI or CABG) and LV dysfunction (intra-aortic balloon pump) in patients with recurrent polymorphic VT despite the use of β-blockers or amiodarone, or both.

Patients with sustained VT or VF occurring late in the hospital course should be considered for long-term prevention and therapy. An ICD provides greater survival benefit than antiarrhythmic drugs in patients with ventricular arrhythmias and can improve survival after acute MI for patients with an ejection fraction of 30% or less, regardless of their rhythm status.[20]

Atrial Fibrillation and Other Supraventricular Tachyarrhythmias

AF occurs in up to 10 to 15% of patients after an acute MI, usually within the first 24 hours (Chapter 64). The incidence of atrial flutter or another supraventricular tachycardia is much lower. The risk for AF increases with age, larger MIs, heart failure, pericarditis, atrial infarction, hypokalemia, hypomagnesemia, hypoxia, pulmonary disease, and hyperadrenergic states. The incidence of AF is reduced by effective early recanalization. Hemodynamic compromise with rapid rates and systemic embolism (in ~2%) are adverse consequences of AF. Systemic embolism can occur on the first day, so prompt anticoagulation with heparin is indicated.

Recommendations for management of AF include the following: electrical cardioversion for patients with severe hemodynamic compromise or ischemia; rate control with intravenous digoxin for patients with ventricular dysfunction (i.e., give 1.0 mg, one half initially and one half in 4 hours), with an intravenous β-blocker (e.g., metoprolol, 5 mg over 2 minutes to a total of 15 mg over 10 to 15 minutes) in those without clinical ventricular dysfunction, or with intravenous diltiazem or verapamil in hemodynamically compensated patients with a contraindication to β-blockers; and anticoagulation with heparin (or LMWH). Amiodarone, which is generally reserved for patients with or at high risk for recurrence, may be continued for 6 weeks if sinus rhythm is restored and maintained.

Bradycardias, Conduction Delays, and Heart Block

Sinus and AV nodal dysfunction is common during acute MI. Sinus bradycardia, a result of increased parasympathetic tone often in association with inferior acute MI, occurs in 30 to 40% of patients. Sinus bradycardia is particularly common during the first hour of acute MI and with recanalization of the right coronary artery (Bezold-Jarisch reflex). Vagally mediated AV block also can occur in this setting. Anticholinergic therapy (atropine, 0.5 to 1.5 mg IV) is indicated for *symptomatic* sinus bradycardia (heart rate generally <50 beats per minute associated with hypotension, ischemia, or escape ventricular arrhythmia), including ventricular asystole, and *symptomatic* second-degree (Wenckebach) or third-degree block at the AV nodal level (narrow QRS complex escape rhythm). Atropine is not indicated and can worsen infranodal AV block (anterior MI, wide complex escape rhythm).

New-onset infranodal AV block and intraventricular conduction delays or bundle branch blocks (BBBs) predict substantially increased in-hospital mortality. Fortunately, their incidence has declined in the recanalization era (from 10 to 20% to ~4%). Mortality is related more to extensive myocardial damage than to heart block itself, so cardiac pacing only modestly improves survival. Prophylactic placement of multifunctional patch electrodes, which allow for immediate transcutaneous pacing (and defibrillation) if needed, is indicated for symptomatic sinus bradycardia refractory to drug therapy, infranodal second-degree (Mobitz II) or third-degree AV block, and new or indeterminate-age bifascicular (LBBB; RBBB with left anterior or left posterior fascicular block) or trifascicular block (bilateral or alternating BBB [any age], BBB with first-degree AV block). Transcutaneous pacing is uncomfortable and is intended for prophylactic and temporary use only. In patients who require a pacemaker to maintain a rhythm or who are at very high risk (>30%) of requiring pacing (including patients with alternating, bilateral BBB, with new or indeterminate-age bifascicular block with first-degree AV block, and with infranodal second-degree AV block) should have a transvenous pacing electrode inserted as soon as possible.

Indications for permanent pacing after acute MI depend on the prognosis of the AV block and not solely on symptoms. Class I indications include even transient second- or third-degree AV block in association with BBB and symptomatic AV block at any level. Advanced block at the AV nodal level (Wenckebach) rarely is persistent or symptomatic enough to warrant permanent pacing.

Heart Failure and Other Low-Output States

Cardiac pump failure is the leading cause of circulatory failure and in-hospital death from acute MI. Manifestations of circulatory failure can include a weak pulse, low blood pressure, cool extremities, a third heart sound, pulmonary congestion, oliguria, and obtundation. However, several distinct mechanisms, hemodynamic patterns, and clinical syndromes characterize the spectrum of circulatory failure in acute MI. Each requires a specific approach to diagnosis, monitoring, and therapy (see Table 73-3).

Left Ventricular Dysfunction

The degree of LV dysfunction correlates well with the extent of acute ischemia or infarction. Hemodynamic compromise becomes evident when impairment involves 20 to 25% of the left ventricle, and cardiogenic shock or death occurs with involvement of 40% or more (Chapter 107). Pulmonary congestion and S_3 and S_4 gallops are the most common physical findings. Early recanalization (with fibrinolytic agents, PCI, or CABG) is the most effective therapy to reduce infarct size, ventricular dysfunction, and associated heart failure. Medical treatment of heart failure related to the ventricular dysfunction of acute MI is otherwise generally similar to that of heart failure in other settings (Chapter 59) and includes adequate oxygenation and diuresis (begun early, blood pressure permitting, and continued on a long-term basis if needed). Morphine sulfate (i.e., 2 to 4 mg IV, with increments as needed after 5 to 15 minutes or more) is useful for patients with pulmonary congestion. Nitroglycerin also reduces preload and effectively relieves congestive symptoms. Titrated oral ACE inhibitor therapy (e.g., captopril, incremented from 3.125 to 6.25 mg three times daily to 50 mg twice daily as tolerated) also is indicated for heart failure and pulmonary edema unless excessive hypotension (systolic blood pressure <100 mm Hg) is present. Treatment can be begun sublingually (0.4 mg every 5 minutes three times), and then the transition can be made to intravenous therapy (initially 5 to 10 μg/minute, incrementing by 5 to 20 μg/minute until symptoms are relieved or until mean arterial pressure falls by 10% in normotensive or 30% in hypertensive patients but not <90 mm Hg or >30 mm Hg lower than baseline). Intravenous vasodilator therapy to reduce preload and afterload, inotropic support, and intra-aortic balloon counterpulsation (IABP), together with urgent recanalization, are indicated in cardiogenic shock (Chapter 107).

Volume Depletion

Relative or absolute hypovolemia is a frequent cause of hypotension and circulatory failure and is easily corrected if it is recognized and treated promptly. Poor hydration, vomiting, diuresis, and disease- or drug-induced peripheral vasodilation can contribute to this condition. Hypovolemia should be identified and corrected with intravenous fluids before more aggressive therapies are considered. An empirical fluid challenge may be tried in the appropriate clinical setting (e.g., for hypotension in the absence of congestion, for inferior or RV infarction, and for hypervagotonia). If filling pressures are measured, cautious fluid administration to a pulmonary capillary wedge pressure of up to about 18 mm Hg may optimize cardiac output and blood pressure without impairing oxygenation.

Right Ventricular Infarction

RV ischemia and infarction occur with proximal occlusion of the right coronary artery (before the take-off of the RV branches). Ten to 15% of inferior acute STEMIs show classic hemodynamic features, and these patients form the highest-risk subgroup for morbidity and mortality (25 to 30% versus <6% hospital mortality). Improvement in RV function commonly occurs over time, a finding suggesting reversal of ischemic stunning and other favorable accommodations, if short-term management is successful.

Hypotension in patients with clear lung fields and elevated jugular venous pressure in the setting of inferior or inferoposterior acute MI should raise the suspicion of RV infarction. Kussmaul's sign (distention of the jugular vein on inspiration) is relatively specific and sensitive in this setting. Right-sided ECG leads show ST segment elevation, particularly in V_{4R} (Chapter 54), in the first 24 hours of RV infarction. Echocardiography is helpful in confirming the diagnosis (RV dilation and dysfunction are observed). When right-sided heart pressures are measured, a right atrial pressure of 10 mm Hg or greater and 80% or more of the pulmonary capillary wedge pressure are relatively sensitive and specific for RV ischemic dysfunction.

Management of RV infarction consists of early maintenance of RV preload with intravenous fluids, reduction of RV afterload (i.e., afterload-only reducing drugs as for LV dysfunction; consider intra-aortic balloon pump), early recanalization, short-term inotropic support if needed, and avoidance of venodilators (e.g., nitrates) and diuretics used for LV failure (they may cause marked hypotension). Volume loading with normal saline solution alone is often effective. If the cardiac output fails to improve after 0.5 to 1 L fluid, inotropic support with intravenous dobutamine (starting at 2 μg/kg/minute and titrating to hemodynamic effect or tolerance, up to 20 μg/kg/minute) is recommended. High-grade AV block is common, and restoration of AV synchrony with temporary AV sequential pacing can lead to substantial improvement in cardiac output. The onset of AF (in up to one third of RV infarcts) can cause severe hemodynamic compromise requiring prompt cardioversion. Early coronary recanalization with fibrinolysis or PCI markedly improves outcomes.

Cardiogenic Shock

Cardiogenic shock (Chapter 107) is a form of severe LV failure characterized by marked hypotension (systolic pressures <80 mm Hg) and reductions in cardiac index (to <1.8 L/minute/m²) despite high LV filling pressure (pulmonary capillary wedge pressure >18 mm Hg). The cause is loss of a critical functional mass (>40%) of the left ventricle. Cardiogenic shock is associated with mortality rates of more than 70 to 80% despite aggressive medical therapy. Risk factors include age, large (usually anterior) acute MI, previous MI, and diabetes. In patients with suspected shock, hemodynamic monitoring and IABP are indicated. Intubation often is necessary. Vasopressors are often needed. Early urgent mechanical revascularization (PCI or CABG), if feasible, affords the best chance for survival, especially in patients younger than 75 years (Chapter 107).

IABP remains useful for patients with medically refractory unstable ischemic syndromes and for cardiogenic shock. The deflated balloon catheter is introduced into the femoral artery and is advanced into the aorta. The ECG triggers balloon inflation during early diastole, thereby augmenting coronary blood flow; deflation then occurs in early systole, thereby reducing LV afterload. Primary IABP therapy for cardiogenic shock associated with acute MI provides temporary stabilization but does not reduce mortality (>80%). IABP is currently recommended in the setting of acute MI as a stabilizing measure for patients undergoing angiography and subsequent PCI or surgery for (1) cardiogenic shock, (2) mechanical complications (acute mitral regurgitation, acute ventricular septal defect), (3) refractory post-MI ischemia, or (4) recurrent intractable VT or VF associated with hemodynamic instability. IABP is not useful in patients with significant aortic insufficiency or severe peripheral vascular disease.

Mechanical Complications

Mechanical complications usually occur within the first weeks and account for approximately 15% of MI-related deaths. Such complications include acute mitral valve regurgitation, ventricular septal defect, free wall rupture, and LV aneurysm. Suspicion and investigation of a mechanical defect should be prompted by a new murmur or sudden, progressive hemodynamic deterioration with pulmonary edema or a low output state. Transthoracic or transesophageal Doppler echocardiography usually establishes the diagnosis. A balloon flotation catheter can be helpful in confirming the diagnosis. Arteriography to identify correctable coronary artery disease is warranted in most cases. Surgical consultation should be requested promptly, and urgent repair is usually indicated.

Acute mitral valve regurgitation (Chapter 75) results from infarct-related rupture or dysfunction of a papillary muscle. Total rupture leads to death in 75% of patients within 24 hours. Medical therapy is initiated with nitroprusside (beginning with 0.1 μg/kg/minute and titrating upward every 3 to 5 minutes to the desired effect, as tolerated by blood pressure response, up to 5 μg/kg/minute), to lower preload and to improve peripheral perfusion, and inotropic support (e.g., dobutamine, titrated from 2 up to 20 μg/kg/minute in normotensive patients; dopamine, titrated from 2 up to 20 μg/kg/minute in hypotensive patients; or combined dobutamine and dopamine). An IABP is used to maintain hemodynamic stability. Emergency surgical repair (if possible) or replacement is then undertaken. Surgery is associated with high mortality (≥25 to 50%), but it leads to better functional and survival outcomes than medical therapy alone.

Post-infarction septal rupture with *ventricular septal defect,* which occurs with increased frequency in elderly patients, in patients with hypertension, and possibly after fibrinolysis, also warrants urgent surgical repair. Because a small post-MI ventricular septal defect can suddenly enlarge and cause rapid hemodynamic collapse, all septal perforations should be repaired. On diagnosis, invasive monitoring is recommended, together with vasodilators (e.g., nitroprusside, initially 0.1 µg/kg/minute, titrated upward every 3 to 5 minutes to desired effect, as tolerated by blood pressure response, up to 5 µg/kg/minute) and, if needed, judicious use of inotropic agents (e.g., dobutamine, titrated from 2 up to 20 µg/kg/minute in normotensive patients; dopamine, titrated from 2 up to 20 µg/kg/minute in hypotensive patients; or combined dobutamine and dopamine). An IABP should be inserted, a surgical consultation promptly obtained, and surgical repair undertaken as soon as feasible.

LV free wall rupture usually causes acute cardiac tamponade with sudden death. In a small percentage of cases, however, resealing or localized containment ("pseudoaneurysm") can allow medical stabilization, usually with inotropic support or an IABP, followed by emergency surgical repair.

An *LV aneurysm* can develop after a large, usually anterior, acute MI. If refractory heart failure, VT, or systemic embolization occurs despite medical therapy and PCI, aneurysmectomy with CABG is indicated.

Thromboembolic Complications

Thromboembolism has been described in approximately 10% of clinical series and 20% of autopsy series, a finding suggesting a high rate of undiagnosed events. Thromboembolism contributed to up to 25% of hospital deaths from acute MI in the past, but the incidence has declined in the recanalization era in association with greater use of antithrombotics, reductions of infarct size, and earlier ambulation. Systemic arterial emboli (including cerebrovascular emboli) typically arise from an LV mural thrombus, whereas pulmonary emboli commonly arise from thrombi in leg veins. Arterial embolism can cause dramatic clinical events, such as hemiparesis, loss of a pulse, ischemic bowel, or sudden hypertension, depending on the regional circulation involved.

Mural thrombosis with embolism typically occurs in the setting of a large (especially anterior) ST segment elevation acute MI and heart failure. The risk for embolism is particularly high when a mural thrombus is detected by echocardiography. Thus, in patients with anterior ST segment elevation acute MI and in other high-risk patients, echocardiography should be performed during hospitalization; if results are positive, anticoagulation should be started (with an antithrombin), if not already initiated, and continued (with warfarin) for 6 months.

Deep vein thrombosis can be prevented by lower extremity compression therapy, by limiting the duration of bedrest, and by the use of subcutaneous unfractionated heparin or LMWH (in patients at risk not receiving intravenous heparin) until patients are fully ambulatory (Chapter 81). Patients with pulmonary embolism are treated with intravenous heparin, then oral anticoagulation for 6 months (Chapter 98).

Risk Stratification after Myocardial Infarction

The goal of risk stratification before and early after discharge for acute MI is to assess ventricular and clinical function, latent ischemia, and arrhythmic risk, to use this information for patient education and prognostic assessment, and to guide therapeutic strategies (see Fig. 73-3).

Cardiac Catheterization and Noninvasive Stress Testing

Risk stratification generally involves functional assessment by one of three strategies: cardiac catheterization, submaximal exercise stress ECG before discharge (at 4 to 6 days), or symptom-limited stress testing at 2 to 6 weeks after discharge. Many or most patients with ST segment elevation acute MI undergo invasive evaluation for primary PCI or after fibrinolytic therapy. Catheterization generally is performed during hospitalization for patients at high risk. In others, predischarge submaximal exercise testing (to peak heart rate of 120 to 130 beats per minute or 70% of the predicted maximum) appears safe when it is performed in patients who are ambulating without symptoms; it should be avoided within 2 to 3 days of acute MI and in patients with unstable post-MI angina, uncompensated heart failure, or serious cardiac arrhythmias. Alternatively or in addition, patients may undergo symptom-limited stress testing at 2 to 6 weeks before they return to work or resume other increased physical activities. Abnormal test results include not only ST segment depression but also low functional capacity, exertional hypotension, and serious arrhythmias. Patients with positive test results should be considered for coronary angiography.

The sensitivity of stress testing can be augmented with radionuclide perfusion imaging (thallium-201 or technetium-99m sestamibi, or both; Chapter 56) or echocardiography (Chapter 55). Supplemental imaging also can quantify the LV ejection fraction and size the area of infarction or ischemia (e.g., by cardiac magnetic resonance imaging; Chapter 56). For patients taking digoxin or for those with ST segment changes that preclude accurate ECG interpretation (e.g., baseline LBBB or LV hypertrophy), an imaging study is recommended with initial stress testing. In others, an imaging study may be performed selectively for those in whom the exercise ECG test result is positive or equivocal. For patients unable to exercise, pharmacologic stress testing can be performed using adenosine, a long-acting bolus analogue of adenosine (e.g., regadenoson) or dipyridamole scintigraphy or using dobutamine echocardiography.

Electrocardiographic Monitoring

Modern telemetry systems capture complete rhythm information during hospital observations and allow for identification of patients with serious arrhythmias, so routine 24- to 48-hour ambulatory ECG (Holter) monitoring

before or after hospital discharge is not recommended. Patients with sustained VT or VF occurring late during hospitalization or provoked during electrophysiologic study with nonsustained VT on monitoring are candidates for an ICD, especially if the ejection fraction is less than 40% (Fig. 73-4) (Chapters 65 and 66). Prophylactic ICD placement at least 1 month after acute MI prevents sudden death for patients with severely depressed function (ejection fraction ≤ 0.30) regardless of the rhythm status.[22]

Secondary Prevention, Patient Education, and Rehabilitation

Secondary Prevention

Advances in secondary prevention have resulted in increasingly effective measures to reduce recurrent MI and cardiovascular death. Secondary prevention should be conscientiously applied after acute MI (Table 73-8).

A fasting *lipid profile* is recommended on admission, and *lipid-lowering therapy*, typically with a statin, is begun in the hospital, generally with an LDL cholesterol goal of less than 70 mg/dL (Chapter 213). Continued smoking doubles the subsequent mortality risk after acute MI, and *smoking cessation* reduces the risk for reinfarction and death within 1 year (Chapter 31). An individualized smoking cessation plan should be formulated, including pharmacologic aids (nicotine gum and patches, bupropion, or varenicline).

Antiplatelet therapy (Chapter 37; Fig. 73-5) should consist of aspirin, given on a long-term basis to all patients without contraindications (maintenance dose, 75 to 162 mg/day). Clopidogrel (75 mg/day) or prasugrel (10 mg/day) is given to patients who received PCI with stenting, and clopidogrel is also appropriate for others at higher risk for recurrent vascular events. Therapy is recommended for a minimum of 1 month after a bare metal stent, for at least 3 months for sirolimus-eluting stents, and for at least 6 months for paclitaxel-eluting stents. If patients are not at high risk for bleeding, therapy is continued for up to 1 year or more.

Anticoagulant therapy (i.e., warfarin, with an international normalized ratio goal of 2.0 to 3.0) is indicated after acute MI for patients unable to take antiplatelet therapy (aspirin or clopidogrel), for those with persistent or paroxysmal AF, for those with LV thrombus, and for those who have suffered a systemic or pulmonary embolism. Anticoagulants also may be considered for patients with extensive wall motion abnormalities and markedly depressed ejection fraction with or without heart failure. Data on the benefits and risks of warfarin added to antiplatelet therapy (Fig. 73-5) are sparse.

ACE inhibitor therapy can prevent adverse myocardial remodeling after acute MI and can reduce heart failure and death; it is clearly indicated for long-term use in patients with anterior acute MI or an LV ejection fraction of less than 40%. ACE inhibitors also reduce recurrent MI in higher-risk patients with an ejection fraction greater than 40%. In contrast, ACE inhibition, when added to other contemporary therapies, provides little additional benefit in reducing cardiovascular events in patients who have stable coronary disease and a low risk (<5%/year) for a coronary event. These data suggest a rationale for the long-term use of ACE inhibitors (e.g., ramipril, 2.5 mg titrated to 10 mg/day, or lisinopril, 2.5 to 5 mg titrated to 10 mg/day) in all patients after MI, except perhaps those at lowest risk (i.e., without heart failure, hypertension, glucose intolerance, or reduced ejection fraction). An ARB (e.g., valsartan, 80 to 160 mg twice daily, or losartan, 50 to 100 mg/day) should be substituted in patients who cannot tolerate an ACE inhibitor; in patients with advanced heart failure, both an ACE inhibitor and an ARB may be complementary (Chapter 59). An aldosterone receptor blocker (e.g., eplerenone, 25 mg/day orally, increased to 50 mg/day after 4 weeks if tolerated, with monitoring of serum potassium levels) also should be added to the ACE inhibitor or ARB (but not both) regimen on a long-term basis in patients with depressed ejection fraction (≤0.40) and clinical heart failure or diabetes, unless this approach is contraindicated.

Long-term β-blocker therapy is strongly recommended for all MI survivors without uncompensated heart failure or other contraindications. Options include metoprolol, 20 to 200 mg per day, or carvedilol, 6.25 to 25 mg twice daily. Long-term therapy in patients at low risk (normal ventricular function, successful recanalization, absence of arrhythmias) is reasonable but not mandatory.

Nitroglycerin (0.4 mg) is prescribed routinely for sublingual or buccal administration for acute anginal attacks. Longer-acting oral therapy (isosorbide mononitrate, 30 to 60 mg orally every morning, or dinitrate, 10 to 40 mg orally two to three times daily) or topical nitroglycerin (e.g., start 0.5 inch, can titrate up to 2 inches, every 6 hours for 2 days) may be added to treatment regimens for angina or heart failure in selected patients.

Calcium-channel blockers are negatively inotropic and are *not* routinely given on a long-term basis; however, they may be given to selected patients without LV dysfunction (ejection fraction > 0.40) who are intolerant of β-blockers and who require these drugs for antianginal therapy (e.g., amlodipine, 5 to 10 mg/day orally, or diltiazem, 120 to 480 mg/day orally as sustained release or divided doses) or for control of heart rate in AF (e.g., diltiazem, 120 to 480 mg/day orally, or verapamil, 180 to 480 mg/day orally, as sustained release or in divided doses). Short-acting nifedipine should be avoided.

Hormone therapy with estrogen with or without progestin is not begun after an acute MI because it increases thromboembolic risk and does not prevent reinfarction. For women already receiving hormone replacement, therapy

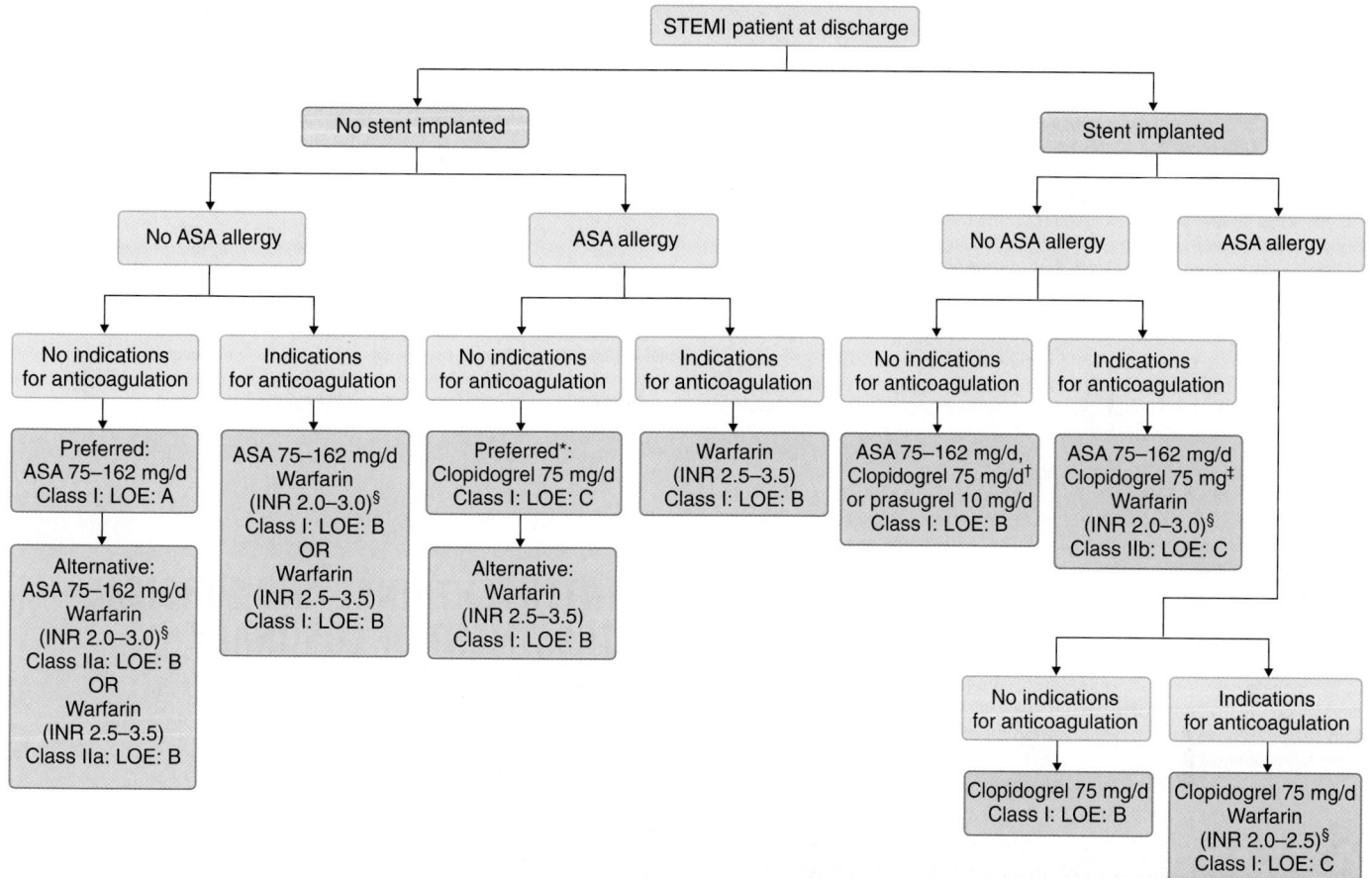

FIGURE 73-5. Long-term antithrombotic therapy at hospital discharge after ST segment elevation myocardial infarction (STEMI). *Clopidogrel is preferred over warfarin because of increased risk of bleeding and low patient compliance in warfarin trials. †For 12 months. ‡Discontinue clopidogrel 1 month after implantation of a bare metal stent or several months after implantation of a drug-eluting stent (3 months after sirolimus and 6 months after paclitaxel) because of the potentially increased risk of bleeding with warfarin and two antiplatelet agents. Continue aspirin (ASA) and warfarin on a long-term basis if warfarin is indicated for other reasons such as atrial fibrillation, left ventricular thrombus, cerebral emboli, or extensive regional wall motion abnormality. §An International Normalized Ratio (INR) of 2.0 to 3.0 is acceptable with tight control, but the lower end of this range is preferable. The combination of antiplatelet therapy and warfarin may be considered in patients younger than 75 years who have a low bleeding risk and who can be monitored reliably. LOE = level of evidence. (Adapted from Antman EM, Anbe DT, Armstrong PW, et al. ACC/AHA guidelines for the management of patients with ST-elevation myocardial infarction—executive summary. A report of the American College of Cardiology/American Heart Association Task Force on Practice Guidelines [Writing Committee to Revise the 1999 Guidelines for the Management of Patients with Acute Myocardial Infarction]. *Circulation.* 2004;110:588-636.)

TABLE 73-8 DISCHARGE MEDICATION CHECKLIST AFTER MYOCARDIAL INFARCTION*

MEDICATION	DOSES	REASONS NOT TO USE	COMMENTS
Aspirin	Initial: 162-325 mg Maintenance: 75-162 mg daily	High bleeding risk	Reduces mortality, reinfarction, and stroke
Clopidogrel	Initial dose: 300-600 mg (75-150 mg after fibrinolysis in patients >75 years old) Maintenance: 75 mg daily	High bleeding risk; suboptimal antiplatelet response	Indicated after PCI for at least 1 yr (shorter time for BMS if high bleeding risk); also reduces vascular events when added to aspirin in non–ST segment elevation acute MI (also useful based on recent clinical trials after ST segment elevation acute MI) Genetic variants (CYP2C19) may reduce response Controversial interaction with PPIs (e.g., omeprazole)
Prasugrel	Initial dose: 60 mg Maintenance: 10 mg daily	High bleeding risk	Avoid with history of prior stroke/TIA Consider 5 mg daily in patients >75 years old or <60 kg
β-Blocker (e.g., metoprolol, carvedilol)	Metoprolol: 25-200 mg daily Carvedilol: 6.25-25 mg bid	Asthma, bradycardia, heart failure	Reduces mortality, reinfarction, sudden death, arrhythmia, hypertension, angina, atherosclerosis progression
ACE inhibitor (e.g., ramipril, lisinopril) or ARB (e.g., valsartan, losartan)	Ramipril: 2.5-10 mg daily Lisinopril: 5-10 mg daily Valsartan: 80-160 mg daily-bid Losartan: 50-100 mg daily	Hypotension, allergy, hyperkalemia	Reduces mortality, reinfarction, stroke, heart failure, diabetes, atherosclerosis progression
Lipid-lowering agent (e.g., a statin) (e.g., atorvastatin, simvastatin)	Atorvastatin: 10-80 mg daily Simvastatin: 20-40 mg daily	Myopathy, rhabdomyolysis, hepatitis	Goal = LDL <100 and preferably <70 (statins also can benefit patients with lower LDL†); consider addition of niacin or fibrate for high non-HDL cholesterol, low HDL
Nitroglycerin sublingual	0.4 mg SL PRN for angina	Aortic stenosis; sildenafil (Viagra) use	Instruct on PRN use and appropriate need for medical attention

*Medications given at hospital discharge improve long-term compliance.
†Heart Protection Study (*Lancet.* 2002;360:7); and PROVE-IT Study (*N Engl J Med.* 2004;350:1495).
ACE, angiotensin-converting enzyme; ARB = angiotensin receptor blocker; bid = twice daily; BMS = bare metal stent; HDL = high-density lipoprotein; LDL = low-density lipoprotein; MI = myocardial infarction; PCI = percutaneous coronary intervention; PRN = as needed; daily = once daily; SL = sublingual; TIA, transient ischemic attack.
Adapted from Kushner FG, Hand M, Antman EM, et al. 2009 Focused updates: ACC/AHA guidelines for the management of patients with ST-elevation myocardial infarction and the ACC/AHA/SCAI guidelines on percutaneous coronary intervention. *Circulation.* 2009;120:2271-2306.

should be discontinued unless it is being given for another compelling indication.

Hypertension (Chapter 67) and diabetes mellitus (Chapter 236) must be assessed and tightly controlled in patients after acute MI. ACE inhibitors or β-blockers as described earlier are usually the first-choice therapies for hypertension, with ARBs indicated when ACE inhibitors are not tolerated. ACE inhibitors and ARBs also can reduce the long-term complications of diabetes.

Antioxidant supplementation (e.g., vitamin E, vitamin C) does not benefit patients after acute MI and is *not* recommended. Folate therapy reduces homocyst(e)ine levels, but it has not been effective in reducing clinical events in large secondary prevention trials. Fish oil supplements showed no benefit in the best randomized trial.

Antiarrhythmic drugs are *not* generally recommended after acute MI, and class I antiarrhythmic agents can increase the risk for sudden death. Class III drugs (amiodarone, sotalol, dofetilide) may be used as part of the management strategy for specific arrhythmias (e.g., AF, VT) (Chapters 64 and 65).

The intracoronary infusion of stem cells has been proposed as a mechanism to reduce infarct size. To date, however, trials have been inconclusive.

Patient Education and Rehabilitation

The hospital stay provides an important opportunity to educate patients about their MI and its treatment, coronary risk factors, and behavioral modification. Education should begin on admission and should continue after discharge. However, the time before hospital discharge is particularly opportune. Many hospitals use case managers and prevention specialists to augment physicians and nurses, to provide educational materials, to review important concepts, to assist in formulating and actualizing individual risk-reduction plans, and to ensure proper and timely outpatient follow-up. This follow-up should include early return appointments with the patient's physician (within a few weeks). Instructions on activities also should be given before discharge. Many hospitals have cardiac rehabilitation programs that provide supervised, progressive exercise.

1. Van't Hof AW, Ten Berg J, Heestermans T, et al. Prehospital initiation of tirofiban in patients with ST-elevation myocardial infarction undergoing primary angioplasty (On-TIME 2): a multicentre, double-blind, randomised controlled trial. *Lancet.* 2008;372:537-546.
2. Stone GW, Witzenbichler B, Guagliumi G, et al. Bivalirudin during primary percutaneous coronary intervention in acute myocardial infarction. *N Engl J Med.* 2008;358:2218-2230.
3. Wijeysundere HC, Vijayaraghavan R, Nallamothu BK, et al. Rescue angioplasty or repeat fibrinolysis after failed therapy for ST-segment myocardial infarction: a meta-analysis of randomized trials. *J Am Coll Cardiol.* 2007;49:422-430.
4. Cantor WJ, Fitchett D, Borgundvaag G, et al. Routine early angioplasty after fibrinolysis for acute myocardial infarction. *N Engl J Med.* 2009;360:2705-2718.
5. DiMario C, Dudek D, Piscione E, et al. Immediate angioplasty versus standard therapy with rescue angioplasty after thrombolysis in the Combined Abciximab REteplase Stent study in acute myocardial infarction (CARESS-in-AMI): an open, prospective, randomised, multicentre trial. *Lancet.* 2008;371:559-568.
6. Keeley EC, Boura JA, Grines CL. Primary angioplasty versus intravenous thrombolytic therapy for acute myocardial infarction: a quantitative review of 23 randomised trials. *Lancet.* 2003;361:13-20.
7. Andersen HR, Nielsen TT, Rasmussen K, et al. A comparison of coronary angioplasty with fibrinolytic therapy in acute myocardial infarction. *N Engl J Med.* 2003;349:733-742.
8. Kushner FG, Hand M, Antman EM, et al. 2009 focused updates: ACC/AHA guidelines for the management of patients with ST-elevation myocardial infarction and the ACC/AHA/SCAI guidelines on percutaneous coronary intervention. *Circulation.* 2009;120:2271-2306.
9. Ellis SG, Tendera M, de Belder MA, et al. Facilitated PCI in patients with ST-elevation myocardial infarction. *N Engl J Med.* 2008;358:2205-2217.
10. Schomig A, Mehilli J, Antoniucci D, et al. Mechanical reperfusion in patients with acute myocardial infarction presenting more than 12 hours from symptom onset: a randomized controlled trial. *JAMA.* 2005;293:2865-2872.
11. Svilass T, Vlaar PJ, vander Horst I, et al. Thrombus aspiration during primary percutaneous coronary intervention. *N Engl J Med.* 2008;358:557-567.
12. Keeley EC, Boura JA, Grines CL. Comparison of primary and facilitated percutaneous interventions for ST-elevation myocardial infarction: quantitative review of randomized trials. *Lancet.* 2006;367:579-588.
13. Sabatine MS, Cannon CP, Gibson M, et al. Addition of clopidogrel to aspirin and fibrinolytic therapy for myocardial infarction with ST-segment elevation. *N Engl J Med.* 2005;352:1179-1189.
14. COMMIT (Clopidogrel and Metoprolol in Myocardial Infarction Trial) Collaborative Group. Early intravenous then oral metoprolol in 45 of 852 patients with acute myocardial infarction: randomised placebo-controlled trial. *Lancet.* 2005;366:1622-1632.
15. Montalescot G, Wiviott SD, Braunwald E, et al. Prasugrel compared with clopidogrel in patients undergoing percutaneous coronary intervention for ST-elevation myocardial infarction (TRITON-TIMI 38): double-blind, randomised controlled trial. *Lancet.* 2009;373:723-731.
16. Antman EM, Morrow DA, McCabe CH, et al. Enoxaparin versus unfractionated heparin with fibrinolysis for ST-elevation myocardial infarction. *N Engl J Med.* 2006;354:1477-1488.
17. Yusuf S, Mehta SR, Chrolavicius S, et al. Effects of fondaparinux on mortality and reinfarction in patients with acute ST-segment elevation myocardial infarction: the OASIS-6 randomized trial. *JAMA.* 2006;295:1519-1530.
18. Mehran R, Lansky AJ, Witzenbichler B, et al. Bivalirudin in patients undergoing primary angioplasty for acute myocardial infarction (HORIZONS-AMI): 1-year results of a randomised controlled trial. *Lancet.* 2009;374:1149-1159.
19. Pitt B, Remme W, Zannad E, et al. Eplerenone, a selective aldosterone blocker, in patients with left ventricular dysfunction after myocardial infarction. *N Engl J Med.* 2003;348:1309-1321.
20. Moss AJ, Zareba W, Hall J, et al. Prophylactic implantation of a defibrillator in patients with myocardial infarction and reduced ejection fraction. *N Engl J Med.* 2002;346:877-883.
21. Steinbeck G, Andresen D, Seidl K, et al. Defibrillator implantation early after myocardial infarction. *N Engl J Med.* 2009;361:1427-1436.
22. Cannon CP, Steinberg BA, Murphy SA, et al. Meta-analysis of cardiovascular outcomes trials comparing intensive versus moderate statin therapy. *J Am Coll Cardiol.* 2006;48:438-445.

SUGGESTED READINGS

Cohen M, Boiangiu C, Abidi M. Therapy for ST-segment elevation myocardial infarction patients who present late or are ineligible for reperfusion therapy. *J Am Coll Cardiol.* 2010;55:1895-1906. *Low-molecular-weight heparin is recommended for patients who have ST segment elevation myocardial infarction but who present late or are ineligible for reperfusion therapy.*

Lambert L, Brown K, Segal E, et al. Association between timeliness of reperfusion therapy and clinical outcomes in ST-elevation myocardial infarction. *JAMA.* 2010;303:2148-2155. *Prompt reperfusion improves outcomes compared with delayed reperfusion.*

Suh HS, Song HJ, Choi JE, et al. Drug-eluting stents versus bare-metal stents in acute myocardial infarction: a systematic review and meta-analysis. *Int J Technol Assess Heatlh Care.* 2011;27:11-22. *Drug-eluting stents provided better 1-year outcomes but equivalent 2-year outcomes.*

74

INTERVENTIONAL AND SURGICAL TREATMENT OF CORONARY ARTERY DISEASE

PAUL S. TEIRSTEIN AND BRUCE W. LYTLE

Percutaneous coronary intervention (PCI) and coronary artery bypass graft (CABG) surgery represent alternative and sometimes complementary approaches to coronary revascularization. Each has its relative indications, advantages, disadvantages, and contraindications.

PERCUTANEOUS CORONARY INTERVENTION

PCI is applicable to most forms of coronary artery disease, including multivessel disease, total occlusions, saphenous vein graft disease, unstable angina (Chapter 72), and acute myocardial infarction (MI) (Chapter 73). An estimated 2 million PCIs are performed worldwide each year, making it one of the most widely used medical procedures. Its popularity is based largely on its simplicity, the need for only local anesthesia, a short (approximately 1 day) hospitalization, and negligible postprocedure recovery time.

Mechanisms and Technical Considerations

Under local anesthesia, a hollow-bore needle is inserted percutaneously into a peripheral artery (usually the femoral or radial artery). A guidewire (approximately 0.038 inch) is placed through this needle and advanced into the aorta. The needle is removed, leaving the guidewire, over which a small-caliber (approximately 3 mm), specially shaped catheter (called a guiding catheter) is advanced under fluoroscope guidance into the ostium of the obstructed coronary artery. By use of radiographic contrast injections that provide fluoroscopic visualization of the coronary artery lumen, a thin (approximately 0.014 inch), highly steerable guidewire is directed down the coronary artery and across the stenotic lesion. This guidewire becomes a "rail" over which therapeutic tools such as inflatable balloons, stents, and atherectomy catheters are passed to the diseased segment (Fig. 74-1).

Balloon catheters (Fig. 74-2) typically have two lumens, one to allow passage over the guidewire and another to carry a mixture of saline and radiographic contrast material to inflate a balloon at the distal catheter tip. Under fluoroscopy, the balloon is centered across the lesion and inflated to 3 to 20 atmospheres of pressure. Balloon inflation widens the narrowed lumen by stretching the vessel and, in most cases, causing a tear (a therapeutic dissection) at the edges of the plaque, where the atheroma meets the nondiseased media. Atherectomy catheters, which also are passed over a guidewire to the diseased segment, remove plaque by a shaving, grinding, slicing, or suction mechanism. Coronary stents are metallic scaffolding devices that are crimped onto a deflated balloon catheter before insertion into the diseased vessel. During balloon inflation, the collapsed stent expands to support the vessel lumen (Fig. 74-3). Whereas balloons and atherectomy devices create an adequate, albeit rough channel through diseased arteries, the supporting structure of the stent can widen the lumen to near its predisease dimensions.

FIGURE 74-1. Schematic view of coronary angioplasty technique. A guide catheter (A) is inserted into the orifice of the coronary artery (in this figure, the left main); a balloon catheter (B) is advanced over a thin guidewire (C) into the lesion. Balloon inflation dilates the stenotic region. (Modified from Baim DS. Percutaneous balloon angioplasty and general coronary intervention. In: Baim DS, ed. *Grossman's Cardiac Catheterization, Angiography, and Intervention,* 7th ed. Philadelphia: Lippincott Williams & Wilkins; 2005.)

FIGURE 74-3. Balloon-expandable coronary stent. The stainless steel stent is crimped onto a balloon catheter to allow low-profile passage through the coronary artery. When it is positioned across the lesion, the balloon is inflated, expanding the stent. After balloon deflation and removal, the stent remains, providing a scaffold that supports the vessel lumen.

FIGURE 74-2. Balloon angioplasty catheter. The catheter consists of two lumens, an inflation lumen and a guidewire lumen. Two radiopaque markers, indicating the lateral balloon margins, aid in positioning of the balloon before inflation.

findings, such as the presence of collateral vessels that supply a different myocardial territory and that originate distal to the target, should be appreciated. For each patient, the benefits of PCI must be weighed against the procedural risk. Characteristics of the patient conveying increased risk include advanced age (i.e., >75 years), diabetes, smaller vessels that are often found in women, prior MI, significant impairment of left ventricular function, and renal insufficiency.

Procedural Success and Complications

With use of modern techniques in appropriately selected patients, most PCI procedures have a greater than 95% success rate. The single exception is a chronic total coronary occlusion (100% obstruction of the lumen), in which the interventional cardiologist's ability to negotiate a guidewire through the blockage is only about 50 to 80%. With the increased use of coronary stents and adjunctive antiplatelet agents (thienopyridines and platelet glycoprotein IIb/IIIa inhibitors), abrupt coronary artery closure is rarely encountered. When PCI is performed by an experienced interventional cardiologist in appropriately selected patients, the risk of in-hospital death is less than 1%; MI (usually small, non–ST segment elevation MI) is approximately 5%; the need for urgent or emergent CABG surgery is less than 1%; the risk of stroke is less than 0.1%; the chance of coronary perforation is less than 1%; and morbidity at the arterial access site (i.e., hematoma, pseudoaneurysm, or arteriovenous fistula) occurs in less than 5%. Balloons and filters deployed within a coronary vessel beyond the target lesion to limit distal embolization of plaque, platelet aggregates, and other "debris" can further reduce ischemic complications in selected, high-risk patients.

Restenosis and Thrombosis

Restenosis is a renarrowing of an artery after a PCI procedure, usually resulting from one of two general mechanisms. The first mechanism, unfavorable remodeling and elastic recoil, is a mechanical renarrowing caused by adventitial constriction and shrinkage of the vessel lumen. The second mechanism, neointimal hyperplasia, is due to the proliferation of smooth muscle cells and matrix in response to the injury caused by balloons, stents, or atherectomy devices. Restenosis occurs in 10 to 50% of PCI patients after balloon angioplasty without stenting, usually within the first 6 months after the procedure. Characteristics associated with higher risk of restenosis include longer lesions, small-diameter vessels, diabetes, and multivessel disease. Treatment with either balloon angioplasty or atherectomy devices results in similar rates of restenosis. Coronary stents provide a semirigid scaffolding within the lumen and reduce restenosis by eliminating the mechanical renarrowing

With a stent, tissue flaps are "pinned" against the wall, and recoil is limited. Most stents are designed so that the metallic struts compose only about 20% of the surface area to allow a rapid endothelialization (during about 2 weeks) and a reduced risk of thrombosis. Because coronary stents are able to obtain a larger and more secure lumen, some resist restenosis, and some elute beneficial medications, they are now used in more than 95% of PCIs.

During the PCI procedure, the interventional cardiologist is able to assess the target vessel fluoroscopically by injections of contrast material through the guiding catheter (Fig. 74-4). When the coronary artery has been opened successfully, all catheters are withdrawn, and the arterial access site is sealed by mechanical pressure, an absorbable plug, or a remote suturing device. Patients without comorbidity ambulate in 3 to 6 hours. Discharge from the hospital usually occurs on the morning after the procedure, after stability of the arterial access site, cardiac biomarkers, and electrocardiogram is confirmed. Selected patients in some medical centers are treated as outpatients and released 6 to 12 hours after the procedure without an overnight stay.

Selection of Patients

Any decision to perform PCI must include a review of the coronary angiogram (Chapter 57) by an experienced interventional cardiologist to assess the lesion's technical suitability for the procedure. The disease must narrow the coronary artery lumen by at least 60%, and the quantity of myocardium subtended by the vessel should not be trivial. High-risk lesion characteristics, such as longer lesion length, vessel tortuosity, lesion calcification, or the presence of thrombus, must be taken into consideration. Subtle angiographic

FIGURE 74-4. Angiographic images before, after, and at late follow-up after placement of a sirolimus-eluting stent. The left anterior descending artery contains a tight stenosis (*arrow, upper left panel*). After stent implantation (*upper right panel*), the stenosis is abolished (*arrow*). Follow-up at 4 and 12 months (*bottom panels*) reveals a completely open lumen, with no evidence of restenosis (*arrows*).

caused by unfavorable remodeling and elastic recoil. In randomized trials, bare metal stents reduce restenosis by about one third, from approximately 30 to 40% in patients randomized to balloon angioplasty to 20 to 30% in patients receiving stents.[1]

Although bare metal stents reduce restenosis, they do not eliminate restenosis because the stent struts that embed into the vessel wall increase the intimal proliferative response to injury. With bare metal stents, the mechanical component of restenosis is eliminated, but the proliferative component is enhanced. Smooth muscle cell division and matrix formation can migrate through the stent struts to renarrow the vessel lumen. Antiproliferative drugs that are embedded into a polymer stent coating are extremely effective for the control of restenosis. However, drug-eluting stents carry a slightly higher risk of thrombosis later (>1 year), especially if patients cannot or do not continue with aspirin plus a thienopyridine. As a result, trials of stents that release the cell cycle inhibitors sirolimus, everolimus, zotarolimus, and paclitaxel have demonstrated a reduced need for early repeated procedures,[2] but have not always found improved long-term outcome compared with bare metal stents.[3,4] Among the drug-eluting stents, the most favorable current data are for everolimus and sirolimus.[5,6]

Choices Related to Stenting
Based on long-term follow-up data, the choice between a bare metal stent and a drug-eluting stent remains controversial. Patients receiving drug-eluting stents must continue dual antiplatelet therapy with aspirin and a thienopyridine for a minimum of 12 months. If a patient is unlikely to be able to adhere to such therapy because of bleeding risks or the need for an invasive or surgical procedure, a bare metal stent is preferable. Atherectomy is rarely used, with the exception of the Rotablator (Boston Scientific, Maple Grove, MN), which pulverizes plaque into microparticles that pass through the coronary microcirculation and is particularly helpful for the treatment of heavily calcified lesions. After plaque debulking with the Rotablator, a drug-eluting stent is usually implanted.

Discharge Issues
Discharge planning after PCI represents an important opportunity to emphasize evidence-based medical treatment of atherothrombotic disease and coronary risk factor modification. All patients should receive aspirin (81 to 325 mg/day) indefinitely. For patients receiving bare metal stents, a minimum 2-week course of a thienopyridine (i.e., clopidogrel 75 mg daily or prasugrel 10 mg daily) is mandatory. If a drug-eluting stent is deployed, this dual antiplatelet therapy must be extended for at least 12 months, and then either aspirin alone or dual antiplatelet therapy must be continued indefinitely if possible.[7] Prolonged use of aspirin, clopidogrel, angiotensin-converting enzyme inhibitors, β-blockers, and lipid-lowering agents should be considered on the basis of randomized trials showing improved long-term outcome, particularly in patients who present with unstable angina syndromes (Chapters 71, 72, and 73). Smoking cessation (Chapter 31), blood pressure control (Chapter 67), stress management, exercise, weight loss, changes in dietary habits, and strict blood glucose control for diabetic patients (Chapter 237) also are important elements of the discharge plan.

Activity restrictions after PCI are modest. If the femoral artery was instrumented, heavy lifting is discouraged for several days. Intense aerobic exercise is usually discouraged for 2 to 4 weeks (especially after stent implantation) because exercise can activate platelets and lead to formation of thrombus at the angioplasty site. Patients may return to work 1 or 2 days after the procedure if their occupation does not include heavy lifting or excessive physical exercise. There is usually no restriction on driving an automobile.

⬤ CORONARY ANGIOPLASTY VERSUS MEDICAL THERAPY
PCI reduces angina and commonly leads to better treadmill exercise performance and improved quality-of-life measurements. However, PCI has not been shown to reduce the risks of death, MI, or other major cardiovascular events compared with modern optimal medical therapy in patients with stable angina (Chapter 71).[8] PCI reduces symptoms for the first 24 months, especially in patients with more severe angina, but symptoms were similarly improved over baseline with both intensive medical therapy and PCI at 36 months.[9] In truly asymptomatic patients, significant ischemia first should be documented by functional testing, or a large quantity of myocardium should be supplied by the stenotic coronary artery. Patients experiencing acute ST elevation MI (Chapter 73) represent an important subgroup in whom PCI has proved beneficial compared with medical therapy (Fig. 74-5). In ST elevation MI, randomized trials consistently have reported a reduction in

FIGURE 74-5. Primary coronary angioplasty for acute myocardial infarction. This 50-year-old man presented at midnight with 70 minutes of crushing substernal chest pressure accompanied by inferior ST segment elevation. Emergency angiography performed 45 minutes after arrival found 100% occlusion of the right coronary artery (**A**, *arrow*). Within 10 minutes, a guidewire was negotiated through the obstruction (presumably caused by fresh thrombus), allowing perfusion into the distal vessel and uncovering a high-grade stenotic lesion (**B**, *arrow*). After deployment of a coronary stent (**C**, *arrow*), the stenosis was abolished and significant myocardial damage aborted.

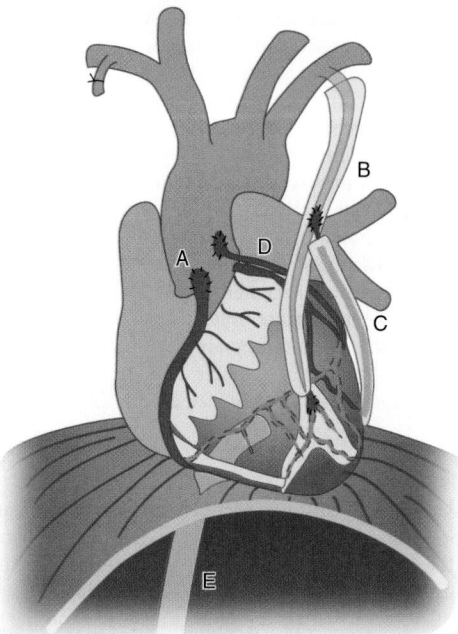

FIGURE 74-6. Types of bypass grafts. Bypass grafts include reversed saphenous vein graft from aorta to right coronary artery (A), in situ left internal mammary artery graft to anterior descending coronary artery (B), Y graft of right internal mammary artery from left internal mammary artery to circumflex coronary artery (C), radial artery graft from aorta to circumflex coronary artery (D), and in situ gastroepiploic graft to posterior descending branch of the right coronary artery (E).

mortality, stroke, subsequent MI, and recurrent ischemia with immediate PCI compared with thrombolytic therapy[10] or with initial thrombolytic therapy followed by rescue PCI as needed,[11] even if immediate PCI requires transfer to another hospital. For non–ST elevation MI and many patients with unstable angina, an early aggressive approach that includes either PCI or CABG in angiographically suitable patients is generally preferable to a conservative strategy,[12,13] except in lower-risk patients (Chapter 72).

CORONARY ARTERY SURGERY

CABG is based on the premise that the morbidity and mortality associated with coronary atherosclerosis are largely related to atherosclerotic coronary stenoses that can be demonstrated by coronary angiography (Chapter 57) and that if grafts are constructed to route blood flow around these stenoses, myocardial blood supply can be improved or preserved, cardiac symptoms relieved, cardiac events diminished, and survival prolonged. Over time, the fundamentals of that concept have been shown to be correct.

The most common types of grafts for coronary artery bypass have been reversed segments of saphenous vein and the internal thoracic arteries. Saphenous vein grafts are anastomosed to the aorta (proximal anastomosis) and to the coronary artery distal to the major obstruction (Fig. 74-6). Saphenous vein grafts have the advantages of availability, larger size than most coronary arteries, and favorable handling characteristics. However, with time, saphenous vein grafts may develop intrinsic pathologic changes, intimal fibroplasia, and vein graft atherosclerosis, each of which may lead to narrowing or occlusions. By 10 years after surgery, approximately 30% of saphenous vein grafts become occluded, and 30 to 35% of those remaining exhibit angiographic evidence of vein graft atherosclerosis. Treatment with platelet inhibitors and statins (Chapter 213) decreases the risk of vein graft failure but does not eliminate it.

Internal thoracic artery grafts, on the other hand, are resistant to the development of late atherosclerosis. When it is used as an in situ (subclavian origin intact) graft to the left anterior descending (LAD) coronary artery, the left internal thoracic artery graft has a more than 90% patency rate up to 20 years after operation. Because the LAD coronary artery has a strong prognostic influence, the left internal thoracic artery to LAD graft is a clinically important part of myocardial revascularization. Patients who receive a left internal thoracic artery to LAD graft with or without saphenous vein grafts have a better long-term survival rate, fewer reoperations, and fewer cardiac events compared with patients receiving only saphenous vein grafts. The right internal thoracic artery may also be used for revascularization as an in situ graft, as an aorta to coronary artery graft, or as a composite arterial graft from the left internal thoracic artery to a coronary artery. Use of both internal thoracic arteries as grafts provides incremental benefit over a single internal thoracic artery graft strategy and produces an improved survival with a lower risk for reoperation. By comparison, radial artery grafts provide outcomes that are essentially equivalent to those with saphenous vein grafts.[14]

Most CABG operations have been performed with a full median sternotomy incision, historically with the aid of cardiopulmonary bypass, aortic cross-clamping, and cardioplegic solution—techniques that allow exposure and arrest of the heart such that detailed microsurgical anastomoses can be constructed while myocardial function is effectively protected. By comparison, strategies for performing operations through smaller incisions (minimally invasive surgery) have had limited application for coronary revascularizations. Although beating heart ("off-pump") surgery without cardiopulmonary bypass has been widely advocated to avoid neurologic complications, it apparently does not provide such protection and leads to lower rates of graft patency compared with traditional on-pump CABG.[15]

Perioperative Risks

The risk of mortality associated with CABG correlates with ischemia at the time of operation, left ventricular function, extent of coronary stenoses, noncardiac atherosclerosis, and comorbid conditions and with the experience, skill, and judgment of the surgeon. Effective myocardial protection has diminished much of the incremental risk based on the severity of cardiac disease. For patients younger than 70 years without serious comorbid conditions, the mortality risk of primary CABG surgery is less than 1% in experienced hands regardless of the number of coronary arteries that are stenotic, and left ventricular dysfunction only slightly increases risk. Nevertheless, CABG surgery in the presence of ongoing myocardial ischemia due to acute myocardial infarction, unstable angina, or acute vessel closure after PCI is still associated with increased risk. National data on primary CABG operations show a 1.7% mortality rate for elective operations, a 2.6% rate for "urgent" operations, a 6% rate for "emergency" procedures, and a 23% rate for "salvage" operations. Noncardiac comorbid conditions (aortic atherosclerosis, renal function, chronic obstructive pulmonary disease, and coagulation system disorders) increase perioperative risk when these conditions are severe.

The most serious postoperative morbidity after CABG is stroke, often related to aortic or cerebrovascular atherosclerosis and atherosclerotic embolization. Heightened awareness of the importance of aortic and carotid atherosclerosis and improved management strategies appear to have decreased the risk of focal stroke in patients previously at high risk. Serious wound complications of median sternotomy are uncommon (1 to 2%). Obesity, diabetes, and bilateral internal thoracic artery grafting (particularly in combination with diabetes) are associated with higher rates of wound complications.

Late Outcomes

The late outcomes after CABG are related to age, severity of cardiac disease before operation, noncardiac comorbid conditions, progression of atherosclerosis, and the operation itself. Many of these factors can be influenced by treatment choices. CABG tends to diminish but not to eliminate long-term survival differences based on the number of diseased coronary vessels, left main stenosis, and different levels of left ventricular function. The achievement of complete revascularization (bypass grafts to all stenotic coronary vessels) and the use of internal thoracic artery grafts improve long-term survival rates and symptomatic status.

Patients often have prolonged survival after CABG; more than 80% of patients are alive more than 10 years after operation. Over the long term, control of the progression of atherosclerosis by lifestyle modifications, pharmacologic treatment of hypertension (Chapter 67) and lipids (Chapter 213), and platelet inhibitors (Chapter 37) appears to extend the benefits of CABG.

● INDICATIONS FOR BYPASS SURGERY

The goals of CABG are to relieve symptoms and to prolong life expectancy. On the basis of randomized trials and the emergence of alternative medical treatments and PCI, the surgical population has evolved toward patients with complex conditions, often involving left main or triple-vessel disease, diffuse coronary stenoses, totally obstructed vessels, abnormal left ventricular function, and diabetes. Surgically treated patients with single-vessel disease usually have LAD stenoses or have failed alternative treatments.

Symptom Relief

If patients who experience angina have severe stenoses in graftable coronary arteries that supply areas of myocardium ischemic at rest or with stress, CABG will reliably relieve angina. Randomized trials have shown that the relief of angina after CABG is more consistent than that achieved with alternative treatments. When intermittent heart failure symptoms represent an "anginal equivalent" that is also caused by ischemia, such symptoms also respond well to relief of that ischemia by CABG. Patients with symptoms of heart failure at rest are more complex, but dobutamine echocardiography (Chapter 55) and positron emission tomography (Chapter 56) can identify segments of viable but hibernating myocardium (ischemic at rest) that may improve with bypass grafting, thus reducing symptoms of heart failure.

Survival
Chronic Stable Angina

In randomized trials of patients with mild to moderate chronic stable angina, an improved survival rate has been documented for patients treated with initial CABG compared with initial medical treatment in the presence of a left main stenosis of more than 50% of the diameter, triple-vessel disease, double-vessel disease with a proximal LAD lesion, abnormal left ventricular function, or a strongly positive exercise test result (Chapter 71). Meta-analysis of these randomized trials also suggests a survival benefit of CABG for any patient with a proximal LAD lesion and myocardial ischemia. These are subgroups of patients for whom bypass surgery should be strongly considered even in the absence of severe symptoms. During these trials, patients with severe angina were not randomized but were included in observational studies that noted improved survival rates with CABG for patients with double- and triple-vessel disease and normal or abnormal left ventricular function. Medical, interventional, and surgical treatments have all advanced substantially since these trials were completed.

Unstable Angina or Non–ST Elevation Myocardial Infarction

Current data suggest an aggressive strategy, including CABG when indicated, in patients with unstable angina or non–ST elevation acute myocardial infarction (Chapter 72).[12]

Ischemic Syndromes without Randomized Trials
ST Elevation Acute Myocardial Infarction

For patients with ST segment elevation acute myocardial infarction, CABG may be indicated in the acute setting when thrombolytic therapy or PCI has not been effective, ischemia is ongoing, and large areas of myocardium remain jeopardized. CABG after a completed MI may be indicated in patients in whom persistent ischemia in noninfarcted areas of myocardium produces post-infarction angina or hemodynamic instability. Mechanical complications of myocardial necrosis, including papillary muscle rupture, ventricular septal rupture, and myocardial free wall rupture, are acute life-threatening situations that usually require urgent operation for repair of the defect, often combined with CABG (Chapter 73).

Failed Percutaneous Coronary Intervention

The availability of intracoronary stents has decreased the need for emergency CABG to treat acute failure of PCIs. Current indications for emergency CABG include closure or threatened closure of a vessel supplying a significant amount of myocardium.

Coronary Bypass Reoperations

Patients in whom new stenoses develop in native arteries or in bypass grafts may have recurrent ischemic syndromes. Observational study of patients with severe vein graft atherosclerosis indicate that this is an unstable lesion often leading to serious cardiac events, particularly if the LAD or multiple vessels are jeopardized; reoperation appears to improve the survival rate of these patients. Reoperations are more difficult and dangerous than primary procedures, but the risk now approaches that for primary procedures in institutions performing a large number of reoperations. PCI is sometimes an alternative for the treatment of vein graft disease.

Coexisting Cardiac Disease

During cardiac operations performed for valvular (Chapter 75) or aortic (Chapter 78) disease, the standard treatment is to perform bypass grafts to major coronary arteries with angiographic stenoses of more than 50% of the luminal diameter. No randomized trials have addressed this issue, and these indications, although logical given the natural history of atherosclerosis, remain practice patterns based on consensus but not on definitive data.

● PERCUTANEOUS CORONARY INTERVENTION VERSUS CORONARY ARTERY BYPASS GRAFTING

The decision between PCI and CABG surgery is largely determined by clinical status and anatomic features but remains controversial. For patients with acute coronary syndromes, PCI is the preferred initial approach and is known to improve the survival rate of patients with ST elevation M. CABG is reserved for patients with failed acute PCI or residual myocardial ischemia. For patients with chronic coronary syndromes, there are currently no data to confirm that PCI prolongs life regardless of anatomy, whereas randomized trials, albeit older trials, demonstrate that CABG prolongs the life expectancy of patients with severe coronary artery disease, particularly patients with left ventricular dysfunction or severe ischemia. Surgery, therefore, is often the initial approach to these patient subsets.

For patients in whom the survival benefit of revascularization is less clear, the decision is often related to anatomic features. For low-risk patients followed for 1 year after revascularization, repeat revascularization is more frequent after PCI (14%) than CABG (6%), stroke is more common after CABG (2.2%) than PCI (0.6%), and the rates of death and MI are similar (Fig. 74-7). Patients with extensive and diffuse coronary stenoses appear to benefit most from surgery, whereas patients with more limited coronary stenoses, including some with left main stenosis, have equivalent outcomes with PCI.[16]

The need for repeated revascularization procedures is consistently higher in patients randomized to PCI.[17] In several randomized trials, diabetic patients with multivessel coronary disease have better outcomes with CABG surgery.[18,19]

*Primary end point

FIGURE 74-7. The SYNTAX trial randomized patients with left main vessel or three-vessel coronary artery disease to coronary artery bypass grafting (CABG) versus percutaneous coronary intervention (PCI). At 12 months, rates of death and myocardial infarction were similar, CABG increased stroke risk (2.2% vs. 0.6%), and PCI resulted in more repeat revascularizations. CVA = cerebrovascular accident, or stroke; MACCE = death, MI, CVA, and repeat revascularization; MI = myocardial infarction; repeat revasc = repeat revascularization. (Data from Serruys PW, Morice MC, Kappetein AP, et al. Percutaneous coronary intervention versus coronary-artery bypass grafting for severe coronary artery disease. N Engl J Med. 2009;360:961-972.)

 Grade A

1. Fischman DL, Leon MB, Baim DS, et al. A randomized comparison of coronary-stent placement and balloon angioplasty in the treatment of coronary artery disease. N Engl J Med. 1994;331:496-501.
2. Moses JW, Leon MB, Popma JJ, et al. Sirolimus-eluting stents versus standard stents in patients with stenosis in a native coronary artery. N Engl J Med. 2003;349:1315-1323.
3. Kastrati A, Mehilli J, Pache J, et al. Analysis of 14 trials comparing sirolimus-eluting stents with bare-metal stents. N Engl J Med. 2007;356:1030-1039.
4. Spaulding C, Daemen J, Boersma E, et al. A pooled analysis of data comparing sirolimus-eluting stents with bare-metal stents. N Engl J Med. 2007;356:989-997.
5. Stone GW, Rizvi, Newman W, et al. Everolimus-eluting versus paclitaxel-eluting stents in coronary artery disease. N Engl J Med. 2010;362:1663-1674.
6. Rasmussen K, Maeng M, Kaltoft A, et al. Efficacy and safety of zotarolimus-eluting and sirolimus-eluting coronary stents in routine clinical care (SORT OUT III): a randomized controlled superiority trial. Lancet. 2010;375:1090-1099.
7. Park SJ, Park DW, Kim YH, et al. Duration of dual antiplatelet therapy after implantation of drug-eluting stents. N Engl J Med. 2010;362:1374-1382.
8. Boden WE, O'Rourke RA, Teo KK, et al. Optimal medical therapy with or without PCI for stable coronary disease. N Engl J Med. 2007;356:1503-1516.
9. Weintraub WS, Spertus JA, Kolm P, et al. Effect of PCI on quality of life in patients with stable coronary artery disease. N Engl J Med. 2008;359:677-687.
10. Keeley EC, Boura JA, Grines CL. Primary angioplasty versus intravenous thrombolytic therapy for acute myocardial infarction: a quantitative review of 23 randomised trials. Lancet. 2003;361:13-20.
11. Di Mario C, Dudek D, Piscione F, et al. Immediate angioplasty versus standard therapy with rescue angioplasty after thrombolysis in the Combined Abciximab REteplase Stent Study in Acute Myocardial Infarction (CARESS-in-AMI): an open, prospective, randomised, multicentre trial. Lancet. 2008;371:559-568.
12. Mehta SR, Granger CB, Boden WE, et al, for the TIMACS Investigators. Early versus delayed invasive intervention in acute coronary syndromes. N Engl J Med. 2009;360:2165-2175.
13. O'Donoghue M, Boden WE, Braunwald E, et al. Early invasive vs. conservative treatment strategies in women and men with unstable angina and non-ST-segment elevation myocardial infarction: a meta-analysis. JAMA. 2008;300:71-80.
14. Goldman S, Sethi GK, Holman W, et al. Radial artery grafts vs saphenous vein grafts in coronary artery bypass surgery: a randomized trial. JAMA. 2011;305:167-174.
15. Shroyer AL, Grover FL, Brack H, et al. On-pump versus off-pump coronary artery bypass surgery. N Engl J Med. 2009;361:1827-1837.
16. Serruys PW, Morice MC, Kappetein AP, et al. Percutaneous coronary intervention versus coronary-artery bypass grafting for severe coronary artery disease. N Engl J Med. 2009;360:961-972.
17. Hlatky Ma, Boothroyd DB, Bravata DM, et al. Coronary artery bypass surgery compared with percutaneous coronary interventions for multivessel disease: a collaborative analysis of individual patient data from ten randomised trials. Lancet. 2009;373;1190-1197.
18. The BARI Investigators. The final 10-year follow-up results from the BARI randomized trial. J Am Coll Cardiol. 2007;49:1600-1606.
19. Frye RL, August P, Brooks MM, et al, for the BARI 2D Study Group. A randomized trial of therapies for type 2 diabetes and coronary artery disease. N Engl J Med. 2009;360:2503-2515.

SUGGESTED READING

Garg S, Serruys PW. Coronary stents: current status. J Am Coll Cardiol. 2010;56:S1-S42. Review.
Magro M, Garg S, Serruys PW. Revascularization treatment of stable coronary artery disease. Expert Opin Pharmacother. 2011;12:195-212. Review.

75

VALVULAR HEART DISEASE
BLASE A. CARABELLO

The cardiac valves permit unobstructed forward blood flow through the heart when they are open while preventing backward flow when they are closed. Most valvular heart diseases cause either valvular stenosis with obstruction to forward flow or valvular regurgitation with backward flow. Valvular stenosis imparts a pressure overload on the left or right ventricle because these chambers must generate higher than normal pressure to overcome the obstruction to pump blood forward. Valvular regurgitation imparts a volume overload on the heart, which now must pump additional volume to compensate for what is regurgitated. When valve disease is severe, these hemodynamic burdens can lead to ventricular dysfunction, heart failure, and sudden death (Table 75-1). In almost every instance, definitive therapy for severe valvular heart disease is mechanical restoration of valve function.

AORTIC STENOSIS

EPIDEMIOLOGY

Bicuspid and Other Congenitally Abnormal Aortic Valves
Approximately 1% of the population is born with a bicuspid aortic valve, with a male preponderance (Chapter 69). Although this abnormality does not usually cause a hemodynamic disturbance at birth, bicuspid aortic valves tend to deteriorate with age. Approximately one third of these valves become stenotic, another third become regurgitant, and the remainder cause only minor hemodynamic abnormalities. When stenosis develops, it usually occurs when patients are in their 40s, 50s, and 60s.

Sometimes, congenital aortic stenosis from a unicuspid, bicuspid, or even abnormal tricuspid valve causes symptoms during childhood and requires correction by adolescence. Occasionally, these congenitally stenotic aortic valves escape detection until adulthood.

Tricuspid Aortic Valve Stenosis
In some patients born with apparently normal tricuspid aortic valves, thickening and calcification develop similar to what occurs in bicuspid valves. When aortic stenosis develops in previously normal tricuspid aortic valves, it usually does so in the 60s to 80s. Although stenosis and calcifications of bicuspid and tricuspid aortic valves were formerly considered to be degenerative processes, it is clear that this type of aortic stenosis arises from an active inflammatory process similar to that of coronary heart disease. This concept is supported by many pieces of evidence. First, the initial lesion of aortic stenosis is similar to the plaque of coronary disease. Second, both diseases have hypertension and hyperlipidemia as risk factors. Third, there is excellent correlation between calcification of the aortic valve and calcification of the coronary arteries. Fourth, patients with the most severe aortic stenosis have the highest levels of C-reactive protein. However, statins, which are so effective in treating coronary disease, have been ineffective in retarding the progression of moderately advanced aortic stenosis.

Rheumatic Valvular Heart Disease
Rheumatic valve disease is now a rare cause of aortic stenosis in developed countries. In virtually every case, the mitral valve is also detectably abnormal.

PATHOBIOLOGY

The normal aortic valve area is 3 to 4 cm², and little hemodynamic disturbance occurs until the orifice is reduced to about one third of normal, at which point a systolic gradient develops between the left ventricle and aorta. Left ventricular (LV) and aortic pressures are normally nearly equal during systole. In aortic stenosis, intracavitary LV pressure must increase above aortic pressure, however, to produce forward flow across the stenotic valve and to achieve acceptable downstream pressure (see Fig. 57-2 in Chapter 57). There is a geometric progression in the magnitude of the gradient as the valve area narrows. Given a normal cardiac output, the gradient rises rapidly from 10 to 15 mm Hg at valve areas of 1.5 to 1.3 cm² to about 25 mm Hg at 1.0 cm², 50 mm Hg at 0.8 cm², 70 mm Hg at 0.6 cm², and 100 mm Hg at

TABLE 75-1 SUMMARY OF SEVERE VALVAR HEART DISEASE

	AORTIC STENOSIS	MITRAL STENOSIS	MITRAL REGURGITATION	AORTIC REGURGITATION
Etiology	Idiopathic calcification of a bicuspid or tricuspid valve Congenital Rheumatic	Rheumatic fever Annular calcification	Mitral valve prolapse Ruptured chordae Endocarditis Ischemic papillary muscle dysfunction or rupture Collagen vascular diseases and syndromes Secondary to LV myocardial diseases	Annuloaortic ectasia Hypertension Endocarditis Marfan syndrome Ankylosing spondylitis Aortic dissection Syphilis Collagen vascular disease
Pathophysiology	Pressure overload on the LV with compensation by LV hypertrophy As disease advances, reduced coronary flow reserve causes angina. Hypertrophy and afterload excess lead to systolic and diastolic LV dysfunction.	Obstruction to LV inflow increases left atrial pressure and limits cardiac output, thus mimicking LV failure. Mitral valve obstruction increases the pressure work of the right ventricle Right ventricular pressure overload is augmented further when pulmonary hypertension develops.	Places volume overload on the LV. Ventricle responds with eccentric hypertrophy and dilation, which allow increased ventricular stroke volume. Eventually, however, LV dysfunction develops if volume overload is uncorrected.	*Chronic:* Total stroke volume causes hyperdynamic circulation, induces systolic hypertension and causes pressure and volume overload. Compensation is by concentric and eccentric hypertrophy. *Acute:* Because cardiac dilation has not developed, hyperdynamic findings are absent. High diastolic LV pressure causes mitral valve preclosure and potentiates LV ischemia and failure.
Symptoms	Angina Syncope Heart failure	Dyspnea Orthopnea PND Hemoptysis Hoarseness Edema Ascites	Dyspnea Orthopnea PND	Dyspnea Orthopnea PND Angina Syncope
Signs	Systolic ejection murmur radiating to the neck Delayed carotid upstroke S_4, soft or paradoxical S_2	Diastolic rumble after an opening snap Loud S_1 Right ventricular lift Loud P_2	Holosystolic apical murmur radiating to the axilla, S_3 Displaced PMI	*Chronic:* Diastolic blowing murmur Hyperdynamic circulation Displaced PMI Quincke pulse de Musset's sign *Acute:* Short diastolic blowing murmur Soft S_1
Electrocardiogram	LAA LVH	LAA RVH	LAA LVH	LAA LVH
Chest radiograph	Boot-shaped heart Aortic valve calcification on lateral view	Straightening of left heart border Double density at right heart border Kerley B lines Enlarged pulmonary arteries	Cardiac enlargement	*Chronic:* Cardiac enlargement Uncoiling of the aorta *Acute:* Pulmonary congestion with normal heart size
Echocardiographic findings	Concentric LVH Reduced aortic valve cusp separation Doppler shows mean gradient ≥40 mm Hg in most severe cases	Restricted mitral leaflet motion Valve area ≤1 cm^2 in most severe cases Tricuspid Doppler may reveal pulmonary hypertension	LV and LAA in chronic severe disease Doppler: large regurgitant jet	*Chronic:* LV enlargement Large Doppler jet PHT <400 msec *Acute:* Small LV Mitral valve preclosure
Catheterization findings	Increased LVEDP Transaortic gradient 50 mm Hg AVA ≤0.7 in most severe cases	Elevated pulmonary capillary wedge pressure Transmitral gradient usually >10 mm Hg in severe cases MVA <1 cm^2	Elevated pulmonary capillary wedge pressure Ventriculography shows regurgitation of dye into LV	Wide pulse pressure Aortography shows regurgitation of dye into LV Usually unnecessary
Medical therapy	Avoid vasodilators Digitalis, diuretics, and nitroglycerin in inoperable cases	Diuretics for mild symptoms Anticoagulation in atrial fibrillation Digitalis, β-blockers, verapamil, or diltiazem for rate control	Vasodilators in acute disease No proven therapy in chronic disease	*Chronic:* Vasodilators may help in chronic asymptomatic disease with normal left ventricular function. *Acute:* Vasodilators
Indications for surgery	Appearance of symptoms in patients with severe disease (see text)	Appearance of more than mild symptoms Development of pulmonary hypertension Appearance of persistent atrial fibrillation	Appearance of symptoms EF <0.60 ESD ≥40 mm	*Chronic:* Appearance of symptoms EF <0.55 ESD ≥55 mm *Acute:* Even mild heart failure Mitral valve preclosure

AVA = aortic valve area; EF = ejection fraction; ESD = end-systolic diameter; LAA = left atrial enlargement; LV = left ventricle; LVEDP = left ventricular end-diastolic pressure; LVH = left ventricular hypertrophy; MVA = mitral valve area; PHT = pressure half-time; PMI = point of maximal impulse; PND = paroxysmal nocturnal dyspnea; RVH = right ventricular hypertrophy.

0.5 cm^2. The rate of progression of aortic stenosis varies widely from patient to patient; it may remain stable for many years or increase by more than 15 mm Hg per year.

A major compensatory response to the increased LV pressure associated with aortic stenosis is the development of concentric LV hypertrophy. The Laplace equation—stress (s) = pressure (p) × radius (r)/2 × thickness (th)—indicates that the force on any unit of LV myocardium (afterload) varies directly with ventricular pressure and radius and inversely with wall thickness. As pressure increases, it can be offset by increased LV wall thickness (concentric hypertrophy). The determinants of LV ejection fraction are contractility, preload, and afterload. By normalizing afterload, the development of concentric hypertrophy helps preserve ejection fraction and cardiac output despite the pressure overload. Although hypertrophy clearly serves a compensatory function, it also has a pathologic role and is in part responsible for the classic symptoms of aortic stenosis.

Angina

In general, angina (Chapter 71) results from myocardial ischemia when LV oxygen (and other nutrient) demand exceeds supply, which is predicated on coronary blood flow. In normal subjects, coronary blood flow can increase five- to eight-fold under maximum metabolic demand, but in patients with aortic stenosis, this reserve is limited. Reduced coronary blood flow reserve may be caused by a relative diminution in capillary ingrowth to serve the needs of the hypertrophied left ventricle or by a reduced transcoronary gradient for coronary blood flow because of the elevated LV end-diastolic pressure. Restricted coronary blood flow reserve appears to be responsible for angina in many patients who have aortic stenosis despite normal epicardial coronary arteries. In other patients, angina is due to increased oxygen demand when inadequate hypertrophy allows wall stress, a key determinant of myocardial oxygen consumption, to increase.

Syncope

Syncope (Chapters 50 and 62) generally occurs because of inadequate cerebral perfusion. In aortic stenosis, syncope is usually related to exertion. It may result when exertion causes a fall in total peripheral resistance that cannot be compensated by increased cardiac output because output is limited by the obstruction to LV outflow; this combination reduces systemic blood pressure and cerebral perfusion. In addition, high LV pressure during exercise may trigger a systemic vasodepressor response that lowers blood pressure and produces syncope. Cardiac arrhythmias, possibly caused by exertional ischemia, also cause hypotension and syncope.

Heart Failure

In aortic stenosis, contractile dysfunction (systolic failure) and failure of normal relaxation (diastolic failure) occur and cause symptoms (Chapter 58). The extent of ventricular contraction is governed by contractility and afterload. In aortic stenosis, contractility (the ability to generate force) is often reduced. The mechanisms of contractile dysfunction may include abnormal calcium handling, microtubular hyperpolymerization causing an internal viscous load on the myocyte, and myocardial ischemia. In some cases, contractile function is normal, but the hypertrophy is inadequate to normalize wall stress and excessive afterload results. Excessive afterload inhibits ejection, reduces forward output, and leads to heart failure.

The increased wall thickness that helps normalize stress increases diastolic stiffness. Even if muscle properties remain normal, higher filling pressure is required to distend a thicker ventricle. As aortic stenosis advances, collagen deposition also stiffens the myocardium and adds to the diastolic dysfunction.

▶ CLINICAL MANIFESTATIONS

The diagnosis of aortic stenosis is usually first suspected when the classic systolic ejection murmur is heard during physical examination (Chapter 50). The murmur is loudest in the aortic area and radiates to the neck. In some cases, the murmur may disappear over the sternum and reappear over the LV apex, thereby giving the false impression that a murmur of mitral regurgitation is also present (Gallavardin's phenomenon). The intensity of the murmur increases with cycle length because longer cycles are associated with greater aortic flow. In mild disease, the murmur peaks in intensity in early systole or mid-systole. As the severity of stenosis worsens, the murmur peaks progressively later in systole. Perhaps the most helpful clue to the severity of aortic stenosis by physical examination is the characteristic delay in the carotid pulse with a diminution in its volume (see Fig. 50-5 in Chapter 50);

in elderly patients, however, increasing carotid stiffness may pseudonormalize the carotid upstrokes. The LV apical impulse in aortic stenosis is not displaced but is enlarged and forceful. The simultaneous palpation of a forceful LV apex beat and a delayed and weakened carotid pulse is a persuasive clue that severe aortic stenosis is present. S_1 in aortic stenosis is generally normal. In congenital aortic stenosis when the valve is not calcified, S_1 may be followed by a systolic ejection click. In calcific disease, S_2 may be single and soft when the aortic component is lost because the valve neither opens nor closes well. In some cases, delayed LV emptying secondary to LV dysfunction may create paradoxical splitting of S_2. An S_4 gallop is common. In advanced disease, pulmonary hypertension and signs of right-sided failure are common.

Because of the dire consequences of missing the diagnosis of aortic stenosis, the physician must have a low threshold for obtaining an echocardiogram whenever aortic stenosis cannot be excluded by physical examination, especially in patients with a history of angina, syncope, or heart failure. In asymptomatic patients with suspicious murmurs, early diagnosis allows the patient and physician to be more vigilant regarding possible early signs and symptoms.

▶ DIAGNOSIS

The electrocardiogram (ECG) in patients with aortic stenosis usually shows LV hypertrophy (Chapter 54). In some cases of even severe aortic stenosis, however, LV hypertrophy is absent on the ECG, possibly because of the lack of LV dilation. Left atrial abnormality is common because the stiff left ventricle increases left atrial afterload and causes the left atrium to dilate.

The chest radiograph in aortic stenosis is generally nondiagnostic. The cardiac silhouette is not usually enlarged but may assume a boot-shaped configuration. In advanced cases, there may be signs of cardiomegaly and pulmonary congestion; aortic valve calcification may be seen in the lateral view.

Echocardiography (Chapter 55) is indispensable to assess the extent of LV hypertrophy, systolic ejection performance, and aortic valve anatomy (Fig. 75-1). Doppler interrogation of the aortic valve makes use of the modified Bernoulli equation (gradient = 4 × velocity^2) to assess the severity of the stenosis (Chapter 55). As blood flows from the body of the left ventricle across the stenotic valve, the flow rate must accelerate for the volume to remain constant. Doppler interrogation of the valve can be performed to detect this increase in velocity for estimation of the valve gradient. The peak aortic flow velocity in patients with preserved LV systolic function is a useful clinical guide to prognosis. In patients with a flow velocity of 3.0 mL/second or less, symptoms are unlikely to develop in the next 5 years; by comparison, in patients with a flow velocity of 4.0 mL/second or greater, symptoms usually develop within 2 years.

Although exercise testing is contraindicated in symptomatic patients with aortic stenosis because of the high risk for complications, cautious exercise

FIGURE 75-1. Doppler echocardiogram from a patient with aortic stenosis. The *left panel* shows thickened aortic valve leaflets that dome into the aorta with restricted opening in systole. The *top right panel* shows a miniaturized apical four-chamber view at the top with a Doppler cursor through the aorta, whereas the *bottom right panel* shows a continuous-wave spectral Doppler signal with a peak velocity of 3 m/sec. The peak valve gradient can be calculated as 4 × 3^2, or 36 mm Hg. AO = aorta; LA = left atrium; LV = left ventricle; RV = right ventricle. (Courtesy of Dr. Anthony DeMaria.)

testing is gaining favor in asymptomatic patients. Such testing often reveals latent symptoms or hemodynamic instability that have gone unrecognized during the patient's normal daily activities. Exercise-induced hypotension or symptoms are indications for aortic valve replacement in patients with severe aortic stenosis; in patients with mild to moderate aortic stenosis, another source of exercise limitation should be sought.

Brain natriuretic peptide levels may be higher in patients who will become symptomatic in a short time span. Levels exceeding 550 pg/mL portend a poor prognosis, but use of this biomarker to indicate the need for valve replacement is still premature.

Cardiac catheterization for performance of coronary arteriography is usually undertaken before surgery because most patients with aortic stenosis are of the age at which coronary disease is common. When echocardiography shows severe aortic stenosis and the patient has one or more of the classic symptoms of the disease, formal invasive documentation of the severity of the stenosis is not necessary, and coronary angiography need not be performed in young adults. When the hemodynamic diagnosis is unclear, however, right-sided and left-sided heart catheterization should be performed to determine the transaortic valvular pressure gradient and cardiac output, which are used to calculate the aortic valve area by the Gorlin formula:

$$A = \frac{CO/SEP \times HR}{44.3\sqrt{h}}$$

where CO is cardiac output (mL/min), SEP is the systolic ejection period (seconds), HR is the heart rate, and h is the mean gradient.

TREATMENT   Rx

Medical Therapy

In asymptomatic patients, no treatment is indicated, nor is any known to be beneficial. Even statins are not useful, despite the similar pathobiology between aortic stenosis and coronary disease.

There also is no accepted effective medical therapy for symptomatic aortic stenosis. In patients with heart failure awaiting surgery, diuretics can be used cautiously to relieve pulmonary congestion. Nitrates may also be used cautiously to treat angina pectoris. Although vasodilators, especially angiotensin-converting enzyme inhibitors, have become a cornerstone of therapy for heart failure, they are not recommended for aortic stenosis. With fixed valvular obstruction to outflow, vasodilation reduces pressure distal to the obstruction without increasing cardiac output and may cause syncope. Statins do not slow the progression of calcific aortic stenosis. When surgery and valvoplasty are unsuccessful or impossible, digitalis and diuretics can be used to improve symptoms with the understanding that they will not improve life expectancy.

Invasive Therapy

Valve Replacement Surgery

The only proven effective therapy for aortic stenosis is aortic valve replacement. Even octogenarians benefit from valve replacement unless other comorbid factors preclude surgery, so aortic valve replacement should not be denied simply on the basis of age. Valve replacement should also not be denied because the ejection fraction is reduced; the excess afterload imposed by the stenotic valve is relieved with valve replacement, and a depressed

ejection fraction usually improves dramatically after surgery. The exception to this rule is a severely reduced ejection fraction in the face of only a small aortic valve gradient; in this case, the severity of the aortic stenosis may be overestimated because the failing left ventricle has difficulty opening a mildly to moderately stenotic valve. In such patients, LV muscle dysfunction either has another cause or is often so severe that it does not recover after valve replacement. Evidence indicates, however, that even some well-selected patients in this category, such as patients who demonstrate increased cardiac output during dobutamine infusion, may benefit from aortic valve replacement.

Percutaneous Aortic Valve Replacement

Percutaneous transcatheter aortic valve implantation reduces 1-year mortality by 45% (from 51 to 31%) in patients who have severe aortic stenosis and are too ill to undergo surgery.[1] It also is not inferior to standard valve replacement in high-risk adults.[2] In this procedure, the native valve is dilated, and then a stented valve is inserted over a balloon into the aortic annulus (Fig. 75-2). The balloon is expanded to secure the valve and its stent, which is intended to help prevent restenosis. Two such valves have been approved in Europe, where thousands of patients have already received successful implants.

Balloon Aortic Valvotomy

In acquired calcific aortic stenosis, leaflet restriction results from heavy calcium deposition in the leaflets themselves and is not due to commissural fusion. Balloon aortic valvotomy is relatively ineffective in improving aortic stenosis; it generally results in a residual gradient of 30 to 50 mm Hg and a valve area of 1.0 cm². Mortality after this procedure is similar to that in untreated patients. The only occasional indication for balloon aortic valvotomy is palliative in cases in which aortic valve replacement is impossible because of comorbidity or is impractical when immediate temporary relief is required because of the demands of other noncardiac conditions.

PROGNOSIS

In asymptomatic patients with normally functioning or minimally dysfunctional bicuspid aortic valves, survival is similar to age-matched controls, and sudden death is rare, occurring in less than 1% of asymptomatic patients. However, 27% of patients require surgery by 20 years after diagnosis. In adults with asymptomatic but hemodynamically significant aortic stenosis, symptoms typically develop within 5 years. A higher peak aortic-jet velocity and high β-type natriuretic peptide levels predict a worse prognosis.

The progression of mild to moderate aortic stenosis to severe disease is the key to the natural history of the disease and is quite variable. Aortic stenosis may remain mild for a decade or more in some patients, whereas in others, it may progress to severe disease in as little as 5 years.

When symptoms develop, survival declines precipitously. Approximately 35% of patients with aortic stenosis are initially evaluated for angina. Of these, 50% are dead in 5 years unless aortic valve replacement is performed. Approximately 15% have syncope; of these, 50% are dead in only 3 years unless the aortic valve is replaced. Of the 50% with symptoms of heart failure, 50% are dead in 2 years without aortic valve replacement. In all, only 25% of patients with symptomatic aortic stenosis survive 3 years in the absence of valve replacement, and the annual risk for sudden death ranges from 10% in patients with angina to 15% with syncope to 25% with heart failure.

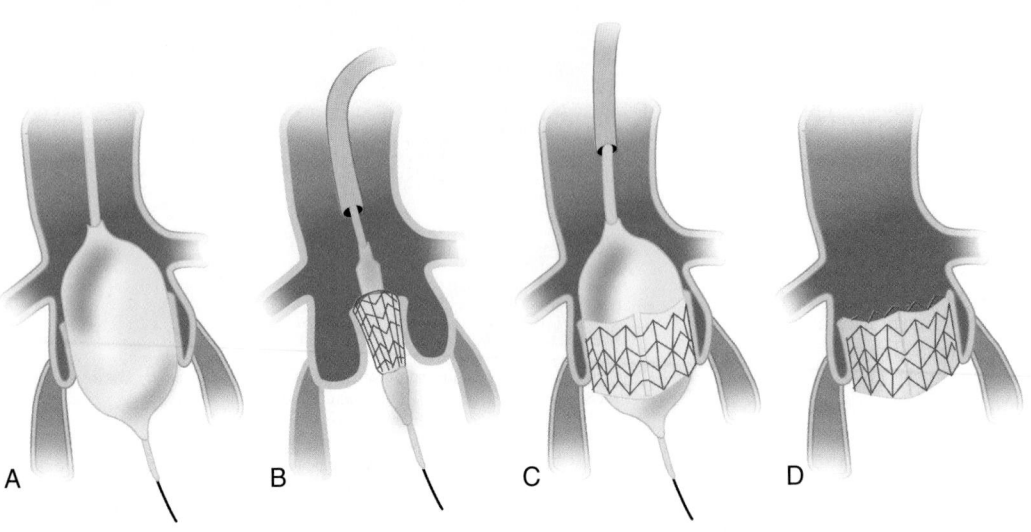

FIGURE 75-2. Steps for percutaneous balloon valvotomy. **A,** Dilation of the native stenotic valve. **B,** A crimped stented valve has been inserted over a guidewire into the aortic annulus. **C,** Inflation of the balloon deploys the valve. **D,** The balloon is deflated and removed with the aortic valve replaced. (Modified from http://my.clevelandclinic.org/heart/percutaneous/percutaneousValve.aspx.)

After valve replacement surgery, prognosis improves to near normal, especially for patients older than 65 years at the time of valve implantation, presumably because older patients have fewer years at risk for valve-related complications.

MITRAL STENOSIS

EPIDEMIOLOGY

In almost all cases of acquired mitral stenosis, the cause is rheumatic heart disease. Occasionally, severe calcification of the mitral annulus can lead to mitral stenosis in the absence of rheumatic involvement. Mitral stenosis is three times more common in women and usually develops in the 40s and 50s. Although the disease has become rare in developed countries because of the waning incidence of rheumatic fever, mitral stenosis is still prevalent in developing nations, where rheumatic fever is common.

PATHOBIOLOGY

At the beginning of diastole, a transient gradient between the left atrium and left ventricle normally initiates LV filling. After early filling, left atrial and LV pressures equilibrate. In mitral stenosis, obstruction to LV filling increases left atrial pressure and produces a persistent gradient between the left atrium and the left ventricle (see Fig. 57-2 in Chapter 57). The combination of elevated left atrial pressure (and pulmonary venous pressure) and restriction of inflow into the left ventricle limits cardiac output. Although myocardial involvement from the rheumatic process occasionally affects LV muscle function, the muscle itself is normal in most patients with mitral stenosis. However, in approximately one third of patients with mitral stenosis, LV ejection performance is reduced despite normal muscle function because of reduced preload (from inflow obstruction) and increased afterload as a result of reflex vasoconstriction caused by reduced cardiac output.

Because the right ventricle generates most of the force that propels blood across the mitral valve, the right ventricle incurs the pressure overload of the transmitral gradient. In addition, secondary but reversible pulmonary vasoconstriction develops, thus further increasing pulmonary artery pressure and the burden on the right ventricle. As mitral stenosis worsens, right ventricular (RV) failure develops.

CLINICAL MANIFESTATIONS

Patients with mitral stenosis usually remain asymptomatic until the valve area is reduced to about one third its normal size of 4 to 5 cm^2. Then the symptoms typical of left-sided failure—dyspnea on exertion, orthopnea, and paroxysmal nocturnal dyspnea—develop. As the disease progresses and RV failure occurs, ascites and edema are common. Hemoptysis, which is common in mitral stenosis but uncommon in other causes of left atrial hypertension, develops when high left atrial pressure ruptures the anastomoses of small bronchial veins. In some cases, a large left atrium may impinge on the left recurrent laryngeal nerve and cause hoarseness (Ortner's syndrome) or may impinge on the esophagus and cause dysphagia.

Physical Examination

Although mitral stenosis produces typical and diagnostic findings on physical examination, the diagnosis is missed frequently because the auscultatory findings may be subtle. Palpation of the precordium finds a quiet apical impulse. If pulmonary hypertension and RV hypertrophy have developed, the examiner notes a parasternal lift. S_1 is typically loud and may be the most prominent physical finding of the disease. A loud S_1 is present because the transmitral gradient holds the mitral valve open throughout diastole until ventricular systole closes the fully opened valve with a loud closing sound. In far-advanced disease, the mitral valve may be so damaged, however, that it neither opens nor closes well, so S_1 may become soft. S_2 is normally split; the pulmonic component is increased in intensity if pulmonary hypertension has developed. Left-sided S_3 and S_4 gallop sounds, which represent the ventricular and atrial components of rapid LV filling, are exceedingly rare in mitral stenosis because obstruction at the mitral valve prevents rapid filling. S_2 is usually followed by an opening snap. The distance between S_2 and the opening snap provides a reasonable estimation of left atrial pressure and the severity of the mitral stenosis. The higher the left atrial pressure, the sooner the left atrial pressure and the falling LV pressure of early ventricular relaxation equilibrate. At this equilibration point, the mitral valve opens, and the opening snap occurs. When left atrial pressure is high, the opening snap closely (0.06 second) follows S_2. Conversely, when left atrial pressure is relatively normal, the snap occurs later (0.12 second) and may mimic the cadence

of an S_3 gallop. The opening snap is followed by the classic low-pitched early diastolic mitral stenosis rumble, which increases in length as the mitral stenosis worsens. This murmur may be inaudible if the patient has a relatively low resting cardiac output. Modest exercise, such as isometric handgrip, may accentuate the murmur's intensity. If the patient is in sinus rhythm, atrial systole may produce a presystolic accentuation of the murmur. If pulmonary hypertension has developed, the pulmonic component of S_2 increases in intensity to become as loud or louder than the aortic component. With pulmonary hypertension, a diastolic blowing murmur of pulmonary insufficiency (Graham Steell's murmur) is often heard, although in many cases, a coexistent murmur of mild aortic insufficiency is mistaken for this murmur. Neck vein elevation, ascites, and edema are present if RV failure has developed.

DIAGNOSIS

If the patient is in sinus rhythm, left atrial abnormality is generally present on the ECG. Atrial fibrillation is common, however. If pulmonary hypertension has developed, there is often evidence of RV hypertrophy.

On the chest radiograph, left atrial enlargement produces straightening of the left heart border and a double density at the right heart border as a result of the combined silhouettes of the right atrium and left atrium. Pulmonary venous hypertension produces increased vascularity. Kerley B lines, which represent thickening of the pulmonary septa secondary to chronic venous engorgement, may also be seen.

The echocardiogram produces excellent images of the mitral valve and is the most important diagnostic tool in confirming the diagnosis (Fig. 75-3). Transthoracic echocardiography or, if necessary, transesophageal echocardiography makes the diagnosis in nearly 100% of cases and accurately assesses severity. Mitral stenosis, similar to aortic stenosis, can be quantified by assessing the transvalvular gradient with the modified Bernoulli principle. The stenosis is considered mild when the calculated or planimetered valve area is more than 1.75 cm^2, moderate at 1.25 to 1.75 cm^2, moderately severe at 1.0 to 1.25 cm^2, and severe at less than 1.0 cm^2.

During echocardiography, the suitability of the valve for balloon valvotomy can also be assessed (see later). If even mild tricuspid regurgitation is present, the systolic gradient across the tricuspid valve can be used to gauge pulmonary artery pressure, which is an important prognostic factor in mitral stenosis because the prognosis worsens as pulmonary pressure increases.

Invasive Evaluation
Cardiac Catheterization
Cardiac catheterization is usually unnecessary to assess the severity of mitral stenosis. Because many patients with mitral stenosis are of an age when coronary disease might be present, however, coronary arteriography is generally performed if cardiac surgery is anticipated or if the patient has coexistent angina. In these cases, it is common to perform left-sided and right-sided heart catheterization to confirm the transmitral gradient and to calculate the valve area from the Gorlin formula (see earlier).

FIGURE 75-3. Mitral stenosis. An en face view of a stenotic mitral valve in the short-axis view of the left ventricle is shown on the *left*. Planimetry for the mitral valve orifice yielded an area of 1.09 cm^2. The M-mode echocardiogram on the *right* has been aligned with the appropriate structures on the *left*. It shows the restricted opening of the mitral valve in diastole associated with the classic diastolic rumbling murmur. RV = right ventricle. (From Assey ME, Usher BW, Carabello BA. The patient with valvular heart disease. In: Pepine CJ, Hill JA, Lambert CR, eds. *Diagnostic and Therapeutic Cardiac Catheterization*, 3rd ed. Baltimore: Williams & Wilkins; 1998:709.)

PREVENTION, TREATMENT, AND PROGNOSIS (Rx)

Mitral stenosis can be prevented by appropriate antibiotic treatment of β-hemolytic streptococcal infections (Chapter 298).

Medical Therapy

Asymptomatic patients with mitral stenosis and sinus rhythm require no therapy. Symptoms of mild dyspnea and orthopnea can be treated with diuretics alone. When symptoms worsen to more than mild or if pulmonary hypertension develops, mechanical correction of the stenosis is preferable to medical therapy because it improves longevity in severely symptomatic patients.

Patients with mitral stenosis in whom atrial fibrillation develops usually decompensate because the rapid heart rate reduces diastolic filling time, increases left atrial pressure, and decreases cardiac output. The heart rate must be controlled promptly, preferably with an infusion of diltiazem or esmolol for acute atrial fibrillation or with a β-blocker, a calcium-channel blocker, or oral digoxin in chronic atrial fibrillation (Chapter 64).

Conversion to sinus rhythm is routinely recommended either pharmacologically or with direct-current countershock (Chapter 64) after anticoagulation is therapeutic. It should be noted that patients with rheumatic atrial fibrillation have been excluded from trials of echocardiogram-guided cardioversion without anticoagulation and trials of rate control versus rhythm control for the chronic management of atrial fibrillation. If sinus rhythm cannot be maintained, mechanical therapy for the mitral stenosis is generally recommended in the hope that sinus rhythm can be restored after the obstruction to atrial outflow is corrected. However, the cause of atrial fibrillation in patients with mitral stenosis probably includes atrial rheumatic inflammation, so restoration of sinus rhythm is unpredictable even after mechanical intervention.

Because patients with concomitant mitral stenosis and atrial fibrillation have an extraordinarily high risk for systemic embolism, they should undergo chronic anticoagulation with warfarin at an international normalized ratio (INR) target of 2.5 to 3.5. Anticoagulation is warranted in all patients unless there is a serious contraindication to its use.

Mechanical Therapy

When symptoms progress past early functional class II, that is, symptoms with more than ordinary activity, or if pulmonary hypertension develops, the prognosis is worse unless the mitral stenosis is relieved. In most instances, an excellent result can be achieved with percutaneous balloon valvotomy. In contrast to aortic stenosis, in mitral stenosis there is fusion of the valve leaflets at the commissures. Balloon dilation produces a commissurotomy and a substantial increase in valve area that appears to persist for at least a decade and provides improvement comparable to that of closed or open commissurotomy in suitable patients. Suitability for balloon valvotomy is determined partially during echocardiography. Patients with pliable valves, little valvular calcification, little involvement of the subvalvular apparatus, and less than moderate mitral regurgitation are ideal candidates. Even when valve anatomy is not ideal, however, valvotomy may be attempted in patients with advanced age or in situations in which comorbid risk factors increase surgical risk. In otherwise healthy patients with unfavorable valve anatomy, surgery to perform an open commissurotomy or valve replacement is undertaken.

MITRAL REGURGITATION

EPIDEMIOLOGY

The mitral valve is composed of the mitral annulus, the leaflets, the chordae tendineae, and the papillary muscles. Abnormalities in any of these structures may lead to mitral regurgitation. The most common cause of mitral regurgitation in the United States is mitral valve prolapse, which is responsible for approximately two thirds of all cases and comprises many diseases, including myxomatous degeneration of the valve. Myocardial ischemia leading to papillary muscle dysfunction or infarction is the next most common cause and accounts for approximately a fourth of all cases. Annular calcification, endocarditis, collagen vascular disease, and rheumatic heart disease are less common causes. Use of the weight loss agents dexfenfluramine and fenfluramine has been implicated in causing valve damage in a few patients who received these drugs.

Mitral regurgitation can be subdivided on the basis of chronicity. Common causes of severe acute mitral regurgitation include ruptured chordae tendineae, ischemic papillary muscle dysfunction or rupture, and infective endocarditis. Chronic severe mitral regurgitation is more likely to be due to myxomatous degeneration of the valve, rheumatic heart disease, or annular calcification.

PATHOBIOLOGY

The pathophysiology of mitral regurgitation can be divided into three phases (Fig. 75-4). In acute mitral regurgitation of any cause, the sudden option for ejection of blood into the left atrium "wastes" a portion of the LV stroke volume as backward rather than forward flow. The combined regurgitant and forward flow causes volume overload of the left ventricle and stretches the existing sarcomeres toward their maximum length. Use of the Frank-Starling mechanism is maximized, and end-diastolic volume increases concomitantly. The regurgitant pathway unloads the left ventricle in systole because it allows ejection into the relatively low-impedance left atrium and thereby reduces end-systolic volume. Although increased end-diastolic volume and decreased

	Preload SL (μ)	Afterload ESS (kdyne/cm^2)	CF	EF	RF	FSV (mL)
N	2.07	90	N	.67	.0	100
AMR	2.25	60	N	.82	.50	70
CCMR	2.19	90	N	.79	.5	95
CDMR	2.19	120	↓	.58	.57	65

FIGURE 75-4. Mitral regurgitation. **A** and **B,** Normal physiology (N) **(A)** is compared with the physiology of acute mitral regurgitation (AMR) **(B).** Acutely, the volume overload increases preload (sarcomere length [SL]), and end-diastolic volume (EDV) increases from 150 to 170 mL. Unloading of the left ventricle by the presence of the regurgitant pathway decreases afterload (end-systolic stress [ESS]), and end-systolic volume (ESV) falls from 50 to 30 mL. These changes result in an increase in the ejection fraction (EF). Because 50% of the total left ventricular (LV) stroke volume (regurgitant fraction [RF]) is ejected into the left atrium (LA), however, forward stroke volume (FSV) falls from 100 to 70 mL. At this stage, contractile function (CF) is normal. **C,** Chronic compensated mitral regurgitation (CCMR). In CCMR, eccentric cardiac hypertrophy has developed, and EDV has increased substantially. Increased EDV, combined with normal contractile function, permits ejection of a larger total stroke volume and a larger forward stroke volume than in the acute phase. Left atrial enlargement permits lower left atrial pressure. Because the radius term in the Laplace equation has increased with increasing LV volume, afterload and ESV return to normal. **D,** Chronic decompensated mitral regurgitation (CDMR). In this stage, contractile dysfunction causes a large increase in ESV with a fall in total and forward stroke volume. Additional LV enlargement leads to worsening mitral regurgitation. The relatively favorable loading conditions in this phase still permit a normal EF, however, despite contractile dysfunction. (From Carabello BA. Mitral regurgitation: basic pathophysiologic principles. *Mod Concepts Cardiovasc Dis.* 1988;57:53-57.)

end-systolic volume act in concert to increase total stroke volume, forward stroke volume is subnormal because a large portion of the total stroke volume is regurgitated into the left atrium. This regurgitant volume increases left atrial pressure, so the patient experiences heart failure with low cardiac output and pulmonary congestion despite normal LV contractile function.

In many cases, severe acute mitral regurgitation necessitates emergency surgical correction. Patients who can be managed through the acute phase may enter the phase of compensation. In this phase, eccentric LV hypertrophy and increased end-diastolic volume, combined with normal contractile function, allow ejection of a sufficiently large total stroke volume to permit forward stroke volume to return toward normal. Left atrial enlargement allows accommodation of the regurgitant volume at a lower filling pressure. In this phase, the patient may be relatively asymptomatic even during strenuous exercise.

Although severe mitral regurgitation may be tolerated for many years, the lesion often causes LV dysfunction, atrial fibrillation, or heart failure within 5 years of the detection of severe mitral regurgitation. The now damaged ventricle has impaired ejection performance, and end-systolic volume increases. Greater LV residual volume at end systole increases end-diastolic volume and end-diastolic pressure, and the symptoms of pulmonary congestion may reappear. Additional LV dilation may worsen the amount of regurgitation by causing further enlargement of the mitral annulus and malalignment of the papillary muscles. Although there is substantial contractile dysfunction, the increased preload and the presence of the regurgitant pathway, which tends to normalize afterload despite ventricular enlargement, augment the ejection fraction and may maintain it in a relatively normal range.

The causes of LV contractile dysfunction in patients with mitral regurgitation may relate to loss of contractile proteins and abnormalities in calcium handling. In at least some cases, contractile dysfunction is reversible by timely mitral valve replacement.

CLINICAL MANIFESTATIONS

In the medical history, the standard symptoms of left-sided heart failure should be sought (Chapter 58). An attempt to discover potential causes should be made by questioning for a prior history of a heart murmur or abnormal findings on cardiac examination (Chapter 50), rheumatic heart disease, endocarditis (Chapter 76), myocardial infarction (Chapter 73), or the use of anorexigenic drugs.

Volume overload of the left ventricle displaces the apical impulse downward and to the left. S_1 may be reduced in intensity, whereas S_2 is usually physiologically split. In severe mitral regurgitation, S_2 is followed by S_3, which does not indicate heart failure but reflects rapid filling of the left ventricle by the large volume of blood stored in the left atrium during systole. The typical murmur of mitral regurgitation is a holosystolic apical murmur that often radiates toward the axilla (Chapter 50). There is a rough correlation between the intensity of the murmur and the severity of the disease, but this correlation is too weak to use in clinical decision making because the murmur may be soft when cardiac output is low. In contrast to aortic stenosis, murmur intensity does not usually vary with the RR interval. In acute mitral regurgitation, the presence of a large v wave may produce rapid equilibration of left atrial and LV pressure, thereby reducing the driving gradient and shortening the murmur. Pulmonary hypertension may develop and produce right-sided signs, including an RV lift, an increased P_2, and if RV dysfunction has developed, signs of right-sided heart failure.

DIAGNOSIS

The ECG usually shows LV hypertrophy and left atrial abnormality. The chest radiograph typically shows cardiomegaly; the absence of cardiomegaly indicates either that the mitral regurgitation is mild or that it has not been chronic enough to allow cardiac dilation to occur.

Echocardiography shows the extent of left atrial and LV enlargement (Chapter 55). Ultrasonic imaging of the mitral valve is excellent and offers clues to the mitral valve abnormalities responsible for the regurgitation. In some patients, three-dimensional echocardiography can add pathoanatomic information of potential use in aiding surgical repair of the valve. Color flow Doppler interrogation of the valve (Fig. 75-5) helps assess the severity of regurgitation, but because this technique images flow velocity rather than actual flow, it is subject to errors in interpretation. The Doppler technique is excellent for excluding the presence of mitral regurgitation and for distinguishing between mild and severe degrees. Although newer techniques may quantify regurgitation more precisely, they are not yet in widespread use, and standard color flow Doppler examination may not be sufficient for exact

FIGURE 75-5. Two-dimensional echocardiogram of mitral regurgitation with Doppler flow mapping superimposed on a portion of the image. The color information is represented in the sector of the imaging plane extending from the apex of the triangular plane to the *two small arrows* at the *bottom* of the image plane. Mitral regurgitation (MR) is indicated (*open arrows*) and extends from the mitral valve leaflets toward the posterior aspect of the left atrium (LA) during systole. The mosaic of colors representing the mitral regurgitant signal is typical of high-velocity turbulent flow. The low-intensity *orange-brown* signal represents flow directed away from the transducer on the chest wall, and the *blue* shades represent blood in the left ventricular outflow tract moving toward the transducer. AO = aorta; LV = left ventricle; RV = right ventricle.

quantification of mitral regurgitation or to determine whether the severity of the lesion is sufficient to cause eventual LV dysfunction. When the severity of mitral regurgitation is in doubt or if mitral valve surgery is being contemplated, cardiac catheterization (Chapter 57) is helpful in resolving the severity of the lesion; coronary arteriography should be included in patients older than 40 years or with symptoms suggesting coronary disease (Chapter 71).

TREATMENT AND PROGNOSIS   Rx

Medical Therapy
Severe Acute Mitral Regurgitation

In severe acute mitral regurgitation, the patient is usually symptomatic with heart failure or even shock. The goal of medical therapy is to increase forward cardiac output while concomitantly reducing regurgitant volume (Chapter 59). Arterial vasodilators reduce systemic resistance to flow and preferentially increase aortic outflow and simultaneously decrease the amount of mitral regurgitation and left atrial hypertension. If hypotension already exists, vasodilators such as nitroprusside lower blood pressure further and cannot be used. In these cases, intra-aortic balloon counterpulsation (Chapter 107) is preferred if the aortic valve is competent. Counterpulsation increases forward cardiac output by lowering ventricular afterload while augmenting systemic diastolic pressure.

Chronic Symptomatic Mitral Regurgitation

In patients with *symptomatic* mitral regurgitation, angiotensin-converting enzyme inhibitors (such as lisinopril, 20 mg per day) reduce LV volume and improve symptoms. Mitral valve surgery rather than medical therapy is generally preferred, however, in most symptomatic patients with mitral regurgitation. When atrial fibrillation is present, long-term anticoagulation should achieve the same INR goal as for mitral stenosis.

Chronic Asymptomatic Mitral Regurgitation

Vasodilators have had little effect in reducing LV volume or improving normal exercise tolerance in patients with mitral regurgitation, perhaps because afterload is not usually increased in those with chronic asymptomatic mitral regurgitation. There is no definitive indication to begin afterload reduction before symptoms appear because no large randomized trials have been performed, and smaller trials have generally shown no benefit from these therapies.

Surgical Therapy

The timing of mitral valve surgery must weigh the risks of the operation and placement of a prosthesis, if one is inserted, against the risk for irreversible LV dysfunction if surgery is delayed unwisely. For most other types of valve diseases, surgical correction usually requires placement of a prosthetic valve, but in patients with mitral regurgitation, the native valve can often be repaired. Because conservation of the native valve obviates the risks associated with a prosthesis, the option of mitral valve repair should influence the patient and physician toward earlier surgery.

Types of Mitral Valve Surgery

Mitral Valve Repair

When feasible, mitral valve repair (Fig. 75-6) is the preferred operation. Repair restores valve competence, maintains the functional aspects of the apparatus, and avoids the insertion of a prosthesis. Repair is most applicable in cases of posterior chordal rupture; anterior involvement and rheumatic involvement make repair more difficult. Currently, the percentage of mitral valve surgeries that are valve repair varies from 0 to 95% at different hospital centers, averaging about 60% across the United States overall. Percutaneous mitral valve repair with implantation of a clip device is less effective than conventional mitral valve repair for reducing the amount of mitral regurgitation but is safer and provides equivalent clinical benefit.**3** In all cases, the feasibility of repair depends on the pathoanatomy that is causing the mitral regurgitation and the skill and experience of the operating surgeon.

Mitral Valve Replacement with Preservation of the Mitral Apparatus

In this procedure, a prosthetic valve is inserted, but continuity between the native leaflets and the papillary muscles is maintained. This procedure has the advantage of ensuring mitral valve competence while preserving the LV functional aspects of the mitral apparatus. Even if only the posterior leaflets and chordae are preserved, the patient benefits from improved postoperative ventricular function and better survival. In many cases, it is possible to preserve the anterior and posterior chordal attachments, although anterior continuity can be associated with LV outflow tract obstruction. Although the patient benefits from restored mitral valve competence and maintenance of LV function, insertion of a prosthesis still carries all prosthesis-associated risks.

Mitral Valve Replacement without Preservation of the Mitral Apparatus

When the native valve cannot be repaired or the chordae preserved, such as in severe rheumatic deformity, the mitral valve leaflets and its apparatus are removed, and a prosthetic valve is inserted. Although this operation almost guarantees mitral valve competence, the mitral valve apparatus is responsible for coordinating LV contraction and for helping maintain the efficient prolate ellipsoid shape of the left ventricle. Destruction of the apparatus leads to a sudden fall in LV function and a decline in postoperative ejection fraction that is often permanent.

Timing of Surgery

Symptomatic Patients

Most patients with symptoms of dyspnea, orthopnea, or fatigue should undergo surgery regardless of which operation is performed because they already have lifestyle limitations from their disease. The mere presence of symptoms may worsen the prognosis despite relatively well-preserved LV function. The onset or worsening of symptoms is a summary of the patient's pathophysiology and may give a broader view of cardiovascular integrity than possible with any single measurement of pressure or function.

Asymptomatic Patients with Normal Left Ventricular Function

Surgery has increasingly been considered in asymptomatic patients who have normal LV function but echocardiographic findings indicating that valve *repair* is likely to be successful. Although these patients are at low risk without surgery, the risk associated with valve repair is less than 1%, and this approach avoids the risks of later valve *replacement*, which may be required if the valvular disease progresses. Valve repair obviates the need for protracted, expensive follow-up and provides a durable correction of the lesion. This approach is sensible, however, only if it is certain that valve repair can be performed because insertion of a prosthesis carries unacceptable risk in this low-risk group.

Asymptomatic Patients with Left Ventricular Dysfunction

The onset of LV dysfunction in patients with mitral regurgitation may occur without causing symptoms. Early surgery is warranted to prevent the muscle dysfunction from becoming severe or irreversible. Regardless of whether valve repair or replacement is eventually performed, survival is prolonged to or toward normal if surgery is performed before the ejection fraction declines to less than 0.60 or before the left ventricle is unable to contract to an end-systolic dimension of 40 mm. Patients with severe mitral regurgitation should be monitored yearly with a history, physical examination, and echocardiographic evaluation of LV function. When the patient reports symptoms or echocardiography shows the onset of LV dysfunction, surgery should be undertaken.

Asymptomatic Elderly Patients

Patients older than 75 years may have poorer surgical results than younger patients, especially if coronary disease is present or if mitral valve replacement rather than repair must be performed. However, results of surgery in older patients with mitral regurgitation have steadily improved during the past decade, and elderly patients with symptoms refractory to medical therapy may benefit from surgery. Nevertheless, there is little compelling reason to commit elderly *asymptomatic* patients to a mitral valve operation.

FIGURE 75-6. The stages of mitral valve repair. (Modified from http://my.clevelandclinic. org/heart/disorders/valve/mvrepair.aspx.)

⬤ MITRAL VALVE PROLAPSE

DEFINITION

Mitral valve prolapse occurs when one or both of the mitral valve leaflets prolapse into the left atrium superior to the mitral valve annular plane during systole. The importance of mitral valve prolapse varies from patient to patient. In some cases, prolapse is simply a consequence of normal LV physiology without significant medical impact, such as in situations that produce a small left ventricle (e.g., the Valsalva maneuver or an atrial septal defect), in which reduction of ventricular volume causes relative lengthening of the chordae tendineae and subsequent mitral valve prolapse. At the other end of the spectrum, severe redundancy and deformity of the valve, which occurs in myxomatous valve degeneration, increases the risk for stroke, arrhythmia, endocarditis, and progression to severe mitral regurgitation.

DIAGNOSIS

History

Most patients with mitral valve prolapse are asymptomatic. In some cases, however, mitral valve prolapse is associated with symptoms, including palpitations, syncope, and chest pain. In some cases, chest pain is associated with a positive thallium scintigram indicating the presence of true ischemia despite normal epicardial coronary arteries, perhaps because excessive tension on the papillary muscles increases oxygen consumption and causes ischemia. Palpitations, syncope, and presyncope, when present, are linked to autonomic dysfunction (Chapters 50, 62, and 427), which appears to be more prevalent in patients with mitral valve prolapse.

Physical Examination

On physical examination, the mitral valve prolapse syndrome produces the characteristic findings of a midsystolic click and a late systolic murmur. The click occurs when the chordae tendineae are stretched taut by the prolapsing mitral valve in mid-systole. As this occurs, the mitral leaflets move past their coaptation point, permit mitral regurgitation, and cause the late systolic murmur (see Table 50-7 in Chapter 50). Maneuvers that make the left ventricle smaller, such as the Valsalva maneuver, cause the click to appear earlier and the murmur to be more holosystolic and often louder (see Table 50-8 in Chapter 50). In some cases of echocardiographically proven mitral valve prolapse, neither the click nor the murmur is present; in other cases, only one of these findings is present.

Noninvasive Evaluation

Echocardiography is useful to prove that prolapse is present, to image the amount of regurgitation and its physiologic effects, and to discern the pathoanatomy of the mitral valve. Although an echocardiogram is not necessary to diagnose prolapse in patients with the classic physical findings, the echocardiogram adds significant prognostic information because it can detect patients who have specifically abnormal valve morphology and in whom most of the complications of the disease occur.

In the 1990s, it became clear that the mitral annulus did not exist in a single plane but had a saddleback shape. Prolapse shown in the four-chamber echocardiographic view should be confirmed in the parasternal long-axis view. Echocardiographic diagnoses made before the understanding that the mitral valve plane was multidimensional (circa 1987) may have been made in error.

TREATMENT   Rx

Because most cases of mitral valve prolapse are asymptomatic, therapy is unnecessary. Although prophylaxis against infective endocarditis was previously recommended in these patients, guidelines no longer recommend antibiotic prophylaxis based on available data (Chapter 76). In patients with palpitations and autonomic dysfunction, β-blockers are often effective in relieving symptoms. Low-dose aspirin therapy has been recommended for patients with redundant leaflets because these patients have a slightly increased risk for stroke. No data from large studies are available to support this contention, however. If severe mitral regurgitation develops, the therapy is the same as for other causes of mitral regurgitation.

PROGNOSIS

Most patients with mitral valve prolapse have a benign clinical course; even for complication-prone patients with redundant and misshapen mitral leaflets, complications are relatively rare. Approximately 10% of patients with thickened leaflets experience infective endocarditis, stroke, progression to severe mitral regurgitation, or sudden death. The progression to severe mitral regurgitation varies with gender and age, and men are approximately twice as likely to progress as women. By 50 years of age, only approximately 1 in 200 men requires surgery to correct mitral regurgitation. By the age of 70 years, the risk increases to approximately 3%.

● AORTIC REGURGITATION

DEFINITION

Aortic regurgitation is caused either by abnormalities of the aortic leaflets or by abnormalities of the proximal aortic root. Leaflet abnormalities causing aortic regurgitation include a bicuspid aortic valve, infective endocarditis, and rheumatic heart disease; anorexigenic drugs have also been implicated. Common aortic root abnormalities that cause aortic regurgitation include Marfan syndrome (Chapter 268), hypertension-induced annuloaortic ectasia, aortic dissection (Chapter 78), syphilis (Chapter 327), ankylosing spondylitis (Chapter 273), and psoriatic arthritis (Chapter 273). Acute aortic regurgitation is usually caused by infective endocarditis (Chapter 76) or aortic dissection.

PATHOBIOLOGY

As with mitral regurgitation, aortic regurgitation imparts a volume overload on the left ventricle because the left ventricle must pump the forward flow entering from the left atrium and the regurgitant volume returning through the incompetent aortic valve. Also as with mitral regurgitation, the volume overload is compensated for by the development of eccentric cardiac hypertrophy, which increases chamber size and allows the ventricle to pump a greater total stroke volume and a greater forward stroke volume. Ventricular enlargement also allows the left ventricle to accommodate the volume overload at a lower filling pressure. In contrast to mitral regurgitation, the entire stroke volume is ejected into the aorta in aortic regurgitation. Because pulse pressure is proportional to stroke volume and elastance of the aorta, the increased stroke volume increases systolic pressure. Systolic hypertension leads to afterload excess, which does not generally occur in mitral regurgitation. Ventricular geometry also differs between mitral and aortic

regurgitation because the afterload excess in aortic regurgitation causes a modest element of concentric hypertrophy, as well as severe eccentric hypertrophy.

In acute aortic insufficiency, such as might occur in infective endocarditis, severe volume overload of the previously unprepared left ventricle results in a sudden fall in forward output while precipitously increasing LV filling pressure. It is probably this combination of pathophysiologic factors that leads to rapid decompensation, presumably because the severely diminished gradient for coronary blood flow causes ischemia and progressive deterioration in LV function. In acute aortic insufficiency, reflex vasoconstriction increases peripheral vascular resistance. In compensated chronic aortic insufficiency, vasoconstriction is absent, and vascular resistance may be reduced and contribute to the hyperdynamic circulation observed in these patients.

CLINICAL MANIFESTATIONS

The most common symptoms from chronic aortic regurgitation are those of left-sided heart failure, that is, dyspnea on exertion, orthopnea, and fatigue. In acute aortic regurgitation, cardiac output and shock may develop rapidly. The onset of symptoms in patients with chronic aortic regurgitation usually heralds the onset of LV systolic dysfunction. Some patients with symptoms have apparently normal systolic function, however, and the symptoms may be attributed to diastolic dysfunction. Other patients may have ventricular dysfunction yet remain asymptomatic.

Angina may also occur in patients with aortic insufficiency but less commonly than in those with aortic stenosis. The cause of angina in aortic regurgitation is probably multifactorial. Coronary blood flow reserve is reduced in some patients because diastolic runoff into the left ventricle lowers aortic diastolic pressure while increasing LV diastolic pressure—these two influences lower the driving pressure gradient for flow across the coronary bed. When angina occurs in aortic regurgitation, it may be accompanied by flushing. Other symptoms include carotid artery pain and an unpleasant awareness of the heartbeat.

DIAGNOSIS

Physical Examination

Aortic regurgitation produces a myriad of signs because a hyperdynamic, enlarged left ventricle ejects a large stroke volume at high pressure into the systemic circulation. Palpation of the precordium finds a hyperactive apical impulse displaced downward and to the left. S_1 and S_2 are usually normal. S_2 is followed by a diastolic blowing murmur heard best along the left sternal border with the patient sitting upright. In mild disease, the murmur may be short and heard only in the beginning of diastole when the gradient between the aorta and the left ventricle is highest. As the disease worsens, the murmur may persist throughout diastole. A second murmur, a mitral valve rumble, is heard at the LV apex in patients with severe aortic insufficiency. Although the cause is still debated, this Austin Flint murmur is probably produced as the regurgitant jet impinges on the mitral valve and causes it to vibrate.

In chronic aortic regurgitation, the high stroke volume and reduced systemic arterial resistance result in a wide pulse pressure, which may generate a number of signs, including Corrigan's pulse (sharp upstroke and rapid decline of the carotid pulse), de Musset's sign (head bobbing), Duroziez's sign (combined systolic and diastolic bruits created by compression of the femoral artery with the stethoscope), and Quincke's pulse (systolic plethora and diastolic blanching in the nail bed when gentle traction is placed on the nail). Perhaps the most reliable of physical signs indicating severe aortic regurgitation is Hill's sign, an increase in femoral systolic pressure of 40 mm Hg or more compared with systolic pressure in the brachial artery.

In contrast to chronic aortic insufficiency with its myriad clinical signs, acute aortic insufficiency may have a subtle manifestation. The eccentric hypertrophy, which compensates for chronic aortic insufficiency, has not yet had time to develop, and the large total stroke volume responsible for most of the signs of chronic aortic insufficiency is absent. The only clues to the presence of acute aortic insufficiency may be a short diastolic blowing murmur and reduced intensity of S_1. This latter sign occurs because high diastolic LV pressure closes the mitral valve early in diastole (mitral valve preclosure) so that when ventricular systole occurs, only the tricuspid component of S_1 is heard.

Noninvasive Evaluation

The ECG in patients with aortic insufficiency is nonspecific but almost always demonstrates LV hypertrophy. The chest radiograph shows an enlarged heart, often with uncoiling and enlargement of the aortic root.

FIGURE 75-7. Echocardiogram of a patient with aortic regurgitation caused by infective endocarditis. The *left panel* shows a linear vegetation (*arrow*) prolapsing into the left ventricular outflow tract from the aortic valve leaflet in diastole. The *right panel* is a color flow Doppler image exhibiting turbulent blood flow filling the left ventricular tract during diastole. AO = aorta; LA = left atrium; LV = left ventricle; RV = right ventricle. (Courtesy of Dr. Anthony DeMaria.)

Echocardiography (Chapter 55) is the most important noninvasive tool for assessing the severity of aortic insufficiency and its impact on LV geometry and function (Fig. 75-7). During echocardiography, the LV end-diastolic dimension, end-systolic dimension, and fractional shortening are determined. Aortic valve anatomy and aortic root anatomy can be assessed and the cause of the aortic regurgitation can often be determined. Color flow Doppler examination of the aortic valve helps quantify the severity of aortic regurgitation by assessing the depth and width to which the diastolic jet penetrates the left ventricle. Another way to assess the severity of aortic regurgitation is the pressure half-time method: continuous-wave Doppler interrogation of the aortic valve displays the decay of the velocity of retrograde flow across the valve. In mild aortic insufficiency, the gradient across the valve is high throughout diastole, and its rate of decay is slow, with production of a long Doppler half-time (the time that it takes the velocity to decay from its peak to that value divided by the square root of 2). In severe aortic regurgitation, there is rapid equilibration between pressure in the aorta and pressure in the left ventricle, and the Doppler half-time is short. If mitral valve preclosure is detected in acute aortic insufficiency, urgent surgery is necessary. In cases in which the severity of aortic insufficiency is in doubt, catheterization to perform aortography is useful in resolving the issue.

TREATMENT AND PROGNOSIS   Rx

Medical Therapy
Asymptomatic Patients with Normal Left Ventricular Function
Because aortic regurgitation increases LV afterload, which decreases cardiac efficiency, afterload reduction with nifedipine and other vasodilators, including angiotensin-converting enzyme inhibitors and hydralazine, improves hemodynamics in the short term. Although initial data suggested that such therapy could delay or reduce the need for aortic valve surgery without any adverse effects when surgery is finally performed, more recent data suggest no benefit from such therapy. These discrepant results from relatively small trials preclude firm recommendations.

Symptomatic Patients or Patients with Left Ventricular Dysfunction
Patients who have symptoms or manifest LV dysfunction should not be treated medically, except for short-term stabilization, but should undergo aortic valve surgery as soon as feasible.

Surgical Therapy
Acute Aortic Regurgitation
When any of the symptoms or signs of heart failure develop, even if mild, medical mortality is high and approaches 75%. Therapy with vasodilators, such as nitroprusside, may temporarily improve the patient's condition before surgery but is never a substitute for surgery. In patients with acute aortic regurgitation caused by bacterial endocarditis (Chapter 76), surgery may be delayed to permit a full or partial course of antibiotics, but persistent, severe aortic regurgitation requires emergency valve replacement. Even when blood cultures have been positive recently and antibiotic therapy has been of brief duration, the valve reinfection rate is low, 0 to 10%, with valve replacement or valve repair. Emergency surgery should not be withheld simply because the duration of antibiotic therapy has been brief.

Chronic Aortic Regurgitation
Asymptomatic patients who manifest evidence of LV dysfunction benefit from surgery. Because loading conditions differ between aortic and mitral regurgitation, the objective markers for the presence of LV dysfunction also differ. In aortic regurgitation, when the ejection fraction is less than 0.55 or the end-systolic dimension is greater than 55 mm, postoperative outcome is impaired, presumably because these markers indicate that LV dysfunction has developed. Surgery should be performed before these benchmarks are reached. A calculated regurgitant orifice above 40 mm² portends a poorer prognosis and also may warrant surgery.

Patients with advanced symptoms are at increased risk for a suboptimal surgical outcome regardless of whether they have evidence of LV dysfunction. Patients should undergo aortic valve replacement before symptoms impair lifestyle.

Although some patients may be able to undergo successful aortic valve repair to restore aortic valve competence, most patients require insertion of an aortic valve prosthesis.

TRICUSPID REGURGITATION

DEFINITION
Tricuspid regurgitation is usually secondary to a hemodynamic load on the right ventricle rather than a structural valve deformity. Diseases that cause pulmonary hypertension, such as chronic obstructive airway disease or intracardiac shunts, lead to RV dilation and subsequent tricuspid regurgitation. Because most of the force that is needed to fill the left ventricle is provided by the right ventricle, LV dysfunction leading to elevated LV filling pressure also places the right ventricle under a hemodynamic load and can eventually lead to RV failure and tricuspid regurgitation. In some instances, tricuspid regurgitation may be caused by pathology of the valve itself. The most common cause of primary tricuspid regurgitation is infective endocarditis, usually stemming from drug abuse and unsterile injections. Other causes include carcinoid syndrome, rheumatic involvement of the tricuspid valve, myxomatous degeneration, RV infarction, and mishaps during endomyocardial biopsy.

DIAGNOSIS
The symptoms of tricuspid regurgitation are those of right-sided heart failure and include ascites, edema, and occasionally right upper quadrant pain. On physical examination, tricuspid regurgitation produces jugular venous distention accentuated by a large v wave as blood is regurgitated into the right atrium during systole. Regurgitation into the hepatic veins causes hepatic enlargement and liver pulsation. RV enlargement is detected as a parasternal lift. Ascites and edema are common.

The definitive diagnosis of tricuspid regurgitation is made during echocardiography. Doppler interrogation of the tricuspid valve shows systolic disturbance of the right atrial blood pool. Echocardiography (Chapter 55) can also be used to determine the severity of pulmonary hypertension, measure RV dilation, and assess whether the valve itself is intrinsically normal or abnormal.

TREATMENT AND PROGNOSIS   Rx

Therapy for secondary tricuspid regurgitation is generally aimed at the cause of the lesion. If LV failure has been responsible for RV failure and tricuspid regurgitation, the standard therapy for improving LV failure (Chapter 59) lowers LV filling pressure, reduces secondary pulmonary hypertension, relieves some of the hemodynamic burden of the right ventricle, and partially restores tricuspid valve competence. If pulmonary disease is the primary cause, therapy is directed toward improving lung function. Vasodilators, so useful in the treatment of left-sided heart failure, are often ineffective in treating pulmonary hypertension itself. Medical therapy directed at tricuspid regurgitation is usually limited to diuretic use.

Surgical intervention for the tricuspid valve is rarely entertained in isolation. However, if other cardiac surgery is planned in a patient with severe tricuspid regurgitation, concomitant ring annuloplasty or tricuspid valve repair is frequently attempted to ensure postoperative tricuspid competence. Since a second operation to address residual tricuspid regurgitation after successful left-sided valve surgery carries an unacceptably high mortality rate, concomitant tricuspid annuloplasty is now entertained for even mild to moderate tricuspid regurgitation during left-sided valve surgery. Tricuspid valve replacement is often not well tolerated and is rarely performed except when severe deformity, as is often seen in endocarditis or carcinoid disease, precludes valve repair.

FIGURE 75-8. Different types of commonly used prosthetic valves. **A,** Starr-Edwards caged ball mitral prosthesis. **B,** Starr-Edwards aortic prosthesis. **C,** St. Jude Medical bileaflet prosthesis. **D,** Medtronic-Hall tilting disc valve. **E,** Carpentier-Edwards bioprosthesis. (From Wernly JA, Crawford MH. Choosing a prosthetic heart valve. *Cardiol Clin.* 1991;9:329-338.)

PULMONIC STENOSIS

DEFINITION

Pulmonic stenosis is a congenital disease resulting from fusion of the pulmonic valve cusps (Chapter 69). It is usually detected and corrected during childhood, but occasionally cases are diagnosed for the first time in adulthood. Symptoms of pulmonic stenosis include angina and syncope. Occasionally, symptoms of right-sided heart failure develop. During physical examination, the uncalcified valve in pulmonic stenosis produces an early systolic ejection click on opening. During inspiration, the click diminishes or disappears because increased flow into the right side of the heart during inspiration partially opens the pulmonic valve in diastole so that systole causes less of an opening sound. The click is followed by a systolic ejection murmur that radiates to the base of the heart. If the transvalvular gradient is severe, RV hypertrophy develops and produces a parasternal lift.

The diagnosis of pulmonic stenosis is confirmed by echocardiography, which quantifies the transvalvular gradient and the degree of RV hypertrophy and dysfunction.

TREATMENT AND PROGNOSIS Rx

In asymptomatic patients with a gradient less than 25 mm Hg, no therapy is required. If symptoms develop or the gradient exceeds 50 mm Hg, balloon commissurotomy is effective in reducing the gradient and relieving symptoms. Although long-term prognosis is not yet established, 90% of patients do not require reintervention 10 years after balloon therapy.

Postoperative Care of Patients with Substitute Heart Valves

After a prosthetic valve has been inserted, a baseline echocardiogram should be obtained to provide a reference point in the event that valve dysfunction is suspected at a later date. Echocardiography does not need to be repeated unless there is a change in clinical status or physical findings. The major causes of valve dysfunction are infective endocarditis, clot, and valve degeneration. Dysfunction is manifested most commonly by valvular regurgitation, but valvular stenosis can also occur with a clot, vegetations, or degeneration, especially degeneration of a bioprosthesis.

Whenever a patient with a prosthetic heart valve has a temperature higher than 100° F, endocarditis must be excluded by blood culture; for fever with signs of sepsis, broad-spectrum antibiotics must be begun while awaiting culture results. For patients with bioprosthetic valves, mechanical prostheses, and homografts, endocarditis prophylaxis should be instituted at the time of procedures that are associated with a high risk for bacteremia (Chapter 76). Whether prophylaxis is necessary for pulmonary autografts is currently unclear, but physicians usually prescribe prophylaxis for these patients.

All patients with a mechanical heart valve require anticoagulation. Recommended INR values range from 2.0 for a young normotensive patient in sinus rhythm with an aortic valve prosthesis to 3.5 for a patient with atrial fibrillation and a mitral valve prosthesis. Aspirin, 325 mg, is recommended in addition to warfarin to reduce the risk for valve thrombosis in patients who have mechanical prosthetic valves that are at higher risk for thromboembolic complications. When thrombosis occurs on a prosthetic valve, about 60% of

patients can have restored valve function after intravenous infusion of a thrombolytic agent.

Choices among Prosthetic Valves

Different types of prosthetic valves (Fig. 75-8) have different advantages and disadvantages (Table 75-2). At long-term follow-up, primary valve failure with resulting need for reoperation is much more common with bioprosthetic valves,[4,5] and bleeding is generally more common with mechanical valves. For mitral valves, long-term survival is similar with bioprosthetic and mechanical valves.[4] Survival after aortic valve replacement is probably better with mechanical valves. Another alternative is to use the patient's own pulmonic valve to replace the diseased aortic valve and then to implant a prosthetic pulmonic valve (the Ross procedure). In a randomized trial, this procedure was superior to homograft valve and root replacement, with a 10-year survival of 97% compared with 83%.[6]

In general, a tissue valve is recommended in patients who have a life expectancy of less than 15 years or who are unable or unwilling to maintain warfarin anticoagulation. A mechanical valve is preferred in patients who already have another indication for anticoagulation or who have a longer life expectancy and want to minimize the risk of reoperation. Because many patients prefer the risk of reoperation to that of anticoagulation, the age at which bioprostheses are implanted has steadily declined, and many 60-year-old patients now request and receive a bioprosthetic valve.

TABLE 75-2 ADVANTAGES AND DISADVANTAGES OF SUBSTITUTE CARDIAC VALVES

TYPE OF VALVE	ADVANTAGES	DISADVANTAGES
Bioprosthesis (Carpentier-Edwards, Hancock)	Avoids anticoagulation in patients with sinus rhythm	Durability limited to 10-15 yr Relatively stenotic
Mechanical valves (St. Jude, Medtronic-Hall, Starr-Edwards)	Good flow characteristics in small sizes Durable	Require anticoagulation
Homografts and autografts	Anticoagulation not required Durability increased over that of bioprostheses	Surgical implantation technically demanding

1. Leon MB, Smith CR, Mack M, et al. Transcatheter aortic-valve implantation for aortic stenosis in patients who cannot undergo surgery. *N Engl J Med.* 2010;363:1597-1607.
2. Smith CR, Leon MB, Mack M, et al, for the PARTNER Trial Investigators. Comparison of transcatheter and surgical aortic valve replacement for aortic stenosis in patients at high risk for operation. *N Engl J Med.* 2011. [Epub ahead of print.]
3. Feldman T, Foster E, Glower DG, et al. Percutaneous repair or surgery for mitral regurgitation. *N Engl J Med.* 2011;364:1395-1406.
4. Hammermeister K, Sethi GK, Henderson WG, et al. Outcomes 15 years after valve replacement with a mechanical versus a bioprosthetic valve: final report of the Veterans Affairs randomized trial. *J Am Coll Cardiol.* 2000;36:1152-1158.
5. Stassano P, Di Tommaso L, Monaco M, et al. Aortic valve replacement: a prospective randomized evaluation of mechanical versus biological valves in patients ages 55 to 70 years. *J Am Coll Cardiol.* 2009;54:1862-1868.

6. El-Hamamsy I, Eryigit Z, Stevens LM, et al. Long-term outcomes after autograft versus homograft aortic root replacement in adults with aortic valve disease: a randomised controlled trial. *Lancet.* 2010;376:524-531.

SUGGESTED READINGS

Foster E. Clinical practice. Mitral regurgitation due to degenerative mitral-valve disease. *N Engl J Med.* 2010;363:156-165. *Review.*

Rahimtoola SH. Choice of prosthetic heart valve in adults an update. *J Am Coll Cardiol.* 2010;55:2413-2426. *Review.*

Siu SC, Silversides CK. Bicuspid aortic valve disease. *J Am Coll Cardiol.* 2010;55:2789-2800. *Review.*

Vaishnava P, Fuster V, Goldman M, et al. Surgery for asymptomatic degenerative aortic and mitral valve disease. *Nat Rev Cardiol.* 2011;8:173-177. *Review suggesting a targeted role for pre-emptive intervention in selected, asymptomatic individuals with AS or MR.*

76

INFECTIVE ENDOCARDITIS

VANCE G. FOWLER JR. AND ARNOLD S. BAYER

DEFINITION

Infective endocarditis is defined as an infection, usually bacterial, of the endocardial surface of the heart. Infective endocarditis affects primarily the cardiac valves, although in some cases the septa between the chambers or the mural endocardium may be involved. Traditionally, infective endocarditis has been categorized as acute or subacute, depending on the duration of symptoms before presentation; however, this distinction is somewhat arbitrary. A classification that considers the causative organism and the valve involved is more clinically relevant.

EPIDEMIOLOGY

The incidence of infective endocarditis is difficult to determine because of the different criteria for diagnosis and methods of reporting. An analysis based on strict case definitions reveals that only a relatively small proportion (about 20%) of clinically diagnosed cases are categorized as definite. Nevertheless, in 10 large surveys, infective endocarditis accounted for approximately 1 case per 1000 U.S. hospital admissions, with a range of 0.16 to 5.4 cases per 1000 admissions. This incidence has not changed appreciably over the past 30 years. Estimates from the American Heart Association place the annual incidence of infective endocarditis in the United States at 10,000 to 20,000 new cases.

Men are more commonly affected than women (mean male-female ratio of 1.7 : 1 in 18 large series). However, in patients younger than 35 years, more cases occur in women. More than 50% of patients with infective endocarditis in the United States are now older than 50 years owing to the low incidence of acute rheumatic fever (Chapter 298) and the low subsequent prevalence of rheumatic heart disease compared with prior eras and with developing countries, as well as a simultaneous rise in the prevalence of degenerative heart disease as the population lives longer.

Although some patients have no clearly definable risk factor for endocarditis, cardiac conditions that cause turbulent flow at the endocardial surface or across a valve (Chapter 75) predispose patients to infective endocarditis (Table 76-1). Historically, rheumatic heart disease with valvular dysfunction was the most common underlying condition, although its contribution has diminished in the antibiotic era, especially in developed countries.

Degenerative valvular disease is also associated with infective endocarditis, particularly in elderly patients; the increasing relevance of senile calcification as a risk factor is reflected in the increasing proportion of aortic valve involvement in infective endocarditis. Most significant congenital heart defects (Chapter 69) confer an increased risk of infective endocarditis, particularly complex cyanotic disease such as single-ventricle states, transposition of the great vessels, and tetralogy of Fallot. Similarly, surgically constructed pulmonary-systemic shunts and ventricular septal defects place patients at high risk for infective endocarditis.

Mitral valve prolapse is currently the most common underlying cardiac condition in infective endocarditis, a statistic that reflects its prevalence in the general population (4%). Notably, mitral valve prolapse is a risk only in patients with thickened mitral leaflets and/or regurgitation, in which case the risk of endocarditis increases by about 10-fold over that of the general population. In addition, patients with hypertrophic cardiomyopathy are at increased risk of infective endocarditis, particularly in the presence of outflow obstruction. Finally, previous endocarditis is among the highest risk factors for infective endocarditis.

Prosthetic cardiac valves represent an important risk factor for infective endocarditis. More than 150,000 heart valves are implanted annually worldwide, and prosthetic valve infective endocarditis develops in 1 to 4% of prosthetic valve recipients in the first year after valve replacement and in approximately 0.8% of recipients annually thereafter. Mechanical prosthetic valves may initially be more susceptible to infective endocarditis, but bioprosthetic valves are more likely to develop infective endocarditis after 1 year; overall, the rate is similar with either type of valve.

The incidence of infective endocarditis in injection drug users (Chapter 33) may be 30 times higher than in the general population and 4 times higher than in adults with rheumatic heart disease. In some areas of the United States, injection drug use is the most common predisposing cause of infective endocarditis in patients younger than 40 years. *Staphylococcus aureus* is the predominant organism, and tricuspid valve involvement is noted in 78% of cases, mitral involvement in 24%, and aortic involvement in 8%. More than one valve is infected in approximately 20% of cases, and some of these infections are polymicrobial.

Health care–associated infective endocarditis arises primarily as a consequence of invasive therapies, including intravenous catheters, hyperalimentation lines, pacemakers, and dialysis shunts. In a recent prospective multinational cohort study of more than 1600 patients with native valve endocarditis and no injection drug use, more than one third of patients had health care–associated endocarditis, and many of these cases were community acquired (e.g., in patients on outpatient hemodialysis). The emerging importance of health care–associated infective endocarditis in industrialized nations has also influenced the microbiology of the disease, with an increasing prevalence of *S. aureus* and a decreasing prevalence of viridans streptococci in much of the industrialized world.

Systemic medical conditions predispose patients to the development of infective endocarditis. For example, HIV infection is an independent risk factor for the development of infective endocarditis in injection drug users, with the risk increasing as the CD4 count decreases. Catheter-related bacteremia is an important risk factor for nosocomial infective endocarditis. Patients with end-stage renal disease—particularly those receiving long-term hemodialysis—and patients with diabetes mellitus are also at increased risk, presumably because of the recurrent vascular access associated with the former and the low-level immunosuppression associated with both conditions.

The mitral valve has classically been the most commonly affected valve, followed by the aortic valve. Although mitral valve relapse remains the most common underlying condition, the decreasing frequency of rheumatic mitral disease and the increasing senescence of the population may account for the increase in aortic valve endocarditis reported in many studies. The next most commonly affected valves in descending order of prevalence are the mitral and aortic valves together, the tricuspid valve, mixed right- and left-sided infection, and the pulmonic valve.

Microbiology

About 90% of community-acquired, native valve infective endocarditis is due to staphylococci, streptococci, or enterococci, each of which is a normal inhabitant of the skin, oropharynx, and urogenital tract with frequent access to the blood stream. These organisms express specific receptors for attachment and adherence to damaged valve surfaces. Streptococcal species (Chapter 298) are the most common cause in community-dwelling patients

TABLE 76-1	PREDISPOSING CONDITIONS ASSOCIATED WITH INCREASED RISK OF ENDOCARDITIS
MORE COMMON	**LESS COMMON**
Mitral valve prolapse	Rheumatic heart disease
Degenerative valvular disease	Idiopathic hypertrophic subaortic stenosis
Intravenous drug use*	Pulmonary-systemic shunts*
Prosthetic valve*	Coarctation of the aorta
Congenital abnormalities (valvular or septal defect)	Previous endocarditis*
	Complex cyanotic congenital heart disease*

*Indicates conditions with highest risk for endocarditis.

with no history of injection drug use or health care contact. In patients with either of these epidemiologic risk factors, *S. aureus* (Chapter 298) is the predominant cause of infective endocarditis. Because of the emergence of health care contact as the predominant risk factor for blood stream infections, *S. aureus* is now the most common cause of infective endocarditis in many regions of the world.

Viridans streptococci (Chapter 298) are the most common streptococci implicated in native valve infective endocarditis. This group of organisms, which normally inhabit the oropharynx, includes species such as *Streptococcus sanguis, Streptococcus mutans,* and *Streptococcus mitis.* Group B streptococci, β-hemolytic organisms that are also normal oropharyngeal and urogenital flora, most frequently cause infective endocarditis in patients with cirrhosis or diabetes mellitus and in injection drug users. By contrast, group A streptococci, although also β-hemolytic, rarely cause infective endocarditis. *Streptococcus bovis,* a group D streptococcus, is now a leading cause of infective endocarditis in some parts of the world; for example, its incidence in France has increased significantly in recent years. Its presence should prompt endoscopic evaluation for adenocarcinoma of the colon or other malignant lesions of the gastrointestinal tract.

Pneumococcal endocarditis is decreasing in incidence but is quite fulminant when present. It may occur as part of Austrian's (or Osler's) triad of endocarditis, meningitis, and pneumonia and is associated with high morbidity and mortality.

S. aureus (Chapter 296) is the pathogen of primary concern among injection drug users or patients with health care contact. The clinical course of *S. aureus* endocarditis is typically acute, with a rapid progression over the course of several days. Because approximately 12% of nonselected patients with *S. aureus* bacteremia have infective endocarditis, the possibility of cardiac involvement should always be considered in any patient with *S. aureus* bacteremia; those with persistent bacteremia or fever, community acquisition, or cutaneous findings are at particular risk for infective endocarditis and other complications. Coagulase-negative staphylococci are an unusual cause of native valve disease but are an important pathogen in prosthetic valve endocarditis; presentation is usually subacute.

Enterococcal bacteremia is far more common, particularly in hospitalized patients, than enterococcal endocarditis; however, enterococci are responsible for a significant number of cases of both community-acquired and nosocomial endocarditis. In most cases, the source of the bacteria is thought to be the genitourinary tract, and the presentation is usually subacute. Enterococcal endocarditis, as opposed to enterococcal bacteremia, is suggested by community acquisition of infection, the absence of a clear source of infection, preexistent valvular heart disease, and the absence of polymicrobial bacteremia. As in most enterococcal infections, the overwhelming majority of cases (>90%) are due to *Enterococcus faecalis.*

The HACEK group of gram-negative organisms (*Haemophilus* spp, *Actinobacillus actinomycetemcomitans, Cardiobacterium hominis, Eikenella corrodens,* and *Kingella* spp) accounts for about 5% of cases of endocarditis. Because these fastidious organisms usually grow in blood cultures within 7 days using current methods, prolonged incubation is no longer required to isolate HACEK strains. Many other gram-negative bacilli have been reported to cause infective endocarditis but are even more unusual. Traditionally, injection drug use has been regarded as the primary risk factor for enteric gram-negative bacterial endocarditis. However, recent experience from large multinational studies shows that health care contact, not injection drug use, is the most common risk factor for enteric gram-negative endocarditis.

Fungal endocarditis is difficult to diagnose and treat; it is most commonly found in patients with a history of injection drug use, recent cardiac surgery, or prolonged use of indwelling vascular catheters, especially those used for total parenteral nutrition. The most common fungi found in infective endocarditis are *Aspergillus* and *Candida* species. *Aspergillus* (Chapter 347) rarely grows in blood cultures and must usually be cultured from a pathologic specimen (either an embolic site or vegetation); by contrast, *Candida* (Chapter 346) frequently grows out of blood cultures. Mortality is very high, and valve replacement surgery is usually necessary.

Special Situations: Health Care–Associated Infective Endocarditis and Prosthetic Valves

Health care–associated infective endocarditis is defined as endocarditis occurring in the presence of extensive health care contact. Traditionally, this definition was synonymous with nosocomial in-hospital acquisition; however, the increased complexity of outpatient therapy and the increase in

TABLE 76-2 CAUSES OF PROSTHETIC VALVE ENDOCARDITIS*

EARLY (<2 MO POSTOPERATIVELY)	LATE (>12 MO POSTOPERATIVELY)
Staphylococcus aureus	Coagulase-negative staphylococci
Coagulase-negative staphylococci	*Staphylococcus aureus*
Gram-negative bacilli	Coagulase-negative staphylococci
Enterococci	Enterococci
Fungi	
Diphtheroids	

*Listed in order of relative frequency.
Adapted from Wang A, Athan E, Pappas PA, et al. Contemporary clinical profile and outcome of prosthetic valve endocarditis. *JAMA.* 2007; 297:1354-1361.

the number of patients in long-term care facilities have resulted in a growing number of nonhospitalized patients with health care–associated bacteremia and infective endocarditis. Such patients have many of the same risk factors (e.g., long-term intravascular catheters, extensive instrumentation) and are infected with the same array of pathogens (e.g., high rates of methicillin-resistant *S. aureus* [MRSA]) as patients with nosocomial infection. Health care–associated infective endocarditis now constitutes about one quarter of all cases and is most frequently associated with indwelling vascular catheters; as a result, the most common organisms implicated in nosocomial infective endocarditis are *S. aureus* and coagulase-negative staphylococci.

Prosthetic valve endocarditis can be classified into one of three groups based on the time between valve surgery and disease onset: early (<2 months after surgery), intermediate (2 to 12 months), and late (>12 months) (Table 76-2). Staphylococci, particularly *S. aureus,* predominate during the early period, when most episodes of infective endocarditis are thought to be related to perioperative infection. The intermediate period has a fairly similar microbiologic spectrum, with unusual gram-negative organisms and diphtheroids decreasing and streptococci increasing. In the late period, 1 year or more after surgery, the spectrum of organisms becomes more akin to that of community-acquired native valve disease, in which *S. aureus* and streptococci predominate. Of note, approximately 50% of prosthetic valve recipients with *S. aureus* bacteremia develop infective endocarditis.

PATHOBIOLOGY

Experimental models of infective endocarditis have demonstrated that the disease follows a predictable sequence: endocardial damage, aggregation of platelets and fibrin to create a sterile vegetation, transient bacteremia resulting in seeding of the vegetation, microbial proliferation on and invasion of the endocardial surface, and metastatic infection to visceral organs and brain.

Most cases of infective endocarditis begin with a damaged endocardial surface. Damage to the endocardium may be caused by a number of factors, ranging from rheumatic disease to senile degeneration and calcification; indeed, any excessive turbulence or high-pressure gradient can cause injury to the nearby endocardium. Next, fibrin-platelet aggregates develop at the site of damage to form sterile vegetations, also termed *nonbacterial thrombotic endocarditis.* Nonbacterial thrombotic endocarditis may occur spontaneously in patients with systemic illnesses (e.g., the marantic endocarditis of malignancy [Chapter 60] or other wasting diseases, or Libman-Sacks endocarditis in systemic lupus erythematosus [Chapter 274]). When transient bacteremia occurs—for example, as a result of distant infection or gingival disease—the previously sterile vegetation may be seeded. Some bacterial species, such as staphylococci and streptococci, are more avidly adherent than others to vegetations and therefore more frequently cause endocarditis. The bacteria then proliferate within the vegetation and may ultimately achieve an organism load of 10^9 to 10^{11} colony-forming units per gram of tissue. The surfaces of cardiac valves and vegetations are avascular, making antibiotic therapy and healing difficult.

CLINICAL MANIFESTATIONS

History

The initial presentation of infective endocarditis varies enormously from patient to patient, so it is sometimes difficult to make the diagnosis. Some cases develop acutely, with symptoms progressing rapidly over several days. Other cases develop insidiously and present with nonspecific symptoms that

TABLE 76-3 PHYSICAL EXAMINATION AND LABORATORY FINDINGS IN INFECTIVE ENDOCARDITIS

FINDING	% OF CASES
Fever	96
Worsening of old murmur	20
New murmur	48
Vascular embolic event	17
Splenomegaly	11
Splinter hemorrhages	8
Osler's nodes	3
Janeway's lesions	5
Roth's spots	2
Elevated ESR	61
Hematuria	26
Positive rheumatoid factor	5
Abnormal CXR (effusion, infiltrate, septic emboli)	67-85 (right-sided infective endocarditis)

CXR = chest x-ray; ESR = erythrocyte sedimentation rate.
Adapted from Murdoch DR, Corey GR, Hoen B, et al. Clinical presentation, etiology, and outcome of infective endocarditis in the 21st century: International Collaboration on Endocarditis—Prospective Cohort Study. *Arch Intern Med.* 2009;169:463-473.

FIGURE 76-1. Petechiae in infective endocarditis.

FIGURE 76-2. Osler's node in infective endocarditis.

have been progressing for weeks or months. In patients suspected of having infective endocarditis, the initial history should include a complete review of systems, a travel history, and a thorough discussion of health-related behaviors such as illicit drug use and sexual activity. Most patients complain of fever and nonspecific constitutional symptoms such as fatigue, malaise, or weight loss. Nearly 50% of patients complain of musculoskeletal symptoms ranging from frank arthritis to diffuse myalgias; 5 to 10% of patients have low back pain as their chief complaint, even in the absence of osteomyelitis or epidural abscess. Many intravenous drug users with endocarditis complain of pleuritic chest pain, because tricuspid valve endocarditis mimics pneumonia. Health care–associated infective endocarditis is more likely to be clinically occult and requires a high index of suspicion.

Physical Examination

A thorough physical examination should be performed, including a search for the peripheral stigmata of infective endocarditis (Table 76-3). Fever is present in nearly 50% of patients in most studies; however, elderly patients and those with renal failure or heart failure may be less likely to mount a febrile response. A widened pulse pressure should alert the clinician to the possibility of acute aortic insufficiency (Chapter 75). The skin and nails should be carefully examined for embolic phenomena such as petechiae, Osler's nodes, Janeway's lesions, and splinter hemorrhages; these findings are uncommon in infective endocarditis in the current era but are extremely helpful diagnostic clues when present. Petechiae are most often found on the conjunctiva, palate, and extremities; like the other peripheral stigmata of infective endocarditis, they are a nonspecific but suggestive finding (Fig. 76-1). Osler's nodes are small, painful nodules found most often on the palmar surfaces of the fingers and toes; they frequently wax and wane (Fig. 76-2). Classically considered to be an immunologic phenomenon, Osler's nodes may have an immune complex–mediated component but are most likely initiated by microemboli. Janeway's lesions (Fig. 50-11 in Chapter 50) are hemorrhagic, nonpainful macules also found primarily on the palms and soles; they are embolic in origin and are less frequently noted than the other cutaneous stigmata. Splinter hemorrhages (see Fig. 50-11 in Chapter 50) are nonblanching, linear, brownish red lesions in the nail beds perpendicular to the direction of nail growth; they are nonspecific and may also be found in a significant percentage of hospitalized patients without infective endocarditis.

Funduscopic examination should be performed to look for Roth's spots (see Fig. 431-28 in Chapter 431), chorioretinitis, or endophthalmitis; the latter two are present in a substantial proportion of cases of fungal endocarditis. A careful cardiac examination should be performed to detect any systolic or diastolic murmurs or evidence of heart failure, which is an ominous sign. Of note, patients with health care–associated infective endocarditis are less likely than others to have a pathologic murmur on initial presentation.

The abdomen should be examined for evidence of splenomegaly (Chapter 171), a finding that is more common in patients with a subacute form of infective endocarditis. Finally, a thorough neurologic examination should be performed, both to assess for any focal neurologic deficits and to serve as a baseline during the patient's hospital stay. The neurologic examination may demonstrate evidence of major vessel embolism, cranial nerve palsies, visual field defects, or generalized toxic-metabolic encephalopathy with altered mental status.

Laboratory Findings

Initial laboratory tests should include a complete blood count with differential, serum electrolytes, measurement of renal function, urinalysis, chest radiograph, and electrocardiogram (ECG). All patients should receive at least three sets of blood cultures as well, and many require an echocardiogram (see later). Most patients with subacute infective endocarditis have anemia of chronic disease. The white blood cell count may or may not be elevated; it is more frequently elevated in cases of acute infective endocarditis, particularly if *S. aureus* or a fungus is the causative organism. Microscopic hematuria is noted in many cases, as is proteinuria. The chest radiograph is abnormal—demonstrating consolidation, atelectasis, pleural effusion, or clear septic emboli—in the overwhelming majority of patients with right-sided endocarditis; in others, it may provide evidence of heart failure. The ECG should be carefully examined for evidence of atrioventricular conduction blocks, especially a prolonged PR interval (see Figs. 64-7 through 64-11 in Chapter 64), suggestive of an aortic ring abscess or frank myocardial infarction (see Figs. 73-1 and 73-2 in Chapter 73). Other ancillary tests might include an erythrocyte sedimentation rate, which is elevated in nearly all cases of infective endocarditis, with a mean value of 57 mm/hour. Rheumatoid factor is positive in about half of cases, particularly in subacute endocarditis.

Complications

The complications of infective endocarditis can be divided into four groups for ease of classification: direct valvular damage and consequences of local invasion, embolic complications, metastatic infections from bacteremia, and immunologic phenomena. Local damage to the endocardium or myocardium is a dreaded complication that can be difficult to diagnose and treat. Infection may directly erode through the involved cardiac valve or adjacent myocardial wall, resulting in hemodynamically significant valvular perforations or cardiac fistulas. Such local complications typically present clinically with the acute onset of heart failure and carry a poor prognosis, even with prompt cardiac surgery. Valve ring abscesses also require surgical intervention and are more frequent in patients with prosthetic valves. Although a conduction defect on ECG may suggest the diagnosis, transesophageal echocardiography (TEE) is the diagnostic technique of choice for paravalvular abscess, valve perforation, or intracardiac fistula. Frank myocardial abscess has been found in up to 20% of cases on autopsy; *Aspergillus* endocarditis invades the myocardium in more than 50% of cases. Pericarditis is rare and is associated with myocardial abscess in most cases. Myocardial infarction, thought to be due to embolism of vegetative material in the coronary arteries, has been found in 40 to 60% of cases on autopsy, although most cases are clinically silent and lack characteristic ECG changes. However, up to 16% of elderly patients may present with clinical evidence of acute myocardial infarction, with potentially disastrous complications if the myocardial infarction is thought to be the primary event and the patient is given thrombolytic therapy. Heart failure is the leading cause of death in infective endocarditis, usually related to direct valvular damage.

Embolic events are less common now than in the preantibiotic era; nevertheless, about 35% of patients have at least one clinically evident embolic event. In fungal endocarditis, the majority of patients have at least one embolic event, frequently with a large embolus. The presence of large (>10 mm), mobile vegetations on the echocardiogram, particularly when the anterior mitral valve leaflet is involved, predicts a high risk of embolic complications. Most of the classic peripheral stigmata of infective endocarditis are probably embolic in nature; in addition, patients may have frank infarction of cutaneous tissue from emboli. In addition to the skin, emboli most commonly lodge in the lungs (in right-sided endocarditis), kidneys, spleen, large blood vessels, or central nervous system (CNS). Vegetations of right-sided endocarditis usually embolize to the lungs, resulting in an abnormality on the chest radiograph.

Renal abscesses are rare in infective endocarditis, but renal infarction is seen in more than 50% of cases at autopsy. Similarly, splenic infarction occurs in up to 44% of autopsy-confirmed cases; although frequently silent, such emboli may cause left upper quadrant pain radiating to the left shoulder, sometimes as the presenting symptom of infective endocarditis. Splenic infarction progressing to abscess may be a cause of persistent fever in patients with infective endocarditis; patients with infective endocarditis and unexplained persistent fever should undergo abdominal computed tomography to exclude this complication. Vascular aneurysms, which frequently occur at bifurcation points, may be clinically silent until they rupture (which may be months to years after apparently successful antibiotic treatment of infective endocarditis) and have been found in 10 to 15% of cases at autopsy. The presence of large emboli occluding major vessels can suggest the presence of fungal infective endocarditis. Peripheral mycotic aneurysms require surgical resection; intracerebral aneurysms should be resected if they bleed or if they are causing a mass effect.

Finally, many patients have evidence of cerebrovascular emboli, which have a predilection for the middle cerebral artery distribution and may be devastating. Most emboli to the CNS occur early in the course of the disease and are evident at the time of presentation or shortly thereafter. Cerebrovascular accidents related to these emboli are prone to catastrophic hemorrhagic transformation. The possibility of right-sided infective endocarditis leading to a paradoxical CNS embolism through a patent foramen ovale (Chapter 69) should not be neglected. Of note, the majority of patients with fungal endocarditis have a CNS embolic event.

Some complications of infective endocarditis are a result of bacteremic seeding causing metastatic infection at a distant site. Patients may present with osteomyelitis, septic arthritis, or epidural abscess. Purulent meningitis (Chapter 420) is a rare complication except in pneumococcal endocarditis, although many patients with *S. aureus* infective endocarditis who undergo lumbar puncture have a pleocytosis. Importantly, the finding of one metastatic complication of infective endocarditis does not exclude the possibility of additional sites of hematogenous infection, particularly in *S. aureus* endocarditis. Thus, the need for additional diagnostic evaluations should be guided by the patient's clinical course. Intracranial abscesses are uncommon in bacterial endocarditis but frequent in *Aspergillus* endocarditis; such a

finding in the setting of culture-negative endocarditis should prompt the consideration of *Aspergillus* as an etiologic agent.

Multiple immunologic phenomena may occur, many of which are directly related to the circulating immune complexes characteristic of the disease. Renal biopsies performed in the setting of active infective endocarditis show some abnormality in nearly all cases. Infective endocarditis classically causes a hypocomplementemic glomerulonephritis. Histopathologically, the glomerular changes may be focal, diffuse, or membranoproliferative, or they may be akin to the immune complex disease found in systemic lupus erythematosus. In addition, many of the musculoskeletal conditions associated with infective endocarditis, including monoarticular and oligoarticular arthritides, are probably immune mediated.

DIAGNOSIS

The "gold standard" for the diagnosis of infective endocarditis is culture of a pathologic organism from a valve or other endocardial surface. However, unless the patient undergoes valve replacement or postmortem examination, the diagnosis is made clinically. As a result, various clinical criteria have been proposed over the years, the most widely accepted of which are the modified Duke criteria (Table 76-4), which have an estimated 76 to 100% sensitivity and 88 to 100% specificity, with a negative predictive value of at least 92%.

TABLE 76-4 MODIFIED DUKE CRITERIA FOR THE DIAGNOSIS OF INFECTIVE ENDOCARDITIS

MAJOR CRITERIA

1. Blood culture positive
   a. Typical organism (α-hemolytic streptococcus, *Streptococcus bovis*, HACEK organisms, or community-acquired *Staphylococcus aureus* or enterococcus without a primary focus) from 2 separate blood cultures
   or
   b. Persistent bacteremia with any organism (2 positive cultures >12 hr apart or 3 positive cultures or a majority of ≥4 cultures positive >1 hr apart)
   or
   c. Bacteremia with *S. aureus*, regardless of whether the bacteremia was nosocomially acquired or whether a removable focus of infection is found
2. Evidence of endocardial involvement
   a. Echocardiographic findings: mobile mass attached to valve or valve apparatus, abscess, or new partial dehiscence of prosthetic valve
   b. New valvular regurgitation
3. Serology: single positive blood culture for *Coxiella burnetii* or antiphase 1 IgG antibody titer >1 : 800

MINOR CRITERIA

1. Predisposing condition: intravenous drug use or predisposing cardiac condition
2. Fever ≥38° C
3. Vascular phenomena: arterial embolism, septic pulmonary emboli, mycotic aneurysm, intracranial hemorrhage, conjunctival hemorrhages, Janeway's lesions
4. Immunologic phenomena: glomerulonephritis, Osler's nodes, Roth's spots, rheumatoid factor
5. Echocardiogram findings consistent with endocarditis but not meeting major criteria
6. Microbiologic evidence: positive blood cultures not meeting major criteria or serologic evidence of active infection consistent with endocarditis

DEFINITIVE INFECTIVE ENDOCARDITIS

1. Pathologically proven infective endocarditis
or
2. Clinical criteria meeting
   a. Two major criteria *or*
   b. One major and one minor criteria *or*
   c. Three minor criteria

POSSIBLE INFECTIVE ENDOCARDITIS

Findings that fall short of definitive infective endocarditis but do not reject it

REJECTED INFECTIVE ENDOCARDITIS

1. Firm alternative diagnosis *or*
2. Resolution of infective endocarditis syndrome with antibiotic therapy for ≤4 days
   or
3. No pathologic evidence of infective endocarditis at surgery or autopsy with antibiotic therapy for ≤4 days

HACEK = *Haemophilus* spp, *Actinobacillus actinomycetemcomitans*, *Cardiobacterium hominis*, *Eikenella corrodens*, and *Kingella* spp; IgG = immunoglobulin G.
Adapted from Li JS, Sexton DJ, Mick N, et al. Proposed modifications to the Duke criteria for the diagnosis of infective endocarditis. *Clin Infect Dis.* 2000;30:633-638.

TABLE 76-5 ORGANISMS CAUSING "CULTURE-NEGATIVE" ENDOCARDITIS*

ORGANISM	EPIDEMIOLOGY	DIAGNOSTIC TESTS
HACEK spp	Mostly oral flora, so often preceded by dental work or history of periodontal disease	Prolonged incubation of standard blood cultures; may need to be subcultured onto blood or chocolate agar
Nutritionally variant streptococci	Slow and indolent course	Supplemented culture media or growth as satellite colonies around *Staphylococcus aureus* streak
Coxiella burnetii (Q fever)	Worldwide; exposure to raw milk, farm environment, or rural areas	Serologic tests (high titers of antibody to both phase 1 and phase 2 antigens); also PCR on blood or valve tissue
Brucella spp	Ingestion of contaminated milk or milk products; close contact with infected livestock	Bulky vegetations usually seen on echocardiography; blood cultures positive in 80% of cases with incubation time of 4-6 wk; lysis-centrifugation technique may expedite growth; serologic tests are available
Bartonella spp	*B. henselae:* transmitted by cat scratch or bite or by cat fleas *B. quintana:* transmitted by human body louse; predisposing factors include homelessness and alcohol abuse	Bulky vegetations usually seen on echocardiography; serologic testing (may cross-react with *Chlamydia* spp); PCR of valve or emboli is best test; lysis-centrifugation technique may be useful
Chlamydia psittaci	Exposure to birds; lawn mowing	Serologic tests available, but must exclude *Bartonella* because of cross-reactivity; monoclonal antibody direct stains on tissue may be useful; PCR now available
Tropheryma whippelii (Whipple's disease)	Systemic symptoms include arthralgias, diarrhea, abdominal pain, lymphadenopathy, weight loss, CNS involvement; however, endocarditis may be present without systemic symptoms	Histologic examination of valve with PAS stain; valve cultures may be done using fibroblast cell lines; PCR on vegetation material
Legionella spp	Contaminated water distribution systems; often nosocomial outbreaks; usually prosthetic valves	Lysis-centrifugation technique; also periodic subcultures onto buffered charcoal yeast extract medium; serologic tests and PCR available
Aspergillus and other noncandidal fungi	Prosthetic valve	Lysis-centrifugation technique; also culture and direct examination of any emboli

*Listed in approximate order of relative frequency.
CNS = central nervous system; HACEK = *Haemophilus* spp, *Actinobacillus actinomycetemcomitans, Cardiobacterium hominis, Eikenella corrodens,* and *Kingella* spp; PAS = periodic acid–Schiff; PCR = polymerase chain reaction.

The Duke criteria rely heavily on the appropriate use of blood cultures and echocardiographic data. At least three sets of blood cultures, with each set consisting of one aerobic and one anaerobic bottle, should be obtained from separate sites, with careful attention to aseptic technique. Ideally, these sets should be collected at least 1 hour apart to document continuous bacteremia; however, when patients are critically ill, this approach may not be feasible.

In most cases of endocarditis, in the absence of prior antibiotic therapy, every blood culture is positive because the bacteremia of endocarditis is continuous. Blood cultures are truly negative in less than 5% of cases of endocarditis; however, prior antibiotic administration may decrease the yield of blood cultures by up to 35%. Accordingly, most "culture-negative" cases of endocarditis occur in patients who have recently received antimicrobial agents. These cases are probably caused by the same organisms responsible for most native valve endocarditis; viridans streptococci and the HACEK organisms are the most likely suspects because they are much more fastidious than staphylococci and enterococci and are therefore more likely to be affected by previous antibiotic administration. Ultimately, however, when blood cultures are negative and endocarditis is suspected, especially when a history of recent antimicrobials is lacking, consideration should be given to fastidious organisms, fungi, and noncultivatable organisms (Table 76-5). This possibility should receive particular attention when the patient's history suggests exposure to farm animals or unpasteurized milk (*Coxiella burnetii, Brucella*), cats (*Bartonella henselae*), or body lice (*Bartonella quintana*) or contact with birds or frequent lawn mowing (*Chlamydia psittaci*). It is important to notify the microbiology laboratory that endocarditis is suspected because special culture techniques can increase the yield for the HACEK species, nutritionally variant streptococci (*Abiotrophia* and *Granulicatella* spp), *Brucella, Legionella,* and some fungi. The traditional practice of "holding" blood cultures for 2 to 4 weeks to investigate culture-negative endocarditis is no longer required routinely. Specific serologic tests can be used to diagnose endocarditis related to *C. burnetii* (the agent of Q fever), *Brucella* species, *Bartonella,* and *C. psittaci. Tropheryma whippelii,* the etiologic agent in Whipple's disease, and multiple other organisms may be diagnosed by polymerase chain reaction. If the search for a causative organism is fruitless, noninfectious causes such as marantic or Libman-Sacks endocarditis and atrial myxoma (Chapter 60) should be considered.

Both transthoracic echocardiography (TTE) and TEE (Chapter 55) are highly specific tests (≈98%) when used as part of the diagnostic evaluation of suspected endocarditis. By contrast, TEE has a sensitivity of 90 to 95% in

this setting, which is significantly better than TTE's usual sensitivity of 48 to 63%. Significant controversy still exists over whether the diagnostic evaluation of suspected infective endocarditis should begin with TTE or TEE. In most cases in which endocarditis is a serious diagnostic consideration, the evaluation should begin with TEE because negative TTE is not sensitive enough to exclude endocarditis (Fig. 76-3). If TEE is unavailable, technically impossible, or considered too invasive by the patient, it is reasonable to begin with TTE.

Some special situations may also dictate whether to begin with TTE or TEE. TEE is the only relatively noninvasive means of detecting perivalvular extension of infection; the esophageal probe's proximity to the aortic root and basal septal wall of the myocardium allows better visualization of these structures, which are most frequently involved in local spread of infection. For this reason, any patient with a new conduction system abnormality or persistent fever—clinical predictors of perivalvular extension—should be evaluated with TEE. Likewise, TEE's heightened sensitivity is especially important in the evaluation of suspected prosthetic valve endocarditis; TEE provides superior definition of prosthetic valve vegetations and valve ring abscesses. Finally, the high sensitivity of TEE in detecting valvular vegetations on native valves may be used in combination with clinical parameters (e.g., prompt resolution of bacteremia and defervescence) to support the clinical decision to abbreviate therapy in patients with vascular catheter–associated *S. aureus* bacteremia.

The combination of negative TTE and negative TEE has a negative predictive value of 95%. Nevertheless, when clinical suspicion of endocarditis is high and the initial TEE is negative, repeat TEE in 7 to 10 days may reveal the diagnosis.

TREATMENT   Rx

Definitive antibiotic treatment of infective endocarditis (Table 76-6) is guided by antimicrobial susceptibility testing of the responsible pathogen isolated from clinical cultures. Although it is often advisable to begin empirical treatment before definitive culture results are available, not all patients admitted to rule out endocarditis need to be treated empirically. Patients who are clinically stable, with a subacute presentation of disease and without evidence of heart failure or other end-organ complications, can be closely observed without antibiotics so that serial blood cultures can be obtained. Likewise, stable patients who were started on empirical antibiotics before

Infective Endocarditis Suspected

*Initial high-risk features include prosthetic heart valves, many congenital heart diseases, previous endocarditis, new murmur, heart failure, or other stigmata of IE.

†High-risk echocardiographic features include large and/or mobile vegetations, valvular insufficiency, suggestions of perivalvular extension, or secondary ventricular dysfunction.

FIGURE 76-3. Algorithm for the diagnostic use of echocardiography in suspected cases of infective endocarditis (IE). TEE = transesophageal echocardiography; TTE = transthoracic echocardiography. (Adapted from Bayer AS, Bolger AF, Taubert KA, et al. Diagnosis and management of infective endocarditis and its complications. *Circulation.* 1998;98:2936-2948.)

hospitalization and before blood was drawn for cultures can discontinue the antibiotics so that blood cultures can be obtained, preferably as long as possible after stopping the antibiotics. By contrast, acutely ill patients, those with evidence of complications of endocarditis, and patients who are at high risk for endocarditis should be treated empirically with antibiotics pending culture results. In most cases of infective endocarditis, it is advisable to seek consultation from an infectious diseases specialist to assist in designing an appropriate antibiotic regimen.

Either of two regimens provides appropriate empirical coverage for patients with suspected native valve endocarditis: nafcillin (or oxacillin)-penicillin-gentamicin or vancomycin-gentamicin (Table 76-7). Nafcillin-penicillin-gentamicin is suitable in most cases of suspected native valve endocarditis, providing optimal coverage for streptococci, staphylococci, enterococci, and HACEK organisms. If MRSA is an important consideration, as it is for injection drug users and those with health care contact, empirical therapy should consist of vancomycin and gentamicin. This regimen is also acceptable for patients with a severe penicillin allergy. Patients with prosthetic valves should be empirically treated with vancomycin, gentamicin, and rifampin for adequate coverage of *S. aureus* (including MRSA), coagulase-negative staphylococci, and gram-negative organisms.

Treatment of Specific Organisms

When the organism is definitively identified, antibiotic treatment must be narrowed accordingly. Standardized regimens have been developed and validated for the most common organisms, and these protocols should be followed assiduously (see Table 76-6). More controversy exists over the treatment of unusual organisms, and consultation with infectious disease specialists is advisable in such circumstances. Of note, these regimens recommend low-dose gentamicin, which reduces the risk of toxicity while providing adequate levels for synergism. In cases in which the risk of aminoglycoside toxicity is significantly increased (e.g., elderly people, patients with preexisting renal disease or hearing impairment, diabetics), exposure to gentamicin should be

minimized or avoided entirely. In fact, for the organisms listed in Table 76-6, gentamicin is critical for cure only in cases of enterococcal endocarditis. As a result, current American Heart Association guidelines classify even low-dose, short-course gentamicin therapy as "optional" for the treatment of native valve *S. aureus* endocarditis. Since the publication of these guidelines, a post hoc analysis of the data from a large randomized trial showed that a decrease in creatinine clearance occurred in 22% of patients receiving initial low-dose gentamicin, compared with 8% of patients not receiving it. Based on these results and on the minimal data supporting its benefit, initial low-dose gentamicin probably should not be used for *S. aureus* bacteremia in patients without prosthetic valves and should not be used for native valve endocarditis except when enterococcal or gram-negative infection is suspected.

In uncomplicated viridans streptococcal endocarditis, outpatient therapy with once-daily ceftriaxone is as effective as more complex regimens, provided the patient has been observed in the hospital for the development of complications.∎ The decision to administer antimicrobial therapy in the outpatient setting must, of course, take into account the patient's social situation, likelihood of compliance, and other risks involved with either an indwelling intravenous line or recurrent peripheral intravenous placement.

Standard therapy for infective endocarditis caused by fully susceptible enterococci includes penicillin or ampicillin plus either streptomycin or gentamicin. Although gentamicin is preferred over streptomycin, the choice of a specific aminoglycoside should be based on in vitro susceptibility testing, and the duration of aminoglycoside therapy can be as short as 2 to 3 weeks in some clinical settings. Although the optimal therapy for infective endocarditis due to ampicillin-sensitive aminoglycoside-resistant enterococci is undefined, in vitro and experimental data suggest the potential efficacy of a combination of ceftriaxone plus ampicillin for such infections.

Optimal therapy for enterococci that are "resistant" (e.g., to aminoglycosides and/or vancomycin) is not well defined. Endocarditis caused by vancomycin-resistant strains of enterococci may be treatable with daptomycin, quinupristin-dalfopristin (7.5 mg/kg intravenously every 8 hours), or linezolid (600 mg

TABLE 76-6 DEFINITIVE THERAPY OF BACTERIAL ENDOCARDITIS

ORGANISM/REGIMEN*	COMMENTS
PCN-SUSCEPTIBLE VIRIDANS STREPTOCOCCI (MIC ≤0.1 µg/mL) AND *STREPTOCOCCUS BOVIS*	
1. PCN 2-3 million units IV q4h × 4 wk	1. Also effective for other PCN-susceptible nonviridans streptococci
2. Ceftriaxone 2 g IV qd × 4 wk	2. Uncomplicated infection with viridans streptococci in a candidate for outpatient therapy; also for those with PCN allergy
3. PCN 2-3 million units IV q4h × 2 wk plus gentamicin 1 mg/kg IV q8h × 2 wk	3. Uncomplicated infection with none of the following features: renal insufficiency, eighth cranial nerve deficit, prosthetic valve infection, CNS complications, severe heart failure, age >65 yr; also not acceptable for nutritionally variant streptococci
4. PCN 2-4 million units IV q4h × 4 wk plus gentamicin 1 mg/kg IV q8h × 2 wk	4. Nutritionally variant strain; for prosthetic valve, give 6 wk of PCN
5. Vancomycin 15-20 mg/kg IV q8-12h × 4 wk	5. For PCN allergy; goal trough level of 15-20 mg/L
RELATIVELY PCN-RESISTANT VIRIDANS STREPTOCOCCI (MIC 0.12-<0.5 µg/mL)	
1. PCN 4 million units IV q4h × 4 wk plus gentamicin 1 mg/kg IV q8h × 2 wk	—
2. Vancomycin 15-20 mg/kg IV q8-12h × 4 wk	2. For PCN allergy or to avoid gentamicin; goal trough level of 15-20 mg/L
ENTEROCOCCI[†] AND PCN-RESISTANT VIRIDANS STREPTOCOCCI (PENICILLIN MIC >0.5 µg/mL)	
1. PCN[‡] 18-30 million units IV per day in divided doses × 4-6 wk or ampicillin 12 g/24 hr IV in 6 equally divided doses plus gentamicin 1 mg/kg IV q8h × 4-6 wk	1. Increase duration of both drugs to 6 wk for prosthetic valve infection or symptoms >3 mo in enterococcal infection
2. Vancomycin 15-20 mg/kg IV q8-12h × 6 wk plus gentamicin 1 mg/kg IV q8h × 6 wk[§]	2. For PCN allergy; PCN desensitization is also an option; high risk of nephrotoxicity with this regimen
STAPHYLOCOCCUS AUREUS	
1. Nafcillin 2 g IV q4h × 4-6 wk with optional addition of gentamicin 1 mg/kg IV q8h × 3-5 days	1. Methicillin-susceptible strain; omit gentamicin if significant renal insufficiency
2. Vancomycin 15-20 mg/kg IV q8-12h × 6 wk	2. PCN allergy (immediate hypersensitivity or anaphylaxis) or MRSA
3. Nafcillin 2 g IV q4h × 2 wk plus gentamicin 1 mg/kg IV q8h × 2 wk	3. Methicillin-susceptible strain; 2-wk regimen only for use in IV drug abusers with only tricuspid valve infection, no renal insufficiency, and no extrapulmonary infection
4. Nafcillin 2 g IV q4h × >6 wk plus gentamicin 1 mg/kg IV q8h × 2 wk plus rifampin 300 mg PO/IV q8h × ≥6 wk	4. Prosthetic valve infection with methicillin-susceptible strain; use vancomycin instead of nafcillin for MRSA
5. Cefazolin 2 g IV q8h × 4-6 wk with optional addition of gentamicin 1 mg/kg IV q8h × 3-5 days	5. PCN allergy other than immediate hypersensitivity
6. Daptomycin 6 mg/kg IV qd × 14-42 days	Daptomycin is FDA-approved for treatment of right-sided *S. aureus* infective endocarditis; for adults, some experts recommend 8-10 mg/kg IV
COAGULASE-NEGATIVE STAPHYLOCOCCI, PROSTHETIC VALVE INFECTION	
Vancomycin 15-20 mg/kg IV q8-12h × >6 wk plus gentamicin 1 mg/kg IV q8h × 2 wk plus rifampin 300 mg PO/IV q8h × >6 wk	Can substitute nafcillin in above doses for vancomycin if isolate is methicillin sensitive
HACEK STRAINS	
1. Ceftriaxone 2 g IV qd × 4 wk; 6 wk for prosthetic valves	—
2. Ampicillin-sulbactam 3 g IV q6h × 4 wk; 6 wk for prosthetic valves	2. HACEK strains increasingly may produce β-lactamase
NON-HACEK GRAM-NEGATIVE BACILLI	
Enterobacteriaceae	
Extended-spectrum PCN or cephalosporin plus aminoglycosides for susceptible strains	Treat for a minimum of 6-8 wk; some species exhibit inducible resistance to third-generation cephalosporins; valve surgery is required for most patients with left-sided endocarditis caused by gram-negative bacilli; consultation with a specialist in infectious diseases is recommended
Pseudomonas aeruginosa	
High-dose tobramycin (8 mg/kg/day IV or IM in once-daily doses) with maintenance of peak and trough concentrations of 15 to 20 µg/mL and ≤2 µg/mL, respectively, in combination with an extended-spectrum penicillin (e.g., ticarcillin, piperacillin, azlocillin); ceftazidime, cefepime, or imipenem in full doses; or imipenem	Treat for a minimum of 6-8 wk; early valve surgery usually required for left-sided *Pseudomonas* endocarditis; consultation with a specialist in infectious diseases is recommended
Fungi	
Treatment with a parenteral antifungal agent (usually an amphotericin B–containing product) and valve replacement	Long-term/lifelong suppressive therapy with oral antifungal agents often required; consultation with a specialist in infectious diseases is recommended

*Dosages are for patients with normal renal function; for those with renal insufficiency, adjustments must be made for all drugs except nafcillin, rifampin, and ceftriaxone. Gentamicin doses should be adjusted to achieve a peak serum concentration of approximately 3 µg/mL 30 min after dosing and a trough gentamicin level of <1 µg/mL.

[†]Enterococci must be tested for antimicrobial susceptibility. These recommendations are for enterococci sensitive to PCN, gentamicin, and vancomycin.

[‡]Ampicillin 12 g/day can be used instead of PCN.

[§]The need to add an aminoglycoside has not been demonstrated for PCN-resistant streptococci.

HACEK = *Haemophilus* spp, *Actinobacillus actinomycetemcomitans*, *Cardiobacterium hominis*, *Eikenella corrodens*, and *Kingella* spp; MIC = minimum inhibitory concentration; MRSA = methicillin-resistant *Staphylococcus aureus*; PCN = penicillin.

Adapted from Baddour LM, Wilson WR, Bayer AS, et al. Infective endocarditis: diagnosis, antimicrobial therapy, and management of complications. *Circulation*. 2005;111:e394-e433.

TABLE 76-7 EMPIRICAL TREATMENT OF ENDOCARDITIS

CHARACTERISTICS OF PATIENTS	TREATMENT REGIMEN*
Native valve, community-acquired infection, MRSA unlikely	Nafcillin 2 g IV q4h plus penicillin 4 million units IV q4h plus gentamicin 1 mg/kg IV q8h
Any of the following: health care–associated infection or other reason to suspect MRSA; severe penicillin allergy	Vancomycin 15-20 mg/kg IV q8-12h[†] plus gentamicin 1 mg/kg IV q8h
Prosthetic valve	Vancomycin 15-20 mg/kg IV q8-12h[†] plus gentamicin 1 mg/kg IV q8h plus rifampin 300 mg PO/IV q8h

*Dosages are for patients with normal renal function; for those with renal insufficiency, adjustments must be made for all drugs except nafcillin.
[†]Goal is trough level of 15-20 mg/L.
MRSA = methicillin-resistant *Staphylococcus aureus*.

orally or intravenously twice daily); however, clinical experience with these agents is limited. In this situation, relapse or failure rates are likely to be high, and many cases require surgical intervention (discussed later).

Data suggest that patients with MRSA endocarditis treated with vancomycin have higher rates of bacteriologic failure than those treated with nafcillin. Therefore, every attempt should be made to treat MRSA endocarditis with an antistaphylococcal β-lactam. In a recent randomized trial, daptomycin 6 mg/kg/day for 10 to 42 days, depending on the severity of infection, was as effective as either semisynthetic antistaphylococcal penicillin or vancomycin for the treatment of *S. aureus* bacteremia and right-sided infective endocarditis,[2] and it is approved by the Food and Drug Administration for these indications.

Fungal endocarditis is usually a consequence of extensive health care contact. Traditionally, fungal endocarditis was regarded as an indication for valvular surgery, and amphotericin B (Chapter 339) was considered the treatment of choice. However, the high mortality associated with fungal endocarditis and the availability of new classes of antifungals suggest that these principles should be re-evaluated. The management of fungal endocarditis should always involve the collaboration of an experienced infectious diseases specialist.

Zoonotic endocarditis is usually culture-negative and most commonly caused by *Bartonella* species (Chapter 323), *C. burnetii* (Chapter 335), or *Brucella* species (Chapter 318). The treatments of choice for these fastidious pathogens are based on limited data, but documented *Bartonella* endocarditis is treated with doxycycline for 6 weeks and gentamicin for 2 weeks.

In cases of presumed culture-negative endocarditis in which unusual organisms (see Table 76-5) and other infections have been reasonably excluded, an empirical course of treatment may be undertaken. In this situation, most authorities recommend a 4- to 6-week regimen of ceftriaxone alone, vancomycin-ceftriaxone, or vancomycin-gentamicin (if the clinical setting suggests enterococci).

Continuing Care of the Patient with Endocarditis

In addition to antibiotics, appropriate inpatient care includes careful surveillance for the development of complications. Repeat echocardiography, as clinically indicated in the acute setting and at the end of antibiotic therapy, and serial ECGs should be obtained to look for the development of conduction system disease that might herald perivalvular extension, especially in patients with prosthetic valves and persistent fever. Widening pulse pressure should alert the clinician to the possible development of acute aortic insufficiency (Chapter 75). Similarly, a careful cardiac examination should be performed on a daily basis to assess for new regurgitant murmurs. Any new neurologic findings should prompt a search for evidence of CNS complications such as embolic events, cerebral hemorrhage, mycotic aneurysm, and brain abscess. Renal function should be closely monitored so that antibiotic doses can be adjusted, if necessary. If gentamicin is used for more than a few days, the patient should be alerted to watch for the signs and symptoms of vestibular or otic toxicity. Audiometric testing at baseline and periodically thereafter should be considered in patients at high risk for aminoglycoside-induced ototoxicity, including the elderly, patients with preexisting renal dysfunction or hearing damage, and patients receiving prolonged courses of gentamicin. Serum gentamicin trough concentrations should also be assayed at regular intervals (e.g., twice weekly, and more often if renal function is changing) and should be less than 1 μg/mL; higher concentrations should lead to lower or less frequent dosing or both. Follow-up blood cultures may be indicated toward the end of the first week of therapy in patients whose infective endocarditis is caused by organisms that commonly fail first-line treatment, such as *S. aureus* and enterococci. Positive cultures in this setting might suggest the need to change therapy or intervene surgically, whereas negative cultures are reassuring.

Patients with infective endocarditis may continue to be febrile for some time after the institution of appropriate antibiotic treatment. About 50% of patients defervesce within 3 days of starting antibiotics, 75% by 1 week, and 90% by 2 weeks. Patients whose endocarditis is caused by *S. aureus,* gram-negative organisms, or fungi tend to defervesce more slowly than patients infected with other organisms. Prolonged fever (>1 week after the institution of appropriate antibiotics) should prompt repeat blood cultures. If such cultures are negative, several possibilities should be considered: myocardial abscess, extracardiac infection (e.g., mycotic aneurysm, psoas or splenic abscess, vertebral osteomyelitis, septic arthritis), immune complex–mediated tissue damage, or a complication of hospitalization and therapy (e.g., drug fever, nosocomial superinfection, pulmonary embolism). Appropriate studies might include TEE, computed tomography of the abdomen, bone scan, and urinalysis with microscopy (to elicit evidence of interstitial nephritis). Intravenous line sites should be carefully examined for evidence of infection, and indwelling central lines should be changed.

Anticoagulation in individuals with infective endocarditis is controversial. Although new anticoagulation in the setting of native valve endocarditis does not appear to provide a benefit, continuing ongoing anticoagulation may be advisable. Some authorities recommend continuing anticoagulation in patients with mechanical prosthetic valve endocarditis. However, discontinuation of all anticoagulation for at least the first 2 weeks of antibiotic therapy is generally advised in patients with *S. aureus* prosthetic valve endocarditis who have experienced a recent CNS embolic event; this allows the thrombus to organize and potentially prevents the acute hemorrhagic transformation of embolic lesions. Reintroduction of anticoagulation in these patients must be cautious, and the international normalized ratio must be monitored carefully. The best option for patients with other indications for anticoagulation, such as deep venous thrombosis, major vessel embolization, or atrial fibrillation, is less clear and should be decided in a multidisciplinary fashion that balances the risks and benefits for each individual patient. Aspirin does not prevent embolic events and tends to increase the incidence of bleeding.[3]

Surgery

Some patients require surgical treatment, either to cure infective endocarditis or to prevent death from it (Table 76-8). Most patients with evidence of direct extension of infection to myocardial structures, prosthetic valve dysfunction, or heart failure from endocarditis-induced valvular damage should undergo surgery. In addition, many cases of endocarditis caused by fungi or by gram-negative or resistant organisms (e.g., vancomycin- or gentamicin-resistant enterococci) require surgical management. Progression of disease or persistence of fever and bacteremia for more than 7 to 10 days in the presence of appropriate antibiotic therapy may indicate the need for surgery; however, a thorough search must first be conducted to exclude other foci of infection. Surgical management should also be considered for patients with recurrent (two or more) embolic events or those with large vegetations (>10 mm) on echocardiography and one embolic event, although the data in these situations are less convincing. The presence of *S. aureus* endocarditis involving the anterior mitral valve leaflet and large vegetations (>10 mm) may be a special circumstance calling for early surgical intervention to reduce the high risk of CNS emboli, especially when mitral valve repair, rather than valve replacement, can be accomplished.

Delaying surgery in patients with deteriorating cardiac function in an attempt to "sterilize" the affected valve is ill advised because the risk of progressive heart failure or further complications usually outweighs the relatively small risk of recurrent infective endocarditis after prosthetic valve implantation. Relative contraindications to valve replacement include recent CNS emboli or bleed (because of the risk of bleeding in the perioperative period, when anticoagulation is required), multiple prior valve replacements (because of the difficulty of sewing a new valve into tissue already weakened from previous surgeries), and ongoing injection drug use. On occasion, patients have both a compelling indication for valve replacement (e.g., acute heart failure) and a recent CNS embolic event. The risk of hemorrhagic transformation of such lesions during cardiac bypass–associated anticoagulation is controversial. However, it appears that the greatest risk of such transformation events is in larger (>2 cm) emboli, especially those that have exhibited a hemorrhagic component. In these latter scenarios, it is prudent to try to delay surgery for at least 2 to 4 weeks to allow organization and resolution of such emboli. It appears that valve replacement can be performed safely without such delays in patients with smaller, nonhemorrhagic CNS emboli.

After definitive surgical treatment, most patients should receive further antibiotic therapy unless a full course of antibiotics was administered before surgery and there is no evidence of ongoing infection. If the patient received antibiotics for less than 1 week before surgery or the culture from the operative site is positive, the patient should receive the equivalent of a full initial course of antibiotics appropriate for the organism. If the patient received antibiotics for 2 weeks or more and the culture from the operative site is negative, the patient should receive whatever remains of the originally planned course of appropriate antibiotic therapy.

TABLE 76-8 INDICATIONS FOR SURGERY IN ENDOCARDITIS

INDICATION	CLASS*
NATIVE VALVE ENDOCARDITIS	
Acute aortic insufficiency or mitral regurgitation with heart failure	I
Acute aortic insufficiency with tachycardia and early closure of the mitral valve on echocardiogram	I
Fungal endocarditis	I
Evidence of annular or aortic abscess, sinus or aortic true or false aneurysm, valvular dehiscence, rupture, perforation, or fistula	I
Evidence of valve dysfunction and persistent infection after a prolonged period (7-10 days) of appropriate therapy, provided there are no noncardiac causes for infection	I
Recurrent emboli after appropriate antibiotic therapy	I
Infection with gram-negative organisms or organisms with a poor response to antibiotics in patients with evidence of valve dysfunction	I
Anterior mitral leaflet vegetation (especially with size >10 mm) or persistent vegetation after systemic embolization	IIa
Increase in vegetation size despite appropriate antimicrobial therapy	IIb
Early infections of the mitral valve that can probably be repaired	III
Persistent fever and leukocytosis with negative blood cultures	III
PROSTHETIC VALVE ENDOCARDITIS	
Early prosthetic valve endocarditis (<2 mo after surgery)	I
Heart failure with prosthetic valve dysfunction	I
Nonstreptococcal endocarditis	I
Evidence of perivalvular leak, annular or aortic abscess, sinus or aortic true or false aneurysm, fistula formation, or new-onset conduction disturbances	I
Persistent bacteremia after 7-10 days of appropriate antibiotic therapy, with no noncardiac causes for bacteremia	IIa
Recurrent peripheral embolus despite therapy	IIa
Vegetation of any size seen on or near the prosthesis	IIb

*Class I = conditions for which there is evidence and/or general agreement that a given procedure or treatment is useful and effective; class II = conditions for which there is conflicting evidence and/or a divergence of opinion about the usefulness or efficacy of a procedure or treatment; class IIa = weight of evidence or opinion is in favor of usefulness or efficacy; class IIb = usefulness or efficacy is less well established by evidence or opinion; class III = conditions for which there is evidence and/or general agreement that the procedure or treatment is not useful and in some cases may be harmful.

Adapted with permission from Bonow RO, Carabello B, de Leon AC, et al. Guidelines for the management of patients with valvular heart disease. *Circulation.* 1998;98:1949-1984.

TABLE 76-9 HIGH-RISK CARDIAC CONDITIONS FOR WHICH ENDOCARDITIS PROPHYLAXIS WITH DENTAL PROCEDURES IS REASONABLE

Prosthetic cardiac valve or prosthetic material used for cardiac valve repair

Previous endocarditis

Complex congenital heart disease involving unrepaired cyanotic congenital heart disease (including palliative shunts and conduits), completely repaired congenital heart disease with prosthetic material within 6 mo of the procedure, or repaired congenital heart disease with residual defects at the site or adjacent to the site of prosthetic material

Cardiac transplantation recipients who develop cardiac valvulopathy

Adapted from Wilson W, Taubert KA, Gewitz M, et al. Prevention of infective endocarditis guidelines from the American Heart Association: a guideline from the American Heart Association Rheumatic Fever, Endocarditis, and Kawasaki Disease Committee, Council on Cardiovascular Disease in the Young, and the Council on Clinical Cardiology, Council on Cardiovascular Surgery and Anesthesia, and the Quality of Care and Outcomes Research Interdisciplinary Working Group. *Circulation.* 2007;116:1736-1754.

TABLE 76-10 RECOMMENDATIONS FOR ENDOCARDITIS PROPHYLAXIS

PROPHYLAXIS IS REASONABLE*

Dental: All dental procedures involving manipulation of gingival tissue or the periapical region of teeth or perforation of the oral mucosa

Respiratory: Procedures involving incision or biopsy of the respiratory mucosa, such as tonsillectomy and adenoidectomy

Other: Infected skin, skin structures, or musculoskeletal tissue

PROPHYLAXIS IS NOT RECOMMENDED

Dental: Routine anesthetic injections through noninfected tissue, dental radiographs, placement of removable prosthodontic or orthodontic appliances, adjustment of orthodontic appliances, placement of orthodontic brackets, shedding of deciduous teeth, bleeding from trauma to the lips or oral mucosa

Respiratory: Procedures not involving incision or biopsy of the respiratory mucosa, including bronchoscopy (unless the procedure involves incision of the respiratory tract mucosa)

Genitourinary: Antibiotic prophylaxis solely to prevent infective endocarditis is not recommended

Gastrointestinal: Antibiotic prophylaxis solely to prevent infective endocarditis is not recommended

*Only in patients with underlying cardiac conditions associated with the highest risk for adverse outcome from endocarditis (listed in Table 76-9).

Adapted from Wilson W, Taubert KA, Gewitz M, et al. Prevention of infective endocarditis guidelines from the American Heart Association: a guideline from the American Heart Association Rheumatic Fever, Endocarditis, and Kawasaki Disease Committee, Council on Cardiovascular Disease in the Young, and the Council on Clinical Cardiology, Council on Cardiovascular Surgery and Anesthesia, and the Quality of Care and Outcomes Research Interdisciplinary Working Group. *Circulation.* 2007;116:1736-1754.

PREVENTION

Although the administration of prophylactic antibiotics to patients with known risk factors for infective endocarditis before undergoing procedures known to cause bacteremia is widespread, the efficacy of this practice has not been established. In 2007 the American Heart Association substantially reduced the situations in which prophylactic antibiotics were recommended. These revised recommendations were based on the following points: (1) endocarditis is much more likely to result from frequent exposure to random bacteremias associated with daily activities than from bacteremia caused by a dental, gastrointestinal tract, or genitourinary tract procedure; (2) prophylaxis may prevent an exceedingly small number of infective endocarditis cases, if any, in individuals who undergo dental, gastrointestinal tract, or genitourinary tract procedures; (3) the risk of antibiotic-associated adverse events often exceeds the benefit, if any, from prophylactic antibiotic therapy; and (4) maintenance of optimal oral health may reduce the incidence of bacteremia from daily activities and is more important than prophylactic antibiotics for a dental procedure to reduce the risk of infective endocarditis.

Prophylaxis is now judged to be reasonable for patients with the highest risk of adverse outcomes from endocarditis (Table 76-9) who must undergo dental procedures that involve manipulation of gingival tissue or the periapical region of teeth or perforation of the oral mucosa; an invasive procedure of the respiratory tract that involves incision or biopsy of the respiratory mucosa, such as tonsillectomy and adenoidectomy; or invasive procedures involving infected skin, skin structures, or musculoskeletal tissue (Table 76-10). The new recommendations focus on single-dose oral regimens in most clinical scenarios.

The antibiotics chosen for pre-procedure prophylaxis should be active against the organisms most likely to be released into the blood stream by the procedure (Table 76-11). Antibiotics that cover primarily oral flora are recommended. For patients with the conditions listed in Table 76-9 who undergo a procedure for infected skin, skin structure, or musculoskeletal tissue, it may be reasonable that the therapeutic regimen administered to treat the infection contain an agent active against staphylococci and β-hemolytic streptococci.

PROGNOSIS

Untreated, infective endocarditis is uniformly fatal. Aggressive medical and surgical management, however, has dramatically improved the outcome. Mortality overall from both native and prosthetic valve endocarditis remains fairly high, ranging from 17 to 36%. Certain subgroups carry a lower risk of death (endocarditis related to viridans streptococci), whereas *S. aureus*, fungal, and zoonotic endocarditis have higher mortalities. Heart failure and CNS events are the most frequent causes of death.

Endocarditis recurs in 12 to 16% of patients and is more common in injection drug users, elderly people, and patients with prosthetic valves. The rate

TABLE 76-11	SUGGESTED ANTIBIOTICS FOR ENDOCARDITIS PROPHYLAXIS FOR DENTAL OR RESPIRATORY TRACT PROCEDURES* IN PATIENTS WITH HIGH-RISK CARDIAC CONDITIONS†
PATIENT CHARACTERISTICS	**REGIMEN‡**
Able to take oral medications	Amoxicillin 2 g PO
Unable to take oral medications	Ampicillin 2 g IV or IM; or cefazolin or ceftriaxone 1 g IM or IV
Allergic to penicillin or ampicillin and able to take oral medications	Cephalexin 2 g PO (or other first- or second-generation oral cephalosporin in equivalent adult doses); clindamycin 600 mg PO; azithromycin 500 mg PO; or clarithromycin 500 mg PO Cephalosporins should not be used in an individual with a history of anaphylaxis, angioedema, or urticaria with penicillin or ampicillin
Allergic to penicillin or ampicillin and unable to take oral medications	Cefazolin or ceftriaxone 1 g IM or IV; or clindamycin 600 mg IM or IV

*For the applicable procedures, see Table 76-10.
†For the applicable conditions, see Table 76-9.
‡All regimens consist of a single dose 30-60 min before the procedure.
Adapted from Wilson W, Taubert KA, Gewitz M, et al. Prevention of infective endocarditis guidelines from the American Heart Association: a guideline from the American Heart Association Rheumatic Fever, Endocarditis, and Kawasaki Disease Committee, Council on Cardiovascular Disease in the Young, and the Council on Clinical Cardiology, Council on Cardiovascular Surgery and Anesthesia, and the Quality of Care and Outcomes Research Interdisciplinary Working Group. *Circulation.* 2007;116:1736-1754.

of relapse also varies depending on the causative organism. Easily treated infections, such as those with α-hemolytic streptococci, have a low rate of relapse (5%), whereas more difficult to eradicate organisms may have significantly higher rates.

FUTURE DIRECTIONS

As cardiac imaging technology continues to improve, the duration of treatment of endocarditis may be dictated in part by the characteristics of visualized vegetations. In addition, now that large vegetations have been demonstrated to cause more embolic events, interventions to remove vegetations (e.g., valve repair, vegectomy) or to introduce agents that prevent the formation or promote the dissolution of vegetations may be feasible. Finally, novel therapeutic approaches (e.g., antibacterial antibodies and cell wall–specific enzymes) that act as adjuncts to antibiotics in facilitating bacteriologic clearance are currently in development.

 Grade A

1. Sexton DJ, Tenenbaum MJ, Wilson WR, et al. Ceftriaxone once daily for four weeks compared with ceftriaxone plus gentamicin once daily for two weeks for treatment of endocarditis due to penicillin-susceptible streptococci. Endocarditis Treatment Consortium Group. *Clin Infect Dis.* 1998;27:1470-1474.
2. Fowler VG Jr, Boucher HW, Corey GR, et al. Daptomycin versus standard therapy for *Staphylococcus aureus* bacteremia and endocarditis. *N Engl J Med.* 2006;355:653-665.
3. Chan KL, Dumesnil JG, Cujec B, et al. A randomized trial of aspirin on the risk of embolic events in patients with infective endocarditis. *J Am Coll Cardiol.* 2003;42:775-780.

SUGGESTED READINGS

Prendergast BD, Tornos P. Surgery for infective endocarditis: who and when? *Circulation.* 2010;121:1141-1152. *Review.*
Snygg-Martin U, Rasmussen RV, Hassager C, et al. Warfarin therapy and incidence of cerebrovascular complications in left-sided native valve endocarditis. *Eur J Clin Microbiol Infect Dis.* 2011;30:151-157. *Data suggesting that patients with native valve endocarditis who are already taking and continue warfarin anticoagulation have fewer cerebrovascular complications than patients who are not.*
Tissari P, Zumla A, Tarkka E, et al. Accurate and rapid identification of bacterial species from positive blood cultures with DNA-based microarray platform: an observational study. *Lancet.* 2010;375:224-230. *The DNA-based microarray platform is more sensitive and faster than the culture-based method.*

77

PERICARDIAL DISEASES

WILLIAM C. LITTLE AND JAE K. OH

The pericardium, which is a relatively avascular fibrous sac that surrounds the heart, has two layers: the visceral and parietal pericardium. The potential space between the two layers normally contains only 10 to 50 mL of fluid, which is an ultrafiltrate of plasma. The pericardium is well innervated, so pericardial inflammation may produce severe pain and trigger vagally mediated reflexes.

As a result of its relatively inelastic physical properties, the pericardium limits acute cardiac dilation and enhances mechanical interactions of the cardiac chambers. In response to long-standing stress, the pericardium dilates to allow a slowly accumulating pericardial effusion to become quite large without compressing the cardiac chambers and to allow left ventricular remodeling to occur without pericardial constriction. Conversely, a scarred or thickened pericardium can limit the filling of the heart, resulting in pericardial constriction. Despite the important functions of the normal pericardium, congenital absence or surgical resection of the pericardium does not appear to have any major untoward effects.

ACUTE PERICARDITIS

EPIDEMIOLOGY AND PATHOBIOLOGY

Acute inflammation of the pericardium, with or without an associated pericardial effusion, can occur as an isolated clinical problem or as a manifestation of systemic disease. Although about 85% of isolated cases of acute pericarditis are idiopathic or viral, the list of other potential causes is quite extensive (Table 77-1). Patients with fever greater than 38° C or a subacute course or who fail to respond promptly to therapy are most likely to have pericarditis caused by a systemic autoimmune disease, malignancy, or viral or bacterial infection.

Pericarditis can occur after an acute myocardial infarction (MI). It occurs 1 to 3 days after a transmural MI, presumably owing to the interaction between the healing necrotic epicardium and the overlying pericardium. Dressler's syndrome, which is another form of pericarditis associated with MI, typically occurs weeks to months after MI. It is similar to the pericarditis that can occur days to months following traumatic pericardial injury, surgical manipulation of the pericardium, or pulmonary infarction. This syndrome is presumed to be mediated by an autoimmune mechanism and is associated with signs of systemic inflammation, including fever and polyserositis.

CLINICAL MANIFESTATIONS

Most patients with acute pericarditis experience sharp retrosternal chest pain (see Table 50-2 in Chapter 50), which can be quite severe and debilitating. In some cases, however, pericarditis is asymptomatic, such as when it accompanies rheumatoid arthritis. Pericardial pain is usually worse with inspiration and when supine, and it is generally relieved by sitting and leaning forward. Typically, pericardial pain is referred to the scapular ridge, presumably owing to irritation of the phrenic nerves, which pass adjacent to the pericardium. The chest pain of acute pericarditis must be differentiated from pulmonary embolism and myocardial ischemia or infarction (Table 77-2).

The pericardial friction rub is the classic finding in patients with acute pericarditis. A friction rub is a high-pitched, scratchy sound that can have one, two, or three components occurring when the cardiac volumes are most rapidly changing: during ventricular ejection, during rapid ventricular filling in early diastole, and during atrial systole. A pericardial rub, which is differentiated from a murmur by its scratchy quality, is sometimes localized to a small area on the chest wall and may come and go spontaneously or with changes in position. To hear a rub, it may be necessary to auscultate the heart with the patient in multiple positions, especially using the diaphragm with the patient learning forward and not breathing. The pericardial friction rub must be differentiated from a pleural rub, which is absent during suspended respiration, whereas the pericardial rub is unaffected.

DIAGNOSIS

Early in the course of acute pericarditis, the electrocardiogram (ECG) typically displays diffuse ST elevation in association with PR depression (Fig. 77-1). The ST elevation is usually present in all leads except for aVR, but the

TABLE 77-1   CAUSES OF PERICARDITIS: INFECTIOUS AND NONINFECTIOUS

INFECTIOUS PERICARDITIS (⅔ OF CASES)

Viral (most common): echovirus and coxsackievirus (usual), influenza, EBV, CMV, adenovirus, varicella, rubella, mumps, HBV, HCV, HIV, parvovirus B19, human herpesvirus 6 (increasing reports)

Bacterial: tuberculosis (4-5%)* and *Coxiella burnetii* (most common); other bacterial causes (rare) include pneumococcosis, meningococcosis, gonococcosis, *Haemophilus*, staphylococci, chlamydia, *Mycoplasma, Legionella, Leptospira, Listeria*

Fungal (rare): histoplasmosis more likely in immunocompetent patients; aspergillosis, blastomycosis, candidiasis more likely in immunosuppressed patients

Parasitic (very rare): *Echinococcus, Toxoplasma*

NONINFECTIOUS PERICARDITIS (⅓ OF CASES)

Autoimmune pericarditis (<10%)*
  Pericardial injury syndromes: post–myocardial infarction syndrome, post-pericardiotomy syndrome, post-traumatic pericarditis, including iatrogenic pericarditis (e.g., after percutaneous coronary interventions, pacemaker insertion, ablation)
  Pericarditis in systemic autoimmune and autoinflammatory diseases: more common in systemic lupus erythematosus, Sjögren's syndrome, rheumatoid arthritis, systemic sclerosis, systemic vasculitides, Behçet's syndrome, sarcoidosis, familial Mediterranean fever
  Autoreactive pericarditis*
Neoplastic pericarditis (5-7%)*
  Primary tumors (rare): pericardial mesothelioma
  Secondary metastatic tumors (common): lung and breast cancer, lymphoma
Metabolic pericarditis: uremia, myxedema (common); others rare
Traumatic pericarditis (rare)
  Direct injury: penetrating thoracic injury, esophageal perforation, iatrogenic
  Indirect injury: nonpenetrating thoracic injury, radiation injury
Drug-related pericarditis (rare): procainamide, hydralazine, isoniazid, and phenytoin (lupus-like syndrome), penicillins (hypersensitivity pericarditis with eosinophilia), doxorubicin, and daunorubicin (often associated with cardiomyopathy; may cause pericardiopathy)

*Percentages refer to unselected cases.
The diagnosis of autoreactive pericarditis is established using the following criteria: (1) increased number of lymphocytes and mononuclear cells >5000/mm³ (autoreactive lymphocytic) or the presence of antibodies against heart muscle tissue (antisarcolemmal) in the pericardial fluid (autoreactive antibody mediated); (2) signs of myocarditis on epicardial or endomyocardial biopsies by ≥14 cells/mm²; and (3) exclusion of infections, neoplasia, and systemic and metabolic disorders.
CMV = cytomegalovirus; EBV = Epstein-Barr virus; HBV = hepatitis B virus; HCV = hepatitis C virus; HIV = human immunodeficiency virus.
From Imazio M, Spodick DH, Brucato A, et al. Controversial issues in the management of pericardial diseases. *Circulation.* 2010;121:916-928.

TABLE 77-2   DIFFERENTIATION OF PERICARDITIS FROM MYOCARDIAL ISCHEMIA OR INFARCTION AND PULMONARY EMBOLISM

FINDINGS	MYOCARDIAL ISCHEMIA OR INFARCTION	PERICARDITIS	PULMONARY EMBOLISM
CHEST PAIN			
Character	Pressure-like heavy, squeezing	Sharp, stabbing, occasionally dull	Sharp, stabbing
Change with respiration	No	Worsened with inspiration	In phase with respiration (absent when the patient is apneic)
Change with position	No	Worse when supine; improved when sitting up or leaning forward	No
Duration	Minutes (ischemia); hours (infarction)	Hours to days	Hours to days
Response to nitroglycerin	Improved	No change	No change
PHYSICAL EXAMINATION			
Friction rub	Absent (unless pericarditis is present)	Present in most patients	Pleural friction rub may occur
ELECTROCARDIOGRAM			
ST segment elevation	Localized convex	Widespread concave	Limited to leads III, aVF, and V₁
PR segment depression	Rare	Frequent	None

Modified from Little WC, Freeman GL. Pericardial disease. *Circulation.* 2006;113:1622-1632.

FIGURE 77-1. Electrocardiogram demonstrating typical features of acute pericarditis on presentation. There is diffuse ST elevation and PR depression except in aVR, where there is ST depression and PR elevation.

changes may be more localized in post-MI pericarditis. Classically, the ECG changes of acute pericarditis evolve over several days; resolution of the ST elevation is followed by widespread T wave inversion that subsequently normalizes. Uremic pericarditis frequently occurs without the typical electrocardiographic abnormalities.

Patients with acute pericarditis usually have evidence of systemic inflammation, including leukocytosis, an elevated erythrocyte sedimentation rate, and increased C-reactive protein level. A low-grade fever is common, but a temperature greater than 38° C is unusual and suggests the possibility of bacterial pericarditis.

About 85% of cases of acute pericarditis are idiopathic or viral. Viral causes include echoviruses and group B coxsackieviruses, but obtaining specific viral titers does not alter patient management. About 6% of cases are neoplastic in origin, about 4% are caused by tuberculosis, about 3% are caused by other bacterial or fungal infections, and about 2% are caused by collagen vascular disease. A targeted evaluation (Table 77-3) can help identify the various causes (Table 77-4).

Troponin levels typically are minimally elevated in acute pericarditis owing to some involvement of the epicardium by the inflammatory process. An elevated troponin level in acute pericarditis usually returns to normal within 1 to 2 weeks and is not associated with a worse prognosis. Although the elevated troponin level may lead to the misdiagnosis of an ST elevation MI (Chapter 73), most patients with elevated troponin levels and acute pericarditis have normal coronary angiograms. An echocardiogram (Chapter 55) can help avoid a misdiagnosis of MI.

Echocardiography may demonstrate a small pericardial effusion in the presence of acute pericarditis, but a normal echocardiogram does not exclude the diagnosis of acute pericarditis. An echocardiogram is critical, however, in excluding the diagnosis of cardiac tamponade (see later). When the diagnosis of acute pericarditis is unclear, cardiac magnetic resonance imaging (MRI) can demonstrate pericardial inflammation as delayed enhancement of the pericardium (Fig. 77-2). Diagnostic pericardiocentesis is indicated in suspected purulent tuberculosis or malignant pericarditis or if the patient has cardiac tamponade.

TABLE 77-3 SELECTED DIAGNOSTIC TESTS IN ACUTE PERICARDITIS

IN ALL PATIENTS

Tuberculin skin test (plus control skin test to exclude anergy)
BUN and creatinine to exclude uremia
Erythrocyte sedimentation rate
Electrocardiogram
Chest radiograph
Echocardiogram

IN SELECTED PATIENTS

Cardiac magnetic resonance imaging
ANA and rheumatoid factor to exclude systemic lupus erythematosus or rheumatoid arthritis in patients with acute arthritis or pleural effusion
TSH and T_4 to exclude hypothyroidism in patients with clinical findings suggestive of hypothyroidism and in asymptomatic patients with unexplained pericardial effusion
HIV test to exclude AIDS in patients with risk factors for HIV disease or a compatible clinical syndrome
Blood cultures in febrile patients to exclude infective endocarditis and bacteremia
Fungal serologic tests in patients from endemic areas or in immunocompromised patients
ASO titer in children or teenagers with suspected rheumatic fever
Heterophil antibody test to exclude mononucleosis in young or middle-aged patients with a compatible clinical syndrome or acute fever, weakness, and lymphadenopathy

AIDS = acquired immunodeficiency virus; ANA = antinuclear antibody; ASO = antistreptolysin O; BUN = blood urea nitrogen; HIV = human immunodeficiency virus; T_4 = thyroxine; TSH = thyroid-stimulating hormone.
Modified from Nishimura RA, Kidd KR. Recognition and management of patients with pericardial disease. In: Braunwald E, Goldman L, eds. *Primary Cardiology*, 2nd ed. Philadelphia: WB Saunders; 2003:625.

TABLE 77-4 PRESENTATION AND TREATMENT OF THE MOST COMMON CAUSES OF PERICARDITIS

TYPE	PATHOGENESIS OR ETIOLOGY	DIAGNOSIS	TREATMENT	COMPLICATIONS	COMMENTS
Viral	Coxsackievirus B Echovirus type 8 Epstein-Barr virus	Leukocytosis Elevated erythrocyte sedimentation rate Mild cardiac biomarker elevation	Symptomatic relief, NSAIDs	Tamponade Relapsing pericarditis	Peaks in spring and fall
Tuberculous	*Mycobacterium tuberculosis*	Isolation of organism from biopsy fluid Granulomas not specific	Triple-drug antituberculosis regimen Pericardial drainage followed by early (4-6 wk) pericardiectomy if signs of tamponade or constriction develop	Tamponade Constrictive pericarditis	1-8% of patients with tuberculosis pneumonia; rule out HIV infection
Bacterial	Group A streptococcus *Staphylococcus aureus* *Streptococcus pneumoniae*	Leukocytosis with marked left shift Purulent pericardial fluid	Pericardial drainage by catheter or surgery Systemic antibiotics Pericardiectomy if constrictive physiology develops	Tamponade in one third of patients	Very high mortality rate if not recognized early
Post–myocardial infarction	12 hr–10 days after infarction	Fever Pericardial friction rub Echo: effusion	Aspirin Prednisone	Tamponade rare	More frequent in large Q wave infarctions Anterior > inferior
Uremic	Untreated renal failure: 50% Chronic dialysis: 20%	Pericardial rub: 90%	Intensive dialysis Indomethacin: probably ineffective Catheter drainage Surgical drainage	Tamponade Hemodynamic instability on dialysis	Avoid NSAIDs About 50% respond to intensive dialysis
Neoplastic	In order of frequency: lung cancer, breast cancer, leukemia and lymphoma, others	Chest pain, dyspnea Echo: effusion CT, MRI: tumor metastases to pericardium Cytologic examination of fluid positive in 85%	Catheter drainage Subxiphoid pericardiectomy Chemotherapy directed at underlying malignant neoplasm	Tamponade Constriction	

CT = computed tomography; HIV = human immunodeficiency virus; MRI = magnetic resonance imaging; NSAIDs = nonsteroidal anti-inflammatory drugs.
Modified from Malik F, Foster E. Pericardial disease. In: Wachter RM, Goldman L, Hollander H, eds. *Hospital Medicine*, 2nd ed. Philadelphia: Lippincott Williams & Wilkins; 2005:449.

FIGURE 77-2. Cardiac magnetic resonance image of a patient with acute pericarditis shows late gadolinium hyperenhancement of the pericardium and epicardium.

TREATMENT   Rx

Acutely ill patients with fever should be hospitalized, as should patients with suspected acute MI (Chapter 73), large effusions, evidence of impending hemodynamic compromise, or a cause other than viral or idiopathic pericarditis, because of the risk of a rapidly accumulating effusion with potential tamponade. Patients without effusions can usually be followed as outpatients (Fig. 77-3).

If acute pericarditis is a manifestation of an underlying disease, it often responds to treatment of the primary condition. Most cases of acute idiopathic or viral pericarditis are self-limited and respond to treatment with aspirin (650 mg every 6 hours) or another nonsteroidal anti-inflammatory drug (NSAID) such as ibuprofen (300 to 800 mg every 6 to 8 hours). The dose of NSAID should be tapered once symptoms or the pericardial effusion have resolved, but the medication should be taken for at least 3 to 4 weeks to minimize the risk of recurrent pericarditis.

If the pericardial pain and inflammation do not respond to NSAIDs or if the acute pericarditis recurs, colchicine (0.6 mg once or twice daily) for 3 months is effective in relieving pain and preventing recurrent pericarditis.**1** Alternatively, colchicine can be started in all patients to increase the likelihood of a favorable response to treatment. A major side effect is diarrhea. Colchicine should be avoided in patients with abnormal renal or hepatic function and in those being treated with macrolide antibiotics, which alter its metabolism.

Although acute pericarditis usually responds dramatically to systemic corticosteroids, observational studies strongly suggest that the use of steroids increases the probability of relapse in patients treated with colchicine. Accordingly, systemic steroids should be considered only in patients with recurrent pericarditis unresponsive to NSAIDs and colchicine or when needed to treat an underlying inflammatory disease. If steroids are used, low-dose prednisone (0.2 to 0.5 mg/kg) appears to be as effective as higher doses and is less likely to be associated with recurrence. Steroids should be continued for at least 1 month prior to slow tapering.

A proton pump inhibitor, such as omeprazole (20 mg/day), should be considered to improve the gastric tolerability of NSAIDs. Warfarin and heparin should be avoided to minimize the risk of hemopericardium, but anticoagulation may be required if the patient is in atrial fibrillation or has a prosthetic heart valve. It is prudent to avoid exercise until after the chest pain completely resolves. If pericarditis reoccurs, the patient can be reloaded with colchicine and intravenous ketorolac (20 mg) and then continued on an oral NSAID and colchicine for at least 3 months. Every effort should be made to avoid the use of steroids, reserving low-dose steroids for patients who cannot tolerate aspirin and other NSAIDs or whose recurrence is not responsive to colchicine and intravenous NSAIDs. Pericardiocentesis is not recommended unless purulent or tuberculous pericarditis is clinically suspected or the patient fails to respond to 2 to 3 weeks of NSAID therapy.

PROGNOSIS

The course of viral and idiopathic pericarditis is usually self-limited, and most patients recover completely. About 25% of patients, however, have recurrent pericarditis weeks to months later, probably due to an immune response, and some patients may have multiple debilitating episodes. Recurrent pericarditis is more common in patients treated with steroids for the acute episode, especially during a rapid steroid taper. In these patients, prolonged high-dose NSAID treatment (e.g., ibuprofen 300 to 600 mg three times a day) plus colchicine (0.6 mg twice daily, declining to once daily after 3 to 6 months) is

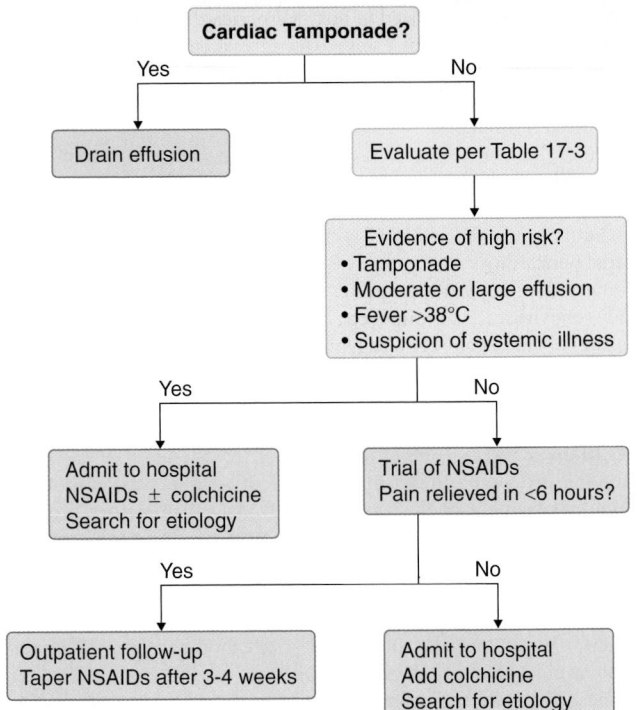

FIGURE 77-3. Initial management of patients with pericarditis. NSAIDs = nonsteroidal anti-inflammatory drugs.

TABLE 77-5   CAUSES OF MODERATE TO LARGE ASYMPTOMATIC PERICARDIAL EFFUSIONS

CAUSE	% OF CASES
Idiopathic/viral	37
Neoplastic	19
Iatrogenic/trauma	13
Tuberculous or purulent	6
Acute myocardial infarction	6
Collagen vascular disease	4
Heart failure	4
Uremia	4
Radiation induced	2
Aortic dissection	2
Hypothyroidism	1
Other	2

Modified from Nishimura RA, Kidd KR. Recognition and management of patients with pericardial disease. In: Braunwald E, Goldman L, eds. *Primary Cardiology,* 2nd ed. Philadelphia: WB Saunders; 2003:625.

recommended.**2** In patients who cannot tolerate colchicine or who have recurrent episodes despite high-dose NSAID treatment (e.g., indomethacin 50 mg three times a day or ibuprofen 800 mg four times a day), oral steroids (e.g., prednisone 0.2 to 0.5 mg/kg/day for 2 to 4 weeks, then slowly tapered over several months) are generally recommended, with pericardiectomy reserved for refractory cases. Patients who have recurrent pericarditis are at increased risk for progression to constrictive pericarditis (see later).

CARDIAC EFFUSION AND TAMPONADE

EPIDEMIOLOGY

A pericardial effusion can be caused by any disease that causes acute pericarditis (see Table 77-1), but a majority of cases are caused by conditions other than viral or idiopathic pericarditis (Table 77-5). For example, tamponade occurs in about 10 to 15% of patients with idiopathic pericarditis, but it develops in more than 50% of patients with malignant, tuberculous, or purulent pericarditis. Tuberculosis and neoplastic disease are typically associated

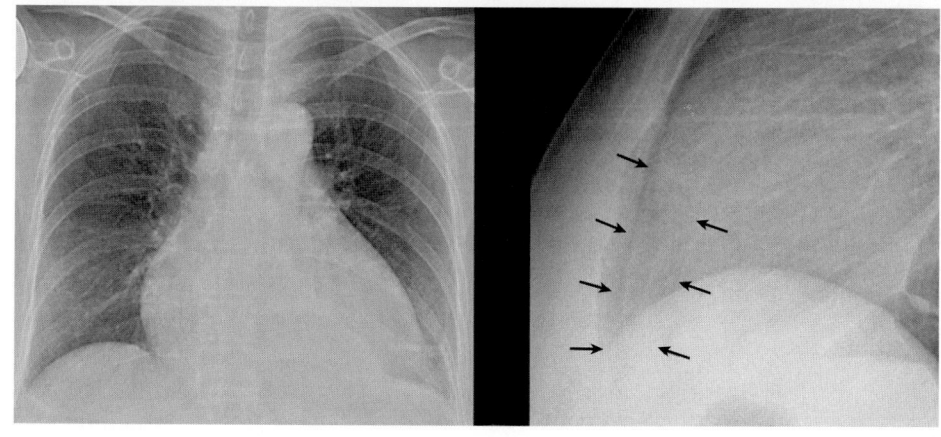

FIGURE 77-4. Chest radiographs in a patient with a large pericardial effusion. The cardiac silhouette on the posteroanterior view *(left)* is enlarged with a "water bag" configuration. The lateral view *(right)* shows a separation between the pericardial and epicardial fat stripes *(arrows)*.

with serosanguineous effusions, but such effusions can also be seen with typical viral or idiopathic pericarditis, with uremia, and after mediastinal irradiation. Hemopericardium is seen most commonly with trauma, myocardial rupture after MI, catheter-induced myocardial or epicardial coronary artery rupture, aortic dissection with rupture into the pericardial space, or primary hemorrhage in patients receiving anticoagulant therapy, often after cardiac valve surgery. Chylopericardium is rare and results from leakage or injury to the thoracic duct.

PATHOBIOLOGY

Under normal conditions, the space between the parietal and visceral pericardium can accommodate only a small amount of fluid before the development of tamponade physiology. The clinical consequences of a pericardial effusion depend on the rate of increase. A rapidly accumulating effusion, as in hemopericardium caused by trauma or aortic dissection, may result in tamponade physiology with just 100 to 200 mL of fluid. It is not surprising, therefore, that cardiac perforation quickly results in tamponade. By comparison, a more slowly developing effusion, as is typical with uremia and hypothyroidism, may allow the gradual stretching of the pericardium, with asymptomatic or minimally symptomatic effusions of 1500 mL or more.

Tamponade physiology occurs when fluid accumulation in the intrapericardial space is sufficient to compress the heart, resulting in impaired cardiac filling. The increased pericardial pressure in cardiac tamponade accentuates the interdependence among the cardiac chambers as the total cardiac volume is limited by the pericardial effusion. With normal inspiration, right ventricular filling is enhanced, the intraventricular septum is displaced toward the left ventricle, and left ventricular filling and the resulting stroke volume are reduced. Because of its lower pressures, the right ventricle is most vulnerable to compression by a pericardial effusion, and abnormal right heart filling is the earliest sign of a hemodynamically significant pericardial effusion. In tamponade, left heart filling occurs preferentially during expiration, when there is less filling of the right heart. The small normal respiratory increase in right ventricular volume, with a concomitant decrease in left ventricular stroke volume and systolic arterial pressure, is markedly accentuated in cardiac tamponade and results in the clinical finding of "paradoxical pulse." A small (<10 mm Hg) pulsus paradoxus, which is a decline in systemic blood pressure during inspiration, is normal and is related to the ventricles being confined within the pericardium and sharing a common septum. In cardiac tamponade, this phenomenon is exaggerated, and systemic blood pressure falls by more than 10 mm Hg during inspiration. A pulsus paradoxus also may be present with hypovolemic shock, chronic obstructive pulmonary disease, and bronchospasm.

CLINICAL MANIFESTATIONS

A slowly accumulating, isolated pericardial effusion is often completely asymptomatic. The physical examination may be normal, but the heart sounds may be muffled. The diagnosis is usually suggested by a chest radiograph that shows cardiomegaly with a globular heart (Fig. 77-4; see also Fig. 53-12 in Chapter 53) or by an echocardiogram, computed tomography (CT) scan, or MRI performed for another indication. Patients with hypothyroidism, uremia, or collagen vascular disease may have asymptomatic effusions discovered during comprehensive evaluations.

Patients with impending or early tamponade are usually anxious and tachycardic, and they may complain of dyspnea, orthopnea, and chest pain. The

FIGURE 77-5. Electrical alternans. Lead V_5 rhythm strip from a patient with a large pericardial effusion and tamponade physiology. Note the relatively low voltage and electrical alternans.

increased venous pressure is usually apparent as jugular venous distention. The x descent (during ventricular systole) is typically the dominant jugular venous wave, with little or no y descent (during early diastole) (Chapter 50). The heart sounds are classically soft or muffled, especially if there is a large pericardial effusion. In rapidly developing cardiac tamponade, especially hemorrhagic cardiac tamponade, the jugular veins may not be distended because the time course has been insufficient for a compensatory increase in venous pressure. Such "low-pressure" tamponade may also occur with uremic pericarditis in volume-depleted patients. The patient may have signs of right heart failure, with peripheral edema, right upper quadrant pain caused by hepatic congestion, or abnormal liver enzymes and serum bilirubin level.

The hallmark of cardiac tamponade is a paradoxical pulse, which is defined as more than a 10 mm Hg drop in systolic arterial pressure during inspiration. When severe, the paradoxical pulse may be apparent as the absence of a palpable brachial or radial pulse during inspiration. A paradoxical pulse can also occur when there are wide swings in intrathoracic pressure, pulmonary embolism (Chapter 98), or hypovolemic shock (Chapter 106). A paradoxical pulse may be difficult to recognize in the presence of severe shock.

DIAGNOSIS

Cardiac tamponade, which is a treatable cause of shock (Chapter 107), can be rapidly fatal if unrecognized. As such, cardiac tamponade should be considered in the differential diagnosis of any patient with shock or pulseless electrical activity.

Cardiac tamponade is usually suspected based on jugular venous distention, sinus tachycardia with hypotension, narrow pulse pressure, elevated (>10 mm Hg) pulsus paradoxus, and distant heart sounds. Pulsus paradoxus may be obvious by palpation; it is more accurately measured with a sphygmomanometer during slow inspiration.

The ECG often shows low voltage and sometimes electrical alternans (Fig. 77-5) when the heart swings within a large pericardial effusion. The chest radiograph shows a globular, enlarged cardiac shadow (see Fig. 53-12 in Chapter 53 and Fig. 77-4) without pulmonary venous congestion.

Echocardiography, which is the key diagnostic test for cardiac tamponade, must be performed without delay in any patient suspected of having this condition. Echocardiography visualizes pericardial effusions as an echo-free space around the heart (Fig. 77-6), demonstrates the presence and size of the pericardial effusion, and reflects its hemodynamic consequences. The inferior vena cava is almost always enlarged, right atrial and right ventricular collapse indicates cardiac compression, and enhanced respiratory variation of ventricular filling is a manifestation of increased ventricular interdependence. Right ventricular collapse is more specific for tamponade than is right atrial

FIGURE 77-6. Two-dimensional echocardiogram from a patient with cardiac tamponade. A large pericardial effusion (PE) is apparent as an echo-free space surrounding the left ventricle (LV) and right ventricle (RV). In diastole, there is collapse of the right ventricle (arrow).

collapse, but the right-sided chambers may not collapse when tamponade occurs in patients with pulmonary hypertension. Cardiac tamponade can result from a loculated pericardial effusion after cardiac surgery or trauma. A loculated effusion may not be apparent on transthoracic echocardiography, but transesophageal echocardiography and thoracic CT or MRI can delineate loculated pericardial effusions.

On Doppler study, mitral inflow velocity (especially early diastolic velocity) normally increases with expiration and decreases with inspiration; the opposite respiratory variation is seen in tricuspid inflow velocity. Doppler findings for tamponade, which are more sensitive than two-dimensional echocardiography, include augmented respiratory variation of mitral and tricuspid inflow velocities as a function of ventricular interdependence. These changes may be seen even before frank hemodynamic compromise due to pericardial effusion. Although Doppler echocardiography provides important information, it must be emphasized that cardiac tamponade is ultimately a clinical diagnosis.

The routine evaluation should include an assessment of renal function, a thyroid-stimulating hormone level, a complete blood count with differential, a platelet count, coagulation parameters, and a tuberculin skin test. Common medications that can cause a pericardial effusion include cromolyn, isoniazid, and phenytoin; hydralazine, procainamide, and reserpine are others. Blood cultures are indicated if an infectious cause is suspected. Complement levels, antinuclear antibodies, and the sedimentation rate can suggest systemic lupus erythematosus (Chapter 274), which rarely presents initially as an isolated pericardial effusion.

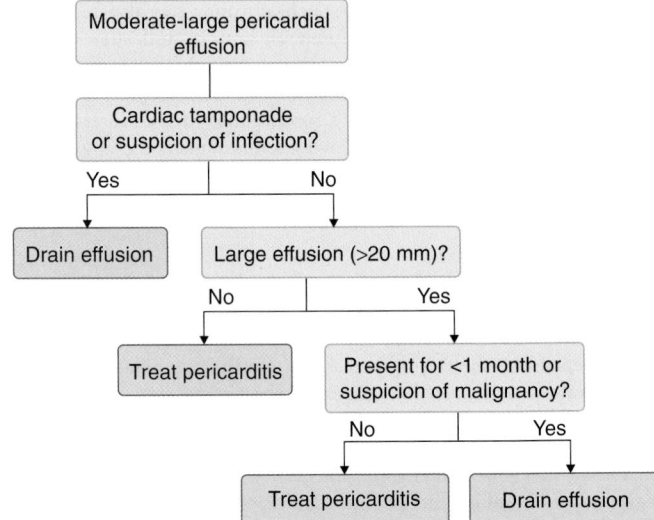

FIGURE 77-7. Algorithm for managing patients with moderate to large pericardial effusions. (Modified from Little WC, Freeman GL. Pericardial disease. *Circulation.* 2006;113:1622-1632.)

TREATMENT   Rx

Pericardial Effusion without Tamponade

Acute pericarditis is often accompanied by a small pericardial effusion that does not produce tamponade. If there is no hemodynamic compromise and the diagnosis can be established by other means, pericardiocentesis is not necessary (Fig. 77-7). Even small pericardial effusions may be related to underlying systemic illnesses such as systemic lupus erythematosus (Chapter 274), cardiac amyloid (Chapter 194), scleroderma (Chapter 275), hypothyroidism (Chapter 233), or AIDS, so it is important to consider and treat associated illnesses. Chylous pericardial effusion, which is usually related to obstruction of the thoracic duct, may require a surgical procedure for relief.

For suspected pericardial effusion, transthoracic echocardiography is the initial test of choice, although loculated effusions may be identified better by CT or MRI. If a small (0.5 to 1 cm) echolucent or "organized" pericardial effusion is observed, a follow-up echocardiogram in 1 to 2 weeks, or sooner if the patient deteriorates, is recommended. If the effusion is getting smaller, subsequent echocardiograms are not necessary unless the patient's clinical condition changes.

For moderate (1 to 2 cm) or large (>2 cm) effusions in patients who are hemodynamically stable and in whom tamponade is not suspected, a follow-up echocardiogram should be performed in 7 days and then every month until the effusion is minimal. If bacterial or malignant pericarditis is suspected, diagnostic pericardiocentesis should be performed immediately, even in the absence of clinical instability or suggestion of tamponade; tuberculous pericarditis is diagnosed best by pericardial biopsy. Anticoagulation with heparin or warfarin should be discontinued unless the patient has a mechanical heart valve or atrial fibrillation.

In hypothyroidism (Chapter 233), the effusion and the coexistent cardiomyopathy respond to hormone replacement, sometimes over several months.

Uremic pericardial effusions often respond to initiation of dialysis or more intensive dialysis (Chapter 132).

Cardiac Tamponade

The treatment of cardiac tamponade is urgent drainage of the pericardial effusion, especially when there is hemodynamic compromise. Fluid resuscitation may be of transient benefit if the patient is volume depleted (hypovolemic cardiac tamponade), but inotropic agents are usually ineffective because there is already intense endogenous adrenergic stimulation. The initiation of mechanical ventilation in a patient with tamponade may produce a sudden drop in blood pressure because the positive intrathoracic pressure further impairs cardiac filling.

Echocardiographic-guided percutaneous pericardiocentesis, which can be performed at the bedside by experienced operators (Fig. 77-8), is indicated if a patient is in dire circumstances and at least 1 cm of fluid is seen anterior to the mid-right ventricular free wall throughout diastole. The ideal entry site (usually the apex) is defined using echocardiography as the minimal distance from skin to pericardial fluid without intervening structures. The pericardial space is entered with a needle and then drained through a catheter. As much fluid as possible should be removed. The pericardial fluid should be sent for pH, glucose, lactate dehydrogenase, protein, cell count, and cytology as well as staining and culture for bacteria, fungi, and tuberculosis. Continued drainage of the pericardial fluid through an indwelling catheter minimizes the risk of recurrent effusion. For hemodynamically significant effusions of less than 1 cm, organized or multiloculated effusions, and focal effusions, a limited thoracotomy-mediastinoscopy and creation of a pericardial window are advised.

Surgical drainage may be the preferred treatment if pericardial tissue is required for diagnosis or in the case of recurrent effusions or bacterial pericarditis. Malignant pericardial effusions frequently reoccur and, like other recurrent pericardial effusions, may necessitate the surgical creation of a pericardial window that allows the effusion to drain into the pleural space, preventing

FIGURE 77-8. Aspiration of pericardial fluid is indicated in cardiac tamponade or to obtain fluid for diagnostic purposes. A wide-bore needle is inserted in the epigastrium below the xiphoid process and advanced in the direction of the medial third of the right clavicle. An alternative site is over the left ventricular apex. The procedure should be performed under echocardiographic guidance, but it may need to be performed emergently for life-saving purposes in other settings. Complications of the procedure include puncture of the heart, arrhythmias, vasovagal attack, and pneumothorax. (From Forbes CD, Jackson WF. *Color Atlas and Text of Clinical Medicine,* 3rd ed. London: Mosby; 2003.)

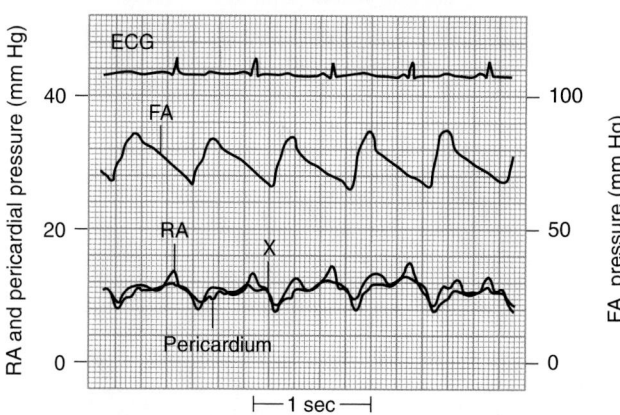

FIGURE 77-9. Right atrial (RA) pressure recording from a patient with constrictive pericarditis. Note the elevation in pressure and the prominent y descent, corresponding to rapid, early diastolic right atrial emptying. ECG = electrocardiogram; FA = femoral artery. (From Lorell BH. Profiles in constriction, restriction and tamponade. In: Baim DS, Grossman W, eds. *Cardiac Catheterization, Angiography, and Intervention,* 6th ed. Philadelphia: Williams & Wilkins; 2000: 832.)

reoccurrence of cardiac tamponade. An attractive alternative in these patients, especially if their overall prognosis is poor from the malignancy, is the percutaneous creation of a pericardial window by balloon dilation. Hemorrhagic effusions related to cardiac trauma or aortic dissection are best managed by emergency surgery.

PROGNOSIS

A pericardial effusion may recur or persist. Symptoms are usually weight loss, fatigue, dyspnea on exertion, and whatever symptoms are associated with the specific cause. Treatment of chronic or recurrent idiopathic effusions is similar to the treatment of recurrent pericarditis. If medical therapy is unsuccessful, creation of a pericardial window is indicated.

A large idiopathic, asymptomatic effusion that persists for 6 months or longer can unpredictably result in tamponade in as many as 30% of patients over long-term follow-up; diagnostic pericardiocentesis occasionally detects a neoplastic or tuberculous cause. Pericardiocentesis with prolonged drainage resolves many chronic large pericardial effusions, but pericardiectomy is often required. Long-term prognosis depends on the cause of the effusion. With pericardial tamponade, the in-hospital mortality rate is less than 10%, but the subsequent mortality rate is about 75% with a malignant effusion, compared with only 3 to 5% subsequent annual mortality for other causes.

PERICARDIAL CONSTRICTION

EPIDEMIOLOGY AND PATHOBIOLOGY

Pericardial constriction, which is usually the result of long-standing pericardial inflammation, occurs when a scarred, thickened, and/or calcified pericardium impairs cardiac filling, thereby limiting the total cardiac volume. The most frequent causes in the developed world are previous cardiac surgery, chronic idiopathic or viral pericarditis, and mediastinal radiation. Constriction may follow cardiac surgery by several weeks to months and may occur decades after chest wall irradiation. In developing countries, tuberculous pericarditis is a more common cause of constrictive pericarditis. Other less common causes include malignant disease, especially lung cancer, breast cancer, or lymphoma; histoplasmosis; rheumatoid arthritis; and uremia. However, a specific cause may not be identified in many patients.

With chronic constriction, the pericardium may thicken from its normal 3 mm or less to 6 mm or more, calcify, and adhere to the epicardium. In subacute constriction, the pericardium may be only minimally thickened and less calcified. Fibrous scarring and adhesions of both pericardial layers obliterate the pericardial cavity. The ventricles are unable to fill because of physical constraints imposed by a thickened, rigid, and sometimes calcified pericardium. The pathophysiologic hallmark of pericardial constriction is the exaggerated interventricular dependence and differential ventricular filling with respiration.

Although both cardiac tamponade and pericardial constriction impair diastolic ventricular filling and elevate venous pressure, the impairment in ventricular filling with constriction is minimal in early diastole until cardiac volume reaches the anatomic limit set by the noncompliant pericardium, at which time diastolic pressure rises abruptly and remains elevated until the onset of systole. This prominent y descent with an elevated plateau of ventricular pressure, which has been termed the "square root" sign (Fig. 77-9), differentiates constriction from tamponade, in which the y descent is absent. Stroke volume and cardiac output are reduced because of impaired filling, but the intrinsic systolic function of the ventricles can be normal.

CLINICAL MANIFESTATIONS

Patients with pericardial constriction typically present with manifestations of elevated systemic venous pressures and low cardiac output. Because there is equalization of all cardiac pressures (including right and left atrial pressures), systemic congestion is much more marked than pulmonary congestion. Typically, patients develop marked jugular venous distention, hepatic congestion, ascites, and peripheral edema, but their lungs remain clear. The limited cardiac output typically presents as exercise intolerance and may progress to cardiac cachexia with muscle wasting. In long-standing pericardial constriction, pleural effusions, ascites, and hepatic dysfunction may be prominent clinical features. Patients with pericardial constriction are much more likely to have left-sided or bilateral pleural effusions than right-sided effusions. Because of the prominent clinical symptoms of ascites and liver enzyme abnormalities, patients may be evaluated for hepatic disease before constrictive pericarditis is recognized.

The jugular veins are distended with prominent x and y descents. The normal inspiratory drop in jugular venous distention may be replaced by a rise in venous pressure (Kussmaul's sign). The classic auscultatory finding of pericardial constriction is a pericardial knock (Chapter 50), which is a high-pitched sound early in diastole when there is the sudden cessation of rapid ventricular diastolic filling, coinciding with the nadir of the y descent.

DIAGNOSIS

Pericardial constriction should be considered in any patient with unexplained systemic venous congestion. Pericardial calcification, seen best on the lateral plain chest radiograph, is a classic finding but is present in only 25% of patients with constrictive pericarditis, mostly in those with long-standing constriction. Similarly, most patients with pericardial constriction have a thickened pericardium (>2 mm) that can be imaged by echocardiography, CT, and MRI (Fig. 77-10). It is important to recognize, however, that pericardial constriction can be present without pericardial calcification and, in about 20% of patients, without any obvious pericardial thickening.

Transesophageal Doppler echocardiography may demonstrate pericardial thickening and calcification, but increased pericardial thickness can be missed on a transthoracic echocardiogram. Echocardiography also differentiates pericardial constriction from right heart failure caused by tricuspid valve disease and/or associated pulmonary hypertension.

FIGURE 77-10. Computed tomography in a patient with constrictive pericarditis shows a thickened pericardium (arrow).

flow velocity during expiration is characteristic of constriction, whereas the reversal flow velocity occurs during inspiration in patients with right heart failure from other causes. Patients with pericardial constriction usually have only minimally elevated (<200 pg/mL) B-type natriuretic peptide (BNP), but BNP levels are typically markedly increased (>600 pg/mL) in patients with restrictive cardiomyopathy.

Confirmation of the diagnosis of constriction may require cardiac catheterization in patients whose noninvasive evaluation is not clear-cut. Traditional invasive hemodynamic findings of equalized end-diastolic pressures in the right and left ventricles and the "dip and plateau" pattern of left ventricular diastolic pressure do not reliably differentiate constriction from restrictive cardiomyopathy. More specific invasive hemodynamic features of constriction and restriction are based on the respiratory variation in ventricular filling; the simultaneous measurement of left and right ventricular pressures demonstrates discordant changes in their systolic pressures with respiration in constrictive pericarditis. By comparison, the direction of these pressures is concordant (both left and right sides increase with expiration and decrease with inspiration) in restrictive cardiomyopathy.

All patients with documented but otherwise unexplained pericardial constriction should be evaluated for potential tuberculosis.

TABLE 77-6 DIFFERENTIATION OF PERICARDIAL CONSTRICTION FROM RESTRICTIVE CARDIOMYOPATHY

FINDINGS	PERICARDIAL CONSTRICTION	RESTRICTIVE CARDIOMYOPATHY
PHYSICAL EXAMINATION		
Pulmonary congestion	Usually absent	Usually present
Early diastolic sound	Pericardial knock	S_3 (low pitched)
ECHO/DOPPLER		
Respiratory variation in E wave	>25%	<20%
Mitral septal annular early diastolic velocity	>7 cm/sec	<7 cm/sec
CT/MRI		
Pericardial thickness	>2 mm (but <2 mm in 20%)	<2 mm
BIOMARKER		
B-type natriuretic peptide	<200 pg/mL	>600 pg/mL
HEMODYNAMICS		
PA systolic pressure	<60 mm Hg	>60 mm Hg
PCW-LV diastolic pressure	Respiratory variation with reduction in inspiration	No variation
Respiratory variation in RV/LV peak systolic pressure	Discordant	Concordant

CT = computed tomography; LV = left ventricular; MRI = magnetic resonance imaging; PA = pulmonary artery; PCW = pulmonary capillary wedge; RV = right ventricular.
Modified from Little WC, Freeman GL. Pericardial disease. *Circulation.* 2006;113:1622-1632.

Differential Diagnosis

The most difficult differentiation is between pericardial constriction and restrictive cardiomyopathy (Chapter 60), the clinical manifestations of which may be very similar to those of pericardial constriction (Table 77-6). Doppler echocardiography is the most useful method to distinguish constriction from restriction. Patients with pericardial constriction usually have pronounced respiratory variation (>25%) of mitral inflow, whereas patients with restrictive cardiomyopathies do not. In some patients with pericardial constriction and markedly elevated venous pressures, the respiratory variation may be present only after head-up tilt. The Doppler measurement of early diastolic septal mitral annular velocity is almost always reduced in patients with myocardial restriction, whereas it remains normal or increased in patients with pericardial constriction. A prominent diastolic reversal of hepatic vein

TREATMENT AND PROGNOSIS Rx

In some patients with pericardial constriction of less than 3 months' duration, the symptoms and constriction may resolve over several weeks with medical therapy consisting of NSAIDs (e.g., ibuprofen 300 to 800 mg every 6 to 8 hours), colchicine (0.6 mg once or twice daily), and the cautious use of diuretics. For more chronic pericardial constriction or cases that do not respond to medical therapy, the definitive treatment is surgical pericardial decortication, with a wide resection of both the visceral and parietal pericardium. This operation is a major undertaking with substantial risk (>6% mortality even in the most experienced centers). In many patients, surgery does not immediately restore normal cardiac function; it may take weeks after removal of the constricting pericardium to return to normal. Empirical treatment of tuberculosis (Chapter 332) may be required in patients with constriction and a high suspicion of tuberculosis, even without a definitive diagnosis.

Effusive-Constrictive Pericarditis

In some patients (<10%) who present with cardiac tamponade, the elevated right atrial pressure and jugular venous distention do not resolve after removal of the pericardial fluid. In these patients, pericardiocentesis converts the hemodynamics from those typical of tamponade to those of constriction. Thus, the restriction of cardiac filling is due not only to pericardial effusion but also to pericardial constriction, predominantly involving the visceral pericardium. Effusive-constrictive pericarditis most likely represents an intermediate transition from acute pericarditis with pericardial effusion to pericardial constriction. Frequently, the symptoms resolve after several weeks of treatment with an NSAID (e.g., ibuprofen 300 to 800 mg every 6 to 8 hours).

● SPECIFIC FORMS OF PERICARDIAL DISEASE

Postcardiotomy Syndrome

Postcardiotomy syndrome is acute pericarditis occurring weeks to months after open heart surgery. Patients have typical symptoms of acute pericarditis, which is associated with antimyocardial antibodies. A similar clinical picture is seen with the postperfusion syndrome caused by cytomegalovirus infection (Chapter 384) in patients who were previously uninfected but were exposed to cytomegalovirus-positive blood during cardiopulmonary bypass or transfusions. Atypical lymphocytes and elevated liver enzymes are often seen. Treatment of postcardiotomy syndrome is similar to the treatment of acute pericarditis.

Some patients who have undergone cardiac surgery develop late pericardial constriction without preceding acute pericarditis owing to bleeding in and around the open pericardium, followed by inflammation, scarring, and fibrosis. If active inflammation is present, a trial of anti-inflammatory agents may be instituted; however, surgical removal of the blood clot, usually accompanied by more extensive pericardiectomy, is typically required.

Post–Myocardial Infarction Pericarditis

Acute pericarditis can develop several days after an acute MI (Chapter 73), usually because of transmural extension of the infarction to the pericardial surface. This syndrome is uncommon in the reperfusion era. Anticoagulation should be temporarily withheld to avoid a bloody effusion that might progress to cardiac tamponade.

A late autoimmune pericarditis, termed *Dressler's syndrome*, can develop weeks to months after MI. Diagnosis and treatment are as for acute pericarditis.

Uremic Pericarditis

Pericardial effusions develop in patients with severe renal failure, especially those on dialysis (Chapter 133). Aggressive dialysis may decrease the pericardial effusion, but sometimes the effusion persists and requires drainage or even pericardiectomy.

Infectious Pericarditis

BACTERIAL PERICARDITIS

Purulent bacterial pericarditis may result from direct extension of bacterial pneumonia, direct extension of pleural empyema, or, rarely, peritonitis or a subphrenic abscess. Most patients are acutely ill with systemic sepsis and develop acute tamponade. The most common organisms are streptococci, pneumococci, and staphylococci. Urgent pericardiocentesis, which is required for both diagnosis and therapy, shows leukocytosis and frank pus, and the fluid glucose level is markedly depressed. Persistent or recurrent drainage with an indwelling catheter or repeated taps combined with antimicrobial therapy lead to a high survival rate, but late constrictive pericarditis requiring pericardiectomy develops in 30 to 40% of patients.

TUBERCULOUS PERICARDITIS

Tuberculous pericarditis is common in developing countries but accounts for less than 5% of cases of acute pericarditis in developed countries, usually in patients who are immunosuppressed. Symptoms are often nonspecific, and acute painful pericarditis is rare. Most patients have an effusive-constrictive physiology or pericardial constriction. The chest radiograph suggests active pulmonary tuberculosis is about 30% of cases, and a pleural effusion is present in 40 to 60% of cases. The echocardiogram typically shows fibrinous strands in the pericardial effusion, with multiple echo densities adherent to the pericardial surface. Pericardiocentesis is mandatory if tuberculous pericarditis is suspected. About 75% of patients have a positive culture, and a pericardial fluid adenosine deaminase level of 40 U/L or greater is seen in 75% of patients. Polymerase chain reaction testing and pericardial biopsy are recommended when tuberculous pericarditis is strongly suspected but not otherwise confirmed.

Aggressive antituberculosis therapy (Chapter 332) yields a cure rate of about 85 to 90%. Empirical treatment may be required in patients with a consistent clinical picture but without a confirmed diagnosis.

Even with prompt treatment, 30 to 60% of patients develop constrictive pericarditis, for which surgical pericardiectomy is the treatment of choice. In cases of suspected tuberculous constriction, antituberculosis therapy (Chapter 332) should be administered before and after pericardial surgery.

FUNGAL PERICARDITIS

The most common fungal pericarditis is histoplasmosis, which usually resolves in several weeks and can be treated successfully with NSAIDs. Specific antifungal therapy (Chapter 340) is recommended only in patients with disseminated histoplasmosis.

Malignant Pericarditis

About 6% of cases of acute pericarditis that initially have no obvious cause and about 20% of cases of moderate to large pericardial effusions are related to malignant diseases; in patients with cardiac tamponade, the percentage is even higher. About 80% of malignant pericarditis is linked to breast cancer (Chapter 204), lymphoma (Chapters 191 and 192), and leukemia (Chapters 189 and 190). Melanoma (Chapter 210) is an uncommon cause of malignant pericarditis, but a large proportion of patients with melanoma have pericardial involvement.

Most patients have direct tumor extension from an adjacent malignant lesion or a tumor from hematogenous or lymphatic spread. Pericardial effusions also may be caused by pericardial irritation or compromised lymphatic drainage in patients with mediastinal lymphoma.

Pericardiocentesis is key to diagnosis and management. Fluid cytology is positive in about 85% of patients. Complete drainage with an indwelling catheter for 2 or 3 days is the treatment of choice; if the effusion does not resolve, pericardiectomy is recommended. The prognosis depends on the treatment of the underlying malignancy, but the 1-year mortality rate is 80% or higher.

Post-Radiation Pericarditis

Post-radiation pericarditis develops in about 2% of patients after mantle radiation for Hodgkin's disease (Chapter 192) and in 0.4 to 5% of patients after irradiation for breast cancer. Pericardial injury occasionally manifests during treatment, but it more commonly appears months or even a decade later. The initial pericarditis and effusion may resolve spontaneously, but constrictive pericarditis, adjacent myocarditis, and even coronary artery damage can develop. Pericardiocentesis is critical to distinguish post-radiation pericarditis from malignant pericardial disease. Pericardiectomy is recommended for recurrent pericarditis and for large recurrent pericardial effusions.

Autoimmune Pericarditis

Up to 50% of patients with systemic lupus erythematosus (Chapter 274) have pericarditis, usually during an acute flare. Patients usually present with acute pericarditis or an asymptomatic effusion; cardiac tamponade is uncommon, and constrictive pericarditis is rare. If purulent pericarditis is not suspected, pericardiocentesis is not usually required. The underlying disease should be treated aggressively.

Acute pericarditis or asymptomatic pericardial effusions can develop in patients with advanced rheumatoid arthritis (Chapter 272), scleroderma (Chapter 275), or mixed connective tissue disease (Chapter 275). The process is usually self-limited or responds to aggressive treatment of the underlying disease, although cardiac tamponade can develop.

Myopericarditis

Concomitant myopericarditis (Chapter 60) may develop in patients with pericarditis, probably owing to direct extension of the inflammatory process. It is often manifested by ECG conduction delays, ventricular arrhythmias, and elevated troponin levels. No specific treatment is available.

Acute ventricular dilation and sudden or progressive heart failure develop in some patients after pericardiectomy for constrictive pericarditis or even after drainage of a large pericardial effusion. The syndrome may be underlying myocarditis.

Congenital Abnormalities

Congenital total absence of the pericardium is asymptomatic and clinically unimportant. However, partial or localized absence of the pericardium around the left atrium can cause focal herniation and lead to strangulation. CT or MRI can establish the diagnosis. Patients may present with atypical chest pain or sudden death. Surgical repair is often recommended for a partial pericardial defect.

Benign Cysts

Benign pericardial cysts are rare and are usually asymptomatic, but they can be associated with chest pain. They are typically seen as rounded or lobulated structures adjacent to the heart on the chest radiograph or adjacent to the right atrium on transthoracic echocardiography (Chapter 55). Thoracic CT and MRI are useful for the diagnosis. Cysts rarely rupture and do not require treatment unless they become symptomatic with chest pain. In this situation, the cyst can be removed surgically or drained percutaneously or with a thoracoscope.

1. Imazio M, Bobbio M, Cecchi E, et al. Colchicine in addition to conventional therapy for acute pericarditis: results of the colchicine for acute pericarditis (COPE) trial. *Circulation*. 2005;112: 2012-2016.
2. Imazio M, Bobbio M, Cecchi E, et al. Colchicine as first-choice therapy for recurrent pericarditis. Results of the CORE (Colchicine for Recurrent Pericarditis) trial. *Arch Intern Med*. 2005;165:1987-1991.

SUGGESTED READINGS

Imazio M, Spodick DH, Brucato A, et al. Controversial issues in the management of pericardial diseases. *Circulation*. 2010;121:916-928. *Review of causes and treatments.*

Khandaker MH, Espinosa RE, Nishimura RA, et al. Pericardial disease: diagnosis and management. *Mayo Clin Proc*. 2010;85:572-593. *Review.*

Mitiku TY, Heidenreich PA. A small pericardial effusion is a marker of increased mortality. *Am Heart J*. 2011;161:152-157. *After adjustment for other characteristics, even a small pericardial effusion is associated with about a 17% higher mortality.*

78

DISEASES OF THE AORTA

ERIC M. ISSELBACHER

The aorta is composed of three tissue layers. The intima is a thin inner layer lined with endothelial cells. The middle layer, or media, is the thickest layer of the aortic wall and is composed of sheets of elastic tissue that give the aorta tremendous tensile strength. The outermost layer, or adventitia, is composed mostly of collagen and carries the vasa vasorum, which nourish the aortic wall.

The ascending aorta is about 3 cm wide and 5 cm long and is located in the anterior mediastinum. Its most proximal portion (just above the aortic valve) is called the *aortic root* and is composed of the three sinuses of Valsalva. In the superior mediastinum, the ascending aorta meets the aortic arch and gives rise to the brachiocephalic arteries. The descending thoracic aorta courses posteriorly and is about 2.5 cm in diameter and 20 cm long. After crossing the diaphragm, it becomes the abdominal aorta, which is normally 2 cm wide and about 15 cm long; it then bifurcates into the two common iliac arteries.

AORTIC ANEURYSMS

DEFINITION

An aortic aneurysm is pathologic dilation of the aorta. Aneurysms are described in terms of their location, size, shape, and cause. The shape of an aneurysm is *fusiform* when there is symmetrical dilation of the aorta and *saccular* when the dilation involves mainly one wall. In addition, there may be a *false aneurysm* or *pseudoaneurysm* when the aorta is enlarged as a consequence of dilation of only the outer layers of the vessel wall, such as occurs with a contained rupture of the aortic wall.

EPIDEMIOLOGY

Aneurysms can involve any part of the aorta, but abdominal aortic aneurysms are much more common than thoracic aneurysms. Abdominal aortic aneurysms are 5 to 10 times more frequent in men than in women and have a prevalence of at least 3% in persons older than 50 years. Among thoracic aortic aneurysms, those of the ascending aorta are most common, followed by aneurysms involving the descending aorta; aneurysms of the aortic arch are uncommon. If a descending thoracic aortic aneurysm extends distally and involves the abdominal aorta, a thoracoabdominal aortic aneurysm is created.

Smoking is the strongest risk factor associated with the development of abdominal aortic aneurysms, followed by age, hypertension, and hyperlipidemia. In addition, there appears to be a genetic predisposition to their development because up to 28% of first-degree relatives of patients with abdominal aortic aneurysms may be similarly affected.

PATHOBIOLOGY

Atherosclerosis has long been considered the common underlying cause of abdominal aortic aneurysms. Indeed, the infrarenal aorta tends to be most severely affected by the atherosclerotic process and is accordingly a common site for aortic aneurysm formation. However, although aortic atherosclerosis clearly contributes to the process, the pathogenesis of abdominal aortic aneurysms is multifactorial, with genetic, environmental, hemodynamic, and immunologic factors all contributing to the development and progressive growth of aneurysms.

The strength of the aortic wall lies in its extracellular matrix, the most important components of which are elastin and collagen. Consequently, degradation of these structural proteins weakens the aortic wall, allowing aneurysms to develop. There is histologic evidence of inflammatory infiltrates—in particular, macrophages and T lymphocytes—within the media and adventitia of aneurysms, and this inflammation may lead to degradation of the extracellular matrix. Furthermore, matrix metalloproteinases—enzymes produced by smooth muscle and inflammatory cells that can degrade elastin and collagen—are significantly elevated in the walls of abdominal aortic aneurysms and probably contribute to their formation. As the wall begins to dilate, tension on the wall increases according to Laplace's law (tension is proportional to the product of pressure and the radius), thereby promoting further expansion of the aneurysm.

Atherosclerosis is also a common cause of aneurysms of the descending thoracic aorta. However, the most important cause of aneurysms of the ascending thoracic aorta is a process known as *cystic medial degeneration*, which histologically appears as smooth muscle cell necrosis and degeneration of elastic layers within the media. Cystic medial degeneration is found in almost all patients with Marfan syndrome (Chapter 268), who are at very high risk for thoracic aortic aneurysms. Among patients without overt evidence of connective tissue disease, a bicuspid aortic valve and familial thoracic aortic aneurysm syndrome are important congenital causes (Chapter 69). A long-standing history of hypertension is a common risk factor in older patients. Syphilis (Chapter 327), once a common cause of thoracic aortic aneurysms, is now rarely a factor. Other uncommon causes of thoracic aortic aneurysms include infectious aortitis (Chapter 76), great vessel arteritis, aortic trauma (Chapter 112), and aortic dissection (see later). Many thoracic aortic aneurysms are idiopathic.

CLINICAL MANIFESTATIONS

The large majority of abdominal and thoracic aortic aneurysms are asymptomatic and are discovered incidentally on routine physical examination or imaging study. When patients with abdominal aortic aneurysms experience symptoms, pain in the hypogastrium or lower part of the back is the most frequent complaint. The pain tends to have a steady, gnawing quality that may last hours or days. Expansion or impending rupture of an aneurysm may be heralded by new or worsening pain, often of sudden onset. With rupture, the pain is frequently associated with hypotension and a pulsatile abdominal mass.

Patients with thoracic aortic aneurysms may have chest pain or, less often, back pain. Vascular complications include aortic insufficiency (sometimes with secondary heart failure), hemoptysis, and arterial thromboembolism. An enlarging aneurysm may produce local mass effects as a result of compression of adjacent mediastinal structures, with symptoms including coughing, wheezing, dyspnea, hoarseness, recurrent pneumonia, or dysphagia.

DIAGNOSIS

Abdominal aortic aneurysms may be palpable on physical examination, although obesity can obscure even large aneurysms. Typically, abdominal aortic aneurysms are hard to size accurately by physical examination alone because adjacent structures frequently make an aneurysm feel larger than it really is. Thoracic aortic aneurysms usually cannot be palpated at all.

Definitive diagnosis of an aortic aneurysm is made by radiographic examination. Abdominal aortic aneurysms can be detected and sized by either abdominal ultrasonography or computed tomography (CT). Ultrasound is extremely sensitive and is the most practical screening method for aortic aneurysms. Screening is recommended in men aged 65 years or older and women aged 65 years or older who have smoked or have a family history. Such ultrasound screening programs are cost-effective and have been shown to reduce mortality in men aged 65 to 79.▮ CT is even more accurate (Fig. 78-1)

FIGURE 78-1. **Abdominal aortic aneurysm on computed tomography.** This sensitive imaging method allows precise measurement of size (point A to point B) and demonstrates the thickened wall of the aneurysm. (From Forbes CD, Jackson WF. *Color Atlas and Text of Clinical Medicine,* 3rd ed. London: Mosby; 2003.)

and can size an aneurysm to within a diameter of 2 mm. Although CT is less practical than ultrasound as a screening tool, it is the preferred modality for monitoring serial changes in size over time after the diagnosis has been made.

Thoracic aortic aneurysms are frequently recognized on chest radiographs; they often produce widening of the mediastinal silhouette, enlargement of the aortic knob, or displacement of the trachea from midline. CT is an excellent modality for detecting and sizing thoracic aneurysms and is particularly useful for monitoring size over time. Transthoracic echocardiography, which generally visualizes the aortic root and ascending aorta well, is useful for screening patients with Marfan syndrome, who are at particular risk for aneurysms involving this portion of the aorta.

TREATMENT ℞

The goal of therapy for patients with aortic aneurysms is to reduce the risk for expansion and rupture of the aneurysm. Although blood pressure control is generally recommended, β-blockers do not reduce the rate of growth of abdominal aortic aneurysms. Nonrandomized data suggest a potential benefit from statins, angiotensin-converting enzyme inhibitors, and even macrolide antibiotics, which may act as matrix metalloproteinase inhibitors. However, no specific medical therapy can be recommended at the current time. Aneurysms should be monitored closely with serial imaging studies (e.g., CT) to detect any progressive enlargement over time, which may indicate the need for surgical repair.

Aortic aneurysms that produce symptoms secondary to expansion, vascular complications, or compression of adjacent structures should be repaired. Substantial evidence confirms a strong correlation between a surgeon's and hospital's aneurysm surgery volume and the outcome of abdominal aortic aneurysm repair.

Size is the major indicator for repair of asymptomatic aortic aneurysms. Abdominal aortic aneurysms larger than 5.5 cm should be repaired,**2·3** as should aneurysms larger than 5 cm in good operative candidates. Abdominal aneurysms of 3.5 to 4.4 cm should be monitored every 12 months, and those 4.5 to 5.4 cm should be monitored every 6 months. Descending thoracic aortic aneurysms larger than 6 cm should undergo surgical repair. Aneurysms of the ascending thoracic aorta should be repaired at 5.5 cm or larger, except that patients with Marfan syndrome or a bicuspid aortic valve should undergo repair when the aneurysm is 5 cm or larger because of the high risk of rupture in these patients.

Open surgical repair consists of insertion of a synthetic prosthetic tube graft. When aneurysms involve branch vessels, such as the renal or mesenteric arteries, the vessels must be reimplanted into the graft. Similarly, when a dilated aortic root must be replaced in the repair of an ascending thoracic aortic aneurysm, the coronary arteries must be reimplanted. An alternative approach for repair of abdominal aortic aneurysms (and some descending thoracic aneurysms) is the percutaneous placement of an expandable endovascular stent graft inside the aneurysm. This endovascular technique is associated with a better short-term outcome,**4·5** but there is no survival advantage after 2 years when compared with open repair.**4-6** In patients who are not candidates for open repair because of comorbid diseases or high surgical risk (Chapter 439), endovascular repair reduces aneurysm-related mortality substantially but does not reduce all-cause mortality compared with conservative medical management.**7**

PROGNOSIS

The chief concern in managing an aortic aneurysm is its tendency to rupture. Most aneurysms expand over time, and the risk for rupture increases with size.

Abdominal aortic aneurysms less than 4.0 cm have only a 0.3% annual risk for rupture, whereas aneurysms 4.0 to 4.9 cm have a 1.5% annual risk for rupture, and aneurysms 5.0 to 5.9 cm have a 6.5% annual risk for rupture. The overall mortality in patients with abdominal aortic aneurysm rupture is 80%, including 50% mortality even among those who reach the hospital.

Thoracic aneurysms smaller than 5 cm typically expand slowly and rarely rupture, but the rate of growth and risk of rupture increase significantly when thoracic aneurysms are 6 cm or larger. Similar to abdominal aneurysms, rupture of thoracic aneurysms has a high early mortality of 76% at 24 hours.

● INTRAMURAL AORTIC HEMATOMA AND AORTIC DISSECTION

DEFINITION

An intramural aortic hematoma occurs when bleeding from the vasa vasorum or a tiny intimal tear causes a hematoma within the aortic media. Aortic

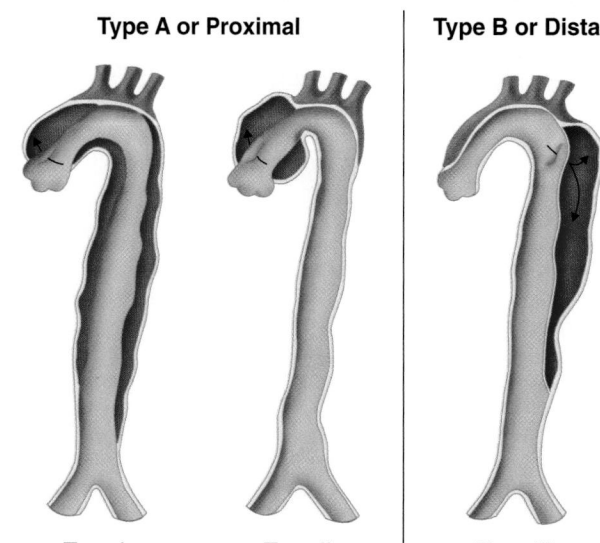

FIGURE 78-2. **Classification systems for aortic dissection.** (From Isselbacher EM. Diseases of the aorta. In: Braunwald E, Zipes DP, Libby P, Bonow RO, eds. *Braunwald's Heart Disease: A Textbook of Cardiovascular Medicine,* 7th ed. Philadelphia: Saunders; 2004:1416.)

dissection occurs when the media of the blood vessel is cleaved longitudinally to form a false lumen that communicates with the true lumen.

The location of an intramural aortic hematoma or dissection may be described according to one of several classification systems (Fig. 78-2). Two thirds of aortic dissections are type A (proximal), and the other third are type B (distal). All the classification schemes serve the same purpose, which is to distinguish dissections that involve the ascending aorta from those that do not. Involvement of the ascending aorta carries a high risk for early rupture and death from cardiac tamponade, so the prognosis and management differ according to the extent of aortic involvement. Hematomas and dissections are also classified according to their duration: less than 2 weeks is considered acute, whereas 2 weeks or more is considered chronic.

The peak incidence of aortic dissection in patients without Marfan syndrome occurs in individuals in their 60s and 70s, and men are affected twice as often as women. A history of hypertension is present in most cases, whereas a bicuspid aortic valve or known preexisting thoracic aortic aneurysm is less common. Rarely, aortic dissection occurs in a young woman during the peripartum period. Iatrogenic trauma from intra-aortic catheterization procedures or cardiac surgery may also cause aortic dissection.

PATHOBIOLOGY

Disease of the aortic media, with degeneration of the medial collagen and elastin, is the most common predisposing factor for aortic dissection. Patients with Marfan syndrome have classic cystic medial degeneration and are at particularly high risk for aortic dissection at a relatively young age. Aortic dissection classically begins either with a tear in the aortic intima, thereby exposing the diseased medial layer to the systemic pressure of intraluminal blood, or with an intramural hematoma and subsequent rupture of the overlying intima. This hematoma may propagate longitudinally along a variable length of the aorta. If the intimal layer remains intact, the hematoma does not communicate with the aortic lumen; however, if open communication occurs, the result is no different than for a dissection that began with an intimal tear. The media cleaves into two layers longitudinally, producing a blood-filled false lumen within the aortic wall. This false lumen propagates distally (or sometimes retrogradely) a variable distance along the aorta from the site of the intimal tear.

CLINICAL MANIFESTATIONS

Pain, which is typically severe and occurs in 96% of cases of both aortic intramural hematoma and dissection, is the most common initial symptom. The pain may be retrosternal, in the neck or throat, interscapular, in the lower part of the back, abdominal, or in the lower extremities, depending on the location of the aortic hematoma or dissection. The pain may migrate as the dissection propagates distally. Thoracic pain is often of sudden onset and most severe at the start. It is sometimes described as "tearing," "sharp," or "stabbing." Although an isolated hematoma rarely causes symptoms other

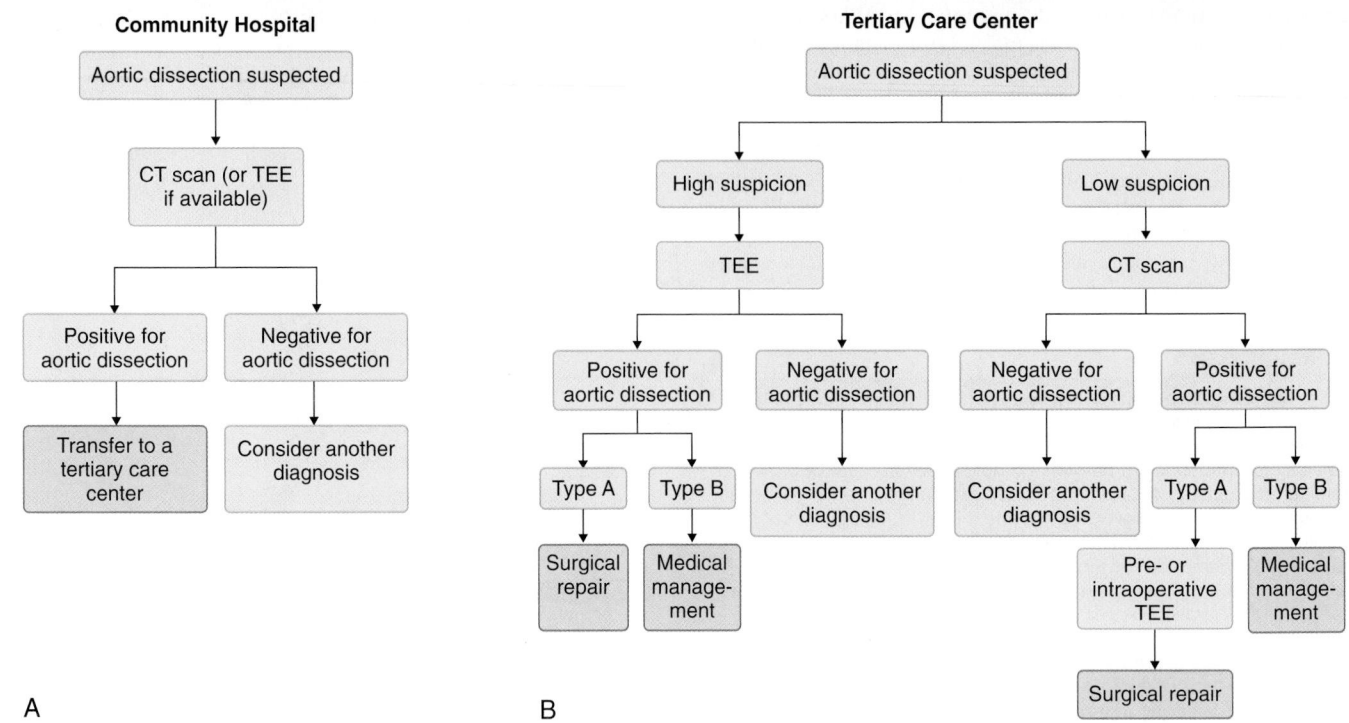

FIGURE 78-3. Algorithms for the evaluation of suspected acute aortic dissection. **A,** This approach is used in many community hospitals where cardiac surgery is not performed. **B,** This approach is used in many tertiary care centers where transesophageal echocardiography (TEE) and cardiac surgery are available. CT = computed tomography.

than pain, a dissection, regardless of how it starts, may also result in acute aortic insufficiency (Chapter 75), right coronary artery occlusion, hemopericardium (Chapter 77), syncope (Chapters 50 and 62), cerebrovascular accident (Chapter 414), mesenteric ischemia (Chapter 145), or ischemic peripheral neuropathy (Chapter 428).

Hypertension is a common finding on physical examination and is present in 70% of patients with distal aortic dissection. Hypotension may also occur, particularly in patients with proximal dissections, and is usually due to rupture into the pericardium or severe aortic insufficiency. Pseudohypotension occurs when a falsely low measure of upper extremity blood pressure is obtained because of involvement of the subclavian artery by the dissection. Similarly, pulse deficits are a common finding on physical examination, particularly in patients with proximal aortic dissections with involvement of the subclavian, carotid, or femoral arteries. Aortic insufficiency occurs in more than a third of patients with a proximal dissection; paradoxically, however, when acute aortic insufficiency is severe, the murmur may not be appreciable, so finding a widened pulse pressure and heart failure should raise suspicion of its presence.

Vascular complications from aortic dissection include compromise of a coronary artery, with subsequent myocardial ischemia or infarction. Involvement of the brachiocephalic arteries may produce a stroke or coma, whereas compromise of the spinal arteries may produce paraplegia. When a dissection extends into the abdominal aorta, flow to one or both renal arteries may be compromised and produce acute renal failure, which may exacerbate the hypertension. Mesenteric ischemia or frank infarction may manifest as abdominal pain. Finally, the dissection may extend distally to the aortic bifurcation and compromise or occlude one of the common iliac arteries and thereby produce a femoral pulse deficit and ischemia of the lower extremities.

An abnormality on a chest radiograph often raises the first suspicion of aortic dissection. The findings on chest radiography are nonspecific, however, and rarely diagnostic. An enlarged mediastinal silhouette is the most common finding, but it may be present in as few as 65% of patients in whom dissection is ultimately diagnosed. A left pleural effusion is commonly seen in patients with involvement of the descending thoracic aorta; when small, this typically represents an exudate from the inflamed aortic wall. A normal chest radiograph does not exclude the diagnosis of aortic dissection. Electrocardiographic findings in aortic dissection are nonspecific.

DIAGNOSIS

When there is clinical suspicion of aortic dissection, it is essential to confirm or exclude the diagnosis promptly with an imaging study (Fig. 78-3). Several

FIGURE 78-4. Transesophageal echocardiogram of the ascending aorta in the long axis in a patient with type A aortic dissection. The aortic valve (AV) is on the left, and the ascending aorta extends to the right. Within the aorta is an intimal flap (I) that originates at the level of the sinotubular junction. The true (T) and the false (F) lumens are separated by the intimal flap. LA = left atrium. (From Isselbacher EM. Diseases of the aorta. In: Braunwald E, Zipes DP, Libby P, Bonow RO, eds. *Braunwald's Heart Disease: A Textbook of Cardiovascular Medicine,* 7th ed. Philadelphia: Saunders; 2004:1423.)

imaging modalities can be used to diagnose the presence of aortic dissection accurately, including aortography, CT (Chapter 56), magnetic resonance imaging (Chapter 56), and transesophageal echocardiography (TEE; Chapter 55). Each institution must determine which of these modalities is most appropriate as an initial diagnostic approach, based on their availability and the skill and experience of the clinicians who perform and interpret the studies.

Nevertheless, when suspicion of aortic dissection is high, TEE (Fig. 78-4) is the most rapid means of providing sufficient detail to proceed directly to the operating room. When clinical suspicion is low (i.e., when the goal is to rule out aortic dissection), contrast-enhanced CT (Fig. 78-5) is preferred because it is entirely noninvasive. If TEE is not readily available, contrast-enhanced CT is the imaging modality of choice in both high-probability and low-probability patients.

FIGURE 78-5. Aortic dissection. Contrast-enhanced computed tomography scan of the chest at the level of the pulmonary artery shows an intimal flap (I) separating the two lumens of the ascending (A) and descending (D) thoracic aorta in a type A aortic dissection.

On cross-sectional imaging, an isolated intramural hematoma appears as a crescentic thickening around the aortic wall rather than true and false lumens separated by an intimal flap (Fig. 78-6). The presence of an intramural hematoma may be missed on aortography.

TREATMENT   **Rx**

The goal of initial medical therapy for acute aortic intramural hematoma or dissection is to halt further progression and reduce the risk for rupture. Acute management of an isolated hematoma should be the same as for dissection because of the risk that the hematoma will propagate.

Whenever there is suspicion of aortic intramural hematoma or dissection, therapy should be instituted immediately while imaging studies are ordered, rather than waiting until the diagnosis is confirmed. The initial goal is to reduce the force of ventricular contraction and reduce systolic blood pressure to 100 to 120 mm Hg or to the lowest level that maintains cerebral, cardiac, and renal perfusion. Intravenous labetalol (20 mg administered over a 2-minute period, followed by additional doses of 20 to 80 mg every 10 to 15 minutes, up to a maximum total dose of 300 mg, and then a continuous infusion at 2 to 8 mg/minute), which acts as an α-blocker and a β-blocker, may be particularly useful in aortic dissection for controlling hypertension and contractile force. After labetalol or a pure β-blocker (e.g., intravenous propranolol at 1-mg boluses every 3 to 5 minutes to start, followed by a continuous infusion at rates up to 20 mg/hour) has been administered, intravenous nitroprusside (0.5 to 8 µg/kg/minute) should be added to titrate blood pressure minute by minute as needed. If β-blockers are contraindicated, calcium-channel blockers (e.g., intravenous diltiazem with an initial bolus of 20 mg over a 2-minute period, followed by a continuous infusion of 5 to 15 mg/hour) may be useful.

When patients have significant hypotension, pseudohypotension should be carefully excluded first. True hypotension may be due to hemopericardium and cardiac tamponade as a result of rupture of the dissection into the pericardium. These patients should be treated with volume expansion and taken to surgery as quickly as possible because early mortality is extremely high. Pericardiocentesis should be performed only as a last resort because it may precipitate hemodynamic collapse and death.

After initial medical therapy has been instituted and the diagnosis of aortic dissection confirmed, definitive therapy must be determined. Whenever an acute dissection involves the ascending aorta, surgical repair is indicated to minimize the risk of life-threatening complications such as rupture, cardiac tamponade, severe aortic insufficiency, or stroke. Patients with acute dissections confined to the descending aorta are at much lower risk for these complications and tend to fare as well with medical therapy as they do with endovascular repair 8 or surgical repair. When a type B dissection is associated with a serious complication, however, such as end-organ ischemia, intervention is indicated with either endovascular techniques or open surgery. Patients

FIGURE 78-6. Intramural aortic hematoma. **A,** Contrast-enhanced computed tomography scan of the chest at the level of the pulmonary artery demonstrates an intramural hematoma (H) of the descending thoracic aorta (D). The hematoma appears as a crescentic thickening of the aortic wall that does not enhance from the contrast within the aortic lumen. The ascending thoracic aorta (A) is unaffected. **B,** Corresponding image from a non-contrast-enhanced computed tomography scan in which the intramural hematoma appears as a bright crescentic thickening of the aortic wall because the density of the hematoma is greater than that of the blood within the aortic lumen. **C,** Corresponding image from a contrast-enhanced computed tomography scan performed 1 week later for surveillance, in which the intramural hematoma has evolved into a classic aortic dissection with an intimal flap (I) and contrast evident within a patent false lumen.

with chronic type A dissections can often be managed medically because they have already survived the early period of high mortality associated with acute proximal dissections.

For an isolated intramural hematoma, the likelihood of progressive dissection or other complications is lower than in patients who initially have a frank dissection, especially those with smaller hematomas and normal aortic dimensions. Although the 25 to 50% risk of progression may warrant early surgery, serial imaging, with surgery reserved for progressive disease, is reasonable in patients at increased risk with surgery. For distal intramural hematomas, management is generally the same as for distal dissection.

PROGNOSIS

Acutely, the mortality rate from untreated aortic dissection is about 1% per hour. Patients with acute aortic dissection who survive the initial hospitalization generally do well thereafter, whether treated medically or surgically. Late complications such as aortic insufficiency, recurrent dissection, aneurysm formation, and aneurysm rupture can occur, however. Medications to control hypertension and reduce ventricular contractility can dramatically reduce the incidence of late complications and should be continued indefinitely. β-Blockers (e.g., metoprolol 25 to 200 mg twice daily or atenolol 25 to 200 mg/day) are the drugs of choice in this setting, but typically a second (e.g., lisinopril 5 to 40 mg/day) or third (amlodipine 2.5 to 10 mg/day or hydrochlorothiazide 12.5 to 50 mg/day) agent needs to be added to achieve the goal of systolic blood pressure less than 120 mm Hg (Chapter 67).

Patients are at highest risk for complications during the first 2 years after an intramural hematoma or aortic dissection. Progressive aortic expansion typically occurs without symptoms, so patients must be observed closely with serial aortic imaging at 6-month intervals for the first 2 years and annually thereafter, provided the anatomy is stable.

● TAKAYASU'S ARTERITIS

DEFINITION

Takayasu's arteritis, which is a chronic inflammatory disease of unknown cause, involves the aorta and its branches. The mean age at onset is 29 years, with women affected eight times as often as men. It occurs more often in Asia and Africa than in Europe or North America. An early stage characterized by active inflammation involving the aorta and its branches progresses at a variable rate to a later sclerotic stage with intimal hyperplasia, medial degeneration, and obliterative changes. Most of the resulting arterial lesions are stenotic, but aneurysms may also occur. The aortic arch and brachiocephalic vessels are affected most often, and the disease tends to be most pronounced at branch points in the aorta. The abdominal aorta is also commonly involved, and the pulmonary artery is sometimes involved. The disease may be diffuse or patchy, with affected areas separated by lengths of normal aorta.

CLINICAL MANIFESTATIONS

Most patients initially have symptoms of a systemic inflammatory process, such as fever, night sweats, arthralgia, and weight loss. There is often a delay of months to years, however, between the onset of symptoms and diagnosis. At the time of diagnosis, 90% of patients have entered the sclerotic phase and have symptoms of vascular insufficiency, typically with pain in the upper (or, less often, lower) extremities. There are often absent pulses and diminished blood pressure in the upper extremities, and the condition has earned the name *pulseless disease*. There may be bruits over affected arteries. Significant hypertension (secondary to renal artery involvement) occurs in more than half the patients, but its presence may be difficult to recognize because of the diminished pulses. Aortic insufficiency may result from proximal aortic involvement. Heart failure may result from either hypertension or aortic insufficiency. Involvement of the ostia of the coronary arteries may cause angina or myocardial infarction. Carotid artery involvement may cause cerebral ischemia or stroke. Abdominal angina may result from mesenteric artery compromise.

The overall 15-year survival rate in patients diagnosed with Takayasu's arteritis is 83%, with most deaths being caused by stroke, myocardial infarction, or heart failure. The survival rate in patients with major complications of the disease is 66%; the survival rate in patients without a major complication is 96%.

DIAGNOSIS

Laboratory abnormalities during the acute phase include an elevated erythrocyte sedimentation rate, elevated C-reactive protein level, mild leukocytosis, anemia, and elevated immunoglobulin levels. The diagnosis is best made by aortography, CT angiography, or magnetic resonance angiography, which reveal stenosis of the aorta and stenosis or occlusion of its branch vessels, often with post-stenotic dilation or associated aneurysms.

TREATMENT   Rx

Corticosteroids (e.g., prednisone 60 to 100 mg/day, often for months and tapered after symptoms or evidence of inflammation subside) are the primary therapy for the acute inflammatory stage and may be effective in improving constitutional symptoms, lowering the erythrocyte sedimentation rate, and

slowing disease progression. Cyclophosphamide (2 mg/kg/day) or methotrexate (15 to 25 mg/week) may be used when corticosteroid therapy alone is ineffective. It is unknown whether medical therapy reduces the risk for major complications or prolongs life.

Percutaneous balloon angioplasty can effectively dilate short stenotic lesions of the aorta and its branch arteries, although restenosis is common. Surgery may be necessary to bypass or reconstruct key segments, such as the coronary, carotid, or renal arteries, or to treat aortic insufficiency. Ideally, surgery should not be performed during the inflammatory phase.

● GIANT CELL ARTERITIS

Giant cell arteritis (Chapter 279) is more common than Takayasu's arteritis. Its cause is also unclear, but it tends to occur in an older population with a mean age of 67 years. It typically affects medium-sized arteries, but in 15% of cases it involves the aorta and branches of the aortic arch. Narrowing of the aorta is rare, but weakening of the ascending aortic wall may lead to localized thoracic aortic aneurysms and secondary aortic insufficiency. Narrowing of the branches of the aortic arch produces symptoms similar to those seen in Takayasu's arteritis. Because the temporal artery is commonly involved, the diagnosis is usually made by temporal artery biopsy. Management involves high-dose corticosteroid therapy (e.g., prednisone 60 to 100 mg/day, often for months and tapered after symptoms or evidence of inflammation subside), to which the disease is usually responsive.

1. Thompson SG, Ashton HA, Gao L, et al. Screening men for abdominal aortic aneurysm: 10 year mortality and cost effectiveness results from the randomised Multicentre Aneurysm Screening Study. *BMJ.* 2009;338:b2307-b2312.
2. United Kingdom Small Aneurysm Trial Participants. Long-term outcomes of immediate repair compared with surveillance of small abdominal aortic aneurysms. *N Engl J Med.* 2002;346:1445-1452.
3. Ashton HA, Buxton MJ, Day NE, et al. The Multicentre Aneurysm Screening Study (MASS) into the effect of abdominal aortic aneurysm screening on mortality in men: a randomised controlled trial. *Lancet.* 2002;360:1531-1539.
4. Lederle FA, Freischlag JA, Kyriakides TC, et al. Outcomes following endovascular vs open repair of abdominal aortic aneurysm: a randomized trial. *JAMA.* 2009;302:1535-1542.
5. United Kingdom EVAR Trial Investigators. Endovascular versus open repair of abdominal aortic aneurysm. *N Engl J Med.* 2010;362:1863-1871.
6. De Bruin JL, Baas AF, Buth J, et al. Long-term outcome of open or endovascular repair of abdominal aortic aneurysm. *N Engl J Med.* 2010;362:1881-1889.
7. United Kingdom EVAR Trial Investigators. Endovascular repair of aortic aneurysm in patients physically ineligible for open repair. *N Engl J Med.* 2010;362:1872-1878.
8. Nienaber CA, Rousseau H, Eggebrecht H, et al. Randomized comparison of strategies for type B aortic dissection: the INvestigation of STEnt Grafts in Aortic Dissection (INSTEAD) trial. *Circulation.* 2009;120:2519-2528.

SUGGESTED READINGS

Braverman AC. Acute aortic dissection: clinician update. *Circulation.* 2010;122:184-188. *Review.*
Hiratzka LF, Bakris GL, Beckman JA, et al. 2010 ACCF/AHA/AATS/ACR/ASA/SCA/SCAI/SIR/STS/SVM Guidelines for the diagnosis and management of patients with thoracic aortic disease: a report of the American College of Cardiology Foundation/American Heart Association Task Force on Practice Guidelines, American Association for Thoracic Surgery, American College of Radiology, American Stroke Association, Society of Cardiovascular Anesthesiologists, Society for Cardiovascular Angiography and Interventions, Society of Interventional Radiology, Society of Thoracic Surgeons, and Society for Vascular Medicine. *Circulation.* 2010;121:e266-e369. *Consensus guidelines.*
Moll FL, Powell JT, Fraedrich G, et al. Management of abdominal aortic aneurysms: clinical practice guidelines of the European Society for Vascular Surgery. *Eur J Vasc Endovasc Surg.* 2011;41:S1-S58. *Consensus guidelines.*

79

ATHEROSCLEROTIC PERIPHERAL ARTERIAL DISEASE

CHRISTOPHER J. WHITE

DEFINITION

Lower extremity atherosclerotic peripheral arterial disease is one subset of a larger group of peripheral vascular diseases that includes all noncoronary vascular disorders that may affect the arterial, venous (Chapter 81), or lymphatic circulation. Atherosclerotic arterial diseases are characterized by arterial narrowing or occlusion caused by the accumulation of atherosclerotic

How to Perform and Calculate the ABI

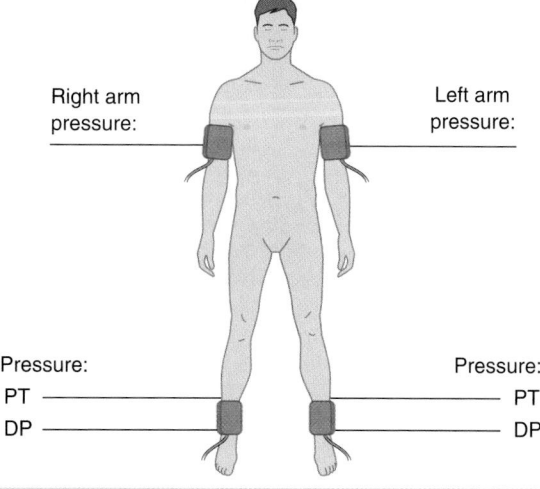

Right arm pressure:

Left arm pressure:

Pressure: PT ——— DP ———

Pressure: PT ——— DP ———

RIGHT ABI

$$\frac{\text{Higher right ankle pressure}}{\text{Higher arm pressure}} = \frac{\text{mm Hg}}{\text{mm Hg}} \_\_\_\_ = \frac{\text{Higher left ankle pressure}}{\text{Higher arm pressure}} = \frac{\text{mm Hg}}{\text{mm Hg}} = \_\_\_\_$$

LEFT ABI

EXAMPLE

$$\frac{\text{Higher ankle pressure}}{\text{Higher arm pressure}} = \frac{92 \text{ mm Hg}}{164 \text{ mm Hg}} = 0.56 \qquad \text{See ABI Chart}$$

FIGURE 79-1. Performing pressure measurements and calculating the ankle-brachial index (ABI). To calculate the ABI, systolic pressures are determined in both arms and both ankles with the use of a handheld Doppler instrument. The highest readings for the dorsalis pedis (DP) and posterior tibial (PT) arteries are used to calculate the index.

plaque elements in the vessel wall (Chapter 70). Atherosclerotic vascular disease can also lead to aneurysm formation, which is the pathologic enlargement of arterial segments, and may result in rupture, dissection, or thromboembolism (Chapter 78).

EPIDEMIOLOGY

The prevalence of lower extremity peripheral arterial disease in the United States, Europe, and Asia continues to increase as the population ages and is exposed to atherosclerotic risk factors (Chapter 51). The presence of peripheral arterial disease is defined as an ankle-brachial index (ABI)—the ratio of the systolic blood pressure in the ankle divided by the systolic blood pressure in the arm (Fig. 79-1)—less than 0.90. Among individuals aged 40 years and older, the prevalence is 4.3% (95% confidence interval [CI] 3.1 to 5.5%), but the prevalence in diabetic individuals ranges from 20 to 30%.

Risk factors for atherosclerosis (Chapter 51) increase the likelihood of developing lower extremity peripheral arterial disease. More than 95% of individuals with peripheral arterial disease have at least one traditional cardiovascular risk factor, and most have multiple risk factors. More than one third of patients with peripheral arterial disease have significant coronary disease, and up to one quarter have carotid artery disease. As a result, the risk of heart attack, stroke, and death are increased several-fold in patients with peripheral arterial disease.

Among conventional atherosclerotic risk factors, cigarette smoking is two to three times more likely to cause lower extremity peripheral arterial disease than to cause coronary artery disease. Hypertension is also associated with lower extremity peripheral arterial disease. The development of peripheral arterial disease is more likely in patients with lipid abnormalities (elevated total and low-density lipoprotein cholesterol, decreased high-density lipoprotein cholesterol, and hypertriglyceridemia), and the risk increases by 5 to 10% for each 10 mg/dL rise in total cholesterol. Increased homocysteine levels are associated with a two- to three-fold increased risk for developing atherosclerotic peripheral arterial disease. Diabetes mellitus increases the risk of lower extremity peripheral arterial disease by two- to four-fold, and the risk of developing lower extremity peripheral arterial disease is proportional to the severity and duration of diabetes. Tight control of diabetes is important, and the risk of developing peripheral arterial disease increases by 28% for every 1% increase in glycosylated hemoglobin (Chapters 236 and 237). Diabetic patients with lower extremity peripheral arterial disease are 7- to 15-fold more likely to undergo a major amputation than nondiabetics with lower extremity peripheral arterial disease.

Peripheral arterial disease disproportionately affects older individuals (Fig. 79-2), non-Hispanic blacks, current smokers, diabetics, and those with abnormal renal function. The overall prevalence of peripheral arterial disease

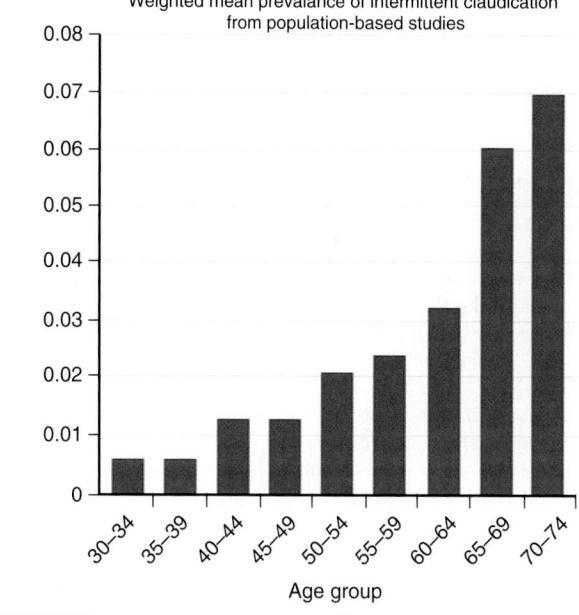

Weighted mean prevalance of intermittent claudication from population-based studies

FIGURE 79-2. Weighted mean prevalence of intermittent claudication. (Modified from Dormandy JA, Rutherford RB. Management of peripheral arterial disease. TransAtlantic Inter-Society Consensus (TASC) Working Group. *J Vasc Surg.* 2000;31:S1-S296.)

in the United States among persons aged 70 years and older is 14.5% (95% CI 10.8 to 18.2%), which corresponds to approximately 4 million individuals.

PATHOBIOLOGY
Acute Limb Ischemia

Acute limb ischemia occurs when blood flow to an extremity is abruptly halted or markedly diminished, resulting in hypoperfusion that threatens the viability of the limb. Acute limb ischemia is most commonly caused by either thrombosis or embolism. Thrombosis of a lower extremity arterial bypass graft is the most common clinical scenario. Most emboli originate from the heart as a mural thrombus from a recent myocardial infarction (Chapter 73) or from the atrial appendage in a patient with atrial fibrillation (Chapter 64). A less common cause of lower extremity emboli is an atherosclerotic or aneurysmal abdominal aorta (Chapter 78) that serves as the source of cholesterol emboli (Chapter 80).

Arterial in situ thrombosis as a result of plaque rupture usually represents the final stage of a chronically diseased artery, most commonly the femoral or popliteal artery. Conditions such as severe dehydration or low-output heart failure promote thrombosis at the site of stenosis. If native artery thrombosis occurs in the absence of a preexisting stenosis, a thorough search for a hypercoagulable state should be undertaken. Acutely thrombosed femoral or popliteal aneurysms may present as acute limb ischemia.

Chronic Limb Ischemia

Chronic, stable lower extremity peripheral arterial disease, manifested by the symptoms of intermittent claudication, may be due to atherosclerosis, thromboembolism, inflammatory disease, trauma, aneurysmal disease, adventitial cysts, entrapment syndromes, or congenital abnormalities. Aneurysms may be associated with atherosclerosis, or they may be due to underlying hereditary (familial) or acquired (e.g., due to smoking or trauma) causes.

Patients with critical limb ischemia have inadequate blood flow to sustain viability in the distal tissue bed. Critical limb ischemia is most often caused by atherosclerosis, but it can also be caused by atheroembolic or thromboembolic disease, vasculitis, in situ thrombosis related to hypercoagulable states, thromboangiitis obliterans, cystic adventitial disease, popliteal entrapment, or trauma. Patients presenting with critical limb ischemia typically have multisegment disease along the length of the limb.

Inflammation plays a fundamental role in the development and progression of atherosclerosis (Chapter 70). Elevated levels of C-reactive protein (CRP) are strongly associated with the development of peripheral arterial disease. Markers of inflammation such as interleukin-6, tumor necrosis factor-α, CRP, and platelet activation are increased compared with normal subjects.

No specific genetic markers have been confirmed for peripheral arterial disease, although one study identified a linkage on chromosome 1p. The proportion of low ABIs attributable to heritability is estimated at 20%. Concordance rates among twins are about 33% for monozygotic pairs and about 31% for dizygotic pairs, suggesting a limited role for heritability. Taken together, these data studies suggest a modest but significant heritability factor for peripheral arterial disease.

CLINICAL MANIFESTATIONS

Acute Limb Ischemia

A patient with acute limb ischemia classically presents with a cool, painful extremity. Typically, the major muscle groups below the level of obstruction are symptomatic. The absence of a pulse may help localize the site of occlusion, but pulses may be normal in cases of microemboli or cholesterol emboli (Chapter 80). Venous and capillary filling is an indicator of the severity of acute limb ischemia. The leg should be carefully examined for color and temperature abnormalities. Pallor is seen early on, but with time, cyanosis is common. Poikilothermia, or coolness, is an important finding, particularly if the opposite limb is warm. A transition level for color and temperature changes, which is often clinically obvious, should be correlated with the

pulses and denoted as a baseline reference at the initial examination for comparison with subsequent examinations.

Sensory changes include numbness and paresthesias. Paralysis indicates advanced, limb-threatening ischemia. The extent of any motor deficit is a good index of the degree of tissue anoxia and correlates well with the prognosis. Motor deficits progress from distal to more proximal muscle groups, so early motor weakness is seen in the intrinsic foot muscles. Complete motor paralysis is a late symptom that suggests impending irreversible injury. In due course, paralysis progresses to rigor when irreversible ischemia has developed.

Chronic Stable Lower Limb Ischemia

Patients with chronic peripheral arterial disease may be clinically stable and report no symptoms, atypical symptoms, or symptoms of exertional discomfort (claudication). If they are clinically unstable with pain at rest or with ulceration or spreading gangrene, they have critical limb ischemia that threatens the limb (Table 79-1). The majority of patients with chronic peripheral arterial disease are asymptomatic and are identified by abnormal pulse examinations, investigation of vascular bruits, or routine measurement of the ABI (see Fig. 79-1). Patients with typical symptoms of intermittent claudication are only the tip of the iceberg, representing no more than 20% of patients with objective evidence of peripheral arterial disease.

Claudication is defined as exertional discomfort, relieved with rest, in specific muscle groups at risk for ischemia during exercise. Symptoms usually begin one segment below the level of the arterial narrowing. For example, vascular blockages (occlusions or stenoses) of the iliac vessels typically cause hip, thigh, and calf pain, whereas femoral and popliteal artery obstructions typically cause symptoms in the calf and foot muscles. Claudication, which is a specific vascular syndrome, must be distinguished from other conditions that cause exertional leg pain, which have been termed *pseudoclaudication* (Table 79-2).

TABLE 79-1   FONTAINE'S AND RUTHERFORD'S CLINICAL CLASSIFICATIONS OF CHRONIC LOWER LIMB ISCHEMIA

	Fontaine		Rutherford	
STAGE	**CLINICAL**	**GRADE**	**CATEGORY**	**CLINICAL**
I	Asymptomatic	0	0	Asymptomatic
IIa	Mild claudication	I	1	Mild claudication
IIb	Moderate to severe claudication	I I	2 3	Moderate claudication Severe claudication
III	Rest pain	II	4	Rest pain
IV	Ulceration or gangrene	III IV	5 6	Minor tissue loss Ulceration or gangrene

Adapted from Norgren L, Hiatt WR, Dormandy JA, et al. Inter-society consensus for the management of peripheral arterial disease (TASC II). *Eur J Vasc Endovasc Surg.* 2007;33:S1-S75.

TABLE 79-2   DIFFERENTIATION OF TRUE CLAUDICATION FROM PSEUDOCLAUDICATION

	INTERMITTENT CLAUDICATION	SPINAL STENOSIS	ARTHRITIS	VENOUS CONGESTION	COMPARTMENT SYNDROME
Character of discomfort	Cramping, tightness, or tiredness	Same as claudication or tingling, weakness, clumsiness	Aching	Tightness, bursting pain	Tightness, bursting pain
Location of discomfort	Buttock, hip, thigh, calf, foot	Buttock, hip, thigh	Hip, knee	Groin, thigh	Calf
Exercise-induced discomfort	Yes	Variable	Variable	After walking	Excessive exercise
Walking distance to discomfort	Reproducible	Variable	Variable	Variable	Excessive exercise
Occurs with standing	No	Yes	Yes, but positional	Yes, but positional	Yes, but positional
Relief of discomfort	Rapid relief with rest	Relief with sitting or changing position	Slow relief with avoidance of weight bearing	Slow relief with leg elevation	Slow relief with leg elevation
Other	Associated with atherosclerosis and decreased pulses	History of lower back problems	Discomfort at joint	History of deep vein thrombosis, signs of venous congestion	Typical in athletes

From White C. Intermittent claudication. *N Engl J Med.* 2007;356:1241-1250.

TABLE 79-3 CLINICAL CATEGORIES OF ACUTE LIMB ISCHEMIA

CATEGORY	DESCRIPTION	SENSORY LOSS	MUSCLE WEAKNESS	DOPPLER ARTERIAL	DOPPLER VENOUS
I. Viable	Not immediately threatened	None	None	Audible	Audible
IIa. Threatened marginally	Salvageable if promptly treated	Minimal or none	None	Inaudible	Audible
IIb. Threatened immediately	Salvageable if immediately treated	More than toes, associated with rest pain	Mild to moderate	Inaudible	Audible
III. Irreversible	Major tissue loss inevitable	Profound, anesthetic	Profound, paralysis, rigor	Inaudible	Inaudible

Adapted from Rutherford RB, Baker JD, Ernst C, et al. Recommended standards for reports dealing with lower extremity ischemia: revised version. *J Vasc Surg.* 1997;26:517-538.

Symptoms in individual patients are remarkably variable despite similar degrees of vascular stenosis, in part owing to collateral vessel formation. A patient with superficial femoral artery occlusion but robust collateral formation via the deep femoral artery and geniculate collaterals, which supply blood to the infrapopliteal vessels, may have minimal or no symptoms. Another patient with similar anatomy but poor collaterals may have severe symptoms.

Chronic Critical Lower Limb Ischemia

Critical limb ischemia develops in about 10% of all patients with peripheral arterial disease; it presents as resting limb pain or impending limb or tissue loss, as manifested clinically by nonhealing lower extremity ulcers or the presence of gangrene. These patients' limbs are in jeopardy, and even the most minor trauma from a poorly fitting shoe or a carelessly clipped toenail may cause a nonhealing wound or infection necessitating amputation. Critical limb ischemia can be exacerbated by conditions that reduce blood flow to the microvascular bed, such as diabetes, severe low cardiac output states, and, rarely, vasospastic diseases.

▶ DIAGNOSIS

Acute Limb Ischemia

In patients with acute limb ischemia, the history and physical examination are important steps not only in assessing the cause and severity of ischemia but also in determining the diagnostic and therapeutic path. Upon completion of the history and physical examination, the physician should be able to answer the following questions about the severity of acute limb ischemia: Is the limb viable? Is its viability immediately threatened? Are there already irreversible changes that may preclude salvage of the limb? Three findings that help differentiate "threatened" from "viable" extremities are the presence of persistent pain, sensory loss, and muscle weakness (Table 79-3).

Chronic Limb Ischemia

The clinical severity of acute and chronic limb ischemia can be semiquantitatively assessed using either the Fontaine or the Rutherford classification (see Table 79-1). The clinician must distinguish intermittent claudication from nonvascular causes that may mimic claudication (i.e., pseudoclaudication), such as neurogenic pain from spinal stenosis or nerve root compression (Chapter 407), musculoskeletal or arthritic pain, or discomfort from venous congestion or a compartment syndrome (see Table 79-2). A typical history of claudication has a low sensitivity but a high specificity for peripheral arterial disease.

Patients presenting with peripheral arterial disease should be assessed for atherosclerotic risk factors (Table 79-4) and undergo a complete vascular physical examination, including measurement of the ABI (see Fig. 79-1). In healthy adults without arterial occlusive disease, ankle systolic pressure is typically 10 to 15 mm Hg greater than arm (brachial) systolic pressure, owing to the effect of pulse wave reflection. A truly normal ABI is greater than 1.10, although peripheral arterial disease is generally defined as a resting ABI of 0.90 or less.

Imaging

Duplex imaging combines ultrasound imaging and Doppler blood velocity measurements to localize vascular obstructions and estimate lesion severity. The sensitivity and specificity of duplex ultrasound for the diagnosis of a 50% or greater stenosis in the lower extremity are 90% or higher. Duplex ultrasound has proved useful for the surveillance of post-surgical vein graft patency in the lower extremities, although the specific utility of ultrasound surveillance after synthetic bypass grafting or after endovascular therapy has not been demonstrated.

TABLE 79-4 INITIAL LABORATORY EVALUATION OF A PATIENT WITH PERIPHERAL ARTERIAL DISEASE

Serum electrolytes, including fasting serum glucose
Renal function (serum creatinine, blood urea nitrogen, estimated glomerular filtration rate)
Complete blood count
Fasting lipid profile
High-sensitivity C-reactive protein
Ankle-brachial index

DSA   CTA   MRA

FIGURE 79-3. Aortography with distal run-off in three different patients by three different methods: digital subtraction angiography (DSA), computed tomography angiography (CTA), and magnetic resonance angiography (MRA). (From White C. Intermittent claudication. *N Engl J Med.* 2007;356:1241-1250.)

Computed tomography angiography (CTA) and magnetic resonance angiography (MRA) obtain cross-sectional images that can be reconstructed into a three-dimensional angiogram (Fig. 79-3). CTA requires iodinated intravenous contrast material and ionizing radiation, whereas MRA uses gadolinium contrast and does not expose the patient to ionizing radiation. The major toxicity of gadolinium is an uncommon but potentially lethal systemic disorder called nephrogenic systemic fibrosis or nephrogenic sclerosing dermopathy (Chapter 275); chronic kidney disease with a glomerular filtration rate of 60 mL/minute or less is the major risk factor for the development of nephrogenic sclerosing dermopathy.

07/14/00   09/12/00   05/10/06   6/26/06

A   B   C   D

FIGURE 79-4. **A,** Baseline angiogram of left leg showing occlusion (arrowheads) of the femoral-popliteal segment. **B,** Post-treatment angiogram after balloon angioplasty and stent placement. **C,** More than 5 years later, the patient returns with claudication and a reduced ankle-brachial index. Follow-up computed tomography angiogram shows narrowing of the superficial femoral artery between the two stents. **D,** Final angiogram following balloon angioplasty and stent placement in the femoral narrowings.

An advantage of CTA over MRA is its ability to visualize metallic stents and stent-grafts (Fig. 79-4). CTA requires only about one fourth the radiation required for invasive digital angiography, and it can be performed more quickly and with less pretreatment planning than MRA. Vascular calcification may be a source of artifact with CTA but is inconsequential with MRA. MRA tends to overestimate lesions at the ostia of arteries owing to turbulent flow, and MRA cannot be performed in patients with ferromagnetic metallic implants. In a randomized trial comparing MRA with CTA for initial imaging in peripheral arterial disease, there was no difference between the two techniques in terms of ease, clinical utility, or patient outcome, but CTA reduced total diagnostic costs.**1**

Invasive digital angiography remains the "gold standard" for the diagnosis and evaluation of peripheral arterial disease (see Fig. 79-3), despite the need for iodinated contrast material and the exposure to ionizing radiation. Another limitation is the two-dimensional nature of the images, given the vascular system's tortuous, three-dimensional structure and detailed morphology, which may be obscured by the overlap of side branches. Invasive angiographic procedures (Chapter 57) are associated with a relatively small but nontrivial rate of complications, including severe contrast allergy in 0.1%, access-related bleeding complications, contrast-induced nephropathy, and, very rarely, infection.

TREATMENT   Rx

The treatment of patients with atherosclerotic lower extremity peripheral arterial disease is directed at salvaging the limb, improving walking distance, and reducing the patient's risk for life-threatening cardiovascular complications of atherosclerosis. The decision to perform a percutaneous or surgical revascularization procedure for the relief of claudication is based on a risk-benefit assessment that weighs the patient's disability and discomfort against the estimated short- and long-term success and risks of the procedure. Because very few patients with claudication are in danger of losing their limbs, the primary goal of revascularization is long-lasting relief of symptoms, not limb salvage.

Revascularization strategies now emphasize percutaneous endovascular treatments rather than traditional open surgical approaches because of their lower morbidity (see Fig. 79-4). Stenting has made catheter-based procedures safer, more durable, and more predictably successful.

Acute Limb Ischemia

Patients with irreversible limb ischemia should not undergo angiography and should be scheduled for amputation (Fig. 79-5). All other patients with acute limb ischemia should undergo emergent angiography. Before angiography, anticoagulation to prevent thrombus propagation and/or embolization (e.g., unfractionated heparin 5000 IU bolus, then 1000 IU/hour infusion) and analgesia (e.g., morphine 2 mg intravenously, as needed) should be initiated, and any underlying medical comorbidities (e.g., heart failure) should be managed aggressively to stabilize the patient. The method used for direct revascularization must be tailored to the patient and to the physician's skills (operative or endovascular).

The options for prompt revascularization consist of endovascular therapies with intra-arterial thrombolysis (e.g., recombinant tissue plasminogen activator 0.5 mg/hour intra-arterially) or thrombectomy, or surgical thrombectomy with or without arterial bypass. In general, endovascular therapy is recommended for patients with an onset of acute symptoms less than 14 days earlier, and surgical revascularization is recommended for patients with a duration of symptoms greater than 14 days. These treatments are often complementary, each with its own advantages and limitations. The less invasive endovascular therapy allows simultaneous angiography to guide reperfusion therapy, but it may be difficult to pass the guidewire across a total occlusion. Surgery offers definitive restoration of blood flow with thrombectomy or bypass surgery, but it carries higher short-term risks. When choosing a treatment, consideration should be given to the location of the occlusion, the type of occlusion (thrombus or embolus), the duration of ischemia, patient-related risks, the type of conduit to be recanalized (artery or graft), and therapy-related risks and outcomes. For example, an in situ thrombus is more amenable to thrombolysis than is an embolus, which may require thrombectomy.

Chronic Stable Lower Limb Ischemia

The treatment of patients with claudication is directed at both improving the walking distance and, perhaps more importantly, reducing the patient's risk for life-threatening cardiovascular complications of atherosclerosis. Risk factor modification (Chapter 51), antiplatelet therapy (Chapter 37), and an exercise prescription are the basic elements of treating peripheral arterial disease.

Exercise Therapy

Improvement in walking distance can often be achieved with pharmacologic management, discontinuation of tobacco use, and a regular, supervised exercise program. Patients should be reassured that exercising, even though it may precipitate their claudication symptoms, is not harmful and is the preferred initial treatment.**2** A meta-analysis of eight randomized trials demonstrated that a supervised, as opposed to unsupervised, exercise program improved symptoms of claudication.**3** Supervised exercise commonly involves walking on a treadmill, with the initial workload set to elicit symptoms within 3 to 5 minutes of walking. The patient is permitted to rest until the symptoms resolve but then resumes exercising. Maximal benefits are associated with programs that require the patient to continue walking until the pain is near maximal and with sessions that last more than 30 minutes, occur three or more times per week, and continue for more than 6 months. It typically takes 1 to 2 months for the patient to begin to notice benefits, which gradually increase over several months.

Pharmacology

Currently, two medications are approved in the United States for the symptomatic treatment of intermittent claudication: pentoxifylline and cilostazol. In randomized clinical trials, pentoxifylline has not consistently improved treadmill walking distance, so it cannot be recommended. Cilostazol (50 to 100 mg twice daily), a phosphodiesterase inhibitor, improves maximal walking distance by 40 to 50% compared with placebo.**4** Cilostazol is contraindicated in patients with heart failure. Oral vasodilating prostaglandins, vitamin E, and chelation therapy with EDTA have not been effective in improving either symptoms or walking distance.

Risk Factor Treatment

Antiplatelet therapy with aspirin (usually 81 mg/day) has an established role in the secondary prevention of cardiovascular events in patients at high risk, based on clinical evidence of either coronary artery disease or stroke (Chapter 414). However, the role of aspirin in other populations, such as those with peripheral arterial disease but no clinical evidence of coronary artery disease or stroke, has not been established. The thienopyridines, such as

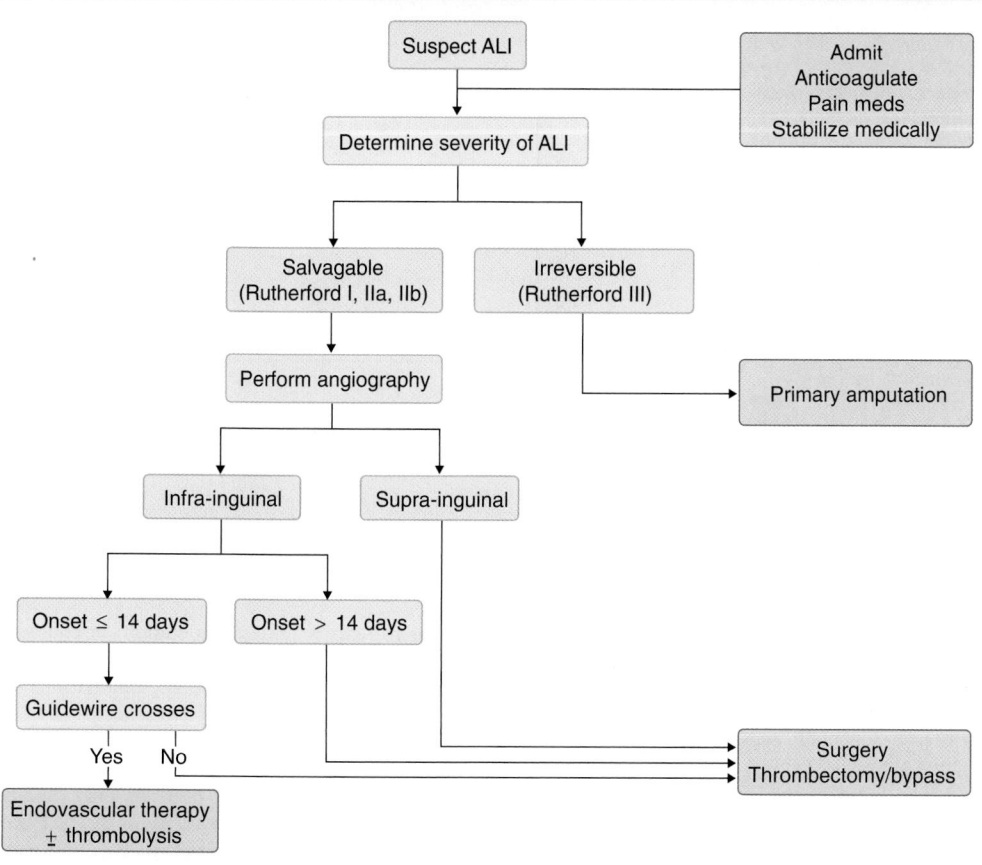

FIGURE 79-5. Treatment algorithm for acute limb ischemia (ALI). (Modified from Gray BH, Conte MS, Dake MD, et al. Atherosclerotic Peripheral Vascular Disease Symposium II: lower-extremity revascularization: state of the art. *Circulation.* 2008;118:2864-2872.)

FIGURE 79-6. Discrete stenosis *(arrows)* of the left superficial femoral artery seen on computed tomography angiography (CTA; left), digital subtraction angiography (middle), and digital angiography after percutaneous transluminal angioplasty (PTA; right). (From White C. Intermittent claudication. *N Engl J Med.* 2007;356:1241-1250.)

clopidogrel (usually 75 mg/day), are indicated only if aspirin is not tolerated, based on clopidogrel's efficacy compared with aspirin among patients with peripheral arterial disease.[5]

Patients with known peripheral arterial disease should be encouraged to modify or eliminate atherosclerotic risk factors such as diabetes (Chapter 237), tobacco use (Chapter 31), hyperlipidemia (Chapter 213), and hypertension (Chapter 67) and to exercise regularly (Chapter 15). Medical therapy, dietary modification, and exercise should all be tailored to meet current guidelines for controlling hyperlipidemia (Chapter 213) and hypertension (Chapter 67).

For patients with severe peripheral arterial disease and elevated CRP levels, statin therapy substantially improves overall survival.[6] This finding in patients with peripheral arterial disease is consistent with findings in other studies of patients with a history of vascular disease, with or without peripheral arterial disease, and with either elevated low-density lipoprotein cholesterol levels or elevated CRP levels. Blood pressure control is very important, especially in patients with coexisting diabetes.[7] β-Blockers are effective antihypertensive therapy and are not contraindicated in peripheral arterial disease. Angiotensin-converting enzyme inhibitors reduce the risk of cardiovascular death in patients with peripheral arterial disease.[8]

Revascularization

Patients selected for revascularization to relieve symptoms of intermittent claudication should have significant lifestyle limitations or be unable to work and should have failed to respond to pharmacologic and exercise therapy. They should also have a favorable risk-benefit ratio and favorable vascular anatomy for the planned revascularization procedure.

Superficial femoral artery stenosis or occlusion is the most common lesion associated with claudication (Fig. 79-6). Revascularization with surgery or percutaneous transluminal angioplasty is indicated for the relief of vocational or lifestyle-limiting claudication in patients who have failed exercise and pharmacologic therapy. Angioplasty with stenting is preferred when possible in patients younger than 50 years, as they have a higher risk of surgical graft failure than do older patients.

Clinical trials comparing medical therapy and percutaneous transluminal angioplasty with and without stenting for patients with claudication and for those with femoral-popliteal arterial disease demonstrate substantially better early relief of symptoms and long-term vessel patency with angioplasty. A meta-analysis comparing exercise therapy with balloon angioplasty in claudicants found no difference in quality-of-life measures at 3 and 6 months, but the ABI and functional capacity improved more with angioplasty than with exercise therapy.[9]

Some randomized trials comparing surgery with percutaneous transluminal angioplasty show similar rates of mortality, amputation, and patency at 4 years in patients with lower extremity ischemia. Percutaneous transluminal angioplasty is preferred in amenable lesions because of its lower periprocedural mortality and morbidity. Percutaneous transluminal angioplasty is more cost-effective than surgery if the expected 5-year patency rate of the treated vessel is 30% or greater. Outcomes following femoral-popliteal percutaneous transluminal angioplasty have improved over time, with current patency rates of 87, 69, and 55% at 1, 3, and 5 years, respectively.

Clinical success for patients with claudication caused by femoral lesions depends on obtaining a durable, long-lasting result. Although one option is angioplasty followed by provisional "bailout" stenting if the angioplasty itself is not successful, primary stenting with nitinol self-expanding stents is superior to provisional stent replacement for longer femoral lesions (7 to 10 cm) in terms of restenosis, improvement in ABI, and longer walking distance.[10] At 2 years follow-up, the benefit of primary stenting remained statistically significant, but the restenosis rate for femoral stents is about 50%. In more discrete femoral lesions (mean, 4.5 cm), a strategy of balloon angioplasty first, with stenting only for bailout, is as good as routine stenting.[11,12] The difference in outcomes for short versus long lesions is because stenting is equally good for long and short lesions, but longer lesions are more prone to restenosis after balloon angioplasty; as a result, stents improve outcomes in longer lesions. For shorter superficial femoral artery lesions, a strategy of percutaneous transluminal angioplasty with bailout stenting is preferable.

Adjunctive angioplasty devices such as atherectomy, cryotherapy, and the cutting balloon have not been meaningfully tested in any population, and there are few data to support their use versus less expensive, more conventional therapies. In randomized trials, laser angioplasty is not superior to conventional percutaneous transluminal angioplasty and/or stent placement in the superficial femoral artery. Given the substantial additional expense associated with these devices, more evidence of their efficacy is needed before widespread adoption can be justified.

Attempts to use drug-eluting stents in the femoral artery to reduce recurrence rates have failed. However, two randomized controlled trials using paclitaxel-coated balloons in femoral lesions showed lower restenosis rates compared with control balloons. Despite the small number of patients tested, these two trials provide reason for optimism.

Chronic Critical Lower Limb Ischemia

Patients with critical limb ischemia who have extensive necrosis or infectious gangrene or who are nonambulatory may best be served by primary amputation. For other patients with critical limb ischemia, the optimal treatment is prompt revascularization. The therapeutic goal is to reestablish pulsatile, straight-line flow to the distal extremity. Establishment of uninterrupted flow to at least one infrapopliteal vessel (i.e., the anterior or posterior tibial or peroneal arteries) is a prerequisite for wound healing. When treating patients with potential tissue or limb loss, transient restoration of flow to the extremity may effectively heal an ulcer. The healed ulcer usually does not recur, even if restenosis occurs after several months, if there is no recurrent injury.

In patients with critical limb ischemia caused by infrainguinal disease, percutaneous transluminal angioplasty and surgery are comparable as first-line therapies, but angioplasty is less costly and is associated with a lower morbidity.[13] Percutaneous transluminal angioplasty should be tried first if a patient is a candidate for either procedure, particularly if the patient's life expectancy is less than 2 years. Primary stenting with a drug-eluting stent may be preferable to regular angioplasty.[14] compared with percutaneous transluminal angioplasty with "provisional" bailout stenting in patients with occlusions and critical limb ischemia.

PROGNOSIS

Peripheral arterial disease is a major cause of acute and chronic illness associated with impaired functional capacity, reduced quality of life, limb loss, and increased risk of death (Fig. 79-7). Approximately two thirds of patients with peripheral arterial disease have at least one severely diseased coronary artery, and up to one quarter of patients have significant carotid artery stenosis. Consequently, patients with peripheral arterial disease face an increased risk of cardiovascular ischemic events such as myocardial infarction, ischemic stroke, and death. It is estimated that coronary and cerebrovascular adverse events occur two- to four-fold more commonly than do limb adverse events in patients with peripheral arterial disease.

The annual mortality for patients with peripheral arterial disease is about 5%, but it is higher for patients with severe disease. For example, the estimated 1-year mortality rate for patients with critical limb ischemia is 25%,

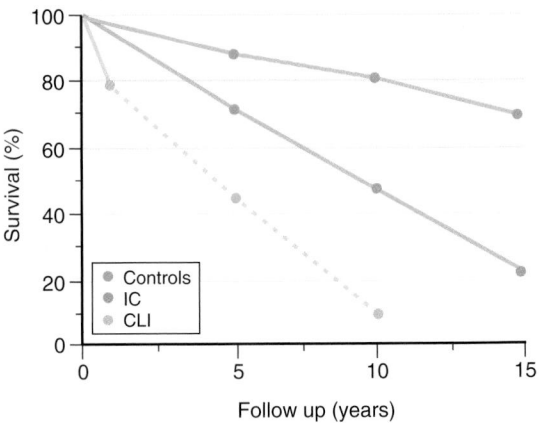

FIGURE 79-7. Survival curve of patients with intermittent claudication (IC) versus critical limb ischemia (CLI). (Modified from Norgren L, Hiatt WR, Dormandy JA, et al. Intersociety consensus for the management of peripheral arterial disease (TASC II). *Eur J Vasc Endovasc Surg.* 2007;33:S1-S75.)

but this can climb to 45% for patients requiring amputation; in contrast, annual mortality for patients with intermittent claudication is only 1 to 2%. For patients presenting with acute limb ischemia, the 30-day amputation rate is as high as 40%, and mortality rates up to 30% have been reported.

Patients with lower extremity claudication should be reassured that the risk of limb loss is low and that claudication usually does not worsen or improve at a rapid rate. Moreover, a history of claudication, by itself, only slightly increases the risk of amputation after 10 years. However, a reduced ABI and diabetes mellitus are associated with the development of ischemic rest pain and ischemic ulceration, which may lead to limb loss. Among patients with peripheral arterial disease, those who have diabetes are 15 times more likely to have an amputation than are patients without diabetes, whose annual amputation rate is about 0.6%.

 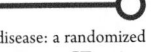

1. Ouwendijk R, de Vries M, Pattynama PM, et al. Imaging peripheral arterial disease: a randomized controlled trial comparing contrast-enhanced MR angiography and multi-detector row CT angiography. *Radiology.* 2005;236:1094-1103.
2. Mazari FA, Gulati S, Rahman MN, et al. Early outcomes from a randomized, controlled trial of supervised exercise, angioplasty, and combined therapy in intermittent claudication. *Ann Vasc Surg.* 2010;24:69-79.
3. McDermott MM, Ades P, Guralnik JM, et al. Treadmill exercise and resistance training in patients with peripheral arterial disease with and without intermittent claudication: a randomized controlled trial. *JAMA.* 2009;301:165-174.
4. Dawson DL, Cutler BS, Hiatt WR, et al. A comparison of cilostazol and pentoxifylline for treating intermittent claudication. *Am J Med.* 2000;109:523-530.
5. A randomised, blinded, trial of clopidogrel versus aspirin in patients at risk of ischaemic events (CAPRIE). CAPRIE Steering Committee. *Lancet.* 1996;348:1329-1339.
6. Schillinger M, Exner M, Mlekusch W, et al. Statin therapy improves cardiovascular outcome of patients with peripheral artery disease. *Eur Heart J.* 2004;25:742-748.
7. Mehler PS, Coll JR, Estacio R, et al. Intensive blood pressure control reduces the risk of cardiovascular events in patients with peripheral arterial disease and type 2 diabetes. *Circulation.* 2003;107:753-756.
8. Yusuf S, Sleight P, Pogue J, et al. Effects of an angiotensin-converting-enzyme inhibitor, ramipril, on cardiovascular events in high-risk patients. The Heart Outcomes Prevention Evaluation Study Investigators. *N Engl J Med.* 2000;342:145-153.
9. Whyman MR, Fowkes FG, Kerracher EM, et al. Is intermittent claudication improved by percutaneous transluminal angioplasty? A randomized controlled trial. *J Vasc Surg.* 1997;26:551-557.
10. Schillinger M, Sabeti S, Loewe C, et al. Balloon angioplasty versus implantation of nitinol stents in the superficial femoral artery. *N Engl J Med.* 2006;354:1879-1888.
11. Kasapis C, Henke PK, Chetcuti SJ, et al. Routine stent implantation vs. percutaneous transluminal angioplasty in femoropopliteal artery disease: a meta-analysis of randomized controlled trials. *Eur Heart J.* 2009;30:44-55.
12. Laird JR, Katzen BT, Scheinert D, et al. Nitinol stent implantation versus balloon angioplasty for lesions in the superficial femoral artery and proximal popliteal artery twelve-month results from the RESILIENT Randomized Trial. *Circulation.* 2010;3:267-276.
13. Conte MS. Bypass versus angioplasty in severe ischaemia of the leg (BASIL) and the (hoped for) dawn of evidence-based treatment for advanced limb ischemia. *J Vasc Surg.* 2010;51:69S-75S.
14. Feiring AJ, Krahn M, Nelson L, et al. Preventing leg amputations in critical limb ischemia with below-the-knee drug-eluting stents: the PaRADISE (PReventinig Amputations using Drug eluting StEnts) trial. *J Am Coll Cardiol.* 2010;55:1580-1589.

SUGGESTED READING

Hamburg NM, Balady GJ. Exercise rehabilitation in peripheral artery disease: functional impact and mechanisms of benefits. *Circulation.* 2011;123:87-97. *Review.*

80

OTHER PERIPHERAL ARTERIAL DISEASES

JEFFREY W. OLIN

LIVEDO RETICULARIS

Livedo reticularis is characterized by a reticular, fishnet, or lacy pattern on the skin of the lower extremities and other parts of the body. This pattern is red or blue and is caused by deoxygenated blood in the surrounding horizontally arranged venous plexus.

Primary or benign livedo reticularis occurs most commonly in young women between the ages of 20 and 40 years. Ulceration generally does not occur with this form of the disease, which may result from vasomotor instability or increased sensitivity (e.g., to cold, stress, tobacco) of the dermal blood vessels. It is intensified by cold exposure and is relieved by rewarming, and it may occur in association with Raynaud's phenomenon. The benign variety of livedo reticularis often needs no treatment other than measures to keep the body as warm as possible.

Secondary livedo reticularis occurs in association with atheromatous embolization (Fig. 80-1), polyarteritis nodosa (Chapter 278), systemic lupus erythematosus (Chapter 274), leukocytoclastic vasculitis (Chapter 278), cryoglobulinemia (Chapter 193), other connective tissue diseases, therapy with amantadine, and various neoplastic, neurologic, or endocrine diseases and in patients receiving large doses of vasopressors such as epinephrine, norepinephrine, and dopamine. Livedo reticularis is also one of the many skin manifestations of the antiphospholipid antibody syndrome (Chapter 179). In patients with secondary livedo reticularis, therapy should be directed at the underlying cause.

Livedoid Vasculopathy

In livedoid vasculopathy or livedoid vasculitis, extensive livedo reticularis surrounds a painful, ischemic-appearing ulceration located on the anterior or posterior portion of the lower leg (Fig. 80-2). Pathologically, thrombosis of the microvasculature occurs, with little or no active inflammatory component. Small doses of tissue plasminogen activator (10 mg intravenously daily for 14 days) may be effective in treating the ulcerations. Atrophie blanche (Fig. 80-3) is a variant of livedoid vasculopathy. These ulcerations generally occur around the ankle or foot. They have a white or yellowish base with poor granulation tissue and are exquisitely painful and difficult to heal.

ATHEROMATOUS EMBOLIZATION

DEFINITION

Atheromatous embolization (cholesterol embolization) refers to the embolization of cholesterol crystals or platelet fibrin aggregates to the extremities or to one or more organs. Atheromatous emboli usually originate from ulcerated or stenotic atherosclerotic plaques or from aneurysms that are primarily in the thoracic or abdominal aorta, iliac artery, or carotid artery.

EPIDEMIOLOGY AND PATHOBIOLOGY

Atheromatous embolization of the kidneys (Chapter 127) is a common histologic finding and may occur in 15 to 30% of patients with severe aortic atherosclerosis or aneurysm of the abdominal aorta. Increasing aortic plaque thickness, protruding aortic atheroma, and mobile aortic atheroma are associated with a high likelihood of atheromatous embolization. Atheromatous embolization may be spontaneous, but it occurs most often after percutaneous coronary, peripheral, or cerebrovascular intervention. Pathologically, biconvex cholesterol crystals lodge in the arterioles and lead to a foreign body reaction in which polymorphonuclear leukocytes, macrophages, and multinucleated giant cells appear several days to several weeks after the inciting event.

CLINICAL MANIFESTATIONS

The most common clinical manifestations are skin changes. These changes occur in more than one third of patients and are generally found in the lower extremities, but they may also be seen in the trunk, over the buttocks, and rarely in the upper extremities. These manifestations include livedo reticularis (embolization to the dermal blood vessels), purple or blue toes (see Fig. 80-1), splinter hemorrhages, gangrenous digits or ulcerations, and nodules in the presence of palpable foot pulses. The pain associated with ischemic lesions is disproportionate to the amount of tissue involvement.

FIGURE 80-2. Livedoid vasculitis. Ischemic ulceration is evident on the posterior portion of the calf, surrounded by a livedoid pattern on the skin.

FIGURE 80-1. Typical livedo reticularis on the lateral portion of the left foot and both heels. The second and fourth toes are cyanotic. These findings are typical of atheromatous embolization, and the fact that both feet are involved indicates a source above the aortic bifurcation. (From Bartholomew JR, Olin JW. Atheromatous embolization. In: Young JR, Olin JW, Bartholomew JR, eds. *Peripheral Vascular Diseases*, 2nd ed. St. Louis: Mosby; 1996.)

FIGURE 80-3. Atrophie blanche. Typical appearance of atrophie blanche. Note the pearly white plaque surrounded by prominent venules and a shallow ulceration. These lesions are quite painful and notoriously difficult to heal.

Atheroembolic renal disease is a small vessel occlusive disease leading to uncontrolled hypertension and advanced or end-stage renal disease. Atheromatous embolization may also involve the gastrointestinal tract and may produce ischemic bowel, with generalized abdominal pain, nausea, vomiting, melena, or hematochezia. Cholesterol emboli to the gallbladder may produce acute gangrenous cholecystitis, whereas emboli to the pancreas can cause acute pancreatitis.

Cardiac manifestations of atheroemboli include angina pectoris (Chapter 71) and myocardial infarction (Chapter 73). Patients may develop amaurosis fugax or blindness caused by retinal artery occlusion. A Hollenhorst plaque (yellow, highly refractile atheromatous material) may be present at the bifurcation of retinal blood vessels. Stroke, headache, confusion, organic brain syndrome, dizziness, and spinal cord infarction can occur. Constitutional signs and symptoms such as fever, weight loss, anorexia, fatigue, myalgia, headache, nausea, vomiting, or diarrhea may suggest necrotizing vasculitis, infection, or malignant disease.

DIAGNOSIS

Atheromatous embolization is frequently overlooked or misdiagnosed. No single laboratory test is diagnostic. Nonspecific findings such as elevation in the erythrocyte sedimentation rate, leukocytosis, or anemia may be present. Increased levels of serum amylase, hepatic transaminases, blood urea nitrogen, or serum creatinine may be noted if the pancreas, liver, or kidney is involved. The urine sediment may be abnormal but is nonspecific. Eosinophilia and eosinophiluria may be present early in the course, and hypocomplementemia has been reported in a small number of series. Biopsy is the most specific way to make the diagnosis, but it is often not required because the clinical findings are so highly suggestive of atheromatous embolization.

A markedly irregular and shaggy aorta may be observed on various imaging techniques. Transesophageal echocardiography may detect mobile, protruding atheroma, which are associated with a very high risk for future embolization.

Atheromatous embolization may mimic vasculitis, such as polyarteritis nodosa or leukocytoclastic vasculitis, or it may suggest an underlying malignant disease, nonbacterial thrombotic endocarditis, subacute bacterial endocarditis, multiple myeloma, antiphospholipid antibody syndrome, or atrial myxoma. A cardiac source of emboli should always be excluded.

TREATMENT   Rx

The treatment of atheromatous embolization has three goals: (1) removal of the source of atheromatous material (by surgical exclusion and bypass, percutaneous transluminal angioplasty, stent implantation, or stent grafting), (2) symptomatic care of the end organs in which the emboli are located, and (3) optimal treatment of cardiovascular risk factors (Chapter 51) to prevent myocardial infarction, stroke, and cardiovascular death.

Pain control and local care of ischemic ulcers are critical to the management of patients with atheromatous embolization. Intravenous prostaglandin analogues (iloprost 0.5 to 2.0 ng/kg/minute continuously for 10 to 14 days, followed by 8-hour infusions three times a week for an additional 2 to 3 weeks) may be useful in the healing of ischemic ulcerations and in controlling pain secondary to atheromatous embolization. Patients should be given antiplatelet therapy with aspirin (81 mg/day) and clopidogrel (75 mg/day). Use of anticoagulants such as heparin or warfarin should be avoided unless a compelling reason exists to use this class of drugs. If a vasospastic component is present, a dihydropyridine calcium-channel blocker (amlodipine 2.5 to 10 mg/day or nifedipine extended release 30 to 120 mg/day) may be effective in relieving some of the symptoms. Chemical or surgical sympathectomy or spinal cord stimulators have been helpful for ulcer healing and pain relief in some patients.

Covered stents or stent grafts, which can be inserted in the thoracic or abdominal aorta for aneurysms or occlusive disease, are now the treatment of choice to prevent future embolic events when such approaches are technically feasible. In other cases, surgical bypass therapy is an alternative, although patients who are poor surgical risks may require ligation of the common femoral arteries followed by extra-anatomic bypass, such as axillobifemoral bypass.

PROGNOSIS

Patients with atheromatous embolization generally have advanced atherosclerosis and a poor prognosis. Patients should receive appropriate risk factor modification (Chapter 71) to slow the progression of atherosclerosis and to improve overall cardiac and cerebrovascular morbidity and mortality. Statins may reduce the risk of embolic events.

● THROMBOANGIITIS OBLITERANS (BUERGER'S DISEASE)

DEFINITION

Thromboangiitis obliterans (Buerger's disease) is a nonatherosclerotic, segmental inflammatory disease that most commonly affects the small and medium-sized arteries and veins in the upper and lower extremities. The origin of Buerger's disease is unknown, but there is an extremely strong association with tobacco use, and progression of the disease is closely linked to continued tobacco use.

EPIDEMIOLOGY

Buerger's disease has a worldwide distribution, but it is more prevalent in the Middle East, Near East, and Far East than in North America and western Europe. The prevalence of Buerger's disease is decreasing as the consumption of tobacco products declines.

PATHOBIOLOGY

Patients with Buerger's disease may be hypercoagulable, and some patients have anti–endothelial cell antibodies, anticollagen antibodies, circulating immune complexes, and/or impaired endothelial-dependent vasorelaxation. Patients with thromboangiitis obliterans also have an increase in cellular sensitivity to type I and III collagen (normal constituents of human arteries).

In the acute phase of thromboangiitis obliterans, a highly inflammatory thrombus may affect both the arteries and the veins. The lesion is characterized by acute inflammation involving all layers of the vessel wall in association with occlusive inflammatory cellular thrombosis. Around the periphery of the thrombus, one may see polymorphonuclear leukocytes with karyorrhexis, the so-called microabscess that may contain one or more multinucleated giant cells. The acute phase lesion is followed by an intermediate phase characterized by progressive organization of the acute occlusive thrombus in the arteries and veins; a prominent, inflammatory cellular infiltrate may persist within the thrombus. The chronic phase or end-stage lesion is characterized by complete organization of the occlusive thrombus, with extensive recanalization, prominent vascularization of the media and adventitia, and perivascular fibrosis.

CLINICAL MANIFESTATIONS

Classically, Buerger's disease occurs in young male smokers, with the onset of symptoms before age 40 to 45 years; however, 20 to 30% of patients with Buerger's disease may be women. Buerger's disease usually begins with ischemia of the toes, feet, fingers, and hands (Fig. 80-4). As the disease progresses, it may involve more proximal arteries, but involvement of large arteries is unusual.

Patients may present with claudication of the feet, the legs, and occasionally the arms and hands. Foot or arch claudication may be the presenting manifestation and is often mistaken for an orthopedic problem. Seventy-five to 80% of patients present with ischemic rest pain and/or ulcerations. Two or more limbs are always involved, and angiographic abnormalities are consistently found in limbs that are not yet clinically involved. Superficial thrombophlebitis and Raynaud's phenomenon each occur in approximately 40% of patients.

A positive Allen test indicates the distal nature of thromboangiitis obliterans and its involvement of the lower and upper extremities, helping to differentiate it from atherosclerosis. In this test, the physician simultaneously occludes both the radial and the ulnar arteries. When pressure is released from either artery, one should note prompt filling from that artery, with the return of color to the hand. A positive test result occurs when color does not return to the blanched hand.

DIAGNOSIS

No specific laboratory tests aid in the diagnosis of Buerger's disease, but tests should exclude vasculitis, connective tissue diseases, hypercoagulable states, and a proximal source of emboli. On arteriography, the proximal arteries are normal, and the disease is most often infrapopliteal in the lower extremities and distal to the brachial artery in the upper extremities. Multiple vascular occlusions with collateralization around the obstruction (corkscrew collaterals) may occur, similar to what may be seen in other small vessel occlusive diseases such as the CREST syndrome (calcinosis cutis, Raynaud's phenomenon, esophageal motility disorder, sclerodactyly, and telangiectasias) or

FIGURE 80-4. Buerger's disease. Ischemic finger of a young male patient (**A**) and ischemic toe of a 28-year-old woman (**B**) with Buerger's disease.

scleroderma (Chapter 275). However, the arteriographic appearance of Buerger's disease may also be similar to that of systemic lupus erythematosus (Chapter 274), rheumatoid vasculitis (Chapter 272), mixed connective tissue diseases (Chapter 275), and antiphospholipid antibody syndrome (Chapter 179), although the diagnosis of these other diseases can usually be established or excluded by other tests. Because cocaine and cannabis use (Chapter 33) may produce a clinical and angiographic picture identical to that of thromboangiitis obliterans, a toxicology screen may be indicated if the diagnosis in not clear-cut. Patients with Takayasu's arteritis (Chapter 78) or giant cell arteritis (Chapter 279) present with proximal vascular involvement and can readily be distinguished from patients with Buerger's disease.

TREATMENT   **Rx**

The cornerstone of therapy for thromboangiitis obliterans is the complete discontinuation of cigarette smoking and tobacco use in any form. Patients who stop using tobacco almost always avoid amputation, whereas 40% or more of patients who continue to use tobacco progress to one or more amputations.

In a randomized trial, intravenous iloprost was superior to aspirin at 28 days in relieving rest pain and in healing ischemic ulcerations. At 6 months, 88% of patients receiving iloprost (0.5 to 2.0 ng/kg/minute, maintaining hemodynamic stability for 6 hours daily for up to 28 days) responded to therapy, compared with 21% in the aspirin-treated group; only 6% underwent amputation in the iloprost-treated group, compared with 18% in the aspirin-treated group.**1** Other treatments such as calcium-channel blockers (amlodipine, 2.5 to 10 mg/day or nifedipine extended release 30 to 120 mg/day), antibiotics, and anticoagulants, as well as sympathectomy, are palliative.

Surgical bypass is not a viable option in most patients because they may not have a distal target vessel with which to bypass. Sympathectomy and implantable spinal cord stimulators may help some patients, but iloprost is more effective than lumbar sympathectomy.**2** Stem cell and gene therapy have helped in healing ischemic ulcers and preventing amputation in patients with Buerger's disease. The use of intermittent pneumatic compression (arterial pump device) enhances blood flow to the foot and is useful in relieving rest pain and healing ulcers in patients with small vessel occlusive disease.

● VASCULAR DISEASES ASSOCIATED WITH CHANGES IN TEMPERATURE
Raynaud's Phenomenon

DEFINITION

Raynaud's phenomenon is the abrupt onset of a triphasic color (white, blue, and red) response: well-demarcated pallor of the digits progresses to cyanosis with pain and often numbness, followed by reactive hyperemia on rewarming. This vasospastic phenomenon is often precipitated by cold exposure or stress. *Primary Raynaud's phenomenon* denotes patients who have no underlying cause, whereas *secondary Raynaud's phenomenon* is associated with or caused by some other systemic illness or disease process (Fig. 80-5).

EPIDEMIOLOGY

Raynaud's phenomenon is common in patients with connective tissue diseases. Approximately 90% of patients with scleroderma (Chapter 275) experience Raynaud's phenomenon, and it may be a presenting manifestation in many of them. Raynaud's phenomenon is also a component of the CREST syndrome. These patients have small vessel occlusive disease that may lead to digital pitting or ulceration and eventual amputation.

FIGURE 80-5. Raynaud's phenomenon in the acute phase, with severe blanching of the tip of one finger. (From Forbes CD, Jackson WF. *Color Atlas and Text of Clinical Medicine,* 3rd ed. London: Mosby; 2003.)

The β-adrenergic receptor antagonists are most commonly associated with Raynaud's phenomenon because they block the vasodilatory β-receptors and thus leave the vasoconstrictive α-receptors unopposed. Ergotamine preparations, polyvinyl chloride, and several cancer chemotherapeutic agents can also cause Raynaud's phenomenon.

Raynaud's phenomenon occurs frequently in individuals who use vibratory tools such as pneumatic hammers, chain saws, sanders, and grinders. This has been termed the *hand-arm vibration syndrome,* and the prevalence of Raynaud's phenomenon may exceed 90% at 10 years in individuals with heavy exposure. Continued use of vibratory tools can lead to chronic occlusive small vessel disease. The syndrome has also been described in typists, pianists, meat cutters, and sewing machine operators.

Trauma to the distal ulnar artery (several centimeters distal to the wrist) may occur with pounding the palm of the hand, karate, or other activities that traumatize the hypothenar eminence and lead to an aneurysm or pseudoaneurysm of the distal ulnar artery (hypothenar hammer syndrome). Thrombus within the aneurysm may then embolize to the fingers, or the distal ulnar artery may thrombose.

PATHOBIOLOGY

The initial manifestation of Raynaud's phenomenon occurs when the digits turn white as a result of the intense vasoconstriction or spasm of the digital arteries. At this point, blood flow ceases totally, and the digits are often numb and painful. As the arterial vasoconstriction abates, subsequent postcapillary venule constriction causes the blood in the capillaries and veins to become deoxygenated, producing the cyanotic appearance. When rewarming occurs, blood flow is markedly increased due to marked vasodilation, producing reactive hyperemia to the digits (red color).

The pathophysiologic factors operative in Raynaud's phenomenon include vascular, neural, and intravascular abnormalities. Vascular factors include small vessel occlusive disease, such as is seen in scleroderma, and functional abnormalities, such as impaired endothelium-dependent (nitric oxide–mediated) and endothelium-independent vasodilation, reduced production of vasodilators, and increased vasoconstriction. Neural abnormalities include impaired sympathetic nervous system activity that disturbs the balance between vasoconstriction and vasodilation. Intravascular factors such as platelet activation, impaired fibrinolysis, white blood cell activation, reduced red blood cell deformability, and oxidative stress may play important roles in some patients.

TABLE 80-1 DIFFERENTIATING PRIMARY FROM SECONDARY RAYNAUD'S PHENOMENON

CHARACTERISTICS	PRIMARY	SECONDARY
Associated diseases	No	Yes
Age at onset	Younger (<30 yr)	Older (>30 yr)
Nail-fold capillaries	Normal	Large, tortuous with "dropout"
Autoantibodies	Negative or low titers	Frequent
Endothelial cell activation	Yes	Yes
Endothelial damage	No	Frequent
Structural occlusion	No	Yes
Digital gangrene	Rare; only superficial	Common
α_2-Adrenergic activity	High	High
Calcitonin gene-related peptide	Low	Low

From Block JA, Sequeira W. Raynaud's phenomenon. *Lancet.* 2001;357:2042-2048.

CLINICAL MANIFESTATIONS

The signs of Raynaud's phenomenon may include pallor (see Fig. 80-5), cyanosis, and rubor. The triphasic color response occurs in 4 to 65% of patients. Exposure to the cold is the typical precipitating factor, but emotional lability may also cause or exacerbate attacks in some patients. Vasospastic attacks usually occur only in the fingers, but vasospasm can occur in the toes, nose, ears, lips, and other body parts.

In primary Raynaud's phenomenon, the physical examination is normal between attacks. However, in secondary Raynaud's phenomenon, pits or ulcerations on the fingertips may be present in patients with scleroderma, CREST syndrome, or thromboangiitis obliterans. An abnormal Allen test on physical examination indicates fixed arterial obstruction.

DIAGNOSIS

The diagnosis of Raynaud's phenomenon is not difficult when it is based on the patient's description of the attacks. Patients with persistent cyanosis or persistent hyperemia generally have some condition other than Raynaud's phenomenon. In primary Raynaud's phenomenon, vasospastic attacks are precipitated by exposure to the cold or emotional stimuli; there is bilateral involvement of the extremities without gangrene; and, after a careful search, no evidence indicates an underlying systemic disease that could be responsible for the vasospastic attacks (Table 80-1).

To evaluate systemic illnesses, a serologic evaluation should include a complete blood cell count, multiphasic serologic analysis, urinalysis, erythrocyte sedimentation rate, C-reactive protein, antinuclear antibody, extractable nuclear antigen (anti-Smith and ribonuclear protein), anti-DNA, cryoglobulins, complement, anticentromere antibodies, and SCL70 scleroderma antibodies. In addition, nail-fold capillaroscopy can be performed to help confirm a diagnosis of CREST syndrome or scleroderma in patients whose symptoms are not clear. Abnormal nail-fold capillaroscopy indicates that the patient does not have primary Raynaud's phenomenon.

The noninvasive vascular laboratory (pulse volume recordings) is useful in identifying the degree of digital arterial occlusive disease (fixed ischemia) and in predicting whether ischemic ulcerations on the digits will heal. Arteriography is not routinely performed.

TREATMENT   Rx

In patients with mild vasospastic attacks, reassurance about the benign nature of the disease and instructions on how to prevent attacks are often all that is needed. Patients should limit their exposure to the cold and should dress warmly and protect not only the extremities but also the entire body. Mittens are better than gloves for keeping the hands warm. Patients need to be especially careful when they handle cold objects. Hand- and foot-warming devices (battery operated or chemical) may be helpful. Smoking should be avoided because nicotine causes intense vasoconstriction. β-Blocking agents may exaggerate the symptoms of Raynaud's phenomenon. Conditioning techniques and biofeedback are sometimes helpful in controlling vasospastic episodes.

The dihydropyridine calcium-channel blockers are the most effective pharmacotherapeutic agents for Raynaud's phenomenon.[3] Patients who have infrequent attacks may benefit from a short-acting calcium-channel blocker such as nifedipine 10 to 20 mg, given 30 minutes to 1 hour before cold exposure. When vasospasm occurs more frequently, the extended-release preparations of nifedipine (30 to 120 mg/day) or amlodipine (2.5 to 10 mg/day) should be used. α_1-Adrenergic receptor antagonists such as prazosin (1 to 10 mg twice daily) or terazosin (2 to 20 mg/day) are also highly effective in decreasing the severity, frequency, and duration of vasospastic attacks. Nitroglycerin or its analogues can be used topically (0.1 to 0.8 mg/hour),[4] whereas prostacyclin can be given intravenously (0.5 ng/kg/minute for 6 hours/day for 21 days).[5] Dual endothelin receptor blockade (e.g., bosentan 62.5 to 125 mg twice daily) has been beneficial in randomized trials.[6] Angiotensin-converting enzyme inhibitors, angiotensin receptor blockers, phosphodiesterase-5 inhibitors, niacin, and papaverine are not of proven benefit. Several reports have suggested a beneficial effect from selective serotonin reuptake inhibitors such as fluoxetine (20 to 40 mg/day). Small case series suggest that cilostazol (100 mg twice daily, 30 minutes before breakfast and 30 minutes before dinner) may improve ulcer healing in patients with secondary Raynaud's phenomenon. L-Arginine (2 to 8 g/day) and sildenafil (50 mg twice daily) have been used with variable success.

Although sympathectomy may be beneficial in the short term, with about a 50% improvement rate, the vasospastic attacks may recur in 6 months to 2 years. Some patients with severe disease have had success with digital sympathectomy.

PROGNOSIS

The prognosis in patients with primary Raynaud's phenomenon is excellent. No mortality is associated with this condition. In a long-term study involving 307 patients with primary Raynaud's phenomenon, 38% had stable disease, 36% were improved, 16% were worsened, and the syndrome disappeared in 10%. The prognosis associated with secondary Raynaud's phenomenon depends on the underlying condition that caused it.

Pernio (Chilblains)

DEFINITION AND EPIDEMIOLOGY

Pernio is a Latin word that means "frostbite"; its synonym *chilblains* is an Anglo-Saxon term that means "cold sore." It is a localized inflammatory lesion of the skin caused by an abnormal response to the cold. Whereas in Raynaud's phenomenon there is acute and readily reversible vasospasm, in pernio the vasospasm is more prolonged. Pernio is frequently encountered in the temperate, humid climates of northwestern Europe and in the northern United States.

PATHOBIOLOGY

Pernio develops in susceptible individuals who are exposed to nonfreezing cold. The pathologic changes include edema of the papillodermis, vasculitis characterized by perivascular infiltration (with lymphocytes) of the arterioles and venules of the dermis, thickening and edema of the blood vessel walls, fat necrosis, and a chronic inflammatory reaction with giant cell formation.

CLINICAL MANIFESTATIONS AND DIAGNOSIS

Pernio most commonly occurs in young women between the ages of 15 and 30 years, but it may occur in older individuals or in children. Acute pernio may develop 12 to 24 hours after exposure to the cold. Single or multiple erythematous, purplish, edematous lesions appear, accompanied by intense itching or burning. These lesions may have a yellowish or brownish discoloration and may be associated with some flaking. They tend to affect the toes and dorsum of the proximal phalanges. The lesions of acute pernio are usually self-limited, although they may lead to recurrent disease. The arterial circulation is normal on physical examination and in the noninvasive vascular laboratory. Chronic pernio occurs when repeated exposure to the cold results in the persistence of lesions, with subsequent scarring and atrophy. Characteristically, the lesions begin in the fall or winter and disappear in the spring or early summer. In advanced cases, the seasonal variation may disappear, and chronic occlusive vascular disease may develop.

In the typical form, the patient develops violet or yellow-brown blisters and shallow toe ulcers that burn and itch (Fig. 80-6). The differential diagnosis of pernio includes recurrent, erythematous, nodular, and ulcerative lesions such as erythema induratum, nodular vasculitis, erythema nodosum, and cold panniculitis. The skin lesions of pernio may resemble those of atheromatous embolization (see earlier).

FIGURE 80-6. **Pernio on the toes of the right foot.** The lesions on the second, third, and fourth toes are the typical red, brown, and yellow scaling lesions. The lesion on the fifth toe can be confused with atheromatous embolization.

FIGURE 80-7. Frostbite of the hand in a mountaineer. On rewarming, the hand became painful, red, and edematous, with signs of probable gangrene in the fifth finger. (From Forbes CD, Jackson WF. *Color Atlas and Text of Clinical Medicine,* 3rd ed. London: Mosby; 2003.)

PREVENTION AND TREATMENT   Rx

Prevention is the best form of therapy. Cold exposure should be minimized as much as possible. In randomized trials, nifedipine (20 to 60 mg/day)[7] and pentoxifylline (400 mg three times daily)[8] reduce pain and facilitate the healing process. The severe itching may be treated with local application of an antipruritic agent.

Acrocyanosis

Acrocyanosis, which is a persistent blue or cyanotic discoloration of the digits, occurs most commonly in the hands and may worsen with exposure to cold and improve with rewarming. The primary form is a benign cosmetic condition, but it may also be seen in patients with connective tissue diseases, thromboangiitis obliterans, and diseases associated with central cyanosis. The exact pathophysiologic abnormality is not clear, but it may be vasospasm in the cutaneous arteries and arterioles, with compensatory dilation and oxygen desaturation in the postcapillary venules.

Ulceration or tissue loss is unusual, and the overall prognosis is excellent. Patients should be advised to keep their entire body and extremities warm. Drugs such as α-adrenergic blocking agents (prazosin 1 to 10 mg twice daily or terazosin, 2 to 20 mg/day) or calcium-channel blockers (amlodipine 2.5 to 10 mg/day or nifedipine extended release 30 to 120 mg/day) may be helpful.

Frostbite

EPIDEMIOLOGY AND PATHOBIOLOGY

Frostbite is the freezing of tissues resulting from exposure to cold. It may occur in above-freezing temperatures under circumstances such as wetness, strong wind, or high altitude.

A person's response to cold is aimed at conserving the core (internal body) temperature as well as the viability of the extremities. Heat loss is reduced by peripheral vasoconstriction caused by sympathetic stimulation and catecholamine release. Maintenance or augmentation of body heat is accomplished by muscular activity such as shivering. However, the heat production from shivering cannot be sustained for more than a few hours because of the depletion of glycogen, which is the source of heat during shivering. The extremities are also protected by the "hunting reaction," which consists of irregular, 5- to 10-minute cycles of alternating vasoconstriction and vasodilation that protect the extremities against excessive sustained vasoconstriction with minimal loss of internal body temperature. However, when the body is exposed to cold of a magnitude or a duration that threatens the internal body temperature, this mechanism fails. Because the disruption of core temperature is more deleterious to the body than is peripheral vasoconstriction, conservation of core temperature takes precedence over rewarming of the extremities, and the hunting response is replaced by continuous and more intense vasoconstriction that promotes frostbite by means of ice crystal formation, cellular dehydration, and thrombosis of the microvasculature.

CLINICAL MANIFESTATIONS AND DIAGNOSIS

Soon after exposure to the cold, pain develops and gradually progresses to numbness; the frozen part turns white because of intense vasoconstriction (Fig. 80-7). With rewarming or thawing, the circulation is restored, and the affected parts become hyperemic. Edema may first occur within hours of

thawing and persist for days or weeks. Blisters appear within the first 24 hours and are reabsorbed within 1 to 2 weeks, after which a black eschar may persist. Overactivity of the sympathetic nervous system is manifested by hyperhidrosis or a burning sensation.

Seventy percent of frostbite victims develop chronic sequelae, including cold sensitivity, pain, and sensory disturbances, often resembling complex regional pain syndrome (Chapter 428). Frostbite arthritis may occur in particularly severe cases.

It is important to establish the depth of the frostbite and determine whether the tissue is viable. This may not be obvious on initial clinical examination; it is usually determined weeks or months after the cold injury, when the demarcation zone appears and the dead tissue is sloughed.

TREATMENT   Rx

In mild cases of frostbite, the only treatment necessary may be daily whirlpool baths and bedrest. However, treatment of deep frostbite should be considered a medical emergency because the early institution of therapy may reduce the amount of tissue loss. Thawing, the mainstay of therapy, should not be implemented if the patient may be exposed to cold again, because refreezing of thawed tissue promotes further tissue damage. Walking on a frozen limb produces substantially less damage than walking on a thawed limb.

After the patient's transfer to a medical facility, frozen tissue should be rapidly rewarmed in a water bath of 40 to 42° C (104 to 108° F) for 15 to 30 minutes until complete thawing has occurred. After thawing, reappearance of normal color signifies the reestablishment of blood flow. Thawing is often a painful process and may require the administration of narcotics.

After thawing, the extremity should be cleansed twice daily in a whirlpool bath with an aseptic solution at 35 to 37° C (95 to 99° F). Care should be taken to prevent and treat secondary infections. Tetanus prophylaxis should be administered. A frostbite protocol consisting of débridement of clear blisters with a topical application of aloe vera, oral ibuprofen, and daily hydrotherapy is highly effective. An important principle is to avoid early débridement or amputation, which is indicated only when infected gangrene or generalized sepsis occurs.

● ERYTHROMELALGIA

DEFINITION AND EPIDEMIOLOGY

Erythromelalgia literally means "red, painful extremities." It may be classified as primary (or idiopathic) or secondary. The primary form may be nonfamilial or familial. Secondary erythromelalgia is associated with other diseases, the most common being myeloproliferative disorders such as polycythemia vera and essential thrombocythemia. Other diseases associated with secondary erythromelalgia include hypertension, diabetes, rheumatoid arthritis, gout, spinal cord disease, multiple sclerosis, systemic lupus erythematosus, cutaneous vasculitis, and viral infection; it also may result from therapy with various drugs (e.g., nifedipine, nicardipine, verapamil, bromocriptine, pergolide).

PATHOBIOLOGY

Families with autosomal dominant erythromelalgia have demonstrated mutations in the sodium channel $Na_v1.7$, which is selectively expressed within the nociceptive dorsal root ganglion and sympathetic ganglion neurons. The histologic features vary from normal findings to arterial occlusion with thrombus formation.

CLINICAL MANIFESTATIONS AND DIAGNOSIS

Erythromelalgia is characterized by the clinical triad of erythema, burning pain, and increased temperature, usually of the extremities. The feet, especially the soles, are more commonly involved than the hands. The peripheral pulses are generally normal in the primary type and variable in secondary erythromelalgia. The symptoms may occur in "attacks" that last for minutes to hours or occasionally days and are precipitated by a warm environment. Exercise and dependency tend to exacerbate symptoms. Patients seek relief by exposing the affected extremity to a cooler environment, such as placing it in cold water, walking on a cold floor barefoot, or running an air conditioner even in the winter. This response often leads to a cold-induced vascular injury superimposed on the erythromelalgia. Erythromelalgia may precede the clinical appearance of a myeloproliferative disorder by several years, so patients older than 30 years should be monitored periodically with blood cell counts.

TREATMENT   Rx

The treatment of erythromelalgia is often difficult and frustrating. Symptoms can be so debilitating that they lead to suicide. In secondary erythromelalgia, treatment of the underlying disease (phlebotomy in patients with polycythemia vera, and normalization of the platelet count in patients with thrombocythemia) may relieve the symptoms. Aspirin (81 to 325 mg/day) is the most effective treatment available, particularly for patients with erythromelalgia secondary to myeloproliferative disorders. Other therapies with variable success in case reports include methysergide, ephedrine, nonsteroidal anti-inflammatory drugs, phenoxybenzamine, nitroglycerin, sodium nitroprusside, corticosteroids, and surgical sympathectomy. Lidocaine transdermal patches (Lidoderm) on the feet and thalamic stimulation have also been used anecdotally.

● POPLITEAL ARTERY ENTRAPMENT SYNDROME

In popliteal artery entrapment syndrome, the popliteal artery is compressed by a congenital anatomic abnormality or an abnormal muscle or fibrous band. In the most common abnormality, the medial head of the gastrocnemius muscle compresses the popliteal artery and causes its medial deviation.

The clinical presentation consists of a healthy, "athletic-type" patient complaining of typical claudication symptoms in the absence of premature atherosclerosis. Disappearance of the pulse with passive dorsiflexion of the foot or active plantar flexion against resistance may suggest the diagnosis. Duplex ultrasound may help, and computed tomography or magnetic resonance imaging can confirm the diagnosis. On arteriography, the characteristic finding is medial deviation of the popliteal artery with post-stenotic dilation. Other diseases that can cause mid-popliteal occlusion include cystic adventitial disease, thrombosed popliteal artery aneurysm, and atherosclerosis of the superficial femoral and popliteal arteries. The primary treatment of popliteal artery entrapment syndrome is surgical resection of the abnormal muscle or fibrous band.

● CYSTIC ADVENTITIAL DISEASE

In cystic adventitial disease, gelatinous fluid accumulates in an arterial wall cyst, and the cyst encroaches on the vessel lumen, with resulting stenosis or occlusion. The cyst arises in the outer portion of the media or subadventitial layer, most commonly in the popliteal artery. Cystic adventitial disease is an isolated lesion not associated with a systemic process, and the precise pathophysiologic mechanism is unknown.

The disease predominates in men, with an approximate male-female ratio of 5 : 1, and the mean age at diagnosis is about 45 years. Claudication is the most frequent symptom. The pulses may disappear on flexion of the knee (Ishikawa's sign). However, if the artery is occluded, no pulses are palpable.

Pulse volume recordings may show the characteristic decrease in blood pressure and the change in waveform configuration in the affected limb. A perivascular cystic structure may be visualized on duplex ultrasound, computed tomography, or magnetic resonance imaging. Computed tomography–guided needle aspiration can partially but usually not completely remove the highly viscous and gelatinous fluid. Surgical resection is indicated when

FIGURE 80-8. Fibromuscular dysplasia. Note the "string of beads" or "accordion" appearance in the external iliac artery. This radiographic appearance is diagnostic of fibromuscular dysplasia of the medial type. Also note the aneurysm proximal to the area of dysplasia.

claudication interferes with a patient's lifestyle or ischemic rest pain is present.

● FIBROMUSCULAR DYSPLASIA OF THE EXTREMITIES

Although fibromuscular dysplasia (in particular, medial fibroplasia) is most common in the renal and carotid arteries (Chapters 67 and 127), it may also occur in peripheral arteries of the extremity (iliac, superficial femoral, popliteal, tibial, subclavian, axillary, radial, and ulnar). These lesions may be asymptomatic, or they may produce a difference in blood pressure between the two limbs, with paresthesias, claudication, or critical limb ischemia.

The typical arteriographic appearance of a "string of beads" is virtually pathognomonic of medial fibroplasia (Fig. 80-8). Long, smooth areas of narrowing are characteristic of intimal fibroplasia, but they may also be seen in Takayasu's arteritis (Chapter 78) and giant cell arteritis (Chapters 78 and 279).

Therapy should be reserved for patients with lifestyle-interfering claudication or critical limb ischemia. Under most circumstances, percutaneous balloon dilation is the treatment of choice.

 Grade **A**

1. Fiessinger JN, Schafer M. Trial of iloprost versus aspirin treatment for critical limb ischaemia of thromboangiitis obliterans: The TAO Study. *Lancet.* 1990;335:555-557.
2. Bozkurt AK, Köksal C, Demirbas MY, et al. A randomized trial of intravenous iloprost (a stable prostacyclin analogue) versus lumbar sympathectomy in the management of Buerger's disease. *Int Angiol.* 2006;25:162-168.
3. Thompson AE, Shea B, Welch V, et al. Calcium-channel blockers for Raynaud's phenomenon in systemic sclerosis. *Arthritis Rheum.* 2001;44:1841-1847.
4. Chung L, Shapiro L, Fiorentino D, et al. MQX-503, a novel formulation of nitroglycerin, improved the severity of Raynaud's phenomenon: a randomized, controlled trial. *Arthritis Rheum.* 2009; 60:870-877.
5. Kawald A, Burmester GR, Huscher D, et al. Low versus high-dose iloprost therapy over 21 days in patients with secondary Raynaud's phenomenon and systemic sclerosis: a randomized, open, single-center study. *J Rheumatol.* 2008;35:1830-1837.
6. Nguyen VA, Eisendle K, Gruber I, et al. Effect of the dual endothelin receptor antagonist bosentan on Raynaud's phenomenon secondary to systemic sclerosis: a double-blind prospective, randomized, placebo-controlled pilot study. *Rheumatology (Oxford).* 2010;49:583-587.
7. Rustin MH, Newton JA, Smith NP, et al. The treatment of chilblains with nifedipine: the results of a pilot study, a double-blind placebo-controlled randomized study and a long-term open trial. *Br J Dermatol.* 1989;120:267-275.
8. Noaimi AA, Fadheel BM. Treatment of perniosis with oral pentoxifylline in comparison with oral prednisone plus topical clobetasol ointment in Iraqi patients. *Saudi Med J.* 2008;29:1762-1764.

SUGGESTED READINGS

Heidrich H. Functional vascular diseases: Raynaud's syndrome, acrocyanosis and erythromelalgia. *Vasa.* 2010;39:33-41. *Review.*

Olin JW, Sealove BA. Diagnosis, management, and future developments of fibromuscular dysplasia. *J Vasc Surg.* 2011;53:826-836. *Comprehensive review of the clinical manifestations and treatment.*
Piazza G, Creager MA. Thromboangiitis obliterans. *Circulation.* 2010;121:1858-1861. *Clinical review.*
Prakash S, Weisman MH. Idiopathic chilblains. *Am J Med.* 2009;122:1152-1155. *Clinical review.*

81

PERIPHERAL VENOUS DISEASE

JEFFREY GINSBERG

DEEP VEIN THROMBOSIS

DEFINITION

Deep vein thrombosis (DVT), which is the most important disease affecting the peripheral veins, has an estimated annual incidence of 0.1% in whites. Most pulmonary emboli (Chapter 98) arise from DVT of the legs. In fact, DVT and pulmonary embolism are usually considered different clinical manifestations of one disease, venous thromboembolism (VTE), because up to 50% of patients who present with proximal (popliteal vein or more proximal) DVT have abnormal lung scans suggestive of clinically silent pulmonary emboli, whereas up to 90% of patients with proven pulmonary emboli have DVT, even though only 15% of them have leg symptoms. For the most part, the cornerstones of management of DVT and pulmonary embolism are the same: immediate and long-term anticoagulation.

Superficial thrombophlebitis consists of thrombosis and inflammation of one or more superficial veins. Provided the associated thrombus has not extended into the deep veins, affected patients have a negligible risk for development of pulmonary emboli and can often be effectively managed conservatively with ice, elevation, and anti-inflammatory medication.

EPIDEMIOLOGY

In nonpregnant patients, DVT usually originates in one of the distal or calf veins, where it has little or no potential to cause clinically important pulmonary emboli. The true incidence of calf vein thrombosis is not known because many affected patients remain asymptomatic while the thrombus forms and spontaneously resolves. On the basis of results of studies of *symptomatic* patients with suspected DVT, about 10 to 25% actually have a diagnosable DVT, of whom about 15% have isolated calf DVT. Approximately one fourth of these thrombi that are initially isolated to a calf vein subsequently extend into the proximal veins, usually within 1 week of presentation, where they *then* have the potential to cause pulmonary emboli.

In pregnancy, most (~90%) thrombi occur in the deep veins of the left leg and frequently involve the ileofemoral veins but not the calf or popliteal veins. These findings suggest an anatomic predisposition to left leg ileofemoral DVT, which may be a result of compression of the left iliac vein by the fetus, an exaggeration of the "obstruction" that occurs where the right iliac artery crosses the left iliac vein, and an increase in venous webs at the left iliac vein (May-Thurner syndrome). These observations strongly suggest that most if not all of the increase in VTE during pregnancy is attributable to the increase in left iliac DVT.

From a clinical perspective, risk factors can be subdivided by duration, that is, transient and finite duration (e.g., fractured fibula treated with plaster immobilization) compared with permanent or long-term duration (e.g., congenital antithrombin deficiency, metastatic cancer), and according to the magnitude of the risk, that is, major (hip or knee replacement surgery) or minor (long-distance air travel, use of oral contraceptives). Classification of patients according to the presence or absence and type of risk factor is predictive of the risk of recurrence after a prolonged (≥3 months) course of anticoagulant therapy and provides key information that helps determine the optimal duration of anticoagulant therapy. Patients in whom DVT develops in association with a major risk factor that has resolved have a much lower risk of recurrence after a 3-month course of anticoagulants than do patients whose DVT was associated with a transient minor risk factor that has resolved or patients whose DVT was apparently idiopathic or associated with an ongoing risk factor.

PATHOBIOLOGY

Virchow's triad of hypercoagulability, venous stasis, and injury to the vessel wall provides a model for understanding many of the risk factors that lead to the formation of thrombosis. For example, in patients who have total hip or knee replacement surgery, there is venous endothelial injury caused by surgery, venous stasis due to perioperative immobilization, and hypercoagulability as a result of postoperative fibrinolytic shutdown. In other patients, an identifiable "thrombophilia" or "tendency to clot," such as congenital antithrombin (formerly antithrombin III) deficiency or the presence of factor V Leiden (Chapter 179), combined with use of oral contraceptives results in DVT in women of childbearing age. However, a relatively high proportion of patients have unexplained DVT without "clinical" risk factors that cause endothelial damage or venous stasis or identifiable thrombophilias that cause hypercoagulability. Undoubtedly, some of these patients have yet to be determined thrombophilias, but the DVT currently is labeled idiopathic.

CLINICAL MANIFESTATIONS

The clinical features of lower extremity DVT include leg pain, tenderness, swelling (Fig. 81-1), palpable cord, discoloration, venous distention, prominence of the superficial veins, and cyanosis. In most patients in whom DVT is clinically suspected, the symptoms and signs are nonspecific, and DVT is confirmed in less than 50% of cases. Conversely, patients with relatively minor symptoms and signs may have extensive DVT.

In some patients, DVT may be asymptomatic, but the patient will present with pulmonary embolism. Conversely, pulmonary embolism occurs in 50% of patients with objectively documented proximal leg vein thrombosis, but many of the emboli are asymptomatic. Usually, only part of the thrombus embolizes, so 50 to 70% of patients with angiographically documented pulmonary emboli have detectable DVT of the legs at the time of initial evaluation.

DIAGNOSIS

By itself, clinical diagnosis of DVT is inaccurate because no individual symptom or sign is sufficiently sensitive or specific for the diagnosis to be made or excluded. Clinical assessment can categorize patients according to their pretest probability of DVT with reasonable accuracy. By combining a validated prediction rule (Table 81-1) to assess this pretest probability with the results of noninvasive tests, diagnostic accuracy can be improved, thereby often limiting or eliminating the need for further investigation (Fig. 81-2).

FIGURE 81-1. **Deep vein thrombosis (DVT) presenting as an acutely swollen left leg.** Note the dilation of the superficial veins. The leg was hot to the touch, and palpation along the line of the left popliteal and femoral veins caused pain. Less than 50% of DVTs present in this way, and other conditions may mimic DVT, so further investigation is always indicated. Note the coincidental psoriatic lesion below the patient's right knee. (From Forbes CD, Jackson WF. *Color Atlas and Text of Clinical Medicine,* 3rd ed. London: Mosby; 2003.)

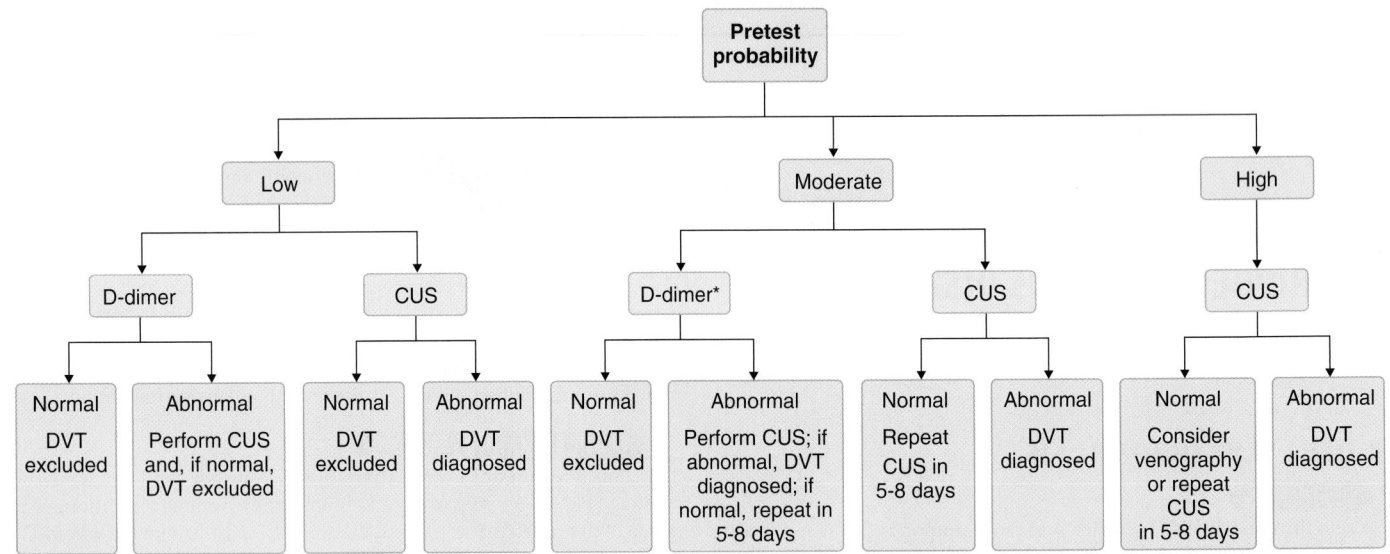

FIGURE 81-2. **Diagnostic algorithm for suspected deep vein thrombosis.** This algorithm uses evaluation of pretest probability based on a clinical prediction rule (see Table 81-1) and D-dimer testing to complement compression ultrasonography (CUS). The *asterisk* indicates use of a highly sensitive (>95%) D-dimer.

TABLE 81-1	PREDICTION RULE FOR DEEP VEIN THROMBOSIS	
CLINICAL CHARACTERISTIC		**SCORE***
Active cancer (treatment ongoing within previous 6 mo or palliative)		1
Paralysis, paresis, or recent plaster immobilization of the lower extremities		1
Recent bed rest of >3 days or major surgery within 3 mo requiring anesthesia		1
Localized tenderness of the deep veins of the leg		1
Entire leg swollen		1
Calf swelling of >3 cm larger than asymptomatic side measured 10 cm below tibial tuberosity		1
Pitting edema confined to the symptomatic leg		1
Collateral superficial veins (not varicosed)		1
Previously documented deep vein thrombosis		1
Alternative diagnosis as likely as or more likely than deep vein thrombosis		−2

*A score of 0 or less indicates low probability, 1 or 2 indicates moderate probability, and 3 or more indicates high probability.
Modified from Wells PS, Anderson DR, Bormanis J, et al. Value of assessment of pretest probability of deep-vein thrombosis in clinical management. *Lancet.* 1997;350:1795-1798.

FIGURE 81-3. Abnormal venogram demonstrates a persistent (two or more different views) intraluminal filling defect in the popliteal vein.

Imaging
Contrast Venography
Ascending contrast venography remains the "gold standard" for diagnosis, but because of its expense, discomfort to the patient, and potential for adverse experiences, venography is currently indicated in symptomatic patients only when diagnostic uncertainty persists after noninvasive testing or if noninvasive testing is unavailable. A constant intraluminal filling defect is diagnostic of acute thrombosis (Fig. 81-3), and DVT can essentially be excluded in patients who have a normal, adequately performed venogram. Minor side effects of local pain, nausea, and vomiting are not uncommon, whereas more serious adverse reactions, such as bronchospasm, are rare; however, venography itself can also induce DVT.

Compression Ultrasonography
Compression venous ultrasonography is currently the most widely used noninvasive test for suspected DVT because of its accuracy in detection of thrombus involving the popliteal or more proximal veins; absence of compressibility (Fig. 81-4) of the proximal leg veins on ultrasonography has a sensitivity of 97% and a specificity of 96% for symptomatic patients with suspected DVT. Thus, the finding of a noncompressible venous segment, particularly in the

popliteal or common femoral vein, has a high positive predictive value for DVT in symptomatic patients and is an indication for treatment. Of patients with symptoms suggestive of DVT but with normal findings on initial ultrasound examination of the proximal veins, about 15% will have undetected isolated calf DVT; progression into the proximal veins occurs in a minority of patients, usually within a week of presentation. Isolated calf DVT that does not extend into the proximal veins is rarely if ever associated with clinically important pulmonary embolus. The sensitivity of ultrasonography for calf DVT is well below 90%, with a wide range of accuracies reported for different populations of patients.

Imaging of the calf veins is time-consuming and potentially inaccurate. Rather, two-point (common femoral and popliteal) or three-point (two-point plus the calf "trifurcation") ultrasonography should be performed and, if the results are normal, repeated in 1 week after the initial examination. This approach will identify the 20 to 25% of patients who have had proximal

FIGURE 81-4. Compression venous ultrasonography demonstrates thrombosis of the popliteal vein. The sonograms in the *top row* demonstrate examination without *(left side)* and with *(right side)* gentle probe compression of the skin overlying the popliteal vein. The lack of compressibility is diagnostic of deep vein thrombosis. The *bottom row* shows analogous views of the femoral vein, which shows partial compressibility.

extension of distal clot in the calf veins. If the repeated ultrasound examination 1 week later also is normal, further investigation and therapy can be safely withheld. In centers with highly skilled operators, however, one normal ultrasound of the proximal and calf veins at presentation may be sufficiently accurate to exclude clinically important DVT and eliminate the need for follow-up testing, especially in patients with either a normal D-dimer test result or a low clinical pretest probability (see later).

Magnetic Resonance Venography

Magnetic resonance venography (MRV), which uses the difference in magnetic resonance signals between flowing blood and stationary clot, has a high sensitivity and specificity for proximal DVT. Recent interest has focused on magnetic resonance for direct imaging of the thrombus because a thrombus produces a positive image without the use of contrast material owing to its methemoglobin content. Although MRV is undoubtedly accurate in diagnosing and excluding DVT, it is expensive and not readily available in most centers outside of the United States.

Laboratory Findings
D-Dimer

D-dimer is a plasma protein specifically produced after lysis of cross-linked fibrin by plasmin. Levels are almost invariably elevated in the presence of acute VTE, so measurement of D-dimer levels is a sensitive test for recent DVT and pulmonary emboli. Unfortunately, numerous nonthrombotic conditions, including sepsis, pregnancy, surgery, and cardiac or renal failure, can also cause elevated levels. As a result of this nonspecificity, the role of D-dimer assays is limited to helping exclude VTE when levels are not raised.

Laboratory tests for D-dimer use enzyme-linked immunosorbent assay (ELISA) or agglutination techniques, both involving specific monoclonal antibodies. Sensitivity and cut points vary among assays, so results cannot be generalized. Highly sensitive tests, consisting of new rapid ELISA or immunoturbidimetric assays, have sensitivities of 95 to 100% for acute VTE but in general have low specificities (20 to 50%). Moderately sensitive tests, of which the SimpliRED red cell agglutination assay is the main example, have a reported sensitivity of approximately 90% but a higher specificity (~75%) for acute VTE. Serial two-point ultrasonography plus D-dimer is as good as whole-leg color-coded Doppler ultrasonography for diagnosing suspected

symptomatic DVT.∎ Highly sensitive D-dimer assays can be employed as "stand-alone tests" for exclusion of DVT, but clinicians must be aware of the accuracy of the assay in their institution before using the D-dimer assay to make management decisions. A point-of-care D-dimer test can help exclude DVT, which is rare in patients with less than four points using the following scale: male sex, use of hormonal contraceptives, active cancer in prior 6 months, surgery in prior month, absence of leg trauma, distention of collateral veins (1 point each); greater than 3-cm difference in calf circumference (2 points), and abnormal D-dimer assay (6 points).

D-dimer measured after a 3-month (or longer) initial treatment with warfarin also appears to be predictive of recurrent or persistent DVT. In addition, an elevated D-dimer level 1 month after stopping warfarin predicts a clinically and statistically significant higher recurrence rate than is seen in patients in whom the D-dimer levels were normal or low.

Algorithms for Diagnosis of Deep Venous Thrombosis

A number of diagnostic algorithms have been tested in prospective management trials (see Fig. 81-2).

Clinical Assessment and Venous Ultrasonography

It is safe to perform only a single ultrasound examination in patients with a low pretest probability by a validated clinical prediction rule (Table 81-2). Other patients require serial ultrasonographic testing if only clinical assessment and ultrasonography are used. Venography should be considered in patients with a high pretest probability and normal compression ultrasonography because the probability of DVT is still approximately 20% in such patients.

Clinical Assessment, D-Dimer Testing, and Venous Ultrasonography

Diagnostic imaging and treatment can be safely withheld in patients who have (1) a low pretest probability based on a validated clinical prediction rule and a negative value on a moderately sensitive D-dimer assay or (2) a low or intermediate pretest probability and a negative value on a highly sensitive D-dimer assay. Patients with a high pretest probability require ultrasonography regardless of the D-dimer result. A normal D-dimer result with use of either a moderately or highly sensitive assay can safely obviate the need for

TABLE 81-2 ALTERNATIVE DIAGNOSES IN 87 CONSECUTIVE PATIENTS WITH CLINICALLY SUSPECTED VENOUS THROMBOSIS AND NORMAL VENOGRAMS*

DIAGNOSIS	PATIENTS (%)
Muscle strain	24
Direct twisting injury to the leg	10
Leg swelling in paralyzed limb	9
Lymphangitis, lymphatic obstruction	7
Venous reflux	7
Muscle tear	6
Baker's cyst	5
Cellulitis	3
Internal abnormality of the knee	2
Unknown	26

*The diagnosis was made once venous thrombosis was excluded by venography.

repeated imaging in patients with normal findings on the initial ultrasound examination.

Differential Diagnosis

A number of conditions can mimic DVT (see Table 81-2), but DVT often can be excluded only by accurate diagnostic testing. In some patients, however, the cause of pain, tenderness, and swelling remains uncertain.

Suspected Recurrent Deep Venous Thrombosis

Approximately 10% of patients with unprovoked VTE will experience recurrent thromboembolism in the first year after ceasing anticoagulant therapy. In addition, many patients will have positional leg swelling and pain early during treatment as a result of venous outflow obstruction or later (≥6 months after diagnosis) because of the post-thrombotic syndrome when venous valvular incompetence is manifested. These and other nonthrombotic disorders can produce symptoms that are similar to acute recurrent DVT, so accurate diagnostic testing to confirm recurrence is mandatory. However, residual venous abnormalities are common after an initial event; persistent abnormalities are seen on compression ultrasonography in approximately 80% of patients at 3 months and 50% of patients at 1 year after a documented proximal DVT. Therefore, comparison with previous ultrasound images is required in patients with suspected recurrence. Although an increase in diameter of 4 mm or more in the compressed vein strongly suggests recurrent DVT, a new noncompressible proximal venous segment is the most reliable criterion for the diagnosis of recurrence. When compression ultrasonography is inconclusive, venography should be considered; a new intraluminal filling defect is diagnostic of acute DVT, and the absence of a filling defect excludes the diagnosis. Nonfilling of venous segments may mask recurrent DVT and is considered a nondiagnostic finding. A normal D-dimer test result is useful in excluding recurrent DVT.

Pregnancy

Symptoms of leg pain or swelling, shortness of breath, and atypical chest pain are common during pregnancy, so objective testing is needed to diagnose VTE. As in nonpregnant patients, compression ultrasonography is the initial test of choice. A normal D-dimer test is also reassuring in excluding DVT. Because isolated iliac and iliofemoral DVT is more common in pregnancy and has the potential to be missed by ultrasonography, venography should be considered when clinical suspicion is high even if the findings of the initial ultrasound examination are normal. MRV, which is sensitive for pelvic DVT, may be useful in this circumstance.

TREATMENT   Rx

Anticoagulant therapy, which is the treatment of choice in most patients with VTE, reduces the extension and recurrence of symptomatic proximal and calf DVT and reduces mortality in patients with pulmonary emboli (Fig. 81-5). Coumarin derivatives (e.g., warfarin) are usually the drugs of choice for long-term anticoagulant therapy, but such drugs have a delayed onset of anticoagulant effect (Chapter 37). Therefore, initial short-term therapy with a

TABLE 81-3 GUIDELINES FOR ANTICOAGULATION WITH LOW-MOLECULAR-WEIGHT HEPARIN AND FONDAPARINUX

INDICATIONS	GUIDELINES
VTE suspected	Obtain baseline aPTT, PT, CBC Check for contraindication to heparin therapy Order imaging study; consider giving IV unfractionated heparin (5000 IU) or LMWH
VTE confirmed	Give LMWH (dalteparin,* enoxaparin,† nadroparin,‡ tinzaparin,§ fondaparinux‖) Start warfarin therapy on day 1 at 5 mg and adjust the subsequent daily dose according to INR Check platelet count between days 3 and 5 Stop LMWH therapy after at least 4 or 5 days of combined therapy when the INR is >2 Anticoagulate with warfarin for at least 3 months at an INR of 2.5, range of 2-3

*Dalteparin sodium, 200 anti-Xa IU/kg/day subcutaneously. A single dose should not exceed 18,000 IU (approved in Canada).
†Enoxaparin sodium, 1 mg/kg q12h subcutaneously, or enoxaparin sodium, 1.5 mg/kg/day subcutaneously. A single daily dose should not exceed 180 mg (approved in both the United States and Canada).
‡Nadroparin calcium, 86 anti-Xa IU/kg two times a day subcutaneously for 10 days (approved in Canada), or nadroparin calcium, 171 anti-Xa IU/kg subcutaneously daily. A single dose should not exceed 17,100 anti-Xa IU.
§Tinzaparin sodium, 175 anti-Xa IU kg/day subcutaneously daily (approved in Canada and the United States).
‖Fondaparinux subcutaneously according to weight: <50 kg, 5 mg once daily; 50-100 kg, 7.5 mg; and >100 kg, 10 mg.
aPTT = activated partial thromboplastin time; CBC = complete blood count; INR = international normalized ratio; LMWH = low-molecular-weight heparin; PT = prothrombin time; VTE = venous thromboembolism.
Modified from Hyers TM, Agnelli G, Hull RD, et al. Antithrombotic therapy for venous thromboembolic disease. *Chest.* 2001;119:176S-193S.

rapid-acting heparin or heparin derivative for approximately 1 week is necessary to provide an immediate antithrombotic effect and to reduce the risk of thrombus growth or embolization in patients with acute DVT. Initial outpatient therapy with a low-molecular-weight heparin (LMWH) or fondaparinux is preferred to inpatient treatment with intravenous unfractionated heparin whenever feasible in patients with DVT. Rarely, medical therapy is unsuccessful or cannot be tolerated; such patients may require procedural therapy.

Initial Treatment

LMWH preparations, which are produced by either enzymatic or chemical depolymerization of unfractionated heparin, have lower mean molecular weights ranging from 4000 to 6000. The reduced molecular size provides a sufficient pentasaccharide moiety to antithrombin to inhibit factor Xa but reduces the ability of LMWH to inhibit thrombin in comparison with unfractionated heparin. Therefore, LMWH has an increased ratio of anti–factor Xa to anti–factor IIa (thrombin) inhibitory activity. The reduced size of LMWH also decreases charge-related nonspecific protein binding, thereby resulting in improved subcutaneous bioavailability, more predictable anticoagulant response, and predominantly dose-independent renal clearance. These qualities have made outpatient management of DVT with unmonitored, weight-based subcutaneous LMWH feasible and preferable.

LMWH products differ in their method of production, molecular weight, and anticoagulant effect. Few trials have directly compared different LMWH preparations for treatment of acute VTE, and definitive conclusions with regard to comparative efficacy and safety cannot be made. Dosage regimens differ for the various LMWH formulations (Table 81-3), but once-daily administration of LMWH is thought to be as safe and effective as twice-daily administration.

Because the antithrombotic response to weight-based dosing of LMWH is predictable, laboratory monitoring during LMWH treatment is usually unnecessary. There are, however, three populations of patients in whom anti–factor Xa monitoring should be considered: (1) patients with renal insufficiency (calculated creatinine clearance of less than 30 mL/minute); (2) obese patients, in whom the volume of distribution of LMWH might be different, so weight-adjusted dosing might not be appropriate; and (3) pregnant women, in whom it is unclear whether the dose should be adjusted according to the woman's weight change. Levels are usually determined on blood samples drawn 4 hours after subcutaneous injection; therapeutic ranges of 0.6 to 1.0 U/mL for twice-daily administration and 1.0 to 2.0 U/mL for once-daily treatment have been proposed.

Meta-analyses have documented that unmonitored, fixed-dose subcutaneous injection of LMWH is as effective and safe as adjusted-dose intravenous administration of unfractionated heparin for the treatment of acute DVT, with a trend toward a significant difference in mortality benefit favoring

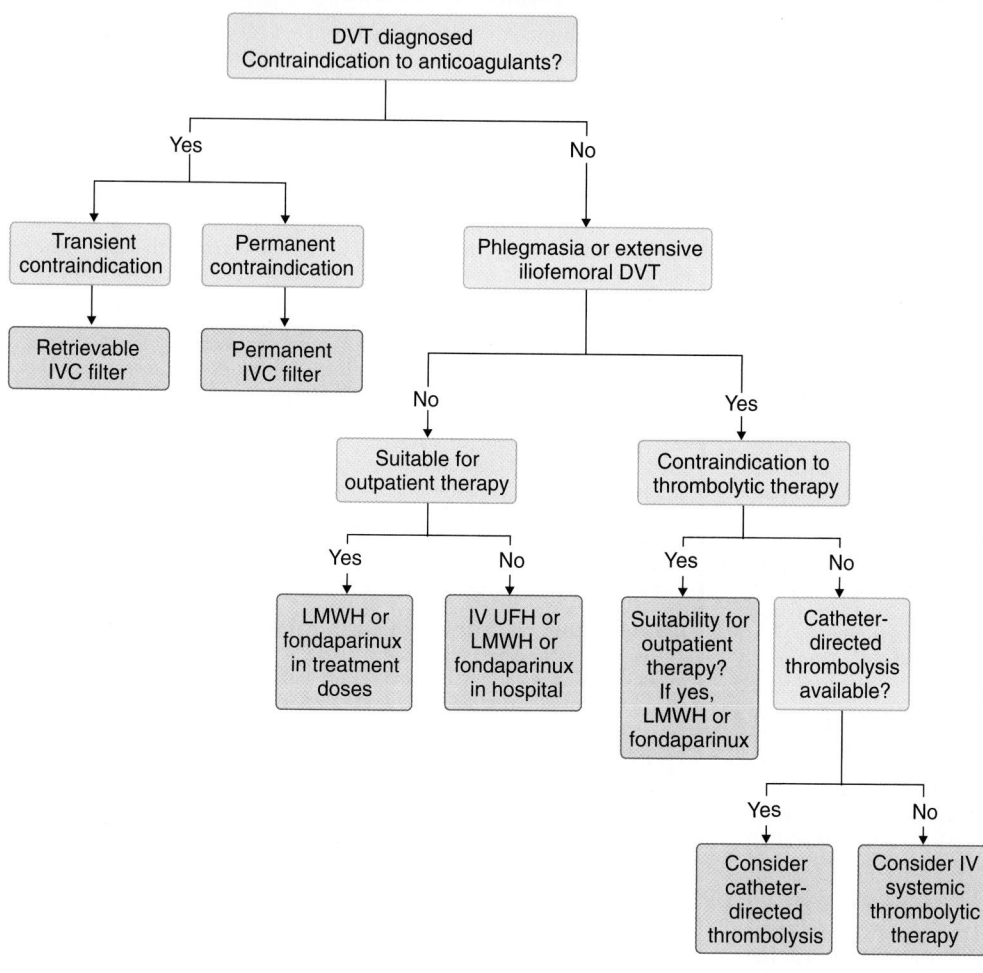

FIGURE 81-5. Guidelines for treatment of deep vein thrombosis (DVT). IVC = inferior vena cava; IV = intravenous; LMWH = low-molecular-weight heparin; UFH = unfractionated heparin.

LMWH, probably because of improved survival in patients with malignant disease.[2] However, patients with extensive iliofemoral DVT have often been excluded from trials of LMWH, and extended-duration (i.e., more than 5 days) intravenous unfractionated heparin therapy is often administered to such patients. Outpatient therapy with LMWH is as good as inpatient treatment, thereby making LMWH more cost-effective than intravenous unfractionated heparin in most health care settings.

Fondaparinux

Fondaparinux is a synthetic analogue of the critical pentasaccharide sequence required for binding of heparin molecules to antithrombin (Chapter 37). Chemically engineered, it has minor modifications from the natural pentasaccharide moiety, thereby improving stability and resulting in enhanced binding to antithrombin. Given subcutaneously, fondaparinux demonstrates 100% bioavailability, with peak plasma concentrations occurring 1.7 hours after dosing. Once-daily subcutaneous administration of fondaparinux (5.0 mg daily if weight is less than 50 kg; 7.5 mg daily if weight is 50 to 100 kg; 10 mg daily if weight is more than 100 kg) is an effective and safe alternative to LMWH for the initial 5 to 10 days of treatment of DVT.[3] Clearance is predominantly renal, with approximately 70% of the initial dose recovered in the urine in an unchanged form. Patients with reduced creatinine clearance, such as elderly patients, have higher peak drug levels and longer drug half-life, so their dose may need to be adjusted downward.

Unfractionated Heparin

Unfractionated heparin is a sulfated glycosaminoglycan that exerts its anticoagulant effect predominantly by binding to antithrombin and inducing a conformational change that accelerates the rate at which antithrombin inhibits coagulation enzymes (Chapter 37). It consists of a heterogeneous group of molecules ranging in molecular weight from 3000 to 30,000, and only one third of unfractionated heparin molecules contain the unique pentasaccharide sequence required for binding to antithrombin. This molecular heterogeneity, along with variable charge-related nonspecific binding of unfractionated heparin to other plasma proteins such as von Willebrand factor and platelet factor 4, contributes to the large variability in the anticoagulant response in individual patients.

Unfractionated heparin is usually administered by continuous intravenous infusion, a route that has been shown to be effective in reducing recurrence and extension of thrombus. The use of validated nomograms (Table 81-4), with either fixed initial dosing or dosing according to a patient's weight, results in more rapid achievement of therapeutic activated partial thromboplastin time

TABLE 81-4	WEIGHT-BASED NOMOGRAM FOR INITIAL INTRAVENOUS HEPARIN THERAPY	
aPTT	**DOSE (IU/kg)**
Initial dose	80 bolus, then 18/h
<35 sec (<1.2×)*	80 bolus, then 4/h
35-45 sec (1.2-1.5×)	40 bolus, then 2/h
46-70 sec (1.5-2.3×)	No change
71-90 sec (2.3-3×)	Decrease infusion rate by 2/h
>90 sec (>3×)	Hold infusion 1 h, then decrease infusion rate by 3/h

*Figures in parentheses show comparison with control.
aPTT = activated partial thromboplastin time. In general, with contemporary aPTT reagents, the target therapeutic range is more than 1.2 to 2.3 times control.
Modified from Raschke RA, Reilly BM, Guidry JR, et al. The weight-based heparin dosing nomogram compared with a "standard care" nomogram: a randomized controlled trial. *Ann Intern Med.* 1993;119:874-881.

(aPTT) levels and improves outcome, although adjustment according to the sensitivity of local aPTT methods is required. The initial aPTT level should be measured 6 hours after therapy is commenced. Up to 25% of patients with acute VTE have resistance to heparin, defined as a requirement for greater than expected doses of unfractionated heparin to achieve a "therapeutic" aPTT. If it is available, anti–factor Xa monitoring is recommended in patients with heparin resistance. Larger doses (front-loaded and weight-adjusted follow-up doses) of subcutaneous, 12-hourly unfractionated heparin are as safe and efficacious as LMWH without requiring monitoring of the aPTT. However, this regimen has not been widely embraced by clinicians because of a bias toward monitoring unfractionated heparin with frequent aPTT adjustments.

Transition to Oral Treatment
Coumarin Derivatives (Warfarin)

Warfarin is a vitamin K antagonist that inhibits the production of clotting factors II (prothrombin), VII, IX, and X as well as the naturally occurring anticoagulants protein C and protein S. In patients with DVT, the drug should be started within 24 to 48 hours of initiation of heparin with a goal of achieving international normalized ratio (INR) results between 2.0 and 3.0 (Chapter 37). A higher target INR of 3.0 to 4.0 is associated with more bleeding but no better efficacy, even in patients with the antiphospholipid antibody syndrome (Chapter 179),[4] and lower intensity warfarin therapy (target INR, 1.5 to 1.9) is significantly less effective at preventing recurrent VTE despite similar rates of major bleeding.[5]

The dose is empirical, but a starting dose of 5 to 10 mg is suitable for most patients. Warfarin doses are adjusted according to the prothrombin time, expressed as the INR, performed daily or every other day until the results are in the therapeutic range for at least 24 hours. After initial dosing, warfarin can be monitored two or three times per week for 1 to 2 weeks and then less frequently, depending on the stability of INR results, up to intervals as long as 4 to 6 weeks. If dose adjustment is needed, such as when medications that can interact with warfarin are introduced, the cycle of more frequent monitoring is repeated until a stable dose response is again achieved.

It is now clear that pharmacogenetics have a large impact on the relatively wide range of warfarin dose requirements among different populations as well as the variability of warfarin requirements over time in any individual patient. Polymorphisms in the gene encoding cytochrome P-450 2C9 enzyme, the enzyme that primarily clears the S-enantiomer of warfarin, contribute to variable responses to warfarin; some genetic variants result in an increased sensitivity to warfarin and a lower required dose of warfarin. Vitamin K epoxide reductase (VKORC1) recycles vitamin K epoxide to the reduced form of vitamin K and is the target of warfarin. Its common genetic variants result in altered sensitivity to warfarin, and *VKORC1* polymorphisms are associated with a need for lower doses of warfarin during long-term therapy. Routine pharmacogenetic testing may ultimately be recommended in candidates for long-term (>3 months) warfarin therapy to identify individuals who are likely to require higher or lower warfarin doses.

Side Effects of Anticoagulants

Bleeding is the most common side effect of anticoagulant therapy. Major bleeding (e.g., intracranial [Chapter 415], gastrointestinal [Chapter 137], or retroperitoneal) leading to hospitalization or transfusion or death occurs in approximately 2% of patients treated with intravenous unfractionated heparin for acute VTE. Factors such as recent surgery, trauma, and concurrent aspirin or thrombolytic therapy increase the risk of bleeding.

The risk of major bleeding with warfarin in doses adjusted to achieve a target INR of 2.0 to 3.0 ranges from 1 to 3% per year and appears to be highest soon after treatment is started or if anticoagulation is difficult to control. The risk of major bleeding increases according to individual characteristics, such as older age, the presence of comorbid conditions (e.g., diabetes, hypertension, renal insufficiency, previous gastrointestinal bleeding, or cancer), and the use of concomitant drugs, in particular antiplatelet therapy.

Heparin-induced thrombocytopenia, which is a relatively common non-hemorrhagic complication of therapy with unfractionated heparin and a very uncommon complication of LMWH, is manifested typically with thrombocytopenia and new thrombosis (Chapter 37). Monitoring of the platelet count is recommended every other day until day 14 in patients receiving therapeutic unfractionated heparin but is not routinely recommended with LMWH or fondaparinux because of the extremely low risk with these newer medications.

Long-Term Treatment

The preferred long-term treatment of DVT for most patients is warfarin or another coumarin derivative (e.g., acenocoumarol), continued until the benefits of treatment for reducing recurrent VTE no longer outweigh its risks of major bleeding. The decision to prolong or to stop anticoagulation should be individualized, and a patient's preferences should be considered.

Patients with symptomatic proximal DVT or pulmonary emboli should be treated for at least 3 months, even if the VTE was associated with a transient risk factor,[6] but the optimal duration of treatment for patients whose VTE is not associated with a transient risk factor is controversial. Three months of treatment is associated with a 10 to 27% risk of a recurrence during the 12 months after anticoagulant therapy is stopped, whereas 6 months of anticoagulant therapy reduces the risk of recurrence in the first year after stopping to about 10%. In patients whose VTE developed in association with minor risk factors (e.g., air travel, pregnancy, within 6 weeks of estrogen therapy, after leg injury or immobilization), the risk of recurrence is probably lower than 10%. Continuation of treatment beyond 6 months reduces the risk of recurrent VTE during the course of therapy, but the benefit is lost after warfarin is discontinued.

The most convincing association of thrombophilia with the risk of recurrent VTE is the antiphospholipid antibody (lupus anticoagulant or anticardiolipin antibody; Chapter 179), which is associated with a two-fold increase in the risk of recurrence. Homozygous factor V Leiden, elevated levels of homocysteine, and deficiencies of antithrombin, protein C, and protein S also have been associated with an increased risk of recurrence in some reports, but other data suggest that testing for heritable thrombophilia does not predict recurrent VTE in the first 2 years after anticoagulant therapy is stopped. In the absence of randomized trials to assess different durations of anticoagulation in patients with VTE and thrombophilia, routine testing for thrombophilias need not be

performed but should be considered in young (<50 years) patients, patients with venous thrombosis in unusual sites, and patients with a strong family history of VTE (i.e., one or more first-degree relatives with a history of VTE).

The decision to extend anticoagulant therapy beyond 3 months must balance the risk of recurrent VTE with the risk of bleeding. The annual risk of major bleeding when warfarin is adjusted to achieve a target INR of 2.0 to 3.0 is 1 to 3%, with a case-fatality rate of 10% when major bleeding occurs in patients who received treatment for more than 3 months. By comparison, the case-fatality rate for recurrent VTE is about 5%. In patients whose VTE is associated with a transient risk factor or who are at high risk of bleeding, treatment for 3 months is generally adequate because the risk of fatal recurrent VTE is lower than the risk of fatal bleeding if warfarin treatment is prolonged. Among patients without a reversible or transient cause, however, prolonged warfarin therapy for more than 6 months can be considered because the risk of fatal hemorrhage is counterbalanced by the risk of fatal recurrence. The argument to prolong therapy is stronger in patients with high-risk thrombophilia (e.g., homozygous factor V Leiden; antiphospholipid antibody; deficiency of antithrombin, protein C, or protein S; or combined heterozygous state for factor V Leiden and the prothrombin gene mutation). Indefinite therapy (preferably with LMWH) should be considered in patients with cancer-related VTE (Chapter 187) if the risk of bleeding is not high because the risk of recurrent VTE is more than 10% in the first year after anticoagulation is stopped. In motivated and capable patients, self-management of warfarin therapy is better than management by a physician or nurse.[7]

Alternatives to Coumarin Derivatives

For patients in whom warfarin is impractical or contraindicated and for those who have recurrent VTE while being treated with appropriate doses of oral anticoagulants, therapeutic doses of LMWH are as effective as warfarin. For patients with cancer-related VTE (DVT, pulmonary embolus, or both), weight-based LMWH that is decreased to 75% of the initial dose after 1 month of treatment reduces the risk of recurrent VTE compared with warfarin, with similar bleeding rates.[8]

Therapeutic strategies to manage patients in whom symptomatic VTE recurs while they are receiving conventional-intensity warfarin include unfractionated heparin, LMWH, higher-intensity warfarin (e.g., INR range of 3.0 to 4.0), and insertion of a vena caval filter. However, the optimal management of such patients is unknown because no randomized studies have been performed.

Thrombolytic Therapy

Although thrombolytic therapy results in increased rates of early patency of leg veins after DVT, it has not been conclusively shown to decrease the subsequent rate of post-thrombotic syndrome or pulmonary emboli. Except for patients who have life-threatening limb ischemia due to massive thrombosis, thrombolysis is not recommended in patients with DVT. An ongoing trial of catheter-directed thrombolysis versus "standard therapy" should provide the definitive evidence about the relative efficacy of catheter-directed thrombolysis for the prevention of post-thrombotic syndrome.

Vena Caval Filters

In a randomized trial of 400 patients with DVT, the incidence of pulmonary emboli at day 12 was lower in patients who received an inferior vena caval filter plus therapeutic anticoagulation than in those who received anticoagulation alone. However, filters did not reduce early or late mortality and are not recommended in patients who can receive therapeutic anticoagulation because this benefit did not persist at 2 years and was offset by an almost doubling of the risk of recurrent DVT. Inferior vena caval filters should be used in patients who have contraindications to anticoagulant therapy or develop major bleeding while receiving it as well as in patients who develop recurrent VTE while receiving appropriate anticoagulation. Retrievable or removable inferior vena caval filters can be retrieved and removed within 14 days to several weeks after insertion or can be left in permanently. These filters are ideal for a patient who has a reversible cause of or the potential for major bleeding (e.g., DVT after craniotomy, DVT late in pregnancy).

Oral Direct Thrombin and Factor Xa Inhibitors

Ximelagatran is an oral direct thrombin inhibitor that does not require anticoagulant monitoring. When it is used for the acute and long-term treatment of patients with acute VTE, ximelagatran is as effective and safe as unfractionated heparin or LMWH followed by warfarin in preventing recurrent VTE. However, elevation in liver enzymes, especially the alanine aminotransferases, has been reported in 5 to 10% of patients with long-term use. Although the clinical implications of these elevated levels, which may decrease to normal with continued treatment, are unclear, the drug has been removed from the market by the manufacturers.

Rivaroxaban, an oral factor Xa inhibitor, is effective at 15 mg twice daily for 3 weeks then 20 mg daily for up to 12 months, but it also is associated with elevated aminotransferase levels. These and other thrombin inhibitors are under development for acute and chronic treatment of VTE. Although none has yet been approved for use in North America for the treatment of DVT and pulmonary embolism, some have already been approved for other indications.

PREVENTION

In one large randomized trial, rosuvastatin reduced the rate of DVT by 55%.[9] It is unknown at present whether this benefit can be achieved with other statins. Despite the plethora of large randomized trials demonstrating the efficacy and safety of mechanical and pharmacologic measures in reducing the risk of VTE in a wide range of hospitalized populations of patients, prophylaxis remains grossly underused. Factors that increase the risk of DVT include surgery (particularly major hip and knee surgery, as well as neurosurgery; Chapters 439 and 441), major trauma (Chapter 112), prolonged bed rest or immobilization, previous episodes of VTE, presence of malignant disease, paralysis, morbid obesity, and increasing age.

Comprehensive consensus guidelines have been developed for the prevention of VTE in different populations of patients (see Table 37-2 in Chapter 37). In general, mechanical prophylaxis (antiembolic stockings and intermittent pneumatic compression) should be used as an adjunct to pharmacologic prophylaxis or in patients with a high risk of bleeding. For general medical patients admitted to the hospital with a major illness and in whom mobility is likely to be reduced for 72 hours or longer, low-dose unfractionated heparin or LMWH (see Table 37-2 in Chapter 37) should be considered. In patients who undergo major hip or knee surgery, warfarin (to an INR of 2.0 to 3.0), subcutaneous LMWH, subcutaneous fondaparinux (2.5 mg once daily), or oral rivaroxaban (10 mg once daily) should be used for at least 7 to 14 days postoperatively. In patients with continued immobility, prophylaxis should be considered until the patient regains preoperative mobility.

Management of Deep Vein Thrombosis in Pregnancy

The management of pregnant women with DVT (Chapter 247) is problematic because all coumarin derivatives cross the placenta and have the potential to cause warfarin embryopathy, consisting of nasal hypoplasia and epiphyseal stippling, if the newborn is exposed to warfarin between 6 and 12 weeks of gestation. Consequently, parenteral unfractionated heparin and LMWH, which do not cross the placenta and are safe for the fetus, are the agents of choice. The easiest approach is to initiate therapy with weight-adjusted "treatment" doses of LMWH (see Table 81-3), continued for the duration of the pregnancy. Although it is not proved, it is likely that the dose of LMWH can be safely decreased to approximately 80% of the therapeutic dose after 3 months of therapy. As pregnancy progresses, women normally gain weight and generally require higher doses of LMWH to achieve an anti–factor Xa level similar to that achieved at the time of diagnosis. The adequacy of the dose can be assessed by measuring a 4-hour postinjection anti–factor Xa level and targeting the dose to achieve a level of 0.5 to 1.0 U/mL for twice-daily LMWH and 0.8 to 1.5 U/mL for once-daily LMWH. Alternatively, the dose of LMWH can simply be adjusted periodically on the basis of the woman's weight.

Unfractionated heparin is less attractive than LMWH because it is associated with a greater reduction of bone density and a higher risk of heparin-induced thrombocytopenia. Unfractionated heparin can be initiated either by continuous intravenous infusion in doses adjusted to maintain an aPTT in the therapeutic range, followed by 12-hourly subcutaneous injections, or simply with 12-hourly subcutaneous injections throughout the course of pregnancy. The dose should be adjusted to target a mid-interval (6-hour postinjection) aPTT in the therapeutic range.

Pregnant women with a DVT should probably be treated for the duration of pregnancy and for at least 6 weeks postpartum. If the DVT occurred early in pregnancy, elective induction of delivery at about 37 weeks with discontinuation of the heparin 24 hours earlier is recommended. If the DVT occurs in the latter part of the third trimester, intravenous heparin should be administered by continuous infusion until approximately 6 hours before the expected time of delivery. Intravenous unfractionated heparin or subcutaneous LMWH should be started postpartum as soon as hemostasis has been achieved. Maternal warfarin therapy is safe for the breast-fed infant because warfarin and its metabolites are not secreted into breast milk in doses sufficient to cause an anticoagulant effect. Consequently, warfarin (with bridging LMWH or unfractionated heparin until the INR is 2.0 or higher) can be used after delivery.

Venous Thrombosis of the Upper Extremities

DVT of the upper extremities (including the arm and the axillary, subclavian, and internal jugular veins as well as the superior vena cava) is much less common than DVT of the legs, but it is not rare. Factors associated with upper extremity DVT include central venous catheters, acquired or hereditary thrombophilias, and anatomic (cervical rib) and physiologic (muscular individuals) impingement of the vein. The incidence of clinically important post-thrombotic syndrome is not high if patients are treated with anticoagulants alone.

Contrast venography is the gold standard for the diagnosis of upper extremity DVT, but venous ultrasonography is accurate and less invasive. Because it is not feasible to test for compression of the subclavian vein, a diagnosis of subclavian DVT by ultrasonography is based on flow abnormalities or direct visualization of thrombus by B-mode ultrasonography. Upper extremity DVT can cause pulmonary emboli, although the exact frequency is not known.

Considerable controversy exists about the management of patients in whom DVT develops in association with a central venous catheter. If the line is not necessary or is nonfunctional, some recommend simply removing the line without subsequent anticoagulant therapy, whereas others treat with full-dose anticoagulants (a heparin-related compound, followed by 1 to 3 months of warfarin). If the line is functional and must stay in place (e.g., no alternative venous access), full-dose anticoagulants should be given. Otherwise, anticoagulant therapy should be given in all patients with upper extremity DVT, with medications, doses, regimens, and durations identical to those for treatment of DVT of the leg.

● SUPERFICIAL THROMBOPHLEBITIS

Superficial thrombophlebitis usually presents with pain, swelling, redness, and tenderness of superficial veins. Varicose veins (Fig. 81-6) can be red, warm, and clustered in a circumscribed area. When superficial thrombophlebitis occurs in the short or long saphenous veins, there is usually redness, tenderness, and often linear induration that follow the course of the involved vein (medial calf or thigh). Superficial thrombophlebitis can also occur at the insertion site of an intravenous catheter. Invariably, superficial thrombophlebitis is associated with thrombosis of the corresponding vein, and particularly when the long saphenous vein is involved, venous ultrasonography should be performed to exclude extension into the deep veins, which occurs in up to 19% of patients.

Nonsteroidal anti-inflammatory drugs and either moderate or full doses of LMWH are each about 70% better than placebo for treating superficial thrombophlebitis.[10] LMWH relieves symptoms more quickly and prevents growth of thrombus more effectively than do nonsteroidal anti-inflammatory drugs. Fondaparinux, 2.5 mg daily for 45 days, reduces the risk of DVT or pulmonary embolism from about 1.3% to 0.2% without adverse effects.[11] Thus, it is reasonable to use moderate doses of LMWH or fondaparinux for the initial treatment of acute, symptomatic superficial thrombophlebitis, particularly for patients with severe symptoms, proximal

FIGURE 81-6. Varicose veins are a risk factor for deep vein thrombosis and may result from it. (From Forbes CD, Jackson WF. *Color Atlas and Text of Clinical Medicine*, 3rd ed. London: Mosby; 2003.)

saphenous vein thrombosis, recurrent disease, or evidence of thrombophilia. Alternatively, and particularly for intravenous catheter-induced superficial thrombophlebitis, a nonsteroidal anti-inflammatory drug can be tried.

POST-THROMBOTIC SYNDROME

The initial pain and swelling in many patients with DVT are due to the venous obstruction or the inflammatory process mediated by the acute thrombus. Once anticoagulant therapy is initiated, the acute obstruction usually resolves during a period of several months as recanalization occurs and collateral venous channels develop, thereby leading to initial improvement in pain and swelling. However, in the long term, probably because of venous valvular incompetence produced when the thrombosed venous segments recanalize and sometimes because of residual chronic obstruction, venous hypertension and sometimes pain and swelling can recur.

This post-thrombotic syndrome develops in up to 50% of patients with proximal DVT, usually within the first 1 to 2 years after DVT. The syndrome is often a chronic, progressive disease with pain, swelling, and occasionally ulceration of the leg in patients with previous DVT.

PREVENTION AND TREATMENT   Rx

The use of below-knee graduated compression stockings for 2 years after acute DVT reduces the risk of the post-thrombotic syndrome by about 50%.[12] Some experts recommend routine stocking therapy in all patients with DVT. Others recommend waiting until the acute inflammatory process and acute outflow obstruction have subsided (usually up to 6 months) and then prescribing stockings if the patient's symptoms persist at that time. The use of graduated compression stockings does not significantly reduce DVT after stroke, however, and results in adverse skin events.[13]

However, stockings are hot in the summer, relatively expensive, difficult for many patients to put on in the morning, and cosmetically unappealing to many patients. In addition, simple lifestyle alteration (such as frequent leg elevation, avoidance of prolonged standing or sitting, and occasional use of analgesics) suffices in relieving symptoms in many patients. If symptoms are severe, it is usually because of extensive thrombus causing massive edema. In such patients, a lightweight stocking (such as support hose) can be helpful until the edema improves. If symptoms persist or worsen despite these measures, or if ulceration seems imminent (as evidenced by severe skin changes), a full-strength stocking (30 to 40 mm Hg of pressure at the ankle) can be prescribed. However, if symptoms subside and the patient remains asymptomatic or has only trivial persistent signs or symptoms with little or no effect on quality of life, stockings can be avoided, and the patient can be observed for clinically important signs and symptoms of the post-thrombotic syndrome.

VENOUS ULCERS

Venous ulcers, which are the most severe complication of post-thrombotic syndrome, typically occur in the perimalleolar area of the leg. The best management is prevention by application of graduated compression stockings either at the time of diagnosis of DVT or, at the latest, when skin changes develop in association with leg swelling. When an ulcer occurs, treatment with an emollient and regular wrapping should be commenced. Once the ulcer heals, the patient should be prescribed graduated compression stockings and watched for recurrent ulceration. Surgical closure or removal of the incompetent saphenous veins plus dressing management in patients with chronic venous ulceration does not reduce healing time of the acute ulcer compared with dressing management alone but significantly reduces the rate of recurrent ulceration for at least the next 4 years.[14]

 Grade A

1. Bernardi E, Camporese G, Büller HR, et al. Serial 2-point ultrasonography plus D-dimer vs whole-leg color-coded Doppler ultrasonography for diagnosing suspected symptomatic deep vein thrombosis: a randomized controlled trial. *JAMA*. 2008;300:1653-1659.
2. Hull RD, Pineo GF, Brant RF, et al. Long-term low-molecular-weight heparin versus usual care in proximal-vein thrombosis patients with cancer. *Am J Med*. 2006;119:1062-1072.
3. Buller HR, Davidson BL, Decousus H, et al. Fondaparinux or enoxaparin for the initial treatment of symptomatic deep venous thrombosis: a randomized trial. *Ann Intern Med*. 2004;140:867-873.
4. Crowther MA, Ginsberg JS, Julian J, et al. A comparison of two intensities of warfarin for the prevention of recurrent thrombosis in patients with the antiphospholipid antibody syndrome. *N Engl J Med*. 2003;349:1133-1138.
5. Kearon C, Ginsberg JS, Kovacs MJ, et al. Comparison of low-intensity warfarin therapy with conventional-intensity warfarin therapy for long-term prevention of recurrent venous thromboembolism. *N Engl J Med*. 2003;349:631-639.
6. Kearon C, Ginsberg JS, Anderson DR, et al. Comparison of 1 month of anticoagulation with 3 months of anticoagulation for a first episode of venous thromboembolism provoked by a transient risk factor. *J Thromb Haemost*. 2003;2:743-749.
7. Bloomfield HE, Krause A, Greer N, et al. Meta-analysis: effect of patient self-testing and self-management of long-term anticoagulation on major clinical outcomes. *Ann Intern Med*. 2011;154:472-482.
8. Lee AY, Levine MN, Baker RI, et al. Randomized comparison of low-molecular-weight heparin versus oral anticoagulant therapy for the prevention of recurrent venous thromboembolism in patients with cancer. *N Engl J Med*. 2003;349:109-111.
9. Glynn RJ, Danielson E, Fonseca FA, et al. A randomized trial of rosuvastatin in the prevention of venous thromboembolism. *N Engl J Med*. 2009; 360:1851-1861.
10. Di Nisio N, Wichers IM, Middeldorp S. Treatment for superficial thrombophlebitis of the leg (Review). *Cochrane Database Syst Rev*. 2007;2:CD004982.
11. Decousus H, Prandoni P, Mismetti P, et al, for the CALISTO Study Group. Fondaparinux in the treatment of lower-limb superficial-vein thrombosis. *N Engl J Med*. 2010;363:1222-1232.
12. Prandoni P, Lensing AW, Prins MH, et al. Below-knee elastic compression stockings to prevent the post-thrombotic syndrome: a randomized, controlled trial. *Ann Intern Med*. 2004;141:249-256.
13. Dennis M, Sandercock PA, Reid J, et al, for the CLOTS Trials Collaboration. Effectiveness of thigh-length graduated compression stockings to reduce the risk of deep vein thrombosis after stroke (CLOTS trial 1): a multicentre, randomised controlled trial. *Lancet*. 2009;373:1958-1965.
14. Gohel MS, Barwell JR, Taylor M, et al. Long term results of compression therapy alone versus compression plus surgery in chronic venous ulceration (ESCHAR): randomised controlled trial. *BMJ*. 2007;335:55-56.

SUGGESTED READINGS

Decousus H, Quéré I, Presles E, et al. Superficial venous thrombosis and venous thromboembolism: a large, prospective epidemiologic study. *Ann Intern Med*. 2010;152:218-224. *About 25% of patients who have superficial venous thrombosis have concurrent deep venous thrombosis at the time of presentation, and about 3% of the others will subsequently develop deep venous thrombosis or pulmonary embolism in the next 3 months.*

Goldhaber SZ, Piazza G. Optimal duration of anticoagulation after venous thromboembolism. *Circulation*. 2011;123:664-667. *Review.*

Kucher N. Clinical practice. Deep-vein thrombosis of the upper extremities. *N Engl J Med*. 2011;364:861-869. *Case-based review.*

Watson HG, Baglin TP. Guidelines on travel-related venous thrombosis. *Br J Haematol*. 2011;152:31-34. *Review.*

82

CARDIAC TRANSPLANTATION

MARIELL JESSUP

Cardiac transplantation is the treatment of choice for suitable patients with refractory heart failure (Chapters 59, 60, and 107). The number of heart transplantation procedures worldwide reached a peak of about 4500 in 1994 but has subsequently declined because the rate of identification of potential donors has not kept pace with the increased number of patients on waiting lists, where the annual mortality is 10 to 20% (Fig. 82-1). Because newer therapeutic options have usually failed and they now lack other alternatives, patients referred for heart transplantation are becoming progressively older and more ill, with increasing medical comorbidities, which have significantly increased the risk of cardiac transplantation. In many institutions, at least one third of patients are sustained on a ventricular assist device while awaiting transplantation. At the same time, the selection criteria for donors have been broadened to increase the number of organs available. As a result, sicker recipients are now receiving less ideal organs than in the past.

POPULATION OF PATIENTS

Evaluation of the Potential Recipient

The purposes of heart transplantation are to prolong life and to improve quality of life, so the referring physician must understand the potential benefits of transplantation as well as comorbidities that may portend an unsatisfactory outcome. Suitable patients for consideration have cardiogenic shock requiring mechanical support or high-dose inotropic or pressor drugs (Chapter 107); stage D heart failure symptoms despite maximal therapy (Chapter 59); recurrent life-threatening arrhythmias despite maximal interventions, including implanted defibrillators (Chapters 63 and 65); or, rarely, refractory angina without the potential for revascularization (Chapter 71) (Table 82-1). The most potent predictor of outcome in ambulatory patients with heart failure is a symptom-limited metabolic stress test to calculate peak oxygen consumption; a peak of less than 12 mL/kg/minute indicates a lower survival with medical therapy than after transplantation.

An extensive medical and psychosocial evaluation must be performed to exclude contraindications to transplantation. In the setting of fixed

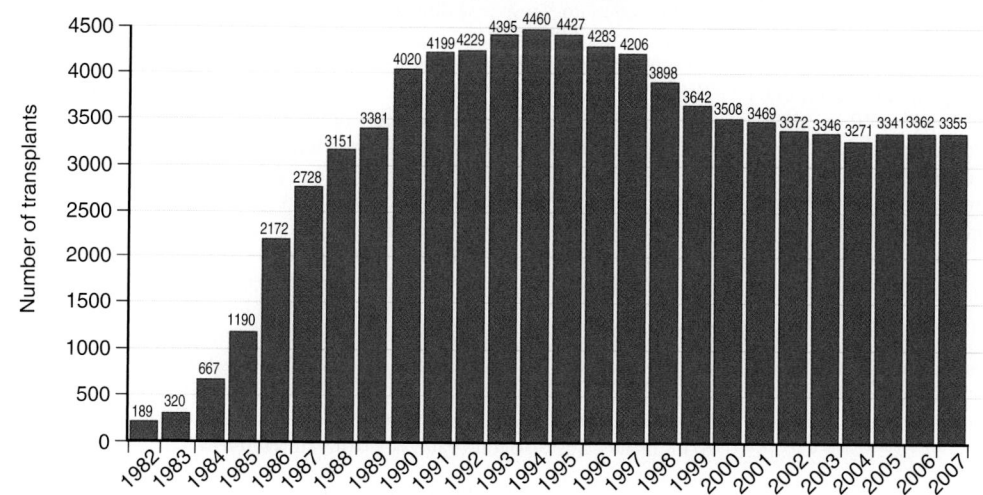

Adult Heart Transplants: January 1982 to June 2007

FIGURE 82-1. The number of heart transplantation procedures by year. (Data from the Registry of the International Society for Heart and Lung Transplantation. Reproduced with permission.)

TABLE 82-1 EVALUATION OF THE POTENTIAL HEART TRANSPLANT RECIPIENT

INDICATIONS FOR HEART TRANSPLANTATION

Cardiogenic shock requiring mechanical support or high-dose inotropic drugs
Stage D heart failure symptoms despite maximal therapy
Recurrent life-threatening arrhythmias despite maximal interventions and implanted defibrillator
Refractory angina without potential for revascularization

CONTRAINDICATIONS TO HEART TRANSPLANTATION

	ALTERNATIVE TREATMENT	OPTIONS
Age > 70 yr	Consider permanent mechanical support	End-of-life considerations or investigational therapy
Active or recent malignant disease	End-of-life considerations or investigational therapy	
Diabetes with severe end-organ damage	Consider permanent mechanical support	End-of-life considerations or investigational therapy
FEV/FVC < 40%	Consider heart-lung transplantation	End-of-life considerations or investigational therapy
BMI < 20 or BMI > 35	Nutritional modification; BMI > 35, consider permanent mechanical support or weight loss	
Irreversible pulmonary hypertension (≥4 Wood units)	Consider heart-lung transplantation	End-of-life considerations or investigational therapy
Other comorbidities: cirrhosis, vascular disease, addictions, hepatitis C, human immunodeficiency virus infection, social or psychiatric disorders	Individual transplantation team decisions	

BMI = body mass index; FEV = forced expiratory volume; FVC = forced vital capacity.

pulmonary hypertension, such patients are occasionally considered for combined heart-lung transplantation.

An immunologic evaluation includes determination of ABO blood type, antibody screen, panel-reactive antibody level, and human leukocyte antigen (HLA) typing. Using virtual crossmatch methods, flow cytometry–based single-antigen bead assays can identify prospective donors with undesirable antigens without the need for a prospective crossmatch, thereby allowing for matches outside the recipient's geographic area.

Management of the Patient Waiting for Cardiac Transplantation

A patient's priority status according to the United Network for Organ Sharing is based on the recipient's acuity status, blood type, body size, and duration of time at a particular status level. Patients who can be managed successfully outside the hospital are the lowest priority. Intermediate priority is given to patients who require hospitalization and some continuous inotropic support. The highest priority, status 1A, is given to patients requiring high-dose inotropic support or mechanical support, such as intra-aortic balloon counterpulsation or ventricular assist device. Hearts are offered geographically, by the location of the donor, and limited by an ischemic time of approximately 4 hours. Patients who are waiting for transplantation are regularly reevaluated for a change in status or the development or worsening of a comorbidity that would preclude transplantation.

THE CARDIAC TRANSPLANTATION PROCEDURE

The Cardiac Donor

Relevant history for the assessment of cardiac donors includes the presence or absence of thoracic trauma, hemodynamic stability, pressor and inotropic requirements, duration of cardiac arrest, need for cardiopulmonary resuscitation, and assessment of hypotensive episodes. In many potential donors, brain death causes hemodynamic deterioration that requires inotropic support and substantial fluid administration. Donors up to the age of 50 to 55 years are considered safe by most centers. The final decision to accept a heart for transplantation is made at the time of harvest, after direct examination for myocardial infarction, trauma, and coronary calcification.

Currently, the acceptable cold ischemia time between explant and implant is approximately 4 hours. One of the main reasons for early graft failure after transplantation is inadequate myocardial protection during prolonged ischemic periods.

Surgical Considerations

The biatrial anastomosis technique consists of four suture lines: left atrium, pulmonary artery, aorta, and right atrium. The bicaval anastomosis technique, introduced to minimize distortion of the heart and to preserve atrial conduction, has five anastomoses: left atrium, pulmonary artery, aorta, inferior vena cava, and superior vena cava. To date, there has been no prospective trial to establish the superiority of either technique. Failure to wean a heart transplant recipient from cardiopulmonary bypass is most commonly the result of right-sided heart failure, which is evidenced by low cardiac output in the face of a rising central venous pressure. Native heart pacemakers and cardiac defibrillators are usually surgically removed at the end of the operation after the chest has been closed.

POSTOPERATIVE MANAGEMENT

Early Postoperative Management

Cardiovascular Issues

Management of the heart transplant recipient early after surgery does not differ substantially from management after other cardiac procedures

(Chapter 74). Cardiac transplant patients typically need chronotropic and inotropic support for a few days in the intensive care unit.

Because the donor heart is denervated, bradycardia is a frequent problem. It is usually treated with titrated isoproterenol to maintain a heart rate above 90 beats per minute for the first several days after transplantation. Temporary pacing leads are necessary for all patients, and as many as 10 to 15% of patients require a permanent pacemaker after transplant surgery.

Inhaled nitric oxide, in a usual dose of 20 to 60 parts per million, is a potent vasodilator that has a selective effect on the pulmonary vasculature, reduces pulmonary vascular resistance, and improves right ventricular function in patients with pulmonary hypertension. Intravenous epoprostenol, an alternative, is typically used at 5 to 50 ng/kg/minute.

Immunosuppression

Most immunosuppressive regimens begin with the simultaneous use of three classes of drugs: glucocorticoids, calcineurin inhibitors, and antiproliferative agents. In addition, patients may receive a variety of drugs during induction therapy (Chapter 48).

Perioperative Induction Therapy

The goal of perioperative induction therapy is to inhibit only those T cells that respond to donor antigen, thus achieving immunologic unresponsiveness to the transplant in the face of a fully functioning immune system, called donor-specific tolerance. Agents include the polyclonal anti-thymocyte antibodies, the interleukin-2 receptor antagonists daclizumab and basiliximab, and, less often, the anti-CD3 antibody OKT3.

Acute and Maintenance Immunosuppression

Patients initially receive high doses of intravenous corticosteroids (e.g., 500 mg of intravenous [IV] methylprednisolone at the end of cardiopulmonary bypass, followed by 150 mg IV every 8 hours for three additional doses), then oral steroids that are gradually tapered during the next 6 months in an attempt to minimize side effects (Chapter 34). Corticosteroids also are usually the drug of first choice to treat acute rejection.

The calcineurin inhibitors tacrolimus and cyclosporine act specifically on the immune system and do not affect other rapidly proliferating cells. In a meta-analysis, tacrolimus was as good as cyclosporine in terms of survival and significantly reduced episodes of acute rejection.[1] Important and often limiting side effects include nephrotoxicity, which occurs in up to 40 to 70% of patients, and hypertension. Target therapeutic levels 2 hours after a dose improve outcome.

Mycophenolate mofetil has replaced azathioprine as the first-line antiproliferative drug, with several randomized trials demonstrating superiority to azathioprine.[2] Mycophenolate mofetil may cause leukopenia, debilitating diarrhea, and nausea.

Sirolimus (often called rapamycin) and everolimus are complementary to calcineurin inhibitors, and both drugs have been used as alternatives to standard maintenance immunosuppression and as rescue drugs for rejection. In one randomized trial using cyclosporine and steroids, addition of sirolimus halved the number of patients with acute rejection and reduced the development of vasculopathy in the donor heart compared with addition of azathioprine.[3]

Other Potential Management Issues

The transplant recipient is often debilitated or malnourished. Depression (Chapter 404) is common, and many patients exhibit a marked emotional lability that is aggravated by high-dose steroids. Successful heart transplantation teams must include dedicated physical therapists, nutritionists, and social workers or psychologists, in addition to the nurses and physicians, so that all these needs may be addressed.

Long-Term Care of the Cardiac Transplant Recipient
Rejection

Rejection is categorized histologically and immunologically into three major types: hyperacute, acute (cellular or humoral), and chronic. Hyperacute rejection, which results when an abrupt loss of allograft function occurs within minutes to hours after circulation is established in the allograft, is rare in modern-day transplantation. The phenomenon is mediated by preexisting antibodies to allogeneic antigens on the vascular endothelial cells of the donor organ. These antibodies fix complement, which promotes intravascular thrombosis, leading to rapid occlusion of graft vasculature and swift rejection.

Acute cellular rejection, which is a predominantly lymphocytic mononuclear inflammatory response directed against the cardiac allograft, commonly occurs from the first week to several years after transplantation. The key event in both the initiation and the coordination of the rejection is T-cell activation. The risk of acute cellular rejection in the first 6 months is 40 to 70%. Acute cellular rejection after 6 months occurs most often in patients who have had substantial rejection early after transplantation, recent reduction in immunosuppression, intercurrent infection, or noncompliance with medication.

Acute humoral rejection occurs days to weeks after transplantation and is initiated by alloantibodies directed against donor HLA or endothelial cell antigens rather than by T cells. Patients at greatest risk for humoral rejection are women and patients with a high panel-reactive antibody screen or a positive crossmatch. It is estimated that significant humoral rejection occurs in about 7% of patients, but the rate may be as high as 20%.

Chronic rejection, or late graft failure, is an irreversible gradual deterioration of graft function occurring in many allografts months to years after transplantation. It is characterized by intimal thickening and fibrosis, which lead to luminal occlusion of the graft vasculature; it is often called cardiac allograft vasculopathy.

DIAGNOSIS

Allograft rejection is most frequent within the first month after cardiac transplantation and declines progressively thereafter. Clinical symptoms of rejection are often vague and relatively late in terms of immune injury to myocytes. Endomyocardial biopsy has been the "gold standard" for the diagnosis of rejection. Biopsies are performed by a transjugular approach weekly for 3 or 4 weeks, then every other week for several months; monthly biopsies continue for 6 to 12 months in many transplant programs. Biopsy grading of cellular rejection is based on the severity of lymphocyte infiltration and myocyte necrosis (Table 82-2). In one randomized trial, gene expression profiling of peripheral blood reduced the number of biopsies and provided equivalent outcomes over a mean follow-up of 19 months among patients who were stable 6 months to 5 years after transplantation.[4]

Humoral rejection is usually suspected clinically when there is evidence of suboptimal graft function but the endomyocardial biopsy specimen shows either no evidence of cellular rejection or only mild rejection. The pathologic markers of humoral rejection identifiable in endomyocardial biopsy tissue include deposits of immunoglobulin M, immunoglobulin G, or complement in the microvasculature or myocytes. In particular, C4d, which is a degradation product of the classic complement pathway and which binds to the endothelial and collagen basement membrane, is increasingly used as a marker of antibody-mediated rejection. Evidence for antibodies in the circulation with specificity for non-HLA antigens on the graft also supports the diagnosis of humoral rejection.

PROGNOSIS

Acute rejection causes approximately 12% of deaths in the first year after transplantation, but cardiac allograft vasculopathy represents a substantial portion of annual mortality beyond 3 years. Moreover, efforts to avert rejection with potent immunosuppressive therapy are responsible for other common complications after cardiac transplantation.

Infection

Infections cause approximately 20% of deaths within the first year after transplant surgery and continue to be a common cause of morbidity and mortality throughout the recipient's life. Infections of any type during the first month after transplantation also increase the risk of a subsequent fatal cytomegalovirus (CMV) infection (Chapter 384).

TABLE 82-2	STANDARDIZED CARDIAC BIOPSY GRADING: ACUTE CELLULAR REJECTION* 2004
Grade 0 R	No rejection
Grade 1 R, mild	Interstitial and/or perivascular infiltrate with up to one focus of myocyte damage
Grade 2 R, moderate	Two or more foci of infiltrate with associated myocyte damage
Grade 3 R, severe	Diffuse infiltrate with multifocal myocyte damage, ± edema, ± hemorrhage, ± vasculitis

*International Society for Heart and Lung Transplantation.

Prophylaxis against CMV infection, *Pneumocystis jiroveci* pneumonia, herpes simplex virus infection, and oral candidiasis is now routine during the first 6 to 12 months after transplantation. As a result, the most common infections seen in the first month after surgery are nosocomial bacterial and fungal infections related to mechanical ventilation, catheters, the surgical site, and residual infections from prior implantation of ventricular assist devices.

The prophylactic use of trimethoprim-sulfamethoxazole, typically for the first year after transplantation, has virtually eliminated *P. jiroveci* pneumonia (Chapter 349) and also prevents nocardial infections and toxoplasmosis. The combination drug is generally reinstituted during subsequent episodes of increased risk, such as enhanced immunosuppression. Aspergillosis and candidiasis (Chapters 346 and 347) are the most common fungal infections after heart transplantation; oral nystatin solution or clotrimazole troches are routinely used in the first 6 to 12 months. Viral infections, especially CMV infection (Chapter 384), can increase immunosuppression, resulting in additional opportunistic infections. Prophylactic intravenous ganciclovir or oral valganciclovir is generally given for variable amounts of time in the CMV-seronegative recipient of a CMV-positive donor.

Health Maintenance

After 5 years, 95% of recipients have hypertension, 81% have hyperlipidemia, and 32% have diabetes. In addition, 25% to 50% have cardiac allograft vasculopathy, and up to 33% have renal insufficiency. Lifelong immunosuppression makes all recipients more susceptible to a number of malignant neoplasms, so careful follow-up is mandatory.

In many centers, recipients are given daily aspirin to reduce vascular disease, but no randomized trial has evaluated the benefits of antiplatelet therapy in heart transplant patients. Likewise, most recipients are given vitamins, stool softeners, iron supplements, and proton pump inhibitors early after surgery on an empirical basis.

Surveillance

New Health Problems

Because osteoporosis (Chapter 251) is a major problem, in part related to use of corticosteroids, prophylaxis with calcium and vitamin D is usually initiated. Depression occurs in up to 25% of recipients. A number of antidepressants may be used, but the potential for adverse drug interactions must be considered. The management of gout is difficult because colchicine may increase the risk of myoneuropathy, nonsteroidal anti-inflammatory drugs often worsen renal insufficiency and hyperkalemia, and allopurinol used with azathioprine can cause life-threatening neutropenia. Minimizing diuretic use and judicious use of colchicine with allopurinol will usually alleviate most patients' symptoms.

Risk factors for malignant disease (Chapter 183) include impaired immunoregulation, a synergistic effect with other carcinogens such as nicotine or ultraviolet light exposure, and oncogenic causes such as Epstein-Barr virus and papillomavirus. The cumulative amount of immunosuppression is positively correlated with risk for malignant change. Lymphoproliferative diseases, skin and lip cancers, and Kaposi's sarcoma are particularly common. Malignant neoplasms account for 24% of deaths after 5 years.

● TRANSPLANT VASCULOPATHY

EPIDEMIOLOGY AND PATHOBIOLOGY

Transplant vasculopathy remains the most daunting long-term complication of heart transplantation, with an annual incidence rate of 5 to 10%. After the first postoperative year, cardiac allograft vasculopathy becomes increasingly important as a cause of death. The risk of transplant vasculopathy increases as the number of HLA mismatches and the number and duration of rejection episodes increase. CMV infection and ischemia-reperfusion injury also increase the risk, as do classic risk factors for atherosclerotic disease (Chapter 51), such as smoking, obesity, diabetes, dyslipidemia, and hypertension. Transplant vasculopathy can develop as early as 3 months after transplantation and is detected angiographically in 20% of grafts at 1 year and in 40 to 50% at 5 years.

CLINICAL MANIFESTATIONS

In contrast to eccentric lesions seen in atheromatous disease, cardiac allograft vasculopathy produces concentric narrowing from neointimal proliferation of vascular smooth muscle cells and affects the entire length of the coronary tree, from the epicardial to the intramyocardial segments, leading to rapid tapering, pruning, and obliteration of third-order branch vessels. Most

patients will not experience anginal symptoms because of denervation of coronary arteries, so the first clinical manifestation may be myocardial infarction, heart failure, ventricular arrhythmia, or sudden death. As a result, most transplantation centers screen patients annually for possible transplant vasculopathy.

DIAGNOSIS

Intravascular ultrasonography, which is currently the most sensitive imaging technique to study early transplant vasculopathy, provides quantitative data on intimal thickness, luminal cross-sectional area, and external elastic membrane cross-sectional area. An increase in intimal thickness of at least 0.5 mm in the first year after transplantation is a reliable indicator of both cardiac allograft vasculopathy and 5-year mortality. However, increased invasiveness and cost of intravascular ultrasonography preclude its widespread application. Dobutamine stress echocardiography (Chapter 55) has a high sensitivity (83 to 95%) and specificity (between 53 and 91%) compared with angiography. Most transplantation centers do one of the screening tests on an annual basis to assess the risk of new cardiac allograft vasculopathy.

TREATMENT Rx

The only definitive treatment of transplant vasculopathy is repeated transplantation. The statins pravastatin and simvastatin repress the induction of class II major histocompatibility complex antigen expression by interferon-γ and thereby inhibit T-cell proliferation and have a direct influence on the expression of genes for growth factors that are essential for the proliferation of smooth muscle cells. Randomized controlled trials have shown that either drug significantly reduces rates of severe rejections and transplant vasculopathy while also significantly reducing cholesterol levels and improving survival (see later).[5] It is not clear whether all statin drugs have the same benefit in this population. Sirolimus and everolimus are also being evaluated to prevent the development or progression of cardiac allograft vasculopathy, but their role has not yet been determined.

Diabetes

Diabetes (Chapter 237) occurs in 32% of transplant recipients, and patients who develop new-onset diabetes mellitus after transplantation are at increased risk for morbidity and mortality. Although impaired B-cell function appears to be the primary mechanism of calcineurin inhibitor-induced new-onset diabetes, impaired peripheral glucose use also appears to contribute to insulin resistance and abnormal glucose metabolism. Risk factors include obesity, increased age, family history of diabetes, abnormal glucose tolerance, and African American or Hispanic descent. Management is generally similar to that of the nontransplant patient.

Hypertension and Renal Insufficiency

The 5-year incidence of hypertension (Chapter 67) in the population of cardiac transplant recipients is 95%. Excess risk of hypertension is attributable primarily to the use of calcineurin inhibitors because of both direct effects and the associated renal insufficiency. Treatment often requires a combination of agents and is generally as in the nontransplant patient.

The risk of chronic renal failure is about 16% at 10 years, largely related to direct calcineurin inhibitor–mediated renal arteriolar vasoconstriction, increased levels of endothelin-1, decreased nitric oxide production, and alterations in the kidney's ability to adjust to changes in serum tonicity. Once early renal insufficiency occurs, no single treatment has yet been shown to be effective.

Hyperlipidemia

Hyperlipidemia (Chapter 213) occurs in more than 80% of cardiac transplant recipients and is associated with the development of cardiac allograft vasculopathy, cerebrovascular disease, and peripheral vascular disease. Characteristically, total cholesterol, low-density lipoprotein cholesterol, apolipoprotein B, and triglyceride levels increase by 3 months after transplantation and then generally fall somewhat after the first year. Corticosteroids, cyclosporine, sirolimus, and mycophenolate mofetil all have unfavorable effects on lipid levels, whereas tacrolimus probably causes less hyperlipidemia.

In heart transplant recipients, pravastatin and simvastatin have been associated with better outcomes, but there are no long-term data in this population demonstrating that lowering of low-density lipoprotein cholesterol levels to less than 100 mg/dL (compared with 100 to 130 mg/dL) with more potent

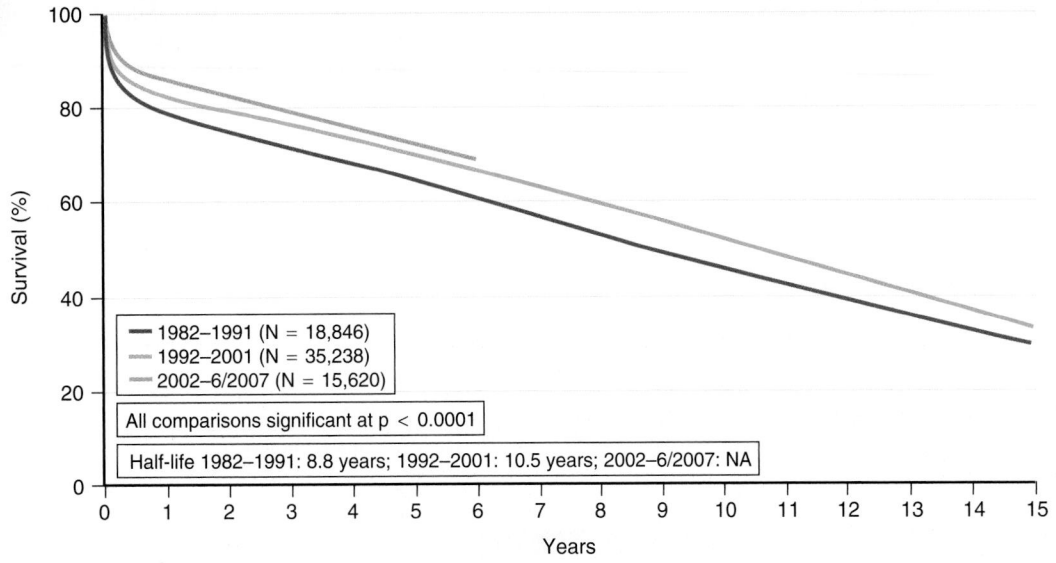

or higher-dose statin therapy improves outcomes. Different statins are metabolized differently, so caution must be exercised in the prescription of statins beyond the doses used in the randomized trials: simvastatin, 20 to 40 mg daily, and pravastatin, 10 to 20 mg daily.

OUTCOME OF TRANSPLANTATION

During the first year after transplantation, early causes of death are graft failure, infection, and rejection, with an overall survival of 87.7% at 1 year and 79.1% at 3 years (Fig. 82-2). The percentage of patients dying of early graft failure, malignant disease, and infection has remained relatively stable during the past decade. After 5 years, cardiac allograft vasculopathy and late graft failure (33% together), malignant disease (23%), and non-CMV infection (11%) are the most prominent causes of death. With advances in immunosuppression, the average half-life of the cardiac allograft increased approximately 15 months (8.8 years to 10.5 years) from 1986-1990 to 1992-2001.

Hemodynamic and Functional Outcomes

The transplanted heart markedly improves cardiac hemodynamics, but there may be a slightly diminished maximal cardiac output during exercise secondary to denervation, limited atrial function, decreased myocardial compliance from rejection or ischemic injury, and donor-recipient size mismatch. Immediately after surgery, a restrictive hemodynamic pattern is frequently observed, but it gradually improves during a few days to weeks. Some 10 to 15% of recipients develop a chronic restrictive cardiomyopathy (Chapter 60) that may produce fatigue and breathlessness during exercise. Because parasympathetic innervation, which normally lowers the heart rate, is absent, the typical resting heart rate of a recipient is 90 to 115 beats per minute.

At 1 year, 90% of surviving patients report no functional limitations, and approximately 35% return to work. Adapting to life after transplantation depends on many factors, including the patient's condition and duration of illness before transplantation and the patient's personality, intelligence, social support, and financial well-being.

Other Key Long-Term Issues for the Nontransplantation Physician
Drug Interactions

The physician outside the transplanting hospital may be reluctant to interact at all with the heart transplant recipient, a fear that complicates the comprehensive care of these patients. Often a phone call placed to the transplantation center to clarify any proposed medications or new symptoms will obviate the need for the recipient to travel to the transplanting hospital. The most common errors made by nontransplantation physicians are the addition of new drugs that result in adverse drug interactions; examples include acyclovir, allopurinol, amlodipine, antacids, antidepressants, cimetidine, clarithromycin, clotrimazole, colchicine, diltiazem, erythromycin, felodipine, ganciclovir, grapefruit juice, iron, ketoconazole, phenobarbital, phenytoin, primidone, rifampin, statin drugs, St. John's wort, trimethoprim-sulfamethoxazole, valganciclovir, and verapamil. In addition, the index of suspicion must be higher in evaluating the possibility of infection in a transplant recipient (Chapter 289).

FUTURE DIRECTIONS IN CARDIAC TRANSPLANTATION

It is not surprising that uniform agreement has not been achieved among transplantation centers regarding the precise indications for and timing of listing for cardiac transplantation. The basic tenet of organ allocation embraces two axioms that are at times contradictory: equity, or equal access of all patients to donor organs, with priority given to patients closest to death; and utility, an allocation policy for organs that maximizes survival of the patient and graft. As newer therapies, such as cell transplantation and better permanent mechanical devices, become available, the role of heart transplantation will need to be redefined.

1. Ye F, Ying-Bin X, Yu-Guo W, et al. Tacrolimus versus cyclosporine microemulsion for heart transplant recipients: a meta-analysis. *J Heart Lung Transplant.* 2009;28:58-66.
2. Eisen HJ, Kobashigawa J, Keogh A, et al. Three-year results of a randomized, double-blind, controlled trial of mycophenolate mofetil versus azathioprine in cardiac transplant recipients. *J Heart Lung Transplant.* 2005;24:517-525.
3. Keogh A, Richardson M, Ruygrok P, et al. Sirolimus in de novo heart transplant recipients reduces acute rejection and prevents coronary artery disease at 2 years: a randomized clinical trial. *Circulation.* 2004;110:2694-2700.
4. Pham MX, Teuteberg JJ, Kfoury AG, et al. Gene-expression profiling for rejection surveillance after cardiac transplantation. *N Engl J Med.* 2010;362:890-900.
5. Kobashigawa JA, Moriguchi JD, Laks H, et al. Ten-year follow-up of a randomized trial of pravastatin in heart transplant patients. *J Heart Lung Transplant.* 2005;24:1736-1740.

SUGGESTED READINGS

Mancini D, Lietz K. Selection of cardiac transplantation candidates in 2010. *Circulation.* 2010;122:173-183. *Review.*

Singh TP, Almond C, Givertz MM, et al. Improved survival in heart transplant recipients in the United States: racial differences in era effect. *Circ Heart Fail.* 2011;4:153-160. *Early survival has improved across all ethnic groups, but long-term survival has improved in white but not black or Hispanic recipients.*

Zimmer RJ, Lee MS. Transplant coronary artery disease. *JACC Cardiovasc Interv.* 2010;3:367-377. *Review of pathogenesis and treatment.*

IX

RESPIRATORY DISEASES

83

APPROACH TO THE PATIENT WITH RESPIRATORY DISEASE

MONICA KRAFT

Respiratory symptoms, which are among the most common reasons why patients seek medical care, are responsible for about 20% of office visits to a primary care physician. Key common respiratory complaints include cough, wheezing, dyspnea, and hemoptysis.

APPROACH TO THE PATIENT WITH COUGH

Cough is the single most common respiratory complaint for which patients seek care. Referrals of patients with persistently troublesome chronic cough of unknown etiology account for 10 to 38% of outpatient visits to respiratory specialists.

For acute cough, defined as coughing that has been present for less than 8 weeks, a careful medical history and physical examination will usually reveal the diagnosis (Table 83-1). Although most acute coughs are of minor consequence, cough can occasionally be a sign of a potentially life-threatening illness, such as pulmonary embolism (Chapter 98), pneumonia (Chapter 97), or heart failure (Chapter 58).

Up to 98% of all cases of chronic cough, defined as a cough that persists for more than 8 weeks, in immunocompetent adults are caused by eight common conditions: postnasal drip syndrome from a variety of rhinosinus conditions (Chapter 259), asthma (Chapter 87), gastroesophageal reflux disease (GERD) (Chapter 140), chronic bronchitis (Chapter 88), eosinophilic bronchitis, bronchiectasis (Chapter 90), use of angiotensin-converting enzyme (ACE) inhibitors, and postinfectious cough. Postinfectious cough is usually nonproductive and lasts for 3 to 8 weeks following an upper respiratory infection; patients have a normal chest radiograph. Uncommon causes of chronic cough include bronchogenic carcinoma (Chapter 197), chronic interstitial pneumonia (Chapter 92), sarcoidosis (Chapter 95), left ventricular failure (Chapter 58), and aspiration (Chapter 94).

DIAGNOSIS

In chronic cough (Fig. 83-1), the character and timing are not of diagnostic help. A chest radiograph should be obtained in all patients, but other tests should not be ordered in current smokers or patients taking ACE inhibitors until the response to smoking cessation or discontinuation of the drug for at least 4 weeks can be assessed. Sinus radiographs, barium esophagography, methacholine challenge, esophageal pH, and bronchoscopy can be ordered as part of the initial evaluation, depending on the history and physical examination (Table 83-2; see Fig. 83-1). If a test points toward a possible diagnosis, a trial of treatment for that condition is needed to confirm the diagnosis.

TREATMENT   Rx

The specific cause of cough can be diagnosed and treated successfully 84 to 98% of the time, so nonspecific therapy aimed to suppress the cough per se is rarely indicated. There is no strong evidence that nonspecific therapies such as antitussives, mucolytics, decongestants, or antihistamine-decongestant combinations are efficacious for acute cough in the setting of an upper respiratory tract infection.[1] For nonspecific persistent cough, effective treatment of chronic gastroesophageal reflux disease with a proton pump inhibitor (Chapter 140) provides no more than modest benefit, with about one in five patients improving.[2]

APPROACH TO THE PATIENT WITH WHEEZING

Wheeze is a continuous musical sound that lasts longer than 80 to 100 msec, likely generated by flow though critically narrowed collapsible bronchi. Although expiratory wheezing is a common physical finding in asthma (Chapter 87), the many causes of wheezing (Table 83-3) (e.g., chronic obstructive pulmonary disease [COPD; Chapter 88], pulmonary edema [Chapter 58], bronchiolitis [Chapter 92], bronchiectasis [Chapter 90], and

less common entities such as carcinoid [Chapter 240] and parasitic infections) often can be distinguished based on the history, physical examination, and pulmonary function testing (Chapter 85).

DIAGNOSIS

On pulmonary function testing, the shape of inspiratory and expiratory flow-volume loops provides key information about the presence of airway obstruction and whether the obstruction is extrathoracic or intrathoracic (Fig. 83-2). An important cause of extrathoracic obstruction is vocal cord lesions (Chapter 196). Variable intrathoracic obstruction can be caused by tracheomalacia, whereas fixed upper airway obstruction can be caused by a proximal tracheal tumor.

TREATMENT   Rx

Treatment of the specific cause will usually lead to complete or at least partial resolution of wheezing. However, treatment of associated asymptomatic or minimally symptomatic gastroesophageal reflux disease is not beneficial.[3]

APPROACH TO THE PATIENT WITH DYSPNEA

Dyspnea is the sensation of difficult, labored, or unpleasant breathing. The word *unpleasant* is very important to this definition because the labored or difficult breathing encountered by healthy individuals while exercising does not qualify as dyspnea because it is at the level expected for the degree of exertion. The sensation of dyspnea is often poorly or vaguely described by the patient. The physiology of dyspnea remains unclear, but multiple neural pathways can be involved in processes that lead to dyspnea.

In acute dyspnea, or shortness of breath of sudden onset, the history, physical examination, and laboratory testing must first focus on potential life-threatening conditions, including pulmonary embolism (Chapter 98), pulmonary edema (Chapters 58 and 59), acute airway obstruction from anaphylaxis or foreign bodies, pneumothorax (Chapter 99), or pneumonia (Chapter 97). For chronic dyspnea, specific conditions to consider include COPD (Chapter 88), asthma (Chapter 87), interstitial lung disease (Chapter 92), heart failure (Chapter 58), cardiomyopathy (Chapter 60), GERD (Chapter 140), other respiratory diseases, or hyperventilation syndrome.

DIAGNOSIS

A chest radiograph, electrocardiogram, pulmonary function testing, and an exercise test with electrocardiographic (ECG) monitoring and pulse oximetry at rest and during exercise are key tests to assess patients with unexplained dyspnea (Fig. 83-3). For acute dyspnea, B-type natriuretic peptide testing can be extremely helpful in distinguishing heart failure from other causes.[4] The utility of more detailed pulmonary testing with maximal inspiratory and expiratory pressures, flow-volume loops, with or without methacholine challenge, computed tomographic screening of the chest, and echocardiography depends on history and physical examination and the results of these tests. When GERD is a suspected cause of dyspnea, a modified barium esophagogram or 24-hour esophageal pH monitoring, or both, should be considered (Chapter 140). Other more invasive tests such as cardiac catheterization or lung biopsy may be indicated when the results of less invasive tests have not been conclusive.

TREATMENT   Rx

Whenever possible, the final determination of the cause of dyspnea is made by observing which specific therapy eliminates it. Because dyspnea may be simultaneously due to more than one condition, it may be necessary to treat more than one condition.

APPROACH TO THE PATIENT WITH HEMOPTYSIS

Hemoptysis is the expectoration of blood from the lung parenchyma or airways. Hemoptysis may be scant, with just the appearance of streaks of bright red blood in the sputum, or massive, with the expectoration of a large volume of blood. Massive hemoptysis, which is defined as the expectoration of at least 600 mL of blood in 24 to 48 hours, may occur in 3 to 10% of patients with hemoptysis. Dark red clots may also be expectorated when the blood has been present in the lungs for days.

Pseudohemoptysis, which is the expectoration of blood from a source other than the lower respiratory tract, may cause diagnostic confusion when patients cannot clearly describe the source of their bleeding.

Pseudohemoptysis can occur when blood from the oral cavity, nares, pharynx, or tongue clings to the back of the throat and initiates the cough reflex, or when patients who have hematemesis aspirate into the lower respiratory tract. When the oropharynx is colonized with *Serratia marcescens*, a red-pigment-producing aerobic gram-negative rod, the sputum can also be red and be confused with hemoptysis.

Hemoptysis can be caused by a wide variety of disorders. Virtually all causes of hemoptysis (Table 83-4) may result in massive hemoptysis, but massive hemoptysis is most frequently caused by infection (e.g., tuberculosis [Chapter 332], bronchiectasis and lung abscess [Chapter 90], and cancer [Chapter 197]). Infections with aspergilloma (Chapter 347) and in patients with cystic fibrosis (Chapter 89) also are associated with massive hemoptysis. Iatrogenic causes of massive hemoptysis include rupture of a pulmonary

TABLE 83-1 SPECTRUM OF CAUSES AND FREQUENCIES OF COUGH IN IMMUNOCOMPETENT ADULTS

COMMON	LESS COMMON
ACUTE COUGH	
Common cold	Asthma
Acute bacterial sinusitis	Pneumonia
Pertussis	Heart failure
Exacerbations of COPD	Aspiration syndromes
Allergic rhinitis	Pulmonary embolism
Environmental irritant rhinitis	Exacerbation of bronchiectasis
CHRONIC COUGH	
Rhinosinus conditions	Bronchogenic carcinoma
Asthma	Chronic interstitial pneumonia
Gastroesophageal reflux	Sarcoidosis
Chronic bronchitis	Left heart failure
Eosinophilic bronchitis	
Bronchiectasis	
ACE inhibitors	
Postinfection	

ACE = angiotensin converting enzyme; COPD = chronic obstructive pulmonary disease.

TABLE 83-2 TESTING CHARACTERISTICS OF DIAGNOSTIC PROTOCOL FOR EVALUATION OF CHRONIC COUGH

TESTS	DIAGNOSIS	POSITIVE PREDICTIVE VALUE, %	NEGATIVE PREDICTIVE VALUE, %
Sinus radiograph	Sinusitis	57-81	95-100
Methacholine inhalation challenge	Asthma	60-82	100
Modified barium esophagography	GERD, esophageal stricture	38-63	63-93
Esophageal pH*	GERD	89-100	<100
Bronchoscopy	Endobronchial mass/lesion	50-89	100

*24-Hour esophageal pH monitoring.
GERD = gastroesophageal reflux disease.

FIGURE 83-1. Algorithm for the management of chronic cough lasting >8 weeks. CT = computed tomography; Rx = prescription.

TABLE 83-3   DIAGNOSIS OF SELECTED WHEEZING ILLNESSES OTHER THAN ASTHMA

	DISTINGUISHING FEATURES
UPPER AIRWAY DISEASES	
Postnasal drip syndrome	History of postnasal drip, throat clearing, nasal discharge; physical exam shows oropharyngeal secretions or cobblestone appearance to mucosa.
Epiglottis	History of sore throat out of proportion to pharyngitis. Evidence of supraglottitis on endoscopy or lateral neck radiographs.
Vocal cord dysfunction syndrome	Lack of symptomatic response to bronchodilators, presence of stridor plus wheeze in absence of increased P(A-a)o₂; extrathoracic variable obstruction on flow-volume loops; paradoxical inspiratory and/or early expiratory adduction of vocal cords on laryngoscopy during wheezing. This syndrome can masquerade as asthma, be provoked by exercise, and often coexists with asthma.
Retropharyngeal abscess	History of stiff neck, sore throat, fever, trauma to posterior pharynx; swelling noted by lateral neck or CT radiographs.
Laryngotracheal injury due to tracheal cannulation	History of cannulation of trachea by endotracheal or tracheostomy tube; evidence of intrathoracic or extrathoracic variable obstruction on flow-volume loops, neck and chest radiographs, laryngoscopy, or bronchoscopy.
Neoplasms	Bronchogenic carcinoma, adenoma, or carcinoid tumor is suspected when there is hemoptysis, unilateral wheeze, or evidence of lobar collapse on chest radiograph or combinations of these; diagnosis is confirmed by bronchoscopy.
Anaphylaxis	Abrupt onset of wheezing with urticaria, angioedema, nausea, diarrhea, and hypotension, especially following insect bite, in association with other signs of anaphylaxis such as hypotension or hives, or administration of drug or IV contrast, or family history.
LOWER AIRWAY DISEASES	
COPD	History of dyspnea on exertion and productive cough in cigarette smoker. Because productive cough is nonspecific, it should only be ascribed to COPD when other cough-phlegm syndromes have been excluded, forced expiratory time to empty more than 80% of vital capacity >4 sec, and there is decreased breath sound intensity, unforced wheezing during auscultation, and irreversible, expiratory airflow obstruction on spirometry.
Pulmonary edema	History and physical exam consistent with passive congestion of the lungs, ARDS, impaired lung lymphatics; abnormal chest radiograph, echocardiogram, radionuclide ventriculography, cardiac catheterization, or combinations of these.
Aspiration	History of risk for pharyngeal dysfunction or gastroesophageal reflux disease; abnormal modified barium swallow and/or 24-hr esophageal pH monitoring.
Pulmonary embolism	History of risk for thromboembolic disease, positive confirmatory tests.
Bronchiolitis	History of respiratory infection, connective tissue disease, transplantation, ulcerative colitis, development of chronic airway obstruction over months to a few years rather than over many years in a nonsmoker; mixed obstructive and restrictive pattern on PFTs and hyperinflation; may be accompanied by fine nodular infiltrates on chest radiograph.
Cystic fibrosis	Combination of productive cough, digital clubbing, bronchiectasis, progressive COPD with *Pseudomonas* species colonization and infection, obstructive azoospermia, family history, pancreatic insufficiency, and two sweat chloride determinations of >60 mEq/L; some patients are not diagnosed until adulthood, in one instance as late as age 69 yr; when sweat test is occasionally normal, definitive diagnosis may require nasal transepithelial voltage measurements and genotyping.
Carcinoid syndrome	History of episodes of flushing and watery diarrhea; elevated 5-hydroxyindoleactic acid level in 24-hr urine specimen.
Bronchiectasis	History of episodes of productive cough, fever, or recurrent pneumonias; suggestive chest radiographs or typical chest CT findings; ABPA should be considered when bronchiectasis is central.
Lymphangitic carcinomatosis	History of dyspnea or prior malignancy; reticulonodular infiltrates with or without pleural effusions; suggestive high-resolution chest CT scan; confirmed by bronchoscopy with biopsies.
Parasitic infections	Consider in a nonasthmatic patient who has traveled to an endemic area and complains of fatigue, weight loss, fever; peripheral blood eosinophilia; infiltrates on chest radiograph; stools for ova and parasites for nonfilarial causes; blood serologic studies for filarial causes.

ABPA = allergic bronchopulmonary aspergillosis; ARDS = acute respiratory distress syndrome; COPD = chronic obstructive pulmonary disease; CT = computed tomography; IV = intravenous; P(A-a)o₂ = alveolar-arterial oxygen tension gradient; PFTs = pulmonary function tests.

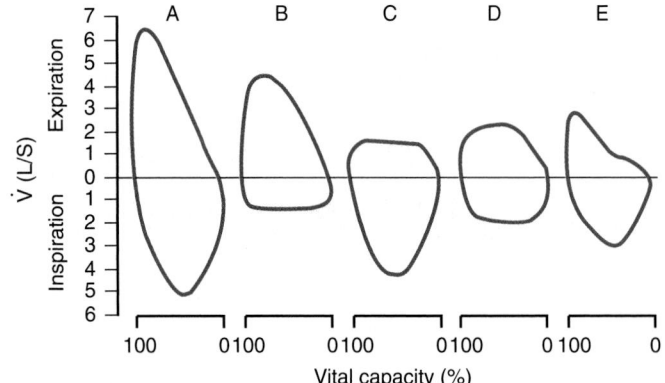

FIGURE 83-2. Schematic flow-volume loop configurations in a spectrum of airway lesions. *A* is normal; *B* is variable extrathoracic upper airway obstruction; *C* is variable intra-thoracic upper airway lesion; *D* is fixed upper airway obstruction; and *E* is small airway obstruction. L/S = liters per second; V̇ = ventilation.

TABLE 83-4   COMMON CAUSES OF MASSIVE HEMOPTYSIS

Cardiovascular
   Arterial bronchial fistula
   Heart failure, especially from mitral stenosis
   Pulmonary arteriovenous fistula
Diffuse intrapulmonary hemorrhage
Diffuse parenchymal disease
Iatrogenic
   Malposition of chest tube
   Pulmonary artery rupture following pulmonary arterial catheterization
   Tracheoarterial fistula
Infections
   Aspergilloma
   Bronchiectasis
   Bronchitis
   Cystic fibrosis
   Lung abscess
   Sporotrichosis
   Tuberculosis
Malignancies
   Bronchogenic carcinoma
   Leukemia
   Metastatic cancer
Trauma

Evaluation of Patients with Subacute or Chronic Dyspnea

FIGURE 83-3. Algorithm outlining the approach to chronic dyspnea. (Modified from Karnani NG, Reisfield GM, Wilson GR. Evaluation of chronic dyspnea. *Am Fam Phys.* 2005;71:1529-1537.)

artery after less than 0.2% of cases of balloon-guided flotation catheterization and tracheal artery fistula as a complication of tracheostomy.

In nonmassive hemoptysis, the etiology is bronchitis in more than one third of cases (Chapter 88), bronchogenic carcinoma (Chapter 197) in one fifth of cases, tuberculosis (Chapter 332) in 7%, pneumonia (Chapter 97) in 5%, and bronchiectasis in 1% (Chapter 90). Using a systematic diagnostic approach (see later), the cause of hemoptysis can be found in 68 to 98% of cases. The remaining 2 to 32% have idiopathic or central hemoptysis, which occurs most commonly in men between the ages of 30 and 50 years. Prolonged follow-up of idiopathic hemoptysis almost always fails to reveal the source of bleeding, even though 10% continue to have occasional episodes of hemoptysis.

DIAGNOSIS

The diagnostic evaluation for hemoptysis begins with a detailed medical history and a complete physical examination. Information on the amount of bleeding should be obtained, as well as details about the frequency, timing, and duration of hemoptysis. For example, repeated episodes of hemoptysis occurring over a period of months to years suggest a bronchial adenoma or bronchiectasis as the cause, whereas small amounts of hemoptysis occurring every day for weeks are more likely to be caused by bronchogenic carcinoma. A travel history can suggest coccidioidomycosis (Chapter 341) and histoplasmosis (Chapter 340) in the United States, paragonimiasis and ascariasis (Chapter 366) in the Far East, and schistosomiasis (Chapter 363) in South America. Orthopnea and paroxysmal nocturnal dyspnea suggest heart failure (Chapter 58), especially from mitral stenosis (Chapter 75). In patients who have occupational exposure to trimellitic anhydride, which occurs when heated metal surfaces are sprayed with a corrosion-resistant epoxy resin, hemoptysis can be part of the postexposure syndrome. In a patient with the triad of upper airway disease, lower airway disease, and renal disease, Wegener's granulomatosis (Chapter 278) should be suspected. Pulmonary

hemorrhage may also be a presenting manifestation of systemic lupus erythematosus (Chapter 274). Goodpasture's syndrome, which typically occurs in young men, is also associated with renal disease (Chapter 123). Diffuse alveolar hemorrhage occurs in 20% of cases during autologous bone marrow transplantation (Chapter 181) and should be suspected in patients who have undergone recent bone marrow transplantation (Chapter 181) when they present with cough, dyspnea, hypoxemia, and diffuse pulmonary infiltrates.

On physical examination, inspection of the skin and mucous membranes may show telangiectasias suggesting heredity hemorrhagic telangiectasia (Chapter 176) or ecchymoses and petechiae, suggesting a hematologic abnormality (Chapter 175). Pulsations transmitted to a tracheostomy cannula should heighten suspicion of a tracheal artery fistula. Inspection of the thorax should show evidence of recent or old chest trauma, and unilateral wheeze or rales may herald localized disease such as a bronchial adenoma or carcinoma. Although pulmonary embolism (Chapter 98) cannot be definitively diagnosed on physical examination, tachypnea, phlebitis, and pleural friction rub suggest this disorder. If rales are heard on the chest examination, heart failure as well as other diseases causing diffuse pulmonary hemorrhage (see earlier) or idiopathic pulmonary hemosiderosis (Chapter 92) should be considered. Careful cardiovascular examination may help diagnose mitral stenosis (Chapter 75), pulmonary artery fistulas, or pulmonary hypertension (Chapter 68).

Routine laboratory studies should include a complete blood count, urinalysis, and coagulation studies. The complete blood count may suggest an infection, hematologic disorder, or chronic blood loss. Urinalysis may reveal hematuria and suggest the presence of a systemic disease (e.g., Wegener's granulomatosis, Goodpasture's syndrome, systemic lupus erythematosus) associated with renal disease. Coagulation studies may uncover a hematologic disorder that is primarily responsible for hemoptysis or that contributes to excessive bleeding from another disease. The ECG may help suggest the presence of a cardiovascular disorder. Although as many as 30% of patients

4. Lam LL, Cameron PA, Schneider HG, et al. Meta-analysis: effect of B-type natriuretic peptide testing on clinical outcomes in patients with acute dyspnea in the emergency setting. *Ann Intern Med.* 2010;153:728-735.

TABLE 83-5 EXAMPLES OF SPECIAL EVALUATIONS FOR HEMOPTYSIS ACCORDING TO CATEGORY OF DISEASE*

TRACHEOBRONCHIAL DISORDERS

Expectorated sputum for TB, parasites, fungi, and cytology
Bronchoscopy (if not done)
Bronchography
High-resolution chest CT scan

LOCALIZED PARENCHYMAL DISEASES

Expectorated sputum for TB, parasites, fungi, and cytology
Chest CT scan
Lung biopsy with special stains

DIFFUSE PARENCHYMAL DISEASES

Expectorated sputum for cytology
Blood for BUN, creatinine, ANA, RF, complement, cryoglobulins, ANCA, anti-GBM antibody
Lung or kidney biopsy with special stains

CARDIOVASCULAR DISORDERS

Echocardiogram
Arterial blood gas on 21% and 100% oxygen
Ventilation-perfusion scans
Pulmonary arteriogram
Aortogram, contrast-enhanced CT scan

HEMATOLOGIC DISORDERS

Coagulation studies
Bone marrow

*This table is not meant to be all inclusive.
ANA = antinuclear antibody; ANCA = antineutrophil cytoplasmic antibody; BUN = blood urea nitrogen; CT = computed tomography; GBM = glomerular basement membrane; RF = rheumatoid factor; TB = tuberculosis.

---

with hemoptysis have a normal chest radiograph, routine chest radiographs may be diagnostically valuable.

Bronchoscopy can localize the bleeding site in up to 93% of patients by fiberoptic bronchoscopy and in up to 86% with rigid bronchoscopy. It may establish sites of bleeding different from those suggested by the chest radiograph. The best results are obtained when bronchoscopy is performed during or within 24 hours of active bleeding, and rates of diagnosis fall to about 50% by 48 hours after bleeding. When there is no active bleeding, bronchoscopy with bronchoalveolar lavage can be helpful in patients thought to have diffuse intrapulmonary hemorrhage. Typical findings include bright red or blood-tinged lavage fluid from multiple lobes in both lungs or a substantial number of hemosiderin-laden macrophages (i.e., at least 20% of the total number of alveolar macrophages).

Depending on the results of the initial evaluation and the likely categories of hemoptysis, additional diagnostic tests can be helpful (Table 83-5). Bronchoscopy may not be needed in patients who have stable chronic bronchitis (Chapter 88) with one episode of blood streaking or who have acute tracheobronchitis (Chapter 88). Bronchoscopy may also not be needed with obvious cardiovascular causes of hemoptysis, such as heart failure and pulmonary embolism.

TREATMENT Rx

Treatment is targeted toward the cause of hemoptysis. Bronchoscopic approaches (Chapter 101) are increasingly used for endobronchial lesions.

1. Smith SM. Over-the-counter medications for acute cough in children and adults in ambulatory settings. *Cochrane Database Syst Rev.* 2008;1:CD001831.
2. Chang AB, Lasserson TJ, Kiljander TO, et al. Systematic review and meta-analysis of randomised controlled trials of gastro-oesophageal reflux interventions for chronic cough associated with gastro-oesophageal reflux. *BMJ.* 2006;332:11-17.
3. Mastronarde JG, Anthonisen NR, Castro M, et al, for the American Lung Association Asthma Clinical Research Centers. Efficacy of esomeprazole for treatment of poorly controlled asthma. *N Engl J Med.* 2009;360:1487-1499.

SUGGESTED READINGS

Benbassat J, Baumal RV. Should teaching of the respiratory physical examination be restricted only to signs with proven reliability and validity? *J Gen Intern Med.* 2010;25:865-872. *Review of value of the full range of respiratory physical findings.*
Burki NK, Lee LY. Mechanisms of dyspnea. *Chest.* 2010;138:1196-1201. *Review.*
Pavord ID, Chung KF. Management of chronic cough. *Lancet.* 2008;371:1375-1384. *Useful review.*
Sakr L, Dutau H. Massive hemoptysis: an update on the role of bronchoscopy in diagnosis and management. *Respiration.* 2010;80:38-58. *Review.*

IMAGING IN PULMONARY DISEASE

PAUL STARK

IMAGING OF THE LUNGS, MEDIASTINUM, AND CHEST WALL

EPIDEMIOLOGY

Worldwide, chest radiography is the most commonly performed imaging procedure; more than 75 million chest radiographs are performed every year in the United States alone. Chest radiographs provide useful information about the patient's anatomy and disease at a minimal monetary cost and with radiation exposure that most experts agree is negligible. Although many novel imaging techniques are available, the plain chest radiograph remains invaluable in the initial assessment of disorders of the lung, pleura, mediastinum, and chest wall.

Imaging Techniques

Chest radiographs, although classically obtained with cassettes and x-ray film, are now commonly acquired by digital imaging with electronic display at workstations and distribution of data through networks. Regardless of the image processing approach used, the standard chest radiograph is performed at 2 m from the x-ray tube focal spot to the image detector, in frontal and lateral projections. If possible, the radiographs should be obtained with the patient inhaling to total lung capacity. These images provide views of the lungs, mediastinum, and chest wall simultaneously.

Portable Radiography

Although bedside or portable radiography accounts for a large number of chest radiographs, the images obtained are generally of lower technical quality, cost more, and are more difficult to interpret. Lung volumes are low, thereby leading to crowding of vascular structures, and the low kilovoltage technique required for the mobile equipment yields radiographs with over-exposed lungs and an underpenetrated mediastinum. The anteroposterior projection and the slightly lordotic angulation of the x-ray beam combine to distort the basal lung structures and magnify the cardiac silhouette. Recumbent studies also make recognition of pleural effusions or pneumothoraces more difficult.

Computed Tomography

Computed tomography (CT) has multiple advantages over conventional radiography. It displays cross-sectional anatomy free of superimposition, with a ten-fold higher contrast resolution. Multislice CT scanners acquire a continuous, volumetric, isotropic data set with possibilities for high-quality two-dimensional or three-dimensional reformatting (volume rendering) in any plane. High-resolution CT of the lung parenchyma is an important application; narrow collimation of the beam combined with an edge-enhancing high spatial frequency algorithm results in exquisite detail of normal and abnormal lungs, and correlation with pathologic anatomy is high.

Magnetic Resonance Imaging

Magnetic resonance imaging (MRI) depends on the magnetic properties of hydrogen atoms. Magnetic coils and radio frequency coils lead to induction,

FIGURE 84-1. **A,** Patient with diffuse alveolar damage. Chest radiograph shows diffuse homogeneous opacification of both lungs with clearly visible air bronchograms. **B,** Patient with acute varicella pneumonia. Chest radiograph demonstrates multiple "acinar" nodules with tendency for confluence, yielding multifocal patchy parenchymal opacification.

excitation, and eventual readout of magnetized protons. The molecular environment of hydrogen atoms will affect the rate at which they release energy; this energy yields a spatial distribution of signals that is converted into an image by computer algorithms, similar to CT. Because of its soft tissue specificity, MRI has applications in the assessment of chest wall invasion, mediastinal infiltration, and diaphragmatic involvement by lung cancer or malignant mesothelioma.

Positron Emission Tomography

Fluorodeoxyglucose positron emission tomography (FDG-PET) uses labeled fluorodeoxyglucose to image the glycolytic pathway of tumor cells or other metabolically active tissues with affinity for glucose. This technique has proved helpful in studying intrathoracic tumors and has facilitated the work-up of solitary pulmonary nodules. Integrated PET-CT scans have improved the diagnosis and staging of intrathoracic tumors.**1**

Ultrasonography

Outside the heart, ultrasonography plays only a limited role in thoracic imaging. Its primary use is to localize pleural effusions and to guide their drainage.

Evaluation of Chest Images

Images of the chest are best evaluated by examining regions of the lung for specific findings and relating these findings to known diagnostic groups. A number of critical radiographic features should be considered, with an appreciation for the known causes of these changes.

Diffuse Lung Disease

Diffuse lung disease is an overall term for a number of related abnormal parenchymal radiographic patterns. Although radiologists have attempted to separate alveolar from interstitial lung disease radiographically, this distinction is no longer recommended because the correlation between the radiographic localization to a compartment and the actual histopathologic findings is relatively poor. For example, nodular patterns can be produced by either interstitial or alveolar disease. Conversely, so-called alveolar disease processes can induce an interstitial reaction. Ground-glass opacities can be induced by either alveolar or interstitial disease. Air bronchograms, the presumed paradigm of air space disease, can be identified in a small percentage of patients with predominantly interstitial lung disease, such as sarcoidosis, pulmonary lymphoma, and pulmonary calcinosis.

Because of such limitations, a graphically descriptive approach that combines analysis of predominant opacities, assessment of lung expansion, and distribution and profusion of disease yields a differential diagnosis. The term *infiltrate* should be avoided; instead, pulmonary opacities are classified as large (i.e., >1 cm in largest dimension) or small (i.e., <1 cm in diameter).

TABLE 84-1 CLASSIFICATION OF LARGE PULMONARY OPACITIES

Diffuse homogeneous
Multifocal patchy
Lobar without atelectasis
Lobar with atelectasis
Perihilar
Peripheral

Large Opacities

Large opacities (Table 84-1) are characterized according to their distribution. Diffuse homogeneous opacities are typical for diffuse alveolar damage (Fig. 84-1A), increased permeability (noncardiogenic) pulmonary edema, diffuse viral pneumonia, or *Pneumocystis jirovecii* pneumonia. Multifocal patchy opacities (see Fig. 84-1B) are found in multifocal bronchopneumonia, recurrent aspiration, or vasculitis. Lobar opacities without atelectasis are typically seen in lobar pneumonia. Lobar opacities with atelectasis often result from obstruction of a lobar bronchus by foreign bodies, tumors, or mucous plugs. Perihilar opacities are seen in hydrostatic pulmonary edema due to left-sided heart failure (Fig. 84-2), renal failure, volume overload, or pulmonary hemorrhage.

Small Opacities

In contrast to the large pulmonary opacities, a number of radiographic patterns characterize small pulmonary opacities in diffuse lung disease. It is helpful to differentiate small nodular, linear, reticular, or combined patterns (Table 84-2). Micronodular opacities, which include nodules 1 mm and smaller in diameter, can result from talc granulomatosis in intravenous drug abusers (Chapter 33), alveolar microlithiasis, rare cases of silicosis, talcosis, coal workers' pneumoconiosis (Chapter 93), and beryllium-induced lung diseases (Chapter 93) as well as from occasional cases of sarcoidosis (Chapter 95) or hemosiderosis. The nodular pattern includes nodules up to 1 cm in diameter. Frequent causes include infections or inflammatory granulomas such as miliary tuberculosis (Chapter 332), sarcoidosis (Chapter 95), fungal diseases, extrinsic allergic alveolitis, and Langerhans cell histiocytosis (Chapter 92).

Linear Patterns

Linear patterns, also called Kerley's lines, are mostly a reflection of thickened interlobular septa. Kerley's A lines, which radiate 2 to 4 cm from the hilum toward the pulmonary periphery and particularly toward the upper lobes (Fig. 84-3), reflect thickening of the axial interstitial compartment and can be a feature of left ventricular failure or allergic reactions. Kerley's B lines,

FIGURE 84-2. Patient with hydrostatic pulmonary edema due to left-sided heart failure. Chest frontal radiograph demonstrates classic "batwing" distribution of pulmonary edema.

FIGURE 84-4. Diffuse reticular lung disease. Chest radiograph in a 94-year-old patient with diffuse reticular opacities due to idiopathic pulmonary fibrosis with honeycombing and traction bronchiectases. The lung volumes are typically reduced by a decreased pulmonary compliance.

Reticular Patterns

Reticular patterns are small polygonal, irregular, or curvilinear opacities on chest radiographs (Fig. 84-4). The differential diagnosis varies according to the timeline of the pathologic change. Acute onset of a reticular pattern can occur in interstitial edema (e.g., due to left-sided heart failure), atypical pneumonitides (e.g., viral or mycoplasmal pneumonia), early exudative changes in a connective tissue disorder (e.g., systemic lupus erythematosus; Chapter 274), and acute allergic reactions (e.g., transfusion reactions [Chapter 180] or reactions to *Hymenoptera* stings). The common chronic processes resulting in a reticular pattern are idiopathic interstitial pneumonias (Chapter 92), connective tissue diseases (particularly scleroderma and rheumatoid lung), asbestosis (Chapter 93), radiation fibrosis (Chapter 92), end-stage hypersensitivity pneumonia (Chapters 92 and 93), drug reactions, lymphangitic spread of cancer, end-stage granulomatous infection, lymphoma in its bronchovascular form, Kaposi's sarcoma in its bronchovascular manifestation, and sarcoidosis.

Honeycombing

Honeycombing, which is an indication of end-stage interstitial lung disease (Chapter 92), reflects a restructuring of pulmonary anatomy accompanied by bronchiolectasis. Honeycombs form a multilayer of small subpleural spaces between 3 and 10 mm in diameter. They can be distinguished from paraseptal emphysema by their thicker wall and multiple layers.

Alveolar Pattern

An alveolar (Chapter 91) or air space pattern is characterized by acinar nodules, 0.6 to 1 cm in diameter. These nodules encompass more than the acinus, in the strict anatomic sense, with surrounding peribronchiolar lung tissue. Other patterns include ground-glass opacities (a reflection of incomplete alveolar filling), coalescent large opacities, consolidation involving whole lobes or segments, opacification in a bronchocentric distribution, air bronchograms, and air alveolograms. These radiographic features are helpful in placing a disease into a particular radiologic category, but the radiographic pattern called *alveolar* does not simply correspond to exclusive histologic alveolar filling because the interstitial compartment is involved as well in most cases. A more accurate description is parenchymal rather than alveolar opacification or consolidation.

FIGURE 84-3. Patient with known transfusion reaction. Chest radiograph displays ground-glass opacification of both lungs and bilateral Kerley's A lines, presenting as long linear structures extending from the hilar regions into the pulmonary periphery.

Bronchial Patterns

Bronchial patterns, as best depicted by diffuse bronchiectasis (Chapter 90), are seen on conventional radiographs as linear, tubular, or cystic lucencies and opacities that follow the expected path of bronchi, so-called tramlines because they resemble tram tracks. Mucoid impaction, as seen in patients with asthma, allergic bronchopulmonary aspergillosis, or plastic bronchitis, leads to opacities described as toothpaste, cluster of grapes, or finger-in-glove. The "dirty lung" pattern seen in smokers with chronic bronchitis (Chapter 88) results from bronchial wall thickening, peribronchial fibrosis, respiratory bronchiolitis, and pulmonary arterial hypertension.

TABLE 84-2   PATTERNS OF SMALL PULMONARY OPACITIES

Micronodular
Acinar
Linear
Reticular
Bronchial
Arterial
Destructive

which reflect thickening of the subpleural interstitial compartment, typically are about 1 cm in length and 1 mm in thickness and usually found in the periphery of the lower lobes, abutting the pleura. The B lines are characteristic of subacute and chronic left ventricular failure (Chapter 58), mitral valve disease (Chapter 75), lymphangitic carcinomatosis, viral pneumonia, and pulmonary fibrosis (Chapter 92). Kerley's C lines, which are rarely diagnosed by radiologists, result from thickening of the lung parenchymal interstitium and form a reticular pattern on chest radiographs.

FIGURE 84-5. Patient with left ventricular failure. Chest frontal radiograph shows cephalization of pulmonary blood flow.

FIGURE 84-7. Patient with **severe emphysema.** Chest radiograph shows hyperexpansion of both lungs with bullous changes at the right lung base and leftward mediastinal shift.

FIGURE 84-6. Patient with **primary pulmonary arterial hypertension.** Chest frontal radiograph shows centralization of flow with pulmonary artery aneurysms and peripheral pulmonary oligemia.

TABLE 84-3	CONDITIONS ASSOCIATED WITH VARIOUS LUNG VOLUMES IN PATIENTS WITH AN UNDERLYING DIFFUSE LUNG DISEASE PATTERN

LARGE LUNG VOLUMES

Emphysema
Chronic asthma
Diffuse bronchiolitis obliterans
Highly trained athletes
Lymphangioleiomyomatosis

SMALL LUNG VOLUMES

End-stage lung fibrosis
Bilateral diaphragmatic paralysis
Massive ascites

NORMAL LUNG VOLUMES

Sarcoidosis
Langerhans cell histiocytosis
Neurofibromatosis
Emphysema with pulmonary fibrosis

Vascular Patterns

Arterial patterns reflect changes in pulmonary perfusion. The term *caudalization* reflects the normal blood flow distribution pattern in an upright person in which the basilar pulmonary vessels are two to three times wider than the upper lobe vasculature. *Cephalization,* in which the ratios of diameters of vessels are reversed, is frequently seen in recumbent persons, in whom it may be considered normal; however, when it is present in individuals imaged in the upright position, it indicates left ventricular failure, mitral valve disease, or basilar emphysema (Fig. 84-5). Equalization, or balanced flow with well-demonstrated vessels to upper and lower lung zones, is found in hyperkinetic circulation due to anemia, obesity, pregnancy, Graves' disease, or left-to-right shunts. Equalization or balanced flow with oligemia can be seen in hypovolemia, diffuse emphysema, or right-to-left shunts. Centralization reflects dilation of central pulmonary vessels, with accompanying normal or diminished peripheral circulation. Typically, it is seen in pulmonary arterial hypertension (Fig. 84-6). Lateralization of flow, favoring one lung over the other, also called *asymmetrical perfusion,* is visible with unilateral emphysema, unilateral bronchiolitis obliterans (Swyer-James-McLeod syndrome), or unilateral obstruction of the pulmonary artery. Locally enlarged vessels occur in patchy emphysema, multiple pulmonary emboli, arteriovenous malformations, and

nonuniform bronchiolitis obliterans. This pattern produces a mosaic perfusion on high-resolution CT scanning.

Lung Volume

Conventional radiographs and CT scans are taken during a breath hold at full inspiration. Low lung volumes are inferred by the high position of the diaphragm and the crowding of basal vascular structures (Table 84-3). Lung volumes larger than expected are commonly found in patients with diffuse emphysema (Fig. 84-7) (Chapter 88), chronic asthma (Chapter 87), or diffuse bronchiolitis and in highly trained athletes. With a few rare exceptions, chronic diffuse infiltrative lung diseases (Chapter 92) lead to loss of volume.

Anatomic Distribution

The anatomic distribution of disease can significantly facilitate the approach to diagnosis (Table 84-4 and Fig. 84-8). Upper-zone lung disease predominates in tuberculosis, fungal disease, sarcoidosis, pneumoconiosis (except asbestosis), Langerhans cell histiocytosis, ankylosing spondylitis, cystic fibrosis, cystic *P. jirovecii* pneumonia, radiation pneumonitis, and end-stage hypersensitivity pneumonia. Basal lung disease is preferentially found in bronchiectases, aspiration, desquamative interstitial pneumonia, nonspecific interstitial pneumonia, usual interstitial pneumonia, drug reactions, asbestosis, scleroderma, and rheumatoid arthritis. However, any diffuse lung

FIGURE 84-8. **A,** Basilar pulmonary disease. Chest radiograph in a 48-year-old patient with known scleroderma. Bibasilar fine reticular opacities and parenchymal bands are visible in both lower lobes. **B,** Apical lung disease. Chest radiograph in a 42-year-old patient with ankylosing spondylitis. Severe architectural distortion with cicatrizing atelectasis of both upper lobes, retraction of both pulmonary arteries cephalad, and bilateral bulla formation containing fungus balls are evident.

TABLE 84-4	CONDITIONS ASSOCIATED WITH DISEASE DISTRIBUTION PATTERNS

UPPER ZONE LUNG DISEASE

Tuberculosis
Fungal disease
Sarcoidosis
Pneumoconioses
Langerhans cell histiocytosis
Cystic fibrosis
End-stage hypersensitivity pneumonitis
Ankylosing spondylitis
Radiation pneumonitis

BASILAR LUNG DISEASE

Bronchiectasis
Aspiration
Drug reactions
Interstitial pulmonary fibrosis, nonspecific interstitial pneumonitis, desquamative interstitial pneumonitis, cryptogenic organizing pneumonia, bronchiolitis obliterans with organizing pneumonia
Asbestosis
Scleroderma

FIGURE 84-9. Multifocal pulmonary opacities. Chest radiograph in a 70-year-old patient with known carcinoma of the thyroid gland widening the superior mediastinum and displacing the cervical trachea to the right. Bilateral large and small pulmonary nodules and masses due to metastatic tumor are present.

process will eventually progress to involve both lungs irrespective of zonal boundaries.

Lymph Nodes

Enlarged lymph nodes that are visible on chest CT scans and, when larger, on chest radiographs can provide diagnostic information (Table 84-5). The following entities can be associated with diffuse lung disease and concurrent enlarged lymph nodes: sarcoidosis (Chapter 95); lymphoma; fungal disease; tuberculosis (Chapter 332); pneumoconioses (Chapter 93), particularly silicosis and beryllium-associated lung disease; lung cancer; and metastatic malignant disease other than lung cancer.

Pulmonary Nodules

Solitary pulmonary nodules are covered in Chapter 197. Most patients with multiple pulmonary nodules larger than 1 cm in diameter have metastatic disease from primary cancers either within or outside the lung (Fig. 84-9). These lesions have a predilection for subpleural lung regions, including the interlobar fissures. In patients with human immunodeficiency virus infection, Kaposi's sarcoma and lymphoma can induce the formation of such nodules. Infectious processes that present with multiple nodules include multiple abscesses from recurrent aspiration (Chapter 94) or septic emboli (Chapter 76); tuberculous and nontuberculous mycobacterial granulomas (Chapters 332 and 333); fungal processes, including histoplasmosis (Chapter 340), coccidioidomycosis (Chapter 341), and cryptococcosis (Chapter 344); and infection with flukes, such as *Paragonimus westermani*

TABLE 84-5	CONDITIONS ASSOCIATED WITH HILAR AND MEDIASTINAL LYMPH NODE ENLARGEMENT

Sarcoidosis
Lymphoma
Fungal disease
Tuberculosis
Metastatic cancer
Silicosis, coal worker's pneumoconiosis, beryllium lung

(Chapter 364). Noninfectious inflammatory conditions that can present with multiple pulmonary nodules include Wegener's granulomatosis (Chapter 278), rheumatoid nodules (Chapter 272), sarcoidosis (Chapter 95), and amyloidosis (Chapter 194).

Pleural Disease

Pleural diseases are covered in Chapter 99. Abnormalities of the pleural space easily can be displayed by conventional radiographic methods supplemented by CT scanning. The volume of pleural effusions can be reliably estimated on standard posteroanterior films: 75 mL obscures the posterior costophrenic sulcus, 150 mL obscures the lateral costophrenic sulcus, 200 mL produces a

FIGURE 84-10. Patient with known prior occupational asbestos exposure. Chest radiograph shows extensive bilateral calcified plaques seen en face, in profile, and along the diaphragmatic contour.

FIGURE 84-11. Patient with spontaneous tension hydropneumothorax. Chest radiograph shows complete atelectasis of the left lung with a large pneumothorax and a left basilar gas-liquid level. The patient had primary tuberculosis.

rind of 1 cm in thickness on decubitus films, 500 mL obscures the diaphragm and is visible on supine radiographs, and 1000-mL effusions reach the level of the fourth anterior rib on upright chest radiographs. An effusion of 200 mL or more can be sampled by thoracentesis. The smallest amount visible on decubitus radiographs is 10 mL. With care, as little as 175 mL of effusion can be detected on supine images. Free layering effusions produce a veil of opacity or filter effect superimposed on the aerated lung; pulmonary vessels are clearly visible through the added opacity generated by the effusion, and air bronchograms are absent.

Subpulmonic Effusions

Subpulmonic effusions elevate the lung base, mimicking a high-riding hemidiaphragm. The highest curvature point of the pseudodiaphragm is shifted laterally. Large effusions can lead to diaphragmatic inversion. Separation of the lung base from the gas-containing stomach is indicative of a subpulmonic effusion, particularly when the stomach gas bubble is displaced inferomedially. Loculated pleural effusions suggest the presence of pleural adhesions. Such encapsulated collections have obtuse angles of interface with the chest wall and have a sharply defined border with the adjacent lung.

Pleural Plaques

Pleural plaques result from parietal pleural accumulation of hyalinized collagen fibers (Fig. 84-10); their presence suggests asbestos exposure (Chapter 93). Plaques preferentially involve the parietal pleura adjacent to ribs six through nine and the diaphragm. They are less pronounced in the intercostal spaces and spare the costophrenic sulci as well as the apices. Calcifications are visible on chest radiographs in 20% and on CT scans in 50% of individuals with plaques. Imaged in profile, pleural plaques produce focal areas of apparent pleural thickening. Over the diaphragm, they appear as curvilinear calcifications or scalloping. Pleural plaques viewed en face can simulate lung disease. Their appearance has been likened to holly leaves, sunburst patterns, "geographic" patterns, or stippled or irregular structures. Rare visceral pleural plaques that occur in interlobar fissures can mimic pulmonary nodules.

Diffuse Pleural Thickening

Diffuse pleural thickening is a response observed after exposure to any of a number of stimuli including infection, inflammation, trauma, tumor, thromboembolism, radiation, and asbestos. Severe involvement results in formation of a generalized pleural peel with smooth margins, usually less than 2 cm in thickness. Radiologically diffuse pleural thickening is characterized by a smooth, noninterrupted pleural opacity involving at least one fourth of the chest wall circumference, obliterating the costophrenic sulci and encompassing also the apices. The CT criteria for diffuse pleural thickening include a thickness of at least 3 mm.

Malignant Disease

Malignant tumors of the pleura are more common than benign ones, and metastatic disease is more frequent than primary pleural mesothelioma. Primary tumors originate from pleural membranes. Pleural invasion by lung cancer, subpleural plaques in lymphoma, hematogenous dissemination to the pleura, and direct pleural seeding are other mechanisms of pleural involvement by tumor. Benign pleural tumors include lipomas, fibrous tumors, and neurogenic tumors. Lipomas are most common; their diagnosis is facilitated by CT scanning. Fibrous tumors of the pleura originate from pluripotent mesenchymal cells found in the visceral pleura or, less commonly, in the parietal pleura. They can induce paraneoplastic syndromes such as hypertrophic osteoarthropathy (Chapter 187) or hypoglycemia and only rarely invade or metastasize. In nearly half of these patients, the tumor can be on a pedicle and be mobile as a patient changes position.

Pneumothorax

Pneumothorax means gas in the pleural space (Chapter 99). The most important radiologic feature of a pneumothorax is a visceral pleural line or edge that is convex or straight toward the chest wall and produces a lucent separation of the visceral and parietal pleura (Fig. 84-11). In most cases, no pulmonary vascular structures are visible beyond the visceral pleura. On upright chest radiographs, gas is primarily found in the apicolateral pleural space. Expiratory chest radiographs are not necessary for the detection of small pneumothoraces because all pneumothoraces are visible on inspiratory films. On supine chest radiographs, pleural gas accumulates in a subpulmonic location; it outlines the costophrenic sulcus, forming the deep sulcus sign. A tension pneumothorax leads to a marked shift of the mediastinum to the contralateral side and to flattening or inversion of the ipsilateral hemidiaphragm.

Imaging of the Mediastinum

The mediastinum encompasses midline thoracic structures that are delineated by mediastinal pleura, the diaphragm, the sternum, the spine, and the thoracic inlet. The mediastinum is commonly divided into an anterior compartment, a visceral middle compartment, and a paraspinal, posterior mediastinal compartment (Table 84-6). Each compartment contains specific pathologic entities.

Imaging Techniques

On well-penetrated chest radiographs, the anterior junction line, the posterior-superior junction line, the azygoesophageal stripe, the pleuroesophageal stripe, the paratracheal stripe, and the para-aortic and the paraspinal stripes or lines should be assessed (Fig. 84-12). Mediastinal masses need to be detected and localized first. Their obtuse angles of interface with the mediastinal pleura, as well as extension into both hemithoraces, indicate the mediastinal origin of such lesions.

CT facilitates localization of a mass to a specific mediastinal compartment. When it is known whether the mass is predominantly fat, cystic, soft tissue, or calcified, the differential diagnosis can be limited. MRI of the mediastinum has a role in diagnosis of vertebral disease or neurogenic tumors with extension into the spinal canal. It is as good as CT in diagnosis of aortic aneurysms and dissections (Chapter 78).

Mediastinal Compartments

The anterior mediastinum is actually a potential space that may contain the fatty replaced thymus and small normal lymph nodes. Space-occupying lesions in this compartment typically include thymomas, lymphomas, teratomas and other germ cell tumors, substernal thyroid goiters, lipomas, and other connective tissue tumors as well as hemangiomas or lymphangiomas (Fig. 84-13A).

The middle mediastinum is subdivided into the subcarinal space, paratracheal region, retrotracheal region, aortic-pulmonic window region, and retrocardiac space. Characteristic lesions are enlarged lymph nodes and bronchopulmonary foregut malformations (see Fig. 84-13B).

FIGURE 84-12. Chest radiograph with superimposed mediastinal stripes. *Yellow:* right paratracheal stripe. *Light blue:* right and left paraspinal stripes. *Red:* azygoesophageal stripe. *Brown:* pleuroesophageal stripe. *Purple:* anterior junction line complex. *Pink:* left subclavian artery border. *Light green:* posterior-superior junction line. *Dark green:* para-aortic line.

TABLE 84-6	CLASSIFICATION OF MEDIASTINAL COMPARTMENTS

ANTERIOR MEDIASTINUM

Retrosternal

MIDDLE MEDIASTINUM—VISCERAL COMPARTMENT

Subcarinal space
Paratracheal region
Retrotracheal space
Aortic-pulmonic window
Retrocardiac space

POSTERIOR MEDIASTINUM

Paraspinal region

FIGURE 84-13. A, Patient with anterior mediastinal teratoma. Chest radiograph shows a mediastinal contour abnormality due to projection of the mass into the right hemithorax. Note the obtuse angle of interface formed by the pleura covering the mass with the mediastinum. **B,** Patient with Castleman's giant lymph node hyperplasia. Chest frontal radiograph shows large subcarinal middle mediastinal mass that projects lateral to the right atrium. **C,** Patient with paraspinal ganglioneuroma. Chest radiograph shows right lower paraspinal contour abnormality widening the right paraspinal region and encompassing the height of three thoracic vertebrae.

In the retrotracheal region, aberrant right subclavian arteries, posterior descending goiters, esophageal tumors, diverticula, or thoracic duct cysts can be found. In the aortic-pulmonic window, ductus diverticula, bronchopulmonary foregut malformations, or aortic or pulmonic artery aneurysms can form compartment-specific space-occupying lesions.

The paraspinal region is considered radiologically to belong to the posterior mediastinum. Important masses in that space include neurogenic tumors that originate from the sympathetic chain or from segmental nerve roots (see Fig. 84-13C). Extramedullary hematopoiesis in patients with severe anemia can result in paravertebral masses formed by hypertrophied bone marrow that extrudes from ribs or vertebral bodies. Enlarged lymph nodes due to lymphoma or metastatic disease are occasionally seen in a paraspinal location. Vertebral disease, including bacterial or tuberculous spondylitis, tumors, and post-traumatic hematomas, can widen the paraspinal region and produce contour abnormalities.

1. Fischer B, Lassen U, Mortensen J, et al. Preoperative staging of lung cancer with combined PET-CT. *N Engl J Med.* 2009;361:32-39.

SUGGESTED READINGS

Oba Y, Zaza T. Abandoning daily routine chest radiography in the intensive care unit: meta-analysis. *Radiology.* 2010;255:386-395. *Chest radiography can be ordered selectively without increasing adverse outcomes.*

Petinaux B, Bhat R, Boniface K, et al. Accuracy of radiographic readings in the emergency department. *Am J Emerg Med.* 2011;29:18-25. *Approximately 3% of radiographs are incorrectly read by the emergency physician, with air-space disease and pulmonary nodules most commonly misread on chest radiographs.*

85

RESPIRATORY STRUCTURE AND FUNCTION: MECHANISMS AND TESTING

HERBERT Y. REYNOLDS

The lungs are designed for oxygen uptake and carbon dioxide elimination through the process of ventilation and molecular diffusion. To maintain health, purified air must be presented to the alveolar epithelial surface to aerate pulmonary capillary blood. Ambient air, which contains environmental debris, microbes, and possibly solubilized toxins and is admixed at times with aspirated oropharyngeal secretions, must be cleansed. Inspired ambient air encounters a system of host defenses that usually removes these contaminants mechanically (by sneezing, rhinorrhea, coughing, and mucociliary clearance), through innate (natural) immunity mechanisms, or immunologically through adaptive (acquired) immunity. This nonventilatory function can be missing (primary host defects) or compromised by systemic illness or the side effects of other medical therapy. Because ventilation and nonventilatory function are so intertwined, both are described together; methods for assessment of clinical function then follow.

RESPIRATORY STRUCTURE AND FUNCTION

Respiratory Tract Structure

Although the respiratory tract is a continuum of branching tubes leading to the air exchange-alveolar surface, it functionally has four distinct anatomic segments: naso-oropharynx or upper airways, conducting airways (larynx, trachea, and bronchi that branch to terminal bronchioles), respiratory bronchioles, and alveolar ducts and alveoli. Vascular and neural structures are integral to each segment; lymphatic channels begin at the level of respiratory bronchioles and flow upward or cephalad into the hilar nodes. But much still remains unknown about various cell lineages contributing to development of the lung, the phenotype and function of perhaps half of the approximately 40 resident cells that compose the human respiratory tract, and the roles of neuroendocrine cells and various progenitor cells that can replenish structural cells after injury.

The airways and their accompanying blood supply develop from an evagination of the foregut and primitive esophagus. The conducting airways form

a continuum of approximately 14 generations of branches, which are extended by another 10 or so branches within the acinar airways, finally ending as alveolar sacs. This anatomic structure has been described as a tree with irregular, dichotomously branching tubes. Later developments in the fetus initiate progressive thinning of the mucosal epithelial layer in distal bronchi and then the respiratory bronchioles to a single cell surface, which defines the beginning of the gas exchange unit within the acinar-alveolar structures. Mechanisms to cleanse inspired air are dispersed along the entire tract.

The *naso-oropharynx* includes the upper airways and associated sinuses (Chapter 434). It begins at the nares and lips and extends back through a richly vascular, undulant mucosal covering of the nasal passage, through the glottis, into the extrathoracic trachea. Nasal hairs and turbinates filter out large particles (>10 μm diameter) as inspired air passes over the nasal surface in a turbulent flow pattern. In this process, air is humidified and warmed as it passes through the nose and over the soft palate; it typically is fully conditioned before it reaches the posterior pharynx. Because sinus and posterior nasal secretions can collect in the posterior pharynx, deglutition and respiration are coordinated exquisitely by the epiglottis and laryngeal musculature to direct fluids and food into the esophagus and air into the subglottic trachea. Control is not perfect, however, and microaspiration can occur in normal persons during sleep. Esophageal reflux can cause cough in normal individuals and asthma symptoms in patients with more hyperreactive airways (Chapters 87 and 140). Mucociliary clearance declines with age, explaining in part the more frequent occurrence of respiratory infections in elderly patients.

The *conducting airways* begin with the trachea, a flexible tube held open by cartilaginous, horseshoe-shaped rings with a posterior muscular face that abuts the esophagus. The trachea is about 10 cm in length and contains about 15 rings. At the carina, it divides into two major bronchi, and thereafter multiple smaller bronchial branches diverge through many generations of smaller divisions. In aggregate, however, the branching creates a much greater overall cross-sectional area that not only reduces resistance to airflow but also decelerates the velocity of air molecules as they prepare to enter the acinar ducts and alveolar sacs. Airflow beyond the conducting airways is largely laminar; the slower movement further cleanses the air by allowing the settling out of any 0.5- to 3-μm particulates that still are present and would be impacted at branching points. This action seems especially important in the respiratory bronchioles, which serve as the transition segment between the conducting airways and alveoli, where several adaptations facilitate further removal of particulates or antigens. Throughout the conducting airways (E-Fig. 85-1), the mucosal surface provides a barrier function because of the tight apical junctions between epithelial cells. About half of the epithelial cells are ciliated; a fluid film and mucus cover the beating cilia, creating the mucociliary apparatus. The thickness of the mucosal surface attenuates as the pseudostratified cell layer flattens to become a single cell layer in the terminal bronchioles. Here the less protected surface may become more vulnerable to injury from inhaled toxins and microbes and more susceptible to ravages of chronic inflammation (bronchiolitis).

The airway layer of pseudostratified epithelial cells creates a physical barrier by forming tight apical junctions that control permeability and promote pericellular ion and fluid flux. About half of the epithelial cells have cilia to propel a covering layer of fluid and admixed mucus that can collect airway debris and eliminate it by a process known as *mucociliary clearance*. These epithelial cells have dynamic turnover of several days, with continuous self-renewal from progenitor stem cells, but the normal replication rate may vary at different locations along the airways. If airway injury has destroyed epithelial cells and denuded the surface, regeneration begins quickly from reservoirs of self-renewing stem cells found in niches in the ducts of submucosal glands in the trachea or bronchi and within the surface epithelium of more distal airways.

The *respiratory bronchioles*, which are positioned between the distal conducting airways and the alveolized air exchange surface, functionally separate the upper and lower respiratory tracts. This segment is a bottleneck for airflow and a last surface to capture small particulates and microbial or antigenic debris before the alveolar space; immune responses can be initiated here. The respiratory bronchioles can be the site of airway obstruction, caused by inflammation; a common form is termed *bronchiolitis obliterans* (Chapter 92) and is associated with several lung diseases, such as chronic graft rejection after lung transplantation (Chapter 101) and lung involvement by collagen vascular diseases (Chapter 92). In this transition region of the airway, several changes occur: the single-layer cuboidal epithelial surface further differentiates into alveolar type I cells that cover the alveolar lining surface;

mucus-secreting cells disappear, although goblet cells can develop in cigarette smokers; and another secretory cell type emerges, the Clara cells. Pulmonary brush cells with a tuft of squat microvilli are dense in this area and may be involved with chemosensing or trapping of inhaled particles and pollutants as well as with regulation of fluid and solute absorption. Also, many dendritic macrophage-like cells, which may constitute 1% of the cells, are present to capture antigens. Surface host defenses change from mucociliary clearance to macrophage phagocytes, inflammatory cells (neutrophils or eosinophils), and opsonins. Lymphatic channels form to collect the lymphatic fluid squeezed up from the interalveolar interstitial spaces into lymphatic capillaries that course along pulmonary capillaries and venules in the alveolar walls. The bronchial arterial circulation supplies the conducting airways, whereas the pulmonary arterial to pulmonary capillary circulation encompasses the alveoli and is the locus for diffusion of oxygen into the blood and carbon dioxide from the blood.

The *air exchange* compartment, or the alveolar space, is composed of about 480 million alveoli supported by a fibrous scaffolding and intertwined with a meshwork of pulmonary artery capillaries that permit air-blood contact. Oxygen uptake and carbon dioxide elimination occur across a thin tissue layer of type I epithelial cells and capillary endothelium that in aggregate creates a large surface area of approximately 130 square feet. To increase the likelihood that respiratory function will support a healthy human lifespan despite pollutants, infections, or systemic diseases that affect the lungs, an intricate system of host defenses has evolved. The system specialized for the alveoli is different from the system described in the proximal airways. Although an alveolus is reasonably protected from airborne debris by aerodynamic filtration that occurs in the upper respiratory tract, small particles (<0.5 μm) can remain suspended in air or toxic gases can gain access to the alveoli directly.

Cellular Host Defenses

Respiratory host defenses balance two mechanisms that eliminate or detoxify microbes and other antigenic materials that enter the airways (E-Fig. 85-2). First is an innate or quick response reaction that produces inflammation as an end point (bronchitis or pneumonitis) with subsequent apoptosis of neutrophils and suppression of inflammation to limit the reaction. Second is a more deliberate approach that stimulates lymphocytic pathways, creating a versatile and adaptive response involving specific T-cell activity or production of immunoglobulins (antibodies).

Microbes can be contained in aspirated fluid or carried intravascularly to the parenchyma (septicemia). A microbe entering an alveolus may encounter an antigen-presenting cell or several opsonins in the epithelial lining fluid, including immunoglobulin (Ig) G antibodies (IgG1 and IgG3 subtypes) and nonimmune substances (type II cell-secreted surfactant proteins A and D, fibrinogen, and complement fragments [C3b]) that can promote receptor-mediated uptake or phagocytosis by macrophages. Alveolar T lymphocytes can stimulate the macrophage with cytokines, such as interleukin (IL)-1 and interferon-γ, that enhance its bactericidal activity or, if microbes are too numerous or too virulent, can create an inflammatory response quickly. Chemokines, derived from macrophages or epithelial cells, including IL-8, leukotriene B_4, and tumor necrosis factor, can attract neutrophils and other inflammatory products from adjacent capillaries into the alveolus. If inflammation, or pneumonitis, is successful in eradicating infection, neutrophils undergo apoptosis, the inflammation resolves, and normal lung tissue function is restored. If the inflammatory process is prolonged, a smoldering, chronic inflammatory response can persist and lead to tissue injury that causes fibrosis and scarring, or depending on the antigen-particle or microbe involved, a granulomatous reaction may develop from IL-2 stimulating T_H1 lymphocytes. If this wound-type healing occurs after substantial injury, respiratory function can be lost permanently.

Epithelial cells have about the same repertoire of proinflammatory chemokines as alveolar macrophages, including IL-8, leukotriene B_4, transforming growth factor-β, monocyte chemotactic protein 1, and RANTES. They also can inhibit or downregulate inflammation. This dual capability to help initiate inflammation and then suppress it makes the epithelium crucial for the pathogenesis of diseases such as asthma (Chapter 87), bronchitis, emphysema (Chapter 88), and pulmonary fibrosis (Chapter 92). Chronic inflammatory changes can cause bronchiectasis (Chapter 90) or cell atypia that leads to endobronchial cancer (Chapter 197).

Dendritic cells or surface macrophages process antigens, using Toll-like receptors such as TLR2 and TLR4, and present them to major histocompatibility complex–compatible but naive CD4+ lymphocytes, a process

facilitated with the stimulatory cytokine IL-12. IL-2 produced by CD4+ T cells subsequently can direct Th1 lymphocytes to develop and proliferate. Th1 cells can produce IL-1 and interferon-γ, which can stimulate macrophages for heightened activity (phagocytic uptake) in the inflammatory pathway. Also, IL-2 can induce clonal expansion of CD4+ lymphocytes that contributes to creating granulomas for containment of certain microbes, such as mycobacteria, or particles (silica or beryllium).

● ASSESSMENT OF PULMONARY VENTILATORY FUNCTION

Pulmonary physiologic function can be measured by examining the relationships between expired airflow and volume or time or by using tests that measure exercise capacity or the distance that can be walked in a prespecified amount of time (typically 6 minutes). These functional tests provide measures of physiologic function and may be used to reproduce clinical symptoms, such as breathlessness or dyspnea, and to correlate these symptoms with the degree of physical limitation. These tests are used to measure baseline status, to monitor treatment, and to estimate prognosis.

Pulmonary Function Tests

Lung function tests (Table 85-1) measure a person's ventilatory capacity in comparison with that of normal subjects. By adjusting for sex, height, ethnicity, and age, the values for a given individual can be compared with those from otherwise normal individuals. Basic tests for preliminary assessment and for monitoring disease progression include spirometry, which is a record of exhaled volume versus time during a forced exhalation (with or without determination of the response to an inhaled bronchodilator for possible reversible airflow); diffusion capacity, which measures the transfer of carbon monoxide to indicate how well inspired gases cross the alveolar-interstitial-capillary endothelial interface into blood; and noninvasive pulse oximetry, for oxygen saturation measured at rest or during ambulation. Pulmonary function tests (PFTs) performed after graduated exercise on a treadmill or a timed walking test on a level surface provides a more dynamic assessment of pulmonary function and correlates well with prognosis in patients with chronic pulmonary conditions such as lung fibrosis and chronic obstructive disease. More specialized tests include body plethysmography to determine total lung volumes and airway resistance as well as maximal cardiopulmonary exercise testing to assess cardiac function and oxygen uptake and consumption. The clinical utility of these tests can be appreciated by understanding how they can be applied to representative types of patients (Table 85-2).

Spirometry

A tracing of the relationship between maximal expiratory airflow and time, termed a *spirogram*, is the most common measure of ventilatory lung

---

TABLE 85-1   PULMONARY FUNCTION TESTS

LUNG VOLUME

TLC	Total lung capacity (volume of gas in lungs at the end of maximal inspiration)
FRC	Functional residual capacity (volume of gas in the lungs when elastic inward pull is balanced by outward pull of the chest wall and diaphragm)
ERV	Expiratory reserve volume (volume of gas expired from FRC to maximal expiration)
RV	Residual volume (FRC − ERV, volume of gas left in lungs after maximal exhalation)

EXPIRATORY FLOW

FEV_1	Forced expiratory volume (in 1 second)
FVC	Forced vital capacity
FEV_1%	FEV_1/FVC ratio (expressed as percentage)

DIFFUSING CAPACITY

D_{LCO}	Diffusing capacity for carbon monoxide

ARTERIAL BLOOD GASES

Pa_{O_2}	Arterial oxygen pressure
Pa_{CO_2}	Arterial carbon dioxide pressure
pH	

TABLE 85-2 CLINICAL EXAMPLES OF TESTING IN REPRESENTATIVE TYPES OF PATIENTS WITH COMMON PULMONARY COMPLAINTS

CLINICAL PRESENTATION	PHYSICAL FINDINGS AND CHEST RADIOGRAPH	PULMONARY FUNCTION TESTS	RESULTS OF VENTILATORY FUNCTION (% PREDICTED)	CHARACTERISTIC ABNORMALITIES	DIAGNOSIS	MONITORING OR PREDICTIVE USE OF TESTS
Young adult with episodic attacks of cough, wheezing, and anxiety	Rapid respiratory rate; Wheezing and prolonged expiration; Thorax hyperresonant; Radiograph normal or hyperinflated	Spirometry (but cough and dyspnea may preclude complete results); Oximetry; Arterial blood gas analysis (only if the episode is prolonged or severe)	PEFR > 60%; FEV_1, 45-75%; MMEFR, 30-50%; ABG (while breathing ambient air): PaO_2, 70 mm Hg, $PaCO_2$, 30 mm Hg	Decreased PEFR, FEV_1, MMEFR to grade as mild, moderate, or severe attack; Hypoxemia, hypocapnia, and pH changes on blood gas analysis during an attack	Asthma exacerbation of moderate intensity	Spirometry after bronchodilator treatment or challenge testing; Daily peak flow measurements (keep diary of results); FEV_1 may return to normal range after episode or therapy
Middle aged, male, former smoker	Abdominal obesity (large waist circumference); BP, 140/85 mm Hg; BMI, 32 kg/m²; Hyperglycemia; Dyslipidemia	Spirometry	FEV_1, 80%; FVC, 84%; FEV_1/FVC, 82%	FEV_1 and FVC decreased; restrictive function	Metabolic syndrome with lung restriction from abdominal obesity	Regular spirometry not indicated
Middle aged, moderate smoker (20 cigarettes per day), mild dyspnea, occasional cough and sputum	Examination findings and radiograph are likely to be normal	Baseline spirometry and oximetry; Optional baseline cardiorespiratory exercise test	FEV_1 > 80%; FEV_1/FVC, 70%; D_LCO, 80%	Slight decrease in FEV_1 and perhaps FVC	Normal smoker with occasional episodes of acute bronchitis; Mild COPD	Spirometry with health maintenance visit/yearly; Daily peak flow monitoring; Reduce or stop smoking
Older middle aged, moderate smoker for 30-40 yr, dyspnea (with moderate exertion), morning cough and phlegm, mild weight loss	Respiratory rate is likely to be increased at rest; Thorax hyperinflated; Breath sounds decreased; Scattered wheezes and crackles; Nail-bed cyanosis; Radiograph normal or hyperinflated; no mass lesions evident	Spirometry and oximetry or arterial blood gas analysis; Timed walk test; Cardiopulmonary exercise testing (especially if heart failure is evident)	FEV_1 > 30% but <50%; FEV_1/FVC < 70%; D_LCO, 30%; TLC and RV ~100%; Timed walk test shows less than predicted for age and sex	Decreased FEV_1 (usually about 40% predicted), FVC, and FEV_1/FVC (<0.70); increased residual volume and total lung capacity; D_LCO decreased; Hypoxemia; CO_2 retention perhaps	COPD of moderate severity	Spirometry yearly and after exacerbations on return to baseline; Daily peak flow monitoring; Blood gas analysis yearly (if FEV_1 < 40% predicted); Echocardiogram with signs of CHF; Chest radiograph yearly; Reduce or stop smoking; Observe nutritional status and weight
Elderly patient, prior smoker, with insidious onset of dyspnea (occurs only with exertion for past 2 years) and mild nonproductive cough, without prior, relevant occupational exposures	Gaunt; Respiratory and heart rates increased; Coarse crackles heard at lung bases; Mild clubbing; Radiograph with diffuse infiltrates, decreased lung volume, and cystic areas at bases	Spirometry; D_LCO; Timed walking, with oximetry and arterial blood gas analysis; Cardiopulmonary exercise test advised; Baseline ABGs	TLC, 65%; FVC, 65%; D_LCO, 45%; PaO_2, 70% (RA); Timed walk test shows values about 50% of predicted	Reduced lung volumes (vital capacity, total lung capacity); FEV_1/FVC ratio increased; D_LCO reduced; Hypoxemia, but normal CO_2; Exercise tolerance limited	Pulmonary fibrosis	Spirometry at each visit every 6-12 mo; Oximetry; Timed velocity walk (with oxygen if O_2 < 88% at rest); Echocardiogram with signs of CHF
Patient above, seemingly stable for past 1 yr, and on no therapy, developed worsening dyspnea over 3 wk	As above; Afebrile; Radiograph with more diffuse ground-glass opacities; No clear etiology	Spirometry; D_LCO; ABG	FVC, 52%; D_LCO, 30%; Tests difficult to obtain because of respiratory distress	As above, but tests may be difficult to obtain; Will find more restriction and worsened gas exchange	Acute exacerbation; Pulmonary fibrosis	Occurs in 10% of patients per year with 70% mortality; Resume tests above, pending recovery
Middle-aged female with scleroderma and diffuse skin thickening disease for 3 yr; now exertional dyspnea; Nonsmoker; Taking prednisone 10 mg/day dose	Thickened skin, has Raynaud's, dry cough; No overt cardiac failure; HRCT with ground-glass opacities; No pulmonary artery enlargement	Spirometry; D_LCO; ABG	TLC, 70% predicted; FVC, 68%; FEV_1/FVC, 83%; FRC, 74%; RV, 70%; D_LCO, 47% (RA)	Ventilatory restriction with FVC between 45% and 80%; D_LCO, 40-50%	Scleroderma-related interstitial lung fibrosis, possible mild pulmonary hypertension	Spirometry and D_LCO with health maintenance exams; FVC decline of about 10%/year expected

ABG = arterial blood gases; CHF = congestive heart failure; COPD = chronic obstructive pulmonary disease; D_LCO = diffusing capacity of lung for carbon monoxide; FEV_1 = forced expiratory volume in 1 second; FVC = forced vital capacity; FRC = functional reserve capacity; MMEFR = maximum mid-expiratory flow rate; PEFR = peak expiratory flow rate; RV = residual volume; TLC = total lung capacity.

TABLE 85-3 BRONCHOALVEOLAR LAVAGE CELL AND FLUID FINDINGS

STATUS OR ILLNESS	CELL PROFILE	NONCELLULAR COMPONENTS	OTHER ILLNESSES IN THE DIFFERENTIAL DIAGNOSIS WITH OVERLAPPING FINDINGS
Normal nonsmokers Mean, 1.3×10^5 cells/mL of recovered BAL fluid (range, 0.6-2.1)	Differential cell count (mean %): AM, 85%; lymphocytes, 7-12%; PMN, 1-2%; eosinophils-basophils, <1%; ciliated cells, 1-5%, 1% dendritic cells Lymphocyte subsets: CD4 helper, 50%; CD8 suppressor or cytotoxic, 30%; CD4/CD8 ratio, 1.5; B lymphocytes (plasma cells), 5%	95% as IgA (40% as IgA2), 90% IgA in dimeric form with secretory component, almost no IgM, IgG (IgG1-3/albumin ratios similar to serum), increased IgG4 Low concentrations of cytokines (IL-6, IL-8) Adhesion molecules detectable Histamine detectable Surfactant present	
Healthy moderate smokers Mean, 3.6×10^5 cells/mL of recovered BAL fluid (range, 2.2-4.8)	Three-fold increase of total cells, 95% AM, 3- to 5-fold increased AM, PMNs approximately 3% Lymphocytes 3% in differential cell count	Increased IgG as IgG/albumin ratio with serum, increased IgG3 and IgG4, decreased FSC, less surfactant recovered (lipid component profile same as that of nonsmoker) Decreased A₁AT elastase inhibitory activity Increased ACE (in AM) may be found	

INTERSTITIAL LUNG DISEASES

STATUS OR ILLNESS	CELL PROFILE	NONCELLULAR COMPONENTS	OTHER ILLNESSES IN THE DIFFERENTIAL DIAGNOSIS WITH OVERLAPPING FINDINGS
Sarcoidosis	Lymphocytes, >30% total cells, increased CD4 cells, increased CD4/CD8 ratio AM-lymphocytes (T cells) form spontaneous rosettes PMNs > 3% may indicate deterioration and need for therapy Considerable increase in T lymphocytes as CD4 or T_H1 cells and a raised CD4/CD8 ratio is a common finding A raised neutrophil count may correlate with more severe disease on chest radiograph	Increased IL-2, IL-6, IL-8, IL-10, IL-12, MCP-1, TNF-α, interferon-γ ACE level can be increased Increased adhesion molecule ICAM-1 Increased fibronectin PPARγ deficient in AM MMP-12 and ADAMDECI gene and protein expression increased	Extrathoracic granulomatous diseases (e.g., Crohn's disease), primary biliary cirrhosis, extrinsic allergic alveolitis, idiopathic pulmonary fibrosis, collagen vascular disease
Extrinsic allergic alveolitis (hypersensitivity pneumonitis) Acute and chronic forms	Increased lymphocytes to >40-60% of total cells, often increased CD8 with slight reversal of CD4/CD8 ratio Foamy cytoplasm of AM Increased plasma cells, sometimes increased mast cells or basophils Striking increase of T lymphocytes with most as CD8 cells is usual	Increased IgM and IgG; IgG fraction may have specific precipitating antibody activity against etiologic antigens (thermophilic microbes) Increased IL-4, IL-10, interferon-γ, MIF, MCP	Drug-induced hypersensitivity Fibrotic form of NSIP
Idiopathic pulmonary fibrosis	Increased PMN; approximately 5-15% of cells Increased eosinophils, approximately 3-6% Increased lymphocytes, 15% in some cases A raised percentage of neutrophils and eosinophils is characteristic An increase of lymphocytes and neutrophils could indicate an NSIP pattern in lung biopsy	Increased IgG, increased monomeric IgA Increased IL-4, IL-6, IL-8, IL-13, TGF-β, MIF, galactin-1, CC Chemokines (CCL 2, CCL 17, CCL 22) Increased collagenase and histamine levels Increased fibronectin, decreased interferon-γ, metalloproteinases MMP7, MMP1, and their genes overexpressed	Usually diagnosis of exclusion (occupational, environmental) Increased lymphocytes may indicate EAA (HP) or NSIP
Bronchiolitis obliterans after lung transplantation	Increased PMNs that persist, CD4 T_H17 cells Persistence of neutrophils >3% in serial BAL cell count samples is a clue	Increased IL-1β, IL-6, IL-8, TNF-α, IL-17, fibronectin, collagenase	Autoimmune response to type V collagen in donor lung
Scleroderma (systemic sclerosis)	Increased PMNs to approximately 3-10% of cells Increased eosinophils to approximately 3% of cells Lymphocytes about 10%, but CD8 cells may be increased Myofibroblasts can be recovered BAL cell eosinophilia > 4% may indicate more severe lung fibrosis	Increased IL-4, IL-8, IL-10, IL-12, MCP-1, PDGF, TGF-β, CTGT, and thrombin activity Interferon-γ increased in 15%	
Langerhans cell histiocytosis	Cell profile similar to that of smokers: increased CD1⁺ cells (>5% AM) Cytoplasmic X body or Birbeck granule on EM		Most patients are smokers
Alveolar lipoproteinosis (pulmonary alveolar proteinosis)	Foamy cytoplasm of AM	Milky, turbid fluid with altered phospholipid proportions; increased surfactant protein A	Extrinsic allergic alveolitis, lipoid pneumonia, drug-induced hypersensitivity (e.g., amiodarone), silicosis
Eosinophilic pneumonia	Increased percentage of eosinophils to 40% of cells	Increased IL-5, IL-18, and VEGF	Churg-Strauss, allergic bronchopulmonary aspergillosis, drug-induced hypersensitivity
Alveolar hemorrhage (Goodpasture's, Wegener's)	Hemosiderin-laden AM		
Inhalation exposure (asbestosis, fiber, silica)	Asbestos bodies or fiber in AM Modest increase in PMNs		Subclinical exposure must be considered in asymptomatic subjects

A₁AT = α₁-antitrypsin protease; ACE = angiotensin-converting enzyme; AM = alveolar macrophages; BAL = bronchoalveolar lavage; CD4 = helper T-lymphocyte subset; CD8 = suppressor T lymphocyte; CTGT = connective tissue growth factor; EM = electron microscopy; FSC = free secretory component; ICAM-1 = intercellular adhesion molecule 1; Ig = immunoglobulin; IL = interleukin; MCP = monocyte chemotactic protein; MIF = macrophage migration inhibition factor; MMP-12 and ADAMDECI = matrix metalloproteinases; NSIP = nonspecific interstitial pneumonia; PDGF = platelet-derived growth factor; PMN = polymorphonuclear neutrophil; PPARγ = peroxisome proliferator-activated receptor γ; TGF-β = transforming growth factor-β; TNF-α = tumor necrosis factor-α; VEGF = vascular endothelial growth factor.

function. It is used to make a preliminary diagnostic assessment or to monitor patients as lung or cardiac disease evolves and responds to treatment. Spirometry is recorded by having a seated subject breathe calmly several times at tidal volume, draw a maximal inhalation, perform a forced exhalation that is continued for at least 6 seconds with sustained vigorous effort (forced vital capacity [FVC]), and finally make a vigorous full inspiration (inspiratory vital capacity). These maneuvers are represented as a volume-time loop or as a flow-volume loop (plotting flow against FVC and inspiratory vital capacity). Flow-volume loops are scrutinized for special patterns that can indicate various clinical or anatomic conditions (E-Fig. 85-3). Considerable physical effort and attentiveness are required for adequate spirometry. Patients, especially during hospitalization, after medical procedures, or if they are deconditioned, often cannot give maximal effort or cooperate or coordinate well, and their test results will not be optimum. PFTs in a patient who is still under treatment for an exacerbation of chronic obstructive pulmonary disease (COPD) or asthma but who is not yet back to pre-illness status will show results that reflect their current status but not their baseline status. Recent treatment with a bronchodilator often improves PFT results and does not reflect intrinsic pulmonary function; about 8 to 12 hours should elapse from the last treatment to provide the most useful data. Reproducibility of several test attempts (at least three) is important and is a criterion for valid interpretation of test results. Other medical problems that can confuse spirometric testing include pulmonary congestion, coughing, thyroid dysfunction, neurologic illness, poor nutrition, and corticosteroid-associated muscle weakness. Serial testing is required to assess improvement, a return to baseline, or the need for intensified treatment in an outpatient.

Among the most common measures made from a spirometric tracing are FVC (liters), forced expiratory volume in the first second of exhalation (FEV_1, liters), ratio of FEV_1 to FVC (percentage), and forced expiratory flow in the middle of expiration ($FEF_{25-75\%}$, liters/second). Residual volume (liters) cannot be determined by spirometry and often is measured by helium dilution or plethysmographic methods. Residual volume is necessary to compute total lung capacity (liters), which is a measure of the air capacity of the maximally inflated lung. FEV_1, although recorded as a volume, is equated with a measure of airflow and is effort dependent.

FEV_1 values, when expressed as a percentage of predicted values, correlate with the amount of physical activity a patient can sustain. Peak flow can be measured from a spirographic tracing or using a portable device made for the outpatient monitoring of lung function; these devices are commonly prescribed for patients with asthma, COPD, or interstitial lung diseases. Encouraging a patient to keep a daily log of peak flow rates to share with the physician or medical staff can improve compliance with therapy and monitor improvement or the lack of it.

Although a healthy young person can produce a peak flow of 500 to 600 L/minute, many people with COPD are unable to achieve a peak flow greater than 200 to 350 L/minute and experience significant exertional dyspnea when peak flow decreases to less than 200 L/minute. Patients whose peak flow is about 150 L/minute are usually sedentary.

Analysis of measured values for FEV_1 and FVC (and their ratio) and total lung capacity allows the physician to make ventilatory diagnosis of the presence of obstructive or restrictive physiology (E-Fig. 85-4). A reduced FEV_1 and low FEV_1/FVC ratio combined with a large total lung capacity indicate obstructive disease of large airways and bronchi, a pattern typically observed in patients with COPD and asthma. FVC is preserved, but the time of exhalation is prolonged. After the administration of bronchodilators, the FEV_1 and FVC may increase by 10 to 15%, especially in asthma, indicating reversibility of airway obstruction. A lesser degree of improvement often is found, however, in patients who are already using inhaled bronchodilators regularly. A decrease in the $FEF_{25-75\%}$ with relatively preserved values of FEV_1 and FVC typically is found in patients with obstruction of small airways. If a person's postbronchodilator FEV_1 is less than 80% of the predicted value and FEV_1/FVC is less than 70%, airflow limitation is not fully reversible—the defining characteristic of COPD (Chapter 88). In patients with restrictive lung disease, the FEV_1 and FVC are reduced, as is total lung capacity, but the FEV_1/FVC ratio is usually normal or increased. Causes of restrictive interstitial lung disease include fibrosis of the lung parenchyma due to many toxic and inhalation exposures and toxic drug reactions (Chapter 94) and idiopathic interstitial lung diseases (Chapter 92). Restrictive physiology with a normal or low FEV_1 may reflect the chest wall habitus, chest wall muscle weakness or deformity, and pleural thickening (Chapter 99).

Diffusion Capacity

Diffusion capacity assesses how well a tracer gas in inspired air can cross from the air into the blood. The test measures the absorption of a low concentration of carbon monoxide in inhaled air by hemoglobin in red blood cells that circulate through pulmonary capillaries. Results must be corrected for reduced lung volumes, anemia, increased carbon monoxide levels in cigarette smokers, and high altitude. The diffusion capacity provides a general assessment of the air-blood interface; reduced values are obtained when interstitial fibrosis is extensive or when the capillary surface is compromised by vascular obstruction or nonperfusion (e.g., pulmonary embolism; Chapter 98) or is destroyed as in emphysema (Chapter 88).

Site-Specific Sampling, Including Bronchoalveolar Lavage

An assessment of airway inflammation can be made by measuring the fraction of nitric oxide in exhaled air or the pH of exhaled air condensates. It is also possible to measure endogenously produced biomarkers of oxidative stress in condensates (i.e., reactive oxygen and nitrogen species or aldehydes of lipid peroxides damaged in cell membranes). Mediators of inflammation can be measured in induced sputum (e.g., IL-8, leukotriene B$_4$, myeloperoxidase, IL-6, and elastase products). For example, as COPD worsens, induced sputum specimens or exhaled breath condensates provide evidence of neutrophilic inflammation with higher concentrations of exhaled nitric oxide, tumor necrosis factor-α, IL-6, transforming growth factor-β, IL-8, and growth-related oncogene-α as well as more leukotriene B$_4$.

Site-specific sampling to detach cells by washing or abrading the mucosal surface, coupled with endobronchial or transbronchial biopsy, can provide contiguous samples containing viable cells, noncellular secretions, and adjacent tissue. Multiple sites can be sampled; mucosal cell function can be compared between the nose and lower airways to assess allergic diseases. Bronchoalveolar lavage retrieves cells and secretions from the distal airways and the alveolar space surface. In combination with a thorough clinical evaluation and lung imaging studies, distinctive cellular patterns sometimes can obviate the need for lung biopsy (Table 85-3). Lung biopsy tissue can be microdissected with laser capture of specific cell types, and cells recovered in bronchoalveolar lavage fluid can be prepared for microarray analysis; gene chips created specifically for gene expression patterns may prove helpful for determining genetic susceptibility, aiding diagnosis, predicting response to certain therapeutic agents, and monitoring clinical activity.

Visit expertconsult.com for e-expanded chapter

SUGGESTED READINGS

Burney PG, Hooper R. Forced vital capacity, airway obstruction and survival in a general population sample from the USA. *Thorax.* 2011;66:49-54. *Forced vital capacity, but not airway obstruction, predicts survival in asymptomatic adults without chronic respiratory diagnoses or symptoms.*

Konishi K, Gibson KF, Lindell KO, et al. Gene expression profiles of acute exacerbations of idiopathic pulmonary fibrosis. *Am J Respir Crit Care Med.* 2009;180:167-175. *Potential for using genomic patterns as early indications of serious impending disease.*

Reynolds HY. Present status of bronchoalveolar lavage in interstitial lung disease. *Curr Opin Pulm Med.* 2009;15:479-485. *An overview of research and clinical uses.*

Woodruff PG, Modrek B, Choy DF, et al. T-helper type 2 driven inflammation defines major subphenotypes of asthma. *Am J Respir Crit Care Med.* 2009;180:388-395. *How gene expression can identify molecular mechanisms that identify clinical types of eosinophilic driven T$_H$2 innate immunity diseases.*

DISORDERS OF VENTILATORY CONTROL

86

ATUL MALHOTRA

DEFINITIONS AND PATHOGENESIS

Ventilatory Control

Ventilation is controlled by complex interactions between central chemoreceptors, which predominantly are responsive to carbon dioxide (CO_2) tensions in arterial blood, and peripheral chemoreceptors, which predominantly are responsive to CO_2 and oxygen (O_2) tensions (Table 86-1). Disorders of ventilatory control are caused by derangements in these control mechanisms.

TABLE 86-1 CLASSIFICATION OF CENTRAL SLEEP APNEA

CENTRAL SLEEP APNEA SYNDROME	MECHANISM	THERAPY
Sleep transition apneas	CO_2 fluctuations during transitions from sleep to wake to sleep	Reassurance, occasionally hypnotics or oxygen
Chronic narcotic therapy	Lack of central drive	Reduce narcotic dose Consider positive-pressure device
Cheyne-Stokes breathing	High loop gain from robust chemosensitivity and ventilatory drive	Optimize medical therapy for heart failure, consider PAP devices
Idiopathic central apnea	Unknown	Supportive, bilevel PAP; consider ventilatory stimulants
Treatment of emergent central apnea or "complex apnea"	Lowering upper airway resistance at CPAP initiation improves efficiency of CO_2 excretion	Reassurance, generally resolves spontaneously
Sleep hypoventilation syndromes	Fall in drive with loss of wakefulness stimulus, loss of accessory muscle activity during REM sleep	Noninvasive ventilation

CPAP = continuous positive airway pressure; PAP = positive airway pressure; REM = rapid eye movement.

TABLE 86-2 CLASSIFICATION OF HYPERCAPNIC DISEASES

HYPERCAPNIC DISEASE	MECHANISM	DIAGNOSIS	TREATMENT
Narcotic overdose	Reduced central drive	History, narcotized pupils, toxicology	Supportive care, naloxone
Acute severe asthma	Severe airflow obstruction, high dead space	Typical history, wheezing on exam, low FEV_1/FVC	Bronchodilators, anti-inflammatories, mechanical ventilation (usually invasive)
Acute exacerbation of COPD	Airflow obstruction, high dead space	History, cigarette smoking, low FEV_1/FVC, infectious etiology	Bronchodilators, anti-inflammatories, noninvasive ventilation
Obesity-hypoventilation syndrome	Low respiratory system compliance, high upper airway resistance, low central drive	High BMI, lack of other diagnoses; blunted CO_2 response	Weight loss, nocturnal bilevel positive airway pressure
Central congenital hypoventilation syndrome	*PHOX2B* mutation, lack of central drive	Genetic testing	Supportive care, mechanical ventilation (usually noninvasive)
Neuromuscular disease (e.g., myasthenia gravis, ALS, polymyositis, GBS/AIDP)	Lack of respiratory muscle force	Immediate orthopnea, low VC, low MIPs/MEPs	Underlying cause; nocturnal noninvasive ventilation; supportive care
Severe parenchymal lung disease, e.g., COPD	Lack of alveolar surface area; high pulmonary dead space and work of breathing	Typical history, smoking, low FEV_1 and FEV_1/FVC	Bronchodilator, anti-inflammatory therapy, possible nocturnal noninvasive ventilation, smoking cessation
Kyphoscoliosis	Low respiratory system compliance	Physical examination	Supportive care, noninvasive ventilation

AIDP = acute inflammatory demyelinating polyneuropathy; ALS = amyotrophic lateral sclerosis; BMI = body mass index; COPD = chronic obstructive pulmonary disease; FEV_1 = forced expiratory volume in 1 second; FVC = forced vital capacity.

HYPOVENTILATION SYNDROMES

Hypoventilation syndromes are defined by a lack of adequate alveolar ventilation to maintain an arterial CO_2 tension of 40 mm Hg. The two most common clinical settings that result in hypoventilation are severe chronic obstructive pulmonary disease (COPD; Chapter 88) and morbid obesity (Chapters 100 and 227); less common etiologies include chronic opiate therapy, neuromuscular weakness (Chapters 429 and 430), and severe kyphoscoliosis (Chapter 99). The epidemiology of these hypoventilation syndromes is poorly studied, but about 15% of patients with severe COPD or morbid obesity have an elevated $Paco_2$. Regardless of the cause, patients with hypoventilation frequently have further worsening of their ventilation at the onset of sleep, owing to loss of the wakefulness stimulus, which is the normal drive to breathe while awake, and some degree of upper airway collapse after the onset of sleep (Chapter 100).

Patients with central sleep apnea (Chapter 100), which is a group of conditions in which cessation of airflow occurs because of a lack of respiratory effort, are classified into those with inadequate ventilatory drive and those with excessive drive. The paradox of how excessive drive leads to central apnea is explained by the concept of loop gain. A system with a high loop gain is prone to instability that leads to periods of excessive breathing followed by periods of apnea (Table 86-2). The prototype of a condition with high loop gain is periodic breathing or Cheyne-Stokes breathing (Fig. 86-1).

Cheyne-Stokes Breathing

Cheyne-Stokes breathing is a waxing and waning pattern of breathing that often includes periods of central apnea. It is seen most commonly during sleep in patients with heart failure.

EPIDEMIOLOGY

Cheyne-Stokes breathing is a form of ventilatory instability that occurs in 30 to 40% of patients with left ventricular systolic dysfunction and heart failure.

Male sex, advanced age, low baseline $Paco_2$, and atrial fibrillation are risk factors for Cheyne-Stokes breathing among patients with heart failure. Controversy remains regarding whether this breathing pattern itself is deleterious or whether it is simply a marker of the underlying severity of cardiac disease. Cheyne-Stokes breathing represents about 5 to 10% of all cases of sleep apnea (Chapter 100) and is uncommon among patients who do not have heart failure.

PATHOBIOLOGY

Individuals with Cheyne-Stokes breathing have robust chemosensitivity as evidenced by marked increases in ventilation with small changes in $Paco_2$. The drive to breathe may be further increased by neural reflexes that are triggered by extravascular lung fluid and an elevated left atrial pressure. Intermittent hypoxemia and catecholamine surges, which are frequent in these patients, contribute to oxidative stress and neuroendocrine activation, both of which are thought to contribute to worsening of the underlying heart failure.

CLINICAL MANIFESTATIONS AND DIAGNOSIS

Patients with Cheyne-Stokes breathing can sometimes be diagnosed at the bedside by careful observation of their breathing pattern. During sleep or exercise, breathing becomes more dependent on metabolic stimuli. Patients may complain of fatigue or sleepiness because arousals from sleep tend to occur during the hyperpneic phase. Paroxysmal nocturnal dyspnea, a classic symptom of heart failure (Chapter 58), most commonly reflects underlying Cheyne-Stokes breathing. Patients often are diagnosed in the sleep laboratory while undergoing investigation for possible obstructive sleep apnea.

The diagnosis of Cheyne-Stokes breathing, if not readily apparent, can be made during overnight polysomnography, when the typical oscillatory pattern of tidal volume is seen in the absence of ventilatory efforts during the apneic periods. When evaluating such recordings, it is important to note that

Cheyne-Stokes Respiration

FIGURE 86-1. Cheyne-Stokes breathing with crescendo-decrescendo pattern of breathing. The thermistor detects air temperature changes at the mouth and nose. Note absences in airflow without respiratory effort seen in the abdominal belts. This breathing pattern leads to intermittent desaturations, arousals from sleep, and bursts of tachycardia. The loop gain concept can be understood by considering the thermostat analogy in which a control system is working to regulate a stable room temperature (e.g., 20° C). By analogy, the respiratory control system is working primarily to maintain a stable $PaCO_2$ of 40 mm Hg and stable pH. Situations in which marked fluctuations in room temperature might occur would include one in which the thermostat is excessively sensitive (i.e., furnace turns on if room temperature falls to 19.999° C); if the furnace is too powerful, a marked overshoot in room temperature will be followed by a prolonged period when the furnace does not run. In the analogy to Cheyne-Stokes breathing, CO_2 is equated to room temperature and would be predicted to be unstable if chemoresponsiveness (i.e., the thermostat) were excessively robust (i.e., a marked increase in ventilation for small change in CO_2), if the efficiency of CO_2 excretion were high (i.e., marked fall in $PaCO_2$ with increased ventilation), or if the end-expiratory lung volume were small. Situations that increase the propensity for CO_2 fluctuations lead to elevated loop gain and thus increase the risk for Cheyne-Stokes breathing.

Cheyne-Stokes breathing usually resolves during rapid eye movement (REM) sleep, that arousals on the electroencephalogram typically occur during the hyperpneic phase, and that Cheyne-Stokes breathing generally does not resolve immediately when nasal continuous positive airway pressure (CPAP) is applied.

TREATMENT   Rx

Medical management of Cheyne-Stokes breathing most often is treatment of the underlying heart failure (Chapter 59). Many patients with clinically significant Cheyne-Stokes breathing are taking inadequate doses of angiotensin-converting enzyme inhibitors, β-adrenergic blockers, or diuretics. After optimization of medical management, the Cheyne-Stokes breathing pattern frequently resolves. By comparison, CPAP is no better than standard medical therapy.[1]

Central Congenital Hypoventilation Syndrome

DEFINITION AND EPIDEMIOLOGY

Central congenital hypoventilation syndrome is a rare congenital condition, previously referred to as Ondine's curse, characterized by a diminished ventilatory response to CO_2. The central congenital hypoventilation syndrome was traditionally diagnosed in neonates, but it is increasingly noted in adults.

PATHOBIOLOGY

The syndrome is now defined by a mutation in the *PHOX2B* gene, located on chromosome 4p12. Because most parents of affected children with the central congenital hypoventilation syndrome do not carry a *PHOX2B* mutation, the mutations are de novo. About 90% of patients are heterozygous for a polyalanine repeat expansion mutation, in which the affected allele has 24 to 33 alanines rather than the normal 20 alanines. The remaining 10% of central congenital hypoventilation syndrome patients have missense, nonsense, or frameshift mutations in the *PHOX2B* gene.

The *PHOX2B* gene is a paired-like homeobox that encodes a highly conserved transcription factor key to autonomic development in mice. Mice that are genetically modified for *PHOX2B* have irregular breathing, do not respond to hypercapnia, and die soon after birth from central apnea. These mice have neuronal loss in the retrotrapezoid nucleus and parafacial region of the brain stem, thereby suggesting the importance of this medullary region in normal breathing. Abnormalities in *PHOX2B* genes have also been associated with Hirschsprung's disease (Chapter 138), neural crest tumors, cardiac asystole (Chapter 63), and other abnormalities of the autonomic nervous system (Chapter 427).

CLINICAL MANIFESTATIONS AND DIAGNOSIS

Neonates can present with cyanosis at birth, recurrent central apneas, or both. Adults can present with idiopathic central sleep apnea, unexplained hypercapnia, or autonomic abnormalities (Chapter 427). Confirmation of the diagnosis requires the demonstration of an abnormality in the *PHOX2B* gene.

TREATMENT   Rx

There are currently no specific therapies for central congenital hypoventilation syndrome beyond supportive care. Genetic counseling is required for afflicted individuals and their families given the autosomal dominant pattern of inheritance. Patients must be cautioned against the use of sedatives, which could precipitate respiratory failure. Mechanical ventilation during sleep either invasively (through tracheostomy) or noninvasively (through bilevel positive airway pressure support [Chapter 100]) is required in most patients. Some patients remain fully ventilator dependent. Alternative treatments, such as ventilatory stimulants and diaphragmatic pacing, are generally ineffective.

Acquired Hypoventilation Syndromes

DEFINITION AND EPIDEMIOLOGY

Patients with hypoventilation syndromes cannot maintain adequate minute ventilation to keep their $PaCO_2$ at 40 mm Hg. Patients can be classified into those who lack central ventilatory drive and those who have a pulmonary mechanical or neuromuscular abnormality that prevents adequate gas exchange. The case frequency is unknown, but hypercapnic respiratory failure is one of the more common admission diagnoses in intensive care units.

PATHOBIOLOGY

Patients with conditions characterized by the lack of central drive have reasonably normal lungs and respiratory muscle function but lack adequate response to CO_2 and hypoxia. In contrast, most patients with mechanical or neuromuscular abnormalities have a larger work of breathing compared with normal individuals; the most common underlying conditions are severe

FIGURE 86-2. A flow chart of a systematic approach to hypercapnia and various causes of hypoventilation. The change in pH can help determine the cause and chronicity. A careful history and physical examination, coupled with pulmonary function testing, can help classify patients into those who "can't breathe" owing to neuromuscular or mechanical abnormalities of the respiratory system as compared with those who "won't breathe" owing to central nervous system pathology. COPD = chronic obstructive pulmonary disease; MEP = maximal expiratory pressure; MIP = maximal inspiratory pressure; P0.1 = the negative mouth pressure generated during the first 100 msec of an occluded inspiration; PFT = pulmonary function test.

COPD (Chapter 88) or morbid obesity (Chapter 227) with the obesity-hypoventilation syndrome. Such individuals have diminished but not absent chemoresponsiveness. Another cause of inadequate gas exchange is neuromuscular disease; common causes include disorders of neuromuscular transmission (Chapter 430), severe muscle weakness (Chapter 429), the residua from poliovirus infection (Chapter 423), Guillain-Barré syndrome (Chapter 428), or acute poisoning (Chapter 110).

CLINICAL MANIFESTATIONS AND DIAGNOSIS

Patients with hypoventilation have a myriad of presentations ranging from asymptomatic abnormalities in laboratory testing (e.g., elevated $Paco_2$, unexplained low Sao_2, or an elevated serum bicarbonate level) to respiratory failure in the intensive care unit (e.g., respiratory infection with laboratory evidence of chronic abnormalities, such as acute-on-chronic respiratory acidosis). Patients who acutely overdose on sedative-hypnotic or narcotic agents may present with acute respiratory acidosis and loss of consciousness. Other patients may present with central sleep apnea-hypopnea or otherwise unexplained oxygen desaturation at night.

Once suspected, the diagnosis of hypoventilation is confirmed by the finding of $Paco_2$ higher than 42 mm Hg on analysis of an arterial blood sample. If the increase in $Paco_2$ is of short duration so that renal compensation has not yet occurred (Chapter 120), the serum bicarbonate level is increased by 1 mEq/liter for every 10-mm Hg rise in $Paco_2$. By comparison, if the respiratory acidosis is of sufficient duration for renal compensation to occur, the serum bicarbonate level will be increased by 4 mEq for every 10-mm Hg rise in $Paco_2$ (Fig. 86-2).

Once an elevated $Paco_2$ is established, it is appropriate to distinguish patients who "can't breathe" from those who "won't breathe." "Can't breathe" implies that a respiratory mechanical problem or neuromuscular weakness is causing the elevation in $Paco_2$. Abnormalities in pulmonary function testing (e.g., a markedly diminished vital capacity) are consistent with a pulmonary parenchymal or chest wall disorder.

Patients who "won't breathe" have central nervous system abnormalities that affect central drive or chemosensitivity, or both.

TREATMENT AND PROGNOSIS   Rx

The treatment of hypoventilation should focus on the underlying cause. Acute poisonings can be managed supportively or, in some cases, with specific antidotes (Chapter 110). Chronic conditions can be treated by addressing the underlying cause, such as weight loss in obesity hypoventilation syndrome or cholinesterase inhibitors in myasthenia gravis (Chapter 430). For parenchymal lung disease, treatment is directed at the underlying cause (Chapters 88 and 92).

Sedative medications should be used cautiously because they can occasionally precipitate acute respiratory failure. Although profound hypoxemia can clearly be deleterious, oxygen occasionally can precipitate severe acute respiratory acidosis, particularly in patients with acute exacerbations of COPD (Chapter 88). As a result, hypoventilating patients with COPD require the careful administration of supplemental oxygen, which should be titrated to an arterial oxygen saturation of 90% or an arterial oxygen tension of 60 mm Hg.

Severe hypoventilation requires mechanical ventilation (Chapter 105), such as noninvasive ventilation for an acute exacerbation of COPD.[2] For other presentations in which the $Paco_2$ is believed to be acutely elevated, endotracheal intubation and mechanical ventilation are frequently used, especially in patients with impaired consciousness. For chronic hypoventilation in hypercapnic COPD, noninvasive bilevel positive airway pressure through a face mask during sleep can maintain alveolar ventilation and improve outcome.[3] However, the considerable difficulty of adhering to nocturnal bilevel therapy in COPD emphasizes the need for discussions with patients and families regarding its risks and benefits. Other chronic hypoventilation syndromes are also commonly treated with bilevel positive airway pressure, although data are less compelling. In some chronic conditions, such as motor neuron disease (Chapter 418), tracheostomy should be discussed, although the impact of such interventions on quality of life should be carefully considered. Regardless of the underlying cause, an elevation in the $Paco_2$ level is considered a poor prognostic sign. End-of-life discussions are also important in such cases because the prognosis of chronic respiratory failure patients is generally poor.

1. Bradley TD, Logan AG, Kimoff RJ, et al. Continuous positive airway pressure for central sleep apnea and heart failure. *N Engl J Med.* 2005;353:2025-2033.
2. Lightowler JV, Wedzicha JA, Elliott MW, et al. Non-invasive positive pressure ventilation to treat respiratory failure resulting from exacerbations of chronic obstructive pulmonary disease: Cochrane systematic review and meta-analysis. *BMJ.* 2003;326:185.
3. McEvoy RD, Pierce RJ, Hillman D, et al. Nocturnal non-invasive nasal ventilation in stable hypercapnic COPD: a randomised controlled trial. *Thorax.* 2009;64:561-566.

SUGGESTED READINGS

Brown LK. Hypoventilation syndromes. *Clin Chest Med.* 2010;31:249-270. *Review of mechanisms and syndromes.*
Pack AI. Central sleep apnea. *Handb Clin Neurol.* 2011;98:411-419. *Review.*
Weese-Mayer DE, Berry-Kravis EM, Ceccherini I, et al. An official ATS clinical policy statement. Congenital central hypoventilation syndrome: genetic basis, diagnosis, and management. *Am J Respir Crit Care Med.* 2010;181:626-644. *Review of the condition, which is defined by the presence of a PHOX2B mutation.*

ASTHMA

JEFFREY M. DRAZEN

DEFINITION

Asthma is a clinical syndrome of unknown etiology characterized by three distinct components: (1) recurrent episodes of airway obstruction that resolve spontaneously or as a result of treatment; (2) exaggerated bronchoconstrictor responses to stimuli that have little or no effect in nonasthmatic subjects, a phenomenon known as *airway hyperresponsiveness*; and (3) inflammation of the airways as defined by a variety of criteria. Although airway obstruction is largely reversible, it is currently thought that changes in the asthmatic airway may be irreversible in some settings.

EPIDEMIOLOGY

Asthma is an extremely common disorder affecting boys more commonly than girls and, after puberty, women slightly more commonly than men; approximately 8% of the adult population of the United States has signs and symptoms consistent with a diagnosis of asthma. Although most cases begin before the age of 25 years, new-onset asthma may develop at any time throughout life.

The worldwide prevalence of asthma has increased more than 45% since the late 1970s. The greatest increases in asthma prevalence have occurred in countries that have recently adopted an "industrialized" lifestyle. Data from many sources now show that children raised in a farming environment have a much lower risk of asthma than their peers raised in an urban environment; the specific exposures responsible for this decreased disease burden are not known.

Asthma is among the most common reasons to seek medical treatment. In the United States, it is responsible for about 15 million annual outpatient visits to physicians and for nearly 2 million annual inpatient hospital days of treatment. The yearly direct and indirect costs of asthma care are more than $25 billion; more than half of these costs are attributable to direct expenditures on medical care encounters or asthma medications.

PATHOBIOLOGY

Genetics

In twin studies, asthma has about 60% heritability, indicating that both genetic and environmental factors are important in its etiology. A locus on chromosome 17q21, at or near the locus for *ORMDL3*, a member of a gene family that encodes endoplasmic reticulum transmembrane proteins, has been associated with childhood-onset asthma. Although the exact functional variant in this region has not been identified, the isolation of a locus for childhood-onset asthma supports the clinical observation that adult- and childhood-onset asthma appear to be distinct disorders. Genetic variants that influence the response to treatment also have been identified and widely replicated.

Pathology

The pathology of mild asthma, as delineated by bronchoscopic and biopsy studies, is characterized by edema and hyperemia of the mucosa and by infiltration of the mucosa with mast cells, eosinophils, and lymphocytes bearing the T_H2 phenotype. Small placebo-controlled trials with daclizumab, an antibody against CD25, in patients with asthma of moderate severity provides solid evidence for the pathobiologic role of lymphocyte activation in asthma. Chemokines such as eotaxin, RANTES, macrophage inflammatory protein 1α, and interleukin-8 (IL-8), produced by epithelial and inflammatory cells, and the loss of the T-cell signaling molecule T-bet serve to amplify and to perpetuate the inflammatory events within the airway. The role of IL-4 and IL-13 as critical signaling molecules has been confirmed through small randomized controlled trials with pitakinra, an agent that inhibits binding of these cytokines to their receptors. As a result of these inflammatory stimuli coupled with the mechanical deformation of the epithelium from airway smooth muscle constriction, the airway wall is thickened by the deposition of type III and type V collagen below the true basement membrane. In addition, in severe chronic asthma, there is hypertrophy and hyperplasia of airway glands and of both surface and glandular secretory cells as well as hyperplasia of airway smooth muscle. Morphometric studies of airways from asthmatic subjects have demonstrated airway wall thickening of sufficient magnitude to increase airflow resistance and enhance airway responsiveness. During a severe asthmatic event, the airway wall is thickened markedly; in addition, patchy airway occlusion occurs by a mixture of hyperviscous mucus and clusters of shed airway epithelial cells.

The episodic airway narrowing that constitutes an asthma attack results from obstruction of the airway lumen to airflow. Although it is now well established that asthma is associated with infiltration of the airway by inflammatory cells, the links between these cells and the pathobiologic processes that account for asthmatic airway obstruction have not been clearly delineated. Three possible but not mutually exclusive links have been postulated: (1) the constriction of airway smooth muscle, (2) the thickening of airway epithelium, and (3) the presence of liquids within the confines of the airway lumen. Among these mechanisms, the constriction of airway smooth muscle due to the local release of bioactive mediators or neurotransmitters is the most widely accepted explanation for the acute reversible airway obstruction in asthma attacks. Several bronchoactive mediators are thought to be the agents that initiate the airway obstruction characteristic of asthma.

Mediators of the Acute Asthmatic Response

Acetylcholine
Acetylcholine released from intrapulmonary motor nerves causes constriction of airway smooth muscle through direct stimulation of muscarinic receptors of the M_3 subtype. The potential role for acetylcholine in the bronchoconstriction of asthma primarily derives from the observation that tiotropium bromide can be used as an effective asthma treatment.

Histamine
Histamine, or β-imidazolylethylamine, was identified as a potent endogenous bronchoactive agent 100 years ago. Mast cells, which are prominent in airway tissues obtained from patients with asthma, constitute the major pulmonary source of histamine. Clinical trials with novel potent antihistamines indicate a minor role for histamine as a mediator of airway obstruction in asthma.

Leukotrienes and Lipoxins
The cysteinyl leukotrienes, namely, LTC_4, LTD_4, and LTE_4, as well as the dihydroxy leukotriene LTB_4, are derived by the lipoxygenation of arachidonic acid released from target cell membrane phospholipids during cellular activation. 5-Lipoxygenase, the 5-lipoxygenase-activating protein, and LTC_4 synthase make up the cellular protein and enzyme content needed to produce the cysteinyl leukotrienes. The production of LTB_4 requires 5-lipoxygenase, the 5-lipoxygenase-activating protein, and LTA_4 epoxide hydrolase. Mast cells, eosinophils, and alveolar macrophages have the enzymatic capability to produce cysteinyl leukotrienes from their membrane phospholipids, whereas polymorphonuclear leukocytes produce exclusively LTB_4, which is predominantly a chemoattractant molecule; LTC_4 and LTD_4 are among the most potent contractile agonists ever identified for human airway smooth muscle. Clinical trials with leukotriene receptor antagonists or synthesis inhibitors have shown significant clinical efficacy in the treatment of chronic persistent

asthma, leading to the conclusion that the leukotrienes are important but not exclusive mediators of the asthmatic response. Lipoxins, which are double lipoxygenase products of arachidonic acid metabolism, have been shown to be endogenous downregulators of the inflammatory response. The amounts of lipoxins are decreased in the airways of patients with severe asthma.

Nitric Oxide

Nitric oxide (NO•) is produced enzymatically by airway epithelial cells and by inflammatory cells found in the asthmatic lung. Free NO• has a half-life on the order of seconds in the airway and is stabilized by conjugation to thiols to form RS-NO. Both NO• and RS-NO have bronchodilator actions and may play a homeostatic role in the airway. Paradoxically, high levels of NO•, when it is coavailable with superoxide anion, may form toxic oxidation products, such as peroxynitrite ($OONO^-$), which could damage the airway. Patients with asthma have higher than normal levels of NO• in their expired air, and these levels decrease consistently after treatment with corticosteroids.

Physiological Changes in Asthma

An increased resistance to airflow is the consequence of the airway obstruction induced by smooth muscle constriction, thickening of the airway epithelium, or free liquid within the airway lumen. Resistance to airflow is manifested by increased airway resistance and decreased flow rates throughout the vital capacity. At the onset of an asthma attack, obstruction occurs at all airway levels; as the attack resolves, these changes are reversed—first in the large airways (i.e., mainstem, lobar, segmental, and subsegmental bronchi) and then in the more peripheral airways. This anatomic sequence of onset and reversal is reflected in the physiological changes observed during resolution of an asthmatic episode (Fig. 87-1). Specifically, as an asthma attack resolves, flow rates first normalize at a high point in the vital capacity and only later at a low point in the vital capacity. Because asthma is an airway disease, not an air space disease, no primary changes occur in the static pressure-volume curve of the lungs. However, during an acute attack of asthma, airway narrowing may be so severe as to result in airway closure, with individual lung units closing at a volume that is near their maximal volume. This closure results in a change of the pressure-volume curve such that for a given contained gas volume within the thorax, elastic recoil is decreased, which in turn further depresses expiratory flow rates.

Additional factors influence the mechanical behavior of the lungs during an acute attack of asthma. During inspiration in an asthma attack, the pleural pressure becomes more negative than the 4- to 6-cm H_2O subatmospheric pressure usually required for tidal airflow. The expiratory phase of respiration also becomes active as the patient tries to force air from the lungs. As a consequence, peak pleural pressures during expiration, which normally are, at most, only a few centimeters of water above atmospheric pressure, may be as high as 20 to 30 cm H_2O above atmospheric pressure. The low pleural pressures during inspiration tend to dilate airways, whereas the high pleural pressures during expiration tend to narrow airways. During an asthma attack, the wide pressure swings, coupled with alterations in the mechanical properties of the airway wall, lead to a much higher resistance to expiratory airflow than to inspiratory airflow.

The respiratory rate is usually rapid during an acute asthmatic attack. This tachypnea is driven not by abnormalities in arterial blood gas composition but rather by stimulation of intrapulmonary receptors with subsequent effects on central respiratory centers. One consequence of the combination of airway narrowing and rapid airflow rates is a heightened mechanical load on the ventilatory pump. During a severe attack, the load can increase the

work of breathing by a factor of 10 or more and can predispose to fatigue of the ventilatory muscles. The patchy nature of asthmatic airway narrowing results in a maldistribution of ventilation (V) relative to pulmonary perfusion (Q). A shift occurs from the normal preponderance of V/Q units, with a ratio of near unity, to a distribution with a large number of alveolar-capillary units, with a V/Q ratio of less than unity. The net effect is to induce arterial hypoxemia. In addition, the hyperpnea of asthma is reflected as hyperventilation with a low arterial P_{CO_2}.

CLINICAL MANIFESTATIONS

History

During an acute asthma attack, patients seek medical attention for shortness of breath accompanied by cough, wheezing, and anxiety. The degree of breathlessness experienced by the patient is not closely related to the degree of airflow obstruction but is often influenced by the acuteness of the attack. Dyspnea may occur only with exercise (exercise-induced asthma), after aspirin ingestion (aspirin-exacerbated respiratory disease), after exposure to a specific known allergen (extrinsic asthma), or for no identifiable reason (intrinsic asthma). Variants of asthma exist in which cough, hoarseness, or inability to sleep through the night is the only symptom. Identification of a provoking stimulus through careful questioning helps establish the diagnosis of asthma and may be therapeutically useful if the stimulus can be avoided. Most patients with asthma complain of shortness of breath when they are exposed to rapid changes in the temperature and humidity of inspired air. For example, during the winter months in less temperate climates, patients commonly become short of breath on leaving a heated house; in warm humid climates, patients may complain of shortness of breath on entering a cold dry room, such as an air-conditioned theater.

An important factor to consider in taking a history from a patient with asthma is the potential for occupational exposures in asthma (Chapter 93). Asthma that is brought on by occupational exposures is termed *occupational asthma*; preexisting asthma that is exacerbated by workplace exposures is termed *workplace-exacerbated asthma*. In reactive airway dysfunction syndrome (RADS), a single large exposure leads to a persistent asthma-like phenotype in a previously normal individual.

Physical Examination

Vital Signs

Common features noted during an acute attack of asthma include a rapid respiratory rate (often 25 to 40 breaths per minute), tachycardia, and pulsus paradoxus (an exaggerated inspiratory decrease in the systolic pressure). The magnitude of the pulsus is related to the severity of the attack; a value greater than 15 mm Hg indicates an attack of moderate severity. Pulse oximetry, with the patient respiring ambient air, commonly reveals an oxygen saturation near 90%.

Thoracic Examination

Inspection may reveal that patients experiencing acute attacks of asthma are using their accessory muscles of ventilation; if so, the skin over the thorax may be retracted into the intercostal spaces during inspiration. The chest is usually hyperinflated, and the expiratory phase is prolonged relative to the inspiratory phase. Percussion of the thorax demonstrates hyperresonance, with loss of the normal variation in dullness due to diaphragmatic movement; tactile fremitus is diminished. Auscultation reveals wheezing, which is the cardinal physical finding in asthma but does not establish the diagnosis (Chapter 83). Wheezing, commonly louder during expiration but heard

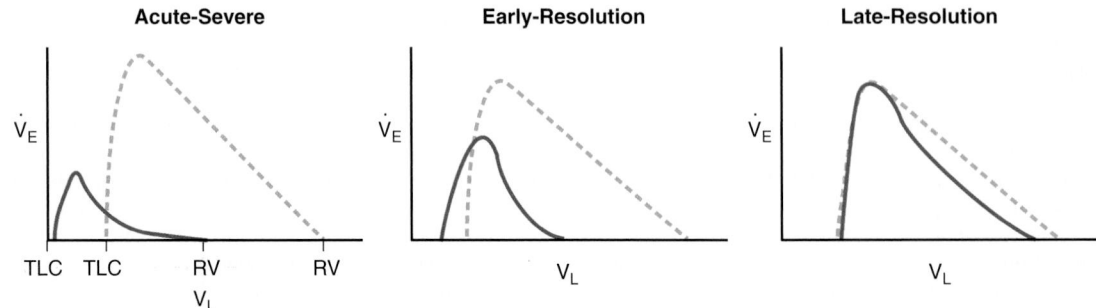

FIGURE 87-1. Schematic flow-volume curves in various stages of asthma. In each figure, the *dashed line* depicts the normal flow-volume curve. Predicted and observed total lung capacity (TLC) and residual volume (RV) are shown at the extremes of each curve. $\dot{V}_E$ = expiratory flow rate; V_L = lung volume.

TABLE 87-1	RELATIVE SEVERITY OF AN ASTHMATIC ATTACK AS INDICATED BY PEFR, FEV₁, AND MMEFR	
TEST	PREDICTED VALUE (%)	SEVERITY OF ASTHMA
PEFR	>80	
FEV₁	>80	No spirometric abnormalities
MMEFR	>80	
PEFR	>80	
FEV₁	>70	Mild asthma
MMEFR	55-75	
PEFR	>60	
FEV₁	45-70	Moderate asthma
MMEFR	30-50	
PEFR	<50	
FEV₁	<50	Severe asthma
MMEFR	10-30	

FEV₁ = forced expiratory volume in the first second; MMEFR = maximal mid-expiratory flow rate; PEFR = peak expiratory flow rate.

during inspiration as well, is characterized as polyphonic in that more than one pitch may be heard simultaneously. A recording of wheezing from a patient with asthma can be heard at *www.expertconsult.com*. Accompanying adventitious sounds may include rhonchi, which are suggestive of free secretions in the airway lumen, or rales, which should raise the suspicion of an alternative diagnosis and are indicative of localized infection or heart failure. The loss of intensity or the absence of breath sounds in a patient with asthma is an indication of severe airflow obstruction.

DIAGNOSIS
Laboratory Findings
Pulmonary Function Findings
A decrease in airflow rates throughout the vital capacity is the cardinal pulmonary function abnormality during an asthmatic episode. The peak expiratory flow rate (PEFR), the forced expiratory volume in the first second (FEV₁), and the maximal mid-expiratory flow rate (MMEFR) are all decreased in asthma (Chapter 85). In severe asthma, dyspnea may be so severe as to prevent the patient from performing a complete spirogram. In this case, if 2 seconds of forced expiration can be recorded, useful values for PEFR and FEV₁ can be obtained. Gradation of attack severity (Table 87-1) *must* be assessed by objective measures of airflow; no other methods yield accurate and reproducible results. As the attack resolves, the PEFR and the FEV₁ increase toward normal together while the MMEFR remains substantially depressed; as the attack resolves further, the FEV₁ and the PEFR may normalize while the MMEFR remains depressed (see Fig. 87-1). Even when the attack has resolved clinically, residual depression of the MMEFR is not uncommon; this depression may resolve during a prolonged course of treatment. If the patient is able to cooperate such that more complete measurements of lung function can be made, lung volume measurements made during an attack demonstrate an increase in both total lung capacity and residual volume; the changes in total lung capacity and residual volume resolve with treatment. Because of the extra cooperation needed for this testing, it is not advised during an acute asthmatic event; such testing is, however, indicated between episodes of asthma.

Exhaled NO·
The fraction of NO· in the exhaled air (Fe_{NO}) is elevated in patients with asthma. Although the exact concentration considered "elevated" will vary with the details of the technique, a concentration of 15 parts per billion is a convenient and reliable level that can be used to distinguish normal subjects from patients with untreated asthma. However, the measurement of exhaled nitric oxide has not been shown to be of value in the day-to-day management of asthma.[1-3]

Arterial Blood Gases
Blood gas analysis need not be undertaken in individuals with mild asthma. If the asthma is of sufficient severity to merit prolonged observation, however, blood gas analysis is indicated; in such cases, hypoxemia and hypocapnia are the rule. With the subject breathing ambient air, the Pa_{O_2} is usually between 55 and 70 mm Hg and the Pa_{CO_2} between 25 and 35 mm Hg. At the onset of the attack, an appropriate pure respiratory alkalemia is usually evident;

with attacks of prolonged duration, the pH returns toward normal as a result of a compensatory metabolic acidemia. A normal Pa_{CO_2} in a patient with moderate to severe airflow obstruction is reason for concern because it may indicate that the mechanical load on the respiratory system is greater than can be sustained by the ventilatory muscles and that respiratory failure is imminent. When the Pa_{CO_2} increases in such settings, the pH decreases quickly because the bicarbonate stores have become depleted as a result of renal compensation for the prolonged preceding respiratory alkalemia. Because this chain of events can take place rapidly, close observation is indicated for asthmatic patients with "normal" Pa_{CO_2} levels and moderate to severe airflow obstruction.

Other Blood Findings
Asthmatic subjects are frequently atopic; thus, blood eosinophilia is common but not universal. In addition, elevated serum levels of immunoglobulin E (IgE) are often documented; epidemiologic studies indicate that asthma is unusual in subjects with low IgE levels. If indicated by the patient's history, specific radioallergosorbent tests, which measure IgE directed against specific offending antigens, can be conducted. In rare instances during severe asthma attacks, serum concentrations of aminotransferases, lactate dehydrogenase, muscle creatine kinase, ornithine transcarbamylase, and antidiuretic hormone may be elevated.

Radiographic Findings
The chest radiograph of a subject with asthma is often normal. Severe asthma is associated with hyperinflation, as indicated by depression of the diaphragm and abnormally lucent lung fields. Complications of severe asthma, including pneumomediastinum or pneumothorax, may be detected radiographically. In mild to moderate asthma without adventitious sounds other than wheezing, a chest radiograph need not be obtained; if the asthma is of sufficient severity to merit hospital admission, a chest radiograph is advised.

Electrocardiographic Findings
The electrocardiogram, except for sinus tachycardia, is usually normal in acute asthma. However, right axis deviation, right bundle branch block, "P pulmonale," or even ST-T wave abnormalities may arise during severe asthma and resolve as the attack resolves.

Sputum Findings
The sputum of the asthmatic patient may be either clear or opaque with a green or yellow tinge. The presence of color does not invariably indicate infection, and examination of a Gram-stained and Wright-stained sputum smear is indicated. The sputum often contains eosinophils, Charcot-Leyden crystals (crystallized eosinophil lysophospholipase), Curschmann's spirals (bronchiolar casts composed of mucus and cells), or Creola bodies (clusters of airway epithelial cells with identifiable cilia that, in fresh samples, can often be seen to beat), which can affect color without the presence of infection.

DIAGNOSIS
Differential Diagnosis
Asthma is easy to recognize in a young patient without comorbid medical conditions who has exacerbating and remitting airway obstruction accompanied by blood eosinophilia. A rapid response to bronchodilator treatment is usually all that is needed to establish the diagnosis. However, in the patient with cryptic episodic shortness of breath, an elevated Fe_{NO} can help establish a diagnosis of asthma. However, in the absence of an elevated Fe_{NO}, other causes of wheezing (see Table 83-3 in Chapter 83) should be investigated.

PREVENTION AND TREATMENT

There is currently no way to prevent a patient from developing an asthmatic diathesis. For example, trials of allergen avoidance in childhood have not been successful. If a patient has such a diathesis with an allergic component, avoidance of allergens can reduce the frequency of asthma attacks. For example, removal of indoor mold can improve symptoms by 25% and reduce medication use by 50%.

The treatment of asthma is directed at the airway obstruction and the propensity for the airways to narrow too much and too easily in response to inhaled bronchoconstrictors. It is not acceptable practice to manage patients with asthma without objective measures of lung function. The best measure is FEV₁, but measures of PEFR can be substituted. Inexpensive and easy-to-use peak flowmeters make the measurement feasible in virtually all cases.

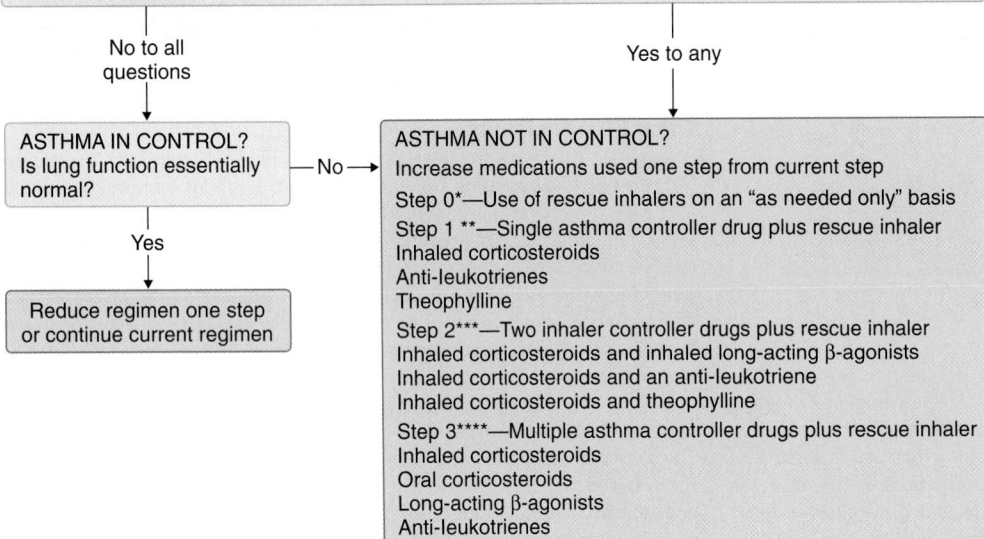

Have your activities of daily life been limited or interrupted because of asthma?

Has asthma caused you to awake from sleep more than one night in two weeks?

Have you had to use your rescue inhaler more than two or three times a day because of asthma symptoms?

Have you had to seek emergent medical care for your asthma since your last visit?

Is the fraction of nitric oxide in the exhaled air greater than 15 parts per billion? (In centers where this test is available)

No to all questions → **ASTHMA IN CONTROL?** Is lung function essentially normal? —No→

Yes to any → **ASTHMA NOT IN CONTROL?**
Increase medications used one step from current step

Step 0*—Use of rescue inhalers on an "as needed only" basis

Step 1 **—Single asthma controller drug plus rescue inhaler
Inhaled corticosteroids
Anti-leukotrienes
Theophylline

Step 2***—Two inhaler controller drugs plus rescue inhaler
Inhaled corticosteroids and inhaled long-acting β-agonists
Inhaled corticosteroids and an anti-leukotriene
Inhaled corticosteroids and theophylline

Step 3****—Multiple asthma controller drugs plus rescue inhaler
Inhaled corticosteroids
Oral corticosteroids
Long-acting β-agonists
Anti-leukotrienes

Yes → Reduce regimen one step or continue current regimen

FIGURE 87-2. Approach to chronic control of asthma as well as to treatment of acute asthma symptoms. *Inhaled albuterol or, in patients predisposed to adverse effects from this treatment, inhaled ipratropium bromide. **The choice between these two agents as first-line therapy is up to the patient and provider. Inhaled corticosteroids are more potent for improving lung function but have adverse effects when used at high doses for extended periods. Efforts should be made to use the lowest doses possible. Although antileukotrienes are less effective, some patients prefer oral to inhaled treatment and wish to avoid the potential side effects of inhaled steroids. If a response to one treatment is not achieved, it makes sense to try the other. ***The best documented combination is a long-acting β-agonist plus an inhaled steroid, but the dose of inhaled steroids should be at least the median dose (see Table 87-2) before long-acting β-agonists are added. ****The use of multiple medications indicates asthma of substantial severity. Unless success is easily achieved, consultation with an asthma specialist may be appropriate.

Treatment of asthma has two components. The first is the use of acute reliever (rescue) agents (i.e., bronchodilators) for acute asthmatic airway obstruction. The second is the use of controller treatments, which modify the asthmatic airway environment so that acute airway narrowing, requiring rescue treatments, occurs much less frequently.

In a given individual, the intensity of asthma treatment is adjusted, for the most part, to achieve five goals:

1. Allow the patient to pursue the activities of his or her daily life without excessive interference from asthma
2. Allow the patient to sleep without awakening because of asthmatic symptoms
3. Minimize the use of rescue bronchodilator treatment
4. Prevent the need for unscheduled medical care
5. Maintain lung function reasonably near normal

A patient who meets these standards is said to be "in control," whereas a patient whose disease activities prevent these goals from being met is said to be "out of control." Treatment is titrated to achieve reasonable control in each patient. The recommendations given herein for chronic control of asthma are based on the Global Initiative for Asthma, 2009 revision (Fig. 87-2), but are not taken verbatim from them. Based on a directed history and physical examination, the patient's current degree of control can be determined, and then recommendations for future treatment can be made.

Rescue Treatments

All patients with asthma should be prescribed a rescue inhaler to use if they develop acute asthmatic airway obstruction.

β-Adrenergic Agents

Short-acting β-adrenergic agents given by inhalation are the mainstay of bronchodilator treatment of asthma. Constricted airway smooth muscle relaxes in response to stimulation of β_2-adrenergic receptors. β-Adrenergic agonists with varying degrees of β_2-selectivity are available for use in inhaled (by nebulizer or metered-dose inhaler; Fig. 87-3), oral, or parenteral preparations. Most patients with mild intermittent asthma should be treated with a short-acting β_2-selective inhaler (such as albuterol) on an as-needed basis. Regardless of the specific type of medication used, rescue treatment should consist of two "puffs" from the inhaler, with the first and second puffs separated by a 3- to 5-minute interval, which is thought to allow enough time for the first puff to dilate narrowed airways, thus giving the agent better access to affected areas of the lung. Patients should be instructed to exhale to a comfortable volume, to breathe in very slowly (such as they would when sipping hot soup), and to actuate the inhaler as they inspire. Inspiration to near total lung capacity is followed by holding the breath for 5 seconds to allow the deposition of smaller aerosol particles in more peripheral airways. This treatment can be repeated every 4 to 6 hours; patients should be instructed to "advance" their asthma treatment as noted in Figure 87-2 if they need to use more than 12 puffs of a β-agonist in a 72-hour period.

FIGURE 87-3. Commonly used inhalers. **A,** A pressurized metered-dose inhaler for a branded form of albuterol. Such inhalers propel the medication by means of a pressurized gas; many inhalers use propellants that do not harm the ozone layer. **B,** One of many types of dry powder inhalers; the one shown is a Flexhaler and dispenses budesonide. When this type of inhaler is activated, the active agent is released as a dry powder into a chamber. The patient creates the energy for airflow by means of an inspiratory effort that is directed through the device and that entrains medication into the inhaled airway.

Patients should receive specific instructions for correct inhaler use. Aerosol "spacers" are available from many manufacturers for patients who have difficulty coordinating their inspiratory effort and inhaler actuation. There is definitive evidence from prospective, randomized, placebo-controlled trials that the regularly scheduled use of prophylactic inhaled β-agonists has no deleterious effects in most patients with asthma.

In 2008, albuterol inhalers containing chlorofluorocarbon propellants were withdrawn from the market and replaced by inhalers powered by hydrofluoroalkanes. These inhalers have a lower velocity aerosol plume, so patients will notice a subjective difference in how the aerosol feels as it is dissipated into the mouth; nevertheless, clinical trials document that most hydrofluoroalkane inhalers will have nearly identical therapeutic effects.

Anticholinergics

Atropinic agents inhibit the effects of acetylcholine released from the intrapulmonary motor nerves that run in the vagus and innervate airway smooth muscle. Ipratropium bromide, the atropinic agent used therapeutically in asthma, is available in a metered-dose inhaler; the recommended dose is two puffs from a metered-dose inhaler every 4 to 6 hours. In adults with uncontrolled asthma, inhaled tiotropium (18 μg every morning) added to an

TABLE 87-2 ESTIMATED EQUIPOTENT DAILY DOSE FOR INHALED GLUCOCORTICOSTEROIDS FOR ADULTS

DRUG	LOW DAILY DOSE (μg)	MEDIAN DAILY DOSE (μg)	HIGH DAILY DOSE (μg)
Beclomethasone dipropionate	200-500	500-1000	>1000-2000
Budesonide*	200-400	400-800	>800-1600
Ciclesonide*	80-160	160-320	>320-1280
Flunisolide	500-1000	1000-2000	>2000
Fluticasone	100-250	250-500	>500-1000
Mometasone furoate*	200-400	400-800	>800-1200
Triamcinolone acetonide	400-1000	1000-2000	>2000

*Once-a-day dosing is acceptable.

Note: Some doses may be outside package labeling. Metered-dose inhaler doses are expressed as the amount of drug leaving the valve, not all of which is available to the patient. Dry powder inhaler doses are expressed as the amount of drug in the inhaler after activation.

Modified from 2010 Global Initiative for Asthma guidelines (*www.ginasthma.com*).

inhaled glucocorticoid is more effective than a double dose of glucocorticoids and similar in effect to salmeterol.[4]

Controller Treatments
Inhaled Corticosteroids

Inhaled corticosteroids (see Fig. 87-3), which have less systemic impact for a given level of therapeutic effect than systemic steroids, are effective controller treatments for improving lung function and preventing asthmatic exacerbations in patients with persistent asthma.[5] Accumulating data[6,7] indicate that treatment of patients whose disease can be categorized as "mild persistent asthma" can be limited to periods when the patients have increased asthma symptoms rather than requiring an inhaled corticosteroid on a regularly scheduled basis. However, inhaled corticosteroids do not change the natural history of asthma. A wide variety of inhaled corticosteroid products are on the market (Table 87-2). All available products are effective treatments of persistent asthma but differ in terms of cost, the magnitude of adrenal suppression, and the potential for systemic effects, including growth retardation in children, loss of bone mineralization, cataracts, and glaucoma. Overall, no convincing data are available to suggest that there is reason to prefer one corticosteroid over the others. Adverse effects common to all inhaled corticosteroids are oral thrush and hoarseness (attributed to myopathy of the laryngeal muscles); the risk and severity can be reduced by aerosol spacers and good oropharyngeal hygiene (i.e., rinsing out the mouth by gargling after dosing).

Antileukotrienes

Agents with the capacity to inhibit the synthesis of the leukotrienes (zileuton—controlled release [Zyflo-CR], 1200 mg twice daily) or the action of leukotrienes at the CysLT$_1$ receptor (montelukast [Singulair], 10 mg once a day; pranlukast [Onon, Ultair], 225 mg twice a day, not available in the United States; and zafirlukast [Accolate], 20 mg twice a day) are effective oral controller medications for patients with mild or moderate persistent asthma. In patients treatment with zileuton, function should be monitored for the first 3 to 6 months of treatment; if levels rise to more than three times the upper limit of normal, the drug should be stopped. Theophylline metabolism is slowed by zileuton, so monitoring of levels is indicated if both are prescribed. These treatments can be used on their own for mild persistent asthma or in combination with inhaled steroids for more severe asthma.

Long-Acting β-Agonists

In contrast to medium-acting β-agonists, long-acting β-agonists currently available in the United States (salmeterol [Serevent, 42 μg per puff; the same dose is labeled 50 μg per puff outside of the United States; one or two puffs should be delivered every 12 hours] and formoterol [Foradil, 12 μg through a proprietary dry powder inhaler every 12 hours]) have a duration of action of nearly 12 hours; they are considered a controller rather than a bronchodilator agent. Randomized controlled trials demonstrate that long-acting β-agonists should not be used as a sole controller agent. Other trials have shown that there are excess asthma deaths (about one for every 650 patient years of treatment) when long-acting β-agonists are used.[8] Therefore, long-acting β-agonists should be used only when they are given in concert with inhaled corticosteroids. Combination products with both inhaled steroids and long-acting β-agonists in the same aerosol device are available. These products prevent patients with asthma from using inhaled long-acting β-agonists without inhaled corticosteroids. When prescribing a combination inhaler, the physician should determine the inhaled dose of corticosteroids (fluticasone, budesonide, or beclomethasone) that the patient requires and then choose a combination product that will deliver a dose of long-acting β-agonist with the inhaled corticosteroid when given as two puffs twice per day. The dose of long-acting β-agonist varies with brand and type of inhaler used.

Theophylline

Theophylline and its more water-soluble congener aminophylline are moderately potent bronchodilators that are useful in both inpatient and outpatient management of asthma. The mechanism by which theophylline exerts its effects has not been established with certainty but is probably related to the inhibition of certain forms of phosphodiesterase. Theophylline is not widely used because of its toxicity and the wide variations in the rate of its metabolism, both in a single individual over time and among individuals in a population. Because blood levels need to be monitored for optimal dosing, most physicians have reserved theophylline for third- or fourth-line therapy. For most preparations, the starting dose should be about 300 mg/day; the frequency will depend on the preparation used.

Acceptable plasma levels for therapeutic effects are between 10 and 20 μg/mL; higher levels are associated with gastrointestinal, cardiac, and central nervous system toxicity, including anxiety, headache, nausea, vomiting, diarrhea, cardiac arrhythmias, and seizures. These last catastrophic complications may occur without antecedent mild side effects when plasma levels exceed 20 μg/mL. Because of these potentially life-threatening complications of treatment, plasma levels need to be measured with great frequency in hospitalized patients receiving intravenous aminophylline and less frequently in stable outpatients receiving one of the long-acting theophylline preparations. Most asthma care providers use dosing amounts and intervals to achieve steady-state theophylline levels of 10 to 14 μg/mL, thereby avoiding the toxicity associated with decrements in metabolism. Treatment with theophylline is recommended only for patients who have moderate or severe persistent asthma and who are receiving controller medications, such as inhaled steroids or antileukotrienes, but whose asthma is not adequately controlled.

Systemic Corticosteroids

Systemic corticosteroids are effective for the treatment of moderate to severe persistent asthma as well as for occasional severe exacerbations of asthma in a patient with otherwise mild asthma, but the mechanism of their therapeutic effect has not been established. No consensus has been reached on the specific type, dose, or duration of corticosteroid to be used in the treatment of asthma. In nonhospitalized patients with asthma refractory to standard therapy, a steroid "pulse" with initial doses of prednisone on the order of 40 to 60 mg/day, tapered to zero during 7 to 14 days, is recommended. For patients who cannot stop taking steroids without having recurrent uncontrolled bronchospasm despite the addition of multiple other controller treatments, alternate-day administration of oral steroids is preferable to daily treatment. For patients whose asthma requires in-hospital treatment but is not considered life-threatening, an initial intravenous bolus of 2 mg/kg of hydrocortisone, followed by continuous infusion of 0.5 mg/kg/hour, has been shown to be beneficial within 12 hours. In attacks of asthma that are considered life-threatening, the use of intravenous methylprednisolone (125 mg every 6 hours) has been advocated. In each case, as the patient improves, oral steroids are substituted for intravenous steroids, and the oral dose is tapered during 1 to 3 weeks; addition of inhaled steroids to the regimen is strongly recommended when oral steroids are started.

Monoclonal Antibody Treatment
Omalizumab

Subcutaneous administration of omalizumab, a humanized murine monoclonal antibody that binds circulating IgE, is associated with decreased serum free (not total) IgE levels. In patients who have moderate to severe allergic asthma with elevated levels of serum IgE and who are receiving inhaled corticosteroids, omalizumab treatment improves asthma control even as doses of inhaled steroids are decreased. Dosing is guided by weight and by pretreatment IgE levels: a monthly subcutaneous dose of 0.016 mg × body weight (kg) × IgE level (IU/mL). For example, in a patient weighing 70 kg with a pretreatment total IgE level of 300 IU/mL, 336 mg of omalizumab would be administered monthly by subcutaneous injection. Dosing calculators can be found online (e.g., *http://www.xolairhcp.com/xolairhcp/determining-the-dose.html*). Anti-IgE antibodies can reduce exacerbations and improve quality of life in patients with severe allergic asthma, but their place in treatment schema has not been established. Because of the potential for anaphylaxis, all patients need to be monitored after injection; the duration of the monitoring period is not specified by the U.S. Food and Drug Administration (FDA), but most physicians monitor for 30 to 60 minutes.

Mepolizumab

Mepolizumab is a monoclonal antibody directed against IL-5. Although it is not approved for clinical use, in small randomized trials it reduced asthma exacerbations among relatively rare patients with moderately severe asthma who still had sputum eosinophilia despite treatment with oral and inhaled corticosteroids. Among patients with more conventional asthma, however, mepolizumab treatment did not have a salutary effect.

Other Controller Drugs

Cromolyn sodium (one or two puffs from a metered-dose inhaler three or four times a day) and nedocromil sodium (two puffs from a metered-dose inhaler three or four times a day) are nonsteroid inhaled treatments that have proved beneficial in the management of mild to moderate persistent asthma. They appear to be most useful in pediatric populations or when an identifiable stimulus (such as exercise or allergen exposure) elicits an asthmatic response.

The use of systemic gold (as in rheumatoid arthritis), methotrexate, or cyclosporine has been suggested as adjunctive treatment of patients with severe chronic asthma who cannot otherwise discontinue high-dose corticosteroid treatment. However, these agents are experimental, and their routine use is not advocated. Despite initial encouraging trials, agents that inhibit the action of tumor necrosis factor-α do not benefit patients with asthma and should not be used.

Based on the concern that asthma could be caused by silent gastroesophageal reflux disease, treatment with a proton pump inhibitor has been advocated in patients with mild to moderate asthma even if in the absence of gastrointestinal symptoms. Adequately powered clinical studies suggest that this approach provides no benefit for asthma control.**9**

Vaccination for Seasonal Influenza and Pneumococcal Disease

Vaccination of patients for seasonal influenza is safe and not associated with enhanced asthma exacerbations. Vaccination against seasonal influenza and pneumococcal disease is recommended in patients with asthma.

Radio Frequency Ablation of Airway Smooth Muscle

A proprietary system to ablate airway smooth muscle by delivering radio frequency energy through a bronchoscopically placed probe has reduced asthma exacerbations in sham controlled trials among patients whose asthma remained out of control despite the use of multiple controller medications. A device for such treatment was recently approved by the FDA.

Control-Driven Asthma Therapy

Because all asthma treatment is symptomatic (i.e., no current treatment changes the disease history), the approach to the management of asthma is to titrate treatment to achieve an adequate level of control. If a patient's asthma is well controlled, treatment can be continued or "stepped down" (see Fig. 87-2).**10** If a patient's asthma is poorly controlled, treatment intensity should be stepped up. At the mild end of the spectrum, a patient who has rare limitations in activities of daily life, has nearly normal lung function, and sleeps without interruption from asthma can be prescribed nothing more than inhaled rescue treatment on an as-needed basis. In general, if a patient can control his or her asthma with the use of a single metered-dose inhaler of rescue treatment dispensed every 7 to 8 weeks or less frequently, there is no need for background controller treatment. If a patient has a requirement for more rescue treatment, has symptoms that interfere with sleeping through the night, or has moderately deranged lung function, controller therapy should be added.

Single-agent controller therapy should consist of an inhaled corticosteroid or an antileukotriene. If control is not achieved with one of these agents, the patient can be switched to the other or have a second agent added. The best studied two-agent combination is inhaled corticosteroids and a long-acting inhaled β_2-adrenergic agonist, available in a single inhaler under the trade names of Symbicort and Advair in the United States. These combinations provide excellent disease control and often allow a reduction in the dose of inhaled corticosteroids. Data indicate that another combination, an antileukotriene and inhaled steroid, is more effective than either treatment alone, but this regimen does not have as substantial an evidence base as the combination of inhaled corticosteroids and a long-acting β-agonist.

Specific Treatment Scenarios

Concurrent Pulmonary Infection

In some patients, acute exacerbations of asthma may be due to concurrent infection, which requires targeted therapy (Chapters 88, 90, and 97).

Aspirin-Exacerbated Respiratory Disease (Previously Termed Aspirin-Induced Asthma)

Approximately 5% of patients with moderate to severe persistent asthma develop asthma when they ingest agents that inhibit cyclooxygenase, such as aspirin and other nonsteroidal anti-inflammatory drugs (Chapter 36). Inhibitors of cyclooxygenase 2 are less likely to cause these reactions, but aspirin-type reactions have been reported in sensitive patients treated with selective cyclooxygenase 2 inhibitors. Although the physiologic manifestations of laboratory-based aspirin challenge can be blocked by leukotriene pathway inhibitors, these agents do not prevent clinical aspirin-exacerbated respiratory disease. Thus, patients with this form of asthma must avoid aspirin and other nonsteroidal anti-inflammatory drugs.

Asthma in the Emergency Department

When a patient with asthma presents for acute emergency care, objective measures of the severity of the attack, including quantification of pulsus paradoxus and measurement of airflow rates (PEFR or FEV$_1$), should be evaluated in addition to the usual vital signs. If the attack has been prolonged and failed to respond to treatment with bronchodilators (e.g., albuterol by metered-dose inhaler, two puffs every 2 to 3 hours) and high-dose inhaled steroids (e.g., more than 2000 µg per day of beclomethasone or half that amount of fluticasone) before arrival at the emergency department, intravenous steroids (40 to 60 mg of methylprednisolone or its equivalent) should be administered. If the patient has not been receiving treatment with a leukotriene receptor antagonist, such agents should be administered (10 mg of montelukast or 20 mg of zafirlukast) as soon as possible.**11** Treatment with inhaled β-agonists (either nebulized albuterol, 0.5 mL of a 0.5% solution—repeated at 20- to 30-minute intervals, or albuterol by metered-dose inhaler, two puffs every 30 minutes) should be used until the PEFR or FEV$_1$ increases to greater than 40% of the predicted values. If this point is not reached within 2 hours, admission to the hospital for further treatment is strongly advocated.

When patients have PEFR and FEV$_1$ values that are greater than 60% of their predicted value on arrival in the emergency department, treatment with inhaled β_2-agonists alone, albuterol (0.5 mL of an albuterol 0.083% solution) or equivalent, is likely to result in an objective improvement in airflow rates. If significant improvement takes place in the emergency department, such patients can usually be treated as outpatients with inhaled β_2-agonists and a controller agent (see Fig. 87-2). A good strategy is to add inhaled corticosteroids if the patient has not been receiving this treatment or has been using a single controller therapy.

For patients whose PEFR and FEV$_1$ values are between 40% and 60% of the values predicted at the time of initial evaluation in the emergency care setting, a plan of treatment varying in intensity between these two plans is indicated. Failure to respond to treatment by objective criteria (PEFR or FEV$_1$) within 2 hours of arrival at the emergency department is an indication for the use of systemic corticosteroids.

Status Asthmaticus

The asthmatic subject whose PEFR or FEV$_1$ does not increase to greater than 40% of the predicted value with treatment, whose PaCO$_2$ increases without improvement of indices of airflow obstruction, or who develops major complications such as pneumothorax or pneumomediastinum should be admitted to the hospital for close monitoring. Frequent treatments with inhaled β-agonists (0.5 mL of an albuterol 0.083% solution every 2 hours), intravenous aminophylline (at doses to yield maximal acceptable plasma levels, that is, 15 to 20 µg/mL; 500- to 1000-mg loading dose given during an hour followed by an infusion of 30 to 60 mg/hour), and high-dose intravenous steroids (methylprednisolone, 40 to 60 mg every 4 to 6 hours) are indicated. Oxygen should be administered by face mask or nasal cannula in amounts sufficient to achieve SaO$_2$ values between 92 and 94%; a higher FIO$_2$ promotes absorption atelectasis and provides no therapeutic benefit. If objective evidence of an infection is present, appropriate treatment should be given for that infection. If no improvement is seen with treatment and if respiratory failure appears imminent, bronchodilator treatment should be intensified to the maximum tolerated by the patient as indicated by the maximum tolerated heart rate, usually 130 to 140 beats per minute. If indicated, intubation of the trachea and mechanical ventilation can be instituted; in this case, the goal should be to provide a level of ventilation just adequate to sustain life but *not sufficient to normalize arterial blood gases*. For example, a PaCO$_2$ of 60 to 70 mm Hg, or even higher, is acceptable for a patient in status asthmaticus.

Asthma in Pregnancy

Asthma may be exacerbated, remain unchanged, or remit during pregnancy (Chapter 247). There need not be substantial departures from the ordinary management of asthma during pregnancy. However, no unnecessary medications should be administered; systemic steroids should be used sparingly to avert fetal complications, and certain drugs should be avoided, including tetracycline (as a treatment of intercurrent infection), ipratropium bromide (which may cause fetal tachycardia), terbutaline (which is contraindicated during active labor because of its tocolytic effects), and iodine containing mucolytics (such as saturated solution of potassium iodide). Moreover, use of prostaglandin F$_2\alpha$ as an abortifacient should be avoided in asthmatic patients.

PROGNOSIS

Asthma is a chronic relapsing disorder. Most patients have recurrent attacks without a major loss in lung function for many years. A minority of patients experience a significant irreversible loss in lung function over and above the normal pulmonary senescence. Methods to distinguish these various clinical phenotypes have not been developed.

Grade A

1. Shaw DE, Berry MA, Thomas M, et al. The use of exhaled nitric oxide to guide asthma management: a randomized controlled trial. *Am J Respir Crit Care Med.* 2007;176:231-237.
2. de Jongste JC, Carraro S, Hop WC, et al, for the CHARISM Study Group. Daily telemonitoring of exhaled nitric oxide and symptoms in the treatment of childhood asthma. *Am J Respir Crit Care Med.* 2009;179:93-97.

3. Szefler SJ, Mitchell H, Sorkness CA, et al. Management of asthma based on exhaled nitric oxide in addition to guideline-based treatment for inner-city adolescents and young adults: a randomised controlled trial. *Lancet.* 2008;372:1065-1072.
4. Peters SP, Kunselman SJ, Icitovic N, et al. Tiotropium bromide step-up therapy for adults with uncontrolled asthma. *N Engl J Med.* 2010;363:1715-1726.
5. Busse WW, Pedersen S, Pauwels RA, et al, for the START Investigators Group. The Inhaled Steroid Treatment As Regular Therapy in Early Asthma (START) study 5-year follow-up: effectiveness of early intervention with budesonide in mild persistent asthma. *J Allergy Clin Immunol.* 2008;121:1167-1174.
6. Boushey HA, Sorkness CA, King TS, et al, for the National Heart, Lung, and Blood Institute's Asthma Clinical Research Network. Daily versus as-needed corticosteroids for mild persistent asthma. *N Engl J Med.* 2005;352:1519-1528.
7. Papi A, Canonica GW, Maestrelli P, et al, for the BEST Study Group. Rescue use of beclomethasone and albuterol in a single inhaler for mild asthma. *N Engl J Med.* 2007;356:2040-2052.
8. Nelson HS, Weiss ST, Bleecker ER, et al, for the SMART Study Group. The Salmeterol Multicenter Asthma Research Trial: a comparison of usual pharmacotherapy for asthma or usual pharmaco-therapy plus salmeterol. *Chest.* 2006;129:15-26.
9. Mastronarde JG, Anthonisen NR, Castro M, et al, for the American Lung Association Asthma Clinical Research Centers. Efficacy of esomeprazole for treatment of poorly controlled asthma. *N Engl J Med.* 2009;360:1487-1499.
10. Peters SP, Anthonisen N, Castro M, et al, for the American Lung Association Asthma Clinical Research Centers. Randomized comparison of strategies for reducing treatment in mild persistent asthma. *N Engl J Med.* 2007;356:2027-2039.
11. Silverman RA, Nowak RM, Korenblat PE, et al. Zafirlukast treatment for acute asthma-evaluation in a randomized, double-blind, multicenter trial. *Chest.* 2004;126:1480-1489.

SUGGESTED READINGS

Gibson PG, McDonald VM, Marks GB. Asthma in older adults. *Lancet.* 2010;376:803-813. *Review.*
Lazarus SC. Emergency treatment of asthma. *N Engl J Med.* 2010;363:755-764. *Review.*
Morjaria JB, Proiti M, Polosa R. Stratified medicine in selecting biologics for the treatment of severe asthma. *Curr Opin Allergy Clin Immunol.* 2011;11:58-63. *An approach to the use of newer biologic agents.*

88

CHRONIC OBSTRUCTIVE PULMONARY DISEASE

DENNIS E. NIEWOEHNER

DEFINITIONS

Chronic obstructive pulmonary disease (COPD) is now the preferred term for a condition that is characterized by progressive, largely irreversible airflow obstruction, usually with clinical onset in middle-aged or elderly persons with a history of cigarette smoking, and which cannot be attributed to another specific disease, such as bronchiectasis (Chapter 90) or asthma (Chapter 87). Commonly used terms for this condition in the past included *chronic bronchitis* and *emphysema*. That terminology is outdated because nearly all patients with a clinical diagnosis of COPD have both air space destruction (i.e., emphysema) and pathologic changes of the conducting airways consistent with chronic bronchitis.

Emphysema is defined pathologically by abnormal enlargement of the air spaces owing to destruction and deformation of alveolar walls. The severity of emphysema may vary widely in COPD patients with similar degrees of airflow obstruction. Chronic bronchitis is defined clinically as persistent cough and sputum production and pathologically as abnormal enlargement of the mucous glands within the central cartilaginous airways. Chronic bronchitis was once thought to be a key element in the pathogenesis of chronic airflow obstruction, but it is now known that increased airflow resistance in COPD can be attributed principally to a variety of pathologic changes within the distal airways of the lung ("small airways disease").

EPIDEMIOLOGY

COPD represents a growing global public health problem, although estimates vary widely according to the definition used. Cigarette smoking (Chapter 31) is the principal risk factor for COPD, so prevalence tends to reflect societal smoking habits with a lag phase of 20 to 30 years. Cigarette consumption has leveled off or decreased in large segments of North America and Europe, but the prevalence of COPD may continue to increase as these populations age. A greater future burden of COPD may be anticipated in Asia and other regions of the world because of rapidly increasing cigarette consumption.

More than 10% of the population older than 45 years in the United States has airflow obstruction of at least moderate severity as judged by spirometric criteria. COPD is the fourth leading cause of death in the United States, with mortality in women now exceeding that in men. COPD is projected to become the third leading cause of death worldwide by 2020. In 2007, medical costs and lost productivity attributable to COPD exceeded $40 billion in the United States. Direct medical costs rise precipitously as COPD becomes more severe, with hospitalization for exacerbations accounting for more than one half of the total.

Cigarette Smoking

Cigarette smoking is the principal cause of COPD, but the relationship between smoking and COPD is complex and incompletely understood. Airflow obstruction is the sentinel physiologic disturbance in COPD, and the forced expiratory volume in the first second (FEV_1) is the single best indicator of severity. Cigarette smoking causes declines in lung function that exceed those expected from aging alone, and the magnitude of loss is dependent on both the intensity and duration of exposure to cigarette smoke. Thus, the cumulative effects of smoking largely account for the increasing prevalence of COPD with advancing age.

Individual losses of lung function vary widely, even after adjustment for smoking intensity. After age 30 years, everyone loses lung function on a yearly basis, but smoking further impacts the rate of lung function loss. The mean annual reduction in the FEV_1 (Chapter 85) in normal nonsmoking white men is about 25 mL per year, but the loss increases to an average of about 40 mL per year among smokers (Fig. 88-1). A small minority of smokers, "susceptible smokers," suffer annual FEV_1 losses of 100 mL or more and may develop clinically significant airflow obstruction in the fourth and fifth decades of life. Factors that distinguish the susceptible smoker from the average smoker remain largely unknown.

Adverse effects of cigarette smoke on lung function may extend as far back as fetal development. Maternal smoking during pregnancy, secondhand cigarette smoke exposure during early childhood, and active smoking during adolescence impair lung growth. As a consequence, the lower lung function in early adulthood constitutes a significant risk factor for COPD later in life.

Other Environmental Exposures

Workers exposed to dust in certain workplace environments, such as mines, cotton mills, and grain-handling facilities, commonly develop respiratory symptoms and may suffer permanent loss of lung function (Chapter 93). In some regions of the world, repeated exposures to biomass combustion in confined living quarters causes airflow obstruction. Current urban air pollution in economically advanced countries appears to have little effect on the prevalence of airflow obstruction, but this factor may be more important in heavily polluted urban centers in industrializing countries.

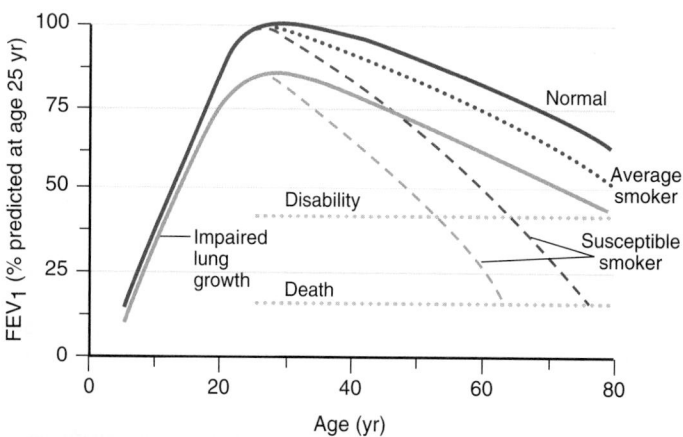

FIGURE 88-1. Lung growth occurs during childhood and adolescence with the forced expiratory volume in one second (FEV_1) reaching a maximum at about 25 years of age. Thereafter, the FEV_1 steadily declines owing to normal aging effects. Lung function declines more rapidly in smokers, but the average effect is so small that clinically significant airflow obstruction would never develop. However, a proportion of "susceptible smokers" lose lung function much faster than the average, so they develop disabling chronic obstructive pulmonary disorder (COPD). If lung growth is impaired, lung function reserve is less as a young adult, and a susceptible smoker will develop disabling COPD at an earlier age.

Respiratory Infections

Recurrent respiratory infections were once thought to be a major factor in the development of airflow obstruction, but longitudinal cohort studies have yielded inconclusive findings. An effect, if present, appears weak relative to cigarette smoking. Whether childhood respiratory infections leave residual effects on adult lung function is similarly unclear.

Airway Responsiveness

Acute bronchoconstriction after inhalation of dilute concentrations of methacholine or histamine, termed *bronchial hyperresponsiveness* (Chapter 87), is a defining feature of asthma but is also present in many COPD patients. Bronchial hyperresponsiveness independently predicts accelerated loss of lung function in persons with mild to moderate COPD, especially among persons who continue to smoke.

Genetic Factors

A severe deficiency of α_1-antitrypsin, which is the only proven genetic risk factor for COPD, is found in about 1-2% of patients with an established diagnosis of COPD. Alpha-1-antitrypsin, which is a serine protease inhibitor that is secreted into the circulation from the liver, is thought to protect lung tissue against digestion by neutrophil elastase and related serine proteinases that have been implicated in the pathogenesis of human emphysema. The most common allele at the α_1-antitrypsin genetic locus is M, and MM homozygotes have what are considered normal levels of α_1-antitrypsin (100 to 300 mg/dL). Numerous variant alleles have been identified, but severe deficiency is most commonly found in persons who are homozygous for the Z allele, in whom serum levels are generally less than 20 to 30% of the lower range of normal. Affected persons are very susceptible to cigarette smoke–induced damage and may develop severe COPD at a relatively early age. The risk for clinically important emphysema appears to be much less if patients with the risk alleles do not smoke. Emphysema associated with severe α_1-antitrypsin deficiency is characteristically of the panacinar type with a predominant basal distribution.

About 2 to 3% of northern European populations possess the MZ heterozygote serum and have α_1-antitrypsin levels about half of normal. Whether these individuals are at greater risk for developing COPD remains unclear. Familial aggregations of COPD not attributed to α_1-antitrypsin deficiency states suggest additional genetic risks. Women with severe COPD appear to have relatively more airway disease and less emphysema compared with men with similar airflow obstruction.

PATHOBIOLOGY

Pathology

Emphysema

Emphysema is characterized by abnormal enlargement of the air spaces distal to the terminal bronchiole, with destruction of the alveolar walls but without obvious fibrosis. The terminal bronchiole, which is the most distal nonalveolated airway within the bronchial tree, supplies ventilation to a lung unit that is termed the *acinus*. Distal to the terminal bronchiole are two or three generations of partially alveolated respiratory bronchioles, and then the alveolar zone, where most gas exchange occurs. Air spaces may enlarge throughout the alveolated zone owing to destruction or rearrangement of their walls.

Human emphysema consists of two major subtypes. Centriacinar emphysema localizes to the respiratory bronchioles just distal to the terminal bronchiole, whereas the remainder of the acinus is largely spared. Individual lesions, which may be up to 10 mm in diameter, tend to be more prominent in the upper lobe. Severe centriacinar emphysema is almost always related to cigarette smoking, but mild centriacinar emphysema can occur from other environmental exposures. Focal areas of inflammation, fibrosis, and carbonaceous pigment are commonly present in adjacent alveolar and bronchiolar walls.

In panacinar emphysema, alveolar ducts are diffusely enlarged; adjacent alveoli may become effaced to the extent that individual units can no longer be identified. With progression of the disease, individual lesions can coalesce to form large bullae. Panacinar emphysema, which is typical of severe α_1-antitrypsin deficiency, also commonly occurs in patients in whom the major risk factor for COPD is cigarette smoking. Most patients with severe COPD appear to have mixed elements of centriacinar and panacinar emphysema, and individual subtypes cannot be reliably distinguished in advanced disease.

Chronic Bronchitis and Bronchiolitis

Mucous glands, located between the epithelial basement membrane and the cartilage plates within the central bronchial tree, and goblet cells in the airway epithelium secrete mucus into the bronchial lumen to aid in host defenses. Enlargement of the bronchial mucous glands and expansion of the epithelial goblet cell population, which occur commonly in COPD, are correlated with clinical symptoms of cough and excess sputum production but not with airflow obstruction. A low-grade inflammatory response, consisting of neutrophils, macrophages, and CD8+ T lymphocytes, may also be seen in the cartilaginous airways of COPD patients.

The principal sites of increased airflow resistance in COPD are the small distal airways that have an internal diameter near the lung's functional residual capacity of less than 2 mm. The earliest pathologic changes identified in young cigarette smokers consist of focal collections of brown-pigmented macrophages in the respiratory bronchiole and a sparse infiltrate of neutrophils and lymphocytes in the walls of the terminal bronchiole. In older patients with established COPD, the inflammatory response is more intense, but still with a similar mix of neutrophils, macrophages, and lymphocytes. Other pathologic changes in the distal airways include fibrosis, goblet cell and squamous cell metaplasia of the lining epithelium, smooth muscle enlargement within the airway walls, and scattered regions of mucous plugging. Compared with normal subjects, distal airways in patients with COPD have thicker airway walls and smaller lumens.

Pulmonary Vasculature

Hypoxemia causes vasoconstriction in small pulmonary arteries and a consequent increase in pulmonary vascular resistance. Vascular remodeling in response to chronic hypoxemia results in irreversible pulmonary hypertension (Chapter 68). Medial smooth muscle enlargement and intimal fibrosis in small pulmonary arteries are the most important vascular changes. Additionally, a substantial portion of the capillary bed may be destroyed by severe emphysema.

Pathogenesis

Emphysema appears to be caused by an elastase-antielastase imbalance in the lung, due either to elastase excess or to antielastase deficiency. Human lungs contain a rich network of elastin-containing fibers and other matrix proteins that confer structural integrity and elasticity to alveolar walls. Intratracheal instillation of proteinases, particularly those capable of hydrolyzing native elastin, induce lesions with morphologic and functional features of human emphysema in experimental animals. Chronic inflammation induced from cigarette smoke increases the burden of inflammatory cell-derived proteinases within lung parenchyma. Severe deficiencies of α_1-antitrypsin, a potent inhibitor of neutrophil elastase and other serine proteinases, is associated with development of severe panacinar emphysema in humans. In addition to neutrophil elastase, other neutrophil-derived serine proteinases, such as proteinase 3 and cathepsin G, and matrix metalloproteinases degrade elastin and other matrix components, including collagen, proteoglycans, and fibronectin. A macrophage-derived metalloproteinase, MMP-12, is essential to the development of cigarette smoke–induced emphysema in an animal model, and genetic studies show a linkage with the region of the genome containing DNA encoding MMP-12.

Relatively less is understood about the pathogenesis of distal airways disease. Particulate matter and toxic gases from inhaled cigarette smoke initiate an inflammatory response composed primarily of macrophages and neutrophils. This early inflammatory response may be mediated by the innate defense system as a response to cell injury. In more advanced disease, inflammation persists even after the patient has stopped smoking. At this stage, humoral and cellular components of the adaptive immune system may predominate, possibly in response to infection or specific antigens from other sources. Infiltration of airway walls with CD4+, CD8+, and B lymphocytes is a prominent feature of more advanced COPD. Repair from either type of immune response might cause airway remodeling by stimulating connective tissue matrix synthesis and smooth muscle formation and by increasing the proportion of mucus-secreting goblet cells within the epithelial layer.

Pathophysiology

Lung and Heart Mechanics

Elastic recoil refers to the lung's intrinsic tendency to deflate following inflation. A dense labyrinth of elastic fibers and other matrix elements within the lung parenchyma, along with surface tension at the alveolar air-liquid interface, confers this important mechanical property. Elastic recoil maintains the patency of small airways through radial alveolar attachments, similar to the way a tent is held up by its guy ropes, and provides a portion of the driving pressure during expiration. Age-related loss of lung elasticity largely explains the normal decline in FEV_1 with advancing age. In emphysema, loss of lung elastic recoil results from damage to elastic fibers and loss of alveolar surface area.

An increase in bronchial airflow resistance is another sentinel feature of lung mechanics in COPD. The increased resistance in COPD is due primarily to changes in the small airways of less than 2 mm diameter. Compared with normal lungs, peripheral airflow resistance of COPD is larger by an order of magnitude or more. In contrast, airflow resistance in the central airways of lungs from COPD patients differs little from that of normal lungs. One of the key physiologic aspects of COPD is limitation of this expiratory airflow (Fig. 88-2) owing to loss of lung elastic recoil and increased viscous resistance to airflow in the small airways (Chapter 85). The severity of emphysema and airflow obstruction is directly related to impaired left ventricular filling, reduced stroke volume, and lower cardiac output without reducing the ejection fraction.

Gas Exchange

Mild hypoxemia may be detected in the early stages of COPD, and hypoxemia often becomes more prominent as airflow obstruction worsens. Hypercapnia usually appears only with severe COPD but is sometimes absent even in late-stage disease. Ventilation-perfusion mismatching, owing to changes in both the airways and pulmonary vessels, is largely responsible for hypoxemia, with uneven ventilation being the primary event. Gas exchange is most efficient when the ratio of ventilation to perfusion is uniform in all lung regions. In COPD, there is "wasted ventilation" because some lung regions have inadequate pulmonary blood flow for the ventilation. The calculated A-a gradient for oxygen is larger than anticipated for the patient's age (Chapter 103). Thus, in most cases of COPD, modest increases in the fraction of inspired oxygen result in a resolution of clinical hypoxemia.

CLINICAL MANIFESTATIONS

History and Physical Examination

COPD should be suspected in all adults who complain of chronic respiratory symptoms, particularly dyspnea (Chapter 83) that limits activities of daily living. Clinical features that increase the likelihood of COPD include older age, current or past cigarette use, insidious onset of dyspnea with slow progression, history of acute bronchitis for which medical care is sought, and symptoms of chronic cough, sputum production, or wheezing. Symptoms of cough and sputum may antedate dyspnea by many years. Some patients date the onset of dyspnea to a respiratory infection, but careful questioning usually elicits some history of impaired exercise tolerance before that event. Absence of cigarette smoking does not preclude a diagnosis of COPD because a few persons develop severe irreversible airflow obstruction without smoking history and even without known genetic predispositions. Some nonsmokers may relate a history of occupational dust or noxious gas exposure (Chapter 94), but sometimes no putative cause can be discerned.

The physical examination is usually normal in patients with mild to moderate disease, and characteristic physical signs may be absent even in severe disease. Physical examination findings commonly present in severe COPD include the appearance of a barrel-shaped chest, low diaphragm detected by percussion, prolonged expiratory phase, and use of accessory muscles of respiration. Heart sounds are usually distant, and auscultation of the chest may reveal diminished breath sounds or a variety of rhonchi, wheezes, and rattles. Auscultatory wheezes may be prominent, particularly during exacerbations, but this physical sign does not reliably differentiate COPD from asthma. With severe hypoxemia, cyanosis may be clinically evident. Clubbing is not associated with COPD, and its presence should suggest another diagnosis. Pedal edema, distended jugular veins, and hepatic congestion are signs of pulmonary hypertension and cor pulmonale (Chapter 68). Patients with advanced COPD may be cachectic, with loss of muscle mass and subcutaneous fat.

Clinical Phenotypes

One of the more enduring efforts to categorize COPD into subtypes is the description of the patients as either "pink puffers" or "blue bloaters." The pink puffer is described as a cachectic individual with unrelenting dyspnea, clinical and radiographic signs of severe lung hyperinflation, and normal or near-normal arterial blood gases at rest. Salient features of the blue bloater are a stout body habitus, chronic cough and sputum, less troubling dyspnea, and severe hypoxemia and hypercapnia resulting in polycythemia and signs of cor pulmonale. In the original description of these phenotypes, the pink puffer phenotype was equated with severe emphysema, whereas the blue bloater was thought to have predominant chronic bronchitis.

Selected COPD patients do fit one or the other of these clinical subtypes, but most cannot be simply categorized. Limited information from clinical and pathologic correlative studies fails to show a consistent association of either clinical subtype with distinguishing pathologic features in lung parenchyma or airways. The blue bloater phenotype may now be less common, possibly because hypoxemia is recognized and treated earlier or because some COPD patients once described as blue bloaters may have had coexisting obstructive sleep apnea (Chapter 100).

COPD patients with similar degrees of airflow obstruction vary greatly with respect to severity of dyspnea, impairment of exercise tolerance, frequency of exacerbations, body habitus, and severity of arterial blood gas disturbances. There is limited understanding about the mechanisms underlying these clinical characteristics.

DIAGNOSIS

Pulmonary Function Tests

Airflow obstruction can be determined only by spirometry. If the ratio of FEV_1 to FVC is less than 0.70 (Chapter 85) after administration of an inhaled bronchodilator, an obstructive defect is present (Table 88-1). A large improvement of perhaps 30 to 40% in FEV_1 after treatment with an inhaled

FIGURE 88-2. Inspiratory and expiratory flow-volume loops at rest, with exercise, and with maximal effort in a normal subject are compared with those in a patient with chronic obstructive pulmonary disorder (COPD). The normal subject can easily increase both tidal volume and breathing frequency to match the metabolic requirements of vigorous exercise. In contrast, the COPD patient exhibits maximal expiratory flow limitation even at rest and must breathe at larger lung volumes to optimize expiratory airflow. Lung hyperinflation requires greater respiratory work because the lung and chest wall become stiffer at larger volumes. This effect is accentuated during exercise, which causes end-expiratory lung volume to increase further. This phenomenon is described as *dynamic hyperinflation* and is an important mechanism in limiting exercise and causing dyspnea.

bronchodilator may help identify a patient with predominant asthma, but the test otherwise has little clinical utility and cannot reliably identify patients who will benefit from any particular form of therapy.

Lung volume measurements may help distinguish obstructive and restrictive lung diseases in selected patients, but they are unnecessary in most COPD patients. The diffusing capacity for carbon monoxide (D_{LCO}; Chapter 85) measures the uptake of carbon monoxide between inspired air and the blood stream. Decreases in the D_{LCO} reflect the loss of alveolar surface area that is available for gas transfer and roughly correspond to the severity of emphysema. However, the test provides information of no practical value in the customary management of COPD.

After the diagnosis is established, follow-up spirometry may help determine whether worsening breathlessness is due to COPD, as indicated by a decrease in FEV_1, or to another cause, such as heart failure (Chapter 58). However, repeated spirometry should not be used as a guide to drug therapy because the background variability of the measurement is large relative to treatment effects.

Oximetry

Hypoxemia and hypercapnia become increasingly common as COPD worsens. Because treatment with supplemental oxygen improves mortality, patients with severe COPD should be tested for hypoxemia at regular intervals. Hypoxemia can be detected and quantified by oximetry or arterial blood gases. Oximetry is generally preferred because it is simpler, cheaper, and causes no discomfort. The added information from a set of arterial blood gases (Chapter 103) is most helpful in COPD patients with severe exacerbations.

Radiographic Studies

Common signs of severe COPD on a chest radiograph include hyperinflated lungs, flattened diaphragms, and increased retrosternal clear space (Fig. 88-3). The walls of large emphysematous bullae may be visualized as thin curvilinear lines, and severe emphysema may appear as regions of relative hyperlucency. Chest radiographs are usually normal in mild to moderate COPD and sometimes in severe COPD. Hence, a chest radiograph is not an adequate diagnostic test for COPD, and it is used mostly to exclude other pulmonary diseases. Chest computed tomography (CT), which is a superior imaging modality to assess the magnitude and distribution of emphysema (Fig. 88-4), is not helpful in the usual management of COPD.

Other Studies

Measurement of the serum level of α_1-antitrypsin deficiency may be considered, particularly if the patient has a strong family history of COPD or if the onset of airflow obstruction occurs at an early age. If the α_1-antitrypsin level is less than 20 to 30% of normal, further testing with specialized phenotyping and genotyping studies is required to confirm the diagnosis.

Differential Diagnosis

COPD is most commonly confused with asthma (Chapter 87), particularly in older patients. Clinical features that favor asthma over COPD include onset of disease at an early age, presence of atopy, lack of a smoking history, substantial variability of symptoms over time, and largely reversible airflow obstruction. However, new onset of asthma may occur in elderly people, some asthmatics smoke, an atopic history is not a requisite for developing asthma, and airflow obstruction may become fixed in patients with severe, long-standing asthma. Because treatment is much the same, distinguishing asthma from COPD may not be so important.

Bronchiectasis (Chapter 90) is characterized by chronic inflammation and abnormal dilation of airways associated with chronic cough and expectoration of purulent sputum. It can be distinguished from COPD with a predominant bronchitis component by chest CT imaging.

Bronchiolitis obliterans is characterized by cicatricial narrowing of the distal airways with severe irreversible airflow obstruction. The condition may occur in association with collagen vascular diseases (Chapters 272 and 274) and is commonly seen after lung transplantation (Chapter 101). A similar

TABLE 88-1	STAGE AND SEVERITY OF COPD ACCORDING TO POSTBRONCHODILATOR SPIROMETRY
STAGE AND SEVERITY	**DEFINITION**
I: Mild	$FEV_1/FVC < 0.70$, $FEV_1 \geq 80\%$ of predicted
II: Moderate	$FEV_1/FVC < 0.70$, $50\% \leq FEV_1 < 80\%$ of predicted
III: Severe	$FEV_1/FVC < 0.70$, $30\% \leq FEV_1 < 50\%$ of predicted
IV: Very severe	$FEV_1/FVC < 0.70$, $FEV_1 < 30\%$ of predicted or FEV_1 < 50% of predicted plus chronic respiratory failure

Data from the Global Initiative for Chronic Obstructive Lung Disease. http://www.goldcopd.com.

FIGURE 88-3. **Posteroanterior (A) and lateral (B) radiographs of the thorax in a patient with emphysema.** The most obvious abnormalities are those associated with increased lung volume. The lungs appear dark because of their increased air relative to tissue. The diaphragms are caudal to their normal position and appear flatter than normal. The heart is oriented more vertically than normal because of caudal displacement of the diaphragm, and the transverse diameter of the rib cage is increased; as a result, the width of the heart relative to the rib cage on the posteroanterior view is decreased. The space between the sternum and heart and great vessels is increased on the lateral view.

disorder has been described with certain industrial inhalants, such as diacetyl, a butter-like flavoring manufactured for use with microwavable popcorn (Chapter 93). In nonsmokers, the diagnosis of bronchiolitis obliterans can be reliably inferred from history, the presence of irreversible airflow obstruction, and the absence of emphysema or other explanatory conditions on chest CT images. Attribution of cause in smokers is more difficult because the airway pathology with diacetyl exposure is similar to that found with cigarette smoke.

TREATMENT   **Rx**

Stable Disease
Smoking Cessation

Smoking cessation (Chapter 31) reduces symptoms of cough and sputum production in many patients with COPD, but it improves lung function to only a small extent (Fig. 88-5). Most important, after smoking cessation, the rate of decline of FEV_1 in patients with mild to moderate disease reverts back to that seen in lifelong nonsmokers, thereby making it unlikely that these former smokers will ever develop severe COPD. Smoking cessation in patients with

FIGURE 88-4. High-resolution axial computed tomography scan of a 1-mm section of the thorax of a patient with emphysema at the level of the tracheal carina. The right lung is on the *left*. Multiple large bullae—black holes—are evident. Many smaller areas of similar tissue destruction are also present in both lungs. The right upper lobe bronchus is seen entering the lung; its walls are thickened, suggesting chronic inflammation. (Courtesy of Dr. Bruce Maycher.)

mild to moderate COPD also improves long-term mortality by reducing both respiratory and cardiovascular deaths.**[1]** It is not known whether smoking cessation slows the decline in lung function or improves mortality in patients with severe COPD.

Limited information indicates that counseling and pharmacotherapy achieve the same low success rates in COPD patients as in the general population. COPD patients tend to quit smoking as the disease progresses, possibly because they have greater awareness of their disease or because cigarette smoke makes their respiratory symptoms worse. Information regarding abnormal spirometry does not motivate patients to quit smoking.

Bronchodilators

Both β_2-adrenergic agonists and anticholinergics are widely used to treat COPD (Table 88-2). Short-acting β_2-adrenergic agonists, such as albuterol and the short-acting anticholinergic ipratropium bromide, can be administered either by oral inhaler devices or by nebulization, with little objective superiority of one delivery device over the other if a spacer is used with oral inhaler devices. Longer-acting bronchodilators have largely replaced shorter-acting drugs, but a short-acting bronchodilator, such as albuterol, is still recommended for "rescue" or "as-needed" use in patients who experience bothersome dyspnea.

The inhaled long-acting bronchodilators widely used for COPD include the β_2-adrenergic agonists salmeterol and formoterol, both administered by one inhalation twice daily, and the anticholinergic tiotropium, administered by one inhalation once or twice daily. Compared with placebo, they consistently provide clinically meaningful improvement in respiratory health status in only about 10 to 15% of patients.**[2]** Tiotropium (18 μg once daily) appears to be superior to salmeterol (50 μg twice daily) for reducing exacerbations.**[3]**

Compared with placebo, both classes of long-acting bronchodilators reduce exacerbation rates by about 15 to 20% in relative terms. Because the average patient with severe COPD has about one serious exacerbation per year, the number of patients that need to be treated to prevent one exacerbation is about six.

Adverse symptomatic events of both classes of long-acting bronchodilators in COPD patients are generally minor. Despite concerns about their long-term safety, the largest and longest trials to date have shown no serious safety issues when long-acting β_2-adrenergic agonists or long-acting anticholinergics are used to treat COPD.

Theophylline is a poor bronchodilator that largely has been replaced with inhaled drugs, but its effect is additive when given along with inhaled bronchodilators. Theophylline may also reduce exacerbations. To be used effectively and safely, it should be started with an oral daily dose of between 150 and 300 mg and titrated to achieve serum levels of 8 to 12 μg/mL. Higher levels are poorly tolerated, especially in older patients. Theophylline interacts with numerous other drugs (e.g., allopurinol, diazepam, cimetidine, ciprofloxacin), and conditions such as heart failure and liver disease may reduce its elimination rates. Patients' drug levels must be monitored on a regular basis, and even a patient on a stable dose can develop toxic levels. Oral roflumilast, a phosphodiesterase-4 inhibitor at 500 μg once daily, can increase FEV_1 by 50 mL and reduce moderate to severe exacerbations of COPD, even in patients already treated with tiotropium.**[4]**

Corticosteroids

Inhaled corticosteroids produce marginal improvements in lung function and respiratory health status in COPD patients, and they reduce COPD exacerbation rates by about 15 to 20% in relative terms.**[5]** Inhaled corticosteroids combined with an inhaled long-acting β_2-agonist provide added benefit over that seen with either monotherapy. However, multiple large trials found little effect of inhaled corticosteroids on FEV_1 loss over periods of several years.

FEV_1, % predicted	80-65%	64-50%	49-30%	<30%

Smoking cessation and avoidance of other risk factors
Influenza and polysaccharide pneumococcal vaccinations
Short-acting bronchodilator when needed

Regular long-acting bronchodilator
Pulmonary rehabilitation

Oxygen therapy if hypoxemic
Inhaled steroids if exacerbation prone
Consider theophylline

Consider surgery

FIGURE 88-5. The flow diagram illustrates step management of stable COPD; more therapies are added as the disease becomes more severe. The percent predicted FEV_1 provides only a rough guide to the severity of the disease so other factors, such as exercise limitations and the frequency of exacerbations, should also be considered in the global assessment.

TABLE 88-2 COMMONLY USED MEDICATIONS FOR STABLE COPD

	MODE OF DELIVERY	DOSE AND FREQUENCY	POSSIBLE ADVERSE REACTIONS
SHORT-ACTING INHALED BRONCHODILATORS			
Albuterol (β_2-adrenergic agonist)	Inhaler	100 µg per inhalation; 1-2 inhalations every 4-6 hours, as needed	Palpitations, tachycardia, tremor, hypersensitivity reaction
	Nebulizer	2.5 mg; every 4-6 hours, as needed	
Ipratropium (anticholinergic)	Inhaler	17 µg per inhalation; 2 inhalations 4 times daily, up to 12 inhalations a day	Dry mouth, cough, blurred vision, hypersensitivity reaction
	Nebulizer	0.5 mg; every 6-8 hours	
Albuterol, ipratropium	Inhaler device	90 µg/18 µg per inhalation; 2 inhalations 4 times daily, up to 12 inhalations per day	All those occurring with either albuterol or ipratropium
	Nebulizer	2.5 mg/0.5 mg; 4 times daily, up to 2 additional doses daily	
LONG-ACTING INHALED BRONCHODILATORS			
Formoterol (β_2-adrenergic agonist)	Inhaler	12 µg; 1 inhalation twice daily	Dizziness, tremor, throat irritation, hypersensitivity reaction
	Nebulizer	20 µg; twice daily	
Salmeterol (β_2-adrenergic agonist)	Inhaler	50 µg; 1 inhalation twice daily	Headache, tremor, throat irritation, hypersensitivity reaction
Tiotropium (anticholinergic)	Inhaler	18 µg; one inhalation each morning	Dry mouth, urinary retention, symptoms of narrow-angle glaucoma, hypersensitivity reaction
INHALED CORTICOSTEROIDS			
Fluticasone powder	Inhaler	250 µg; 1-2 inhalations twice daily	Sore throat, dysphonia, headache, hypersensitivity reaction
Budesonide	Inhaler	160 µg; 1-2 inhalations twice daily	Nasopharyngitis, thrush, hypersensitivity reactions
COMBINATION β-ADRENERGIC AGONIST BRONCHODILATOR AND INHALED CORTICOSTEROID			
Fluticasone/salmeterol	Inhaler	250 µg/50 µg; 1 inhalation twice daily	All those occurring with either fluticasone or salmeterol
Budesonide/formoterol	Inhaler	160 µg/4.5 µg; 2 inhalations twice daily	All those occurring with either budesonide or formoterol
METHYLXANTHINES			
Theophylline (24-hour sustained release)	Pill	200-800 mg, once daily; start with daily dose of 150-300 mg and titrate to blood level of 8-12 µg/mL	Nausea and vomiting, seizures, tremor, insomnia, multifocal atrial tachyarrhythmia, hypersensitivity reaction

The most common adverse effects of inhaled corticosteroids are dysphonia and upper airway thrush. Observational studies suggest that inhaled corticosteroids may cause osteoporosis (Chapter 251) and cataracts (Chapter 431).

A few COPD patients are prescribed systemic corticosteroids on a regular basis, usually in doses of 10 to 15 mg per day of prednisone or its equivalent. These patients are sometimes considered "prednisone dependent" because it is frequently difficult to wean them completely off drug. There are no proven benefits of chronic, low-dose prednisone in COPD, and adverse effects involving bone, eyes, and other organs are well documented (Chapter 34). Consequently, efforts should be made to reduce or discontinue chronic systemic corticosteroids while optimizing other treatment.

Oxygen

Chronic hypoxemia in patients with COPD can induce irreversible pulmonary hypertension and cor pulmonale (Chapter 68). Long-term oxygen therapy extends life in patients who are persistently hypoxemic.[6] The principal qualifying criteria are an arterial PaO_2 of less than 56 mm Hg or an arterial oxygen saturation of less than 89%, both while breathing ambient air at rest in a stable clinical state. Patients should also be considered for home oxygen if their PaO_2 is less than 60 mm Hg in the presence of right heart failure or polycythemia. Treatment should consist of home oxygen to be used for at least 18 hours daily, to include sleep time. To determine an appropriate prescription, the oxygen flow rate should be adjusted in 1-L/minute increments at 15-minute intervals until the resting oxygen saturation remains above 90%. In qualifying patients, long-term oxygen may also decrease polycythemia and pulmonary hypertension and improve neuropsychiatric function. Oxygen does not improve mortality in patients with similarly severe airflow obstruction but milder hypoxemia.

Many patients with severe COPD may be normoxemic at rest while breathing ambient air but exhibit oxygen desaturation with exercise. Physicians commonly prescribe ambulatory oxygen in this setting, with the expectation that it will improve exercise tolerance and increase daily activity. Ambulatory oxygen modestly improves exercise endurance for such patients in a laboratory setting, but efforts to show benefit during activities of daily living have been mostly unsuccessful. It is also unclear whether COPD patients with isolated nocturnal hypoxemia benefit from oxygen therapy.

Immunizations

An annual influenza vaccination (Chapter 17) is recommended for all patients with COPD, although few trials have targeted this patient population. Observational studies suggest that influenza vaccination substantially reduces hospitalization and mortality rates in COPD patients. Polysaccharide pneumococcal vaccination (Chapter 17) is also recommended, although supporting evidence is weak.

Pulmonary Rehabilitation

COPD patients become increasingly sedentary as their disease progresses. Lack of physical activity causes muscular and cardiovascular deconditioning, which further complicates the ability to perform routine tasks. The principal goal of pulmonary rehabilitation is to reverse this process with a program of exercise endurance training. Educational and behavior modification elements are usually included in an effort to improve coping skills and psychological functioning. Most programs are hospital based and consist of 3- to 4-hour sessions, three times a week, over a 6- to 12-week period. Patients who become breathless with minimal activity or who have exercise limiting comorbidities are not suitable candidates.

Numerous randomized, controlled trials have shown that pulmonary rehabilitation confers substantial improvements in respiratory health status and in walking distance and possibly in reduction of health care use.[7] Unfortunately, the benefits of pulmonary rehabilitation erode rapidly in the absence of a continuation plan after completion of the initial program. Pulmonary rehabilitation is also not accessible to most patients for a variety of reasons.

Surgical Options

In lung volume reduction surgery (Chapter 101), severely emphysematous tissue is resected from the upper lobes of both lungs to permit less diseased portions of unresected lung to expand and function more normally. Patients who are severely disabled from COPD and who have no other major comorbid conditions may be candidates for this procedure if CT imaging shows that severe emphysema is mostly localized to the upper lobes. Compared with controls receiving no surgical treatment, lung volume reduction surgery improves lung function, exercise capacity, and respiratory health status in COPD patients with severe emphysema.[8] There is no mortality benefit from this procedure, with a possible exception in the subset of patients with both predominant upper lobe emphysema and low exercise capacity.

Lung transplantation is an option for patients who are severely incapacitated from COPD and have no major comorbid conditions (Chapter 101). Median survival after lung transplantation is only about 5 years, primarily because of the development of bronchiolitis obliterans, a form of chronic graft rejection causing severe airflow obstruction in the peripheral airways. It is unclear whether lung transplantation extends survival in patients with COPD, but patients who are fortunate enough to avoid complications are able to resume normal daily activities.

Exacerbations

Exacerbations represent an important element in the natural history of COPD. An exacerbation is defined as some combination of dyspnea, cough, and productive sputum, each of which has worsened from the stable state or has newly appeared. Exacerbations may also be associated with symptoms of rhinorrhea, sore throat, fever, and chest congestion. A symptom-based clinical event, as described previously, coupled with administration of an antibiotic or a systemic corticosteroid or admission to a hospital, is a definition that has been widely used in clinical trials.

Patients with severe COPD experience an average of about one such exacerbation per year along with additional milder exacerbations that meet the symptomatic definition but do not require a medical intervention. Exacerbations are acute in onset, but recovery may require several weeks. Severe exacerbations have a major adverse impact on health status and may cause permanent loss of lung function. Hospitalization for exacerbations consumes more than half of total medical costs for COPD. For poorly understood reasons, some patients suffer frequent exacerbations, whereas others have very few, despite similar degrees of airflow obstruction. Independent risk factors include low lung function, older age, history of frequent exacerbations and hospitalizations, presence of productive cough, and presence of cardiovascular comorbidities.

Respiratory infections are thought to cause most exacerbations, although many of these implicated microorganisms may be recovered from sputum during periods of stable disease. Bacteria commonly implicated include *Haemophilus influenzae* (Chapter 308), *Streptococcus pneumoniae* (Chapter 297), and *Moraxella catarrhalis* (Chapter 308). *Pseudomonas aeruginosa* (Chapter 314) and enteric gram-negative bacilli (Chapters 312 and 313) are less common but are seen in patients with very severe COPD who were recently hospitalized or intubated. Putative viral pathogens include rhinoviruses (Chapter 369), influenza (Chapter 372), parainfluenza (Chapter 371), and respiratory syncytial virus (Chapter 370). Periods of increased airborne pollution with diesel particulates, sulfur dioxide, ozone, and nitrogen dioxide are associated with more COPD hospitalizations, but no cause can be assigned to many exacerbations.

Evaluation and management of a patient with a suspected exacerbation varies according to severity. Mild exacerbations encountered in an office setting can be diagnosed and treated on the basis of a brief history and physical examination. Patients seen in emergency department or hospital settings generally are sicker and require a more extensive evaluation (Table 88-3). A chest radiograph should be obtained to look for signs of pneumonia (Chapter 97), pneumothorax (Chapter 99), and heart failure (Chapter 58). If pulmonary embolism (Chapter 98) is suspected, spiral CT of the chest is the test of choice. Arterial blood gases should be measured if there is any suspicion of hypercarbia because this information influences subsequent therapy. Sputum cultures need not be done routinely because they are unproven guides to antibiotic therapy. During seasonal outbreaks of influenza (Chapter 372), type A and B viruses can be identified with rapid commercially available assays. However, the sensitivity of these assays is only about 50 to 70%, so they should not be relied on to withhold antiviral therapy if there is a strong clinical suspicion of influenza.

Cardiac disease is a common comorbidity in COPD patients, and distinguishing a COPD exacerbation from left ventricular failure (Chapter 58) by history and physical examination alone is often problematic. Dyspnea (Chapter 83) is common to both conditions. Peripheral edema (Chapter 50) and elevated jugular venous pressure may occur with either left ventricular failure or with cor pulmonale secondary to COPD. Echocardiography (Chapter 55) and serum brain natriuretic peptide (BNP) levels (Chapter 58) are very useful in this clinical setting, although echocardiography is more difficult to perform in patients with severe COPD. BNP levels may be modestly elevated in both stable and exacerbated COPD in the absence of left ventricular dysfunction. A normal BNP level excludes a diagnosis of left heart failure with a high level of confidence, but an elevated level does not confirm its presence unless markedly elevated.

Decisions about the need for hospitalization rely mostly on clinical judgment because there are no well-validated guidelines. Clinical assessment should consider intensity of dyspnea, use of accessory muscles of respiration, arterial blood gas disturbances, hemodynamic stability, and mental alertness.

TABLE 88-3 GUIDELINE RECOMMENDATIONS FOR HOSPITAL MANAGEMENT OF COPD EXACERBATIONS

	GLOBAL INITIATIVE FOR CHRONIC OBSTRUCTIVE LUNG DISEASE*	AMERICAN THORACIC SOCIETY/ EUROPEAN RESPIRATORY SOCIETY[†]	NATIONAL INSTITUTE FOR CLINICAL EXCELLENCE[‡]
Date of statement	2010	2004	2010
Diagnostic testing	Chest radiograph, oximetry, ABGs, and ECG. Other testing as warranted by clinical indication.	Chest radiograph, oxygen saturation, ABGs, ECG, sputum Gram stain and culture.	Chest radiograph, ABG, ECG, complete blood count, sputum smear and culture, blood cultures if febrile.
Bronchodilator therapy	Inhaled short-acting β_2-agonist is recommended. Consider ipratropium if inadequate clinical response. Consider theophylline or aminophylline as second-line intravenous therapy.	Inhaled short-acting β_2-agonist and/or ipratropium with spacer or nebulizer, as needed.	Administer inhaled drugs by nebulizer or hand-held inhaler. Specific agents and dosing regimens not specified. Consider theophylline if inadequate response to inhaled bronchodilators.
Antibiotics	Recommended if (1) increases in dyspnea, sputum volume, and sputum purulence all are present; (2) increase in sputum purulence along with increase in either dyspnea or sputum volume; or (3) need for assisted ventilation. See original document for complex treatment algorithm.	Base choice on local bacterial resistance patterns. Consider amoxicillin/clavulanate or respiratory fluoroquinolones. If *Pseudomonas* species and/or other Enterobacteriaceae are suspected, consider combination therapy.	Administer only if history of purulent sputum. Initiate with an aminopenicillin, a macrolide, or a tetracycline, taking into account local bacterial resistance patterns. Adjust therapy according to sputum and blood cultures.
Systemic corticosteroids	Daily prednisolone 30-40 mg (or its equivalent) orally for 7-10 days.	Daily prednisone 30-40 mg orally for 10-14 days. Equivalent dose intravenously if unable to tolerate oral intake. Consider inhaled corticosteroids.	Daily prednisolone 30 mg (or its equivalent) orally for 7-14 days.
Supplemental oxygen	Maintain oxygen saturation >90%. Monitor ABGs for hypercapnia and acidosis.	Maintain oxygen saturation >90%. Monitor ABGs for hypercapnia and acidosis.	Maintain oxygen saturation within the individualized target range. Monitor ABGs.
Assisted ventilation	Indications for NPPV include severe dyspnea, acidosis (pH ≤ 7.35) and/or hypercapnia (P_{CO_2} > 45 mm Hg), and respiratory rate >25 breaths/min. Contraindications to NPPV include respiratory arrest, hemodynamic instability, impaired mental status, copious bronchial secretions, and extreme obesity. Intubate if contraindication to NPPV or failure of NPPV (worsening ABGs or clinical status). Consider likelihood of recovery and patient's wishes and expectations before intubation.	Consider with pH < 7.35 and P_{CO_2} > 45-60 mm Hg and respiratory rate > 24 breaths/min. Institute NPPV in a controlled environment, unless there are contraindications (e.g., respiratory arrest, hemodynamic instability, impaired mental status, copious bronchial secretions, and extreme obesity). Intubate if contraindication to NPPV or failure of NPPV (worsening ABGs or clinical status).	NPPV treatment of choice for persistent hypercapnic respiratory failure. Consider functional status, body mass index, home oxygen, comorbidities, prior ICU admissions, age, and FEV_1 when assessing suitability for intubation and ventilation.

*Data from http://www.goldcopd.com.
[†]Data from MacNee W. Standards for the diagnosis and treatment of patients with COPD: a summary of the ATS/ERS position paper. *Eur Respir J.* 2004;23:932-946.
[‡]Data from http://www.nice.org.uk.

ABGs, arterial blood gases; ECG, electrocardiogram; ICU, intensive care unit; NPPV, noninvasive positive pressure ventilation.

Guideline recommendations (see Table 88-3) for treatment of patients hospitalized for COPD exacerbations emphasize that antibiotics hasten recovery.**9** Antibiotics are most effective when cough and purulent sputum are present, but there are no well-validated methods for determining which patients should be treated. If patients are sufficiently ill to seek medical attention for an exacerbation, most should probably receive an antibiotic.

Most randomized placebo-controlled trials evaluated first-generation antibiotics, such as amoxicillin, trimethoprim-sulfamethoxazole, and tetracyclines, and it is unclear whether newer classes of antibiotics, such as macrolides and fluoroquinolones, are more effective. Choice of an antibiotic should be made with considerations to cost, safety, and local patterns of antibiotic resistance among the bacterial species commonly isolated from sputa during exacerbations. Doxycycline, 100 mg twice daily for 7 to 10 days, or trimethoprim/sulfamethoxazole, 160–800 mg twice daily for 7 to 10 days, would be reasonable choices for initial therapy in many locales.

Systemic corticosteroids improve lung function, shorten the recovery period, and prevent relapse when given to patients who are hospitalized or present to an emergency department with a COPD exacerbation.**10** Severely symptomatic patients seen in other clinical settings are also likely to benefit. Prednisone, 40 mg once daily for 10 to 14 days, is appropriate for most patients. Longer courses of systemic corticosteroid therapy are strongly discouraged because they are no more effective and they increase the likelihood of adverse effects. Parenteral corticosteroids should be given if gastrointestinal absorption is thought to be impaired. The major adverse effect of systemic corticosteroids is transient hyperglycemia, which may require treatment, particularly in patients with known diabetes mellitus (Chapter 237).

Patients should be encouraged to increase their use of short-acting bronchodilators during outpatient treatment of an exacerbation. For hospitalized patients, a short-acting bronchodilator should be administered on a regular schedule, every 4 to 6 hours and more frequently as needed. Anticholinergic and β₂-agonist agents are similarly effective, and a few small trials found no significant additive effect during exacerbations. Some patients express a preference for a nebulizer delivery system, although equivalent objective results can be achieved when inhalers are used with a spacer.

Sufficient oxygen should be provided to maintain arterial oxygen saturations just above 90%, usually with oxygen flow rates of 2 to 3 L/minute delivered through a nasal cannula. Even at low flow rates, oxygen therapy can be expected to increase $PaCO_2$ by an average of about 5 to 10 mm Hg in patients with chronic hypercapnia. It is prudent to use the lowest flow of oxygen that achieves the desired result. If oxygen is prescribed for hypoxemia during an exacerbation, it is important to retest the patient several weeks later after recovery to determine when long-term oxygen is needed.

The introduction of noninvasive positive-pressure ventilation (NIPPV) has significantly improved the care of patients with severe COPD exacerbations who have respiratory failure. With NIPPV, the patient wears a tightly fitting nasal or full facial mask that is attached to a positive-pressure ventilator, avoiding the need for an endotracheal tube or a tracheostomy (Chapter 105). Compared with usual care, treatment with NIPPV is associated with fewer intubations, a shorter hospital stay, and improved all-cause mortality.

PROGNOSIS

Severe COPD is associated with excess mortality, and lung function, usually expressed as the percent of predicted FEV_1, is the single strongest predictor of death. Only about one half of patients with an FEV_1 that is about 40% of predicted will survive 5 years. Additional risk factors include the severity of dyspnea, weight loss, limited walking distance, hospitalization for exacerbation, hypoxemia, hypercapnia, and impaired quality of life. The only interventions shown to reduce mortality are smoking cessation in patients with mild to moderate COPD and home oxygen therapy for the subset of patients with chronic hypoxemia.

1. Anthonisen NR, Skeans MA, Wise RA, et al. The effects of a smoking cessation intervention on 14.5-year mortality: a randomized clinical trial. *Ann Intern Med.* 2006;142:233-239.
2. Tashkin DP, Celli B, Senn S, et al. A 4-year trial of tiotropium in chronic obstructive pulmonary disease. *N Engl J Med.* 2008;359:1543-1554.
3. Vogelmeier C, Hederer B, Glaab T, et al. Tiotropium versus salmeterol for the prevention of exacerbations of COPD. *N Engl J Med.* 2011;364:1093-1103.
4. Calverley PM, Rabe KR, Goehring UM, et al. Roflumilast in symptomatic chronic obstructive pulmonary disease: two randomized clinical trials. *Lancet.* 2009;374:685-694.
5. Drummond MB, Dasenbrook EC, Pitz MW, et al. Inhaled corticosteroids in patients with stable chronic obstructive pulmonary disease: a systematic review and meta-analysis. *JAMA.* 2008;300:2407-2416.
6. Cranston JM, Crockett A, Moss J, et al. Domiciliary oxygen for chronic obstructive pulmonary disease. *Cochrane Database Syst Rev.* 2005;4:CD001744.
7. Lacasse Y, Goldstein R, Lasserson TJ, et al. Pulmonary rehabilitation for chronic obstructive pulmonary disease. *Cochrane Database Syst Rev.* 2006;4:CD003793.
8. National Emphysema Treatment Trial Research Group. A randomized trial comparing lung volume reduction surgery with medical therapy for severe emphysema. *N Engl J Med.* 2003;348:2059-2073.
9. Ram FSF, Rodriguez-Roisin R, Granados-Navarrete A, et al. Antibiotics for exacerbations of chronic obstructive pulmonary disease. *Cochrane Database Syst Rev.* 2006;2:CD004403.
10. Walters JA, Gibson PG, Wood-Baker R, et al. Systematic corticosteroids for acute exacerbations of chronic obstructive pulmonary disease. *Cochrane Database Syst Rev.* 2009;1:CD001288.

SUGGESTED READINGS

Hurst JR, Vestbo J, Anzueto A, et al. Susceptibility to exacerbation in chronic obstructive pulmonary disease. *N Engl J Med.* 2010;363:1128-1138. *Exacerbations become more frequent as COPD progresses.*
Moullec G, Laurin C, Lavoie KL, et al. Effects of pulmonary rehabilitation on quality of life in chronic obstructive pulmonary disease patients. *Curr Opin Pulm Med.* 2011;17:62-71. *Rehabilitation provides modest benefits.*
Niewoehner DE. Clinical practice: outpatient management of severe COPD. *N Engl J Med.* 2010;362:1407-1416. *Case-based review.*
Salvi SS, Barnes PJ. Chronic obstructive pulmonary disease in non-smokers. *Lancet.* 2009;374:733-743. *Review emphasizing indoor and outdoor air pollution and occupational exposures.*

89

CYSTIC FIBROSIS

FRANK J. ACCURSO

DEFINITION

Cystic fibrosis is an autosomal recessive disease largely caused by mutations in the gene that encodes the cystic fibrosis transmembrane conductance regulator (CFTR) protein. Cystic fibrosis affects the lungs, pancreas, intestines, liver, sweat glands, sinuses, and vas deferens, and it results in substantial morbidity and premature mortality, with progressive lung disease as the cause of death in 90% of patients.

EPIDEMIOLOGY

The incidence of cystic fibrosis in the United States, Europe, and Australia is 1 in 3000 to 5000 births. Cystic fibrosis is most common in the non-Hispanic white population but also occurs in significant numbers in Hispanics (1 in 7000), African Americans (1 in 12,000), and some Native American populations. It also occurs rarely in individuals of Asian origin.

Approximately 30,000 persons in the United States have cystic fibrosis, so the prevalence is approximately 1 in 10,000. Worldwide, an estimated 100,000 individuals are affected. Exacerbations, particularly those requiring hospitalization, are associated with enormous social and monetary costs.

PATHOBIOLOGY

Lung and Sinus

The pathobiology of cystic fibrosis is based on the ion transport functions of the CFTR, which is a membrane glycoprotein that functions as a chloride channel but is also involved in the regulation of transepithelial sodium and bicarbonate transport. In the airway, CFTR dysfunction reduces chloride secretion from the epithelial lining cell into the airway lumen. In addition, sodium absorption from the lumen into the cell is markedly increased. The net effect is a thinning of the airway surface's liquid lining layer, thereby crucially impairing mucociliary clearance. The subsequent chronic infection leads to an intense neutrophil-dominated inflammatory response. Neutrophil products, including proteolytic enzymes and oxidants, are thought to mediate the subsequent pathologic changes in the airway, including bronchiectasis, bronchiolectasis, bronchial stenosis, and fibrosis. Mucous plugging of airways, likely from chronic infection and inflammation, is another prominent feature of airway disease. Because CFTR is expressed in relatively high concentration in the ductal portions of submucosal glands, speculation exists that mucus is abnormal in cystic fibrosis, but no abnormality has been identified.

The origin of sinus disease is believed to be similar to that in the lung. Impaired mucociliary clearance leads to chronic infection and inflammation. Nasal and sinus polyps are common, but their cause is poorly understood.

Pancreas

Pathologic studies of the pancreas in infants demonstrate ductal obstruction and dilation as well as acinar dilation. The CFTR is expressed in ductal tissue, suggesting that impairment of chloride and bicarbonate secretion into the lumen of the ducts leads to the viscous secretions that obstruct the ducts and cause acinar dilation. The exposure of pancreatic tissue to proteolytic enzymes of acinar origin leads to a cystic and fibrotic pancreas in the first few years of life. Unlike the lung, injury to the exocrine pancreas does not involve infection. Almost complete exocrine pancreatic insufficiency is seen in 85% of patients and is related to genotype.

Intestine and Liver

CFTR is expressed throughout the intestine. In approximately 15% of cases, cystic fibrosis is accompanied by meconium ileus as a manifestation of severe intestinal obstruction at birth. The incidence of jejunal and ileal stenoses and atresias is greatly increased compared with normal individuals. It is unclear how these severe abnormalities arise, but mucous obstruction in intestinal crypts is frequently seen at birth and suggests that abnormalities in CFTR lead to viscous meconium that interferes with normal intestinal development.

In the liver, bile duct obstruction is the first pathologic change noted. Focal areas of sclerosis ensue, probably owing to obstructed bile ducts. Infection is not involved in hepatic injury.

Sweat Gland

In the sweat gland, CFTR dysfunction leads to a failure of chloride absorption from the lumen into the sweat ductal lining cell. In contrast, the abnormality in the lung involves chloride secretion. The failure to absorb chloride and, by electroneutrality, sodium results in marked elevations in the chloride and sodium content of sweat. This abnormality is not accompanied by tissue destruction. The histology of the sweat gland is normal.

Male Reproductive Tract

The vas deferens appears to be the organ that is most sensitive to CFTR dysfunction. It often becomes obstructed in the fetus or in infancy. Resorption of the vas deferens occurs very early in life, and the vas is ultimately not identifiable in most males.

Other Organ Involvement

The primary abnormalities in cystic fibrosis result in secondary involvement of a number of other systems. Diabetes (Chapters 236 and 237), which is increasingly common in adolescents and adults, is thought to result when extensive scarring of the exocrine pancreas extends to the islets of Langerhans. Osteopenia and osteoporosis (Chapter 251), which are common in adults, result from a combination of malnutrition and chronic infection. Delayed puberty (Chapters 242 and 243) is also common. Patients can experience recurrent vasculitis and/or arthralgias that are believed to be caused by the host response to chronic infection. Exocrine pancreatic insufficiency leads to impaired growth and to a multitude of potential nutritional complications, including deficiencies in fat-soluble vitamins and trace elements (Chapter 225).

Genetics

The gene that encodes the CFTR spans more than 250,000 base pairs on the long arm of chromosome 7. The CFTR (ABCC7), which is a protein of 1480 amino acids, belongs to the ATP-binding cassette transporter family. More than 1500 mutations of five different classes have been described (Table 89-1). In the United States, only five mutations are present in more than 1% of cases. The F508δ mutation is by far the most common and is present in approximately 90% of patients in the United States. The next most common mutation, G542X, is present in only 4 to 5% of patients.

In class 1 mutations, protein is not produced because of nonsense mutations. Class II mutations lead to defective protein processing; in the case of 508δF, protein trafficking to the cell membrane is disrupted because the protein is recognized as being defective by cellular quality-control mechanisms, which direct it to the proteasome for degradation. In class III mutations, a protein is produced and processed correctly, but the channel remains closed in response to physiologic stimuli. Class IV mutations are present in the membrane and result in a channel that opens only partially in response to stimuli. In class V mutations, normal CFTR is produced, but in reduced amounts because of defective splicing.

Different mutations lead to differing levels of CFTR dysfunction. Severe mutations may reduce CFTR activity to 1 to 3% of normal, whereas mild mutations may be associated with CFTR activity that is 10 to 20% of normal. An important clinical correlation of CFTR activity is in the exocrine pancreas: patients with severe mutations almost always have pancreatic insufficiency, whereas some patients with milder mutations may retain pancreatic sufficiency. Patients with mild mutations tend, on average, to have less severe lung disease as well.

The clinical course of cystic fibrosis is variable, however, even after controlling for the type of mutation in CFTR, suggesting additional heritable and environmental influences. The genes that code for transforming growth factor-β, mannose-binding lectin, and interferon-related developmental regulator 1 have been identified as modifier genes. Each appears to modify the host response to infection and/or the development of fibrosis, rather than modifying the ion transport function of CFTR.

CLINICAL MANIFESTATIONS

Without specific supportive care, most patients succumb in infancy or early childhood because of malnutrition or lung disease. With the use of pancreatic enzyme replacement therapy, better pulmonary care, and the establishment of specialized centers of expertise, most patients live into the third or fourth decade of life.

CLASS	MECHANISM	GENETIC AND MOLECULAR ABNORMALITIES	REPRESENTATIVE GENOTYPE
I	Defective protein production	Unstable mRNA Truncated protein Premature stop mutations Frameshift Splicing variants	W1282X Del394TT 1717-1G to A
II	Defective protein processing	Trafficking abnormality Protein degraded in proteasome Deletion	F508del
III	Defective regulation	Protein at membrane Failure of gating Amino acid substitution	G551D
IV	Defective conductance	Protein at membrane Decreased gating Amino acid substitution	R117H
V	Decreased active CFTR	CFTR has normal activity at membrane but is decreased in amount Splice variant Substitution	3849+10kb C to T A455E

TABLE 89-1 CLASSES OF CFTR MUTATIONS

LUNG DISEASE

Cough, often persistent after viral infections, is the most prominent early feature of the disease. Viral infection may require more frequent hospitalization in children with cystic fibrosis than in normal children.

Although the lung disease begins in infancy, pulmonary function is often preserved until adolescence, when a steep decline frequently begins; at this time, pulmonary exacerbations become common. Most patients with cystic fibrosis have a daily productive cough by late adolescence or young adulthood.

Cystic fibrosis causes obstructive lung disease, initially with decreased flows at low lung volumes. Forced expiratory volume in 1 second (FEV_1) (Chapter 85) is the best correlate of outcome and starts to differ markedly from normal during adolescence. The rate of decline in FEV_1 often predicts the clinical course.

Early in the disease, the chest radiograph demonstrates hyperinflation and peribronchial thickening. Computed tomography can demonstrate bronchiectasis (Chapter 90) early in the course of the disease.

Airway infection, which is the key clinical manifestation, can be detected by sputum culture or bronchoalveolar lavage. *Pseudomonas aeruginosa* (Chapter 314) is the primary pathogen, although its prevalence is decreasing in the United States, likely owing to improved treatment. *Staphylococcus aureus* (Chapter 296), which is another prominent pathogen, can be methicillin resistant and exist in a small-colony variant form that makes antibiotic treatment difficult.

Most infections remain endobronchial and rarely cause invasive disease, although *Burkholderia* infection can result in sepsis that leads to death. *Burkholderia* infection can also lead to an accelerated decline in lung function and result in death over months to years. Nontuberculous mycobacterial infection can cause granulomatous disease in the airway. *Aspergillus* (Chapter 347) and other fungal species, which are often identified in sputum samples, can cause allergic bronchopulmonary mycoses, but whether they contribute to endobronchitis apart from allergy is unknown.

The polymicrobial nature of airway disease is increasingly appreciated. *Stenotrophomonas maltophilia*, *Achromobacter xylosoxidans*, and *Inquilinus limosus* are frequently identified serially in airway cultures. Anaerobic infection may also be important.

Individuals with cystic fibrosis are subject to acute exacerbations characterized by cough, dyspnea, decreased exercise tolerance, fatigue, increased sputum production, and change in sputum color that may last days to weeks. Frequently crackles are increased on physical examination, and both the resting oxygen saturation and lung function may decline. Increasing evidence suggests that the permanent loss of lung function is accelerated during periods of exacerbation.

Pulmonary complications can also include pneumothorax (Chapter 99), hemoptysis (Chapter 83), and pulmonary hypertension (Chapter 68). Some patients with more advanced disease exhibit acute ventilatory failure with infection.

GASTROINTESTINAL DISEASE

Exocrine pancreatic insufficiency, which is apparent in the first year of life in most patients, results in impaired growth and lifelong difficulty in maintaining normal weight. Patients at all ages may exhibit signs of malabsorption, including bulky, foul-smelling stools and flatulence. Fat-soluble vitamin and trace element deficiencies are not uncommon and are difficult to diagnose without regular laboratory monitoring.

About 15% of patients retain exocrine pancreatic sufficiency, most of whom have mild mutations associated with 10 to 20% of CFTR function. About one sixth of these patients are subject to recurrent episodes of pancreatitis (Chapter 146) that can lead to pancreatic pseudocysts or ultimately result in exocrine pancreatic insufficiency.

Intestinal obstruction can occur at any age. Frequently the blockage is at the ileocecal valve, but generalized chronic constipation (Chapter 138) is even more common. Intussusception of the appendix can also occur. Inflammatory bowel disease (Chapter 143) and gastrointestinal malignancies (Chapters 198 and 199) appear to be more common than in the general population. Chronic abdominal pain can occur at any time of life, and its cause is often difficult to identify.

Most patients who develop liver disease do so in childhood or adolescence. Liver abnormalities are often first appreciated when a physical examination reveals splenomegaly or a palpable, firm liver. Occasionally, hematemesis leads to the identification of esophageal or gastric varices that are indicative of portal hypertension. Splenic sequestration can lead to neutropenia or thrombocytopenia. Decreased hepatic production of clotting factors can also contribute to bleeding. Occasionally, jaundice is a presenting sign of hepatobiliary disease. Except for γ-glutamyl transpeptidase (GGT) levels, liver enzymes are frequently normal, even in patients with advanced disease. Gallstones (Chapter 158) are common and may or may not lead to symptoms. The hepatopulmonary syndrome (Chapter 157) can occur.

OTHER ORGAN INVOLVEMENT

Although most patients have radiographic evidence of sinus disease, acute or chronic sinusitis occurs in only a minority of individuals. Sinusitis can be accompanied by debilitating headache and anosmia. Nasal or sinus polyposis can lead to obstructed breathing during sleep.

Hypoelectrolytemia can occur at any age. Symptoms range from nausea, vomiting, and decreased appetite to seizures and circulatory collapse with fatal consequences. Sweat electrolyte loss is often an underappreciated problem in cystic fibrosis.

Almost all males are sterile because of the changes in the vas deferens. Spermatogenesis is normal, however.

Cystic fibrosis–related diabetes (Chapter 236) increases in frequency with age. By 30 years of age, approximately one third of patients have diabetes. Although patients rarely develop ketoacidosis, the microvascular and macrovascular complications of diabetes can occur. In addition, patients with diabetes appear to have an accelerated decline in lung function. Osteoporosis (Chapter 251), osteopenia, and increased fractures also increase in frequency with age. Vasculitis accompanied by rash or arthralgia can occur at any time of life. Chronic pain and depression are other important complications that increase with age.

DIAGNOSIS

Newborn Screening and Diagnosis

In the United States, all 50 states require newborn screening to allow early diagnosis and immediate treatment. All newborn screening programs currently measure immunoreactive trypsinogen, a marker of pancreatic injury, from a dried blood spot taken during the first few days of life as the first step in the screening process. This biochemical screen identifies a large number of infants, only a fraction of whom have cystic fibrosis. Most programs perform genetic mutation analysis as the next step. Sweat testing is required to establish the diagnosis if suspected patients carry only one identifiable mutation, but most programs perform confirmatory sweat testing even if two mutations are present.

Sweat testing measures the chloride concentration in sweat that is stimulated by pilocarpine iontophoresis. The result is considered abnormal in adults and children when the concentration of chloride in the sweat is greater than 60 mmol/L; in infants, a concentration greater than 40 mmol/L is considered diagnostic. A family history of cystic fibrosis also provides supportive evidence. In parts of the world where genetic testing is not readily available, the appearance in infancy or childhood of intestinal obstruction or recurrent pulmonary problems should prompt sweat testing.

Diagnosis in Adulthood

Five percent of patients are diagnosed after 18 years of age, mostly on the basis of recurrent pancreatitis, nasal polyposis, chronic sinusitis, bronchiectasis, male infertility, allergic bronchopulmonary mycoses, and nontuberculous mycobacterial infection (Table 89-2). If the predominant symptoms are respiratory, the differential diagnosis includes primary ciliary dyskinesia, immune deficiency, or postinfectious bronchiectasis (Chapter 90). If the predominant symptom is recurrent pancreatitis (Chapter 146), the differential diagnosis includes hereditary pancreatitis with abnormalities in the *SPINK* gene. Transepithelial potential differences are altered in cystic fibrosis because of abnormal transport of sodium and chloride. The measurement of nasal potential difference, therefore, can sometimes be used as a diagnostic tool, particularly in adults.

It is increasingly recognized that some patients appear to have cystic fibrosis on clinical grounds but do not meet the criteria for diagnosis, usually because their sweat test is in the normal range or two genetic mutations cannot be identified. These patients are sometimes diagnosed as having atypical cystic fibrosis, nonclassical cystic fibrosis, or variant cystic fibrosis. Full analysis of the CFTR coding and flanking regions may be helpful in making the diagnosis. Such patients should be followed at a cystic fibrosis center so that their lung disease can be treated and they can be monitored for other complications of cystic fibrosis.

TABLE 89-2	APPROACH TO DIAGNOSIS OF CYSTIC FIBROSIS IN ADULT PATIENTS

CONDITIONS SUGGESTING THE DIAGNOSIS OF CYSTIC FIBROSIS IN ADULTS

Recurrent pancreatitis
Male infertility
Chronic sinusitis
Nasal polyposis
Nontuberculous mycobacterial infection
Allergic bronchopulmonary mycosis
Bronchiectasis

RECOMMENDED DIAGNOSTIC STUDIES

Sweat electrolyte determination
Extended CFTR mutation analysis
Nasal potential difference
High-resolution CT scan to identify bronchiectasis
CT scan of sinuses for polyposis
Sputum induction or bronchoalveolar lavage to identify bacterial and fungal pathogens

CFTR = cystic fibrosis transmembrane conductance regulator; CT = computed tomography.

TREATMENT Rx

The general consensus is that treatment is best conducted at specialized centers that use a team approach. Much of their success is based on the education of patients and families with regard to the range of symptoms and complications, as well as the close monitoring of pulmonary function and rapid intervention for any detected abnormalities.

Pulmonary Infections

Pulmonary infections can be treated with oral, inhaled, or systemic antibiotics. Increase in cough or other respiratory symptoms should be addressed with the introduction of antibiotics or a change in antibiotics within a few days. Nebulized antibiotics (4 weeks of either aztreonam 75 mg two or three times a day [1] or tobramycin 300 mg twice daily [2]), alone or in combination with oral antibiotics, improve lung function and decrease exacerbations in patients with chronic *Pseudomonas* infection. [3] Chronic oral macrolide treatment (e.g., azithromycin 5 to 15 mg/kg/day, 500 mg three times per week, or 1250 mg once per week [4,5]) can reduce exacerbations for up to 6 months. It is not yet clear whether the chronic use of antibiotics in this setting leads to the development of more resistant organisms.

More severe changes in symptoms or an acute fall in lung function requires intravenous antibiotics aimed at the cultured pathogen (Chapter 97). Nontuberculous mycobacterial infections are treated for 6 months or longer using multiple antibiotic agents (Chapter 333). Allergic bronchopulmonary mycoses are treated with corticosteroids and antifungal agents (Chapter 339).

Agents to alter the viscosity of respiratory secretions include inhaled hypertonic (7%) saline, which can increase pulmonary function and reduce exacerbations. [6] Daily use of inhaled rhDNase (2.5 mg) is associated with improvement in lung function and fewer exacerbations. [7] Conversely, nebulized thiol derivatives do not appear to be beneficial. [8]

Many patients have hyper-reactive airways and may benefit from inhaled bronchodilators (Chapter 87). Inhaled corticosteroids are controversial and do not have proven benefit. [9] Oral corticosteroid "bursts" (e.g., 5 days of prednisone, 1 mg/kg twice a day in children and 30 mg/kg twice a day in adults) are often useful, but chronic administration of oral corticosteroids can result in severe complications, including diabetes and stunted growth. Most patients perform physical means of airway secretion clearance one or more times a day.

Even passive smoke exposure is deleterious. Oxygen therapy is often required to maintain saturation and prevent the development of pulmonary hypertension. Noninvasive ventilation is used mainly in patients with more advanced disease. Pneumothorax almost always requires pleurodesis. Persistent or recurrent hemoptysis is treated with bronchial artery embolization. Occasionally, lobectomy is required. Patients in acute ventilatory failure should receive mechanical ventilation unless they have decided against such treatment. The possible need for ventilation should be addressed in patients with advanced disease before the need arises.

Lung transplantation (Chapter 101) is an option for many adult patients. Individuals with cystic fibrosis have survival rates after transplantation comparable to or better than those of other patients.

Gastrointestinal Diseases

Pancreatic enzyme replacement (Chapter 146) is the mainstay of treatment for exocrine pancreatic insufficiency. Because gastric acid decreases enzyme activity, H₂-blockers (e.g., ranitidine 150 mg twice daily in children weighing >30 kg and in adults) or proton pump inhibitors (e.g., lansoprazole 30 mg orally once daily in children weighing >30 kg and in adults) are often used.

Children and adolescents frequently use multiple nutritional supplements every day to maintain weight. Fat-soluble vitamin replacement therapy is necessary in most patients. Between 10 and 20% of patients may require gastrostomy feeding to aid growth or maintain weight.

To prevent intestinal obstruction, dietary fiber should be increased, and polyethylene glycol at varying doses (e.g., 17 mg orally with 8 ounces of water one to three times per day) is frequently used on a daily basis. Acute obstructions can be treated with more intensive use of polyethylene glycol or Gastrografin enema. Occasionally, refractory constipation (Chapter 138) requires surgical approaches that can result in loss of intestine.

Other Organ Systems

A combination of nasal rinses and topically applied corticosteroids and antibiotics is used to treat sinus disease (Chapter 434). Surgery is often required, however, especially for polyps.

Many pediatric patients receive daily salt supplementation. Adults should be counseled on the symptoms of salt depletion and encouraged to increase the amount of salt in their diet if there are no medical contraindications to doing so.

Regular screening for the onset of impaired glucose homeostasis or frank diabetes is required in all patients older than 10 years. Diabetes is treated with insulin (Chapter 236) because the safety and efficacy of oral antihyperglycemic agents have not been demonstrated in cystic fibrosis. Bone health is addressed through vitamin D supplementation, calcium supplementation, and oral bisphosphonate therapy (Chapter 251). Delayed puberty and short stature require consultation with endocrinologists and sometimes hormonal administration. Most clinics believe that both aerobic exercise and strength training can have beneficial effects, although the implementation of exercise programs has been difficult in clinical practice. Males with cystic fibrosis can father children through the use of epididymal aspiration to retrieve sperm, followed by in vitro fertilization.

General Care

Given all the pulmonary, nutritional, and other therapies prescribed for individuals with cystic fibrosis, their care amounts to several hours a day. This burden has a major influence on the quality of life in patients and their families and may contribute to the increasing incidence of depression observed in this population.

End-of-life care encompasses many complex issues. Patients are often depressed and experience chronic pain. They are asked to perform increasingly intense therapeutic regimens. They may have changed locations to await transplantation. Family, medical, and professional relationships are disrupted. Excellent communication with caregivers about advance directives and other planning is necessary.

PREVENTION

Prenatal carrier screening, which is offered in many countries, can decrease the incidence of cystic fibrosis by approximately 25%. Newborn screening programs may also help decrease the incidence by influencing the future reproductive decisions of parents of an affected child.

PROGNOSIS

Prognosis is now greatly improved compared with the natural history of the disease. The median expected survival in the United States is 37 years, but the peak age at death is 26 years, demonstrating that some patients are particularly vulnerable to devastating lung disease. Late adolescence and early adulthood are high-risk times for pulmonary insufficiency. Patients who survive to their 30s and beyond are often more stable, with a very slow decline in lung function.

This variability in prognosis is related to patients' ability to sustain lung function, recognizing that those with severe mutations succumb in adolescence or young adulthood, whereas patients with "milder" mutations often live longer.

Grade A

1. McCoy KS, Quittner AI, Oermann CM, et al. Inhaled aztreonam lysine for chronic airway *Pseudomonas aeruginosa* in cystic fibrosis. *Am J Respir Crit Care Med.* 2008;178:921-928.
2. Ramsey BW, Pepe MS, Quan JM, et al. Intermittent administration of inhaled tobramycin in patients with cystic fibrosis. *N Engl J Med.* 1999;340:23-30.
3. Langton Hewer SC, Smyth AR. Antibiotic strategies for eradicating *Pseudomonas aeruginosa* in people with cystic fibrosis. *Cochrane Database Syst Rev.* 2009;7:CD004197.
4. Kabra Sk, Pawaiya R, Lodha R, et al. Long-term daily high and low doses of azithromycin in children with cystic fibrosis: a randomized controlled trial. *J Cyst Fibros.* 2010;9:17-23.
5. Steinkamp G, Schmitt-Grohe S, Doring G, et al. Once-weekly azithromycin in cystic fibrosis with chronic *Pseudomonas aeruginosa* infection. *Respir Med.* 2008;102:1643-1653.

6. Elkins MR, Robinson M, Rose BR, et al. A controlled trial of long-term inhaled hypertonic saline in patients with cystic fibrosis. *N Engl J Med.* 2006;354:229-240.
7. Fuchs HJ, Borowitz DS, Christiansen DH, et al. Effect of aerosolized recombinant human DNase on exacerbations of respiratory symptoms and on pulmonary function in patients with cystic fibrosis. *N Engl J Med.* 1994;331:637-642.
8. Nash EF, Stephenson A, Ratjen F, et al. Nebulized and oral thiol derivatives for pulmonary disease in cystic fibrosis. *Cochrane Database Syst Rev.* 2009;21:CD007168.
9. Balfour-Lynn IM, Welch K. Inhaled corticosteroids for cystic fibrosis. *Cochrane Database Syst Rev.* 2009;21:CD001915.

SUGGESTED READINGS

Accurso FJ, Rowe SM, Clancy JP, et al. Effect of VX-770 in persons with cystic fibrosis and the G551D-CFTR mutation. *N Engl J Med.* 2010;363:1991-2003. *In a safety/efficacy trial of adults with cystic fibrosis, VX-770 at various doses improved CFTR function and also improved forced expiratory volume in one second by about 9%.*
Sears EH, Gartman EJ, Casserly BP. Treatment options for cystic fibrosis: state of the art and future perspectives. *Rev Recent Clin Trials.* 2011. [Epub ahead of print.] *Review.*
Simmonds NJ, Macneill SJ, Cullinan P, et al. Cystic fibrosis and survival to 40 years: a case-control study. *Eur Respir J.* 2010;36:1277-1283. *Survival is better in patients with a higher body mass index and forced vital capacity and no history of pneumothorax or* Pseudomonas *infection.*

90

BRONCHIECTASIS, ATELECTASIS, CYSTS, AND LOCALIZED LUNG DISORDERS

ANNE E. O'DONNELL

BRONCHIECTASIS

DEFINITION

Bronchiectasis is an abnormal permanent dilatation of the bronchi and bronchioles caused by repeated cycles of airway infection and inflammation. The distal airways become thickened; the mucosal surfaces develop edema, inflammation, and suppuration; ultimately, there is neovascularization of the adjacent bronchial arterioles. Bronchiectasis, which can be focal or diffuse, is triggered by a variety of genetic, anatomic, and systemic processes. Abnormalities of cilia, mucus clearance, mucus rheology, airway drainage, and host defenses can result in bronchiectasis. Regardless of the cause, patients with bronchiectasis develop chronic infections, which may lead to progressive lung destruction.

EPIDEMIOLOGY

Based on insurance claims reviews, it is estimated that there are at least 110,000 persons in the United States receiving treatment for bronchiectasis that is not related to cystic fibrosis (Chapter 89). The prevalence in the United States has been reported as 4.2 per 100,000 persons age 18 to 34 years and 272 per 100,000 among those older than 75 years. In the older age category, women are disproportionally represented. In Hong Kong, bronchiectasis results in a hospital admission rate of 14.4 per 100,000 persons. Other epidemiologic surveys suggest that there is increased risk for the development of bronchiectasis in individuals with reduced access to health care and higher rates of pulmonary infection in childhood.

PATHOBIOLOGY

In up to one third of cases, the cause of bronchiectasis is not identified. Other cases are related to pulmonary infections, genetic causes, anatomic abnormalities, and immune and autoimmune diseases.

Pulmonary Infections

Approximately one third of patients with bronchiectasis have an infectious trigger, usually years before the onset of the disease. Childhood viral infections, such as pertussis (Chapter 321) and bacterial infection, can cause permanent damage to the airways, leading to bronchiectasis years after the initial infection. Mycobacterial tuberculosis with its resultant granulomatous inflammation of the airway, lung parenchyma, and lymph nodes can cause subsequent bronchiectasis (Chapter 332), and *Mycobacterium avium-intracellulare* (MAI) infections have been recognized as an increasing cause and complication of bronchiectasis, particularly in white women older than

55 years (Chapter 333). MAI-related bronchiectasis typically involves the right middle lobe and lingula and can be associated with the "tree-in-bud" pattern of bronchiolar infection as well.

Genetics

Cystic fibrosis (Chapter 89) is characterized by bilateral diffuse bronchiectasis. Although many cystic fibrosis patients are diagnosed in childhood with multisystem disease, older patients may present with only pulmonary or pulmonary and sinus manifestations.

In primary ciliary dyskinesia, abnormalities in the dynein arms prevent normal ciliary beating. Patients with primary ciliary dyskinesia generally have significant sinopulmonary disease and infertility, and approximately half of these patients have Kartagener's syndrome with situs inversus (Chapter 69). Patients with α_1-antitrypsin deficiency also may develop bronchiectasis.

Anatomic Causes

Patients with chronic abnormalities of their swallowing mechanism or with esophageal dysfunction may develop focal or diffuse bronchiectasis with lower lobe predominance (Chapter 140). Direct lung injury due to acid or particulate matter aspiration or recurrent pneumonia may lead to bronchiectasis.

Chronic obstructive pulmonary disease is sometimes complicated by bronchiectasis (Chapter 88). Patients with chronic lower airway bacterial colonization and increased airway inflammation may develop areas of bronchiectasis. Rarely, patients with asthma (Chapter 87) have been found to have bronchiectasis. Allergic bronchopulmonary aspergillosis (Chapter 347) can cause a distinct "finger-in-glove" central bronchiectasis owing to chronic inflammation and mucous plugging. Airway abnormalities such as endobronchial tumors (Chapter 197), extrinsic compression by lymph nodes (right middle lobe syndrome), and foreign bodies are also rare causes of focal bronchiectasis. Tracheobronchomegaly (Mounier-Kuhn syndrome) is associated with distal bronchiectasis.

Immune and Autoimmune Diseases

Primary hypogammaglobulinemia (Chapter 258) leads to recurrent pulmonary infections that may result in bronchiectasis. Patients with immunoglobulin G subclass deficiencies may develop bronchiectasis if the deficiency leads to reduction in antibody production. Defects of neutrophil adhesion and chemotaxis (Chapter 172) have been found to cause bronchiectasis. Patients with human immunodeficiency virus infection (Chapter 394) have a higher prevalence of bronchiectasis than individuals with a normally functioning immune system.

Bronchiectasis is an increasingly recognized complication of collagen vascular diseases, particularly rheumatoid arthritis (Chapter 272) and Sjögren's syndrome (Chapter 276). The airway injury is likely due to chronic inflammation or esophageal dysfunction. Inflammatory bowel disease (Chapter 143) also causes bronchiectasis by undetermined mechanisms.

CLINICAL MANIFESTATIONS

Patients present with chronic cough and usually have mucopurulent or purulent sputum production. Occasionally, a dry nonproductive cough is the primary manifestation. Other symptoms include dyspnea, intermittent hemoptysis, and pleuritic chest pain. Weight loss, malaise, and fatigue sometimes develop. When patients have infectious exacerbations, they may develop fever as well as an increase in their baseline symptoms. Physical findings in patients with bronchiectasis are nonspecific: an abnormal chest examination with wheezing or crackles, or both. Clubbing of the digits is rare.

The clinical course of patients with bronchiectasis is variable. Some patients have few to no symptoms, others have daily cough with sputum production, and some patients have occasional to frequent exacerbations. A slow decline in pulmonary function is seen with bronchiectasis; decline is more rapid in patients infected with *Pseudomonas aeruginosa* (Chapter 314) and in patients who have more frequent exacerbations.

DIAGNOSIS

Imaging Studies

Although the diagnosis may be suspected by plain chest radiography, high-resolution computed tomography (HRCT) is the current "gold standard" for confirming bronchiectasis. The characteristic computed tomography (CT) findings are lack of bronchial tapering, bronchi visible in the peripheral 1 cm of the lungs, and an internal bronchial diameter greater than the diameter of the accompanying bronchial artery. Other associated HRCT findings are

FIGURE 90-1. A and B, High-resolution computed tomographic images of bilateral bronchiectasis in a patient with primary ciliary dyskinesia.

FIGURE 90-2. High-resolution computed tomographic image of nodular bronchiectasis due to nontuberculous mycobacterium infection.

cysts off the end of a bronchus, tree-in-bud irregular branching lines indicating mucus impaction, and occasionally associated consolidation (Fig. 90-1). The location of the bronchiectatic airways may suggest the cause: upper lobe predominance is seen in cystic fibrosis; lower lobe predominance in aspiration syndromes. Right middle lobe and lingula involvement suggests the presence of nontuberculous mycobacterial infection (Fig. 90-2), whereas central bronchiectasis is seen with allergic bronchopulmonary aspergillosis (Fig. 90-3).

Pulmonary function testing, which should be performed on all patients with suspected bronchiectasis, usually shows airflow obstruction as measured by the ratio between the forced expiratory volume in 1 second (FEV_1) and forced vital capacity (FVC) (Chapter 85). The severity of the airflow obstruction and the rate of decline correlate with radiographic extent of disease and frequency of exacerbation. Bronchoscopy will detect airway abnormalities including tumors, structural deformities, and foreign bodies and hence should be considered in the evaluation of localized bronchiectasis.

Cultures of sputum and of bronchoalveolar lavage when expectorated sputum is not available have an important role in assessing the infectious complications of bronchiectasis. The presence of *P. aeruginosa* portends a worse prognosis and more frequent exacerbations. Patients with no identifiable pathogens have the mildest disease. The presence of *Staphylococcus aureus* in the airway may suggest cystic fibrosis as the cause of the bronchiectasis. Nontuberculous mycobacteria are found with increasing frequency in the airways of patients with bronchiectasis, usually as a complication of preexisting bronchiectasis but occasionally as its primary cause. The laboratory evaluation of patients with bronchiectasis should be individualized. All patients should have sputum cultures for bacterial and mycobacterial testing. Other tests that should be considered include measurement of serum immunoglobulin levels and screening for genetic diseases, particularly in patients with diffuse bronchiectasis. Cystic fibrosis (Chapter 89) is diagnosed by elevated sweat chloride levels and by genetic testing. Primary ciliary dyskinesia is confirmed by electron microscopic evaluation of airway mucosal cilia. α_1-Antitrypsin deficiency is diagnosed by measuring levels and performing phenotyping (Chapter 88). Screening for rheumatoid arthritis (Chapter 272) or Sjögren's syndrome (Chapter 276) also may be reasonable in patients with diffuse bronchiectasis.

TREATMENT   Rx

The goals of treatment are to reduce the numbers of exacerbations and potentially to improve quality of life, reduce symptoms, and alter the natural history of the disease (Table 90-1). Currently, maintenance treatment is considered for patients with more advanced disease or more frequent exacerbations. Exacerbations are treated based on clinical acuity. Because patients are heterogeneous and therapeutic trials are few, therapy is commonly individualized in patients with bronchiectasis.

Preventing Exacerbations

The 23-valent pneumococcal vaccination is recommended for patients with bronchiectasis. Routine seasonal influenza vaccination is also standard. At present, no vaccines are available for prevention of the other infectious complications of bronchiectasis.

Treatment of the Underlying Etiology

For treatable conditions, such as immunoglobulin deficiency, replacement therapy (Chapter 258) should be considered even though there are few data on whether that alters the natural history of the lung disease. Patients with allergic bronchopulmonary aspergillosis (Chapter 347) should be treated with steroids to mitigate the inflammatory process that leads to the bronchiectasis.

Antimicrobial Therapy

Nebulized gentamicin (80 mg twice daily) for 12 months can provide sustained bacteriologic and clinical benefit.[1] Clinical trials have demonstrated microbiologic benefits with inhaled tobramycin, 300 mg twice per day as a 4-week trial for one cycle and a 2-week-on/2-week-off trial for three cycles,[2] but clinical benefit was not firmly established, and some patients experienced unacceptable respiratory side effects. Antimicrobial resistance is also a concern. In a retrospective study, radiographic stability was achieved in a limited number of patients who received cycles of alternating antibiotics, including a quinolone, over 6 to 84 months. At present, there is no firm evidence to support the use of routine maintenance antibiotics, although such therapy may be considered in patients with frequent exacerbations and progressive lung destruction. When mycobacterial species are cultured from patients with bronchiectasis, decisions regarding whether to treat and which antimicrobial agents to use are based on published guidelines (Chapters 332 and 333).

Reduction of Airway Inflammation

In two randomized trials of patients treated for 3 and 12 months, inhaled fluticasone, 500 μg twice daily, improved clinical status compared with placebo.[3,4] Small pilot trials of twice- or thrice-weekly oral erythromycin

FIGURE 90-3. A and B, High-resolution computed tomographic images of finger-in-glove central bronchiectasis due to allergic bronchopulmonary aspergillosis.

TABLE 90-1	POTENTIAL THERAPIES FOR BRONCHIECTASIS

Treat underlying condition, if possible
Antimicrobial therapy
    Pathogen specific
Anti-inflammatory therapy
    Inhaled steroids
    Macrolides
Mobilization of secretions
    Pharmacologic
    Mechanical
Surgery
    Localized or refractory disease
Transplantation
    End-stage disease

Reprinted with permission from O'Donnell A. *Chest.* 2008;134:815-823.

(500 mg twice daily for 8 weeks) and azithromycin (500 mg twice weekly for 6 months) suggest that macrolide therapy can be beneficial in bronchiectasis, but these agents should not be used alone in the presence of infection because they may result in resistant nontuberculous mycobacterial organisms. Oral steroids, although sometimes used in bronchiectasis, have never been tested in a clinical trial setting.

Other Medical Treatments

Chest physiotherapy and the use of devices to aid mucociliary clearance appear to be beneficial in non–cystic fibrosis bronchiectasis. In a randomized trial, twice daily use of an oscillatory positive expiratory pressure device (Acapella) improved sputum volume and quality of life end points compared with no routine physiotherapy.**5** Other techniques that may also have a role for airway clearance include traditional chest physical therapy with postural drainage and the use of chest wall oscillator vests. At least one clinical trial**6** has demonstrated improvement in overall clinical status for bronchiectasis patients enrolled in a pulmonary rehabilitation program.

Inhaled therapy with nebulized hypertonic saline (7%) may enhance airway clearance and decrease exacerbations, but long-term clinical trials have not been performed in patients with non–cystic fibrosis bronchiectasis. Preliminary data suggest that inhalation of mannitol may enhance secretion clearance by improving sputum physical properties. Although recombinant human DNase is efficacious in cystic fibrosis bronchiectasis, a large clinical trial showed it had deleterious effects in patients with non–cystic fibrosis bronchiectasis when given as maintenance therapy, so it should not be used.

No randomized trials support the use of routine β-agonist or anticholinergic bronchodilators in bronchiectasis. However, a subset of patients with airway reactivity likely benefit from use of these agents (Chapter 87).

Surgery and Transplantation

Resectional surgery may have a role for patients who have focal disease or for patients who have hemoptysis that cannot be controlled by embolization of the bleeding vessels (Chapter 101). Surgical resection can also benefit some patients who have diffuse bronchiectasis unresponsive to conventional therapy and some patients infected with nontuberculous mycobacteria.

Double-lung transplantation (Chapter 101) has been successfully performed in patients with end-stage lung disease due to non–cystic fibrosis bronchiectasis, and the clinical outcomes parallel those seen with transplantation for other end-stage lung diseases.

Treatment of Acute Exacerbations of Bronchiectasis

When the bronchiectasis patient experiences an acute exacerbation, antimicrobial treatments should be targeted to the known infecting organisms. Mild to moderate exacerbations can be treated with oral antibiotics, targeted to the results of the sputum culture, for 2 to 3 weeks. More severe exacerbations or exacerbations due to resistant organisms generally require intravenous antibiotics administered in hospital or at home. No benefit has yet been demonstrated by adding an inhaled antibiotic to systemic therapy for an acute exacerbation. Patients experiencing an acute exacerbation likely benefit from airway clearance modalities and the other nonantibiotic therapies discussed previously.

PROGNOSIS

Non–cystic fibrosis bronchiectasis is a heterogeneous disease with a widely variable prognosis. Patients with more severe obstructive and restrictive findings on pulmonary function tests, poor gas transfer, and chronic pseudomonal infection have the worst prognosis. Radiographic extent of disease, hypoxemia, hypercapnia, and evidence of right heart failure are also predictors of outcome. Bronchiectasis patients who are admitted to an intensive care unit for respiratory failure have been reported to have a 60% 4-year survival rate.

ATELECTASIS

DEFINITION

Atelectasis, or collapse, is due to hypoventilation of lung units. Atelectasis may involve an entire lung or a lobe, segment, or subsegment. Atelectasis can be caused by intrinsic obstruction of an airway or external compression from lymph nodes, parenchymal masses, or other entities. When lung units are atelectatic, ventilation-perfusion mismatch leads to hypoxemia. Infection may result from sustained atelectasis.

EPIDEMIOLOGY AND PATHOBIOLOGY

The lung bases and posterior segments are vulnerable to dependent atelectasis, which is caused by inadequate ventilation, particularly in the immobilized or postoperative patient. Patchy atelectasis is caused by alveolar filling processes, such as hemorrhage and edema (Chapter 91). Passive, relaxation, or compression atelectasis occurs when the lung recoils to a smaller volume because of fluid or air in the adjacent pleural space.

Obstructive or resorptive atelectasis is due to bronchial block to the entry of air, with resultant retractile consolidation. Intrinsic airway obstruction may be caused by mucous plugs, foreign bodies, or tumors in the airway. Extrinsic airway obstruction results from compression of the airway owing to peribronchial lymph node enlargement or other masses impinging on the airway.

Rounded atelectasis is caused by pleural thickening that invaginates and traps adjacent lung. Any chronic pleural disease can cause rounded atelectasis, particularly asbestos-related pleural disease.

CLINICAL MANIFESTATIONS AND DIAGNOSIS

Atelectasis is typically asymptomatic and diagnosed on chest imaging, but it may cause dyspnea and tachypnea and result in hypoxemia. In postoperative patients, atelectasis may be a cause of low-grade fever. Plain chest radiography shows loss of lung volume and the displacement of the lobar fissure, mediastinum, or diaphragm toward the involved lung unit (Figs. 90-4 and 90-5). Platelike or discoid atelectasis manifests as horizontal or curvilinear lines on plain chest radiography. Rounded atelectasis is an ovoid masslike density abutting the pleura. The type and cause of atelectasis can sometimes be elucidated by CT or ultrasonography. Bronchoscopy is required to confirm intrinsic versus extrinsic compression in obstructive-resorptive atelectasis and to determine the exact pathology of the obstruction. An oxygen saturation concentration can help assess the severity of the atelectasis and overall lung dysfunction.

FIGURE 90-4. Plain chest radiograph demonstrating right upper lobe atelectasis (due to endobronchial tumor).

FIGURE 90-5. Computed tomographic image of rounded atelectasis.

PREVENTION AND TREATMENT

Incentive spirometry is commonly prescribed to prevent or treat atelectasis in patients with limited mobility due to recent surgery, neuromuscular weakness, or any prolonged immobilization, but there are no randomized controlled trials that prove its effectiveness. Preoperative inspiratory muscle training reduces atelectasis in patients undergoing upper abdominal surgery,[7] and prophylactic use of noninvasive ventilation may reduce pulmonary dysfunction after lung resection surgery.[8] Other modalities such as positive expiratory pressure devices and high-frequency chest wall oscillation airway clearance are of uncertain benefit.

Patchy atelectasis is treated by addressing the underlying disease process in the lung parenchyma. Compression atelectasis is treated by alleviating the pleural space process.

Obstructive or resorptive atelectasis often requires bronchoscopy for diagnosis and treatment. In patients with obstruction owing to retained secretions, multiple bronchoscopies are sometimes required, but the mucus often rapidly reaccumulates and will resolve only when the patient's overall status improves.

Rounded atelectasis does not require treatment. CT is helpful in distinguishing rounded atelectasis from parenchymal tumor.

● CONGENITAL CYSTIC DISEASES OF THE THORAX

Thoracic cysts, which are exceedingly rare, develop because of abnormal development or branching of the foregut. Cysts may develop in the mediastinum at an early stage of gestation or in the lung parenchyma at a later stage. Abnormalities include bronchogenic cysts (mediastinal and parenchymal), congenital pulmonary airway malformation, and pulmonary sequestrations. The cysts are lined with airway and alveolar epithelium but do not communicate in a normal fashion with the airways or lung tissue.

Most patients with thoracic cysts present in childhood, but the cysts can remain asymptomatic and unnoticed until adulthood. In the absence of symptoms, these cystic lesions sometimes present as an incidental finding on chest imaging performed for another indication. Congenital cystic diseases can cause recurrent pneumonia, hemoptysis, or compression of normal structures.

CT scanning with CT angiography can usually detect congenital cystic lesions of the thorax, but pulmonary or bronchial angiography is sometimes necessary to define the blood flow to the lesion.

Bronchogenic cysts are usually found in the right paratracheal or subcarinal areas of the mediastinum but are occasionally seen in the lung parenchyma. These cysts are often asymptomatic, but they can cause wheezing, dyspnea, and cough when they compress adjacent structures. Secondary infection may develop in the cysts, and there are a few case reports of malignant transformation. Complete surgical resection is generally recommended, but partial excision with de-epithelization of the cysts has also been performed. Observation is also an option when the cysts are asymptomatic.

Congenital pulmonary airway malformation, previously called *congenital cystic adenomatoid malformation of the lung*, is an exceedingly rare abnormality with reported incidence of 1 in every 25,000 to 35,000 pregnancies. The abnormality is caused by arrested development of the bronchial tree. Most patients are diagnosed prenatally by ultrasound, but a few adults have first presented with complications, including pneumothorax and air embolism. Treatment is anatomic surgical resection.

Pulmonary sequestrations are areas of nonfunctioning pulmonary parenchyma with no communication to the tracheobronchial tree and abnormal arterial supply and venous drainage (Fig. 90-6). Intralobar sequestration, which accounts for about 75% of cases, does not have visceral pleura and is generally found in a lower lobe, left more frequently than right. Extralobar sequestrations have their own visceral pleura, are separate from the normal lobes, and may even be found below the diaphragms. Sequestrations usually have a feeding vessel that arises from the aorta. Patients with sequestrations may be asymptomatic but sometimes develop recurrent infections and or hemoptysis. Surgical excision with special care for the management of the feeding vessel is curative. Embolization of the feeding vessel is sometimes a successful treatment option.

Hyperlucent lungs are diagnosed by a paucity of vascular and interstitial markings noted on chest imaging. Lung parenchymal air collections can be caused by congenital parenchymal cysts, congenital lobar emphysema (almost exclusively diagnosed in infancy), giant bullous emphysema (vanishing lung syndrome), or Swyer-James syndrome. Lung parenchymal cysts may be a bullous alveolar type or may contain bronchial wall elements such as

FIGURE 90-6. Pulmonary sequestration. **A,** Computed tomographic image of pulmonary sequestration in right lower lobe. **B,** Feeding vessel visible arising from the aorta.

cartilage, smooth muscle, and glands. They may become infected and may rupture to cause pneumothorax. Surgical resection is generally recommended unless the lesions are small. Congenital lobar emphysema, otherwise known as *congenital large hyperlucent lobe*, may cause severe respiratory distress in infants owing to compression of surrounding lung tissue. Giant bullous emphysema is a rare condition that usually affects the upper lobes of young male smokers. Compression of normal lung parenchyma from these overdistended lobes may require surgical resection.

Swyer-James-Macleod syndrome, which is characterized by unilateral lucency of an entire lung, is caused by childhood bronchiolitis obliterans owing to viral or bacterial infection or toxic inhalation. CT shows air trapping and hyperlucency of the affected lung, with a normal contralateral lung. No therapy is required.

1. Murray MP, Govan JR, Doherty CJ, et al. A randomized controlled trial of nebulised gentamicin in non-cystic fibrosis bronchiectasis. *Am J Respir Crit Care Med.* 2011;183:491-499.
2. Scheinburg P, Shore E. A pilot study of the safety and efficacy of tobramycin solution for inhalation in patients with severe bronchiectasis. *Chest.* 2005;127:1420-1426.
3. Martinez-Garcia MA, Perpina-Tordera M, Roman-Sanchez P, et al. Inhaled steroids improved quality of life in patients with steady state bronchiectasis. *Respir Med.* 2006;100:1623-1632.
4. Tsang KW, Tan KC, Lam WK, et al. Inhaled fluticasone in bronchiectasis: a 12 month study. *Thorax.* 2005;60:239-243.
5. Murray MP, Pentland JL, Hill AT. A randomized crossover trial of chest physiotherapy in non-cystic fibrosis bronchiectasis. *Eur Respir J.* 2009;34:1086-1092.
6. Newall C, Stockley RA, Hill SL. Exercise training and inspiratory muscle training in patients with bronchiectasis. *Thorax.* 2005;60:943-948.
7. Guimaraes MM, El Dib R, Smith AF, et al. Incentive spirometry for prevention of postoperative pulmonary complications in abdominal surgery. *Cochrane Database Syst Rev.* 2009;3:CD0006058.
8. Perrin C, Jullien V, Venissac N, et al. Prophylactic use of noninvasive ventilation in patients undergoing lung resectional surgery. *Respir Med.* 2007;101:1572-1578.

SUGGESTED READINGS

Gursoy S, Ozturk AA, Ucvet A, et al. Surgical management of bronchiectasis: the indications and outcomes. *Surg Today.* 2010;40:26-30. *Review of surgery for bronchiectasis.*

King PT. The pathophysiology of bronchiectasis. *Int J COPD.* 2009;4:411-419. *Overview of pathobiology.*

Lai PS, Cohen DW, DeCamp MM, et al. A 40 year old woman with an asymptomatic cystic lesion in her right lung. *Chest.* 2009;136:622-627. *Review of congenital pulmonary airway abnormality.*

Pasteur MC, Bilton D, Hill AT. British Thoracic Society guideline for non-CF bronchiectasis. *Thorax.* 2010;65(Suppl 1):i1-i58. *Consensus guidelines.*

91

ALVEOLAR FILLING DISORDERS

STEPHANIE M. LEVINE

DEFINITION

Alveolar filling disorders (Table 91-1) are characterized by chest radiographic findings of alveolar involvement ranging from a ground-glass appearance to

TABLE 91-1 ALVEOLAR FILLING DISORDERS

DISEASES	PATHOPHYSIOLOGY	RADIOGRAPHIC FINDINGS
Pulmonary alveolar proteinosis	Impaired processing of surfactant by alveolar macrophages due to defects in GM-CSF signaling	Bilateral alveolar infiltrates with "crazy paving" and diffuse areas of ground-glass attenuation on CT scan
Acute interstitial pneumonia	Diffuse alveolar damage with temporal uniformity	Diffuse alveolar filling process similar to the acute respiratory distress syndrome
Diffuse alveolar hemorrhage	Bleeding from the pulmonary microcirculation, usually from the capillaries	Acute development of bilateral alveolar infiltrates
Bronchioloalveolar cell carcinoma	Cancer cells growing along the alveolar septa	Pneumonic infiltrate or nodules (either solitary or multiple)

CT = computed tomographic; GM-CSF = granulocyte-macrophage colony-stimulating factor.

consolidation; the pathologic process shows primary involvement of the alveolar air spaces distal to the terminal bronchioles. For example, in pulmonary alveolar proteinosis, the alveoli are filled by proteinaceous fluid; in bronchioloalveolar cell cancer, the alveolar walls are lined by adenocarcinoma cells. In acute interstitial pneumonia, exudative organizing fibroproliferative infiltrates fill the alveolar space; in the alveolar hemorrhage disorders, blood fills the alveolar space. Alveolar spaces filled with acute inflammatory cells, as in bacterial pneumonia (Chapter 97), or water, as in cardiogenic or hydrostatic pulmonary edema (Chapter 58), or high-protein fluid, as in noncardiogenic or increased permeability pulmonary edema (Chapter 104), are also part of the radiographic differential diagnosis of alveolar filling disorders and must be excluded.

A general approach to these suspected alveolar filling diseases (Fig. 91-1) can be stratified by time since the onset of symptoms. The typical patient may present with the onset of cough (usually dry) and dyspnea of variable duration, depending on the disease process. Hemoptysis is a frequent presenting symptom in the alveolar hemorrhagic disorders. With the exception of acute interstitial pneumonia, acute infectious symptoms such as fever, leukocytosis, and productive cough are usually absent. If the initial chest radiograph or chest computed tomographic (CT) scan is consistent with a possible alveolar filling process (Chapter 84), and acute pneumonia and pulmonary edema are excluded, bronchoscopy with bronchoalveolar lavage (Chapter 85) and transbronchial biopsy should be performed, particularly if pulmonary alveolar proteinosis, bronchioloalveolar cell cancer (Chapter 197), or alveolar hemorrhage is suspected. When these tests are nondiagnostic and in most cases of suspected acute interstitial pneumonia, a surgical lung biopsy obtained by thoracoscopy or an open surgical procedure is indicated.

PULMONARY ALVEOLAR PROTEINOSIS

EPIDEMIOLOGY

Pulmonary alveolar proteinosis is a rare alveolar filling disease caused by the accumulation of phospholipoproteinaceous material in the alveoli. The

FIGURE 91-1. A general approach to the alveolar filling disorders. *See Chapter 58. †See Chapter 97. ARDS = acute respiratory distress syndrome; BAL = bronchoalveolar lavage; PAS = periodic acid–Schiff; TBBX = transbronchial biopsy.

incidence is estimated to be 3.7 cases per million people. Pulmonary alveolar proteinosis in adults is an acquired primary disorder in more than 90% of cases, but similar histopathologic features may be found with identifiable causes, such as acute silicosis (silicoproteinosis; Chapter 93), aluminum dust exposure (Chapter 93), immunodeficiency disorders (e.g., immunoglobulin G monoclonal gammopathy and severe combined immunodeficiency syndrome), hematologic malignant neoplasms (particularly myeloid leukemias; Chapters 189 and 190), and certain infections (e.g., *Pneumocystis* pneumonia). Pulmonary alveolar proteinosis has also been described after bone marrow transplantation (Chapter 181).

PATHOBIOLOGY

The pathogenesis of pulmonary alveolar proteinosis is related to impaired processing of surfactant by alveolar macrophages due to defects in granulocyte-macrophage colony-stimulating factor (GM-CSF) signaling. This impairment may be due to autoantibodies against GM-CSF or GM-CSF receptor gene mutations, but it is not thought to be due to a problem with GM-CSF production. An autosomal recessive congenital form of pulmonary alveolar proteinosis, caused by a mutation in the genes encoding surfactant protein B or C, results in abnormal surfactant function and severe respiratory distress in homozygous infants. The result of this impairment is accumulation of surfactant-rich material and progressive dysfunction in phagocytosis due to excessive production or diminished clearance of surfactant by alveolar macrophages.

Histologic examination in pulmonary alveolar proteinosis reveals alveoli filled with lipoproteinaceous material that stains pink (positive reaction) with periodic acid–Schiff stain. Classically, there is no destruction of alveolar architecture. Electron microscopy reveals lamellar (phospholipid-containing) myelin bodies.

CLINICAL MANIFESTATIONS

Pulmonary alveolar proteinosis presents in patients in the third to fourth decade with a 2:1 male predominance. Most patients (72%) are smokers. Patients present with the insidious onset of dyspnea and cough, which may be dry or occasionally productive of grayish material. The duration of symptoms before diagnosis is typically 6 weeks to 6 to 8 months. Low-grade fevers, malaise, and weight loss may also be present. Hemoptysis is unusual. On physical examination, rales are present in 50% of cases. Clubbing is an unusual finding until later stages of disease.

DIAGNOSIS

Mildly elevated leukocyte counts and mildly to moderately elevated lactate dehydrogenase levels may be found in more than 80% of patients; lactate dehydrogenase levels may correlate with the severity of disease. The chest radiograph (Fig. 91-2) and chest CT scans demonstrate a diffuse symmetrical alveolar filling process with predominance in the lower two thirds of the lung fields; the radiographic appearance may mimic pulmonary edema. The

FIGURE 91-2. A chest radiograph showing bilateral alveolar infiltrates in a patient with pulmonary alveolar proteinosis.

characteristic CT pattern is often described as "crazy paving," which is due to scattered or diffuse areas of ground-glass attenuation with thickening of intralobular structures and interlobular septa in polygonal shapes (Fig. 91-3). This radiographic pattern is not specific for this disorder and can be seen with acute respiratory distress syndrome (ARDS; Chapter 104), *Pneumocystis jirovecii* pneumonia (Chapter 349), bronchioloalveolar cell carcinoma (Chapter 197), lipoid pneumonia (Chapter 94), sarcoidosis (Chapter 95), organizing pneumonia (Chapter 92), drug reactions, and pulmonary hemorrhage as well as with cardiogenic pulmonary edema (Chapter 59) and acute interstitial pneumonias. Pulmonary function tests often but not always show a restrictive pattern, with a reduced diffusing capacity. Arterial blood gas analyses reveal hypoxemia.

Bronchoscopy should be the initial procedure when pulmonary alveolar proteinosis is suspected. The diagnosis of pulmonary alveolar proteinosis can be established in most cases by the recovery of milky white to sandy-colored or light brown fluid on bronchoalveolar lavage. When it is subjected to microscopic analysis, the bronchoalveolar lavage fluid has a positive reaction on periodic acid–Schiff staining. Transbronchial biopsy or thoracoscopic biopsy can confirm the diagnosis by providing tissue that has similar staining characteristics.

TREATMENT ℞

About 8 to 30% of cases of pulmonary alveolar proteinosis resolve spontaneously, and smoking cessation may contribute to spontaneous resolution. A second group of patients will progress to respiratory failure. The remainder will have stable disease. Superinfection with *Nocardia* species, atypical mycobacteria, and other opportunistic organisms can occur in more than 15% of patients as a result of macrocyte phagocytic dysfunction.

Therapy begins with multistage or sequential whole lung lavage performed under general anesthesia with a double-lumen endotracheal tube. This procedure may have to be repeated at variable intervals. A small open-label trial using GM-CSF resulted in improved quality of life, oxygenation, pulmonary function, and exercise capacity in 48% of patients studied. Lung transplantation can be performed, but recurrent pulmonary alveolar proteinosis has been reported.

Survival rates at 5 years approach 75%.

TREATMENT   Rx

Treatment includes supportive intensive care unit management. In small case series, corticosteroids at doses of 1 g of methylprednisolone intravenously per day for three consecutive days followed by prednisone or equivalent at 1 mg/kg/day with a taper during several weeks to months, with or without cyclophosphamide, may be of benefit, but mortality remains higher than 60% during the subsequent 6 months. Patients also can have recurrences in months to years. Some cases of acute interstitial pneumonia may resolve without sequelae, but in some series, more than 50% of survivors may be left with residual fibrosis.

● ACUTE INTERSTITIAL PNEUMONIA

DEFINITION

Acute interstitial pneumonia, also referred to as the *Hamman-Rich syndrome*, is a rare and often fatal disease that mimics ARDS (Chapter 104). The etiology is unknown, and acute interstitial pneumonia is sometimes defined as the development of ARDS in the absence of known triggers. A similar acute presentation may be seen in patients with idiopathic pulmonary fibrosis (Chapter 92), but most investigators believe that acute interstitial pneumonia is a separate disease process.

PATHOBIOLOGY

The pathogenesis of acute interstitial pneumonia is damage to the epithelium of the alveolar membranes by a neutrophil-mediated mechanism; the result is pouring of exudate into the air space in the initial exudative phase of disease. Histologic examination reveals diffuse alveolar damage with intra-alveolar hyaline membrane formation, interstitial and intra-alveolar edema, acute inflammation, and epithelial cell necrosis with a nonspecific distribution and temporal uniformity. This process progresses to the organizing phase, characterized by alveolar septal thickening, type II pneumocyte hyperplasia, and fibroblast proliferation along the interstitium and alveolar spaces. In situ thrombi of small pulmonary arteries may be present. Finally comes a fibrotic phase with alveolar septal thickening from organizing fibrosis. One of the key pathologic findings in acute interstitial pneumonia is the temporal uniformity of the diffuse alveolar damage and of organizing and proliferating connective tissue. This uniformity supports a single acute injury at a particular point in time. Long-standing fibrosis is not a typical pathologic finding in acute interstitial pneumonia.

CLINICAL MANIFESTATIONS

Acute interstitial pneumonia manifests with equal frequency in men and women, typically in previously healthy individuals in the 50- to 55-year age range. It develops acutely to subacutely during a few days to a few weeks. The mean duration of symptoms is 15 days. Dry cough, shortness of breath, malaise, and fever (in 50% of patients) are typical clinical findings. A virus-like prodrome period has been described. Pulmonary rales are heard on physical examination, and hypoxemia is characteristic. Acute interstitial pneumonia often progresses to hypoxemic ventilatory failure, and intensive care unit admission with mechanical ventilation is usually required. Early mortality is high. Radiographic features of acute interstitial pneumonia are diffuse alveolar infiltrates and air space consolidation similar to the appearance of ARDS; CT scans reveal bilateral air space consolidation with areas of ground-glass opacities with little honeycombing. Septal thickening and a subpleural distribution of the opacities may also be present.

DIAGNOSIS

The diagnosis of acute interstitial pneumonia is made in the appropriate clinical setting in a patient who has a clinical presentation compatible with ARDS but without a clear etiology. The differential diagnosis histologically and clinically includes other causes of ARDS (Chapter 104), such as severe infection, trauma, and sepsis, and other causes of acute lung injury (Chapter 94), such as drug toxicity, inhalation injury, and collagen vascular diseases. The presentation is clinically and radiographically similar to that of diffuse alveolar hemorrhage, acute hypersensitivity pneumonitis, acute exacerbation of pulmonary fibrosis, acute eosinophilic pneumonia, and cryptogenic organizing pneumonia. Bronchoscopy with bronchoalveolar lavage is often performed to exclude alveolar hemorrhage, eosinophilic pneumonias, and infectious causes of lung injury. In a small number of cases, transbronchial biopsy may yield the diagnosis, but definitive diagnosis in most cases of acute interstitial pneumonia requires a surgical lung biopsy.

● DIFFUSE ALVEOLAR HEMORRHAGE

DEFINITION

The alveolar hemorrhage syndromes cause alveolar filling disease, usually with an acute onset and often with life-threatening severity. They can be associated with vasculitides, such as microscopic polyangiitis (Chapter 278) and c-ANCA-associated (Wegener's) vasculitis (Chapter 278); immunologic diseases, such as Goodpasture's syndrome (anti–glomerular basement membrane antibody disease; Chapter 123); collagen vascular diseases, such as systemic lupus erythematosus (Chapter 274); cocaine inhalation (Chapter 33); drugs (including penicillamine, mitomycin C, trimellitic anhydride, all-*trans* retinoic acid, propylthiouracil, and isocyanates); bone marrow transplantation (Chapter 181); coagulopathy (Chapter 177); and mitral stenosis (Chapter 75). A small percentage of idiopathic and recurrent cases are termed *idiopathic pulmonary hemosiderosis*. In Goodpasture's syndrome, there is a strong association with tobacco use and a male predominance, with young men most frequently affected. A viral syndrome and exposure to hydrocarbons may simulate Goodpasture's disease. Idiopathic pulmonary hemosiderosis most often occurs in children and young adults.

PATHOBIOLOGY

Alveolar hemorrhage is caused by bleeding from the pulmonary microcirculation, including the capillaries, arterioles, and venules. It may be associated with injury or neutrophilic inflammation of the capillaries or a capillaritis, usually when it is associated with collagen vascular or vasculitic processes. In Goodpasture's syndrome, for example, the circulating anti–glomerular basement membrane antibodies are directed against the α_3 chain of type IV collagen in the glomerular basement membrane, where they cause glomerulonephritis; these core antibodies can cross-react with the alveolar capillary basement membranes, resulting in alveolar hemorrhage. Alternatively, alveolar hemorrhage may be associated with relatively bland pathologic changes with red blood cells in the alveolar spaces. Idiopathic pulmonary hemosiderosis is an example of bland hemorrhage.

CLINICAL MANIFESTATIONS

Patients present acutely (usually in hours to a week) with dyspnea, shortness of breath, hemoptysis (which may not be present in all patients), and cough. Some patients also have low-grade fever. Lung examination reveals rales.

Laboratory examination may reveal anemia. In Goodpasture's syndrome and the ANCA-associated vasculitides, hematuria and renal insufficiency due to glomerulonephritis are typically present.

Radiographic features include the acute development of bilateral alveolar filling disease similar to pulmonary edema but without cardiomegaly or pleural effusions. Rapid remission and recurrences are seen with repeated episodes of bleeding, which also may result in chronic interstitial changes on the chest radiograph. Pulmonary function testing may reveal an increase in the diffusion capacity for carbon monoxide because of the presence of hemoglobin in the alveolar spaces.

DIAGNOSIS

The diagnosis of alveolar hemorrhage is usually made in the appropriate clinical setting by the triad of diffuse alveolar infiltrates (see Fig. 91-3), hemoptysis (in two thirds of patients), and anemia. Bronchoalveolar lavage typically demonstrates the return of progressively more bloody aliquots of fluid, and cytologic analysis reveals that more than 20% of the macrophages are hemosiderin laden. Goodpasture's syndrome is diagnosed by circulating anti–glomerular basement membrane antibodies, which are present in more than 90% of patients, or by the demonstration of linear deposition

FIGURE 91-3. A chest computed tomographic scan showing the "crazy paving" pattern characteristic of pulmonary alveolar proteinosis.

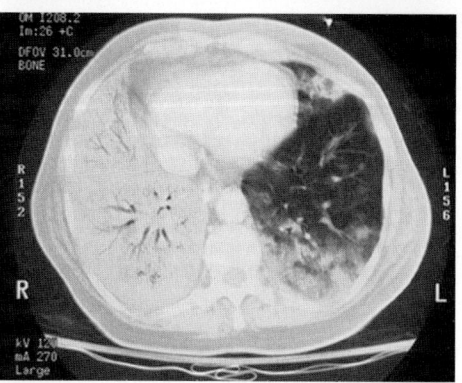

FIGURE 91-4. A chest computed tomographic scan in a patient with bronchioloalveolar cell cancer revealing the pneumonic form of the disease.

of immunoglobulin G antibodies along the alveolar or renal capillary basement membrane tissue when it is viewed by direct immunofluorescence. c-ANCA-associated vasculitis causes a focal, segmental, necrotizing glomerulonephritis and is associated with the presence of proteinase 3 antineutrophilic cytoplasmic antibodies in 90% of active cases (Chapter 278). Necrotizing granulomatous inflammation is often found in the upper airway in addition to the lungs and kidneys. A perinuclear myeloperoxidase antineutrophilic antibody is often present in association with microscopic polyarteritis (Chapter 278). Patients with systemic lupus erythematosus usually have antinuclear antibodies (Chapter 274). Idiopathic pulmonary hemosiderosis is a diagnosis of exclusion after other causes of diffuse alveolar hemorrhage have been eliminated.

TREATMENT ℞

Treatment of alveolar hemorrhage varies according to its underlying cause. Massive hemoptysis from any cause of alveolar hemorrhage should be managed as needed. In the case of drug- or toxin-related alveolar hemorrhage, the offending agent should be withdrawn, and supportive care is indicated. In Goodpasture's syndrome, the ANCA-associated vasculitides, and other vasculitides (Chapter 278), treatment typically includes immunosuppressant agents such as corticosteroids (methylprednisolone, 500 to 2000 mg/day in divided doses for 3 to 5 days followed by a prednisone taper beginning at 1 mg/kg/day during the next 6 to 9 months) and cyclophosphamide (2 mg/kg/day orally or 0.75 g/m² intravenously for one dose). In Goodpasture's syndrome, plasmapheresis is also a mainstay of therapy to remove the offending circulating antibody. Plasmapheresis (3 to 14 exchanges) may also be used in some cases of alveolar hemorrhage from ANCA-associated vasculitis and systemic lupus erythematosus.

PROGNOSIS

Recurrent alveolar hemorrhage from any cause, such as idiopathic pulmonary hemosiderosis, can be associated with the development of pulmonary fibrosis. Alveolar hemorrhage related to collagen vascular disease, vasculitides, and idiopathic pulmonary hemosiderosis can have mortality rates ranging from 25 to 50%. With Goodpasture's syndrome, renal failure is common, and the degree of renal impairment may correlate with outcome.

BRONCHIOLOALVEOLAR CELL CARCINOMA

DEFINITION

Bronchioloalveolar cell carcinoma, which is a subtype of bronchogenic adenocarcinoma, is characterized by well-differentiated, malignant cells lining the alveolar cell wall (Chapter 197). Of bronchogenic carcinomas, bronchioloalveolar cell carcinoma is the least strongly associated with tobacco use, and patients are more likely to be nonsmokers. Unlike other non–small cell lung cancers, the female-to-male ratio approaches 1:1, and younger patients may be affected. Using the strict pathologic definition described later, the prevalence of bronchioloalveolar carcinoma among the non–small cell carcinomas is less than 5%.

PATHOBIOLOGY

Bronchioloalveolar cell carcinoma usually arises in the periphery of the lung and is characterized by pure lepidic growth, which means contiguous growth along the intact alveolar septa, without stromal, pleural, vascular, or lymphatic invasion and without a known primary adenocarcinoma elsewhere. Bronchioloalveolar cell carcinoma can be categorized into mucinous and nonmucinous forms histologically; the mucinous type is thought to derive from respiratory goblet cells, and the nonmucinous type from type II pneumocytes or Clara cells.

CLINICAL MANIFESTATIONS

Patients present with the gradual onset of shortness of breath and cough. The duration of symptoms is usually several months. Constitutional symptoms such as malaise and weight loss may be present. An unusual but unique clinical finding is bronchorrhea, with patients reporting the production of copious amounts of clear sputum daily. This finding is more common in the pneumonic form of disease. Nodal involvement and extrathoracic metastases are less frequent than in other forms of non–small cell lung cancer.

DIAGNOSIS

Radiographic patterns vary and can include localized disease with peripheral solitary or multiple nodules or masses in 60% of cases or a persistent pneumonic pattern in 40% of cases (Fig. 91-4). The radiographic findings are often thought to be consistent with pneumonia, and a typical clinical presentation is that of a nonresolving peripheral density on chest radiograph. In addition, computed tomography may show areas of ground-glass attenuation. Positron emission tomography may be normal because of the low glucose uptake of this lesion. The diagnosis of bronchioloalveolar cell carcinoma is most often made by bronchoscopy with transbronchial biopsy.

TREATMENT ℞

For staging and treatment, bronchioloalveolar cell carcinoma is approached like other types of non–small cell lung cancers (Chapter 197), although bronchioloalveolar carcinoma may respond to epidermal growth factor receptor (EGFR) agents. Bilateral lung transplantation has been performed, but recurrence in the transplanted lungs has been reported.

PROGNOSIS

Prognosis correlates with disease stage and probably with the histologic and radiographic patterns. Patients with a single focus of disease (i.e., a solitary nodule) who undergo surgical resection have a prognosis better than that of patients with nonbronchioloalveolar adenocarcinomas of like stage. Multinodular, pneumonic, and diffuse forms of disease have a worse prognosis, as does the mucinous histologic subtype.

SUGGESTED READINGS

Das M, Salzman GA. Pulmonary alveolar proteinosis: an overview for internists and hospital physicians. *Hosp Pract (Minneap)*. 2010;38:43-49. *Overview*.

Lara AR, Schwarz MI. Diffuse alveolar hemorrhage. *Chest*. 2010;137:1164-1171. *Review*.

Luisetti M, Kadija Z, Mariani F, et al. Therapy options in pulmonary alveolar proteinosis. *Ther Adv Respir Dis*. 2010;4:239-248. *Emphasizes utility of whole lung lavage and of approaches to supplement GM-CSF or reduce autoantibodies against it*.

Perlman CE, Lederer DJ, Bhattacharya J. Micromechanics of alveolar edema. *Am J Respir Cell Mol Biol*. 2011;44:34-39. *Overview of the causes and implications*.

Suzuki T, Maranda B, Sakagami T, et al. Hereditary pulmonary alveolar proteinosis caused by recessive CSF2RB mutations. *Eur Respir J*. 2011:37:201-204. *Gene that can be responsible for adult onset hereditary disease*.

92

INTERSTITIAL LUNG DISEASE

GANESH RAGHU

DEFINITION

In an apparently immunocompetent host, interstitial lung disease (ILD) is a clinical term for a heterogenous group of lower respiratory tract disorders with many potential causes. However, clinical and physiologic features common to all ILDs include exertional dyspnea, a restrictive pattern on pulmonary function testing (Chapter 85), coexistent airflow obstruction, decreased diffusing capacity (D_{LCO}), increased alveolar-arterial oxygen difference (P_{AO_2}-P_{aO_2}) (Chapter 103) at rest or during exertion, and absence of pulmonary infection or neoplasm. ILDs comprise several acute and chronic lung disorders with variable degrees of pulmonary fibrosis (Table 92-1). The term *interstitial* is a misnomer because the pathologic processes are not restricted to the interstitium, which is the microscopic space bounded by the basement membranes of epithelial and endothelial cells. Rather, all of the several cellular and soluble constituents that make up the gas exchange units (alveolar wall, capillaries, alveolar space, and acini) and the bronchiolar lumen, terminal bronchioles, and pulmonary parenchyma beyond the gas exchange units (as well as the pleura, lymphatics, and sometimes the lymph nodes) are involved in the pathogenesis and manifestations of ILD.

EPIDEMIOLOGY

Among persons 18 years or older, the prevalence of all ILDs in the United States is about 81 per 100,000 men and 67 per 100,000 women. The overall incidence is also higher in men (31.5 per 100,000 per year) than in women (26.1 per 100,000 per year). Moreover, the prevalence of undiagnosed or early ILD is estimated to be 10 times that of clinically recognized disease; as physicians' awareness of these entities increases, it is expected that the frequency of the diagnosis of ILD will rise. Among the ILDs, the most common is idiopathic pulmonary fibrosis, which represents at least 30% of incident cases; in the United States, its annual incidence is estimated to be 6.8 to 16.3 per 100,000, with a prevalence of 14.0 to 42.7 per 100,000.

PATHOBIOLOGY

ILDs are thought to result from an unknown tissue injury and attempted repair in the lung of a genetically predisposed person. Genetic variants within the *hTERT* or *hTR* components of the telomerase gene and surfactant protein gene have been associated in a subset of familial pulmonary fibrosis and in some sporadic cases. An *MUC5B* promotor polymorphism is associated with familial interstitial pneumonia and idiopathic pulmonary fibrosis.

In *idiopathic pulmonary fibrosis*, varying degrees of acute, subacute, and chronic fibroproliferation are present in the lungs at the time of diagnosis. Ultimately, progressive fibrosis results in honeycombing, an end-stage finding that is often associated with increased pulmonary vascular resistance and secondary pulmonary hypertension. As a reflection of these dynamic processes, histopathologic examination of lung tissue often reveals highly heterogeneous findings; for example, a single biopsy specimen may show normal alveoli adjacent to abnormal areas of inflammation and fibrosis, with or without granulomas, vasculitis, or secondary vascular changes within the pulmonary parenchyma.

CLINICAL MANIFESTATIONS

ILDs are typically characterized by progressive dyspnea. Nonproductive cough and fatigue are also common complaints. Pleuritic chest pain may

TABLE 92-1 CLINICAL CLASSIFICATION OF INTERSTITIAL LUNG DISEASE

IDIOPATHIC INTERSTITIAL PNEUMONIAS

Idiopathic pulmonary fibrosis
Nonspecific pulmonary fibrosis
Respiratory bronchiolitis–associated interstitial lung disease
Desquamative interstitial pneumonia
Acute interstitial pneumonia
Cryptogenic organizing pneumonia
Lymphoid interstitial pneumonia

INTERSTITIAL LUNG DISEASE ASSOCIATED WITH COLLAGEN VASCULAR DISEASE

Progressive systemic sclerosis
Rheumatoid arthritis
Systemic lupus erythematosus
Dermatomyositis and polymyositis
Sjögren's syndrome
Mixed connective tissue disease
Ankylosing spondylitis

HYPERSENSITIVITY PNEUMONITIS

Occupational and environmental factors (e.g., farmer's lung; bird fancier's lung)
Iatrogenic

DRUG-INDUCED AND IATROGENIC INTERSTITIAL LUNG DISEASE

See Table 92-2

ALVEOLAR FILLING DISORDERS (CHAPTER 91)

Goodpasture's syndrome
Pulmonary alveolar proteinosis
Pulmonary hemosiderosis
Alveolar hemorrhage syndromes
Chronic eosinophilic pneumonia

INTERSTITIAL LUNG DISEASE ASSOCIATED WITH PULMONARY VASCULITIS

Pulmonary capillaritis
Wegener's granulomatosis
Churg-Strauss syndrome

OTHER SPECIFIC FORMS OF INTERSTITIAL LUNG DISEASE

Sarcoidosis
Langerhans cell histiocytosis (histiocytosis X)
Lymphangioleiomyomatosis

INHERITED FORMS OF INTERSTITIAL LUNG DISEASE

Familial idiopathic pulmonary fibrosis
Familial pulmonary fibrosis or interstitial pneumonia
Tuberous sclerosis
Neurofibromatosis
Gaucher's disease
Niemann-Pick disease
Hermansky-Pudlak syndrome

occur with certain collagen vascular or drug-induced ILDs, whereas acute pleuritic chest pain with dyspnea may represent a spontaneous pneumothorax (Chapter 99) in association with lymphangioleiomyomatosis, tuberous sclerosis (Chapter 426), neurofibromatosis, or Langerhans cell histiocytosis. Hemoptysis suggests a diffuse alveolar hemorrhagic syndrome, systemic lupus erythematosus (Chapter 274), lymphangioleiomyomatosis, Wegener's granulomatosis (Chapter 283), or Goodpasture's syndrome (Chapter 123); it is rare in other ILDs. In patients with existing ILD, new hemoptysis should prompt consideration of a superimposed malignancy, pulmonary embolus, or infection such as aspergillosis.

In some patients, the first and the only clue to the presence of an ILD may be the finding of coarse rales (crackles) on auscultation of the lungs. These coarse crackles must be distinguished from the finer rales typical of heart failure (Chapter 58) or noncardiogenic pulmonary edema (Chapter 104). Unlike patients with obstructive lung disease, wheezes are not common. A history of wheezing suggests the coexistence of occult hyperactive airways and airflow obstruction and raises the possibility of allergic bronchopulmonary aspergillosis (Chapter 347), Churg-Strauss syndrome (Chapter 278), chronic eosinophilic pneumonia (see later), or parasitic infection (Chapter 352). In some patients, the initial presentation may be with peripheral cyanosis, clubbing, or the signs and symptoms of an underlying systemic disease (see later).

DIAGNOSIS

The first key in patients with an ILD is to establish the syndromic diagnosis and then pursue the differential diagnosis of its specific cause (Fig. 92-1). However, a conclusive cause often may not be identified despite an exhaustive medical history and invasive diagnostic interventions, including sufficiently large and multiple lung biopsy specimens. Thus, the cause of several of the ILDs, even when diagnosed as specific entities, remains unknown.

History

The patient's age, sex, and cigarette smoking history may provide useful clues to the diagnosis. Idiopathic pulmonary fibrosis is an adult disorder that usually occurs in patients older than 50 years. Pulmonary sarcoidosis (Chapter 95), in contrast, is more common in young adults and middle-aged persons. Pulmonary Langerhans cell histiocytosis (previously known as pulmonary histiocytosis X or eosinophilic granuloma) characteristically occurs in young cigarette-smoking men, whereas lymphangioleiomyomatosis occurs exclusively in women of childbearing age. Respiratory bronchiolitis-associated interstitial lung disease is seen almost exclusively in cigarette smokers but occurs in both men and women of all ages.

The medical history also should focus on environmental factors, especially changes in environmental exposure (domestic, recreational, hot tub, whirlpool baths, indoor swimming pool, ventilation system at home, automobiles, and workplace), occupational exposure, medications, and drug use (Chapters 93 and 94). A family medical history should address possible familial ILD. Environmental risk factors that may suggest the diagnosis of hypersensitivity pneumonitis include farming or exposure to avian antigens ("bird fancier's lung" or "pigeon breeder's lung"), visible molds, water leaks, or humidifiers in the domestic environment (hypersensitivity to thermophilic actinomycetes). Other at-risk occupations include mining (pneumoconioses), machine tool grinding, sandblasting and working with granite (silicosis), welding and working in a shipyard (asbestosis), and working in the aerospace or electronic industries (berylliosis) (Chapters 93 and 94). Because of the long interval between the exposure and the onset of symptoms in many occupations associated with ILD, it is important to take a lifelong occupational history (Chapter 18) as well as to establish the interval between exposure and the onset of symptoms. Because the list of medications known to cause ILD is long and continues to grow (Table 92-2), a careful history regarding recent use of prescription and over-the-counter products is essential. Risk factors for immunosuppression, including infection with human immunodeficiency virus, raise the possibility of opportunistic lung infections (Chapter 398), neoplasm (Chapter 197), and transplant-related pulmonary complications.

Particular attention should be paid to the onset and duration of symptoms, the rate of disease progression, and association with hemoptysis, fever, or extrathoracic symptoms. Symptoms that persist 4 weeks or less and the presence of fever suggest cryptogenic organizing pneumonia, drug-induced pulmonary injury, or acute hypersensitivity pneumonitis, whereas idiopathic pulmonary fibrosis, ILD associated with connective tissue diseases, and Langerhans cell histiocytosis tend to have a more subacute onset. Extrapulmonary symptoms suggests that the ILD may be associated with systemic disorders (e.g., sarcoidosis; Chapter 95), and symptoms such as dysphagia, dry eyes or mouth, skin rashes, or arthritis may suggest a collagen vascular disorder (Chapters 274 and 278). Proximal muscle aches or weakness suggests the possibility of polymyositis or dermatomyositis (Chapter 277), and recurrent sinusitis suggests Wegener's granulomatosis (Chapter 278). Extrathoracic manifestations present in tuberous sclerosis (Chapter 426) include hematuria, epilepsy, and mental retardation.

Physical Examination

Physical examination of the respiratory system is rarely helpful in the diagnostic evaluation of ILD because findings such rhonchi and rales on auscultation and digital clubbing are nonspecific. Findings on cardiac examination, such as an accentuated P₂, a right ventricular heave, or tricuspid insufficiency, are suggestive of pulmonary hypertension (Chapter 68) and cor pulmonale in patients with advanced lung disease. However, extrathoracic findings such as skin abnormalities, peripheral lymphadenopathy, and hepatosplenomegaly may be more specifically associated with underlying sarcoidosis (Chapter 95); muscle tenderness and proximal muscle weakness may point to coexisting polymyositis (Chapter 277); and signs of arthritis may indicate collagen vascular disease (Chapters 272, 274, and 278) or sarcoidosis (Chapter 95).

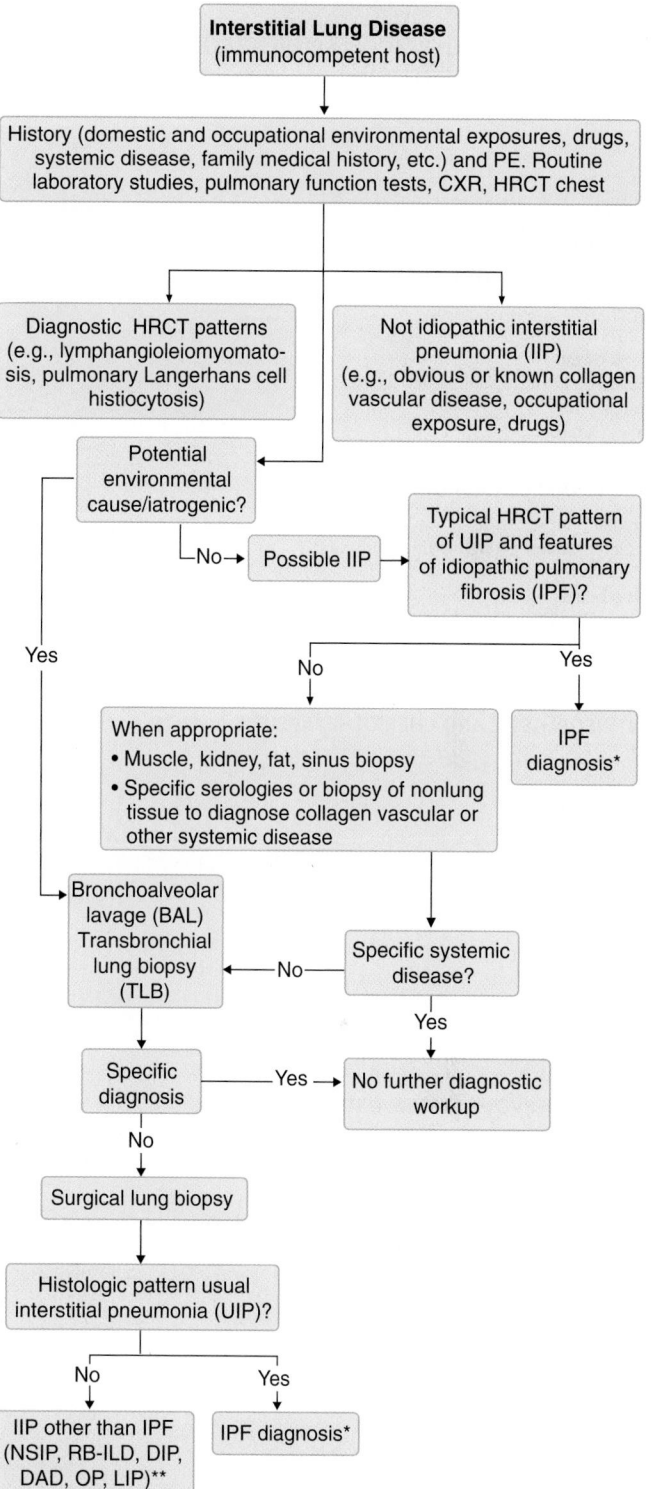

FIGURE 92-1. An approach to interstitial lung disease. DAD = diffuse alveolar damage; DIP = desquamative interstitial pneumonia; HRCT = high-resolution computed tomography; LIP = lymphoid interstitial pneumonia; NSIP = nonspecific interstitial pneumonia; OP = organizing pneumonia; PE = physical examination; RB-ILD = respiratory bronchiolitis–associated interstitial lung disease; UIP = usual interstitial pneumonia. *Adapted from American Thoracic Society/European Respiratory Society: International multidisciplinary consensus classification of idiopathic interstitial pneumonias. *Am J Respir Crit Care Med.* 2002;165:277-304 and Raghu G, Collard HR, Egan JJ, et al. An official ATS/ERS/JRS/ALAT statement: idiopathic pulmonary fibrosis: evidence-based guidelines for diagnosis and management. *Am J Respir Crit Care Med.* 2011;183:788-824.

Characteristic rashes occur in several collagen vascular diseases, disseminated Langerhans cell histiocytosis, tuberous sclerosis, and neurofibromatosis. Ophthalmologic findings (Chapter 431) such as iridocyclitis, uveitis, or conjunctivitis may be a clue to the diagnosis of sarcoidosis or a collagen vascular disease, whereas central nervous system abnormalities may be present in sarcoidosis, systemic lupus erythematosus, Langerhans cell histiocytosis, or tuberous sclerosis.

TABLE 92-2 DRUG-INDUCED AND IATROGENIC INTERSTITIAL LUNG DISEASE*

ANTIMICROBIAL AGENTS

Cephalosporins
Isoniazid
Nitrofurantoin
Penicillins
Sulfonamides

ANTI-INFLAMMATORY AGENTS

Aspirin
Gold
Methotrexate
Nonsteroidal anti-inflammatory agents
Penicillamine
Phenylbutazone
Zafirlukast

CARDIOVASCULAR DRUGS

Amiodarone
Angiotensin-converting enzyme inhibitors
β-Blockers
Hydralazine
Hydrochlorothiazide
Procainamide
Protamine sulfate
Tocainide

ANTINEOPLASTIC AND CHEMOTHERAPEUTIC AGENTS

Bleomycin
Busulfan
Chlorambucil
Cyclophosphamide
Erlotinib
Gefitinib
Gemcitabine
Imatinib
Melphalan
Mercaptopurine
Methotrexate
Mitomycin
Nitrosoureas
Procarbazine

CENTRAL NERVOUS SYSTEM DRUGS

Carbamazepine
Chlorpromazine
Imipramine
Phenytoin

ORAL HYPOGLYCEMIC AGENTS

Chlorpropamide
Tolazamide
Tolbutamide

ILLICIT DRUGS

Cocaine
Heroin
Methadone
Propoxyphene

OTHER AGENTS

Antithymocyte globulin
All-*trans*-retinoic acid
Colony-stimulating factors
Interferon-α and -β
Irradiation
Mycophenolate mofetil
Tumor necrosis factor-α modulating agents
High fraction of inspired oxygen (FIO_2) with mechanical ventilation

*This list contains examples only and is not meant to be exhaustive.

Laboratory Testing

Routine laboratory testing should include a complete blood count, leukocyte differential, erythrocyte sedimentation rate, chemistry panel (calcium, liver enzymes, electrolytes, creatinine), and urinalysis. Although these data rarely yield a specific diagnosis, they may provide helpful clues. When appropriate,

patients should be screened for systemic lupus erythematosus (e.g., antinuclear antibodies), rheumatoid arthritis (rheumatoid factor, anticitrullinated peptide antibody), scleroderma (ScL 70), dermatomyositis or polymyositis (creatine kinase, aldolase, and anti-Jo-1 antibody), Wegener's granulomatosis (antineutrophil cytoplasmic antibodies), and Goodpasture's syndrome (anti–basement membrane antibodies).

Mild hypoxemia is typically present on arterial blood gas analysis because of abnormal ventilation-perfusion ratios, especially in moderate to severe cases of ILD. However, carbon dioxide retention is rare and suggests possible coexisting emphysema (Chapter 88) or a hypoventilatory disorder (Chapter 86).

Noninvasive Evaluation

Chest Radiograph

The distribution and appearance of radiographic abnormalities (Chapter 84) may prove useful in differentiating the clinicopathologic syndromes in patients with ILD (Table 92-3). Comparison of previous chest radiographs with the current one is important in establishing the rate of progression of the patient's disease. A diffuse ground-glass pattern is often observed early in the course of ILD, followed by progression to reticular (linear) infiltrates with nodules (reticulonodular infiltrates) or, in the case of alveolar filling disorders, ill-defined nodules (acinar rosettes) with air bronchograms. Most ILDs cause infiltrates in the lower lung zones, but upper lobe predominance is typically present in sarcoidosis, berylliosis, Langerhans cell histiocytosis, silicosis, chronic hypersensitivity pneumonitis, cystic fibrosis, and ankylosing spondylitis, whereas the middle and lower lung zones show the most prominent abnormalities in lymphangitic carcinomatosis, idiopathic pulmonary fibrosis, subacute eosinophilic pneumonia, asbestosis, and pulmonary fibrosis caused by rheumatoid arthritis or progressive systemic sclerosis. Hilar adenopathy and mediastinal adenopathy are not common in ILDs; their presence should suggest sarcoidosis, berylliosis, silicosis, lymphocytic interstitial pneumonia, amyloidosis, or Gaucher's disease. A pattern of peripherally located pulmonary infiltrates in the upper and middle lung zones with relatively clear perihilar and central zones is a clue to chronic eosinophilic pneumonia. Recurrent infiltrates raise the possibility of cryptogenic organizing pneumonia, chronic eosinophilic pneumonia, or drug- or radiation-induced pneumonitis, whereas fleeting or migratory infiltrates may occur in Churg-Strauss syndrome (allergic angiitis), allergic bronchopulmonary aspergillosis, tropical eosinophilic pneumonia, or Löffler's syndrome. Localized pleural plaques may indicate asbestosis, whereas diffuse pleural thickening can result from asbestosis, rheumatoid arthritis, progressive systemic sclerosis, radiation pneumonitis, nitrofurantoin, or malignancy. In the absence of left ventricular failure, the presence of a pleural effusion (Chapter 99) raises the possibility of rheumatoid arthritis, systemic lupus erythematosus, acute hypersensitivity pneumonitis, sarcoidosis, asbestosis, amyloidosis, lymphangioleiomyomatosis, or lymphangitic carcinomatosis. Reduction of lung volumes is typical in most ILDs; the presence of preserved lung volumes or hyperinflation should raise suspicion for chronic hypersensitivity pneumonitis, Langerhans cell histiocytosis, lymphangioleiomyomatosis, neurofibromatosis, sarcoidosis, or tuberous sclerosis. However, plain chest radiographs may be normal in about 10% of patients with ILD.

High-Resolution Computed Tomography

Because of its increased sensitivity and ability to distinguish ground-glass changes, which are generally considered to be reversible areas of lung disease, from irreversible fibrotic and honeycomb changes, high-resolution computed tomography (HRCT) is essential in both the diagnosis and staging of ILD. Although microscopic ILD cannot be excluded by a normal HRCT, HRCT allows recognition of abnormalities not apparent in plain chest radiographs and may lead to an earlier diagnosis, help narrow the differential diagnosis patterns (Table 92-4), aid in selecting the site or sites for bronchoalveolar lavage and lung biopsy, and assist in choosing among therapeutic options and in estimating the response to treatment. The presence of patchy subpleural reticular and basilar septal fibrosis, traction bronchiectasis, and honeycombing increases the level of diagnostic confidence for the pattern of usual interstitial pattern, which is characteristic of idiopathic pulmonary fibrosis. The finding of bilateral cysts, including their size, configuration, distribution, and appearance, helps differentiate among lymphangioleiomyomatosis, tuberous sclerosis, and pulmonary Langerhans cell histiocytosis. HRCT can detect ILD despite normal chest radiographs in patients with asbestosis, silicosis, sarcoidosis, and scleroderma. Patients with respiratory bronchiolitis-associated interstitial lung disease typically have patchy ground-glass

TABLE 92-3 CHARACTERISTIC CHEST RADIOGRAPHIC PATTERNS IN PATIENTS WITH INTERSTITIAL LUNG DISEASE

PATTERN	SUGGESTED DIAGNOSES*
Decreased lung volumes	Idiopathic pulmonary fibrosis, nonspecific interstitial pneumonia, desquamative interstitial pneumonia, collagen vascular disease, chronic eosinophilic pneumonia, asbestosis, chronic hypersensitivity pneumonitis, or drug-induced interstitial lung disease (ILD)
Increased or preserved lung volumes	Idiopathic pulmonary fibrosis with emphysema, respiratory bronchiolitis-associated ILD, cryptogenic organizing pneumonia, hypersensitivity pneumonitis, lymphangioleiomyomatosis, Langerhans cell histiocytosis, sarcoidosis, neurofibromatosis, tuberous sclerosis
Micronodules	Infection, hypersensitivity pneumonitis, sarcoidosis, respiratory bronchiolitis-associated ILD
Septal thickening	Malignancy, infection, chronic congestive heart failure, pulmonary veno-occlusive disease
Honeycombing	Idiopathic pulmonary fibrosis, fibrotic nonspecific interstitial pneumonia, collagen vascular disease, asbestosis, chronic hypersensitivity pneumonitis, sarcoidosis
Recurrent infiltrates	Cryptogenic organizing pneumonia, chronic eosinophilic pneumonia, drug- or radiation-induced ILD
Migratory or fleeting infiltrates	Cryptogenic organizing pneumonia, hypersensitivity pneumonitis, Churg-Strauss syndrome, Löffler's syndrome, allergic bronchopulmonary aspergillosis
Pleural disease	Collagen vascular disease, asbestosis, malignancy, radiation-induced ILD, amyloidosis, sarcoidosis, lymphangioleiomyomatosis, nitrofurantoin-induced ILD
Pneumothorax	Langerhans cell histiocytosis, lymphangioleiomyomatosis, tuberous sclerosis, neurofibromatosis
Mediastinal and/or hilar adenopathy	Lymphocytic interstitial pneumonia, collagen vascular disease, silicosis, chronic berylliosis, malignancy, infection, sarcoidosis, amyloidosis, Gaucher's disease
Normal (rare)	Cellular nonspecific interstitial pneumonia, respiratory bronchiolitis–associated interstitial lung disease, collagen vascular disease, hypersensitivity pneumonitis, sarcoidosis

LOCATION OF RADIOGRAPHIC ABNORMALITY	SUGGESTED DIAGNOSES*
Mid to upper lung zone	Hypersensitivity pneumonitis, chronic berylliosis, ankylosing spondylitis, silicosis, Langerhans cell histiocytosis, sarcoidosis, cystic fibrosis
Lower lung zone	Idiopathic pulmonary fibrosis, nonspecific interstitial pneumonia (fibrotic), collagen vascular disease, asbestosis, chronic hypersensitivity pneumonitis
Peripheral	Idiopathic pulmonary fibrosis, nonspecific interstitial pneumonia (fibrotic), cryptogenic organizing pneumonia, chronic eosinophilic pneumonia

*This list is not intended to be comprehensive.
Adapted from Raghu G, Brown K. Clinical issues: patient evaluation. In: Baughman RP, du Bois RM, eds. *Diffuse Lung Disease: A Practical Approach*. New York: Oxford University Press; 2004.

TABLE 92-4 RADIOGRAPHIC FEATURES OF IDIOPATHIC INTERSTITIAL PNEUMONIAS

CLINICAL DIAGNOSIS	USUAL RADIOGRAPHIC FEATURES	TYPICAL FINDINGS ON HRCT
Idiopathic pulmonary fibrosis	Basal-predominant reticulation abnormality with volume loss	Peripheral, basal, subpleural reticulation with honeycombing, traction bronchiectasis, and focal ground-glass attenuation
Nonspecific interstitial pneumonia	Ground-glass and reticular opacification	Peripheral, basal, subpleural, symmetrical ground-glass attenuation with irregular lines and consolidation
Cryptogenic organizing pneumonia	Patchy bilateral consolidation	Subpleural or peribronchial patchy consolidation and/or nodules
Acute interstitial pneumonia	Diffuse ground-glass density/consolidation	Diffuse consolidation and ground-glass opacification, often with lobular sparing and late traction bronchiectasis
Desquamative interstitial pneumonia	Ground-glass opacity	Peripheral, lower lung zone ground-glass attenuation with reticulation and/or small cysts
Respiratory bronchiolitis-associated interstitial lung disease	Bronchial wall thickening, ground-glass opacification	Diffuse bronchial wall thickening with poorly defined centrilobular nodules and patchy ground-glass opacification
Lymphocytic interstitial pneumonia	Reticular opacities and nodules	Diffuse centrilobular nodules, ground-glass attenuation, septal and bronchovascular wall thickening, and thin-walled cysts

HRCT = high-resolution computed tomography.
Adapted from American Thoracic Society/European Respiratory Society. International multidisciplinary consensus classification of the idiopathic interstitial pneumonias. *Am J Respir Crit Care Med*. 2002;165:277-304.

(Chapter 85). Forced expiratory volume in 1 second (FEV_1) and forced vital capacity (FVC) are decreased proportionally such that the ratio of the two remains normal or may even be increased. Both total lung capacity and lung volumes measured by body plethysmography are reduced. Pulmonary function tests (PFTs) may be useful in monitoring the progression of disease and prognosis; significant changes in FVC, D_{LCO} (corrected to hemoglobin), and physiologic measurements (FVC, D_{LCO}) at 1 year portend a worse survival in patients with idiopathic pulmonary fibrosis.

Certain PFT findings may also aid in the differential diagnosis. A mixed obstructive-restrictive pattern occurs in patients with Churg-Strauss syndrome, allergic bronchopulmonary aspergillosis, endobronchial sarcoidosis, hypersensitivity pneumonitis, cryptogenic organizing pneumonia, tropical pulmonary interstitial eosinophilia, coexisting chronic obstructive pulmonary disease or asthma, or secondary bronchiectasis. Diseases associated with respiratory muscle weakness, such as polymyositis, progressive systemic sclerosis, and systemic lupus erythematosus, may exhibit a decrease in maximal voluntary ventilation and increased residual volume out of proportion to the decrease in FEV_1.

Exercise Testing

The magnitude of the increase in P_{AO_2}-P_{aO_2} on exercise correlates well with the severity of disease and the degree of pulmonary fibrosis in patients with idiopathic pulmonary fibrosis. Other exercise-induced physiologic abnormalities in ILD include a decrease in work rate and maximal oxygen consumption, abnormally high minute ventilation at submaximal work rates, decreased peak minute ventilation, and failure of tidal volumes to increase at submaximal levels of work while the respiratory rate increases disproportionately. The 6-minute walk test, performed on a flat surface, can provide quantitative data on exercise capacity and oxygen desaturation with exercise.

attenuation on HRCT in concert with bilateral interstitial prominence, fine nodular radiographic infiltrates, and normal lung volumes. Images obtained in the supine and prone positions and on deep inspiration and exhalation sometimes help to differentiate fibrosis from atelectasis.

Pulmonary Function Tests

The most characteristic physiologic abnormalities in patients with ILD, regardless of etiology, are a restrictive lung defect and decreased D_{LCO}

Invasive Evaluation

A collegial interaction and multidisciplinary discussions among the pulmonary clinician, chest radiologist, thoracic surgeon, and pathologist can help determine the best diagnostic approach for an individual patient (see Fig. 92-1).

Findings on bronchoalveolar lavage (BAL) can be diagnostic in some patients with ILD and can narrow the differential diagnosis in others (see Table 85-3 in Chapter 85). For example, a lymphocyte-predominant cellular pattern raises the possibility of sarcoidosis or hypersensitivity pneumonitis in the appropriate clinical setting. Eosinophils are seen in pulmonary Langerhans cell granulomatosis, an asbestos body count greater than 1 fiber per milliliter of BAL fluid is seen in asbestosis, and specially staining surfactant material is seen in pulmonary alveolar proteinosis. A transbronchial lung biopsy may reveal noncaseating granulomas in sarcoidosis, "loose" noncaseating granulomas in hypersensitivity pneumonitis, giant cell granulomas in hard metal pneumoconiosis, or smooth muscle proliferation in lymphangioleiomyomatosis. However, failure to establish a diagnosis on BAL and transbronchial lung biopsy does not exclude these entities.

Video-assisted thoracoscopic biopsy (Chapter 101) or open lung biopsy may be required to obtain an adequate sample for histologic evaluation of a patient with unexplained signs and symptoms when other studies have failed to establish a diagnosis, but most patients with idiopathic pulmonary fibrosis do not need to have a biopsy to confirm the diagnosis. The mortality rate for the procedure is generally less than 1%, and the morbidity is less than 3%.

TREATMENT   Rx

When the cause of the ILD is clearly known (e.g., acute or subacute hypersensitivity pneumonitis, occupational ILD, iatrogenic), further avoidance of the inciting agent or agents is essential (Chapter 93). Although systemic corticosteroids are generally indicated and are associated with a favorable response in some ILDs, the dosage and duration are unclear and essentially based on anecdotal experience (Table 92-5).

Supportive oxygen supplementation is dictated by clinical needs. For selected patients with end-stage ILDs, such as those associated with significant pulmonary fibrosis and pulmonary hypertension, lung transplantation (Chapter 101) may be a feasible and viable option. Treatments for pulmonary hypertension (Chapter 68) are generally recommended, although their utility for ILD patients is unproved.

● SPECIFIC TYPES OF INTERSTITIAL LUNG DISEASE

Idiopathic Interstitial Pneumonias

Idiopathic interstitial pneumonias, which are a subset of acute or chronic ILDs of unknown etiology, are characterized by the presence of varying degrees of interstitial and alveolar inflammation and fibrosis. Distinct clinicopathologic forms of idiopathic interstitial pneumonia include idiopathic pulmonary fibrosis, nonspecific interstitial pneumonia, respiratory bronchiolitis-associated ILD, desquamative interstitial pneumonia, acute interstitial pneumonia, cryptogenic organizing pneumonia, and lymphocytic interstitial pneumonia.

Although clinical severity may vary, the idiopathic interstitial pneumonias tend to manifest as an insidious onset of exertional dyspnea and a nonproductive cough. Chest pain and systemic symptoms such as weight loss and fatigue may be present. Bibasilar end-inspiratory crackles are often heard on auscultation. Clubbing, although not specific, is found in 25 to 50% of patients with idiopathic pulmonary fibrosis. Findings on the chest radiograph are most often nonspecific, and the presence of normal lung markings on the chest radiograph does not exclude ILD. On HRCT, many pathologic entities have characteristic image patterns that have greatly aided diagnosis (see Table 92-4).

IDIOPATHIC PULMONARY FIBROSIS

EPIDEMIOLOGY AND CLINICAL MANIFESTATIONS

Idiopathic pulmonary fibrosis accounts for 50 to 60% of all idiopathic interstitial pneumonias. Idiopathic pulmonary fibrosis occurs in adult men and women with a mean age at onset of 62 years. It is a distinct entity limited to the lungs in adults, usually older than 50 years, and generally occurs in men

---

TABLE 92-5 INTERSTITIAL LUNG DISEASE: CLINICAL RESPONSE TO SYSTEMIC CORTICOSTEROIDS ALONE*

GENERALLY RESPONSIVE	UNRESPONSIVE[†]
Sarcoidosis	Idiopathic interstitial pneumonia
Acute hypersensitivity pneumonitis	Idiopathic pulmonary fibrosis (usual interstitial pneumonia)
Drug induced	
Environmental causes (some)	Desquamative interstitial pneumonia (subset)
Idiopathic interstitial pneumonia	Chronic secondary and advanced pulmonary fibrosis
Cryptogenic organizing pneumonia	
Nonspecific interstitial pneumonia (cellular)	Chronic hypersensitivity pneumonitis (subset)
	Chronic radiation fibrosis
Respiratory bronchiolitis-associated ILD	Cryptogenic organizing pneumonia (subset)
Lymphocytic interstitial pneumonia	Acute interstitial pneumonia (?)
	Chronic pulmonary hemorrhage syndromes
Desquamative interstitial pneumonia (subset)	Pulmonary veno-occlusive disease
Acute interstitial pneumonia (?)	Environmental (e.g., asbestosis, pneumoconiosis)
Acute pulmonary capillaritis	
Eosinophilic pneumonia (acute and chronic)	End-stage ILDs, pulmonary fibrosis coexisting or associated with pulmonary hypertension
Acute radiation pneumonitis[‡]	Pulmonary Langerhans cell granulomatosis
Organizing pneumonia associated with collagen vascular diseases	Lymphangioleiomyomatosis
	ILD in inherited disorders (?)

*The dosage plus duration of corticosteroids used is variable and based on anecdotal experience, individual expert opinion, clinical judgment, and response as judged by objective measurements (clinical, radiologic, and/or physiologic). Oral prednisone/prednisolone is the most common corticosteroid used. Most patients who respond during the first few weeks of 20 to 60 mg of prednisone per day require maintenance low-dose oral prednisone at 5 to 10 mg/day beyond 6 months. Some patients who require maintenance of oral prednisone doses higher than 20 mg/day beyond 4 to 6 months may tolerate lower doses of prednisone if other immune-modulating agents (e.g., azathioprine, mycophenolate) are used in combination. There is no evidence to recommend a specific regimen. Patients should be monitored carefully and regularly for known side effects of corticosteroid use (e.g., osteoporosis, glucose intolerance), and preventive and therapeutic measures must be undertaken appropriately.
†Some patients unresponsive to oral corticosteroids alone may respond to combined treatment with corticosteroids and other immune-modulating drugs (e.g., azathioprine, mycophenolate).
‡Although most patients respond to modest doses of oral prednisone (initially, 40 to 60 mg/day), it is important to taper the prednisone very slowly to reach a maintenance dose of 5 to 10 mg/day beyond 6 months; rapid taper of oral prednisone has been associated with "rebound"—an exaggerated lung injury beyond the irradiated segment of the lung and in the contralateral lung.
ILD = interstitial lung disease.

---

with a history of cigarette smoking. Typical manifestations include a gradual onset and progression of exertional dyspnea, restrictive abnormalities on PFTs (Chapter 85), and a distinct pattern of bilateral pulmonary fibrosis on HRCT. Most often patients have otherwise been in good health and have no known collagen vascular disease or exposure to drugs or environmental factors known to cause pulmonary fibrosis, although patients with significant cigarette smoking history may have coexisting emphysema.

The natural course of idiopathic pulmonary fibrosis in most patients is a slow and steady decline with a median survival of 3 to 5 years after the diagnosis. A small subset of patients decline at a rapid rate over several months. Another subset of patients remain stable over several years before declining. About 5 to 10% of patients experience acute exacerbation that requires hospitalization and intensive care. There are no known risk factors or biomarkers that accurately identify which patients will have various clinical courses.

DIAGNOSIS

Chest radiographs typically show basal-predominant reticular abnormalities with low lung volumes. The diagnostic features on HRCT are peripheral, predominantly basilar patchy intralobular reticulation, often with subpleural honeycomb cysts, traction bronchiectasis, and traction bronchiolectasis as the disease becomes more advanced (Fig. 92-2A). Reticulation may progress to honeycombing, although neither alveolar consolidation nor parenchymal nodules are present. When compared with the other idiopathic interstitial pneumonias, the HRCT appearance of idiopathic pulmonary fibrosis is distinguished by a greater extent of fibrotic abnormality, by its hallmark honeycombing, and by a notable absence of extensive ground-glass opacification, micronodules, cysts, consolidation, and extensive mediastinal adenopathy, all of which are typical of *usual interstitial pneumonia*.

PFTs usually show a progressive restrictive pattern. However, patients with milder disease may have normal lung volumes and a small decrease in Dlco; rarely, PFTs may be normal.

The cellular pattern in BAL fluid, which is nonspecific, is marked by an excess of neutrophils in proportion to the extent of reticular change on HRCT; the percentage of eosinophils may be mildly increased. The histopathologic pattern of usual interstitial pneumonia consists of patchy interstitial changes alternating with zones of honeycombing, fibrosis, minimal inflammatory cells, collagen deposition, and normal lung (see Fig. 92-2B). Subepithelial fibroblastic foci, small aggregates of myofibroblasts, and fibroblasts within myxoid matrix are invariably present and represent areas of active fibrosis. The presence of temporal heterogeneity, or areas at different stages of fibrosis transitioning with normal areas and honeycomb cysts, along with fibrotic foci within the lung, is an essential feature of usual interstitial pneumonia that distinguishes it from other processes such as nonspecific interstitial pneumonia. Interstitial cellular inflammation is minimal in usual interstitial pneumonia. Although usual interstitial pneumonia characterizes the microscopic abnormality in idiopathic pulmonary fibrosis, the same histologic and radiologic pattern can also be seen in patients with rheumatologic lung diseases and asbestosis (Chapter 93).

In the appropriate clinical setting (and after exclusion of other known clinical conditions associated with ILD) (see later), a definitive diagnosis of idiopathic pulmonary fibrosis is based on the presence of a pattern of usual interstitial pneumonia on HRCT and/or surgical lung biopsy (Table 92-6).

TABLE 92-6 DIAGNOSIS OF IDIOPATHIC PULMONARY FIBROSIS: CRITERIA

The diagnosis of idiopathic pulmonary fibrosis requires the presence of usual interstitial pneumonia (UIP) in the absence of other causes of interstitial lung disease (e.g., domestic, occupational, and environmental exposures, connective tissue disease, and drug toxicity) AND

a. The presence of a UIP pattern on HRCT of the chest in the absence of a lung biopsy or
b. Specific combinations* of patterns on HRCT of the chest (UIP, possible UIP, inconsistent with UIP) and histopathologic features (UIP, probable UIP, possible UIP, not UIP) on surgical lung biopsy

HRCT FEATURES OF UIP	HISTOPATHOLOGIC FEATURES OF UIP
• Subpleural, basal predominance • Reticular abnormality • Honeycombing with or without traction bronchiectasis • Absence of peribronchovascular predominance, extensive ground-glass abnormality, diffuse micronodules, discrete cysts, diffuse mosaic attenuation, or consolidation	• Evidence of marked fibrosis/architectural distortion, +/− honeycombing in a predominantly subpleural/paraseptal distribution • Presence of patchy involvement of lung parenchyma by fibrosis • Presence of fibroblast foci • Absence of features against a diagnosis of UIP suggesting an alternate diagnosis*

*From Raghu G, Collard HR, Egan JJ, et al. An official ATS/ERS/JRS/ALAT statement: idiopathic pulmonary fibrosis: evidence-based guidelines for diagnosis and management. *Am J Respir Crit Care Med.* 2011;183:788-824.
HRCT = high-resolution computed tomography.

TREATMENT Rx

Because no treatment to date has been proved to improve survival or other clinically relevant outcomes, all treatments for idiopathic pulmonary fibrosis should be considered experimental. Physicians are urged to enroll their patients with idiopathic pulmonary fibrosis into one of the many ongoing clinical trials. The physician must spend adequate time to tailor treatment to individual patients' preferences and values.

A recent clinical trial demonstrated better preservation of PFT results after 1 year of treatment with combined oral prednisone (initiated at 0.5 mg/kg ideal body weight per day during the first month and tapered to a maintenance dose of 0.1 to 0.2 mg/kg of ideal body weight per day, or about 10 mg/day, over the subsequent 3 to 4 months), azathioprine (maintenance dose of 2 mg/kg of ideal body weight per day, or 100 to 150 mg/day), and N-acetylcysteine (600 mg three times daily) than with prednisone and azathioprine.[1] However, no randomized trials have compared the results of a triple-drug regimen with no treatment at all.

Pirfenidone (1800 mg daily for 1 year), a novel antifibrotic agent, reduced the loss of lung function and improved progression-free survival in one randomized trial in Japan, where it is approved for the treatment of idiopathic pulmonary fibrosis.[2] Interferon-γ1b,[3] cyclophosphamide, colchicine, D-penicillamine, and oral corticosteroids as monotherapy or in combination with immunosuppressive agents are not beneficial.

Despite the absence of data, patients who require hospitalization and intensive care for an acute exacerbation with loss of respiratory function in the absence of infection or other complications are usually treated with empirical intravenous corticosteroids (e.g., methylprednisolone 1.0 g intravenously as a pulse dose once a day for 3 days and followed by hydrocortisone, 125 mg every 6 hours for another 3 to 5 days), with further dosing dependent on the clinical response. Ancillary treatment measures, including supplemental oxygen (based on clinical and physiologic needs), prompt detection and treatment of respiratory tract infections and pulmonary embolism (Chapter 98), pulmonary rehabilitation, and immunization for influenza, herpes zoster, and pneumococcus, are all appropriate. Pulmonary hypertension, if present, may be treated (Chapter 68). Lung transplantation (Chapter 101) is indicated in selected patients, but about two thirds of patients with idiopathic pulmonary fibrosis are older than 60 to 65 years, which is a relative contraindication to lung transplantation. Gastroesophageal reflux, which is more common in patients with idiopathic pulmonary fibrosis, should receive appropriate treatment (Chapter 140). It is important to initiate discussion of palliative care measures before patients reach the terminal stages of the disease.

FIGURE 92-2. Diagnosis of idiopathic pulmonary fibrosis. **A,** The usual interstitial pneumonia pattern of idiopathic pulmonary fibrosis in the lower lobes on high-resolution computed tomography consists of (1) subpleural fibrotic changes with (2) traction bronchiectasis and (3) honeycomb cysts in the lower lobes. **B,** Usual interstitial pneumonia pattern of idiopathic pulmonary fibrosis. Note the presence of (1) subpleural fibrosis with (2) traction emphysema, (3) fibroblastic foci, and temporal heterogeneity of microscopic abnormalities at low magnification. (Courtesy of Dr. Kevin Leslie.)

PROGNOSIS

The usual clinical course is progressive impairment of lung function and gas exchange with a fatal outcome, unless the patient undergoes lung transplantation. Median survival is 3 to 5 years after diagnosis. Patients who survive longer generally have less fibrosis on HRCT, less functional impairment, no evidence of pulmonary hypertension, and no significant oxygen desaturation during a modified version of the 6-minute walk test. Patients with coexisting emphysema, pulmonary hypertension, or episodes of acute exacerbation have even shorter survival times.

NONSPECIFIC INTERSTITIAL PNEUMONIA

Nonspecific interstitial pneumonia is an ILD that is often associated with collagen vascular diseases or hypersensitivity pneumonitis; it may also occur as an idiopathic entity. Two subgroups have been described: cellular and fibrotic. Because the average age at onset is about 10 years earlier in nonspecific interstitial pneumonia than in idiopathic pulmonary fibrosis, and because the clinical features of idiopathic fibrotic nonspecific interstitial pneumonia are very similar to early cases of idiopathic pulmonary fibrosis, questions persist as to whether idiopathic fibrotic nonspecific interstitial pneumonia is a separate clinical entity or represents an early form of idiopathic pulmonary fibrosis.

DIAGNOSIS

Chest radiographs show bilateral patchy pulmonary infiltrates with a lower lung zone predominance in all forms of nonspecific interstitial pneumonia. HRCT reveals a predominant ground-glass pattern of attenuation, usually bilateral and often associated with subpleural reticulation and loss of volume in the lower lobe. In cellular nonspecific interstitial pneumonia, HRCT shows ground-glass opacification, consolidation or both, whereas the biopsy shows mild to moderate lymphoplasmacytic interstitial chronic inflammation. The major differential diagnosis to consider as an alternative to cellular nonspecific interstitial pneumonia is acute or subacute hypersensitivity pneumonitis, so a thorough history regarding environmental exposures is crucial. In contrast, fibrotic nonspecific interstitial pneumonia has a bilateral lower lobe distribution with architectural derangement on HRCT; histopathologically, it has uniformly dense interstitial fibrosis and may sometimes be difficult to distinguish from idiopathic pulmonary fibrosis and usual interstitial pneumonia in the early clinical stages. In these circumstances, the diagnosis of fibrotic nonspecific interstitial pneumonia can be ascertained only by the histologic features in a surgical lung biopsy specimen.

TREATMENT AND PROGNOSIS   Rx

Patients with cellular nonspecific interstitial pneumonia usually respond to treatment with corticosteroids (see Table 92-5), and their prognosis is generally better than that of patients with idiopathic pulmonary fibrosis. Given its similarities with idiopathic pulmonary fibrosis, treatment approaches to fibrotic nonspecific interstitial pneumonia have been extrapolated from studies in idiopathic pulmonary fibrosis. However, no clinical trials document this approach.

RESPIRATORY BRONCHIOLITIS–ASSOCIATED INTERSTITIAL LUNG DISEASE

This ILD is almost invariably associated with chronic and current cigarette smoking, and it usually manifests clinically during the fourth or fifth decade of life. However, it may also be detected incidentally on radiographs in relatively younger and asymptomatic persons with a previous history of cigarette smoking or in people passively exposed to chronic cigarette smoke.

DIAGNOSIS

PFTs show varying degrees of airway obstruction, mildly decreased or preserved total lung capacity, and decreased DLCO. The chest radiograph typically reveals bronchial wall thickening and areas of ground-glass attenuation. HRCT reveals centrilobular nodules with an upper lobe predominance, patchy ground-glass attenuation, and peribronchial alveolar septal thickening (Fig. 92-3A). Areas of hypoattenuation (mosaic attenuation) represent air trapping as a result of small airways disease. The characteristic finding on BAL is numerous brown-pigmented alveolar macrophages, often with a modest increase in neutrophils. The hallmark histopathologic feature on biopsy is the accumulation of pigmented alveolar macrophages with glassy eosinophilic cytoplasm and granular pigmentation within respiratory bronchioles, typically with a chronic inflammatory cell infiltrate in the bronchioles and surrounding alveolar walls (see Fig. 92-3B). Fibroblastic foci and honeycomb change are not present, but centrilobular emphysema is frequent.

TREATMENT AND PROGNOSIS   Rx

Progression to honeycomb lung and end-stage fibrosis seldom occurs, and the prognosis is good with cessation of smoking. Discontinuation of cigarette smoking is essential, and patients may benefit from low-dose corticosteroids (e.g., prednisone, 10 to 20 mg/day) for a few months.

DESQUAMATIVE INTERSTITIAL PNEUMONIA

Desquamative interstitial pneumonia is a rare entity (<3% of all ILDs) that may represent a more extensive form of respiratory bronchiolitis-associated ILD. Although most affected individuals are cigarette smokers, the histologic pattern of desquamative interstitial pneumonia may also occur in pneumoconiosis, rheumatologic disease, and drug-associated ILD. Patients are often initially seen with advanced disease and striking hypoxemia.

DIAGNOSIS

PFTs reveal a restrictive lung defect and decreased DLCO with or without coexisting airway obstruction. The chest radiograph shows patchy basal consolidation with a lower lobe and peripheral predominance. HRCT shows bilateral symmetrical ground-glass opacities with a predominantly basal and peripheral distribution as well as diffuse alveolar septal thickening (Fig. 92-4A). Irregular linear opacities, typically associated with traction bronchiectasis, may be noted. The finding of small discrete cysts, believed to represent trapped air in dilated bronchioles, within areas of ground-glass

FIGURE 92-3. Respiratory bronchiolitis–associated interstitial lung disease. **A,** Ground-glass attenuation with a mosaic pattern on high-resolution computed tomography. **B,** Note the dense aggregates of (1) pigmented macrophages present in the air spaces around the terminal airways with (2) variable bronchiolar metaplasia and (3) interstitial fibrosis.

FIGURE 92-4. **Desquamative interstitial pneumonia. A,** Ground-glass attenuation with (1) cystic spaces on high-resolution computed tomography. **B,** Note that the alveolar spaces are densely filled with macrophages *(arrowheads).*

changes and intervening normal lung parenchyma is highly suggestive of desquamative interstitial pneumonia. Fluid recovered from BAL quite often shows increased numbers of pigmented alveolar macrophages, frequently with increased neutrophils. Histopathologic findings on biopsy include diffuse alveolar septal thickening, hyperplasia of type II pneumocytes, and intense accumulation of intra-alveolar granular pigmented macrophages in a uniform manner (see Fig. 92-4B); fibrosis is minimal.

TREATMENT AND PROGNOSIS **Rx**

Therapeutic outcomes are generally good, particularly with cessation of smoking and administration of oral corticosteroid therapy (see Table 92-5); the estimated overall survival rate is 70% at 10 years. However, a subset of patients may progress despite cessation of cigarette smoking, and a trial of corticosteroid therapy and lung transplantation is an appropriate consideration for selected patients.

ACUTE INTERSTITIAL PNEUMONIA

Acute interstitial pneumonia is seen in otherwise healthy persons immediately after an apparent viral upper respiratory infection (Fig. 92-5). The syndrome, historically known as Hamman-Rich syndrome (Chapter 91), mimics the acute respiratory distress syndrome.

CRYPTOGENIC ORGANIZING PNEUMONIA

Cryptogenic organizing pneumonia, previously referred to as bronchiolitis obliterans organizing pneumonia of unknown cause (BOOP), is an idiopathic pneumonia that most commonly manifests as a flulike illness with a nonproductive cough, followed by exertional dyspnea.

DIAGNOSIS

PFTs show a restrictive defect, but 20% of patients, most of whom are current or past smokers, also have an obstructive defect. Chest radiography reveals patchy unilateral or bilateral alveolar opacities that may be peripheral or migratory; small nodular opacities are seen in 10 to 50% of cases. In about 90% of patients, HRCT shows areas of air space consolidation with lower lung zone predominance, frequently in a subpleural or peribronchial distribution; other features include small nodules along bronchovascular bundles and ground-glass attenuation. BAL is nonspecific; increased lymphocytes, neutrophils, and eosinophils may be seen. On biopsy, key histologic features are excessive proliferation of granulation tissue within the small airways and alveolar ducts as well as chronic inflammation in the surrounding alveoli.

FIGURE 92-5. **Acute interstitial pneumonia with diffuse alveolar damage histologically.** Note the dense air space consolidation.

TREATMENT AND PROGNOSIS **Rx**

Most patients recover rapidly and completely when treated with oral corticosteroids (see Table 92-5) for 6 months but may relapse after discontinuation and require oral corticosteroids indefinitely, often with adjunct immunosuppressive agents such as azathioprine. A small subset of patients in whom pulmonary fibrosis develops despite corticosteroids and azathioprine behave similarly to patients with idiopathic pulmonary fibrosis. Spontaneous remissions are known to occur.

LYMPHOID AND LYMPHOCYTIC INTERSTITIAL PNEUMONIA

This condition is more common in women, especially in the fifth decade of life, but it may occur at any age. Concurrent collagen vascular disease or an autoimmune disorder (especially Sjögren's syndrome) should be sought because idiopathic lymphocytic interstitial pneumonia is very rare. Symptoms are nonspecific and include a gradual onset of cough and exertional dyspnea.

DIAGNOSIS

Chest radiographs show a reticular or reticulonodular pattern predominantly involving the lower lung zones. HRCT reveals bilateral ground-glass attenuation, small or large nodules, and scattered cysts; perivascular honeycombing and reticular abnormalities may also be seen. Increased numbers of lymphocytes are found on BAL, and biopsy reveals a dense interstitial lymphocytic infiltrate.

TREATMENT AND PROGNOSIS

Some patients respond to or stabilize with oral corticosteroids (see Table 92-5). The prognosis is variable, with more than one third of patients progressing to diffuse pulmonary fibrosis.

Interstitial Lung Disease Associated with Collagen Vascular Disease

Many of the collagen vascular diseases, including progressive systemic sclerosis (Chapter 275), rheumatoid arthritis (Chapter 272), systemic lupus erythematosus (Chapter 274), dermatomyositis and polymyositis (Chapter 277), Sjögren's syndrome (Chapter 276), and mixed connective tissue disorder (Chapter 275), may have ILD as one of their manifestations. In fact, up to 20% of patients with collagen vascular disease may initially be thought to have an ILD alone. Therefore, these diagnoses must be considered in patients with ILD, even in the absence of extrathoracic findings. Conversely, because pulmonary involvement is a major cause of death in patients with collagen vascular disease, the presence of ILD should be carefully sought in affected patients. All forms of idiopathic interstitial pneumonia can occur in patients with collagen vascular disease. The natural history of ILD complicating collagen vascular diseases is variable, especially because coexisting pulmonary vascular disease or nonparenchymal pulmonary involvement may be present.

PROGRESSIVE SYSTEMIC SCLEROSIS

Of the collagen vascular diseases, progressive systemic sclerosis is most frequently associated with ILD. Pulmonary symptoms may antedate cutaneous or digital manifestations of the disease by several years. Most patients affected have nonspecific interstitial pneumonia, with a minority having a usual interstitial pneumonia pattern, and DLCO levels correlate with mortality. Pulmonary hypertension, which can occur in the absence of pulmonary fibrosis, may result in cor pulmonale. The chronic pulmonary fibrosis also increases the risk for bronchogenic carcinoma, usually either bronchoalveolar cell carcinoma or adenocarcinoma. In a controlled trial, treatment with cyclophosphamide (50 to 100 mg/day orally) for 1 year stabilized the PFT findings and improved health-related quality of life in patients with scleroderma-related interstitial lung disease.■

RHEUMATOID ARTHRITIS

Although rheumatoid arthritis is more common in women (2:1 to 4:1 ratio), ILD associated with rheumatoid arthritis is more common in men (3:1 ratio). Most cases occur at 50 to 60 years of age, and pulmonary symptoms follow the onset of arthritis in about 75% of cases. Lung involvement in rheumatoid arthritis may take many forms, but bronchiectasis, bronchiolitis, idiopathic interstitial pneumonias, and pleural effusions or pleural thickening are some of the most common. Early in the course, the histologic changes are similar to those of idiopathic interstitial pneumonias, including pulmonary fibrosis, but are distinguished by a prominent lymphocytic infiltrate that may contain germinal follicles adjacent to vessels and airways. As the disease progresses, the infiltration becomes less pronounced and is replaced by fibrous tissue, honeycomb changes, or both. Other pulmonary manifestations include pulmonary nodules, vasculitis, pulmonary hypertension, and Caplan's syndrome (progressive upper lobe nodular pulmonary fibrosis in a coal miner with rheumatoid arthritis) but are relatively rare. Treatment is directed at the underlying rheumatoid arthritis (Chapter 272).

SYSTEMIC LUPUS ERYTHEMATOSUS

Pulmonary abnormalities complicating systemic lupus erythematosus (Chapter 274) may vary greatly. Pleural disease or pleural effusions (or both) are commonly present in lung disease that complicates systemic lupus erythematosus. Acute lupus pneumonitis may mimic acute interstitial pneumonia, with widespread ground-glass attenuation admixed with consolidation, or it may manifest as diffuse alveolar hemorrhage. Chronic ILD may also occur. Infection must always be considered in acutely ill patients who have received steroids or other immunosuppressive therapy. Rarely, the restrictive lung defect, which may be predominantly a result of diaphragmatic weakness, leads to a chest radiographic pattern of small-appearing lungs that may look progressively smaller over time. This so-called shrinking lung is generally resistant to corticosteroids or other immunosuppressive agents used to treat systemic lupus erythematosus. Otherwise, treatment of the ILD is similar to treatment of the underlying systemic lupus erythematosus.

DERMATOMYOSITIS AND POLYMYOSITIS

In contrast to progressive systemic sclerosis, the pattern of lung involvement in dermatomyositis and polymyositis is more heterogeneous. Usual interstitial pneumonia, nonspecific interstitial pneumonia, and organizing pneumonia have all been reported. Most patients have anti-Jo-1 antibody, and the disease is typically progressive over time. An acute interstitial pneumonia–like syndrome occurs in a subset of patients and is associated with high mortality rate despite aggressive immunosuppressive agents and high-dose corticosteroids. ILD may precede the muscular manifestations by months to years or be superimposed on established muscle disease. The severity of the muscular disease does not correlate with that of the ILD. Treatment is directed at the underlying disease (Chapter 277).

SJÖGREN'S SYNDROME

ILD is seen in patients with Sjögren's syndrome, particularly those with the primary form of the disease. Lymphocytic interstitial pneumonia is the most frequent subtype, but cryptogenic organizing pneumonia may also be present. Respiratory infections and bronchiectasis are common in advanced stages, perhaps because of inspissated mucus. Response to corticosteroid or immunosuppressive therapy is usually good (Chapter 275).

MIXED CONNECTIVE TISSUE DISEASE

This overlap syndrome (Chapter 275) combines features of progressive systemic sclerosis, systemic lupus erythematosus, rheumatoid arthritis, and polymyositis or dermatomyositis. Pulmonary disease is common, but it is most often subclinical and identified only radiographically. Treatment includes corticosteroids and other immune-modulating agents for the underlying disease.

ANKYLOSING SPONDYLITIS

The most common pulmonary manifestation of ankylosing spondylitis (Chapter 273) is upper lobe, bilateral reticulonodular infiltrates with cyst formation as a result of parenchymal destruction. There is no known effective therapy for this apical fibrobullous disease.

Hypersensitivity Pneumonitis

EPIDEMIOLOGY AND PATHOBIOLOGY

Hypersensitivity pneumonitis, also known as extrinsic allergic alveolitis, is a syndrome caused by repeated inhalation of specific antigens from occupational or environmental exposure (Chapters 93 and 94) in sensitized individuals. Within a short period after inhalation of an inciting agent, patients develop a nonspecific diffuse pneumonitis with inflammatory cell infiltration of the bronchioles, alveoli, and interstitium. In the subacute and chronic stages, loosely formed, noncaseating, epithelioid cell granulomas may be dispersed in the interstitium. Hypersensitivity pneumonitis can occur with exposure to a wide range of inhaled antigens (Chapters 93 and 94). Some of the more common exposures are farmer's lung, bird fancier's lung, parakeet keeper's lung, and pigeon breeder's lung. Hobbies (woodworker's lung) and recreational activities (sauna taker's lung) may be implicated as well as occupations (Chapter 93).

CLINICAL MANIFESTATIONS

The clinical features and severity of symptoms vary according to the frequency and intensity of exposure. A history of exposure to potential agents or changes in the domestic and other environments (or both) is essential to diagnosis and treatment (Chapters 18 and 93). The interval between exposure to the antigen and the clinical manifestations of lung disease is unknown, although symptoms can occur as soon as 4 to 12 hours after exposure. In such cases, fever and chills are common symptoms, are often temporally related to the workplace or to hobbies, and may actually disappear on vacations or during absence from the site of exposure, only to recur when exposure is resumed. In more chronic and low-level exposures, however, the onset is insidious.

DIAGNOSIS

Findings on chest radiography are diverse, with focal patchy consolidation or a diffuse ground-glass appearance in acute hypersensitivity pneumonitis, micronodular and reticular shadowing in subacute forms, and diffuse, predominantly upper lung zone reticulation with honeycombing in the chronic form. Chest radiographs may be normal in up to 30% of patients with significant physiologic abnormalities.

On HRCT, small centrilobular ill-defined nodules of ground-glass densities are seen, along with evidence of mosaic attenuation (trapped air) as a result of concomitant bronchiolitis. Chronically, findings of lung fibrosis may be indistinguishable from the patterns seen in usual interstitial pneumonia and idiopathic pulmonary fibrosis.

BAL may be quite helpful by showing the most marked increase in lymphocytes of any of the ILDs as well as increased numbers of plasma cells. The characteristic histologic triad in hypersensitivity pneumonitis is cellular nonspecific interstitial pneumonia, cellular bronchiolitis, and granulomatous inflammation; however, this triad is seen in no more than 75% of affected patients. Differentiation from cellular nonspecific interstitial pneumonia may be challenging.

Precipitating serum antibodies for potential causes of hypersensitivity pneumonitis confirm exposure but not cause and effect, and the absence of antibodies does not exclude hypersensitivity pneumonitis. In some cases, a thorough investigation of the patient's home and workplace by an industrial hygienist may reveal molds, spores, thermoactinomycetes species, and other precipitating causes.

TREATMENT AND PROGNOSIS   Rx

Further avoidance of exposure to the antigen or antigens and treatment with corticosteroids (see Table 92-5) are important if improvement is to be obtained. Continued exposure to the unidentifiable antigens or prolonged exposure to antigens, or both, can lead to chronic hypersensitivity pneumonitis and irreversible fibrosis that may not respond to any treatment regimen. In the fibrotic stages, the prognosis may be similar to that for idiopathic pulmonary fibrosis.

Occupational Interstitial Lung Diseases

ILDs associated with specific occupations generally involve the inhalation and deposition of dust in the lungs, followed by a tissue reaction that ultimately results in fibrosis. Examples include silicosis (inhalation of silica in crystalline form or silicon dioxide as quartz, cristobalite, or tridymite; at-risk occupations include sandblasting and working with granite), coal workers' pneumoconiosis (inhalation of coal dust), asbestosis (deposition of fibers during mining, milling, or other handling of asbestos; welding and working in a shipyard are two at-risk occupations), berylliosis (seen in aerospace workers and in electronic industries), and hard metal disease (Chapter 93). Radiographic features vary depending on the inciting inhalant. Cessation of the exposure is important, but the fibrosis is generally irreversible.

Drug-Induced Interstitial Lung Disease

More than 300 drugs, biomolecules, or homeopathic remedies (see Table 92-2) can cause acute, subacute, or chronic ILD, and the list continues to increase as new medications are introduced. The clinical and radiographic manifestations are quite varied. Examples of known syndromes include chronic nitrofurantoin-induced ILD that mimics idiopathic pulmonary fibrosis (and is fatal in approximately 8% of cases), granulomatous pneumonitis secondary to methotrexate (<5%), sarcoid-like granulomatous ILD induced by interferon-α and tumor necrosis factor modulating agents, nonspecific bilateral alveolar and interstitial inflammatory and fibrotic abnormalities caused by bleomycin and other chemotherapeutic agents, and alveolar and interstitial abnormalities and nodular densities in acute and chronic amiodarone pulmonary toxicity. Most drug-induced ILD is reversible if recognized early and if use of the responsible drug is discontinued. In addition to discontinuing the implicated drug, treatment with corticosteroids (see Table 92-5) is indicated in patients with moderate to severe functional impairment.

Alveolar Filling Disorders

In alveolar filling disorders (Chapter 91), air spaces distal to the terminal bronchioles are filled with blood, lipid, protein, water, or inflammatory cells. The radiographic appearance is that of an alveolar infiltrate with small nodular densities and ill-defined margins; hence, the radiographic picture is similar to an ILD, and virtually all the alveolar filling disorders may result in ILD, including Goodpasture's syndrome, pulmonary alveolar proteinosis (primary and secondary), alveolar hemorrhage syndromes (Chapter 91), acute interstitial pneumonia, and bronchoalveolar cell carcinoma (Chapter 197).

IDIOPATHIC PULMONARY HEMOSIDEROSIS

This rare disorder of children and young adults is characterized by intermittent, diffuse alveolar hemorrhage without evidence of vasculitis, inflammation, granulomas, or necrosis. The etiology is poorly understood. Anemia and hepatosplenomegaly may be present. Hemosiderin-laden macrophages in BAL fluid and lung tissue are part of the diagnostic picture. The chest radiograph reveals diffuse, bilateral alveolar infiltrates. A chronic interstitial infiltrate may develop after repeated episodes, infrequently with hilar and mediastinal adenopathy. Systemic corticosteroids (see Table 92-5) may be beneficial in treating acute disease.

CHRONIC EOSINOPHILIC PNEUMONIA

The clinical manifestation of chronic eosinophilic pneumonia varies over a wide spectrum, from asymptomatic to respiratory failure. The disease often occurs in women in the second to fourth decades of life; such women often manifest constitutional symptoms of fevers, sweats, weight loss, fatigue, dyspnea, and cough. Peripheral blood eosinophilia (Chapter 173), usually at levels of 10 to 40%, is common but may be absent in up to one third of affected patients at initial evaluation. On chest radiography and HRCT, the cardinal feature is peripheral multifocal consolidation, predominantly in the upper and mid lung zones. These dense peripheral infiltrates, which have sometimes been called the "photographic negative of pulmonary edema," often resolve dramatically after treatment with corticosteroids. Ground-glass attenuation commonly accompanies the consolidation. BAL fluid may show greater than 40% eosinophils during exacerbations. Treatment with corticosteroids (see Table 92-5) results in rapid response, frequently within hours; in fact, such a dramatic resolution of symptoms with radiographic clearance of infiltrates shortly after initiation of corticosteroid therapy is considered "diagnostic." However, the rate of relapse is high, so most patients require prolonged treatment with low-dose corticosteroids (prednisone, 5 to 10 mg/day) to stay in remission.

Interstitial Lung Disease Associated with Pulmonary Vasculitides

Wegener's Granulomatosis

Wegener's granulomatosis (Chapter 278) is the most common form of vasculitis that involves the lung. The systemic necrotizing granulomatous inflammation and small-vessel vasculitis are often manifested first in the upper respiratory tract as chronic rhinitis or sinusitis (or both), epistaxis, oropharyngeal ulcerations, gingival hyperplasia with clefting, or serous otitis media. Destruction of the nasal cartilage may lead to septal perforation or a saddle nose deformity. Ulcerative lesions of the tracheobronchial tree, cavitating nodules within the lung parenchyma, and diffuse alveolar hemorrhage caused by pulmonary capillaritis are lower respiratory tract manifestations. Focal segmental necrotizing glomerulonephritis is the most common extrathoracic manifestation, although pulmonary involvement may occur without renal disease. Chest radiography usually reveals multiple nodular or cavitating infiltrates, but single nodules may be found as well. The diagnosis is most commonly made serologically, with demonstration of antineutrophil cytoplasmic antibodies, although a negative test does not exclude the disease. Treatment is usually with cyclophosphamide (50 to 100 mg/day or 2 mg/kg of ideal body weight per day, but not more than 150 mg/day) in conjunction with oral corticosteroids (prednisone, 10 to 40 mg/day). Initial remission occurs in more than 90% of patients, but most patients require treatment for several years. Relapses may occur in up to 30% of patients, especially when treatment is tapered; such patients may need treatment indefinitely. Rituximab is an alternative if cyclophosphamide is unsuccessful or not tolerated (Chapter 278). Prophylaxis for *Pneumocystis carinii* infection is indicated in patients receiving chronic treatment.

CHURG-STRAUSS SYNDROME (ALLERGIC ANGIITIS)

This systemic necrotizing vasculitis (Chapter 291) affects both the upper and lower respiratory tracts and is almost invariably preceded by allergic disorders such as asthma, allergic rhinitis, sinusitis, or a drug reaction. Peripheral and lung eosinophilia, bronchospasm, increased immunoglobulin E levels, and rashes are common manifestations. The pulmonary radiographic findings are bilateral patchy, fleeting infiltrates, diffuse nodular infiltrates, or diffuse reticulonodular disease. Histopathologic examination of lung tissue is generally diagnostic with features of granulomatous angiitis or vasculitis. Although treatment with corticosteroids is indicated, the dosage and duration are unclear (see Table 92-5).

IDIOPATHIC PULMONARY CAPILLARITIS

Idiopathic pulmonary capillaritis may involve the pulmonary vasculature within the alveolar walls and be manifested as ILD. Patients may also have subclinical alveolar hemorrhage, often associated with the presence of perinuclear antineutrophilic cytoplasmic antibodies. Corticosteroids are the mainstay of treatment, but the doses and duration of treatment are unclear. Frequently, patients need adjunctive treatment with cyclophosphamide or rituximab, similar to patients with vasculitis and Wegener's granulomatosis (Chapter 278).

Other Forms of Interstitial Lung Disease
Sarcoidosis
See Chapter 95.

PULMONARY LANGERHANS CELL HISTIOCYTOSIS

This condition, previously known as pulmonary histiocytosis X or eosinophilic granuloma of the lung, is an idiopathic, granulomatous ILD that typically occurs in the second or third decade of life; there is a male preponderance. The currently accepted term is *Langerhans cell histiocytosis*. Pulmonary Langerhans cell histiocytosis is rare, with an estimated incidence of two to five cases per million population. The large majority (~90%) of affected individuals are smokers, and current evidence suggests that the disorder results from an abnormal immune response to a component or derivative of cigarette smoke.

CLINICAL MANIFESTATIONS

The clinical findings are variable and range from an abnormal chest radiograph in an asymptomatic patient to progressive dyspnea with a nonproductive cough. Systemic symptoms of malaise, fever, and weight loss may be present. Hemoptysis is rare. Spontaneous pneumothorax, which occurs in approximately 25% of patients and is due to rupture of subpleural cysts, may be an initial finding. Langerhans cell histiocytosis may be confined to the lung or may be a component of a multisystem disease that includes painful cystic bone lesions and diabetes insipidus (Chapter 232).

DIAGNOSIS

The chest radiograph shows diffuse symmetrical reticulonodular opacities superimposed on multiple small cysts in the upper and mid lung zones. HRCT reveals subpleural nodules, scattered ground-glass densities, and irregular cysts of varying number, size, and configuration in both lungs, with sparing of the lung bases; in the appropriate clinical setting, this pattern may be pathognomonic. As the disease progresses, the increase in fibrosis and cysts may lead to honeycombing of the lung. PFTs are characterized by a mixed restrictive and obstructive pattern, including a reduction in diffusing capacity. Vital capacity is disproportionately reduced compared with total lung capacity because of air trapping within the cysts; the result is an increased residual volume. BAL reveals Langerhans cells (atypical histiocytes) that have the characteristic "x body" (i.e., Birbeck granule) on electron microscopy; immunostaining shows CD1 antigen on the cell surface and S-100 protein in the cytoplasm. However, the absence of these findings does not exclude the diagnosis. The diagnosis is usually made by transbronchial biopsy or open lung biopsy, which reveals interstitial and peribronchiolar collections of histiocytes, eosinophils, and lymphocytes; peribronchiolar nodules; and cysts with areas of central stellate fibrosis.

LYMPHANGIOLEIOMYOMATOSIS

This rare interstitial lung disease is limited to women, primarily of childbearing age. Proliferation of abnormal smooth muscle around bronchioles leads to bilateral small cysts, which give an appearance of ILD on chest radiographs, and progressive impairment of lung function. Hemoptysis, pneumothorax (from rupture of subpleural cysts), and chylothorax (from lymphatic obstruction) may be initial symptoms that distinguish this disorder from other diffuse lung diseases. Although lymphangioleiomyomatosis is usually limited to the lungs, an association with angiomyolipomas of the mediastinal and retroperitoneal lymph nodes and kidney has been described, so the disease may mimic the manifestations of tuberous sclerosis (Chapter 426). Coarse reticulonodular infiltrates, often with cysts or bullae, are typically seen on chest radiographs. In contrast to most other ILDs, increased lung volumes may be present and should prompt consideration of this diagnosis in a nonsmoking woman of reproductive age. HRCT shows characteristic diffuse thin-walled cysts, generally less than 2 cm in diameter. BAL may show occult alveolar hemorrhage. Lung biopsy reveals abnormal smooth muscle cells lining the airways, lymphatics, and blood vessels, with concurrent airflow obstruction and replacement of the lung parenchyma with cysts.

TREATMENT AND PROGNOSIS   Rx

In a randomized trial, sirolimus, an inhibitor of rapamycin signaling, initially at 2 mg per day and titrated to maintain trough levels between 5 and 15 ng/mL, was safe and stabilized lung function. Treatment with progesterone or tamoxifen has been tried, but no randomized trials support the use of interventions to alter the estrogen-progesterone balance. Although lung transplantation is indicated as the patient reaches severe functional impairment, the disease may recur in the transplanted lung. Most patients currently die of respiratory failure about 10 years after the onset of symptoms.

Inherited Disorders

Several rare genetic disorders are associated with ILD and pulmonary fibrosis. Inheritance is autosomal dominant with variable penetrance for most cases of familial idiopathic pulmonary fibrosis and idiopathic interstitial pneumonia and for tuberous sclerosis (Chapter 426), neurofibromatosis (Chapter 426), and familial hypocalciuric hypercalcemia (Chapter 253). Inheritance is autosomal recessive for Gaucher's disease (Chapter 215), Niemann-Pick disease (Chapter 215), and Hermansky-Pudlak syndrome (Chapter 215). The congenital form of the alveolar filling disorder pulmonary alveolar proteinosis also is inherited in an autosomal recessive manner.

Tuberous sclerosis (Chapter 426), an autosomal dominant disease of variable penetrance, is characterized pathologically by the presence of hamartomas in multiple organs. The most well-known clinical manifestations include epilepsy, mental retardation, adenoma sebaceum, and renal angiomyolipomas. ILD occurs in only 1% of patients with tuberous sclerosis, usually in women older than 30 years with little or no mental retardation. The pulmonary involvement, which is indistinguishable from lymphangioleiomyomatosis both radiographically and histopathologically, may be manifested as exertional dyspnea, recurrent pneumothorax, and hemoptysis. HRCT reveals thin-walled cysts and a diffuse reticulonodular infiltrate. Recurrent parenchymal hemorrhage may lead to hemosiderin deposition and interstitial pulmonary fibrosis. There is no cure, and treatment is supportive.

Neurofibromatosis (Chapter 426) may affect all age groups and both sexes. Type 1 (von Recklinghausen's disease) is characterized by cafe au lait spots, neurofibromas, optic glioma, and bony lesions; the more rare type 2 is associated with bilateral acoustic neuromas. Diffuse ILD is manifested as bilateral lower lobe fibrosis as well as bullae or cystic changes. Interstitial fibrosis and alveolitis with thickening of the alveolar septa, accompanied by a cellular infiltrate, are seen on lung biopsy. Management is as for idiopathic pulmonary fibrosis.

Gaucher's disease (Chapter 215), a lysosomal glycolipid storage disorder, has a predilection for the Ashkenazi Jewish population. Pulmonary manifestations, which occur most frequently in type 2 disease, may be a result of interstitial infiltration by Gaucher cells with fibrosis, alveolar consolidation, and filling of alveolar spaces; capillary plugging by Gaucher cells may cause secondary pulmonary hypertension. Treatment is as for the systemic disease, and the general approaches for idiopathic interstitial pneumonias and pulmonary arterial hypertension may be followed for these patients.

TREATMENT AND PROGNOSIS   Rx

Although definitive regression after discontinuation of smoking has not been proved, small series report improvement, so patients should be encouraged to discontinue smoking. The prognosis in pulmonary Langerhans cell histiocytosis is usually favorable, with approximately 75% of patients improving or stabilizing, especially with cessation of smoking; some patients, however, may progress to end-stage lung disease. In patients with progressive disease, corticosteroids (see Table 92-5) with or without vincristine, cyclosporine, cyclophosphamide, and azathioprine have been used with some anecdotal reports of success. Lung transplantation has been performed, but recurrent disease has been reported in the allograft.

Niemann-Pick disease (Chapter 215) is a rare lipid storage disease that may cause infiltration of the characteristic "foam cell" throughout the pulmonary lymphatics, the pulmonary arteries, and the pulmonary alveoli. Patients with type B may survive into adulthood. Treatment is as for the systemic disease.

Hermansky-Pudlak syndrome (Chapter 215) is characterized by oculocutaneous albinism, a bleeding diathesis, and ceroid inclusions in macrophages. Most patients are of Puerto Rican ancestry, and women are affected more frequently than men. Pulmonary fibrosis, with onset in the third or fourth decade, is slowly progressive. Treatment principles and interventions are largely supportive and extrapolated from other related conditions, especially idiopathic pulmonary fibrosis.

1. Demedts M, Behr J, Buhl R, et al. High dose acetyl cysteine in idiopathic pulmonary fibrosis. *N Engl J Med.* 2005;353:2229-2242.
2. Taniguichi H, Ebina M, Kondoh Y, et al. Pirfenidone in idiopathic pulmonary fibrosis. *Eur Respir J.* 2010;35:821-829.
3. King TE Jr, Albera C, Bradford WZ, et al. Effect of interferon gamma-1b on survival in patients with idiopathic pulmonary fibrosis (INSPIRE): a multicentre, randomised, placebo-controlled trial. *Lancet.* 2009;374:222-228.
4. Tashkin DP, Elashoff R, Clements PJ, et al. Cyclophosphamide versus placebo in scleroderma lung disease. *N Engl J Med.* 2006;354:2655-2666.
5. McCormack FX, Inoue Y, Moss J, et al. Efficacy and safety of sirolimus in lymphangioleiomyomatosis. *N Engl J Med.* 2011;364:1595-1606.

SUGGESTED READINGS

Chan AL, Rafil R, Louie S, et al. Therapeutic update in idiopathic pulmonary fibrosis. *Clin Rev Allergy Immunol.* 2011. [Epub ahead of print.] *Review.*
Fernández Pérez ER, Daniels CE, Schroeder DR, et al. Incidence, prevalence, and clinical course of idiopathic pulmonary fibrosis: a population-based study. *Chest.* 2010;137;129-137. *Median survival was about 4 years.*
Raghu G, Collard HR, Egan JJ, et al. An official ATS/ERS/JRS/ALAT statement: idiopathic pulmonary fibrosis: evidence-based guidelines for diagnosis and management. *Am J Respir Crit Care Med.* 2011; 183:788-824. *Consensus guidelines.*

93

OCCUPATIONAL LUNG DISEASE

SUSAN M. TARLO

Occupational lung diseases include a wide spectrum of respiratory disorders with symptoms, signs, and diagnostic test results that often present with features similar to nonoccupational diseases (Table 93-1). For example, adult-onset asthma (Chapter 87) may be occupational asthma, presumed sarcoidosis (Chapter 95) may actually be chronic beryllium disease, apparent idiopathic pulmonary fibrosis may be asbestosis, or a suspected viral pneumonia (Chapter 97) may be hypersensitivity pneumonitis from an occupational cause such as contaminated metal-working fluid.

When evaluating any respiratory disease, the clinician should consider the possibility of an occupational cause or contribution (see E-Fig. 18-1 in Chapter 18; see Table 93-1). The onset of disease after an occupational exposure may occur with a short latency period, as for an acute toxic inhalation injury, or over a period of months to years, as for occupational asthma or hypersensitivity pneumonitis. Latency can be 20 years or more in chronic beryllium disease or lung cancer from chromium, asbestos, or other carcinogens. The most relevant job and occupational exposure history will therefore depend in part on the type of lung disease: for acute syndromes, the recent job exposure is most relevant; for asthma or hypersensitivity pneumonitis, the exposures at the onset of symptoms and ongoing exposures are most relevant; but for chronic diseases or diseases that may result from a long latency exposure, a full working history is essential. Consideration also should be given to potentially relevant exposures that may be related to a patient's hobbies or avocations (e.g., woodworking, model building, or insect collecting).

The clinical relevance of a correct occupational attribution is most apparent for diseases with a close temporal relationship between exposure and the onset of symptoms because intervention to reduce or remove exposure

may reverse the disease or prevent progression. In addition, interventions in the workplace may reduce or prevent disease in other workers. However, even for diseases with a potential long latency, such as chronic beryllium disease, identification of disease in one worker should be regarded as a sentinel event that can lead to investigation of the workplace exposures and introduction of preventive measures. With the assistance of their physicians, workers with occupational lung diseases also often can qualify for workers' compensation.

EPIDEMIOLOGY

No reliable figures exist for the total incidence or prevalence of occupational lung diseases, and regional variation in occupations and exposures is substantial. Work-related asthma has become the most common chronic occupational lung disease in developed countries, where occupational asthma (asthma caused by work) accounts for about 15% of all adult-onset asthma, and work-exacerbated asthma occurs in 25 to 52% of asthmatic workers. The occupational contribution of workplace dusts, fumes, and gases to chronic obstructive pulmonary disease (COPD) is estimated at 15%.

In contrast, pneumoconiosis from silica or coal dust, although still important in developing countries, is declining in incidence in developed countries (E-Fig. 93-1) as a result of occupational hygiene measures. For example, approximately 100,000 Americans received benefits from the Federal Black Lung Program in 2005, compared with about 500,000 in 1980, and the percentage of coal miners with pneumoconiosis has fallen from 11% in the mid-1970s down to 3%. However, newer exposures that lead to silicosis include the textile industry's use of jet silica blasting of denim jeans, reported from Turkey. Newly recognized asbestos-related diseases continue to occur, owing to the long latency period between exposure and clinical disease, despite the declining exposure to asbestos in developed countries. Although annual deaths from asbestosis have now reached a plateau in North America and will likely decline, new cases of mesothelioma, which has a latency of up to 35 years or more, are not estimated to plateau until 2020.

Chronic beryllium disease declined in frequency and severity after the elimination of beryllium from fluorescent lightbulbs in the 1950s, but then increased because of the increasing use of beryllium in nuclear facilities, aerospace, electronics, dental ceramics, metal alloys, recycling of metals, and products such as golf clubs and bicycles. The beryllium lymphocyte proliferation test can identify beryllium sensitization, which can be found in up to 10% of exposed workers and facilitates earlier diagnosis of chronic beryllium disease.

SPECIFIC OCCUPATIONAL LUNG DISORDERS

Occupational lung diseases are often misdiagnosed as other common nonoccupational diseases, but a careful history and appropriate investigations can lead to a correct diagnosis. For many occupational lung diseases, the diagnosis can significantly improve prognosis and lead to measures to prevent illness in other workers.

Work-Related Asthma

Work-related asthma includes both occupational asthma that is caused by work and asthma that is not caused by work but is exacerbated by work exposures.

SENSITIZER-INDUCED OCCUPATIONAL ASTHMA

EPIDEMIOLOGY

Occupational asthma is most commonly associated with a specific immune response to a high- or low-molecular-weight sensitizer (Table 93-2). Sensitizer-induced occupational asthma usually affects no more than 5 to 10% of workers exposed to the sensitizing agent, but exposure to complex platinum salts or detergent enzymes may result in symptoms in about 50% of highly exposed workers. In most studies, higher levels of exposure are associated with higher rates of sensitization in the exposed populations, but there is no clear threshold exposure below which all workers are protected from the risk of sensitization.

PATHOBIOLOGY

Genetic factors increase the risk of sensitization, but the risks appear to be polygenic and may differ for different allergens and sensitizers. Underlying atopy, as exemplified by a history of allergy or positive skin tests to common environmental allergens (Chapter 257), carries an increased risk of

TABLE 93-1 EXAMPLES OF OCCUPATIONAL RESPIRATORY DISEASES THAT COULD BE MISDIAGNOSED AS COMMON NONOCCUPATIONAL RESPIRATORY DISEASE

DISEASE THAT IS MIMICKED	POSSIBLE OCCUPATIONAL DISEASE	EXAMPLES OF SUGGESTIVE FEATURES LEADING TO A CORRECT DIAGNOSIS
Asthma	Occupational asthma from a work sensitizer	Asthma symptoms begin and are worse during a working period, with some improvement on days or weeks off work. Exposure to a high- or low-molecular-weight workplace sensitizer
	Occupational asthma—irritant-induced, including reactive airways dysfunction syndrome	Asthma begins within days after a high-level (accidental) workplace exposure
	Work-exacerbated asthma	Asthma usually began before starting the job or exposure, but severity is worse on days of work, or work exposures to expected asthma triggers or common allergens at work
COPD	Occupational COPD	Prolonged exposure at work to dusts, fumes, or gases
Pneumonia	Acute hypersensitivity pneumonitis	Symptoms typically resolve within days and recur on re-exposure to the same work trigger (e.g., metal-working fluid, moldy hay, humidifiers)
Acute viral respiratory illness or pneumonia	Humidifier fever, organic dust toxic syndrome, metal fume fever, polymer fume fever, cotton dust fever	Exposure triggers the episodes
Sarcoidosis	Chronic beryllium disease	History of exposure to beryllium dust or fumes up to 30 years or more before onset of disease
	Silicosis	History of exposure; typical radiographic findings of rounded opacities with upper lobe predominance and progressive massive fibrosis, biopsy
Idiopathic pulmonary fibrosis	Asbestosis	History of moderate or high previous asbestos exposure and appropriate latency period, often with other markers of asbestos exposure, such as radiographic evidence of pleural plaques
	Chronic hypersensitivity pneumonitis	± Work exposure to a known trigger, ± improvement during periods away from exposure
	Flock-worker's lung	Lymphocytic bronchiolitis and interstitial lung disease from nylon/synthetic textile microfibers
Idiopathic pulmonary fibrosis or hypersensitivity pneumonitis	Hard metal disease	History of exposure to hard metal (tungsten, cobalt), and histologic findings of giant cell pneumonitis on lung biopsy
Chest infections	Occupational causes of chest infections, e.g., SARS or TB in health care workers, histoplasmosis in construction workers, anthrax in wool workers or farmers	History of occupation and exposures
Pleural effusion	Asbestos-related benign pleural effusion	Previous asbestos exposure with appropriate latency; pleural plaques commonly present
Incidental pulmonary nodule	Rounded atelectasis from asbestos	Previous asbestos exposure with appropriate latency; pleural plaques commonly present
Multiple nodules	Silicosis or pneumoconiosis	History of exposure, distribution of nodules, presence of progressive massive fibrosis
Lung cancer	Occupational lung cancer	History of exposure to carcinogens at work, with an appropriate latency period (e.g., asbestos, radon, chromium)
Bronchiolitis obliterans	Popcorn lung	History of working with microwave popcorn or flavorings

COPD = chronic obstructive pulmonary disease; SARS = severe acute respiratory syndrome; TB = tuberculosis.

sensitization to the high-molecular-weight allergens, and smoking (Chapter 31) has been reported as a risk factor for sensitization to complex platinum salts. Currently, no host factors are sufficiently specific to justify exclusion of workers from settings with exposure to potential sensitizers.

Occupational asthma from a high-molecular-weight allergen is associated with specific immunoglobulin E (IgE) antibody production. Low-molecular-weight sensitizers may act as haptens or may induce neoantigens by reacting with proteins in vivo, but specific IgE antibodies have been demonstrated with only a few low-molecular-weight sensitizers, such as complex platinum salts and acid anhydrides used in epoxy compounds.

CLINICAL MANIFESTATIONS

Sensitizer-induced occupational asthma has a latency period ranging from weeks to several years before it develops, but most patients develop symptoms within the first few years of exposure. Once a patient has become sensitized and has developed asthma, even very small subsequent exposures can trigger asthma, sometimes including exposures that may be below the limit of measurable detection. Pulmonary function and histologic changes are similar to those in nonoccupational asthma (Chapter 87). Sensitizer-induced occupational asthma from a high-molecular-weight agent sensitizer typically causes a prompt asthmatic response within minutes after exposure with or without a late asthmatic response starting 4 to 6 hours after exposure. By comparison, responses to low-molecular-weight sensitizers typically start 4 to 6 hours after exposure.

DIAGNOSIS

The diagnosis of sensitizer-induced occupation asthma is clinically suspected by history and should be considered in all cases of new-onset asthma in patients who work. Supportive features include symptomatic improvement when away from work, such as weekends off work or holidays, but not necessarily in the evenings after a work shift, when symptoms from a late asthmatic response may occur. In patients who are exposed to high-molecular-weight sensitizers, allergic rhinitis or conjunctivitis associated with work frequently appears before the development of asthma. A detailed occupational history (Chapter 18) or review of material safety data sheets or occupational hygiene reports may reveal a known occupational sensitizer. However, more than 300 occupational respiratory sensitizers are currently known, and new agents or exposures are reported each year; as a result, the absence of a recognized sensitizer does not exclude occupational asthma.

Although the history can be very helpful, the evaluation should always include objective pulmonary function testing (Chapter 85) to confirm asthma, either when the patient has symptoms or within 24 hours of the typical suspected work exposure (Fig. 93-1). Allergy skin-prick tests, blood samples, or both should be obtained to test for specific IgE antibodies to any relevant sensitizer if feasible. Serial monitoring of peak expiratory flow rates, symptom diaries, or use of rescue inhalers can provide supportive information. The results of a methacholine challenge test (Chapter 87) toward the

TABLE 93-2 COMMON CAUSES OF SENSITIZER-INDUCED OCCUPATIONAL ASTHMA

OCCUPATION	ALLERGEN BY SETTING
Bakers	Wheat, rye, fungal amylase in flour
Laboratory workers	Animal allergens, e.g., proteins in rat urine, mouse or rabbit dander
Detergent-making, medical instrument cleaning, pharmaceuticals or laboratory workers	Enzymes: e.g., *Bacillus subtilis*, pancreatic enzymes
Farmers	Grains, plant, and animal allergens; mites
Greenhouse workers and florists	Pollen, fungi, mites
Food workers	Airborne food allergens, e.g., powdered milk or eggs and vegetables
Some office workers	Fungal allergens in moldy or "sick" buildings
Health care workers	Latex allergens from gloves, glutaraldehyde, orthophthaldehyde, aerosolized medications
Factory or other industrial workers	Chemicals in spray paints, glues, polyurethane, coatings and spray insulation, adhesives
Electronic workers	Soldering flux with colophony

end of a typical work week can help when compared with results after 10 days or more without exposure. A comparison of eosinophil counts in induced sputum at work and after a period away from exposure, showing higher levels when exposed, provides supportive diagnostic information. If the diagnosis is still in doubt, a carefully controlled specific inhalation challenge with the suspected workplace sensitizer can be performed. Each investigation can be falsely positive or negative, so a combination of investigations is advised while the patient continues to work until the diagnosis is confirmed. Given the specialized nature of many of these studies, consultation with a specialist is recommended. The main differential diagnosis for patients with confirmed asthma is the coincidental onset of asthma with subsequent work-exacerbated asthma. Other conditions, such as vocal cord dysfunction, may explain symptoms or may coexist with asthma and confound the diagnosis.

TREATMENT AND PREVENTION — Rx

The optimal management of patients with sensitizer-induced occupational asthma includes complete removal from further exposure to the sensitizer and cross-reacting agents combined with the usual pharmacologic approach to the treatment of asthma (Chapter 87) and advocacy for appropriate workers' compensation. Consideration of the other exposed workers typically includes communication with the workplace or public health officials, in the hope that measures may be instituted to protect other workers from similar exposures and symptoms. Recommendations for primary prevention have been to reduce exposures to occupational sensitizers as far as possible, removing unnecessary sensitizing agents (e.g., removing high-powdered and high-protein latex gloves) and limiting exposures to sensitizers with occupational hygiene measures. Ongoing medical surveillance measures in the workplace may also be of value.

PROGNOSIS

Outcome is best if an early diagnosis results in removal from further exposure while asthma is relatively mild. Improvement may continue to occur up to 10 years after removal from exposure, but asthma does not completely resolve in most patients. For patients with occupational asthma from natural rubber latex, use of powder-free, low-protein latex gloves by coworkers and direct avoidance of natural rubber products by the sensitized worker results in improvement that is similar to the improvement in patients who are completely removed from work.

Work-Exacerbated Asthma

EPIDEMIOLOGY AND CLINICAL MANIFESTATIONS

Work-exacerbated asthma is defined as asthma that is not caused by work but is aggravated or exacerbated by work conditions. Asthma may have been present before starting employment or may begin coincidentally during employment, but it is not caused by work. Work exposures that commonly exacerbate asthma include extreme temperature or humidity, exertion, dusts, fumes, and gases. Patients may be exposed at work to common environmental allergens (e.g., fungal allergens in an office setting or dust mites or animals in domestic settings) that exacerbate asthma in patients who are sensitized to these allergens. Symptoms of work-exacerbated asthma may occur transiently with an unusual work exposure (e.g., during renovation in a work building) or may occur on a daily basis (e.g., daily exposure to fumes while performing physical exertion in an industrial setting).

DIAGNOSIS AND TREATMENT — Rx

Transient work-exacerbated asthma is commonly diagnosed on the basis of the history of work exposures and the associated increase in asthmatic symptoms, medication requirements, or unscheduled physician visits. The recommended evaluation of patients with daily or frequent work exacerbations of asthma is similar to that for patients with suspected occupational asthma. Work-related changes in serial peak flow recordings mimic those seen in occupational asthma, but sputum eosinophil counts typically show less of a work-related increase than is observed with occupational asthma. If the workplace exposure includes a potential work sensitizer, immunologic testing or a controlled challenge exposure may confirm whether respiratory sensitization has occurred.

Management includes the same pharmacologic measures as for non-work-related exacerbations, including the optimization of pharmacologic asthma management (Chapter 87) and, when needed, adjusting the work exposures to avoid ongoing exacerbations. Occupational hygiene measures can reduce exposures, but some patients require a change in job description or work area. Workers' compensation may be available for some patients who miss work owing to work-exacerbation of asthma.

IRRITANT EXPOSURE AND REACTIVE AIRWAYS DYSFUNCTION SYNDROME

A high level of usually accidental exposure to an irritant agent can cause asthma. Although the clinical manifestations can be dramatic, irritant-induced occupational asthma represents a relatively small proportion of all occupational asthma. The most definitive criteria for this condition are those applied to the term *reactive airways dysfunction syndrome*: the onset of asthma symptoms within 24 hours of the exposure, generally severe enough to lead to an unscheduled physician visit; exposure to a single high-level irritant; asthma symptoms that persist for at least 3 months; pulmonary function testing that confirms asthma with a significant beneficial response to bronchodilators or a bronchoconstrictor response to a methacholine challenge; and the lack of preexisting lung disease or other conditions to explain the symptoms. When these criteria are not completely met (e.g., symptoms start later than 24 hours after exposure or resolve within weeks after exposure), the term *irritant-induced asthma* is commonly applied, recognizing that this diagnosis is less certain than reactive airways dysfunction syndrome.

Irritant-induced asthma and reactive airways dysfunction syndrome may clear after weeks or months. Management is the same as for other causes of asthma (Chapter 87), although these patients are often less responsive to the usual pharmacologic treatment.

Occupational hygiene measures at the workplace should be improved to prevent similar future exposures. Affected patients may need a modified work environment to prevent subsequent exacerbations of asthma.

OCCUPATIONAL CHRONIC OBSTRUCTIVE PULMONARY DISEASE

Chronic exposure to dusts, fumes, and gases can cause occupationally induced COPD, with pathophysiologic changes essentially identical to those seen in COPD that is related to smoking (Chapter 88). Symptoms of chronic bronchitis, including chronic cough and sputum production, may occur with or without changes on pulmonary function testing. Causes include mineral dusts such as silica and organic dust exposures such as those of farmers and woodworkers; particulate matter in diesel exhaust fumes; and nitrogen oxides, ozone, and ultrafine particles in welding fumes.

FIGURE 93-1. Clinical evaluation and management of work-related asthma. IgE = immunoglobulin E; MSDS = Material Safety Data Sheets; PEFR = peak expiratory flow rates; SIC = specific inhalation challenge. (From American College of Chest Physicians. Consensus statement: diagnosis and management of work-related asthma. *Chest.* 2008;134:1S-41S.)

No specific diagnostic tests distinguish an occupational from a nonoccupational cause of COPD. The history of exposure, with objective documentation, is helpful. Confirmation of the absence of a smoking history can assist in determining probability of an occupational cause, but a positive smoking history does not exclude an occupational contribution.

Management is the same as for patients with nonoccupational COPD (Chapter 88). In addition, however, further exposure to dusts, fumes, and gases that are likely to worsen disease should be minimized.

HYPERSENSITIVITY PNEUMONITIS

Many exposures that lead to hypersensitivity pneumonitis (Chapter 92) occur in the workplace, and several bear the name of the occupation or job associated with them: farmer's lung; maple bark stripper's lung; cheese washer's lung; thatcher's lung; mushroom worker's lung, and metal-working fluid hypersensitivity pneumonitis (Table 93-3). Occupational causes also include exposure to contaminated humidifiers (with protozoa or fungi) in factories

TABLE 93-3 EXAMPLES OF OCCUPATIONAL CAUSES OF HYPERSENSITIVITY PNEUMONITIS

OCCUPATION	CAUSE
Farmer	Thermophilic actinomycetes in moldy hay
Metal worker	Contamination of metal-working fluids with microorganisms such as *Mycobacteria immunogens* or fungi
Worker exposed to humidifiers	Contamination with microorganisms such as protozoa or fungi
Sugarcane worker	Moldy sugarcane (bagassosis)
Maple bark stripper	Fungi
Chicken or turkey worker	Avian proteins
Pharmaceutical worker	Penicillin
Food handler	Soybeans
Office worker	Microorganisms contaminating air conditioners or humidifiers
Swimming pool attendant	Fungal contamination in sprays around pool area
Animal worker	Rat proteins
Mushroom worker	Fungi
Wheat farmer or handler	Weevil-infested flour
Greenhouse worker	Fungi
Workers spraying urethane paint or adhesives/sealants (or less often, other workers using diisocyanate)	Methylene diphenyl diisocyanate, hexamethylene diisocyanate, toluene diisocyanates
Chemical worker using plastics, resins, paints	Trimellitic anhydride

or office buildings (humidifier lung), as well as lifeguards exposed to sprays of water from pool fountains contaminated with microorganisms. Metal workers or machinists can develop hypersensitivity pneumonitis from recirculated coolants that can become contaminated with gram-negative bacteria or atypical mycobacteria, which then are aerosolized in the coolant mist and inhaled.

PATHOBIOLOGY

Most antigenic exposures that lead to hypersensitivity pneumonitis are organic, especially thermophilic actinomycetes (Chapter 337), fungi, atypical mycobacteria (Chapter 333), and protozoa. Other common antigens include avian and rat proteins. Less commonly, hypersensitivity pneumonitis can be induced by low-molecular-weight chemical antigens, such as penicillin or methylene diphenyl diisocyanate (MDI), which is used as a sealant or binder. Small particles, commonly 3 to 5 μm in mass median aerodynamic diameter, reach the small airways and alveoli, where the immune response leads to hypersensitivity pneumonitis. This immune response is associated with specific IgG antibodies and T lymphocytes, and it recurs with repeated exposures.

CLINICAL MANIFESTATIONS AND DIAGNOSIS

The acute form of disease manifests as cough, dyspnea, chills, and malaise, typically 4 to 8 hours after exposure and clearing by 12 to 24 hours. On examination, patients typically are febrile and tachypneic, with reduced chest expansion and basal crackles. Neutrophilia is common, and the chest radiograph shows acute infiltrates. Pulmonary function testing may show a restrictive pattern, with a reduced diffusing capacity, and arterial blood gases may show hypoxemia owing to ventilation-perfusion mismatch.

Chronic hypersensitivity pneumonitis may follow repeat acute episodes or start de novo. It causes a chronic dry cough, progressive dyspnea, and often significant weight loss. The physical examination typically reveals reduced chest expansion and basal crackles. Results on pulmonary function testing and radiographic findings may be similar to nonspecific idiopathic pulmonary fibrosis (Chapter 92), and ground-glass opacities are often seen on a computed tomography (CT) scan of the chest. Bronchoalveolar fluid typically shows an increase in the lymphocyte count, and there may be a predominance of CD8 T lymphocytes (Chapter 85).

The specific occupational cause for hypersensitivity pneumonitis may be suspected from a temporal relationship to work exposures. The differential diagnosis in the chronic form includes idiopathic pulmonary fibrosis, although clubbing is less common in hypersensitivity pneumonitis. Radiographic and pulmonary function test findings may also mimic idiopathic pulmonary fibrosis, but a distinguishing finding is often a bronchoalveolar lavage that shows lymphocytes as high as 60 to 80% of the cells, usually with a predominance of CD8$^+$ T lymphocytes, but sometimes with CD4$^+$ cells in chronic forms of disease.

Laboratory investigations include determining the presence of serum IgG antibodies to the suspected antigen. However, IgG antibodies may also be present in exposed individuals who do not have disease and are therefore not specific to the diagnosis. Conversely, failure to demonstrate specific antibodies is not uncommon in hypersensitivity pneumonitis because the limited number of antigens used for testing may not include the relevant occupational antigen. Specific challenge with the suspected antigen in a laboratory setting is occasionally needed if the diagnosis is in doubt.

Some patients can safely undergo "work challenge" that monitors changes in symptoms, fever, blood neutrophil count, radiographic findings, and pulmonary function with and without exposure to the suspected agent. Lung biopsy, if performed, may show granulomas and foreign body giant cells. If other findings are supportive of hypersensitivity pneumonitis, however, open biopsy and challenges usually are not needed.

TREATMENT AND PROGNOSIS — Rx

Treatment principles are the same as for nonoccupational hypersensitivity pneumonitis (Chapter 94). Removal from exposure to the causative agent is the primary treatment measure. As with occupational asthma from a sensitizer, the removal must be complete and often requires a change in work if the causative agent cannot be removed. Reduction of exposure by use of respiratory protective devices is generally not practical and not effective, with the exception of air-supplied helmet respirators for occasional short-term exposures. Patients with acute hypersensitivity pneumonitis may not require any medications in addition to removal from antigen exposure, but if acute episodes are severe, they may need supportive measures, including corticosteroids (e.g., 20 to 60 mg of prednisone orally per day), supplemental oxygen, and intensive care (Chapter 94). Chronic hypersensitivity pneumonitis may require additional oral corticosteroid treatment (e.g., 5 to 10 mg of prednisone orally per day) as for nonoccupational chronic hypersensitivity pneumonitis, and severe end-stage fibrosis may lead to need for lung transplantation. Prognosis is better with early diagnosis and complete removal from exposure to the causative agent. Preventive measures include occupational hygiene measures to avoid contamination of aerosolized fluid or dusts with bio-organisms and use of appropriate respiratory protective devices.

● CHRONIC BERYLLIUM DISEASE

EPIDEMIOLOGY AND PATHOBIOLOGY

Acute toxic pneumonitis was described in workers who had high exposure to beryllium in the manufacture of fluorescent lightbulbs in the 1940s, and a hypersensitivity response causing chronic beryllium disease was described in the 1950s. Acute toxic effects are now rare, but chronic beryllium disease remains a problem because of the expanded use of beryllium (Table 93-4) and better recognition of sensitization by development of an immunologic blood test.

Chronic beryllium disease is a hypersensitivity disease with a strong genetic association with HLA-DPB1 gene variants that code for Glu69 and that have been identified in 83 to 97% of patients with disease. However, this gene variant occurs in 30 to 48% of the general population and, as a result, is not useful as a screening test.

CLINICAL MANIFESTATIONS

The pulmonary clinical features of chronic beryllium disease are similar to those of sarcoidosis (Chapter 95), ranging from asymptomatic histologic or radiographic findings, to potential progression, to severe granulomatous restrictive lung disease. Onset can occur up to 20 years or more after exposure to beryllium, even if the patient no longer is exposed. The clinical history in all patients with apparent sarcoidosis must include inquiry about possible beryllium exposure, even many years ago.

DIAGNOSIS AND TREATMENT

The chest radiograph shows changes that appear identical to sarcoidosis with enlarged hilar or mediastinal lymph nodes or multiple lung nodules, or both (Fig. 93-2). Sensitization to beryllium can be detected by a beryllium lymphocyte proliferation test that demonstrates the presence of sensitized lymphocytes in blood or bronchoalveolar lavage fluid. This test also can detect sensitization to beryllium among asymptomatic exposed workers, who can then be evaluated to assess possible chronic beryllium disease and provided with advice for reducing or eliminating further work exposures.

After disease develops, removal from exposure is advised, but the disease may still worsen. Progressive deterioration in lung function is treated similarly to sarcoidosis (Chapter 95), with oral corticosteroids and supportive measures.

● ASBESTOS-RELATED DISEASES

Although the use of asbestos has declined, and better protective equipment has been mandated, asbestos-related disease has continued to occur owing to the long latency between exposure and disease. Chrysotile asbestos has less effect on the lungs than other forms of asbestos, that is, amphiboles. Effects of exposure include benign and malignant disease.

Benign asbestos disease is often asymptomatic and identified on chest imaging. Pleural thickening and pleural plaques, commonly with calcification, can occur 20 to 30 years after first exposure and may initially appear on the chest radiograph as calcified linear opacities over the hemidiaphragms and cardiac border (see Fig. 84-10 in Chapter 84). If extensive, it may be difficult to exclude intrapulmonary opacities except by CT scan. Pleural plaques are a marker of asbestos exposure but do not occur in all workers with significant asbestos exposure. They generally do not cause significant changes in lung function, except diffuse pleural thickening may result in exertional dyspnea and extrapulmonary restrictive lung disease. Pleural thickening may cause rounded atelectasis (Chapter 90) when encasement of a portion of the peripheral lung tissue by thickened pleura causes an apparent lung nodule, typically with a "comet sign" showing the thickened pleura. Benign pleural effusion can develop, typically about 10 to 15 years after asbestos exposure. It requires further investigation because the differential diagnosis includes malignant pleural effusion (Chapter 99).

Asbestosis is the term for interstitial lung disease caused by asbestos. The clinical presentation is usually with dry cough and dyspnea on exertion. Physical examination usually reveals digital clubbing and basal crackles on lung auscultation. Chest imaging shows basal interstitial lung disease, with or without additional pleural changes as described earlier. Pulmonary function testing shows restrictive lung disease (Chapter 85), and histologic findings are the same as in usual interstitial pneumonia (Chapter 92). Findings supporting the diagnosis of asbestosis rather than usual interstitial pneumonia include a significant duration and level of exposure to asbestos, an appropriate latency of usually 20 to 40 years after first exposure, and the finding of ferruginous asbestos bodies in sputum or lung tissue (Fig. 93-3). Unfortunately, pharmacologic treatment is not effective, and the lung disease may progress to end-stage fibrosis. Management is supportive, including supplemental oxygen and consideration for lung transplantation (Chapter 101). As with the other diseases of long latency, preventing exposure is paramount.

Mesothelioma (Chapter 197), a malignant tumor of the pleura, peritoneum, or both, is the one complication of asbestos exposure that can occur after even relatively minor exposure, such as second-hand exposure from dust on clothing in the families of those working with exposure. It typically occurs 30 to 40 years after exposure to asbestos and may present incidentally on chest imaging or with chest pain or weight loss. Radiographs show pleural thickening, and a pleural effusion may be present. Mesothelioma often is difficult to distinguish from benign pleural thickening without a biopsy. No treatment has proved effective (Chapter 197), so routine screening to detect mesothelioma in exposed persons is not currently recommended. The risk of lung cancer (Chapter 197) increases after significant exposure to asbestos, with a usual latency period of 20 to 30 years. Smoking and asbestos exposure have multiplicative effects on the risk of lung cancer.

TABLE 93-4 POTENTIAL EXPOSURES TO BERYLLIUM
OCCUPATIONAL EXPOSURES
Metal and alloy production (alloys of aluminum, copper, and nickel; recently includes golf clubs and metal pen clips)
Ceramic manufacturing
Metal casting, including dental technicians (crowns, bridges)
Electronics, including computer components, transistors, microwave and x-ray windows, heat sinks, telecommunications
Aerospace and atomic engineering (rocket fuels, heat shields, nose cones, and metal parts)
Aircraft manufacture and repair
Nuclear reactors, nuclear weapons and defense industry
Coating of cathode ray tubes for radar and similar installations
Laboratories
Extraction from ore
Metal reclamation and recycling
NONOCCUPATIONAL EXPOSURES
Family members exposed to dust from workers' clothing
Breakage of old fluorescent lamps (made before 1950 in North America)
Downwind exposure from industrial accidents (e.g., from a nuclear processing plant in Kazakhstan, in the former Soviet Union in 1990)

From Tarlo SM, Rhee K, Powell E, et al. Marked tachypnoea in siblings with chronic beryllium disease due to copper-beryllium alloy. *Chest.* 2001;119:647-650.

FIGURE 93-2. Posteroanterior chest radiograph (A) and high-resolution computed tomography scan (B) from patients with chronic beryllium disease. The chest radiograph demonstrates hilar adenopathy and infiltrates, and the scan shows air space destruction and infiltrates.

FIGURE 93-3. Histology from a lung biopsy showing asbestos bodies. Ferruginous bodies consisting of asbestos fibers coated by iron-protein-mucopolysaccharide material with typical golden-brown, beaded appearance. The two longest asbestos bodies at the centre of the figure are present within a multinucleated giant cell. (Hematoxylin and eosin stain, × 400). (Courtesy of Dr. David Hwang, Toronto General Hospital.)

FIGURE 93-4. Posteroanterior chest radiographs from two patients with silicosis. **A**, Small nodules and eggshell calcification of hilar lymph nodes. **B**, Progressive massive fibrosis of the upper lung zones with compensatory emphysema.

SILICOSIS AND OTHER PNEUMOCONIOSES

The incidences of silicosis and other inorganic dust diseases of the lungs (Table 93-5) have declined substantially in recent decades owing to better worksite protection in mines, sandblasting, and other settings. There is an association between silicosis and the development of collagen-vascular disease, especially rheumatoid arthritis. Patients with pneumoconiosis and rheumatoid arthritis may be at higher risk of developing rheumatoid nodules in the lung, so-called Caplan's syndrome, and mycobacterial infections.

Patients may initially be identified incidentally during a medical surveillance program or by a chest radiograph that shows multiple small lung nodules, often with enlarged mediastinal lymph nodes that can mimic sarcoidosis (Fig. 93-4). Nodules can coalesce and lead to progressive massive fibrosis, especially in the upper lungs, with compensatory emphysema in the lower lung fields. On chest imaging, mediastinal lymph nodes may have a characteristic "eggshell" calcification in silicosis. Treatment is supportive. Patients with exposure to silica or coal dust may develop COPD from the dust exposure. Patients who develop end-stage lung disease may be considered for lung transplantation.

ACUTE FEBRILE SYNDROMES

A variety of occupational exposures can cause acute febrile respiratory syndromes that may mimic acute viral respiratory illnesses (Table 93-6). The mechanism of these syndromes is incompletely understood, but they are

TABLE 93-5 JOBS THAT CAN LEAD TO SILICOSIS
Mining: surface or underground mining (tunneling)
Milling: ground silica for abrasives and filler
Quarrying
Sandblasting: e.g., of buildings, preparing steel for painting
Pottery; ceramic or clay work
Grinding, polishing using silica wheels
Stone work
Foundry work: grinding, molding, chipping
Refractory brick work
Glass making: to polish and as an abrasive
Boiler work: cleaning boilers
Manufacture of abrasives

associated with systemic neutrophilia and cytokine activation, often with increased interleukin-6 (IL-6) and IL-8.

CLINICAL MANIFESTATIONS AND DIAGNOSIS

Typically, chills, fever, malaise, dry cough, and chest tightness start about 6 to 8 hours after onset of an exposure at work and generally resolve by the next day. Occasionally, shortness of breath and other respiratory symptoms are

TABLE 93-6 OCCUPATIONAL CAUSES OF AN ACUTE FEBRILE SYNDROME

SYNDROME	CAUSE
Polymer fume fever or Teflon fever	Polytetrafluoroethylene and other fluorocarbon polymer fumes
Metal fume fever	Zinc fumes from welding of galvanized steel, less commonly other metal fumes
Cotton mill fever	Dust and endotoxins from bacterial contamination of unprocessed cotton, flax, and hemp
Humidifier fever	Microorganisms found in reservoirs, e.g., humidifiers, air conditioners, aquariums
Organic dust toxic syndrome	Grain dust, moldy wood chips

severe enough for patients to seek emergency medical attention. Infiltrates on the chest radiograph can occur with neutrophilia and hypoxemia that can mimic acute pneumonia or acute hypersensitivity pneumonitis. Symptoms and signs generally resolve in 24 to 48 hours without antibiotics and recur with further exposures, although the clinical manifestations generally become milder with repeated daily exposures (e.g., Monday morning fever in cotton mill workers). Workers are often familiar with the syndrome because it commonly affects up to 30% of exposed workers. If the diagnosis is not provided by the patient, however, careful elicitation of potential work exposures is needed.

TREATMENT

Treatment is supportive. If the causative exposure can be removed (e.g., cleaning a contaminated humidifier), symptoms can be prevented. If the cause cannot be removed and symptoms are severe, the patient may need reduction or change of the work exposure.

OCCUPATIONAL LUNG CANCER

A significant duration and level of exposure to a recognized carcinogen such as asbestos, hexavalent chromium (as in chromate production and the pigment industry), soluble radon compounds or radon gas, polycyclic aromatic hydrocarbons, chloromethyl ethers, arsenic, or silica can increase the risk of lung cancer (Chapter 197). Such a history should be elicited in all patients. The International Agency for Research on Cancer provides a listing of occupational lung carcinogens and the likelihood of their association with cancer (*http://monographs.iarc.fr/ENG/Monographs/PDFs/index.php*).

SUGGESTED READINGS

CDC NIOSH Work-Related Lung Disease (WoRLD) Surveillance System. http://www2.cdc.gov/drds/WorldReportData. Accessed Oct. 27, 2010. *Information on the prevalence of occupational lung diseases in the United States.*

Peden DB, Bush RK. Advances in environmental and occupational respiratory diseases in 2009. *J Allergy Clin Immunol.* 2010;125:559-562. *Review.*

Sawyer RT, Maier LA. Chronic beryllium disease: an updated model interaction between innate and acquired immunity. *Biometals.* 2011;24:1-17. *Review of how beryllium drives chronic inflammation and granuloma formation.*

94

PHYSICAL AND CHEMICAL INJURIES OF THE LUNG

DAVID C. CHRISTIANI

SUBMERSION INCIDENTS: DROWNING

DEFINITION

Drowning is defined as "the process of experiencing respiratory impairment from submersion/immersion in liquid." The term *near-drowning* was previously used to describe individuals who survived a submersion incident, at least temporarily, but it has been abandoned on the basis of recommendations of the First World Congress of Drowning in Amsterdam in 2002.

EPIDEMIOLOGY

The estimated annual number of deaths worldwide due to drowning is 500,000. About 4200 persons are treated per year for nonfatal drowning in U.S. emergency departments, and about another 3400 suffer fatal drowning. Alcohol use, age younger than 4 years, and male gender are associated with increased rates of both nonfatal and fatal drowning.

PATHOBIOLOGY

The initial response to submersion/immersion is apnea, followed almost invariably by aspiration. Laryngospasm may result in aspiration of a variable quantity of liquid medium into the lungs. Hypoxemia, hypercapnia, and acidemia develop acutely. Aspiration of either fresh or salt water results in occlusion of the airway, reduced surfactant activity, direct alveolar injury, and bronchospasm. Acute lung injury or the acute respiratory distress syndrome (ARDS), associated with noncardiogenic pulmonary edema and severe hypoxemia, may develop hours or days after the incident. Mortality is primarily due to cardiovascular effects as a result of severe early or late hypoxia. The most serious secondary consequence of hypoxia is anoxic brain injury. Acute renal failure may also occur. Alcohol consumption also increases the risk for hypothermia. Changes to serum electrolytes with drowning in either fresh water or salt water are not clinically significant.

CLINICAL MANIFESTATIONS

The initial presentation of a drowning victim varies widely. Hypothermia, which is common in drowning victims, may be associated with bradycardia or cardiac arrest due to asystole or ventricular fibrillation. Tachypnea, tachycardia, and low-grade fever are typical in nonhypothermic patients. Cyanosis may be present, and a coughing patient may produce pink frothy sputum. Neurologic evaluation may reveal agitation with or without intoxication or coma. The patient should be examined carefully for signs of associated trauma.

Expected laboratory findings include mild electrolyte abnormalities independent of whether submersion occurs in salt water or fresh water, moderate leukocytosis, slight decrease in hematocrit in the first 24 hours or slight increase in free hemoglobin with a stable hematocrit in fresh water submersion due to hemolysis, severe hypoxemia, and metabolic acidosis. Evidence of disseminated intravascular coagulation may occur. Initial electrocardiographic changes include sinus tachycardia and nonspecific ST segment and T wave changes, which revert to normal within hours. Life-threatening ventricular arrhythmias, complete heart block, or evidence of myocardial infarction can occur early or late in the course. Chest radiographs may initially be normal, despite severe respiratory impairment. Bilateral patchy alveolar infiltrates indicating progression to acute lung injury or ARDS may develop.

DIAGNOSIS

The diagnosis of drowning is made on clinical history of submersion in liquid medium with resulting respiratory impairment. Patients with unusual presenting circumstances should be carefully examined for evidence of trauma or assault.

PREVENTION

Drowning incidents are largely preventable, particularly in children. Pool fencing is a proven, effective strategy to prevent drowning. The primary cause of drowning of infants and toddlers is lack of adult supervision, and supervision of all young children near any form of water is strongly recommended. The role of alcohol in teenage and adult drowning incidents is substantial, and all individuals participating in water-based activities should restrict alcohol intake. The use of personal flotation devices is recommended for children and adults.

TREATMENT

Once the victim has been recovered from submersion, treatment should focus on basic life support algorithms, including notification of emergency response personnel and establishment of an adequate airway and cardiopulmonary resuscitation, if necessary (Chapter 63). If the victim is apneic, rescue breathing should occur immediately, even before removal from the water. Cervical spine stabilization is needed if there is a history of diving, use of a water slide, signs of injury, or signs of alcohol intoxication. Spinal cord injury

(Chapter 406) is otherwise unlikely, and cervical spine stabilization techniques and equipment may impede timely and effective treatment. Attempts to remove water from the airway are unnecessary. Cardiac arrhythmias should be treated with Advanced Cardiac Life Support (ACLS) protocols, including the use of automated external defibrillators when appropriate (Chapter 63). Most drowning victims who receive cardiopulmonary resuscitation or rescue breathing will vomit; if vomiting occurs, the head should be turned to the side and the vomitus removed with a finger. When vomiting occurs in patients who may have spinal cord injury, log rolling techniques are recommended for turning the patient to the side.

All victims of a submersion incident should be transported to a hospital for further evaluation, treatment of potential respiratory failure (Chapter 104), and monitoring for up to 24 hours. Bronchoscopy may be required to evaluate localized wheezing or persistent atelectasis. Prophylactic antibiotics are not useful, but evidence of pneumonia (Chapter 97) should be treated with appropriate antibiotics. Because unusual microorganisms may be isolated from the lower airways, efforts should be made to identify specific microbial flora pertinent to the locus of the drowning incident.

Treatment of neurologic injury is focused on supportive care while the extent of cerebral edema is minimized. To decrease cerebral edema and intracranial pressure, intravenous 23% hypertonic saline (30 mL initially then 75 to 100 mL/hour; goal serum sodium level of 155 mM/L) through a central line may be preferred to mannitol (1 g/kg bolus of 20% solution initially, with repeated doses of 0.25 to 0.5 g/kg every 6 to 8 hours). Hyperventilation to a $PaCO_2$ of 34 to 36 mm Hg may be helpful. Intracranial pressure may increase in response to shivering or purposeless movements, which should be reduced. Induced therapeutic hypothermia improves neurologic outcome after cardiac arrest (Chapter 109), and current recommendations for drowning victims who remain comatose after rescue are to avoid rewarming to core or tympanic temperatures above 34° C and to maintain temperature of 32° to 34° C for 24 to 48 hours. Hyperthermia should be avoided at all times.

PROGNOSIS

The mortality rate for drowning victims who present alive to an emergency department is about 25%. Long-term neurologic deficits persist in approximately 6% of nonfatal drowning victims. Although prolonged duration of submersion is associated with a worse prognosis, young children who are hypothermic when they are rescued after submersion times of up to 60 minutes have recovered without neurologic damage. Other factors associated with poor prognosis include hypotension, persistent apnea, coma, more than a 10-minute delay in receiving basic life support, and duration of resuscitation of more than 25 minutes.

DISEASES OF HIGH ALTITUDE

DEFINITION

Neurologic and pulmonary disturbances, primarily due to direct tissue effects of hypoxia, occur in individuals who either ascend to or reside at altitudes of 7000 feet (2133 meters) or more (Table 94-1).

EPIDEMIOLOGY

Acute mountain sickness is the most common high-altitude syndrome. It occurs in approximately 20% of individuals who ascend to altitudes of 7000 to 9000 feet, 40% at 10,000 to 14,000 feet, and more than 50% above 14,000 feet. The incidence of chronic mountain sickness, also known as Monge's disease, is thought to be between 5 and 18%. More severe neurologic

disturbances due to high-altitude cerebral edema are rare, occurring in approximately 1 to 2% of individuals who ascend to altitudes above 15,000 feet. High-altitude pulmonary edema occurs in approximately 2 to 6% of otherwise healthy individuals who ascend to altitudes of 8000 to 15,000 feet. However, the incidence in individuals with a prior history of high-altitude pulmonary edema may be as high as 60%, or higher during rapid ascents. The occurrence of high-altitude retinal hemorrhage is approximately 33% among individuals who ascend to very high altitudes (up to 19,000 feet) and is thought to be common at lower altitudes as well. High-altitude retinal hemorrhage is not associated with high-altitude cerebral edema or long-term visual consequences.

PATHOBIOLOGY

Clinically significant hypoxemia is the underlying factor in all high-altitude diseases. The decrease in barometric pressure during an ascent to altitude causes a decrease in the alveolar pressure of oxygen (PaO_2). For example, PaO_2 drops from 105 mm Hg at sea level to 60 mm Hg at 10,000 feet and to 40 mm Hg at 18,000 feet. Below 60 mm Hg, oxygen dissociates from hemoglobin more readily (see Fig. 161-2 in Chapter 161), thereby decreasing oxygen saturation and oxygen delivery to tissues. The effect is even more noticeable in individuals with impaired diffusion capacity, for example, emphysema, interstitial lung diseases, or heart failure. Furthermore, increased ventilatory drive induces an acute respiratory alkalosis. In the brain, hypoxia causes cerebral vasodilation, whereas hypobaria causes cerebral vasoconstriction. In severe hypoxia, vasodilation is the likely cause of cerebral edema in susceptible individuals. The response to hypoxia in the lungs is primarily increased pulmonary arterial pressures due to hypoxic pulmonary vasoconstriction, which results in reversible injury to pulmonary capillaries, increased capillary permeability, and eventually pulmonary edema. Reduced oxygen consumption also occurs, perhaps from impaired mitochondrial function in the presence of hypoxia. Periodic breathing during sleep is also noted but has minimal if any clinical significance.

CLINICAL MANIFESTATIONS

Symptoms of acute mountain sickness begin 2 to 3 hours after ascent and include breathlessness, lightheadedness, fatigue, nausea, anorexia, headache, and insomnia. Most symptoms resolve within 2 to 3 days, although insomnia may persist. Chronic symptoms of headache, fatigue, sleep disturbances, dyspnea, and digestive complaints are seen with chronic mountain sickness in individuals residing at higher elevations. Chronic mountain sickness may be associated with polycythemia (hemoglobin concentrations above 21 g/dL). Severe neurologic symptoms with high-altitude cerebral edema include ataxia and confusion that may progress to coma or death. Symptoms of high-altitude pulmonary edema that usually begin 2 to 4 days after ascent to higher altitudes include dyspnea, cough, and tachycardia. Funduscopic changes of flame-shaped hemorrhages are seen with high-altitude retinal hemorrhage.

DIAGNOSIS

Diagnosis of most high-altitude disease is made on the basis of clinical manifestations at high altitude. Diagnosis of chronic mountain sickness, and a milder form often called subacute mountain sickness, is more challenging because it may mimic other cardiopulmonary, neurologic, or psychiatric disease. Individuals with chronic mountain sickness typically have higher hemoglobin concentrations, higher serum erythropoietin levels, higher nocturnal heart rates, lower nocturnal oxygen saturation, and higher systolic and diastolic arterial pressure than normal individuals living at similar altitude.

PREVENTION

Prevention of high-altitude disease can be achieved by avoidance in high-risk individuals, such as young children and persons with a history of high-altitude disease. Gradual ascent and acclimatization are crucial to prevention of high-altitude illness, particularly at extreme altitudes. At altitudes up to 10,000 feet, 2 to 3 days or more may be needed for adjustment to the effects of hypoxia. For mountaineers, current recommendations are to ascend no more than approximately 984 feet (300 m) per day at altitudes higher than 9843 feet (3000 m).

When rapid ascent is unavoidable, such as flights to high-altitude locales, the carbonic anhydrase inhibitor acetazolamide (250 mg orally once or twice daily) provides effective prophylaxis of acute mountain sickness, and 125 mg at night may improve sleep.[1] Dexamethasone (given in doses of 4 mg twice daily)[2] and prednisolone (20 mg daily) have been shown to decrease the

TABLE 94-1 HIGH-ALTITUDE SYNDROMES

SYNDROME	CLINICAL DESCRIPTION
Acute mountain sickness	Recent ascent to altitudes above 7000 feet; headache, anorexia, and malaise; common
Chronic mountain sickness	Dwelling above 10,000 feet; headache, fatigue, dyspnea, and digestive disturbances; incidence: 5-18%
High-altitude cerebral edema	Above 15,000 feet; confusion, ataxia, hallucinations, coma, or death; rare
High-altitude pulmonary edema	Above 9500 feet; dyspnea, cough, and tachycardia; incidence: 2-6%
High-altitude retinal hemorrhage	Above 15,000 feet; asymptomatic or reversible vision changes; common

severity of acute mountain sickness. The long-acting β-adrenergic agonist salmeterol (125 μg inhaled twice daily) also reduces the risk for high-altitude pulmonary edema.**3** Sumatriptan, 50 mg, after ascent is useful for reducing symptoms.**4** The calcium-channel blocker nifedipine (20 mg of slow-release formulation) is useful for preventing recurrent high-altitude pulmonary edema in individuals with previous episodes.

TREATMENT   Rx

For acute, life-threatening symptoms such as high-altitude pulmonary edema and high-altitude cerebral edema, the best treatment is immediate descent, if possible, combined with supplemental oxygen therapy and, if needed, use of a portable hyperbaric chamber. For individuals who develop less severe symptoms, sildenafil (50 mg) can increase exercise capacity at altitude by 10 to 35%.**5** Increasing inspired oxygen concentrations in high-altitude working facilities also improves productivity and quality of sleep. Sustained-release theophylline (375 mg twice daily) significantly reduces the symptoms of acute mountain sickness compared with placebo.**6** Acetazolamide (250 mg or 500 mg once daily) is also useful in treating symptoms of chronic mountain sickness.**7** Milder forms of acute mountain sickness, such as headache, can be treated with typical doses of nonsteroidal anti-inflammatory medications, including aspirin and acetaminophen.

PROGNOSIS

Symptoms of high-altitude disease respond rapidly to immediate descent. However, high-altitude cerebral edema and high-altitude pulmonary edema can be fatal, particularly at extreme altitudes and weather when descent may be impossible.

● DECOMPRESSION ILLNESS: DECOMPRESSION SICKNESS, BAROTRAUMA, AND ARTERIAL GAS EMBOLISM

DEFINITION

Exposures to changes in ambient pressure cause a spectrum of illness, either (1) by increasing or decreasing the volume of gas in air-filled body cavities, or (2) by causing the release of inert gas bubbles from solution in tissues or blood vessels. Symptoms associated with decreasing ambient pressure, which occur most commonly with ascent from depth during recreational or occupational diving, are known as decompression illness. The most common form of decompression illness is decompression sickness, which is classified as either type I (mild symptoms, such as general fatigue or joint pain) or type II (more severe neurologic or cardiopulmonary disturbances). Life-threatening forms of decompression illness include pulmonary barotrauma and arterial gas embolism syndromes. During the descent of a dive, increasing ambient pressure may cause mild symptoms of facial or sinus pain, often called "the squeezes."

EPIDEMIOLOGY

In addition to the approximately 9 million recreational divers in the United States, aviators, astronauts, and compressed air workers are also exposed to changes in ambient pressure that may cause decompression illness. Among recreational divers, the annual incidence rate for either type I or type II decompression sickness is estimated at 1 case per 5000 to 10,000 dives. Approximately 1000 episodes of decompression illness severe enough to warrant recompression therapy occur each year, up to 10% of which are fatal. Well-recognized risk factors for decompression illness include long duration of dives, deep dives, repetitive dives, heavy exertion at depth, cold water, and rapid ascent. Additional risk occurs in individuals who experience further decreases in ambient pressure after the dive, such as on commercial or private aircraft or driving over mountainous areas.

PATHOBIOLOGY

The principles of Boyle's law and Henry's law describe the properties of gases during changes in ambient pressure. Boyle's law states that the volume of a gas varies inversely to changes in pressure, $P_1V_1 = P_2V_2$. During the descent of a dive, pain due to the "squeezes" is caused by increasing ambient pressures that are not equalized by an increase in gas volume. The resulting negative pressure causes a vacuum effect in the mask associated with engorgement of the blood vessels in adjacent tissues, such as periorbital and ocular vessels, and may result in swelling, pain, and subconjunctival hemorrhages. Facial sinuses, the middle ear, and the external auditory canal may also be affected.

Barotrauma in sinus, otic, or pulmonary tissues may be due to changes in ambient pressures and the resulting increase or decrease in the volume of gas. During descent, the decreasing volume of gas causes vascular engorgement in the sinuses and otic compartments and may result in rupture of the tympanic or inner ear membranes. During ascent, breath-holding, particularly with compressed air devices (SCUBA diving), and the presence of obstructive lung disease with delayed exhalation times and air trapping impair equilibration and increase the risk for pulmonary barotrauma. If the expanding volume of gas causes a pressure gradient between the alveoli and pulmonary interstitium that exceeds the compliance of the lung, alveolar disruption will lead to pulmonary interstitial emphysema. Further extension of gas along pulmonary tissues may cause additional barotrauma, leading to pneumothorax, mediastinal emphysema, pneumopericardium, and soft tissue emphysema.

Arterial gas embolism, which is a serious consequence of pulmonary barotrauma, results in the development of free gas in the pulmonary arterial circulation. The resulting bubbles may then enter the systemic circulation by overwhelming the filtering mechanism of the pulmonary capillaries or through a right-to-left intracardiac shunt (Chapter 69), such as a patent foramen ovale. Bubbles may then migrate to the brain, spinal cord, heart, lung, or kidney and lead to tissue ischemia or infarct.

Henry's law states that the solubility of a gas in liquid is proportional to the partial pressure of that gas above the liquid. An increase in partial pressure of gases during descent will therefore cause the amount of gas dissolved in the pulmonary capillaries to increase. Dissolved oxygen is used during normal body metabolism; however, inert nitrogen, which is abundant in inspired air, becomes dissolved in the blood and tissues, particularly in fat, where it is five-fold more soluble than in water. During ascent, decreasing ambient pressure causes tissues to become supersaturated with nitrogen, and nitrogen is subsequently released into blood vessels and tissues as gas bubbles. Decompression-induced gas bubbles cause decompression illness by either mechanical compression of tissues or embolization through blood vessels to end organs. Bubbles that obstruct capillaries or venules damage the endothelium and cause tissue ischemia, which leads to activation of inflammatory mediators or tissue reperfusion injury. Although not well understood, toxic effects due to increased partial pressure of gases also are likely to contribute to symptoms of decompression illness, possibly by denaturing of proteins and release of fatty acids from cell membranes.

CLINICAL MANIFESTATIONS AND DIAGNOSIS

Symptoms of decompression illness can occur within minutes and up to 24 hours or more after exposure to changes in ambient pressure associated with dives of 20 feet in depth or more. The severity of symptoms depends on the rate and the magnitude of the change of ambient pressure and can vary among individuals. Diagnosis is based on clinical manifestations, which can be classified according to whether they are caused by formation of inert nitrogen gas bubbles or the localized toxic effects of gas (associated with decompression sickness), barotrauma associated with descent (sinus or otic barotrauma), barotrauma associated with ascent (pulmonary barotrauma), or more severe arterial gas embolism syndromes.

Symptoms vary according to location of bubble formation. For example, type I decompression sickness, also known as the bends or caisson disease, is typically associated with pain in the joints, from mild to severe, and numbness of the extremities. Rashes and lymphedema may also occur. Symptoms of type II decompression sickness may be systemic (fatigue, hypovolemic shock), cardiopulmonary (cough, substernal chest pain, tachypnea, asphyxia), otic (vertigo, hearing loss), or neurologic (ataxia, aphasia, speech disturbances, incontinence, confusion, personality changes, depression, paralysis, and loss of consciousness).

Otic barotrauma, which typically occurs during descent, can affect the external, middle, or inner ear (Chapter 434). External ear symptoms, such as a sensation of ear fullness or otalgia, are caused by a blockage of the canal, for example, with the use of ear plugs or presence of cerumen. Middle ear symptoms of otalgia, vertigo, tinnitus, transient conductive hearing loss, and facial nerve palsy occur when inadequate equalization of pressures results from blocked eustachian tubes, typically in association with allergic rhinitis or upper respiratory infections. Inner ear barotrauma, which is a more serious form of otic barotrauma, is associated with elevated intracranial pressure and rupture of the inner ear membrane. Inner ear barotrauma causes symptoms of sensorineural deafness, tinnitus, vertigo, nausea, and vomiting. Sinus barotrauma typically occurs during descent, is associated with facial pain and epistaxis, and occurs more frequently in individuals with mucosal inflammation from allergies or infection.

Pulmonary barotrauma, which is the second leading cause of death among divers, should be suspected in postdive individuals, particularly at-risk individuals, with symptoms of sudden pleuritic pain, dyspnea, or coughing. Physical examination findings include tachypnea, subcutaneous emphysema, and dullness to percussion or decreased breath sounds over a pneumothorax. Development of tension pneumothorax (Chapter 99) or severe pneumomediastinum may lead to decreased venous return of systemic blood and reduced cardiac preload, a situation that is characterized by hypotension and may lead to refractory shock or cardiac arrest. Chest and neck radiographs are recommended for diagnosis, particularly because pneumothoraces must be treated with chest tube thoracostomy before recompression therapy.

Because arterial gas embolism syndromes are caused by pulmonary barotrauma, careful neurologic assessment is critical. The neurologic findings are similar to those of an acute stroke (Chapter 414), with manifestations of focal or unilateral motor deficits, visual disturbances, sensory deficits, speech difficulties, and cognitive disturbances, including loss of consciousness. Symptoms typically occur within 10 minutes after ascent. Delayed neurologic symptoms are more likely to be due to type II decompression sickness.

PREVENTION

Education is the most effective method of preventing decompression illness. Before participation in diving-related activities, all individuals should undergo a thorough and intensive training program. Instruction of proper pressure equalization techniques is critical in the prevention of decompression illness. Persons with asthma who wish to dive should be assessed by a physician (preferably knowledgeable in the field of diving medicine), have no wheezing on physical examination, and have normal spirometry before and after exercise. The presence of structural lung disease (e.g., lung cysts or bullae) is associated with a significant increase in the risk for pneumothorax and is a contraindication to diving. Presence of a known right-to-left intracardiac shunt, such as a patent foramen ovale, is not an absolute contraindication to diving, although conservative diving is recommended, and patients should be cautioned that they are at increased risk for decompression illness.

TREATMENT Rx

Symptoms of decompression illness at altitude should be treated with supplemental oxygen and return to the lowest attainable altitude. Serious decompression illness associated with diving requires immediate medical evaluation by emergency personnel, including basic and advanced life support (Chapter 63) when hemodynamic instability is present. Pneumothorax (Chapter 99) should be treated immediately with needle decompression or chest tube thoracostomy. Symptoms that persist for more than 2 hours or increase in intensity require recompression therapy, preferably with 100% oxygen or transfer to a facility with a hyperbaric chamber, where standard protocols should be followed. Tenoxicam (20 mg daily) decreases the number of recompression treatments needed in divers with decompression illness.[8]

PROGNOSIS

Survival of patients with decompression illness depends on prompt medical evaluation and treatment. Immediate hyperbaric oxygen therapy per standard protocols is associated with resolution of symptoms in 95% of cases. However, symptoms of decompression illness, even neurologic deficits, may respond to recompression therapy after delays of 24 hours or more.

● SMOKE INHALATION
Smoke Inhalation and Thermal Injury

DEFINITION

Pulmonary complications, largely caused by smoke inhalation, occur in a large proportion of burn victims (Chapter 112) and account for a substantial number of deaths in these patients. Even patients who do not sustain surface burns in a fire can inhale sufficient smoke to result in injury to the lungs or airways.

EPIDEMIOLOGY

Modern building codes and the widespread presence of firefighting personnel in communities have decreased the importance of fire as a cause of death in the United States. However, fire continues to cause several thousand deaths annually. Also, larger-scale fires with mass casualties and wildfires that affect large geographic areas still occur occasionally.

PATHOGENESIS

Smoke loses heat rapidly as it traverses the upper airway, so direct thermal injury is often limited to the mucosa of the supraglottic airway. A notable exception is steam inhalation, which can produce thermal injury throughout the airways. Smoke inhalation injury affects the entire respiratory tract. The pathogenesis of smoke inhalation is complicated by the wide variety of pulmonary irritants in smoke, many of which are directly toxic to respiratory epithelial or alveolar cells: aldehydes such as acrolein, acetaldehyde, and formaldehyde; acids such as hydrochloric, hydrofluoric, and hydrocyanic acid; and ammonia, nitrogen oxides, and phosgene.

Irritants can rapidly induce intense neutrophilic inflammation, which evolves during 12 to 24 hours after injury and is characterized by mucosal edema and ulceration, abnormally increased permeability of pulmonary capillaries with resultant capillary leak, and epithelial, alveolar, and immune cellular dysfunction. Bronchospasm or bronchorrhea may occur, and the processes may result in ARDS. In addition, because oxygen is consumed in fires, breathing of hypoxic air for prolonged periods may potentiate other injuries or cause clinically significant hypoxia in its own right.

CLINICAL MANIFESTATIONS

Thermal injury to upper airway mucosa can cause airway compromise, particularly due to laryngeal edema, sometimes rapidly and sometimes after 12 to 24 hours. Burns to the face, mouth, and neck can externally damage and distort structures of the upper airway and cause airway compromise, both subacutely and late in the course. Inhalation injury manifests primarily with bronchospasm and bronchorrhea, which cause cough, dyspnea, or wheezing and may progress rapidly to respiratory failure. Accumulation of secretions, failure of mucociliary clearance and immune mechanisms, and epithelial necrosis predispose to pulmonary infection, particularly 3 to 5 days after injury. Late pulmonary complications can also be caused indirectly by eschar formation and restriction of thoracic motion.

DIAGNOSIS

Patients with apparent or suspected burn injuries (Chapter 112) should be assessed emergently for airway patency. Head or neck burns, respiratory distress, stridor, or visibly erythematous or edematous oral mucosa should prompt immediate laryngoscopic evaluation of the oropharynx and supraglottic airway. Hypoxemia may develop and may be severe enough to meet criteria for ARDS. Chest radiography should be performed serially to detect the evolution of lung injury or superinfection.

TREATMENT Rx

If airway patency is threatened, endotracheal intubation should be performed immediately. Delay can result in increased edema and greater technical difficulty of intubation. Patients who cannot be intubated should have emergent tracheostomy performed surgically. Because of the risk for ARDS, mechanical ventilation with a goal tidal volume of 3 to 6 mL/kg of ideal body weight should be considered. All patients should receive supplemental oxygen with the goal of providing a high fractional concentration of inspired oxygen (FIO_2) to reverse the effects of hypoxia and carbon monoxide inhalation (see later).

Pulmonary toilet is essential to clear secretions in the face of bronchorrhea and epithelial sloughing. Because of the risk for superinfection, surveillance for infection should be vigilant, including diagnostic bronchoscopy if ventilator-associated pneumonia is suspected.

PROGNOSIS

Patients who survive burns and recover generally do not have long-term pulmonary sequelae. Tracheostomies placed at the time of injury can usually be removed later, unless airway structures are damaged or distorted. Impaired pulmonary function is uncommon but may be manifested as airway hyperresponsiveness that has been termed *reactive airway dysfunction syndrome*.

Carbon Monoxide Poisoning

DEFINITION AND EPIDEMIOLOGY

Carbon monoxide is a colorless, odorless gas produced by the combustion of carbon-based fuels. Because of the ubiquity of these substances, carbon monoxide inhalation is often coincident with smoke inhalation in fires or may occur accidentally in association with malfunctioning equipment or improper venting of emissions from heaters, stoves, combustion motors, or other similar devices. In addition, intentional inhalation of carbon monoxide is a method commonly used in suicide attempts (404). Carbon monoxide inhalation is the leading cause of death from poisoning (Chapter 110) worldwide.

PATHOBIOLOGY

Carbon monoxide readily diffuses across the alveolar-capillary interface and binds to hemoglobin with extremely high affinity. When the resulting carboxyhemoglobin molecule undergoes an allosteric change at oxygen-binding sites, the ability of bound oxygen to dissociate and to be delivered to peripheral tissues is greatly reduced. This tissue hypoxia can cause severe functional impairment and ischemic injury of oxygen-sensitive tissues, particularly in the brain and heart.

CLINICAL MANIFESTATIONS

Mild carbon monoxide intoxication may go unrecognized because the symptoms are nonspecific and may include headache, nausea, malaise, fatigue, and dizziness. With more severe intoxications, neuropsychiatric symptoms may range from minor disturbances in attention and cognition to agitation, confusion, hallucination, or, in the worst intoxications, seizures or frank coma. Physical findings, which are generally nonspecific, can include tachycardia or hyperthermia. The classic cherry-red skin thought to be associated with carbon monoxide intoxication is rarely seen. Other manifestations of severe intoxications may include lactic acidosis, cardiac dysfunction with arrhythmia or ischemia, pulmonary edema, and rhabdomyolysis.

DIAGNOSIS

A high index of suspicion is required for diagnosis because clinical findings are nonspecific. All patients known to have been involved in fires, suicide attempts, or other scenarios compatible with exposures should have arterial carboxyhemoglobin levels checked by co-oximetry. Although levels do not correlate well with clinical findings or risk for complications, symptoms generally occur at carboxyhemoglobin concentrations of 10% or higher.

TREATMENT   Rx

All patients should be treated with 100% supplemental oxygen, which competes with carbon monoxide for hemoglobin-binding sites and gradually eliminates it from the blood. If patients require mechanical ventilation because of depressed neurologic status or respiratory problems, 100% oxygen should be administered by endotracheal tube. Treatment with hyperbaric oxygen at a pressure of 2.5 to 3.0 atm can increase the dissolved oxygen content of blood by more than ten-fold, and at least one treatment of approximately 2 hours should be considered in severe cases to reverse the effects of acute intoxication; three hyperbaric oxygen treatments within 24 hours of diagnosis reduce neurocognitive sequelae. A small, but intriguing, randomized trial of seven healthy volunteers examined normocapnic hyperpnea and CO elimination and showed that persons randomized to normocapnic hyperpnea (compared with those getting 100% O₂ at normal minute ventilation) had a significantly faster half-time of decrease in carboxyhemoglobin.

PROGNOSIS

The mortality rate is highly variable according to the severity of intoxication but can approach 30% in severe cases. Approximately two thirds of patients who survive acute intoxication will recover without sequelae. Many of the remainder will suffer from long-term neuropsychiatric symptoms including cognitive dysfunction, abnormal mood or affect, memory disturbances, and other motor or sensory abnormalities, which can often occur within the first month but may be delayed for up to 6 to 9 months.

Cyanide and Other Gases

PATHOBIOLOGY

In addition to carbon monoxide and pulmonary irritants, cyanide gas may be formed when a number of commonly found substances, particularly plastics and textiles, are combusted. This gas is highly toxic and can rapidly cause morbidity and death by binding to cytochrome enzymes and inhibiting cellular respiration.

Other inhaled gases that can injure the lungs in occupational settings include ammonia, chlorine, nitrogen dioxide, organic dust, paraquat,

phosgene (which has also been used as a chemical weapon), sulfur dioxide, and toxic metal fumes such as cadmium and mercury.

CLINICAL MANIFESTATIONS AND DIAGNOSIS

Cyanide intoxication typically includes shock, lactic acidosis, and coma; it can rapidly lead to death before results of laboratory studies are available. In the setting of possible exposure, an elevated venous oxygen saturation indicates that cyanide is preventing cells from extracting oxygen from arterial blood.

Other inhaled gases that can produce potent irritant responses include ammonia, chlorine, and nitrogen dioxide ("silo-filler's lung"). Phosgene is notable for its propensity to cause delayed symptoms, up to 24 hours after exposure. Other inhalants may produce an acute chemical pneumonitis with respiratory distress (Chapter 93). A diverse group of inhaled toxins can cause syndromes of inhalational fever, including heavy metal fumes, polymer fumes, and organic dust aerosols that contain thermophilic bacteria, gram-negative bacteria and their associated endotoxins, and fungal elements. These inhalations are characterized by fever and malaise with mild respiratory symptoms and are also notable for tachyphylaxis with repeated exposure (and thus referred to as Monday morning fever in some professions).

TREATMENT   Rx

Cyanide intoxication is treated by use of a Taylor Cyanide Antidote Package (Taylor Pharmaceuticals) that contains amyl nitrite gas ampules (one 0.3-mL ampule each minute until sodium nitrite infusion begins) for inhalation. This treatment is followed by intravenous administration of sodium nitrite (300 mg), which acts by converting hemoglobin to methemoglobin. Finally, patients are treated with intravenous sodium thiosulfate (12.5 g), which converts cyanide to less harmful thiocyanate ions. If carboxyhemoglobinemia is present, sodium thiosulfate should be used alone because of the additive toxicity of this condition with methemoglobinemia.

Hydroxocobalamin, which directly binds cyanide, can be used in conjunction with sodium thiosulfate. It is thought to be safer than the amyl nitrate gas ampules because it does not cause methemoglobinemia and is better suited to prehospital care.

The mainstay for treatment of other irritating inhalations is to remove the patient immediately from the toxic environment and to provide supportive care for respiratory injury. Depending on the intensity and duration of exposure, most patients will recover completely without sequelae.

OXYGEN TOXICITY

DEFINITION

Hypoxic respiratory failure often requires treatment with supplemental oxygen to maintain tissue oxygenation. In some settings, such as ARDS, patients may require high F_{IO_2} for prolonged periods to combat severe hypoxia. However, it has long been recognized that oxygen may be toxic to the lungs when it is present in concentrations higher than those found in ambient air.

PATHOBIOLOGY

When the concentration of oxygen in the airways is high, formation of reactive oxygen species and free radicals is increased. Under normal circumstances, innate antioxidant mechanisms in airway epithelia and alveoli are sufficient to abrogate the effect of these molecules. However, under conditions of critical illness, prolonged exposure to increased concentrations of these toxins may overwhelm these defenses. Superoxide, hydrogen peroxide, and hydroxyl radicals may directly oxidize cellular components. Cellular damage potentiates inflammation and may be synergistic with inflammatory processes already under way in the diseased lung; the result can be alveolar edema, formation of hyaline membranes, hypoxemia, and progression to fibrosis and obliteration of alveolar and capillary structures. In addition, washout of nitrogen from air spaces can result in absorptive atelectasis if oxygen is removed by the circulation faster than it can be replenished by ventilation (especially in the setting of ventilation-perfusion mismatch). Hyperoxia can also worsen hypercapnia through multiple mechanisms, as occurs in patients with chronic obstructive pulmonary disease who suffer from carbon dioxide retention.

CLINICAL MANIFESTATIONS AND DIAGNOSIS

Although the exact levels of hyperoxia that cause lung injury are unclear, it appears to occur with exposure to F_{IO_2} of 50 to 60% after exposures as short as 6 hours in duration. Because of the high flow of supplemental oxygen required to deliver this FIO_2, oxygen toxicity is observed primarily in mechanically ventilated patients being treated for hypoxic respiratory failure. This level of exposure can cause a clinically detectable tracheobronchitis, demonstrable by symptoms of cough and dyspnea, as well as airway erythema that is visible macroscopically on bronchoscopy. This syndrome may impair mucociliary clearance and result in impaction of secretions, especially in conjunction with absorptive atelectasis.

Patients who may be susceptible to oxygen toxicity generally already have a significant degree of parenchymal injury from other processes. Thus, although some patients may appear to display a syndrome of worsening air space disease, atelectasis, consolidation, hypoxia, and diffuse alveolar damage, it is not clear when these changes are related to oxygen therapy or merely occur as part of the acute lung injury from other causes.

TREATMENT

Because the threshold level for oxygen toxicity is unknown, a general guideline for treatment of hypoxemic respiratory failure (Chapter 104) is that patients be ventilated with the lowest possible FIO_2 that is required to restore an acceptable oxygen saturation. An SaO_2 of 90%, corresponding to PaO_2 of 55 to 60 mm Hg, is generally considered the minimum acceptable level. Unfortunately, under conditions of severe hypoxia, as in ARDS, patients often require an FIO_2 approaching 100% to achieve this oxygen level. Maneuvers to improve oxygenation without increasing FIO_2 include red blood cell transfusions to improve the delivery of oxygen; alternative ventilatory strategies, such as high-frequency oscillatory ventilation, airway pressure-release ventilation, inverse-ratio ventilation, and prone positioning; and alveolar recruitment maneuvers using positive end-expiratory pressure or transiently increased inflation pressures (Chapter 105).

PROGNOSIS

Patients who sustain oxygen toxicity in the setting of prior bleomycin exposure may be left with residual pulmonary fibrosis. In other patients, the incremental impact of oxygen toxicity on prognosis is unknown.

LUNG INJURY
Radiation Lung Injury
DEFINITION

Accidental or occupational radiation exposures (Chapter 19) are generally characterized by systemic toxicity that outweighs any injury to the lungs. As such, radiation lung injury refers to a pneumonitis that can progress to pulmonary fibrosis and that results from therapeutic use of ionizing radiation, usually in the treatment of malignant neoplasms.

EPIDEMIOLOGY

As many as 50% of patients receiving thoracic radiation will display radiographic abnormalities after treatment; duration and dose of therapy affect the odds for development of lung injury. However, most of these patients will never have clinically significant radiation lung injury. For unclear reasons, the incidence of lung injury appears to vary by the type of underlying malignant disease and modality of treatment. The highest frequency appears to be found in patients with lung cancer (10 to 15%).

PATHOBIOLOGY AND CLINICAL MANIFESTATIONS

The pathogenesis of radiation lung injury is often divided into three or four phases on the basis of time course. Typically, the early phase occurs immediately after exposure and is characterized by injury to alveolar cells, resulting in mild alveolitis, recruitment of inflammatory cells, capillary leak, and pulmonary edema. These changes are usually asymptomatic; patients do not usually come to clinical attention, although the chest radiograph will be abnormal if it is performed. In most patients, these changes resolve without progression within 1 to 3 months.

A minority of patients will progress to the next phase, in which alveolar cells desquamate and the air spaces fill with protein-rich fluid. In this phase, referred to as radiation pneumonitis, patients complain of cough, dyspnea, and occasionally fever or pleuritic chest pain. Severe cases may present with hypoxemic respiratory failure. This phase generally resolves within 3 to 6 months after exposure and is followed by an organizing phase, in which alveolar edema resolves and the damaged alveoli heal. Clinically, patients generally show improvement in symptoms during this period. However, this phase is also characterized by fibroblast proliferation and deposition of collagen in the lung. In a minority of patients, this process will proceed unchecked and result in clinically significant fibrosis, with progressive loss of alveolar-capillary surface and development of restrictive lung disease.

DIAGNOSIS

Clinical history and radiographic evaluation are often sufficient for diagnosis of radiation lung injury because patients typically present with respiratory symptoms and opacities on chest radiography after undergoing radiation therapy. Radiography may show air space disease with alveolar filling or consolidation during the pneumonitis phase, which may progress to an interstitial pattern and eventual honeycombing with parenchymal distortion in the chronic phase. Because radiation characteristically causes injury only within directly affected lung tissue, radiography may show opacities that are well delineated and form straight lines that cross anatomically distinct regions of lung. This finding is rarely if ever seen in other conditions.

The differential diagnosis may include pneumonia, recurrence, and metastatic malignant disease. On occasion, invasive evaluation with bronchoalveolar lavage or even biopsy is required to exclude these possibilities if the clinical history and imaging do not provide a diagnosis.

TREATMENT AND PREVENTION

Corticosteroids such as prednisone, 1 mg/kg body weight/day followed by a slow taper over several weeks or months, are the mainstay of therapy. Patients often show a dramatic response to treatment, and symptoms may recur after treatment is discontinued. Other immunosuppressive agents have been used successfully in case reports of patients who failed to respond to corticosteroids. Prophylactic amifostine, a cytoprotective agent (340 mg/m² given 15 minutes before irradiation), significantly reduces the risk for radiation pneumonitis in patients who receive radiation treatment for lung cancer.[9]

PROGNOSIS

Within 2 years after initial exposure, progression will usually slow, and symptoms and lung function will stabilize and improve. After this time, further improvement or worsening is uncommon. In severe cases that become chronic, patients may develop features of advanced interstitial lung disease, including pulmonary hypertension and hypoxic respiratory failure.

Aspiration Injury
DEFINITION

Aspiration, which is defined as the inhalation of any nongaseous foreign substance into the lungs, generally refers specifically to the inhalation of gastric contents or secretions from the oropharynx. Aspiration is a common occurrence, and in most cases it resolves spontaneously without clinical manifestations. Clinically significant aspiration can range from acute pneumonitis and respiratory failure caused by a single massive aspiration to chronic symptoms of respiratory disease caused by recurrent small-scale aspiration. These syndromes may overlap with pneumonia that occurs when the lungs are exposed to bacteria from the gastrointestinal tract (Chapter 97).

PATHOBIOLOGY

The common element of clinically significant aspiration is impairment of normal airway protective mechanisms. Under normal circumstances, the airway is protected by the normal swallowing mechanism, the cough reflex, and the anatomy of the supraglottic airway. However, even healthy individuals experience microaspiration despite having functional protective mechanisms. These secretions are handled by normal pulmonary clearance mechanisms.

Any disturbance of these protective mechanisms can result in aspiration injury to the lungs. An altered level of consciousness can impair normal swallowing and suppress the cough reflex. Even in patients who are alert, neurologic injury can result in dysphagia and concomitant aspiration, as in patients who have bulbar neurologic deficits in association with ischemic stroke. Patients with altered airway or oropharyngeal anatomy, such as patients who have received surgical or radiation therapy for head and neck malignant neoplasms, may also be highly susceptible to aspiration of oral secretions.

The nature of the aspirated material is also important in determining whether an injury occurs. Materials with a pH lower than 2.5, such as acidic gastric contents, are much more likely to cause a significant chemical pneumonitis.

Particulate matter also increases the likelihood for development of clinically significant inflammation. A large-volume aspiration with distribution throughout the lungs is more likely to produce an acute, severe pneumonitis.

Once material has been aspirated into the lungs, the injury that occurs is similar to a chemical burn. Acid rapidly injures airway epithelial and alveolar cells; within hours, cells become dysfunctional and capillary leak occurs, resulting in profound noncardiogenic pulmonary edema. In severe cases, diffuse alveolar damage may result.

CLINICAL MANIFESTATIONS

The classic eponym applied to aspiration pneumonia is Mendelsohn's syndrome, which refers to a single, large-volume aspiration of gastric contents followed by rapidly progressive hypoxemic respiratory failure that develops within hours. Patients may suffer from cough, dyspnea, fever, and respiratory distress. Physical examination may reveal diffuse crackles, wheezing, cyanosis, and hypotension. Chest radiography may show a pattern of alveolar filling with diffuse bilateral involvement or involvement of dependent regions, particularly the right lower lobe. In many patients, this period of acute deterioration is followed by stabilization and resolution within 2 or 3 days. In other patients, deterioration may continue, and patients may meet clinical criteria for ARDS. If the volume of aspirated material is large enough, the initial aspiration may be sufficient to cause tracheal obstruction and asphyxiation.

In patients who initially improve, a small percentage will show further deterioration after 2 or 3 days. This deterioration should prompt an investigation for bacterial superinfection.

DIAGNOSIS

The clinical history and presentation are generally sufficient for diagnosis of aspiration pneumonitis. Bacterial pneumonia and other causes of ARDS also should be considered, as should cardiogenic pulmonary edema. Airway erythema and edema on bronchoscopy can be suggestive of aspiration. Bronchoalveolar lavage may help evaluate for the presence of bacterial infection.

PREVENTION

Prevention should focus on identification of patients who are at risk for aspiration and then use of strategies to minimize the risk. Patients with swallowing dysfunction or airway abnormalities can work with speech pathologists to learn effective strategies for swallowing. Patients who are unsuccessful or not suitable for this approach may benefit from tracheostomy or enteral tube feedings, which do not prevent microaspiration but can prevent large-volume aspiration. In hospitalized patients, particularly patients with an altered mental status due to illness or sedation, simple strategies such as avoidance of oral feeding and semirecumbent positioning can effectively reduce the risk for aspiration. Use of histamine-2 blockers or proton pump inhibitors (Chapter 141) can alter gastric pH to reduce the risk for injury from acidic secretions.

TREATMENT   Rx

Because of the acuity and severity of aspiration pneumonitis, immediate attention should be paid to maintaining a patent airway. The oropharynx and trachea should be suctioned to clear any potentially obstructing material, and endotracheal intubation should be performed if necessary (Chapter 105). Bronchoscopy is often performed to clear residual particulate or solid matter, but it cannot remove acidic secretions, which damage airways and parenchyma quickly and then are rendered neutral. Oxygen supplementation should be provided as needed for hypoxia. Corticosteroids have not been shown to be beneficial. Antibiotics should be reserved for patients who appear to have developed bacterial superinfection (Chapter 97).

PROGNOSIS

For patients with severe respiratory failure or ARDS, mortality can be high. In others, improvement should be expected within days. If the underlying factor that led to aspiration is irreversible, patients have an increased likelihood of recurrent episodes.

Lipoid Pneumonia

DEFINITION

Lipoid pneumonia is a chronic inflammatory reaction of the lungs to the presence of lipid substances. Exogenous lipoid pneumonia results from the aspiration of vegetable, animal, or (most commonly) mineral oils.

PATHOBIOLOGY

The most frequently implicated agent is mineral oil used as a laxative and to reduce dysphagia, either in clear liquid form or as petroleum jelly. Mineral oil is bland and, when introduced into the pharynx, can enter the bronchial tree without eliciting the cough reflex. It also mechanically impedes the ciliary action of the airway epithelium. The risk for mineral oil aspiration is increased in debilitated or senile patients, in those with neurologic disease that interferes with deglutition, and in patients with esophageal disease. Mineral oil taken as nose drops to relieve nasal dryness can also cause lipoid pneumonia. Inhalation of mineral oil mist by airplane and automobile mechanics has also been implicated as a cause.

Mineral oils, which cannot be hydrolyzed in the body, provoke a chronic inflammatory reaction that may not become clinically overt until years later. In the alveolar spaces, macrophages accumulate and phagocytose the emulsified oil. Some macrophages disintegrate, releasing their lysosomal enzymes and oil. The alveolar septa become thickened and edematous, containing lymphocytes and lipid-laden macrophages. Oil droplets are seen in the pulmonary lymphatics and hilar nodes. Later, fibrosis develops, and the normal lung architecture is effaced. A single pathologic specimen may include both the early inflammatory and the later fibrotic picture, in keeping with repetitive aspirations during many months or years. Nodular lesions may grossly resemble tumor and be called paraffinomas.

CLINICAL MANIFESTATIONS

Most patients are asymptomatic and come to the physician's attention because of an abnormal chest radiograph. When patients are symptomatic, cough and exertional dyspnea are the most frequent complaints. Chest pain (sometimes pleuritic), hemoptysis, fever (usually low grade), chills, night sweats, and weight loss may occur. Findings on physical examination may be completely normal, but fever, tachypnea, dullness on percussion of the chest, bronchial or bronchovesicular breath sounds, rales, and rhonchi may be found. Clubbing and cor pulmonale are rare.

DIAGNOSIS

In mild lipoid pneumonia, arterial blood gas values may be normal with the patient at rest but may show hypoxemia after exercise. In more severe disease, resting hypoxemia, hypocapnia, and mild respiratory alkalosis develop. Pulmonary function testing reveals a restrictive ventilatory defect; lung compliance is decreased. The only specific laboratory finding is the presence in sputum of macrophages with clusters of vacuoles that are 5 to 50 μm in diameter and that stain deep orange with Sudan IV; extracellular droplets may stain similarly.

On radiographic examination, the earliest abnormalities are air space infiltrates, most often in the dependent portions of the lung. The infiltrates may be unilateral or bilateral, localized or diffuse. Air bronchograms may be seen. Hilar adenopathy and pleural reaction are rare. As fibrosis develops, volume loss occurs, and linear and nodular infiltrates appear. A solid lesion that closely resembles bronchogenic carcinoma may develop. High-resolution computed tomography usually shows consolidated areas of low attenuation and "crazy paving" (Fig. 94-1).

The differential diagnosis is extensive, particularly in the late phase, when multiple other causes of pulmonary fibrosis must be considered. The key to the correct diagnosis before biopsy is the history of chronic oral or intranasal use of an oil- or a lipid-based product or an occupational exposure to oil mists. The presence of lipid-laden macrophages in sputum or bronchoalveolar lavage fluid also can be used to confirm the diagnosis, particularly in conjunction with typical findings on high-resolution computed tomography.

TREATMENT AND PREVENTION   Rx

Once the diagnosis has been made and the aspiration stopped, the subsequent course is variable. Because the only way the lung can dispose of mineral oil is by expectoration, the patient should be instructed in coughing exercises to be performed many times each day for months. Expectorants have not been shown to help. In some uncontrolled case reports, systemic corticosteroids at varying doses and durations have been associated with a successful outcome, but they cannot be routinely recommended for treatment.

FIGURE 94-1. Lipoid pneumonia on a computed tomographic scan.

Transfusion-Related Acute Lung Injury

DEFINITION

The syndrome of transfusion-related acute lung injury (TRALI; Chapter 180) involves the rapid onset of respiratory distress within minutes to hours after the transfusion of blood products (fresh-frozen plasma, platelets, and red blood cells). The initial clinical picture is indistinguishable from acute lung injury or ARDS due to other causes, such as sepsis, multiple trauma, and lung injury. TRALI may similarly be confused with pulmonary edema due to volume overload (Chapter 58).

EPIDEMIOLOGY

The true incidence of TRALI is unknown; incidence rates are underestimated because of the difficulty in distinguishing TRALI from other causes of acute respiratory failure and the labor-intensive and costly diagnostic evaluation required. Reported incidences range from 1 in 1000 to 1 in 100,000 units of blood products transfused. The risk for TRALI varies according to the type of blood product transfused, with pooled products associated with a higher incidence. Only 8 to 21 TRALI-related deaths are reported to the U.S. Food and Drug Administration annually, and even liberal estimates accounting for under-reporting suggest the number may be only as high as 300 per year of an estimated 25 million transfusions in the United States.

PATHOBIOLOGY

The physiologic manifestations of TRALI are caused by alveolar filling with fluid and protein. This alveolar process is the result of increased microvascular permeability due to pulmonary endothelial damage mediated by either leukocyte antibodies or the priming and activation of neutrophils in the pulmonary circulation by bioactive substances.

TRALI most commonly occurs when human leukocyte antigen (HLA) type I or II or neutrophil-specific antigen antibodies from the donor attach to the recipient's leukocytes, leading to the release of injurious oxidative and nonoxidative products. Development of HLA antibodies occurs commonly in women during pregnancy, and increasing parity in female blood donors is associated with an increased risk for TRALI.

Episodes of TRALI occurring in patients without HLA or neutrophil-specific antigen antibodies in either the donor or recipient are thought to be caused by a two-hit process of neutrophil priming and activation. Neutrophils are primed and sequestered in the lung by conditions that often occur in patients requiring blood products, such as multiple trauma, surgery, or sepsis. Primed neutrophils are then activated by bioactive lipids and cytokines stored in the blood products, thereby leading to lung injury and alveolar damage. Levels of these bioactive lipids or cytokines may increase after prolonged storage of blood products.

CLINICAL MANIFESTATIONS

Although most cases of TRALI present within 1 to 2 hours after the transfusion of blood products, tachypnea, hypoxemia, cyanosis, dyspnea, and fever can develop during the transfusion or up to 6 hours later. Hypertension or hypotension commonly occurs, depending on the severity of the reaction. Copious amounts of pink, frothy edema fluid may be present. Lung auscultation generally reveals bilateral crackles and decreased breath sounds in dependent lung zones.

DIAGNOSIS

Bilateral patchy infiltrates consistent with alveolar edema are found on plain chest radiographs, typically without effusions. Arterial blood gas analysis demonstrates reduced Po_2, and further laboratory testing may reveal thrombocytopenia or a transient leukopenia. Diagnosis of TRALI requires the presence of the following: acute onset of hypoxemia with Pao_2/Fio_2 of 300 or less, or room air oxygen saturation less than 90% during or within 6 hours after a transfusion; bilateral infiltrates on the chest radiograph; no evidence of left atrial hypertension; no preexisting acute lung injury before transfusion; and no temporal relationship to an alternative risk factor for acute lung injury.

The diagnosis of "possible TRALI" is made in patients who have a concurrent diagnosis of another risk factor for acute lung injury, including (1) direct lung injury due to aspiration, pneumonia, toxic inhalation, lung contusion, or nonfatal drowning; and (2) indirect lung injury due to severe sepsis, shock, multiple trauma, burn injury, acute pancreatitis, cardiopulmonary bypass, or drug overdose. Absolute confirmation of the diagnosis requires testing for HLA and neutrophil-specific antigen antibodies, usually performed first in female donors, then in male donors, and finally in the recipient.

TREATMENT

Most cases are self-limited and resolve within hours to days with supplemental oxygen and supportive care. Volume resuscitation, with or without vasopressors, is required for hypotension. Mechanical ventilation should be managed as for any other case of acute lung injury, with the implementation of a low tidal volume ventilation strategy to prevent further ventilator-induced lung injury. Diuresis should be attempted cautiously and may even be detrimental because intravascular filling pressures are often low.

PROGNOSIS

The mortality rate of TRALI is approximately 5%. If an implicated donor can be identified, the recipient should not receive any further transfusions from that donor, but patients are not at increased risk for further episodes of TRALI from nonimplicated donor transfusions.

1. van Patot MC, Leadbetter G 3rd, Keyes LE, et al. Prophylactic low-dose acetazolamide reduces the incidence and severity of acute mountain sickness. *High Alt Med Biol.* 2008;9:289-293.
2. Fischler M, Maggiorini M, Dorschner L, et al. Dexamethasone but not tadalafil improves exercise capacity in adults prone to high-altitude pulmonary edema. *Am J Respir Crit Care Med.* 2009;180:346-352.
3. Sartori C, Allemann Y, Duplain H, et al. Salmeterol for the prevention of high-altitude pulmonary edema. *N Engl J Med.* 2002;346:1631-1636.
4. Jafarian S, Gorouhi F, Salimi S, et al. Sumatriptan for prevention of acute mountain sickness: randomized clinical trial. *Ann Neurol.* 2007;62:273-277.
5. Ghofrani HA, Reichenberger F, Kohstall MG, et al. Sildenafil increased exercise capacity during hypoxia at low altitudes and at Mount Everest base camp: a randomized, double-blind, placebo-controlled crossover trial. *Ann Intern Med.* 2004;141:169-177.
6. Küpper TE, Strohl KP, Hoefer M, et al. Low-dose theophylline reduces symptoms of acute mountain sickness. *J Travel Med.* 2008;15:307-314.
7. Richalet JP, Rivera-Ch M, Maignan M, et al. Acetazolamide for Monge's disease: efficiency and tolerance of 6-month treatment. *Am J Respir Crit Care Med.* 2008;177:1370-1376.
8. Bennett MH, Lehm JP, Mitchell SJ, et al. Recompression and adjunctive therapy for decompression illness: a systematic review of randomized controlled trials. *Anesth Analg.* 2010;111:757-762.
9. Sasse AD, Clark LG, Sasse EC, et al. Amifostine reduces side effects and improves complete response rate during radiotherapy: results of a meta-analysis. *Int J Radiat Oncol Biol Phys.* 2006;64:784-791.

SUGGESTED READINGS

Divers Alert Network. Available at *http://www.diversalertnetwork.org/index.asp. This website includes a link to a 24-hour hotline for diving emergencies.*
Nasrullah M, Muazzam S. Drowning mortality in the United States, 1999-2006. *J Community Health.* 2011;36:69-75. *About 3500 Americans drown annually, with males and minorities most at risk.*
Sololovic M, Pastores SM. Transfusion therapy and acute lung injury. *Expert Rev Respir Med.* 2010;4:387-393. *Review.*

95

SARCOIDOSIS

MICHAEL IANNUZZI

DEFINITION

Sarcoidosis, a systemic granulomatous disease of unknown cause, is characterized by a variable clinical presentation and course. More than 90% of patients exhibit thoracic involvement with mediastinal and hilar lymph node enlargement or parenchymal lung disease, but any organ may be involved. The presentation and course vary from asymptomatic disease with spontaneous resolution to organ system failure and even death.

EPIDEMIOLOGY

Sarcoidosis occurs worldwide, affects people of all racial and ethnic groups, and may present at any age. Sarcoidosis usually develops before the age of 50 years with the incidence peaking at 20 to 39 years. The incidence of sarcoidosis fluctuates throughout the world, most likely because of differences in the presentation of the disease and the surveillance methods used. The annual incidence of sarcoidosis is highest in northern European countries, where it is 5 to 40 cases per 100,000 people. The incidence in Japan is about 1 to 2 cases per 100,000 people. In the United States, the adjusted annual incidence among black Americans is about 3.5 times higher than among white Americans (35.5 cases per 100,000 compared with 10.9 per 100,000). Regardless of ethnic or racial group, sarcoidosis affects women more often. The reportedly low incidence in certain regions such as Africa, China, India, and Russia may be due to decreased access to health care, minimal surveillance, and misdiagnosis of sarcoidosis as tuberculosis or leprosy.

Black women in the United States have the highest lifetime risk of developing sarcoidosis (2.7%). In both black men and women, sarcoidosis occurs later in life, peaks in the fourth decade, and is more likely to be chronic and fatal. Socioeconomic status does not affect the incidence of sarcoidosis, but low income and other financial barriers to care are associated with more severe sarcoidosis, even after adjustment for age, sex, and race or ethnic group.

Sarcoidosis clusters in families and monozygotic twins are more often concordant for disease than are dizygotic twins. Familial sarcoidosis occurs in 10% of cases from the Netherlands, 7.5% from Germany, 6% from the United Kingdom, 4.7% from Finland, and 0.8% from Spain. In the United States, sarcoidosis patients are five times as likely to have siblings or parents with sarcoidosis as control subjects. However, less than 1% of the first-degree relatives of patients with sarcoidosis are affected, so screening for disease in asymptomatic relatives is ineffective.

PATHOBIOLOGY

The development and accumulation of granulomas represent the basic pathologic abnormality in sarcoidosis. Sarcoidal granulomas are tightly organized collections of macrophages and macrophage-derived epithelioid cells encircled by lymphocytes. Fused epithelioid cells, which become multinucleated giant cells, are often found scattered throughout the granuloma. This appearance suggests that the granuloma is meant to contain an inciting agent, but no such agent has been identified.

Granuloma formation begins with HLA-mediated processing of antigens by macrophages. T-cell activation follows, with oligoclonal expansion of CD4$^+$ (helper-inducer) lymphocytes. These CD4$^+$ cells, primarily of the T_H1 phenotype, produce interleukin-2 (IL-2) and interferon-γ (IFN-γ). A complex interplay of cytokines, along with macrophage-derived tumor necrosis factor-α, organizes the inflammatory cells into granulomas. In some cases, fibroblasts and collagen encase the granulomas with subsequent fibrosis. Fibrosis has been associated with a shift in the involved lymphocytes from the T_H1 (IL-2 and IFN-γ) to the T_H2 phenotype (IL-4, -10, and -13). This fibrotic process irreversibly alters organ architecture and function. Increased 1-α hydroxylase activity in macrophages within granulomas and the alveoli converts 25-hydroxyvitamin D to the biologically active form 1,25-dihydroxyvitamin D (calcitriol), thereby resulting in increased intestinal absorption of calcium.

In sarcoidosis, an immune paradox exists: patients often develop anergy as indicated by a suppressed response to tuberculin, despite active granulomatous inflammation. This anergy results in part from an expansion of CD25^{bright} regulatory T cells, which are a subgroup of CD4$^+$ T lymphocytes and which can abolish production of IL-2 and inhibit T-cell proliferation. Although sarcoidosis is predominantly a T-cell-driven disease, the presence of polyclonal hyperglobulinemia indicates that B lymphocytes may also play a role.

Multiple inciting agents rather than a single pathogen are likely to cause sarcoidosis. Airborne antigens are suspected because the lungs, followed by the eyes and skin, are the most commonly involved organs. A microbial origin of the antigens is favored because sarcoidosis occurs sporadically in clusters and is worldwide. Furthermore, sarcoidosis may recur in transplanted organs and can develop in recipients of tissues from donors with sarcoidosis.

Several environmental exposures are modestly associated with the risk for sarcoidosis, each with odds ratios of about 1.5: mold or mildew, musty odors at work, agricultural employment, and pesticide-using industries. Highly sensitive methods for detecting microbial DNA and proteins, such as polymerase chain reaction and mass spectrometry, have yielded potential etiologic agents. One promising candidate of microbial origin is the mycobacterial KatG protein.

Major histocompatibility complex (MHC) genes and non-MHC genes located on the short arm of chromosome 6p have been implicated as genetic risk factors for sarcoidosis. HLA-DQB1*0201 and HLA-DRB1*0301 alleles are strongly associated with acute disease and good prognosis. The HLA-DRB1*1501/DQB1*0602 haplotype predicts a chronic course and severe pulmonary sarcoidosis. Genome-wide scans have identified the gene candidates BTNL2 (butyrophilin-like 2 gene) and ANXA11 (annexin A11).

CLINICAL MANIFESTATIONS

Patients may present with any organ involved, with or without concomitant intrathoracic involvement. The severity of symptoms and organ dysfunction also varies, and as many as 30 to 50% of patients have no symptoms at the time of diagnosis. Clinical manifestations also vary by ethnicity, race, and sex as well as by the particular organ system predominantly affected.

Sarcoidosis often first comes to attention during routine screening when enlarged mediastinal and hilar lymph nodes are detected on a chest radiograph (Fig. 95-1). Symptomatic individuals commonly experience fatigue, night sweats, and weight loss. Fatigue often remains a prominent problem and can lead to impaired quality of life.

Symptomatic sarcoidosis may present insidiously or as an acute illness. Löfgren's syndrome, an acute form of the disease, consists of erythema nodosum (see Fig. 448-23 in Chapter 448), arthritis, and bilateral hilar adenopathy. Fever and uveitis may also accompany Löfgren's syndrome. Erythema nodosum occurs predominantly in women, whereas arthritis predominates in men.

FIGURE 95-1. Chest radiograph demonstrating a stage I disease with enlarged mediastinal and hilar lymph nodes.

Respiratory System Disease

More than 90% of patients have respiratory tract involvement, sometimes with symptoms and sometimes with asymptomatic radiographic abnormalities. The most common respiratory symptoms are dry cough and dyspnea. Chest pain, when present, is vague and nonspecific.

Upper respiratory tract involvement occurs in from 2 to 6% of patients, with most having nasal mucosal involvement. Severe upper respiratory tract disease may lead to anosmia, erosion of septal cartilage, and nasal deformity. Supraglottic and glottic involvement can lead to stridor, dysphonia, cough, and dysphagia.

Examination of the chest often reveals few or no findings. Localized wheezing suggests endobronchial granulomatous disease, whereas diffuse wheezing suggests hyperreactive airways disease. Crackles may be heard when bronchiectasis and fibrosis are present. Hemoptysis may occur with bronchiectasis or cavitary disease.

The most common radiographic finding is intrathoracic lymph node enlargement with or without parenchymal lung involvement. Mediastinal lymphadenopathy without hilar adenopathy is extremely rare. Hilar lymph node enlargement is usually symmetrical, and less than 3% of patients have unilateral enlargement. Concurrent enlargement of right paratracheal and aortic-pulmonary window lymph nodes is common.

The chest radiograph is traditionally categorized into five stages (Table 95-1), but these stages do not necessarily denote the severity or chronologic progression of disease, particularly when extrathoracic involvement is present. Furthermore, 50 to 94% of patients will have hilar or mediastinal lymphadenopathy on computed tomographic (CT) scans irrespective of their stage on a plain chest radiograph.

Chest CT may demonstrate nodules, ground-glass opacities, bronchiectasis, cysts, and thickening of the pleural surface (Fig. 95-2). CT scanning, however, generally adds little to diagnosis and management, particularly for those with a stage I chest radiograph. CT scanning can be justified when atypical clinical and chest radiographic findings are present, a normal chest radiograph is found during the evaluation of suspected extrathoracic disease, or complications are suspected.

Endobronchial sarcoidosis may lead to bronchial stenosis and recurrent obstructive pneumonias. Pleural effusions on plain radiography are uncommon (1 to 3% of patients). Pulmonary hypertension (Chapter 68) may complicate sarcoidosis, particularly when pulmonary fibrosis is present.

Skin Disease

Skin involvement occurs in 25 to 35% of patients, but lesions are commonly misdiagnosed because they can present as macules, papules, plaques, subcutaneous lesions, areas of increased or decreased pigmentation, and ulcerations. Lesions are commonly found on the upper back, the nape of the neck, and extremities (Fig. 95-3) and have a predilection for scars and tattoos. The most common skin manifestation is a maculopapular eruption, consisting of firm, flesh-colored to violaceous lesions that have a predilection for the eyelids and perioral area. Scalp involvement with alopecia may occur. Skin lesions in black American patients frequently leave scars and pale or depigmented areas.

Erythema nodosum occurs in about 10% of patients and commonly occurs as part of Löfgren's syndrome. It presents as raised, red, hot, tender subcutaneous nodular lesions, most commonly on the shins, but sometimes also on the arms and buttocks (see Fig. 448-3 in Chapter 448). Lesions persist for 1 to 3 weeks and may recur. The lesions of erythema nodosum typically show nonspecific septal panniculitis without sarcoidal granulomas, so biopsy is not usually helpful. Erythema nodosum portends a good prognosis, with up to 85% of patients resolving their sarcoidosis within 2 years.

Lupus pernio (Fig. 95-4) consists of chronic, lumpy, violaceous, indurated plaques and nodules distributed around the nose, cheeks, lips, and ears; it is specific to sarcoidosis. Patients with lupus pernio more commonly have a chronic course, fibrotic lung disease, and upper respiratory tract involvement.

FIGURE 95-3. Skin lesions of sarcoidosis. Sarcoidal lesions may occur at any site. This patient's papules have a waxy appearance and are located on the upper part of the back.

TABLE 95-1	CHEST RADIOGRAPHIC STAGING

Stage 0: Normal
Stage 1: Bilateral hilar adenopathy, often with right paratracheal adenopathy
Stage 2: Bilateral hilar adenopathy and parenchymal infiltration
Stage 3: Parenchymal infiltration without lymphadenopathy
Stage 4: Advanced parenchymal disease demonstrating fibrosis and may include honeycombing, cysts, bullae, and traction bronchiectasis

FIGURE 95-2. High-resolution chest computed tomography scan demonstrating numerous small nodules in a predominantly bronchovascular distribution.

FIGURE 95-4. Lupus pernio is the term used to describe infiltrative skin lesions affecting the nose, cheeks, and ears in chronic sarcoidosis.

Eye Disease

More than 25% of patients have ocular involvement (Chapter 431), and any part of the eye and adnexa may be involved. Lacrimal gland enlargement and conjunctival involvement are common. Conjunctival involvement consists of pale yellow nodules, which demonstrate granulomas on biopsy. Corneal involvement is rare. Acute anterior uveitis presents with pain, photophobia, lacrimation, and redness. Chronic anterior uveitis, which is more common than acute uveitis, may have minimal symptoms. Posterior uveitis, which occurs in about 30% of patients with ocular sarcoidosis, is frequently accompanied by central nervous system involvement. Choroidal lesions may occur anywhere in the fundus and may be multifocal. In 10 to 15% of patients with uveitis, both the anterior and posterior segments are affected.

Uveitis can herald the nonocular signs of sarcoidosis and may precede the diagnosis of sarcoidosis by decades. Chronic anterior uveitis may lead to cataracts and glaucoma. Heerfordt's syndrome consists of anterior uveitis accompanied by parotid gland enlargement and fever.

Cardiac Disease

Cardiac granulomas are found in about 25% of sarcoidosis patients who are examined at autopsy, but cardiac sarcoidosis is suspected in only about 5% of patients. In cardiac sarcoidosis (Chapter 60), granulomas most often infiltrate the left ventricular free wall. Next most frequently, sarcoidal granulomas infiltrate the intraventricular septum, where they often involve the conduction system. Cardiac manifestations include atrioventricular block, ventricular arrhythmias, left ventricular dysfunction, and sudden death.

Neurologic Disease

Nervous system granulomas are found in up to 25% of sarcoidosis patients who undergo autopsy, but only 10% of patients present with neurologic symptoms (Table 95-2). In patients with neurologic involvement, the neurologic signs or symptoms precede the diagnosis of sarcoidosis in up to 75% of patients and may be the only manifestation of sarcoidosis.

Neurosarcoidosis has a predilection for the base of the brain, hypothalamus, and pituitary gland. Myelopathy may occur anywhere in the spinal cord and carries a poor prognosis. Peripheral neuropathy (Chapter 428) may manifest as mononeuropathy or polyneuropathy.

Liver and Spleen

Liver involvement is twice as common in black Americans as in white Americans. Symptoms due to liver disease are infrequent, but abdominal pain and pruritus are the most common symptoms. Fever, weight loss, and jaundice are present in less than 5% of those with liver involvement. About 20% of patients will have hepatomegaly on physical examination, and 35% will have an elevated serum aminotransferase or alkaline phosphatase level. Sarcoidosis can rarely (<1%) cause progressive liver disease that leads to portal hypertension with variceal bleeding; the hepatopulmonary syndrome, with refractory hypoxemia, cirrhosis, and liver failure, may also occur.

Splenomegaly is found on physical examination in 5 to 15% of patients with sarcoidosis. Massive splenomegaly is rare.

Bone and Joint

Most patients complain of arthralgias, but only about 35% develop arthritis. Acute sarcoid arthritis (Chapter 283) consists of large joint periarthritis, particularly involving the ankles and knees, and commonly occurs with

TABLE 95-2   NEUROSARCOIDOSIS

Cranial neuropathies
  VII—Facial nerve palsy (unilateral, bilateral)
  II—Optic nerve (unilateral and bilateral)
  VIII—Hearing loss
  Other cranial neuropathies
Myelopathy (sensory and motor)
Seizure
Basilar meningitis
Central diabetes insipidus
Panhypopituitarism
Intraparenchymal mass
Hydrocephalus
Peripheral neuropathy

Löfgren's syndrome. These patients often report difficulty walking related to joint pain. Acute sarcoid arthritis usually persists for up to 3 months but is self-limited. Chronic sarcoid arthritis with direct granulomatous synovial infiltration is rare. Osseous sarcoidosis usually does not produce symptoms.

Calcium Metabolism

Aberrant calcium and vitamin D metabolism occurs in up to 50% of patients and may result in renal stones (Chapter 128), nephrocalcinosis with renal insufficiency, and hypercalciuria (urine calcium > 300 mg/24 hours) with or without hypercalcemia (Chapter 253). In chronic sarcoidosis, 10 to 14% of patients have at least one symptomatic renal stone.

Renal Involvement

Renal involvement, other than as a result of dysregulated calcium metabolism, occurs in less than 1% of patients. Renal disease may include granulomatous interstitial nephritis, glomerular disease, renal tubular dysfunction, renal vascular disease, and obstructive uropathy. Granulomatous interstitial nephritis is more common in white men.

DIAGNOSIS

The diagnosis of sarcoidosis should be based on compatible clinical and radiographic findings supported by histologic evidence of noncaseating granulomas in one or more organs in the absence of any foreign particles or organisms. An occupational history consistent with beryllium exposure (Chapter 93), such as employment in the aerospace, automotive, ceramic, or computer industries, requires further investigation because chronic beryllium disease cannot be clinically or histologically distinguished from sarcoidosis.

A diagnosis of sarcoidosis is reasonably certain even without histologic confirmation in patients who present with Löfgren's syndrome. In all other cases, a biopsy specimen from an involved organ should be obtained. The organ for which biopsy is safest, such as the skin, peripheral lymph nodes, lacrimal glands, or conjunctiva, should be sampled.

If diagnosis requires intrathoracic sampling, transbronchial biopsy by means of bronchoscopy has a diagnostic yield of at least 85%. Even when pulmonary parenchymal involvement is not visible on plain chest radiography, transbronchial lung biopsy has an excellent diagnostic yield when multiple lung segments are sampled. Bronchoalveolar lavage sampling demonstrates lymphocytosis with normal or low granulocyte counts in more than 85% of patients (Chapter 85). The CD4/CD8 ratio is increased in bronchoalveolar lavage in about 50% of patients with sarcoidosis, but bronchoalveolar lavage findings are nonspecific and should not be used to diagnose sarcoidosis. Bronchoalveolar lavage findings also cannot predict prognosis or responsiveness to corticosteroid therapy.

Fine-needle aspiration of enlarged intrathoracic lymph nodes guided by endobronchial ultrasound has an 80% diagnostic yield and is significantly more likely to make the diagnosis than in unguided transbronchial biopsy.[1] Endobronchial ultrasound allows visualization of mediastinal structures, including the subcarinal region, paraesophageal space, and aortopulmonary window. Bronchoscopy and endobronchial ultrasound-guided fine-needle aspiration generally make the need for more invasive approaches, such as mediastinoscopy or video-assisted thoracoscopic surgical biopsies, unnecessary.

Sarcoidal granulomas produce angiotensin-converting enzyme (ACE). Although serum ACE levels are elevated in 60% of patients with sarcoidosis, the value of a serum ACE level in diagnosing sarcoidosis remains limited because positive and negative predictive values are only about 84% and 74%, respectively.

Patients should routinely undergo pulmonary function testing, which often does not correlate with the chest radiographic stage. For example, pulmonary function tests may be abnormal even in patients with a normal chest radiograph. Diffusion capacity for carbon monoxide (D_{LCO}) is usually the first abnormality detected and the last to normalize on remission. A D_{LCO} of less than 50% of predicted is associated with exercise-induced oxygen desaturation and should prompt formal oxygen saturation testing with exercise.

About two thirds of patients have airflow limitation at presentation. Spirometry usually indicates restrictive ventilatory dysfunction with a reduced forced vital capacity (FVC) and reduced forced expiratory volume in 1 second (FEV_1). At least 50% of patients have concurrent obstructive airways disease. Airway hyperreactivity, as measured by increased responsiveness to methacholine, occurs in up to 83% of patients. In patients with abnormal spirometric findings at diagnosis, spirometry returns to normal in 80%.

Alterations in cardiopulmonary exercise testing have been reported in nearly 50% of patients with sarcoidosis. Abnormalities, including a ventilatory limitation with exercise and a widened alveolar-arterial O_2 gradient, may be present. FVC is the single best test for following respiratory involvement and correlates well with FEV_1, total lung capacity, and D_{LCO}.

Because ocular involvement is common and vision loss may occur, complete ocular evaluation with slit lamp and funduscopic examinations should be routinely performed during the initial evaluation and then annually in patients with active systemic disease.

An electrocardiogram (ECG) should be performed at the initial encounter. Screening for cardiac symptoms (palpitations, dizziness, and syncope) should be performed during the initial evaluation and routinely during follow-up visits if the disease is active. Any cardiac symptoms or abnormalities on the ECG should prompt further cardiac event monitoring (Chapter 62) and testing by echocardiography (Chapter 55). Endomyocardial biopsy has less than 20% diagnostic yield because cardiac involvement is patchy and is usually most dense in the left ventricle and basal ventricular septum where endomyocardial biopsies are avoided. If cardiac involvement is suspected, positron emission tomography (PET) or cardiac magnetic resonance imaging (MRI) with contrast should be performed. For significant symptoms, such as arrhythmias, decreased ventricular function, or septal involvement detected on MRI or PET, electrophysiologic studies should be considered and the need for an automatic implantable cardioverter-defibrillator (AICD) should be evaluated (Chapters 65 and 66).

The criteria for the diagnosis of neurosarcoidosis in the absence of histologic confirmation are not established. Compatible MRI findings, a characteristic presentation, and exclusion of other neurologic diseases are required. Histologic confirmation of disease elsewhere supports the diagnosis of neurosarcoidosis. Cerebrospinal fluid (CSF) analysis typically demonstrates nonspecific lymphocytic inflammation (Chapter 420). The CSF glucose can be as low as 14 mg/dL, with a white blood cell count as high as 350 cells/μL and a protein concentration as high as 670 mg/dL. CSF ACE levels are neither sensitive nor specific. CSF oligoclonal immunoglobulin bands are elevated in one third of patients, thereby making it difficult to differentiate sarcoidosis from multiple sclerosis (Chapter 419).

Up to 65% of patients will have granulomas on liver biopsy, but hepatic granulomas (Chapter 154) occur commonly with other disorders such as infection and drug-induced hepatitis. As a result, the diagnosis of sarcoidosis should not be based solely on detection of hepatic granulomas.

On plain radiographic images, most skeletal lesions of sarcoidosis are seen in the small bones of the hands and feet. MRI and PET scanning show much greater involvement of the axial skeleton and long bones, and osseous sarcoidosis may appear similar to metastatic disease on a PET scan.

Sarcoidosis Complicating Type 1 Interferon Therapy

Type 1 interferons, IFN-α and IFN-β, used to treat viral hepatitis (Chapter 151), multiple sclerosis (Chapter 419), and autoimmune and malignant disease may increase the T_H1 cytokines, IFN-γ, and IL-2 and rarely (<1 to 5%) result in sarcoidosis. Most reported cases of interferon-induced sarcoidosis occur within 6 months of therapy and manifest primarily with lung and skin involvement.

PREVENTION AND TREATMENT (Rx)

Because the inciting agent has not yet been identified nor genetic risk factors firmly established, no means exist to prevent sarcoidosis. Most patients with sarcoidosis are not disabled by their illness, so the decision to recommend treatment should weigh the risks of using corticosteroids (Chapter 34), which are the most common treatment, against potential benefits (Table 95-3). Hypercalcemia, cardiac disease, and neurologic disease are indications for treatment, and immediate treatment is appropriate whenever organ function is threatened or when symptoms are severe. Detection of granulomatous inflammation on physical examination, biopsy, or imaging or the presence of an elevated serum ACE level is not a mandate to provide treatment.

Oral prednisone at a dose of 20 to 40 mg per day for 3 months is usually the initial recommended therapy. Response to treatment is indicated by improvement in symptoms or objective measures, such as decreased size and number of skin lesions, increased FVC, or a reduction of detectable cardiac or brain lesions. For pulmonary involvement, steroids improve symptoms, pulmonary function test results, and chest radiographic findings.[2] If a response is noted at 3 months, the prednisone dose should be tapered to 10 to 15 mg per day for an additional 6 to 9 months and then tapered off. Because recurrence may occur, patients should be followed closely for 1 to 2 years after discontinuing treatment. The indications for restarting treatment are the same as those used to begin treatment. Lack of response after a 3-month trial suggests nonadherence to therapy, an inadequate dose of prednisone, or irreversible fibrotic disease. Inhaled corticosteroids should be used only in patients with bronchial hyperreactivity or persistent cough.

Cytotoxic and immunosuppressive drugs have been used to treat patients who do not respond to corticosteroid therapy or who cannot tolerate it (see Table 95-3), but data on their benefit are inconclusive,[3] and no large randomized trials confirm an optimal agent. Generally, 3 to 6 months of cytotoxic and immunosuppressive treatment is required to determine whether a response has occurred. For patients who respond, the duration of treatment should be 9 to 12 months. In patients who are steroid dependent but have ongoing extrapulmonary disease, the addition of infliximab, 3 to 5 mg/kg for 24 weeks, can be efficacious.[4]

Moderate doses of corticosteroids (15 to 20 mg prednisone) reduce the elevated serum and urinary calcium within a few days of starting treatment. Failure of serum calcium to normalize within 2 weeks should alert the clinician to an alternative diagnosis such as hyperparathyroidism or malignancy (Chapter 253). With treatment, most patients with granulomatous interstitial nephritis regain renal function but are often left with chronic kidney disease of varying severity.

Less than 1% of heart and liver and about 3% of lung transplantations are performed in patients with sarcoidosis. The 1- and 5-year graft survival rates for lung, liver, and heart transplantations in patients with sarcoidosis compare favorably with the results obtained for patients with other disorders.

TABLE 95-3 TREATMENT

ORGAN	CLINICAL FINDINGS	TREATMENT
Respiratory	Dyspnea, persistent cough, FVC < 70%	Prednisone, 20-40 mg/day
	Mild cough, wheezing	Inhaled corticosteroid
Skin	Lupus pernio	Prednisone, 20-40 mg/day Hydroxychloroquine, 400 mg/day Methotrexate, 10-15 mg/wk Infliximab, 3-5 mg/kg every 2-4 weeks
	Maculopapular eruptions	Topical corticosteroid Hydroxychloroquine, 400 mg/day Prednisone, 20-40 mg/day
	Erythema nodosum	NSAID*
Eyes	Anterior uveitis	Topical corticosteroid
	Posterior uveitis	Prednisone, 20-40 mg/day
Cardiac	Complete heart block, ventricular arrhythmias	AICD, prednisone, 20-40 mg/day
	Decreased LVEF (<35%)	AICD, prednisone, 20-40 mg/day
Central nervous system	Cranial nerve palsies	Prednisone, 20-40 mg/day
	Myelopathy	Prednisone, 40-60 mg/day, and azathioprine, 150 mg/day (or mycophenolate mofetil, or cyclophosphamide)
	Intracerebral involvement	Prednisone, 40-60 mg/day, and azathioprine, 150 mg/day (or mycophenolate mofetil, or cyclophosphamide)
Liver	Cholestatic hepatitis	Prednisone, 20-40 mg/day
Bone and joint	Arthralgias	NSAID
	Granulomatous arthritis	Prednisone, 20-40 mg/day Methotrexate, 10-15 mg/wk
	Bone destruction/pain	Prednisone, 20-40 mg/day Methotrexate, 10-15 mg/wk
Hypercalciuria and hypercalcemia	Kidney stones	Prednisone, 20-40 mg/day Hydroxychloroquine, 400 mg/day

*For example, ibuprofen, 200-800 mg three times a day.
AICD = automatic implantable cardioverter-defibrillator; FVC = forced vital capacity; LVEF = left ventricular ejection fraction; NSAID = nonsteroidal anti-inflammatory drug.

PROGNOSIS

Patients with Löfgren's syndrome have a good prognosis characterized by spontaneous resolution with few consequences. Overall, spontaneous remission with few or no consequences occurs in more than 50% of patients within 3 years of diagnosis and in two thirds of patients within a decade. After one or more years of remission without treatment, recurrence occurs in fewer than 5% of patients. Up to one third of patients have unrelenting disease that leads to significant organ impairment, but less than 5% of patients die from sarcoidosis. Black Americans tend to have a worse prognosis with more chronic disease and more extrathoracic involvement of the eyes, liver, bone marrow, extrathoracic lymph nodes, and skin. Patients with neurologic and cardiac involvement have a poorer prognosis.

 Grade A

1. Tremblay A, Stather DR, Maceachern P, et al. A randomized controlled trial of standard vs endobronchial ultrasonography-guided transbronchial needle aspiration in patients with suspected sarcoidosis. *Chest.* 2009;136:340-346.
2. Paramothayan NS, Lasserson TJ, Jones PW. Corticosteroids for pulmonary sarcoidosis. *Cochrane Database Syst Rev.* 2000;18:CD001114.
3. Paramothayan S, Lasserson TJ, Walters EH. Immunosuppressive and cytotoxic therapy for pulmonary sarcoidosis. *Cochrane Database Syst Rev.* 2006;3:CD003536.
4. Judson MA, Baughman RP, Costabel U, et al. Efficacy of infliximab in extrapulmonary sarcoidosis: results from a randomized trial. *Eur Respir J.* 2008;31:1189-1196.

SUGGESTED READINGS

Dubrey SW, Falk RH. Diagnosis and management of cardiac sarcoidosis. *Prog Cardiovasc Dis.* 2010;52:336-346. *Review of clinical manifestations, diagnosis, and treatment.*
Iannuzzi MC, Fontana JR. Sarcoidosis: clinical presentation, immunopathogenesis, and therapeutics. *JAMA.* 2011;305:391-399. *Review.*
Jones N, Mochizuki M. Sarcoidosis: epidemiology and clinical features. *Ocul Immunol Inflamm.* 2010;18:72-79. *Review with emphasis on eye involvement.*
Kollert F, Geck B, Suchy R, et al. The impact of gas exchange measurement during exercise in pulmonary sarcoidosis. *Respir Med.* 2011;105:122-129. *Impaired gas exchange during exercise reflects disease activity and a prolonged need for immunosuppressive treatment.*

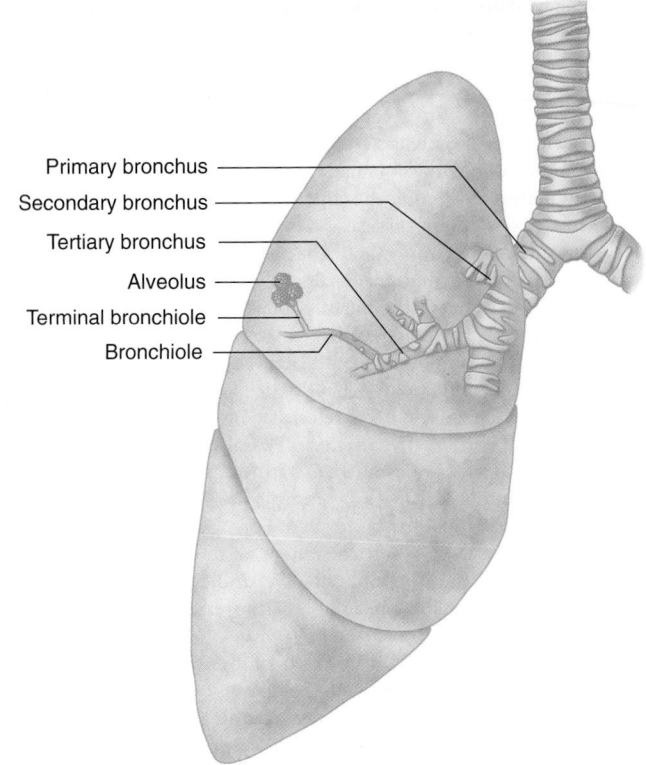

Primary bronchus
Secondary bronchus
Tertiary bronchus
Alveolus
Terminal bronchiole
Bronchiole

FIGURE 96-1. Many infecting agents that cause bronchitis and tracheitis can infect both large and small airways of the lung and occasionally the alveoli. Not surprisingly, a wide spectrum of signs and symptoms are associated with bronchitis, including cough, wheezing, and shortness of breath.

96

ACUTE BRONCHITIS AND TRACHEITIS

RICHARD P. WENZEL

DEFINITION

The term *acute bronchitis and tracheitis* defines a self-limited (1 to 3 weeks) inflammation of the large airways of the lung that extends to the tertiary bronchi (Fig. 96-1). In patients with a primary symptom of cough (Chapter 83), the diagnosis is made if there is no clinical or radiologic evidence of pneumonia. At the bedside, the absence of criteria for systemic inflammatory response syndrome (SIRS) (Chapter 108) suggests bronchitis and tracheitis and makes a diagnosis of pneumonia (Chapter 97) unlikely. The SIRS criteria are met if the patient has more than two of the following: temperature lower than 36° C or higher than 38° C, pulse greater than 90 beats/minute, respiratory rate higher than 20 breaths/minute, or white blood cell count less than 4000 cells/mm³ or higher than 12,000 cells/mm³ or with greater than 10% bands.

The definition of acute bronchitis and tracheitis also seeks to differentiate the illness from acute inflammation of the small airways (bronchiolitis), even though the accompanying symptoms with the former may include sputum production, wheezing, and shortness of breath. Among patients with primarily small airways disease, some might be expected to have prominently decreased breath sounds in the areas involved. Acute bronchitis and tracheitis is also different from bronchiectasis (Chapter 90), which is associated with permanent dilation of bronchi and a chronic cough. Furthermore, a diagnosis of chronic bronchitis (Chapter 88) is reserved for patients who have prolonged cough and sputum production: at least 3 months of the year for 2 consecutive years.

EPIDEMIOLOGY

Occurring at a rate of 44 per 1000 adults per year, acute bronchitis and tracheitis affects approximately 5% of adults annually. A higher incidence is observed in the winter and fall than in the summer and spring. In the United States, acute bronchitis and tracheitis is the ninth most common illness in outpatients as reported by physicians.

The disorder is thought to be viral in origin almost all the time. However, viruses have been isolated in only 8 to 37% of patients. Thus, the true causes of the illness are unknown in most cases. Nevertheless, at least 70% of patients with acute bronchitis and tracheitis in the United States receive antibacterial antibiotics after visiting a physician. Importantly, although the same bacteria that are commonly implicated in community-acquired pneumonia are also isolated from the sputum in half the patients, their role in the pathobiology of acute bronchitis and tracheitis or its attendant symptoms is unclear, and bronchial biopsies have not shown bacterial invasion.

PATHOBIOLOGY

Infections of the epithelium of the bronchi and trachea are thought to incite an inflammatory response. Pathologically, there is an accompanying microscopic thickening of bronchial and tracheal mucosa corresponding to the inflamed areas. Such pathologic findings are also consistent with the occasional case report of upper airway inflammation confined to the bronchi and trachea detected by ¹⁸F-labeled fluorodeoxyglucose positron emission tomography (FDG-PET).

In human experimental rhinovirus infections (Chapter 369), virus was detected in all subjects in induced sputum samples and also in approximately one third of bronchial biopsy specimens, almost one fourth of bronchoalveolar lavage samples, and more than one third of biopsy and brushing samples. Such data indicating viral infection of the lower airways may help explain the relationship observed between rhinovirus infection and exacerbations of asthma (Chapter 87). Furthermore, pathologic islands of inflammation have been found in the trachea with rhinovirus infection, thus supporting the idea of a patchy distribution. The viruses implicated in acute bronchitis and tracheitis include influenza A and B (Chapter 372), parainfluenza (Chapter 371), respiratory syncytial virus (Chapter 370), coronavirus (Chapter 374), adenovirus (Chapter 373), and rhinoviruses (Chapter 369), usually in this order from the most to the least common. However, a recent French study of influenza-vaccinated adults found a viral cause in 37% of 164 cases of acute bronchitis, 21% of which were rhinovirus. Thus, at least three variables can influence the yield of specific pathogens: the presence of epidemics, the season of the year, and the population's influenza vaccination status. More recently, human metapneumovirus (Chapter 369) has been identified as an etiologic agent.

Up to 10% of cases of acute bronchitis and tracheitis may be due to "atypical" bacteria: *Bordetella pertussis* (Chapter 321), *Chlamydophila (Chlamydia) pneumoniae* (Chapter 325), and *Mycoplasma pneumoniae* (Chapter 326). Severe bronchiolitis has also been reported with *M. pneumoniae,* even though this pathogen is usually associated with either pneumonia or acute bronchitis and tracheitis in adults. In children, bronchiolitis has been associated with respiratory syncytial virus, influenza virus, parainfluenza virus, and metapneumovirus (Chapter 369). Thus, there are probably wide variations in the anatomic distribution of all pathogens causing acute bronchitis and tracheitis, extending from the nasal mucosa to the bronchiolar epithelium.

CLINICAL MANIFESTATIONS

The cardinal clinical symptom is cough (Chapter 83) of recent onset. Because most upper respiratory infections resolve within 1 week, a more extended period of cough is useful for considering the diagnosis of acute bronchitis. Patients usually seek care from their physician after 4 to 7 days of coughing that is not resolving. With acute bronchitis, there is often a continued cough and sometimes a worsened cough that lasts an initial 1 to 3 weeks. Associated symptoms vary and include sputum production, fever, malaise, wheezing, and dyspnea. Adults with pertussis may exhibit paroxysms of coughing, whooping, or vomiting, although less commonly than seen in children with this infection.

DIAGNOSIS

Acutely ill patients may not be able to distinguish their early symptoms from those accompanying very mild upper respiratory infections. However, with acute bronchitis and tracheitis, a protracted phase of coughing persists beyond 1 to 5 days, during which time pulmonary function tests may become abnormal. A substantial proportion of patients will have significant declines in forced expiratory volume in the first second (FEV$_1$) (Chapter 85).

Rapid diagnostic tests exist for most viruses linked to acute bronchitis and tracheitis. However, their value lies in identifying a virus for which there is therapy or avoiding antibacterial antibiotics if any virus is identified. Not all rapid tests are widely available, and they are expensive and rarely cost-effective in an outpatient setting.

When "atypical" bacteria are identified by culture or serology, patients tend to be seen later in the course of their illness than patients with viral causes and more often have wheezing. In some studies, 12 to 32% of patients with coughing that persists for longer than 1 week had pertussis. In other studies, however, pertussis has been confirmed in only 1% of such patients.

Polymerase chain reaction (PCR) testing of nasopharyngeal swabs or aspirates is the easiest and most sensitive way to diagnose infections by *B. pertussis, M. pneumoniae,* and *C. pneumoniae;* most experts recommend calcium alginate swabs for pertussis because cotton inhibits growth. Dacron swabs with aluminum handles are preferred for specimens used to diagnose *Chlamydophila* because cotton, calcium alginate, and the wooden shaft can all inhibit growth of the organism. Cultures for *M. pneumoniae* are slow and insensitive. In general, testing for atypical organisms should not be done because of the cost of PCR and both the insensitivity and slowness of cultures. However, if the clinician suspects an outbreak in the community or the likelihood of pertussis, rapid testing with PCR may be quite beneficial.

TREATMENT   Rx

In a meta-analysis of nine randomized trials of antibacterial antibiotics for acute bronchitis, patients receiving antibiotics were significantly less likely to have a cough, but their 0.58 fewer days with cough, 0.52 fewer days of productive cough, and 0.58 fewer days of feeling ill were not statistically significant.[1] A large clinical trial in a population with a high prevalence of human immunodeficiency virus infection found that amoxicillin for 7 days was no better than placebo.[2]

These results are not surprising because, at most, about 50% of cases are probably caused by bacterial pathogens. Nevertheless, antibiotics are used in 50 to 85% of cases worldwide.

Antibiotics may be used in patients with known atypical pathogens, but even then their effect on outcomes is not clear except to limit the spread of pertussis, especially during a defined outbreak. In adults suspected of having pertussis, erythromycin, 500 mg four times a day for 14 days, is thought to be most effective. However, many patients cannot tolerate erythromycin, and either doxycycline, 100 mg every 12 hours, or a newer macrolide such as

azithromycin, 500 mg on day 1 and 250 mg/day thereafter, is effective. The latter two drugs are also active against *C. pneumoniae* and *M. pneumoniae,* although the optimal duration of therapy for acute bronchitis is unknown. A useful range is 5 to 14 days.

During influenza season, anti-influenza agents may be useful in decreasing symptoms by approximately 1 day and may lead to a 0.5-day earlier return to normal activity in patients with influenza. The first-generation drugs amantadine and rimantadine are ineffective against H3N2 influenza A viruses and are not recommended. Second-generation drugs such as zanamivir (two inhalations of 5 mg each, twice a day) or oseltamivir (75 mg twice a day) can be given for 5 days. Up to 20% of patients given oseltamivir will have nausea or vomiting.

Antihistamines and over-the-counter antitussives and expectorants have no apparent value. Subsets of patients with bronchial hyperresponsiveness may benefit from β-agonists, but no data support the use of inhaled steroids. Mucolytic agents may be of small benefit.[3]

In experimental rhinovirus colds, nonsteroidal drugs, alone or in combination with antihistamines, reduce the severity of symptoms, including cough. However, the widespread use of either type of drug alone or as a combination in naturally occurring, community-acquired bronchitis and tracheitis has not been evaluated. In patients with acute bronchitis, a meta-analysis of four placebo-controlled clinical trials suggested that *Pelargonium sidoides* (a herbaceous perennial widely used in Europe) reduced bronchitis symptom scores by day 7.[4]

PROGNOSIS

Coughing usually lasts 10 to 14 days, during which time the illness causes significant transient decrements in vitality and social functioning. Limited data on short- and long-term outcomes show that up to 20% of patients have persistent or recurrent symptoms for a month. Antibiotics may reduce symptoms by a fraction of a day, but side effects, the emergence of antibiotic resistance, and cost must be weighed against their modest benefits. The mean duration of an office visit for adults in the United States with upper respiratory tract infections is 14.2 minutes when patients are prescribed antibiotics versus 15.2 minutes without prescription of antibiotics, but antibiotic use is not an independent predictor of visit length. Future widespread use of rapid diagnostic tests for specific bacterial and viral pathogens will be useful in targeting effective therapies.

Grade **A**

1. Smucny J, Fahey T, Becker L, et al. Antibiotics for acute bronchitis. In: The Cochrane Collaboration. New York: J Wiley & Sons; 2005:1-26. Available at *http://www.cochrane.org/reviews/en/ab000245.html.*
2. Nduba VN, Mwachari CW, Margaret AS, et al. Placebo found equivalent to amoxicillin for treatment of acute bronchitis in Nairobi, Kenya: a triple-blind randomized, equivalence trial. *Thorax.* 2008;63:999-1105.
3. Poole P, Black PN. Mucolytic agents for chronic bronchitis or chronic obstructive pulmonary disease. *Cochrane Database Syst Rev.* 2010;2:CD001287.
4. Agbabiaka TB, Guo R, Edzard E. *Pelargonium sidoides* for acute bronchitis: a systematic review and meta-analysis. *Phytomedicine.* 2008;15:378-385.

SUGGESTED READINGS

Fahy JV, Dickey BF. Airway mucus function and dysfunction. *N Engl J Med.* 2010;363:2233-2247. *Review.*
Sethi S. Antibiotics in acute exacerbations of chronic bronchitis. *Expert Rev Anti Infect Ther.* 2010;8:405-417. *Review of guidelines.*

97

OVERVIEW OF PNEUMONIA

ANDREW H. LIMPER

It is a useful distinction to separate pneumonias, which are infections of the lung parenchyma and thus distinct from infections limited to the trachea or large bronchi (Chapter 96), into those acquired in the community (community-acquired pneumonia) and those arising in institutional settings, with the second group being composed of hospital-acquired pneumonia, ventilator-associated pneumonia, and health care–associated pneumonia. These two major pneumonia categories are considered separately in this chapter. Additional consideration should be given to pneumonia caused by recurrent aspiration of oropharyngeal contents.

The term *pneumonia* itself, however, includes other causes of inflammation of the lower respiratory air spaces, particularly the alveoli, such as acute or chronic eosinophilic pneumonia, cryptogenic organizing pneumonia, and usual interstitial pneumonia, all of which are presented in more detail elsewhere (Chapter 92).

COMMUNITY-ACQUIRED PNEUMONIA

DEFINITION

Community-acquired pneumonia includes cases of infectious pneumonia in patients living independently in the community. Patients who have been hospitalized for other reasons for less than 48 hours before the development of respiratory symptoms are also considered to have community-acquired pneumonia because it is likely that the inoculation had occurred before admission. However, patients who have previously been hospitalized for at least 2 days within the 90 days before infection; patients from nursing homes who received intravenous antibiotic therapy, chemotherapy, or wound care within the past 30 days; and patients from hemodialysis centers are considered to have health care–associated pneumonia and are therefore excluded from the case definition of community-acquired pneumonia. Patients contracting pneumonia more than 48 hours after the institution of endotracheal intubation and mechanical ventilation are also excluded inasmuch as they are considered to have ventilator-associated pneumonia. These distinctions are important because they help define the most likely infectious agents and hence strongly influence appropriate choices for the initial antibiotic therapy.

EPIDEMIOLOGY

More than 10 million cases of infectious pneumonia occur annually in the United States and result in more than 1 million hospitalizations. Pneumonia is a leading cause of death worldwide, the sixth leading cause of death in the United States, and the most common lethal infectious disease. The mortality rate associated with community-acquired pneumonia ranges from less than 5% in mildly ill outpatients to somewhat greater than 12% overall in patients who are admitted to a hospital. Mortality is even greater in patients who have severe invasive disease, which is often associated with bacteremia, and in elderly nursing home patients. Mortality from pneumonia can exceed 40% in patients who require management in the intensive care unit (ICU). It costs approximately $7000 to manage an uncomplicated case of pneumonia in the hospital, or about 20-fold more than treating it in the outpatient setting.

PATHOBIOLOGY

Aspiration of Oropharyngeal Contents

The most common mechanism by which the lung is inoculated with pathogenic organisms is through microaspiration of oropharyngeal contents, a process that occurs in otherwise healthy individuals during sleep (Chapter 94). Colonization of the oral pharynx with pathogenic organisms, such as *Streptococcus pneumoniae* (Chapter 297), can thereby lead to delivery of sufficient quantities of organisms to infect the lung. In contrast, gross aspiration normally occurs only in individuals with altered sensorium, depressed consciousness, abnormalities in protective cough or gag reflexes, or substantial gastroesophageal reflux. Gross aspiration, which can also deliver large numbers of anaerobic bacteria to the lower respiratory tract, is a major contributing factor to anaerobic lung infection and abscess formation (Chapter 90).

Inhalation of Aerosolized Droplets

The second most frequent mechanism of lung infection is the inhalation of small, suspended aerosolized droplets ranging in size from 0.5 to 1 μm that may contain microorganisms. In view of the limited number of organisms delivered in such a manner, only relatively aggressive pathogenic organisms such as *Mycobacterium tuberculosis* (Chapter 332), *Legionella pneumophila* (Chapter 322), *Yersinia pestis* (plague; Chapter 320), *Bacillus anthracis* (anthrax; Chapter 302), and some viral infections can be transmitted in this manner.

Blood Stream Infection

Less commonly, the lung may become infected as a consequence of a blood stream infection. Blood-borne pneumonia is seen especially in staphylococcal sepsis (Chapter 296) or right-sided endocarditis (Chapter 76), both of which are more common in intravenous drug users (Chapter 33), and in

gram-negative bacteremias, particularly in an immunocompromised host. The lung may also rarely be inoculated directly by penetrating chest trauma or by local spread from a nearby infected organ (bacterial or amoebic liver abscess or paragonimiasis; Chapters 360 and 364) or a contiguous soft tissue infection.

Fortunately, the lung is well equipped to defend against inoculation with most microbes. When large droplets of infected material reach the airways, they are removed by the mucociliary escalator, which sweeps entrapped contents up to the oropharynx, where they are swallowed or expectorated. Smaller particles, in the range of 0.5 to 2.0 μm, are deposited in the alveoli, where alveolar macrophages phagocytize and destroy most pathogens. These macrophages are further activated to release potent cytokines and chemokines, including tumor necrosis factor-α, interleukin-8, and leukotriene B$_4$, which help recruit neutrophils from the blood stream into the alveolar spaces, where they participate in the uptake and degradation of microorganisms. For many microorganisms such as *S. pneumoniae* (Chapter 297), clearance of infection is greatly facilitated by the development of specific immunoglobulin G that binds the surface of the organisms or their polysaccharide capsule. These specific antibodies, which act as immune opsonins, greatly augment the ability of neutrophils and macrophages to phagocytize and destroy the bacteria. In addition, pattern recognition receptors and other nonimmune opsonins, including surfactant proteins A and D, fibronectin, and vitronectin, also bind to specific epitopes on the surface of organisms that reach the lower respiratory tract and assist in their recognition and elimination. Only when organisms overwhelm or evade these multiple host defense systems does inoculation of the lung result in clinically significant pneumonia.

CLINICAL MANIFESTATIONS

The possibility of pneumonia should be considered in any patient who has new respiratory symptoms, including cough, sputum, or dyspnea, particularly when these symptoms are accompanied by fever or abnormalities on physical examination of the chest, such as rhonchi and rales. The initial manifestation is frequently more subtle in patients who are elderly or have an altered immunologic status; in such patients, nonspecific symptoms, including loss of appetite, confusion, dehydration, worsening of symptoms or signs of other chronic illnesses, or failure to thrive, may be the initial manifestation of pneumonia. Pneumonia is also increasingly prevalent in patients with specific comorbid conditions, including smoking, chronic obstructive pulmonary disease (COPD; Chapter 88), diabetes mellitus, malignancy, heart failure, neurologic diseases, narcotic and alcohol use, and chronic liver disease.

The initial symptoms and signs are often variable from patient to patient and cannot be reliably used to establish a specific (microbiologic) diagnosis. The classic physical findings in lobar pneumonia include evidence of consolidation with altered transmission of breath sounds, egophony, crackles, and changes in tactile fremitus. However, in many patients, the physical findings are subtler and may be limited to scattered rhonchi. A thorough physical examination, posteroanterior and lateral chest radiographs, and a blood leukocyte count with a differential cell count should be performed when pneumonia is suspected. An assessment of gas exchange (oximetry or arterial blood gas determination) should be obtained for all patients who are admitted to the hospital. The clinician needs to be mindful of competing diagnoses that can mimic the findings of pneumonia, such as pulmonary embolism (Chapter 98), bronchogenic and bronchoalveolar carcinoma (Chapter 197), drug-induced lung diseases (Chapter 94), and idiopathic interstitial lung diseases (Chapter 92).

DIAGNOSIS

Even with intensive laboratory investigation, the specific microbiologic cause can be established with certainty only in approximately 50% of patients with pneumonia. The probable predominant organism varies with the host's epidemiologic factors, the severity of illness, and which laboratory approach is used to establish the diagnosis.

Bacterial Pneumonia

S. pneumoniae (Chapter 297) is the organism most frequently detected by culture of sputum or blood. In contrast, *Mycoplasma pneumoniae* (Chapter 325) is frequently detected with serologic tests. Additional bacterial agents include *Haemophilus influenzae* (Chapter 308), *Staphylococcus aureus* (Chapter 296), enteric gram-negative bacilli (Chapters 290 and 314), and *L. pneumophila* (Chapter 322). *Chlamydia* and respiratory viruses have also been implicated in up to 10% of cases. The so-called atypical pathogens,

TABLE 97-1 HOST FACTORS ASSOCIATED WITH SPECIFIC PATHOGENIC CAUSES OF PNEUMONIA

UNDERLYING CONDITION	ASSOCIATED MICROORGANISM
Active smoking/chronic obstructive lung disease	*Streptococcus pneumoniae, Haemophilus influenzae, Legionella pneumophila, Moraxella catarrhalis, Pseudomonas aeruginosa, Chlamydophila pneumonia*
Nursing home residents	*S. pneumoniae,* gram-negative bacilli, *H. influenzae, Staphylococcus aureus, Chlamydophila pneumoniae,* anaerobes, *Mycobacterium tuberculosis*
Alcoholism	*S. pneumoniae* (including drug-resistant strains), gram-negative bacilli, anaerobes, *Mycobacterium tuberculosis, Klebsiella pneumoniae, Acinetobacter* species
Gross aspiration/poor dentition	Anaerobes, gram-negative enteric pathogens
Travel to southwestern United States	*Coccidioides immitis*
Exposure to bats	*Histoplasma capsulatum*
Exposure to birds	*Cryptococcus neoformans, Chlamydia psittaci, H. capsulatum*
Exposure to rabbits	*Francisella tularensis*
Exposure to farm animals	*Coxiella burnetii* (Q fever)
Viral influenza	Influenza, *S. aureus, S. pneumoniae, H. influenzae*
Bronchiectasis, cystic fibrosis	*Pseudomonas aeruginosa, Burkholderia cepacia, S. aureus, Aspergillus* species, *Mycobacterium avium* complex
Lung abscess	CA-MRSA, oral anaerobes, endemic fungal pneumonia, *M. tuberculosis,* atypical mycobacteria
Intravenous drug use	*S. aureus,* anaerobes, *M. tuberculosis, S. pneumoniae*
Endobronchial obstruction	Anaerobes
Recent antibiotic therapy	Drug-resistant *S. pneumoniae, P. aeruginosa*
HIV (early)	*S. pneumoniae, H. influenza, M. tuberculosis*
HIV (late)	The pathogens listed for early HIV infection, plus *Pneumocystis jirovecii, Cryptococcus, Histoplasma, Aspergillus,* atypical mycobacteria (especially *M. kansasii* and *M. avium* complex), *P. aeruginosa, H. influenza*
In the context of bioterrorism	*Bacillus anthracis* (anthrax), *Yersinia pestis* (plague), *Francisella tularensis* (tularemia)

CA-MRSA = community-acquired methicillin-resistant *Staphylococcus aureus*; HIV = human immunodeficiency virus.
Adapted from Infectious Diseases Society of America/American Thoracic Society. Consensus guidelines on the management of community acquired pneumonia in adults. *Clin Infect Dis.* 2007;44:S27-S72.

including *M. pneumoniae, Chlamydia pneumoniae,* and *Legionella* species, are increasingly being recognized as important and prevalent causes of pneumonia. Mixed infections, particularly those related to coinfection with these "atypical" pathogens in addition to the usual bacterial pathogens, have been reported in up to one third of patients with lower respiratory tract infection.

Specific host factors also influence the relative risk for infection with specific microorganisms (Table 97-1). For instance, smokers and those with COPD are at increased risk for invasive *S. pneumoniae,* as well as *H. influenzae, Moraxella catarrhalis* (Chapter 308), and *Legionella* species. Alcoholism is associated with increased risk for drug-resistant *S. pneumoniae,* anaerobic lung infection, and tuberculosis.

The clinician also should solicit information about household and workplace exposure, such as to other ill persons. The clinician should ask about recent travel to specific geographic regions, such as the central United States, where histoplasmosis is endemic (Chapter 340), the Southwest, where coccidioidomycosis is found (Chapter 341), and selected northern and central regions of the United States, where blastomycosis is found (Chapter 342). Recent travel to regions with epidemic viral respiratory infections, including seasonal influenza, avian influenza, H1N1 (swine) influenza, and severe acute respiratory syndrome (SARS), or travel to Asia, Africa, and central and eastern Europe, which are highly endemic for tuberculosis, should be

considered (Chapter 332). In addition, environmental exposure, such as to birds (psittacosis), bird droppings (histoplasmosis), bats (histoplasmosis), rabbits (tularemia, Chapter 319), and farm animals (Q fever, Chapter 335), is additional data that should be obtained during the history.

Viral Pneumonia

Although most attention traditionally focuses on bacterial causes of severe community-acquired pneumonia, viruses can also cause serious lower respiratory tract infections. The predominant respiratory viruses that can cause severe pneumonia include various influenza viruses and respiratory syncytial virus (RSV) (Chapter 370). Both influenza virus and RSV can be detected in respiratory secretions, which should be obtained in suspected cases. It is estimated that influenza infections are responsible for in excess of 36,000 respiratory- and circulatory-related deaths annually in the United States, predominantly in elderly patients and those with underlying cardiopulmonary or metabolic disease. Influenza-associated pneumonia should be considered in the differential diagnosis of respiratory infections in high-risk patients with underlying disease and in residents of nursing homes or other chronic care facilities during the season of October through May, especially in patients who have not received appropriate vaccination.

It is also increasingly being appreciated that RSV and parainfluenza (Chapter 371) viruses, although formerly considered mainly infections of pediatric populations, can lead to serious lower respiratory tract infections in adults during the winter season. Host immunity to RSV infection in childhood is incomplete, and recurrent infections can occur in both immune-competent and immune-impaired adults, particularly in elderly patients. It is estimated that RSV is associated with more than 11,000 deaths each year in the United States, with most deaths occurring in elderly people and in patients with chronic cardiopulmonary disease.

Emerging influenza infections must also be considered. Although typical seasonal influenza tends to occur in North America during the months of October to May, novel influenza viruses do not always follow that epidemiology. In particular in the spring and summer of 2009, a novel H1N1 (swine) influenza virus occurred in epidemic proportions in Mexico and rapidly spread over the world. In contrast to many other influenza outbreaks, the virus continued to circulate over the summer months in both the northern and southern hemispheres. H1N1 generally produced a typical syndrome with fever, headaches, cough, malaise, and myalgias. Most cases were mild or self-limited. However, excess hospitalization and mortality from H1N1 infection has been observed in infants, children, and adults younger than 24 years. Pregnant women and children, in particular those who are immunosuppressed, are at particular risk.

Avian influenza A (H5N1; Chapter 372) generally infects wild birds, which carry the H5N1 virus in their intestines, but usually are not made very sick by the virus. However, avian influenza can be highly contagious and fatal among domesticated birds, including chickens, turkeys, and ducks. Transmission to humans has been relatively uncommon, despite the lack of immunity against the virus, but human outbreaks have occurred from contact with infected birds (e.g., domesticated chicken and turkeys) or with secretions or excretions from infected birds.

SARS emerged as an additional form of life-threatening atypical pneumonia that was first detected in the Guangdong Province of China in late 2002, with major outbreaks in Hong Kong, Guangdong, Singapore, and Toronto and Vancouver, Canada. The disease is caused by a novel coronavirus (Chapter 374) with an incubation period of 2 to 10 days. The initial source of the infection remains uncertain, although palm civet cats and Chinese ferret badgers harbor a coronavirus with greater than 99% similarity to human SARS isolates. Worldwide, however, the illness is largely a nosocomial disease, with health care workers representing a significant fraction of the infected individuals. SARS is characterized by an insidious onset of fever, chills, headache, cough, malaise, and dyspnea, with radiologic evidence of pneumonia. Although upper respiratory symptoms are uncommon, voluminous watery diarrhea without mucus or blood develops in up to 70% of patients. SARS is believed to be principally transmitted by respiratory droplets. Current treatment is supportive, with no antiviral agent yet having been proved to be efficacious. SARS pneumonia tends to resolve slowly and spontaneously, usually by the third week of illness. However, the estimated case-fatality rate remains approximately 10%. SARS is highly contagious, and lethal transmission to health care workers has been documented. Isolation procedures and equipment appropriate for SARS include standard, contact, and airborne isolation precautions such as scrupulous hand hygiene, gowning, disposable gloves, the use of N95 respirators, and eye protection. Suspected cases of SARS require notification of local public health departments and the Centers for Disease Control and Prevention.

Agents of Bioterrorism

Physicians should also be vigilant for clues of pneumonia related to agents of bioterrorism (Chapter 20). These clues can include outbreaks of severe illness and pneumonia in multiple, otherwise healthy individuals or the isolation of unusual organisms in patients with pneumonic illness. The microorganisms most likely to be associated with severe pneumonia during bioterrorism-related inhalation exposure include *B. anthracis* (Chapter 302), *Francisella tularensis* (Chapter 319), and *Y. pestis* (Chapter 320). Inhalational anthrax always indicates a bioterrorism threat, whereas pneumonic plague or tularemia may or may not be associated with bioterrorism.

Radiography

Clinical suspicion of pneumonia should prompt standard posteroanterior and lateral chest radiography. Although the pattern of infiltration can rarely establish a specific microbiologic etiology, chest films are most useful for providing essential information on the distribution and extent of involvement, as well as potential pneumonic complications. Many bacterial pneumonias result in localized alveolar infiltrates and consolidation. Even though pneumococcal pneumonia is classically described as having a lobar distribution, the pattern can be multilobar (Fig. 97-1) or bilateral. The "bulging" fissure sign, which represents lobar filling and consolidation, has traditionally been attributed to *Klebsiella pneumoniae*, but this finding is not specific and can be observed with *S. pneumoniae* and other bacteria and even with bronchoalveolar carcinoma. Diffuse interstitial and alveolar infiltrates should suggest viral infections (cytomegalovirus, influenza virus, or RSV), *L. pneumophila*, or enteric gram-negative pneumonia, particularly in neutropenic patients. These diffuse pulmonary infiltrations can be indistinguishable from other causes of acute respiratory distress syndrome. Diffuse alveolar and interstitial infiltration can also be observed in patients with *Pneumocystis jirovecii* pneumonia (Chapter 349) related to immune suppression, such as in those with acquired immunodeficiency syndrome. Cavitary lesions often indicate a necrotizing infection related to *S. aureus*, *M. tuberculosis* (Fig. 97-2), and certain endemic fungi such as *Coccidioides immitis*, *Aspergillus* species infection in an immunocompromised patient (Chapter 347), or anaerobic lung infection with abscess formation. Mediastinal adenopathy and widening have been observed in inhalational anthrax infections.

The chest radiograph provides further important information about potential infectious complications of pneumonia. Pleural effusions (Chapter 99), which occur in a variety of respiratory infections, are best documented with lateral decubitus views or with computed tomography (CT) imaging of the thorax. The discovery of any pleural effusion greater than 10 mm in thickness on a lateral decubitus film or any loculated effusion should prompt thoracentesis to aid in the identification of a complicated parapneumonic effusion or empyema, which may require definitive drainage (Chapter 99). Enlargement of mediastinal and hilar lymph nodes, which is rare in acute bacterial infection, suggests fungal or mycobacterial infection or an underlying lung cancer. Loss of volume of a lung segment or lobe should raise suspicion of

postobstructive pneumonia distal to an endobronchial lesion caused by a neoplasm, occult foreign body, or broncholithiasis.

Laboratory Findings

Sputum Gram Stain and Culture

Considerable controversy exists over the appropriate microbiologic evaluation of patients with suspected pneumonia. Despite intensive microbiologic evaluation, a specific organism may not be discovered in half the patients with pneumonia. Furthermore, most patients with pneumonia satisfactorily respond to simple, relatively nontoxic antibiotic regimens based on the most likely organisms causing infection. Thus, the necessity to document the precise cause of the process remains uncertain.

Debate continues over the need to perform a sputum examination with Gram staining in every patient with community-acquired pneumonia. An American Thoracic Society consensus panel has recommended that a sputum Gram stain and culture be obtained primarily if an organism that is resistant to the usual empirical treatment regimens is suspected. To be useful, sputum should contain fewer than 10 squamous cells and more than 25 leukocytes per low-power field; a well-performed Gram stain may reveal a single, predominant organism such as encapsulated gram-positive cocci (pneumococci) or small pleomorphic gram-negative coccobacilli (*Haemophilus*). However, current data have not clearly correlated Gram stain findings with the results of culture of alveolar materials in large numbers of patients with community-acquired pneumonia. Nevertheless, sputum examination can strongly support the diagnosis of certain specific infections, including *M. tuberculosis* (acid-fast stain), endemic fungi (KOH preparations), *P. jirovecii* (methenamine silver or fluorescent antibody stain), or *Legionella* species (direct fluorescent antibody staining). In most cases of community-acquired pneumonia, the general intent of sputum Gram stain examination, if it is performed, should be to detect additional or unusual pathogens and hence to expand rather than narrow the initial antibiotic therapy. All too often, an adequate sputum specimen cannot be obtained, and the Gram stain interpretation may be equivocal. Therefore, the initial therapeutic plan must be based on the most likely pathogens responsible for the pneumonia.

If unusual or drug-resistant pathogens are suspected, sputum specimens should be sent for culture before antibiotic therapy is initiated. When the culture results are available, they should be compared with the predominant organisms observed on Gram stain. Unfortunately, the sensitivity and specificity of sputum culture are not optimal, each being roughly 50%. Antibiotic susceptibility information on an isolated pathogenic organism can, however, be useful both for epidemiologic surveillance and for management of patients who do not respond to initial empirical therapy.

Other Bacterial Cultures

Cultures of normally sterile body fluids such as blood, pleural fluid, or occasionally cerebrospinal fluid (CSF) are highly specific when positive.

FIGURE 97-1. Radiologic diagnosis of pneumonia. A standard posteroanterior radiograph in a 70-year-old woman demonstrates chronic obstructive pulmonary disease complicated by right multilobar *Streptococcus pneumoniae* pneumonia and empyema.

FIGURE 97-2. Cavitary lesions. A posteroanterior radiograph in a 54-year-old man with cough and fever shows a right upper lobe cavitary process caused by *Mycobacterium tuberculosis* infection.

Approximately one fourth of patients with bacterial pneumonia have demonstrable bacteremia. Blood should be drawn for culture before administration of antibiotics in patients with serious illness attributable to pneumonia, and diagnostic thoracentesis should be performed if an effusion is large enough to be aspirated safely. CSF examination is generally reserved for patients with additional signs and symptoms of meningeal irritation (Chapter 420) or abnormalities on neurologic examination.

Testing for Suspected Bioterrorism
Recommended testing for suspected anthrax includes blood culture and chest CT scanning. For the diagnosis of pneumonic plague, blood culture as well as sputum Gram stain and culture are advised. For tularemic pneumonia, cultures should be obtained from blood, sputum, and the pharynx. Culture of these extremely virulent organisms should be undertaken in a level 3 (BL3) biocontainment laboratory.

Immunologic Studies
Immunologic techniques such as immunofluorescence, enzyme-linked immunosorbent assay, antigen detection, polymerase chain reaction, and DNA hybridization may be considered when specific organisms are strongly suspected on clinical grounds, but these tests are not routinely indicated in most cases of community-acquired pneumonia. For example, *Legionella* urinary antigen screening and acute and convalescent serologic evaluation may be helpful when *L. pneumophila* pneumonia is suspected (Chapter 322). *Legionella* urinary antigen testing may underdiagnose infections caused by organisms other than *Legionella* serogroup 1. Furthermore, the judicious use of fungal serology can detect endemic mycoses, particularly histoplasmosis and coccidioidomycosis (Chapters 340, 341, and 342). Histoplasmosis can also be confirmed by urinary antigen testing with high sensitivity. The measurement of *Aspergillus galactomannan* antigen in serum can be a useful adjunct in the diagnosis of invasive *Aspergillus* pneumonia in various immunocompromised patients. Bronchoscopy with lavage for immunostaining may, in selected circumstances, provide enhanced sensitivity, such as in the diagnosis of *P. jirovecii* pneumonia (Chapter 349).

Viral Studies
Rapid antigen detection tests are now available, with tests that distinguish between influenza A and B being preferred. These tests are currently recommended for epidemiologic purposes in the community and also help direct individual therapy. RSV antigen detection tests are likewise available, but they are relatively less sensitive when applied to sputum in adult patients. A variety of other assays, including polymerase chain reaction (PCR) and specialized antigen testing, are available in reference laboratories for detection of diagnosis of novel H1N1 (swine) influenza, H5N1 (avian) influenza, and the SARS coronavirus.

Bronchoscopy
Invasive sampling of respiratory secretions is not usually necessary in patients with community-acquired pneumonia. Flexible fiberoptic bronchoscopy with a protected catheter brush and bronchoalveolar lavage (BAL) sampling has largely supplanted transtracheal and transthoracic needle aspiration. Bronchoscopy is indicated in selected clinical situations in which a delay in accurate diagnosis may have serious consequences, such as in immunocompromised hosts or patients whose condition has worsened despite initial antimicrobial therapy. Other indications for bronchoscopy in the setting of apparent community-acquired pneumonia include either lung abscess detected on a chest radiograph (Chapter 84) or evidence of volume loss and distal consolidation suggesting endobronchial obstruction.

PREVENTION
In light of the significant morbidity and potential mortality of pneumonia, appropriate measures should be instituted to reduce the possibility of lung infection. Important but often neglected interventions include smoking cessation (Chapter 31) and avoidance of illicit drugs (Chapter 33) or excess alcohol (Chapter 32), which may impair consciousness. Optimizing the patient's nutritional status is also important in that markedly underweight or obese patients are at increased risk. Finally, the appropriate and consistent use of vaccines can strongly reduce the risk for pneumonia in appropriate patient populations (Chapter 17). The current pneumococcal vaccine contains 23 purified capsular polysaccharides from the serotypes of *S. pneumoniae* that are responsible for more than 85% of invasive pneumococcal infections. Overall, this vaccine is approximately 50 to 80% effective in

preventing death from invasive infection. Accordingly, current recommendations are that it should be administered to all patients older than 65 years and to patients younger than 65 years who have chronic pulmonary disease, heart disease, diabetes mellitus, alcoholism, chronic liver disease, CSF leaks, or asplenia and to patients who live in certain settings, including Alaskan natives, high-risk Native American populations, and patients in long-term care facilities. Current pneumococcal vaccines have little toxicity, limited mainly to local site irritation. Individuals generally receive one dose of vaccine, but a single revaccination 5 years later should be considered in those who received their vaccination before 65 years of age or who are at increased risk for severe pneumonia. Pneumococcal vaccine can safely be administered at the time of hospitalization for community-acquired pneumonia.

Vaccination (Chapter 17) should also be considered for viral influenza (Chapter 372). Although usually manifested as an upper respiratory tract infection, influenza can itself cause pneumonia in both immunocompetent and immunosuppressed individuals. More commonly, influenza may precipitate a subsequent bacterial infection, often with *S. aureus*, *H. influenzae*, and *S. pneumoniae*. Influenza vaccines are developed annually against the current influenza strains, so annual revaccination is necessary (Chapter 17). Influenza vaccines are estimated to be roughly 80% effective in preventing mortality related to influenza. The vaccine should be considered in all patients older than 50 years; residents of nursing homes and chronic care facilities; persons with chronic pulmonary, cardiac, or other diseases requiring ongoing medical care; pregnant women in the second or third trimester during influenza season; and all health care workers with direct patient contact. A weakened virus vaccine, which is administered through a nasal application, does not cause influenza and is approved for healthy people 2 years to 49 years of age who are not pregnant. An inactivated vaccine containing killed virus, administered by injection, is approved for people 6 months of age and older, including healthy people, people with chronic medical conditions, and pregnant women. Both have demonstrated efficacy in preventing influenza and its related complications, including pneumonia.

Contraindications to influenza vaccine include allergy to raw eggs or thimerosal. Side effects are generally self-limited and include injection site soreness, myalgias, mild fever, and malaise. Seasonal influenza vaccination does not lead to exacerbations of asthma. The vaccine should be administered in the fall of the year, but it can also be administered during local epidemics.

TREATMENT
Oversight agencies are increasingly focused on objective measures of optimal care for community-acquired pneumonia, particularly in the hospital setting. Although recommendations are evolving and sometimes vary, current recommendations are that hospitalized patients with community-acquired pneumonia should undergo assessment of oxygenation, initiation of antibiotic therapy in the emergency department, drawing of blood for culture before antimicrobial initiation, smoking cessation intervention, and review and update of immunization status. Most experts also advise chest radiography at the time of admission. The use of biomarkers for bacterial infection, such as levels of procalcitonin, may prove to be helpful when determining which patients can avoid immediate antibiotics or discontinue initial empirical antibiotics because of a low likelihood of bacterial infection.**1**

Initial Empirical Therapy
Because the microbiologic etiology of community-acquired pneumonia is determined in only approximately 50% of cases and the diagnosis may take a day or two, the clinician must institute appropriate empirical therapy based on the most likely agents contributing to the lung infection (Table 97-2). When possible, empirical therapy should be initiated as soon as possible after the diagnosis is established—immediately in the outpatient setting and in the emergency department if the patient is hospitalized. Empirical antimicrobial therapy is based on the severity of illness (inpatient or outpatient setting) and should broadly cover the most likely organisms. The most common bacterial pathogens are *S. pneumoniae* (Chapter 297) and *H. influenzae* (Chapter 308); however, the so-called atypical pathogens, including *M. pneumoniae*, *C. pneumoniae*, and *Legionella* species (Chapters 325, 326, and 322, respectively), can be the primary or coinfecting agents in up to 40% of community-acquired pneumonia and must be covered in empirical antibiotic regimens. Therapy can be narrowed later after any relevant culture information is obtained.

Guidelines for Hospital and Intensive Care Unit Admission and Treatment
Under current guidelines, patients are stratified with respect to where treatment is initiated (outpatient, inpatient, or ICU setting), the presence of underlying cardiopulmonary disease, and other modifying factors, such as whether

TABLE 97-2   MOST COMMON MICROBIOLOGIC CAUSES OF COMMUNITY-ACQUIRED PNEUMONIA IN APPROXIMATE ORDER OF FREQUENCY

OUTPATIENTS	HOSPITALIZED PATIENTS	SEVERE PNEUMONIA/ICU
Streptococcus pneumoniae	S. pneumoniae	S. pneumoniae
Mycoplasma pneumoniae	M. pneumoniae	Staphylococcus aureus
Haemophilus influenzae	C. pneumoniae	Legionella species
Chlamydophila pneumoniae	H. influenzae	Gram-negative bacilli
Respiratory viruses	Legionella species Aspiration Respiratory viruses	H. influenzae

Adapted from Infectious Diseases Society of America/American Thoracic Society. Consensus guidelines on the management of community acquired pneumonia in adults. *Clin Infect Dis.* 2007;44:S27-S72.

TABLE 97-3   TRIAGE GUIDELINES FOR COMMUNITY-ACQUIRED PNEUMONIA

DECISION TO ADMIT TO THE HOSPITAL

Follow CURB-65 Guidelines and admit patients who have two or more of the following:
Confusion
Uremia (with blood urea nitrogen ≥20 mg/dL)
Respiratory rate >30 breaths/min
Blood pressure ≤90 mm Hg systolic or <60 mm Hg diastolic
Age ≥65 yr

INDICATIONS FOR ICU ADMISSION (1 MAJOR AND ≥3 MINOR)

Major Criteria

Hypotension requiring vasopressors
Respiratory compromise requiring mechanical ventilation

Minor Criteria

Respiratory rate >30 breaths/min
PaO_2/FIO_2 ratio ≤250
Multilobar infiltrate
Confusion/disorientation
Uremia (blood urea nitrogen ≥20 mg/dL)
Leukopenia (white blood cell count ≤4000 cells/mm^3)
Thrombocytopenia (platelets ≤100,000 cells/mm^3)
Hypothermia (≤36° C)
Hypotension requiring aggressive fluid resuscitation

the patient is likely to be infected with drug-resistant *S. pneumoniae,* gram-negative enteric bacilli, or *Pseudomonas aeruginosa.* Following these guidelines reduces the number of hospital admissions without adversely affecting outcomes.

The decision to admit a patient to the hospital must be made on clinical grounds. Patients can be effectively and safely managed as outpatients if they are mildly ill, are younger than 65 years, and do not have coexisting cardiopulmonary disease, malignancy, immune compromise, or renal, liver, or other significant systemic diseases (Table 97-3).

In general, outpatients who are mildly ill and do not have any underlying cardiopulmonary disease or other modifying factors are usually infected with *S. pneumoniae, M. pneumoniae, C. pneumoniae, H. influenzae,* respiratory viruses, or *Legionella* species. These uncomplicated outpatient cases can be managed with an oral advanced-generation macrolide, such as azithromycin or clarithromycin, both of which are better tolerated and provide better coverage of *Haemophilus* species than erythromycin.[2] Alternatively, doxycycline may be used in patients who are intolerant of macrolides, although this option is less optimal because of increasing levels of tetracycline resistance in *S. pneumoniae* isolates. Outpatients who have underlying comorbidities (e.g., chronic heart, lung, liver, or renal disease, diabetes mellitus, alcoholism, asplenia, immunosuppressive conditions or drugs, use of antibiotics within the past 3 months, or exposure to a child in a daycare center) are at higher risk of having drug-resistant *S. pneumoniae.* If their pneumonia is not sufficiently severe to warrant admission, and any comorbid illnesses are stable and compensated, patients can be treated either with respiratory fluoroquinolones (e.g., moxifloxacin, gemifloxacin, or levofloxacin) or with a β-lactam plus a macrolide (e.g., high-dose amoxicillin or amoxicillin-clavulanate is preferred; alternatives

TABLE 97-4   EMPIRICAL TREATMENT GUIDELINES FOR COMMUNITY-ACQUIRED PNEUMONIA

OUTPATIENT MANAGEMENT

1. Previously healthy patients without comorbidities and no use of antimicrobials within the prior 3 months
   A macrolide (preferred) (e.g., clarithromycin, extended release, 1000 mg orally each day for at least 5 days, or azithromycin, 500 mg orally on day 1, followed by 250 mg orally each day on days 2-5)
   Doxycycline, 100 mg orally twice daily for at least 5 days
2. Presence of comorbidities such as chronic cardiopulmonary, liver, or renal disease; diabetes mellitus; alcoholism; malignancies; asplenia; immunosuppressive conditions or drugs; or use of antimicrobials in the prior 3 months (if so, select an alternative agent from a different class)
   A respiratory fluoroquinolone (oral moxifloxacin, 400 mg/day, or gemifloxacin, 320 mg/day, or levofloxacin, 750 mg daily for at least 5 days), *or*
   A β-lactam (e.g., ceftriaxone, 1-2 g IM each day for at least 5 days) *plus* a macrolide (e.g., azithromycin, 500 mg orally on day 1, followed by 250 mg orally each day on days 2-5)
3. In regions with a high rate (>25%) of infection with high-level (MIC ≥16 mg/mL) macrolide-resistant *Streptococcus pneumoniae,* consider an alternative agent as noted under (2) for patients without comorbidities.

INPATIENTS, NON-ICU MANAGEMENT

1. A respiratory fluoroquinolone (moxifloxacin, 400 mg/day, or gemifloxacin, 320 mg/day, or levofloxacin, 750 mg IV for 2 days followed by oral for at least 5 days total), *or*
2. A β-lactam (e.g., ceftriaxone 1-2 g IV daily for at least 1-2 days, followed by 1-2 g IM daily for at least 5 days total), *plus*
   A macrolide (azithromycin, 500 mg IV each day for at least 2 days, followed by 500 mg orally each day for a total of at least 5 days)

INPATIENTS—ICU MANAGEMENT

1. A β-lactam (cefotaxime, 1-2 g IV every 6-8 hr, or ceftriaxone, 1-2 g IV each day, or ampicillin-sulbactam, 1.5-3 g IV every 6 hours, up to maximum of 4 g of sulbactam/day, for 7-14 days, *plus*
   Either azithromycin, 500 mg IV each day for at least 2 days, followed by 500 mg orally each day for a total of at least 5 days, or a respiratory fluoroquinolone (e.g., moxifloxacin, 400 mg/day, or gemifloxacin, 320 mg/day, or levofloxacin, 750 mg IV daily for 7-14 days)
2. For penicillin-allergic individuals, a respiratory fluoroquinolone (e.g., moxifloxacin, 400 mg/day, or gemifloxacin, 320 mg/day, or levofloxacin, 750 mg IV daily for 7-14 days) and aztreonam, 2 g IV every 6-8 hr for 7-14 days, are recommended.

SPECIAL CONCERNS

If *Pseudomonas* species infection is a concern:
1. An antipneumococcal, antipseudomonal β-lactam (piperacillin-tazobactam, 3.375 g IV every 6 hr, or cefepime, 1-2 g every 12 hr, or imipenem, 500 mg every 6 hr or 1 g every 8 hr, or meropenem, 1 g IV every 8 hr), *plus* either ciprofloxacin, 400 mg IV every 8 hr, or levofloxacin, 500-750 mg IV every day, for 7-14 days, *or*
2. The above β-lactam plus an aminoglycoside (e.g., gentamicin, 7 mg/kg/day in three divided doses, with monitoring to maintain trough levels lower than 1 µg/mL, or tobramycin, 7 mg/kg/day in three divided doses, with monitoring to maintain trough levels lower than 1 µg/mL) and azithromycin (500 mg IV each day for at least 2 days, followed by 500 mg orally each day) for 7-14 days, *or*
3. The above β-lactam plus an aminoglycoside (as described above) and an antipneumococcal fluoroquinolone (ciprofloxacin, 400 mg IV every 8 hr, or levofloxacin, 500-750 mg IV every day) for 7-14 days
   For penicillin-allergic patients, use aztreonam, 2 g IV every 6-8 hr for 7-14 days, instead of the β-lactam.
If community-acquired methicillin-resistant *Staphylococcus aureus* is a consideration, add vancomycin, 15 mg/kg every 12 hr with monitoring to maintain trough at 15-20 µg/mL, or linezolid, 600 mg every 12 hr, for 7-14 days.

Adapted from Infectious Diseases Society of America/American Thoracic Society. Consensus guidelines on the management of community acquired pneumonia in adults. *Clin Infect Dis.* 2007;44:S27-S72.

include ceftriaxone, cefpodoxime, and cefuroxime; doxycycline is an alternative to the macrolide) (Table 97-4). In regions that have a high incidence of macrolide-resistant (>25%) *S. pneumoniae,* the alternative agents should be used. When pneumonia is treated on an outpatient basis, patients require careful monitoring to be certain that they respond over the first 72 hours of therapy. The clinician must maintain vigilance about the need to hospitalize patients who deteriorate or fail to respond to the initial empirical therapy.

Patients who have more severe respiratory illnesses, significant unstable or uncompensated comorbid illnesses, or a poor initial response to otherwise appropriate outpatient therapy generally should be admitted to the hospital promptly. Patients who require hospitalization but not intensive care should be treated initially with either an intravenous respiratory fluoroquinolone, such as levofloxacin or moxifloxacin,**3** or with the combination of an intravenous β-lactam plus a macrolide.

Patients who have respiratory insufficiency, septicemia, shock, or significant multiorgan dysfunction, with or without the need for mechanical ventilatory support, require management in an ICU and evaluation to exclude infection with *P. aeruginosa* (Chapter 314). ICU admission should also be considered for patients who exhibit three or more of the minor criteria for severe community-acquired pneumonia (see Table 97-3).

Among patients with severe community-acquired pneumonia, those at increased risk for *P. aeruginosa* infection include patients with structural lung disease (particularly bronchiectasis), greater than 10 mg/day of previous corticosteroid therapy, neutropenia, malnutrition, or previous broad-spectrum antibiotics for more than 7 days in the past month. ICU patients who are *not* considered at risk for *P. aeruginosa* infection can be treated initially with a β-lactam (cefotaxime, ceftriaxone, or ampicillin-sulbactam) plus either azithromycin or a respiratory fluoroquinolone (moxifloxacin or levofloxacin) (see Table 97-4). In penicillin-allergic patients, a respiratory fluoroquinolone and aztreonam is a reasonable regimen. Fluoroquinolone monotherapy is not considered appropriate in the setting of severe community-acquired pneumonia. In the ICU population considered to be at risk for *P. aeruginosa* infection, combination antipseudomonal therapy should be used, including an antipneumococcal, antipseudomonal β-lactam (piperacillin-tazobactam, cefepime, imipenem, or meropenem) plus either ciprofloxacin or levofloxacin or a β-lactam plus an aminoglycoside and azithromycin. If community-acquired methicillin-resistant *S. aureus* (MRSA) infection is a consideration, vancomycin or linezolid should be added to the regimen.

Suspected or Proven Viral Infection

Therapies for suspected and proven viral infection are relatively limited when compared with those for bacterial infections. Early treatment of influenza A or B within the first 48 hours of symptoms with oseltamivir (75 mg orally taken twice daily for 5 days), or zanamivir (two inhalations of 5 mg per inhalation every 12 hours for 5 days) is effective in reducing symptoms and the duration of illness (Chapter 368). Both agents have been used for novel H1N1 swine influenza, and oseltamivir may also have activity against H5N1 bird flu. Empirical antibiotic treatment of possible bacterial superinfection in addition to influenza should include agents effective against *S. pneumoniae* (Chapter 297), *S. aureus* (Chapter 296), and *H. influenzae* (Chapter 308). In these considerations, amoxicillin-clavulanate, cefpodoxime, cefprozil, cefuroxime, or a respiratory fluoroquinolone would be appropriate. Pneumonias caused by varicella-zoster and herpes simplex virus should be treated with parenteral acyclovir (10 mg/kg intravenously every 8 hours for 7 days) (Chapters 382 and 383). No antiviral agents have established efficacy against RSV in adults, parainfluenza virus, adenovirus, metapneumovirus, the SARS coronavirus, or hantavirus. Treatment is largely supportive, with oxygen and ventilator therapy as necessary.

Duration of Therapy

Most patients respond to empirical antibiotic regimens over the first 3 days of therapy. In general, it is not advisable to alter the antibiotic program in the first 72 hours unless the patient is deteriorating or culture results indicate alternative therapy. Patients initially begun on parenteral therapy may be switched to an oral regimen when they are afebrile (temperature less than 38° C [100° F] on two occasions 8 hours apart) and demonstrate improvement in cough, dyspnea, and leukocytosis.

Patients with community-acquired pneumonia should be treated for at least 5 days,**4** should be afebrile for at least 48 to 72 hours, and should not show signs of clinical instability before discontinuation of antibiotic therapy. Accordingly, the total duration of antimicrobials should be individualized to the patient's clinical response. Initial multiagent regimens of a β-lactam with the addition of macrolides for the coverage of *Legionella* and *Mycoplasma* can frequently be de-escalated after several days to the β-lactams alone if *Legionella* urinary antigen and *Mycoplasma* serology prove negative. The clinical caveat remains, however, that macrolides may still be required in clinical situations in which a strong clinical suspicion for *Legionella* persists because urinary antigen testing does not detect organisms other than *Legionella* serogroup 1. Furthermore, in situations in which a causative organism is isolated from a normally sterile site, such as blood or pleural fluid, antibiotic therapy should be simplified and directed by susceptibility testing. Finally, when alternative clinical diagnoses other than pneumonia are proved to be the cause of the respiratory symptoms and all cultures remain negative over the first 72 hours, antibiotic therapy may be safely discontinued.

Treatment Failure

Treatment failures occur in approximately 10% of patients with community-acquired pneumonia, and complications occur in roughly 25% of patients. Adherence to treatment guidelines, such as those described earlier, increases the likelihood of a good outcome.

For patients who do not respond to initial empirical coverage, an aggressive search should be undertaken to detect unusual pathogens, alternative diagnoses such as pulmonary embolism (Chapter 98), or complications of pneumonia such as a complicated pleural effusion (Chapter 99), empyema, or lung abscess (Chapter 90). Additional diagnostic testing may include a chest CT scan, sampling of pleural fluid, and bronchoscopy with collection of respiratory secretions, brushings, and BAL fluid for microbiologic analysis.

Follow-Up after Treatment

Even when the patient appears to respond to the initial antibiotic regimen, the chest radiograph signs resolve more slowly (over a period of 6 to 8 weeks) than other clinical signs and symptoms. The physician must document that abnormalities on the chest radiograph have resolved completely or, in some cases, have led to the formation of a fibrotic scar. Usual practice includes performing repeat radiography 6 to 8 weeks after completion of the antibiotic regimen. Persistence of abnormalities on the chest radiograph or the development of recurrent pneumonia in a similar distribution should prompt a careful search for an underlying endobronchial obstruction such as an occult neoplasm (Chapter 197), foreign body, bronchostenosis, or broncholithiasis. Follow-up CT scanning is usually the prelude to formal pulmonary consultation for consideration of bronchoscopy and other further diagnostic tests.

ASPIRATION PNEUMONIA

EPIDEMIOLOGY AND PATHOBIOLOGY

Although microaspiration is the mechanism underlying most cases of pneumonia, the clinician is occasionally confronted with recurrent bacterial pneumonia in a patient experiencing repeated gross aspiration of oropharyngeal contents. Most of these patients have difficulty swallowing related to either underlying neuromuscular disorders or altered sensorium as a result of medications, drugs or alcohol, or underlying neurologic diseases. Common clinical scenarios associated with recurrent aspiration pneumonia include tracheobronchial fistulas secondary to esophageal or tracheal malignancies, esophageal obstruction related to esophageal cancer and its treatment (Chapter 198), and a wide variety of neurologic disorders, including amyotrophic lateral sclerosis (Chapter 418), multiple sclerosis (Chapter 419), stroke (Chapter 414), and other myopathic processes. Other patients with severe esophageal reflux (Chapter 140) may also experience significant aspiration during sleep despite apparently normal deglutition mechanisms and protective reflexes during wakefulness. Patients with neuromuscular disorders tend to have greater difficulty swallowing thin or liquid materials, whereas patients with obstruction from either malignancy or benign strictures tend to have the greatest difficulty swallowing solid food.

CLINICAL MANIFESTATIONS

Aspiration pneumonias tend to have a less acute manifestation than the usual bacterial pneumonias, with the onset of fever, dyspnea, purulent sputum, malaise, and other systemic symptoms, including loss of appetite, evolving over a number of days. Physical examination of the chest generally reveals only coarse rhonchi in the lower lobes or dependent lung regions.

DIAGNOSIS

The diagnosis of aspiration pneumonia relies foremost on maintaining a high clinical index of suspicion. Recovery of tracheal secretions containing food particles or lipid-laden macrophages strongly supports the diagnosis. In patients receiving tube feedings, the respiratory secretions should be tested for glucose because these secretions normally contain low levels of glucose. Alternatively, methylene blue or similar tracer dyes can be added to tube feeding materials to confirm the presence of aspiration. Additional diagnostic modalities include the use of cineradiographic swallowing studies with thin liquid water-soluble contrast agents to confirm the aspiration event. Radionuclide imaging studies may also document aspiration in adults whose neurologic status precludes them from cooperating fully with the cineradiographic studies. Overnight esophageal pH monitoring may be undertaken in individuals who are suspected of having recurrent esophageal reflux and aspiration events at night. However, except in the most severe cases, it remains difficult to predict which patients with gastroesophageal reflux will actually experience aspiration pneumonia.

Chest radiographs should be reviewed in light of the patient's probable position during aspiration. The lower lobes, particularly the superior segments of the right lower lobe, and the posterior segments of the upper lobes are frequently involved. However, unilateral aspiration or aspiration into virtually any pulmonary segment has been reported, depending on the patient's position during the aspiration event. The radiographic appearance usually reflects a parenchymal bronchopneumonia process. Pleural involvement is uncommon initially, unless aggressive anaerobic infection is present. Nonresolving or inadequately treated aspiration pneumonia can result in lung abscess and empyema formation.

Bronchoscopy, although not routinely necessary, can confirm the presence of aspiration by recovering food particles or lipid-laden macrophages derived from fats present in the aspirated food. Bronchoscopy with BAL can be useful in providing quantitative counts of aerobic bacteria, and protected specimen brush sampling can document anaerobic organisms, although negative cultures do not exclude the presence of anaerobes.

Microbiology

Oropharyngeal secretions contain massive numbers of microorganisms, with counts of aerobic bacteria ranging between 10^6 and 10^8 and anaerobic organisms being as high as 10^9 per milliliter of saliva. Accordingly, aspiration pneumonia should be viewed as a polymicrobial infection, with the clinical manifestations being driven by the predominant and most aggressive organisms in the mixture. Oropharyngeal colonization is strongly influenced by the clinical setting in which the patient was dwelling at the time of aspiration (outpatient versus hospital or institutional). In otherwise healthy outpatients, aggressive organisms such as *S. pneumoniae*, *S. aureus*, and *H. influenzae* may also be present. In contrast, the oropharyngeal secretions of hospitalized patients and residents of long-term care facilities include aerobic gram-negative bacteria and *P. aeruginosa*. Anaerobic organisms, which are a major consideration in both settings, include anaerobic and microaerophilic streptococci, *Bacteroides* species, *Fusobacterium nucleatum*, and *Prevotella* species. Cultures of sputum and tracheal secretions probably document such mixed flora.

TREATMENT   Rx

Empirical antibiotic therapy should be initiated rapidly once the diagnosis of aspiration pneumonia is made; the regimen can be modified later after culture information from sputum, tracheal secretions, or bronchoscopic sampling is available. Otherwise healthy individuals with isolated aspiration pneumonia related to trauma, seizures, or oversedation may be treated initially with either oral amoxicillin-clavulanate (amoxicillin, 875 mg, and clavulanate acid, 125 mg, orally every 12 hours for at least 5 days), intravenous clindamycin (600 mg intravenously [IV] every 8 hours for at least 5 days), or intravenous piperacillin-tazobactam (3.375 g IV every 6 hours for at least 5 days), depending on the severity of illness. In uncomplicated mild to moderate aspiration pneumonia in elderly patients, intravenous clindamycin is as effective, less expensive, and associated with a lower rate of post-treatment occurrence of MRSA. For patients with underlying chronic diseases, intravenous piperacillin-tazobactam (3.375 g IV every 6 hours for 7 to 14 days) or intravenous fluoroquinolones that cover anaerobes, such as moxifloxacin (400 mg IV each day for 7 to 14 days), can be considered. In seriously ill individuals, particularly patients requiring intubation and mechanical ventilation, as well as patients experiencing aspiration in the hospital or long-term care setting, coverage must be extended to aerobic gram-negative bacteria and *Pseudomonas* species; treatment considerations would include extended-spectrum β-lactam/β-lactamase inhibitor combinations such as piperacillin-tazobactam (3.375 g IV every 6 hours for 7 to 14 days) or ticarcillin-clavulanate (3 g of ticarcillin, and 0.1 g of clavulanic acid IV every 4 to 6 hours for 7 to 14 days), or carbapenems such as imipenem (500 mg IV every 6 to 8 hours for 7 to 14 days). Intravenous clindamycin (600 mg IV every 8 hours) can also be added in these settings, or alternatively, intravenous clindamycin can be given in combination with ciprofloxacin (400 mg IV every 8 hours for 7 to 14 days) or aztreonam (2 g IV every 6 to 8 hours for 7 to 14 days). In patients with concern about organisms with high levels of antibiotic resistance, such as *P. aeruginosa*, an antipseudomonal β-lactam such as ceftazidime (2 g IV every 8 hours for 7 to 14 days) or cefepime (1 to 2 g every 12 hours for 7 to 14 days) can be combined with an antipseudomonal fluoroquinolone such as ciprofloxacin or an aminoglycoside (e.g., gentamicin 7 mg/kg/day in three divided doses IV for 7 to 14 days, measuring drug levels and adjusting doses to achieve a trough level of <1 µg/mL). Again, addition of extended anaerobic coverage with clindamycin should be considered. Finally, if the patient is known or suspected to harbor MRSA, intravenous vancomycin (15 mg/kg every 12 hours IV and measuring drug level and adjusting doses to achieve trough levels of 15 to 20 µg/mL) or linezolid (600 mg IV every 12 hours) for 10 to 14 days should be added to the regimen.

Surgical Therapy

Adequate nutrition is a concern in patients with multiple episodes of aspiration pneumonia and underlying neurologic disease or malignancy.

Endoscopic or surgical placement of a gastrostomy or jejunostomy feeding tube can be considered to aid in providing nutrition, fluids, and medications in the palliation of such patients. Of greater challenge are patients who continue to have pneumonia related to aspiration of saliva, sometimes around cuffed endotracheal and tracheostomy tubes. If aggressive therapy is considered appropriate, ligation of the submaxillary and parotid salivary ducts can decrease the production of saliva.

● HOSPITAL-ACQUIRED PNEUMONIA, VENTILATOR-ASSOCIATED PNEUMONIA, AND HEALTH CARE–ASSOCIATED PNEUMONIA

EPIDEMIOLOGY

Hospital-acquired pneumonia, ventilator-associated pneumonia, and health care–associated pneumonia represent the second most common nosocomial infections in the United States. Hospital-acquired pneumonia on average increases the length of hospital stay from 7 to 9 days, at an additional cost of more than $40,000 per patient; it is responsible for one fourth of all ICU infections and half of all antibiotic use. Early-onset hospital-acquired pneumonia and ventilator-associated pneumonia, defined as infections occurring within the first 4 hospital days, tend to be caused by antibiotic-susceptible bacteria, whereas late-onset infections are more frequently caused by multidrug-resistant (MDR) organisms (Table 97-5), which are associated with greater morbidity and mortality. The overall mortality attributed to hospital-acquired pneumonia may be as high as 30 to 50%.

PATHOBIOLOGY

Gram-negative bacterial pneumonias are fairly uncommon in previously healthy outpatients, except in patients with impaired immunity or underlying structural lung disease such as chronic obstructive pulmonary disease. However, aerobic gram-negative bacilli, including *P. aeruginosa*, *Escherichia coli*, *K. pneumoniae*, and *Acinetobacter* species, play major roles in patients with hospital-acquired pneumonia, ventilator-associated pneumonia, and health care–associated pneumonia. Many cases are polymicrobial, and gram-positive agents such as *S. aureus*, particularly MRSA strains, are also increasingly common. The frequency of MDR bacteria varies by the patient population, hospital, ICU, and local use of antimicrobial agents, so routine surveillance and monitoring of local pathogens and drug susceptibilities are key to adjusting antibiotic use appropriately.

P. aeruginosa, *Acinetobacter* species, *Stenotrophomonas maltophilia*, and *Burkholderia cepacia* complex are of particular concern because these organisms rapidly become resistant to multiple classes of antibiotics. MDR organisms are most commonly found in patients with severe underlying chronic disease, in patients with health care–associated pneumonia, and in those with late-onset hospital-acquired pneumonia and ventilator-associated pneumonia. Although considerable emphasis is placed on gram-negative bacteria in the hospital setting, more traditional bacterial pathogens such as *S. pneumoniae* and *H. influenzae* must also be considered as potential causes.

TABLE 97-5	HOST RISK FACTORS ASSOCIATED WITH DEVELOPMENT OF MULTIDRUG-RESISTANT INFECTION DURING HAP, VAP, AND HCAP

Antibiotic therapy in the past 90 days
High incidence of antibiotic resistance in the community or in the specific hospital unit
Current hospitalization for 5 or more days
Immunosuppressive disease or therapy
Presence of risk factors for HCAP
    Hospitalization for 2 or more days in the past 90 days
    Resident in a nursing home or extended care facility
    Home infusion therapy (including antibiotics)
    Chronic dialysis within the past 30 days
    Home wound care
    Family member with an MDR pathogen

HAP = hospital-associated pneumonia; HCAP = health care-associated pneumonia; MDR = multidrug resistant; VAP = ventilator-associated pneumonia.
Adapted from American Thoracic Society and Infectious Diseases Society of America. Guidelines for management of adults with hospital-acquired, ventilator-associated, and health care–associated pneumonia. *Am J Respir Crit Care Med.* 2005;171:388-416.

L. pneumophila also occasionally occurs as a nosocomial infection, particularly where there is contaminated water or during construction.

CLINICAL MANIFESTATIONS

Hospital-acquired pneumonia, ventilator-associated pneumonia, and health care–associated pneumonia are often first suspected with the demonstration of new or worsening radiographic infiltrates along with other clinical signs of infection, including fever, leukocytosis, and purulent sputum. Oxygenation may have also worsened. In general, two of the three major clinical features (fever, leukocytosis, purulent sputum) should be present. In patients with acute respiratory distress syndrome, however, a single clinical factor alone should prompt additional investigation and microbiologic culture.

DIAGNOSIS

All patients with suspected hospital-acquired pneumonia, ventilator-associated pneumonia, and health care-associated pneumonia should receive a comprehensive history and physical examination to define the severity of disease and potential sources of infection. Chest radiography is essential to determine the extent of pneumonia, particularly whether it is focal or multilobar. Some patients without new or evolving radiographic infiltrates but with other signs of infection may have purulent tracheobronchitis (Chapter 96), which may require antibiotic therapy if clinical signs of infection are present. Arterial blood gases, complete blood count, electrolytes, and liver and renal function should also be evaluated. Blood should be obtained for culture, although it is positive in only a minority of patients, before instituting new antibiotics whenever possible.

Lower respiratory tract secretions should be obtained for culture from all patients by endotracheal aspiration, BAL, or protected specimen brush whenever possible before changes in antibiotic therapy; a reliable Gram stain can help direct initial empirical therapy. A sterile culture of lower respiratory tract secretions in the absence of a new antibiotic in the past 72 hours essentially excludes most bacterial pneumonias with a 94% negative predictive value, although *Legionella* and viral infection are still possible in this situation. The quantitative diagnostic threshold for significant bacterial infection, in the absence of recent (<72 hours) changes in antibiotic regimens, is as follows: greater than 10^6 colony-forming units (cfu)/mL for tracheal aspirates, greater than 10^4 or 10^5 cfu/mL for quantitative BAL fluid, and greater than 10^3 cfu/mL for protected specimen brushings. The use of bronchoscopically obtained specimens and quantitative bacterial culture in directing therapy reduces the 14-day mortality in suspected ventilator-associated pneumonia.

TREATMENT Rx

Initial Empirical Therapy

If the patient is unstable or has evidence of sepsis, or if there is a high suspicion for hospital-acquired pneumonia, ventilator-associated pneumonia, or health care–associated pneumonia, prompt antibiotic therapy is required regardless of whether bacteria are found on the initial microscopic examination of lower respiratory tract samples because delays in antimicrobial therapy increase mortality. The choice of initial empirical therapy is based on several factors, including whether the pneumonia is early onset, whether there are risk factors for MDR bacterial infections (Table 97-6), and local surveillance data on bacterial prevalence and susceptibilities.

Suspected or Early-Onset Disease

For patients with suspected hospital-acquired or ventilator-associated pneumonia, with early-onset disease, and with no identifiable risk factors for MDR organisms, initial empirical therapy can include either ceftriaxone, an intravenous fluoroquinolone (levofloxacin, moxifloxacin, or ciprofloxacin), ampicillin/sulbactam, or ertapenem. These options will cover *S. pneumoniae*,

---

TABLE 97-6 EMPIRICAL ANTIBIOTIC TREATMENT OF HOSPITAL-ACQUIRED PNEUMONIA, VENTILATOR-ASSOCIATED PNEUMONIA, AND HEALTH CARE–ASSOCIATED PNEUMONIA

GROUP A: PATIENTS WITH EITHER HAP OR VAP, WITHOUT RISK FACTORS FOR MDR PATHOGENS, AND WITH EARLY-ONSET PNEUMONIA

POTENTIAL PATHOGENS	RECOMMENDED THERAPY
Streptococcus pneumoniae *Haemophilus influenzae* Methicillin-sensitive *Staphylococcus aureus* Antibiotic-sensitive enteric gram-negative bacilli *Escherichia coli* *Klebsiella pneumoniae* *Enterobacter* species *Proteus* species *Serratia marcescens*	Ceftriaxone, 1-2 g IV/IM every 12-24 hr, maximum of 4 g/day, with duration dependent on clinical response and individualized, as discussed in text *or* Levofloxacin, 500-750 mg IV every day, with duration dependent on clinical response and individualized; or ciprofloxacin, 400 mg IV every 8 hr, with duration dependent on clinical response and individualized; or moxifloxacin, 400 mg IV or orally every 24 hr, with duration dependent on clinical response and individualized *or* Ampicillin-sulbactam, 1.5-3 g (1-2 g ampicillin and 0.5-1 g sulbactam) IV/IM every 6 hr, maximum of 4 g sulbactam/day, depending on type and severity of infection, with duration dependent on clinical response and individualized *or* Ertapenem, 1 g IV/IM once a day, with duration dependent on clinical response and individualized

GROUP B: PATIENTS WITH HAP, VAP, OR HCAP AND WITH LATE-ONSET PNEUMONIA OR WITH RISK FACTORS FOR MDR PATHOGENS

ORGANISMS	THERAPY
Streptococcus pneumoniae *Haemophilus influenzae* Methicillin-sensitive *S. aureus* Antibiotic-sensitive enteric gram-negative bacilli *E. coli* *K. pneumoniae* *Enterobacter* species *Proteus* species *S. marcescens* MDR pathogens *Pseudomonas aeruginosa* *K. pneumoniae* (extended spectrum β-lactamase producing) *Acinetobacter* species Methicillin-resistant *S. aureus* *Legionella pneumophila*	Antipseudomonal cephalosporin (ceftazidime, 2 g IV every 8 hr, or cefepime, 1-2 g every 8-12 hr, with duration dependent on clinical response and individualized) *or* Antipseudomonal carbapenems (meropenem, 1 g every 8 hr, or imipenem, 500 mg every 6 hr or 1 g every 8 hr, with duration dependent on clinical response and individualized) *or* β-Lactam/β-lactamase inhibitor (piperacillin-tazobactam, 4.5 g IV every 6 hr, with duration dependent on clinical response and individualized) *plus* Antipseudomonal fluoroquinolone (levofloxacin, 750 mg IV every day, or ciprofloxacin, 400 mg IV q8h, with duration dependent on clinical response and individualized) *or* Aminoglycoside (amikacin, 15-20 mg/kg/day, divided every 8-12 hours, with monitoring to maintain trough lower than 4-5 µg/mL; or gentamicin, 7 mg/kg/day as a single daily dose, with monitoring to maintain trough levels lower than 1 µg/mL; or tobramycin, 4-7 mg/kg/day as a single daily dose, with monitoring to maintain trough levels lower than 1 µg/mL and duration dependent on clinical response and individualized) *plus* Vancomycin (15 mg/kg IV every 12 hr, with monitoring to maintain trough at 10-15 µg/mL and duration dependent on clinical response and individualized) or linezolid (600 mg IV every 12 hr, with duration dependent on clinical response and individualized)

HAP = hospital-associated pneumonia; HCAP = health care–associated pneumonia; MDR = multidrug resistant; VAP = ventilator-associated pneumonia.
Adapted from American Thoracic Society. Guidelines for management of adults with hospital-acquired ventilator associated, and healthcare-associated pneumonia. *Am J Respir Crit Care Med.* 2005:171:388-416.

H. influenzae, MRSA, and most antibiotic-sensitive gram-negative bacilli, including *E. coli, K. pneumoniae, Proteus* species, *Enterobacter* species, and *Serratia marcescens.*

Late-Onset Disease

In contrast, with late-onset hospital-acquired pneumonia, ventilator-associated pneumonia, or health care–associated pneumonia, or when risk factors for MDR infection have been identified, multiagent regimens should be used initially. Options include an antipseudomonal cephalosporin such as ceftazidime or cefepime, an antipseudomonal carbapenem (meropenem or imipenem), or a β-lactam/β-lactamase inhibitor agent such as piperacillin-tazobactam; in addition, either an antipseudomonal fluoroquinolone (ciprofloxacin or levofloxacin) or an aminoglycoside such as amikacin, gentamicin, or tobramycin should be used. In combination, these agents should empirically address most MDR pathogens, including *P. aeruginosa, Acinetobacter* species, and *K. pneumoniae* strains with extended-spectrum β-lactamase production. Most *L. pneumophila* isolates will also be covered, but if *Legionella* is strongly suspected, a macrolide such as azithromycin should be included. Finally, either vancomycin or linezolid should be added for coverage of MRSA if risk factors are present or the risk for MRSA is high locally.

Duration of Treatment

The initiation of empirical antibiotic therapy mandates careful daily reassessment. If the patient improves over the first 48 to 72 hours, strong consideration should be given to de-escalating antibiotic therapy based on culture results. If lower respiratory cultures remain negative but the patient has not improved, an extrapulmonary site of infection should be considered. Additional radiographic imaging and cultures from the lung, pleura, and other sites may be helpful. The total duration of therapy, therefore, must be individualized. In general, aminoglycoside use should be limited to 5 to 7 days. Overall antibiotic therapy can be as short as 7 days if the patient has improved, but patients with sluggish improvement may require 14 to 21 days of therapy.

PREVENTION

Sources of pathogens for hospital-acquired pneumonia include the environment, health care devices, and transfer of microbes by patients, staff, and visitors. Thus, scrupulous hand hygiene is essential for reducing these infections. Colonization plus aspiration of oropharyngeal pathogens or leakage of secretions around endotracheal tubes is the usual route of inoculation. The stomach and sinuses may be additional sites harboring pathogens. Infected biofilms on endotracheal tubes may also serve as an important reservoir for these infections. In this light, aggressive measures should be enforced to reduce the risk for hospital-acquired pneumonia and ventilator-associated pneumonia. Prevention centers first on staff education and compliance with alcohol-based hand disinfection, which must be used before and after each patient interaction. In addition, patients with documented MDR organisms should be isolated to reduce the risk for patient cross-contamination. Microbiologic surveillance within the hospital environment is also necessary to identify MDR organisms and determine antibiotic use and susceptibility patterns. Within the ICU, intubation and reintubation rates should be monitored and reduced as feasible, the duration of mechanical ventilation should be minimized to reduce the risk for ventilator-associated pneumonia, and methods known to reduce infection rates should be followed (Chapter 105). Ventilator-associated pneumonia can be reduced by elevation of the head of the patient's bed, daily "sedation vacations," daily assessment of the patient's readiness for extubation, peptic ulcer disease prophylaxis, and deep vein thrombosis prophylaxis. In addition, continuous aspiration of subglottic secretions is a safe procedure that also reduces the use of antimicrobial agents and the incidence of ventilator-associated pneumonia in patients who are at risk.[6]

1. Schuetz P, Albrich W, Christ-Crain M, et al. Procalcitonin for guidance of antibiotic therapy. *Expert Rev Anti Infect Ther.* 2010;8:575-587.
2. Paris R, Confalonieri M, Dal Negro R, et al. Efficacy and safety of azithromycin 1 g once daily for 3 days in the treatment of community-acquired pneumonia: an open-label randomized comparison with amoxicillin-clavulanate 875/125 mg twice daily for 7 days. *J Chemother.* 2008;20:77-86.
3. Vardakas KZ, Siempos II, Grammatikos A, et al. Respiratory fluoroquinolones for the treatment of community-acquired pneumonia: a meta-analysis of randomized controlled trials. *CMAJ Can Med Assoc J.* 2008;179:1269-1277.
4. Shorr AF, Zadeikis N, Xiang JX, et al. A multicenter, randomized, double-blind, retrospective comparison of 5- and 10-day regimens of levofloxacin in a subgroup of patients aged > or = 65 years with community-acquired pneumonia. *Clin Ther.* 2005;27:1251-1259.
5. Kadowaki M, Demura Y, Mizuno S, et al. Reappraisal of clindamycin IV monotherapy for treatment of mild-to-moderate aspiration pneumonia in elderly patients. *Chest.* 2005;127:1276-1282.
6. Bouza E, Perez MJ, Munoz P, et al. Continuous aspiration of subglottic secretions in the prevention of ventilator-associated pneumonia in the postoperative period of major heart surgery. *Chest.* 2008;134:938-946.

SUGGESTED READINGS

Fung HB, Monteagudo-Chu MO. Community-acquired pneumonia in the elderly. *Am J Geriatr Pharmacother.* 2010;8:47-61. *Review.*
McCabe C, Kirchner C, Zhang H, et al. Guideline-concordant therapy and reduced mortality and length of stay in adults with community-acquired pneumonia: playing by the rules. *Arch Intern Med.* 2009;169:1525-1531. *Compliance with the current IDSA and ATS community-acquired pneumonia guidelines improves mortality and length of hospitalization.*
Mortensen EM, Copeland LA, Pugh MJ, et al. Diagnosis of pulmonary malignancy after hospitalization for pneumonia. *Am J Med.* 2010;123:66-71. *About 9% of patients hospitalized with pneumonia were diagnosed with a pulmonary malignancy within the next year.*
Ruuskanen O, Lahti E, Jennings LC, et al. Viral pneumonia. *Lancet.* 2011;377:1264-1275. *Review.*

98

PULMONARY EMBOLISM

JEFFREY I. WEITZ

DEFINITIONS

Pulmonary embolism (PE) refers to an obstruction of a pulmonary artery by material that has traveled to the lungs from elsewhere in the body through the blood stream. Thrombus from the deep veins of the legs or arms represents the most common type of material to embolize to the lungs—a process known as venous thromboembolism (VTE). In addition to thrombotic pulmonary emboli, nonthrombotic material also can embolize to the lungs. Such material includes fat, air, amniotic fluid, tumor cells, talc in intravenous drug users, and various medical devices. Regardless of the type of embolic material, blockage of blood flow through the lungs and the resultant increased pressure in the right ventricle are responsible for the symptoms and signs of PE.

THROMBOTIC PULMONARY EMBOLISM

EPIDEMIOLOGY

VTE, which includes deep vein thrombosis (DVT; Chapter 81) and PE, represents the third most common cause of cardiovascular death after myocardial infarction and strokes. A first episode of VTE occurs in about 1 person per 1000 each year in the United States. The incidence rises exponentially with age, with 5 cases per 1000 persons per year by the age of 80 years. Although men and women are affected equally, the incidence is higher in whites and African Americans than in Hispanic persons and Asian-Pacific Islanders.

Approximately one third of patients with symptomatic VTE present with PE, whereas the remainder present with DVT alone. Up to half of the patients with a first episode of VTE have no identifiable risk factors and are described as having unprovoked or idiopathic VTE. The remainder develop VTE secondary to well-recognized, transient risk factors, such as surgery or immobilization. PE accounts for an estimated 15% of deaths in hospitalized patients, with at least 100,000 deaths from PE each year in the United States.

PATHOBIOLOGY

PE and DVT are part of the spectrum of VTE and share the same genetic and acquired risk factors, which determine the intrinsic risk of VTE for each individual (Fig. 98-1). Genetic risk factors include abnormalities associated with hypercoagulability of the blood (Chapter 174), the most common of which are factor V Leiden and the prothrombin 20210 gene mutation. Acquired risk factors include advanced age, history of previous VTE, obesity, and active cancer, all of which limit mobility and may be associated with hypercoagulability. Superimposed on this background risk, VTE often occurs in the presence of a triggering factor, which increases the risk above the critical threshold. The triggering factors, including surgery and pregnancy or estrogen therapy, lead to vascular damage, stasis, and hypercoagulability, which are the components of Virchow's triad.

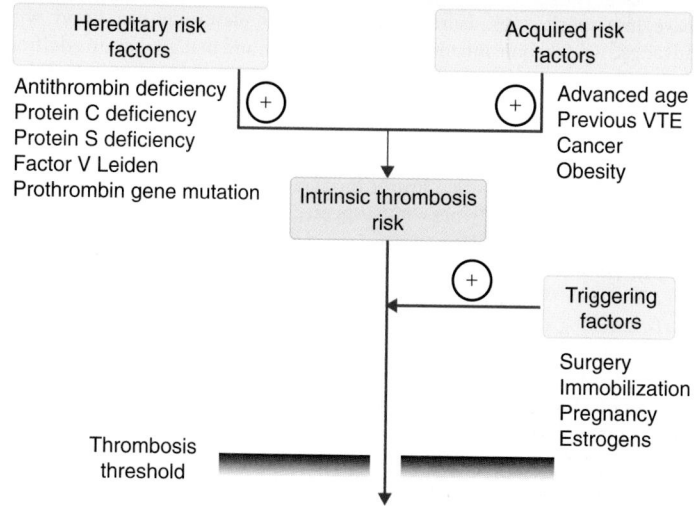

FIGURE 98-1. Thrombosis threshold. Hereditary and acquired risk factors combine to create an intrinsic risk of thrombosis for each individual. This risk is increased by extrinsic triggering factors. If the intrinsic and extrinsic forces exceed a critical threshold where thrombin generation overwhelms protective mechanisms, thrombosis occurs. VTE = venous thromboembolism.

In at least 90% of patients, PE originates from DVT in the lower limbs, and up to 70% of patients with proven PE still have demonstrable DVT on presentation. Thrombi usually start in the calf veins. About 20% of these calf vein thrombi then extend into the popliteal and more proximal veins of the leg, from which they are more likely to embolize. Although often asymptomatic, PE can be detected in about 50% of patients with proximal DVT (Chapter 81). Upper extremity DVT involving the axillary or subclavian veins also can give rise to PE, but only 10 to 15% of such patients develop PE. Upper extremity DVT most often occurs in patients with cancer (Chapter 187), particularly those with indwelling central venous catheters. Unprovoked upper extremity DVT, usually involving the dominant arm, can occur with strenuous effort—the so-called Paget-Schroetter syndrome.

PE often involves both lungs, with the lower lobes affected more frequently than the upper. Larger emboli tend to lodge in the main pulmonary artery or its branches, whereas smaller emboli occlude in more peripheral arteries. Peripheral PE can lead to pulmonary infarction, which is characterized by intra-alveolar hemorrhage and necrosis that may be pleura based. Because the circulation to the lungs arises from bronchial as well as pulmonary arteries, pulmonary infarction occurs in only about 10% of patients without underlying cardiopulmonary disease. In contrast, pulmonary infarction occurs in up to 30% of patients who have compromised oxygenation of the affected areas of lung because of preexisting disorders such as airways disease or increased pulmonary venous pressure because of left ventricular dysfunction.

The clinical impact of PE depends on the extent of reduction in pulmonary blood flow, the time frame over which vascular obstruction occurs, and the absence or presence of underlying cardiopulmonary disease. With acute PE, most patients develop tachypnea and some degree of hypoxemia. Stimulation of irritant receptors in the lungs likely accounts for the increase in respiratory rate. Obstruction of pulmonary arteries contributes to the hypoxemia and the increase in alveolar-arterial oxygen tension gradient, which reflects inefficient oxygen transfer across the lungs. These abnormalities result mainly from the increase in alveolar dead space that occurs because ventilation to alveoli exceeds blood flow in the adjacent capillaries in parts of the lung affected by PE. Other contributing factors to the hypoxemia include ventilation-perfusion mismatch because of relative overperfusion of normal areas of the lung, and shunting of blood through nonventilated atelectatic or collapsed areas of lung that retain at least some perfusion.

Pulmonary vascular resistance increases with PE because of vascular occlusion by thrombi. In addition, humoral mediators, such as serotonin and thromboxane, are released from activated platelets and may trigger vasoconstriction in unaffected areas of lung. Consequently, the increase in pulmonary vascular resistance may be disproportionate to the extent of pulmonary vascular occlusion. With obstruction of less than 50% of the pulmonary vascular bed, the mean pulmonary artery pressure rarely exceeds 25 mm Hg. Under these circumstances, the right ventricle maintains its output, so cardiac output and systemic blood pressure remain normal.

With acute occlusion of more than 50% of the pulmonary circulation, the pulmonary artery systolic pressure increases, thereby increasing right ventricular afterload. The pulmonary artery systolic pressure rarely exceeds 55 mm Hg with sudden occlusion because of insufficient time for right ventricular hypertrophy to occur. If the thin-walled right ventricle fails to maintain output in the face of the increased pulmonary artery pressure, it dilates, and right heart failure ensues. Right ventricular end-diastolic and right atrial pressures increase as the right ventricle fails. Dilation of the right ventricle may result in tricuspid regurgitation, which can compromise left ventricular filling and lead to reduced cardiac output and subsequent hypotension. Rightward bulging of the interventricular septum may also contribute to left ventricular diastolic dysfunction. The decrease in aortic pressure, together with the increase in right ventricular pressure, can produce right ventricular ischemia because of decreased perfusion of the right coronary artery despite increased demand by the dilated right ventricle. If this process occurs over a rapid time frame, syncope or sudden death, often associated with electromechanical dissociation, may be the first manifestation of severe PE.

With multiple pulmonary emboli over an extended period of time, the right ventricle has an opportunity to adapt to the increased pulmonary vascular resistance. The subsequent increase in right ventricular systolic pressure results in less right heart failure than occurs with acute large PE. Patients with multiple smaller PEs over an extended period of time often have increasing dyspnea with progressively decreasing exercise tolerance. With maintained cardiac output, hypotension does not develop. Additional emboli, however, may convert the clinical picture to one of severe acute PE.

Patients who have underlying cardiopulmonary disease or who are elderly, frail, and debilitated will be more sensitive to the effects of PE than patients who were previously healthy. Consequently, even a small PE may be fatal in patients with limited reserve.

CLINICAL MANIFESTATIONS

Patients with PE most often present with a history of dyspnea, which may be sudden in onset and tends to progress in severity over time. Dyspnea may be associated with pleuritic chest pain, cough, and hemoptysis, particularly in patients with pulmonary infarction. Although the symptoms and signs of PE can be nonspecific, the diagnosis should be suspected in patients with risk factors for VTE, such as prolonged immobility, recent surgery, or active malignancy. Patients with associated DVT (Chapter 81) may present with recent onset of leg pain or with swelling and tenderness along the course of the deep veins. The superficial veins of the leg may be dilated, and the affected leg may be warm to touch, with skin that is red or dusky blue in color.

Most patients with PE have tachypnea and tachycardia associated with hypoxemia, but these findings also can occur with disorders such as heart failure, pneumonia, or chronic obstructive pulmonary disease. Other nonspecific symptoms include palpitations, anxiety, and lightheadedness.

Patients with acute severe PE often complain of dyspnea at rest or with minimal exertion, and they may present with syncope (Chapters 50 and 62) because of hypoxemia and low cardiac output. The combination of hypotension, hypoxemia, and increased cardiac work load may trigger angina (Chapter 72) or overt myocardial infarction (Chapter 73).

Central and peripheral cyanosis can occur, and a gallop rhythm may develop as a consequence of heart failure. The jugular veins may be distended if right heart failure develops. The second heart sound can be widely split, with a loud pulmonic component because of delayed emptying of the right ventricle. A right ventricular heave may be present with massive PE and acute pulmonary hypertension.

DIAGNOSIS

Most patients with PE will have one or more of the following clinical features: dyspnea, often of sudden onset; tachypnea, with a respiratory rate of more than 20 breaths per minute; and chest discomfort, which is usually substernal and often pleuritic in nature. When patients present with these features, the differential diagnosis includes pulmonary disorders, such as pneumonia (Chapter 97), an exacerbation of chronic obstructive lung disease (Chapter 88), or asthma (Chapter 87); pleurisy secondary to connective tissue disease (Chapter 99); cardiac disorders, such as heart failure (Chapter 58), acute coronary syndrome (Chapter 72), or pericarditis (Chapter 77); and musculoskeletal disorders, such as rib fracture.

Because the clinical features are nonspecific, the diagnosis of PE requires objective testing. Patients who require such testing can be identified by their pretest likelihood of PE using validated clinical prediction rules (Table 98-1) that include components of the clinical assessment, presence of risk factors for VTE, and absence of an alternative diagnosis to explain the symptoms and signs. Some clinical prediction rules also include the results of simple tests, such as the electrocardiogram (ECG) and the chest radiograph.

Based on the results of such an assessment, the pretest likelihood of PE can be designated as low, moderate, or high, and this likelihood then guides the subsequent selection of blood tests, such as the D-dimer assay, and non-invasive or invasive tests for diagnosis of PE or DVT (Fig. 98-2) (Chapter 81). Tests for diagnosis of DVT are relevant because a diagnosis of DVT in patients with suspected PE provides sufficient grounds for initiation of treatment, and the treatment of DVT and PE is usually the same. Noninvasive tests include computed tomography (CT) pulmonary angiography or ventilation-perfusion lung scanning for diagnosis of PE and venous compression ultrasound for diagnosis of DVT. These tests have largely replaced pulmonary angiography to diagnose PE and venography to diagnose DVT.

Diagnostic Tests
D-Dimer

A plasmin-derived degradation product of cross-linked fibrin, D-dimer can be measured in whole blood or plasma to provide an indirect index of ongoing activation of the coagulation system. An elevated D-dimer level has an 85% to 98% sensitivity for the diagnosis of PE, but all available D-dimer assays have low specificities. False-positive D-dimer elevations can occur with advanced age, chronic inflammatory conditions, and malignancy. In addition, hospitalized patients are more likely to have an elevated D-dimer level than outpatients. Because of this lack of specificity, the value of the D-dimer assay resides with its high negative predictive value and the ability of a normal D-dimer to reduce the probability of PE sufficiently to avoid further diagnostic testing in patients with a low or moderate pretest likelihood,[1] who represent up to 30% of patients with suspected VTE.

Computed Tomography Pulmonary Angiography

Multidetector CT pulmonary angiography has largely replaced ventilation-perfusion lung scanning for PE diagnosis because of its wide availability and the rapidity of its results. In contrast to lung scanning, CT pulmonary angiography not only permits direct visualization of thrombi in the pulmonary arteries of patients with PE (Fig. 98-3) but also provides an alternative diagnosis in many of those who prove not to have PE. With the evolution from single-detector to multidetector CT scanners, the sensitivity and specificity of CT pulmonary angiography are sufficient for its use as a stand-alone test: a CT pulmonary angiogram showing thrombus in pulmonary arteries up to

TABLE 98-1	WELLS' CLINICAL PREDICTION RULE FOR LIKELIHOOD OF PULMONARY EMBOLISM	
VARIABLE		**POINTS**
PREDISPOSING FACTORS		
Previous VTE		1.5
Recent surgery or immobilization		1.5
Cancer		1
SYMPTOMS		
Hemoptysis		1
SIGNS		
Heart rate over 100 beats/min		1.5
Clinical signs of DVT		3
CLINICAL JUDGMENT		
Alternative diagnosis less likely than PE		3
CLINICAL PROBABILITY		**TOTAL POINTS**
Low		<2
Moderate		2-6
High		>6

DVT = deep vein thrombosis; PE = pulmonary embolism; VTE = venous thromboembolism.
Adapted from Wells PS, Ginsberg JS, Anderson DR, et al. Use of a clinical model for safe management of patients with suspected pulmonary embolism. *Ann Intern Med.* 1998;129:997-1005.

FIGURE 98-3. Computed tomographic pulmonary arteriogram demonstrating a pulmonary embolus.

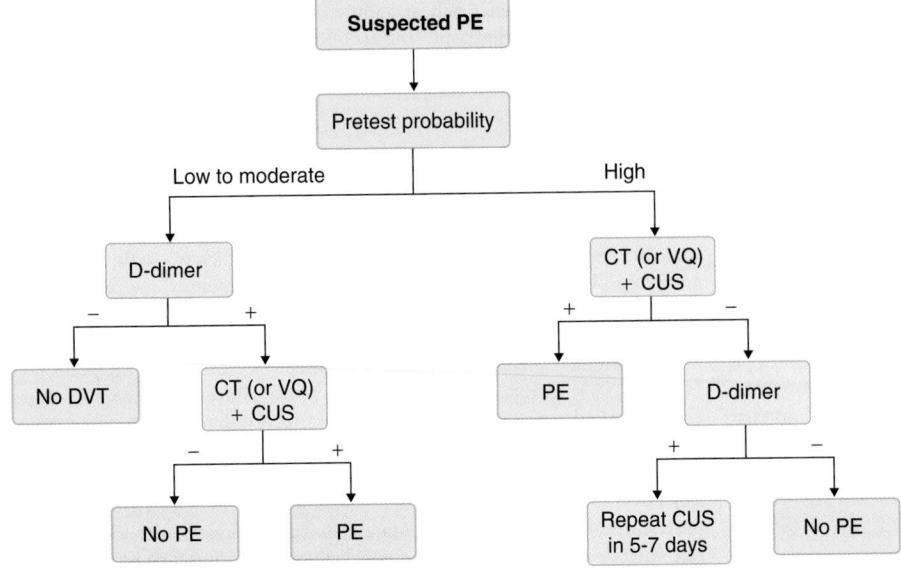

FIGURE 98-2. Clinical management of patients with suspected pulmonary embolism (PE). CT = computed tomography; CUS = venous compression ultrasound; DVT = deep vein thrombosis; VQ = ventilation-perfusion lung scan.

FIGURE 98-4. Ventilation-perfusion lung scan demonstrating pulmonary emboli.

the segmental level provides evidence of PE, whereas a negative CT pulmonary angiogram excludes PE with subsequent clinical outcomes at least as good as with lung scanning.[2] Compared with lung scanning, CT pulmonary angiography detects more isolated subsegmental thrombi in about 1 to 5% of patients, but the importance of such thrombi is unclear because patients with isolated subsegmental defects have uneventful outcomes despite withholding treatment. A negative D-dimer or a normal venous compression ultrasound examination may help to exclude the possibility of VTE in this setting.

Ventilation-Perfusion Lung Scanning

In this two-part test; the ventilation phase involves inhalation of an aerosol form of xenon or technetium to assess air delivery to the various parts of the lung, whereas the perfusion phase involves the intravenous injection of technetium-labeled macroaggregates of albumin, which enables assessment of blood flow within the lungs once the aggregates lodge in the pulmonary microcirculation. Images for both parts of the test are acquired using a gamma counter. Areas of lung affected by PE do not light up on the perfusion scan because the macroaggregates of albumin fail to reach sites where the pulmonary arteries are occluded (Fig. 98-4). In contrast, areas with abnormal perfusion ventilate normally yielding a ventilation-perfusion mismatch.

A normal lung scan effectively excludes the diagnosis of PE, but only 25% of patients with suspected PE have a normal scan. One or more segmental or larger perfusion defects that ventilate normally characterize a high probability lung scan, which establishes the diagnosis of PE, but even use of single-photon emission CT technology identifies only about 10% of patients with suspected PE as having a high probability lung scan. The remaining 65% of lung scans exhibit smaller areas of mismatch or matched defects and fall within the non-high-probability category. Because up to 40% of patients with non-high-probability scans have PE, such patients require additional investigations to exclude the diagnosis.

Although CT pulmonary angiography has largely replaced lung scanning, the lung scan remains the diagnostic test of choice for patients with renal impairment or a history of allergy to angiographic contrast media. For diagnosis of PE in pregnancy, lung scanning produces less maternal and fetal radiation exposure and is preferred over CT pulmonary angiography.

Magnetic Resonance Imaging

In contrast to CT pulmonary angiography, gadolinium-enhanced magnetic resonance imaging (MRI) does not subject patients to ionizing radiation, and gadolinium can safely be given to patients with a history of allergy to contrast dye. Although originally promoted as the test of choice to diagnose PE in patients with renal impairment, the emergence of nephrogenic systemic fibrosis (Chapter 275) as a complication of gadolinium administration in patients with renal impairment has tempered enthusiasm for the test. The accuracy of MRI for the detection of PE appears to be similar to that of CT pulmonary angiography, but magnetic resonance (MR) pulmonary angiography is more technically demanding. The combination of MR pulmonary angiography with MR venography has a higher sensitivity than MR pulmonary angiography alone for the diagnosis of PE. With these limitations, MRI should be used to diagnose PE only in centers with experience with the test and in patients for whom standard tests are contraindicated.

Pulmonary Angiography

Pulmonary angiography requires direct contrast injection into the pulmonary arteries, followed by imaging using digital subtraction technology to provide high-quality images. Presence of a thrombus, which appears as a filling defect or as a sudden cutoff of blood flow in a pulmonary arterial branch, establishes the diagnosis of PE. Although direct angiography allows visualization of small thrombi in subsegmental pulmonary arteries, high interobserver variability in the interpretation of isolated findings at this level limits the specificity of this finding. As an invasive test, the mortality rate associated with pulmonary angiography is 0.2%, with deaths usually occurring in patients with hemodynamic compromise or respiratory failure. Because of its associated risks and because CT pulmonary angiography offers similar or better information, direct pulmonary angiography is now rarely performed, except in the patient who may undergo pulmonary embolectomy.

Diagnostic Strategies

The diagnosis of DVT (Chapter 81) is usually based on venous compression ultrasound, which has a sensitivity and specificity of about 95% for the diagnosis of proximal DVT. In patients with suspected PE, the venous compression ultrasound examination can be limited to the proximal veins, which are the sources of most PE.

CT venography can be combined with CT pulmonary angiography as a simple test to diagnose DVT because both tests require only one injection of contrast dye. Compared with CT pulmonary angiography alone, the combination of CT pulmonary angiography and CT venography increases the sensitivity from 83 to 90%, but the specificity remains unchanged, thereby resulting in only a modest increase in negative predictive value. CT venography adds significant radiation exposure and only marginally increases the overall detection rate, so venous compression ultrasound is preferred because it provides the same information without exposing patients to ionizing radiation. Standard venography is not recommended in patients with suspected PE.

In summary, patients with a low to moderate pretest likelihood should undergo D-dimer testing (see Fig. 98-2). A negative D-dimer test excludes the diagnosis of PE in these patients, whereas a positive test should prompt multidetector CT pulmonary angiography. Patients with a high pretest likelihood of PE should be sent directly for multidetector CT pulmonary angiography. A positive CT pulmonary angiogram establishes the diagnosis of PE, whereas a negative test excludes it.

The role of venous compression ultrasound remains controversial. Because of the suboptimal sensitivity of single-detector CT pulmonary angiography for the diagnosis of PE, bilateral venous compression ultrasound should also be performed if multidetector technology is not available. Although a negative multidetector CT pulmonary angiogram safely excludes PE, at least in patients with low to moderate pretest likelihood, bilateral venous compression ultrasound can still be helpful. For example, the finding of proximal DVT obviates the need for further testing, a result that can be particularly helpful in patients who are poor candidates for CT pulmonary angiography, such as those with renal impairment or a history of allergy to contrast dye. Patients with a non-high-probability lung scan or with equivocal CT pulmonary angiographic findings should undergo serial venous compression ultrasound examination to exclude the possibility of calf DVT, which then extends into the proximal veins.

Other Tests

Blood markers of right ventricular dysfunction, which is seen in more severe pulmonary emboli, include brain natriuretic peptide (BNP) or its precursor, N-terminal proBNP, which are released in response to myocardial stretching. Although elevated levels of these markers in patients with PE are associated with a worse prognosis, their positive predictive value is low.

Elevated levels of troponin I or T and fatty acid–binding protein provide evidence of myocardial injury in PE patients with right ventricular infarction. In PE patients without hemodynamic compromise, elevated levels of these markers are associated with increased mortality.

The ECG may show new changes suggestive of right ventricular strain, such as T wave inversion in leads V_1 to V_4; the classic S1, Q3, T3 pattern (Fig. 98-5); and complete or incomplete right bundle branch block. However, these ECG changes have limited sensitivity and are seen predominantly in patients with more severe pulmonary emboli.

Echocardiography findings suggestive of right ventricular dysfunction include right ventricular dilation or hypokinesis, increased right ventricular diameter relative to that of the left ventricle, and increased velocity of the jet of tricuspid regurgitation. Echocardiography can also detect a right-to-left shunt through a patent foramen ovale and may provide evidence of right ventricular thrombus, both of which are associated with increased mortality in patients with PE. With no universal criteria for the diagnosis of right ventricular dysfunction, however, the utility of routine echocardiography remains uncertain. In general, routine echocardiography is recommended only in patients with severe hypoxia or other evidence to suggest hemodynamic compromise.

Other routinely ordered tests should include a complete blood count, platelet count, and international normalized ratio (INR) to help guide anticoagulation. A creatinine level and blood urea nitrogen level provide useful baseline information, as do serum electrolytes and liver enzymes.

TREATMENT   Rx

Although anticoagulant therapy remains the mainstay of treatment of PE, patients with severe PE may require reperfusion therapy to increase blood flow quickly to the pulmonary arteries and to reduce pulmonary artery pressure.**3** Therefore, rapid risk stratification is crucial to help guide treatment. PE patients who have contraindications to anticoagulant therapy may require insertion of a filter.

Severe Pulmonary Embolism

High-risk patients can be identified at the bedside (Table 98-2) based on the presence or absence of hemodynamic compromise, right ventricular dysfunction, and elevated biomarkers. Patients with severe PE usually die because they develop acute right ventricular failure, which causes low systemic output. Patients with severe PE require hemodynamic and respiratory support and may require reperfusion therapy. Patients with right ventricular failure often require modest fluid expansion and may need inotropic agents, such as

dobutamine (starting at a dose of 0.5 to 1.0 μg/kg/minute and then titrated according to the blood pressure), dopamine (starting at a dose of 5 μg/kg/minute and then increased gradually in 5- to 10-μg/kg/minute increments, according to the blood pressure, up to 20 to 50 μg/kg/minute) or norepinephrine (starting at a dose of 2 to 4 μg/minute and then titrated according to the blood pressure) for severe hypotension or shock. Emerging data raise the possibility that endothelin antagonists and phosphodiesterase-5 inhibitors may attenuate the pulmonary hypertension in patients with severe PE, but these drugs are not currently approved for use in PE.

Patients with PE frequently have hypoxemia and hypocapnia. Hypoxemia can usually be reversed with nasal oxygen. Measures to reduce fever and agitation with acetaminophen and mild sedation may help minimize oxygen consumption. In patients who have severe PE and who require mechanical ventilation, low tidal volumes should be used, and positive end-expiratory pressure should be applied with caution because it can reduce venous return and worsen right ventricular failure (Chapter 105).

Reperfusion Therapy

Patients with severe PE associated with hypotension or shock may benefit from pharmacologic, mechanical, or surgical reperfusion therapy. Pharmacologic reperfusion therapy involves the systemic administration of a fibrinolytic agent (Table 98-3), preferably within 48 hours of the onset of symptoms, but later treatment may still be of benefit. Up to 13% of patients who receive fibrinolytic therapy experience a major bleed, and the rate of intracranial or fatal bleeding can reach 1.8%. Consequently, fibrinolytic therapy currently is justified only in patients who have severe PE and no contraindications (Table 98-4). It remains unclear whether the benefits of fibrinolytic therapy outweigh the risks in patients at intermediate risk.

Mechanical reperfusion includes percutaneous catheter embolectomy with thrombus fragmentation, an approach that avoids the need for fibrinolytic drugs altogether, or catheter-directed fibrinolytic therapy, which requires lower doses of fibrinolytic agents than used for systemic administration. In some centers, surgical pulmonary embolectomy may be an option for patients who have severe PE and who are at high risk for bleeding with systemic fibrinolytic therapy or who have failed such treatment. Mechanical techniques require skilled operators but provide useful alternatives to systemic fibrinolytic therapy for patients who have severe PE and who are at high risk for bleeding.

Anticoagulation Therapy

Anticoagulation therapy is the cornerstone of PE treatment and should be initiated immediately with parenteral anticoagulants, such as heparin, low-molecular-weight heparin (LMWH), or fondaparinux, even while patients with suspected PE are awaiting the results of confirmatory tests. Patients with severe PE should be treated with heparin because neither LMWH nor fondaparinux has been extensively evaluated in this setting. Heparin should be used in patients with severe renal impairment (creatinine clearance < 30 mL/minute) because LMWH and fondaparinux are cleared by the kidneys. If LMWH or fondaparinux is used in patients with moderate renal impairment (creatinine clearance of 30 to 50 mL/min), anti–factor Xa levels should be measured at trough to ensure there is no accumulation.

FIGURE 98-5. Classic electrocardiogram of pulmonary embolus. Note the "S1, Q3, T3" pattern.

TABLE 98-3	APPROVED REGIMENS FOR FIBRINOLYTIC THERAPY FOR TREATMENT OF SEVERE PULMONARY EMBOLISM

AGENTS	RECOMMENDED REGIMENS
Streptokinase	250,000 IU as a loading dose over 30 min, followed by 100,000 IU/hr over 12 to 24 hr
Tissue plasminogen activator	100 mg over 2 hr, or 0.6 mg/kg over 10 to 15 min (maximal dose of 50 mg)

TABLE 98-2	RISK STRATIFICATION OF PATIENTS WITH PULMONARY EMBOLISM AND TREATMENTS IN ADDITION TO ANTICOAGULATION			
CLASSIFICATION	**HEMODYNAMIC COMPROMISE**	**RIGHT VENTRICULAR DYSFUNCTION**	**INCREASED TROPONIN AND/OR BNP LEVELS***	**TREATMENT**
Severe	Yes	Yes	Yes	Fibrinolytic therapy
Moderate	No	Yes	Yes	May consider fibrinolytic therapy if very symptomatic
Mild	No	No	No	Consider outpatient treatment

*Blood markers include troponin, brain natriuretic peptide (BNP), and N-terminal proBNP.

TABLE 98-4 CONTRAINDICATIONS TO FIBRINOLYTIC THERAPY

ABSOLUTE CONTRAINDICATIONS

Any hemorrhagic stroke or stroke of unknown origin
Central nervous system damage or neoplasm
Major trauma, surgery, or head injury in past 3 weeks
Gastrointestinal bleeding in past month
Significant ongoing bleeding

RELATIVE CONTRAINDICATIONS

Ischemic stroke or transient ischemic attack in past 6 months
Treatment with a vitamin K antagonist
Pregnancy or within 1 week of delivery
Noncompressible puncture site
Traumatic resuscitation
Advanced liver disease
Infective endocarditis
Active peptic ulcer disease

TABLE 98-5 LOW-MOLECULAR-WEIGHT HEPARIN AND FONDAPARINUX REGIMENS FOR TREATMENT OF PULMONARY EMBOLISM

AGENT	DOSE	INTERVAL
Enoxaparin	1 mg/kg	Twice daily
	1.5 mg/kg	Once daily
Dalteparin	100 U/kg	Twice daily
	200 U/kg	Once daily
Tinzaparin	175 U/kg	Once daily
Fondaparinux	5 mg (weight < 50 kg)	Once daily
	7.5 mg (weight 50-100 kg)	Once daily
	10 mg (weight > 100 kg)	Once daily

Heparin should be administered by continuous intravenous infusion and dosed using weight-based nomograms (see Table 81-4 in Chapter 81). Typically, an 80 U/kg bolus is followed by an infusion at the rate of 18 U/kg per hour, and subsequent doses are adjusted based on the results of the activated partial thromboplastin time (aPTT). Rapid achievement and maintenance of a therapeutic aPTT are important to reduce the risk of recurrent PE. In addition to monitoring the aPTT, the platelet count should be measured frequently because of the risk of heparin-induced thrombocytopenia (Chapter 37).

LMWH or fondaparinux can be used for intermediate- or low-risk PE patients (see Table 98-2) using the regimens illustrated in Table 98-5.[4,5] Unlike heparin, these agents do not require coagulation monitoring. In addition, the risk of heparin-induced thrombocytopenia is lower with LMWH than with heparin, and the risk is minimal with fondaparinux. Outpatient management of PE is safe for low-risk PE patients. In PE patients at intermediate risk (see Table 98-2), outpatient management can be considered, but brief admission to hospital may be a safer approach.

After initial treatment with a parenteral anticoagulant, most patients with PE receive extended therapy with a vitamin K antagonist, such as warfarin (Chapter 81), to prevent recurrent DVT and PE. In PE patients at low or intermediate risk (see Table 98-2), warfarin can be started on the same day that parenteral anticoagulant therapy is initiated. Parenteral anticoagulant therapy should be continued for at least 5 days and should only be stopped when the INR has been within the therapeutic range of 2 to 3, which is needed for long-term therapy, for 2 consecutive days. Initiation of warfarin therapy should be delayed in patients with severe PE; such patients should receive heparin until they have stabilized.

An emerging option is unmonitored, fixed-dose dabigatran etexilate (150 mg twice daily) for patients with VTE, including PE. The rates of recurrent VTE and bleeding are similar with dabigatran and warfarin, but dabigatran is superior to warfarin for preventing stroke in patients with atrial fibrillation.[6] This agent and oral factor Xa inhibitors (e.g., rivaroxaban, apixaban, and edoxaban) have the potential to replace warfarin, thereby simplifying long-term anticoagulant treatment.

Patients who develop PE as a complication of a reversible risk factor, such as surgery, trauma, or medical illness, have a low risk of recurrence when anticoagulant therapy is stopped. Consequently, a 3-month course of warfarin therapy represents adequate treatment in such patients provided that their risk factors have resolved. Women who develop PE with estrogen therapy also can be treated for 3 months, provided that hormonal treatment is withdrawn. In contrast, patients with unprovoked PE have a higher rate of recurrent VTE

when anticoagulant therapy stops and require longer treatment; some experts recommend indefinite anticoagulant therapy provided that the risk of bleeding remains low. One month after stopping anticoagulant therapy, an elevated D-dimer level or residual venous compression ultrasound abnormalities identify patients at higher risk for recurrence who require indefinite anticoagulation therapy.[7,8] After a minimum 3-month course of usual-intensity warfarin (target INR between 2 and 3), a lower-intensity regimen (target INR between 1.5 and 2.0) may simplify management by decreasing the frequency of INR monitoring and reducing the risk of bleeding,[9] but the risk of recurrent VTE is slightly higher with this lower-intensity warfarin regimen.[10]

Caval Filters

Filters, which are inserted percutaneously, are usually placed below the level of the renal veins but can be placed higher for thrombus in the inferior vena cava. Both permanent and retrievable filters reduce the risk of recurrent PE but have not been shown to prolong survival, in part because permanent filters can be associated with long-term complications, including inferior vena cava occlusion because of thrombus, recurrent DVT, and post-thrombotic syndrome.[11] Retrievable filters, designed to be removed within 2 to 4 weeks of implantation, can circumvent these long-term complications, but device migration or thrombosis occurs in up to 10% of patients with temporary filters because most are not removed. Because of these potential problems, caval filters should be restricted to patients who have high risk for recurrent PE and an absolute contraindication for anticoagulation, such as patients who develop a PE after major surgery, patients who experience major bleeding with anticoagulant therapy, and pregnant women who have a PE shortly before delivery. Retrievable filters should be used in these cases, and the devices should be removed as soon as anticoagulant therapy can safely be administered. Permanent filters are suitable for patients who have ongoing contraindications to anticoagulation.

Specific Patient Subgroups

Patients with PE in the setting of active cancer, women who suffer a PE during pregnancy, and patients with chronic thromboembolic pulmonary hypertension (Chapter 68) require special treatment.

Cancer

Active cancer and its treatment with chemotherapy, radiation therapy, and growth factors or other biological agents increase the risk of VTE (Chapter 187). Patients with advanced cancer often have limited mobility, which adds to their risk of VTE. In addition, indwelling central venous access catheters can trigger upper extremity DVT, which can lead to PE. Therefore, the index of suspicion should be high in cancer patients who present with symptoms and signs suggestive of PE or DVT, or both. With advances in diagnostic imaging, incidental PE may be discovered on CT scans performed for staging purposes or for monitoring response to treatment. Although 20% of patients with VTE have an underlying malignancy, patients with PE should not undergo routine extensive screening for cancer.

Like patients without cancer, initial treatment of PE in cancer patients involves administration of a rapidly acting parenteral anticoagulant. For extended treatment, however, LMWH reduces the risk of recurrent VTE to a greater extent than warfarin. In addition, in the face of poor nutritional intake, severe nausea and vomiting, transient thrombocytopenia, or invasive procedures, LMWH is easier to manage than warfarin.

Cancer patients who develop PE after curative surgery or with adjuvant chemotherapy for limited-stage disease should be treated for at least 3 months or until they have completed their chemotherapy. Those with PE on the background of advanced cancer have a risk of recurrence of at least 20% in the first year after stopping anticoagulant therapy, so they require lifelong treatment.

Pregnancy

Treatment of PE in pregnancy (Chapter 247) centers mainly on heparin or LMWH because, unlike warfarin, these agents do not cross the placenta. Although both agents can be given subcutaneously, weight-adjusted LMWH has advantages over heparin because it can be given once daily without routine monitoring and because the risks of heparin-induced thrombocytopenia and osteoporosis are lower with LMWH than with heparin. Anti–factor Xa monitoring of LMWH should be considered in women at extremes of body weight and in those with renal impairment. Fondaparinux should be considered for pregnant women who have a history of heparin-induced thrombocytopenia or who develop injection-site reactions to heparin or LMWH.

Heparin or LMWH should be continued throughout pregnancy. Warfarin must be avoided because it crosses the placenta and can cause bone and central nervous system abnormalities, fetal hemorrhage, or placental abruption. During labor and delivery, epidural analgesia should be avoided unless prophylactic LMWH has been stopped at least 12 hours before insertion of the epidural catheter and therapeutic LMWH has been stopped at least 24 hours before. Treatment can be resumed within 6 hours of catheter withdrawal. After delivery, anticoagulation therapy should be continued for at least 3 months; warfarin can be used because it does not appear in breast milk.

Fibrinolytic agents have been used successfully for treatment of severe PE in pregnancy but can cause bleeding, usually from the genital tract. If PE develops late in pregnancy, a retrievable filter may prevent recurrence during delivery when anticoagulant therapy must be withheld.

Chronic Thromboembolic Pulmonary Hypertension

A complication of PE, chronic thromboembolic pulmonary hypertension develops in 0.5 to 5% of patients over the course of months or years when emboli in major pulmonary arteries are replaced by fibrous tissue that becomes incorporated into the vessel wall, thereby narrowing or obstructing it. Chronic obstruction of the pulmonary vascular bed increases pulmonary arterial resistance and can lead to right heart failure. Although patients initially may be asymptomatic, they experience increasing dyspnea on exertion and hypoxemia as the disease progresses. Chronic thromboembolic pulmonary hypertension should be suspected in patients with pulmonary hypertension (Chapter 68), and the diagnosis can be established with a combination of echocardiography and lung scanning or CT pulmonary angiography.

Medical therapy focuses on treatment of right heart failure and the use of prostacyclin, endothelin receptor antagonists, or phosphodiesterase-5 inhibitors, or a combination of these, to lower pulmonary artery pressure (see Table 68-2 and Fig. 68-7 in Chapter 68). These agents may be of limited utility, however, because of the fibrotic nature of the obstructing material. Definitive treatment involves surgical thromboendarterectomy to remove the occluding material from the pulmonary arteries. This procedure is associated with a perioperative mortality rate that can be as high as 4%, depending on the severity of the disease, and a 3-year survival rate of about 80%.

PREVENTION

At least half of the outpatients with newly diagnosed VTE have a history of recent hospitalization, and most failed to receive thromboprophylaxis during their hospital stay; as a result, PE is the most common preventable cause of death in hospitalized patients in the United States. Guidelines for primary prophylaxis are available and should be followed (see Tables 37-2 and 37-3 in Chapter 37).

PROGNOSIS

With the diagnosis established and adequate anticoagulant therapy initiated, most patients with PE survive. Case-fatality rates 1 month after diagnosis of DVT or PE are 6% and 12%, respectively. Patients with severe PE who present with shock have the highest mortality rate, and many die within an hour of presentation. Although the case-fatality rate in patients with PE is twice that in those with DVT, many of the deaths are the result of comorbid conditions rather than the PE itself. Factors associated with early mortality after VTE include presentation as PE, advanced age, cancer, and underlying cardiovascular disease. The most serious long-term complication of PE is chronic thromboembolic pulmonary hypertension (Chapter 68), a rare condition associated with significant morbidity and mortality.

Despite anticoagulant therapy, recurrent VTE occurs in about 6% of patients during the first 6 months. While on anticoagulation treatment, patients with unprovoked VTE and those with secondary VTE have similar risks of recurrence. In contrast, when anticoagulant therapy is stopped, patients with unprovoked VTE have a risk of recurrence of 10% at 1 year and 30% at 5 years, whereas those with secondary VTE have recurrence rates of 3% at 1 year and 10% at 5 years. Recurrent events often mirror the index events; after an initial PE, about 60% of recurrences are PE. Because of the high risk of recurrence in patients with unprovoked VTE, many experts recommend indefinite anticoagulant therapy for such patients. In contrast, because of the lower risk of recurrence, anticoagulation therapy can be stopped after 3 months in patients with secondary VTE whose risk factors have resolved.

● NONTHROMBOTIC PULMONARY EMBOLISM

DEFINITION

Nonthrombotic material that can embolize to the lungs includes fat, air, amniotic fluid, tumor cells, talc in intravenous drug abusers, and medical devices.

Fat Embolism Syndrome

EPIDEMIOLOGY

Fat embolism syndrome usually occurs in the setting of trauma, particularly after fracture of long bones or the pelvis. The risk increases with the number of fractured bones, and the syndrome occurs more often with closed fractures than with open ones. Fat embolism also can complicate orthopedic surgery or trauma to tissues rich in fat, such as may occur with liposuction.

PATHOBIOLOGY

Characterized by a combination of respiratory, neurologic, hematologic, and cutaneous manifestations, fat embolism syndrome reflects a combination of vascular obstruction by fat globules, as well as the deleterious effects of free fatty acids released from these fat globules by the action of lipoprotein lipases. These free fatty acids increase vascular permeability, induce a capillary leak syndrome, and can trigger platelet aggregation.

CLINICAL MANIFESTATIONS

Symptoms typically develop 24 to 72 hours after trauma or surgery. Patients often complain of vague chest pain and shortness of breath. Tachypnea and fever associated with disproportionate tachycardia are common. The syndrome can rapidly progress to severe hypoxemia that requires mechanical ventilation. Neurologic manifestations, which often start after the respiratory distress, include drowsiness, confusion, decreased level of consciousness, and seizures. Patients may have petechiae, particularly involving the conjunctiva, oral mucosa, and upper half of the body.

DIAGNOSIS

Fat embolism syndrome should be suspected when respiratory distress occurs a day or more after major trauma or orthopedic surgery, particularly when there are associated neurologic defects and petechiae. The chest radiograph may reveal diffuse alveolar infiltrates. Although fat droplets may be found in bronchoalveolar lavage fluid, this finding lacks specificity for the fat embolism syndrome.

PREVENTION, TREATMENT, AND PROGNOSIS (Rx)

Early stabilization of long bone fractures reduces the risk of fat embolization. Supportive treatment should be provided, including oxygen and mechanical ventilation. The utility of corticosteroids remains controversial.

Although mortality rates as high as 10% have been reported, the prognosis is generally good.

Venous Air Embolism

EPIDEMIOLOGY

Venous air embolism, which involves entrapment of environmental air or exogenous gas in the venous system, requires direct communication between the air and a vein, as well as a pressure gradient that favors entry of the air into the vein. Air can be introduced through indwelling central venous catheters as a consequence of invasive surgical or medical procedures or after barotrauma.

PATHOBIOLOGY

Large venous air emboli obstruct the right ventricular pulmonary outflow tract, whereas mixtures of air bubbles and fibrin thrombi can obstruct pulmonary arterioles. In either case, right ventricular failure can result. With a patent foramen ovale (Chapter 69), venous air emboli can enter the coronary, cerebral, or systemic circulation.

CLINICAL MANIFESTATIONS

Symptoms and signs depend on the volume of air and the rapidity of its entry into the circulation. Large, rapid boluses of air are tolerated less well than slow entry of smaller amounts. Small air emboli may be asymptomatic. With larger emboli, patients often complain of dyspnea and retrosternal chest discomfort, and they may feel lightheaded. Physical findings include tachypnea, tachycardia, and evidence of respiratory distress. Patients may have signs of right heart failure. A continuous, drumlike, mill-wheel murmur, which reflects air in the right ventricle, may be heard.

DIAGNOSIS

Patients may present with ECG evidence of right ventricular dysfunction associated with elevated levels of troponin, indicative of myocardial injury. Echocardiography or chest CT may reveal air in the right ventricle. Patients may have hypoxemia and hypercapnia, and the platelet count may be low.

PREVENTION AND TREATMENT

All catheters should be removed using techniques that minimize air embolism, air should be removed from syringes before injection, and care should be taken during surgery to ensure that air bubbles do not form in blood vessels. To avoid air embolism associated with barotrauma, divers require training in how to dive and surface safely (Chapter 94).

The source of any air embolism should be identified so that further embolism can be prevented. Left lateral decubitus positioning may benefit patients who have a large air bubble trapped in the right ventricular outflow tract; such positioning places the outflow tract below the right ventricular cavity, thereby allowing the air bubble to migrate into a nonobstructing position. Aspiration of the right ventricle through a central venous catheter may also be of benefit. Patients should receive high-flow supplemental oxygen, and hyperbaric oxygenation should be considered for patients with cardiac or neurologic dysfunction.

PROGNOSIS

The outcome depends on the extent of air embolism. With good supportive care, the mortality rate can be less than 10%, even in patients with major air emboli. However, residual neurologic defects often persist.

Amniotic Fluid Embolism

EPIDEMIOLOGY AND PATHOBIOLOGY

Amniotic fluid embolism is a rare but catastrophic complication of pregnancy, occurring in about 1 in 8000 to 1 in 80,000 pregnancies. The syndrome develops when amniotic fluid and fetal cells enter the maternal blood stream through small tears in the uterine veins during labor. Emboli to the heart and lungs cause cardiac dysfunction and respiratory distress. In addition, amniotic fluid and other debris activate the coagulation system, and the resultant thrombin then triggers fibrin formation and platelet activation to induce disseminated intravascular coagulation.

CLINICAL MANIFESTATIONS AND DIAGNOSIS

The syndrome often starts with the abrupt onset of dyspnea, cyanosis, and hypotension that can rapidly progress to cardiovascular collapse and death. Patients who survive this stage often develop manifestations of disseminated intravascular coagulation (Chapter 178) characterized by diffuse bleeding, petechiae, and ecchymoses.

The diagnosis should be suspected in women late in pregnancy, often in labor, who present with sudden onset of respiratory distress followed by cyanosis, hypotension, and shock. These findings are often associated with confusion or reduced level of consciousness, seizures, and evidence of a consumptive coagulopathy.

TREATMENT

Supportive measures include oxygen, mechanical ventilation, and hemodynamic support. Fresh-frozen plasma, cryoprecipitate, and platelets transfusion can be given to replace consumed clotting factors and platelets. Heparin, often in low therapeutic doses, may be useful in some cases. If amniotic fluid embolism occurs before or during delivery, the fetus often has a poor outcome. As soon as the mother stabilizes, therefore, every attempt should be made to deliver the fetus.

PROGNOSIS

Although rare, amniotic fluid embolism remains the leading cause of maternal death during labor and the first few hours after delivery. Despite advances in critical care management, maternal and fetal mortality rates continue to be about 60% and 20%, respectively, with up to half of the survivors, both mother and baby, suffering from permanent hypoxia-induced neurologic dysfunction.

Other Embolic Material

Many substances, such as talc, starch, and cellulose are used as fillers in the manufacture of drugs. Some of these drugs are ground up by drug users (Chapter 33), mixed in liquids, and then injected intravenously. The filler particles can then be trapped in the pulmonary vasculature, where they can induce granuloma formation.

Tumor emboli (Chapter 179) in the lung can mimic pneumonia, tuberculosis, or interstitial lung disease on the chest radiograph. Cancers of the prostate and breast are the most common sources of such emboli, followed by hepatoma and cancers of the stomach and pancreas. Although found in up to 26% of autopsies in patients with advanced cancer, tumor emboli are infrequently identified before death.

Various types of intravascular devices can embolize to the lungs, including vena cava filters, broken catheter tips, guidewires, stent fragments, and coils used for embolization. Many of these devices lodge in the right atrium, right ventricle, or pulmonary arteries. Intravascular retrieval can recover most of these devices; open surgery may be required for the remainder.

1. Kearon C, Ginsberg JS, Douketis J, et al, for the Canadian Pulmonary Embolism Diagnosis Study (CANPEDS) Group. An evaluation of D-dimer in the diagnosis of pulmonary embolism: a randomized trial. *Ann Intern Med.* 2006;144:812-821.
2. Anderson DR, Kahn SR, Rodger MA, et al. Computed tomographic pulmonary angiography vs ventilation-perfusion lung scanning in patients with suspected pulmonary embolism: a randomized controlled trial. *JAMA.* 2007;298:2743-2753.
3. Wan S, Quinlan DJ, Agnelli G, et al. Thrombolysis compared with heparin for the initial treatment of pulmonary embolism: a meta-analysis of the randomized controlled trials. *Circulation.* 2004;110:744-749.
4. Quinlan DJ, McQuillan A, Eikelboom JW. Low-molecular-weight heparin compared with intravenous unfractionated heparin for treatment of pulmonary embolism: a meta-analysis of randomized, controlled trials. *Ann Intern Med.* 2004;140:175-183.
5. Büller HR, Davidson BL, Decousus H, et al, for the Matisse Investigators. Subcutaneous fondaparinux versus intravenous unfractionated heparin in the initial treatment of pulmonary embolism *N Engl J Med.* 2003;349:1695-1702.
6. Schulman S, Kearon C, Kakkar AK, et al, for the RE-COVER Study Group. Dabigatran versus warfarin in the treatment of acute venous thromboembolism. *N Engl J Med.* 2009;361:2342-2352.
7. Palareti G, Cosmi B, Legnani C, et al, for the PROLONG Investigators. D-dimer testing to determine the duration of anticoagulation therapy. *N Engl J Med.* 2006;355:1780-1789.
8. Prandoni P, Prins MH, Lensing AW, et al, for the AESOPUS Investigators. Residual thrombosis on ultrasonography to guide the duration of anticoagulation in patients with deep venous thrombosis: a randomized trial. *Ann Intern Med.* 2009;150:577-585.
9. Ridker PM, Goldhaber SZ, Danielson E, et al, for the PREVENT Investigators. Long-term, low-intensity warfarin therapy for the prevention of recurrent venous thromboembolism. *N Engl J Med.* 2003;348:1425-1434.
10. Kearon C, Ginsberg JS, Kovacs MJ, et al, for the Extended Low-Intensity Anticoagulation for Thrombo-Embolism Investigators. Comparison of low-intensity warfarin therapy with conventional-intensity warfarin therapy for long-term prevention of recurrent venous thromboembolism. *N Engl J Med.* 2003;349:631-639.
11. The PREPIC Study Group. Eight year follow-up of patients with permanent vena cava filters in the prevention of pulmonary embolism. *Circulation.* 2005;112:416-422.

SUGGESTED READINGS

Agnelli G, Becattini C. Acute pulmonary embolism. *N Engl J Med.* 2010;363:266-274. *Review.*
Bourjeily G, Paidas M, Khalil H, et al. Pulmonary embolism in pregnancy. *Lancet.* 2010;375:500-512. *Review.*
Ceylan N, Tasbakan S, Bayraktaroglu S, et al. Predictors of clinical outcome in acute pulmonary embolism: correlation of CT pulmonary angiography with clinical, echocardiography and laboratory findings. *Acad Radiol.* 2011;18:47-53. *Neither CT pulmonary angiographic findings nor echocardiography predicts in-hospital mortality.*
Jakobsson C, Jimenez D, Gomez V, et al. Validation of a clinical algorithm to identify low-risk patients with pulmonary embolism. *J Thromb Haemost.* 2010;8:1242-1247. *Validates an easy-to-use risk scoring system to identify low-risk patients whose pulmonary emboli might be treated on an outpatient basis.*
Piazza G, Goldhaber SZ. Management of submassive pulmonary embolism. *Circulation.* 2010;122:1124-1129. *Review.*

99

DISEASES OF THE DIAPHRAGM, CHEST WALL, PLEURA, AND MEDIASTINUM

F. DENNIS MCCOOL

DIAPHRAGM

The diaphragm is a dome-shaped structure that separates the thorax from the abdomen. It consists of a central tendon and a peripheral muscular component that inserts into the rib cage laterally along the inner surface of the lower six ribs, the costal cartilages anteromedially, and the upper three lumbar vertebral bodies posteriorly. The diaphragm is innervated by the phrenic nerve, which originates from cervical nerve roots 3 through 5.

DIAPHRAGMATIC WEAKNESS AND PARALYSIS

EPIDEMIOLOGY AND PATHOBIOLOGY

When the diaphragm is activated, it contracts and descends caudally. The downward descent of the diaphragm expands the lower rib cage and lowers pleural pressure, thereby resulting in lung inflation. It is the major muscle of inspiration, and its action accounts for approximately 70% of the inspired tidal volume in the normal individual. Diaphragm function can be impaired by disorders that affect the brain (Chapter 411), spinal cord (Chapter 407), phrenic nerve (Chapter 428), neuromuscular junction (Chapter 430), and muscle itself (Chapter 429). The incidence and prevalence of diaphragm paralysis and weakness are unknown.

CLINICAL MANIFESTATIONS

Diaphragmatic weakness or paralysis can involve either one or both hemidiaphragms. With unilateral diaphragmatic paralysis, patients are generally asymptomatic at rest but may have dyspnea with exertion or when supine. If they are asymptomatic, the abnormality may be discovered as an incidental finding of an elevated hemidiaphragm on chest radiography.

Bilateral diaphragmatic paralysis is not as common as unilateral paralysis. Generally, the disability with bilateral paralysis is more dramatic than with unilateral paralysis. Orthopnea is an especially prominent symptom, and patients are often unable to sleep in the supine position. These individuals also experience significant dyspnea with exertion and are at an increased risk to hypoventilate during sleep, especially during rapid eye movement (REM) sleep. Consequently, initial symptoms of individuals with bilateral or unilateral diaphragm weakness or paralysis may be related to nocturnal hypoventilation and include frequent nocturnal awakenings, nocturia, vivid nightmares, night sweats, daytime hypersomnolence, depression, and morning headaches.

The physical examination is remarkable for use of accessory muscles of inspiration and paradoxical inward motion of the abdominal wall during inspiration, which is especially noticeable when these individuals are asked to lie flat. Percussion during inspiration and expiration can detect the absence of diaphragmatic movement.

DIAGNOSIS

Disorders that can cause unilateral diaphragmatic weakness or paralysis (Table 99-1) include traumatic phrenic nerve injury, herpes zoster (Chapter 383), cervical spinal disease (Chapter 407), compressive tumors, and phrenic nerve injury related to cardiac or thoracic surgery. Diagnosis is often suggested by elevation of a hemidiaphragm on a chest radiograph. The diagnosis can be confirmed by performing a "sniff test" using fluoroscopy, in which paradoxical (cephalad) movement of the hemidiaphragm occurs during a sniff maneuver.

The presence of bilateral diaphragmatic paralysis can be much more difficult to ascertain than unilateral paralysis. Chest radiography, which typically shows elevation of both hemidiaphragms, may be interpreted as a "poor inspiratory effort" or "low lung volumes."

Tests that can support or refute the diagnosis include pulmonary function testing (Chapter 85), which typically shows a moderate to severe reduction of vital capacity (VC) and total lung capacity (TLC) (30 to 60% predicted). The restriction becomes more severe (10 to 30% further decrease for unilateral and 30 to 50% further decrease for bilateral paralysis) when the individual assumes the supine position. Maximal static inspiratory pressure measured at the airway opening (PI_{max}) is reduced to 20 to 30% of predicted in individuals with bilateral diaphragmatic paralysis. The diagnosis can be confirmed if measurements of transdiaphragmatic pressure (the pressure difference between the thoracic and abdominal cavity) do not change with inspiration. Diaphragm electromyography and phrenic nerve conduction studies may be useful to distinguish neuropathy or myopathy. Unlike unilateral diaphragmatic paralysis, a sniff test is not helpful in individuals with bilateral diaphragmatic paralysis because it can yield both false-negative and false-positive results. Using two-dimensional ultrasound, the normal thickening of the diaphragm during inspiration will not be observed. If the diagnosis of bilateral diaphragmatic paralysis is confirmed, an evaluation for nocturnal hypoventilation (Chapter 86) should be undertaken.

TREATMENT AND PROGNOSIS Rx

Bilateral diaphragmatic paralysis may not be reversible unless the underlying cause is treatable. For example, myopathies (Chapter 429) related to metabolic disturbances may be improved by correcting electrolyte imbalances or

TABLE 99-1	CAUSES OF DIAPHRAGMATIC WEAKNESS AND PARALYSIS

TRAUMA

Cardiac surgery with cold cardioplegia
Blunt trauma
Spinal cord injury
Cervical manipulation
Scalene and brachial nerve block

TUMOR COMPRESSION

Lung cancer
Metastatic mediastinal tumor

METABOLIC

Diabetes
Vitamin deficiency (B_6, B_{12}, folate)
Hypothyroidism
Acid maltase deficiency

INFLAMMATORY NEURITIS

Neuralgic amyotrophy (Parsonage-Turner)
Mononeuritis multiplex
Vasculitis
Paraneoplastic

MUSCULAR DYSTROPHIES

Limb-girdle
Duchenne's and Becker's

MISCELLANEOUS

Amyloidosis
Malnutrition
Radiation injury
Cervical spondylosis
Poliomyelitis
Amyotrophic lateral sclerosis

IDIOPATHIC

replacing thyroid hormone. Toxic or metabolic disturbances related to diabetes, alcohol, or viral infections may resolve with treatment of the underlying disease. Idiopathic diaphragmatic paralysis or paralysis due to neuralgic amyotrophy (brachial plexus neuritis) may spontaneously improve or resolve completely in approximately 60% of individuals, but recovery can take 18 months to 3 years. Phrenic nerve damage related to cardiac surgery usually resolves spontaneously. For a high spinal cord injury, in which the phrenic nerve roots remain intact (injury above C-3), phrenic nerve pacing can provide ventilation.

As in sleep-disordered breathing (Chapter 100), noninvasive positive-pressure ventilation (NPPV) is the preferred method of treatment for patients with diaphragmatic paralysis because it can improve both symptoms and physiologic derangements.

Nocturnal positive-pressure ventilation is associated with a number of benefits in patients with neuromuscular disease (Table 99-2). The improvement in ventilation may be related to resting the diaphragm during periods of mechanical ventilation; this reduced work appears to reverse chronic respiratory muscle fatigue and improve daytime function. Other benefits may be related to changes in the control of breathing by reversing the brain's adaptation to high levels of CO_2 by "resetting" the central controller toward normal. When patients with unilateral paralysis have severe symptoms, surgical plication of the paralyzed hemidiaphragm may improve vital capacity.

MISCELLANEOUS DIAPHRAGMATIC DISORDERS

Diaphragmatic eventration results from localized atrophy of the diaphragm muscle or from part of the diaphragm being replaced with fibroelastic tissue. Eventration most often results in an elevation of the right anteromedial portion of the diaphragm. Metastatic tumors to the diaphragm usually are related to direct extension of lung cancer. Primary tumors of the diaphragm are very rare. Lipomas are the most common benign tumor, and fibrosarcomas are the most common malignant neoplasm.

CHEST WALL

The chest wall is a key component of the "inspiratory pump" and allows for maintenance of normal alveolar ventilation. It consists of the bony structures

TABLE 99-2	THERAPEUTIC BENEFITS OF NONINVASIVE MECHANICAL VENTILATION IN PATIENTS WITH CHEST WALL AND NEUROMUSCULAR DISORDERS*	
GAS EXCHANGE INDICES		
PaO_2	Increase	
$PaCO_2$	Decrease	
Bicarbonate	Decrease	
RESPIRATORY MECHANICS		
MIP, MEP	No change or slight increase	
HEMODYNAMIC PARAMETERS		
PAP	Decrease	
VENTILATORY CONTROL		
Hypercapnic ventilatory response	Increase	
SLEEP		
Epworth sleepiness score	Decrease	
OTHER PARAMETERS		
Quality of life	Improvement	
Survival	Increase	

*Efficacy data derived from mostly nonrandomized, noncontrolled studies.
MEP = maximal expiratory pressure; MIP = maximal inspiratory pressure; PAP = pulmonary artery pressure.

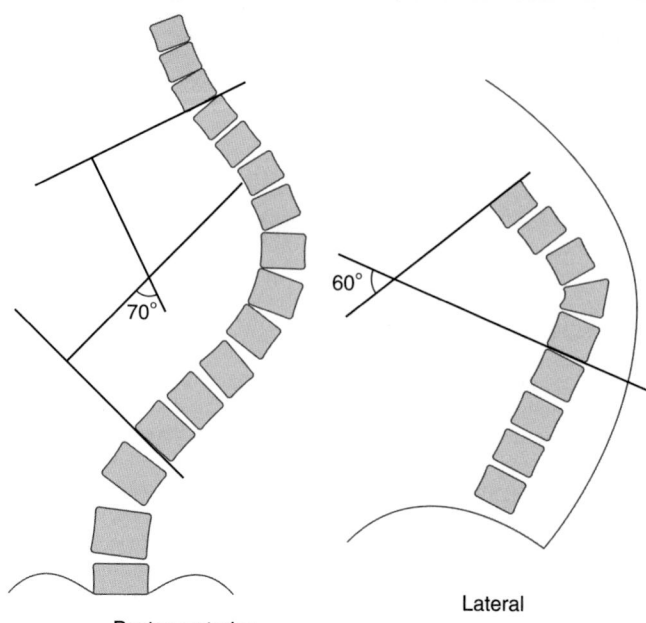

FIGURE 99-1. Schematic drawings of the spine illustrating the lines constructed to measure the Cobb angle of scoliosis and kyphosis. The angle can be calculated either from the intersection of the lines parallel to the vertebrae (as shown for kyphosis, on the *right*) or from the intersection of lines perpendicular to these lines (as shown for scoliosis, on the *left*).

of the rib cage, the articulations between the ribs and the vertebrae, the diaphragm, intercostal muscles, and the abdomen. Disorders that affect any of the components of the chest wall can result in impaired breathing.

KYPHOSCOLIOSIS

EPIDEMIOLOGY AND PATHOBIOLOGY

Kyphoscoliosis, which is a common spinal disorder, affects approximately 1 in 1000 individuals, and about 1 in 10,000 affected individuals has a severe spinal deformity. Deformities include excessive spinal curvature in the coronal (scoliosis) and sagittal (kyphosis) planes as well as rotation of the spinal axis. Kyphoscoliosis can be idiopathic or can be secondary (paralytic) and associated with neuromuscular diseases, such as muscular dystrophy and polio (Chapters 423 and 429).

Idiopathic kyphoscoliosis, in which there may be a familial predominance, usually manifests in late childhood or early adolescence and involves females more than males with a ratio of 4:1. Although a defect in the chromatin-remodeling gene family (*CHD7*) has been associated with idiopathic kyphoscoliosis, other genes have also been identified.

Kyphoscoliosis produces one of the most severe restrictive impairments of all the chest wall diseases. Total lung capacity and vital capacity may be reduced to as low as 30% of predicted values. This restrictive pathology becomes most severe as the degree of spinal angulation increases. The patient's age, degree of spinal rotation, presence of respiratory muscle weakness, and involvement of the thoracic vertebrae are all factors that promote the restrictive process. Respiratory failure is a common cause of morbidity and mortality in patients with kyphoscoliosis.

CLINICAL MANIFESTATIONS

Individuals with mild to moderate kyphoscoliosis may have complaints of back pain and have psychosocial problems as a result of their deformity. Adolescents with mild idiopathic kyphoscoliosis usually have normal exercise capacity, whereas those with moderate idiopathic kyphoscoliosis have reduced exercise capacity with additional exercise limitation due to deconditioning. With severe deformities, patients may experience dyspnea with minimal exertion or at rest.

Severe kyphoscoliosis can be readily diagnosed on physical examination. Typical findings are the dorsal hump, which is due to the angulated ribs and shoulder asymmetry, as well as the hip tilt that is related to the spinal rotation. In younger individuals with milder spinal deformities, the initial changes may be subtle. The Adams forward bend test, in which the examiner observes for thoracic or lumbar region asymmetry while the patient bends forward at the waist until the spine becomes parallel to the floor, can help detect minor deformities. With severe kyphoscoliosis, signs of right heart

failure (Chapter 58) may be present such as cyanosis, distended neck veins, peripheral edema, and hepatomegaly.

Individuals with kyphoscoliosis are particularly prone to hypoventilation during sleep, especially REM sleep. Because sleep-related abnormalities and their effects on cardiorespiratory function are potentially treatable, individuals with kyphoscoliosis should be evaluated for nocturnal hypoventilation well in advance of the development of daytime hypercapnia.

DIAGNOSIS

Although spinal deformity is often readily apparent on physical examination, the degree of spinal deformity should be assessed by calculation of the angle of spinal curvature (the Cobb angle) from radiographs. This angle is formed by the intersection of lines parallel to the top and bottom vertebrae of the scoliotic or kyphotic curves (Fig. 99-1). Angles more than 100 degrees are usually associated with respiratory symptoms, and angles more than 120 degrees with respiratory failure. Factors associated with progression of the spinal deformity include inspiratory muscle weakness, a large spinal curvature at the time of presentation, skeletal immaturity, and a thoracic location of the curve apex. Individuals with inspiratory muscle weakness and kyphoscoliosis are more prone to develop respiratory failure than those with normal inspiratory muscle strength.

TREATMENT

Patients should be encouraged to remain physically active to minimize peripheral muscle deconditioning. In addition, general supportive measures including immunizations against influenza and pneumococci (Chapter 17), smoking cessation (Chapter 31), maintenance of a normal body weight (Chapter 227), and treatment of respiratory infections in a timely fashion should be instituted. Patients with severe kyphoscoliosis and Cobb angles of more than 100 degrees should be monitored closely for respiratory complications. Respiratory failure may be precipitated by respiratory infections or by medications that produce central nervous system depression.

Nocturnal hypoventilation typically precedes findings of daytime hypercapnia and hypoxemia and should be treated with NPPV. Indications for instituting NPPV include symptoms of nocturnal hypoventilation or signs of cor pulmonale (Chapter 68) with either an elevated daytime $PaCO_2$ or nocturnal oxygen saturation of less than 89% for 5 consecutive minutes. Supplemental oxygen will be needed if hypoxemia persists despite correction of hypoventilation. NPPV can reduce the number and duration of hospitalizations and improve gas exchange, daytime blood gases, quality of life, and survival (see Table 99-2).

Surgical and nonsurgical (back-brace) treatments have been used in skeletally immature patients with idiopathic kyphoscoliosis in an effort to correct or prevent progression of the spinal deformity. Braces have been used for growing children with Cobb angles between 25 and 40 degrees, whereas surgery has been used for adolescents with a Cobb angle of more than 45 degrees. The overall role of surgical management in restoring function to that of nonscoliotic individuals and minimizing the possibility of respiratory failure is not clear.

PROGNOSIS

Idiopathic kyphoscoliosis has a better prognosis than kyphoscoliosis secondary to neuromuscular diseases. In general, individuals with mild idiopathic kyphoscoliosis have an overall benign course. Patients with moderate or severe deformities are at higher risk of developing respiratory complications.

In secondary kyphoscoliosis, factors such as an early age of onset, rapid curve progression during growth, progression of scoliosis after skeletal maturity, large curves at the time of presentation, and a thoracic rather than a thoracolumbar or lumbar location of the curve apex are risk factors for respiratory complications. Respiratory failure may occur in individuals with mild or moderate kyphoscoliosis owing to concurrent respiratory muscle dysfunction. Muscle strength should be evaluated in individuals with respiratory failure and Cobb angles of less than 100 degrees. When cor pulmonale develops (Chapter 68), the prognosis is poor, and death may occur within 1 year without therapy.

PECTUS EXCAVATUM

EPIDEMIOLOGY AND PATHOBIOLOGY

Pectus excavatum, a chest wall deformity that occurs in approximately 0.5 to 2% of the population, is characterized by excessive depression of the sternum and its adjacent costal cartilages. The ratio of affected males to females is 4:1, and a family history is common. Pectus excavatum produces minimal functional impairment of the respiratory system. Occasionally, a restrictive defect will be present with mild reductions in VC and TLC. Individuals with the most severe pectus deformities may exhibit a mild reduction in maximal exercise capacity.

CLINICAL MANIFESTATIONS

Cosmetic concerns are the usual reason for seeking medical attention. Dyspnea with activity or exercise may be present but is usually out of proportion to any measurable abnormality in cardiopulmonary function. On physical examination, sternal depression is readily apparent, and there is normal excursion of the rib cage during inspiration. A mild degree of scoliosis may be present in 40 to 60% of individuals.

DIAGNOSIS

Chest computed tomography (CT) is the best means of assessing the sternal deformity. The anteroposterior diameter of the rib cage and the transverse diameter of the rib cage are measured at the level of the deepest sternal depression. Normally, the transverse-to-anteroposterior diameter ratio is 2.5. A ratio of greater than 3.5 signifies a significant pectus deformity.

TREATMENT AND PROGNOSIS **Rx**

Surgical correction of the deformity is considered for patients with a CT ratio of more than 3.5 in conjunction with symptoms of dyspnea or laboratory evidence of cardiac or pulmonary restriction. However, there is no convincing evidence that correction of the deformity improves either cardiopulmonary function or exercise capacity. Invasive surgical approaches include resecting costal cartilage and repositioning the sternum. Sternal necrosis and infection may complicate invasive surgical procedures, and sternal osteotomy should be avoided in early childhood because it may be complicated by arrested growth of the rib cage. Minimally invasive approaches insert curved metal rods into the sternum through small incisions on each side of the rib cage; over time, the rod is rotated to force the sternum outward. After approximately 2 years, the rods are removed. The prognosis is excellent in individuals who have only mild deformity and patients who have undergone minimally invasive surgical correction of more severe deformities.

FLAIL CHEST

EPIDEMIOLOGY AND PATHOBIOLOGY

Flail chest occurs following trauma in which there have been either double fractures of three or more contiguous ribs or combined sternal and rib fractures. The result is an unstable segment of the chest wall, which moves paradoxically inward with inspiration and outward with expiration. In adults, flail chest is most commonly a consequence of blunt chest wall trauma owing to automobile accidents or falls (Chapter 112).

With a flail chest, inspiratory capacity is limited, and VC may be reduced by 50% or more. Reductions in lung compliance, owing to concomitant pulmonary contusion or microatelectasis, will worsen the restrictive dysfunction and impair gas exchange. The most common location for a flail segment is the lateral chest wall, and this location is generally associated with more clinical derangement. By contrast, a posterior flail segment has less impact on the respiratory system because of splinting provided by the paraspinal muscles.

Hypoventilation and flail-induced changes in respiratory muscle function are key factors to the development of respiratory failure in individuals with flail chest (E-Fig. 99-1). Excessive shortening of the inspiratory muscles related to the flail segment increase the work of breathing. The increased work, in concert with reduced oxygen supplies due to pulmonary contusion or hypoventilation, predisposes these individuals to developing respiratory muscle fatigue. Pain associated with the rib fractures and the disordered motion of the flail segment during expiration impair cough.

DIAGNOSIS

Bedside inspection and gentle palpation of the rib cage and abdomen can reveal the characteristic paradoxical movement of the flail segment during spontaneous breathing. Chest radiographs will confirm the presence of multiple rib fractures, but a three-dimensional reconstruction of a thoracic CT can provide better visualization of thoracic injuries, including lung contusion. The diagnosis may be less apparent in a sedated mechanically ventilated patient, in whom paradoxical motion of a segment of the rib cage may not occur because the positive alveolar and pleural pressures act as a "pneumatic splint" and allow for uniform inflation of the chest wall. However, after withdrawal of sedation, spontaneous breathing should reveal the flail segment.

TREATMENT **Rx**

Nonsurgical management of flail chest consists of adequate analgesia, clearance of bronchial secretions, and mechanical ventilatory assistance if needed. Pain relief (Chapter 29) can be accomplished by oral medications, patient-controlled analgesic pumps, intercostal nerve blocks, or epidural anesthesia. These interventions often produce a successful outcome with avoidance of respiratory failure and mechanical ventilation, and as the rib cage heals, function is restored. If respiratory failure ensues, not only will mechanical ventilation enhance gas exchange, but also the positive pleural pressure provided by the ventilator during inspiration will stabilize the flail segment. Ventilation delivered by a nasal or face mask to patients who are spontaneously breathing improves gas exchange and may allow for early mobilization and access to physical therapy.

Surgical techniques, none of which is supported by randomized clinical trial evidence, include open thoracotomy with stabilization of the fractured ribs. The indications for operative fixation are not fully defined, but patients who are unable to wean from mechanical ventilation owing to chest wall instability or patients who are undergoing thoracotomy for concomitant injuries may be candidates for surgical fixation.

PROGNOSIS

The overall mortality from chest wall trauma is high, ranging from 7 to 14%. If concomitant lung contusion is present, the mortality rate increases further and may be as high as 70%. The associated high mortality rate is also partly due to the coexistence of other injuries, such as fractures of the long bones, head trauma, or rupture of major vascular structures (Chapter 112). Older age is another poor prognostic factor.

In patients with flail chest without lung contusion, the restrictive impairment can resolve, and the VC can return to baseline values within 6 months after the acute injury. By contrast, individuals with flail chest and concomitant lung contusion often have persistent impairment of pulmonary function, which may persist for up to 4 years after injury. Operative fixation of the chest wall may reduce long-term respiratory dysfunction in these individuals.

ANKYLOSING SPONDYLITIS

EPIDEMIOLOGY AND PATHOBIOLOGY

Ankylosing spondylitis (Chapter 273) is an inflammatory disease that involves the ligamentous structures of the spine, sacroiliac, and large peripheral joints. It affects men more than women, with the most common age of onset between 15 and 25 years. There is a genetic predisposition, with the HLA-B27 antigen present in 95% of whites with ankylosing spondylitis. Chronic inflammation of the spine and peripheral joints may cause fibrosis and ossification of structures adjacent to the spine. Fusion of the costovertebral and sternoclavicular joints produces relative fixation of the rib cage in an inspiratory position, with limited motion of the rib cage during inspiration and a mild restrictive respiratory impairment. The degree of restriction is proportional to disease activity and duration as well as to the degree of spinal and rib cage immobility. Concomitant kyphosis, which may occur in advanced disease or be secondary to osteoporosis, will further impair respiratory function. Because the rib cage is less distensible, the diaphragm shortens to a greater degree for a given tidal volume, thereby increasing the work performed by the diaphragm. Intercostal muscle atrophy secondary to decreased rib cage mobility may cause inspiratory muscle weakness.

About 1 to 4% of patients with ankylosing spondylitis develop fibrobullous upper lobe disease. The cause of this apical disease is unknown, but its presence may impair gas exchange. Occasionally, individuals with ankylosing spondylitis develop nonapical interstitial lung disease (Chapter 92).

CLINICAL MANIFESTATIONS AND DIAGNOSIS

Ankylosing spondylitis is diagnosed when there is a history of low back pain and stiffness for more than 3 months, limited chest wall expansion, limited lumbar spine motion in the sagittal and frontal planes, and radiographic evidence of sacroiliitis. Radiographic findings include calcifications and ossifications of the vertebrae and paravertebral tissues.

Low back pain and spinal stiffness are the most common presenting symptoms. Dyspnea may be present as the disease progresses and chest wall expansion becomes more restricted. Physical examination may reveal loss of lateral flexion of the lumbar spine, tenderness over the sacroiliac joints, and kyphosis.

TREATMENT AND PROGNOSIS Rx

Exercise and physiotherapy programs can enhance cardiorespiratory fitness and spinal mobility. Ankylosing spondylitis is treated with nonsteroidal anti-inflammatory agents and biological agents, such as tumor necrosis factor antagonists that relieve symptoms, reduce spinal inflammation, and improve quality of life. These agents also are associated with improvements in rib cage expansion. Corticosteroids do not prevent the progression of fibrobullous disease, which can be complicated by major hemoptysis. Thoracic surgery may be indicated for hemoptysis, but surgical intervention carries major risk, with 50 to 60% of patients developing bronchopleural fistulas. Ankylosing spondylitis rarely leads to disability unless individuals develop fibrobullous disease.

OBESITY

PATHOBIOLOGY

The degree of obesity (Chapter 227) can be assessed by measuring the body mass index (BMI), which is the ratio of body weight (BW) in kilograms to the square of the height (Ht) in meters (BW/Ht^2). Individuals with a BMI between 18.5 and 24.9 kg/m² are normal, whereas those with a BMI greater than 40 kg/m² are considered morbidly obese.

Obesity can be accompanied by changes in pulmonary function or alterations in respiratory control. Obesity characteristically reduces end-expiratory lung volume or functional reserve capacity (FRC) and expiratory reserve volume (ERV). TLC and VC may be normal or only mildly reduced except in the most severe cases. Obesity can be accompanied by alterations in respiratory control resulting in elevated levels of $Paco_2$ (Chapter 86).

Dyspnea and exercise intolerance, which are the most frequent respiratory complaints of obese individuals, may be related to disordered chest wall mechanics, restrictive pulmonary dysfunction, altered respiratory control, or the presence of inflammatory mediators, such as those linking obesity to airway hyper-responsiveness. Weight loss (Chapter 227) is the optimal therapy, and it improves lung volumes, respiratory muscle performance, gas exchange, dyspnea, and sleep apnea. In individuals with obesity-hypoventilation

syndrome (Chapter 100), nocturnal positive-pressure ventilation can reverse gas exchange abnormalities.

PLEURA

The pleura, which is a thin membrane that covers the inner surfaces of the thoracic cavity, consists of a layer of mesothelial cells supported by a network of connective and fibroelastic tissue. The visceral pleura lines the lung, whereas the parietal pleura lines the rib cage, diaphragm, and mediastinal structures. The closed space between the visceral and parietal pleura is referred to as the pleural space. The vascular supply of the parietal pleural surface is from the systemic circulation, and it contains sensory nerves and lymphatics. By contrast, the visceral pleura is supplied with blood vessels from the pulmonary circulation and has no sensory nerves.

PLEURAL EFFUSION

EPIDEMIOLOGY AND PATHOBIOLOGY

The overall frequency of pleural effusion on a chest radiograph ranges from 0.3 to 1% but varies widely depending on the underlying disease. Pleural effusions occur most frequently in patients with pneumonia (Chapter 97) or heart failure (Chapter 58).

Normally, a small amount of fluid in the pleural space forms a thin layer between the visceral and parietal pleural surfaces and acts as a lubricant to minimize friction between the chest wall and lung as they move against each other during inspiration and expiration. There is continual movement of fluid into and out of the pleural space. This flux of fluid depends on the oncotic and hydrostatic pressures within the parietal and visceral pleura as well as the pressure within the pleural space itself. Hydrostatic pressure in the parietal pleura is similar to systemic circulation (30 cm H_2O), whereas that of the visceral pleura is similar to the pulmonary circulation (10 cm H_2O). Accordingly, most fluid in the pleural space is filtered from the higher-pressure vascular structures in the parietal pleura. Because the pressure within the pleural space itself is more subatmospheric at the apex than at the base, most of the fluid filters in from the less dependent upper lung zones. Fluid is drained out primarily through lymphatics in the parietal pleura. The fluid enters through lymphatic stomas on the surface of the parietal pleura, which are located beneath the mesothelial monolayer. The normal turnover of fluid within the pleural space is 10 to 20 mL/day, with only 0.2 to 1 mL remaining in the pleural space.

Under abnormal circumstances, fluid can accumulate within the pleural space. An increase in hydrostatic pressure, a decrease in oncotic pressure, decreased pressure in the pleural space, increased pleural membrane permeability, or obstruction of pleural lymphatics will promote pleural fluid accumulation (Table 99-3).

An increase in hydrostatic pressure or decrease in oncotic pressure will result in a low-protein collection of pleural fluid characterized as transudates (Table 99-4). For example, heart failure (Chapter 58) can produce transudates by increasing hydrostatic pressure in the pulmonary venous system, atelectasis (Chapter 90) can promote transudates by making pleural pressure more subatmospheric, and occasionally, oncotic pressure may be sufficiently reduced to cause transudates (e.g., with hypoalbuminemia). Changes in pleural membrane permeability can produce high-protein effusions, which are characterized as exudates and can be seen in inflammatory states such as pneumonia, tuberculosis, or rheumatoid arthritis. Tumors can disrupt the

TABLE 99-3 MECHANISMS PROMOTING PLEURAL FLUID ACCUMULATION

MICROVASCULAR CIRCULATION

Increased hydrostatic pressure (heart failure)
Decreased oncotic pressure (severe hypoalbuminemia)
Increased permeability (pneumonia)

PLEURAL SPACE

Decreased pressure (lung collapse)

LYMPHATICS

Impaired lymphatic drainage (malignant effusion)

DIAPHRAGM

Movement of fluid from the peritoneal space (hepatic hydrothorax)

TABLE 99-4 CONDITIONS THAT CAUSE PLEURAL EFFUSION

TRANSUDATES

Heart failure
Nephrotic syndrome
Hepatic hydrothorax
Superior vena cava syndrome
Peritoneal dialysis
Atelectasis
Urinothorax

EXUDATES

Parapneumonic effusions
   Simple
   Complicated
   Empyema
Other infections
   Tuberculosis
   Fungal
   Parasites
   Nocardia
Esophageal rupture
Malignancy
   Carcinoma
   Lymphoma
   Mesothelioma
   Metastatic disease

INFLAMMATORY DISORDERS

Connective tissue disease
   Rheumatoid arthritis
   Systemic lupus erythematosus
   Churg-Strauss syndrome
   Wegener's granulomatosis
   Familial Mediterranean fever
Abdominal disease
   Subdiaphragmatic abscess (hepatic, splenic)
   Pancreatitis, pancreatic pseudocyst
   Postoperative
Iatrogenic
   Drug induced
   Misplacement of enteral feeding tube
   Esophageal endoscopic interventions
Miscellaneous
   Asbestos exposure
   Atelectasis
   Cholesterol effusion
   Chylothorax
   Dressler's syndrome
   Meigs' syndrome
   Pulmonary embolus
   Radiation
   Sarcoidosis
   Trapped lung
   Uremia
   Yellow nail syndrome

integrity of the mesothelial layer or the integrity of the capillary epithelium, thereby resulting in exudative effusions, or they may block lymphatic drainage either through interference with stomal openings into the pleural space or obstruction of lymphatic channels.

CLINICAL MANIFESTATIONS

Patients with pleural effusions may be asymptomatic or may experience dyspnea. When the parietal pleura is actively inflamed, pain can be present, and it is generally unilateral, sharp, and worsens with inspiration. At times, effusions may be sufficiently large to contribute to respiratory failure. Physical findings include dullness to percussion in the area of the effusion, along with diminished breath sounds and absent tactile fremitus.

DIAGNOSIS

Chest radiography is often the first imaging method used to detect an effusion (Fig. 99-2). The volume of fluid in the pleural space needs to exceed 250 mL to be visualized on the chest radiograph. When an effusion is present, there is blunting of the costophrenic angle on the posteroanterior chest radiograph (Fig. 99-3), and a meniscus can be seen posteriorly on the lateral chest radiograph (see Fig. 99-2B). Fluid may also collect in either the minor or major fissures. Occasionally, pleural fluid collections in the major or minor fissures may appear as a pulmonary mass and are referred to as *pseudotumors*. A lateral decubitus chest radiograph can be obtained to determine whether fluid is free flowing or loculated. Chest CT provides much better characterization of pleural and parenchymal abnormalities by better defining loculated effusions, distinguishing between atelectasis and effusion, and distinguishing loculated effusion from lung abscess (Fig. 99-4).

FIGURE 99-3. Chest computed tomography showing pleural effusion in the same patient as in Fig. 99-2.

FIGURE 99-2. Patient with bilateral pleural effusions as seen on the posteroanterior radiograph of the chest (A) and lateral radiograph of the chest (B).

FIGURE 99-4. Computed tomographic angiogram of the chest in a patient with mesothelioma. There is diffuse thickening of the pleura and pericardium on the right with a rindlike appearance.

TABLE 99-6	CORRELATION OF THE CHARACTERISTICS OF PLEURAL EXUDATES WITH SPECIFIC DISEASE
TEST	**DISEASE**
pH < 7.2	Empyema, malignancy, esophageal rupture; rheumatoid, lupus, and tuberculous pleuritis
Glucose (<60 mg/dL)	Infection, rheumatoid pleurisy, tuberculous and lupus effusions, esophageal rupture
Amylase (>200 μg/dL)	Pancreatic disease, esophageal rupture, malignancy, ruptured ectopic pregnancy
RF, ANA, LE cells	Collagen vascular disease
↓ Complement	SLE, RA
RBCs (>5000/μL)	Trauma, malignancy, pulmonary embolus
Chylous effusion (triglycerides > 110 mg/dL)	Tuberculosis, disruption of thoracic duct (trauma, malignancy)
Cytology or biopsy (+)	Malignancy
ADA (>50 μg/L)	Tuberculosis

ADA = adenosine deaminase; ANA = antinuclear antibody; RA = rheumatoid arthritis; RBC = red blood cell; RF, rheumatoid factor; SLE = systemic lupus erythematosus.

TABLE 99-5	PLEURAL FLUID CHARACTERISTICS OF EXUDATES
LIGHT'S CRITERIA	
Protein	>0.5 pleural fluid/serum value
LDH	>0.6 pleural fluid/serum value
LDH	>2/3 upper limit of normal serum value
TWO-TEST RULE	
LDH	>0.45 upper limit of normal serum value
Cholesterol	>45 mg/dL
THREE-STEP CRITERIA	
LDH	>0.45 upper limit of normal serum value
Cholesterol	>45 mg/dL
Protein	>2.9 g/dL

LDH = lactate dehydrogenase.

A sample of fluid from the pleural space by thoracentesis is the key to determining the etiology of a pleural effusion. The tests needed to make a diagnosis require a relatively small amount of fluid (30 to 50 mL). Larger volumes of fluid can be removed (1 to 1.5 L) in an attempt to alleviate symptoms. Removing volumes greater than 1.5 L may result in re-expansion pulmonary edema. Most thoracenteses can be performed at the bedside, using ultrasound guidance to enhance the procedure's safety. In instances when the effusion is small or fluid is loculated, a CT scan can help direct the thoracentesis catheter into fluid that would otherwise be difficult to drain. Relative contraindications to a diagnostic thoracentesis include a bleeding diathesis, a very small volume of pleural fluid, and a low benefit-to-risk ratio.

Once fluid is obtained, a definitive diagnosis may be achieved, and the fluid can be classified as either a transudate or exudate (Table 99-5). To differentiate an exudate from a transudate, the pleural fluid needs to be analyzed for protein and lactate dehydrogenase (LDH). Simultaneous serum values of protein and LDH also need to be obtained. A pleural fluid exudate is characterized by a pleural fluid–to–serum protein ratio greater than 0.5, a pleural fluid–to–serum LDH ratio greater than 0.6, and a pleural fluid LDH greater than two thirds the normal serum value for LDH. An exudate can also be defined if the pleural fluid cholesterol is higher than 45 mg/dL, protein higher than 2.9 g/dL, or LDH higher than 0.45 upper limit of normal serum value.

Transudates

Effusions that accumulate owing to changes in osmotic and hydrostatic forces usually form transudates. Transudative effusions are most commonly due to heart failure, in which the effusions are often bilateral or, if unilateral, preferentially involve the right hemithorax. Transudates may also be seen in cirrhosis (Chapter 156), nephrotic syndrome (Chapter 123), myxedema (Chapter 233), pulmonary embolism (Chapter 98), superior vena caval obstruction, and peritoneal dialysis (Chapter 133). With cirrhosis, ascites may cross from the peritoneum into the pleural space through small defects in the diaphragm (hepatic hydrothorax) (see Table 99-4). Unusual causes of transudates include peritoneal dialysis and atelectasis. Although malignancy typically causes an exudate, it can occasionally produce a transudate. Urinothorax, which is a rare cause of transudate, results from obstruction of the urinary system.

Exudates

An effusion is characterized as an exudate if it meets one of the following criteria: pleural fluid–to–serum protein ratio higher than 0.5, pleural fluid–to–serum LDH ratio higher than 0.6, or a pleural fluid LDH concentration higher than two thirds the normal serum value. Cholesterol levels also may be increased in exudates (>45 mg/dL). The pleural fluid analysis helps distinguish among the causes of pleural exudates (Table 99-6).

Parapneumonic Effusions

Parapneumonic effusions, which are the most common type of exudative pleural effusion, occur in up to 40% of patients with pneumonia. They typically occur in patients with bacterial pneumonia (Chapter 97) and can be classified as uncomplicated or complicated. With uncomplicated parapneumonic effusion, the pH is generally greater than 7.3, the glucose content more than 60 mg/dL, and the pleural fluid LDH less than 1000 IU/L. Uncomplicated parapneumonic effusions are usually free flowing, do not require drainage, and will respond to the same antibiotic therapy as the pneumonia itself. However, uncomplicated parapneumonic effusions can, at times, transition to complicated effusions. Complicated effusions are characterized by a pH of less than 7.2 and often have a low glucose content. These effusions generally will not respond to antibiotic therapy alone but require drainage to prevent formation of an empyema or a thick pleural peal.

Empyema

An empyema is present when frank pus is aspirated from the pleural space or when the Gram stain of the fluid is positive for bacteria. Pneumonia due to *Streptococcus pneumoniae* (Chapter 297) or *Staphylococcus aureus* (Chapter 296) infection can cause empyema. Individuals who aspirate are at high risk for empyema caused by anaerobic organisms, and patients with tuberculosis (Chapter 332) can develop a tuberculous empyema. Methicillin-resistant staphylococci, *Klebsiella* species pneumonia, and *Pseudomonas* species infections may cause an empyema that is difficult to treat. Uncommon infectious causes of effusions include *Actinomyces* species (Chapter 337), *Nocardia* species (Chapter 338), amebiasis (Chapter 360), *Echinococcus* species (Chapter 362), and paragonimiasis (Chapter 364).

Individuals with empyema often complain of pleuritic chest pain and have refractory fevers several days or more into the course of their pneumonia, but immunocompromised patients may develop empyema sooner and more rapidly. When an empyema is present, it requires prompt chest tube drainage. If chest tube drainage is unsuccessful in resolving the empyema, video-assisted thoracic surgery (Chapter 101) is preferred, with intrapleural streptokinase reserved for patients who are poor candidates for video-assisted thoracic surgery or are in situations in which it is not available.[3]

Tuberculous Effusions

Tuberculosis (Chapter 332) can cause pleural effusion in up to 30% of patients who reside in endemic locations for tuberculosis. The pleural effusion typically is not due to direct mycobacterial infection itself, but rather to increased vascular permeability of the pleural membrane because of a hypersensitivity reaction to mycobacterial proteins. The pleural fluid is generally lymphocyte predominant and culture negative for acid-fast bacilli. Adenosine deaminase levels higher than 50 U/L may be helpful in identifying tuberculous pleural effusions. A tuberculous empyema, which is distinct from a tuberculous effusion, is characterized by direct extension of the infection from thoracic lymph nodes or hematogenous spread of tuberculosis into the pleural space.

Malignancy

Malignant effusions are the second most common cause of exudative pleural effusions. Rarely, a malignant effusion may be transudative. Lung cancer (Chapter 197) is the most frequent cause of malignant pleural effusion, and other malignancies that can involve the pleural space include breast cancer (Chapter 204), ovarian cancer (Chapter 205), gastric cancer (Chapter 198), and lymphoma (Chapters 191 and 192). When malignancy involves the pleural space, the prognosis is poor. However, the finding of a pleural effusion in an individual with underlying malignancy does not necessarily imply that there is a metastatic malignant process involving the pleural space. Benign effusions in patients with underlying malignancy may be due to atelectasis, postobstructive pneumonia, hypoalbuminemia, pulmonary emboli (Chapter 98), lymphatic obstruction, and complications from radiation (Chapter 19) or chemotherapy. For this reason, it is important to obtain a sample of pleural fluid in these individuals. The diagnosis of malignant pleural effusion is established by demonstrating malignant cells in the pleural fluid. Approximately 60% of malignant pleural effusions can be diagnosed with one thoracentesis, and the yield increases to 80% with repeat thoracenteses. If needed, a biopsy of the pleura may be useful in identifying the malignancy. Pleural biopsies are optimally obtained either by medical or surgical thoracoscopy (Chapter 101) rather than in a blind fashion (e.g., using a Cope or Abrams needle).

Systemic Inflammatory Disorders

Effusions may be seen in as many as 15% of patients with rheumatoid arthritis (Chapter 272), with a male preponderance to the development of effusions. Effusions typically appear within 5 years after the onset of disease but occasionally occur before the onset of joint disease. Rheumatoid factor in the pleural fluid is often greater than 1:320, and pleural fluid glucose is low (<60 mg/dL, or the pleural fluid–to–serum glucose ratio is <0.5). Other causes of low pleural fluid glucose include complicated parapneumonic effusions or empyema, malignant effusions, tuberculous pleurisy, lupus pleuritis, and esophageal rupture. Pleural effusions can be seen in 15 to 50% of patients with systemic lupus erythematosus (SLE). Lupus erythematosus cells and low levels of complement (C3 and C4) can be seen in effusions due to SLE. Wegener's granulomatosis, Sjögren's syndrome, and sarcoidosis are less common causes of pleural effusions.

Pancreatitis

Patients with pancreatitis or pancreatic pseudocysts (Chapter 146) may develop exudative pleural effusions that often involve the left hemithorax. A pleural fluid amylase concentration that is greater than the upper limits of normal for serum amylase is consistent with acute or chronic pancreatitis as a cause of the effusion. Amylase also may be seen in the pleural fluid with an esophageal rupture or malignancy. Pancreatic disease is associated with pancreatic isoenzyme amylase, whereas malignancy and esophageal rupture are characterized by a predominance of salivary amylase isoenzymes.

Chylothorax

A chylothorax has a milky-white appearance and is characterized by high levels of triglycerides (>110 mg/dL) and chylomicrons. A chylothorax is caused by leakage of lymph from the thoracic duct into the pleural space, most commonly related to mediastinal malignancy but also occurring after trauma to the thoracic duct. Major complications from a chylothorax are malnutrition and immunologic compromise when fat, protein, and lymphocytes are depleted by repeated thoracentesis or chest tube drainage. Chylous effusions must be distinguished from pseudochylous effusions,

which have a white appearance but are devoid of chylomicrons, and are indicative of a chronic long-standing effusion.

Hemothorax

Blood in the thorax is easily recognized during a thoracentesis. A hemothorax has a pleural fluid hematocrit that is at least half that of the circulating hematocrit. By contrast, a bloody pleural effusion will appear red but have a lower hematocrit. A bloody effusion often suggests a malignant process. Other causes include trauma, pulmonary infarction (Chapter 98), tuberculosis (Chapter 332), collagen vascular disease (Chapters 272 and 274), and hematologic disorders. Generally, blood removed from the pleural space does not clot, whereas blood due to the trauma of the thoracentesis itself will clot when collected. Because blood in the pleural space does not clot, it can be removed by lymphatics if the volume is small. Larger hemothoraces may require chest tube drainage.

Asbestos Exposure

Pleural effusion may occur following exposure to asbestos. The effusion is often small, unilateral, and serosanguineous, with fewer than 6000 cells/mL. The effusion tends to resolve within a year, resulting in pleural plaques that may calcify over time. Malignant mesothelioma should be excluded in these individuals.

Other Causes of Pleural Exudates

Meigs' syndrome is the triad of ovarian tumor (Chapter 205), ascites, and pleural effusion. The effusion, which is usually large and on the right side, is formed when fluid moves from the abdomen to the pleural space through diaphragmatic defects. Meigs' syndrome usually occurs in postmenopausal women and resolves following removal of the tumor.

Dressler's syndrome may occur from 3 to 30 days following open heart surgery or myocardial infarction. The patient usually experiences pleuritic pain and has a small to moderate left-sided effusion. Treatment is as for the accompanying pericardial effusion (Chapter 77).

Uremia (Chapter 132), which can cause a polyserositis with effusion, must be distinguished from the transudate that commonly is seen in the nephrotic syndrome (Chapter 123). Subdiaphragmatic processes, such as hepatic or splenic abscesses (Chapter 154), may cause effusions. Trapped lung occurs when a lobe or segment is unable to re-expand owing to a restrictive visceral pleural peel or an endobronchial mass. Increased negative intrapleural pressures associated with trapped lung promote the formation of an effusion. A number of drugs, including amiodarone, bleomycin, dantrolene, hydralazine, isoniazid, methotrexate, methysergide, mitomycin, procainamide, and procarbazine, can cause pleural effusions. Treatment consists of discontinuing the offending agent, although treatment with oral corticosteroids may be needed (Chapter 262).

TREATMENT AND PROGNOSIS   Rx

Empyemas and complicated parapneumonic effusions require drainage by tube thoracostomy in concert with appropriate antibiotic therapy. Treatment options for malignant pleural effusion include observation, chemical pleurodesis with talc or tetracycline derivatives, ambulatory drainage catheter, and treatment of underlying malignancy. A complete response occurs in perhaps 50% of patients. A low pleural fluid pH (<7.2) tends to impart a poor response to chemical pleurodesis. Malignant effusions with a tendency to respond to generalized chemotherapy include those related to breast cancer (Chapter 204) and small cell carcinoma of the lung (Chapter 197). Malignant effusions related to lymphomas and obstruction of lymphatic drainage of the pleural space may also respond to treatment of the underlying disease. Treatment of inflammatory effusions centers on the use of anti-inflammatory agents and corticosteroids (Chapters 272 and 274). Treatment of chylous effusions may involve chest tube drainage, although fat malnutrition may ensue. Attempts to decrease chyle formation can be accomplished by intravenous hyperalimentation, decreased oral fat intake, and the intake of medium- and light-chain fatty acids, which are absorbed directly into the portal circulation. Ligation of the thoracic duct should be considered for traumatic chylous effusions.

MESOTHELIOMA

EPIDEMIOLOGY AND PATHOBIOLOGY

Malignant mesotheliomas are neoplasms arising from the serosal membrane of body cavities. Eighty percent of mesotheliomas originate in the pleural space, and most others arise from the peritoneum. Individuals are usually older than 55 years and often have a history of asbestos exposure in the distant past (frequently, 30 to 40 years ago). Smoking is not a risk factor for developing mesothelioma, but smoking in concert with asbestos exposure increases the risk of lung cancer. Approximately 3000 cases of mesothelioma occur in the United States each year. The annual incidence is decreasing in the United States owing to better control of occupational exposure, but it may still be increasing in other countries where there are fewer regulations.

CLINICAL MANIFESTATIONS AND DIAGNOSIS

Patients with mesothelioma often complain of dyspnea, weight loss, and pain. Malignant mesothelioma may present as an extremely large mass or pleural effusion occupying the entire hemithorax at times. Chest CT may demonstrate either localized or circumferential pleural thickening associated with various amounts of calcified pleural plaque (see Fig. 99-4). Thoracoscopy is the most efficient means of obtaining the diagnosis. Elevated levels of hyaluronic acid in the pleural fluid, as well as special stains and electron microscopy of biopsy tissue, may help to make the difficult distinction between metastatic adenocarcinoma and mesothelioma.

A fraction of mesotheliomas are benign. Benign mesotheliomas are usually large and often pedunculated at the time of diagnosis.

TREATMENT AND PROGNOSIS   Rx

Unfortunately, no particular therapy, surgical or chemotherapy, has met with great success in malignant mesothelioma, and median survival is only 8 to 12 months after diagnosis.◢ Pleurodesis with talc or pleurectomy is usually performed for palliation and control of symptoms related to any pleural effusion. In highly selected patients with localized disease and no comorbid illnesses, surgical resection or radical extrapleural pneumonectomy may be attempted. Radiation therapy can provide symptom palliation and has been used following attempts at curative surgery. Treatment of benign mesothelioma involves surgical resection.

● PNEUMOTHORAX

Pneumothorax refers to the accumulation of air in the pleural space. Normally, the pressure within the pleural space is slightly subatmospheric. However, when more than a very small amount of air accumulates within the pleural space, pressure within it becomes positive, and there is compression of underlying lung.

EPIDEMIOLOGY AND PATHOBIOLOGY

Pneumothorax is often associated with blunt or penetrating trauma. With penetrating trauma, air may leak into the pleural space through the injured chest wall or into the pleural space from the injured lung. Patients with underlying lung disease undergoing mechanical ventilation may acutely develop a pneumothorax when high local pressures disrupt lung tissue, thereby leading to a leak (Chapter 105).

Pneumothorax also may occur spontaneously or be secondary to underlying lung disease. Typically, spontaneous pneumothorax occurs in tall, young, thin men, presumably as a result of rupture of preexisting apical blebs. Diseases that are associated with pneumothorax include emphysema (Chapter 88), cystic fibrosis (Chapter 89), granulomatous inflammation, necrotizing pneumonia, pulmonary fibrosis (Chapter 92), eosinophilic granulomatous disease, sarcoidosis (Chapter 95), and endometriosis (Chapter 244).

CLINICAL MANIFESTATIONS AND DIAGNOSIS

Symptoms typically include acute shortness of breath and sharp chest pain. Physical examination is characterized by tachycardia, decreased breath sounds, decreased tactile fremitus, a pleural friction rub, subcutaneous emphysema, hyper-resonance to percussion, and a tracheal shift toward the uninvolved hemithorax.

Air within the pleural space will separate the visceral from parietal pleura and appears as an area of lucency on the chest radiograph (Fig. 99-5). With a small pneumothorax, the lucency is best appreciated at the lung apex when the patient is upright (see Fig. 84-11 in Chapter 84). An end-expiratory radiograph is particularly helpful in diagnosing a small pneumothorax. During expiration, the density of the lung will increase because of a reduction in volume, thereby highlighting the difference between lung parenchymal and pleural gas. When a portable chest radiograph is obtained with the patient in the supine position, such as a patient in an intensive care unit, the lucent area may be most noticeable over the lower rib cage (superior sulcus sign).

FIGURE 99-5. A portable anteroposterior chest radiograph demonstrating a right-sided pneumothorax. Note that the right lung has collapsed to less than half the size of the right hemithorax. In addition, there is a pneumoperitoneum best seen as a collection of air under the right hemidiaphragm.

A tension pneumothorax is defined as a pneumothorax associated with a mediastinal shift and hemodynamic compromise, usually because high intrathoracic pressures compress the vena cava and atrium. This physiology implies an ongoing leak of air into the pleural space.

TREATMENT AND PROGNOSIS   Rx

If the pneumothorax is small and the patient is not in distress, tube thoracostomy is not needed, and observation alone may be sufficient. If a pneumothorax occupies more than 50% of the hemithorax, the patient develops symptoms, or a tension pneumothorax develops, tube thoracostomy and suction followed by water-seal drainage are indicated. If there is a continuing leak despite tube thoracostomy, a bronchopleural fistula may be suspected. In this instance, chemical pleurodesis or surgical correction, usually by video-assisted thorascopic surgery, may be necessary (Chapter 101).

● MEDIASTINUM

The mediastinum, which is the central part of the thoracic cavity, lies between the right and left lung. It contains the heart and aorta, esophagus, trachea, lymph nodes, thymus, and great vessels. It is bordered by the two pleural cavities laterally, the diaphragm inferiorly, and the thoracic inlet superiorly.

● MEDIASTINAL MASSES

PATHOBIOLOGY

For clinical purposes, the mediastinum has been divided into three compartments: anterior, middle, and posterior (E-Fig. 99-2). The anterior compartment contains the thymus, substernal extensions of the thyroid, blood vessels, pericardium, and lymph nodes. The middle compartment contains the heart, great vessels, trachea, main bronchi, lymph nodes, and the phrenic and vagal nerves. The posterior compartment contains the vertebrae, descending aorta, esophagus, thoracic duct, azygous and hemizygous veins, lower portion of the vagus, sympathetic chain, and lymph nodes.

CLINICAL MANIFESTATIONS

Mediastinal masses usually are not accompanied by symptoms, and most masses are incidentally found on either a chest radiograph or a chest CT scan. If present, however, symptoms include chest pain, cough, hoarseness, stridor, dysphasia, and dyspnea. One third of patients with a mediastinal thymoma have symptoms or weakness owing to myasthenia gravis (Chapter 430), and individuals with mediastinal lymphoma (Chapters 191 and 192) may have systemic symptoms such as fever, night sweats, and weight loss. Occasionally, a mass may produce superior vena cava obstruction with resultant facial edema and dilated neck and chest veins (Fig. 99-6).

DIAGNOSIS

Once a mass is identified by chest radiography or chest CT, further evaluation is mandatory. If a benign process is suspected, a follow-up CT may be

FIGURE 99-6. Superior vena cava obstruction in bronchial carcinoma. Note the swelling of the face and neck and the development of collateral circulation in the veins of the chest wall.

FIGURE 99-7. Chest computed tomography of a patient with an anterior mediastinal mass that proved to be a substernal goiter.

TABLE 99-7 CAUSES OF MEDIASTINAL MASSES

ANTERIOR	MIDDLE	POSTERIOR
Teratoma	Pericardial cyst	Neurogenic tumor
Thymoma	Lymph node hyperplasia	Esophageal tumor
Thyroid tumor	Bronchogenic tumor	Bronchogenic tumor
Goiter	Bronchogenic cyst	Bronchogenic cyst
Aneurysm	Aneurysm	Aneurysm
Lymphoma	Lymphoma	Lymphoma
Parathyroid tumor		Meningocele
Lipoma		Enteric cyst
Morgagni's diaphragm hernia		Esophageal diverticula
		Bochdalek's diaphragm hernia

indicated. If a malignant process is suspected, radiologic evaluation may include angiography, positron emission tomography, or magnetic resonance imaging. Biopsies can be obtained either with mediastinoscopy, mediastinotomy, or ultrasound-guided transbronchial needle aspiration biopsy. Direct sampling by transthoracic CT-guided needle aspiration may be useful in evaluating anterior or posterior mediastinal masses. The evaluation and differential diagnosis of mediastinal masses are guided by the compartment in which they arise (Table 99-7). The *anterior mediastinal compartment* includes lesions such as thymomas, germ cell tumors (teratomas), lymphomas, and intrathoracic thyroid tissue. Thymomas make up about 20% of mediastinal neoplasms in adults, in whom they are the most common anterior mediastinal primary neoplasm. Patients with systemic lymphoma often have involvement of the mediastinum, but only 5 to 10% of patients with lymphoma present with primary mediastinal lesions. Teratomas, which account for 10% of mediastinal tumors, may contain squamous cells, hair follicles, sweat glands, cartilage, and linear calcifications; about one third are malignant. Intrathoracic goiters (Chapter 233) (Fig. 99-7) may compress the trachea and cause stridor, cough, dyspnea, and, occasionally, superior vena cava obstruction. Anterior masses in the right cardiophrenic angle, which are rare and may be associated with pericardial defects or obesity, may be due to herniation of liver or intestinal contents through the foramina of Morgagni.

In the posterior mediastinum, neurogenic tumors are the most common lesions. Many of these tumors are benign and originate in the nerve sheath or sympathetic ganglion cells (ganglioneuroma). Posterior mediastinal masses also include cysts, meningocele, lymphoma (Chapter 191 and 192), aortic aneurysm (Chapter 78), and esophageal disorders (Chapter 140) such as diverticula and neoplasm. Herniation of abdominal contents into the thorax can result in posterior mediastinal masses. Herniation of abdominal contents through the foramina of Bochdalek results in a mass in the posterolateral area of the diaphragm, usually on the left side; it is the most common congenital hernia and may contain spleen or kidney. Herniation of the stomach through the esophageal hiatus (Chapter 140), which is the most common type of diaphragmatic herniation, produces a mass posterior to the heart, often with an air-fluid level.

Benign cysts can occur in the anterior, middle, or posterior compartments. Pericardial cysts, which are often located in the cardiophrenic angle, contain clear liquid. Bronchogenic cysts occur in the middle or posterior compartments and are filled with liquid and lined with respiratory epithelium; they often develop around the paratracheal area or carina and do not communicate with the tracheal bronchial tree.

TREATMENT

The treatment of a mediastinal mass depends on the underlying pathology. Some lesions, such as thymomas, teratomas, cysts, neurogenic tumors, and hernias, require surgical resection. Others, such as lymphoma, are treated with radiation or chemotherapy. Some can be monitored over time.

MEDIASTINITIS

Acute mediastinitis is most commonly caused by bacterial infection. Mediastinal infections may be iatrogenic after sternotomy or invasive procedures involving the esophagus or tracheobronchial tree. Rupture of the esophagus or trachea from trauma or tissue necrosis can cause mediastinitis. Treatment of acute mediastinitis requires antibiotics, pleural drainage, and evacuation of necrotic tissue. Chronic mediastinitis (fibrosing mediastinitis) is a progressive illness that may be idiopathic or can be caused by granulomatous infection, neoplasm, radiotherapy, or drugs (such as methysergide). Patients with chronic mediastinitis remain asymptomatic until vascular or neurologic structures are affected, and the diagnosis and treatment often require surgical exploration.

PNEUMOMEDIASTINUM

Pneumomediastinum occurs when air infiltrates the mediastinal structures after a rupture of the esophagus, trachea, or lung dissects into the mediastinum. Loss of esophageal or tracheal integrity often results from trauma, whereas leaks from alveoli may result from trauma, occur spontaneously, or be a complication of mechanical ventilation. The diagnosis can be made by seeing thin columns of hyperlucency between mediastinal structures on chest radiography or CT scan. Pneumomediastinum may present as a sore throat, neck pain, or shortness of breath. Often, the mediastinal air dissects into the subcutaneous tissues of the neck and chest wall, where it results in subcutaneous emphysema. A characteristic crepitus is palpable when subcutaneous emphysema is present. Spontaneous pneumomediastinum generally resolves without treatment. When more severe collections of subcutaneous air occur, surgical decompression is often warranted.

1. Consensus Conference. Clinical indications for noninvasive positive pressure ventilation in chronic respiratory failure due to restrictive lung disease, COPD, and nocturnal hypoventilation—a consensus conference report. *Chest.* 1999;116:521-534.

2. van der Heijde D, Kivitz A, Schiff MH, et al. Efficacy and safety of adalimumab in patients with ankylosing spondylitis: results of a multicenter, randomized, double-blind, placebo-controlled trial. *Arthritis Rheum.* 2006;54:2136-2146.
3. Maskell N, Davies C, Nunn A, et al. U.K. controlled trial of intrapleural streptokinase for pleural infection. *N Engl J Med.* 2005;351:865-874.
4. Muers MF, Stephens RJ, Fisher P, et al. Symptom control with or without chemotherapy in the treatment of patients with malignant pleural mesothelioma (MS01): a multicentre randomized trial. *Lancet.* 2008;371:1685-1694.

SUGGESTED READINGS

Mishra EK, Davies RJ. Advances in the investigation and treatment of pleural effusions. *Expert Rev Respir Med.* 2010;4:123-133. *Review.*
Uzbeck MH, Almeida FA, Sarkiss MG, et al. Management of malignant pleural effusions. *Adv Ther.* 2010;27:334-347. *Review of pharmaceutical and nonpharmaceutical approaches.*
Volpicelli G. Sonographic diagnosis of pneumothorax. *Intensive Care Med.* 2011;37:224-232. *Ultrasound can accurately diagnose or exclude pneumothorax at the bedside in most patients.*

OBSTRUCTIVE SLEEP APNEA

ROBERT C. BASNER

DEFINITION

Obstructive sleep apnea (OSA) is a chronic condition of cyclic obstruction of the upper airway during sleep, combined with associated symptoms or signs of disturbed sleep (Chapter 412), the most common being excessive daytime sleepiness and loud snoring. A frequency of at least five obstructive events per hour of sleep is a minimal criterion for diagnosing OSA in adults, although a higher frequency of obstructive events is more consistently correlated with an increased risk of cardiovascular and neurocognitive disorders.

EPIDEMIOLOGY

OSA is underrecognized by clinicians and underreported by patients. It is estimated that most adults with moderate to severe OSA remain undiagnosed. In adults, OSA is characteristically found in overweight persons, although other anatomic (primarily upper airway and craniofacial) and ventilatory abnormalities may also predispose to development of the syndrome. The presence of at least five obstructive events per hour of sleep has been found in 9 to 28% of persons without specific risk factors for, or symptoms of, OSA. Its overall prevalence appears to be much greater in men than in women, but postmenopausal and obese women are at increased risk. Populations with a particularly high prevalence of OSA include those older than 60 years; patients with systemic hypertension, particularly those with poorly controlled hypertension (Chapter 67); patients who have had strokes (Chapter 414); patients with heart failure (Chapter 58); and patients with medically refractory epilepsy (Chapter 410). African Americans, particularly those younger than 25 and older than 65 years; adult Hispanics; and Asians have a higher incidence and/or greater severity of OSA than whites. There is a strong familial disposition to OSA, such that the presence of OSA in a given patient more than doubles the chance of family members having the disorder when compared with controls. Mean annual medical costs for patients with untreated OSA are almost double those of otherwise normal people, and the costs increase in proportion to the severity of the OSA.

PATHOBIOLOGY

Genetics

Most identified candidate genes linked to OSA share linkages to body mass index (BMI). Similarly, most polymorphic DNA sequences related to expression of OSA appear to be linked to characteristics that predispose to the disorder, including obesity, serotonin transport, and craniofacial structure, or to correlates of the disorder, such as elevated blood pressure. Thus, no specific genes or genetic loci for OSA have been identified to date.

Pathogenesis

OSA involves complete or partial closure of the collapsible segments of the pharynx, including the velopharynx, oropharynx, and hypopharynx.

Obstructive apnea is defined by absent airflow for at least 10 seconds associated with continued ventilatory effort. Partial obstruction is referred to as *hypopnea* and is recognized functionally by a discrete decrease in rather than cessation of airflow for at least 10 seconds, associated with either a pathologic decrease in the oxygen saturation of hemoglobin (SaO_2) or an abrupt arousal from sleep, typically with progressive ventilatory effort and/or crescendo snoring. Respiratory effort–related arousal occurs when such limitations of airflow and decrease in SaO_2 are not severe enough to cause hypopnea but the progressive ventilatory effort is nevertheless associated with abrupt arousal from sleep.

Both excess weight and increasing weight are closely linked to the development of OSA and the worsening of existing OSA in adults. Conversely, weight loss, both surgical and nonsurgical, has been associated with improvement in OSA (see Treatment). Anatomic and physiologic explanations of how excess weight contributes to OSA include restriction of chest wall movement, with resultant mechanical and reflex upper airway narrowing; increased compliance and narrowing of the upper airway; ventilatory instability; and impaired ability to compensate for increased upper airway resistance at sleep onset.

The final common pathway in each obstructive event is attainment of a critical pharyngeal closing pressure. Once collapsed, the pharynx is more difficult to expand during the next inspiratory effort, resulting in the characteristic generation of progressively more forceful inspiratory efforts against the obstructed upper airway and increasingly negative intrathoracic pressure excursions. The subsequent arousal is usually associated with reopening of the airway. After several hyperpneic breaths, re-transition into sleep generally occurs. The cycling of blood gases and the recurrent awake-to-asleep transitions interfere with the respiratory controllers' need to find a set point during sleep. Hypopnea or outright apnea followed by hyperpnea is the hallmark of OSA.

The pathogenic importance of respiratory periodicity in OSA varies by sleep stage (Chapter 412). The transition into "light" stages of sleep, termed *stages N1 and N2 non–rapid eye movement* (NREM) *sleep*, is characterized by a tendency for arousal and sleep-wake cycling. These stages are most likely to demonstrate the periodic obstructive events characteristic of OSA. In contrast, "deep" NREM sleep, termed *stage N3* or *slow-wave sleep*, is characteristically a time of relatively regular central nervous system output, with a decreased tendency for arousal, a regularization of breathing, and a relative paucity of obstructive events, even with generally increased upper airway resistance when compared with N1 and N2 sleep. During rapid eye movement (REM) sleep, descending neural inhibition of accessory respiratory muscles may lead to severe alveolar hypoventilation. Severe hypoxemia, caused by a combination of obstructive events and ventilation-perfusion mismatch, is characteristic of REM sleep in patients with OSA.

Pathophysiology

With each obstructive event, the combination of progressive asphyxia, increasingly negative intrathoracic pressure, and sudden autonomic and behavioral arousal leads to acute cardiac and cerebrovascular perturbations, including increased afterload of both the left and right ventricles, decreased left ventricular compliance, increased pulmonary artery pressure, decreased coronary artery blood flow, and increased myocardial oxygen demand (Chapter 52). The abrupt arousal at the termination of the majority of obstructive events is associated with sympathetic discharge, leading to peripheral vasoconstriction and an abrupt increase in the heart rate and in systolic and diastolic blood pressure, even as cardiac output continues to fall when ventilation resumes with the airway reopened. Accordingly, systemic blood pressure characteristically fluctuates; it is relatively low during apnea and acutely elevated at termination of the obstructive event (Chapter 67). Electrocardiographic abnormalities include sinus bradycardia during obstructive events and acceleration at arousal; in REM sleep, which is a time of increased vagal tone, sinoatrial and atrioventricular block may be seen. Ventricular and supraventricular ectopy and atrial fibrillation occur with OSA. At the termination of obstructive apnea, cerebral blood flow and oxygenation are decreased. The recurrent abrupt, transient arousal from sleep at the termination of each obstructive event is associated with fragmented sleep and a decreased ability to consolidate restorative sleep.

CLINICAL MANIFESTATIONS

Symptoms and Signs

The cardinal manifestations of OSA include loud, chronic snoring; excessive daytime somnolence; and apneas witnessed by third parties. Snoring in OSA reflects vibratory noise from partially occluded pharyngeal soft tissue, usually

FIGURE 100-1. Polysomnographic tracing of a patient with obstructive sleep apnea during 2 minutes of non–rapid eye movement sleep. Displayed are airflow in the upper airway ("nasal flow"), recorded with a nasal pressure transducer; respiratory effort ("abdomen"), recorded by inductance plethysmography; and oxygen saturation of hemoglobin (SpO$_2$), recorded with pulse oximetry.

with the mouth open, and it typically occurs in a crescendo pattern, with a burst of louder noise at resolution of the event. Loud snoring without OSA may progress to OSA, particularly if the patient gains weight.

In the hospital setting, OSA may be detected because of apnea or refractory decreases in SaO$_2$ during surgical or endoscopic procedures that require sedation or anesthesia. In other cases, the diagnosis may be suspected when hospital staff note nocturnal heart block or dysrhythmias during sleep.

Excessive Daytime Somnolence
Patients with excessive daytime somnolence (Chapter 412) fall asleep unexpectedly; this is typically microsleep rather than sustained sleep episodes. Excessive daytime somnolence may be quantified by laboratory tests that monitor the propensity to fall asleep during the day or by questionnaires or subjective scales that assess sleepiness or decrements in quality of life. Resolution of OSA does not necessarily resolve excessive daytime somnolence, suggesting the possibility of sustained neurologic perturbation from chronic intermittent hypoxemia. However, many patients with significant OSA do not complain of excessive daytime somnolence, nor are patients typically aware of their degree of sleep fragmentation. Mood disorders, including depression and irritability, as well as perturbations in visual memory and working memory appear to be related to the severity of sleep fragmentation and hypoxemia.

Obstructed Breathing
The bed partners of OSA patients often describe breathing cessation rather than obstructed breathing; close questioning usually elicits the obstructive nature of the breathing. Patients may be aware of their own snoring or complain of choking or dyspnea, particularly in relation to an inability to sleep supine. Morning dry mouth is a common symptom, as is morning headache.

Insomnia and Parasomnia
Insomnia, which is the subjective complaint of difficulty falling asleep or staying asleep (Chapter 412), is associated with the consistent sleep interruption characteristic of OSA. Transient arousals during N3 sleep may result in confusional parasomnias, such as sleep walking and sleep talking. Arousals and increased work of breathing may result in restless sleep and night sweats. Nocturia, possibly mediated via atrial natriuretic receptors, may resolve with treatment of OSA.

Upper Airway Abnormalities
Nasal congestion, rhinitis, chronic sinusitis, and nasopharyngeal anatomic abnormalities are often associated with OSA, as are craniofacial abnormalities such as micrognathia and retrognathia. Large tonsils, redundant soft palate tissue, and a large tongue may all be associated with a "crowded" oropharynx, but the precise role of these upper airway abnormalities in the pathogenesis of adult OSA is unclear.

DIAGNOSIS
The spectrum of sleep-related breathing disorders other than OSA includes hypoventilation and gas exchange disorders that may worsen with sleep, including nocturnal asthma (Chapter 87), chronic obstructive pulmonary disease (Chapter 88), neuromuscular and chest wall disorders (Chapter 99), and obesity-hypoventilation syndrome (Chapter 227), as well as other disorders in which central apnea (Chapter 412) is prominent, such as idiopathic central apnea, Cheyne-Stokes breathing, and central alveolar hypoventilation

(Chapter 86). Patients with OSA alone characteristically do not hypoventilate while awake, unlike patients with other disorders of hypoventilation. Disorders associated with hypersomnia, such as narcolepsy, insufficient sleep, poor sleep hygiene, periodic limb movement disorder, and circadian rhythm disorders such as shift work sleep disorder, must also be considered in patients with suspected OSA (Chapter 412).

Polysomnography
The definitive diagnostic study is polysomnography (Fig. 100-1), which generally involves all-night monitoring in a sleep laboratory via electroencephalography, electro-oculography (primarily to determine rapid eye movements characteristic of REM sleep), electrocardiography, leg and chin electromyography, and measures of respiratory effort, airflow, SaO$_2$, and alveolar or arterial carbon dioxide (usually end-tidal or transcutaneous CO$_2$). Audiovisual recordings can identify crescendo snoring and thoracoabdominal paradoxical breathing efforts to help differentiate obstructive from nonobstructive hypopnea.

The severity of OSA is usually described by the apnea-hypopnea index (AHI), which is the number of obstructive apneas plus hypopneas per hour of sleep (Fig. 100-2). The term *respiratory disturbance index* includes obstructive apneas and hypopneas, as well as obstructive events that do not meet the threshold for hypopnea but nevertheless result in a discrete arousal that appears to be associated with abnormal indices of oxygen desaturation. Oxygen desaturation more directly reflects the chronic intermittent hypoxia that has been increasingly linked to adverse cardiovascular effects and outcomes.

It is possible to diagnose OSA by means of unattended home studies that include cardiorespiratory monitoring and/or use of an autotitrating positive airway pressure (PAP) machine, which continuously self-adjusts the level of positive pressure delivered to the airway on a breath-to-breath basis in response to upper airway impedance changes. Such autotitration allows the immediate diagnosis and treatment of a patient suspected of having severe OSA.

TREATMENT   Rx

The goal of treatment is to decrease sleep fragmentation and repetitive asphyxia, the resultant cardiovascular and cerebrovascular stress, and the increased work of breathing associated with OSA.

Mechanical Therapy
Positive Airway Pressure
PAP, which is the current first-line therapy for OSA, consistently lowers the AHI, decreases oxygen desaturation, decreases diurnal and nocturnal blood pressure, and improves sleep efficiency, daytime sleepiness, and quality of life at a reasonable cost compared with oral appliances or no treatment,[1] especially in patients with an AHI greater than 30/hour. For patients with less severe OSA, continuous positive airway pressure (CPAP) is generally recommended in those with prominent oxygen desaturation, daytime sleepiness, or concurrent respiratory, cardiovascular, or cerebrovascular disease. CPAP improves cognitive function, improves left ventricular function in patients with heart failure and decreases the risk of motor vehicle accidents.

The major equipment required to administer PAP includes an interface with appropriate headgear, anchoring straps, and hosing and a compact airflow generator (Fig. 100-3). With CPAP, the fixed level of positive pressure delivered to the upper airway acts as a physiologic splint throughout the respiratory cycle, allowing the patient to achieve normal ventilation as well as more continuous and deeper sleep. CPAP does not supply ventilation above this

FIGURE 100-2. Continuous 10-minute polysomnographic tracing in a patient with severe obstructive sleep apnea. The 14 repetitive obstructive apneas constitute an apnea-hypopnea index of 84/hour. Each obstructive event is associated with a cyclic waxing-waning respiratory effort (seen in the thoracic and abdominal effort tracings), absent airflow (in the nasal pressure transducer), electroencephalographic arousal (C3-A2, top tracing), oxygen desaturation, and increased end-tidal PCO_2.

A   B   C

FIGURE 100-3. Positive airway pressure–patient interfaces. **A**, Subject wearing a nasal mask and headgear with positive airway pressure being delivered. Positive pressure is delivered only to the nasal airway; opening of the mouth may cause air to leak and decrease the efficacy of the positive-pressure regimen. **B**, Subject wearing nasal pillows. Positive pressure is delivered directly into the nares rather than covering the nose or mouth; only minimal headgear is necessary to anchor the interface in place. **C**, Subject wearing a full face mask. Positive pressure is delivered to both the nose and the mouth based on the subject's own breath-to-breath partitioning of nasal and oral airflow.

splinting; the positive end-expiratory pressure may, however, result in improved oxygenation.

Prescribing PAP

PAP is typically prescribed after therapeutic titration in the sleep laboratory, beginning with CPAP of 2 to 4 cm H_2O and increasing by 1- to 2-cm H_2O increments to the minimum level that eliminates obstructive events in all sleep stages. Such a level should reduce other evidence of increased upper airway resistance and increased work of breathing (e.g., snoring, use of accessory inspiratory muscles, thoracoabdominal paradoxical respiration), while improving sleep. Although CPAP is typically prescribed in the 8- to 12-cm H_2O range, it is not uncommon for patients with severe OSA to need pressures up to 20 cm H_2O. However, as pressures increase above 12 to 14 cm H_2O, the likelihood of air leak and discomfort rises. When laboratory titration is not available, starting CPAP at a level of 10 cm H_2O is reasonable. Short-term outcomes, including AHI, symptomatic sleepiness, and quality of life, are similar, regardless of whether CPAP is guided by titration at a sleep center or use of an autotitrating machine at home to determine a fixed pressure.[2,3] Adding a feature that decreases expiratory pressure ("pressure relief") does not improve outcomes or adherence or reduce side effects.[4]

The first night of CPAP is generally associated with a "rebound" of slow-wave NREM sleep and REM sleep, along with amelioration of acute fluctuations in heart rate and blood pressure. Daytime sleepiness and vigilance consistently improve with chronic use of CPAP; diurnal and nocturnal blood pressure and catecholamine levels decrease, and left ventricular ejection fraction and diastolic function improve. However, OSA returns when CPAP is removed, so CPAP must be used nightly throughout sleep. The term *complex sleep apnea* refers to the commonly noted emergence of central apneas during initial CPAP titration; the significance of this phenomenon remains to be elucidated.

Bilevel PAP

In some cases, a more ventilatory mode of pressure delivery—generally, bilevel PAP, wherein inspiratory pressure is set higher than expiratory pressure—may be helpful after the degree of expiratory positive pressure necessary to prevent closure of the airway during expiration is established. Bilevel PAP may be delivered with a backup rate, similar to assist/control mode ventilation. Bilevel PAP should be considered in those with hypoventilation syndromes that overlap OSA, such as obese patients who continue to have significant hypoventilation or ventilation-perfusion mismatch–related hypoxemia despite CPAP. For most OSA patients beginning treatment, however, no high-quality data show improved outcomes or cost-effectiveness of bilevel PAP compared with CPAP, even when bilevel PAP is used as secondary therapy when CPAP is unsuccessful; numerous randomized controlled trials have demonstrated similar adherence with CPAP and bilevel PAP.[5]

Autotitrating PAP

Both CPAP and bilevel PAP can be delivered so that the pressure automatically adjusts to the patient's breathing, based on either breath-to-breath detection of changes in airway resistance or the pattern of breathing. However, autotitrating PAP does not improve adherence or outcomes compared with fixed-pressure CPAP.[5]

PAP-Patient Interface

The choice of interface is important for achieving optimal efficacy and adherence. Aside from many different shapes, sizes, and consistencies of nasal masks (Fig. 100-3A), flexible nasal "pillows" or "prongs" (Fig. 100-3B) can fit directly into the nares, avoiding the discomfort of a mask over the nose and pain and pressure at the bridge of the nose and over the upper teeth. Although nasal PAP is most commonly used, nasal delivery is often ineffective because of nasal congestion, nasopharyngeal anatomic abnormalities, or inability to keep the mouth closed, allowing air to leak from the mouth so that ineffective pressure is delivered to the collapsible airway. Soft "hybrid" interfaces, which have a mouthpiece and nasal prongs to permit both mouth and nose breathing, are often used in such settings. Full face masks (Fig. 100-3C) may also improve CPAP efficacy in such situations, but gastrointestinal bloating secondary to air swallowing is a common side effect, and the risks of vomiting and aspiration are a concern. Regardless of the interface used, the patient must be vigilant to maintain the interface throughout sleep, particularly after changes in position. Cold or heated humidification may be added directly to the circuit to improve comfort and adherence, but contamination of the humidifier with pathogenic organisms must be avoided.

Adherence and Outcome

Adherence to PAP is generally similar to that for treatments of other chronic medical disorders, although most studies suggest that CPAP is not used optimally for maximizing restorative sleep. Adherence may be improved by systematic cognitive behavioral and educational strategies, as well as strategies that address the specific issues of individual patients.[6] Treatment with PAP should be objectively monitored by tracking the amount of time that physiologically successful PAP levels are delivered.

Oxygen

Although supplemental oxygen alone during sleep may ameliorate hypoxemia and improve sleep quality in OSA, such treatment alone may lengthen apneas, cause paradoxical worsening of SaO_2, and fail to improve sleep fragmentation. Therefore, oxygen alone should not be used as first-line treatment for suspected or proven OSA without nocturnal monitoring.

When sleep SaO_2 remains low despite otherwise optimal levels of CPAP or bilevel PAP, oxygen can be added directly to the mask, to an adapter near the mask, or beneath the mask via nasal cannulae. Higher flow rates of oxygen may be necessary as PAP levels increase, particularly if bilevel PAP is used.

Other Ways to Relieve or Bypass Obstruction

Oral appliances, usually in the form of mandibular advancement devices fitted by an expert, improve symptoms in patients with mild to moderate OSA, particularly with predominantly supine OSA. However, such devices are generally less effective than CPAP in improving AHI and oxygen desaturation during sleep,[7] and they are currently recommended only for patients with mild or moderate OSA who do not benefit from CPAP or who prefer such an appliance over CPAP.

General Measures

Sleep Positioning and Nasal Treatments

Sleep positioning may benefit many patients who have OSA predominantly in the supine position, although such positioning does not appear to be as effective as CPAP in decreasing the AHI.[8] Treatment of chronic nasal congestion and inflammation with nasal steroids, saline washes, and systemic antihistamine-decongestant regimens may ameliorate OSA in many cases. Otolaryngologic consultation can be useful to identify treatable nasopharyngeal disorders, including the rare nasopharyngeal neoplasm.

Weight Loss

Weight loss is a primary treatment in an overweight patient with OSA. It not only affects the severity of the breathing disorder during sleep but also may contribute to regression of the deleterious metabolic and cardiovascular perturbations associated with OSA. In obese diabetic patients with a mean BMI greater than 35 kg/m², an intensive lifestyle intervention resulting in a mean weight loss of 10.8 kg produced a significantly greater decrease in the number of apneic-hypopneic events per hour, less oxygen desaturation during sleep, and a better resolution rate of OSA than was achieved in a control group with a mean weight loss of 0.6 kg.[9] Non–morbidly obese patients who achieve nonsurgical weight loss also have significantly greater improvements in OSA than do controls without such weight loss. In severely obese patients with marked OSA, weight loss achieved with bariatric surgery significantly ameliorates but usually does not resolve OSA.[10]

Treatment of Other Underlying Conditions

It is important to treat underlying conditions such as diabetes (Chapter 237) and heart failure (Chapter 59) in patients with OSA, but such treatment does not substitute for treating the OSA itself. For example, in patients with OSA and heart failure, cardiac atrial overdrive pacing provides small improvements in the AHI and sleep-related oxygen desaturation, but it is not as effective as CPAP.

Surgery

Tracheostomy

Tracheostomy, which bypasses the site of upper airway obstruction, decreases morbidity and mortality and improves blood gas abnormalities in OSA. However, tracheostomy makes speech difficult and is reserved for only the most severe cases and for patients with concomitant hypoventilation syndromes that do not respond to noninvasive forms of PAP.

Uvulopalatopharyngoplasty

Procedures to reduce uvular or palatal tissue, which were once widely recommended, have not shown a consistent benefit in high-quality studies.[11] As a result, surgical uvulopalatopharyngoplasty, radio frequency volumetric tissue reduction of the palate or tongue (or both), and laser-assisted uvuloplasty are not recommended as first-line therapy to treat symptomatic OSA patients.

Medical Therapy

At this time, there is no acceptably efficacious pharmacologic therapy for OSA. Respiratory stimulants, including medroxyprogesterone and acetazolamide, have not proved effective in patients with normal $PaCO_2$ levels. Selective serotonin re-uptake inhibitors, including fluoxetine and paroxetine, have been associated with a decreased apnea index during NREM but not REM sleep in a small number of patients. Tricyclic antidepressants have shown some utility in predominantly REM sleep–associated OSA by decreasing REM volume, although side effects have hindered the use of such agents. Hormone replacement therapy may ameliorate the breathing disorder in postmenopausal women.

PROGNOSIS

Population studies show an increased risk of all-cause and cerebrovascular and coronary mortality in patients with untreated severe OSA and in patients with AHIs of 30 or more per hour, independent of other major risk factors. When patients with severe OSA are prescribed CPAP, 5-year survival rates are significantly higher in those with good CPAP adherence (>6 hours/day) than in those with poor adherence. Like other patients with sleep disorders (Chapter 412), patients with OSA are at greater risk for morbidity and mortality from motor vehicle accidents compared with drivers without OSA.

 Grade **A**

1. Giles T, Lasserson TJ, Smith BH, et al. Continuous positive airways pressure for obstructive sleep apnoea in adults. *Cochrane Database Syst Rev.* 2006.1.CD001106.
2. Mulgrew AT, Fox N, Ayas NT, et al. Diagnosis and initial management of obstructive sleep apnea without polysomnography: a randomized validation study. *Ann Intern Med.* 2007;146:157-166.
3. Berry RB, Hill G, Thompson L, et al. Portable monitoring and autotitration versus polysomnography for the diagnosis and treatment of sleep apnea. *Sleep.* 2008;31:1423-1431.
4. Nilius G, Happel A, Domanski U, et al. Pressure-relief continuous positive airway pressure vs constant continuous positive airway pressure: a comparison of efficacy and compliance. *Chest.* 2006;130:1018-1024.
5. Smith I, Lasserson TJ. Pressure modification for improving usage of continuous positive airway pressure machines in adults with obstructive sleep apnoea. *Cochrane Database Syst Rev.* 2009.4.CD003531.
6. Smith I, Nadig V, Lasserson TJ. Educational, supportive and behavioural interventions to improve usage of continuous positive airway pressure machines for adults with obstructive sleep apnoea. *Cochrane Database Syst Rev.* 2009.4.CD007736.
7. Lim J, Lasserson TJ, Fleetham J, et al. Oral appliances for obstructive sleep apnoea. *Cochrane Database Syst Rev.* 2006.1.CD004435.
8. Skinner MA, Kingshott RN, Filsell S. Efficacy of the "tennis ball technique" versus nCPAP in the management of position-dependent obstructive sleep apnoea syndrome. *Respirology.* 2008;5:708-715.
9. Foster GD, Borradaile KE, Sanders MH, et al. A randomized study on the effect of weight loss on obstructive sleep apnea among obese patients with type 2 diabetes. The Sleep Ahead Study. *Arch Intern Med.* 2009;169:1619-1626.
10. Greenburg DL, Lettieri CJ, Eliasson AH. Effects of surgical weight loss on measures of obstructive sleep apnea: a meta-analysis. *Am J Med.* 2009;122:535-542.
11. Aurora RN, Casey KR, Kristo D, et al. Practice parameters for the surgical modifications of the upper airway for obstructive sleep apnea in adults. *Sleep.* 2010;33:1408-1413.

SUGGESTED READINGS

Kasai T, Bradley TD. Obstructive sleep apnea and heart failure: pathophysiologic and therapeutic implications. *J Am Coll Cardiol.* 2011;57:119-127. *Review.*
Pack AI, Pien GW. Update on sleep and its disorders. *Annu Rev Med.* 2011;62:447-460. *Review focusing on obstructive sleep apnea.*

101

INTERVENTIONAL AND SURGICAL APPROACHES TO LUNG DISEASE

ARMIN ERNST AND MALCOLM M. DECAMP

Currently available interventional and surgical procedures can provide diagnostic and staging information and sometimes definitively treat or effectively palliate patients with benign, infectious, and malignant lung diseases.

BRONCHOSCOPY

Bronchoscopy affords a direct view of the major airways and access to lung parenchyma for blind biopsy. Endobronchial therapy has conventionally been used for the management of central airway obstruction, but newer technologic developments permit minimally invasive diagnosis and staging of lung cancer with endobronchial ultrasound (US) and endoscopic approaches to diseases such as emphysema.

Bronchoscopy for Central Airway Obstruction

Airway disorders that cause central airway obstruction of the trachea, mainstem bronchi, and bronchus intermedius are a common indication for therapeutic bronchoscopy. The airway obstruction may be caused by malignant

FIGURE 101-1. Three-dimensional reconstruction of a computed tomographic scan in a 20-year-old woman status after bilateral lung transplantation. The image clearly shows the high-grade stenosis at the level of the left mainstem anastomosis. The right-sided airways are normal.

FIGURE 101-2. Bronchoscopic view of the proximal trachea in a 54-year-old man with shortness of breath and stridor. Significant circumferential narrowing is noted in the subglottic space, consistent with gastric reflux–induced subglottic stenosis.

conditions (e.g., bronchogenic carcinoma or metastatic malignancy to the bronchi) and benign disorders (e.g., sarcoidosis, amyloidosis, goiters). The reduction in the airway lumen may remain asymptomatic until a critical airway diameter (5 to 8 mm) is reached or a new event (infection, bleeding, or mucous plugging) exacerbates the underlying narrowing.

CLINICAL MANIFESTATIONS AND DIAGNOSIS

A high index of suspicion is mandatory because patients with central airway obstruction often do not have specific symptoms. Stridor is usually a sign of impending respiratory failure that requires urgent intervention.

Hemoptysis may be prominent in patients with malignancies. Some patients may present with a postobstructive pneumonia that responds poorly to antibiotic treatment or recurs. Most patients, however, present with nonspecific symptoms, including dyspnea and cough.

Patients who have risk factors for chronic airway obstruction and present with symptoms consistent with obstruction unresponsive to conventional therapy should undergo airway imaging by computed tomography (CT) scanning (Fig. 101-1) and flexible bronchoscopy (Fig. 101-2). Because loss of airway patency can be lethal, evaluation of these patients must be performed by individuals experienced in the management of critical airway disorders.

TREATMENT

Removal of obstructing tissue is a key objective in the relief of airway obstruction. Mechanical débridement, which is accomplished by "coring-out" the tissue with the barrel of the rigid bronchoscope, is the safest approach to patients with chronic airway obstruction. Although laser and electrocautery can be used to vaporize tumor tissue, the preferred technique is to use electrocautery or argon plasma coagulation before mechanical débridement, in a fashion known as *heat-assisted mechanical debulking.*

Airway stenting is the primary treatment for airway obstruction caused by extrinsic compression, as may be seen by patients with large malignant mediastinal masses. However, airway stenting is associated with long-term complications, including stent and airway fractures, secondary airway occlusion, infection, and migration, so it should be considered primarily as a palliative procedure for malignant diseases.

For malignant disease, local débridement may temporize the clinical situation while extirpative options are considered. If the lesion or patient is deemed inoperable, such procedures, with or without stenting, are usually a complement to definitive radiation therapy. Patients with endoscopically relieved malignant airway obstruction usually experience a significant improvement in their of quality of life and are more likely to succumb to distant disease than to a local recurrence.

Endobronchial Ultrasound

Bronchoscopy is a standard component of the evaluation and staging of patients with thoracic tumors. Endobronchial US incorporated into the tip of special endoscopes provides ultrasonographic visualization of peri-airway abnormalities and allows transbronchial needle biopsies to be targeted at abnormal areas instead of being taken blindly. Endobronchial ultrasound with biopsy of enlarged nodes has largely obviated the need for mediastinoscopy for the biopsy of mediastinal lymph nodes for staging or diagnosis of cancer and can be useful for the diagnosis of sarcoidosis (Chapter 95). For example, adding endobronchial ultrasound to surgical staging improves the sensitivity for finding nodal metastases and can reduce the unnecessary thoracotomy rate from 18 to 7%.[1]

Surgical Approaches
Open Approaches

Thoracotomy has been the standard approach to evaluate the contents of the pleural space, lung parenchyma, pulmonary hilum, and ipsilateral mediastinum and diaphragm. Selective lung ventilation, achieved by use of a double-lumen endotracheal tube or mainstem bronchial blocker, allows one lung to be collapsed and visualized. Given the precision and accuracy of contemporary preprocedure CT and magnetic resonance imaging (MRI), many procedures can be performed using smaller targeted incisions, with a muscle-sparing technique that allows specific access to regional pathology. Many lung processes can also be approached through a median sternotomy, which affords access to both lungs, although access to the left lower lobe through this approach can be challenging.

Video-Assisted Thoracoscopic Surgery

Thoracoscopy, or video-assisted thoracoscopic surgery (VATS), requires two or three incisions, termed *ports,* to place instruments in any intercostal space. A common configuration is to place one port for the video thoracoscope and two ports for endoscopic instrumentation. With the VATS approach, recovery is shorter than following an open thoracotomy because little if any muscle is divided and no mechanical rib spreading retractors are used.

The size of the surgical incisions depends on the goals of the procedure and the anatomic findings at the time of exploration. Unexpected pleural symphysis or incomplete lobar fissures may require extension of the incision to facilitate visualization. In patients undergoing anatomic resection, such as segmentectomy or lobectomy, at least one of the port incisions is extended to 4 to 8 cm in length to permit extraction of the resected lung from the hemithorax.

⬤ SURGERY FOR BENIGN LUNG DISEASE

A variety of benign lung diseases present as focal parenchymal lesions that require a tissue biopsy for diagnosis. Thoracoscopy has essentially replaced a limited thoracotomy and wedge resection for this purpose. VATS provides a more complete view of the ipsilateral hemithorax, including the visceral, parietal, and mediastinal pleura. In addition, subpleural nodules that are too small to be visualized by preoperative radiography can be identified so that representative biopsy samples can be obtained.

Spontaneous Pneumothorax

Although most spontaneous pneumothoraces (Chapter 99) are uncomplicated, up to 20% of patients with pneumothoraces experience complications such as tension pneumothorax, persistent air leak despite tube

drainage, or recurrent pneumothoraces either ipsilaterally or contralaterally. Patients in whom a second pneumothorax develops have a 70 to 80% chance of a third recurrence within 2 years. The current surgical approach to the treatment of recurrent pneumothoraces is VATS resection of the subpleural blebs responsible for the pneumothorax, usually combined with mechanical abrasion of the parietal pleura or chemical pleurodesis with insufflated talc to cause an inflammatory reaction that will allow the lung to adhere to the chest wall.

Giant Bullae

Most patients with chronic obstructive pulmonary disease (COPD) have diffuse parenchymal disease, but a small number of patients with COPD have dominant or giant bullae that may occupy 50% or more of the volume of the hemithorax and that compress relatively preserved lung parenchyma. The indications for bullectomy include progressive symptoms with demonstrated disability, obstructive spirometry (Chapter 85), and a single or dominant bullous lesion with radiographic demonstration of compression of the surrounding preserved lung parenchyma. Either excision or plication can remove the bullous lesion.

Malignant Lung Disease
Solitary Pulmonary Nodules

Most small pulmonary nodules (see Fig. 197-5 in Chapter 197) present in the periphery of the lung beyond the reach of diagnostic bronchoscopy. For such lesions, VATS excisional biopsy of a small pulmonary nodule leads to a definitive diagnosis in almost all cases and is generally preferred over transthoracic needle biopsy. Furthermore, thoracoscopy can allow concurrent nodal staging should a primary malignancy (Chapter 197) be confirmed. In the absence of regional adenopathy, patients with primary malignant lesions can undergo definitive resection at the same time.

Primary Lung Cancer

In patients with node-negative primary lung cancer and adequate pulmonary reserve, lobectomy or pneumonectomy is indicated to obtain optimal survival and to decrease the risk of local recurrence. Lobectomy can be achieved by thoracotomy or VATS with similar outcomes. Although VATS wedge resection of primary lung cancer has not been specifically studied in randomized trials, available evidence suggests that an open wedge resection may not be as good as lobectomy for staging or for tumor-free prognosis.

Metastatic Cancer

The lung is a frequent site of metastatic recurrence. Common histologies include colorectal cancer (Chapter 199), renal cell carcinoma (Chapter 203), sarcoma (Chapter 209), melanoma (Chapter 210), breast cancer (Chapter 204), and head and neck cancer (Chapter 196). VATS is often the diagnostic procedure of choice to detect and locate nodules too small for reliable percutaneous biopsy.

The role of pulmonary metastectomy as therapy for advanced disease remains controversial. Five-year survival rates of 20 to 30% have been reported for selected patients, especially if the disease-free interval from original diagnosis to lung metastasis is greater than 3 years. These cases often require resection of bilateral lung nodules, which in turn mandate either a median sternotomy, clamshell incision, or staged, bilateral VATS.

⬤ SURGERY FOR ADVANCED LUNG DISEASES: LUNG VOLUME REDUCTION SURGERY

Emphysema (Chapter 88) is the most common chronic progressive disabling lung disease treated by pulmonologists and thoracic surgeons. In eligible patients (Table 101-1), lung volume reduction surgery confers durable symptomatic, physiologic, and survival benefits compared with medical therapy (Fig. 101-3) for patients who have severe emphysema but who do not have a forced expiratory volume in 1 second (FEV_1) measure of less than 20% of predicted with either a homogeneous distribution of emphysema on CT or a diffusing capacity of less than 20% of predicted.[2] However, subgroup analyses suggest that the benefit is mainly in patients with upper lobe predominant disease.

For eligible patients, most programs require a 6- to 10-week preoperative pulmonary rehabilitation followed by a cardiopulmonary exercise test to assess the risks and benefits of surgery. Patients with upper lobe predominant emphysema and a low preoperative exercise capacity have a nearly 50% lower risk of death after lung volume reduction surgery compared with continued

TABLE 101-1 INCLUSION AND EXCLUSION CRITERIA FOR LUNG VOLUME REDUCTION SURGERY

INCLUSION CRITERIA

Radiographic evidence of emphysema, especially involving upper lobes
Hyperinflation evidenced by TLC > 100% predicted and RV > 150% predicted
FEV_1 > 20 and < 45% predicted (after bronchodilator)
D_{LCO} > 20% predicted
Severe dyspnea
Restricted activities of daily living
Decreased quality of life
Abstinence from tobacco

EXCLUSION CRITERIA

Active smoking
Bronchiectasis
Pulmonary nodule requiring evaluation
Excessive daily sputum production
Previous thoracotomy
Obvious pleural disease
Active or inducible coronary ischemia
Pulmonary hypertension
Depressed LVEF (<45%)
Obesity (BMI > 32)
Unable or unwilling to participate in pulmonary rehabilitation
Systemic steroids, ≥20 mg prednisone/day

BMI = body mass index; D_{LCO} = diffusion capacity for carbon monoxide; FEV_1 = first second forced expiratory volume; LVEF = left ventricular ejection fraction; RV = residual capacity; TLC = total lung capacity.
Adapted from DeCamp MM Jr, McKenna RJ Jr, Deschamps CC, et al. Lung volume reduction surgery: technique, operative mortality and morbidity. *Proc Am Thorac Soc.* 2008;5:442-446; and DeCamp MM Jr, Lipson D, Krasna M, et al. The evaluation and preparation of the patient for lung volume reduction surgery. *Proc Am Thorac Soc.* 2008;5:427-431.

TABLE 101-2 DECISION GUIDE FOR SELECTION OF LUNG VOLUME REDUCTION SURGERY VERSUS TRANSPLANTATION FOR SEVERE CHRONIC OBSTRUCTIVE PULMONARY DISEASE

FACTORS FAVORING LVRS	FACTORS FAVORING TRANSPLANTATION
Age > 65 yr	$FEV_1 \leq 20\%$ predicted
Upper lobe predominant disease	$D_{LCO} \leq 20\%$ predicted
Chronic medical conditions	Homogeneous or lower lobe distribution
Hepatitis B and/or C	of disease
HIV infection	TLC < 100% predicted
Renal insufficiency	RV < 150% predicted
Cirrhosis	Pa_{CO_2} > 60 mm Hg
Neuropathy	Pa_{O_2} < 45 mm Hg
Poorly controlled diabetes	6 MWD < 140 m or
Osteoporosis	< 3 min unloaded pedaling cycle ergometer
Severe GERD	Pulmonary hypertension
Poor esophageal motility	Bronchiectasis
Malignancy	Recurrent pulmonary infections
Unable to maintain long-term follow-up	
Psychiatric issues limiting compliance	
Insufficient social support	

6 MWD = six-minute walk distance; D_{LCO} = diffusion capacity of carbon monoxide; FEV_1 = first second forced expired volume; GERD = gastroesophageal reflux disease; HIV = human immunodeficiency virus; LVRS = lung volume reduction surgery; RV = residual volume; TLC = total lung capacity.
Adapted from Patel N, DeCamp M, Criner GJ. Lung transplantation and lung volume reduction surgery versus transplantation in chronic obstructive pulmonary disease. *Proc Am Thorac Soc.* 2008;5:447-453.

FIGURE 101-3. Long-term mortality of all patients treated with lung volume reduction surgery (LVRS) versus maximal medical therapy in the National Emphysema Treatment Trial. Note the statistically significant (*P* = .02) reduction in relative risk of death (RR = 0.85) for the surgical cohort. (Adapted from Naunheim KS, Wood DE, Mohsenifar Z, et al, for the National Emphysema Treatment Trial Research Group. Long-term follow-up of patients receiving lung-volume-reduction surgery versus medical therapy for severe emphysema in the National Emphysema Treatment Trial. *Ann Thorac Surg.* 2006;82:431-443.)

medical therapy. High-risk patients with severe airflow obstruction (FEV_1 < 20%) should be assessed for lung transplantation evaluation unless their disease is localized to the upper lobes and their gas exchange as defined by diffusing capacity is preserved (Table 101-2).

In experienced centers, bilateral stapled resection approaches yield nearly twice the physiologic benefit of unilateral lung volume reduction surgery without adversely affecting operative morbidity or mortality. Bilateral lung volume reduction surgery using the VATS approach reduces hospital length of stay and increases the likelihood of living independently 60 days after surgery. **3**

ENDOSCOPIC MANAGEMENT OF EMPHYSEMA

Endoscopic approaches to lung volume reduction include airway valves, blockers, stents, sealants, and implants. Unlike lung volume reduction surgery, which causes peridiaphragmatic pleural scarring and can restrict diaphragmatic movement when lower lobe emphysema is treated, endobronchial lung volume reduction does not cause such scarring and may result in better postoperative functional outcomes. Endobronchial lung volume reduction may permit stepwise and gradual therapy that may facilitate weaning of COPD patients from ventilators. Furthermore, some endobronchial lung volume reduction modalities, such as endobronchial valves, are reversible and can be removed if they are not beneficial or if complications arise.

Endobronchial valves are designed to exclude the most affected emphysematous regions from ventilation and reduce dynamic air trapping. If segmental or lobar atelectasis can be induced, a physiologic effect similar to lung volume reduction surgery can be obtained. In a randomized trial, bronchoscopic implantation of endobronchial valves to allow air to escape from but not enter emphysematous lung areas resulted in a 7% relative improvement in FEV_1 but at the expense of more hemoptysis, pneumonia, and exacerbations of COPD. **4** Endobronchial valve therapy for emphysema is safer than lung volume reduction surgery, with a reported mortality rate of approximately 1% and with most patients being discharged within 2 to 4 days. Postobstructive pneumonia has not been a commonly reported complication.

The bronchoscopic creation of extra-anatomic bronchial fenestrations allows trapped air to escape by bypassing obstructed airways, thereby partially deflating emphysematous lung segments through enhanced collateral ventilation.

Biological sealants induce localized irreversible atelectasis by sealing off highly damaged areas of lung. Unlike endobronchial valves or bypass, sealants work at the alveolar level, where air space inflammation and remodeling leads to scarring and contraction of lung parenchyma. Within 6 to 8 weeks, a mature scar and functional lung volume reduction reduce dead space and residual volume to a degree similar to what can be achieved with lung volume reduction surgery.

LUNG TRANSPLANTATION

About 150 worldwide lung transplant centers perform more than 2700 transplantations per year. Lung transplantation is now an accepted therapy for all forms of advanced lung disease.

TABLE 101-3 INDICATIONS AND CONTRAINDICATIONS FOR LUNG TRANSPLANTATION

SINGLE-LUNG TRANSPLANT	PATIENTS (%)	DOUBLE-LUNG TRANSPLANT	PATIENTS (%)
INDICATIONS			
COPD	49	CF, bronchiectasis	31
Pulmonary fibrosis, sarcoid	31	Emphysema	26
α_1-Antitrypsin deficiency	6	α_1-Antitrypsin deficiency	8
PPH, Eisenmenger's	1.2	PPH, Eisenmenger's	6
CF, bronchiectasis	2.4	Pulmonary fibrosis, sarcoid	17
Retransplantation	3	Retransplantation	2
Other*	7	Other*	10

ABSOLUTE CONTRAINDICATIONS

Untreatable advanced extrapulmonary organ dysfunction (e.g., heart, liver, kidney)
    CAD not amenable to PCI or bypass
    Poor LV function (could consider heart-lung transplantation)
Malignancy within 2 years (excludes cutaneous squamous or basal cell carcinoma)
    5-year disease-free interval preferred
Noncurable extrapulmonary infection
    Infection with human immunodeficiency virus
    Hepatitis B antigen positivity
    Hepatitis C with histologic evidence of active liver disease
Active substance abuse (including cigarettes)
Severe musculoskeletal disease affecting the thorax
Documented noncompliance
Untreatable psychiatric condition which impairs compliance
Absence of consistent and reliable social support

RELATIVE CONTRAINDICATIONS

Physiologic age > 65 years
Poor nutritional status (<70% ideal body weight)
Severe obesity (BMI > 30 kg/m)
Symptomatic osteoporosis
Colonization with highly virulent and/or highly resistant fungi, mycobacteria, or bacteria
Requirement for invasive ventilation and/or circulatory support
Uncontrolled chronic medical conditions (e.g., diabetes, hypertension, GERD)
Severely limited functional status with poor rehabilitation potential
Psychosocial problems likely to affect the outcome adversely
High-dose (>20 mg of prednisone daily) corticosteroid use

*Other includes lymphangioleiomatosis, non-retransplantation-related obliterative bronchiolitis, and miscellaneous indications.
BMI = body mass index; CAD = coronary artery disease; CF = cystic fibrosis; COPD = chronic obstructive pulmonary disease; GERD = gastroesophageal reflux disease; LV = left ventricle; PCI = percutaneous coronary intervention; PPH = primary pulmonary hypertension.
Adapted from Registry of the International Society for Heart and Lung Transplantation. Twenty-second official adult lung and heart-lung transplant report—2009. *J Heart Lung Transplant.* 2009;28:989-1049; and Orens JB, Estenne M, Arcasoy S, et al. International guidelines for the selection of lung transplant candidates: 2006 update. A consensus report from the Pulmonary Scientific Council of the International Society for Heart and Lung Transplantation. *J Heart Lung Transplant.* 2006;25:745-755.

The most common indications for transplantation (Table 101-3) are diseases or conditions that share the following features: they produce extreme disability in affected patients, they are unresponsive to medical therapy, and they are responsible for limited life expectancy in affected patients. With the exception of a small number of cases of sarcoidosis and lymphangioleiomyomatosis, the original lung disease does not usually recur after lung transplantation.

Types of Procedures

Currently, four types of lung transplantation procedures are performed. *Single-lung transplantation*, which is typically performed through a posterolateral thoracotomy incision, requires three anastomoses: the mainstem bronchus, pulmonary artery, and pulmonary veins and left atrium. The contralateral lung is not removed, so single-lung transplantation is not performed in patients with bilaterally infected lungs (e.g., patients with cystic fibrosis or bronchiectasis) (see Table 101-3).

Bilateral lung transplantation is performed in a sequential fashion that is functionally equivalent to two single-lung transplantations completed during a single operation, most commonly through a transverse sternotomy ("clamshell") incision. It requires six anastomoses: both mainstem bronchi, both pulmonary arteries, and both sets of pulmonary veins. It is the procedure of choice for patients with bilaterally infected lungs and is also performed in certain patients with emphysema, primary pulmonary hypertension, and other diseases (see Table 101-3). Bilateral transplantations are preferred for nearly all indications because a double-lung recipient can expect a half-life of 6.6 years compared with 4.6 years for a single-lung recipient.

Heart-lung transplantation is now performed in only about 75 cases per year. It is an en bloc procedure with right atrial, aortic, and distal tracheal anastomoses. It is performed in patients with advanced lung disease and coexistent irreparable cardiac disease, usually associated with fixed pulmonary hypertension, and Eisenmenger's syndrome (Chapter 69).

Living donor lobar transplantation involves the removal of a lower lobe from each of two living donors. One is implanted into each hemithorax of the recipient in a manner similar to bilateral lung transplantation.

Evaluation of Potential Transplant Recipients

The ideal candidate for lung transplantation has lung disease unresponsive to medical therapy but is in otherwise good health. Patients who experience critical illness as a result of lung disease often have poor nutritional status, coexistent major organ dysfunction, refractory infection, or other contraindications to transplantation. The specific evidence-based recommendations for referral for transplant evaluation vary with the underlying disease.

In the United States, the lung allocation system is based on expected disease-specific and patient-specific survival during the waiting period and following engraftment, thereby reflecting net transplant benefit. Early evaluations of the system, which was introduced in 2005, indicate shorter waiting times, an increase in the total number of transplantations performed, a decreased waitlist mortality, and an unchanged overall survival after transplantation.

Post-transplantation Issues

Most of the medical issues that patients and physicians face after lung transplantation are the consequence of the transplantation and post-transplantation medication rather than the underlying disease for which the transplantation was performed. Examples include immunosuppression, infections and their prophylaxis, acute allograft rejection, chronic allograft rejection, and nonpulmonary complications of transplantation.

Immunosuppression

The standard chemotherapeutic regimen for immunosuppression after lung transplantation consists of a calcineurin inhibitor such as cyclosporine or tacrolimus, azathioprine or mycophenolate mofetil, and corticosteroids. Some centers add an antilymphocyte antibody preparation in the first days after transplantation, although this addition has not been demonstrated to improve outcome.

Infections and Prophylaxis after Lung Transplantation

Lung transplant recipients are at high risk for bacterial, viral, fungal, and protozoal infections; infections are the leading causes of death during the early post-transplantation period. In the first 3 months after transplantation, bacterial infections are responsible for most deaths. In approximately one third of patients, pneumonia is diagnosed in the first weeks after transplantation, with gram-negative organisms as the cause in 75% of cases. Colonization and recurrent infections, usually with *Pseudomonas* species, often develop in patients with chronic rejection.

Among potential viral pathogens, *cytomegalovirus* (CMV; Chapter 384) is the most important in lung transplant recipients. Seronegative patients who receive an allograft from a seropositive donor are at particularly high risk for the development of a clinically significant CMV infection. Seronegative patients who have a seronegative donor are at low risk for infection if they are treated with seronegative blood products. Epstein-Barr virus (EBV) has been associated with the development of post-transplantation lymphoproliferative disorder.

Aspergillus species are the most common cause of invasive fungal infection (Chapter 347). Colonized patients and those deemed at risk may receive prophylactic inhaled amphotericin B.

Because of the nature of the immunosuppressive chemotherapeutic regimen used, patients are at high risk for infection by the protozoan *Pneumocystis jirovecii* (Chapter 349). The use of trimethoprim-sulfamethoxazole prophylaxis (typically 1 double-strength tablet three times weekly indefinitely) has virtually eliminated *Pneumocystis* pneumonia.

Acute Rejection

Histologically, the initial manifestation of acute rejection is a lymphocyte-predominant inflammatory response, usually centered around blood vessels, airways, or both. By convention, acute rejection is graded histologically from 0 (normal) to 4 (severe), with subclasses defined by the presence or absence of airway inflammation.

The risk for acute allograft rejection is highest in the early months after transplantation and declines with time. Multiple episodes of acute rejection are the major risk factor for the subsequent development of chronic rejection.

Clinically, patients may have fever, cough, and exertional dyspnea. Evaluation may demonstrate rales or rhonchi on chest examination, a decline in pulmonary function by spirometry, leukocytosis, opacities on chest radiography, and exertional desaturation. The clinical manifestation is often indistinguishable from infectious pneumonia, and the clinical impression is accurate in only 50% of cases.

Treatment of acute rejection most often consists of high-dose corticosteroids (typically, 1 g/day of methylprednisolone administered intravenously for 3 days).

Chronic Rejection

PATHOBIOLOGY

The bronchiolitis obliterans syndrome is thought to be a manifestation of chronic rejection. Risk factors for development of the syndrome include the number of acute rejection episodes and, in some series, previous symptomatic CMV infection. Pathologically, "early" lesions demonstrate inflammation and disruption of the epithelium of small airways, followed by growth of granulation tissue into the airway lumen and subsequent complete or partial obstruction. The granulation tissue then organizes in a stereotypical pattern with resultant fibrosis that obliterates the lumen of the airway.

CLINICAL MANIFESTATIONS

Clinically, bronchiolitis obliterans is accompanied by nonspecific symptoms. Progressive exertional breathlessness typically develops, and pulmonary function testing usually demonstrates evidence of progressive airflow obstruction (Chapter 85). Bronchiolitis obliterans is classified according to the FEV_1: 0 (no significant abnormality) if FEV_1 is greater than 80% of baseline; 1 (mild) if FEV_1 is 65 to 80% of baseline; 2 (moderate) if FEV_1 is 50 to 65% of baseline; and 3 (severe) if FEV_1 is 50% or less of baseline. In early stages, chest radiography is notable only for hyperinflation, but it may show bronchiectasis as the syndrome progresses. Later stages of bronchiolitis obliterans may include a syndrome of bronchiectasis with chronic productive cough and airway colonization with *Pseudomonas* species.

DIAGNOSIS

The diagnosis of bronchiolitis obliterans is made on both clinical and pathologic grounds. Transbronchial biopsy has a low yield for demonstrating histologic evidence of bronchiolitis obliterans, but when such evidence is seen, it is diagnostic. In patients with a compatible clinical syndrome, exclusion of anastomotic stenosis and occult pulmonary infection is sufficient to establish the diagnosis.

TREATMENT (Rx)

A variety of therapies have been tried, including pulse corticosteroids, antilymphocyte antibodies, total lymphoid irradiation, photopheresis, and nebulized cyclosporine, but none has been clearly established as effective. Most patients with bronchiolitis obliterans experience a progressive decline in pulmonary function despite immunosuppression.

PROGNOSIS

Bronchiolitis obliterans is the leading cause of late mortality after lung transplantation. Half of lung transplant recipients surviving to 5 years will have either biopsy-proven bronchiolitis obliterans or the clinical diagnosis of bronchiolitis obliterans syndrome.

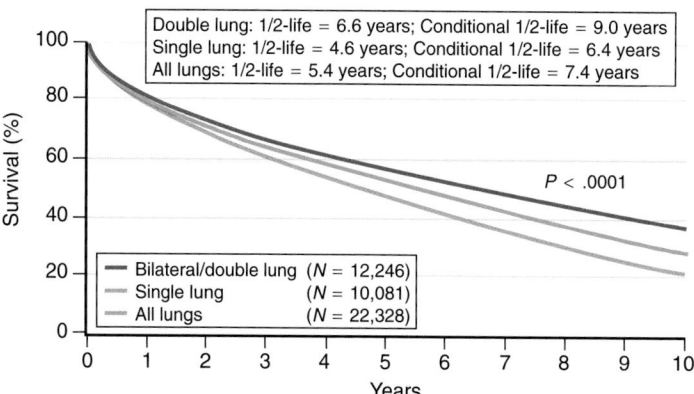

Adult Lung Transplantation
Kaplan-Meier Survival (transplants: January 1994-June 2007)

Double lung: 1/2-life = 6.6 years; Conditional 1/2-life = 9.0 years
Single lung: 1/2-life = 4.6 years; Conditional 1/2-life = 6.4 years
All lungs: 1/2-life = 5.4 years; Conditional 1/2-life = 7.4 years

$P < .0001$

Bilateral/double lung (N = 12,246)
Single lung (N = 10,081)
All lungs (N = 22,328)

FIGURE 101-4. Kaplan-Meier survival estimates for all lung transplantations reported to the International Registry for Heart and Lung Transplantation from 1994 to 2007. Note the highly statistically significant survival advantage conferred by double lung grafts. (Adapted from Registry of the International Society for Heart and Lung Transplantation. Twenty-second official adult lung and heart-lung transplant report—2009. *J Heart Lung Transplant.* 2009;28:989-1049.)

Nonpulmonary Medical Complications of Lung Transplantation

Most of the nonpulmonary medical complications that arise in patients after lung transplantation are the result of immunosuppressive therapy. One or more of these complications develop in virtually all lung transplant recipients.

Osteoporosis (Chapter 251) is common because of the long-term use of corticosteroids and cyclosporine. Bone density should be monitored periodically, and pharmacologic therapy should be instituted if excessive bone loss is identified.

Chronic renal insufficiency (Chapter 132) is common and is the result of therapy with the calcineurin inhibitors cyclosporine or tacrolimus, both of which affect afferent vascular tone in the kidneys and result in an average 50% drop in the glomerular filtration rate in the first 12 months after lung transplantation. Systemic arterial hypertension is also common and is caused by corticosteroids and cyclosporine. Calcium-channel blockers, which are often used to treat hypertension, raise serum cyclosporine levels; appropriate monitoring and dose adjustment are needed when starting such therapy. Both corticosteroids and tacrolimus contribute to the development of diabetes mellitus and hyperlipidemia.

Solid organ transplantation is associated with an increased incidence of malignancy, thought to be due to pharmacologic immunosuppression and alteration in immune surveillance. Patients are at increased risk for lymphoproliferative malignancies and other types of cancers. Post-transplantation lymphoproliferative disorders occur in about 4% of patients after organ transplantation; most are associated with EBV. These syndromes can be polyclonal or monoclonal. Reduction in immunosuppression is sometimes therapeutic in those with polyclonal disease. The prognosis in patients with monoclonal disease is poor, with little response to modification of immunosuppression or antineoplastic chemotherapy. Patients are also at increased risk for skin, cervical, anogenital, and hepatobiliary malignancy after solid organ transplantation.

Outcomes after Lung Transplantation

Currently, the annual mortality following lung transplantation is 8 to 10% per year, largely owing to bronchiolitis obliterans syndrome. The median survival after lung transplantation is about 5.4 years (Fig. 101-4).

1. Annema JT, van Meerbeeck JP, Rintoul RC, et al. Mediastinoscopy vs endosonography for mediastinal nodal staging of lung cancer: a randomized trial. *JAMA.* 2010;304:2245-2252.
2. Naunheim KS, Wood DE, Mohsenifar Z, et al, for the National Emphysema Treatment Trial Research Group. Long-term follow-up of patients receiving lung-volume-reduction surgery versus medical therapy for severe emphysema in the National Emphysema Treatment Trial. *Ann Thorac Surg.* 2006;82:431-443.

3. National Emphysema Treatment Trial Research Group. Safety and efficacy of median sternotomy versus video-assisted thoracic surgery for lung volume reduction surgery. *J Thorac Cardiovasc Surg.* 2004;127:1350-1360.

4. Sciurba FC, Ernst A, Herth FJF, et al: A randomized study of endobronchial valves for advanced emphysema. *N Engl J Med.* 2010;363:1233-1244.

SUGGESTED READINGS

Ernst A, Anantham D. Endoscopic management of emphysema. *Clin Chest Med.* 2010;31:117-126. Review.

Floreth T, Bhorade SM. Current trends in immunosuppression for lung transplantation. *Semin Respir Crit Care Med.* 2010;31:172-178. Review.

Kreisel D, Krupnick AS, Puri V, et al. Short- and long-term outcomes of 1000 adult lung transplant recipients at a single center. *J Thorac Cardiovasc Surg.* 2011;141:215-222. *Five-year survival is improving but is limited by the development of bronchiolitis obliterans.*

X

CRITICAL CARE MEDICINE

APPROACH TO THE PATIENT IN A CRITICAL CARE SETTING

DEBORAH J. COOK

THE INTENSIVIST-LED MULTIDISCIPLINARY TEAM

Patients with critical illness in the intensive care unit (ICU) usually require advanced life support such as mechanical ventilation, inotropic agents, or dialysis. Morbidity associated with critical illness includes complications of both acute and chronic diseases, nosocomial and iatrogenic consequences, and impaired quality of life among survivors. Critically ill patients are at a higher risk of death than any other hospital population. Accordingly, the goals of critical care are to reduce morbidity and mortality, maintain organ function, and restore health. Unlike many other specialties, critical care medicine is not limited to a particular population, disease, diagnosis, or organ system.

Staffing of ICUs with critical care physicians, often referred to as *intensivists*, who provide mandatory consultations or principal ongoing care is associated with a significantly reduced ICU and hospital mortality and reduced ICU and hospital lengths of stay. These findings emphasize the value of the on-site availability of trained physicians who are dedicated to appropriate triaging, prevention, diagnosis, monitoring, treatment, and palliation of critically ill patients.

In addition, daily rounds by an ICU physician who leads a multidisciplinary team appear to improve outcomes. Emerging evidence suggests that leadership, communication, and organizational culture can streamline the process of critical care. These favorable findings may be due to the intensivist-coordinated teamwork of physicians, nurses, respiratory therapists, dieticians, and pastoral care workers to meet the needs of patients and families.

FLUID RESUSCITATION

Intravenous fluids to maintain or restore intravascular volume are an important component of ICU therapy. Both crystalloid and colloid solutions are in widespread use. Crystalloids are readily available and inexpensive, whereas colloids generally require less volume to achieve a specific physiologic goal. Albumin is a naturally occurring protein colloid that increases intravascular oncotic pressure, but its use also carries a small risk of transmitting infection.

In a large randomized trial of fluid replacement with either normal saline or 4% albumin, mortality was the same (21%) in both groups, and there were no differences in organ failure, duration of mechanical ventilation, renal replacement therapy, or length of ICU or hospital stay[1]; however, crystalloid resulted in lower mortality for the pre-specified subgroup of patients with traumatic brain injury. Based on these data, either crystalloid- or albumin-based fluid resuscitation is recommended for most critically ill patients, but crystalloids are recommended for head-injured patients.

Intravenous hydroxyethyl starch, which, like albumin, draws extravascular fluid into the intravascular space, appears to be associated with an increased risk of adverse outcomes, especially in the setting of severe sepsis and septic shock[2] Although starch has not been shown to increase overall mortality, it should be avoided in patients with severe sepsis and septic shock pending ongoing randomized trials.

SEDATION, ANALGESIA, AND SPONTANEOUS BREATHING TRIALS

Endotracheal intubation, central venous catheterization, postoperative pain management, and other ICU procedures require that most patients receive sedation, analgesia, or both. Continuous infusion of sedatives and analgesics is preferable to intermittent boluses, because infusions ensure ongoing tolerance to mechanical ventilation and provide consistent relief of pain and anxiety.

Daily interruption of the infusion of sedatives and analgesics, using protocols that provide an opportunity for the patient to be observed in a less sedated state, is associated with a shorter duration of mechanical ventilation and ICU length of stay.[3] A standardized approach to sedation and analgesia, combining a drug titration protocol with a sedation scale, can favorably impact ICU outcomes and resource consumption.

Discontinuation of ventilatory support is affected by sedation and analgesic infusions, and vice versa. A daily sedation vacation followed by a spontaneous breathing test increases the days of breathing without assistance and shortens ICU stay and hospital stay compared with usual sedation management plus a daily spontaneous breathing test.[4] Although sedation vacations may theoretically increase the risk of self-extubation, the number of patients requiring reintubation does not appear to be increased. In the year after enrollment, patients who were treated with a "wake up and breathe" protocol, which linked daily sedation vacation periods with daily spontaneous breathing trials, had a 32% better survival rate. Based on these data, a nurse-implemented sedation and analgesic management scale with daily drug interruption and daily spontaneous breathing trials are recommended for mechanically ventilated critically ill patients.

LONG-TERM OUTCOMES FOR SURVIVORS

For survivors of critical illness, triggers for ICU discharge are restoration of hemodynamic stability, ability to protect the airway, and spontaneous breathing. However, biomarkers of inflammation, residual organ dysfunction, and functional disabilities persist in most ICU survivors. Treatments administered in the ICU also have serious sequelae. For example, neuromuscular blockers and corticosteroids may contribute to critical illness polyneuropathy. These problems have particularly serious adverse consequences for elderly critically ill patients who are deconditioned before hospitalization.

In addition, anxiety, post-traumatic stress, and major mood disorders are common among patients and their caregivers during recovery. Therefore, although ICU discharge and hospital discharge are milestones in a patient's trajectory, sequelae of critical illness have rarely resolved completely when patients are on the regular hospital floor or at home. Accordingly, multidimensional rehabilitation may optimize the long-term outcomes of survivors of critical illness and their families.

Sedative-induced immobility is now understood to be a preventable contributor to ICU-acquired weakness and functional impairment in the recovery phase of critical illness. This concept has prompted multifaceted interventions to improve long-term outcomes. In a randomized trial of previously independent patients who received mechanical ventilation for 72 hours or less, the addition of graduated, individualized, early physical therapy and occupational therapy during daily sedation vacation periods improved functional capacity at hospital discharge, reduced the duration of delirium, and reduced the number of ventilator days during the 28-day follow-up.[5] Discontinuation of therapy as a result of patient instability, usually patient-ventilator asynchrony, occurred in only 4% of all sessions. This trial highlights how the recovery of critically ill patients can be improved by coordinated multidisciplinary care, including the interruption of sedation, physical therapy, and occupational therapy in the early days of critical illness.

APPLYING EVIDENCE TO PREVENT COMPLICATIONS OF CRITICAL ILLNESS

Considerable evidence of effective preventive and therapeutic ICU interventions has emerged in randomized trials over the past decade. However, barriers to applying this evidence in fast-paced ICUs can lead to a lack of responsibility and decisional authority and to errors of omission.

Analysis of most clinical practices has shown that passive dissemination of information, whether written or verbal, is generally ineffective in modifying physicians' behavior. More effective strategies to encourage the implementation of evidence-based recommendations are interactive education, audit and feedback, reminders (written or computerized), involvement of local opinion leaders, and multifaceted approaches. In the high-acuity ICU setting, preprinted physician orders may help guide (but never dictate) management (Table 102-1). Highlights of evidence-based management include low tidal volume ventilation, high positive end-expiratory pressure,[6] inotrope or vasopressor infusion, low-dose corticosteroids, early enteral small bowel nutrition, head of bed elevation, oral antisepsis, stress ulcer prophylaxis, thromboprophylaxis, and insulin therapy aimed at avoiding marked hyperglycemia but not achieving normoglycemia (Chapters 104 and 105).[7,8] Another useful management strategy is oral decontamination with nonabsorbable antiseptic agents such as chlorhexidine, which decreases the risk of pneumonia. This antiseptic approach is favored over using antibiotics

TABLE 102-1 ICU ADMISSION ORDERS: EXAMPLE FOR A PATIENT WITH UROSEPSIS AND ARDS

MANAGEMENT STRATEGY	ORDERS	REEVALUATE
ACUTE PHASE		
Mechanical ventilation	Target TV 5-7 mL/kg of ideal body weight, PC 16 cm, rate 12, F$_{IO_2}$ 0.7, PEEP 18 cm, plateau pressure <30 cm	PRN
Maintenance fluid	Ringer's lactate 75 mL/hr IV	PRN
Norepinephrine	Titrate to mean arterial pressure >65 mm Hg	PRN
Corticosteroids	Hydrocortisone 50 mg IV q6h while vasopressor dependent	Daily
Sedation	Midazolam 2-8 mg/hr IV, bolus 2-4 mg PRN	PRN
Analgesia	Morphine 1-4 mg IV PRN	PRN
Antibiotics	Ampicillin 2 g IV q6h	Daily
Head of bed	45-degree elevation from horizontal	PRN
Oral antisepsis	Chlorhexidine 15 mL q6h	Daily
Small bowel enteral nutrition	10 mL/hr of a commercial balanced feed containing about 1 kcal/mL; increase by 10 mL q6h to 70 mL/hr	Daily
Stress ulcer prophylaxis	Ranitidine 50 mg IV q8h	Daily
Thromboprophylaxis	Unfractionated heparin 5000 U SC q12h	Daily
Intensive insulin therapy if glucose >180 mg/dL	50 U insulin in 50 mL NS; start at 0.5 U/hr, repeat glucose q1h for 4 hr, and reassess; target 110-150 mg/dL	Daily
Glucometer calibration	Calibrate glucose from glucometer and central laboratory every morning	Daily
Tests	Glucose q4h when stable, ABG with each ventilator change, other tests as per ICU team	PRN
Monitoring	Arterial catheter for systolic blood pressure, central venous catheter for central venous pressure and mixed venous oxygen saturation, ECG, oximetry, ABGs, sedation scale, Foley catheter, others as per ICU monitoring protocols	PRN
RECOVERY PHASE		
Sedation vacation	Daily interruption of sedation from 0700 h until 0900 h; restart at half prior infusion at 0900 h as tolerated	Daily
Spontaneous breathing trials	Spontaneous breathing trial when weaning readiness criteria met	Daily
Early mobility	Physiotherapy and occupational therapy when able	Daily

ABG = arterial blood gas; ARDS = acute respiratory distress syndrome; ECG = electrocardiogram; F$_{IO_2}$ = fraction of inspired oxygen; ICU = intensive care unit; IV = intravenous; NS = normal saline; PC = pressure control; PEEP = positive end-expiratory pressure; PRN = as needed; SC = subcutaneous; TV = tidal volume.

for conventional selective digestive tract decontamination, given concerns about global microbial antibiotic resistance.[9] In mechanically ventilated adults, chest radiographs on demand provide equivalent clinical outcomes as do routine radiographs, despite about one-third fewer radiographs.[10] Later during the recovery phase of critical illness, evidence-based management includes daily interruption of sedation infusions, daily spontaneous breathing trials, and early mobilization.

For example, in a statewide study, the creation and coaching of local safety teams to lead multidisciplinary education, central venous catheter carts stocked with necessary equipment, a five-step procedural checklist to decrease blood stream infections (handwashing, full barrier precautions for catheter insertion, chlorhexidine skin cleansing, avoidance of the femoral site, and removal of unnecessary catheters), and periodic site-specific feedback on infection rates decreased catheter-related blood stream infections from 7.7 per 1000 catheter-days at baseline to 1.4 at 18 months' follow-up.[11]

PREDICTIONS, PREFERENCES, AND END-OF-LIFE CARE

As the population ages and new technologies are developed, the use of basic and advanced life support will increase. Since demand for ICU beds is outstripping supply, the selection of patients to receive critical care is challenging. Three common but not mutually exclusive approaches to rationing ICU beds are admitting the sickest patients; admitting on a first-come, first-served basis; and triaging on the grounds of likely relative benefit. When ICU beds are rationed, patients who are refused ICU admission owing to a perceived minimal potential to benefit have a three-fold higher hospital mortality than those admitted. However, when ICU beds are reduced because of bed closures, admitted patients are sicker, are less frequently admitted for monitoring, and have shorter stays without adverse effects.

Once in the ICU, the prognosis of many critically ill patients improves. For others, treatment responsiveness is delayed or not realized, organ dysfunction evolves but does not resolve, and complications arise. Despite best efforts of the multidisciplinary ICU team, critical illness proves fatal to between 5 and 40% of adults. When a therapeutic trial of critical care is started, and particularly when it is failing, it is crucial to discuss prognosis

openly with families. Families bring key information about the patients' prior function and preferences. In the shared decision-making model that dominates today, these exchanges often result in plans to withhold or withdraw basic or advanced life support.

Mechanical ventilation is the most frequent life support administered to, and withdrawn from, critically ill patients. Ventilator withdrawal very often precedes death in the ICU. Patients undergoing ventilator withdrawal or who die while mechanically ventilated have a shorter ICU stay than patients successfully weaned from the ventilator. Such withdrawal may be guided by the severity of the illness and other physiologic characteristics, but it is more heavily influenced by the contemporary life support model that is attentive to a patient's values and the physician's predictions about future quality of life. This complexity underscores the need for ICU teams to be expert communicators, sensitive in eliciting patients' preferences, timely in relieving suffering, and compassionate in providing dignity to the dying while administering culturally competent, family-centered end-of-life care.

1. The SAFE Study Investigators. A comparison of albumin and saline for fluid resuscitation in the intensive care unit. *N Engl J Med.* 2004;350:2247-2256.
2. Zarychanski R, Turgeon AF, Fergusson DA, et al. Renal outcomes following hydroxyethyl starch resuscitation in critically ill patients: a meta-analysis of randomized trials. *Open Med.* 2009;3:196-209.
3. Kress JP, Pohlman AS, O'Connor MF, et al. Daily interruption of sedative infusions in critically ill patients undergoing mechanical ventilation. *N Engl J Med.* 2000;342:1471-1477.
4. Girard T, Kress JP, Fuchs BD, et al. Efficacy and safety of a paired sedation and ventilator weaning protocol for mechanically ventilated patients in intensive care (Awakening and Breathing Controlled trial): a randomised controlled trial. *Lancet.* 2008;371:126-134.
5. Schweickert WD, Pohlman MC, Pohlman AS, et al. Early physical and occupational therapy in mechanically ventilated, critically ill patients: a randomised controlled trial. *Lancet.* 2009;373: 1874-1882.
6. Briel M, Meade M, Zhou Q, et al. Higher versus lower positive end-expiratory pressure in patients with acute lung injury and acute respiratory distress syndrome: systematic review and individual patient data meta-analysis. *JAMA.* 2010;303:865-873.
7. The NICE-SUGAR Study Investigators. Intensive versus conventional glucose control in critically ill patients. *N Engl J Med.* 2009;360:1283-1297.
8. Soylemez Wiener R, Wiener DC, Larson RJ. Benefits and risks of tight glucose control in critically ill adults: a meta-analysis. *JAMA.* 2008;300:933-944.
9. Chaney E, Ruest A, Meade MO, et al. Oral decontamination for prevention of pneumonia in mechanically ventilated adults: systematic review and meta-analysis. *BMJ.* 2007;334:889.

10. Hejblum G, Chalumeau-Lemoine L, Ioos V, et al. Comparison of routine and on-demand prescription of chest radiographs in mechanically ventilated adults: a multicentre, cluster-randomized, two-period crossover study. *Lancet.* 2009;374:1687-1693.
11. Pronovost P, Needham D, Berenholtz S, et al. An intervention to decrease catheter-related bloodstream infections in the ICU. *N Engl J Med.* 2006;355:2725-2732.

SUGGESTED READINGS

Magder S. Hemodynamic monitoring in the mechanically ventilated patient. *Curr Opin Crit Care.* 2011;17:36-42. *Review.*

Pronovost PJ, Goeschel CA, Colantuoni E, et al. Sustaining reductions in catheter related bloodstream infections in Michigan intensive care units: observational study. *BMJ.* 2010;340:c309. *Multi-modality intervention to reduce bloodstream infections showed continued benefit 18 months after the intervention ended.*

Scales DC, Dainty K, Hales B, et al. A multifaceted intervention for quality improvement in a network of intensive care units. *JAMA.* 2011;305:363-372. *In community ICUs, a multifaceted quality improvement intervention improved adoption of beneficial care practices.*

Wunsch H, Guerra C, Barnato AE, et al. Three-year outcomes for Medicare beneficiaries who survive intensive care. *JAMA.* 2010;303:849-856. *Survivors of the ICU had a higher mortality rate than controls, especially if they required mechanical ventilation.*

RESPIRATORY MONITORING IN CRITICAL CARE

103

JAMES K. STOLLER AND NICHOLAS S. HILL

Monitoring the respiratory system involves a broad array of assessment techniques, ranging from low-technology approaches like a careful physical examination to using very sophisticated technologies to monitor oxygenation and ventilation.

PHYSICAL EXAMINATION

The physical examination can provide important information regarding the patient's ventilation and oxygenation. Ventilation can be assessed by recording the respiratory rate (normally 12 to 20 breaths/minute in adults) as well as by closely inspecting the pattern of chest wall movement during inspiration and by noting the use of accessory inspiratory muscles (e.g., the scalene, trapezius, and sternocleidomastoid muscles). Hypopnea (shallow or slow breathing) or a slowed respiratory rate (bradypnea) can indicate decreased ventilation. Shallow breathing may relate to muscle weakness (Chapter 429) or increased lung stiffness, which is commonly accompanied by a compensatory increase in the ratio of the respiratory rate to maintain ventilation. Bradypnea may relate to a suppressed respiratory drive (e.g., excessive use of narcotics, slowing the respiratory rate). Conversely, sustained tachypnea (e.g., >35 breaths/minute in an adult) can indicate ongoing increased work of breathing, impending respiratory failure, and the need for mechanical assistance, such as noninvasive ventilation or intubation and mechanical ventilation, depending on the etiology of the respiratory failure.

Contraction of the sternocleidomastoid muscles or scalene muscles, often with a seated, bent posture, is called the *tripod sign* (E-Fig. 103-1). This response indicates inadequate diaphragmatic function, most commonly in the setting of emphysema with associated diaphragmatic flattening, which causes a mechanical disadvantage of diaphragmatic contraction. In this circumstance, patients may demonstrate Hoover's sign, which is inspiratory retraction of the rib cage at the level of the zone of apposition, where the diaphragm inserts on the chest wall.

The physical examination of the nail beds and lips may also reveal cyanosis, which suggests hypoxemia. Cyanosis occurs when saturation falls, but it requires the presence of 5 g of desaturated hemoglobin. As such, polycythemic patients may show cyanosis with relatively high oxyhemoglobin saturation values, whereas patients with profound anemia may not demonstrate cyanosis even in the face of low values of oxyhemoglobin saturation.

SYSTEMIC ARTERIAL BLOOD GAS ANALYSIS

Sampling arterial blood, either through a percutaneous arterial puncture or by withdrawing blood from an indwelling arterial catheter, provides important information about the patient's oxygenation and ventilation status as well as the acuity of and compensation for derangements. The partial pressure of carbon dioxide ($Paco_2$) reflects ventilation, the elimination of carbon dioxide. In many but not all cases, $Paco_2$ is close to the mixed alveolar Pco_2.

The $Paco_2$ in the arterial blood is closely related to the ratio of metabolic CO_2 production to alveolar ventilation:

$$Paco_2 = (K)(CO_2 \text{ production rate})/(\text{alveolar ventilation}[V_A]) \quad (1)$$

The partial pressure of oxygen (Pao_2) reflects the level of oxygenation, with normal levels of oxygenation defined by the alveolar-arterial oxygen gradient, $P(A\text{-}a)o_2$, which is calculated as:

$$P(A\text{-}a)o_2 = Fio_2(P_B - P_{H_2O \text{ at standard pressure and body temperature}}) - (Pao_2 + Paco_2/\text{respiratory quotient}) \quad (2)$$

where the respiratory quotient equals the number of moles of CO_2 produced for each mole of oxygen consumed (generally ~0.8 under normal metabolic conditions at rest, but variable with dietary intake and metabolic rate). The normal value of the alveolar-arterial oxygen gradient varies with age and position and can be approximated by the simple equation:

$$P(A\text{-}a)o_2 = (\text{age}/4) + 4 \quad (3)$$

Normal age-related values of Pao_2 in the sitting position can be determined by the equation:

$$Pao_2 \text{ sitting} = 104.2 - (0.27 \times \text{age in years}) \quad (4)$$

Normal values of Pao_2 are generally in the range of 70 to 95 mm Hg, depending on the patient's age.

The $Paco_2$ helps assess the adequacy of the patient's ventilation. At sea level, normal values of $Paco_2$ range from 35 to 45 mm Hg. Values of $Paco_2$ below 35 mm Hg indicate hyperventilation, either as a primary respiratory event (e.g., with anxiety) or in response to another insult (e.g., hypoxemia, sepsis, liver disease). Similarly, values of $Paco_2$ exceeding 45 mm Hg indicate hypoventilation, hypercapnia, and respiratory acidosis, which may result either from suppression of the ventilatory drive (Chapter 86) (e.g., excess narcotics; Chapter 33) or from respiratory insufficiency (e.g., respiratory muscle weakness; Chapter 429).

Assessment of the patient's bicarbonate level (HCO_3^-) helps define the chronicity of changes in the patient's Pco_2, where the value of bicarbonate is defined by the Henderson-Hasselbalch equation:

$$pH = 6.1 + \log_{10}[HCO_3^-]/0.003 \, Paco_2 \quad (5)$$

Acute increases in $Paco_2$ drive the normal kidney to retain bicarbonate (Chapter 120), whereas acute decreases in $Paco_2$, as in hyperventilation from anxiety or liver disease, would be expected to cause the normal kidney to waste bicarbonate in order to preserve the body's pH (normally 7.35 to 7.45).

The clinician can also assess whether the patient's ventilatory response to metabolic acidosis is appropriate or inadequate by using the Winter equation, which predicts the expected $Paco_2$ in the face of a decreased bicarbonate from a metabolic acidosis (Equation 6). Specifically, a measured $Paco_2$ above the expected value indicates an inadequate ventilatory response, whereas a value of $Paco_2$ that falls within the expected range indicates an expected, appropriate ventilatory response to the metabolic derangement (i.e., the acidosis).

$$Paco_2 = (1.5[HCO_3^-] + 8) \pm 2 \quad (6)$$

When the patient is hypercapnic and hypoxemic, a useful step is to calculate the ambient air $P(A\text{-}a)o_2$ and to determine whether it is normal or increased for the patient's age. Of the six mechanisms of hypoxemia, only two (hypoventilation and breathing decreased ambient oxygen, as at altitude or from a hypoxic gas mixture) are associated with a preserved $P(A\text{-}a)o_2$ (Table 103-1). Under clinical circumstances at sea level, hypoxemia in the face of a normal $P(A\text{-}a)o_2$ indicates that the patient's hypoxemia is caused by hypoventilation and should prompt the clinician to consider the various etiologies of suppressed respiratory drive (Chapter 86) or respiratory insufficiency that interferes with a normal ventilatory response (e.g., respiratory muscle weakness; Chapter 429).

PULSE OXIMETRY

Pulse oximetry is a noninvasive method to assess arterial blood oxygenation. The percentage of hemoglobin that is oxygenated is measured by passing light of two different wavelengths (660 nm [for deoxyhemoglobin] and 940 nm [for oxyhemoglobin]) through a blood-carrying tissue (e.g., finger, earlobe, forehead), identifying the pulsatile component (which contains arterial blood and background tissue elements), and subtracting the nonpulsatile component to isolate the arterial component. The device can estimate the percent of oxygenated hemoglobin over the range of 100% to about 75%. Most clinicians regard the output of pulse oximeters to be inaccurate for percent saturation values of less than 70%, although the probability of a low saturation should not be discounted (Fig. 103-1). Pulse oximetry measurements may help identify significant drops in Pao_2 below 60 to 65 mm Hg but are relatively insensitive to changes in Pao_2 from 90 to 65 mm Hg.

CARBON DIOXIDE MONITORING: CAPNOMETRY AND TRANSCUTANEOUS CARBON DIOXIDE MEASUREMENT

The fraction of CO_2 in exhaled air can be measured in real time by infrared capnometry. Partial pressures can then be calculated based on knowledge of atmospheric pressure. The expiratory capnogram (see Fig. 103-1) represents a continuous plot of exhaled Pco_2 versus time or exhaled volume and reflects the sequential appearance of gas from various compartments (e.g., the endotracheal tube, central airways, and finally the alveoli, where the Pco_2 is in equilibrium with end-capillary blood). The shape of the capnogram provides clues to the presence of chronic obstructive pulmonary disease, in that emptying of areas of lung with increased dead space (see later) can cause the capnogram to have a rising contour (see Fig. 103-1A), whereas the attainment of a so-called alveolar plateau on the normal capnogram (see Fig. 103-1B) indicates that alveolar gas is composed of a mix with a relatively small contribution from areas of increased dead space. The value of P_ECO_2

measured at the end of expiration on the capnometer (i.e., the highest value recorded) represents the end-tidal $P_{ET}CO_2$. Notably, the value of $P_{ET}CO_2$ is always below the $Paco_2$ because there is a normal component of dead space ventilation (V_D/V_T) related to the anatomic dead space of the conducting airways (i.e., the trachea and airways to the level of gas-exchanging alveolar ducts and alveoli). The numerical difference between the $Paco_2$ and the mixed exhaled CO_2 tension (P_ECO_2, defined as the partial pressure of carbon dioxide that would be measured in a balloon in which the entire exhaled volume is gathered) is related to the magnitude of dead space ventilation (i.e., areas of the lung that are ventilated without accompanying blood flow, normally ~0.3 to 0.4) as defined by the Bohr equation:

$$V_D/V_T = (Paco_2 - P_ECO_2)/Paco_2 \qquad (7)$$

The difference between $Paco_2$ and P_ECO_2 may be as low as several millimeters of mercury, but changing conditions of ventilation-perfusion matching (e.g., with pulmonary embolism [Chapter 98], atelectasis [Chapter 90]) may change the gradient over time. Measurement of the $P_{ET}CO_2$ can be clinically useful to assess trends, to help detect esophageal intubation, to detect disconnection from the ventilator, and to detect perfusion during cardiopulmonary resuscitation, but it is not a reliable surrogate for $Paco_2$. Furthermore, measurement of the dead space fraction has prognostic value in patients with early acute respiratory distress syndrome (Chapter 104), in whom rising dead space is linearly related to increased mortality risk.

Measurement of transcutaneous Pco_2 using heated probes applied to the skin represents an alternative noninvasive method for estimating $Paco_2$. This approach is less widely used clinically, at least in adults, because of technical requirements, such as site rotation for the probes and repetitive calibration, and its generally lower accuracy in estimating $Paco_2$.

ARTERIAL OXYGEN CONTENT AND SYSTEMIC OXYGEN DELIVERY

Arterial (Cao_2) and venous oxygen content (Cvo_2) are used to calculate cardiac output using the Fick equation (Equation 8), which is an alternative to determining cardiac output by the thermodilution method using a flow-directed pulmonary artery (Swan-Ganz) catheter (Chapter 57). The Fick equation is:

$$\text{Oxygen consumption}\,(\text{mL O}_2/\text{min}) = \text{cardiac output} \times (Cao_2 - Cvo_2) \quad (8)$$

where oxygen content has the units of mL O_2/100 mL of blood and is calculated as:

$$\text{Oxygen content} = 1.34(\text{hemoglobin})(\%\,\text{saturation}) + 0.0031(Pao_2) \quad (9)$$

Under normal conditions (with, for example, an arterial percent saturation of 95% and a hemoglobin of 15 g/100 mL and an oxygen consumption of 250 mL/minute), arterial oxygen content is about 20 mL/100 mL and, because mixed venous oxygen saturation is about 75%, central venous oxygen content is about 15 mL/100 mL, making the normal arteriovenous oxygen content difference with a normal cardiac output about 5 mL/100 mL.

Systemic oxygen transport defines the amount of oxygen delivered to the tissues and multiplies the arterial oxygen content by the cardiac output:

$$\text{Systemic oxygen transport}\,(\text{mL/min}) = \text{cardiac output} \times Cao_2 \quad (10)$$

where the normal value is about 1000 mL/minute.

TABLE 103-1	PHYSIOLOGIC MECHANISMS OF HYPOXEMIA AND ACCOMPANYING VALUES OF THE ALVEOLAR-ARTERIAL OXYGEN GRADIENT BREATHING ROOM AIR	
MECHANISM/ PHYSIOLOGIC PROCESS	**EXAMPLE**	**ALVEOLAR-ARTERIAL OXYGEN GRADIENT ON ROOM AIR**
Ventilation-perfusion mismatch	Pneumonia	Increased
Diffusion impairment	Interstitial lung disease	Increased
Anatomic right-to-left shunt	Pulmonary arteriovenous malformation	Increased
Hypoventilation	Neuromuscular weakness	Normal
Breathing decreased ambient oxygen (from either hypobaric conditions [e.g., altitude] or breathing a gas mixture with decreased inspired oxygen fraction)	Altitude exposure	Normal
Diffusion-perfusion impairment	Hepatopulmonary syndrome	Increased

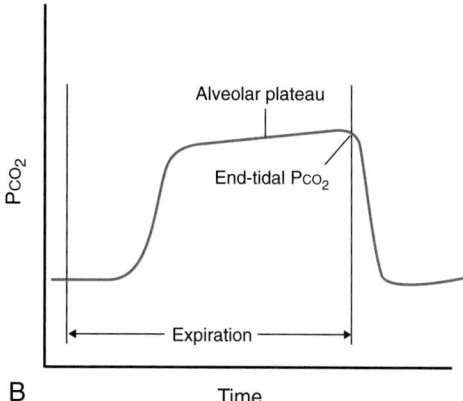

FIGURE 103-1. Abnormal and normal end-tidal capnograms. **A,** Illustration of a capnogram from a patient with chronic obstructive pulmonary disease in which the end-tidal Pco_2 rises throughout expiration as CO_2 excretion varies from different parts of the lung. **B,** Illustration of a normal capnogram in which the end-tidal Pco_2 reaches a plateau with more uniform CO_2 excretion. The end-tidal Pco_2 ($P_{ET}CO_2$) is the highest point of the alveolar plateau.

MEASURING VENTILATION: MINUTE VENTILATION AND ALVEOLAR VENTILATION

Minute ventilation ($\dot{V}E$), which is the amount of gas exhaled from the airway per minute, is the product of the respiratory rate times the exhaled tidal volume, measured at body temperature and standardized to barometric pressure at sea level, saturated with water vapor (BTPS). The BTPS is a standard condition under which many measurements for most pulmonary function equipment and mechanical ventilators are made. These devices use an airflow meter to measure exhaled airflow and integrate the signal to derive tidal volume. An alternative way to measure tidal volume in an intensive care setting is respiratory impedance plethysmography, which uses calibrated magnetic coils in belts strapped around the chest and abdomen to monitor respiratory frequency and changes in thoracic volume.

Alveolar ventilation is the rate of gas delivery in liters per minute to gas-exchanging areas of the lung (i.e., the alveoli and alveolar ducts). The portion of minute ventilation that fails to undergo gas exchange is dead space ventilation ($\dot{V}D$) and is determined by Equation 7 above. Minute, alveolar ($\dot{V}A$), and dead space ventilation are related as follows:

$$\dot{V}E = \dot{V}A + \dot{V}D \qquad (11)$$

It follows that conditions such as acute lung injury or acute respiratory distress syndrome (ARDS; Chapter 104) that are associated with very high dead space ratios require high $\dot{V}E$ to achieve a sufficient $\dot{V}A$. Conversely, conditions that cause neuromuscular weakness (Chapter 429) are associated with small tidal volumes and have a high VD/VT ratio because the anatomic dead space is fixed and constitutes a higher fraction of the diminished tidal volume.

MEASURING CARBON DIOXIDE PRODUCTION

Measurement of CO_2 production is sometimes referred to as *indirect calorimetry* because it provides an index of metabolic rate and permits estimation of caloric requirements. Metabolic "carts" that simultaneously measure not only CO_2 production but also O_2 consumption and respiratory quotient are commonly used clinically to estimate metabolic needs in order to prescribe nutritional repletion (Chapter 223). The normal baseline CO_2 production is in the range of 200 mL/minute but is subject to wide variation because of hypermetabolic states commonly encountered in critically ill patients, such as sepsis or the systemic inflammatory response syndrome. A high CO_2 production might be used as an indication to increase caloric delivery.

The respiratory quotient also gives insight into the composition of feedings because carbohydrates yield a respiratory quotient of 1, whereas fatty acids yield a ratio of 0.8 and amino acids a ratio of 0.7. Thus, balanced nutrition should yield a respiratory quotient of approximately 0.85. A respiratory quotient of 1 in combination with a high CO_2 production suggests that the dietary proportion of carbohydrates is excessive.

MEASURING RESPIRATORY COMPLIANCE

Respiratory compliance is the change in respiratory system volume induced by a change in applied pressure (i.e., inspiratory pressure) and is the inverse of elastance. Compliance diminishes in conditions like lung injury and ARDS (Chapter 104) or pulmonary fibrosis (Chapter 92), in which diffuse inflammation and scarring alter lung structure and contribute to increased lung "stiffness." Static respiratory compliance is measured in patients receiving volume-limited mechanical ventilation by imposing a brief inspiratory hold at end inspiration. Assuming the patient has no spontaneous breathing effort, the airway pressure measured when airflow ceases is referred to as the plateau pressure ($P_{plateau}$). The difference between this pressure and the positive end-expiratory pressure (PEEP) is taken as the driving pressure required to deliver the tidal volume (Fig. 103-2). Static respiratory system compliance (CRS) is then calculated as:

$$C_{RS} = \Delta V(\text{exhaled tidal volume})/\Delta P(P_{plateau} - PEEP) \qquad (12)$$

This compliance not only reflects the status of the lung but also includes contributions of the chest wall and abdomen. Thus, patients with chest wall deformities or morbid obesity have lower values of respiratory compliance even in the absence of lung abnormalities (Chapter 99). The normal respiratory compliance is in the range of 50 to 70 mL/cm H_2O, and patients with ARDS usually have values of CRS of less than 30 cm H_2O. If respiratory compliance is below 20 to 25 cm H_2O, weaning from mechanical ventilation (Chapter 105) is unlikely because of the high work of breathing requirements (see later).

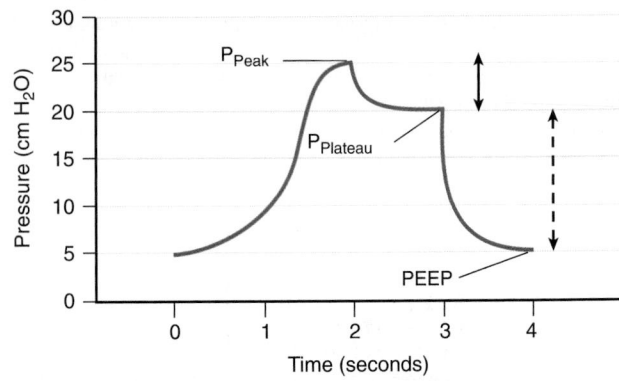

FIGURE 103-2. Illustration of inspiratory hold maneuver to determine plateau pressure ($P_{plateau}$). Airway pressure during volume-targeted mechanical ventilation rises as the tidal volume is delivered and reaches a peak. An inspiratory hold is initiated at peak pressure that prevents exhalation, so pressure falls to a "plateau" of about 20 cm H_2O. The drop in pressure reflects the pressure needed to overcome airway resistance. After slightly more than 1 second, the inspiratory hold is released, and airway pressure falls to positive end-expiratory pressure (PEEP). The difference between ($P_{plateau}$) and PEEP is used to calculate static compliance by dividing the difference into the tidal volume.

MEASURING RESPIRATORY DRIVE

The respiratory center, located in the pons and medulla, regulates respiratory drive. Hypercapnia is a strong stimulus to ventilation (Chapter 86). This response may be blunted by chronic CO_2 retention or by drugs like narcotics. Hypoxemia is a weaker ventilatory stimulus that is potentiated by hypercapnia and blunted by hypocapnia.

Thus, respiratory drive can be assessed as the response to CO_2 in the blood in the hypercapnic ventilatory response. In one technique to measure respiratory drive, the patient rebreathes his or her exhaled air while minute ventilation and $P_{ET}CO_2$ are monitored; a graph relating $P_{ET}CO_2$ with minute ventilation is used to measure respiratory drive. However, this technique is impractical in an intensive care unit (ICU) setting. Another technique is to measure the negative swing in airway pressure during the first 100 msec of inspiration (P_{100}). This technique avoids the problem of diminished ventilatory response due to airway obstruction, but it is still subject to blunting by some drugs and still underestimates drive in patients with respiratory muscle weakness, a very common problem in the ICU. In patients who are failing to wean from mechanical ventilation, a practical way to assess the integrity of respiratory drive is to determine whether the respiratory rate increases, usually into the 30s or 40s, as $PaCO_2$ rises after the patient is removed from ventilatory support.

MEASURING RESPIRATORY MUSCLE STRENGTH

Respiratory muscle weakness has long been recognized as a contributor to respiratory failure and failure to wean from mechanical ventilation in the ICU (Chapter 105). This recognition has intensified in recent years with the increased awareness of ICU-acquired weakness following critical illness. However, measurement of respiratory muscle strength remains challenging because of the need to differentiate between actual weakness and reduced muscle performance owing to inability to cooperate or to exert a full inspiratory effort.

The most commonly used measures of respiratory muscle strength are the maximal inspiratory and expiratory pressures (PI_{max} or MIP and PE_{max} or MEP). These values are obtained by measuring the pressure change with a manometer when the patient inhales with maximal force from residual volume and exhales with maximal force from total lung capacity. Normal MIP is usually more negative than −75 cm H_2O, and normal MEP is usually more positive than 125 cm H_2O. When the value for MIP is less negative than −20 or −30 cm H_2O, weaning may be difficult, and values less positive than 60 cm H_2O suggest cough insufficiency. However, these values have poor predictive value in mechanically ventilated patients because many of these patients are unable to cooperate. This problem may be addressed by attaching a one-way valve to the end of endotracheal tube that permits exhalation but not inhalation and then measuring the inspiratory pressure efforts for 20 to 25 seconds.

MEASURING WORK OF BREATHING

Work of breathing is the product of pressure and volume for each breath (Fig. 103-3). The components include work needed to overcome elastic recoil of

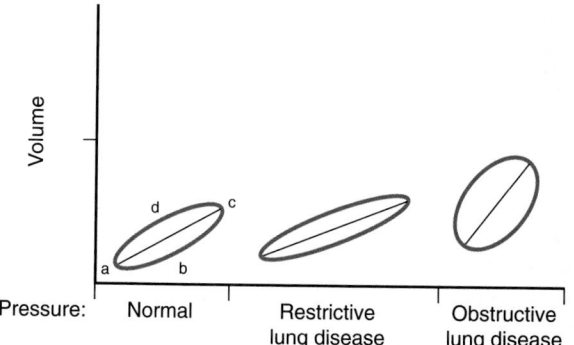

FIGURE 103-3. Pressure-volume curves illustrating components of work in a normal subject and in patients with restrictive or obstructive disease. The line between **a** and **c** represents elastic work as the lung expands, but this work is a net zero because static forces return the lung to its neutral position. The restrictive curve is flatter than normal because the lung is stiffer and volume changes less for a given unit change in pressure. The obstructive curve has a greater slope because (e.g., in emphysema) the lung is more compliant and starts inhalation from a higher volume. The **abc** curve represents resistive work during inspiration, and **cda** represents resistive work during exhalation. Resistive work during exhalation is greater in patients with obstructive lung disease.

the lung and to displace the chest wall and abdomen as well as work needed to overcome airway resistance and lung viscosity and work needed to overcome inertia. With restrictive lung diseases, the inspiratory work of breathing is increased because of the decreased lung elasticity. With obstructive diseases, the work of breathing is increased because of increased airway resistance.

In clinical settings, a more practical way to assess the inspiratory work of breathing is to calculate the pressure-time product (PTP) in cm H_2O-seconds. The PTP can be calculated using the decrease in airway pressure during inspiration, esophageal pressure (measured using an esophageal balloon manometer), or transdiaphragmatic pressure (measured using esophageal and gastric balloon manometers)—as an index of diaphragmatic work. The work can be calculated as work of breathing per breath or as work of breathing per minute by multiplying the work per breath by the respiratory frequency. Commercially available devices using esophageal manometry automatically calculate the inspiratory work of breathing, which may be of some value in assessing the likelihood of weaning from mechanical ventilation. If the drop in inspiratory pressure necessary to achieve an adequate tidal volume is too large, the calculated work of breathing will be high, and the likelihood of successful weaning will be reduced.

SUGGESTED READINGS

De Wit M, Miller K, Green D, et al. Ineffective triggering predicts increased duration of mechanical ventilation. *Crit Care Med.* 2009;37:2740-2745. *Graphic waveforms from the mechanical ventilator are correlated with the duration of mechanical ventilation.*

Gattinoni L, Carlesso E, Cressoni M. Assessing gas exchange in acute lung injury/acute respiratory distress syndrome: diagnostic techniques and prognostic relevance. *Curr Opin Crit Care.* 2011;17:18-23. *Dead space and CO_2 retention are most closely associated with outcome.*

See KC, Phua J, Mukhopadhyay A. Monitoring of extubated patients: are routine arterial blood gas measurements useful and how long should patients be monitored in the intensive care unit? *Anaesth Intens Care.* 2010;38:96-101. *Data suggesting that blood gases at 1 and 3 hours are not useful predictors of successful extubation.*

104

ACUTE RESPIRATORY FAILURE

LEONARD D. HUDSON AND ARTHUR S. SLUTSKY

ACUTE RESPIRATORY FAILURE

DEFINITION

Acute respiratory failure occurs when dysfunction of the respiratory system results in abnormal gas exchange that is potentially life-threatening. Each element of this definition is important to understand. The term *acute* implies

a relatively sudden onset (from hours to days) and a substantial change from the patient's baseline condition. Dysfunction of the respiratory system indicates that the abnormal gas exchange may be caused by abnormalities in any element of the respiratory system (e.g., a central nervous system abnormality affecting the regulation of breathing or a musculoskeletal thoracic abnormality affecting ventilation; Chapter 83), in addition to abnormalities of the lung itself. The term *respiration* refers, in a broad sense, to the delivery of oxygen (O_2) to metabolically active tissues for energy usage and the removal of carbon dioxide (CO_2) from these tissues (Table 104-1). Respiratory failure is a failure of the process of delivering O_2 to the tissues and/or removing CO_2 from the tissues. Abnormalities in the periphery (e.g., cyanide poisoning, pathologic distribution of organ blood flow in sepsis) can also lead to tissue

TABLE 104-1	ABBREVIATIONS COMMONLY USED IN ACUTE RESPIRATORY FUNCTION
ABG	Arterial blood gas or arterial blood gas analysis
ALI	Acute lung injury
ARDS	Acute respiratory distress syndrome
ARF	Acute respiratory failure
cm H_2O	Centimeters of water
Cao_2	Content of oxygen in arterial blood
Cco_2	Content of oxygen in end-capillary blood
CO_2	Carbon dioxide
COPD	Chronic obstructive pulmonary disease
CPAP	Continuous positive airway pressure (used when positive pressure during exhalation is applied with spontaneous ventilation)
Cvo_2	Content of oxygen in mixed venous blood
Fio_2	Fraction of inspired oxygen
g/dL	Grams per deciliter
HbO_2	Saturation of hemoglobin by oxygen
L/min	Liters per minute
mL/kg	Milliliters per kilogram
mL/min	Milliliters per minute
mm Hg	Millimeters of mercury
NIPPV	Noninvasive positive-pressure ventilation
O_2	Oxygen
$P(A-a)o_2$	Difference of partial pressure of oxygen between mean alveolar gas and arterial blood (alveolar-to-arterial oxygen difference)
$Paco_2$	Partial pressure of carbon dioxide in alveolar gas
$Paco_2$	Partial pressure of carbon dioxide in arterial blood
Pao_2	Partial pressure of oxygen in alveolar gas
Pao_2	Partial pressure of oxygen in arterial blood
Pao_2/Fio_2	Ratio of partial pressure of oxygen in arterial blood to fraction of inspired oxygen
PBW	Predicted body weight
$Pcco_2$	Partial pressure of carbon dioxide in end-capillary blood
Pco_2	Partial pressure of oxygen in end-capillary blood
PEEP	Positive end-expiratory pressure (used when positive pressure during exhalation is applied with mechanical ventilation)
P/F	Pao_2/Fio_2 ratio
Pio_2	Partial pressure of oxygen in inspired gas
Po_2	Partial pressure of oxygen
$Pvco_2$	Partial pressure of carbon dioxide in mixed venous blood
Pvo_2	Partial pressure of oxygen in mixed venous blood
Q	Blood flow or perfusion
RR	Respiratory rate
Sao_2	Percentage of saturation of hemoglobin by oxygen in arterial blood
$\dot{V}$	Ventilation
$\dot{V}/\dot{Q}$	Ventilation-to-perfusion ratio
V_T	Tidal volume

TABLE 104-2 SYSTEMS TO CLASSIFY ACUTE RESPIRATORY FAILURE

HYPOXIC VERSUS HYPERCAPNIC-HYPOXIC ARF	ARF WITH AND WITHOUT CHRONIC LUNG DISEASE
Causes of Hypoxic ARF	**With Chronic Lung Disease**
Acute lung injury/ARDS Pneumonia Pulmonary thromboembolism Acute lobar atelectasis Cardiogenic pulmonary edema Lung contusion Acute collagen vascular disease (Goodpasture's syndrome, systemic lupus erythematosus)	COPD Asthma Parenchymal lung diseases Restrictive lung/chest wall diseases
	Without Chronic Lung Disease‡
	Acute lung injury/ARDS Pneumonia Pulmonary thromboembolism
Causes of Hypercapnic-Hypoxic ARF	**ARF BY ORGAN SYSTEM INVOLVED**

Pulmonary disease
   COPD
   Asthma: advanced, acute, severe asthma
Drugs causing respiratory depression
Neuromuscular
   Guillain-Barré syndrome
   Acute myasthenia gravis
Spinal cord tumors
Metabolic derangements causing weakness (including hypophosphatemia, hypomagnesemia)
Musculoskeletal
   Kyphoscoliosis
   Ankylosing spondylitis
Obesity hypoventilation syndrome (often with additional acute, superimposed abnormality as cause of ARF)
	Respiratory (Lungs and Thorax)

	Airway/airflow obstruction
	   COPD
	   Asthma
	Pulmonary parenchyma
	   Pneumonia
	   Acute lung injury/ARDS
	   Acute flare of chronic collagen vascular disease (e.g., Goodpasture's syndrome, systemic lupus erythematosus)

	Central Nervous System

	Respiratory depression
	   Increased sedatives, tranquilizers with respiratory effect; opiates; alcohol
	Brain stem and spinal cord involvement
	   Tumors, trauma, vascular accidents

ETIOLOGIC MECHANISMS OF HYPOXEMIA	**Neuromuscular**
Normal $P(A-a)_{O_2}$*	Guillain-Barré syndrome Myasthenia gravis

$\downarrow P_{IO_2}$
   High altitude; inadvertent administration of low F_{IO_2} gas mixture
Hypoventilation
   See causes of hypercapnic-hypoxic ARF above
	Cardiovascular

	Cardiogenic pulmonary edema Pulmonary thromboembolism
Increased $P(A-a)_{O_2}$*	**Renal/Endocrine**

Ventilation-perfusion ($\dot{V}/\dot{Q}$) mismatch
   Airway disease
   Vascular disease, including pulmonary thromboembolism
Shunt
   Acute lung injury/ARDS
   Pneumonia
   Parenchymal lung disease
   Cardiogenic pulmonary edema
   Pulmonary infarction
Diffusion limitation†
	Volume overload
	Metabolic abnormalities

*Calculated using the alveolar-air equation; see text for description.
†See text for discussion.
‡These can also be superimposed on chronic disease.
ARDS = acute respiratory distress syndrome; ARF = acute respiratory failure; COPD = chronic obstructive pulmonary disease; F_{IO_2} = fraction of inspired oxygen; $P(A-a)_{O_2}$ = alveolar-to-arterial oxygen difference; P_{IO_2} = partial pressure of inspired oxygen; $\dot{V}/\dot{Q}$ = ventilation-to-perfusion ratio.

hypoxia; although these conditions represent forms of respiratory failure in the broadest terms, this chapter focuses on respiratory failure resulting from dysfunction of the lungs, chest wall, and control of respiration.

PATHOBIOLOGY

Abnormal gas exchange is the physiologic hallmark of acute respiratory failure, which can be classified in several ways (Table 104-2). Although gas exchange can be abnormal for either oxygenation or CO_2 removal, significant hypoxemia is nearly always present when patients with acute respiratory failure breathe ambient air. If CO_2 is retained at a potentially life-threatening level, this is usually accompanied by significant hypoxemia (see later). The *life-threatening* aspect of the condition places the degree of abnormal gas exchange in a clinical context and calls for urgent treatment.

The diagnosis of acute respiratory failure requires a significant change in blood gases from baseline. Many patients with chronic respiratory problems can function with blood gas tensions that would be alarming in a physiologically normal individual. Over time, these patients with so-called chronic respiratory failure or chronic respiratory insufficiency develop mechanisms to compensate for inadequate gas exchange. Conversely, this chronic condition makes patients vulnerable to insults that could be easily tolerated by a previously healthy individual.

In acute respiratory failure, the O_2 content in the blood (available for tissue use) is reduced to a level at which the possibility of end-organ dysfunction

increases markedly. The value of the partial pressure of O_2 in the arterial blood (Pa_{O_2}) that demarcates this vulnerable zone is the point of the oxyhemoglobin dissociation relationship at which any further decrease in the Pa_{O_2} results in sharp decreases in the amount of hemoglobin saturated with O_2 (Sa_{O_2}) and in the arterial blood O_2 content (Ca_{O_2}). Although arbitrary, acute respiratory failure is often defined in practice as occurring when the Pa_{O_2} is less than 55 mm Hg (Fig. 104-1). In general, the locus on the curve that indicates the partial pressure at which O_2 is being unloaded to the tissues is the most important determinant of how much O_2 is available for the cells and their mitochondria. Usually, the ability to unload O_2 at the tissue level more than compensates for small decreases in the amount of O_2 picked up in the lungs when the oxyhemoglobin dissociation curve is shifted rightward. With a leftward shift in the curve, O_2 is bound more tightly to hemoglobin, so less O_2 is available for tissue delivery.

These clinical considerations imply that any definition of acute respiratory failure based on an absolute level of Pa_{O_2} is arbitrary. A healthy, young, conditioned individual climbing at high altitude may have a Pa_{O_2} of less than 50 mm Hg because of the reduction in inspired O_2 pressure. This individual is not in acute respiratory failure, even though the Pa_{O_2} may be in the low 40s. A patient who has chronic obstructive pulmonary disease (COPD) and whose usual range of Pa_{O_2} is 50 to 55 mm Hg would not be considered to be in acute respiratory failure if the Pa_{O_2} was 50 mm Hg. However, if a patient's usual Pa_{O_2} was 60 to 70 mm Hg, a Pa_{O_2} of 50 mm Hg would be associated

FIGURE 104-1. Oxyhemoglobin association-dissociation curve. The axis for oxygen saturation in the arterial blood (SaO_2) is on the left, and the axis for arterial content of oxygen (CaO_2) is on the right. CaO_2 is the sum of the oxygen dissolved in plasma (denoted as "Dissolved" in the figure) plus the oxygen bound to hemoglobin. At a normal hemoglobin, most of the oxygen is carried in combination with hemoglobin, with only a relatively small amount of oxygen dissolved in plasma. When the value of the arterial partial pressure of oxygen (PaO_2) is on the "flat" portion of the curve ($PaO_2 \geq 60$ to 65 mm Hg, normal partial pressure of carbon dioxide [PCO_2], and normal pH), raising the PaO_2 further has relatively little effect on total oxygen content. Increases in temperature, PCO_2, hydrogen ion concentration, or 2,3-diphosphoglycerate cause a rightward shift in the oxyhemoglobin association-dissociation curve.

with a substantial risk for a further life-threatening reduction in oxygenation; this patient should be considered to have acute respiratory failure.

Traditionally, the level of arterial CO_2 partial pressure ($PaCO_2$) that defines acute respiratory failure has been 50 mm Hg or greater, if accompanied by arterial acidosis with a pH of 7.30 or less. The $PaCO_2$ is linked to pH because it is generally thought that acidosis leads to tissue dysfunction and symptoms. Patients with severe COPD may have chronic CO_2 retention, but renal compensation for the respiratory acidosis protects them against abnormalities related to the elevation in CO_2. A further acute rise in $PaCO_2$ can precipitate symptoms and other organ dysfunction; however, even severe respiratory acidosis (pH 7.1) seems to be better tolerated than metabolic acidosis of the same pH in most previously healthy individuals if arterial and tissue oxygenation is adequate.

Pathophysiology

Five mechanisms can lead to a reduction in PaO_2: (1) decreased inspired partial pressure of O_2 (PIO_2) (e.g., at high altitude or when breathing a reduced percentage O_2 mixture); (2) hypoventilation; (3) ventilation-perfusion ($\dot{V}/\dot{Q}$) mismatch; (4) shunting of blood from the pulmonary to systemic circulation, bypassing the alveoli anatomically or functionally; and (5) abnormal diffusion of O_2 from the alveoli into the capillary blood. In essence, a shunt is an extreme $\dot{V}/\dot{Q}$ mismatch in which blood perfuses alveoli with *no* ventilation; it is differentiated clinically from other $\dot{V}/\dot{Q}$ mismatching by the response to breathing supplemental O_2 (see later).

For clinical purposes, diffusion abnormalities are not an important cause of hypoxemia at sea level because there is sufficient time for adequate diffusion of O_2 during the transit of a red blood cell through the pulmonary capillary bed, even in the presence of severe lung disease. Even when diffusion abnormalities are present and contribute to hypoxemia, $\dot{V}/\dot{Q}$ mismatch and shunting nearly always coexist and are quantitatively more important causes of hypoxemia. Except at high altitude or when a subject is breathing a gas mixture low in O_2, hypoventilation, $\dot{V}/\dot{Q}$ mismatch, and shunting are the dominant causes of acute respiratory failure.

If only hypoventilation is present, the resulting hypoxemia is associated with a normal difference between the calculated alveolar and the measured arterial oxygenation levels ($P(A-a)O_2$). In this setting, an elevated $PaCO_2$ suggests disease processes that affect nonpulmonary respiratory function (e.g., central respiratory depression resulting from drug overdose, neuromuscular

diseases such as Guillain-Barré syndrome, or chest wall disease such as flail chest; Chapter 86). In contrast, $\dot{V}/\dot{Q}$ mismatch and shunting are associated with an elevated $P(A-a)O_2$, which may or may not coexist with hypoventilation. The normal value for $P(A-a)O_2$ varies as a function of the fraction of inspired O_2 (FIO_2), increasing as FIO_2 increases.

When $\dot{V}/\dot{Q}$ mismatch or shunting is the cause of hypoxemia, some alveolar regions have increased $PACO_2$ and reduced PAO_2; the blood in the vessels perfusing these alveoli reflects these abnormal gas tensions. The increased $PACO_2$ usually can be reversed by increasing overall ventilation, but hyperventilation does not correct the decreased PaO_2.

$\dot{V}/\dot{Q}$ mismatch is distinguished from shunting by assessing the PaO_2 response to enhanced O_2 administration. Hypoxemia caused by $\dot{V}/\dot{Q}$ mismatch can be corrected to a nearly complete O_2 saturation of the hemoglobin in most patients by a relatively small increase in FIO_2, such as from 0.24 to 0.28 by face mask or 1 to 2 L/minute O_2 by nasal prongs, in patients with acute exacerbations of COPD. If the airways to poorly ventilated alveoli remain open and the enriched O_2 mixture is administered for an adequate length of time (ranging from a few minutes to 20 minutes, depending on the degree of $\dot{V}/\dot{Q}$ inequality), the increased PIO_2 is reflected by an increased PAO_2 and an increased PaO_2. When a shunt is present (no ventilation but continued perfusion), a relatively small increase in the FIO_2 has little or no effect on the PaO_2, and even large increases in FIO_2 up to 1.0 result in only modest increases in PaO_2 (Fig. 104-2).

CLINICAL MANIFESTATIONS

The hallmark of acute respiratory failure is the inability to maintain adequate oxygenation or the inability to maintain an appropriate $PaCO_2$. Patients are typically dyspneic and tachypneic, unless progressive respiratory failure causes fatigue—sometimes leading to respiratory arrest—or a drug overdose or neuromuscular condition prevents an appropriate respiratory response to hypoxia and/or the hypercapnic acidosis. Neurologic function may deteriorate, and myocardial ischemia or even infarction may be precipitated by the hypoxemia. In addition, each cause has its own specific manifestations (see later).

DIAGNOSIS

As part of the diagnosis of acute respiratory failure, the physician has three objectives: (1) confirm the clinical suspicion that acute respiratory failure is present, (2) classify the type of acute respiratory failure (e.g., hypoxemia caused by hypoventilation vs. hypoxemia caused by $\dot{V}/\dot{Q}$ mismatch or shunting), and (3) determine the specific cause (e.g., acute lung injury secondary to sepsis or decompensated COPD because of acute bronchitis). Defining the type of acute respiratory failure and determining the specific cause are prerequisites to optimal management.

The initial approach to diagnosis consists of considering information from four sources: (1) clinical history and physical examination; (2) physiologic abnormalities, particularly arterial blood gas derangements, which help establish the pathophysiologic mechanisms of hypoxemia; (3) chest radiographic findings; and (4) other tests aimed at elucidating specific causes. In many cases, the clinical picture from the history is so clear that the presumptive type of acute respiratory failure (and sometimes the cause) is obvious, so treatment can be started while confirmatory laboratory studies are ordered. In other cases, a clinician may be asked to see a patient because of an abnormal chest radiograph or abnormal arterial blood gases ordered by someone else and may elicit the pertinent history based on these clues. When the degree of hypoxemia is life-threatening, therapeutic decisions must be made quickly, even if data are limited. The clinician must obtain updated information continually and should view most therapeutic decisions as therapeutic trials, with careful monitoring to assess desired benefits and possible detrimental effects.

Clinical Evaluation

The presentation often reflects one of three clinical scenarios: (1) the effects of hypoxemia and/or respiratory acidosis, (2) the effects of primary (e.g., pneumonia) or secondary (e.g., heart failure) diseases involving the lungs, and (3) the nonpulmonary effects of the underlying disease process. The clinical effects of hypoxemia and/or respiratory acidosis manifest mainly in the central nervous system (e.g., irritability, agitation, changes in personality, depressed level of consciousness, coma) and the cardiovascular system (e.g., arrhythmias, hypotension, hypertension) (Table 104-3). In patients with underlying COPD (Chapter 88) with a gradual onset of acute respiratory failure, central nervous system abnormalities may be the major presenting

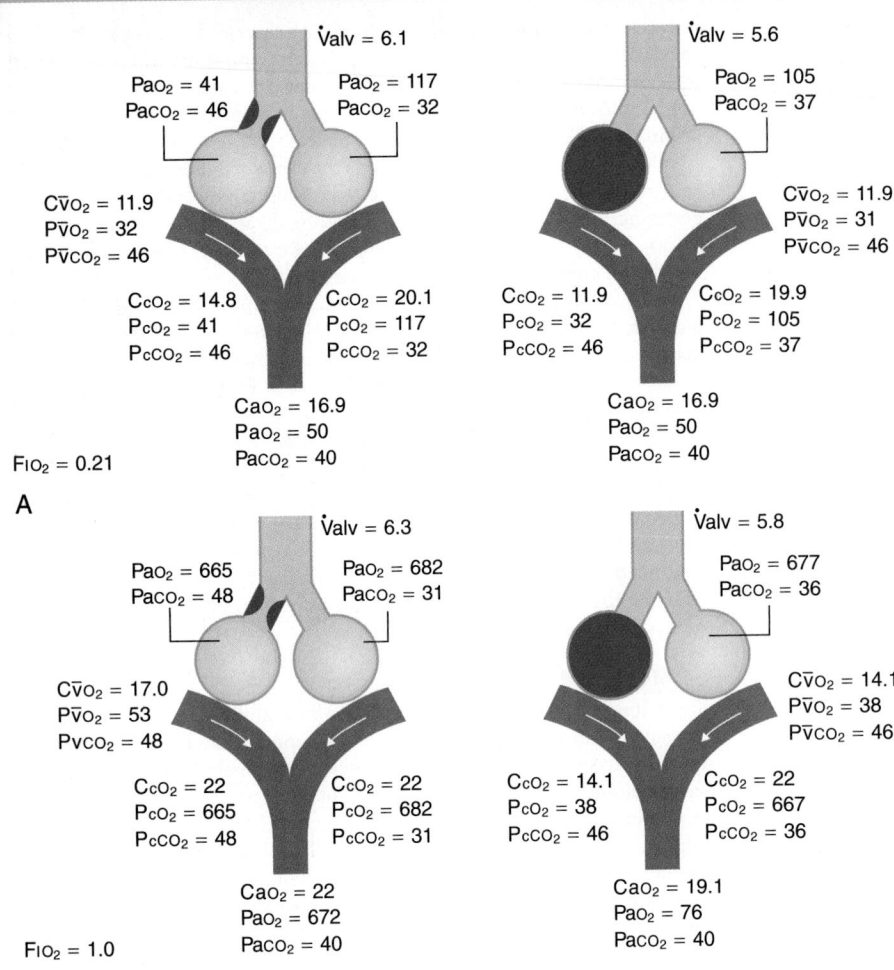

FIGURE 104-2. Arterial oxygenation. Comparison of the effect on arterial oxygenation of increasing the fraction of inspired oxygen (FiO_2) from breathing ambient air ($FiO_2 = 0.21$) **(A)** and breathing 100% oxygen ($FiO_2 = 1.0$) **(B)** with a low ventilation-to-perfusion ratio ($\dot{V}/\dot{Q}$) (left) and a shunt (right), using a two-compartment lung model. Shunting and decreased $\dot{V}/\dot{Q}$ can lead to identical arterial blood gases (partial pressure of oxygen in arterial blood [PaO_2] = 50 mm Hg; partial pressure of carbon dioxide in arterial blood [$PaCO_2$] = 40 mm Hg). The response to supplemental oxygen administration is markedly different. Hypoxemia is only partially corrected by breathing 100% oxygen when a shunt is present because arterial oxygenation represents an average of the end-capillary oxygen content (CcO_2) from various parts of the lung, not an average of the partial pressures of oxygen (partial pressure of carbon dioxide in the end-capillary blood [$PcCO_2$]). When the CcO_2 values are mixed, the PaO_2 is determined from the resultant content of oxygen in the arterial blood (CaO_2) by the oxyhemoglobin association-dissociation relationship (see Fig. 104-1). With low $\dot{V}/\dot{Q}$ (as is often the case in patients with chronic obstructive pulmonary disease), an increase in FiO_2 increases the alveolar partial pressure of oxygen (PO_2) of the low $\dot{V}/\dot{Q}$ unit and leads to a marked increase in arterial PO_2. The values in this figure were generated from modeling to result in the same $PaCO_2$ (40 mm Hg) for all four situations shown; this is the reason for slight changes in alveolar ventilation ($\dot{V}/\dot{Q}$ alv) for some of the conditions. Several assumptions are made: (1) no diffusion limitation is present; (2) oxygen consumption = 300 mL/minute, and CO_2 production = 240 mL/minute; (3) cardiac output = 6.0 L/minute; (4) the low $\dot{V}/\dot{Q}$ regions in the left panels represent 60% of the cardiac output perfusing alveoli with a $\dot{V}/\dot{Q}$ 25% of normal; and (5) the shunts in the right panels represent a 37% shunt (i.e., 37% of the cardiac output is perfusing alveoli with no ventilation).

TABLE 104-3	CLINICAL MANIFESTATIONS OF HYPOXEMIA AND HYPERCAPNIA
HYPOXEMIA	**HYPERCAPNIA**
Tachycardia	Somnolence
Tachypnea	Lethargy
Anxiety	Restlessness
Diaphoresis	Tremor
Altered mental status	Slurred speech
Confusion	Headache
Cyanosis	Asterixis
Hypertension	Papilledema
Hypotension	Coma
Bradycardia	Diaphoresis
Seizures	
Coma	
Lactic acidosis*	

*Usually requires additional reduction in oxygen delivery because of inadequate cardiac output, severe anemia, or redistribution of blood flow.

findings. Cyanosis, which requires at least 5 g/dL of unsaturated hemoglobin to be detectable, may not be seen before serious tissue hypoxia develops, especially in patients with underlying anemia.

Pulmonary symptoms and signs often reflect the respiratory disease causing the acute respiratory failure. Examples include cough and sputum with pneumonia (Chapter 97) or chest pain from pulmonary thromboembolism with infarction (Chapter 98). Dyspnea and respiratory distress are nonspecific reflections of the respiratory system's difficulty in meeting the increased demands from pulmonary and nonpulmonary diseases.

Physical findings may be associated with a particular pathologic lung process, such as pneumonia, causing bronchial breathing and crackles on auscultation, or the crackles (rales) of cardiogenic pulmonary edema (Chapter 58). Abnormal findings may be minimal or absent in patients with acute lung injury or pulmonary thromboembolism.

In some patients, the clinical picture is dominated by the underlying disease process, particularly with diseases that cause acute lung injury, such as sepsis (Chapter 108), severe pneumonia (Chapter 97), aspiration of gastric contents (Chapter 94), and trauma. In these conditions the physical examination is often nonspecific, with no obvious clues except, for example, fever with sepsis or pneumonia and hypotension with septic shock.

Assessment of Physiologic Abnormalities

The clinical suspicion of acute respiratory failure must be addressed by arterial blood gas analysis to answer several questions.

1. *Is hypoxemia present?* The answer is based largely on the value of the PaO_2 or SaO_2, and the degree of the hypoxemia not only confirms the diagnosis of acute respiratory failure but also helps define its severity.
2. *Is hypoventilation present?* If the $PaCO_2$ is elevated, alveolar hypoventilation is present.
3. *Does the degree of hypoventilation explain the hypoxemia?* If the $P(A-a)O_2$ is normal, hypoventilation explains the presence and degree of hypoxemia. In this case, the most likely causes of acute respiratory failure are central nervous system abnormalities and a chest wall abnormality. If the $P(A-a)O_2$ is increased but hypoventilation does not explain the hypoxemia, another condition must be present; common diagnoses include COPD, severe asthma, and early-stage acute respiratory distress syndrome (ARDS).
4. If hypoxemia exists without hypoventilation, an elevated $P(A-a)O_2$ should be confirmed, and the response to breathing an enhanced O_2 mixture would answer this question: *Is the increase in $P(A-a)O_2$ the result of a $\dot{V}/\dot{Q}$ abnormality or of shunting?* If hypoxemia is primarily the result of a $\dot{V}/\dot{Q}$ abnormality, the likely cause is an airway disease, either COPD or acute severe asthma, or a vascular disease, such as pulmonary

FIGURE 104-3. Chest radiographs (left) and computed tomography (CT) scans (right) of the three most common findings in diseases causing acute respiratory failure. **A,** Relatively clear chest, consistent with an acute exacerbation of airway disease (e.g., asthma, chronic obstructive pulmonary disease) or a central nervous system or neuromuscular disease as the cause of acute respiratory failure. **B,** Localized alveolar filling opacity, most commonly seen with acute pneumonia. **C,** Diffuse bilateral alveolar filling opacities consistent with acute lung injury and acute respiratory distress syndrome. The CT scan in **C** shows a small left pneumothorax and cavities or cysts that are not apparent on the anteroposterior chest radiograph.

thromboembolism. If shunting is the major explanation for the hypoxemia, processes that fill the air spaces (e.g., cardiogenic pulmonary edema, noncardiogenic pulmonary edema in acute lung injury or ARDS, or purulent pulmonary secretions in acute pneumonia) or, less commonly, an intracardiac or anatomic intrapulmonary shunt is the likely cause. Conditions that fill air spaces should be confirmed by an abnormal chest radiograph; if the radiograph is normal, an intracardiac shunt should be considered and confirmed by echocardiography.

Chest Radiography

The chest radiograph in acute respiratory failure is likely to show one of three patterns (Fig. 104-3): (1) normal (or relatively normal), (2) localized alveolar filling opacities, or (3) diffuse alveolar filling opacities. Diffuse interstitial opacities are also possible, but diseases that cause this pattern usually have a more gradual onset and are associated with chronic respiratory failure. If the chest radiograph is normal (i.e., it is clear or relatively clear), airway diseases, such as COPD and asthma, or pulmonary vascular diseases, such as thromboembolism, are more likely. If a localized alveolar filling abnormality is present, pneumonia is the major consideration, but pulmonary embolism and infarction should also be considered. When diffuse (bilateral) alveolar filling abnormalities are present, cardiogenic pulmonary edema, acute lung injury (e.g., as seen in sepsis, trauma, or aspiration of gastric contents), and diffuse pneumonia are the major considerations. The combination of the chest radiograph and the arterial blood gas interpretation can be helpful. The finding of a significant shunt may suggest acute lung injury in a patient in whom this diagnosis was not clinically obvious; the chest radiograph should help to confirm that possibility.

Other Evaluations

All patients with acute respiratory failure should have a complete blood count, including a platelet count; routine blood chemistry tests; prothrombin time; and urinalysis to screen for possible underlying causes and comorbid conditions. Other blood tests should be guided by the clinical picture. Examples include a serum amylase level if pancreatitis is a possible cause of ARDS and thyroid indices if severe hypothyroidism is a possible cause of hypoventilation. Blood cultures are recommended whenever sepsis is suspected.

Any abnormal fluid collections, especially pleural effusion (Chapter 99), should be aspirated for diagnostic purposes. Sputum Gram stain and culture are indicated when pneumonia is suspected.

Other specific tests should be directed by the history, physical examinations, arterial blood gas levels, and chest radiograph. An abdominal computed tomography (CT) scan may be indicated to search for the source of infection in a patient with sepsis and acute lung injury. A chest CT scan may help define pulmonary disease if the chest radiograph is not definitive. A CT arteriogram of the pulmonary circulation may diagnose pulmonary thromboembolism (Chapter 98). A head CT scan may be indicated if a stroke involving the respiratory center is suspected. Routine blood chemistry studies can detect diabetic ketoacidosis or renal failure as contributing causes.

TREATMENT   Rx

General Measures

The management of acute respiratory failure depends on its cause, its clinical manifestations, and the patient's underlying status. Certain goals apply to all patients: (1) improvement of the hypoxemia to eliminate or markedly reduce the acute threat to life, (2) improvement of the acidosis if it is considered life-threatening, (3) maintenance of cardiac output or improvement if cardiac output is compromised, (4) treatment of the underlying disease process, and (5) avoidance of predictable complications.

The precise methods for improving hypoxemia depend on the cause of the acute respiratory failure. An increase in the inspired O_2 concentration is a cornerstone of treatment for nearly all patients, however.

The level of acidosis that requires treatment other than for the underlying disease process is not clear. Although normalization of the arterial pH was suggested in the past, respiratory acidosis is apparently well tolerated in many patients with severe ARDS, so a patient with a pH of 7.15 or greater may not require bicarbonate therapy. If the acidemia coexists with clinical complications, such as cardiac arrhythmias or a decreased level of consciousness, that have no other obvious cause, treatments to increase pH should be considered. The therapeutic goal is alleviation or reduction of the accompanying complications by improving the level of acidosis; it usually is not necessary to normalize the pH (Chapter 120).

The maintenance of cardiac output is crucial for O_2 delivery in acute respiratory failure, especially because mechanical ventilation and positive end-expiratory pressure (PEEP) may compromise cardiac output. Placement of a pulmonary artery catheter allows measurement of cardiac output and filling pressures, but patients who have these catheters do no better than similar patients managed without them.[1]

Many therapeutic interventions that improve short-term physiologic variables may worsen long-term, clinically important outcomes. Transfusing all patients to maintain a hemoglobin greater than 10 g/dL increases mortality in critically ill patients who have not had an acute myocardial infarction and do not have unstable angina, even though the O_2 carrying capacity of the blood is acutely increased. Use of a relatively large tidal volume (e.g., 12 mL/kg predicted body weight, which is equivalent to approximately 10 to 10.5 mL/kg measured body weight in patients who are somewhat overweight) increases mortality in patients with ARDS when compared with a lower tidal volume (6 mg/kg predicted body weight), even though it raises PaO_2 more in the short term than does a lower tidal volume. Conservative use of fluids improves lung function and shortens the duration of mechanical ventilation and intensive care.[2]

Improvements in oxygenation, acid-base status, and cardiac output are of no more than temporary benefit unless the underlying disease processes are diagnosed and treated properly. In patients with acute lung injury, sepsis may worsen injury to the lung and other organs despite optimal supportive care. Similarly, if the precipitating cause of acute respiratory failure in a patient with COPD is not identified and treated, supportive care is likely to be futile. Complications may arise from the physiologic effects of the gas exchange abnormality, from the disease processes causing the acute respiratory failure, from being critically ill and its associated incursions on homeostasis (e.g., sleep deprivation), or from iatrogenic complications of therapy.

Mechanical Therapy to Improve Oxygenation

A PaO_2 greater than 60 mm Hg is usually adequate to produce an SaO_2 in the low to middle 90s. The PaO_2 can be increased by the administration of supplemental O_2, by pharmacologic manipulations, by continuous positive airway pressure (CPAP), by mechanical ventilation with or without maneuvers such as PEEP, and by the prone position. PEEP, pharmacologic manipulations, and positioning are used primarily in patients with acute lung injury (see later).

The initial choice of the concentration and amount of supplemental O_2 is based on the severity of the hypoxemia, the clinical diagnosis, the likely mechanism causing the hypoxemia, and the O_2 delivery systems available. For the tracheal FIO_2 to be the same as the delivered FIO_2, the O_2 delivery system must deliver a flow that matches the patient's peak inspiratory flow rate with gas of a known FIO_2. High-flow O_2 blenders can achieve this goal by delivering gas at 80 L/minute or greater to a nonintubated patient. These systems require a large flow of O_2 (from a wall unit or tank), however, and are not universally available. Other systems for nonintubated patients (including nasal prongs, simple face masks, and non-rebreather and partial rebreather masks) use a simple regulator that mixes room air with O_2 at 12 L/minute from a wall unit or tank, with resulting flows that are frequently unable to match the patient's peak inspiratory flow rate. The patient entrains more air from the environment, and the resulting tracheal FIO_2 or partial pressure of oxygen in inspired gas (PIO_2) is unknown. The amount of air entrained depends on the patient's inspiratory pattern and minute ventilation. Although the resulting FIO_2 is unknown, these systems are satisfactory if the delivery is constant and if they result in adequate arterial O_2 saturation, as monitored by arterial blood gases or oximetry. Nasal prongs can deliver a tracheal FIO_2 of approximately 0.50, and non-rebreather masks can deliver 50 to 100% O_2; in both cases, this depends on the inspiratory pattern and flow rate. If only hypoventilation or $\dot{V}/\dot{Q}$ mismatch is present, only a small increment in FIO_2 (e.g., an FIO_2 of 0.24 or 0.28 delivered by a Venturi principle face mask or by mechanical ventilation; or 1 to 2 L/minute O_2 delivered by nasal prongs) is likely to be required. By comparison, if marked shunting or many lung units with low but not zero $\dot{V}/\dot{Q}$ are the cause of hypoxemia, a considerably higher FIO_2 (e.g., >0.7) may be required, and even this high FIO_2 may not reverse the hypoxemia. A common practice when a significant shunt is suspected is to give an FIO_2 of 1.0, then adjust the FIO_2 downward as guided by the resulting PaO_2 or SaO_2.

The O_2 concentration that is toxic to the lungs in critically ill patients is not known, but prior injury may provide tolerance to O_2 toxicity, whereas other conditioning agents, such as bleomycin, may enhance oxidative injury. An FIO_2 of 0.7 or higher is generally considered injurious to the normal human lung. Because it is unknown what lower concentration is safe, however, patients should be given the lowest FIO_2 that provides an adequate SaO_2 (≥90%). If an FIO_2 equal to or greater than 0.5 to 0.7 is required for adequate oxygenation, other measures, especially PEEP or CPAP, should be considered. Even a lower FIO_2 of about 0.5 may be associated with impaired ciliary action in the airways and impaired bacterial killing by alveolar macrophages, but the clinical importance of these effects is not known.

A low concentration of supplemental O_2 can be administered by nasal prongs or nasal cannula, which most patients find comfortable and allows them to cough, speak, eat, and drink while receiving O_2. When the nasal passages are open, the PIO_2 does not depend too much on whether the patient breathes through the nose or the mouth because O_2 is entrained from the posterior nasal pharynx during a breath taken through the mouth. The level of O_2 can be adjusted by the flow rate to the nasal prongs. In patients with COPD, flows as low as 0.5 to 2 L/minute are usually adequate unless an intrapulmonary shunt is contributing to the hypoxemia, as usually occurs in acute pneumonia. At flows greater than approximately 6 L/minute, only a small further augmentation in the PIO_2 can be achieved. Because gas flow through the nose has a drying and irritating effect, a face mask should be considered at high flow rates. O_2 face masks using the Venturi principle allow the regulation of FIO_2 and can be particularly useful when COPD is suspected, and it is important to avoid the CO_2 retention that can be associated with the unregulated administration of O_2. A higher FIO_2 of 0.5 to nearly 1.0 can be administered through a non-rebreathing face mask with an O_2 reservoir. If an FIO_2 equal to or greater than 0.70 is required for more than several hours, particularly in an unstable patient, endotracheal intubation should be considered so O_2 can be administered by a closed system with reliable maintenance of the patient's SaO_2. Indications for placing an artificial airway in a patient with acute respiratory failure include airway protection against massive aspiration of gastric contents, delivery of an increased FIO_2, facilitation of prolonged mechanical ventilation, and to aid in the control of respiratory secretions (Chapter 105).

Ventilatory maneuvers that may increase arterial oxygenation include mechanical ventilation itself and the administration of PEEP or CPAP, all of which allow ventilation of areas of the lung that were previously poorly ventilated or unventilated. Although large tidal volumes with mechanical ventilation may open areas of atelectasis and may improve oxygenation initially, these higher tidal volumes can cause lung injury, particularly if the lung is already injured (Chapter 105).

CPAP refers to the maintenance of positive pressure during the respiratory cycle while breathing spontaneously. PEEP refers to the maintenance of positive pressure throughout the expiratory cycle when it is applied together with mechanical ventilation (Chapter 105). CPAP and PEEP can result in recruitment of microatelectatic regions of the lung that are perfused but were not previously ventilated, thus contributing substantially to hypoxemia. CPAP and PEEP have the theoretical advantage of keeping some of these regions open during exhalation, thus preventing cyclic closure and reopening of lung units, which can result in alveolar wall stress and injury.

Supportive Measures

Every patient with acute respiratory failure is at risk for deep vein thrombosis, pulmonary thromboembolism, and gastric stress ulceration. Prophylactic anticoagulation is recommended in patients who are not at high risk for bleeding complications; sequential leg compression therapy may be preferred for high-risk patients (Chapter 81).

The best means of preventing stress ulceration is not known, but current evidence indicates that the use of an H_2-blocker is superior to the gastric administration of sucralfate, based on a large randomized, controlled trial that found a higher incidence of significant bleeding in patients receiving sucralfate than in those receiving ranitidine. Evidence also indicates that proton pump inhibitors may be useful in the acute care setting. There is little firm evidence to guide nutritional management in patients with acute respiratory failure (Chapters 221 and 224).

Current evidence supports maintaining the head of the bed at a 45-degree angle to reduce aspiration in critically ill patients. Attempts should be made to ensure a normal day-night sleep pattern, including minimizing activity and reducing direct lighting at night. The patient should change position frequently, including sitting in a chair and walking short distances if possible, even while receiving mechanical ventilatory support. Mobilization can enhance the removal of secretions, help maintain musculoskeletal function, reduce the risk of deep vein thrombosis, and provide psychological benefits.

⬤ SPECIFIC ACUTE RESPIRATORY FAILURE SYNDROMES
Chronic Obstructive Pulmonary Disease

EPIDEMIOLOGY AND PATHOBIOLOGY

The epidemiology and pathobiology of COPD are discussed in Chapter 88.

CLINICAL MANIFESTATIONS

When COPD causes acute respiratory failure, patients commonly have a history of increasing dyspnea and sputum production. Acute respiratory failure may manifest in more cryptic ways, however, such as changes in mental status, arrhythmias, or other cardiovascular abnormalities. Acute respiratory failure must be considered whenever patients with COPD have significant nonspecific clinical changes.

DIAGNOSIS

The diagnosis can be confirmed or excluded by arterial blood gas analysis. The pH is helpful in assessing whether the hypoventilation is partly or exclusively acute: The pH drops by approximately 0.08 for each 10 mm Hg rise in the $PaCO_2$ in acute respiratory acidosis without renal compensation. By comparison, in chronic respiratory acidosis with normal renal compensation, the pH drops only about 0.03 for each 10 mm Hg rise in the $PaCO_2$.

TREATMENT   (Rx)

General Care

As soon as acute respiratory failure is confirmed in a patient with COPD, attention must focus on detecting any precipitating events (Table 104-4), including decreased ventilatory drive, commonly because of oversedation; decreased muscle strength or function, often related to electrolyte abnormalities, including hypophosphatemia and hypomagnesemia; decreased chest wall elasticity, possibly related to rib fracture, pleural effusion, ileus, or ascites; atelectasis, pneumonia, or pulmonary edema; increased airway resistance, caused by bronchospasm or increased secretions; or increased metabolic O_2 requirements, such as with systemic infection. Many of these abnormalities can impair the cough mechanism, diminish the clearance of airway secretions, and precipitate acute respiratory failure.

Infection

The most common specific precipitating event is airway infection, especially acute bronchitis. The role played by viral agents, *Mycoplasma pneumoniae*, chronic contaminants of the lower airway such as *Haemophilus influenzae* and *Streptococcus pneumoniae*, and other acute pathogens is difficult to determine on a clinical or even microbiologic basis. Acute exacerbations of COPD commonly result from new infections rather than re-emergence of an infection from preexisting colonization. Antibiotics modestly shorten the duration of the exacerbation, with no significant increase in toxicity, compared with placebo; the impact of antibiotics on the subsequent emergence of resistant organisms is not known. It is standard practice to use antibiotics to treat a patient with COPD who has an exacerbation severe enough to cause acute respiratory failure and who has evidence consistent with acute tracheobronchitis (Chapters 88 and 96). Pneumonia may account for 20% of cases of acute respiratory failure in patients with COPD. Compared with the physiologically normal population, patients with COPD who have community-acquired pneumonia are more likely to have gram-negative enteric bacteria or *Legionella* infections and are more likely to have antibiotic-resistant organisms.

Other Precipitating Causes

Other common precipitating causes of acute respiratory failure include heart failure and worsening of the underlying COPD, often related to noncompliance with medications. Less common and often difficult to diagnose in this setting is pulmonary thromboembolism.

TABLE 104-4 KEY PRINCIPLES IN THE MANAGEMENT OF CHRONIC OBSTRUCTIVE PULMONARY DISEASE PATIENTS WITH ACUTE RESPIRATORY FAILURE

1. Monitor and treat life-threatening hypoxemia (these measures should be performed virtually simultaneously).
   a. Assess the patient clinically, and measure oxygenation by arterial blood gases and/or oximetry.
      (1) If the patient is hypoxemic, initiate supplemental oxygen therapy with nasal prongs (low flows [0.5-2. L/min] are usually sufficient) or by Venturi face mask (24 or 28% oxygen delivered).
      (2) If the patient needs ventilatory support, consider noninvasive ventilation.
      (3) Determine whether the patient needs to be intubated; this is almost always a clinical decision. Immediate action is required if the patient is comatose or severely obtunded.
   b. A reasonable goal in most patients is PaO_2 of 55-60 mm Hg or SaO_2 of 88-90%.
   c. After changes in FIO_2, check blood gases and check regularly for signs of carbon dioxide retention.
2. Start to correct life-threatening acidosis.
   a. The most effective approach is to correct the underlying cause of ARF (e.g., bronchospasm, infection, heart failure).
   b. Consider ventilatory support, based largely on clinical considerations.
   c. With severe acidosis, the use of bicarbonate can be considered, but it is often ineffective, and there is little evidence of a clinical benefit.
3. If ventilatory support is required, consider noninvasive mechanical ventilation.
   a. The patient must have intact upper airway reflexes and be alert, cooperative, and hemodynamically stable.
   b. Careful monitoring is required; if the patient does not tolerate the mask, becomes hemodynamically unstable, or has a deteriorating mental status, consider intubation.
4. Treat airway obstruction and the underlying disease process that triggered the episode of ARF.
   a. Treat airway obstruction with pharmacologic agents: systemic corticosteroids and bronchodilators (ipratropium and/or β-adrenergic agents).
   b. Improve secretion clearance: encourage the patient to cough, administer chest physical therapy if cough is impaired and a trial appears effective.
   c. Treat the underlying disease process (e.g., antibiotics, diuretics).
5. Prevent complications of the disease process and minimize iatrogenic complications.
   a. Pulmonary thromboembolism prophylaxis: use subcutaneous heparin if no contraindications exist.
   b. Gastrointestinal complications: administer prophylaxis for gastrointestinal bleeding.
   c. Hemodynamics: if the patient is ventilated, monitor and minimize auto-PEEP.
      (1) Treat the underlying obstruction.
      (2) Minimize minute ventilation; use controlled hypoventilation.
      (3) Use small tidal volumes; increase the inspiratory flow rate to decrease the inspiratory time and lengthen the expiratory time.
   d. Cardiac arrhythmias: maintain oxygenation and normalize electrolytes.

ARF = acute respiratory failure; FIO_2 = fraction of inspired oxygen; PaO_2 = partial pressure of oxygen in arterial blood; PEEP = positive end-expiratory pressure; SaO_2 = oxygen saturation.

Site of Care

Many patients with COPD and acute respiratory failure can be managed on a general medical hospital floor rather than in an intensive care unit if the precipitating cause of acute respiratory failure has been diagnosed and is potentially responsive to appropriate therapy, if any blood gas abnormalities respond to O_2 therapy and are not life-threatening, if the patient can cooperate with the treatment, and if appropriate nursing and respiratory care can be provided (Chapter 88). An unstable patient who requires closer observation and monitoring should be admitted to an intensive care unit.

Mechanical Therapy

The decision to use mechanical ventilation in patients with COPD and acute respiratory failure must be made on clinical grounds and is not dictated by any particular arterial blood gas values. In general, if the patient is alert and is able to cooperate with treatment, mechanical ventilation is unlikely to be necessary. If ventilatory support is required (Chapter 105), the decision is whether to use noninvasive positive-pressure ventilation therapy (without endotracheal intubation) or endotracheal intubation with positive-pressure ventilation. Many studies have demonstrated that noninvasive positive-pressure ventilation is preferred for patients with COPD and can decrease mortality if applied in appropriate patients with no factors that are likely to lead to complications. **3**

TABLE 104-5 DISORDERS ASSOCIATED WITH ACUTE LUNG INJURY AND ACUTE RESPIRATORY DISTRESS SYNDROME

COMMON

Sepsis (gram-positive or gram-negative bacterial, viral, fungal, or parasitic infection)
Diffuse pneumonia (bacterial, viral, or fungal)
Aspiration of gastric contents
Trauma (usually severe)

LESS COMMON

Near-drowning (fresh or salt water)
Drug overdose
    Acetylsalicylic acid
    Heroin and other narcotic drugs
Massive blood transfusion (likely a marker of severe trauma, but also seen with severe gastrointestinal bleeding, especially in patients with severe liver disease)
Leukoagglutination reactions
Inhalation of smoke or corrosive gases (usually requires high concentrations)
Pancreatitis
Fat embolism

UNCOMMON

Miliary tuberculosis
Paraquat poisoning
Central nervous system injury or anoxia (neurogenic pulmonary edema)
Cardiopulmonary bypass

PROGNOSIS

Acute respiratory failure in patients with severe COPD is associated with an in-hospital mortality of 6 to 20%. The severity of the underlying disease and the severity of the acute precipitating illness are important determinants of hospital survival. Hospital mortality is higher if the respiratory failure is associated with a pH less than 7.25. The pH, the $PaCO_2$, and other clinical characteristics are not very reliable in predicting a particular patient's chances of survival.

Acute Lung Injury/Acute Respiratory Distress Syndrome

DEFINITION

ARDS was first described in 1967 as the abrupt onset of diffuse lung injury characterized by severe hypoxemia (shunting) and generalized pulmonary infiltrates on the chest radiograph in the absence of overt cardiac failure. In the early 1990s the term *acute lung injury* was officially introduced to include traditional ARDS and less severe forms of lung injury. Both acute lung injury and ARDS, by definition, require bilateral pulmonary infiltrates compatible with pulmonary edema in the absence of clinical heart failure (usually determined by the lack of elevated left atrial pressures). The two are differentiated by the degree of abnormal oxygenation: Patients are defined as having acute lung injury if the PaO_2 divided by the FIO_2 (PaO_2/FIO_2, also called the P/F ratio) is less than or equal to 300. When the PaO_2/FIO_2 is less than or equal to 200, the patient meets the criteria for ARDS.

EPIDEMIOLOGY

Acute lung injury and ARDS are major public health problems and major causes of death. The annual incidence of acute lung injury is about 80 cases per 100,000 adult population. Case-fatality rates are 30 to 50% and are highly dependent on disease severity and the underlying predisposing condition.

ETIOLOGY

Acute lung injury is a clinical syndrome triggered by some other cause (Table 104-5). This underlying precipitating factor may affect and injure the lungs directly, such as in diffuse pneumonia or aspiration of gastric contents, or it may affect the lungs indirectly, such as in severe sepsis (Chapter 108) or severe nonthoracic trauma (Chapter 112). Severe sepsis is the most common precipitating cause of acute lung injury worldwide. The organisms vary widely, ranging from gram-negative and gram-positive bacteria and viruses (e.g., H1N1 influenza in 2009) to leptospiral infections or malaria. It may be difficult to determine whether pneumonia is diffuse, with endobronchial spread involving most of the lungs, or whether localized pneumonia has precipitated a sepsis syndrome, with secondary injury to other parts of the lung.

PATHOBIOLOGY

Pathology

Despite the variety of underlying disease processes leading to acute lung injury, the response to these insults in the lung is monotonously characteristic, with similar clinical findings, physiologic changes, and morphologic abnormalities. The pathologic abnormalities in acute lung injury and ARDS are nonspecific and are described as *diffuse alveolar damage* by pathologists. The initial process is inflammatory, with neutrophils usually predominating in the alveolar fluid. Hyaline membranes develop, similar to those seen in premature infants with infant respiratory distress syndrome, presumably related to the presence of large-molecular-weight proteins that have leaked into the alveolar space. Alveolar flooding leads to impairment of surfactant, which is abnormal in quantity and quality. The result is microatelectasis, which may be associated with impaired immune function. Cytokines and other inflammatory mediators are usually markedly elevated, although with different patterns over time in the bronchoalveolar lavage fluid and the systemic blood. Lung repair is also disturbed; early evidence of pro-fibrotic processes includes the appearance of breakdown products of pro-collagen in the bronchoalveolar lavage fluid, followed by scarring. The pulmonary fibrosis observed on lung biopsy or at autopsy is identical to that seen in patients with idiopathic pulmonary fibrosis (Chapter 92). Because lung function improves over time in survivors of ARDS, however, it has been assumed that this scarring is often reversible.

Pathophysiology

The physiologic abnormalities are dominated by severe hypoxemia with shunting, decreased lung compliance, decreased functional residual capacity, and increased work of breathing. Initially, the $Paco_2$ is low or normal, usually associated with increased alveolar ventilation. The initial abnormalities in oxygenation are thought to be related to alveolar flooding and collapse. As the disease progresses, especially in patients who require ventilatory support, fibroproliferation develops; the lungs (including alveoli, blood vessels, and small airways) remodel and scar, with a loss of microvasculature. These changes may lead to pulmonary hypertension and increased dead space; marked elevations in minute ventilation are required to achieve a normal $Paco_2$, even as oxygenation abnormalities are improving.

CLINICAL MANIFESTATIONS

In most cases of acute lung injury, the onset either coincides with or occurs within 72 hours of the onset of the underlying disease process; the mean time from onset of the underlying cause to onset of acute lung injury is 12 to 24 hours. The presenting picture is dominated by respiratory distress and the accompanying laboratory findings of severe hypoxemia and generalized infiltrates or opacities on the chest radiograph. Alternatively, it may be dominated by manifestations of the underlying disease process, such as severe sepsis with hypotension and other manifestations of systemic infection.

DIAGNOSIS

The key to diagnosis is to distinguish ARDS from cardiogenic pulmonary edema (Table 104-6). No specific biochemical test exists to define ARDS. Certain blood or bronchoalveolar lavage (Chapter 85) abnormalities are frequent but are not sufficiently specific to be useful clinically.

TREATMENT   Rx

Treatment for acute lung injury and ARDS consists predominantly of respiratory support and treatment of the underlying disease (Fig. 104-4). Although sepsis is a common predisposing condition for the development of acute lung injury, a small study examining the usefulness of activated protein C in patients with acute lung injury did not demonstrate any beneficial effects in terms of ventilator-free days or mortality.

Mechanical Therapy

Current recommendations for mechanical ventilation via endotracheal intubation (Table 104-7) emphasize lower tidal volumes based on the patient's predicted body weight (Chapter 105).**4** PEEP is a mainstay in the ventilatory strategy for acute lung injury; although the method for determining the optimal level of PEEP has not been established, higher PEEP levels appear to benefit patients with ARDS.**4,5** PEEP may allow a lower FIO_2 to provide adequate oxygenation, thus avoiding O_2 toxicity. It also may prevent the cyclic collapse and reopening of lung units, a process that is thought to be a major

TABLE 104-6   FEATURES ASSOCIATED WITH NONCARDIOGENIC AND CARDIOGENIC PULMONARY EDEMA*

NONCARDIOGENIC EDEMA (ARDS)	CARDIOGENIC EDEMA/VOLUME OVERLOAD
PRIOR HISTORY	
Younger	Older
No history of heart disease	Prior history of heart disease
Appropriate fluid balance (difficult to assess after resuscitation from shock or trauma)	Hypertension, chest pain, new-onset palpitations; positive fluid balance
PHYSICAL EXAMINATION	
Flat neck veins	Elevated neck veins
Hyperdynamic pulses	Left ventricular enlargement, lift, heave, dyskinesis
Physiologic gallop	S_3 and S_4; murmurs
Absence of edema	Edema: flank, presacral, legs
ELECTROCARDIOGRAM	
Sinus tachycardia, nonspecific ST-T wave changes	Evidence of prior or ongoing ischemia, supraventricular tachycardia, left ventricular hypertrophy
CHEST RADIOGRAPH	
Normal heart size	Cardiomegaly
Peripheral distribution of infiltrates	Central or basilar infiltrates; peribronchial and vascular congestion
Air bronchograms common (80%)	Septal lines (Kerley's lines), air bronchograms (25%), pleural effusion
HEMODYNAMIC MEASUREMENTS	
Pulmonary artery wedge pressure <15 mm Hg, cardiac index >3.5 L/min/m^2	Pulmonary capillary wedge pressure >18 mm Hg, cardiac index <3.5 L/min/m^2 with ischemia, may be >3.5 L/min/m^2 with volume overload

*These features are neither highly sensitive nor specific. Although the findings are more commonly associated with the type of pulmonary edema as listed, they do not have high positive or negative predictive value.
ARDS = acute respiratory distress syndrome.

cause of ventilator-induced lung injury, even when adequate oxygenation can be obtained at relatively low levels of FIO_2. The early use of cisatracurium besylate (15 mg rapid infusion followed by 37.5 mg/hr for 48 hours), a neuromuscular blocker, can reduce ARDS mortality rates by about 25%.**6** In patients with severe ARDS who do not respond to standard therapy but otherwise have a reasonable life expectancy, extracorporeal membrane oxygenation can improve the 6-month survival from 47 to 63% at an acceptable cost of about $35,000 per quality-adjusted year of life saved.**7**

Acute Respiratory Failure without Lung Disease

Acute respiratory failure without pulmonary abnormalities (see Table 104-2) is seen in patients with depressed ventilatory drive secondary to central nervous system dysfunction and in patients with severe neuromuscular disease. The prototypical patient with suppressed ventilatory drive has taken an overdose of a sedative or tranquilizing medication (Chapter 110). The prototypical patient with neuromuscular disease has Guillain-Barré syndrome (Chapter 428). The treatment for both types of patients is supportive. In the case of a patient with a sedative overdose, the threshold for intubation with mechanical ventilatory support should be low because this temporary condition is quickly reversible when the responsible drug is eliminated. Such a patient may require intubation for airway protection against aspiration of gastric contents.

Patients with Guillain-Barré syndrome or other forms of progressive neuromuscular disease should be monitored with serial measurements of vital capacity. In general, when the vital capacity decreases to less than 10 to 15 mL/kg body weight, intubation and mechanical ventilatory support should be considered without regard to the patient's $Paco_2$.

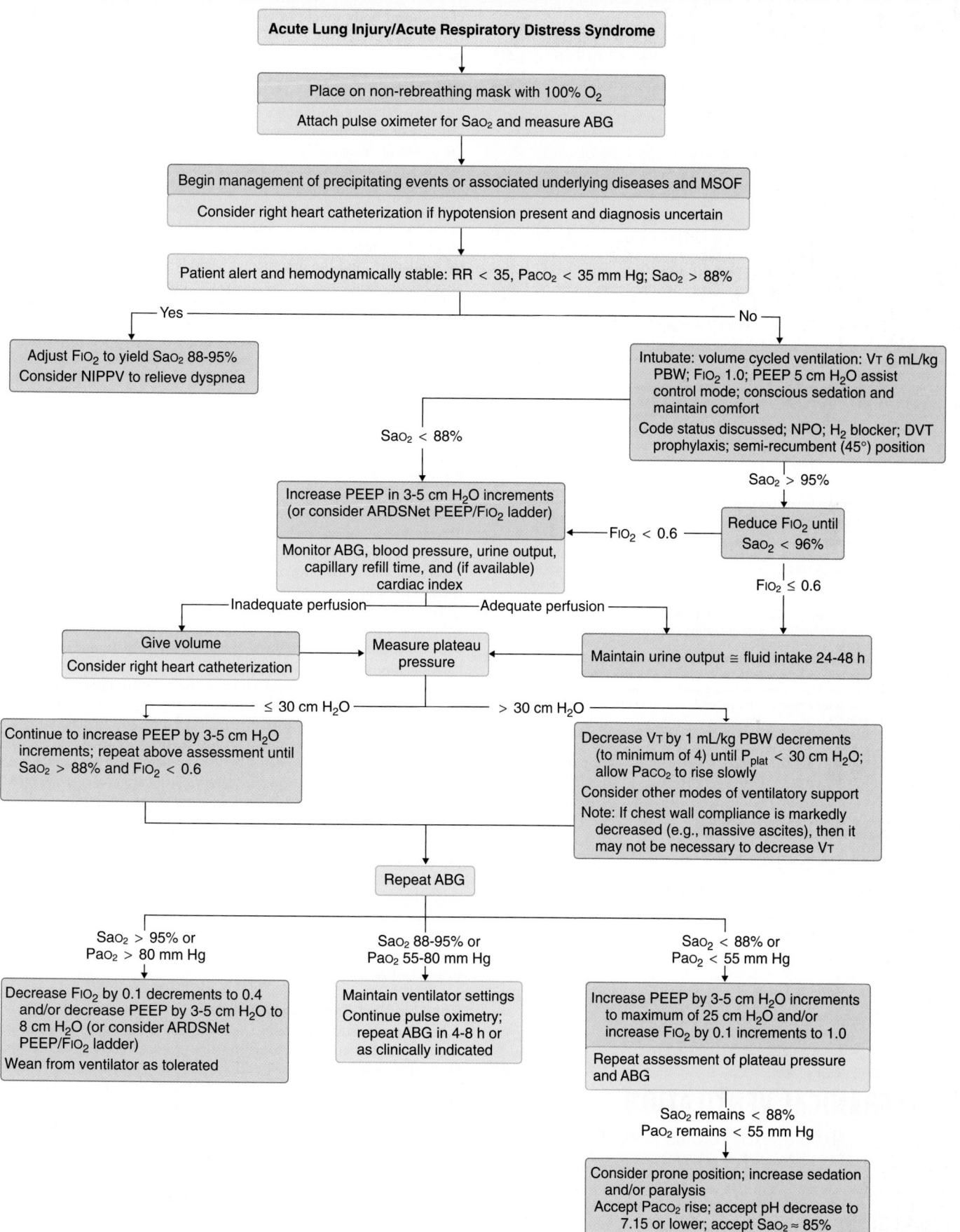

FIGURE 104-4. Algorithm for the initial management of acute respiratory distress syndrome. ABG = arterial blood gas analysis; CO_2 = carbon dioxide; DVT = deep vein thrombosis; FIO_2 = inspired oxygen concentration; MSOF = multisystem organ failure; NIPPV = noninvasive intermittent positive-pressure ventilation; O_2 = oxygen; $PaCO_2$ = arterial partial pressure of carbon dioxide; PaO_2 = arterial partial pressure of oxygen; PBW = predicted body weight; PEEP = positive end-expiratory pressure; P_{plat} = plateau pressure; RR = respiratory rate; SaO_2 = arterial oxygen saturation; V_T = tidal volume.

TABLE 104-7 ARDSNet VENTILATORY MANAGEMENT PROTOCOL FOR TIDAL VOLUME AND PLATEAU PRESSURE

Calculate PBW:

Male PBW: $50 + 2.3$ (height in inches -60) or $50 + 0.91$ (height in centimeters -152.4)

Female PBW: $45.5 + 2.3$ (height in inches -60) or $45.5 + 0.91$ (height in centimeters -152.4)

Select assist control mode

Set initial V_T at 8 mL/kg PBW

Reduce V_T by 1 mL/kg at intervals < 2 hr until $V_T = 6$ mL/kg PBW

Set initial RR to approximate baseline minute ventilation (maximum RR = 35/min)

Set inspiratory flow rate higher than patient's demand (usually > 80 L/min)

Adjust V_T and RR further to achieve P_{plat} and pH goals

If $P_{plat} > 30$ cm H_2O: decrease V_T by 1 mL/kg PBW (minimum = 4 mL/kg PBW)

If pH ≤ 7.30, increase RR (maximum = 35)

If pH < 7.15, increase RR to 35; consider sodium bicarbonate administration or increase V_T

PBW = predicted body weight; P_{plat} = plateau pressure (airway pressure at the end of delivery of a tidal volume breath during a condition of no airflow); RR = respiratory rate; V_T = tidal volume.

See the ARDSNet website (*http://www.ardsnet.org*) for further details about the protocol, including the approach for setting positive end-expiratory pressure and fraction of inspired oxygen.

1. Wheeler AP, Bernard GR, Thompson BT, et al. National Heart, Lung, and Blood Institute Acute Respiratory Distress Syndrome (ARDS) Clinical Trials Network: pulmonary-artery versus central venous catheter to guide treatment of acute lung injury. *N Engl J Med.* 2006;354:2213-2224.
2. The National Heart, Lung, and Blood Institute Acute Respiratory Distress Syndrome (ARDS) Clinical Trials Network. Comparison of two fluid-management strategies in acute lung injury. *N Engl J Med.* 2006;354:2564-2575.
3. Ram FS, Lightowler JV, Wedzicha JA. Non-invasive positive pressure ventilation for treatment of respiratory failure due to exacerbations of chronic obstructive pulmonary disease. *Cochrane Database Syst Rev.* 2004.3.CD004104.
4. Putensen C, Theuerkauf N, Zinserling J, et al. Meta-analysis: ventilation strategies and outcomes of the acute respiratory distress syndrome and acute lung injury. *Ann Intern Med.* 2009;151:566-576.
5. Briel M, Meade M, Mercat A, et al. Higher vs lower positive end-expiratory pressure in patients with acute lung injury and acute respiratory distress syndrome: systematic review and meta-analysis. *JAMA.* 2010;303:865-873.
6. Papazian L, Forel JM, Gacouin A, et al. Neuromuscular blockers in early acute respiratory distress syndrome. *N Engl J Med.* 2010;363:1107-1116.
7. Peek GJ, Mugford M, Tiruvoipati R, et al. Efficacy and economic assessment of conventional ventilator support versus extracorporeal membrane oxygenation for severe adult respiratory failure (CESAR): a multicentre randomized controlled trial. *Lancet.* 2009;374:1351-1363.

SUGGESTED READINGS

Del Sorbo L, Slutsky AS. Acute respiratory distress syndrome and multiple organ failure. *Curr Opin Crit Care.* 2011;17:1-6. Review.

Esan A, Hess DR, Raoof S, et al. Severe hypoxemic respiratory failure: part 1—ventilatory strategies. *Chest.* 2010;137:1203-1216. Review.

Raoof S, Goulet K, Esan A, et al. Severe hypoxemic respiratory failure: part 2—nonventilatory strategies. *Chest.* 2010;137:1437-1448. Review.

105

MECHANICAL VENTILATION

ARTHUR S. SLUTSKY AND LEONARD D. HUDSON

DEFINITION

Mechanical ventilation, a life-sustaining therapy for patients with respiratory failure (Chapter 104), is provided partially or fully by external sources through a variety of mechanical strategies termed *modes of ventilation.* In addition to providing ventilation, the treating physician can also alter the inspired oxygen tension, the pressure at the airway opening at the end of a breath, and other facets of the volume or pressure time pattern imposed on the patient. Current approaches focus on ventilatory strategies that minimize iatrogenic injury through the use of tidal volumes on the order of 6 mL/kg

of predicted body weight or end-inspiratory airway pressures of 25-30 cm H_2O or less, even if the arterial blood gases achieved are not in the "normal range."

TYPES OF MECHANICAL VENTILATORS

Negative-Pressure Ventilators

Delivery of gas to the lungs requires a hydrostatic pressure gradient between the airway opening and the airways and alveoli. During spontaneous breathing, this pressure gradient is generated by development of a negative pleural pressure as a result of contraction of the respiratory muscles. Some ventilators operate by generating negative pressure around the chest wall (e.g., cuirass) or the entire body below the neck (e.g., iron lung). Such ventilators have two major advantages: there is no need to intubate the patient to apply mechanical ventilation, and the detrimental hemodynamic consequences are minimized if the ventilators generate negative pressure solely around the chest wall. However, these ventilators have several difficulties. First, the device around the chest wall or the patient's body used to apply the negative pressure must have an adequate seal so that the negative pressure is not dissipated to the room—a task that is not always easy to accomplish in a manner that is comfortable for the patient. Second, the nursing care of patients in such ventilators can be difficult, especially with iron lungs, which enclose the entire patient from the neck down. Although this type of ventilator was widely used during the polio epidemic of the mid-1950s, its only current use is for patients who have relatively normal lungs but who require long-term ventilation for neuromuscular problems.

Positive-Pressure Ventilators

The most widely used mechanical ventilation approach is to deliver gas to the lung using positive-pressure ventilation (PPV) applied through an endotracheal tube, a tracheostomy, or a tight-fitting mask. The approach using a mask is considered noninvasive ventilation (NIV) and is considered separately.

The most basic mode of PPV is *controlled ventilation,* in which a preset tidal volume at a predetermined rate is delivered to the patient regardless of the patient's requirements or efforts. This form of ventilation is usually used in patients who cannot initiate spontaneous breaths (e.g., heavily sedated or paralyzed patients) or in those who need full ventilatory support because of extremely severe pulmonary or cardiovascular disease (e.g., severe shock). This mode is not routinely used in patients who are able to make spontaneous ventilatory efforts because it can lead to asynchrony between the patient's efforts and the breaths generated by the ventilator. *Assisted ventilation* is the term used when spontaneous ventilatory efforts are present; the onset of a breath is triggered by the patient's respiratory efforts, rather than being based strictly on the time between breaths.

Mechanical ventilation can be applied using either volume-controlled or pressure-controlled modes. In volume-controlled ventilation, the desired tidal volume and respiratory rate are set by the user, and the airway pressure is the dependent variable that changes with the mechanical properties of the patient's respiratory system and with the flow settings on the ventilator. In pressure-controlled ventilation, the pressure imposed at the airway opening and the respiratory rate are set by the user, and the tidal volume becomes the dependent variable.

Positive End-Expiratory Pressure

A key characteristic that can be used with any of the modes of ventilation is the level of the end-expiratory pressure. Positive end-expiratory pressure (PEEP) is used in patients with diffuse pulmonary diseases (e.g., pulmonary edema, acute respiratory distress syndrome [ARDS]) to recruit collapsed alveolar regions and to maintain them in a recruited state, to reopen collapsed airways, to redistribute fluid in the lung, to increase functional residual capacity, and to redistribute ventilation to dependent regions. All these changes can improve the ratio of ventilation to perfusion as well as oxygenation, thereby allowing the fractional inspiratory concentration of oxygen (FIO_2) to be reduced. PEEP does not usually improve alveolar ventilation and, in fact, may increase dead space by overdistending alveoli, with a concomitant decrease in alveolar capillary blood flow in certain regions of the lung. PEEP can also be administered to spontaneously breathing subjects by using a technique termed *continuous positive airway pressure.* Continuous positive airway pressure and PEEP can be used in patients with exacerbations of chronic obstructive pulmonary disease (COPD) to overcome auto-PEEP (see later) and to minimize the work of breathing, provided the magnitude of the PEEP is low enough that it does not cause additional hyperinflation.

Volume-Controlled Ventilation

The term *volume-controlled ventilation* (or *volume-limited ventilation*) refers to mechanical ventilation in which the tidal volume is preset. The major advantage is that the delivered tidal volume is maintained even if lung mechanics change, thereby ensuring a more constant partial pressure of arterial carbon dioxide ($Paco_2$). The potential disadvantage is that if lung mechanics deteriorate, higher pressures may be required to achieve the tidal volume goal, and regions of overinflation with lung injury may result. Although controlled ventilation as described earlier can be either volume limited (preset tidal volume) or pressure limited (preset peak airway pressure), clinicians usually use the term *controlled mechanical ventilation* to refer to volume-limited ventilation with a set rate. In volume-controlled ventilation, an upper limit to applied airway pressure is commonly included for safety reasons.

The most common form of volume-controlled ventilation is one in which the patient assists the ventilator, thus triggering at least some of the breaths. The term *assisted mechanical ventilation* can refer either to volume-limited ventilation or to pressure-limited ventilation when the patient triggers some or all of the breaths, but the ventilator will always deliver a minimum number of breaths if apnea occurs. This mode is also referred to as *assist/control* (A/C).

Intermittent Mandatory Ventilation

The term *intermittent mandatory ventilation* (IMV) refers to a mode in which the patient is allowed to breathe spontaneously through an endotracheal tube or tracheostomy but also receives some preset (and thus mandatory) volume-limited breaths from the ventilator. In current ventilators, the mandatory breaths are triggered by the patient and thus are synchronized (synchronized IMV); however, if the patient ceases spontaneous ventilatory efforts, breaths at the rate set on the ventilator will still be delivered. Synchronized IMV is a form of partial ventilatory support because some breaths are spontaneous, rather than full ventilatory support, in which all breaths are delivered by the ventilator. This mode allows the patient to do a variable amount of the respiratory work but with the security of a set minimal backup rate should spontaneous ventilatory efforts stop.

Pressure-Control Ventilation

Pressure-control ventilation is a type of ventilation in which the ventilator delivers pressure-limited breaths to the patient; delivered volume becomes a dependent variable. The initiation of each breath may be triggered by the patient (assisted breaths) or may be initiated by the ventilator (controlled breaths). The delivered tidal volume depends on the preset pressure, the ventilatory rate, the inspiratory-to-expiratory ratio, and the patient's respiratory mechanics (resistance, compliance, and auto-PEEP). At a fixed preset pressure and inspiratory-to-expiratory ratio, tidal volume decreases as respiratory frequency increases. In patients with COPD, the tidal volume at low frequencies is relatively high but decreases substantially as the respiratory rate is increased, whereas in patients with stiff respiratory systems (e.g., ARDS), the tidal volume does not change much with respiratory frequency because the lung fills with gas quickly.

Pressure-Support Ventilation

Pressure-support ventilation is a pressure-limited, patient-triggered ventilatory mode. Once the patient triggers the ventilator, by creating either a small negative pressure or a low inspiratory flow at the airway, the ventilator switches to inspiratory mode and provides the airflow needed to maintain a preset level of pressure. In contrast to pressure-control ventilation, inspiration terminates when the inspiratory airflow decreases to a threshold level (the specific algorithm varies from ventilator to ventilator). This mode provides flexibility for the patient with respect to tidal volume, inspiratory flow, and ratio of time allowed for inspiration as compared with expiration. Tidal volume depends on patient-related factors (effort), respiratory system mechanics, and the level of pressure set for support. Pressure-support ventilation is a form of partial ventilatory support in which the size of each breath is determined partially by the patient's muscular effort and partially by the ventilator. This mode can compensate for the added work of breathing imposed by the resistance of the endotracheal tube compared with the natural airway. Pressure-support ventilation has largely been used to wean patients from ventilatory support because it provides a simple way to reduce the magnitude of mechanical support while the patient assumes a larger fraction of the ventilatory work than with most other modes of assisted ventilation.

High-Frequency Ventilation

The term *high-frequency ventilation* refers to certain ventilatory modes that have the common feature of providing ventilation using frequencies that are substantially greater than those used during normal breathing. Several different approaches are used for the delivery of high-frequency ventilation: high-frequency PPV, high-frequency jet ventilation, and high-frequency oscillatory ventilation. During high-frequency ventilation, tidal volumes may be less than the dead space, so adequate gas transport takes place by various convective and diffusive mechanisms. Interest in using these modes of ventilation has waxed and waned over the past 2 decades. In recent years, interest in high-frequency ventilation has had a resurgence, based on the concept that it may be the ideal way to minimize ventilator-induced lung injury because the small tidal volumes make it easier to avoid both overdistention of lung units and injury that occurs during ventilation at low lung volumes. Animal data in support of this approach are very strong in models of acute lung injury. Recent data in infants with respiratory distress syndrome and in adults with ARDS suggest that high-frequency ventilation may be as effective as conventional mechanical ventilatory assistance.

Proportional Assist Ventilation and Neurally Adjusted Ventilatory Assist

One of the difficulties when providing assisted ventilation to patients is ensuring that there is adequate synchrony between the patient's respiratory drive and the delivery of each breath from the ventilator. This issue is particularly problematic for patients with severe obstructive airways disease, especially if they have significant auto-PEEP. Two newer modes of ventilation, proportional assist ventilation (PAV) and neurally adjusted ventilatory assist (NAVA), have been developed and implemented on some ventilators in part to address this concern. Both these modes deliver ventilation in proportion to the instantaneous effort of the patient, but the underlying principles are different. Although both of these modes improve patient-ventilator synchrony, data are insufficient to know whether either will improve clinically important outcomes.

PAV is based on the mathematical relationships between airway pressure and airflow; these state that the pressure applied by the respiratory muscles is used to overcome the elastic forces (i.e., compliance) and the resistive forces of the respiratory system. With PAV, the pressure that is applied during inspiration varies based on the patient's inspiratory effort and respiratory system mechanics. This form of ventilation is not in widespread use currently, in part because of its complexity and the need to estimate the patient's compliance and resistance on a regular basis. This latter issue has been addressed in new versions of the technique in which intermittent measurements of compliance and resistance are automatically measured repeatedly.

By contrast, NAVA makes use of the electrical activity of the diaphragm (Edi) as measured by an array of electrodes attached to a nasogastric tube inserted into the esophagus. Pressure is then delivered by the ventilator in direct proportion to the (virtually) instantaneous Edi. Because the initiation and delivery of the breath by the ventilator is not dependent on measurement of pressures in the lung, patient-ventilator synchrony is improved in patients with auto-PEEP. The mode is relatively easy to use; the only parameter to set is the proportionality factor linking the Edi and the pressure delivered by the ventilator.

Noninvasive Positive-Pressure Ventilation

Since the mid-1990s, interest in providing PPV through a mask rather than through an endotracheal tube has increased. This method has been termed *noninvasive* because the patient is not intubated. This approach, although conceptually simple, requires appropriate implementation and monitoring for its successful application. Of particular importance are the selection of patients and the appropriate training of hospital personnel. Patients must be alert, cooperative, and hemodynamically stable. Patients must also have intact upper airway reflexes, so they do not aspirate upper airway materials into the lung, and they must not have any facial trauma that would preclude the use of a mask. Once patients are started on NIV, they should be carefully monitored, and NIV should be discontinued if the patient does not tolerate the mask, if it becomes clear from clinical examination that the patient may aspirate, if cardiovascular instability exists, or if the patient's mental status is deteriorating. NIV can also be delivered through a "helmet" that avoids some of the problems associated with the use of face masks.

NIV has certain potential advantages compared with invasive ventilation. It is relatively easy to apply and can be used for short intervals because it can be started and stopped very easily. The major advantages are that it avoids the complications associated with intubation, it is usually more comfortable for the patient, and it reduces the need for sedation. Patients receiving NIV are able to communicate verbally with medical staff and family members, are likely able to sleep better, and are able to eat if they are sufficiently stable to remove the mask for short periods of time.

However, NIV has several disadvantages. Implementation of NIV takes more time from caregivers at the bedside initially, and the time course of correction of blood gases is slower than usually occurs in patients who are intubated and ventilated. Gastric distention is an unusual occurrence; medical staff should be aware of this complication and should watch for signs of abdominal distention. Data strongly support the use of NIV for patients with COPD (see later), and it is preferred in cardiogenic pulmonary edema,█ but whether it provides better outcomes in other forms of respiratory failure is uncertain.

● COMPLICATIONS

Intubation
Endotracheal intubation can be used to secure a patient's airway, to act as a conduit to deliver gas from the ventilator to the patient, to prevent aspiration, and to help with pulmonary toilet when secretions are increased. However, intubation can be associated with certain complications, including upper airway trauma, disruption of normal host defense mechanisms, and the risk of aspiration during insertion of the endotracheal tube. Pressure from the cuff of the tube that provides a pneumatic seal between the tube and trachea can lead to regions of tracheal ischemia and may eventually cause tracheal stenosis as a result of injury repair processes. The endotracheal tube causes an increase in airway resistance because its diameter is smaller than the airway into which it is inserted. The magnitude of the increase depends on the length, diameter, and shape of the tube as well as the buildup of secretions and mucus that narrow the tube's diameter. Furthermore, the upper airway is normally a very effective means of heating and humidifying inspiratory gases. This natural system is bypassed by an endotracheal tube; inadequately humidified inspiratory gases can reduce mucociliary clearance and can lead to inspissation of tracheal secretions.

Cough is impaired in patients in whom an endotracheal tube has been placed. Normally, cough involves an increase in airway pressure as respiratory muscles are contracted against a closed glottis. When the glottis opens, expiratory flow sharply increases, resulting in dynamic compression of major airways. The presence of an endotracheal tube limits the buildup of airway pressure and alters the dynamics of expiratory flow, thereby greatly impairing the efficacy of the patient's cough.

A cuffed endotracheal tube helps to prevent gross aspiration, but pharyngeal secretions that pool at the top of the cuff often seep into the lungs and increase the probability of developing nosocomial pneumonia (Chapter 97). Endotracheal tubes also make swallowing and communication difficult. Silver-coated tubes reduce the risk of ventilator-associated pneumonia but are considerably more expensive than conventional endotracheal tubes and are unlikely to be used routinely for initial intubation. Endotracheal tubes with a port that allows suctioning of secretions above the cuff may also reduce the incidence of ventilator-associated pneumonia, although results of studies have been mixed.

Hemodynamic Compromise
The major mechanical determinants of cardiovascular hemodynamics during mechanical ventilation are intrathoracic pressure, changes in lung volume, and the patient's circulatory volume status. An increase in lung volume can cause a beneficial decrease in pulmonary vascular resistance, if lung units that had been closed are opened as a result of mechanical ventilation, or it can lead to a detrimental increase in pulmonary vascular resistance related to overdistention of the lung with concomitant compression and lengthening of alveolar vessels.

PPV can have a major impact on cardiovascular hemodynamics through its effect on pleural pressure, an effect that is directly related to changes in lung volume and not necessarily directly reflected in measurements of airway pressure; the relation between alveolar pressure and lung volume depends on respiratory system mechanics. For example, in a patient with stiff lungs (e.g., ARDS), a given increase in plateau pressure (Pplat) will lead to much less of an increase in lung volume than in a patient with COPD, so the increase in pleural pressure will be much less in the patient with ARDS. As a result, patients with ARDS tolerate relatively high PEEP levels, whereas similarly high levels in patients with normal lungs (e.g., in a drug overdose) or in

patients with COPD would markedly reduce cardiac output. At very high lung volumes, a direct effect of the pressure of the lung on the heart can increase pericardial pressure and can thereby decrease cardiac filling.

Auto-PEEP and Dynamic Hyperinflation
A key factor that affects cardiovascular hemodynamics and other physiologic variables during mechanical ventilation is the development of *auto-PEEP*, defined as the difference between alveolar pressure and airway pressure at the end of expiration. Auto-PEEP leads to dynamic hyperinflation, which is an increase in the end-expiratory lung volume higher than the value that would be obtained if there were complete exhalation to the static functional residual capacity. This phenomenon occurs whenever time is insufficient for a complete exhalation to occur; the respiratory system is thus prevented from reaching its static end-expiratory volume. The major determinants of auto-PEEP and hence dynamic hyperinflation are increased expiratory airway resistance, high minute ventilation, increased respiratory system compliance, and decreased expiratory time.

Auto-PEEP is more likely to occur in patients with airway obstruction. Avoidance of high levels of auto-PEEP using approaches such as controlled hypoventilation is a fundamental principle when ventilating patients with airways obstruction.

Auto-PEEP may not be detected by routine measurements of pressure at the airway opening because the major pressure drop occurs across the airways. Moreover, measurements of auto-PEEP are difficult to make in spontaneously breathing patients. When patients are not making spontaneous breathing efforts, auto-PEEP can be assessed as the difference in pressure between the set PEEP and the pressure obtained when the airway opening is occluded at the end of expiration (Fig. 105-1). It can also be assessed using the change in Pplat after a prolonged pause during volume cycle ventilation. If it is considered safe for the patient, a rapid estimate of the effect of auto-PEEP on cardiovascular hemodynamics can be obtained by transiently disconnecting the ventilator and allowing the auto-PEEP to approach zero during a long expiration. If the auto-PEEP is less than 5 cm H_2O, it is unlikely to cause clinically important changes in the measured intravascular pressures.

If auto-PEEP is not considered in the interpretation of respiratory mechanics, measurements of respiratory system compliance will be falsely low.

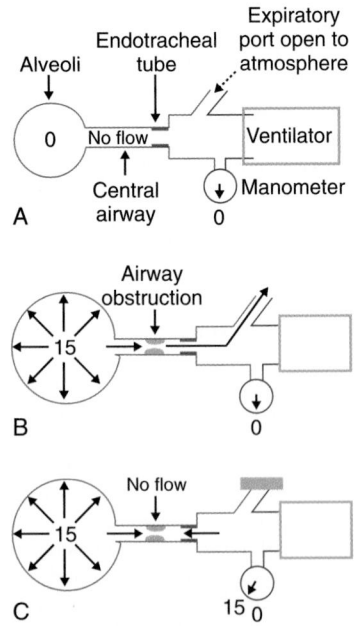

FIGURE 105-1. The relationships among alveolar, central airway, and ventilator circuit pressure at the end of exhalation under the following conditions: **A,** Normal conditions (no auto–positive end-expiratory pressure [auto-PEEP]). **B,** Severe dynamic airway obstruction with the expiratory port open. **C,** Severe dynamic airway obstruction with the expiratory port occluded at the end of exhalation. The auto-PEEP level is identified by creating an end-expiratory hold, thereby allowing the alveolar, central airway, and ventilator circuit pressures to equilibrate because there is no flow in the circuit. During equilibration, the level of auto-PEEP can be read on the manometer in the ventilator circuit (Adapted from Pepe PE, Marini JJ. Occult positive end-expiratory pressure in mechanically ventilated patients with airflow obstruction: the auto-PEEP effect. *Am Rev Respir Dis.* 1982;126: 166-170.)

Dynamic hyperinflation can be measured as the volume of gas that is released when the expiratory time of a given breath is lengthened by 20 to 30 seconds. These techniques are based on the assumptions that no respiratory efforts are made and that the alveoli communicate with the airway opening, thereby allowing equilibration of pressures or exhalation of trapped gas. However, this assumption is not necessarily correct in patients with very severe airways obstruction (e.g., status asthmaticus).

Auto-PEEP should be suspected whenever flow at the end of expiration is detectable or when a patient fails to trigger the ventilator consistently with inspiratory efforts. This failure to trigger the ventilator occurs because the patient must generate sufficient pressure to overcome the level of auto-PEEP before a negative deflection of pressure or generation of inspiratory flow (either of which may be used by the ventilator to detect the onset of inspiration) is sensed at the airway opening.

Auto-PEEP and dynamic hyperinflation have numerous detrimental consequences. In a patient who is not breathing spontaneously, the dynamic hyperinflation increases pleural pressure and right atrial pressure, thereby leading to a decrease in the driving pressure for venous return, with a concomitant decrease in cardiac output. This effect can be magnified in the patient with airway obstruction immediately after intubation and initiation of mechanical ventilation because compensatory mechanisms to enhance venous return are impaired by pharmacologic agents that are often used to prepare the patient for endotracheal tube insertion and that also reduce venous and arterial tone. In such patients, auto-PEEP can also lead to gross misinterpretation of vascular pressures. For example, the absolute value of capillary wedge pressure will be directly affected by the increase in intrathoracic pressure during auto-PEEP. The clinician may interpret this high (absolute) capillary wedge pressure as indicating adequate ventricular filling, when, in fact, transmural capillary wedge pressure is low because intrathoracic pressure is also high. This misinterpretation, coupled with the decreased cardiac output related to the high intrathoracic pressure, may suggest the diagnosis of cardiogenic shock, rather than the correct diagnosis of auto-PEEP.

Treatment of the detrimental hemodynamic consequences of auto-PEEP include decreasing the level of auto-PEEP by increasing the expiratory time, decreasing airway resistance (e.g., bronchodilators, when appropriate), or decreasing minute ventilation. The last approach is usually the most effective ventilatory maneuver but results in an increase in the $Paco_2$. Cardiovascular hemodynamics can also usually be restored by infusion of fluids.

In a spontaneously breathing patient, dynamic hyperinflation can markedly increase the oxygen cost of breathing for two reasons. First, because the respiratory system is stiffer at higher lung volumes, more energy is required to complete each ventilatory cycle. Second, to initiate flow into the lung, the patient must generate a pressure in the alveolar zone that is lower than atmospheric pressure. However, if dynamic hyperinflation is present, the patient first has to generate an inspiratory effort sufficient to overcome the (positive) end-expiratory alveolar pressure before he or she begins to lower alveolar pressure to less than atmospheric pressure to initiate airflow. The increase in lung volume associated with dynamic hyperinflation also has an impact on the effectiveness of the ventilatory muscles: at high lung volumes, the diaphragm is relatively flat, so it is at a mechanical disadvantage in producing changes in pleural pressure. Mechanical ventilation for just 18 to 69 hours causes extensive atrophy of diaphragmatic muscle fibers.

Ventilator-Induced Lung Injury

Mechanical ventilation itself can lead to numerous types of lung injuries (Fig. 105-2). The term *barotrauma* refers to large pulmonary air leaks, such as pneumothorax and pneumomediastinum. However, a much more subtle injury, *diffuse alveolar damage* presenting as pulmonary edema, also occurs. For both types of injuries, the critical factor is the degree of overdistention of the lung, best assessed by the transpulmonary pressure (Ptp, the airway opening minus pleural pressure). The esophageal pressure, measured using an esophageal balloon, estimates pleural pressure (Ppl), although this measurement has not been routinely performed in clinical practice.

The usual pressures measured during mechanical ventilation are airway pressures referenced to atmospheric pressure. The peak inspiratory pressure (PIP) is easy to measure, but its interpretation is not always simple. PIP represents the sum of the pressure required to inflate the lungs plus the pressure needed to overcome the resistance to flow. Thus, a high PIP does not necessarily indicate an increased propensity to the development of ventilator-induced lung injury. For example, if inspiratory flow is constant and a smaller endotracheal tube is used, PIP will increase even though the danger of pulmonary overdistention is no greater than would be present with

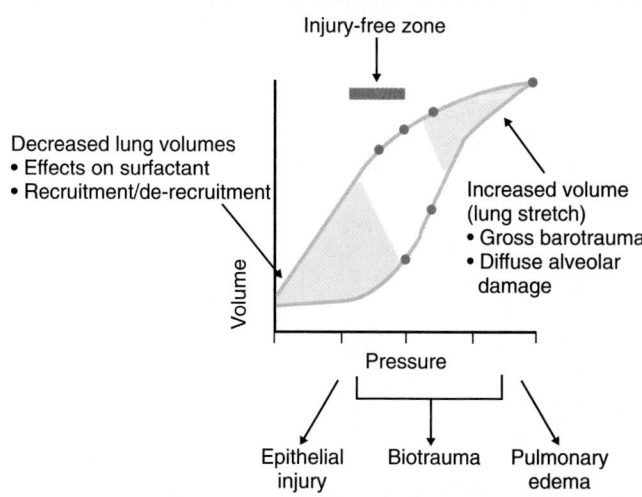

FIGURE 105-2. Schematic representation of the pressure-volume curve of a lung with diffuse alveolar edema. Mechanical ventilation can induce or worsen lung injury by numerous mechanisms when ventilation occurs at high lung volumes or when ventilation occurs at low lung volumes. Lung-protective strategies during ventilation of patients with acute respiratory distress syndrome should try to keep the ventilatory pattern in the *injury-free zone*. Data in patients confirm the benefit of ensuring that overdistention does not occur.

ventilation using a larger-bore tube. The Pplat, which is the airway pressure at the end of an end-inspiratory pause (>0.5 second), is the pressure that can be most easily measured at the bedside and that bears some relationship, depending on Ppl, to the development of overdistention; however, there is no single value of Pplat that is "dangerous" from a lung injury perspective because Ppl can vary so much. However, based on the ARDS Clinical Network (ARDSNet) study, a reasonable maximal value of Pplat in patients with acute lung injury is 30 cm H_2O. Certain caveats should be noted in interpreting Pplat and PIP, related to associated changes in Ppl. If the patient is breathing spontaneously, Ppl will be negative, and overdistention may occur even with a Pplat lower than 30 cm H_2O. Conversely, in a patient who is either paralyzed or not making ventilatory efforts and who has a very stiff chest wall (e.g., due to ascites, obesity, pregnancy), as airway pressure increases, most of the pressure drop will be dissipated across the chest wall, thus leading to values of Ppl that are positive. In this setting, a high Pplat may not be indicative of a high Ptp and hence may not indicate increased lung distention. Thus, the physician caring for a patient receiving mechanical ventilatory support must analyze the measured airway pressures within their clinical context. Measurement of Ppl, as noted earlier, may help resolve these difficulties.

During mechanical ventilation, some areas of the lung may undergo cyclic recruitment and derecruitment. This process, which is of particular importance in patients who have acute lung injury or ARDS, has been termed *atelectrauma* and can cause significant lung injury. The precise mechanisms of injury are not entirely clear but are thought to result from shear stress owing to opening and closing of lung units, regional hypoxia in atelectatic lung units, and effects on surfactant. Prevention of this type of injury provides part of the rationale for the use of PEEP to maintain recruitment of lung units during tidal ventilation.

Finally, evidence suggests that mechanical ventilation strategies that promote overdistention and atelectrauma can lead to an inflammatory response in the lung, a mechanism of injury termed *biotrauma*, through the release of certain pro-inflammatory cytokines and chemokines. To the extent that these mediators can translocate from the lung into the systemic circulation, they could potentially lead to dysfunction of other organs (Fig. 105-3). This concept suggests that optimal ventilatory strategies are important not only for maintenance of lung function but also for preventing the development of multiple-organ dysfunction (Chapter 104) that commonly occurs in this setting. This hypothesis may explain the decreased mortality recently observed with a strategy designed to avoid overdistention in a large randomized trial of mechanical ventilation in patients with ARDS.

● SPECIFIC COMMON TREATMENT SCENARIOS

Initiation of Mechanical Ventilation

The initiation of mechanical ventilation involves several steps in clinical decision making (Table 105-1). Despite the utility of such guidelines, each

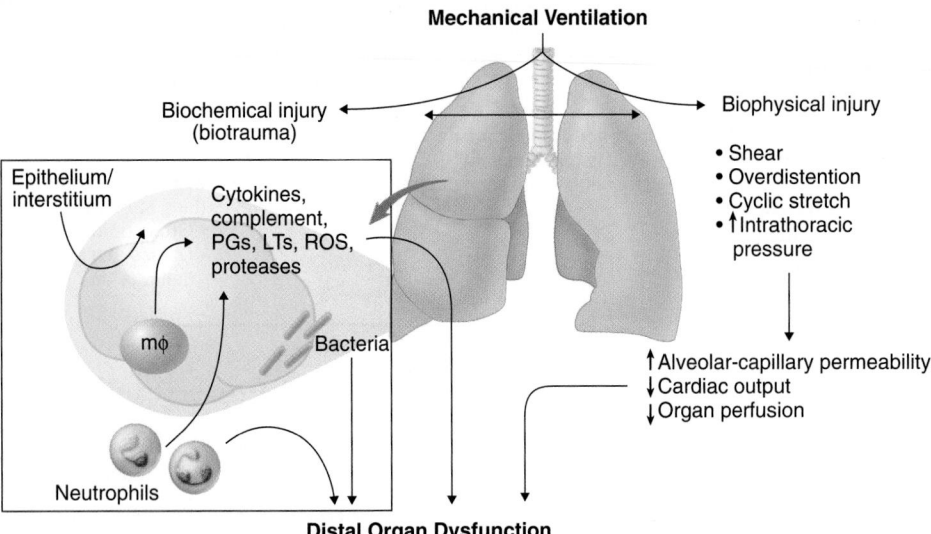

FIGURE 105-3. Mechanisms by which mechanical ventilation may lead to distal organ dysfunction. LTs = leukotrienes; mø = macrophages; PGs = prostaglandins; ROS = reactive oxygen species. (Adapted from Slutsky AS, Tremblay LN. Multiple system organ failure: is mechanical ventilation a contributing factor? *Am J Respir Crit Care Med.* 1998;157:1721-1725.)

TABLE 105-1   STEPS AND GUIDELINES FOR INITIATING MECHANICAL VENTILATION*

1. Ventilatory mode
   Unintubated patients:
   - NIV for patients with COPD and acute hypercapnic respiratory failure if alert, cooperative, and hemodynamically stable
   - NIV not routinely recommended for acute hypoxemic respiratory failure
   Intubated patients:
   - Assist/control with volume-limited ventilation as initial mode
   - Consider specific indications for PCV or HFOV (see text) in acute lung injury
   - SIMV: consider if some respiratory effort, dyssynchrony
   - PSV: consider if patient's effort good, ventilatory needs moderate to low, and patient more comfortable during PSV trial
2. Oxygenation
   - If infiltrates on chest radiograph, then
     F_{IO_2}: begin with 0.8-1.0, reduce according to SpO_2
     PEEP: begin with 5 cm H_2O, increase according to PaO_2 or SpO_2, F_{IO_2} requirements, and hemodynamic effects; consider PEEP/F_{IO_2} "ladder" (see Fig. 105-4); goal of SpO_2 >90%, F_{IO_2} ≤ 0.6
   - No infiltrates on chest radiograph (COPD, asthma, PTE),
     F_{IO_2}: start at 0.4 and adjust according to SpO_2 (consider starting higher if pulmonary embolism is strongly suspected)
3. Ventilation
   - Tidal volume: begin with 8 mL/kg PBW (see Fig. 105-4 for formulas); decrease to 6 mL/kg PBW over a few hours if acute lung injury present (see Fig. 105-4)
   - Rate: begin with 10-20 breaths/min (10-15 if not acidotic; 15-20 if acidotic); adjust for pH; goal pH > 7.3 with maximal rate of 35; may accept lower goal if minute ventilation high
4. Secondary modifications
   - Triggering: in spontaneous modes, adjustment of sensitivity levels to minimize effort
   - Inspiratory flow rate of 40-80 L/min; higher if tachypneic with respiratory distress or if auto-PEEP present, lower if high pressure in ventilator circuit leads to a high-pressure alarm
   - Assessment of auto-PEEP, especially in patients with increased airways obstruction (e.g., asthma, COPD)
   - I/E ratio: 1:2, either set or as function of flow rate; higher (1:3 or more) if auto-PEEP present
   - Flow pattern: decelerating ramp reduces peak pressure
5. Monitoring
   - Clinical: blood pressure, ECG, observation of ventilatory pattern including assessment of dyssynchrony, effort or work by the patient; assessment of airflow throughout expiratory cycle
   - Ventilator: tidal volume, minute ventilation, airway pressures (including auto-PEEP), total compliance
   - Arterial blood gases, pulse oximetry

*Decisions within this algorithm will be influenced by the specific conditions of the individual patient.
COPD = chronic obstructive pulmonary disease; ECG = electrocardiogram; F_{IO_2} = fraction of inspired oxygen; HFOV = high-frequency oscillatory ventilation; I/E ratio = inspiratory-to-expiratory ratio; NIV = noninvasive ventilation; PaO_2 = partial pressure of oxygen in arterial blood; PBW = predicted body weight; PCV = pressure control ventilation; PEEP = positive end-expiratory pressure; PSV = pressure support ventilation; PTE = pulmonary thromboembolism; SIMV = synchronized intermittent mandatory ventilation; SpO_2 = arterial oxygen saturation by pulse oximetry.

patient must be evaluated for specific factors that could modify the recommendation or mandate an alternative.

Acute Respiratory Distress Syndrome

Patients with ARDS (Chapter 104) have noncardiogenic pulmonary edema, with a reduced functional residual capacity and a mortality rate of 30 to 60%. Although therapy may be available for the underlying disease process that led to the development of ARDS (e.g., antibiotics for a predisposing pneumonia), no effective therapy is directly aimed at the diffuse alveolar damage. These patients require mechanical ventilation as supportive therapy to improve oxygenation and to decrease the oxygen cost of breathing until their lungs recover from the primary insult that led to the alveolar damage.

The lungs in a patient with ARDS are stiff and are characterized on computed tomographic scans by patchy, heterogeneous infiltrates that consist of airless atelectatic or consolidated regions. Many patients have a dependent region that is consolidated, atelectatic, or fluid filled; a nondependent region that looks relatively normal; and a middle region that has some areas that look like the dependent regions but can be recruited to resemble the nondependent regions if high enough tidal volumes or increased levels of airway pressure are used transiently; these latter approaches are called *recruitment maneuvers.*

The challenge in ventilating patients with ARDS is to provide adequate gas exchange while at the same time not causing further lung injury (see earlier), an approach termed *lung protective ventilation strategy.* Arterial oxygen saturation can often be increased by high tidal volumes but at the expense of regional overdistention of those lung units that were not affected by the disease process itself, thereby improving oxygen saturation initially but, over time, worsening lung injury and clinical outcome.

The injury caused by mechanical ventilation can be reduced by using ventilatory strategies that avoid or minimize regional lung overdistention: limiting inspiratory pressure to some "safe" level or using smaller tidal volumes to limit end-inspiratory stretch, or both. However, in some patients, this lower "dose" of ventilation results in higher levels of $PaCO_2$ (so-called permissive hypercapnia) and a lower pH. Higher tidal volumes (12 mL/kg predicted body weight) yielded more normal blood gases, but lower tidal volumes (6 mL/kg predicted body weight) decreased mortality by 22% (from an absolute value of 40 to 31%) in a large clinical trial (Fig. 105-4).

Data also suggest that limiting tidal volume in ventilated patients who are intubated for reasons other than acute lung injury prevents injury later in the course of their intensive care unit stay. A lung protective strategy with limitation of tidal volume should be considered in ventilated patients who are at high risk of developing acute lung injury or ARDS.

Positive End-Expiratory Pressure

PEEP has been used traditionally to improve oxygenation while at the same time allowing reduction in F_{IO_2} to relatively nontoxic levels. Within the context of the current paradigm of trying to minimize iatrogenic complications of mechanical ventilation, PEEP is viewed as a therapy that potentially can abrogate or minimize the injury caused by ventilation at low lung volumes, by recruiting lung units and keeping them open. No definitive answer exists regarding how PEEP levels should be set in patients with ARDS; outcomes

Ventilatory Strategy for Patients with ARDS*

Goal 1: Low Vt/Pplat
Initiation:
Calculate PBW
—Male:
50 + 2. 3 (height [inches] − 60)
—Female:
45.5 + 2.3 (height [inches] − 60)
Initiate volume assist control
—start with 8 mL/kg, and ↓ to 6 mL/kg over a few hours

↓

Keep Pplat (based on 0.5-sec pause) <35 cm H_2O
If Pplat > 30 cm H_2O, ↓ Vt by 1 mL/kg to 5 or 4 mL/kg
If Pplat < 25 AND Vt < 6 mL/kg, ↑Vt by 1 mL/kg until Pplat > 25 cm H_2O OR Vt = 6 mL/kg
If patient severely distressed and/or breath stacking, consider ↑Vt to 7 or 8 mL/kg, as long as Pplat ≤ 30 cm H_2O†

Goal 2: Adequate Oxygenation
Specific goal:
Pao_2 55-80 mm Hg
or
Spo_2 88-95%
Use only Fio_2 /PEEP combinations shown below to achieve this target
• if oxygenation is low, choose Fio_2 /PEEP combination (from Fio_2 /PEEP table) to the right
• if oxygenation is high, choose Fio_2 /PEEP combination to the left

Goal 3: Arterial pH
Goal:
pH: 7.30–7.45
Acidosis algorithm
If pH 7.15–7.30
• ↑ set rate until pH > 7.30 or $Paco_2$ < 25 mm Hg (max RR = 35)
• if RR = 35 & pH < 7.30 $NaHCO_3$ may be given
If pH < 7.15
• ↑ set RR to 35
• if set RR = 35 & pH < 7.15, Vt may be ↑ in 1 mL/kg steps until pH > 7.15
(Pplat target may be exceeded)
Alkalosis algorithm
If pH > 7.45
• ↓ set RR until patient RR > set RR
(minimum set RR = 6/min)

Fio_2/PEEP Table

Fio_2	0.3	0.4	0.4	0.5	0.5	0.6	0.7	0.7	0.7	0.8	0.9	0.9	0.9	1.0
PEEP	5	5	8	8	10	10	10	12	14	14	14	16	18	20–24

*Based on ARDS Network Algorithm

† If compliance of the chest wall is markedly decreased (e.g., massive ascites), it may not be reasonable or necessary (if the patient is very hypoxemic) to allow a Pplat >30 cm H_2O.

FIGURE 105-4. Ventilatory strategy for patients with the acute respiratory distress syndrome (ARDS). Several caveats should be considered when using the low tidal volume strategy: (1) tidal volume (Vt) is based on predicted body weight (PBW),**1** not actual body weight; PBW tends to be about 20% lower than actual body weight; (2) the protocol mandates decreases in the Vt lower than 6 mL/kg of PBW if the plateau pressure (Pplat) is greater than 30 cm H_2O and allows for small increases in Vt if the patient is severely distressed and/or if there is breath stacking, as long as Pplat remains at 30 cm H_2O or lower; (3) because arterial carbon dioxide (CO_2) levels will rise, pH will fall; acidosis is treated with increasingly aggressive strategies dependent on the arterial pH; (4) the protocol has no specific provisions for the patient with a stiff chest wall, which in this context refers to the rib cage and abdomen; in such patients, it seems reasonable to allow Pplat to increase to more than 30 cm H_2O, even though it is not mandated by the protocol; in such cases, the limit on Pplat may be modified based on analysis of abdominal pressure, which can be estimated by measuring bladder pressure. RR = respiratory rate; Spo_2 = oxygen saturation based on pulse oximeter.

appear to be similar with the routine use of higher (≈13 cm H_2O) and lower (≈8 cm H_2O) levels of PEEP. The critical issues are how to assess the level of PEEP in an individual patient and how to determine whether the procedures to recruit the lung units and keep them open are less harmful than allowing the lung units to remain de-recruited. One experimental option is chest computed tomography to assess whether areas of the lung are recruited, but this technique is not practical for routine assessment. A second approach is to measure the mechanical properties of the respiratory system by generating a pressure-volume curve (see Fig. 105-2). Investigators have suggested that the optimal strategy is to set PEEP just higher than the lower inflection point, which is thought to represent the opening pressure of the lung, and to adjust tidal volume so that Pplat is just lower than the upper inflection point, at which compliance decreases. Although lung continues to be recruited well above the lower inflection point, and the upper inflection point may not indicate over-distention, two clinical studies that based their lung protection strategies on the pressure-volume curve demonstrated reductions in mortality; however, both studies also included other features to reduce lung injury, so use of the pressure-volume curve to set PEEP levels and tidal volume (or pressure limits) cannot be recommended at this time. In the trial that demonstrated the benefit of lower tidal volumes, PEEP levels were individualized based on a PEEP/Fio_2 table (see Fig. 105-4); a subsequent trial using PEEP about 5 cm H_2O higher found no additional benefit. Higher PEEP (to achieve a plateau pressure of 28 to 30 cm of H_2O) can reduce the duration of ventilation and organ failure but not mortality compared with moderate PEEP (5 to 9 cm H_2O).**2** Multifaceted ventilation therapy protocols using low tidal volumes, recruitment maneuvers, and high PEEP can improve oxygenation but not reduce barotrauma or mortality compared with conventional therapy.**3** PEEP guided by esophageal pressure measured by an intraesophageal balloon may result in significantly higher PO_2 levels and better respiratory compliance than treatment guided by a standard protocol.**4** Pooled results of all trials suggest higher PEEP improves survival only in patients with ARDS.**5**

Obstructive Airways Diseases

The major pathophysiologic abnormality in patients with obstructive airways diseases is an increase in airway resistance leading to expiratory

airflow limitation; patients may also have a concomitant increase in minute ventilation. These factors may lead to dynamic hyperinflation, which is associated with numerous complications, including respiratory muscle compromise, an increased oxygen cost of breathing, and hemodynamic compromise. Thus, the main goals in the ventilatory support of patients with obstructive airway diseases (COPD, asthma) are to minimize auto-PEEP, to rest the respiratory muscles, to maintain adequate gas exchange, and to decrease the oxygen cost of breathing while simultaneously minimizing the iatrogenic complications of mechanical ventilation and allowing time for the successful diagnosis and treatment of the primary cause of the exacerbation and the resulting increase in airway obstruction (Chapters 87 and 88).

Noninvasive Ventilation

For patients with acute respiratory failure resulting from an exacerbation of COPD, the preferred approach is NIV if the patient is hemodynamically stable, alert, and cooperative and does not need to be intubated to protect the airway. It is important to choose a comfortable mask and to reassure the patient because some patients find the mask difficult to tolerate. This strategy may be applied using several ventilation modes, including pressure support or bilevel positive airway pressure. The ventilation settings are adjusted to improve gas exchange and to ensure the patient's comfort. Despite this approach, some patients with COPD require intubation and ventilation because of cardiac or respiratory arrest, agitation, increased sputum, or other concomitant severe disorders.

Intubation and Ventilation

The key goal after intubation is to minimize the detrimental effects of dynamic hyperinflation. The most effective way to minimize dynamic hyperinflation is to decrease the minute ventilation, even if this means an increase in $Paco_2$, a strategy known as *permissive hypercapnia* or *controlled hypoventilation*. Judicious use of sedation may decrease carbon dioxide production and improve patient-ventilator synchrony, although the avoidance of sedation can reduce the duration of ventilation and hospitalization.**6** In a randomized study, no difference was found between dexmedetomidine and midazolam in time at targeted sedation level, but dexmedetomidine resulted in less time on mechanical ventilation, less delirium, and less hypertension and with less tachycardia but more bradycardia. [7] Care must be taken in the use of paralytic agents, especially when patients with asthma are also receiving corticosteroids. However, early neuromuscular blockade using cisatracurium besylate (15 mg rapid infusion followed by 37.5 mg/hr for 48 hours) can reduce mortality by 25% in patients with ARDS. [8]

Increasing expiratory time by using a higher peak inspiratory flow may be somewhat helpful, but it is not nearly as effective as decreasing minute ventilation. What level of $Paco_2$ (and pH) should be tolerated is not known with certainty, but maintaining pH higher than approximately 7.15 is a reasonable target, although much lower values have been reported in clinical studies.

In patients with COPD who are spontaneously breathing, the addition of external (set) PEEP at a level that is just less than what is necessary to overcome the auto-PEEP fully may not increase Pplat and may decrease the inspiratory effort that the patient needs to generate to initiate inspiratory airflow. This strategy does not appear to be as effective in patients with status asthmaticus, in whom it may cause an increase in Pplat. Measurements of auto-PEEP by airway occlusion may be inaccurate in some patients with status asthmaticus, likely because of gas trapping at the end of expiration with closed-off lung regions that do not communicate with the central airways.

ADJUNCTS

Tracheal gas insufflation involves washing out the carbon dioxide–rich gas in the anatomic dead space with fresh gas through a special catheter or endotracheal tube, thereby allowing a reduction in tidal volume while maintaining the same $Paco_2$. A clinically significant outcome benefit has not yet been demonstrated with tracheal gas insufflation.

The prone position compared with the supine position in patients with acute lung injury results in improved oxygenation in approximately 70% of patients and has a rationale (through more even distribution of pleural pressure) for preventing ventilator-induced lung injury and decreasing Fio_2. Trials in adults, however, have not demonstrated an outcome benefit, including a trial of prone positioning for 16 hours per day with all patients ventilated with the so-called lung-protective ventilation strategy used in the ARDSNet trial. Based on current studies, the prone position cannot be recommended for routine use but should be considered in patients with severe gas exchange abnormalities (e.g., $P/F \le 100$) who require high PEEP and high Fio_2.

Inhaled nitric oxide is a potent vasodilator and bronchodilator that can enhance arterial oxygenation. It has not been shown to improve outcome in clinical trials, however, so its routine use cannot be recommended.

DISCONTINUATION OF MECHANICAL VENTILATION

To minimize the iatrogenic consequences of intubation and mechanical ventilation, discontinuation of ventilatory support and extubation should occur as expeditiously as possible. However, if discontinuation is attempted too early, patients may deteriorate and require urgent reintubation.

From the moment that mechanical ventilation is instituted, it is important for the clinician to start planning for eventual discontinuation of ventilatory support. A key aspect of this approach is serial evaluation, with aggressive treatment of the factors contributing to the patient's ventilatory dependence, including respiratory systems factors (e.g., respiratory muscles), cardiovascular factors (e.g., myocardial ischemia), neurologic factors (e.g., respiratory muscle weakness), and metabolic factors (e.g., increased oxygen consumption).

Two major types of weaning strategies have been used historically: (1) a ventilatory mode thought to hasten the weaning process and (2) daily monitoring of the patient for criteria to suggest the likelihood of successful weaning and a trial of spontaneous breathing for those deemed likely to succeed. Studies of ventilatory modes of weaning have included trials in which patients are allowed to breathe spontaneously from a fresh gas supply delivered to the endotracheal tube (a so-called T-tube), trials of IMV, and studies of pressure-support ventilation. With all approaches, the level of support is gradually decreased until extubation is tolerated by the patient. These methods have been compared in randomized controlled trials, with mixed results, although weaning with IMV appeared less favorable in most trials. Likewise, using ventilatory criteria to predict weaning success has been disappointing, mainly because some patients who fail to meet the criteria will be successfully weaned if they are given the opportunity to breathe spontaneously. The

Approach to Discontinuing Ventilation/Extubation

FIGURE 105-5. Algorithm for assessing whether a patient is ready to be liberated from mechanical ventilation and extubated. ECG = electrocardiogram; HR = heart rate; P/F = Pao_2/Fio_2 ratio; PSV = pressure support ventilation; RR = respiratory rate; SBP = systolic blood pressure; Spo_2 = oxygen saturation based on pulse oximeter; WOB = work of breathing.

criterion with the greatest predictive accuracy is the so-called rapid shallow breathing index, in which the respiratory rate is divided by tidal volume (in liters), with a value less than 105 suggesting the ability to wean; however false-negative and false-positive test results occur.

More recently, the approach to weaning has been based on the concept that a patient is ready to be removed from ventilatory support when the underlying disease process that led to the intubation has resolved or improved substantially. Rather than applying rigorous ventilatory criteria, the only requirements are that the patient be clinically stable (i.e., has shown improvement in the underlying process), be hemodynamically stable, and have oxygen requirements that can be met by face mask once the patient is extubated. If the patient meets these general criteria, a spontaneous breathing trial is recommended (Fig. 105-5); if the patient passes the trial, the patient can be extubated. A corollary is that a gradual weaning is not necessary; instead, patients should be assessed on a daily basis regarding their suitability to be removed from ventilatory support, and, if they are not ready, a comfortable, nonfatiguing form of mechanical ventilation should be used between the assessments. Assisted modes of ventilation are preferred between the spontaneous breathing trials.

An important recommendation in relation to weaning or discontinuing mechanical ventilation relates to evidence that intensive care units should develop weaning or discontinuation protocols that are designed to be implemented by health care professionals other than physicians. Three large randomized trials demonstrated that protocols implemented by health care professionals other than physicians improved care and were associated with substantial savings in costs compared with standard management approaches, even though the specifics of the protocols were different. More recently, a strategy that paired spontaneous awakening, based on the interruption of sedatives, with spontaneous breathing trials improved extubation rates, reduced intensive care length of stay, and decreased mortality by 32%.[9]

A major issue to assess before extubation is the patency of the patient's airway and whether the patient will be able to clear secretions after extubation. Assessment of the likely patency of the upper airway can be achieved using the *cuff-leak volume,* which is the difference between the inspiratory and expiratory tidal volume when the cuff of the endotracheal tube is deflated. If this volume is greater than 110 mL, it is usually an indication that major upper airway obstruction will not occur after extubation. Although this test is not required before extubation, a low *cuff-leak volume* warrants added precautions, such as the availability of equipment and personnel for managing a difficult intubation, when extubating the patient. In patients who have been ventilated for more than 36 hours, methylprednisolone (20 mg intravenously) started 12 hours before a planned extubation and repeated every 4 hours until tube removal substantially reduces postextubation laryngeal edema and reduces the need for reintubation by 50%.[10]

Despite the use of all these techniques, approximately 5 to 25% of patients will have to be reintubated and have mechanical ventilation reinstituted. Once a patient is reintubated, it is again necessary to reevaluate the respiratory and nonrespiratory reasons for the failure.

The choice of the specific weaning protocol should be left to the individual institution and should be individualized to the specific group of patients considered. In instituting such protocols, several key issues should be recognized. First, protocols are guides that should not replace clinical judgment. If a clinician does not follow some aspect of the protocol, there should be a mechanism in place for keeping track of what recommendations were not accepted, with an explanation of the rationale; these data should be collated and used to reassess the protocol. Second, protocols should be viewed as dynamic structures that are open to change and should be reevaluated on a regular basis. Third, implementation of a protocol requires adequate resources, and an institution must make a commitment not only to develop protocols but also to implement and assess them.

Grade A

1. Gray A, Goodacre S, Newby DE, et al. Noninvasive ventilation in acute cardiogenic pulmonary edema. *N Engl J Med.* 2008;359:142-151.
2. Mercat A, Richard JC, Vielle B, et al. Positive end-expiratory pressure setting in adults with acute lung injury and acute respiratory distress syndrome: a randomized controlled trial. *JAMA.* 2008;299:646-655.
3. Meade MO, Cook DJ, Guyatt GH, et al. Ventilation strategy using low tidal volumes, recruitment maneuvers, and high positive end-expiratory pressure for acute lung injury and acute respiratory distress syndrome: a randomized controlled trial. *JAMA.* 2008;299:637-645.
4. Talmor D, Sarge T, Malhotra A, et al. Mechanical ventilation guided by esophageal pressure in acute lung injury. *N Engl J Med.* 2008;359:2095-2104.
5. Briel M, Meade M, Mercat A, et al. Higher vs lower positive end-expiratory pressure in patients with acute lung injury and acute respiratory distress syndrome: systematic review and meta-analysis. *JAMA.* 2010;303:865-873.
6. Strom T, Martinussen T, Toft P. A protocol of no sedation for critically ill patients receiving mechanical ventilation: a randomized trial. *Lancet.* 2010;375:475-480.
7. Riker RR, Shehabi Y, Bokesch PM, et al. Dexmedetomidine vs midazolam for sedation of critically ill patients: a randomized trial. *JAMA.* 2009;301:489-499.
8. Papazian L, Forel JM, Gacouin A, et al. Neuromuscular blockers in early acute respiratory distress syndrome. *N Engl J Med.* 2010;363:1107-1116.
9. Girard TD, Kress JP, Fuchs BD, et al. Efficacy and safety of a paired sedation and ventilator weaning protocol for mechanically ventilated patients in intensive care (Awakening and Breathing Controlled trial): a randomised controlled trial. *Lancet.* 2008;371:126-134.
10. Francois B, Bellisant E, Gissot V, et al. 12-h Pretreatment with methylprednisolone versus placebo for prevention of postextubation laryngeal oedema: a randomised double-blind trial. *Lancet.* 2007;369:1083-1089.

SUGGESTED READINGS

Bouferrache K, Viellard-Baron A. Acute respiratory distress syndrome, mechanical ventilation, and right ventricular function. *Curr Opin Crit Care.* 2011;17:30-35. *The up to 25% incidence of acute cor pulmonale may be prevented by keeping the plateau pressure below 27-28 cm H$_2$O, controlling hypercapnia, avoiding intrinsic PEEP, and keeping the applied PEEP low.*
Burns KE, Adhikari NK, Keenan SP, et al. Use of non-invasive ventilation to wean critically ill adults off invasive ventilation: meta-analysis and systematic review. *BMJ.* 2009;338:b1574. *Review of data to support this approach.*
Magder S. Hemodynamic monitoring in the mechanically ventilated patient. *Curr Opin Crit Care.* 2011;17:36-42. *A practical approach.*
Phoenix SI, Paravastu S, Columb M, et al. Does a higher positive end expiratory pressure decrease mortality in acute respiratory distress syndrome? A systematic review and meta-analysis. *Anesthesiology.* 2009;110:1098-1105. *Evidence favors the use of high PEEP when ventilating patients with severe ARDS syndrome.*

106

APPROACH TO THE PATIENT WITH SHOCK

EMANUEL P. RIVERS

DEFINITION

The key feature of shock is tissue hypoperfusion, not a specific level of systemic arterial blood pressure. The clinical picture may be cryptic or obvious.

EPIDEMIOLOGY

More than 1 million patients present in shock or develop shock in U.S. hospitals each year, at an annual cost of more than $100 billion. Shock can be categorized as hypovolemic, cardiogenic (Chapter 107), extracardiac/obstructive, distributive, or dissociative.

PATHOBIOLOGY

The delivery and utilization of oxygen are essential for cellular viability, and the failure to deliver or utilize oxygen is central to the concept of shock and its pathogenesis (Fig. 106-1). Systemic oxygen delivery—that is, the amount of oxygen delivered to tissues by the arterial blood—depends on the concentration of hemoglobin in the blood, the fractional saturation of the hemoglobin with oxygen (SaO_2), the amount of oxygen dissolved in the blood (PaO_2), and cardiac output. Cardiac output is a product of stroke volume and heart rate. Stroke volume is determined by ventricular preload and afterload, as well as contractility of the right or left heart. Systemic vascular resistance (SVR), the force resisting cardiac contraction, can be calculated using equation 1:

$$SVR = (MAP - CVP) * 80 / CO \qquad (1)$$

$$MAP = Diastolic\ blood\ pressure + (Systolic - Diastolic\ blood\ pressure)/3 \qquad (2)$$

MAP denotes the mean systemic arterial blood pressure, CVP denotes central venous pressure, and CO denotes cardiac output. SVR is determined primarily by the degree of vasomotor tone in the precapillary smooth muscle sphincters.

The systemic circulation is normally autoregulated, so that when systemic arterial pressure increases, vessel diameter decreases to maintain flow at a steady level. The clinical significance of these relationships is apparent when

FIGURE 106-1. The hemodynamic, oxygen transport, and oxygen utilization components of shock management. Systemic oxygen delivery is impacted by cardiac output (CO) and arterial oxygen content. The cardiac, pulmonary, and blood determinants of systemic oxygen delivery are shown. CVP = central venous pressure; MAP = mean arterial pressure; PAOP = pulmonary artery occlusion pressure.

a patient presents with a decrease in cardiac output, but a compensatory increase in systemic vascular resistance maintains a near-normal mean arterial blood pressure. Despite the near-normal blood pressure, however, the patient is in "cryptic shock" because of tissue hypoperfusion. Compensatory mechanisms are organ specific. Blood flow to organs such as the heart and brain is carefully regulated and maintained over a wide range of blood pressures. In other organs, however, such as the intestine or liver, autoregulation is not as tightly maintained.

Systemic oxygen consumption, which is the amount of oxygen consumed by the body per minute, is calculated as the systemic oxygen delivery multiplied by the systemic oxygen extraction ratio. Oxygen demand is the amount of oxygen required by the tissues to avoid anaerobic metabolism. Normally, systemic oxygen delivery is sufficient so that systemic oxygen consumption is not altered by or dependent on changes in delivery. However, if systemic oxygen delivery drops below a critical value, a compensatory increase in the oxygen extraction ratio maintains systemic oxygen consumption at adequate levels to meet systemic oxygen demands. When this compensatory response in the oxygen extraction ratio is inadequate to meet systemic oxygen demands, a switch occurs from aerobic metabolism to the less efficient anaerobic metabolism. The result is depletion of adenosine triphosphate (ATP) and intracellular energy reserves. Intracellular acidosis occurs, and anaerobic glycolysis leads to the production of lactate. Below this critical value of systemic oxygen delivery, systemic oxygen consumption is dependent on systemic oxygen delivery, a relationship termed *physiologic oxygen supply dependency.*

A pathologic oxygen delivery dependency exists in patients with sepsis, trauma, and acute respiratory distress syndrome (ARDS) and after resuscitation from prolonged cardiac arrest. These patients have systemic oxygen delivery in the normal or elevated range but an impairment of oxygen utilization. This condition of cytopathic tissue hypoxia is a result of maldistribution of blood flow or a defect in the utilization of substrate at the microcirculatory or subcellular level. This pathologic supply dependency is accompanied by very high mixed venous oxygen saturation levels or venous hyperoxia, as well as by elevated lactate levels. This process is believed to be an important mechanism of cellular damage in various forms of shock.

Compensatory Responses

Minor decreases in arterial blood pressure and systemic oxygen delivery activate the baroreceptor reflex via stretch receptors or sensing mechanisms located in the carotid sinus, splanchnic vasculature, aortic arch, right atrium, and juxtaglomerular apparatus of the kidney, as well as chemoreceptors sensitive to concentrations of carbon dioxide or oxygen located in the central nervous system, mostly in the medulla. These compensatory responses mediated by activation of the sympathetic nervous system include (1) release of

cortisol, aldosterone, and epinephrine; (2) activation of the renin-angiotensin system; (3) release of arginine vasopressin (AVP) from the posterior pituitary; (4) augmentation of myocardial contractility and heart rate; (5) constriction of arterial and venous capacitance vessels, particularly in the splanchnic bed, thereby augmenting venous return; (6) redistribution of blood flow away from skeletal muscle beds and the splanchnic viscera; and (7) creation of a local tissue environment to enhance the unloading of oxygen to tissues and improve its extraction because of acidosis, pyrexia, and increased red blood cell 2,3-diphosphoglycerate.

Noncompensatory Responses

Noncompensatory responses develop when physiologic adjustments are exaggerated or lead to pathologic results. Vasodilatory shock results from many sources, including unregulated nitric oxide synthesis, inadequate ATP synthesis in vascular smooth muscle cells, activation of the enzyme poly (ADP ribosyl) polymerase (PARP)-1, lipid mediators, and opening of ATP-sensitive potassium channels in vascular smooth muscle cells. This multifaceted insult leads to interstitial fluid and cellular edema, which impairs oxygen diffusion from capillary to cell, causing a failure of energy-dependent ion transport, the production of lactate, and the inability to maintain normal transmembrane gradients of potassium, chloride, and calcium. Cells lose their ability to utilize available oxygen as a result of mitochondrial dysfunction, abnormal carbohydrate metabolism, and failure of many energy-dependent enzyme reactions.

Acidosis commonly accompanies shock. When a molecule of ATP is hydrolyzed to adenosine diphosphate (ADP) and inorganic phosphate, the reaction also generates a proton. The net yield of protons is positive when ATP is hydrolyzed in the cell and then regenerated only by the anaerobic breakdown of glucose. Thus, during anaerobic glycolysis, the use of ATP to power cellular processes, coupled with the anaerobic production of ATP by substrate-level phosphorylation reactions, results in the development of acidosis.

Cells in organs such as the kidneys, liver, and brain can convert lactate into glucose via gluconeogenesis or oxidize lactate to pyruvate and then, ultimately, to carbon dioxide and water.

Lactate levels are a reflection of tissue hypoxia, clearance, and alternative sources of production. When the splanchnic circulation is compromised in shock, hepatic lactate clearance is impaired, contributing to the buildup of lactate levels in the circulation. In sepsis, however, the rate of glycolysis increases even in the absence of tissue hypoxia. This phenomenon, which has been termed *accelerated aerobic glycolysis,* may reflect a change in the ratio of the active to the inactive form of pyruvate dehydrogenase, which is the rate-limiting step for the entry of substrate into the mitochondrial tricarboxylic acid cycle.

When systemic oxygen delivery continues to fail to meet systemic oxygen demands, the oxygen debt accumulates. Three stages of shock can ensue. The first stage, which is called early, reversible, or compensated shock, is characterized by compensatory responses to minimize tissue injury. This stage of shock can be self-limited, with full recovery and minimal residual morbidity, if the cause is recognized and treated early. If substantial oxygen debt persists without timely repayment or resolution, inflammation and cellular and microvascular injury define the second stage of shock, which is associated with a prolonged recovery and is typically complicated by organ failure, including acute lung injury and acute tubular necrosis. The third stage is late, irreversible, or decompensated shock. In this situation, the oxygen debt is large, and repayment is slow to nonexistent. When shock reaches this point, cellular and tissue injury is extensive and largely irreversible. Progression to multisystem organ failure and/or death is inevitable, regardless of therapy.

CLINICAL MANIFESTATIONS

The five general types of shock are cardiogenic, distributive, hypovolemic, obstructive, and dissociative. The distinction among these five shock syndromes can be made by combining the history, clinical picture, and hemodynamic measurements. Cardiogenic shock (Chapter 107) and shock syndromes related to sepsis (Chapter 108) are covered in detail elsewhere.

The clinical manifestation of shock is variable and depends on the initiating cause and the response of multiple organs. Shock typically presents as absolute or relative systemic arterial hypotension and evidence of end-organ dysfunction (Table 106-1). The extremities are cool and pale if shock is associated with peripheral vasoconstriction, which is typical of hypovolemic, cardiogenic, and obstructive shock, but they are typically warm and pink with the peripheral vasodilation of distributive shock and dissociative shock (cyanide poisoning).

The most frequent neurologic finding in shock is alteration in the level of consciousness, ranging from confusion to coma. Many of the clinically apparent manifestations of cardiac involvement in shock result from sympathoadrenal stimulation, with tachycardia being the most sensitive indicator that shock is present. Acute lung injury causes impaired gas exchange; the work of breathing is increased, and respiratory muscle fatigue and ventilatory failure require mechanical ventilation. Hypovolemia with or without acute tubular necrosis results in oliguria, although polyuria may be seen in early shock.

Typical clinical manifestations of gut involvement during shock include abdominal pain, ileus, erosive gastritis, pancreatitis, acalculous cholecystitis, and submucosal hemorrhage. If the integrity of the gut barrier is compromised, bacteria and their toxins are translocated into the blood stream. The most common manifestation of liver involvement in shock is a mild increase in serum levels of aminotransferases and lactate dehydrogenase. With severe hypoperfusion, shock liver may manifest with massive aminotransferase elevations and extensive hepatocellular damage.

Thrombocytopenia may result from dilution during volume repletion or from immunologic platelet destruction, which is especially common during septic shock. Activation of the coagulation cascade can lead to disseminated intravascular coagulation (Chapter 178), which results in thrombocytopenia, decreased fibrinogen, elevated fibrin split products, and microangiopathic hemolytic anemia.

Hypovolemic Shock

Hemorrhagic shock, be it from internal or external bleeding, is the most common cause of hypovolemic shock (Table 106-2). Nonhemorrhagic hypovolemic shock can be caused by severe dehydration owing to massive urinary or gastrointestinal fluid losses. Such losses are common in conditions such as diabetic ketoacidosis (Chapters 236) or diarrhea from some infectious diseases, such as cholera (Chapter 310). Massive insensible losses of water or perspiration can precipitate shock in patients with major burn injuries (Chapter 112) or heatstroke (Chapter 109). Sequestration of fluid in the extravascular compartment, commonly referred to as "third spacing," can cause shock in patients as a result of surgery, bowel obstruction, hepatic failure (Chapter 157), systemic inflammation, acute pancreatitis (Chapter 146), or thermal injuries (Chapter 112). Regardless of whether hypovolemic shock is due to hemorrhage or fluid losses, the rate of loss is a critical component of the presentation. If volume is lost at a slow rate, compensatory mechanisms are usually effective, and any given amount of volume depletion is often better tolerated than if the same volume were lost acutely. In addition, underlying diseases, especially those that limit cardiac reserve, can substantially influence the clinical severity of a hypovolemic insult.

TABLE 106-1	PHYSICAL EXAMINATION AND SELECTED LABORATORY SIGNS IN SHOCK
Central nervous system	Acute delirium, restlessness, disorientation, confusion, and coma, which may be secondary to decreased cerebral perfusion pressure (mean arterial pressure minus intracranial pressure). Patients with chronic hypertension or increased intracranial pressure may be symptomatic at normal blood pressures. Cheyne-Stokes respirations may be seen with severe decompensated heart failure. Blindness can be a presenting complaint or complication.
Temperature	Hyperthermia results in excess tissue respiration and greater systemic oxygen delivery requirements. Hypothermia can occur when decreased systemic oxygen delivery or impaired cellular respiration decreases heat generation.
Skin	Cool distal extremities (combined low serum bicarbonate and high arterial lactate levels) aid in identifying patients with hypoperfusion. Pallor, cyanosis, sweating, and decreased capillary refill and pale, dusky, or clammy extremities indicate systemic hypoperfusion. Dry mucous membranes and decreased skin turgor indicate low vascular volume. Low toe temperature correlates with the severity of shock.
General cardiovascular	Neck vein distention (e.g., heart failure, pulmonary embolus, pericardial tamponade) or flattening (e.g., hypovolemia), tachycardia, and arrhythmias. Decreased coronary perfusion pressures can lead to ischemia, decreased ventricular compliance, and increased left ventricular diastolic pressure. A "mill wheel" heart murmur may be heard with an air embolus.
Heart rate	Usually elevated. However, paradoxical bradycardia can be seen in patients with preexisting cardiac disease and severe hemorrhage. Heart rate variability is associated with poor outcomes.
Systolic blood pressure	May actually increase slightly when cardiac contractility increases in early shock and then fall as shock advances. A single episode of undifferentiated hypotension with a systolic blood pressure <80 mm Hg carries an in-hospital mortality of 18%.
Diastolic blood pressure	Correlates with arteriolar vasoconstriction and may rise early in shock and then fall when cardiovascular compensation fails.
Pulse pressure	Defined as systolic minus diastolic pressure and related to stroke volume and the rigidity of the aorta. Increases early in shock and decreases before systolic pressure decreases.
Pulsus paradoxus	An exaggerated change in systolic blood pressure with respiration (systolic blood pressure declines >10 mm Hg with inspiration) seen in asthma, cardiac tamponade, and air embolus.
Mean arterial blood pressure	Diastolic blood pressure + [pulse pressure/3]
Shock index	Heart rate/systolic blood pressure. Normal = 0.5 to 0.7. A persistent elevation of the shock index (>1.0) indicates impaired left ventricular function (as a result of blood loss and/or cardiac depression) and is associated with increased mortality.
Respiratory	Tachypnea, increased minute ventilation, increased dead space, bronchospasm, hypocapnia with progression to respiratory failure, acute lung injury, and adult respiratory distress syndrome.
Abdomen	Low-flow states may result in abdominal pain, ileus, gastrointestinal bleeding, pancreatitis, acalculous cholecystitis, mesenteric ischemia, and shock liver.
Renal	Because the kidney receives 20% of cardiac output, low cardiac output reduces the glomerular filtration rate and redistributes renal blood flow from the renal cortex toward the renal medulla, leading to oliguria. Paradoxical polyuria in sepsis may be confused with adequate hydration.
Metabolic	Respiratory alkalosis is the first acid-base abnormality, but metabolic acidosis occurs as shock progresses. Hyperglycemia, hypoglycemia, and hyperkalemia may develop.

TABLE 106-2 CLASSIFICATION OF HEMORRHAGIC SHOCK*

	CLASS I	CLASS II	CLASS III	CLASS IV
Blood loss (mL)	Up to 750	750-1500	1500-2000	>2000
% Volume	Up to 15	15-30	30-40	>40
Pulse rate (per min)	<100	>100	>120	>140
Blood pressure	Normal	Normal	Decreased	Decreased
Pulse pressure	Normal or increased	Decreased	Decreased	Decreased
Respiratory rate (per min)	14-20	20-30	30-40	>35
Urine output (mL/hr)	>30	20-30	5-15	Negligible
Mental status	Slightly anxious	Mildly anxious	Anxious, confused	Confused, lethargic
Fluid replacement	Crystalloid	Crystalloid	Crystalloid and blood	Crystalloid and blood

*Estimates based on a 70-kg patient.
From Committee on Trauma of the American College of Surgeons. *Advanced Trauma Life Support for Doctors*. Chicago: American College of Surgeons; 1997:108.

Distributive Shock

The most important and prevalent cause of distributive shock is septic shock (Chapter 108), but anaphylaxis (Chapter 261), drug overdose (Chapter 33), neurogenic insults, and addisonian crisis (Chapter 234) can also produce vasodilatory shock. Sepsis can be a combination of hypovolemia, vasodilation, myocardial suppression, and impaired tissue oxygen use (dissociative shock). In approximately 10 to 15% of septic shock patients, myocardial dysfunction results in a low-cardiac-output form of shock. Early interventions (Chapter 108) can improve outcomes substantially.

Cardiogenic Shock

Cardiogenic shock (Chapter 107) is defined by a decrease in systemic oxygen delivery caused by an acute or chronic deterioration of cardiac function owing to myocardial, valvular, structural, toxic, or infectious causes. The clinical picture of cardiogenic shock is variable, depending on which structural component of the ventricle is impaired.

Extracardiac Obstructive Shock

This form of shock results from acute obstruction to flow in the circulation. Examples include impaired diastolic filling of the right ventricle (e.g., superior vena cava syndrome; Chapter 187), obstruction of right ventricular output (e.g., massive pulmonary embolism; Chapter 98), or an air embolus from cardiopulmonary bypass or central line placement (Chapter 98). Systemic arterial hypertension (Chapter 67) severe enough to impair left ventricular function or acute pericardial tamponade or constrictive pericarditis (Chapter 77) can also produce an obstructive shock pattern.

Dissociative Shock

Dissociative shock results from microvascular abnormalities, with maldistribution or shunting of blood flow, or cytopathic tissue hypoxia. Dissociative shock includes disorders that inhibit oxygen utilization, such as cyanide poisoning, sodium nitroprusside use, and sepsis.

Mixed Shock States

Shock may arise from multiple causes. For example, a patient with pneumonia and a history of ischemic cardiomyopathy may present in a hypodynamic rather than a hyperdynamic state when combined with sepsis. Thus, a mixture of hypovolemic, distributive, and cardiogenic shock can be seen in the same patient.

DIAGNOSIS

A key element in the approach to shock is a problem-directed history and physical examination. Some patients present with few symptoms other than generalized weakness, lethargy, or altered mental status. A discussion with the patient and family members should specifically address symptoms that suggest volume depletion, including bleeding, vomiting, diarrhea, excessive urination, insensible losses due to fever, or orthostatic lightheadedness. The history should also inquire about prior or current evidence of cardiovascular disease, especially episodes of chest pain (Chapter 50) or symptoms of heart failure (Chapter 58). Prior neurologic diseases can render patients more

susceptible to complications from hypovolemia. Medication use, both prescribed and nonprescribed, must be ascertained. Some medications cause volume depletion (e.g., diuretics), whereas others depress myocardial contractility (e.g., β-blockers, calcium-channel blockers). The possibility of an anaphylactic reaction to a new medication or cardiovascular depression owing to drug toxicity should be considered. A recent or remote history of steroid use may suggest adrenal insufficiency (Chapter 34).

Findings on the physical examination can provide critical information to aid in the diagnosis (see Table 106-1). Traditionally, shock is defined by a systolic blood pressure less than 90 mm Hg or 40 mm Hg less than the baseline systolic blood pressure if the patient has a history of hypertension.

Acidosis

A common theme in shock is that tissue hypoxia leads to acidosis (Chapter 120), which develops as a consequence of anaerobic metabolism and generally parallels the severity of shock. Laboratory manifestations may include a base deficit, low arterial and venous pH levels, and an elevated serum lactate level. Base deficit is the absolute decrease in the serum concentration of bicarbonate (normal minus the patient's bicarbonate). A mild base deficit is −2 to −5, moderate is −6 to −14, and severe is −15 mM/L or greater. When patients are resuscitated using large volumes of normal saline, the large fluid load can cause a dilutional acidosis, and the large chloride load can induce metabolic acidosis even in the absence of tissue hypoxia and anaerobic metabolism. Base deficit can also be caused by cocaine, alcohol, and diabetic ketoacidosis. Despite its limitations, base deficit provides the clinician with a quick indicator to assess the severity of tissue hyperfusion and the adequacy of resuscitation in relieving anaerobic metabolism and oxygen debt.

The low pH of metabolic acidosis can result from different acids. Acidosis caused by lactate and unidentified anions produces an ion gap. The blood lactate concentration rises with increased anaerobic metabolism, as is seen in shock but also in diabetic ketoacidosis (Chapter 236) , total parenteral nutrition (Chapter 224), seizures (Chapter 410), thiamine deficiency (Chapter 225), treatment of HIV infection with protease inhibitors (Chapter 396), and administration of metformin, salicylate, isoniazid, propofol, and cyanide (Chapter 110). A lactate concentration greater than 4 mmol/L is unusual in normal and non–critically ill hospitalized patients and warrants concern. A lactate concentration greater than 4 mmol/L is associated with an in-hospital mortality exceeding 25%, regardless of the cause, and failure to decrease lactate levels over the first 6 hours of shock is associated with an increased inflammatory response, the development of organ failure, and mortality.

Urine Output

The kidneys normally receive 20% of the systemic oxygen delivery, and because of this large amount of blood flow per gram of tissue, they are highly sensitive to changes in renal blood flow. Urine output is a valuable indicator of renal perfusion and vital organ blood flow. Although a significant drop in urine output indicates reduced renal blood flow, an adequate urine output does not always indicate successful resuscitation. Other factors that may affect urine output include the use of mannitol or diuretics. Preexisting conditions, such as renal failure, may also limit the ability of this measure to reflect the adequacy of resuscitation.

TREATMENT Rx

The goal of initial management is to restore global and microvascular perfusion to levels that sustain aerobic cellular respiration. Multiple randomized trials have shown significant and consistent reductions in mortality when shock is reversed aggressively before organ failure develops. Once this initial management is accomplished, the definitive diagnosis leads to more specific therapy based on the cause of shock.

Markers of shock serve not only as diagnostic tools for risk stratification but also as targets or end points for the early restoration of adequate tissue perfusion. Clinical monitoring of tissue oxygenation and organ function commonly involves measuring traditional end points of resuscitation, such as heart rate, blood pressure, mentation, urine output, and skin perfusion. Many clinicians continue to use these parameters as indicators that systemic oxygenation imbalances have been corrected. However, there is increasing evidence that clinical parameters may be poor indicators of the ongoing tissue hypoxia that is associated with increased mortality.

Initial Management

The initial management of shock requires immediate diagnostic and therapeutic interventions, including attention to airway, breathing, circulation, and definitive diagnosis and treatment (Chapter 63). The first step to optimize systemic oxygen delivery is to provide supplemental oxygen to increase arterial oxygen content. If any doubt exists about the patency of the airway or the adequacy of ventilation, endotracheal intubation should be performed and mechanical ventilation initiated (Chapter 105). Mechanical ventilation helps provide adequate oxygenation and carbon dioxide elimination and decreases oxygen utilization by the respiratory muscles, which may be responsible for up to 40% of systemic oxygen consumption and lactate production.

Although endotracheal intubation and mechanical ventilation may be critical for patients in shock, the sudden increase in airway pressure can lead to a series of deleterious hemodynamic complications, especially in patients who are hypovolemic or vasodilated or have compromised cardiac function. In such patients, the resulting decreased venous return, increased pulmonary vascular resistance, and decreased ventricular compliance may lead to hypotension and cardiovascular collapse. Furthermore, when sedatives, anxiolytics, or induction agents are used during and after intubation, the decrease in catecholamine levels, peripheral vascular resistance, and cortisol levels may result in hypotension. If possible, preparations should be made to monitor physiologic variables, ensure adequate fluid administration, and provide rapid access to vasopressors should systemic arterial pressure fall to dangerously low levels.

Upon initial presentation, it is good practice to place one or two large-bore (≥16 gauge) peripheral intravenous catheters and to administer a crystalloid solution (normal saline or Ringer's lactate solution). If MAP is less than 60 to 65 mm Hg, systolic blood pressure is less than 90 mm Hg, or evidence of tissue hypoperfusion is present, an intravenous fluid challenge (20 to 40 mL/kg crystalloid or colloid) should be given rapidly. A bolus of 500 mL every 30 minutes titrated to MAP or measurement of preload is recommended. In an 80-kg person, the average intravascular volume is 5 L. In shock states, such as septic shock, in which intravascular hypovolemia is a predominant feature, 5 to 6 L of fluid over the first 6 hours is considered an average volume resuscitation. If hemorrhage is the likely cause of shock, blood should be used to replace volume. Fluids should not be withheld, even in patients with end-stage renal disease.

Central venous access and arterial blood pressure monitoring should be established to monitor hemodynamics and venous and arterial blood gases, respectively. Electrocardiographic monitoring and continuous measurement of oxygen saturation by pulse oximetry are useful adjuncts. Because the Trendelenburg position may impair gas exchange and promote aspiration, an alternative is to raise the patient's legs above the level of the heart with the patient in the supine position.

If the patient remains hypotensive, vasopressors such as norepinephrine, dopamine, or Neo-Synephrine (Table 106-3) should be administered to restore adequate systemic arterial pressure while the diagnostic evaluation is ongoing. Treatment with vasopressors should not be postponed while trying to achieve euvolemia by using fluid boluses, because patients with cerebrovascular and coronary artery disease may be intolerant of the hypotensive interval. However, vasopressors may also mask hypovolemia when they increase blood pressure. If the volume status remains undefined or the hemodynamic condition requires repeated fluid challenges or vasopressor treatment, a central venous

catheter should be placed to determine central venous oxygen saturation, ventricular filling pressures, and intravascular volume status while echocardiography is performed. Based on these data, patients can usually be classified and managed according to their hemodynamic and oxygen transport patterns (Figs. 106-2 and 106-3).

Fluid Replacement

Rapid and appropriate restoration of vascular volume decreases the need for vasopressor therapy, adrenal replacement therapy, and invasive monitoring; in addition, it modulates the inflammation that arises when a patient progresses to severe shock. The goal of fluid resuscitation is not merely to achieve a predetermined volume but rather to titrate fluid to optimize systemic oxygen delivery and meet tissue oxygen demands.

To assess the adequacy of cardiac preload during the resuscitation of a patient with shock, a central venous catheter is as good as a pulmonary artery catheter.[1] However, the CVP does not correlate well with left ventricular enddiastolic volume: although a low CVP indicates hypovolemia, a "normal" CVP does not exclude inadequate preload as a cause of shock. A fluid challenge in a volume-responsive patient increases cardiac output by about 20% for each 2 cm H_2O change in CVP; by comparison, cardiac output does not change if the CVP is raised in a patient with adequate left ventricular volume.

When intrathoracic pressure increases during the application of positive airway pressure in a mechanically ventilated patient, venous return decreases and, as a consequence, left ventricular stroke volume also decreases. The variation in pulse pressure or stroke volume during a positive-pressure breath can also predict the responsiveness of cardiac output to changes in preload. Pulse pressure variation is defined by equation 3:

$$100 \times (PPmax - PPmin)/[(PPmax + PPmin)/2] \qquad (3)$$

PPmax and PPmin are the maximal and minimal pulse pressures, respectively, in a respiratory cycle. Pulse pressure variation values of 13 to 15% suggest that hypovolemia is present and that the cardiac index will increase by at least 15% after the rapid infusion of 500 mL of crystalloid. Pulse pressure variation is generally the best predictor of volume status and response to fluids, although atrial arrhythmias can interfere with the usefulness of this technique.

Types of Fluids

The two most commonly used crystalloid solutions are 0.9% sodium chloride solution (normal saline) and Ringer's lactate solution. Although these two solutions have been regarded as essentially interchangeable, accumulating data suggest that large volumes of normal saline, but not Ringer's lactate solution, promote the development of hyperchloremic metabolic acidosis and coagulopathy (Table 106-4).

Colloids are higher-molecular-weight solutions that increase plasma oncotic pressure; they are classified as natural (albumin) or artificial (starches, hetastarch, pentastarch, dextrans, and gelatins). Colloids are dissolved in either normal saline or a balanced salt solution. There are no clinically significant differences among the various colloid solutions when they are used for shock resuscitation. When compared with saline-based solutions, hetastarch dissolved in a calcium-containing, low-chloride, balanced salt solution may be

TABLE 106-3 VASOPRESSOR AGENTS

AGENT	DOSE RANGE	Peripheral Vasculature		Cardiac Effects			TYPICAL USE
		VASOCONSTRICTION	VASODILATION	HEART RATE	CONTRACTILITY	DYSRHYTHMIAS	
Dopamine	1-4 µg/kg/min	0	1+	1+	1+	1+	"Renal dose" does not improve renal function; may be used with bradycardia and hypotension
	5-10 µg/kg/min	1-2+	1+	2+	2+	2+	
	11-20 µg/kg/min	2-3+	1+	2+	2+	3+	Vasopressor range
Vasopressin	0.04-0.1 units/min	3-4+	0	0	0	1+	Septic shock, post–cardiopulmonary bypass shock state, no outcome benefit in sepsis
Phenylephrine	20-200 µg/min	4+	0	0	0	1+	Vasodilatory shock, best for supraventricular tachycardia
Norepinephrine	1-20 µg/min	4+	0	2+	2+	2+	First-line vasopressor for septic shock, vasodilatory shock
Epinephrine	1-20 µg/min	4+	0	4+	4+	4+	Refractory shock, shock with bradycardia, anaphylactic shock
Dobutamine	1-20 µg/kg/min	1+	2+	1-2+	3+	3+	Cardiogenic shock, septic shock
Milrinone	37.5-75 µg/kg bolus followed by 0.375-0.75 µg/min	0	2+	1+	3+	2+	Cardiogenic shock, right heart failure, dilates pulmonary artery; caution in renal failure

FIGURE 106-2. General hemodynamic management. aPTT = activated partial thromboplastin time; BNP = brain natriuretic peptide; bpm = beats per minute; CVP = central venous pressure; DO_2 = (systemic) oxygen delivery; ECG = electrocardiogram; HR = heart rate; INR = international normalized ratio; MAP = mean arterial pressure; PAOP = pulmonary artery occlusion pressure; pHi = intestinal mucosal pH; PPV = pulse pressure variation; PT = prothrombin time; SBP = systolic blood pressure; SVR = systemic vascular resistance; SVV = stroke volume variation; VO_2 = (systemic) oxygen eonsumption; WBC = white blood cell.

associated with less acidosis and less use of blood products, but its use in severe sepsis and septic shock has been associated with increased renal failure and mortality.[2]

Colloids stay in the intravascular space significantly longer than crystalloids do, with an intravascular half-life of 16 hours for albumin versus 30 to 60 minutes for normal saline and lactated Ringer's. When titrated to the same volume status, colloids and crystalloids restore tissue perfusion to the same magnitude, but a two to four times greater volume of crystalloids is required to achieve the same end point. Various types of fluids have potential advantages and disadvantages, but the outcomes of patients with hypovolemic shock are equivalent for crystalloids and albumin (see Table 106-4).[3]

Fluid Management Strategies

Initial aggressive fluid resuscitation usually occurs within 6 hours of presentation, but different strategies are needed for the longer-term management

of fluid status, especially in patients with acute lung injury. For example, conservative volume therapy (euvolemia) beginning an average of 47 hours after admission to the intensive care unit (ICU) and 24 hours after the establishment of acute lung injury results in significantly better lung and central nervous system function and a decreased need for sedation, mechanical ventilation, and ICU care.[4] However, patients who receive conservative volume replacement transiently may need more vasopressor support.

Optimal Hemoglobin

In hemorrhagic shock, the rapid administration of packed red blood cells and, if indicated, platelets and thawed fresh-frozen plasma can be life-saving. Whenever possible, fully cross-matched packed red blood cells are preferable, but type-specific blood can often be given safely when immediate therapy is warranted (Chapter 180). In dire emergencies, type O Rh-negative blood can be administered to women of childbearing potential, and type O

Shock

Definition

Hypovolemic
Blood or fluid loss, both leading to a decreased circulating blood volume, diastolic filling pressure, and volume.

Cardiogenic
Severe reduction in cardiac function resulting from direct myocardial damage or a mechanical abnormality of the heart.

Extracardiac/ Obstructive
Obstruction to flow in the cardiovascular circuit that leads to inadequate diastolic filling or decreased systolic function because of increased afterload.

Distributive
Arterial and venous dilation leads to a decrease in preload, with decreased, normal, or elevated cardiac output, depending on the presence of myocardial depression. Inflammatory causes produce micro-circulatory dysfunction, hypotension, and multiple organ system dysfunction without a decrease in cardiac output.

Dissociative
Impairment of oxygen utilization or impairment of the cellular machinery.

Etiologies

Hemorrhagic:
Trauma
Gastrointestinal
Retroperitoneal
Postoperative surgical procedures

Fluid depletion (nonhemorrhagic):
External fluid loss
Dehydration
Vomiting
Diarrhea
Polyuria

Interstitial fluid redistribution:
Thermal injury
Trauma
Anaphylaxis

Increased vascular capacitance (venodilation):
Sepsis
Anaphylaxis
Toxins/drugs

Myopathic:
Myocardial infarction
Left ventricle
Right ventricle

Myocardial contusion (trauma):
Myocarditis
Cardiomyopathy
Postischemic myocardial stunning
Septic myocardial depression
Pharmacologic
Anthracycline
cardiotoxicity
Calcium-channel blockers

Mechanical:
Valvular failure (stenotic or regurgitant)
Hypertrophic cardiomyopathy
Ventricular septal defect

Arrhythmias:
Bradycardia
Tachycardia

Impaired diastolic filling (decreased ventricular preload):
Direct venous obstruction (vena cava)
Intrathoracic obstructive tumors

Increased intrathoracic pressure:
Tension pneumothorax
Mechanical ventilation (with excessive pressure or volume depletion)
Asthma

Decreased cardiac compliance:
Constrictive pericarditis
Cardiac tamponade

Impaired systolic contraction (increased ventricular afterload):
Right ventricle
Pulmonary embolus (massive)
Air embolus
Acute pulmonary hypertension
Left ventricle occlusion or aortic dissection

Septic (bacterial, fungal, viral, rickettsial)
Toxic shock syndrome
Anaphylactic anaphylactoid
Neurogenic (spinal shock)
Endocrinologic
Adrenal crisis
Thyroid storm

Toxic (e.g., nitroprusside, bretylium, cyanide)
End-stage sepsis
Catecholamine toxicity

FIGURE 106-3. Definitions, etiologies, and therapies of various shock states. CI = cardiac index; CO = cardiac output; CT = computed tomography; CVP = central venous pressure; DO₂ = systemic oxygen delivery; ECG = electrocardiogram; IABP = intra-aortic balloon pumping; LV = left ventricular; MAP = mean arterial pressure; MRI = magnetic resonance imaging; PA = pulmonary artery; PAOP = pulmonary artery occlusion pressure; RA = right atrial; RV = right ventricular; SVR = systemic vascular resistance; US = ultrasonography; VSD = ventricular septal defect.

Continued

Hemodynamic Characterization

	Box 1	Box 2	Box 3	Box 4	Box 5
CVP/RA	↓	↑	↑↑	↓ early, normal later	↓ early, normal to ↑ later
PAOP	↓	↓ early ↑ later	↓	↓ early, normal later	↓ early, normal to ↑ later
CO/CI/DO₂	↓	↓↓	↔	↓ early ↑ later	↓ early ↑ later
SVR	↑	↑	↑	↑ early ↓ later	↑ early ↓ later
SvO₂/ScvO₂	↓	↓	↓	↓ early ↑ later	↑ early ↓ later

Box 1 Comments: Preexisting heart disease may alter the filling pressures

Box 2 Comments: If there is a VSD, there may be ScvO₂/SvO₂ or a step up from the right atrium to right ventricle to the pulmonary artery. Large V wave is seen on PA catheter with mitral regurgitation.

Box 3 Comments: Equalization of intracardiac diastolic pressure is consistent with pericardial tamponade. A rapid x and blunted y descent on CVP wave form indicates the inability of the heart to fill.

Box 4 Comments: In the early stage, filling pressures are low, leading to low to normal cardiac output and variable ScvO₂/SvO₂. If myocardial depression accompanies, then a similar profile of cardiogenic shock is seen. After resuscitation a hyperdynamic circulation is seen.

Box 5 Comments: Filling pressures can be variable, depending on stage of the disease. Cardiac output is generally increased. SVR is decreased and ScvO₂/SvO₂ and lactate are increased.

Therapy

Box 1:
Rapid replacement of blood, colloid or crystalloid
Identify source of blood/fluid loss
Replace deficient coagulation factors
Consider factor VIIa
Endoscopy/colonoscopy
Angiography
CT/MRI/US or other

Box 2:
LV infarction:
  intra-aortic balloon pump (IABP) coronary angiography
Recanalization:
  thrombolytic therapy, angioplasty, coronary bypass surgery
RV infarction:
  fluids and inotropes with PA catheter
Mechanical abnormality:
  echocardiography, cardiac catheterization
Corrective surgery:
  mechanical assist devices, transplantation

Box 3:
Pericardial tamponade:
  pericardiocentesis, surgical drainage (if needed)
Pneumothorax:
  chest tube
Pulmonary embolism:
  heparin
  ventilation-perfusion lung scan
  pulmonary angiography
  consider thrombolytic therapy, embolectomy
Severe hypertension:
  afterload reduction

Box 4:
Identify site of infection
Antimicrobial agents
Early goal-directed therapy
  fluids
  vasopressors
  inotropic agents
Goals:
  ScO₂ > 70%
  CVP > 8 mm Hg
  MAP > 65 mm Hg
Improving organ function
Decreasing lactate levels
Consider activated protein C
Requiring vasopressors, consider corticosteroids

Box 5:
Toxin antidote or remove agent, hyperbaric oxygen therapy
Recombinant activated protein C
Nitroglycerin (speculative)
Prostacyclin (speculative)

FIGURE 106-3, cont'd.

TABLE 106-4	FLUID THERAPY
Normal saline	Normal saline is a slightly hyperosmolar solution containing 154 mEq/L of both sodium and chloride. Owing to the relatively high chloride concentration and low pH, normal saline carries a risk of inducing hyperchloremic metabolic acidosis when given in large amounts.
Lactated Ringer's solution (LR)	Lactate is metabolized to carbon dioxide (CO_2) and water by the liver, leading to the release of CO_2 in the lungs and excretion of water by the kidneys. LR is preferred over normal saline and buffers acidemia. Because LR contains a very small amount of potassium, there is a small risk of inducing hyperkalemia in patients with renal insufficiency or renal failure. LR may be incompletely metabolized in severe hepatic failure.
Albumin	Albumin is a protein derived from human plasma and is available in varying concentrations from 4 to 25%. A study comparing fluid resuscitation with albumin versus saline found similar 28-day mortalities and secondary outcomes in each arm.[3] However, a post-hoc subset analysis of patients with sepsis and acute lung injury resuscitated with albumin showed a trend toward a decrease in mortality. There was a significant increase in mortality in trauma patients, particularly those with head injury.
Hydroxyethyl starch (HES)	HES, which is a synthetic colloid derived from hydrolyzed amylopectin, causes renal impairment at recommended doses and impaired long-term survival at high doses. HES can also cause coagulopathy and bleeding complications from reduced factor VIII and von Willebrand factor levels, as well as impaired platelet function. HES increases the risk of acute renal failure and reduces the probability of survival in patients with sepsis.
Dextrans	Dextrans are artificial colloids synthesized by *Leuconostoc mesenteroides* bacteria grown in sucrose media. Dextrans are used more frequently to lower blood viscosity than for rapid plasma expansion. They can cause renal dysfunction as well as anaphylactoid reactions.
Gelatins	Gelatins are produced from bovine collagen. Because they have a small molecular weight, they are not very effective at expanding plasma volume, but they cost less than other options. They have been reported to cause renal impairment as well as allergic reactions ranging from pruritus to anaphylaxis. Gelatins are not currently available in North America.

Rh-negative or Rh-positive blood can be given to men or postmenopausal women.

The appropriate hemoglobin level in shock remains controversial, but a value of 10 mg/dL is often recommended as long as the patient has increased lactate levels, decreased venous oxygen saturation, or evidence of systemic hypoperfusion. A more conservative transfusion strategy (hemoglobin value of 7 to 10 mg/dL) is appropriate when the patient is in the more convalescent phase of critical illness.

Vasopressor Therapy

To optimize end-organ perfusion, the second phase of intervention after adequate fluid resuscitation is to maintain perfusion pressure. A specific MAP goal has not been established for all shock states, but a MAP of at least 60 to 65 mm Hg is a reasonable target.

The most common vasopressors are agonists at various adrenergic receptors. Receptors include peripheral α-adrenergic receptors that lead to vasoconstriction, cardiac β_1 receptors with both chronotropic and inotropic effects, β_2 receptors located in the circulation and airways that mediate vasodilation and bronchodilation, and dopaminergic receptors located throughout the cardiovascular, mesenteric, and renal circulations. Based on these mechanisms, therapy can be tailored to a specific circumstance. For example, a patient with severe tachycardia would be best served by an agent with more α-selective activity and less β activity to avoid tachycardia and increased myocardial oxygen consumption (see Table 106-3).

Norepinephrine, which is a vasoconstrictor and an inotrope, provides better splanchnic oxygen utilization compared with dopamine. It is generally considered the first-line vasopressor for treating persistent hypotension in septic patients despite adequate resuscitation,[5] and it may be superior to dopamine in treating cardiogenic shock. For example, a randomized trial comparing dopamine with norepinephrine in patients with shock showed no significant difference in mortality for hypovolemic and septic shock but a significant benefit of norepinephrine in cardiogenic shock.[5] In addition, there was a significant two-fold increase in arrhythmic events with dopamine compared with norepinephrine (24.1 vs. 12.4%).

Dopamine's effects result from transduction at dopaminergic receptors in the renal, mesenteric, coronary, and systemic circulations. The positive chronotropic and inotropic effects of dopamine can lead to tachycardia and tachyarrhythmias; this effect frequently limits its dosing because the increased myocardial oxygen requirements promote the development of myocardial ischemia, especially in the presence of coronary artery disease.

Phenylephrine is a synthetic catecholamine that is a selective α-adrenergic agonist and is ideal in patients with tachycardia. However, the resulting increase in myocardial oxygen consumption, decrease in splanchnic blood flow, and decrease in cardiac output can be detrimental for patients with septic shock.

Epinephrine, which is a potent α-, β_1-, and β_2-adrenergic agonist, increases peripheral arteriolar tone as well as cardiac contractility. It is the first-line agent for the treatment of anaphylactic shock and is used to support myocardial contractility following cardiac surgery. Epinephrine increases the white blood cell count and the blood lactate concentration because of accelerated aerobic glycogenolysis and/or maldistribution of blood flow.

Vasopressin deficiency accompanies vasodilatory shock. Vasopressin is not a potent vasopressor in normal subjects, but very low doses (0.04 unit/minute) markedly increase arterial blood pressure in septic patients with intractable hypotension. In addition, vasopressin enhances the pressor response to catecholamines.

Adrenal Dysfunction

Beyond their metabolic functions, glucocorticoids are required to maintain responsiveness to vasopressors, intravascular volume, vascular permeability, and myocardial contractility. If the hypothalamic-pituitary-adrenocortical axis is depressed in shock, clinical findings can include unexplained fever, hypoglycemia, metabolic acidosis, hypotension refractory to fluid resuscitation, and eosinophilia. Cortisol levels and the results of cosyntropin stimulation testing may not be clinically helpful. If adrenal insufficiency is strongly suspected, or if patients have refractory hypotension despite vasopressors and hemodynamic optimization, stress doses of intravenous hydrocortisone (e.g., 50 mg every 6 hours) are recommended.[6]

 PROGNOSIS

Clinical characteristics associated with a poor outcome include the severity of shock; its temporal duration, underlying cause, and reversibility; and pre-existing vital organ dysfunction. Direct noninvasive measurement of maximal oxygen uptake predicts outcome in patients who have cardiogenic shock. Persistently elevated lactate levels are prognostic in trauma, septic shock, and after cardiac arrest, and an anion gap acidosis is associated with significantly higher hospital mortality than is hyperchloremic acidosis. Regional measurements of pH are highly predictive of outcome; for example, if the gastric mucosal pH remains below 7.3 for 24 hours, the hospital mortality rate is about 50%. The severity of the base deficit correlates with the development of multisystem organ failure in trauma. The mortality for an undiagnosed patient who is sent to a general medical floor and develops shock is three times higher than for a patient who is admitted directly to the ICU.

Grade
A

1. The National Heart, Lung, and Blood Institute Acute Respiratory Distress Syndrome (ARDS) Clinical Trials Network. Pulmonary-artery versus central venous catheter to guide treatment of acute lung injury. *N Engl J Med.* 2006;354:2213-2224.
2. Brunkhorst FM, Engel C, Bloos F, et al. Intensive insulin therapy and pentastarch resuscitation in severe sepsis. *N Engl J Med.* 2008;358:125-139.
3. Finfer S, Bellomo R, Boyce N, et al. A comparison of albumin and saline for fluid resuscitation in the intensive care unit. *N Engl J Med.* 2004;350:2247-2256.
4. The National Heart, Lung, and Blood Institute Acute Respiratory Distress Syndrome (ARDS) Clinical Trials Network. Comparison of two fluid-management strategies in acute lung injury. *N Engl J Med.* 2006;354:2564-2575.
5. De Backer D, Biston P, Devriendt J, et al. Comparison of dopamine and norepinephrine in the treatment of shock. *N Engl J Med.* 2010;362:779-789.
6. Sprung CL, Annane D, Keh D, et al. Hydrocortisone therapy for patients with septic shock. *N Engl J Med.* 2008;358:111-124.

SUGGESTED READINGS

Barbee RW, Reynolds PS, Ward KR. Assessing shock resuscitation strategies by oxygen debt repayment. *Shock.* 2010;33:113-122. *Incorporates the concept of the oxygen supply and delivery relationship with that of oxygen debt and shows the relevance to shock and resuscitation.*
Greer R. The temporal evolution of acute respiratory distress syndrome following shock. *Eur J Anaesthesiol.* 2010;27:3:226-232. *Comprehensive overview.*
Groeneveld AB, Navickis RJ, Wilkes MM. Update on the comparative safety of colloids: a systematic review of clinical studies. *Ann Surg.* 2011;253:470-483. *Among colloids, albumin is safer than hydroxyethyl starch solutions.*

Strehlow MC. Early identification of shock in critically ill patients. *Emerg Med Clin North Am.* 2010; 28:57-66. *Reviews the physiologic definition, the importance of early intervention, and the clinical and diagnostic signs clinicians can use to identify patients in shock.*

107

CARDIOGENIC SHOCK

STEVEN HOLLENBERG

DEFINITION

Cardiogenic shock is the syndrome that ensues when the heart is unable to deliver enough blood to maintain adequate tissue perfusion. The hemodynamic picture includes sustained systemic hypotension, pulmonary capillary wedge pressure (PCWP) greater than 18 mm Hg, and cardiac index less than 2.2 L/minute/m^2 (Table 107-1). Although systolic blood pressure less than 90 mm Hg is a commonly accepted threshold for shock, a decrease of 30 mm Hg from baseline can also be used. The diagnosis of cardiogenic shock is often made on clinical grounds—hypotension combined with signs of poor tissue perfusion, including oliguria, clouded sensorium, and cool extremities, all in the setting of myocardial dysfunction. To make the diagnosis, it is important to document myocardial dysfunction and to exclude or correct factors such as hypovolemia, hypoxemia, and acidosis.

EPIDEMIOLOGY

The predominant cause of cardiogenic shock (Fig. 107-1) is left ventricular failure secondary to acute myocardial infarction (MI)—an extensive first acute MI, cumulative loss of myocardial function in a patient with previous MI or cardiomyopathy, or a mechanical complication of MI (Chapter 73). However, any cause of severe left ventricular (LV) or right ventricular (RV) dysfunction can lead to cardiogenic shock, including end-stage cardiomyopathy (Chapter 60), prolonged cardiopulmonary bypass, valvular disease (Chapter 75), myocardial contusion (Chapter 112), sepsis with unusually profound myocardial depression (Chapter 108), and fulminant myocarditis (Chapter 60) (Table 107-2). Stress-induced (takotsubo) cardiomyopathy (Chapter 60), a syndrome of acute apical LV dysfunction that occurs after emotional distress, may also present with cardiogenic shock. Acute valvular regurgitation, most often caused by endocarditis (Chapter 76) or chordal rupture (Chapter 75), can lead to shock, as can physiologic stress in the setting of severe valvular stenosis. Cardiac tamponade (Chapter 77) and massive pulmonary embolism (Chapter 98) with acute RV failure can cause shock without pulmonary edema.

The incidence and mortality associated with cardiogenic shock appear to be declining. In the past 30 years the incidence has fallen from about 8% to 6% of MIs, largely because of the benefit of early perfusion strategies (Chapter 73). In parallel, mortality from cardiogenic shock has decreased from 70 to 80% to 50% or less, suggesting that increasingly effective early treatment and more widespread adoption of early revascularization have improved the outcomes of patients in whom shock has already developed.

Risk factors for the development of cardiogenic shock in MI parallel those for LV dysfunction and the severity of coronary artery disease. Patient characteristics include older age, anterior MI, diabetes, hypertension, multivessel coronary artery disease (CAD), previous MI, and peripheral vascular and cerebrovascular disease. Clinical risk factors include decreased ejection fractions, larger infarctions, and lack of compensatory hyperkinesis in myocardial territories remote from the infarction. Clinical harbingers of impending shock include the degree of hypotension and tachycardia at hospital presentation. The factors that predict mortality reflect the severity of the acute insult as well as comorbid conditions.

FIGURE 107-1. Causes of cardiogenic shock in patients with myocardial infarction in the SHOCK trial registry. LV = left ventricular; MR = mitral regurgitation; RV = right ventricular; VSD = ventricular septal defect. (Adapted from Hochman JS, Boland J, Sleeper LA, et al. Current spectrum of cardiogenic shock and effect of early revascularization on mortality. Report of an international registry. SHOCK registry investigators. *Circulation.* 1995;91:873-881.)

TABLE 107-1 DIAGNOSIS OF CARDIOGENIC SHOCK

CLINICAL SIGNS

Hypotension
Oliguria
Clouded sensorium
Cool and mottled extremities

HEMODYNAMIC CRITERIA

Systolic blood pressure < 90 mm Hg or > 30 mm Hg decrease from baseline for > 30 min
Cardiac index < 2.2 L/min/m^2
Pulmonary capillary wedge pressure > 18 mm Hg

OTHER

Documented myocardial dysfunction
Exclusion of hypovolemia, hypoxia, and acidosis

TABLE 107-2 CAUSES OF CARDIOGENIC SHOCK

ACUTE MYOCARDIAL INFARCTION

Pump failure
    Large infarction
    Smaller infarction with preexisting left ventricular dysfunction
    Infarct extension
    Reinfarction
    Infarct expansion
Mechanical complications
    Acute mitral regurgitation due to papillary muscle rupture
    Ventricular septal defect
    Free wall rupture
    Pericardial tamponade
Right ventricular infarction

CARDIOMYOPATHY

Myocarditis
Peripartum cardiomyopathy
End-stage low-output heart failure
Hypertrophic cardiomyopathy with outflow tract obstruction
Stress cardiomyopathy

VALVULAR HEART DISEASE

Acute mitral regurgitation (chordal rupture)
Acute aortic regurgitation
Aortic or mitral stenosis with tachyarrhythmia or other comorbid condition causing decompensation
Prosthetic valve dysfunction

TACHYARRHYTHMIA

OTHER CONDITIONS

Prolonged cardiopulmonary bypass
Septic shock with severe myocardial depression
Penetrating or blunt cardiac trauma
Orthotopic transplant rejection
Massive pulmonary embolism
Pericardial tamponade

Coronary angiography most often demonstrates multivessel CAD. About 30% of patients have a left main coronary artery occlusion, about 60% have three-vessel coronary disease, and only about 20% have single-vessel disease. Multivessel CAD helps explain the failure to develop compensatory hyperkinesis in remote myocardial segments, because of either previous infarction or high-grade coronary stenoses.

Only one fourth of patients who develop cardiogenic shock are in shock when they initially present to the hospital; in the others, shock usually evolves over several hours, suggesting that early treatment may prevent shock. Comparison of the clinical characteristics of patients with early and late shock shows similar demographic, historical, clinical, and hemodynamic characteristics, but shock tends to develop earlier in patients with single-vessel CAD than in those with triple-vessel disease. This finding suggests that early shock in the setting of acute MI may be more amenable to revascularization of the culprit vessel via thrombolysis or angioplasty (Chapter 73), whereas shock developing later may require more complete revascularization with multivessel percutaneous coronary intervention (PCI) or coronary artery bypass graft (CABG) surgery (Chapter 74).

PATHOBIOLOGY

Cardiogenic shock is characterized by a downward cascade in which myocardial dysfunction reduces stroke volume, cardiac output, and blood pressure; these changes compromise myocardial perfusion, exacerbate ischemia, and further depress myocardial function, cardiac output, and systemic perfusion. Concomitant diastolic dysfunction increases left atrial pressure, which leads to pulmonary congestion and hypoxemia and exacerbates myocardial ischemia and impairs ventricular performance.

Compensatory mechanisms include sympathetic stimulation, which increases heart rate and contractility, and renal fluid retention, which increases preload. Increases in heart rate and contractility increase myocardial oxygen demand and exacerbate ischemia. Another compensatory mechanism, vasoconstriction to maintain blood pressure, increases myocardial afterload, further impairing cardiac performance and increasing myocardial oxygen demand. In the face of inadequate perfusion, this increased demand can worsen ischemia and perpetuate a vicious circle that, if unbroken, may culminate in death. Interrupting this circle of myocardial dysfunction and ischemia is the basis for therapeutic regimens for cardiogenic shock.

In cardiogenic shock, LV dysfunction is not always severe. In one large study, the mean LV ejection fraction was 30%, indicating that mechanisms other than primary pump failure were operative. Furthermore, systemic vascular resistance is not always elevated, suggesting that compensatory vasoconstriction is not universal. Inflammatory responses may contribute to the vasodilation and myocardial dysfunction in cardiogenic shock.

Patients in cardiogenic shock may have areas of nonfunctional but viable myocardium owing to stunning or hibernation. Myocardial stunning represents postischemic dysfunction that persists despite restoration of normal blood flow. Hibernating myocardial segments have persistently impaired function at rest owing to severely reduced coronary blood flow; function in these segments might be normalized by improving blood flow. Although hibernation is conceptually different from stunning, the two conditions may not differ much clinically. Repetitive episodes of myocardial stunning can occur in areas of viable myocardium subtended by a critical coronary stenosis. Such episodes can recapitulate the hibernation phenotype, blurring the distinction between myocardial stunning and hibernation. Regardless of the degree of overlap, the therapeutic implications make distinguishing the two conditions vital in patients with cardiogenic shock. The contractile function of hibernating myocardium improves with revascularization, whereas stunned myocardium retains inotropic reserve and can respond to inotropic stimulation. In addition, the severity of the antecedent ischemic insult determines the intensity of stunning, providing a rationale for reestablishing the patency of occluded coronary arteries in patients with cardiogenic shock. Finally, the notion that some myocardial tissue may recover function emphasizes the importance of measures to support the patient hemodynamically and minimize myocardial necrosis in patients with shock.

CLINICAL MANIFESTATIONS

The physical examination should be geared toward evaluating congestion and systemic perfusion to characterize the patient's hemodynamic profile (Table 107-3). An assessment of whether the patient is "wet" or "dry" and "cold" or "warm" is integral to management. Signs of congestion (Chapter 58) include jugular venous distention (see Fig. 50-3 in Chapter 50) and pulmonary rales

TABLE 107-3	CLINICAL SIGNS OF VOLUME STATUS AND PERFUSION

SIGNS AND SYMPTOMS OF CONGESTION

Orthopnea, paroxysmal nocturnal dyspnea
Jugular venous distention
Abdominojugular reflux
Rales
Hepatomegaly
Edema
Right upper quadrant tenderness

POSSIBLE EVIDENCE OF LOW PERFUSION

Narrow pulse pressure
Obtundation
Cool extremities
Cachexia, muscle loss
Decreased exercise tolerance
Renal/hepatic dysfunction
Hypotension with angiotensin-converting enzyme inhibition

and may include peripheral edema and ascites. Whether the patient is "cold" or "warm" is an indication of systemic perfusion.

The majority of the cardiogenic shock patients present "wet" and "cold." Patients with shock are usually ashen or cyanotic, and they have cool skin and mottled extremities. Cerebral hypoperfusion may cloud the sensorium. Pulses, which are rapid and faint, may be irregular in the presence of arrhythmias. Jugular venous distention and pulmonary rales are usually present, although their absence does not exclude the diagnosis. A precordial heave resulting from LV dyskinesis may be palpable. The heart sounds may be distant, and third and/or fourth heart sounds are usually present. A systolic murmur of mitral regurgitation or a ventricular septal defect may be heard, but either complication can occur without an audible murmur (Chapter 73).

DIAGNOSIS

After recognizing the clinical manifestations of apparent cardiogenic shock, the clinician must confirm its presence and assess its cause while simultaneously initiating supportive therapy before there is irreversible damage to vital organs. The clinician must balance overzealous pursuit of an etiologic diagnosis before achieving stabilization with overzealous empirical treatment without establishing the underlying pathophysiology.

An electrocardiogram (ECG) should be performed immediately. In cardiogenic shock caused by acute MI, the ECG most commonly shows ST elevation, but ST depression or nonspecific changes are found in 25% of cases. If RV infarction is suspected, ST elevation in modified right-sided leads may be diagnostic (Chapter 73). The ECG may also provide information on previous MIs and rhythm abnormalities. A relatively normal ECG or one showing only diffuse, nonspecific changes in a patient with clinical cardiogenic shock should suggest myocarditis (Chapter 60), especially if the patient has arrhythmias. In end-stage heart failure, the ECG may show Q waves and/or bundle branch block, indicative of extensive disease.

Other initial diagnostic tests include a chest radiograph, complete blood count, and measurement of arterial blood gases, electrolytes, and cardiac biomarkers. A high-quality chest film can assess signs of pulmonary edema and is helpful when signs suggest an alternative diagnosis, such as a widened mediastinum indicative of aortic dissection (Chapter 78).

Echocardiography

Echocardiography should be performed as early as possible, preferably with color flow Doppler, to provide an expeditious assessment of cardiac chamber size, LV and RV function, valvular structure and motion, atrial size, and the pericardium (Chapter 55). Echocardiography can also assess or diagnose overall and regional systolic function, diastolic function, papillary muscle rupture, acute ventricular septal defect, free wall rupture, degree of mitral regurgitation, presence of RV infarction, cardiac tamponade, and valvular stenosis.

Right Heart Catheterization

If the history, physical examination, chest radiograph, and echocardiogram demonstrate systemic hypoperfusion, low cardiac output, and elevation of venous pressures, right heart catheterization may not be necessary for diagnosis. However, therapy with vasopressors and inotropic agents is best optimized using hemodynamic measurements. Right heart catheterization can exclude other causes of shock such as volume depletion and sepsis, and it helps diagnose mechanical complications. A step-up in oxygen saturation between the right atrium and pulmonary artery can indicate a ventricular septal defect (Chapter 69), and large "V" waves in the PCWP waveform can reflect acute severe mitral regurgitation. RV infarction should be suspected when the PCWP is normal but right-sided filling pressures are notably elevated.

Right heart catheterization is most useful, however, to optimize therapy in unstable patients. In such patients, clinical estimates of filling pressures can be unreliable, and changes in myocardial performance or therapeutic interventions can change cardiac output and filling pressures precipitously. Although patients with a low cardiac index (<2.2 L/minute/m^2) and a PCWP greater than 18 mm Hg meet the definition of cardiogenic shock, optimal filling pressures may be even higher in individual patients with LV diastolic dysfunction.

TREATMENT   Rx

Initial Management

Initial stabilization of the patient with suspected cardiogenic shock consists of venous access, supplemental oxygen, and continuous ECG monitoring (Fig. 107-2). Many patients require endotracheal intubation and mechanical ventilation (Chapter 105), if only to reduce the work of breathing and facilitate sedation and stabilization before cardiac catheterization. Electrolyte abnormalities should be corrected. Morphine (1 to 2 mg every 5 minutes) relieves pain and anxiety, reduces excessive sympathetic activity, and decreases oxygen demand, preload, and afterload. Atrial bradyarrhythmias or tachyarrhythmias (Chapter 64) or ventricular tachyarrhythmias can reduce

cardiac output and should be corrected promptly with antiarrhythmic drugs (see Table 64-7 in Chapter 64), cardioversion, or pacing (Chapter 66).

If the cause is likely an acute MI, aspirin and heparin should be given immediately (Chapter 73). Some therapies routinely used in acute MI (e.g., nitrates, β-blockers, angiotensin-converting enzyme inhibitors) have the potential to exacerbate hypotension in cardiogenic shock and should be avoided in patients with a tenuous hemodynamic status until they stabilize.

An initial assessment of fluid status and systemic perfusion should be performed. Patients are commonly diaphoretic, and relative hypovolemia may be present. Ischemia produces diastolic dysfunction, so high filling pressures may be necessary to maintain stroke volume in some patients. Some patients may benefit from judicious fluid replacement with predetermined rapid infusions of 100 to 200 mL of normal saline titrated to clinical end points. Patients who do not respond rapidly to initial treatment should be considered for invasive hemodynamic monitoring to identify the filling pressure at which cardiac output is maximized. Maintenance of adequate preload is particularly important in patients with RV infarction.

Following initial stabilization and restoration of adequate blood pressure, tissue perfusion should be assessed. If tissue perfusion is adequate but significant pulmonary congestion remains, low-dose diuretics may be used, taking care not to remove too much fluid. If tissue perfusion remains inadequate, inotropic support or an intra-aortic balloon pump (IABP) should be initiated.

Vasopressors and Inotropes

Maintenance of adequate blood pressure is essential to break the vicious circle of progressive hypotension and further myocardial ischemia. When arterial pressure remains inadequate, therapy with vasopressor agents, titrated not only to blood pressure but also to clinical indices of perfusion and mixed venous oxygen saturation, may be required. Norepinephrine and dopamine are considered first-line drugs for hypotension in this situation. Dopamine acts as both an inotrope (particularly at 3 to 10 µg/kg/minute) and a vasopressor (10 to 20 µg/kg/minute). Norepinephrine (0.02 to 1.0 µg/kg/minute) acts primarily as a vasoconstrictor, has a mild inotropic effect, and increases

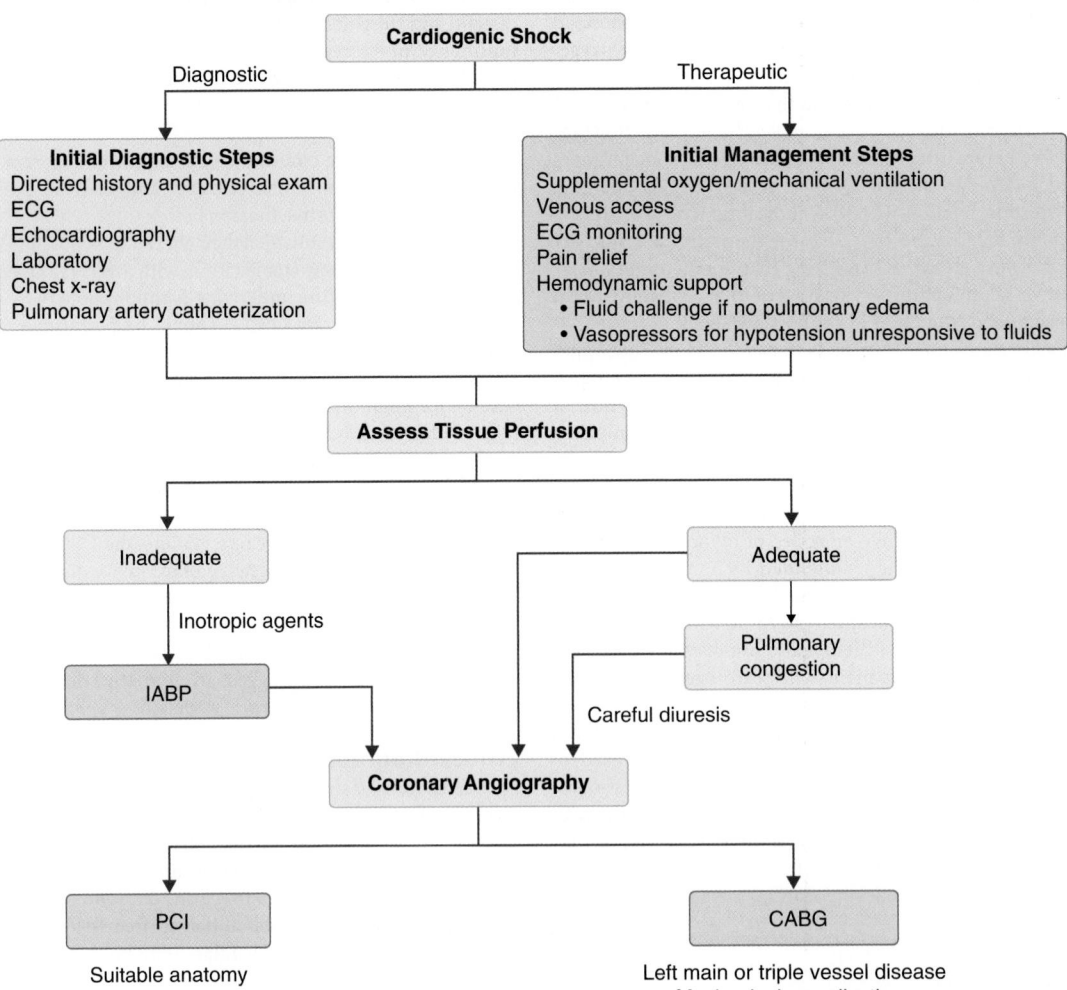

FIGURE 107-2. Approach to the diagnosis and treatment of cardiogenic shock caused by myocardial infarction. Right ventricular infarction and mechanical complications are discussed in the text. CABG = coronary artery bypass graft; ECG = electrocardiogram; IABP = intra-aortic balloon pump; PCI = percutaneous coronary intervention. Adapted from Hochman JS, Boland J, Sleeper LA, et al. Current spectrum of cardiogenic shock and effect of early revascularization on mortality: results of an International Registry. SHOCK Registry Investigators. *Circulation.* 1995;91:873-881.

coronary flow. In a randomized trial of patients with shock, there was no significant difference overall in 28-day mortality between those receiving dopamine and those receiving norepinephrine, but norepinephrine reduced mortality in a prespecified subgroup of patients with cardiogenic shock.[1] Vasopressor infusions need to be titrated carefully in patients with cardiogenic shock to maximize coronary perfusion pressure with the least possible increase in myocardial oxygen demand. Invasive hemodynamic monitoring with an arterial line and right heart catheterization are advisable during the initial titration of vasoactive agents.

If tissue perfusion remains inadequate despite norepinephrine, inotropic therapy should be initiated. Dobutamine (2.5 to 20 μg/kg/minute), a selective β₁-adrenergic receptor agonist, can improve myocardial contractility and increase cardiac output, and it is the initial agent of choice in patients with a low-output syndrome and systolic blood pressures greater than 90 mm Hg. Dobutamine may exacerbate hypotension in some patients owing to its vasodilatory effects, and it can precipitate tachyarrhythmias. Milrinone (0.125 to 0.75 μg/kg/minute), a phosphodiesterase inhibitor, has fewer chronotropic and arrhythmogenic effects than catecholamines, but it has a long half-life and can cause hypotension; in patients whose clinical status is tenuous, it is usually reserved for situations in which other agents have proved ineffective. Levosimendan (0.05 to 0.2 μg/kg/minute) is a calcium sensitizer that has both inotropic and vasodilatory properties and does not increase myocardial oxygen consumption. Levosimendan is more effective than dobutamine in treating low-output heart failure,[2] but it may cause hypotension, and it must be used with caution in patients with cardiogenic shock. Attempts to inhibit nitric oxide synthase have not been beneficial.

Intra-aortic Balloon Counterpulsation

An IABP reduces systolic afterload and augments diastolic perfusion pressure. In contrast to the effects of inotropic or vasopressor agents, these benefits occur without an increase in oxygen demand. IABPs do not, however, produce a significant improvement in blood flow distal to a critical coronary stenosis; thus, they act as a bridge, helping patients through a critical period of shock, but they are not definitive therapy.

An IABP should be used for MI patients when cardiogenic shock is not quickly reversed with pharmacologic therapy. Although it has not been shown to improve mortality when used alone, use of an IABP in cardiogenic shock complicating acute MI improves survival at 30 days and 1 year,[3] suggesting its efficacy as a stabilizing measure before angiography and prompt revascularization in appropriately selected patients.

Reperfusion

Supportive therapy may improve blood pressure and cardiac output in cardiogenic shock, but it does not interrupt the vicious circle of myocardial dysfunction and ischemia. Rapid restoration of myocardial blood flow is the cornerstone of therapy for patients with cardiogenic shock due to MI (Chapter 73). Fibrinolytic therapy (see Table 73-5 in Chapter 73) restores patency of the infarcted artery and decreases the likelihood of progression to cardiogenic shock. After cardiogenic shock has already developed, however, fibrinolytic therapy is less effective at achieving and maintaining reperfusion, likely due to a combination of hemodynamic, mechanical, and metabolic factors that prevent the achievement and maintenance of patency in the infarct-related artery.

Prompt revascularization is the only intervention that consistently reduces mortality rates in patients with cardiogenic shock. In a randomized trial of patients with LV failure complicating ST elevation MI, cardiac catheterization with PCI or CABG within 48 hours of presentation reduced all-cause mortality marginally at 30 days (47% in the revascularization group vs. 56% in the medical therapy group; P = 11) and significantly at 6 months, 1 year,[4] and 6 years[5] compared with optimal medical management, including IABP, in 86% of patients. Subgroup analyses also revealed benefits in patients younger than 75 years, those with prior MI, and those randomized less than 6 hours from the onset of infarction. Another trial with a similar design was terminated early owing to difficulties in patient recruitment, but it also showed a trend toward reduced 30-day and 1-year mortality. Together, these trials suggest that for each 100 patients treated, 9 lives will be saved at 30 days and 13.2 lives will be saved at 1 year.

On the basis of these results, emergent coronary revascularization, most often with PCI and stents, is the standard of care for cardiogenic shock due to pump failure in acute MI. Outcomes are best when PCI is performed within 6 hours after the onset of symptoms, but survival benefits are still demonstrable up to 48 hours after the onset of MI and 18 hours after the onset of shock. Elderly patients who are suitable for aggressive therapy also appear to benefit.

CABG surgery is more likely to provide complete revascularization and achieves long-term survival rates comparable to PCI, often despite worse coronary anatomy and a higher prevalence of diabetes. In practice, however, emergency CABG is performed less than 10% of the time.

When cardiogenic shock results from mechanical complications of MI (Chapter 73), surgery is recommended when feasible. For acute mitral regurgitation owing to papillary muscle rupture, supportive therapy with an IABP and vasoactive agents is a temporizing measure; definitive therapy requires expeditious surgical valve repair or replacement (Chapter 75). Although

mortality is 20 to 40%, survival and ventricular function are improved compared with medical therapy.

Timely surgery is also critical in patients whose cardiogenic shock is caused by ventricular septal or free wall rupture. Because perforations are exposed to shear forces, the rupture site can expand abruptly. Repair can be technically difficult owing to the need to suture in areas of necrosis. Surgical mortality is 20 to 50% and is especially high for serpiginous inferoposterior ruptures, which are typically less well circumscribed than anteroapical ruptures. RV function is an important determinant of outcome in this setting. Timing of surgery has been controversial, but guidelines now recommend that operative repair be undertaken early, within 48 hours of the rupture. Placement of a septal occluding device may be helpful in selected patients.

Circulatory Support

Mechanical support with a left ventricular assist device (LVAD; Chapter 73) can interrupt the downward spiral of myocardial dysfunction, hypoperfusion, and ischemia in cardiogenic shock, allowing time for stunned or hibernating myocardium to recover. In cardiogenic shock after acute MI, percutaneous LVADs can be placed in the catheterization laboratory. These devices provide short-term support and are usually intended as a bridge to recovery or, occasionally, as a bridge to transplantation. Extracorporeal support has been used in selected patients.

Management of Special Conditions

At the end stage of a dilated or restrictive cardiomyopathy (Chapter 60), low cardiac output can result in cardiogenic shock. A search for reversible precipitating causes should be undertaken. Some patients will respond to inotropic therapy and will have a brief period of relative improvement. Appropriate candidates should be referred for evaluation for possible cardiac transplantation (Chapter 82). In selected patients, a surgically placed LVAD, such as a continuous-flow device, can provide 45% two-year survival free of device surgery or disabling stroke.[6] LVADs can be used either as a bridge to transplantation or as destination therapy. A discussion about end-of-life care is also warranted.

Acute myocarditis (Chapter 60) can have a fulminant course leading to shock in 10 to 15% of cases. Patients with acute myocarditis are typically younger than those with cardiogenic shock due to MI, and they present more commonly with dyspnea rather than chest pain. Echocardiography usually shows global LV dysfunction. Supportive therapy is indicated; some patients may require circulatory support and even consideration of cardiac transplantation. Immunosuppressive therapy does not improve outcome in this setting.

Patients with hypertrophic cardiomyopathy (Chapter 60) may present with severe outflow tract obstruction and shock. Recognition of this condition is important, because diuretic and inotropic therapy may worsen the obstruction. Careful volume resuscitation and use of a pure α-agonist, such as phenylephrine (0.1 to 0.3 mg/kg/minute), can increase afterload and cavity size. β-Blockers (esmolol 0.05 to 0.2 mg/kg/minute; metoprolol 2.5 to 5 mg IV every 2 to 5 minutes, up to 15 mg) and/or calcium blockers with negative inotropic properties (e.g., diltiazem 5 mg IV every 2 minutes, up to 20 mg) can also be helpful.

Some patients with stress (takotsubo) cardiomyopathy (Chapter 60) may have LV dysfunction severe enough to produce shock. Because the presentation is similar to that of acute MI, with chest pain and ECG changes, the diagnosis is usually made in the catheterization laboratory, when significant coronary obstruction is excluded and the characteristic apical hypokinesis or dyskinesis is documented. Treatment is supportive and may include an IABP. Most patients have recovery of LV function within days to weeks, and the long-term prognosis is excellent.

Acute valvular regurgitation (Chapter 75) presents with pulmonary edema and decreased forward cardiac output. The regurgitant murmur may be soft or inaudible, and the diagnosis is best made by echocardiography. Acute ischemic mitral regurgitation is usually associated with rupture of the posterior papillary muscle, which has a single blood supply. Other causes include spontaneous chordal rupture, infective endocarditis (Chapter 76), rheumatic fever (Chapter 298), and trauma (Chapter 112). Immediate management includes afterload reduction (Chapter 59) and an IABP as temporizing measures. Inotropic or vasopressor therapy may also be needed to support cardiac output and blood pressure. Definitive therapy, however, consists of surgical valve repair or replacement (Chapter 75).

Acute aortic regurgitation most commonly results from infective endocarditis (Chapter 76) with leaflet destruction, but it may also be due to traumatic injury (Chapter 112) or acute aortic dissection (Chapter 78). The pulse pressure is usually narrow, indicating decreased forward stroke volume, and the bounding pulsations seen with chronic aortic regurgitation are usually absent. Temporizing measures include afterload reduction, with vasopressor and inotropic support as needed. IABP is contraindicated, and excessive slowing of the heart rate may worsen hemodynamics by prolonging diastole. Definitive therapy is surgical.

PROGNOSIS

Cardiogenic shock is still the most common cause of death in acute MI. Survival rates are improving, however, coincident with the increasing use of reperfusion therapy in appropriately selected patients. Hemodynamics predict short-term but not long-term mortality. Among patients undergoing revascularization, age, time to revascularization, and restoration of coronary blood flow independently predict survival, but the benefits of revascularization are seen at every level of risk, with an average 1-year survival of 50 to 55%. Encouragingly, the survival benefit of early revascularization is maintained at 6-year follow-up, with 5-year survival approaching 45%. The quality of life in survivors is usually excellent, with 83% either asymptomatic or having only mildly symptomatic heart failure. For patients with end-stage nonischemic myocardial disease, the prognosis is very poor in the absence of heart transplantation.

1. De Backer D, Biston P, Devriendt J, et al. Comparison of dopamine and norepinephrine in the treatment of shock. *N Engl J Med*. 2010;362:779-789.
2. Follath F, Cleland JGF, Just H, et al. Efficacy and safety of intravenous levosimendan compared with dobutamine in severe low-output heart failure (the LIDO study): a randomised double-blind trial. *Lancet*. 2002;360:196-202.
3. Stone GW, Marsalese D, Brodie BR, et al. A prospective, randomized evaluation of prophylactic intra-aortic balloon counterpulsation in high-risk patients with acute myocardial infarction treated with primary angioplasty: Second Primary Angioplasty in Myocardial Infarction (PAMI-II) Trial Investigators. *J Am Coll Cardiol*. 1997;29:1459-1467.
4. Hochman JS, Sleeper LA, White HD, et al. One-year survival following early revascularization for cardiogenic shock. *JAMA*. 2001;285:190-192.
5. Hochman JS, Sleeper LA, Webb JG, et al. Early revascularization and long-term survival in cardiogenic shock complicating acute myocardial infarction. *JAMA*. 2006;295:2511-2515.
6. Slaughter MS, Rogers JG, Milano CA, et al. Advanced heart failure treated with continuous-flow left ventricular assist device. *N Engl J Med*. 2009;361:2241-2251.

SUGGESTED READINGS

Goldstein D, Neragi-Miandoab S. Mechanical bridge to decision: what are the options for the management of acute refractory cardiogenic shock? *Curr Heart Fail Rep*. 2011;8:51-58. *Review*.
Sarswat N, Hollenberg SM. Cardiogenic shock. *Hosp Pract (Minneap)*. 2010;38:74-83. *Review*.

108

SHOCK SYNDROMES RELATED TO SEPSIS

JAMES A. RUSSELL

DEFINITION

Sepsis is defined by presence of at least two of the four signs of the systemic inflammatory response syndrome (SIRS): (1) fever (>38°C) or hypothermia (<36°C); (2) tachycardia (>90 beats/minute); (3) tachypnea (>20 breaths/minute), hypocapnia (partial pressure of carbon dioxide <32 mm Hg), or the need for mechanical ventilatory assistance; and (4) leukocytosis (>12,000 cells/mm³), leukopenia (<4000 cells/mm³), or a left shift (>0% immature band cells) in the circulating white cell differential and suspected or proven infection. *Bacteremia* is defined as the growth of bacteria in blood cultures, but infection does not have to be proved to diagnose sepsis at the onset. *Severe sepsis* is sepsis in addition to dysfunction of one or more organ systems (e.g., hypoxemia, oliguria, lactic acidosis, thrombocytopenia, decreased Glasgow Coma Scale score). *Septic shock* is defined as severe sepsis in addition to hypotension (systolic blood pressure <90 mm Hg or a >40 mm Hg decrease from baseline) despite adequate fluid resuscitation.

EPIDEMIOLOGY

Approximately 750,000 cases of severe sepsis or septic shock occur every year in the United States. Sepsis causes as many deaths as acute myocardial infarction, and septic shock and its complications are the most common causes of death in noncoronary intensive care units (ICUs). The medical care costs associated with sepsis are approximately $16.7 billion a year in the United States alone. The frequency of septic shock is increasing as physicians perform more aggressive surgery, as more resistant organisms are present in the environment, and as the prevalence of immune compromise resulting from disease and immunosuppressive drugs increases. Recent studies suggest that African Americans have a higher incidence of severe sepsis than whites (6.0 vs. 3.6 per 1000 population) and a higher mortality in ICUs (32.1 vs. 29.3%; *P* < .0001), even after adjusting for poverty levels. The mechanisms of this apparent difference in risk for and mortality from sepsis are not known.

Gram-positive or gram-negative bacteria, fungi, and, very rarely, protozoa or rickettsiae can cause septic shock. Increasingly common causes of septic shock are gram-positive bacteria, especially methicillin-resistant *Staphylococcus aureus*, vancomycin-resistant enterococci, penicillin-resistant *Streptococcus pneumoniae*, and resistant gram-negative bacilli.

The common infections causing septic shock are pneumonia, peritonitis, pyelonephritis, abscess (especially intra-abdominal), primary bacteremia, cholangitis, cellulitis, necrotizing fasciitis, and meningitis. Nosocomial pneumonia is the most common cause of death from nosocomial infection.

PATHOBIOLOGY

At onset, septic shock activates inflammation, leading to enhanced coagulation, activated platelets, increased neutrophils and mononuclear cells, and diminished fibrinolysis (Table 108-1). After several days, a compensatory anti-inflammatory response with immunosuppression may contribute to death. Several pathways amplify one another: inflammation triggers coagulation, and coagulation triggers inflammation, resulting in a positive feedback loop that is pro-inflammatory and pro-coagulant. Tissue hypoxia in septic shock also amplifies inflammation and coagulation. Many mediators that are critical for the homeostatic control of infection may be injurious to the host (e.g., tumor necrosis factor-α [TNF-α]), so therapies that fully neutralize such mediators are largely ineffective.

Widespread endothelial injury is an important feature of septic shock; an injured endothelium is more permeable, so the flux of protein-rich edema fluid into tissues such as the lung increases. Injured endothelial cells release nitric oxide, a potent vasodilator that is a key mediator of septic shock. Septic shock also injures epithelial cells of the lung and intestine. Intestinal epithelial injury increases intestinal permeability; this leads to epithelial translocation of intestinal bacteria and endotoxin, which further augments the inflammatory phenotype of septic shock.

Early Infection, the Innate Immune Response, Inflammation, and the Endothelium

Host defense is organized into innate and adaptive immune responses. The innate immune system responds by using pattern recognition receptors (e.g., Toll-like receptors [TLRs]) to pathogen-associated molecular patterns, which are extremely well-conserved molecules of microorganisms. Surface molecules of gram-positive and gram-negative bacteria (peptidoglycan and lipopolysaccharide, respectively) bind to TLR-2 and TLR-4, respectively (Fig. 108-1). TLR-2 and TLR-4 binding initiates an intracellular signaling cascade that culminates in nuclear transport of the transcription factor nuclear factor kappa B (NFκB), which triggers transcription of cytokines such as TNF-α and interleukin (IL)-6. Cytokines upregulate adhesion molecules of neutrophils and endothelial cells, and neutrophil activation leads to bacterial killing. However, cytokines also directly injure host endothelial cells, as do activated neutrophils, monocytes, and platelets. Inhibition of early cytokine mediators of sepsis, such as TNF-α and IL-1β, has not proved successful, likely because TNF-α and IL-1β peak and then decline quickly, before these antagonist therapies can be applied clinically.

After the early cytokine inflammatory response, immune cells, including macrophages and neutrophils, release later mediators, such as high-mobility group box-1 (HMGB-1). HMGB-1 activates neutrophils, monocytes, and endothelium. Unlike TNF-α antagonists, inhibitors of HMGB-1 decrease mortality even when they are given 24 hours after the induction of experimental peritonitis.

Adaptive Immunity Adds Specificity and Amplifies the Immune Response

Microorganisms stimulate specific humoral and cell-mediated adaptive immune responses that amplify innate immunity. B cells release immunoglobulins that bind to microorganisms and thereby facilitate delivery of microorganisms to natural killer cells and neutrophils. In sepsis, type 1 helper T (T$_H$1) cells generally secrete pro-inflammatory cytokines (TNF-α, IL-1β),

TABLE 108-1 PATHWAYS; MEDIATORS; AND POSITIVE, NEGATIVE, AND POTENTIALLY ATTRACTIVE TRIALS IN SEPTIC SHOCK

PATHWAYS	MEDIATORS	POSITIVE RCTs*	NEGATIVE RCTs	EXAMPLES OF POTENTIAL THERAPIES
Organism features	Superantigens: TSST-1 Streptococcal exotoxins (pyrogenic exotoxin A) Lipopolysaccharide (endotoxin)		Anti-lipopolysaccharide	Anti-TSST1 Polymyxin B hemoperfusion† Anti-exotoxins
Innate immunity	TLR-2, TLR-4 Monocytes, macrophages Neutrophils			TLR agonists; TLR antagonists GM-CSF, interferon-γ G-CSF‡
Adaptive immunity	B cells, plasma cells, immunoglobulin T cells: CD4, T_H1, T_H2			Immunoglobulin G
Pro-inflammatory pathway	TNF-α IL-1β IL-6 Prostaglandins, leukotrienes Bradykinin Platelet-activating factor Proteases (e.g., elastase) Oxidants Nitric oxide		Anti–TNF-α IL-1 receptor antagonist Ibuprofen, high-dose corticosteroids Bradykinin antagonist Platelet-activating factor acetylhydrolase Elastase inhibitor§ Nitric oxide synthase inhibitor	IL-6 antagonist Antioxidants (e.g., N-acetylcysteine)
Pro-coagulant pathway	↓ Protein C ↓ Protein S ↓ Antithrombin ↓ Tissue factor pathway inhibitor ↑ Tissue factor ↑ Plasminogen activator inhibitor (PAI-1)	Activated protein C [14]	Antithrombin Tissue factor pathway inhibitor Heparin‖	Protein S Tissue factor antagonist Tissue plasminogen activator
Anti-inflammatory pathway	IL-10 TNF-α receptors		IL-10¶ TNF-α receptors	
Tissue hypoxia	HIF-1α, VEGF	Early goal-directed therapy [3]	Supernormal oxygen delivery Epinephrine, norepinephrine, dobutamine††	Erythropoietin**
Immunosuppression/apoptosis	Lymphocyte apoptosis Intestinal epithelial cell apoptosis			Anti-caspases Anti-caspases
Endocrine dysfunction	Adrenal insufficiency Vasopressin deficiency Hyperglycemia		Corticosteroids‡‡	Corticosteroids§§ Vasopressin‖‖ Intensive insulin¶¶
Renal dysfunction	Metabolites with renal clearance		Intensive renal support***	

*Positive RCTs are pivotal randomized controlled trials powered for mortality as the primary end point.
†In a small RCT, polymyxin B hemoperfusion decreased mortality compared with usual care.
‡G-CSF is effective in septic patients with profound neutropenia.
§Elastase inhibitor was ineffective in a phase II trial in acute lung injury.
‖Unfractionated heparin did not decrease mortality in acute sepsis.
¶IL-10 was ineffective in a phase II trial in acute lung injury.
**Erythropoietin does not decrease red blood cell transfusions in the critically ill and may increase the risk of thrombotic events.
††In an RCT of norepinephrine plus dobutamine versus epinephrine alone, there was no difference in mortality.
‡‡In a randomized placebo-controlled trial, corticosteroids did not change mortality in septic shock, regardless of whether there was an abnormal corticotropin stimulation test.
§§Corticosteroids, which have no effect on overall 28-day mortality, decreased mortality in a subgroup of nonresponders to corticotropin in one study [12] but not another. [2]
‖‖In an RCT, vasopressin compared with norepinephrine did not change overall mortality, but it was associated with decreased mortality in patients who had less severe septic shock (norepinephrine infusion 5-15 μg/min).
¶¶Intensive insulin (compared with conventional insulin) did not change mortality in one RCT and increased mortality in another.
***In an RCT, intensive renal support (six times/wk) compared with conventional renal support (three times/wk) did not change mortality in critically ill patients with acute kidney injury (many of whom had sepsis).
↑ = increased; ↓ = decreased; G-CSF = granulocyte colony-stimulating factor; GM-CSF = granulocyte-macrophage colony-stimulating factor; HIF-1α: hypoxia-inducing factor-1α; IL = interleukin; RCT = randomized controlled trial; T_H1 and T_H2 = type 1 and 2 helper T cell, respectively; TNF-α = tumor necrosis factor-α; TLR = Toll-like receptor; TSST-1 = toxic shock syndrome toxin-1; VEGF = vascular endothelial growth factor.

and type 2 helper T (T_H2) cells secrete anti-inflammatory cytokines (IL-4, IL-10).

Coagulation Response to Infection

Septic shock activates the coagulation system (Fig. 108-2) and ultimately converts fibrinogen to fibrin, which is bound to platelets to form microvascular thrombi. Microvascular thrombi further amplify endothelial injury by the release of mediators and by tissue hypoxia because of obstruction to blood flow.

Normally, natural anticoagulants (protein C, protein S, antithrombin, and tissue factor pathway inhibitor) dampen coagulation, enhance fibrinolysis, and remove microthrombi. Thrombin-α binds to thrombomodulin, which activates protein C when protein C is bound to the endothelial protein C receptor (EPCR). Activated protein C dampens the pro-coagulant phenotype

because it inactivates factors Va and VIIIa and inhibits the synthesis of plasminogen activator inhibitor-1 (PAI-1). Activated protein C also decreases apoptosis, leukocyte activation and adhesion, and the production of cytokines.

Septic shock decreases the levels of the natural anticoagulants protein C, protein S, antithrombin, and tissue factor pathway inhibitor. Furthermore, lipopolysaccharide and TNF-α decrease thrombomodulin and EPCR, thereby limiting the activation of protein C. Lipopolysaccharide and TNF-α also increase levels of PAI-1, inhibiting fibrinolysis.

Tissue Hypoxia in Septic Shock

Tissue hypoxia independently activates inflammation (by activation of NFκB and cytokines, synthesis of nitric oxide, and activation of HMGB-1), induces coagulation (through tissue factor and PAI-1), and activates neutrophils,

FIGURE 108-1. Inflammatory responses to sepsis. Gram-positive and gram-negative bacteria, viruses, and fungi have unique cell wall molecules called pathogen-associated molecular patterns that bind to pattern recognition receptors (called Toll-like receptors [TLRs]) on the surface of immune cells. The lipopolysaccharide (LPS) of gram-negative bacilli binds to LPS-binding protein–CD14 complex. The peptidoglycan of gram-positive bacteria and the LPS of gram-negative bacteria bind to TLR-2 and TLR-4, respectively. TLR-2 and TLR-4 binding activates intracellular signal transduction pathways that lead to the activation of the cytosolic transcription factor nuclear factor kappa B (NFκB). Activated NFκB moves from the cytoplasm to the nucleus, binds to transcription start sites, and increases the transcription of cytokines such as tumor necrosis factor-α (TNF-α), interleukin-1β (IL-1β), and interleukin-10 (IL-10). TNF-α and IL-1β are pro-inflammatory cytokines that activate the adaptive immune response but also cause both direct and indirect host injury. IL-10 is an anti-inflammatory cytokine that inactivates macrophages and has other anti-inflammatory effects. Sepsis increases the activity of inducible nitric oxide synthase (iNOS), which increases the synthesis of nitric oxide (NO), a potent vasodilator. Cytokines activate endothelial cells by upregulating adhesion receptors such as intercellular adhesion molecule (ICAM), and they injure endothelial cells by the activation and binding of neutrophils, monocytes, macrophages, and platelets to endothelial cells. These effector cells release mediators such as proteases, oxidants, prostaglandins, and ICAM leukotrienes. Cytokines also activate the coagulation cascade.

FIGURE 108-2. Pro-coagulant response in sepsis. Sepsis initiates coagulation by activating the endothelium to increase tissue factor. Activation of factors Va and VIIIa leads to the formation of thrombin-α, which converts fibrinogen to fibrin. Fibrin binds to platelets that adhere to endothelial cells, forming microvascular thrombi. Microvascular thrombi amplify injury by the release of mediators and by microvascular obstruction, which causes distal ischemia and tissue hypoxia. Normally, natural anticoagulants—protein C (PC), protein S (PS), antithrombin, and tissue factor pathway inhibitor (TFPI)—dampen coagulation, enhance fibrinolysis, and remove microthrombi. Thrombin-α binds to thrombomodulin on endothelial cells and thus activates the binding of PC to endothelial PC receptor (EPCR). PC forms a complex with its cofactor PS. PC binding to EPCR increases the activation of PC to activated PC (APC). APC proteolytically inactivates factors Va and VIIIa and decreases the synthesis of plasminogen activator inhibitor-1 (PAI-1). Sepsis decreases levels of PC, PS, antithrombin, and TFPI. Lipopolysaccharide and tumor necrosis factor-α (TNF-α) decrease thrombomodulin and EPCR, thus decreasing the activation of PC. Lipopolysaccharide and TNF-α also inhibit PAI-1, so fibrinolysis is inhibited. HIFα = hypoxia-inducing factor-α; NO = nitric oxide; tPA = tissue plasminogen activator; VEGF = vascular endothelial growth factor.

monocytes, and platelets. Hypoxia induces hypoxia-inducing factor-1α (HIF-1α), which upregulates erythropoietin, and vascular endothelial growth factor (VEGF). Erythropoietin is protective to brain and other tissues. VEGF inhibits fibrinolysis and increases inducible nitric oxide synthase, which augments nitric oxide–induced vasodilation. Nitric oxide has a further injurious effect: excessive nitric oxide inhibits the beneficial actions of HIF-1α (e.g., upregulating synthesis of erythropoietin) during hypoxia.

Late Septic Shock, Immunosuppression, and Apoptosis of Immune and Epithelial Cells

After about 1 week of septic shock, death can result from immunosuppression, which is suggested by anergy, lymphopenia, hypothermia, and nosocomial infection. Multiple organ dysfunction may be an anti-inflammatory

phenotype because of the apoptosis of immune, epithelial, and endothelial cells. Activated CD4+ T cells evolve into either a T$_H$1 pro-inflammatory (TNF-α, IL-1β) or a T$_H$2 anti-inflammatory (IL-4, IL-10) phenotype. Sepsis leads to migration from a T$_H$1 to a T$_H$2 phenotype; for example, persistent elevation of IL-10 is associated with an increased risk of death. Immunosuppression also develops because of apoptosis of lymphocytes. Pro-inflammatory cytokines, activated B and T cells, and glucocorticoids induce lymphocyte apoptosis, whereas TNF-α and endotoxin induce apoptosis of lung and intestinal epithelial cells. The fact that glucocorticoids also stimulate apoptosis could be the biologic explanation for the observation that patients with septic shock who are treated with hydrocortisone have more superinfections than do patients treated with placebo. ∎

Death from infectious disease appears to be highly heritable. Sepsis is a prime example of a polygenic disease related to the interaction of multiple

TABLE 108-2 HEMODYNAMIC VARIABLES, ABBREVIATIONS, AND NORMAL VALUES

Arterial pressure: systolic pressure (SAP) (>100 mm Hg), diastolic pressure, pulse pressure, mean arterial pressure (MAP) (>65 mm Hg)

Central venous pressure (CVP): normal 6-12 mm Hg

Pulmonary artery pressure (PAP): normal 25/15 mm Hg

Pulmonary vascular resistance (PVR): normal 150-250 dynes/sec/cm

$$\left(\equiv \frac{PAP - PAOP}{CO} \times 80\right)$$

Pulmonary artery occlusion pressure (PAOP) or pulmonary artery wedge pressure (PAWP): normal 8-15 mm Hg

Systemic vascular resistance (SVR): normal 900-1400 dynes/sec/cm

$$\left(\equiv \frac{MAP - CVP}{CO} \times 80\right)$$

Cardiac output (CO): normal 5 L/min

Left ventricular stroke work index (LVSWI): normal (60-100 grams × meters/beats) = (SV × [MAP − PAWP] × 0.0136)

Oxygen delivery (DO_2): normal 1 L/min (= CO × [Hg × 1.38 × SaO_2] + [0.003 × PO_2])

Oxygen consumption (VO_2): normal 250 mL/min (= CO × Hg × 1.38 × [$SaO_2 - SvO_2$] + [0.003 × ($PaO_2 - PvO_2$)])

Oxygen extraction ratio: normal 0.23-0.32 (= VO_2/DO_2)

Hemodynamic variables are often normalized to account for different body mass by dividing by body surface area (BSA):

Pulmonary vascular resistance index (PVRI): normal (= PVR/BSA)

Systemic vascular resistance index (SVRI): normal (= SVR/BSA)

Cardiac index (CI): normal 2.5-4.2 L/min/m² (= CO/BSA)

Left ventricular stroke work index (LVSWI): normal (= LVSW/BSA)

Oxygen delivery index (DO_2I): normal 460-650 mL/min/m² (= DO_2/BSA)

Oxygen consumption index (VO_2I): normal 95-170 mL/min/m² (= VO_2/BSA)

---

genes and an environmental insult (infection). Single nucleotide polymorphisms of cytokines (TNF-α, IL-6, IL-10), coagulation factors (protein C, fibrinogen-β), the catecholamine pathway (β-adrenergic receptor), and innate immunity genes (CD14, TLR-1, TLR-2) have been variably associated with an increased risk of death from sepsis.

Cardiovascular Dysfunction

Inadequate tissue perfusion and tissue hypoxia are the cardinal features of all types of shock. Early in septic shock, most patients have sinus tachycardia and, by definition, decreased blood pressure (<90 mm Hg systolic, a decrease of ≥40 mm Hg from baseline systolic pressure, or mean arterial pressure <65 mm Hg; Table 108-2). Septic shock is the classic form of distributive shock (Chapter 106), characterized by increased pulse pressure (bounding pulses), decreased systemic vascular resistance (warm, flushed skin), and functional hypovolemia (low jugular venous pressure). Distributive shock means that the distribution of systemic blood flow is abnormal, such that areas of both low flow (and low venous oxygen saturation) and high flow (and increased venous oxygen saturation) are present. Nevertheless, about one third of patients with septic shock initially present with findings more typical of hypovolemic shock (low central venous pressure and low central venous oxygen saturation), because the clinical features depend on the stage and severity of septic shock as well as on the degree of fluid resuscitation that has occurred. After fluid resuscitation, patients typically develop the characteristic clinical and hemodynamic features of classic distributive shock.

Ventricular preload is commonly decreased in early septic shock, for several reasons. First, patients may be volume depleted because of decreased fluid intake and because of increased fluid losses as a result of fever, vomiting, and diarrhea if gastrointestinal disease is present. Second, fluid loss from the intravascular to the interstitial space (capillary leak) is caused by mediators that induce widespread endothelial injury, which increases capillary permeability. Increased capillary permeability leads to loss of protein-rich edema fluid into the interstitial space. In the lung, increased permeability is a key component of acute lung injury. A third reason that ventricular preload is decreased in septic shock is venodilation induced by mediators such as nitric oxide. Venodilation increases venous capacitance, leading to relative volume depletion, which compounds the absolute volume depletion. Ventricular afterload is decreased because of excessive release of potent vasodilators such as nitric oxide, prostaglandin I₂, adenosine diphosphate, and other vasodilators.

In addition to abnormal vasodilation, patients have concurrent microvascular vasoconstriction. Microvascular vasoconstriction may not be apparent

clinically or hemodynamically, but it can lead to tissue hypoxia, detected by increased arterial lactate concentrations. Microvascular vasoconstriction is caused by increased norepinephrine, thromboxanes, and other local vasoconstrictors. Microvascular vasoconstriction causes focal hypoxia, which is exacerbated by microvascular obstruction by platelets and leukocytes.

The abnormal mismatch of oxygen delivery to oxygen demand can disturb the global relationship of oxygen delivery to oxygen consumption. Normally, oxygen consumption is independent of oxygen delivery over a wide range. When oxygen delivery decreases to less than the critical oxygen delivery level, oxygen consumption decreases and leads to a state in which oxygen consumption depends on oxygen delivery. At levels lower than the critical oxygen delivery level, arterial lactate increases as a result of tissue hypoxia. The clinical implication is that oxygen delivery should be increased (e.g., by increasing cardiac output by volume resuscitation, infusion of dobutamine, or transfusion of erythrocytes) to more than the critical level.

Cardiovascular function is further compromised in septic shock because of decreased ventricular contractility. Decreased ventricular contractility may be difficult to detect clinically and may be diagnosed only by hemodynamic or echocardiographic assessment. Numerous circulating mediators of sepsis, including endotoxin, cytokines (e.g., IL-6, TNF-α), and nitric oxide (locally released into the coronary circulation), decrease contractility. Endotoxin signals via TLRs to upregulate the expression of proteins such as S110A8 and S100A9 to cause a receptor for advanced glycation end products (RAGE)–dependent decrease in calcium flux, which decreases the ejection fraction. Coronary ischemia resulting from microvascular obstruction by leukocytes and oxygen free radicals, which are released by neutrophils adherent to the coronary capillary endothelium, is another mechanism of decreased contractility.

Early in septic shock, patients who survive have increased left ventricular end-diastolic volume, which likely allows them to maintain cardiac output despite decreased contractility. In contrast, nonsurvivors do not have increased left ventricular end-diastolic volume, so their cardiac output is compromised. In some patients with septic shock, concurrent acute lung injury and secondary pulmonary hypertension increase right ventricular afterload, with a secondary shift of the interventricular septum from right to left. This septal shift decreases left ventricular end-diastolic volume and can also limit cardiac output.

CLINICAL MANIFESTATIONS

Cardiovascular dysfunction in septic shock is characterized by decreased preload (because of decreased intake, fluid losses, third spacing resulting from increased permeability, and venodilation), decreased afterload, and often decreased ventricular contractility. Decreased ventricular volume is detected clinically by low jugular venous pressure and hemodynamically by decreased central venous pressure. Left ventricular resistance, or afterload, is also commonly decreased and is detected clinically by warm, flushed skin and hemodynamically by decreased systemic vascular resistance.

DIAGNOSIS

Even as the diagnostic evaluation is beginning, the initial assessment of a critically ill patient must focus immediately on the airway (need for intubation), breathing (respiratory rate, respiratory distress, pulse oximetry), circulation (heart rate, blood pressure, jugular venous pressure, skin perfusion), and rapid initiation of resuscitation (Fig. 108-3). Vital signs and the leukocyte count quickly establish whether the patient has SIRS (two of the four criteria). Arterial blood gases and lactate levels are useful complementary tests. A secondary survey is designed to determine the likely source of infection and the status of organ function. Pneumonia (Chapter 97) is suggested by cough, sputum, and respiratory distress; empyema (Chapter 99) is suggested by pleuritic chest pain. Signs of peritonitis, an abdominal mass, and right upper quadrant tenderness suggest abdominal sepsis. Pyelonephritis (Chapter 292) is likely in patients with dysuria and costovertebral angle tenderness. Integumentary assessment for erythema (cellulitis), line site erythema (line sepsis), tenderness (necrotizing fasciitis), crepitus (anaerobic myonecrosis), and petechiae and purpura (meningococcemia) can be illuminating. Headache, stiff neck, and signs of meningismus raise the suspicion of meningitis (Chapter 420). Focal neurologic signs suggest brain abscess (Chapter 421).

Laboratory investigations that are helpful to identify the source of infection include appropriate cultures and Gram stains (blood, sputum, urine, fluids, and cerebrospinal fluid). Blood cultures are positive in 40 to 60% of patients who have septic shock. The chest radiograph aids in the diagnosis of

Clinical Evaluation	Laboratory Evaluation	Management

FIGURE 108-3. Algorithm for the clinical and laboratory evaluation and management of septic shock. ABGs = arterial blood gases; AlkPhos = alkaline phosphatase; APACHE II = Acute Physiology and Chronic Health Evaluation II; APC = activated protein C; AST = aspartate aminotransferase; BP = blood pressure; BUN = blood urea nitrogen; C&S = culture and sensitivity; CBC = complete blood count; CNS = central nervous system; CSF = cerebrospinal fluid; CT = computed tomography; CV = cardiovascular; CVP = central venous pressure; CXR = chest radiograph; Hct = hematocrit; HR = heart rate; IBW = ideal body weight; INR = international normalized ratio; JVP = jugular venous pressure; LOC = level of consciousness; MAP = mean arterial pressure; PaCO₂ = partial pressure of carbon dioxide; PTT = partial thromboplastin time; RR = respiratory rate; ScvO₂ = central venous oxygen saturation; SIRS = systemic inflammatory response syndrome; T = temperature; U/S = ultrasound; WBC = white blood cell count.

pneumonia, empyema, and acute lung injury. Abdominal ultrasound and computed tomography are indicated if abdominal sepsis is suspected.

Hemodynamic assessment of the patient includes insertion of a central venous or pulmonary artery catheter. In early septic shock, central venous pressure is usually low and increases in response to volume resuscitation. Central venous oxygen saturation, cardiac output, and ventricular filling pressures may be determined continuously. Pulmonary artery pressure is usually normal but may be increased because septic shock can cause pulmonary hypertension. Pulmonary artery occlusion (or wedge) pressure is usually low before resuscitation, but it may be normal or increased if the patient has underlying preexisting heart disease (e.g., heart failure or coronary artery disease with prior myocardial infarction) or if left ventricular contractility is decreased by sepsis. Cardiac output may be low or normal before fluid resuscitation and typically increases to higher than normal after fluid resuscitation. If fluid resuscitation increases central venous pressure and pulmonary artery occlusion pressure but cardiac output does not increase, left ventricular dysfunction is presumably present.

Echocardiographic features of decreased ventricular contractility include decreased right and left ventricular ejection fractions and increased end-diastolic and end-systolic volumes. Early in septic shock, the left ventricular ejection fraction is decreased, and it remains low in nonsurvivors. In survivors, the left ventricular ejection fraction usually returns to normal over 5 to 10 days.

Renal, hepatic, and coagulation function tests are helpful to evaluate organ function. After determining the source of sepsis, it is crucial to address that source by draining abscesses and empyemas; radiologically or surgically

correcting urinary tract obstruction; and surgically managing peritonitis, bowel infarction, cholecystitis, cholangitis, necrotizing fasciitis, and gas gangrene.

Differential Diagnosis

The major differential diagnoses of classic septic shock are other nonseptic causes of SIRS, such as acute pancreatitis (Chapter 146), acute respiratory distress syndrome (Chapter 104), aspiration pneumonitis (Chapter 94), multiple trauma (Chapter 112), and recent major surgery without infection (Chapter 441). Other causes of distributive shock are anaphylactic shock (suggested by angioedema and hives; Chapter 448), spinal shock (recent trauma and paraplegia; Chapter 406), acute adrenal insufficiency ("tanned skin," hyperkalemia, metabolic alkalosis; Chapter 234), and acute or acute-on-chronic hepatic failure (jaundice, ascites, encephalopathy; Chapter 157).

The differential diagnosis of septic shock must include the other causes of shock: hypovolemic, cardiogenic, and obstructive shock (Chapters 106 and 107). Patients with hypovolemic shock (from internal or external fluid losses, hemorrhage) present with a suggestive history and signs of hypovolemia (low jugular venous pressure) and skin hypoperfusion (cool, clammy, cyanotic extremities). Cardiogenic shock (resulting from myocardial infarction or acute-on-chronic congestive heart failure or occurring after cardiovascular surgery) is suggested by the history, signs of increased filling pressure (increased jugular venous pressure, crackles, S₃, pulmonary edema, cardiomegaly), and skin hypoperfusion (Chapter 107). Some patients who have acute myocardial infarction and cardiogenic shock have features of SIRS

TABLE 108-3 RELEVANT RANDOMIZED CONTROLLED TRIALS IN SEVERE SEPSIS, SEPTIC SHOCK, AND ACUTE LUNG INJURY

PATIENT GROUP	INTERVENTION	CONTROL	INTERVENTION MORTALITY (%)*	CONTROL MORTALITY (%)*	NNT
ALI/ARDS[†][2]	Low tidal volume (6 mL/kg)	High tidal volume (12 mL/kg)	31	40	11
Sepsis and septic shock[3]	Early goal-directed therapy	Usual therapy	33	49	6
Severe sepsis and septic shock[14]	Activated protein C	Placebo	25	31	16
Severe sepsis and septic shock at increased risk of death[‡][14]	Activated protein C	Placebo	31	44	7.7
Septic shock[12]	Hydrocortisone and fludrocortisone	Placebo	53[§]	63[§]	10

*28-day mortality.
†Many also had sepsis.
‡As defined by Acute Physiology and Chronic Health Evaluation (APACHE) II quartiles 3 and 4, APACHE II ≥ 25.
§Nonresponders to a 250-µg corticotropin stimulation test.
ALI/ARDS = acute lung injury/acute respiratory distress syndrome; NNT = number needed to treat to save one life.

without infection. Obstructive shock (from pulmonary thromboembolism, cardiac tamponade, pneumothorax) manifests similarly to cardiogenic shock.

PREVENTION

Measures to prevent sepsis include handwashing, elevation of the head of the bed, scrupulous sterile techniques for the insertion of catheters, and possibly the use of antibiotic-impregnated catheters. New catheter insertion sites for catheter changes, isolation of patients who have resistant organisms, and isolation of significantly immunocompromised patients may also prevent infection.

Preventing the progression from sepsis to septic shock requires early diagnosis and aggressive resuscitation. Early goal-directed therapy, lung-protective ventilation, antibiotics, and consideration of activated protein C are critical therapies in early septic shock (Table 108-3).

TREATMENT   Rx

Respiratory Therapy

All patients in septic shock require oxygen initially, and many require mechanical ventilation. Mechanical ventilation is required in most patients who have septic shock because acute lung injury is the most common complication. Lung-protective ventilation (mechanical ventilation that minimizes lung injury by using a relatively low tidal volume, such as <6 mL/kg of predicted body weight) decreases mortality from acute lung injury and acute respiratory distress syndrome (Chapter 105).[2]

Patients who require ventilation need adequate but not excessive sedation, which can worsen hemodynamic instability, prolong ventilation, and increase the risk of developing nosocomial pneumonia. Sedation should be titrated using objective assessment. Daily interruption of sedation decreases the duration of mechanical ventilation and intensive care. Neuromuscular blocking agents should be avoided because of the risk of prolonged neuromuscular dysfunction.

Circulatory Therapy

Early goal-directed therapy is the cornerstone of emergency management, and this approach decreases hospital, 28-day, and 60-day mortality rates dramatically (see Table 108-3).[3] In general, the goal of resuscitation is to increase tissue oxygen delivery by increasing profoundly low blood pressure, increasing inadequate blood flow, increasing low arterial oxygen saturation, and increasing mixed venous oxygen saturation. Although oxygen delivery is higher in survivors than in nonsurvivors, it is not clear that a specific oxygen delivery target is more beneficial than clinical end points. Several trials have shown that supernormal global oxygen delivery does not decrease mortality rates in sepsis and septic shock. Goal-directed therapy requires continuous monitoring of central venous oxygen saturation, with resuscitation directed to increase and then maintain central venous oxygen saturation greater than 70%.

In patients who have acute lung injury, no difference in outcomes is seen with management using a pulmonary artery catheter versus a central venous catheter; this finding suggests that there is no advantage to using a pulmonary catheter to guide the hemodynamic management of acute lung injury.[4] Patients whose acute lung injury is managed after 24 to 48 hours with a conservative fluid strategy (compared with a liberal fluid strategy) have significantly improved lung function and shorter duration of ventilation and ICU stay.[5]

Fluids should be used to maintain central venous pressure at 8 to 12 mm Hg; at present, no convincing data indicate that albumin is better than normal saline solution.[6] In patients with severe sepsis, modified Ringer's lactate is preferred over 10% hetastarch (a colloid) because of lower rates of both acute kidney injury and the need for renal replacement therapy.[7] If central venous oxygen saturation is less than 70%, packed red cell transfusions should be used to maintain a hematocrit greater than 30%.

Vasopressors (e.g., norepinephrine 1 to 50 µg/minute; epinephrine 1 to 30 µg/minute) should be added if the mean arterial pressure is less than 65 mm Hg. Dobutamine (2.5 to 20 µg/kg/minute) is required if central venous pressure, mean arterial pressure, and hematocrit are optimized but the central venous oxygen saturation remains less than 70%. In a randomized trial of patients with septic shock, the combination of norepinephrine plus dobutamine resulted in a similar mortality as epinephrine alone, with no differences in organ dysfunction, time to resolution of shock, or adverse events.[8] In another randomized trial, norepinephrine was slightly but not significantly better than dopamine for reducing mortality when used as the first-line vasopressor for patients with septic shock[9]; however, norepinephrine was associated with a lower rate of arrhythmias, especially atrial fibrillation. These accumulated data suggest that norepinephrine may be preferable to dopamine as the first vasopressor in septic shock.

Clinicians can use epinephrine alone, norepinephrine alone, or norepinephrine plus dobutamine in patients with low cardiac output.

As a strategic approach to persistent hypotension despite adequate fluid resuscitation, a vasopressor such as norepinephrine (1 to 50 µg/minute) can be added first. If the cardiac index is low or if the mixed venous oxygen saturation is low (<70%) despite an adequate central venous pressure, an inotropic agent such as dobutamine should be added, initially at approximately 2 to 5 µg/kg/minute and increasing until the mixed venous oxygen saturation is adequate. In some patients in septic shock, the cardiac index is inadequate, as reflected by a low mixed venous oxygen saturation despite a high central venous pressure (>12 mm Hg) and/or pulmonary artery wedge pressure (>18 mm Hg), because of underlying cardiovascular dysfunction or because of acute left ventricular dysfunction resulting from sepsis. In such patients, earlier use of an inotropic agent such as dobutamine should be considered to increase left ventricular contractility. The overall goal is to achieve an adequate mean arterial pressure (>65 mm Hg), central venous pressure, and mixed venous oxygen saturation while other indices of adequate perfusion are monitored, such as hourly urine output (>0.5 mL/kg/hour), arterial lactate levels (<2 mmol/L), mental status, and skin perfusion. To assess the adequacy of early resuscitation of severe sepsis and septic shock and to guide ongoing therapy, a central venous oxygen saturation goal greater than 70% or a lactate clearance of at least 10% is an equally good measure.[10]

Transfusion of Erythrocytes and Erythropoietin

Anemia is common in septic shock, but the optimal hemoglobin level for resuscitation is controversial. Goal-directed therapy aims for a hematocrit of 30%, whereas a randomized trial of transfusion in critically ill patients found that a hemoglobin range of 7 to 9 g/dL was equivalent to or better than a higher hemoglobin (10 to 12 g/dL), except possibly in patients with acute myocardial infarction or unstable angina. A reasonable approach is to use a hematocrit level of 30% as the threshold for erythrocyte transfusion for the first 6 hours and then to lower the threshold to a hemoglobin of 7 to 9 g/dL for the rest of the hospital course, except in patients with underlying cardiac disease. Recombinant erythropoietin decreases the need for transfusion in critically ill patients, but it does not decrease mortality.

Drugs
Antibiotics

The infected site and infecting organisms of septic shock are often not known initially. After appropriate cultures are obtained, intravenous broad-spectrum antibiotics should be administered on an emergency basis (within 1 hour) while considering host factors such as immune and allergic status (Chapters 288 and 289; see Fig. 108-3). Outcomes in patients with septic shock are worse if the organisms causing the sepsis are not sensitive to the initial antibiotic regimen.

Emergency, empirical antibiotic therapy (Table 108-4) should be guided by the greater frequency of gram-positive bacteria, the possibility of resistant organisms, and local bacteriologic features. If a causative organism is identified (<20% of septic patients have negative cultures), the antibiotic regimen should be narrowed to decrease the emergence of resistant organisms. Empirical fluconazole treatment does not result in better outcomes in critically ill, non-neutropenic patients at risk for invasive candidiasis.[11] The duration of antibiotics should be guided by the cause of septic shock, but patients generally require 10 to 14 days of therapy.

Corticosteroids

High-dose corticosteroids do not improve outcomes in the full spectrum of patients with sepsis or acute respiratory distress syndrome, but the evidence supporting the use of low-dose corticosteroids in septic shock is controversial. In one trial, corticosteroids (hydrocortisone 50 mg intravenously every 6 hours, plus fludrocortisone 50-μg tablet/day per nasogastric tube or orally for 7 days) increased survival in septic patients whose serum cortisol response after stimulation with an intravenous infusion of 250 μg corticotropin was 9 μg/dL or less.[12] In a subsequent randomized trial of hydrocortisone (50 mg every 6 hours intravenously for 5 days) versus placebo, however, mortality was not improved, regardless of the patient's response to corticotropin stimulation.[2] Adding fludrocortisone to hydrocortisone does not appear to be better than hydrocortisone alone, and aggressive insulin therapy to address the hyperglycemia that often accompanies corticosteroid treatment is no better than usual glucose control.[13] Hydrocortisone treatment is often associated with a shorter duration of septic shock but can increase the risk of superinfec-

tions. Current sepsis guidelines suggest that corticosteroids should be considered only in patients who are poorly responsive to vasopressors.

Corticosteroids administered before antibiotics also decrease the neurologic sequelae of bacterial, especially pneumococcal, meningitis (Chapter 420). Enthusiasm for corticosteroid therapy must be tempered by the risk of complications such as superinfection, neuromyopathy, hyperglycemia, immune suppression, and impaired wound healing.

Recombinant Human Activated Protein C

Activated protein C infusion (24 μg/kg/hour for 96 hours) decreases mortality, improves organ dysfunction, and decreases biomarkers of inflammation and coagulation in severe sepsis and septic shock.[14] Activated protein C is approved for patients who have severe sepsis and a high risk of death, as defined by an Acute Physiology and Chronic Health Evaluation (APACHE) II score of 25 or higher and/or two or more dysfunctional organs (see Fig. 108-3). By comparison, activated protein C is not beneficial in low-risk patients.[15] Activated protein C has not been tested in patients with major trauma, recent surgery (within 12 hours), active hemorrhage, coagulopathy, thrombocytopenia, or recent stroke because of the increased risk of hemorrhage. Even in patients without these risk factors, treatment increases the risk of serious hemorrhage nearly two-fold, and about 0.5% of treated patients develop intracranial hemorrhage. Activated protein C should not be used in surgical patients who have severe sepsis with single-organ dysfunction. If patients are receiving subcutaneous low-dose heparin prophylaxis and activated protein C is to be used, discontinuation of heparin should be weighed carefully: although its discontinuation while using activated protein C reduces bleeding, discontinuation also increases the risk of stroke[16] and may increase the risk of death. The use of activated protein C in septic shock is being reevaluated in

TABLE 108-4 POTENTIAL ANTIBIOTIC REGIMENS FOR PATIENTS WITH SEPTIC SHOCK*		
SOURCE OF SEPSIS	**INITIAL ANTIBIOTIC REGIMEN**	**ALTERNATIVE ANTIBIOTIC REGIMEN**
Community-acquired pneumonia	Third-generation cephalosporin: cefotaxime 2 g IV q6h; ceftriaxone 2 g IV q12h; ceftizoxime 2 g IV q8h PLUS Fluoroquinolone (e.g., ciprofloxacin 400 mg IV q12h, levofloxacin 750 mg IV q24h, moxifloxacin 400 mg IV q24h) OR Macrolide (azithromycin 500 mg IV q24h)	Piperacillin-tazobactam 3.375 g IV q6h PLUS Fluoroquinolone OR Macrolide
Hospital-acquired pneumonia	Imipenem 0.5 g IV q6h OR Meropenem 1 g IV q8h	Fluoroquinolone (ciprofloxacin 400 mg IV q12h) PLUS Vancomycin 1.5 g IV q12h OR Piperacillin-tazobactam 3.375 g IV q6h PLUS Tobramycin 1.5 mg/kg q8h PLUS Vancomycin
Abdominal (mixed aerobic/anaerobic)	Piperacillin-tazobactam 3.375 g IV q6h OR Imipenem 0.5 g IV q6h (or meropenem 1 g IV q8h)	Ampicillin 2 g IV q4h PLUS Metronidazole 500 mg IV q8h PLUS Fluoroquinolone (ciprofloxacin 400 mg IV q12h)
Urinary tract	Fluoroquinolone (ciprofloxacin 400 mg IV q12h)	Ampicillin 2 g IV q4h PLUS Gentamicin 1.5 mg/kg IV q8h OR Third-generation cephalosporin (cefotaxime 2 g IV q6h, ceftriaxone 2 g IV q12h, OR ceftizoxime 2 g IV q8h)
Necrotizing fasciitis	Imipenem 0.5 g IV q6h	Penicillin G (if confirmed group A streptococci)
Primary bacteremia (normal host)	Piperacillin-tazobactam 3.375 g IV q6h PLUS Vancomycin 1.5 g IV q12h	Imipenem 0.5 g IV q6h PLUS Vancomycin 1.5 g IV q12h
Primary bacteremia (intravenous drug user)	Vancomycin 1.5 g IV q12h PLUS Fluoroquinolone (ciprofloxacin 400 mg IV q12h)	Piperacillin-tazobactam 3.375 g IV q6h PLUS Vancomycin 1.5 g IV q12h
Febrile neutropenia	Cefepime 2 g IV q8h PLUS Vancomycin 1.5 g IV q12h	Piperacillin-tazobactam 3.375 g IV q6h PLUS Gentamicin 1.5 mg/kg q8h OR Imipenem 0.5 g IV q6h PLUS Gentamicin 1.5 mg/kg q8h
Bacterial meningitis	Ceftriaxone 2 g IV q12h PLUS Ampicillin 3 g IV q6h PLUS Vancomycin 1.5 g IV q12h PLUS Dexamethasone 0.15 mg/kg IV q6h for 2-4 days	Gram-positive cocci: Vancomycin PLUS Ceftriaxone 2 g IV q12h Gram-negative diplococci: Cefotaxime 2 g IV q4-6h Gram-positive bacilli: Ampicillin 3 g IV q6h PLUS Gentamicin Gram-negative bacilli: Ceftazidime 2 g IV q8h PLUS Gentamicin 1.5 mg/kg IV q8h All above PLUS Dexamethasone
Cellulitis	Ciprofloxacin 400 mg IV q12h PLUS Clindamycin 900 mg IV q8h	Imipenem 0.5 g IV q6h

*Most antibiotic doses must be adjusted if there is hepatic or renal dysfunction. Some antibiotics require adjustment based on levels (e.g., gentamicin). When selecting a drug, carefully consider the patient's history of antibiotic (especially penicillin) allergy.

a large, multicenter, randomized controlled trial; until that study is completed, activated protein C is still recommended for patients who meet the criteria and have no contraindications to its use.

Controversial Therapies in Septic Shock
Vasopressin Deficiency and Use of Vasopressin

Vasopressin deficiency and downregulation of vasopressin receptors are common findings in septic shock. Vasopressin selectively dilates renal afferent but not efferent glomerular arterioles, and it also dilates pulmonary, cerebral, and coronary arterioles. Low-dose vasopressin infusion (0.03 to 0.04 U/minute) increases blood pressure, urine output, and creatinine clearance while dramatically decreasing the dosage of norepinephrine required to maintain blood pressure in patients with septic shock. In a randomized trial, low-dose vasopressin added to norepinephrine was not significantly better than as-needed norepinephrine alone,[17] although added vasopressin may be useful in patients with less severe shock. Complications of vasopressin include gastrointestinal ischemia, decreased cardiac output, skin or digital necrosis, and cardiac arrest (especially at doses >0.04 U/minute).

Hyperglycemia and Intensive Insulin Therapy

Hyperglycemia and insulin resistance are common in septic shock. Hyperglycemia is a pro-coagulant and pro-apoptotic stimulus; it impairs neutrophil function, increases the risk of infection, impairs wound healing, and is associated with increased mortality. However, the risks of unrecognized hypoglycemia and cerebral injury may be increased in septic shock because of unstable endocrine function and the use of sedation. In addition, brain ischemia and hypoxia increase sensitivity to even transient hypoglycemia. At present, the appropriate glucose range and insulin doses are controversial. Intensive insulin therapy to control hyperglycemia is not beneficial in patients in medical ICUs because of significantly higher rates of hypoglycemia[7,18] and perhaps increased mortality.[18] Therefore, intensive insulin therapy cannot be recommended for patients with septic shock.

Renal Dysfunction and Dialysis

Acute renal failure is an important complication of septic shock because of its associated morbidity, mortality, and resource use (Fig. 108-4). Continuous renal replacement therapy induces less hemodynamic instability compared with intermittent hemodialysis, but no conclusive evidence indicates that continuous renal replacement therapy or more intensive dialysis changes the mortality of acute renal failure. In critically ill patients who have acute kidney injury, hemodialysis six times per week is no better than conventional hemodialysis, and intensive renal replacement therapy is no better than standard therapy overall or in patients who have sepsis.[19]

Low-dose dopamine (2 to 4 µg/kg/minute) does not decrease the need for renal support, does not improve outcomes, and is not recommended. Lactic acidosis is a common complication of septic shock, but administration of sodium bicarbonate in the setting of lactic acidosis does not improve hemodynamics or the response to vasopressors.

A small randomized controlled trial evaluated the use of polymyxin B hemoperfusion in patients with abdominal sepsis to reduce blood endotoxin levels. Polymyxin B hemoperfusion increased blood pressure, decreased vasopressor requirements, improved organ dysfunction, and reduced mortality by one third.[20] However, this intervention requires further evaluation before it can be recommended.

Other Therapies

Deep vein thrombosis prophylaxis using low-dose heparin, which can be administered in combination with activated protein C, is recommended for patients who do not have active bleeding, coagulopathy, or a contraindication to heparin (see Fig. 108-4). Stress ulcer prophylaxis using H₂-receptor antagonists decreases the risk of gastrointestinal hemorrhage. Proton pump inhibitors may also be effective, but they have not been fully evaluated in septic shock.

Enteral nutrition is generally safer and more effective than total parenteral nutrition, but total parenteral nutrition is sometimes required in patients with abdominal sepsis, surgery, or trauma. The use of sedation, neuromuscular blocking agents, and corticosteroids should be minimized because they can exacerbate septic encephalopathy and the polyneuropathy or myopathy of sepsis. Neutropenic patients may benefit from granulocyte colony-stimulating factor (Chapter 170). The risk of nosocomial infection is decreased by narrow-spectrum antibiotics, early weaning from ventilation, and periodic removal and replacement of catheters (Chapter 290).

B. Breathing—Oxygen, with a tidal volume 6 mL/kg IBW if ventilated. Wean according to ARDSNet protocol (Chapters 105 and 106)

C. Circulation
- Fluids, vasopressors, inotropes, transfusion; goals include:
  - MAP > 65 mm Hg
  - CVP 8-12 mm Hg
  - Hg 70-90 g/L
  - ScvO₂ > 70%

  Consider pulmonary artery catheter or echocardiogram especially if known cardiovascular disease; goals include:
  - Wedge pressure 8-15 mm Hg
    - Cardiac index: normal or increased

D. Drugs:
- Antibiotics: Narrow spectrum to cause of infection
- APC (if indicated): 24 µg/kg/hour infusion for 96 hours
- Hydrocortisone (if evidence of relative adrenal insufficiency [see text]): hydrocortisone 50 mg intravenously every 6 hours and fludrocortisone 50-µg tab orally or per NG tube daily for 7 days

Other Organ Support
- Renal function: Continuous renal replacement
- DVT prophylaxis: Low-dose heparin 5000 IU subcutaneously every 12 hours
- Stress ulcer prophylaxis: H₂-receptor antagonist (e.g., ranitidine 50 mg intravenously every 8 hours)
- Nutrition: Enteral preferred
- Sedation: Intermittent with daily awakening

FIGURE 108-4. Ongoing critical care support and management in septic shock. APC = activated protein C; CVP = central venous pressure; DVT = deep vein thrombosis; Hg = hemoglobin; IBW = ideal body weight; MAP = mean arterial pressure; NG = nasogastric; ScvO₂ = central venous oxygen saturation.

PROGNOSIS

The 28-day mortality of septic shock is 40 to 70%. Early deaths (in the first 72 hours) are usually the result of refractory, progressive shock despite escalating life support. Later deaths from septic shock (after day 3) are usually secondary to multiple organ dysfunction. The number of dysfunctional organs and the progression or lack of improvement of organ dysfunction are indicators of increased risk of death. Other factors that portend a poor prognosis are increased age, underlying medical conditions, high APACHE II score, increased arterial lactate concentrations, and lack of response to vasopressors. Furthermore, recent evidence indicates that a delay in achieving the goals of early goal-directed therapy is associated with increased mortality. Survivors of sepsis who also had acute lung injury (Chapter 104) can have weakness, fatigue, and dyspnea on exertion after hospital discharge owing to pulmonary dysfunction, neuromuscular dysfunction, or other persistent organ dysfunction.

1. Sprung CL, Annane D, Keh D, et al. Hydrocortisone therapy for patients with septic shock. *N Engl J Med.* 2008;358:111-124.
2. Acute Respiratory Distress Syndrome Network. Ventilation with lower tidal volumes as compared with traditional tidal volumes for acute lung injury and the acute respiratory distress syndrome. *N Engl J Med.* 2000;342:1301-1308.
3. Rivers E, Nguyen B, Havstad S, et al. Early goal-directed therapy in the treatment of severe sepsis and septic shock. *N Engl J Med.* 2001;345:1368-1377.
4. Wheeler AP, Bernard GR, Thompson BT, et al. National Heart, Lung, and Blood Institute Acute Respiratory Distress Syndrome (ARDS) Clinical Trials Network: pulmonary-artery versus central venous catheter to guide treatment of acute lung injury. *N Engl J Med.* 2006;354:2213-2224.
5. Wiedemann HP, Wheeler AP, Bernard GR, et al. Comparison of two fluid management strategies in acute lung injury. *N Engl J Med.* 2006;354:2564-2575.
6. SAFE. A comparison of albumin and saline for fluid resuscitation in the intensive care unit. *N Engl J Med.* 2004;350:2247-2256.
7. Brunkhorst FM, Engel C, Bloos F, et al. Intensive insulin therapy and pentastarch resuscitation in severe sepsis. *N Engl J Med.* 2008;358:125-139.
8. Annane D, Vignon P, Renault A, et al. Norepinephrine plus dobutamine versus epinephrine alone for management of septic shock: a randomized trial. *Lancet.* 2007;370:676-684.
9. De Backer D, Biston P, Devriendt J, et al. Comparison of dopamine and norepinephrine in the treatment of septic shock. *N Engl J Med.* 2010;362:779-789.
10. Jones AE, Shapiro NI, Trzeciak S, et al. Lactate clearance vs. central venous oxygen saturation as goals of early sepsis therapy: A randomized clinical trial. *JAMA.* 2010;303:739-746.
11. Schuster MG, Edwards JE Jr, Sobel JD, et al. Empirical fluconazole versus placebo for intensive care unit patients: a randomized trial. *Ann Intern Med.* 2008;149:83-90.
12. Annane D, Sebille V, Charpentier C, et al. Effect of treatment with low doses of hydrocortisone and fludrocortisone on mortality in patients with septic shock. *JAMA.* 2002;288:862-871.

13. The COIITS Study Investigators. Corticosteroid treatment and intensive insulin therapy for septic shock in adults: a randomized controlled trial. *JAMA.* 2010;303:341-348.

14. Bernard GR, Vincent JL, Laterre PF, et al. Efficacy and safety of recombinant human activated protein C for severe sepsis. *N Engl J Med.* 2001;344:699-709.

15. Abraham E, Laterre PF, Garg R, et al. Drotrecogin alfa (activated) for adults with severe sepsis and a low risk of death. *N Engl J Med.* 2005;353:1332-1341.

16. Levy M, Levy M, Williams M, et al. Prophylactic heparin in patients with severe sepsis treated with drotrecogin alfa (activated). *Am J Resp Crit Care Med.* 2007;176:483-490.

17. Russell JA, Walley KR, Singer J, et al. Vasopressin versus norepinephrine infusion in patients with septic shock. *N Engl J Med.* 2008;358:877-887.

18. NICE SUGAR. Intensive versus conventional glucose control in critically ill patients. *N Engl J Med.* 2009;360:1283-1297.

19. VA/NIH Network. Intensity of renal support in critically ill patients with acute kidney injury. *N Engl J Med.* 2008;359:7-20.

20. Cruz DN, Antonelli M, Fumagalli R, et al. Early use of polymyxin B hemoperfusion in abdominal septic shock. *JAMA.* 2009;301:2445-2452.

SUGGESTED READINGS

Angus DC. Management of sepsis: a 47-year-old woman with an indwelling intravenous catheter and sepsis. *JAMA.* 2011;305:1469-1477. *Case-based review.*

Funk DJ, Kumar A. Antimicrobial therapy for life-threatening infections: speed is life. *Crit Care Med.* 2011;27:53-76. *Emphasizes that early recognition of life-threatening infection and rapid initiation of appropriate antimicrobial therapy is the critical element in reducing mortality.*

Levy MM, Dellinger RP, Townsend SR, et al. The Surviving Sepsis campaign: results of an international guidelines-based performance improvement program targeting severe sepsis. *Crit Care Med.* 2010;38:367-374. *Suggests that the use of guidelines improves quality of care and may decrease mortality of severe sepsis and septic shock.*

Winters BD, Eberlein M, Leung J, et al. Long-term mortality and quality of life in sepsis: a systematic review. *Crit Care Med.* 2010;38:1276-1283. *Survivors have increased mortality and impaired quality of life for at least 2 years.*

109

DISORDERS DUE TO HEAT AND COLD

WILLIAM WINKENWERDER JR. AND MICHAEL N. SAWKA

TEMPERATURE REGULATION

Body temperature is regulated through two parallel processes that modify body heat balance: behavioral (clothing, shelter, physical activity) and physiologic (skin blood flow, sweating, shivering). Both peripheral (skin) and central (core) thermal receptors provide afferent input to a central nervous system integrator (hypothalamic thermoregulatory center), and any deviation between the controlled variable (body temperature) and a reference variable ("set point" temperature) results in a heat loss or conservation response (Fig. 109-1).

Humans normally regulate body (core) temperature at about 37° C (98.6° F), and fluctuations within the narrow range of 35 to 41° C (95 to 105.8° F) can be tolerated by healthy acclimatized persons; core temperatures outside this range can induce morbidity and mortality. There is no single core temperature because it varies at different deep body sites and during rest and physical exercise. Arterial blood temperature provides the best invasive measurement of core temperature. The most accurate noninvasive index of core temperature is esophageal temperature, followed in order of preference by rectal, gastrointestinal tract (telemetry pill), and oral temperature. Ear (tympanic and auditory meatus) or scanned temporal artery temperature should not be relied on for clinical judgment.

HEAT ILLNESS

DEFINITIONS

Minor heat-related illnesses include miliaria rubra, heat syncope, and heat cramps. Serious heat illness represents a continuum from heat exhaustion to heat injury and heatstroke.

EPIDEMIOLOGY

Body temperature can increase from exposure to environmental heat (impeded heat dissipation), physical exercise (increased heat production), and fever (elevated set point). Febrile persons have accentuated elevations in core temperature when exposed to high ambient temperature, physical exercise, or both. Serious heat illness is associated with a variety of individual factors, health conditions, drugs, and environmental factors (Table 109-1). Anticholinergic and sympathomimetic poisoning (Chapter 110) can induce hyperthermia. Malignant hyperthermia (Chapter 440) is caused by rapid and massive skeletal muscle contraction from exposure to anesthesia. Neuroleptic malignant syndrome (Chapter 442) is hyperthermia caused by skeletal muscle rigidity from treatment with neuroleptic medications (e.g., antipsychotics, antidepressants, antiemetics).

Heat illness can also occur in low-risk individuals who have taken appropriate precautions relative to situations they have been exposed to in the past. Historically, such unexpected cases were attributed to dehydration (which impairs thermoregulation and increases hyperthermia and cardiovascular strain), but it is now suspected that a previous heat exposure or event (e.g., sickness or injury) might make these individuals more susceptible to serious heat illness. One theory is that previous heat injury or illness primes the acute phase response and augments the hyperthermia of exercise, inducing unexpected serious heat illness. Another theory is that previous infection produces pro-inflammatory cytokines that deactivate the cells' ability to protect against heat shock.

PATHOBIOLOGY

Environmental and exercise heat stress challenges the cardiovascular system to provide high blood flow to the skin, where blood pools in warm, compliant vessels such as those found in the extremities. When blood flow is diverted to the skin, reduced perfusion of the intestines and other viscera can result in ischemia, endotoxemia, and oxidative stress. In addition, excessively high

FIGURE 109-1. Control of human thermoregulation. (From Sawka MN, Young AJ. Physiological systems and their responses to conditions of heat and cold. In: Tipton CM, Sawka MN, Tate CA, Terjung RL, eds. *ACSM's Advanced Exercise Physiology.* Baltimore: Lippincott Williams & Wilkins; 2005:535-563.)

TABLE 109-1   FACTORS PREDISPOSING TO SERIOUS HEAT ILLNESS

INDIVIDUAL FACTORS

Lack of acclimatization
Low physical fitness
Excessive body weight
Dehydration
Advanced age
Young age

HEALTH CONDITIONS

Inflammation and fever
Viral infection
Cardiovascular disease
Diabetes mellitus
Gastroenteritis
Rash, sunburn, and previous burns to large areas of skin
Seizures
Thyroid storm
Neuroleptic malignant syndrome
Malignant hyperthermia
Sickle cell trait
Cystic fibrosis
Spinal cord injury

DRUGS

Anticholinergic properties (atropine)
Antiepileptic (topiramate)
Antihistamines
Glutethimide (Doriden)
Phenothiazines
Tricyclic antidepressants
Amphetamines, cocaine, "Ecstasy"
Ergogenic stimulants (e.g., ephedrine, ephedra)
Lithium
Diuretics
β-Blockers
Ethanol

ENVIRONMENTAL FACTORS

High temperature
High humidity
Little air motion
Lack of shade
Heat wave
Physical exercise
Heavy clothing
Air pollution (nitrogen dioxide)

TABLE 109-2   COMPARISON OF CLASSIC AND EXERTIONAL HEATSTROKE

PATIENT CHARACTERISTICS	CLASSIC	EXERTIONAL
Age	Young children or elderly	15-55 yr
Health	Chronic illness	Usually healthy
Fever	Unusual	Common
Prevailing weather	Frequent in heat waves	Variable
Activity	Sedentary	Strenuous exercise
Drug use	Diuretics, antidepressants, anticholinergics, phenothiazines	Ergogenic stimulants or cocaine
Sweating	Often absent	Common
Acid-base disturbances	Respiratory alkalosis	Lactic acidosis
Acute renal failure	Uncommon	Common (≈15%)
Rhabdomyolysis	Uncommon	Common (≈25%)
CK	Mildly elevated	Markedly elevated (500-1000 U/L)
ALT, AST	Mildly elevated	Markedly elevated
Hyperkalemia	Uncommon	Common
Hypocalcemia	Uncommon	Common
DIC	Mild	Marked
Hypoglycemia	Uncommon	Common

ALT = alanine aminotransferase; AST = aspartate aminotransferase; CK = creatine kinase; DIC = disseminated intravascular coagulation.

Heat exhaustion is a mild to moderate illness characterized by an inability to sustain cardiac output with moderate (>38.5° C [101° F]) to high (>40° C [104° F]) body temperatures. It is frequently accompanied by sweaty hot skin, dehydration, and collapse. Heat injury is a moderate to severe illness characterized by organ (e.g., liver, renal) and tissue (e.g., gut, muscle) injury with high body temperatures, usually but not always greater than 40° C (104° F).

Heatstroke is a severe illness characterized by mental status changes with high body temperatures, usually but not always greater than 40° C (104° F). However, patients with a core temperature higher than 40° C do not universally have a heat injury or heatstroke, and the entire clinical picture, including mental status and laboratory results, must be considered. Heatstroke is often categorized as classic or exertional, with the former observed primarily in otherwise sick and compromised individuals and the latter observed primarily in apparently healthy and physically fit individuals (Table 109-2). Heatstroke victims have profound neuropsychiatric impairments that develop early and universally. In addition, heatstroke can be complicated by liver damage, rhabdomyolysis, disseminated intravascular coagulation, water and electrolyte imbalance, and renal failure.

PREVENTION, TREATMENT, AND PROGNOSIS (Rx)

Heat illness can be prevented by heat acclimatization and acquired thermal tolerance, maintenance of adequate hydration, and avoidance of overwhelming heat exposure. Adequate fluid intake is critical, and oral rehydration solutions may be preferable to other forms of hydration.▉

Management of serious heat illness includes cooling, rehydration, and monitoring (Table 109-3). Body cooling should be initiated immediately and continued until the core temperature falls below 38.8° C (102° F). Body cooling lowers tissue temperatures and reduces cardiovascular stress by causing vasoconstriction in the skin. Immersion or soaking the skin in cool or iced water with skin massage is the most effective method, but other effective methods include soaking the skin followed by accelerated evaporation with fans or the use of ice sheets or ice packs. Cooling can induce shivering, which is usually not sufficient to increase body temperature, so shivering need not be treated.

Fluid and electrolyte deficits should be corrected; restoration of plasma volume with isotonic fluids sufficient to sustain adequate perfusion, as judged by urine output, is a priority. Rapid overcorrection of serum electrolytes (e.g., sodium) should be avoided. If rhabdomyolysis (Chapter 115) and myoglobinuria are present, maintaining urine flow helps minimize renal injury. Patients should be monitored for cardiac arrhythmia and acute respiratory failure. Medications to be avoided include antipyretics and sedatives with hepatic toxicities. Lorazepam (1 to 2 mg administered intravenously over a

tissue temperatures (heat shock: >41° C [105.8° F]) can produce direct tissue injury; the magnitude and duration of the heat shock influence whether cells respond by adaptation (acquired thermal tolerance), injury, or death (apoptotic or necrotic). Heat shock, ischemia, and systemic inflammatory responses can result in cellular dysfunction, disseminated intravascular coagulation, and multiorgan dysfunction syndrome. In addition, reduced cerebral blood flow, combined with abnormal local metabolism and coagulopathy, can lead to dysfunction of the central nervous system.

CLINICAL MANIFESTATIONS AND DIAGNOSIS

Mild heat illness is common and can be recognized by its clinical features. Miliaria rubra (heat rash) results from the occlusion of eccrine sweat gland ducts and can be complicated by secondary staphylococcal infection. Heat syncope (fainting) is caused by temporary circulatory insufficiency as a result of blood pooling in the peripheral veins, especially the cutaneous and lower extremity veins. Heat cramps (skeletal muscles cramps) occur during and after intense exercise and are believed to result from excessive loss of sodium in sweat.

Serious heat illness is often not apparent at the initial evaluation. Patients who exhibit symptoms (e.g., dizziness, unsteady gait, ataxia, headache, confusion, weakness, fatigue, nausea, vomiting, diarrhea) should have an immediate assessment of their mental status, core (rectal) temperature, and other vital signs. Heatstroke should be the working diagnosis in anyone who is a heat casualty and has an altered mental status.

TABLE 109-3 MANAGEMENT OF HEAT ILLNESS

HEAT EXHAUSTION

Rest and shade
Loosen and remove clothing
Supine position and elevate legs
Actively cool skin
Fluids by mouth
Monitor core temperature
Monitor mental status

HYPERTHERMIA

Protect the airway
Insert at least two large-bore intravenous lines
Monitor core temperature; options include pulmonary artery, rectal probe, esophageal probe
Actively cool the skin until core temperature reaches 39° C (102.2° F)
Ice baths or cool water (≈22° C [71.6° F]) immersion
Wetting with water (avoid alcohol rubs)
Continuous fanning
Exposure to cool environment
Axillary or perineal ice packs and ice sheets
Infusion of room-temperature saline
Gastric or colonic iced saline lavage
Peritoneal lavage with cool saline
Monitor electrocardiogram for arrhythmia
Obtain serial diagnostic studies*

*Electrocardiogram, chest radiograph, complete blood count with differential, platelet count, urinalysis, aminotransferases, alkaline phosphatase, bilirubin, creatine kinase, blood urea nitrogen, creatinine, phosphate, calcium, glucose, electrolytes, uric acid, prothrombin time and partial thromboplastin time, fibrin split products, fibrinogen, arterial blood gases, toxicology screen.

2- to 5-minute period, repeated if necessary) is a safe sedative because of its low hepatotoxicity and rapid metabolism.

A single episode of heat exhaustion does not imply a predisposition to heat illness, and most patients recover within several hours after cooling and rehydration. In contrast, heat injury and heatstroke patients should not be reexposed to heat until recovery is complete, and about 10% of heatstroke patients remain intolerant of heat. The long-term consequences of heatstroke likely include sustained organ damage, which presumably explains why patients have a higher long-term mortality from cardiovascular, liver, and digestive diseases.

COLD INJURY

DEFINITIONS

Cold injuries are classified as hypothermia and peripheral cold injuries. Hypothermia is whole body cooling, whereas peripheral cold injuries are localized to the extremities and exposed skin. Peripheral cold injuries can be divided into nonfreezing (chilblain, trench foot) and freezing (frostbite). Both hypothermia and peripheral cold injuries often occur simultaneously.

EPIDEMIOLOGY

A variety of individual factors, health conditions, medications, and environmental factors are associated with a predisposition to cold injury (Table 109-4). In trauma patients (Chapter 112), hypothermia is associated with increased morbidity and mortality.

PATHOBIOLOGY

Cold exposure elicits peripheral vasoconstriction to reduce heat transfer between the body's core and shell (skin, subcutaneous fat). If sufficiently cold, the underlying tissues (e.g., muscle) constrict to thicken the isolative shell while reducing the body's core area. This vasoconstrictor response defends core temperature, but at the expense of declining peripheral tissue temperatures, which contribute to peripheral cold injuries. Hypothermia depresses enzymatic activity, interferes with physiologic functions (e.g., clotting, respiration, cardiac conduction and rhythm), impairs the expression of cytokines, and can induce cellular injury and death.

CLINICAL MANIFESTATIONS AND DIAGNOSIS

Hypothermia is a core temperature below 35° C (95° F), and clinical manifestations are related to the core temperature achieved (Table 109-5). The

TABLE 109-4 FACTORS PREDISPOSING TO COLD INJURY

INDIVIDUAL FACTORS

Inadequate clothing and shelter
Lean and low body fat
Low physical fitness
Advanced age
Young age
Black race (men and women)

HEALTH CONDITIONS

Burns
Diabetes mellitus
Hypoglycemia
Neurologic lesions
Dementia
Hypoadrenalism, hypopituitarism, hypothyroidism
Prior frostbite or trench foot
Raynaud's phenomenon
Sickle cell trait
Trauma
Spinal cord injury

DRUGS

Alcohol
Anesthetics
Antidepressants
Antithyroid agents
Sedatives and narcotics

ENVIRONMENTAL FACTORS

Cold temperatures
High air motion
Rain and immersion
Skin contact with metal and fuels
Repeated cold exposure
Physical fatigue
Immobility
High-altitude and low-oxygen-tension environments

TABLE 109-5 HYPOTHERMIA: STAGES AND ASSOCIATED CLINICAL MANIFESTATIONS

STAGE	Core Temperature °F	Core Temperature °C	CLINICAL MANIFESTATIONS
Normothermia	98.6	37.0	
Mild hypothermia	95.0	35.0	Cold diuresis, maximal shivering
	93.0	33.8	Ataxia, poor judgment, J wave
	91.0	32.7	Amnesia, blood pressure difficult to measure
Moderate hypothermia	89.0	31.6	Stupor, pupils dilated
	87.0	30.5	Shivering ceases
	85.0	30.0	Cardiac arrhythmias, insulin inactive
	82.0	27.8	Unconsciousness, ventricular fibrillation likely
	80.0	26.6	No muscle reflexes
Profound hypothermia	78.0	25.5	Acid-base disturbances, no response to pain
	75.0	23.8	Pulmonary edema, hypotension
	73.0	22.7	No corneal reflexes
	66.0	18.8	Heart standstill
	62.0	16.6	Isoelectric electrocardiogram
	57.6	14.2	Lowest infant survival from accidental hypothermia
	48.2	9.0	Lowest adult survival from accidental hypothermia

classic J wave on the electrocardiogram (Fig. 109-2) appears at a core temperature below about 33.8° C (93° F).

Chilblain (Chapter 80) appears as localized inflammatory lesions of the skin most often involving the dorsal surface of fingers, but the ears, face, and exposed shins are other common areas. Trench foot is caused by prolonged

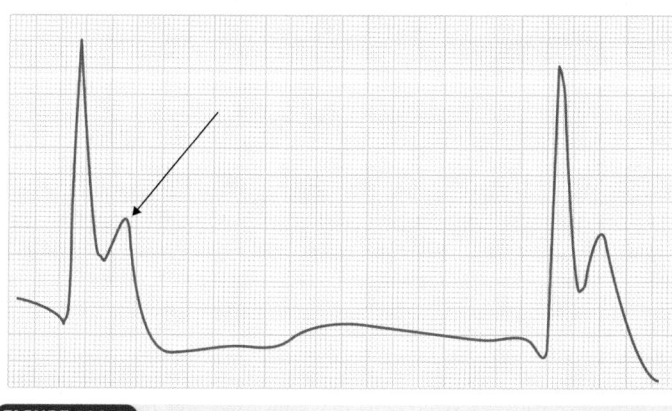

FIGURE 109-2. J (Osborne) wave.

TABLE 109-6	TREATMENT OF HYPOTHERMIA	
STAGE	**MANAGEMENT**	**BODY REWARMING**
Mild hypothermia	Monitor vital signs Warm intravenous saline Oxygen Monitor electrocardiogram for arrhythmia	Insulate Shivering Warm bath Active warming blanket
Moderate hypothermia	Diagnostic studies* Intensive care Anticipate infection and multiorgan dysfunction	Prevent extra heat loss by supplementing with airway rewarming Colonic irrigation Peritoneal dialysis
Profound hypothermia	Diagnostic studies*	Central rewarming

*See Table 109-3. Also lactate dehydrogenase, serum lactate, cortisol, thyroid-stimulating hormone, T_3, and T_4.

cold, wet exposure (e.g., wet socks or gloves), which can cause skin breakdown and nerve damage. Trench foot is often accompanied by infection and increased sensitivity to pain. Frostbite is the freezing of tissues and can be categorized as first degree (superficial, "frostnip"), second degree (full skin), third degree (subcutaneous tissue), and fourth degree (extensive tissue and bone). It may take many days to weeks to determine the severity of frostbite. Frostbite requires early surgical consultation once the diagnosis is made.

PREVENTION, TREATMENT, AND PROGNOSIS Rx

Humans demonstrate minimal cold acclimatization, so prevention depends primarily on avoiding cold exposure and having adequate protection and caloric intake to support metabolism. Management of hypothermia depends on the core temperature (Table 109-6). Patients' wet clothing should be removed, and they should be provided with dry insulation. Shivering is an effective physiologic rewarming mechanism and should not be pharmacologically suppressed. Moderately and profoundly hypothermic patients require active rewarming. Rewarming at a rate of 0.5 to 1.0° C (0.9 to 1.8° F) per hour is acceptable in most cases, except that aggressive rewarming is warranted in patients with significant trauma (because coagulation is hindered by hypothermia) or cardiac arrest.

Patients should be warmed gently because ventricular fibrillation is easily precipitated. When ventricular fibrillation is present, repeated electrical shocks should not be attempted until the patient has been rewarmed to a core temperature higher than 30° C (86° F); instead, cardiopulmonary resuscitation should be maintained during this period. Arrhythmias can be treated with lidocaine, propranolol, or bretylium (Chapter 63). Body cooling induces cold diuresis, so plasma volume needs to be reestablished to support adequate perfusion: patients should receive an intravenous infusion of 250 to 1000 mL of heated (40 to 42° C [104 to 108° F]) 5% dextrose in normal saline. Lactated Ringer's solution should be avoided because the liver cannot metabolize lactate efficiently during hypothermia. Patients should be monitored for disturbances in potassium and glucose. If hypoglycemia, alcohol, or opiate intoxication is contributing to hypothermia, intravenous glucose (10 to 25 g), thiamine (100 mg), or naloxone (1 to 2 mg), respectively, may be indicated.

Frostbitten tissues should be protected from friction or trauma and gently rewarmed in a water bath (38 to 43° C [100 to 108° F]). Frostbitten tissues should not be thawed until there is confidence in the ability to maintain warmth, because refreezing causes more injury. Patients should receive ibuprofen, antibiotics if infection is suspected, and possibly an analgesic.

Hypothermic Syndromes

Exercise-induced bronchospasm (Chapter 87) can be triggered by exercise in cold air, particularly in patients with asthma. Livedo reticularis (Fig. 80-2 in Chapter 80) is patchy mottling of the limbs with cold exposure. Cryoglobulinemia (Chapter 193) occurs when immunoglobulins (IgM, IgG) reversibly precipitate after being cooled and contribute to impaired capillary blood flow in hypothermic tissues. Cold urticaria (Chapters 260 and 448) is the development of localized and general erythema and wheals in skin exposed to cold. Paroxysmal hypothermia is periodic lowering of the thermoregulatory set point and is often associated with hypothalamic abnormalities. Raynaud's phenomenon (Fig. 80-5 in Chapter 80) is intense vasoconstriction with sensitivity to pain in limbs exposed to cold.

Trauma Hypothermia

In trauma patients (Chapter 112), unintended hypothermia (<34° C [93° F]) is associated with increased morbidity and mortality due to impaired coagulation, peripheral vasoconstriction, respiratory depression, and increased risk for cardiac arrhythmias. Shivering aggravates perfusion problems by requiring blood flow to support increased metabolism in contracting muscles. Trauma patients become hypothermic because of heat loss from exposed cavities, environmental exposure, infusion of cool fluids, and ischemia, which depletes cell energy stores. Body temperature should be measured, and appropriate actions should be taken to restore normothermia during the early treatment of trauma patients.

● THERAPEUTIC HYPOTHERMIA AND HYPERTHERMIA

Therapeutic Hypothermia

Therapeutic hypothermia provides benefits by suppressing metabolism, free radical production, lipid peroxidation, inflammatory products, excitatory amino acid release, and calcium release. Induction of mild hypothermia (32 to 34° C [89 to 93° F]) for 12 to 24 hours provides long-term benefits to patients after a cardiac arrest (Chapter 63). **2** It is being tested for spinal cord injury but has not consistently shown a benefit in neonates with traumatic brain injury or hypoxic-ischemic encephalopathy. **3,4** Mild hypothermia may be beneficial for patients suffering from hemorrhagic shock, brain injury, or stroke.

Therapeutic hypothermia should be initiated as soon as possible by either skin cooling (e.g., cooling packs to the axilla, groin, head, and neck while simultaneously treating the patient with a cooling blanket, water mattress, or fan), endovascular cooling, or both. Endovascular cooling can be achieved either by the infusion of cool fluids (e.g., 30 mL/kg crystalloids at 4° C [40° F]) or by indwelling heat transfer devices. Cooling by peritoneal and pleural lavage is not generally used. Endovascular cooling provides a more rapid and better-controlled cooling than skin cooling. Thermoregulatory responses (shivering and peripheral vasoconstriction) will resist induced hypothermia and elevate blood pressure and should therefore be pharmacologically blunted. Low-dose meperidine (e.g., 12.5 mg intravenously) can blunt shivering without excessive toxicity.

Hyperthermia Treatment

Hyperthermia treatment (whole body or regional) is an experimental technique used as an adjunct to chemotherapy or radiation therapy in advanced cancer patients. Hyperthermia (40 to 43° C [104 to 109° F]) alone can damage or kill cancer cells, but more importantly, hyperthermia might potentiate the effectiveness of chemotherapy and radiation by softening the tumor tissue, thus reducing its interstitial pressure.

Whole body hyperthermia is usually induced by externally applied radiant heat, microwaves, or extracorporeal circulation. Target temperatures are usually achieved over 1 to 2 hours and then maintained for approximately 1 hour, followed by a 1-hour cooling phase. Patients are usually sedated while core and skin temperatures are monitored. In regional hyperthermia, the part of the body where the tumor is located is heated while being perfused or bathed by a warmed solution containing anticancer drugs.

Grade A

1. Ishikawa T, Tamura H, Ishiguro H, et al. Effect of oral rehydration solution on fatigue during outdoor work in a hot environment: a randomized crossover study. *J Occup Health*. 2010;52:209-215.
2. Janata A, Holzer M. Hypothermia after cardiac arrest. *Prog Cardiovasc Dis*. 2009;52:168-179.
3. Azzopardi DV, Strohm B, Edwards AD, et al. Moderate hypothermia to treat perinatal asphyxia encephalopathy. *N Engl J Med*. 2009;361:1349-1358.
4. Hutchison JS, Ward RE, Lacroix J, et al. Hypothermia therapy after traumatic brain injury in children. *N Engl J Med*. 2008;358:2447-2456.

SUGGESTED READINGS

Holzer M. Targeted temperature management for comatose survivors of cardiac arrest. *N Engl J Med*. 2010;363:1256-1264. *Review*.
Metzger KB, Ito K, Matte TD. Summer heat and mortality in New York City: how hot is too hot? *Environ Health Perspect*. 2010;118:80-86. *Risk rises abruptly at a heat index between 95 and 100° F*.
Nelson NG, Collins CL, Comstock RD, et al. Exertional heat-related injuries treated in emergency departments in the U.S. 1997-2006. *Am J Prev Med*. 2011;40:54-60. *Review of about 55,000 cases*.

110

ACUTE POISONING

MARSHA D. FORD

EPIDEMIOLOGY

Each year, more than 4 million poisoning cases, suspected or verified, and 300,000 related hospital admissions occur in the United States. Poisoning-related deaths total more than 30,000 per year and are increasing. Unintentional poisonings are now the second leading cause of injury-related death in the United States, and they exceed motor vehicle accidents as the leading cause of injury-related death in adults 34 to 56 years of age. Ninety-two percent of these deaths involve drugs, predominantly prescription opioid analgesics. The incidence of recurrent, purposeful self-poisoning is 12 to 18%, with most events occurring within 3 months of the original attempt. These facts emphasize the need for regulatory measures to improve the safety of opioid analgesic drugs, including appropriate prescribing, and aggressive treatment of poisoned patients, including early psychiatric intervention for suicidal behavior, to reduce fatalities and repeat attempts (Chapter 404).

DIAGNOSIS

Diagnosis and management of poisoned patients require knowledge and skill in five areas to identify and treat the factors that contribute to the risk for death or long-term disability: (1) history taking; (2) physical examination, with recognition of specific toxic syndromes, or *toxidromes*; (3) appropriate use of diagnostic tests; (4) treatment, including initial stabilization and critical care, decontamination, and administration of antidotes for specific poisonings; and (5) use of methods to enhance the elimination of specific toxicants.

History

Details elicited about toxic exposures should include the involved drugs and other toxicants, their estimated or known amounts, the time and routes of exposure, the patient's symptoms and signs, and any treatment already administered. Intoxication may result from acute, chronic, or acute-on-chronic exposure. A *toxicant* is defined as a chemical capable of harming a biologic organism; this definition encompasses toxins, which are derived from living organisms, as well as drugs and industrial and other chemicals. Determination of chronicity is important because signs and symptoms of chronic intoxication (Chapter 21) can differ from those of acute and acute-on-chronic intoxication. For example, a history of acute collapse narrows the toxicant possibilities to a few gases, chemicals, and drugs. A listing of available medications (e.g., medications of the patient, spouse, relatives, or friends); use of nonprescription medications, herbal or dietary supplements, or ethnic remedies; and occupational and avocational activities should be obtained. Occupational and avocational histories should include present and all past jobs and hobbies, with a focus on chemicals, metals, and gases. Known medical conditions may suggest classes of medications available to the patient. The patient's history, which may be incomplete if the patient is confused or suicidal, should be correlated with the clinical manifestations and course. Further history from relatives and friends and findings from the scene as reported by the transporting emergency medical services personnel may be relevant.

Physical Examination

The physical examination should focus on vital signs; the eye, ear, nose, and throat examination; and the neurologic, cardiopulmonary, gastrointestinal, and dermatologic systems. Findings can suggest certain toxidromes, which are clusters of signs and symptoms typical of poisoning with adrenergic, anticholinergic, cholinomimetic, opioid, and sedative-hypnotic agents (Table 110-1). Patients may have some or all of these signs and symptoms; an incomplete clinical picture does not exclude a particular toxidrome, but it can still assist the clinician in identifying the correct category of toxicant involved.

TABLE 110-1 TOXIDROMES AND ASSOCIATED DRUGS AND TOXICANTS

TOXIDROME	Syndrome Features		COMMON DRUGS/TOXICANTS
	VITAL SIGNS	**END ORGAN**	
Adrenergic	Hypertension, hyperthermia, tachycardia, tachypnea	Agitation, arrhythmias, diaphoresis, mydriasis, seizures	Amphetamines, caffeine, cathinone derivatives, cocaine, ephedrine, pseudoephedrine, *Ephedra* sp, phenylpropanolamine,* theophylline
Anticholinergic	Hyperthermia, tachycardia	Agitation, delirium, decreased or absent bowel sounds, dry flushed skin and mucous membranes, mydriasis or blurred vision, seizures, urinary retention	First-generation H_1-receptor antagonists (e.g., classic antihistamines), belladonna alkaloids (e.g., scopolamine, hyoscyamine) from plants (e.g., *Datura* sp—deadly nightshade, henbane), benztropine, cyclic antidepressants, dicyclomine, muscle relaxants (e.g., orphenadrine, cyclobenzaprine), trihexyphenidyl
Cholinomimetic	Tachycardia or bradycardia[†]	Agitation, delirium, coma; bronchorrhea; bronchospasm; diaphoresis; fasciculations; lacrimation; miosis; urination; diarrhea; vomiting; seizures	Carbamates, cholinesterase inhibitors (e.g., physostigmine, neostigmine, edrophonium), *Inocybe* or *Clitocybe* mushroom sp, nerve gases (e.g., soman, sarin), organophosphorus compounds
Opiate, opioid	Bradycardia, bradypnea or apnea, hypotension (rare), hypothermia	CNS depression; hypotonia; miosis; mydriasis (dextromethorphan, meperidine, pentazocine)	Codeine, fentanyl, designer fentanyls, heroin, opioids (e.g., hydrocodone, oxycodone, meperidine, morphine), propoxyphene, central α_2-agonists (e.g., clonidine, imidazolines)
Sedative-hypnotic	Bradypnea or apnea, hypotension, hypothermia	Ataxia, CNS depression, hyporeflexia, slurred speech, stupor, or coma	Barbiturates, benzodiazepines, bromides, chloral hydrate, ethanol, ethchlorvynol, etomidate, glutethimide, meprobamate, methaqualone, methyprylon, propofol, zolpidem

*Reflex bradycardia can occur as a result of a pure α-adrenergic agonist effect.
†Tachycardia can occur early as a result of a preganglionic nicotinic effect; as toxicity progresses, postganglionic muscarinic effects predominate, and bradycardia develops.
CNS = central nervous system.

Vital Signs

Tachycardia can occur with numerous toxicants and with anxiety and other nontoxicologic conditions and is not a helpful finding. The limited differential diagnosis for toxicant-induced *bradycardia* includes baclofen, β-adrenergic receptor antagonists, L-type calcium-channel antagonists (diltiazem or verapamil), cardiac glycosides, α-adrenergic receptor agonists (e.g., phenylpropanolamine, whose effects are mediated by baroreceptor reflexes), γ-hydroxybutyric acid, opioids, some sedative-hypnotics, central α_2-agonists, organophosphorus compounds, carbamates, cyanide, muscarine-containing mushrooms (*Clitocybe, Inocybe* sp), plant- and animal-derived toxins (aconitine, andromedotoxin, ciguatoxin, veratridine), therapeutic cholinesterase inhibitors (e.g., physostigmine), cyclic antidepressants (bradycardia is a preterminal sign), and some antiarrhythmic drugs (e.g., procainamide, flecainide, other class IA and IC drugs such as amiodarone, sotalol).

Many toxicants cause *hypotension* (Chapter 7). The primary mechanisms are decreased peripheral vascular resistance, decreased myocardial contractility, hypovolemia secondary to vomiting or loss of intravascular volume, and, occasionally, arrhythmias. Common causes of *hypertension* (Chapter 67) include amphetamines, cocaine, ephedrine and similar agents, ergots, phencyclidine, nicotine, phenylpropanolamine, thyroid hormones, chronic yohimbine use, and chronic lead toxicity. Blood pressure can rise early in poisoning with cyclic antidepressants, central α_2-adrenergic agonists, and monoamine oxidase inhibitors.

Hyperthermia (Chapter 109) occurs with toxicants that cause agitation or excessive motor activity (e.g., cocaine, phencyclidine, monoamine oxidase inhibitors, strychnine), uncouple oxidative phosphorylation (e.g., salicylates, 2,4-dinitrophenol), increase the metabolic rate (thyroid hormones), impair sweating (e.g., first-generation antihistamines, anticholinergics, cocaine, phenothiazines, zonisamide), cause vasoconstriction (e.g., amphetamines, ephedrine), or impair vasodilation and alter perception of heat (cocaine). Other toxicant-induced states associated with hyperthermia include malignant hyperthermia, neuroleptic malignant syndrome, serotonin syndrome, metal fume fever, and hydrocarbon aspiration. Toxicant-induced *hypothermia* is typically due to sedative-hypnotics, opioids, barbiturates, ethanol, phenothiazines, or hypoglycemic agents such as insulin, sulfonylureas, meglitinides, or unripe akee fruit. Oxygen saturation (Figure 161-2 in Chapter 161) as measured by *pulse oximetry*, decreases with true hypoxemia (Figure 104-1 in Chapter 104) or methemoglobinemia (Chapter 161) but remains normal or may be increased in carbon monoxide poisoning (Chapter 94).

Eyes, Ears, Nose, and Throat

Toxicant-induced bilateral miosis (Fig. 110-1) has a limited differential diagnosis that includes central α_2-agonists such as clonidine, guanfacine, and the imidazolines; olanzapine; opioids; organophosphorus compounds or carbamates; therapeutic cholinesterase inhibitors (e.g., physostigmine); topical miotic ophthalmic drugs (e.g., pilocarpine, carbachol); and, variably, phencyclidine, phenothiazines, ethanol, and some sedative-hypnotics (Chapter 432). Pontine hemorrhage is the major nontoxicologic diagnosis to consider in a comatose patient with miotic pupils (Chapter 415). Mydriasis is a nonspecific finding. A unilateral dilated pupil may be due to topical ocular application of sympathomimetics (e.g., phenylephrine), antihistamines, or anticholinergic agents (e.g., inhaled anticholinergics such as ipratropium or tiotropium, dust or sap from *Datura* sp) and can be caused by a postauricular scopolamine patch. Failure of topical 4% pilocarpine ophthalmic drops to constrict the pupil supports the diagnosis of pupillary dilation from a topical mydriatic agent. Visual disturbances, including partial or total blindness as a result of systemic toxicity, have been reported with anticholinergic agents, carbon monoxide, digitalis, ethambutol, methanol, methyl bromide, quinine, and agents that are associated with pseudotumor cerebri, including antimicrobials (e.g., ampicillin, metronidazole, nalidixic acid, nitrofurantoin, sulfa drugs, tetracycline), glucocorticosteroids, lead, lithium, oral contraceptives, phenothiazines, phenytoin, and vitamin A. Nonarteritic anterior ischemic optic neuropathy has developed after the use of sildenafil and other related drugs (Chapter 242); the causal relationship is unknown.

Acute hearing loss (Chapter 436) can occur as a toxic effect of aminoglycosides, bromates, chloroquine, cisplatin, carboplatin, high-dose loop diuretics, nitrogen mustard, quinine, salicylates, vinblastine, and vincristine. Nasal septal erosions and perforations may be due to chronic exposure to intranasal cocaine (Chapter 33) or inhalation of fumes from chromium and nickel (Chapters 93 and 94).

Neurologic Signs

Many toxicants affect the central nervous system (CNS) and can produce agitated delirium, depression, or seizures (Table 110-2). Distinguishing features of various toxicants may assist in making the correct diagnosis. Patients withdrawing from opioids are alert and oriented, whereas patients withdrawing from alcohol, barbiturates, benzodiazepines, and other sedative-hypnotics can be disoriented. Initial CNS depression can also develop with large ingestions of acetaminophen or ibuprofen. Isoniazid and theophylline are noted for producing seizures refractory to the usual doses of benzodiazepines and barbiturates. Pyridoxine treats isoniazid-induced seizures by increasing CNS γ-aminobutyric acid; phenytoin is relatively ineffective for theophylline-induced seizures. Plant or mushroom ingestion can also produce CNS depression (e.g., *Rhododendron* sp, *Solanum* [bittersweet], *Taxus* [yew], *Sophora* [mescal bean]), CNS stimulation (e.g., *Catha edulis* [khat], *Strychnos nux vomica* [contains strychnine], *Cicuta* sp [water hemlock], *Ephedra* [Mormon tea]), atropine-like effects (e.g., *Atropa belladonna* [deadly

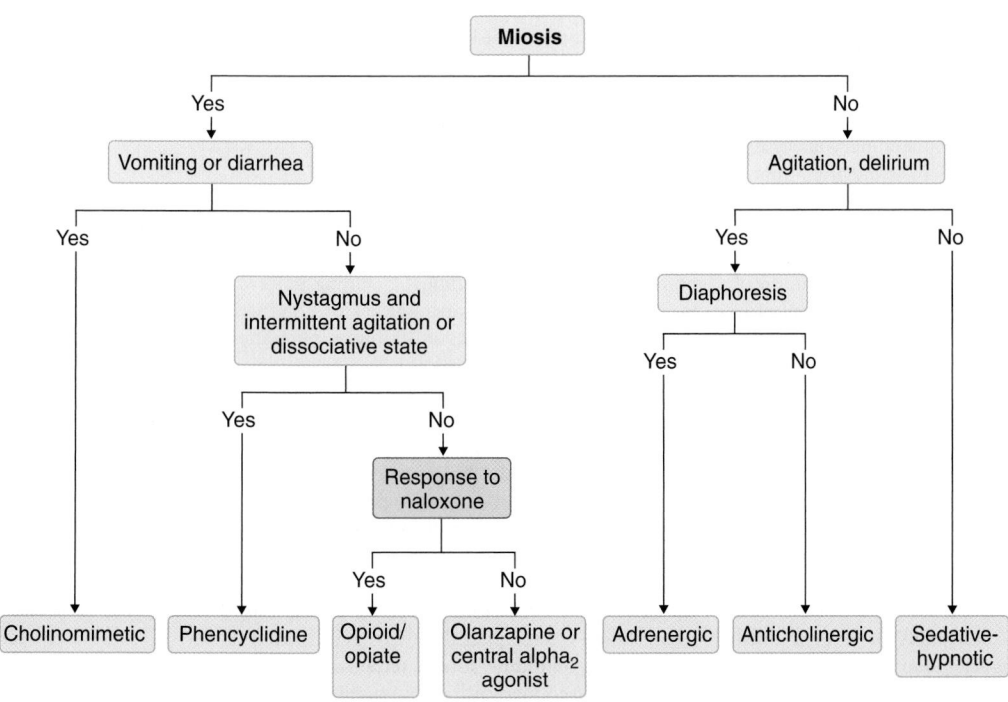

FIGURE 110-1. Diagnostic algorithm using the size of the pupils.

TABLE 110-2 CENTRAL NERVOUS SYSTEM EFFECTS OF TOXICANTS

TOXICANT CATEGORIES/AGENTS	CNS Effects		
	AGITATED DELIRIUM	DECREASED LEVEL OF CONSCIOUSNESS	SEIZURES
CATEGORIES			
Adrenergic agonists	•		•
Anticholinergic agents	•	•	•
Anticonvulsants		•	• (paradoxical with some agents)
Antipsychotic drugs	•	•	•
β-Adrenergic receptor antagonists		•	•
Hallucinogenic agents	•		•
Monoamine oxidase inhibitors	•	•	•
Opioids	• (propoxyphene, normeperidine, tramadol)	•	• (propoxyphene, normeperidine, tramadol)
Sedative-hypnotics		•	• (rare)
Serotonin agonists	•	•	•
AGENTS			
Amphetamines, cocaine	•		•
Antidepressants	•	•	• (can be delayed with bupropion)
Antihistamines (first generation, e.g., diphenhydramine)	•	•	
Barbiturates		•	
Benzodiazepines		•	
Cytochrome oxidase inhibitors (e.g., carbon monoxide, cyanide, hydrogen sulfide, azides)		•	•
Ephedra alkaloids and similar agents			•
Ethylene glycol, methanol	•	•	
γ-Hydroxybutyrate and precursors		•	• (rare)
Lithium		•	•
Organophosphorus compounds, carbamates (e.g., diazinon, malathion, fenthion, carbaryl)		•	
Salicylates	•	•	•
SSRIs/SRIs	•	•	• (uncommon)
Withdrawal from alcohol, barbiturates, benzodiazepines, other sedative-hypnotics	•		•
Withdrawal from opioids			• (reported only in neonates)

CNS = central nervous system; SRIs = serotonin re-uptake inhibitors; SSRIs = selective serotonin re-uptake inhibitors.

nightshade], *Datura* sp [jimsonweed]), and cholinomimetic effects (e.g., *Nicotiana* genus [tobacco], *Conium maculatum* [poison hemlock], *Inocybe* and *Clitocybe* mushrooms). Seizures can also occur with many of these plants and with mushrooms that contain gyromitrins (e.g., *Gyromitra* sp) and muscimol (e.g., *Amanita muscaria, Amanita pantherina*).

Distal axonopathy, a primary degeneration of peripheral nervous system axons with secondary degeneration of the myelin sheath, is the predominant type of toxicant-induced peripheral neuropathy. Common causative agents include acrylamide monomer, allyl chloride, arsenic (inorganic), capsaicin, carbon disulfide, chloramphenicol, cisplatin, colchicine, cyanate, dapsone, dideoxycytidine (ddC), dideoxyinosine (ddI), disulfiram, ethambutol, ethanol, ethylene oxide, gold salts, hexachlorophene, *n*-hexane, hydralazine, interferon, isoniazid, lead, linezolid, mercury, methyl bromide, methyl *n*-butyl ketone, metronidazole, nitrofurantoin, nitrous oxide, some organophosphorus compounds, phenol, platinum, podophyllotoxin, polychlorinated biphenyls, pyridoxine, tacrolimus, taxoids, thalidomide, thallium, vidarabine, vinca alkaloids, and vinyl chloride. Amiodarone, arsenic, and trichloroethylene can produce a demyelinating neuropathy, whereas pyridoxine can produce a sensory neuronopathy.

Neuronal transmission can be altered by aminoglycosides; the venom of *Latrodectus* species (widow spiders), scorpions (only the bark scorpion, *Centruroides exilicauda*, in the United States), and crotaline (e.g., rattlesnakes) and elapid snakes; brevetoxin (shellfish) and ciguatoxin (various fish); neuromuscular blocking drugs; nicotine and related alkaloids; paralytic shellfish toxins; saxitoxin (shellfish); organophosphorus compounds and carbamates; tetrodotoxin (puffer fish [fugu], blue-ringed octopus, salamanders, newts, and others); and veratridine (e.g., false hellebore). Cranial nerves can be affected by carbon disulfide, ciguatoxin, domoic acid (shellfish), elapid venom, ethylene glycol metabolites, paralytic shellfish toxins, bark scorpion, saxitoxin, tetrodotoxin, thallium, and trichloroethylene. Mononeuropathies and vasculitic neuropathies are unlikely to be induced by toxicants (Chapters 113 and 114).

Cardiopulmonary Effects

The examination should focus on blood pressure, heart rate, electrocardiographic abnormalities (e.g., rhythm, conduction, depolarization, repolarization), and pulmonary findings, including pulse oximetry. Drugs and other toxicants that can cause arrhythmias or conduction abnormalities include β-adrenergic receptor antagonists, butyrophenones (e.g., droperidol), L-type calcium-channel antagonists, cardiac glycosides (e.g., digoxin; bufadienolides, found in toxic toad venom and incorporated into some illicit aphrodisiacs; cardenolides, found in plants such as oleander and lily of the valley), chloral hydrate, chloroquine, cocaine, cyclic antidepressants, ethanol, halogenated hydrocarbons (e.g., halothane, trichloroethylene), magnesium, potassium, propoxyphene, thioridazine or mesoridazine, and antiarrhythmics and other agents that affect the myocardial voltage-gated sodium channels (e.g., bupivacaine, chloroquine, cocaine, cyclic antidepressants, flecainide, mexiletine, quinidine, procainamide, propafenone) and potassium channels (e.g., astemizole, cisapride, citalopram, erythromycin [especially when taken concomitantly with cytochrome P-450 A inhibitors; see Chapter 28], quinidine, sotalol, terfenadine). Bedside echocardiography may reveal depressed myocardial contractility as a result of agents that block the myocardial voltage-gated sodium channel, β-adrenergic receptor antagonists, calcium-channel antagonists, cyclic antidepressants, magnesium, arsenic, ciguatoxin, cyanide, ethanol, iron, scorpion venom, and tetrodotoxin.

Toxicants can produce myriad pulmonary effects, including airway irritation; parenchymal, pleural, and vascular diseases; and barotrauma. Immediate life-threatening toxic effects include acute lung injury and pulmonary edema, acute respiratory distress syndrome (ARDS; Chapter 104), and rapidly developing pulmonary fibrosis or bronchiolitis obliterans. Typical syndromes and etiologic agents include pulmonary edema (β-adrenergic receptor antagonists, calcium-channel antagonists, antiarrhythmics, daunorubicin, doxorubicin), acute lung injury or ARDS (amphetamines, cadmium, chlorine, cocaine, ethchlorvynol, methotrexate, opioids, heroin, paraquat, salicylates; inhalation of smoke, zinc chloride, methyl bromide, methyl chloride), and rapidly developing pulmonary fibrosis or bronchiolitis obliterans (nitrogen dioxide, paraquat).

Gastrointestinal Effects

Symptoms of nausea, vomiting, diarrhea, and abdominal pain are nonspecific and must be interpreted in the context of other findings. Agents that produce severe or life-threatening toxicity with early gastrointestinal findings include acid or large alkali ingestions; cardiac glycosides, colchicines, and other microtubular toxicants; iron; metals such as arsenic, acute high-level lead, mercury salts, or thallium; mushrooms containing amanitine (*Amanita phalloides, Amanita virosa, Amanita verna, Lepiota chlorophyllum*), gyromitrins (*Gyromitra esculenta*), orellanines (*Cortinarius orellanus*), or allenic norleucine (*Amanita smithiana*); nicotine; organophosphorus compounds; and theophylline. Severe abdominal pain and rigidity can occur with envenomation by *Latrodectus* species (widow spiders). Right upper quadrant tenderness develops with toxic hepatitis. Hepatotoxicity can occur as an adverse effect of the therapeutic use of many drugs; in the United States, acetaminophen and ethanol are the most common causes of toxicant-induced hepatotoxicity (Chapter 152). Other notable hepatotoxicants include aflatoxins (in food contaminated with *Aspergillus flavus*), arsenicals, carbon tetrachloride, copper sulfate, cyclopeptide mushrooms (e.g., *Amanita phalloides*), *Ephedra* species (e.g., ma huang), iron, methamphetamine, pennyroyal oil, pyrrolizidine alkaloids (various plant species used in herbal teas), and vitamin A in chronic excessive doses.

Dermatologic Signs

The skin, hair, nails, and mucous membranes should be examined for evidence of intravenous drug use; the presence or absence of skin and mucous membrane moisture; abnormal skin coloration, including erythema and cyanosis; alopecia; and nail abnormalities. Bullous skin lesions have been reported with chronic barbiturate use, glutethimide, carbon monoxide, meprobamate, methadone, and valproic acid. Cyanosis may reflect hypoxemia or methemoglobinemia. Commonly used agents that can cause methemoglobinemia include aniline dyes, benzocaine and other amide anesthetics, dapsone, naphthalene, nitrates, nitrites, phenazopyridine, rifampin, and sulfonamides. Skin erythema or flushing occurs with anticholinergic agents, boric acid ingestion, monosodium glutamate, niacin, scombroid toxicity as a result of the ingestion of inadequately refrigerated fish with a high histidine content (e.g., tuna, mahi-mahi, amberjack), vancomycin, and interactions between ethanol and numerous agents that produce disulfiram or disulfiram-like reactions (e.g., carbon disulfide, some cephalosporins, *Coprinus atramentarius* mushroom, disulfiram, griseofulvin, metronidazole, thiuram herbicides, trichloroethylene).

Specific Toxicants

Some common toxicants can be suspected from their characteristic manifestations (Table 110-3). These suspicions should guide specific diagnostic and therapeutic strategies that complement general decontamination and supportive treatments.

Diagnostic Tests

Drug testing should be guided by the history and physical examination, with emphasis on tests that can influence management. Rapid qualitative urine drug screening tests are readily available in most hospitals, but their clinical value is limited by the number of drugs that can be tested and the reliability of the tests themselves. A positive test result may be unrelated to the patient's condition because drug analytes may be detectable within hours to more than 30 days after drug use, depending on the drug, dose, and frequency of use. False-positive and false-negative results occur (Table 110-4), and the

screening result must be verified with a second method, such as gas chromatography–mass spectrometry. The type of drug use in a population should be considered when determining the drugs to be screened to decrease the incidence of false-positive results. A test with 99% specificity for a drug with a prevalence of 0.1% in a population would produce 10 false-positive results for every true-positive result. Clinically irrelevant true-positive findings also occur, such as when poppy seeds produce a positive opiate test. Failure to consider these limitations of drug screens can result in misdiagnosis.

For a limited number of drugs and toxicants, levels in blood or urine are useful for diagnosis, therapy, or monitoring (Table 110-5). Threshold levels of certain toxicants indicate the need for specific therapies: acetaminophen (*N*-acetylcysteine), ethylene glycol (fomepizole and hemodialysis), iron (deferoxamine), methanol (fomepizole and hemodialysis), methemoglobin (methylene blue), salicylates (urine alkalinization and hemodialysis), and theophylline (hemoperfusion or hemodialysis). In chronic poisoning with some drugs, such as salicylates or theophylline, these therapies may be indicated at lower drug levels. In general, any end-organ toxicity that is evident or anticipated (based on the toxicant, amount ingested, and time required to produce toxic effects) is more important than a specific level in determining the need for treatment.

Occult acetaminophen ingestion with toxic serum levels occurs in 0.3 to 1.9% of intentional ingestions. Given that these patients may be asymptomatic until hepatotoxicity develops and that administration of an antidote can prevent this hepatotoxicity, the current recommendation is to test for acetaminophen in all patients with intentional ingestions.

Other Blood Tests

Anion gap metabolic acidosis resulting from primary lactic acidosis can be caused by cyanide, hydrogen sulfide, iron, isoniazid, metformin, nucleoside reverse transcriptase inhibitors, phenformin, sodium azide, and, rarely, acetaminophen with high serum levels. Anion gap metabolic acidosis not related to lactic acidosis occurs with diethylene glycol, ethylene glycol, nonsteroidal anti-inflammatory drugs (NSAIDs), methanol, salicylates, theophylline, and toluene. In poisonings resulting from ibuprofen, methanol, propylene glycol, and salicylates, lactic acid can also be produced, but the level is insufficient to account for the anion gap. Anion gap metabolic acidosis can also develop in patients with ongoing agitation, hyperthermia, and muscle rigidity, such as in neuroleptic malignant syndrome (Chapter 442), or in some cases of rhabdomyolysis (Chapter 115) secondary to toxicants such as doxylamine, phencyclidine, strychnine, cocaine, and amphetamines. Elevated serum creatinine and blood urea nitrogen levels indicative of declining renal function may be seen with numerous toxicants. Direct toxicity occurs with acetaminophen, aminoglycosides, cadmium, Chinese weight-loss botanicals (containing *Stephania tetrandra* or *Magnolia officinalis*), chromium, *Crotalus durissus* venom, diethylene glycol, diquat, ethylene glycol, fluorinated anesthetics, gold, heroin, lithium (diabetes insipidus), mercury salts, mushrooms (*Amanita smithiana* and *Cortinarius* sp), paraquat, radiocontrast agents, solvents (e.g., carbon tetrachloride, trichloroethylene, tetrachloroethylene, toluene), and sulfonamides. Agents that decrease glomerular perfusion by reducing renal blood flow include amphotericin, angiotensin-converting enzyme inhibitors, angiotensin receptor blockers, cocaine, cyclosporine, mannitol (excessive chronic doses), methotrexate, and NSAIDs.

Imaging

A computed tomographic scan of the head can detect life-threatening cerebral edema secondary to toxicant-induced hepatic failure, ethylene glycol, and methanol. It also detects intracranial bleeding caused by anticoagulant drugs and rodenticides, scorpion venom, and sympathomimetics (e.g., amphetamines, cocaine, phenylpropanolamine). An abdominal radiograph can reveal radiopaque ferrous sulfate tablets or metals such as arsenic, lead, mercury, and thallium.

Diagnostic Syndromes

Given the myriad combinations of signs, symptoms, and laboratory findings, making the correct diagnosis in a noncommunicative patient can be daunting. A thorough history from bystanders, friends, and prehospital medical personnel may yield crucial information. Additionally, the diagnostic possibilities can be narrowed by noting a finding to limit that list. For example, consider a patient with sudden loss of consciousness, anion gap metabolic acidosis, and bradycardia without hypoxemia. Among the possible causes of anion gap metabolic acidosis (see earlier) and sudden loss of consciousness

TABLE 110-3 PATHOPHYSIOLOGY, CLINICAL EFFECTS, AND MANAGEMENT OF SPECIFIC DRUGS AND TOXICANTS

DRUG OR TOXICANT	PATHOPHYSIOLOGY	CLINICAL EFFECTS	LABORATORY	SPECIFIC THERAPY
Acetaminophen	NAPQI (toxic metabolite) binds hepatic and renal tubular cells; acetaminophen itself induces transient decrease in functional factor VII	Initial: nausea, vomiting, coma, lactic acidosis in severe cases Days 1-3: elevated INR, aminotransferase, and bilirubin levels; RUQ tenderness; increased creatinine level in severe cases Days 4-14: gradual recovery or continued increase in INR and creatinine, lactic acidosis, coma, cerebral edema, death	Potentially toxic level ≥ 150 µg/mL 4 hr after ingestion* INR may be transiently elevated in first 24 hr because of decrease in functional factor VII; further increases indicate hepatic necrosis; elevated aminotransferase and bilirubin levels not predictive of hepatic failure Creatinine elevated in severe cases	NAC (see dosing guidelines in Table 110-6); NAC can increase INR but not aPTT[†]
Amphetamines	Increased release of presynaptic norepinephrine and dopamine Increased serotonin release (especially MDMA, PMA, DOB, other synthetic amphetamines)	Mild: euphoria, decreased appetite, repetitive behavior Moderate: vomiting, agitation, hypertension, tachycardia, mydriasis, bruxism, diaphoresis Severe: hypertension or hypotension, arrhythmias, hyperthermia, seizures, coma, hepatotoxicity, rhabdomyolysis, DIC, hyponatremia (SIADH), renal failure, cerebral infarction or hemorrhage	Not helpful; many false-positives and false-negatives on screening tests (see Table 110-4)	IV crystalloids External cooling Benzodiazepines or barbiturates to control agitation or seizures Benzodiazepines or nitroprusside for hypertension See SSRIs/SRIs for features and treatment of serotonin syndrome
β-Adrenergic receptor antagonists	Blocks catecholamines from β-adrenergic receptors α- and β-adrenergic receptor antagonism: carvedilol, labetalol Delayed rectifier potassium-channel blockade: sotalol	Bradyarrhythmias, decreased myocardial contractility, hypotension, respiratory depression, decreased consciousness with seizures or coma (lipophilic agents, e.g., propranolol), prolonged QT interval (sotalol)	ECG No specific tests	IV glucagon, 3.5-5 mg over 2-min period; if no increase in BP or HR, can repeat up to 10 mg; if effective, immediately start continuous infusion at 2-10 mg/hr; if still unstable, options include (1) regular insulin, 1 U/kg by IV bolus, followed by 1 U/kg/hr, plus dextrose to maintain euglycemia; (2) norepinephrine or dobutamine infusion titrated to desirable BP and HR; (3) IV milrinone, 50 µg/kg over 10-min period, then 0.375-0.75 µg/kg/min based on hemodynamic status[†] Electrical pacing and IABP in refractory cases
L-type calcium-channel antagonists	Blocks L-type voltage-sensitive calcium channels, thereby decreasing calcium entry into myocardial and vascular smooth muscle cells Decreases pancreatic insulin release and increases insulin resistance	Bradyarrhythmias (verapamil, diltiazem), hypotension, hyperglycemia	ECG No specific tests	IV 10% calcium chloride, 10-20 mg/kg (0.1-0.2 mL/kg); can repeat once; if BP improves, continuous infusion at 0.2-0.5 mL/kg/hr (20-50 mg/kg/hr) Ionized Ca²⁺ levels should not exceed 2× normal (severe cases will be refractory to calcium therapy) Glucagon, high-dose insulin and dextrose, catecholamines, and milrinone (as for β-adrenergic antagonists)

Cardiac glycosides, including digoxin, bufadienolides (toxic toad venom), or cardenolides (e.g., oleander, lily of the valley, dogbane)	Inhibits Na⁺,K⁺-ATPase
	Decreased CNS sympathetic output
	Decreased baroreceptor sensitivity
	Increased vagal acetylcholine discharge
		Bradyarrhythmias, including second- and third-degree AV block and asystole
		Ventricular ectopy, tachycardia, fibrillation
		Junctional tachycardia, paroxysmal atrial tachycardia with block
		Weakness, visual disturbances, nausea, vomiting
			Serum digoxin level
			Serum potassium (hyperkalemia occurs in acute poisoning; hypokalemia may be present in chronic poisoning), magnesium, and creatinine levels
				Correct hypokalemia and hypomagnesemia; do not give calcium
				Digoxin-specific antibody fragments (Fab) indicated if patient has hemodynamically significant arrhythmias, serum potassium ≥5 mg/L, Mobitz II or third-degree AV block, ingestion of bufadienolide- or cardenolide-containing agents, or renal insufficiency
				Empirical dose
				  Chronic: 2-5 vials
				  Acute: 10-20 vials
				Calculated dose
				  Chronic: number of vials = 2 × serum digoxin level (ng/mL) × 5.6 × weight (kg)/1000
				  Acute: number of vials = 2 × oral digoxin dose (mg) × 0.8

Cyclic antidepressants	Myocardial sodium- and potassium-channel blockade Blockade of α-adrenergic and cholinergic muscarinic receptors Inhibition of norepinephrine re-uptake	Decreased level of consciousness (can develop rapidly), myoclonus, seizures, coma Anticholinergic toxidrome (see Table 110-1) Sinus tachycardia, ventricular conduction delays, ventricular arrhythmias, asystole Hypotension	Serum levels not helpful in management	Intermittent IV boluses of NaHCO₃ (1 mEq/kg) to maintain arterial pH at 7.5 because acidemia can worsen cardiovascular complications Intubation and neuroparalytic drugs may be useful to ameliorate acidemia from muscular hyperactivity while seizures are being treated Contraindicated drugs: types IA and IC antiarrhythmic agents, physostigmine, flumazenil

TABLE 110-3 PATHOPHYSIOLOGY, CLINICAL EFFECTS, AND MANAGEMENT OF SPECIFIC DRUGS AND TOXICANTS—cont'd

DRUG OR TOXICANT	PATHOPHYSIOLOGY	CLINICAL EFFECTS	LABORATORY	SPECIFIC THERAPY
Ethylene glycol, methanol (e.g., antifreeze, window cleaners, camping stove fuels)	Ethylene glycol: toxic metabolites produce cytotoxicity in CNS, kidneys, lungs, heart, liver, muscles; metabolic acidosis is due to glycolate accumulation; oxalate complexes with calcium, so hypocalcemia can develop Methanol: metabolized to formic acid, which is responsible for metabolic acidosis and inhibition of cytochrome aa₃; target organs include retina, optic nerve, CNS	Ethylene glycol: CNS depression, cerebral edema, seizures, anion gap metabolic acidosis, renal failure with acute tubular necrosis, pulmonary edema, myositis Methanol: nausea, vomiting; cerebral edema, hemorrhage, infarcts; necrosis of thalamus and putamen; anion gap metabolic acidosis; visual disturbances, papilledema, hyperemic optic disc, nonreactive pupils	Serum ethylene glycol and methanol levels; levels may be low or undetectable if significant metabolism has occurred Ethylene glycol: serum calcium, creatinine, BUN levels; examine urine for calcium oxalate crystals; false hyperlactatemia occurs with certain analyzers using L-lactate oxidase, which cross-reacts with glycolic and glyoxylic acids	For both: fomepizole (which inhibits alcohol dehydrogenase and blocks formation of toxic metabolites), 15 mg/kg IV loading dose, then 10 mg/kg IV for 4 doses during the next 48 hr, then 15 mg/kg for subsequent doses; interval dosing is q12h (q4h during hemodialysis, with dosing interval adjustments at start and finish); continue until ethylene glycol or methanol is no longer detectable Use of ethanol is no longer recommended Hemodialysis: initiate if level is ≥50 mg/dL or metabolic acidosis with end-organ toxicity; continue until acidosis resolves and serum level of ethylene glycol or methanol is undetectable Monitor for cerebral edema with possible herniation Ethylene glycol: IV calcium for symptomatic hypocalcemia Methanol: folinic acid, 50 mg IV q4h until methanol not detectable and acidosis cleared
γ-Hydroxybutyrate (GHB) and its precursors (γ-butyrolactone and 1,4-butanediol [1,4-BD])	Agonist effect on CNS GHB receptors; indirect action with opioid receptors (may increase proenkephalins); metabolized to GABA, interacts with GABAᴮ receptors; decreases dopamine release	CNS: rapid loss of consciousness, with recovery typical within 2-4 hr; myoclonus (possible seizures) Respiratory depression; bradycardia; nausea, vomiting	No specific tests	Supportive care, including respiratory support as needed Withdrawal resembles sedative-hypnotic withdrawal and can be treated with benzodiazepines or pentobarbital
Lithium	Decreases brain inositol; alters CNS serotonin, dopamine, and norepinephrine; inhibits adenylate cyclases, including those that mediate vasopressin-induced renal concentration and thyroid function	Chronic toxicity usually more severe than acute toxicity: tremor, hyperreflexia, drowsiness, incoordination, clonus, confusion, ataxia; in severe cases, seizures, coma, death; recovery may take weeks, and CNS deficits may persist Sinus node dysfunction, QT prolongation, T wave abnormalities, U waves Nephrogenic diabetes insipidus, hypothyroidism, hyperthyroidism, hypercalcemia, pseudotumor cerebri Acute toxicity: nausea, vomiting, diarrhea, and milder neurologic findings	Peak serum levels: Normal dose 2-3 hr; up to 5 hr for sustained-release lithium Acute overdose Peak may be delayed ≥4-12 hr	Replenish intravascular volume, maintain urinary output at 1-2 mL/kg/hr Consider GI decontamination with oral polyethylene glycol electrolyte solution within 1-2 hr after acute overdose of sustained-release drug Hemodialysis§ in patients with altered mental status, ataxia, seizures, or coma or in patients with mild symptoms in the setting of acute overdose or renal insufficiency Ineffective or contraindicated therapies include oral activated charcoal, diuretics, and aminophylline
Opioids (e.g., heroin, morphine, oxycodone, fentanyl)	Agonist effect at CNS μ, κ, and δ opioid receptors; result is cell hyperpolarization and decreased neurotransmitter release	CNS depression, respiratory depression, miosis (see Table 110-1) Dextromethorphan increases CNS serotonin and inhibits NMDA receptors, which causes hallucinations Propoxyphene and its metabolite norpropoxyphene block sodium channels and can cause seizures and wide-complex arrhythmias similar to cyclic antidepressants; NaHCO₃ treats arrhythmias Seizure risk with tramadol, meperidine, propoxyphene Rapid, powerful heroin-like effect when sustained-release oxycodone is crushed before ingestion, snorting, or smoking QTc prolongation and torsades de pointes with methadone	Rapid urine drug screens detect morphine and codeine but may not detect semisynthetic and synthetic opioids; some interferents/irrelevants (see Table 110-4)	IV naloxone, 0.4-2 mg; can repeat up to 10 mg if no response Continuous infusion for recurrent symptoms or sustained-release opioid ingestion; give 50% of dose that produces desired effect 15 min after initial effect is obtained, then infuse two thirds of this dose every hr; infusion rate can be increased or decreased to maintain normal respiration and avoid withdrawal symptoms Contraindicated therapies: nalmefene and naltrexone should not be used for acute opioid reversal

TABLE 110-3 PATHOPHYSIOLOGY, CLINICAL EFFECTS, AND MANAGEMENT OF SPECIFIC DRUGS AND TOXICANTS—cont'd

DRUG OR TOXICANT	PATHOPHYSIOLOGY	CLINICAL EFFECTS	LABORATORY	SPECIFIC THERAPY
Organophosphorus compounds and carbamates (e.g., diazinon, mevinphos, fenthion, aldicarb)	Inhibits acetylcholinesterase, resulting in excessive acetylcholine stimulation of nicotinic and muscarinic receptors in autonomic and somatic motor nervous systems and CNS	Nicotinic-mediated effects: tachycardia, mydriasis, hypertension, delirium, coma, seizures, muscle weakness, fasciculations Muscarinic-mediated effects: salivation, lacrimation, urination, vomiting, defecation, miosis, bronchorrhea, bronchospasm, bradycardia	Serum (butyrylcholinesterase) or RBC (acetylcholinesterase) activity <50% of normal (see Table 110-6) Clinical recovery occurs before serum cholinesterase levels normalize	Atropine, 1-2 mg by initial IV bolus; double the dose every 5 min (2 mg, 4 mg, 8 mg, 16 mg, etc) until drying of bronchial secretions, adequate oxygenation, pulse >80 bpm, systolic blood pressure >80 mm Hg achieved; continuous infusion at 10- 20% of total stabilizing dose per hr; stop infusion if patient develops any signs or symptoms of anticholinergic toxidrome (see Table 110-1); restart infusion at lower rate when signs or symptoms abate Pralidoxime‖ chloride 30 mg/kg (maximum 2 g) IV bolus over 30 min, then 8-10 mg/kg/hr (maximum 650 mg/hr) continuous infusion; administer as soon as possible after poisoning; continue 12-24 hr after atropine no longer required and symptoms resolve🄋
Salicylates	Inhibits cyclooxygenase; decreases formation of prostaglandins and thromboxane A₂; stimulates CNS medullary respiratory receptor and chemoreceptor trigger zone; impairs platelet function; disrupts carbohydrate metabolism; uncouples oxidative phosphorylation; increases vascular permeability	Acute toxicity Mild: nausea, vomiting, diaphoresis, tinnitus, decreased hearing, hyperpnea, tachypnea Moderate–severe: confusion, delirium, coma, seizures, hyperthermia, ALI; death can occur within hours of overdose Chronic toxicity: same as acute, but may not have diaphoresis or vomiting Consider diagnosis in patients with new-onset confusion, anion gap metabolic acidosis, or ALI	Serum salicylate level: toxic ≥30 mg/dL; level ≥100 mg/dL indicates life-threatening toxicity with possible sudden, rapid clinical deterioration; in chronic toxicity, levels may be minimally elevated (>30 mg/dL), and clinical evaluation is more reliable for gauging degree of toxicity Arterial blood gases: respiratory alkalosis with metabolic acidosis Anion gap metabolic acidosis Prolonged PT and PTT, ketonuria, ketonemia	Multidose activated charcoal q2-3h in acute overdose with progressive symptoms or rising salicylate level
SSRIs/SRIs	Inhibits re-uptake of serotonin SRIs have additional effects (e.g., duloxetine inhibits norepinephrine re-uptake, nefazodone inhibits serotonergic 5-HT2 receptors, trazodone inhibits peripheral α-adrenergic receptors, venlafaxine inhibits norepinephrine and dopamine re-uptake)	Vomiting, blurred vision, CNS depression, tachycardia Seizures and coma rare Torsades de pointes reported with citalopram Serotonin syndrome: clonus, agitation, tremor, diaphoresis, hyperreflexia; hyperthermia and hypertonicity in severe cases	No specific tests If serotonin syndrome suspected: electrolytes, BUN, glucose, liver enzymes, coagulation panel, blood gases, chest radiograph	Respiratory support as needed Benzodiazepines for agitation or seizures Serotonin syndrome: consider cyproheptadine, 12 mg PO initial dose, then 2 mg PO q2h (to a maximum of 32 mg/day) until symptoms resolve Critical care therapies for hyperthermia, rhabdomyolysis, DIC, ARDS, renal and hepatic dysfunction, torsades de pointes

*A nomogram to evaluate the potential toxicity of levels drawn more than 4 hours after ingestion is provided in Rumack BH, Matthew H. Acetaminophen poisoning and toxicity. *Pediatrics.* 1975;55:871-876. The nomogram is valid only for levels drawn after a single acute ingestion.

†NAC can be discontinued in patients with uncomplicated disease after a loading dose plus six maintenance doses if hepatic aminotransferase levels are normal and acetaminophen is not detected; otherwise, the full regimen should be administered.

‡Adjust infusion for reduced renal function.

§Continue hemodialysis until the serum lithium level is less than 1 mEq/L. Recheck the level 8 hours after dialysis, and restart hemodialysis if the level is higher than 1 mEq/L. Repeat this cycle until the serum lithium level remains lower than 1 mEq/L.

‖A double-blind, randomized, placebo-controlled trial of pralidoxime in acute organophosphorus poisoning found no significant difference in mortality rates or need for intubation.🄋

ALI = acute lung injury; aPTT = activated partial thromboplastin time; ARDS = acute respiratory distress syndrome; AV = atrioventricular; BP = blood pressure; bpm = beats per minute; BUN = blood urea nitrogen; CNS = central nervous system; DIC = disseminated intravascular coagulation; DOB = 4-bromo-2,5-dimethoxyamphetamine; ECG = electrocardiogram; GABA = γ-aminobutyric acid; GI = gastrointestinal; HR = heart rate; IABP = intra-aortic balloon counterpulsation; INR = international normalized ratio; IV = intravenous; MDMA = 3,4-methylenedioxymethamphetamine; Na⁺,K⁺-ATPase = sodium, potassium adenosine triphosphatase; NAC = N-acetylcysteine; NAPQI = N-acetyl-p-benzoquinone imine; NMDA = N-methyl-D-aspartate; PMA = paramethoxyamphetamine; PT = prothrombin time; PTT = partial thromboplastin time; RBC = red blood cell; RUQ = right upper quadrant (abdomen); SIADH = syndrome of inappropriate antidiuretic secretion; SRI = serotonin re-uptake inhibitor; SSRI = selective serotonin re-uptake inhibitor.

are hydrogen sulfide, cyanide, and severe poisoning with sodium azide; however, sinus bradycardia in the absence of acute ischemic injury is typical only of cyanide poisoning.

TREATMENT   Rx

Initial Stabilization

Intubation and Respiratory Support

Appropriate airway management should be instituted to correct hypoxemia and respiratory acidosis and to protect against pulmonary aspiration (Fig. 110-2); intubation should be considered if the patient has depressed consciousness and a decreased gag reflex. Rapid-sequence intubation facilitates airway management. Anatomic difficulties should be anticipated in patients with caustic ingestions (hypopharyngeal burns that may perforate); angioedema caused by angiotensin-converting enzyme inhibitor therapy or envenomation by some rattlesnakes, such as the canebrake (*Crotalus horridus atricaudatus*) and eastern diamondback (*Crotalus adamanteus*) (Chapter 113); and swelling secondary to direct tissue injury (e.g., huffing Freon, snakebite on the tongue) or secondary to anaphylactoid and anaphylactic reactions. Endotracheal intubation via flexible fiberoptic nasopharyngoscopy may be indicated in these cases. Hypoxemia can occur with toxicants that produce CNS depression, such as antidepressants, barbiturates, sedative-hypnotics, and central α₂-adrenergic receptor agonists (clonidine), or agents causing peripheral neuromuscular impairment, such as nicotine, organophosphorus

TABLE 110-4 QUALITATIVE URINE DRUG SCREENS: CAUSES OF ERRONEOUS RESULTS*

DRUG/TOXICANT	INTERFERENTS/IRRELEVANTS†	COMMENTS
Amphetamines	Amantadine, bupropion, chlorpromazine, ephedrine, pseudoephedrine, desoxyephedrine, *Ephedra* sp, mexiletine, phenylephrine, phenylpropanolamine, selegiline, trazodone	Vicks nasal inhaler (desoxyephedrine) and selegiline also cause positive GC-MS findings; chiral confirmation is required; newer immunoassays have eliminated false-positive results from desoxyephedrine Interferents in older assays include labetalol and ranitidine
Benzodiazepines	Oxaprozin, sertraline	Poor detection of parent drugs with absent or low concentration of oxazepam metabolite (e.g., alprazolam, lorazepam, triazolam)
Cocaine	Coca leaf teas	Urine is most reliable for detecting true positives
Opiates, opioids	Dextromethorphan, poppy seeds, quinine, quinolones, rifampin	Does not detect semisynthetic or designer opioids (e.g., fentanyls, meperidine, methadone, propoxyphene)
Phencyclidine	Dextromethorphan, diphenhydramine, doxylamine, ibuprofen, ketamine, meperidine, mesoridazine, thioridazine, tramadol, venlafaxine	
Tetrahydrocannabinol	Dronabinol, efavirenz, proton pump inhibitors	Positive result is seldom clinically relevant; synthetic cannabinomimetics are not detected
Tricyclic antidepressants	Carbamazepine, cyclobenzaprine, cyproheptadine, diphenhydramine, phenothiazines, quetiapine	

*Advances in drug screening and variability in immunoassay results should be considered by the clinician when interpreting qualitative drug screening results. Consultation with the testing laboratory is advised. Positive screening results are considered presumptive and should be verified by GC-MS.
†Irrelevants are agents causing true-positive but clinically irrelevant results on laboratory screening tests; they vary, depending on the screening method.
GC-MS = gas chromatography–mass spectrometry.

TABLE 110-5 CLINICALLY IMPORTANT QUANTITATIVE DRUG LEVELS

DRUG OR TOXICANT	Levels	
	THERAPEUTIC	TOXIC
SOURCE: BLOOD OR SERUM		
Acetaminophen*	10-30 µg/mL	≥150 g/mL 4 hr after ingestion†
Carbamazepine	4-12 µg/mL	>15 g/mL
Carboxyhemoglobin	Nonsmoker: 0.5-1.5% Smoker: 4-9%	>20%‡
Cholinesterase§		
Serum (butyrylcholinesterase)	3100-6500 U/L	<50% of normal value
Red blood cell (acetylcholinesterase)	26.7-49.2 U/g of hemoglobin	<50% of normal value
Digoxin (≥12 hr after dose for long-term therapy)	0.8-2.0 ng/mL‖	>2.0 ng/mL
Ethanol	None measured	>80-100 mg/dL
Ethylene glycol	None measured	>25 mg/dL
Iron	50-175 µg/dL	>350 g/dL
Lead	<10 µg/dL	>25 g/dL
Lithium	0.6-1.2 mEq/L	>1.2 mEq/L§
Methanol	None measured	>20 mg/dL
Methemoglobin	1-2%	>15%
Phenobarbital	15-40 µg/mL	>40 g/mL
Phenytoin	10-20 µg/mL	>20 g/mL
Salicylates	≤30 mg/dL	>30 mg/dL
Theophylline	8-20 µg/mL	>20 g/mL
Valproic acid	50-100 µg/mL	>100 g/mL
SOURCE: URINE		
Arsenic	None measured	>100 g/24-hr urine¶
Mercury	None measured	>20 g/L¶
Thallium	None measured	>200 g/L¶

*False-positive levels of 16-28 µg/mL have been reported in patients with bilirubin levels greater than 17 mg/dL.
†Levels drawn more than 4 hours after ingestion should be plotted on the nomogram provided by Rumack and Matthew (Rumack BH, Matthew H. Acetaminophen poisoning and toxicity. *Pediatrics.* 1975;55:871-876) to assess the potential for toxicity.
‡Lower levels may be toxic in pregnant patients and in those with prolonged exposure to carbon monoxide.
§Consult a reference laboratory for normal values; results are assay dependent.
‖Some patients may require levels above the therapeutic range to control symptoms.
¶Lower values may indicate toxicity if appropriate clinical findings are present.

FIGURE 110-2. Algorithm for the management of acute poisoning. AC = activated charcoal; ALS = advanced life support; BARAs = β-adrenergic receptor antagonists; CCAs = L-type calcium-channel antagonists; HF = hydrofluoric acid; MDAC = multidose activated charcoal; NS = 0.9% saline solution; PEG = nonabsorbable polyethylene glycol solution.

compounds, strychnine, tetrodotoxin (puffer fish, blue-ringed octopus), botulinum, or envenomation from elapids (coral snake), Mojave rattlesnakes, or certain coelenterates (box jellyfish, Portuguese man-of-war) (Chapters 113 and 114).

Respiratory acidosis can rapidly worsen the toxicities of cyclic antidepressants and salicylates; sedation of these patients should be accompanied by immediate airway support. Intoxicated patients may have an increased risk for pulmonary aspiration because of concomitant CNS depression, attenuated airway reflexes, full stomachs, and delayed gastric emptying.

Succinylcholine can cause prolonged paralysis in patients with organophosphorus poisoning and can exacerbate hyperkalemia from cardiac glycosides, hydrofluoric acid, or rhabdomyolysis (Chapter 115). Rhabdomyolysis has been reported with adrenergic agents, doxylamine, phencyclidine, heroin, *Tricholoma equestre* mushrooms, and envenomation by crotaline snakes,

scorpions, or widow spiders (*Lactrodectus* sp); short-acting nondepolarizing agents, such as vecuronium and rocuronium, are preferable in these cases.

Advanced Life Support

Standard emergency cardiovascular care algorithms (Chapter 63) must be modified for effects caused by specific poisons. Atropine often does not reverse bradycardia secondary to β-adrenergic receptor antagonists, L-type calcium-channel antagonists, or cardiac glycosides. In these cases, more specific therapy with intravenous calcium (calcium-channel antagonists), high doses of glucagon (β-adrenergic receptor antagonists, calcium-channel antagonists), or digoxin-specific Fab antibody (cardiac glycosides) is indicated. High-dose insulin-glucose therapy can successfully reverse myocardial depression and conduction abnormalities in humans poisoned with β-adrenergic receptor antagonists and calcium-channel antagonists. Intravenous sodium bicarbonate may reverse cardiac conduction delays caused by antiarrhythmic drugs with sodium-channel blockade recovery rates of greater than 1 second (Vaughn-Williams classification IA and IC), cocaine, cyclic antidepressants, diphenhydramine, propoxyphene, and quinine. β-Adrenergic receptor antagonists are contraindicated in patients with cocaine-induced myocardial syndromes, but phentolamine can reverse the agonistic effects of cocaine on α-adrenergic receptors. Benzodiazepines can reverse significant sinus tachycardia from sympathomimetic agents. Calcium may also be life-saving in systemic hydrofluoric acid poisoning and severe hypermagnesemia, and it is indicated for symptomatic hypocalcemia caused by ethylene glycol toxicity. Drug-induced hypertension may be transitory; nitroprusside should be used if treatment is clinically indicated. In patients with toxicant-induced circulatory collapse refractory to maximal therapy, including vasopressors, circulatory assist devices may support the patient until sufficient toxicant is eliminated (Chapter 107).

Decontamination
Activated Charcoal
Single-dose activated charcoal without prior gastric emptying has been the preferred method of treatment for the ingestion of substances that have the potential to cause moderate to life-threatening toxicity and are known to adsorb to activated charcoal. The absence of clinical signs and symptoms does not preclude administering activated charcoal, because drug absorption and toxicity can be delayed. Activated charcoal can also be administered when the ingested toxicant cannot be identified but significant toxicity is a concern. Activated charcoal consists of pyrolysis products that have been specially cleaned to produce an internal pore structure to which substances can reversibly adsorb, thus preventing their absorption by the gastrointestinal tract. Activated charcoal can be administered with antiemetic drugs or given through a nasogastric tube, when necessary. The oral dose is approximately 1 g/kg body weight, with a maximum single dose of 100 g. Efficacy in preventing toxicant absorption declines with time, so activated charcoal should be given as soon as possible after ingestion. A large randomized trial in Sri Lankan hospitals showed no benefit of activated charcoal in reducing mortality,[1] but 87% of the study patients had ingested a pesticide or yellow oleander (which contains a cardiac glycoside); the applicability of this study's findings to populations in which other toxicants are more commonly ingested is unknown. Activated charcoal should not be used in patients with CNS depression until the airway is secure to minimize aspiration; the patient's head should also be elevated unless contraindicated. Activated charcoal is contraindicated in patients with a perforated bowel, functional or mechanical bowel obstruction, ingestion of a pure aliphatic hydrocarbon such as gasoline or kerosene (no benefit and increased risk for aspiration), and ingestion of caustic acid and alkali (no benefit and obscures endoscopy). Certain agents, such as lithium, iron, metals, and ethanol, do not adsorb significantly to activated charcoal, but its use is not precluded if the patient has ingested other toxicants that do adsorb to activated charcoal. Pulmonary aspiration and bowel obstruction from inspissated activated charcoal are the most common complications; both occur more frequently when multidose activated charcoal is administered, but they can be avoided by withholding treatment in patients who have suboptimal bowel function or decreased fecal elimination.

Gastric Emptying
Two methods of gastric emptying, syrup of ipecac and orogastric lavage via a large-bore tube, are no longer routinely used. Both are relatively ineffective therapies that potentially increase the risk for aspiration. No well-designed study has documented any benefit of gastric emptying, either by lavage or by syrup of ipecac, when compared with the use of activated charcoal alone. Gastric emptying via lavage or, rarely, by syrup of ipecac may be of benefit and should be performed in patients who have ingested toxicants that do not adsorb to activated charcoal and are known to produce significant morbidity, or for which aggressive decontamination may offer the best chance for survival (e.g., colchicine, sodium azide, sodium fluoroacetate). Removal of a liquid toxicant, such as ethylene glycol, may be accomplished by aspiration of gastric contents via a nasogastric tube. Contraindications to gastric emptying include those for activated charcoal, a bleeding diathesis, and the ingestion of sharp objects. Placement of an endotracheal tube before gastric lavage may be necessary to protect the airway in patients who have a decreased level of consciousness and impaired gag reflex; major complications of gastric emptying include pulmonary aspiration, esophageal tears and perforations, and laryngospasm (with lavage).

Whole Bowel Irrigation
Whole bowel irrigation with a nonabsorbable polyethylene glycol solution has been recommended for iron and sustained-release medications, for agents not adsorbed to activated charcoal, and for body packers (smugglers who swallow packets of illicit drugs). The most common complication is vomiting, and whole bowel irrigation is contraindicated in patients with bowel perforation, obstruction, hemorrhage, or hemodynamic or respiratory instability. The initial recommended dose is 500 mL/hour given orally or via nasogastric tube, with titration to 2000 mL/hour as tolerated; treatment continues until the rectal effluent clears. Rarely, surgery may be necessary to remove packets in smugglers who have symptoms of drug toxicity; endoscopic removal of these packets should never be attempted because of the risk of packet rupture.

Antidotes
Few toxicants have specific therapies (Table 110-6). Although antidotes may be essential in treating patients exposed to certain toxicants, their use does not preclude the need for ongoing supportive care and, in some cases, extracorporeal elimination.

Enhanced Elimination
Three methods are used to accelerate the elimination of toxicants or drugs from the body: (1) multiple doses of oral activated charcoal, (2) urinary alkalinization, and (3) extracorporeal removal. A fourth method using the oral ion exchange resins sodium polystyrene sulfonate and cholestyramine has experimentally enhanced the elimination of lithium, digoxin, digitoxin, and organochlorines but has limited clinical usefulness.

Multiple Doses of Oral Activated Charcoal
The rationale for administering multiple doses of oral activated charcoal includes the adsorption of any toxic agent remaining in the gastrointestinal tract (e.g., sustained-release drugs, drugs that retard their absorption); interference with the enterohepatic and enteroenteric recirculation of toxicants; and enhancement of the elimination of drugs with a long half-life, a volume of distribution less than 1 L/kg body weight, and low protein binding. The existing evidence shows enhanced elimination of carbamazepine, dapsone, phenobarbital, quinine, salicylates, and theophylline, but multiple doses of activated charcoal may also be effective for amitriptyline,

Text continues on p. 684

TABLE 110-6	ANTIDOTES AND INDICATIONS FOR USE			
ANTIDOTE	**INDICATION FOR USE**	**DOSE***	**TREATMENT END POINT**	**COMMENTS**
Antivenom (Fab)[†]	Crotalines	4-6 vials; repeat for persistent or worsening clinical condition; repeat doses of 2 vials at 6, 12, and 18 hr after initial antivenom dose(s) are recommended	Halt in progression of circumferential and proximal swelling Resolving systemic effects	Better safety profile than equine-derived antivenom Repetitive dosing indicated for recurrent soft tissue swelling
Antivenom, *Latrodectus* (equine)[†]	Black widow spider (*Latrodectus* sp)	1 vial diluted in 100 mL NS, infused over 1 hr; can repeat	Resolution of symptoms, vital signs normal	Dilution and slow infusion rate are **critical** to avoid anaphylactoid reaction Indications include severe pain unresponsive to opioids and severe hypertension Serum sickness can occur IV calcium is ineffective
Atropine	Carbamates Nerve agents Organophosphorus compounds	2 mg IV; double the dose every 5 min to achieve atropinization and hemodynamic stability; then start continuous infusion of 10-20% of total stabilizing dose per hr	Cessation of excessive oral and pulmonary secretions, >80 bpm, systolic blood pressure >80 mm Hg	Doubling of the dose every 5 min (e.g., 2 mg, 4 mg, 8 mg, 16 mg) estimated to achieve atropinization within 30 min Stop infusion if patient develops any signs or symptoms of anticholinergic toxidrome (see Table 110-1); restart infusion at lower rate when signs or symptoms abate

TABLE 110-6 ANTIDOTES AND INDICATIONS FOR USE—cont'd

ANTIDOTE	INDICATION FOR USE	DOSE*	TREATMENT END POINT	COMMENTS
Calcium[†]	Calcium-channel antagonists	Calcium chloride 10%, 20-50 mg (0.2-0.5 mL)/kg/hr	Reversal of hypotension; may not reverse bradycardia	*All indications:* Monitor ionized calcium levels IV extravasation causes tissue necrosis, especially with calcium chloride Can administer at faster than stated rates for immediate life-threatening conditions Taper infusions and monitor for relapse of toxicity when discontinuing therapy Calcium chloride contains three times more elemental calcium than calcium gluconate does Calcium-channel antagonists: may be ineffective in severe toxicity
	Hydrofluoric acid	Systemic toxicity: calcium gluconate 10%, 1-3 g (10-30 mL) per dose IV over 10-min period; repeat as needed every 5-10 min	Reversal of life-threatening manifestations of hypocalcemia and hyperkalemia	Can dilute and give intra-arterially or IV with a Bier block for extremity exposures and burns
	Hyperkalemia (except cardiac glycosides)	Calcium gluconate 10%, 1 g (10 mL) per dose IV over 10-min period; repeat as needed every 5-10 min	Reversal of myocardial depression and conduction delays	May precipitate ventricular arrhythmias
	Hypermagnesemia	Calcium gluconate 10%, 1-2 g (10-20 mL) per dose IV over 10-min period; repeat as needed every 5-10 min	Reversal of respiratory depression, hypotension, and cardiac conduction blocks	Simultaneous therapies to increase magnesium elimination should be instituted
	Hypocalcemia (e.g., ethylene glycol)	Calcium gluconate 10%, 0.5-1.0 g (5-10 mL) per dose over 10-min period; repeat as needed every 10 min	Reversal of tetany	Correct symptomatic hypocalcemia; avoid excessive administration that may increase production of calcium oxalate crystals in ethylene glycol poisoning
L-Carnitine	Valproate-induced hyperammonemia or hepatotoxicity	100 mg/kg (maximum 6 g) IV over 30 min, then 15 mg/kg IV over 30-min period q4h (max 6 g/day)	Treat until clinical improvement occurs	Levocarnitine is active form Adjust dose for end-stage renal disease
Cyanide antidote kit Amyl nitrite Sodium nitrite Sodium thiosulfate	Cyanide	Amyl nitrite: 0.3-mL pearls, crush and inhale over 30-sec period Sodium nitrite 3%: 10 mL IV over 10-min period Sodium thiosulfate 25%: 50 mL (12.5 g) IV over 10-min period	Resolution of lactic acidosis and moderate to severe clinical signs and symptoms: seizures, coma, dyspnea, apnea, hypotension, bradycardia	Coordinate amyl nitrite with continued oxygenation and give only until sodium nitrite infusion is begun; nitrites may produce hypotension and excess methemoglobinemia Sodium nitrite dose must be adjusted if patient has hemoglobin <12 g/dL Sodium thiosulfate dosing can be repeated
Deferoxamine	Iron	15 mL/kg/hr IV (max 8 g/day) Mild to moderate: administer for 6-12 hr Severe toxicity: administer 24 hr	Resolution of clinical signs and symptoms Do not use urine color, which is an unreliable marker for iron clearance	Indications: symptomatic patients with lethargy, severe abdominal pain, hypovolemia, acidosis, shock; any symptomatic patient with peak serum iron level >350 g/dL Prolonged therapy can cause pulmonary toxicity
Digoxin-specific antibody fragments (Fab)	Digoxin Digitalis Other cardiac glycosides (e.g., bufodienalides [Bufo toads], oleander)	Unknown digoxin dose or serum level or for plant or toad source: acute toxicity—10-20 vials; chronic toxicity—3-6 vials Digoxin dose known: number of vials = (mg ingested × 0.8) ÷ 0.5 Digoxin serum level known: number of vials = [serum level (ng/mL) × weight (kg)] ÷ 100	Resolution of hyperkalemia, symptomatic bradydysrhythmias, ventricular arrhythmias, Mobitz II or third-degree heart block	Each vial binds 0.5 mg of digoxin or digitoxin Monitor ECG and potassium levels Digoxin serum levels unreliable after antidote administered unless test is specific for free serum digoxin

TABLE 110-6 ANTIDOTES AND INDICATIONS FOR USE—cont'd

ANTIDOTE	INDICATION FOR USE	DOSE*	TREATMENT END POINT	COMMENTS
Dimercaprol (BAL)	Arsenic Lead Mercury, elemental and inorganic salts	Arsenic: 3-5 mg/kg IM q4h Lead: 75 mg/m² (4 mg/kg) IM q4h for 5 days Inorganic mercury: 5 mg/kg IM, then 2.5 mg/kg IM q12h for 10 days or until patient clinically improved	Arsenic: 24-hr urinary arsenic <50 µg/L Lead: encephalopathy resolved, blood lead level <100 µg/dL, and succimer therapy can be started Mercury, elemental and inorganic: 24-hr urinary mercury <20 µg/L	Maximum adult dose is 3 g/day BAL started 4 hr before initiation of concomitant CaNa₂EDTA for lead encephalopathy Dosing not well established for arsenic and elemental or inorganic mercury toxicity; not used for organic mercury poisoning Adverse effects: painful injections, fever, diaphoresis, agitation, headache, salivation, nausea and vomiting, hemolysis in G6PD-deficient patients, chelation of essential metals Check essential metal levels if chelation is prolonged Succimer is replacing BAL for many indications except lead encephalopathy Treatment end points for arsenic and mercury include improving clinical condition
Edetate calcium disodium (CaNa₂EDTA)	Lead	1500 mg/m²/24 hr (max 3 g) by continuous infusion	Treat for 5 days, followed by 2-day hiatus; repeat until encephalopathy resolved, lead level <100 µg/dL, and succimer therapy can be started	Use in patients with lead encephalopathy or lead level >100 g/dL Administer BAL 4 hr before initiating CaNa₂EDTA Hydrate patient and establish good urinary output before starting therapy Avoid thrombophlebitis by diluting in NS or D₅W to a concentration ≤0.5% Substitution of Na₂EDTA can cause fatal hypocalcemia
Flumazenil	Benzodiazepines Venlafaxine	0.1 mg/min IV to a total dose of 1 mg	Reversal of respiratory depression	Limit use to reversal of inadequate respiration in benzodiazepine-toxic patients Increases intracranial pressure and risk for seizures in presence of underlying seizure disorder or ingestion of seizure-producing toxicants Monitor for resedation up to 2 hr after last dose
Folinate (tetrahydrofolic acid [leucovorin])	Methanol Methotrexate	Methanol: 50 mg IV q4h Methotrexate: 100 mg/m² IV q3-6h	Methanol: methanol undetectable, metabolic acidosis cleared Methotrexate: serum level <1 × 10⁻⁸ mol/L	Essential therapy for both toxicants Methotrexate: large ingestions may require increased dose Glucarpidase administered 2-4 hr before or after folinate
Fomepizole	Ethylene glycol Methanol	Dose 1: 15 mg/kg IV Doses over next 48 hr: 10 mg/kg IV All subsequent doses: 15 mg/kg IV Administer q12h, except when HD performed: HD initiation: ½ next dose if >6 hr since last dose HD ongoing: q4h End of HD (based on time of last dose): <1 hr, no dose; 1-3 hr, ½ next dose; >3 hr, next dose	For both: serum level <20 mg/dL and metabolic acidosis resolved	Start immediately if toxic alcohol suspected, without waiting for confirmatory levels Dose amount is not affected by interval timing of doses
Glucagon	β-Adrenergic receptor antagonists Calcium-channel antagonists	Bolus of 3.5-5 mg IV; can repeat to achieve clinical effect, then infusion of 2-10 mg/hr	Reversal of hypotension and bradycardia; taper infusion	Can precipitate vomiting; be prepared to protect airway Mild hyperglycemia occurs Maximum dosing amounts unknown; bolus doses up to 30 mg reported Duration of effect is 15 min; thus infusion must be started immediately

Hydroxocobalamin	Cyanide	Initial: 5 g IV over 15-min period
		Second dose: 5 g IV over 15 min-2 hr; maximum total dose is 10 g
		Follow each hydroxocobalamin dose with sodium thiosulfate 25%: 50 mL (12.5 g) IV over 10-min period
			Resolution of lactic acidosis and moderate to severe clinical signs and symptoms: seizures, coma, dyspnea, apnea, hypotension, bradycardia	Can be administered IV push if patient is in cardiac arrest
				Do not give hydroxocobalamin and sodium thiosulfate through the same IV line
				Adverse effects: red discoloration of plasma, urine, mucous membranes, skin; transient hypertension
				Interference with laboratory colorometric assays:
				    Levels increased: bilirubin; creatinine; glucose; hemoglobin; magnesium; co-oximetry total Hb, COHb%, MetHb%
				    Levels decreased: AST, ALT, creatinine, co-oximetry O₂Hb%

TABLE 110-6 ANTIDOTES AND INDICATIONS FOR USE—cont'd

ANTIDOTE	INDICATION FOR USE	DOSE*	TREATMENT END POINT	COMMENTS
Hyperbaric oxygen (HBO)	Carbon monoxide Experimental: carbon tetrachloride, cyanide, hydrogen sulfide	3.0 atm pressure for 60 min (25 min O₂, 5 min air, 25 min O₂, 5 min air), then 2.0 atm for 65 min (30 min O₂, 5 min air, 30 min O₂), then "surface" to 1.0 atm	One treatment Second treatment rarely administered (controversial)	Carbon monoxide: treatment protocols may vary HBO indicated for loss of consciousness; seizures; cerebellar dysfunction; impaired cognition; headache, nausea/vomiting persisting after 4 hr O₂ therapy regardless of carboxyhemoglobin level Experimental indications: treatment protocols not established
Insulin-glucose	Calcium-channel antagonists β-Adrenergic receptor antagonists	Regular insulin, 1 U/kg bolus, followed by 0.5-1 U/kg/hr Titrate 50% dextrose IV to avoid hypoglycemia	Reversal of myocardial depression	Beneficial in case series and reports Initiate if glucagon and vasopressor or inotropic drugs fail to reverse myocardial depression; more effective if used before onset of cardiogenic shock Monitor glucose and potassium; hypoglycemia can occur during and after therapy Hyperglycemia results from toxicant-induced insulin resistance, and initial dextrose requirements may be less than anticipated. Recovery may be heralded by normalization of glucose levels, with increased dextrose required to avoid hypoglycemia
Intralipid	Cardiac toxicity from local anesthetics (e.g., bupivacaine, ropivacaine) Experimental: verapamil, diltiazem, tricyclic antidepressants, bupropion, propranolol	Use 20% formulation Initial bolus: 1.5 mL/kg IV over 1 min, followed immediately by infusion of 0.25 mL/kg/min for 30-60 min Can repeat bolus for asystole	Return of hemodynamic stability	Use based on animal experiments and human case reports; numerous dosing regimens have been used Use if advanced life support measures fail; continue CPR as needed during drug administration
Methylene blue	Methemoglobin-producing agents	1-2 mg/kg body weight (0.1-0.2 mL/kg) of 1% methylene blue is administered over 5-min period; repeat dose for persistent or recurrent symptoms or signs	Resolution of dyspnea and altered mental status	Use if patient is symptomatic (i.e., dyspneic, altered mental status) Maximum dose should not exceed 7 mg/kg (0.7 mL/kg) Contraindicated in G6PD-deficient patients; may cause hemolysis Some toxicants (e.g., dapsone) may require prolonged therapy
N-acetylcysteine (NAC)	Acetaminophen Experimental: carbon tetrachloride, chloroform, pennyroyal oil	Oral: Load—140 mg/kg Maintenance (starting 4 hr after load)—70 mg/kg q4h IV: Load—150 mg/kg over 1-hr period Maintenance infusion—12.5 mg/kg over 4-hr period, then 6.25 mg/kg per hour as continuous infusion	Administer 24 hr of NAC and repeat AST and APAP levels: if AST normal and APAP not detected, stop NAC; if AST normal and APAP detected, continue NAC for 12 hr, then reassess AST and APAP levels; if AST elevated, continue NAC for total of 72 hr of therapy After 72 hr of therapy, if INR <2.0, stop NAC After patient has received 72 hr of therapy, if INR ≥2.0 or severe hepatotoxicity present, continue NAC until INR <2.0	Most effective if initiated within 8 hr after ingestion; may be started any time after ingestion and is beneficial in severe hepatotoxic states Use IV in patients unable to tolerate PO or with severe hepatotoxicity; the dose and timing differ from the oral regimen Dosage and administration of FDA-approved IV formulation assumes early treatment of acute overdose without hepatotoxicity; longer duration of treatment required in patients with hepatotoxicity Treatment end points simplified for ease of use INR result not valid indicator if FFP recently administered
Naloxone	Opioids	Bolus: 0.4-2 mg via IV, sublingual injection, or endotracheal instillation; 0.4-0.8 mg SC Continuous infusion: establish bolus dose required to reverse respiratory depression Begin infusing two thirds of reversal dose every hour, and titrate to maintain adequate respirations Rebolus with half of reversal dose 15 min after reversing respiratory depression	Initial: reversal of respiratory depression with resolution of hypoxia and hypercapnia Final: resolution of CNS and respiratory depression	Preventilate patients with respiratory depression by bag-valve mask or intubation before administration Use smaller doses in opioid-dependent patients; some opioids (e.g., propoxyphene, pentazocine, fentanyls) may require larger doses of naloxone; use continuous infusion for recurrent symptoms and prolonged action of some formulations (e.g., sustained-release morphine, methadone) Resedation can occur Do not use nalmefene or naltrexone to reverse acute toxicity
Octreotide	Sulfonylureas	50 mg SC q6h	Resolution of hypoglycemia and dextrose not required	Maintain dextrose infusion as needed

TABLE 110-6 ANTIDOTES AND INDICATIONS FOR USE—cont'd

ANTIDOTE	INDICATION FOR USE	DOSE*	TREATMENT END POINT	COMMENTS
Physostigmine	Anticholinergic agents (e.g., diphenhydramine, jimsonweed [*Datura* sp], scopolamine)	1-2 mg IV over 5-min period; can repeat once after 10-15 min if no effect	Reversal of anticholinergic effects	Duration of effect is 60-90 min Benzodiazepine used for subsequent treatment of agitation and seizures; additional physostigmine used rarely (e.g., refractory seizures or agitation) Adverse effects include seizures, excessive oral secretions, bradyarrhythmias; contraindicated in cyclic antidepressant toxicity
Pralidoxime chloride	Organophosphorus compounds Nerve agents—sarin, VX	30 mg/kg IV bolus (max 2 g) over 30 min, followed by continuous infusion of 8-10 mg/kg/hr (max 650 mg/hr)	Resolution of signs and symptoms, atropine no longer required	Can give initial dose over 2-min period for life-threatening clinical effects Administer early when diagnosis known or strongly suspected Efficacy variable, depending on the organophosphate Fat-soluble organophosphates may require prolonged treatment
Pyridoxine	Ethylene glycol (theoretical efficacy) Isoniazid Monomethylhydrazine mushrooms	100 mg IV 5 g IV, repeat for refractory seizures	One dose Resolution of seizures	Efficacy theoretical Pyridoxine may stop seizures, but patient can remain comatose (isoniazid, mushrooms); use benzodiazepines and phenobarbital concomitantly to manage seizures Excessive dosing can cause neuropathy
Sodium bicarbonate ($NaHCO_3$)	Reversal of myocardial sodium-channel blockers (e.g., cyclic antidepressants, cocaine, propoxyphene, sodium-channel-blocking antiarrhythmics with $\tau_{recovery}$ >1 sec, piperidine phenothiazines (thioridazine, mesoridazine)	1-2 mEq $NaHCO_3$/kg via intermittent bolus; repeat as needed	Narrowing of prolonged QRS, resolution of ventricular arrhythmias, reversal of hypotension	Monitor blood pH (optimal pH approximately 7.50); avoid pH > 7.55
	Altered tissue distribution or enhanced elimination of salicylates; may be used in chlorophenoxy herbicides, chlorpropamide, formic acid, methotrexate, phenobarbital	1-2 mEq $NaHCO_3$/kg, followed by 3 ampules (150 mL) $NaHCO_3$ (44 mEq per 50 mL) in 850 mL of D_5W, infused at 2-3 times normal maintenance fluid rate	Serum salicylate <30 mg/dL and patient clinically stable	Monitor urinary pH hourly; adjust infusion to maintain urine pH of 7.5-8.0 (avoid blood pH >7.55) Monitor ABGs Maintain normokalemia
Succimer (DMSA)	Arsenic Lead Mercury, all forms	10 mg/kg/dose q8h for 5 days, followed by q12h for 14 days Drug holiday for 2 wk; repeat if treatment end point not reached	Arsenic: 24-hr urinary arsenic <50 µg/L Lead: resolution of encephalopathy, gastrointestinal symptoms, neuropathy, nephropathy, arthralgias, myalgias, and blood lead level <70 µg/dL Mercury, elemental and inorganic: 24-hr urinary mercury <20 µg/L Mercury, organic: end point not well established	Oral chelator; adverse effects include rash, transient AST and alkaline phosphatase elevations, and gastrointestinal distress; minimal chelation of essential metals occurs Dosing for arsenic and mercury not well established Therapeutic end point for organic mercury not established; neurotoxicity not responsive to chelation therapy; suggest chelation until blood mercury level within normal value range for reference laboratory
Vitamin K	Anticoagulants (e.g., warfarin, long-acting anticoagulant rodenticides [LAARs])	Subcutaneous: AquaMEPHYTON (K_1), 10-25 mg, repeat every 6-12 hr until oral vitamin K_1 started Oral: 25-50 mg q6h; larger doses may be required	INR is normal 48-72 hr after stopping vitamin K_1 therapy Can also monitor factor VII activity	Anaphylactoid reaction can occur with IV administration Severe bleeding may also require FFP or factor concentrates Base decision to treat on finding of elevated INR; do not administer prophylactic vitamin K_1 Oral therapy has been required for months with LAAR poisoning because of lipophilicity of toxicant, with slow body clearance

*Dose concentrations and infusion times are not given. Drug dosages may require adjustment in patients with renal or hepatic failure.

†Administer antivenom in a monitored setting; antivenom must be reconstituted and then diluted; initially infuse at a rate of 2 to 5 mL/hr, and double the infusion rate every 5 minutes as tolerated to administer antivenom over a 1-hour period.

‡Ten percent calcium chloride solution = 100 mg/mL (27.2 mg/mL elemental calcium); 10% calcium gluconate solution = 100 mg/mL (9 mg/mL elemental calcium).

ABG = arterial blood gas; ALT = alanine aminotransferase; APAP = acetyl-para-aminophenol (acetaminophen); AST = aspartate aminotransferase; BAL = British antilewisite; bpm, beats per minute; CNS = central nervous system; COHb% = percent carboxyhemoglobin; CPR, cardiopulmonary resuscitation; D_5W = 5% dextrose in water; DMSA = 2,3-dimercaptosuccinic acid; ECG = electrocardiogram; FDA = Food and Drug Administration; FFP = fresh-frozen plasma; G6PD = glucose-6-phosphate dehydrogenase; Hb = hemoglobin; HD = hemodialysis; IM = intramuscular; INR = international normalized ratio; IV = intravenous; MetHb% = percent methemoglobinemia; NS = normal saline; PO = per os (by mouth); SC = subcutaneous ; $\tau_{recovery}$ = drug blockade recovery rate.

TABLE 110-7   COMMON TOXICANTS REMOVED BY HEMODIALYSIS

TOXICANT	INDICATIONS	COMMENTS
Ethylene glycol	Serum level ≥50 mL/dL, or lower levels with concomitant metabolic acidosis and evidence of end-organ toxicity	May not be required in a patient with normal creatinine clearance and acid-base status who is receiving fomepizole
Lithium*	Clinical indications	Clinical indication is CNS toxicity (e.g., decreased mental status, ataxia, coma, seizures) Use dialysate containing bicarbonate to decrease Na^+/K^+ antiporter intracellular sequestration of lithium
Methanol	Serum level ≥50 mL/dL, or lower levels with concomitant metabolic acidosis and evidence of end-organ toxicity	Usually required because of slow elimination half-life in presence of fomepizole (mean, 52 hr; range, 22-87 hr), even in patients with no metabolic acidosis or evidence of end-organ toxicity
Phenobarbital	Clinical indications	Rarely necessary except when a patient is hemodynamically unstable despite aggressive support
Salicylates	Acute toxicity: serum level ≥100 mL/dL or <100 mg/dL in the presence of a clinical indication Chronic toxicity: any clinical indication	Serum protein binding decreases with increasing toxic levels, increasing the amount of free salicylate available for HD removal; clinical indications are one or more of the following: altered mental status, seizures, pulmonary edema, intractable acidosis, renal failure
Theophylline	Acute toxicity: serum level ≥90 μg/mL or <90 μg/mL plus any clinical indication Chronic toxicity: serum level ≥40 μg/dL and not declining despite MDAC; any clinical indication	Clinical indications for HD: seizures, hypotension, ventricular arrhythmias
Valproic acid	Severe intoxication with serum concentration >850 mg/L	Clinical indications include hepatic dysfunction; coma, especially with hyperammonemia; deteriorating clinical status despite aggressive support

*Hemodiafiltration removes lithium; the clinical benefit of this technique is unknown.
CNS = central nervous system; HD = hemodialysis; MDAC = multidose activated charcoal.

dextropropoxyphene, digitoxin, digoxin, disopyramide, nadolol, phenylbuta-zone, phenytoin, piroxicam, and sotalol. Whether enhanced elimination trans-lates into decreased morbidity and mortality has not been examined in controlled clinical trials. The usual recommendations are an average dose of 12.5 g of activated charcoal (after the initial dose) administered every 1, 2, or 4 to 6 hours after the previous dose. The contraindications to single-dose activated charcoal also apply to multidose activated charcoal. Reported com-plications include pulmonary aspiration, bowel obstruction, and fluid and electrolyte imbalance from multiple doses of a simultaneously administered cathartic.

Urinary Alkalinization

Alkalinization of the urine, which increases the renal elimination of weak acids, is used primarily to enhance the elimination of salicylates, but the elimi-nation of chlorpropamide, 2,4-dichlorophenoxyacetic acid, formic acid, meth-otrexate, and phenobarbital may be increased with this method. Urinary alkalinization is accomplished by an intravenous bolus of 1 to 2 mEq of sodium bicarbonate per kilogram body weight, followed by three ampules (150 mL) of sodium bicarbonate (44 mEq/50 mL) in 850 mL of 5% dextrose in water infused at two to three times the normal maintenance fluid rate. Urinary pH should be checked hourly, and the infusion should be adjusted to maintain a urine pH of 7.5 to 8.0. Potassium should be administered simultaneously to avoid hypokalemia, which would result in urinary acidification because the distal tubule excretes hydrogen ion in exchange for potassium (Chapter 112). Serum pH should be monitored to avoid excessive alkalemia. Contraindica-tions to this therapy include volume overload and cerebral or pulmonary edema. Urinary acidification is no longer recommended to enhance the elimi-nation of weak bases, such as amphetamines, because of the danger of pre-cipitating tubular myoglobin in patients with rhabdomyolysis.

Extracorporeal Removal

Extracorporeal techniques enhance the elimination of a few drugs and toxi-cants that exhibit single-compartment kinetics, a volume of distribution less than 1 L/kg, and endogenous clearance of less than 4 mL/minute/kg (Table 110-7). For hemodialysis, the toxicant must be water soluble, have a molecular weight less than 500 D, and exhibit low protein binding. For hemoperfusion, the toxicant must adsorb to activated charcoal. For continuous renal replace-ment therapy, the toxicant must have a molecular weight less than the perme-ability limit of the filter membrane. Rarely, extracorporeal removal has been used for aminoglycosides, atenolol, bromide, carbamazepine, diethylene glycol, isopropanol, magnesium, metformin, methotrexate, N-acetylprocain-amide, phenobarbital, procainamide, sotalol, and trichloroethanol (chloral hydrate).

1. Eddleston M, Juszczak E, Buckley NA, et al. Multiple-dose activated charcoal in acute self-poisoning: a randomised controlled trial. *Lancet.* 2008;371:579-587.
2. Eddleston M, Eyer P, Worek F, et al. Pralidoxime in acute organophosphorus insecticide poisoning—a randomized controlled trial. *PLOS Med.* 2009;6:e1000104.

SUGGESTED READINGS

Brent J. Fomepizole for ethylene glycol and methanol poisoning. *N Engl J Med.* 2009;360:2216-2223. *Review.*
Eddleston M, Buckley NA, Eyer P, et al. Management of acute organophosphorus pesticide poison-ing. *Lancet.* 2008;371:597-607. *Clinical review.*
Hill GE, Ogunnaike B, Nasir D. Patients presenting with acute toxin ingestion. *Anesthesiol Clin.* 2010;28:117-137. *Review.*
Miech R, Koester S, Dorsey-Holliman B. Increasing U.S. mortality due to accidental poisoning: the role of the baby boom cohort. *Addiction.* 2011;106:806-815. *Emphasizes the need to bolster overdose preven-tion programs and policies.*
Yarema MC, Johnson DW, Berlin RJ, et al. Comparison of the 20-hour intravenous and 72-hour oral acetylcysteine protocols for the treatment of acute acetaminophen poisoning. *Ann Emerg Med.* 2009;54:606-614. *In this retrospective study, the relative risk of hepatotoxicity was lower in the 20-hour group when acetylcysteine was started within 12 hours of ingestion.*

111

ELECTRIC INJURY

BASIL A. PRUITT JR.

ELECTRIC CURRENT INJURY

DEFINITION

The tissue damage caused by electric current ranges from a transient increase in cell membrane permeability to immediate coagulation necrosis of large volumes of tissue. The clinical consequences include disturbances in the physiologic electrical conduction systems, which may cause cardiopulmo-nary arrest; tetanic muscle contractions, with resulting compression fractures of vertebrae; and delayed tissue damage, such as cataract formation.

EPIDEMIOLOGY

As the use of electricity has increased worldwide, the number of electric injuries has increased. The precise incidence of electric injury is unknown,

PROGNOSIS

Almost all patients who reach the hospital alive survive with appropriate care. Inpatient mortality rates are 0.2 to 0.5%.

but the National Centers for Health and Centers for Disease Control and Prevention have estimated that each year in the United States there are 52,000 trauma admissions for electric injuries. During a recent 86-month period, 5.3% of patients admitted to the U.S. Army Burn Center had an electric injury; at other burn centers, the percentage of admissions related to electric injury ranges from 0.04 to 6.7% in developed countries and as high as 32 to 42% in developing countries.

PATHOBIOLOGY

Environmental conditions, duration of contact, pathway of the current, type of current (and, if alternating current, its frequency), and voltage all influence the effects of electricity on tissue. Voltage greater than 40 is potentially dangerous, and the likelihood of sudden death and remote tissue injury increases as voltage increases to 1000. Voltages greater than 1000 are considered to be high tension and are associated with immediate severe tissue damage. Alternating current is more dangerous than direct current because of its likelihood to produce cardiac arrest or cessation of respiration and its tetanic effect, which may prevent the patient from breaking contact with the source of electricity. As the frequency of alternating current increases to greater than 60 cycles per second, tissue injury decreases. The path of the current through the body between the points of contact is important in determining tissue damage; a course through the heart or the respiratory center of the brain is especially dangerous. Ventricular fibrillation can be produced by current flow of only 100 mA from a hand to the feet. Rapid separation from the source of electricity is crucial, because tissue damage increases in proportion to the duration of contact. Resistance to current flow at the point of contact is influenced by environmental conditions; dry and thickened palmar or plantar skin is more resistant to the passage of current than is skin moistened by perspiration or other liquid.

Heat is the principal mediator of tissue damage in electric injury, the severity of which is related to voltage and duration of contact. Tissue-specific differences in resistance to the flow of current (neural tissue least; blood vessels, muscle, and skin intermediate; bone greatest) may explain differences in tissue injury caused by low-voltage current. Because all body tissues and fluids are conductive, the soft tissues between bone and skin can be viewed as a volume conductor. Heat is produced in tissues as a function of voltage drop and current flow per unit of cross-sectional area (i.e., density of the current). The inverse relationship between the density of the current and the tissue's cross-sectional area accounts for the frequency of severe injury to the digits and extremities and the rarity of major injury to the trunk in patients with high-tension electric injury (Fig. 111-1). Contact with less than 1000 V causes injuries that are self-limited because at the contact points, where the density of the current is greatest, the skin is severely injured and chars, which results in a rapid increase in resistance and reduction in the passage of current. When the source is greater than 1000 V, arcing is so intense that tissue destruction is increased markedly as relatively constant levels of current are maintained. Arcing, which may occur across the flexor surfaces of joints, can

char the skin in these areas and ignite the patient's clothing. After cessation of the flow of current, the heated tissue acts like a volume radiator and cools unevenly, with the superficial portions cooling more rapidly than the deeper portions; deeper tissues are therefore more prone to severe injury.

Tissue damage can also be caused by low-voltage direct current (e.g., contact with automobile battery terminals or with defective or inappropriately used medical equipment, such as electrosurgical devices, external pacing devices, or defibrillators). Direct-current injuries are reportedly common during laparoscopy with high-voltage coagulation.

CLINICAL MANIFESTATIONS AND DIAGNOSIS

Cardiopulmonary arrest can be caused by low-voltage electric injury but is more common with high-voltage electric injury. Extensive tissue necrosis may also liberate enough potassium to cause cardiac dysfunction. Because cardiac arrhythmias may recur after resuscitation or develop 24 to 48 hours after injury, all patients who have sustained high-voltage electric injury should undergo continuous electrocardiogram (ECG) monitoring for at least 48 hours after the last ECG-documented arrhythmia. Early imaging of the heart with technetium-99m tetrofosmin has been proposed as a means of detecting myocardial perfusion defects requiring cardiac monitoring and predicting the possibility of long-term cardiac effects. Renal failure may occur in patients with high-voltage electric injury if inapparent deep tissue injury with accompanying occult edema results in an underestimation of fluid requirements, inadequate resuscitation, and oliguria. Additionally, the destruction of muscle and red blood cells liberates hemochromes, which may precipitate in the renal tubules unless adequate urinary output is maintained (Chapter 122).

Muscle Damage

High-voltage electric injury commonly causes edema beneath the investing fascia of the involved muscle compartments, thereby compromising nutrient blood flow to muscles within the compartments and to distal unburned tissue. Clinical indications for the surgical release of intracompartmental pressure by fasciotomy and surgical exploration of a limb include impaired capillary refilling of distal unburned skin or nails, cyanosis of distal unburned skin, stony hardness of a muscle compartment on palpation, and diminished or absent pulsatile flow in the distal arteries as assessed by Doppler ultrasound. Tissue pressures 30 mm Hg or higher above atmospheric pressure, as measured by a catheter placed in the compartment, indicate the need for immediate decompression. If clinical signs are consistent with deep tissue injury but large-vessel pulses are intact, arteriography can determine the need for operative intervention, including amputation of the affected limb. "Pruning" of the arterial tree, with a decrease in the density of nutrient branches in the muscles of an involved limb, identifies the level of amputation required to remove muscle that has been irreversibly damaged. Muscle blood flow of 1 mL/minute/100 g of tissue, as determined by xenon-133 "washout," has been proposed as the minimum level required for ultimate tissue viability. In patients with high-voltage electric injury, myoglobinemia and elevation of serum creatine phosphokinase reflect significant muscle damage, and myoglobinuria is a strong predictor of the need for fasciotomy in the first 24 hours after injury.

Neurologic Examination

On admission and at scheduled intervals thereafter, a detailed neurologic examination must be performed on all patients with high-voltage electric injury; all nerve deficits should be documented fully. Central nervous system or peripheral nerve dysfunction may be apparent immediately after electric injury or may appear later. Recovery of function after direct electrical nerve damage is rare. Conversely, the spontaneous resolution of immediate and early functional deficits of nerves not injured directly (motor nerves are more sensitive to nondestructive injury than are sensory nerves) is common. A polyneuritic syndrome of relatively late onset can cause deficits in the function of peripheral nerves far removed from the points of contact. Direct nerve damage of the spinal cord causes immediate deficits, which are more likely to be transient than are deficits with a later onset. Delayed-onset spinal cord deficits can manifest as quadriplegia, hemiplegia, localized nerve deficits with signs of ascending paralysis, transverse myelitis, and even an amyotrophic lateral sclerosis–like syndrome. The cause of delayed paresthesias and nerve dysfunction after electric injury is unknown, but an increase in permeability of the cell membrane and an associated loss of cell contents induced by exposure to a millivoltage electric field (electroporation) have been implicated. Children have greater improvement in neurologic function than adults do, owing to their greater neurologic plasticity. Children with electric injuries

FIGURE 111-1. Charring at the contact site in the first web space and at the site of arcing in the antecubital space *(black arrows)* of a victim of electric injury. The fixed flexion deformity of the thumb and other digits is characteristic of severe high-voltage injury to the hand and forearm. The severity of the injury is indicated by the marked edema of the forearm muscles, bulging above the cut edges of the fasciotomy incision, and by patchy dark discoloration of the muscles of the arm and the forearm, particularly the deeper muscle exposed in the central portion of the forearm incision *(white arrow)*.

that cause full-thickness destruction of the calvaria may have direct brain injury, with affective and/or cognitive difficulties that can persist for a year or longer.

Remote Organ Injury

Direct liver injury, focal pancreatic and gallbladder necrosis, and intestinal perforation have been reported after electric injury, but all are uncommon. Delayed hemorrhage from moderate to large blood vessels has been ascribed to an arteritis caused by the electric injury, but this hemorrhage seems to be related to inadequate débridement of injured tissue or to vascular wall necrosis as a consequence of exposure after débridement.

Compression fractures of vertebral bodies may be produced by tetanic contractions of the paraspinous muscles. Fractures of the skull and the long bones of both the upper and lower extremities may be caused by falls after the electric shock.

TREATMENT   Rx

Cardiopulmonary arrest must be treated by immediate institution of cardiopulmonary resuscitation (Chapter 63). In patients with high urinary hemochrome concentrations, a urinary output of 75 to 100 mL/hour should be maintained (Chapter 115). If the hemochromes do not clear promptly or the patient remains oliguric despite the administration of resuscitation fluids at more than twice the required rate, as estimated based on the extent of the burn and the patient's weight (Chapter 112), 25 g of mannitol should be given as an intravenous bolus, and 12.5 g of mannitol should be added to each liter of intravenous fluid until the pigment has cleared from the urine. Hyperkalemia is treated as in any other patient (Chapter 119).

If the electric injury is limited to the skin and subcutaneous tissue, an antibacterial cream such as Sulfamylon should be applied twice daily to the burned tissue until débridement is performed. The antimicrobial (mafenide acetate) in Sulfamylon readily diffuses into the nonviable tissue to limit microbial proliferation. As soon as resuscitation has restored hemodynamic stability, severely damaged limbs or other areas of tissue necrosis should be surgically explored. The viability of vital structures and the extent of deep tissue damage are assessed to determine the need for amputation. If amputation is not required, all necrotic tissue is débrided to eliminate the source of hyperkalemia and reduce the risk for infection. It is imperative to examine the periosteous muscles, which may be necrotic because of delayed heat dissipation but overlain by more superficial viable muscles. After débridement or amputation, the operative wound is dressed but not surgically closed, and the patient is scheduled for re-exploration of the wound 24 to 72 hours later. At that time, residual necrotic tissue is débrided, and the wound is closed by skin grafts, tissue transfer, or biologic dressings, depending on the condition, extent, and site of the wound. An exception to early excision of questionably viable tissue is the conservative removal of only obviously necrotic tissue from low-voltage oral commissure wounds that result from a child's biting or sucking on exposed wires or house current outlets (Fig. 111-2).

PROGNOSIS

Cardiopulmonary and fluid resuscitation combined with monitoring of limb tissue pressure and wound care have maximized tissue salvage, reduced renal failure, and increased the survival of patients with electric injuries. Overall, current treatment is associated with a 96% survival rate.

Among the patients with serious high-voltage electric injuries hospitalized at the U.S. Army Burn Center over the past decade or so, about 8% died and another 22% had permanent neurologic deficits at discharge. High-voltage electric injury has been associated with the subsequent formation of cataracts, most frequently when the contact site was on the head or neck. Cataracts may form rapidly, but they more commonly develop 3 years or more after the injury. Rarely, exfoliative debris may be evident in the anterior chamber of the eye immediately after injury. Cholelithiasis and gastrointestinal dysfunction have been reported after high-voltage injury, but they appear to be rare.

Most patients with low-voltage injuries, many caused by electric flash burns, develop long-term sequelae. The neurologic symptoms (memory loss, numbness, headache, chronic pain, weakness), psychological symptoms (depression, insomnia, post-traumatic stress syndrome, nightmares, anxiety), and musculoskeletal symptoms (pain, reduced range of motion, contracture) often have a delayed onset (1.6 to 29.5 months), persist on average for 300 days after injury, and limit return to work in more than 40% of patients.

● LIGHTNING INJURY

An estimated 300 to 350 persons are struck by lightning each year, and about 30% of them die. The duration of a lightning bolt is $\frac{1}{100}$ to $\frac{1}{1000}$ of a second, but it may have a voltage of approximately 1 billion V and induce currents ranging from 12,000 to 200,000 A. The temperature in a lightning bolt, which may be 30,000 K, dissipates in a few microseconds.

CLINICAL MANIFESTATIONS

Cardiopulmonary arrest, which can be secondary to either asystole or ventricular fibrillation, is common in patients struck by lightning. Cardiopulmonary resuscitation (Chapter 63) must be instituted immediately; recovery has been reported in some patients who were apparently without life signs for 15 minutes or longer. Although signs of acute myocardial damage may become evident later, persistent or recurrent ECG abnormalities are uncommon. Coma is common immediately after injury and typically resolves in a few hours. Abdominal signs of peritonitis with free air in the peritoneal cavity should alert one to the possibility of intestinal perforation, which must be treated by prompt primary closure. Keraunoparalysis (lightning paralysis), which is characterized by paresthesias and paralysis, usually involves the lower limbs, often develops over a period of several days after lightning injury, is typically associated with vasomotor disorders, and is usually transient. Myoglobinuria is uncommon; when present, it is treated as described earlier for other electric injuries. Tympanic membrane rupture and hearing loss may

FIGURE 111-2. **A,** This child sustained a potentially disfiguring injury by biting on wires carrying house current. **B,** Note the extent of the injury, with black areas of necrotic tissue on each lip and the white plaque of nonviable tissue on the upper surface of the tongue. **C,** Spontaneous separation and removal of only unequivocally dead tissue minimizes disfigurement and reduces the magnitude of surgical reconstruction required to restore lip function.

FIGURE 111-3. The arborescent current markings on the face, neck, and anterior trunk of this young patient, which are characteristic of lightning injury, healed without the need for grafting. Note the focal lesions on the right arm, indicating the spread of the current that produced the marks on the right anterolateral aspect of the chest wall.

also be caused by lightning injury. Cutaneous burns of the trunk and proximal areas of the limbs caused by lightning injury, called *Lichtenberg figures*, typically have a "splashed on" arborescent and spidery appearance and are generally superficial (Fig. 111-3). Small, circular, full-thickness burns of the tips of the toes are also common and have been termed the *tiptoe sign*. Mottling of the skin and other signs of vasoconstriction previously considered specific to lightning injury generally resolve with adequate resuscitation.

TREATMENT AND PROGNOSIS   **Rx**

Current treatment, which emphasizes immediate cardiopulmonary resuscitation, has decreased mortality significantly, and two thirds of lightning-injured patients now survive. Persistent nerve deficits and long-term problems are relatively uncommon in survivors. However, Guillain-Barré syndrome, with neurologic deficits persisting beyond hospital discharge, has been reported.

SUGGESTED READINGS

Li AL, Gomez M, Fish JS. Effectiveness of pain management following electrical injury. *J Burn Care Res.* 2010;31:73-82. *Review emphasizing the chronic need for pain medications in many patients.*

Ritenour AE, Morton MJ, McManus JG, et al. Lightning injury: a review. *Burns.* 2008;34:585-594. *Describes the epidemiology, treatment, and sequelae.*

Vierhapper MF, Lumenta DB, Beck H, et al. Electrical injury: a long-term analysis with review of regional differences. *Ann Plast Surg.* 2011;66:43-46. *Review of 56 hospitalized cases, with mean burn surface area of 26% and a 4% mortality rate.*

112

MEDICAL ASPECTS OF TRAUMA AND BURN CARE

ROBERT H. DEMLING AND JONATHAN D. GATES

MEDICAL ASPECTS OF TRAUMA

EPIDEMIOLOGY

Trauma is the third leading cause of death in people of all ages in the United States, surpassed only by cancer and atherosclerosis. Trauma is the leading cause of death in children, adolescents, and young adults aged 1 to 44 years.

More than 140,000 deaths and twice as many permanent disabilities occur annually in the United States from injuries. Fatal injuries have a trimodal distribution. Half of all fatalities occur within minutes of the injury as a result of massive hemorrhage from the heart, lacerations of large blood vessels, or catastrophic neurologic injury. In such cases, there is insufficient time for medical intervention to alter the outcome; the only method to reduce this category of trauma-related morbidity and mortality is through prevention and education programs. Of the fatalities, 30% occur within a few hours after injury from airway obstruction, shock, or neurologic dysfunction. This interval represents an opportunity during which appropriate and timely medical or surgical intervention is most likely to influence outcome. Fatalities within this second peak occur as a result of epidural and subdural hematomas, chest injuries, liver lacerations, splenic rupture, pelvic fractures, or the accumulation of multiple injuries resulting in significant blood loss. The third peak of trauma fatalities is due to multisystem organ dysfunction or overwhelming infection weeks later. This delayed systemic response is related to the degree of the initial insult, the individual response to the injury, and the cumulative effect of any additional complications that arise after injury.

Motor vehicle crashes, firearms, and falls are major contributors to injury in the United States. In 2008, an estimated 2.35 million people were injured in motor vehicle traffic crashes, which resulted in approximately 38,000 fatalities. About 50% of all traffic deaths in 15- to 34-year-olds are alcohol related (Chapter 32). About 35,000 gun-related deaths, unintentional and intentional, occur annually. Of all injury deaths, 8% are related to falls, and fall from a height is responsible for one third of all injury-related hospitalizations.

PATHOBIOLOGY

Mechanism of Injury

Trauma produces a structural or physiologic alteration as a result of an external force, whether it is mechanical, chemical, electrical, or thermal energy. The force that initiated the motion of an object must be absorbed or dissipated in an effort to decelerate that object. When an automobile traveling at a given speed strikes an immobile object, a tremendous amount of energy in the moving vehicle is transmitted to the immobile object and the structure of the vehicle, deforming both until the automobile stops. These same forces are imparted to the occupants of the vehicle with potentially dire consequences. In a head-on impact, the driver continues to move forward until impeded by objects inside the automobile or until the energy is dissipated by the restraint of a seat belt or air bag. Deceleration forces are imparted to individual organs. These same physical principles apply to injury after a fall from a height. Compression, shear, and overpressure from these and other forces injure internal organs.

Penetrating injuries, which are described as either low velocity or high velocity, result from the kinetic energy of the missile. In the case of a bullet discharged from a gun, the tissue immediately contacted by the bullet is crushed to create a permanent cavity. Transfer of energy farther away from the bullet path creates a temporary cavity beyond the boundary of the permanent tract, the so-called blast effect. A simple stab wound from a knife or sharp object is considered a low-velocity injury in which the wound is confined to the tract itself. Virtually no temporary cavity is created, but the consequences may be just as devastating as a high-velocity injury if a vital structure is affected.

Pathophysiology of Injury

Shock (Chapter 106) results in inadequate organ perfusion and subsequent failure to deliver sufficient oxygen to maintain aerobic metabolism. Poor peripheral perfusion results in cellular hypoxia and slowing of oxidative phosphorylation, with the accumulation of H^+ ion in the extracellular fluid, resulting in metabolic acidosis. The initial step in managing shock associated with trauma is to recognize inadequate organ perfusion. The second step is to identify and treat the probable cause. The four general categories of shock in trauma are hemorrhagic, compressive, neurogenic, and cardiogenic; however, most shock is hypovolemic in nature. Adrenal insufficiency (Chapter 234), anaphylaxis (Chapter 261), and septic shock (Chapter 108) are less common but may occur during the recovery period. The goal of treatment is restoration of cellular and organ perfusion with adequately oxygenated blood volume.

Hemorrhagic Shock

Hemorrhagic shock results from a decline in cardiac filling pressure as blood is lost (Chapter 106). Cardiac output is preserved through compensatory mechanisms when the loss of blood is about 10% of blood volume. Endogenous neurogenic and endocrine responses result in peripheral vasoconstriction and shunting of blood from the nonessential areas of skin, muscle, and abdominal viscera to maintain perfusion to the heart and brain. Cardiac output decreases with a blood volume loss of 20 to 40%, with a resultant decrease in systolic blood pressure. Additional compensatory mechanisms to maintain perfusion pressure in the face of a sudden decrease in intravascular volume result in a shift of proteins and fluids from the extracellular space to the intravascular compartment. The relative decrease in volume and increase in osmolarity of the extracellular space stimulate movement of fluid out of the cells to replace it.

It is imperative to identify a patient in shock or compensated shock. A normal systemic arterial blood pressure or absence of tachycardia may lead an inexperienced physician to believe that the patient is hemodynamically stable when in fact the patient may be in the precarious situation of partially compensated shock. A high index of suspicion and early aggressive diagnostic evaluation and treatment minimize the possibility that occult blood loss may be missed and lead to appropriate volume resuscitation and possible surgical correction.

Compressive Shock

Compressive shock arises when external compression of the lungs or heart from air, fluid, or blood either compromises diastolic filling of the right ventricle or prevents adequate ventilation and oxygenation. The two most notable forms of compressive shock are tension pneumothorax (Chapter 99) and pericardial tamponade (Chapter 77).

In tension pneumothorax, air within the pleural space impedes expansion of the ipsilateral lung and shifts the mediastinum. Compression of the inferior and superior vena cava leads to inadequate filling of the right atrium and ventricle, which decreases cardiac output. Identification of the injury is paramount; typical findings include absence of breath sounds in the ipsilateral chest, jugular venous distention, and tracheal deviation to the opposite side. Appropriate intervention involves release of air under tension in the pneumothorax by means of needle or tube thoracentesis.

Cardiac tamponade occurs because of extrinsic compression of the chambers of the heart from blood within the pericardial space, which is normally a potential space filled with less than 50 mL of pericardial fluid (Chapter 77). An external chest wound that penetrates the pericardium and the heart may create a rent in the pericardium too small to vent the accumulated blood; as a result, blood collects in the noncompliant pericardial sac, and pressure is directed inward toward the hollow chambers of the heart. The external compression inhibits diastolic filling of the chambers and reduces stroke volume. Pericardial tamponade should be suspected in patients who have wounds in the vicinity of the precordium and epigastrium, hypotension, tachycardia, jugular venous distention, and muffled heart sounds. Treatment is immediate evacuation of the pericardial space by needle pericardiocentesis, followed by sternotomy or left thoracotomy.

Neurogenic Shock

Complete injury to the cervical or upper thoracic spinal cord may result in sympathetic denervation manifested as loss of vasomotor tone in the periphery. Neurogenic shock should be considered in any trauma patient who is hypotensive but not actively bleeding. Only about 20% of patients with a complete high spinal cord injury have neurogenic shock, however, and patients with incomplete motor or sensory deficits (or both) rarely have hypotension directly caused by neurologic injury.

Cardiogenic Shock

Cardiogenic shock (Chapter 107) implies inadequate peripheral perfusion as a result of pump failure. It may be caused by arrhythmias, valvular dysfunction, or failing myocardial contraction. The latter may be seen with cardiac contusion or ischemic dysfunction of a previously damaged myocardium with marginal reserve.

DIAGNOSIS AND TREATMENT Rx

An organized approach to a trauma patient is mandatory to avoid confusion or missing life-threatening injury. A randomized trial found no benefit in advanced prehospital life support, whereby paramedics in the field perform endotracheal intubation and administer intravenous therapy, compared with basic prehospital life support and rapid transfer to a trauma center.[1] The American College of Surgeons Advanced Trauma Life Support (ATLS) guidelines divide management into the primary survey for rapid diagnosis and treatment of life-threatening injuries and the secondary survey for a more complete, in-depth evaluation of the whole patient for definitive therapy.

The initial management of a trauma patient requires immediate intravenous access for volume resuscitation. The type and rapidity of solution delivered are determined by the patient's hemodynamic stability, as reflected by the degree of intravascular depletion or blood loss. Four classes of hemorrhage are widely accepted (Table 112-1). Intravenous access also allows the administration of analgesics, sedatives, and antibiotics. The rapidity of volume resuscitation with isotonic crystalloid and blood products is determined by the initial degree or class of shock. The guidelines are based on the "three-to-one" rule, which derives from the empirical observation that most patients in hemorrhagic shock require 300 mL of electrolyte solution for each 100 mL of blood loss because crystalloid equilibrates in the entire extracellular space.

More recently, the experience of the U.S. military had led to the concept of damage control resuscitation, which focuses on the strategy of transfusing blood products (red cells, plasma, and platelets) early and often in the exsanguinating patient while limiting the use of crystalloids to avoid hemodilution of coagulation products. Despite the absence of randomized trials, a 1:1 ratio of plasma and platelets to packed red blood cells appears to result in higher survival among patients with exsanguinating injury. Use of leukoreduced blood provides no advantage over standard blood products.[2] Tranexamic acid (loading dose 1 g over 10 minutes then infusion of 1 g over 8 hours), which inhibits thrombolysis, beginning within 8 hours of injury reduces mortality by 9% in trauma patients who require blood transfusions.[3]

Primary Survey

The primary survey (airway, breathing, circulation) is the same whether the mechanism of injury was blunt, penetrating, or thermal. Evaluation of the airway is paramount. Supplemental oxygen is given to all trauma patients to maximize delivery of oxygen to the periphery. If the patient is hemodynamically unstable or is unable to maintain a patent airway because of mental status changes or airway debris, endotracheal intubation should be performed. There is little role for the use of oral airways or nasal trumpets in a trauma patient. Care must be taken to avoid movement of the cervical spine during intubation so that exacerbation of an undiagnosed cervical spine fracture or ligamentous disruption is avoided. Inability to perform endotracheal intubation in a trauma patient should lead to rapid surgical control of the airway by cricothyroidotomy. Tracheostomy is a poor second choice because

TABLE 112-1 CATEGORIZATION AND INITIAL TREATMENT OF HEMORRHAGIC SHOCK*

	CLASS I	CLASS II	CLASS III	CLASS IV
Blood loss (mL)	≤750	750-1500	1500-2000	≥2000
Blood loss (% of blood volume)	≤15	15-30	30-40	≥40
Pulse rate	<100	>100	>120	≥140
Blood pressure	Normal	Normal	Decreased	Decreased
Capillary refill test	Normal	Positive	Positive	Positive
Respiratory rate	14-20	20-30	30-40	>35
Urine output (mL/hr)	≥30	20-30	5-15	Negligible
Mental status	Slightly anxious	Mildly anxious	Anxious and confused	Confused and lethargic
Fluid replacement (3:1 rule)	Crystalloid	Crystalloid	Crystalloid + blood	Crystalloid + blood

*Based on a 70-kg adult.

it is more time-consuming and potentially bloody, especially if the landmarks are obscured by trauma.

The primary survey should observe the symmetry of chest wall movement, determine whether breath sounds are equal bilaterally and adequate, and assess the chest wall for crepitus, instability, or tenderness. If a tension pneumothorax or massive hemothorax is suspected (and the findings are not caused by intubation of the right mainstem bronchus), a large-bore chest tube is placed in the ipsilateral anterolateral fifth intercostal space. Chest tube insertion is diagnostic and therapeutic. Return of greater than 1500 mL of blood suggests a significant injury within the ipsilateral hemothorax; this magnitude of initial output or ongoing hourly blood loss of 200 to 250 mL through the chest tube may warrant urgent thoracic surgical exploration.

Adequacy of the circulation is determined clinically by noting the presence of carotid, radial, and femoral pulses. Brisk capillary refill, as elicited by transient compression of the nail bed, and a warm, well-perfused patient suggest good peripheral perfusion. A patient in extremis may have a barely palpable carotid pulse, mental status changes, and mottled, cold, clammy skin. During this evaluation, simultaneous insertion of short, large-caliber intravenous catheters into the antecubital veins is recommended for the initial administration of lactated Ringer's solution.

The primary survey should include an evaluation of neurologic function. The Glasgow Coma Scale (Chapter 406) grades the patient's eye movement, best motor response, and best verbal response on a scale from 1 to 5, with a total score of 15 indicating the best function. For patients with brain trauma (Chapter 406), resuscitation with a saline solution provides better outcomes than using albumin.▪

The patient should be assessed for all evidence of traumatic injury. This assessment should include an examination of the back with the patient logrolled under cervical spine precautions.

Secondary Survey

The secondary survey is the head-to-toe physical examination of the patient to evaluate the airway, reassess the adequacy of breathing and circulation, and look for any injuries or underlying conditions that were not immediately apparent during the primary survey. At this stage, pertinent radiographs, blood tests, and other tests (e.g., an electrocardiogram) are obtained, and a Foley catheter can be inserted if needed.

Head and Neck

Evaluation of neurologic function should determine whether there is evidence of closed head injury (Chapter 406). Physical examination should assess for skull and facial fractures and eye and ear injuries. The physician should have a low threshold for performing computed tomography (CT) of the head, which is preferred over magnetic resonance imaging in this situation.

The management of neck injuries that penetrate the platysma is dependent on the anatomic level of injury. The neck is divided into threes zones. Zone I injury, including the thoracic inlet up to the level of the cricothyroid membrane, is treated as an upper thoracic injury. In a stable patient, injuries in zone I require an arteriogram or CT angiography to define the injury and plan the surgical approach; hemodynamically unstable patients should undergo immediate surgical exploration.

Zone III injury, from the angle of the mandible to the base of the skull, is treated as a head injury. Most patients with injuries in this region are hemodynamically stable. Arteriography, bronchoscopy, esophagoscopy, and sometimes direct laryngoscopy should be performed to evaluate the type and extent of injury.

Zone II injuries, which are in the most exposed area of the neck between the other two zones, must be evaluated locally to determine whether the platysma muscle has been penetrated. Both selective operative management and mandatory exploration of penetrating injuries to zone II of the neck appear to be equally justified and safe. Selective operative management of a patient with penetrating wounds deep to the platysma requires nonoperative evaluation with arteriography and diagnostic upper endoscopy and bronchoscopy, with operative intervention reserved for situations in which the evaluation reveals pathology. Spiral CT with intravenous contrast material can define arterial injuries and has replaced angiography except where CT cannot define the arterial anatomy. Hemodynamically unstable patients should be resuscitated and explored surgically without further testing.

Chest

Life-threatening injuries of the chest include tension pneumothorax, massive hemothorax, cardiac tamponade (see earlier), flail chest, open pneumothorax, and disruption of the thoracic aorta. Flail chest implies an unstable segment of the chest wall as a result of multiple rib fractures. The negative pleural pressure required for inspiration pulls the unstable segment of the chest wall inward while the remainder of the chest moves in the opposite direction. An open pneumothorax implies air entering the pleural space through an external chest wound. The wound should be covered with a partially occlusive dressing, and a chest tube should be inserted to prevent the accumulation of air and the development of tension pneumothorax. Large open chest wounds require endotracheal intubation, operative débridement,

FIGURE 112-1. **Chest evaluation.** A chest computed tomographic scan shows bilateral pulmonary contusions *(arrow a)* and effusions with a small pneumothorax on the left *(arrow b).*

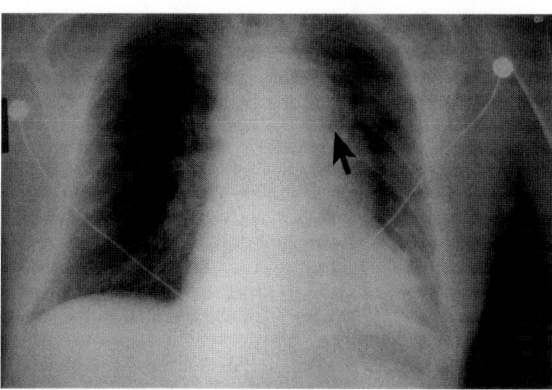

FIGURE 112-2. Widened superior mediastinum on an upright chest radiograph. Note the loss of normal contour of the aortic knob *(arrow).*

chest tube drainage, chest wall stabilization, and closure. Although not usually considered life-threatening, there are a myriad of chest injuries, including simple pneumothorax, pulmonary contusions (Fig. 112-1), rib fractures, and minor to moderate hemothorax, that may play a major role in the duration of lung dysfunction or the need for ventilatory support, or both.

All trauma patients should have a supine chest radiograph taken to examine the lung fields, the mediastinal contour, and the chest wall. Thoracic aortic injury, which is a feared complication of severe acceleration-deceleration injury, results in the immediate death of 90% of persons with this injury. Survivors who reach medical care often have a contained mediastinal hematoma that appears as a widened superior mediastinum or loss of the aortic contour on the chest radiograph, or both (Fig. 112-2). These patients have historically been evaluated by arteriography (Fig. 112-3), but now chest CT is used to screen for this injury. A contained mediastinal hematoma is an unstable condition that demands timely evaluation and possible endovascular or open operative intervention.

Myocardial Injury

Myocardial contusion results from transmission of force to the myocardium in the form of compression, blast, or sudden deceleration. The true incidence is difficult to define given the absence of consensus on a reliable test to identify myocardial contusion. A high degree of suspicion is needed because there are no specific clinical signs of myocardial injury. Sternal fracture, anterior rib fractures, and aortic injuries are all examples of trauma that may suggest underlying cardiac contusion. Life-threatening myocardial contusion (5%) is manifested within the first 6 to 12 hours after injury as malignant arrhythmias or, if enough of the left ventricle is damaged, cardiogenic shock. Myocardial rupture is uncommon and typically involves the right ventricle because of the thin muscular wall and close proximity to the sternum. More commonly, arrhythmias or conduction disturbances may occur with elevation of cardiac biomarkers. Electrocardiographic findings include ST-T wave anomalies, supraventricular and ventricular arrhythmias, and atrioventricular nodal dysfunction. The echocardiogram may show left ventricular wall motion abnormalities, valvar dysfunction, or pericardial effusion. There is no evidence to support prophylactic treatment of arrhythmias, and emergency surgery for other injuries does not appear to carry a risk for increased morbidity or mortality in the presence of minor abnormalities.

FIGURE 112-3. Arteriography of the chest. An arteriogram shows thoracic aortic disruption *(arrow)* beyond the left subclavian artery in the patient depicted in Fig. 112-2.

FIGURE 112-4. Abdominal injury. An abdominal computed tomographic scan shows an injury to the right lobe of the liver *(arrow)*.

Commotio cordis is sudden cardiac arrest after acute blunt trauma to the chest. The so-called concussion to the heart is one of the more common causes of sudden death in youth sports. By definition, there is no preexisting cardiac disease or identifiable morphologic change in the heart. The precordial impact, most commonly from softballs, baseballs, and hockey pucks, presumably occurs during an electrically vulnerable period between 30 and 15 msec before the T wave peak and produces ventricular fibrillation. The mortality rate is 90%, and nearly all survivors require resuscitation (Chapter 63) initiated within 1 minute of the insult. Education, improved chest protective equipment, and personnel competent in the use of automatic external defibrillators at youth sporting events may reduce the incidence of this infrequent but feared injury.

Injuries to the coronary arteries are uncommon. Potential vascular injuries include laceration, intimal disruption with dissection, and vasospasm. The sequelae and treatment are similar to those for myocardial ischemia from atherosclerotic occlusion (Chapter 73).

Back

Palpation of the thoracic and lumbar spine combined with a thorough history is sufficient to exclude a thoracolumbar spine fracture in an alert patient. Ongoing back discomfort or a mechanism suggestive of the possibility of injury should lead to radiographic examination of the spine.

Abdomen

The abdominal contents may be injured by blunt or penetrating mechanisms. The ability to identify intra-abdominal injury is limited on physical examination. If the patient is hemodynamically stable, has a normal abdominal examination, and has sustained no other injuries that warrant operative repair, serial abdominal examination, a complete blood count, and amylase and lipase levels suffice. If there is any question about the normality of the abdominal examination or the ability to monitor the patient reliably, further evaluation is warranted.

Abdominal CT has proved a reliable determinant of intra-abdominal injury in a stable patient (Fig. 112-4). It identifies both intraperitoneal and retroperitoneal injury (Fig. 112-5). CT evaluation can identify sources of blood loss and help decide whether the problem requires operative exploration.

The most frequently injured intra-abdominal organ is the spleen. Left-sided rib fractures, left upper quadrant pain or tenderness, and pain referred to the left shoulder secondary to diaphragmatic irritation are suggestive of splenic injury. CT allows definition of the grade of splenic injury and detection of free intraperitoneal blood. Hemodynamic instability, ongoing blood loss, and CT findings of a high-grade injury to the spleen are all indications for splenectomy or, preferably, splenorrhaphy for salvage of the damaged spleen with preservation of splenic function.

Blunt injury to the liver is often associated with right-sided rib fractures and right upper quadrant tenderness with or without peritonitis. An abdominal CT scan with intravenous contrast material allows classification of the liver injury according to the location, depth, and extent of the hematoma or laceration. Currently, most (85%) blunt liver injuries are managed successfully nonoperatively if other intra-abdominal injuries do not require surgery.

Focused abdominal sonography in trauma (FAST) has a sensitivity of 95% for detecting free blood in the abdomen (Fig. 112-6). FAST sequentially surveys for the presence or absence of blood in the pericardial sac and dependent abdominal regions, including the right upper quadrant, left upper quadrant, and pelvis. Evaluation of the pericardial sac also allows the operator to identify tamponade physiology (Chapter 77). FAST is limited in its ability to identify the

FIGURE 112-5. Intraperitoneal and retroperitoneal injury. An abdominal computed tomographic scan shows blood in the retroperitoneum surrounding a shattered left kidney, with pooling of contrast *(arrow)* in the kidney parenchyma. These findings are consistent with a pseudoaneurysm of a branch of the left renal artery.

FIGURE 112-6. Positive focal abdominal sonography in trauma (FAST) study. There is a collection of fluid that shows up as a black strip between the liver and kidney. The white appearance is fat around the kidney. These findings are consistent with a fluid collection in Morrison's pouch.

source of bleeding and the retroperitoneal structures. It is effective in a pregnant trauma patient and allows evaluation of the fetus.

An alternative to FAST is diagnostic peritoneal aspiration or lavage. In this approach, a small midline infraumbilical incision is made in the peritoneum to allow sampling of fluid in the peritoneal cavity. If blood is found, laparotomy is necessary to identify and correct the source.

Wounds that penetrate the anterior abdominal region are further divided into low-velocity stab wounds and gunshot wounds, each of which has a different management algorithm. Because mandatory laparotomy for stab wounds results in a high number of negative explorations, many institutions have adopted a selective approach. An unstable victim of an abdominal stab wound should be explored immediately in the operating room. In contrast, a stable patient can undergo local exploration of the wound to determine the depth of penetration. If the wound is superficial, it is irrigated and the patient is observed; if the wound extends beneath the fascia, the patient should undergo exploratory laparotomy to exclude intra-abdominal injury. All gunshot wounds to the anterior abdominal region, except injuries with tangential trajectories, are now routinely explored, but this approach may change in the future.

In an unstable patient or a patient with clinical signs of peritonitis, penetrating wounds to the flanks and posterior abdominal region require exploratory laparotomy. In a stable patient without peritoneal signs, a CT scan with oral, intravenous, and occasionally rectal contrast material may help identify injury to retroperitoneal structures, the ascending and descending colon, the duodenum, the pancreas, and the kidneys.

Pelvis, Perineum, and Buttocks

Clinical evaluation of the pelvis is accomplished through compression of the lateral and anterior aspect of the pelvis to elicit tenderness or bony instability. Rectal examination is essential to exclude bony fragments or blood. Bladder catheterization can identify hematuria and monitor urinary output as a reflection of intravascular volume. Scrotal hematoma, meatal blood, or a high-riding boggy prostate indicates potential urethral injury and requires a urethrogram before insertion of a Foley catheter. All patients with major trauma require an anteroposterior plain film of the pelvis to exclude pelvic or hip fractures. A wound in the perineum in the presence of a pelvic fracture represents an open fracture until proven otherwise.

Penetrating wounds of the buttocks should not be overlooked or underestimated. The likelihood of concomitant peritoneal penetration is 25%, with a mortality rate of 5%. Structures at risk include the retroperitoneal rectum, bladder, ureters, and major arterial and venous structures within the pelvis.

Extremities

Palpation of the long bones is performed to determine whether there is any tenderness or deformity. Range of motion should be assessed in all joints of the upper and lower extremities. Areas of concern on examination should be evaluated radiographically. If there is any suspicion of vascular injury, angiographic examination should be performed.

The compartments of the lower part of the leg are most prone to intracompartmental swelling from direct trauma, long bone fracture, or arterial injury with ischemia or bleeding. Palpation of rigid compartments suggests elevated compartment pressures, which may be measured directly; if pressures are elevated, four-compartment fasciotomies should be performed.

Penetrating wounds to an extremity require operative exploration if they are associated with an enlarging hematoma, active arterial bleeding, or absent arterial pulses. Penetrating wounds resulting in diminished or fluctuating pulses require arteriography to document arterial injury. Otherwise, extremity wounds in proximity to major arterial structures do not require an arteriogram, but the vascular territory should be observed for 24 hours.

MEDICAL ASPECTS OF BURNS

EPIDEMIOLOGY

The National Fire Prevention and Control Administration estimates that 2.6 million fires are reported annually in the United States. About 500,000 burn injuries occur per year and result in about 4000 deaths. About 75% of these deaths occur at the scene of the incident or during initial transport. The most common age groups involved are toddlers (2 to 4 years), for whom scalding is the most common cause, and young adults (17 to 25 years), usually male, for whom the most common cause is a flammable liquid. Structural fires account for less than 5% of hospital admissions but are responsible for more than 45% of burn-related deaths.

Burns can be categorized as scalds, contact burns, and flame burns. Scald burns are the predominant injury in children, whereas contact and flame burns are most common in adults. The major cause of the injury to the skin is exposure to high temperature, which destroys surface tissue. Flames result in temperatures of several thousand degrees Fahrenheit, especially in a closed space. Because water can conduct heat 1000 times better than air, a much

lower temperature (about 48 to 55° C, or 120 to 130° F) is required to produce a deep burn from hot liquid.

Chemical and electrical burns (Chapter 111), although often severe, account for less than 5% of burn admissions. The mechanism of a chemical burn is protein coagulation of skin caused by the acid or alkali. The injury progresses until the chemical is removed by aggressive water lavage. An electrical burn produces tissue coagulation along the course of passage of the current. This deeper injury is hidden from view and must be anticipated to make an early diagnosis and initiate effective treatment.

PATHOBIOLOGY

The skin is the largest organ of the body and ranges from 0.25 m^2 in a newborn to more than 2 m^2 in an adult (Chapter 443). The outermost layer of the epidermis is composed of dead, cornified cells that act as a tough protective barrier against the environment. The second, thicker layer, the corneum (0.06 to 0.12 mm), is composed chiefly of fibrous connective tissue. The dermis contains the blood vessels and nerves to the skin and the epithelial appendages of specialized function. The nerve endings that mediate pain are found in the dermis. Partial-thickness injuries are extremely painful because the nerve endings are exposed. Full-thickness burns are usually anesthetic because of destruction of the nerves.

The skin is also the barrier that prevents loss of body heat and fluids by evaporation. Sweat glands help maintain body temperature by controlling the amount of heat lost by evaporation. Increased loss of water and heat through burned skin is a major problem early after a burn. In addition, the skin is the primary protective barrier against invasive infection. The skin also detects the sensations of touch, pressure, pain, cold, and heat; loss of this function leads to long-term impairment.

TREATMENT   Rx

A burned patient undergoes many dramatic physiologic and metabolic changes over the course of the injury. The burn injury is divided into four phases, each of which has many different physiologic and metabolic characteristics: (1) resuscitation phase (0 to 36 hours), (2) postresuscitation phase (2 to 6 days), (3) inflammation and infection phase (7 days to wound closure), and (4) rehabilitation and wound-remodeling phase (admission to 1 year afterward).

Resuscitation Phase (0 to 36 hours)

Life-threatening airway and breathing problems are of major immediate concern, with the effects of smoke inhalation injury being the most concerning problem (Chapter 94). The initial phase is also characterized by hypovolemia as plasma volume is lost into the burned tissue. The burn itself is of less immediate concern except for initial assessment regarding its severity and depth and the selected need for escharotomy. Wound management becomes a higher priority in later phases. The adequacy of initial treatment of pulmonary and circulatory abnormalities sets the stage for subsequent management.

Smoke Inhalation Injury

The first priority in managing a burn victim is recognition and treatment of smoke exposure. Inhalation injury can be divided into three components based on the onset of symptoms and pathophysiology (Table 112-2).

Carbon Monoxide Toxicity

Carbon monoxide and sometimes cyanide toxicity is evident immediately, with peak symptoms occurring at the scene of the inhalation (Chapter 94). Carbon monoxide rapidly displaces oxygen from hemoglobin and produces carboxyhemoglobin, which impairs oxygen delivery to tissues. The peak level

TABLE 112-2   SMOKE INHALATION COMPLEX

CARBON MONOXIDE (CYANIDE) TOXICITY

Onset of peak symptoms is immediate
Symptoms are systemic

SUPRAGLOTTIC INJURY

Onset of peak symptoms is delayed (hours)
Problem is upper airway edema

INFRAGLOTTIC INJURY

Onset of peak symptoms is delayed (days)
Problem is lower airway mucosal injury

of carboxyhemoglobin also occurs at the scene of the burn; its half-life is about 20 minutes. Treatment is 100% oxygen. Symptoms, which range from confusion to coma, resolve with oxygen therapy unless the patient also suffered severe anoxic injury. The use of hyperbaric oxygen remains controversial in this situation.

Cyanide, which is present in smoke, is absorbed rapidly through the lung and causes systemic toxicity. Cyanide levels are difficult to obtain, but an unexplained base deficit can be assumed to be due to cyanide mitochondrial toxicity; treatment consists of oxygen along with sodium thiosulfate and hydroxocobalamin.

Supraglottic Injury

Smoke injures the mucosa above the glottis because of the combination of superheated air and the toxins in smoke. Mucosal edema, which usually develops over a period of several hours, impedes and potentially obstructs the upper airway. Early endotracheal intubation is indicated if significant edema is evident on direct laryngoscopy, especially if the edema is increasing on subsequent examinations. Upper airway edema generally resolves in 3 to 4 days.

Infraglottic Injury

Toxins in the inhaled air or coating the inhaled soot particles damage the tracheobronchial mucosa, but heat does not usually reach this level. The extent of damage depends on the toxicity of the chemicals and the duration of exposure. Symptoms vary from transient bronchospasm to sloughing of the airway mucosa, which results in plugging and infection. Bronchoscopic evidence of erythema and edema indicates that an injury has occurred but does not predict the degree of injury or time course to recovery.

Endotracheal intubation and positive-pressure ventilation are indicated if symptoms increase, especially if there is an early and progressive impairment in gas exchange. Aggressive pulmonary toilet is necessary to avoid respiratory failure. The time course to resolution may be days or weeks.

Burn Shock and Resuscitation

Adequate volume resuscitation is crucial to survival of the victim of a major body burn. Hypovolemia can also rapidly lead to conversion of viable burned tissue to a nonviable, full-thickness burn, thus further increasing mortality. With modern treatment in burn centers, the failure rate of initial volume restoration is less than 5%, even for large burns involving greater than 85% of the total body skin surface.

Two processes lead to postburn hypovolemia: an increase in microvascular permeability in the burn wound and an increase in the osmolarity of surface burn tissue. A large intravascular-to-extravascular plasma shift occurs. The phase of rapid loss of intravascular fluid persists for about 24 to 36 hours.

Isotonic crystalloid, preferably lactated Ringer's solution, is used in the first 24 hours. Normal saline in large amounts predictably leads to hyperchloremic metabolic acidosis. A volume of 4 mL/kg is given for each percent of body surface burned, with 50% given in the first 8 hours and 50% in the subsequent 16 hours. Isotonic crystalloid is used for the first 24 hours in view of the change in skin capillary permeability for protein. Albumin can be added to the resuscitation fluid to maintain a serum albumin level greater than 2.5 g/dL. After the acute injury, the major fluid loss is water from the injured skin surface, which is no longer able to act as a barrier to the evaporation of water.

Burn Wound

The initial management of a burn wound is based on knowledge of the anatomy of the skin and the functional losses with injury. The major objectives are to decrease the potential for further local damage and the systemic abnormalities that can be produced by loss of the barrier function. Early treatment focuses on neutralizing the source of burn injury, avoiding excess heat loss, determining the extent of the injury, cleaning and débriding the wound, controlling infection with topical antibiotics, and maintaining tissue perfusion.

Assessment of Burn Depth and Size

Burns are categorized as partial thickness or full thickness. A partial-thickness burn is defined by destruction of the epidermis and a portion of the dermis; a superficial partial-thickness burn is confined to the upper third of the dermis, a mid partial-thickness burn involves the middle third, and a deep partial-thickness burn leaves only a portion of the dermis viable. For management purposes, a deep partial-thickness burn is managed similarly to a full-thickness burn: wound excision and skin grafting are required. The approach to superficial partial-thickness burns is to provide for optimal healing, which is initiated by the remaining viable epidermal cells in the hair follicles. Burn size in older children and adults is determined by the percentage of total skin surface area that is involved by the burn (Fig. 112-7).

Postresuscitation Phase (2 to 6 days)

The early postresuscitation phase is a period of transition from the shock phase to the hypermetabolic phase. In general, cardiopulmonary stability is optimal during this period because wound inflammation and infection have not yet developed. Early wound excision and grafting are initiated during this period. Operative risks, especially blood loss and septicemia, are substantially less than later, when inflammation and infection are common.

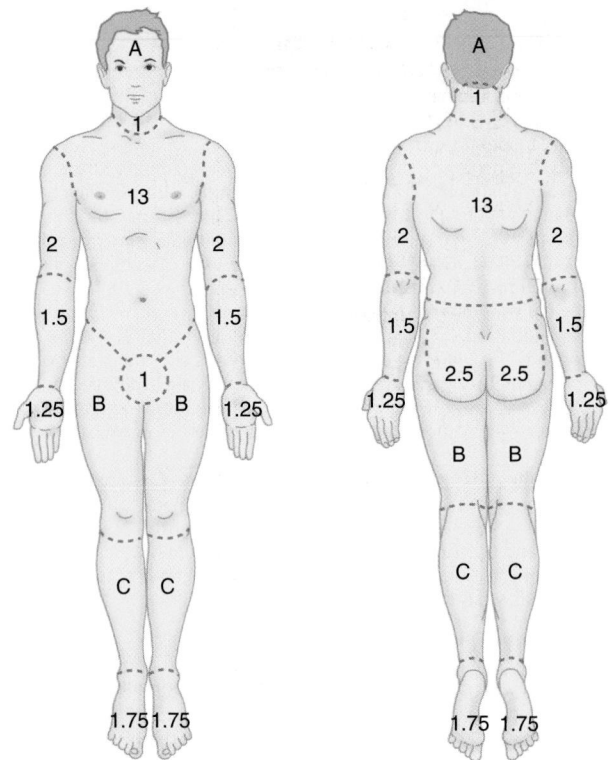

Relative percentages of areas affected by growth			
	Age		
Area	10	15	Adult
A = half of head	5.5	4.5	3.5
B = half of one thigh	4.25	4.5	4.75
C = half of one leg	3	3.25	3.5

FIGURE 112-7. Assessment tool for assessing burn size as a percentage of total body surface area.

Pulmonary Support

Continued upper airway maintenance with an endotracheal tube may be required. Placement of the patient with the head elevated 30 to 45 degrees allows faster resolution of edema. Deciding when to extubate is difficult, and the degree of lower airway injury dictates the timing. Laryngoscopy to determine the presence of cord edema is helpful. Extubation should not be performed unless reintubation is feasible. Lower airway injury is managed by aggressive pulmonary toilet for increased sputum production and microbial overgrowth. Progressive tracheobronchitis and bronchopneumonia are common. The predicted extravascular-to-intravascular fluid shift results in an increased risk for pulmonary edema. Increased levels of antidiuretic stress hormones can prevent appropriate diuresis.

Hemodynamic Stability

The postresuscitation period is characterized by major fluid shifts mainly from the extravascular to the intravascular fluid space. Edema in burned tissue is maximum between 24 and 30 hours after injury in patients with well-controlled fluid resuscitation. The red blood cell mass continues to decrease. Electrolyte and acid-base changes are prominent.

Evaporation from the surface of the burn is a major source of water loss that persists until the wound is closed. The loss is measured in terms of water vapor pressure at the surface. In normal skin, vapor pressure is 2 to 3 mm Hg, whereas the pressure is about 32 mm Hg in a full-thickness burn in which the eschar is soft and hydrated. The rate of loss is increased with increasing surface blood flow. A reasonable estimate of the average loss per hour can be obtained from the following formula: evaporative water loss (mL/hr) = (25 + % total body surface burn) × body surface area (m^2).

Burn Wound

The wound undergoes dramatic changes during the next several days as inflammation develops. Of particular importance is the potential for change in the zone of injured, but still viable, tissue. Changes in local wound microcirculatory blood flow as a result of vasoactive inflammatory agents or local infection can convert this zone of ischemia to a zone of necrosis.

TABLE 112-3 MOST COMMON ORGANISMS IN BURN INFECTIONS

	STAPHYLOCOCCUS AUREUS	PSEUDOMONAS AERUGINOSA	CANDIDA ALBICANS
Wound appearance	Loss of wound granulation	Surface necrosis, patchy black	Minimal exudates
Course	Slow onset, 2-5 days	Rapid onset, 12-36 hr	Slow onset, days
Central nervous system	Disorientation	Modest changes	Often no change
Temperature	Marked increase	High or low	Modest changes
White blood cells	Marked increase	High or low	Modest changes
Hypotension	Modest	Often severe	Minimal change
Mortality	5%	20-30%	30-50%

Hypermetabolic-Sepsis Phase (7 Days to Recovery)

The generalized inflammation of the final phase alters organ function and magnifies any preexisting organ dysfunction. The burn wound is now colonized with bacteria, so wound sepsis is of prominent concern. Infection, whether in the lung or burn wound, becomes increasingly difficult to diagnose because of the continued presence of a non-infection-induced hyperdynamic state. Multisystem organ failure, if it is to occur, is seen during this period.

Burn Wound Infection

Burn wounds are never sterile, even with the administration of topical agents or systemic antibiotics. The presence of bacteria just on the wound surface is termed *colonization*. Colonization may be with a single type of organism or with multiple types. Infection of the wound (Table 112-3) indicates invasion of the underlying viable tissue; this process is diagnosed by eschar biopsy and quantitative culture showing greater than 10^5 organisms per gram of tissue. With progression, viable tissue and its blood vessels are invaded, and septicemia develops. Wound infections require systemic antibiotics. Because all patients have a hyperdynamic state with an elevated temperature and leukocytosis, it is difficult to make a diagnosis of infection based on systemic symptoms. Optimally, most of the eschar should be removed in the first week to avoid burn wound sepsis. *Staphylococcus aureus* is the most common organism isolated from the burn, especially during the first week.

Hypermetabolic State

Beginning at day 5 or 6, there is a gradual increase in the metabolic rate from a normal of 35 to 40 cal/m^2/hr (25 cal/kg/day) to levels twice this value at about 10 days. The increase in metabolic rate after burns is far in excess of that seen after any other severe injury, including sepsis. The magnitude of the increase is related to the size of the burn. The hypermetabolic state is characterized by increased oxygen consumption, increased heat production, increased body temperature, and increased protein catabolism. Body temperature increases from normal to 38 to 38.5° C (100 to 101° F) because of resetting of the hypothalamic temperature center as a result of the altered hormonal environment (Chapter 288).

Marked and sustained increases in circulatory catecholamines lead to hypermetabolism, and treatment with β-blockers (e.g., propranolol titrated to reduce the resting heart rate by 20%)[5] may reduce muscle catabolism. Sustained increases in glucagon and glucocorticoids result in excessive gluconeogenesis and an insulin-resistant state. Increased glucocorticoids also lead to a severe catabolic state, especially because anabolic hormones (growth hormone and testosterone) are decreased after a burn injury.

Nutritional Support

Optimal nutritional support is essential and can decrease net catabolism by about 50%. Currently, there is no recognized ideal nutritional program because of evolving changes with new research findings on postburn nutrient processing. Decreasing stress by wound closure and control of pain, heat loss, and hypovolemia further controls the hypermetabolism. Caloric requirements can be measured with indirect calorimetric techniques. Because more than 95% of the energy generated requires oxygen, there is a direct relationship between oxygen consumption and the metabolic rate. Caloric needs can be estimated by the formula whereby energy requirements = basal metabolic rate × 1.25 × stress factor; the stress factor is 1.2 for a 10% burn, 1.5 for a 20% burn, 1.7 for a 30% burn, 1.8 for a 40% burn, and 2.0 for a 50% or greater burn. If the activity level is increased markedly or additional stress (e.g., severe pain) is present, the metabolic rate can be increased further.

Nutrients Required

Carbohydrate is the preferred fuel for most tissues, but there is a limit to the amount that is used, especially in a hypermetabolic or septic patient (Chapters 221, 223, and 224). Current recommendations are that carbohydrate infusions not exceed 5 to 7 mg/kg per minute, or approximately 1800 to 2200 carbohydrate calories per day. Excess carbohydrate results in the formation of fat, which requires energy rather than produces energy. Approximately 50% of the estimated calorie requirements is usually given as glucose to spare nitrogen. Fat is used as a calorie source, but fat should account for no more than 30%

of the total calories. Protein represents 20 to 25% of infused calories. A standard estimate of 1.5 to 2 g of protein per kilogram of body weight can be used for all major burns. Necessary vitamins and trace elements should be provided in the form of high-potency multivitamin-mineral pills or liquid.

Route of Administration of Nutrition

Nutritional support is best managed during this period by the enteral route, generally through a combination of balanced tube feeding and voluntary intake (Chapter 223). Parenteral hyperalimentation (Chapter 224) through a central vein is occasionally required if for some reason the gastrointestinal tract is not functioning adequately, as sometimes occurs in a patient on a ventilator or a patient with sepsis.

Use of Anabolic Agents

An increase in anabolic activity can decrease the catabolic response to burns, thereby preserving lean body mass, which improves all aspects of wound healing. Glutamine, a conditionally essential amino acid, is invariably deficient several days after a burn because of increased utilization and decreased intake. Glutamine supplementation in major burns, at a dose of 0.4 g/kg body weight, improves wound healing and decreases infections and mortality.[6] Endogenous levels of anabolic human growth hormone and testosterone are decreased after burn surgery, and insulin resistance often develops. These intrinsic changes are all detrimental to wound healing. Supplemental human growth hormone significantly decreases the rate of muscle loss and increases wound healing.[7] Similarly, insulin infusion with glucose in burn patients increases lean mass loss and improves outcome.

The only anabolic steroid approved by the U.S. Food and Drug Administration to treat weight loss and catabolism is oxandrolone, which is given orally (10 mg twice a day), is excreted by the kidney, and has no effects on metabolism other than protein synthesis. Oxandrolone acts on androgenic receptors in lean mass, especially on skin fibroblasts. A number of studies have demonstrated its ability to preserve lean mass after burn injury and thereby improve local healing.[8] In addition, several recent studies have demonstrated direct wound-healing properties.

Rehabilitation after burns is critical to recovery. An augmented exercise program can effectively treat deconditioning and improve subsequent aerobic capacity.[9]

Grade A

1. Stiell IG, Nesbitt LP, Pickett W, et al. The OPALS Major Trauma Study: impact of life-support on survival and morbidity. *CMAJ.* 2008;178:1141-1152.
2. Watkins TR, Rubenfeld GD, Martin TR, et al. Effects of leukoreduced blood on acute lung injury after trauma: a randomized controlled trial. *Crit Care Med.* 2008;36:1493-1499.
3. Shakur H, Roberts R, Bautista R, et al, for the CRASH-2 Trial Collaborators. Effects of tranexamic acid on death, vascular occlusive events, and blood transfusion in trauma patients with significant haemorrhage (CRASH-2): a randomised, placebo-controlled trial. *Lancet.* 2010; 376:23-32.
4. SAFE Study Investigators, Australian and New Zealand Intensive Care Society Clinical Trials Group, Australian Red Cross Blood Service, et al. Saline or albumin for fluid resuscitation in patients with traumatic brain injury. *N Engl J Med.* 2007;357:874-884.
5. Herndon DN, Hart DW, Wolf SE, et al. Reversal of catabolism by beta-blockade after severe burns. *N Engl J Med.* 2001;345:1223-1229.
6. Garrel D, Patenaude J, Nedelec B, et al. Decreased mortality and infectious morbidity in adult burn patients given enteral glutamine: a prospective controlled randomized clinical trial. *Crit Care Med.* 2003;10:2444-2449.
7. Ramirez R, Wolf S, Herndon D. Growth hormone treatment in pediatric patients: a safe therapeutic approach. *Ann Surg.* 1998;4:439-448.
8. Demling R, Orgil D. The anticatabolic and wound-healing effects of the testosterone analog oxandrolone after severe burn injury. *J Crit Care.* 2000;15:12-17.
9. de Lateur BJ, Magyar-Russell G, Bresnick MG, et al. Augmented exercise in the treatment of deconditioning from major brain injury. *Arch Phys Med Rehabil.* 2007;88:S18-S23.

SUGGESTED READINGS

Milia DJ, Brasel K. Current use of CT in the evaluation and management of injured patients. *Surg Clin North Am.* 2011;91:233-248. *Review.*

Moore CL, Copel JA. Point-of-care ultrasonography. *N Engl J Med.* 2011;364:749-757. *Review emphasizing its utility in the emergency department and in seriously ill patients.*

Rafla K, Tredget EE. Infection control in the burn unit. *Burns.* 2011;37:5-15. *Review of epidemiology, diagnosis, management, and prevention.*

Roppolo LP, Wigginton JG, Pepe PE. Intravenous fluid resuscitation for the trauma patient. *Curr Opin Crit Care.* 2010;16:283-288. *Review including evidence for plasma and factor VIIa.*

Wolf SJ, Bebarta VS, Bonnett CJ, et al. Blast injuries. *Lancet.* 2009;374:405-415. *Review.*

113

VENOMOUS SNAKE BITES

STEVEN A. SEIFERT, JAMES O. ARMITAGE, AND
G. RALPH COREY

About 500 of the approximately 2900 species of snakes are venomous, and more than 200 species have caused fatal envenomation in humans. It has been estimated that, worldwide, there are up to 5 million snake bites annually, causing up to 125,000 deaths.

EPIDEMIOLOGY

The incidence of venomous snake bites varies enormously throughout the world. Snake-free areas consist primarily of islands, and Europe continues to be the continent with the lowest incidence of venomous snake bites. In the United States, it is estimated that up to 8000 venomous bites by native species occur each year, mostly by pit vipers (rattlesnakes, copperheads, cottonmouths), with fewer than 100 bites by coral snakes, the only native elapid. Fortunately, the number of fatalities, primarily caused by rattlesnakes, is less than 10 per year. Children and possibly pregnant women are at highest risk for complications. In addition, there are approximately 50 venomous snake bites a year in the United States by non-native (exotic) species; most of these snakes are in private collections, but also in zoos and academic institutions. In the past 10 years, human envenomation by more than 90 different non-native species has occurred. The majority of bites are by viperids, with about 40% by elapids, mostly cobras. The case-fatality rate of exotic envenomation is an order of magnitude higher than that of native species, because of both the number of highly venomous animals that are kept and the logistical issues of management. Most bites occur on extremities when snakes are threatened by being trod on, by someone reaching without looking, or by intentional handling of venomous snakes. Because the crotaline antivenom in the United States is effective against all U.S. crotaline species (and because coral snakes are easily identifiable), there is no need to capture or kill the offending snake for purposes of genus or species identification; such actions only increase the risk of a second envenomation or additional victims. Prevention of snake bite is better than therapy.

Venomous snakes belong to one of five families: Viperidae, with its two subfamilies—Viperinae, or Old World vipers, and Crotalinae, or pit vipers (e.g., rattlesnakes, copperheads, cottonmouths [water moccasins]); Elapidae (e.g., cobras, mambas, kraits, coral snakes); Hydrophiidae (e.g., sea snakes); Atractaspididae (e.g., asps); and Colubridae (e.g., garter snakes, corn snakes, boomslangs). Although all five families contain venomous species, the two responsible for more than 90% of venomous bites are Viperidae and Elapidae. In North America, pit vipers, named for the heat-sensitive organ between the eye and nostril used for hunting warm-blooded prey, are responsible for the majority of venomous snake bites. Fatalities are rare because of a well-developed health care system and the ready availability of antivenom.

In Europe, the only snake of importance is the adder, a viperid snake. Bites are uncommon and rarely fatal. Australia is home to numerous very dangerous Elapidae, including the taipan, death adder, tiger snake, and eastern brown snake. As a result, there are many serious bites each year, despite the low-density population. Fatalities are infrequent, however.

In Central and South America, pit vipers are the primary subfamily responsible for human envenomation; rattlesnakes (Crotalinae, *Sistrurus*) and the *Bothrops* species (*Bothrops jararaca*, fer-de-lance) are responsible for the high morbidity and mortality. The largest venomous snake in the Americas is the bushmaster (*Lachesis muta muta*).

Africa is home to a large number of venomous species. Elapids (cobras and mambas) and the Old World vipers (e.g., saw-scaled viper, puff adder) are among the most prevalent and dangerous of all the world's snakes.

Asia produces the largest number of fatalities from snake envenomation. In India and its eastern neighbors, elapids and viperids are prominent. Cobras, kraits, pit vipers, saw-scaled vipers, and Russell's viper inflict most of the injuries. Although antivenoms are available for most African and Asian snakes of clinical importance, mortality remains high because the health care system is less well developed in these regions.

PATHOBIOLOGY

Snake venoms are complex poisons and often consist of dozens of components that immobilize and digest prey. The effects of venom may be neurotoxic, cardiotoxic, hemotoxic, or myotoxic. Particular species generally produce a characteristic envenomation profile, but the presence or absence of particular components may be variable even within a single species.

Local swelling and bruising after a bite are caused by increased vascular permeability as a result of endothelial cell damage and are mediated by hydrolases, proteases, phospholipase A_2, polypeptide toxins, metalloproteinases, and the release of endogenous autacoids such as bradykinin and histamine. Snakes from the Viperidae and Elapidae families are primarily responsible for these effects.

Hemostatic abnormalities are frequent and varied. Pro-coagulants activate factors V, IX, and X, protein C (Russell's viper), and prothrombin (vipers) and cleave fibrinopeptide A from fibrinogen. Fibrinolytic activators result in a disseminated intravascular coagulation (DIC)–like picture, although there are key differences from true DIC, including the absence of thrombin formation and the failure of heparin therapy in snake envenomation. Snake venom hemorrhagins damage endothelium and increase the potential for serious bleeding, especially after viper bites. Intravascular hemolysis, which can occur after bites by *Bothrops* (e.g., fer-de-lance) and other species, results in severe anemia and acute renal failure.

Paralysis is the primary function of many types of venom of the Elapidae and Hydrophiidae families and of some Viperidae snakes. Presynaptic neurotoxins (e.g., β-bungarotoxins, crotoxin, taipoxin) prevent acetylcholine release, and postsynaptic toxins (e.g., α-bungarotoxins, cobrotoxin) bind to acetylcholine receptors on the motor end plate.

Rhabdomyolysis (Chapter 115) occurs most commonly from the presynaptic neurotoxins of sea snakes, but myotoxins have also been found in Australasian elapids, Russell's viper, and selected rattlesnakes. Acute renal failure, hyperkalemia, and death often result. Other mechanisms of renal failure after envenomation include a direct renal toxin, hemoglobinuria after massive intravascular hemolysis, hypotension, and DIC-like defects.

Toxins that do not immobilize prey through neurotoxins may immobilize by causing hypotension. Some snakes (primarily vipers) produce an acute hypotensive syndrome within minutes after envenomation through the release of vasodilating autacoids. *Bothrops* species inhibit the breakdown of bradykinin and angiotensinogen (angiotensin-converting enzyme inhibitors). Vasodilation, diffuse vascular permeability, myocardial depression, and atrioventricular block all play roles in the hypotension caused by crotalines and elapids. Individuals who handle snakes or who have been bitten previously may develop an immunoglobulin (Ig) E–mediated anaphylactic reaction. A non-IgE-mediated anaphylactoid response may be seen with the rapid introduction of foreign proteins into circulation; nonspecific effects, such as vagal reactions and hypovolemia secondary to massive tissue fluid accumulation as a result of local venom injury, may also produce hypotension.

CLINICAL MANIFESTATIONS
Pit Viper Envenomation

Swelling and pain are the first and most important findings of early pit viper envenomation. These symptoms often occur within minutes and are followed by progressive proximal swelling and ecchymosis in the bitten extremity, although onset of the latter may be delayed for hours. Local swelling, usually extracompartmental, may be massive, and elevated tissue or compartment pressures may occur from tension created by the skin's limited elasticity. Necrosis may develop as a consequence of direct venom-related tissue injury or possibly as a result of pressure-mediated vascular compromise. Necrosis typically occurs over a period of several days, with the potential for permanent tissue loss. Progression of local injury usually ceases within 24 to 36 hours. Secondary infection of snake bites is rare, but the presence of necrosis increases its likelihood. The development of systemic symptoms such as nausea, diaphoresis, paresthesias, metallic taste, and dizziness may indicate more severe envenomation. Hypotension and bleeding manifestations (e.g., distant petechiae; hematuria; gingival, gastrointestinal, central nervous system bleeding) may also occur early and pose the greatest risk for death. During the first 24 hours, the white blood cell count is often increased. Various coagulation abnormalities, alone or in combination, may be seen, including thrombocytopenia; elevated D-dimer or fibrin-fibrinogen degradation products, with or without hypofibrinogenemia; and prolongation of the international normalized ratio or activated partial thromboplastin time. Hematologic effects are more common with rattlesnake bites but can occur with copperhead or cottonmouth envenomation as well. Spontaneous bleeding is more likely with combined and severe coagulation system abnormalities. In patients with persistent hypotension, the presence of coma, acidosis, and oliguric renal failure presages death.

Progression of local injury may recur in the first 24 hours, particularly in patients treated with a Fab antivenom. This occurs as protective levels of circulating antivenom decline rapidly secondary to their larger volume of distribution compared with IgG or $F(ab')_2$ antivenoms and the renal clearance of unbound antivenom. This recurrence is not associated with a recurrence of detectable blood venom antigens and appears to be the result of a lack of adequate amounts of neutralizing antivenom at the leading margin of envenomated tissue. Coagulation system disorders may persist despite antivenom and may also recur. Recurrence of coagulation defects typically occurs several days after treatment with a Fab antivenom and is associated with the loss of protective circulating antivenom secondary to renal clearance, thereby allowing unneutralized venom still entering the circulation to exert its toxic effects. This recurrence is associated with detectable blood venom antigens. The specific hematologic abnormalities (e.g., thrombocytopenia) seen early in the course tend to recur, with similar degrees of severity ("like predicts like in kind and degree"). The ultimate severity of envenomations treated within 1 to 2 hours may have been masked, and such patients are also at risk of severe recurrence, despite apparently mild early effects. Recurrent coagulation abnormalities may persist or continue to recur following additional treatment, for up to 3 weeks.

Coral Snake Envenomation

Unlike the pit vipers, local symptoms after coral snake bites are often confined to paresthesias around the bite and mild swelling in a minority of patients. Systemic symptoms are often delayed for 1 to 6 hours. Because of species differences, coral snake bites in Florida (*Micrurus fulvius*) tend to be more severe than those in Texas (*Micrurus tener*). In the bordering states (Louisiana, Alabama), which may have either species, the risk of toxicity may be difficult to determine. Coral snake bites in Arizona and New Mexico (*Micruroides euryxanthus*) do not produce significant clinical effects. With severe envenomation, perioral paresthesias, nausea, vomiting, hypersalivation, and euphoria give way to cranial nerve paralysis (e.g., ptosis, diplopia, dysphagia) and respiratory failure. Respiratory failure may develop within minutes of the onset of neurologic signs.

TREATMENT ℞

Expert assistance in managing a snake bite of any kind can be obtained by contacting the regional poison center at 1-800-222-1222.

Snake bite is primarily a medical rather than a surgical condition. On a patient's arrival at an emergency care facility, primary attention should be given to assessing and establishing the airway, breathing, and circulation. Management might include antivenom administration, management of type I hypersensitivity reactions to snake venom or antivenom (e.g., epinephrine, H_1- and H_2-blockers), intravenous fluids, tetanus toxoid, airway protection, mechanical ventilation, pressors, pain medications, radiographs of the wound to rule out retained foreign bodies (fangs or teeth), and, later, physical therapy. Late surgical débridement of necrotic tissue, if any, may be required. Surgical treatment of elevated tissue or compartment pressures is very rarely indicated. Because of the inability of prophylactic antibiotics to prevent infection[1] and the potential of an adverse drug reaction occurring simultaneously with venom toxicity, antibiotics should be reserved for documented infection, a clinical appearance that cannot be easily distinguished from infection, or frank tissue necrosis.

A wide variety of ineffective and potentially harmful therapies for snake bite have been and, in some cases, continue to be popular (Table 113-1). Use of these methods in true envenomations may contribute to venom injury and could result in tragedy if they delay or supplant effective therapy.

TABLE 113-1 INEFFECTIVE OR POTENTIALLY HARMFUL REMEDIES FOR SNAKE BITE

LOCAL WOUND MEASURES

Aloe vera leaves
Cold
Electricity
Heat
Incision
Kerosene
Pineapple concentrate
Suction
Tourniquets (arterial or venous)

SYSTEMIC OR LOCAL MEASURES

Castor oil
Chinese herbs
Colloidal silver
Drinking water
Echinacea
Ethanol
Euphorbia
Grape juice
Impatiens
Lantana
Turmeric
Vitamin C

Pit Viper Envenomation

Prehospital

Appropriate care consists of immobilization of a bitten extremity, consideration of the need to slow systemic absorption by dependent positioning or lymphatic obstruction, and, most important, rapid transit to a hospital emergency department. Any treatment that increases or prolongs the local concentration of venom may result in greater local injury and should be used only when life-threatening systemic effects (e.g., profound hypotension, anaphylaxis, severe bleeding) are occurring. The application of a lymphatic constriction band (15 to 25 mm Hg) or a pressure immobilization bandage requires training and proper equipment and is rarely required. Popular prehospital treatments such as arterial or venous tourniquets, incision, suction, heat, cold, and electric shock are not helpful, can delay definitive treatment, and can cause additional trauma.

Hospital

The chance of a North American crotaline bite resulting in envenomation is around 80%. The onset of symptoms of pit viper envenomation is usually rapid and obvious but may be delayed for many hours. Potentially "dry" bites should be observed for at least 10 to 12 hours.

The ultimate severity of envenomation becomes apparent only over time, and "mild" envenomation may progress to "severe," depending on the venom load, venom components, and host factors. Definitive therapy for systemic symptoms of snake bite, including hypotension and coagulation abnormalities, is antivenom, which should be used for any significant or progressive envenomation. The starting dose is based on the severity of symptoms or signs and the rapidity of progression. Administration of blood product components is usually futile in the absence of adequate venom neutralization. With neutralization, the body replenishes platelets, fibrinogen, and clotting factors on its own. Blood products should be reserved for life-threatening bleeding and should be given in conjunction with additional antivenom.

The crotaline snake antivenom available in the United States, CroFab, consists of Fab antibodies to specific crotaline venoms that were raised in sheep. It is indicated and efficacious for all North American crotaline snakes.[2] Because antivenom contains foreign proteins, type I (immediate) hypersensitivity reactions are possible, including anaphylaxis. With Fab antivenom, predominantly mild type I hypersensitivity reactions have been reported to date in less than 7% of patients. Cutaneous sensitivity testing before administration is not recommended and does not adequately predict the likelihood of a type I reaction in other settings. Type I hypersensitivity reactions are managed by stopping or slowing the rate of infusion and by administering H_1-blockers (e.g., diphenhydramine 50 mg IV), H_2-blockers (e.g., ranitidine 50 mg IV or cimetidine 300 mg IV), and epinephrine (0.3 mg SC as a 1:1000 dilution) as needed. It is usually possible to restart the infusion at a slower rate after treatment and to give the complete dose, although a risk-benefit reassessment should be made regarding the ongoing need for antivenom. Means of treating anaphylaxis should always be immediately available.

The initial dose of Fab antivenom is 4 to 6 vials, regardless of the patient's weight, because the objective is to neutralize a specific quantity of injected venom. Children may, in fact, require higher doses because of higher serum venom levels (a larger venom dose relative to weight) and particular

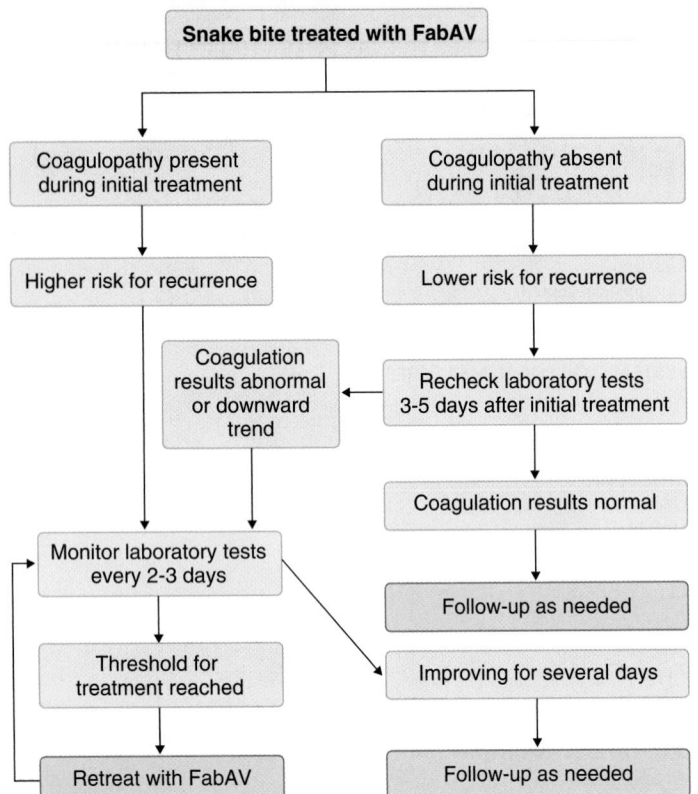

FIGURE 113-1. Monitoring for coagulopathy in patients treated with Crotalidae polyvalent immune Fab (ovine) (FabAV).

TABLE 113-2	RECOMMENDATIONS FOR RETREATMENT WITH ANTIVENOM FOR PERSISTENT OR RECURRENT HEMATOLOGIC ABNORMALITIES

Active, significant bleeding (in conjunction with blood products as needed)
Fibrinogen < 50 µg/mL
Platelet count < 25,000/mm³
INR > 3.0 sec or aPTT > 50 sec
Multicomponent effects with lesser abnormalities
Worsening trend in a patient at risk for severe recurrence
High-risk behaviors for trauma in a patient with lesser abnormalities
Comorbid conditions that increase bleeding risk

aPTT = adjusted partial thromboplastin time; INR = international normalized ratio.

days after treatment) are usually mild with Fab antivenom but occur in up to 5% of cases. For management of mild type III hypersensitivity reactions, treatment is with nonsteroidal anti-inflammatory drugs (e.g., ibuprofen 200 to 800 mg orally four times a day as needed for arthralgia, myalgia, and fever) and antihistamines (e.g., diphenhydramine 25 to 50 mg orally four times a day as needed for urticaria). For more severe reactions, corticosteroids (e.g., prednisone 20 to 40 mg/day orally, with a taper over 2 weeks if treatment is needed for more than 5 days) are recommended. Type III reactions are self-limited and typically have a duration of 2 to 10 days, rarely lasting more than 3 to 4 weeks.

Coral Snake Envenomation
Prehospital
Appropriate care consists of immobilization of a bitten extremity and efforts to slow systemic absorption with the use of a pressure immobilization bandage. Proper application of this bandage requires training, and it is frequently misapplied by untrained providers; therefore, a lymphatic constriction band (blood pressure cuff inflated to 15 to 25 mm Hg) may be safer but possibly less effective. Most important is rapid transit to a hospital emergency department. Because local effects are minimal and neurologic toxicity may progress rapidly, there is little risk in the use of a properly applied pressure immobilization bandage or lymphatic constriction band. Popular prehospital treatments such as tourniquets, incision, suction, heat, cold, and electric shock are not helpful, can delay definitive treatment, and can cause additional trauma.

Hospital
The chance of a bite from an eastern coral snake resulting in envenomation is around 75%. The onset of neurologic symptoms may be quickly evident, but it may also be delayed for many hours. Because of minimal local effects and potentially delayed neurotoxicity, envenomation and the seriousness of such bites can easily be underestimated. The snake bite severity score is not valid for these snake bites. Potentially "dry" bites should be closely observed for at least 24 hours.

In the United States, the Food and Drug Administration–approved monovalent, equine IgG antivenom (manufactured by Wyeth) should be given at the first signs of envenomation by bites of the eastern coral snake (*Micrurus fulvius*) or the Texas coral snake (*Micrurus tener*). However, Wyeth ceased production in 2006, and supplies are limited and dwindling in endemic areas. It is estimated that replacement supplies will no longer be available in 2010 or 2011, after which remaining antivenom stocks, currently distributed primarily to hospitals in endemic areas, will gradually be consumed.

Skin testing is suggested by the manufacturer, although such testing is not adequately predictive of the risk for type I (immediate) hypersensitivity reactions, and an expert consensus panel has concluded that skin testing should not be performed. Regardless, testing should not delay administration in the event of life-threatening effects. When available, the initial dose is 3 to 6 vials, repeated as needed until progression of signs and symptoms ceases. Rarely are more than 10 vials required. Type III hypersensitivity reactions ("serum sickness") may occur; management is as described earlier.

If fresh Wyeth antivenom is not available, some advocate using expired Wyeth antivenom, despite medicolegal concerns. Neostigmine (infants, 0.025 to 0.1 mg/kg/dose; children, 0.025 to 0.08 mg/kg/dose; adults, 0.5 to 2.5 mg/dose, total dose not to exceed 5 mg) is efficacious against the neurotoxicity of other elapids, including several South American species of coral snake; doses can be repeated as needed to maintain reversal of blockade. Neostigmine may be considered a temporizing measure, adjunctive therapy, or monotherapy; however, there are no published reports on its use in U.S. coral snake envenomations. If neostigmine is used, atropine (0.4 mg per 1 mg of neostigmine) should be given several minutes before the neostigmine to counter unwanted cholinergic effects. Foreign antivenoms, which may have efficacy against U.S. coral snakes, can be located and obtained through the Antivenom Index, which can be accessed via the regional poison center (1-800-222-1222). If respiratory compromise results in intubation, days to weeks of respiratory support may be required.

vulnerabilities, such as smaller airway size and the increased proportion of vascular volume lost into tissues. Additional antivenom doses may be administered as needed to obtain initial control of the signs and symptoms of envenomation. Initial control includes reversal of systemic symptoms, cessation of progression of proximal swelling or a reduction in circumferential swelling and tissue pressures, and cessation of worsening or evidence of improvement in coagulation components. Repeated dosing of Fab antivenom after initial control (2 vials every 6 hours for three doses) is recommended to prevent the recurrence of local effects (Fig. 113-1). Additional doses (2 vials) may be required for breakthrough local recurrences.

Management of elevated tissue or compartmental pressures (Chapter 115) is controversial. Dermotomy may be considered in areas without true compartments (e.g., fingers) if the degree of swelling compromises circulation; however, additional antivenom and elevation may reduce the swelling, making this procedure unnecessary. In practice, dermotomy is very rarely required. If there is concern about significantly elevated tissue or compartmental pressures, they should be measured directly. In general, additional antivenom and elevation are recommended for increased pressure (>30 mm Hg). Elevation is controversial because it decreases local tissue perfusion in the typical compartment syndrome. After snake bites, however, elevated compartmental pressures may be entirely secondary to subcutaneous edema and may respond to elevation with a proximal redistribution of tissue fluid and a reduction in tissue pressures. Conversely, in true compartment syndrome, owing to either direct intracompartmental injection of venom or lymphatic drainage of venom into the compartment, elevation may be harmful. Nevertheless, judicious elevation seems reasonable to see whether a reduction in pressures can avoid fasciotomy, which does not appear to be beneficial in compartment syndrome caused by venom injection.

Patients with early, severe coagulopathic abnormalities are at risk for recurrence of severe abnormalities of the same kind; about 70% of those with early coagulation defects return with late recurrences. Optimal management of severe recurrence is undetermined, but patients with severe abnormalities in multiple coagulation systems (e.g., platelets and fibrinogen) or with comorbid conditions (e.g., advanced age, hypertension, bleeding diathesis, risk-taking behavior) are at increased risk for significant bleeding and are candidates for repeat dosing of Fab antivenom (Table 113-2). Two vials should be given intravenously, and the patient should be monitored and possibly treated daily until a clear improving trend is observed (see Fig. 113-1).

Postacute Phase
In an effort to improve functional outcome, physical therapy should begin as soon as the acute phase of local injury has subsided, usually in 36 to 48 hours. Type III hypersensitivity reactions ("serum sickness," occurring 5 to 21

Bites by Non-native Species

Management of bites by non-native species is challenging because of both their unfamiliarity and potential delays in obtaining appropriate antivenom, which is usually kept by zoos that have specimens of the biting species. Poison centers have access to information about zoo supplies of antivenom through an online listing, the Antivenom Index. Assistance in locating and obtaining species-specific antivenom and clinical case management can be obtained through the regional poison center (1-800-222-1222).

PROGNOSIS

In general, the prognosis is good if timely access to antivenom is possible. For coral snake bites, the mortality rate before the introduction of antivenom in 1967 was between 10 and 15%. Age and underlying disease can increase morbidity, particularly if hemorrhage and hypotension develop.

1. Kularatne SA, Kumarasiri PV, Pushpakumara SK, et al. Routine antibiotic therapy in the management of the local inflammatory swelling in venomous snakebites: results of a placebo-controlled study. *Ceylon Med J.* 2005;50:151-155.
2. Dart RC, Seifert SA, Boyer LV, et al. A randomized multicenter trial of crotalinae polyvalent immune Fab (ovine) antivenom for the treatment of crotaline snakebite in the United States. *Arch Intern Med.* 2001;161:2030-2036.

SUGGESTED READINGS

Kasturiratne A, Wickremasinghe AR, de Silva N, et al. The global burden of snakebite: a literature analysis and modelling based on regional estimates of envenoming and deaths. http://www.plosmedicine.org/article/info:doi/10.1371/journal.pmed.0050218. *Review of the worldwide morbidity and mortality burden of snake bite.*

Warrell D. Snake bite. *Lancet.* 2010;375:77-88. *Review of management.*

Weinstein SA, Dart RC, Staples A, et al. Envenomations: an overview of clinical toxinology for the primary care physician. *Am Fam Phys.* 2009;80:793-802. *Management of envenomation.*

VENOMS AND POISONS FROM MARINE ORGANISMS

JAY W. FOX

The term *envenomation* implies penetration of a target by an organism for delivery of venom containing one or more toxins. In contrast, poisons are toxins acquired from the environment by mechanisms such as absorption, inhalation, and ingestion. In the marine environment, both forms of intoxication cause effects ranging from mild irritation and discomfort to death (Table 114-1). Severe outbreaks of poisoning can result from the ingestion of marine organisms that contain toxins, and such outbreaks have become more frequent as microorganisms in coastal waters increase, owing to a combination of global sea warming, eutrophication, aquaculture, and discharge of organisms from ship ballasts. Encroachment on the marine environment for recreation, living space, and food sources increases the frequency of adverse encounters with venomous and poisonous marine organisms.

VENOMOUS MARINE ORGANISMS

Venomous marine organisms deliver their venom by bites and stings. Envenomation involves penetration of the skin and may be complicated by secondary bacterial infections, especially after deep puncture wounds and bites.

Chordata

Sea Snakes

Sea snakes, which are members of the family *Hydrophiidae*, are generally found in tropical and subtropical waters, especially the coastal waters of Thailand, Indonesia, the Persian Gulf, Australia, and India. One species, the yellow-bellied sea snake (*Pelaramis platurus*), is found in the Pacific coastal waters of Central America. Sea snakes, which are very capable swimmers and are relatively immobile on land, inject their venom with two small maxillary fangs (2 to 4 mm long) that contain ducts connected to venom glands located

posterior and ventral to the maxillary bone. The relatively short length of the fangs prevents effective envenomation through most protective clothing such as dive suits. If the subject reacts to envenomation by forceful retraction, the fangs are often dislodged from the maxillary bone of the snake and may remain in the site—a condition that imposes an additional risk for infection.

Because of the nature of the venom and the size of the fangs, the sea snake bite itself is not generally painful. One or two small prick marks are present at the envenomation site, occasionally with additional marks from the other teeth in the snake's mouth. The primary toxin in sea snake venom is a postsynaptic peptide neurotoxin that functions by blocking the acetylcholine receptor at neuromuscular junctions (Fig. 114-1). Ptosis, dysphagia, and nonrigid paralysis, which are the most common symptoms of sea snake envenomation, typically appear within 30 minutes to 2 hours after the bite. In severe cases, respiratory failure may develop, and respiratory support may be necessary. Antivenom is available.

Weeverfish, Lionfish, Scorpionfish, and Stonefish

Weeverfish belong to the *Trachinidae* family, whereas scorpionfish, stonefish, and lionfish all belong to the family *Scorpaenidae*. Members of the *Scorpaenidae* family are found mostly in tropical and subtropical waters, but weeverfish are in European and African waters. All of these fish sting by using dorsal spines. The anal spines of *Scorpaenidae* fish and the opercular spines of *Trachinidae* fish can also deliver venom. The spines are encased in an integumentary sheath that is torn when the spine punctures the victim's skin. Venom glands are located at the base of the spine.

Few details are known regarding the biochemistry and pharmacology of the toxins in weeverfish venom. The sting of the weeverfish is extremely painful and may produce systemic effects such as aphonia, fever, chills, dyspnea, cyanosis, nausea, syncope, hypotension, and arrhythmias. The wound is edematous, erythematous, and ecchymotic. Bacterial infection is typical, and gangrene has developed in severe cases of infection. The venom may be somewhat heat labile, and soaking in tolerably hot water may reduce pain and attenuate the effects of the venom. Death from an untreated weeverfish sting is rare.

Scorpaenidae envenomation symptoms are generally less severe for lionfish (*Pterois*), more severe for scorpionfish (*Scorpaena*), and most severe for stonefish (*Synanceia*). Lionfish (turkey fish, dragon fish, butterfly cod), which are found worldwide, have long thin spines. Scorpionfish have shorter, thicker spines and are primarily found in tropical and subtropical waters and the Mediterranean. The local consequences of edema and erythema from stings of these fish are very similar to those of the weeverfish. Immersion in hot water is generally effective to alleviate pain associated with envenomation.

The stonefish (*Synanceja*) group has short strong spines and is found throughout the Indo-Pacific area, China, Australia, and the Indian Ocean. Their toxins are high-molecular-weight, multimeric, heat-labile proteins. Symptoms of envenomation are similar to those from the stings of members of the other groups. A lethal toxin, stonustoxin, from the venom of *Synanceja horrida* causes muscle relaxation by producing nitric oxide and also causes hemolysis, platelet aggregation, and inhibition of neuromuscular function. Trachynilysin, a pore-forming neurotoxin from *Synanceja trachynis*, causes massive presynaptic release of acetylcholine. Soaking of the wound site in hot water (45° C) is recommended. In cases of severe blistering, the blisters should be excised to flush residual active venom from the blister fluid to ameliorate dermal necrosis. As with all fish stings, care should be taken to ensure that no broken portions of the spines remain in the wound; vigilance against bacterial infections is imperative. Antivenom should be used only if it is clear that envenomation has occurred.

Stingrays

Stingrays (family Dasyatidae) are found in most seas but are predominant in the Indo-Pacific area. Some members of the family are also found in fresh water. Venom containing serotonin is delivered by stings from spines (one or more) on the tail of the stingray. Stingray spines are retroserrated on the margins and are covered by an integumentary sheath. Venomous glandular tissue is located at the base of the spines. On puncture of the skin, the sheath is torn by the serrated spine, and venom flows along the two ventrolateral grooves of the spine into the surrounding tissue. The spines are often deeply embedded in the tissue and difficult to extract because of the retroserration. Care must be taken to remove all spine and sheath fragments. Depending on the location of the spine and the depth of penetration, specialized care may

TABLE 114-1 SIGNIFICANT VENOMOUS AND POISONOUS MARINE ORGANISMS

ORGANISM	MECHANISM OF INTOXICATION (EVENOMING/POISONING)	PRIMARY TOXINS	ANTIVENOM AVAILABLE (SOURCE)
Sea snakes (Hydrophiidae)	Bite	Postsynaptic neurotoxins	Yes (CSL, Ltd.)
Blue-ringed octopus (Octopodidae)	Bite	Tetrodotoxin (neurotoxin)	No
Cone shell (Conidae)	Sting	Presynaptic and postsynaptic neurotoxins	No
Box jellyfish (*Chironex fleckeri, Chiropsalmus quadrigatus*)	Sting	Hemolysins, proteinases, cardiotoxin, necrotoxins	Yes (CSL, Ltd.)
Portuguese man-of-war (*Physalia physalis*)	Sting	Hemolysins, proteinases, cardiotoxin, necrotoxins	No
Sea nettles (*Chrysaora quinquecirrha, Cyanea capillata*)	Sting	Hemolysins, proteinases, cardiotoxin, necrotoxins	No; generally no need
Sea anemone (*Anemonia sulcata*)	Sting	Neurotoxins	No; generally no need
Scorpionfish (Scorpaenidae)	Sting puncture	Hemolysins, necrotoxins?	Yes (CSL, Ltd.)
Lionfish (Scorpaenidae)	Sting puncture	Hemolysins, necrotoxins?	No
Stonefish (Scorpaenidae)	Sting puncture	Hemolysins, necrotoxins?	Yes (CSL, Ltd)
Weeverfish (Trachinidae)	Sting puncture	Hemolysins, necrotoxins?	No
Stingrays (Rajiformes)	Sting puncture	Uncertain	No
Dinoflagellates	Ingestion (found in seafood)	Ciguatera poisoning	No
Gambierdiscus toxicus	Ingestion (found in fish)	Ciguatoxins, maitotoxin (neurotoxins)	No
Ptychodiscus brevis	Ingestion (found in shellfish)	Neurotoxic shellfish poisoning, neurotoxins	No
Gonyaulax species	Ingestion (found in shellfish)	Paralytic shellfish poisoning	No
Pyrodinium species	Ingestion (found in shellfish)	Saxitoxin, neosaxitoxin, and gonyautoxin	No
Jania species	Ingestion (found in shellfish)	Okadaic acid (phosphatase inhibitors)	No
Pufferfish (Tetraodontiformes)	Ingestion	Tetrodotoxin (neurotoxin)	No
Porcupinefish (Tetraodontiformes)	Ingestion	Tetrodotoxin (neurotoxin)	No
Sunfish (*Mola* species)	Ingestion	Tetrodotoxin (neurotoxin)	No

FIGURE 114-1. Schematic representation of a motor axon synapse and the sites of action of various marine neurotoxins.

be necessary to extract the spine and cleanse the wound. A sting produces severe pain and edema, which in extreme cases is accompanied by hemorrhage, syncope, vomiting, hypotension, and cardiac arrhythmias. In rare cases, death can occur, especially if the pericardial, peritoneal, or pleural cavities are penetrated. Soaking the wound in hot water inactivates some of the heat-labile toxins in the venom.

Mollusca

Cone Snails

Cone snail (Conidae) venom is injected into victims through a hollow, harpoon-like tooth. The venom, which is primarily neurotoxic, causes paresthesias, hypotension, and respiratory impairment or failure. Fourteen superfamilies of conopeptide toxins have been identified in cone snail venom:

A, I, M, O, P, S, T, I2, J, L, O2, O3, V, and Y. All of the conopeptides are short polypeptides that demonstrate a variety of neurotoxic actions by targeting specific subtypes of ion channels, neurotransmitter receptors, or transporters (see Fig. 114-1). The bite is very painful and may be followed by systemic symptoms such as dysphagia, aphonia, pruritus, blurred vision, syncope, muscular paralysis, and respiratory and cardiac failure. Treatment is supportive; in cases of severe envenomation, preparation for cardiovascular and respiratory support should be made. Rare cases of coagulopathy have been reported, and fatal envenomation has occurred.

Octopuses

The two species of blue-ringed octopuses (*Hapalochlaena maculosa* and *Hapalochlaena lunulata*), found in Australian waters, inject their venom by a relatively painless bite that produces two small puncture wounds. Hemorrhage at the site may occur. The major toxic component in the venom is tetrodotoxin, a neurotoxin that blocks action potentials of voltage-activated sodium channels and causes perioral and intraoral paresthesias, dysphagia, nausea, ataxia, aphonia, flaccid muscular paralysis, and respiratory distress or failure. Fatal envenomation has occurred, and urgent respiratory support may be required in severe cases.

Cnidaria
Jellyfish and Anemones

Jellyfish and anemones belong to the Cnidaria phylum, so named because of their venomous organelles called *cnidae*. The cnidae found in jellyfish and anemones (called *nematocysts* and *spirocysts*, respectively) are located on exposed tentacles. On tactile stimulation, the tentacles send forth a tethered projectile to deliver venom through the dermis. As the victim's surrounding musculature contracts, the venom is disseminated. Hemolysins, DNAase, and histamine releasers have been identified in some venoms. A number of peptide toxins of sea anemones mostly function by binding to sodium channel receptor site 3 to delay the inactivation phase of the channel. Other peptide toxins from anemones target the Kv3 potassium channel.

Stings by jellyfish and anemones typically produce immediate pain at the site of envenomation, followed by erythematous and urticarial lesions. Anaphylaxis is not common unless the patient has previously been sensitized. Depending on the severity of the sting, wheals and whiplike patterns may appear at the sites of envenomation within a few minutes or be delayed by several hours, followed in some cases by dermal necrosis. Eruptions sometimes recur days after the envenomation. Systemic reactions may include muscle spasms and cramps, vomiting, nausea, diarrhea, diaphoresis, and, in rare cases, cardiorespiratory failure.

Unfired nematocysts on tentacles adhering to the skin may be neutralized by vinegar or baking soda, depending on the species of jellyfish. Vinegar appears to be most useful for Australian blue bottle (*Physalia utriculus*) stings, whereas baking soda appears more efficacious for sea nettle (*Chrysaora quinquecirrha*) stings.

The box jellyfish (*Chironex fleckeri*) found in Australian waters is perhaps the most venomous jellyfish; it produces very severe stings that may cause death from hypotension, muscular and respiratory paralysis, and ultimately, cardiac arrest. Treatment of box jellyfish stings may require respiratory support and administration of antivenom.

The Portuguese man of war (*Physalia physalis*) is not a true jellyfish, and its venom differs from true jellyfish. It stings through nematocysts that cause intense pain and, occasionally, an allergic reaction. Flushing with salt water (sea water) followed by application of heat may ease the pain.

Sponges

Some sponges colonized by coelenterates produce toxins that can cause a pruritic, allergic dermatitis or an irritant dermatitis. These toxins are delivered by the sharp spicules, which penetrate the dermis. The toxins can cause the typical sponge diver's disease, which is characterized by local burning and itching and may be accompanied by soft tissue edema and purulent vesiculation. Serious illness is rare.

Corals

Fire coral (*Millepora alcicornis*) is found in shallow tropical waters. Stings are a common consequence of brushing or rubbing against the coral. Envenomation produces a burning or stinging sensation, followed by severe pruritus. Edematous wheals may develop but generally dissipate over the course of several days. The site of envenomation should be soaked in vinegar (5% acetic acid) or 70% isopropanol to relieve pain.

Annelida
Bristle worms

Bristle worms are segmented invertebrates found in tropical Pacific waters and the Gulf of Mexico. The bristles can penetrate the skin and produce severely painful envenomation, with pruritus and burning that may persist for several days. Local paresthesia is typical and may linger for weeks. Treatment is symptomatic, with consideration of possible tetanus infection (Chapter 304). Little is known regarding the chemistry of bristle worm venom.

Echinodermata
Sea Urchins

Of the echinoderms, sea urchins and sea stars are responsible for most stings in humans. The venom is delivered by the long spines and pedicellaria protruding from the sea urchin body. The spines are covered at the tips with a venom sac that is broken when it penetrates the skin. The pedicellaria, present on some species of sea urchins, are pincer-like appendages carrying venom glands. The toxins of sea urchin venom are not well characterized. Stings can produce pain, hemorrhage, aphonia, paresthesias, paralysis, hypotension, nausea, syncope, and respiratory distress. Immersion in hot water helps inactivate heat-labile toxins in the venom. Attached pedicellaria and embedded spines must be removed to prevent additional envenomation and infection.

● POISONOUS MARINE ORGANISMS

Unlike envenomation, marine poisoning nearly always results from consumption of fish or shellfish that have accumulated various toxins from dinoflagellates. Most marine poisonings cause neurologic and gastrointestinal effects associated with the specific toxins found in the food source. Diagnosis is clinical, based on the type of fish ingested and the clinical symptoms presented. Neurotoxic marine poisoning is generally caused by one of six different toxins.

Neurotoxic Marine Toxins
Ciguatoxins

Ciguatoxins are occasionally found in reef fish of the Caribbean and Pacific. These toxins are cyclic polyethers that act as excitatory agents by binding to sodium channels. Maitotoxin, from the same dinoflagellate, is a water-soluble polyether that acts by enhancing calcium entry through L-type calcium channels. Symptoms of ciguatera poisoning generally appear within 2 to 12 hours after the ingestion of contaminated fish. Gastrointestinal symptoms, including diarrhea, abdominal pain, nausea, and vomiting, appear first, followed by neurologic and cardiovascular symptoms. Neurologic symptoms include aphonia, dental dysesthesias, fatigue, tremor, ataxia, pruritus, extremity and perioral dysesthesia, vertigo, headache, myalgia, arthralgia, temperature reversal, and hyporeflexia. Cardiovascular symptoms, such as bradycardia and hypotension, are less common. Treatment of ciguatera poisoning is supportive, with symptom-based therapy as indicated. Death from ciguatera poisoning is rare.

Tetrodotoxin

Pufferfish (i.e., blowfish, balloonfish, and toadfish), porcupinefish, and sunfish (*Mola* species) have a very potent toxin, tetrodotoxin, in their livers, gonads, intestines, and skin. The flesh of the fish (fugu) is a delicacy in Japan, where it is prepared by specially trained chefs to avoid serving significant amounts of toxins. Tetrodotoxin is a heterocyclic compound that binds at voltage-sensitive sodium channels to block sodium-channel conduction, thereby preventing nerve and muscle action potentials and resulting in paralysis. Symptoms occur rapidly (several minutes to several hours), beginning with circumoral paresthesias and progressing to descending widespread paresthesias. After the initial paresthesias, additional symptoms soon follow, including ataxia, weakness, aphonia, diaphoresis, excess salivation, dyspnea, dysphagia, weakness, and respiratory distress or failure. Gastrointestinal symptoms include nausea, vomiting, and diarrhea. Coagulopathies also may develop. Respiratory intervention is crucial because of the potential for complete flaccid paralysis. Without respiratory assistance, death is not unusual with severe intoxication.

Palytoxin

Palytoxin is an extremely potent toxin produced in sea anemones (*Palythoa* species) and accumulated in sharks, crabs, and marine turtles. The toxin functions by targeting sodium-potassium ion pumps, thereby disrupting ion gradients. Symptoms include tachycardia, hemolysis, and angina-like chest pain. Treatment is generally symptomatic and supportive.

Saxitoxin and Gonyautoxin

Paralytic shellfish poisoning is typically associated with the ingestion of mussels, clams, and oysters. The two toxins associated with this poisoning, saxitoxin and gonyautoxin, are produced by marine microalgae dinoflagellates that are associated with harmful algal blooms, such as "red tides," and are then accumulated in bivalve shellfish to give rise to "paralytic" shellfish poisoning. The primary paralytic shellfish poisoning toxins are heterocyclic compounds that block nerve and muscle action potentials by binding to sodium channels at the same site as tetrodotoxin, thereby resulting in paralysis.

Paralytic shellfish poisoning, which is significantly more severe than neurotoxic shellfish poisoning, predominantly involves neurologic symptoms with less pronounced nausea, vomiting, or diarrhea. Symptoms appear soon after the consumption of contaminated shellfish (minutes to hours), beginning with circumoral and extremity paresthesias. Additional neurologic symptoms such as ataxia, arthralgia, dysphagia, dysmetria, diaphoresis, and tachycardia soon follow the initial paresthesias. Respiratory depression or failure can result in death, usually within 12 hours of the onset of symptoms. As with other shellfish poisoning, therapy is supportive, with close attention to potential respiratory distress or failure.

Brevetoxins

Neurotoxic shellfish poisoning is caused by eating shellfish that contain brevetoxins, which are produced by the annual blooms of the red tides that are associated with the dinoflagellate *Karenia brevis*. Brevetoxins are cyclic polyethers that function similarly to ciguatoxins. Gastrointestinal and neurologic symptoms of intoxication appear within 3 hours after toxic shellfish is eaten and are similar to those of ciguatera poisoning. Treatment is supportive. No deaths have been reported after neurotoxic shellfish poisoning.

Domoic Acid

Domoic acid is a neurotoxin produced by the algae *Nitzschia* during harmful algae blooms and causes amnesic shellfish poisoning following ingestion of contaminated shellfish. The toxin disrupts neuron function by altering calcium influx into cells. Symptoms include headaches, dizziness, loss of short-term memory, confusion, seizures, and coma. After about 24 hours, gastrointestinal symptoms may include diarrhea, vomiting, and abdominal cramping. Death is rare.

Non-neurotoxic Poisoning
Histamine

Scrombroid fishes, such as mackerel, bonito, and tuna, can contain an inordinate amount of histamines in their tissues as a result of bacterial destruction of fish proteins associated with spoilage. Ingestion of spoiled fish with high histamine concentrations can result in pseudoallergic symptoms such as diarrhea, flushing, headache, rash, and vomiting. A metallic taste in the mouth may be reported by some patients. Treatment usually is not necessary for scombrotoxic fish poisoning, and the symptoms usually resolve in several hours. For more severe cases, antihistamines or epinephrine have been reported to be effective.

SUGGESTED READINGS

James KJ, Carey B, O'Halloran J, et al. Shellfish toxicity: human health implications of marine algal toxins. *Epidemiol Infect.* 2010;138:927-940. *Review.*

Shiomi K. Novel peptide toxins recently isolated from sea anemones. *Toxicon.* 2009;54:1112-1118. *A review of peptide toxins found in sea anemones and their structures.*

Stewart I, Lewis RJ, Eaglesham GK, et al. Emerging tropical diseases in Australia. Part 2. Ciguatera fish poisoning. *Ann Trop Med Parasitol.* 2010;104:557-571. *Review.*

RHABDOMYOLYSIS

115

FRANCIS G. O'CONNOR AND PATRICIA A. DEUSTER

DEFINITION

Rhabdomyolysis, an acute, potentially fatal clinical syndrome, reflects the dissolution and disintegration of striated muscle, with the release of muscle cell contents into the systemic circulation. Myoglobinemia and myoglobinuria are common. Skeletal muscle destruction can cause systemic effects mediated by substances released from affected muscle cells (e.g., myoglobin, calcium, potassium). Prerenal azotemia, complicated by the toxicity of free myoglobin on the renal tubules, may lead to acute renal failure, which exacerbates other metabolic abnormalities. At the extreme, arrhythmias, caused by the release of intracellular potassium and organic acids, coupled with hypocalcemia may be fatal.

EPIDEMIOLOGY

Approximately 26,000 hospitalized cases of rhabdomyolysis are reported each year in the United States. Rhabdomyolysis, which precipitates acute kidney injury in 13 to 67% of affected individuals, accounts for 5 to 10% of all cases of acute renal failure in the United States.

ETIOLOGY

Rhabdomyolysis is a complex and multifactorial clinical disorder, with multiple potential inherited and acquired causes (Table 115-1). In urban adults, alcohol (and other drug) abuse, muscle compression, and status epilepticus are common causes of rhabdomyolysis. In pediatric patients, the most common cause is trauma, followed by nonketotic hyperosmolar coma, viral myositis, dystonia, and malignant hyperthermia. However, exercise-induced rhabdomyolysis from repetitive exercise is also a concern in children. Importantly, children and adolescents with recurrent rhabdomyolysis are increasingly being recognized as possibly having inherited metabolic disorders.

Drugs and Intoxications

Among intoxications, which are a common cause of rhabdomyolysis, the most frequent illegal drug-associated causes are cocaine and heroin (Chapter 33), with nearly 20% of cocaine overdoses complicated by rhabdomyolysis. Other substances that can induce rhabdomyolysis include ethanol (Chapter 32), amphetamines, phenylalkylamine derivatives, caffeine, and statins. Statins (Chapter 213) may result in myalgias in up to 10% of patients receiving treatment, but reported rates of statin-induced rhabdomyolysis are only 0.1 to 0.2 cases per 1000 person years.

Exertional Rhabdomyolysis

Rhabdomyolysis can also be a consequence of excessive exertion, prolonged heat exposure (Chapter 109), coexisting sickle cell trait (Chapter 166), and the use of dietary supplements (e.g., ephedra). In one series, 35 of 225,000 emergency department visits to an urban tertiary care center were for exertional rhabdomyolysis. The average creatine kinase (CK) level was 40,000 U/L, but no patient developed acute renal failure. In another series, 57% of participants in an ultramarathon had evidence of myoglobinemia, but none progressed to acute renal failure. Rhabdomyolysis has also been diagnosed in other sports settings (e.g., baseball, football, track, wrestling), but none with a higher frequency than that seen with endurance events.

In the military, acute exertional rhabdomyolysis occurs in 2 to 40% of individuals undergoing basic training, usually within the first 6 days. Resolution of myoglobinuria typically occurs within 2 to 3 days, with clinical improvement within 1 week. Consistent risk factors are low levels of physical fitness and early introduction of repetitive exercises (e.g., squats, push-ups, sit-ups). Although most cases are self-limited, with no long-term evidence of renal or muscle injury, patients who demonstrate systemic signs, generalized clinical findings, or acute renal failure often have an underlying metabolic myopathy. Importantly, 25% of all cases of heatstroke in the military between 1980 and 2000 were associated with rhabdomyolysis; acute renal failure developed in 33%. A retrospective review of deaths in a military basic trainee

TABLE 115-1 INHERITED AND ACQUIRED CAUSES OF RHABDOMYOLYSIS

INHERITED	ACQUIRED
Glycolytic/glycogenolytic, e.g., McArdle's disease (myophosphorylase deficiency)	Exertion, e.g., exercise, status epilepticus, delirium, electrical shock, status asthmaticus, cardiopulmonary resuscitation (see also Table 115-2)
Fatty acid oxidation, e.g., carnitine palmitoyltransferase II deficiency	Crush, e.g., external weight, prolonged immobility, bariatric surgery
Krebs cycle, e.g., aconitase deficiency	Ischemia, e.g., arterial occlusion, compartment syndrome, sickle cell disease, disseminated intravascular coagulation
Pentose phosphate pathway, e.g., glucose-6-phosphate dehydrogenase deficiency	Extremes of body temperature, e.g., fever, exertional heatstroke, burns, malignant hyperthermia, hypothermia, lightning
Purine nucleotide cycle, e.g., myoadenylate deaminase deficiency	Metabolic, e.g., hypokalemia, hypernatremia or hyponatremia, hypophosphatemia, pancreatitis, diabetic ketoacidosis, renal tubular acidosis, hyperthyroidism or hypothyroidism, nonketotic hyperosmolar states
Mitochondrial respiratory chain, e.g., succinate dehydrogenase deficiency	Drugs or toxins, e.g., anticholinergics, amphetamines, antihistamines, arsenic, ethanol, opiates, statins, cocaine, succinylcholine, halothane, corticosteroids, cyclosporine, itraconazole, phenothiazines
Malignant hyperthermia susceptibility, e.g., familial malignant hyperthermia (*RyR1*) mutations, myotonic dystrophy, Duchenne's and Becker's dystrophies	Infections, e.g., Epstein-Barr virus, human immunodeficiency virus, herpes simplex, influenza A and B, *Borrelia burgdorferi*, tetanus
Other, e.g., familial recurrent myoglobinuria	Inflammatory and autoimmune disorders, e.g., polymyositis, dermatomyositis

Adapted and reproduced with permission from Warren JD, Blumbergs PC, Thompson PD. Rhabdomyolysis: a review. *Muscle Nerve.* 2002;25:332-347.

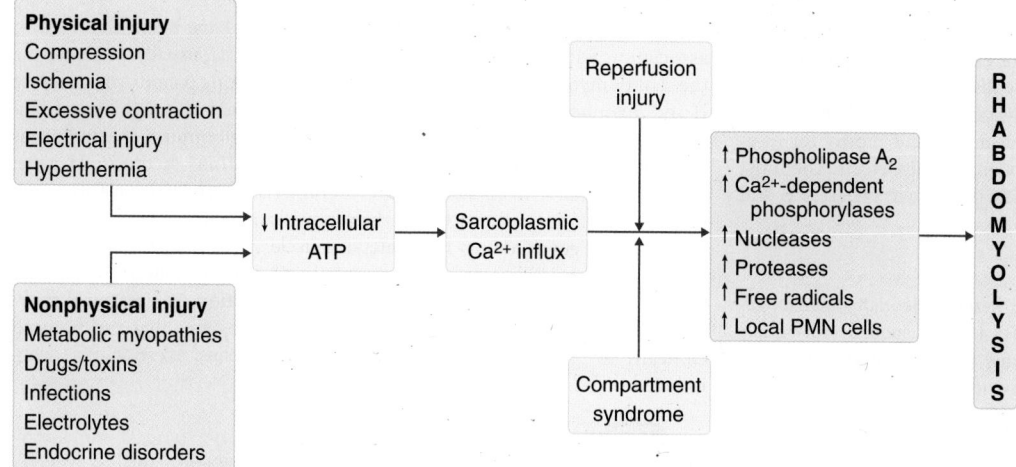

FIGURE 115-1. A, Pathogenesis of rhabdomyolysis. **B,** Vicious circle of rhabdomyolysis. ATP = adenosine triphosphate; PMN = polymorphonuclear.

population found an increased risk for nontraumatic exertional sudden death in African Americans with sickle cell trait.

The extreme exertion characteristics of military service carry over to the population of correctional inmates and civil servants. Reports indicate that unsupervised repetitive exercise in prison populations has led to exertional rhabdomyolysis. Among New York City firefighters, 32 of 16,506 candidates (0.2%) were hospitalized for rhabdomyolysis after a physical fitness test, with 4 requiring hemodialysis. In a group of 50 prospective police officers from Massachusetts, 13 trainees were hospitalized with rhabdomyolysis and CK levels greater than 32,000 U/L; 6 required dialysis, and 1 died 44 days later as a result of complications of heatstroke, rhabdomyolysis, and renal and hepatic failure.

PATHOBIOLOGY

Pathophysiology

The final common pathway for all cases of rhabdomyolysis is destruction of muscle cells as a result of direct or indirect injury, with displacement of their intracellular contents into extracellular fluid, the circulation, or both (Fig. 115-1). Cell function is critically dependent on the relationship between intracellular calcium (Ca^{2+}) and sodium (Na^+) concentrations. Sarcolemmal Na^+, K^+-ATPase regulates extracellular Ca^{2+} concentrations by exchanging Na^+ for Ca^{2+} across the sarcolemma. A low intracellular Na^+ concentration creates a gradient that actively results in efflux of Ca^{2+} as it is exchanged for Na^+ ions. This process maintains intracellular Ca^{2+} levels at several orders of magnitude lower than extracellular Ca^{2+}.

When the cell is subjected to mechanical stress, stretch-activated channels in the sarcolemma can open and cause an influx of Na^+ and Ca^{2+}. With excessive intracellular Ca^{2+}, several pathologic processes begin. Excessive intracellular Ca^{2+} results in persistent contraction of myofibers, depletion of adenosine triphosphate (ATP), production of free radicals, activation of vasoactive molecules, release of proteases, and, ultimately, cell death. Cell death is followed by an invasion of neutrophils, which amplify the damage by further release of proteases and increased production of free radicals. Rather than simple necrosis, a self-sustaining, inflammatory myolytic reaction develops.

Rhabdomyolysis can be further complicated by reperfusion injury and compartment syndrome. In reperfusion injury, ischemia for a prolonged period is followed by restoration of vascular flow. The increase in blood flow results in the delivery of activated neutrophils in combination with an abundance of oxygen, which contributes to the development of highly reactive free radicals. Because most muscle groups are contained within rigid fascial compartments, rhabdomyolysis can quickly precipitate a secondary acute compartment syndrome. The swelling associated with traumatized tissue can also lead to increased intracompartmental pressure, which can provoke additional damage by compromising both venous and arterial blood flow. Thus, compartment syndrome can also lead to rhabdomyolysis.

Inherited and Acquired Rhabdomyolysis

Rhabdomyolysis can be classified into two major categories: inherited and acquired (see Table 115-1). Metabolic myopathies, though not the most common cause, should be carefully considered in patients who have recurrent episodes triggered by low levels of stress or exertion. A number of pathways that lead to the formation of ATP can be disrupted by genetic defects (e.g., inherited disorders of glycogenolysis, glycolysis, and lipid and purine metabolism). In one series of 77 patients who underwent biopsy for idiopathic myoglobinuria, 47% were found to have enzymatic defects. The most common disorders were deficiencies of carnitine palmitoyltransferase II and myophosphorylase.

Inherited Rhabdomyolysis

Malignant hyperthermia is a potentially fatal, heterogeneous, pharmacogenetic disorder triggered by volatile anesthetics in predisposed individuals (Chapter 440). The disorder is most commonly inherited in an autosomal dominant pattern. Evidence from molecular studies indicates that 25% of patients who are susceptible to malignant hyperthermia have mutations in the ryanodine receptor (*RyR1*) gene, which is responsible for coding proteins for one of the primary Ca^{2+} release channels involved in triggering muscle contraction. When a susceptible patient is exposed to a triggering agent, excessive release of Ca^{2+} into the myoplasm leads to a hypermetabolic state manifested by hypercapnia, tachycardia, and metabolic acidosis. Whether the genetic predisposition to malignant hyperthermia is related to exertional rhabdomyolysis and exercise-induced heat injury has not been proved.

Acquired Rhabdomyolysis

DRUGS AND TOXINS. Drugs and toxins, also common causes of rhabdomyolysis, operate through a number of mechanisms, including direct membrane toxicity (e.g., herbicides), indirect metabolic derangements (e.g., anticholinergics), ischemia (e.g., cocaine), and agitation (e.g., hemlock). The most commonly cited drugs precipitating rhabdomyolysis are alcohol, statins, cocaine, amphetamines, and phenothiazines. Alcohol can induce rhabdomyolysis through a combination of mechanisms, including immobilization, direct myotoxicity, and electrolyte abnormalities. Statins, which inhibit 3-hydroxy-3-methylglutaryl-coenzyme A (HMG-CoA) reductase, can be directly myotoxic and appear to trigger sustained increases in intracellular Ca^{2+}. Although the precise mechanisms underlying statin-induced myopathy are currently incompletely understood, it can be aggravated by the concomitant administration of cytochrome P-450 3A4 inhibitors (e.g., itraconazole, erythromycin, cyclosporine, danazol) and fibrates, as well as by physical exercise, excessive alcohol intake, and preexisting comorbid medical conditions. Amphetamines and phenothiazines may lead to a clinical picture of rhabdomyolysis through the serotonin syndrome (Chapter 442) and the neuroleptic malignant syndrome (Chapter 427), respectively.

INFECTIONS. Both viral and bacterial infections can trigger rhabdomyolysis. Either cellular invasion or generation of various toxins may precipitate infection-induced rhabdomyolysis by the virus or bacterium. Influenza A and B (Chapter 372) are the most common viral causes, followed by human immunodeficiency virus (Chapter 394), coxsackievirus (Chapter 387), and Epstein-Barr virus (Chapter 385). The most common bacterial organisms that induce rhabdomyolysis are *Legionella* species (Chapter 322), followed by *Francisella tularensis* (Chapter 319) and *Streptococcus pneumoniae* (Chapter 297). Acute renal failure develops in approximately 57% (33 to 100%) of bacterial cases and 34% (0 to 100%) of viral cases of rhabdomyolysis.

TRAUMA. Trauma is traditionally thought of as the principal cause of rhabdomyolysis. Wars, natural disasters, and traffic and occupational accidents are frequent causes of trauma-induced "crush injury syndrome" (Chapter 112). Other less common causes of trauma- or compression-induced rhabdomyolysis include struggling against restraints, direct blows, child abuse, torture, prolonged immobilization (e.g., anesthesia, coma, drug- or alcohol-induced stupor), and bariatric and other forms of surgery. The primary mechanism of crush syndrome and compression-induced rhabdomyolysis is reperfusion of damaged tissue after a period of ischemia.

Exertional rhabdomyolysis can result from excessive exercise in fit and unfit individuals, particularly eccentrically based activities (lengthening contractions, such as lowering a weight), but it can also be triggered by exertion in combination with thermal stress, sickle cell trait, altitude, or the use of medications (e.g., anticholinergics) or ergogenic substances (e.g., caffeine, ephedra). Exertional rhabdomyolysis may also reveal or provide evidence of an underlying inherited disorder in certain individuals. The spectrum of exertional rhabdomyolysis is broad and can range from a subclinical event to catastrophic collapse and death. The underlying mechanisms may be either mechanical or metabolic in nature, but exertional rhabdomyolysis is associated with elevated myoplasmic Ca^{2+} concentrations.

A number of genetic mutations (Table 115-2) have been identified in association with metabolic myopathies, with exercise usually precipitating the rhabdomyolysis. Multiple mutations in the carnitine palmitoyltransferase II and myophosphorylase genes have been found, and although each mutation has been associated with exercise-induced myoglobinuria, the mutations alone may not explain the clinical episodes. Mutations in the *RyR1* gene, which are common in malignant hyperthermia (Chapter 440), have also been noted in persons with exertional rhabdomyolysis. Two single-point mutations in the gene coding for skeletal muscle myosin light chain kinase (*C37885A* and *C49T*) have been associated with an exaggerated CK response to an exercise challenge, but the role of these mutations in exertional rhabdomyolysis is not known. Yet to be identified are genes that can be used clinically to predict susceptibility to infection-, toxin-, exertion-, or drug-induced rhabdomyolysis.

CLINICAL MANIFESTATIONS

The classic manifestation of rhabdomyolysis includes acute myalgia and pigmenturia as a result of myoglobinuria in association with elevated serum muscle enzymes (CK in particular). Many clinical features are nonspecific, however, and the course and initial signs, symptoms, and laboratory abnormalities are clearly dependent on the underlying cause and severity of the event.

TABLE 115-2 GENETIC MUTATIONS ASSOCIATED WITH EXERTIONAL RHABDOMYOLYSIS

GENE	
Ryanodine receptor 1	*RyR1*
Myoadenylate deaminase	*AMPDA1*
Carnitine palmitoyltransferase II	*CPT2*
Myophosphorylase	*PYGM*
Phosphofructokinase	*PFKM*
Phosphorylase b kinase	*PHKA1*
Very long chain acyl coenzyme-A dehydrogenase	*ACAD9*
Phosphoglycerate mutase	*PGAMM*
Phosphoglycerate kinase	*PGK1*
Lactate dehydrogenase	*LDHA*
Cytochrome c oxidase	*COX I, II,* and *III*
Cytochrome b (complex III)	*CYTB*
Mitochondrial tRNA	*Mt-tRNA*
β-Sarcoglycan	*SGCB*

Rhabdomyolysis can be accompanied by both local and systemic features. Local features, generally noted in the area of the traumatized muscle groups, can occur within hours of the trauma and include muscle pain, tenderness, and swelling. Systemic features include tea-colored urine, chills, fever, and malaise. In extreme cases, patients complain of nausea and vomiting and demonstrate confusion, agitation, or delirium. Whenever systemic features such as chills, fever, malaise, or generalized muscular involvement are observed, an underlying metabolic myopathy should be considered.

Clinical findings may also include compartment syndrome, which can occur in muscle groups encased by fascia, especially the lower leg, forearm, and thigh muscle groups. Sensory abnormalities caused by nerve compression are an early manifestation of compartment syndrome; the loss of a pulse as a result of vascular compromise is a later finding. If compartment syndrome is not addressed within 6 to 8 hours, irreversible ischemic muscle and nerve damage may occur.

Laboratory findings are related to the degree of muscle involvement. Early findings include elevated blood levels of CK, myoglobin, potassium, urea, and phosphorus. CK levels typically peak 2 to 5 days after the initial insult; levels higher than 16,000 U/L are more likely to be associated with renal failure than are lower levels. Hypocalcemia, caused by the influx and deposition of Ca^{2+} in damaged muscle tissue, may accompany rhabdomyolysis. Moreover, an anion gap metabolic acidosis may develop because of the release of organic acids from damaged muscle. With resolution of rhabdomyolysis, sequestered Ca^{2+} may be released back into the circulation and cause hypercalcemia.

DIAGNOSIS

Creatine Kinase Levels

A diagnosis of rhabdomyolysis is made when there is clinical evidence of myonecrosis and release into the systemic circulation of muscle cell contents, including myoglobin, creatinine, CK, organic acids, potassium, aldolase, lactate dehydrogenase, and hydroxybutyrate dehydrogenase. The skeletal muscle subtype CK-MM is abundantly present in skeletal muscle and released as a result of muscle destruction. Serum levels exceeding 100,000 U/L are not uncommon with rhabdomyolysis. Because CK remains in the circulation longer than myoglobin does and can be detected clinically both easily and efficiently, it is the most frequently used marker to diagnose rhabdomyolysis. No universally accepted clinical or laboratory definition of rhabdomyolysis currently exists, but CK elevations ranging from more than 5 times to more than 50 times the upper limits of normal, as well as varying requirements for serum creatinine elevation, have been proposed. Importantly, gender, ethnicity, and baseline physical activity levels all affect individual baseline CK levels. African American males and young athletic men have the highest baseline CK levels, and non–African American women have the lowest. Thus, gender, ethnicity, and prior activity must be considered when using CK for the diagnosis of rhabdomyolysis. In general, CK levels in excess of 5 times normal, with the appropriate clinical presentation, are accepted as evidence of muscle breakdown, which may be consistent with a diagnosis of rhabdomyolysis.

Myoglobin Testing

Because myoglobinuria does not occur in the absence of rhabdomyolysis, myoglobin should be the best marker and the diagnostic cornerstone. However, testing for serum or urine myoglobin is problematic and is not always consistent. Myoglobin is normally bound to plasma globulins; therefore, only a small fraction reaches the glomeruli. In the presence of severe muscle damage, blood levels of myoglobin overwhelm the binding capacity of the circulating proteins, so free myoglobin reaches the glomeruli and eventually the renal tubules. Elevations in serum myoglobin occur before the rise in serum CK, but the elimination kinetics of serum myoglobin is more rapid than that of CK, which makes the often evanescent rise in serum myoglobin a less reliable marker of muscle injury. Furthermore, the liver can quickly metabolize myoglobin. Diagnostic tests for urine myoglobin are often not readily available; in addition, it may take more than 24 hours to obtain results, and urine myoglobin is not an accurate predictor of acute kidney injury. Nevertheless, urine screening for rhabdomyolysis may be performed by dipstick if the urine sediment is also examined. The orthotoluidine portion of the dipstick turns blue in the presence of hemoglobin or myoglobin, so if the urine sediment does not contain erythrocytes, one can assume, in the appropriate clinical setting, that a positive dipstick reading reflects the presence of myoglobin. Other associated laboratory findings in acute rhabdomyolysis can include hypocalcemia or hypercalcemia, hyperphosphatemia, metabolic (lactic) acidosis, thrombocytopenia, and disseminated intravascular coagulation.

Differential Diagnosis

The clinical findings of acutely swollen muscles or muscle weakness (or both) with reddish brown urine are not always the result of rhabdomyolysis, and the examining clinician must be careful to scrutinize all information. The differential diagnosis includes disorders that may indirectly affect myocytes, such as Guillain-Barré syndrome and periodic paralysis. Guillain-Barré syndrome (Chapter 428) is distinguished from rhabdomyolysis in that it is characterized as a fulminant polyneuropathy, usually after an antecedent viral infection. Periodic paralysis (Chapter 429) is frequently associated with transient electrolyte disturbances and is distinguished from rhabdomyolysis in that most cases follow periods of rest or sleep.

Myoglobinuria causes the urine to be reddish brown, but tea-colored (or cola-colored) urine does not necessarily indicate the presence of myoglobin. Other conditions associated with discoloration of urine include hemoglobinuria from hemolysis, intrinsic renal disease, porphyria, acute glomerulonephritis, "athletic pseudonephritis," or external factors such as ingestion of beets and various drugs (e.g., phenytoin, rifampin, vitamin B_{12}).

The diagnosis of rhabdomyolysis is complete when the clinician determines the cause. This step, though frequently established during the history and physical examination, may require further diagnostic assessment after initiating clinical treatment during the acute phase. Clinical issues that are both controversial and poorly defined include which patients warrant further testing and what tests to perform. Individuals with recurrent rhabdomyolysis, a positive family history of rhabdomyolysis or malignant hyperthermia, low exercise tolerance, no apparent cause, or a fulminant or explosive form of rhabdomyolysis appear to warrant further testing.

Testing may include a nonischemic forearm test, which involves isometric exercise at 70% of maximal voluntary contraction for 30 seconds under nonischemic conditions; electromyography; blood tests for muscle enzymes (e.g., mitochondrial myopathies [Chapter 429], fatty acid transport defects [Chapter 429], glycogen storage diseases [Chapter 214], diseases associated with myoglobinuria); muscle biopsy to investigate specific metabolic myopathies and other enzyme or genetic defects; or any combination of such testing. The forearm exercise test may help identify metabolic and genetic causes of rhabdomyolysis. Patients who have had an episode of malignant hyperthermia or exertional heat illness may be candidates for a caffeine halothane contracture test, which evaluates the force produced in small muscle biopsy samples after exposure to caffeine and separate exposure to halothane in the laboratory. Isolated, perfused muscle fibers must show an increase in tension of at least 0.2 g when exposed to 2 mM of caffeine or at least 0.7 g of tension after exposure to 3% halothane. Additionally, genetic investigation for mutations of the *RyR1* receptor gene may be warranted.

PREVENTION

Approaches for preventing rhabdomyolysis induced by infections, medications, toxins, heat stress, or exercise may emerge in the future, but no definitive guidelines can be presented at this time. To prevent further muscle injury, blood flow to ischemic areas must be promptly restored to minimize ischemia-reperfusion damage. Administration of free radical scavengers to prevent rhabdomyolysis may prove useful in the future.

TREATMENT Rx

Treatment of rhabdomyolysis begins with a careful history and physical examination to identify and manage any underlying illness; it then focuses on preserving renal function. All patients require aggressive early management because it is difficult to stratify risk initially (Table 115-3). Careful observation plus treatment of potential early and late complications is critical. Accordingly, vital signs, urine output, serial electrolyte levels, and CK levels should be obtained as soon as possible. Intensive care monitoring may be required, depending on the clinical situation.

Hydration

Hydration is the cornerstone of preserving renal function in patients with rhabdomyolysis. Providing fluids addresses the early threats to survival: hypovolemic shock and hyperkalemia. Currently, there is no way to accurately predict or stratify overall risk or risk of acute renal failure among patients with rhabdomyolysis, but CK levels greater than 15,000 U/L are thought to portend an increased risk. Patients with mild symptoms and serum CK levels less than 3000 U/L are considered to be at low risk and may be treated as outpatients with hydration, limited physical activity, and careful follow-up. Victims of collapse, trauma, or exertional heat injury, or patients who demonstrate moderate early symptoms with more than mild elevations in CK or abnormal

TABLE 115-3 STEPS IN THE PREVENTION AND TREATMENT OF RHABDOMYOLYSIS-INDUCED ACUTE KIDNEY INJURY

Check for extracellular volume status, central venous pressure, and urine output.*

Measure serum creatine kinase levels. Measurement of other muscle enzymes (myoglobin, aldolase, lactate dehydrogenase, alanine aminotransferase, aspartate aminotransferase) adds little information relevant to diagnosis or management.

Measure levels of plasma and urine creatinine, potassium, and sodium; blood urea nitrogen; total and ionized calcium, magnesium, and phosphorus; and uric acid and albumin. Evaluate acid-base status, blood cell count, and coagulation.

Perform a urine dipstick test, and examine the urine sediment.

Initiate volume repletion with normal saline promptly at a rate of approximately 400 mL/hr (200-1000 mL/hr, depending on the setting and severity), and monitor the clinical course or central venous pressure.

Target urine output of approximately 3 mL/kg body weight/hr (200 mL/hr).

Check serum potassium levels frequently.

Correct hypocalcemia only if symptomatic (e.g., tetany, seizures) or if severe hyperkalemia occurs.

Investigate the cause of rhabdomyolysis.

Check urine pH: if it is <6.5, alternate each liter of normal saline with 1 L 5% dextrose or 0.45% saline plus 100 mmol bicarbonate. Avoid potassium- and lactate-containing solutions.

Consider treatment with mannitol (up to 200 g/day; cumulative dose up to 800 g). Check for plasma osmolality and plasma osmolal gap. Discontinue if diuresis (>20 mL/hr) is not established.

Maintain volume repletion until myoglobinuria is cleared (as evidenced by clear urine or urine dipstick test that is negative for blood).

Consider renal replacement therapy if there is resistant hyperkalemia (>6.5 mmol/L) that is symptomatic (as assessed by electrocardiography), rapidly rising serum potassium levels, oliguria (<0.5 mL of urine/kg/hr for 12 hr), anuria, volume overload, or resistant metabolic acidosis (pH < 7.1).

*In the case of the crush syndrome (e.g., earthquake, building collapse), institute aggressive volume repletion promptly before evacuating the patient.
From Bosch X, Poch E, Grau JM. Rhabdomyolysis and acute kidney injury. *N Engl J Med.* 2009;361:62-72.

metabolic panels, should be treated with intravenous hydration in an inpatient setting. Hydration is accomplished by aggressive intravenous fluid therapy with isotonic fluids at a rate that results in a urine output of 200 mL/hour until CK levels begin to decrease. When fluid resuscitation fails to correct intractable hyperkalemia and acidosis, renal replacement therapy should be considered (Chapter 122).

Specific Therapeutic Measures

Several retrospective clinical studies and case reports, as well as animal models, promote the addition of bicarbonate and mannitol, but no prospective clinical trials have been conducted to support or refute their benefit in patients with rhabdomyolysis. Alkalinization of the urine decreases cast formation, minimizes the toxic effects of myoglobin on the renal tubules, inhibits lipid peroxidation, and decreases the risk for hyperkalemia. However, this approach can cause Ca^{2+} to precipitate and be deposited in the soft tissues, as well as contributing to a hyperosmolar state. Mannitol serves as an osmotic diuretic, volume expander, and free radical scavenger; it should be used very carefully in patients with marginal cardiac function, and only after adequate renal function is established.

Despite the absence of definitive evidence in humans, both mannitol and a forced alkaline diuresis are recommended for rhabdomyolysis caused by crush syndrome when CK levels are greater than 20,000 U/L. The treatment goals are to (1) achieve a urine output of 200 mL/hour, (2) maintain urine pH between 6 and 7, (3) keep serum pH below 7.50, and (4) achieve hemodynamic stability and prevent volume overload. Fluid resuscitation begins with a bolus of 1 L of 5% dextrose plus 0.22% NaCl and 100 mEq $NaHCO_3$ over a 30-minute period, followed by an infusion at 2 to 5 mL/kg/hour. A 20% mannitol infusion at a dose of 0.5 g/kg is given over a 15-minute period, followed by an infusion at 0.1 g/kg/hour. Adjustments are made to maintain urine output above 200 mL/hour. Urinary and serum pH levels should be monitored, with acetazolamide added if the serum pH exceeds 7.45 or urinary pH remains below 6.0. However, the use of mannitol and forced alkaline diuresis in patients with crush syndrome, as well as other clinical manifestations of rhabdomyolysis, has not been tested in randomized trials.

Management of Metabolic Abnormalities

Deposition of Ca^{2+}, which occurs early in rhabdomyolysis, is directly related to the degree of muscle destruction and administration of Ca^{2+}. Reversal of hypocalcemia may in fact worsen ectopic calcification and exacerbate hypercalcemia during the resolution phase. Accordingly, hypocalcemia should be treated only when clinical symptoms, signs of tetany, or severe hyperkalemia develops.

Management of Compartment Syndrome

Compartment syndrome (Chapter 112) is a well-described late complication as well as a potential cause of rhabdomyolysis. Compartment syndrome can occur as a direct consequence of muscle injury with increased vascular permeability, aggressive fluid resuscitation, or restoration of reperfusion. When a compartment syndrome is suspected, such as when the muscles are tense and swollen or there is evidence of neurovascular compromise, compartment pressures should be measured; in the proper clinical setting, pressures in excess of 30 mm Hg should prompt consideration of fasciotomy. However, late fasciotomy (>12 hours after the onset of symptoms) may be counterproductive by converting a closed injury to an open wound, with an increased risk of uncontrollable infection. Accordingly, late fasciotomy is relatively contraindicated.

Management of Crush Injury

Management of crush injury victims (Chapter 112) is unique, in that many individuals have the opportunity to receive treatment before extrication and reperfusion. Current recommendations for on-site management of trauma victims before extrication include aggressive hydration with intravenous normal saline. In the event of massive damage, amputation of the extremity may be required to protect the patient's overall health. A Mangled Extremity Severity Score (MESS) may be used to identify nonsalvageable extremities prospectively. The MESS is a grading system based on four groups of clinical criteria, including the degree of skeletal and soft tissue injury, rating of blood pressure (shock) and pulse (ischemia), and age. Scores from each group are added to obtain a total score that ranges from 0 to 14; higher scores indicate more severe involvement, and a score of 7 or greater has a positive predictive value of nearly 100% for amputation. It is hoped that ongoing clinical trials in this population will elucidate the roles of *N*-acetylcysteine, continuous renal replacement therapy, and deferoxamine in reducing the direct toxic effects of myoglobin on the kidneys.

Malignant Hyperthermia

One cause of rhabdomyolysis that requires rapid and aggressive management is malignant hyperthermia (Chapter 440). Episodes of malignant hyperthermia occur most commonly in the operating room and are recognized by the anesthesiologist. The typical clinical features represent an uncontrolled, exaggerated, hypermetabolic state; an increase in end-tidal carbon dioxide during ventilation is the most sensitive sign. With the clinical recognition of impending malignant hyperthermia, anesthetics should be discontinued, and the patient should be treated with dantrolene sodium. The usual initial dose is 2.5 to 4 mg/kg, followed by about 1 mg/kg every 4 hours for up to 48 hours to avoid recrudescence.

PROGNOSIS

The most serious consequence of rhabdomyolysis is acute renal failure, which occurs in up to 67% of all cases, regardless of cause. Although acute renal failure may be relatively benign, the mortality rate from myoglobinuric renal failure reportedly ranges from 3 to 80%. Various clinical factors are used to predict the risk for acute renal failure, including serum CK, creatinine, potassium, and Ca^{2+}, as well as the urine myoglobin level, but no single parameter has been established. However, mortality appears to be significantly higher in patients with CK values in excess of 75,000 U/L and in those with hyperkalemia or hypocalcemia. For compartment syndrome, a poor prognosis is associated with an ischemic period lasting longer than 6 hours.

The prognosis of patients with rhabdomyolysis improves markedly when treatment is started soon after the diagnosis is made. With mild episodes, the prognosis is customarily excellent, and the patient can typically resume usual activities within several weeks after CK levels have normalized. However, some patients do not return to normal and continue to experience extreme fatigue and muscle pain on exertion. These patients require additional testing (nonischemic forearm test, electromyography, muscle disease enzyme panel, muscle biopsy) to determine whether an underlying metabolic myopathy exists. The results of these tests will help determine future recommendations, but the patient's tolerance of and response to light and more strenuous exercise are important factors.

For patients with statin-induced myopathy, deciding when to discontinue statin therapy remains controversial. However, most authorities agree that suspension should occur with either intolerable muscle symptoms or evidence of rhabdomyolysis.

FUTURE DIRECTIONS

Although a number of genetic mutations have already been defined, the prevalence of such mutations is unknown. Moreover, a genetic linkage in individuals susceptible to exertional or drug-induced rhabdomyolysis (or both) has not been thoroughly investigated. It is likely that the greatest progress will come from prospective trials that evaluate both diagnostic and treatment modalities for myoglobinuric renal failure.

SUGGESTED READINGS

Bosch X, Poch E, Grau JM. Rhabdomyolysis and acute kidney injury. *N Engl J Med*. 2009;361:62-72. *A comprehensive review*.

Cervellin G, Comelli I, Lippi G. Rhabdomyolysis: historical background, clinical, diagnostic and therapeutic features. *Clin Chem Lab Med*. 2010;48:749-756. *Review*.

Graziani G, Calvetta A, Cucchiari D, et al. Life-threatening hypercalcemia in patients with rhabdomyolysis-induced oliguric acute renal failure. *J Nephrol*. 2011;24:128-131. *Review of this unusual but serious complication*.

Joy TR, Hegele RA. Narrative review: statin-related myopathy. *Ann Intern Med*. 2009;150:858-868. *Rhabdomyolysis remains rare*.

XI

RENAL AND GENITOURINARY DISEASES

116

APPROACH TO THE PATIENT WITH RENAL DISEASE

DONALD W. LANDRY AND HASAN BAZARI

DIAGNOSIS

The prominent functions of the kidney include the excretion of nitrogenous waste; the regulation of the excretion of sodium, potassium, and acid; and the synthesis of a variety of hormones, including 1,25-dihydroxyvitamin D, erythropoietin, and renin. A patient can have an isolated failure in a particular function, such as in acid excretion (Chapter 120), in which case the "approach to the patient" is distinct for the isolated defect. First and foremost, however, the kidney is a filtration organ, and acute kidney injury (Chapter 122) and chronic kidney disease (Chapter 132) refer specifically to defects in the filtration function of the kidney. In the context of impaired filtration, many of the individual functions may fail.

The approximately 2 million renal glomeruli normally filter about 180 L/day. The renal glomerulus is not simply a filter, but rather a size- and charge-dependent ultrafilter that excludes not only cells but also proteins larger than 60 kD from the ultrafiltrate. Smaller proteins are variably filtered at the glomerulus and endocytosed in the proximal tubule, so that the protein concentration of the urine is normally quite low. Kidney disease reflects a failure in the quantity or quality of the glomerular ultrafiltrate.

The normal glomerular filtration rate (GFR) may decline in hours or a few days in acute kidney injury or over months and years in chronic kidney disease. An acute decline in glomerular filtration is the necessary and sufficient condition for the diagnosis of acute kidney injury, but abnormal urinary findings can assist with elucidating of the etiology of the injury. Proteinuria, ranging from microscopic to the nephrotic range (Chapter 123), and urinary findings, from a few cells per microscopic high-power field to gross hematuria or pyuria, may be the only evidence of the earliest stages of chronic kidney disease. As chronic kidney disease advances, the decline in the GFR progresses until dialysis or transplantation (Chapter 133) is required to forestall or treat the syndrome of uremia.

Serum creatinine is, to a first approximation, neither secreted nor reabsorbed, so the amount appearing in the urine per unit time is a measure of the amount that was filtered at the glomerulus during that period. As a result, the rate of creatinine clearance is, at first approximation, equivalent to the GFR. A decrement in the GFR diminishes creatinine clearance but has no immediate effect on creatinine production by muscle; as a result, the serum creatinine concentration rises. The change in serum creatinine over time indicates the tempo of the renal disease and can distinguish acute injury from chronic kidney disease. Advanced chronic kidney disease (Chapter 132) is commonly associated with anemia, renal osteodystrophy, and a small kidney size on ultrasonography, although kidney size may be normal or increased with amyloidosis or diabetes mellitus. Hyperphosphatemia, which develops within 1 or 2 weeks after acute kidney injury, is less useful as a discriminator of acute versus chronic renal injury.

The serum creatinine level is elevated in both acute and chronic kidney disease, but an actively rising serum creatinine level confirms an acute or acute-on-chronic insult to kidney function. As a blood filtration organ, the kidney is susceptible to an acute compromise of renal arterial perfusion (Chapter 127), such as prerenal kidney injury, or blockage in urine outflow, such as urinary obstruction owing to benign prostatic hypertrophy (Chapter 131). The intrarenal causes of acute kidney injury (Chapter 122) include acute tubular necrosis, acute interstitial nephritis, acute glomerulonephritis, and acute vasculitis and vascular disease. Dysmorphic red blood cells in the urine or clumps of cells in the form of the renal tubules, so-called tubular casts, suggest the site of the lesion and narrow the range of potential etiologies.

Most of the diagnoses of renal disease can be made with a careful history and physical examination supplemented by review of basic laboratory tests, especially the urinary sediment. The specificity of the diagnosis can be improved by the use of serologic analysis, imaging, and, occasionally, invasive procedures such as angiography and renal biopsy.

History

The history reviews potential factors that contribute to the development of renal disease and identifies the systemic features of diseases that may affect the kidney. These factors include the following:

- Medication use
- Family history of renal disease
- The time of onset of symptoms of renal dysfunction
- Changes in bladder function, including nocturia, polyuria, and hesitancy
- Fatigue and weakness
- Dyspnea on exertion, a manifestation of fluid overload or acidosis
- Systemic features of vasculitis

A systemic vasculitis may present in a variety of ways, with skin manifestations including petechial rash, purpura, digital gangrene, and splinter hemorrhages. Otitis, sinusitis, epistaxis, hemoptysis, and nasal septal ulcers are common manifestations of Wegener's granulomatosis (Chapter 278). Pulmonary hemorrhage can be a catastrophic manifestation of Goodpasture's syndrome (Chapter 123) or anti–glomerular basement membrane (anti-GBM) disease. Abdominal distention may be seen in nephrotic syndrome with ascites, as well as in autosomal polycystic kidney disease (Chapter 129). Abdominal pain and tenderness and gastrointestinal hemorrhage may be observed in Henoch-Schönlein purpura and classic polyarteritis nodosa (Chapter 278). Lower extremity edema is common in cirrhosis (Chapter 156), heart failure (Chapter 58), and nephrotic syndrome (Chapter 123). Neurologic symptoms may be a manifestation of vasculitis, such as microscopic polyangiitis (Chapter 278) and cryoglobulinemia (Chapter 193).

Physical Examination

The vital signs are crucial. A patient with a "normal blood pressure" may be relatively hypotensive in the setting of renovascular disease. Orthostatic hypotension may explain the acute decompensation of kidney function in a patient with chronic kidney disease (Chapter 132). Pulsus paradoxus may reflect cardiac tamponade (Chapter 77).

The eyes may exhibit conjunctivitis, episcleritis, or uveitis. In the abdomen, ascites may be seen in cirrhosis, nephrosis, and heart failure. Hepatomegaly is seen in passive congestion and amyloidosis (Chapter 194). Splenomegaly may be seen in amyloidosis, endocarditis (Chapter 76), and lymphoma (Chapters 191 and 192). Kidney and liver enlargement may be seen in autosomal dominant polycystic kidney disease. Lower extremity edema can be seen in cirrhosis, nephrotic syndrome, and heart failure. Splinter hemorrhages, as well as Osler nodes and Janeway lesions, may represent bacterial endocarditis. Rashes can be seen in many of the vasculitides.

Cardiovascular Signs

Assessment of the jugular venous pressure (Chapter 50) can play a crucial role in the bedside evaluation of volume status. The presence of a pericardial friction rub can be observed in the serositis associated with systemic lupus erythematosus (SLE; Chapter 274) or the pericarditis associated with uremia (Chapter 132). Infiltrative diseases, such as amyloidosis and sarcoidosis (Chapter 95), can lead to restrictive cardiomyopathy with associated heart failure. The presence of a fourth heart sound (S_4) may be a sign of cardiac hypertrophy, and S_3 may be a sign of heart failure. Vascular bruits reflect generalized atherosclerosis, and the presence of an abdominal bruit may be an important clue to the presence of renovascular disease (Chapter 127).

Neurologic Signs

Peripheral neuropathy may be seen in vasculitis with involvement of the nerves as mononeuritis multiplex. Frank cerebrovascular accidents may be seen in SLE and in the antiphospholipid antibody syndrome (Chapter 179).

The signs and symptoms of chronic renal failure are shown in Figure 116-1.

Laboratory Findings

Measurement of Renal Function

Renal function is routinely assessed in clinical practice by the measurement of serum creatinine. Creatine is released as a waste product from myocytes and converted to creatinine in the liver. The normal range of serum creatinine is 0.6 to 1.5 mg/dL, and the value for a given patient is relatively fixed in the absence of a change in renal function. About 90% of the daily production of creatinine is excreted through glomerular filtration and the remainder by tubular secretion. Mild elevations of the plasma creatinine concentration can

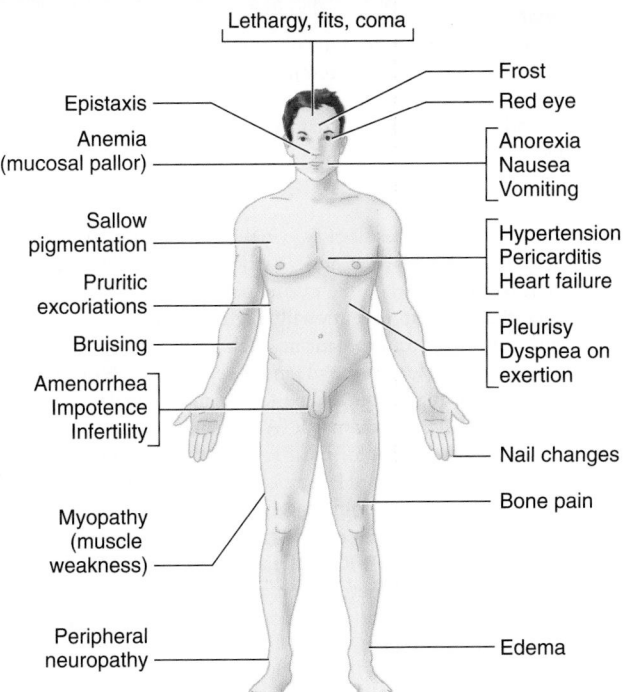

FIGURE 116-1. Common symptoms and signs of chronic renal failure. (Redrawn from Forbes CD, Jackson WF. *Color Atlas and Text of Clinical Medicine*, 3rd ed. London: Mosby; 2003.)

occur during treatment with cimetidine or trimethoprim, both of which interfere with the tubular secretion of creatinine, but neither is likely to cause significant elevations of the plasma creatinine level. Ketoacids (Chapter 236) can cause an artifactual increase in the plasma creatinine by interfering with the creatinine assay. The reciprocal relationship between the GFR and the serum creatinine level explains why the serum creatinine concentration will rise but still remain in the normal range despite a substantial loss of renal function. The concentration of blood urea nitrogen (BUN), which is a product of protein catabolism, is about ten-fold higher than the creatinine concentration; because the BUN-to-creatinine ratio commonly rises with arterial underfilling, the BUN typically is used as a marker of effective volume status. The BUN may be inappropriately high in other circumstances, however, such as gastrointestinal bleeding or the use of steroids or tetracyclines. The BUN may be low in patients who have a poor dietary intake of protein or who have liver disease.

The creatinine clearance can be estimated from the serum creatinine concentration by the Cockcroft-Gault formula:

$$\text{GFR} = \frac{(140 - \text{age}) \times \text{weight [in kg]}}{72 \times \text{serum creatinine}} (\times 0.85 \text{ if female})$$

Creatinine clearance often is calculated using a 24-hour urine collection for measurement of the creatinine concentration. The patient must be instructed to discard the first-morning urine before initiating the collection and to conclude the collection by including the next morning void. The formula for calculating creatinine clearance is as follows:

$$\text{CCr} = (\text{urine Cr} \times \text{V})/(\text{plasma Cr})$$

where *CCr* is creatinine clearance, *urine Cr* is urine creatinine concentration, *V* is urine flow rate, and *plasma Cr* is plasma creatinine. The creatinine clearance overestimates GFR by about 10% owing to tubular secretion of creatinine. This secretion can be modified by the use of cimetidine, which is a competitive inhibitor of tubular creatinine secretion.

Inulin, a 5200-D uncharged polymer of fructose, is an ideal marker for the measurement of GFR because it is not reabsorbed, secreted, synthesized, or metabolized. It is not available for routine clinical assessment, however. Iothalamate clearance is an accurate measurement of GFR and is available as a diagnostic tool in clinical studies. Other agents that are used for the measurement of GFR include technetium-99m diethylenetriaminepentaacetic acid (^{99m}Tc-DTPA) and chromium 51-labeled ethylenediaminetetraacetic acid.

Urine Tests

The following aspects of the assessment of the urine are important in the approach to the patient with renal disease.

Twenty-Four-Hour Urine Collection for Protein Excretion

Proteinuria (as albuminuria) of greater than 3.5 g in 24 hours generally indicates glomerular disease (Chapter 123). Lesser quantities do not preclude glomerular disease, and electrophoresis gives valuable insight into the composition of the proteinuria (Chapter 193). Occasionally, overflow proteinuria of a low-molecular-weight protein, such as light chains in Bence Jones proteinuria, can be greater than 3.5 g/day without any of the manifestations or implications of the nephrotic syndrome; a urine protein electrophoresis study is important in making the distinction. Collection must be done by discarding the first morning void and collecting all urine output for the next 24 hours, including the first morning void the next day.

Protein-to-Creatinine Ratio

The 24-hour urine collection for protein excretion is cumbersome and subject to inaccuracies. Instead, a spot urine sample for protein and creatinine can be used to estimate the amount of protein excreted. A protein-to-creatinine ratio of 3 estimates that the 24-hour protein excretion is about 3 g. The ratio may be inaccurate in patients with orthostatic proteinuria.

Urine for Microalbumin

The excretion of abnormal quantities of albumin below the level detectable by the urine dipstick is called *microalbuminuria*. Normal albumin excretion, which is less than 30 mg/day, is best detected by radioimmunoassay or enzyme immunoassay. Microalbuminuria is the earliest clinically detectable stage of diabetic nephropathy (Chapter 126).

Fractional Excretion of Sodium

The excretion of sodium in the setting of oliguria and acute kidney injury (Chapter 122) often gives insight into the appropriateness of tubular function. The fractional excretion of sodium (Fe_{Na}) is calculated as follows:

$$\text{Fe}_{\text{Na}} = (\text{urine Na}/\text{plasma Na})/(\text{urine Cr}/\text{plasma Cr}) \times 100$$

where *Na* is the sodium concentration (in millimoles per liter [mmol/L]), and *Cr* is the creatinine concentration (in mmol/L). In the setting of oliguria, an Fe_{Na} of less than 1% often denotes prerenal azotemia, whereas an Fe_{Na} of greater than 1% denotes intrinsic renal damage. Although this measurement is generally useful, an Fe_{Na} of less than 1% may be seen without evidence of a prerenal component, including contrast nephropathy, hepatorenal syndrome (Chapter 157), obstructive uropathy (Chapter 125), interstitial nephritis (Chapter 124), glomerulonephritis (Chapter 123), and rhabdomyolysis (Chapter 115). Conversely, a high Fe_{Na} can be seen in cases in which there is a prerenal component, including diuretic use, adrenal insufficiency, cerebral salt wasting, and salt-wasting nephropathy (Chapter 118). The Fe_{Na} must be evaluated in the context of the clinical situation because it can be low or high in a normal patient or in a patient with chronic kidney disease. Ultimately, volume assessment is done best by assessing the patient at the bedside and cannot be deduced from a measurement of electrolytes.

Fractional Excretion of Urea

Urea reabsorption varies with volume status, increasing in the setting of volume depletion. A fractional excretion of urea less than 30% indicates a state of decreased effective circulating volume. The formula for calculation of the fractional excretion of urea is as analogous to that of Fe_{Na}.

Twenty-Four-Hour Urine for Calcium, Uric Acid, Oxalate, and Citrate

These studies are performed in the evaluation of the patient with recurrent kidney stones (Chapter 128). Depending on the laboratory, the calcium measurement may be made on a different collection from the others. These measurements should be conducted with the patient on a normal diet and with normal activity, and they should not be done during a hospitalization. Often these tests need to be repeated before therapeutic decisions are made. The 24-hour urine creatinine excretion should be determined with each measurement to ensure an adequate collection.

Urine Potassium Excretion

Potassium is handled differently than sodium. Potassium is completely reabsorbed and then secreted in a flow-dependent manner. Secretion depends on adequate distal sodium delivery and reabsorption to provide a sufficient electrochemical gradient for tubular potassium excretion (Chapter 119). The excretion of less than 15 mmol/day of potassium in the face of hyperkalemia suggests an inadequate renal response. The transtubular potassium gradient (TTKG) is an approximation of the gradient of potassium before the effect of antidiuretic hormone on the concentration of potassium in the urine. The formula for the measurement of the TTKG is as follows:

$$TTKG = (urine\ K / plasma\ K) / (urine\ Osm / plasma\ Osm)$$

where *K* is the potassium concentration and *Osm* is osmolality. A TTKG ratio of less than 4 in the setting of hyperkalemia implies either inadequate distal sodium delivery or inadequate distal potassium excretion system. A TTKG ratio of greater than 10 in the setting of hypokalemia supports the presence of renal potassium wasting, and further elucidation of the exact stimulus for potassium loss is warranted.

Urine Net Charge
Urine net charge measures the ability of the kidney to synthesize ammonia (NH_4^+) and to excrete acid in non–anion gap metabolic acidosis. The difference between the concentration of urine cations (Na^{++} and K^{++}) and that of urine anions (mainly Cl^-) represents the urine net charge:

$$Urine\ net\ charge = (urine\ Na^+ + urine\ K^+) - (urine\ Cl^-)$$

A negative urine net charge indicates NH_4^+ in the urine. This formula does not apply when an unmeasured anion is present in the urine in a patient with an anion gap metabolic acidosis (Chapter 120).

Urinalysis
The analysis of the urine sample involves simple observation and separate measurements using specific tools or commercially available dipsticks.

Appearance and Color
The normal color of the urine is derived from urochromes, which are pigments excreted in the urine. Abnormal color or appearance of the urine may be explained by many conditions (Table 116-1).

TABLE 116-1   MACROSCOPIC APPEARANCE OF URINE

APPEARANCE	CAUSE
Milky	Acid urine: urate crystals Alkaline urine: insoluble phosphates Infection: pus Spermatozoa Chyluria
Smoky pink	Hematuria (>0.54 mL blood/L urine)
Foamy	Proteinuria
Blue or green	*Pseudomonas* urinary tract infection Bilirubin Methylene blue
Pink or red	Aniline dyes in sweets Porphyrins (on standing) Blood, hemoglobin, myoglobin Drugs: phenindione, phenolphthalein Anthocyaninuria (beetroot, "beeturia")
Orange	Drugs: anthraquinones (laxatives), rifampicin Urobilinogenuria
Yellow	Mepacrine Conjugated bilirubin Phenacetin Riboflavin
Brown or black	Melanin (on standing) Myoglobin (on standing) Alkaptonuria
Green or black	Phenol Lysol
Brown	Drugs: phenazopyridine, furazolidone, L-dopa, niridazole Hemoglobin and myoglobin (on standing) Bilirubin

From Forbes CD, Jackson WF. *Color Atlas and Text of Clinical Medicine,* 3rd ed. London: Mosby; 2003.

Specific Gravity
The specific gravity of the urine generally is related linearly with osmolality. However, it can be raised by the presence of molecules with relatively high molecular weight, such as glucose or contrast dye. A fixed specific gravity of 1.010, so called isosthenuria, is characteristic of chronic kidney disease (Chapter 132).

pH
Urine pH typically is 5 as a result of daily net acid excretion. An alkaline pH often is noted after meals, when an "alkaline tide" to balance gastric acid excretion increases urine pH. A high urine pH also is seen in patients who are on a vegetarian diet. An exceptionally high urine pH is indicative of an infection with a urea-splitting organism, such as *Proteus* species (Chapter 292). An inappropriately high urine pH in the setting of systemic non–anion gap metabolic acidosis may be seen in certain forms of renal tubular acidosis (RTA; Chapter 130). In a proximal RTA, the urine pH is high until the tubular reabsorption threshold for bicarbonate, which is abnormally low, is reached. At this point, the urine pH decreases to 5. In distal RTA, the inability to create a sufficient gradient for hydrogen ions results in a urine pH that is always higher than 5.5; the urine net charge gives complementary and confirmatory information. In type 4 RTA, the urine pH is often 5, and the urine net charge is often positive, thereby confirming the absence of significant amounts of ammonium in the urine; this defect is exacerbated by the accompanying hyperkalemia.

Glucose
Glucose in the urine is detected by an assay using dipsticks impregnated with the enzyme glucose oxidase. Glycosuria is seen in diabetes mellitus (Chapter 236), when pregnancy causes the tubular threshold for glucose reabsorption to change, and in tubular diseases that affect the proximal convoluted tubule and cause tubular glycosuria. Evidence for pan-proximal tubular dysfunction (e.g., glycosuria, aminoaciduria, phosphaturia) indicates that Fanconi's syndrome is present.

Protein
The dipstick for protein is a sensitive assay based on color change induced by the presence of proteins at a given pH. It is most sensitive to the presence of albumin and is much less sensitive to other proteins, such as the light chains of Bence Jones protein (Chapter 193). The presence of 1+ protein correlates with about 30 mg/dL of albuminuria, and 3+ protein correlates with greater than 500 mg/dL of proteinuria. Because the dipstick is not a quantitative measurement, small amounts of proteinuria in an oliguric patient may give the false appearance of high-grade proteinuria.

Heme
The dipstick for heme uses the peroxidase-like activity of hemoglobin and myoglobin molecules to detect the presence of heme pigment. The reaction occurs on exposure to hemoglobin, myoglobin, or intact red blood cells (RBCs). The presence of myoglobin, which is found in patients with rhabdomyolysis (Chapter 115), or free hemoglobin, which is seen in patients with intravascular hemolytic anemias (Chapter 163), is suspected if the heme reaction is intensely positive and there is a paucity of cellular elements in the sediment.

Leukocytes
The dipstick detection of leukocytes depends on the presence of leukocyte esterase. Leukocyte esterase is usually present in infections (Chapter 292) and in inflammatory conditions.

Urine Sediment
Cells
RBCs, white blood cells (WBCs), tubular cells, transitional cells, and squamous epithelial cells may be seen in the urine. Casts are formed in tubules and may contain cells or cellular debris, or may be acellular.

RBCs may originate from intrarenal vessels, glomeruli, tubules, or anywhere in the urogenital tract. Dysmorphic RBCs are cells that have been deformed by transit through the glomerulus and through the medullary interstitium, as opposed to RBCs from the remainder of the genitourinary tract (Figs. 116-2 and 116-3); these cells are often lysed and less refractile than nonglomerular RBCs. Dysmorphic RBCs often fragment with poikilocytosis and with blebs, forming so-called Mickey Mouse RBCs. Phase contrast microscopy aids in the identification of dysmorphic RBCs. The presence of

FIGURE 116-2. Dysmorphic erythrocytes. These dysmorphic erythrocytes vary in size, shape, and hemoglobin content and reflect glomerular bleeding. (From Johnson RJ, Feehally J. *Comprehensive Clinical Nephrology*. London: Mosby; 2000.)

FIGURE 116-3. Isomorphic erythrocytes. These erythrocytes are similar in size, shape, and hemoglobin content. Isomorphic cells reflect nonglomerular bleeding from lesions such as calculi or papillomas or hemorrhage from cysts in polycystic renal disease. (From Johnson RJ, Feehally J. *Comprehensive Clinical Nephrology*. London: Mosby; 2000.)

FIGURE 116-4. Hyaline cast of the type seen in small numbers in normal urine. (From Johnson RJ, Feehally J. *Comprehensive Clinical Nephrology*. London: Mosby; 2000.)

FIGURE 116-5. Number and type of granules and their density in the cast vary in different casts. The presence of erythrocytes in this cast may mean that the granules are derived partly from disrupted erythrocytes. (From Johnson RJ, Feehally J. *Comprehensive Clinical Nephrology*. London: Mosby; 2000.)

FIGURE 116-6. A cast composed entirely of erythrocytes reflects heavy hematuria and active glomerular disease. Crescentic nephritis is likely to be present if erythrocyte cast density is greater than 100/mL. (From Johnson RJ, Feehally J. *Comprehensive Clinical Nephrology*. London: Mosby; 2000.)

a majority of dysmorphic RBCs in a urine sediment points to a glomerular origin of the hematuria. The presence of RBC casts is often conclusive evidence for the presence of glomerulonephritis.

WBCs are seen most commonly in urinary tract infections, but they also can be seen in acute interstitial nephritis, with *Legionella* (Chapter 322) and *Leptospira* (Chapter 331) species infections, chronic infections such as tuberculosis (Chapter 332), allergic interstitial nephritis (Chapter 124), atheroembolic diseases (Chapter 127), and granulomatous diseases such as sarcoidosis (Chapter 95) and tubulointerstitial nephritis uveitis syndrome. Mononuclear cells often appear with transplant rejection. Tubular cells, which are seen in many conditions involving tubulointerstitial diseases, also are seen in ischemic and nephrotoxic injury, such as with myeloma kidney (Chapter 193) or cast nephropathy. Eosinophils require special stains, with the Giemsa stain being much less sensitive than the Hansel stain (Chapter 124). Urine eosinophils classically are seen in allergic interstitial nephritis (Chapter 124), but they also are seen in atheroembolic disease (Chapter 127), prostatitis (Chapter 131), and vasculitis.

Other Elements
Bacteria may be seen in the urine sediment. A spun urine sediment may show rods or cocci in chains, but bacteria are identified best by Gram staining of the urine sediment. Budding yeast forms, which are highly refractile, trichomonads, and spermatozoa also may be seen in the urinary sediment.

Casts
Casts, which are formed in tubules, are characterized by the arrangement of the cells in a clearly formed matrix composed of Tamm-Horsfall protein. Because casts are formed in the renal parenchyma, they may give a clue to the origin of accompanying cellular elements.

Hyaline casts are composed of Tamm-Horsfall proteins that are formed normally and are seen in increased numbers after exercise (Fig. 116-4). *Granular casts* are degenerated tubular cell casts that are seen in the setting of tubular injury (Fig. 116-5). *Pigmented granular casts* are seen in rhabdomyolysis (Chapter 115) with myoglobinuria or, rarely, hemoglobinuria. *RBC casts* (Fig. 116-6) are rarely seen in allergic interstitial nephritis and diabetic nephropathy, but they are frequently seen in acute glomerulonephritis (Chapter 123). The presence of RBC casts in a patient with microscopic hematuria can narrow the focus of the evaluation to a glomerular lesion. *WBC casts* are seen commonly in pyelonephritis (Chapter 292) and in acute and chronic nonbacterial infections. They also are seen in other conditions in which WBCs are associated with parenchymal renal processes, such as allergic interstitial nephritis (Chapter 124), atheroembolic diseases (Chapter

FIGURE 116-7. Typical hexagonal cystine crystal. A single crystal provides a definitive diagnosis of cystinuria. (From Johnson RJ, Feehally J. *Comprehensive Clinical Nephrology*. London: Mosby; 2000.)

FIGURE 116-8. Oxalate crystals. A pseudocast of calcium oxalate crystals accompanied by crystals of calcium oxalate dehydrate. (From Johnson RJ, Feehally J. *Comprehensive Clinical Nephrology*. London: Mosby; 2000.)

FIGURE 116-9. Coffin-lid crystals of magnesium ammonium phosphate (struvite). (From Johnson RJ, Feehally J. *Comprehensive Clinical Nephrology*. London: Mosby; 2000.)

FIGURE 116-10. Urate crystals. Complex crystals suggestive of acute urate nephropathy or urate nephrolithiasis. (From Johnson RJ, Feehally J. *Comprehensive Clinical Nephrology*. London: Mosby; 2000.)

127), and granulomatous diseases such as sarcoidosis (Chapter 95). Rarely, WBC casts can be a dominant feature of many diseases that traditionally are thought of as glomerular diseases, such as SLE (Chapter 274) and Wegener's granulomatosis (Chapter 278). *Tubular cell casts* are seen with any acute tubular injury and are the dominant cellular casts in ischemic acute tubular necrosis (Chapter 122). They also can be seen with nephrotoxic injury, such as with aminoglycosides and cisplatin. Some casts may contain both leukocytes and tubular cells or be difficult to distinguish.

Crystals

Crystals can be a normal finding in the urine or serve as clues to pathophysiologic processes. Certain crystals, such as the hexagonal crystals seen with cystinuria (Chapter 130), are always abnormal (Fig. 116-7). Others, such as the octahedral calcium oxalate crystals (Fig. 116-8), may be a normal finding or may be evidence for ethylene glycol intoxication (Chapter 110). Triple phosphate crystals, which are composed of ammonium magnesium phosphate and are coffin shaped (Fig. 116-9), are seen in urinary tract infections with urea-splitting organisms (Chapter 292). Uric acid crystals, sodium urate crystals (Fig. 116-10), and calcium phosphate amorphous crystals are common and do not have pathologic significance.

Serologies for the Evaluation of Renal Disease

The evaluation of renal dysfunction has to follow a stepwise progression from noninvasive serologic evaluation to a definitive or confirmatory diagnostic evaluation, such as a renal biopsy. Sometimes an expeditious diagnosis is needed, and a biopsy may be done relatively early in the evaluation. Serologic diagnostic markers for certain diseases, such as Wegener's granulomatosis (Chapter 278), can sometimes avoid the need for a diagnostic renal biopsy in patients with renal insufficiency.

Antinuclear Antibody

An antinuclear antibody (ANA) can be useful to evaluate glomerular disease, especially the nephrotic syndrome. A high ANA titer (e.g., 1:320), especially if it is accompanied by a more specific finding such as anti-double-stranded DNA (anti-dsDNA) antibody or anti-Smith antibody, can be highly specific for the diagnosis of SLE renal disease (Chapter 274), which usually requires a renal biopsy. Lower titers (e.g., 1:80 or 1:40) are nonspecific.

Rheumatoid Factor

A rheumatoid factor titer will usually be elevated in patients with rheumatoid arthritis, but vasculitis is a relatively late and rare event. Rheumatoid factor can be detected in cryoglobulinemia (Chapter 193); immunoglobulin M (IgM), which is present in type II and type III cryoglobulinemia, has rheumatoid factor activity. Rheumatoid factor also can be seen as a nonspecific finding in bacterial endocarditis (Chapter 76) and systemic vasculitis (Chapter 278).

Complement

The levels of complement components C3 and C4 and the 50% hemolyzing dose of complement (CH_{50}) usually are measured in the evaluation of suspected rapidly progressive glomerulonephritis (Chapter 123). Complement levels are usually low in active SLE (Chapter 274), poststreptococcal glomerulonephritis (Chapter 123), endocarditis (Chapter 76), membranoproliferative glomerulonephritis, cryoglobulinemia (Chapter 193), shunt nephritis, and glomerulonephritis associated with visceral abscesses. A particularly depressed C4 compared with C3 should raise the suspicion of cryoglobulinemia.

Serum and Urine Immunoelectrophoresis and Bence Jones Protein

Elevated polyclonal IgA levels are seen in about 50% of cases of IgA nephropathy (Chapter 123) and Henoch-Schönlein purpura (Chapter 123). Polyclonal elevation of IgG may occur in a variety of systemic diseases and is a nonspecific finding. The presence of a monoclonal protein in the serum should raise the suspicion for a monoclonal gammopathy–associated disease (Chapter 193). The differential diagnosis includes monoclonal gammopathy of uncertain significance, myeloma kidney, lymphomas (Chapter 191), amyloidosis (Chapter 194), light chain deposition disease, heavy chain deposition disease, immunotactoid glomerulonephritis, and cryoglobulinemia. The concentration of the monoclonal protein is higher when the diagnosis of multiple myeloma is made, but even small quantities of Bence Jones proteins in the serum can have clinical significance. Because a substantial fraction of multiple myelomas can have no heavy chain excretion and small quantities of light chains may be hard to detect by serum immunoelectrophoresis, a urine immunoelectrophoresis always should be obtained concomitantly to ensure a complete evaluation. A new, more sensitive assay for serum free light chains and an assessment of the ratio of kappa to lambda lights chains increase the sensitivity for detecting monoclonal gammopathies.

A urine test for Bence Jones protein complements the serum immunoelectrophoresis. Patients may have Bence Jones proteinuria even in the absence of an M component in the serum immunoelectrophoresis. Bence Jones proteinuria may be present in myeloma kidney, amyloidosis, light chain deposition disease, lymphoma, or, occasionally, monoclonal gammopathy of uncertain significance. However, many patients with systemic amyloidosis have a normal serum immunoelectrophoresis and no Bence Jones proteinuria (Chapter 193).

Antineutrophil Cytoplasmic Antibody

The antineutrophil cytoplasmic antibody (ANCA) assay has allowed for earlier and more definitive recognition of one of the most common causes of rapidly progressive glomerulonephritis. The ANCA test, when confirmed by enzyme-linked immunosorbent assay (ELISA), is highly sensitive and specific for a group of vasculitides (Chapter 278). The antibodies are present in the serum of the affected patient and cause two different patterns of staining: perinuclear staining (p-ANCA) and cytoplasmic staining (c-ANCA). Both antigens actually have a cytoplasmic distribution, and the former pattern is an artifact of the fixation method. The antigen for p-ANCA is myeloperoxidase, and the antigen for c-ANCA is proteinase-3. p-ANCA is associated with microscopic polyangiitis, idiopathic crescentic glomerulonephritis, or Churg-Strauss syndrome (Chapter 278). The c-ANCA serology result often correlates with the classic disease of Wegener's granulomatosis (Chapter 278). Immunofluorescence is highly sensitive but is not specific, unless used with ELISA and Western blotting. In the appropriate clinical setting, it can avoid the need for renal biopsy. Anti-GBM antibody staining also may occur in the presence of a positive ANCA, the significance of which is unclear. It is speculated that exposure of the Goodpasture antigen, as a result of the glomerular injury, leads to anti-GBM antibody formation as a secondary process.

Anti–Glomerular Basement Membrane Antibody

Anti-GBM antibodies are autoantibodies to the Goodpasture antigen, which resides in a domain of the α chain of type 4 collagen. An early and accurate diagnosis of Goodpasture's syndrome can be made by immunofluorescence and confirmed by Western blot analysis.

Cryoglobulins

Cryoglobulins (Chapter 193) are thermolabile immunoglobulins of single monoclonal type (type I cryoglobulinemia); in type II and type III cryoglobulinemia, the mixture of immunoglobulins includes one with rheumatoid factor activity against IgG. Type I and type II cryoglobulins are more likely to be associated with clinical disease, especially at higher titers. In type II cryoglobulinemia, the monoclonal component has rheumatoid factor activity and is often an IgM κ M component. Type III cryoglobulinemia is often of less clinical significance. Type I cryoglobulinemia is seen with Waldenström's macroglobulinemia and multiple myeloma (Chapter 193); type II, with hepatitis C infection (Chapters 150 and 151), Sjögren's syndrome (Chapter 276), lymphomas (Chapters 191 and 192), and SLE (Chapter 274); and type III, with hepatitis C (Chapters 150 and 151),

chronic infections, and inflammatory conditions. When cryoglobulinemia is associated with hepatitis C, the hepatitis C virus (HCV) RNA is concentrated in the cryoprecipitate; the diagnosis can be made by an RNA assay of the cryoprecipitate at 37° C.

Other Serologies

Membranous nephropathy is associated with chronic hepatitis B infection with hepatitis B surface antigenemia (Chapter 151). Classic polyarteritis nodosa (Chapter 278) occasionally is seen with chronic hepatitis B infection, often with surface antigenemia and hepatitis B e-antigenemia.

Hepatitis C serology is associated with a variety of renal entities, including cryoglobulinemia, membranoproliferative glomerulonephritis, and membranous nephropathy. The evaluation may include the antibody test and an assay for HCV RNA. Occasionally, the HCV RNA analysis may have to be conducted on the cryoprecipitate at 37° C.

Human immunodeficiency virus (HIV)-associated nephropathy (Chapter 123) is associated with nephrotic syndrome and acute kidney injury. In the appropriate clinical setting, HIV serology and viral titers are appropriate tests for both clinical syndromes.

Streptococcal infection can be confirmed as the cause of postinfectious glomerulonephritis (Chapter 123) with an anti-DNase or antistreptolysin assay. Acute and convalescent serology assays are used to confirm recent infection.

Erythrocyte Sedimentation Rate

The erythrocyte sedimentation rate (ESR) is a relatively nonspecific test in the evaluation of renal disease. However, a high ESR often points to systemic vasculitis (Chapter 278), multiple myeloma (Chapter 193), or malignancy as the underlying cause. However, the ESR often is elevated in the nephrotic syndrome (Chapter 123), including diabetic nephropathy (Chapter 126).

Noninvasive Imaging

A variety of renal imaging techniques can assist in the evaluation of diseases of the kidney. Of note is that plain films and intravenous pyelography largely have been replaced by renal ultrasonography and computed tomography (CT) for the evaluation of renal size and the detection of stones and masses.

Renal Ultrasonography

Ultrasonography, which is the most commonly used renal imaging study (Fig. 116-11), provides reliable information regarding obstruction, renal size, the presence of masses, and renal echotexture. The study has only 90% sensitivity for the detection of hydronephrosis, however, and is not sufficient to exclude obstruction with certainty. Additionally, its inability to detect stones in the ureters and bladder limits its utility in the evaluation for kidney stones. Doppler imaging permits evaluation of the renal vessels and resistive index.

Computed Tomography

A stone protocol CT scan of the kidneys, ureter, and bladder has become the study of choice for the detection of kidney stones (Chapter 128) because of its ability to detect stones of all kinds, including uric acid stones and nonobstructing stones in the ureters (Fig. 116-12). Masses in the kidney can be evaluated using either contrast CT or a renal ultrasound. CT angiography with iodinated contrast material can assess possible renal artery stenosis

FIGURE 116-11. Normal sagittal renal ultrasound. The cortex is hypoechoic compared with the echogenic fat containing the renal sinus. (From Johnson RJ, Feehally J. *Comprehensive Clinical Nephrology.* London: Mosby; 2000.)

FIGURE 116-12. Delayed excretion in the left kidney secondary to a distal calculus. Contrast-enhanced computed tomography scan shows dilated left renal pelvis. (From Johnson RJ, Feehally J. *Comprehensive Clinical Nephrology*. London: Mosby; 2000.)

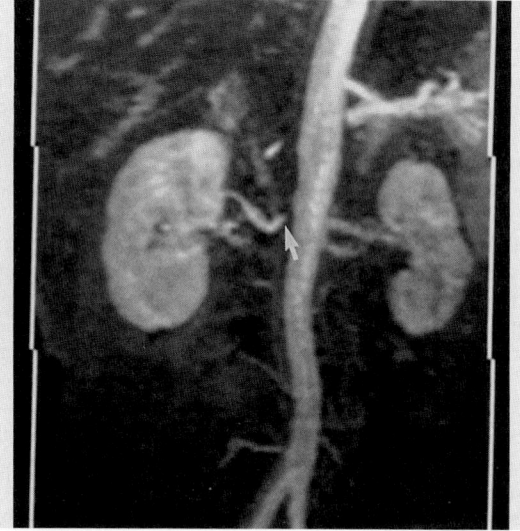

FIGURE 116-13. Magnetic resonance angiography. Coronal three-dimensional image shows right renal artery stenosis *(arrow)*. (From Johnson RJ, Feehally J. *Comprehensive Clinical Nephrology*. London: Mosby; 2000.)

(Chapter 127) with an accuracy comparable to magnetic resonance (MR) angiography.

Magnetic Resonance Imaging with Magnetic Resonance Angiography

Magnetic resonance imaging (MRI) with MR angiography (Fig. 116-13) is highly sensitive for detecting atherosclerotic renovascular disease (Chapter 127), but it tends to overestimate the degree of stenosis. Its accuracy in detecting fibromuscular dysplasia, however, is less well validated. MRI also can be used to evaluate renal masses. MRI does not require iodinated contrast material, but gadolinium-based contrast agents for vascular studies are associated with the syndrome of nephrogenic systemic fibrosis in patients with renal failure (Chapter 275).

Renography

The uptake by the kidneys of ^{99m}Tc-DTPA, as a marker of GFR, and mercaptoacetyl triglycine, as a marker of renal blood flow, can help evaluate patients with suspected renovascular disease. However, neither is commonly used now that CT angiography and MR angiography are widely available.

Invasive Evaluation
Renal Angiography

Renal arteriography, which is the gold standard in the evaluation of renal artery stenosis (Chapter 127), also is used for the evaluation of arteriovenous

FIGURE 116-14. Systemic lupus erythematosus. This renal biopsy specimen shows proliferative change and crescent formation in both glomeruli (hematoxylin and eosin stain; magnification, 116×). (From Johnson RJ, Feehally J. *Comprehensive Clinical Nephrology*. London: Mosby; 2000.)

FIGURE 116-15. Renal amyloidosis. The glomerulus shows amyloid deposition, stained by Congo red, in the glomerular capillaries (magnification, 330×). (From Johnson RJ, Feehally J. *Comprehensive Clinical Nephrology*. London: Mosby; 2000.)

malformations, polyarteritis nodosa, and other vascular lesions of the kidneys. This invasive study uses iodinated contrast material and incurs a small risk for atheroembolic disease (Chapter 127). Therapeutic angioplasty and stenting can be done at the time of the angiogram.

Renal Biopsy

Renal biopsy usually is performed percutaneously with real-time ultrasound or CT guidance. The risk for bleeding that requires a transfusion is 1 to 2% in patients without coagulopathy. The transjugular approach can be used in patients in whom the risks for bleeding are high. Current indications for renal biopsy include the following:

1. Rapidly progressive glomerulonephritis. Biopsy is generally indicated for ANCA-related vasculitis unless the case is classic, such as red blood cell casts and renal dysfunction. For patients with cryoglobulinemia and SLE, biopsy is recommended to stratify patients before therapy.
2. SLE with renal involvement to categorize the degree of nephropathy, which cannot be assessed based on clinical criteria (Fig. 116-14). A repeat biopsy is indicated if a change in immunosuppressive therapy is planned and the clinical picture is at all ambiguous (e.g., serum creatinine, urine sediment, and proteinuria are in good control but anti-DNA antibody titers remain high).
3. Nephrotic syndrome without an obvious cause. In childhood nephrotic syndrome, empirical steroid therapy is used routinely because of the high prevalence of steroid-responsive minimal change disease. In adults, the approach generally is to use the biopsy to guide appropriate therapy (Fig. 116-15).
4. Unexplained renal failure of any cause, especially if immunosuppressive therapy is contemplated. Patients with hospital-acquired renal failure rarely require renal biopsy.
5. Unexplained proteinuria below the nephrotic range to exclude nephrosis in evolution. Biopsy is recommended if proteinuria exceeds 1 g per 24 hours or occurs in the setting of a reduced GFR.

6. Renal transplantation with acute and chronic renal failure, in which the biopsy information can be crucial in guiding diagnosis and treatment.

● MAJOR RENAL SYNDROMES

Renal disease can be divided logically into major overlapping categories, which are used to characterize the most common renal syndromes.

Acute Kidney Injury

Acute kidney injury (Chapter 122) is a syndrome in which glomerular filtration declines over a period of hours to days. The patient with acute renal failure is approached best by evaluation for prerenal, renal, and postrenal causes. Most cases of acute renal failure in the hospital have hemodynamic or toxic etiologies. The careful and systematic evaluation of the patient should start with a thorough history and physical examination, which should be followed by selected laboratory tests and often an imaging test, such as renal ultrasonography.

Nephritic Syndrome

The acute nephritic syndrome is an uncommon but dramatic presentation of an acute glomerulonephritis (Chapter 123). The hallmark of the acute nephritic syndrome is the presence of dysmorphic RBCs and RBC casts, but their absence does not exclude the syndrome. The acute nephritic syndrome can be caused by any of the rapidly progressive glomerulonephropathies, all of which warrant urgent and usually inpatient evaluation.

Nephrotic Syndrome

The nephrotic syndrome (Chapter 123) is characterized by the presence of proteinuria of greater than $3.5 \text{ g/day}/1.73 \text{ m}^2$, with accompanying edema, hypertension, and hyperlipidemia. Other consequences include a predisposition to infection and hypercoagulability. In general, the diseases associated with nephrotic syndrome do not cause acute kidney injury, although acute kidney injury may be seen with minimal change disease, HIV-associated nephropathy, and bilateral renal vein thrombosis (Chapter 127). The causes of primary idiopathic nephrotic syndrome, in decreasing order of prevalence, are focal and segmental glomerulosclerosis, membranous nephropathy, minimal change disease, and membranoproliferative glomerulonephritis. Secondary causes of the nephrotic syndrome include diabetic nephropathy (Chapter 126), amyloidosis (Chapter 194), and SLE (Chapter 274) with membranous nephropathy.

Tubulointerstitial Diseases

Tubulointerstitial diseases (Chapter 124) vary in presentation from acute kidney injury to chronic kidney dysfunction that manifests as asymptotic mild renal insufficiency (Table 116-2). The urine sediment often contains small-to-moderate amounts of proteinuria, usually less than 1 g/day, as well as WBCs, RBCs, tubular cells, and WBC casts. RBC casts are rare in acute interstitial nephritis and are more characteristic of glomerular disease.

Vascular Diseases of the Kidney

Vascular diseases of the kidney can be divided into large-vessel obstruction and medium- to small-vessel diseases (Chapter 127). Renovascular disease is a common cause of hypertension, heart failure, and renal insufficiency. About 90% of renal artery stenosis is atherosclerotic in origin, with most of the remaining caused by fibromuscular dysplasia, which is more common in women 20 to 50 years of age. Medium-sized arterial vessel diseases include polyarteritis nodosa, which is seen in patients with hepatitis B, HIV infection,

or, rarely, hepatitis C. Symptoms include abdominal pain, hypertension, and mild renal insufficiency, often with a benign sediment; diagnostic findings include microaneurysms at the bifurcation of medium-sized arteries. Other diseases involving small vessels include atheroembolic disease (Chapter 127), which is seen either spontaneously or after arteriography or surgery; this syndrome typically affects the kidneys, gastrointestinal tract, and lower extremities, but it can also involve the central nervous system when the aortic arch is affected.

The thrombotic microangiopathies include hemolytic-uremic syndrome and thrombotic thrombocytopenic purpura (Chapter 174). Thrombocytopenic purpura is associated with an acquired inhibitor to, or the congenital inherited absence of, a protease that cleaves large-molecular-weight von Willebrand multimers. Hemolytic-uremic syndrome is caused by endothelial injury induced by Shiga toxin from *Escherichia coli* O157:H7 infection. The antiphospholipid antibody syndrome (Chapter 179) can cause large vessel thrombosis and stenosis as well as a thrombotic microangiopathy with proteinuria, hypertension, and renal insufficiency. Scleroderma renal crisis, which is a manifestation of systemic sclerosis (Chapter 275), often leads to an inexorable progression to end-stage renal insufficiency if it is untreated.

Papillary Necrosis

Acute necrosis of the renal papilla is associated with sickle cell anemia (Chapter 166), analgesic nephropathy (Chapter 124), diabetic nephropathy (Chapter 126), and obstructive pyelonephritis (Chapter 125). In sickle cell disease (Chapter 166), the hypoxic and hypertonic milieu of the inner medulla promotes sickling, and chronic sickling at the vasa recta results in medullary ischemia. Massive and prolonged consumption of analgesics, particularly the combination of aspirin, caffeine, and acetaminophen, is associated with chronic interstitial nephritis and a predisposition to papillary necrosis (Chapter 124); medullary ischemia is thought to be caused by inhibition of synthesis of vasodilatory prostaglandins by aspirin, and direct toxicity is attributed to metabolites of phenacetin. Similarly, medullary perfusion is thought to be compromised in diabetic nephropathy (Chapter 126) and obstructive pyelonephritis (Chapter 125).

The clinical manifestations of papillary necrosis can include flank pain and hematuria. If the papilla is sloughed, obstruction may occur at the renal pelvis or ureter of the affected kidney, with referred pain migrating from the flank to the groin. A sloughed papilla may precipitate frank renal failure if the function of the contralateral kidney is impaired or if obstruction occurs at the level of the bladder or urethra (Chapter 125).

Classically, papillary necrosis is diagnosed on an excretory pyelogram as a calyceal defect after sloughing of a papilla, but CT with contrast is as good for advanced lesions. If the necrotic papilla is retained, however, the defect will be more subtle. Transitional cell carcinoma (Chapter 203) can occur in the setting of papillary necrosis or can mimic its appearance. Obstruction, if present, must be relieved, but treatment otherwise is limited to pain control and hydration.

Chronic Kidney Disease

Chronic kidney disease, which is defined as either kidney damage or a GFR of less than $60 \text{ mL/min}/1.73 \text{ m}^2$ for longer than 3 months, includes five stages (Table 116-3). Kidney damage is defined as pathologic abnormalities or markers of kidney damage, including abnormalities in the composition of blood or urine or abnormalities on imaging tests. The excretion of 30 to 300 mg of albumin in a 24-hour period defines microalbuminuria. An estimated 12% of the adult U.S. population has abnormal albumin excretion in the urine, and the frequency increases with age. Kidney failure is defined as either a GFR of less than $15 \text{ mL/min}/1.73 \text{ m}^2$ that is accompanied by signs and symptoms of uremia or a need for initiation of kidney replacement therapy for treatment of complications of decreased GFR. End-stage renal disease includes all cases requiring treatment by dialysis or transplantation regardless of the level of GFR.

Patients with chronic kidney disease warrant referral to a nephrologist. Care of these patients should focus on efforts to slow disease progression, optimize medical management, and make a seamless transition to renal replacement therapy (Chapter 132). The care should include optimal blood pressure control, use of angiotensin-converting enzyme inhibitors and angiotensin receptor blockers if indicated, dietary counseling, careful management of calcium and phosphorus levels, control of the parathyroid hormone level, and management of anemia with the use of erythropoietin and iron supplements. Early referral for placement of access for dialysis and initiation of

TABLE 116-2	MAJOR CAUSES OF TUBULOINTERSTITIAL DISEASE

Ischemic and toxic acute tubular necrosis
Allergic interstitial nephritis
Interstitial nephritis secondary to immune complex–related collagen vascular disease, such as Sjögren's disease or systemic lupus erythematosus
Granulomatous diseases: sarcoidosis, tubulointerstitial nephritis with uveitis
Pigment-related tubular injury: myoglobulinuria, hemoglobinuria
Hypercalcemia with nephrocalcinosis
Tubular obstruction: drugs such as indinavir, uric acid in tumor lysis syndrome
Myeloma kidney or cast nephropathy
Infection-related interstitial nephritis: *Legionella*, *Leptospira* species
Infiltrative diseases, such as lymphoma

TABLE 116-3	STAGES OF CHRONIC KIDNEY DISEASE*	
STAGE	**DESCRIPTION**	**GFR (mL/min/1.73 m²)**
1	Kidney damage with normal or ↑GFR	≥90
2	Kidney damage with mild or ↓GFR	60-89
3	Moderate ↓GFR	30-59
4	Severe ↓GFR	15-29
5	Kidney failure	<15 (or dialysis)

*Chronic kidney disease is defined as either kidney damage or GFR <60 mL/min/1.73 m² for ≥3 months. Kidney damage is defined as pathologic abnormalities or presence of markers of damage, including abnormalities in blood or urine tests or image studies.
GFR = glomerular filtration rate.
From http://www.kidney.org/kidneydisease/ckd/knowGFR.cfm. Accessed Jan. 31, 2010.

transplant evaluation (Chapter 133) are important components of the care of patients with chronic kidney disease.

SUGGESTED READINGS

Abboud H, Henrich WL. Stage IV chronic kidney disease. *N Engl J Med.* 2010;362:56-65. *Treatment guidelines to slow the progression of advanced kidney disease and prepare for renal replacement therapy.*
James MT, Hemmelgarn BR, Tonelli M. Early recognition and prevention of chronic kidney disease. *Lancet.* 2010;375:1296-1309. *Review.*
Kidney Foundation Disease Outcomes Quality Initiative (DOQI) Guidelines. http://www.kidney.org/professionals/KDOQI/index.cfm. Accessed Dec. 13, 2010. *A periodically updated source of consensus guidelines for the management of chronic kidney disease.*
Poff JA, Hecht EM, Ramchandani P. Renal imaging in patients with renal impairment. *Curr Urol Rep.* 2011;12:24-33. *Suggestions for choosing studies to minimize the adverse effects of contrast media.*
Tonelli M, Muntner P, Lloyd A, et al. Using proteinuria and estimated glomerular filtration rate to classify risk in patients with chronic kidney disease: a cohort study. *Ann Intern Med.* 2011;154:12-21. *The combination of proteinuria and estimated GFR is effective for risk stratification.*

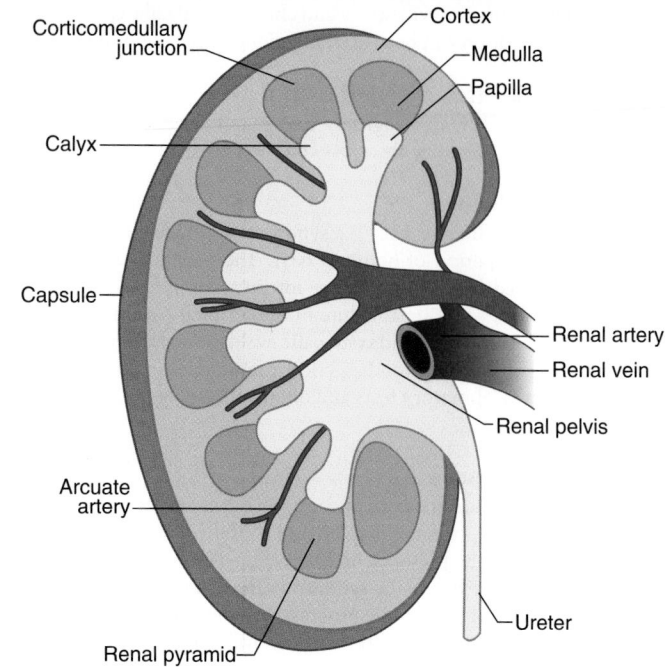

FIGURE 117-1. Sagittal section of the human kidney depicting gross anatomy and organization.

117

STRUCTURE AND FUNCTION OF THE KIDNEYS

QAIS AL-AWQATI AND JONATHAN BARASCH

The kidney regulates the ionic composition and volume of body fluids, the excretion of nitrogenous waste, the elimination of exogenous molecules (e.g., many drugs), the synthesis of a variety of hormones (e.g., erythropoietin), and the metabolism of low-molecular-weight proteins (e.g., insulin). Befitting such an array of responsibilities, the kidney receives 25% of the cardiac output. The gross anatomy of the kidney is notable for a weight of approximately 150 g and a characteristic bean shape with approximate dimensions of 11 × 6 × 2.5 cm. On bisection, a simple gross structure is evident with an outer cortex and a more central medulla that narrows to multiple papillae at the apices of so-called pyramids (Fig. 117-1).

Understanding the kidney, however, requires an appreciation of the intricate microstructure that underlies its complex functions. The kidney is a composite organ comprising approximately 1 million essentially identical functional units termed *nephrons*. All the functions of the kidney are performed by each individual nephron, and at a first approximation, all nephrons are independent of each other because they have their own innervation and blood supply. The nephron is made up of two functional subunits, the glomerulus and the following tubules and ducts (Fig. 117-2). The glomerulus begins with the branching of the afferent arteriole, an end artery of the corresponding renal artery, to a tuft of capillaries. The glomerular capillaries invaginate an epithelium with the visceral epithelial cells adjacent to the capillary and the parietal epithelial cells outside this tuft. The space between the epithelial layers is the urinary space. The fenestrated glomerular capillary endothelium, the intervening basement membrane, and the foot processes of the visceral epithelium, so-called podocytes, make up the glomerular filtration barrier. The balance of hydrostatic and oncotic pressures drives the extrusion of a protein-free filtrate through this barrier into the urinary space. The urinary space then leads to a series of tubules and ducts: the proximal tubule, the thin limb of the loop of Henle, the thick limb of the loop of Henle,

the distal convoluted tubule, the cortical collecting duct, and the medullary collecting duct. The papillary collecting duct empties through the renal papilla into the renal pelvis and then to the ureter. The glomerular capillary bed coalesces to form the efferent arteriole, a vessel that is exquisitely sensitive to angiotensin II, and then to the peri (proximal) tubular capillaries. This system allows efferent arteriole constriction to regulate proximal tubule reabsorption, as described later.

The nephron regulates homeostasis by three actions. First, in the glomerulus, nephrons produce as much as 120 mL/minute of an ultrafiltrate of blood. Second, in different segments of the nephron, the composition of the filtrate is altered by the transfer of nearly 99% of its components (e.g., glucose, NaCl, water) from the lumen to the blood. Third, additional electrolytes (e.g., NH_4^+, K^+, HCO_3^-) are secreted from the blood into the lumen.

To perform these functions, each nephron segment, with the exception of the collecting ducts, is composed of a single epithelial cell type whose luminal or apical surface (facing the urine) and basolateral surface (facing the blood) differentially express various proteins and lipids. For example, the apical membrane often has microvilli or cilia, whereas the basolateral membrane does not. Apical polarized endocytosis and exocytosis are often important in the regulation of the number of transport proteins on the apical surface. In addition, epithelia are connected to one another by tight junctions, which confer a characteristic ionic permeability on the epithelial sheet. Transepithelial transport occurs largely through the cell, but transport through the tight junction (the *paracellular pathway*) can also be important in different segments of the tubule. For instance, Na transport begins with entry at the luminal surface down an electrochemical gradient, whereas its exit at the basolateral surface is uphill and requires adenosine triphosphate (ATP) hydrolysis. The Na^+, K^+-ATPase is located at the basolateral surface of all epithelia, and all "active" energy-consuming transport is coupled directly or indirectly to it with the exception of H^+ transport. Each segment has a distinct composition of channels, carriers, and ATPases, and each segment is regulated by different chemical and physical sensors, so the "final urine" contains the components that must be discarded to maintain constancy of body composition.

THE KIDNEY REGULATES EXTRACELLULAR FLUID VOLUME BY REGULATING ITS SODIUM CONTENT

Filtration of 180 L/day containing 24,000 mEq of Na^+ is followed by the reabsorption of more than 99% of the filtered Na^+. Na^+ reabsorption accounts for more than 90% of oxygen consumed by the kidney. Na^+ reabsorption is regulated by volume receptors, which are located in the carotid artery and

FIGURE 117-2. Structure of the nephron. **A,** Components of the cortical and juxtaglomerular nephrons. **B,** Anatomy of the glomerulus. **C,** Light micrograph of a human glomerulus. E = endothelial cell; M = mesangial cell; P = parietal epithelial cell; V = visceral epithelial cell. (**C,** Courtesy of Dr. Glen Markowitz.)

increase β-sympathetic output, which in turn release renin, an aspartate protease from the granular cells of the juxtaglomerular apparatus. The renin-releasing cells are close to the afferent arterioles, where renin cleaves angiotensinogen to angiotensin I, which is then converted locally to angiotensin II. Angiotensin II binds to angiotensin receptors and constricts the efferent arteriole, thereby affecting glomerular hemodynamics. The increased hydrostatic pressure within the glomerular capillaries drives the formation of an ultrafiltrate of plasma. As filtration progresses, a protein-rich, oncotically active solution in the capillary opposes the glomerular capillary hydrostatic pressure until a pressure equilibrium is achieved before the efferent arteriole is reached. Consequently, angiotensin II may not change glomerular filtration rate (GFR) markedly, but it can increase proximal reabsorption by reducing the hydrostatic pressure and increasing the oncotic pressure in the peritubular capillaries that surround the proximal tubule in a plexus, thereby favoring reabsorption of water and solutes such as urea.

The glomerular filtrate next enters the tubular portion of the nephron, where Na^+ traverses the cell by entering the apical membrane either through a cotransporter or countertransporter or through an Na^+ channel, depending on the specific mechanisms of different segments. In the apical membrane of

the proximal tubule, an Na^+/H^+ (NHE_3) exchanger, an Na-coupled glucose carrier, and an Na^+-coupled amino acid and phosphate cotransporter are present. Subsequently, Na^+ is actively transported by the basolateral Na^+, K^+-ATPase into the paracellular space, thereby resulting in local hypertonicity, which causes osmosis through low-resistance tight junctions of the initial segments of the proximal tubule (Fig. 117-3).

In the thick ascending limb of Henle, Na^+ is absorbed by an NaK-2Cl cotransporter. The driving force for this neutral carrier allows Na^+ and Cl^- to enter the cell, but K^+ is then recycled across the apical membrane, thereby resulting in depolarization of the transepithelial membrane potential. In the distal convoluted tubule, Na^+ is absorbed by a thiazide-sensitive cotransporter, which conducts Na^+ and Cl^- in a strict 1:1 stoichiometry. Na^+ exits as usual by the Na^+, K^+-ATPase, but there is also a basolateral Na/Ca exchanger. In this short segment, the macula densa helps control the GFR by regulating renin release through secretion of adenosine and prostaglandins.

In the principal cells of the collecting duct, aldosterone, derived from the zona glomerulosa of the adrenal cortex, increases reabsorption of the final 50 to 100 mEq/day of Na^+ remaining in the lumen by increasing the number of open Na^+ channels (ENac), by activating expression of α-subunits, and by

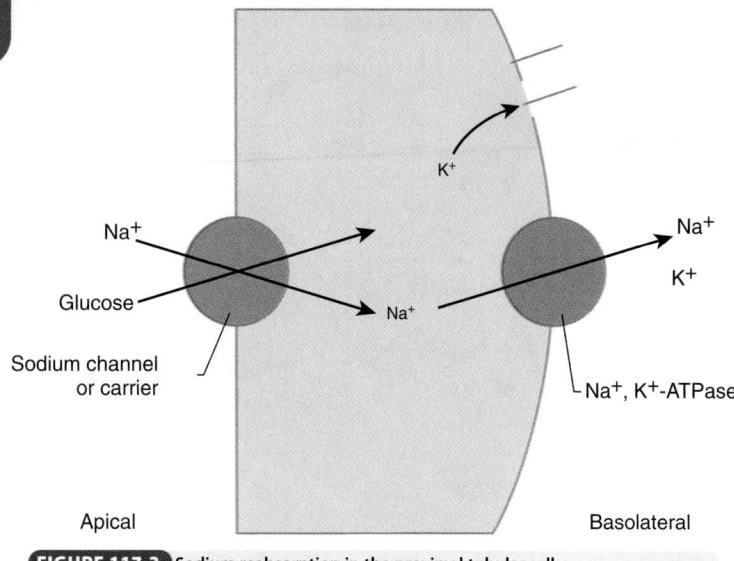

FIGURE 117-3. Sodium reabsorption in the proximal tubular cell.

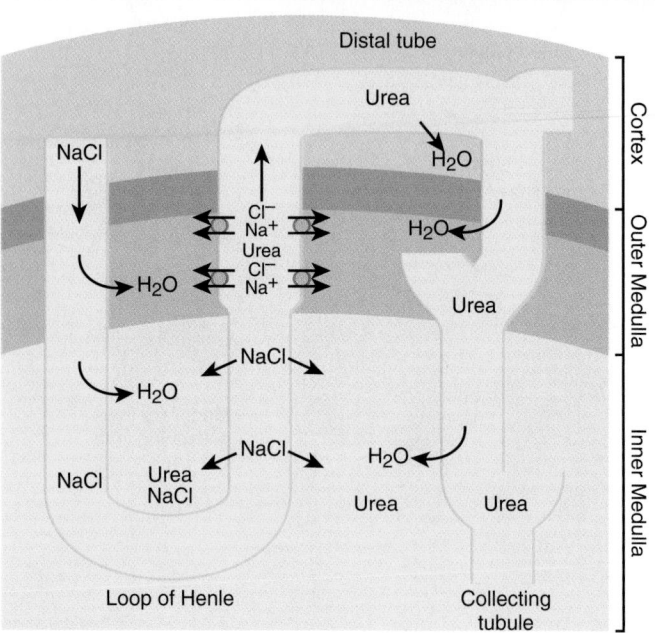

FIGURE 117-4. Regulation of water content.

increasing the activity of the basolateral Na⁺, K⁺-ATPase. Aldosterone is the final critical regulator of Na⁺ balance.

A number of the steps that regulate Na⁺ reabsorption can be counteracted by atrial natriuretic peptide (ANP), which is released from the atria in response to volume overload. ANP increases filtration in the glomerulus by dilating the afferent arteriole, thereby increasing glomerular capillary pressure and lowering the oncotic pressure. Additionally, ANP increases Na⁺ excretion by inhibiting the release of renin, the production of aldosterone, and the tubular reabsorption of Na⁺ in the terminal collecting duct.

● THE KIDNEY REGULATES BODY FLUID OSMOLARITY BY REGULATING ITS WATER CONTENT

Water moves freely among all cells and compartments of the body, and its concentration, or osmolarity, is strictly regulated to prevent cells from swelling or contracting. The kidney regulates water content by varying the osmolarity of urine. It can dilute the urine by absorbing Na⁺ without water in the thick ascending limb, the distal tubule, and the collecting duct. Conversely, the absorbed NaCl and urea provide a hyperosmotic region in the medulla, where the limited blood flow maintains an osmotic gradient. To concentrate the urine, water is removed from the filtrate by this osmotic gradient as it passes through the cortical and medullary collecting tubules.

Antidiuretic hormone (ADH), also called *vasopressin*, is a critical component of water reclamation. The neurohypophysis releases ADH as a result of activation of Trvp1 channels, which are responsive to cell shrinkage caused by changes in osmolarity of as little as 1%. In the kidney, ADH binds to the V2R receptor Trvp1 on collecting tubules and increases water permeability by reversibly inserting a water channel, called *aquaporin-2*, in the apical membrane by the fusion of vesicles. During states of water deprivation, the dilute urine generated by the thick ascending limb enters vasopressin-sensitive segments in the cortical collecting tubule, where the bulk of the water is absorbed into the cortex to increase the osmolarity of the urinary filtrate to 300 mOsm, which is the osmolarity of plasma. Subsequently, the urine becomes concentrated when it equilibrates with the osmolarity of the medulla as the urine courses down the medullary collecting duct (Fig. 117-4).

● THE KIDNEY REGULATES PLASMA pH BY REGULATING HCO₃ CONTENT

The concentration of free H⁺ in the intracellular and extracellular fluids is maintained at about 40 nM (pH 7.4) by the daily excretion of acid or base in amounts equal to what is generated by dietary intake and by cellular activity. The complete oxidation of carbohydrates and fats generates approximately 15 to 20 mol/day of the volatile acid CO_2, and nonvolatile acids generated by the metabolism of protein-rich diets account for 60 to 80 mEq/day. HCO_3^- is the most important buffer not only because it is consumed by metabolic acid, thereby producing CO_2 that can be exhaled, but also because it can be regenerated by the kidney. The overall relationship of this buffer system is described by the Henderson-Hasselbalch equation: $pH = pKa + \log [HCO_3^-]/\alpha\, PCO_2$, where pKa is 6.1 and α represents the solubility coefficient of PCO_2 (which is 0.03). Because all the body buffers (e.g., bone, intracellular proteins) are in equilibrium, changes in the concentration of HCO_3^- regulate the pH of body fluids.

Although one task of the kidney is to replace the HCO_3^- that is lost as a consequence of the production of acid by oxidative metabolism, it must first reabsorb the 5000 mEq/day HCO_3^- that is filtered every day. The proximal tubule reabsorbs luminal HCO_3^- by secreting H⁺ through an apical Na⁺/H⁺ exchanger, which is directly stimulated by angiotensin II to secrete H⁺ in strict 1:1 exchange for Na⁺, thereby mediating both sodium absorption and H⁺ secretion. An H⁺-ATPase is also present in the microvilli and apical endocytic vesicles that fuse with the apical membrane in response to elevated blood PCO_2. H⁺ secretion titrates filtered HCO_3 and, catalyzed by carbonic anhydrase, converts it to CO_2 and water, thereby allowing CO_2 reabsorption. H⁺ secretion leads to an excess of OH⁻ in the cell, where it combines with this CO_2 to produce cellular HCO_3^-, which then exits across the basolateral membrane through an Na-HCO_3^- cotransporter (Fig. 117-5).

Given that the proximal tubule regulates bicarbonate reabsorption, the collecting duct must produce "new" HCO_3 to replace what is lost during titration by nonvolatile acids. The cortical and medullary collecting tubules contain intercalated cells that mediate H⁺-HCO_3 transport; α- and β-cell types are present in the cortex, whereas only α cells are present in the medulla. H⁺ secretion is mediated by the α-intercalated cell, where the H⁺-ATPase is delivered to the apical membrane by fusion of apical vesicles as stimulated by ambient PCO_2 (Fig. 117-6).

In a reaction catalyzed by carbonic anhydrase II, the excess OH⁻ is carboxylated by CO_2 to form HCO_3^-. HCO_3^- is subsequently transported across the basolateral surface in exchange for Cl⁻ by an alternately spliced form of the red cell anion exchanger (band 3). In contrast, β cells secrete HCO_3^- by an apical Cl/HCO_3 exchanger (pendrin) and a basolateral H⁺-ATPase. An H⁺, K⁺-ATPase in the collecting tubule also may play a role in K absorption and perhaps in H⁺ secretion.

The collecting tubule is a "tight epithelium" that can maintain electrical and concentration gradients. Secretion of H⁺ reduces the pH of the filtrate; the maximal gradient is 3 pH units or 180 mV, but both the size of the pH gradient and its transepithelial membrane potential can be modified to regulate H⁺ secretion. For example, Na⁺ absorption by the principal cell hyperpolarizes the membrane and can drive H⁺ transport. Aldosterone can stimulate not only Na⁺ absorption but also independently H⁺ secretion—hence, it is the major hormone that stimulates acid secretion in the collecting tubule. Finally, chronic metabolic acidosis converts the β-intercalated cells into α-intercalated cells, thereby increasing the number of acid-secreting cells and reducing the amount of HCO_3^- secretion in this segment.

The secreted H⁺ titrates urinary NH₃, and HPO₄²⁻. NH₃, which is synthesized by the conversion of glutamine to α-ketoglutarate, is secreted into the proximal lumen. In the loop of Henle and distal segments, the protonated ammonium ion is transferred into the interstitium, from where it reenters the nephron as ammonia gas. Once in the lumen, ammonia gas becomes reprotonated to ammonium, thus trapping a proton. The amount of NH_3 generated from glutamine increases up to four- to five-fold in the setting of metabolic acidosis. Net acid secretion is consequently urinary NH_4^+ plus titratable weak acids (such as HPO_4^{2-}) minus urinary HCO_3^-. Each of these components is regulated by the kidney.

THE KIDNEY REGULATES PLASMA POTASSIUM BY EXCRETION AND THE CONTROL OF EXTRACELLULAR PH

Because the membrane potential of most cells is governed by the ratio of intracellular to extracellular K, the plasma K concentration must be heavily regulated. Most dietary K^+ is pumped into the cell by the Na/K-ATPase, but about 90% of ingested K^+ eventually must be excreted into the urine. K^+ is filtered but is then reabsorbed by the proximal tubule and loop of Henle. K^+ is then secreted by the distal convoluted tubule and the principal cells through apical potassium inwardly rectifying (ROMK) and potassium large conductance calcium-activated (BK) channels. K^+ is secreted in response to a gradient, with cell K^+ greater than lumen K^+, which drives K^+ into the lumen. Secretion is enhanced by the increased entry of K^+ into the principal cell as a result of high extracellular concentration, by metabolic alkalosis, and by aldosterone. Aldosterone increases the synthesis of Na^+, K^+-ATPase and increases the probability that the ROMK channels will be open. Aldosterone also enhances Na^+ reabsorption by ENaC and thereby hyperpolarizing the transepithelial membrane potential, which increases the driving force for K secretion. High urinary flow rates deliver a large volume of fluid that is essentially K^+ free, thereby providing a concentration gradient. However, the flow rate also activates mechanosensory flagella that lead to an increase in cell calcium, which in turn activates BK channels. K^+ reabsorption is not regulated to the same extent as Na^+ retention, and profound K^+ depletion may be required for K^+ excretion by the kidneys to be eliminated completely.

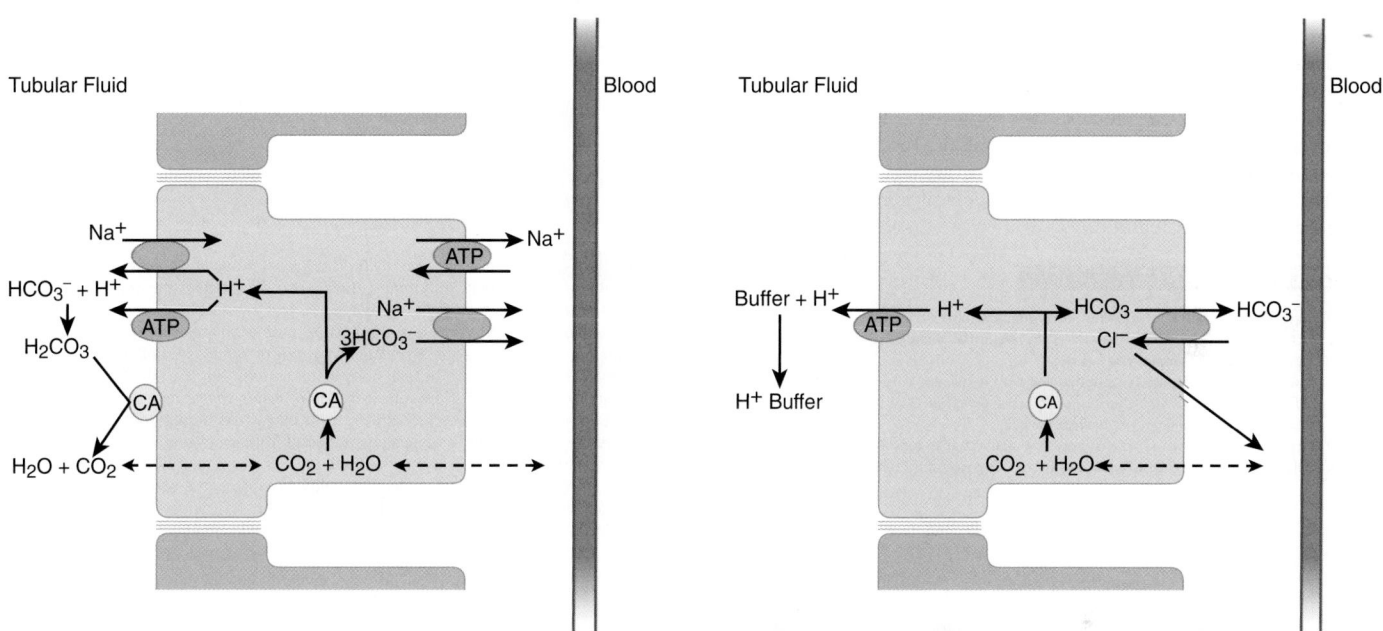

FIGURE 117-5. **Ion transport in the proximal tubule.** ATP = adenosine triphosphate; CA = carbonic anhydrase.

FIGURE 117-6. **Mechanism of acid secretion in the collecting duct.** ATP = adenosine triphosphate; CA = carbonic anhydrase.

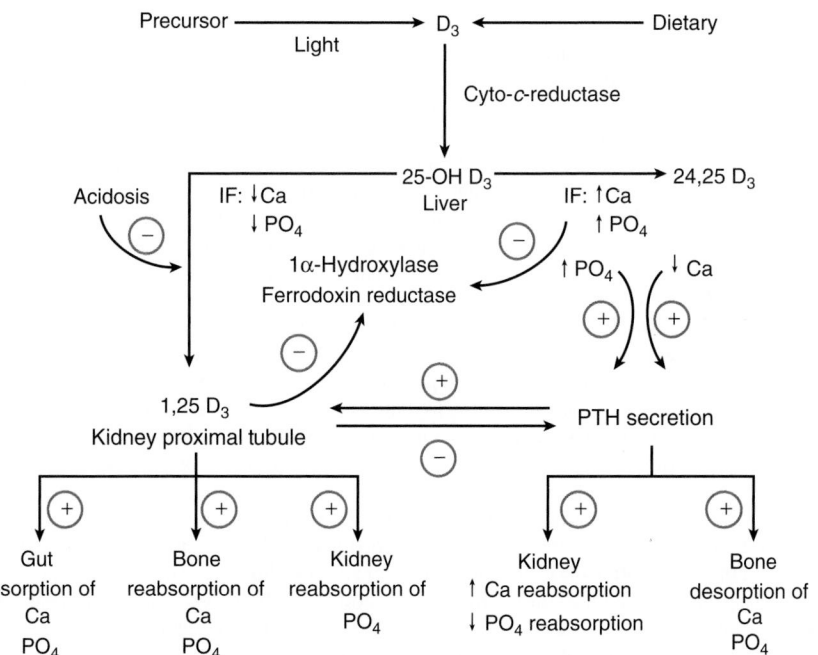

FIGURE 117-7. **Calcium and phosphate metabolism.** PTH = parathyroid hormone.

THE KIDNEY REGULATES PLASMA PO₄ AND CA²⁺ BY EXCRETION AND BY SYNTHESIZING VITAMIN D₃

The level of PO_4 also critically regulates serum Ca^{2+} because their plasma concentrations are close to their saturation, at which point crystallization occurs. Thus, any significant increase in PO_4 results in precipitation of $CaPO_4$.

The level of PO_4 is regulated by glomerular filtration. Initially, about 85% is reabsorbed by the proximal tubule NaPi-2a/c cotransporter. Parathyroid hormone and the heteromeric receptor FGFR/Klotho, which binds FGF23, inhibit the expression of NaPi and hence increase excretion of PO_4. Conversely, the proximal tubule generates vitamin D_3 [1,25-$(OH)_2$ cholecalciferol] by capturing 25-OH cholecalciferol, bound to its filtrable transport protein with brush boarder megalin (Fig. 117-7), after which 1α-hydroxylation is stimulated by low Ca^{2+} and PO_4. 1,25-vitamin D_3 inhibits parathyroid hormone and stimulates PO_4 reabsorption in gut and kidney, thereby counteracting parathyroid hormone and FGF23-Klotho. Nonetheless, Klotho signaling blocks 1,25-vitamin D_3 synthesis, thereby suggesting that it dominates the control of PO_4.

The level of serum calcium is also regulated by the kidney. Approximately 60% of serum Ca^{2+} is filtered, after which it follows Na^+ reabsorption in the proximal tubule and in the loops of Henle, where Ca^{2+} absorption is driven by the positive membrane potential generated by the Na-K-2Cl/K recycling transporter. In contrast, Ca^{2+} and Na^+ are regulated independently in the distal convoluted tubule by parathyroid hormone and Klotho, which increase reabsorption. Phosphate and calcium metabolism are regulated by Na^+ reclamation, parathyroid hormone, 1,25-$(OH)_2$ cholecalciferol, and Klotho in different segments of the nephron.

SUGGESTED READINGS

Hamm LL, Feng Z, Hering-Smith KS. Regulation of sodium transport by ENaC in the kidney. *Curr Opin Nephrol Hypertens.* 2010;19:98-105. *A review of the role of the amiloride-sensitive epithelial sodium channel in regulating sodium transport and balance.*

Riccardi D, Brown EM. Physiology and pathophysiology of the calcium-sensing receptor. *Am J Physiol Renal Physiol.* 2010;298:F485-F499. *Overview of the role of the extracellular calcium-sensing receptor in calcium regulation, kidney physiology, and pathophysiology.*

Toda N, Okamura T. Modulation of renal blood flow and vascular tone by neuronal nitric oxide synthase–derived nitric oxide. *J Vasc Res.* 2011;48:1-10. *Overview of the control of renal blood flow.*

FIGURE 118-1. Composition of body fluid compartments. **A**, Schematic representation of body fluid compartments in humans. The *shaded areas* depict the approximate size of each compartment as a function of body weight. The figures indicate the relative sizes of the various fluid compartments and the approximate absolute volumes of the compartments (in liters) in a 70-kg adult. **B**, Relative volumes of various body fluid compartments. In a normally built individual, the total body water content is roughly 60% of body weight. Because adipose tissue has a low concentration of water, the relative water-to-total body weight ratio is lower in obese individuals. Intracellular electrolyte concentrations are in millimoles per liter and are typical values obtained from muscle. ECF = extracellular fluid; ICF = intracellular fluid; ISF = interstitial fluid; IVF = intravascular fluid; TBW = total body water. (**A**, From Verbalis JG. Body water osmolality. In: Wilkinson B, Jamison R, eds. *Textbook of Nephrology.* London: Chapman & Hall; 1997:89-94. Reproduced with permission of Hodder Arnold.)

118

DISORDERS OF SODIUM AND WATER HOMEOSTASIS

KARL SKORECKI AND DENNIS AUSIELLO

SODIUM AND WATER HOMEOSTASIS

EPIDEMIOLOGY

Disturbances in sodium and water balance or distribution, with attendant perturbations in the volume or solute composition of body fluid compartments, are among the most frequently encountered abnormalities in clinical medicine. The principal clinical manifestations of these disturbances are *hypovolemia, hypervolemia, dysnatremia (hyponatremia* or *hypernatremia),* and *polyuria.* Disturbances in body tonicity, reflected by hyponatremia or hypernatremia, are estimated to affect up to 15 to 20% of hospitalized patients, with severe disturbances (>10% deviation from normal values) affecting 1 to 2% of patients. Prevalence rates for these abnormalities in ambulatory populations are lower, and elderly individuals and patients treated with multiple medications are the most susceptible.

PATHOBIOLOGY

Approximately 60% of body mass is composed of solute-containing fluid solutions that are divided into extracellular fluid (ECF) and intracellular fluid (ICF) compartments. Water flows freely across cell membranes through specific water channels (aquaporin family of transmembrane proteins) according to the dictates of osmotic forces, thereby maintaining near equality of the solute-to-water ratio (osmolality) in the ICF and ECF. However, the composition of the major solutes differs between the ECF and ICF (Fig. 118-1). Sodium and potassium are the major cations in the ECF and ICF, respectively. Chloride and bicarbonate are the major accompanying anions in the ECF, and negative charges on organic molecules maintain electroneutrality with potassium in the ICF. The difference in cationic solute composition between these two compartments is maintained by a pump-leak mechanism involving the activity of Na^+, K^+-adenosine triphosphate (ATPase) operating in concert with cell membrane sodium and potassium conductance pathways. The free movement of water ensures that the sodium concentration in ECF is nearly equivalent to the potassium concentration in ICF. *Osmolality* refers to the concentration of all solutes, whereas *tonicity* refers to the concentration of solutes that are "effective" in eliciting a water shift between body fluid compartments. Addition or removal of solutes causes a sustained shift of water to restore the near equality of concentrations, and they are thus considered effective solutes that contribute to body fluid tonicity. The restriction of sodium to the ECF compartment by virtue of the pump-leak mechanism, together with maintenance of osmotic equilibrium between the ECF and ICF, ensures that ECF volume is determined principally by the total body fluid sodium content and governs the partitioning of fluid between the ECF and ICF compartments. In contrast, solutes that permeate across most cell membranes, such as urea, do not elicit a sustained shift in water and therefore do not contribute to the steady-state partitioning of fluid volumes across body compartments. However, urea and glucose do contribute to the laboratory measurement of fluid osmolality. The addition or removal of water without solutes results in a proportionate reduction or increase, respectively, in both osmolality and tonicity of all body fluid compartments.

The mechanisms that govern body fluid homeostasis preserve near constancy of the volumes of the ECF and ICF compartments despite variations in dietary intake and extrarenal losses of sodium and water and adjust this balance in response to variations in the capacity of these compartments. Thus, the overriding principle of body fluid and solute homeostasis is mass balance of total body intake and output of water as well as balance of osmotically active particles. Even the slightest perturbations in these parameters activate neural and hormonal mediators for restoration of balance. This restoration of balance is achieved through adjustments in the urinary excretion of sodium and water in response to perceived changes in ECF or ICF volume. Constancy of ECF volume, together with control of vascular capacitance, ensures a high degree of circulatory stability.

Sodium Balance

Sodium balance refers to the difference between intake and excretion. In the nonclinical setting, sodium intake is controlled by dietary habits. In the clinical setting, prescribed adjustments in sodium intake or the administration of sodium-containing medications or solutions cause variation to overall sodium intake. Although nonrenal loss is under some regulatory influence (e.g., aldosterone-mediated regulation of sodium concentration in stool and sweat), the fine adjustment of sodium balance in response to changes in intake is mediated by regulation of urinary sodium excretion. In the steady state, urinary excretion of sodium is closely matched to dietary salt intake. This balance depends on a series of afferent mechanisms that sense the volume of the ECF compartment relative to its capacitance and trigger effector mechanisms that modify the rate of renal sodium excretion to maintain ECF volume homeostasis. Normal functioning of these mechanisms in turn is impacted by the partitioning of the ECF into two subcompartments: intravascular and extravascular (interstitial) (see Fig. 118-1). The composition and concentration of small, noncolloid electrolyte solutes in these two ECF subcompartments are nearly equivalent, but there is a higher concentration of colloid osmotic particles, mostly molecules of albumin and globulin proteins, in the intravascular compartment. Opposing transcapillary hydraulic and colloid osmotic (oncotic) pressure gradients (Starling forces) favor the net transudation of fluid from the intravascular to the interstitial compartment. At the same time, lymphatic fluid movement from interstitial sites back to the circulation through the thoracic duct ensures that the intravascular subcompartment is replenished and maintains a nearly constant proportion of approximately 25% of the overall ECF, which corresponds to 3.5 L of plasma. The remaining approximately 75% of ECF volume (equivalent to 10.5 L in a normal 70-kg male) is contained in the interstitial spaces. Because intravascular volume is one of the key determinants of circulatory integrity, preservation of the constancy of ECF volume, and appropriate partitioning of the ECF volume between the intravascular and interstitial subcompartments are critical for hemodynamic stability.

Effective Arterial Blood Volume

The circulatory network is composed of central and peripheral venous compartments as well as renal and extrarenal arterial compartments. Each compartment reflects a unique characteristic of overall circulatory function (e.g., cardiac filling, tissue perfusion, renal perfusion, and transudation of fluid into the interstitial space) (Table 118-1).

The concept of effective arterial blood volume (EABV) is crucial to understanding the afferent mechanisms that govern the regulation of sodium homeostasis. Unlike ICF, ECF, and intravascular volume, EABV is not measurable as an anatomically defined space but rather is best understood in functional terms as an integration of hemodynamic parameters that emanate from specific sites in the arterial circuit that monitor tissue perfusion and trigger appropriate changes in urinary sodium excretion. These sites include the carotid baroreceptor and intrarenal mechanisms located at the glomerular afferent arterioles, the juxtaglomerular apparatus, and peritubular capillaries. EABV often, but not always, varies directly with actual ECF volume.

TABLE 118-1	MECHANISMS FOR SENSING REGIONAL CHANGES IN BODY FLUID VOLUME

Cardiopulmonary volume sensors
  Atria (neural and humoral pathways)
  Ventricular and pulmonary sensing sites
Arterial volume sensors
  Carotid and aortic arch baroreceptors
  Renal volume sensors
Central nervous system sensors
Hepatic and gastrointestinal tract sensors

Low-pressure sensors (e.g., cardiac atrial transmural stretch and tension receptors) respond to the state of cardiac filling and tend to protect against overfilling of the ECF compartment, but they also have a role in renal sodium retention in states of perceived underfilling. Taken together, the integrated ECF volume-sensing signals elicit an appropriate renal response for modulating sodium excretion in an effort to maintain a constant ECF volume.

The filtered load of sodium vastly exceeds net intake, so tubular reabsorption usually serves as the principal modulator of urinary sodium excretion, the preservation of sodium balance, and the maintenance of a constant ECF volume. Specific luminal membrane sodium transporters or channels at each tubular segment mediate movement of sodium from the luminal fluid into the cell in a carefully regulated manner, followed by extrusion of sodium across the basolateral surface through Na^+, K^+-ATPase and other sodium transporters. Among many others, these regulated luminal transporters include the Na/H exchanger (proximal tubule), the Na-K-2Cl (NKCC2) cotransport pathway (loop of Henle), the NaCl cotransporter (NCCT) along the distal convoluted tubule, and the apical sodium channel (ENaC) along the connecting and cortical collecting tubule. At some nephron sites, sodium reabsorption is isotonic (e.g., proximal tubule), whereas at other sites, sodium reabsorption exceeds water resorption, so tubular fluid has a sodium concentration less than that of plasma (e.g., thick ascending limb of the loop of Henle). Sodium reabsorptive transport pathways are subject to a series of regulatory influences that sense EABV, including the renin-angiotensin-aldosterone pathway, natriuretic peptides, endothelium-derived endothelins and nitric oxide, the eicosanoid-prostaglandin system, guanylin peptides of gut origin, and urotensins. This redundancy of multiple hormonal mediators, which act together with the sympathetic nervous system, renal neural stimulation, and intrarenal physical factors (e.g., peritubular capillary Starling forces, tubule lumen sodium chloride delivery, and tubuloglomerular feedback), underscores the evolutionary importance of regulating urinary sodium excretion to maintain volume homeostasis.

Water Balance

Water balance refers to the difference between intake (oral, enteral, or parenteral) and excretion (insensible, gastrointestinal, perspiratory, and renal). Maintaining equivalency of intake and excretion of water ensures constancy of body fluid tonicity (osmoregulation). Osmoregulation ensures that the content of effective solutes in each body fluid compartment determines the volume of that compartment. Positive water balance or negative water balance and the corresponding changes in tonicity and cell volume are sensed by osmoreceptor and thirst center cells in the hypothalamus. The osmoreceptors are situated in the supraoptic and paraventricular nuclei of the hypothalamus; the thirst center is situated in the organum vasculosum of the anterior hypothalamus. Just a 2% change in effective osmolality or tonicity elicits a change in release of the hormone arginine vasopressin (AVP) from the posterior pituitary gland and the perception of thirst. Endothelin-1 also is released from the posterior pituitary in response to water deprivation and increases plasma AVP levels. Stimulation of thirst depends on centrally produced angiotensin II. A reduction of more than approximately 8% of ECF volume serves as an overriding afferent signal (carried by the ninth and tenth cranial nerves) for the nonosmotically driven release of AVP and also stimulates thirst by means of angiotensin II, even when body tonicity is not elevated (Fig. 118-2A).

The urinary excretion of water depends on the delivery of isotonic sodium-containing filtrate to the thick ascending limb of the loop of Henle, reabsorption of sodium and accompanying electrolytes in the thick ascending limb of the loop of Henle and the distal tubule, and the AVP-regulated reabsorption of the appropriate volumes of solute-free water through aquaporin-2 water channels in the cells of the collecting tubule. The hydro-osmotic movement of water from the collecting tubule lumen to the hyperosmotic milieu of the renal medulla minimizes urinary excretion of the hypotonic fluid generated in the thick ascending limb of the loop of Henle and the distal tubule, thereby promoting positive water balance. In the *absence* of AVP, this hypotonic fluid is excreted, and negative water balance ensues. Typical levels of urine osmolality that can be achieved in the human kidney by fluctuations in AVP action range between 50 and 1200 mOsm/kg, but this range narrows at the extremes of age or in the presence of intrinsic renal disease. Laboratory measurement of urine osmolality reflects overall renal concentrating ability, including the hydro-osmotic action of AVP. However, not all solutes that contribute to the laboratory measurement of urine osmolality correspond to effective solutes in terms of body fluid tonicity. Thus, excretion of urine with high concentrations of urea and low concentrations of sodium, potassium, and chloride

FIGURE 118-2. Relationship between arginine vasopressin (AVP) and osmolality. **A,** Comparative sensitivity of AVP secretion in response to increases in plasma osmolality versus decreases in blood volume or blood pressure in human subjects. The *arrow* indicates the low plasma AVP concentrations found at basal plasma osmolality. Note that AVP secretion is much more sensitive to small changes in blood osmolality than to changes in volume or pressure. **B,** The relationship between the osmolality of plasma and the concentration of AVP in plasma is modulated by blood volume and pressure. The line labeled N shows plasma AVP concentrations across a range of plasma osmolality in an adult with normal intravascular volume (euvolemic) and normal blood pressure (normotensive). The lines to the left of N show the relationship between plasma AVP concentration and plasma osmolality in adults whose low intravascular volume (hypovolemia) or blood pressure (hypotension) is 10%, 15%, and 20% below normal. Lines to the right of N are for volumes and blood pressure 10%, 15%, and 20% above normal. Note that hemodynamic influences do not disrupt the osmoregulation of AVP but rather raise or lower the set point and possibly also the sensitivity of AVP secretion in proportion to the magnitude of the change in blood volume or pressure.

indicates a strong renal concentrating capacity but contributes less to positive water balance than does excretion of urine with the same measured osmolality and higher concentrations of these electrolytes.

PATHOPHYSIOLOGY

Disturbances in sodium balance primarily affect ECF volume, and disturbances in water balance primarily affect body fluid tonicity. A cumulative negative balance of sodium (sodium deficit) in the absence of a change in tonicity results in ECF volume contraction (hypovolemia), whereas a cumulative positive balance of sodium (sodium surfeit) results in ECF volume expansion (hypervolemia). In contrast, a cumulative positive body water balance (water surfeit) results in volume expansion of all the body fluid compartments, whereas negative water balance (water deficit) results in volume contraction of all the body fluid compartments. However, because ICF volume is double that of ECF at baseline, the more prominent expansion or contraction in absolute volume terms involves the ICF compartment. Furthermore, maintenance of a surfeit or deficit of water relative to solutes results in a uniform decrease or increase in body fluid tonicity in all fluid compartments. Because the solute composition of the plasma component of the ECF compartment is sampled, a disturbance in tonicity is most commonly detected as an abnormality in plasma sodium concentration (hyponatremia for water surfeit and hypernatremia for water deficit). Frequently,

TABLE 118-2 PATHOGENIC PROCESSES LEADING TO DISORDERS OF BODY SODIUM AND FLUID HOMEOSTASIS

CLINICAL STATE	EXTRACELLULAR FLUID VOLUME	BODY FLUID TONICITY	PATHOGENIC PROCESS
Normal	↔	↔	
Hypervolemic normonatremia	↑	↔	Isotonic net gain of sodium and water
Hypervolemic hyponatremia	↑	↓	Hypotonic net gain of sodium and water
Hypervolemic hypernatremia	↑	↑	Hypertonic net gain of sodium and water
Normovolemic hyponatremia	↔	↓	Net water gain ± sodium loss
Normovolemic hypernatremia	↔	↑	Net water loss ± sodium gain
Hypovolemic hypernatremia	↓	↑	Net loss of water in excess of sodium
Hypovolemic normonatremia	↓	↔	Isotonic net loss of sodium and water
Hypovolemic hyponatremia	↓	↓	Net loss of sodium in excess of water

↔ = Unchanged.

disturbances in water and sodium balance occur together, and all combinations of surfeit or deficit can occur (Table 118-2). The clinical approach to a patient with a sodium or water balance disturbance (or both) can be facilitated by careful consideration of which states apply.

SODIUM BALANCE DISORDERS
Hypovolemia

DEFINITION

Hypovolemia is a reduction in the volume of the ECF compartment in relation to its capacitance. In states of absolute hypovolemia, a deficit in sodium reflects past or ongoing negative sodium balance. The volume of the ECF intravascular and extravascular (interstitial) subcompartments may vary in the same or opposite directions. ICF volume is reflected by the measurement of plasma osmolality and sodium concentration and may be concomitantly disturbed (see Table 118-2).

EPIDEMIOLOGY

Causes of absolute and relative hypovolemia (Table 118-3) can be categorized into extrarenal and renal causes. Bleeding is the most frequent and direct cause of a reduction in the absolute volume of the intravascular subcompartment of the ECF (Chapters 106 and 137). Other causes of absolute hypovolemia include fluid loss from the kidney or from the gastrointestinal, integumentary, or respiratory systems. Infectious diarrhea remains a leading cause of death from hypovolemia in many areas of the world. Burns allow the loss of large volumes of plasma and interstitial fluid and can rapidly lead to profound hypovolemia similar to what is seen with bleeding (Chapter 112). Enhanced evaporative water loss from the respiratory tract can occur with exercise, in response to heat stress (Chapter 109), in febrile states, and in patients undergoing mechanical ventilation with inadequate humidification.

ECF also can be sequestered into compartments within the body without an evident history of loss. Such pathologic conditions are often referred to as third space loss and include gastrointestinal obstruction, sequestration of fluids in subcutaneous tissue after trauma or burns (Chapter 112), and sequestration in the retroperitoneal or peritoneal space in patients with pancreatitis (Chapter 146) or peritonitis (Chapter 144), respectively. The accumulation of ascites may also compromise intravascular volume.

In any form of kidney disease in which tubular reabsorption of the filtered sodium load does not match the sum of this filtered load plus dietary intake, a renal sodium-wasting state may ensue. Most of the widely used diuretic medications inhibit specific pathways for sodium reabsorption at various sites along the nephron and should more properly be referred to as natriuretic medications. Loop diuretics (furosemide, bumetanide, torsemide, and ethacrynic acid) are the most potent diuretics, and their potential to induce renal reabsorption causes absolute ECF volume depletion. The composition of the fluid and electrolyte loss differs according to the cause and source of gastrointestinal fluid loss (Chapters 134 and 142).

Given its large surface area, it is not surprising that fluid losses from the integumentary system can be an important cause of hypovolemia. In the absence of medical intervention, hemoconcentration and hypoalbuminemia ensue; however, because of the isotonic composition of the lost fluid, no changes in plasma osmolality or sodium concentration are expected. Exertion in hot environments increases thermoregulatory fluid losses from the skin in the form of sweat. Fluid loss through perspiration can reach 1 L/hour or more, depending on exertion and environment. The sodium concentration in sweat varies among individuals (range of approximately 20 to 50 mmol/L). Thus, although the fluid loss is hypotonic, a significant sodium deficit and ECF volume contraction can ensue. The extent of hypovolemia and the resulting body fluid composition (plasma osmolality and sodium concentration) will depend on fluid replacement, which is determined primarily by thirst and availability.

All extrarenal causes of hypovolemia are expected to invoke a renal response, whose hallmark is sodium and fluid conservation. Obviously, this expected response is absent when the kidney itself is responsible for sodium loss, whether owing to the effect of pharmacologic or hormonal influences or to intrinsic renal disease.

Renal Causes of Hypovolemia

When the glomerular filtration rate (GFR) and plasma sodium concentration are normal, approximately 24,000 mmol of sodium are filtered per day. Even when the GFR is markedly impaired, the quantities of sodium filtered far exceed normal dietary intake. Thus, the small quantities of sodium excreted in urine relative to the filtered load depend on the integrity of tubular sodium reabsorptive mechanisms to match urinary sodium excretion to dietary intake through volume sensing and effector mechanisms. Impairment in the integrity of one or more of these sodium reabsorptive mechanisms can result in a profound sodium deficit and absolute volume depletion.

An underappreciated but frequent clinical setting for renal sodium loss occurs after the iatrogenic administration of high volumes of volume-expanding, salt-containing solutions to hospitalized patients. Such patients are usually in the postoperative or post-trauma setting and are frequently administered many liters of saline or other sodium-containing maintenance intravenous fluids for several consecutive days, during which tubule reabsorption of sodium is downregulated. There may be a lag in the restoration of full tubule reabsorptive capacity, when intravenous fluids are discontinued, and high volumes of urine rich in sodium continue to be excreted. During this lag phase, the patient may become mildly, but transiently, hypovolemic. This scenario can be avoided by a graduated reduction in administered sodium-containing fluids, at a pace that allows sodium reabsorptive tubular pathways to be upregulated and restored to their normal reabsorptive levels.

Diabetes insipidus represents a spectrum of conditions resulting from deficiency or tubular resistance to the action of AVP. However, because it is the tubular reabsorption of water and not solutes that is impaired, the impact on ECF volume is generally a minor consideration in comparison to the impact on ICF and body fluid tonicity.

CLINICAL MANIFESTATIONS

The clinical manifestations of hypovolemia depend on the magnitude and rate of volume loss, the solute composition of the net fluid loss (taking into account ingested or administered fluids), and vascular and renal responses. A detailed history is often helpful in assessing bleeding, vomiting, diarrhea, polyuria, medications, and diaphoresis.

However, the absence of symptoms does not exclude mild to moderate hypovolemia, especially if the volume loss has occurred gradually. Intravascular volume contraction of less than 5% does not usually elicit symptoms and readily escapes detection by physical examination. With greater degrees of absolute hypovolemia (corresponding to intravascular volume contraction in the 5 to 15% range), symptoms and signs begin to appear. Patients may exhibit nonspecific symptoms related to end-organ hypoperfusion, including weakness, muscle cramps, and postural lightheadedness. Thirst may be an early manifestation but more likely reflects a concomitant hypertonic state.

A number of clinical scenarios illustrate the relationship of clinical manifestations to causes of hypovolemia. For example, a patient with an acute *gastrointestinal hemorrhage* (Chapter 137) of 0.5 L of whole blood can experience tachycardia, postural hypotension, peripheral vasoconstriction with cool extremities, lightheadedness, and oliguria, with high urine osmolality

sodium loss is augmented when they are combined with other classes of diuretic agents (thiazides, carbonic anhydrase inhibitors, aldosterone antagonists, and distal epithelial sodium-channel blockers).

Natriuretic medications often are used to treat hypervolemic states, but their overuse or inappropriate use can result in hypovolemia. Tubular sodium reabsorption also may be disrupted by inherited or acquired renal tubulopathies, such as various forms of proximal tubulopathy and different forms of Bartter's and Gitelman's syndromes (Chapter 130).

Impairment of renal tubule sodium reabsorption may also occur with nonoliguric acute kidney injury and the recovery phase after oliguric acute kidney injury or after release of urinary obstruction (Chapters 122 and 125). Interstitial renal disease (Chapter 124) may result in fluid and electrolyte abnormalities, which can include renal sodium wasting. Nonelectrolyte urinary solutes such as glucose (in severe hyperglycemia) and mannitol cause polyuria and hypovolemia. Mineralocorticoid deficiency and resistance, including adrenal insufficiency (Chapter 234), should always be considered in a patient with evidence of urinary sodium loss in the face of hypovolemia. In cerebral salt wasting (also referred to as renal salt wasting), tubular sodium reabsorption is impaired in the setting of acute head injury (Chapter 406) or intracranial hemorrhage.

In *relative hypovolemia*, ECF volume is not reduced in absolute terms, but the capacitance of the ECF or intravascular compartment is expanded, thereby leading to clinical manifestations that mimic those of absolute hypovolemia. Relative hypovolemic states can be classified into two categories: states of vasodilation and states of generalized edema. Vasodilation occurs in response to endogenous endothelial substances (e.g., nitric oxide) and to exogenous agents that induce vasodilation (e.g., vasodilator drugs). Peripheral vasodilation occurs in sepsis (Chapter 108) and in normal pregnancy. Relative hypovolemia also occurs in patients with a positive sodium and water balance and generalized edema but a reduced intravascular volume. Examples include heart failure (Chapters 58 and 59), decompensated cirrhosis with ascites (Chapter 156), and the nephrotic syndrome (Chapter 123).

PATHOBIOLOGY

Extrarenal Causes of Absolute Hypovolemia

The immediate effect of bleeding is a proportionate net loss in plasma and erythrocytes and hence an isotonic reduction in ECF volume. Compensatory hemodynamic responses include tachycardia and vasoconstriction, followed by a shift of fluid from the interstitial to the intravascular compartment because of altered transcapillary Starling hydraulic forces. Additional neural and hormonal responses result in renal sodium and water retention, with the aim of restoring intravascular volume and stabilizing the circulation.

Besides dietary intake, approximately 7 L of isotonic fluid enters the gastrointestinal tract on a daily basis, the bulk of which is reabsorbed to minimize fecal fluid loss. Because these fluids contain varying concentrations of sodium and accompanying anions, enhanced secretion or impaired and low urine sodium concentration. Hemoglobin and albumin will probably remain constant initially, and then a drop in hemoglobin will ensue after movement of ECF from the interstitial to the intravascular compartment. The plasma solute composition (sodium and potassium concentration, acid-base parameters) is not likely to change initially. The plasma concentration of urea may rise somewhat as a result of increased proximal tubular reabsorption of urea, increased proximal reabsorption of salt and water, and the increased nitrogen load from the destruction of erythrocytes in the gastrointestinal tract. Jugular venous pressure is expected to fall, and central venous pressure (CVP) will generally be less than 5 cm H_2O in the absence of confounding factors. Urine output is expected to be low, with a high specific gravity and osmolality and a low urine sodium concentration.

In another scenario, a patient inappropriately receiving potent *loop diuretics* over a period of many days for localized peripheral edema may suffer a cumulative net ECF loss of 3 L, or about 20%; approximately one third of this lost volume will have originated from the intravascular compartment, with the remainder coming from the interstitial compartment. This degree of intravascular loss usually induces weakness, tachycardia, low jugular venous pressure, and hypotension. However, because the deficit may have accumulated over time, a degree of adaptation would attenuate the severity of these clinical manifestations and lead the clinician to underestimate the extent of hypovolemia. The plasma sodium concentration may remain unaltered because disruption of the urine-concentrating mechanism by loop diuretics attenuates the tendency to water retention, and an intact thirst mechanism prevents hypertonicity. Because loop diuretics enhance urinary potassium and ammonium excretion, hypokalemic metabolic alkalosis is expected. The ongoing effect of the loop diuretic would mitigate oliguria and lead to inappropriately high concentrations of solutes including sodium and potassium in urine. After cessation of the loop diuretic, the appropriate renal response of oliguria, high urine osmolality, and sodium concentration would be expected.

A third scenario is a patient with relative hypovolemia owing to the vasodilation that typically accompanies *bacteremic sepsis* (Chapter 108). No source of fluid loss would be identified in the history, but the patient would usually manifest symptoms of weakness and even prostration, accompanied tachycardia and hypotension. The extremities may be warm, but reduced tissue perfusion may reduce the level of consciousness and cause oliguria, elevated plasma urea and creatinine levels, and lactic acidosis.

DIAGNOSIS

The most readily appreciated physical findings related to contraction of the intravascular compartment include tachycardia, orthostatic hypotension, and reduced jugular venous pressure. Although low CVP often reliably reflects intravascular volume contraction, an elevated CVP does not necessarily exclude hypovolemia because of the possible confounding influence of cardiac or lung disease. Severe degrees of hypovolemia (corresponding to intravascular volume contraction exceeding 10 to 20%) cause hypotension (even in the supine position), peripheral cyanosis, cold extremities, and reduced levels of consciousness (extending even to coma) as a result of end-organ and cerebral hypoperfusion. Hemodynamic collapse (hypovolemic shock; Chapter 106) also can occur with more rapid volume loss, comorbid conditions, and greater degrees of hypovolemia. When the source of volume loss is purely extrarenal, oliguria is expected. Physical findings such as reduced skin or eyeball turgor and dry mucous membranes are not reliable indicators of hypovolemia.

Laboratory Findings

Laboratory measurements are an adjunct to clinical assessment but do not replace symptoms and physical examination findings as a primary diagnostic tool. Decreases in *hemoglobin* indicate past or ongoing bleeding, but a normal or stable hemoglobin does not exclude acute bleeding. Hemoconcentration is often observed when hypovolemia is not the consequence of bleeding, but comorbid disease processes that produce anemia may mitigate this rise.

The *albumin* concentration may rise with gastrointestinal, urinary, or skin losses of albumin-free fluids. Conversely, fluid losses that are accompanied by albumin loss (e.g., proteinuria, protein-losing enteropathy) may mitigate this rise or even result in hypoalbuminemia. Similarly, burns and hepatic disease are often accompanied by hypoalbuminemia as a result of the loss or third spacing of protein-rich fluid.

Serum levels of *sodium* and *other electrolytes* also can vary widely. Even subtle and subclinical degrees of hypovolemia trigger urinary water retention and result in a hypotonic hyponatremic plasma composition if the patient is exposed to solutions that are more hypotonic than that of the fluid lost. In

contrast, loss of hypotonic fluids with inadequate water ingestion or replacement results in a hypertonic plasma composition and hypernatremia.

Acid-base (Chapter 120) and *potassium* (Chapter 119) changes point to specific causes. For example, hypokalemia with metabolic alkalosis frequently accompanies vomiting and some causes of diarrhea (e.g., a villous adenoma). More often, diarrheal fluid loss is associated with a non–anion gap metabolic acidosis. Loop and thiazide diuretic-induced hypovolemia is often associated with hypokalemic metabolic alkalosis, as are the inherited tubulopathies (Bartter's and Gitelman's syndromes) (Chapter 130), which disrupt sodium reabsorptive mechanisms at the loop of Henle and distal convoluted tubule, respectively. Severe hypovolemia with circulatory compromise and tissue hypoperfusion is often accompanied by lactic acidosis.

Increases in *plasma urea* and *creatinine* concentrations are frequently observed in hypovolemic states and reflect reduced renal plasma flow. If acute tubule injury does not supervene, the rise in plasma urea concentration is often disproportionate to the rise in plasma creatinine concentration (see Prerenal Azotemia in Chapter 122). The rise in plasma urea and creatinine concentrations is particularly common when hypovolemia is a consequence of urinary fluid losses. In such conditions, the patient is not oliguric, even though renal plasma flow and GFR are compromised. Other forms of urinary sodium loss, such as occur with adrenal insufficiency or aldosterone unresponsiveness, are accompanied by a tendency toward hyperkalemia and mild metabolic acidosis.

Urinary biochemical parameters may also help in the clinical assessment of hypovolemic states. When fluid loss is extrarenal, the expected renal response of water and sodium conservation results in oliguria with an elevated urine specific gravity (>1.020) and osmolality (>400 mOsm/kg) and a sodium concentration less than 20 mmol/L because of enhanced renal tubule reabsorptive activity. More complex indices of the appropriate renal response to hypovolemia include fractional excretion of sodium less than 1% and fractional excretion of urea less than 30 to 35%. Intrinsic renal injury confounds the diagnostic value of these urinary indices.

Differential Diagnosis

Relative hypovolemia secondary to arterial vasodilation mimics some of the clinical manifestations of absolute hypovolemia. With vasodilation, as seen for example in sepsis (Chapter 108), tachycardia and hypotension are common, but the extremities may be warm. However, tissues are actually underperfused, as reflected by reduced renal and cerebral function and lactic acidosis.

TREATMENT   Rx

Absolute Hypovolemia

The major goal in treatment of hypovolemia is to restore hemodynamic integrity and tissue perfusion. The treatment approach includes treatment of the underlying disease state when possible, replacement of the volume deficit, and fluid administration to maintain ECF volume in the event of continuing losses. Beyond the specific treatments, the mainstay of therapy involves fluid administration. The important issues are the volume, rate of administration, and composition of the replacement and maintenance fluids. These decisions may vary during different stages of treatment and should be adjusted according to the patient's response as determined by closely monitored clinical parameters.

The choice of oral or intravenous replacement fluids (or both) for hypovolemic states is dictated principally by the disturbances in other electrolyte and acid-base parameters. The rate of replacement is a function of the urgency of the threat to circulatory integrity and consideration of complications related to overzealous or too rapid correction.

Fluid therapy for hypovolemic states sometimes begins with a diagnostic fluid challenge. In situations in which clinical parameters do not permit a firm diagnosis of hypovolemia, the response to a fluid challenge can be informative and serve as the initial treatment step. For example, a patient with known long-standing compensated heart failure who is being maintained on a therapeutic regimen that includes diuretics may have tachycardia, a reduction in blood pressure from baseline values, poor cognition, and renal dysfunction. Such a clinical scenario could have a number of different explanations, including superimposed volume depletion with inadequate left ventricular filling volume. CVP, whether measured directly or assessed by jugular venous pressure, may be misleading in the face of right ventricular dysfunction, but direct measurement of pulmonary capillary wedge pressure does not significantly improve clinical outcomes.∎ In such a case, a carefully monitored diagnostic fluid challenge can minimize the risk for fluid overload. Such monitoring should include clinical assessment of parameters indicating pulmonary venous hypertension (pulmonary congestion or edema by physical examination or chest radiograph). Reversal of the disturbed clinical parameters would support the diagnosis of volume depletion.

Another example is a patient with hyponatremia in the setting of suspected volume depletion. Often the degree of volume depletion is too subtle to be detected by clinical examination, and a therapeutic challenge with fluid of the appropriate composition can be informative.

The initial volume and rate of therapeutic replacement fluid should be determined by ongoing monitoring of clinical parameters rather than a priori estimates of volume deficit. In some settings, the clinical state will dictate rapid fluid replacement, as in a patient with unambiguous hypovolemic shock and life-threatening circulatory collapse. In such cases, fluids can be administered at the most rapid rate possible, limited only by intravenous access, until blood pressure and tissue perfusion are restored. However, in most cases, much slower rates are indicated, especially in elderly patients, patients whose medical background is unclear, or those with known comorbid conditions. It is important to note that replacement fluids of different compositions have quite disparate volumes of distribution in the body fluid compartments and therefore differ in their efficiency of restoring ECF volume. *Crystalloid solutions* with sodium as the principal cation are the mainstay in fluid replacement therapy for hypovolemic states and are indicated primarily for hypovolemic states that are caused by renal, gastrointestinal, or sweat-based sodium losses. These solutions also are useful initial agents and adjuncts to therapy for the hypovolemia of hemorrhage and burns. *Isotonic saline* is confined to the ECF compartment (except in cases of severe dysnatremia). Thus, retention of 1 L of infused isotonic saline increases plasma volume by about 300 mL, with the remaining portion distributed in the interstitial subcompartment of the ECF. In contrast, a solution of *5% dextrose in water (D_5W)* is equivalent to administering solute-free water and distributes uniformly throughout all body fluid compartments (one third of the retained volume of infusate remains in the ECF compartment and only approximately 10 to 15% in the intravascular compartment). Infusing a given volume of *half isotonic saline (0.45% sodium chloride plus 5% glucose)* can be considered equivalent to infusing half that volume as solute-free water (distributed throughout body fluid compartments) and the other half as isotonic saline (confined to the ECF compartment). The retained solute-free volume reduces body tonicity and the plasma sodium concentration, potential benefit in the follow-up treatment of patients whose hypovolemia is accompanied by hypertonicity and hypernatremia, but a detriment for patients with normotonic or hypotonic hyponatremia.

When hypovolemia is accompanied by hypobicarbonatemia (metabolic acidosis), it may be appropriate to design a solution in which a portion of the sodium is accompanied by bicarbonate (Chapter 120). For example, it is possible to add a given quantity of hypertonic sodium bicarbonate to a solution of half isotonic saline (in which chloride is the anion accompanying sodium) to obtain an isotonic replacement fluid appropriate for the given acid-base status of the patient. Similarly, in patients with concomitant potassium depletion (Chapter 119), especially when accompanied by metabolic alkalosis, addition of potassium chloride to the replacement solution may be indicated. A number of crystalloid solutions with predetermined concentrations of potassium, lactate (converted to bicarbonate by the liver), and other electrolytes are commercially available, but it is more appropriate to begin with a sodium chloride–containing solution at a concentration appropriate to body tonicity, then to add other solutes as indicated or at a separate intravenous administration site. This approach provides maximal flexibility in tailoring individualized fluid replacement therapy to patient needs.

Colloid-containing solutions include albumin or high-molecular-weight carbohydrate molecules (e.g., hydroxyethyl starch or dextran) at concentrations that exert a colloid osmotic pressure equal to or greater than that of plasma. Banked human plasma is also considered a colloid solution. Because large molecules such as albumin and high-molecular-weight carbohydrates do not readily cross the transcapillary barrier, they are thought to expand the intravascular compartment more rapidly and efficiently than crystalloid solutions. However, a randomized trial showed no benefit of colloids compared with crystalloids for fluid resuscitation.[2] Nevertheless, albumin-containing solutions may be useful in hypovolemia associated with burns (Chapter 112), when cutaneous protein losses are appreciable. Furthermore, because of the capacity for rapid intravascular volume expansion with just a small volume of replacement fluid, colloid-containing solutions are frequently used when rapid intravascular expansion is desired, such as at trauma sites outside of the hospital setting. Some large-molecular-weight carbohydrates are nephrotoxic and should be used with caution in patients with renal impairment. In patients with multiorgan system failure and capillary leakage, albumin is both rapidly catabolized and redistributed into the interstitial compartment, so it can aggravate interstitial edema without providing an intravascular volume repletion benefit. It is for these reasons that crystalloid-containing solutions remain the mainstay of volume replacement therapy.

Blood products can be used for volume replacement in hypovolemic states, and a unit of packed red blood cells remains entirely in the vascular compartment. However, erythrocytes are actually considered part of the intracellular compartment and do not contribute to organ plasma flow. The role of packed red cells in the treatment of hemorrhage is to restore the principal function of the erythrocyte in oxygen carriage and delivery, not as a means of ECF volume replacement.

In addition to replacement fluids, maintenance fluids must be provided to counteract ongoing losses. Such ongoing losses may be a continuation of the underlying disease state (e.g., continued vomiting, diarrhea, polyuric states, or severe burns). The volume, rate of administration, and composition of these replacement fluids are best determined by actual measurements of the corresponding ongoing fluid losses, with appropriate adjustments for the patient's clinical assessment parameters.

Relative Hypovolemia

The treatment approach to relative hypovolemia is more complex than for absolute hypovolemia. When relative hypovolemia is the result of peripheral vasodilation, therapy should be directed toward reversal of the underlying cause and restoration of normal vascular reactivity. Bridging to maintain circulatory integrity until the underlying cause is successfully reversed can be achieved by infusion of an *isotonic crystalloid solution* such as normal saline. In such situations, selection of volumes and rates must be done with extreme caution because there is no absolute deficit and the administered volume will have to be excreted or removed once systemic vascular resistance and vascular capacitance are restored to normal. Furthermore, it is more difficult to estimate an increase in vascular capacitance than it is to estimate an absolute volume deficit. Occasionally, it is appropriate to consider the use of vasoconstrictor agents. When relative hypovolemia occurs in the setting of an edema state, therapy must take into account the fact that the patient actually has a total body sodium surfeit with excess ECF volume, but a maldistribution of that volume away from the EABV. When crystalloid solutions are provided to such patients, a variable, but usually substantial, proportion of administered fluid is distributed into the interstitial compartment and consequently does not contribute to restoration of EABV. This vicious cycle emphasizes the importance of treatment directed at the underlying disease state.

Hypervolemia

DEFINITION

Hypervolemia refers to expansion of ECF volume, which varies, even in normal individuals, with dietary sodium intake. Thus, an individual in steady state with low daily dietary sodium intake (e.g., 20 mmol/day, corresponding to approximately 1.2 g of table salt per day) will have correspondingly low urinary sodium excretion, equivalent to dietary intake minus extrarenal losses. A shift to much higher sodium intake (e.g., 200 mmol/day, corresponding to approximately 12 g of table salt per day) will bring the individual to a new steady state characterized by a correspondingly higher urinary sodium excretion rate. This shift is accompanied by an increase in ECF volume, which triggers the sensor and effector mechanisms for increased urinary sodium excretion (described earlier). In most individuals, this increase in ECF volume is not clinically detectable and does not have pathologic consequences. In some individuals, however, this upward shift in ECF volume increases systemic arterial blood pressure. When the sodium surfeit expands the ECF volume beyond the range necessary for the adjustment needed to restore sodium balance, a state of pathologic hypervolemia ensues.

EPIDEMIOLOGY

Primary and secondary renal sodium retention (Table 118-4) can lead to hypervolemia. Patients with oliguric renal failure of any cause (Chapters 122 and 132) have a limited ability to excrete both sodium and water. Urinary sodium retention can be one of the cardinal manifestations of primary glomerular diseases (Chapter 123), even when the GFR is well preserved. States of *mineralocorticoid excess* (Chapter 234) or enhanced activity are associated with a phase of sodium retention; however, because of the phenomenon of "mineralocorticoid escape," the clinical manifestation is generally that of hypertension rather than hypervolemia. Both heart failure (Chapter 58) and cirrhosis (Chapter 156) are associated with renal sodium retention.

PATHOBIOLOGY

Two pathophysiologic mechanisms can lead to sodium retention with ECF volume expansion. The first involves renal sodium retention that is primary and unrelated to the activation of afferent sensor mechanisms. This category includes primary renal diseases and endocrine disorders characterized by excess mineralocorticoid action. In the second category, EABV is reduced, and afferent sensory mechanisms activate effector responses that drive renal sodium retention. In these conditions, ECF volume is expanded; intravascular volume may be expanded, normal, or contracted; but the volume homeostatic mechanisms of the body mimic those of hypovolemia because of the perception of reduced EABV. The degree of solute-free water retention that

TABLE 118-4	PRIMARY AND SECONDARY RENAL SODIUM-RETAINING STATES

Oliguric renal failure
Chronic kidney disease
Glomerular disease, including nephrotic syndrome
Severe bilateral renovascular obstruction
Mineralocorticoid excess
Inherited sodium-retaining tubulopathies
Cardiac failure
Cirrhosis
Idiopathic edema

accompanies the sodium surfeit has a relatively small influence on the extent of hypervolemia but influences the accompanying tonicity state and determines whether the hypervolemia is hypotonic or isotonic.

When the ECF volume is expanded, the relative distribution between the intravascular and extravascular (interstitial) compartments depends on a number of factors. When cardiac and hepatic functions are normal and peripheral transcapillary Starling forces are intact, the excess ECF volume is evenly distributed between the intravascular and interstitial fluid compartments. In such cases, edema does not occur until there is a substantial surfeit of sodium, and hypertension is expected. In contrast, concomitant disruption of transcapillary Starling forces in a given microcirculatory bed would favor the accumulation of retained fluid at one or more such interstitial locations (e.g., dependent edema progressing to anasarca, ascites, pleural effusion, pulmonary congestion).

Primary Renal Sodium Retention

Patients who retain ingested or administered sodium and water loads expand their ECF volume. In patients with chronic kidney disease, the filtered load of sodium remains well above dietary intake until very late stages of severely reduced GFR: even when the GFR is decreased by as much as 90%, the daily filtered load of approximately 2400 mmol still greatly exceeds dietary intake. Nevertheless, the relationship between tubular reabsorption and filtered load may be disrupted in kidney disease.

Monogenic disorders that cause or mimic enhanced mineralocorticoid activity or are associated with enhanced activity of the distal nephron sodium reabsorptive pathways include Liddle's syndrome and pseudohypoaldosteronism type II (Chapters 67, 119, and 130). In these conditions and in other causes of mineralocorticoid excess, the only clue to mild hypervolemia may be hypertension, which can be severe. Mineralocorticoid excess, glucocorticoid remediable hypertension, apparent mineralocorticoid excess, and Liddle's syndrome are associated with hypokalemia, whereas pseudohypoaldosteronism type II or Gordon's syndrome are often accompanied by hyperkalemia.

Secondary Renal Sodium Retention

With both low-output and high-output heart failure, and both systolic and diastolic dysfunction, sodium retention is typical (Chapter 58). Low cardiac output, diversion of cardiac output away from arterial intravascular volume-sensing sites, or a high cardiac output that still is not sufficient to meet tissue demands appears to be a necessary and sufficient condition for initiating renal sodium retention. In the case of cirrhosis with ascites (Chapter 156), hepatic intrasinusoidal hypertension is a sufficient and necessary condition for initiating renal sodium retention. These pathophysiologic disturbances in cardiac or hepatic function disrupt afferent signals that govern normal sodium homeostasis and trigger effector mechanisms that lead to enhanced tubular reabsorption of sodium at multiple nephron sites. At the very earliest stages of disease, sodium retention occurs independently of any measurable or detectable reduction in the volume of the intravascular compartments or any of its measurable subcompartments. At more advanced stages of disease, reduced intravascular volume serves as the overriding stimulus for renal sodium retention and thereby leads to a decompensated state of intractable ECF volume accumulation. The more advanced stages, which often are accompanied by a disproportionate degree of positive water balance and consequent hyponatremia, herald imminent compromise of the GFR. Among the many neuronal and humoral abnormalities that characterize the sodium retention associated with heart failure and cirrhosis are endothelial dysfunction, enhanced sympathetic nerve activity, activation of the renin-angiotensin-aldosterone axis, and resistance to natriuretic peptides. In cirrhosis with ascites (Chapter 156), portosystemic shunting together with

translocation of intravascular volume to the splanchnic and venous circulation further compromise EABV. In addition, synthetic dysfunction with resulting hypoalbuminemia favors transudation of fluid into the interstitial compartment. At the level of intrahepatic hemodynamics, intrasinusoidal hypertension results in enhanced hepatic lymph formation. When the rate of enhanced hepatic lymph formation exceeds the capacity for return to the intravascular compartment through the thoracic duct, hepatic lymph accumulates in the form of ascites, and the intravascular compartment is further compromised.

CLINICAL MANIFESTATIONS

In addition to the clinical manifestations of the underlying disease, the clinical manifestations of *hypervolemia* depend on the amount and relative distribution of accumulated fluid in the various ECF subcompartments, including the venous and arterial components of the intravascular compartment (jugular venous distention and hypertension), the interstitial spaces of the extremities, subcutaneous tissues of the lower back and the periorbital region (peripheral pitting edema, whose predominant location depends on the patient's position), the peritoneal and pleural spaces (ascites and pleural effusion, respectively), and the alveolar space (pulmonary edema). When cardiac and hepatic function is normal and the transcapillary Starling forces are not disrupted, the excess volume is distributed proportionately throughout the ECF compartment. *Hypertension* may be an early manifestation depending on cardiac function and the state of systemic vascular resistance. Jugular venous distention (see Fig. 50-3 in Chapter 50) and peripheral edema (see Fig. 50-7 in Chapter 50) may be present. Clinically detectable pitting peripheral edema usually signifies the accumulation of at least 3 L of excess interstitial volume. Because intravascular plasma volume is itself only 3 L, any state of generalized peripheral edema must signify ECF volume expansion and therefore past or ongoing renal sodium retention, or both.

When cardiac function is impaired because of myocardial disease, valvular disease, or pericardial disease, pulmonary and systemic venous hypertension predominates, and systemic arterial pressure may be low as a result of disproportionate accumulation of intravascular volume in the venous as opposed to the arterial circulation (Chapter 58). The presence of transudative ascites (see Fig. 148-5 in Chapter 148) signifies the substantial accumulation of excess ECF volume in the peritoneal cavity, most commonly secondary to disruption of intrahepatic hemodynamics in the setting of liver disease. Pleural effusions can also be a manifestation of hypervolemia, particularly in the setting of heart failure or advanced cirrhosis with ascites.

DIAGNOSIS

Hypervolemia usually is easily detected by findings of generalized edema, ascites, elevated jugular venous pressure, inspiratory pulmonary crackles, or evidence of the presence of pleural effusion. The prevailing systemic arterial blood pressure often provides a clue about whether the hypervolemic state is secondary to reduced EABV or instead due to primary renal sodium retention. The history and physical examination are often sufficient to yield the diagnosis of an underlying secondary cause of sodium retention, such as heart failure or cirrhosis. Adjunctive laboratory tests providing evidence of cardiac dysfunction or liver disease may be helpful. The presence of glomerular-range proteinuria with hypoalbuminemia indicates a glomerular cause of the sodium retention and hypervolemia. Elevated creatinine points to renal failure, which can be intrinsic or may occur in association with advanced stages of some of the aforementioned conditions, such as heart failure or hepatic cirrhosis (hepatorenal failure). Hypoalbuminemia is characteristic of both cirrhosis and nephrotic syndrome.

A low urine sodium concentration and low fractional excretion of sodium confirm renal sodium retention secondary to a perceived decrease in EABV in the edema states, even in the face of overall hypervolemia. More recently, elevated concentrations of brain natriuretic peptide have been used to support the diagnosis of hypervolemia, particularly in the setting of cardiac failure and renal disease.

TREATMENT   Rx

Recognition and treatment of the underlying disease is the most important step in ameliorating renal sodium retention. Optimization of hemodynamic parameters in heart failure (Chapter 59), improvement of liver function (Chapter 157), or remission of nephrotic syndrome (Chapter 123) improves or reverses sodium retention. Therapeutic intervention to reduce ECF volume without addressing the underlying disease is often met by complications, especially when ECF volume expansion is associated with decreased intravascular volume or EABV. Nevertheless, three treatment modalities are available to reduce ECF volume directly by inducing negative sodium balance: dietary sodium restriction, diuretics, and extracorporeal fluid removal by ultrafiltration. The modality and the desired rate of sodium removal vary with the clinical setting and depend on the relative distribution of the sodium surfeit and excess volume in the body fluid compartments. Therefore, before initiating any treatment, the clinician should identify the specific disturbances that are harmful to the patient in clinical parameters and monitor the improvement in these parameters during the course of treatment. Harmful manifestations of hypervolemia include hypertension, pulmonary congestion and edema or pleural effusions with compromised respiratory function, hepatic congestion and ascites, and degrees of peripheral edema that compromise skin integrity and predispose the patient to cellulitis. Once ECF volume reduction has removed these threats to the patient's well-being, rates of sodium removal should be slowed significantly. Thus, a patient with mild peripheral edema, small pleural effusions, minimal ascites, jugular venous distention, and normal blood pressure might be managed with sodium restriction and limited use of natriuretic medications to induce a gradual negative sodium balance over a period of many days to weeks. In contrast, a patient with limb- or life-threatening anasarca, pulmonary congestion, or hypervolemia-induced hypertension might require the continuous intravenous infusion of natriuretics or in some cases extracorporeal ultrafiltration therapy.

Sodium Restriction

Other modalities are futile if not accompanied by restriction of sodium intake because renal sodium avidity results in the reaccumulation of ECF fluid as soon as the influence of diuretics has ceased. Dietary sodium restriction in the range of 20 to 40 mmol/day is often recommended and requires abstention from added salt as well as from foods rich in sodium. Sodium substitutes can be useful, although caution needs to be exercised in patients with a tendency to hyperkalemia because some salt substitutes contain potassium. Caloric intake and nutritional parameters should be monitored to ensure that an overly draconian diet does not induce protein-energy malnutrition. In hospitalized patients, it is particularly important to ensure that the sodium content of administered intravenous fluids and sodium-containing medications is monitored and reduced to the minimum possible. The practice of infusing sodium-containing solutions on the one hand and simultaneously treating with diuretics has no sound physiologic or therapeutic basis. Furthermore, water restriction is not appropriate in hypervolemic edema states unless severe (plasma sodium concentration <135 mmol/L) or symptomatic hyponatremia supervenes.

Diuretics

Diuretics and other natriuretic medications (Table 118-5) enhance the urinary excretion of sodium-containing fluid by inhibiting tubule reabsorption at specific nephron sites (Fig. 118-3).

Proximal Tubule Natriuretics

The cardinal example of a proximal tubule natriuretic is acetazolamide, a carbonic anhydrase inhibitor that blocks proximal reabsorption of sodium bicarbonate. Consequently, prolonged use of acetazolamide may lead to

hyperchloremic acidosis, in contrast to all other natriuretics, which act at loci before the late distal nephron. Metolazone, a congener of the thiazide class of natriuretics, blocks sodium chloride absorption in the proximal tubule as well as the early distal tubule. Because the major locus for phosphate absorption is in the proximal nephron, the phosphaturia accompanying metolazone administration considerably exceeds that observed with other thiazide-class diuretics. Proximal tubule natriuretics rarely are used as primary therapy but are used as supplements to loop natriuretics when loop natriuretics alone are ineffective.

Loop Natriuretics

Loop natriuretics, such as furosemide, bumetanide, torsemide, and ethacrynic acid, induce natriuresis by inhibiting the coupled entry of Na^+, Cl^-, and K^+ across apical plasma membranes in the thick ascending limb of the loop of Henle, which is responsible for the reabsorption of approximately 25% of filtered sodium. Loop diuretics, which are the most potent diuretics, continue to be effective even in patients with relatively compromised kidney function.

Distal Tubule Natriuretics

Distal tubule natriuretics, such as hydrochlorothiazide, chlorthalidone, and metolazone, interfere primarily with sodium chloride absorption in the earliest segments of the distal convoluted tubule, where they block the sodium chloride cotransport mechanism across apical plasma membranes. Distal tubule natriuretics generally are used in the same conditions as loop natriuretics, but not in chronic kidney disease and in disorders of calcium metabolism. Whereas loop natriuretics are calciuretic and are valuable for managing acute hypercalcemia (Chapter 253), thiazide natriuretics promote hypocalciuria and calcium retention and are useful in managing hypercalciuric states. With the exception of acetazolamide, which impairs bicarbonate absorption, tubule natriuretics can cause hypokalemia and metabolic alkalosis.

Collecting Duct Natriuretics

Spironolactone and eplerenone compete with aldosterone and inhibit sodium absorption in the collecting duct, while concomitantly suppressing potassium and proton secretion. Triamterene and amiloride directly block sodium uptake by collecting duct cells and concomitantly suppress potassium and proton secretion. These agents are used in combination with thiazide and loop natriuretics to offset hypokalemia. However, hyperkalemia and hyperchloremic metabolic acidosis may complicate the injudicious use of any of these agents. Spironolactone and eplerenone are useful in managing disorders characterized by secondary hyperaldosteronism, such as cirrhosis with ascites, in promoting natriuresis in hypokalemic patients, and in competitively blocking nonepithelial mineralocorticoid receptors in patients with left ventricular dysfunction (Chapter 59).

Nesiritide is the recombinant version of a naturally occurring brain natriuretic peptide with unique vasodilator and natriuretic actions. Nesiritide may compromise renal function, especially when high levels are achieved after an initial bolus, so its usefulness appears to be quite limited and to require frequent monitoring of urine output, plasma urea, and creatinine concentrations.

Patients with severe degrees of renal sodium avidity can be resistant to conventionally recommended doses of individual classes of diuretic agents. In such patients, combinations of diuretic agents acting at different sites along the nephron may overcome this resistance and induce a natriuretic response.

TABLE 118-5 DIURETICS AND OTHER NATRIURETIC MEDICATIONS

DIURETICS IN COMMON USE	DAILY DOSE RANGE	ADVERSE REACTIONS	COMMENTS
Thiazides (oral)		Rash, neutropenia, thrombocytopenia, hyperglycemia, hyperuricemia	Usually not effective below GFR of 30-40 mL/mm (metolazone 20-30 mL/mm)
Hydrochlorothiazide	25-100 mg		
Metolazone	2.5-5 mg		
Chlorthalidone	20-50 mg		
Loop diuretics (oral or intravenous)			Rapid onset, short duration: split doses in normal renal function, give intravenously in acute situations or if reduced GI absorption; can use up to 500 mg furosemide (or equivalent) in severe renal insufficiency
Furosemide	20-320 mg	Ototoxicity at high doses	
Bumetanide	1-8 mg		
Torsemide	20-200 mg		
Potassium sparing		Hyperkalemia	Not very potent
Spironolactone	25-400 mg		
Triamterene	25-100 mg		
Amiloride	5-20 mg		
Eplerenone	25-50 mg		

GI = gastrointestinal; GFR = glomerular filtration rate.

FIGURE 118-3. Major transport processes along the nephron segment and primary sites of action of diuretics. The numbers next to the diuretics in the insert refer to the site of action along the nephron. ADH = antidiuretic hormone. (From Kokko JP. Diuretics. In: Alexander RW, Schlant RC, Fuster V, eds. *The Heart*, 9th ed. New York: McGraw-Hill; 1998.)

The continuous intravenous infusion of furosemide, sometimes in conjunction with intermittent bolus infusions of albumin, also can overcome natriuretic resistance in some hospitalized patients. Monitoring of plasma sodium, potassium, magnesium, calcium, and phosphate concentrations is mandatory in patients treated with high or frequent doses or continuous infusions of natriuretic agents. Besides body tonicity and electrolyte disturbances, other potential adverse consequences include a reduction in GFR. Drug-specific idiosyncratic adverse responses such as allergic cutaneous reactions, interstitial nephritis, pancreatitis, and blood dyscrasias are much less common.

Extracorporeal Ultrafiltration

In a small subset of patients, either superimposed renal impairment or extreme resistance to natriuretic action requires the direct removal of excess ECF volume by hemofiltration or peritoneal dialysis (Chapter 133). Chronic ambulatory peritoneal dialysis has been used for the symptomatic relief of pulmonary congestion and anasarca in some patients with chronic heart failure who are unresponsive to other therapeutic modalities and are not candidates for cardiac transplantation.

WATER BALANCE DISORDERS

Water balance disorders generally come to medical attention because of one or more of three clinical manifestations: hyponatremia, hypernatremia, or polyuria.

Hyponatremia

DEFINITION

Hyponatremia, which is defined as a plasma sodium concentration less than 136 mmol/L, is the most frequently encountered electrolyte abnormality in hospitalized patients.

EPIDEMIOLOGY AND PATHOBIOLOGY

Hyponatremia does not necessarily signify a hypotonic state. *Hypertonic hyponatremia* occurs when there is an accumulation in the ECF compartment of non-sodium-containing effective solutes such as very high concentrations of glucose in diabetic patients or exogenously administered mannitol or glycerol. These hypertonic hyponatremic states are characterized by a shift of water from the ICF to the ECF compartments, with ICF shrinkage rather than swelling. The accumulation of a solute such as urea, which contributes to the measured plasma osmolality but is not an osmotically effective solute in terms of transcellular water shift, should not be included in the category of hypertonic hyponatremic states. *Isotonic hyponatremia* signifies the laboratory finding of hyponatremia in patients with no disturbances in body fluid tonicity and almost always reflects the interference of marked hyperlipidemia or marked hyperglobulinemia with certain laboratory techniques for the measurement of the plasma sodium concentration; these situations are termed *pseudohyponatremia* and should not prompt diagnostic or therapeutic measures to alter water balance or body tonicity.

True *hypotonic hyponatremia* always reflects an important underlying disorder that leads to abnormal body water balance, and the hypotonic state indicates either past or ongoing expansion of ICF volume. Even in chronic hypotonic hyponatremic states, in which cell volume has been restored to normal by osmotic adaptive mechanisms, the compensation occurs at the price of loss of intracellular solutes and compromised cell function.

Heart failure (Chapter 59) and cirrhosis with ascites (Chapter 156) are examples of hypervolemic hyponatremia. In these conditions, reduced EABV stimulates the release of AVP and also may limit the delivery of glomerular ultrafiltrate to the diluting segments of the nephron.

Most fluid lost from the body is hypotonic compared with plasma, so sweat, most gastrointestinal losses, and even many cases of urinary fluid loss do not cause hyponatremia. However, if the replacement fluid that is ingested or administered is more hypotonic than the lost fluid (e.g., ingestion of water or intravenous administration of D$_5$W), the net result is to decrease body tonicity. Another important consideration is the potassium concentration in the lost fluid. For example, diarrheal fluid and natriuretic-medication-induced polyuric urine are often rich in potassium as well as sodium; even if the concentration of sodium alone is less than that in the ECF, combined loss of sodium plus potassium can cause hypotonicity.

CLINICAL MANIFESTATIONS

The finding of hyponatremia is often incidental on routine laboratory testing, on laboratory testing of patients with nonspecific complaints, or as part of the investigation of other clinical syndromes. The symptoms of hypotonic hyponatremia depend on its duration. In the first hours to days, the major clinical manifestations are neurologic and are due to acute brain swelling or cerebral edema. Symptoms include headache, lethargy, seizures, and a progressively decreased level of consciousness that can progress to coma and death. The severity of these neurologic manifestations depends more on the rate of the hypotonic decline in plasma sodium concentration than on the absolute concentration. In addition, women between menarche and menopause are particularly susceptible to the life-threatening neurologic manifestations of acute hyponatremia, even of relatively mild degree. If a patient survives the acute hyponatremia, osmotic adaptation tends to mitigate the symptoms of cerebral edema.

DIAGNOSIS

After immediate assessment of the clinical urgency of the situation, the first step in the diagnostic approach to a patient with the laboratory finding of hyponatremia is to confirm the presence of true hypotonic hyponatremia. A repeat set of plasma determinations, including electrolytes, osmolality, urea, and glucose, allows comparison of the measured with the calculated plasma osmolality according to the following equation:

$$\text{Plasma osmolality (mOsm/kg)} = 2Na^{+}(\text{mmol/L}) +$$
$$(\text{blood urea nitrogen [mg/dL]}/2.8) + (\text{glucose [mg/dL]}/18)$$

A careful history, including a search of the medical record for previous measured concentrations of plasma sodium, is critical. The history, together with the physical examination, usually provides important clues to underlying disorders, disease states, or medication exposures that can inform the diagnosis. A history of weight gain or loss also can be helpful in the assessment of recent fluid mass balance. The physical examination should focus on attempts to establish the state of ECF volume. The presence of generalized edema with jugular venous distention and ascites, especially in the setting of heart or liver disease, points quite clearly to hypervolemic hyponatremia. Orthostatic hypotension and tachycardia, particularly in the setting of a history of natriuretic medication use or gastrointestinal fluid losses, suggests hypovolemia, but the absence of these findings does not exclude hypovolemia.

Laboratory tests should include a repeat set of plasma electrolyte concentrations, including potassium and chloride levels, which together with determination of acid-base parameters (pH, Pco_2, and bicarbonate) can point to processes not always elicited in the history, such as vomiting, diarrhea, or natriuretic medication exposure. Other laboratory tests should include liver function tests and measurement of plasma urea, creatinine, uric acid, thyroid-stimulating hormone, cortisol concentrations, and, if indicated, an adrenocorticotropic hormone stimulation test. High levels of both urea and creatinine point to intrinsic renal disease, whereas a disproportionate elevation of urea over creatinine might support hypovolemia with a tendency to prerenal azotemia (Chapter 122). In contrast, very low levels of urea and uric acid are typical of both the syndrome of inappropriate antidiuretic hormone secretion (SIADH) and the cerebral salt-wasting syndrome.

Marked elevation in the plasma glucose concentration increases both measured and calculated plasma osmolality and indicates a state of hypertonic hyponatremia that should be approached as a state of body fluid hypertonicity with cell shrinkage (see later) rather than hypotonicity. The plasma sodium concentration declines by approximately 1.6 mmol/L for each 100-mg/dL (5.5-mmol/L) increase in plasma glucose concentration. However, the value of approximately 1.6 is quite variable and is greater in states of progressively severe hyperglycemia. In contrast to hyperglycemia, an elevated urea concentration should not be considered as contributing to plasma or ECF tonicity, even though urea does contribute to the laboratory measurement of plasma osmolality. Thus, a hyponatremic patient with a normal or elevated laboratory measurement of plasma osmolality, which can be fully attributed to an increased urea concentration, should be considered as having hypotonic hyponatremia. A discrepancy in which measured plasma osmolality exceeds calculated plasma osmolality and cannot be attributed to either glucose or urea indicates the presence of an unidentified small solute (osmolar gap), including alcohols (e.g., ethanol, methanol, ethylene glycol, and isopropyl alcohol), and the organic anions of weak acids, which raise the plasma anion gap. Because these small solutes are not effective solutes in terms of water movement, the water balance and tonicity status of the patient is determined by the plasma sodium concentration. Just as for urea, a patient with hyponatremia and normal or elevated measured plasma osmolality as a result of one of these small solutes should be approached as having a true hypotonic hyponatremia, notwithstanding the normal or elevated plasma osmolality measurement. However, the finding of such an osmolar gap should prompt a thorough investigation for poisoning, intoxication, or an organic acidosis (Chapter 120).

Once a state of true hypotonic hyponatremia has been established, determination of the cause and further diagnostic approach follows a classification into one of three categories based on assessment of the volume status of the patient (Fig. 118-4). Abnormal liver function test results can provide adjunctive support for hepatic disease and a hypervolemic hyponatremic state. The diagnosis of heart failure should be made clinically, but it can be assisted by a brain natriuretic peptide level, chest radiograph, or echocardiograph (Chapter 58). A radiograph or chest computed tomography (CT) scan may help identify intrathoracic lesions that are associated with SIADH.

Approximately 85% of hyponatremic inpatients have true hypotonic hyponatremia; among these patients, about 25% are hypovolemic, about 25% have an edema state, about one third are normovolemic, and most of the remainder have renal failure.

In the absence of a clinically obvious edema state, a low urine sodium concentration (<20 mmol/L) or a low fractional excretion of sodium (<1%) supports the diagnosis of hypovolemic hyponatremia secondary to extrarenal losses or past renal losses that have since abated. If hypovolemia is due to ongoing renal losses, the urine sodium concentration may remain high in the face of hypovolemia, but a low fractional excretion of urea (<35%) may still be evident. High urinary concentrations of potassium point to persistent vomiting or the ongoing effect of potassium-depleting natriuretic drugs. In

FIGURE 118-4. Diagnostic approach to hyponatremia. RTA = renal tubular acidosis; SIADH = syndrome of inappropriate antidiuretic hormone secretion. (Modified from Halterman R, Berl T. Therapy of dysnatremic disorders. In: Brady H, Wilcox C, eds. *Therapy in Nephrology and Hypertension*. Philadelphia: Saunders; 1999:256.)

SIADH, the urine sodium concentration often reflects sodium intake, as well as mild volume expansion, and is therefore most often greater than 40 mmol/L and frequently higher than 100 mmol/L. The combination of hypotonic hyponatremia in a patient without evidence of either hypovolemia or hypervolemia, together with low plasma urea and uric acid concentrations without hypothyroidism or adrenal insufficiency, strongly suggests SIADH. If there is any doubt about the presence of hypovolemia, a carefully monitored volume challenge can be of diagnostic as well as therapeutic benefit (see later). Lack of sustained improvement after an adequate salt-containing volume challenge lends further support to the diagnosis of SIADH. Once the diagnosis of SIADH has been established in this manner, the cause should be sought, including a thorough review of medication exposure, review of the history for symptoms and signs of malignancy, and magnetic resonance imaging (MRI) or CT of the brain and chest (see Table 118-5).

Hypervolemic Hyponatremia

A patient with hypervolemic hyponatremia suffers from a surfeit of both sodium and water, but the surfeit of water is disproportionate to that of sodium. As for any hypervolemia, the clinical approach is to establish that the patient is hypervolemic and to determine the cause of the sodium surfeit. The most frequently diagnosed causes are heart failure, decompensated cirrhosis with ascites, and renal failure. The occurrence of hyponatremia in any of these conditions often signifies either advanced disease or overzealous sodium deprivation and natriuretic medications. Patients who have heart failure or cirrhosis with ascites experience avid renal sodium retention with urine sodium concentrations less than 20 mmol/L and fractional sodium excretion less than 1% in the face of clear-cut clinical evidence of ECF volume expansion, usually with generalized edema. However, these urine parameters can be masked by the ongoing influence of medications. The edema state of the nephrotic syndrome is less commonly associated with hyponatremia, unless the patient has been exposed to severe salt restriction and natriuretic therapy. Water retention with hyponatremia is a feature of renal failure only in its more advanced stages (stages IV and V chronic kidney disease; Chapter 132).

Normovolemic and Hypovolemic Hyponatremia

It is often difficult to distinguish normovolemic from hypovolemic hyponatremia because mild hypovolemia can easily escape clinical detection. The initial history and physical examination should try to establish or exclude a cause of hypovolemia. In extrarenal hypovolemia, a low urine sodium concentration and low fractional excretion of sodium are characteristic. When the hypovolemia is due to urinary loss, the urine sodium concentration is usually elevated rather than decreased.

Hypovolemic hyponatremia always signifies past or ongoing sodium loss (often with potassium), accompanied by a degree of net water loss that does not match the electrolyte loss and hence leaves the patient hypotonic. The high levels of AVP that are associated with hypovolemic hyponatremia are usually an appropriate response to the physiologic stimulus of hypovolemia. The most common extrarenal causes of hypovolemia leading to hyponatremia are gastrointestinal fluid losses and excessive sweating. In gastrointestinal fluid losses, any concomitant nausea and vomiting may be independent triggers for the central release of AVP. Clues to vomiting may include the characteristic plasma and urine biochemical parameters of metabolic alkalosis (Chapter 120), often with higher than expected urinary concentrations of sodium and bicarbonate. Hyponatremia is a more common complication of diarrhea when the diarrheal fluid is secretory and rich in electrolytes. Sweating-induced hyponatremia occurs when individuals ingest high volumes of hypotonic fluid, often pure water, while losing sodium in sweat.

The renal causes of hyponatremic hypovolemia (see Fig. 118-4) include thiazide-induced hyponatremia, which occurs when patients with impaired urinary diluting capacity excrete concentrated urine because thiazides do not affect the ability of the renal medulla to concentrate urine. Thiazide-treated patients are particularly susceptible to hyponatremia when they ingest or receive hypotonic solutions that exceed their maximal capacity to excrete electrolyte-free water in their urine. In cerebral salt wasting (also known as renal salt wasting), patients who have suffered a head injury or intracranial hemorrhage experience a state of negative sodium balance because urinary fluid loss stimulates the release of AVP, coupled with the ingestion or administration of hypotonic fluids. In these patients, urine sodium concentrations can be impressively high, and the syndrome can be difficult to distinguish from hyponatremia caused by the syndrome of inappropriate secretion of AVP (see later). Persistent uricosuria, even after correction of the hyponatremia, remains an unexplained distinguishing feature of this syndrome.

TABLE 118-6	CAUSES OF THE SYNDROME OF INAPPROPRIATE ANTIDIURETIC HORMONE SECRETION

MALIGNANT NEOPLASIA

Carcinoma: bronchogenic, pancreatic, duodenal, ureteral, prostatic, bladder
Lymphoma and leukemia
Thymoma and mesothelioma

CENTRAL NERVOUS SYSTEM DISORDERS

Trauma
Infection
Tumors
Porphyria

PULMONARY DISORDERS

Tuberculosis
Pneumonia
Fungal infections
Lung abscesses
Mechanical positive-pressure ventilation

DRUG INDUCED

Carbamazepine
Desmopressin
Oxytocin
Vincristine
Chlorpropamide
Nicotine
Cyclophosphamide
Morphine
Amitriptyline
Selective serotonin reuptake inhibitors

In normovolemic hypotonic hyponatremia, there is neither an osmolar nor a volume stimulus to the release of AVP. Thus, concentrated urine, usually containing high concentrations of sodium (often >40 mmol/L as a result of dietary intake plus the effects of mild ECF volume expansion), indicates either inappropriate secretion or an augmented renal response to AVP. Conditions that can result in inappropriate AVP secretion or responsiveness include tumors, central nervous system lesions or disorders, intrathoracic or chest wall disease, and numerous drugs and medications (Table 118-6). All syndromes in which AVP levels or the kidney's responsiveness are inappropriately high and not attributable to osmolar or volume stimuli are known collectively as SIADH (Chapter 232). Patterns of abnormal AVP secretion (Fig. 118-5) include erratic release of AVP from the neurohypophysis without any apparent coordination with incoming volume or osmotic stimuli (type A pattern), a constant low-level leak of AVP from the neurohypophysis (type B pattern), a reduced threshold for osmotic release of AVP at a lower than normal plasma osmolality (type C pattern), or an abnormal renal response to circulating AVP in patients whose neurohypophysial regulation is intact (type D pattern). However, no consistent correlation between these various patterns and an underlying cause has emerged. A specific monogenic disorder involves a mutation in which the V_2 AVP receptor is constitutively active in the absence of ligand. Hypothyroidism (Chapter 233) and adrenal glucocorticoid insufficiency (Chapter 234) can be associated with hypotonic hyponatremia without clinically evident hypovolemia and with a clinical and biochemical profile that mimics SIADH; abnormal regulation of the aquaporin-2 water channel may be involved. Pregnancy, which also is associated with a reduction in both the osmotic threshold for AVP release and thirst, results in mild hyponatremia (Chapter 247). Another unusual setting for normovolemic hyponatremia is the "beer potomania" syndrome. Because the minimal urine osmolarity, even in the absence of AVP, is 30 to 50 mOsm/L, the upper limit of solute-free water excretion depends on total obligate solute excretion. A paucity of available urinary solutes sets an upper limit on the total water intake that can be tolerated without inducing hyponatremia. For example, when patients consume large volumes of beer (rich in carbohydrates and water, but poor in sodium and electrolytes), the absence of protein intake limits urea production and excretion, thereby limiting non-electrolyte urinary solutes and hence urinary water excretion. Together with the large volumes of beer ingested, the result is the unusual combination of a normovolemic hypotonic hyponatremic state with low urine osmolality.

FIGURE 118-5. Patterns of serum antidiuretic hormone (ADH) abnormalities in the syndrome of inappropriate ADH secretion (SIADH). The *shaded areas* indicate the normal relationship between increases in effective extracellular osmolality and ADH levels; the normal osmotic threshold is lower than the normal serum osmolality. The *three shaded areas* indicate ADH patterns in SIADH. (Adapted from Zerbe R, Strope L, Robertson G. Vasopressin function in the syndrome of inappropriate diuresis. *Annu Rev Med.* 1980;31:315-327.)

FIGURE 118-6. Treatment of severe normovolemic hyponatremia. (From Thurman J, Halterman R, Berl T. Therapy of dysnatremic disorders. In: Brady H, Wilcox C, eds. *Therapy in Nephrology and Hypertension*, 2nd ed. Philadelphia: Saunders; 2003.)

TREATMENT   (Rx)

Treatment of hyponatremia varies depending on the category and underlying diagnosis (Fig. 118-6). The overall treatment approach can be divided into the immediate approach to newly appreciated hypotonic hyponatremia and the long-term management of chronic persistent hyponatremia.

The first principle is the importance of identifying and treating any underlying disorder. Thus, in a patient with hypervolemic hyponatremia associated with heart failure, measures to optimize cardiac function are the most appropriate and effective means of restoring normal sodium concentration. Indeed, restoration of normal sodium concentration provides one of the most reassuring indices for successful management of this underlying disorder.

Another principle common to all causes of hypotonic hyponatremia, irrespective of the underlying cause, is that the sodium concentration and the rate of correction should be guided by the patient's age, gender, neurologic status, and any information about recent past plasma sodium concentrations or osmolality values. Delayed correction of hyponatremia can perpetuate cerebral edema and result in irreversible neurologic damage and death, especially in women of reproductive age and in patients whose hyponatremia developed at a rapid pace that outstripped the rate of osmotic adaptation by brain cells. In contrast, too rapid correction or correction to a sodium concentration that is above the level needed to safeguard the patient from the neurologic sequelae of cerebral edema can result in the *osmotic demyelination syndrome*. This devastating and often irreversible syndrome is characterized by fluctuating levels of consciousness, pseudobulbar palsy, ataxia, dysarthria, difficulty swallowing, and characteristic MRI abnormalities in the region of the brain stem. Osmotic demyelination syndrome can be fatal, and recovery in nonfatal cases is either slow or incomplete, often with irreversible residual neurologic sequelae.

Hypotonic Hyponatremia

Current guidelines suggest that if the hyponatremia is known to be acute (<24 to 48 hours) and is accompanied by severe neurologic symptoms such as seizures or decreased level of consciousness, correction should be rapid and should reach a target sodium concentration based on amelioration of neurologic symptoms. However, even under these circumstances, the desired rise in sodium concentration should not exceed 2 mmol/L/hour, and the total increase in sodium concentration during the first 12 to 24 hours of treatment should not exceed 12 mmol/L. The only exceptions to these guidelines would be an unusual patient who has suffered documented severe acute water intoxication, such as occurs during the inadvertent instillation of a glycine-containing irrigation solution during prostate surgery or the administration of hypotonic solutions to a patient who is anuric.

Chronic Hyponatremia

If the rate of decline in plasma sodium concentration has been slow, brain cells have the opportunity to undergo osmotic adaptation by extruding or eliminating intracellular solutes. It is this subgroup of patients who are most susceptible to osmotic demyelination after too rapid or overzealous correction

of hyponatremia. Patients in whom there is no previous record of sodium concentration or osmolality should be considered in the same category and treated accordingly. In such cases, the targeted rate of increase in sodium concentration should not exceed 0.5 mmol/L/hour, and the total rise in sodium concentration should not exceed 8 mmol/L in the first 24 hours, even (and especially) if the initial sodium concentration is extremely low (<110 mmol/L), provided that the hyponatremia is not accompanied by severe neurologic symptoms. Patients with severe degrees of chronic hyponatremia in the setting of malnutrition, alcoholism, or chronic illness are particularly susceptible to osmotic demyelination. Frequent monitoring of the plasma sodium concentration and osmolality is crucial, and osmotic demyelination can be prevented by slowing the rate of correction, or even returning to a lower plasma sodium concentration by the judicious readministration of hypotonic solutions or administration of vasopressin analogues (see later).

Having established a target goal and rate of correction, the specific approach varies with the underlying diagnosis. Mild degrees of hyponatremia can be tolerated over long periods, and only symptomatic hyponatremia or sodium concentrations below 125 to 130 mmol/L require specific additional treatment. In hypervolemic hyponatremia, there is a surfeit of both sodium and water, but in tonicity terms, the excess water is disproportionate to the excess sodium. Thus, the goal of treatment is to remove both sodium and water, but to replace proportionately less water than sodium. Water restriction is helpful but is often inadequate or impractical because patients are thirsty, and their adequate nutrition requires caloric intake that is accompanied by obligate water ingestion and metabolic water production. The AVP V_2-receptor antagonist tolvaptan (starting at 15 mg once daily, with a maximal dose of 60 mg once daily)▣ ameliorates hyponatremia and improves symptoms and outcomes in patients with hypervolemic hyponatremic syndromes, including decompensated heart failure and hepatic cirrhosis. It is useful in normovolemic hyponatremic states, such as SIADH (see later), but should be assiduously avoided in hypovolemic hyponatremic states. Two related oral drugs, lixivaptan and conivaptan, have not been proved to be as effective in reducing symptoms of heart failure.

Hypovolemic Hypotonic Hyponatremia

A frequent diagnostic dilemma is the distinction between hypovolemic and normovolemic hypotonic hyponatremia. When hypovolemia is clearly evident (appropriate clinical history, orthostatic hypotension, low urine sodium concentration in the setting of extrarenal fluid losses, elevated plasma urea and uric acid concentrations), administration of volume repletion in the form of isotonic saline is the treatment of choice. The salutary effect of saline derives mostly from the effect of volume repletion to remove the hypovolemic stimulus to release of AVP, thereby inducing a water diuresis, with a minor contribution of the osmolar effect of the infused solute. However, great caution should be exercised in the administration of isotonic saline to these patients because sometimes the administration of small volumes of isotonic saline can induce a brisk and rapid decrease in urine osmolality and an accompanying water diuresis, with an overly rapid correction of hyponatremia. Accordingly, whenever isotonic saline or other forms of volume repletion therapy are administered to patients with known or suspected hypovolemic hyponatremia, careful hour-by-hour monitoring of urine output, urine osmolality, the plasma concentration of sodium, and plasma osmolality are required. A rapid drop in urine osmolality accompanied by water diuresis should prompt cessation of volume repletion and, in some cases, administration of hypotonic solutions or even analogues of AVP itself (see later) to halt or reverse the rapid rise in sodium concentration to within the recommended guidelines so as to prevent osmotic demyelination. When hypovolemia is not clearly evident but cannot be excluded, a brisk drop in urine osmolality in response to a saline challenge confirms the suspicion of hypovolemia and simultaneously initiates therapy. In contrast, failure to induce such a response lends support to the diagnosis of normovolemic hyponatremia.

Normovolemic Hyponatremia

In patients with normovolemic hyponatremia, the appropriate therapeutic approach is to address the underlying disease. Hypothyroidism (Chapter 233) and adrenal insufficiency (Chapter 234) should be corrected with appropriate hormonal replacement therapy. Medication-induced SIADH mandates identification and cessation of the offending medication when possible. If the underlying disease cannot be identified or reversed, treatment is aimed at removing the water surfeit. The therapeutic outcome depends on the minimal urine osmolality that can be achieved, which in turn depends on the severity of SIADH. In many cases, when urine osmolality cannot be suppressed below certain high levels, the severity of water restriction required would not be consistent with the need for caloric intake nor compatible with reasonable expectations for patient adherence. Therefore, maneuvers to generate a gradual net negative water balance are required. In such cases, titrated dose oral tolvaptan (beginning at 15 mg once daily and increasing to a maximum of 60 mg once daily) and reliance on an intact thirst mechanism are crucial to avoid polyuria or hypernatremia. In rare cases with an urgent need to correct the hyponatremia because of a neurologic emergency or definitive documentation that the sodium concentration has decreased acutely over a 24- to 72-hour period, intravenous conivaptan (20 mg loading dose followed by 40 to 80 mg/day by continuous infusion)🔢 can be used cautiously to avoid overly rapid correction of hyponatremia. When in doubt about volume status, however, these agents are better avoided until the possibility of hypovolemic hyponatremia has been addressed. Hemodialysis, which can rapidly raise the plasma sodium concentration, should be reserved for the most extreme cases of acute-life threatening hyponatremia for which no other solution is available (Chapter 133).

Hypernatremia

DEFINITION

Hypernatremia, defined as a plasma sodium concentration greater than 144 mmol/L, always reflects a state of hypertonicity, with an increase in the ratio of the concentration of osmotically active solutes to water throughout all body fluid compartments because sodium is an osmotically effective ECF solute.

EPIDEMIOLOGY AND PATHOBIOLOGY

Hypernatremic patients have undergone a process whereby water has moved from the ICF to the ECF compartment, accompanied by a reduction in ICF volume and cell shrinkage. Cell shrinkage in the brain is associated with intracerebral hemorrhage, which often punctates but sometimes disrupts blood vessels, particularly at the brain surface and arachnoid interface. In an effort to restore their cell volume, brain cells undergo osmotic adaptation by accumulating sodium and other electrolytes and then subsequently producing nonelectrolyte small solutes (osmolytes) such as inositol, taurine, glutamine, and glutamate, among others. This process partially reverses cell shrinkage, but at the price of an altered intercellular solute composition with consequent perturbations in neuronal function.

Hypernatremia is the most frequent but not the only hypertonicity state in clinical medicine. Glucose, mannitol, and glycerol can produce hypertonicity states that may not be accompanied by hypernatremia and, in fact, are frequently accompanied by hyponatremia (see earlier). In hypertonicity states, the measured plasma osmolality is always high, but the converse is not necessarily true because a number of solutes that contribute to the measured plasma osmolality are not osmotically effective in terms of movement of water from the ICF to the ECF compartment. Thus, patients with high concentrations of urea or small alcohols (e.g., methanol, ethylene glycol, ethanol) often have elevated plasma osmolality but should not be considered to have a hypertonicity state.

TABLE 118-7	CAUSES OF HYPERNATREMIA CLASSIFIED BY TOTAL BODY SODIUM CONTENT
Hypervolemia	Hypertonic saline excess
	Hypertonic sodium bicarbonate solutions
Hypertonicity with near normovolemia	Diabetes insipidus
	Febrile fluid loss
Hypovolemia	Gastrointestinal loss (diarrhea, vomiting)
	Skin fluid loss (burn, sweat)
	Loop diuretics
	Osmotic diuresis
	Impaired thirst perception

Although hypernatremia can be diagnosed as an incidental laboratory abnormality, it most commonly occurs in the setting of a severe underlying disease with other accompanying disturbances in body fluid homeostasis (Table 118-7).

In *hypervolemic hypernatremia*, a disproportionate excess of sodium as opposed to water expands ECF volume, but ICF volume is decreased because cells shrink. Hypervolemic hypernatremia usually occurs in the hospital setting because inadvertent or overzealous administration of hypertonic saline, the administration of hypertonic sodium bicarbonate solutions during cardiopulmonary resuscitation, or dialysis against a hypertonic dialysate can lead to hypervolemic hypernatremia in the clinical setting.

In *normovolemic hypernatremia*, a pure water deficit with no disturbance in body sodium content does not generally result in a clinically perceptible decrease in ECF volume because the predominant (approximately two thirds) origin of the water deficit is in the ICF rather than the ECF compartment. Thus, for example, a 3-L pure net water deficit will reduce ECF volume by only 1 L, approximately 300 mL of which emanates from plasma water. Yet a 3-L or greater deficit certainly increases body fluid tonicity and the measured plasma sodium concentration. Therefore, such pure net water deficits with no change in body sodium content often are considered to be approximately normovolemic. Clinical conditions that fit this category require a source of fluid loss that has a relatively low content of osmotically effective solutes (principally sodium and potassium and their accompanying anions), such as the various forms of diabetes insipidus or use of vaptan drugs without adequate monitoring. In these conditions, profuse volumes of low osmolality urine are excreted. However, hypernatremia is actually uncommon as long as thirst perception and availability of water remain intact. The principal clinical manifestation is polyuria and polydipsia (see later). Insensible evaporative losses from the skin and respiratory tract also are a source of hypotonic fluid loss. Increased fluid loss can occur in febrile patients (skin and respiratory tract), patients on mechanical ventilation (respiratory tract), and patients with profuse sweating. The sweat sodium concentration decreases with increasing volumes of perspiration. These conditions will lead to hypernatremia with body fluid hypertonicity only if the thirst mechanism or access to water is impaired.

Hypovolemic hypernatremia is by far the most common hypertonicity state. Patients with hypovolemic hypernatremia have lost both sodium and water, but the net loss of water is disproportionately greater than the net loss of sodium. The actual plasma sodium concentration resulting from loss of hypotonic fluid depends not only on the sodium concentration of the fluid lost but also on the concentration of other osmotically active solutes, such as potassium, and on the solute composition of concomitantly ingested or administered fluids. The extrarenal and renal causes of such fluid losses are similar to those of hypovolemia. Among gastrointestinal causes of hypovolemic hypernatremia, diarrhea is more common than vomiting, and osmotic diarrheas result in disproportionately greater loss of water than electrolytes, with a greater propensity to hypernatremia than for secretory diarrheas. Among the renal sources of sodium and water loss, the two most common causes are loop natriuretic medications and osmotic diuresis. Loop natriuretic agents interfere with the countercurrent mechanism and generate large volumes of urine with an iso-osmolar composition. Because some of the solutes are nonelectrolyte (urea), the impact on body tonicity may be to increase tonicity, unless there is concomitant intake or administration of hypotonic fluids. In contrast, thiazides do not interfere with the countercurrent mechanism and therefore rarely promote hypernatremia. The presence of nonelectrolyte solutes in urine causes an osmotic diuresis. Such solutes can be of either endogenous origin (e.g., urea or glucose) or exogenous origin (e.g., mannitol or glycerol). The presence of these solutes in tubular fluid impairs both sodium and water reabsorption, but the excretion of urine that is relatively rich in nonelectrolyte solutes tends to promote body fluid hypertonicity, unless sufficient hypotonic fluids are ingested or administered concomitantly.

Failure to replace hypotonic fluid losses generally reflects either impairment in thirst, disability, or infirmity that prevents the patient from responding to thirst, or failure of the clinician to recognize the need for hypotonic fluid replacement. Rarely, impaired thirst in patients who are awake and alert can be caused by damage to the hypothalamic osmoreceptors that control thirst perception and response, a condition known as *primary hypodipsia*. Usually this condition tends to be associated with an abnormality in the osmotic regulation of AVP secretion. However, cases have been described in which the osmotic regulation of AVP secretion has been dissociated from the osmotic regulation of thirst. Such patients suffer hypernatremia only when extrarenal fluid losses exceed their habitual water intake, as might occur in settings of thermal stress or exercise.

CLINICAL MANIFESTATIONS

The clinical features of patients with hypernatremia can be divided into those associated with the underlying disease state, those associated with a concomitant disturbance in ECF volume, and those associated with an increase in body fluid tonicity. The main clinically relevant consequence of increased body fluid tonicity is decreased brain cell volume, with the attendant risk for intracerebral hemorrhage. Thus, the major symptoms are neurologic and include confusion, seizures, focal neurologic deficits, and a progressively decreasing level of consciousness that can progress to coma. In the absence of an underlying neurologic problem or disturbance in the thirst mechanism, the patient would be expected to complain of thirst unless the neurologic injury has disturbed consciousness.

In patients with hypernatremia of sufficient duration to enable brain cells to undergo osmotic adaptation, the risk for intracerebral hemorrhage from cell shrinkage is decreased, but a hypertonic intracellular environment with the accumulation of new intracellular solutes can perturb normal cellular function.

DIAGNOSIS

The diagnosis of hypernatremia is made by laboratory testing of the sodium concentration, which always should be repeated to confirm its accuracy, corroborated by measurement of plasma osmolality, which is expected to be elevated in all cases. The underlying cause of the hypernatremia is usually evident from the history and physical examination. The history should include a review of recent and current medication use and questions regarding exercise, heat exposure, sweating, vomiting, diarrhea, urine output, recent fluid intake, and the presence of thirst. Physical examination should include an assessment of ECF volume and a complete neurologic evaluation. Urine volume should be monitored, urine osmolality should be measured in several spot urine samples, and 24-hour urine osmolar excretion should be measured if polyuria is present. In the less common situation of hypervolemic hypernatremia, there is often an antecedent history of the administration of sodium-containing solutions, and the findings on physical examination are consistent with ECF volume expansion. In the absence of underlying intrinsic renal disease or diuretic action, urine osmolality should be high because of the hypertonic stimulus to AVP release, which overrides the attenuating effect of hypervolemia. In such patients, the urine sodium concentration should be elevated in response to hypervolemia.

In the more common condition of hypovolemic hypernatremia with extrarenal fluid loss, urine output should be reduced to less than 500 mL/day, and urine osmolality should be the maximum expected for age (urine osmolality >1000 mOsm/kg in young adulthood and decreasing to >600 mOsm/kg by the seventh decade of life and beyond). Polyuria with a submaximal urine osmolality in the presence of hypernatremia suggests impaired urine-concentrating ability, such as occurs with preexisting or underlying intrinsic renal disease or exposure to diuretic agents. A spot urine osmolality measurement less than 100 to 200 mOsm/kg or polyuria (>3 L/day), together with 24-hour urine solute excretion less than 600 mOsm/day in the face of hypernatremia, suggests diabetes insipidus. In contrast, daily solute excretion exceeding 800 to 1000 mOsm/day suggests an osmotic diuresis, which can be confirmed by measuring glucose and urea in urine.

TREATMENT Rx

The main components of treatment are to treat the underlying disorder, correct the abnormality in ECF volume, replace the water deficit, and provide maintenance fluids to match continuing ongoing fluid losses if they persist.

The therapeutic approach to serious symptomatic hypovolemic hypernatremia is challenging and often controversial. It is best to divide the therapeutic approach into two separate phases: rapid correction of the depleted ECF volume, followed by gradual replacement of the water deficit, including provision for ongoing fluid losses. When ECF volume contraction is severe, as evidenced by tissue hypoperfusion and shock, administered fluid should have a sodium concentration as close as possible to that of the patient and should distribute to the ECF or even the intravascular compartment. Isotonic saline is generally the fluid of choice, and the volume and rate of administration should be guided by clinical parameters related to reversal of hypovolemia. After the patient's tissue perfusion has been restored, further fluid replacement should be aimed at correcting the estimated water deficit. This estimate begins with a simple calculation of the percent deficit based on the measured sodium concentration:

$$\text{Total body water deficit} = 0.6 \times \text{premorbid weight} \times (1 - [140/\text{Na}^+])$$

Total body water is used because the sodium concentration reflects tonicity in all body fluid compartments, including the ICF. Unlike the isotonic fluid replacement for ECF volume, the water replacement should be administered gradually over a period of hours to days, unless there is clear documentation that the hypernatremia has itself evolved over minutes to hours. The necessity for gradual replacement is dictated by the process of osmotic adaptation described previously, and ideally, the rate of water replacement should match the rate at which brain intracellular solutes can be adaptively extruded or removed. More rapid rates of administration could result in brain cell swelling with attendant dangerous neurologic consequences. It is recommended that the estimated volume of the water deficit be replaced at a rate that will lead to an approximately 0.5 to 1.0 mmol/L reduction in measured plasma sodium concentration per hour. In addition to the estimated water deficit, the estimated ongoing water loss during replacement should include at least 1 L per 24 hours of insensible fluid losses (greater volumes in patients who are febrile or mechanically ventilated), supplemented with any ongoing water losses (renal or gastrointestinal) resulting from continuation of the underlying disease process. Because of the need to distribute replacement of the initial water deficit, which can amount to several liters over a number of days during which ongoing water losses continue, it is not unusual for patients to require large volumes of water, sometimes reaching 5 to 10 L, over the duration of the correction period. This water deficit, together with ongoing losses, can be replaced by the dietary ingestion of tap water if the patient's condition is suitable or by an enteral feeding tube. If a gastrointestinal or other disease process precludes these preferred routes, a hypotonic intravenous solution such as D₅W or half-normal saline can be used. When D₅W is used, the glucose is either stored as glycogen or fat or metabolized into carbon dioxide and water, thus effectively providing the patient with solute-free water replacement. In the case of half-normal saline, for any given liter administered, only half can be considered as replacement of the water deficit, and the sodium content will either replace any remaining sodium deficit that has not been fully corrected in the first phase of treatment or be excreted if there is no impairment in urinary sodium excretion. In elderly patients with known or possible underlying cardiac, hepatic, or renal disease, caution should be exercised in the provision of excessive volumes of salt-containing solutions. In any case, the sodium concentration should be monitored at regular intervals of no less than every 4 hours to avoid too slow or too rapid correction, and ECF volume parameters should be monitored to avoid hypervolemic complications.

Special considerations apply for hypertonic states in the setting of uncontrolled diabetes with hyperglycemia (Chapters 236 and 237). The unusual cases of patients with hypervolemic hypernatremia in the hospital setting also need special attention and sometimes require continuous infusions of loop diuretics together with the administration of hypotonic solutions or, in some cases, extracorporeal means to remove both the sodium and water excess in a controlled and safe manner under careful monitoring, often in the intensive care unit.

The route of administration should change in accordance with the patient's response. Although an initial parenteral or nasogastric enteral route might be appropriate when the patient's neurologic status is compromised, subsequent therapy can consist of simple dietary intake of water. Once a patient is awake and alert and if thirst mechanisms are intact, the patient will generally correct the hypertonic state by spontaneous oral fluid intake.

Polyuria

Polyuria (Table 118-8), which is defined as a urine output greater than 3 L/day, should be distinguished from urinary frequency, which can occur with frequent voiding of small volumes totaling less than this amount per day. Polyuria occurs when urine-concentrating mechanisms are not being used at any time during the day (water diuresis) or urine solute excretion is excessive (solute diuresis).

SOLUTE DIURESIS

Solute diuresis is defined as the excretion of greater than 800 to 1000 mOsm of urinary solute per day. The composition of these excess solutes can be electrolyte or nonelectrolyte. Electrolyte solute diuresis usually occurs in response to the iatrogenic administration of high volumes of electrolyte-containing solutions, which are disposed by the kidney through normal physiologic mechanisms. Nonelectrolyte solute diuresis is equivalent to osmotic diuresis in which the presence of a nonreabsorbable nonelectrolyte solute in the tubule fluid prevents reabsorption of sodium and other electrolytes as well as water. The result is the excretion of large volumes of urine with a urine osmolality close to that of plasma osmolality.

WATER DIURESIS

When polyuria is associated with 24-hour urine solute excretion greater than 600 mOsm/day, a defect in urine concentrating ability is generally suggested. In some cases, this defect occurs in association with a more general state of intrinsic renal injury and can be part of the spectrum of interstitial injury in chronic renal disease. More specific defects in urine-concentrating ability fall into the category of the diabetes insipidus disorders (Chapter 232).

TABLE 118-8 REASONS FOR POLYURIA

WATER DIURESIS

Diabetes insipidus
  Central (neurogenic)
    Inherited
    Acquired (e.g., tumors, trauma, hypoxia)
  Nephrogenic
    Hypercalcemia
    Amyloidosis
    Drugs (e.g., lithium, foscarnet, cidofovir, vaptans)
    Sjögren's syndrome
    Sickle cell disease
    Inherited
Polydipsia
  Primary (e.g., hypothalamic)
  Psychogenic

SOLUTE DIURESIS

Sodium
  Excess sodium intake (oral, enteral, parenteral)
  Renal sodium wasting (e.g., inherited tubulopathies, interstitial nephritis, natriuretic drugs)
Anion-based (usually sodium is the associated cation)
  Chloride excretion (e.g., Bartter's syndrome, loop diuretic)
  Bicarbonate excretion (e.g., exogenous bicarbonate, carbonic anhydrase inhibition)
Glucose/ketoacids
  Diabetic ketoacidosis
  Hyperglycemic-hyperosmolar syndrome
  Renal glycosuria
Sugar alcohols
  External loading (e.g., mannitol, glycerol)
Urea
  Exogenous loading (e.g., urea, protein, amino acids)
  Diuretic phase of acute kidney injury
  Post-obstructive diuresis
  Hypercatabolic states
  Hemoglobin/myoglobin driven (post-rhabdomyolysis or reabsorption of a hematoma)
Other
  Radiocontrast agents

TREATMENT

Once a patient with polyuria has been classified as having abnormally increased excretion of solute (solute diuresis) or water (water diuresis) (see Table 118-8), the clinical manifestations and treatment will be those of the underlying disease, and the consequences of changes in ECF volume and tonicity are the same as discussed earlier. Depending on the nature of fluid intake and medication used at the onset of polyuria, a significant percentage of polyuric patients will have alterations in serum sodium and ECF volume and will need attention to the underlying disease, as well as correction of fluid and electrolyte abnormalities. Thus, for example, although antihyperglycemic treatment effectively corrects the solute diuresis and polyuric state of uncontrolled diabetes mellitus, initial correction of the concomitant electrolyte and ECF volume disorders takes precedence (Chapters 236 and 237).

1. Wheeler AP, Bernard GR, Thompson BT, et al. for the National Heart, Lung, and Blood Institute Acute Respiratory Distress Syndrome (ARDS) Clinical Trials Network. Pulmonary-artery versus central venous catheter to guide treatment of acute lung injury. *N Engl J Med.* 2006;354: 2213-2224.
2. The Saline versus Albumin Fluid Evaluation (SAFE) study investigators. A comparison of albumin and saline for fluid resuscitation in the intensive care unit. *N Engl J Med.* 2004;350:2247-2256.
3. Schrier RW, Gross P, Gheorghiade M, et al. Tolvaptan, a selective oral vasopressin V2-receptor antagonist, for hyponatremia. *N Engl J Med.* 2006;355:2099-2012.
4. Zeltser D, Rosansky S, van Rensburg H, et al. Assessment of the efficacy and safety of intravenous conivaptan in euvolemic and hypervolemic hyponatremia. *Am J Nephrol.* 2007;27:447-457.

SUGGESTED READINGS

Elhassan EA, Schrier RW. Hyponatremia: diagnosis, complications, and management including V2 receptor antagonists. *Curr Opin Nephrol Hypertens.* 2011;20:161-168. *Review.*
King JD, Rosner MH. Osmotic demyelination syndrome. *Am J Med Sci.* 2010;339:561-567. *Review of clinical manifestations and of potential role of corticosteroids and the reintroduction of hyponatremia in preventing the syndrome.*
Neville KA, Sandeman DJ, Rubinstein A, et al. Prevention of hyponatremia during maintenance intravenous fluid administration: a prospective randomized study of fluid type versus fluid rate. *J Pediatr.* 2010;156:313-319. *The risk of hyponatremia was decreased by isotonic saline solution but not fluid restriction.*
Sterns RH, Hix JK, Silver S. Treatment of hyponatremia. *Am J Kidney Dis.* 2010;56:774-779. *Review including newer vasopressin antagonists.*

119

POTASSIUM DISORDERS

JULIAN L. SEIFTER

DEFINITION

Potassium is ubiquitous in both plant and animal sources of nutrition, so it is difficult to avoid eating potassium in a normal diet. Plant cells have cytosolic potassium concentrations of approximately 80 mmol/L, whereas animal cells may have as much as 140 mmol/L.

EPIDEMIOLOGY

Maintenance of a normal and narrow range of serum potassium, usually on the order of 3.5 to 5.0 mmol/L, is vital for health. The actual concentration may vary during the day, according to a circadian rhythm of decreased excretion in the morning and dietary intake. Insulin-deficient diabetic patients have a greater tendency to develop hyperkalemia, especially if other factors, such as a high-potassium diet, renal disease, or treatment with medications that interfere with renal excretion also are at work. Athletes may have chronically mild decreases in serum potassium. β-blockers may be associated with increased potassium during exercise, particularly in patients with renal failure.

PATHOBIOLOGY

Potassium Balance

Within the human body, potassium is not equally distributed in the total body water. Approximately two thirds of body water is intracellular, and within that compartment, potassium is the major cation. Most cells express sodium-potassium adenosine triphosphatase (Na$^+$, K$^+$-ATPase) on the cell plasma membranes and by this enzyme utilize metabolic energy in the form of adenosine triphosphate (ATP) to establish gradients of potassium and sodium. As a result, the potassium concentration of the cell may reach 140 mmol/L, compared with the extracellular potassium concentration of approximately 4 mmol/L. These established ion gradients, and the associated electrical gradients that follow, provide the essential mechanisms for electrical activity in excitable cells such as muscle and neural tissue, cellular nutrient uptake, and transcellular solute transport in polarized epithelial cells in the kidney and intestine.

If there is a ratio of 35:1 intracellular-to-extracellular potassium and a 2:1 ratio of intracellular-to-extracellular water, it is apparent that more than 98% of potassium resides within cells. The total amount of potassium is usually on the order of 50 mmol/kg of body weight, so a 70-kg individual has a store of about 3500 mmol of potassium. In the entire extracellular fluid, which is approximately 20% of body weight, or 14 L in a 70-kg person, the total potassium content is 50 to 60 mmol.

From these calculations, several important issues of potassium homeostasis emerge. First, total body potassium balance may be poorly reflected by the extracellular or serum potassium concentration. This fact dissociates hypokalemia from potassium depletion or hyperkalemia from potassium excess. Changes in the distribution between the cells and extracellular fluid can occur rapidly, within minutes, in contrast to the matching of dietary intake of potassium to potassium elimination from the body, which occurs within hours. It is also apparent that potassium ingestion at the time of a meal may be equal to a large fraction of the total extracellular potassium. An average daily consumption may be on the order of 50 to 100 mmol. Because this potassium cannot be eliminated instantaneously, there is the potential danger of rapid rises in extracellular potassium concentration after meals. Protection against this eventuality comes from the ability of potassium to distribute from the extracellular to intracellular spaces. The intracellular space, given its large volume and potassium content, can accommodate, or buffer, an extra load of potassium without significant changes in concentration. Distribution of potassium from extracellular to intracellular spaces is known as *internal balance*, and the matching of intake to losses from the body is known as *external balance*.

Importance of Potassium

Potassium is essential for a number of critical body functions, including enzymatic reactions that regulate protein synthesis, glycogen synthesis, cell growth, and cell division. The ability of cells to take up or extrude potassium contributes to the regulation of cell volume during periods of osmotic stress. In excitable cells, such as cardiac myocytes, the relationship of intracellular to extracellular potassium concentrations is critical in establishing the resting membrane potential, which normally may approach the Nernst equilibrium potential for potassium. Because larger percentage changes can occur in the extracellular potassium concentration compared with the intracellular concentration, changes in extracellular potassium have the greatest impact on the electrical potential difference across cell membranes. The serum potassium itself has effects on conductance of potassium through specific K$^+$ channels.

Potassium is also an important local mediator of vascular tone in muscle beds. During exercise, local extracellular potassium concentrations may rise to as high as 10 mmol/L, thereby causing local vasodilation to allow more blood supply to the exercising muscle. Very little of that potassium remains within the total extracellular fluid, so severe hyperkalemia does not usually occur with exercise. The trained athlete develops an adaptive increase in Na$^+$, K$^+$-ATPase to allow for efficient reuptake of potassium into muscle cells. The importance of adequate potassium stores to muscle function is well known to experienced marathoners, and overexertion of muscles in a state of potassium depletion can lead to rhabdomyolysis.

Renal Potassium Handling

In the kidney, potassium excretion begins with filtration. Because the extracellular potassium concentration is approximately 4 mmol/L, and that of sodium is 140 mmol/L, far less potassium is filtered than sodium (about 3%). The renal proximal tubule reabsorbs potassium in the process of reabsorbing sodium and water. In the thick ascending limb of the loop of Henle,

potassium is reabsorbed both by the apical sodium-potassium-2-chloride cotransporter (NKCC) and, like calcium and magnesium, by paracellular reabsorption of the cation. The latter mechanism is a consequence of the luminal electropositivity created by recycling of potassium through K$^+$ channels from the cell to the lumen. Luminal ammonium (NH$_4^+$) can substitute for potassium on the NKCC cotransporter; the resulting increase in medullary interstitial fluid NH$_4^+$ concentrations enhances medullary collecting duct net acid excretion. In hyperkalemic states, less NH$_4^+$ appears in the urine because the high concentration of luminal potassium competes with NH$_4^+$ for reabsorption in the thick limb. As a consequence, a renal mechanism exists for metabolic acidosis to develop in hyperkalemic states, and this in part accounts for the success in treating acidosis by lowering the elevated serum potassium level.

In hypokalemia, whether through proximal tubule intracellular acidosis or other mechanisms, glutaminase enzymes are increased, and more ammonia is produced. This ammonia leads to greater medullary interstitial fluid concentrations and therefore to enhanced net acid elimination. Ammonium production in hypokalemia could be considered an adaptation to allow for potassium to be reabsorbed as NH$_4^+$ accompanies excreted anions into the urine. The increase in ammonia production can have a deleterious effect in that it may contribute to the chronic tubulointerstitial nephritis of chronic hypokalemia.

By the time the tubular fluid reaches the distal tubule and collecting duct, more than 90% of potassium has been reabsorbed. In potassium depletion, an increase in the apical membrane hydrogen-potassium H$^+$, K$^+$-ATPase of the collecting duct intercalated cell allows near-complete removal of potassium from the urine. However, potassium reabsorption is seldom as complete as that of sodium. It is unusual to see potassium concentrations in the urine lower than 5 to 10 mmol/L.

When dietary potassium is abundant, the reabsorption of 90% of filtered potassium by the proximal and distal nephron is followed by net potassium secretion. The urinary potassium most closely reflects potassium secreted by the distal nephron. The major regulatory site for potassium secretion resides in the principal cells of the cortical collecting duct. Three major mechanisms control overall potassium secretion (Fig. 119-1), which may vary depending on the need by as much as 400%: (1) development of a lumen-negative transepithelial potential difference that provides the driving force for potassium secretion into the lumen, (2) adequacy of a variety of apical membrane secretory potassium channels, and (3) flow-dependent movement of fluid through the lumen.

Mechanism of Potassium Secretion

First, sodium must be delivered in ample amounts (depending on the flow rate and sodium concentration of the tubular fluid) to result in sodium reabsorption through the apical epithelial sodium channel (ENaC) in the principal cell. In severely prerenal states of avid sodium reabsorption, sodium delivery may become rate limiting for potassium secretion. Low urinary sodium concentrations limit K$^+$ secretion in the hepatorenal syndrome or severe heart failure. Assuming that sodium delivery is not limiting, reabsorption of the sodium cation creates a lumen-negative transepithelial potential difference. The reabsorption of sodium in turn is dependent on the low intracellular sodium concentrations resulting from the energy-requiring Na$^+$, K$^+$-ATPase on the basolateral membrane. Although K$^+$ secretion is increased by Na$^+$ reabsorption, most of the potassium that enters the principal cell from the extracellular fluid through the Na$^+$, K$^+$-ATPase is recycled back to the extracellular fluid by basolateral potassium transport mechanisms.

Extracellular potassium is also a regulator of potassium secretion in the kidney. As plasma potassium increases, Na$^+$, K$^+$-ATPase increases, bringing more potassium into the cells for transepithelial secretion.

Another determinant of the transepithelial potential difference is the effect of anions in the collecting duct lumen. Non-reabsorbable anions maximize lumen negativity. To the extent that anions such as chloride are reabsorbed, the effect on luminal negativity will be reduced as sodium is reabsorbed. As a consequence, there will be less driving force for potassium (and hydrogen) secretion.

Aldosterone affects the transepithelial potential difference in several ways. The intracellular mineralocorticoid receptor functions to increase the density of ENaC and of basolateral Na$^+$, K$^+$-ATPase enzymes. Cortisol, which is normally present in higher concentrations than aldosterone, has equal affinity for the aldosterone receptor and therefore could lead to enhanced potassium secretion. However, the enzyme 11β-hydroxysteroid dehydrogenase type 2 is present in the collecting duct cells and converts cortisol to inactive cortisone.

A   Principal cell

B   α-Intercalated cell

FIGURE 119-1. Two cell types in the cortical collecting duct. **A,** The principal cells mediate sodium (Na^+) reabsorption energized by the basolateral Na^+, K^+ pump. Entry from the lumen is through the epithelial Na^+ channel (ENaC), which renders the lumen negatively charged (^-mv). This transepithelial voltage stimulates secretion of potassium (K^+) through K^+ channels. Reabsorbable anions such as chloride (Cl^-) lessen the luminal negativity and decrease K^+ secretion. Bicarbonate (HCO_3^-) has an effect to increase K^+ secretion. High flow rates increase net K^+ secretion by preventing development of high lumen K^+ concentrations. The effects of the renin-angiotensin-aldosterone axis are shown: increased mineralocorticoid receptor (MR) activation increases ENaC, the Na^+, K^+ pump, and K^+ channels, thereby increasing Na^+ reabsorption and K^+ secretion. Cortisol would also increase MR activity, but it is inactivated by the enzyme, 11β-hydroxysteroid dehydrogenase (11β-HSD). AI = angiotensin I; AII = angiotensin II; ACE = angiotensin-converting enzyme; mv = millivolts. **B,** Intercalated cells are carbonic anhydrase–rich cells that secrete acid and reabsorb HCO_3^-. The H^+-ATPase secretes H^+ in a way favored by the negatively charged lumen in conjunction with the aldosterone-stimulated effect on Na^+ reabsorption in neighboring principal cells. The K^+, H^+-ATPase is an electroneutral pump. The K^+/H^+ exchanger, reabsorbing K^+, is important in states of K^+ depletion when urinary K^+ is decreased. ADP = adenosine diphosphate; ATP = adenosine triphosphate.

Role of Potassium Secretory Channels

The second mechanism for collecting duct potassium secretion is adequate function of several types of potassium secretory channels on the luminal membrane of the principal cell. Among many factors regulating these channels, antidiuretic hormone (ADH) and intracellular pH are likely of most significance. The increase in K^+ channel activity in response to ADH, combined with an ADH effect to increase ENaC, allows for the highest possible potassium concentration in the urine under circumstances of low flow that accompanies increased water reabsorption. Cellular acidification, as occurs in metabolic acidosis, inhibits potassium secretion through an effect on potassium secretory channels, thereby contributing to potassium retention in metabolic acidosis.

Flow Rate Dependence of Potassium Secretion

The third mechanism for regulating K^+ secretion in the collecting duct is the flow rate of urine. Increasing flow allows for greater sodium delivery and, hence, greater sodium reabsorption through ENaC; it also maintains optimal K^+ gradients for further secretion into the lumen. Conversely, in conditions of water diuresis, the decreased ADH diminishes the net amount of potassium secreted. Yet, because the urine cannot fully be free of potassium, polyuria over a prolonged period is likely to lead to significant potassium losses.

Because potassium excretion is highly dependent on flow rate, conditions in which high urine flow rates are accompanied by high aldosterone levels may result in substantial potassium losses. Such is the case with diuretic use

(e.g., acetazolamide, thiazide, and loop diuretics). Increased urinary flow rates contribute to the hypokalemia in osmotic diuresis, Fanconi's syndrome, and metabolic alkalosis from vomiting. Conversely, low urinary flow rates make potassium excretion difficult and may contribute to hyperkalemic states. The increase in aldosterone and ADH that accompanies prerenal states may offset the K^+ retention that would otherwise accompany oliguria.

Excretion Mechanisms and Normal Function

Taken together, three feedback loops are relevant to normal function. First, drinking excessive water does not acutely lead to large losses of potassium because there is a simultaneous decrease in ADH. Second, expansion of the extracellular fluid with isotonic sodium chloride does not necessarily result in potassium depletion because the renin-angiotensin-aldosterone axis is suppressed. Third, in metabolic acidosis, intracellular acidification limits potassium secretion, favoring more acid secretion to compensate for the acidosis.

Diuretics such as furosemide and thiazides are well known and common causes of hypokalemia. The potassium-losing effects of thiazides are greater than those of loop diuretics.

Proximal tubule disorders associated with Fanconi's syndrome increase the delivery of solute, with an osmotic diuresis and bicarbonaturia that increase potassium secretion The volume depletion increases renin and aldosterone. Increased bicarbonate delivery from the proximal tubule overwhelms the capacity to reabsorb bicarbonate by the collecting duct. Bicarbonate acts as a non-reabsorbable anion that stimulates potassium secretion. For example, marked potassium wasting associated with vomiting is caused by renal losses when the urine is alkaline, not by lost potassium from the gastrointestinal tract.

The feedback mechanism coupling aldosterone with serum potassium is important in regulating the degree of potassium losses in the urine. For example, hyperaldosteronism results in K^+ loss, and then the resulting hypokalemia reduces aldosterone production and subsequent K^+ losses. Hyperkalemia has the opposite effect: it is an important stimulus of aldosterone synthesis and release. Thus, with volume expansion and low angiotensin II, the rise in K^+ stimulates aldosterone release from the zona glomerulosa of the adrenal cortex, thereby allowing for K^+ to be secreted into the urine.

Potassium Depletion and Excess

Potassium has critical effects on excitable tissues, especially cardiac and skeletal muscle. Low serum potassium not only hyperpolarizes most cells, thereby leading to an increase in the resting potential, but also alters potassium channels required for repolarization. Thus, hypokalemia decreases or slows potassium conductance.

Because of an increased potassium conductance, hyperkalemia antagonizes the normal slow depolarization of pacemaker tissue that is usually associated with a decrease in potassium conductance. Certain muscle-depolarizing anesthetic agents, such as succinylcholine, may potentiate effects of hyperkalemia, as may gentamicin, particularly in patients with renal failure.

Potassium is as important a body fluid osmole as sodium, and losses of potassium obligate sodium to replace it in the intracellular space, thereby resulting in hyponatremia. Hypokalemia contributes to the hyponatremia associated with thiazide diuretics. Isoosmotic losses of combined potassium and sodium salts in watery diarrhea may result in isotonic extracellular volume depletion. Similarly, if potassium chloride is added to isotonic saline, a hypertonic solution results, and potassium may enter cells as sodium exits, thereby contributing to hypernatremia.

Internal Potassium Balance

Because of the delay in hours before renal excretion matches dietary intake and because potassium first enters the extracellular fluid from the gastrointestinal tract, it is critical that the process of cellular buffering be effective (Table 119-1). Essentially, increases in postprandial blood potassium are minimized before potassium is eliminated from the body. A major factor in this regulation after meals is the feedback loop involving insulin and potassium. An increase in serum potassium stimulates insulin release from the β cells of the pancreatic islets. Insulin increases potassium uptake into cells, primarily muscle, independent of its effect on glucose uptake. Potassium uptake is chiefly the result of increased Na^+, K^+-ATPase trafficking to the plasma membranes in these cells.

Another important mechanism of regulating the distribution of potassium between extracellular and cellular spaces involves the sympathoadrenal system. β-Adrenergic activation, particularly through the $β_2$-receptor,

TABLE 119-1	FACTORS REGULATING INTERNAL POTASSIUM BALANCE
Insulin	
β-Adrenergic activity	
Acid-base balance	
Magnesium	
Osmolality	
Thyroid hormone	
Potassium	

increases potassium uptake into muscle and fat cells. As with insulin, potassium uptake is the consequence of increased Na^+, K^+-ATPase activity associated with increased intracellular cyclic adenosine monophosphate (AMP). The adrenergic effect is important in regulating the serum potassium concentration during exercise and is independent of the additional effect that catecholamines may have on blood sugar with the expected increases in insulin. In the trained athlete, a chronic increase in Na^+, K^+-ATPase on cell membranes may cause a transient lowering of the serum potassium concentration after exertion. Conversely, a severe stress may contribute to hypokalemia, through both direct β_2 effects and insulin action secondary to the blood sugar rise.

Phenylephrine, an α-adrenergic agonist, increases serum potassium. Importantly, epinephrine, which also has α-adrenergic effects, is associated with a transient increase in potassium release from the liver before a more prolonged period of decreased serum potassium mediated by the β_2-receptor.

Metabolic acidosis raises the potassium level more than does respiratory acidosis; both metabolic alkalosis and respiratory alkalosis lower the potassium level. Anion gap acidosis does not raise the potassium level, probably because of the movement of the organic anion (e.g., lactate) from cells into the extracellular space with an accompanying proton, whereas the ingestion of chloride salts has the most profound effect on the potassium level because chloride is restricted to the extracellular space and protons enter cells in exchange for the exit of the potassium cation. The ingestion of excessive chloride salts of arginine and lysine is associated with hyperkalemic acidosis. ε-Aminocaproic acid has also been associated with hyperkalemia and is hypothesized to exchange for cellular potassium, much like the other cationic amino acids.

Just as multiple simultaneous acid-base disturbances lead to a single blood pH level, many processes that affect potassium can be simultaneously present. Metabolic acidosis may be associated with diarrheal or urinary losses of potassium, so that the potassium concentration is low, not high. Metabolic acidosis in diabetes can also be associated with insulin deficiency and renal failure, in which case the serum potassium level might be elevated despite osmotically driven urinary losses of potassium and total body potassium depletion.

Other hormonal effects on potassium include thyroid and growth hormone, but patients with disorders of these hormones do not usually have significant changes in their blood potassium levels. Some patients with hyperthyroidism may have mild hypokalemia, perhaps related to increased sympathetic activity. Growth states are associated with a greater need for potassium; for example, in normal pregnancy, the maternal potassium concentration may fall as the developing fetus grows.

Hypomagnesemia frequently accompanies hypokalemia. Both magnesium and potassium are found predominantly in cells, but Na^+, K^+-ATPase requires magnesium for function. If magnesium is deficient, potassium distributes more to the extracellular fluid, thereby masking the degree of potassium deficiency. Moreover, magnesium deficiency leads to renal potassium wasting, so potassium depletion is hard to correct until magnesium is repleted.

External Potassium Balance and Associated Disorders

Normally, no more than 10 to 20% of total potassium excretion is accomplished by the gastrointestinal tract, but colonic excretion is increased in renal failure, primarily through potassium-induced increases in epithelial Na^+, K^+-ATPase activity and aldosterone. In renal failure, the normal mechanisms to distribute potassium acquire increased importance.

Some conditions that cause the greatest losses of gastrointestinal potassium include secretory diarrheas of the colon, the result of infection or laxative abuse. Disorders of the small intestine, which may lead to large quantities of liquid stool with a low potassium concentration, engender favorable

gradients for marked potassium secretion by the colon. A syndrome of watery diarrhea and hypokalemia is associated with neuroendocrine tumors (Chapter 211) that secrete vasoactive intestinal peptide. Rectosigmoid secretion of potassium may result in particularly high potassium losses, and potassium deficiency is seen in patients who have ureterosigmoidostomies. Potassium can be lost from a variety of other sources, including excess sweat or salivation, vomiting, and diarrhea.

Potassium can be depleted by vomiting or diarrhea. Urinary losses may exceed intake in renal tubular disorders, when excessive quantities of osmotic or anionic products are excreted in the urine, or in patients who take diuretics.

It is unusual for hyperkalemia to be caused by excessive potassium intake unless the patient has renal dysfunction. However, patients who have brisk hemolysis, internal hemorrhage, or rhabdomyolysis, particularly if the hemoglobinuria or myoglobinuria also results in acute kidney injury, can quickly develop life-threatening hyperkalemia owing to rapid release of cellular potassium stores.

CLINICAL MANIFESTATIONS

Hypokalemia

Clinical manifestations of potassium depletion include hypertension, decreased growth, and muscle symptoms such as weakness, cramps, fasciculations, and even paralysis. In severe cases, the diaphragm may be paralyzed, leading to respiratory failure. Cardiac arrhythmias are a critical component of low potassium states and are usually seen when the serum potassium falls below 3 mmol/L or when ischemia, hypercalcemia, or drugs such as digoxin are simultaneously present. A patient who has a chronically low potassium level (e.g., from diuretic use) may be particularly vulnerable to supraventricular and ventricular tachyarrhythmias during periods of stress, such as head trauma, or during the acute coronary syndrome, to which cardiac ischemia also contributes. The prolonged cardiac repolarization phase of hypokalemia accounts for the characteristic electrocardiographic findings of broad, flattened T waves. U waves are also indicative of this delay in repolarization (Fig. 119-2). In the intestine, hypokalemia may result in paralytic ileus, which may interfere with oral replacement. Hypokalemia may result in acute skeletal muscle weakness and even paralysis.

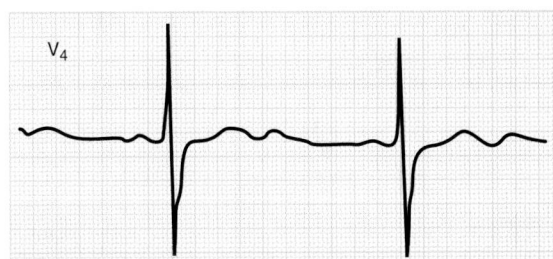

FIGURE 119-2. The electrocardiographic manifestations of hypokalemia. The serum potassium concentration was 2.2 mEq/L. The ST segment is prolonged, primarily because of a U wave following the T wave, and the T wave is flattened.

In addition to these systemic effects of potassium imbalance, the kidney is particularly sensitive to depletion of potassium. Structural changes in the glomeruli and tubules lead to a decreased glomerular filtration rate (GFR), increased proximal tubule ammoniagenesis, increased sodium bicarbonate reabsorption, and net acid excretion. A condition of nephrogenic diabetes insipidus results when potassium depletion decreases expression of vasopressin-dependent water channels (aquaporin-2) in the collecting duct luminal plasma membranes. Hypokalemia diminishes insulin secretion and may be associated with glucose intolerance.

Hyperkalemia

In hyperkalemia, the depolarizing effect on the resting membrane potential and increased potassium channel conductance lead to the classic electrocardiographic changes of hyperacute peaked T waves associated with rapid repolarization (Fig. 119-3). Hyperkalemia commonly results in sinus bradycardia. Heart block, loss of P waves on the electrocardiogram, and prolonged QRS intervals are all seen in cases of severe hyperkalemia, usually in excess of 6 mmol/L. The electrocardiogram, however, is not a sensitive indicator of severe hyperkalemia, and cardiac arrest may occur without warning. Like hypokalemia, severe hyperkalemia can cause skeletal muscle paralysis; unlike hypokalemic paralysis, it is often ascending in nature.

Lead V$_3$

A

B

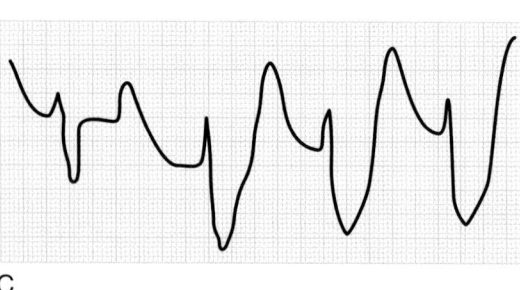

C

FIGURE 119-3. The effects of progressive hyperkalemia on the electrocardiogram. All of the illustrations are from lead V$_3$. **A,** Serum potassium concentration ([K$^+$]) = 6.8 mEq/L; note the peaked T waves together with normal sinus rhythm. **B,** Serum [K$^+$] = 8.9 mEq/L; note the peaked T waves and absent P waves. **C,** Serum [K$^+$] = >8.9 mEq/L; note the classic sine wave with absent P waves, marked prolongation of the QRS complex, and peaked T waves.

DIAGNOSIS

The first clue to a disorder in potassium balance usually is an abnormal serum potassium concentration obtained as part of a laboratory evaluation, not because an abnormal potassium level itself is suspected. When the potassium is elevated above normal, it is imperative to exclude common artifacts, known as pseudohyperkalemia. Hemolysis in the test tube is a common artifact; in cases of cold-induced hemolysis (Chapter 164), it is important to collect the blood and allow it to clot in a warm environment. Some patients have pseudohyperkalemia resulting from high platelet counts, usually in excess of 1 million/μL, or myelogenous leukemia (Chapters 189 and 190); in such cases, plasma potassium levels should be within the normal range. Sometimes the serum potassium level may be elevated because of local ischemia related to application of the tourniquet and clenching of the fist.

A detailed medical history should focus on medications, family history, and sources of potassium excess or loss. The physical examination should pay particular attention to blood pressure, extracellular volume status, heart rate and rhythm, and muscle strength and reflexes.

Laboratory testing should include a complete blood count as well as serum levels of sodium, chloride, bicarbonate, creatinine, and blood urea nitrogen. In more serious cases, arterial blood gases and levels of creatine kinase and magnesium should be obtained. A 12-lead electrocardiogram also should be obtained.

A low urinary potassium level is expected in hypokalemia. In a hypokalemic patient, a urinary potassium concentration greater than 30 mEq/L suggests renal potassium wasting, whereas extrarenal losses are usually reflected by concentrations lower than 20 mEq/L. In a state of potassium excess, urinary potassium excretion should exceed about 35 mEq/L, unless urinary underexcretion was the cause of the hyperkalemia. A high aldosterone level causes a high urinary potassium-to-sodium ratio, whereas hypoaldosteronism may cause the opposite. Another way to determine the appropriateness of urinary potassium content is to calculate the transtubular potassium gradient (TTKG) as follows:

$$TTKG = (urinary\ potassium\ concentration \div plasma\ potassium$$
$$concentration) / (urine\ osmolality \div plasma\ osmolality)$$

Correct use of the TTKG requires the urine Na$^+$ to be greater than 25 mEq/L and the urine osmolality as high as or higher than the serum osmolality.

In a hyperkalemic patient, a TTKG of more than 7 to 8 would be expected. Lower values suggest renal underexcretion as the cause of the hyperkalemia. In a hypokalemic patient, a healthy kidney should conserve potassium, so the TTKG should be less than 2 to 3; if it is more than 3, urinary potassium wasting would be suspected as the cause of the hypokalemia.

Hypokalemic Disorders

The most common cause of hypokalemia (Table 119-2) in medical practice is the use of thiazide diuretics or loop diuretics. Patients may have low, normal, or high blood pressures depending on their volume status and whether the diuretics were prescribed for hypertension or heart failure. The most common acute causes of hypokalemia are diarrhea or vomiting.

Hypokalemic Hypertensive Syndromes

If the renal collecting duct cells develop a transepithelial electrical gradient that is more lumen negative than is needed to maintain potassium balance, urinary potassium wasting, inappropriate to the blood potassium level, occurs. Because a parallel increase in H$^+$ secretion will occur, it is common to see an accompanying metabolic alkalosis. If the abnormality is related to a primary increase in sodium reabsorption, hypertension or extracellular volume expansion also will develop.

Evaluation of plasma renin and aldosterone levels can help distinguish among specific diagnoses (see Table 119-2). Primary hyperaldosteronism is associated with low renin levels owing to volume expansion. If corrected for serum potassium, an aldosterone-to-renin ratio of 30:1 suggests a primary adrenal cortical tumor (aldosteronoma) or hyperplasia (Chapter 234). The tubular delivery of large amounts of sodium chloride in a setting of volume expansion and nonsuppressible aldosterone results in hypokalemia, which improves after sodium restriction and worsens with the administration of intravenous saline. In congenital adrenal hyperplasia (Chapter 234), such as 11β-hydroxylase deficiency, hypokalemic alkalosis is associated with excessive androgen production. In patients with renin-secreting tumors or unilateral renal artery stenosis, high renin levels stimulate angiotensin and then

TABLE 119-2 CAUSES OF HYPOKALEMIA AND INCREASED POTASSIUM EXCRETION

CAUSES OF INCREASED K⁺ EXCRETION AND HYPOKALEMIA	RENIN	ALDOSTERONE	EXTRACELLULAR VOLUME OR BLOOD PRESSURE	ACID-BASE STATUS
Increased ENaC: Liddle's syndrome	Low	Low	High	Alkalosis
Decreased β-OH steroid dehydrogenase: apparent mineralocorticoid excess, licorice	Low	Low	High	Alkalosis
Adrenal tumor or hyperplasia	Low	High	High	Alkalosis
Ectopic ACTH; Cushing's syndrome	Low	Low	High	Alkalosis
Congenital adrenal hyperplasia	Low	High	High	Alkalosis
Unilateral renal artery stenosis	High	High	High	Alkalosis
Renin-secreting tumor	High	High	High	Alkalosis
Diuretics:				
Acetazolamide	High	High	Variable	Acidosis
Furosemide, thiazides	High	High	Low	Alkalosis
Bartter's syndrome	High	High	Low	Alkalosis
Gitelman's syndrome	High	High	Low	Alkalosis
Fanconi's syndrome	High	High	Low	Acidosis
Distal RTA	High	High	Low	Acidosis

ACTA = adrenocorticotropic hormone; β-OH = β-hydroxy; ENaC = epithelial Na⁺ channel; RTA = renal tubular acidosis.

aldosterone secretion, with a resulting increase in sodium reabsorption, hypertension, and hypokalemic metabolic alkalosis.

In some patients with overproduction of adrenocorticotropic hormone (ACTH), as in ectopic production from lung and other malignancies (Chapter 187), cortisol may overwhelm the aldosterone receptor and result in hypertensive hypokalemic alkalosis. The patient may not show signs of Cushing's syndrome, unless the syndrome is prolonged. In glucocorticoid-remediable aldosteronism, which is a familial disorder in which episodes of hypokalemia and hypertension develop, a chimeric gene duplication couples the ACTH-responsive 11β-hydroxylase promoter to the coding region of aldosterone synthase.

Glycyrrhizic acid, which is found in licorice or anisette, inhibits the renal enzyme 11β-hydroxysteroid dehydrogenase and thereby causes hypokalemia, metabolic alkalosis, and hypertension. A rare genetic disorder known as apparent mineralocorticoid excess syndrome produces the same effect owing to deficiency of 11β-hydroxysteroid dehydrogenase. The syndrome produces a high ratio of cortisol to cortisone; as a result, renin and aldosterone are suppressed by the volume expansion.

Activating mutations of ENaC cause increased Na⁺ reabsorption (Liddle's syndrome; Chapter 130). The syndrome can be distinguished from primary or secondary hyperaldosteronism by a decrease in renin and aldosterone levels.

Hypokalemic Hypotensive Syndromes

In contrast to the hypokalemic hypertensive syndromes, in which an increased sodium reabsorption is a primary event, many hypokalemic alkaloses are associated with extracellular volume depletion. With a physiologic response to volume depletion, the K⁺ losses may be a result of appropriate Na⁺ reabsorption; signs of hypotension or extracellular volume depletion will be observed. Secretory diarrheas, whether associated with hypochloremic alkalosis or hyperchloremic acidosis, lead to extracellular volume depletion and secondary increases in renin and aldosterone; the result is both gastrointestinal and urinary K⁺ losses.

Diuretic use, Bartter's syndrome (Chapter 130), and Gitelman's syndrome (Chapter 130) are renal tubular causes of extracellular volume depletion, hypotension, and hypokalemic alkalosis; sodium and chloride are lost in the urine, and secondary rises in renin and aldosterone occur. Increased urinary flow rates are important contributors to the increased potassium losses in each of these examples. Bartter's syndrome affects the function of the thick ascending limb through mutations in NKCC or in K⁺ or Cl⁻ channels, whereas Gitelman's syndrome is characterized by inactivating mutations or dysregulation of the sodium-chloride cotransporter (NCC) in the distal tubule. The hypokalemia in Gitelman's syndrome may be caused by secondary hyperaldosteronism, bicarbonaturia, and, hypomagnesemia.

Classic type 1 distal renal tubular acidosis (Chapter 130) is often associated with hypokalemia, which may improve with correction of the acidemia. In contrast, proximal renal tubular acidosis, when corrected with bicarbonate,

often results in worsening of the hypokalemia owing to greater bicarbonate wasting associated with increases in the filtered bicarbonate load.

Acetazolamide, when given to an alkalotic patient, is a particularly potent kaliuretic agent. Volume depletion and hyperaldosteronism contribute to the potassium losses, as does the bicarbonate wasting, which appears to have a direct effect on potassium secretion. Whenever the urine is alkaline, potassium will usually be present in significant amounts.

Tubular toxins that may be associated with severe potassium losses include aminoglycosides, cisplatinum, and ifosfamide. Amphotericin B results in significant potassium wasting accompanied by renal tubular acidosis. In many of these conditions, simultaneous use of amiloride may diminish potassium losses by as much as 50%.

Patients who present with unexplained hypokalemia and alkalosis with volume depletion should have urinary electrolytes measured to determine whether the urine chloride is low, as with vomiting or laxative abuse. If the urine contains chloride, a diuretic screen should be considered; Gitelman's syndrome and Bartter's syndrome are other possibilities.

Hyperkalemic Disorders

In clinical practice, acute hyperkalemia is seen most commonly with renal failure (Chapter 133), with acidosis (Chapter 120), and with acute muscle damage from rhabdomyolysis (Chapter 115) (Table 119-3). Chronic hyperkalemia is most commonly seen with medications that reduce potassium secretion and with renal tubular disorders.

Hyperkalemic Hypotensive or Normotensive Syndromes

Type IV renal tubular acidoses (Chapter 130) that are associated with an inability to acidify the urine are caused by diseases that disrupt distal nephron function, including systemic lupus erythematosus (Chapter 274), urinary tract obstruction (Chapter 125), amyloidosis (Chapter 194), the nephropathy associated with kidney and bone marrow transplantation (Chapters 133 and 181), and sickle cell nephropathy (Chapter 127). Males who present with hyperkalemia and renal insufficiency of unknown cause should be evaluated for possible prostatic obstruction (Chapter 131). Each of these conditions may also be associated with failure to concentrate the urine (nephrogenic diabetes insipidus) or with a hyperchloremic metabolic acidosis caused by abnormalities in acid secretion.

Primary selective hypoaldosteronism or complete adrenal cortical deficiency (Chapter 234) is associated with elevated renin and low aldosterone. Secondary hypoaldosteronism may be seen in hyporenin states caused by β-blockers, renin antagonists, or nonsteroidal anti-inflammatory drugs (NSAIDs). Angiotensin-converting enzyme inhibitors and angiotensin receptor blockers increase renin and decrease aldosterone. Heparin, including low-molecular-weight and fractionated forms (Chapter 37), can lead to hyperkalemia even in small subcutaneous doses.

Disorders that affect the transepithelial potential difference and can result in hyperkalemia, acidosis, and extracellular volume depletion include

TABLE 119-3 CAUSES OF HYPERKALEMIA AND DECREASED POTASSIUM EXCRETION

CAUSE OF DECREASED K⁺ EXCRETION AND HYPERKALEMIA	RENIN	ALDOSTERONE	EXTRACELLULAR VOLUME OR BLOOD PRESSURE	ACID-BASE STATUS
Decreased ENaC: Drugs: amiloride, triamterene, trimethoprim, lithium Pseudohypoaldosteronism type 1 autosomal recessive ENaC mutation	High	High	Low or normal	Normal or acidosis
Pseudohypoaldosteronism type 1 autosomal dominant MR mutation	High	High	Low	Acidosis
MR blockade: spironolactone, eplerenone, progesterone	High	High	Low	Acidosis
Hypoaldosteronism: Adrenal insufficiency	High	Low	Low	Acidosis
Hyporenin-hypoaldosteronism: NSAIDs, β-blockers, autonomic neuropathy	Low	Low	Low	Acidosis
Pseudohypoaldosteronism type 2	Low	Low	High	Acidosis

ENaC = epithelial Na⁺ channel; MR = mineralocorticoid receptor; NSAIDs = nonsteroidal anti-inflammatory drugs.

inactivating mutations of ENaC (autosomal recessive pseudohypoaldosteronism type 1), which may be accompanied by high renin and aldosterone levels. The ENaC may also be inhibited by the potassium-sparing diuretics (i.e., amiloride and triamterene) and certain medications secreted by the proximal tubule organic cation transporters, such as trimethoprim and pentamidine, as well as by lithium. Inhibition of the aldosterone receptor may be the result of antagonists such as spironolactone and eplerenone.

Hyperkalemic Hypertensive Syndromes

NSAIDs can cause hyperkalemia, particularly in patients with renal disease, by decreasing sodium delivery, increasing water reabsorption, and decreasing renin and aldosterone. Hypertension with the NSAIDs is most likely caused by renal salt and water retention.

Cyclosporine or tacrolimus may produce a hyperkalemic acidosis. The mechanism may involve inhibition of cyclooxygenase 2 (COX2) and therefore hyporenin-hypoaldosteronism. There may also be a decrease in apical potassium secretion in the collecting duct. Gordon's syndrome is a genetic disorder (pseudohypoaldosteronism type 2) associated with hyperkalemia, volume expansion, and metabolic acidosis; it is highly responsive to thiazide diuretics.

TREATMENT   Rx

It may be difficult to determine the exact state of total body potassium stores from the serum potassium level because as much as 100 to 300 mmol of potassium may be lost from the body with a fall in serum potassium of only 1 mmol/L.

Hypokalemia

The goal of acute therapy for hypokalemia is to prevent or manage potentially life-threatening arrhythmias or paralysis. Patients at greatest risk are elderly patients, patients with known liver disease or cardiac disturbances, and patients who have had an abrupt fall in serum K⁺ to less than 2.5 mEq/L. Potassium must traverse the extracellular space before repleting intracellular stores, so it is dangerously easy to replete potassium too quickly. Oral potassium should be given, if possible. If the K⁺ is greater than 3 mEq/L, increasing dietary K⁺ can be considered, along with removing the underlying cause of hypokalemia. Usual oral replacement is with KCl at a dose of 40 to 100 mmol per day. The Cl salt has the advantage of treating concomitant metabolic alkalosis, but other available forms include K citrate (in the acidotic patient) and K phosphate (in patients with a phosphate deficit). Giving potassium with a nonreabsorbable anion, such as gluconate, may not replace the potassium deficit adequately. Intravenous potassium is reserved for patients who are unable to take enteral potassium and patients with symptomatic hypokalemia, paralysis, or cardiac arrhythmias. It is usually given as a solution of 20 to 40 mmol of K⁺ in 1 L of solution at a rate that does not exceed 10 to 20 mmol/hour. In some cases of severe hypokalemia (<2.5 mEq/L) and in symptomatic patients, higher concentrations (up to 40 mmol in 100 mL) have been used. If the potassium level is less than 3 mmol/L or if more than 10 mmol/hour is to be delivered, it may be best to treat the patient in a monitored setting to observe for cardiac complications. A central venous catheter may be required for these higher concentrations. In these unusual circumstances, it is best to consult with a renal specialist and the pharmacy.

In patients who have prerenal azotemia associated with hyperglycemia or severe metabolic alkalosis, volume expansion with sodium chloride solutions alone can result in life-threatening potassium losses, despite improvement in the extracellular volume. Potassium must be given in anticipation of such events.

In a hypokalemic patient, care must be exercised when glucose-containing solutions are given because the resulting increase in insulin may further decrease the blood potassium level. Attention to the urine output and ongoing losses is crucial. If ongoing losses of potassium are severe, it may be necessary to provide a potassium-sparing diuretic (e.g., amiloride, 5 to 10 mg orally) and to treat the cause of the ongoing losses (e.g., diarrhea). Magnesium should be measured and replaced, if necessary, in any hypokalemic patient.

In the outpatient setting, hypokalemia is a common side effect of diuretic therapy. The serum potassium level should be maintained within the normal range (>3.5 mEq/L), especially in high-risk patients. Addition of 40 to 100 mmol of K⁺ per day as the chloride salt is the usual treatment, depending on the patient's response.

Hyperkalemia

If hyperkalemia is severe, the goal is to achieve a rapid reduction in potassium concentration. If hyperkalemia is associated with cardiac arrhythmias, however, the cardiac effects of the hyperkalemia require interim treatment in a monitored setting, before the serum potassium can be expected to decline, even with aggressive therapy. Calcium gluconate, 10 mL of a 10% solution (8.9 mg calcium) over 10 to 20 minutes, is often indicated to stabilize electrical effects on cardiac excitation. Calcium chloride (3 to 4 mL of a 10% solution) is used as another alternative, but it should be administered through a central access line because extravasation of the chloride salt may result in tissue necrosis.

However, calcium does not lower the potassium concentration. Nebulized or inhaled β-agonists and intravenous insulin and glucose, either alone or the two in combination, are the best treatments.[1] To lower the potassium within 15 minutes, 10 units of regular insulin should be given, with glucose given as a 10% solution over 1 hour for a total of 30 to 50 g in the normoglycemic patient. The blood glucose level should be monitored. Albuterol by nebulizer (10 to 20 mg in 4 mL saline over 10 minutes) can redistribute potassium acutely but should not be the sole treatment because some patients are not responsive. In some cases, intravenous β-adrenergic agonists (e.g., albuterol, 0.5 mg in 100 mL of 5% dextrose over 15 minutes) have been used to lower the serum potassium level by about 1 mmol/L within minutes to hours. Sodium bicarbonate, as an isotonic mixture calculated to correct acid-base status, should be reserved for acidemic patients who otherwise require alkalinization, while being careful to avoid hypocalcemia; complications of sodium bicarbonate infusions include hypernatremia, volume expansion, and decreased ionized calcium, potentially resulting in tetany. Diabetic patients may be potassium depleted even though they present with hyperkalemia; as they are volume repleted, they typically require potassium replacement (Chapter 236).

Over the longer term, potassium loss can be sustained by using cation exchange resins such as sodium polystyrene sulfonate, given orally or as an enema (Chapter 133). A dose of 30 to 50 g can reduce potassium levels over several hours. This resin will also provide a sodium load and bind calcium, thereby resulting in volume expansion and hypocalcemia. These resins may interfere with the absorption of lithium and thyroxine. A serious complication of sodium polystyrene sulfonate resins when used in combination with sorbitol is colonic ulceration and necrosis. These resins also should not be given in combination with aluminum-based antacids because the resulting concretions can obstruct the gastrointestinal tract. If the patient is volume expanded, furosemide (40 to 100 mg), chlorothiazide (500 mg) or, if the patient is also alkalotic, acetazolamide (250 to 500 mg) may enhance renal potassium clearance. If the patient is volume depleted, isotonic saline expansion may improve urine output and, with it, potassium excretion.

Specific Clinical Syndromes
Hypokalemia

Patients with pernicious anemia who receive vitamin B_{12} to stimulate erythropoiesis may deplete extracellular potassium and suffer from hypokalemia as a cost of producing new red blood cells. Leukemias with rapid growth rates (Chapter 189) also may cause a drop in the serum potassium level, and some forms of myelogenous leukemia are associated with a high level of lysozyme, which leads to urinary potassium loss as well (Chapter 190).

Familial hypokalemic periodic paralysis is caused by a variety of mutations in a cellular calcium channel, with resulting reduced activity of an ATP-regulated K^+ channel that extrudes potassium from skeletal muscle cells. Without the ability to recycle potassium to the extracellular space, the hypokalemic effect of the Na^+, K^+-ATPase is unopposed. The presentation is usually in the teenage years or early adulthood. In some cases, a progressive proximal myopathy may develop. A form is seen in Asian patients with hyperthyroidism; it manifests as episodic paralysis brought out by high-carbohydrate meals (insulin secretion). Another aggravating factor is rest after exercise, a time when blood potassium falls owing to reuptake of potassium by the ATPase pumps. The condition is treated by a high potassium diet as well as with β_2-blockers (e.g., propranolol, 20 to 40 mg twice daily) and carbonic anhydrase inhibitors (e.g., acetazolamide, 125 to 500 mg), which in part work by creating a hyperchloremic acidosis that offsets the urinary potassium wasting they cause.

Hyperkalemia

The abnormal distribution of potassium between cells and the extracellular space results in the hyperkalemia that is associated with acidosis, insulin-deficient states, and β_2-adrenergic blockade. Although it is not always possible, it is best to know the levels of serum glucose and potassium in an unconscious diabetic patient before infusing concentrated glucose solutions, because of the risk for aggravating an already elevated potassium concentration.

Familial hyperkalemic periodic paralysis is a myopathy caused by a genetic defect in voltage-gated Na^+ channels in skeletal muscle. Exercise or dietary increases in plasma potassium result in mild depolarization of skeletal muscle that then unmasks the sodium channel defect, rendering the cells unexcitable. Treatment is frequent meals and acetazolamide (125 to 500 mg).

Potassium competes with digoxin-binding sites on the Na^+, K^+-ATPase, so that, if hypokalemia coexists, digoxin will have an intensified effect and may lead to drug toxicity. In extreme cases of digitalis overdose, severe hyperkalemia develops owing to generalized blockade of Na^+, K^+-ATPase.

PROGNOSIS

The prognosis of patients with hypokalemia and hyperkalemia depends on the severity and underlying illness. Most hypokalemic cases are mild (K^+, 3 to 3.5 mEq/L). However, mortality of hospitalized patients with hypokalemia is increased ten-fold. Hyperkalemia is reported in 1 to 10% of hospitalized patients, of whom 10% have severe hyperkalemia (K^+, >6.0 mEq/L). Hyperkalemia is associated with increased mortality (14 to 41%), and it accounts for 2 to 5% of deaths in patients with end-stage renal disease.

1. Mahoney BA, Smith WA, Lo DS, et al. Emergency interventions for hyperkalemia. *Cochrane Database Syst Rev.* 2005;2:CD003235.

SUGGESTED READINGS

Einhorn LM, Zhan M, Hsu VD, et al. The frequency of hyperkalemia and its significance in chronic kidney disease. *Arch Intern Med.* 2009;169:1156-1162. *Emphasizes the association of hyperkalemia with adverse outcomes.*

Khanna A, White WB. The management of hyperkalemia in patients with cardiovascular disease. *Am J Med.* 2009;122:215-221. *Review.*

Lippi G, Favaloro EJ, Montagnana M, et al. Prevalence of hypokalaemia: the experience of a large academic hospital. *Intern Med J.* 2010;40:315-316. *Review.*

Sterns RH, Rojas M, Bernstein P, et al. Ion-exchange resins for the treatment of hyperkalemia: are they safe and effective? *J Am Soc Nephrol.* 2010;21:733-735. *Review of usefulness and potential complications when used with sorbitol or aluminum-based antacids.*

ACID-BASE DISORDERS

JULIAN L. SEIFTER

DEFINITION

The pH is defined as the negative log of the hydrogen ion concentration. At a pH of 7.40, the hydrogen ion concentration is 40 nanoequivalents (nEq) per liter, a very small concentration in comparison to serum sodium at 140 mEq/L. The hydrogen ion concentration of body fluids is in equilibrium with each of multiple buffers, such as proteins, phosphate, and hemoglobin (the isohydric principle), but acid-base equilibria in the body are often analyzed by using the CO_2/HCO_3^- system and the relationship of the proton concentration (thus pH) to the ratio of HCO_3^- to CO_2. The Henderson-Hasselbalch equation is a logarithmic expression of the relationship.

$$CO_2 + H_2O \rightarrow H_2CO_3 \rightarrow H^+ + HCO_3^-$$

$$pH = pK + \log[HCO_3^-]/0.03(P_{CO_2})$$

In this equation, pK, or the dissociation constant, is 6.1; 0.03 (mM/mm Hg) is the solubility factor for CO_2 in solution. The product of $0.03 \times P_{CO_2}$ represents dissolved CO_2; the "total CO_2" in plasma is the sum of HCO_3^-, normally about 25 mM, and $0.03 \times P_{CO_2}$, normally about 1.2 mM. It is important to note that pH is a function of the *ratio* of HCO_3^- to P_{CO_2}. The HCO_3^- concentration in the numerator is regulated by the kidney, and P_{CO_2} is regulated by the lung, the major organ systems involved in acid-base balance.

EPIDEMIOLOGY

If the production of acid exceeds elimination, a state of acidosis exists, whereas if elimination exceeds production, alkalosis will develop. In metabolic acidosis, production could exceed excretion through a marked excess in the production rate, as might be seen with diabetic ketoacidosis (Chapter 236) or lactic acidosis, or it could develop even with a normal rate of metabolic acid production if the kidney were unable to eliminate acid normally, as in kidney failure (Chapters 122 and 132).

In most humans, particularly those who eat animal protein or an acid-ash diet, the requirement for net acid excretion dominates. However, vegetarians can have an overall alkaline-ash diet, for which net alkali must be excreted to match intake.

Hypochloremic alkalosis might be anticipated in a patient with a history of vomiting or the use of thiazide or loop diuretics. Metabolic acidosis might be anticipated in hypotensive shock, sepsis, diarrhea, and renal failure. Chronic lung disease can be associated with respiratory acidosis, whereas fever, infection, stroke, or acute pulmonary disease may be a cause of acute respiratory alkalosis.

PATHOBIOLOGY

Normal Acid-Base Physiology

Many of the body's metabolic and physiologic functions are pH dependent or pH sensitive. The range of normal arterial pH is 7.38 to 7.42. Intracellular pH is lower than extracellular pH because cells are electronegative with respect to extracellular fluid and metabolically produced acids are constantly being transported to extracellular fluid for eventual elimination from the body. Net acid production must equal net acid excretion. When the diet calls for excretion of acids, urine pH will fall to a value as low as 5.0, and the urine will become nominally free of bicarbonate. When there is an alkaline load, the kidney will reject the excess filtered HCO_3^-, and urine pH may approach a maximal value of 8.0 to 8.5.

In severe disease states, arterial pH may fall as low as 6.8 and rise as high as 7.8. Strenuous exercise with the metabolic production of lactate may transiently but severely lower pH, even in normal healthy individuals.

Production of Acids and the Elimination of CO_2 by the Lung

Volatile acid is the term used for the carbon dioxide produced by metabolic processes in all tissues, an amount that approximates 20,000 mmol/day. This CO_2 is carried from tissues to the lung, where it is eliminated by alveolar ventilation. Steady-state P_{CO_2} is normally 38 to 42 mm Hg.

Nonvolatile acid is a term used to describe acids other than carbonic acid that are formed primarily from protein metabolism. The usual amount of formation is approximately 1 to 2 mEq of H^+ per kilogram of body weight per day. Most diets that contain animal protein have a net positive quantity of nonvolatile acids, primarily from the sulfur-containing amino acids cysteine and methionine; phosphates from phosphoproteins, phospholipids, and phosphonucleotides; nonmetabolizable organic acids, such as uric acid, and inorganic sources; and HCl derived from chloride salts of lysine, arginine, and histidine. The addition of protons to body fluids by these acid end products consumes bicarbonate, which then must be replenished by the kidney as it eliminates the proton. The kidney must excrete any nonvolatile acid or alkali load to maintain a steady-state serum HCO_3^- concentration in the 22- to 28-mM range.

Oxidation of carbohydrates and fats results in the production of water and CO_2, but not nonvolatile acids. To maintain a steady state, any acid or base produced per day must be equivalent to what is excreted. If CO_2 production exceeds CO_2 excretion by the lungs, respiratory acidosis characterized by a high PCO_2 will develop. If the rate of CO_2 excretion exceeds production, respiratory alkalosis develops. By the equation,

$$\text{alveolar ventilation} \sim CO_2 \text{ elimination} \div PCO_2$$

the inverse relationship of alveolar ventilation to PCO_2 is obvious. At steady state, CO_2 production by tissues must equal CO_2 elimination by the lungs for a constant PCO_2 to be maintained. The changes in PCO_2 are almost always caused by changes in alveolar ventilation rather than production of CO_2. Thus, respiratory acidosis is nearly always a consequence of decreased pulmonary ventilation because of lung or central nervous system (CNS) disease and not a consequence of increased production of CO_2. Similarly, respiratory alkalosis develops because of hyperventilation rather than decreased CO_2 production. In either case, when the elimination rate of CO_2 (alveolar ventilation × PCO_2) again equals CO_2 production, a new steady state will prevail, with no net retention or loss of carbonic acid.

Bicarbonate and the Kidney in Acid-Base Balance

The first role of the kidney in acid-base balance is to reabsorb all filtered HCO_3^- (Fig. 120-1). At a normal glomerular filtration rate (i.e., ~180 L/day

in an adult) and serum HCO_3^- concentration of 25 mEq/L, about 4500 mEq of HCO_3^- is filtered in 1 day. Loss of even a small fraction of that amount would result in metabolic acidosis if not replaced by intake.

The Proximal Tubule

About 80 to 90% of HCO_3^- reabsorption is accomplished in the proximal tubule by a proton secretory process. The brush border membranes facing the lumen of the proximal tubule cell contain transporters known as Na/H exchangers (NHE3 is the abundant isoform). Through the normal function of basolateral membrane Na^+,K^+-adenosine triphosphatase (ATPase), cell Na^+ is kept at low concentration so that filtered Na^+ in the lumen will be favored to enter the cell in exchange for H^+ secreted into the lumen. This H^+ rapidly combines with filtered HCO_3^- to form H_2CO_3, which then dehydrates in the lumen to form CO_2 and H_2O. This last process is greatly facilitated by luminal carbonic anhydrase (CA_{IV}). The CO_2 diffuses into the proximal cell, where it reforms HCO_3^-, a reaction catalyzed by intracellular carbonic anhydrase (CA_{II}). The HCO_3^- is then transported back to the blood by a sodium bicarbonate cotransporter (NBC), which couples 1Na and 3HCO_3^-, thereby completing net Na^+ and HCO_3^- reabsorption. The entire process requires a mitochondrial source of adenosine triphosphate (ATP) for the Na/K pump, intact NHE3 and NBC, and two isoforms of carbonic anhydrase. Additionally, there must be favorable ion gradients for luminal Na^+ entry, H^+ secretion, and basolateral HCO_3^- transport. A disturbance in any of these factors may disrupt proximal HCO_3^- reabsorption enough to cause loss of HCO_3^- in urine. Another 10 to 15% of HCO_3^- is reabsorbed in the thick ascending limb of Henle through a similar mechanism so that only small amounts of the filtered HCO_3^- are normally delivered to more distal nephron segments.

The Cortical Collecting Duct

The cortical connecting tubule and collecting duct reabsorb less than 10% of the filtered HCO_3^-. In principal cells, Na^+ is reabsorbed from lumen to cell by the epithelial Na^+ channel (ENaC), driven by the inwardly directed Na^+ gradient and favorable electrical potential. With the reabsorption of Na^+, the lumen becomes electronegative, thus favoring the secretion of both K^+, through K^+ channels, and H^+, through vacuolar H^+-ATPases on the luminal

FIGURE 120-1. Renal acidification mechanisms. ATP = adenosine triphosphate; CA = carbonic anhydrase.

surface of neighboring α-intercalated cells, which are acid-secreting cells. The secreted H^+ will combine with the remaining HCO_3^- in the lumen to generate CO_2, with subsequent reabsorptive diffusion of CO_2, re-formation of cellular HCO_3^- with the help of cellular carbonic anhydrase (CA_{II}), and then exchange of HCO_3^- from cell to blood for entry of Cl^- through Cl/HCO_3 exchangers. It is at this distal site that tubular fluid pH starts to fall to levels below pH 6.0.

Some collecting duct cells have reverse polarity and secrete HCO_3^- into the lumen in exchange for Cl^- entry into the cell. In these cells, the H^+-ATPase faces the blood side of the cell (β-intercalated cells). An elevated extracellular HCO_3^- concentration, as seen with an alkaline-ash diet or alkalosis, will increase HCO_3^- secretion by these cells.

The Medullary Collecting Duct

The medullary collecting duct continues to secrete protons into the luminal fluid, where the pH reaches its lowest values of close to 5.0. The mechanism is based on continued function of H^+-ATPases with an additional role of an ATP-dependent K/H exchanger, a member of the family of K^+, H^+-ATPases found in the stomach and colon.

Once the filtered HCO_3^- is fully reabsorbed, the kidney is still required to eliminate an additional net amount of acid equivalent to that produced in metabolism. Most of this net acid excretion is in the form of ammonium (NH_4^+), which is derived from the renal synthesis of ammonia from glutamine in the proximal tubule and the titration of filtered phosphate to acid phosphate (titratable acidity).

$$NH_3 + H^+ \rightarrow NH_4^+ \; pK \; 9.1, \text{ and}$$

$$HPO_4^{2-} + H^+ \rightarrow H_2PO_4^- \; pK \; 6.8$$

Urinary Buffers

As the collecting duct cells continue to secrete H^+ into urine with a diminishing luminal HCO_3^- concentration and decreasing pH, H^+ is captured by the urinary buffers. The resulting alkalinization of the cells after H^+ leaves results in the formation of HCO_3^- ready for transport into blood. This process generates "new" HCO_3^- that is not a result of the reabsorption of filtered HCO_3^-. The amount of new HCO_3^- matches the amount of net acid eliminated and is also equal to each of the following: the amount of acid produced, the amount of body buffer consumed by that acid, and the amount of fixed acid anions, such as sulfate, phosphate, and Cl^-, that accompanied the H^+. The result is maintenance of normal acid-base equilibrium.

The ability of the kidney to lower urinary pH to values as low as 5.0 enables the buffers to capture a proton. Net acid excretion in urine is accomplished not simply by a decrease in urine pH but mostly by titration of these important urinary buffers. For example, a typical daily urine volume of 1 liter at pH 5.0 contains only 10^{-5} molar hydrogen ion, or 0.01 mmol, a trivial amount compared with the amount of produced acid (~1 mmol/kg/day). In chronic kidney disease, it is the failure to produce enough ammonium that leads to a poorly buffered, though acid, urine and an inability to excrete enough net acid to stay in normal balance.

Regulation of Urinary Acid Secretion

Renal mechanisms of urinary acidification are adaptable. Transport processes such as H^+-ATPases, Na/H exchange, and Cl/HCO_3 exchange can increase or decrease their capacity to handle acid-base equivalents, depending on the challenge presented. Renal ammoniagenic mechanisms are also critically regulated to serve the acid-base needs of the individual. Metabolic acidosis and respiratory acidosis increase the capacity to reabsorb HCO_3^-, including increased expression of the transporters involved in acidifying the urine. At the same time, increased glutamine uptake into proximal cells and ammonia production enables increased acid excretion and the generation of new HCO_3^- in the distal nephron. Metabolic alkalosis and respiratory alkalosis have the opposite effects.

Carbonic anhydrase is important in acid-secreting epithelia as well as in other cells, such as red blood cells, in which rapid interconversion of large quantities of CO_2 to HCO_3^- is required. In the proximal tubule, carbonic anhydrase exists not only within cells but also on the luminal brush border membrane, where it accelerates the dehydration of carbonic acid to CO_2, thereby allowing the large amount of HCO_3^- reabsorption in that segment. The distal nephron, which has a smaller requirement for bicarbonate reabsorption, lacks luminal carbonic anhydrase. However, intracellular carbonic anhydrase is present in all cells that transport CO_2 and HCO_3^-.

In acid-secreting cells, bicarbonate exits back to blood across the basolateral membrane as protons exit across the apical membrane. These processes are reversed in bicarbonate-secreting cells. In addition, the mechanisms of proton secretion and bicarbonate reabsorption may vary in different cell types.

Ammoniagenesis, which is a key element in urinary acid excretion, provides the major acceptor for protons. Ammonia is produced predominantly in the proximal tubule cell by mitochondrial glutaminase enzymes. Production is increased by increasing the metabolic acid load in the body, respiratory acidosis, and hypokalemia. NH_4^+ can preserve potassium in the hypokalemic state by serving as a counter-ion for anion excretion. Similarly, in response to metabolic acidosis, the kidney would ideally excrete chloride with ammonium and preserve Na^+ and K^+.

Ammonia can be secreted by nonionic diffusion into the proximal fluid, where it will pick up a proton and form ammonium (NH_4^+), or it could form ammonium within the proximal tubule cell and be secreted by Na/NH_4 exchange, a mode of operation of the Na/H exchanger. Ammonium may be reabsorbed by the thick ascending limb of Henle on the Na/K/2Cl transporter, where it can substitute for K^+. By countercurrent multiplication, NH_4^+ concentrates in the medullary interstitial fluid rather than remaining in the ascending limb fluid as it reaches the highly perfused renal cortex, where it could otherwise dissipate into renal venous blood. The countercurrent mechanism also allows for ammonia to diffuse into the lumen of the medullary collecting duct, where it will be trapped as ammonium in the acid tubular fluid. Collecting duct cells also secrete NH_3 by way of glycoproteins that are in the family of the Rh factor, red blood cell ammonia transporters.

Regulation is accomplished at a number of levels. Hormones such as angiotensin II and catecholamines stimulate Na^+ reabsorption in the proximal tubule by increasing Na/H exchange. Aldosterone increases H^+-ATPase in the distal collecting duct cell and stimulates Na^+ reabsorption, thereby increasing proton secretion. Low extracellular fluid volume increases proximal HCO_3^- reabsorption, as does hypokalemia and high P_{CO_2}. Hyperkalemia (Chapter 119) may limit urinary acidification by several mechanisms, including decreased ammonia synthesis, decreased NH_3 entering the countercurrent multiplier in the loop of Henle, and decreased H^+ secretion by ATPases in the collecting duct as the need to secrete K^+ predominates.

CLINICAL MANIFESTATIONS AND DIAGNOSIS

An acid-base disturbance never should be considered an isolated problem but always should alert the clinician to the possible presence of an important underlying condition. Anion gap acidoses usually represent important underlying metabolic conditions, ranging from sepsis (Chapter 108) to uremia (Chapter 132) to diabetic ketoacidosis (Chapter 236) to serious poisonings (Chapter 110). Specific renal abnormalities as well as diarrhea (Chapter 142) can cause hyperchloremic acidosis (Table 120-1). Metabolic alkaloses are commonly caused by renal abnormalities or the loss of acid from the stomach owing to vomiting or nasogastric suction (Table 120-2). Respiratory acidosis and alkalosis are related to ventilation, which is increased by conditions such as sepsis (Chapter 108) and anxiety and decreased in many pulmonary conditions (Chapter 86).

Assessment of clinical acid-base disturbances usually begins with measurement of arterial blood gases (Fig. 120-2 and Table 120-3). In some situations, venous blood can be used as an alternative, accounting for the fact that the normal venous pH is approximately 0.05 pH units more acid than arterial pH, and P_{CO_2} is 5 to 6 mm Hg higher than that of arterial blood. Venous bicarbonate concentrations are normally greater than arterial concentrations.

If arterial pH is below 7.35, acidemia is said to exist. If pH is greater than 7.45, alkalemia exists. However, several processes may simultaneously drive the pH upward or downward; these individual processes are known as *acidoses* or *alkaloses*. Because multiple processes may coexist, an abnormal pH is not always noted in acid-base disturbances. Because pH is related to the ratio of HCO_3^- to P_{CO_2}, the finding of an abnormal bicarbonate level alone also cannot define acidemia or alkalemia.

It is customary to define acid-base balance in terms of the hydrogen ion concentration, bicarbonate, and P_{CO_2}, where

$$CO_2 + H_2O <\rightarrow H_2CO_3 <\rightarrow H^+ + HCO_3^-$$

The addition of CO_2, as in respiratory acidosis, will increase the hydrogen and bicarbonate concentrations. Removal of CO_2, as in respiratory alkalosis, will decrease CO_2, protons, and bicarbonate. The addition of protons with an anion other than HCO_3^-, as in metabolic acidosis, will lead to increased

TABLE 120-1   CAUSES OF HYPERCHLOREMIC ACIDOSIS

TYPE	CAUSE
Renal with hypokalemia	Proximal RTA, type 2 Distal RTA, type 1 Some anion gap acidoses with high anion clearance
Renal with hyperkalemia	Type 4 RTA; hyporenin-hypoaldosteronism
Nonrenal with hypokalemia	Diarrhea Urinary diversions: ureteroileostomy, ureterosigmoidostomy
Nonrenal with hyperkalemia	$NaCl$, KCl, NH_4Cl, $CaCl_2$, Arg-HCl, Lys-HCl

RTA = renal tubular acidosis.

TABLE 120-2   CAUSES OF METABOLIC ALKALOSIS

TYPE	CAUSES
Renal, hypochloremic alkalosis: Cl responsive with urine Cl > 20	Loop and distal tubule diuretics Bartter's syndrome Gitelman's syndrome Posthypercapnic status
Nonrenal, hypochloremic alkalosis: Cl responsive with urine Cl < 20	Vomiting, nasogastric suction Chloridorrhea Villous adenoma
Renal, alkalosis with extracellular expansion: Cl unresponsive with urine Cl > 20	Hyperaldosteronism, primary and secondary Liddle's syndrome
Nonrenal alkalosis, Cl unresponsive	$NaHCO_3$, acetate, citrate, lactate
Other causes of metabolic alkalosis	Excessive non-reabsorbable anion excretion Hypoproteinemia

FIGURE 120-2. Evaluation of acidemia.

TABLE 120-3   LABORATORY STEPS IN IDENTIFYING ACID-BASE DISORDERS

EVALUATE pH	ACIDEMIC	ALKALEMIC
Elevated PCO_2	Respiratory acidosis	Metabolic alkalosis
Elevated HCO_3	Respiratory acidosis	Metabolic alkalosis
Decreased PCO_2	Metabolic acidosis	Respiratory alkalosis
Decreased HCO_3	Metabolic acidosis	Respiratory alkalosis

EVALUATE FOR EXPECTED COMPENSATION

Meets expectation: simple disorder with compensation or could be offsetting metabolic alkalosis and acidosis

Does not meet expectation: complex disorder, but pH indicates whether acidosis or alkalosis is dominant

If a metabolic disorder is dominant, a PCO_2 greater than predicted indicates an additional respiratory acidosis. A PCO_2 less than predicted indicates an additional respiratory alkalosis.

If a respiratory disorder is dominant, an HCO_3 concentration greater than predicted indicates additional metabolic alkalosis. An HCO_3 concentration less than predicted indicates an additional metabolic acidosis.

ASSESS ANION GAP

Elevated: metabolic acidosis is present whether acidemic or alkalemic. If alkalemic, an additional metabolic or respiratory alkalosis is present.

If the gap is greater than the fall in HCO_3, consider an additional metabolic alkalosis or respiratory acidosis.

If the gap is less than the fall in HCO_3, consider an additional nongap acidosis or respiratory alkalosis.

concentration. Metabolic alkalosis might be caused by the addition of $NaHCO_3$ with a resulting decrease in the proton concentration or by removal of H^+ with chloride, thereby leading to a decreased proton concentration and increased HCO_3^-.

Compensatory Changes

Few patients have an isolated acid-base disturbance. In nearly all cases, a respiratory or renal compensation (or both) occurs in response to counteract a primary acid-base disturbance.

With normal organ function, the lungs may maintain a normal pH and PCO_2 during changes in volatile acid production. The kidneys will also help maintain normal acid-base balance during changes in fixed acid production. Only excesses beyond the capacity to eliminate an acid or alkali load will lead to clinical disturbances. It follows that patients with renal or lung disease may do less well in response to metabolic and respiratory disorders.

When an acid-base disturbance develops, the initial response to modulate its severity depends on the titration of various body buffer pairs. For example, phosphate, hemoglobin, and albumin change their protonated and unprotonated concentrations. The body will then further attempt to correct the extracellular pH toward normal but usually not to normal. For metabolic disturbances caused by increased or decreased nonvolatile acid, the response is respiratory; for primary respiratory acidosis and alkalosis, the compensation is renal (Table 120-4). The direction of change in HCO_3^- and PCO_2 is the same when the primary disturbance is compensated; the ratio of HCO_3^- to PCO_2 and thus pH becomes more normal. These compensations tend to take time, so acid-base disturbances, particularly the respiratory conditions, are classified as acute (lasting less than 24 to 48 hours) or chronic.

Peripheral blood does not demonstrate complete compensation for most acid-base disturbances, with the occasional exception of chronic respiratory alkalosis. Yet the CNS closely regulates its pH, with nearly full correction within 1 to 2 days. Before this compensation occurs, acute alkalemia may be associated with cerebral vasoconstriction and ischemia, whereas acidemia may result in vasodilation and cerebral edema. Rapid changes in PCO_2 affect the CNS chemosensors more quickly than do changes in HCO_3^- because of the more rapid movement of nonionic CO_2 across the blood-brain barrier. Increases in CNS CO_2 lead to acidification of the medullary center interstitial fluid and an increased ventilatory drive. Decreases in CNS CO_2 lead to hypoventilation.

In metabolic acidosis, peripheral chemosensors in the carotid body stimulate the CNS to increase ventilation to reduce PCO_2. The fall in peripheral PCO_2 will lead to dissolved CO_2 leaving the CNS ahead of HCO_3^-; the alkalinization of the medullary center interstitial fluid will then slow the hyperventilatory response until a new steady state of hypocapnia is achieved.

concentrations of protons and a decreased bicarbonate concentration. This increase in CO_2 can be rapidly removed by the lungs because it constitutes a small additional amount of CO_2 over the usually produced quantities. Removal of HCO_3^- with a cation such as Na^+, also a cause of metabolic acidosis, will increase the proton concentration and lower the HCO_3^-

TABLE 120-4 EXPECTED DEGREES OF COMPENSATION IN ACID-BASE DISORDERS

DISORDER	EXPECTED COMPENSATION
Metabolic acidosis	Steady state in 12-36 hr Expected P_{CO_2} = 1.5 (measured HCO_3) + 8 ± 2
Metabolic alkalosis	Less predictable Expected P_{CO_2} increases 0.5 mm Hg per 1-mEq/L increase in HCO_3
Respiratory acidosis	
Acute	Expected 1-mEq/L increase in HCO_3 per 10-mm Hg rise in P_{CO_2}
Chronic, 24-36 hr	Expected 3- to 5-mEq/L increase in HCO_3 per 10-mm Hg rise in P_{CO_2}
Respiratory alkalosis	
Acute	Expected 1- to 2-mEq/L fall in HCO_3 per 10-mm Hg fall in P_{CO_2}
Chronic, after 24-36 hr	Expected 5-mEq/L fall in HCO_3 per 10-mm Hg fall in P_{CO_2}

Patients may sense dyspnea or air hunger acutely with rapid and shallow respirations. In severe cases of metabolic acidemia, the respirations are deep and gasping, typical of Kussmaul breathing.

When the bicarbonate concentration increases as a result of metabolic alkalosis, a hypoventilatory response, signaled from the peripheral chemosensors, raises P_{CO_2}. As P_{CO_2} rises, the dissolved CO_2 will enter the cerebrospinal fluid (CSF) and will acidify the medullary respiratory center. The stimulus to breathe will, in part, antagonize the peripheral signal until a steady state of hypoventilation is reached.

The acute stimulus of hypercapnia to increase net renal acid excretion disappears in chronic respiratory acidosis when, at the elevated P_{CO_2}, carbonic acid production and elimination are again equal. However, the hypochloremia, brought about by the compensatory early excretion of NH_4Cl, and elevated serum HCO_3^-, maintained by the high P_{CO_2}, persist.

In respiratory alkalosis, the primary event is a fall in P_{CO_2} because of increased alveolar ventilation. Upon transition from acute to chronic respiratory alkalosis, the compensatory mechanisms that initially helped maintain a more normal systemic pH are no longer required as CO_2 production and elimination become equal. Thus, the initial compensatory decrease in renal acid excretion brought about by increased loss of filtered $NaHCO_3$ ceases, but low serum HCO_3^- and high serum Cl^- concentrations are still maintained.

In identifying whether an acid-base disturbance is simple (a single disturbance with its compensation) or complex (multiple processes simultaneously present), it is useful to compare the expected compensation with the observed parameters of the blood gases (see Table 120-3). For example, if P_{CO_2} is lower than would be predicted in a patient with a simple, compensated metabolic acidosis, an additional respiratory alkalosis must be driving the P_{CO_2} down. If P_{CO_2} is higher than what would be predicted for a low bicarbonate level in a patient with metabolic acidosis, a coexistent respiratory acidosis is present.

METABOLIC ACIDOSIS

EPIDEMIOLOGY AND PATHOBIOLOGY

In metabolic acidosis, the primary change is a fall in serum bicarbonate. The compensatory response is to increase ventilation to reduce P_{CO_2}. Worsening acidosis elicits increasing alveolar ventilation.

Primary metabolic acidosis results from an imbalance between net acid production and net acid excretion (NAE) in the form of urinary ammonium and acid phosphate. Consider the following relationship, where U_x represents the urinary concentration and $\dot{V}$ the urinary flow rate:

$$NAE = (U_{NH_4^+} \dot{V}) + (U_{phos} \dot{V}) - (U_{bicarb} \dot{V})$$

In a normal steady-state condition, the rate of excretion of net acid must be equal to the rate of production. The normal production rate depends on diet. If net acid production is normal, metabolic acidosis could occur because of a failure to reabsorb bicarbonate or a failure to elaborate enough urinary buffers, as is the case in renal failure and renal tubular acidosis. An inequality also could develop if net acid production were excessive or if large extrarenal bicarbonate losses were unable to be matched by maximal adaptive increases

in net acid excretion. Endogenous sources of acid include ketoacidosis and lactic acidosis, whereas exogenous sources are metabolic products of ingested ethylene glycol or methanol. On occasion, strong inorganic acids may be ingested. When net acid is retained in body fluids, the serum bicarbonate concentration falls. However, maintenance of a constant serum HCO_3^- concentration does not guarantee that there is a new steady state in which net acid production is equal to net acid excretion because body buffers such as carbonate salts of bone may become depleted by relentless acid retention, as in renal failure and distal renal tubular acidosis.

The causes of metabolic acidosis are usually categorized according to the presence of either a normal or an elevated serum anion gap. The serum anion gap is the net charge difference when the sum of chloride and bicarbonate is subtracted from the serum sodium concentration.

$$Anion\ gap = Na^+ - (Cl^- + HCO_3^-)$$

The normal anion gap is due to the unmeasured anionic charge associated predominantly with albumin. When acidemia is present, albumin is in a more protonated form, which lowers the normal gap. In alkalemia, the effect of pH is to increase the gap attributed to albumin. Each 1 g/dL of albumin contributes approximately 2.8 mEq/L to the normal anion gap. The anion gap may be low with hypoalbuminemia or with an increase in unmeasured cations, such as immunoglobulin G myeloma paraproteins, calcium, lithium, or magnesium. When the anion gap is increased above the normal value of approximately 10 to 12 mEq/L by a nonchloride acid anion, an anion gap metabolic acidosis exists. The accompanying proton is responsible for lowering the serum bicarbonate concentration. The degree of increase in the anion gap, sometimes referred to as the *gap delta*, may be estimated by the difference between the observed anion gap and a normal value of 10 to 12 mEq/L. A similar calculation for a change in serum HCO_3^- can be made by subtracting the observed HCO_3^- from the normal value of about 25 mEq/L. Comparison of the two values (the *delta-delta*) may help identify more complicated acid-base disorders. If the increase in the anion gap is larger than the decrease in serum HCO_3^-, a process is raising the HCO_3^- level. The patient may have a coexisting metabolic alkalosis or be compensating for chronic respiratory acidosis. If the decreases in serum HCO_3^- are larger than the increases in the anion gap, a sign that another process is lowering the HCO_3^- level, the patient may have an additional hyperchloremic acidosis or respiratory alkalosis.

CLINICAL MANIFESTATIONS

The effects of metabolic acidosis depend on its rapidity of onset and severity. Patients often complain of fatigue and dyspnea, particularly on exertion. Nausea and vomiting are common. On examination, deep respirations, often labored with the use of accessory muscles, may be detected acutely, but hyperventilation may be less notable with long-standing metabolic acidemia. Metabolic acidemia also may be associated with vasodilation, tachycardia, and hypotension (Chapter 106). The negative inotropic effect of acidemia on the heart can exacerbate septic shock (Chapter 108). The stress of either an underlying illness or an increase in adrenergic and corticosteroid activity associated with acidemia may elevate the peripheral white blood cell count and cause hyperglycemia. Other laboratory findings include variable degrees of hyperkalemia, hyperphosphatemia, and hyperuricemia, as well as hypocalcemia as a result of decreased renal synthesis of 1,25-dihydroxyvitamin D.

Anion Gap Metabolic Acidoses

A variety of abnormalities can cause anion gap acidosis (Table 120-5). Other organic anions that may be detectable by special screening include hereditary disorders of methylmalonic aciduria or 5-oxoprolinuria. In patients who ingest acetaminophen and deplete intracellular glutathione, acquired 5-oxoprolinuria anion gap acidosis may occur.

UREMIC ACIDOSIS

The metabolic acidosis of advanced chronic kidney disease (Chapter 132) may be due to tubular leakage of HCO_3^-, but it is often present when inadequate ammonia production is unable to facilitate excretion of the normal metabolic acid load. Many patients with renal failure can acidify their urine, but the lack of buffering capacity diminishes net acid excretion. Many organic and inorganic anions, such as phosphate and sulfates, are retained at glomerular filtration rates of less than 25 mL/minute and constitute an increased anion gap in association with the metabolic acidosis. The magnitude of the gap is usually less than 20 mEq/L.

The systemic acid-base disturbance in renal diseases that particularly target the renal tubules is attributable to the kidney's inability to secrete hydrogen

TABLE 120-5	CAUSES OF INCREASED ANION AND OSMOLAL GAPS	
ANION GAP METABOLIC ACIDOSIS		**OSMOLAL GAP**
Uremia		No
Lactic acidosis		Variable/no
D-Lactic acidosis		No
Diabetic ketoacidosis		No
Starvation ketoacidosis		No
Alcoholic ketoacidosis		If ethanol is present
Ethylene glycol		Yes
Methanol		Yes
Salicylates		No
5-Oxoprolinuria (acetaminophen)		No

and to reabsorb and generate HCO_3^-. It is particularly pronounced in oliguric acute renal failure and is exacerbated by hypercatabolic states such as infection. A significant metabolic acidosis in a patient with chronic kidney disease of unknown cause should raise the possibility of urinary tract obstruction (Chapter 125) or chronic tubulointerstitial diseases (Chapter 124), including amyloidosis (Chapter 194), myeloma (Chapter 193), autoimmune disorders and analgesic nephropathy (Chapter 124).

The presentation and approach to uremia are discussed in Chapters 132 and 133. It is important to treat the metabolic acidosis of chronic kidney disease. Maintaining the serum HCO_3^- concentration above 20 to 22 mEq/L, by administering $NaHCO_3$ at a rate of 1 mEq HCO_3^-/kg/day, will slow the progression of chronic kidney disease, delay end-stage renal failure, and improve nutritional state.[1]

OVERPRODUCTION OF ENDOGENOUS ACIDS
Lactic Acidosis

EPIDEMIOLOGY AND PATHOBIOLOGY

Lactic acidosis is caused by an imbalance in the rates of lactate production and its clearance, primarily in the liver. Lactic acidosis, which increases the anion gap, is most often due to impaired lactate clearance owing to circulatory failure, hypoxia, and mitochondrial dysfunction that increase anaerobic glycolysis and the rate of conversion of pyruvate to lactate. Other causes are thiamine deficiency (Chapter 221), hypophosphatemia (Chapter 121), isoniazid toxicity (Chapter 110), and hypoglycemic states (Chapter 238). Metformin may cause lactic acidosis, particularly in elderly patients with cardiac, hepatic, or renal dysfunction. Nucleoside antivirals (Chapter 396), including zidovudine, may cause lactic acidosis and abnormal liver function as a result of toxic mitochondrial effects. Abnormal mitochondrial function is also a feature of aspirin overdose (Chapter 36) or toxicity with hypoglycin from ingestion of the unripe akee fruit (Jamaican vomiting sickness).

Lactic acidosis can also be caused by the overproduction of lactate, which may occur with severe exertion and malignancies, particularly with a large tumor burden from lymphoma or widely metastatic cancer. Malignant cells can upregulate glycolytic activity, which may increase their uptake of glucose and decrease their dependence on mitochondrion-derived energy.

Lactate, the final product in the anaerobic pathway of glucose metabolism, is produced from pyruvate by the following reaction catalyzed by lactate dehydrogenase:

$$NADH + pyruvate + H^+ \rightarrow lactate + NAD$$

CLINICAL MANIFESTATIONS

Symptoms and signs are related to the underlying cause as well as to the metabolic acidosis itself (see earlier). Sepsis (Chapter 108) is associated with an elevated lactate level because of poor clearance and impaired gluconeogenesis. Lactic acidosis can also result from seizure activity (Chapter 410) when lactate is released from muscle cells that have sustained a period of anaerobic metabolism.

A high reduced nicotinamide adenine dinucleotide (NADH)/NAD ratio will favor lactate formation. Conversion of ethanol to acetaldehyde and conversion of β-hydroxybutyrate to acetoacetate uses NAD and

produces NADH. Alcohol metabolism may be associated with excessive β-hydroxybutyrate and lactic acidosis.

DIAGNOSIS

In any patient with an anion gap acidosis, the serum lactate level should be directly measured. Glucose, creatinine, and blood urea nitrogen levels also should be obtained. In cases in which a toxic ingestion is suspected (see Table 120-5), a screen for such toxins in the serum should be performed.

TREATMENT

Treatment of lactic acidosis is aimed at correcting the underlying cause. Tissue perfusion and ventilation should be restored if possible. Sodium bicarbonate therapy should be considered when the arterial pH is below 7.0 or when acidemia has resulted in decreased cardiac inotropy or systemic vasodilation and shock. It is preferable to give $NaHCO_3$ as an isotonic mixture in 5% dextrose and water, rather than as a hypertonic bolus, because the latter carries the risk of pulmonary edema and hypernatremia. The quantity of administered sodium bicarbonate to raise arterial pH to 7.2 should be estimated by multiplying the desired minus observed bicarbonate concentration by the estimated total body water. Full correction should be avoided. Bicarbonate treatment of less severe lactic acidosis is controversial. In a randomized trial of patients with lactic acidosis (pH 6.9 to 7.2 and an average 7.8-mM lactate level) in an intensive care unit, sodium bicarbonate infused at a rate of 2 mEq/kg per 15 minutes did not improve hemodynamics, despite improvement in pH, but adversely lowered ionized serum calcium compared with saline.[2] In patients with a metabolic acidosis after seizures (Chapter 410), the lactate is quickly metabolized to HCO_3^- by the liver and kidneys, and the acidosis often resolves within 60 minutes. The administration of HCO_3^- is usually unnecessary and may precipitate an overshoot metabolic alkalosis as the lactate is metabolized, which lowers the seizure threshold.

In patients with intestinal bacterial overgrowth (Chapter 142), a syndrome of disorientation, ataxia, and anion gap metabolic acidosis may develop after a carbohydrate meal because of bacterial production of D-lactate. This isomer of the mammalian L-lactate can be measured only by a specific D-lactate assay. The condition is treated with oral antibiotics and appropriate diet.

PROGNOSIS

Lactic acidosis when severe is associated with a high early mortality. When the pH is less than 7.2, only 17% of patients who are admitted to an intensive care unit are ultimately discharged from the hospital.

Diabetic Ketoacidosis

EPIDEMIOLOGY AND PATHOBIOLOGY

Diabetic ketoacidosis is defined as hyperglycemia with metabolic acidosis resulting from generation of the acid anions β-hydroxybutyrate and acetoacetate in response to insulin deficiency and elevated counter-regulatory hormones such as glucagon. It is most commonly seen in cases of type 1 diabetes mellitus (Chapter 236) but can occasionally be seen in type 2 diabetes mellitus (Chapter 237).

The lack of insulin increases lipolysis in adipose tissue; free fatty acids are transported to the liver, where hepatic mitochondria produce ketone bodies, including acetoacetate, from acetyl coenzyme A. In the presence of high NADH/NAD ratio, the more reduced form of β-hydroxybutyrate is produced.

CLINICAL MANIFESTATIONS

Symptoms include nausea, vomiting, anorexia, polydipsia, and polyuria. Patients often exhibit Kussmaul respirations and volume depletion. Neurologic symptoms include fatigue and lethargy with depression of the sensorium. CSF exhibits a change in acid-base status with treatment of diabetic ketoacidosis. Even without bicarbonate administration, CSF pH falls as a result of the ventilatory response to the correction of acidosis and the sudden rise in PCO_2. However, no correlation between decreased CSF pH and depression of sensorium has been established. Ketoacidosis is also seen in cases of starvation, in which it is generally mild and not associated with hyperglycemia.

Ketoacids in the urine may be accompanied by cations, including sodium and potassium, thereby contributing to volume depletion, potassium depletion, relative chloride retention, and a mixed anion gap and hyperchloremic acidosis. The "delta HCO_3^-" will exceed the "delta anion gap," especially if the glomerular filtration rate and the filtered load of ketoacids are high. The serum anion gap in general will be greatest when renal failure is present because the additional anions cannot be cleared from extracellular fluid.

DIAGNOSIS

The urinary dipstick nitroprusside test for ketones may underestimate the degree of ketosis because it does not detect β-hydroxybutyrate; in fact, the ketone test may become more positive as treatment helps metabolize β-hydroxybutyrate to acetoacetate. This problem should be addressed by direct measurement of serum β-hydroxybutyrate. Diabetic patients also are more prone to lactic acidosis because an increase in NADH favors the formation of lactate from pyruvate, and pyruvate dehydrogenase is inhibited in the absence of insulin.

TREATMENT   Rx

Treatment of diabetic ketoacidosis (Chapter 236) consists of volume repletion, insulin administration with dextrose if necessary to avoid hypoglycemia, and potassium replacement (Chapter 119). Bicarbonate administration should be considered only if ketoacidosis is accompanied by shock or if arterial pH is less than 7.0 or 7.1, and bolus infusion should be avoided. The administration of bicarbonate occasionally results in cerebral edema significant enough to lead to loss of consciousness and even death.

PROGNOSIS

Most patients with diabetic ketoacidosis recover. In the less than 0.5% of patients who present with coma from cerebral edema, the mortality rate ranges from 20% to as high as 90%. The cerebral edema may be exacerbated by bicarbonate administration, which is discouraged in this situation.

Salicylate Intoxication

EPIDEMIOLOGY AND PATHOBIOLOGY

Salicylate intoxication can be caused by accidental overdose, therapeutic overdose, or a suicide attempt (Chapters 36 and 110). Salicylate functions as an uncoupler of oxidative phosphorylation and consequently results in increased oxygen consumption and CO_2 production. However, the increase in alveolar ventilation resulting from stimulation of central chemoreceptors overcomes this increase in CO_2.

CLINICAL MANIFESTATIONS AND DIAGNOSIS

The most common clinical manifestation is a combined anion gap metabolic acidosis and respiratory alkalosis, although the condition also can be manifested as either one or the other only. Children are often seen with metabolic acidosis, whereas adults often have predominant respiratory alkalosis. Hypoglycemia, ketoacidosis, and lactic acidosis may result. Other manifestations of intoxication include hemorrhage, fever, nausea and vomiting, hyperventilation, diaphoresis, tinnitus, and occasionally polyuria followed by oliguria. Severe cases may lead to seizures, respiratory depression, and coma. Noncardiogenic pulmonary edema is sometimes seen in adults.

Respiratory alkalosis is the result of a direct stimulatory effect of salicylate on the medullary respiratory control center. Salicylate intoxication also increases the metabolic rate. Diagnosis is suspected by the clinical presentation and confirmed by the salicylate level (Chapters 36 and 110).

Treatment of salicylate intoxication (Chapter 110) is aimed at correcting the metabolic acidosis and removing salicylate. Bicarbonate as a sodium salt should be administered according to an estimated calculation of the deficit if metabolic acidosis predominates. Salicylates are removed by alkaline diuresis because the less reabsorbable salicylate anion will predominate when the urine pH increases. Urinary alkalinization with acetazolamide is not advised because carbonic anhydrase inhibition may impair CO_2 transport from tissue to blood and potentially worsen acidosis in the respiratory center. In severe intoxication (salicylate concentrations greater than 35 mg/dL) or when renal failure is present, dialysis may be required.

PROGNOSIS

The prognosis of salicylate toxicity is better with early diagnosis and prompt management, in which case most patients do well. Patients who ingest oil of wintergreen (methylsalicylate) may have more severe deterioration because of the highly lipid soluble form of the drug.

Alcoholic Ketoacidosis

EPIDEMIOLOGY AND PATHOBIOLOGY

Alcoholic ketoacidosis occurs in a patient who has been drinking very heavily without eating. The pathophysiology is based on the overproduction of β-hydroxybutyrate and, to a lesser extent, acetoacetate because of an increased production of free fatty acids. Alcohol inhibits the conversion of lactate to glucose in the liver. The oxidation of ethanol increases the ratio of NADH to NAD^+ and favors the production of β-hydroxybutyrate. Damage to mitochondria by alcohol can further elevate the ratio of β-hydroxybutyrate to acetoacetate by preventing reoxidation of NADH to NAD. The oxidative metabolism of ethanol favors the reaction of dehydrogenase enzymes to form β-hydroxybutyrate and lactate (opposing glucose production).

CLINICAL MANIFESTATIONS

Alcoholic ketoacidosis usually follows binge drinking and may be associated with withdrawal symptoms (Chapters 32 and 425) and the associated hyperadrenergic state. Alcoholic ketoacidosis is associated with abdominal pain, vomiting, starvation, and volume depletion. In contrast to diabetic ketoacidosis, coma is rare. Blood glucose levels are generally low or normal, and the insulin level is frequently low, with elevated glucagon and cortisol levels. Some patients have hyperglycemia because of the increased catecholamine response.

DIAGNOSIS

Patients typically have a high osmolal gap initially (defined as the difference between the measured and the calculated serum osmolality).

$$\text{Calculated osmolality} = 2(Na^+) + (\text{Glucose }[\text{mg/dL}] \div 18) + (\text{Blood urea nitrogen }[\text{mg/dL}] \div 2.8)$$

Blood alcohol levels may be absent or elevated on initial evaluation. A clue to the diagnosis of toxic alcohol ingestion is the simultaneous presence of an anion gap metabolic acidosis and an osmolal gap. This osmolal gap, if secondary to ethanol, should be equal to the ethanol concentration in milligrams per deciliter divided by 4.6. If this calculation does not yield the expected gap based on the ethanol concentration, ingestion of another alcohol such as methanol, isopropanol, or ethylene glycol should be suspected (see Table 120-2).

The serum osmolality should be measured by a freezing point depression technique and compared with the calculated osmolality. If possible, ethanol, ethylene glycol, propylene glycol, and methanol levels should be measured directly; each is associated with a metabolic acidosis. In contrast, isopropanol metabolizes to acetone and causes ketosis without acidosis.

TREATMENT   Rx

Treatment of alcoholic metabolic acidosis consists of volume repletion with normal saline in dextrose; the administration of thiamine (50 to 100 mg intravenously) and enough glucose to treat hypoglycemia; and the correction of any hypophosphatemia (Chapter 121), hypokalemia (Chapter 119), and hypomagnesemia (Chapter 121) that may be present. The acid-base disturbance usually resolves after several hours. Both hypophosphatemia and thiamine deficiency, which may not be apparent until 12 to 24 hours after the initiation of treatment in an undernourished patient, are exacerbated by glucose administration.

PROGNOSIS

The prognosis of alcoholic ketoacidosis is usually favorable. The long-term outlook is more closely tied to other complications of continued alcohol abuse.

Ethylene Glycol

Ethylene glycol (Chapter 110) is commonly found in antifreeze and is used as an industrial solvent. It has a sweet taste, and patients occasionally ingest it as a substitute for ethanol. Although ethylene glycol itself is not particularly damaging, its highly toxic metabolites include glyoxylate, glycolate, oxalic acid, and ketoaldehydes. Glycolic acid appears to be primarily responsible for the metabolic acidosis observed in this condition.

Intoxication is characterized by profound CNS symptoms, including seizures and coma, severe metabolic acidosis, and cardiac, pulmonary, and renal failure. Patients are often dehydrated because of osmotic diuresis from the renal excretion of the alcohol.

An increased anion gap is attributable to ethylene glycol metabolites. A high osmolal gap will also be present because of the uncharged alcohol. However, an osmolal gap may not be present if all of the alcohol has been converted to the toxic anionic forms. Calcium oxalate crystals in the urine may cause intratubular obstruction and acute renal failure. Treatment is aimed at rehydration with saline and correction of acidosis with $NaHCO_3$ based on an estimate of the bicarbonate deficit. When an osmolal gap exists, competitive inhibition of alcohol dehydrogenase should be initiated with fomepizole at a loading dose of 15 to 20 mg/kg intravenously in 100 mL normal saline over 30 minutes to 1 hour, followed by a maintenance dose of 10 mg/kg every 12 hours (Chapter 110). If ethanol is used, a solution of 10% ethanol in 5% dextrose can be given as a loading dose of 0.6 g/kg intravenously followed by a maintenance dose of 150 mg/kg per hour in alcoholic patients, or 65 mg/kg per hour in nonalcoholic patients. The ethanol level should be maintained at a 100 to 200 mg/dL. The goal of therapy is early recognition to prevent metabolism of the uncharged glycol to acidic products. Hemodialysis is required in severe cases. If the diagnosis is made promptly and appropriate therapy is instituted, outcomes are favorable. Renal failure may be reversible.

Methanol

Methanol, wood alcohol, is a component of shellac and windshield wiper fluid and is highly toxic to the CNS after metabolism to formaldehyde and formic acid. Optic papillitis may cause blindness. Treatment consists of competitive inhibitors for alcohol dehydrogenase, including ethanol or fomepizole, in similar amounts as for ethylene glycol poisoning, to reduce the formation of acid anions and the anion gap while maintaining a higher level of methanol in the blood (Chapter 110). Hemodialysis may be necessary to increase elimination.

Early diagnosis and treatment are associated with a favorable outcome, but visual loss may be permanent. Late presentation is associated with a poor prognosis, particularly if the amount consumed exceeds 30 mL. As with ethylene glycol, the simultaneous presence of ethanol on presentation may help slow the metabolism of methanol and improve outcome.

Isopropyl Alcohol

Toxic ingestion of isopropyl alcohol, as in rubbing alcohol, does not cause an increased anion gap or ketoacidosis because the metabolite is acetone, but tests for ketones are positive and a high osmolal gap will be present.

Propylene Glycol

Occasionally, patients in the intensive care unit setting are given high doses of intravenous benzodiazepines, such as lorazepam or diazepam, that contain propylene glycol as a diluents. Other intravenous medications that also contain this diluent include phenobarbital, phenytoin, nitroglycerine, and esmolol. Propylene glycol has also been used as a less toxic substitute for methanol in windshield wiper fluid. A high osmolal gap may develop because of the propylene glycol and lead to a clinical picture of sedation, failure to wean from the respirator, and an increased lactate level. Propylene glycol metabolites include lactate and pyruvate. Treatment, which consists of early recognition and withdrawal of the offending agent, usually results in a favorable prognosis.

Hyperchloremic (Normal Anion Gap) Acidosis

Hyperchloremic metabolic acidoses (see Table 120-1) can be caused by renal or nonrenal mechanisms and can be associated with an elevated, normal, or low serum potassium level.

Hyperchloremic Metabolic Acidosis of Nonrenal Origin Associated with Normal or Increased Potassium

Hyperchloremic metabolic acidoses with a normal or elevated potassium concentration can develop as a result of the addition of chloride salts such as $NaCl$, KCl, $CaCl_2$, NH_4Cl, arginine and lysine hydrochlorides, or HCl itself. If the quantity of Cl^- introduced exceeds the ability of the kidney to eliminate Cl^- salts in urine, hyperchloremia will develop. Electroneutrality is maintained by a decrease in the serum HCO_3^- concentration, and a hyperchloremic acidosis ensues. Renal production of NH_3 increases in an attempt to improve HCl excretion. Hyperkalemia can occur because the acidemia favors the exit of K^+ from cells. Hyperkalemia also inhibits K^+ secretion in the renal collecting duct.

Hyperchloremic Metabolic Acidosis of Nonrenal Origin Associated with Hypokalemia

Hypokalemic, hyperchloremic acidosis may result from loss of a body fluid that is low in Cl^- relative to Na^+ and K^+ when compared with the ratio of Cl^- to Na^+ in extracellular fluid. For example, stool losses of Na^+, K^+, and HCO_3^- in small bowel diarrhea or organic acid anions of bacterial origin in colonic diarrhea lead to hyperchloremic acidosis (Chapter 142). Pancreatic secretions (Chapter 201) or heavy losses from ileostomy sites may lead to loss of bicarbonate-containing fluids. Secretagogues such as vasoactive intestinal peptide (VIP), which is associated with neoplasms of the pancreas or sympathetic chain (Chapter 201), cause large losses of HCO_3^- in stool, with a resulting hypokalemic, hyperchloremic metabolic acidosis. Concomitant gastric achlorhydria is part of the syndrome known as *watery diarrhea, hypokalemic, hypochlorhydric acidosis*. Urinary diversions, such as ureterosigmoidostomies and ileal loops, may increase chloride absorption in exchange for bicarbonate in the intestinal segment and lead to hyperchloremic acidosis.

RENAL TUBULAR ACIDOSIS TYPES 1 AND 2
Proximal Renal Tubular Acidosis

Renal tubular acidosis causes the cations Na^+ and K^+ to be lost in the urine with HCO_3^- rather than Cl^-, thereby leading to hyperchloremia. Proximal renal tubular acidosis (type 2) is characterized by a decreased threshold for bicarbonate reabsorption. HCO_3^- wasting and concomitant urinary losses of potassium occur until a lower level of serum bicarbonate reduces the filtered HCO_3^- to a level that the renal tubule can completely reabsorb.

Isolated proximal renal tubular acidosis may result from mutations of specific transporters of the proximal tubule, such as the $NaHCO_3$ cotransporter, or from hereditary deficiency of carbonic anhydrase. More commonly, proximal renal tubular acidosis is associated with generalized proximal tubule dysfunction. Causes (Table 120-6) include genetic diseases such as glucose-6-phosphatase deficiency (Chapter 164), cystinosis (Chapter 130), hereditary fructose intolerance (Chapter 212), and Wilson's disease (Chapter 218). Multiple myeloma (Chapter 193) and Sjögren's syndrome (Chapter 276) should be considered in an adult patient. Primary hyperparathyroidism (Chapter 253) results in proximal renal tubular acidosis and hypophosphatemia secondary to inhibition of Na/H exchange and sodium phosphate cotransport in the proximal tubule. Drug toxicity with aminoglycosides, tenofovir, cisplatin, and ifosfamide may cause proximal tubule dysfunction. The syndrome also may be seen after kidney transplantation (Chapter 133).

Distal Renal Tubular Acidosis

In distal renal tubular acidosis (type 1), failure to produce ammonia leads to an inability to excrete net acid, thereby leading to continuous retention of acid in the body. The degree of acidemia is often severe, with pH reaching values as low as 7.2, whereas urine pH usually exceeds 5.3.

Kindreds have been described in which mutations in genes for the distal vacuolar H^+-ATPase cause an autosomal recessive distal renal tubular acidosis with deafness. Mutations resulting in defective Cl/HCO_3 exchange protein (AE1) have been linked to an autosomal dominant form of distal renal tubular acidosis.

Distal renal tubular acidosis (see Table 120-6) is also associated with autoimmune disorders, including systemic lupus erythematosus (Chapter 274) and Sjögren's syndrome (Chapter 276), and genetic diseases, including sickle cell anemia (Chapter 166), Wilson's disease (Chapter 218), Fabry's disease (Chapter 215), cystic kidney diseases (Chapter 129), and hereditary elliptocytosis (Chapter 164). Hypercalciuria and hyperoxaluria may cause distal renal tubular acidosis; nephrocalcinosis may be present. Amyloidosis (Chapter 194) may be manifested as severe acidemia and other tubular dysfunction, including nephrogenic diabetes insipidus. Tubulointerstitial disease of the kidney (Chapter 124), including reflux nephropathy and urinary obstruction, may result in renal tubular acidosis with hypokalemia or hyperkalemia. Drugs such as amphotericin B can cause hypokalemic distal renal tubular acidosis.

HYPERCHLOREMIC METABOLIC ACIDOSIS OF RENAL ORIGIN ASSOCIATED WITH HYPERKALEMIA

Hyperkalemic, hyperchloremic acidosis (type 4) suggests dysfunction of the cortical collecting duct, where acidification of urine and disorders in potassium secretion may occur. Some patients with high blood potassium and hyperchloremic acidosis can lower urinary pH below 5.3, whereas others appear to have defects in both potassium balance and urinary acidification. Hyperkalemia itself may worsen metabolic acidosis by decreasing NH_3 accumulation by countercurrent multiplication in the medullary interstitium.

TABLE 120-6 CAUSES OF RENAL TUBULAR ACIDOSIS*

HYPOKALEMIC DISTAL (TYPE 1) RTA

Hereditary tubule disorders
  Vacuolar H^+/ATPase β-subunit gene mutations
  Carbonic anhydrase type II deficiency
  Cl/HCO_3 exchanger (AE-1) mutations
Genetic causes
  Sickle cell
  Fabry's disease
  Wilson's disease
  Elliptocytosis
  Paroxysmal nocturnal hemoglobinuria
  Medullary cystic kidneys
Autoimmune disorders
  Systemic lupus erythematosus
  Sjögren's syndrome
Multiple myeloma and amyloidosis
Drugs: amphotericin, cisplatinum, aminoglycosides
Nephrocalcinosis and hypercalcemic disorders
Tubulointerstitial diseases
  Acute tubulointerstitial nephritis
  Reflux nephropathy
  Analgesic nephropathy

PROXIMAL (TYPE 2) RTA

Hereditary tubule disorders
  Na HCO_3 cotransport (NBC) mutations
  Carbonic anhydrase deficiency
Generalized proximal tubular dysfunction
  Hereditary Fanconi's syndrome
  Genetic diseases: cystinosis, glycogen storage disease (glucose-6-phosphatase deficiency), Wilson's disease
  Hormonal: hyperparathyroidism, vitamin D deficiency
  Multiple myeloma, lysozymuria
  Sjögren's syndrome
  Renal transplantation
  Heavy metals: cobalt, mercury, lead
  Drugs: ifosfamide, outdated tetracycline, tenofovir, tacrolimus, aminoglycosides

HYPERKALEMIC (TYPE 4) RTA

Renal diseases-aldosterone resistance
  Diabetes mellitus
  Amyloidosis
  Systemic lupus erythematosus
  Urinary tract obstruction
Hyporeninism
  Autonomic neuropathy (diabetic)
  Sickle cell anemia
Primary hypoaldosteronism
Adrenal insufficiency: Addison's disease,
Tubular mutations: pseudohypoaldosteronism
Drugs: K-sparing diuretics, amiloride, triamterene, spironolactone, nonsteroidal anti-inflammatory drugs, lithium, trimethoprim, cyclosporine, tacrolimus, renin inhibitors, angiotensin-converting enzyme inhibitors, angiotensin II receptor antagonists

*Type 3 renal tubular acidosis (RTA) is not listed separately because it is an overlap of proximal and distal dysfunction.

Causes include hyporenin-hypoaldosteronism, as seen in diabetic renal disease (Chapter 126); other tubulointerstitial diseases (Chapter 124), usually with some renal impairment; sickle cell anemia (Chapter 166); or the use of drugs such as β-blockers and nonsteroidal anti-inflammatory drugs. Low renin and aldosterone levels can also be found in cases of volume expansion with hypertension. Cyclosporine and tacrolimus may lead to decreased electrical driving forces for K^+ and H^+ secretion. Hyperkalemic acidosis with elevated renin and low aldosterone is found in adrenal insufficiency (Chapter 234), isolated hypoaldosteronism (Chapter 234), and the use of angiotensin-converting enzyme inhibitors, renin inhibitors, and angiotensin II receptor blockers. High renin and aldosterone levels are anticipated when the renal collecting duct cell is insensitive to aldosterone, as in urinary tract obstruction, sickle cell anemia, amyloidosis, and systemic lupus erythematosus. Inhibition of aldosterone action with spironolactone or eplerenone may cause hyperkalemic acidosis, as does ENaC inhibition by amiloride and triamterene.

Pseudohypoaldosteronism type 1 is due to autosomal recessive, inactivating mutations of the Na^+ channel ENaC, whereas autosomal dominant

pseudohypoaldosteronism type 1 is due to mutations of the mineralocorticoid receptor. Both cause hypovolemia, metabolic acidosis, and hyperkalemia with secondary increases in renin and aldosterone. In Gordon's syndrome (pseudohypoaldosteronism type 2), increases in Na^+ and Cl^- reabsorption through increased activity of the distal thiazide-sensitive NaCl transporter lead to hypertension, hyperkalemic acidosis, volume expansion, and consequently, low renin and aldosterone. Type 3 renal tubular acidosis is the syndrome of combined proximal and distal renal tubular acidosis.

CLINICAL MANIFESTATIONS AND DIAGNOSIS

The urinary anion gap helps distinguish renal tubular acidosis from extrarenal bicarbonate loss (e.g., from diarrhea). Because the normal renal response to metabolic acidosis is an increase in ammoniagenesis, the urine should contain large amounts of NH_4Cl while the kidney retains sodium and potassium; the urinary anion gap, which is $(Na^+ + K^+) - Cl^-$, should be strongly negative because of the unmeasured NH_4^+.

In renal diseases such as distal renal tubular acidosis, however, the urinary anion gap will be zero or positive because of either the failure of ammoniagenesis or the excretion of sodium plus potassium with bicarbonate. With type 2 (proximal) renal tubular acidosis, patients often have Fanconi's syndrome with glycosuria, phosphaturia, aminoaciduria, and uricosuria. In proximal renal tubular acidosis, the steady-state urine pH is usually less than 5.3, the acidosis is not severe (i.e., HCO_3^- usually not less than 16), and acid excretion may balance acid production at this new steady state.

In contrast to proximal renal tubular acidosis, distal renal tubular acidosis (type I) is generally a more severe metabolic disorder that may be accompanied by hypercalciuria, nephrocalcinosis, calcium phosphate kidney stones (Chapter 128), and bone disease that includes rickets in children and osteomalacia in adults. Although rarely necessary to perform, the NH_4Cl loading test can confirm the diagnosis of distal renal tubular acidosis. In this test, the plasma bicarbonate is lowered by an acid challenge. If urine pH remains above 5.3, a distal abnormality is suspected. Proximal and distal renal tubular acidoses usually can be distinguished by a careful clinical evaluation (Fig. 120-3). Helpful findings include the presence of a urine pH greater than 5.3 in distal but not proximal renal tubular acidosis during acidemia; a fractional excretion of bicarbonate as high as 10 to 15% in proximal renal tubular acidosis; and the lowering of serum potassium upon correction of proximal but not distal tubular acidosis.

In patients with an elevated serum anion gap, unmeasured anions such as ketoacids and lactate, rather than NH_4^+, are present in urine, so a positive urinary anion gap does not indicate renal tubular acidosis. On occasion, however, the prompt renal excretion of organic anions with sodium and potassium may minimize the increase in the serum anion gap. In the metabolic acidosis of glue sniffers, hippurate, which is a product of toluene, is rapidly excreted, thus giving the appearance of a nongap metabolic acidosis with a positive urinary anion gap.

TREATMENT   Rx

If possible, treatment of metabolic acidosis should focus on correcting the underlying cause and permitting the body's homeostatic mechanisms to correct the acid-base disturbance. Patients whose pH is less than 7.2 are typically treated with infusions of sodium bicarbonate, guided by the estimated base deficit in milliequivalents, calculated using the serum HCO_3^- concentration in milliequivalents per liter:

$$\text{Amount of } HCO_3^- = (25 - [HCO_3^-]) \times \text{wt (kg)}/2$$

In general, the correction of metabolic acidemia should be based on a calculated amount, with not more than 50% of the estimate given before recalculation. Moreover, this equation is used for deficit correction only; the ongoing losses of 1 to 2 mEq/kg per day, equivalent to the daily acid load, should be replaced in distal renal tubular acidosis with $NaHCO_3$, $KHCO_3$, or citrate salts in divided doses. Hypokalemia may accompany distal renal tubular acidosis and may improve with treatment.

Proximal renal tubular acidosis in children may affect growth and require large quantities of bicarbonate in excess of 1 to 2 mEq/kg per day to correct the acidosis because ingested alkali is promptly excreted in alkaline urine. In adults, treatment is often deferred because the steady state acidosis allows for a normal acid excretion rate. Hypokalemia may worsen with bicarbonate treatment of proximal renal tubular acidosis.

In type 4 renal tubular acidosis, treatment of hyperkalemia with a low potassium diet, thiazide, or loop diuretics or sodium polystyrene sulfonate often improves urinary acidification without the use of bicarbonate salts.

FIGURE 120-3. Diagnosis of renal tubular acidosis (RTA). FE = fractional excretion; NaHCO₃ = sodium bicarbonate.

PROGNOSIS

The prognosis of renal tubular acidosis generally depends on the presence of an underlying systemic disease, such as myeloma (Chapter 193). In children, disorders such as medullary cystic kidney disease (Chapter 129) or cystinosis (Chapter 130) usually result in renal failure by the teenage years. These patients are candidates for renal replacement therapy, including transplantation. Chronic metabolic acidosis in children, if not well treated, is associated with rickets (Chapter 252) and short stature.

● METABOLIC ALKALOSIS

EPIDEMIOLOGY AND PATHOBIOLOGY

In metabolic alkalosis, the primary event is elevation of the plasma bicarbonate concentration. In response to increased systemic pH, alveolar ventilation is decreased to increase Pco_2 and thereby decrease pH. However, respiratory compensation is generally less effective in cases of metabolic alkalosis than in cases of metabolic acidosis. Contributing factors may include the fact that hypoventilation also decreases Po_2, which is a potent stimulus for the peripheral chemoreceptors to increase alveolar ventilation when Po_2 falls below about 60 mm Hg. A second mechanism that may blunt respiratory compensation is intracellular acidosis in the brain in the setting of hypokalemia. In acute metabolic alkalosis, an initial paradoxical acidotic shift in CSF pH secondary to a sudden increase in Pco_2, similar to the alkaline shift in CSF pH in acute metabolic acidosis, may activate central chemoreceptors and increase ventilatory drive despite peripheral stimulation to decrease alveolar ventilation. In chronic metabolic alkalosis, CSF pH may return to normal, so respiratory drive is controlled entirely by the peripheral chemoreceptors. The result is that the ventilatory response to metabolic alkalosis is highly varied: many patients with metabolic alkalosis maintain nearly normal Pco_2 levels, and the level rarely rises above 60 mm Hg.

Metabolic alkalosis requires a generation phase, in which new HCO_3^- is added to the extracellular fluid, and a maintenance phase, in which the new elevated serum HCO_3^- concentration is sustained. Without the latter phase, a kidney with normal filtration and tubular function has a high capacity to excrete HCO_3^-, thereby preventing alkalosis. Maintenance of a high HCO_3^- concentration usually occurs because of volume depletion, a reduced glomerular filtration rate, hypokalemia, or low chloride levels.

Metabolic Alkalosis of Renal Origin Associated with Volume Depletion

Metabolic alkalosis of renal origin may be the result of excessive urinary chloride excretion, most commonly related to diuretics that inhibit reabsorption of Cl^-. The Cl^- loss results in hypochloremia, with a compensatory increase in plasma HCO_3^- to maintain electroneutrality. Extracellular volume depletion stimulates the renin-angiotensin-aldosterone pathway, and high aldosterone levels superimposed on increased distal urinary flow rates results in increased K^+ excretion and hypokalemia. The volume depletion and hypokalemia enhance proximal HCO_3^- reabsorption, thereby maintaining the alkalosis, and the prerenal fall in the glomerular flow rate limits HCO_3^- filtration.

Important but rare genetic syndromes characterized by urinary chloride wasting include Bartter's syndrome and Gitelman's syndrome. Bartter's syndrome is an autosomal recessive salt-losing state associated with extracellular volume depletion and excessive urinary chloride loss that results in hypokalemia and hypochloremic metabolic alkalosis. Secondary increases of plasma renin and aldosterone occur, as does renal juxtaglomerular cell hyperplasia. The syndrome resembles the effects of furosemide on the thick ascending limb of Henle; gene mutations in the Na-K-2Cl cotransporter, K^+ channel, and Cl^- channels have been described. Because calcium reabsorption occurs in the thick ascending limb of Henle, Bartter's syndrome, like furosemide, causes hypercalciuria as well as polyuria.

Gitelman's syndrome is an autosomal recessive cause of extracellular volume depletion, urinary chloride wasting, and hypokalemic metabolic alkalosis. It is due to inactivating mutations in the SLC12A3 gene encoding the thiazide-sensitive NaCl cotransporter of the renal distal tubule. Urinary concentrating ability is preserved, and patients are hypocalciuric because decreased NaCl reabsorption in the distal tubule is associated with a decrease in calcium excretion. Hypomagnesemia may also be severe.

Metabolic Alkalosis of Nonrenal Origin with Extracellular Volume Depletion

Metabolic alkalosis may develop as a result of gastrointestinal Cl^- loss from vomiting, nasogastric suctioning, or secretory diarrhea. In such cases, extracellular volume is usually contracted, hypochloremia develops, and the urinary chloride level is usually less than 20 mEq/L.

In Zollinger-Ellison syndrome (Chapter 201), excessive gastrin-induced gastric acid secretion may result in an acidic stool with high chloride content. Diarrhea does not cause metabolic alkalosis unless the stool electrolytes $[(Na^+ + K^+) - Cl^-]$ are less than plasma HCO_3^-.

Infectious gastroenteritis, congenital chloridorrhea, and villous adenomas also cause chloride losses in stool. Congenital chloridorrhea is an autosomal recessive disorder of defective colonic, apical Cl/HCO_3 exchange associated with the downregulated adenoma *(DRA)* gene.

With vomiting, the initiating event is loss of HCl. This secretion of HCl into the stomach lumen by the parietal cell is coupled to the absorption of HCO_3^- in exchange for chloride at the basolateral membrane. When gastric acid is normally secreted, a mild increase in serum HCO_3^- spills into urine and causes an "alkaline tide." With vomiting, however, the net loss of HCl generates the alkalosis. Initially, this increased HCO_3^- is filtered by the glomeruli and excreted in urine accompanied by Na^+ and K^+; volume depletion begins to develop. As vomiting continues, extracellular volume depletion worsens, glomerular filtration falls, HCO_3^- filtration is limited, volume depletion increases the renin-angiotensin II–aldosterone system, proximal fluid and HCO_3^- reabsorption increase, distal Na^+ reabsorption increases under the influence of aldosterone, and greater H^+ secretion enhances HCO_3^- reabsorption. These effects reduce renal Na^+ loss but at the expense of maintaining the metabolic alkalosis. Significant K^+ losses, which occur as a result of the bicarbonaturia and hyperaldosteronism, lead to hypokalemia, which is actually due to renal, not gastrointestinal, losses as a consequence of attempts to maintain extracellular volume. The hypokalemia further increases proximal $NaHCO_3$ reabsorption, distal H^+ secretion, and K^+ reabsorption, all at the expense of further reabsorption of HCO_3^-. At the new steady state after vomiting or nasogastric suctioning ceases, the paradoxical aciduria of metabolic alkalosis develops as HCO_3^- reabsorption is complete, and the urine contains low levels of Na^+, K^+, and Cl^-. The patient may be hypovolemic, hypokalemic, and alkalemic, but because Na^+, K^+, and acid-base balance are intrinsically linked, life-threatening volume depletion, K^+ depletion, and alkalemia are usually avoided.

Most nonrenal metabolic alkaloses with volume depletion are due to gastrointestinal losses. However, some patients with cystic fibrosis (Chapter 89) may develop hypochloremic alkalosis as a consequence of excessive sweat chloride content related to the *CFTR* gene mutation.

Metabolic Alkalosis of Renal Origin with Volume Expansion and Hypertension

The renal conditions that cause metabolic alkalosis and volume expansion are due to a proportionately greater increase in Na^+ reabsorption above what is required to maintain a steady state of Na^+ balance, rather than primary loss of the Cl^- anion. As Na^+ is reabsorbed, electroneutrality is maintained by an increase in plasma HCO_3^-. The plasma Na^+ concentration may be increased, and Cl^- balance is normal; Cl^- appears in urine, and hypochloremia is not present. In the kidney, the loss of net acid as NH_4Cl in excess of the acid produced generates a metabolic alkalosis, in which the new bicarbonate generated is due to proton secretion by the distal nephron through H^+-ATPases. The H^+ then combines with NH_3 to form NH_4^+ in urine.

Na^+ is reabsorbed independently of Cl^- in the cortical collecting duct through the aldosterone-sensitive cells containing the ENaC. When Na^+ is reabsorbed by the principal cells of the cortical collecting duct, the tubule lumen becomes electronegative and stimulates both K^+ and H^+ secretion by the electrogenic H^+-ATPases. To the extent that HCO_3^- remains in the lumen, the secreted protons complete HCO_3^- reabsorption. Additional secreted protons combine with NH_3 and phosphates and lead to net acid excretion. Any increase in the distal H^+ secretory mechanism will produce more urinary net acid; more "new" HCO_3^- will be generated and returned to the now expanded extracellular fluid, and metabolic alkalosis will develop. The increased plasma HCO_3^- will be filtered, but in the absence of a stimulus to increase proximal HCO_3^- reabsorption, the HCO_3^- will flow distally to be reabsorbed by the increased H^+ secretion of the collecting duct. At first, the alkalosis is mild, but increased cortical collecting duct Na^+ reabsorption will also lead to increased K^+ secretion and hypokalemia. Hypokalemia increases the capacity for proximal HCO_3^- reabsorption, thereby opposing the effect of volume expansion, so that distal delivery of HCO_3^- decreases. The higher than normal distal H^+ secretion titrates urinary buffers so further "new" HCO_3^- is formed and the alkalosis worsens. Metabolic alkaloses in the hypermineralocorticoid syndromes are sustained by hypokalemia.

Metabolic Alkalosis of Nonrenal Origin Associated with Normal or Expanded Volume

If an alkalotic patient is not hypochloremic, electroneutrality must be maintained either by depletion of an alternative anion or by an excessive concentration of a cation. An example of a metabolic alkalosis associated with depletion of a nonchloride anion is hypoproteinemic alkalosis, with hypoalbuminemia and a small anion gap. Chloride balance is normal and chloride appears in urine.

Alkalosis also may result from the addition of alkali salts of organic anions. The normal response to the ingestion of $NaHCO_3$ is rapid urinary alkalinization because of an unaltered threshold for HCO_3^- reabsorption. However, a marked excess of HCO_3^-, as may be administered in an attempt to alkalinize a patient's urine, expands volume and causes an alkalemia, especially in the presence of volume depletion or low glomerular filtration. Milk-alkali syndrome, usually seen when patients in renal failure ingest milk or calcium antacids, is associated with hypercalcemia, alkalemia, and normal Cl^-.

Other situations in which intake of alkali salts results in metabolic alkalosis include infusion of large quantities of sodium salts of metabolizable organic compounds such as acetate, citrate, lactate, or bicarbonate; hyperalimentation with acetate salts; chronic peritoneal dialysis with acetate or lactate dialysate; or excessive transfusions or plasmapheresis, in which large quantities of citrate, used as an anticoagulant, are delivered.

CLINICAL MANIFESTATIONS

Mild metabolic alkalosis up to a pH of 7.50 *is* usually asymptomatic. When the pH exceeds 7.55, however, the alkalosis itself and the compensatory hypoventilation are frequently associated with metabolic encephalopathy. Symptoms include confusion, obtundation, delirium, and coma. The seizure threshold is lowered; tetany, paresthesias, muscular cramping, and other symptoms of low calcium are seen. In patients with hypocalcemia, these signs may be seen at pH values above 7.45. Other findings include cardiac tachyarrhythmias and hypotension. Lactate production increases as a result of the increased anaerobic glycolysis.

DIAGNOSIS

In diagnosing the cause of metabolic alkalosis, it is important to distinguish whether the condition is chloride responsive or chloride unresponsive. Metabolic alkalosis is generally divided into two categories based on its responsiveness to chloride (see Table 120-2). Chloride-responsive metabolic alkalosis is associated with extracellular fluid and chloride depletion and is seen in cases of gastric fluid loss and diuretic use. A diagnostic clue comes from the serum electrolytes. HCO_3^- is increased with a corresponding fall in serum chloride (hypochloremic alkalosis). Chloride-unresponsive metabolic alkalosis is seen in patients with extracellular fluid expansion in conditions such as primary aldosteronism and hypokalemia. Entry of hydrogen ions into cells can also lead to metabolic alkalosis in patients with hypokalemia.

Vomiting, nasogastric suction, and diarrhea are usually obvious sources of metabolic alkalosis. However, the Zollinger-Ellison syndrome (Chapter 201), villous adenomas (Chapter 199), and VIPomas (Chapter 201) may be more difficult to diagnose unless the index of suspicion is high.

Patients who present with hypokalemic metabolic alkalosis with normal or low blood pressure and have urinary chloride concentrations above 25 mEq/L may be taking diuretics such as furosemide or thiazides surreptitiously; a diuretic screen can document the presence of the drug. If the screen is negative, Bartter's or Gitelman's syndrome (Chapter 130) should be considered. Bartter's syndrome is less common, usually more severe, and presents in young patients. The presence of hypercalciuria favors Bartter's syndrome, whereas hypocalciuria suggests Gitelman's syndrome.

Specific causes of renal alkalosis with volume expansion and hypertension can be classified according to levels of renin and aldosterone. Primary increases in renin with secondary increases in aldosterone can be seen in patients with unilateral renal artery stenosis (Chapter 127), renin-secreting tumors of the kidney (Chapter 67), and malignant hypertension (Chapter 67). Low renin and elevated aldosterone levels are characteristic of primary hyperaldosteronism from adrenal adenoma or hyperplasia (Chapter 235). A high cortisol level with volume expansion is seen in hypercortisolism (Chapter 234) and adrenocorticotropic hormone-secreting tumors (Chapter 186). Inhibition of the intracellular enzyme 11β-hydroxysteroid dehydrogenase, which normally inactivates cortisol to form cortisone in the cortical collecting duct, will also result in low renin levels, low aldosterone levels, and hypokalemic alkalosis. Both genetic mutations (the apparent mineralocorticoid excess syndrome) and an excess consumption of glycyrrhizic acid found in licorice or anisette are causes of this enzyme block. Another cause of hypertension with hypokalemic alkalosis but with low renin and aldosterone levels is Liddle's syndrome (Chapter 130), in which an activating mutation in the cortical collecting duct Na^+ channel (ENaC) leads to increased Na^+ reabsorption.

Metabolic alkalosis may also develop without volume expansion when a non-reabsorbable anion is presented to the cortical collecting duct lumen. Nitrates, sulfates, and certain antibiotics such as nafcillin, carbenicillin, and ticarcillin may obligate K^+ and H^+ secretion as Na^+ is reabsorbed. Topical administration of silver nitrate to burn victims may result in alkalosis.

TREATMENT

In chloride-responsive patients (see Table 120-2), treatment is directed at increasing urinary excretion of bicarbonate. In patients with mild to moderate alkalosis, liberalizing salt intake and administering potassium chloride is effective in increasing renal HCO_3^- excretion. The K deficit is likely to be at least 100 mEq for every 1 mEq/L decrease in serum potassium. Unless KCl is also replenished, the improvement in filtration and proximal reabsorption will result in severe K^+ wasting as bicarbonaturia develops and aldosterone's effects remain. In addition, complete resolution of alkalosis will not occur until K^+ is normalized. In a patient with renal failure and vomiting, the elevation in HCO_3^- may be more severe because of poor HCO_3^- filtration. In cases of volume expansion and alkalosis, acetazolamide may be administered carefully while monitoring its potential for losing K^+. If this agent fails to work, dilute solutions of HCl (0, 1N HCl) may be cautiously administered. The amount of H^+, in milliequivalents, to be given may be calculated as the product of the desired change in serum HCO_3^- concentration (mEq/L) times the estimated total body water (L). It is likely that the this calculation will overestimate the amount of acid needed for correction, so no more than one third of the amount should be given before recalculating to avoid metabolic acidosis. Full correction of HCO_3^- should not be the goal. In the absence of renal failure, intravenous acetazolamide (250 to 500 mg every 8 hours) may be effective but may greatly increase K^+ losses.

Chloride-unresponsive patients (see Table 120-2) include those with mineralocorticoid excess. In these patients, the metabolic alkalosis can be lessened by potassium replacement or by blocking Na^+ reabsorption with aldosterone antagonists such as spironolactone, starting with 25 mg orally, or amiloride, beginning with 5 mg orally. Indomethacin effectively treats Bartter's syndrome (Chapter 130) by interfering with prostaglandin E_2 to allow greater Na-Cl reabsorption in the thick ascending limb. Gitelman's and Bartter's syndromes are best treated with combinations of KCl, a potassium-sparing diuretic, and magnesium if needed.

● RESPIRATORY ACIDOSIS

Respiratory acidosis is characterized by a primary elevation in Pco_2 as reflected by reduced arterial pH with variable elevation in the HCO_3^- concentration. It is most frequently caused by a decrease in alveolar ventilation owing to pulmonary disease (Chapter 104), respiratory muscle fatigue (Chapter 99), or abnormalities in ventilatory control (Chapter 86).

CLINICAL MANIFESTATIONS

Clinical findings in respiratory acidosis are related to the degree and duration of the respiratory acidosis and whether hypoxemia is present. A precipitous rise in Pco_2 can lead to confusion, anxiety, psychosis, asterixis, seizures, and myoclonic jerks, with progressive depression of the sensorium and coma at an arterial Pco_2 greater than 60 mm Hg (CO_2 narcosis). Hypercapnia, which increases cerebral blood flow and volume, can lead to symptoms and signs of elevated intracranial pressure, including headaches and papilledema. Other findings in acute respiratory acidosis include signs of catecholamine release, such as skin flushing, diaphoresis, and increased cardiac contractility and output. Symptoms of chronic hypercapnia include fatigue, lethargy, and confusion, in addition to the findings seen in acute hypercapnia.

The slow time course of many of these diseases allows the kidney to compensate adequately as the disease progresses by increasing its excretion of hydrogen ion as ammonium and generating and reabsorbing bicarbonate to restore systemic pH toward normal values. This compensatory process is not maximal until 3 to 5 days after the onset of respiratory acidosis.

DIAGNOSIS

Disorders that cause a respiratory acidosis include central effects of drugs, stroke, and infection; airway obstruction; primary parenchymal processes

such as chronic obstructive pulmonary disease (Chapter 88) and acute respiratory distress syndrome (Chapter 104); disorders of ventilation (Chapter 105); and neuromuscular diseases such as myasthenia gravis (Chapter 430) and muscular dystrophies (Chapter 429). Permissive hypercapnia has been used clinically in patients with acute respiratory distress syndrome to limit pulmonary damage secondary to mechanical ventilation (Chapter 105).

It can be difficult to distinguish the signs of hypercapnia from those of hypoxemia because the two often appear together. If correction of the hypoxemia does not improve the clinical picture, however, it can be surmised that hypercapnia is responsible.

TREATMENT **Rx**

Treatment of both chronic and acute respiratory acidosis is aimed primarily at correcting the underlying cause and ensuring adequate ventilation. In acute respiratory acidosis, measures to relieve severe hypoxemia and acidemia should be instituted immediately, including intubation and assisted mechanical ventilation (Chapter 105) if necessary.

In patients with chronic respiratory acidosis, however, ventilation may be driven by hypoxemia; oxygen must be carefully titrated because correction of the hypoxemia can worsen the hypercapnia. In patients with compensated chronic respiratory acidosis, rapid and complete correction of hypercapnia can also result in posthypercapnic metabolic alkalosis. Patients recovering from an acute-on-chronic respiratory acidosis should be monitored carefully to correct hypokalemia, hypochloremia, and hypovolemia so that adequate renal excretion of bicarbonate can occur.

Bicarbonate therapy is not indicated for respiratory acidosis unless the pH falls below 7.0 and the patient is about to be intubated. There is a role for bicarbonate therapy in patients with renal failure (Chapter 132), in whom adequate compensatory acid excretion cannot take place.

● RESPIRATORY ALKALOSIS

EPIDEMIOLOGY AND PATHOBIOLOGY

In respiratory alkalosis, a primary decrease in Pco_2 is reflected by increases in arterial pH and variable decreases in plasma bicarbonate concentration. The most common cause is alveolar hyperventilation, not underproduction of CO_2.

Acute hypocapnia results in an initial increase in the pH of both the CSF and the brain's intracellular environment. However, this increase is quickly offset by a decrease in bicarbonate levels. In acute respiratory alkalosis, one of the primary mechanisms of this fall in bicarbonate appears to be the generation of lactate as a result of vasoconstriction, hypoxia, and increased hemoglobin affinity for oxygen. The combination of increased oxygen demand and decreased oxygen delivery may contribute to adverse clinical outcomes in hypocapnic alkalosis.

Cerebral blood flow is significantly decreased by hypocapnia, which is a potent vasoconstrictor. As in respiratory acidosis, the CNS is immediately affected by decreases in systemic Pco_2 because of the blood-brain barrier's permeability to CO_2. In addition, as in respiratory acidosis, CSF and intracellular pH show an initial short-lived response that parallels the systemic increase in pH.

Renal compensation for sustained hypocapnia is complete in 36 to 72 hours. The mechanism rests primarily in the kidney's net reduction of hydrogen ion excretion, which it accomplishes largely by decreasing ammonium and titratable acid excretion. The threshold for bicarbonate excretion is also lowered, and bicarbonaturia develops. As a result, systemic bicarbonate levels decrease, and arterial pH returns toward normal values.

CLINICAL MANIFESTATIONS

The clinical manifestations of respiratory alkalosis depend on the degree and duration of the condition but are primarily those of the underlying disorder. Chronic hypocapnia does not appear to be associated with any significant clinical symptoms.

Symptoms of acute hypocapnia are largely attributable to the alkalemia and include dizziness, perioral or extremity paresthesias, confusion, asterixis, hypotension, seizures, and coma. Most symptoms, which are manifested only when the Pco_2 falls below 25 or 30 mm Hg, can be related to decreased cerebral blood flow or reduced free calcium because alkalosis increases calcium's protein-bound fraction. Shortness of breath and chest wall pain, which frequently may be seen when patients hyperventilate because of pain or anxiety, do not appear to be related to hypocapnia.

Adaptation to High Altitude

Acute exposure to high altitude (Chapter 94) results in hypoxia-induced hyperventilation. Compensation requires at least several days and is characterized by a gradual further increase in hyperventilation, a steadily decreasing Pco_2, and an increasing Po_2. The effect of the hypoxic stimulus to ventilate is initially modulated by the effects of alkalosis, both peripherally and centrally. However, as HCO_3^- in CSF falls, inhibition of the central stimulus to ventilate decreases. Once a steady state is achieved, the drive to ventilate is determined by the effects of hypoxemia and alkalemia on the peripheral chemoreceptors.

DIAGNOSIS

Alveolar hyperventilation leading to respiratory alkalosis is seen with hypoxemia from pulmonary disease (Chapter 83), heart failure (Chapter 58), high altitudes (Chapter 94), or anemia. Mechanical ventilation (Chapter 105) is also a common cause of respiratory alkalosis.

Another common cause of respiratory alkalosis is primary stimulation of the central chemoreceptor, as seen in sepsis (Chapter 108), hepatic cirrhosis (Chapter 156), salicylate intoxication (Chapters 36 and 110), correction of metabolic acidosis, hyperthermia (Chapter 109), and pregnancy, as well as cortical hyperventilation from anxiety and pain. In these situations, central signals override peripheral chemoreceptors until the primary stimulus is removed.

Primary neurologic diseases that can stimulate alveolar hyperventilation include acute stroke, infection, trauma, and tumors. Two patterns of respiration are seen: central hyperventilation and Cheyne-Stokes respiration (Chapter 86). Central hyperventilation, which is associated with lesions at the pontine-midbrain level, is regular, but with an increased rate and tidal volume. Cheyne-Stokes breathing, which is characterized by periods of hyperventilation alternating with apnea, is seen in patients with bilateral cortical and upper pontine lesions and in patients with heart failure.

TREATMENT   Rx

Treatment of respiratory alkalosis must address the underlying cause of the disturbance. Hyperventilation syndrome is a diagnosis of exclusion, but patients who exhibit symptoms, such as tetany and syncope, and who do not have more serious causes of hyperventilation can be treated with a rebreathing mask. Hypophosphatemia can be seen in these patients, but it usually improves with treatment of the alkalosis. Patients with respiratory alkalosis associated with mountain sickness can be pretreated with acetazolamide to induce a metabolic acidosis, thereby preventing extreme elevations in pH (Chapter 94).

Grade **A**

1. de Brito-Ashurst I, Varagunam M, Raftery MJ, et al. Bicarbonate supplementation slows progression of CKD and improves nutritional status. *J Am Soc Nephrol.* 2009;20:1869-1870.
2. Cooper DJ, Walley KR, Wiggs BR, et al. Bicarbonate does not improve hemodynamics in critically ill patients who have lactic acidosis: a prospective, controlled clinical study. *Ann Intern Med.* 1990;112:492-498.

SUGGESTED READINGS

Karet FE. Disorders of water and acid-base homeostasis. *Nephron Physiol.* 2011;118:28-34. *Review.*
Yaqoob MM. Acidosis and progression of chronic kidney disease. *Curr Opin Nephrol Hypertens.* 2010;19:489-492. *Review of data supporting the concept that correction of acidosis by sodium bicarbonate in patients with advanced CKD attenuates the decline of renal function.*
Yunos NM, Bellomo R, Story D, et al. Bench-to-bedside review: chloride in critical illness. *Crit Care.* 2010;14:226. *Review.*

121

DISORDERS OF MAGNESIUM AND PHOSPHORUS

ALAN S. L. YU

MAGNESIUM METABOLISM

Magnesium is an important mineral component of the bony skeleton, a cofactor for many metabolic enzymes, and a regulator of ion channels and transporters in excitable tissues.

Normal Magnesium Metabolism

The majority of total body magnesium is intracellular or in bone, with only 1% in extracellular fluid. The normal serum magnesium concentration is 1.8 to 2.3 mg/dL (1.5 to 1.9 mEq/L). The average daily intake of magnesium is 300 mg, the main sources of which are green vegetables, nuts, whole grain cereals, milk, and seafood. Magnesium is absorbed mainly in the jejunum and ileum. In the kidney, 70 to 80% of serum magnesium is filtered at the glomerulus, with the majority being reabsorbed along the length of the tubule, particularly in the thick ascending limb of Henle. In states of magnesium deficiency or excess, renal tubule reabsorption is tightly regulated so that magnesium excretion is adjusted accordingly.

Magnesium Deficiency

PATHOBIOLOGY

Magnesium deficiency is usually detected when hypomagnesemia becomes evident. However, because magnesium is stored primarily intracellularly, substantial depletion of total body magnesium can occur before serum magnesium levels drop appreciably.

Magnesium deficiency may be due to nutritional deficiency, intestinal malabsorption, redistribution into bone, or losses via cutaneous, lower gastrointestinal, or renal routes (Table 121-1). The recommended daily allowance of magnesium is 420 mg for males and 320 mg for females. Approximately 25% of alcoholics are chronically hypomagnesemic because of a combination of poor nutritional intake and increased renal loss. Magnesium deficiency can rarely occur in protein-calorie malnutrition and may be associated with acute hypomagnesemia during refeeding because of rapid cellular magnesium

TABLE 121-1   CAUSES OF MAGNESIUM DEFICIENCY

Nutritional deficiency
  Alcoholism*
  Malnutrition
  Refeeding syndrome
Intestinal malabsorption*
Proton pump inhibitors
Lower gastrointestinal losses
  Colonic diarrhea*
  Intestinal fistula
  Laxative abuse
Cutaneous losses
  Burns*
  Exercise-induced sweating
Redistribution into bone
  Hungry bone syndrome
Renal losses
  Polyuria (including diabetes mellitus)*
  Volume expansion
  Hyperaldosteronism
  Bartter's and Gitelman's syndromes
  Hypercalcemia
  Loop and thiazide diuretics*
  Nephrotoxins (cisplatin, amphotericin, aminoglycosides, pentamidine, cyclosporine)*
Epidermal growth factor monoclonal antibodies (cetuximab, panitumumab)*

*Common causes.

uptake. Fat malabsorption in conditions such as celiac disease, Crohn's disease, and small intestinal resection causes magnesium deficiency because free fatty acids accumulate in the intestinal lumen, where they combine with magnesium to form insoluble soaps. Proton pump inhibitors can also cause hypomagnesemia, which is thought to be due to inhibition of intestinal absorption. Lower gastrointestinal secretions are rich in magnesium, so diarrhea of colonic origin is a common cause of hypomagnesemia. Sweat contains significant amounts of magnesium, and transient hypomagnesemia can occur after prolonged, intense exercise such as marathon runs. Magnesium is also lost from burned skin surfaces, and 40% of patients with severe burns (Chapter 112) are hypomagnesemic.

In patients with severe hyperparathyroidism (Chapter 253) and high bone turnover, continued sequestration of minerals within bone may continue for several days after parathyroidectomy and cause transient hypocalcemia, hypomagnesemia, and hypophosphatemia. Renal magnesium losses can occur in any polyuric state, including the recovery phase of acute tubular necrosis or urinary tract obstruction. Hypomagnesemia is common in diabetes mellitus (Chapters 236 and 237), where it is thought to be due to a combination of poor intestinal absorption owing to autonomic neuropathy, osmotic diuresis, and decreased renal tubule reabsorption. Failure of sodium reabsorption in the thick ascending limb of Henle as a result of the use of loop diuretics and in the distal convoluted tubule as a result of thiazide diuretics inhibits tubular magnesium reabsorption and leads to urinary magnesium wasting. Drugs that are tubular toxins are also common causes of renal magnesium wasting. Such drugs include cisplatin, amphotericin B, and aminoglycosides, which are commonly associated with hypokalemia and rarely with renal tubule acidosis, as well as calcineurin inhibitors such as cyclosporine and tacrolimus, which also cause hyperkalemia. Antibodies to the epidermal growth factor receptor, such as cetuximab and panitumumab, which are used to treat metastatic colorectal cancer, downregulate a distal tubule magnesium channel and are an increasing cause of isolated severe hypomagnesemia.

Inherited hypomagnesemia is usually caused by renal magnesium loss and can be subdivided into three main types, depending on the coexistence of other electrolyte disturbances: Bartter's and Gitelman's syndromes, which are associated with renal salt wasting and hypokalemic metabolic alkalosis; familial hypomagnesemia with hypercalciuria and nephrocalcinosis; and isolated hypomagnesemia, which is usually associated with hypocalcemia.

CLINICAL MANIFESTATIONS

Mild to moderate hypomagnesemia or magnesium deficiency is frequently asymptomatic. Manifestations of increased neuronal excitability are the most common symptoms, including paresthesias, tetany, and seizures. These may be associated with Chvostek's sign (twitching of the cheek muscles in response to tapping the facial nerve in front of the ear) or Trousseau's sign (carpal spasm induced by compressing the upper arm with a tourniquet or blood pressure cuff). Cardiac disturbances may also occur and range in severity from mild electrocardiographic abnormalities (nonspecific T wave changes, U waves, prolonged QT interval, and repolarization alternans) to ventricular tachycardia, torsades de pointes, and ventricular fibrillation (Chapter 65).

Coexistent hypokalemia is very common, for two reasons: many of the causes of hypomagnesemia are also causes of potassium loss, and hypomagnesemia itself causes renal potassium wasting. Severe hypomagnesemia also impairs parathyroid hormone secretion and induces tissue resistance to its actions, thereby leading to hypocalcemia.

DIAGNOSIS

The cause of the magnesium deficiency is often obvious from the history. In difficult diagnostic cases, 24-hour urinary magnesium excretion should be measured. With extrarenal magnesium loss (usually malabsorption or laxative abuse), urinary magnesium excretion is appropriately suppressed (<25 mg/day). Higher urinary magnesium levels indicate renal magnesium wasting, often secondary to surreptitious diuretic use or one of the familial magnesium-wasting disorders.

TREATMENT   Rx

It is unclear whether mild, asymptomatic hypomagnesemia needs to be treated. Magnesium repletion is recommended in hypomagnesemic patients if they are symptomatic, have underlying cardiac or seizure disorders, exhibit concurrent severe hypocalcemia or hypokalemia, or have severe hypomagnesemia (<1.4 mg/dL). In mild cases or in the outpatient setting, oral magnesium salts such as magnesium oxide (250 to 500 mg four times daily) can be used for repletion, but these substances frequently cause diarrhea, particularly at high doses. In the inpatient setting, intravenous magnesium sulfate (1 to 2 g every 6 hours) can be used for repletion. Because the redistribution of magnesium from extracellular to intracellular compartments is relatively slow, the serum magnesium concentration may normalize before total body magnesium stores are replete. It is therefore prudent to continue intravenous magnesium for an additional 1 to 2 days after restoration of normomagnesemia. In patients with normal renal function, any excess magnesium is simply excreted renally. Adverse effects from intravenous magnesium administration are primarily due to transient hypermagnesemia and include flushing, hypotension, and flaccid paralysis. Amiloride (10 to 20 mg orally once daily) abrogates renal magnesium wasting in some patients with this problem, but the mechanism is unknown.

PROGNOSIS

In patients with a self-limited cause of magnesium deficiency, repletion is easily accomplished. However, in patients with persistent magnesium wasting, such as in Gitelman's syndrome (Chapter 119), it can be difficult to keep up with the ongoing losses with oral therapy. Fortunately, these individuals tend to adapt to their chronic hypomagnesemia and tolerate it fairly well.

Hypermagnesemia

Transient hypermagnesemia can occur in patients given large doses of intravenous magnesium, for example, in the setting of preeclampsia. It has also been reported in individuals taking large doses of magnesium-containing antacids or cathartics, particularly in settings in which intestinal absorption is enhanced, such as inflammatory bowel disease and intestinal obstruction. However, the kidney has a very large capacity to excrete excess magnesium. Thus, persistent hypermagnesemia is seen almost exclusively in patients who have chronic renal insufficiency (Chapter 132) who are also taking excessive amounts of magnesium in the form of antacids, cathartics, or enemas.

CLINICAL MANIFESTATIONS

Magnesium toxicity is a serious and potentially fatal condition. Mild hypermagnesemia (serum magnesium level >4 to 6 mg/dL) causes hypotension, nausea, vomiting, facial flushing, urinary retention, and ileus. Above serum levels of 8 to 12 mg/dL, flaccid skeletal muscle paralysis and hyporeflexia may ensue, along with bradyarrhythmias, respiratory depression, coma, and cardiac arrest. A low or even negative serum anion gap is sometimes seen.

TREATMENT   Rx

Mild hypermagnesemia in a patient with good renal function usually requires no treatment because renal clearance is rapid and the normal serum half-life of magnesium is about 1 day. In the event of serious toxicity, the effects of magnesium can be temporarily antagonized by the administration of intravenous calcium salts (5 to 10 mL of 10% calcium chloride). Renal magnesium excretion can be enhanced by administering furosemide (20 to 40 mg every 4 hours) together with a saline infusion (0.9% NaCl at 150 mL/hour, titrated to replace urinary losses). In patients with advanced renal insufficiency, the most effective method of magnesium removal is hemodialysis.

PROGNOSIS

Severe hypermagnesemia is potentially fatal. Lesser degrees of hypermagnesemia usually respond well to treatment.

⬤ PHOSPHORUS METABOLISM

Phosphorus has many critical roles. It is a major component of bone mineral, of phospholipids in cell membranes, and of nucleic acids. It forms high-energy phosphate bonds in compounds such as adenosine triphosphate (ATP), is post-translationally bound to proteins as an intracellular signal, and acts as a major pH buffer in serum and urine.

Normal Phosphorus Metabolism

Of the total body phosphorus content, 85% is in bone, 14% is in intracellular compartments, and only 1% is in extracellular fluid. The normal concentration of phosphorus in plasma is 3 to 4.5 mg/dL (1 to 1.5 mM). Daily intake of phosphorus is 800 to 1500 mg. Phosphorus is present in many foods, including dairy products, meats, and grains, and it is absorbed in the small intestine. The kidneys excrete excess phosphorus, which is the principal mechanism by which the body regulates extracellular phosphate balance. Ninety percent of serum phosphate is filtered at the glomerulus, of which 80 to 97% is reabsorbed along the nephron, primarily in the proximal tubule. Parathyroid hormone increases renal phosphate excretion by inhibiting the sodium-phosphate cotransporter in the proximal tubule, whereas vitamin D enhances intestinal phosphate absorption.

Hypophosphatemia

PATHOBIOLOGY

Hypophosphatemia may be caused by decreased intake, impaired intestinal absorption, redistribution into cells or bone, and renal losses (Table 121-2). Phosphate is frequently depleted in alcoholism (Chapter 32) because of the intake of a carbohydrate-rich, phosphate-poor diet, as well as renal phosphate wasting. Divalent cation-containing antacids bind phosphate in the intestinal lumen to form insoluble salts, thereby preventing their absorption. Vitamin D deficiency also leads to decreased intestinal phosphate absorption and hence to hypophosphatemia. Respiratory but not metabolic alkalosis (Chapter 120) may cause transient hypophosphatemia. In this disorder, intracellular pH is increased, thereby stimulating glycolysis, which depletes the intracellular inorganic phosphate pool and leads to a shift of phosphate into cells.

Insulin is also a strong stimulus for shifting phosphate into cells. Patients with diabetic ketoacidosis (Chapter 120) are often hyperphosphatemic because of a shift of phosphate out of cells under insulinopenic conditions, but their total body phosphate is actually depleted as a result of urinary losses. Subsequent treatment with insulin may uncover severe hypophosphatemia. Similarly, in malnourished patients (Chapter 222), whose total body phosphate stores may be depleted, overzealous intravenous refeeding with carbohydrate-rich fluids may stimulate insulin release and cause acute hypophosphatemia. The tyrosine kinase inhibitors imatinib and sorafenib, which are used in the treatment of various cancers (Chapter 190), can cause profound hypophosphatemia, which appears to be due to inhibition of bone resorption.

Renal phosphate wasting is usually due to impaired proximal tubule phosphate reabsorption. In primary hyperparathyroidism (Chapter 253), hypercalcemia is typically associated with hypophosphatemia. Fanconi's syndrome is a generalized proximal tubule disorder characterized by hypophosphatemia in association with glycosuria, aminoaciduria, hypokalemia, and type II renal tubular acidosis; it can be caused by a variety of inherited metabolic disorders, multiple myeloma (Chapter 193), heavy metal intoxication (Chapter 21), and drugs such as ifosfamide, cidofovir, and tenofovir. Phosphaturia can also occur with diuretics, particularly carbonic anhydrase inhibitors, and with antimicrobial agents such as pentamidine and foscarnet.

Oncogenic osteomalacia is a paraneoplastic syndrome (Chapter 187) associated primarily with mesenchymal tumors that secrete a variety of phosphaturic factors collectively known as phosphatonins. A similar phenotype is found in X-linked and autosomal dominant hypophosphatemic rickets; these inherited disorders are characterized by an increase in a circulating phosphatonin called fibroblast growth factor-23. Phosphatonins inhibit both renal tubular phosphate reabsorption and 1α-hydroxylation of 25-hydroxycholecalciferol, thereby leading to hypophosphatemia, rickets or osteomalacia (Chapter 252), and inappropriately low serum levels of 1,25-dihydroxycholecalciferol.

CLINICAL MANIFESTATIONS

Clinical complications, which are usually observed only with severe hypophosphatemia (<1 mg/dL), are thought to be due to the disruption of cell membrane composition, depletion of ATP (which particularly affects high energy-consuming tissues such as skeletal and cardiac muscle), and depletion of 2,3-diphosphoglycerate in erythrocytes, with impaired tissue oxygen delivery. Manifestations of severe hypophosphatemia include encephalopathy, dilated cardiomyopathy, generalized muscle weakness that can lead to respiratory failure, rhabdomyolysis, and hemolysis. Hypophosphatemia also impairs renal ammoniagenesis and reduces the availability of urinary buffer, thereby impairing renal acid excretion and causing metabolic acidosis. Chronic hypophosphatemia leads to resorption of bone and osteomalacia.

DIAGNOSIS

The cause of hypophosphatemia is often evident from the history and physical examination. If not, measurement of either 24-hour urinary phosphate excretion or fractional excretion of phosphate (F_EPO_4) in a spot urine sample is often helpful.

$$F_EPO_4 = \frac{\text{Urine phosphate} \times \text{Serum creatinine}}{\text{Serum phosphate} \times \text{Urine creatinine}}$$

In the setting of hypophosphatemia, the normal response of the kidney is to reduce urinary phosphate excretion to less than 100 mg/day or to reduce F_EPO_4 to less than 5%. Higher values suggest one of the causes of renal phosphate wasting.

TREATMENT — Rx

Patients with asymptomatic mild to moderate hypophosphatemia, normal total body phosphorus stores, and minimal ongoing phosphorus losses (e.g., a patient with hypophosphatemia as a result of acute respiratory alkalosis) do not require treatment. Phosphate should be repleted in patients who are symptomatic, are suspected of having severely depleted intracellular phosphorus stores (malnourished or alcoholic patients), have ongoing gastrointestinal or renal losses, or have severe hypophosphatemia (<1 mg/dL). Oral repletion can be accomplished with sodium or potassium phosphate salts (1 to 2 g/day) or with skimmed milk. Intravenous phosphorus repletion at a dose of 0.16 to 0.64 mmol/kg over 4 to 8 hours is recommended for severe hypophosphatemia but is contraindicated in patients with renal insufficiency or hypercalcemia. Complications of phosphate therapy include hypocalcemia, metastatic calcification, hypotension, acute renal failure, and arrhythmias, as well as concomitant hypernatremia or hyperkalemia, depending on which salt is administered.

PROGNOSIS

Most patients with hypophosphatemia respond well to treatment.

Hyperphosphatemia

PATHOBIOLOGY

Pseudohyperphosphatemia may occur in blood specimens that are hemolyzed or hyperglobulinemic, such as in multiple myeloma (Chapter 193). True hyperphosphatemia is caused by excessive phosphate intake, increased intestinal absorption, redistribution from intracellular stores, or impaired renal excretion (Table 121-3). Overzealous phosphate repletion can obviously cause hyperphosphatemia. The phosphorus in some laxatives and enemas may be absorbed and cause hyperphosphatemia. Intoxication with vitamin D or its analogues increases intestinal absorption of both calcium and phosphorus. Conditions associated with massive cell lysis, such as rhabdomyolysis (Chapter 115) and tumor lysis syndrome (Chapter 182), cause the release of intracellular phosphate into the extracellular fluid. Patients with diabetic ketoacidosis (Chapters 236 and 237) are often hyperphosphatemic at initial evaluation because of the redistribution of phosphate out of cells in the insulin-deficient state. Decreased phosphate excretion is most commonly

---

TABLE 121-2 CAUSES OF HYPOPHOSPHATEMIA

Nutritional deficiency
   Alcoholism*
Impaired intestinal absorption
   Antacids
   Vitamin D deficiency*
Redistribution into cells
   Respiratory alkalosis*
   Insulin*
   Refeeding syndrome
   Burns*
Redistribution into bone
   Hungry bone syndrome
Tyrosine kinase inhibitors (imatinib, sorafenib)
Renal losses
   Hyperparathyroidism*
   Renal tubulopathy
     Fanconi's syndrome
     Drugs (pentamidine, foscarnet, acetazolamide)
   Phosphatonin excess syndrome
     Oncogenic osteomalacia
     Familial hypophosphatemic rickets

*Common causes.

TABLE 121-3   CAUSES OF HYPERPHOSPHATEMIA

Phosphate intake
    Phosphate repletion
    Phosphate-containing laxatives and enemas*
Increased intestinal absorption
    Vitamin D toxicity
Redistribution from intracellular stores
    Rhabdomyolysis
    Tumor lysis syndrome
    Diabetic ketoacidosis
Decreased renal excretion
    Renal failure*
    Hypoparathyroidism

*Common causes.

TABLE 121-4   MEDICATIONS FOR HYPERPHOSPHATEMIA

MEDICATION	USUAL DOSE WITH EACH MEAL	COMMENTS
CALCIUM SALTS		
Calcium acetate	1334 mg	Calcium level will increase about 0.5 mg/dL
Calcium carbonate	500-1000 mg	Calcium level will increase about 0.5 mg/dL
MAGNESIUM SALTS		
Magnesium hydroxide	311-622 mg	Can cause diarrhea or hypermagnesemia
Magnesium carbonate	63-126 mg	Can cause diarrhea or hypermagnesemia
ALUMINUM SALTS		
Aluminum hydroxide	300-600 mg	Encephalopathy and osteomalacia with prolonged use
OTHERS		
Sevelamer hydrochloride	800-1600 mg	Gastrointestinal side effects
Sevelamer carbonate	800-1600 mg	Gastrointestinal side effects
Lanthanum carbonate	250-500 mg	Monitor serum bicarbonate and chloride levels as well as folic acid and vitamin D, E, and K levels

due to acute or chronic renal failure (Chapter 132). With a normal diet, serum phosphate levels can be maintained within the normal range until the glomerular filtration rate falls below 25 mL/minute. However, even mild degrees of renal insufficiency may predispose to hyperphosphatemia if there is a concurrent excessive intake of phosphate-containing compounds such as laxatives. Finally, because parathyroid hormone stimulates proximal tubule phosphate excretion, primary hypoparathyroidism (Chapter 253) is often associated with mild hyperphosphatemia together with hypocalcemia.

CLINICAL MANIFESTATIONS

Acute hyperphosphatemia increases the risk of precipitation of calcium phosphate and subsequent metastatic calcification in soft tissues, including the kidney, where it can cause acute renal failure. The resultant hypocalcemia (Chapter 253) can cause tetany, hypotension, seizures, and cardiac arrhythmias. In the chronic hyperphosphatemia of chronic renal insufficiency, patients with a serum phosphate concentration greater than 6.5 mg/dL have higher mortality. Hyperphosphatemia in this setting is a risk factor for coronary and other vascular calcification, which is associated with increased mortality.

TREATMENT   **Rx**

Acute hyperphosphatemia in an asymptomatic patient with normal renal function often resolves spontaneously as excess phosphate is excreted. In symptomatic patients and those with impaired renal function, phosphate should be removed by extracorporeal therapy. Because of the slow rate of phosphate mobilization from intracellular stores, continuous venovenous hemodiafiltration is considerably more effective than intermittent hemodialysis. Chronic hyperphosphatemia (Chapter 132) can be managed by minimizing dietary phosphorus intake and administering oral phosphate binders such as calcium salts (e.g., calcium acetate 1334 mg with each meal), lanthanum carbonate (500 mg with each meal), or sevelamer (800 to 1600 mg with each meal) (Table 121-4). Aluminum hydroxide (300 to 600 mg with meals) is also a very effective phosphate binder, but prolonged use leads to aluminum accumulation and results in encephalopathy and osteomalacia. Cinacalcet (30 to 180 mg/day), a calcimimetic used in patients with chronic renal insufficiency to treat secondary hyperparathyroidism, also reduces the serum phosphate concentration and calcium-phosphate product.

PROGNOSIS

Severe acute hyperphosphatemia can be life-threatening owing to metastatic calcification and multiorgan failure, but it generally responds well to prompt therapy. Chronic hyperphosphatemia in patients with chronic kidney failure (Chapter 132) is often fairly resistant to treatment, particularly in poorly compliant individuals, and is associated with increased long-term mortality.

SUGGESTED READINGS

Geerse DA, Bindels AJ, Kuiper MA, et al. Treatment of hypophosphatemia in the intensive care unit: a review. *Crit Care.* 2010;14:147. *Review.*
Musso CG. Magnesium metabolism in health and disease. *Int Urol Nephrol.* 2009;41:357-362. *Review.*
Tonelli M, Pannu N, Manns B. Oral phosphate binders in patients with kidney failure. *N Engl J Med.* 2010;362:1312-1324. *Review suggesting that calcium carbonate, calcium acetate, magnesium hydroxide, and magnesium carbonate are as good as sevelamer or lanthanum and much less expensive.*
Zeki S, Culkin A, Gabe SM, et al. Refeeding hypophosphataemia is more common in enteral than parenteral feeding in adult in patients. *Clin Nutr.* 2011. [Epub ahead of print.] *Refeeding hypophosphatemia may occur in up to one third of patients.*

122

ACUTE KIDNEY INJURY

BRUCE A. MOLITORIS

DEFINITION

Acute kidney injury (AKI) describes the clinical syndrome formerly called acute renal failure (ARF). This nomenclature defines AKI as a functional or structural abnormality of the kidney that manifests within 48 hours, as determined by blood, urine or tissue tests or by imaging studies. Diagnostically, the reduction in kidney function in AKI is associated with either an absolute increase in serum creatinine of 0.3 mg/dL or a percentage increase in serum creatinine of 50%. In addition, a reduction in urine output with oliguria (<0.5 mL/kg/hour) for more than 6 hours also fulfills the diagnostic criteria for AKI.

EPIDEMIOLOGY

Most episodes of AKI occur in the hospital, with an incidence ranging from 5 to 7% among all hospitalized patients and 15 to 40% among patients in intensive care units (ICUs). By contrast, the incidence of community-acquired AKI is no more than 1%.

Both conceptually and diagnostically, the various causes of AKI are divided broadly into three anatomic categories: prerenal, intrarenal or intrinsic, and postrenal (Fig. 122-1). Each of the categories represents a unique pathophysiologic process with distinctive diagnostic parameters and prognosis.

Prerenal Azotemia

Prerenal azotemia, which is the most common cause of AKI, accounts for approximately 60 to 70% of community-acquired and 40% of hospital-acquired cases. Decreased renal perfusion is seen in disease states that reduce intravascular volume, such as sepsis (Chapter 108), heart failure (Chapter 58), or liver failure (Chapter 157). Additionally, medications that reduce glomerular capillary perfusion, such as angiotensin-converting enzyme (ACE) inhibitors, angiotensin-receptor blockers (ARBs), and nonsteroidal anti-inflammatory drugs (NSAIDs), can also cause prerenal AKI.

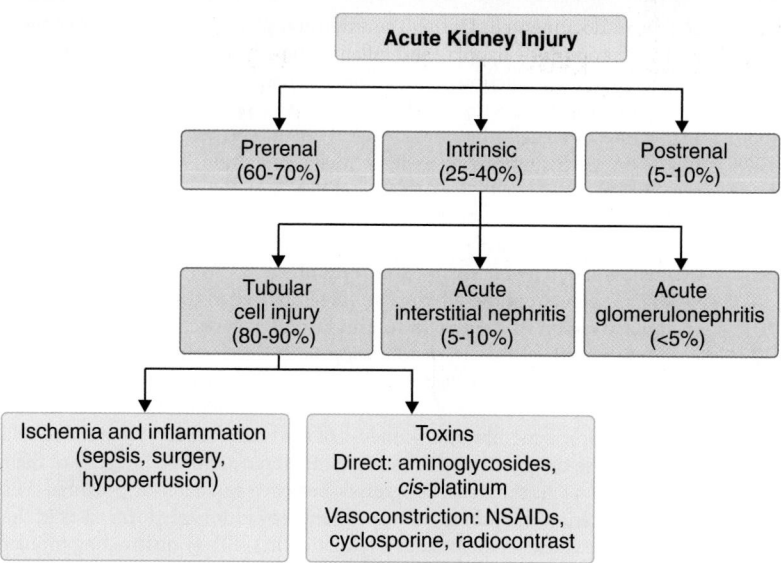

FIGURE 122-1. Main categories of acute kidney injury. NSAIDs = nonsteroidal anti-inflammatory drugs.

FIGURE 122-2. Mechanisms of prerenal and intrinsic acute renal injury. See text for descriptions.

TABLE 122-1	COMMON RENAL TUBULAR TOXINS
Aminoglycosides	
Radiocontrast agents	
Acyclovir	
Cisplatin	
Sulfonamides	
Methotrexate	
Cyclosporine	
Tacrolimus	
Amphotericin B	
Foscarnet	
Pentamidine	
Ethylene glycol	
Toluene	
Cocaine	
HMG-CoA reductase inhibitors	

HMG-CoA = 3-hydroxy-3-methylglutaryl coenzyme A.

TABLE 122-2	MEDICATIONS ASSOCIATED WITH ACUTE INTERSTITIAL NEPHRITIS
β-LACTAM ANTIBIOTICS	
Penicillin	
Cephalosporins	
Ampicillin	
Methicillin	
Nafcillin	
DIURETICS	
Furosemide	
Hydrochlorothiazide	
Triamterene	
OTHER ANTIBIOTICS	
Sulfonamides	
Vancomycin	
Rifampin	
Acyclovir	
Indinavir	
NSAIDS	
Ibuprofen	
Naproxen	
Indomethacin	

NSAIDs = nonsteroidal anti-inflammatory drugs.

Intrinsic Acute Kidney Injury

Intrarenal AKI is often the result of untreated or untreatable prerenal azotemia that leads to ischemic AKI. The diverse causes of intrinsic AKI can involve any portion of the renal vasculature, nephron, or interstitium (Fig. 122-2). Ischemic and septic injury are major causes. Renal toxins also can damage tubules both directly and indirectly (Table 122-1). Fortunately, AKI does not develop in every patient exposed to these agents, but elderly patients with diabetes mellitus, hypotensive patients, and patients with a reduced effective arterial volume (heart failure, burns, cirrhosis, hypoalbuminemia) are the most susceptible to toxic renal injury. In fact, the incidence of aminoglycoside antibiotic nephrotoxicity increases from 3 to 5% to 30 to 50% in these high-risk patients.

AKI secondary to injury to the renal interstitium is termed *acute interstitial nephritis*. Commonly implicated medications for interstitial nephritis include penicillins, cephalosporins, sulfonamides, and NSAIDs (Table 122-2) (Chapter 124). Bacterial and viral infections can be the causative agents. Interstitial nephritis is also associated with a kidney-confined or systemic autoimmune process, such as systemic lupus erythematosus (Chapter 274), Sjögren's syndrome (Chapter 276), cryoglobulinemia (Chapter 193), and primary biliary cirrhosis (Chapter 156).

Postrenal Acute Kidney Injury

Postrenal AKI can occur in the setting of bilateral urinary outflow obstruction or in a patient with a solitary kidney when a single urinary outflow tract is obstructed (Chapter 125). Most commonly, this type of outflow obstruction is observed in patients with prostatic hypertrophy (Chapter 131), prostatic or cervical cancer (Chapter 205), or retroperitoneal disorders. A functional obstruction can be observed in patients with a neurogenic bladder. In addition, intraluminal obstruction can be seen in patients with bilateral renal calculi (Chapter 128), papillary necrosis, blood clots, and bladder carcinoma, whereas extraluminal obstruction can develop in connection with retroperitoneal fibrosis, colon cancer, and lymphomas. Finally, intratubular crystallization of compounds such as uric acid, calcium oxalate, acyclovir, sulfonamide, and methotrexate, as well as myeloma light chains, can result in tubular obstruction.

PATHOBIOLOGY

The etiology of AKI is diverse, and it can arise from a number of physiologic insults that injure the kidney and reduce the glomerular filtration rate (GFR). Decreased kidney perfusion and a reduced GFR can occur with or without cellular injury; toxic, ischemic, or obstructive injury to the renal tubule; inflammation and edema of the tubulointerstitium; and a primary glomerular disease process.

Prerenal Acute Kidney Injury

The precipitating event for prerenal AKI is renal hypoperfusion (see Fig. 122-2), which can be caused by a reduction in the volume of extracellular fluid or disease states associated with normal or even increased extracellular fluid volumes but decrements in effective arterial volume, such as in sepsis, heart failure, and advanced cirrhosis. Prerenal azotemia is also divided functionally into volume responsive and nonresponsive azotemia, based on the etiology. For example, in severe heart failure (Chapter 58), additional intravascular volume may not improve kidney perfusion, whereas afterload reduction may. Early in the course of prerenal AKI, the renal parenchyma remains intact and functional. During this initial phase, the GFR remains largely intact because renal hypoperfusion initiates a neurohormonal cascade that results in afferent arteriolar dilation and efferent arteriolar constriction. Because prerenal azotemia is often easily reversible and mortality rates are low, early diagnosis and correction of the underlying pathophysiology are of critical importance. However, without early medical corrective intervention, prerenal azotemia progresses, ischemia worsens, and the resulting injury to tubular epithelial cells further decreases the GFR. This progression from prerenal azotemia to ischemic AKI is a continuum that depends on the severity and duration of the physiologic insult.

Intrarenal Acute Kidney Injury

Intrinsic AKI is classified according to the primary histologic site of injury: tubules, interstitium, vasculature, or glomerulus. Renal tubular epithelial cell injury, commonly termed *acute tubular necrosis* (ATN), occurs more commonly in the setting of ischemia, although the renal tubules can also be damaged by specific renal toxins. Ischemia can arise from a number of different clinical scenarios, but the common underlying pathogenesis is reduced renal blood flow (Table 122-3) with progression from prerenal azotemia to ischemic AKI in four distinct clinical and cellular phases: initiation, extension, maintenance, and recovery. Each of these phases encompasses distinct cellular events and declines in GFR as the kidneys respond to the insult and attempt to maintain and reestablish function (Fig. 122-3). The initiation phase, which marks the transition from prerenal to tubular cell injury and dysfunction, is characterized by severe cellular depletion of adenosine triphosphate. Renal tubular epithelial cell injury is a prominent feature during this phase; however, endothelial and vascular smooth muscle cell injury has

also been documented. During the extension phase, microvascular congestion with continued hypoxia and inflammation are most pronounced in the corticomedullary junction of the kidney, where reperfusion is limited owing to endothelial dysfunction at the capillary and postcapillary venule levels, with white blood cell adhesion. The GFR is at its ebb during the maintenance phase, but cells continue to undergo repair, migration, and proliferation, as the kidney attempts to reestablish cellular and tubular integrity. Finally, during the recovery phase, the GFR begins to improve as cellular differentiation continues and normal cellular and organ function returns. This last phase is often heralded by increasing urine output.

The S3 segment of the proximal tubule is located in the outer stripe of the medullary region of the nephron. This region is particularly susceptible to continued reduced perfusion following injury, and ongoing or worsening hypoxia results in continued cellular injury. Proximal tubular cell injury during the initiation phase of renal ischemia is first manifested as bleb formation in the apical membranes, with loss of the brush border. Proximal tubule cells also lose the polarity of the surface membrane and the integrity of their tight junctions. As the injury progresses, both live and necrotic proximal cells detach and enter the tubular lumen, where they ultimately form casts in the distal tubule. Casts contribute to a reduction in GFR by obstructing tubular urine flow, thereby preventing further filtration into that nephron. In addition, loss of the epithelial cell barrier and cell tight junctions allows backleak of the glomerular filtrate into the interstitium, thus further compromising GFR (see Fig. 122-2).

Common agents that can cause direct tubular cell toxicity (see Table 122-1) include the aminoglycoside antibiotics, intravenous radiocontrast agents, and cisplatin. Other agents such as radiocontrast dyes, NSAIDs, and cyclosporine induce vasoconstriction and reduce renal perfusion. Cocaine and the 3-hydroxy-3-methylglutaryl coenzyme A (HMG-CoA) reductase inhibitors can damage skeletal muscle and cause *rhabdomyolysis* (Chapter 115), which results in the release of myoglobin that is toxic to the tubular epithelium. Finally, the precipitation of some compounds or their metabolites can cause intratubular obstruction; agents in this category include acyclovir, sulfonamides, ethylene glycol (calcium oxalate metabolite; Chapter 110), methotrexate, and the light chains of multiple myeloma (Chapter 193).

In AKI caused by the interstitial injury, a mixed inflammatory infiltrate composed of T lymphocytes, monocytes, and macrophages, is seen. These inflammatory lesions can be diffuse or patchy in distribution. Granulomas can also occasionally be observed, especially in drug hypersensitivity reactions. Acute interstitial nephritis that persists and becomes chronic is characterized by interstitial fibrosis and tubular atrophy, although foci of inflammatory cells can persist. This process can lead to chronic and even end-stage kidney disease requiring chronic dialysis.

Vascular causes of intrinsic AKI can include microvascular and macrovascular processes. Classic microvascular disorders, which include thrombotic thrombocytopenic purpura (Chapter 175), sepsis (Chapter 108), hemolytic-uremic syndrome (Chapter 127), and the HELLP syndrome (*h*emolysis, *e*levated *l*iver enzymes, and *l*ow *p*latelet count; Chapter 153), cause AKI as a

TABLE 122-3	CONDITIONS THAT LEAD TO ISCHEMIC ACUTE RENAL FAILURE
MECHANISM	**CONDITION**
Intravascular volume depletion and hypotension	Hemorrhage; gastrointestinal, renal, and dermal losses
Decreased effective intravascular volume	Heart failure, cirrhosis, hepatorenal syndrome, peritonitis
Systemic vasodilation, renal vasoconstriction	Sepsis, hepatorenal syndrome
Large-vessel renal vascular disease	Renal artery thrombosis or embolism, intraoperative arterial cross-clamping, renal artery stenosis, cholesterol emboli
Small-vessel renal vascular disease	Sepsis, vasculitis, atheroembolism, hemolytic-uremic syndrome, malignant hypertension, scleroderma, preeclampsia, sickle cell anemia, hypercalcemia, transplant rejection
Impaired renal blood flow	Cyclosporine, tacrolimus, ACEIs, ARBs, NSAIDs, radiocontrast agents

ACEIs = angiotensin-converting enzyme inhibitors; ARBs = angiotensin-receptor blockers; NSAIDs = nonsteroidal anti-inflammatory drugs.

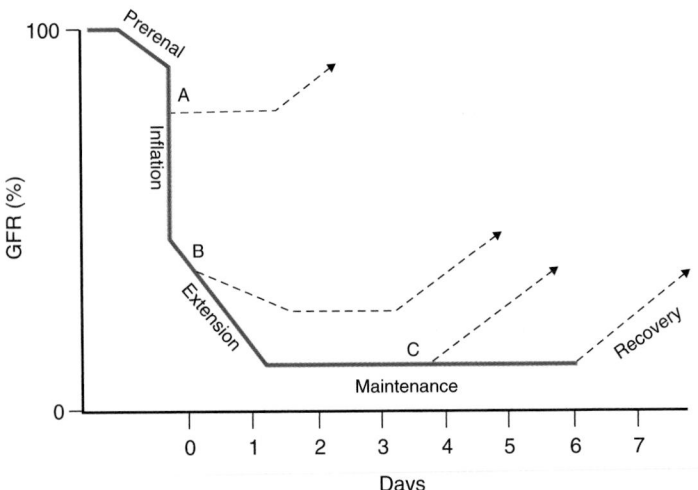

FIGURE 122-3. Phases of acute kidney injury. GFR = glomerular filtration rate. (From Sutton TA, Fisher CJ, Molitoris BA. Microvascular endothelial injury and dysfunction during ischemic acute renal failure. *Kidney Int.* 2002;62:1539-1549.)

result of glomerular capillary thrombosis and microvascular occlusion. Macrovascular disease such as atherosclerosis can cause AKI secondary to atheroembolization (Chapter 126), especially during or after an invasive or interventional vascular procedure in a patient with preexisting atherosclerotic disease.

A less common cause of AKI is glomerulonephritis (Chapter 123), which can be seen in systemic lupus nephritis (Chapter 274), Wegener's granulomatosis (Chapter 278), polyarteritis nodosa (Chapter 278), Goodpasture's syndrome (Chapter 123), Henoch-Schönlein purpura (Chapter 278), and hemolytic-uremic syndrome (Chapter 176). AKI in this setting is termed *rapidly progressive glomerulonephritis* and results from direct inflammatory glomerular or vascular injury.

Postrenal Acute Kidney Injury

Postrenal AKI is caused by obstruction to luminal flow of the glomerular filtrate. This obstruction results in a relatively complex pathophysiology that begins with transmission of backpressure to Bowman's space of the glomerulus. Intuitively, this backpressure would be expected to reduce the GFR. However, by dilation of the glomerular afferent arteriole, the GFR remains largely preserved. Unfortunately, such compensation is only transient, and the GFR will begin to attenuate if the obstruction is not rapidly relieved. With continued obstruction for more than 12 to 24 hours, renal blood flow and intratubular pressure decline, and large unperfused and underperfused areas of the renal cortex result in a reduction in GFR.

CLINICAL MANIFESTATIONS

AKI, even when advanced, frequently is first diagnosed by abnormalities observed in a patient's laboratory studies and not by any specific symptom or sign. The clinical manifestations associated with AKI are frequently protean, occur late in the course, and are often not apparent until the renal dysfunction has become severe. The clinical findings of AKI also depend on the stage at which it is diagnosed. Patients with AKI may report symptoms such as anorexia, fatigue, nausea and vomiting, and pruritus, as well as a decline in urine output or dark-colored urine. Furthermore, if the patient has become volume overloaded, shortness of breath and dyspnea on exertion may be noted.

A thorough physical examination with special emphasis on determination of volume status and effective arterial volume is essential. If volume overload is present, jugular venous distention, pulmonary crackles, and peripheral edema may be found (Chapter 58). Findings such as asterixis, myoclonus, or a pericardial rub may be seen in severe AKI.

DIAGNOSIS

A systematic approach that considers each of the three major categories in the pathogenesis of AKI will ensure that an accurate diagnosis and an appropriate therapeutic plan will be achieved. An appropriate diagnostic strategy is to exclude prerenal and postrenal causes first and then, if needed, begin an evaluation for possible intrinsic causes.

Laboratory analysis of blood and urine samples of patients with AKI reveals the level of dysfunction, will frequently suggest a cause, and may also direct the rapidity with which a specific therapy needs to be instituted. All patients with clinical findings of AKI should be evaluated with serum measurements of electrolytes, creatinine, calcium, and phosphorus; a blood urea nitrogen level; and complete blood count with differential. In addition, urine studies, including sodium, potassium, chloride, and creatinine (Cr) determinations for calculation of the fractional excretion of sodium (FE$_{Na}$), are important. The formula for calculating FE$_{Na}$ is as follows:

$$FE_{Na} = \frac{Urine\ Na \times Plasma\ Cr}{Plasma\ Na \times Urine\ Cr} \times 100$$

The numerical value of FE$_{Na}$ can be helpful in determining the potential cause of the AKI (Table 122-4). In some cases, it is better to use FE$_{Cl}$ because urinary sodium can be elevated during systemic alkalosis when a high urinary bicarbonate level obligates the loss of sodium. Urine dipstick and microscopy (Table 122-5) should be performed on a fresh urine sample because important cellular elements that could indicate potential causes degrade rapidly with time. Finally, renal ultrasound to determine the presence or absence of outlet obstruction should also be included in the initial evaluation. Measurement of serum levels of structural biomarkers, such as kidney injury molecule 1 (KIM-1) and neutrophil gelatinase-associated lipocalin (NGAL), may aid in the diagnosis of AKI, although the data are not yet conclusive.

TABLE 122-4	FE$_{Na}$ VALUES FOR THE VARIOUS CAUSES OF ACUTE KIDNEY INJURY	
ETIOLOGY OF ACUTE KIDNEY INJURY	**FE$_{Na}$**	**BUN-TO-SERUM CREATININE RATIO**
Prerenal	<1%	>20
Intrarenal		<10-15
Tubular necrosis	≥1%	
Interstitial nephritis	≥1%	
Glomerulonephritis (early)	<1%	
Vascular disorders (early)	<1%	
Postrenal	≥1%	>20

TABLE 122-5	COMMON URINALYSIS FINDINGS IN ACUTE KIDNEY INJURY
CAUSE OF ACUTE KIDNEY INJURY	**URINALYSIS**
Prerenal	Normal or hyaline casts
Intrarenal	
Tubular cell injury	Muddy-brown, granular, epithelial casts
Interstitial nephritis	Pyuria, hematuria, mild proteinuria, granular and epithelial casts, eosinophils
Glomerulonephritis	Hematuria, marked proteinuria, red blood cell casts, granular casts
Vascular disorders	Normal or hematuria, mild proteinuria
Postrenal	Normal or hematuria, granular casts, pyuria

PRERENAL AZOTEMIA

Prerenal azotemia, which is the most common cause of renal dysfunction, can often be determined by the patient's history. Common historical features in patients with prerenal azotemia include vomiting, diarrhea, and poor oral intake. Heart failure can suggest a possible prerenal cause of reduced renal perfusion from overdiuresis or as exacerbation of the heart failure itself. Other medications that can attenuate renal perfusion, such as NSAIDs, ACE inhibitors, and ARBs, can cause prerenal azotemia. Common physical examination findings include tachycardia, systemic or orthostatic hypotension (or both), and dry mucous membranes.

Laboratory studies in patients with prerenal azotemia demonstrate elevated serum creatinine and blood urea nitrogen (BUN) levels. FE$_{Na}$ is typically less than 1%. However, in a patient taking diuretics such as furosemide, FE$_{Na}$ may be greater than 1% even though the patient has prerenal azotemia because of diuretic-induced natriuresis. For these clinical situations, the fractional excretion of urea can be used and is calculated in similar fashion:

$$FE_{urea} = \frac{Urine\ urea \times Plasma\ Cr}{Plasma\ urea \times Urine\ Cr} \times 100$$

FE$_{urea}$ less than 35% suggests prerenal AKI. Other causes of an FE$_{Na}$ greater than 1% include the presence of a non-reabsorbable solute such as bicarbonate, glucose, or mannitol. Chronic kidney disease, ATN, and late obstructive nephropathy are also associated with FE$_{Na}$ greater than 1%. Therefore, in these disease states, FE$_{Na}$ cannot provide reliable diagnostic information regarding AKI unless the FE$_{Na}$ is less than 1%. Moreover, FE$_{urea}$ has not been validated for these clinical entities.

Another laboratory parameter to assist in diagnosing prerenal AKI is the ratio of BUN to serum creatinine. Commonly, a patient with prerenal azotemia will have a BUN-to–serum creatinine ratio of greater than 20:1.

INTRARENAL ACUTE KIDNEY INJURY

A history of hypotension or exposure to a nephrotoxin or medication is a common finding in patients with intrarenal AKI. The nephrotoxin can be a specific tubular toxin that causes ATN or a medication that causes an allergic reaction as in acute interstitial nephritis (see Tables 122-1 and 122-2). Physical examination may reveal signs and symptoms of fluid overload. Rash may accompany acute interstitial nephritis. Cholesterol embolism in patients with severe atherosclerotic disease (Chapter 127) may manifest classically as cyanotic digits and AKI; this finding is frequently seen after invasive vascular surgery or an interventional study.

Laboratory studies will demonstrate elevated serum creatinine and BUN levels in intrarenal AKI. ATN and acute interstitial nephritis are frequently associated with FE_{Na} greater than 1, whereas FE_{Na} is typically less than 1 in glomerulonephritis and vascular disorders. Peripheral eosinophilia and urinary eosinophils may be present in acute interstitial nephritis, although the latter are neither sensitive nor specific for this type of AKI. Urinary eosinophils are also associated with cholesterol microembolic disease (Chapter 127). Intrarenal AKI has specific urinalysis findings that can be helpful in making diagnostic and therapeutic decisions (see Table 122-5).

POSTRENAL ACUTE KIDNEY INJURY

A history of prostatic hypertrophy (Chapter 131), prostate cancer (Chapter 207), lymphoma (Chapter 191), cervical cancer (Chapter 205), or retroperitoneal disease can often be found in patients with postrenal AKI. Postrenal AKI should always be in the differential diagnosis of patients with severe oliguria (urine output < 450 mL/day) or anuria (urine output < 100 mL/day). However, many patients with postrenal AKI are neither oliguric nor anuric. Beyond an elevation in a patient's serum creatinine and BUN levels, laboratory studies generally yield benign results. Bladder catheterization can be both diagnostic and therapeutic in postrenal AKI. However, renal ultrasound is the diagnostic test of choice, although it may be falsely negative early in postrenal AKI.

A Vicious Cycle

FIGURE 122-4. A vicious cycle exists between acute kidney injury (AKI) and chronic kidney disease (CKD), with CKD increasing the risk of developing AKI, and AKI accelerating progression of CKD.

TREATMENT ℞

The cornerstones of therapy for AKI are rapid recognition and correction of reversible causes, avoidance of any further renal injury, and correction and maintenance of a normal electrolyte and fluid volume milieu. Preventive therapy or medical interventions performed during the initiation and extension phases of AKI provide the greatest chance for minimizing the extent of injury (see Fig. 122-3, lines A and B) and hastening renal recovery (see Fig. 122-3, line B); interventions provided during the maintenance phase of AKI have not proved beneficial (see Fig. 122-3, line C). If prerenal AKI is not addressed early in a patient's course or if the patient is seen late in the course, ATN may occur and markedly increase morbidity and mortality.

Prerenal azotemia in its early stages often can be rapidly corrected by aggressive normalization of effective arterial volume, although more care must be taken during volume resuscitation in patients with a history of heart failure. Key approaches include administering volume (e.g., normal saline) to achieve euvolemia, improving cardiac output by afterload reduction (Chapter 59), or normalizing systemic vascular resistance.

Postrenal AKI secondary to prostatic hypertrophy can frequently be corrected by placement of a bladder catheter. However, outlet obstruction from a neoplastic process will usually require urologic consultation for consideration of ureteral stenting or placement of a percutaneous nephrostomy tube.

Intrarenal AKI can be the most complex and difficult to treat. AKI caused by glomerulonephritis (Chapter 123) or vasculitis (Chapters 274 and 278) will frequently require immunosuppressive therapy. For suspected acute interstitial nephritis, the offending medication must be determined and discontinued; a 2-week tapering course of glucocorticoids, beginning with 1 mg/kg of prednisone for 3 days, is commonly recommended despite the absence of definitive data.

General supportive measures include avoiding any further nephrotoxins and paying careful attention to the patient's fluid balance by monitoring weight and daily input and output. In addition, serum electrolytes, creatinine, and BUN should be monitored at least daily, more frequently if the patient's renal function appears to be tenuous. Patients with AKI should also receive a low sodium, potassium, and protein diet, which can be liberalized as the patient's renal function improves. A phosphate binder (e.g., calcium acetate [1334 mg], lanthanum carbonate [500 mg], sevelamer [300 to 1000 mg], or aluminum hydroxide [300 to 600 mg] with each meal; see Table 121-4) is also usually helpful in controlling the serum phosphate level by minimizing the absorption of dietary phosphate.

Early nephrology consultation will ensure that the patient receives optimal care. Some patients will warrant urgent hemodialysis because of marked metabolic acidosis unresponsive to sodium bicarbonate infusions; electrolyte abnormalities, such as hyperkalemia that is unresponsive to medical management; pulmonary edema not responding to diuretic therapy; and uremic symptoms of encephalopathy, seizures, and pericarditis. In the absence of acute indications, however, when to initiate dialysis in AKI remains unresolved.

For AKI, intensive dialytic renal support therapy is no better than standard dialytic therapy,[1] and intermittent hemodialysis and continuous renal replacement therapy lead to similar clinical outcomes in acute renal failure.[2] Neither furosemide[3] nor low-dose dopamine[4] improve outcome, even though low-dose dopamine may temporarily improve metrics of renal physiology.

PREVENTION

Given the marked increase in morbidity and mortality associated with AKI, especially for critically ill patients, potential measures to prevent AKI are essential. The first step in prevention, however, is being aware of patients who are at highest risk for AKI because of known kidney disease or comorbid medical conditions, such as diabetes, hypertension, nephrotic syndrome, heart failure, and peripheral vascular disease.

Of all the risk factors for acquiring AKI, the presence of preexisting chronic kidney disease is the most predictive. Recent data document a vicious cycle involving AKI and CKD (Fig. 122-4). Appropriate hospital surveillance measures include avoiding nephrotoxic medications (e.g., NSAIDs and aminoglycosides); minimizing diagnostic procedures that require radiocontrast material, especially in the prerenal patient; and careful monitoring of urinary output with daily determination of serum electrolytes and creatinine levels after any procedures known to induce AKI. Additionally, educating the patient regarding common nonprescription nephrotoxins such as NSAIDs can reduce the risk for AKI in outpatients.

Before a potentially nephrotoxic exposure, early consultation with a nephrologist is warranted for this high-risk group to advise whether a specific medication or intervention may reduce the risk of AKI or whether an alternative medication or procedure, such as magnetic resonance imaging instead of computed tomography with intravenous radiocontrast agents, may be preferred. All potential nephrotoxins, such as NSAIDs, should be discontinued before a potentially nephrotoxic procedure and avoided after it. The patient's volume and hemodynamic status must be maximized.

In high-risk patients, a renal protective intervention is often instituted before exposure to the agent. Interventions that may be useful for preventing AKI associated with intravenous radiocontrast agents include sodium bicarbonate[5] (e.g., 15 mEq/L infused at 3 mL/kg/hour for 1 hour before the procedure and at 1 mL/kg/hour for 6 hours after it) and N-acetylcysteine[6] (usually 600 mg orally or intravenously 4 hours before the procedure), although the data for each individually or even the two together remain controversial.[7]

PROGNOSIS

Typically, AKI secondary to prerenal causes, if diagnosed and treated early, has the best prognosis for renal recovery. Patients with prerenal AKI commonly return to their baseline level of renal function and have a mortality rate of less than 10%. Similarly, patients with postrenal AKI also have a good prognosis for renal recovery if the outlet obstruction is promptly diagnosed and definitively treated.

In contrast, patients with intrarenal AKI have a less predictable renal outcome, and mortality in this group varies between 30 and 80%, depending on the severity of injury. Higher mortality rates occur in older patients with hospital-acquired AKI admitted to ICUs. Furthermore, mortality in patients with AKI is incremental, and seemingly modest increases in serum creatinine can result in marked increases in the mortality rate. Even a rise in serum creatinine of only 0.3 mg/dL results in a significantly increased risk of mortality.

The clinical course after recovery from ATN is subsequent tubular regeneration with recovery of renal function. However, this outcome is less ensured in patients with preexisting kidney disease. In addition, given the frequent systemic nature of their illness, patients with ATN, glomerulonephritis, and vasculitic causes of AKI may not fully recover to their baseline renal function. Patients who have a severe episode of AKI requiring hemodialysis may not recover their renal function and may need hemodialysis indefinitely (Chapter 133), especially if they have a preexisting history of chronic kidney disease. AKI hastens progression of chronic kidney disease to end-stage kidney disease and is often the major factor that causes such progression.

1. Palevsky PM, Zhang JH, et al. VA/NIH Acute Renal Failure Trial Network. Intensity of renal support in critically ill patients with acute kidney injury. *N Engl J Med.* 2008;359:7-20.
2. Pannu N, Klarenbach S, Wiebe N, et al. Renal replacement therapy in patients with acute renal failure: a systematic review. *JAMA.* 2008;299:793-805.
3. Ho KM, Sheridan DJ. Meta-analysis of furosemide to prevent or treat acute renal failure. *BMJ.* 2006;333:420.
4. Friedrich JO, Adhikary N, Herridge MS, et al. Meta-analysis: low-dose dopamine increases urine output but does not prevent renal dysfunction or death. *Ann Intern Med.* 2005;142:510-524.
5. Zoungas S, Ninomiya T, Huxley R, et al. Systematic review: sodium bicarbonate treatment regimens for the prevention of contrast-induced nephropathy. *Ann Intern Med.* 2009;151:631-638.
6. Trivedi H, Daram S, Szabo A, et al. High-dose N-acetylcysteine for the prevention of contrast-induced nephropathy. *Am J Med.* 2009;122:874.
7. Brown JR, Block CA, Malenka DJ, et al. Sodium bicarbonate plus N-acetylcysteine prophylaxis: a meta-analysis. *JACC Cardiovasc Interv.* 2009;2:1116-1124.

SUGGESTED READINGS

Anderson S, Eldadah B, Halter JB, et al. Acute kidney injury in older adults. *J Am Soc Nephrol.* 2011;22:28-38. *Review.*

Brochard L, Abroug F, Brenner M, et al. An Official ATS/ERS/ESICM/SCCM/SRLF Statement: prevention and management of acute renal failure in the ICU patient. An international consensus conference in intensive care medicine. *Am J Respir Crit Care Med.* 2010;181:1128-1155. *Review.*

Devarajan P. Biomarkers for the early detection of acute kidney injury. *Curr Opin Pediatr.* 2011;23:194-200. *Overview including the potential usefulness of neutrophil gelatinase-associated lipocalin (NGAL).*

Solomon P, Dauerman HL. Contrast-induced acute kidney injury. *Circulation.* 2010;122:2451-2455. *Review recommending hydration with normal saline or sodium bicarbonate.*

123

GLOMERULAR DISORDERS AND NEPHROTIC SYNDROMES

GERALD B. APPEL AND JAI RADHAKRISHNAN

GLOMERULAR DISORDERS

DEFINITION

Each *glomerulus,* the basic filtering unit of the kidney, consists of a tuft of anastomosing capillaries formed by the branching of the afferent arteriole. Approximately 1 million glomeruli comprise about 5% of the kidney weight and provide almost 2 m² of glomerular capillary filtering surface. The glomerular basement membrane provides both a size- and charge-selective barrier to the passage of circulating macromolecules. Renal pathology involving all glomeruli is called *diffuse* or *generalized;* if only some glomeruli are involved, the process is called *focal.* When dealing with the individual glomerulus, a process is *global* if the whole glomerular tuft is involved and *segmental* if only part of the glomerulus is involved. The modifying terms *proliferative, sclerosing,* and *necrotizing* are often used (e.g., focal and segmental glomerulosclerosis; diffuse global proliferative lupus nephritis). Extracapillary proliferation or crescent formation is caused by the accumulations of macrophages, fibroblasts, proliferating epithelial cells, and fibrin within Bowman's space. In general, crescent formation in any form of glomerular damage conveys a serious prognosis. Scarring of the tissue between the tubules and glomeruli, interstitial fibrosis, is also a poor prognostic sign in every glomerular disease.

EPIDEMIOLOGY

At present, about 17% of the U.S. population has proteinuria or renal dysfunction, and many, if not most, cases are caused by glomerular diseases. More than 500,000 Americans are in end-stage renal disease (ESRD) programs, and chronic kidney disease costs about $60 billion per year and accounts for about 28% of all Medicare spending, largely as a result of renal involvement by glomerular diseases. Diabetic renal damage alone affects many millions of persons and is the major cause of ESRD in the United States (Chapter 126). Worldwide, glomerular diseases associated with infectious agents such as malaria (Chapter 353) and schistosomiasis (Chapter 363) are still major health problems. The emergence of glomerular diseases linked to human immunodeficiency virus (HIV) and the hepatitis B and C viruses (Chapter 151) has focused new attention on the patterns and mechanisms of glomerular injury. Manifestations of glomerular injury range from asymptomatic microhematuria and albuminuria to rapidly progressive oliguric renal failure. Some patients develop massive fluid retention and edema at onset of their glomerular disease, whereas others present with only the slow insidious signs and symptoms of chronic renal failure (Chapter 132).

PATHOBIOLOGY

Common mechanisms such as breaks in the glomerular capillary wall and loss of the selective barrier to particles based on size and charge underlie the proteinuria and hematuria that are characteristic of glomerular diseases. Nevertheless, the nature of the initiating processes varies among different glomerular diseases. In some glomerular disorders, such as diabetes and amyloidosis, structural and biochemical alterations are present in the glomerular capillary wall. In others, immune-mediated renal injury is caused by deposition of circulating immune complexes, the localized effects of anti–glomerular basement membrane (anti-GBM) antibodies, or other mechanisms.

CLINICAL MANIFESTATIONS

Findings indicative of a glomerular origin of renal disease include erythrocyte casts and dysmorphic red blood cells (RBCs) in the urinary sediment as well as large amounts of albuminuria. Persistent urinary excretion of more than 500 to 1000 erythrocytes per milliliter (or greater than two RBCs per high-power field on microscopy) is abnormal. Dysmorphic RBCs, which are deformed as a result of their passage through the glomerular capillary wall and tubules, and red blood cell casts, which are formed when these erythrocytes become enmeshed in a proteinaceous matrix in the lumen of the tubules, are also indicative of glomerular disease.

In a normal person, the urinary excretion of albumin is less than 30 mg/day, and the total urinary excretion of protein is less than 150 mg/day. Although increases in urinary protein excretion may come from the filtration of abnormal circulating proteins (e.g., light chains in multiple myeloma) or from the deficient proximal tubular reabsorption of normal, filtered low-molecular-weight proteins (e.g., β_2-microglobulin), the most common cause of proteinuria, and specifically albuminuria, is glomerular injury. Proteinuria associated with glomerular disease may range from several hundred milligrams to more than 30 g daily. In some diseases, such as minimal change nephrotic syndrome, albumin is the predominant protein in the urine. In others, such as focal sclerosing glomerulonephritis and diabetes, the proteinuria, although still largely composed of albumin, is nonselective and contains many higher-molecular-weight proteins.

DIAGNOSIS

Some patients have asymptomatic microhematuria or proteinuria discovered by routine evaluations. Microscopic hematuria associated with deformed RBCs or RBC casts is likely to be glomerular in origin. Subnephrotic levels of proteinuria may arise from orthostatic proteinuria, hypertension, tubular disease, or glomerular damage.

In patients with asymptomatic urinary abnormalities of glomerular origin, the underlying glomerular lesion may represent the early phase of one of the progressive glomerular diseases or may be due to a benign, nonprogressive glomerular lesion. In general, if patients have less than 1 g of proteinuria daily or glomerular microhematuria but a normal glomerular filtration rate (GFR) and no evidence of systemic disease based on a careful history, physical examination, and serologic tests, it is not necessary to proceed to a renal biopsy to establish a diagnosis, because most of these patients need no immunosuppressive therapy. The patient can be followed closely, and biopsy need be performed only in patients with progressively increasing proteinuria or evidence of a decreasing GFR.

TABLE 123-1 TYPICAL FINDINGS OF NEPHROTIC SYNDROME VERSUS NEPHRITIS

NEPHROTIC SYNDROME	NEPHRITIS
RENAL INSUFFICIENCY	
Uncommon	Common at presentation
PROTEINURIA	
Typically high (>3 g/day)	Variable
URINE RBCs	
Few	Prominent
URINE RBC CASTS	
Unlikely	Likely

RBCs = red blood cells.

TABLE 123-2 CAUSES OF IDIOPATHIC NEPHROTIC SYNDROME IN ADULTS

	INCIDENCE (%)
Minimal change disease	5-10
Focal segmental glomerulosclerosis	20-25
Membranous nephropathy	25-30
Membranoproliferative glomerulonephritis	5
Other proliferative and sclerosing glomerulonephritides	15-30

TABLE 123-3 NEPHROTIC SYNDROME ASSOCIATED WITH SPECIFIC CAUSES ("SECONDARY" NEPHROTIC SYNDROME)

SYSTEMIC DISEASES

Diabetes mellitus
Systemic lupus erythematosus and other collagen diseases
Amyloidosis (amyloid AL- or AA-associated)
Vasculitic-immunologic disease (mixed cryoglobulinemia, Wegener's granulomatosis, rapidly progressive glomerulonephritis, polyarteritis, Henoch-Schönlein purpura, sarcoidosis, Goodpasture's syndrome)

INFECTIONS

Bacterial (post-streptococcal, congenital and secondary syphilis, subacute bacterial endocarditis, cerebral ventriculoatrial shunt nephritis)
Viral (hepatitis B, hepatitis C, HIV infection, infectious mononucleosis, cytomegalovirus infection)
Parasitic (malaria, toxoplasmosis, schistosomiasis, filariasis)

MEDICATION RELATED

Gold, mercury, and the heavy metals
Penicillamine
Nonsteroidal anti-inflammatory drugs including COX2 inhibitors
Lithium
Paramethadione, trimethadione
Captopril
"Street" heroin
Others: probenecid, chlorpropamide, rifampin, tolbutamide, phenindione, pamidronate

ALLERGENS, VENOMS, AND IMMUNIZATIONS

NEOPLASMS

Hodgkin's lymphoma and leukemias/lymphomas (with minimal change lesion)
Solid tumors (with membranous nephropathy)

HEREDITARY AND METABOLIC DISEASE

Alport's syndrome
Fabry's disease
Sickle cell disease
Congenital (Finnish type) nephrotic syndrome
Familial nephrotic syndrome
Nail-patella syndrome
Partial lipodystrophy

OTHER

Pregnancy related (includes preeclampsia)
Transplant rejection
Serum sickness
Accelerated hypertensive nephrosclerosis
Unilateral renal artery stenosis
Massive obesity–sleep apnea
Reflux nephropathy

THE NEPHROTIC SYNDROME

DEFINITION

The nephrotic syndrome (Table 123-1) is defined by albuminuria in amounts of more than 3 to 3.5 g/day accompanied by hypoalbuminemia, edema, and hyperlipidemia. In practice, many clinicians refer to "nephrotic range" proteinuria regardless of whether their patients have the other manifestations of the full syndrome, which is a consequence of the proteinuria.

EPIDEMIOLOGY

Many cases of the nephrotic syndrome are idiopathic (Table 123-2), but others are caused by known underlying conditions (Table 123-3). Although minimal change disease is the most common cause of nephrotic syndrome in children, idiopathic membranous nephropathy and focal segmental glomerular sclerosis are the most common causes in adults. In England, men account for about 58% of hospitalizations for nephrotic syndrome, and the mean hospital length of stay for nephrotic syndrome is about 6 days.

PATHOBIOLOGY

Hypoalbuminemia is largely a consequence of urinary protein loss. It also can be due to the catabolism of filtered albumin by the proximal tubule, the redistribution of albumin within the body, and the reduced hepatic synthesis of albumin. As a result, the relationship among urinary protein loss, the level of the serum albumin, and other secondary consequences of heavy albuminuria is inexact.

The salt and volume retention in the nephrotic syndrome may occur through at least two different major mechanisms. The classic teaching is that hypoalbuminemia reduces the oncotic pressure of plasma, the resulting intravascular volume depletion leads to activation of the renin-angiotensin-aldosterone axis, and this activation increases the retention of renal sodium and fluid. However, primary salt retention in the distal nephron also may occur independently of the renin-angiotensin-aldosterone axis.

CLINICAL MANIFESTATIONS

Patients may present with weight gain, peripheral edema, and periorbital edema. Hypertension is common. The urinalysis shows more than 3+ of proteinuria and varying degrees of hematuria, depending on the cause. A 24-hour urine usually shows 3 to 5 mg/kg/day of proteinuria.

Nephrotic patients often have a hypercoagulable state and are predisposed to deep vein thrombosis (Chapter 81), pulmonary emboli (Chapter 98), and renal vein thrombosis (Chapter 127). Patients with the nephrotic syndrome have increased risk of atherosclerotic complications. Most nephrotic patients have elevated levels of total and low-density lipoprotein (LDL) cholesterol with low or normal high-density lipoprotein (HDL) cholesterol. Lipoprotein(a) levels are elevated as well and return to normal with remission of the nephrotic syndrome.

DIAGNOSIS

Initial evaluation of the nephrotic patient includes laboratory tests to define whether the patient has primary idiopathic nephrotic syndrome (see Table 123-2) or a secondary cause related to a systemic disease, toxin, or medication (see Table 123-3). Common screening tests include the fasting blood sugar and glycosylated hemoglobin tests for diabetes, an antinuclear antibody test for collagen vascular disease, and a serum complement level, which screens for many immune complex–mediated diseases (Table 123-4). In selected patients, cryoglobulins, hepatitis B and C serologies, HIV testing, antineutrophil cytoplasmic antibodies (ANCAs), anti-GBM antibodies, serum protein electrophoresis, and other tests may be useful.

After exclusion of secondary causes, a renal biopsy is often required in the adult nephrotic patient. Biopsy results in patients with heavy proteinuria and the nephrotic syndrome are likely to provide a specific diagnosis, determine prognosis, and guide therapy.

TABLE 123-4	SERUM COMPLEMENT LEVELS IN GLOMERULAR DISEASES

DISEASES WITH A REDUCED COMPLEMENT LEVEL

Post-streptococcal glomerulonephritis
Subacute bacterial endocarditis, visceral abscess, shunt nephritis
Systemic lupus erythematosus
Cryoglobulinemia
Idiopathic membranoproliferative glomerulonephritis

DISEASES ASSOCIATED WITH A NORMAL SERUM COMPLEMENT

Minimal change nephrotic syndrome
Focal segmental glomerulosclerosis
Membranous nephropathy
Immunoglobulin A nephropathy
Henoch-Schönlein purpura
Anti–glomerular basement disease
Pauci-immune rapidly progressive glomerulonephritis
Polyarteritis nodosa
Wegener's granulomatosis

FIGURE 123-1. Unremarkable light microscopic appearance of minimal change disease glomerulopathy. Glomerular basement membranes are thin, and there is no glomerular hypercellularity.

TREATMENT Rx

Treatment varies by the specific cause. Elevated lipid levels should be treated (Chapter 213). Anticoagulation is not recommended routinely but is needed if any thrombotic complications occur. Edema is treated with diuretics, and the combination of furosemide plus albumin is more effective than furosemide alone for patients with refractory edema. **1**

Idiopathic Nephrotic Syndrome
MINIMAL CHANGE DISEASE

Minimal change disease, which is the most common pattern of nephrotic syndrome in children, accounts for only about 5 to 10% of cases of idiopathic nephrotic syndrome in adults. A similar histologic pattern may be seen as an adverse reaction to certain medications (nonsteroidal anti-inflammatory drugs [NSAIDs], lithium) or in association with certain tumors (e.g., Hodgkin's disease).

CLINICAL MANIFESTATIONS

Patients typically present with weight gain and periorbital and peripheral edema related to the proteinuria, which is usually well into the nephrotic range. Additional findings in adults are hypertension and microscopic hematuria, each in about 30% of patients. However, active urinary sediment with RBC casts is not found. Many adult patients have mild to moderate azotemia, which may be related to hypoalbuminemia and intravascular volume depletion. Complement levels and serologic test results are normal.

DIAGNOSIS

In true minimal change disease, histopathology typically reveals no glomerular abnormalities on light microscopy (Fig. 123-1). The tubules may show lipid droplet accumulation from absorbed lipoproteins (hence the older term *lipoid nephrosis*). Immunofluorescence staining and electron microscopy (Fig. 123-2) show no immune-type deposits. By electron microscopy, the GBM is normal, and effacement or "fusion" of the visceral epithelial foot processes is noted along virtually the entire distribution of every capillary loop.

FIGURE 123-2. Minimal change disease. Electron micrograph shows widespread effacement of foot processes with microvillous transformation of the visceral epithelium. No electron-dense deposits are present (uranyl acetate, lead citrate stain; ×6000).

TREATMENT Rx

The course of minimal change nephrotic syndrome is often one of remissions, relapses, and responses to additional treatment. When treated with corticosteroids for 8 weeks, 85 to 95% of children experience a remission of proteinuria. In adults, the response rate is somewhat lower, with 75 to 85% of patients responding to regimens of daily (1 mg/kg, maximum 80 mg) or alternate-day (2 mg/kg, maximum 120 mg) prednisone therapy, tapered after 2 months of treatment for a total of 5 to 6 months of therapy. The time to clinical response is slower in adults, and they are not considered steroid resistant until they have failed to respond in 16 weeks of treatment. Tapering of the steroid dose after remission should be gradual over 1 to 2 months. Approximately 40% of adults relapse by 1 year and 50% by 5 years. Most clinicians treat the first relapse similarly to the initial episode. Patients who relapse a third time or who become corticosteroid dependent (unable to decrease the prednisone dose without proteinuria recurring) may be treated with a 2- to 3-month course of the alkylating agent cyclophosphamide at a dose of up to 2 mg/kg/day. Up to 50% of patients will have a remission of at least 5 years, but the response rate is lower in corticosteroid-dependent patients. Other alternative treatments for patients who frequently relapse or are steroid resistant include low-dose cyclosporine (3 to 5 mg/kg/day in divided doses for 4 months), tacrolimus (0.05 to 0.1 mg/kg/day in divided doses), and mycophenolate mofetil (750 to 1000 mg twice daily). All provide approximately equivalent remission and relapse rates, but cyclosporine and tacrolimus increase the risk of nephrotoxicity, so their blood levels must be carefully monitored.

PROGNOSIS

The prognosis of minimal change disease is excellent in terms of kidney function, and most patients who have a decline in kidney function have focal segmental glomerulosclerosis on a subsequent kidney biopsy. However, more than 50% of patients have relapses, and 10 to 20% may become steroid dependent.

FOCAL SEGMENTAL GLOMERULOSCLEROSIS

About 20 to 25% of adults with idiopathic nephrotic syndrome are found on biopsy to have focal segmental glomerulosclerosis (FSGS). The incidence of FSGS is increasing in all races, but it is especially common in African Americans. FSGS may be either idiopathic or secondary to a number of different causes (e.g., heroin abuse, HIV infection, sickle cell disease, obesity, reflux of urine from the bladder to the kidneys, and lesions associated with single or remnant kidneys). FSGS can occur in multiple family members owing to genetic defects in components of the visceral epithelial cell: an autosomal recessive pattern caused by mutations in the structural protein podocin; and autosomal dominant forms, caused by mutations in the structural protein α-actinin 4, the TRPC6 glomerular slit diaphragm-associated channel, or INF2, which encodes a formin (actin-regulating protein). The predisposition of African Americans to FSGS is related to alleles in the genes for myosin heavy chain 9 (MYH9) and apolipoprotein L1.

CLINICAL MANIFESTATIONS

Patients with idiopathic FSGS typically present with either asymptomatic proteinuria or edema. Although criteria for the nephrotic syndrome are met in two thirds of patients at presentation, proteinuria may vary from less than 1 to more than 30 g/day. Hypertension is found in 30 to 50% of patients, and microscopic hematuria occurs in about one half of all patients. The GFR is decreased at presentation in 20 to 30% of patients. Complement levels and other serologic test results are normal.

DIAGNOSIS

By light microscopy, only some glomeruli initially have areas of segmental scarring (Fig. 123-3). As renal function declines, repeat biopsy specimens show more glomeruli with segmental sclerosing lesions and increased numbers of globally sclerotic glomeruli. By immunofluorescence staining, immunoglobulin M (IgM) and C3 commonly are trapped in the areas of glomerular sclerosis. Electron microscopy shows no deposits and only visceral epithelial cell foot process effacement. The histopathologic variants of

FIGURE 123-3. Focal segmental glomerulosclerosis. **A,** Light micrograph of classic focal segmental glomerulosclerosis. **B,** Silver stain of collapsing focal segmental glomerulosclerosis showing collapse of the glomerular tufts.

FSGS are associated with epidemiologic, clinical, and prognostic differences. For example, the "tip lesion" variant has a relatively benign course, whereas the collapsing variant progresses more rapidly to renal failure.

TREATMENT   Rx

For primary (idiopathic) FSGS, corticosteroids are used as initial therapy (e.g., prednisone, 1 mg/kg/day, maximum 80 mg, or 2 mg/kg every other day, maximum 120 mg, as tolerated) for a minimum of 3 to 4 months and slowly tapered over the next 3 to 6 months if remission is achieved. A complete or partial remission may be seen in up to 40 to 60% of patients, with preservation of long-term renal function. In patients who relapse after initial therapy, oral cyclophosphamide (2 to 2.5 mg/kg/day for 12 weeks) or cyclosporine (4 mg/kg/day in divided doses) is used for 12 to 24 months, with slow tapering thereafter. With cyclosporine, careful monitoring of renal function and cyclosporine levels are necessary to avoid nephrotoxicity. In patients who are steroid resistant after 4 months of high-dose prednisone, the dose of prednisone should be tapered and patients should be treated with cyclosporine (3.5 mg/kg/day in divided doses adjusted to serum levels 125 to 225 μg/L) plus prednisone (0.15 mg/kg/day in divided doses, maximum 15 mg/day) for 6 months. **2**

PROGNOSIS

The course of untreated FSGS is usually one of progressive proteinuria and declining GFR. Only a minority of patients experiences a spontaneous remission of proteinuria, and most untreated patients eventually develop ESRD within 5 to 20 years from presentation. Patients with a sustained remission of their nephrotic syndrome are unlikely to progress to ESRD, whereas those with unremitting nephrotic syndrome are likely to progress.

In general, patients with genetic forms of the disease are steroid resistant, have a progressive course, and do not experience recurrences of the FSGS when they receive a renal transplant. Overall, however, focal sclerosis recurs in the transplanted kidney in up to 30% of cases, often in association with elevated levels of a circulating permeability factor. Younger patients, those with a rapid course to renal failure, and those with a prior recurrence are more likely to have recurrence in the allograft.

MEMBRANOUS NEPHROPATHY

Membranous nephropathy is the most common pattern of idiopathic nephrotic syndrome in white patients. It may also be associated with infections (syphilis [Chapter 327] and hepatitis B and C [Chapter 151]), systemic lupus erythematosus (SLE; Chapter 274), medications (gold salts, NSAIDs), and certain tumors (solid tumors and lymphomas). In many cases of what was previously classified as idiopathic membranous nephropathy, the antigen is the M-type phospholipase A₂ receptor in the podocyte.

CLINICAL MANIFESTATIONS

Membranous nephropathy typically presents as proteinuria and edema. Hypertension and microhematuria are not infrequent findings, but renal function and GFR are usually normal at presentation. Despite the finding of complement in the glomerular immune deposits, serum complement levels are normal. Membranous nephropathy is the most common pattern of the nephrotic syndrome to be associated with a hypercoagulable state and renal vein thrombosis (Chapter 127). The presence of sudden flank pain, deterioration of renal function, or symptoms of pulmonary disease in a patient with membranous nephropathy should prompt an investigation for renal vein thrombosis and pulmonary emboli.

DIAGNOSIS

On light microscopy, the glomerular capillary loops often appear rigid or thickened (Fig. 123-4), but there is no cellular proliferation. Immunofluorescence staining and electron microscopy show subepithelial immune dense deposits all along the glomerular capillary loops (Fig. 123-5). The presence of circulating antibodies to the M-type phospholipase A₂ receptor are 75% sensitive and 100% specific for idiopathic membranous nephropathy.

TREATMENT   Rx

Studies using corticosteroids to treat membranous nephropathy have given conflicting results, and proof of their benefit is lacking. By comparison, corticosteroid therapy (methylprednisolone, 1 g intravenously daily for 3 days, then oral prednisone, 0.5 mg/kg/day for 27 days, in months 1, 3, and 5) and oral cytotoxic therapy (chlorambucil, 0.2 mg/kg/day, or cyclophosphamide,

FIGURE 123-6. Membranoproliferative glomerulonephritis with lobulation of the glomerular tuft and splitting of the basement membrane as seen by silver stain.

FIGURE 123-4. **Membranous nephropathy. A,** Light micrograph of membranous nephropathy demonstrating thickening of the glomerular capillary wall but no hypercellularity. **B,** Silver stain of idiopathic membranous nephropathy showing spike formation along the outer aspect of the glomerular basement membrane corresponding to projections of the basement membrane between the epimembranous deposits.

2.5 mg/kg/day, for 30 days in months 2, 4, and 6) given in alternating months over 6 months results in more total remissions and better preservation of renal function compared with symptomatic therapy.**3** The combination of cyclosporine (3.5 mg/kg/day adjusted to serum levels of 125 to 225 μg/L) plus prednisone (0.15 mg/kg/day up to a maximum of 15 mg/day) for 6 months also is more likely to induce remission of the nephrotic syndrome compared with placebo or prednisone alone.**4** Other agents used successfully in uncontrolled or small controlled trials in membranous nephropathy include mycophenolate mofetil, adrenocorticotropic hormone, and the monoclonal anti-CD20 antibody, rituximab.

PROGNOSIS

In most large series, renal survival is more than 75% at 10 years, with a spontaneous remission rate of 20 to 30%. In general, older patients, males, and those with heavy persistent proteinuria are most likely to progress to renal failure and hence to benefit from therapy.

Membranoproliferative Glomerulonephritis

Idiopathic type I membranoproliferative or mesangiocapillary glomerulonephritis (MPGN) is an uncommon primary glomerular disease that represents only a small percentage of renal biopsy results. However, by light microscopy, similar patterns of glomerular damage commonly have been seen in association with hepatitis C (Chapter 151), SLE (Chapter 274), monoclonal gammopathies, and thrombotic microangiopathy associated with antiphospholipid antibodies (Chapter 179). All these stimuli have been proposed to incite the glomerular mesangial cells to grow out along the capillary wall and split the glomerular basement membrane.

Type II MPGN, or dense deposit disease, is an even less common disease that is associated with uncontrolled systemic activation of the alternative complement pathway. The cause may be C3 nephritic factor, which is an autoantibody directed against the C3 convertase of the alternate complement pathway, deficiencies of factor H or I or other inhibitors of the alternate complement cascade. Dense deposit disease may be associated with partial lipodystrophy. Because the histology of dense deposit disease may show patterns other than what are typical in MPGN (e.g., mesangial proliferation, sclerosis, crescents) and its pathogenesis is unique, many investigators feel it should be categorized independently of the other forms of MPGN.

CLINICAL MANIFESTATIONS AND DIAGNOSIS

Most patients with idiopathic MPGN are children or young adults who present with proteinuria or the nephrotic syndrome. A low serum complement level is found intermittently in type I MPGN, whereas the C3 level is usually reduced in dense deposit disease. The diagnosis of type II MPGN requires a renal biopsy that shows complement C3 in a characteristic ribbon-like pattern around the capillary loop by light microscopy (Fig. 123-6).

FIGURE 123-5. **Membranous glomerulopathy.** On ultrastructural examination, there are numerous, closely apposed epimembranous electron-dense deposits separated by basement membrane spikes (uranyl acetate, lead citrate stain; ×2500).

FIGURE 123-7. Immunoglobulin A (IgA) nephropathy with mesangial cell proliferation by light microscopy and IgA deposition on immunofluorescence.

TREATMENT AND PROGNOSIS Rx

Attempts to treat idiopathic type I MPGN have included corticosteroids, other immunosuppressive medications, anticoagulants, and antiplatelet agents. No therapy has been proved effective in a randomized trial in adults, but corticosteroids have had some success in children at a dose of 40 mg/m^2 every other day for a mean period of 41 months. Most studies have found a similar course and prognosis for the various patterns of MPGN, with half of the patients progressing to ESRD within 10 years of diagnosis.

ACUTE GLOMERULONEPHRITIS AND THE NEPHRITIC SYNDROME

EPIDEMIOLOGY AND PATHOBIOLOGY

Known inciting causes of acute glomerulonephritis include infectious agents, such as type 12 and type 49 "nephritogenic" strains of group A streptococci and endocarditis caused by *Staphylococcus aureus* and *Streptococcus viridans*. Acute glomerulonephritis can also be caused by the deposition of immune complexes in autoimmune diseases such as SLE (Chapter 274), and the damaging effect of circulating antibodies directed against the GBM, as in Goodpasture's syndrome.

Invading neutrophils and monocytes, as well as resident glomerular cells, can damage the glomerulus through a number of mediators, including oxidants, chemoattractant agents, proteases, cytokines, and growth factors. Some factors, such as transforming growth factor-β, have been related to eventual glomerulosclerosis and chronic glomerular damage.

CLINICAL MANIFESTATIONS AND DIAGNOSIS

Patients with acute glomerulonephritis often present with a nephritic picture characterized by a decreased GFR, azotemia, oliguria, hypertension, and an active urinary sediment (see Table 123-1). Hypertension is common and is caused by intravascular volume expansion, although renin levels may not be appropriately suppressed for the degree of volume expansion. Patients may note dark, smoky, or cola-colored urine in association with an active urinary sediment, which is composed of erythrocytes, leukocytes, and a variety of casts, including RBC casts. Although many patients with acute glomerulonephritis have proteinuria, sometimes even in the nephrotic range, most patients have lesser degrees of albumin leakage into the urine, especially when the GFR is markedly reduced. Regardless of the inciting cause, acute glomerulonephritis is characterized on light microscopy by hypercellularity of the glomerulus, which may be composed of infiltrating inflammatory cells, proliferation of resident glomerular cells, or both.

Immunoglobulin A Nephropathy

EPIDEMIOLOGY AND PATHOBIOLOGY

IgA nephropathy, which is now recognized as the most frequent form of idiopathic glomerulonephritis worldwide, represents 15 to 40% of primary glomerulonephritides in parts of Europe and Asia. In geographic areas where renal biopsies are commonly performed for milder urinary findings, a higher incidence of IgA has been noted. In the United States, some centers report this diagnosis in up to 20% of all primary glomerulopathies. Affected males outnumber females, and the peak occurrence is in the second to third decades of life.

In IgA nephropathy, the predominant antibody is composed of polymeric IgA1, but the antigen—whether infectious, dietary, or other—to which it is directed is unknown in most cases. The pathogenesis may involve abnormal O-linked galactosylation of the IgA molecule at the hinge region, with resultant abnormal binding of IgA complexes to the glomerular mesangial cells.

CLINICAL MANIFESTATIONS AND DIAGNOSIS

IgA nephropathy often presents either as asymptomatic microscopic hematuria with or without proteinuria (the most common presentation in adults) or as episodic gross hematuria following an upper respiratory tract infection or exercise (the most common presentation in children and young adults). Hypertension is present in 20 to 50% of all patients. Increased serum IgA levels, noted in one third to one half of cases, do not correlate with the course of the disease. Serum complement levels are normal. The diagnosis of IgA nephropathy is established by finding glomerular IgA deposits as either the dominant or the codominant immunoglobulin on immunofluorescence microscopy (Fig. 123-7). Deposits of C3 and IgG also are often found. The light microscopy picture varies from the most common picture of mild mesangial proliferation to severe crescentic glomerulonephritis. By electron microscopy, immune-type dense deposits are typically found in the mesangial and paramesangial areas.

TREATMENT Rx

Because the pathogenesis of IgA nephropathy is thought to involve abnormal antigenic stimulation of mucosal IgA production and subsequent immune complex deposition in the glomeruli, treatment has been directed at these sites. Efforts to treat the disease by preventing antigenic stimulation, including broad-spectrum antibiotics (e.g., doxycycline), tonsillectomy, and dietary manipulations (e.g., gluten elimination), generally have been controversial or unsuccessful. Most physicians choose to treat only patients at high risk for progression to renal failure. Trials using fish oils to decrease proteinuria and slow progressive disease have given conflicting results. Controlled studies suggest that glucocorticoids (e.g., pulse methylprednisolone, 1 g daily for three doses in months 0, 2, and 4, followed by prednisone, 0.5 mg/kg every other day for 6 months) may decrease proteinuria and progressive renal failure in some patients.⑤ The benefit of immunosuppressive agents (e.g., cyclophosphamide, azathioprine, mycophenolate mofetil) is far from clear. For the few patients with crescentic IgA nephropathy, cytotoxic agents have been used. Angiotensin-converting enzyme (ACE) inhibitors and angiotensin receptor blockers (ARBs) have reduced proteinuria and the progression of renal disease in small randomized studies and appear to have incremental benefit when added to glucocorticoid therapy.

PROGNOSIS

The course is variable, with some patients showing no decline in GFR over decades and others developing the nephrotic syndrome, hypertension, and renal failure. Factors predictive of a poor outcome in IgA nephropathy include older age at onset, absence of gross hematuria, hypertension, persistent proteinuria greater than 1 g/day, male gender, an elevated serum creatinine level, and the histologic features of severe proliferation and sclerosis or tubulointerstitial damage and crescent formation. Renal survival rates are estimated at 75 to 85% at 10 years and 70 to 75% at 20 years. A significant percentage of transplant recipients have a morphologic recurrence in the allograft, but graft loss owing to the disease is uncommon.

Henoch-Schönlein Purpura

Henoch-Schönlein purpura (HSP; Chapter 278) is characterized by a small-vessel vasculitis with arthralgias, skin purpura, and abdominal symptoms as well as a proliferative acute glomerulonephritis. HSP is predominantly a disease of childhood, although cases occur in adults. Despite the finding of circulating IgA-containing immune complexes, no infectious agent or allergen has been defined as causative, and serum complement levels are normal.

CLINICAL MANIFESTATIONS AND DIAGNOSIS

The clinical manifestations of HSP (Chapter 278) include dermatologic, gastrointestinal, rheumatologic, and renal findings. Skin involvement typically starts with a macular rash that coalesces into purpuric lesions (see Fig. 278-2 in Chapter 278) on the ankles, legs, and occasionally arms and buttocks. Gastrointestinal symptoms include cramps, diarrhea, nausea, and vomiting, with melena and bloody diarrhea in the most severely involved cases. Although arthralgias of the knees, wrists, and ankles are common, true arthritis is uncommon. Symptoms of different organ system involvement may occur concurrently or separately, and recurrent episodes during the first year are not uncommon. The renal histopathology of HSP is similar to that of IgA nephropathy. In the skin, there is a small-vessel leukocytoclastic angiitis with immune deposition of IgA.

TREATMENT AND PROGNOSIS (Rx)

Like IgA nephropathy, HSP has no proven therapy. Episodes of rash, arthralgias, and abdominal symptoms usually resolve spontaneously. Some patients with severe abdominal findings have been treated with short courses of high doses of corticosteroids. Patients with severe glomerular involvement may benefit by modalities used to treat patients with severe IgA nephropathy. Although most patients with HSP recover fully, patients with a more severe nephritic or nephrotic presentation and more severe glomerular damage on renal biopsy have an unfavorable long-term prognosis.

Post-streptococcal Glomerulonephritis

Acute post-streptococcal glomerulonephritis may occur in either an epidemic form or as sporadic cases after infection with nephritogenic strains of group A β-hemolytic streptococci (Chapter 298). Post-streptococcal glomerulonephritis is largely a disease of childhood, but severe disease in adults has been well documented. The disease is most common after episodes of pharyngitis, but it can follow streptococcal infections at any site, and subclinical cases greatly outnumber clinical cases. Post-streptococcal glomerulonephritis is an acute immune complex disease characterized by the formation of antibodies against streptococci with the localization of immune complexes with complement in the kidney.

CLINICAL MANIFESTATIONS AND DIAGNOSIS

Most cases are diagnosed by detecting hematuria, proteinuria, hypertension, and the nephritic syndrome (see Table 123-1) 10 days to several weeks after a streptococcal infection. Throat cultures and skin cultures of suspected sites of streptococcal involvement often may not be positive for group A β-hemolytic streptococci. A variety of antibodies (e.g., antistreptolysin O [ASLO], antihyaluronidase [AHT]) and a streptozyme panel of antibodies against streptococcal antigens (which includes ASLO, AHT, antistreptokinase, and anti-DNase) often show high titers, but a change in titer over time is more indicative of a recent streptococcal infection. More than 95% of patients with post-streptococcal glomerulonephritis secondary to pharyngitis and 85% of patients with streptococcal skin infections have positive antibody titers. The serum total hemolytic complement levels and C3 levels are decreased in more than 90% of patients during the episode of acute glomerulonephritis.

In a patient with a classic acute nephritic episode after a documented streptococcal infection, a change in streptococcal antibody titer, and a

FIGURE 123-8. Post-streptococcal glomerulonephritis with hypercellular glomerulus filling Bowman's space and infiltrated by polymorphonuclear and other cells.

depressed serum complement level, a renal biopsy adds little to the diagnosis. In other cases, a biopsy may be necessary to confirm or refute the diagnosis. On light microscopy (Fig. 123-8), glomeruli are markedly enlarged and often fill Bowman's space. Glomeruli exhibit hypercellularity owing to an infiltration of monocytes and polymorphonuclear cells and a proliferation of the glomerular cellular elements. The capillary lumens often are compressed by the glomerular hypercellularity. Some cases demonstrate extracapillary proliferation with crescent formation. On immunofluorescence microscopy, there is coarse granular deposition of IgG, IgM, and complement, especially C3, along the capillary wall. Electron microscopy shows large dome-shaped, electron-dense subepithelial deposits resembling the humps of a camel at isolated intervals along the GBM.

TREATMENT AND PROGNOSIS (Rx)

Therapy is symptomatic and directed at controlling the hypertension and fluid retention with antihypertensive agents (see Tables 67-5 and 67-7 in Chapter 67) and diuretics. In most patients, post-streptococcal glomerulonephritis is a self-limited disease, with recovery of renal function and disappearance of hypertension in several weeks. However, the presence of underlying renal disease, especially diabetic nephropathy, is associated with a worse prognosis. Proteinuria and hematuria may resolve more slowly over months.

Glomerulonephritis with Endocarditis and Visceral Abscesses

Various glomerular lesions are found in patients with acute and chronic bacterial endocarditis (Chapter 76). Although embolic phenomena can lead to glomerular ischemia and infarcts, a common finding is an immune complex glomerulonephritis. With *S. viridans* endocarditis, both focal and diffuse proliferative glomerulonephritides are common. With the increased incidence of *S. aureus* endocarditis, 40 to 80% of patients with endocarditis have clinical evidence of an immune complex proliferative glomerulonephritis. Glomerulonephritis is now more common with acute than subacute bacterial endocarditis, and the duration of illness is not an important determinant of the renal disease.

Patients often have hematuria and RBC casts in their urinary sediment, proteinuria ranging from less than 1 g/day to nephrotic levels, and progressive renal failure. Serum total complement and C3 levels are usually reduced. Renal insufficiency may be mild and reversible with appropriate antibiotic therapy, or it may be progressive and lead to dialysis and irreversible renal failure.

A proliferative immune complex glomerulonephritis can occur in patients with deep visceral bacterial abscesses and infections, such as empyema of the lung (Chapter 99) and osteomyelitis (Chapter 296). Immune complex forms of acute glomerulonephritis also have been noted in patients with bacterial pneumonias, including *Mycoplasma* (Chapter 325), and patients with chronically infected cerebral ventriculoatrial shunts for hydrocephalus. Many patients have nephrotic-range proteinuria and only mild renal dysfunction. With appropriate antibiotic therapy, most patients' glomerular lesions heal, and renal function recovers.

TABLE 123-5 CLASSIFICATION OF RAPIDLY PROGRESSIVE ("CRESCENTIC") GLOMERULONEPHRITIS

PRIMARY

Type I: Anti–glomerular basement membrane antibody disease, Goodpasture's syndrome (with pulmonary disease)
Type II: Immune complex mediated
Type III: Pauci-immune (usually antineutrophil cytoplasmic antibody-positive)

SECONDARY

Membranoproliferative glomerulonephritis
Immunoglobulin A nephropathy, Henoch-Schönlein purpura
Post-streptococcal glomerulonephritis
Systemic lupus erythematosus
Polyarteritis nodosa, hypersensitivity angiitis

TABLE 123-6 COMMON RENAL DISEASES WITH ASSOCIATED PULMONARY DISEASES

DISEASE	MARKER
Goodpasture's syndrome	+Anti–glomerular basement membrane antibodies
Wegener's granulomatosis, polyarteritis	+Antineutrophil cytoplasmic antibodies
Systemic lupus erythematosus	+Anti-DNA antibodies, low complement
Nephrotic syndrome, renal vein thrombosis, pulmonary embolus	+Lung scan or +CT angiography
Pneumonia with immune complex glomerulonephritis	Low complement, circulating immune complexes
Uremic lung	Elevated creatinine level

CT = computed tomography.

Rapidly Progressive Glomerulonephritis

Rapidly progressive glomerulonephritis (RPGN) represents a variety of glomerular diseases that are notable for progression to renal failure in a matter of weeks to months (Table 123-5). Patients with primary RPGN can be divided into three patterns as defined by immunologic pathogenesis: type I, with anti-GBM disease (e.g., Goodpasture's syndrome); type II, with immune complex deposition (e.g., SLE, Henoch-Schönlein purpura, post-streptococcal); and type III, without immune deposits or anti-GBM antibodies (so-called pauci-immune, usually ANCA-positive RPGN). The renal biopsy in all RPGN shows extensive extracapillary proliferation, that is, crescent formation.

ANTI–GLOMERULAR BASEMENT MEMBRANE DISEASE

The disease has two peaks of occurrence: in the third decade of life in men and in women after 60 years of age. Anti-GBM disease (Table 123-6) is caused by circulating antibodies that are directed against the noncollagenous domain of the α_3 chain of type IV collagen and that damage the GBM. The result is an inflammatory response, breaks in the GBM, and the formation of a proliferative and often crescentic glomerulonephritis. If the anti-GBM antibodies cross-react with and damage the basement membrane of pulmonary capillaries, the patient develops pulmonary hemorrhage and hemoptysis, an association called *Goodpasture's syndrome*.

CLINICAL MANIFESTATIONS AND DIAGNOSIS

Patients present with a nephritic picture (see Table 123-1). Renal function may deteriorate from normal to dialysis-requiring levels in a matter of days to weeks. Patients with pulmonary involvement may have life-threatening hemoptysis with dyspnea and with diffuse alveolar infiltrates on chest radiograph.

The pathology of anti-GBM disease shows a proliferative glomerulonephritis, often with severe crescentic proliferation in Bowman's space. There is linear deposition of immunoglobulin (usually IgG) along the GBM by immunofluorescence (Fig. 123-9), but electron microscopy does not show any electron-dense deposits.

Although the treatment of this rare disease has not been studied in large controlled trials, intensive immunosuppressive therapy with cyclophosphamide (e.g., 2 mg/kg/day as tolerated) and corticosteroids (e.g., pulse methylprednisolone, 15 to 30 mg/kg to a maximum of dose of 1000 mg intravenously daily for three doses, followed by oral prednisone, 1 mg/kg per day to a maximum of 60 to 80 mg/day and slowly tapered after achieving clinical remission) to reduce the production of anti-GBM antibodies, combined with daily plasmapheresis to remove circulating anti-GBM antibodies, has been successful in many patients. Rapid treatment is recommended to prevent irreversible renal damage and is necessary in patients with pulmonary hemorrhage. The optimal duration of therapy is uncertain, but daily plasmapheresis should be performed, preferably until anti-GBM antibody is undetectable, and corticosteroids and cyclophosphamide should be continued until clinical remission is achieved, typically between 3 and 6 months. Patients who already require dialysis at the time of treatment generally do not regain renal function despite aggressive therapy.

IMMUNE COMPLEX RAPIDLY PROGRESSIVE GLOMERULONEPHRITIS

Type II RPGN, which is associated with immune complex–mediated damage to the glomeruli, may occur with idiopathic glomerulopathies, such as IgA nephropathy and MPGN, or with postinfectious glomerulonephritis and SLE. The therapy for IgA nephropathy and MPGN was discussed earlier.

FIGURE 123-9. Anti–glomerular basement membrane (GBM) glomerulonephritis. An immunofluorescence micrograph of a portion of a glomerulus with anti-GBM glomerulonephritis shows linear staining of GBM for immunoglobulin G (IgG) (fluorescein isothiocyanate anti-IgG stain, ×600). (From Falk RJ, Jennette JC, Nachman PH. Primary glomerular disease. In: Brenner BM, ed. Brenner and Rector's The Kidney. 7th ed. Philadelphia: Elsevier; 2004.)

Many cases of crescentic postinfectious glomerulonephritis resolve with successful treatment of the underlying infection. For the treatment of severe SLE, see later.

PAUCI-IMMUNE AND VASCULITIS-ASSOCIATED RAPIDLY PROGRESSIVE GLOMERULONEPHRITIS

Pauci-immune type III RPGN includes patients with and without evidence of systemic vasculitis. Most patients have circulating ANCAs that are directed against components of neutrophil primary granules.

CLINICAL MANIFESTATIONS AND DIAGNOSIS

Patients often present with progressive renal failure and a nephritic picture (see Table 123-1). Patients who are perinuclear ANCA positive (antibodies usually directed against granulocyte myeloperoxidase) more often have a clinical picture akin to that of microscopic polyangiitis (Chapter 278) with arthritis, leukocytoclastic angiitis, and constitutional and systemic signs. Patients who are cytoplasmic ANCA positive (antibodies usually directed against a granulocyte serine proteinase, anti-PR3) more often have Wegener's granulomatosis (Chapter 278) associated with their glomerulonephritis. However, there is considerable overlap among these groups, and some patients have both ANCA and anti-GBM antibodies (Fig. 123-10). Although there is no direct correlation between ANCA titers and disease activity, patients with high titers (especially high anti-PR3 titers) and those with a four-fold increase in titers are more likely to have flares of their disease.

TREATMENT AND PROGNOSIS   **Rx**

For induction therapy, combination therapy with corticosteroids (e.g., pulse methylprednisolone, 10-15 mg/kg/day up to a maximum of 500-1000 mg intravenously daily, for 3 days, followed by oral prednisolone, 1 mg/kg/day)

FIGURE 123-10. Crescentic glomerulonephritis typical of both anti–glomerular basement membrane disease and antineutrophil cytoplasmic antibody–positive pauci-immune glomerulonephritis.

FIGURE 123-11. Diffuse proliferative lupus nephritis with involvement of all glomeruli.

and cyclophosphamide (e.g., 15 mg/kg intravenously every 2 to 3 weeks or 1.5 to 2 mg/kg/day orally), with or without plasmapheresis, has markedly improved renal and patient survival rates in patients with Wegener's granulomatosis (Chapter 278) and microscopic polyangiitis (Chapter 278). Methotrexate (20 to 25 mg per week orally for 12 months) is as effective as cyclophosphamide in achieving remission but leads to a higher relapse rate, so it should be limited to non-organ- or non-life-threatening disease, in which it is a less toxic alternative to cyclophosphamide. In severe renal vasculitis, renal survival, but not patient survival, is improved with the addition of plasmapheresis.[6] Rituximab (375 mg/m² weekly for 4 weeks) is as effective as cyclophosphamide at 6-month follow-up.[7] Maintenance regimens using azathioprine (1.5 mg/kg/day) or methotrexate (20 to 25 mg/week) should be administered for 12 to 18 months after achieving remission.[8] Corticosteroids should be slowly tapered off, as determined by the presence of clinical symptoms. Ongoing trials include the comparison of mycophenolate mofetil to azathioprine for maintenance therapy of ANCA-positive vasculitis.

As in all forms of RPGN, renal function may deteriorate rapidly. In pauci-immune RPGN, high-risk patients include older patients, patients with severe pulmonary involvement, and patients with severe renal failure. Analyses have found no difference in prognosis in patients with or without documented true arterial vasculitis or with crescentic or focal segmental necrotizing glomerulonephritis.

● GLOMERULAR DISEASES ASSOCIATED WITH GENETIC DEFECTS

Some patients, often with a history of similar findings in siblings and other relatives, have a hereditary nephritis.

Alport syndrome is a hereditary form of glomerulonephritis that often presents with asymptomatic urinary findings. In approximately 85% of cases, it is an X-linked condition with hematuria and proteinuria, often in association with high-pitched hearing loss and abnormalities of the lens of the eye (lenticonus). The defect in most of these cases is localized to a mutation in the α_5 chain of type IV collagen (COL4A5). Other families have different patterns of inheritance, more often with mutations in the α_3 and α_4 chains of type IV collagen (COL4A3, COL4A4). Although the light microscopy findings vary from mild mesangial proliferative to advanced sclerosing lesions depending on the stage of biopsy, electron microscopy typically shows areas of GBM thinning and areas of basement membrane splitting with lamellations. Some patients with mutations in the collagen IV gene have microhematuria and proteinuria with areas of extreme basement membrane thinning on electron microscopy. In males, Alport's syndrome often leads to progressive glomerulosclerosis and ESRD.

Fabry's disease (Chapter 215), which is caused by an X-linked recessive genetic defect of α-galactosidase, leads to the deposition of ceramide trihexose in the kidneys and other organs. It may cause progressive proteinuria and renal insufficiency in males and in some female carriers. It also is associated with telangiectasias of the skin, typically in the bathing suit area; acroparesthesias; cardiac abnormalities; and eye changes.

Nail-patella syndrome, associated with skeletal and nail deformities, is a rare cause of the nephrotic syndrome in children. It is due to an autosomal dominant mutation in the LMX1B transcription factor that regulates collagen, nephrin, and podocin gene expression.

TABLE 123-7 CLASSIFICATION OF LUPUS NEPHRITIS

CLASS	CLINICAL FEATURES
I. Minimal mesangial LN	No renal findings
II. Mesangial proliferative LN	Mild clinical renal disease; minimally active urinary sediment; mild to moderate proteinuria (never nephrotic) but may have active serology
III. Focal proliferative LN < 50% glomeruli involved A. Active A/C. Active and chronic C. Chronic	More active sediment changes; often active serology; increased proteinuria (about 25% nephrotic); hypertension may be present; some evolve into class IV pattern; active lesions require treatment, chronic do not
IV. Diffuse proliferative LN (>50% glomeruli involved); all may be with segmental or global involvement (S or G) A. Active A/C. Active and chronic C. Chronic	Most severe renal involvement with active sediment, hypertension, heavy proteinuria (frequent nephrotic syndrome), often reduced glomerular filtration rate; serology very active. Active lesions require treatment
V. Membranous LN glomerulonephritis	Significant proteinuria (often nephrotic) with less active lupus serology
VI. Advanced sclerosing LN	More than 90% glomerulosclerosis; no treatment prevents renal failure

LN = lupus nephritis.

Systemic Lupus Erythematosus

Renal involvement may greatly influence the course and therapy of SLE (Chapter 274). Although the incidence of clinical renal disease in SLE varies from 15% to 75%, histologic evidence of renal involvement is found in most biopsy specimens.

The International Society of Nephrology classification of lupus nephritis uses light microscopy, immunofluorescence, and electron microscopy to classify each biopsy in order to separate milder mesangial lesions and bland membranous lupus nephritis from true proliferative lupus nephritis (Table 123-7). In general, class I and II patients have mild lesions that require no therapy directed at the kidney. All patients with class IV lesions on biopsy deserve some form of vigorous therapy for their lupus nephritis. Many class III patients, especially those with active necrotizing lesions and large amounts of subendothelial deposits (Fig. 123-11), also benefit from therapy. For class V patients, the optimal therapy is less clear, and recommendations vary from vigorous treatment of all patients with membranous lupus nephritis to reserving such therapy for those with serologic activity or more severe nephrotic syndrome. Vigorous therapy of lupus nephritis now emphasizes monthly high-dose intravenous cyclophosphamide therapy (0.5 to 1 g/m²) for 6 months combined with intravenous methylprednisolone (1000 mg/m²) as the best regimen for preventing flares of disease or progression to renal failure. Daily oral mycophenolate mofetil (target dose, 1500 mg twice daily) appears to be equally effective in inducing remissions of severe lupus nephritis.[9] Maintenance therapy with mycophenolate mofetil (500 to 1000 mg twice daily) or azathioprine (1 to 3 mg/kg/day) is more effective and less toxic than continued intravenous cyclophosphamide therapy after the 6-month induction period. Rituximab, an anti-CD20 monoclonal antibody, has not proved beneficial when added to full doses of other immunosuppressive agents in controlled trials of patients with SLE renal disease. Other agents under investigation include blockers of T- and B-cell costimulatory molecules, and anti-B LyS therapy.

Many patients with lupus nephritis (40 to 50%) produce autoantibodies against certain phospholipids, including anticardiolipin antibodies. If these patients experience clotting in the glomeruli and arterioles, they require anticoagulation or antiplatelet agents, or both, as well as immunosuppressive medications.

Diabetes Mellitus

Diabetic nephropathy, which is the most common form of glomerular damage seen in developed countries, is discussed in detail in Chapter 126.

Amyloidosis

Renal amyloid deposits, whether due to AL or to AA amyloid, are predominantly found within the glomeruli, where they often appear as amorphous eosinophilic extracellular nodules (Chapter 194) that stain positively with Congo red and display apple-green birefringence under polarized light. By electron microscopy, amyloid appears as nonbranching rigid fibrils 8 to 10 nm in diameter.

Although almost 80% of patients with AL amyloid have renal disease, amyloidosis is a disease with multisystem involvement. Renal manifestations include albuminuria and renal insufficiency. Approximately 25% of patients with AL amyloid present with the nephrotic syndrome, which eventually is diagnosed in up to one half of patients. Patients may present with symptoms referable to cardiac involvement (Chapter 60) or neuropathy (Chapter 428), as well as with renal symptoms. Diagnosis may be made from organ biopsy other than the kidney (e.g., gingival biopsy, rectal biopsy, or fat pad biopsy). Treatment strategies for renal AL amyloidosis are similar to those for multiple myeloma and other plasma cell dyscrasias (Chapter 193).

AA amyloid is usually associated with chronic inflammatory conditions such as rheumatoid arthritis (Chapter 272), familial Mediterranean fever (Chapter 269), inflammatory bowel disease (Chapter 143), osteomyelitis (Chapter 296), and other chronic infections. Treatment is directed at the underlying inflammatory process. Specific therapy against the primary inflammatory disease (e.g., anti–tumor necrosis factor therapy in rheumatoid arthritis and colchicine in familial Mediterranean fever) can prevent fibrillogenesis in AA amyloid patients. Eprodisate, a compound that inhibits polymerization and deposition of amyloid fibrils (800 to 2400 mg/day based on renal function), can slow the progression of renal disease in patients with AA amyloidosis. [10]

Light Chain Deposition Disease

Light chain deposition disease, like AL amyloidosis, is a systemic disease caused by the overproduction and extracellular deposition of a monoclonal immunoglobulin light chain (Chapter 193). However, the deposits do not form β-pleated sheets, do not stain with Congo red, and are granular rather than fibrillar. Most patients with light chain deposition disease have a lymphoplasmacytic B-cell disease similar to multiple myeloma (Chapter 193).

Albuminuria is common, and the nephrotic syndrome is found in one half of patients at presentation, often accompanied by hypertension and renal insufficiency. On light microscopy, most glomeruli contain eosinophilic mesangial glomerular nodules. Some biopsies show associated light chain cast nephropathy with eosinophilic laminated casts obstructing the tubules, as seen in myeloma. By immunofluorescence, a single class of immunoglobulin light chain (κ in 80% of cases) stains in a diffuse linear pattern along the GBM, in the nodules, and along the tubular basement membranes. The treatment for most patients with light chain deposition disease is chemotherapy similar to that for myeloma (Chapter 193).

Fibrillary Glomerulopathy-Immunotactoid Glomerulopathy

Some patients with renal disease have glomerular lesions with deposits of nonamyloid fibrillar proteins ranging in size from 12 to more than 50 nm. Patients with these lesions have been divided into two groups: those with fibrillary glomerulonephritis with fibrils of 20 nm in diameter, and those with immunotactoid glomerulonephritis, a much rarer disease often associated with lymphoproliferative disorders, in which the fibrils are much larger (30 to 50 nm). Proteinuria is found in almost all patients, and hematuria, the nephrotic syndrome, and renal insufficiency eventually develop in most. There is no proven therapy for fibrillary glomerulopathy at this time.

Human Immunodeficiency Virus–Associated Nephropathy

Infection with human immunodeficiency virus (HIV) (Chapter 394) is associated with a number of patterns of renal disease, including acute renal failure and a unique form of glomerulopathy now called HIV-associated nephropathy. HIV-associated nephropathy is characterized by heavy proteinuria and rapid progression to renal failure. On light microscopy, findings on renal biopsy include diffuse global collapse of the glomerular tufts, severe tubulointerstitial changes with interstitial inflammation, edema, microcystic dilation of tubules, and severe tubular degenerative changes. On electron microscopy, tubuloreticular inclusions can be seen in the glomerular endothelium. The use of ACE inhibitors, in doses needed to achieve a target systolic blood pressure of 120 mm Hg or lower as tolerated (see Table 67-5 in Chapter 67), and highly active antiretroviral therapy (HAART) may slow the progression to renal failure and decrease proteinuria. Corticosteroids (e.g., prednisone, 1 mg/kg for 1 month followed by a taper over several months) may be beneficial in selected patients with HIV-associated nephropathy.

Mixed Cryoglobulinemia

Cryoglobulinemia (Chapter 193) is caused by the production of circulating immunoglobulins that precipitate on cooling and resolubilize on warming. Cryoglobulinemia may be found in association with many types of diseases, including infections, collagen-vascular disease, and lymphoproliferative diseases such as multiple myeloma and Waldenström's macroglobulinemia. Many patients with what was originally described as glomerulonephritis due to essential mixed cryoglobulinemia have been found to have hepatitis C–associated renal disease. Some patients develop an acute nephritic picture with acute renal insufficiency. Most patients have proteinuria, and about 20% present with the nephrotic syndrome. Most patients with renal disease have a slow, indolent course characterized by proteinuria, hypertension, hematuria, and renal insufficiency. Hypocomplementemia, especially of the early components C1q to C4, is a characteristic finding in cryoglobulinemic glomerulonephritis whether hepatitis C–related or idiopathic. Treatment of hepatitis C–associated cryoglobulinemia includes antiviral therapy (Chapter 151). When significant renal disease is present, various combinations of corticosteroids with or without rituximab or cyclophosphamide or plasmapheresis can be tried.

Thrombotic Microangiopathies

A number of systemic diseases, including hemolytic-uremic syndrome (Chapters 127 and 175), thrombotic thrombocytopenic purpura (TTP; Chapter 175), and the antiphospholipid syndrome (Chapter 179), as well as microangiopathy associated with drugs such as mitomycin and cyclosporine, are characterized by microthromboses of the glomerular capillaries and small arterioles. The renal findings may be dominant or only part of a more generalized picture of microangiopathy.

Renal manifestations of the thrombotic microangiopathies may include gross or microscopic hematuria, proteinuria that is typically less than 2 g/day but may reach nephrotic levels, and renal insufficiency. Patients may have oliguric or nonoliguric acute renal failure. The histologic findings in all of the microangiopathies resemble each other and include glomerular capillary thromboses, areas of ischemic damage, and intimal proliferation with luminal narrowing by thrombi of arterioles and small arteries. In all thrombotic microangiopathies, treatment includes correcting hypovolemia, controlling hypertension, and the use of dialytic support for those with severe renal failure. In TTP associated with an acquired or hereditary deficiency of the von Willebrand's convertase ADAMTS-13 and in some other cases, plasmapheresis with fresh-frozen plasma is beneficial (Chapter 175). In the antiphospholipid syndrome, anticoagulation with heparin and then warfarin is useful (Chapter 37).

1. Dharmaraj R, Hari P, Bagga A. Randomized cross-over trial comparing albumin and frusemide infusions in nephritic syndrome. *Pediatr Nephrol.* 2009;24:775-782.
2. Cattran DC, Appel GB, Hebert LA, et al. A randomized trial of cyclosporine in patients with steroid-resistant focal segmental glomerulosclerosis. North America Nephrotic Syndrome Study Group. *Kidney Int.* 1999;56:2220-2226.

3. Ponticelli C, Altieri P, Scolari F, et al. A randomized study comparing methylprednisolone plus chlorambucil versus methylprednisolone plus cyclophosphamide in idiopathic membranous nephropathy. *J Am Soc Nephrol.* 1998;9:444-450.
4. Cattran DC, Appel GB, Hebert LA, et al. Cyclosporine in patients with steroid-resistant membranous nephropathy: a randomized trial. *Kidney Int.* 2001;59:1484-1490.
5. Samuels JA, Strippoli GF, Craig JC, et al. Immunosuppressive treatments for immunoglobulin A nephropathy: a meta-analysis of randomized controlled trials. *Nephrology (Carlton).* 2004;9:177-185.
6. Jayne DR, Gaskin G, Rasmussen N, et al. Randomized trial of plasma exchange or high dosage methyl-prednisolone as adjunctive therapy for severe renal vasculitis. *J Am Soc Nephrol.* 2007;18:2180-2188.
7. Stone JH, Merkel PA, Spiera R, et al, for the RAVE-ITN Research Group. Rituximab versus cyclophosphamide for ANCA-associated vasculitis. *N Engl J Med.* 2010;363:221-232.
8. Jayne D, Rasmussen N, Andrassy K, et al, for the European Vasculitis Study Group. A randomized trial of maintenance therapy for vasculitis associated with ANCA. *N Engl J Med.* 2003;349:36-44.
9. Kamanamool N, McEvoy M, Attia J, et al. Efficacy and adverse events of mycophenolate mofetil versus cyclophosphamide for induction therapy of lupus nephritis: systematic review and meta-analysis. *Medicine (Baltimore).* 2010;89:227-235.
10. Dember LM, Hawkins PN, Hazenberg BP, et al. Eprodisate for the treatment of renal disease in AA amyloidosis. *N Engl J Med.* 2007;356:2349-2360.

SUGGESTED READINGS

Ayodele OE, Okpechi IG, Swanepoel CR. Predictors of poor renal outcome in patients with biopsy-proven lupus nephritis. *Nephrology (Carlton).* 2010;15;482-490. *Baseline serum creatinine, no-remission following therapy, and higher blood pressure predict poor renal outcome.*

Beck LH Jr, Salant DJ. Membranous nephropathy: recent travels and new roads ahead. *Kidney Int.* 2010;77:765-770. *Circulating antibodies to the M-type phospholipase A2 receptor are 75% sensitive and 100% specific for idiopathic membranous nephropathy.*

Eison TM, Ault BH, Jones DP, et al. Post-streptococcal acute glomerulonephritis in children: clinical features and pathogenesis. *Pediatr Nephrol.* 2011;26;165-180. *Review.*

Kaufman L, Collins SE, Klotman PE. The pathogenesis of HIV-associated nephropathy. *Adv Chronic Kidney Dis.* 2010;17:36-43. *Review.*

Peto P, Salama AD. Update on antiglomerular basement membrane disease. *Curr Opin Rheumatol.* 2011;23:32-37. *Review.*

124

TUBULOINTERSTITIAL DISEASES

ERIC G. NEILSON

TUBULOINTERSTITIAL NEPHRITIS

DEFINITION

Interstitial nephritis can be primary and begin in the tubulointerstitium or appear as a secondary event and spread from blood vessels, including the glomerular capillaries. Although injury to the tubulointerstitial compartment can be the result of autoimmunity, a toxic insult, an infection, or exposure to a drug, the inflammatory process always has an immunologic component that leads to the release of tissue cytokines, which eventually convert tubular epithelia into fibroblasts to produce fibrosis.

Tubulointerstitial nephritis can be arbitrarily divided into acute and chronic types. The acute form of interstitial nephritis often begins abruptly. When inciting events subside, so does the nephritis, and the glomerular filtration rate tends to normalize, with little residual damage except in patients with preexisting disease. Chronic interstitial nephritis is persistent and over time reduces the number of functioning nephrons by encasing and dismantling them, with irreversible fibrosis. So-called toxic nephropathy is similar to this form of nephritis. Sometimes acute and chronic injury are difficult to distinguish because global destruction of the tubulointerstitium can occur within a matter of weeks.

EPIDEMIOLOGY

Acute interstitial nephritis appears unexpectedly in otherwise healthy individuals from a variety of causes. About 1% of patients with hematuria and proteinuria have acute interstitial nephritis, and it is seen in 1 to 15% of autopsy series.

The development of acute interstitial nephritis is largely due to the use of pharmaceuticals. Other important causes include infection and idiopathic autoimmune diseases (Table 124-1). Penicillin moieties (less so nafcillin and piperacillin), cephalosporins, sulfa-like drugs, and nonsteroidal anti-inflammatory drugs (NSAIDs) top the list. NSAIDs cause both acute interstitial nephritis and chronic analgesic nephropathy. Diphtheria in children

TABLE 124-1 CAUSES OF ACUTE INTERSTITIAL NEPHRITIS

DRUGS

Antibiotics
  Penicillins
  Rifampin, ethambutol
  Sulfa
  Vancomycin
  Ciprofloxacin
  Cephalosporins
  Erythromycin
  Trimethoprim-sulfamethoxazole
  Acyclovir
Nonsteroidal anti-inflammatory drugs
  Selective and nonselective cyclooxygenase-2 inhibitors
Diuretics
  Thiazides
  Furosemide
  Triamterene
Miscellaneous
  Captopril
  Ranitidine
  Omeprazole
  Phenobarbital
  Phenytoin
  Sodium valproate
  Carbamazepine
  Allopurinol
  Interferon
  Interleukin-2
  All-*trans*-retinoic acid

INFECTIONS

Bacteria
  Legionella
  Brucella
  Diphtheria
  Streptococcus
  Staphylococcus
  Yersinia
  Salmonella
  Escherichia coli
  Campylobacter
Viruses
  Epstein-Barr virus
  Cytomegalovirus
  Hantaan virus
  Human immunodeficiency virus (HIV)
  Herpes simplex virus
  Hepatitis B virus
Other
  Mycoplasma
  Rickettsia
  Leptospira
  Mycobacterium tuberculosis
  Schistosoma mekongi
  Toxoplasma
  Chlamydia

AUTOIMMUNE DISEASES

Anti–tubular basement membrane disease
Tubulointerstitial nephritis and uveitis (TINU) syndrome
Kawasaki disease

(Chapter 300), legionellosis (Chapter 322), leptospirosis (Chapter 331), histoplasmosis (Chapter 340), tuberculosis (Chapter 332), and DNA viruses such as cytomegalovirus (Chapter 384) and Epstein-Barr virus (Chapter 385) are well-recognized agents of acute interstitial nephritis. Anti–tubular basement membrane disease is a rare cause of autoimmune interstitial nephritis. Although sarcoidosis or the tubulointerstitial nephritis and uveitis (TINU) syndrome can manifest as acute interstitial nephritis on biopsy, they often quickly evolve into chronic disease.

All forms of injury to the kidney, regardless of origin, progress to end-stage renal disease through a terminal phase of chronic interstitial nephritis. In addition to glomerulonephrites (Chapter 123), cystic diseases (Chapter 129), and diabetes (Chapters 236 and 237), a wide variety of renal conditions start slowly in the tubulointerstitium and often go unrecognized until late in the course, when biopsy shows chronic interstitial nephritis.

TABLE 124-2 CAUSES OF CHRONIC INTERSTITIAL NEPHRITIS

HEREDITARY DISEASES

Mitochondrial mutations

METABOLIC DISTURBANCES

Hypercalcemia, nephrocalcinosis
Hyperoxaluria
Hypokalemia
Hyperuricemia
Cystinosis
Methylmalonicacidemia

DRUGS AND TOXINS

Analgesics
Cadmium
Lead
Health food botanicals, herbs
Lithium
Cyclosporine, tacrolimus
Cisplatin, methotrexate
Nitrosoureas

AUTOIMMUNE DISEASES

Renal allograft rejection
Wegener's granulomatosis
Sjögren's syndrome
Systemic lupus erythematosus, vasculitis
Progressive glomerular disease
Sarcoidosis

HEMATOLOGIC DISTURBANCES

Multiple myeloma, light chains
Lymphoma
Sickle cell disease

INFECTIONS

Complicated pyelonephritis
Human immunodeficiency virus (HIV)
Epstein-Barr virus
Malacoplakia
Xanthogranulomatous pyelonephritis

OBSTRUCTIVE NEPHROPATHY

Tumors
Stones
Outlet obstruction
Vesicoureteral reflux

MISCELLANEOUS

Age-related vascular disease
Hypertension
Ischemia
Balkan (endemic) nephropathy
Radiation nephritis

Primary chronic interstitial nephritis can be caused by a variety of toxic, metabolic, hematologic, obstructive, and infectious processes. Ingestion of six or more tablets per day of acetaminophen, aspirin, or NSAIDs, alone or together, for at least 3 years puts patients at risk for analgesic nephropathy. A careful history of drug or toxin exposure, previous renal images, and a family history often point to a probable diagnosis (Table 124-2).

PATHOBIOLOGY

Pathophysiology

Regardless of the origin of renal inflammation, the kidneys do not fail until interstitial nephritis, fibrosis, and tubular atrophy develop. Interstitial nephritis is the pathologic equivalent of clinical progression because it is the final common pathway to permanent tissue damage. The degree of reduction in the glomerular filtration rate correlates with the degree of interstitial injury. Urinary flow is impeded by tubular obstruction. Increased vascular resistance causes progressive tubular injury and fibrosis. A net reduction in the cross-sectional area of peritubular vessels increases postglomerular resistance to the extent that the compensatory increase in glomerular hydrostatic pressure cannot fully restore filtration to normal levels. Tubuloglomerular feedback assumes increasing importance in the transition from acute to chronic glomerulonephritis when autoregulation of renal blood flow is disrupted by tubulointerstitial fibrosis. Loss of autoregulation by tubuloglomerular feedback results from the absence or insensitivity of the afferent arteriole. Perhaps more significant is the effect of interstitial pressure on the sensitivity of the feedback mechanism. Tubular atrophy may disrupt the normal renal osmotic gradient by decreasing sodium chloride transport along the proximal tubule or thick ascending loop of Henle. The result is poor abstraction of water from the filtrate, with hyposthenuria and polyuria. Such an increase in solute and water within the tubular fluid results in adaptive downregulation of the glomerular filtration process.

The antigen targets for the immune system in interstitial nephritis are poorly understood. Drugs act as haptens, mimic endogenous structures in the interstitium, alter regulation of the immune system, or function in some combination of the foregoing. Bacteria, fungi, and viruses can infect the kidney and cause mononuclear cell infiltration or activate Toll-like receptors on tubular epithelia, which subsequently educate the adaptive immune response to events in the interstitium. Autoimmune diseases such as anti–tubular basement membrane disease or spontaneous interstitial nephritis remain confined to the kidney, whereas systemic diseases spread to the kidney where they cause persistent, chronic interstitial nephritis.

Although the adaptive immune response is similar to that of other tissues, T-cell activation figures prominently in interstitial nephritis. Antibodies (anti–tubular basement membrane disease) and immune complex deposition along the tubular basement membrane (systemic lupus erythematosus) are rarely seen. Antigens presented by class II major histocompatibility complex molecules on macrophages, dendritic cells, and adjacent tubular epithelia, in conjunction with associative recognition molecules, engage the CD4/CD8 T-cell repertoires. The resultant cytokine and protease activity injures tubular nephrons and basement membranes and causes fibroblasts to form locally by epithelial-mesenchymal transition. Transforming growth factor-β (TGF-β), fibroblast growth factor 2, and platelet-derived growth factor are particularly active in this transition. If the nephritis persists, fibrogenesis dismantles nephrons and causes tubular atrophy; in late stages, the inflammatory reaction outgrows its survival factors, and lymphocytes and fibroblasts disappear by apoptosis and leave an acellular fibrotic scar.

Viruses, including Epstein-Barr virus, have long been suspected of contributing to idiopathic, chronic interstitial nephritis. Malacoplakia and xanthogranulomatous pyelonephritis are probably not defects in nephrogenesis but rather are destructive responses to bacterial inflammation in the interstitium. Focal abnormalities in kidney structure can be a nidus for infections associated with perinephric, psoas, or peritoneal abscesses. Children with vesicoureteral reflux can have chronic or repeating episodes of pyelonephritis, but whether the reflux or the infection is more important to progression to renal failure is unclear. There is also no agreement on whether recurrent pyelonephritis by itself produces chronic interstitial nephritis in adults.

Pathology

Both kidneys are typically involved, except in cases of unilateral infection, obstruction, or trauma. The inflammatory reaction in acute interstitial nephritis consists mainly of T lymphocytes and monocytes, but neutrophils, plasma cells, and eosinophils can be present. The T cells are of a mixed phenotype with a distinct preference for CD4+ lymphocytes. The infiltrative process is associated with interstitial edema, which displaces tubules away from one another and causes the kidneys to swell. The tubular basement membrane may be disrupted in more severe cases, but immune deposits are rarely found by immunofluorescence.

In chronic interstitial nephritis, the kidney assumes an irregular or contracted appearance. The tubular epithelia sit on thickened or disrupted tubular basement membranes and are often effaced against dilated lumens, and the tubules eventually dismantle and atrophy. *Chronic* is a relative term, because fibrotic changes can be seen within 7 to 10 days of continuing inflammation. Normal glomeruli in primary interstitial nephritis are eventually surrounded by periglomerular fibrosis and subsequently undergo segmental or global sclerosis. Chronic vascular thickening and glomerular changes are present in advanced stages of disease, so pathologic determination of the primary cause may be difficult in some biopsy samples. Progressive glomerular sclerosis also occurs with aging and must be factored in when interpreting the biopsy findings.

A third pathologic category, granuloma formation, can be seen in either acute or chronic interstitial nephritis. In acute granulomatous interstitial nephritis, granulomas are sparse and non-necrotic, and giant cells are rare. The granulomas in chronic interstitial nephritis contain an abundance of giant cells, and those caused by tuberculosis may become necrotic. Drugs are a common cause of this lesion in the acute setting, and most of the drugs associated with acute interstitial nephritis have been reported to cause granuloma formation. In the absence of drug exposure, sarcoidosis (Chapter 95), Wegener's granulomatosis (Chapter 278), histoplasmosis (Chapter 340), or tuberculosis (Chapter 332) should be considered, depending on the context, when numerous granulomas are present. The renal granulomas seen in Wegener's granulomatosis are almost always accompanied by glomerular and vascular pathology.

ACUTE INTERSTITIAL NEPHRITIS

CLINICAL MANIFESTATIONS

Most patients present with an asymptomatic rise in the serum creatinine level or an abnormal urinalysis, and it is important to consider acute interstitial nephritis in any patient with an unexplained precipitous diminution in renal function. Because injury is often asymptomatic, patients may already have substantial renal failure on initial presentation. Patients may also present with nonspecific symptoms such as lethargy or weakness, and many patients have fever and oliguria owing to severe acute kidney injury (Chapter 122).

Several features can distinguish acute interstitial nephritis from acute tubular necrosis (Chapter 122) or glomerulonephritis (Chapter 123) (Table 124-3). Fever and occasional flank pain over the kidneys occur in infection or with drug-induced acute interstitial nephritis. Lumbar pain, sometimes unilateral, is due to distention of the renal capsule. Allergic reactions are associated with maculopapular rash, fever, and eosinophilia, but the entire triad is seen in less than 33% of patients, and such signs are uncommon when NSAIDs cause acute interstitial nephritis.

The course of renal failure in acute interstitial nephritis takes several days to weeks and follows the kinetics of the primary immune response. However, renal failure can be precipitous, especially in patients re-exposed to a previous agent. Rarely, the course can be protracted, with the glomerular filtration rate declining over a period of months if the diagnosis is not recognized. This protracted course is more common with diuretic-induced interstitial nephritis. The onset of drug-induced nephritis ranges from days to weeks after the initiation of therapy, and a previous allergic history is rare. The classic setting for a drug reaction is a febrile patient with an infectious process and who defervesces while taking antibiotics but then develops recurrent fever several days later.

DIAGNOSIS

Urinalysis is particularly helpful. Mild to moderate proteinuria and hematuria are seen in most cases, and gross hematuria is observed occasionally. The sediment typically shows red and white blood cells, and white blood cell casts are commonly seen. Conversely, red blood cell casts suggest a glomerular diagnosis. The finding of eosinophils in the urine supports the diagnosis of allergic interstitial nephritis, but the absence of eosinophiluria does not exclude the diagnosis of acute interstitial nephritis.

An elevated serum creatinine level is usually the first abnormal laboratory result in renal injury. The normal serum creatinine of 0.6 to 1.3 mg/dL varies with muscle mass, age, and gender. Early recognition of acute interstitial nephritis requires a high degree of clinical suspicion because the serum creatinine level may be only mildly elevated even after the kidneys lose half their function.

The magnitude of proteinuria in acute interstitial nephritis is nearly always less than 3 g/24 hours and is typically less than 1 g/24 hours. Nephrotic-range proteinuria is not seen unless there is a coexisting glomerular lesion, such as a concurrent minimal-change lesion, or after exposure to NSAIDs. Many patients with acute interstitial nephritis also have a fractional excretion of sodium (FE_{Na}) greater than 1, but occasionally they are oliguric.

Imaging is of little diagnostic value. The kidney in acute interstitial nephritis is usually normal or slightly increased in size on echographic or tomographic images. Increased cortical echogenicity may correlate with diffuse interstitial infiltrates on renal biopsy. Gallium scanning is not particularly useful because a variety of other renal processes can cause gallium uptake, including minimal change glomerulonephritis, cortical necrosis, and acute tubular necrosis; in addition, acute interstitial nephritis can be found on biopsy in those with a normal scan.

Differential Diagnosis

It is sometimes difficult to distinguish among nonoliguric acute tubular necrosis, acute interstitial nephritis, and glomerulonephritis without a biopsy. Selective tubular defects and tubular syndromes such as proximal acquired Fanconi's syndrome (bicarbonaturia with a plasma carbon dioxide [CO_2] content <20 mEq/L, aminoaciduria, phosphate wasting, uricosuria, and glycosuria) or distal renal tubular acidosis type 1 (urine pH >5.6, plasma CO_2 content <20 mEq/L, with low or high potassium) can be seen in subacute or chronic interstitial nephritis but argue against acute interstitial nephritis.

Biopsy

Ultimately, the diagnosis can be established with certainty only by renal biopsy, which confirms and assesses the extent of acute interstitial inflammation. A biopsy should be performed in patients with acute renal failure who have suggestive signs or symptoms of an interstitial process and in whom prerenal azotemia and obvious acute tubular necrosis cannot be excluded on clinical grounds (Table 124-4). In primary acute interstitial nephritis, the biopsy demonstrates inflammatory cells that typically spare the glomeruli until late in the course (Fig. 124-1A). Lesions that reduce renal function are usually diffuse, but drug-induced interstitial injury is often patchy, beginning deep in the cortex before spreading.

TREATMENT   **Rx**

Biopsy is important to confirm acute interstitial nephritis, because chronic interstitial fibrosis rarely responds to aggressive treatment. The principal intervention for acute interstitial nephritis is to remove the inciting drug or treat the infection. Switching to different derivatives of a suspected drug is unwise. Concomitantly, or if the serum creatinine concentration does not fall after a few days, steroids (prednisone 0.75 to 1.0 mg/kg orally) can be given daily for approximately 1 week. If no further improvement occurs, oral cyclophosphamide (1 to 2 mg/kg/day) can be added for several more weeks. In patients who respond, cyclophosphamide can be steroid sparing, particularly in those with persistent sarcoidosis. It is important not to continue high-dose immunosuppression without some evidence of benefit because immunosuppressive drugs in patients with azotemia can lead to serious infection and even death. It is better to reserve these drugs for use with kidney transplantation if the primary disease does not respond.

PROGNOSIS

The prognosis for acute interstitial nephritis is good if it is recognized early. Early removal of offending agents or prompt treatment with antibiotics or immunosuppressive drugs can be renoprotective.

CHRONIC INTERSTITIAL NEPHRITIS

CLINICAL MANIFESTATIONS

Patients with primary chronic interstitial nephritis typically have elevated levels of serum creatinine and signs and symptoms of renal failure, including

---

TABLE 124-3	TYPICAL CLINICAL MANIFESTATION OF ACUTE INTERSTITIAL NEPHRITIS

History of drug hypersensitivity or recent infection and taking antibiotics
Sudden onset of fever lasting several days to weeks
Variable degrees of hypertension
Rise in creatinine with FE_{Na} >1.0; no expected acute tubular necrosis or glomerulonephritis
Kidney size normal or increased
Hematuria with mild proteinuria (<1.0 g)
Presence of WBC casts and WBCs on urinalysis; rarely eosinophils

FE_{Na} = fractional excretion of sodium; WBC = white blood cell.

TABLE 124-4	WHEN TO CONSIDER A RENAL BIOPSY TO DIAGNOSE NEPHRITIS

The setting, history, or clinical findings do not support a diagnosis of acute tubular necrosis or volume depletion
The clinical setting warrants a tissue diagnosis to determine the type of lesion, the extent of involvement, or the degree of fibrosis
The patient is stable enough to undergo biopsy and receive immunosuppressive drugs
The physician believes that the choice of therapy or the length of treatment is partially determined by the type of tissue injury

FIGURE 124-1. Tubulointerstitial nephritis on biopsy. **A,** Acute interstitial nephritis can be most aggressive when the interstitium is crowded with mononuclear cells and giant cells that destroy nearly all tubular nephrons (hematoxylin-eosin). **B,** Chronic interstitial nephritis is a slower process, with substantial collagen deposition (blue color; trichrome), tubular dropout, and fibroblasts in the interstitial spaces widened by fibrosis.

hematuria, hyposthenuria, nocturia, fatigue, and nausea. Urinalysis shows a fixed specific gravity of about 1.010, occasional glycosuria, and non-nephrotic–range proteinuria (often <1 g/L), with red and white blood cells and granular casts. Pyuria and positive urine cultures for bacteria are seen occasionally, and varying degrees of metabolic acidosis and hyperphosphatemia may be present. Before the glomerular filtration rate falls below 25 to 30 mL/minute, tubular acidosis is common. Anemia is often out of proportion to the degree of renal failure, and many patients have hypertension but only minimal edema until advanced stages of renal failure. Acquired Fanconi's syndrome can be seen in patients with a serum creatinine level less than 2.5 mg/dL in the setting of drug exposure, myeloma, human immunodeficiency virus (HIV) infection, lead exposure, and herbal nephropathy.

DIAGNOSIS

A careful dietary history is critical. As for any patient with evidence of renal failure, the evaluation includes laboratory tests to determine possible causes and severity. These tests include measures of renal function(serum creatinine level and blood urea nitrogen level), as well as levels of serum electrolytes, calcium, phosphate, uric acid, and albumin. Urinalysis shows a fixed specific gravity of about 1.010, occasional glycosuria, proteinuria (often <1 g/L), and red cells, white cells, and granular casts. Depending on the clinical situation, the search for specific causes may include serum and urine protein electrophoresis, blood cultures, and serologic tests for autoimmune diseases (e.g., cryoglobulin level, antinuclear antibodies [see Table 265-1 in Chapter 265], anti–neutrophil cytoplasmic antibody, and anti–glomerular basement membrane antibody levels).

Classic images of analgesic nephropathy on tomography are quite specific (Fig. 124-2) and show a decrease in overall kidney size, with atrophic scars and an irregular cortical contour, sometimes accompanied by papillary necrosis.

On biopsy (see Table 124-4), chronic interstitial nephritis is manifest by a cellular infiltrate that is eventually replaced by tubulointerstitial fibrosis (Fig. 124-1B). Infiltrates of lymphocytes and rare neutrophils are scattered and less abundant than in acute interstitial nephritis.

Specific Causes

Analgesics
Aspirin, acetaminophen, and NSAIDs alone or together are a source of toxic metabolites and can induce medullary ischemia and papillary necrosis, sometimes with papillary calcification. The likelihood of analgesic nephropathy from taking acetaminophen alone is much less than with the others. Uroepithelial malignancies also occur with increased frequency in this group of patients.

Aristolochic Acid Nephropathy
Aristolochic acid has been implicated as a cause of Balkan nephropathy and so-called Chinese herbal nephropathy. A growing number of people are taking vitamins and herbal preparations purchased from health food stores (Chapter 38). Some of these remedies contain botanicals that produce chronic interstitial nephritis. Patients who are dieting often use these remedies and are first seen when they already have late-stage disease, which increases the risk for uroepithelial malignancies.

Vascular Disease
Chronic renal ischemia from vascular injury can lead to interstitial nephritis, nephrosclerosis, and fibrosis. This is the classic renal lesion of untreated essential hypertension (Chapter 67). Similar injury is seen with aging, diabetes (Chapter 126), sickle cell disease (Chapter 166), and radiation nephritis (Chapter 19). This tubulointerstitial injury from the vascular diseases just mentioned is quite different from the aggressive necrosis seen with acute vasculitis. In patients taking calcineurin inhibitors such as cyclosporine or tacrolimus, renal ischemia from vasoconstriction can cause interstitial fibrosis that is sometimes difficult to distinguish from chronic allograft rejection.

Obstruction
Significant urinary obstruction (Chapter 125) owing to occlusion of both ureters by bladder tumors, cervical carcinoma, ureteral valve disease, or bladder outlet obstruction is an important cause of chronic interstitial nephritis. Complete or partial urinary tract obstruction is accompanied by a decline in glomerular filtration and classic tubular abnormalities, including diminished reabsorption of solutes, impaired excretion of H^+ and K^+, and a vasopressin-resistant concentrating defect in the medulla. Obstruction is associated with a fall in the glomerular filtration rate because of reduced plasma flow and hydraulic pressure associated with the release of angiotensin II, leukotrienes, and nitric oxide, a process leading to mononuclear cell infiltration. Growth factors such as TGF-β, released by infiltrating cells, may contribute to the interstitial and glomerular fibrosis. Obstruction is more common in men than in women and is part of the routine assessment of renal failure by renal ultrasound (Chapters 122 and 125). Almost all obstructed kidneys eventually become infected if the obstruction is not relieved.

Hypercalcemia
Hypercalcemia can decrease glomerular filtration through renal vasoconstriction, a decrease in the glomerular ultrafiltration coefficient, and volume depletion as a result of a vasopressin-resistant concentrating defect associated with nephrocalcinosis and calcium deposition around the basement membranes of the distal tubules and collecting ducts. Such deposition secondarily leads to mononuclear cell infiltration and tubular death. Nephrocalcinosis also occurs in normocalcemic disorders of augmented calcium absorption through the gut (sarcoidosis [Chapter 95], vitamin D intoxication [Chapter 253]), skeletal breakdown (neoplasms or multiple myeloma [Chapter 193]), or classic distal renal tubular acidosis.

Myeloma
The chronic renal failure of multiple myeloma (Chapter 193) is caused by several mechanisms, including cast nephropathy ("myeloma kidney"), coexistent volume depletion, hypercalcemia (Chapter 253), nephrocalcinosis (Chapter 253), and uric acid nephropathy. Proteinaceous casts form in dilated, atrophic distal nephron segments that are surrounded by multinucleated giant cells in interstitial infiltrates. The casts typically contain both Tamm-Horsfall protein and a pathologic light chain. Interstitial plasma cells and mononuclear infiltrates, calcifications in the interstitium, and amyloid deposits in the vessels and glomeruli are often present. Light chains are nephrotoxic by direct injury to tubular cells or through intrarenal obstruction from cast formation. In the setting of excess light chain production, the proximal tubule reabsorptive capacity is overwhelmed, leading to their urinary excretion as Bence Jones

FIGURE 124-2. Renal changes in analgesic nephropathy seen by tomographic imaging. Structural changes, including reduced volume, nodularity, and calcifications, are seen on computed tomography. RA = right artery; RV = right vein; SP = spinal vertebra. (From Elseviers MM, De Schepper A, Corthouts R, et al. High diagnostic performance of CT scan for analgesic nephropathy in patients with incipient to severe renal failure. *Kidney Int.* 1995;48:1316.)

proteins. An elevated intratubular pressure partly accounts for the decline in glomerular filtration in experimental cast nephropathy.

Lead Toxicity

Epidemiologic analyses support the association between excess lead burden (Chapter 21) and chronic renal failure. Blood lead levels reflect only recent, not chronic, exposure and can be normal in patients with a significant lead burden. Lead preferentially deposits in the proximal tubule, and nuclear inclusions within proximal tubular cells are characteristic of lead nephropathy.

Ingestion of moonshine liquor, with its high lead content, can be an important historical clue to the diagnosis. In adults, lead nephropathy produces chronic interstitial nephritis, fibrosis, and nephrosclerosis. Proximal tubular dysfunction may produce isolated tubule defects or a full Fanconi's syndrome. Patients often have recurrent gout, and hyperuricemia and hypertension may be present. Some laboratories can measure δ-aminolevulinic acid dehydratase, which is inhibited by lead. Although chelation studies may document lead burden, this test is difficult to perform in patients with renal failure. X-ray fluorescent measurements of in vivo skeletal lead stores correlate well with ethylenediaminetetraacetic acid (EDTA) chelation tests and have the advantage of being rapid and noninvasive.

Cadmium Toxicity

Cadmium nephropathy (Chapter 21) is seen in regions with contamination from smelters that result in prolonged low-level exposure. Cadmium is bound to metallothionein, and proximal tubular cells take up these complexes. The liver and kidney are the two major organs in which cadmium accumulates. Its half-life in the body is longer than 10 years. Like blood levels of lead, blood levels of cadmium fall after acute exposure because of extensive tissue deposition. Once a threshold of renal deposition is exceeded, excess cadmium is excreted in urine. Cadmium intoxication produces irreversible proximal tubular dysfunction, hypercalciuria, nephrolithiasis, and metabolic bone disease with pain (called "ouch-ouch" disease in Japan).

Hyperuricemia

Hyperuricemia, especially in acutely treated myeloproliferative disease, can cause acute renal failure. Many patients with chronic renal failure have serum uric acid levels higher than 10 mg/dL, attributable to diminished glomerular filtration and the effects of diuretics. However, most studies have not demonstrated an independent association of hyperuricemia with chronic interstitial disease that could not otherwise be attributed to hypertension, vascular disease, calculi, or aging.

TREATMENT **Rx**

Chronic interstitial nephritis tends to progress slowly. Inciting factors such as obstruction, infection, drugs, or toxins should be removed whenever possible. Angiotensin-converting enzyme inhibitors or angiotensin II receptor blockers (see Table 67-5 in Chapter 67) are used early to slow disease progression, with a systolic blood pressure goal of 130 mm Hg or less (Chapters 67 and 132), except when hyperkalemia limits their use. Early treatment of acidosis with oral sodium bicarbonate, starting at 600 mg three times daily. Anemia with erythropoietin (e.g., darbepoetin alfa 0.45 μg/kg weekly to keep the hemoglobin concentration between 10 and 12 g/L), hyperphosphatemia with oral phosphate binders (see Table 121-4 in Chapter 121), and hyperparathyroidism with calcitriol (starting at 0.25 μg/day) can improve performance status and protect against bone loss (Chapters 132 and 133). There is no clear role for immunosuppressive drugs in the treatment of chronic interstitial nephritis, except perhaps in early sarcoidosis (Chapter 95).

For certain specific causes of chronic interstitial nephritis, specific therapeutic approaches are warranted. For analgesic nephropathy, stopping analgesic use can help reduce progression. For hypercalcemia (Chapter 253), therapy is directed toward the primary disease: reduction of the serum calcium concentration, when appropriate, and correction of acid-base disturbances.

Appropriate therapy for presumed cast nephropathy in multiple myeloma includes chemotherapy to ameliorate excess light chain production (Chapter 193); treatment of hypercalcemia (Chapter 253); alkalinization of the urine with the addition of bicarbonate to hypotonic fluids; and avoidance of radiocontrast agents, which may enhance the nephrotoxicity of light chains. Loop diuretics should be used with caution, particularly in the setting of volume depletion.

EDTA is advocated as chelation therapy for lead toxicity (Chapter 21). The goal of chelation is to normalize the EDTA mobilization test. In occasional patients, this may arrest or reverse the progression of the renal failure.

PROGNOSIS

The prognosis for chronic interstitial nephritis is highly variable and depends on the underlying condition and on comorbid conditions, including cardiovascular disease and diabetes mellitus, which become increasingly common in these patients over time.

Grade A ————————————————————O

1. de Brito-Ashurst I, Varagunam M, Raftery MJ, et al. Bicarbonate supplementation slows progression of CKD and improves nutritional status. *J Am Soc Nephrol.* 2009;20:2075-2084.

SUGGESTED READINGS

Perazella MA, Markowitz GS. Drug-induced acute interstitial nephritis. *Nat Rev Nephrol.* 2010;6:462-470. *Review, including the potential role for corticosteroids.*

Praga M, González E. Acute interstitial nephritis. *Kidney Int.* 2010;77:956-961. *Review suggesting a role for early corticosteroid therapy.*

Tanaka T, Nangaku M. Pathogenesis of tubular interstitial nephritis. *Contrib Nephrol.* 2011;169:297-310. *Review.*

125

OBSTRUCTIVE UROPATHY

MARK L. ZEIDEL

DEFINITION

Each day in the average adult, 1.5 to 2 L of urine flows from the kidneys to the end of the urethra, a process that requires proper functioning of each renal pelvis, the ureters, bladder, and urethra. *Obstructive uropathy* occurs when a defect (structural or functional) in the urinary tract blocks or reduces urine flow. When obstructive uropathy impairs renal function, *obstructive nephropathy* ensues. Increased hydrostatic pressure from obstruction downstream may cause dilation of upstream elements of the urinary tract, or *hydronephrosis*. Because recovery of renal function is inversely related to the duration and severity of the obstruction, prompt recognition and treatment of obstructive uropathy can preserve renal function in this condition.

EPIDEMIOLOGY

Although there are few studies of unselected populations, autopsy series reveal a 3.1% frequency of hydronephrosis in all subjects (2.9% in females, 3.3% in males). Autopsy series of children younger than 16 years reveal hydronephrosis in 2.2% of boys and 1.5% of girls; 80% of hydronephrosis occurs in children younger than 12 months. In adults, hydronephrosis occurs with equal frequency in both sexes in those younger than 20 years, but owing to pregnancy and uterine cancer, it is more common in women than in men between the ages of 20 and 60 years. In those older than 60 years, obstructive uropathy is more common in men because of prostate disease. The annual frequency of hospitalization for obstructive uropathy in the United States is 166 per 100,000. Each year, about 2000 patients with a presumed diagnosis of obstructive nephropathy begin treatment for end-stage renal disease (ESRD), representing 2% of ESRD patients. Among these patients, 4% are younger than 20 years, 44% are aged 20 to 64 years, and the balance are older than 64 years.

PATHOBIOLOGY

Normal urine flow from the renal papilla requires the orderly contraction of the renal pelvis, which "milks" the urine into the proximal end of the ureter. The ureter drives the urine to the bladder by rhythmic peristalsis coupled with periodic opening of the ureterovesical junction. As the bladder fills, stretch is detected in the wall and possibly the urothelium, thereby activating relaxation reflexes that suppress contraction of the bladder wall musculature and tighten the urethral sphincter to allow the bladder to expand without large increases in intravesicular pressure (Fig. 125-1; Chapter 25). When filling reaches a critical level, the voiding reflex is initiated. Suppression of detrusor muscle contraction ends, and stimulation begins, while the urethral sphincter is relaxed, leading to the buildup of pressure needed for voiding. Obstructive uropathy may occur as a result of functional or mechanical defects. Functional failures include an inability to open the ureteropelvic or ureterovesical junction, failure to open the urethrovesical junction, or failure of bladder reflexes. Partial or complete mechanical blockade of the urinary tract at any level can lead to obstruction.

Obstruction can occur at any point along the urinary tract from the renal pelvis and proximal urethra to the end of the urethra (phimosis). Because diagnosis and treatment depend heavily on the location of the obstruction, disorders are classified by anatomic location and whether the obstruction is due to factors within the urinary tract (intrinsic obstruction) or factors outside the tract (extrinsic obstruction) (Table 125-1). Intrinsic obstruction

FIGURE 125-1. Neural circuits controlling continence and micturition. **A,** Reflexes mediating urine storage and continence. As the bladder fills, distention stimulates low-level firing of vesical afferents (pelvic nerve), which in turn stimulate sympathetic outflow to the bladder outlet (hypogastric nerve to contract the internal sphincter and inhibit detrusor activity) and pudendal outflow to the external urethral sphincter. These responses occur by spinal reflex pathways that promote continence. The pontine storage center in the rostral pons augments pudendal nerve firing to enhance external urethral sphincter activity. **B,** Voiding reflexes. As the bladder becomes fuller, afferents fire more intensely and activate spinobulbospinal reflex pathways passing through the pontine micturition center. These reflexes stimulate parasympathetic outflow to the bladder and urethral smooth muscle (hypogastric nerve) and inhibit sympathetic and pudendal outflow to the urethral outlet. Ascending afferent input from the spinal cord may pass through the periaqueductal gray (PAG) matter before reaching the cortex, leading to the sensation of urgency. (Modified from DeGroat WC. Integrative control of the lower urinary tract: a preclinical perspective. *Br J Pharmacol.* 2006;147[Suppl 2]:S25-S40.)

TABLE 125-1 CAUSES OF URINARY TRACT OBSTRUCTION

INTRARENAL

Uric acid nephropathy
Sulfonamide precipitates
Acyclovir, indinavir precipitates
Multiple myeloma

URETERAL

Intrinsic

Intraluminal
    Nephrolithiasis
    Papillary necrosis
    Blood clots
    Fungus balls
Intramural
    Ureteropelvic junction dysfunction
    Ureterovesical junction dysfunction
    Ureteral valve, polyp, or tumor
    Ureteral stricture
        Schistosomiasis
        Tuberculosis
        Scarring from instrumentation
        Drugs (e.g., nonsteroidal anti-inflammatory agents)

Extrinsic

Vascular system
    Aneurysm: abdominal aorta or iliac vessels
    Aberrant vessels: ureteropelvic junction
    Venous: retrocaval ureter
Gastrointestinal tract
    Crohn's disease
    Diverticulitis
    Appendiceal abscess
    Colon cancer
    Pancreatic tumor, abscess, or cyst
Reproductive system
    Uterus: pregnancy, prolapse, tumor, endometriosis
    Ovary: abscess, tumor, ovarian remnants
    Gartner's duct cyst, tubo-ovarian abscess
Retroperitoneal disease
    Retroperitoneal fibrosis: radiation, drugs, idiopathic
    Inflammatory: tuberculosis, sarcoidosis
    Hematoma
    Primary tumor (e.g., lymphoma, sarcoma)
    Metastatic tumor (e.g., cervix, ovarian, bladder, colon)
    Lymphocele
    Pelvic lipomatosis

BLADDER

Neurogenic bladder
    Diabetes mellitus
    Spinal cord defect
    Trauma
    Multiple sclerosis
    Stroke
    Parkinson's disease
    Spinal anesthesia
    Anticholinergics
Bladder neck dysfunction
Bladder calculus
Bladder cancer

URETHRA

Urethral stricture
Prostate hypertrophy or cancer
Obstruction from instrumentation

may be due to intraluminal or intramural causes. Intraluminal causes include stones or sludging of material, such as sloughed papillae or clots in papillary necrosis. Intramural causes may be anatomic (e.g., tumors or strictures) or functional (e.g., uncoordinated ureteral peristalsis or failure to open the ureteropelvic or ureterovesical junction). Extrinsic causes of obstruction are grouped according to the organ system causing the obstruction.

PATHOLOGY AND PATHOPHYSIOLOGY

Acute obstruction of urine flow out of the nephron reversibly alters renal blood flow, glomerular filtration, and tubular function. Acute unilateral obstruction may cause minimal clinical disturbance because, in the absence of other disease, the contralateral kidney compensates for the loss of function in the affected kidney. Obstructive uropathy is most often partial and of prolonged duration; this chronic obstruction leads to fibrosis and permanent damage.

In acute complete obstruction, glomerular filtration ceases and tubular transport is markedly reduced. Immediately after the onset of complete ureteral obstruction, blockage of urine flow markedly increases tubular intraluminal pressure, which is transmitted back to the glomerulus. Initial dilation of the afferent arteriole maintains glomerular filtration. However, local production of the potent vasoconstrictors angiotensin II and thromboxane A_2 soon decreases the renal blood flow, glomerular filtration pressure, and glomerular filtration rate. Angiotensin and thromboxane also contract glomerular mesangial cells, reducing the glomerular capillary bed surface area available for filtration. At the same time, prostaglandin E_2 and I_2 levels rise and attenuate the level of vasoconstriction.

Obstruction also disrupts the ability of renal tubules (including the proximal tubule, the medullary thick ascending limb of Henle, and the cortical and medullary collecting ducts) to absorb sodium, secrete potassium and acid, and concentrate and dilute the urine. Reduced tubular transport results from the local release of mediators, such as prostaglandin E_2, that inhibit transport, the local accumulation of macrophages, and the release of inflammatory mediators, as well as mechanisms intrinsic to tubular epithelial cells. When urine flow is halted or markedly slowed, reduced delivery of solutes to tubular cells slows the rate of apical sodium entry, resulting in reduced synthesis and deployment to the plasma membrane of crucial transporter proteins, such as Na^+, K^+-ATPase, and apical sodium entry pathways, such as the epithelial sodium channel and Na/K/Cl cotransporter. As obstruction becomes more prolonged, renal fibrosis and permanent damage ensue. In addition to attenuation of salt reabsorption, reduced solute reabsorption in the thick ascending limb leads to loss of high solute concentrations in the medullary interstitium. Obstruction also markedly reduces the synthesis and membrane trafficking of aquaporins, especially aquaporin 2. The combined impact of the absence of medullary solute accumulation and reduced aquaporin activity leads to an inability to concentrate and dilute the urine.

With bilateral complete obstruction, the loss of function of both kidneys leads to the accumulation of salt, water, and uremic toxins; acidosis; and hyperkalemia. Accumulation of salt and water leads to elevated levels of salt-wasting hormones, such as atrial natriuretic peptide, kinins, and prostaglandins, and reduced levels of salt-retaining hormones, such as angiotensin II, catecholamines, and aldosterone. These hormonal changes act synergistically with the postobstructive state of the kidneys to enhance glomerular filtration and reduce tubular salt reabsorption.

Obstructive nephropathy markedly attenuates the ability of distal nephron segments to secrete potassium and acid, leading to hyperkalemia and a non–anion gap metabolic acidosis. With acidemia, failure to acidify the urine may be revealed by a high urine pH (>5.5) and a positive urine anion gap (urine sodium and potassium higher than urine chloride), which indicates distal nephron failure to excrete ammonium in urine. In elderly patients, especially those with azotemia, chronic partial obstruction is associated with hyporeninemic hypoaldosteronism. In this condition, hyperkalemia and non–anion gap metabolic acidosis result from a combination of inadequate aldosterone production for the level of potassium and blood pH and an inadequate tubular response to aldosterone secondary to tubular dysfunction.

Chronic partial urethral obstruction, such as that caused by prostatic hypertrophy in men, can lead to dilation and remodeling of the bladder. Under normal circumstances, as the bladder fills, stretch receptors in the bladder wall and possibly in the epithelium sense the filling. Signaling via afferents to brain stem centers transmits efferent impulses to inhibit bladder wall contraction, permitting the bladder to fill with a modest increase in hydrostatic pressure (see Fig. 125-1). These bladder-filling reflexes also tighten the internal urethral sphincter and allow the maintenance of continence without the need for voluntary contraction of the external sphincter. However, bladder filling to volumes of 200 to 300 mL in women and 300 to 400 mL in men activates additional stretch receptors, stimulating brain stem micturition centers (see Fig. 125-1). Efferents from these centers augment reflex contraction of the bladder detrusor musculature, relax the internal sphincter, and alert the cortex of the need to void. As the bladder fills further, the micturition reflex becomes stronger, the urge to void becomes uncomfortable and urgent, and the bladder begins to contract against the voluntary, external sphincter, rendering it difficult to maintain continence.

With chronic urethral obstruction, micturition requires higher contractile pressure, resulting in detrusor muscle hypertrophy. The bladder empties less completely, and residual volumes increase. Initially, retained urine owing to incomplete emptying diminishes the volume capacity of the bladder between micturitions, thereby resulting in frequency and nocturia. Over time, with bladder remodeling and changes in autonomic reflexes, the transition from bladder accommodation to the micturition reflex may be delayed and occur at increasingly higher bladder-filling volumes. When the micturition reflex is suddenly activated in patients whose bladders are dilated, urgency, dribbling, and frank incontinence ensue. Some of these same features occur in women with pelvic floor disturbances that impede normal bladder function. Bladder wall remodeling and elevated pressures on voiding may increase back pressure up the ureters and result in the physiologic changes of chronic obstruction, including diminished ability to acidify and concentrate the urine, as well as reduced glomerular filtration.

The renal response to the release of obstruction depends on several factors, including whether the obstruction is unilateral or bilateral and the extent and duration of the obstruction. Release of acute unilateral obstruction leads to gradual reversal of renal vasoconstriction and rapid recovery of the glomerular filtration rate. Because tubular transport mechanisms may still be inhibited, postobstructive salt wasting, inability to secrete potassium and acid, and inability to concentrate and dilute the urine persist and lead to the production of a high quantity of isosthenuric urine (urine with a tonicity similar to that of plasma) from the affected kidney. However, the normal contralateral kidney compensates for these abnormalities in tubular transport. Release of an acute bilateral obstruction can lead to high volumes of urine output and striking salt wasting.

CLINICAL MANIFESTATIONS

The clinical appearance of obstructive uropathy depends on the extent (partial or complete), duration (acute or chronic), and location of the obstruction, as well as on whether one or both kidneys are affected (Table 125-2). Patients may be asymptomatic even with severe obstruction, especially when the obstruction has developed gradually.

Symptoms

In patients with acute obstruction, bladder distention caused by the inability to relax the urethral sphincter (e.g., postoperatively) gives rise to sharp pain. By contrast, significant bladder stretching may occur without pain in the setting of gradual urethral obstruction from prostatic enlargement.

Renal colic from the abrupt distention of the ureter is a common manifestation of the passage of a renal calculus (Chapter 128), with or without acute ureteral obstruction. Renal colic is a severe, stabbing pain localized to the flank (when the stone is in the upper third of the ureter) or radiating to the

groin or pelvic structures (when the stone is located in the lower two thirds of the ureter).

Patients with chronic partial obstruction may have no symptoms or may have intermittent pain. Chronic partial ureteral obstruction may cause intermittent flank pain. Abdominal pain that radiates to the flank during voiding may indicate vesicoureteral reflux. Increasing the urine volume with the administration of fluid loads or diuretics may elicit pain in patients with partial obstruction by stretching the ureteral wall.

Symptoms such as reduced force and caliber of the urine stream, urinary frequency, hesitancy, incontinence, nocturia, postvoid dribbling, and urgency often arise with urethral obstruction. A neurogenic bladder may alter micturition and result in frequency, urgency, and incontinence. Incontinence may occur because an inadequate sensation of bladder fullness or an inability to void properly leads to overfilling of the bladder and reflex emptying (overflow incontinence).

In patients with complete bilateral ureteral obstruction, complete obstruction of a solitary functioning kidney, or complete obstruction to urine flow beyond the bladder, anuric acute renal failure occurs. Patients with partial obstruction may have normal urine volumes or polyuria. In some cases, partial obstruction prevents urinary concentration, leading to polyuria, increased thirst, and sometimes hypernatremia. Although unusual, a history of oligoanuria alternating with polyuria or the sudden onset of anuria strongly suggests obstructive uropathy.

Bilateral complete obstruction or complete obstruction of a single functioning kidney may cause signs, symptoms, and laboratory evidence of acute renal failure (Chapter 122), with volume overload, hypertension, and metabolic disturbances. By contrast, unilateral obstruction with a functioning contralateral kidney usually does not lead to manifestations of renal failure because the functioning kidney may compensate in large part for the failure of filtration and tubular transport in the obstructed kidney. If the obstruction affects both kidneys, patients may have symptoms of impaired renal function, including nocturia and polyuria from failure to concentrate the urine and increased levels of potassium, phosphate, creatinine, and blood urea nitrogen (Chapter 122).

Physical Examination

In patients with acute ureteral obstruction, the physical examination may be normal or it may reveal flank tenderness. Flank tenderness can denote obstruction or pyelonephritis. Renal colic may cause abdominal distention and evidence of reduced peristalsis with diminished bowel sounds. Kidneys enlarged by chronic hydronephrosis may be palpable on the abdominal examination or may cause costovertebral angle tenderness and flank rigidity. In patients with acute obstruction below the bladder, acute bladder distention may be detectable as a suprapubic mass, and the bladder may be tender. In the setting of bladder distention, the rectal examination in men may reveal prostatic enlargement, whereas the pelvic examination in women may reveal pelvic masses. Obstructive uropathy may cause hypertension owing to salt and water retention. Examination of the sensory and reflex pathways of the sacral nerves may reveal neurologic causes of urinary retention.

Hematuria
Laboratory Findings

Patients with obstruction may exhibit gross hematuria, especially in the setting of ureteral stones, which may cause bleeding by abrading the ureteral epithelium (urothelium) as they pass. Microscopic examination of the urine reveals round, regular red cells; this is different from hematuria from glomerular disease, in which red cells (because they cross the glomerulus and remain for prolonged periods in the tubules) appear dysmorphic. Gross hematuria from any cause may lead to clots, which themselves can cause obstruction.

A urinary tract infection in a younger man or repeated urinary tract infections without apparent cause suggest a structural lesion in the urinary tract and are often associated with partial or complete obstruction. Infection occurs more commonly in patients with obstruction involving the bladder or urethra, likely due to disruption of normal defenses against bacterial access and adherence to the bladder urothelium. The finding of unusual organisms (e.g., *Pseudomonas* or *Proteus* species) in noninstrumented patients suggests the disruption of normal defense mechanisms and possible obstruction.

Depending on the extent and duration of obstruction, obstructive uropathy impairs renal function. Hyperkalemia and a nonanion acidosis, owing to distal renal tubular acidosis (Chapter 130), commonly develop. Chronic and

---

TABLE 125-2   CLINICAL MANIFESTATIONS AND LABORATORY FINDINGS IN URINARY TRACT OBSTRUCTION

No symptoms (chronic hydronephrosis)
Intermittent pain (chronic hydronephrosis)
Elevated levels of blood urea nitrogen and serum creatinine with no other symptoms (chronic hydronephrosis)
Renal colic (usually caused by ureteral stones or papillary necrosis)
Changes in urinary output
   Anuria or oliguria (acute renal failure)
   Polyuria (incomplete or partial obstruction)
   Fluctuating urinary output
Hematuria
Palpable masses
   Flank (hydronephrotic kidney, usually in infants)
   Suprapubic (distended bladder)
Hypertension
   Volume dependent (usually caused by chronic bilateral obstruction)
   Renin dependent (usually caused by acute unilateral obstruction)
Repeated urinary tract infections or infection refractory to treatment
Hyperkalemic, hyperchloremic acidosis (usually caused by defective tubular secretion of hydrogen and potassium)
Hypernatremia (seen in infants with partial obstruction and polyuria)
Polycythemia (increased renal production of erythropoietin)
Lower urinary tract symptoms: hesitancy, urgency, incontinence, postvoid dribbling, decreased force and caliber of the urinary stream, nocturia

TABLE 125-3	DIAGNOSTIC TESTS FOR OBSTRUCTIVE UROPATHY

UPPER URINARY TRACT OBSTRUCTION

Sonography (ultrasound)
Plain films of the abdomen (KUB)
Excretory or intravenous pyelography
Retrograde pyelography
Isotopic renography
Computed tomography*
Magnetic resonance imaging*
Pressure flow studies (Whitaker test)

LOWER URINARY TRACT OBSTRUCTION

Tests marked with an asterisk above
Cystoscopy
Voiding cystourethrography
Retrograde urethrography
Urodynamic tests
Cystometrography
Electromyography
Urethral pressure profile

KUB = kidneys, ureter, bladder.
From Klahr S. Obstructive uropathy. In: Jacobson HR, Striker GE, Klahr S, eds. *The Principles and Practice of Nephrology*. Toronto: BC Decker; 1991:432-441.

FIGURE 125-2. **A,** Renal ultrasound of a normal kidney. The outline of the kidney is clearly seen, and the calyces (darker areas) are small and somewhat indistinct. **B,** Renal ultrasound of an obstructed kidney. The arrow points directly at a dilated renal calyx. Other dilated calyces are seen as large, round, dark areas adjacent to the calyx pointed out by the arrow. For orientation, the tail end of the arrow overlies the margin of the renal cortex. (Courtesy Jonathan Kruskal, MD.)

more complete obstruction causes permanent renal damage and can lead to ESRD. Any patient with no previous history of kidney disease who has significant renal impairment should be evaluated for obstructive uropathy, especially if the urinary sediment is bland (Chapter 122). In addition, obstruction should be considered as a potential cause of accelerating deterioration of renal function in patients with underlying disease. In some obstructed kidneys, vasoconstriction may reduce cortical blood flow and oxygen tension, leading to increased erythropoietin production and polycythemia, which reverses with relief of the obstruction.

DIAGNOSIS

Because obstructive uropathy may be asymptomatic or may manifest in many different ways, the diagnosis may not be apparent. However, early diagnosis (Table 125-3) and prompt treatment reduce the extent of long-term renal damage.

Age, gender, and concomitant conditions often help identify the cause of obstruction. In children, congenital sources of obstruction at the ureteropelvic or ureterovesical junction are a major cause of ESRD. In adult women, complications of pregnancy or reproductive malignancies such as cervical or uterine cancer may cause obstruction due to compression of the ureters or ureterovesical junction. In older men, prostatic hypertrophy or cancer often causes urethral obstruction.

In outpatients, a history of renal colic, flank pain, or hematuria may suggest stone disease leading to ureteral obstruction. Changes in the volume or frequency of urination, including anuria, polyuria, or swings from oligoanuria to polyuria, may suggest obstruction. Bladder dysfunction is suggested by symptoms of frequency, urgency, and nocturia. In addition, a history of conditions that predispose to obstructive uropathy, such as sickle cell disease, chronic ingestion of high levels of pain relievers (papillary necrosis), previous stone disease, or abdominal cancer (which may lead to ureteral obstruction), should raise the suspicion of obstruction. Finally, the presence of a single functioning kidney should raise the possibility that unilateral obstruction may be causing azotemia. In the inpatient setting, monitoring the pattern of urine output may reveal oligoanuria or polyuria.

Laboratory Studies

Initial laboratory evaluation includes a careful urinalysis and standard chemistry panel. The urine may reveal hematuria in the case of stones, bacteriuria, numerous granulocytes in the setting of obstruction and infection, or a urine pH greater than 7.5 in the case of chronic infection with urea-splitting organisms. Serum chemistries may reveal hyperkalemia, non–anion gap acidosis, and, more rarely, hypernatremia. Corresponding urine chemistry evaluation may reveal a pH higher than 5.5, lack of a negative anion gap (see earlier), and isosthenuria. The urine sediment may also reveal evidence of crystals

(uric acid or calcium oxalate), suggestive of stone disease. In addition, laboratory measurements should include blood urea nitrogen and creatinine to assess the adequacy of glomerular filtration.

Diagnostic Testing

When obstructive uropathy is suspected, ultrasonography is the best screening modality because it is highly sensitive, safe, and inexpensive and does not expose the patient to contrast material or ionizing radiation. Because of its safety and low cost, ultrasonography is often used in patients with acute renal failure to rule out obstruction. Ultrasound may reveal dilation of the calyces, renal pelvis, and, on occasion, proximal ureter (Fig. 125-2). It is also the preferred test to diagnose a renal calculus (Chapter 128; see Fig. 125-2). False-positive findings (dilation in the absence of obstruction) occur in patients with congenital anomalies, during diuresis, and in many patients with ileal conduits. False-negative findings may occur because the pelvis and calyces fail to dilate despite obstruction, as may occur with retroperitoneal fibrosis or volume depletion. Because of the possibility of false-negative ultrasound results, computed tomography (CT) is warranted when the clinical setting strongly suggests obstruction and the ultrasound findings are negative. CT scanning may define the anatomic location of obstruction in patients found to have hydronephrosis on ultrasound, or it may identify obstruction in patients with negative ultrasound studies. In the setting of cancer or other structural lesions obstructing the ureters or invading the bladder, CT may help identify the cause of obstruction.

Diffusion-weighted magnetic resonance imaging (MRI) can noninvasively detect changes in renal perfusion and in tissue density that occur during acute ureteral obstruction, but the role of MRI in patients with suspected obstructive uropathy remains unclear. MRI is limited by the risk of nephrogenic systemic fibrosis in azotemic patients, especially if the glomerular filtration rate is below 30 mL/minute. Definitive diagnosis of the location of obstruction can be obtained by retrograde pyelography, in which contrast material is injected directly into the ureters via catheters inserted into the urethra and bladder, or by antegrade pyelography, in which the contrast material is injected into the renal pelvis via a percutaneous catheter. Retrograde pyelography is performed when obstruction has been diagnosed or is strongly suggested. This procedure precisely localizes the site of obstruction and guides the urologist in the placement of stents to clear the obstruction.

When bladder dysfunction or lesions in the bladder have been identified, retrograde cystograms may define bladder anatomy. In addition, cystometrography with urodynamic testing can define the force of detrusor function, determine whether the detrusor and sphincter act in a coordinated fashion (lack of coordination is referred to as *dyssynergy*), and define the extent to which pressure within the bladder is elevated and is causing obstruction to urine flow (Chapter 25).

Differential Diagnosis

Because obstructive uropathy may have subtle manifestations that mimic many other conditions, the differential diagnosis depends on the initial clinical symptoms and signs. Though suggestive of obstructive uropathy, anuria and acute renal failure (Chapter 133) may result from intrarenal diseases such as glomerulonephritis or acute tubular necrosis. Patients with polyuria, hypernatremia, and dilute urine may have nephrogenic or central diabetes insipidus (Chapters 236 and 237). Obstructive uropathy is a rare cause of nephrogenic diabetes insipidus. Patients with hyperkalemic hyperchloremic metabolic acidosis may have hyporeninemic hypoaldosteronism, which is associated with chronic mild obstruction or other tubular disorders (Chapter 124). Renal colic may resemble abdominal pain secondary to diseases of the gastrointestinal or reproductive tract, such as appendicitis (Chapter 144) or an ovarian cyst (Chapter 243), especially when the colic is associated with nausea, vomiting, and diaphoresis.

TREATMENT (Rx)

Once obstructive nephropathy has been identified, therapy focuses on the rapid restoration of normal urine flow, treatment of any accompanying infection, and management of postobstructive complications. The degree to which renal function recovers depends on several factors, including the extent and duration of the obstruction and the extent of previous renal dysfunction.

Acute Obstruction

Complete obstruction causes acute renal failure. Because the extent and rate of recovery of renal function depend on the speed of relief, prompt resolution of obstruction obviates the complications of uremia and the need for acute dialysis in patients with bilateral obstruction or obstruction of a single functioning kidney. In the setting of antecedent renal disease, partial obstruction may lead to permanent renal damage, so prompt relief can salvage significant renal function. In all cases of obstruction, the urine should be examined and cultured to identify and treat infections (Chapter 292). In patients with urinary sepsis and obstruction, the sepsis cannot be treated successfully until the obstruction is relieved; in such patients, it is also crucial to look for perinephric abscesses and drain them if present.

The site of the obstruction and its cause determine the therapeutic approach. Obstruction in the urethra or owing to bladder dysfunction may be relieved by placement of a urethral catheter. If catheters cannot be passed through the urethra, urgent suprapubic cystotomy is needed, followed by a more permanent approach, such as surgical diversion or ileal conduits, to prevent recurrent obstruction. If the obstruction is in the upper urinary tract, retrograde ureteral catheters with stents or nephrostomy tubes may be needed to relieve the obstruction. Retrograde catheters have the advantage that internal stents can be left in place to restore normal voiding, avoiding the need to maintain percutaneous drainage tubes.

Acute Obstruction Caused by Calculi

Calculi (Chapter 128) are the most common cause of ureteral obstruction. The cornerstones of therapy include analgesia, relief of the obstruction, and treatment of concomitant infections (Chapter 292). Stones smaller than 6 mm often pass without procedural intervention, but larger (7 to 15 mm) stones are more likely to cause complete obstruction and are unlikely to pass without intervention. If the stone is above the pelvic brim and is less than 15 mm,

extracorporeal shock wave or ultrasonic lithotripsy is 90% effective, with passage of the fragments within 3 months. It is important to increase the volume of urine flow after these approaches to help the patient pass the fragments. For stones located below the pelvic brim or for larger stones, endoureteroscopy with direct removal may be performed via catheters passed through the urethra. In all patients with stone disease, it is crucial to identify the cause and initiate appropriate measures to prevent further stones (Chapter 128). The common practice of routinely placing a ureteral stent after ureteroscopy increases irritative lower urinary symptoms without any demonstrable clinical benefit.**1**

Chronic Partial Obstruction

Although patients with chronic partial obstruction may do well for prolonged periods, the obstructive process should be relieved because it poses a long-term threat to renal function. Prompt relief is mandatory when partial obstruction progresses to frank urinary retention, the obstruction is accompanied by urinary sepsis or repeated urinary tract infections, the obstruction is causing renal damage, or the patient has symptoms such as voiding dysfunction, flank pain, or dysuria. Most often, chronic partial obstruction results from lesions in the lower urinary tract, including urethral blockage from prostate enlargement (Chapter 131). In men, benign prostatic hypertrophy, which may remain stable for long periods, usually responds to medications, but therapeutic decisions, including surgery, depend on symptoms, the presence of infection, and the risk for permanent bladder or renal dysfunction (Chapter 131). The possibility of prostate cancer also must be assessed (Chapter 207).

Chronic obstruction at the bladder neck or urethra can lead to bladder dilation and remodeling, with attendant persistence of dysfunction and symptoms even after relief of the obstruction. On this basis, it may be appropriate to relieve the obstruction before infection, major symptoms, or renal dysfunction occurs. Urethral strictures can be treated by dilation or urethrotomy.

Postobstructive Diuresis

Though usually self-limited, postobstructive diuresis can last several days to a week and may result in clinically important depletion of sodium, potassium, and chloride. Because postobstructive diuresis is prolonged and promoted by excessive fluid replacement, administration of volume is justified only when excessive losses result in clear volume depletion. Proper replacement is guided by measurement of urine chemistries and osmolality. Because the urine is generally isosthenuric, with relatively high sodium levels as a result of residual tubular dysfunction, appropriate replacement fluid is often 0.45% saline given at a rate somewhat slower than that of urine output. By careful monitoring of vital signs, volume status, urine output, and serum and urine chemistry and osmolality, coupled with judicious fluid replacement, the diuresis can be limited and will not cause serious volume or electrolyte abnormalities.

PROGNOSIS

The recovery of renal function depends on the duration and completeness of the obstruction. If the obstruction involves only one kidney and the other kidney has relatively normal function, the preserved kidney will compensate for the loss of function in the obstructed kidney. If obstruction is of relatively short duration and is partial, renal function will likely improve, leaving the patient with no symptoms of renal failure. However, if obstruction is bilateral, complete, or near-complete and persists for a week or more, significant permanent renal damage ensues, particularly if renal function was impaired before the onset of obstruction. Following restoration of urine flow, it may take weeks for renal function to recover, and recovery may be partial or negligible. In these cases, patients may need chronic renal replacement therapy (Chapter 133).

1. Nabi G, Cook J, N'Dow J, et al. Outcomes of stenting after uncomplicated ureteroscopy: systemic review and meta analysis. *BMJ.* 2007;334:572-584.

SUGGESTED READINGS

Chung DE, Sandhu JS. Overactive bladder and outlet obstruction in men. *Curr Urol Rep.* 2011;12:77-85. *Review.*

Rodrigues P, Hering F, Meller A, et al. Outline of 3830 male patients referred to urodynamic evaluation for lower urinary tract symptoms: how common is infravesical outlet obstruction? *Urol Int.* 2009;83:404-409. *Infravesical obstruction explains less than 50% of lower urinary tract symptoms in men.*

Swartz, RD. Idiopathic retroperitoneal fibrosis: a review of the pathogenesis and approaches to treatment. *Am J Kidney Dis.* 2009;54:546-553. *Review.*

126

DIABETES AND THE KIDNEY

RAYMOND C. HARRIS

EPIDEMIOLOGY

In the industrialized world, diabetes mellitus is the single leading cause of end-stage renal disease (ESRD). Both the incidence and the prevalence of ESRD secondary to diabetes continue to rise. In the United States, more than 30% of patients undergoing either dialysis or renal transplantation have ESRD as a result of diabetic nephropathy, and 40% of the new (incident) cases of ESRD are attributable to diabetes.

In the United States, Europe, and Japan, more than 90% of patients with diabetes have type 2 (Chapter 237) rather than type 1 (Chapter 236) (insulinopenic) diabetes. Correspondingly, more than 80% of the ESRD secondary to diabetes is also seen in patients with type 2 diabetes. Although it was previously supposed that ESRD was less common in type 2 diabetes than in type 1 diabetes, when cohorts of patients with both types are monitored for an extended period, the incidence of renal disease is equivalent. The demographics of ESRD secondary to type 2 diabetes mirror the prevalence of type 2 diabetes in the U.S. population, with a higher incidence in females and in African Americans, Hispanic Americans, Native Americans, and Asian Americans and a peak incidence in the fifth to seventh decades of life. Given the global epidemic of obesity in developed countries, an increasing incidence of diabetic nephropathy is being widely appreciated.

PATHOBIOLOGY

Hyperglycemia

Increasing evidence implicates the metabolic sequelae of hyperglycemia as the most important causative factor in the development of diabetic nephropathy. Nearly 20 years ago, randomized clinical trials first demonstrated that aggressive control of blood sugar decreases the development of nephropathy, as well as other microvascular complications, in type 1 diabetes. Furthermore, repeat renal biopsies have documented that the renal lesions of diabetic nephropathy may reverse after long-term (10 years) functioning pancreas transplantation. Hyperglycemia leads to increased generation of reactive oxygen species; depletion of the reduced form of nicotinamide dinucleotide (phosphate); activation of the polyol pathway, which can lead to de novo synthesis of diacylglycerol and increased protein kinase C activity; alterations in the hexosamine pathway; and nonenzymatic protein glycation (advanced glycosylation end products), all of which have been implicated in development of diabetic nephropathy as well as other diabetic microvasculopathies.

Hemodynamics

Patients with type 1 and, to a lesser extent, type 2 diabetes exhibit an increased glomerular filtration rate (GFR)—so-called hyperfiltration—that is mediated by proportionally greater relaxation of the afferent arteriole than the efferent arteriole; such hyperfiltration leads to increased glomerular blood flow and elevated glomerular capillary pressure. With poorly controlled diabetes, patients develop glomerular hypertrophy, with an increased glomerular capillary surface area. These intraglomerular hemodynamic and structural alterations may contribute to the beginning or progression (or both) of diabetic renal injury. Because angiotensin-converting enzyme (ACE) inhibitors and decreased dietary protein reduce intraglomerular capillary pressure in experimental animals, the hyperfiltration hypothesis provides one rationale for the success of these interventions in resisting the progression of diabetic nephropathy (see later).

Hormones and Cytokines

Studies in experimental animals have implicated a number of cytokines, hormones, and intracellular signaling pathways in either the development or the progression of diabetic nephropathy, notably transforming growth factor-β (TGF-β), connective tissue growth factor, angiotensin II, vascular endothelial growth factor (VEGF), endothelin, prostaglandins, and nitric oxide. Because these factors have also been implicated in a variety of nondiabetic kidney diseases, it is likely that they are not specific for diabetic nephropathy. However, agents that interrupt angiotensin II production and signaling are very effective in slowing the progression of diabetic nephropathy. Furthermore, agents that interrupt intracellular pathways activated by these factors or by other consequences of hyperglycemia may provide future therapeutic opportunities.

Genetics

At present, it is impossible to predict in which patients diabetic nephropathy will develop. Although poor glycemic and blood pressure control undoubtedly contributes, nephropathy may or may not develop in an individual patient even after many years of hypertension and hyperglycemia. Type 1 diabetics with siblings who have diabetic nephropathy have a greater than 70% lifetime risk of developing diabetic nephropathy. There also appears to be a hereditary predisposition for the development of diabetic nephropathy in patients with type 2 diabetes.

Diabetic nephropathy is likely to be a polygenic disease. Various genetic linkage analyses have provided conflicting results, likely owing to genetic heterogeneity and the relatively small number of cases examined in individual studies. For example, in some (but not all) studies, an ACE insertion (I)/deletion (D) polymorphism has been associated with an increased incidence of the D allele, which predisposes to increased levels of ACE and the development or greater severity of a variety of nondiabetic renal diseases. Similarly, some but not all linkage studies have suggested the involvement of angiotensinogen polymorphisms and angiotensin II type 1 (AT1) receptor polymorphisms in the development of diabetic nephropathy.

Endothelial dysfunction in diabetes is associated with impaired vascular nitric oxide synthesis. Linkage studies have suggested that polymorphisms in endothelial nitric oxide synthase (eNOS) are associated with nephropathy in Pima Indians with type 2 diabetes, and some but not all linkage studies in other populations with diabetic nephropathy have identified eNOS polymorphisms. Polymorphisms in apolipoprotein E have also been linked to a predisposition to develop diabetic nephropathy in some studies. A variety of other genes, including those for the receptor for advanced glycosylation end products (RAGE), the glucose transporter Glut1, plasminogen activator inhibitor 1 (PAI-1), TGF-β, the B2 bradykinin receptor paroxonase, the homocysteine metabolism-related enzyme methylenetetrahydrofolate reductase, atrial natriuretic peptide, RANTES (regulated on activation, T-cell expressed and secreted), superoxide dismutase, lipoprotein lipase, decorin, VEGF, and peroxisome proliferator-activated receptor-γ (PPAR-γ), have also been linked in some but not all studies.

CLINICAL MANIFESTATIONS

Natural History

Although a minority of patients with diabetic nephropathy have type 1 diabetes, the natural history of the disease is best exemplified in this population. This is true because the onset of diabetes is more clearly definable, and initially, patients with type 1 diabetes usually do not have the comorbid conditions often associated with type 2 diabetes, including essential hypertension, atherosclerotic cardiovascular disease, and obesity, which may independently produce chronic renal injury. Furthermore, the relatively advanced age of onset of type 2 diabetes and the increased cardiovascular mortality in this population may preclude the development of all manifestations of diabetic nephropathy. In type 1 diabetes, diabetic nephropathy progresses in four relatively distinct stages (Fig. 126-1).

Stage I

In stage I, which commences soon after the overt manifestations of diabetes, the kidney undergoes hypertrophy of both the glomeruli and the tubules in comparison with age- and weight-matched normal control subjects. Despite up to a 50% increase in renal blood flow and GFR, macroalbuminuria is not yet detectable, but transient microalbuminuria (measurable by radioimmunoassay, enzyme-linked immunosorbent assay, or special dipsticks) is occasionally evident, especially when induced by stress, physical exertion, concurrent illness, or poor glycemic control. Hypertension is usually absent in the early stages of type 1 diabetes but is often present in type 2 diabetes at its initial detection.

Stage II

Approximately 30% of type 1 diabetic patients progress to clinically silent stage II, characterized by fixed microalbuminuria of at least 30 mg/24 hours, after having diabetes for a median of 10 years. Although the GFR remains elevated or is within the normal range, abnormal renal histology manifests as glomerular and tubular basement membrane thickening and expansion of the

	Stage I	Stage II	Stage III	Stage IV
Median year of onset	0	10	15-17	18-20
% of diabetics	100	30-35	30	30
Urinary protein	Occasional and transient microalbuminuria	Fixed microalbuminuria	Proteinuria (>500 mg/24 hr) and microalbuminuria (200 mg/24 hr)	Nephrotic-range proteinuria (3.5 g/24 hr)
Systemic manifestations	Hypertension: absent in type 1, often present in type 2		Hypertension: absent in type 1, and worsening in type 2	Manifestations of chronic renal insufficiency
Renal morphology and history	Kidney hypertrophy	Glomerular basement membrane thickening and mesangial matrix expansion	Focal glomerulosclerosis (± nodular or Kimmelstiel-Wilson lesions) Microvascular hyalinosis and tubulointerstitial fibrosis	Kidney may still be inappropriately large for level of renal insufficiency Global glomerulosclerosis and tubulointerstitial fibrosis

FIGURE 126-1. Stages of diabetic nephropathy. GFR = glomerular filtration rate.

mesangial matrix. Microalbuminuria is more likely to develop in patients with other microvascular insults, especially proliferative retinopathy. Microalbuminuria is more likely to be caused by diabetic nephropathy in type 1 than in type 2 diabetes, in which hypertension itself may lead to microalbuminuria.

Stage III

The great majority of patients who initially have fixed microalbuminuria progress within 5 to 7 years to overt nephropathy (stage III), with proteinuria (>500 mg of total protein per 24 hours) and macroalbuminuria (>200 mg/24 hours) detectable on a routine urinary protein dipstick. Blood pressure begins to rise in type 1 patients and becomes more problematic in type 2 patients.

Renal biopsy reveals diffuse or nodular (Kimmelstiel-Wilson) glomerulosclerosis. Although the Kimmelstiel-Wilson lesion is considered pathognomonic of advanced diabetic nephropathy, only about 25% of patients manifest this lesion. A nodular pattern of glomerulopathy mimicking Kimmelstiel-Wilson lesions may also be seen in light chain nephropathy (Chapter 193), amyloidosis (Chapter 194), and membranoproliferative glomerulonephritis type II (Chapter 123). Also pathognomonic of diabetic nephropathy is the finding of both afferent and efferent arteriolar hyalinosis; this differs from the arteriolar lesion of essential hypertension, which is restricted to the afferent arteriole. In overt diabetic nephropathy, progressive tubulointerstitial fibrosis correlates most closely with the decline in renal function. The GFR begins to fall from the normal range, but the serum creatinine level may remain in the normal range.

Stage IV

Stage IV, or advanced diabetic nephropathy, is characterized by a relentless decline in renal function to end-stage disease. Patients manifest nephrotic-range proteinuria (>3.5 g/24 hours) and systemic hypertension but have no evidence of inflammatory glomerular (red blood cell casts) or tubulointerstitial (white blood cells, white blood cell casts) lesions. The kidneys may be inappropriately large for the observed degree of renal insufficiency.

Other Renal Complications

Type IV (hyporeninemic, hypoaldosteronemic) renal tubular acidosis (Chapter 124) with hyperkalemia is commonly encountered in patients with diabetes and mild to moderate renal insufficiency. These patients should be carefully monitored for the development of severe hyperkalemia (Chapter 119) in response to volume depletion or after the initiation of drugs that

interfere with the renin-angiotensin system, such as ACE inhibitors, angiotensin receptor blockers (ARBs), β-adrenergic blockers, both nonselective and selective cyclooxygenase 2 nonsteroidal anti-inflammatory agents, and heparin, as well as potassium-sparing diuretics.

Patients with diabetes have an increased incidence of bacterial and fungal infections of the genitourinary tract (Chapter 292), as well as an increased risk for developing intrarenal and perinephric abscesses. Unilateral or bilateral renal artery stenosis (Chapter 127) is more frequent in type 2 diabetes and should be considered if a diabetic patient has intractable hypertension or a rapidly rising serum creatinine level immediately after initiation of therapy with an ACE inhibitor or AT1 receptor blocker. Other causes of acute deterioration in renal function include papillary necrosis with ureteral obstruction owing to sloughing of a papilla, obstructive uropathy (Chapter 125) caused by bladder dysfunction as a result of autonomic neuropathy, and contrast media–induced acute tubular necrosis (Chapter 124). In addition, prerenal azotemia or acute tubular necrosis may develop in diabetic patients as a result of heart failure or volume depletion owing to vomiting induced by gastroparesis (Chapter 236) or diarrhea from autonomic neuropathy.

PREVENTION

Tight glycemic control (Chapter 236) significantly lessens but does not completely eliminate the incidence of diabetic nephropathy.**1** Elevated blood pressure is an important risk factor for the progression of diabetic nephropathy, and blood pressure targets for patients with diabetes are lower (130/80 mm Hg) than those for those without diabetes. However, blood pressure control does not prevent the development of microalbuminuria.**2**

TREATMENT

Latent (Stage II) and Overt (Stage III) Diabetic Nephropathy

Tight glycemic control in type 1 diabetes may not prevent progression to macroalbuminuria, but it prevents other microvascular complications such as retinopathy and peripheral neuropathy (Fig. 126-2). It also slows the progression of nephropathy in type 2 as well as type 1 diabetic patients (Chapter 236).**3,4**

Optimal blood pressure control does not retard the progression of renal disease in patients without macroalbuminuria,**5** but it does retard the progression of frank diabetic nephropathy. In addition to lowering systemic blood pressure, both ACE inhibitors and ARBs have the additional benefit of delaying

Stage I	Tight glucose control BP control—consider use of ACEI or ARB
Stage II	Tight glucose control ACEI or ARB BP control Smoking cessation Weight reduction Exercise Annual eye examination
Stage III	ACEI or ARB BP control Restriction of dietary protein (to 0.8g/kg of ideal body weight/day) Antihyperlipidemic medications
Stage IV	Treat manifestations of nephrotic syndrome and chronic renal insufficiency Prepare for renal replacement therapy, including prevention of abnormalities in calcium/phosphorus metabolism and prevention of anemia by early use of erythropoietin

FIGURE 126-2. Treatment of diabetic nephropathy. ACEI = angiotensin-converting enzyme inhibitor; ARB = angiotensin receptor blocker; BP = blood pressure.

the progression of nephropathy in both type 1 and type 2 patients.**6,7** The combination of a direct renin inhibitor and an ARB may further decrease proteinuria in patients with diabetic nephropathy.**8**

When administering ACE inhibitors or ARBs to patients with diabetic nephropathy, serum potassium and creatinine levels should be monitored closely for the first week because of the possibility of associated type IV renal tubular acidosis or renal artery stenosis. If blood pressure control is not achieved with these agents, diuretics and other antihypertensive agents, including cardioselective β-blockers, α-blockers, and nondihydropyridine calcium-channel blockers (CCBs), can be added (Chapter 67). Although dihydropyridine CCBs may increase intraglomerular capillary pressure, control of systemic blood pressure is essential, and both dihydropyridine and nondihydropyridine CCBs can effectively treat hypertension in these patients without accelerating renal injury.

Judicial restriction of dietary protein (to 0.8 g/kg of ideal body weight per day) is recommended. Although further dietary protein restriction may retard the progression of diabetic nephropathy, an individual's nutritional requirements must be considered. Smoking cessation (Chapter 31) and the use of antihyperlipidemic medications in patients with documented lipid abnormalities (Chapter 213) should be encouraged.

The efficacy of treatment can be determined by monitoring albuminuria and/or total proteinuria. For patients with deteriorating renal function, GFR determined by creatinine clearance and plots of the reciprocal of serum creatinine versus time (1/sCr) are effective indicators of whether interventions are slowing the progression of nephropathy.

Renal Replacement Therapy

In general, management of a diabetic patient nearing ESRD is similar to that of a nondiabetic patient. The patient should be under the care of a nephrologist, and planning for dialysis should be initiated. Although dialysis is generally started when the GFR declines to approximately 10 to 15 mL/minute, early initiation of dialysis is sometimes necessary in diabetic patients when either volume-dependent hypertension or hyperkalemia is not manageable by nondialytic therapy or when uremia, combined with gastroparesis, leads to anorexia, malnutrition, or uncontrollable emesis. Ultimately, more than 80% of patients with end-stage diabetic nephropathy require dialysis (Chapter 133), with about six times as many undergoing hemodialysis as peritoneal dialysis. Approximately 25% of the renal transplant recipients (Chapter 133) in the United States are diabetic patients. The vast majority (>90%) are type 1 diabetics, given their younger age and less severe macrovascular comorbidities in comparison with type 2 patients. Pancreas or combined kidney-pancreas transplantation has a significant effect on quality of life among patients with diabetic nephropathy by improving autonomic neuropathy, either retarding or possibly correcting retinopathy, and avoiding the potential complications of insulin administration. However, all transplantation options remain limited by organ availability.

PROGNOSIS

Because of the associated macrovascular complications (cardiovascular, cerebrovascular, peripheral vascular) and the increased risk for infection, the mortality of diabetic patients who receive either type of dialysis is 1.5 to 2.0

times that of nondiabetic patients, with a 5-year survival rate of less than 20%. The survival of diabetic patients is slightly worse with peritoneal dialysis than with hemodialysis, although it is not clear whether this is related to the type of dialysis or reflects the severity of illness among patients treated with peritoneal dialysis.

Long-term survival and quality of life are generally superior in patients undergoing transplantation compared with those receiving only dialysis. However, the other microvascular complications (retinopathy, neuropathy) are not improved by renal transplantation alone.

1. The Diabetes Control and Complications Trial Research Group. The effect of intensive treatment of diabetes on the development and progression of long-term complications in insulin-dependent diabetes mellitus. *N Engl J Med.* 1993;329:977-986.
2. Bilous R, Chaturvedi N, Sjølie AK, et al. Effect of candesartan on microalbuminuria and albumin excretion rate in diabetes: three randomized trials. *Ann Intern Med.* 2009;151:11-20.
3. UKPDS Group. Intensive blood-glucose control with sulphonylureas or insulin compared with conventional treatment and risk of complications in patients with type 2 diabetes. *Lancet.* 1998;352:837-852.
4. Writing Team for the Diabetes Control and Complications Trial/Epidemiology of Diabetes Interventions and Complications Research Group. Sustained effect of intensive treatment of type 1 diabetes mellitus on development and progression of diabetic nephropathy: the Epidemiology of Diabetes Interventions and Complications (EDIC) study. *JAMA.* 2003;290:2159-2167.
5. Mann JF, Schmieder RE, Dyal L, et al. Effect of telmisartan on renal outcomes: a randomized trial. *Ann Intern Med.* 2009;151:1-10.
6. Strippoli GF, Bonifati C, Craig M, et al. Angiotensin converting enzyme inhibitors and angiotensin II receptor antagonists for preventing the progression of diabetic kidney disease. *Cochrane Database Syst Rev* 2006.4.CD006257.
7. Brenner BM, Cooper ME, de Zeeuw D, et al. RENAAL Study Investigators: Effects of losartan on renal and cardiovascular outcomes in patients with type 2 diabetes and nephropathy. *N Engl J Med.* 2001;345:861-869.
8. Parving HH, Persson F, Lewis JB, et al. Aliskiren combined with losartan in type 2 diabetes and nephropathy. *N Engl J Med.* 2008;358:2433-2446.

SUGGESTED READINGS

Decleves E, Sharma K. New pharmacological treatments for improving renal outcomes in diabetes. *Nat Rev Nephrol.* 2010;6:371-380. *Review.*
Matheson A, Willcox MD, Flanagan J, et al. Urinary biomarkers involved in type 2 diabetes: a review. *Diabetes Metab Res Rev.* 2010;26:150-171. *Potential of newer, more sensitive biomarkers to monitor the development and progression of diabetic nephropathy.*
Van Buren PN, Toto R. Hypertension in diabetic nephropathy: epidemiology, mechanisms, and management. *Adv Chronic Kidney Dis.* 2011;18:28-41. *Review.*

127

VASCULAR DISORDERS OF THE KIDNEY

THOMAS D. DUBOSE JR. AND RENATO M. SANTOS

Vascular disorders that significantly alter renal perfusion can impact the glomerular filtration rate (GFR), tubular function, and, ultimately, kidney function. Stenosis, thrombosis, emboli, atherosclerosis, inflammation, or hypertension may involve the renal arteries, arterioles, microvasculature, and renal veins.

ARTERIES
Renal Artery Stenosis

DEFINITION

Renal artery stenosis, which is a narrowing of the renal arteries, leads to hypoperfusion of one or both of the kidneys. The two most common forms of renal artery stenosis are atherosclerotic disease and fibromuscular dysplasia. The two differ in prevalence, pathophysiology, clinical presentation, prognosis, and management.

EPIDEMIOLOGY

Atherosclerotic disease, which is much more common than fibromuscular dysplasia, accounts for 90% of renal artery stenosis. The prevalence of renal artery stenosis in the Medicare population is only 0.5%, but it is 2 to 4% in patients with hypertension (Chapter 67) and about 5.5% in patients with chronic kidney disease. Atherosclerotic disease is also more common in the elderly and in patients with typical cardiovascular risk factors such as coronary artery disease, heart failure, carotid or peripheral vascular disease, and dyslipidemia. In patients with established coronary artery disease or peripheral vascular disease and hypertension, the prevalence of some degree of renal artery stenosis may be as high as 20 to 40%.

Fibromuscular dysplasia is 2 to 10 times more common in women than in men. It is an important cause of treatable hypertension in young patients without cardiovascular risk factors, and it is pathologically and angiographically distinct from atherosclerotic disease. Although the cause is unknown, there appears to be a genetic predisposition to fibromuscular dysplasia. Other possible pathogenetic factors include hormonal influences (most patients are women of childbearing age), mechanical factors, and ischemia of the vessel wall.

PATHOBIOLOGY

The pathobiology of atherosclerotic renal artery stenosis is identical to that of atherosclerotic disease in other arterial beds (Chapter 70). Fibromuscular dysplasia includes four distinct histopathologic types: medial fibroplasia, which is the most common type and accounts for 75 to 80% of cases; perimedial fibroplasia, with irregular thickening of the media; medial hyperplasia, with smooth muscle hyperplasia without fibrosis; and intimal fibroplasia. Unlike atherosclerotic disease, which localizes at the ostial and proximal segments of the renal arteries, fibromuscular dysplasia more commonly involves the middle and distal arterial segments.

Models of renovascular hypertension using renal artery clips in animals have elegantly demonstrated that activation of the renin-angiotensin-aldosterone system by renal hypoperfusion causes an increase in systemic blood pressure. This mechanism is further supported by the ability of angiotensin-converting enzyme (ACE) inhibitors and angiotensin receptor blockers (ARBs) to control the resulting hypertension in animals and in patients with fibromuscular dysplasia. The mechanism for the development of hypertension with renal artery stenosis, however, appears to be more complex. Although atherosclerotic renal activation of the renin-angiotensin-aldosterone system by renal hypoperfusion is essential for initiating the pressor response, it is transient. Over time, the pathobiology transitions to pressor mechanisms independent of angiotensin II, including vasoconstriction owing to oxidative stress, endothelial dysfunction, endothelin release, and sympathetic activation. Confounding risks including smoking, advanced age, dyslipidemia, diabetes, and hypertension itself, which can contribute to vascular injury. The uncertain cause-and-effect relationship of these confounding risks may explain the inconsistent blood pressure response to renal revascularization for atherosclerotic renal artery stenosis compared with fibromuscular dysplasia.

Renal artery stenosis leads to ischemic nephropathy, defined as an impairment of renal function beyond the occlusive disease in the main renal arteries. However, the pathophysiologic basis of renal injury is likely multifactorial. Unlike cardiac or cerebral tissue, perfusion of the kidneys is determined by glomerular ultrafiltration and the autoregulation of the GFR and renal blood flow rather than metabolic needs. Less than 10% of renal blood flow is required to meet the oxygen demands of the kidneys. Therefore, a severe reduction in perfusion to the entire renal parenchyma is necessary to affect kidney function materially. This relationship is supported by the observation that hemodynamically significant lesions of fibromuscular dysplasia are rarely associated with renal dysfunction. Conversely, a decline in kidney function is common in atherosclerotic renal artery stenosis. Atherogenic stimuli such as hypercholesterolemia can magnify oxidative stress and activate pro-inflammatory and pro-fibrogenic pathways. Repetitive bouts of hypoperfusion in atherosclerotic disease may lead to renal tubular injury and, over time, can lead to tubulointerstitial fibrosis. Thus, a combination of repetitive perfusion insults superimposed on atherogenic risk factors contributes to renal dysfunction.

CLINICAL MANIFESTATIONS

The clinical features of renal artery stenosis are related primarily to renovascular hypertension and ischemic nephropathy (Table 127-1). A significant percentage of patients has resistant hypertension that is unresponsive to high doses of multiple antihypertensive agents. Malignant phase hypertension, though rarely seen with contemporary antihypertensive drugs, still occurs.

Hemodynamically significant renal artery stenosis can also lead to end-organ manifestations remote from the kidneys. A common association is

TABLE 127-1	CLINICAL FEATURES OF RENAL ARTERY STENOSIS

Onset of hypertension before 30 or after 50 years of age
Absence of a family history of hypertension
Short duration or recent worsening of hypertension
Severe hypertension or retinopathy
Resistance to antihypertensive therapy
Signs of other cardiovascular disease
Deterioration of renal function with angiotensin-converting enzyme inhibitor or angiotensin receptor blocker therapy
Abdominal bruit
Unexplained hypokalemia with or without metabolic alkalosis
Unexplained progression of kidney disease or failure
Neurofibromatosis

FIGURE 127-1. Magnetic resonance angiogram of the abdominal aorta showing bilateral renal artery stenosis. Significant iliac stenosis is also demonstrated.

"flash" pulmonary edema (Chapter 58) that cannot be explained by other cardiac problems, particularly if left ventricular function is preserved. Severe hypertension can also precipitate the acute coronary syndrome (Chapter 72), stroke (Chapter 414), transient ischemic attack (Chapter 414), intracranial hemorrhage (Chapter 415), encephalopathy, or papilledema.

DIAGNOSIS

There are no universally accepted guidelines for routine screening for renal artery stenosis (see Table 67-4 in Chapter 67), but the decision to perform diagnostic imaging studies depends on the likelihood that revascularization would be beneficial. Incidental renal artery stenosis is a common finding on noninvasive imaging tests obtained for unrelated reasons.

Preferred imaging modalities include renal duplex ultrasonography, computed tomography (CT) angiography, and magnetic resonance angiography (MRA) (Fig. 127-1). Captopril renal scintigraphy is no longer recommended owing to its poor sensitivity and specificity in the presence of renal insufficiency, bilateral disease, or disease in a solitary functioning kidney.

Renal Doppler ultrasonography is an excellent noninvasive screen for either type of renal artery stenosis and is the preferred initial test for fibromuscular dysplasia. However, it is not available in all centers, is highly operator dependent, and is affected by body habitus and bowel gas; therefore, multiple views, such as oblique and flank approaches, may be required to visualize the cortical branches.

In patients with suspected atherosclerotic renal artery stenosis, the choice among ultrasonography, CT angiography, and MRA depends in part on the availability of the technology, the experience of the vascular imaging department, and the preferences and expertise of the institution. CT angiography is rapid and has good spatial resolution but has the distinct disadvantage of requiring a large contrast load. MRA avoids the need for iodinated contrast

FIGURE 127-2. Renal angiograms from an elderly patient with heart failure. Cardiac catheterization revealed normal coronary arteries, but after initiation of therapy with an angiotensin-converting enzyme inhibitor and spironolactone, progressive kidney disease with hyperkalemia and poor blood pressure control ensued. Renal Doppler ultrasonography suggested bilateral renal artery stenosis, as confirmed by angiography (**A** and **B**). The patient underwent successful percutaneous revascularization in stages, leading to a return to normal left ventricular function and improved blood pressure control (**C**).

and can accurately visualize the proximal segment of the renal artery, although motion artifact and spatial resolution limit the ability to image the middle and distal segments. MRA requires gadolinium enhancement, which may precipitate a rare but severe condition called nephrogenic systemic fibrosis (Chapter 275), especially when the linear gadolinium chelate gadodiamide is used in patients with advanced chronic kidney disease or acute kidney injury. Clearly, the risk of nephrogenic systemic fibrosis limits the applicability of enhanced MRA for patients with advanced renal dysfunction. When the diagnosis remains unclear or when renal artery revascularization is being considered, invasive digital subtraction renal angiography (Fig. 127-2), the "gold standard" test, may be required. In addition to providing anatomic information, the translesion gradient can be measured. Although the complication rates are low, the usual risks of catheterization should be considered, including access site trauma, contrast reactions, and contrast nephropathy.

TREATMENT Rx

The goals of therapy are to control blood pressure, stabilize renal function, and reduce cardiovascular complications.

Atherosclerotic renal artery stenosis reflects a high atherosclerotic burden and is a strong predictor of subsequent cardiovascular events and cardiac mortality. Efforts to optimize medical therapy for secondary prevention include aspirin (81 mg/day), statins to treat dyslipidemia (Chapter 213), management of diabetes (Chapter 236), and control of blood pressure (Chapter 67). Medical therapy for blood pressure control should include ACE inhibitors or ARBs because of their proven benefit in renal protection (see Table 67-6 in Chapter 67). The serum creatinine and GFR should be monitored for the first weeks after initiating ACE inhibitor or ARB therapy, particularly in the elderly. An increase in creatinine of 1.0 mg/dL or greater is an indication to discontinue ACE inhibitor or ARB therapy; it suggests bilateral renal artery stenosis, renal artery stenosis in a unilateral functional kidney, or, in a kidney transplant recipient, renal artery stenosis in the allograft. Smoking cessation, weight control, and increased exercise should be universally recommended.

Renal artery revascularization for atherosclerotic renal artery stenosis remains controversial. In a large trial that randomized more than 800 patients with atherosclerotic renal artery stenosis to medical therapy or renal stenting, no difference was found in blood pressure control or recovery of renal function.**1** Similarly, smaller randomized trials of balloon angioplasty or stenting versus medical therapy showed no benefit of revascularization.**2** The potential utility of renal revascularization for atherosclerotic renal artery stenosis remains poorly defined, and the challenge is to identify patients with ischemic nephropathy and viable renal parenchyma who might improve from revascularization—perhaps those with a recent deterioration in blood pressure control, a sudden decline in renal function, a resistive index of less than 0.8, resistant hypertension, or episodes of malignant hypertension.

In patients with fibromuscular dysplasia, medical treatment alone is usually ill-advised because the stenosis can progress to renal artery occlusion despite adequate blood pressure control. Fibromuscular dysplasia responds well to balloon angioplasty; stenting is rarely needed, and restenosis rates are generally low. Close follow-up with serial blood pressure measurements and evaluation of renal function should be performed every 3 to 4 months.

PROGNOSIS

When adjusted for baseline variables, atherosclerotic renal artery stenosis remains an independent predictor of cardiovascular mortality, with a 4-year adjusted mortality rate of 25 to 40%. Factors associated with higher mortality include an elevated baseline creatinine level, more severe renal artery stenosis, worsening renal function, age, diabetes, other cardiovascular disease, and heart failure. Improvement of blood pressure control or renal function after revascularization is associated with improved survival, even though revascularization does not affect overall survival.

For fibromuscular dysplasia, angioplasty cures hypertension in about 45% of patients. Younger age, milder hypertension, and shorter duration of hypertension are associated with successful outcomes. An atrophic kidney (<8 cm), however, is unlikely to recover with revascularization.

Thromboembolic Occlusion of the Renal Arteries

EPIDEMIOLOGY AND PATHOBIOLOGY

Acute occlusion of the renal arteries and segmental branches may arise as a result of intrinsic pathology of the renal arteries, abdominal trauma, or embolization of thrombi arising in the heart or proximal aorta (Table 127-2). Thrombosis can occur as a complication of progressive atherosclerosis, in which case it may be an important cause of progressive renal insufficiency. In other patients, thrombosis may be associated with thrombophilic states (Chapter 179), such as the antiphospholipid antibody syndrome. Thrombosis also may occur as a consequence of inflammatory disorders, including Takayasu's arteritis (Chapter 78), syphilis (Chapter 327), thromboangiitis obliterans (Chapter 80), and systemic vasculitides, especially Wegener's granulomatosis (Chapter 278). In situ thrombosis has been observed in structural lesions of the renal arteries, such as fibromuscular dysplasia or renal artery aneurysms. In patients younger than 60 years, traumatic thrombosis is the most common cause. Blunt trauma and deceleration injuries can cause acute thrombosis as a result of intimal tears, contusion against the vertebral column, or compression from a retroperitoneal hematoma. Iatrogenic causes include diagnostic angiography or arterial intervention in the renal arteries or vessels proximal to the kidneys.

Embolization, which is a more common cause of renal artery occlusion than in situ thrombosis, is generally unilateral but is bilateral in 15 to 30% of cases. Total infarction of the kidney is much less common than segmental infarction or ischemia. Approximately 90% of thromboemboli to the renal arteries originate in the heart. Atrial fibrillation with embolization of atrial thrombus is the most common cause, but left ventricular thrombus, valvular heart disease (Chapter 75), bacterial endocarditis (Chapter 76), nonbacterial (aseptic) endocarditis (Chapter 76), and atrial myxoma (Chapter 60) are other causes. Noncardiac sources include aortic atheroma and mural thrombus, as well as paradoxical emboli through an atrial septal defect or patent foramen ovale (Chapter 69).

TABLE 127-2 CAUSES OF RENAL ARTERY OCCLUSION

THROMBOSIS

Progressive atherosclerosis
Trauma, blunt
Aortic or renal artery aneurysm
Aortic or renal artery dissection
Aortic or renal artery angiography
Superimposed on inflammatory disorders
    Vasculitis
    Thromboangiitis obliterans
    Syphilis
Superimposed on structural lesions
    Fibromuscular dysplasia

THROMBOEMBOLISM

Atrial fibrillation
Mitral stenosis
Mural thrombus
Atrial myxoma
Prosthetic valve
Septic or aseptic valvular vegetations
Paradoxical emboli
Tumor emboli
Fat emboli

ATHEROEMBOLI (CHOLESTEROL EMBOLIZATION)

Elderly patients with advanced atherosclerosis
Abdominal aortic surgery
Trauma, blunt
Angiographic catheters
Angioplasty or stent placement
Excessive anticoagulation

FIGURE 127-3. Computed tomography demonstrating a clot in the main renal artery and segmental renal infarction.

CLINICAL MANIFESTATIONS

The clinical presentation of renal vascular disease can be variable, and the diagnosis is often confused with more common disorders such as renal colic. Occlusion of a primary or secondary branch of the renal artery in a patient with preexisting disease and established collateral circulation, such as in long-standing renal artery stenosis, may produce little or no infarction and minimal symptoms. Acute thrombosis and infarction may cause the sudden onset of flank pain, fever, nausea, vomiting, and, on occasion, hematuria. Pain may be localized to the abdomen, back, or even the chest, but pain is absent in more than 50% of cases. Hypertension, which occurs with infarction as a result of the release of renin from the ischemic renal parenchyma, may be severe.

Anuria suggests bilateral involvement or occlusion of the artery to a solitary kidney. Urinalysis usually, but not always, reveals microscopic hematuria, and mild proteinuria may be seen.

If infarction occurs, leukocytosis usually develops, and serum enzyme levels of aspartate aminotransferase, lactate dehydrogenase, and alkaline phosphatase may be elevated. These laboratory findings are nonspecific, but elevation of the urinary lactate dehydrogenase level is more specific because its concentration should be normal in extrarenal disorders. Blood urea nitrogen and creatinine levels typically increase transiently with unilateral infarction, but more severe and protracted renal dysfunction may follow bilateral renal infarction or infarction of a solitary kidney.

DIAGNOSIS

The diagnosis of renal artery occlusion is most reliably established by CT with and without contrast. CT is accurate, can be performed rapidly, and can identify associated traumatic injury. Findings may include filling defects in the main or segmental renal arteries, as well as the absence of enhancement of renal tissue, indicating a lack of perfusion (Fig. 127-3). The complication of contrast nephropathy is a major concern in patients with a creatinine level of 2.0 mg/dL or greater or an estimated GFR less than 60 mg/dL. Alternatives to contrast administration should be considered in patients with chronic kidney disease, acute renal failure, or diabetes mellitus and in elderly patients. MRA has a high diagnostic accuracy and may be preferable to contrast CT in the elderly or in patients with diabetes mellitus, although it is contraindicated in patients with renal insufficiency. Radioisotope renograms, excretion urograms, and duplex ultrasound scanning are not recommended for the diagnosis of acute occlusions. Invasive angiography carries inherent risks but is occasionally required if the diagnosis remains uncertain or if percutaneous reperfusion is considered.

In patients with suspected embolic renal artery occlusion, echocardiography is indicated to search for a possible intracardiac thrombus. In nontraumatic thrombotic occlusion, evaluation for thrombophilia (Chapter 179), vasculitides (Chapter 278), or progressive atherosclerosis (Chapter 70) should be considered.

TREATMENT Rx

The human kidney can tolerate 60 to 90 minutes of warm ischemia, although the presence of collateral circulation may permit longer ischemic times. As a result, acute renal artery thrombosis requires urgent treatment in an attempt to reopen the artery. Treatment options for nontraumatic renal artery occlusion include systemic anticoagulation with unfractionated heparin (see Table 81-4 in Chapter 81) or low-molecular-weight heparin (see Table 37-3 in Chapter 37 and Table 81-3 in Chapter 81), followed by oral warfarin (Coumadin) to maintain an international normalized ratio of 2.0 to 3.0, or intra-arterial thrombolytic therapy. Surgical revascularization has been associated with higher mortality than medical therapy, without improved renal salvage rates; it is not recommended as primary therapy but can be considered for patients with bilateral renal artery occlusion or occlusion of the renal artery of a solitary kidney. Percutaneous endovascular therapies (e.g., local thrombolysis, thrombectomy, stent placement) have also been successful in acute renal artery occlusion. For iatrogenic occlusion of the renal artery as a result of angiographic manipulations or angioplasty, intra-arterial stent placement may be considered. For traumatic renal artery thrombosis, surgery is the treatment of choice, but it typically can salvage renal function only if accomplished immediately.

Patients with renal artery thrombosis also require close medical care, often with multiple parenteral agents (see Table 67-8 in Chapter 67), to control their hypertension and achieve a blood pressure between 140/90 and 110/70 mm Hg. Adequate hydration is also imperative.

PROGNOSIS

Mortality is high, especially in patients who require hemodialysis, and it correlates with the severity of underlying conditions. For patients undergoing surgical revascularization for complete acute renal artery occlusion, the mortality rate is 11 to 25%. The risk of losing renal function is variable, and rates of 0 to greater than 50% have been reported. Hypertension, which may develop as a late sequela of renal artery occlusion, is preferably treated with ACE inhibitors, ARBs, or nondihydropyridine calcium-channel blockers (see Table 67-5 in Chapter 67).

ARTERIOLES AND MICROVASCULATURE
Atheroembolic Disease of the Renal Arteries

EPIDEMIOLOGY AND PATHOBIOLOGY

Cholesterol crystal embolization is a potential complication of widespread atherosclerosis. The risk factors are similar to those for all atherosclerotic disease (Chapter 51), including smoking, hypertension, hyperlipidemia, diabetes, and age. Atheroembolic disease appears to be more common in whites, but the condition may be underdiagnosed in African Americans owing to the difficulty of assessing livedo reticularis in this population.

The most common triggering events are manipulation of a thrombus or of the abdominal aorta or renal arteries during angiography or transluminal angioplasty. It is therefore not unusual for cholesterol crystal embolization to be mistaken for contrast-induced nephropathy. Atheroemboli can also be associated with anticoagulant or thrombolytic therapy and may be accompanied by the finding of a cyanotic toe on physical examination. Spontaneous atheroembolism after detachment of a mural plaque is uncommon. Cholesterol crystals typically do not occlude arterial flow but induce an inflammatory response and subsequent endothelial proliferation, so the clinical manifestations may occur some time after the initial insult.

CLINICAL MANIFESTATIONS

Although all organ systems can be affected (Chapter 80), the kidneys are most commonly involved, followed by the spleen and gastrointestinal tract. Renal insufficiency, hypertension, or both typically occur. Nonspecific complaints may include fever, myalgias, headaches, and weight loss. Evidence of cholesterol embolization may be present in the retina, muscles, or skin, where livedo reticularis (see Fig. 80-1 in Chapter 80) or blue toes may be seen. Embolization can also result in cerebrovascular events, acute pancreatitis, ischemic bowel, and gangrene of the extremities (Chapter 79).

DIAGNOSIS

Although most atheroembolic events are diagnosed because of an acute clinical change, clinically silent, chronic, low-grade embolization may be overlooked because patients at risk for this complication often have other chronic illnesses associated with renal failure, hypertension, and atherosclerosis. Urinalysis may not be helpful because cholesterol crystals often are not present, although mild proteinuria, eosinophiluria, and increased cellularity are frequently observed. Transient eosinophilia is common, and an elevated erythrocyte sedimentation rate, hypocomplementemia, anemia, and leukocytosis may also be present. As many as 80% of patients may have a serum creatinine level exceeding 2 mg/dL.

Although the demonstration of cholesterol crystals in the renal microvasculature with subsequent vessel occlusion is considered a diagnostic feature, a kidney biopsy generally is not necessary for patients with typical clinical features, including livedo reticularis and violaceous mottling of the toes, eosinophilia, and an elevated erythrocyte sedimentation rate. When uncertainty exists, noninvasive biopsy of the skin of the lower extremity, muscle of the calf or thigh, or gastric mucosa can be diagnostic in up to 80% of patients.

TREATMENT **Rx**

There is no curative therapy for atheroembolic disease, so supportive care is often all that can be offered. Aggressive control of dyslipidemia with statins (Chapter 213) is recommended and may have the added benefit of stabilizing the endothelial surface. Anticoagulants are of no value and may delay the healing of ulcerating atherosclerotic lesions; if possible, anticoagulant therapy should be discontinued. Adequate hydration is important to sustain renal perfusion. Hypertension should be treated (see Table 67-5 in Chapter 67) with angiotensin II antagonists and vasodilators, and volume should be controlled with diuretics, while being careful not to cause hypotension. Intravascular radiologic procedures and vascular surgery should be avoided if possible.

PROGNOSIS

Recent series suggest up to 80% survival at 1 year. Most patients die of cardiovascular complications. With adequate blood pressure control for several months or years, renal function may recover sufficiently to avoid dialysis. Patients who develop end-stage renal disease have a significantly higher mortality.

Hypertensive Arteriolar Nephrosclerosis

EPIDEMIOLOGY

The risk of nephrosclerosis among hypertensive patients is a function of the severity and duration of hypertension (Chapter 67). Although only a small percentage of patients with hypertensive nephrosclerosis progress to end-stage renal disease, the high prevalence of this condition makes it an important cause. The availability of effective antihypertensive medications has sharply reduced the occurrence of this devastating disorder. However, both benign and malignant hypertensive renal disease and the sequelae of these disorders appear to be more prevalent in African Americans.

PATHOBIOLOGY

The renal vasculature is exquisitely sensitive to damage caused by systemic hypertension when elevated blood pressure is transmitted to the glomerular capillary bed. Unopposed or sustained increases in glomerular capillary hydrostatic pressure eventually result in sclerosis. In benign nephrosclerosis, the kidney is the victim of the adverse effects of chronic hypertension. In malignant or accelerated hypertension, intimal changes in the renal arterial vessels lead to ischemia, increased production of renin, and exacerbation of hypertension, potentially resulting in acute renal failure that, if not treated successfully, will result in end-stage renal disease. Renal vascular lesions similar to those seen in malignant hypertension are also observed in scleroderma (Chapter 275), thrombotic microangiopathy (Chapter 123), and renal transplant rejection (Chapter 133). *MYH9* (myosin, heavy chain 9, nonmuscle) gene polymorphisms are associated with a spectrum of kidney diseases in African Americans with essential hypertension and nephropathy attributed to hypertension, focal segmental glomerulosclerosis, or HIV-associated nephropathy; these data suggest that much of the excess risk of end-stage renal disease in African Americans is linked to genetic susceptibility.

CLINICAL MANIFESTATIONS AND DIAGNOSIS

Typically, patients with benign hypertensive nephrosclerosis have been hypertensive for more than 10 to 15 years. Kidney size is usually reduced, and the urine sediment is unremarkable except for proteinuria, which is generally less than 1.5 g/day. The sudden development of malignant or accelerated hypertension (Chapter 67), either in patients with previously established mild to moderate hypertension or in patients with no previous diagnosis of hypertension, manifests as an abrupt increase in blood pressure (diastolic usually >130 mm Hg). Hypertensive retinopathy (see Fig. 67-1 in Chapter 67) is common, papilledema (see Fig. 431-27) may develop, and renal function may decline rapidly. The kidneys may be enlarged, the urinary sediment may show gross or microscopic hematuria, and proteinuria is often in the nephrotic range. Microangiopathic hemolytic anemia may be present. Abnormalities in the central nervous system are usually evident and include headaches, cerebrovascular accidents, generalized seizures, and coma.

TREATMENT **Rx**

In benign hypertensive nephrosclerosis, the renal outcome depends on the timely initiation of effective therapy, patient adherence, and careful follow-up. The primary goal is a blood pressure of 130/80 mm Hg or less (Chapter 67). Medications that provide renal protection include ACE inhibitors and ARBs (see Table 67-5 in Chapter 67). Nondihydropyridine calcium-channel blockers do not afford protection from progression of renal insufficiency and should be used only in patients who cannot tolerate ACE inhibitor or ARB therapy. For malignant hypertension, more aggressive therapy is required (see Table 67-8 in Chapter 67).

PROGNOSIS

With the skillful selection of renal-specific antihypertensive agents and control of blood pressure, progression of kidney disease can usually be avoided. Unfortunately, such measures may not be initiated sufficiently early or may not be successful in preventing progression to end-stage renal disease.

SYSTEMIC DISORDERS AFFECTING THE RENAL MICROVASCULATURE

Hemolytic-Uremic Syndrome and Thrombotic Thrombocytopenic Purpura

Renal failure is a common consequence of both hemolytic-uremic syndrome (HUS) and thrombotic thrombocytopenic purpura (TTP) (Chapter 175). These conditions are characterized by platelet and fibrin thrombi within the renal microvasculature, accompanied by thrombocytopenia and microangiopathic hemolytic anemia.

TTP is suggested by the co-occurrence of hemolysis, thrombocytopenia, fever, purpura, and alternating mental status changes. HUS may be associated with acute renal failure, thrombocytopenia, and microangiopathic hemolytic anemia, most commonly in children after an acute diarrheal illness. Either disorder may be observed in the setting of cancer and infection and while administering chemotherapeutic agents. In addition to specific therapies (Chapter 175), acute implementation of renal replacement therapy has significantly improved survival.

Scleroderma

The clinical features and progression of scleroderma are highly variable, but mild proteinuria without loss of renal function or evidence of glomerular disease is the most common sign of renal disease (Chapter 275). Significant renal involvement, which has been reported in 50% of patients with systemic sclerosis of 20 or more years' duration, is the most dreaded complication and has the poorest prognosis. A renal crisis may be associated with the use of corticosteroids and can be precipitated in situations that compromise renal blood flow (e.g., dehydration). An increase in vasomotor tone at the level of the renal vasculature contributes to a reduction in renal blood flow, hypertension, and progressive impairment in renal function. The resulting increase in renin and angiotensin II contributes to the development of worsening hypertension and hypertensive nephrosclerosis. Once azotemia develops, hypertension may become more difficult to manage, and dialysis is required within 1 to 2 years. Conversely, patients may initially come to medical attention with a "renal crisis" manifested by the abrupt onset of malignant hypertension and renal failure, commonly associated with heart failure and microangiopathic hemolytic anemia. This manifestation is seen in approximately 2.8% of all patients with scleroderma but in 14 to 18% of those with diffuse cutaneous disease.

TREATMENT   Rx

Therapy should be directed primarily toward controlling hypertension, which may require several drugs in combination, such as ACE inhibitors or ARBs, nondihydropyridine calcium-channel blockers, vasodilators (e.g., minoxidil), and other agents (see Table 67-5 in Chapter 67). Renal crisis is an emergency that usually requires intravenous antihypertensive therapy (see Table 67-8 in Chapter 67). Some patients follow a progressive course despite blood pressure control. Patients with an initial serum creatinine level of 3.0 mg/dL or greater have a poorer prognosis. If dialysis is required, aggressive management of hypertension may allow a small but significant percentage of patients to regain sufficient renal function to allow cessation of renal replacement therapy.

Sickle Cell Nephropathy

PATHOBIOLOGY

The hypoxemic and hypertonic environment of the renal medulla (vasa recta) encourages the sickling of red blood cells circulating through this region (Chapter 166). When sickle hemoglobin desaturates, polymerization of hemoglobin can impair or interrupt capillary flow. The major manifestations of sickle cell nephropathy can all be explained by the development of papillary infarction.

CLINICAL MANIFESTATIONS

A defect in urinary concentration results in a tendency toward volume depletion in sickle cell disease and in sickle cell trait. A defect in urinary acidification is common and is manifested as distal renal tubular acidosis with hyperkalemia and hyperchloremic metabolic acidosis (type 4 renal tubular acidosis; Chapter 120). The acidification defect is usually not observed in patients with sickle trait. Microscopic hematuria occurs in most patients with sickle cell anemia. Painless gross hematuria occurs in up to 50% of patients with sickle cell nephropathy and also occurs in patients with hemoglobin SC disease. With recurrent papillary infarction, papillary necrosis can occur and progress. Sickle cell "crisis," dehydration, hypoxemia, and the use of nonsteroidal anti-inflammatory drugs predispose to papillary necrosis. Renal papillary necrosis is often silent, but it may progress to chronic renal insufficiency and predispose the patient to repeated urinary tract infections. Nephrotic syndrome may develop in approximately 4% of patients with sickle glomerulopathy. Findings on renal biopsy usually indicate membranoproliferative glomerulopathy (Chapter 123) with segmental and global sclerosis. As this disorder progresses, glomerulopathy results in sclerosis and progressive loss of glomerular function. In contrast, papillary infarction can result in persistent hematuria.

TREATMENT   Rx

Volume depletion should be corrected by the intravenous administration of isotonic or hypotonic saline, as dictated by the serum sodium concentration. Hyperkalemia may require potassium exchange resin (sodium polystyrene [Kayexalate] 50 g in 70% sorbitol) per rectum or orally (15 g in water or 70% sorbitol). When acidosis accompanies the hyperkalemia, alkali may help correct both. Long-term administration of Shohl solution (15 mL two or three times daily) or sodium bicarbonate tablets (two 650-mg [7.6-mEq] tablets orally twice a day) may be necessary, and loop diuretics may be helpful. Potassium-sparing diuretics, nonsteroidal anti-inflammatory drugs, and potassium supplements should be strictly avoided. Rarely, small doses of ε-aminocaproic acid may be necessary for life-threatening hematuria, but this can result in thrombosis or ureteral obstruction.

RENAL VEINS
Renal Vein Thrombosis

EPIDEMIOLOGY

Unilateral or bilateral thrombosis of the major renal veins or their segments is often a subtle disorder that can develop in a variety of conditions (Table 127-3), but especially with nephrotic syndrome (Chapter 123) or renal malignancies (Chapter 203). Cases have also been associated with trauma, oral contraceptive use, hypovolemia, renal transplantation (Chapter 133), and thrombophilic states (Chapter 179). The reported incidence of renal vein thrombosis ranges from 5 to 62% in patients with nephrotic syndrome, including those with membranous nephropathy, membranoproliferative glomerulonephritis, focal glomerular sclerosis, sickle cell nephropathy, amyloidosis, diabetic nephropathy, renal vasculitis, and lupus nephritis. Spontaneous renal vein thrombosis is unusual in patients without underlying risk factors.

PATHOBIOLOGY

The precipitating factors are apparently abnormalities in coagulation or fibrinolysis. Antithrombin III and plasminogen levels may be depressed as a result of urinary excretion of antithrombin III in patients with nephrotic syndrome. Thrombocytosis, increased platelet activation, hyperfibrinogenemia, inhibition of plasminogen activation, and altered circulating levels of proteins S and C in nephrotic syndrome contribute to thromboembolic complications.

Extrinsic compression of the renal veins from retroperitoneal sources such as lymph nodes, fibrosis, abscess, aortic aneurysm, or tumor may cause renal vein thrombosis as a result of sluggish renal venous flow. Acute pancreatitis, trauma, and retroperitoneal surgery also may predispose to renal vein thrombosis. Renal cell carcinoma characteristically invades the renal vein and compromises venous flow, resulting in renal vein thrombosis. Renal vein thrombosis in the setting of severe volume depletion and impaired renal blood flow has been described in young adults.

CLINICAL MANIFESTATIONS

The manifestations of renal vein thrombosis depend on the extent and rapidity of the development of the occlusion. Patients with acute renal vein thrombosis may have nausea, vomiting, flank pain, leukocytosis, hematuria, compromised renal function, and an increase in kidney size. These features may be confused with renal colic or pyelonephritis. Adult patients with nephrotic syndrome and chronic renal vein thrombosis may have more subtle findings, such as a dramatic increase in proteinuria or evidence of tubular dysfunction, including glycosuria, aminoaciduria, phosphaturia, and impaired urinary acidification. Chronic renal vein thrombosis may first present in association with a pulmonary embolus.

TABLE 127-3   CAUSES OF RENAL VEIN THROMBOSIS

Nephrotic syndrome
Renal cell carcinoma with renal vein invasion
Pregnancy or estrogen therapy
Volume depletion (especially in infants)
Extrinsic compression (lymph nodes, tumor, retroperitoneal fibrosis, aortic aneurysm)
Corticosteroids

DIAGNOSIS

For acute renal vein thrombosis, which is typically associated with thrombophilia, contrast-enhanced CT shows an enlarged kidney, stretching of the calyces, and notching of the ureters. A venogram is rarely required but can be considered in cases of acute renal failure in which thrombectomy or thrombolysis is considered. In chronic renal vein thrombosis, an incidentally noted renal vein thrombus may be seen on imaging studies ordered for other reasons. Routine screening for thrombus is not recommended for those with nephrotic syndrome, but contrast-enhanced CT is recommended in patients with suggestive clinical manifestations.

TREATMENT   **Rx**

The most widely accepted form of therapy for both acute and chronic renal vein thrombosis is anticoagulation with low-molecular-weight heparin (see Table 81-3 in Chapter 81) or unfractionated heparin (see Table 81-4 in Chapter 81), which can be converted to oral warfarin after 7 to 10 days and should continue for at least 1 year and to an international normalized ratio of 2.0 to 3.0. In patients with ongoing risk factors, such as persistent nephrotic syndrome, or recurrent thrombosis, anticoagulation should be continued indefinitely. Fibrinolytic therapy may be considered in patients with acute renal vein thrombosis associated with acute renal failure.

PROGNOSIS

The prognosis of renal vein thrombosis depends entirely on the underlying condition causing or associated with it. Renal vein thrombosis associated with membranous glomerulonephritis and nephrotic syndrome (Chapter 123) usually resolves if the underlying condition responds to therapy or spontaneously resolves. In contrast, renal vein thrombosis associated with renal cell carcinoma (Chapter 203) has a very poor prognosis. Renal vein thrombosis associated with trauma or hypovolemia may resolve after appropriate therapy.

 Grade **A** ———————————○

1. Wheatley K, Ives N, Gray R, et al. Revascularization versus medical therapy for renal artery stenosis. *N Engl J Med.* 2009;361:1953-1962.
2. Bax L, Woittiez AJ, Kouwenberg HG, et al. Stent placement in patients with atherosclerotic renal artery stenosis and impaired renal function: a randomized trial. *Ann Intern Med.* 2009;150:840-848.

SUGGESTED READINGS

Colyer WR Jr, Cooper CJ. Management of renal artery stenosis: 2010. *Curr Treat Options Cardiovasc Med.* 2011;13:103-113. *Review.*
Dworkin LD, Cooper CJ. Renal-artery stenosis. *N Engl J Med.* 2009;361:1972-1978. *Review.*
Fries C, Roos M, Gaspert A, et al. Atheroembolic disease—a frequently missed diagnosis: results of a 12-year matched-pair autopsy study. *Medicine (Baltimore).* 2010;89:126-132. *Review emphasizing an association with intravascular procedures.*
Scolari F, Ravani P. Atheroembolic renal disease. *Lancet.* 2010;375:1650-1660. *Review recommending treatment with a statin and perhaps corticosteroids.*

128

NEPHROLITHIASIS

GARY C. CURHAN

DEFINITION

A kidney stone is a crystalline mass that is formed in the kidney and that is of sufficient size to be clinically detectable, either by symptoms or by imaging. The composition of different types of kidney stones determines the clinical evaluation, treatment, and prognosis. The most common component is calcium oxalate; other types are calcium phosphate, uric acid, struvite, and cystine stones (Fig. 128-1). Infrequently, stones may be composed of medications, including acyclovir, indinavir, and triamterene.

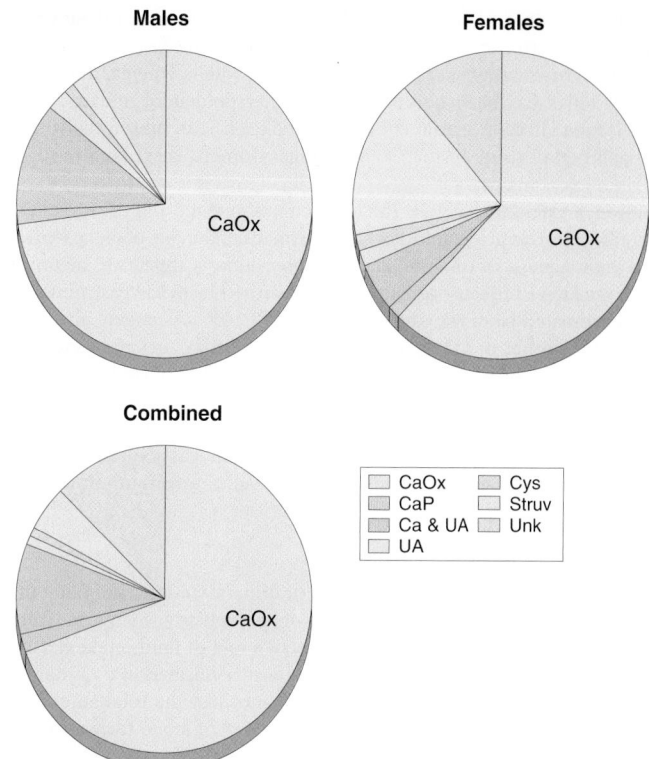

Males   **Females**   CaOx   CaOx

Combined   CaOx

☐ CaOx ☐ Cys
☐ CaP ☐ Struv
☐ Ca & UA ☐ Unk
☐ UA

FIGURE 128-1. Types of stones and frequency in adults. Ca & UA = calcium and uric acid; CaOx = calcium oxalate; CaP = calcium phosphate; Cys = cystine; Struv = struvite; UA = uric acid; Unk = unknown. (From Coe F, Parks J, eds. *Nephrolithiasis: Pathogenesis and Treatment.* Chicago: Year Book; 1988. Reprinted in Greenberg A, Cheung AK. *Primer on Kidney Diseases.* Philadelphia: Elsevier; 2005.)

EPIDEMIOLOGY

The prevalence of a history of kidney stone disease increased between the early 1970s and 1990 in both men and women and in whites and blacks. Nephrolithiasis accounts for nearly 2 million physician office visits with estimated annual health care costs of approximately $2 billion. The lifetime risk of stone formation in the United States is approximately 12% in men and 6% in women. The risk in blacks is one fourth that of whites.

Among men who have never had a stone, the incidence is 3 to 4 cases per 1000 men per year between the ages of 30 and 60 years and then slowly declines with age. For women, the incidence is 2 cases per 1000 women per year between the ages of 20 and 30 and then declines to approximately 1 per 1000 women per year for the next four decades.

The risk of recurrent stone formation in untreated patients after the first stone remains uncertain. Earlier studies reported stone recurrence rates ranging from 30 to 50% at 5 years. However, control groups in recent randomized controlled trials of incident calcium oxalate stone formers experienced substantially lower rates of first recurrence (2 to 5 per 100 person years). Unfortunately, no information on sex-specific rates is available from these trials.

Risk Factors
Dietary Factors
Nutrients

Dietary factors that appear to increase the risk for nephrolithiasis include animal protein, oxalate, sodium, sucrose, fructose, and vitamin C. Higher intake of potassium and phytate reduces the risk.

Low dietary calcium intake increases the risk for stone formation. Although the mechanism is uncertain, low calcium intake increases the gastrointestinal absorption and urinary excretion of oxalate. It is also possible that other factors in dairy products, the major source of dietary calcium, may reduce the risk for stone formation. In contrast, calcium supplements appear to increase the risk of incident stone formation. Thus, they should be used with caution in individuals with a history of calcium stone disease.

Higher animal protein intake may raise urinary excretion of calcium and uric acid and decrease urinary excretion of citrate, thereby increasing the risk for stone formation. Higher sodium or sucrose intake increases urinary calcium excretion, and potassium supplementation decreases calcium excretion. In prospective studies, an increased risk for stone formation has been observed in men with higher intakes of animal protein, whereas a decreased risk for stones has been observed with higher potassium intake. Phytate, which is found in cold cereals, dark bread, and beans, can substantially reduce the likelihood of stone formation in younger women. These studies suggest that risk factors may vary by age and gender.

Although calcium oxalate is the most common stone and urine oxalate is clearly an important risk factor for stone formation, the role of dietary oxalate in the pathogenesis of calcium oxalate nephrolithiasis appears to be limited. The proportion of dietary oxalate that is absorbed from the gastrointestinal tract is estimated to range from 10 to 50%. Factors influencing absorption likely include other dietary components (e.g., calcium), genetic factors, and possibly intestinal flora. In addition, the bioavailability of oxalate in food is unknown. Urinary oxalate is also derived from the endogenous metabolism of glycine, glycolate, hydroxyproline, and vitamin C. Individuals who have Crohn's disease (Chapter 143) or who have had gastrointestinal bypass surgery often have very high urinary oxalate values owing to an increased absorption of dietary oxalate.

Fluid Intake

Fluid intake is the primary determinant of urinary volume, and daily urine volume is a crucial factor in stone formation, particularly when urine output is less than 1 L/day. The important protective role of fluid intake has been demonstrated in observational studies and was confirmed in a randomized controlled trial. Because the concentrations, not just the total amounts, of relevant urinary factors are the key determinants of stone formation, fluid intake and subsequent urinary volume are critical.

Systemic Conditions

Systemic conditions that increase the risk for formation of calcium-containing stones include primary hyperparathyroidism (Chapter 253) and renal tubular acidosis (Table 128-1). Primary hyperparathyroidism is found in less than 5% of stone formers. Obesity, gout, and diabetes mellitus are independently associated with stone formation, as are Crohn's disease and surgical treatments for obesity, such as gastric bypass surgery.

PATHOBIOLOGY
Genetics

Individuals with a family history of stone disease have a two-fold higher risk of becoming stone formers. Rare monogenic causes of nephrolithiasis include Dent's disease and cystinuria (Chapter 130). A recent genome-wide association study suggested that a single nucleotide polymorphism in the claudin-14 gene is associated with a higher risk of stone formation. Conversely, studies of specific genes involved in calcium metabolism, such as the calcium-sensing receptor and the vitamin D receptor, have not been conclusive in humans.

Pathogenesis
Supersaturation

Stone formation is the result of a complex physicochemical process that leads to crystallization. Although normal individuals can have crystalluria and not actual stones, the presence of crystalluria substantially increases the likelihood of stone formation. Formation of crystals in urine is largely a function of supersaturation, a concentration above a material's solubility in water.

Evidence suggests that the initial crystal nidus of calcium oxalate stones forms in the *medullary interstitium* and is composed of calcium phosphate. The calcium phosphate crystals then erode through the papilla, forming the classic Randall's plaque, where they act as a nidus for the deposition of calcium oxalate.

TABLE 128-1	SYSTEMIC DISORDERS ASSOCIATED WITH A HIGHER RISK FOR STONE FORMATION

Crohn's disease
Primary hyperparathyroidism
Gout
Diabetes mellitus
Obesity
Gastric bypass procedure
Renal tubular acidosis

Most stones do not contain one single type of crystal but rather are a mixture with one or two types that predominate. Furthermore, kidney stones also contain protein in the stone matrix.

Modifiable factors that influence supersaturation include pH, volume, and inhibitors. Crystallization of uric acid and calcium phosphate is strongly influenced by urinary pH, which has little effect on calcium oxalate. For all types of stones, supersaturation is dependent on urinary volume; increasing daily urine volume (ideally to greater than 2 L) is of practical benefit in reducing the supersaturation and incidence of stones.

The urine of most individuals is supersaturated with respect to calcium oxalate and calcium phosphate. The remarkable ability of urine to inhibit crystallization prevents most of the population from continuously forming stones. The compounds that stabilize and prevent crystallization within the tubules and the urinary tract are incompletely characterized but include citrate and urinary proteins.

Hypercalciuria

The common definition of hypercalciuria is urine calcium excretion greater than 300 mg/day in men, greater than 250 mg/day in women, or greater than 4 mg/kg/day on a 1000-mg/day calcium diet. Although this higher cutoff for men is reasonable from a calcium balance perspective, it is not relevant for stone formation because urine volumes in men and women are similar. Second, a definition based on weight is problematic. For example, if an individual gains 20 kg in weight, the amount of calcium that that person would be "allowed" to excrete would increase by 80 mg, but the risk of forming stones would rise.

Hyperoxaluria

Hyperoxaluria is often defined as urinary oxalate excretion of more than 45 mg/day, but the risk of stone formation begins well below this level. Elevated urinary oxalate excretion may be present in up to 40% of male and 10% of female stone formers, but hyperoxaluria is also frequently found in individuals who do not have a history of stone disease.

Hyperuricosuria

Persons with gout (Chapter 281) have an increased frequency of stone disease, and a double-blind trial about 25 years ago showed that allopurinol successfully decreased recurrence rates of calcium stones in patients with hyperuricosuria, often defined as more than 800 mg/day in men or more than 750 mg/day in women. However, a large study did not find a correlation of 24-hour urine uric acid excretion with an increased risk of calcium oxalate stone formation. Although hyperuricosuria is a risk factor for uric acid stones, its role in calcium oxalate stones is uncertain, and any protective benefit of allopurinol may be through a mechanism other than the lower urine urate.

Hypocitraturia

Citrate inhibits the growth and aggregation of crystals, and individuals with hypocitraturia (<320 mg/day for men and women) are at increased risk for stone formation. It is likely that an increase of urinary citrate above the normal range provides additional protection against stones. Although citrate in normal individuals is influenced by foods that are high in alkali (e.g., fruits, vegetables) or that generate acid (e.g., nondairy animal protein), they do not completely account for the higher renal tubular reabsorption of citrate in patients who have hypocitraturia and idiopathic calcium stones.

Formation of Non-Calcium-Containing Stones
Uric Acid Stones

Although uric acid excretion is important, the major driver of uric acid supersaturation and subsequent uric acid stone formation is low urinary pH. Many patients who form uric acid stones do not have markedly elevated urinary uric acid excretion (defined previously), but they do have persistently acid urine with the urinary pH typically below 5.5 throughout the day. Factors that contribute to lower urinary pH include obesity, type 2 diabetes mellitus, and high nondairy animal protein intake.

Struvite Stones

Struvite stones, also known as infection or triple-phosphate stones, form only when the upper urinary tract is infected with urease-producing bacteria such as *Proteus mirabilis, Klebsiella pneumoniae,* or *Providencia* species. Hydrolysis of urea by urease results in a supraphysiologic urine pH higher than 8.0 and the formation of struvite $[(NH_4)MgPO_4 \cdot 6(H_2O)]$. If the infection is inadequately treated, struvite stones may grow quickly, fill the renal collecting system, and result in a staghorn calculus.

Cystine Stones

Cystine stones form in individuals with an uncommon autosomal recessive disorder of defective proximal renal tubular reabsorption of filtered dibasic amino acids. Cystine is clinically significant because of its poor solubility in urine. Normal cystine excretion is less than 18 mg/day, but heterozygotes with hypercystinuria (Chapter 130) may excrete up to 100 mg/day, and homozygotes may excrete more than 1 g/day. Cystine solubility is about 250 mg/L, so heterozygotes typically do not form cystine stones. Cystine stones are visible on plain radiographs and will often be manifested as staghorn calculi or multiple bilateral stones.

CLINICAL MANIFESTATIONS

A kidney stone takes weeks to months (and often much longer) to grow to a clinically detectable size. Although the passage of a stone is a dramatic event, a stone's formation and growth are typically clinically silent. A stone can remain asymptomatic in the kidney for years or even decades. Signs (e.g., hematuria) and symptoms may not become apparent until years after the stone has formed. Thus, it is important to remember that onset of symptoms, typically attributable to a stone moving into the ureter, does not provide insight into when the stone actually formed. The precipitants of movement of a stone are unknown.

Acute Renal Colic

When a stone moves from the renal pelvis into the ureter, the typical symptom is the sudden onset of unilateral flank pain of sufficient severity that the individual eventually seeks medical attention, often at an emergency department. Although the term *colic* is used, the pain does not completely remit but rather waxes and wanes. The pain, which is often accompanied by nausea and occasionally by vomiting, may radiate differently, depending on the location of the stone. If the stone lodges in the upper part of the ureter, pain may radiate anteriorly; if the stone is in the lower part of the ureter, pain can radiate to the ipsilateral testicle in men or the ipsilateral labium in women; and if lodged at the ureterovesical junction, the major symptoms may be urinary frequency and urgency. Occasionally, a patient will have gross hematuria without pain.

DIAGNOSIS

Physical examination alone will rarely make the diagnosis, but it may uncover clues to guide the evaluation. The patient will typically be in obvious pain and unable to find a comfortable position. Ipsilateral costovertebral tenderness is common. If the stone causes urinary obstruction, signs of infection and sepsis may be found. Occasionally, the examination may reveal findings associated with stone formation, such as tophi, but the physical examination rarely is diagnostic for stone disease.

Serum chemistry findings are typically normal, but the white blood cell count may be elevated. Urinalysis will classically reveal red and white blood cells and occasionally crystals. The absence of hematuria does not exclude a stone because no urine will be flowing from a ureter that is completely obstructed by a stone.

The diagnosis often is so clear, based on the history, physical examination, and urinalysis, that urgent radiographic confirmation is not required for acute care to be started. When such stable patients respond to analgesic therapy, imaging studies can be deferred for 2 to 3 weeks and performed only in patients whose stones do not pass or symptoms resolve.**1**

Diagnosis is confirmed by an appropriate imaging study (Fig. 128-2), preferably helical computed tomography (CT) because of its high sensitivity, ability to visualize uric acid stones (traditionally considered "radiolucent"), and ability to avoid radiocontrast. Helical CT detects stones as small as 1 mm, thus identifying small stones that may be missed by intravenous urography. Typically, helical CT will reveal a ureteral stone or evidence of recent passage (e.g., perinephric stranding or hydronephrosis), whereas a plain abdominal radiograph (kidney-ureters-bladder) can miss a stone in the ureter or kidney, even if radiopaque, and provides no information on obstruction. Although abdominal ultrasound has the advantage of avoiding radiation, this technique can image only the kidney and possibly the proximal segment of the ureter, so it misses most ureteral stones.

Differential Diagnosis

Because stone disease is common, a stone in the renal pelvis does not alone confirm the diagnosis in a patient with acute abdominal or flank pain.

FIGURE 128-2. High-resolution helical computed tomographic (CT) scan of the upper part of the abdomen demonstrating a stone in the right renal pelvis and a smaller stone in the left kidney *(arrowheads)*. There is no hydronephrosis. (From Curhan GC. Clinical crossroads: a 44-year-old woman with kidney stones. *JAMA.* 2005;293:1107-1114.)

A stone lodged at the right ureteropelvic junction may mimic acute cholecystitis (Chapter 158), a stone in the distal right ureter may mimic acute appendicitis (Chapter 144), a stone at the ureterovesical junction may mimic acute cystitis (Chapter 292), and a stone in the distal left ureter may mimic diverticulitis (Chapter 144). An obstructing stone with proximal infection may mimic acute pyelonephritis (Chapter 292). Infection in the setting of ureteral obstruction is a medical emergency ("pus under pressure") that requires immediate drainage by placement of either a ureteral stent or a percutaneous nephrostomy tube. Other conditions to consider in the differential diagnosis include muscular or skeletal pain, herpes zoster (Chapter 383), duodenal ulcer (Chapter 141), abdominal aortic aneurysm (Chapter 144), gynecologic causes, ureteral stricture, and ureteral obstruction by materials other than a stone, such as a blood clot or sloughed papilla. Although extraluminal processes, such as extensions of gynecologic malignancies (Chapter 205) or retroperitoneal fibrosis (Chapter 284), can lead to ureteral obstruction, patients with these conditions tend not to have colic because of the usually gradual onset of the obstruction.

Chronic Nephrolithiasis

Among individuals with a documented history of nephrolithiasis, chronic back or flank pain is not infrequently encountered. Clinically, patients with an asymptomatic renal stone often have microscopic hematuria. Because stone disease itself is rarely a cause of chronic pain, the goal should be to determine the source of the pain. The differential diagnosis includes musculoskeletal pain, other intra-abdominal and pelvic conditions, and drug seeking. A thorough urologic evaluation, including appropriate radiologic studies, may curtail the long-term use of narcotics and avert frequent trips to the emergency room.

TREATMENT Rx

Medical Therapy

Renal colic can cause excruciating pain, so pain control is a priority after the definitive diagnosis has been made (Fig. 128-3). Nausea and vomiting often prevent the use of oral medication, so parenteral medication is typically required. Narcotics and parenteral nonsteroidal anti-inflammatory drugs (NSAIDs) have been demonstrated to be equally effective, and NSAIDs are preferred because of fewer side effects.**2** Ketorolac, 30 mg given intravenously (IV), is the usual adult dose. If oral NSAIDs are selected, ibuprofen is the most common choice. Morphine (5 to 10 mg IV) and hydromorphone (1 to 2 mg IV) are the most commonly used parenteral narcotics in adults. Oral oxycodone may be given for pain control after discharge. If antiemetics are required, ondansetron (2 to 4 mg IV) is often used because it is not sedating. However, the risk of parenteral NSAIDs may be increased in the setting of dehydration, decreased renal function, or the use of radiocontrast. Alkalinization of urine may be effective for the acute treatment of ureteral uric acid stones, but these are not nearly as common as calcium stones. Intravenous

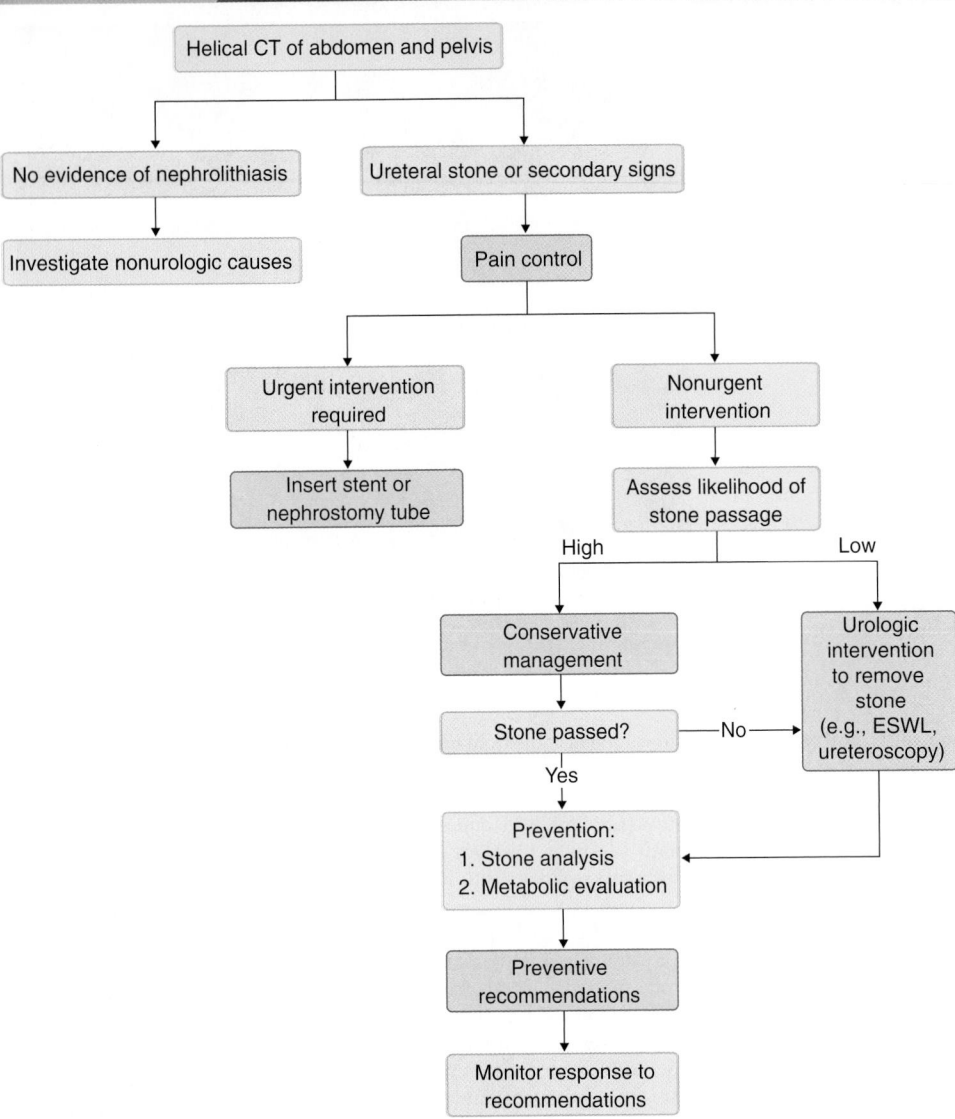

FIGURE 128-3. Algorithm for evaluation of suspected renal colic. ESWL = extracorporeal shock wave lithotripsy.

fluids are routinely given in the hope that increased ureteral flow will increase the likelihood that the stone will pass, but hydration status has little, if any, impact on stone passage.[3] Maintenance intravenous fluid replacement, such as half-normal saline with dextrose at 50 to 75 mL/hour, is reasonable for patients who are not able to take fluids orally.

A patient who is able to tolerate oral analgesics does not require admission, but instructions should be given to return if fever or uncontrollable pain develops. A urologist should be involved if infection is suspected, if the patient has persistent or uncontrollable pain, if the stone is not passed within 1 week, if urinary extravasation is detected by imaging, if there is high-grade obstruction with a large stone, or if the patient has a solitary kidney or is pregnant. For distal ureteral stones, meta-analysis suggests that oral calcium-channel blockers (e.g., nifedipine, 30 mg slow-release daily) or α-blockers (e.g., tamsulosin, 0.4 mg daily) administered for up to 28 days can increase the rate of spontaneous stone passage by 65%.[4]

Surgical Therapy

Most urologists usually wait several days before intervening unless there is evidence of urinary tract infection, a low probability of spontaneous stone passage (e.g., stone >6 mm or an anatomic abnormality), or intractable pain. Relief of obstruction is critical. A ureteral stent may be placed cystoscopically, but general anesthesia is typically required. Although the stent can be quite uncomfortable and may cause gross hematuria, it may help with stone passage.

The approach to removing a stone is dictated by its size, location, and composition; urinary tract anatomy; availability of technology; and the experience of the urologist. The least invasive approach is extracorporeal shock wave lithotripsy (ESWL). The ESWL procedure uses shock waves that are generated outside the body and that are focused on the stone using fluoroscopy or ultrasound. The shock waves fragment the stone into smaller pieces that then can be passed more easily. The strength of the shock waves, which is determined by the model of lithotripter machine used, determines the type of anesthesia required. ESWL can be used in the acute setting for upper tract

stones,[5] but the success rate depends on the size, location, and composition of the stone. Cystoscopic stone removal, either by basket extraction or by laser fragmentation, is more invasive than ESWL but has a higher success rate, especially for ureteral stones, and is as good as ESWL for removing lower pole renal caliceal stones less than 1 cm in diameter.[6] Percutaneous nephrostolithotomy has the highest likelihood of making a patient stone free but is more invasive than cystoscopic methods. These endoscopic approaches have virtually eliminated the need for open surgical procedures such as ureterolithotomy or pyelolithotomy.

Asymptomatic Stones

With the increasing use of imaging, more incidental stones are being found. The best approach for asymptomatic renal stones is unsettled. Slightly less than 50% of individuals with radiologically documented asymptomatic stones will become symptomatic over a 5-year period. Most urologists would not consider removal of a stone that is 6 mm or smaller. For stones that are 10 mm or larger, many would recommend "prophylactic lithotripsy," but there are no data to support this approach.

Struvite Stones

Struvite stones require urologic intervention to ensure complete removal. The recommended approach is a combination of percutaneous nephrolithotomy and extracorporeal shock wave lithotripsy. Prolonged use of antibiotics alone may slow stone growth but rarely eradicates the infection. Although the medication acetohydroxamic acid inhibits bacterial urease, it is rarely used because of frequent and serious side effects.

PREVENTION

Evaluation after the First Stone

A complete history should include the pace and severity of all prior stone episodes as well as information regarding previous imaging studies (to

TABLE 128-2 LABORATORY EVALUATION

Spot urinalysis	Measure pH and examine the sediment for RBC, WBC, and crystals
24-Hour urine collection	Perform at least two at baseline; measure total volume, calcium, oxalate, citrate, uric acid, sodium, potassium, and creatinine If patient with cystine stones, also measure cystine
Blood	Electrolytes, calcium, phosphorus, BUN, creatinine If urine calcium or serum calcium is high, then measure PTH; if PTH is elevated, measure 25-hydroxyvitamin D to rule out secondary hyperparathyroidism If history of gout or considering use of a thiazide, measure serum uric acid If history of cystine stones, CBC and liver function tests should be performed before starting tiopronin

BUN = blood urea nitrogen; CBC = complete blood count; PTH = parathyroid hormone; RBC = red blood cells; WBC = white blood cells.

TABLE 128-3 DIETARY PRESCRIPTION FOR CALCIUM STONE PREVENTION ACCORDING TO URINARY RISK FACTOR

URINARY ABNORMALITY	DIETARY CHANGES
High calcium	Adequate dietary calcium intake Reduce nondairy animal protein intake (5-7 servings of meat, fish, or poultry/week) Reduce sodium intake to <2.4 g/day Reduce sucrose intake
High uric acid	Reduce purine intake
High oxalate	Avoid high-oxalate foods Avoid vitamin C supplements Adequate dietary calcium intake
Low citrate	Increase fruit and vegetable intake Reduce nondairy animal protein intake
Low volume	Increase total fluid intake to maintain urine volume to >2 L/day

Taylor EN, Curhan GC. Diet and fluid prescription in stone disease. *Kidney Int.* 2006;70:835-839.

distinguish stone passage events from actual new stone formation), surgical interventions, urinary tract infections, bowel disease or surgery, diarrhea or laxative abuse, family history of stone disease, and signs or symptoms suggestive of hyperparathyroidism (Chapter 253). In addition, information should be collected on dietary intake and the use of vitamins (e.g., C and D), minerals, and other supplements, as well as medications (e.g., carbonic anhydrase inhibitors, diuretics). The evaluation should also include appropriate clinical and laboratory evaluation to identify derangements and predict the likelihood of recurrence. Advice should be deferred until after the evaluation is complete; specifically, patients should be encouraged to resume their usual dietary habits while laboratory studies are completed.

Metabolic Evaluation

Every effort should be made to recover a stone that has passed or was removed, and its chemical composition should be analyzed by modern crystallographic methods. Even if the content of the stone is known, the metabolic evaluation for first-time and recurrent stone formers (Table 128-2) should include a serum chemistry profile and two 24-hour urine collections (because of substantial day-to-day variability).

Blood studies should include measurements of creatinine, calcium, phosphorus, albumin, uric acid, potassium, and total CO_2. Measurement of plasma parathyroid hormone level is recommended if serum or urine calcium levels are elevated.

The 24-hour urinary studies should be performed at least 6 weeks after the stone episode to ensure that patients have resumed their usual diet. The 24-hour measurements should include calcium, oxalate, uric acid, citrate, sodium, total volume, and creatinine. The urinary sediment should be examined for crystalluria in a freshly voided sample.

The 24-hour urine composition provides important prognostic information and directs recommendations for stone prevention. Traditionally, patients have been categorized into "normal" and "abnormal" with respect to the amount of lithogenic substances excreted. However, the measured values for the urinary factors are continuous variables, so dichotomization into normal and abnormal is somewhat artificial and potentially misleading. Second, stone formation is a disease of *concentration*, not just absolute amounts. Although a patient may have a normal amount of calcium in the urine over 24 hours, if the volume is low, the concentration of calcium would be abnormally high.

Patients with hypercalciuria can be divided into those with *absorptive* hypercalciuria (increased gastrointestinal calcium absorption), *resorptive* hypercalciuria (increased bone resorption), or *renal* hypercalciuria. However, a substantial proportion of patients do not fit into one category, an individual's classification may change over time, low bone mineral density may not be causally related to stone formation, and this classification approach rarely affects therapy.

All Stones
Dietary Modification

The observed increasing prevalence of nephrolithiasis and the physiologic impact of dietary factors have focused attention on the role of diet in stone formation (Table 128-3). In addition, the strong associations found in prospective studies of diet and initial stone formation (see earlier) suggest that dietary factors play an important role.

Fluid Intake

Stone formation is strongly influenced by urinary concentration, so the risk for stone formation decreases with increasing urine output. A general target is to encourage patients to drink enough fluid to produce more than 2 L of urine each day. The composition of the fluid ingested may be important, and observational studies suggest that higher intakes of coffee, tea, or alcoholic beverages are associated with a decreased risk for stone formation, perhaps because of the known diuretic action of these beverages.

Dietary Measures
Calcium Stones

The most controversial topic in dietary intervention for patients with nephrolithiasis is calcium intake. A low-calcium diet is often inappropriately recommended despite evidence that a low-calcium diet may in fact be *harmful* by increasing oxalate absorption from the intestine and also by leading to negative calcium balance and bone mineral loss. For example, in a randomized trial in men with hypercalciuria and recurrent calcium oxalate stones, a diet containing 1200 mg of calcium with a low intake of sodium and animal protein significantly reduced subsequent stone formation compared with a low-calcium diet (400 mg day).[7] The protective role for adequate dietary calcium intake does not extend to calcium from supplements, which either have no effect or slightly increase the risk of stone formation, and a very high calcium intake (>2 to 3 g/day) should be discouraged. Although the bioavailability of calcium is the same in dairy and calcium supplements, it is possible that dairy products, the major source of dietary calcium, contain some unidentified protective factor.

Other Dietary Factors

Restriction of nondairy animal protein (e.g., meat, chicken, seafood) is a reasonable option and may result in higher excretion of citrate and lower excretion of uric acid and calcium. For patients with high oxalate excretion, restriction of dietary oxalate may be beneficial. Reliable and complete data on the oxalate content of many commonly consumed foods are now available (*https://regepi.bwh.harvard.edu/health/Oxalate/files*). Spinach should be avoided because it is the highest oxalate-containing food. Reducing sodium intake to less than 3 g/day may decrease the obligatory, concurrent urinary excretion of calcium and may be particularly important for patients prescribed a thiazide. Sucrose intake, which may increase urinary calcium excretion, should be minimized. In contrast, potassium-rich foods should be encouraged. Dietary recommendations should be tailored to the patient's urinary chemistry profile, and the impact of the recommendations can be monitored by repeating the urine collections.

Uric Acid Stones

The mainstay of treatment to prevent uric acid stones is increasing urine pH by dietary modification, which should focus on decreasing acid production by reducing the intake of animal flesh and increasing the intake of alkali-rich foods, specifically fruits and vegetables. If dietary modification is unsuccessful, alkalinization with oral bicarbonate, typically requiring 20 to 30 mEq three times per day, or a bicarbonate precursor (e.g., potassium citrate, 20 to 30 mEq three times per day) should be started. The pH goal is 6 to 7 throughout the day and night. Alkali three or four times a day is typically needed to match the endogenous acid production of approximately 1 mEq/kg per 24 hours. However, a urine pH greater than 7 should be avoided to minimize the likelihood of inducing calcium phosphate crystallization. Allopurinol (100 to 300 mg/day) should be prescribed for patients in whom alkalinization fails.

Cystine Stones

The total amount of cystine excreted cannot be easily modified, so treatment is directed at decreasing the urinary cystine concentration below the limit of solubility. Increasing urinary volume is the first approach, but some patients would need more than 4 L of urine per day, which is impractical. Increasing urine pH above 7.5 using oral alkali, such as 20 to 30 mEq of potassium citrate twice daily, will slightly increase cystine solubility, but this pH is often difficult to maintain in the long term. Tiopronin, typically 300 mg orally three times per day, will bind cystine and reduce urine supersaturation. Although side effects are common, tiopronin is first-line therapy in patients with recurrent cystine stone formation because there are no other alternatives.

Medical Prevention

Although nephrolithiasis is a common disease, surprisingly few well-designed prospective double-blind controlled trials have been conducted. Some medications may improve the urinary chemistry profile but not cure the underlying abnormality. Thus, the decision to start medication requires consideration of efficacy, side effects, cost, and adherence of the patient. Certainly, if new stone formation occurs despite dietary recommendations, medication should be prescribed. If urine calcium levels are elevated, a thiazide diuretic is recommended. For patients with hypocitraturia or hyperuricosuria as a sole finding, potassium citrate and allopurinol can be used, respectively. Unfortunately, the optimal duration of treatment is unclear, and long-term adherence remains suboptimal.

Thiazides

Thiazide diuretics, such as hydrochlorothiazide and chlorthalidone, increase calcium reabsorption in the proximal convoluted tubule and distal tubule and effectively lower urinary calcium excretion by 20 to 50%. In some patients, urine calcium levels may rise after a year despite continued therapy. Thiazides can also increase the mineral content of bone. About 30 years ago, two trials showed that thiazides reduced the risk of recurrent calcium oxalate stones in otherwise unclassified patients. The doses required for urinary calcium reduction (25 to 100 mg/day) are higher than those needed for treating hypertension. Side effects are reported in 8 to 35% of patients. Thiazide-induced hypokalemia can be treated with potassium citrate (20 mEq per day) or amiloride (2.5 to 5.0 mg per day). Because of its potential to precipitate in the urine, triamterene should be avoided in these patients. Indapamide (2.5 mg per day), although not strictly a thiazide, will also reduce urine calcium. Monitoring the urine calcium response with subsequent dosage adjustment is recommended.

Allopurinol

Allopurinol (300 mg per day) can reduce urine uric acid excretion by up to 50%, and it was shown 25 years ago to reduce stone recurrence in individuals with hyperuricosuric calcium oxalate stone disease. In patients without hyperuricosuria, allopurinol has no benefit when compared with placebo.

Potassium Citrate

Systemic alkalinization of the urine with bicarbonate (typically 30 mEq twice daily) or citrate (typically 30 mEq twice daily) will lead to an increase in urinary citrate excretion. The most commonly used salt is potassium citrate, which avoids the calciuric effect of a sodium load and restores any potassium deficiency. Citrate supplementation reduces recurrent calcium oxalate stones compared with placebo, but adherence to prescribed dosing is suboptimal.[8]

Magnesium

Oral magnesium from supplements may reduce stone risk by forming soluble complexes with oxalate in the bowel or urine. However, in a 3-year double-blind trial, magnesium was no more effective than placebo. Thus, the role of magnesium supplementation remains uncertain.

Other Genitourinary Stones

Stones can form in other parts of the genitourinary tract, including the bladder and rarely the prostate. In the United States, the most common type of bladder stone is uric acid. Bladder stones are much more common in men because the primary risk factors are urinary stasis owing to bladder outlet obstruction and a persistently low urine pH. As with uric acid stones that form in the kidney, hyperuricosuria is not always present, but the low urine pH dramatically reduces the solubility of uric acid in the urine. Patients with bladder stones often pass stones frequently, sometimes on a daily basis. The stones can range in size from "sand" or "gravel" to several centimeters. Stones of sufficient size are characteristically round because of the rolling that can occur in the bladder. Bladder stones do not cause renal colic but can cause partial or complete acute urinary retention by obstructing the urethra. The rate of stone formation can be dramatically reduced or even halted by improving urine flow by medications or surgery (Chapter 131) or through alkalinization of the urine. Potassium citrate, typically 20 to 30 mEq three times daily, is sufficient to stop stone formation.

Grade A

1. Lindqvist K, Hellstrom M, Holmberg G, et al. Immediate versus deferred radiological investigation after acute renal colic: a prospective randomized study. *Scand J Urol Nephrol*. 2006;40:119-124.
2. Holdgate A, Pollock T. Systematic review of the relative efficacy of non-steroidal anti-inflammatory drugs and opioids in the treatment of acute renal colic. *BMJ*. 2004;328:1401.
3. Springhart WP, Marguet CG, Sur RL, et al. Forced versus minimal intravenous hydration in the management of acute renal colic: a randomized trial. *J Endourol*. 2006;20:713-716.
4. Hollingsworth JM, Rogers MAM, Kaufman SR, et al. Medical therapy to facilitate urinary stone passage: a meta-analysis. *Lancet*. 2006;368:1171-1179.
5. Kravchick S, Bunkin I, Stepnov E, et al. Emergency extracorporeal shockwave lithotripsy for acute renal colic caused by upper urinary-tract stones. *J Endourol*. 2005;19:1-4.
6. Pearle MS, Lingeman JE, Leveillee R, et al. Prospective, randomized trial comparing shock wave lithotripsy and ureteroscopy for lower pole caliceal calculi 1 cm or less. *J Urol*. 2005;173:2005-2009.
7. Borghi L, Schianchi T, Meschi T, et al. Comparison of two diets for the prevention of recurrent stones in idiopathic hypercalciuria. *N Engl J Med*. 2002;346:77-84.
8. Ettinger B, Pak CY, Citron JT, et al. Potassium-magnesium citrate is an effective prophylaxis against recurrent calcium oxalate nephrolithiasis. *J Urol*. 1997;158:2069-2073.

SUGGESTED READINGS

Kenny JE, Goldfarb DS. Update on the pathophysiology and management of uric acid renal stones. *Curr Rheumatol Rep*. 2010;12:125-129. *Review*.
Moe OW, Pearle MS, Sakhaee K. Pharmacotherapy of urolithiasis: evidence from clinical trials. *Kidney Int*. 2011;79:385-392. *Comprehensive review*.
Worcester EM, Coe FL. Calcium kidney stones. *N Engl J Med*. 2010;363:954-963. *Clinical review*.

129

CYSTIC KIDNEY DISEASES

M. AMIN ARNAOUT

DEFINITION AND EPIDEMIOLOGY

The term *cystic kidney diseases* refers to a heterogeneous group of hereditary and acquired disorders characterized by the presence of unilateral or bilateral renal cysts. When acquired singly or in small numbers and in the absence of any other pathology, renal cysts are termed *simple cysts*, which are present in approximately 50% of individuals older than 40 years, are usually not loculated, and tend to bulge out from the renal surface (Fig. 129-1). The *polycystic kidney diseases* (PKDs), by comparison, constitute a clinically important group of genetically mediated disorders characterized by prominent, expanding, bilateral renal cysts. PKDs are classified as dominant, recessive, or X-linked, based on their pattern of inheritance. Autosomal dominant PKD (ADPKD), with a prevalence rate between 1:400 and 1:1000, is the most common monogenic disease in humans and accounts for about 10% of all end-stage renal disease (ESRD) in the United States. ADPKD develops in an age-dependent manner and affects mainly adults. Autosomal recessive PKD (ARPKD), by contrast, is a relatively rare childhood disorder that appears in 1 in every 6000 to 50,000 live births. Renal cysts are also seen in several other rare hereditary kidney diseases and in several syndromic PKDs (Table 129-1). Collectively, the hereditary PKDs generally affect both genders and all races equally and cost more than $1 billion annually to manage in the

FIGURE 129-1. **Gross pathology of selected cystic kidney diseases. A,** Photograph of a kidney with multiple simple cysts. The cysts bulge out from the surface of a normal-sized kidney. **B,** Sagittal cross section of a kidney from an adult with autosomal dominant polycystic kidney disease (ADPKD). Multiple macroscopic cysts have resulted in an enlarged but still reniform kidney (note the evidence of prior hemorrhage within some of the cysts). **C,** Sagittal cross section of a kidney segment from a neonate with autosomal recessive polycystic kidney disease (ARPKD). The kidney is enlarged, with numerous small cysts. (Courtesy Dr. Robert Colvin, Massachusetts General Hospital.)

United States alone. *Acquired cystic kidney disease* refers to the multiple bilateral renal cysts that develop in patients who already have kidney disease. Cysts occur in 90% of patients who have been receiving renal replacement therapy for 8 years or longer and are associated with increased rates of renal cell carcinoma.

AUTOSOMAL DOMINANT POLYCYSTIC KIDNEY DISEASE

PATHOBIOLOGY

ADPKD is a systemic disorder characterized by cyst formation in multiple organs, including the kidneys, other ductal organs, and the cardiovascular system. Renal cysts originate as outpouchings of tubules and may affect any portion of the nephron, with up to 1% of nephrons involved. The outpouchings expand and eventually separate from the parent tubules, yielding cysts (Fig. 129-2). Expansion of cysts is caused by proliferation of the cyst lining cells, by chloride-driven fluid secretion that outpaces absorption, and by remodeling of the extracellular matrix. The kidneys become massively enlarged.

Genetics

Heterogeneous mutations in two genes, *PKD1* and *PKD2,* cause ADPKD. Mutations in *PKD1* account for approximately 85% of cases of ADPKD. Heterogeneous mutations in *PKD2* contribute an additional 10 to 15% of cases. The onset and severity of the disease are dramatically affected by the developmental stage at which gene inactivation occurs. In a minority of ADPKD cases, no demonstrable *PKD1* or *PKD2* mutations are found, suggesting that a third gene may be involved.

PKD1 is 54 kb long and is located on chromosome 16p13.3, adjacent to the tuberous sclerosis 2 (*TSC2*) gene. *PKD1* has 46 exons, generates a 14-kb transcript, and encodes a 4302- residue protein called polycystin-1, the first described member of an expanding group of polycystins. The 5′ region of human *PKD1* (to exon 33) is replicated on the same chromosome, resulting in approximately six copies of *PKD1*-like pseudogenes, which must be distinguished from the *PKD1* gene in direct mutational analysis. To date, more than 330 truncating mutations have been identified throughout the gene, but especially in the 3′ half. Mutations in the 5′ half of the gene are associated with more severe disease, with only 19% of patients retaining adequate renal function at 60 years of age (vs. 40% of those with 3′ mutations), and they are more likely to be associated with intracerebral aneurysms and aneurysm rupture.

The 68-kb *PKD2* gene is located on chromosome 4q13-23, transcribes 15 exons, and generates a 5-kb transcript, which encodes a protein of 968 residues called polycystin-2. Ninety-five heterogeneous mutations in *PKD2* have been identified to date.

Large intrafamilial variability in the onset and severity of ADPKD may be caused by bilineal inheritance of *PKD1* and *PKD2* mutant alleles or of hypomorphic variants of either gene. Mosaicism in a parent in whom a mutation has arisen de novo could result in one sibling having the disease while another is disease free, despite sharing the identical inherited haplotype at the *PKD* gene. Concomitant mutations affecting other genes can also result in ADPKD in infancy. Because cysts appear from a small number of nephrons, somatic inactivation of the normal allele has been proposed as the main mechanism of disease. *PKD1* or *PKD2* haplo-insufficiency and gene dose effects are associated with a high frequency of genomic instability, which likely increases the incidence of somatic second hits in ADPKD. Genomic instability may also explain the increased rate of apoptosis and the low incidence of renal cell carcinoma in this disease.

PATHOGENESIS

Polycystin-1 comprises a large extracellular modular ectodomain, followed by an 11-pass transmembrane segment and a short cytoplasmic carboxyl terminus (E-Fig. 129-1). The polycystin-1 ectodomain contains multiple functional motifs, suggesting a role in cell-cell and/or cell-matrix adhesion. Polycystin-2 is a six-membrane spanner that acts as a nonselective voltage-dependent, calcium-permeable ion channel with cytoplasmic amino and carboxyl termini. Its six-transmembrane segment bears a topologic and sequence similarity to the carboxyl terminal six-transmembrane segment of polycystin-1. The coiled-coil domains within the carboxyl termini of polycystin-1 and polycystin-2 interact to stabilize the channel activity of polycystin-2 and facilitate its translocation to the plasma membrane. In addition, polycystin-1 interacts with intermediate filaments, E-cadherin, focal adhesion proteins, β-catenin, and tuberin. Polycystin-1 and polycystin-2 also interact with a number of other proteins, and each of these interactions could serve as a modifier of the polycystins' functions.

Polycystin-1 and polycystin-2 are widely expressed in tissues, with some overlap consistent with their direct interaction. Polycystin-1 is found at multiple membrane sites, including adherens junctions, desmosomes and focal adhesions, primary cilia, and intracellular vesicles. Polycystin-2 is found in primary cilia as well as the basolateral membrane, endoplasmic reticulum, centrosome, and mitotic spindles in dividing cells. Both polycystin-1 and polycystin-2 are also found in urinary vesicles. Levels of polycystin-1 expression are highest in fetal tissue and progressively decline thereafter, whereas polycystin-2 levels are maintained throughout development.

Cyst Formation

Both polycystin-1 and polycystin-2 localize to primary cilia, which are found on the apical surface of all renal cells except intercalated cells. The primary cilium consists of an axoneme comprising nine microtubular doublets surrounded by a cell membrane. It is assembled during the interphase from the mother centriole (basal body), which serves as a microtubule-organizing center just beneath the plasma membrane. Transition fibers associated with the basal body regulate protein entry and exit into the cilium. Because cell division requires both centrioles to form the mitotic spindle, the cell is unable to divide until its cilium is resorbed, linking the structural integrity of the cilium to cell cycle regulation. A mechanosensitive cilium is normally deflected by the tubular flow of urine, thereby activating polycystin-1– and polycystin-2–mediated calcium influx, which is amplified by calcium released from internal stores. How this process translates into regulation of tube diameter (cyst formation) is still unclear. It is proposed that calcium influx through normal primary cilia favors the noncanonical Wnt pathway (also known as planar cell polarity) over the mitogenic canonical (β-catenin–dependent) Wnt pathway, thereby maintaining cell polarity and suppressing proliferation. Planar cell polarity couples polarized cell movement and cell division for proper control of tube diameter size during tube elongation. Loss of polycystin-1 or polycystin-2 disrupts this structural link, causing cysts.

Regulation of calcium influx by polycystin-1 and polycystin-2 may not be restricted to the cilium. For example, polycystin signaling also activates the JAK/STAT pathway. Polycystin-1– and polycystin-2–mediated calcium influx suppresses intracellular cyclic adenosine monophosphate (cAMP) signaling by inhibiting adenylyl cyclase and stimulating cAMP phosphodiesterase (E-Fig. 129-2). Loss of the polycystin-1 and polycystin-2 calcium signal may lead to a buildup of cAMP, promoting cell proliferation.

TABLE 129-1 COMPARISON OF CLINICAL FEATURES OF CYSTIC KIDNEY DISEASES

DISEASE	INHERITANCE	FREQUENCY	GENE PRODUCT	AGE OF ONSET	CYST ORIGIN	RENOMEGALY	CAUSE OF ESRD	OTHER MANIFESTATIONS
ADPKD	AD	1:400–1000	Polycystin-1 Polycystin-2	20s and 30s	Anywhere (including Bowman's capsule)	Yes	Yes	Liver cysts Cerebral aneurysms Hypertension Mitral valve prolapse Kidney stones UTIs
ARPKD	AR	1:6000–10,000	Fibrocystin/ polyductin	First year of life	Distal nephron, CD	Yes	Yes	Hepatic fibrosis Pulmonary hypoplasia Hypertension
ACKD	No	90% of ESRD patients at 8 yr	None*	Years after onset of ESRD	Proximal and distal tubules	Rarely	No	None
Simple cysts	No	50% in those older than 40 yr	None*	Adulthood	Anywhere (usually cortical)	No	No	None
Nephronophthisis	AR	1:80,000	Nephrocystins (NPHP1–9)	Childhood or adolescence	Medullary DCT	No	Yes	Retinal degeneration; neurologic, skeletal, hepatic, cardiac malformations
MCKD	AD	Rare	Uromodulin, others	Adulthood	Medullary DCT	No	Yes	Hyperuricemia, gout
MSK	No	1:5000–20,000	None*	30s	Medullary CD	No	No	Kidney stones Hypercalciuria
Tuberous sclerosis	AD	1:10,000	Hamartin (TSC1), tuberin (TSC2)	Childhood	Loop of Henle, DCT	Rarely	Rarely	Renal cell carcinoma Tubers, seizures Angiomyolipoma Hypertension
VHL syndrome	AD	1:40,000	VHL protein	20s	Cortical nephrons	Rarely	Rarely	Retinal angioma, CNS hemangioblastoma, renal cell carcinoma, pheochromocytoma
Oral-facial-digital syndrome-1	XD	1:250,000	OFD1 protein	Childhood or adulthood	Renal glomeruli	Rarely	Yes	Malformation of the face, oral cavity, and digits; liver cysts; mental retardation
Bardet-Biedl syndrome	AR	1:65,000–160,000	BBS 1-14	Adulthood	Renal calyces	Rarely	Yes	Syn- and polydactyly, obesity, retinal dystrophy, male hypogenitalism, hypertension, mental retardation

*No known genetic susceptibility.
ACKD = acquired cystic kidney disease; AD = autosomal dominant; ADPKD = autosomal dominant polycystic kidney disease; AR = autosomal recessive; ARPKD = autosomal recessive polycystic kidney disease; CD = collecting duct; CNS = central nervous system; DCT = distal convoluted tubule; ESRD = end-stage renal disease; MCKD = medullary cystic kidney disease; MSK = medullary sponge kidney; UTI = urinary tract infection; VHL = von Hippel-Lindau; XD = X-linked dominant.

CLINICAL MANIFESTATIONS

ADPKD has a highly variable presentation, even within families. The clinical features of *PKD2*-associated ADPKD are indistinguishable from those of *PKD1*-associated disease. However, *PKD2* disease is milder, with an older average age of onset—74 years versus about 54 years for *PKD1*-associated disease—owing to the development of fewer cysts at an early age rather than to a slower cyst growth rate.

Despite an estimated 100% penetrance by age 90 years, only half the individuals with heterozygous mutations in *PKD1* or *PKD2* are ever diagnosed clinically with ADPKD. Of these patients, the majority present in the third or fourth decade of life with symptoms referable to renal cystic disease. However, ADPKD can develop at any age, including infancy, and it can have a nonrenal presentation. Renomegaly may predominate the clinical picture, with abdominal distention, discomfort, or pain; however, renomegaly can also be discovered incidentally on physical examination or after radiographic studies of the abdomen.

Nocturia, which is one of the earliest signs of abnormal renal function in ADPKD, reflects the early impairment in urinary concentration. The urinary pH is typically low, with hypocitric aciduria. Hematuria is typical, but proteinuria is less prominent than in many other renal diseases. Anemia features less prominently than in other renal diseases, probably because of the relatively well-preserved erythropoietin secretion. Recurrent cyst infection, usually by common urinary tract–infecting organisms, is characterized by flank or abdominal pain, fever, rigors, leukocytosis, and occasionally sepsis. Cyst hemorrhage and sometimes rupture, which can occur spontaneously or after trauma, present as sharp pain and hematuria.

Arterial hypertension is present in approximately 70% of cases before renal dysfunction is detected. Enhanced vascular smooth muscle contractility, reduced endothelial-dependent vasorelaxation, lower constitutive nitric oxide synthase activity, activation of the intrarenal renin-angiotensin system, and increased sympathetic nerve activity are likely causes of the accompanying arterial hypertension. Development of hypertension at a young age is associated with a four-fold increased risk of ESRD and increased cardiovascular morbidity. The risk for preeclampsia is also higher than in the general population.

An estimated 4 to 15% of individuals with ADPKD develop saccular cerebral aneurysms (Chapter 415), a prevalence rate that is 4 to 10 times greater than in the general population. These aneurysms tend to segregate in families, making ADPKD one of a group of diseases characterized by autosomal dominant inheritance of cerebral aneurysms. ADPKD-associated aneurysms tend to rupture at a smaller size and in younger individuals—on average, 10 years younger than among the general population. Although usually clinically silent, intact cerebral aneurysms can present with focal neurologic symptoms and headaches. By contrast, aneurysms that rupture lead to subarachnoid hemorrhage (Chapter 415) and have dramatic presentations that include severe headaches, seizures, altered sensorium, and death. Aortic and coronary

FIGURE 129-2. **A** to **D**, Steps involved in cyst formation in autosomal dominant polycystic kidney disease. Note that this process occurs hundreds or thousands of times during the natural history of the disease. ECM = extracellular matrix.

A, Initially normal nephron

B, Focal hyperproliferation and apoptosis / Alterations in ECM

C, Secretion into lumen with cyst expansion

D, Interstitial fibrosis / Obliteration of nephrons

FIGURE 129-3. **A**, Ultrasound images of a kidney from a patient with autosomal dominant polycystic kidney disease. **B**, Ultrasound images of a kidney from a patient with autosomal recessive polycystic kidney disease. (Courtesy Dr. Javier M. Romero and Jennifer A. McDowell, Massachusetts General Hospital.)

artery aneurysms are also more prevalent in patients with ADPKD, and the frequency of aortic insufficiency is increased.

Although almost never severe enough to cause end-stage liver disease, age-dependent hepatic cysts occur in 30 to 80% of patients with ADPKD and can lead to signs and symptoms of mass effect, infection, hemorrhage, and rupture. Estrogen intake and multiparity in women are risk factors in developing larger and more symptomatic cysts. The cysts that occasionally form in other organs, such as the pancreas, spleen, brain, ovaries, epididymis, and prostate, are usually asymptomatic. Sperm abnormalities and defective motility may occur but rarely cause male infertility. Bronchiectasis (Chapter 90) is three-fold more common, inguinal hernias may be more prevalent, and colonic diverticulosis and diverticulitis are more common in ESRD patients with ADPKD.

DIAGNOSIS

The specific diagnosis of ADPKD requires a consideration of associated extrarenal manifestations, age at presentation, and family history. Because only about 60% of individuals give a family history of PKD, ultrasound screening of asymptomatic parents or grandparents may be required to uncover diagnostically relevant silent PKD. To account for the common age-dependent appearance of simple cysts, ADPKD is diagnosed if at least three renal cysts (distributed in one or both kidneys) are present in individuals 15 to 39 years old, if at least two renal cysts are present in each kidney in individuals aged 40 to 59 years, or if at least four renal cysts are present in each kidney in individuals 60 years and older (Fig. 129-3A). Fewer than two renal cysts in an individual aged 40 years or older from an ADPKD family with an unknown genotype, or the absence of renal cysts in such an individual aged 30 to 39 years, is sufficient to exclude the disease, with negative predictive values of 100 and 99.3%, respectively. A negative ultrasound is less accurate in excluding disease in individuals younger than 30 years, so computed tomography (CT) or magnetic resonance imaging (MRI) is recommended. When a young relative is being considered as a potential kidney donor to a family member with end-stage ADPKD, contrast-enhanced, three-dimensional CT or magnetic resonance angiography (MRA) is required because these tests can detect 3-mm cysts, compared with ultrasound's ability to detect 10-mm cysts.

DNA-based diagnosis of ADPKD by means of direct sequencing is commercially available and detects mutations in more than 90% of affected individuals. Such testing is expensive, however, and the marked allelic heterogeneity of the *PKD1* and *PKD2* mutations, as well as the paucity of phenotype-genotype correlations, contributes to the complexity of DNA-based diagnostics. Testing is recommended when imaging studies are equivocal, in a young transplant donor from an ADPKD family when imaging studies are negative, or to facilitate preimplantation genetic diagnosis.

Monitoring Disease Progression

Despite ongoing renal cyst expansion, the glomerular filtration rate (GFR) and the serum creatinine level are generally maintained within the normal range in ADPKD patients until the fourth to sixth decade of life. As a result, these markers are insensitive for monitoring disease progression, especially in the young. Estimating kidney volume from measurements of kidney length, width, and thickness using MRI, CT, or ultrasonography can reliably monitor disease progression in the early stages of ADPKD, when the GFR is still in the normal range. Although gadolinium-enhanced MRI provides excellent detail of kidney structures, MRI without gadolinium is recommended to monitor kidney volume, especially in ADPKD patients with a reduced GFR, because of concern about nephrogenic systemic fibrosis (Chapter 275) and further impairment of renal function associated with its use. The combined kidney volume in ADPKD patients progressively increases in most cases, but at widely differing rates, ranging from less than 1% to more than 10%. Combined kidney volumes greater than 1500 mL are frequently associated with a decreased GFR and gross hematuria and invariably with arterial hypertension.

PREVENTION AND TREATMENT   Rx

Management strategies are aimed at monitoring for complications of ADPKD and treating them, as well as providing counseling. Frequent blood pressure monitoring is recommended because hypertension accelerates the decline in renal function. The goals of blood pressure control are the same as for other patients with renal disease, including the attainment of a symptom-free blood pressure of 125/75 mm Hg or less. Although all available antihypertensive agents have been used with roughly equivalent success, theoretical considerations and preliminary data suggest that angiotensin-converting enzyme (ACE) inhibitors or angiotensin receptor blockers (ARBs) combined with salt restriction may be more efficient in slowing the rate of progression to ESRD (see Tables 67-5 and 67-7 in Chapter 67). If these drugs fail to lower blood pressure sufficiently owing to the associated plasma volume expansion, thiazides or loop diuretics may be added (see Table 67-5 in Chapter 67).

Treatment of urinary tract infection (Chapter 292) and prevention of nephrolithiasis (Chapter 128) are the same as in the general population and include standard antimicrobial therapy and increased fluid intake, respectively. Renal or hepatic cyst infections are optimally treated with lipophilic antibiotics that possess cyst-penetrating capabilities, including ciprofloxacin, trimethoprim, clindamycin, and vancomycin. Blood or urine cultures and sensitivities are used to guide the choice of antibiotic therapy.

Cyst hemorrhage and rupture, with resultant pain and hematuria, are usually managed conservatively with rest and analgesics; nonsteroidal anti-inflammatory drugs (NSAIDs) are avoided, owing to their antiplatelet action and potential renal toxicity. Alternatives include acetaminophen 500 mg up to every 4 hours for mild to moderate pain, nonopiates such as tramadol 50 mg up to every 4 hours for moderate to severe pain, and the addition of an oral or transdermal opioid (see Table 29-4 in Chapter 29) as needed. Patients with enlarged kidneys should be advised to avoid playing contact sports, and those with massively enlarged kidneys should refrain from wearing belts and seatbelts. Some patients with unusually painful cysts respond to cyst fluid aspiration, cyst deroofing, or ethanol-induced sclerosis.

Nephrectomy is rarely indicated before the onset of ESRD. Renal replacement therapies, including renal transplantation (Chapter 133), are at least as effective as in other causes of ESRD.

The massive cystic enlargement of the liver commonly seen by midlife in women with ADPKD makes it prudent to avoid estrogen intake and repeated pregnancies. Partial hepatectomy has been successful in improving the quality of life in patients with massive liver enlargement.

Screening MRA is not routinely recommended for asymptomatic patients without a family history of cerebral aneurysm or subarachnoid hemorrhage, but it is recommended for patients with a positive family history and may be considered in those with high-risk occupations, such as airline pilots, or with incapacitating anxiety. The risk of a patient with a positive family history developing a new aneurysm after an initially negative magnetic resonance angiogram is 2.6% at a mean follow-up of 9.8 years, so rescreening every 5 to 10 years in such cases may be appropriate, especially in patients with early-onset hypertension or a history of heavy smoking. Individuals shown to have cerebral aneurysms should be referred to a neurosurgeon for consideration of clipping (Chapter 415). Annual MRA screening is recommended in all patients with untreated aneurysms to assess for aneurysmal growth.

Patients should be advised that their children have a 50% probability of inheriting a disease-causing germline mutation. DNA-based diagnostics are most useful in identifying the germline mutation prenatally or preimplantation. As DNA-based diagnostics become more widely available and less expensive, and as promising new treatment options are developed, counseling will become an increasingly important component of prevention.

Experimental Therapies

The better understanding of the pathobiology of ADPKD raises the hope of directed therapies to halt or slow the progression of disease. The metabolically stable somatostatin analogue octreotide (at a dose of 40 mg intravenously every 28 days) halted the expansion of renal cysts but did not have a beneficial effect on the GFR in a small trial of ADPKD patients.[1] Neither sirolimus[2] nor everolimus[3] slowed the decline of renal function in ADPKD patients, although everolimus slowed the increase in kidney volume. These data suggest that cyst growth may not be the key determinant of renal function decline. ACE inhibitors and ARBs are currently being tested in large clinical trials, and the vasopressin V2 receptor inhibitor tolvaptan is being evaluated in phase III clinical trials.

PROGNOSIS

The rate of progression of renal disease is highest in men with poorly controlled hypertension, an early age at diagnosis, and mutations in *PKD1*. The presence of one affected family member who developed ESRD by age 60 years is highly predictive of PKD1 disease (positive predictive value, 100%; sensitivity, 75%), whereas the development of ESRD after age 70 years in a family member is highly predictive of PKD2 disease (positive predictive value, 95%; sensitivity, 75%). Approximately 5% of all ADPKD patients with cerebral aneurysms die from aneurysmal rupture.

AUTOSOMAL RECESSIVE POLYCYSTIC KIDNEY DISEASE

DEFINITION AND EPIDEMIOLOGY

ARPKD is a multisystem childhood disorder characterized by severe and early PKD dominated by dilation of the kidney collecting ducts, biliary ductal plate dysgenesis in neonates, and portal tract fibrosis in older children.

PATHOBIOLOGY

ARPKD has been linked to heterogeneous mutations in a single gene, *PKHD1* (polycystic kidney and hepatic disease 1). Located on chromosome 6q21, *PKHD1* has 67 exons and spans a genomic region of approximately 470 kb, the longest open reading frame of which is 12,222 base pairs long. *PKHD1* encodes a unique type I membrane protein, fibrocystin/polyductin, comprising 4074 amino acids, with a large extracellular segment and a short cytoplasmic carboxyl terminus. The precise physiologic function of fibrocystin/polyductin in collecting duct and biliary duct epithelium is not clear, but its domains are known to mediate cell motility and invasion, extracellular protein and carbohydrate binding, and catalysis of polysaccharide hydrolysis. Alternatively-spliced transcripts of *PKHD1* encode a membrane protein with variable extracellular domains, as well as forms lacking the transmembrane segment. Homozygous truncating mutations in *PKHD1* are associated with perinatal renal disease, whereas patients with homozygous missense mutations present later because some functional protein is produced.

PKHD1 messenger RNA is detected mostly in the cortical and medullary collecting ducts and the thick ascending limbs of Henle, but it is also found to a lesser degree in the pancreas, liver, and lungs, which are also affected in ARPKD. In common with many cystogenic proteins, the fibrocystin/polyductin protein is found in basal bodies and primary apical cilia, suggesting that it is important in maintaining the structural integrity of cilia.

Loss of the fibrocystin/polyductin protein downregulates polycystin-2, which is the deficient protein in one form of ADPKD. Fibrocystin/polyductin–polycystin-2 interactions may regulate calcium influx mediated by polycystin-2. These findings suggest that cystogenesis in ADPKD and ARPKD share a common mechanism, with the variability in the ARPKD phenotype traced to the degree of polycystin-2 expression among patients. However, renal cysts can originate from any part of the nephron and are detached from the nephron proper in ADPKD, whereas they originate from and remain attached to the distal nephron in ARPKD, suggesting that additional signaling pathways specific for each disease and gene product likely explain these anatomic differences.

CLINICAL MANIFESTATIONS

Although ARPKD can present as renal cysts discovered radiographically either antenatally or during adulthood, it usually manifests as bilateral abdominal masses and renal insufficiency in infancy. It carries a 30% mortality owing to severe pulmonary hypoplasia; oligohydramnios, presumably linked to in utero renal disease, likely accounts for the pulmonary hypoplasia. Hypertension is almost universal, typically develops before renal impairment is apparent, and probably accelerates the decline in renal function. Findings related to renal tubular dysfunction may be present and include polyuria, enuresis, hyponatremia, and hyperchloremic metabolic acidosis. Cystic complications related to infection and rupture also occur, although hematuria is an infrequent finding. ESRD can take up to 20 years to develop, and in rare instances, it never occurs.

Hepatic fibrosis, secondary to dilation of the intrahepatic and extrahepatic bile ducts, manifests as recurrent ascending cholangitis (Chapter 158) and portal hypertension with splenomegaly and esophageal varices. Pancreatic fibrosis is rarely a clinical concern.

DIAGNOSIS

The demonstration by abdominal ultrasound (Fig. 129-3B) or CT of symmetrically enlarged polycystic kidneys that retain their reniform shape (owing to uniform microcystic dilation of collecting ducts) and hepatic fibrosis is sufficient to diagnose ARPKD. In contrast to ADPKD cysts, ARPKD cysts tend to retain their connections with the originating nephron. Aside from an occasional affected sibling, a family history is often not elicited. Distinguishing ARPKD from ADPKD, especially in patients presenting in childhood or adulthood, may require a liver biopsy to document otherwise undetectable hepatic fibrosis. Gene-based diagnostics in ARPKD are helpful in making a firm diagnosis, especially in patients with late-onset disease, and they are useful in preimplantation and in prenatal diagnosis.

PREVENTION AND TREATMENT Rx

In the absence of specific therapy for ARPKD, management goals focus on early detection and treatment of the complications of hypertension, urinary tract or cyst infection, ESRD, and portal hypertension. Kidney transplantation may be necessary in late childhood in ARPKD patients who present with renal disease perinatally. Treatment of portal hypertension may require liver transplantation or portosystemic shunting (Chapter 157). Treatment of hypertension begins with ACE inhibitors and ARBs (see Tables 67-5 and 67-7 in Chapter 67), which are generally effective. As in all children with ESRD, attention to nutrition and renal osteodystrophy is paramount (Chapter 132). With improving sensitivity of gene-based diagnostics, genetic counseling will play a more active role in prevention.

PROGNOSIS

For patients with ARPKD, the highest mortality rates occur during the first year of life. Approximately 50 to 80% of patients survive to 15 years of age.

● NEPHRONOPHTHISIS

DEFINITION AND EPIDEMIOLOGY

The autosomal recessive disorder nephronophthisis is characterized pathologically by renal interstitial fibrosis, tubular atrophy with basement membrane thickening and disruption, and renal cysts and diverticula that are largely restricted to the loops of Henle and distal tubules at the corticomedullary junctions. Nephronophthisis is the most common genetic cause of ESRD in childhood and adolescence, accounting for 5 to 15% of cases. Kidney size is generally normal or reduced, except in the rare infantile form of nephronophthisis that leads to ESRD by 5 years of age.

Patients exhibit extrarenal anomalies, with missense mutations causing a milder phenotype and truncating mutations causing severe disease. The most frequently associated extrarenal abnormalities are retinal degeneration secondary to photoreceptor cell defects (Senior-Loken syndrome), seen in 15% of cases; cerebellar ataxia (Joubert's syndrome and related diseases), observed in 10 to 15% of cases; and hepatic fibrosis (Boichis disease), seen in 5% of cases.

The clinical syndrome of nephronophthisis is caused by recessively acquired homozygotic and compound heterozygotic mutations in nine known genes (*NPHP1* through *NPHP9*), which account for only about 30% of cases, indicating the presence of yet-to-be-discovered genes. Expression of the encoded proteins, called nephrocystins, at extrarenal sites accounts for the associated retinal, neural, liver, and skeletal abnormalities. Each of the nine genes is associated with a somewhat different phenotype, although some share common phenotypes, explained by protein-protein interactions between two or more gene products. Most of the encoded proteins localize to centrosomes or cilia, but some also localize to adherens junctions and/or focal adhesions in epithelia.

CLINICAL MANIFESTATIONS

Presenting symptoms include polyuria, growth failure, and anemia. Polyuria occurs early, owing to reduced urinary concentrating ability and to salt wasting. Decreased growth rate is related to chronic dehydration, and growth failure and anemia occur with the onset of ESRD. Blood pressure is normal and edema is absent before the onset of renal failure. Hematuria and proteinuria are absent or minimal. Patients with mutations in specific nephronophthisis genes may also present with eye defects, oculomotor apraxia, congenital amaurosis, retinitis pigmentosa, neural anomalies, cerebellar ataxia, seizures, liver fibrosis, skeletal defects, scoliosis, cleft palate, and situs inversus.

DIAGNOSIS

Diagnosis relies on clinical suspicion of the disorder in a pediatric or adolescent patient who presents with ESRD and extrarenal manifestations such as abnormal eye movements, blindness, mental retardation, and polydactyly. Abdominal ultrasound, MRI (without gadolinium), electroretinogram, and full neurologic and ophthalmologic evaluations should assess the patient's renal, liver, retinal, and neurologic status. A renal ultrasound showing loss of corticomedullary differentiation, increased parenchymal echogenicity, and occasionally small medullary or corticomedullary cysts in normal-sized or moderately small kidneys is highly suggestive of juvenile nephronophthisis in a child with severe uremia. Genetic testing may be required for a conclusive diagnosis. A renal biopsy showing evidence of chronic tubulointerstitial nephritis may be necessary to confirm the diagnosis if genetic testing is not available.

PREVENTION AND TREATMENT Rx

Treatment is largely supportive, focusing on the progressive renal failure and the need for dialysis and transplantation. Vasopressin V2 receptor antagonists and rapamycin show promise in animal models, but clinical trials are needed to assess these treatments in patients.

Prenatal genetic testing in families with a genetic diagnosis of nephronophthisis is feasible. DNA-based diagnostics are most useful in identifying the germline mutation prenatally or preimplantation.

● MEDULLARY CYSTIC KIDNEY DISEASE

Medullary cystic kidney disease is an autosomal dominant interstitial kidney disease that results in renal failure after the fourth decade of life. It is rarer than autosomal recessive nephronophthisis, with which it shares a number of histologic features, including tubular basement membrane disintegration, tubular cyst formation, and tubulointerstitial inflammation and fibrosis.

At least two genes, *MCKD1* and *MCKD2*, cause medullary cystic kidney disease. *MCKD2* encodes an 85-kD nonciliary protein, uromodulin, which is secreted by the thick ascending limb of the loop of Henle and is the most abundant protein in human urine. The *MCKD1* gene has not yet been identified, but some studies have linked it to chromosome 1q21.

Mutations in *MCKD1* and *MCKD2* result in a similar clinical picture, except for an earlier onset of ESRD and precocious gout with mutations in *MCKD2*. Polyuria and anemia are usually not clinically present in the early stages, and renal failure generally occurs after the fourth decade of life. Hypertension is likely secondary to renal failure.

Corticomedullary cysts, which are present in most adult patients, cannot always be recognized on ultrasonography or CT because they tend to be very small. Except for the treatment of gout (Chapter 281), management is similar to that of patients with nephronophthisis.

● MEDULLARY SPONGE KIDNEY

Medullary sponge kidney, which is a rare disorder of unknown pathogenesis, is characterized by congenitally acquired inner medullary and papillary collecting duct dilations, hypercalciuria, and a mild defect in urinary concentration and acidification owing to tubular dysfunction. Patients present with hematuria and recurrent kidney stones, usually by the second or third decade of life. Medullary sponge kidney may also be an incidental finding on an intravenous pyelogram that shows the characteristic pooling of contrast material within the cystic collecting ducts. ESRD is uncommon, and the long-term prognosis is excellent.

OTHER INHERITED CYSTIC SYNDROMES

Bardet-Biedl syndrome is an autosomal recessive disorder characterized by obesity, hypertension, and dystrophy of the hands, eyes, kidneys, and male genitalia. Mutations in 14 different genes encoding proteins that localize to basal bodies have been identified. Calyceal cysts and calyceal clubbing predominate the renal lesion and are best diagnosed by intravenous urography rather than ultrasound. Renal impairment is frequent and is an important cause of death.

Oral-facial-digital syndrome is characterized by malformations of the face, oral cavity, and digits. It is inherited in an X-linked pattern and is caused by defects in the *OFD1* gene, which encodes OFD1 protein expressed in basal bodies but otherwise has an undetermined function. Renal (primarily glomerular) cysts are found in as many as 50% of patients, all of whom are females; males carrying the mutation die in utero. ESRD has been reported in affected females ranging in age from 11 to 72 years.

Autosomal dominant renal cyst formation is also seen in tuberous sclerosis and von Hippel-Lindau syndrome (Chapter 426). In tuberous sclerosis, cyst formation is commonly associated with hypertension; this disorder can resemble ADPKD and is associated with about a 5% incidence of renal cell carcinoma. In von Hippel-Lindau syndrome, cyst formation can also lead to features of ADPKD; more importantly, the syndrome is associated with a 25% incidence of renal cell carcinoma.

ACQUIRED CYSTIC KIDNEY DISEASE

Acquired cystic kidney disease is largely confined to the ESRD population on dialysis (Chapter 133). Cysts arise from proximal and distal tubule dilations in small end-stage kidneys regardless of cause, mode of dialysis, or presence of a functioning kidney transplant. Identifiable risk factors include duration of ESRD, older age, large cysts, male gender, black race, and chronic hypokalemia.

CLINICAL MANIFESTATIONS AND DIAGNOSIS

Acquired cystic kidney disease is usually asymptomatic, but it occasionally leads to enlarged kidneys with associated abdominal discomfort and pain. Cyst hemorrhage, which is more common than cyst infection, presents with flank pain, anemia, or hematuria. The most significant complication of acquired cystic kidney disease is malignant conversion of cysts into renal cell carcinoma (Chapter 203). Carcinomas commonly present as hematuria and are 2 to 200 times more common in patients with acquired cystic kidney disease than in the general dialysis population.

Acquired cystic kidney disease is diagnosed by ultrasound or CT demonstrating multiple and bilateral renal cysts in a patient with preexisting chronic renal failure or ESRD. In contrast to ADPKD and ARPKD, the kidneys are usually not enlarged, and there is no family history of PKD. Renal CT or MRI is preferable to detect cysts in small kidneys and to assess for malignant conversion.

PREVENTION AND TREATMENT **Rx**

There are no strategies to prevent the appearance or delay the expansion of renal cysts in patients on hemodialysis, but cysts may stabilize or regress following successful renal transplantation. New or frank hematuria raises the concern of renal cell carcinoma (Chapter 203), which should be assessed using ultrasound and contrast-enhanced CT. Any evidence of septa formation, solid material, or contrast enhancement within a cyst is suspicious for renal cell carcinoma and warrants consideration of nephrectomy.

PROGNOSIS

Asymptomatic acquired cystic kidney disease does not affect survival. The incidence of renal cell carcinoma in patients with acquired cystic kidney disease is approximately 0.18% per year. Although metastasis is less common at the time of diagnosis in patients with acquired cystic kidney disease than in other patients with renal cell carcinoma, the 5-year mortality rates are higher, likely related to the almost invariable coexistence of ESRD.

Grade **A**

1. Hogan MC, Masyuk TV, Page LJ, et al. Randomized clinical trial of long-acting somatostatin for autosomal dominant polycystic kidney and liver disease. *J Am Soc Nephrol.* 2010;21:1052-1061.
2. Serra AL, Poster D, Kistler AD, et al. Sirolimus and kidney growth in autosomal dominant polycystic kidney disease. *N Engl J Med.* 2010;363:820-829.
3. Walz G, Budde K, Mannaa M, et al. Everolimus in patients with autosomal dominant polycystic kidney disease. *N Engl J Med.* 2010;363:830-840.

SUGGESTED READINGS

Barua M, Pei Y. Diagnosis of autosomal-dominant polycystic kidney disease: an integrated approach. *Semin Nephrol.* 2010;30:356-365. *Review of imaging and molecular-based diagnostic tests.*
Harris PC, Rossetti S. Molecular diagnostics for autosomal dominant polycystic kidney disease. *Nat Rev Nephrol.* 2010;6:197-206. *Review of molecular testing methods to detect mutations in ADPKD.*
Hildebrandt F. Genetic kidney diseases. *Lancet.* 2010;375:1287-1295. *Review.*
Kyongtae T, Bae KT, Grantham JJ. Imaging for the prognosis of autosomal dominant polycystic kidney disease. *Nat Rev Nephrol.* 2010;6:96-106. *Supports imaging as an invaluable tool to monitor the onset and progression of ADPKD.*
Pei Y. Practical genetics for autosomal dominant polycystic kidney disease. *Nephron Clin Pract.* 2011;118:19-30. *Review of clinical predictors of gene types, imaging, and molecular-based diagnostic tests.*

130

HEREDITARY NEPHROPATHIES AND DEVELOPMENTAL ABNORMALITIES OF THE URINARY TRACT

LISA M. GUAY-WOODFORD

HEREDITARY NEPHROPATHIES

The proximal tubule is responsible for reclaiming most of the filtered glucose, amino acids, uric acid, phosphate, bicarbonate, and low-molecular-weight proteins. The loop of Henle and the distal nephron reabsorb approximately 30% of the filtered sodium chloride and 50% of the filtered divalent cations. The collecting duct, under the regulatory control of aldosterone, fine-tunes sodium reabsorption and secretes hydrogen and potassium ions. In the terminal collecting duct, antidiuretic hormone regulates water reabsorption and urinary concentration.

Inherited renal tubular disorders are a group of conditions in which the normal renal tubular reabsorption of ions, organic solutes, and water (Chapter 118) is disrupted. These defects can be categorized by the nephron segment affected (Table 130-1).

Disorders of Proximal Tubule Function

CYSTINURIA

Cystinuria is characterized by defective proximal tubular reabsorption of cystine and dibasic amino acids, resulting in the formation of urinary calculi (Chapter 128). This autosomal recessive trait has an estimated prevalence of 1 in 7000 individuals. Two cystinuria genes have been identified: *SLC7A9*, which encodes the luminal transport channel itself, and *SLC3A1*, which encodes the transporter regulatory subunit. Several large studies indicate that mutations in *SLC3A1* are more common than mutations in *SLC7A9*. Mutations in *SLC3A1* cause cystinuria type A, mutations in *SLC7A9* cause cystinuria type B, and mutations in both genes (compound heterozygotes) cause cystinuria type AB.

Although the severity of the disease is similar in all types of cystinurias, the clinical presentation can be quite variable, and the onset of disease may occur from infancy to the seventh decade of life. Affected children can be identified by elevated urinary cystine levels, but testing must be performed after tubular transport has fully matured (at age 2 years). Cystine stones are radiopaque and often form the nidus for secondary calcium oxalate stones. Symptoms include renal colic, which may be associated with urinary tract obstruction and/or infection. Conservative therapy with high urine volume and urinary alkalinization is sufficient for many patients with cystinuria, but recurrent stone formation may cause renal damage and warrants treatment with thiol agents (e.g., D-penicillamine: pediatric dose, 15 to 20 mg/kg/day; adult dose, 2 g/day in four divided doses) or α-mercaptopropionylglycine

TABLE 130-1 HEREDITARY NEPHROPATHIES BY NEPHRON SEGMENT

DISORDER	INHERITANCE	OMIM*	MAJOR RENAL FEATURES
PROXIMAL TUBULE			
Renal glucosuria	AR	233100	Isolated glucosuria
Proximal renal tubular acidosis	AR	604278	Hyperchloremic, hypokalemic metabolic acidosis
Carbonic anhydrase II deficiency	AR	259730	Mixed proximal and distal renal tubular acidosis
Hartnup disease	AR	234500	Neutral aminoaciduria
Cystinuria	AR	Type A: 220100 Type B: 604144	Urinary calculi
Cystinosis	AR	Infantile: 219800 Late-onset: 219900 Non-nephropathic: 219750	Renal Fanconi's syndrome
Dent disease	X-linked	Dent disease 1: 300009 Dent disease 2: 300555	Nephrocalcinosis, urinary calculi, low-molecular-weight proteinuria
Lowe syndrome	X-linked	309000	Renal Fanconi's syndrome
Hereditary fructose intolerance	AR	229600	Renal Fanconi's syndrome
Tyrosinemia type I	AR	276700	Renal Fanconi's syndrome
Wilson disease	AR	277900	Renal Fanconi's syndrome
LOOP OF HENLE			
Bartter's syndrome	AR	Type I: 601678 Type II: 241200 Type III: 607364 Type IV: 602522	Hypokalemic, hypochloremic metabolic alkalosis
	AD	Type V: 601199	
DISTAL TUBULE			
Gitelman's syndrome	AR	263800	Hypokalemic, hypochloremic metabolic alkalosis
Familial hypomagnesemia with hypercalciuria	AR	248250, 248190	Severe renal magnesium and calcium wasting
Isolated hypomagnesemia	AD	154020	Renal magnesium wasting
COLLECTING DUCT			
Liddle's syndrome	AD	177200	Low-renin hypertension
Glucocorticoid-remediable hyperaldosteronism	AD	103900	Low-renin hypertension
Apparent mineralocorticoid excess	AR	218030	Low-renin hypertension
Pseudohypoaldosteronism type I	AR, AD	AR: 264350 AD: 177735	Hyponatremic, hypokalemic metabolic acidosis
Pseudohypoaldosteronism type II (Gordon's syndrome)	AD	114300	Low-renin hypertension with hyperkalemia
Distal renal tubular acidosis	AR, AD	AR: 602722, 605239 AD: 179800, 611590	Hyperchloremic, hypokalemic metabolic acidosis
Carbonic anhydrase II deficiency	AR	259730	Mixed proximal and distal renal tubular acidosis
Nephrogenic diabetes insipidus	X-linked, AR, AD	X-linked: 304800 AR and AD: 125800	Urinary concentrating defect

*Entries in Online Mendelian Inheritance in Man (OMIM), available at www.ncbi.nlm.nih.gov/omim. Accessed Dec. 15, 2009.
AD = autosomal dominant; AR = autosomal recessive.

(pediatric dose, 10 to15 mg/kg/day; adult dose, 1 to 2 g/day in two divided doses) to form soluble mixed disulfides with cystine and maintain free urine cystine levels below 200 mg/g of creatinine.

CYSTINOSIS

Cystinosis is the most common inherited cause of renal Fanconi's syndrome; it also affects the eyes, muscles, central nervous system, lungs, and various endocrine organs. Cystinosis is an autosomal recessive disorder caused by mutations in the gene *CTNS*, which encodes cystinosin, a lysosomal cystine transporter. Defects in this transporter lead to the accumulation of intralysosomal cystine crystals and widespread cellular destruction.

Three clinical presentations have been described. The most severe is infantile (classic) cystinosis, which manifests in the first year of life with renal tubular acidosis, impaired growth, and evidence of renal Fanconi's syndrome, including aminoaciduria, glucosuria, phosphaturia, and low-molecular-weight proteinuria. Progressive renal failure reaches end-stage renal disease in childhood. A less severe, late-onset (juvenile or intermediate) form causes renal dysfunction in adolescence and involves cystine deposits in the cornea. The mildest form, an ocular, non-nephropathic form, features photophobia but no renal problems.

The mainstay of cystinosis therapy is oral cysteamine (adult dose, 500 mg four times daily), an aminothiol that can lower intracellular cystine content by 90%. In well-treated adolescent and young adult patients, cysteamine delays renal glomerular deterioration, enhances growth, prevents hypothyroidism, and lowers muscle cystine content. Therefore, early diagnosis and prompt, proper treatment are critical for preventing or significantly delaying the complications of cystinosis.

Disorders of Loop of Henle and Distal Tubule Function

THE BARTTER-GITELMAN DISORDERS

The Bartter-Gitelman syndromes are a group of disorders characterized by markedly reduced salt transport in the thick ascending limb of Henle (Bartter's syndrome) or in the distal convoluted tubule (Gitelman's syndrome).

Most patients with Gitelman's syndrome have defects in *SLC12A3*, the gene encoding the sodium-chloride cotransporter NCCT. However, a minority of patients with the Gitelman phenotype have mutations in *CLCNKB*.

Bartter's syndrome can be caused by mutations in one of four genes— *SLC12A2*, encoding the sodium-potassium-chloride cotransporter NKCC2;

TABLE 130-2 FEATURES OF THE INHERITED RENAL TUBULAR ACIDOSES (RTAs)

DISORDER	RENAL TRANSPORT DEFECT	MINIMAL URINE pH DURING ACIDOSIS	ALKALI SUPPLEMENTATION (HCO₃⁻)	UAG DURING ACIDOSIS*
Proximal RTA	↓Proximal bicarbonate reabsorption	<5.5	Children: 10-15 mEq/kg/day	0 or +
Carbonic anhydrase II deficiency	↓Proximal bicarbonate reabsorption and ↓distal acidification	Variable	Variable	0 or +
Distal RTA	↓Distal acidification	>5.5	Adults: 1-3 mEq/kg/day Children: 3-6 mEq/kg/day	0 or +

*In RTA, the UAG is usually 0 or positive, whereas in metabolic acidosis associated with diarrheal illness, the UAG is negative.
HCO_3^- = bicarbonate; UAG = urinary anion gap ($[Na^+] + [K^+] - [Cl^-]$).

KCNJ1, encoding the ROMK1 potassium ion channel; *CLCNKB*, encoding the ClC-Kb basolateral chloride ion channel; and *BSND*, encoding barttin, a regulatory subunit required for basolateral chloride channel targeting to the membrane. These mutations cause autosomal recessive Bartter's syndrome types I, II, III, and IV, respectively. Defects in any of these genes disrupt salt transport in the thick ascending limb, causing a furosemide-like effect (E-Fig. 130-1). In addition, severe gain-in-function mutations in *CASR*, the gene encoding the extracellular calcium ion–sensing receptor CaSR, can cause a Bartter-like phenotype (referred to as Bartter's type V) that is distinguished from the others by autosomal dominant transmission and associated hypocalcemic hypercalciuria.

Individuals with Bartter's syndrome exhibit renal salt wasting, lowered blood pressure, polyuria, hypokalemic metabolic alkalosis, and hypercalciuria with a variable risk of nephrocalcinosis. In comparison, individuals with Gitelman's syndrome exhibit milder renal salt wasting, normal blood pressure, hypokalemic metabolic alkalosis, hypomagnesemia, and hypocalciuria. This clinical disorder resembles the effects of long-term thiazide administration. Clinical differences between Bartter's and Gitelman's syndromes relate to the severity of salt wasting, whereas phenotypic differences among Bartter's types I through V correlate with the specific physiologic roles played by the individual transporters or channels in the kidney and other organs.

The mainstay of treatment includes replacing salt and water losses and providing potassium supplementation to maintain serum levels greater than 3 mEq/dL. In patients with perinatal (type I or II) Bartter's syndrome, cyclooxygenase inhibitors (e.g., indomethacin 2-4 mg/kg/day in two to four divided doses) may be beneficial. In patients with Gitelman's syndrome and some patients with Bartter's syndrome type III, oral magnesium supplementation may be required to maintain serum levels above 1.2 mg/dL.

Disorders of Collecting Duct Function
LIDDLE'S SYNDROME (PSEUDOALDOSTERONISM)
Liddle's syndrome, which is an autosomal dominant form of salt-sensitive hypertension (Chapter 67), is caused by mutations in the α, β, or γ subunits of the epithelial sodium channel, which is expressed at the apical surface of collecting duct cells and plays a critical role in maintaining salt balance and blood pressure. Both the β and the γ subunits regulate the channel activity of the α subunit. Mutations in either of these regulatory subunits result in increased epithelial sodium channel activity and Liddle's syndrome.

Severe hypertension typically manifests in childhood, with features of hypokalemic metabolic alkalosis that resemble primary aldosteronism. However, renin and aldosterone secretion is suppressed in this disorder. The clinical abnormalities can be ameliorated by a low-salt diet plus a potassium-sparing diuretic (e.g., amiloride 5 to 10 mg/day), which acts as an antagonist of the epithelial sodium channel.

DISTAL RENAL TUBULAR ACIDOSIS
Distal renal tubular acidosis (dRTA) results from failure of the collecting duct α-intercalated cells to excrete fixed acids (see Fig. 120-1 in Chapter 120). Both autosomal dominant and autosomal recessive forms of dRTA have been described. These heritable disorders include mutations in genes encoding carbonic anhydrase II, the chloride-bicarbonate exchanger AE1, and subunits of the hydrogen–adenosine triphosphatase (H⁺-ATPase) proton pump. Mutations in the *SLC4A1* gene encoding AE1 cause autosomal dominant dRTA and are rarely associated with recessive forms of the disease. Mutations in subunits of H⁺-ATPase are the primary causes of autosomal recessive

dRTA. Vacuolar H⁺-ATPases (V-type ATPases) are ubiquitous, multi-subunit protein complexes that mediate the ATP-dependent transport of protons. In the kidney, V-type ATPases are the major proton-secreting pumps in the distal nephron and are involved in net proton secretion (bicarbonate generation) or proton reabsorption (net bicarbonate secretion). Defects in two genes, *ATP6B1* and *ATP6N1B*, cause dRTA with or without associated sensorineural deafness.

Clinical consequences include hypokalemic, hyperchloremic metabolic acidosis; impaired growth; hypercalciuria; hypocitraturia; nephrocalcinosis; nephrolithiasis; rickets in children; and osteomalacia in adults. Classic dRTA can be distinguished from other metabolic acidoses by an inappropriately high urine pH (>5.5), diminished net acid excretion, positive urinary anion gap, and low urinary ammonium concentration (Table 130-2). Treatment with alkali supplementation (1 to 3 mEq/kg/day in adults and 3 to 6 mEq/kg/day in children) is usually effective in correcting the acidosis. In contrast to proximal RTA, urinary potassium wasting can be ameliorated with alkali therapy alone.

⬤ DEVELOPMENT OF THE KIDNEY AND URINARY TRACT
The human kidney and urogenital tract develop from three principal embryonic structures: the metanephric mesenchyme, the mesonephric (wolffian) duct, and the cloaca (Fig. 130-1). At 4 to 5 weeks of gestation, the ureteric bud originates as a diverticulum of the mesonephric duct. Reciprocal interactions between the branching ureteric bud and the metanephric mesenchyme induce kidney development, with the metanephros undergoing an epithelial transformation to form the glomeruli and the proximal and distal tubules. The ureteric bud branches give rise to the collecting ducts, the renal pelvis, the ureter, and the bladder trigone. Nephrogenesis is completed by 34 weeks of gestation.

Concurrent with the initial nephrogenic events, the urorectal fold divides the cloaca into the urogenital sinus and the future rectum. The mesonephric duct opening into the bladder becomes the vesicoureteric orifice of the trigone. Between 5 and 6 weeks of gestation, the second genital duct (müllerian duct) appears and runs in parallel with the wolffian duct. In males, the müllerian duct subsequently regresses, the wolffian duct proceeds to form the epididymis, the vas deferens, the seminal vesicle, and the ejaculatory duct. In females, the wolffian duct regresses, and the müllerian ducts fuse to form the ureterovaginal primordium, which merges with the urogenital sinus and eventually gives rise to the uterus, the oviducts, and the proximal vagina. The remnants of the allantois form the urachus, a fibrous cord that connects the bladder to the umbilicus.

Congenital abnormalities of the kidney and urinary tract occur in 1 in 500 newborns and account for approximately 20 to 30% of all anomalies identified in the prenatal period. Some urinary tract anomalies are asymptomatic and inconsequential, but many renal tract malformations are important causes of infant mortality as well as morbidity in older children and adults, including the progression to renal failure.

⬤ ABNORMALITIES OF THE URINARY TRACT
Renal Parenchymal Malformations
Congenital defects in renal development may result in the absence of a kidney (agenesis) or abnormalities in kidney size, structure, or position. Irregularities in the renal contour may arise from the persistence of fetal lobulation or

FIGURE 130-1. Key events in the development of the urinary tract. In the 4-week embryo, the ureteric bud emerges from the wolffian duct (A). Reciprocal interactions between the branching ureteric bud and the metanephric mesenchyme induce kidney development. Concurrently, the cloaca is divided by the urorectal fold into the urogenital sinus and the future rectum (B). In the 8-week male embryo, the wolffian duct begins to give rise to the epididymis, the seminal vesicles, and the caudal part of the vas deferens (C). By 9 weeks, axial growth of the fetal spine prompts the developing kidney to ascend from the pelvis to its final lumbar position. The external genitalia develop between 8 and 16 weeks, and testicular descent begins in month 7 of gestation (D).

a depression in the midpole of the left kidney caused by the spleen (a "dromedary hump"). Neither irregularity impairs renal function.

RENAL AGENESIS

Renal agenesis reflects a complete failure of nephrogenesis. Unilateral agenesis can occur as an isolated abnormality or as a component of syndromic disorders, such as Turner's syndrome (Chapter 241). As an isolated entity, the complete absence of one kidney occurs in 1 in 5000 individuals. The incidence is higher in males and occurs somewhat more frequently on the left side; in about half the patients, the ipsilateral ureter and hemitrigone are also absent. The remaining kidney is usually enlarged owing to compensatory hypertrophy, but it may be ectopic or malrotated. Vesicoureteral reflux is observed on the contralateral side in about 30% of patients.

Renal agenesis is commonly associated with genital anomalies, suggesting that it represents a developmental field defect. In females, absence of the ipsilateral oviduct and malformation of the uterus and vagina result from maldevelopment of the müllerian duct, whereas in males, wolffian duct–derived structures, such as the vas deferens and the seminal vesicles, are often absent. Other associated anomalies can include cardiovascular malformations, vertebral defects, and imperforate anus.

Bilateral renal agenesis has an estimated incidence of 1 in 10,000 births and is associated with the Potter phenotype, which includes pulmonary hypoplasia, a characteristic facies, and deformities of the spine and limbs. At birth, these neonates have a critical degree of pulmonary hypoplasia that is incompatible with survival. The familial association of unilateral and bilateral renal agenesis, renal dysplasia, and congenital hydronephrosis occurs in hereditary renal adysplasia syndrome (Online Mendelian Inheritance in Man entry 191830), a rare autosomal dominant disorder with variable penetrance.

RENAL HYPOPLASIA

The term *renal hypoplasia* describes small kidneys with normally differentiated nephrons that are reduced in number. *Oligomeganephronia* describes a form of bilateral renal hypoplasia with a marked reduction in nephron number and associated hypertrophy of individual glomeruli and tubules. This abnormality occurs sporadically as an isolated developmental defect that must be differentiated from acquired renal atrophy and the nephronophthisis–

medullary cystic disease complex. Renal function declines slowly, with progression to end-stage renal failure in the second to third decade of life.

RENAL DYSPLASIA

Renal dysplasia, which can be associated with various abnormalities of kidney size, results from abnormal metanephric differentiation that causes anomalous and/or incompletely differentiated renal elements. Small dysplastic kidneys are commonly referred to as *aplastic*. Large dysplastic kidneys are often cystic; the most extreme type is referred to as *multicystic dysplastic kidney.*

Unilateral dysplasia may be asymptomatic well into adult life. Small aplastic and large multicystic dysplastic kidneys are nonfunctioning and can be distinguished from renal agenesis by imaging studies. The ipsilateral ureter is typically atretic. Contralateral malformations, including obstruction and vesicoureteral reflux, are common. Unilateral multicystic kidneys involute over time and often disappear. Unilateral aplasia and multicystic dysplasia may be manifestations of the hereditary renal adysplasia syndrome. Bilateral multicystic dysplastic kidneys are incompatible with neonatal survival.

Renal and Ureteral Structural Abnormalities

RENAL MALROTATION AND ECTOPIA

Metanephric kidney development begins caudally. By 9 weeks of gestation, the kidney has ascended to its normal level (L1-L3), and the renal pelvis has rotated 90 degrees toward the midline. Anomalies of ascent and/or failure of rotation are common. Bilateral renal ectopia is often associated with kidney fusion. The most common fusion anomaly is the horseshoe kidney, which occurs in 1 in 500 newborns with a 2 : 1 male predominance. Renal ascent is prevented by the root of the inferior mesenteric artery (Fig. 130-2A). Crossed renal ectopia can occur with or without fusion. Supernumerary (extra) kidneys are typically ectopic and vary in location. Although almost one third of patients with renal ectopia remain asymptomatic, the associated malrotation of the renal pelvis increases the risk of hydronephrosis, infection, and stone formation.

PELVIURETERAL ABNORMALITIES

Obstruction of the ureteropelvic junction impedes the flow of urine from the renal pelvis into the ureter. It is one of the most frequently occurring urinary

Megaureter

Prostate

Posterior
urethral valve

FIGURE 130-2. Developmental abnormalities of the urinary tract. **A,** Horseshoe kidney. **B,** Ectopic ureter associated with a ureterocele. **C,** Megaureter with the aperistaltic segment (arrow). **D,** Bladder outlet obstruction caused by posterior urethral valves.

tract anomalies in children and is the most common cause of collecting system dilation in the fetal kidney. In congenital obstruction of the ureteropelvic junction, urologic anomalies in the contralateral system are common, including renal agenesis, renal dysplasia, multicystic dysplasia, ureteropelvic junction obstruction, and vesicoureteral reflux. Ureteropelvic junction obstruction may occur in adults secondary to external compression, kinking, or stenosis of the proximal ureter. Surgical intervention is indicated if there is associated renal function impairment, pyelonephritis, stones, or pain.

Hydrocalyx or *hydrocalycosis* refers to dilation of a major calyx that occurs in the context of intrinsic obstruction, as in infundibular stenosis, or in the context of extrinsic compression of the pelvis, as caused by a vessel or a parapelvic cyst. In comparison, *megacalycosis* represents a nonobstructive, dysplastic lesion seen primarily in males, in which the calyces are dilated and usually increased in number. Associated renal medullary hypoplasia causes malformation of the renal papillae.

Calyceal diverticula are cystic structures connected by a narrow channel to an adjacent minor calyx. In imaging studies, these diverticula typically fill with contrast material, which distinguishes them from renal parenchymal cysts.

Partial duplication of the renal pelvis and ureter is a common anomaly that occurs more frequently in females, is typically unilateral, and is clinically insignificant.

URETERIC ANOMALIES

Ectopic ureters usually reflect complete ureteric and renal duplication. Approximately 10% are bilateral. The ectopic ureter typically drains the dysplastic upper pole of a duplex kidney and inserts below the normal vesicoureteral junction into the lower trigone or the proximal urethra. Ectopic ureters occur much more frequently in females, and the insertion sites can include the vagina and the vulva, with resulting incontinence. An ectopic ureter is often associated with a ureterocele, a cystic dilation of the terminal ureter (Fig. 130-2B). In children, ureteroceles can be associated with urinary tract infection and obstruction of the bladder neck or even of the contralateral ureter. In adults, the clinical presentation usually involves an associated infection, ureteric stones, or both.

A megaureter, or grossly dilated ureter, has multiple potential causes, including intrinsic ureteric obstruction by a stone, bladder outflow obstruction, vesicoureteral reflux, and external compression of the distal ureter. In contrast, primary megaureter results from a functional obstruction of the distal ureter caused by an aperistaltic segment (Fig. 130-2C).

VESICOURETERAL REFLUX

In the normal urinary tract, urinary reflux from the bladder into the ureters is prevented by a functional valve-like mechanism at the vesicoureteral junction. The competence of this valve is dependent on several critical factors, such as the intramural length of the ureter, the position of the ureteric orifice in the bladder, and the integrity of the bladder wall musculature. Primary vesicoureteral reflux, with an estimated incidence of 1 to 2% in children, results from incompetence of the vesicoureteral junction owing to the shortened length of the ureter's submucosal segment and the lateral, ectopic position of its orifice. Genetic factors appear to contribute to the pathogenesis of primary vesicoureteral reflux, as there is a 30- to 50-fold increased risk in immediate relatives of an index case. As the intramural ureter lengthens with age, primary vesicoureteral reflux tends to remit or disappear. Vesicoureteral reflux can also occur secondary to obstructive maldevelopment of the lower urinary tract, such as in triad syndrome and posterior urethral valves.

In both primary and secondary vesicoureteral reflux, intrarenal reflux can lead to the development of reflux nephropathy, a tubulointerstitial lesion associated with gross scarring at the renal poles. In addition, the development of a glomerular lesion consistent with focal and segmental glomerulosclerosis can cause proteinuria, hypertension, and progressive loss of renal function.

In children younger than 18 years with prior urinary tract infections, daily treatment with trimethoprim (2 mg/kg/day) plus sulfamethoxazole (10 mg/kg/day) reduces recurrent infections by about 40%,**1** but the value of long-term suppression is less clear.**2** Although surgical correction is the current standard of care for severe grades of vesicoureteral reflux, particularly secondary forms associated with maldevelopment of the lower urinary tract, the long-term benefit of either endoscopic or surgical intervention appears to be small and is unlikely to prevent renal damage.**3**

Lower Urinary Tract Abnormalities
TRIAD SYNDROME (PRUNE-BELLY SYNDROME, EAGLE-BARRETT SYNDROME)

Triad syndrome, also referred to as prune-belly syndrome or Eagle-Barrett syndrome, involves a constellation of anomalies including congenital absence or deficiency of the abdominal wall musculature, gross ureteral dilation, bladder wall thickening, prostatic hypoplasia, and bilateral undescended testes (cryptorchidism). The full syndrome is expressed only in males, and surviving individuals are typically infertile. Patients with an incomplete syndrome can have anomalies of the abdominal wall musculature, bladder, and upper urinary tract; 3% of these patients are females. Although the specific molecular events have yet to be defined, defects in mesenchymal development appear to cause poor prostate and bladder differentiation, ureteral smooth muscle aplasia with consequent ureteral aperistalsis, and varying degrees of renal dysplasia. Three fourths of patients with triad syndrome have associated malformations in the cardiopulmonary system, gastrointestinal tract, and skeleton. In the immediate postnatal period, prognosis depends on the severity of extragenitourinary anomalies. Long-term outcome is based on the degree of renal dysplasia and the success of urodynamic management.

BLADDER ABNORMALITIES

Bladder exstrophy results from a midline closure defect involving the lower anterior abdominal wall, the bladder, and the external genitalia. These abnormalities have been attributed to a primary defect in the differentiation of the cloacal membrane, but the precise molecular events are unclear. In severe cases, bladder exstrophy may be associated with imperforate anus and rectal atresia. However, other congenital anomalies are rarely associated. Clinical studies indicate that there is a correlation between the success of bladder reconstruction and long-term preservation of renal function.

In adults, neuropathic or neurogenic bladder (Chapter 25) has numerous etiologic contributors, including central nervous system trauma, stroke, disorders such as Parkinson's disease, spinal trauma, multiple sclerosis, and peripheral nerve damage caused by trauma or surgery. In children, myelomeningocele (spina bifida) is the most common cause of neurogenic bladder dysfunction. Other forms of myelodysplasia, such as spinal dysraphism (spina bifida occulta) and sacral agenesis, are less common causes.

POSTERIOR URETHRAL VALVES

In male infants, posterior urethral valves are the most common cause of bladder outflow obstruction, with resulting bilateral hydronephrosis and megaureters. However, among all infants with hydronephrosis, only 10% have posterior urethral valves. The urethral obstruction results from defective reabsorption of mucosal folds in the posterior urethra, just distal to the verumontanum. As a result, dilation of the proximal urethra, bladder wall hypertrophy and trabeculation, associated vesicoureteral reflux, and varying degrees of renal dysplasia are present (Fig. 130-2D). Surgical management

strategies are dictated by the age of the child and the degree of associated renal insufficiency. Survival and long-term renal outcome depend on the severity of the associated renal dysplasia.

1. Craig JC, Simpson JM, Williams GJ, et al. Antibiotic prophylaxis and recurrent urinary tract infection in children. *N Engl J Med.* 2009;361:1748-1759.
2. Garin EH, Olavarria F, Garcia Nieto V, et al. Clinical significance of primary vesicoureteral reflux and urinary antibiotic prophylaxis after acute pyelonephritis: a multicenter, randomized, controlled study. *Pediatrics.* 2006;117:626-632.
3. Hodson EM, Wheeler DM, Vimalchandra D, et al. Interventions for primary vesicoureteric reflux. *Cochrane Database Syst Rev.* 2007.3.CD001532.

SUGGESTED READINGS

Hildebrandt F. Genetic kidney disease. *Lancet.* 2010;375:1287-1295. *Review.*
Jeck N, Seyberth HW. Loop disorders: insights derived from defined genotypes. *Nephron Physiol.* 2011;118:7-14. *Review.*
Tiselius HG. New horizons in the management of patients with cystinuria. *Curr Opin Urol.* 2010;20:169-173. *Review.*

131

BENIGN PROSTATIC HYPERPLASIA AND PROSTATITIS

MICHAEL J. BARRY AND MARY MCNAUGHTON COLLINS

The prostate gland, the largest accessory gland in the male reproductive system, surrounds the prostatic urethra below the bladder. Superiorly, its base is contiguous with the bladder neck; inferiorly, its apex adjoins the urogenital diaphragm. The prostatic urethra is angulated at the verumontanum, the union with the two ejaculatory ducts. In younger men, the prostate weighs about 20 g. As men age, the prostate enlarges and develops a characteristic zonal anatomy (Fig. 131-1). Its acini, which communicate with the urethra via prostatic ducts, supply about 20% of semen volume. Prostatic fluid is rich in citrate, zinc, and polyamines, although their roles in reproduction are poorly defined.

BENIGN PROSTATIC HYPERPLASIA
DEFINITION

Benign prostatic hyperplasia (BPH) is defined histologically by hyperplasia of both epithelial and stromal cells, beginning in the periurethral area. With aging, multiple small hyperplastic nodules grow, coalesce, and compress normal tissue outward against the true prostatic capsule, creating a surgical capsule that bounds the expanding adenoma.

EPIDEMIOLOGY

The hyperplastic process often begins in the third decade of life; by age 80 years, 85% of men have BPH. The age-specific prevalence of BPH at autopsy is remarkably similar among men of different ethnicities. Aging and functioning testes are the dominant risk factors. The onset of clinical manifestations of BPH before age 65 in a first-degree relative is also a risk factor. The prevalence of clinical manifestations is uncertain because of a lack of consensus on a working definition. Nevertheless, in the United States, about one third of men aged 40 to 79 years have moderate to severe lower urinary tract symptoms, a majority of which are attributable to BPH.

PATHOBIOLOGY

Testosterone is converted by the 5α-reductase enzyme into dihydrotestosterone, the major intraprostatic androgen. BPH does not develop in men who are castrated before puberty or who have 5α-reductase deficiency. Although the type 2 isoenzyme predominates in the prostate, the type 1 isoenzyme predominates elsewhere. An array of peptide growth factors, along with dihydrotestosterone, mediates stromal-epithelial interactions that alter the balance of cell proliferation and apoptosis and thereby lead to BPH. The mechanisms are poorly understood.

The genetics of BPH are also unclear. An autosomal dominant hereditary form may account for less than 10% of cases.

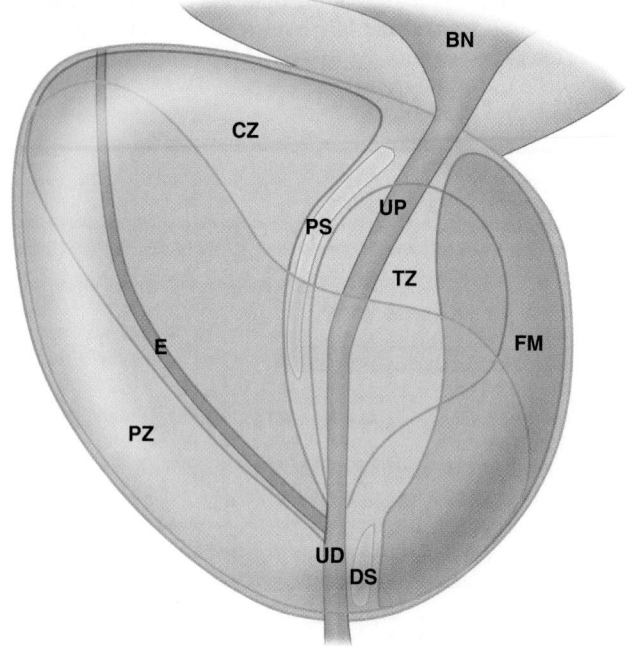

FIGURE 131-1. Anatomy of the prostate. Sagittal diagram of the distal prostatic urethral segment (UD), proximal urethral segment (UP), and ejaculatory ducts (E), showing their relationships to a sagittal section of the anteromedial nonglandular tissues: the bladder neck (BN), anterior fibromuscular stroma (FM), preprostatic sphincter (PS), and distal striated sphincter (DS). These structures are shown in relation to a three-dimensional representation of the glandular prostate: central zone (CZ), peripheral zone (PZ), and transitional zone (TZ). (From McNeal J. Normal histology of the prostate. *Am J Surg Pathol.* 1988;12:619-633.)

CLINICAL MANIFESTATIONS

The morbidity of BPH is conferred through bothersome lower urinary tract symptoms. Traditionally, voiding symptoms such as hesitancy, straining, a sense of incomplete emptying, intermittency, a weak stream, and postvoid dribbling were considered a consequence of mechanical bladder outlet obstruction. Filling symptoms, such as frequency, nocturia, urgency, and urge incontinence (Chapter 25), were thought to be caused by secondary uninhibited detrusor contractions. However, poor correlations among the severity of symptoms, prostatic size, degree of obstruction, and detrusor instability suggest that the pathophysiology is more complex. The key lower urinary tract symptoms of BPH can be quantified by asking the seven symptom questions in the International Prostate Symptom Score (IPSS) (Fig. 131-2).

Bladder outlet obstruction owing to BPH has both static and dynamic components. The static component is due to the enlarged prostate, whereas the dynamic component is due to increased adrenergic tone in the prostate, where α_2-adrenoreceptors predominate.

In the setting of obstruction, increased detrusor pressure can result in detrusor hypertrophy and, eventually, fibrosis. Complications of BPH include acute urinary retention, which may result from prostatic infarction. Postvoid residual urine probably increases the risk of urinary tract infection or stone formation. With long-standing obstruction, hydroureter and hydronephrosis may develop, and renal failure may eventually ensue. Men with BPH may have hematuria because of the complex of veins stretched over the enlarged prostate; however, other causes, especially malignancy (Chapter 203), need to be considered.

DIAGNOSIS

History

Symptoms are commonly attributed to BPH when an older man presents with lower urinary tract symptoms. IPSSs of 0 to 7 represent mild symptoms;

	Not at all	Less than 1 time in 5	Less than half the time	About half the time	More than half the time	Almost always
1. Over the past month or so, how often have you had a sensation of not emptying your bladder completely after you finished urinating?	0	1	2	3	4	5
2. Over the past month or so, how often have you had to urinate again less than two hours after you finished urinating?	0	1	2	3	4	5
3. Over the past month or so, how often have you found you stopped and started again several times when you urinated?	0	1	2	3	4	5
4. Over the past month or so, how often have you found it difficult to postpone urination?	0	1	2	3	4	5
5. Over the past month or so, how often have you had a weak urinary stream?	0	1	2	3	4	5
6. Over the past month or so, how often have you had to push or strain to begin urination?	0	1	2	3	4	5

7. Over the past month, how many times did you most typically get up to urinate from the time you went to bed at night until the time you got up in the morning?

0	none	1	1 time	2	2 times	3	3 times	4	4 times	5	5 or more times

Total IPSS Score = sum of questions 1–7 = _____

Quality of life due to urinary symptoms

If you were to spend the rest of your life with your urinary condition just the way it is now, how would you feel about that?

Delighted	Pleased	Mostly satisfied	Mixed—about equally satisfied and dissatisfied	Mostly dissatisfied	Unhappy	Terrible
0	1	2	3	4	5	6

FIGURE 131-2. International Prostate Symptom Score (IPSS). The seven symptom questions constitute a scale initially developed by the American Urological Association. The eighth question about quality of life is scored separately. (From Barry MJ, Fowler FJ Jr, O'Leary MP, et al. The American Urological Association symptom index for benign prostatic hyperplasia: the Measurement Committee of the American Urological Association. *J Urol.* 1992;148:1549.)

8 to 19, moderate symptoms; and 20 to 35, severe symptoms (see Fig. 131-2). When frequency and nocturia are the dominant symptoms, a voiding diary, in which the patient records the times and amounts of each void over several days, may be helpful. For example, if the diary documents nocturnal polyuria alone, causes other than BPH should be strongly considered. Men with BPH tend to have a balance of voiding and filling symptoms that slowly progress with age. A complete list of medications should be obtained because many drugs, especially over-the-counter antihistamines, sympathomimetics, and anticholinergics, can affect the urinary tract.

Differential Diagnosis
Although lower urinary tract symptoms in older men are often due to BPH, the differential diagnosis includes systemic diseases that cause frequency and nocturia, such as diabetes (Chapter 236 and 237), hypercalcemia (Chapter 253), bladder outlet obstruction due to urethral strictures, and neurologic diseases affecting the bladder (Chapter 25). Rapid onset of symptoms, presentation before age 50, or filling symptoms without voiding symptoms are "red flags" that suggest these alternative causes. Older men can have over-active bladders either primarily or secondary to outlet obstruction. A general medical history and the pattern of symptoms should provide clues to systemic diseases. Men with strictures usually have undergone genitourinary instrumentation or have had sexually transmitted diseases (Chapter 293). Primary bladder problems should be suspected in men with previous stroke (Chapter 414), Parkinson's disease (Chapter 416), or diabetic neuropathy (Chapter 428).

Physical Examination
The physical examination should include a digital rectal examination and a focused neurologic examination to look for evidence of peripheral neuropathy or saddle-area anesthesia (the S2-S4 segments innervate the bladder), which might suggest an underlying neuropathic bladder. The digital rectal examination should assess the size and consistency of the prostate. Classically, BPH causes a symmetrically enlarged, firm prostate, with a consistency similar to that of the tip of the nose. Asymmetry or frank nodules suggest prostate cancer (Chapter 207), but prostate cancer can be present even when the prostate feels normal. Physicians tend to underestimate the prostate's size; if the prostate feels enlarged, it usually is.

Laboratory Findings
Urinalysis should assess possible pyuria or hematuria. Optional studies include measurement of the serum creatinine and prostate-specific antigen (PSA) levels. Peak urinary flow is often measured in urologists' offices, but results are unreliable with low voided volumes (<150 mL). Peak flows less than 10 mL/second are more suggestive of outlet obstruction, whereas peak flows greater than 15 mL/second are less suggestive. Unfortunately, men can have good flows with forceful bladder contractions despite obstruction, and they can have poor flows with weak bladder contractions in the absence of obstruction.

PSA results must be interpreted with caution. Generally, a level greater than 4 ng/mL should trigger an ultrasonography-guided prostate biopsy. About 50% of men with PSA levels greater than 10 ng/mL have prostate cancer at biopsy, about 25% with levels of 4.1 to 10 ng/mL have cancer, and 15% with levels of 4 ng/mL or less have cancer. Most authorities doubt the value of early detection of nonpalpable prostate cancer in men with a life expectancy of less than 10 years or those older than 75 years with average comorbidities. However, for medicolegal reasons, it is wise to discuss the possibility of an underlying prostate cancer with any older man who presents with lower urinary tract symptoms. A PSA level, probably by serving as a proxy for prostate size, can also help stratify the future risk of progression to surgery or acute urinary retention, with higher values predicting greater risk.

The "gold standard" test for the diagnosis of bladder outlet obstruction (Chapter 25) is the documentation of increased bladder pressure relative to urinary flow. Pressure-flow studies should be considered in men who have atypical presentations, diseases that increase their risk of primary bladder problems, or no response to adequate medical therapy.

PREVENTION
There are no documented effective strategies for the prevention of BPH. For the prevention of adverse outcomes from prostate cancer, which may present similarly to BPH, data are still evolving. A PSA level may detect prostate cancer in patients evaluated for suspected BPH, but the PSA level has relatively poor specificity in this situation. Early detection of prostate cancer with routine PSA testing may reduce prostate cancer–specific mortality somewhat, but at the expense, morbidity, and inconvenience of substantial false-positive and overtreatment rates (Chapter 207).**[1]**

TREATMENT ℞

Men with IPSSs in the mild range are rarely bothered enough by their symptoms to warrant treatment. Similarly, an enlarged prostate alone is not an indication for treatment. The key step in decision making for men with moderate or severe symptoms is to assess the degree to which the patient is bothered. The last IPSS question—"If you were to spend the rest of your life with your urinary condition just the way it is now, how would you feel about that?"—can serve as an entrée to this discussion.

For men whose symptoms cause little inconvenience, "watchful waiting" is appropriate. The patient's situation should be reassessed periodically. Avoidance of offending medications is also wise. Self-managed lifestyle changes, including fluid management (daily intake of 1500 to 2000 mL and fluid restriction before long journeys and within 2 hours of bedtime), avoiding caffeine, and the use of voiding techniques (double voiding, urethral milking, and bladder retraining) can improve symptoms and decrease the need for medical or surgical intervention substantially, at least over the short term.**[2]**

Medical Therapy
Most men with bothersome symptoms initially choose medical therapy. α_1-Adrenergic blockers and 5α-reductase inhibitors are the prescription options in the United States. When men present with symptomatic BPH, an α-blocker is a reasonable first choice for medical therapy. Finasteride or dutasteride can also be offered to men with palpably enlarged prostates or higher PSA levels for added preventive benefit. Combination α_1-adrenergic blocker and antimuscarinic therapy, though not yet approved by the Food and Drug Administration (FDA), may be effective for men with BPH symptoms related to overactive bladder; however, men need to be monitored closely for acute urinary retention, particularly during the first month of therapy.

α-Blockers (Table 131-1), which attack the dynamic component of BPH, reduce symptoms significantly, independent of prostate size, but they do not significantly reduce the risks of acute retention or progression to surgery over 4 years.**[3]** In general, doses should be increased toward the maximum until the therapeutic effect is optimal, unless side effects, including orthostatic hypotension, dizziness, and asthenia, are limiting. Tamsulosin, alfuzosin, and silodosin, which appear to be more specific for the α_{1a}-receptor subtype that dominates in the prostate, have little or no effect on blood pressure. However, because α-blocker-related dizziness and asthenia are not mediated primarily through hypotension, it is unclear whether these agents have advantages other than a lower risk of orthostatic hypotension. An intraoperative floppy iris syndrome can complicate cataract surgery in patients taking tamsulosin and other α_1-blockers; preoperative risk assessment (Chapter 439) should consider the use of these medications, but it is unclear whether discontinuation before surgery reduces the occurrence rate.

Finasteride and dutasteride are 5α-reductase inhibitors (see Table 131-1) that block the conversion of testosterone to dihydrotestosterone by the type 2 isoenzyme (finasteride) or both isoenzymes (dutasteride). Prostate size decreases by 15 to 20% over 1 year of treatment with either agent. Compared with placebo, finasteride and dutasteride reduce lower urinary tract symptoms for at least 2 to 4 years.**[4]** Although relief of symptoms may be more modest than with α-blockers in some men, dutasteride monotherapy produces more symptom relief than tamsulosin alone in men with larger prostate glands.**[5]** In addition, 5α-reductase inhibitors reduce the rate of progression to surgery or to acute urinary retention in men with larger prostates. The "number needed to treat" for 4 years to prevent an episode of acute retention or surgery is about 30 for men with PSA levels less than 1.4 ng/mL, about 20 for those with PSA levels of 1.4 to 3.2 ng/mL, and about 10 for those with PSA levels greater than 3.2 ng/mL. Given the different mechanisms of α-blockers and 5α-reductase inhibitors, it is not surprising that combination therapy is more effective than monotherapy in preventing progression of symptoms and disease.**[5]**

The main side effect of finasteride and dutasteride is sexual or ejaculatory dysfunction, which occurs in about 5% of men. Both agents lower PSA levels by about 50% but do not appear to interfere with the detection of prostate cancer if the physician mentally doubles the measured PSA and then interprets this higher value as usual. Finasteride reduces the 7-year cumulative incidence of prostate cancer from 24 to 18% in men who are heavily screened, including routine end-of-study biopsies. However, concerns about the higher risk of high-grade prostate cancer observed in this trial have not been completely allayed.**[6]**

Some short-term trials have suggested that daily use of a 5-phosphodiesterase inhibitor can reduce lower urinary tract symptoms, but these agents are not FDA approved for this purpose, and their role in the management of lower urinary tract symptoms due to BPH has yet to be defined. Although a variety of plant extracts, such as saw palmetto, have been suggested for the relief of lower urinary tract symptoms, recent results from a high-quality trial were disappointing.**[7]**

Surgical Therapy

Transurethral prostatectomy (TURP) reduces symptoms significantly more than watchful waiting or any form of medical therapy, without any greater risk of sexual dysfunction or incontinence.[8] Standard TURP, which uses a wire electrode to resect obstructing tissue, generally requires a brief hospital stay and an indwelling catheter for a few days or a week. Newer variations use a rolling electrode or laser energy to vaporize or resect prostate tissue. These procedures appear to result in less short-term bleeding and good short-term symptom improvement, but their long-term effectiveness is undefined.

Minimally invasive transurethral microwave thermotherapy (TUMT) heats and coagulates prostate tissue by using a microwave antenna surrounded by a cooling jacket to protect the urethra. Transurethral needle ablation (TUNA) uses radio frequency needles placed directly into the prostate to generate heat and cause coagulation. The mechanisms by which these treatments work are poorly understood. However, they appear to produce an initial level of symptom relief intermediate between drug therapy and TURP. Their long-term effectiveness remains unclear.

PROGNOSIS

Lower urinary tract symptoms attributable to BPH generally progress slowly over time, but individual experience varies. For example, in one study of men with symptom scores in the moderate range who elected watchful waiting, after 4 years of follow-up, 13% had only mild symptoms, 46% still had moderate symptoms, 17% had severe symptoms, and 24% had opted for surgery. The risk of acute urinary retention for such men is 1 to 2% per year. More serious complications appear to be exceedingly rare.

TABLE 131-1 MEDICATIONS USED IN THE TREATMENT OF MEN WITH LOWER URINARY TRACT SYMPTOMS ATTRIBUTED TO BENIGN PROSTATIC HYPERPLASIA

DRUG	TABLET/CAPSULE SIZE (mg)	RECOMMENDED DOSE STEPS
α-BLOCKERS		
Alfuzosin ER	10	10 mg qd
Doxazosin	1, 2, 4, 8	1, 2, 4, 8 mg qd
Doxazosin XL	4, 8	4, 8 mg qd
Silodosin	4,8	8 mg qd (4 mg qd for moderate renal impairment)
Tamsulosin	0.4	0.4, 0.8 mg qd
Terazosin	1, 2, 5, 10	1, 2, 5, 10 mg qd
5α-REDUCTASE INHIBITORS		
Finasteride	5	5 mg qd
Dutasteride	0.5	0.5 mg qd

PROSTATITIS

DEFINITION

The validity of the traditional etiology-based classification of prostatitis has never been confirmed. The current National Institutes of Health prostatitis classification system incorporates the term *chronic pelvic pain syndrome* to reflect uncertainty about whether chronic nonbacterial prostatitis and prostatodynia are actually related to the prostate (Table 131-2).

EPIDEMIOLOGY

Two million outpatient visits for prostatitis are made annually in the United States. The histologic prevalence ranges widely from 6 to 98%. The prevalence of current prostatitis-like symptoms or a previous physician's diagnosis of prostatitis is about 10%.

PATHOBIOLOGY

Both type I (acute bacterial) and type II (chronic bacterial) prostatitis account for 5 to 10% of cases. Like urinary tract infections, 80% are due to strains of *Escherichia coli*; 10 to 15% are due to *Pseudomonas aeruginosa*, *Serratia*, *Klebsiella*, and *Proteus* species; and 5 to 10% are due to enterococci. The remaining cases (>90%) are type III (chronic abacterial/chronic pelvic pain syndrome) prostatitis, for which the pathogenesis remains uncertain. Type III prostatitis is further divided into inflammatory (type IIIA) and noninflammatory (type IIIB) subtypes, based on the presence of leukocytes in expressed prostatic secretions and prostatic urine. Because there appears to be no correlation between the presence of leukocytes and symptoms, the subdivision into types IIIA and IIIB is controversial; many experts believe that both inflammatory and noninflammatory chronic prostatitis/chronic pelvic pain syndrome are the same noninfectious condition, which may or may not be related to the prostate gland.

Theories about the cause of type III prostatitis include infectious agents such as *Mycoplasma hominis*, *Ureaplasma urealyticum*, *Trichomonas vaginalis*, *Chlamydia trachomatis*, viruses, anaerobic bacteria, and coagulase-negative staphylococci; pro-inflammatory cytokines; autoimmune mechanisms; neurogenic processes; increased prostate tissue pressure; chemical irritation; and increased tension in the muscles of the bladder neck and prostatic urethra or from a tension myalgia of the pelvic floor. Psychological factors have also been implicated.

CLINICAL MANIFESTATIONS

Type I prostatitis is characterized by the acute onset of fever, chills, malaise, low back or perineal pain, and urinary symptoms, particularly dysuria, frequency, and urgency. The presentation is generally dramatic, and the patient may appear toxic. Digital rectal examination often reveals a markedly tender gland.

Type II prostatitis generally occurs in older men in association with recurrent urinary tract infections (Chapter 292). The presentation is less dramatic but involves similar lower urinary tract symptoms, pelvic pain, and sexual dysfunction. On digital rectal examination, the prostate may be normal, swollen, firm, or tender.

TABLE 131-2 CLASSIFICATION AND DEFINITION OF PROSTATITIS

Traditional Classification		National Institute of Diabetes and Digestive and Kidney Diseases Classification	
CATEGORY	DEFINITION	CATEGORY	DEFINITION
Acute bacterial prostatitis	Recovery of bacteria from prostatic fluid, purulence of fluid, and systemic signs of infectious illness (fever, chills, myalgia)	Type I (acute bacterial prostatitis)	Acute infection of the prostate
Chronic bacterial prostatitis	Recovery of bacteria in significant numbers from prostatic fluid in the absence of concomitant urinary infection or significant systemic signs (as in acute bacterial prostatitis)	Type II (chronic bacterial prostatitis) Type III (chronic abacterial prostatitis/chronic pelvic pain syndrome)	Recurrent infection of the prostate No demonstrable infection
Nonbacterial prostatitis	No recovery of significant numbers of bacteria from prostatic fluid, but the fluid consistently reveals microscopic purulence	Type IIIA (inflammatory chronic pelvic pain syndrome)	Leukocytes in semen, expressed prostatic secretions, or post–prostatic massage urine
Prostatodynia	No recovery of significant bacteria or purulence in the prostatic fluid, but patients have persistent pelvic pain and lower urinary tract symptoms	Type IIIB (noninflammatory chronic pelvic pain syndrome) Type IV (asymptomatic inflammatory prostatitis)	No leukocytes in semen, expressed prostatic secretions, or post–prostatic massage urine No subjective symptoms; detected by prostate biopsy or by the presence of leukocytes in expressed prostatic secretions or semen during evaluation for other disorders

NIH-Chronic Prostatitis Symptom Index (NIH-CPSI)

Pain or Discomfort

1. In the last week, have you experienced any pain or discomfort in the following areas?

	Yes	No
a. Area between rectum and testicles (perineum)	☐ 1	☐ 0
b. Testicles	☐ 1	☐ 0
c. Tip of the penis (not related to urination)	☐ 1	☐ 0
d. Below your waist, in your pubic or bladder area	☐ 1	☐ 0

2. In the last week, have you experienced:

	Yes	No
a. Pain or burning during urination?	☐ 1	☐ 0
b. Pain or discomfort during or after sexual climax (ejaculation)?	☐ 1	☐ 0

3. How often have you had pain or discomfort in any of these areas over the last week?

☐ 0 Never
☐ 1 Rarely
☐ 2 Sometimes
☐ 3 Often
☐ 4 Usually
☐ 5 Always

4. Which number best describes your AVERAGE pain or discomfort on the days that you had it, over the last week?

☐ ☐ ☐ ☐ ☐ ☐ ☐ ☐ ☐ ☐ ☐
0 1 2 3 4 5 6 7 8 9 10
NO PAIN   PAIN AS BAD AS YOU CAN IMAGINE

Urination

5. How often have you had a sensation of not emptying your bladder completely after you finished urinating, over the last week?

☐ 0 Not at all
☐ 1 Less than 1 time in 5
☐ 2 Less than half the time
☐ 3 About half the time
☐ 4 More than half the time
☐ 5 Almost always

6. How often have you had to urinate again less than two hours after you finished urinating, over the last week?

☐ 0 Not at all
☐ 1 Less than 1 time in 5
☐ 2 Less than half the time
☐ 3 About half the time
☐ 4 More than half the time
☐ 5 Almost always

Impact of Symptoms

7. How much have your symptoms kept you from doing the kinds of things you would usually do, over the last week?

☐ 0 None
☐ 1 Only a little
☐ 2 Some
☐ 3 A lot

8. How much did you think about your symptoms, over the last week?

☐ 0 None
☐ 1 Only a little
☐ 2 Some
☐ 3 A lot

Quality of Life

9. If you were to spend the rest of your life with your symptoms just the way they have been during the last week, how would you feel about that?

☐ 0 Delighted
☐ 1 Pleased
☐ 2 Mostly satisfied
☐ 3 Mixed (about equally satisfied and dissatisfied)
☐ 4 Mostly dissatisfied
☐ 5 Unhappy
☐ 6 Terrible

Scoring the NIH-Chronic Prostatitis Symptom Index Domains

Pain: Total of items 1a, 1b, 1c,1d, 2a, 2b, 3, and 4   = _____

Urinary Symptoms: Total of items 5 and 6   = _____

Quality of Life Impact: Total of items 7, 8, and 9   = _____

FIGURE 131-3. National Institutes of Health Chronic Prostatitis Symptom Index.

Type III prostatitis is characterized by pelvic pain, often associated with lower urinary tract symptoms and pain during or after ejaculation. Digital rectal examination findings also vary. Type IV prostatitis is, by definition, asymptomatic.

The hallmark of chronic prostatitis is a complex of symptoms that wax and wane. A brief, self-administered questionnaire (Fig. 131-3) has been developed and validated to quantify symptoms for clinical practice and research protocols.

DIAGNOSIS

Whereas acute prostatitis is relatively straightforward to diagnose, chronic prostatitis is more challenging. The symptom complexes of chronic prostatitis and BPH overlap, and BPH may be misdiagnosed in older men with chronic prostatitis. Although men can and do get both conditions, pain generally distinguishes chronic prostatitis from BPH. A PSA test is not indicated for the evaluation of chronic prostatitis; however, if a PSA test is performed and the level is found to be elevated, this should not be ascribed to chronic prostatitis/chronic pelvic pain syndrome.

Type I prostatitis is diagnosed primarily by clinical findings and a positive urine culture. Prostate massage is not recommended because of concern for precipitating bacteremia.

Type II and type III prostatitis are traditionally diagnosed with the four-glass test. This segmented, quantitative culture technique involves culturing initial-stream urine, midstream urine, expressed prostatic secretions after massage, and post–prostate massage urine. The simplified two-glass test involves culture and microscopic examination of urine obtained before and after prostate massage; it is easier for all concerned, with similar sensitivity and specificity. Type II prostatitis is characterized by the presence of uropathogenic bacteria, whereas type III prostatitis is defined by the absence of uropathogens in the setting of genitourinary pain. Type IV prostatitis is usually diagnosed incidentally by prostate biopsy or by the finding of leukocytes in prostatic secretions collected for infertility evaluations.

Differential Diagnosis

The diagnosis of type III prostatitis is challenging because it is a diagnosis of exclusion; therefore, a careful evaluation is necessary to rule out other causes of pelvic pain that may be associated with lower urinary tract symptoms and sexual dysfunction. The differential diagnosis for type III prostatitis includes BPH and prostate cancer. The patient's sexual history may suggest a sexually transmitted disease (Chapter 293), and a medical history of genitourinary instrumentation or sexually transmitted disease may suggest a urethral stricture. The physical examination may detect a hernia (Chapter 144) or a scrotal mass (Chapter 206). A urinalysis revealing hematuria should prompt evaluation for a kidney stone (Chapter 128) or bladder cancer (Chapter 203). A urine culture is important to exclude urinary tract infection (Chapter 292).

PREVENTION AND TREATMENT   **Rx**

There is no proven preventive strategy for any type of prostatitis.

Type I prostatitis is relatively easy to treat. Antibacterial agents that normally diffuse poorly into prostatic fluid work well, probably because intense inflammation enhances penetration. The choice of antimicrobial is driven by culture results. Parenteral antibiotics (e.g., ciprofloxacin 400 mg IV every 12 hours) are necessary for sicker patients, but oral fluoroquinolones (e.g., ciprofloxacin 500 mg orally every 12 hours or levofloxacin 500 mg orally daily) or trimethoprim-sulfamethoxazole (one double-strength tablet orally every 12 hours) is adequate for outpatients. Treatment for 4 weeks is generally recommended. Modification of the dosing of fluoroquinolones is advised in patients with renal impairment.

Type II prostatitis is more difficult to treat because prostatic fluid becomes alkaline with chronic inflammation, reducing antibiotic penetration. The fluoroquinolones (e.g., ciprofloxacin 500 mg orally every 12 hours or levofloxacin 500 mg orally daily) and trimethoprim-sulfamethoxazole (one double-strength tablet orally every 12 hours) penetrate the prostate, but the penicillins, cephalosporins, aminoglycosides, and nitrofurantoin do not. The duration of treatment is generally 4 weeks.

Type III prostatitis often engenders frustration on the part of the physician and confusion and dissatisfaction on the part of the patient. Because the cause is unknown, affected men receive various empirical therapies. Antibiotics, α-blocker therapy, and pregabalin have not been beneficial.[9,10]

For type IV prostatitis, no treatment is recommended.

PROGNOSIS

The untreated natural history of all types of prostatitis is poorly defined. Most patients with type I prostatitis respond well to antibiotics, but some may progress to chronic prostatitis. Complications of type I prostatitis include prostatic abscess, acute urinary retention, septicemia, and, rarely, vertebral osteomyelitis. Type II prostatitis can cause repeated urinary tract infections. Both type II and type III prostatitis have been associated with decreased fertility, although this relationship is not certain.

Grade A

1. Schröder FH, Hugosson J, Roobol MJ, et al. Screening and prostate-cancer mortality in a randomized European study. *N Engl J Med.* 2009;360:1320-1328.
2. Brown CT, Yap T, Cromwell DA, et al. Self management for men with lower urinary tract symptoms: randomised controlled trial. *BMJ.* 2007;334:25-28.
3. Djavan B, Chapple C, Milani S, et al. State of the art on the efficacy and tolerability of alpha-1 adrenoreceptor antagonists in patients with lower urinary tract symptoms suggestive of benign prostatic hyperplasia. *Urology.* 2004;64:1081-1088.
4. McConnell JD, Roehrborn CG, Bautista OM, et al. The long-term effect of doxazosin, finasteride, and combination therapy on the clinical progression of benign prostatic hyperplasia. *N Engl J Med.* 2003;349:2385-2396.
5. Roehrborn CG, Siami P, Barkin J, et al. The influence of baseline parameters on changes in international prostate symptom score with dutasteride, tamsulosin, and combination therapy among men with symptomatic benign prostatic hyperplasia and an enlarged prostate: 2-year data from the CombAT study. *Eur Urol.* 2009;55:461-471.
6. Thompson IM, Goodman PJ, Tangen CM, et al. The influence of finasteride on the development of prostate cancer. *N Engl J Med.* 2003;349:215-224.
7. Bent S, Kane C, Shinohara K, et al. Saw palmetto for benign prostatic hyperplasia. *N Engl J Med.* 2006;354:557-566.
8. Wasson JH, Reda DJ, Bruskewitz RC, et al. A comparison of transurethral surgery with watchful waiting for moderate symptoms of benign prostatic hyperplasia. *N Engl J Med.* 1995;332:75-79.
9. Alexander RB, Propert KJ, Schaeffer AJ, et al. Ciprofloxacin or tamsulosin in men with chronic prostatitis/chronic pelvic pain syndrome: a randomized, double-blind trial. *Ann Intern Med.* 2004;141:581-589.
10. Nickel JC, Krieger JN, McNaughton-Collins M, et al. Alfuzosin and symptoms of chronic prostatitis-chronic pelvic pain syndrome. *N Engl J Med.* 2008;359:2663-2673.

SUGGESTED READINGS

Anothaisintawee T, Attia J, Nickel JC, et al. Management of chronic prostatitis/chronic pelvic pain syndrome: a systematic review and network meta-analysis. *JAMA.* 2011;305:78-86. *Antibiotics and alpha blockers give the best results.*
AUA Practice Guidelines Committee. AUA guideline on management of benign prostatic hyperplasia (2010). http://www.auanet.org/guidelines-and-quality-care/clinical-guidelines.cfm?sub=bph. *Consensus guidelines.*
Lipsky BA, Byren I, Hoey CT. Treatment of bacterial prostatitis. *Clin Infect Dis.* 2010;50:1641-1652. *Review.*

132

CHRONIC KIDNEY DISEASE

WILLIAM E. MITCH

DEFINITION

Chronic kidney disease (CKD) refers to the many clinical abnormalities that progressively worsen as kidney function declines. CKD results from a large number of systemic diseases that damage the kidney or from disorders that are intrinsic to the kidney (Table 132-1). A glomerular filtration rate (GFR) persistently below 60 mL/minute/1.73 m², which is below the level of kidney function expected to occur with aging, defines clinically significant CKD.

In CKD, the damage is rarely repaired, so loss of function persists. This distinguishes CKD from acute kidney damage (Chapter 122), which can be repaired to permit the return of kidney function. The chronic loss of kidney function generates even more kidney damage and more severe clinical abnormalities. As a result, CKD progressively worsens even if the disorder that caused it becomes inactive.

CKD describes a spectrum of clinical dysfunction that ranges from abnormalities detectable only by laboratory testing to uremia. *Uremia*, which literally means "urine in the blood," results from the accumulation of unexcreted waste products and the metabolic abnormalities they induce. When the kidney fails to perform most of its functions, the clinical state is called *end-stage renal disease* (ESRD), and dialysis or transplantation is required to sustain life (Chapter 133). However, the progressive and chronic nature of CKD permits the institution of treatment strategies that can slow the loss of kidney function. In addition, many symptoms of uremia can be ameliorated or eliminated, thereby postponing ESRD.

EPIDEMIOLOGY

The increase in the number of patients with ESRD in the United States and other industrialized countries has features of an epidemic. In the United States, the prevalence of CKD continues to increase (Table 132-2). An estimated 13.1% of the U.S. population, representing about 26 million noninstitutionalized individuals older than 20 years, has stages 1 through 4 CKD, and 65% of these have stage 3 or 4 CKD. The prevalence of albuminuria is nearly 10%, representing approximately 19 million adults. Notably, the prevalence of ESRD (stage 5 CKD) has increased by 82% over the past decade or two, from nearly 800 per million persons in the U.S. population to more than 1400 persons per million.

Two disorders account for more than 70% of all new ESRD patients in the United States: 45% of patients have diabetes mellitus (Chapters 236 and 237), and 27% have hypertension-induced kidney damage (Chapter 67). The increasing prevalence of CKD is due in part to the increasing prevalence of diabetes and obesity, plus the aging of the population and an increase in the proportion of minority populations, who seem to be more susceptible to developing CKD. Other epidemiologic factors that increase the risk of progressive CKD include cardiovascular disease, smoking, albuminuria, hyperlipidemia, and a family history of CKD.

PATHOBIOLOGY

The intact nephron hypothesis helps explain the importance of GFR as a measure of remaining kidney function. The nephron consists of the glomerulus, proximal tubule, loop of Henle, distal tubule, and collecting duct. Individuals are born with 0.75 million to 1.25 million nephrons per kidney. If nephrons are lost, new ones are not regenerated. The intact nephron hypothesis maintains that each nephron functions as an independent unit, so the sum of the function of all remaining nephrons determines the whole kidney's GFR, the most accurate estimate of remaining kidney function.

Physiologic and metabolic functions of the kidney include the regulation of blood pressure, several endocrine functions, and ion concentrations in the extracellular and intracellular fluids, as well as the excretion of waste products (Table 132-3). The breadth of these functions yields several direct and derivative consequences of CKD. For example, a limitation in the ability to excrete acid causes hyperventilation and a decrease in PCO_2. In muscle, acidosis activates the ubiquitin-proteasome enzymatic process to degrade muscle protein, causing loss of muscle mass. In bone, acidosis causes loss of calcium and phosphates; this response, plus the secretion of parathyroid hormone (PTH) and decreased activation of vitamin D, demineralizes bone and makes it susceptible to fracture.

Balance and Steady-State Considerations

Metabolic balance is the state in which the intake or production of a substance equals its elimination. For example, a loss of functioning units (nephrons) impairs the ability to excrete sodium, but remaining nephrons adjust to excrete a greater fraction of the sodium filtered by each glomerulus. Similar phenomena occur in the excretion of other ions and substances, allowing the patient with CKD to avoid their accumulation. The ability to achieve balance has a limit, however; if the intake of sodium or other ions or molecules destined for excretion by the kidney is not regulated, complications of CKD will arise.

A related concept is that of steady state. A patient is in steady state when intake and production equal output and metabolism. A single parameter that integrates input and output may, if stable, be taken as indicative of a steady state. Thus, constant weight indicates that sodium intake is balancing sodium output. A steady state does not, however, indicate a normal state; for example, a patient who is grossly edematous may have a stable weight.

The Tradeoff Hypothesis

Another important principle, the tradeoff hypothesis, refers to the activation of pathophysiologic responses that produce adverse consequences. A classic example in CKD patients involves the responses activated to achieve sodium balance. Kidney damage initially reduces salt excretion, leading to sodium retention, expansion of extracellular fluid, and a rise in blood pressure.

TABLE 132-1 CAUSES OF CHRONIC RENAL FAILURE

Diabetic glomerulosclerosis*
Hypertensive nephrosclerosis
Glomerular disease
   Glomerulonephritis
   Amyloidosis, light chain disease*
   Systemic lupus erythematosus, Wegener's granulomatosis*
Tubulointerstitial disease
   Reflux nephropathy (chronic pyelonephritis)
   Analgesic nephropathy
   Obstructive nephropathy (stones, benign prostatic hypertrophy)
   Myeloma kidney*
Vascular disease
   Scleroderma*
   Vasculitis*
   Renovascular renal failure (ischemic nephropathy)
   Atheroembolic renal disease*
Cystic disease
   Autosomal dominant polycystic kidney disease
   Medullary cystic kidney disease

*Systemic disease involving the kidney.

TABLE 132-3 FUNCTIONS OF THE KIDNEY AND IMPAIRMENT OF KIDNEY FUNCTION IN PATIENTS WITH CHRONIC KIDNEY DISEASE

KIDNEY FUNCTION	CONSEQUENCES OF DYSFUNCTION
Maintain concentration and body content of electrolytes and fluid volume	Hyponatremia, hyperkalemia, low total potassium content, hypocalcemia, hyperphosphatemia, decreased tolerance to electrolyte or mineral loading
Regulate blood pressure	Hypertension, cardiovascular disease
Endocrine mediator	Anemia (low erythropoietin), hypertension (renin system activation), bone disease (secondary hyperparathyroidism), low vitamin D activation, prolonged half-lives of peptide hormones (e.g., insulin)
Waste product excretion	Anorexia, nausea, soft tissue deposition of oxalates and phosphates, neurologic dysfunction, loss of muscle protein

---

TABLE 132-2 PREVALENCE OF STAGES OF CHRONIC KIDNEY DISEASE AND FREQUENCY OF COMPLICATIONS

STAGE	DESCRIPTION	GFR* (mL/min/1.73 m²)	ADULT PREVALENCE (MILLIONS)†	SYMPTOMS OR SIGNS
1	Chronic kidney damage; normal or increased GFR	>90	3.6	Anemia 4% Hypertension 40% 5-yr mortality 19%
2	Mild GFR loss	60-89	6.5	Anemia 4% Hypertension 40% 5-yr mortality 19%
3	Moderate GFR loss	30-59	15.5	Anemia 7% Hypertension 55% 5-yr mortality 24%
4	Severe GFR loss	15-29	0.7	Hyperphosphatemia 20% Anemia 29% Hypertension 77% 5-yr mortality 46%
5	Kidney failure†	<15 or dialysis	0.5	Hyperphosphatemia 50% Anemia 69% Hypertension >75% 3-yr mortality 14%

*The formula for estimating the glomerular filtration rate (GFR) of adults with chronic kidney disease (CKD) is derived from data obtained during the National Institutes of Health Modification of Diet in Renal Diseases trial: GFR = 186 × [serum creatinine]$^{-1.154}$ × [age]$^{0.203}$ × [0.742 if patient is female] × [1.212 if patient is black].
†Rate prevalent end-stage renal disease/million; United States Renal Data System Annual Report 2008.
Results based on the CKD Surveillance 2009 Report from the Centers for Disease Control and Prevention (unpublished).

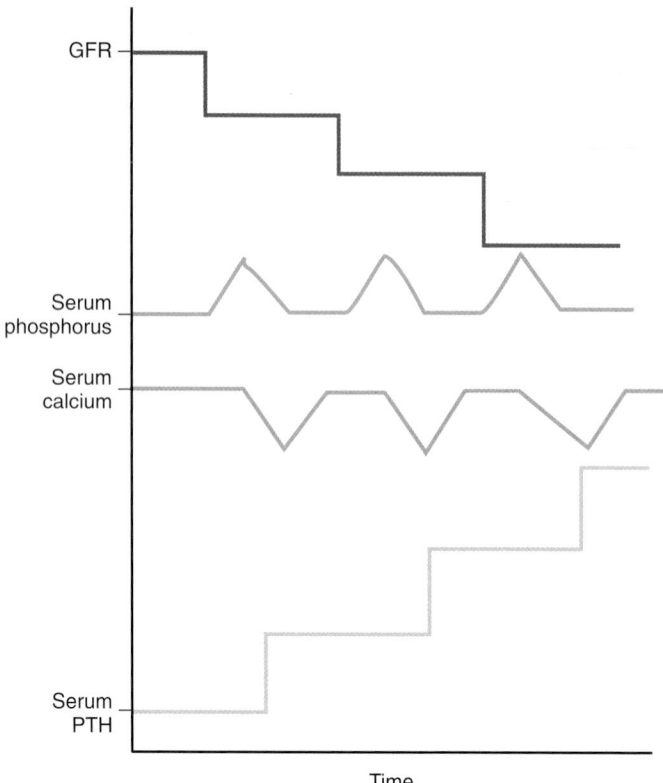

FIGURE 132-1. A decrease in glomerular filtration rate (GFR) is followed by an increase in serum phosphorus and a decrease in serum calcium. An increase in serum parathyroid hormone (PTH) returns phosphorus and calcium to normal levels.

Although a higher blood pressure initially is beneficial because it increases the filtration and excretion of sodium, the tradeoff for maintaining sodium balance is volume-dependent hypertension. Another proposal is that this increased sodium excretion is mediated by an increase in circulating Na^+, K^+-ATPase inhibitors, which increase the sodium concentration in tubular cells, reducing the cells' ability to reabsorb filtered sodium. Thus, the tradeoff for the increased ability to excrete sodium despite a loss of kidney function is that the patient loses the ability to reduce sodium excretion rapidly when salt intake is abruptly reduced. Inappropriately high salt excretion leads to loss of extracellular volume, impaired kidney perfusion, and a decrease in the GFR.

The most extensively studied tradeoff is the adaptation that stimulates secondary hyperparathyroidism (Fig. 132-1). When CKD impairs the kidney's ability to excrete phosphates, they accumulate in extracellular and intracellular fluids and lead to the physicochemical formation of calcium-phosphate complexes that reduce the level of ionized calcium. This process, in turn, stimulates the calcium-sensing receptor to increase the production and release of PTH. PTH release is beneficial because it suppresses the reabsorption of phosphates by the proximal tubule and thereby increases phosphate excretion. As the accumulation of phosphates decreases because of their excretion by the kidney, the ionized calcium rises to suppress PTH production. The tradeoff, however, is that the new steady-state levels of ionized calcium and phosphate can be maintained only as long as the circulating PTH concentration is increased (see Fig. 132-1). This higher level of PTH stimulates osteoclastic activity and leads to renal bone disease (see later).

Hypertension

Hypertension, like anemia, is almost universal in CKD patients and is often the first clinical indication of CKD. The coincidence of CKD and high blood pressure is particularly important because hypertension contributes to the development of cardiovascular disease, which is the leading cause of morbidity and mortality in CKD patients. Hypertension in CKD patients largely reflects an expanded extracellular volume owing to a salt-rich diet plus an impaired capacity to excrete sodium; activation of the renin-angiotensin-aldosterone system also plays a role. The normal response to retained sodium is an increase in extracellular volume, which raises blood pressure and increases sodium excretion, leading to a balance between sodium intake and

the excretion of salt. In the renewed steady state, however, salt balance can be maintained only as long as blood pressure is high. Two practical implications arise from these relationships. First, treatment of hypertensive patients with vasodilating drugs alone is frequently unsuccessful; when vasodilator drugs reduce blood pressure, the initial decrease in sodium excretion leads to sodium retention, expansion of extracellular volume, and a rise in blood pressure. Second, hypertension in CKD patients may not respond to diuretic therapy because a salt-rich diet can cancel the benefits of diuretics even in normal adults.

Another mechanism for hypertension in CKD patients is activation of the renin-angiotensin-aldosterone system and the sympathetic nervous system, as evidenced by circulating levels of renin and aldosterone that are too high for individuals who are hypertensive. Inhibitors of the renin-angiotensin-aldosterone system slow the loss of kidney function. Evidence for activation of the sympathetic nervous system includes higher circulating levels of norepinephrine, which not only causes vasoconstriction but also suppresses the production of nitric oxide.

Endocrine Disorders

CKD, even in patients with serum creatinine values as low as 2.5 mg/dL, reduces the ability of insulin to stimulate glucose uptake by muscle and other organs, an abnormality known as *insulin resistance* (Chapter 237). The result is a transient increase in blood glucose that causes a compensatory increase in insulin release to maintain blood glucose levels near normal. In insulin-resistant CKD patients, the failure is due to a post-receptor defect in cell signaling, including an impaired ability to activate phosphatidylinositol 3-kinase and its downstream kinase Akt. The importance of this abnormality is that the reduced function of these enzymes in muscle cells impairs the metabolism of both glucose and protein, causing loss of muscle protein. Insulin resistance in nondiabetic CKD patients is generally associated with blood glucose values within the normal range; blood glucose levels rarely exceed 200 mg/dL.

One possible cause of insulin resistance in CKD is metabolic acidosis (Chapter 120). Acidosis also activates the degradation of muscle protein, impairs the ability of growth hormone to stimulate insulin-like growth factor-I (IGF-I), depresses circulating levels of thyroxine (T_4) and triiodothyronine (T_3), and increases levels of thyroid-stimulating hormone (Chapter 233). Fortunately, most of these adverse metabolic changes can be reversed simply by treating CKD patients with sodium bicarbonate or other alkalizing agents.

Another mechanism that affects endocrine status in CKD patients is the kidney's impaired ability to degrade small proteins, including several hormones. For example, diabetic CKD patients can progressively lose the ability to degrade insulin and may even develop hypoglycemia if they are treated with their usual dose of insulin. Impaired degradation of peptides by the damaged kidney can also affect the interpretation of the circulating PTH concentration because PTH is not fully degraded when the kidney is damaged; the PTH immunoassay may recognize one or more PTH fragments, which may be misinterpreted as representing excessively high levels of PTH.

In patients with stage 4 CKD, normochromic, normocytic anemia (Chapter 161) is almost universal, principally owing to impaired production of erythropoietin by interstitial cells in the kidney. However, anemia may be detected even in patients with stage 2 CKD and serum creatinine values just above the normal range. Other factors contributing to anemia in CKD patients include a shortened half-life of erythrocytes and deficiencies of vitamins and iron.

Renal Bone Disease

Renal bone disease, also called *renal osteodystrophy,* afflicts virtually all CKD patients to different degrees. Bone biopsies of patients with renal bone disease range from features indicative of increased bone turnover (i.e., greater numbers of osteoclasts, osteoblasts, and osteocytes) to abnormalities reflecting low bone turnover (i.e., reduced numbers of osteoclasts and osteoblasts and the accumulation of demineralized matrix). Patients with high bone turnover have high circulating PTH levels, whereas those with low bone turnover exhibit only a mild increase in circulating PTH. A third type of pathology is mixed uremic osteodystrophy, which has features of hyperparathyroidism and defective mineralization, presumably because increased PTH activates osteoclasts to reduce bone mass, while abnormalities in mineralization of bone result in an increase in fibrosis. Specifically, CKD produces hyperphosphatemia (see Fig. 132-1) because the intake of phosphates exceeds their excretion. Hyperphosphatemia stimulates the development of renal bone disease in two ways. First, the physicochemical interaction between phosphates and "free" or ionized calcium lowers the level of ionized calcium and reduces the interaction between calcium and the calcium receptor. Decreased activation of the calcium receptor causes the parathyroid gland to hypertrophy and PTH production to rise; it also stimulates osteoclast activity, resulting in loss of bone mass. Second, hyperphosphatemia acts directly on the parathyroid glands to stimulate PTH production. Other factors that contribute to CKD-induced bone disease include defects in cellular signaling by the calcium receptor and changes in vitamin D metabolism.

A G protein–coupled plasma membrane protein present in chief cells of the parathyroid gland and in certain renal tubular cells responds directly to calcium ions. The interaction of this receptor with calcium or with cinacalcet, which is a small, orally available molecule that activates the calcium receptor, suppresses the expression and release of PTH from parathyroid chief cells. In contrast, hyperphosphatemia and a decreased level of circulating ionized calcium increase the production and release of PTH (see Fig. 132-1). These responses can be negated by cinacalcet because it effectively suppresses the production and release of PTH even when there is hyperphosphatemia and decreased ionized calcium. Consequently, use of this drug requires careful monitoring to avoid hypoparathyroidism and even hypocalcemia.

Another factor that regulates the circulating calcium level and plays a role in the development of renal bone disease is vitamin D. The activation of vitamin D proceeds by repeated hydroxylation of the parent molecule, cholecalciferol (vitamin D_3). The initial hydroxylation occurs in the liver, where 25-hydroxyvitamin D_3 is formed. This form of vitamin D stimulates the absorption of calcium and phosphates from the intestines and is believed to change the function and metabolism of muscle and possibly other organs by mechanisms that are poorly defined. Moreover, recent evidence indicates that CKD patients who have low circulating values of 25-hydroxyvitamin D_3 experience an increase in the risk of all-cause mortality, thereby supporting the conjecture that the function of 25-hydroxyvitamin D_3 extends beyond serving as a precursor for the most active vitamin D, calcitriol.

Calcitriol is produced when a 25-hydroxycholecalciferol 1α-hydroxylase in the proximal tubules of the kidney hydroxylates 25-hydroxyvitamin D_3. The activity of 1α-hydroxylase changes in response to factors that regulate mineral metabolism: for example, its activity is decreased by hyperphosphatemia, and the decrement in calcitriol decreases the intestinal absorption of calcium and phosphates. However, the β-glucuronidase klotho confers the tissue specificity of fibroblast growth factor-23 (FGF-23), a hormone that increases the renal excretion of phosphates. Both klotho and FGF-23 are involved in the regulation of calcitriol production, but exactly how these factors influence the development of renal bone disease has not been defined.

Because the 1α-hydroxylase enzyme is expressed mainly in proximal tubule cells, progressive loss of kidney function causes calcitriol deficiency. This deficiency, in turn, results in impaired absorption of both calcium and phosphates from the intestine; the resulting decrease in calcium should stimulate 1α-hydroxylase activity to produce more calcitriol. If this is not possible because of a decrease in proximal tubular function, serum calcium decreases, thereby increasing PTH production. Depressed calcitriol production also can augment PTH production by reducing the level of vitamin D receptor in the parathyroid gland, promoting the development of hyperparathyroidism even before hypocalcemia has developed.

Soft tissue calcification, which is the deposition of calcium phosphate crystals and inflammation in the vessels and soft tissues, is common when the product of the concentrations of serum calcium and phosphorus exceeds 60 mg^2/dL^2, but it can occur with lower levels. The deposition of crystals seems to be linked most closely to an increase in the local concentration of phosphates, emphasizing why the serum phosphorus level should be kept in the normal range.

Accumulation of Uremic Toxins

In diets containing protein-rich foods, protein is metabolized to amino acids that can be used to build body protein stores (Fig. 132-2). Alternatively, the amino acids are metabolized to form urea or potentially toxic products that are excreted when kidney function is normal. The serum creatinine level is determined by the degree of renal insufficiency and the rate of creatinine production, which is proportionate to lean body mass. As a result, a serum creatinine concentration of 1.4 mg/dL in an adult with a small muscle mass signifies a much greater loss of kidney function than it does in an individual with a large muscle mass. In addition, the amount of creatinine excreted in 24-hour urine collections can vary by up to 25%, making creatinine clearance of limited use in determining the degree of kidney damage in CKD patients.

FIGURE 132-2. The breakdown of dietary protein enlarges the pool of essential and nonessential amino acids that can be used to synthesize body protein. Protein breakdown also increases the production of urea and other nitrogenous waste products, and it is accompanied by the increased intake of inorganic ions that must be excreted.

Because creatinine is formed from creatine, which is highly concentrated in muscle, extensive cooking of dietary meat converts creatine to creatinine. Consequently, eating a meal containing a large amount of well-cooked meat raises the amount of creatinine excreted. Even if meat and high-protein foods are eliminated from the diet of CKD patients, at least 4 months are required to reach a new steady state. In terms of extrarenal creatinine clearance, the degradation rate of creatinine, presumably by bacteria in the gut, is so small that it is virtually undetectable in patients with normal kidney function; when serum creatinine rises above 5 mg/dL, however, degradation can contribute to creatinine clearance.

With CKD, the accumulation of peptides (also known as *middle molecules*) is associated with disorders that range from the induction of anorexia to neurologic abnormalities. Another potential toxin is indoxyl sulfate, a product of tryptophan metabolism; it has been linked to progressive kidney damage and the symptoms of uremia. High uric acid levels, which are related to excess protein intake, can cause gout (Chapter 281) and may be linked to the development of hypertension and inflammatory responses in blood vessels. Besides generating potentially toxic metabolites, diets containing protein-rich foods also increase the intake of phosphates, sodium, potassium, acid, and other ions that must be eliminated.

Ideally, circulating levels of uremic toxins should be monitored, but measuring these levels is not practical. The blood urea nitrogen (BUN), however, provides an index of the level of uremic toxins because the production of urea is directly proportional to the metabolism of proteins and hence the production of other unexcreted waste products (see Fig. 132-2). Thus, the load of waste product production can be approximated from the 24-hour excretion of urea nitrogen as long as the patient is in the steady state (i.e., BUN concentration and body water are stable). In general, the ratio of BUN to serum creatinine is 10 : 1 in normal adults or CKD patients. When the BUN concentration is below this ratio, it can be concluded that the patient is eating a protein-restricted diet. If the BUN concentration exceeds 10 times the serum creatinine concentration, three possibilities should be considered. First, the patient may have gastrointestinal bleeding or may be suffering from a severely catabolic condition (e.g., trauma or high-dose glucocorticoid administration). Second, the patient may be eating excessive amounts of protein, yielding more urea than the impaired kidney can excrete. Finally, there may be extracellular volume depletion with active proximal tubular reabsorption of sodium and fluid and concomitant passive reabsorption of urea; the result is a rise in BUN. The corollary is that a decrease in urea production is associated with a decrease in the load of uremic toxins. For this reason, the production of urea should be kept to a minimum that is consistent with maintaining body protein stores. To accomplish this goal, the dietary content of protein should be monitored and manipulated to decrease urea production (see later).

Progression of Chronic Kidney Disease

Persistence of diseases affecting the kidney (e.g., diabetes or inflammatory conditions such as systemic lupus erythematosus) is not the only factor that determines the rapidity of the loss of kidney function. Even when the disease that initially damaged the kidney is no longer active, kidney function continues to decline, probably because systemic hypertension, hemodynamic injury

TABLE 132-4   ANGIOTENSIN II RESPONSES IN CHRONIC KIDNEY DISEASE*

Hemodynamic responses
  Systemic hypertension
    Vasoconstriction
    Salt retention (aldosterone)
    Intraglomerular hypertension
    Efferent arteriolar vasoconstriction
Nonhemodynamic responses in the kidney
  Macrophage infiltration and inflammation
  Interstitial matrix accumulation
    Increased transforming growth factor-β
    Increased plasminogen activator inhibitor type 1
    Increased aldosterone

*Includes the proposed actions of angiotensin II that can contribute to the development of cardiovascular disease and progressive loss of kidney function.

TABLE 132-5   COMPLICATIONS OF CHRONIC KIDNEY DISEASE

AFFECTED SYSTEM	CAUSE OR MECHANISM	CLINICAL SYNDROME
Systemic symptoms	Anemia, inflammation	Fatigue, lassitude
Skin	Hyperparathyroidism, calcium-phosphate deposition	Rash, pruritus, metastatic calcification
Cardiovascular disease	Hypertension, anemia, homocysteinemia, vascular calcification	Atherosclerosis, heart failure, stroke
Serositis	Unknown	Pericardial or pleural pain and fluid, peritoneal fluid
Gastrointestinal	Unknown	Anorexia, nausea, vomiting, diarrhea, gastrointestinal tract bleeding
Immune system	Leukocyte dysfunction, depressed cellular immunity	Infections
Endocrine	Hypothalamic-pituitary axis dysfunction	Amenorrhea, menorrhagia, impotence, oligospermia, hyperprolactinemia
Neurologic	Unknown	Neuromuscular excitability, cognitive dysfunction progressing to coma, peripheral neuropathy (restless leg syndrome or sensory deficits)

to the kidney, proteinuria, and accumulation of nephrotoxins all contribute to progressive damage.

The belief that hypertension causes progressive loss of kidney function is based on several observations. First, hypertension alone can damage the kidney; malignant hypertension damages the endothelial cells of the afferent arteriole and the glomerulus and may even cause thrombosis in these vessels. Second, chronic hypertension is frequently associated with ischemic injury to glomeruli owing to transmission of the blood pressure into the afferent arteriole and glomerulus, causing glomerulosclerosis. Third, the degree of hypertension is directly correlated with the rate of loss of kidney function. Fourth, effective treatment of hypertension slows the progression of CKD. Although it is sometimes difficult to determine the extent to which hypertension is a cause or an effect of CKD in an individual patient, hypertension is strongly associated with progressive kidney injury and with the development of cardiovascular disorders.

Experimentally, angiotensin II–related, progressive glomerular damage (Table 132-4) arises from preferential constriction of the glomerular efferent arteriole to a greater extent than in the afferent arteriole. The imbalance in arteriolar vasoconstriction increases intracapillary pressure and tends to raise glomerular filtration (the hyperfiltration mechanism), but the tradeoff for any increase in GFR is damage to glomerular capillaries. Because angiotensin II is the mediator of preferential efferent arteriolar constriction, angiotensin-converting enzyme (ACE) inhibitors and angiotensin receptor blockers (ARBs) may prevent both hyperfiltration and damage to the kidney.

The benefits of treatment with ACE inhibitors or ARBs may extend beyond reducing hyperfiltration. Angiotensin II has growth factor properties, and it activates transforming growth factor-β, plasminogen activator inhibitor type 1, and other cytokines, thereby aggravating interstitial damage to the kidney (see Table 132-4). Aldosterone may also contribute to the development of interstitial damage and collagen deposition in the kidney. However, blocking the actions of aldosterone can cause hyperkalemia.

Patients receiving ACE inhibitor or ARB treatment experience a reduction in albuminuria, presumably because of a decrease in the pressure within glomeruli. Experimental evidence suggests that albumin or some component of albumin (e.g., lipids or molecules bound to albumin) may injure kidney cells; therefore, reducing albuminuria may be directly beneficial. Because the degree of albuminuria is related to the rapidity of the loss of kidney function, reducing albuminuria is a treatment goal.

CLINICAL MANIFESTATIONS

Unfortunately, progressive loss of kidney function produces no clinically distinct signs or symptoms. Findings that should raise the possibility of CKD include urinary abnormalities, such as hematuria or repeated urinary infections, or the appearance of hypertension and/or edema. The possibility of CKD should also be considered in patients with chronic hypertension, diabetes, or albuminuria and those with a family member with CKD.

As the GFR declines, clinical abnormalities become more frequent. Even when CKD is advanced (stage 4; see Table 132-2), however, the symptoms are mostly nonspecific. Some patients complain only of exercise intolerance, fatigue, or anorexia. If these symptoms are present, serum creatinine and BUN levels should be measured, and the urine should be examined for albuminuria. As CKD progresses, patients frequently have anemia, metabolic acidosis, hyperkalemia, hyperphosphatemia, hypocalcemia, and

hypoalbuminemia, each of which can be associated with specific symptoms (Table 132-5).

Specific syndromes are associated with proteinuria and CKD. For example, severe albumin losses (>3 g/day) plus edema and hypercholesterolemia define the nephrotic syndrome (Chapter 123), which can lead to the loss of the relatively small (59 kD) vitamin D–binding protein plus the attached 25-hydroxyvitamin D_3, thereby aggravating bone disease. Advanced proteinuria can also be associated with losses of clotting factors IX, XI, and XII, causing coagulation defects (Chapter 177). Conversely, urinary losses of antithrombin III can result in thrombosis (Chapter 174), especially when inflammation-induced increases in the levels of acute phase reactant proteins lead to hyperfibrinogenemia.

Bone Disease and Extraosseous Calcification

Some patients with renal bone disease complain of vague, ill-defined pain in the lower back, hips, knees, and other locations. Advanced bone disease can cause such severe pain that it impairs the ability to exercise, aggravating the tendency to lose muscle mass. With advanced renal bone disease, minimal trauma may produce fractures.

Another clinical syndrome related to renal bone disease is the development of vascular calcification, which causes vascular stiffness and increases systolic blood pressure, thereby participating in the development of left ventricular hypertrophy. A more disabling manifestation is the development of calcifications in the tunica media of blood vessels (i.e., Mönckeberg's sclerosis) as well as calcifications that impair the function of multiple organs, including the lungs, myocardium, and skin. Calcification of the skin and cutaneous vessels is seen in the syndrome of calciphylaxis.

DIAGNOSIS

If CKD is suspected, emphasis should be placed on eliciting a history of hypertension, urinary abnormalities, and treatment with drugs that might affect kidney function (Chapter 122). The family history should focus on the presence of family members with kidney diseases, kidney stones, or surgery involving the urinary tract, as well as diabetes and hypertension. The physical examination should include lying and standing blood pressure measurements in both arms and a search for findings associated with CKD, such as skin abnormalities, persistent itching, a palpable polycystic kidney (Chapter 129), evidence of decreased lean body mass, peripheral edema, and neurologic abnormalities.

Staging

The severity of CKD is divided into five stages according to persistent reductions in estimated GFR (see Table 132-2). Two assessments of impaired kidney function are necessary: GFR and degree of albuminuria. Generally, the GFR can be estimated based on the serum creatinine level, age, body weight, gender, and race (see Table 132-2). The serum creatinine concentration is influenced by both kidney function and creatinine production, and the latter is directly proportional to lean body mass plus a small contribution from dietary meat. Notably, the serum creatinine concentration can remain in the nominally normal range until as much as 50% of kidney function is lost. Consequently, an elevated serum creatinine level means that both kidneys are functioning inadequately and that more than 50% of nephrons and nearly 50% of kidney function have been lost. By itself, the serum creatinine level is too variable to be used as a measure of GFR, but repeated values can be used to assess how rapidly changes in GFR are occurring. For example, changes in the reciprocal of the creatinine level (1/serum creatinine) yield a linear relationship with the rate of GFR loss (Fig. 132-3). Deviations from linearity signal a change in the course of CKD.

Other methods of estimating kidney function are not as accurate. For example, the BUN concentration is determined not only by the remaining kidney function but also by the amount of protein in the diet.

A careful microscopic examination of the urine is critical. Erythrocytes and erythrocyte casts in urine sediment are consistent with glomerulonephritis (Chapter 123), fine granular casts plus protein suggest diabetic kidney disease (Chapter 126), leukocytes plus fine and coarse granular casts suggest interstitial nephritis (Chapter 124), and eosinophils in the urine suggest a drug reaction with interstitial damage (Chapter 124).

Microalbuminuria is defined as 30 to 300 mg albumin/24 hours or 30 to 300 mg albumin/g creatinine in an initial morning urine specimen. Albuminuria is defined as excretion rates that are greater than those of microalbuminuria. The measured magnitude of albuminuria in a 24-hour urine collection depends on a full collection. An equally accurate alternative is to measure the ratio of albumin to creatinine concentrations in the first morning urine specimen on 3 separate days.

The urea nitrogen content of the 24-hour urine collection also allows calculation of the amount of dietary protein, which is composed of 16% nitrogen (see Fig. 132-2; Table 132-6). When the amount of urea nitrogen excreted in the steady state (i.e., when weight and BUN are stable) is added to the nonurea nitrogen excreted daily—which can accurately be estimated as 0.031 g nitrogen/kg ideal body weight/day—total daily nitrogen excretion can be calculated. If the total amount of nitrogen excreted exceeds the nitrogen contained in the prescribed diet, possibilities include dietary nonadherence, gastrointestinal bleeding, or a catabolic illness.

Other Laboratory Tests

Blood chemistries that evaluate the consequences of CKD include concentrations of sodium, potassium, chloride, bicarbonate, calcium, and phosphorus, as well as uric acid levels. The blood glucose level and hemoglobin A_{1c} level should be monitored in diabetics, and serum complement levels should be measured in patients with inflammatory diseases of the kidney. The hematocrit and/or hemoglobin level should be assessed and monitored because anemia often appears with even mild renal dysfunction and tends to progress as CKD progresses, owing to reduced erythropoietin production and/or iron deficiency. Iron deficiency can be recognized if the serum iron level is low, the serum ferritin concentration is less than 200 ng/mL, and the transferrin saturation level is less than 20% (Chapter 162). To detect CKD-induced bone disease, levels of PTH, alkaline phosphatase, calcium, and phosphorus should be obtained.

Imaging

The initial evaluation should include an ultrasound examination of the kidney and bladder to ensure that there is no obstruction of urine flow (Chapter 125). Enlarged kidneys suggest that CKD is due to diabetes, HIV-associated nephropathy, or infiltrative diseases (e.g., amyloidosis). Small kidneys, especially with a shrunken kidney cortex, suggest chronic glomerular or interstitial diseases (Chapter 124). If the size of the two kidneys differs substantially, stenosis of the renal artery (Chapter 127) of the smaller kidney should be considered, especially in hypertensive patients.

TABLE 132-6	ESTIMATION OF DIETARY PROTEIN FROM 24-HOUR UREA NITROGEN EXCRETION

ASSUMPTIONS

The patient is in the steady state, and neither the serum urea nitrogen concentration nor body weight is changing; there is no edema.

The patient is in nitrogen balance, so that nitrogen intake equals nitrogen excretion. Protein is 16% nitrogen.

The nonurea nitrogen excretion (the nitrogen in urinary creatinine, uric acid, and peptides plus feces) is 0.031 g nitrogen/kg/day.

CASE 1

A 50-year-old patient with a stable weight of 70 kg is prescribed a diet containing 0.8 g protein/kg/day. His 24-hr urea nitrogen excretion is 6.8 g nitrogen/day. How much protein is he eating?

His diet should contain 70 kg × 0.8 protein/kg, or 56 g protein. His intake of nitrogen from this diet is approximately 9 g (56 g protein × 0.16 = 8.96 g nitrogen). His nitrogen excretion is 6.8 g urea nitrogen + 2.17 g nonurea nitrogen/day (70 × 0.031 g nonurea nitrogen/kg/day). The total nitrogen excretion is 8.97 g, so the patient is compliant with the prescribed diet.

CASE 2

A 40-year-old woman weighing 60 kg is confident that she is eating a diet containing 0.6 g protein/kg/day. Her 24-hr urea nitrogen excretion is 10 g nitrogen/kg/day. Does she require additional investigation?

Her diet should contain 60 kg × 0.6 g protein/kg, or 36 g protein. Therefore, her intake of nitrogen is approximately 5.8 g (36 g protein × 0.16 = 5.76 g nitrogen). Her nitrogen excretion is 10 g urea nitrogen + 1.86 g nonurea nitrogen (60 kg × 0.031 g nonurea nitrogen/kg/day). Her total nitrogen excretion is 11.9 g/day, far in excess of the amount of protein she believes she is eating. Consequently, the patient requires investigation for gastrointestinal bleeding.

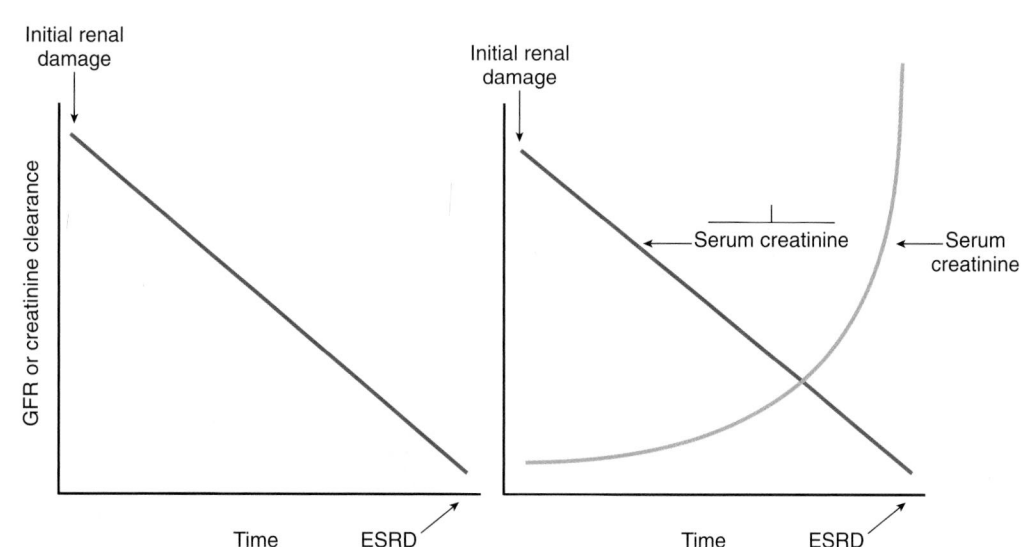

FIGURE 132-3. The course of renal insufficiency from initial renal damage to end-stage renal disease (ESRD; left panel). The course is estimated most easily by the reciprocal of serum creatinine (right panel). (Reprinted, with permission, from *Annual Review of Medicine* 35. ©1984 by Annual Reviews, www.annualreviews.org.)

TREATMENT Rx

Because the risk of developing cardiovascular disorders is increased in CKD, the first goal of treatment is to reduce blood pressure to reduce mortality.[1] Therapy with an ACE inhibitor or ARB should be started to slow the loss of kidney function.[2-4] The preferred strategy is to begin at the lower recommended doses (see Table 67-5 in Chapter 67) and titrate upward until blood pressure is controlled (usually to a goal of 130/80 mm Hg) and albuminuria is decreased. In patients with type 2 diabetes, a systolic blood pressure goal of 135 to 140 mm Hg is preferable to a goal of less than 120 mm Hg, and a blood pressure of about 140/85 mm Hg is as good as 130/80 mm Hg for reducing the progression of hypertensive renal disease.[5,6] Combining an ACE inhibitor and an ARB provides no additional benefit in terms of protecting the kidney and is associated with more frequent adverse events,[6] so this combination is not recommended. Adverse effects of ACE inhibitors or ARBs include an increase in the serum creatinine level and/or hyperkalemia, especially in patients with bilateral renal artery stenosis. In these cases, the fall in GFR is due to a lowering of intraglomerular blood pressure, which reduces albuminuria and slows the loss of GFR, not to additional kidney damage; therefore, an increase in serum creatinine concentration after starting therapy should not trigger an automatic discontinuation of ACE inhibitor or ARB therapy. However, any unexpected changes in the serum creatinine level should stimulate the consideration of progressive CKD from an increase in blood pressure, infection, drugs that adversely affect kidney function, or exacerbation of the underlying renal disease. If no other reason for a decrease in kidney function is uncovered, the ACE inhibitor or ARB treatment should be continued, but with a 50% reduction in dose.

Hyperkalemia occurs with ACE inhibitors and ARBs because reduced angiotensin II decreases the release of aldosterone. Other causes of an increase in serum potassium should be considered (e.g., treatment with nonsteroidal anti-inflammatory drugs or potassium-sparing diuretics, or an increase in

potassium-rich foods) and addressed. If needed, the addition of a loop diuretic (e.g., 40 mg furosemide when the serum creatinine level is <3 mg/dL and higher doses for more advanced CKD) may treat hyperkalemia successfully.

The blood pressure goal of 130/80 mm Hg almost always requires additional therapy, including dietary salt restriction to 2 g sodium/day. This goal is equivalent to 86 mEq sodium/day and is achievable if patients avoid salt-rich foods. For patients who develop problems with inhibitors of the renin-angiotensin system, other vasodilators, such as nondihydropyridine calcium-channel blockers (e.g., diltiazem, verapamil), seem to have fewer side effects than dihydropyridine drugs (e.g., amlodipine). Despite their ability to combat hypertension, vasodilators other than ACE inhibitors and ARBs are not as effective for reducing albuminuria, and they can cause peripheral edema. The loop diuretics are preferred for patients with more advanced CKD because they maintain renal blood flow, have few adverse effects, and, unlike thiazide diuretics, remain effective even at GFRs below 25 mL/minute. As renal insufficiency advances, high daily doses of loop diuretics (e.g., 80 to 160 mg furosemide orally) may be required to reduce extracellular volume. The dose-response relationship of loop diuretics is sigmoidal, so once a dose is identified as being effective in producing loss of edema and body weight, it should not be reduced or given in divided doses.

Stage 1 and Stage 2 Chronic Kidney Disease

In patients with stage 1 or 2 CKD, uremic symptoms are unusual because there is sufficient kidney function to control the levels of potential uremic toxins. Therapy therefore emphasizes reducing blood pressure to 130/80 mm Hg, intensive treatment of the underlying disease (e.g., normalization of blood glucose concentration in diabetic patients), and monitoring changes in albuminuria and loss of GFR (Fig. 132-4).

Dietary salt restriction is routinely recommended, and many patients require a diuretic (see Table 67-5 in Chapter 67) because an ACE inhibitor or ARB rarely controls hypertension unless steps are taken to avoid salt

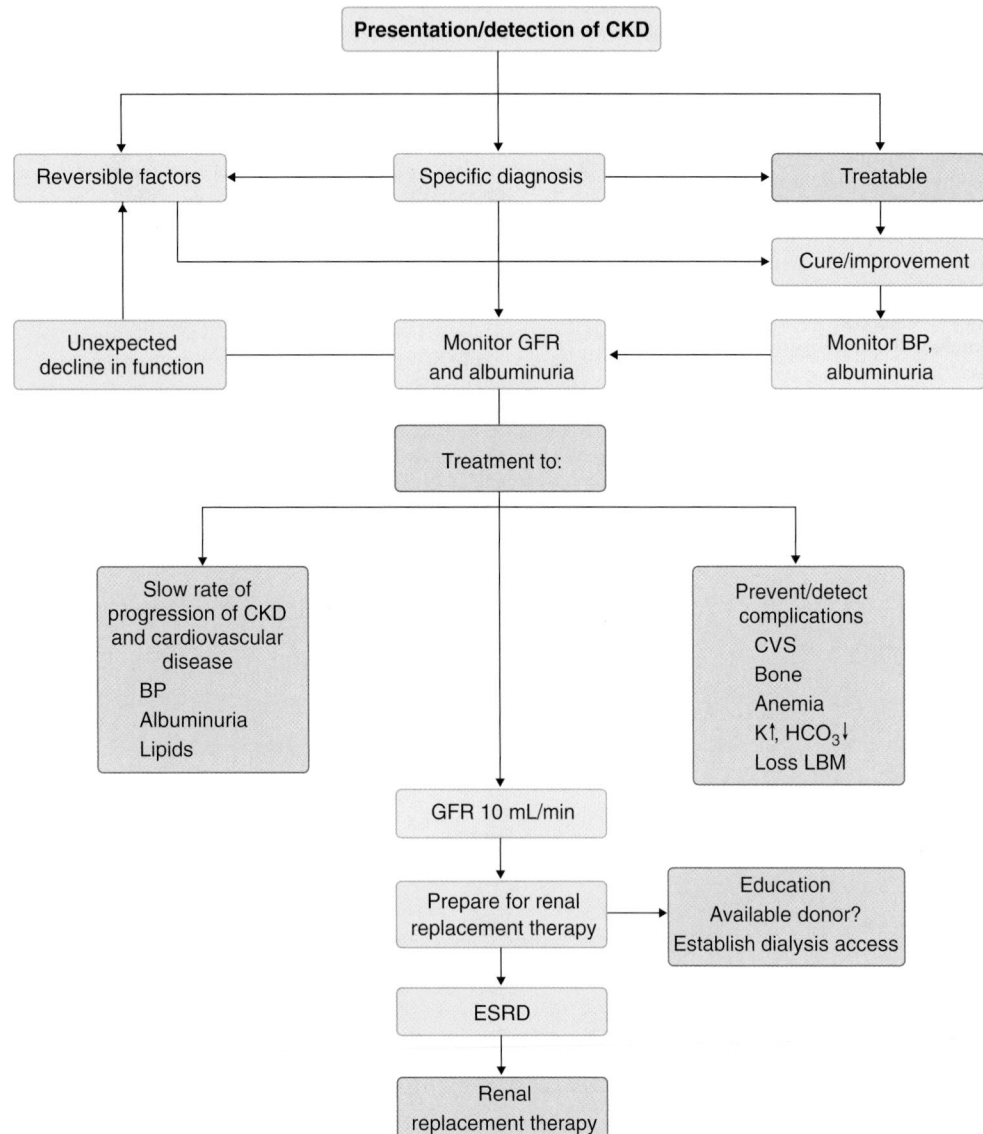

FIGURE 132-4. Management of patients in the various stages of chronic kidney disease (CKD). BP = blood pressure; CVS = cardiovascular system; ESRD = end-stage renal disease; GFR = glomerular filtration rate; LBM = lean body mass.

accumulation. A critical tactic is to monitor body weight; if weight and edema increase, it signifies salt retention. Conversely, a rapid loss of weight and edema would be the first clue that the diuretic dose should be reduced.

Stage 3 and Stage 4 Chronic Kidney Disease

Patients with stage 3 CKD should be referred to a nephrologist to maximize preventive measures and to search for remediable disorders. When stage 4 CKD is reached, a nephrologist should instruct patients about the advantages of therapies such as dialysis or transplantation (Chapter 133).

In stage 3 and stage 4 CKD, the doses of many renally excreted drugs must be adjusted downward to prevent overdosing. Treatable complications of CKD, including hypertension, secondary parathyroidism, acidosis, and uremic symptoms must be addressed. Radiologic tests with nephrotoxic contrast dye should be avoided if possible.

The development of many CKD complications (see Table 132-5) requires modification of the diet. An unrestricted high-protein diet contains an excess of salt, acid precursors, and phosphates and can lead to the development of metabolic acidosis, hyperphosphatemia, edema, hypertension, and uremic symptoms. CKD patients with any of these complications should initiate a diet consisting of 0.8 g protein/kg ideal body weight/day to maintain body protein stores and reduce the likelihood of developing other complications. Calorie intake should be limited to 30 kcal/kg ideal body weight/day for largely sedentary patients, with more for those who still exercise vigorously. If CKD-induced uremic symptoms persist, dietary protein can be restricted to a minimum of 0.6 g protein/kg/day, with a calorie intake of 30 kcal/kg/day. With either diet, successful implementation requires the advice, guidance, and close monitoring of a dietitian to take advantage of the patient's food preferences. Compliance can be monitored by measuring the 24-hour excretion of urea nitrogen (see Table 132-6), and the adequacy of protein stores should be assessed regularly by measuring body weight and serum protein levels. Although low-protein diets may not slow the loss of kidney function, they reduce uremic symptoms and can delay the need for dialysis without compromising the maintenance of protein stores.[7] Most patients on a protein-restricted diet should receive a multivitamin to sustain levels of water-soluble vitamins, but they should take fat-soluble vitamins only for documented deficiencies.

Renal Bone Disease

Treatment of renal bone disease relies on correcting the principal disorder, which is the accumulation of phosphates. This is best detected by measuring the serum phosphorus level after a normal meal. In patients with more advanced CKD (e.g., late stage 3 or stage 4) and an increased PTH level, treatment is directed at reducing the serum phosphorus level to the normal range. Because kidney damage limits the capacity to excrete phosphates, the dietary content of phosphates must be reduced to less than 1000 mg/day. If dietary restriction proves insufficient to control serum phosphorus, "phosphate binders" (see Table 121-4 in Chapter 121) should be added to the treatment regimen to promote the formation of poorly absorbed complexes of phosphates in the gastrointestinal tract. Once complexed, the phosphates are poorly absorbed by the intestine. Aluminum hydroxide binders should be avoided because they are associated with aluminum deposition in bone, where they inhibit normal bone formation and have been associated with neurotoxicity. Other phosphate binders include calcium carbonate (initially one or two 500-mg tablets with each meal), calcium acetate (initially one or two 667-mg tablets with each meal), sevelamer hydrochloride (400- to 800-mg tablets, initially 2 g/day in divided doses), or lanthanum carbonate (750 mg to 1 g/day with meals). Calcium-containing binders must be used cautiously to avoid hypercalcemia and the deposition of calcium phosphate in soft tissues. Conversely, calcium-containing agents are preferred for hyperphosphatemia in association with hyperkalemia (Chapter 119) or neuromuscular irritability, as demonstrated by a positive Trousseau's sign (Chapter 253). The non-calcium-containing phosphate binder sevelamer decreases the progression of aortic and coronary artery calcification when compared with calcium-containing binders. Lanthanum carbonate is a newer binder, and experience with this agent is more limited. For patients with serum phosphorus levels less than 6 mg/dL, calcium-based binders are generally recommended, but the dose should not exceed 2 g calcium/day to reduce the risk of soft tissue calcification. When the serum phosphorus level is higher or higher doses are required, sevelamer is the preferred phosphate binder. If the serum phosphorus level exceeds 7 mg/dL, aluminum-based binders (600 mg of concentrated aluminum hydroxide solution with each meal) can rapidly decrease the serum phosphorus level, but use of this drug should be limited to a week to avoid aluminum toxicity. In all cases, the cornerstone of therapy is to reduce phosphate intake, which generally requires dietary protein restriction because protein-rich foods contain excess phosphates.

Calcitriol, which increases the intestinal absorption of both calcium and phosphates, has the unique ability to suppress the development of hyperparathyroidism. However, calcitriol should not be given to patients who have increased circulating levels of phosphates. Low serum levels of 25-hydroxyvitamin D_3 in CKD patients are associated with increased mortality; patients with low levels of calcitriol and 25-hydroxyvitamin D_3 can be treated with

cholecalciferol 1000 units/day. Careful monitoring is needed to avoid hypercalcemia or urinary calcium values above 250 mg/day.

In a patient who develops calciphylaxis, treatment options are few and are directed mainly at reducing serum phosphorus with phosphate binders and aggressively restricting dietary phosphate. If the disorder persists despite correcting the serum phosphorus level, a trial of cinacalcet (initial dose 30 mg, increasing as needed to achieve a reduction in PTH) is warranted. With advanced calciphylaxis, successful treatment requires parathyroidectomy.

Anemia

Because of the decreased absorption of oral iron in patients with advanced CKD, ferumoxytol (two 500-mg IV injections separated by 3 to 8 days) provides a better response than oral iron supplements, with a low risk of side effects.[8] In pre-dialysis patients, treatment with erythropoietin (e.g., weekly injections of darbepoetin alfa 0.45 µg/kg) corrects anemia and improves quality of life.[9] Caution is necessary, however, because fully correcting the hemoglobin concentration has been associated with an increased risk of stroke.[10] Consequently, erythropoietin-stimulating agents should be used to maintain the hemoglobin concentration between 10 and 12 g/dL.

Atherosclerosis

The increased risk of cardiovascular complications is linked, in part, to high circulating levels of homocysteine and low-density-lipoprotein cholesterol (Chapter 51). However, interventions to reduce homocysteine have not decreased the risk of cardiovascular complications in patients with CKD. Statins have not benefited patients on dialysis but appear to benefit patients with stage 2 or early stage 3 CKD,[11] and possibly those with the nephrotic syndrome.

PROGNOSIS

Because the rate of loss of kidney function varies widely, even in patients who have the same type of kidney disease, it is critical to monitor the course of declining kidney function in each CKD patient by plotting the estimated GFR or 1/serum creatinine versus time (see Fig. 132-3). If the serum creatinine level remains unchanged after 4 months, it is likely that the rate of loss of kidney function has been slowed. Monitoring albuminuria provides additional information about the progressive loss of GFR, because the decline in GFR increases with rising degrees of albuminuria; in addition, persistent microalbuminuria, and especially albuminuria, is associated with an increased risk of cardiovascular disease and a more rapid loss of kidney function. Diabetic patients who decrease their albuminuria reduce their risk of major cardiovascular events and slow their rate of loss of kidney function.

Although population data are of limited value for the individual patient with CKD, epidemiologic studies indicate that one third of patients with stage 4 CKD (see Table 132-2) will progress to ESRD within 3 years. Dialysis or transplantation is generally required when the serum creatinine reaches 10 mg/dL; however, patients should be informed about treatment options well before this stage of CKD because the frequency of complications rises sharply when dialysis is initiated on an emergency basis.

Cardiovascular disease is the most common cause of mortality in CKD. It is present in many patients even in the early stages of kidney disease. Other contributors to the high mortality of CKD include diabetes, anemia, increased low-density-lipoprotein cholesterol levels, vascular calcification, and perhaps increased cysteine levels.

Grade **A**

1. Heerspink HJ, Ninomiya T, Zoungas S, et al. Effect of lowering blood pressure on cardiovascular events and mortality in patients on dialysis: a systematic review and meta-analysis of randomised controlled trials. *Lancet.* 2009;373:1009-1015.
2. Jafar TH, Schmid CH, Landa M, et al. Angiotensin-converting enzyme inhibitors and progression of non-diabetic renal disease: a meta-analysis of patient-level data. *Ann Intern Med.* 2001;135:73-87.
3. Hou FF, Zhang X, Zhang GH, et al. Efficacy and safety of benazepril for advanced chronic renal insufficiency. *N Engl J Med.* 2006;354:131-140.
4. Brenner BM, Cooper ME, De Zeeuw D, et al. Effects of losartan on renal and cardiovascular outcomes in patients with type 2 diabetes and nephropathy. *N Engl J Med.* 2001;345:861-869.
5. Cushman WC, Evans GW, Byington RP, et al. Effects of intensive blood-pressure control in type 2 diabetes mellitus. *N Engl J Med.* 2010;362:1575-1585.
6. Appel LJ, Wright JT, Greene T, et al. Intensive blood-pressure control in hypertensive chronic kidney disease. *N Engl J Med.* 2010;363:918-929.
7. Fouque D, Laville M. Low protein diets for chronic renal failure in non-diabetic adults. *Cochrane Database Syst Rev.* 2009;3:CD001892.
8. Lu M, Cohen MH, Rieves D, et al. FDA report: ferumoxytol for intravenous iron therapy in adult patients with chronic kidney disease. *Am J Hematol.* 2010;85:315-319.
9. Cody J, Daly C, Campbell M, et al. Recombinant human erythropoietin for chronic renal failure anaemia in pre-dialysis patients. *Cochrane Database Syst Rev.* 2001;4:CD003266.

10. Palmer SC, Navaneethan SD, Craig JC, et al. Meta-analysis: erythropoiesis-stimulating agents in patients with chronic kidney disease. *Ann Intern Med.* 2010;153:23-33.
11. Tonelli M, Keech A, Shepherd J, et al. Effect of pravastatin in people with diabetes and chronic kidney disease. *J Am Soc Nephrol.* 2005;16:3748-3754.

SUGGESTED READINGS

James MT, Hemmelgarn BR, Tonelli M. Early recognition and prevention of chronic kidney disease. *Lancet.* 2010;375:1296-1309. *Review.*
Tangri N, Stevens LA, Griffith J, et al. A predictive model for progression of chronic kidney disease to kidney failure. *JAMA.* 2011;305:1553-1559. *A predictive model incorporating age, sex, estimated GFR, albuminuria, and serum levels of calcium, phosphate, bicarbonate, and albumin effectively identifies patients who will progress to kidney failure.*

TREATMENT OF IRREVERSIBLE RENAL FAILURE

NINA TOLKOFF-RUBIN

Therapeutic options for irreversible end-stage renal disease (ESRD) include hemodialysis, peritoneal dialysis, and renal transplantation. Each of these approaches to renal replacement therapy has its unique risks and benefits. Currently, approximately 350,000 patients are on dialysis in the United States, and the ESRD population is projected to grow by about 7% per year.

The physician and the patient should recognize that these treatment modalities also can be complementary, thereby allowing flexibility of care under different clinical circumstances. The key is early identification of patients with progressive renal failure to enable them to make an educated choice that fits their lifestyle and medical situation. Careful planning can decrease emergency hospitalizations, complications, and costs. Early evaluation also enables identification of potential living donors so that preemptive transplantation can be performed.

INDICATIONS FOR RENAL REPLACEMENT THERAPY

The decision as to when to institute dialysis depends on the patient's signs and symptoms rather than an absolute level of blood urea nitrogen (BUN) or serum creatinine (Table 133-1). The benefits of early initiation of dialysis include the avoidance of malnutrition, fluid overload, and the deleterious effects of prolonged exposure to the accumulation of phosphorus, β_2-microglobulin, and other uremic toxins. However, early initiation of dialysis is no better than standard care.∎

Hyperkalemia (Chapter 119) unresponsive to diuretics, ion exchange resins, and dietary restriction in the face of electrocardiographic (ECG) changes is an absolute indication for dialysis to avoid life-threatening arrhythmias. Volume overload refractory to intravenous diuretics, increasing lethargy, difficulty concentrating, nausea, and anorexia may be manifestations of the uremic syndrome requiring dialytic therapy. Intervention should occur before the progression of uremic encephalopathy, seizures, and coma or the development of pericarditis or pericardial tamponade (Chapter 77). Emergency hemodialysis is more costly because such patients typically lack vascular access, are sicker, and often require prolonged hospitalization.

TABLE 133-1	INDICATIONS FOR DIALYSIS IN CHRONIC KIDNEY DISEASE

Uremic encephalopathy or neuropathy
Pericarditis or pleuritis
Bleeding attributable to uremia
Fluid overload refractory to diuretics
Hypertension poorly responsive to medication
Persistent hyperkalemia, metabolic acidosis, hypercalcemia, hypocalcemia, or hyperphosphatemia refractory to medical therapy
Malnutrition or weight loss
Persistent nausea and vomiting

HEMODIALYSIS

Dialysis substitutes two major renal functions: *solute removal* and *fluid removal.* In hemodialysis, solute removal occurs predominantly by diffusive clearance, which is the movement of solutes from the blood compartment to the dialysate compartment across a semipermeable membrane. Several basic principles apply. Clearance is higher for smaller molecules. The greater the concentration gradient between the blood and the dialysis solution, the more rapidly diffusion occurs. The net transfer of solute increases as membrane surface area increases. Membrane permeability is determined by the specific characteristics of the membrane, such as pore size, charge, and quaternary conformation. Higher flow rates allow greater solute removal, especially if the flow of dialysate is countercurrent to blood flow, thereby maximizing the gradient across the membrane.

Solute removal can also occur by the process of convection, the movement of solutes by bulk flow in association with fluid removal (solvent drag). Although the convective mass transfer of solutes may not play a dominant role in conventional hemodialysis, convection does play a significant role in high-flux dialysis and in continuous venovenous hemofiltration (CVVH).

Fluid removal in hemodialysis occurs by the process of ultrafiltration. The ultrafiltration rate is determined by the hydrostatic pressure gradient across the dialysis membrane, called the *transmembrane pressure.* Ultrafiltration increases if positive pressure is applied to the blood compartment or if negative pressure is applied to the dialysate side of the dialysis membrane. During dialysis, the ultrafiltration rate is adjusted to obtain the desired fluid loss.

The hemodialysis machine has three main components: (1) the dialyzer (i.e., the dialysis membrane); (2) a pump that regulates blood flow; and (3) a dialysate solution delivery system. In addition, the machine has many safety devices to monitor arterial and venous pressures, concentration of ions and temperature in the dialysate, and air and blood leaks (Fig. 133-1).

Under most circumstances, solute removal and fluid removal occur simultaneously. However, if vigorous ultrafiltration is attempted during conventional hemodialysis, patients frequently complain of muscle cramping, nausea, and vomiting. Moreover, during aggressive fluid removal systemic vascular resistance may decrease, thereby reducing blood pressure. Separating ultrafiltration from dialysis enables efficient fluid removal with greater hemodynamic stability. Osmotic changes are minimized with isolated ultrafiltration (i.e., fluid removal in the absence of solute removal). As a result, vascular resistance is well maintained, and, consequently, less hypotension occurs despite large fluid shifts.

Performing Hemodialysis
Hemodialyzers

The hollow-fiber dialyzer is composed of thousands of parallel capillary tubes. Blood flows through the capillary tubes, and dialysate flows in a countercurrent direction, bathing the outside of the capillary tubes (see Fig. 133-1). Dialysis membranes made of polycarbonate, polysulfones, polyacrylonitrile, or polymethylmethacrylate are less proinflammatory, provide better filtration rates, and improve survival compared with earlier cellulose-based membranes.

Access

To perform hemodialysis on a repetitive basis, access to the circulation is essential. An arteriovenous fistula involves anastomosis of the radial or brachial artery to the cephalic or basilic veins, with subsequent "arterialization" of the superficial forearm veins to enable blood flow rates up to 400 mL/minute. The most frequent problem is failure of the fistula to mature, particularly in patients with peripheral vascular disease or diabetes. In patients with progressive chronic kidney disease, the nondominant arm should be spared from venipuncture and a fistula should be placed in advance of the need of hemodialysis because the fistula usually takes 6 to 8 weeks to mature. Guidelines recommend elective placement of a fistula when the serum creatinine exceeds 4 mg/dL, the creatinine clearance falls to less than 25 mL/minute, or the initiation of hemodialysis is anticipated within 1 year.

Synthetic arteriovenous grafts, which can be used when a native fistula cannot be placed, have higher rates of thrombosis and infection. A third option is percutaneous dual-lumen catheters, which are placed preferentially in the internal jugular vein with a segment of the line tunneled under the skin.

Anticoagulation

Contact of patient's blood with the dialysis membrane and the tubing leads to activation of the coagulation cascade. Thrombus within the catheter can

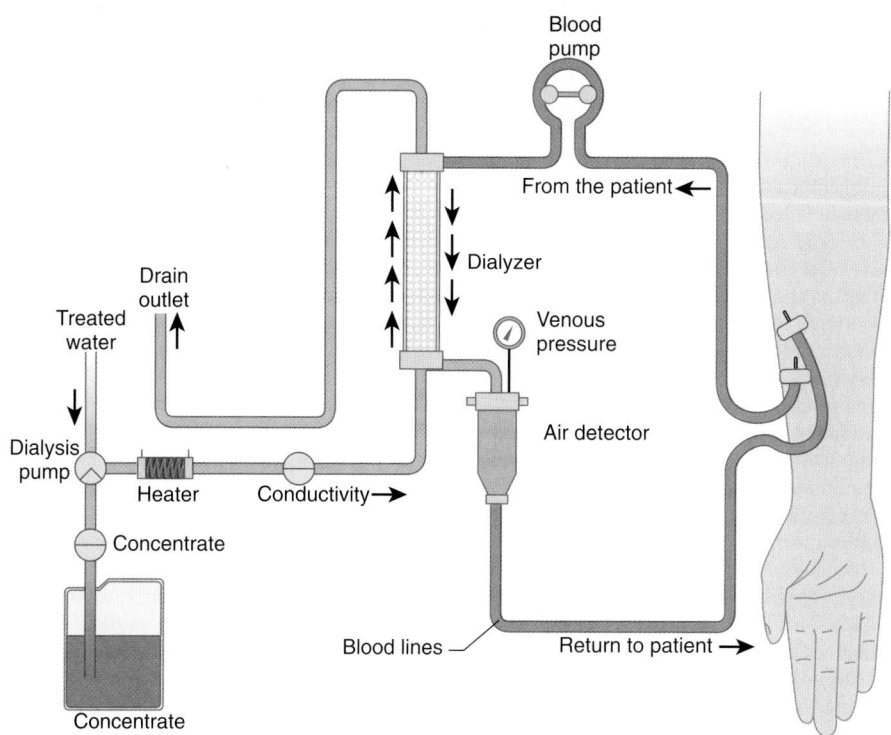

FIGURE 133-1. Hemodialysis. Treated water is mixed with concentrated dialysate. The dialysate solution flows around the fibers of the hollow-fiber dialyzer counter-current to the blood flow through the dialyzer. A computerized ultra-filtration control device regulates fluid removal (Modified from http://www.gml-dialyza.cz/Obrazky/hemodialysis.jpg.)

obstruct blood flow and also serve as a nidus for pathogens. Heparin (dosed at 500 to 1000 units/hour) is usually required to prevent clotting, but it may cause bleeding or heparin-induced thrombocytopenia (Chapter 175).

In patients at high risk for bleeding, hemodialysis can be performed without anticoagulation. Heparin-free dialysis requires a high blood flow rate and frequent flushing of the system with normal saline. Many patients also develop a procoagulant state caused by the development of anticardiolipin (Chapter 177), lupus anticoagulant antibodies, or high homocysteine levels, which may contribute to the tendency for clotting in the dialyzer and vascular access systems.

Dialysate Solution
The dialysate is a balanced solution of sodium, potassium, calcium, magnesium, chloride, and dextrose, with bicarbonate as a buffer. During dialysis, the sodium concentration is usually maintained at 135 to 140 mEq/L. A higher sodium dialysate concentration helps prevent hypotension, muscle cramps, nausea, vomiting, headaches, and seizures during hemodialysis; the sodium concentration can be programmed to return to normal range by the end of hemodialysis. Mannitol can also be used to prevent dialysis disequilibrium syndrome. The potassium concentration in the dialysate can be adjusted from 0 to 4 mEq/L but is generally maintained at 2 mEq/L in chronic outpatient dialysis centers with central delivery systems. The calcium concentration is usually 2.5 mEq/L.

Because patients are exposed to large volumes of water during each hemodialysis treatment, purity of the water is essential. A charcoal filter removes organic toxins such as chloramines, whereas reverse osmosis or de-ionization of the water effectively removes aluminum, fluoride, and copper. Chronic exposure to aluminum can lead to dialysis dementia, bone disease, and erythropoietin-resistant anemia.

Complications
Complications during Hemodialysis
In addition to vascular access problems, the most common complications during hemodialysis are hypotension, muscle cramps, nausea, vomiting, headache, and chest pain. Although excessive fluid removal is the most frequent cause of hypotension, other potential causes if the hypotension persists after fluid replacement include sepsis, myocardial ischemia, pericardial tamponade, arrhythmias, and active bleeding. Antihypertensive agents may need to be withheld before dialysis to avoid hypotension.

Air embolus, which is the most dreaded technical complication of the hemodialysis procedure (Chapter 98), presents with agitation, cough, dyspnea, and chest pain. As soon as the diagnosis is suspected, the patient

should be positioned with the left side down in an attempt to trap air in the right ventricle. One hundred percent oxygen should be administered.

Vascular Access Infections
Although tunneled lines provide immediate and convenient access to the circulation, the surrounding skin and the catheter hubs are the primary sources of bacteria. Infectious complications of the vascular access account for nearly 75% of all cases of bacteremia in the ESRD population. If a patient presents with possible catheter-related bacteremia, blood cultures should be obtained both from the catheter and from a peripheral vein.

Because most vascular access infections are caused by staphylococcal organisms (Chapter 296), which carry high rates of mortality, recurrence, and metastatic complications, empirical vancomycin, 1 g every 3 days for at least 2 weeks while monitoring blood levels, is usually used in institutions with an increased incidence of methicillin-resistant staphylococci. However, the indiscriminate and prolonged use of vancomycin should be avoided to prevent the emergence of vancomycin-resistant organisms, especially *Enterococcus* species. If the patient has any evidence of systemic sepsis with hemodynamic instability, the line should be pulled promptly and reinserted only after blood cultures are negative for at least 48 hours and the patient has defervesced. In the interim, dialysis can be performed femorally or through a temporary nontunneled catheter.

In patients with a prompt response to antibiotic therapy, antimicrobial agents should be administered for at least 2 to 3 weeks. A prolonged course of antibiotic therapy (4 to 8 weeks) is recommended if there is persistent bacteremia or fungemia after catheter removal or if there is evidence of endocarditis (Chapter 76), septic arthritis (Chapter 280), osteomyelitis (Chapter 296), epidural abscess (Chapter 421), or other metastatic infection.

Long-Term Complications in Hemodialysis
Anemia
The development of a normochromic normocytic anemia (Chapter 161) parallels the progression of chronic kidney disease, and almost two thirds of patients who start dialysis have hematocrit levels less than 30% and hemoglobin levels less than 10 g/dL. Decreased erythropoietin production is the major cause, but contributing factors include a shortened life span of red blood cells, uremic inhibitors of erythropoiesis, iron deficiency owing to poor iron absorption, gastrointestinal bleeding, loss of blood with frequent blood sampling, and losses during hemodialysis. Folic acid is removed by dialysis, so folate replacement is necessary. Infection, inflammation, malignancy, and high parathyroid hormone levels can also inhibit red blood cell maturation. Aluminum toxicity, either from aluminum contamination of the

water supply or through the use of aluminum-containing phosphate binders, has been associated with microcytic anemia in dialysis patients with normal iron stores.

Erythropoietin

The administration of erythropoietin (50 to 100 U/kg intravenously three times weekly depending on the baseline hemoglobin level), together with repletion of iron stores, folic acid supplementation, and treatment of concomitant infection, is effective in correcting the anemia of chronic renal disease. The target hemoglobin level, with or without the use of erythropoietin, should be no higher than 12 g/dL because a number of studies have shown that higher levels are associated with increased mortality rates, particularly due to cardiovascular events and strokes.[2] Failure to provide an adequate supply of iron is the most common cause of erythropoietin treatment failure. The best way to replenish the iron stores in dialysis patients is intravenous iron (Chapter 162). A transferrin saturation level (serum iron ÷ total iron-binding capacity × 100%) of less than 20% and a ferritin level of less than 100 ng/mL are indications for intravenous iron therapy in dialysis patients. Erythropoietin resistance also occurs in the presence of ongoing infection, inflammation, hyperparathyroidism, or aluminum toxicity.

Malnutrition

Hypoalbuminemia is associated with an increased mortality among patients undergoing dialysis. Patients with an albumin level of less than 3.0 g/dL have a 2-year mortality rate of up to 40%, in comparison with the expected mortality rate of 20%. Marked catabolism, anorexia, and severe diet limitations during the predialysis period lead to loss of lean weight. After the initiation of dialysis, patients usually have an improved appetite, and their protein intake should be at least 1.2 g/kg per day for a total caloric intake of 35 cal/kg/day. Water-soluble vitamins, including folic acid, need to be replaced because they are depleted during dialysis.

Chronic Kidney Disease and Cardiovascular Disease

Cardiovascular disease, which is the most important cause of death among patients with chronic kidney disease, accounts for approximately 50% of the deaths among patients on dialysis and among recipients of renal allografts. Two thirds of patients with chronic kidney disease have diabetes mellitus or hypertension, but the rates of cardiovascular disease and mortality are also elevated among patients with primary renal diseases such as glomerulonephritis. Among patients younger than 45 years of age, cardiac mortality is 100 times greater than in the general population.

In patients initiating dialysis, the main cardiac abnormality is left ventricular hypertrophy. A number of studies have shown a direct correlation between an elevated serum phosphorus concentration (>5.5 mg/dL), a calcium-phosphorus product (Ca × P) greater than 56, and mortality in hemodialysis patients. A striking degree of coronary and aortic calcification has been demonstrated in young adults with ESRD using electron-beam tomography (Chapter 56). These findings have led to a decrease in the use of calcium-versus non-calcium-containing phosphate binders, such as sevelamer and lanthanum carbonate.

Decreased synthesis of the active principal form of vitamin D (1,25-[OH]$_2$D$_3$) contributes to the secondary hyperparathyroidism of dialysis patients, and pulse-dose intravenous activated vitamin D is used to suppress synthesis of parathyroid hormone (PTH) directly and to prevent skeletal complications. However, randomized trials are needed because the aggressive use of vitamin D analogues may also increase vascular calcification or ossification. Recent retrospective studies suggest that therapy with pulse-dose activated vitamin D improves the survival of patients undergoing chronic hemodialysis and that paricalcitol in particular may provide a survival advantage over calcitriol.

Renal Osteodystrophy

Three forms of bone disease are seen in patients with renal failure. *Osteitis fibrosa cystica* is a condition in which there is increased bone turnover owing to secondary hyperparathyroidism. *Osteomalacia* (Chapter 252) is characterized by an increase in unmineralized bone (widened osteoid seam) as well as low bone turnover. *Adynamic bone disease* is a condition in which there is low bone turnover. Although bone biopsy remains the gold standard for determining the form of renal-associated bone disease, the diagnosis is typically made chemically, guided by serum PTH, calcium, phosphorus, and alkaline phosphatase, as well as the clinical scenario.

At present, adynamic bone disease is the principal bone lesion in dialysis patients, mostly as a result of oversuppression of PTH with overzealous use of calcium-containing binders and vitamin D analogues. Fractures and hypercalcemia can occur. Adynamic bone disease, defined by bone biopsy or intact serum PTH less than 100 picograms/mL, is treated by allowing the PTH to rise by avoiding calcium-containing binders and vitamin D analogues and by using non-calcium-containing phosphate binders, such as sevelamer or lanthanum, to control hyperphosphatemia.

Dialysis Dose

The time-averaged concentration of urea and nutritional status, as determined by protein catabolic rate, is an important determinant of morbidity and mortality in hemodialysis. It is better for patients to be dialyzed longer and be well nourished than to have a low BUN value and be dialyzed for shorter periods. The prescription of hemodialysis is tailored to the patient's size and protein intake. The best method for determining the adequacy of hemodialysis is urea kinetic modeling, a dimensionless formula that determines the fractional urea clearance per treatment normalized to the volume of urea distribution. K is the dialyzer clearance, t is the time (duration) of dialysis therapy, and V is the volume of distribution of urea, which is approximately equal to the total body water. When supplied with simple clinical information (predialysis and postdialysis weights, ultrafiltration volume, hematocrit, and predialysis and postdialysis BUN, as well as the dialyzer clearance), computer software programs perform the calculation. Guidelines recommend a single pool Kt/V greater than 1.2 to minimize uremic complications and hospitalizations. Increasing the chronic dose of dialysis beyond a Kt/V of 1.4 does not appear to increase survival,[3] but chronic hemodialysis six times per week generally improves outcomes compared with conventional hemodialysis three times per week.[4] Similarly, nocturnal hemodialysis, performed six or seven nights a week at home for 6 to 8 hours, improves solute clearance, controls serum phosphate, and provides excellent blood pressure control with a reduction in medication requirements.[5] It also can improve kidney-specific measures of quality of life.[6] A family member can help perform the treatment, or the patient can be monitored at a central station through closed-circuit television. This intensive dialysis modality may be a bridge to transplantation or a long-term option when the patient is not a transplantation candidate.

Continuous Renal Replacement Therapy

Critically ill patients with renal failure are frequently hemodynamically unstable, are hypercatabolic (e.g., sepsis, severe burns, brain injury, liver failure, trauma), and require large amounts of fluids (e.g., nutrition, antibiotics). Standard hemodialysis may be complicated by hypotension, in part owing to rapid fluid and solute removal. Slow, low-efficiency hemodialysis performed with low blood flows for 6 to 8 hours daily is one alternative for unstable dialysis patients with renal failure. However, patients with liver failure, traumatic brain injury, or coma do not tolerate the rapid osmolarity changes produced by hemodialysis, which can cause severe brain edema and herniation. In contrast, during CVVH, the rate of fluid removal through venovenous filtration is slower, and solute clearance relies on convection (solvent drag) rather than diffusion, which does not cause such acute changes in osmolarity.

CVVH requires central venous access (double-lumen catheter) and blood flows between 150 and 200 mL/minute. Blood under pressure passes down one side of a highly permeable membrane, thereby allowing both water and solutes up to a molecular weight of about 60 kD to pass across the membrane. In contrast to hemodialysis, urea, creatinine, and phosphate are cleared at similar rates (convective clearance) during hemofiltration. The filtrate is discarded, and the fluid lost is partially replaced with a solution containing the major crystalloid components of the plasma at physiologic levels. However, if further clearance is needed in highly catabolic patients, diffusive dialysis (CVVH) can be added by passing dialysis solution through the dialysate compartment.

Heparin anticoagulation (500 to 1000 U/hour) is usually required to maintain the patency of the CVVH circuit, except in patients who are at high risk for bleeding. An effective method of regional anticoagulation is the use of a calcium-free citrate replacement fluid administered in a separate central line before filtration; citrate chelates calcium in the blood, thereby preventing clotting of the hemofilter. If the patient cannot metabolize citrate, usually because of liver failure, an anion gap metabolic acidosis will develop. The presence of a low ionized calcium and a high total calcium level also is a clue indicating citrate toxicity. Patients who have liver failure and contraindications to heparin often can tolerate CVVH without anticoagulation using bicarbonate-containing replacement solution.

Presently, there is no evidence from randomized trials that demonstrates that CVVH offers a survival advantage compared with intermittent hemodialysis in patients with acute renal failure, despite the advantages of CVVH in enabling the removal of large amounts of fluid with improved hemodynamic stability and excellent metabolic and acid-base control. Increasing the dose of CVVH (ultrafiltration rates of >35 mL/kg/hour versus 25 mL/kg/hour) does not improve survival in critically ill patients with acute renal failure.[7,8]

PERITONEAL DIALYSIS

Approximately 10% of patients with ESRD in the United States and more than 50% of those in the United Kingdom, Mexico, Canada, and Australia receive continuous ambulatory peritoneal dialysis (CAPD), which provides survival rates comparable to those of hemodialysis, when adjusted for patient age and comorbid conditions. CAPD obviates the need for vascular access, which is a major challenge in diabetic patients, young children, and patients with severe vascular disease. Moreover, peritoneal dialysis can be performed without anticoagulation, thereby decreasing the possible risk for bleeding. Because peritoneal dialysis is a slow, continuous process, it avoids the marked hemodynamic and osmotic shifts associated with hemodialysis. Patients can be taught to do the procedure at home, thereby giving them a sense of control and independence. Also, peritoneal dialysis enables greater liberalization of diet with respect to salt, potassium, protein, and fluid. Peritoneal dialysis, when feasible, is the treatment modality of choice in children because it avoids frequent needle sticks, and, most importantly, allows children to grow.

Performing Peritoneal Dialysis

Peritoneal dialysis uses the patient's own peritoneal membrane for removal of waste products and fluid (Fig. 133-2). During chronic peritoneal dialysis in an adult, 2 to 3 L of dialysate solution containing electrolytes in physiologic concentrations (to correct acid-base and electrolyte disturbances) and varying concentrations of glucose are infused into the peritoneal cavity through a peritoneal catheter. After a specified dwell time varying between 3 and 6 hours per exchange, the fluid is drained, and the process is repeated. The removal of solute from the body, which depends on a concentration gradient between the blood and peritoneal fluid, occurs by diffusion across the peritoneal membrane. Osmotic ultrafiltration is achieved by the addition of increasing concentrations of glucose to the dialysate solution. The osmotic pressure generated by the glucose draws water from the extracellular fluid and the tissues into the peritoneal fluid. However, the net ultrafiltration rate decreases during the exchange, because of glucose absorption.

In peritoneal dialysis, membrane characteristics vary from one individual to another. The peritoneal equilibration test (PET) is a semiquantitative clinical test commonly used to characterize the transport functions of the peritoneal membrane. The standardized PET procedure consists of a 4-hour dwell

using 2 L of 2.5% glucose-containing dialysate solution; equilibration ratios are then determined between plasma and dialysate for creatinine at 0, 2, and 4 hours. The PET also enables measurement of net fluid removal by examining the ratio of dialysate glucose at 4 hours to dialysate glucose at time zero.

Patients who have a high dialysate-to-plasma creatinine ratio and achieve rapid equilibration of creatinine and urea across the peritoneal membrane tend to lose their osmotic gradient for fluid removal. Therefore, high or rapid transporters tend to have excellent solute clearance but have difficulty with ultrafiltration. They do well with frequent exchanges and short dwell times that can be achieved with the automated cycler machine, commonly at night while the patient sleeps.

Patients who have low dialysate-to-plasma ratios for creatinine and urea tend to do best with long dwells and high volumes of dialysate to maximize diffusion. These patients usually have excellent ultrafiltration and excellent fluid removal.

Peritoneal Dialysis Dose

Clearance of small solutes is a key predictor of survival in patients undergoing peritoneal dialysis, and residual renal function also plays a critical role. Current guidelines advocate a minimal target Kt/V urea of at least 1.7 per week. Every effort should be made to maintain residual renal function as long as possible by avoiding nephrotoxins such as nonsteroidal anti-inflammatory drugs, iodinated contrast agents, and aminoglycosides. As residual renal function diminishes over time, the peritoneal dialysis prescription needs to be adjusted accordingly.

Complications

Infection

Infection remains the most common problem in patients undergoing CAPD, and it represents the most frequent cause for catheter removal and discontinuation of therapy. Infection can occur at the exit site, with purulent or bloody drainage, erythema, tenderness, or induration; around the subcutaneous tunnel of the catheter, with redness, swelling, or tenderness; or in the peritoneal cavity (peritonitis). The diagnosis of peritonitis should be entertained if a patient presents with abdominal pain and cloudy dialysate; patients frequently have fever, nausea, and vomiting. Abdominal tenderness, often with rebound, is frequently found on physical examination. The major diagnostic criterion is the cell count in the peritoneal fluid. Patients with peritonitis typically show a white blood cell count higher than 100/mm^3 with a predominance of neutrophils. Lymphocytes may predominate with fungal or mycobacterial infections. Prompt recognition and treatment are critical to avoid relapsing or refractory infections that require catheter removal.

For exit site and tunnel infections, *Staphylococcus aureus* is the most common responsible organism. Initial empirical oral or intravenous therapy therefore should cover gram-positive organisms. Oral penicillinase-resistant penicillins (e.g., dicloxacillin, 250 to 500 mg twice daily for 14 days), fluoroquinolones (e.g., ciprofloxacin, 250 to 500 mg twice daily for 14 days), trimethoprim-sulfamethoxazole (e.g., 40/800 mg for 14 days), or cephalosporins (e.g., cephalexin, 500 mg twice daily for 14 days) are recommended. Vancomycin should be avoided as first-line therapy except for methicillin-resistant *S. aureus*. *S. aureus* nasal carriage is a recognized risk factor for exit site and tunnel infections. Mupirocin nasal ointment used twice daily for 5 days every 4 weeks, or mupirocin ointment applied to the exit site, significantly reduces the incidence of *S. aureus* exit site infections.

In patients with peritonitis, *Staphylococcus epidermidis* (Chapter 296) is the most common organism, usually the result of contamination, such as in the introduction of skin bacteria due to breaks in sterile technique. The introduction of disconnect systems has led to a reduction in the overall rate of *S. epidermidis* peritonitis. *Pseudomonas* species infection (Chapter 314) accounts for 5 to 8% of the episodes of CAPD peritonitis; it is often difficult to eradicate because of the development of a biofilm on the catheter, and the catheter often needs to be removed. Fungal infections are extremely difficult to eradicate despite appropriate antifungal therapy because of the development of biofilm, so many institutions remove the peritoneal dialysis catheter as soon as the diagnosis of fungal peritonitis is made.

Another major cause of peritonitis (Chapter 144) is intra-abdominal pathology such as a perforated diverticulum (Chapter 144), ruptured appendix (Chapter 144), ischemic bowel (Chapter 145), incarcerated hernia (Chapter 144), pancreatitis (Chapter 146), or gynecologic conditions (Chapters 205, 243, and 244). The major diagnostic clue is the presence of polymicrobial enteric organisms on culture, particularly the presence of anaerobic organisms in the dialysate. An abdominal computed tomography

Understanding Fluid Management
Pathways for solute and water transport

Blood in peritoneal capillaries

Urea creatinine — Macromolecules — Water

Endothelium

Glucose — Crystalloid osmosis — Colloid osmosis

Mesothelium

Dialysate-filled peritoneal cavity

FIGURE 133-2. Solute and water transport in peritoneal dialysis. Various pore systems in the vascular wall. The small interendothelial pores are involved in the transport of low-molecular-weight solutes and in water transport. Large pores allow the passage of macromolecules. Crystalloid osmosis induces water transport partly across the small pores, but also through ultrasmall transcellular water channels. Colloid osmosis induces fluid transport only across the small pore system. The mesothelium is not an osmotic barrier. (From Andreucci VE, Fine LG. *International Yearbook of Nephrology*, 1997. Oxford, UK: Oxford University Press; 1998.)

(CT) scan may help identify the anatomic site of the lesion. Although free air may be seen in asymptomatic patients undergoing peritoneal dialysis, the presence of free air should raise the possibility of a perforated viscus, which requires emergency surgery.

For the treatment of CAPD-related peritonitis, current guidelines recommend intravenous or intraperitoneal vancomycin (e.g., 1 g every 5 to 7 days, as guided by serum levels, for at least 2 weeks) or a cephalosporin (e.g., cefazolin, 15 mg/kg in one exchange per day) together with intravenous or intraperitoneal administration of a third-generation cephalosporin with antipseudomonal activity (e.g., ceftazidime, 1 to 1.5 g in one exchange per day) or gentamicin (0.6 mg/kg in one exchange per day or 80 mg IV) as initial empirical therapy. Once culture and sensitivities results are available, the antibiotic prescription should be tailored to avoid gentamicin, if possible, to preserve residual renal function. Therapy should be continued for at least 2 weeks.

Other Complications

Mechanical problems of CAPD include catheter malfunction owing to omental wraps and blood or fibrin clots in the catheter lumen, catheter migration, and abdominal hernias caused by increased intra-abdominal pressure with large volumes of dialysate. Metabolic complications include hyperglycemia and hypertriglyceridemia from high glucose loads, weight gain, and protein loss, especially during an episode of peritonitis. Because peritoneal dialysis requires daily multiple exchanges, it is essential to assess for compliance on an ongoing basis and to ensure that the patient has an adequate support system to avoid "burnout."

The high glucose concentration of the standard CAPD dialysate not only contributes to metabolic abnormalities but also inhibits the function of leukocytes and affects the long-term function of the peritoneal membrane. A dialysate that contains 7.5% icodextrin is a safe and effective substitute for hypertonic glucose and is effective in patients with ultrafiltration failure. This alternative may decrease the metabolic consequences of long-term glucose use and help preserve peritoneal membrane function.

PROGNOSIS

Although dialysis acutely prevents death from uremic complications, the mortality rate among patients undergoing chronic dialysis therapy remains high, at about 20% per year in the United States. Age and comorbid conditions such as diabetes, cardiovascular disease, nutritional status, and infection all contribute significantly to the high mortality in this population.

● RENAL TRANSPLANTATION

Successful renal transplantation offers patients the best quality of life. They are liberated from potassium and fluid restrictions, are free to travel and work, and achieve correction of metabolic abnormalities and anemia with restoration of normal renal function. Moreover, in comparison with hemodialysis, renal transplantation also improves long-term survival in both diabetic and nondiabetic patients.

Because renal transplantation offers patients the best chance for quality as well as quantity of life, it is essential to evaluate candidates early and, if possible, proceed directly to preemptive transplantation if a living donor can be identified. The ideal form of renal transplantation for patients with type 1 diabetes mellitus (Chapter 236) and nephropathy is from a living related donor, followed by pancreas or islet cell transplantation from a deceased donor. If a living donor is unavailable, simultaneous pancreas and kidney transplantation should be pursued from a deceased donor. Although successful pancreas transplantation does not reverse the established macrovascular and microvascular complications of long-standing diabetes mellitus, it improves blood glucose control and quality of life and may prevent the progression of retinopathy and autonomic neuropathy. Islet cell transplantation after renal transplantation is presently under investigation.

Pretransplantation Evaluation of the Recipient

The potential renal transplant recipient must have irreversible ESRD and no evidence of active infection or malignancy. In addition to a careful history and physical examination, the evaluation must address the likelihood of compliance and exclude unmanageable patients with psychosis, substance abuse, or alcohol abuse.

Systemic Diseases

A careful cardiovascular evaluation is critical, including stress testing with imaging (Chapters 56 and 71) and a coronary angiogram if any evidence of ischemia is demonstrated, particularly in diabetic patients. In view of the increasing recognition of calcific aortic stenosis (Chapter 75) and hypertension in patients with ESRD, an echocardiogram (Chapter 55) should be obtained to assess valve area as well as systolic and diastolic function.

Likewise, a careful evaluation of carotid and peripheral vessels should be undertaken because the new kidney will be anastomosed to the iliac vessels. The new kidney's ureter may be implanted into the recipient's bladder, or the patient's own ureter may be used. Further urologic testing may be needed if a neurogenic bladder is suspected or if there is a history of obstructive uropathy (Chapter 125). Bilateral nephrectomies are required if there is persistent, smoldering infection unresponsive to chronic suppressive antimicrobial therapy or there is severe polycystic kidney disease.

It is recommended that patients with Goodpasture's syndrome (Chapter 123), systemic lupus erythematosus (Chapter 274), or antineutrophil cytoplasmic antibody–positive vasculitis (Chapter 278) become clinically and serologically quiescent before transplantation. A number of primary glomerular diseases (Chapter 123) have been shown to recur in the renal allograft, including focal segmental glomerulosclerosis, membranous glomerulonephritis, membranoproliferative glomerulonephritis, and immunoglobulin A (IgA) nephropathy. Diabetic nephropathy also may recur after transplantation and can be prevented by combined kidney-pancreas transplantation. Combined kidney-liver transplantation can cure oxalosis (Chapter 212).

Infectious Diseases

Serologic determination of human immunodeficiency virus (HIV; Chapter 394) and hepatitis B and C virus infection (Chapter 151) status should be obtained. In this era of highly active antiretroviral therapy, HIV positivity is no longer an absolute contraindication to transplantation. Although patients with hepatitis C do better with renal transplantation than dialysis, with time liver failure is the major cause of morbidity and mortality. It is therefore critical to stage patients with hepatitis C before transplantation, by means of liver biopsy, viral load determination, measurement of the α-fetoprotein level, and a CT scan looking for hepatocellular carcinoma (Chapter 202) and portal hypertension (Chapter 157). The possibility of a combined kidney and liver transplantation needs to be explored. Combined therapy with pegylated interferon and ribavirin may be indicated after transplantation but requires cautious monitoring and usually is not well tolerated. Post-transplantation interferon therapy may trigger allograft rejection, possibly by upregulation of genes for the major histocompatibility complex and various cytokines. Severe hemolytic anemia may occur with ribavirin administration and should be avoided in dialysis patients.

All patients waiting for renal transplantation should be vaccinated against hepatitis B, although the response rate appears to be less than 50%. If a patient is positive for hepatitis B surface antigen, a DNA viral load determination and liver biopsy should be obtained for staging. Lamivudine or entecavir therapy may be initiated either before or after transplantation. Once again, if there is significant cirrhosis (Chapter 156), consideration should be given to combined kidney-liver transplantation.

Patients with a newly positive purified protein derivative (PPD) skin test (Chapter 332) should ideally be treated before transplantation. A patient with positive PPD and negative chest radiograph before transplantation may be closely monitored. If the patient has a positive PPD and a history of previous disease or a positive chest radiograph, treatment with isoniazid is indicated starting 1 to 2 months after transplantation.

Patients also should be evaluated for previous exposure to varicella. If the varicella titer is negative before transplantation, an attempt at vaccination may be undertaken. If the patient remains varicella antibody negative or has not been vaccinated, varicella-zoster immune globulin should be given on exposure to patients with chickenpox or herpes zoster (Chapter 383) because the immunosuppressed host is at risk for fulminant varicella with pulmonary infiltrates, pancreatitis, and liver disease.

Special attention needs to be directed to patients from tropical areas, where *Strongyloides stercoralis* (Chapter 365) is endemic. A *Strongyloides* titer should be obtained; if it is positive, the infection should be treated before immunosuppression because fulminant disease can occur after transplantation. If a patient comes from an area where schistosomiasis (Chapter 363) is endemic, diagnosis and treatment should be initiated before transplantation.

Identifying Donors
Living Donors

The demand for deceased donors far exceeds the supply of organs, and the waiting list for cadaver renal transplants is now 4 to 5 years in all blood groups throughout most of the United States. As a result, living organ donation

FIGURE 133-3. Histology of renal allograft with acute cellular rejection (A and B) and acute humoral rejection (C and D). **A,** Interstitial mononuclear infiltrate. The *arrow* points to an area with tubulitis. **B,** Arteritis. Note the accumulation of inflammatory cells beneath the intima, which is characteristic of acute cellular rejection type 2 (Banff classification). **C,** Acute humoral rejection. The peritubular space is occupied by an inflammatory infiltrate with the presence of polymorphonuclear neutrophils *(arrows).* **D,** Positive C4d staining in the peritubular capillaries by immunofluorescence, a hallmark of humoral rejection.

accounts for more than 50% of the transplantations now being performed. Living donation is generally safe, and both the short- and long-term outcomes for the recipient are better with a living donor. Results from a living unrelated donor transplant are equivalent to a one-haplotype parental match, with a 1-year graft survival rate of 92%, thereby suggesting that the quality of the organ is as important as or more important than the closeness of the genetic "match." Donors require a complete medical examination and a psychological evaluation by physicians and psychiatrists independent of the recipient to ascertain their health and the voluntary, altruistic nature of the donor's decision.

For the donor, the immediate risk of surgery is a mortality rate of 0.05%, in addition to the pain, time out of work, and possibility of phlebitis or pulmonary embolus, urinary tract infection, wound infection, or pneumonia. Laparoscopic donor nephrectomy in carefully selected patients allows for a faster recovery and more rapid return to work.

The long-term risks of having one kidney include the slightly increased risk of proteinuria, chance of trauma, and development of cancer in the one remaining kidney. Although isolated cases of chronic renal failure have been reported after donation, for the most part long-term mortality is not affected by kidney donation. Nevertheless, all donors must be carefully monitored long term.

Deceased Donors

The shortage of deceased organs for transplantation has led to the increased use of kidneys from donors older than 55 years of age or with a history of hypertension or cerebrovascular accident. In these situations, a donor kidney biopsy is performed to assess the degree of fibrosis, sclerosis, and vascular disease; if deemed appropriate, these kidneys are then offered with informed consent to older potential recipients or patients with multiple access problems. Although there may be a 10% difference in survival between these kidneys and standard deceased donor kidneys at 3 years, the potential benefit to the recipient is the opportunity to terminate dialysis without waiting on the list for 4 years or longer.

Another alternative is the use of organs from donors who die from traditional cardiac death, known as donation after cardiac death donors. Once the patient's family and the attending physician have decided that life support will be discontinued, the patient is taken to the operating room, the ventilator is discontinued, and cardiac arrest occurs. The patient is pronounced dead only after all signs of respiration have ceased. Patient and graft survival rates are not statistically different from rates with traditional brain death donors.

Tissue Typing

A key element in the evaluation for transplantation is tissue typing. The recipient must receive a transplant from a blood group–compatible donor to avoid hyperacute rejection and immediate irreversible graft loss on the operating table. The donor and recipient need not share the same Rh factor.

HLA typing is performed on all potential recipients and donors. It is critical to determine the recipient's sensitization (i.e., the level of preformed HLA antibodies in the serum of the recipient). These antibodies typically result from previous transplantations, pregnancies, or blood transfusions. The critical test before renal transplantation is the final crossmatch: a complement-dependent cytotoxicity assay performed using the cells of the donor and serum of the recipient. If the crossmatch is positive, the transplantation should not be performed. Another option to increase the availability of organs is the donor exchange program, whereby an incompatible live donor-recipient pair in one institution finds a compatible match at another institution through computerized matching.

Rejection

Allograft rejection is initiated by the recipient's recognition of donor major histocompatibility complex antigens, thereby leading to activation of humoral and cellular immunity (Chapter 48). *Hyperacute humoral rejection,* which is rare, usually causes immediate irreversible necrosis of the allograft on the operating table. Hyperacute rejection is caused by preformed alloantibodies in the recipient directed against donor HLA or ABO antigens, and this form of antibody-mediated rejection can usually be prevented by careful crossmatching techniques.

The clinical manifestations of *acute cellular rejection* (Fig. 133-3), which can occur any time but are generally seen within the first 3 months, may be minimal with the use of newer immunosuppressive agents but may include fever, allograft swelling and tenderness, or oliguria. The BUN and creatinine concentrations are usually elevated. A Doppler ultrasound study should be performed to exclude obstruction or vascular thrombosis (Chapter 127). The diagnosis of acute rejection can be reliably made only with an allograft biopsy (Table 133-2).

Acute humoral rejection (see Fig. 133-3) usually occurs within the first 3 months but can occur at any time, particularly if the patient is noncompliant with medications. It occurs when the recipient develops de novo donor-reactive cytotoxic antibodies after transplantation (i.e., positive crossmatch after but negative before transplantation). These alloantibodies may be reactive with HLA class I or II antigens. Early detection and treatment of acute humoral rejection with plasmapheresis, pooled human immune globulin (e.g., 0.4 to 0.6 g/kg), and rituximab (e.g., 1 g) in addition to tacrolimus (to maintain a level of 8 to 10), mycophenolate mofetil (e.g., 750 to 1000 mg twice daily), and steroids has led to dramatic reversal of the acute allograft dysfunction in approximately 90% of cases. Protocols using plasma exchange, rituximab, and intravenous immune globulin also have been used before transplantation in an attempt to lower the levels of preformed HLA antibody

TABLE 133-2	DIFFERENTIAL DIAGNOSIS OF RENAL ALLOGRAFT DYSFUNCTION

IMMEDIATE/DELAYED GRAFT FUNCTION (1-3 DAYS)

Acute tubular necrosis
Hyperacute humoral rejection
Urinary leak or obstruction
Renal artery or vein thrombosis
Recurrence of disease (e.g., FSGS)

EARLY POST-TRANSPLANTATION PERIOD (FIRST MONTH)

Acute cellular rejection
Acute humoral rejection
Calcineurin inhibitor toxicity
Urinary tract obstruction
Volume depletion
Recurrence of disease

LATE ACUTE DYSFUNCTION

Acute rejection
Cyclosporine or tacrolimus toxicity
Recurrence of primary disease
Tubulointerstitial nephritis, drug-induced
Renal artery stenosis
Infection (bacterial UTI, cytomegalovirus, BK virus)
Hemodynamic (volume; use of ACEI, AIIRB)

CHRONIC DYSFUNCTION

Chronic rejection
Cyclosporine or tacrolimus toxicity
Recurrent renal disease
De novo renal disease
Urinary tract obstruction
Bacterial UTI
Hypertensive nephrosclerosis

ACEI = angiotensin-converting enzyme inhibitor; AIIRB = angiotensin II receptor blocker; FSGS = focal segmental glomerulosclerosis; UTI = urinary tract infection.

in highly sensitized patients. Such protocols often convert a previously positive crossmatch to a negative one, thus enabling transplantation from a living donor.

Another promising approach to the treatment of acute humoral rejection focuses on the depletion of plasma cells with the proteasome inhibitor bortezomib, which is also used in the treatment of multiple myeloma. Long-term studies are needed to determine whether the successful treatment of acute antibody-mediated rejection and chronic humoral rejection will improve long-term graft survival.

Induction Immunosuppression

The goal of immunosuppression therapy (Chapter 48) is to prevent allograft rejection but still allow the immune system to fight infection and malignancy. The multiagent strategy allows for a synergistic effect and reduction of specific drug toxicity (Fig. 133-4). Immunosuppression is initiated at high doses (induction) during the initial period after transplantation, when the risk of rejection is highest, and is reduced over time (maintenance immunosuppression). In recipients with a high risk of rejection (children, retransplant recipients, delayed graft function, multiparous women, and multitransfused patients), induction immunosuppression is often used, consisting of a course of polyclonal antilymphocyte-antithymocyte globulin (ATG) or antilymphocyte globulin; monoclonal anti-CD3 antibodies (OKT3); or anti-interleukin-2 (anti-IL-2) receptor monoclonal antibodies (basiliximab or daclizumab). Appropriate antiviral prophylaxis is essential to reduce the risk of severe cytomegalovirus (CMV) infection and Epstein-Barr virus (EBV)-associated post-transplantation lymphoproliferative disease (PTLD). Likewise, prophylaxis with trimethoprim-sulfamethoxazole has been effective in preventing urinary tract infections as well as *Pneumocystis jirovecii* infection in these highly immunosuppressed patients.

Polyclonal Antibodies

Polyclonal antibodies are raised in various animals (rabbits, goats, horses) using different antigenic preparations (thymocytes, lymphocytes). The polyclonal antilymphocyte antibodies (1.5 mg/kg for three doses) are used for

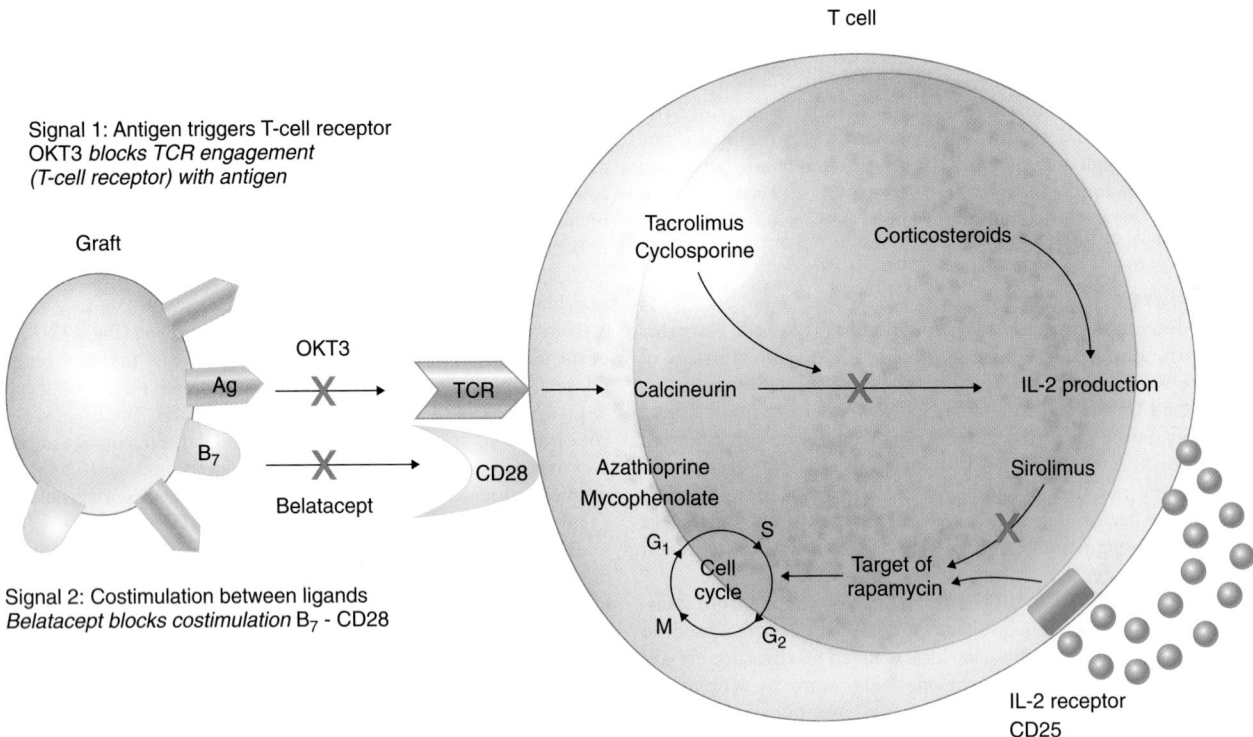

Targets of Immunosuppressive Agents

Signal 1: Antigen triggers T-cell receptor
OKT3 *blocks TCR engagement*
(T-cell receptor) with antigen

Signal 2: Costimulation between ligands
Belatacept blocks costimulation B₇ - CD28

Signal 3: Cytokines trigger receptors
IL-2 receptor blockers: Basiliximab and
daclizumab: humanized monoclonal antibodies

FIGURE 133-4. Targets of immunosuppressive agents. G_1, S, G_2, and M are stages of the cell cycle. Ag = antigen; AZA = azathioprine; B_7 = costimulatory molecule; CsA = cyclosporine; IL = interleukin; MMF = mycophenolate mofetil; SRL = sirolimus; TAC = tacrolimus; TCR = T-cell receptor; TOR = target of rapamycin.

induction therapy in high-risk recipients (i.e., those with high panel-reactive antibodies and those undergoing retransplantation) at the onset of transplantation, for treatment of steroid-resistant acute cellular rejection, and as a calcineurin inhibitor–sparing agent in recipients with delayed graft function. The polyclonal antibodies can cause serum sickness, bone marrow suppression, and hemolysis. The use of these agents also may trigger a potent cytokine response. Most side effects are related either to the degree of purity of the antigenic preparation used to immunize the animals or to the purification of the serum. Serum sickness (Chapter 46) and anaphylactic reactions (Chapter 261) are related to previous exposure to the animal species used to raise the antibody.

OKT3

OKT3, which is a mouse monoclonal antibody directed against the CD3 antigen, is used primarily for treatment of steroid-resistant acute cellular rejection and occasionally as an induction agent. OKT3 can cause myriad side effects, including fever, rigors, nausea, vomiting, diarrhea, severe headache (aseptic meningitis), hypotension, chest pain, dyspnea, wheezing, and, infrequently, pulmonary edema. These symptoms are secondary to massive cytokine release after OKT3 engages the TCR. OKT3 is associated with a higher incidence of severe CMV infections and PTLD, so CMV prophylaxis (Chapter 384) is essential.

Interleukin-2 Receptor Blockers

IL-2 receptor blockers are engineered monoclonal antibodies against the α-chain of the IL-2 receptor. Daclizumab is a humanized molecule consisting of a human IgG1 with antigen-binding regions from a mouse antibody. Basiliximab is a chimeric construct with a murine variable region and human constant regions. Daclizumab and basiliximab are used only as induction agents to prevent rather than treat rejection. They both have a safe side-effect profile, largely because of their human origin.

New Agents

Alemtuzumab is an anti-CD52 monoclonal antibody used as an induction agent at the time of transplantation. Alemtuzumab appears to facilitate minimization of maintenance immunosuppressive protocols (with either sirolimus or low-dose tacrolimus). The dose and frequency of administration remain to be determined.

Maintenance Immunosuppression

Many immunosuppressive agents are available for prevention of rejection in the maintenance phase (Table 133-3). Common regimens consist of low-dose steroids, mycophenolate mofetil, or azathioprine plus a calcineurin inhibitor (either cyclosporine or tacrolimus). Corticosteroids (Chapter 34), which have nonspecific immunosuppressive and anti-inflammatory actions, are used for induction therapy, for maintenance immunosuppression, and in high doses (pulse) for the treatment of acute cellular rejection. Corticosteroids cause many metabolic changes, including diabetes, hypercholesterolemia, osteoporosis, increased risk of cardiovascular events, obesity, and hypertension, and they can cause significant mood swings, irritability, and depression.

The calcineurin inhibitors cyclosporine and tacrolimus inhibit the translocation of nuclear factor of activated T lymphocyte (NFAT) from the cytoplasm to the nucleus. Cyclosporine and tacrolimus levels must be closely monitored to avoid toxicity as well as rejection. The most important nonimmune toxicity of the calcineurin inhibitors is nephrotoxicity, with three distinct patterns. First is an acute hemodynamic effect, which is caused by afferent arteriolar constriction and which may exacerbate ischemic injury and delay graft function, with a reversible decrease in the glomerular filtration rate that improves when the dose of the drug is adjusted. Second is subacute to chronic nephrotoxicity, which may be evidenced by tubular lesions, hyalinosis of small arterioles, or striped fibrosis in the more chronic phase. Third is a thrombotic microangiopathy, which can present a picture similar to the hemolytic-uremic syndrome (Chapter 175) with intimal proliferation, fibrin deposition, and thrombotic occlusion of the arcuate and intralobular arteries. The peripheral smear may show evidence of schistocytes, and thrombocytopenia may or may not be present. Switching from cyclosporine to tacrolimus or vice versa sometimes may be beneficial. Other side effects of the calcineurin inhibitors include neurotoxicity (tremors, mental status changes, irritability, and seizures), hypertension, hyperglycemia, hyperkalemia, hyperuricemia, gout, and an increased incidence of EBV-related B-cell lymphomas (PTLD). Both cyclosporine and tacrolimus are metabolized by the cytochrome P-450 system and excreted by the liver. Therefore, drugs that interact with the P-450 system, such as macrolide antibiotics, diltiazem, imidazole, and triazole antifungals may raise the levels of calcineurin inhibitors. In contrast, agents such as rifampin, phenobarbital, and phenytoin that induce cytochrome P-450 enzymes increase the catabolism of calcineurin inhibitors. Many other significant interactions need to be recognized, including the risk of rhabdomyolysis with statins and interaction with most nephrotoxic agents.

Azathioprine, which was a cornerstone of transplant immunosuppression until the introduction of mycophenolate mofetil, is still useful. Azathioprine inhibits DNA synthesis; its main side effect is bone marrow suppression (see Table 133-3). Azathioprine has also been associated with malignancies, especially skin cancers, and papillomavirus infection. Azathioprine is metabolized by xanthine oxidase, so concomitant administration of allopurinol, a xanthine oxidase inhibitor, should be avoided because significant bone marrow toxicity may occur.

Mycophenolate mofetil, which selectively inhibits lymphocyte proliferation (see Table 133-3), reduces the incidence of acute cellular rejection by 50% and allows for a significant reduction in the use of OKT3/ATG. Gastrointestinal symptoms (e.g., nausea, epigastric discomfort, diarrhea) are the main side effects and usually can be improved by dose reduction. The effect of mycophenolate mofetil on the prevention of chronic rejection is currently under study.

Sirolimus binds to the same immunophilin as tacrolimus but does not affect calcineurin activity (see Table 133-3). Inhibition of mTOR by sirolimus suppresses alloantigen and cytokine-driven T-cell proliferation when it inhibits the cell cycle. Regimens using sirolimus have reduce the incidence of acute cellular rejection. Sirolimus causes hyperlipidemia and also is associated with thrombocytopenia. Sirolimus also interacts with calcineurin inhibitors and may cause an increase in calcineurin inhibitor toxicity.

PROGNOSIS

Since 1975, the 1-year deceased donor kidney survival rate has dramatically improved, from approximately 50% to 90% in 2010. The 1-year allograft survival for kidneys from living donors has increased from 88 to 93%. The acute rejection rates are only about 11% with new immunosuppressive regimens, and 1-year allograft survival rates have improved. However, the initial projected long-term improvement in the survival of grafts from living as well as deceased donors has not been realized.

Patients benefit from aggressive control of coronary risk factors because coronary disease is a major cause of death in these patients (Chapters 51 and 73). The ultimate goal of transplantation is tolerance to donor antigens while maintaining the ability to respond to third-party antigens in the absence of

TABLE 133-3 IMMUNOSUPPRESSIVE AGENTS

AGENT	MECHANISM OF ACTION	SIDE EFFECTS
Corticosteroids	Multiple anti-inflammatory actions, blockade of IL-1, IL-6, TNF-α	Infection, hypertension, glucose resistance, osteoporosis, hyperlipidemia, glaucoma, adrenal suppression
Azathioprine	Blockade of purine synthesis, which affects DNA and RNA synthesis	Bone marrow suppression
Cyclosporine	Binds to cyclophilin, causing calcineurin inhibition, which prevents NFAT activity on IL-2 gene; stimulates production of TGF-β	Hypertension, glucose intolerance, nephrotoxicity, hirsutism, gingival hyperplasia
Tacrolimus	Binds to FKBP-12, causing calcineurin inhibition, which prevents NFAT activity on IL-2 gene	Neurotoxicity, increased incidence of diabetes mellitus (≈20%)
Mycophenolate mofetil	Blocks de novo pathway of purine synthesis by inhibition of IMPDH, selective for lymphocytes	Gastrointestinal symptoms (diarrhea), leukopenia
Sirolimus	Binds to FKBP-12 and mTOR, blocking cell cycle progression	Hyperlipidemia, leukopenia, thrombocytopenia, impaired wound healing

FKBP-12 = FK506-binding protein 12; IL = interleukin; IMPDH = inosine monophosphate dehydrogenase; NFAT = nuclear factor of activated T lymphocyte; TGF-β = transforming growth factor-β; TNF-α = tumor necrosis factor-α; mTOR = mammalian target of rapamycin.

ongoing immunosuppression. The induction of mixed hematopoietic chimerism, using nonmyeloablative conditioning, has been successfully accomplished in rodents, miniature swine, and nonhuman primates. These observations now are being extended to patients with multiple myeloma and ESRD.

1. Cooper BA, Branley P, Bulfone L, et al. A randomized, controlled trial of early versus late initiation of dialysis. *N Engl J Med.* 2010;363:609-619.
2. Singh AK, Szczech L, Tang KL, et al. Correction of anemia with epoetin alfa in chronic kidney disease. *N Engl J Med.* 2006;355:2085-2098.
3. Eknoyan G, Beck GJ, Cheung AK, et al. Effect of dialysis dose and membrane flux in maintenance hemodialysis. *N Engl J Med.* 2002;347:2010-2019.
4. The FNH Trial Group. In-center hemodialysis six times per week versus three times per week. *N Engl J Med.* 2010;363:2287-2300.
5. Culleton BF, Walsh M, Klarenbach SW, et al. Effect of frequent nocturnal hemodialysis vs conventional hemodialysis on left ventricular mass and quality of life: a randomized controlled trial. *JAMA.* 2007;298:1291-1299.
6. Manns BJ, Walsh MW, Culleton BF, et al. Nocturnal hemodialysis does not improve overall measures of quality of life compared to conventional hemodialysis. *Kidney Int.* 2009;75:542-599.
7. Palevsky PM, Zhang JH, O'Connor TZ, et al. for the VA/NIH Acute Renal Failure Trial Network. Intensity of renal support on critically ill patients with acute kidney injury. *N Engl J Med.* 2008;359:7-20.
8. Renal Replacement Study Investigators. Intensity of continuous renal replacement therapy in critically ill patients. *N Engl J Med.* 2009;361:1627-1638.

SUGGESTED READINGS

Gupta G, Unruh ML, Nolin TD, et al. Primary care of the renal transplant patient. *J Gen Intern Med.* 2010;25:731-740. *Review.*

Himmelfarb J, Ikizler TA. Hemodialysis. *N Engl J Med.* 2010;363:1833-1845. *Review.*

Mehrotra R, Chiu YW, Kalantar-Zadeh K, et al. Similar outcomes with hemodialysis and peritoneal dialysis in patients with end-stage renal disease. *Arch Intern Med.* 2011;171:110-118. *Patients who begin treatment with hemodialysis or peritoneal dialysis now have similar outcomes.*

Nankivell BJ, Alexander SI. Rejection of the kidney allograft. *N Engl J Med.* 2010;363:1451-1462. *Comprehensive review.*

http://www.kidney.org/professionals/kdoqi/guidelines.cfm. Accessed Jan. 2010. *Guidelines for the care of patients with end-stage renal failure—anemia, dialysis adequacy, bone metabolism.*

XII

§ GASTROINTESTINAL DISEASES

134

APPROACH TO THE PATIENT WITH GASTROINTESTINAL DISEASE

KENNETH MCQUAID

The luminal gastrointestinal (GI) tract (esophagus, stomach, duodenum, small and large intestine, and anus) and pancreas are responsible for digestion, for the absorption of nutrients and fluids, and for the temporary storage and excretion of undigested waste. The GI tract has an epithelial lining with an enormous surface area that provides nutrient absorption and serves as a barrier to microorganisms. In addition, the GI tract has a large innate and adaptive immune system that interfaces with luminal food antigens, host proteins, commensal and pathogenic bacteria, and parasites and must decide which antigens to tolerate and which require immune activation. The GI tract also contains an extensive enteric endocrine system that regulates food intake, weight control, and glucose homeostasis, as well as secretions from the stomach, intestine, and pancreas. Finally, it has an enteric nervous system that is integrated with the autonomic and central nervous systems to control gastric emptying, intestinal motility, and defecation.

Numerous diseases within and outside the GI tract may alter normal function by causing structural damage (erosion, ulceration, perforation, stenosis, or obstruction), bleeding, inflammation, abnormal absorption or secretion of nutrients and electrolytes, or abnormal motility. Despite its anatomic and physiologic complexity, the GI system has only a limited repertoire of symptoms and signs to express conditions that may be either serious or clinically insignificant: abdominal pain, heartburn, regurgitation, dysphagia, odynophagia, dyspepsia, nausea and vomiting, gas and bloating, weight loss, diarrhea, constipation, overt or occult gastrointestinal bleeding, and incontinence.

GENERAL APPROACH TO PATIENTS WITH GASTROINTESTINAL SIGNS AND SYMPTOMS

An appropriate history and physical evaluation usually can narrow the differential diagnosis of GI complaints. A specific diagnosis can almost always be established thereafter by the judicious use of laboratory, endoscopic, or imaging studies (Table 134-1).

Clinical History

The clinician should elicit the nature of the complaint, including its acuity, severity, location, radiation, duration, pattern (steady vs. colicky; abrupt vs. gradual onset), and relationship to food, meals, and bowel movements. Symptoms that arise from the GI tract are almost always improved or worsened by eating or by bowel movements. For symptoms of recent onset, it is important to elicit recent dietary intake, a medication history, potential exposure to enteric infections or sexually transmitted diseases (Chapter 293), and recent travel. It is also useful to establish whether there are signs or symptoms that suggest a systemic illness, including fever, weight loss, arthralgias, fatigue, weakness, or skin rash.

Most nonsurgical GI diseases manifest with mild to moderate symptoms that develop gradually and do not require immediate attention. Acute symptoms that require urgent assessment are severe abdominal pain and overt GI bleeding (Chapter 137) that manifests by hematemesis, melena, or large-volume hematochezia. Severe or dramatic abdominal pain that develops acutely over minutes to hours requires urgent evaluation to determine whether surgical intervention is required. Severe vomiting or diarrhea with signs of dehydration also warrants urgent attention.

Mild to moderate chronic or intermittent symptoms that have been present for a long period can be evaluated in a deliberate fashion. A substantial proportion of chronic GI complaints have no obvious organic or biochemical basis and ultimately are classified as *functional* GI disorders (Chapter 139). Complaints that have been ongoing for years rarely are attributable to readily remedied structural disorders. In patients with chronic GI symptoms, it is important to elicit and address the current reason for seeking evaluation, which may include concern for underlying serious illness (especially cancer), a change in the character or severity of symptoms, life stressors, or depression. Asking the patient what he or she thinks or fears may provide insights into the proportion of the complaint attributable to these amplifying issues, regardless of whether the problem is functional or structural in origin.

A dietary history (Chapter 221) should be obtained. For acute symptoms of nausea, vomiting, diarrhea, or abdominal pain, intake over the previous 24 to 48 hours should be reviewed for clues to a food-borne illness, including possible exposure to a contaminated food or water source and similar symptoms in other people (Chapter 291). For chronic or intermittent complaints, a recall of meals and types of foods eaten over the previous 1 to 2 days provides insight into eating habits and the amounts and types of fruits and vegetables, whole grains, fiber, protein, fat, and dairy products ingested. A relationship between specific foods and symptoms may be found. For example, pain, flatulence, or diarrhea may be caused by dairy products (lactose intolerance), whole grains, legumes or cruciferous vegetables, or fatty meals (malabsorption), and chronic constipation may be due to a low-fiber diet. Recent and long-term changes in body weight should be elicited. Involuntary loss of greater than 5% of body weight over the prior 12 months is worrisome for serious disease and significant malnutrition (Chapter 222).

The number and consistency of bowel movements should be elicited, and any change in bowel habits must be explored. Signs of acute GI bleeding (melena or hematochezia) or inflammatory colitis (blood, mucus, or pus) should be elicited. Improvement in symptoms after passage of flatus or a bowel movement suggests a disorder of the colon or anorectum.

Past Medical History

The past medical history should be reviewed for conditions that may cause acute or chronic GI symptoms, including endocrine disorders such as diabetes (Chapter 237) or thyroid dysfunction (Chapter 233), cardiovascular diseases such as heart failure (Chapter 58) or peripheral vascular disease (Chapter 81), chronic liver disease and portal hypertension (Chapter 156), neurologic conditions such as Parkinson's disease (Chapter 416) or neuromuscular disorders (Chapter 403), and rheumatologic and collagen vascular disorders (Chapter 264). In addition to their impact on GI tract function, the severity of these conditions must be considered when weighing the risks of diagnostic studies, especially endoscopy. Patients with symptomatic or advanced respiratory insufficiency (Chapter 83), sleep apnea (Chapter 100), valvular heart disease (Chapter 75), coronary artery disease (Chapter 50), heart failure (Chapter 58), cirrhosis (Chapter 156), cerebrovascular disease (Chapter 413), neuromuscular disease (Chapter 430), or dementia (Chapter 409) have an increased risk of sedation-related complications during endoscopy.

A list of prescription and nonprescription medications, vitamins, minerals, and other nutritional supplements should be obtained, paying particular attention to any that were recently initiated or changed. Herbal supplements (Chapter 38) are commonly used but are seldom reported without direct questioning. Medications are potential causes of odynophagia, dyspepsia, nausea or vomiting, abdominal pain, diarrhea, and constipation. The use of antiplatelet agents, including aspirin and anticoagulants, should be determined. The risks of stopping versus continuing these medications must be weighed in patients who have acute or chronic GI bleeding or in whom a therapeutic procedure is to be performed.

Social History

The patient's personal relationships, employment history, quality of life, alcohol intake (Chapter 32), and smoking (Chapter 31) history should be determined. It can be very informative to observe both verbal and nonverbal interactions between the patient and a partner or caregiver during an interview. Alcohol may cause heartburn, dyspepsia, nausea, diarrhea, or chronic liver disease. Many patients are reluctant to disclose the full extent of their alcohol intake on direct questioning; therefore, in addition to asking how often they imbibe (days/week and drinks/day), it may be revealing to inquire about their preferred beverage and how it is purchased (location, volume, and frequency). Cigarette smoking is associated with an increased risk of heartburn, peptic ulcer disease, Crohn's disease, and GI malignancies.

Clinicians should inquire about the degree to which GI symptoms are disrupting a patient's life. GI illness may affect dietary and bowel habits, sleep, and sense of vitality. Concerns about dietary intolerances, inability to eat, inability to have comfortable bowel movements, uncontrolled diarrhea or gas, fecal urgency, or fecal incontinence may affect a patient's social life, personal and sexual relationships, employment, and sense of optimism.

The social history should also be reviewed for recent stressors that may precipitate or exacerbate GI symptoms, including marital or interpersonal discord, personal or family illness, bereavement, financial pressures, job loss, or change in employment. To elicit such information, it may be helpful to tell the patient that stress worsens many conditions and to inquire whether they believe stress may be contributing to their problem.

For elderly, disabled, or marginally housed patients, it is important to elicit how they obtain and prepare their meals and how they access toilet facilities. For patients undergoing GI procedures, it is important to determine whether they have mental, physical, or social barriers that would make it difficult to comply with pre-procedure instructions (including bowel preparation) and whether they have an able-bodied adult who can accompany them to the procedure and observe them at home, if necessary, afterward.

Family History

The family history should be reviewed for GI disorders with a heritable component, especially celiac disease (Chapter 142), inflammatory bowel diseases (Chapter 143), and GI, gynecologic, and genitourinary neoplasms.

Physical Examination
Nonabdominal Examination

The nonabdominal examination should assess nutritional status (Chapter 221) and any signs of systemic conditions that may cause GI symptoms or that must be considered when weighing the risks and benefits of further testing, especially endoscopy. Vital signs should be obtained in all patients. Low-grade fever (<100.5° F) is common in inflammatory conditions, including gastroenteritis, inflammatory bowel disease, appendicitis, cholecystitis, and diverticulitis. High fever (>102° F) suggests sepsis, pelvic, or intra-abdominal infections (e.g., cholangitis, pelvic inflammatory disease, pyelonephritis) or peritonitis. Hemodynamic instability (hypotension or tachycardia) suggests intravascular depletion due to poor oral intake, acute GI or intra-abdominal bleeding, severe diarrhea, or peritonitis. A body mass index less than 18 suggests malnourishment.

A general survey should be performed to assess for signs of weight loss (fat and muscle wasting), malnutrition (dry or thin skin, hair loss, edema, ana-sarca), and vitamin deficiencies (pellagra, scurvy). Skin lesions may provide clues to systemic conditions such as liver disease (jaundice, spider telangiec-tasias, palmar erythema), inflammatory bowel disease (erythema nodosum, pyoderma gangrenosum), celiac disease (dermatitis herpetiformis), vasculitis, and rare gastrointestinal malignancies, polyposis syndromes, and pancreatic endocrine tumors (Chapters 198, 199, and 201). An oral examination looks for mucocutaneous candidiasis (which may reflect immunosuppression), ulcerations (which may reflect inflammatory bowel disease, vasculitis, viral infection, or vitamin deficiencies), and glossitis or angular cheilitis (which may reflect vitamin deficiencies). With the exception of supraclavicular lymph nodes, peripheral lymph nodes are uninvolved with GI diseases but should be examined when systemic infection or advanced malignancy is suspected (Chapter 171). Examination of the lungs and cardiovascular system should focus on evidence of conditions that might increase the risk of moderate sedation in the event endoscopy is required (respiratory insufficiency, heart failure) and for conditions that increase the risk of intestinal ischemia (atrial fibrillation, valvular heart disease, peripheral vascular disease) (Chapter 145). The extremities should be evaluated for edema and peripheral pulses. Finally, a brief neurologic assessment should be performed to screen for intracranial mass lesions or other neurologic disorders that may present with GI symptoms.

Abdominal Examination

The abdominal examination begins with a visual inspection of the abdomen and inguinal region for scars (due to prior surgeries or trauma), asymmetry (suggesting a mass or organomegaly), distention (due to obesity, ascites, or intestinal ileus or obstruction), prominent periumbilical veins (suggesting portal hypertension), or hernias (umbilical, ventral, inguinal). The examination proceeds with auscultation followed by percussion, and it ends with light and deep palpation.

In patients *without* abdominal pain, auscultation of bowel sounds to assess intestinal motility has limited usefulness and may be omitted. Percussion may be performed before or in conjunction with light and deep palpation. Initial cursory light percussion across the upper, mid-, and lower abdomen is useful to denote areas of dullness and tympany, as well as to elicit unanticipated areas of pain or tenderness before palpation. More extensive percussion provides limited but useful information about the size of the liver and spleen, gastric or intestinal distention, bladder distention, and ascites (Chapters 148 and 156). Gentle, light palpation promotes abdominal relaxation and allows

the detection of muscular resistance (guarding), abdominal tenderness, and superficial masses of the abdominal wall or abdomen. Deeper palpation of the abdominal organs (liver, spleen, kidneys, aorta) and abdominal cavity may detect enlargement or abnormal masses. Superficial or deep masses should be assessed for size, location, mobility, content (solid, liquid, or air), and the presence or absence of tenderness. The consistency of a patient's response to palpation with and without distraction is particularly useful in those with suspected chronic functional abdominal discomfort. Superficial masses include hernias, lymph nodes, subcutaneous abscesses, lipomas, and hematomas. Deep abdominal masses may be caused by neoplasms (liver, gallbladder, pancreas, stomach, intestine, kidney), abscesses (appendicitis, diverticulitis, Crohn's disease), or aortic aneurysms.

Examination of the right upper quadrant should assess the liver size, contour, texture, and tenderness. Liver size is crudely estimated by percussion of the upper and lower borders of liver dullness in the midclavicular line. Liver contour and tenderness are best assessed during held inspiration by deep palpation along the costal margin. Examination of the left upper quadrant is useful to detect splenomegaly (Chapter 171), although a normal-sized or even an enlarged spleen often cannot be detected. Percussion in the left upper quadrant near the tenth rib (posterior to the midaxillary line) may detect splenic dullness that is distinct from gastric or colonic tympany. The tip of an enlarged spleen may be palpated during inspiration if the examiner supports the left costal margin with the left hand while palpating below the costal margin with the right hand. Ascites should be suspected in a patient with a protuberant abdomen and bulging flanks. To screen for ascites, percussion of the flanks should be performed to assess the level of dullness. If the level of flank dullness appears to be increased, the most sensitive test for ascites is to check for "shifting" dullness when the patient rolls from the supine to the lateral position.

Digital Rectal and Pelvic Examinations

The digital rectal examination is intrusive and uncomfortable and should be performed only when necessary, such as in patients with perianal or rectal symptoms, incontinence, difficult defecation, suspected inflammatory bowel disease, and acute abdominal pain. The digital examination, with or without fecal occult blood testing, is not a useful screening test for colorectal cancer (Chapter 199). However, in patients with acute or chronic GI bleeding (Chapter 137), it is a rapid means of assessing the stool for color and occult blood. The perianal area should be visually inspected for rashes, soilage (suggesting incontinence or fistula), fistulas, fissures, skin tags, external hemorrhoids, and prolapsed internal hemorrhoids (Chapter 147). After gentle digital insertion, the anal canal should be assessed for resting tone and voluntary squeeze. The distal rectal vault should be swept circumferentially to palpate for mass lesions, tenderness, or fluctuance.

Laboratory Studies
Blood Tests

Blood tests routinely obtained in the evaluation of patients with GI symptoms include a complete blood count, liver tests (Chapter 149), serum chemistries, and, in selected cases, pancreatic enzymes and markers of inflammation. GI causes of anemia include acute or chronic GI blood loss, inflammatory bowel disease, nutrient malabsorption (folate, iron, or vitamin B_{12}), and chronic liver disease. Microcytosis suggests iron deficiency due to chronic GI blood loss or malabsorption. Macrocytosis may be attributable to folate or B_{12} malabsorption, medications (e.g., immunomodulators used for inflammatory bowel disease), or chronic liver disease. An elevated platelet count suggests chronic inflammation (e.g., inflammatory bowel disease) or GI blood loss with compensatory marrow production. A low platelet count may be attributable to portal hypertension with splenic sequestration. Low serum albumin may be caused by chronic GI disorders that result in weight loss, nutrient malabsorption, chronic inflammation, loss of protein across abnormal GI mucosa (i.e., protein-losing enteropathy), or decreased hepatic synthesis (e.g., chronic liver disease). Abnormal liver tests may be due to acute or chronic liver diseases, disorders of the pancreas or biliary tract, and medications (Chapter 149). Serum amylase and lipase are obtained to screen for pancreatitis (Chapter 146) in patients with acute abdominal pain. Increased levels of inflammatory markers, such as an elevated erythrocyte sedimentation rate and C-reactive protein, are nonspecific but useful in the management of patients with inflammatory bowel disease (Chapter 143).

Serum ferritin reflects total body iron and may be decreased in patients with chronic GI blood loss or intestinal malabsorption (e.g., celiac disease).

TABLE 134-1 APPROACH TO COMMON GASTROINTESTINAL SIGNS AND SYMPTOMS

	ABDOMINAL PAIN	GI BLEEDING	DIARRHEA	STEATORRHEA	CONSTIPATION
History (ascertain the following)	Duration: acute vs. chronic Onset: sudden vs. 1-2 hr vs. gradual Character: visceral (vague or dull, steady or cramping, diffuse) or parietal (severe, well localized, worse with movement) Location: upper, middle, or lower; radiation Associated symptoms: vomiting, hematemesis, diarrhea, hematochezia, melena, constipation, obstipation, jaundice Previous episodes Other diseases	Acute vs. chronic (duration); intermittent vs. continuous; quantity; hematemesis, melena, or hematochezia; associated pain and location; symptoms of anemia (e.g., dyspnea, chest pain, lightheadedness); medication use (especially aspirin, NSAIDs, anticoagulants); previous episodes; risk factors for chronic liver disease (alcohol, hepatitis)	Acute (<2 wk) vs. chronic (duration); fever, weight loss, or abdominal pain; stool character: number per 24 hr, watery or bloody, large vs. small volume, change in volume with eating, greasy; dietary history (especially lactose); history of IBD, pancreatic disease, intestinal surgery, DM; recent change in medications or antibiotic use; community outbreak or similar symptoms in family members; potential exposure to contaminated food; elderly immunosuppressed host; risk of HIV or sexually transmitted disease	Duration; weight loss; stool number, consistency (greasy), presence of blood; abdominal pain; flatulence; history of excessive alcohol, chronic liver disease, pancreatitis, intestinal dysmotility, surgery, DM; history of easy bruising, night blindness, bone pain, osteoporosis, dermatitis herpetiformis	Acute vs. chronic (duration); age; number of stools per wk; difficulty with defecation (straining, incomplete evacuation, digital manipulation); bloating or discomfort; blood on stools, weight loss; dietary fiber and fluid intake; chronic illness (DM, neuromuscular, endocrine); abdominal surgeries; medications, impaired mobility
Physical findings (evaluate for the following)	Fever, HR, BP Appearance: calm, restless, motionless Inspect: skin, distention, hernias Bowel sounds: present, absent, roaring Percussion and palpation: organomegaly, mass (abscess), focal tenderness, guarding Peritoneal signs: sharp pain with cough, shaking, percussion, light palpation	HR, BP, orthostatic findings; abdominal pain present or absent; signs of chronic liver disease and portal hypertension (which may indicate varices); jaundice, spider angiomas, hepatosplenomegaly; ascites; examine nasogastric aspirate for blood ("coffee grounds" vs. bright red); examine stool for blood (Hemoccult) and color (melena, maroon, or bright red)	HR, BP, orthostatic findings; fever; wasting; presence of abdominal tenderness or mass; perianal disease; extraintestinal symptoms of IBD (e.g., oral ulcers, arthritis, erythema nodosum)	Wasting, presence or absence of abdominal mass or tenderness; rash (vitamin deficiencies) or excessive bruising (vitamin K deficiency); jaundice or signs of chronic liver disease	Assess mobility and chronic medical conditions; abdominal distention; palpable stool within bowel in left lower quadrant; rectal examination— impacted stool, anal fissure, rectal prolapse, pelvic floor descent with straining, rectocele
Laboratory tests	CBC, BUN, Cr, glucose, amylase, lipase, liver tests (ALT, AST, bilirubin, alkaline phosphatase), albumin, INR, U/A, urine β-HCG	CBC BUN, Cr, liver tests, INR, type and cross	CBC, BUN, Cr, glucose, electrolytes, liver tests, albumin, C-reactive protein Selected cases: consider serum chromogranin A, VIP, calcitonin, gastrin, glucagon, urinary 5-HIAA; stool for culture, ova, parasites; consider fecal weight, fat, electrolytes, laxative screen	CBC, glucose, liver tests, albumin, electrolytes, celiac disease antibodies (anti-tTG or antiendomysial); assessment of vitamin and mineral absorption (A, D) and INR (K is fat soluble), folate, iron, calcium, phosphate, B_{12}; qualitative or quantitative stool for fecal fat; H_2 breath test for bacterial overgrowth	CBC, Chem-7, calcium, magnesium, phosphate, TFTs; selected patients with severe constipation may undergo colonic transit studies and/or anal manometry with balloon expulsion

NAUSEA AND VOMITING	DYSPHAGIA	ODYNOPHAGIA	HEARTBURN AND REGURGITATION	ANOREXIA	WEIGHT LOSS
Nausea with or without emesis; acute vs. chronic (duration); intermittent vs. constant; presence or absence of severe abdominal pain, comorbid illnesses, especially peptic ulcer, endocrine (DM), cardiac, psychiatric; medications; history of excessive alcohol	Oropharyngeal vs. esophageal dysphagia; solids vs. liquids; acute vs. chronic (duration); intermittent vs. progressive; GERD symptoms present or absent; weight loss; history of food impactions, allergies, atopic conditions, skin changes, cold hands (Raynaud's phenomenon)	Duration of pain with swallowing; underlying immunosuppression (e.g., HIV infection, DM); caustic ingestion; use of medications that cause topical injury (especially NSAIDs, KCl, bisphosphonates, iron, antibiotics, zidovudine)	Duration of symptoms; location; relation to meals or specific foods; nocturnal symptoms; dysphagia or chest pain; extraesophageal manifestations: cough, hoarseness, asthma	Acute vs. chronic (duration); association with different foods; psychiatric disease (e.g., depression, dementia); chronic or undiagnosed medical conditions (e.g., DM, thyroid or adrenal disease, COPD, advanced heart failure, renal insufficiency, malignancy, HIV infection); medication use	Acute vs. chronic (duration); age; total amount (>5% is significant); intentional vs. unintentional; appetite increased or decreased; rapid vs. gradual; change in physical activity; documented vs. undocumented; fever or sweats; anorexia, nausea, vomiting, diarrhea, steatorrhea, blood in stool; abdominal pain; history or symptoms of chronic medical, neurologic, or psychiatric illness; medications; alcohol and substance abuse
Acute with severe abdominal pain: evaluate for GI obstruction, pancreatitis, mesenteric ischemia, biliary colic, appendicitis, or other conditions causing peritonitis Acute without abdominal pain: evaluate for pregnancy, medications, food poisoning, infectious gastroenteritis, hepatitis, CNS disease, postoperative ileus Chronic: evaluate for medications, chronic gastric outlet obstruction (due to ulcer disease or malignancy), impaired GI motility (gastroparesis), other chronic medical conditions, intracranial disorders, psychiatric disease (bulimia)	Usually normal; examine oropharynx and neck for lymphadenopathy and masses; evaluate the skin for sclerodermatous changes	Usually normal; evaluate oropharynx for thrush, herpetic lesions, caustic injury; general exam for signs of underlying immunosuppression	Usually normal, unless extraesophageal manifestations are present	Wasting; fever; signs of bulimia (e.g., loss of tooth enamel, knuckle ulcerations and calluses); abdominal masses; enlarged lymph nodes	Wasting; malnutrition; poor dentition or poorly fitting dentures; thyromegaly; COPD or heart failure; abdominal masses; enlarged lymph nodes; pelvic masses in women; diabetic neuropathy; signs of depression, dementia, or bulimia
β-HCG, CBC, serum electrolytes, BUN, Cr, glucose, HbA$_{1c}$, liver tests, albumin, TFTs, cortisol	CBC; eosinophilia or elevated IgE in some patients with eosinophilic esophagitis	CBC, HIV test, fasting glucose	Usually normal	CBC, Chem-7, liver tests, albumin, HIV test, TFTs	CBC, Chem-7, HbA$_{1c}$, TFTs, liver tests, C-reactive protein or ESR, calcium, phosphate, albumin, HIV test, morning cortisol

TABLE 134-1 APPROACH TO COMMON GASTROINTESTINAL SIGNS AND SYMPTOMS—cont'd

	ABDOMINAL PAIN	GI BLEEDING	DIARRHEA	STEATORRHEA	CONSTIPATION
Endoscopy	EGD, colonoscopy	EGD, colonoscopy, enteroscopy, wireless capsule study	Colonoscopy (including ileal inspection) with biopsies; EGD with duodenal biopsies; wireless capsule study	EGD with duodenal biopsies	Colonoscopy if recent change in bowel habits
Imaging	CT scan or ultrasound; angiography; small bowel enterography	Tagged RBC scan, angiography	Small bowel enterography: CT, MRI, or barium (Crohn's disease); somatostatin scintigraphy	CT of the abdomen (pancreatic calcifications; biliary dilation)	Usually not necessary; MRI or defecography

ALT = alanine transaminase; AST = aspartate transaminase; BP = blood pressure; BUN = blood urea nitrogen; CBC = complete blood count; CNS = central nervous system; COPD = chronic obstructive pulmonary disease; Cr = creatinine; CT = computed tomography; DM = diabetes mellitus; EGD = esophagogastroduodenoscopy; ESR = erythrocyte sedimentation rate; GERD = gastroesophageal reflux disease; GI = gastrointestinal; HCG = human chorionic gonadotropin; 5-HIAA = 5-hydroxyindoleacetic acid; HIV = human immunodeficiency virus; HR = heart rate; IBD = inflammatory bowel disease; INR = international normalized ratio; MRI = magnetic resonance imaging; NSAIDs = nonsteroidal anti-inflammatory drugs; RBC = red blood cell; TFTs = thyroid function tests; tTG = tissue transglutaminase; U/A = urinalysis; VIP = vasoactive intestinal polypeptide.

Adapted from Proctor DD. Approach to the patient with gastrointestinal disease. In: Goldman L, Ausiello D, eds. *Cecil Textbook of Medicine*, 23rd ed. Philadelphia: Saunders-Elsevier; 2008.

Disorders of malabsorption that result in steatorrhea may lead to deficiencies in the fat-soluble vitamins (A, D, E, K) (Chapter 142). The serum international normalized ratio may be elevated in patients with cholestasis owing to malabsorption of vitamin K or in patients with chronic liver disease due to decreased hepatic synthetic function. Serum B_{12} may be decreased in patients with autoimmune gastritis (pernicious anemia), gastric bypass surgery, or malabsorption due to small bowel bacterial overgrowth or disease of the terminal ileum (e.g., Crohn's).

Specialized laboratory tests that are useful for the diagnosis of specific diseases include antibodies to *Helicobacter pylori* in patients with peptic ulcer disease or dyspepsia, antibodies to tissue transglutaminase in celiac disease, antibodies to microbial antigens or autoimmune markers in inflammatory bowel disease (anti–*Saccharomyces cerevisiae* [ASCA], perinuclear antineutrophil cytoplasmic antibody [pANCA]), and CA-19-9 in pancreaticobiliary malignancy. Owing to their limited sensitivity and specificity, these tests are not useful for screening but may be helpful in circumscribed situations in which the results may shift the diagnostic probability.

Stool Examination

Fecal occult blood testing is useful to evaluate iron deficiency anemia and acute or chronic GI blood loss. In patients with acute diarrhea, assessment of fecal leukocytes or culture of common pathogens is routine, and in selected patients, testing for parasites (*Giardia, Entamoeba histolytica*), *Clostridium difficile, Escherichia coli* O157:H7, or other specific organisms may be warranted. To distinguish among the causes of chronic diarrhea (Chapter 142), stool samples may be sent for assessment of electrolytes, leukocytes, and fecal fat.

Endoscopy and Radiology

Endoscopy (Chapter 136) and radiographic studies (Chapter 135) play a major role in the evaluation and management of many GI disorders. Esophageal manometry and esophageal pH and impedance monitoring can be useful for the evaluation of heartburn, reflux, and other esophageal symptoms (Chapter 140). Anorectal manometry may be useful in some patients with fecal incontinence and defecatory dysfunction (Chapter 147). Breath tests are commonly used to diagnose *H. pylori* infection (Chapter 141), lactose intolerance, and small bowel bacterial overgrowth (Chapter 142).

The diagnosis of a functional GI disorder is made after organic disorders have been excluded by clinical evaluation and limited, directed diagnostic testing. "Overtesting" should be avoided. Thereafter, the emphasis should switch from finding a "cause" of the symptoms to implementing successful coping and adaptive behaviors.

ABDOMINAL PAIN

Abdominal pain, which is a frequent complaint among outpatients in the office setting and emergency department, may be benign and self-limited or the presenting symptom of severe, life-threatening disease. Chronic abdominal pain that has been present for months or years in the absence of other organic illness is almost always functional in origin and does not require urgent evaluation. By contrast, most patients with severe acute abdominal pain require a thorough but emergent evaluation, which may quickly reveal an acute surgical illness.

PATHOBIOLOGY

Stimulation of hollow abdominal viscera is mediated by splanchnic afferent fibers within the muscle wall, visceral peritoneum, and mesentery that are sensitive to distention and contraction. Visceral afferent nerves are loosely organized, innervate several organs, and enter the spinal cord at several levels. Thus, visceral pain is vague or dull in character and diffuse; patients attempting to localize the pain often move their entire hand over the upper, middle, or lower abdomen. Most visceral pain is steady, but cramping, intermittent pain or "colic" results from peristaltic contractions caused by partial or complete obstruction of the small intestine, ureter, or uterine tubes. In contrast to visceral innervation, the parietal peritoneum is innervated unilaterally by a dense network of nerve fibers that follow a spinal T6 to L1 somatic distribution. Pain fibers of the parietal peritoneum are stimulated by stretch or distention of the abdominal cavity or retroperitoneum; direct irritation from infection, pus, or secretions (e.g., caused by a ruptured viscus); or inflammation caused by contact between the parietal peritoneum and an adjacent inflamed organ (e.g., appendicitis). Parietal pain is sharp, well characterized, and localized by the patient to a precise location on the abdomen, often by pointing with one finger.

The gastrointestinal viscera (liver, biliary system, pancreas, and GI tract) arise during embryology from midline structures that have bilateral innervation. Thus, GI visceral pain is typically localized to the abdominal midline.

Acute Abdominal Pain

CLINICAL MANIFESTATIONS
History

The history should determine the time course, character, and location and radiation pattern of the pain (Table 134-2). Severe abdominal pain that begins suddenly over seconds to minutes indicates a catastrophic event such as esophageal rupture, perforated peptic ulcer or viscus, ruptured ectopic pregnancy, ruptured aortic aneurysm, acute mesenteric ischemia, or myocardial infarction. Pain that progresses within 1 to 2 hours is consistent with a rapidly progressive inflammatory disorder (e.g., cholecystitis, appendicitis, pancreatitis), acute obstruction of a viscus (small intestinal obstruction, ureteral colic), or organ ischemia caused by a strangulated blood supply (volvulus, strangulated hernia, ovarian torsion). Pain that is less severe and develops over several hours is more commonly caused by a medical rather than a surgical condition, including upper GI disorders (dyspepsia), intestinal disorders (gastroenteritis, inflammatory bowel disease), liver disorders (hepatitis, abscess), urinary disorders (cystitis, pyelonephritis), or gynecologic infections; however, the slow evolution of surgical disorders such as cholecystitis (Chapter 158), appendicitis or diverticulitis (Chapter 144), and intra-abdominal abscesses must not be overlooked.

The character of the pain provides important information about whether the symptoms are due to visceral stimulation or parietal stimulation

NAUSEA AND VOMITING	DYSPHAGIA	ODYNOPHAGIA	HEARTBURN AND REGURGITATION	ANOREXIA	WEIGHT LOSS
EGD to exclude gastric outlet obstruction	EGD with biopsies and/or dilation, esophageal motility study, 24-hr pH probe	EGD with biopsies	EGD (to detect erosive esophagitis or Barrett's esophagus); 24-hr pH probe	Directed at detecting underlying disease, e.g., if a GI cause is suspected, EGD and/or colonoscopy with biopsies may be helpful	Directed at detecting underlying disease, e.g., if a GI cause is suspected, EGD and/or colonoscopy with biopsies may be helpful
CT of the abdomen; if chronic, also consider head CT, gastric emptying study, small bowel enterography	Esophagogram (barium swallow) will show stricture, Schatzki's ring, mass, etc.	Usually not necessary	Usually not necessary	Directed at detecting underlying disease, e.g., if a GI cause is suspected, abdominal CT may be helpful	Directed at detecting underlying disease, e.g., chest or abdominal CT may be helpful

(peritonitis). Patients with peritonitis may report severe localized pain or irritation with activities or maneuvers that stretch or move the parietal peritoneum, such as walking, moving in bed, and coughing; as a result, they tend to lie quietly to avoid painful stimulation. By contrast, patients with visceral pain may move or walk restlessly or attempt a bowel movement in an effort to relieve their symptoms.

The location of pain in the upper, middle, or lower abdomen is a crude but important indicator of the diagnosis (Fig. 134-1). Visceral pain arising from the foregut (esophagus, stomach, proximal duodenum, bile duct, gallbladder, pancreas) most often manifests in the epigastrium. Pain derived from the midgut (small intestine, appendix, ascending colon, proximal transverse colon) presents in a periumbilical location. Pain derived from the hindgut (distal transverse colon, left colon, rectum) localizes to the lower midline between the umbilicus and symphysis pubis. Paired intra-abdominal organs such as the kidneys, ureters, ovaries, and fallopian tubes have unilateral innervation that localizes pain to the side of the involved organ. As some surgical conditions progress, the character and location of the pain shift from a visceral to a parietal pain pattern. Thus, early cholecystitis (Chapter 158) may present with vague midline epigastric pain that progresses to sharp right upper quadrant pain as localized peritoneal irritation develops. Likewise, appendicitis (Chapter 144) commonly begins with vague, diffuse periumbilical pain that evolves to sharp, well-localized right lower quadrant pain as peritonitis ensues.

Anorexia, vomiting, diarrhea, distention, and constipation are commonly seen with abdominal pain caused by both medical and surgical disorders. Although nonspecific, the *absence* of any of these symptoms is evidence against an emergent surgical or medical disorder because severe illness usually leads to reflex stimulation or inhibition of gastric and intestinal peristalsis. Vomiting is common in medical and surgical disorders involving the upper GI tract, including acute gastroenteritis, pancreatitis, gastric and small intestinal obstruction, and biliary tract disease. Pain that precedes the onset of vomiting is typical of surgical conditions, whereas the reverse is true of medical conditions (e.g., food poisoning, gastroenteritis). Abdominal pain with prominent diarrhea is most commonly caused by a medical condition (e.g., gastroenteritis, inflammatory bowel disease). Although constipation alone is a nonspecific complaint, the absence of stool passage and flatus is consistent with complete bowel obstruction or paralytic ileus.

Jaundice accompanying acute abdominal pain virtually always indicates a hepatobiliary disorder (Chapter 149), including obstruction of the biliary duct (choledocholithiasis, pancreatic carcinoma, cholangiocarcinoma), complications of acute cholecystitis, acute hepatitis (viral, ischemic), or hepatic malignancies. The possibility of cholangitis should be considered and excluded in all patients with acute abdominal pain and jaundice, especially if the patient has fever, chills, hypotension, altered mental status, or leukocytosis. Hematemesis with upper abdominal pain suggests a Mallory-Weiss tear, alcoholic gastritis, or peptic ulcer disease. Hematochezia with abdominal pain is most commonly caused by medical conditions such as infectious gastroenteritis or inflammatory bowel disease, but it also may be caused by ischemic colitis or mesenteric ischemia. Gross hematuria may be due to

cystitis (Chapter 292) or a ureteral stone (Chapter 125). Abdominal pain with weight loss may be due to inflammatory bowel disease, chronic mesenteric ischemia, or advanced GI malignancies. In women, a missed menstrual period, adnexal pain, spotting, or cramping may suggest pregnancy, ectopic pregnancy, or spontaneous abortion. Acute pain between cycles may be caused by ovarian follicles or ruptured corpus luteum cysts. Pelvic pain with fever, chills, or cervical discharge suggests pelvic inflammatory disease.

The past medical history and review of systems can provide clues about systemic and extra-abdominal conditions that may present with abdominal pain. Acute coronary syndromes (Chapter 72), heart failure (Chapter 58), pneumonia (Chapter 97), or empyema may cause dyspepsia, epigastric or right or left upper quadrant pain, nausea, and vomiting. Metabolic conditions such as uremia (Chapter 132), diabetes with hyperglycemia or ketoacidosis (Chapter 236), hypercalcemia (Chapter 253), or acute adrenocortical insufficiency (Chapter 234) may cause pain, nausea, vomiting, and diarrhea. Acute intermittent porphyria (Chapter 217) and familial Mediterranean fever (Chapter 283) may cause recurrent episodes of severe pain and peritonitis that may be misdiagnosed, leading to unnecessary surgeries. Other causes of acute abdominal pain include narcotic withdrawal (Chapter 33), insect or reptile bites (Chapter 113), and lead or arsenic poisoning (Chapter 21).

Physical Examination

The physical examination must identify life-threatening illnesses that require urgent surgical evaluation. Nevertheless, the examination must be orderly, careful, and complete. If the examiner immediately palpates the site of maximal pain, the patient is unlikely to relax and cooperate for the remainder of the examination.

First, the patient should be observed and the abdomen inspected. Most patients remain calm, cooperative, and freely capable of moving during the examination. Patients who are writhing or restless may have pain due to visceral distention (e.g., renal colic, intestinal obstruction), whereas patients who lie motionless may have peritonitis. Gentle shaking of the bed or having the patient cough may elicit sharp, well-localized pain in patients with parietal but not visceral pain. Auscultation should be performed before percussion or palpation so that intestinal activity is undisturbed. An abdomen that is quiet except for infrequent squeaks or tinkles suggests peritonitis or ileus. Loud peristaltic rushes that occur in synchrony with abdominal pain suggest small bowel obstruction. Light percussion across the upper, middle, and lower abdomen can determine any site of focal tenderness suggestive of peritonitis. Light palpation should be performed with one or two fingers (not the whole hand), beginning away from where the patient localizes the pain and gradually moving to the site of pain. Thereafter, gentle, deeper palpation of the entire abdomen is performed gradually, including the region of tenderness. An attempt should be made to palpate for an abdominal aortic aneurysm (Chapter 78). Examination also should include the inguinal and femoral canals, umbilicus, and surgical scars for evidence of incarcerating hernias. The presence of focal tenderness indicates parietal peritoneal irritation. Voluntary or involuntary tightening of the muscle wall ("guarding") may occur during

TABLE 134-2 TYPICAL MANIFESTATIONS OF KEY CAUSES OF ACUTE AND CHRONIC ABDOMINAL PAIN

CONDITION	LOCATION	QUALITY	ONSET	AGGRAVATING OR RELIEVING FACTORS	ASSOCIATED SYMPTOMS OR SIGNS	DIAGNOSTIC STUDIES
Peptic ulcer disease (Chapter 141)	Epigastric, occasionally RUQ, rarely LUQ	Dyspepsia: mild to moderate aching discomfort, pain, burning, gnawing, postprandial fullness	Days	Variable relief with antacids; may be relieved by, worsened by, or unrelated to meals	Recurrent; associated factors (e.g., *Helicobacter pylori*, aspirin, NSAIDs)	Anemia, upper endoscopy, *H. pylori* testing
Acute pancreatitis (Chapter 146)	Epigastric, radiates to midback (occasionally RUQ or LUQ)	Diffuse, steady, stabbing, penetrating	1-2 hr	Aggravated by food; better when lying still and with narcotics	Severe nausea and vomiting; reduced or absent bowel sounds; associated factors (e.g., alcohol, gallstones)	Elevated amylase and lipase, CT
Acute cholecystitis (Chapter 158)	Epigastric, then moves to RUQ; may radiate to right scapula	Gradual, steady increase, moderate to severe	Hours	May follow a fatty meal; better with narcotics and surgery	Nausea, some vomiting, fever	Elevated WBC count, US or CT
Acute appendicitis (Chapter 144)	Periumbilical, then moves to RLQ	Vague initially; gradual, steady increase to intense, localized, pain	Hours	Unprovoked; better with narcotics and surgery	Anorexia, nausea, obstipation; occasional vomiting, fever late	Elevated WBC count, US or CT
Diverticulitis (Chapter 144)	LLQ or suprapubic	Moderate to severe, steady or cramping, sharp or aching, localized	Hours to days	Unprovoked; better with narcotics and antibiotics or surgery	Anorexia, nausea, distention, constipation or loose stools; partial relief with passage of flatus or BM; fever late	Elevated WBC count, CT
Ruptured viscus and peritonitis (Chapter 144)	Diffuse	Intense	Minutes to hours	Worse with cough or movement; better when lying still or with narcotics or surgery	Fever, anorexia, nausea, vomiting; lack of bowel sounds; tenderness with percussion, light touch, rebound; guarding and rigidity (late); loath to move	Elevated WBC count, CT
Intestinal ischemia (Chapter 145)	Small intestine—periumbilical; proximal (right) colon—periumbilical or RLQ; distal colon—LLQ	Severe, stabbing pain out of proportion to physical findings	Minutes	Chronic ischemia—occurs after eating; acute ischemia—usually unprovoked; better with narcotics, thrombus dissolution, stenting, surgical resection	Nausea, bloody diarrhea; associated factors (e.g., hypotension, cardiac arrhythmias)	Elevated WBC count, angiography or colonoscopy (colonic ischemia)
Strangulated hernia (Chapter 144)	Localized	Sharp, localized, intense; crampy or steady	Minutes to hours	Previous hernia history; unprovoked; better with narcotics and decompression, including surgery	Anorexia, nausea, vomiting, no stool or flatus passage if obstruction; bowel sounds variable—hyperactive early if obstruction present, but absent bowel sounds late, especially with peritonitis	Elevated WBC count, CT, US
Small or large bowel obstruction (Chapter 144)	Small intestine—periumbilical; proximal (right) colon—periumbilical or right abdomen; distal (left) colon—LLQ	Early—diffuse, colicky, crampy; late—steady and better localized	Hours to days	Aggravated by food; better with narcotics, NGT decompression, and/or surgery	Distention, anorexia, nausea, vomiting; no stool or flatus passage; small intestine—increased hyperperistaltic (rushes) bowel sounds (early) or quiet abdomen (late); large intestine—bowel sounds variable; associated factors (e.g., hernia, previous surgery)	CT

TABLE 134-2 TYPICAL MANIFESTATIONS OF KEY CAUSES OF ACUTE AND CHRONIC ABDOMINAL PAIN—cont'd

CONDITION	LOCATION	QUALITY	ONSET	AGGRAVATING OR RELIEVING FACTORS	ASSOCIATED SYMPTOMS OR SIGNS	DIAGNOSTIC STUDIES
Abdominal abscess (Chapter 144)	Located over the abscess, usually LLQ or RLQ	Insidious, intense, constant	Days	May be aggravated by movement; better with abscess drainage	Fever, anorexia, nausea, abdominal mass	Elevated WBC count, CT
Acute hepatitis (Chapter 150)	RUQ	Dull or intense; localized	Days	Worse with deep inspiration	Jaundice, anorexia, nausea; liver enlarged and tender to palpation; associated factors (e.g., alcohol, infection)	Abnormal liver tests
GERD (Chapter 140)	Substernal or epigastric	Burning, gnawing	Days to years	Provoked by large or fatty meals or recumbency; relief with antacids	Recurrent; may have regurgitation, dysphagia, or extraesophageal manifestations (e.g., asthma, chronic cough, laryngitis)	Upper endoscopy (usually normal), 24-hr pH probe
Nonulcer (functional) dyspepsia (Chapter 139)	Epigastric	Mild to moderate discomfort, pain, burning, gnawing, postprandial fullness	Years	May be worsened by meals; cannot be reliably distinguished from ulcer disease by history alone	Other symptoms of functional disorders (IBS, fibromyalgia, pelvic pain)	Normal EGD
IBS (Chapter 139)	Variable; usually lower abdomen	Vague, crampy, sense of urgency	Years	Pain may be precipitated by dietary factors or stress; associated with change in bowel characteristics (e.g., frequency, form, difficulty with passage); relieved with stool passage	Bloating and abdominal distention	Normal sigmoidoscopy, colonoscopy, and CT, but these are usually not necessary for diagnosis
Chronic pancreatitis (Chapter 146)	Epigastric or periumbilical, radiates to midback	Intense, localized	Days to years	Aggravated by food; better with narcotics	Anorexia, nausea, vomiting; associated factors (e.g., alcohol)	Amylase and lipase may be normal; CT may show calcifications, dilated pancreatic duct, pseudocyst
Inflammatory or infectious enterocolitis (Chapters 142 and 291)	Small intestine—periumbilical; large intestine—right or left side of the abdomen over the colon; rectum—tenesmus	Crampy	Hours to days	Better with stool passage and treatment of underlying cause	Nausea, vomiting, bloody diarrhea; associated factors (e.g., infectious—food transmission, IBD—prolonged duration, family history)	Stool studies for culture, colonoscopy with biopsies
Malignancy (Chapter 199)	Variable, depending on cancer location	Variable; intense and crampy if bowel obstruction; steady and vague if local invasion	Days	Better with narcotics and cancer therapy	Primary vs. metastatic disease	CT and biopsies, PET
Pneumonia/pleurisy (Chapters 97 and 99)	Upper abdomen: epigastric, RUQ, or LUQ	Localized; worse with deep breathing	Hours to days	Painful breathing; better with antibiotics	Cough, fever, dyspnea	CXR
Angina and myocardial infarction (Chapters 71-73)	Retrosternal or epigastric	Pressure, squeezing, heaviness, or intense	Minutes	Worse with exertion; relief with nitroglycerin	Dyspnea, diaphoresis	ECG, cardiac enzymes, stress testing
Genitourinary disorders (Chapters 128 and 293)	Bladder—suprapubic; renal colic—abrupt, excruciating LLQ or RLQ pain radiating to the groin; prostate—dull, suprapubic; kidney—CVA	Constant or colicky; stone passage—restless, cannot find a comfortable position	Minutes to days	Better with antibiotics and pain medications (pyelonephritis or nephrolithiasis)	Hematuria, dysuria, prostate tenderness, fever	Urinalysis, urine culture, CT for stone disease

TABLE 134-2   TYPICAL MANIFESTATIONS OF KEY CAUSES OF ACUTE AND CHRONIC ABDOMINAL PAIN—cont'd

CONDITION	LOCATION	QUALITY	ONSET	AGGRAVATING OR RELIEVING FACTORS	ASSOCIATED SYMPTOMS OR SIGNS	DIAGNOSTIC STUDIES
Ovarian cysts or torsion (Chapters 205 and 243)	LLQ or RLQ	Constant, intense	Minutes	Better with NSAIDs or surgery (torsion)	Nausea, vomiting; may be recurrent	US
Ruptured ectopic pregnancy (Chapter 247)	LLQ or RLQ	Constant, intense, stabbing	Minutes	Better with surgery	Rebound and guarding present, abnormal menses or amenorrhea	Acute anemia, elevated β-HCG, US
Musculoskeletal disorders	Specific muscle groups	Aching	Days	Better with heat or NSAIDs; aggravated by movement	History of muscle injury or exertion	Normal laboratory results
Herpes zoster (Chapter 383)	Dermatomal distribution	Burning, itching, neuropathic, constant	Days	Aggravated by touching the dermatome; better with pain or antiviral medications	Recurrent; rash may or may not be present	Skin culture or biopsy
Metabolic disorders (e.g., DM; Chapter 236)	Epigastric or generalized	Intense, constant	Hours to days	Worse with poor metabolic control (e.g., poor glucose control)	Recurrent; nausea, vomiting, diabetic neuropathy	Specific metabolic parameters abnormal (e.g., elevated glucose in DM)
Abdominal epilepsy (Chapter 410)	Epigastric or umbilical	Constant	Hours to days	Unprovoked; better with antiseizure therapy	Recurrent; may have associated seizure disorder	EEG
Dissecting or leaking abdominal aortic aneurysm (Chapter 78)	Over the aneurysm, radiates to the back or groin	Severe, searing, constant	Minutes to hours to days	History of HTN or CAD	Shock, pulsatile mass; bruit *not* usually present	Acute anemia, CT, angiography

BM = bowel movement; CAD = coronary artery disease; CT = computed tomography; CVA = costovertebral angle; CXR = chest x-ray; DM = diabetes mellitus; ECG = electrocardiogram; EEG = electroencephalogram; EGD = esophagogastroduodenoscopy; GERD = gastroesophageal reflux disease; HCG = human chorionic gonadotropin; HTN = hypertension; IBD = irritable bowel disease; IBS = irritable bowel syndrome; LLQ = left lower quadrant; LUQ = left upper quadrant; NGT = nasogastric tube; NSAIDs = nonsteroidal anti-inflammatory drugs; PET = positron emission tomography; RLQ = right lower quadrant; RUQ = right upper quadrant; US = ultrasonography; WBC = white blood cell.

Adapted from Proctor DD. Approach to the patient with gastrointestinal disease. In: Goldman L, Ausiello D, eds. *Cecil Textbook of Medicine*, 23rd ed. Philadelphia: Saunders-Elsevier; 2008.

FIGURE 134-1. Differential diagnosis of abdominal pain by its initial location. IBD = inflammatory bowel disease; TOA = tubo-ovarian abscess.

palpation. With gentle, steady compression of the abdomen with one hand, voluntary guarding usually subsides, allowing the examination to proceed. Persistent involuntary guarding indicates peritonitis with reflex muscle wall contraction. Testing for "rebound tenderness" in patients with suspected peritonitis is not recommended because it causes significant pain and is usually not necessary to establish the diagnosis. When the presentation strongly suggests a nonserious GI disorder but the patient has significant tenderness with palpation, it is useful to use the stethoscope ostensibly to listen for bowel sounds but actually to reproduce the pressure of palpation. A significant discrepancy in the tenderness elicited by the stethoscope and by digital palpation may be seen in patients who are anxious, have functional complaints, or are seeking secondary gain. A digital rectal examination should be performed in most patients with acute abdominal pain to evaluate for tenderness or fluctuance that suggests a perirectal abscess and to assess the stool for signs of overt or occult blood. Women with lower abdominal pain should have a pelvic examination by a skilled examiner to evaluate for gynecologic pathology. Some specific and dramatic findings point to particular diagnoses (Table 134-3).

Special Populations

Increased diligence is required in the evaluation of patients in whom abdominal signs and symptoms may be minimal until the disease process is far advanced. Such patients include the elderly (Chapter 24) and patients who have dementia (Chapter 409), psychiatric disturbances (Chapter 404), or spinal cord injuries. An admitting diagnosis of "altered mental status," "failure to thrive," "obstipation," or "fever of unknown origin" may stem from serious intra-abdominal conditions. Disorders that may be overlooked in the elderly include bowel perforation, bowel obstruction, cholecystitis, diverticulitis, volvulus, mesenteric ischemia, and abdominal aortic aneurysm. In patients with chronic liver disease, the presence of ascites may mask the signs and symptoms of serious surgical conditions such as cholecystitis, appendicitis, and diverticulitis. Even in the presence of perforation, signs of peritonitis may be lacking because the ascites fluid separates the visceral peritoneum and parietal peritoneum. Likewise, immunocompromised populations, who are at risk for infectious, drug-related, and iatrogenic complications, may manifest few physical findings or laboratory abnormalities. Owing to the limitations of the clinical evaluation in these vulnerable populations, there should be a low threshold for the use of abdominal imaging.

Abdominal Pain Developing in the Hospital

When pain develops as a new problem in a hospitalized patient, it is usually caused by a limited number of conditions. Postprocedural complications may cause perforation, infection, or bleeding (intraperitoneal, retroperitoneal, or within solid organs). Shunting of splanchnic blood flow in severely ill medical or surgical patients may cause stress gastritis, nonocclusive mesenteric ischemia, or acalculous cholecystitis. Adynamic ileus or acute colonic pseudo-obstruction is common in critically ill or postoperative patients and manifests as diffuse abdominal pain and distention. *Clostridium difficile* (Chapter 304) colitis is a common cause of pain, diarrhea, and distention, especially in patients on antibiotics. Constipation (Chapter 138), which is a common problem in hospitalized patients, may go unnoticed until pain and distention develop. Finally, many medications can cause dyspepsia and abdominal pain.

DIAGNOSIS

Patients with acute abdominal pain should have a complete blood count with differential; leukocytosis is present in most acute surgical conditions (Fig. 134-2). A pregnancy test is required in women of childbearing age. Serum electrolytes, glucose, blood urea nitrogen, and creatinine levels assess hydration, acid-base status, and renal function. Liver chemistries and pancreatic enzymes should be obtained in most patients, but especially in those with upper abdominal pain, jaundice, or vomiting. An elevation in aspartate or alanine aminotransferase levels may reflect choledocholithiasis with acute biliary obstruction (Chapter 158), acute gallstone pancreatitis (Chapter 146), or a hepatocellular process (Chapter 150). Painful jaundice with a significant rise in the alkaline phosphatase level usually reflects cholestasis caused by extrahepatic biliary obstruction (Chapter 158). Amylase and lipase levels are elevated in most patients with acute pancreatitis, but minor amylase elevations also occur with a perforated viscus or mesenteric ischemia (Chapter 145). Urinalysis may demonstrate pyuria, hematuria, or bacteriuria owing to ureteral calculi (Chapter 128) or urinary tract infection (Chapter 292).

Imaging

Ultrasound is preferred in suspected pregnancy and to evaluate for other acute gynecologic disorders such as tubo-ovarian abscess, ruptured corpus luteum cyst, or ovarian torsion; it is also preferred for the initial evaluation of suspected acute cholecystitis (Chapter 158) and ureteral stones with hydronephrosis (Chapter 125) and for the bedside evaluation of unstable patients. In most other settings, abdominal computed tomography (CT) with oral and intravenous contrast (when possible) is preferred and can provide a definitive diagnosis in up to 90% of patients with acute severe abdominal pain (Chapter 135). Abdominal CT may be falsely negative early in the course of acute pancreatitis, mesenteric ischemia, cholecystitis, appendicitis, and diverticulitis, especially if performed without contrast.

TREATMENT   Rx

Once the diagnosis is clear, treatment of the underlying condition is initiated. In patients with nonspecific acute abdominal pain and no clear diagnosis, early laparoscopy is useful for diagnosis, but outcomes such as complication rates, readmission rates, and length of hospitalization are no better than with a strategy of active observation.[1]

Chronic Abdominal Pain

Chronic or recurrent abdominal pain that has been present for months to years may be caused by structural (organic) disease, but the majority of patients have a functional disorder such as irritable bowel syndrome (Chapter 139). Common organic causes of chronic abdominal pain include medications with GI side effects, peptic ulcer disease (Chapter 141), inflammatory bowel disease (Chapter 143), chronic pancreatitis (Chapter 146), biliary tract disease (Chapter 158), GI cancers (Chapters 198 and 199), and endometriosis (Chapter 244). The clinician should attempt to distinguish patients with symptoms or signs of organic disease, in whom further diagnostic investigation is warranted, from those with probable functional disease (Fig. 134-3). Although functional disorders occur in all age groups, the symptoms usually begin before age 40. "Alarm" features that suggest a structural disorder and are inconsistent with a functional disorder are fever, severe pain, significant weight loss, jaundice, progressive dysphagia, recurrent vomiting, nocturnal pain or diarrhea, and stools that are bloody or positive for fecal occult blood. Laboratory studies should be normal with functional disorders; therefore, an unrevealing evaluation for anemia, leukocytosis, and levels of iron, albumin, C-reactive protein, and vitamins A, D, or B_{12} argues against structural or organic disease.

TABLE 134-3	PHYSICAL SIGNS IN PATIENTS WITH ACUTE ABDOMINAL PAIN	
SIGN	**DESCRIPTION**	**DIAGNOSIS**
Murphy's sign	Cessation of inspiration during right upper quadrant examination	Acute cholecystitis
McBurney's sign	Tenderness located midway between anterior superior iliac spine and umbilicus	Acute appendicitis
Cullen's sign	Periumbilical bluish discoloration	Retroperitoneal hemorrhage Pancreatic hemorrhage Ruptured abdominal aortic aneurysm
Grey Turner's sign	Bluish discoloration of flanks	Retroperitoneal hemorrhage Pancreatic hemorrhage Ruptured abdominal aortic aneurysm
Kehr's sign	Severe left shoulder pain	Splenic rupture Ectopic pregnancy rupture
Obturator sign	Pain with flexed right hip rotation	Appendicitis
Psoas sign	Pain with straight leg raising against resistance (right side)	Appendicitis

Approach to the Patient with Acute Abdominal Pain

FIGURE 134-2. Approach to the patient with acute abdominal pain. CBC = complete blood count; CT = computed tomography; EEG = electroencephalography; EGD = esophagogastroduodenoscopy; RUQ = right upper quadrant; U/A = urinalysis; US = ultrasonography.

In patients younger than 50 years with a suspected functional disorder and no alarm features (e.g., family history of colon cancer or inflammatory bowel disease or abnormalities on screening blood tests), further testing should be minimized, and the emphasis should be shifted to managing symptoms, coping, and making lifestyle changes (Chapter 139). In patients who may have organic disease, testing often includes a combination of upper GI endoscopy, colonoscopy, and ultrasound or CT imaging.

GAS AND BLOATING

Belching

Belching (eructation), which is the involuntary or voluntary release of gas from the esophagus or stomach, commonly occurs during or after a meal. Virtually all belching is caused by swallowed air, which may be increased by eating quickly, drinking carbonated beverages, chewing gum, and smoking. Gas also may be produced within the stomach by antacids, especially sodium bicarbonate, which rapidly neutralize gastric acid and release carbon dioxide. Belching seldom reflects serious GI dysfunction but may be increased in patients with gastroesophageal reflux (Chapter 140), functional dyspepsia (Chapter 139), or gastroparesis (Chapter 138). Chronic, excessive, repetitive belching is a functional disorder caused by habitual aerophagia (air swallowing) and is treated with behavioral modification.

Flatus

Flatus or "gas" is a normal byproduct of digestion. Otherwise healthy adults pass flatus 10 to 20 times daily and excrete up to 1500 mL. Thus, it is difficult to distinguish patients with abnormal or excessive gas production from those with only a heightened awareness of or sensitivity to normal production. Increased flatulence with diarrhea may be symptomatic of disorders of malabsorption, including celiac disease (Chapter 142), pancreatic insufficiency (Chapter 146), and small intestinal bacterial overgrowth (Chapter 142).

In normal adults, flatus is derived from two sources: swallowed air and colonic bacterial fermentation of carbohydrates that results in the production of carbon dioxide or methane. Carbohydrates that may be incompletely absorbed in the small intestine and pass into the colon include lactose (dairy products), fructose, sorbitol, trehalose (mushrooms), and the α-galactosyl oligosaccharides raffinose, stachyose, and verbascose. The latter are found in increased amounts in cruciferous vegetables (cabbage, broccoli, cauliflower, brussels sprouts, turnips, rutabagas), legumes (beans, soy, lentils, peas), pasta, and whole grains. Fructose is present in fruits, especially apples and pears, and is a major component of corn syrups that are used widely as sweeteners. Sorbitol is a natural sugar in stone fruits (peaches, apricots, plums, prunes) and is a common sweetener in sugar-free candies.

TREATMENT ℞

Patients with long-standing flatulence in the absence of other symptoms or signs of GI disease can be treated conservatively. Avoidance of carbonated beverages, chewing gum, sorbitol- and fructose-containing sweeteners, and gas-producing vegetables improves symptoms in most patients. Lactase deficiency may be confirmed by a lactose breath test. Underlying GI illness is suggested by the recent onset of flatulence with other symptoms of organic disease, including weight loss, abdominal pain, diarrhea, distention, and abnormal laboratory studies (Chapter 142). A positive fecal fat analysis confirms malabsorption and merits further investigation (see Table 142-4 in Chapter 142). Suspected small bowel bacterial overgrowth may be confirmed by carbohydrate breath tests or treated empirically with antibiotics.

Bloating and Distention

Bloating and distention are common complaints among patients with functional GI disorders (Chapter 139). As chronic, isolated symptoms, they are almost never caused by serious structural disease. Functional bloating may be caused by heightened sensitivity to minor increases in intestinal gas or impaired transit of gas, even though the total volume of intestinal gas is within normal limits. The acute onset of distention in conjunction with alarm symptoms such as cramping pain, weight loss, nausea, vomiting, obstipation, or diarrhea warrants further evaluation for disorders that cause intestinal

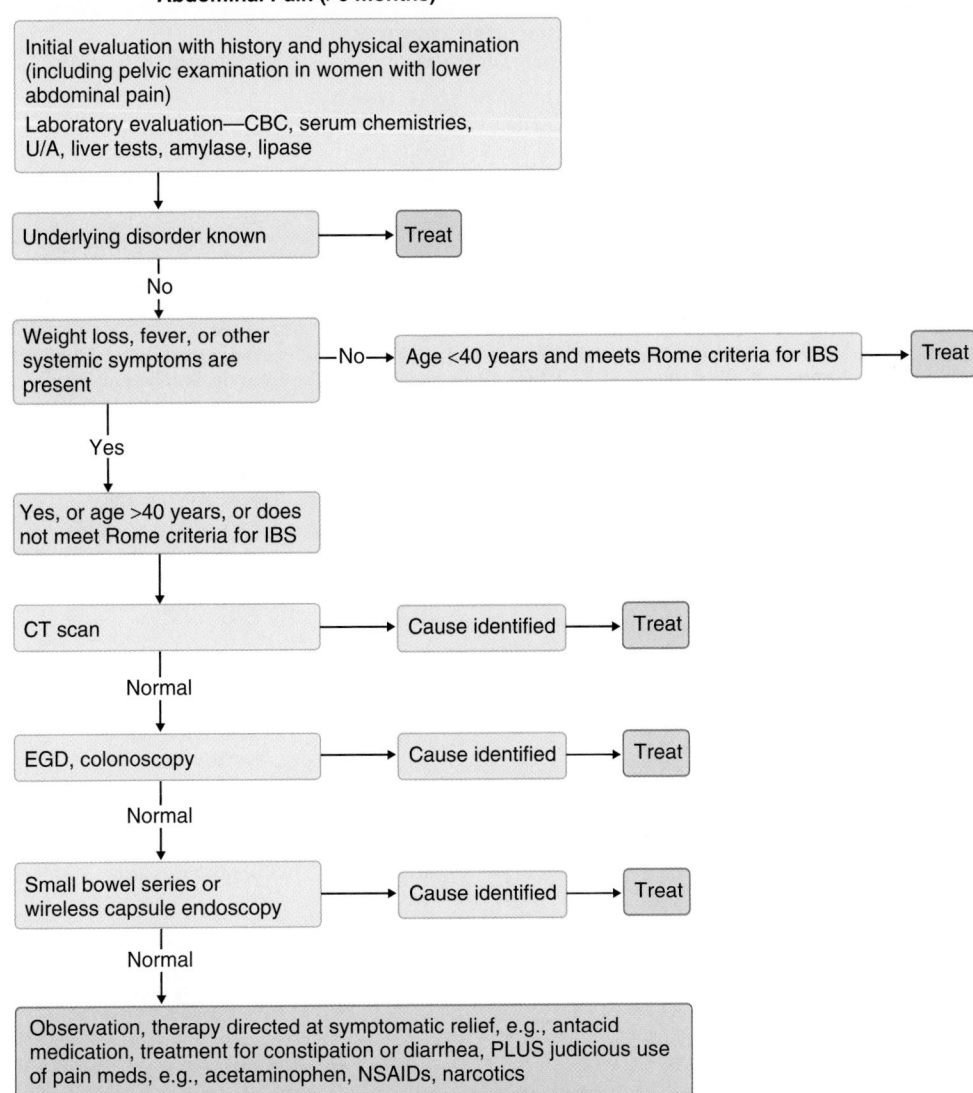

Approach to the Patient with Chronic Abdominal Pain (>6 months)

Initial evaluation with history and physical examination (including pelvic examination in women with lower abdominal pain)
Laboratory evaluation—CBC, serum chemistries, U/A, liver tests, amylase, lipase

↓

Underlying disorder known → Treat

↓ No

Weight loss, fever, or other systemic symptoms are present —No→ Age <40 years and meets Rome criteria for IBS → Treat

↓ Yes

Yes, or age >40 years, or does not meet Rome criteria for IBS

↓

CT scan → Cause identified → Treat

↓ Normal

EGD, colonoscopy → Cause identified → Treat

↓ Normal

Small bowel series or wireless capsule endoscopy → Cause identified → Treat

↓ Normal

Observation, therapy directed at symptomatic relief, e.g., antacid medication, treatment for constipation or diarrhea, PLUS judicious use of pain meds, e.g., acetaminophen, NSAIDs, narcotics
Further evaluation as suggested by symptoms with gallbladder ultrasound, gastric emptying study, ERCP, endoscopic ultrasound, or angiogram and/or consultation with gynecology, surgery, or psychiatry. If ascites is present, paracentesis.

FIGURE 134-3. Approach to the patient with chronic abdominal pain. CBC = complete blood count; CT = computed tomography; EGD = esophagogastro-duodenoscopy; ERCP = endoscopic retrograde cholangiopancreatography; IBS = irritable bowel syndrome; NSAIDs = nonsteroidal anti-inflammatory drugs; U/A = urinalysis.

obstruction (Chapter 144) or malabsorption (Chapter 142). Rifaximin (550 mg three times daily for 2 weeks) is effective for functional bloating, pain, and loose or watery stools;[2] but dietary and behavioral changes and reassurance may also be useful.

INVOLUNTARY WEIGHT LOSS

The unintentional loss of more than 5% of baseline weight within a 12-month period is frequently due to a serious underlying medical or psychiatric illness. Weight loss is seldom the sole presenting sign of medical disorders, but it is often revealed during the clinical evaluation of other complaints. Chronic weight loss in the elderly is commonly caused by depression, dementia, difficulty chewing or swallowing, malignancy, medications, alcoholism, or physical and social limitations to procuring, preparing, and eating meals (Table 134-4) (Chapter 23). Gradual, mild weight loss occurs in some elderly patients owing to the loss of lean body mass. In young patients, weight loss is more commonly caused by eating disorders (Chapter 226), endocrine disorders (Chapters 233 and 234), or chronic GI conditions such as inflammatory bowel disease (Chapter 143) or celiac disease (Chapter 142). In chronic medical conditions, involuntary weight loss is usually caused by a combination of decreased appetite (anorexia) and varying degrees of cachexia; examples include advanced malignancy, chronic infections (HIV, tuberculosis), heart failure, chronic kidney or liver disease, end-stage lung disease, and adrenal insufficiency. Weight loss that occurs in the presence of normal or increased appetite suggests increased metabolism and energy expenditure caused by endocrine disorders such as poorly controlled diabetes (Chapter 236) or hyperthyroidism (Chapter 233) or GI disorders that result in food malabsorption (Chapter 142). Chronic GI disorders that cause progressive narrowing or obstruction of the esophagus (cancer, achalasia), stomach (cancer, peptic ulcer disease with gastric outlet obstruction), small intestine (Crohn's disease), or arterial circulation (chronic mesenteric ischemia) may cause weight loss owing to dysphagia, vomiting, or postprandial pain that limits the ability to ingest sufficient calories.

DIAGNOSIS

The cause of weight loss (see Table 134-4) is usually evident from the history, physical examination, and routine laboratory studies, including complete blood count, electrolytes, liver chemistries, thyroid-stimulating hormone, urinalysis, and, when appropriate, HIV serology (Fig. 134-4). A chest radiograph should be obtained in patients who smoke, have any respiratory symptoms, or are older than 40 years. Signs of dehydration or severe malnutrition may require an assessment for nutritional deficiencies (Chapter 221) and nutritional support (Chapters 223 and 224).

The need for further diagnostic testing is determined by other symptoms and signs. Weight loss with increased appetite merits an assessment of thyroid function (Chapter 233), glucose intolerance (Chapter 237), and malabsorption (Chapter 142). Suspected malabsorption may be confirmed by a positive fecal fat analysis. GI symptoms suggesting obstruction or occult GI malignancy can be evaluated with upper GI endoscopy, upper GI radiographic series, colonoscopy, or abdominal CT. Psychiatric evaluation may be

TABLE 134-4 CAUSES OF INVOLUNTARY WEIGHT LOSS

CONDITION	QUALITY	DURATION	AGGRAVATING OR RELIEVING FACTORS	ASSOCIATED SYMPTOMS OR SIGNS	DIAGNOSTIC STUDIES
WEIGHT LOSS SECONDARY TO GASTROINTESTINAL CAUSES					
GI, pancreatic, or hepatobiliary malignancy (Chapters 198-202)	Progressive, fast	Months	Better with cancer therapy (e.g., surgery, XRT, chemotherapy)	Dysphagia (esophageal); anorexia, nausea, vomiting (gastric, small or large bowel obstruction); visible or occult blood in stool; altered bowel habits; jaundice or hepatomegaly (biliary obstruction, hepatic tumor, metastatic disease); iron deficiency anemia	CBC, FOBT, ferritin, CEA, CA19-9, AFP, EGD, colonoscopy, abdominal CT, PET
Malabsorption (Chapter 142) (poor absorption of nutrients due to pancreatic insufficiency, small intestinal mucosal disorders, or bacterial overgrowth)	Progressive, slow	Months to years	Diarrhea or steatorrhea, excessive flatulence; worse with eating and resolves with NPO status	Usually associated with increased appetite; may have anemia (iron, B_{12}, folate), osteoporosis, or osteomalacia (vitamin D, calcium, phosphorus); easy bruising (vitamin K), night blindness (vitamin A)	72-hr stool for fecal fat; vitamins A and D and INR; calcium, ferritin, B_{12}, albumin; celiac disease antibodies (e.g., anti-tTG, antiendomysial antibodies); EGD with small bowel biopsy; breath test for bacterial overgrowth
Inflammatory bowel disease (especially Crohn's disease) (Chapter 143)	Progressive, slow	Months	Eating causes pain, cramps, increased diarrhea and urgency; improved by low-residue diet or NPO status	Bloody stools, abdominal cramps and pain, perianal disease, extraintestinal manifestations (e.g., oral ulcers, uveitis, erythema nodosum, arthralgias)	CBC, albumin, ESR, CRP, colonoscopy with biopsies, CT or MR enterography, wireless capsule study
GI motility disorders (Chapter 138)	Intermittent, slow	Years	Worse with eating	Nausea, vomiting, distention, diarrhea, or constipation may be present	EGD and colonoscopy, gastric emptying study, CT or MR enterography, surgical full-thickness intestinal biopsies
Cirrhosis (Chapter 156)	Muscle wasting with edema, so weight may increase	Months to years	Worse with salt or fluid intake	Ascites, peripheral edema	Liver biopsy
Chronic intestinal ischemia (Chapter 145)	Progressive	Months to years	Worse with eating	Afraid to eat; postprandial abdominal pain, nausea; associated atherosclerotic disease	CT or MR angiography
WEIGHT LOSS SECONDARY TO NONGASTROINTESTINAL CAUSES					
Poor or inadequate caloric intake due to social factors	Intermittent or progressive, acute (hospitalized) or chronic	Days to months to years	Common in elderly, teenagers; exacerbated by poor dentition or poorly fitting dentures	Will eat if food is made available	Review dietary log and how food is obtained and prepared
Medications	Intermittent or progressive	Months	Worse with medication; resolves with discontinuation of offending drug	Anorexia, nausea, vomiting	Review drug profile
Non-GI malignancy	Progressive	Months	Better with cancer therapy (e.g., surgery, XRT, chemotherapy)	Anorexia, nausea, vomiting; pain; metastatic disease	Calcium, cortisol; CT for underlying disease, PET
Endocrine disorders: DM, hyperthyroidism, adrenal insufficiency (Chapters 233-237)	DM—appetite increased or decreased, early satiety; hyperthyroidism—increased appetite	Months to years	Worse with disease chronicity	DM: gastroparesis, neuropathy, retinopathy, nephropathy Adrenal insufficiency: nausea, vomiting, diarrhea, abdominal pain	Serum glucose, TFT, cortisol
Chronic infections, including HIV and TB (Chapters 332 and 397)	Progressive, fast	Months	Better with directed therapy, megestrol acetate (Megace)	Nausea, anorexia, other infections	HIV test, PPD, cultures, biopsies if necessary
Systemic inflammatory disorders	Progressive, moderate	Months to years	Better with directed therapy, megestrol acetate (Megace)	Arthritis, rash, vasculitis	ANA, RF, ESR, CRP
Chronic renal failure (Chapter 132)	Progressive, slow; edema may increase weight	Months to years	Better with dialysis, megestrol acetate (Megace)	Nausea, anorexia, weight gain	BUN, Cr, 24-hr creatinine clearance
Advanced COPD or heart failure (Chapters 58 and 88)	Progressive, slow	Months to years	Better with oxygen and specific treatment	Fatigue, dyspnea, edema, wasting	Pulmonary function testing or two-dimensional echocardiography
Psychiatric illness: depression, manic-depressive illness (Chapter 404)	Progressive, slow	Months to years		Depression common in elderly; flat affect; manic phase associated with hyperactivity and decreased intake	Psychological testing

TABLE 134-4 CAUSES OF INVOLUNTARY WEIGHT LOSS—cont'd

CONDITION	QUALITY	DURATION	AGGRAVATING OR RELIEVING FACTORS	ASSOCIATED SYMPTOMS OR SIGNS	DIAGNOSTIC STUDIES
Psychogenic eating disorders—anorexia nervosa, bulimia (Chapter 226)	Intermittent or progressive	Months to years	Worse with stressors	Refusal to eat, loss of tooth enamel, calluses and healing ulcerations of hand	Psychiatric testing
Substance abuse (alcohol, opiates, CNS stimulants)	Intermittent or progressive	Months	Resolves with discontinuation	Anorexia, nausea, vomiting	Careful interview; patients may deny or minimize

AFP = α-fetoprotein; ANA = antinuclear antibody; BUN = blood urea nitrogen; CBC = complete blood count; CEA = carcinoembryonic antigen; CNS = central nervous system; COPD = chronic obstructive pulmonary disease; Cr = creatinine; CRP = C-reactive protein; CT = computed tomography; DM = diabetes mellitus; EGD = esophagogastroduodenoscopy; ESR = erythrocyte sedimentation rate; GI = gastrointestinal; FOBT = fecal occult blood test; GI = gastrointestinal; HIV = human immunodeficiency virus; INR = international normalized ratio; MR = magnetic resonance; NPO = nothing orally; PET = positron emission tomography; PPD = purified protein derivative; RF = rheumatoid factor; TB = tuberculosis; TFT = thyroid function test; tTG = tissue transglutaminase; XRT = x-ray therapy.
Adapted from Proctor DD. Approach to the patient with gastrointestinal disease. In: Goldman L, Ausiello D, eds. *Cecil Textbook of Medicine*, 23rd ed. Philadelphia: Saunders-Elsevier; 2008.

FIGURE 134-4. Approach to the patient with unintentional weight loss greater than 5%. CBC = complete blood count; COPD = chronic obstructive pulmonary disease; CRP = C-reactive protein; CT = computed tomography; CXR = chest radiograph; EGD = esophagogastroduodenoscopy; EUS = endoscopic ultrasound; GI = gastrointestinal; HIV = human immunodeficiency virus; PPD = purified protein derivative; PTH = parathyroid hormone; TFTs = thyroid function tests; tTG = tissue transglutaminase; U/A = urinalysis.

warranted in patients with signs of depression, early dementia, or eating disorders. In up to 25% of patients, no cause of weight loss is found.

NAUSEA AND VOMITING

Nausea is an unpleasant feeling of the impending need to vomit. *Vomiting* is the forceful oral expulsion of gastric contents as a result of retrograde contraction of the duodenum and antrum with compression of the thoracoabdominal musculature. Nausea and vomiting may be caused by a number GI and non-GI disorders, but they are best categorized according to chronicity and the presence of abdominal pain. The acute onset of vomiting *with* severe abdominal pain suggests a serious illness potentially requiring surgical intervention, including GI obstruction (Chapter 144), mesenteric ischemia (Chapter 145), pancreatitis (Chapter 146), biliary colic (Chapter 158), or conditions causing peritonitis (Chapter 144), such as appendicitis

FIGURE 134-5. Approach to the patient with vomiting. CNS = central nervous system.

or a perforated viscus. Acute vomiting *without* abdominal pain is most commonly caused by medications (including chemotherapy), motion sickness (Chapter 436), food poisoning (Chapter 291), infectious gastroenteritis (Chapter 291), hepatitis (Chapters 150 and 151), upper GI bleeding, postoperative ileus, or acute central nervous system disease. Chronic or recurrent nausea and vomiting *with* abdominal pain are commonly caused by GI disorders that result in the partial or intermittent obstruction of the stomach or small intestine. Chronic nausea and vomiting *without* abdominal pain may be caused by disorders that impair gastric emptying or small intestine motility and by non-GI causes including medications, pregnancy, intracerebral disorders, cardiac disease, endocrine disease, labyrinth disorders, psychiatric disease (including bulimia), and functional disorders. Vomiting of undigested food eaten hours earlier suggests gastric obstruction or gastroparesis. Abdominal distention or feculent emesis suggests obstruction of the small intestine.

DIAGNOSIS

Most cases of acute vomiting without abdominal pain are self-limited and require no evaluation (Fig. 134-5). Medication-related symptoms and pregnancy should be excluded. With severe vomiting, serum electrolytes should be obtained. Hyperglycemia may cause acute gastroparesis. Increased liver chemistries or pancreatic enzymes suggest hepatobiliary or pancreatic disease. In patients with acute abdominal pain and vomiting, abdominal plain radiographs or CT is obtained to look for evidence of GI obstruction, a perforated viscus, or pancreaticobiliary disease. In patients with chronic vomiting of uncertain cause, the goal is to distinguish structural GI disorders, GI motility disorders, and non-GI disorders. Esophagogastroduodenoscopy, enterography, abdominal cross-sectional imaging, GI motility studies, and head CT or magnetic resonance imaging may all be indicated.

TREATMENT   Rx

The approach to the medical treatment of nausea and vomiting depends on the cause (Table 134-5). Patients who are receiving moderately emetogenic chemotherapy are frequently managed with a 5-HT$_3$-receptor antagonist and dexamethasone[3]; aprepitant is added for highly emetogenic regimens. For patients with mildly emetogenic regimens or vomiting from other causes, treatment with single or combinations of anti-cholinergic agents, dopamine-receptor antagonists, or 5-HT$_3$-receptor antagonists usually provides symptomatic relief.[4,5]

OTHER GASTROINTESTINAL COMPLAINTS

Heartburn, esophageal regurgitation, dysphagia, odynophagia, and noncardiac chest pain suggest esophageal disease (Chapter 140). *Dyspepsia*, which refers to bothersome, intermittent, mild to moderate upper abdominal or epigastric symptoms, can be caused by peptic ulcer disease (Chapter 141) or esophageal disease (Chapter 140), or it can be functional in origin (Chapter 139). An orderly diagnostic approach (Fig. 134-6) can help distinguish among the various causes, avoid unnecessary testing, and minimize symptoms.

Diarrhea, which is defined pathophysiologically as an increase in stool weight to greater than 200 g/day, can be caused by malabsorption of osmotically active substances or by increased intestinal secretion of electrolytes and water. In clinical practice, however, stool weight is seldom quantified, and the term *diarrhea* refers to an increase in stool liquidity and/or frequency (more than three bowel movements/day). Acute and chronic diarrhea should be distinguished because the evaluation and treatment are different (Chapter 142).

Constipation (Chapter 138), which is the most common digestive symptom, occurs in 15% of the population. Constipation may refer to fewer than three bowel movements per week; hard or lumpy stools; or difficulty during defecation, characterized by straining, a sensation of obstruction or incomplete evacuation, or the need to engage in manual manipulations to promote evacuation. Constipation may be caused by systemic conditions that slow colonic transit, including neuromuscular disease, endocrine disorders, and electrolyte abnormalities, or by lesions that obstruct the passage of stool through the distal colon or anorectum, such as neoplasms, strictures, prolapse, and agangliosis (Hirschsprung's disease). Most patients, however, do not have an apparent cause and are deemed to have functional constipation.

GI bleeding (Chapter 137) may be acute and clinically apparent (overt) or chronic, slow, and clinically inapparent (occult). The location of acute GI bleeding is described as either upper or lower, according to whether the source is proximal or distal to the ligament of Treitz (distal duodenum). Upper GI bleeding, which is three times more common than lower GI bleeding, is manifested by bloody emesis (hematemesis), coffee ground emesis, and, in most cases, black stools (melena). Common causes of significant bleeding are peptic ulcer disease, esophageal varices, Mallory-Weiss tears, erosive gastritis or esophagitis, and vascular ectasias. Major lower GI bleeding

TABLE 134-5 MEDICAL TREATMENT OF NAUSEA AND VOMITING

DRUG	USUAL INDICATIONS	USUAL DOSE (RANGE)	ROUTE	COMMENTS
ANTICHOLINERGIC-ANTIHISTAMINE AGENTS				Side effects: sedation, dizziness, delirium, blurred vision, glaucoma, bronchospasm, tachycardia, urinary retention. Avoid concomitant alcohol or CNS depressants; use with caution in elderly patients
Scopolamine patch	MS	1.5 mg/72 hr	Patch	
Dimenhydrinate	MS	50 mg (50-100 mg) q4-6h	PO, IM, IV	Maximum 400 mg/24 hr
Cyclizine	MS, GIDz	50 mg q8h	PO, IM	Maximum 200 mg/24 hr
Meclizine	MS, V	25-50 mg q24h	PO	
Diphenhydramine	GIDz	25-50 mg q6h / 50-100 mg q6h	PO, IV / IM	
Promethazine	GIDz, PONV, MS	25 mg (12.5-25 mg) q6-12h / 25 mg (12.5-50 mg) q4-6h	PO, PR / IV, IM	Phenothiazine derivative, but lacks significant antidopaminergic effects. Avoid perivascular extravasation or subcutaneous injection (severe tissue necrosis)
Trimethobenzamide	GIDz, PONV	200 mg q6-8h	IM	
DOPAMINE RECEPTOR ANTAGONISTS				Side effects: neuromuscular (extrapyramidal) symptoms—agitation, restlessness, involuntary movements, dystonia, torticollis, laryngospasm, Parkinson-like features
Prochlorperazine	GIDz, PONV, CTX	5-10 mg q6-8h / 25 mg q12h	PO, IV, IM / PR	Maximum dose 20-40 mg/24 hr; avoid subcutaneous injection (irritation)
Metoclopramide	GIDz / CTX	10 mg (10-20 mg) q6-8h / 1-2 mg/kg before and 2 hr after CTX	PO, IV, IM / IV	Modest efficacy at these doses. High doses infrequently used owing to availability of safer, more effective CTX regimens; use with diphenhydramine to reduce adverse side effects
Droperidol	PONV	2.5 mg (1.25-5 mg) pre-induction and q4-6h as needed	IV, IM	May cause QTc prolongation and torsades de pointes; use is restricted to patients who fail to respond to other agents
CORTICOSTEROIDS				
Dexamethasone	PONV / CTX	4-8 mg once pre-induction / 8-20 mg on day 1; 8 mg on days 2-4	PO, IV / PO, IV	Most beneficial when used with other agents (e.g., 5-HT$_3$ RA, neurokinin-1 RA)
BENZODIAZEPINES				Used to reduce anxiety and anticipatory vomiting
Lorazepam	CTX	1-2 mg q4-6h	PO, IV	
CANNABINOIDS				May stimulate appetite; adverse side effects (sedation, dizziness, dysphoria, dry mouth) limit use
Dronabinol	GIDz, CTX	5-10 mg q6-8h	PO	
Nabilone	GIDz, CTX	1-2 mg q12h	PO	
5-HT$_3$ RECEPTOR ANTAGONISTS	PONV, CTX			PONV prevention: give IV immediately before anesthesia induction. Prevention of CTX-induced vomiting: give 30 min (IV) to 1 hr (PO) before chemotherapy
Ondansetron	PONV / CTX, RadTx	4 mg once / 4-8 mg / Moderately emetogenic CTX: 8 mg twice daily / Highly emetogenic CTX: 24 mg once	IV / PO / IV or PO / IV or PO	
Granisetron	CTX, RadTx	1-2 mg once daily / 1 mg once daily	PO / IV	
Dolasetron	CTX, PONV	100 mg once daily	PO, IV	
Palonosetron	CTX / / PONV	0.25 mg / 0.5 mg / 0.075 mg	IV / PO / IV	
NEUROKININ-1 RECEPTOR ANTAGONISTS	Highly emetogenic CTX			Used exclusively in combination with a 5-HT$_3$ RA and/or dexamethasone
Aprepitant		125 mg on day 1 / 80 mg on days 2-3	PO	
Fosaprepitant		115 mg on day 1	IV	Aprepitant 80 mg PO on days 2-3
ANTIEMETIC REGIMENS FOR CHEMOTHERAPY				
Mildly emetogenic CTX	Option 1 / Option 2	Dexamethasone 8 mg / Dopamine receptor antagonist	IV or PO	One dose only / One dose only

TABLE 134-5   MEDICAL TREATMENT OF NAUSEA AND VOMITING—cont'd

DRUG	USUAL INDICATIONS	USUAL DOSE (RANGE)	ROUTE	COMMENTS
Moderately emetogenic CTX		Day 1: 5-HT₃ RA plus dexamethasone 8 mg	IV or PO	Days 2-3: continue oral 5-HT₃ RA or dexamethasone 8 mg to reduce delayed emesis
Highly emetogenic CTX		Day 1: 5-HT₃ RA plus dexamethasone 12 mg plus neurokinin-1 RA	IV or PO	Give aprepitant 80 mg PO days 2-3 and dexamethasone 8 mg PO days 2-4 to reduce delayed emesis

CNS = central nervous system; CTX = chemotherapy; GIDz = gastrointestinal disorders associated with nausea and vomiting; 5-HT₃ = serotonin 5-hydroxytryptamine₃; MS = motion sickness; PONV = postoperative nausea and vomiting; RA = receptor antagonist; RadTx = radiation therapy–induced nausea and vomiting; V = vertigo.

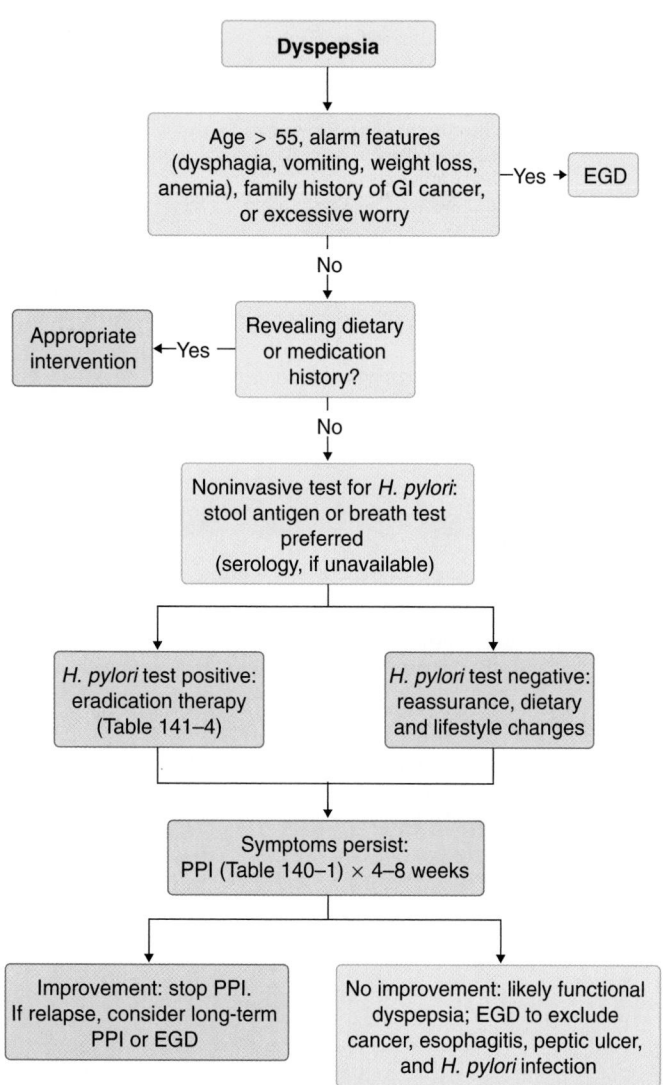

FIGURE 134-6. Approach to the patient with dyspepsia. EGD = esophagogastroduodenoscopy; GI = gastrointestinal; PPI = proton pump inhibitor.

is manifested by large-volume maroon or bright red bloody stools (hematochezia). Although 80 to 90% of patients with hematochezia have a lower source of bleeding, massive upper GI bleeding also may cause hematochezia. Approximately 95% of major lower GI bleeding arises from the colon and 5% from the small intestine. Lower GI bleeding is increased in patients older than 50 years, in whom diverticulosis accounts for 60% of cases; the remainder are due to ischemia, neoplasms, ulcers, vascular ectasias, or hemorrhoids. In patients younger than 50, bleeding is more commonly attributable to inflammatory bowel disease, hemorrhoids, or infectious colitis.

Occult GI bleeding refers to GI blood loss that is small in volume and not apparent to the patient but is detectable by tests for fecal occult blood. Chronic occult bleeding may result in iron deficiency anemia. Both upper endoscopy and colonoscopy should be performed to look for a source of occult bleeding, most commonly gastroesophageal or colonic neoplasia, erosive esophagitis or gastritis, ulcer disease, or vascular ectasia. In patients with recurrent iron deficiency and occult blood loss in whom no source is found on upper and lower endoscopy, video capsule endoscopy or enteroscopy is performed to look for a small bowel source (vascular ectasia, ulcer, or neoplasm).

Fecal incontinence (Chapter 147) is dependent on a number of factors, including a solid or semisolid stool, a compliant and distensible rectal reservoir, the ability to sense rectal fullness, an intact internal anal sphincter (an involuntary muscle innervated by the enteric nervous system), an intact external anal sphincter and puborectalis (voluntary muscles innervated by the pudendal nerve), and the mental and physical ability to reach a toilet facility when needed. Minor incontinence, which occurs in 10% of people older than 70 years, is characterized by the inability to control flatus or by the seepage of fecal matter that results in soiling of the perianal area and undergarments. It tends to be intermittent, occurring after bowel movements; when coughing, lifting, or passing flatus; or when stools are loose. Major incontinence is characterized by the partial or complete inability to reliably control bowel movements, resulting in gross, involuntary loss of feces and the need to wear a diaper. It occurs in less than 1% of the population and is virtually always caused by a central nervous system disorder that results in diminished awareness of bowel needs, neuropathy, or damage to the anal sphincters.

1. Maggio AQ, Reece-Smith AM, Tang TY, et al. Early laparoscopy versus active observation in acute abdominal pain: systematic review and meta-analysis. *Int J Surg.* 2008;6:400-403.
2. Pimentel M, Lembo A, Chey WD, et al. Rifaximin therapy for patients with irritable bowel syndrome without constipation. *N Engl J Med.* 2011;364:22-32.
3. Billio A, Morello E, Clarke MJ. Serotonin receptor antagonists for highly emetogenic chemotherapy in adults. *Cochrane Database Syst Rev.* 2010.1.CD006272.
4. Davis MP, Hallerberg G. Palliative Medicine Study Group of the Multinational Association of Supportive Care in Cancer. A systematic review of the treatment of nausea and vomiting in cancer unrelated to chemotherapy or radiation. *J Pain Symptom Manage.* 2010;39:756-767.
5. Apfel CC, Korttila K, Abdalla M, et al. A factorial trial of six interventions for the prevention of postoperative nausea and vomiting. *N Engl J Med.* 2004;350:2441-2451.

SUGGESTED READINGS

Metalidis C, Knockaert DC, Bobbaers H, et al. Involuntary weight loss. Does a negative baseline evaluation provide reassurance? *Eur J Intern Med.* 2008;19:345-349. *Organic causes were found in 56%, including malignancy in 22%, a psychiatric disorder in 16%, and no cause in 28%.*

Roila F, Herrstedt J, Gralla RJ, et al. Prevention of chemotherapy- and radiotherapy-induced nausea and vomiting: guideline update and results of the Perugia consensus. *Support Care Cancer.* 2011;19:S63-S65. *Consensus guidelines.*

Stoker J, van Randen A, Lameris W. Imaging patients with acute abdominal pain. *Radiology.* 2009;253:31-46. *Abdominal CT scan is recommended, except that ultrasonography is preferred for patients with suspected cholecystitis.*

Strate LL, Naumann CR. The role of colonoscopy and other procedures in the management of lower gastrointestinal bleeding *Clin Gastroenterol Hepatol.* 2010;8:333-343. *Review of lower GI bleeding and the controversies surrounding optimal initial management.*

135

DIAGNOSTIC IMAGING PROCEDURES IN GASTROENTEROLOGY

DAVID H. KIM AND PERRY J. PICKHARDT

A wide range of diagnostic imaging modalities is available for evaluating diseases of the gastrointestinal (GI) tract and the hepatopancreaticobiliary system. Once the workhorse of GI radiology, conventional radiography and fluoroscopy are still relevant but have largely given way to more advanced cross-sectional imaging studies such as ultrasonography, computed tomography (CT), and magnetic resonance imaging (MRI). Many of the visceral vascular evaluations undertaken by conventional angiography have been replaced by these noninvasive modalities as well. These cross-sectional technologies have become the preferred methods of evaluation, allowing more precise and accurate diagnoses. In addition, cross-sectional techniques can be used to guide a wide variety of interventional procedures. With the emergence of molecular imaging, there has been renewed interest in nuclear medicine, most notably positron emission tomography (PET).

CONVENTIONAL RADIOGRAPHY

Conventional radiographs, often referred to as "plain films," remain useful for a limited number of abdominal indications but are generally much less sensitive and specific for pathology compared with techniques such as CT. Advantages of radiography include its wide availability, low cost, and portability, allowing the acquisition of images in acute clinical situations. Supine and upright frontal abdominal radiographs can assess rapidly for bowel obstruction or perforation in the setting of an acute abdomen (Fig. 135-1). Serial abdominal radiographs remain a practical approach for following patients with an abnormal bowel gas pattern suggestive of either evolving small bowel obstruction or adynamic ileus. Conventional radiographs can demonstrate abnormal abdominal calcifications and radiopaque foreign bodies. In each of these cases, however, cross-sectional modalities such as CT have increased sensitivity and provide better delineation of disease processes. CT is often undertaken when the initial plain film evaluation is negative or to provide better information when conventional radiography is positive.

FLUOROSCOPIC PROCEDURES

Standard double-contrast barium examinations that depict the mucosa, particularly of the stomach, duodenum, and colon, have largely been supplanted by endoscopy (Chapter 136) and advanced radiologic techniques. However, a variety of single-column fluoroscopic contrast studies remain quite useful because of their relatively noninvasive nature and their low cost. Real-time fluoroscopic contrast studies can provide a valuable physiologic evaluation, serve as a problem-solving tool when endoscopy is equivocal or contraindicated, and evaluate for suspected leaks, perforations, or fistulas. Depending on the specific indication, either barium or water-soluble iodinated contrast material may be used.

The videofluoroscopic swallowing study and barium esophagram are effective noninvasive means of excluding significant pathology in patients with dysphagia. Endoscopy is generally indicated when an esophageal stricture or mass is encountered on fluoroscopic examination, but it can be avoided in many cases that lack concerning findings. Fluoroscopic contrast evaluation may also avoid the need for endoscopy in symptomatic patients with suspected esophagitis from *Candida* or herpes infection. In the setting of gastroesophageal reflux disease, the barium esophagram is effective for excluding significant complications such as peptic stricture and adenocarcinoma, but it is insensitive to the changes of Barrett's esophagus (Chapter 140).

Although the double-contrast barium upper GI series can identify mucosal abnormalities of the stomach and duodenum, such as erosions, ulcers, polyps, and masses (Fig. 135-2), this function is now largely the domain of esophagogastroduodenoscopy (EGD). Gastroduodenal barium studies still play an important diagnostic role in evaluating for sliding hiatal and/or paraesophageal hernias and in pediatric evaluations for malrotation and hypertrophic pyloric stenosis.

For evaluation of the mesenteric small bowel, capsule endoscopy, CT enterography, and magnetic resonance (MR) enterography have largely replaced barium studies. Although fluoroscopic studies can still provide an anatomic roadmap, assess transit time, and detect fold thickening, the evaluation of unexplained GI bleeding (Chapter 137) or possible Crohn's disease (Chapter 143) is better performed using CT, MRI, or capsule endoscopy.

The single-contrast barium enema remains an important diagnostic tool in such settings as suspected sigmoid volvulus, colonic obstruction, postoperative leak or fistula, and ileocolic intussusception in children (Chapter 144). Many practices continue to perform fluoroscopic defecography to help delineate functional abnormalities in patients with evacuation disorders (Chapter 147), although dynamic MR cine series have replaced defecography at some institutions.

ULTRASONOGRAPHY

The introduction of harmonic and compound imaging, advances in high-resolution transducers, and improvements in color Doppler evaluation have all combined to enhance the diagnostic capabilities of portable ultrasound.

FIGURE 135-1. **Pneumoperitoneum from bowel perforation on conventional radiographs. A,** Supine abdominal radiograph shows abnormal lucency surrounding multiple bowel loops and the liver. Both sides of the bowel wall *(arrowheads)* are outlined by gas in areas (Rigler's sign), which typically requires a large amount of free peritoneal air to be visible on supine films. **B,** Upright radiograph centered over the diaphragm *(arrowheads)* shows the large amount of free intraperitoneal air (lucent area just inferior to the diaphragm) to better advantage. This view is more sensitive for the detection of pneumoperitoneum.

FIGURE 135-2. Metastatic melanoma on barium upper GI study. **A,** Fluoroscopic spot film image shows a filling defect *(arrows)* within the second portion of the duodenum that has a "bull's-eye" or "target" appearance due to the collection of barium in the center of the lesion. This appearance is characteristic of a submucosal mass with central ulceration and is typical of hematogenous metastatic disease from melanoma. **B,** Digital photograph from EGD confirms the presence of an ulcerated submucosal mass within the duodenum.

In general, ultrasound is useful for imaging solid organs and fluid-filled structures, but it is unable to penetrate gas-filled structures. For example, overlying bowel gas often precludes a complete sonographic evaluation of the pancreas. Ultrasound is a relatively versatile imaging technique, in that it can be performed via many different routes, including transabdominal, endoscopic (as part of EGD), transrectal, intravascular, and endovaginal approaches. In addition, it is excellent for many image-guided interventions because of its real-time evaluation.

With regard to GI pathology, ultrasonography is used most frequently to evaluate the liver and biliary system. Suspected acute cholecystitis (Chapter 158) is a common indication for right upper quadrant sonography; classic findings include cholelithiasis, gallbladder wall thickening, and a sonographic Murphy's sign (reproducible pain when the transducer is pressed over the gallbladder) (Fig. 135-3). The sensitivity for detecting gallstones with ultrasonography exceeds 95%. Acalculous cholelithiasis can be a more challenging diagnosis because the findings overlap with nonspecific gallbladder wall thickening in critically ill patients. Ultrasound is typically the first imaging test obtained in patients with new-onset jaundice or cholestatic laboratory findings because it offers a rapid, noninvasive evaluation of the biliary tree to differentiate obstruction from other causes. If biliary ductal dilation is present, the level and cause of the obstruction can sometimes be demonstrated on ultrasound; common causes include choledocholithiasis and pancreatic head masses. In most cases of biliary obstruction, additional imaging tests will be necessary, consisting of CT, MR cholangiopancreatography (MRCP), endoscopic retrograde cholangiopancreatography (ERCP), or percutaneous transhepatic cholangiography (PTC), depending on the specific circumstances.

Ultrasonography can be used to detect or further characterize focal liver lesions (Chapter 154), although it is typically less sensitive and specific than CT or MRI. Ultrasound is quite capable of distinguishing cystic from solid lesions. Although not approved for use in the United States, intravenous contrast agents for ultrasound have been studied fairly extensively in other countries and appear to offer similar advantages seen with CT and MRI contrast agents.

In diffuse disease, ultrasound is being used with increased frequency to screen patients with viral hepatitis for cirrhosis and hepatocellular carcinoma (Chapters 156 and 202). Sonographic findings in cirrhosis include a heterogeneously coarsened parenchymal echotexture, nodular surface contour, predominantly right-sided volume loss, and evidence of portal hypertension, including ascites, splenomegaly, and portosystemic collaterals. Focal hepatic lesions in the setting of cirrhosis are concerning for hepatocellular carcinoma, but they may also represent regenerative or dysplastic nodules. In non-cirrhotic patients with elevated liver enzymes, ultrasonography can often

FIGURE 135-3. Acute cholecystitis on ultrasound. Image from right upper quadrant sonography shows diffuse gallbladder wall thickening and a shadowing impacted gallstone *(arrow)*. A sonographic Murphy's sign was present. These findings are diagnostic for acute calculous cholecystitis.

suggest the diagnosis of hepatic steatosis (fatty liver; Chapter 155) when the parenchyma demonstrates increased echogenicity and decreased penetration of the sound beam. The findings of steatosis can be focal, multifocal, or diffuse; MRI is more specific and can confirm the diagnosis.

Color and power Doppler evaluation allows the noninvasive sonographic assessment of vascular patency. Doppler evaluation of the liver is commonly performed in patients with end-stage liver disease (Chapter 157) to evaluate the portal system and search for portosystemic collaterals. Abnormal portal vein findings include hepatofugal flow and thrombosis (Fig. 135-4). Doppler ultrasound is also used for the evaluation of transjugular intrahepatic portosystemic shunts (TIPS), both before and after stent placement. In orthotopic liver transplant recipients, Doppler evaluation is frequently performed to assess the hepatic vasculature, with particular attention to the hepatic arterial supply.

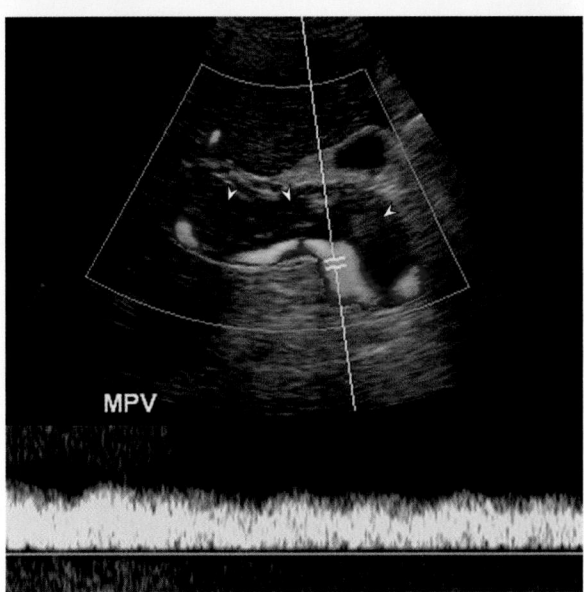

FIGURE 135-4. **Portal vein thrombosis on ultrasound.** Ultrasound gray-scale image with both power color Doppler and spectral Doppler interrogation shows a tubular hypoechoic structure *(arrowheads)* consistent with nonocclusive thrombus filling the majority of the main portal vein (MPV). Flow patency is seen in the deep peripheral aspect of the vessel.

FIGURE 135-5. **Multiple hypervascular liver lesions on CT.** Dynamic contrast-enhanced CT image obtained during the arterial phase shows multiple hypervascular liver lesions *(arrowheads)*, which proved to be hepatic adenomas in a patient with von Gierke's disease.

COMPUTED TOMOGRAPHY

CT has revolutionized the imaging of abdominal pathology, providing a rapid, reproducible, and comprehensive evaluation. The introduction of single-detector helical or spiral CT, followed by multidetector scanners, has resulted in improved resolution and faster acquisition of true volumetric data. High-resolution scans of the entire abdomen and pelvis can now be easily acquired in a single short breath-hold. With the automated, high-rate injection of intravenous contrast materials and advanced processing, specialized CT examinations are replacing many traditional modalities. A major challenge, however, is to minimize radiation doses as CT use increases. The clinical indications for abdominal CT are very broad. One common use is the diagnostic evaluation of a nontraumatic acute abdomen (Chapter 144). Common inflammatory conditions such as appendicitis and diverticulitis are readily diagnosed by CT. Other common indications include evaluation for intra-abdominal abscess, pancreatitis, and small bowel obstruction. In cases of relatively high-grade bowel obstruction, CT can often localize the transition point, elucidate the underlying cause, and evaluate for vascular compromise. In the setting of an acute abdomen due to blunt trauma (Chapter 112), CT has become invaluable for the prompt detection of significant abdominal injury.

In the nonacute setting, multiphase CT with intravenous contrast can characterize lesions and often results in a noninvasive diagnosis, particularly in combination with the clinical history (Fig. 135-5). Primary abdominal malignancies, such as pancreatic cancer and hepatocellular carcinoma, are often first detected on CT. Abdominal staging for metastatic disease, including hematogenous, lymphatic, peritoneal, and local spread, is commonly performed with CT, as is assessing the response to various therapies.

CT is increasingly being used for primary bowel evaluation, often replacing traditional fluoroscopy because of its increased sensitivity and specificity. CT enterography protocols often combine neutral (i.e., water density) oral contrast with dynamic, high-resolution imaging that provides detailed multiplanar evaluation of the small bowel. Dedicated CT enterography and capsule endoscopy yield a complementary and comprehensive evaluation of the small bowel. CT colonography, also referred to as virtual colonoscopy, combines two- and three-dimensional evaluation of the prepared and distended colon for the detection of colorectal polyps and masses (Fig. 135-6). CT colonography is a promising tool for colorectal evaluation, particularly if it can improve adherence rates associated with screening. Optical colonoscopy is still required for polypectomy.

Visceral CT angiography is largely replacing conventional diagnostic angiography. For example, in many institutions, evaluation of the vascular anatomy before hepatic transplantation (Chapter 157) is now undertaken by CT rather than by catheter angiography (Fig. 135-7).

MAGNETIC RESONANCE IMAGING

The advantages of MRI over CT for abdominal evaluation include superior soft tissue contrast resolution and lack of ionizing radiation. However, for many institutions, MRI remains primarily a problem-solving tool for the abdomen because of several drawbacks, including decreased spatial resolution, longer examination times, increased expense, decreased availability, and inability to scan some patients owing to claustrophobia or implanted devices such as cardiac pacemakers. Imaging artifacts can also make MRI interpretation more difficult and less uniform across different readers.

Contrast-enhanced MRI offers a dynamic evaluation comparable to CT for the solid abdominal organs. In addition, intravenous gadolinium-based agents with hepatocyte-specific uptake increase MRI's diagnostic capabilities in evaluating focal hepatic lesions (Fig. 135-8). The high accuracy of MRI in diagnosing hepatic steatosis (Chapter 155) can sometimes prevent unnecessary biopsy, particularly in cases of nodular focal fatty infiltration that simulates metastatic disease. MRI is also sensitive for detecting iron overload within the liver and other organs related to primary hemochromatosis (Chapter 219) and secondary hemosiderosis (most often due to multiple transfusions). Similar to CT, MRI can provide quality arterial and venous angiographic imaging, such that conventional angiography is generally reserved for therapeutic interventions.

In the past, contrast MRI was considered an alternative to CT in patients with decreased renal function. However, the newly recognized condition of nephrogenic systemic fibrosis (Fig. 135-9) argues against this strategy. Nephrogenic systemic fibrosis, characterized by involvement of the skin, eyes, joints, and internal organs, is associated with intravenous gadolinium administration. Patients with impaired renal function are at risk of developing this rare but often fatal condition related to heavy metal toxicity from free gadolinium that has been dissociated from its chelate. Currently, there is no curative treatment.

Two specialized MR examinations have significantly changed practice patterns in recent years. MRCP, a heavily T2-weighted imaging technique for the noninvasive diagnostic evaluation of the biliary and pancreatic ductal systems, relies not on contrast administration but on the presence of static fluid. MRCP can be a useful screening tool to select appropriate candidates for more invasive therapeutic procedures such as ERCP and PTC. MRCP is useful for diagnosing biliary and pancreatic ductal obstruction, choledocholithiasis, primary sclerosing cholangitis, and cystic conditions such as Caroli's disease (Fig. 135-10). T1-weighted MR cholangiography with intravenous contrast agents that undergo biliary excretion can be useful in evaluating for bile leaks, analogous to hepatobiliary scintigraphy.

MR enterography is increasingly used to monitor patients with Crohn's disease (Chapter 143). Given the lack of ionizing radiation, it is particularly

FIGURE 135-6. Pedunculated polyp (tubulovillous adenoma) on virtual colonoscopy (CT colonography). **A,** Three-dimensional endoluminal image shows a large polyp on a prominent stalk. This view simulates conventional colonoscopy and allows the reliable detection of such lesions. **B,** Transverse two-dimensional image confirms that the lesion is composed of soft tissue *(arrow)*. **C,** Colon map generated by the virtual colonoscopy software system allows precise localization of the polyp (red dot in sigmoid colon). The green line represents the centerline for automated navigation.

advantageous in young patients who require multiple examinations over a lifetime. Oral contrast agents such as polyethylene glycol are given to distend the small bowel; spasmolytics are typically administered to decrease bowel peristalsis. Similar to CT, fast breath-held imaging with intravenous contrast administration allows the evaluation of mucosal and wall enhancement or thickening, suggesting active disease. Unlike CT, MRI can assess intrinsic signal characteristics on T2-weighted images to improve specificity and distinguish active inflammation from chronic fibrostenotic disease (Fig. 135-11). Other emerging applications include MR staging for rectal cancer to assess the need for neoadjuvant chemoradiation.

INTERVENTIONAL PROCEDURES

Ultrasound, CT, fluoroscopy, and even MR techniques have been used for guidance when performing a wide variety of abdominal interventional procedures. Percutaneous image-guided biopsy, whether by fine-needle aspiration or core biopsy, is a relatively safe procedure that is commonly performed for tissue diagnosis and has drastically reduced the need for open surgical biopsy. Other common nonvascular procedures that use image guidance include abscess drainage, biliary interventions, gastrostomy, and tumor

ablation. In the case of peridiverticular and periappendiceal abscesses, CT-guided drainage can often simplify the ultimate operative approach and turn high-risk emergent surgery into a safer elective procedure. Biliary interventions include transhepatic access of an obstructed system for stenting or external drainage, as well as cholecystostomy tube placement. Percutaneous CT- or ultrasound-guided tumor ablation is a rapidly evolving technique that is particularly useful in poor operative candidates or in conjunction with surgical resection of other lesions. A variety of ablation methods have been employed, including radio frequency, alcohol, microwave, and cryoablation.

Diagnostic conventional angiography has been largely replaced by noninvasive CT and MR techniques, but direct catheter angiography remains an important procedure for directing various therapies. Vascular interventions include angioplasty, stenting, embolization, and thrombolysis. TIPS placement (Chapter 157) is a commonly performed angiographic procedure in patients with portal hypertension complicated by variceal bleeding or intractable ascites. Placement of a TIPS stent creates a low-pressure communication between the portal and hepatic venous systems. Chemoembolization can provide palliation for those with advanced hepatic malignancy, whether primary or metastatic.

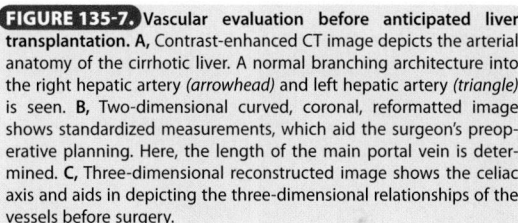

FIGURE 135-7. Vascular evaluation before anticipated liver transplantation. **A,** Contrast-enhanced CT image depicts the arterial anatomy of the cirrhotic liver. A normal branching architecture into the right hepatic artery *(arrowhead)* and left hepatic artery *(triangle)* is seen. **B,** Two-dimensional curved, coronal, reformatted image shows standardized measurements, which aid the surgeon's preoperative planning. Here, the length of the main portal vein is determined. **C,** Three-dimensional reconstructed image shows the celiac axis and aids in depicting the three-dimensional relationships of the vessels before surgery.

FIGURE 135-8. Hepatic cavernous hemangiomas on MRI. Contrast-enhanced fat-suppressed gradient echo MRI shows the characteristic findings of cavernous hemangiomas, including a giant left hepatic lobe lesion *(arrowheads)* and a smaller right hepatic lobe lesion *(arrow)*. Note the peripheral enhancement of the lesions, which matches the signal intensity of the aortic blood pool. These findings are diagnostic, and tissue biopsy is unnecessary.

NUCLEAR MEDICINE (RADIONUCLIDE SCINTIGRAPHY)

Owing to the emergence of PET-CT for oncologic evaluation, nuclear medicine is more relevant now than ever before in abdominal imaging. PET-CT is a powerful diagnostic tool that combines functional and anatomic imaging. PET is useful for both initial staging and evaluating the response to therapy for a wide range of primary malignant tumors, especially when combined with CT (Fig. 135-12). Currently, clinical PET imaging most often utilizes F^{18}-fluorodeoxyglucose, but other positron-emitting agents may be used for specific purposes.

Several other nuclear medicine studies are used to evaluate GI and hepatobiliary diseases. Injection of red blood cells labeled with technetium-99m provides a useful test for GI bleeding. Advantages of performing this as the initial diagnostic imaging study include its noninvasive nature, high sensitivity for active bleeding, and ability to rescan the patient hours later without the need for repeat injection. Disadvantages include relatively poor anatomic localization and lack of therapeutic ability. The use of tagged red blood cell scintigraphy for the diagnosis of hepatic cavernous hemangioma has decreased significantly owing to advances in CT and MRI. Hepatobiliary scintigraphy remains a useful tool in equivocal cases of cholecystitis, particularly acalculous disease, and it can confirm suspected biliary leaks. Scintigraphic imaging with In^{111}-octreotide is valuable for the diagnosis, staging,

FIGURE 135-9. Nephrogenic systemic fibrosis (NSF). Digital photograph of the upper extremities in a patient with NSF shows vague fibrotic plaques that are difficult to visualize but easily palpated. In the skin, NSF presents as bilateral, symmetrical, and variably erythematous fibrotic plaques beginning distally and progressing proximally, often with a reticulated advancing edge. (Courtesy of Dr. Molly A. Hinshaw.)

FIGURE 135-10. Pancreatic intraductal papillary mucinous neoplasm on MRCP. Heavily T2-weighted MR image shows a lobulated cystic lesion in the pancreatic head region *(arrows)* that represents a side branch intraductal papillary mucinous neoplasm. Note the mild focal irregularity of the gallbladder *(arrowhead)*, consistent with the fundal form of adenomyomatosis. The intra- and extrahepatic biliary ducts are normal.

FIGURE 135-11. Active Crohn's disease on MR enterography. **A,** Coronal three-dimensional volume-acquired breath-hold, T1-weighted, gradient-echo image with dynamic gadolinium administration and fat saturation shows wall thickening and enhancement *(arrowhead)* of an abnormal segment of terminal ileum. **B,** Coronal two-dimensional single-shot, fast spin-echo, T2-weighted image shows increased signal in this area *(arrow)*, signifying edema and active disease.

and follow-up of GI neuroendocrine tumors, such as carcinoid and pancreatic islet cell tumors.

SUGGESTED READINGS

American College of Radiology, Expert Panel on Gastrointestinal Imaging. ACR Appropriateness Criteria. http://www.acr.org/s_acr/sec.asp?CID=1207&DID=15048. *Recommended imaging approaches for various clinical presentations.*

Currie GM, Kiat H, Wheat JM. Scintigraphic evaluation of acute lower gastrointestinal hemorrhage: current status and future directions. *J Clin Gastroenterol.* 2011;45:92-99. *Review.*

Mellinger JD, Bittner JG 4th, Edwards MA, et al. Imaging of gastrointestinal bleeding. *Surg Clin North Am.* 2011;91:93-108. *Review.*

Singh JP, Steward MJ, Booth TC, et al. Evolution of imaging for abdominal perforation. *Ann R Coll Surg Engl.* 2010;92:182-188. *Emphasizes the role of CT.*

FIGURE 135-12. Metastatic gastrointestinal stromal tumor (GIST) on fused PET-CT. Transverse fused PET-CT image shows a dominant hypermetabolic mass *(arrow)* representing a gastric GIST. Multiple smaller peritoneal and hepatic hypermetabolic foci are consistent with metastatic deposits. Note the utility of combining the functional information from PET with the anatomic localization provided by CT.

136

GASTROINTESTINAL ENDOSCOPY

PANKAJ JAY PASRICHA

IMPORTANCE AND USE OF ENDOSCOPY

Technologic advances in radiologic and endoscopic imaging have transformed medicine in the past few decades. With its remarkable accessibility, the gastrointestinal tract has benefited from the endoscopic approach perhaps more than any other organ system. The major advantages of endoscopy over contrast radiography in evaluating diseases of the alimentary tract include direct visualization, resulting in a more accurate and sensitive evaluation of mucosal lesions; the ability to obtain biopsy specimens from superficial lesions; and the ability to perform therapeutic interventions. These advantages make endoscopy the procedure of choice in most cases in which mucosal lesions or growths are suspected. Conversely, computed tomography (CT) or, occasionally, contrast radiography may be indicated when extrinsic or intrinsic distortions of anatomy are suspected, such as volvulus, intussusceptions, subtle strictures, or complicated postsurgical changes (Chapter 135).

INSTRUMENTS AND PROCEDURES (TABLE 136-1)

Luminal Endoscopy: Conventional and Wireless

The vast majority of endoscopic procedures are intraluminal in nature. The endoscopic shaft not only carries the optical elements for imaging but also contains channels that enable various functions such as air insufflation, water irrigation, suction, and passage of diagnostic and therapeutic devices.

A relatively recent innovation is capsule endoscopy, with a disposable plastic capsule that measures 11 mm by 26 mm and contains a chip camera, batteries, and a radio transmitter that wirelessly sends images to a device that the patient wears as a belt. At the end of the procedure, the information is downloaded to a computer, and the capsule itself passes harmlessly in the stool. Variations of this instrument have been developed for esophageal and colonic imaging, but these are not yet recommended for routine clinical use.

Ancillary Organ Imaging: Endoscopic Retrograde Cholangiography and Pancreatography

Endoscopic retrograde cholangiopancreatography (ERCP) uses a side-viewing endoscope that accesses the second part of the duodenum, where a small catheter is introduced into the bile or pancreatic duct to inject radiographic contrast medium under fluoroscopic monitoring. Successful cannulation and imaging can be achieved in up to 95% of cases. In some instances, a fine-caliber endoscope can also be introduced into the duct of interest (cholangioscopy or pancreaticoscopy) for direct visualization of intraductal disease.

Mural and Transmural Imaging: Endoscopic Ultrasound

An ultrasonic transducer in the tip of a flexible endoscope or a stand-alone ultrasound probe inserted through the channel of a regular endoscope can image lesions within the wall of the gut and beyond. Endoscopic ultrasonography (EUS) can guide fine-needle aspiration more accurately than abdominal ultrasonography or CT.

COMPLICATIONS AND PRE-ENDOSCOPY PREPARATION

Diagnostic endoscopy is usually a remarkably safe and well-tolerated procedure. It can be performed under conscious sedation with a combination of benzodiazepines and narcotics or with propofol, which provides faster and deeper sedation with rapid recovery (Chapter 440). However, potential complications (Table 136-2) must be carefully explained to the patient as part of the informed consent process. In general, routine blood tests, radiographs, or electrocardiograms are not necessary before endoscopy unless a careful history and physical examination suggest possible hematologic, cardiovascular, or pulmonary or airway problems. Women of childbearing age should be questioned about the possibility of pregnancy and tested if there is any doubt.

Diagnostic endoscopies, including those with mucosal biopsies, are considered low risk and do not warrant discontinuation of anticoagulant medication. Similarly, aspirin or other nonsteroidal anti-inflammatory agents can be continued by patients undergoing screening colonoscopy. In high-risk elective procedures, anticoagulants and antiplatelet agents may be discontinued,

TABLE 136-1 ENDOSCOPIC PROCEDURES AND GENERAL APPLICATIONS

ENDOSCOPIC PROCEDURES	THERAPEUTIC APPLICATIONS
LUMINAL ENDOSCOPY	
Common procedures	Hemostasis
Esophagogastroduodenoscopy	Luminal restoration (dilation, ablation, stenting)
Colonoscopy	Lesion removal (e.g., polypectomy, mucosal ablation)
Flexible sigmoidoscopy	Provision of access (percutaneous endoscopic gastrostomy and jejunostomy)
Less common procedures	Barrier strengthening (antireflux procedures)
Enteroscopy	
Capsule endoscopy	
PANCREATOBILIARY IMAGING	
Endoscopic retrograde cholangiopancreatography	Lesion (stone) removal
	Luminal restoration (dilation, stenting)
	Provision of access (sphincterotomy)
	Drainage (bile, pancreatic pseudocyst)
TRANSLUMINAL IMAGING	
Endoscopic ultrasonography	Analgesic block
	Delivery of therapeutic agents (experimental)

TABLE 136-2 COMPLICATIONS OF ENDOSCOPY

ENDOSCOPIC COMPLICATIONS	INCIDENCE (%)	SPECIFIC PROPHYLAXIS
GENERAL COMPLICATIONS		
Complications related primarily to sedation (cardiovascular and respiratory depression, aspiration)	0.6-0.7	Airway protection with massive upper gastrointestinal bleeding Preprocedure medical evaluation, intraprocedure and postprocedure monitoring Anesthesiology consultation for high-risk patients
Perforation	0.14-0.25 (colonoscopy) 0.1-0.3 (upper endoscopy)	None (except careful technique)
Bleeding	0.7-2.5 (polypectomy) 0.3 (upper endoscopy)	Carefully balance risk and benefits Discontinue or reduce anticoagulant use before high-risk procedures
Bacteremia and infectious complications (endocarditis, bacterial ascites)	<0.1	Antibiotics for patients at risk for endocarditis (patients with artificial valves, pulmonary-systemic shunts, previous history of endocarditis), with synthetic vascular grafts, and with bacterial ascites (cirrhotics)
Death	0.2 (colonoscopy) 0.6 (upper endoscopy)	
COMPLICATIONS ASSOCIATED WITH SPECIALIZED PROCEDURES		
Pancreatitis (ERCP)	3-20	Not well established; experimental
Cholangitis (ERCP)	0.1-2	Preprocedure antibiotics
Wound infections (PEG)	3-4	Preprocedure antibiotics

ERCP = endoscopic retrograde cholangiopancreatography; PEG = percutaneous endoscopic gastrostomy.

in consultation with both the prescribing specialist and the gastroenterologist (Chapter 439). For patients with acute bleeding, reversal therapy or platelet replacement may be considered (Chapters 174 through 178).

ERCP is associated with the highest risk of serious complications, and about 1 to 5% of patients develop pancreatitis. Risk factors include young age, female gender, underlying sphincter of Oddi dysfunction, and previous history of pancreatitis. Despite a variety of trials, no pharmacologic prophylaxis has been unequivocally successful. However, most experts place a short-term pancreatic stent in high-risk cases as a reasonable preventive measure.

● SPECIFIC INDICATIONS

Most indications for gastrointestinal endoscopy are based on the patient's presenting symptoms (e.g., dysphagia, bleeding, diarrhea). In other instances, endoscopy is required to evaluate specific lesions found by other diagnostic imaging, such as a gastric ulcer or colon polyp discovered by barium radiography. Finally, screening endoscopy is often performed in asymptomatic individuals on the basis of their risk for commonly occurring and preventable conditions, such as colon cancer (see later).

Implicit in the decision to perform endoscopy is the assumption that it will have a bearing on future management strategy. When evaluating gastrointestinal symptoms, several questions need to be addressed by the referring physician and the endoscopist: Which patients need endoscopy? When should the endoscopy be done? What is the endoscopist looking for? What endoscopic therapy, if any, should be planned?

Gastroesophageal Reflux and Heartburn (Chapters 140 and 141)

Gastroesophageal reflux disease (GERD) is an extremely common condition in the general population. The fact that its cardinal symptom, heartburn, is relatively specific for this condition justifies an empirical approach to treatment by a combination of lifestyle modifications and over-the-counter or even prescription drugs. Endoscopy is therefore not necessary to make the diagnosis of GERD. Indeed, normal findings on endoscopy do not rule out the diagnosis because the overall sensitivity of endoscopy in GERD is only about 70%. If necessary, further evaluation with ambulatory esophageal manometry and pH monitoring can establish the diagnosis. However, there are several circumstances in which endoscopy should be considered for patients with reflux, including those with warning symptoms ("red flags") such as dysphagia, odynophagia, regurgitation, weight loss, gastrointestinal bleeding, or frequent vomiting (Fig. 136-1). These symptoms imply either the development of a GERD-related complication (erosive esophagitis, stricture, or adenocarcinoma) or another disorder masquerading as GERD (esophageal cancer or a gastric-duodenal lesion such as cancer or peptic ulcer). Other candidates for endoscopy are those with severe, persistent, or frequently recurrent symptoms that suggest significant esophagitis and hence a risk for complications, such as stricture or Barrett's esophagus, which is intestinal metaplasia of the esophageal epithelium.

If a significant length of Barrett's esophagus (especially >3 cm) is discovered (see Fig. 136-1), most experts recommend some form of periodic surveillance endoscopy because of the increased risk for the development of

adenocarcinoma. Control of reflux by either pharmacologic or surgical means does not generally lead to regression of established Barrett's esophagus (Chapter 140). Furthermore, endoscopic techniques to reduce reflux have not resulted in long-term benefits, despite promising initial results.

For patients in whom high-grade dysplasia associated with Barrett's esophagus poses a serious risk for cancer, endoscopic ablation or resection provides a potentially curative alternative to surgical esophagectomy. Ablation can be achieved by a variety of modalities, including radio frequency, cryotherapy, electrical cautery, argon plasma coagulation, and photodynamic therapy. An alternative to ablation is endoscopic mucosal resection, which is en bloc resection of the mucosa to allow complete pathologic analysis and minimize the risk for regrowth of the abnormal mucosal lining.

Heartburn in immunocompromised patients often indicates an esophageal infection. The most common causes in patients with human immunodeficiency virus (HIV) infection are *Candida albicans,* cytomegalovirus, herpesvirus, and idiopathic esophageal ulcers. Because most patients with acquired immunodeficiency syndrome (AIDS) and esophagitis have candidiasis, an empirical 1- to 2-week course of antifungal therapy may be justified. Patients who do not respond to this approach should almost always have endoscopy and biopsy so that more specific therapy can be instituted.

Dysphagia (Chapter 140)

Dysphagia can often be categorized as oropharyngeal on the basis of the clinical features of nasal regurgitation, laryngeal aspiration, or difficulty moving the bolus out of the mouth. These symptoms are usually associated with a lesion in the central or peripheral nervous system. Although endoscopy is often performed in these patients, videofluoroesophagography (modified barium swallow or cine-esophagogram) is the procedure of choice because it allows a frame-by-frame evaluation of the rapid sequence of events involved in transfer of the bolus from the mouth to the esophagus. Common causes of esophageal dysphagia include malignant as well as benign processes (peptic strictures secondary to reflux, Schatzki's rings) and motility disturbances of the esophageal body or the lower esophageal sphincter. Endoscopic examination is considered mandatory in all patients with esophageal dysphagia. However, contrast esophagography may also be helpful; it can provide guidance in cases in which endoscopy is anticipated to be difficult (e.g., a patient with a complex stricture), suggest a disturbance in motility, and occasionally detect subtle stenoses that are not appreciated on endoscopy (the scope diameter is typically ≤10 mm, whereas some symptomatic strictures can be considerably wider).

Endoscopic treatment options are available for many causes of esophageal dysphagia. Tumors may be dilated mechanically, ablated by thermal means (cautery or laser), or stented with prosthetic devices. Metallic expandable stents have become the palliative procedure of choice for most patients with symptomatic esophageal cancer. Benign lesions of the esophagus, such as strictures or rings, can also be dilated endoscopically, usually with excellent results. Finally, some motility disturbances, such as achalasia, are best approached endoscopically with the use of large balloon dilators for the lower esophageal sphincter or the local injection of botulinum toxin.

Dyspepsia (Chapter 139)

Dyspepsia, which is chronic or recurring pain or discomfort centered in the upper abdomen, is a common condition that can be caused by a variety of disorders, including peptic ulcer, reflux esophagitis, gallstones, gastric dysmotility, and, rarely, gastric or esophageal cancer. However, up to 60% of patients with chronic (>3 months) dyspepsia have a so-called functional disorder in which there is no definite structural or biochemical explanation for the symptoms. Although *Helicobacter pylori* gastritis is found frequently in these patients, there is no evidence of a cause-and-effect relationship between these two findings. If a diagnostic test is to be performed, endoscopy, sometimes with biopsies to detect *H. pylori,* is clearly the procedure of choice (see Fig. 141-2 in Chapter 141); it has an accuracy of about 90%, compared with about 65% for double-contrast radiography. Because dyspepsia is a recurrent condition and patients who do not respond to empirical therapy almost always undergo endoscopy, many gastroenterologists opt for early endoscopy, if only for the reassurance that a normal examination provides.

Upper Gastrointestinal Bleeding (Chapter 137)

Acid peptic disease (including ulcers, erosions, and gastritis), variceal bleeding, and Mallory-Weiss tears account for most cases of upper gastrointestinal bleeding. Other less common but important lesions are angioma, gastric vascular ectasia ("watermelon" stomach), and the rarer Dieulafoy's lesion (a

FIGURE 136-1. Severe reflux esophagitis. **A,** Mucosal erythema and linear ulcers with yellow exudates (asterisks). **B,** It is thought that such changes eventually lead to Barrett's esophagus, in which the normal white squamous epithelium (*SE*) is replaced by red columnar epithelium (*BE*). These examples are from different patients.

superficial artery that erodes through the gut mucosa). Finally, upper gastrointestinal cancers are occasionally associated with significant bleeding. Endoscopy is mandatory in all patients with upper gastrointestinal bleeding, with the rare exception being a terminally ill patient in whom the outcome is unlikely to be affected. Endoscopy can detect and localize the site of bleeding in 95% of cases and is clearly superior to contrast radiography (with an accuracy of only 75 to 80%). The endoscopic appearance of bleeding lesions can also help predict the risk of rebleeding, thus facilitating the triage and treatment process. Bleeding can be effectively controlled during the initial endoscopic examination itself in the majority of cases. The risk of recurrent bleeding is diminished, resulting in a shorter hospital stay as well as a reduction in the need for surgery.

In general, endoscopy should be performed only after adequate stabilization of hemodynamic and respiratory parameters. The role of gastric lavage before endoscopy is controversial; some endoscopists prefer that it be done, occasionally even with a large-bore tube, whereas others avoid such preparation for fear of producing artifact. The timing of subsequent endoscopy depends on two factors: the severity of the hemorrhage, and the risk status of the patient. Patients with active, persistent, or severe bleeding (>3 units of blood) require urgent endoscopy. In these patients, endoscopy is best performed in the intensive care unit because of the risk for aspiration and the occasional need for emergent intubation to provide respiratory protection and ventilation. Patients with slower or inactive bleeding can be evaluated by endoscopy in a "semielective" manner (usually within 12 to 20 hours), but a case can be made for early endoscopy even in these stable patients (perhaps in the emergency department itself) to allow more confident triage and more efficient resource management.

Most bleeding from upper gastrointestinal lesions can be effectively controlled endoscopically. The endoscopist considers factors such as age (older patients have a higher risk of rebleeding), severity of the initial hemorrhage (which has a direct correlation to the risk of rebleeding), and appearance of the lesion in determining the need for endoscopic therapy. Nonvariceal bleeding vessels can be treated by a variety of means, including injections of various substances (epinephrine, saline, sclerosants), thermal coagulation (laser or electrocautery), and mechanical means (clipping). In the United States, the most popular approach to a bleeding peptic ulcer lesion is a combination of injection with dilute epinephrine and electrocoagulation. Initial hemostasis can be achieved in 90% or more of cases; rebleeding, which may occur in up to 20% of cases, responds about half the time to a second endoscopic procedure. Patients who continue to bleed (typically those with large ulcers in the posterior wall of the duodenal bulb) are usually managed angiographically (with embolization of the bleeding vessel) or surgically.

Variceal bleeding can also be effectively managed endoscopically, with a success rate similar to that for bleeding ulcers (Fig. 136-2) (Chapter 156). Hemostasis is achieved by band ligation (Fig. 136-3), sclerotherapy, or a combination of both. Increasingly, patients who do not respond to endoscopic treatment are considered candidates for a transjugular intrahepatic portosystemic shunt (TIPS); traditional shunt surgery for bleeding varices is rarely performed. Even if initial endoscopic hemostasis is successful, long-term prevention of rebleeding requires a program of ongoing endoscopic sessions until variceal obliteration is complete. Ligation is the preferred approach in this setting because it is associated with fewer side effects. In patients whose large esophageal varices have never bled, β-blockers are considered first-line treatment, but endoscopic band ligation may be useful in selected patients.

Acute Lower Gastrointestinal Bleeding (Chapter 137)

The most common cause of acute lower gastrointestinal bleeding is angiodysplasia, followed by diverticulosis, neoplasm, and colitis. In about 10% of patients presenting with hematochezia, a small bowel lesion may be responsible. In contrast to upper gastrointestinal bleeding, there is no single best test for acute lower gastrointestinal bleeding. In patients younger than 40 years with minor bleeding, findings that are highly suggestive of anorectal origin (e.g., blood on the surface of the stool or on the wipe) may warrant only flexible sigmoidoscopy. Conversely, patients presenting with hemodynamic compromise may need upper endoscopy first to exclude a lesion in the upper gastrointestinal tract (typically postpyloric) that is bleeding so briskly it presents as hematochezia. Colonoscopy was traditionally recommended after bleeding slowed or stopped and the patient had been given an adequate bowel purge. However, a disadvantage of delaying endoscopy is that when a

FIGURE 136-2. Esophageal varices. **A,** Endoscopic view of esophageal varices in the wall of the esophagus (V). **B,** Varix that has been endoscopically ligated with a band.

FIGURE 136-3. Endoscopic variceal ligation technique. **A,** The endoscope, with an attached ligating device, is brought into contact with a varix just above the gastroesophageal junction. **B,** Suction is applied, drawing the varix-containing mucosa into the dead space created at the end of the endoscope by the ligating device. **C,** The trip wire is pulled, releasing the band around the aspirated tissue. **D,** Completed ligation.

FIGURE 136-4. Mucosal telangiectasia (arteriovenous malformation) in the colon. The patient presented with hematochezia. The lesion was subsequently cauterized endoscopically.

FIGURE 136-5. Endoscopic polypectomy. **A,** A snare (S) has been passed through the endoscope and positioned around the polyp (P). **B,** Cautery was applied, and the polyp was guillotined, leaving behind a clean mucosal defect.

pathologic lesion such as an arteriovenous malformation (Fig. 136-4) or diverticulum is found, it may be impossible to implicate it confidently as the site of bleeding (complementary information by radiography or scintigraphy becomes particularly important in this situation). Some experts therefore recommend urgent diagnostic endoscopy with little or no preparation for acute lower gastrointestinal hemorrhages and have reported significant diagnostic as well as therapeutic success rates. However, such recommendations have not been universally accepted and remain logistically difficult to implement in most hospital settings.

It is not uncommon for gastrointestinal bleeding to develop or to be discovered in hospitalized patients who have had a recent myocardial infarction. In many cases, the bleeding is of a microscopic nature, and endoscopic evaluation can be deferred until the patient has fully recovered from the cardiac event. In other cases, however, the bleeding is more significant, and its risks outweigh the potential adverse effects of endoscopic intervention. In patients with recent myocardial infarction, upper endoscopy and colonoscopy are associated with a higher risk of cardiovascular complications, but they are usually transient and minor.

Occult Gastrointestinal Bleeding or Iron Deficiency Anemia (Chapter 137)

Normal fecal blood loss is usually less than 2 to 3 mL/day. Most standard fecal occult blood tests detect only blood loss of 10 mL/day or more. Therefore, even if this test result is negative, patients with iron deficiency anemia and no other obvious source of blood loss should always undergo aggressive gastrointestinal evaluation, which uncovers a gastrointestinal lesion in the majority of cases. Although most lesions that cause overt gastrointestinal bleeding can also cause occult blood loss, occult bleeding should almost never be ascribed to diverticulosis or hemorrhoids. Endoscopy is always preferable to radiographic studies for the evaluation of occult blood loss or iron deficiency anemia because of its ability to detect flat lesions, particularly vascular malformations, which may be found in 6% or more of patients. If the findings on both upper and lower endoscopy are normal, the next test is capsule endoscopy, which may be helpful to detect small bowel lesions such as erosions, tumors, or angiomas. Although it is relatively contraindicated in patients with suspected narrowing or strictures of the small bowel, capsule endoscopy has become the diagnostic procedure of choice in patients with obscure gastrointestinal bleeding (with normal findings on upper and lower endoscopies) and when mucosal lesions of the small bowel are suspected. Findings on capsule endoscopy may prompt the consideration of enteroscopy (using specialized double- or single-balloon endoscopes), which can theoretically access the entire small bowel and permit biopsy and/or therapy of suspected lesions.

Colorectal Neoplasms (Chapter 199)

Colonoscopy is the most accurate test for detecting mass lesions of the large bowel or colon that are suspected on clinical or radiologic grounds. However, endoscopy's greatest impact on colorectal neoplasia may be in the area of screening and prevention. The adenoma to carcinoma sequence of progression in colorectal cancer provides a unique opportunity for prophylaxis. Thus, if screening programs can identify patients with polyps, and if these polyps are removed, cancer can largely be prevented. Various techniques are available for safe and effective polypectomy, depending on the size, presence of a stalk,

and location (Fig. 136-5). Colonoscopy is currently recommended for screening patients at average risk—that is, anyone older than 50 years. Adenomatous polyps should be removed, and patients should then enter a surveillance program with follow-up colonoscopies every 3 to 10 years, depending on the nature and number of initial lesions. Patients with no polyps generally do not require follow-up colonoscopies more than every 10 years.

More aggressive screening strategies are required for patients considered at high risk for colorectal cancer, including patients with well-defined hereditary syndromes as well as those with a history of colorectal cancer in a first-degree relative. In addition, patients with ulcerative colitis (Chapter 143) with long-standing (>8 years) disease affecting the entire colon have an increased risk for the development of colon cancer, about 0.5 to 3% after 20 years. Periodic colonoscopic surveillance (every 1 to 2 years with biopsies) is recommended for patients with long-standing disease (8 years with pancolitis, 12 to 15 years with left-sided colitis); the discovery of high-grade dysplasia or cancer is an indication for colectomy.

"Virtual colonoscopy" (Chapter 135), which involves the digital construction of an endoluminal view of the colon on the basis of data from abdominal CT, is fast emerging as a viable alternative to colonoscopy, particularly in patients who have failed previous endoscopic attempts or for whom colonoscopy is a high-risk procedure. Alternative screening techniques, including devices that can be used by nonphysicians, electronically mapped and driven instruments, and even completely self-propelled devices, are currently undergoing clinical trials.

Chronic Diarrhea (Chapter 142)

Endoscopy may be a valuable aid in the evaluation of patients with persistent diarrhea. The timing of the endoscopy in these patients often depends on the clinical features of the illness. Patients with bloody diarrhea should have lower endoscopy as part of an initial evaluation to determine whether inflammatory bowel disease is present (Chapter 143). In most patients with chronic diarrhea, endoscopy is often done when routine testing does not yield a specific diagnosis. Both upper and lower endoscopies may be performed, depending on the clinical presentation. Thus, a patient suspected of having a malabsorptive process may require upper endoscopy with jejunal or duodenal biopsies to look for celiac sprue or rarer lesions such as lymphoma or Whipple's disease; endoscopic biopsy has largely replaced blind intestinal biopsy for these conditions. Conversely, a patient thought to have a secretory cause of diarrhea requires a colonoscopy with biopsies to look for overt inflammatory bowel disease or more subtle variants such as microscopic or lymphocytic colitis, in which case the diagnosis requires careful examination of the biopsy specimens.

The endoscopic approach to diarrhea in immunocompromised patients, such as those with HIV infection, is guided by the degree of immunosuppression and the need to find treatable infections. When the results of routine stool tests are negative, patients with CD4 counts less than 100/mm^3 should undergo endoscopic evaluation to detect pathogens such as cytomegalovirus, *Mycobacterium avium* complex, and microsporidia. Small-volume stools with tenesmus suggest proctocolitis, for which sigmoidoscopy (rather than full colonoscopy) with biopsies is usually adequate. In patients with upper gastrointestinal symptoms (large-volume diarrhea, bloating, and dyspepsia), upper endoscopy with small bowel biopsy may be attempted first.

FIGURE 136-6. Impacted food bolus in a young male patient who was found to have a ringed esophagus on endoscopy. This presentation is characteristic and may be either congenital or acquired secondary to reflux-induced or eosinophilic esophagitis.

FIGURE 136-7. Large malignant mass at the gastroesophageal junction, as seen endoscopically.

Miscellaneous Indications

The upper endoscope has provided a relatively quick and noninvasive means of removing accidentally or deliberately ingested foreign bodies. Timing is critical for removal, however, because objects are usually beyond endoscopic retrieval when they reach the small bowel. Any foreign object that is causing symptoms should be removed, as should all potentially dangerous devices such as batteries and sharp objects. In general, objects larger than 2.5 cm wide or 13 cm long are unlikely to leave the stomach and should be removed. On occasion, patients with food impacted in the esophagus require endoscopic removal (Fig. 136-6). This condition almost always indicates an underlying functional or structural problem (Chapter 140) and should prompt a thorough diagnostic evaluation after the acute problem has been addressed.

Because of the relatively poor correlation between oropharyngeal lesions and more distal visceral injury, upper endoscopy is usually recommended urgently in patients with corrosive ingestion (Chapter 110). Endoscopy allows patients to be divided into high- or low-risk groups with regard to complications, with the institution of appropriate monitoring and therapy. Among the myriad causes of nausea and vomiting, a few, such as mucosal lesions and unsuspected reflux disease, are amenable to endoscopic diagnosis.

Malignant obstruction of the gastrointestinal lumen, including the esophagus (Fig. 136-7), pylorus or duodenum, and colon, can now be safely and effectively palliated endoscopically by expandable metal stents, thereby avoiding surgery. Colonoscopy is also useful in patients with pseudo-obstructive (nonobstructive) colonic dilation or Ogilvie's syndrome (Chapter 138); such patients are at risk for colonic rupture at diameters greater than 9 to 12 cm, and colonoscopic decompression is often required, sometimes on an emergent basis.

A major advance in enteral feeding has been the introduction of percutaneous endoscopic gastrostomy (PEG), a relatively quick, simple, and safe endoscopic procedure that has virtually eliminated the surgical placement of gastric tubes. A variation of PEG is percutaneous endoscopic jejunostomy (PEJ), in which a long tube is passed through the gastric tube, past the pylorus, and into the jejunum. PEJ does not prevent aspiration, but it is effective in patients with a significant impairment of gastric emptying. Retrograde tube migration with PEJ is common, however, and PEJ may require frequent replacement. The most common indication for these procedures is the need for sustained nutrition in patients with neurologic impairment of swallowing or with head and neck cancers. Patients with a short life expectancy are not suitable candidates for PEG and can be managed by nasoenteral tubes. Further, despite its intuitive appeal, there is little or no evidence that PEG feeding alters clinical or nutritional outcomes or significantly improves quality of life.

● PANCREATOBILIARY ENDOSCOPY

Suspected Biliary Disease (Chapters 148 and 158)

The diagnostic approach to patients with cholestasis begins with an attempt to differentiate obstructive from hepatocellular causes. The most common causes of obstructive jaundice are common bile duct stones and tumors of the pancreatic and bile ducts. Less invasive conventional imaging with ultrasonography, CT, or magnetic resonance imaging (MRI) demonstrates dilated bile ducts and mass lesions; however, it is not sensitive or specific in the detection or delineation of pathologic change in the distal common bile duct and pancreas, two regions where the majority of obstructing lesions are found. Furthermore, some biliary diseases, such as sclerosing cholangitis, do not result in dilated ducts but have a characteristic appearance on cholangiography. Finally, the ability to use devices such as cytology brushes and biopsy forceps during cholangiography provides an additional aid in the diagnosis of biliary lesions. Both percutaneous and endoscopic cholangiographic techniques are associated with a high rate of success in experienced hands, but the endoscopic approach allows visualization of the ampullary region and the performance of sphincterotomy; it also avoids the small risk of a biliary leak associated with puncture of the liver capsule.

In the past few years, magnetic resonance cholangiopancreatography (MRCP), a digital reconstruction technique based on an abdominal MRI scan, has become a popular imaging modality for the pancreatobiliary system, with excellent sensitivity and specificity. Because of its relative safety, many experts now advocate this procedure for screening patients with a low likelihood of disease. In those with a higher probability, ERCP is still the procedure of choice because of its therapeutic options.

Of the approximately 600,000 patients undergoing cholecystectomy in the United States, 5 to 10% may present with bile duct stones before or after surgery. Endoscopic stone removal is successful in 90% or more of these cases and usually requires a sphincterotomy (Fig. 136-8). The sphincter of Oddi is a band of muscle that encircles the distal common bile duct and pancreatic duct in the region of the ampulla of Vater; cutting of this muscle, or sphincterotomy, is one of the mainstays of endoscopic biliary treatment and is accomplished with a special tool called a papillotome or sphincterotome. This procedure is often sufficient for the treatment of small stones in the bile ducts, but larger stones may require additional procedures such as mechanical, electrohydraulic, or laser lithotripsy, which can be performed endoscopically. In addition, sphincterotomy may be curative for patients with papillary stenosis or muscle spasm (sphincter of Oddi dysfunction). Finally, by enlarging the access to the bile duct, sphincterotomy facilitates the passage of stents and other devices into the bile duct. Sphincterotomy carries an additional small risk of bleeding, but its associated morbidity is about one third that of surgical exploration.

Endoscopic therapy has also revolutionized the palliative approach to malignant biliary obstruction. This technique, which requires the placement of indwelling stents, is superior to both radiologic and surgical techniques. Plastic stents have been the mainstay of treatment, but metal stents last longer and may be preferred in patients with longer life expectancies.

Pancreatic Neoplasms

EUS is probably the single best test for the diagnosis of pancreatic tumors (Chapter 201), particularly the small endocrine varieties, with a sensitivity approaching 95% (Fig. 136-9). It is also the procedure of choice for imaging submucosal and other mural lesions of the gastrointestinal tract (overall accuracy of 65 to 70%) as well as for staging a variety of gastrointestinal tumors (overall accuracy of 90% or more), especially esophageal and pancreatic cancer.

FIGURE 136-8. Biliary sphincterotomy and stone removal from the bile duct. **A,** Endoscopic retrograde cholangiographic image showing stones (arrow) in the distal common bile duct. **B,** Endoscopic image of a sphincterotome in the bile duct, with the wire cutting the roof of the ampulla (sphincter). **C,** A stone is being removed from the bile duct by an endoscopically passed basket.

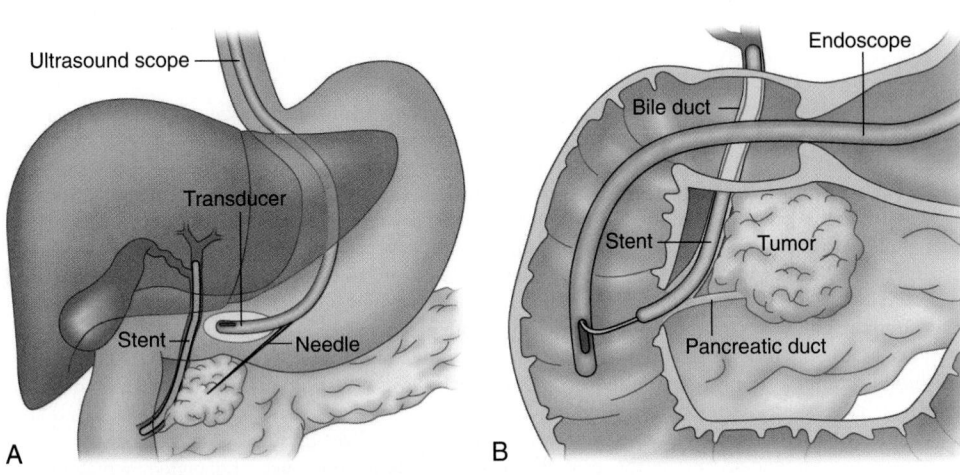

FIGURE 136-9. Diagram of biopsy of a pancreatic mass and stent placement. The biopsy is guided by endoscopic ultrasonography (**A**), and placement of the stent into a malignant bile duct stricture is accomplished with endoscopic retrograde cholangiopancreatography (**B**). (From Brugge WR, Van Dam J. Pancreatic and biliary endoscopy. *N Engl J Med.* 1999;341:1808-1816. Copyright 1999 Massachusetts Medical Society. All rights reserved.)

FIGURE 136-10. High-grade intraepithelial neoplasia. **A,** Confocal microscopy shows high-grade intraepithelial neoplasia of a colorectal polyp during endoscopy. Acriflavine was used as a contrast agent (0.02%), highlighting the cellular and nuclear architecture. **B,** Histologic picture from the same polyp. (Courtesy of Dr. Ralph Kiesselich, University of Mainz.)

EUS-directed celiac plexus neurolysis appears to be effective for the treatment of pain in patients with pancreatic cancer, although it does not work as well in patients with chronic pancreatitis.

Nonmalignant Pancreatic Disease (Chapter 146)

ERCP is indicated for patients with acute or recurrent pancreatitis without any obvious risk factors based on history or routine laboratory evaluation. Imaging of the pancreatic duct may delineate anatomic abnormalities responsible for the pancreatitis, such as congenital variants (pancreas divisum, annular pancreas), intraductal tumors, or possibly sphincter of Oddi dysfunction. In such cases, bile can be collected from the bile duct for microscopic examination for crystals (so-called microlithiasis) that can cause pancreatitis in some patients even in the absence of macroscopic stones. In patients with chronic pancreatitis, which is most often due to excessive alcohol intake, pancreatography can confirm the diagnosis, provide useful information about disease severity, and identify ductal lesions that may be amenable to therapy by either endoscopic or surgical means. In more subtle cases, collection and analysis of pancreatic juice after stimulation with secretin may be useful in establishing exocrine impairment and hence confirming chronic pancreatic injury.

ERCP also has a role in some patients with acute pancreatitis caused by obstructing biliary stones. Patients presenting with severe biliary pancreatitis may benefit from urgent ERCP early in the course of the disease, with the intention being to detect and remove stones from the common bile duct. Similarly, patients with smoldering acute pancreatitis that is not improving satisfactorily with conservative treatment may require ERCP for the identification and treatment of any obstructing lesions in the pancreatic or distal biliary duct.

Therapeutic endoscopy for chronic pancreatic disease is still evolving. Relief of ductal obstruction (e.g., by endoscopic removal of pancreatic stones or dilation of strictures) can provide short- to intermediate-term pain relief in some patients with chronic pancreatitis, although it is probably not as effective as surgery in the long term.[2] Endoscopic pseudocyst drainage by a variety of techniques is now technically feasible, with results that appear to be comparable to those of surgical or radiologic techniques. Patients with ductal disruptions (e.g., pancreatic ascites) can often be treated successfully with endoscopic stent placement. Pancreatic papillotomy may also be useful in some patients with recurrent pancreatitis, such as when pancreas divisum is thought to play a role. Although the ability to approach these difficult clinical entities by less invasive endoscopic techniques represents a major accomplishment, the treatment of pancreatic diseases remains a multidisciplinary effort, with important and in some cases dominant roles played by surgeons and interventional radiologists.

EVOLVING TECHNIQUES AND FUTURE DIRECTIONS

Promising innovations include endoscopic optical coherence tomography, different forms of spectroscopy, and confocal microscopy (Fig. 136-10). These and a variety of other so-called optical biopsy techniques have the ability to provide microscopic images of cells at the surface as well as within deeper layers, thereby providing virtual real-time histology. Further, using targeted probes, it is possible to image function as well as form (E-Fig. 136-1). Innovations in endoscopic therapy include natural orifice transluminal endoscopic surgery (NOTES), by which the endoscopist or surgeon introduces an endoscope through a natural orifice (mouth, vagina, anal canal), traverses the wall of the viscus, and accesses the peritoneal cavity to perform diagnostic and therapeutic procedures.

1. Shaheen NJ, Sharma P, Overholt BF, et al. Radiofrequency ablation in Barrett's esophagus with dysplasia. *N Engl J Med.* 2009;360:2277-2288.
2. Cahen DL, Gouma DJ, Nio Y, et al. Endoscopic versus surgical drainage of the pancreatic duct in chronic pancreatitis. *N Engl J Med.* 2007;356:676-684.

SUGGESTED READINGS

ASGE Technology Committee, Kaul V, Adler DG, Conway JD, et al. Interventional EUS. *Gastrointest Endosc.* 2010;72:1-4. *Consensus guidelines.*
The DAVE (Digital Atlas of Video Education) Project. www.daveproject.org. *This website is devoted to videos and other educational material on a variety of endoscopic procedures.*
Laine L, Sahota A, Shah A. Does capsule endoscopy improve outcomes in obscure gastrointestinal bleeding? Randomized trial versus dedicated small bowel radiography. *Gastroenterology.* 2010;138:1655-1688. *Raises questions about whether the improved diagnostic accuracy of capsule endoscopy translates into better outcomes.*
Leighton JA. The role of endoscopic imaging of the small bowel in clinical practice. *Am J Gastroenterol.* 2011;106:27-36. *Review.*

137

GASTROINTESTINAL HEMORRHAGE AND OCCULT GASTROINTESTINAL BLEEDING

DENNIS M. JENSEN

GASTROINTESTINAL HEMORRHAGE

Background

Gastrointestinal (GI) hemorrhage, which is a common clinical problem, has an annual hospitalization rate of 350 per 100,000 population in the United States, thereby resulting in more than 1 million hospitalizations annually. It can manifest clinically as overt bleeding from the upper GI tract (esophagus, stomach, and duodenum) or lower GI tract (colon), or it can emanate from obscure locations, usually in the small intestine. Alternatively, it can present as occult bleeding that is detected by the presence of iron deficiency anemia (Chapter 162) or a positive fecal occult blood test (Chapter 199).

Upper Gastrointestinal Bleeding

CLINICAL MANIFESTATIONS

Upper GI bleeding, which occurs proximal to the ligament of Treitz, accounts for approximately 50% of hospitalizations for GI bleeding. Upper GI bleeding usually presents as either hematemesis (vomiting of blood or coffee-ground

material) or melena (black, tarry stool), but about 15 to 20% of patients who present with hematochezia, which is passage of red blood or clots per rectum, have an upper GI source of brisk bleeding. The most common causes are peptic ulcer disease , esophageal or gastric varices (Fig. 137-1), and erosive esophagitis (see Fig. 136-1 in Chapter 136). Variceal bleeding, which occurs in the setting of portal hypertension, is discussed in Chapter 156. Other causes of severe upper GI bleeding include tumors, vascular ectasias, Mallory-Weiss tears (Fig. 137-2), and erosions (Table 137-1). Depending on the severity of bleeding, patients may otherwise be asymptomatic, may present with fatigue or dizziness, or may have hypovolemic shock (Chapter 106).

DIAGNOSIS

Initial assessment includes a medical history, vital signs, and a comprehensive physical examination, including a digital rectal examination. Patients should be asked questions that may help determine the source of the bleeding. For example, peptic ulcer bleeding (Chapter 141) should be suspected in patients taking daily aspirin or nonsteroidal anti-inflammatory drugs (NSAIDs). For patients with known or suspected liver disease, bleeding from varices or gastropathy related to portal hypertension (Chapter 156) should be strongly considered. Heavy alcohol intake or vomiting should suggest a Mallory-Weiss tear (Chapter 140). The presence of a feeding tube or a chronic nasogastric

FIGURE 137-1. Bleeding esophageal varix at the gastroesophageal junction. (Courtesy of Pankaj Jay Pasricha, MD.)

FIGURE 137-2. Retroflexed endoscopic image of a Mallory-Weiss tear at the gastroesophageal junction.

tube or a history of gastroesophageal reflux disease raises the suspicion for erosive esophagitis.

On the vital signs, special attention should be paid to signs of hypovolemia such as hypotension and tachycardia. Evidence of postural tachycardia or hypotension may reveal severe volume depletion that is not appreciated on a supine examination. It is important to examine the skin for petechiae, purpura, spider angiomas, and palmar erythema (see Fig. 148-2 in Chapter 148), and the abdomen for ascites (see Fig. 148-5 in Chapter 148), hepatomegaly, or splenomegaly, which may indicate portal hypertension. Tenderness or a mass may indicate an intra-abdominal tumor.

Placement of a nasogastric or orogastric tube can help localize bleeding to the upper GI tract, determine whether red blood or coffee-ground material is present, and assess how brisk, persistent, and recurrent the bleeding is. However, the sensitivity of nasogastric aspiration for upper GI bleeding is only about 80%, usually because blood in the duodenum is not refluxed into the stomach. Guaiac testing of nasogastric tube aspirates for unseen blood is not useful because the trauma of tube placement often may cause scant bleeding and false-positive results. Patients who have witnessed coffee-ground emesis or fresh bloody emesis do not require a nasogastric tube for diagnostic purposes but may need one to help clear the gastric blood for better endoscopic visualization and to minimize the risk of aspiration.

Blood should be sent for standard hematology, chemistry, liver, and coagulation studies, and the patient should be typed and crossmatched for the potential infusion of packed red blood cells (Chapter 180). The hemoglobin concentration and the hematocrit level may not accurately reflect blood loss because equilibration with extravascular fluid requires 24 to 72 hours. A low platelet count suggests chronic liver disease, dilution, drug reaction, or a hematologic disorder. In upper GI bleeding, the blood urea nitrogen level typically increases to a greater extent than the creatinine level because of increased intestinal absorption of urea after breakdown of blood proteins, but this phenomenon may not be seen in the setting of renal insufficiency or rapid transit of blood. An elevated international normalized ratio (INR) can be seen in chronic liver disease or with the use of warfarin.

Endoscopy

Patients with evidence of active bleeding (red blood by nasogastric lavage or hypotension) should undergo emergency endoscopy as soon as possible after medical resuscitation. Other patients should have endoscopic evaluation within 24 hours of their presentation (Chapter 136). Endoscopy can identify the site of bleeding with a sensitivity of about 92% and a specificity of nearly 100%, and it also can provide therapeutic hemostasis in most patients. An intravenous prokinetic agent (either erythromycin, 250 mg, or metoclopramide, 10 mg) 30 to 60 minutes before endoscopy may help move blood out of the stomach and into the small intestine, thereby improving endoscopic visualization.

In addition to localizing and treating the bleeding source, endoscopic evaluation can provide prognostic information and stratification for the risk of rebleeding, based on the presence or absence of stigmata of recent hemorrhage (Table 137-2). Other poor prognostic factors include older age, bleeding onset in the hospital, medical comorbidities, shock, coagulopathy, fresh blood in the nasogastric lavage, and the need for multiple blood transfusions. Clinical scoring systems, such as the Rockall score (Table 137-3), use clinical information and endoscopic findings to predict clinical outcomes. Similarly a Glasgow-Blatchford bleeding score of zero (urea < 6.5 mmol/L [18.3 g/dL], hemoglobin > 13 g/dL in men or >12 g/dL in women, systolic blood pressure ≥ 110 mm Hg, pulse < 100/minute, and no melena, syncope, heart failure, or liver disease) can identify patients whose upper GI hemorrhage can be treated on an outpatient basis.

Pre-endoscopic proton pump inhibitor therapy has not been shown to alter clinical outcomes, but it may downstage the severity of the lesion and decrease the need for endoscopic intervention. Therefore, in patients with suspected ulcer bleeding, intravenous proton pump inhibitors (e.g., pantoprazole, 80 mg bolus, followed by 8 mg/hour for 72 hours) may be considered while waiting for the endoscopy, but this therapy is no substitute for endoscopy and should not delay it.∎

TREATMENT ®x

Resuscitation efforts should be initiated simultaneously with the initial assessment. Large-bore (14- or 16-gauge) intravenous catheters are recommended for essentially all patients so that normal saline can be infused as fast as necessary to maintain hemodynamic stability (Chapter 106). Blood products should be considered as needed to keep the hemoglobin above 8 g/dL, the platelet count above 50,000/mm^3, and the INR below 2. Endotracheal intubation should be considered in patients with active hematemesis or with altered mental status to prevent aspiration, which can cause considerable morbidity and mortality.

The goal of endoscopic therapy is to stop acute bleeding and reduce the risk of recurrent bleeding. Most endoscopic therapies were designed for peptic ulcer hemorrhage, but they can be used for other causes of nonvariceal upper GI bleeding, in which underlying arteries are the source of bleeding. Available treatments include injection (epinephrine or sclerosant), thermal coagulation (with multipolar, bipolar, or heater probe), and mechanical compression (hemostatic clips). Epinephrine injection therapy is effective, safe, and inexpensive, but it should be combined with either thermal coagulation or hemoclips to achieve hemostasis in more than 95% of patients with active bleeding and to reduce the risk of rebleeding. Endoscopic therapy is reserved for lesions that have high-risk stigmata for rebleeding (e.g., active arterial bleeding, nonbleeding visible vessel, or adherent clot) or moderate-risk stigmata, such as oozing blood without associated clot or a nonbleeding visible vessel; it is not warranted for low-risk stigmata (clean-based ulcer or flat pigmented spot), which have the lowest risk of rebleeding (Fig. 137-3). Repeat or "second-look" endoscopy, usually about 24 hours after the initial endoscopy, may occasionally be useful to confirm adequate hemostasis in high-risk patients but is not generally recommended. Some causes of upper GI bleeding, such as gastric or duodenal erosions and neoplasms, generally are not amenable to endoscopic treatment and require appropriate medical or surgical therapy, or both.

TABLE 137-1 CAUSES OF SEVERE UPPER GASTROINTESTINAL BLEEDING IN A LARGE SERIES

DIAGNOSIS	%
Gastric or duodenal ulcer	38
Gastric or esophageal varices	16
Erosive esophagitis	13
No UGI cause found*	8
UGI tumor	7
UGI angioma[†]	6
Mallory-Weiss tear	4
Gastric or duodenal erosions	4
Dieulafoy's lesion	2
Other[‡]	2

*No cause found in esophagus, stomach, or duodenum, but 25% of these patients (2% of all patients) had mouth, nose, or pharyngeal bleeding sites.
[†]Upper gastrointestinal (UGI) angiomas include single or multiple angiectasias, watermelon stomach, or Osler-Weber-Rendu telangiectasia.
[‡]Other lesions were surgical anastomoses, Cameron ulcers, aortoenteric fistulas, and hemobilia.

TABLE 137-2 ENDOSCOPIC STIGMATA OF RECENT ULCER HEMORRHAGE AND THEIR ASSOCIATED FREQUENCIES, RISKS OF REBLEEDING, AND REDUCTION IN BLEEDING RISKS AFTER SUCCESSFUL ENDOSCOPIC HEMOSTASIS

ENDOSCOPIC APPEARANCE	FREQUENCY (%)	RISK OF REBLEEDING (%)	REBLEEDING RISK AFTER ENDOSCOPIC HEMOSTASIS (%)*
Active arterial bleeding	12	80-90	15-30
Nonbleeding visible vessel	22	40-50	15-30
Adherent clot	10	30-35	0-5
Oozing without other stigmata	14	10-20	0-5
Flat spot	10	5-10	—[†]
Clean ulcer base	32	3	—[†]

*Reduction in the risk of rebleeding is based on the administration of a proton pump inhibitor and successful endoscopic hemostasis.
[†]Endoscopic hemostasis is not recommended for these stigmata.

TABLE 137-3 COMPLETE ROCKALL SCORING SYSTEM FOR UPPER GASTROINTESTINAL BLEEDING

VARIABLE	0 POINTS	1 POINT	2 POINTS	3 POINTS
Age (yr)	<60	60-79	>80	—
Shock				
Pulse rate (beats/min)	<100	>100	—	—
Systolic blood pressure	>100	>100	<100	—
Comorbidity	None	—	Ischemic heart disease, cardiac failure, other major illness	Renal failure, hepatic failure, metastatic cancer
Endoscopic stigmata of recent hemorrhage	No stigmata or dark spot in ulcer base	—	Blood in upper GI tract, adherent clot, visible vessel, active bleeding	—
Diagnosis	Mallory-Weiss tear or no lesion seen	All other diagnoses	Malignant lesions	—

PRE-ENDOSCOPY SCORE	MORTALITY (%)	POSTENDOSCOPY SCORE	REBLEED RATE (%)	MORTALITY (%)
0	0.2	0	4.9	0
1	2.4	1	3.4	0
2	5.6	2	5.3	0.2
3	11	3	11.2	2.9
4	24.6	4	14.1	5.3
5	39.6	5	24.1	10.8
6	48.9	6	32.9	17.3
7	50	7	43.8	27
—	—	8+	41.8	41.1

Rockall TA, Logan RFA, Devlin HB, Northfield TC, for the Steering Committee and Members of the National Audit of Acute Upper Gastrointestinal Haemorrhage. Risk assessment after acute upper gastrointestinal haemorrhage. *Gut.* 1996;38:316-321.

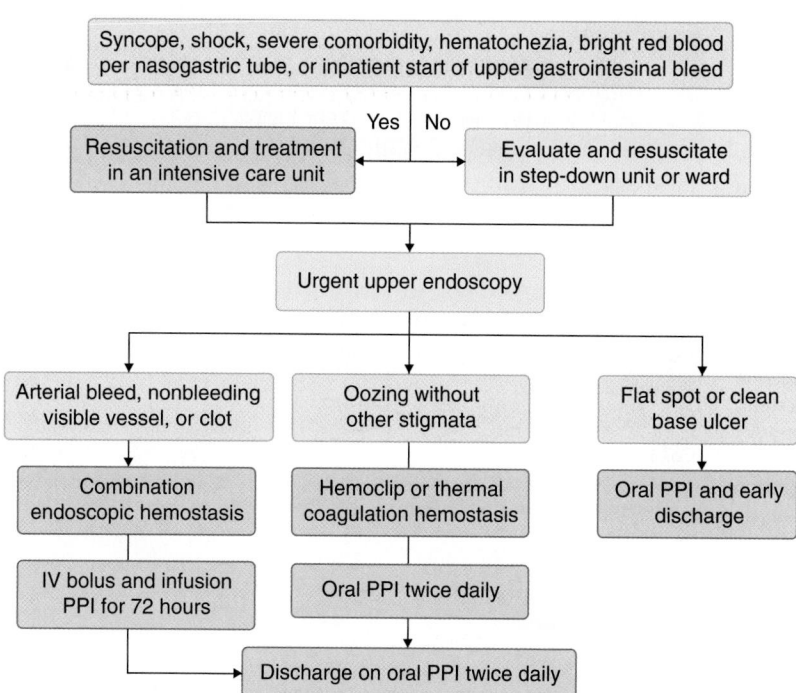

FIGURE 137-3. Management algorithm for nonvariceal upper gastrointestinal hemorrhage. IV = intravenous; PPI = proton pump inhibitor.

Medical Therapy

The most common cause of upper GI bleeding is peptic ulcer disease (Chapter 141), and the most common cause of bleeding peptic ulcers is the use of NSAIDs. Aspirin and other NSAIDs should be discontinued in patients with bleeding peptic ulcers, unless there is a contraindication to doing so (e.g., secondary prophylaxis for stroke). Patients with documented *Helicobacter pylori* infection should be treated with combination antibiotics (see Table 141-4 in Chapter 141) and proton pump inhibitors (see Table 140-1 in Chapter 140). *H. pylori* eradication does not help ulcers heal but reduces the risk of future peptic ulcer disease.

Proton pump inhibitors are the mainstay of medical therapy for hemostasis and healing of peptic lesions. Acid suppression can promote platelet aggregation and clot formation and reduce the risk of rebleeding. High-dose intravenous proton pump inhibitors (e.g., pantoprazole, 80 mg bolus followed by

8 mg/hour for 72 hours) after successful endoscopic hemostasis can reduce rebleeding rates and mortality in patients with high-risk stigmata of recent hemorrhage.[2] Patients with high-risk stigmata should receive proton pump inhibitor infusion for 72 hours before converting to oral proton pump inhibitor therapy. Patients with low-risk or no stigmata can be treated with high-dose oral proton pump inhibitor therapy (see Table 140-1 in Chapter 140) twice daily for 4 to 6 weeks and considered for early discharge. For patients who have upper GI bleeding and who require an NSAID, a proton pump inhibitor combined with a cyclooxygenase-2 inhibitor (e.g., celecoxib; Chapter 36) is preferred to reduce rebleeding. Patients with upper GI bleeding who require secondary cardiovascular prophylaxis should start receiving aspirin plus proton pump inhibitor therapy again as soon as cardiovascular risks outweigh GI risks, usually within 7 days.

Of nonulcer causes of upper GI bleeding, varices (see Fig. 137-1) are the most common cause. Variceal bleeding is treated with a combination of pharmacotherapy (octreotide, somatostatin), endoscopy (band ligation, sclerotherapy), and balloon tamponade (Chapter 156).

A Mallory-Weiss tear (Chapter 140) at the gastroesophageal junction usually stops bleeding spontaneously, but persistent bleeding should be treated similarly to bleeding from peptic ulcers.**3** Bleeding from erosive esophagitis (see Fig. 136-1 in Chapter 136) and gastritis (see Fig. 141-1 in Chapter 141) is generally treated in the same way as ulcer bleeding, although oral liquid sucralfate (1 g twice daily) is another alternative (Chapter 140). Dieulafoy's lesion, which is an aberrant submucosal artery that erodes into the lumen of the stomach, and tumors (Chapter 199) are rare causes of acute upper gastrointestinal bleeding. Vascular lesions commonly present as chronic, low-grade blood loss rather than as acute bleeding. Critically ill patients can bleed from diffuse gastric erosions, which usually do not respond to endoscopy therapy, but may respond to proton pump inhibitors (see Table 140-1 in Chapter 140).

PROGNOSIS

Despite progressive advances in diagnosis, the mortality rate from acute upper intestinal bleeding requiring hospitalization remains about 4% for young patients and has been reported to be as high as 15% for elderly patients.

Lower Gastrointestinal Bleeding

DEFINITION AND EPIDEMIOLOGY

Lower GI hemorrhage generally refers to bleeding from the colon and ano-rectum. Severe lower GI bleeding occurs with an annual incidence of 20 per 100,000 population, a rate that is much less than upper GI bleeding. Patients are usually older and present with painless hematochezia, typically without orthostasis. If orthostasis is present, a brisk upper GI bleed, which occurs in 15 to 20% of patients with severe hematochezia, should be considered. Among colorectal causes of severe lower GI bleeding, diverticulosis is the most common. Other frequent causes include internal hemorrhoids, neoplasms, and ischemic colitis (Table 137-4).

DIAGNOSIS

Patients with hematochezia should have a careful history, physical examination, and laboratory evaluation as for upper GI bleeding. A history of diverticulosis (see Figs. 144-4 and 144-5 in Chapter 144) should raise the suspicion for a diverticular bleed (Chapter 144). Abdominal cramping followed by bloody diarrhea suggests ischemic colitis (see Fig. 145-2 in Chapter 145). A recent polypectomy makes a postpolypectomy bleed more likely.

After medical resuscitation, most patients need endoscopic evaluation. Flexible sigmoidoscopy or anoscopy, or both, may be performed more rapidly than full colonoscopy in patients who are highly likely to be bleeding from the anorectum or distal colon. Colonoscopy allows for the identification of a luminal source of bleeding as well as for hemostasis of amenable lesions, but urgent colonoscopy may be no better than elective colonoscopy for improving outcomes.**4** To cleanse the colon and see the colonic mucosa adequately, a bowel purge with 6 L or more of a polyethylene glycol solution must be administered.

If colonoscopy does not reveal the source of bleeding, an upper GI endoscopic evaluation should be performed. If both are negative, capsule endoscopy (Chapter 136) can be used to look for a small intestinal source, such as angiectasias. Alternatively, if bleeding persists or is too rapid to perform a colonoscopy, a tagged red blood cell nuclear scan or angiography can localize the bleeding. A red blood cell scan is useful only if bleeding is at a rate of at least 0.1 mL/minute, whereas angiography requires an even faster bleeding rate of at least 0.5 mL/minute. Neither red blood cell scan nor angiogram identifies nonbleeding stigmata, and neither usually yields an etiologic diagnosis.

TREATMENT

Medical resuscitation is similar as for upper GI bleeding. Colonoscopic treatment (Fig. 137-4) of focal bleeding sources with stigmata of recent hemorrhage relies on the same methods (epinephrine with either thermocoagulation or hemoclips) as for upper GI bleeding. Colonic angiodysplasias (see Fig. 145-5 in Chapter 145) may be a challenge to diagnose, and some patients who are bleeding from them may have their bleeding mistakenly blamed on diverticula. In addition, coagulation of angiectasias and bleeding biopsy sites is feasible during urgent colonoscopy.

Angiographic embolization or the infusion of vasoconstrictors is about 80% successful for treating rapidly bleeding vessels that are diagnosed at angiography, but with a 10% or so risk of causing local ischemia. Surgical management is rarely required for hemostasis of lower GI bleeding because most bleeding is either self-limited or easily managed with medical or endoscopic therapy. The main indications for surgery are malignant lesions (Chapter 199); diffusely bleeding lesions, such as ischemic colitis (Chapter 145) that fail medical therapy; and recurrent diverticular hemorrhage (Chapter 144). If the bleeding source can be localized preoperatively, a segmental colonic resection rather than a subtotal colectomy can be performed.

TABLE 137-4   MOST COMMON COLONIC SOURCES OF SEVERE HEMATOCHEZIA (486 CASES) (EXPRESSED AS PERCENTAGE OF COLONIC SOURCES)*

Diverticulosis	32%
Internal hemorrhoids	13%
Ischemic colitis	12%
Rectal ulcers	8%
Colonic angiodysplasia, angiectasia, angiomas, or radiation telangiectasias	7%
Ulcerative colitis, Crohn's colitis, other colitis	6%
Postpolypectomy ulcer	5%
Ulcerated polyps	4%
Colorectal cancer	3%

*Less common causes include surgical anastomotic ulcers or sutures, nonsteroidal anti-inflammatory agent colopathy, metastases, portal hypertensive colopathy, lymphoma, and endometriosis.

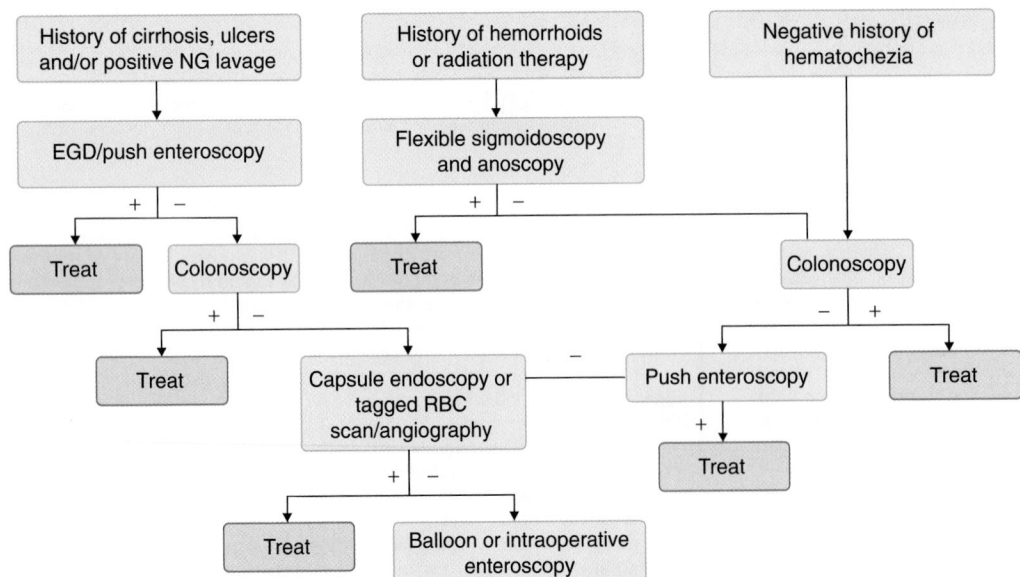

FIGURE 137-4. Management algorithm for severe hematochezia. EGD = esophagogastroduodenoscopy; NG = nasogastric; RBC = red blood cell.

PROGNOSIS

In most patients, the lower GI bleeding stops spontaneously and does not recur. The overall mortality rate from lower GI bleeding is 2 to 4%.

● OBSCURE AND OCCULT GASTROINTESTINAL BLEEDING

DEFINITIONS AND EPIDEMIOLOGY

Obscure GI bleeding is persistent or recurrent bleeding, despite a negative initial GI evaluation, including upper endoscopy, colonoscopy, and radiologic evaluation of the small intestine with a small bowel follow-through. Obscure GI bleeding can be classified as either overt bleeding, with melena, maroon stool, or hematochezia, or occult bleeding, with a positive fecal occult blood test, usually in the setting of iron deficiency anemia.

In most large series of hospitalized patients, 5% of overt GI bleeding cases are considered to be obscure, and 75% of these patients have bleeding from the small intestine that is beyond the reach of an upper endoscope or colonoscope. Angiectasias (see Fig. 136-4 in Chapter 136) are the most common source of small intestinal bleeding, followed by ulcers and tumors (Table 137-5). Other causes of obscure GI bleeding include lesions that are within reach of standard endoscopes but that were not recognized as the bleeding site (e.g., a large hiatal hernia with lesions known as Cameron's ulcers on endoscopy, or internal hemorrhoids on colonoscopy) and intermittently bleeding lesions such as a Dieulafoy's lesion (Fig. 137-5), which is an aberrant submucosal vessel without an ulcer.

Iron deficiency (Chapter 162), which has a prevalence of 2 to 5% among adult men and postmenopausal women, can result from overt or occult blood loss (e.g., GI tract lesions, menorrhagia), iron malabsorption (celiac disease, atrophic gastritis), and chronic red blood cell destruction (hemolysis). It should be suspected in patients with low mean corpuscular volume, low ferritin level, or low transferrin saturation.

DIAGNOSIS

The approaches to overt and occult obscure GI bleeding are similar (Fig. 137-6). In cases with recurrent overt bleeding, upper endoscopy and colonoscopy should be repeated, with the type of bleeding dictating which endoscopic procedure to do first; about 30% of cases will be diagnosed by these repeat tests. Colonoscopy with anoscopy should be done first in patients with hematochezia. If there is melena, a push enteroscopy—a long upper-type endoscope that can be passed well beyond the duodenum and into the jejunum—should be

FIGURE 137-5. Dieulafoy's lesion.

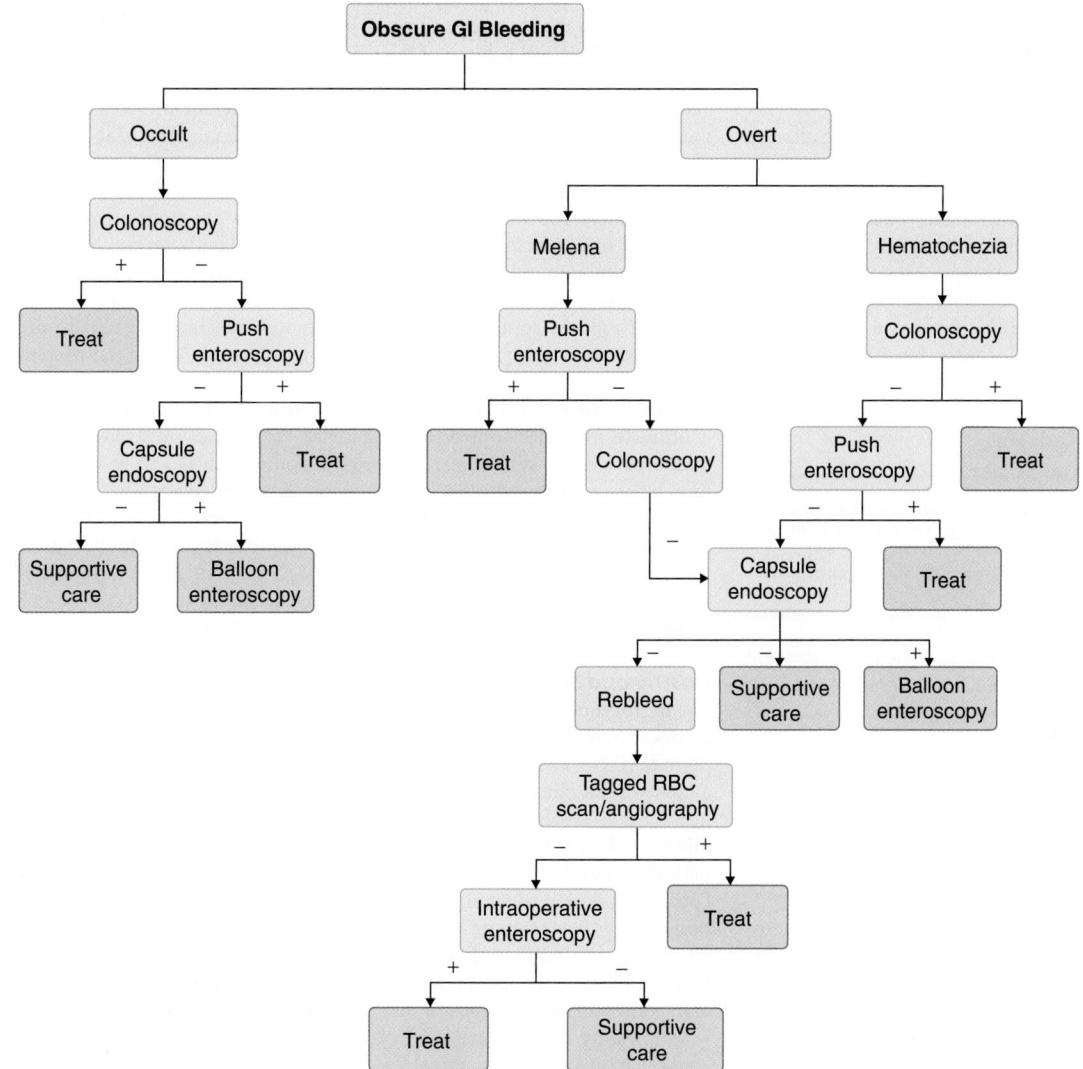

FIGURE 137-6. Management algorithm for obscure gastrointestinal bleeding. GI = gastrointestinal; RBC = red blood cell.

TABLE 137-5	SMALL INTESTINAL LESIONS FOUND DURING DOUBLE-BALLOON ENTEROSCOPY FOR OBSCURE GASTROINTESTINAL BLEEDING IN 488 PATIENTS
LESION	**FREQUENCY (RANGE)**
None	40% (0-57)
Angiectasias	31% (6-55)
Ulcerations	13% (2-35)
Malignancy	8% (3-26)
Other	6% (2-22)

Rajir GS, Gerson L, Das A, Lewis B. American Gastroenterological Association (AGA) Institute technical review on obscure gastrointestinal bleeding. *Gastroenterology.* 2007;133:1697-1717.

performed. If the first procedure is unremarkable, evaluation should be undertaken from the opposite end. If the second test is negative, capsule endoscopy should be performed. If bleeding from the small intestine is observed on capsule endoscopy, further attempts to diagnose and treat the bleeding should be performed with either balloon enteroscopy, which uses a balloon overtube to slide much farther into the small intestine, or intraoperative enteroscopy. All these long enteroscopes facilitate diagnosis and hemostasis. If the capsule endoscopy is negative, a tagged red blood cell scan or angiography may be used if rebleeding is rapid enough for these tests to be useful.

For occult GI bleeding, colonoscopy should be performed first because fecal occult blood testing was designed to screen for colorectal cancer (Chapter 199). Among patients over age 60 years with positive occult fecal blood tests, about 25 to 35% will have a significant colonic polyp and about 3 to 5% will have a colorectal cancer. Upper endoscopy should follow if the colonoscopy is unremarkable. Afterward, the approach is the same as for overt bleeding; if the capsule endoscopy is negative, however, efforts should be focused toward providing supportive care rather than further invasive evaluation.

Iron Deficiency Anemia

GI evaluation of iron deficiency anemia (Chapter 162) is indicated in all adult men, regardless of age, and all postmenopausal women. Women who have not reached menopause may warrant a GI evaluation after obvious or potential causes of iron deficiency, such as chronic menorrhagia, have been excluded. Colonoscopy should be performed first, followed by upper endoscopy if the colonoscopy was negative. Duodenal biopsies should be taken to look for evidence of celiac disease (Chapter 142). If both endoscopic procedures are unrevealing, capsule endoscopy should be performed. If the capsule study is negative, investigation into non-GI causes for iron deficiency (Chapter 162) may be pursued.

1. Barkun AN, Bardou M, Kuipers EJ, et al. International consensus recommendations on the management of patients with nonvariceal upper gastrointestinal bleeding. *Ann Intern Med.* 2010;152: 101-113.
2. Lau JY, Leung WK, Wu JC, et al. Omeprazole before endoscopy in patients with gastrointestinal bleeding. *N Engl J Med.* 2007;356:1631-1640.
3. Sung JJ, Barkun A, Kuipers EJ, et al. Intravenous esomeprazole for prevention of recurrent peptic ulcer bleeding. *Ann Intern Med.* 2009;150:455-464.
4. Laine L, Shah A. Randomized trial of urgent vs. elective colonoscopy in patients hospitalized with lower GI bleeding. *Am J Gastroenterol.* 2010;105:2636-2641.

SUGGESTED READINGS

Halland M, Young M, Fitzgerald MN, et al. Characteristics and outcomes of upper gastrointestinal hemorrhage in a tertiary referral hospital. *Dig Dis Sci.* 2010;55:3430-3435. *The most common nonvariceal causes were ulcers (33%), Mallory-Weiss tear (11%), esophagitis (8%), and malignancy (4%); mortality rate was 4%.*

Kohn A, Ancona C, Belleudi V, et al. The impact of endoscopy and specialist care on 30-day mortality among patients with acute non-variceal upper gastrointestinal hemorrhage: an Italian population-based study. *Dig Liver Dis.* 2010;42:629-634. *Data supporting the benefit of early endoscopy and specialty care.*

Lanas A, Garcia-Rodriguez LA, Polo-Tomás M, et al. The changing face of hospitalisation due to gastrointestinal bleeding and perforation. *Aliment Pharmacol Ther.* 2011;33:585-591. *Hospitalizations due to peptic ulcer bleeding and perforation have decreased significantly, whereas colonic diverticular and angiodysplasia bleeding have increased.*

Riccioni ME, Urgesi R, Spada C, et al. Unexplained iron deficiency anaemia: is it worthwhile to perform capsule endoscopy? *Dig Liv Dis.* 2010;42:560-566. *Lesions were found in about two thirds of patients after negative upper and lower endoscopies.*

138
DISORDERS OF GASTROINTESTINAL MOTILITY

MICHAEL CAMILLERI

DEFINITION

Motility disorders result from impaired control of the neuromuscular apparatus of the gastrointestinal tract. Associated symptoms include recurrent or chronic nausea, vomiting, bloating, abdominal discomfort, and constipation or diarrhea in the absence of intestinal obstruction.

PATHOBIOLOGY
Normal Physiology
Neuroenteric Control

Motor function of the gastrointestinal tract depends on the contraction of smooth muscle cells and their integration and modulation by enteric and extrinsic nerves and by the interstitial cells of Cajal. Extrinsic neural control of gastrointestinal motor function consists of the cranial and sacral parasympathetic outflow (excitatory to nonsphincteric muscle) and the thoracolumbar sympathetic supply (excitatory to sphincters, inhibitory to nonsphincteric muscle). The cranial outflow is predominantly through the vagus nerve, which innervates the gastrointestinal tract from the stomach to the right colon. Parasympathetic innervation of the colon is provided by the vagal fibers coursing along the ileocolonic branches of the superior mesenteric artery and the S2 to S4 parasympathetic supply to the distal colon. Sympathetic fibers to the stomach and small bowel arise from T5 to T10 levels of the intermediolateral column of the spinal cord. Sympathetic innervation of the colon arises from T11 to L3 levels of the spinal cord. The prevertebral ganglia play an important role in the integration of afferent impulses between the gut and the central nervous system and in the reflex control of abdominal viscera.

The enteric nervous system is an independent nervous system comprising approximately 100 million neurons organized into ganglionated plexuses. The larger myenteric or Auerbach's plexus is situated between the longitudinal and circular muscle layers of the muscularis externa; this plexus contains neurons responsible for gastrointestinal motility. The submucosal or Meissner's plexus controls absorption, secretion, and mucosal blood flow. The enteric nervous system also plays an important role in visceral afferent function.

The interstitial cells of Cajal are spontaneously active pacemaker cells that coordinate muscular contraction and sense distortion. They form a nonneural pacemaker system at the interface of the circular and longitudinal muscle layers of the intestine and function as intermediaries between the neurogenic enteric nervous system and the myogenic control system, which regulates the electrical activity generated by gastrointestinal smooth muscle cells. Electrical control activity spreads through the contiguous segments of the gut through neurochemical activation by excitatory (e.g., acetylcholine, substance P) and inhibitory (e.g., nitric oxide, somatostatin) transmitters.

Gastric and Small Bowel Motility

The motor functions of the stomach and small intestine are characterized by distinct manometric patterns of activity in the fasting and postprandial periods (Fig. 138-1). The fasting or interdigestive period is characterized by a cyclic motor phenomenon, the interdigestive migrating motor complex. In healthy individuals, one cycle of this complex is completed every 60 to 90 minutes. The complex has three phases: a period of quiescence (phase I), a period of intermittent pressure activity (phase II), and an activity front (phase III) during which the stomach and small intestine contract at highest frequencies (3 per minute in the stomach, 12 per minute in the duodenum, 8 per minute in the ileum). Another characteristic motor pattern in the distal small intestine is the giant migrating complex, or power contraction, which empties residue from the ileum into the colon in bolus transfers.

With eating, the proximal stomach accommodates food by a vagally mediated reduction in its tone, thereby facilitating the ingestion of food without

FIGURE 138-1. Fasting and postprandial gastroduodenal manometric recordings in a healthy volunteer. A 535-kcal meal is ingested during the study. Note the cyclic interdigestive migrating motor complex (**A**) and the sustained, high-amplitude but irregular pressure activity after a meal (**B**). (From Coulie B, Camilleri M. Intestinal pseudo-obstruction. *Annu Rev Med.* 1999;50:37-55.)

an increase in pressure. Liquids empty from the stomach in an exponential manner. The half-emptying time for non-nutrient liquids in healthy individuals is usually less than 20 minutes. Solids are retained selectively in the stomach, where they undergo acid and peptic digestion as well as "churning" or trituration by high liquid shearing forces in the antrum. Digestible food particles are emptied after their size is reduced by trituration to less than 2 mm. Gastric emptying of solids is characterized by an initial lag period followed by a linear postlag emptying phase. Secretion of hormones that mediate the motor and digestive process (e.g., gastrin for acid secretion; cholecystokinin for gallbladder contraction and bile and pancreatic secretion; and insulin, glucagon, and incretins such as glucagon-like peptide [GLP] 1 for glucose regulation) is integrated with the arrival of food or chyme at different levels of the gut to ensure optimal digestion.

The small intestine transports solids and liquids at approximately the same rate. As a result of the lag phase for the transport of solids from the stomach, liquids typically arrive in the colon before solids. Chyme moves from ileum to colon intermittently in boluses.

In the postprandial period, the interdigestive migrating motor complex is replaced by an irregular pattern of variable amplitude and frequency. This pattern, which enables mixing, digestion, and absorption, is observed in the gastrointestinal regions in contact with food. The maximum frequency of contractions is lower than during phase III of the interdigestive motor complex, and the duration of this postprandial contractile activity is proportional to the number of calories consumed (about 1 hour for each 200 kcal ingested). Segments of the small intestine that are not in contact with food continue with interdigestive motor patterns.

Vomiting is characterized by a stereotypic sequence of motor events, including contractions of the stomach, abdominal muscles, and diaphragm. This sequence is followed immediately in the proximal small bowel by a propagated, rhythmic contractile response similar to the migrating motor complex.

Colonic Motility

The normal colon displays short-duration (phasic) contractions and a background contractility or tone. Nonpropagated phasic contractions have a role in segmenting the colon into haustra, which compartmentalize the colon and facilitate mixing, retention of residue, and formation of solid stool. High-amplitude propagated contractions, which are characterized by an amplitude greater than 75 mm Hg, propagation over a distance of at least 15 cm, and a propagation velocity of 0.15 to 2.2 cm/second contribute to the mass movements in the colon. In health, these contractions occur on average five or six times per day, most often postprandially and between 6 AM and 2 PM.

Colonic transit is a discontinuous process, slow most of the time and rapid at other times. Residue may be retained for prolonged periods in the right colon, and a mass movement may deliver the contents to the sigmoid colon in seconds. Movement of colonic content is stimulated by feeding (gastrocolonic response). In health, the average mouth-to-cecum transit time is about 6 hours, and transit times through the right colon, left colon, and sigmoid colon are about 12 hours each. As dietary fiber is increased, mean colonic transit time decreases, stool frequency increases, and stool consistency

becomes softer. Decreased caloric intake slows colonic transit, whereas a meal (typically >500 kcal) stimulates colonic motor function and propulsion of colonic content. Outlet obstruction in patients with pelvic floor dysfunction or voluntary suppression of defecation often is associated with slow colonic transit and decreased motor response to feeding.

Fluid reabsorption influences gastrointestinal transit. Approximately 9 L of fluid enters the gut from oral intake and endogenous secretions. The small intestine delivers about 1.5 L of fluid to the colon, where most is reabsorbed, leaving a maximum of 200 mL of water excreted in normal stool. Up to 3 L of fluid can be reabsorbed by the colon in a 24-hour period, unless the rate of ileocolonic flow or colonic motility overwhelms the colon's capacity or reabsorptive ability.

Defecation and Continence

Normal defecation requires a series of coordinated actions of the colon, rectum, pelvic floor, and anal sphincter muscles (Fig. 138-2). Filling of the rectum by a volume of 10 mL may be sensed, although the rectum can accommodate 300 mL before a sense of fullness and urge to defecate develop. Distention of the rectum results in the relaxation of the internal anal sphincter (rectoanal inhibitory reflex) and simultaneous contraction of the external anal sphincter to maintain continence. The anal transition zone can sense the difference between solid or liquid stool and gas.

⬤ DISEASES OF SLOW TRANSIT THROUGH THE STOMACH AND SMALL BOWEL

PATHOBIOLOGY

Gastrointestinal motility disturbances (Table 138-1) result from disorders of the extrinsic nervous system, enteric nervous system, interstitial cells of Cajal (or intestinal pacemakers), or smooth muscle. Neuropathic patterns are characterized by normal amplitude but incoordinated contractions, whereas myopathies are characterized by low-amplitude contractions (average of less than 40 mm Hg in the antrum and less than 10 mm Hg in the small bowel). Combined disorders occur in systemic sclerosis (Chapter 275), amyloidosis (Chapter 194), and mitochondrial cytopathy (Chapter 429), which initially can manifest with neuropathic patterns and later display myopathic characteristics with disease progression.

Genetic defects that result in congenital dysmotilities include abnormalities of *RET*, the gene that encodes the tyrosine kinase receptor, and abnormalities in the endothelin B system. Neural crest cells migrate from the vagal and sacral crest to the developing gut and, over time, colonize the entire alimentary canal and its appendages. Endothelin B serves to retard maturation of migrating neural crest cells, thus facilitating colonization of the entire gut with nerve cells. Other abnormalities resulting in congenital dysmotility involve other transcription factors, such as Sox10, which enhances maturation of neural precursors, and *KIT,* a marker for the interstitial cells of Cajal. Defects of *RET*, endothelin B, and Sox10 are associated with the phenotypic picture recognized as Hirschsprung's disease, whereas *KIT* defects have been associated with idiopathic hypertrophic pyloric stenosis and congenital megacolon.

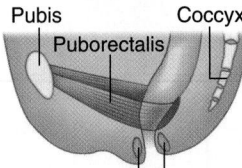

Resting

Pubis   Coccyx

Puborectalis

External anal
sphincter

Straining

Pubis   Coccyx

Puborectalis

External anal
sphincter

Continence requires:
Contraction of puborectalis
Maintenance of anorectal angle
Normal rectal sensation
Contraction of sphincter

Defecation requires:
Relaxation of puborectalis
Straightening of anorectal angle
Relaxation of sphincter

A   B

FIGURE 138-2. Pelvic floor and anorectal functions during continence and defecation. Sagittal view through the pelvis in the resting (**A**) and straining (**B**) postures. Coordinated functions of pelvic floor (puborectalis) and anal sphincter are essential for continence and defecation.

TABLE 138-1   CLASSIFICATION OF GASTROPARESIS AND PSEUDO-OBSTRUCTION

TYPE	NEUROPATHIC	MYOPATHIC
Infiltrative	Progressive systemic sclerosis Amyloidosis	Progressive systemic sclerosis Amyloidosis Systemic lupus erythematosus Ehlers-Danlos syndrome Dermatomyositis
Familial	Familial visceral neuropathies	Familial visceral myopathies Metabolic myopathies
Idiopathic	Sporadic hollow visceral myopathy	Idiopathic intestinal pseudo-obstruction
Neurologic	Porphyria Heavy metal poisoning Brain stem tumor Parkinson's disease Multiple sclerosis Spinal cord transection	Myotonia Other dystrophies
Infectious	Chagas' disease Cytomegalovirus Norwalk virus Epstein-Barr virus	
Drug induced	Tricyclic antidepressants Narcotic agents Anticholinergic agents Antihypertensives Dopaminergic agents Vincristine Laxatives	
Paraneoplastic	Small cell lung cancer Carcinoid syndrome	
Postsurgical	Postvagotomy with or without pyloroplasty or gastric resection	
Endocrine	Diabetes mellitus Hypothyroidism or hyperthyroidism Hypoparathyroidism	

Extrinsic Neuropathic Disorders

Extrinsic neuropathic processes include vagotomy, trauma, Parkinson's disease (Chapter 416), diabetes (Chapter 236), amyloidosis (Chapter 194), and a paraneoplastic syndrome usually associated with small cell carcinoma of the lung (Chapter 197). Another common "neuropathic" problem in clinical practice results from the effect of medications, such as α_2-adrenergic agonists, GLP-1 analogues, opiates, and anticholinergics, on neural control.

Damage to the autonomic nerves by trauma, infection, neuropathy, and neurodegeneration may lead to motor, secretory, and sensory disturbances,

most frequently resulting in constipation. Patients with spinal cord injury (Chapter 406) above the level of the sacral segments have delayed proximal and distal colonic transit attributable to parasympathetic denervation. In these patients, fasting colonic motility and tone are normal, but the response to feeding generally is reduced or absent. Spinal cord lesions involving the sacral segments and damage to the efferent nerves from these segments disrupt the neural integration of rectosigmoid expulsion and anal sphincter control. In patients with these injuries, there is loss of contractile activity in the left colon and decreased rectal tone and sensitivity, which may lead to dilation and fecal impaction. Parkinson's disease (Chapter 416) and multiple sclerosis (Chapter 419) frequently are associated with constipation.

Enteric and Intrinsic Neuropathic Disorders

Disorders of the enteric nervous system are usually the result of a degenerative, immune, or inflammatory process. Virus-induced gastroparesis (e.g., rotavirus, Norwalk virus [Chapter 388], cytomegalovirus [Chapter 384], or Epstein-Barr virus [Chapter 385]) is associated with infiltration of the myenteric plexus with inflammatory cells. In idiopathic chronic intestinal pseudo-obstruction, in which there is no disturbance of the extrinsic neural control, degeneration of the interstitial cells of Cajal, inflammation, or herpesvirus infection may contribute.

Smooth Muscle Disorders

Disturbances of smooth muscle may result in significant disorders of gastric emptying and of transit through the small bowel and colon. These disturbances include, in descending order of prevalence, systemic sclerosis (Chapter 275), amyloidosis (Chapter 194), dermatomyositis (Chapter 277), myotonic dystrophy (Chapter 429), and metabolic muscle disorders (Chapter 429). Motility disturbances may be the result of metabolic disorders, such as hypothyroidism (Chapter 233) and hyperparathyroidism (Chapter 233), but these patients more commonly present with constipation. Scleroderma may result in focal or general dilation, wide-mouthed diverticula in the small bowel and colon, and delayed transit. The amplitude of contractions is reduced, and bacterial overgrowth may result in steatorrhea or pneumatosis intestinalis. Mitochondrial neurogastrointestinal encephalomyopathy, or familial visceral myopathy type II, is an autosomal recessive condition that may present with hepatic failure in neonates, seizures or diarrhea in infants, and hepatic failure or chronic intestinal pseudo-obstruction in adults.

Gastroparesis and Pseudo-obstruction

CLINICAL MANIFESTATIONS

The clinical features of gastroparesis and chronic intestinal pseudo-obstruction are similar and include nausea, vomiting, early satiety, abdominal discomfort, distention, bloating, and anorexia. In severe cases, there may be considerable dilation, as well as weight loss, with depletion of mineral and vitamin stores. Diarrhea and constipation indicate that the motility disorder extends beyond the stomach. Vomiting may be complicated by aspiration pneumonia or Mallory-Weiss esophageal tears, and patients with a generalized motility disorder may have abnormal swallowing or delayed colonic transit.

A careful family and medication history is essential. Review of systems may reveal an underlying collagen vascular disease (e.g., scleroderma) or disturbances of extrinsic autonomic neural control, including orthostatic dizziness, difficulties with erection or ejaculation, recurrent urinary tract infections, dry mouth, dry eyes, dry vagina, difficulties with visual accommodation in bright lights, and absence of sweating.

On physical examination, a succussion splash indicates stasis, typically in the stomach. The hands and mouth may reveal signs of Raynaud's phenomenon (Chapter 275) or scleroderma. Testing of pupillary responses (to light and accommodation), external ocular movements, blood pressure in the lying and standing positions, and general features of a peripheral neuropathy can identify patients with an associated neurologic disturbance (e.g., diabetic neuropathy) or with the oculogastrointestinal dystrophy that typically is found with mitochondrial cytopathies (see under Smooth Muscle Disorders).

The differential diagnosis includes mechanical obstruction, functional gastrointestinal disorders, anorexia nervosa, and the rumination syndrome. The rumination syndrome is a relatively common, underdiagnosed condition that presents with early (0 to 30 minutes) postprandial, effortless regurgitation of undigested food after virtually every meal.

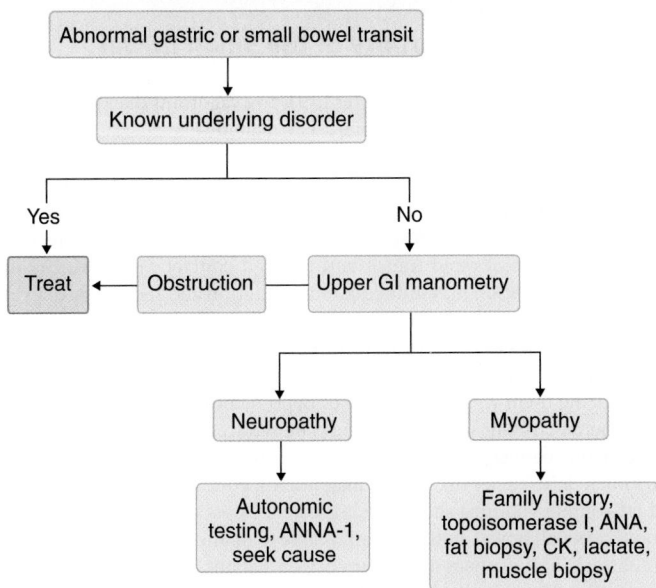

FIGURE 138-3. **Flow diagram outlines steps in diagnosis of idiopathic gastroparesis and intestinal pseudo-obstruction.** ANA = antinuclear antibody; ANNA-1 = type 1 antineuronal nuclear antibody; CK = creatine kinase; GI = gastrointestinal.

FIGURE 138-4. Micrographs showing both types of T lymphocytes, CD4 (**A**) and CD8 (**B**), detectable within the myenteric plexus of the small intestine (proximal ileum) of a 20-year-old man with chronic intestinal pseudo-obstruction. Note the intense CD4 and CD8 immunoreactivities that represent the predominant component of the immune infiltrate observed in cases of lymphocytic ganglionitis. Alkaline phosphatase anti-alkaline phosphatase immunohistochemical technique (×120) in **A** and **B**. (From De Giorgio R, Camilleri M. Human enteric neuropathies: morphology and molecular pathology. *Neurogastroenterol Motil.* 2004;16:515-531.)

DIAGNOSIS

A motility disorder of the stomach or small bowel should be suspected whenever large volumes are aspirated from the stomach, particularly after an overnight fast, or when undigested solid food or large volumes of liquids are observed during esophagogastroduodenoscopy. The clinician should assess the acuity of the symptoms and the patient's state of hydration and nutrition. The goals of the evaluation are to determine what regions of the digestive tract are malfunctioning and whether the symptoms are due to a neuropathy or a myopathy (Fig. 138-3). Key steps include the following:

1. *Suspect and exclude mechanical obstruction.* In symptomatic patients with pseudo-obstruction, plain radiographs of the abdomen typically show dilated loops of small bowel with associated air-fluid levels. Mechanical obstruction should be excluded by upper gastrointestinal endoscopy and small bowel imaging studies, including a small bowel follow-through or computed tomographic enterography. Barium studies may suggest the presence of a motor disorder, particularly if there is gross dilation, dilution of barium, or retained solid food within the stomach. These studies rarely identify the cause, however, except for systemic sclerosis or mitochondrial cytopathy, which are characterized by megaduodenum, multiple small bowel diverticula, and pneumatosis intestinalis.

2. *Assess gastric and small bowel motility.* After mechanical obstruction and alternative diagnoses such as Crohn's disease (Chapter 143) have been excluded, a transit profile of the stomach or small bowel should be performed. In a gastric emptying study, ingestion of a radiolabeled meal is followed by scanning at 0, 1, 2, 3, 4, and 6 hours. If the cause of the motility disturbance is obvious, such as gastroparesis in a patient with long-standing diabetes mellitus, it is usually unnecessary to pursue further diagnostic testing. If the cause is unclear, gastroduodenal manometry by use of a multilumen tube with sensors in the distal stomach and proximal small intestine can differentiate a neuropathic process (normal-amplitude contractions but abnormal patterns of contractility) from a myopathic process (low-amplitude contractions in the affected segments).

3. *Identify the pathogenesis* (see Table 138-1). In patients with neuropathic causes of uncertain origin, tests should assess autonomic dysfunction (Chapter 427), measure type 1 antineuronal nuclear autoantibodies and other autoantibodies associated with paraneoplastic syndromes, and consider the possibility of a brain stem lesion. In patients with a myopathic disorder of unclear cause, the evaluation should consider amyloidosis (immunoglobulin electrophoresis, fat aspirate, or rectal biopsy; Chapter 194), systemic sclerosis (topoisomerase I; Chapter 275), and thyroid disease (Chapter 233). In appropriate settings, porphyria (Chapter 217) and Chagas' disease (Chapter 355) may need to be excluded. In refractory cases, referral to a specialized center may result in genetic testing or full-thickness biopsy of the small intestine (Fig. 138-4) to identify metabolic muscle disorders and mitochondrial cytopathies.

Diabetes mellitus (Chapter 236) is associated with gastroparesis, pylorospasm, intestinal pseudo-obstruction, diarrhea, constipation, and fecal incontinence. All of these manifestations may be caused by autonomic dysfunction, although more recent evidence points to acute changes in glycemia and, more important, to changes in the structure and function of the interstitial cells of Cajal and enteric nervous system. The prevalence of constipation is 22% among diabetic patients with neuropathy but only 9.2% in diabetic patients without neuropathy, a rate that is not significantly different from that of healthy controls.

4. *Identify complications of the motility disorder, including bacterial overgrowth, dehydration, and malnutrition.* In patients presenting with diarrhea, it is important to assess nutritional status and to exclude bacterial overgrowth by culture of small bowel aspirates (Chapter 142). Bacterial overgrowth is relatively uncommon in neuropathic disorders but is found more often in myopathic conditions, such as scleroderma, that are associated more often with dilation or low-amplitude contractions. An empirical trial of antibiotics (see later) often is used instead of formal testing.

TREATMENT Rx

Rehydration, electrolyte repletion, and nutritional supplementation are particularly important during acute exacerbations of gastroparesis and chronic intestinal pseudo-obstruction. Initial nutritional measures include low-fiber supplements with the addition of iron, folate, calcium, and vitamins D, K, and B_{12} at the usually recommended daily levels. In patients with more severe symptoms, enteral or parenteral supplementation may be required. If it is anticipated that enteral supplementation may be needed for more than 3 months, a jejunostomy tube is recommended. Gastrostomy tubes should be avoided in patients with gastroparesis except for venting purposes. The rumination syndrome is treated using behavioral approaches such as diaphragmatic breathing in the early postprandial period.

Medical Therapy

Medications increasingly are being used to treat neuromuscular motility disorders, but there is little evidence of effectiveness in myopathic disturbances except for the rare case of dystrophia myotonica affecting the stomach and for small bowel systemic sclerosis. Small randomized trials demonstrate symptomatic benefit of metoclopramide and domperidone over placebo. Metoclopramide is a dopamine antagonist with prokinetic and antiemetic properties. Antiemetic effects are due in part to its anti-5-hydroxytryptamine type 3 (HT_3) antagonist actions. Long-term use of metoclopramide is limited by the side effects of tremor and parkinsonian-like symptoms. It is available in tablet or elixir form or as a parenteral preparation and, typically, is taken orally 30 minutes before meals and at bedtime. Usual doses are 5 to 10 mg four times daily, but patients may experience side effects (changes in affect, anxiety) at relatively low doses (even 30 to 40 mg/day). The U.S. Food and Drug Administration (FDA) recommends its use only in patients who do not respond to other treatments and for periods of less than 3 months.

Domperidone (10-20 mg, three times per day before meals) is another dopamine antagonist that is approved in some countries but not in the United States, where it is available through an application to the FDA and local Institutional Review Board. Its efficacy appears similar to metoclopramide, with a lower incidence of somnolence and much lower incidence of involuntary movements.

Erythromycin, a macrolide antibiotic that stimulates motilin receptors at higher doses (250 to 500 mg) and cholinergic mechanisms at lower doses (40 to 80 mg), results in the dumping of solids from the stomach. It accelerates gastric emptying in gastroparesis, increases the amplitude of antral contractions, and improves antroduodenal coordination. Erythromycin is most effective when it is used intravenously (3 mg/kg every 8 hours by slow infusion) during acute exacerbations of gastroparesis. For oral erythromycin, tolerance and gastrointestinal side effects often prevent use for longer than 1 month, but sometimes liquid erythromycin can be tolerated at 40 to 80 mg three times daily before meals.

Octreotide (50 μg subcutaneously at bedtime), a cyclized analogue of somatostatin, induces small intestinal activity that mimics phase III of the interdigestive migrating motor complex. It retards gastric emptying, decreases postprandial gastric motility, and inhibits small bowel transit. Octreotide appears to be useful in the treatment of dumping syndromes associated with accelerated transit. Octreotide may be used at night to induce migrating motor complex activity and to avoid bacterial overgrowth. If it is required during the daytime, octreotide often is combined with oral prokinetic to "normalize" the gastric emptying rate.

Antiemetics, including diphenhydramine (25 mg orally up to two times per day for up to 3 months), prochlorperazine (orally or by suppository 25 mg up to two times per day), and metoclopramide (5 to 10 mg orally up to three times per day for up to 3 months), can treat nausea and vomiting in patients with gastroparesis and intestinal pseudo-obstruction. The more expensive serotonin 5-HT$_3$ antagonists (e.g., ondansetron) have not proved to be of greater benefit than these less expensive alternatives in these patients.

Antibiotic therapy is indicated in patients with documented, symptomatic bacterial overgrowth. Although formal clinical trials have not been conducted, it is common practice to use different antibiotics for 7 to 10 days each month, in an attempt to avoid bacterial resistance. Common antibiotics include doxycycline, 100 mg twice daily; metronidazole, 500 mg three times daily; ciprofloxacin, 500 mg twice daily; double-strength trimethoprim-sulfamethoxazole, two tablets twice daily; or rifaximin, 275 mg twice daily. Use of antibiotics in patients with diarrhea and fat malabsorption secondary to bacterial overgrowth results in significant symptomatic relief.

Surgical Therapy

Surgical decompression is rarely necessary in patients with chronic pseudo-obstruction. Venting enterostomy (jejunostomy) is effective, however, in relieving abdominal distention and bloating and in reducing the frequency with which nasogastric intubations and hospitalizations are required for acute exacerbations relative to the period before vent placement. Access to the small intestine by enterostomy also provides nutrients and should be considered in patients with intermittent symptoms. Surgical treatment should be considered whenever the motility disorder is localized to a resectable portion of the gut: completion gastrectomy for patients with post–gastric surgical stasis syndrome, and colectomy with ileorectostomy for intractable constipation associated with chronic colonic pseudo-obstruction.

Gastric electrical stimulation, an approved treatment for humanitarian use, may improve gastric emptying and symptoms in patients with severe gastroparesis, but data on efficacy are inconclusive. Small bowel transplantation currently is limited to patients with intestinal failure who have reversible liver disease induced by total parenteral nutrition or who have life-threatening or recurrent catheter-related sepsis. Isolated transplantation of the small intestine is associated with higher graft and patient survival and fewer complications related to rejection and infection.

● DISEASES OF RAPID TRANSIT THROUGH STOMACH AND SMALL BOWEL
Dumping Syndrome and Accelerated Gastric Emptying

Dumping syndrome and accelerated gastric emptying typically follow truncal vagotomy and gastric drainage procedures (Chapter 141) or fundoplication for gastric esophageal reflux disease (Chapter 140). With the widespread use of highly selective vagotomy and the advent of effective antacid secretory therapy, these problems are becoming rare. A high calorie (usually carbohydrate) content of the liquid phase of the meal evokes a rapid insulin response with secondary hypoglycemia. These patients also may have impaired antral contractility and gastric stasis of solids, which paradoxically may result in a clinical picture of gastroparesis (for solids) and dumping (for liquids).

The management of dumping syndrome and accelerated gastric emptying emphasizes dietary maneuvers, such as avoidance of high-nutrient liquid drinks and possibly addition of guar gum or pectin to retard gastric emptying of liquids. Rarely, pharmacologic treatment with octreotide, 25 to 100 μg subcutaneously before meals, is needed to retard intestinal transit and to inhibit the hormonal responses that lead to hypoglycemia.

Rapid Transit Dysmotility of the Small Bowel

Rapid transit of material through the small bowel may occur in the setting of the irritable bowel syndrome (Chapter 139), postvagotomy diarrhea (Chapter 142), short bowel syndrome (Chapter 142), diabetic diarrhea (Chapter 142), and carcinoid diarrhea (Chapter 240). With the exception of irritable bowel syndrome, these conditions may cause severe diarrhea and result in significant losses of fluid and electrolytes. Ileal resection or disease and idiopathic bile acid malabsorption may represent an inability of the distal ileum to reabsorb bile acids because of rapid transit and reduced contact time with the ileal mucosa; this condition may induce colonic secretion and secondary diarrhea. Accelerated transit may be confirmed by scintigraphic studies.

Treatment goals are to restore hydration and nutrition and to slow small bowel transit. Dietary interventions include avoiding hyperosmolar drinks and replacing them with iso-osmolar or hypo-osmolar oral rehydration solutions. The fat content in the diet should be reduced to approximately 50 g/day to avoid delivery of unabsorbed fat to the colon. All electrolyte and nutritional deficiencies of calcium, magnesium, potassium, and water-soluble and fat-soluble vitamins should be corrected. In patients with less than 1 m of residual small bowel, it may be impossible to maintain fluid and electrolyte homeostasis without parenteral support. In patients with a longer residual segment, oral nutrition, pharmacotherapy, and supplements are almost always effective.

The opioid agent loperamide (4 mg 30 minutes before meals and at bedtime for a total dose of 16 mg/day) suppresses the motor response to feeding and improves symptoms but may be ineffective or cause side effects (e.g., hypotension). Bile acid binding (e.g., with cholestyramine (4 g three times daily) or colesevelam (1.875 g twice daily) is indicated for patients with suspected or proven bile acid malabsorption. Verapamil (40 mg twice daily) or clonidine (0.1 mg twice daily), or both, may be used in addition to loperamide. Octreotide (50 μg subcutaneously three times daily before meals) may be used in patients for whom the oral agents are ineffective or poorly tolerated. 5-HT$_3$ antagonists (e.g., alosetron, 0.5-1 mg orally up to two times per day) may be efficacious in the treatment of carcinoid diarrhea and diarrhea-predominant irritable bowel syndrome, but it should be reserved for patients with severe, unresponsive diarrhea.

● COLONIC MOTILITY DISORDERS
Constipation

EPIDEMIOLOGY

Constipation is a common clinical problem, reported by about 20% of the population, and 40% of Americans report needing to strain excessively to pass their bowel movements.

PATHOBIOLOGY

In functional constipation, transit is normal, and there is no evacuation disorder. These patients may have pain in association with constipation, and there is overlap with constipation-predominant irritable bowel syndrome (Chapter 139). In patients with acquired slow-transit constipation, unassociated with colonic dilation, the number of interstitial cells of Cajal in the different layers of the colon is reduced compared with controls.

Idiopathic megarectum and megacolon can be either congenital or acquired; an enteric nervous system defect is suspected. In megacolon, the dilated segment shows normal phasic contractility but decreased colonic tone, with smooth muscle hypertrophy and fibrosis of the muscularis mucosa, circular muscle, and longitudinal muscle layers.

Acquired defects in the enteric nervous system may result in constipation in Chagas' disease (Chapter 355), which is caused by infection with *Trypanosoma cruzi* and results in the destruction of myenteric neurons. Acquired aganglionosis also has been reported with circulating antineuronal antibodies, with or without associated neoplasm.

DIAGNOSIS

It is essential to distinguish an evacuation disorder, also called functional outlet obstruction (Table 138-2), from constipation resulting from slow transit or other causes. In one study in a tertiary center, 50% of 70 patients with severe, unresponsive constipation had impaired evacuation, and the remainder had constipation associated with either normal transit (also called functional constipation) or delayed colonic transit (also called slow-transit constipation). Characterization of constipated patients (Fig. 138-5) relies on the measurement of transit with radiopaque markers or scintigraphy.

TABLE 138-2 CLINICAL CLUES SUGGESTIVE OF AN EVACUATION DISORDER

HISTORY

Prolonged straining to expel stool
Taking up unusual postures on the toilet to facilitate stool expulsion
Support of perineum or digitation of rectum or vagina to facilitate rectal emptying
Inability to expel enema fluid
Constipation after subtotal colectomy for constipation

RECTAL EXAMINATION (WITH PATIENT IN LEFT LATERAL POSITION)

Inspection

Anus "pulled" forward during attempts to simulate strain during defecation
Anal verge descends <1 cm or >4 cm during attempts to simulate strain during defecation
Perineum balloons down during straining, and rectal mucosa prolapses through anus

Palpation

High anal sphincter tone at rest precludes easy entry of examining finger (in absence of painful perianal condition, e.g., anal fissure)
  Anal sphincter pressure during voluntary squeeze is minimally higher than tone at rest
  Perineum descends <1 cm or >4 cm during attempts to simulate strain during defecation
  Puborectalis muscle palpable through posterior rectal wall is tender
  Palpable mucosal prolapse during straining
  "Defect" in anterior wall of the rectum, suggestive of rectocele

ANORECTAL MANOMETRY AND BALLOON EXPULSION (WITH PATIENT IN LEFT LATERAL POSITION)

Average anal sphincter resting tone >80 cm H_2O or squeeze pressure >240 cm H_2O
Failure of balloon expulsion despite addition of 200 g weight

TREATMENT Rx

The average daily fiber intake is around 12 g/day. In patients with normal-transit constipation, 12 to 30 g/day is effective in relief of constipation. In patients with slow-transit constipation, drug-induced constipation, or evacuation disorders, however, supplementation of 30 g of fiber per day does not result in any improvement in constipation. A second step is to add an osmotic laxative, such as a magnesium salt or polyethylene glycol solution, to enhance the retention of fluid within the lumen by osmotic forces, to increase the fluidity, and to ease aboral transport of colonic content. Polyethylene glycol solutions (such as GoLYTELY, NuLYTELY, MiraLAX, OCL solution) are used frequently as a first-line therapy.**1** If these measures do not suffice, a prokinetic or stimulant agent, such as bisacodyl (5 to 10 mg every 1 to 2 days) may be added.

Newer medications that accelerate colonic transit include prucalopride (2 mg daily), which is beneficial in chronic constipation,**2** and lubiprostone (24 µg twice daily), a chloride channel activator that induces fluid secretion. Methylnaltrexone (0.15 mg/kg subcutaneously every other day for 2 weeks) is 33% more effective than placebo in patients with opiate-induced constipation as a complication of advanced illness.**3** Linaclotide, a guanylate cyclase-C receptor activator that results in fluid secretion, improves bowel habits, global symptoms, and quality of life in patients with chronic constipation, but it is not currently approved for use in the U.S.**4**

When these approaches do not work, the patient should be reassessed to exclude an evacuation disorder. For evacuation disorders, a biofeedback treatment program with muscle relaxation of the anal sphincters and pelvic floor results in a 70% or greater cure rate for the constipation. The response to this treatment program is influenced by comorbidity, such as the coexistence of eating disorders or a psychological or psychiatric diagnosis.

Surgical Therapy

In patients whose constipation is not associated with an evacuation disorder and does not respond to aggressive medical therapies (including combinations described earlier), subtotal colectomy with ileorectostomy is effective in relieving constipation. Laparoscopic colectomy with ileorectostomy achieves the same success rate with less morbidity compared with open colectomy with ileorectostomy.

Hirschsprung's Disease

DEFINITION

Hirschsprung's disease occurs in 1 in 5000 live births. It is characterized by a localized segment of narrowing of the distal colon as a result of failure of local development of intrinsic nerves in the myenteric plexus.

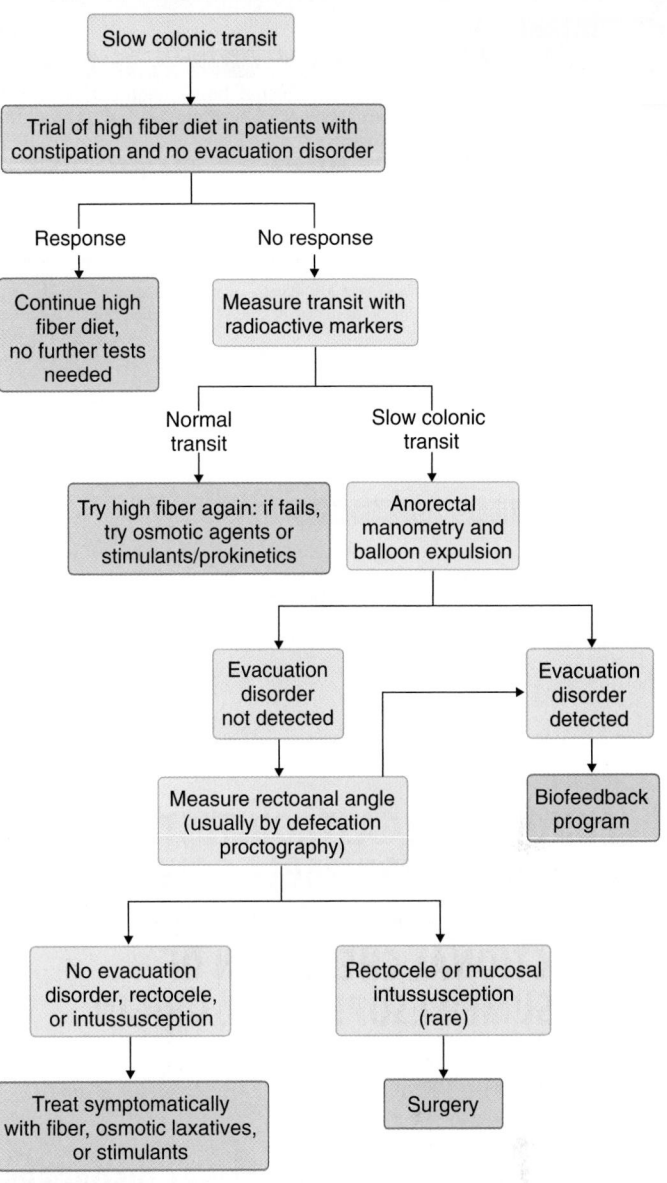

FIGURE 138-5. Flow diagram outlines steps in the management of constipation.

PATHOBIOLOGY

A relative deficiency of *KIT*-positive interstitial cells of Cajal has been reported in Hirschsprung's disease and chronic intestinal pseudo-obstruction. Hirschsprung's disease is well characterized histologically by the absence of ganglion cells in the myenteric and submucosal plexus and the presence of hypertrophied nerve trunks in the space normally occupied by the ganglion cells. The lack of nerve growth factor receptors in the muscle layers of the colon involved with Hirschsprung's disease has been shown. The narrowing and failure of relaxation in the aganglionic segment are thought to be due to the lack of neurons containing nitric oxide synthase.

CLINICAL MANIFESTATIONS

Hirschsprung's disease is usually diagnosed at birth because of failure to pass meconium or the presence of megacolon, although it may be identified in childhood as a result of fecal retention, constipation, or abdominal distention. Onset of symptoms or diagnosis after the age of 10 years is rare.

DIAGNOSIS

Diagnosis is based on the typical focal narrowing of the colon, the absence of the rectoanal inhibitory reflex (relaxation of anal sphincter pressure at rest during distention of a balloon in the rectum depends on natural preservation and maturation of intrinsic nerves in the distal bowel), and a deep rectal biopsy specimen showing absence of submucosal neurons with hypertrophied nerve trunks.

TREATMENT

Treatment involves excision of the affected bowel segment or a pull-through procedure by which normal bowel is anastomosed to the cuff of the rectum, just above the anal sphincters.

1. Dipalma JA, Cleveland MV, McGowan J, et al. A randomized multicenter, placebo-controlled trial of polyethylene glycol laxative for chronic treatment of chronic constipation. *Am J Gastroenterol.* 2007;102:1436-1441.
2. Camilleri M, Kerstens R, Rykx A, et al. A placebo-controlled trial of prucalopride for severe chronic constipation. *N Engl J Med.* 2008;358:2344-2354.
3. Thomas J, Karver S, Cooney GA, et al. Methylnaltrexone for opioid-induced constipation in advanced illness. *N Engl J Med.* 2008;358:2332-2343.
4. Lembo AJ, Kurtz CB, Macdougall JE, et al. Efficacy of linaclotide for patients with chronic constipation. *Gastroenterology.* 2010;138:886-895.

SUGGESTED READINGS

Camilleri M, Bharucha AE, Farrugia G. Epidemiology, mechanisms, and management of diabetic gastroparesis. *Clin Gastroenterol Hepatol.* 2011;9:5-12. *Review.*
Rao SS, Camilleri M, Hasler WL, et al. Evaluation of gastrointestinal transit in clinical practice: position paper of the American and European Neurogastroenterology and Motility Societies. *Neurogastroenterol Motil.* 2011;23:8-23. *Consensus recommendations.*

139

FUNCTIONAL GASTROINTESTINAL DISORDERS: IRRITABLE BOWEL SYNDROME, DYSPEPSIA, AND FUNCTIONAL CHEST PAIN OF PRESUMED ESOPHAGEAL ORIGIN

EMERAN A. MAYER

FUNCTIONAL GASTROINTESTINAL DISORDERS

DEFINITIONS

Irritable bowel syndrome (IBS), functional dyspepsia, and functional chest pain of presumed esophageal origin are characterized by chronic, recurrent symptoms of pain and discomfort referred to the lower abdomen, the epigastrium and upper abdomen, and the retrosternum, respectively. They belong to the family of functional gastrointestinal (GI) disorders that comprise a wide spectrum of chronic GI disorders common in both the adult and pediatric populations. In the absence of disease-specific biomarkers, each syndrome is classified by symptoms and the absence of other conditions that can account for the symptoms. Despite the benign prognoses, functional GI diseases can affect health-related quality of life at least as much as organic diseases.

PATHOBIOLOGY

The pathophysiology of functional GI diseases remains incompletely understood, but these diseases are characterized by alterations in bidirectional interactions between the brain and the gut (brain-gut axis; E-Fig. 139-1), with variable contributions of enhanced perception of visceral signals by the central nervous system (visceral hypersensitivity) and altered signaling from the nervous system to the GI tract, through autonomic nervous system activity. Each diagnostic category of functional GI disease is defined by symptomatic criteria that include different subsets of patients who exhibit different patterns of the brain-gut axis dysregulation and that result in varying abnormalities in GI motility, secretion, immune function, or visceral sensitivity. Despite this heterogeneity, however, functional GI diseases all share certain features, including enhanced sensitivity to stress, the frequent coexistence of psychiatric and chronic pain disorders, an enhanced perception of visceral events, and a greater prevalence in women.

Enhanced Perception of Visceral Pain

About 30 to 70% of patients with functional GI diseases have an altered perception of visceral afferent stimuli ("visceral hypersensitivity"), in which normally innocuous stimuli, such as physiologic contractions, distentions, or chemical stimulation of the intestine, stomach, or esophagus, lead to the sensation of pain or discomfort. The stimulus may be spontaneous peristaltic activity or result from distention by luminal contents, such as ingested food, liquids, gas, or feces. Visceral hypersensitivity may be associated with aberrant referral of visceral sensations to a particular body area, and this referral is often atypical in location and larger compared with most individuals.

Altered Stress Responsiveness

Abnormal autonomic and neuroendocrine responses to psychosocial stressors are a key feature of functional GI disease and may play an important role in both its cause and its exacerbation. For example, stressful events are more likely to lead to abdominal pain and a change in stool pattern in patients with IBS compared with healthy controls, and stress has been correlated with bowel symptoms and physician visit. Data also support an association between stress and functional dyspepsia. Patients with functional GI disease report more lifetime stressful events than healthy controls, and this early life stress may interact with a genetic predisposition to determine the vulnerability of an individual to adult stressors and the subsequent development of functional GI diseases.

IRRITABLE BOWEL SYNDROME

DEFINITION

IBS is defined as chronic, recurring abdominal pain or discomfort that is associated with defecation or a change in bowel habits; the diagnosis also requires the absence of detectable organic disease that may explain the symptoms (Table 139-1). Given the high prevalence of IBS in the general population, comorbid organic GI syndromes may coexist with IBS, including ulcerative colitis (Chapter 143), microscopic and collagenous colitis (Chapter 142), and celiac disease (Chapter 142). As a result, some patients may continue to have GI symptoms after their inflammatory bowel disease or other types of colitis have been treated successfully because at least some of their original symptoms were due to comorbid IBS. For example, a small subset of ulcerative colitis patients exhibit IBS-like symptoms and have demonstrable changes in colonic motility when they are in clinical remission.

IBS is further subdivided into IBS with diarrhea, IBS with constipation, or IBS with mixed bowel habits depending on the predominant bowel habit. Another subset is postinfectious IBS, which includes patients who develop persistent IBS symptoms despite the resolution of an episode or episodes of bacterial gastroenteritis. When patients do not fulfill criteria for these subtypes, they are classified as unspecified IBS.

TABLE 139-1	ROME III DIAGNOSTIC CRITERIA FOR IRRITABLE BOWEL SYNDROME

Recurrent abdominal pain or discomfort at least 3 days per month in the last 3 months (but with symptom onset for at least 6 months) associated with 2 or more of the following:
  Improvement with defecation
  Onset associated with a change in frequency of stool
  Onset associated with a change in form (appearance) of stool

Symptoms that cumulatively support the diagnosis of irritable bowel syndrome
  Abnormal stool frequency: ≤3 bowel movements per week or >3 bowel movements per day
  Abnormal stool form: lumpy/hard stool or loose/watery stool
  Defecation straining
  Urgency
  Feeling of incomplete bowel movement
  Passing mucus
  Bloating or feeling of abdominal distention

Absence of alarm symptoms
  Weight loss
  Bloody stool
  Anemia
  Family history of inflammatory bowel disease
  Colon cancer
  Celiac disease

EPIDEMIOLOGY

IBS is a common disorder, with a worldwide prevalence that ranges between 10 and 20%. As is the case with many related functional pain disorders, it is more common in women, with a female-to-male ratio of 2:1 to 2.5:1. It is generally assumed that IBS most commonly presents between the ages of 30 and 50 years, but IBS is also common in the pediatric population, in which such symptoms have traditionally been referred to as recurrent abdominal pain.

The socioeconomic burden of IBS is substantial, with patients taking three times as many days of sick leave compared with individuals without IBS; about 8% of patients retire early because of their symptoms. IBS is estimated to account for about 12% of primary care visits and 19% of GI specialty visits. In the United States, IBS is estimated to account for $1.6 billion in direct costs and $19.2 billion in indirect costs annually.

PATHOBIOLOGY

Although IBS is the most common and best studied functional GI disease, there is no general agreement on its pathophysiology. However, brain-imaging studies in IBS patients strongly suggest enhanced responses to both expected and delivered visceral pain stimuli, including in brain regions concerned with sensory processing, emotional arousal, and cognitive modulation.

Autonomic Nervous System

Converging results from experimental animal and human studies suggest that stress-induced activation of central autonomic circuits plays an important role in the regulation of gut motility, secretion, and immune modulation. Acute stress-induced activation of contractions and secretions of the hindgut is mediated by sacral parasympathetic pathways, and IBS patients have increased activation of these pathways in response to severe laboratory stressors. Tonic upregulation of sympathetic and sacral parasympathetic activity may result in neuroplastic changes in peripheral target mechanisms within the gut, including the enteric nervous system. For example, increased tonic sympathetic influences on the gut may play a role in the development of constipation.

Altered Gastrointestinal Motility and Secretion

GI motility is quantitatively but not qualitatively different in 25 to 75% of IBS patients compared with healthy controls, but these measured differences are not sufficiently reliable to be used as diagnostic markers. Colonic transit is accelerated in IBS with diarrhea, and high-amplitude propagating contractions occur more frequently in such patients than in controls. These high-amplitude propagating contractions correlate with abdominal pain and may be the mechanism underlying urgency, diarrhea, and associated fecal incontinence in this patient subgroup. By contrast, slowed colonic transit is observed in a subgroup of patients with IBS with constipation. Exaggerated or prolonged colonic motility responses to food intake (gastrocolonic response) may be present in approximately 30% of patients who report an exacerbation of abdominal pain after food intake. Secretory abnormalities and alterations in fluid handling by the intestine may also contribute to alterations in bowel habits.

Hypothalamic-Pituitary-Adrenal Axis

Alterations in neuroendocrine responses in IBS patients may be reflected by altered plasma levels of adrenocorticotropic hormone and cortisol. However, the exaggerated cortisol responses in IBS may be more related to a history of adverse early life events rather than to the IBS itself.

Mucosal Immune Activation

In some patients with postinfectious IBS, symptoms persist after the infective gastroenteritis has resolved. Even after resolution of the initial infection, changes in intestinal permeability, as well as small increases in intraepithelial lymphocytes and enterochromaffin cells, can be detected in postinfectious IBS. However, mucosal changes cannot fully account for the pathogenesis because clinical symptoms do not correlate with the observed mucosal inflammatory changes, most patients with bacterial gastroenteritis do not develop IBS symptoms after infection, and the prevalence of IBS is not greater in countries with endemic GI infections. Psychological stress, female gender, a history of other somatic symptoms (somatization), and the duration of the infection all increase the probability of developing postinfectious IBS.

Patients who meet the current diagnostic criteria for IBS but who do not have a prior history of gastroenteritis may have increased inflammatory cells on mucosal biopsy specimens. Fecal calprotectin, which is a surrogate marker of inflammation and which is increased in most patients with proven organic GI disease, has also been detected in a small subset of IBS patients.

Evidence suggests an increased number of mucosal mast cells in the colon and distal small bowel in IBS patients and a closer proximity of these mast cells with enteric nerves. Mast cell degranulation, in response to increased autonomic nervous system activity, and release of histamine, tryptase, and serotonin may increase nerve activity and contribute to symptoms, but a causative role for mast cells remains unproved.

Altered Intestinal Flora

Some data suggest that the intestinal bacterial flora may be altered in patients with IBS and that these alterations may differ among IBS groups according to predominant bowel habits. Small bowel bacterial overgrowth may contribute to IBS symptoms, especially in patients with predominant bloating-type symptoms, in whom treatment with nonabsorbable antibiotics may reduce symptoms. Qualitative changes in colonic flora, such as a decrease in bifidobacteria, have been described in IBS patients.

Genetics

Familial aggregation has been demonstrated in several studies of IBS patients, and the genetic heritability of functional GI diseases has been estimated to be between 22 and 57%. Candidate gene association studies suggest possible association of IBS with polymorphisms in genes related to the serotonin signaling system.

CLINICAL MANIFESTATIONS

Symptoms

The location of abdominal symptoms in IBS is highly variable, but pain is most typically referred to the lower abdomen. Pain and discomfort are frequently aggravated by emotion or stress, poor sleep, and intake of food, but these aggravating factors cannot be elicited in all patients. By definition, abdominal symptoms are relieved by defecation, but this relief may be temporary.

IBS symptoms occur mainly during wakefulness but may also awaken patients from sleep.

If symptoms are unrelated to defecation or food intake and if patients indicate that symptoms are constant and not relievable by any physiologic intervention, other diagnoses should be considered. Weight loss is uncommon in IBS except in patients with depression (Chapter 404) or eating disorders (Chapter 226), and its presence mandates investigation of an underlying organic cause.

IBS symptoms vary widely, from mild to very severe. Most patients seen by primary care physicians have mild symptoms, whereas most patients seen by gastroenterologists have moderate to severe symptoms.

Psychiatric Comorbidity

Psychiatric disorders (Chapter 404), such as anxiety disorders (e.g., generalized anxiety disorder, panic disorder, and posttraumatic stress syndrome), depression, somatization, hypochondriasis, and phobias, are more common in patients with IBS, even mildly symptomatic patients. The prevalence of coexisting psychiatric disorders can be as high as 40% to more than 90% in patients seen in tertiary referral centers but is lower in patients seen in primary care practices. However, stress plays an important role in exacerbating IBS symptoms in patients seen in all settings.

Comorbid Conditions and Extra-intestinal Manifestations

Patients with IBS have a three-fold or higher prevalence of fibromyalgia (Chapter 282) and migraine headaches (Chapter 405) compared with patients without IBS. IBS also frequently coexists with the chronic fatigue syndrome, and 60% or more of patients with chronic fatigue syndrome have IBS symptoms. Interstitial cystitis, chronic prostatitis (Chapter 131), and chronic pelvic pain are also common in IBS patients.

These associations of IBS with comorbid conditions and other symptoms are more common in female patients, but all patients with IBS on average see primary care physicians for non-GI complaints three times more frequently than do healthy subjects. IBS patients also often complain of extra-intestinal symptoms such as dyspareunia, fatigue, loss of energy, impotence, urinary frequency, backache, and dysmenorrhea.

DIAGNOSIS

Clinical Examination

The Rome III criteria (see Table 139-1) can establish the diagnosis of IBS without additional extensive testing. Alarm features raising concern for an

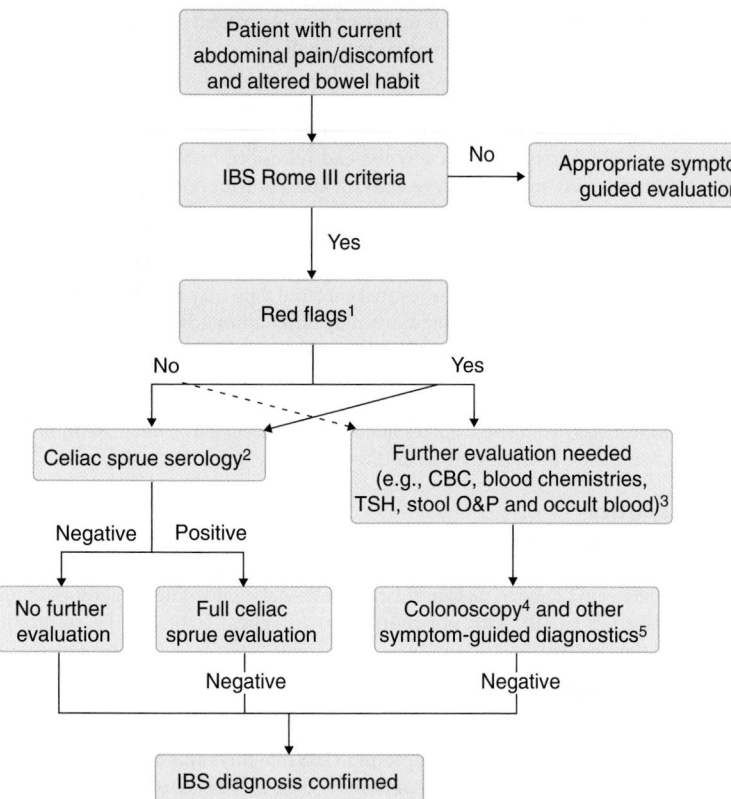

FIGURE 139-1. Diagnostic algorithm for irritable bowel syndrome. (1) Red flags include rectal bleeding, anemia, weight loss, fever, family history of colon cancer, first symptom onset after age 50 years, or major symptom change. (2) Testing for celiac sprue may be useful in patients meeting Rome criteria, in particular in irritable bowel syndrome (IBS) with diarrhea, if there are red flags, and in populations in which the background prevalence of celiac sprue is high. (3) In the absence of red flags, basic complete blood count (CBC), serum biochemistry, stool testing for occult blood and ova and parasites (O&P), and thyroid-stimulating hormone (TSH) levels are only indicated in cases of a supportive clinical history. (4) Colonoscopy is only recommended in the patient with positive red flags. However, according to colon cancer screening guidelines, routine colonoscopy should be performed in irritable bowel syndrome patients at age 50 years or older regardless of irritable bowel syndrome symptoms. (5) If there has been a major qualitative change in the pattern of chronic symptoms, a new comorbid condition producing these symptoms should be suspected and a more comprehensive diagnostic approach is warranted. (From Mayer EA. Clinical perspectives: irritable bowel syndrome. *N Engl J Med.* 2008;358:1692-1699.)

alternative diagnosis include weight loss, bloody stool, anemia, and a family history of inflammatory bowel disease, colon cancer, or celiac disease.

Careful review of medications and dietary supplements may reveal an etiologic agent because many prescribed medications can cause constipation and some diet supplements can lead to the inadvertent ingestion of laxatives. Although specific dietary agents are rarely the cause of IBS symptoms, the presence of lactose malabsorption can be determined by history or by a short trial of a lactose-free diet (Chapter 142). A brief psychosocial assessment is useful in identifying risk factors for chronic pain, such as traumatic early life events or somatization, as well as potential symptom triggers or exacerbating factors, such as anxiety, depression, and life stress.

The physical examination in IBS is usually normal but may reveal abdominal tenderness (most often in the left lower quadrant) or a tender, palpable sigmoid colon. In patients with constipation-predominant IBS and associated defecatory dysfunction, rectal examination may reveal paradoxical contraction of the puborectalis muscle or decreased descent of the pelvic floor when simulating a bowel movement.

Diagnostic Testing

In an otherwise healthy person who is younger than 50 years and who fulfills the ROME III criteria, further diagnostic testing should be minimal and guided by the individual presentation (Fig. 139-1). It remains controversial when to order a complete blood count, sedimentation rate, or thyroid studies, but most agree that it is not cost-effective to obtain these tests in all patients with presumed IBS. Serologic screening for celiac sprue (Chapter 142) should be pursued in patients with diarrhea-predominant or mixed bowel habits and in those with a family history of celiac disease. Colonic biopsies for collagenous or microscopic colitis (Chapter 142) should be considered in the setting of severe persistent diarrhea. The onset of symptoms after age 50 years and the presence of rectal bleeding or unexpected weight loss are indications for colonoscopy to assess for colorectal cancer (Chapter 199). Lower abdominal discomfort occurring with menses or with associated weight loss should trigger gynecologic evaluation. If the duration of diarrhea symptoms is short, it may be useful to assess for giardiasis (Chapter 359) or *Campylobacter* species infection (Chapter 311), but routine stool testing of all patients with diarrhea is not indicated.

Differential Diagnosis

Differential diagnosis for IBS with diarrhea predominance or mixed bowel habit includes inflammatory bowel diseases (e.g., Crohn's disease, ulcerative colitis, collagenous or microscopic colitis) (Chapters 142 and 143), celiac disease (Chapter 142), infection, small bowel bacterial overgrowth (Chapter 142), malabsorptive syndromes (including lactose intolerance) (Chapter 142), bile salt malabsorption (Chapter 142), and pancreatic insufficiency (Chapter 146) or malignancy (including neuroendocrine tumors [Chapter 239] and colorectal adenocarcinoma [Chapter 199]). The differential diagnosis for constipation-predominant IBS includes colonic inertia, pseudo-obstruction, paradoxical pelvic floor contraction, or pelvic outlet obstruction from structural causes such as rectal prolapse, rectocele, or short-segment Hirschsprung's disease (Chapter 138).

TREATMENT   Rx

General Principles

Symptomatic treatment attempts to normalize bowel habits and decrease abdominal pain in part by reassurance that the symptoms are real and the prognosis is benign. Dietary intervention can be helpful, and specific medications can be targeted to the management of individual symptoms, such as constipation, diarrhea, and abdominal pain (Table 139-2).

Physician-Patient Relationship and Patient Education

The doctor-patient relationship is of utmost importance in the treatment of IBS and other functional GI diseases. Many patients have been told previously that their symptoms are "all in their head" and have had their concerns dismissed. The physician must listen to and determine the patient's understanding of the illness and related concerns because patients frequently seek validation from the physician that their symptoms are real. Patients with functional GI disease typically visit a physician because of a flare of their usual symptoms, and it is important to identify such triggering factors, in particular various psychosocial stressors or, less commonly, a gastroenteric infection.

A thorough explanation of the symptoms and relationship to functional GI disease should be provided to the patient, including the natural history and benign prognosis of the disorder. Patients who are not properly informed tend to have more health care visits, whereas symptoms generally are reduced when diagnostic and prognostic information is explained. The physician must then set realistic short-term and long-term goals, including methods of adapting to symptoms that are not amenable to treatment. Patients often benefit from being involved in their treatment, and the maintenance of a symptom diary is one such example. Apart from providing the patient with a sense of empowerment, the symptom diary can help identify erroneous beliefs as well as lifestyle or dietary factors that may exacerbate symptoms; lifestyle modifications based on this information may provide symptomatic relief.

TABLE 139-2 MEDICATIONS USED IN THE TREATMENT OF IRRITABLE BOWEL SYNDROME*

SYMPTOMS AND MEDICATION	INITIAL DOSE (mg/day)†	TARGET DOSE (mg/day)†	COMMON OR SERIOUS SIDE EFFECTS	Degree of Evidence		FDA Approved	
				OF THE SYMPTOM	OF IBS	FOR THE SYMPTOM	FOR IBS
CONSTIPATION							
Laxatives‡ and Secretory Stimulators							
Polyethylene glycol 3350 (MiraLAX)	17,000	70,000	Diarrhea, bloating, cramping	+++	–		
Lactulose (Kristalose)	10,000-20,000	20,000-40,000	Diarrhea, bloating, cramping	+++	–		
Lubiprostone (Amitiza)		24, twice a day	Nausea, diarrhea, headache, abdominal pain and discomfort	+++	–	Yes§	No
Prokinetics							
Tegaserod (Zelnorm)		6, twice a day	Initial diarrhea, abdominal pain, cardiovascular ischemia (rare)	+++	+++	Yes‖	Yes‖
DIARRHEA							
Loperamide (Imodium)	2	2-8	Constipation	+++	–	Yes	No
Alosetron (Lotronex)			Constipation, ischemic colitis (rare)	–	+++	No	Yes¶
BLOATING							
Antibiotics							
Rifaximin		400, three times a day	Abdominal pain, diarrhea, bad taste	–	+	No	No
Probiotics**							
Bifidobacterium infantis 35624		1 capsule per day	None	+	+	No	No
PAIN							
Tricyclic Antidepressants††			Dry mouth, dizziness, weight gain				
Amitriptyline (Elavil)	10, at bedtime	10-75, at bedtime		++	+	No	No
Desipramine (Norpramin)	10, at bedtime	10-75, at bedtime		++	+	No	No
Selective Serotonin Reuptake Inhibitors††			Sexual dysfunction, headache, nausea, sedation, insomnia, sweating, withdrawal symptoms				
Paroxetine (Paxil CR)		10-60		–	+	No	No
Citalopram (Lexapro)		5-20		+	+	No	No
Fluoxetine (Prozac)		20-40	Somnolence, dizziness, headaches, insomnia	+	–	No	No

*This list is not exhaustive but includes major medications for which there is evidence from well-designed clinical trials of effectiveness for global irritable bowel syndrome (IBS) symptoms or for individual symptoms (e.g., constipation, diarrhea, or abdominal pain and discomfort). In the column about evidence, + denotes some evidence from at least one controlled trial; ++, moderate evidence from several controlled trials or from meta-analysis of such trials; +++, strong evidence from well-designed, controlled clinical trials; and –, no evidence. FDA denotes U.S. Food and Drug Administration.
†Dosages are in milligrams per day unless otherwise noted.
‡A wide range of osmotic and irritant laxatives, including fiber products, are available over the counter.
§Lubiprostone is FDA approved for the treatment of chronic constipation.
‖Zelnorm was suspended by the FDA in March 2005 because of rare cardiovascular side effects but is now available as part of a restricted-access program for women who have constipation-predominant IBS or chronic idiopathic constipation, without known or preexisting heart problems, that is unresponsive to other medications.
¶Lotronex use is restricted for women with severe diarrhea-predominant IBS, unresponsive to other medications, because of side effects.
**Many probiotics are available over the counter and are not listed. Align is a probiotic for which a beneficial effect for IBS symptoms has been shown in a high-quality, randomized, controlled trial.
††A wide range of tricyclic antidepressants with various side effects and side-effect profiles are available. Two commonly prescribed tricyclic antidepressants are listed.
‡‡Many selective serotonin reuptake inhibitors are available. Only those that have been evaluated in IBS trials are listed. Also not listed are serotonin-norepinephrine reuptake inhibitors.

Dietary Modification

Patients with functional GI disease, especially patients with IBS and functional dyspepsia, often complain that certain types of food exacerbate their symptoms. Perceived food sensitivity may be related to a variety of factors, including conditioned fear responses related to anticipatory anxiety, food intake in general, volume of the meal, or sensitivities to certain food items. For example, some IBS patients report an exacerbation of symptoms with high-fat food, gas-producing food, alcohol, and caffeine. It is important to inform the patient that there is no universal diet that is successful for IBS. A therapeutic trial of a lactose-free diet may be beneficial in some patients. Others may benefit from a low-carbohydrate, high-protein diet. It is essential, however, for patients to realize that if the dietary changes are not effective in reducing symptoms, they can resume consumption of the eliminated foods.

Pharmacologic Therapy

Antispasmodics

Antispasmodic medications, which include anticholinergic agents, calcium-channel blockers, and opioid receptor antagonists, may reverse or attenuate tonic contractions of the sigmoid colon or high-amplitude contractions of the colon, thereby relieving contractility. A meta-analysis of several low-quality studies reported a short-term benefit of the smooth muscle relaxants otilonium and hyoscine over placebo, but these agents are not available in the United States.**1** Antispasmodic medications have been combined with anxiolytic agents (e.g., clidinium bromide, 2.5 mg, and chlordiazepoxide, 5 mg, 1 to 2 tablets every 8 to 12 hours), but evidence supporting their benefit is lacking.

Medications for Bowel Habit Abnormalities and Bloating

In IBS patients with constipation, osmotic laxatives, such as polyethylene glycol or lactulose, or secretory stimulants, such as lubiprostone,**2** can be useful. Dietary fiber supplements (see Table 139-2) (e.g., psyllium fiber supplement starting at 3 to 6 g per day and increasing slowly every 1 to 2 weeks up to a total of 15 to 20 g per day in divided doses two or three times per day) may be effective**3** in some patients but often increase symptoms of gas, bloating, and flatulence.

In the IBS patient with diarrhea, loperamide is generally effective in reducing urgency and uncontrollable bowel movements. Several 5-HT₃ receptor antagonists and 5-HT₄ agonists are effective.**4** For example, alosetron (0.5 to 1 mg orally twice per day) or tegaserod (6 mg orally twice per day)**4** are beneficial, but alosetron should be considered only in patients who have severe bloating and diarrhea and who have failed all other therapies because of its infrequent but potentially serious side effects.

Manipulation of the intestinal flora with antibiotics (rifaximin 550 mg three times daily for 2 weeks),[5] and probiotics[6] may be effective in some patients, particularly patients with abdominal bloating symptoms. Herbal laxatives such as aloe, rhubarb root products, and peppermint oil may be of use in some patients.

Antidepressants and Psychological Therapies

Low doses of tricyclic antidepressants (e.g., nortriptyline or amitriptyline, 10 to 50 mg at bedtime) are frequently used to treat IBS based on data that about one patient in four may benefit.[7] Doses should be started as low as 5 mg once daily and gradually advanced to a maximum of 75 mg once daily. The therapeutic effect should be expected within days to 2 weeks of initiating therapy; if no beneficial effect is observed at 75 mg once daily or if significant side effects are experienced, the drug should be discontinued. Amitriptyline may be most useful in patients with prominent abdominal pain and diarrhea symptoms and in patients with sleep problems.

To maximize compliance and reduce side effects, the patient should be informed about the rationale of the treatment choice (i.e., the goal is the treatment of pain and not psychiatric symptoms) and informed about the much lower risk for side effects at the low dose range compared with full psychiatric doses.

If the treatment goal is aimed at comorbid depression or anxiety disorders, a selective serotonin reuptake inhibitor (SSRI) generally has fewer side effects than tricyclic antidepressants and appears to be beneficial in patients with IBS.[7] In patients with psychiatric comorbidity, a low-dose tricyclic antidepressant and a full therapeutic dose of an SSRI should also be considered, or a nonselective uptake inhibitor such as duloxetine or venlafaxine may be used.

Cognitive-behavioral therapy, which involves relaxation, change in beliefs, and self-management, can reduce gastrointestinal symptoms in at least 50% of patients,[8] although patients with coexisting depression do not respond as well as other patients. Hypnotherapy also has been reported to improve symptoms.

PROGNOSIS

The natural history of IBS is periods of exacerbation followed by periods of remission, but about 50% of IBS patients become asymptomatic. Patients with coexisting psychiatric disorders are less likely to have their IBS symptoms resolve.

FUNCTIONAL DYSPEPSIA

As with other functional GI diseases, the diagnosis of functional dyspepsia is based on specific symptoms (Tables 139-3 and 139-4). Functional dyspepsia is thought to originate from the upper gastrointestinal tract, but no detectable organic disease can explain the symptoms. Symptoms may include epigastric pain, epigastric burning, postprandial fullness, and early satiation. Abdominal bloating and nausea also may be experienced, but they are less specific and are not considered cardinal symptoms of functional dyspepsia. Symptoms overlap with atypical manifestations of gastroesophageal reflux disease (GERD; Chapter 140), and previous studies on functional dyspepsia may have inadvertently included patients with atypical GERD symptoms.

In the current Rome III criteria, symptoms have been divided into meal-related (postprandial distress syndrome) and meal-unrelated (epigastric pain syndrome) symptoms (see Table 139-4). The clinical utility of these subgroups is controversial because there is considerable overlap between them. Moreover, the concept of distinct pathophysiologies correlating with distinct symptom patterns has not been confirmed.

EPIDEMIOLOGY

Functional dyspepsia is a common disorder, with an estimated prevalence of 15 to 20%. Unlike IBS, there does not appear to be a sex-related difference in prevalence. The socioeconomic burden of functional dyspepsia is substantial; patients with functional dyspepsia take three times as much sick leave as patients with duodenal ulcers. In the United Kingdom, an estimated 2 to 5% of primary care visits and more than 10% of primary care drug expenditures are related to functional dyspepsia. Approximately 1 of 2 individuals with functional dyspepsia seeks health care for symptoms at some time in his or her life. It is therefore not surprising that in the United Kingdom, the annual indirect and direct cost of dyspepsia to society are U.S. $1.46 billion and U.S. $730 million, respectively.

Comorbidity with Irritable Bowel Syndrome

Pain or discomfort in the upper abdomen may at first be assumed to be related to the upper GI tract, but on detailed questioning, the "dyspepsia"

TABLE 139-3 ROME III DIAGNOSTIC CRITERIA FOR FUNCTIONAL DYSPEPSIA*

1. One or more of the following:
   Bothersome postprandial fullness
   Early satiation
   Epigastric pain
   Epigastric burning
   and
2. No evidence of structural disease (including at upper endoscopy) that is likely to explain the symptoms

*The criteria must be fulfilled for the last 3 months with symptom onset at least 6 months before diagnosis.

TABLE 139-4 ROME III DIAGNOSTIC CRITERIA FOR SUBGROUPS OF PATIENTS WITH FUNCTIONAL DYSPEPSIA*

POSTPRANDIAL DISTRESS SYNDROME

One or both of the following:
1. Bothersome postprandial fullness, occurring after ordinary sized meals, at least several times per week
2. Early satiation that prevents finishing a regular meal, at least several times per week

Supportive Criteria

1. Upper abdominal bloating or postprandial nausea or excessive belching can be present.
2. Epigastric pain syndrome may coexist.

EPIGASTRIC PAIN SYNDROME

One or more of the following:
1. Pain or burning localized to the epigastrium of at least moderate severity at least once per week
2. Intermittent pain
3. Pain not generalized or localized to other abdominal or chest regions
4. Pain not relieved by defecation or passage of flatus
5. Pain not fulfilling criteria for gallbladder and sphincter of Oddi disorders

Supportive Criteria

1. The pain may be of a burning quality but without a retrosternal component.
2. The pain is commonly induced or relieved by ingestion of a meal but may occur while fasting.
3. Postprandial distress syndrome may coexist.

*The criteria must be fulfilled for the last 3 months with symptom onset at least 6 months before diagnosis.

---

may be related to bowel disturbances. One third of patients with functional dyspepsia have concurrent symptoms of IBS, and approximately 40% of IBS patients also report symptoms of functional dyspepsia. Moreover, transitions between the two syndromes in the same patient over time are common. In a 1-year follow-up of patients with IBS or dyspepsia, 22% of IBS patients reported a change in their symptom profile to that of functional dyspepsia, and 16% of patients with functional dyspepsia reported a change to an IBS symptom profile. This transition of patients between different diagnostic categories questions the concept that these symptom-based entities are really distinct pathophysiologic syndromes. Compared with patients with non-life-threatening organic GI disease, patients with functional dyspepsia have higher anxiety but not depression or neuroticism scores.

PATHOBIOLOGY

The pathobiology of functional dyspepsia is not fully understood, and both central and peripheral mechanisms have been proposed. Although enhanced perception of gastric stimuli may be a key central mechanism, the roles of gastric acid, acute and chronic gastric mucosal infections, and gastroduodenal dysmotility remain to be determined. Attempts to classify subtypes of functional dyspepsia based on pathophysiologic abnormalities have been unsuccessful.

As with IBS patients, visceral hypersensitivity is common in functional dyspepsia, and 34 to 65% of patients with functional dyspepsia report pain and discomfort at lower volumes of gastric distention than healthy control subjects or patients with dyspepsia from organic causes. Chemical sensitivity to capsaicin also has been reported. Central pain amplification also is likely to contribute to the observed gastric hypersensitivity. For example, the presence of lipids in the duodenum increases the sensitivity of patients with functional dyspepsia to gastric balloon distention compared with controls. This abnormal modulation of gastric perception thresholds to distention by lipid in a distant site supports the concept of a centrally mediated mechanism. Furthermore, about 50% of patients with functional dyspepsia experience altered viscerosomatic referral patterns in response to gastric balloon distention.

Several large multicenter studies have demonstrated that only 10 to 15% of patients with functional dyspepsia benefit from acid suppression therapy. This finding suggests that such patients are hypersensitive to either intraduodenal or intra-antral acid or that they suffer from atypical manifestations of GERD. Chronic *Helicobacter pylori* infection may be related to dyspeptic symptoms in patients with functional dyspepsia.

Some data suggest the presence of alterations in gastroduodenal motility in patients with functional dyspepsia, but the low concordance between symptoms and altered motility findings argues against such testing except in highly selected patients. For example, about 40% of patients with functional dyspepsia have evidence of impaired gastric accommodation, which may cause rapid transit of food from the proximal stomach, thereby resulting in early antral distention, which in turn results in dyspeptic symptoms. In addition, postprandial antral hypomotility can be demonstrated by manometric studies in about 50% of patients with functional dyspepsia, and this abnormality correlates with delayed gastric emptying, which has been demonstrated in one third of patients with functional dyspepsia. A correlation between delayed gastric emptying and dyspeptic symptoms of postprandial fullness has been reported. About 20% of patients with functional dyspepsia develop their symptoms after an acute episode of presumed viral or bacterial gastroenteritis or *Giardia* species infection.

DIAGNOSIS

Clinical Examination

Dyspepsia can be suspected to be functional based on a clinical history consistent with the ROME III criteria (see Tables 139-3 and 139-4) and the absence of alarm features (see Table 139-1). The presence of anxiety, in particular symptom-related anxiety and comorbid IBS, increases the likelihood of functional dyspepsia.

The physical examination is generally normal, although epigastric tenderness may be present. In contrast to gastroparesis, a succussion splash is typically absent. Although confirmation of the functional dyspepsia diagnosis, as noted in the Rome III criteria, requires a normal upper endoscopic examination, invasive testing in the absence of alarm features should be considered only in a minority of symptomatic patients, such as patients older than 50 years with new-onset or changing symptoms or a poor response to initial therapy (see Fig. 134-6 in Chapter 134). Evaluation for *H. pylori* (Chapter 141) should be performed by stool antigen, urea breath test, or gastric biopsy. If present, the infection should be eradicated, and then symptoms should be reassessed. Young patients who respond well to a trial of proton pump inhibitor therapy or *H. pylori* eradication do not require further investigation unless alarm features are identified. Nonsteroidal anti-inflammatory medications, dietary supplements, and other prescription or over-the-counter medications can trigger dyspeptic symptoms. The patient's medication list should be reviewed, and nonessential treatments should be discontinued. As in the evaluation of IBS, a psychosocial history may reveal underlying stressors that contribute to symptoms.

Differential Diagnosis

Common organic causes of dyspepsia include peptic ulcer disease (Chapter 141) and gastroesophageal reflux disease (Chapter 140). Delayed gastric emptying is present in a small number of patients with functional dyspepsia but is characteristic and more pronounced in patients with diabetic or idiopathic gastroparesis (Chapter 138). Vomiting of undigested food is characteristic of these forms of gastroparesis, but not of dyspepsia. Gastric and esophageal cancers (Chapter 198) may also present with symptoms of dyspepsia but are much less common. Pancreaticobiliary disorders (Chapters 146 and 158) (including sphincter of Oddi dysfunction, chronic pancreatitis, or pancreatic cancer) also occasionally mimic dyspepsia.

TREATMENT Rx

Acid suppression therapy is safe and may have a beneficial effect over placebo in approximately 10% of patients, who presumably have either atypical GERD (Chapter 140) or duodenal hypersensitivity to gastric acid. The choice of acid suppressive agents is open to debate (see Table 140-1 in Chapter 140), and both histamine (H_2)-receptor antagonists (e.g., famotidine, 20 mg twice per day) and proton pump inhibitors (e.g., omeprazole, 20 mg per day) have been reported to be more effective than placebo. A proton pump inhibitor (e.g., omeprazole, 20 mg/day, or lansoprazole, 30 mg/day) is superior to placebo or an H_2 antagonist in functional dyspepsia, especially in patients with epigastric pain. In a randomized study of step-up and step-down treatment with antacids, H_2-receptor antagonists, and proton pump inhibitors in patients with new-onset dyspepsia, the two treatments were equally successful (about 70%), but the step-up approach was more cost-effective.[9]

A subset of patients with functional dyspepsia improve after eradication of *H. pylori* (Chapter 141), and the likelihood of a positive response is comparable to that with acid suppression.[10] This short-duration treatment also can reduce the risk of subsequent peptic ulcer disease, atrophic gastritis, and gastric cancer, and it currently is recommended by consensus guidelines.

The use of prokinetic drugs such as metoclopramide or domperidone, 10 mg three times per day, before meals is of uncertain benefit. Low-dose tricyclic antidepressant therapy has not been as extensively evaluated in functional dyspepsia compared with IBS, but small studies reported a beneficial effect. The benefits of psychological therapy for functional dyspepsia are not well established, but it may be a reasonable option in patients who do not respond to pharmacotherapy.

PROGNOSIS

As with all functional disorders, functional dyspepsia has a benign prognosis, although symptoms can be persistent.

FUNCTIONAL CHEST PAIN OF PRESUMED ESOPHAGEAL ORIGIN

DEFINITION

Functional chest pain of presumed esophageal origin (Table 139-5) is a chronic, unexplained midline chest pain that is thought to be of esophageal origin. To make the diagnosis, cardiac causes, gastroesophageal reflux, and well-defined motility disorders (achalasia, scleroderma) must be excluded.

EPIDEMIOLOGY

Most patients who present to a physician with acute chest pain (see Table 50-2 in Chapter 50) have a noncardiac cause, and many are cases of functional chest pain. Most of these are cases of functional chest pain. Despite its frequency, however, the prevalence of functional chest pain and its natural course are not well understood, likely because most patients undergo a cardiac evaluation but then may have no further evaluation of their symptoms.

Functional chest pain is quite common, with prevalence rates as high as 25%, evenly divided between men and women. Its prevalence appears to decline with advancing age. Risk factors for developing functional chest pain are not well defined but include younger age, adversity in childhood, and a history of other functional gastrointestinal conditions. Once symptoms occur, more than 50% of patients have persisting symptoms for longer than 6 months. Even after the initial diagnosis, however, many patients with chronic pain undergo repeated and unnecessary diagnostic cardiac evaluations. Patients with functional chest pain may have comorbid anxiety or panic attacks, but formal referral for psychological treatment is infrequent. When

---

TABLE 139-5	ROME III DIAGNOSTIC CRITERIA FOR FUNCTIONAL CHEST PAIN OF PRESUMED ESOPHAGEAL ORIGIN*

Must include all of the following:
- Midline chest pain or discomfort that is not of burning quality
- Absence of evidence that gastroesophageal reflux is the cause of symptoms
- Absence of histopathology-based esophageal motility disorders

*The criteria must be fulfilled for the last 3 months with symptom onset at least 6 months before diagnosis.

compared with patients who have known cardiac chest pain, patients with functional chest pain report greater impairment of health-related quality of life in the domains of mental health and vitality. These findings suggest a link between psychological disturbance and functional chest pain, at least in a subgroup of patients.

PATHOBIOLOGY

Visceral hypersensitivity, altered esophageal motility, and psychological factors have all been implicated in the pathophysiology of functional chest pain. A substantial proportion of patients show enhanced sensitivity to esophageal distention by a balloon. These same patients will often also have increased perceptual responses to intraesophageal acid infusion. The origin of such findings is not clear, although alterations in central processing of pain signals (central pain amplification) has been implicated. In addition, altered esophageal motility can be observed in a subset of patients with functional chest pain, with or without visceral hypersensitivity. Increased contraction of the esophageal muscle has long been considered a source of chest pain, although reproducible studies to prove this hypothesis are lacking.

CLINICAL MANIFESTATIONS

Patients may complain of pain that is typical for myocardial ischemia or of pain with a variety of characteristics that would be considered atypical for ischemia (Chapters 50 and 71). The location of pain is typically substernal, but radiation to the arm and neck can be described. The pain typically is not precipitated by exertion and may persist for hours. Nitroglycerin may sometimes be helpful acutely in patients with coexisting esophageal spasm. Patients may describe the discomfort using a variety of adjectives, and those descriptions may be indistinguishable from angina.

DIAGNOSIS

Patients who present with chest pain suspicious for angina should undergo prompt cardiac evaluation (Chapters 50 and 71). In patients with an initial negative cardiac evaluation, causes of functional chest pain can be categorized based on historical features (Table 139-6), and repeated cardiac evaluation for recurrent pain is of low yield. Patients with prominent chest wall pain and tenderness on palpation or with changes in pain with movement usually have musculoskeletal rather than an esophageal pain.

The remaining patients may have an esophageal source of pain (Chapter 140) and should be divided into patients with and without alarm symptoms, such as weight loss, progressive dysphagia, or anemia. Upper endoscopy is useful in patients with alarm features but is of lower yield in patients without them.

Many patients with functional chest pain will have underlying GERD. Because clinical features, such as association with certain foods or pain location, do differentiate well between acid-induced versus non-acid-related causes, evaluation for atypical GERD is best performed by a proton pump inhibitor trial (e.g., omeprazole, 20 mg daily). Patients who respond to a 1- to 2-week trial of daily proton pump inhibitor likely have acid-related symptoms and should be treated for GERD (Chapter 140). In patients whose response is equivocal, a longer proton pump inhibitor trial of 4 to 8 weeks, endoscopy, or 24-hour pH testing (Chapter 140) can be considered.

For patients who do not respond to a proton pump inhibitor, a disorder of esophageal motility or visceral hypersensitivity may be present. Esophageal motility disorders such as high-amplitude contractions ("nutcracker esophagus") or diffuse esophageal spasm can be identified by esophageal manometry (Chapter 140), but the low concordance between symptoms and manometric findings suggests that such testing should be performed only in highly selected patients based on the advice of a gastroenterologist.

TABLE 139-6	DIFFERENTIAL DIAGNOSIS OF FUNCTIONAL CHEST PAIN

ORGANIC ESOPHAGEAL CAUSES

Gastroesophageal reflux disease
Achalasia
Virus- or pill-induced esophagitis

NONGASTROINTESTINAL CAUSES

Cardiac chest pain
Chest wall pain
Pulmonary disease
Panic attack

TREATMENT   Rx

All patients benefit from reassurance regarding the benign course of functional chest pain. Fears of cardiac disease should be addressed explicitly, and the significance of a negative cardiac evaluation must be reinforced. If the functional chest pain is responsive to a proton pump inhibitor trial, patients should be continued on such therapy or treated with alternative acid-suppressing medications. The optimal duration of treatment is unclear, but it is reasonable to attempt withdrawal of medication and observe patients who have remained asymptomatic for several months. Although evidence from well-designed clinical trials is lacking, low-dose tricyclic antidepressants (e.g., desipramine, 10 to 75 mg per day) may be useful, particularly in patients suspected to have visceral hypersensitivity.

Comorbid psychological symptoms should be addressed with either pharmacologic or cognitive behavioral therapy. Even in the absence of a specific psychiatric diagnosis, relaxation therapy or cognitive behavioral therapy may be of benefit for functional chest pain.

PROGNOSIS

Functional chest pain has a benign prognosis, although symptoms may persist and continue to diminish quality of life.

Grade A

1. Ford AC, Talley NJ, Spiegel BM, et al. Effect of fibre, antispasmodics, and peppermint oil in the treatment of irritable bowel syndrome: systematic review and meta-analysis. *BMJ.* 2008;337:a2313.
2. Drossman DA, Chey WD, Johanson JF, et al. Clinical trial: lubiprostone in patients with constipation-associated irritable bowel syndrome—results of two randomized, placebo-controlled studies. *Aliment Pharmacol Ther.* 2009;29:329-341.
3. Bijkerk CJ, de Wit NJ, Muris JW, et al. Soluble or insoluble fibre in irritable bowel syndrome in primary care? Randomised placebo controlled trial. *BMJ.* 2009;339:b3154.
4. Ford AC, Brandt LJ, Young C, et al. Efficacy of 5-HT3 antagonists and 5-HT4 agonists in irritable bowel syndrome: systematic review and meta-analysis. *Am J Gastroenterol.* 2009;104:1831-1843.
5. Pimentel M, Lembo A, Chey WD, et al. Rifaximin therapy for patients with irritable bowel syndrome without constipation. *N Engl J Med.* 2011;364:22-32.
6. Nikfar S, Rahimi R, Rahimi F, et al. Efficacy of probiotics in irritable bowel syndrome: a meta-analysis of randomized, controlled trials. *Dis Colon Rectum.* 2008;51:1775-1780.
7. Ford AC, Talley NJ, Schoenfeld PS, et al. Efficacy of antidepressants and psychological therapies in irritable bowel syndrome: systematic review and meta-analysis. *Gut.* 2009;58:367-378.
8. Lackner JM, Mesmer C, Morley S, et al. Psychological treatments for irritable bowel syndrome: a systematic review and meta-analysis. *J Consult Clin Psychol.* 2004;72:1100-1113.
9. van Marrewijk CJ, Mujakovic S, Fransen GA, et al. Effect and cost-effectiveness of step-up versus step-down treatment with antacids, H2-receptor antagonists, and proton pump inhibitors in patients with new onset dyspepsia (DIAMOND study): a primary-care-based randomised controlled trial. *Lancet.* 2009; 373:215-225.
10. Moayyedi P, Soo S, Deeks J, et al. Eradication of Helicobacter pylori for non-ulcer dyspepsia. *Cochrane Database Syst Rev* 2006;2:CD002096.
11. Cremonini F, Wise J, Moayyedi P, et al. Diagnostic and therapeutic use of proton pump inhibitors in non-cardiac chest pain: a meta-analysis. *Am J Gastroenterol.* 2005;100:1226-1232.

SUGGESTED READINGS

Chang JY, Talley NJ. Current and emerging therapies in irritable bowel syndrome: from pathophysiology to treatment. *Trends Pharmacol Sci.* 2010;31:326-334. *Review.*
Olafsdottir LB, Gudjonsson H, Jonsdottir HH, et al. Natural history of functional dyspepsia: a 10-year population-based study. *Digestion.* 2010;81:53-61. *Patients are generally stable but continue to have an increased intensity and frequency of gastrointestinal pain.*
Sperber AD, Drossman DA. Review article: the functional abdominal pain syndrome. *Aliment Pharmacol Ther.* 2011;33:514-524. *Comprehensive review.*

140

DISEASES OF THE ESOPHAGUS

GARY W. FALK AND DAVID A. KATZKA

NORMAL ANATOMY AND PHYSIOLOGY

The esophagus, which averages about 27 cm in length, is a hollow muscular tube consisting of mucosa, submucosa, and muscularis layers and the absence of a serosal layer. The mucosa is a stratified squamous nonkeratinized epithelium that transitions to a columnar epithelium at the gastroesophageal junction. The muscular layer of the esophagus is composed of striated muscle in the upper one third and smooth muscle in the lower two thirds. These muscular components are arranged as an inner circular and an outer longitudinal layer. Located between the circular and longitudinal muscle layers is Auerbach's (myenteric) plexus, whereas Meissner's plexus is located within the submucosa and innervates the muscularis mucosae. The esophagus is bounded by an upper esophageal sphincter proximally and the lower esophageal sphincter distally. The upper esophageal sphincter contains functional contributions from the inferior pharyngeal constrictor proximally and the cricopharyngeus distally. By contrast, the lower esophageal sphincter is anatomically and histologically indistinguishable from the lower esophagus. Blood supply for the cervical portion is derived from branches of the inferior thyroid artery. The intrathoracic segment of the esophagus receives its blood supply from bronchial arteries and direct branches from the aorta, and the short abdominal portion of the esophagus is supplied by the left gastric and the inferior phrenic arteries. Venous drainage follows the arterial supply in the cervical and abdominal portions, whereas the thoracic esophagus drains into the azygous and hemiazygos system. Likewise, the lymphatic drainage of the esophagus is segmental, with the cervical portion draining into deep cervical lymph nodes, the thoracic portion into the superior and posterior mediastinal lymph nodes, and the abdominal portion into the gastric and celiac lymph nodes.

The motor functions of the esophagus are to transport a food bolus from the oropharynx into the stomach and then to keep food from returning to the esophagus after it has entered the stomach. The upper esophageal sphincter and the proximal third of the esophagus compose the first portion of the esophagus. The upper esophageal sphincter, which is approximately 2 to 4 cm in length, is controlled by the recurrent laryngeal nerve inferiorly and a pharyngeal plexus superiorly. The muscle layers close the esophageal lumen and shorten the esophagus to facilitate forward transport through the proximal esophagus. After food traverses the proximal esophagus, it moves into the distal two thirds of the esophagus, where peristalsis is achieved by sequential muscular contraction mediated by an interplay of inhibitory and excitatory neurotransmitters. Peristalsis may be primary, that is, initiated by a swallow, or secondary, that is, stimulated by refluxed gastric contents. Although local mechanisms control most esophageal motor function, vagal input is important in the distal esophagus, where smooth muscle myopathies and autonomic neuropathies can cause dysfunction. The distal esophagus is separated from the stomach by the lower esophageal sphincter, which is 4 to 5 cm in length and is functionally distinct because it maintains a tonic high-pressure zone. This sphincter relaxes nearly completely upon swallowing to allow the passage of food and then regains its tone to provide a barrier against reflux. It also relaxes transiently during normal functions, such as belching and vomiting. The vagus nerve, acetylcholine, and nitric oxide influence tone, but the lower esophageal sphincter tone also is influenced by the crural diaphragm as the esophagus traverses the diaphragmatic hiatus.

Esophageal Functional Testing

Options for esophageal functional testing include barium esophagography, esophageal manometry, and esophageal impedance testing. Barium esophagography (Chapter 135) reveals both anatomic and physiologic information about endoluminal lesions, such as malignancies, ulceration, diverticula, hiatal hernia, and strictures; intramural lesions, such as leiomyomas; and extrinsic lesions, such as occur from vascular (aorta, right atrium, subclavian artery) impingement or solid lesions (pulmonary malignancy, adenopathy) that compress the esophagus. Radiography is also an excellent tool for studying motility patterns, such as peristalsis with either liquid or solid contrast material, while precisely visualizing how the esophagus handles a bolus rather than by implying function from pressure or impedance changes.

Esophageal manometry measures pressure changes generated by esophageal wall contraction using multiple ports that simultaneously measure pressure from the pharynx to the lower esophageal sphincter. Esophageal impedance testing measures conductance between catheter-based electrodes based on the substance that is in contact with each electrode. Air, which is a poor conductor of electric current, will yield high impedance, whereas swallowed or refluxed liquids, which are excellent conductors of electricity, will generate a low impedance signal. From these measurements, the direction and velocity of the transport of air and bolus can help assess peristaltic function and measure reflux of acid and nonacid gastric contents.

Symptoms of Esophageal Disease

The most common symptom of esophageal disease is heartburn, which is defined as a sensation of substernal burning. Chest pain without typical heartburn may occur in a variety of esophageal disorders, including gastroesophageal reflux and motor disorders such as in achalasia. However, esophageal pain and even heartburn can be indistinguishable from cardiac angina (Chapter 50), so care must be taken when a patient at risk for coronary artery disease complains of heartburn for the first time.

Dysphagia, or difficulty swallowing, is another cardinal symptom of esophageal disease. Dysphagia with only solid food tends to occur with structural lesions, which cause esophageal constriction, whereas dysphagia with both liquids and solids occurs more often with motility disorders. Patients with oropharyngeal dysphagia will commonly complain of a feeling of food "sticking" in the throat or the inability to propel the bolus from the mouth to the pharynx; they may also complain of the need for multiple swallowing motions to clear the bolus. Because the cranial nerves that generally control the initial phases of swallowing are responsible for other functions as well, symptoms that may be associated with oropharyngeal dysphagia include drooling, dysarthria (due to tongue dysfunction), nasal regurgitation (due to failure to seal off the nasal passage), or coughing and aspiration (due to failure to elevate and cover the laryngeal vestibule). Dysphagia that results from abnormalities in the body of the esophagus may be referred to the chest or the neck, so the location of pain does not predict the location of the disease. Dysphagia may also lead to a variety of behavioral accommodations, including maneuvers such as slow eating, food aversion, avoidance of hard solid food, and drinking of large amounts of liquids with solid meals.

Regurgitation, which is another typical esophageal symptom, may be described as the feeling of food coming up into the chest or, more dramatically, into the mouth. When regurgitation occurs early in the meal, it suggests a proximal lesion. Regurgitation later in the meal suggests a motility abnormality such as achalasia.

Food impaction is an extreme esophageal symptom. When impaction occurs in the oropharynx, patients may develop a "steakhouse" syndrome, in which an impacted food bolus leads to tracheal impaction or compression. With more distal esophageal lesions, impaction may occur any time during the meal, almost always from a mechanical cause. Patients experience the sudden onset of chest pain and the sensation of food sticking, typically after solids such as meats, raw vegetables, and sometimes sticky rice. With complete impaction, patients who cannot handle secretions because of the obstructing bolus are at risk of aspiration.

GASTROESOPHAGEAL REFLUX DISEASE

DEFINITION

Gastroesophageal reflux disease (GERD) develops when the reflux of stomach contents into the esophagus causes troublesome symptoms or complications.

EPIDEMIOLOGY

It is estimated that GERD, defined as at least weekly heartburn or acid regurgitation, has a prevalence ranging from 10 to 20% in the Western world and less than 5% in Asia. The prevalence also tends to be higher in North America than Europe and higher in northern Europe than in southern Europe. Risk factors for developing GERD include obesity and possibly increasing age. A genetic component may also play a role because GERD is more common in patients with a positive family history and in a monozygotic than in a dizygotic twin.

PATHOBIOLOGY

The esophagus is protected from the harmful effects of refluxed gastric contents by the antireflux barrier at the gastroesophageal junction, by esophageal clearance mechanisms, and by epithelial defensive factors. The antireflux barrier consists of the lower esophageal sphincter, crural diaphragm, phrenoesophageal ligament, and the angle of His, which causes an oblique entrance of the esophagus into the stomach. The attachment of the lower esophageal sphincter to the crural diaphragm results in increased pressure during inspiration and when intra-abdominal pressure increases. Disruption of normal defense mechanisms leads to pathologic amounts of reflux.

Reflux of gastric contents from the stomach into the esophagus occurs in healthy individuals, but refluxed gastric contents are normally cleared in a two-step process: volume clearance by peristaltic function and neutralization of small amounts of residual acid by weakly alkaline swallowed saliva. In normal healthy individuals, physiologic reflux occurs primarily when the lower esophageal sphincter transiently relaxes in the absence of a swallow because of a vagally mediated reflex that is stimulated by gastric distention.

In GERD patients, transient relaxation of the lower esophageal sphincter or a low resting lower esophageal sphincter pressure can result in regurgitation, especially when intra-abdominal pressure is increased.

A hiatal hernia, which results in spatial separation between the augmenting effects of the crural diaphragm and the lower esophageal sphincter, predisposes to reflux events by widening the opening of the gastroesophageal junction and decreasing the pressure of the lower esophageal sphincter. The result is an increased exposure of the esophagus to acid, with increased reflux events during transient physiologic relaxation of the lower esophageal sphincter. Hernias also act as a reservoir for gastric contents when normal esophageal clearance mechanisms result in trapping of fluids in the hernia sac; these contents can reflux into the esophagus when the lower esophageal sphincter relaxes during subsequent swallowing.

Obesity results in an increase in intragastric pressure, which increases the gastroesophageal pressure gradient and the frequency of transient lower esophageal sphincter relaxation, thereby predisposing gastric contents to migrate into the esophagus. In addition, obesity enhances the spatial separation of the crural diaphragm and the lower esophageal sphincter, thereby predisposing obese individuals to a hiatal hernia.

The normal defense mechanisms based on peristalsis and saliva can also be impaired. Peristaltic dysfunction is associated with an increasing severity of esophagitis, and ineffective peristaltic clearance may occur when the amplitude of esophageal contractions is less than 30 mm Hg. Saliva production may be impaired by a variety of mechanisms, such as smoking and Sjögren's syndrome (Chapter 276).

The esophageal mucosa contains several lines of defense. A pre-epithelial barrier is composed of a small unstirred water layer combined with bicarbonate from swallowed saliva and from the secretions of submucosal glands. A second epithelial defense is composed of cell membranes and tight intercellular junctions, cellular and intercellular buffers, and cell membrane ion transporters. The postepithelial line of defense is composed of the blood supply to the esophagus. Acid and acidified pepsin in the refluxate are the key factors that damage the intercellular junctions, increase intracellular permeability, and dilate intercellular spaces. If sufficient quantities of refluxate diffuse into the intercellular spaces, cellular damage may occur. Signs and symptoms of GERD occur when defective epithelium comes into contact with refluxed acid, pepsin, or other noxious gastric contents. In addition to the direct noxious effects of refluxed acid, pepsin, and bile, refluxed gastric juice stimulates esophageal epithelial cells to secrete chemokines that attract inflammatory cells into the esophagus, thereby damaging the esophageal mucosa.

CLINICAL MANIFESTATIONS

The classic symptoms of GERD are heartburn and acid regurgitation; atypical symptoms include chest pain, dysphagia, and odynophagia. Extraesophageal manifestations of reflux disease can include cough (Chapter 83), laryngitis (Chapter 437), asthma (Chapter 87), and dental erosions, but these symptoms can be reliably attributed to reflux only if they are accompanied by classic signs and symptoms of reflux disease. Other proposed associations that are not clearly established include pharyngitis, sinusitis, otitis media, and idiopathic pulmonary fibrosis (Fig. 140-1).

When excessive gastric contents overwhelm the mucosal protective factors in the esophagus, esophagitis may be manifest as erosions or ulceration of

the esophagus and may also lead to fibrosis with stricturing, columnar metaplasia (Barrett's esophagus) or esophageal adenocarcinoma (Chapter 198). However, approximately two thirds of individuals with reflux symptoms have no evidence of esophageal damage by endoscopy.

DIAGNOSIS

When GERD presents with typical signs and symptoms, such as heartburn or acid regurgitation, that are responsive to antisecretory therapy, no diagnostic evaluation is warranted. Diagnostic endoscopy is warranted in individuals who fail to respond to therapy or have alarm symptoms or signs such as dysphagia (see Fig. 134-6 in Chapter 134), weight loss, anemia, gastrointestinal bleeding, or persistent heartburn (Fig. 140-2). Endoscopy permits the detection of erosive esophagitis and complications such as a peptic stricture (Fig. 140-3) and Barrett's esophagus (Fig. 140-4); mucosal biopsy, which is crucial in these settings, also excludes conditions that can mimic GERD, such as eosinophilic esophagitis. However, most patients have no mucosal damage seen on endoscopy, regardless of whether they are on or off antisecretory therapy.

Esophageal manometry is useful to exclude achalasia in patients with suggestive symptoms. Esophageal reflux testing by 24-hour transnasal pH monitoring, by 48-hour devices attached to the esophageal lumen, or by 24-hour combined impedance and pH monitoring, may be performed while patients are not on therapy to detect pathologic acid and nonacid reflux as well to correlate reflux events with atypical symptoms, especially in patients with normal endoscopies. Barium radiography has no role in the diagnostic evaluation of patients with reflux disease.

TREATMENT Rx

Although avoidance of foods or beverages that may provoke symptoms, such as alcohol, coffee, spicy foods, and late meals, makes physiologic sense, data from clinical trials to support these maneuvers are lacking. Similarly, elevation of the head of the bed for patients with nocturnal regurgitation or heartburn also is logical. Given the association of obesity and GERD symptoms, weight loss should be part of any treatment program for obese patients.

Inhibition of gastric acid secretion (Table 140-1) is the cornerstone of the acute treatment of GERD, and proton pump inhibitors (PPIs) are superior to histamine (H₂)-receptor antagonists for both the healing of esophagitis and the control of symptoms.[1] However, the healing of esophagitis is more predictable than improvement in heartburn symptoms, even with PPIs.[2] There are no major differences in treatment efficacy among the various PPIs, and once-daily dosing is adequate.

Given the chronicity of reflux symptoms, long-term maintenance therapy with PPIs is typically required, with dosing titrated to the lowest dose necessary to control symptoms. Data to support the use of PPIs in the management of extraesophageal GERD syndromes are weak, although selected patients may benefit. The safety profile of PPIs is excellent, but short-term adverse events such as headaches and diarrhea may occur. Recent epidemiologic studies suggest that long-term PPI use may be associated with an increased risk of *Clostridium difficile* infection, community-acquired pneumonia, hip fracture, and vitamin B₁₂ deficiency.

Although PPIs are superior to H₂-receptor antagonists for long-term maintenance therapy as well as for short-term relief, H₂-receptor antagonists are

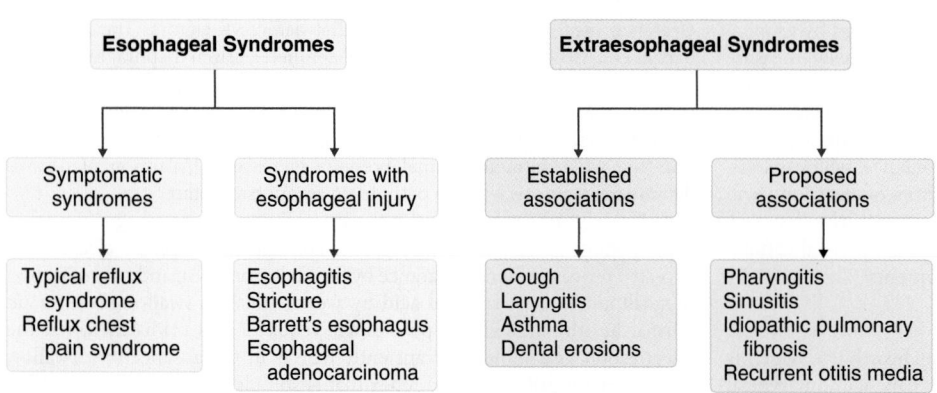

GERD is a condition that develops when the reflux of gastric content causes troublesome symptoms or complications

Esophageal Syndromes

- Symptomatic syndromes
  - Typical reflux syndrome
  - Reflux chest pain syndrome
- Syndromes with esophageal injury
  - Esophagitis
  - Stricture
  - Barrett's esophagus
  - Esophageal adenocarcinoma

Extraesophageal Syndromes

- Established associations
  - Cough
  - Laryngitis
  - Asthma
  - Dental erosions
- Proposed associations
  - Pharyngitis
  - Sinusitis
  - Idiopathic pulmonary fibrosis
  - Recurrent otitis media

FIGURE 140-1. Montreal classification of gastroesophageal reflux disease (GERD). (From Vakil N, van Zanten S, Kahrilas P, et al. The Montreal definition and classification of gastroesophageal reflux disease: a global evidence-based consensus. *Am J Gastroenterol.* 2006;101:1900-1920.)

Heartburn or Acid Regurgitation

↓

Alarm symptoms
Dysphagia
Weight loss

↓

Immediate endoscopy

Yes   No

Rational lifestyle changes
Avoid dietary excess
Avoid late meals
Weight loss if overweight

Not successful   Successful

Trial of antisecretory therapy
(PPIs superior to H₂RAs, which are superior to placebo)

Continue

No response to therapy
   Endoscopy
   If endoscopy negative, manometry
   If endoscopy and manometry negative,
   reflux testing
      pH
      pH/impedance
      Wireless pH

Response to therapy
   Titrate to lowest dose to
   control symptoms
   (see Table 140-1)

FIGURE 140-2. Algorithm for the management of heartburn or regurgitation symptoms. Surgery is indicated only for patients who are intolerant of antisecretory therapy or who have ongoing symptoms, especially regurgitataion if reflux is well documented. H₂RA = histamine-2 receptor antagonist; PPI = proton pump inhibitor. (Based on Kahrilas PJ, Shaheen NJ, Vaezi MF. American Gastroenterological Association Institute technical review on the management of gastroesophageal reflux disease. *Gastroenterology.* 2008;135:1392-1413.)

FIGURE 140-3. Barium radiograph of a peptic stricture. (Image courtesy of Marc Levine, MD.)

FIGURE 140-4. Endoscopic appearance of Barrett's esophagus. Note the white-appearing normal squamous mucosa displaced above the true end of the esophagus. The intervening mucosa appears salmon-pink.

TABLE 140-1   DRUG THERAPY FOR ESOPHAGEAL DISORDERS

AGENT	DOSE
ANTACIDS: LIQUID (TO BUFFER ACID AND INCREASE LESP)	
For example, Mylanta II/Maalox TC (acid-neutralizing capacity, 25 mEq/5 mL)*	15 mL qid 1 hour after meals and at bedtime or as needed
GAVISCON (TO DECREASE REFLUX VIA A VISCOUS MECHANICAL BARRIER AND BUFFER ACID)	
Al(OH)$_3$, NaHCO$_3$, Mg trisilicate, alginic acid	2-4 tablets qid at bedtime or as needed
H$_2$-RECEPTOR ANTAGONISTS (TO DECREASE ACID SECRETION)	
Cimetidine	800 mg bid, 400 mg qid, ≈13 mL bid
Ranitidine	150 mg qid or 10 mL qid; maintenance dose, 150 mg bid, 10 mL bid
Famotidine	20-40 mg bid or 2.5-5 mL bid
Nizatidine	150 mg bid
PROTON PUMP INHIBITORS (TO DECREASE ACID SECRETION AND GASTRIC VOLUME)†	
Omeprazole	20 mg/day; maintenance dose, 20 mg/day
Lansoprazole	30 mg/day; maintenance dose, 15 mg/day
Pantoprazole	40 mg/day; maintenance dose, 40 mg/day
Rabeprazole	20 mg/day; maintenance dose, 20 mg/day
Esomeprazole	20-40 mg/day; maintenance dose, 20 mg/day
Dexlansoprazole	30-60 mg/day; maintenance dose, 30 mg/day

*Patients with reflux are not generally hypersecretors of gastric acid, so the therapeutic doses of antacids are based on their capacity to buffer (normal) basal acid secretion rates of approximately 1 to 7 mEq/hr (mean, 2 mEq/hr) and peak meal-stimulated acid secretion rates of about 10 to 60 mEq/hr (mean, 30 mEq/hr).
†High-dose therapy is a twice-daily administration of the usually daily dose.
LESP = lower esophageal sphincter pressure.

superior to placebo, are useful in patients who are intolerant of PPIs, and can be used at bedtime[3] to supplement PPIs in patients who have persistent symptoms. No high-quality data exist to support the common practice of using metoclopramide as either monotherapy or an adjunct to acid suppression therapy[2]; furthermore, its significant adverse effects argue against the use of this drug in any GERD patients.

Antireflux surgery is an option for patients who have documented esophagitis and who are intolerant of PPIs or unresponsive to them. For the healing of esophagitis, laparoscopic fundoplication yields results comparable to continued PPI therapy.[4] However, surgery has a number of serious complications that may affect quality of life, including dysphagia, vagal nerve injury, gas bloat syndrome, and diarrhea. There are inadequate data to support any of the many proposed endoscopic approaches to GERD at present.

PROGNOSIS

Patients with GERD generally do well with conservative antireflux measures and PPI therapy. When surgery is required, the outcome is usually excellent.

Peptic Strictures

Esophageal strictures are a well-recognized complication of GERD, especially in older patients with long-standing reflux symptoms, but population-based studies suggest that the incidence of new and recurrent strictures is declining. Peptic strictures are thought to be a consequence of severe inflammation, which leads to fibrosis, scarring, esophageal shortening, and loss of compliance of the lumen.

CLINICAL MANIFESTATIONS AND DIAGNOSIS

Symptoms are typically dysphagia to solids with or without antecedent symptoms of heartburn or acid regurgitation. Strictures may be diagnosed by barium radiography or with upper endoscopy, but barium esophagrams (see Fig. 140-3) have a higher sensitivity for detecting subtle lesions, especially if

performed with a solid challenge such a barium-impregnated pill. However, peptic strictures must be distinguished from a wide variety of other causes of luminal narrowing, including pills, prior nasogastric tube intubation, neoplasia, infection, radiation, surgical anastomosis, systemic diseases, caustic substances, and extrinsic compression. As a result, endoscopic biopsy and cytology are critical for differentiating benign from malignant causes of strictures.

TREATMENT

Endoscopic dilation, which remains the cornerstone of therapy, should be done gradually to achieve a luminal diameter that is sufficiently large to relieve symptoms—typically a diameter of 13 mm or greater. After dilation is accomplished, patients should receive chronic PPI therapy (see Table 140-1). For recalcitrant peptic strictures, injection of triamcinolone into the stricture is superior to sham injection in patients who receive balloon dilation and postprocedure PPIs.[5]

PROGNOSIS

Endoscopic dilation will usually alleviate symptoms, but repetitive dilation is required in a significant minority of patients.

Barrett's Esophagus

Barrett's esophagus, which is an acquired condition that results from severe esophageal mucosal injury, is a metaplastic change in the lining of the distal tubular esophagus, where the normal squamous epithelium is replaced by columnar epithelium. Barrett's esophagus would be of little importance if not for its well-recognized association with adenocarcinoma of the esophagus (Chapter 198). However, the risk of cancer in an individual patient with Barrett's esophagus is low.

EPIDEMIOLOGY

It is estimated that Barrett's esophagus is found in approximately 5 to 15% of patients who undergo endoscopy for symptoms of GERD. Population-based studies suggest that the prevalence of Barrett's esophagus is approximately 1.3 to 1.6%, but about 45% of affected patients do not have reflux symptoms. Barrett's esophagus is predominantly a disease of middle-aged white men, but about 25% of patients are women or are less than 50 years of age. The prevalence of Barrett's esophagus increases until a plateau is reached between the seventh and ninth decades. Risk factors include frequent and long-standing reflux episodes, smoking, male gender, older age, and central male pattern obesity.

PATHOBIOLOGY

Barrett's esophagus results from severe esophageal mucosal injury. Patients who develop Barrett's esophagus typically have more esophageal acid exposure, based on 24-hour pH monitoring, and almost always have a hiatal hernia, which is typically longer and associated with larger defects than in patients without Barrett's. However, why some patients with GERD develop Barrett's esophagus whereas others do not remains unclear, as does the cell of origin of columnar metaplasia. Candidates include dedifferentiation of squamous epithelium into columnar epithelium or stimulation of stem cells from either the basal layer of the esophageal epithelium, the esophageal submucosal glands, or the bone marrow. The transcription factor CDX2, which can be induced by both acid and bile salts, appears to play a role in promoting the development of the columnar epithelium. A small subset of patients may have an inherited predisposition, perhaps with an autosomal dominant pattern.

CLINICAL MANIFESTATIONS

The development of reflux symptoms at an earlier age, an increased duration of reflux symptoms, an increased severity of nocturnal reflux symptoms, and prior complications of GERD such as esophagitis, ulceration, stricture, and bleeding may raise the likelihood of Barrett's esophagus. Nevertheless, patients with Barrett's esophagus are difficult to distinguish clinically from patients whose GERD is uncomplicated by a columnar-lined esophagus. Patients with Barrett's esophagus may paradoxically have impaired sensitivity to esophageal acid perfusion compared with patients with uncomplicated GERD.

DIAGNOSIS

Endoscopically, Barrett's esophagus is characterized by displacement of the squamocolumnar junction so that it is now proximal to the gastroesophageal junction, which is defined by the proximal margin of gastric folds (Fig. 140-4). The diagnosis of Barrett's esophagus is established if a biopsy determines that the squamocolumnar junction is displaced proximal to the gastroesophageal junction and if intestinal metaplasia, which is characterized in part by acid mucin-containing goblet cells, is detected.

The precise junction of the stomach and the esophagus may be difficult to determine endoscopically owing to the presence of a hiatal hernia, inflammation, and the dynamic nature of the gastroesophageal junction. If the squamocolumnar junction is above the level of the esophagogastric junction, as defined by the proximal margin of the gastric folds, biopsy specimens should be obtained for confirmation of columnar metaplasia.

Intestinal metaplasia may be seen in the cardia of normal individuals as well as in persons with chronic reflux disease, and the prevalence of intestinal metaplasia at a normal-appearing gastroesophageal junction varies from 5 to 36%. Dysplasia and an increased risk of carcinoma have been reported in patients who have intestinal metaplasia of the gastroesophageal junction or cardia, but the magnitude of that risk appears to be less than that of short-segment Barrett's esophagus.

TREATMENT Rx

Patients who are diagnosed with Barrett's esophagus require surveillance endoscopy at regular intervals (Fig. 140-5). They characteristically worry about cancer risk, which they typically overestimate, face higher life insurance premiums, and may receive conflicting information on how best to treat their condition.

PPIs (see Table 140-1), which are the cornerstone of medical therapy for Barrett's esophagus, consistently relieve symptoms and heal esophagitis. However, PPIs, even at high doses, provide no more than modest regression of Barrett's histology, perhaps because alleviation of reflux symptoms is not necessarily equivalent to normalization of esophageal acid exposure. In fact, abnormal acid exposure persists in approximately 25% of Barrett's esophagus patients despite twice-daily PPIs. The importance of complete control of esophageal acid exposure in patients with Barrett's esophagus remains unknown. Antireflux surgery also effectively alleviates GERD symptoms in these patients, and the indications for surgery are the same as those for patients with GERD without Barrett's esophagus. Surgery should not, however, be viewed as a cancer prevention tool.

Current practice guidelines, based on observational data, recommend endoscopic surveillance of patients with documented Barrett's esophagus in an attempt to detect dysplasia and cancer at an early and potentially curable stage. Before entering into a surveillance program, patients should be advised about risks and benefits, including the limitations of surveillance endoscopy as well as the importance of adhering to appropriate surveillance intervals. Other considerations include age, likelihood of survival over the next 5 years, and ability to tolerate either endoscopic or surgical interventions for early esophageal adenocarcinoma.

Systematic four-quadrant biopsies should be obtained at 2-cm intervals along the entire length of the Barrett's segment after inflammation related to GERD is controlled with antisecretory therapy. Mucosal abnormalities, especially in the setting of high-grade dysplasia, should be resected endoscopically. Surveillance intervals, determined by the presence and grade of dysplasia, are based on a limited understanding of the biology of esophageal adenocarcinoma. Surveillance initially should be annual in patients with metaplasia, but surveillance every 3 years is adequate after two negative examinations. If low-grade dysplasia is found, the diagnosis should be confirmed by an expert gastrointestinal pathologist because of the marked interobserver variability in the interpretation of these biopsies. If confirmed, aggressive PPI therapy (see Table 140-1) is recommended to decrease inflammation and regeneration, which may make pathologic interpretation difficult. A repeat endoscopy

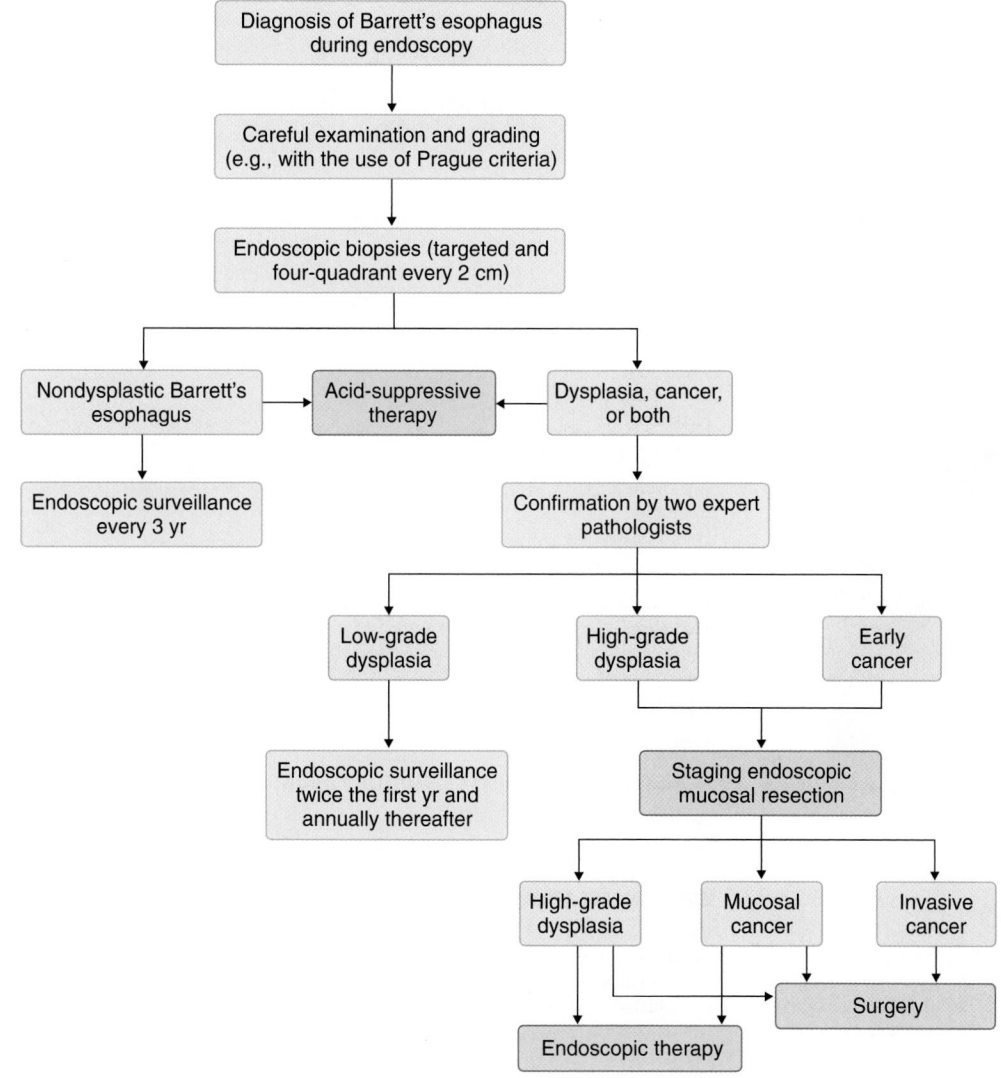

FIGURE 140-5. Proposed treatment algorithm for patients with Barrett's esophagus. (From Sharma P. Barrett's esophagus. *N Engl J Med.* 2009;361:2548-2556, Fig. 3).

should then be performed within 6 months of the initial diagnosis. If low-grade dysplasia is confirmed, annual surveillance is recommended until two consecutive examinations are negative for dysplasia.

If high-grade dysplasia is found, the diagnosis should be confirmed by an experienced gastrointestinal pathologist. Treatment options include continued surveillance, endoscopic therapy by a variety of different methods, or esophagectomy. Factors to consider include the available surgical and endoscopic expertise, age, length of Barrett's epithelium that would require biopsy to eliminate sampling error, compliance with endoscopic surveillance, future need for multiple surveillance endoscopies, and suspicious lesions such as plaque, nodules, and strictures. Currently, endoscopic mucosal resection and radiofrequency ablation[6] are the most promising of the endoscopic methods.

PROGNOSIS

The risk that a patient with Barrett's esophagus will develop esophageal adenocarcinoma is approximately 0.5% to 0.7% annually. These data also emphasize that most patients with Barrett's esophagus will never develop esophageal cancer.

● ESOPHAGITIS
Eosinophilic Esophagitis

Eosinophilic esophagitis is probably caused by an aberrant immune or antigenic response to food and aeroallergens that trigger chronic inflammation in the esophageal mucosa. The disease is most common in children and adolescents, but adults are commonly affected as well. Patients often have a personal and family history of other allergic disorders. A genetic predisposition is suggested by the finding of an abnormal eotaxin gene in almost 50% of children with this disorder.

CLINICAL MANIFESTATIONS AND DIAGNOSIS

Children present with dyspeptic symptoms, whereas adults classically present with solid food dysphagia, food impaction, or chest pain. Diagnosis is made by classic findings on endoscopy, such as linear furrowing and multiple rings (Fig. 140-6), accompanied by biopsies demonstrating eosinophilic infiltration (Table 140-2).

FIGURE 140-6. Endoscopic corrugated (ringed) appearance of esophagus in eosinophilic esophagitis.

TABLE 140-2	GUIDELINES FOR DIAGNOSIS OF EOSINOPHILIC ESOPHAGITIS

Clinical symptoms of esophageal dysfunction
>15 Eosinophils in 1 high-power field
Lack of responsiveness to high-dose proton pump inhibition (see Table 140-1) or normal pH monitoring of the distal esophagus

TREATMENT AND PROGNOSIS   Rx

Treatment is a 2-month course of topical steroids, such as swallowed fluticasone (440-880 μg twice daily) or budesonide suspension (1 mg twice daily, for 15 days, followed by 0.25 mg twice daily)[7] or occasionally a 1-month course of systemic steroids (e.g., prednisone, starting at 40 mg and then tapering). Patients also should undergo a formal allergy evaluation (Chapter 257) to determine whether any food trigger can be identified and avoided. Another option is an empirical six-food elimination diet that eliminates cow's milk protein (casein), soy, wheat, egg, peanut/tree nuts, and seafood. Most patients do well after treatment.

Pill-Induced Esophagitis

Pills (Table 140-3) can induce esophageal injury by producing a caustic acid solution (e.g., ascorbic acid and ferrous sulfate), producing a caustic alkaline solution (e.g., alendronate, button batteries), placing a hyperosmolar solution in contact with the esophageal mucosa (e.g., potassium chloride), or causing direct drug toxicity to the esophageal mucosa (e.g., tetracycline). Because prolonged contact is an essential part of the injury, predisposing factors for pill-induced injury include anatomic barriers, such as a stricture, a prominent aortic arch that compresses the esophagus, or improper ingestion of the pill because of inadequate fluid or improper positioning (i.e., lying down directly after taking the pill). The most common medications are tetracycline and its derivatives, but other commonly implicated medications include nonsteroidal anti-inflammatory drugs (NSAIDs), bisphosphonates, ferrous sulfate, quinidine, and potassium chloride.

Patients usually complain of the acute onset of severe odynophagia. Radiographic or endoscopic findings may range from a discrete ulceration to diffuse esophagitis. Treatment is generally supportive with discontinuation of the medication until the injury resolves. Although acid suppression is commonly recommended, there is no proven evidence for its benefit. Patients should be given careful instructions to avoid lying down immediately after ingesting

TABLE 140-3	MEDICATIONS COMMONLY ASSOCIATED WITH ESOPHAGITIS OR ESOPHAGEAL INJURY

ANTIBIOTICS

Tetracycline
Doxycycline
Clindamycin
Penicillin
Rifampin

ANTIVIRAL AGENTS

Zalcitabine
Zidovudine
Nelfinavir

BISPHOSPHONATES

Alendronate
Etidronate
Pamidronate

CHEMOTHERAPEUTIC AGENTS

Dactinomycin
Bleomycin
Cytarabine
Daunorubicin
5-Fluorouracil
Methotrexate
Vincristine

NONSTEROIDAL ANTI-INFLAMMATORY DRUGS

Aspirin
Naproxen
Ibuprofen

OTHER MEDICATIONS

Quinidine
Potassium chloride
Ferrous sulfate
Ascorbic acid
Multivitamins
Theophylline

medication and to drink adequate fluids helps prevent injury. Rarely, pill-induced injury may lead to strictures and even fistulas.

Caustic Injury

Potentially devastating caustic esophageal injuries may be caused by highly alkaline solutions, such as sodium hydroxide, or highly acidic solutions, such as sulfuric acid. The most common products that contain these substances are drain cleaners and industrial strength cleaners, but other corrosive substances include hair relaxers, oven and toilet bowl cleaners, and button batteries. Patients require emergent endoscopy to determine the degree of injury, which helps predict long-term prognosis. No clear evidence supports routine steroids or antibiotics. Many patients will have lifelong disease marked by chronic strictures that require frequent dilation and even esophageal reconstruction. In patients with a severe initial injury, the risk of esophageal cancer is significantly increased.

● ESOPHAGEAL MOTOR DISORDERS
Oropharyngeal Dysfunction

The cricopharyngeus and inferior pharyngeal constrictor are composed of striated muscle and innervated by upper motor neurons, the brain stem, and the cerebral cortex. Both primary myopathic and neuropathic disorders can result in dysfunction. The most common neurologic cause of oropharyngeal dysphagia is a cerebrovascular accident (Chapter 414). Other neuropathic disorders that may also affect function include myasthenia gravis (Chapter 430), brain stem tumors (Chapter 195), amyotrophic lateral sclerosis (Chapter 418), Parkinson's disease (Chapter 416), Alzheimer's disease (Chapter 409), postpolio syndrome (Chapter 423), Guillain-Barré syndrome (Chapter 428), and botulism (Chapter 304). Myogenic disorders that cause dysfunction include paraneoplastic antibody-mediated syndromes (Chapter 187), thyroid disease (Chapter 233), primary myopathies (Chapter 429) such as dermatomyositis, and drugs that cause myopathy such as statins and amiodarone.

Patients with oropharyngeal abnormalities experience dysphagia, often accompanied by postprandial coughing, hoarseness, and aspiration pneumonia. Treatment focuses on the underlying myopathic or neurologic cause, but prognosis is often poor owing to limited treatment options.

Achalasia

Achalasia, which is the prototypic esophageal motility disorder, is characterized by a hypertensive lower esophageal sphincter with incomplete relaxation upon swallowing, accompanied by aperistalsis of the esophageal body.

EPIDEMIOLOGY AND PATHOBIOLOGY

Achalasia can occur in patients of almost any age, from infants to nonagenarians, but it most commonly presents between 25 and 60 years of age. The prevalence is 10 per 100,000 in the United States, with all races affected and an equal distribution in men and women. The pathophysiology of achalasia most likely reflects an antibody-mediated autoimmune myenteric plexopathy in the lower esophageal sphincter and a generalized neuropathy in the esophageal body. The triggering event is unclear, but a viral cause is suggested. Injury to the lower esophageal sphincter neurons leads to a relative selective deficiency of nitric oxide. With this loss of the main functional inhibitory neurotransmitter, the sphincter becomes hypertensive and loses its ability to relax. The neurochemical process that leads to aperistalsis is unclear.

CLINICAL MANIFESTATIONS AND DIAGNOSIS

The cardinal symptoms of achalasia are dysphagia to both liquids and solids, regurgitation, and chest pain. Some patients may have more subtle symptoms, including heartburn, presumably caused by esophageal stasis of acidic food content, weight loss, and aspiration pneumonia; in these settings, diagnosis is often delayed.

The diagnosis of achalasia relies on esophageal manometry and barium radiography. The classic radiographic appearance is esophageal dilation, stasis of contrast material, and a "bird's beak" appearance to the lower esophageal sphincter (Fig. 140-7). Manometry demonstrates high residual pressures of the lower esophageal sphincter and either simultaneous contractions or complete absence of peristaltic contractions. Endoscopy is recommended to exclude secondary causes of achalasia, such as cancer of the gastroesophageal junction. Occasional patients present with a massively dilated esophagus and marked persistent food retention. Radiographically, these patients develop a "sigmoid" esophagus with a radiographic picture similar to a sigmoid colon.

FIGURE 140-7. **Esophagogram of a patient with idiopathic achalasia.** Note the dilated esophagus with an air-fluid level and distal tapering providing a "bird's beak" deformity in the area of the lower esophageal sphincter. (From Feldman M, Friedman LS, Sleisenger MH, eds. *Sleisenger and Fordtran's Gastrointestinal and Liver Disease: Pathophysiology, Diagnosis, Management,* 7th ed. Philadelphia: Saunders; 2002.)

Achalasia may represent a paraneoplastic presentation of some malignancies, particularly small cell carcinoma of the lung (Chapter 197); in these patients, the tumor produces an antineuronal antibody (anti-Hu) that mediates the autoimmune lower esophageal sphincter plexopathy and produces a syndrome identical to primary achalasia. Some tumors, such as proximal gastric cancer, may also metastasize to or directly extend into the lower esophageal sphincter and produce an achalasia-like picture, possibly owing to extrinsic compression or tumor infiltration.

TREATMENT Rx

Treatment options to decrease the functional obstruction at the level of the lower esophageal sphincter include the intrasphincteric injection of botulinum toxin, pneumatic dilation, and cardiomyotomy. Injection of botulinum toxin during endoscopy reduces symptoms and improves esophageal emptying in up to 90% of patients.⑧ Because symptoms typically recur within 1 to 2 years, this treatment is best for patients who are not candidates for more definitive therapies or to confirm the diagnosis of achalasia when clinical, radiographic, and manometric criteria are not conclusive.

In pneumatic dilation, a 30- to 40-mm pneumatic balloon is placed fluoroscopically to straddle the lower esophageal sphincter; the balloon is then inflated to tear the muscle fibers of the lower esophageal sphincter. In general, one dilation will achieve 5 years of symptomatic remission in 40% of patients, and three dilations will succeed in 90% of patients. The downside of this procedure is the risk of perforation, which occurs in up to 5% of patients.

The third approach is a Heller myotomy, which is now typically performed laparoscopically. This long myotomy starts at least 2 cm below the lower esophageal sphincter and extends for about 6 cm upward past the sphincter; a loose fundoplication is performed to prevent gastroesophageal reflux. The 5-year success rate approaches 90%.

In patients with massive dilation, esophageal dysfunction may warrant total esophagectomy because of life-threatening symptoms such as continued weight loss, recurrent aspiration pneumonia, or tracheal compression. In patients with underlying malignancy, treatment of the tumor may be helpful, and botulinum toxin has been tried with anecdotal success.

PROGNOSIS

No treatment approach is curative, and all are palliative. Recurrent symptoms may be related to an incomplete myotomy, herniation or unwrapping of the fundoplication, esophageal strictures, Barrett's esophagus, or just the natural history of the disease. Achalasia patients may also be predisposed to squamous cell carcinoma of the esophagus, and some recommend yearly screening for patients who have a chronically large dilated esophagus.

Diffuse Esophageal Spasm

Diffuse esophageal spasm is found in less than 5% of patients who undergo manometry for symptoms of chest pain, dysphagia, or both. The pathophysiology of diffuse esophageal spasm is not well understood, but a deficiency of nitric oxide in the esophageal body may lead to a loss of control of esophageal peristalsis, high pressures, and rapid velocity contractions.

CLINICAL MANIFESTATIONS AND DIAGNOSIS

Classically, patients have symptoms of intermittent chest pain (Chapter 139), dysphagia, or both. On endoscopic ultrasound, patients may demonstrate thickening of the circular and longitudinal muscle layers. Diffuse esophageal spasm is defined manometrically by simultaneous contractions in at least 20% of all swallows, accompanied by normal peristalsis. Other manometric features include repetitive contractions, high-amplitude contractions with multiple peaks, and variable relaxation of the lower esophageal sphincter. Radiographically, diffuse esophageal spasm is characterized by a "corkscrew" esophagus with multiple simultaneous contractions that obliterate the lumen (Fig. 140-8).

TREATMENT AND PROGNOSIS   Rx

Treatment of these patients is challenging, and clinical trials have not demonstrated efficacy of any therapy. Empirical therapy may be tried with agents that relax smooth muscle or augment the nitric oxide content, such as hyoscyamine (0.125 mg sublingually), calcium-channel antagonists (nifedipine, 10 mg sublingually), nitroglycerin (0.3 mg sublingually), and sildenafil (50 mg orally). Injection of botulinum toxin into the esophageal body has had equivocal results. Antidepressants, particularly low-dose tricyclics (e.g., imipramine, 10 to 50 mg before bedtime), have had some success. For patients with dysphagia, sphincter options include botulinum toxin injection and pneumatic dilation, but surgery is not indicated unless there is evidence of achalasia. In general, these disorders can be difficult to manage but are not life-threatening.

Other Motility Disorders

Nutcracker esophagus, which is a manometric diagnosis characterized by high-amplitude contractions, likely represents a manometric epiphenomenon of little clinical significance. Antisecretory therapy with PPIs (see Table 140-1) is often warranted.

A hypertensive lower esophageal sphincter is of unknown significance, but isolated incomplete relaxation of the lower esophageal sphincter may represent an achalasia variant and should be treated as such. Patients with manometric findings of low-amplitude contractions, failed contractions, or prolonged nonpropagated contractions have hypotensive peristalsis, which is typically seen in patients with severe underlying GERD.

● STRUCTURAL ABNORMALITIES

Cricopharyngeal Bars

A cricopharyngeal bar, which is caused by a prominent impression of the cricopharyngeus, reflects an inability to relax the upper esophageal sphincter maximally during the flow of barium, with a sustained increase in pressure. The decrease in cross-sectional area of the upper esophageal sphincter is likely caused by fibrosis. This condition may be asymptomatic or accompanied by symptoms of oropharyngeal dysphagia to solids. Treatment of symptomatic patients is usually surgical, and the response is generally excellent.

Esophageal Diverticula

Esophageal diverticula are encountered in less than 1% of upper gastrointestinal radiographic studies and account for less than 5% of cases of dysphagia. Esophageal diverticula may occur in one of three locations: above the upper esophageal sphincter, in the mid-esophagus, and just above the lower esophageal sphincter.

Zenker's diverticulum is a pouch that protrudes posteriorly above the upper esophageal sphincter (Fig. 140-9). This protrusion occurs through a triangular region known as Killian's triangle, which is bordered above by fibers of the inferior constrictor muscle and below by the cricopharyngeal muscle. It is thought to be caused by increased hypopharyngeal pressure that results from decreased compliance and impaired opening of the upper esophageal sphincter. Small diverticula may be asymptomatic, but increasing size is associated with such symptoms as globus, dysphagia to solids or liquids, regurgitation of undigested food, halitosis, and aspiration. Although no treatment is needed for asymptomatic patients, open or endoscopic surgery is indicated when symptoms occur. Prognosis after surgery is excellent.

Mid-esophageal diverticula, which are focal outpouchings of the middle of the esophagus, are thought to be related to an underlying abnormality of esophageal motility. Symptoms typically include dysphagia with or without regurgitation, and diagnosis is usually made with barium contrast radiography. Surgical diverticulectomy with myotomy is reserved for patients with symptoms.

Epiphrenic diverticula are herniations of mucosa and submucosa through the muscular layers of the distal 10 cm of the esophagus. They may be caused by functional obstruction, owing to underlying motility abnormalities, such as achalasia or diffuse esophageal spasm, or a mechanical obstruction, owing to a leiomyoma, prior surgery, stenosis, stricture tumor, or web. Epiphrenic diverticula may be asymptomatic or cause dysphagia, regurgitation,

FIGURE 140-8. Barium esophagogram showing a "corkscrew" esophagus in a patient with diffuse esophageal spasm. The patient had dysphagia, chest pain, and normal endoscopic findings. (From Feldman M, ed. *Gastroenterology and Hepatology: The Comprehensive Visual Reference,* New York: Churchill Livingstone; 1997.)

FIGURE 140-9. Barium radiograph of Zenker's diverticulum *(arrow).* (From Feldman M, ed. *Gastroenterology and Hepatology: The Comprehensive Visual Reference,* New York: Churchill Livingstone; 1997.)

odynophagia, chest pain, heartburn, or aspiration. Diagnosis is typically made by barium radiography (Fig. 140-10), but endoscopy is recommended to exclude a structural cause of obstruction, and esophageal manometry is recommended to evaluate for underlying motility abnormalities. No therapy is warranted in asymptomatic patients, but symptomatic patients generally do well with surgical diverticulectomy, repair of the defect in the esophageal wall, and relief of the underling obstruction, usually with a myotomy and partial fundoplication.

Rings and Webs

Esophageal rings are concentric areas of narrowing, usually in the distal esophagus. *Schatzki's ring* (Fig. 140-11) is a thin, fixed, circumferential membrane-like narrowing at the gastroesophageal junction, typically at the proximal border of a hiatal hernia. The cause may be congenital, secondary to a pleat of redundant mucosa, or related to gastroesophageal reflux. Symptoms typically occur if the ring results in a lumen that is 13 mm or less in diameter. Classic symptoms are intermittent dysphagia to solids or impaction of solid food. Diagnosis is best accomplished with barium radiography, especially for rings larger than 13 mm in diameter, which may be missed at the time of endoscopy. Treatment involves use of large caliber dilators at least

18 mm in diameter, and long-term therapy with PPIs (see Table 140-1) may prevent relapses. Most patients relapse after a single dilation.

Muscular rings, which are located several centimeters above the squamocolumnar junction, are composed of mucosa, submucosa, and muscle. Barium radiography and endoscopy reveal a focal constriction of variable diameter. Optimal therapy is unclear. Dilation leads to only partial or temporary relief. Other treatment modalities include injection of botulinum toxin and anticholinergic agents.

Esophageal webs are thin, eccentric, membranous areas of narrowing that may be found anywhere in the esophagus but most commonly are in the proximal region (Fig. 140-12). The pathogenesis of webs is unknown, but they are associated with a number of systemic diseases, including bullous skin disorders, chronic graft-versus-host disease, and iron deficiency anemia.

Hiatal Hernia

A hiatal hernia involves herniation of elements of the abdominal cavity through the diaphragmatic hiatus. A sliding, or type I hernia, in which the gastroesophageal junction is displaced above the diaphragmatic hiatus, is the most common type. Type I hiatal hernias are typically asymptomatic or present with symptoms of heartburn or acid regurgitation. Treatment is as for GERD (see earlier).

In a type II or true paraesophageal hernia, which is uncommon, the gastroesophageal junction is in its normal location, but the fundus and parts of the greater curvature of the stomach herniate into the mediastinum alongside the esophagus. With type III or mixed paraesophageal hernia, the gastroesophageal junction and a large part of the stomach herniate into the mediastinum. Both types of paraesophageal hernias present with symptoms of postprandial distress, such as epigastric pain, chest pain, substernal fullness, shortness of breath, nausea, or vomiting. Iron deficiency anemia may be seen with large hiatal hernias in which at least one third of the stomach is in the chest; linear gastric erosions at the top of gastric folds at the level of the diaphragm have been implicated as a cause of chronic blood loss. Asymptomatic paraesophageal hernias do not require surgery. Symptomatic paraesophageal hernias warrant surgical therapy because of the risk of strangulation, bleeding, perforation, or obstruction.

⬤ THE ESOPHAGUS IN SYSTEMIC DISEASES
Scleroderma

Up to 90% of patients with scleroderma (Chapter 275) have esophageal involvement, thereby making it the most common gastrointestinal abnormality in the disease. The classic manometric and radiologic findings are aperistalsis of the distal two thirds of the esophagus, initially because of neuropathy and later because of the myopathy. The main clinical manifestation is severe gastroesophageal reflux that may cause Barrett's esophagus in up to 20% of patients and often causes esophageal strictures. Delayed gastric emptying

FIGURE 140-10. Barium radiograph of an esophageal epiphrenic diverticulum. (Image courtesy of Marc Levine, MD.)

FIGURE 140-11. Barium radiograph of Schatzki's ring. (From Feldman M, ed. *Gastroenterology and Hepatology: The Comprehensive Visual Reference.* New York: Churchill Livingstone; 1997.)

FIGURE 140-12. Barium radiograph of an esophageal web. (Image courtesy of Marc Levine, MD.)

may also occur. Marked esophageal stasis may also lead to candidal esophagitis. The diagnosis is confirmed by a patulous (on radiography) or hypotensive (on manometry) lower esophageal sphincter. PPI therapy (see Table 140-1) is the cornerstone of treatment. Lifestyle changes, including small frequent meals and avoiding nighttime meals, may reduce the gastric symptoms. Antireflux surgery can exacerbate dysphagia by creating a functional high-pressure zone in the distal esophagus and is thus contraindicated. Unfortunately, many patients suffer from chronic GERD and are at risk of developing Barrett's esophagus, recurrent strictures, and adenocarcinoma.

Amyloidosis

Amyloidosis (Chapter 194) may lead to smooth muscle and autonomic nervous system dysfunction that involves the esophagus in a pattern similar to scleroderma. Patients will have both dysphagia and severe reflux because of esophageal aperistalsis and a hypotensive lower esophageal sphincter. Dysphagia may result not only from the motility changes but also from diffuse esophageal rigidity and loss of compliance owing to amyloid infiltration of the esophageal wall. Rarely, an achalasia-like pattern may develop. No treatment improves the esophageal manifestations of amyloidosis, other than treatment for the underlying disease and high-dose PPIs given twice daily.

Other Systemic Diseases

Dermatomyositis (Chapter 277) principally involves the striated muscle of the oropharynx and proximal esophagus, but sometimes the distal esophagus may lose normal peristaltic function. Symptoms can be oropharyngeal or esophageal depending on the site of greatest muscular involvement. Dysphagia may be an early presenting symptom of dermatomyositis, and the esophagus may be involved in 10 to 50% of patients. Treatment is directed at the generalized myositis because there are no specific treatments for the esophagus. Swallowing therapy may sometimes be helpful. Return of swallowing commonly lags behind recovery of other striated muscle symptoms.

Esophageal involvement in *systemic lupus erythematosus* (Chapter 274) is not as prominent as in scleroderma, dermatomyositis, or mixed connective tissue disease. Dysphagia occurs in less than 15% of patients and may be caused by decreased salivation from secondary Sjögren's syndrome or reduced esophageal peristalsis. Other causes of esophageal symptoms in patients with systemic lupus erythematosus include GERD, esophageal ulcers, esophageal infection, and medication-induced esophagitis. *Behçet's disease* (Chapter 278) causes esophageal ulcers in less than 15% of affected patients. Ulcers are typically located in the middle third of the esophagus and are often associated with ulcers in the stomach, ileum, or colon. Rare esophageal lesions include strictures, varices, and fistulas connecting with the trachea. These complications can be severely debilitating.

Esophageal involvement in *Crohn's disease* (Chapter 143) is uncommon but has been described in up to 1 to 2% of patients. Occasionally, isolated esophageal disease may occur. Ulceration is the most common manifestation, but strictures, fissures, esophagobronchial fistulas, mediastinal abscesses, and aphthoid lesions have been described. Patients typically complain of dysphagia and odynophagia. Treatment and prognosis are as for the underlying Crohn's disease.

In the *Ehlers-Danlos syndrome* (Chapter 268), hiatal hernias are common, and structural esophageal defects, such as giant epiphrenic diverticula, megaesophagus, and spontaneous esophageal rupture may also be seen.

Skin Disorders that Involve the Esophagus

Lichen planus (Chapter 446) involves the esophagus. Patients generally present in the fourth to seventh decade of life. Histologically, the lesions in up to 25 to 50% of patients show a characteristic lymphohistiocytic inflammatory infiltrate and apoptotic basal keratinocytes. Lesions classically occur on the buccal mucosa and the tongue, but the disease may also involve other areas of the oral cavity and the esophagus, conjunctiva, nose, larynx, stomach, bladder, and anus. Most patients are asymptomatic or have only minor symptoms, but patients with severe esophageal lichen planus often develop strictures and may present with dysphagia, odynophagia, and weight loss. Strictures are typically proximal but may be variable in length, sometimes involving most of the esophageal body. Rare patients may present with esophageal lichen planus in the absence of extraesophageal disease. Endoscopic findings, which can be subtle and nonspecific, include peeling mucosa, hyperemic focal abnormalities, and submucosal plaque or papules. High-dose systemic steroids, starting with at least 40 mg prednisone and then tapering over 1 to 2 months, are often successful, but relapse is common when steroids are tapered. Dilation and intralesional steroids can alleviate the

symptoms associated with strictures, but symptoms frequently recur in less than a year and necessitate repeat dilations. The esophageal lesions of lichen planus may have malignant potential.

Pemphigus vulgaris (Chapter 447) patients who experience acute flares may have upper gastrointestinal symptoms (dysphagia, odynophagia, or retrosternal burning) in 80% of cases and biopsy-proven esophageal pemphigus lesions in nearly 50% of cases. Pemphigus vulgaris may rarely be isolated to the esophagus. Paraneoplastic pemphigus (Chapter 447), most commonly reported with lymphoreticular disease, also may involve the esophagus. Like lesions on the skin, esophageal lesions may be flaccid blisters or erosions, but they may also appear as red longitudinal lines along the entire esophagus. Like cutaneous and oral pemphigus, esophageal pemphigus is generally treated with corticosteroids.

In *mucous membrane pemphigoid* (cicatricial pemphigoid, Chapter 447), the esophagus is the most common site of gastrointestinal involvement, but esophageal disease occurs in less than 15% of patients. The esophageal disease can present as many as 10 years after disease onset and may be the only presentation of the disease. Patients complain of dysphagia and odynophagia. Imaging typically shows erosions, strictures, bullae, or webs. Treatment generally is as for the skin disease.

In *dystrophic epidermolysis bullosa* (Chapter 447), approximately 70 to 95% of patients develop esophageal stenosis or strictures. Strictures are especially common in children with recessive dystrophic epidermolysis bullosa, whereas fewer than 10% of patients with dominant dystrophic epidermolysis bullosa develop strictures by age 50 years.

● ESOPHAGEAL INFECTIONS

Herpes Simplex Virus

Herpes simplex virus (HSV; Chapter 382) esophagitis, which is usually caused by HSV-1, is a well-recognized disease in immunocompromised patients but may also occur in immunocompetent hosts. HSV typically presents as severe odynophagia. Endoscopy and radiology characteristically demonstrate multiple ulcers and friable mucosa, predominantly involving the distal esophagus. Mucosal biopsies demonstrate typical intranuclear inclusion bodies. Depending on the severity of the esophageal disease and the underlying health of the patient, treatment options may include intravenous acyclovir, 5 mg/kg every 8 hours for 7 days, or oral acyclovir, 800 mg five times daily for 7 days, combined with symptomatic treatment.

Candidiasis

Esophageal candidiasis is common in patients with HIV infection or with impaired cellular immunity owing to hematologic malignancies, immunosuppressive therapy, or diabetes mellitus. Esophageal candidiasis is also occasionally seen in immunocompetent patients with marked esophageal stasis, such as patients with advanced achalasia or scleroderma. Esophageal candidiasis characteristically presents with symptoms of odynophagia, dysphagia, and chest pain. Endoscopy demonstrates scattered or coalescent yellowwhite mucosal plaques (Fig. 140-13). Given the high prevalence of esophageal candidiasis in HIV patients, some recommend treating symptomatic HIV patients empirically and reserving endoscopy for refractory symptoms. Mild oropharyngeal candidiasis may be treated with topical clotrimazole (10 mg troche five times daily for 7 to 14 days) or nystatin (600,000 units four times daily for 7 to 10 days), whereas oral fluconazole (100 mg daily for 7 to 14 days) is needed for moderate to severe oropharyngeal and esophageal candidiasis. Intravenous fluconazole or amphotericin B deoxycholate (Chapter 339) are appropriate options for severe esophageal candidiasis or for patients who cannot tolerate oral therapy.

Cytomegalovirus

Cytomegalovirus (CMV) infection of the esophagus is exclusively found in immunocompromised patients. Patients infected with the HIV virus with low CD4 counts are most commonly affected, but CMV also occurs in transplant recipients on immunosuppressive therapy and in immunosuppressed patients with malignancy. Patients typically have severe odynophagia with evidence of radiographic or endoscopic esophageal ulcers. Treatment is usually with intravenous ganciclovir (5 mg/kg once or twice daily for 10 to 14 days) or foscarnet (90 mg/kg every 8 to 12 hours until healing occurs).

Bacterial Esophagitis

Bacterial infection of the esophagus is uncommon but can occur in immunosuppressed patients, typically those with neutropenia and malignancy.

FIGURE 140-13. Candidal esophagitis.

Patients present with chest pain or odynophagia, or both, and endoscopy reveals extensive erosions, usually in the distal esophagus. Biopsy and Gram stain reveal acute and chronic inflammation and bacteria, commonly gram-positive organisms, especially Viridans-group streptococci, *Staphylococcus aureus*, *Staphylococcus epidermidis*, and *Bacillus* species. Treatment is with the appropriate antibiotics administered parenterally.

Human Papillomavirus

Esophageal infections with HPV are typically asymptomatic. HPV lesions are most frequently found in the mid to distal esophagus as erythematous macules, white plaque, nodules, or exuberant frondlike lesions. The diagnosis is made by histologic demonstration of koilocytosis (an atypical nucleus surrounded by a ring), giant cells, or immunohistochemical stains. Treatment is usually not necessary, although large lesions may require endoscopic removal. Other treatments, such as interferon, bleomycin, and etoposide, have yielded varying results. HPV infection is a risk factor for esophageal squamous cell carcinoma, but the value of endoscopic surveillance is not known.

● MISCELLANENOUS ESOPHAGEAL CONDITIONS

Esophageal Emergencies

BOERHAAVE'S SYNDROME

Boerhaave's syndrome, or spontaneous rupture of the esophagus, is a transmural full-thickness tear of the esophageal wall. A sudden rise in intraesophageal pressure during forceful vomiting is the cause in most cases. The tear is most commonly in the lower third of the esophagus, 2 to 3 cm proximal to the gastroesophageal junction.

CLINICAL MANIFESTATIONS AND DIAGNOSIS

The classic presentation is vomiting, lower thoracic pain, and subcutaneous emphysema. Other findings may include pleural effusions, especially left sided, tachypnea, abdominal rigidity, fever, and hypotension. Because the condition is rare and classic antecedent vomiting is not always reported, rupture is often recognized only after the development of mediastinitis.

The chest radiograph may demonstrate mediastinal widening, a unilateral pleural effusion, hydropneumothorax, and pneumomediastinum. The esophagram, typically with a water-soluble agent, reveals extravasation, although false-negative results may be encountered. Computed tomography (CT) scanning with an oral contrast agent, which is perhaps the best diagnostic option, typically demonstrates air in the mediastinum.

TREATMENT AND PROGNOSIS **Rx**

Successful therapy depends on early recognition and the underlying condition of the patient. The classic approach is operative repair in conjunction with broad-spectrum antibiotics and nutritional support, especially if the diagnosis is made within the first 24 hours. Aggressive conservative therapy with percutaneous drains, broad-spectrum parenteral antibiotics, and nutrition has also been successful. In selected individuals, endoscopic insertion of self-expanding covered metallic stents is an option. The mortality rate can be as high as 100% without treatment.

MALLORY-WEISS TEAR

A Mallory-Weiss tear (see Fig. 137-2 in Chapter 137) is a mucosal tear, often at the gastroesophageal junction, usually caused by severe vomiting or retching. The syndrome is more common in alcoholic patients. In about 85% of patients, it is associated with acute upper gastrointestinal bleeding, which requires transfusion in about 70% of patients and urgent intervention in about 10% of cases (Chapter 137). Most tears heal spontaneously within about 48 hours.

IATROGENIC PERFORATION

Esophageal perforation may occur as a result of a variety of iatrogenic causes, including endoscopy, dilation, endosonography, or surgery as well as with foreign body ingestion. Typical symptoms include chest pain with or without abdominal pain, subcutaneous emphysema, and fever. Diagnosis may be made immediately at the time of endoscopy or radiography. Chest radiographs may show pneumomediastinum, subcutaneous emphysema, hydrothorax, or hydropneumothorax. A Gastrografin swallow may show a leak, and chest CT may show mediastinal air. Acute perforations are life-threatening emergencies that warrant immediate closure before contamination of the mediastinum. For acute perforation caused by endoscopy, endoscopic clips or stents are an option. Conservative therapy also is an option for well-contained perforations with minimal mediastinal, pleural, or peritoneal contamination and no obvious signs of sepsis. Prognosis is generally good if the perforation is recognized and treated early, preferably within 12 to 24 hours.

FOREIGN BODIES

Impaction of food or foreign bodies is a common gastrointestinal emergency. Meat impaction is most commonly seen in adults, but other foreign objects that also may be ingested accidentally or by design include batteries, coins, or bones. Many patients have an underlying esophageal abnormality, such as a Schatzki's ring, stricture, eosinophilic esophagitis, tumor, or achalasia. The clinical presentation includes dysphagia, odynophagia, foreign body sensation, chest pain, excessive salivation, and difficulty handling secretions. Immediate endoscopic extraction with concomitant airway protection is recommended because prolonged impaction may result in penetration into the esophageal wall followed by perforation and mediastinitis.

ESOPHAGEAL VARICES

Esophageal varices are described in Chapter 137.

ESOPHAGEAL FISTULAS

Tracheoesophageal fistulas may arise from a variety of different causes, including trauma, infectious esophagitis, necrosis after prolonged endotracheal intubation, esophageal cancer, and radiation therapy. Patients are often critically ill and may not tolerate surgery. Metallic stents are a treatment option.

Atrial-esophageal fistulas are a rare complication after radiofrequency ablation (Chapter 66) for atrial fibrillation. The clinical presentation is nonspecific and includes features such as dysphagia, fever, leukocytosis, bacteremia, massive intestinal bleeding, and septic shock. Diagnosis requires a high index of suspicion and is aided by a chest CT scan. Surgery is required; the prognosis is excellent with early recognition and treatment but can be dire if treatment is delayed.

Congenital Abnormalities

ESOPHAGEAL ATRESIA AND TRACHEOESOPHAGEAL FISTULA

Children with congenital esophageal anomalies commonly survive into adulthood after successful surgery. As adults, these patients commonly have gastroesophageal reflux that warrants PPI therapy. Strictures at prior surgical anastomoses are common, and patients may require periodic endoscopic dilation.

HETEROTOPIC GASTRIC MUCOSA (INLET PATCH)

Inlet patches, which are areas of gastric columnar epithelium, are present in up to 4.5% of adults, and are usually found incidentally at the time of routine endoscopy. Typically, a red columnar patch varying in size from a few millimeters to a few centimeters is seen just below the cricopharyngeus. Inlet patches can be associated with hoarseness, sore throat, and globus sensation. Strictures, ulcers, and rare malignant transformation have also been described. Treatment options include PPIs (see Table 140-1) and endoscopic ablation.

OTHER CONGENITAL ESOPHAGEAL DISORDERS

Duplication cysts, which may be located anywhere in the esophagus, may be in continuity with or separate from the esophageal lumen. Symptoms, which may present initially in adulthood, include dysphagia owing to luminal compression, chest pain, and regurgitation. Treatment is surgical.

Dysphagia lusoria is caused by an aberrant right subclavian artery that originates from the right aortic arch and causes partial compression of the esophagus as it crosses over to the left side. Patients may complain of dysphagia. This condition is most commonly detected incidentally during barium radiography, where it is visualized as a crossing diagonal impression at the junction of the proximal and middle thirds of the esophagus. Surgery is rarely indicated because of the complexity of the operation and the difficulty in establishing a clear relationship between the radiographic findings and symptoms.

1. Khan M, Santana J, Donnellan C, et al. Medical treatments in the short term management of reflux oesophagitis. *Cochrane Database Syst Rev.* 2007;2:CD003244.
2. van Pinxteren B, Sigterman KE, Bonis P, et al. Short-term treatment with proton pump inhibitors, H2-receptor antagonists and prokinetics for gastro-oesophageal reflux disease-like symptoms and endoscopy negative reflux disease. *Cochrane Database Syst Rev.* 2006;3:CD002095.
3. Wang Y, Pan T, Wang Q, et al. Additional bedtime H2-receptor antagonist for the control of nocturnal gastric acid breakthrough. *Cochrane Database Syst Rev.* 2009;7:CD004275.
4. Lundell L, Miettinen P, Myrvold HE, et al, for the Nordic GEORD Study Group. Seven-year follow-up of a randomized clinical trial comparing proton-pump inhibition with surgical therapy for reflux oesophagitis. *Br J Surg.* 2007;94:198-203.
5. Ramage JI Jr, Rumalla A, Baron TH, et al. A prospective, randomized, double-blind, placebo-controlled trial of endoscopic steroid injection therapy for recalcitrant esophageal peptic strictures. *Am J Gastroenterol.* 2005;100:2419-2425.
6. Shaheen NJ, Sharma P, Overholt BF, et al. Radiofrequency ablation in Barrett's esophagus with dysplasia. *N Engl J Med.* 2009;360:2353-2355.
7. Straumann A, Conus S, Degen L, et al. Budesonide is effective in adolescent and adult patients with active eosinophilic esophagitis. *Gastroenterology.* 2010;139:1526-1537.
8. Leyden JE, Moss AC, MacMathuna P. Endoscopic pneumatic dilation versus botulinum toxin injection in the management of primary achalasia. *Cochrane Database Syst Rev.* 2006;4:CD005046.

SUGGESTED READINGS

Becher A, Dent J. Systematic review: ageing and gastro-oesophageal reflux disease symptoms, oesophageal function and reflux oesophagitis. *Aliment Pharmacol Ther.* 2011;33:442-454. *Review.*

Cook IJ. Oropharyngeal dysphagia. *Gastroenterol Clin N Am.* 2009;38:411-431. *Review.*

Rees JR, Lao-Sirieix P, Wong A, et al. Treatment for Barrett's oesophagus. *Cochrane Database Rev Syst.* 2010;1:CD004060. *Review of evidence for medical and interventional therapies.*

Rothenberg ME. Biology and treatment of eosinophilic esophagitis. *Gastroenterology.* 2009;137:1238-1249. *Review.*

141

ACID PEPTIC DISEASE

ERNST J. KUIPERS AND MARTIN J. BLASER

Acid peptic diseases can involve the esophagus (Chapter 140), the stomach, and the duodenum. Dyspeptic symptoms also can occur in patients who have no endoscopic abnormalities, in whom it is termed *nonulcer dyspepsia* (Chapter 139).

DEFINITIONS

Gastric and duodenal ulcers usually occur in an area of inflamed mucosa. This inflammation, termed *gastritis, duodenitis, or bulbitis,* can sometimes be recognized during endoscopy by signs of edema, reddening, and swelling of the mucosa, but microscopic evaluation of endoscopic biopsy specimens is required for a definitive diagnosis of mucosal inflammation.

Gastritis is categorized by endoscopic and histologic criteria, with granulocytes predominating in active gastritis and mononuclear cells in chronic gastritis. Gastritis is also classified by the segment of involved stomach: antral-predominant gastritis, corpus-predominant gastritis, or pangastritis. Finally, the absence or presence of premalignant stages of damage to the mucosa as a result of long-standing inflammation defines the categories of nonatrophic and atrophic gastritis, respectively. Endoscopic findings are usually nonspecific, unless the gastric mucosa has either a typical miniature

FIGURE 141-1. Endoscopic view of uncomplicated erosive gastritis. The erosion appears as a small, superficial mucosal break with a black base *(arrow)*.

FIGURE 141-2. Endoscopic view of an ulcer at the anterior wall of the duodenal bulb. The ulcer has a clean base, with a visible vessel appearing as a dark red protruding spot close to the lower ulcer rim. The surrounding mucosa is inflamed and swollen.

cobblestone appearance, termed *nodular gastritis* (a lesion found particularly in children colonized by *Helicobacter pylori*), or grossly enlarged folds without evidence of cancer, termed *hypertrophic gastritis.*

A *peptic ulcer* is a mucosal defect at least 0.5 cm in diameter that penetrates the muscularis mucosae. Smaller mucosal defects are called *erosions* (Fig. 141-1). Gastric ulcers are subdivided into proximal ulcers, located in the body of the stomach, and distal ulcers, located in the antrum and angulus of the stomach. Gastric ulcers are located mainly along the lesser curvature, in particular at the transitional zone of corpus- to antral-type mucosa. This transitional zone is often in the area of the angulus but may shift proximally. Duodenal ulcers usually are located on the anterior or posterior wall of the duodenal bulb (Fig. 141-2), or occasionally at both sites ("kissing" ulcers). Lesions distal to the duodenal bulb are termed *postbulbar ulcers.* Patients who previously underwent a distal gastric resection (Billroth I or II procedure) can develop ulceration at the gastroduodenal anastomosis (anastomotic ulcer). However, ulcers occurring after Billroth II resection are located predominantly in the jejunal mucosa at the junction between the afferent and efferent loops. Other peptic ulcers can occur at sites of metaplastic or heterotopic gastric mucosa, for example, in Meckel's diverticulum, the rectum, or Barrett's esophagus. Patients with a large hiatal hernia can develop gastric ulceration, known as *Cameron's ulcers,* at the level of the herniation. *Dieulafoy's ulcers,* which are small mucosal defects over an intramural arteriole, can lead to severe bleeding. Although these lesions can occur throughout the gastrointestinal tract, two thirds occur in the stomach.

EPIDEMIOLOGY

The worldwide prevalence of gastritis reflects the prevalence of *H. pylori*. Colonization with this bacterium is virtually always associated with chronic active gastritis, which persists as long as an individual remains colonized and only slowly disappears 6 to 24 months after the eradication of *H. pylori*. In developing countries and among first-generation immigrants from these countries, the prevalence of *H. pylori* gastritis is high (often ≥80%) in all age groups, including children. In Western countries, the prevalence of *H. pylori* gastritis increases with age; it is currently less than 20% in young adults but 40 to 60% in elderly persons.

Although peptic ulcer disease is strongly related to *H. pylori* gastritis and duodenitis, the epidemiology of ulcer disease has shown secular variations even when *H. pylori* was ubiquitous. The incidence of peptic ulcer disease rose steeply in Western countries in the late 19th and early 20th centuries and has decreased over the past 30 years, yet peptic ulceration remains a common disorder. The decline in incidence, associated with a decrease in hospital admissions and surgery for ulcer disease, is believed to reflect mainly the decreasing prevalence of gastric colonization with *H. pylori*. The declining incidence of ulcer disease is also the result of the widespread application of eradication therapy, which strongly reduced recurrent ulcers in *H. pylori*–positive patients. Other factors may include the widespread use of acid suppressive medication. Nevertheless, hospital admissions for complications of ulcers and mortality from ulcer disease have remained relatively stable in both the United States and other countries, as the reduction in *H. pylori*–associated ulcers in younger persons has been counterbalanced by an increase in ulcers related to nonsteroidal anti-inflammatory drugs (NSAIDs) in older persons.

In Western countries, duodenal ulcers occur more frequently than gastric ulcers. The predominant age at which duodenal ulcers occur is between 20 and 50 years, whereas gastric ulcers most commonly occur in patients older than 40 years. The incidence of gastroduodenal ulcer disease is approximately 1 to 2 per 1000 inhabitants per year. Two thirds of patients with ulcers are male, and the disease is more common in smokers. The risk of recurrent disease after initial healing is high; more than 50% of patients have a recurrent ulcer within 12 months of healing in the absence of treatment. Maintenance acid suppressive therapy reduces this recurrence rate, but only therapeutic measures that remove the underlying cause of the ulcer can prevent most ulcer recurrences.

PATHOBIOLOGY

Helicobacter pylori

Most peptic ulcers are associated with colonization with *H. pylori* (Fig. 141-3). Initial clinical studies of the association between *H. pylori* and ulcer disease reported that approximately 85% of patients with gastric ulcer disease and 95% of patients with duodenal ulcer disease were colonized by *H. pylori*. Most persons who are *H. pylori* positive do not have any specific complaints, nor do they develop ulcer disease. The estimated risk for the development of ulcer disease during persistent *H. pylori* colonization is 5 to 15%—that is, three- to eight-fold higher than the risk for patients who are *H. pylori* negative. The risk for the development of an ulcer in the presence of *H. pylori* is determined by a combination of host- and bacteria-related factors. Host factors include immune response, smoking, and stress. Bacterial factors that increase

the risk of ulcer include a high production of the *VacA* product, which reflects the presence of the s1m1 genotype; a high level of cytokine induction, owing to the presence of genes in the *cag* pathogenicity island; and enhanced adherence, resulting from *babA*.

Nonsteroidal Anti-inflammatory Drugs and Aspirin

The other common cause of gastroduodenal ulcer disease is the use of NSAIDs. At least 2 to 4% of the population in many countries use acetylsalicylic acid, acetic acid derivatives (diclofenac, indomethacin, sulindac), or propionic acid derivatives (ibuprofen, ketoprofen, naproxen) on a daily basis. Within 14 days after the start of such treatment, about 5% of patients develop mucosal breaks, that is, erosions and ulcers. In patients who continue therapy for 4 weeks or longer, this proportion increases to 10%. The concomitant presence of *H. pylori* infection increases the incidence of NSAID-related ulcers. The risk of developing an ulcer during NSAID use is also higher in patients who are older than 60 years, those with a previous ulcer, patients who use corticosteroids or high-dose NSAIDs, and those with major comorbid diseases. In patients who use anticoagulants, such as warfarin, or who have severe comorbid disease, an NSAID-induced ulcer is more likely to lead to life-threatening gastroduodenal hemorrhage.

On the basis of their activities, NSAIDs are divided into cyclooxygenase 1 (COX1) and COX2 inhibitors (Chapter 36). The COX1 enzyme is involved in the production of prostaglandins, which play a role in normal cell regulation. The COX2 enzyme, which is also involved in the production of prostaglandins, is induced by inflammatory responses. Most NSAIDs have a nonselective COX inhibitory effect; selective COX2 inhibitors are associated with fewer gastroduodenal ulcers, but their use is limited by their adverse coronary effects (Chapter 36). Because of the strong association between NSAIDs and ulcer disease and the risk for recurrence of ulcers with their continued use, patients with ulcers must be thoroughly assessed for the use of NSAIDs.

Helicobacter pylori–Negative, Non-NSAID Ulcer Disease

In most series, *H. pylori* and NSAID use account for 80 to 95% of cases of ulcer disease. The remaining cases are often referred to as *idiopathic* or *H. pylori–negative, non-NSAID* acid peptic disease. The proportion of ulcer disease that is idiopathic is increasing throughout the world as the prevalence of *H. pylori* decreases. Further, it is likely that some ulcers in *H. pylori*–positive patients were not caused by *H. pylori*. Consistent with this notion is the fact that some *H. pylori*–positive patients develop recurrent ulcers after successful bacterial eradication, so presumably their ulcer disease was idiopathic. It is not known whether the increase in idiopathic ulcer disease is simply proportional to the decrease in *H. pylori*–associated ulcers or whether it reflects a true increase in the incidence of idiopathic ulcers.

In patients with idiopathic ulcer disease, specific clues to the underlying cause are often provided by the medical history, including comorbidity and drug use; the endoscopic appearance of the ulcer; and the histologic features of the ulcer's margins and surroundings. In most cases, these initial data can direct further diagnostic studies (Table 141-1).

Malignant Ulcer Disease

Gastroduodenal ulcers can result from underlying malignant disease. In the stomach, these tumors are related to gastric adenocarcinoma and, rarely, to mucosa-associated lymphoid tissue (MALT) lymphomas (Chapter 198). Malignant ulcers in the duodenum may result from primary duodenal carcinomas or from penetrating pancreatic cancers. Duodenal cancers have an association with polyposis syndromes, especially familial adenomatous polyposis and, to a much lesser extent, MUTYH-associated polyposis and Peutz-Jeghers syndrome (Chapter 199). In both the stomach and the duodenum, ulcer disease can also be caused by metastatic tumors, including cancers of the breast, colon, thyroid, or kidney, or by melanoma, disseminated lymphoma, or Kaposi's sarcoma. Malignant ulcers are characteristically irregular in shape with heaped borders, but they may also be flat or depressed lesions. Current high-resolution and magnification endoscopes allow visualization of the altered mucosal structure surrounding an ulcer, including changes in the microvascular pattern. For a definite diagnosis of malignancy, multiple biopsy specimens are needed, usually from the ulcer margins.

Systemic Inflammatory Disorders

A few gastroduodenal ulcers are caused by systemic inflammatory diseases, in particular, Crohn's disease (Chapter 143). Patients with Crohn's disease affecting the proximal gastrointestinal tract often have multiple ulcers

FIGURE 141-3. Gastric mucosa colonized with *Helicobacter pylori* appearing as curved bacilli on the mucosal surface.

TABLE 141-1   DIFFERENTIAL DIAGNOSIS OF PEPTIC ULCER DISEASE

ORIGIN	CONDITION	FREQUENCY*	DIAGNOSTIC TEST	FINDINGS
Microbes	Helicobacter pylori	Very common	Helicobacter pylori tests	Bacteria, enzymes, antigens, antibodies
			Histology	Gastritis
	Helicobacter heilmannii	Rare	Histology	Spiral bacteria, gastritis
	Treponema pallidum	Very rare	Serology	Antibodies
	Mycobacterial infection	Very rare	Histology, immune response testing, chest radiograph	Acid-fast bacteria, granuloma, immune response, pulmonary infiltrate
	Cytomegalovirus, herpes simplex virus type 1	Rare	Histology, serology	Virus inclusions, antibodies
Drug use	NSAIDs, aspirin	Very common	History, urine test	NSAID use
	Bisphosphonates	Rare	History	Bisphosphonate use
	Corticosteroids	Rare	History	Corticosteroid use, comorbidity
	Amphetamines, cocaine	Rare	History, drug testing	Drug use
	Anticoagulants, coagulopathy	Rare	Endoscopy	Ulcer after intramural bleed
Malignancy	Gastric cancer	Common	Histology	Malignancy
	Duodenal cancer	Rare	Histology, CT	Malignancy
	Pancreatic cancer	Common	Histology, CT	Malignancy
	Mucosa-associated lymphoid tissue lymphoma	Rare	Histology	Malignancy
	Metastatic cancer	Rare	Histology	Malignancy
Gastritis syndromes	Eosinophilic gastritis	Rare	Histology	Eosinophilic infiltration
	Lymphocytic gastritis	Rare	Histology, celiac disease screening	Lymphocytic infiltration, villous atrophy
Hyperacidic syndromes	Zollinger-Ellison syndrome	Rare	Serum gastrin, secretin test	Extreme hypergastrinemia, positive secretin test
	Antral G-cell hyperfunction	Very rare	Serum gastrin, secretin test	Moderate hypergastrinemia, negative secretin test
	Retained gastric antrum	Very rare	Medical history, gastrin	Billroth II resection, hypergastrinemia
	Systemic mastocytosis	Very rare	Histology of affected sites	Mast cell infiltration
	Chronic myelogenous leukemia	Very rare	Leukemia evaluation	Leukemia
Ischemia	Mesenteric vascular occlusion	Common	Angiography	Vascular disease
	Polycythemia vera	Rare	Blood counts	Polycythemia
Specific ulcer types	Cameron's ulcer	Common	Endoscopy	Ulcer in large hiatal hernia
	Marginal ulcer	Common	Endoscopy	Ulcer at anastomosis
	Dieulafoy's ulcer	Common	Endoscopy	Singular bleeding focus with minimal mucosal disruption
Systemic inflammation	Crohn's disease	Common	Histology, ileocolonoscopy	Inflammation, granulomas
	Vasculitides	Rare	Histology, systemic evaluation	Vasculitis, signs of systemic disease
	Gastric amyloidosis	Very rare	Histology	Amyloid deposition
Other conditions	Stress ulcer	Fairly common in patients in intensive care units	Endoscopy	—
	Radiation therapy, chemotherapy	Rare	Endoscopy, history	—

*Frequency as a cause of gastroduodenal ulcer disease.
CT = computed tomography; NSAID = nonsteroidal anti-inflammatory drug.

characterized by irregular longitudinal shapes. Ulcers in the duodenum occur atop Kerckring's folds. Patients with gastroduodenal ulcers from Crohn's disease do not invariably have evidence of disease elsewhere in the digestive tract, nor do blood tests always suggest an active inflammatory bowel disorder. The demonstration of ulcerative inflammation elsewhere in the digestive tract, in particular in the terminal ileum and colon, strongly supports the diagnosis of Crohn's disease, as do granulomas on a biopsy specimen. However, the absence of granulomas does not exclude Crohn's disease, and these lesions are not specific for Crohn's disease; they are also associated with H. pylori gastritis and other conditions, particularly sarcoidosis (Chapter 95). Sarcoidosis can also lead to gastroduodenal ulcer disease.

Other inflammatory disorders that can cause gastritis or gastroduodenal ulcers include various forms of vasculitis affecting the mesenteric system, in particular Behçet's disease (Chapter 278), Henoch-Schönlein purpura (Chapter 278), Takayasu's arteritis (Chapter 278), polyarteritis nodosa (Chapter 278), systemic lupus erythematosus (Chapter 274), Churg-Strauss syndrome (Chapter 278), and Wegener's granulomatosis (Chapter 278). Lymphocytic gastroduodenitis, which is strongly associated with celiac disease (Chapter 142), may lead to duodenal ulceration and subsequent stenotic web formation. Ulcer disease also may occur in patients with polycythemia vera (Chapter 169), possibly in relation to reduced mucosal blood flow. Vasculitis underlying ulcer disease should be considered in patients with chronic or recurrent ulceration in whom other causes have been excluded. Lymphocytic phlebitis, which is a rare vasculitic inflammatory disorder affecting the mesenteric veins, may cause gastric ulcer disease. Systemic

amyloidosis (Chapter 194) affecting the stomach wall may lead to gastric ulcer disease. Rare cases of duodenal ulceration have been described in the presence of annular pancreas or congenital bands obstructing the descending duodenum.

Hypergastrinemic Syndromes

Peptic ulcers can result from chronic gastric hyperacidity related to hypergastrinemia. The most important hypergastrinemic disorder is Zollinger-Ellison syndrome (Chapter 201), a condition of marked hyperacidity leading to severe peptic ulcer disease caused by a gastrin-producing endocrine tumor. These patients usually have multiple therapy-resistant bulbar and postbulbar duodenal ulcers. The diagnosis can be confirmed by the presence of a high fasting serum gastrin level (often but not always ≥10-fold increased and >1000 pg/mL). Similar gastrin levels are sometimes seen in patients treated for chronic ulcer disease with high-dose proton pump inhibitors. For clarification, secretin testing can be performed: in patients with Zollinger-Ellison syndrome, the injection of secretin (1 U/kg) increases serum gastrin levels by more than 50%, or 120 pg/mL or greater in those with fasting gastrin levels less than 10-fold above normal. Imaging techniques, such as computed tomography (CT), magnetic resonance imaging, isotope scanning, endoscopic ultrasonography, videocapsule endoscopy, and balloon-assisted enteroscopy, may be used to detect the primary tumor, which is often located in either the pancreas or the proximal small bowel. In some patients, Zollinger-Ellison syndrome occurs as part of multiple endocrine neoplasia (Chapter 239), particularly in association with hyperparathyroidism. Other

FIGURE 141-4. Endoscopic view of an irregular gastric ulcer at the posterior wall and smaller curvature in a patient with chronic mesenteric ischemia due to subtotal stenosis of the celiac trunk.

hypergastrinemic hyperacidity syndromes are the retained gastric antrum syndrome (see later) and antral G-cell hyperfunction. In the latter, fasting serum gastrin levels are only modestly increased and do not rise after the injection of secretin, but they respond in an exaggerated way to meals, thereby leading to hyperacidity. When the condition occurs in an *H. pylori*–positive patient, bacterial eradication therapy may be curative. However, some patients with G-cell hyperfunction are *H. pylori* negative.

Ischemia

Stenosis or occlusion of the celiac trunk or the superior mesenteric artery (Chapter 145) also can lead to ulceration in the mucosa of the proximal digestive tract (Fig. 141-4). These ulcers typically occur in elderly patients with risk factors for atherosclerosis, but they can also occur in younger subjects with mesenteric obstruction due to other causes. Ischemic ulcers tend to heal slowly and recur. Pallor of the mucosa, consistent with decreased mucosal blood flow, may be noted at endoscopy. Upper mesenteric ischemia is often associated with upper abdominal pain, which can be elicited by a meal or by physical activity. These symptoms may cause patients to decrease their food intake, leading to weight loss before their clinical presentation. The prevalence of upper mesenteric ischemia with secondary ulcer disease is unknown, in part owing to its variable presentation, often with a history of gradual symptoms; the lack of standardized and reliable diagnostic tests; and clinicians' unfamiliarity with the condition. Diagnostic evaluation includes a duplex ultrasound scan for vascular flow and conventional or CT angiography of the affected arteries. Validated functional tests for gastroduodenal mucosal perfusion are not widely available, but a technique for directly measuring mucosal oxygen saturation during endoscopy is investigational.

Stress Ulcers

Patients with severe medical conditions, such as major trauma, sepsis, extensive burns, head injury, or multiorgan failure, can develop stress ulcers in the stomach or duodenum. Major risk factors for stress ulceration in severely ill patients include mechanical ventilation, coagulopathy, and hypotension, but factors such as hepatic and renal failure and the use of ulcerogenic medications may contribute. Stress ulcers occur independently of *H. pylori* colonization. Ulcers associated with head injury are known as Cushing's ulcers, and ulcers associated with extensive burns are known as Curling's ulcers. Stress ulcers were once common in patients in intensive care units, but improvements in overall management, including respiratory and hemodynamic care, acid inhibition, and emphasis on adequate feeding, have reduced the incidence of these ulcers, which currently affect 1 to 2% of these patients. Stress ulcers may be asymptomatic, but they can also cause complications, especially bleeding.

Other Factors
Cameron's Ulcer

Patients with large hiatal hernias (Chapter 140) may present with proximal gastric ulcers, termed *Cameron's ulcers,* at the level of the hiatus, where the stomach is compressed. These ulcers are usually asymptomatic but may cause

occult or overt bleeding. During upper gastrointestinal endoscopy, patients with large hiatal hernias and iron deficiency anemia should be carefully examined in normal and retroverted positions for the presence of Cameron's ulcers.

Anastomotic or Marginal Ulceration

Patients who have undergone partial gastrectomy sometimes develop recurrent ulcers, often located at the anastomosis or within the jejunum immediately opposite the anastomosis. Ischemia and chronic inflammation resulting from *H. pylori* and biliary reflux may cause such ulcers, as may underlying cancer. If biopsy excludes cancer, treatment includes acid suppression and *H. pylori* eradication, if needed. Ulcer disease can be caused by the retained gastric antrum syndrome after partial gastrectomy when the antrum is not completely excised from the detached duodenum. Because it then lacks exposure to acid and is thus not physiologically downregulated, it continues to secrete gastrin despite normal or even high acid levels. Marginal ulcers can also occur after bariatric Roux-en-Y gastric bypass surgery.

Other Microbes

Colonization with *Helicobacter heilmannii* (formerly known as *Gastrospirillum hominis*), which is probably a zoonotic organism, is associated with mild gastritis and sometimes with transient ulcer disease. Ulcer disease also may be infectious, resulting from secondary syphilis (Chapter 327), mycobacterial infection (Chapter 332), infection with herpes simplex virus type 1 (Chapter 382), or cytomegalovirus infection (Chapter 384).

Alcohol

Short-term heavy alcohol use or long-term moderate to heavy alcohol use can lead to signs of acute and chronic gastritis. No evidence indicates that this gastritis is associated with a significant risk for peptic ulceration, although alcohol use increases the risk of bleeding in patients with peptic ulcer disease.

Hyperhistaminic Syndromes

Similar to the hypergastrinemic syndromes, persistent elevation of histamine can lead to hyperacidity as a result of the chronic stimulation of parietal cells. Elevated histamine levels are observed in two rare syndromes. *Systemic mastocytosis* (Chapter 263) is characterized by a proliferation of mast cells in the bone marrow, skin, liver, spleen, and gastrointestinal tract, often associated with both spontaneous and trigger-induced (e.g., alcohol) release of histamine and other vasoactive substances. Patients with systemic mastocytosis often have gastrointestinal symptoms, including pain, diarrhea, and blood loss. Ulceration results from chronic gastric acid hypersecretion. Clues to the diagnosis include symptoms of pruritus, urticaria, or rash. The bone marrow and affected organ mast cell infiltrates carry a specific *C-kit* mutation and express CD2 and CD25. Histamine hypersecretion leading to peptic ulcer disease can also occur in *chronic myelogenous leukemia* (Chapter 190) with basophilia.

Other Drugs

Treatment with oral bisphosphonates, widely used for osteoporosis (Chapter 251), is complicated by gastric erosions and ulceration in an estimated 3 to 10% of treated patients. The risk for ulcer disease may be synergistically increased by NSAID use but is probably independent of *H. pylori* colonization. Although corticosteroid treatment can be complicated by peptic ulcer disease, the relative risk is only slightly increased, except in patients with serious comorbid diseases, using long-term or high-dose therapy, or with prior ulcers. Other patients who use corticosteroids are not at serious risk for ulcer disease and therefore do not require measures to prevent ulcers.

Persons who use amphetamines and crack cocaine (Chapter 33) frequently develop ulcer disease, often with perforation, possibly as a result of vascular insufficiency. Chemotherapy, particularly when given selectively as a high-dose intra-arterial infusion in the celiac system, can be complicated by ulcer disease. Patients on anticoagulant therapy and those with other coagulopathies may rarely develop intramural hematoma of the gastrointestinal tract. Depending on the location, these hematomas may cause obstruction, but they can also leave large ulcers when they rupture into the lumen. Radiation therapy of the upper abdomen is sometimes complicated by chronic ischemic ulceration, especially in long-term follow-up.

CLINICAL MANIFESTATIONS

The clinical manifestations of acid peptic disease (Table 141-2) do not always predict the various morphologic presentations found at endoscopy. Indeed,

TABLE 141-2 KEY SYMPTOMS AND SIGNS OF PEPTIC ULCER

UNCOMPLICATED ULCER

No symptoms ("silent ulcer" in up to 40% of cases)
Epigastric pain
    Pain may radiate to the back, thorax, other parts of abdomen (cephalad most likely, caudad least likely)
    Pain may be nocturnal (most specific), "painful hunger" relieved by food, or continuous (least specific)
Nausea
Vomiting
Heartburn (mimics or associated with gastroesophageal reflex)

COMPLICATED ULCER

Acute perforation
    Severe abdominal pain
    Shock
    Abdominal board-like rigidity (and rebound and other signs of peritoneal irritation)
    Free intraperitoneal air
Hemorrhage
    Hematemesis and/or melena
    Hemodynamic changes, anemia
    Previous history of ulcer symptoms (80%)
Gastric outlet obstruction
    Satiation, inability to ingest food, eructation
    Nausea, vomiting (and related disturbances)
    Weight loss

TABLE 141-3 DIAGNOSTIC PATHS AND TOOLS IN ULCER DISEASE

PATH 1: MORPHOLOGIC DIAGNOSIS

Gastroduodenoscopy
Barium contrast (inferior alternative)
Endoscopic ultrasound (selected cases only)
Computed tomography (useful in selected cases)

PATH 2: ETIOLOGIC DIAGNOSIS

Helicobacter pylori **Testing**

Histologic examination of gastric mucosa
Stool antigen test
Carbon-13 urea breath test
Serum antibodies

Ulcer Associated with Nonsteroidal Anti-inflammatory Drug Use

History of drug ingestion
Decreased platelet adherence
Molecular identification (complex, expensive)

Acid Hypersecretory Syndromes

Serum gastrin elevation
Gastrin provocative tests (intravenous secretin, meal)
Gastric analysis

a silent ulcer may be recognized only when it presents abruptly with a complication, most commonly hemorrhage or perforation, or it may be discovered incidentally when a diagnostic test is performed for other reasons. Nevertheless, the typical presentation of acid peptic disease is recurrent episodes of pain. The pain is almost invariably located in the epigastrium and may radiate to the back or, less commonly, to the thorax or other regions of the abdomen (see Table 141-2). Some patients describe the pain as burning or piercing, whereas others describe it as an uncomfortable feeling of emptiness of the stomach, referred to as *painful hunger*. Indeed, the pain may improve with the ingestion of food, only to return in the postprandial period. The timing of the pain in relation to meals and the soothing effects of food are nonspecific, however, and may also occur in patients with functional dyspepsia without ulcer. Nocturnal epigastric pain that awakens a patient several hours after a late meal is more likely to represent ulcer pain.

Besides the pain during symptomatic episodes, patients may complain of retrosternal burning (heartburn) or acidic regurgitation into the throat, symptoms that reflect associated gastroesophageal reflux (Chapter 140), which is aggravated by hyperacidity or delayed gastric emptying. Nausea and vomiting may also occur but are nonspecific. The presence of significant diarrhea should raise the possibility of Zollinger-Ellison syndrome (Chapter 201), but diarrhea also may result from the heavy use of magnesium-containing antacids. In untreated patients, symptoms tend to be intermittent, with flares of daily pain lasting 2 to 8 weeks, separated by prolonged asymptomatic intervals. During periods of remission, patients may feel well and may be able to eat even heavy or spicy meals without apparent discomfort.

Physical Examination

The physical examination is usually unrevealing. If significant bleeding has occurred (Chapter 137), the patient may present with pallor and may be hypovolemic (Chapter 106). It is always useful to inquire about the characteristics of the stool, because ulcer-related bleeding may manifest not only obviously in the form of hematemesis but also insidiously as melena (black feces). In the case of massive ulcer bleeding with the rapid bowel passage of blood, patients may also present with red rectal blood loss. When a patient has acute perforation, severe epigastric and abdominal pain develops, and the patient appears distressed. Characteristically, intense contracture of the abdominal muscles is apparent on palpation, together with rebound tenderness and other signs of peritoneal irritation. With large amounts of intra-abdominal air, percussion may reveal hypertympany over the liver.

DIAGNOSIS

In a patient who presents with symptoms consistent with ulcer disease, the diagnostic evaluation should proceed along two different but complementary paths: confirmation of the anatomic abnormality and investigation of its cause (Table 141-3). In most patients, it is advisable to follow both diagnostic paths simultaneously, but sometimes it is reasonable to skip the anatomic verification as a cost-saving strategy and proceed to management based on the probable cause.

Anatomic Diagnosis

Endoscopy (Chapter 136) is the primary investigative tool in patients suspected of having acid peptic disease. This technique can detect erosive gastritis (see Fig. 141-1) or an ulcer in the gastric wall or duodenal bulb (see Fig. 141-2). Because of the high prevalence and the often spontaneous improvement of dyspeptic symptoms, endoscopy usually should not be performed immediately; rather its use should be restricted to patients with persistent or recurrent symptoms. However, immediate endoscopy is indicated in patients with alarm symptoms such as weight loss, dysphagia, anorexia, considerable vomiting, anemia, or signs of overt bleeding.

Endoscopy is both highly sensitive and highly specific for the detection of ulcer disease. The most common locations for a peptic ulcer are the stomach and duodenal bulb, but peptic ulcers sometimes occur in the esophagus, the small bowel, and a Meckel's diverticulum lined with heterotopic gastric mucosa. Endoscopic ultrasound may detect an unsuspected submucosal component or enlarged lymph nodes, such as may occur in gastric neoplasia, especially lymphoma and linitis plastica (Chapter 198). Ulcers in the dorsal wall of the duodenal bulb, especially at the transition from the bulb to the postbulbar descending portion of the duodenum, are most difficult to visualize, and they sometimes require a side-viewing endoscope, particularly when endoscopic treatment is needed. Other regions where gastroduodenal ulcers can be easily missed are the cardia and the gastric angulus. Dieulafoy's lesions may be difficult to diagnose because of their small mucosal defects and intermittent bleeding. Some patients require more than one endoscopy, preferably during acute bleeding, to localize the lesion. Endoscopy is also useful for ascertaining the presence of concomitant disorders, including esophagitis and duodenitis, or complications, such as bleeding or a visible vessel (see Fig. 141-2); obtaining biopsy specimens, such as for histologic examination and to assess for H. pylori (see Fig. 141-3); and performing therapeutic interventions.

In rare cases, such as stenosis that blocks the advancing endoscope, conventional barium contrast radiographs (Chapter 135) are indicated. Additional investigations by endosonography or CT are needed when an underlying malignant disease is suspected. The endoscopist should obtain biopsy samples from all gastric ulcers, especially those with a suspicious appearance, to exclude potential malignant disease. Because duodenal ulcers are less likely to be malignant, biopsies are usually not required unless malignancy is specifically suspected.

Etiologic Diagnosis

Diagnosis also must focus on establishing the cause of the ulcer. The first step is to determine whether *H. pylori* or NSAID use is present, because these are the major risk factors for peptic ulcers and can be contributing factors in ulcers with other precipitating causes.

Testing for Helicobacter pylori

In populations with a high prevalence of *H. pylori,* nearly all patients with peptic ulcer disease are positive for *H. pylori,* so diagnostic testing has little value except when antimicrobial susceptibility testing is needed. The prevalence of *H. pylori* remains high in immigrants from developing countries, where most people become *H. pylori* positive in youth. In Western countries, approximately 50% of individuals who are older than 65 years are colonized with *H. pylori,* but the prevalence is less than 20% in those younger than 30 years. In these younger persons, the proportion of patients with ulcers who are *H. pylori* negative is higher than in older patients, making diagnostic testing for *H. pylori,* followed by targeted therapy in those who are positive for the bacterium, more attractive than empirical therapy.

The presence of *H. pylori* can be ascertained by four possible approaches. *Histologic examination* of gastric mucosal biopsies, which is the standard procedure when diagnostic endoscopy is initially performed, is quite sensitive and specific for *H. pylori.* However, the accuracy of this technique may be affected by sampling error, improper orientation of the specimen, and recent therapy with proton pump inhibitors or antibiotics.

A second option is *serology,* which is a relatively simple, inexpensive test that has reduced predictive value in areas where the prevalence of *H. pylori* is low. Serology is not helpful to verify whether *H. pylori* has been eradicated with antibiotics because it may take many months or even years for *H. pylori* antibodies to fall to undetectable levels. None of the diagnostic tests that do not involve endoscopy can determine whether an ulcer is present.

A third option is a *stool antigen test,* which is more accurate than serology. Finally, the *carbon-13 or carbon-14 urea breath test,* which relies on the detection of *H. pylori* urease activity, is a noninvasive and relatively simple test, but it is more expensive than stool or blood testing. Although the test becomes negative as soon as *H. pylori* is eradicated, a minimum interval of 4 to 6 weeks after antibiotic treatment is recommended to reduce false-negative results.

Nonsteroidal Anti-inflammatory Drugs

NSAIDs are usually established as the putative cause of an ulcer based on information obtained from the patient. Assessment of NSAID use in an individual patient presenting with ulcer disease can be difficult, both because NSAID use is common and often intermittent and because many different NSAIDs are widely available over the counter in most countries. NSAID use is usually evaluated by detailed medical history, focusing not only on current and recent drug use but also on symptoms of pain, including musculoskeletal complaints. Further information from family members, family practitioners, and pharmacists is sometimes helpful. If surreptitious use of NSAIDs is suspected, direct serum and urine testing for aspirin and NSAID derivatives is feasible, or aspirin use can be assessed indirectly by a platelet adherence assay; however, these tests are not commonly used in clinical practice.

Hypersecretory Syndromes

Hypersecretory syndromes not related to *H. pylori* or NSAIDs are rare causes of ulcer disease and are diagnosed by special tests (see Table 141-3). Zollinger-Ellison syndrome should be strongly considered in patients with multiple ulcers, particularly in atypical locations such as distal to the duodenal bulb, and when diarrhea is present, because these finding are uncommon in *H. pylori*–related peptic ulcer disease. Hypergastrinemic syndromes (e.g., Zollinger-Ellison syndrome, antral G-cell hyperplasia) are best diagnosed by a determination of serum gastrin levels, both basal and after stimulation with intravenous secretin (gastrinoma detection) or a test meal (antral G-cell hyperplasia detection). When detected early, gastrinomas may be resectable (Chapter 201).

Gastric analysis, which is performed by placing a nasogastric tube to aspirate gastric juice and to quantify gastric acid output (both basal and after stimulation with subcutaneous pentagastrin), is indicated in only two rare circumstances: patients with elevated serum gastrin levels suggestive of Zollinger-Ellison syndrome or antral G-cell hyperplasia, but with equivocal responses to standard gastric provocative tests, and patients with indirect signs of gastric hypersecretion (e.g., enlarged folds and abundant clear fluid at endoscopy), normal gastrin levels, and negative provocative gastrin tests

but who may still be hypersecretors, such as patients with recurrent ulcer disease despite a prior vagotomy with or without antrectomy. A basal acid output greater than 15 mEq/hour or greater than 5 mEq/hour in a postoperative patient is considered a positive test result.

The diagnosis of Zollinger-Ellison syndrome is best confirmed by gastric analysis showing a basal acid output greater than 15 mEq/hour in conjunction with a fasting serum gastrin level exceeding 1000 pg/mL in the presence of gastric pH less than 2. To skip the cumbersome gastric analysis, a gastric pH determination showing a fasting pH of 2 or less is adequate. For serum gastrin levels in the range 100 to 1000 pg/mL and intragastric pH greater than 2, an increase in the serum gastrin to more than 200 pg/mL after a secretin stimulation test is suggestive of the diagnosis. An elevated serum gastrin level alone is not sufficient to diagnose Zollinger-Ellison syndrome, because serum gastrin levels tend to increase over time with atrophic gastritis and are also increased in patients receiving proton pump inhibitor therapy.

Other Causes

In patients in whom a gastroduodenal ulcer cannot be ascribed to colonization with *H. pylori,* use of NSAIDs, or a hypersecretory syndrome, the establishment of a definite etiologic diagnosis may require a more thorough evaluation, starting with a medical history that focuses on the use of other ulcerogenic agents and the presence of symptoms that could suggest an underlying systemic disease. The next step is to evaluate biopsy samples from ulcer borders and from the antrum, corpus, and duodenum. The ulcer specimens may reveal overt or suspicious signs of malignancy, in particular adenocarcinoma (Chapter 198) or lymphoma. In these cases, further diagnostic evaluation should include staging of the malignancy. Alternatively, the biopsies may provide evidence of other infectious conditions, specific types of gastritis, celiac disease, ischemia, amyloidosis, or a systemic inflammatory condition. These data can be combined with clues provided by the endoscopic evaluation, including the character and location of the ulcer, signs of ischemia, and signs of inflammation at other locations. Further evaluation should focus on the presence of systemic disorders and may include a chest radiograph, angiography, ileocolonoscopy, and abdominal CT.

Differential Diagnosis

The differential diagnosis of ulcer-like symptoms includes many disorders of the upper abdominal organs, including malignant diseases of the stomach (Chapter 198), duodenum (Chapter 199), pancreas (Chapter 200), or bile ducts (Chapter 202). The differential diagnosis of upper abdominal symptoms also includes liver and gallstone disease (Chapter 158), pancreatitis (Chapter 146), and motility disorders (Chapter 138). In many patients with upper abdominal dyspeptic complaints, no underlying cause can be identified. In this "nonulcer" or functional dyspepsia group, complaints characteristic of gastroesophageal reflux, ulcer symptoms, or dysmotility symptoms may be prominent. A few of these patients (generally 5%) benefit from eradication of *H. pylori,* with a slow decrease of dyspeptic complaints over 12 to 24 months, but functional dyspepsia is not a proven or widely accepted indication for treatment of *H. pylori.* If such treatment is considered, both the patient and the physician should be prepared for persistent symptoms despite eradication of *H. pylori.*

Diagnostic Scenarios: Acute or Initial Clinical Presentation

Younger (≤45 years old) patients without alarm symptoms or signs such as anemia, rapid weight loss, or other evidence of serious disease do not necessarily require endoscopy, and evidence indicates that malignant gastric disease is unlikely. When a generalist physician is treating a patient who lives in an area of the world with a relatively high prevalence of *H. pylori* infection (>10% of the population is positive), a test-and-treat approach can begin with an *H. pylori* stool antigen determination, urea breath test, or *H. pylori* serologic examination. If the test is positive, the patient can be treated with the appropriate *H. pylori* eradication drugs (see later) and observed for 4 to 6 weeks. If the patient is also taking an NSAID, either orally or parenterally, the same approach is appropriate, but the NSAID should be discontinued. If the *H. pylori* test is negative in a person taking NSAIDs, these drugs should be discontinued, and the patient should be treated with a proton pump inhibitor for 4 to 6 weeks. In patients who are not taking NSAIDs or who do not improve after these drugs are discontinued, endoscopy is indicated to determine whether an ulcer is present.

Conversely, gastroenterologists more commonly proceed directly to endoscopy. If no abnormalities are apparent or the endoscopic study shows only "gastritis" without an overt ulcer, a biopsy should be obtained to ascertain by histologic examination or urease testing whether *H. pylori* is present. If *H. pylori* is found by endoscopic biopsy, eradication treatment may be given; however, the effect of *H. pylori* eradication on relief of functional dyspeptic symptoms is only about 5% greater than with placebo.[1]

If endoscopic examination shows an ulcer, its location determines the subsequent approach. An ulcer in the duodenal bulb has only a remote chance of representing a malignant lesion and need not routinely be examined by biopsy. By contrast, biopsy is mandatory for a gastric ulcerative lesion identified at endoscopy, because malignant gastric disease may present with similar clinical manifestations and may resemble benign ulcer disease morphologically; even if histologic assessment does not identify a malignant process, repeat endoscopy is recommended about 1 month after therapy to verify complete healing and for biopsy of the scar.

TREATMENT   Rx

Helicobacter pylori Infection

H. pylori–associated ulcers often heal spontaneously, but acid suppressive therapy accelerates healing and ameliorates symptoms. Four weeks of acid suppressive therapy heals 70 to 80% of ulcers, and this number increases to more than 90% after 8 weeks of therapy. If *H. pylori* infection persists, however, ulcers recur in 50 to 90% of patients within 12 to 24 months; this rate can be reduced to 20 to 30% with maintenance acid suppression and to less than 5% with *H. pylori* eradication.[2] Eradication treatment is therefore mandatory (Table 141-4). Treatment for 10 to 14 days has about a 5 to 10% advantage over 7- to 10-day therapy,[3] and quadruple drug therapy is probably better than triple therapy.[4] Nevertheless, 7-day treatment may be acceptable in regions where local studies have shown that a particular treatment is very effective, and it is probably the most economical option in countries with low health care budgets. For patients in whom such therapy fails, a 4- to 10-day course of quadruple therapy is advised. This second-line regimen eradicates *H. pylori* in an additional 80 to 90% of patients. Resistance of *H. pylori* to metronidazole varies between 10 and 80% throughout the world. Clarithromycin resistance is increasing and is now estimated to be 5 to 10% in the United States because of the widespread use of macrolides to treat upper respiratory infections. Resistance to amoxicillin and tetracycline is rare and is not usually relevant in clinical practice. Sequential therapy may be superior to standard triple therapy and is a good alternative for both first- and second-line treatment.

Continuation of acid suppressive therapy after antibiotic treatment is needed only when symptoms persist[5] or in cases of complicated ulcer disease until eradication of *H. pylori* has been confirmed. Ascertainment of therapeutic efficacy must be delayed at least 1 month after the end of treatment to prevent false-negative results related to the organism's temporary suppression but not eradication. When repeat endoscopy is needed (e.g., a gastric ulcer requires repeated histologic examination to exclude underlying malignancy), repeat screening for *H. pylori* can be performed using the gastric biopsy specimens for histologic examination, culture, or urease testing. If no clinical indication exists for repeat endoscopy, *H. pylori* status can be determined by a carbon-13 urea breath test, stool *H. pylori* antigen, or repeated serology. Serologic determination is based on a more than 40 to 50% decrease in immunoglobulin G antibody levels in the first 6 months after treatment compared with pretreatment levels in that patient.

After successful *H. pylori* eradication, the risk of recurrent infection in most populations is small. In a minority of patients, ulcers recur either owing to re-infection or in the presence of another ulcerogenic factor, particularly NSAID use.

Disease Related to Nonsteroidal Anti-inflammatory Drug Use

In patients who are diagnosed with acid peptic disease while they are taking NSAIDs or aspirin, the first step is to stop such therapy. Acid suppression with a proton pump inhibitor (in doses similar to those used for *H. pylori*) leads to healing of 85% of NSAID-induced gastric ulcers and more than 90% of duodenal ulcers within 8 weeks of therapy, whereas acid suppression with an H_2-blocker, equivalent to ranitidine 300 mg twice daily, heals approximately 70% of ulcers within 8 weeks. The mucosal protective drug misoprostol (200 mg four times daily) has a similar effect. Treatment must be continued for at least 8 weeks, and maintenance therapy is needed in patients who continue to take NSAIDs. Gastric ulcers, larger lesions, and recurrent lesions heal more slowly.

Ulcer occurrence during NSAID therapy suggests a causative relationship, but patients should also be tested for *H. pylori*. In patients who are *H. pylori* positive, eradication therapy should be considered because there are no clear clinical parameters distinguishing between these etiologic factors. In patients who continue to take NSAIDs, maintenance therapy with a proton pump inhibitor is superior to *H. pylori* eradication for the prevention of recurrent ulcer,[6] except in patients who use aspirin, for whom *H. pylori* eradication alone may be curative.

Idiopathic Ulcer Disease

Patients with idiopathic ulcer disease despite a thorough assessment for underlying causes are treated primarily with an acid suppressant, usually a proton pump inhibitor, because they are at considerable risk for recurrent ulcer disease. After the underlying cause is identified and adequately treated, acid suppressive therapy can be withdrawn if there are no additional risk factors for ulcer disease, such as NSAID therapy or *H. pylori* infection.

PREVENTION

Primary Prevention

A test-and-treat strategy for *H. pylori* colonization may be considered for patients with dyspeptic symptoms, but there is no specific way to prevent *H. pylori*–associated ulcer disease. In contrast, primary prevention of NSAID-associated ulcer disease is widely advocated for patients at high risk because of a prior ulcer, severe concomitant disease, use of warfarin or high-dose corticosteroids, or older age (>65 years). H_2-blockers (at a dose equivalent to ranitidine 300 mg twice daily) partially prevents duodenal ulcer disease during NSAID therapy but has no effect on preventing gastric ulcers unless a higher dose (equivalent to famotidine 40 mg twice daily) is given. Proton

TABLE 141-4	OVERVIEW OF ANTIBIOTICS USED FOR *HELICOBACTER PYLORI* ERADICATION			
DRUG CLASS	**DRUG**	**TRIPLE THERAPY* DOSE**	**QUADRUPLE THERAPY† DOSE**	**SEQUENTIAL THERAPY‡ DOSE**
Acid suppression	Proton pump inhibitor	20-40 mg bid§	20-40 mg bid§	20-40 mg bid§
Standard antimicrobials	Bismuth compound‖	2 tablets bid	2 tablets bid	
	Amoxicillin	1 g bid		1 g bid
	Metronidazole¶	500 mg bid	500 mg tid	500 mg bid
	Clarithromycin	500 mg bid		500 mg bid
	Tetracycline		500 mg qid	
Salvage antimicrobials	Levofloxacin	300 mg bid	300 mg bid	
	Rifabutin	150 mg bid		
	Furazolidone	100 mg bid		
	Doxycycline		100 mg bid	
	Nitazoxanide		1 g bid	

*Triple therapy consists of a proton pump inhibitor or bismuth compound, together with two of the listed antibiotics, usually given for 7-14 days.
†Quadruple therapy consists of a proton pump inhibitor plus either the combination of a bismuth compound, metronidazole, and tetracycline given for 4-10 days, or the combination of levofloxacin, doxycycline, and nitazoxanide for 10 days.
‡Sequential therapy consists of 10 days of proton pump inhibitor treatment, plus amoxicillin during days 1-5 and a combination of clarithromycin and an imidazole (when available, tinidazole; otherwise, metronidazole) during days 6-10.
§Proton pump inhibitor dose equivalent to omeprazole 20 mg bid.
‖Bismuth subsalicylate or subcitrate.
¶An alternative is tinidazole 500 mg bid.

pump inhibitors (at a dose equivalent to omeprazole 20 mg once daily) and misoprostol (in doses varying between 400 and 800 mg/day) partially protect against both gastric and duodenal ulcers during NSAID use. Misoprostol and proton pump inhibitors are equally effective,[7] but adherence with therapy is lower with misoprostol owing to its side effects. Patients should be advised of the importance of adherence because less than 80% adherence to gastroprotection is associated with a more than two-fold increased risk for ulcer disease compared with those who are fully adherent. During low-dose aspirin therapy, primary prevention of ulcers is advocated for the same risk groups, using a proton pump inhibitor or an H_2-receptor antagonist.[8]

Secondary Prevention

Secondary prevention of *H. pylori*–associated ulcer disease is mandatory and consists of successful bacterial eradication. Testing to ascertain *H. pylori* status after eradication therapy is indicated in patients with prior complicated ulcer disease or with persistent or recurrent symptoms after therapy, as well as in patients who fail to complete the therapeutic course.

Secondary prevention of NSAID-related ulcer disease is preferentially achieved by the withdrawal of NSAIDs. In patients who must continue taking NSAIDs, a change to a selective COX2 inhibitor in combination with a proton pump inhibitor at a dose equivalent to esomeprazole 20 mg twice daily is advocated, especially for patients with complicated ulcer disease.[9] This combination is associated with a lower risk of secondary peptic ulcer complications than treatment with a COX2 inhibitor alone.

Secondary prevention of recurrent ulcers in patients who use aspirin may depend on *H. pylori* status. In *H. pylori*–positive patients, *H. pylori* eradication is as effective as a proton pump inhibitor for the prevention of recurrent ulcers.[6] In *H. pylori*–negative patients, additional acid suppressive therapy at a dose equivalent to esomeprazole 20 mg twice daily should be prescribed. Secondary prevention of idiopathic ulcer disease consists primarily of maintenance therapy with a proton pump inhibitor and treatment of the underlying condition.

PROGNOSIS

The majority of peptic ulcers heal spontaneously within weeks to months. However, if the underlying condition is not adequately treated, a large proportion of ulcers recur. Both initial and recurrent ulcers can give rise to complications. The four major complications are intractability, perforation, hemorrhage, and stenosis. Each distinct situation requires specific management approaches. Patients with complicated ulcer disease are at particular risk for recurrent complications and need careful assessment for secondary prevention.

Hemorrhage

Hemorrhage (Chapter 137), which is the most common complication of peptic ulcer disease, occurs in about one in six patients with ulcers over the course of their ulcer activity. Ulcers caused by NSAIDs account for a larger proportion of these hemorrhages. Peptic ulcer is thus the most common cause of nonvariceal upper gastrointestinal bleeding, accounting for 40 to 60% of cases in most populations. Bleeding is associated with a 5 to 15% risk of rebleeding and up to a 10% risk of mortality. Hemorrhage may occur along a continuum from a serious acute event associated with hemodynamic shock and high mortality to slow or intermittent blood loss leading to chronic anemia. Approximately 80% of patients with bleeding ulcers describe a prior history of symptomatic disease, and about 20 to 30% have suffered a previous hemorrhage. Assessment of the magnitude of bleeding is of paramount importance in determining the need for transfusion and subsequent management (Table 141-5). Initial hematocrit levels may be misleading and are likely to fall because of hemodilution. Rapid bleeding is usually apparent on the basis of clinical signs (pallor, systolic blood pressure ≤100 mm Hg, pulse ≥100/minute); immediate fluid resuscitation and transfusions are indicated to prevent circulatory collapse. Mortality is particularly related to complications of the bleed, such as aspiration, and exacerbation of underlying disease, such as pulmonary, cardiovascular, renal, and hepatic disease. On rare occasions, patients may actually bleed to death, especially when a larger artery is affected, such as when an ulcer in the posterior wall of the duodenal bulb perforates the gastroduodenal artery.

Initial treatment aims at hemodynamic stabilization. Endoscopy is the mainstay of therapy and should be performed within 24 hours of presentation in high-risk cases, especially patients who are hemodynamically unstable, require transfusion, or have more severe comorbidities. Endoscopy can be

TABLE 141-5 BLATCHFORD SCORING SYSTEM TO DETERMINE THE NEED FOR INTERVENTION IN PEPTIC ULCER BLEEDING

VARIABLE	VALUE AT ADMISSION	SCORE COMPONENT VALUE
Blood urea (mmol/L)	6.5-7.9	2
	8.0-9.9	3
	10.0-24.9	4
	≥25.0	6
Hemoglobin (g/L)		
Men	120-129	1
	100-119	2
	<100	6
Women	100-119	1
	<100	6
Systolic blood pressure (mm Hg)	100-109	1
	90-99	2
	<90	3
Other markers	Pulse ≥100/min	1
	Presentation with melena	1
	Presentation with syncope	2
	Hepatic disease	2
	Cardiac failure	2

Data from Stanley AJ, Ashley D, Dalton HR, et al. Outpatient management of patients with low-risk upper gastrointestinal haemorrhage: multicentre validation and prospective evaluation. *Lancet.* 2009;373:42-47. Intervention (endoscopic hemostasis, surgery, transfusion) is rarely needed for patients with an admission score ≤2 but is required in more than 40% of patients with a score ≥6.

TABLE 141-6 ENDOSCOPY RESULTS IN PATIENTS WITH BLEEDING ULCERS

ENDOSCOPY RESULT	ULCER CHARACTERISTICS*	RISK OF RECURRENT BLEEDING (%)
Active bleeding	Arterial bleeding	80-90
	Oozing bleeding	10-30
Stigmata of recent bleeding	Nonbleeding visible vessel	50-60
	Adherent clot	25-35
	Flat pigmented spot	0-8
No signs of bleeding	Clean ulcer base	0-12

*The ulcer characteristics determine the risk of recurrent bleeding during follow-up.

performed to ascertain the origin of the bleeding, and, if necessary, provide therapy to stop the bleed and reduce the risk of rebleeding.

The appearance of the ulcer determines the need for endoscopic treatment and the risk of rebleeding (Table 141-6) and mortality. "Clean base" ulcers and those with flat pigmented spots carry a low risk of rebleeding and do not require endoscopic treatment. In contrast, ulcers with active bleeding or stigmata of recent bleeding, in particular a visible vessel or adherent clot, require treatment to stop the bleed and reduce the otherwise high risk of recurrence.

Endoscopic therapy may lead to a three-fold reduction in episodes of recurrent bleeding and in the need for surgical intervention, as well as a 40% reduction in mortality.[10] Treatment modalities include injection therapy with epinephrine or a sclerosant, thermocoagulation, and mechanical pressure by means of clips. Thermocoagulation can be performed by direct contact, such as with a heater probe, or by a noncontact method, such as argon plasma coagulation. The efficacy of these methods is generally comparable, except that epinephrine injection alone is inferior to the other modalities but can be useful when combined with any of the others.[10,11] If an adherent clot is found, an attempt should be made to remove it by water flushing or snaring to allow an assessment of the underlying ulcer base and the treatment of any underlying visible vessels to reduce the risk of rebleeding.[12]

The pre-endoscopy administration of intravenous proton pump inhibitor therapy (at a dose equivalent to a bolus of 80 mg esomeprazole, followed by a continuous infusion of 8 mg/hour until endoscopy) reduces bleeding and the need for emergent endoscopic treatment, but it has no effect on the need

TABLE 141-7 ROCKALL SCORING SYSTEM FOR THE RISK OF MORTALITY FOLLOWING PEPTIC ULCER BLEEDING

VARIABLE	Score 0	1	2	3
Age (yr)	<60	60-79	80	—
Shock	Not present	Pulse >100	Systolic BP <100 mm Hg	—
Comorbidity	None		Cardiac failure Coronary insufficiency Other serious illness	Renal insufficiency Liver failure Metastatic malignancy
Diagnosis	Mallory-Weiss syndrome or no identifiable cause	Ulcer Varices	Malignancy of proximal digestive tract	—
Endoscopy	No signs of recent bleeding		Bleeding, clot, or visible vessel	—

BP = blood pressure.
Data from Rockall TA, Logan RFA, Devlin HB, et al. Risk assessment after acute upper gastrointestinal haemorrhage. *Gut.* 1996;38:316-321.

FIGURE 141-5. Plain chest radiograph in an upright patient with a perforated ulcer. The radiograph shows free air under the diaphragm.

for transfusion or the occurrence of rebleeding or death. For patients with active bleeding or stigmata of recent bleeding, endoscopic treatment should be followed by an intravenous proton pump inhibitor given as a bolus at a dose equivalent to 80 mg esomeprazole over 30 minutes, followed by a continuous infusion at a dose equivalent to esomeprazole 8 mg/hour for 72 hours, to reduce rebleeding and the need for further intervention.[13] Other therapies, including tranexamic acid, vasopressin, somatostatin, and octreotide, should be considered experimental (Chapter 137). Second-look endoscopy is not routinely indicated but can be considered in very high-risk cases, particularly when there is doubt about the adequacy of initial visualization or treatment.

About 70 to 80% of rebleeds occur within the first 3 days and generally should be managed by repeat endoscopy. If endoscopy fails to stop the bleed or prevent further rebleeding, surgery and interventional radiology are equivalent options. Surgery includes stitching of the ulcer and occlusion of the feeding artery, usually the gastroduodenal artery. Interventional radiology uses angiography to insert a coil in the culprit vessel at the site of the bleed. Single-center observational experience suggests that each of these methods is equally effective in the hands of experienced clinicians, and the choice depends on local availability and expertise.

The risk for a fatal outcome of an upper gastrointestinal hemorrhage can be estimated based on five clinical and endoscopic parameters (Table 141-7). In several studies, mortality in patients with a bleeding peptic ulcer was less than 2% among those with a score of 2 points or less, 10% in those with 3 to 5 points, and up to 46% in those with 6 points or more. Management of patients who recover after a peptic ulcer hemorrhage is similar to the treatment of patients with uncomplicated ulcers. Eradication of *H. pylori* provides excellent protection against both recurrence and rebleeding of *H. pylori*–related ulcers. NSAID-induced ulcers are preferentially managed by the withdrawal of NSAIDs or, if this is not feasible, by the combination of a COX2 inhibitor and a proton pump inhibitor at a dose equivalent to esomeprazole 20 mg twice daily. In patients with a history of ulcer bleeding and concomitant cardiovascular disease requiring antiplatelet therapy, the combination of low-dose aspirin and a proton pump inhibitor at a dose equivalent to esomeprazole 20 mg twice daily is associated with a lower risk of complicated ulcer than is clopidogrel monotherapy.[14] If a patient who requires antiplatelet therapy presents with a bleeding ulcer, antiplatelet therapy should be continued or restarted as soon as possible if the risk of a cardiovascular event outweighs the risk of recurrent bleeding.[15]

Perforation

Perforation may manifest as an acute event, whereby gastric contents spill into the peritoneal cavity, or more insidiously as the ulcer slowly penetrates into surrounding tissues. Acute free perforation typically causes abrupt and severe abdominal pain associated with abdominal muscular spasm that produces board-like rigidity of the abdomen and other manifestations of peritoneal irritation. Secondary hemodynamic shock is common. The clinical diagnosis can be confirmed in approximately 80% of patients by a plain chest radiograph with the patient standing (Fig. 141-5); a CT scan can be obtained if doubt persists. Leukocytosis and elevated C-reactive protein levels develop rapidly, and mild hyperamylasemia may occur. Treatment begins by correcting hemodynamic, fluid, and electrolyte imbalances. Nasogastric suction is helpful, and prophylactic antibiotics (e.g., amoxicillin-clavulanic acid 1 g every 8 hours intravenously) are usually administered. Unless a specific contraindication exists, emergency surgery is usually indicated, although more conservative approaches are sometimes appropriate. Given the success in achieving the long-term cure of ulcer disease through the eradication of *H. pylori* and the withdrawal of NSAIDs, suturing of the perforated ulcer may be adequate, permitting the patient to avoid a more radical vagotomy with or without gastric resection.

Intractability

Intractability is a term strictly applied to an ulcer that persists even after intensive and prolonged proton pump inhibitor therapy. Symptoms may or may not be present. These rare cases may result from poor compliance with recommended treatment, surreptitious use of ulcerogenic drugs, or other diseases (e.g., Crohn's disease, ischemia, infection with bacteria other than *H. pylori*, viral infection). If these issues are recognized and these diagnoses are pursued, further complications and interventions such as surgical vagotomy and pyloroplasty can almost always be avoided.

Acid peptic disease related to alcohol or bisphosphonates should be addressed by discontinuing the precipitating agent. Treatment of Zollinger-Ellison syndrome requires high-dose proton pump inhibitors and/or surgery (Chapter 201). Those rare ulcers caused by Crohn's disease (Chapter 143), vasculitis (Chapter 278), sarcoidosis (Chapter 95), polycythemia vera (Chapter 169), amyloidosis (Chapter 194), and other rare disorders should be addressed by treating the underlying condition. Stress ulcers and Cameron's ulcers are treated by potent acid suppression therapy (e.g., omeprazole 20 mg twice daily).

Stenosis

Gastric outlet obstruction is now a rare complication of ulcer disease because of the early detection and treatment of most ulcers. Most patients who develop clinically relevant gastric outlet obstruction have had an ulcer in the duodenal bulb and/or pyloric channel. Edema and inflammation play an important role, and occasionally a patient with active disease presents with symptoms of outlet obstruction as manifested by nausea, vomiting, and gastric stasis without a tight, chronic stenosis. Management therefore involves three key steps. This first is nasogastric tube aspiration and gastric lavage to clean the stomach of retained debris, followed by early endoscopy.

This step facilitates an accurate diagnosis. Nasogastric suction may need to be maintained for several days if vomiting resumes when the tube is clamped. The second step consists of intense antisecretory therapy using intravenous proton pump inhibitors in a dose equivalent to a bolus of 80 mg esomeprazole over 30 minutes, followed by a continuous infusion of 8 mg/hour. Finally, the cause of the ulcer needs to be addressed, usually by eradicating *H. pylori* and withdrawing NSAIDs. If the initial treatment resolves the clinical situation and the patient can resume eating, it is often not necessary to undertake further treatment of the outlet stenosis; however, tight, fibrous scarring may require endoscopic balloon dilation or surgery.

1. Moayyedi P, Soo S, Deeks J, et al. Eradication of *Helicobacter pylori* for non-ulcer dyspepsia. *Cochrane Database Syst Rev.* 2006;2:CD002096.
2. Ford AC, Delaney BC, Forman D, et al. Eradication therapy for peptic ulcer disease in *Helicobacter pylori*-positive patients. *Cochrane Database Syst Rev.* 2006;2:CD003840.
3. Fuccio L, Minardi ME, Zagari RM, et al. Meta-analysis: duration of first-line proton-pump inhibitor based triple therapy for the *Helicobacter pylori* eradication. *Ann Intern Med.* 2007;147:553-562.
4. Malfertheiner P, Bazzoli F, Delchier JC, et al. *Helicobacter pylori* eradication with a capsule containing bismuth subcitrate potassium, metronidazole, and tetracycline given with omeprazole versus clarithromycin-based triple therapy: a randomised, open-label, non-inferiority, phase 3 trial. *Lancet.* 2011;377:905-913.
5. Gisbert JP, Pajares JM. Systematic review and meta-analysis: is 1-week proton pump inhibitor-based triple therapy sufficient to heal peptic ulcer? *Aliment Pharmacol Ther.* 2005;21:795-804.
6. Chan FK, Chung SC, Suen BY, et al. Preventing recurrent upper gastrointestinal bleeding in patients with *Helicobacter pylori* infection who are taking low-dose aspirin or naproxen. *N Engl J Med.* 2001;344:967-973.
7. Graham DY, Agrawal NM, Campbell DR, et al. NSAID-Associated Gastric Ulcer Prevention Study Group. Ulcer prevention in long-term users of non-steroidal anti-inflammatory drugs: results of a double blind, randomized, multicenter, active- and placebo-controlled study of misoprostol versus lansoprazole. *Arch Intern Med.* 2002;162:169-175.
8. Taha AS, McCloskey C, Prasad R, et al. Famotidine for the prevention of peptic ulcers and oesophagitis in patients taking low-dose aspirin (FAMOUS): a phase III, randomised, double-blind, placebo-controlled trial. *Lancet.* 2009;374:119-125.
9. Barkun A, Bardou M, Kuipers EJ, et al. International consensus recommendations on the management of patients with non-variceal upper gastrointestinal bleeding. *Ann Intern Med.* 2010;152:101-113.
10. Barkun AN, Martel M, Toubouti Y, et al. Endoscopic hemostasis in peptic ulcer bleeding for patients with high-risk lesions: a series of meta-analyses. *Gastrointest Endosc.* 2009;69:786-799.
11. Laine L, McQuaid KR. Endoscopic therapy for bleeding ulcers: an evidence-based approach based on meta-analyses of randomized controlled trials. *Clin Gastroenterol Hepatol.* 2009;7:33-47.
12. Kahi CJ, Jensen DM, Sung JJ, et al. Endoscopic therapy versus medical therapy for bleeding peptic ulcer with adherent clot: a meta-analysis. *Gastroenterology.* 2005;129:855-862.
13. Sung JJ, Barkun A, Kuipers EJ, et al. Intravenous esomeprazole for prevention of recurrent peptic ulcer bleeding: a randomized trial. *Ann Intern Med.* 2009;150;455-464.
14. Chan FK, Ching JY, Hung LC, et al. Clopidogrel versus aspirin and esomeprazole to prevent recurrent ulcer bleeding. *N Engl J Med.* 2005;352:238-244.
15. Sung JJ, Lau YW, Ching JYL, et al. Continuation of low-dose aspirin in peptic ulcer bleeding: a randomized, controlled trial. *Ann Intern Med.* 2010;152:1-9.

SUGGESTED READINGS

Lanza FL, Chan FL, Quigley EM, et al. Guidelines for prevention of NSAID-related ulcer complications. *Am J Gastroenterol.* 2009;104:728-738. *International consensus guidelines on the prevention of NSAID-related ulcer disease.*
Madanick RD. Proton pump inhibitor side effects and drug interactions: much ado about nothing? *Cleve Clin J Med.* 2011;78:39-49. *Review.*
Malfertheiner P, Chan FK, McColl KE. Peptic ulcer disease. *Lancet.* 2009;374:1449-1461. *Review.*
McColl KE. *Helicobacter pylori* infection. *N Engl J Med.* 2010;362;1597-1604. *Review.*

142

APPROACH TO THE PATIENT WITH DIARRHEA AND MALABSORPTION

CAROL E. SEMRAD

DEFINITIONS

Normal stool frequency ranges from three times a week to three times a day. As a symptom, diarrhea can be described as a decrease in stool consistency (increased fluidity), stools that cause urgency or abdominal discomfort, or an increase in the frequency of stool. Consistency is defined as the ratio of fecal water to the water-holding capacity of fecal insoluble solids, which are composed of bacterial mass and dietary fiber. Because it is difficult to measure stool consistency and because stool is predominantly (60 to 85%) water, stool weight becomes a reasonable surrogate of consistency.

As a sign, diarrhea is defined by the weight or volume of stool measured over a 24- to 72-hour period. Daily stool weights of children and adults are less than 200 g, and greater stool weights are an objective definition of diarrhea; however, this definition misses 20% of diarrheal symptoms in patients who have loose stools that are less than this daily weight.

Acute diarrheas persist for less than 2 to 3 weeks or, rarely, 6 to 8 weeks. The most common cause of acute diarrhea is infection. Chronic diarrheal conditions persist for at least 4 weeks and, more typically, 6 to 8 weeks or longer. There are four mechanisms of diarrhea: osmotic, secretory, exudative, and altered motility. Because many diarrheal diseases are due to more than one of these mechanisms, it is clinically useful to categorize diarrhea as malabsorptive (fatty), watery, and inflammatory.

EPIDEMIOLOGY

Diarrhea is the second leading cause of mortality worldwide and is particularly problematic for elderly people and for children younger than 5 years of age in developing nations. Infectious diarrheal conditions cause 1.8 million childhood deaths annually, despite the improved use of oral rehydration solutions, zinc, and vitamin A supplements. About one third of these deaths have been due to rotavirus infection (Chapter 388), but the recently introduced oral monovalent rotavirus vaccination has diminished its incidence and mortality in developing and developed nations.

In the United States, about 48 million people suffer from food-borne illness each year, with 128,000 hospitalizations and 3000 deaths, most in elderly people. The complaint of diarrhea accounts for more than 7 million outpatient visits per year. Total costs for diarrheal diseases are about $1.2 billion in direct (health care) costs and $5.4 billion in indirect costs (days lost from work).

PATHOBIOLOGY

Abnormalities of Fluid and Electrolyte Transport

To understand the osmotic, secretory, and inflammatory mechanisms of diarrhea, it is necessary to understand how the normal intestine handles fluid and solutes in health and disease. Whether a hypotonic meal, such as a steak and water, or a hypertonic meal, such as milk and a doughnut, is consumed, the volume of the meal is augmented by gastric, pancreatic, biliary, and duodenal secretions. The permeable duodenum then renders the meal approximately isotonic with an electrolyte content similar to that of plasma by the time it reaches the proximal jejunum. As the intestinal slurry moves toward the colon, the Na^+ concentration in the luminal fluid remains constant, but Cl^- is reduced to 60 to 70 mmol/L, and bicarbonate (HCO_3^-) is increased to a similar concentration as the result of Cl^- and HCO_3^- transport mechanisms in the enterocyte and HCO_3^- secretion in the ileum (Fig. 142-1B and C). In the colon, K^{++} is secreted, and the Na^+ transport mechanism of the colonocyte, together with the low epithelial permeability, extracts Na^+ and fluid from the stool. As a result, the Na^+ content of stool decreases to 30 to 40 mmol/L; K^{++} increases from 5 to 10 mmol/L in the small bowel to 75 to 90 mmol/L; and poorly absorbed divalent cations, such as Mg^{2++} and Ca^{2++}, are concentrated in stool to values of 5 to 100 mmol/L. The anion concentrations in the colon change drastically because bacterial degradation of carbohydrate (i.e., unabsorbed starches, sugars, and fiber) creates short-chain fatty acids that attain concentrations of 80 to 180 mmol/L; at colonic pH, organic anions, such as acetate, propionate, and butyrate, are present. In the setting of carbohydrate malabsorption, the generation of high concentrations of these short-chain fatty acids may decrease stool pH to 4 or lower. The osmolality of the stool is approximately that of plasma (280 to 300 mOsm/kg H_2O) when it is passed.

At the cellular level Na^{++} transport by the epithelium from lumen to blood (by Na^{++}-coupled sugar and amino acid transport in the small intestine, by Na^{++}/H^{++} exchange proteins in the small intestine and proximal colon, and by aldosterone-regulated $^+Na^{++}$ channels in the distal colon) creates a favorable osmotic gradient for absorption (see Fig. 142-1A and B). Chloride transport by the epithelium from blood to lumen (by cystic fibrosis transmembrane conductance regulator [CFTR] and the calcium-activated chloride channel in the small intestine and colon) creates an osmotic gradient for secretion (see Fig. 142-1C). Normally, the intestine is in a net absorptive state, regulated by extrinsic adrenergic nerves and proabsorptive neuropeptides and hormones (see Fig. 142-1D). Stimulation of secretion by neurotransmitters, hormones, and inflammatory mediators (Table 142-1; see Fig. 142-1D) can offset this balance.

FIGURE 142-1. Mechanisms of intestinal transport of water and electrolytes. **A,** Intestinal sodium absorption. Sodium is actively absorbed in villus cells of the small intestine and surface cells of the colon. The sodium-potassium adenosine triphosphatase (Na^{++},K^{++}-ATPase) present on the cell basolateral membrane maintains a low intracellular Na^{+++} concentration and an electronegative cell interior favoring Na^{+++} movement across the apical membrane from lumen into cell. In the small intestine, glucose and galactose are taken up with sodium and water at the apical membrane by the sodium-glucose ligand transporter (SGLT1). Several different sodium-dependent amino acid carriers, some with overlapping substrate specificities, transport cationic, anionic, and neutral amino acids into villus cells. Dipeptides and tripeptides are transported by a hydrogen-coupled oligopeptide carrier, PepT1, that is driven by luminal hydrogen ions generated by the epithelial Na^+/H^+ exchanger. Fructose is taken up by the facilitative glucose transporter (GLUT5). **B,** Sodium also is absorbed by nutrient-independent transport processes in the small intestine and colon. The Na^{++}/H^{++} (NHE) and Cl^-/HCO_3^- (DRA) exchangers are inhibited by agents that elevate intracellular cyclic adenosine monophosphate (cAMP), cyclic guanosine monophosphate (cGMP), or calcium. **C,** Chloride secretion by intestinal crypt cells. Chloride can be secreted actively throughout the small intestine and colon. Intracellular mediators of secretion (cAMP, cGMP, Ca^{2+}) open apical Cl^- channels (cystic fibrosis transmembrane conductance regulator [CFTR], calcium-activated chloride channel [TMEM16]) and basolateral K^{++} channels. Chloride moves from crypt cells into the intestinal lumen, favoring movement of Cl^- from the blood into cells by the $Na^{++}/K^{++}/2Cl^-$ cotransporter (NKCC1). Bicarbonate (HCO_3^-) also may be secreted via the CFTR channel. **D,** Regulation of intestinal water and electrolyte transport. Normally, the intestine is in a net absorptive state under the control of extrinsic adrenergic nerves from the sympathetic nervous system. Guanylin, the natural ligand for the *Escherichia coli* stable-toxin receptor (membrane-bound guanylyl cyclase [GC-C]), may be important in regulating local chloride secretion. The normal tone of the intestine is modified by the enteric nervous system, endocrine and inflammatory cells in the intestinal mucosa, and circulating hormones. The enteric nervous system releases a variety of neurotransmitters, some that stimulate chloride secretion (e.g., vasoactive intestinal peptide [VIP], acetylcholine) and others that promote sodium absorption (e.g., enkephalins, neuropeptide Y). Hormones produced locally from enterochromaffin cells (ECC) in the intestinal epithelium and inflammatory mediators released from immune cells directly affect enterocytes and nearby nerves. Circulating hormones (e.g., aldosterone, glucocorticoids) enhance sodium absorption in the intestine. Glucocorticoids also inhibit release of arachidonic acid and production of prostaglandin by inflammatory cells.

Diarrhea is due primarily to alterations of intestinal fluid and electrolyte transport and less to smooth muscle function. Each 24 hours, 8 to 10 L of fluid enters the duodenum. The diet supplies 2 L of this fluid; the remainder comes from salivary, gastric, hepatic, pancreatic, and intestinal secretions. The small intestine normally absorbs 8 to 9 L (80%) of this fluid and presents 1.5 L to the colon for absorption. Of the remaining fluid, the colon absorbs all but approximately 100 mL. Diarrhea can result from increased secretion by the small intestine or the colon if the maximal daily absorptive capacity of the colon (4 L) is exceeded. Alternatively, if the colon is diseased so that it cannot absorb even the 1.5 L normally presented to it by the small intestine, diarrhea results.

Watery diarrheas may be due to osmotic, secretory, or inflammatory mechanisms. With ingestion of a poorly absorbed (e.g., Mg^{2++}) or unabsorbable (polyethylene glycol, lactulose or, in lactase-deficient individuals, lactose) solute, the osmotic force of the solute pulls water and secondarily sodium and chloride ions into the intestinal lumen. A considerable proportion of the osmolality of stool results from the nonabsorbed solute. This gap between stool osmolality and the sum of the electrolytes in the stool causes osmotic diarrhea.

Active chloride secretion or inhibited sodium absorption, which also create an osmotic gradient favorable for the movement of fluids from blood to lumen, explains the pathophysiology of the secretory diarrheas. Agents that increase enterocyte cyclic adenosine monophosphate (cAMP) (e.g., cholera toxin, prostaglandins), cyclic guanosine monophosphate (cGMP) (e.g., *Escherichia coli* stable toxin), or intracellular ionized calcium (Ca^{2+}) (e.g., acetylcholine) (see Table 142-1) inhibit non-nutrient Na^{++} absorption and stimulate Cl^- secretion (see Table 142-1 and Fig. 142-1C and D).

Inflammatory diarrheas, which may be watery or bloody, are characterized by enterocyte damage, villus atrophy, and crypt hyperplasia. The damaged enterocyte membrane of the small intestine has decreased disaccharidase and peptide hydrolase activity, reduced or absent Na^{++}-coupled sugar or amino acid transport mechanisms, and reduced or absent sodium chloride absorptive transporters. Conversely, the hyperplastic crypt cells maintain their ability to secrete ⁻ Cl^- (and perhaps HCO_3^-). If the inflammation is severe, immune-mediated vascular damage or ulceration allows blood, pus, and protein to leak (exudate) from capillaries and lymphatics and contribute to the diarrhea. Activation of lymphocytes, phagocytes, and fibroblasts releases various inflammatory mediators that induce intestinal chloride secretion (see Fig. 142-1D). Interleukin-1 (IL-1) and tumor necrosis factor, which also are released into the blood, cause fever, anorexia, and malaise.

ACUTE DIARRHEA

CLINICAL MANIFESTATIONS

Approximately 80% of acute diarrheas are due to infections with viruses, bacteria, and parasites. The remainder is due to medications that have an osmotic force, stimulate intestinal fluid secretion, or contain poorly or nonabsorbable sugars (e.g., sorbitol), or less commonly to fecal impaction, pelvic inflammation (e.g., acute appendicitis [Chapter 144]), or intestinal ischemia (Chapter 145).

Food-Borne and Water-Borne Infectious Diarrhea

Most infectious diarrheas are acquired through fecal-oral transmission from water, food, or person-to-person contact (Table 142-2). Patients with infectious diarrhea often complain of nausea, vomiting, and abdominal cramps that are associated with watery, malabsorptive, or bloody diarrhea and fever (dysentery) (Chapters 310 through 320, 344, 345, 358 to 360, 364, 365, 387, and 388). As documented using polymerase chain reaction methods of diagnosis, most outbreaks of nonbacterial acute gastroenteritis in the United States and other countries are caused by noroviruses (Norwalk agent; Chapter 388). Rotavirus (Chapter 388) predominantly causes diarrhea in infants, usually in the winter months, but also may cause nonseasonal acute diarrhea in adults, particularly in elderly people. Mechanisms for diarrhea include decreased fluid absorption due to destruction of villus enterocytes and stimulation of fluid secretion by NSP4 rotatoxin and viral activation of the enteric nervous system.

Food-borne bacterial diseases in the United States are primarily due to *Salmonella* (Chapter 316), *Campylobacter jejuni* (Chapter 311), and *E. coli* O157:H7 (Chapter 312), and less commonly *Shigella* (Chapter 317). Outbreaks of *E. coli* O157:H7 have been associated with petting zoos, uncooked ground beef, and green leafy vegetables. These bacteria most often invade the distal small bowel and colon, where they multiply intracellularly and damage the epithelium. Diarrhea is due to the stimulation of intestinal secretion by inflammatory mediators, decreased absorption across the damaged epithelium, and exudation of protein into the lumen. *Shigella* species and enterohemorrhagic *E. coli* produce a similar toxin, the "Shiga toxin," which is cytotoxic to intestinal epithelial cells and causes inflammation, cell damage, and diarrhea with blood and pus.

Outbreaks of *Cryptosporidium* (Chapter 358) have been reported in water parks. This parasite causes diarrhea by adhering and fusing to the epithelial cell membrane in the small bowel, thereby causing cell damage. Organisms that are specific for seafood include *Vibrio parahaemolyticus* (Chapter 310),

TABLE 142-1 STIMULI OF INTESTINAL SECRETION

AGENT	INTRACELLULAR MEDIATOR	RELATED DIARRHEAL ILLNESS
Enterotoxins		
Cholera, *E. coli* heat labile toxin, *Salmonella, Yersinia*	cAMP	Travelers, endemic
E. coli heat stable toxin	cGMP	
Rotatoxin (NSP4)	?	Viral gastroenteritis
Serotonin, PAF	Ca	Inflammatory, allergic
PG, leukotrienes	cAMP, Ca	Invasive enteric bacteria*
PG	cAMP	Villous adenoma
Histamine	Ca	Intestinal allergies, mastocytosis, scombroid poisoning
VIP	cAMP	VIPoma, ganglioneuromas
5-HT, substance P, bradykinin	Ca	Malignant carcinoid
Calcitonin	?	Medullary carcinoma thyroid
Acetylcholine	Ca	Insecticides, nerve gas poisoning, cholinergic drugs
Ricinoleic acid	cAMP, Ca	Laxative abuse†
Caffeine	cAMP	Coffee, sodas, tea

Shigella species, *Clostridium difficile*, enteroinvasive *E. coli*, *Vibrio parahaemolyticus*, *Clostridium perfringens*.
†Also phenolphthalein, anthraquinones, bisacodyl, dioctyl sodium sulfosuccinate, and senna.
5-HT = 5-hydroxytryptamine; Ca = calcium; cAMP = cyclic adenosine monophosphate; cGMP = cyclic guanosine monophosphate; PAF - platelet-activating factor; PG = prostaglandin; VIP = vasoactive intestinal peptide.

TABLE 142-2 EPIDEMIOLOGY OF ACUTE INFECTIOUS DIARRHEA AND INFECTIOUS FOOD-BORNE ILLNESS

VEHICLE	CLASSIC PATHOGENS
Water (including foods washed in such water)	*Vibrio cholerae*, caliciviruses (Norwalk agent), *Giardia, Cryptosporidium*
Food	
Poultry	*Salmonella, Campylobacter, Shigella* species
Beef, unpasteurized fruit juice	Enterohemorrhagic *Escherichia coli*
Pork	Tapeworm
Seafood and shellfish (including raw sushi and gefilte fish)	*V. cholerae, Vibrio parahaemolyticus*, and *Vibrio vulnificus; Salmonella* and *Shigella* species; hepatitis A and B viruses; tapeworm; anisakiasis
Cheese, milk	*Listeria* species
Eggs	*Salmonella* species
Mayonnaise-containing foods and cream pies	Staphylococcal and clostridial food poisonings
Fried rice	*Bacillus cereus*
Fresh berries	*Cyclospora* species
Canned vegetables or fruits	*Clostridium* species
Sprouts	Enterohemorrhagic *E. coli, Salmonella* species
Animal-to-person (pets and livestock) contact	*Salmonella, Campylobacter, Cryptosporidium*, enterohemorrhagic *E. coli*, and *Giardia* species
Person-to-person (including sexual) contact	All enteric bacteria, viruses, and parasites
Daycare center	*Shigella, Campylobacter, Cryptosporidium*, and *Giardia* species; viruses; *Clostridium difficile*
Hospitalization, antibiotics, or chemotherapy	*C. difficile*
Swimming pool	*Giardia* and *Cryptosporidium* species
Foreign travel	*E. coli* of various types; *Salmonella, Shigella, Campylobacter, Giardia*, and *Cryptosporidium* species; *Entamoeba histolytica*

Adapted from Powell DW. Approach to the patient with diarrhea. In: Yamada T, Alpers DH, Owyang C, et al, eds. *Textbook of Gastroenterology*, 3rd ed. Philadelphia: Lippincott-Raven; 1999.

which causes either watery or bloody diarrhea, and *Vibrio vulnificus,* which causes watery diarrhea and, especially in patients with liver disease, a fatal septicemia. Ingestion of meat contaminated by anthrax (Chapter 302) causes fever, diffuse abdominal pain, and bloody stool or vomitus. Anthrax invades the intestinal mucosa; the organism, or anthrax toxin, causes inflammation, ulceration, and necrosis.

In addition to enteric infections, certain systemic infections (e.g., viral hepatitis [Chapter 150], listeriosis [Chapter 301], legionellosis [Chapter 322]) and emerging infections (e.g., Hanta virus [Chapter 389], severe acute respiratory syndrome [SARS, Chapter 374], avian influenza [Chapter 372]) may cause or manifest with substantial diarrhea.

Environmental and Food Poisonings

Food poisoning refers to the accumulation of toxin in food owing to the growth of toxin-producing organisms, most commonly *Staphylococcus aureus* (Chapter 296), *Bacillus cereus, Clostridium perfringens* (Chapter 304), and *Clostridium botulinum* (Chapter 304). Diarrhea is usually of rapid onset, as early as 4 hours after ingestion, and is often associated with vomiting. Natural toxins also are responsible for mushroom (*Amanita*) poisoning (Chapter 110), which can also cause acute liver and kidney failure.

Environmental poisonings may be caused by heavy metals (arsenic from rat poison, gold, lead, mercury) that impair cell energy production. Arsenic (Chapter 21) also induces cardiovascular collapse at high doses. Insecticide (organophosphates and carbamates) poisoning occurs most commonly in field workers or from the ingestion of contaminated herbs or teas (Chapter 110); diarrhea, excessive saliva, and pulmonary secretions are caused by acetylcholine-stimulated chloride secretion in intestine and other epithelia. Patients often have associated vomiting and abdominal cramps.

Seafood is a common source of food poisoning, particularly fin fish and bivalve shellfish. Most of these toxins cause varying combinations of gastrointestinal (nausea, vomiting, diarrhea) and neurologic symptoms (tingling and burning around the mouth, facial flushing, sweating, headache, palpitations, and dizziness) within hours of seafood ingestion (Chapter 114). Similar symptoms are reported in patients with scombroid poisoning, which is caused by ingestion of decaying flesh of blood fish (tuna, mahi-mahi, marlin, or mackerel) that release large amounts of histamine (Chapter 114).

Marine dinoflagellates (algae) produce toxins that can cause paralytic shellfish poisoning, diarrhetic shellfish poisoning, and ciguatera (Chapter 114). Sporadic outbreaks of diarrhetic shellfish poisoning "red tides" occur when bivalve mollusks ingest dinoflagellates that produce saxitoxins (voltage-sensitive sodium-channel blocker) and okadaic acid (a lipid-soluble toxin that inhibits serine and threonine protein phosphatases 1 and 2A). Ingestion of contaminated mollusks by humans results in diarrhea and neurologic symptoms. Saxitoxins cause predominantly neurologic symptoms (paralytic, neurotoxic, or amnestic shellfish poisonings) and okadaic acid gastrointestinal symptoms (diarrhetic shellfish poisoning).

Food-chain passage of another dinoflagellate species (*Gambierdiscus toxicus*) to fin fish (mackerel, amberjack, snapper, grouper, or barracuda) results in the accumulation of ciguatoxin (Chapter 114) that causes a seafood poisoning called ciguatera. Ciguatoxin activates voltage-sensitive sodium channels and causes neurologic and gastrointestinal symptoms. Fish from the Albemarle-Pamlico estuary (eastern United States) ingest toxic dinoflagellates that cause *Pfiesteria piscicida* poisoning. The dinoflagellate toxins cause nausea, vomiting, abdominal pain, diarrhea, and neurologic symptoms such as fatigue, myalgias, pruritus, circumoral paresthesias, reversal of hot and cold sensation, psychiatric abnormalities, and memory loss. The neurologic symptoms may persist for months to years. Puffer fish poisoning by tetrodotoxin, a voltage-sensitive sodium-channel blocker produced by the fish, causes neurologic symptoms, respiratory paralysis, and death.

Traveler's Diarrhea

North American travelers to developing countries and travelers on airplanes and cruise ships are at high risk for acute infectious diarrhea. Most traveler's diarrhea (85%) is due to enterotoxic *E. coli. E. coli* heat-stable toxin binds to guanylate cyclase in the enterocyte brush-border membrane, where it results in elevation of intracellular cGMP. *E. coli* heat-labile toxin, similar to cholera toxin, binds to the monosialoganglioside GM_1 in the brush-border membrane, thereby resulting in the activation of adenylate cyclase and the elevation of intracellular cAMP. Cyclic AMP and cGMP stimulate intestinal chloride secretion (see Fig. 142-1C) and inhibit the nutrient-independent absorption of sodium and chloride (see Fig. 142-1B). Sodium-glucose

absorption is not affected, hence the basis for oral rehydration therapy. Cholera toxin permanently binds to adenylate cyclase until the natural turnover of the intestinal epithelium in 5 to 7 days, thereby resulting in persistent secretion and severe diarrhea. Of the 10 to 15 cases of cholera reported in the United States each year, about 60% are travel associated.

Antibiotic-Associated Diarrheas

Antibiotics are a common cause of hospital-acquired diarrheas that occur in about 20% of patients receiving broad-spectrum antibiotics; about 30% of these diarrheas are due to *Clostridium difficile* (Chapter 304). Hypervirulent, fluoroquinolone-resistant strains that produce increased levels of toxins A and B and a binary toxin have emerged. These strains are associated with an increase in the incidence and severity of *C. difficile* infections, including fulminant *C. difficile* colitis that can lead to colectomy or even death. The A and B toxins produced by *C. difficile* can cause diarrhea. In animal models, IL-8, substance P, and leukotriene B$_4$ were found to mediate toxin A–stimulated intestinal fluid secretion. *C. difficile* can cause severe diarrhea, pseudomembranous colitis, or toxic megacolon. Patients may have a relapsing course after seemingly successful therapy with metronidazole or vancomycin.

Nosocomial Hospital Diarrhea

Diarrhea is the most common nosocomial illness among hospitalized patients and residents in long-term care facilities. Common causes include antibiotic-associated diarrhea, *C. difficile* infection, medications, fecal impaction, tube feeding, and underlying illness. Magnesium-containing laxatives, antacids, and lactulose cause osmotic diarrheas. Bisacodyl laxatives cause secretory diarrhea. Colchicine, neomycin, methotrexate, and para-aminosalicylic acid damage the enterocyte membrane. Cholestyramine, colestipol, and colesevelam bind bile salts and can result in malabsorption. Gold therapy causes intestinal inflammation and diarrhea. Liquid formulations of medications cause diarrhea (elixir diarrhea) because of the high content of sorbitol or other nonabsorbable sugars (e.g., mannitol) used to sweeten the elixir; patients prescribed liquid medications through feeding tubes may receive more than 20 g of sorbitol daily. An important but poorly understood cause of diarrhea is enteral (tube) feeding (Chapter 223), particularly in critically ill patients, who often develop diarrhea. Dysmotility, increased intestinal permeability, and low sodium content in enteral formulas may be contributing factors.

Patients in mental health institutions and nursing homes have a high incidence of nosocomial infectious diarrhea (e.g., *C. difficile* and less commonly *Shigella, Salmonella,* hemorrhagic *E. coli, Giardia, Entamoeba histolytica*). Infectious diarrhea, 50% or more of which is caused by *C. difficile,* is also common in acute-care hospitals. Severe *C. difficile* infection has also been reported among peripartum women. If outside foods are not brought to hospitalized patients, the likelihood of a nosocomial infection caused by *Salmonella* or *Shigella* is extremely rare. Immunosuppressed patients are also susceptible to nosocomial viral infections (rotavirus, norovirus, adenovirus, and coxsackievirus).

Cancer Treatment–Related Diarrhea

Abdominal or whole body radiation virtually always causes an increased frequency of bowel movements that are often watery. Cancer chemotherapy with amsacrine, azacitidine, cytarabine, dactinomycin, daunorubicin, doxorubicin, floxuridine, 5-fluorouracil, 6-mercaptopurine, methotrexate, plicamycin, IL-2, and resveratrol may cause mild to moderate diarrhea. Irinotecan (CPT-11) and the combination of 5-fluorouracil plus leucovorin are frequent causes of severe watery diarrhea.

Daycare Diarrhea

More than 7 million children in the United States attend daycare, where diarrhea is extremely common, and secondary infection of family members occurs in 10 to 20% of cases. Most outbreaks of diarrhea are due to rotavirus or norovirus; less common causes are *Shigella* (Chapter 317), *Giardia* (Chapter 359), and *Cryptosporidium* (Chapter 358).

Runner's Diarrhea

Diarrhea occurs in 10 to 25% of individuals who exercise vigorously, especially women marathon runners and triathletes. Some athletes have associated abdominal cramps, urgency, nausea, or vomiting. The pathophysiology of runner's diarrhea is unknown. Release of intestinal secretogogues, especially prostaglandins, hormones, or ischemia, may be involved.

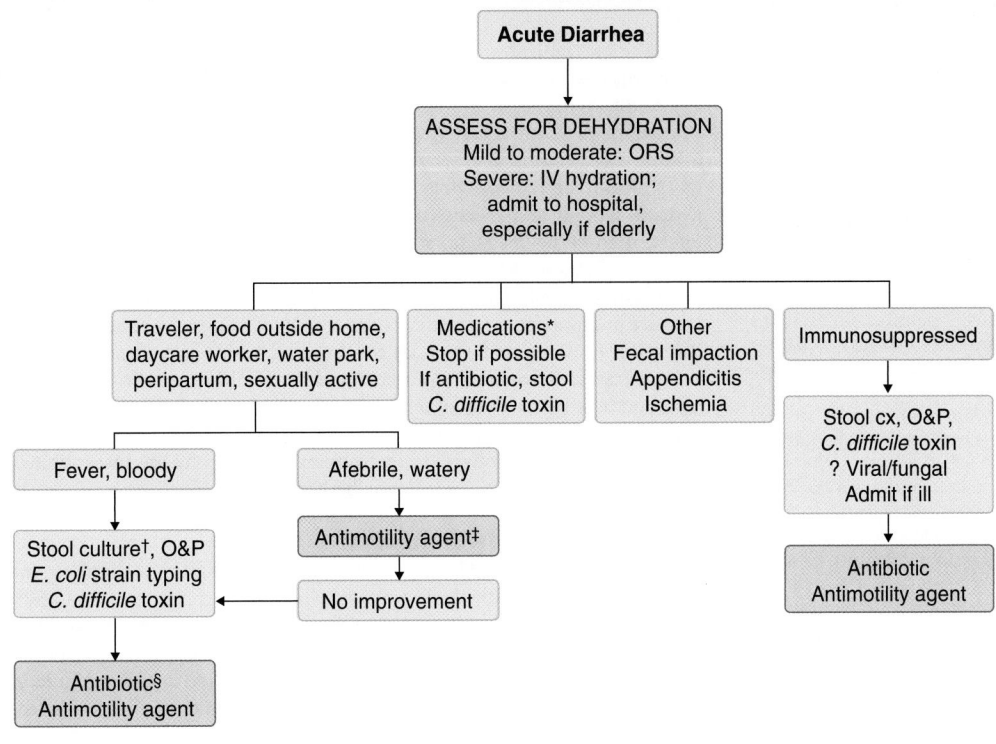

FIGURE 142-2. Approach to the diagnosis of acute diarrhea. *More than 700 medications cause diarrhea, including furosemide, caffeine, protease inhibitors, thyroid preparations, metformin, mycophenolate mofetil, sirolimus, cholinergic drugs, colchicine, theophylline, selective serotonin reuptake inhibitors, proton pump inhibitors, histamine-2 blockers, 5-ASA derivatives, angiotensin-converting enzyme inhibitors, bisacodyl, senna, aloe, anthraquinones, and magnesium- or phosphorus-containing medications. †Specifically request culture for *Yersinia*, *Plesiomonas*, enterohemorrhagic *Escherichia coli* serotype O157:H7, and *Aeromonas* if suspected. ‡If high suspicion for *Clostridium difficile* or invasive bacterial infection, wait for stool culture and toxin studies before starting. Racecadotril has antisecretory effects without paralyzing intestinal motility and can be used if available. §Not recommended for patients with bloody diarrhea due to *E. coli* O157:H7. CX = culture; IV therapy = intravenous rehydration; O&P = ova and parasites; ORS = oral rehydration solution.

DIAGNOSIS

Acute watery diarrhea may be due to infections, food toxins, or medications, or the acute diarrhea may signal the onset of a chronic disease (Fig. 142-2; see Tables 142-1 and 142-2) (Chapters 310 through 320, 344, 345, 359, 360, 364, 365, 387, and 388). The diagnostic approach in patients with fever and watery or bloody diarrhea should focus on stool cultures for *Campylobacter*, *Salmonella*, and *Shigella* species. Routine stool culture is not indicated when diarrhea occurs after 3 to 5 days of hospitalization, except in patients with neutropenia, human immunodeficiency virus infection, or signs of enteric infection. In patients with a history of recent antibiotic use, hospitalization, or peripartum, stools for *C. difficile* toxin should be obtained. Organisms that cause diarrhea but are not routinely tested by clinical microbiology laboratories include *Yersinia*, *Plesiomonas*, enterohemorrhagic *E. coli* serotype O157:H7, *Aeromonas*, *Cyclospora*, microsporidia, and noncholera *Vibrio*. Parasites such as *Giardia*, *Cryptosporidium*, and *Strongyloides* can be difficult to detect in stool but may be diagnosed by stool antigen testing or intestinal biopsy. Despite all testing techniques available, 20 to 40% of acute infectious diarrheas remain undiagnosed.

TREATMENT   Rx

Goals for the treatment of diarrhea include fluid replacement, antidiarrheal agents, nutritional support, and antimicrobial therapy when indicated. Because death in patients with acute diarrhea is caused by dehydration, the first task is to assess the degree of dehydration and to replace fluid and electrolyte deficits.

Fluid Replacement

Severely dehydrated patients should be treated with intravenous Ringer's lactate or saline solution, with additional potassium and bicarbonate as needed. Oral rehydration solutions, which are used extensively to replace diarrheal fluid and electrolyte losses, are effective because they contain sodium, sugars, and, often, amino acids that use nutrient-dependent sodium uptake transporters. In alert patients with mild to moderate dehydration, oral rehydration solution is equally effective as intravenous hydration in repairing fluid and electrolyte losses. Oral rehydration solutions can be given to infants and children in volumes of 50 to 100 mL/kg over 4 to 6 hours; adults may need to drink 1000 mL/hr. Reduced-osmolarity solutions (Na^{++} 75 mmol/L, osmolarity 245 mmol/L versus Na^{++} 90 mmol/L, osmolarity 311 mmol/L in standard solutions) are better tolerated and effective in noncholera diarrhea but may cause hyponatremia in patients with high-volume diarrhea, particularly children. Glucose-based solutions, although effective in rehydrating the patient, may worsen the diarrhea. In contrast to glucose-based solutions, polymeric

rice-based solutions decrease diarrhea in cholera victims; rice is digested to many glucose monomers that aid in the absorption of intestinal secretions. These solutions may not decrease stool output in acute diarrhea, but they will effectively rehydrate the patient despite continued diarrhea. After rehydration has been accomplished, oral rehydration solutions are given at rates equaling stool loss plus insensible losses until the diarrhea ceases.

Reducing Diarrhea

Bismuth subsalicylate (Pepto-Bismol, 525 mg orally every 30 minutes to 1 hour for five doses, may repeat on day 2) is safe and efficacious in bacterial infectious diarrheas. Opiates and anticholinergic drugs are not recommended for invasive bacterial infectious diarrheas because these drugs paralyze intestinal motility and predispose to increased colonization, invasion, and prolonged excretion of infectious organisms. The opiate loperamide is safe in acute or traveler's diarrhea, provided that it is not given to patients with dysentery (high fever, with blood or pus in the stool), and especially when administered concomitantly with effective antibiotics. A combination of loperamide (2 mg orally four times a day) plus simethicone (125 mg orally four times a day) may reduce the abdominal cramps and duration of traveler's diarrhea. Racecadotril (100 mg orally three times a day in adults, 1.5 mg/kg of body weight orally three times a day in children), an intestinal enkephalinase inhibitor that is antisecretory but does not paralyze intestinal motility, is effective in the treatment of acute diarrhea in children and adults. The diarrhea associated with enteral nutrition (Chapter 223) often can be managed with pectin (4 g/kg body weight daily) or, if there are no contraindications, with loperamide (2 mg orally four times a day for 3 to 7 days, maximal dose 16 mg daily), and diarrhea is not a reason to stop tube feeding unless stool volumes exceed 1 L/day.

Anxiolytics (e.g., diazepam 2 mg orally two to four times daily) and antiemetics (e.g., promethazine 12.5 to 25 mg orally once or twice daily) that decrease sensory perception may make symptoms more tolerable and are safe. Some foods or food-derived substances (green bananas, pectins [amylase-resistant starch], zinc) lessen the amount or duration of diarrhea in children. Unabsorbed amylase-resistant starches are metabolized in the colon to short-chain fatty acids that enhance fluid absorption. Zinc supplementation (20 mg of elemental zinc orally once a day) is effective in preventing recurrences of diarrhea in malnourished children; copper deficiency is a potential complication of prolonged zinc therapy.

Probiotics may be of benefit in children with acute diarrhea, predominantly that due to rotavirus infection. *Lactobacillus* GG (10^{10} colony-forming units [CFU]/250 mL daily until diarrhea stops) added to an oral rehydration solution decreases the duration of diarrhea.

Antibiotics

While the clinician is awaiting stool culture results to guide specific therapy (Chapter 295), the fluoroquinolones (e.g., ciprofloxacin, 500 mg orally twice a day for 1 to 3 days, or levofloxacin, 500 mg orally daily for 1 to 3 days) are the treatment of choice when antibiotics are indicated (see Fig. 142-2). Trimethoprim-sulfamethoxazole (one double-strength tablet orally twice a day for 5 days or two single-strength tablets orally twice a day for 5 days) is second-line therapy. If the symptom complex suggests *Campylobacter* infection, azithromycin (500 mg orally once a day for 3 days) should be added. Regardless of the cause of infectious diarrhea, patients should be treated with antibiotics if they are immunosuppressed; have valvular, vascular, or orthopedic prostheses; have congenital hemolytic anemias (especially if salmonellosis is involved); or are extremely young or old.

Certain infectious diarrheas should be treated with antibiotics, including those associated with shigellosis (Chapter 317), cholera (Chapter 310), pseudomembranous enterocolitis (Chapter 304), parasitic infestations (Chapters 358 to 360 and 365), and sexually transmitted diseases (Chapter 293). Treatment of *E. coli* serotype O157:H7 infection is not recommended at present because current antibiotics do not appear to be helpful and the incidence of complications (hemolytic-uremic syndrome) may be greater after antibiotic therapy. Antibiotics are not effective for viral diarrhea or cryptosporidiosis.

For traveler's diarrhea, ciprofloxacin (500 mg orally two times a day for 3 days) is an effective treatment. The nonabsorbable antibiotic rifaximin (200 mg taken orally three times a day or 400 mg two times a day for 3 days) is safe and effective for treatment of traveler's diarrhea in Mexico, but it may not be effective against *Campylobacter* and *Shigella* infections.

Fluoroquinolone-resistant and trimethoprim-sulfamethoxazole-resistant strains of *Shigella, E. coli, Salmonella, Campylobacter,* and *C. difficile* have emerged. Azithromycin, 500 mg orally on day 1 and 250 mg orally once a day for 4 days, may be an effective alternative treatment for resistant strains of *Shigella* and *Campylobacter* and for traveler's diarrhea acquired in Mexico.

If *C. difficile* is suspected on an epidemiologic basis, metronidazole (250 mg orally four times a day or 500 mg orally three times a day for 10 days) or oral vancomycin (125 to 250 mg orally four times a day for 10 days) should be prescribed. In patients with recurrent *C. difficile* infection that is associated with low serum antibody titers to toxin A, immunotherapy with monoclonal antibodies against toxin A and B**1** or fecal bacteriotherapy may decrease recurrence rates. Non–*C. difficile* antibiotic-induced diarrhea is generally mild and self-limited, and it usually clears spontaneously or in response to cholestyramine therapy (4 g orally four times a day for 2 weeks).

Treatment for chemotherapy-induced and radiation-induced mild to moderate diarrhea includes loperamide (2 mg orally four times a day) and nonsteroidal anti-inflammatory drugs (NSAIDs) (e.g., naproxen, 250 to 500 mg orally twice daily). Octreotide may be an effective treatment in those with severe diarrhea in doses up to 700 µg administered subcutaneously daily.

PREVENTION

Rotavirus vaccination (Chapter 388) reduces the risk of infection and generally results in milder symptoms among those infected.**2,3** Travelers to high-risk countries (Central America and parts of Latin America, Africa, Asia, the Middle East) should avoid ingestion of tap water and ice and of raw meat, raw seafood, and raw vegetables. An oral cholera vaccine against recombinant toxin B subunit and killed whole-cell (rBS-WC) is effective in preventing infection from the O1 El Tor strain and partially effective against enterotoxigenic *E. coli* strains.**4** Cholera vaccination is recommended for relief workers and health professionals who work in endemic countries and for individuals who are immunocompromised or have chronic illnesses or hypochlorhydria. Rifaximin (200 mg orally per day for 2 weeks) is safe and effective for preventing traveler's diarrhea in Mexico,**5** and the combination of rifaximin plus loperamide is better than either one alone. Bismuth subsalicylate (525 mg orally four times a day for up to 3 weeks) is also effective. Loperamide and NSAIDs are taken prophylactically by many runners who are susceptible to runner's diarrhea, but it is not clear whether they are effective.

CHRONIC DIARRHEA

An estimated 5% of the U.S. population suffers from chronic diarrhea, and about 40% of these individuals are older than 60 years of age. In 25 to 50% of cases, expert history and physical examination may be sufficient to make a definitive diagnosis (Fig. 142-3). The addition of stool culture and examination for ova and parasites, determination of stool fat, and flexible sigmoidoscopy or colonoscopy with biopsy raises the diagnostic rate to about 75%. The remaining 25% of patients with chronic diarrhea may need extensive testing and perhaps hospitalization to make a diagnosis.

Prolonged, Persistent Infectious Diarrheas

Prolonged infectious diarrheas (>2 weeks) may be due to persistent or recurrent infections. These diarrheas occur most commonly in children exposed to unsafe drinking water in developing countries, patients who have acquired immunodeficiency syndrome (AIDS) or are immunosuppressed for other reasons, and recent travelers. The most common causes in children in developing countries are enteropathogenic and enteroadherent *E. coli* infections (Chapter 312). Other common organisms include *Giardia* (Chapter 359), *Cryptosporidium* (Chapter 358), *Entamoeba* (Chapter 360), *Isospora* (Chapter 361), and microsporidia (Chapter 358). Recurrent or prolonged infectious diarrhea may lead to severe malnutrition and death (mortality rate, 50%). Treatment includes nutrition support with supplemental vitamin A (200,000

FIGURE 142-3. Initial approach to chronic diarrhea. *Fecal occult blood testing (FOBT) is a sensitive test for underlying bowel inflammation. †Perform stool culture in those who are immunosuppressed; perform laxative screen if laxative abuse is suspected. CBC = complete blood count; CRP = C-reactive protein; EGD = esophagogastroduodenoscopy; IV = intravenous; O&P = ova and parasites; PT = prothrombin time; WBC = white blood cells.

IU twice yearly) and zinc (20 mg elemental daily for 14 days). Severe disease may require total parenteral nutrition.

In AIDS patients, protracted diarrhea may be caused by treatable agents such as *Entamoeba histolytica, Giardia,* or *Strongyloides* or by organisms such as *Cryptosporidium, Isospora belli,* and microsporidia that are difficult to treat or untreatable. The most effective treatment is retroviral therapy to improve the immune system (Chapter 396).

Up to 10% of travelers returning from developing countries have infectious diarrhea that persists for longer than 3 to 4 weeks. Stool should be examined for culture and for ova and parasites; in patients with a recent history of antibiotic use, stool should also be sent for *C. difficile* toxin. Any specific organisms that are identified should be treated. If treatment with trimethoprim-sulfamethoxazole or a fluoroquinolone has been unsuccessful, tetracycline (250 mg orally four times a day for 7 to 10 days) or metronidazole (250 mg orally three times a day for 7 to 10 days) can be tried. After documented infectious diarrhea, 25% of patients experience pain, bloating, urgency, a sense of incomplete evacuation, and loose stools for 6 months or longer; some of these patients have celiac disease, so screening (see later) is warranted in this setting. When no other cause is found, these patients are deemed to have postinfectious irritable bowel syndrome (Chapter 139).

Sporadic outbreaks of severe, prolonged diarrhea, often greater than 1 year in duration, occasionally have been reported. This form of prolonged diarrhea is called *Brainerd's diarrhea.* The organism has yet to be identified. The diarrhea is difficult to treat; cholestyramine (4 g orally three times a day) may be helpful.

Malabsorptive Syndromes

Malabsorption is caused by many different diseases, drugs (e.g., the lipase inhibitor orlistat; Chapter 227), and nutritional products (the nonabsorbable fat olestra) that impair intraluminal digestion, mucosal absorption, or delivery of the nutrient to the systemic circulation (Fig. 142-5; Table 142-3). Dietary fat is the nutrient most difficult to absorb. Fatty stools (steatorrhea) are the hallmark of malabsorption; a stool test for fat is the best screening test. Malabsorption does not always cause diarrhea. Clinical signs of vitamin or mineral deficiencies may occur in the absence of diarrhea. A careful history is crucial in guiding further testing to confirm the suspicion of malabsorption and to make a specific diagnosis (see Fig. 142-4). The goals of treatment are to correct or treat the underlying disease and to replenish losses of water, electrolytes, and nutrients.

Conditions That Impair Intraluminal Digestion

Most digestion and absorption of nutrients occur in the small intestine (Fig. 142-5). Carbohydrates and most dietary proteins are water soluble and readily digested by pancreatic enzymes. Pancreatic proteases (trypsinogen, chymotrypsinogen, procarboxypeptidases) are secreted from acinar cells in inactive forms. The cleavage of trypsinogen to trypsin by the duodenal brush-border peptidase enteropeptidase (enterokinase) allows trypsin to cleave the remaining trypsinogen and other proteases to their active form.

Most dietary lipids (long-chain triglycerides, cholesterol, and fat-soluble vitamins) are water insoluble and must undergo lipolysis and incorporation into mixed micelles before they can be absorbed across the intestinal mucosa. Pancreatic lipase, in the presence of its cofactor, colipase, cleaves long-chain triglycerides into fatty acids and monoglycerides. The products of lipolysis interact with bile salts and phospholipids to form mixed micelles, which also incorporate cholesterol and fat-soluble vitamins (D, A, K, and E) in their hydrophobic centers. Bicarbonate secreted from pancreatic duct cells is physiologically important because pancreatic enzyme activity and bile salt micelle formation are optimum at a luminal pH of 6 to 8.

IMPAIRED MIXING

Surgical alterations, such as partial gastrectomy with gastrojejunostomy (Billroth II anastomosis) or gastrointestinal bypass surgeries for obesity, result in the release of biliary and pancreatic secretions into the intestine at a site remote from the site of entry of gastric contents. This imbalance can result in impaired lipolysis and impaired micelle formation, with subsequent fat malabsorption. Bypass of the duodenum also impairs absorption of iron, folate, and calcium. Rapid transit through the jejunum contributes to the malabsorption of nutrients. Individuals with these conditions also have surgical anastomoses that predispose to bacterial overgrowth.

DUMPING SYNDROME

After esophageal (distal esophagectomy, myomectomy for achalasia), gastric (Nissan wrap, hiatal hernia repair, gastrojejunostomy), and bariatric (Roux-en-Y and duodenal switch gastric bypass) surgeries, the unregulated delivery of concentrated sugars and food into the duodenum and jejunum results in altered insulin regulation, maldigestion, osmotic movement of fluid into the intestinal lumen, and rapid transit such that intestinal contact time is insufficient for absorption of nutrients.

FIGURE 142-4. Approach to the diagnosis of malabsorption. DM = diabetes mellitus.

TABLE 142-3 CAUSES OF MALABSORPTION

MECHANISM OF MALABSORPTION	CONDITIONS
Impaired mixing	Partial/total gastrectomy Gastric bypass surgery
Impaired lipolysis	Chronic pancreatitis Pancreatic cancer Congenital pancreatic insufficiency Congenital colipase deficiency Gastrinoma
Impaired micelle formation	Severe chronic liver disease Cholestatic liver disease Bacterial overgrowth Crohn's disease Ileal resection Gastrinoma
Impaired mucosal absorption	Lactase deficiency Congenital enterokinase deficiency Abetalipoproteinemia Giardiasis Celiac disease Tropical sprue Agammaglobulinemia Amyloidosis AIDS-related (infections, enteropathy) Radiation enteritis Graft-versus-host disease Whipple's disease Eosinophilic gastroenteritis Megaloblastic gut Collagenous sprue Ulcerative jejunitis Lymphoma Bacterial overgrowth Short-bowel syndrome Mastocytosis
Impaired nutrient delivery	Congenital lymphangiectasia Lymphoma Tuberculosis Constrictive pericarditis Severe congestive heart failure
Unknown	Hypoparathyroidism Adrenal insufficiency Hyperthyroidism Carcinoid syndrome

AIDS = acquired immunodeficiency syndrome.

IMPAIRED LIPOLYSIS

A deficiency in pancreatic lipase may be caused by the congenital absence of pancreatic lipase or by destruction of the pancreatic gland due to alcohol-related pancreatitis, cystic fibrosis, or pancreatic cancer. Pancreatic lipase also can be denatured by excess secretion of gastric acid (e.g., Zollinger-Ellison syndrome; Chapter 201).

CHRONIC PANCREATITIS

Chronic pancreatitis (Chapter 146) is the most common cause of pancreatic insufficiency and impaired lipolysis. In the United States, chronic pancreatitis most commonly results from alcohol abuse; in contrast, tropical (nutritional) pancreatitis is most common worldwide. Malabsorption of fat does not occur until more than 90% of the pancreas is destroyed.

CLINICAL MANIFESTATIONS

Individuals with pancreatic causes of malabsorption typically present with bulky, fat-laden stools (usually >30 g of fat per day), abdominal pain, and diabetes, although some present with diabetes in the absence of gastrointestinal symptoms. Stools usually are not watery because undigested triglycerides form large emulsion droplets with little osmotic force and, in contrast to fatty acids, do not stimulate water and electrolyte secretion in the colon. Deficiency of fat-soluble vitamins is seen only rarely, presumably because gastric and residual pancreatic lipase generates enough fatty acids for some micelle formation. In severe disease, subclinical protein malabsorption, manifested by the presence of undigested meat fibers in the stool, and subclinical carbohydrate malabsorption, manifested by gas-filled, floating stools, can occur. Weight loss, when it occurs, is most often caused by decreased oral intake to avoid abdominal pain or diarrhea and less commonly by malabsorption.

In the dumping syndrome, patients may present with severe diarrhea, malabsorption, abdominal cramping, gas, and weight loss. Some have associated sweatiness, dizziness, and altered cognition due to postprandial hypoglycemia.

DIAGNOSIS

Between 30 and 40% of individuals with alcohol-related chronic pancreatitis have calcifications on abdominal radiographs. A qualitative or quantitative test for fecal fat is positive in individuals whose pancreas is more than 90% destroyed. Noninvasive tests of pancreatic function are not sensitive enough to detect mild to moderate insufficiency, so the secretin stimulation test is preferred (Table 142-4) if it can be obtained. A modified oral glucose tolerance test that shows late (120 to 180 minutes) hypoglycemia and an early (30 minutes) rise in hematocrit with an increased pulse rate suggests the dumping syndrome in patients with consistent symptoms. Small bowel barium study to assess transit time may be helpful in the diagnosis.

FIGURE 142-5. Phases of intestinal digestion and absorption of dietary fat, protein, and carbohydrate. a.a. = Amino acids; ApoB, A = apolipoproteins B and A; Chol = cholesterol; FA = fatty acids; MG = monoglycerides; TG = triglycerides.

TABLE 142-4 TESTS FOR THE EVALUATION OF MALABSORPTION*

TEST	COMMENTS
GENERAL TESTS OF ABSORPTION	
Quantitative stool fat test	Gold standard test of fat malabsorption, with which all other tests are compared. Requires ingestion of a high-fat diet (100 g) for 2 days before and during the collection. Stool is collected for 3 days. Normally, <7 g/24 hr is excreted on a high-fat diet. Borderline abnormalities of 8-14 g/24 hr may be seen in secretory or osmotic diarrheas that are not caused by malabsorption. There are false-negative findings if fat intake is inadequate. False-positive results can occur if mineral oil laxatives or rectal suppositories (e.g., cocoa butter) are given to the patient before stool collection.
Qualitative stool fat test	Sudan stain of a stool sample for fat. Many fat droplets per medium-power field (×40) constitute a positive test result. The nuclear magnetic resonance method determines the percentage of fat in the stool (normal, <20%). The test depends on an adequate fat intake (100 g/day). There is high sensitivity (90%) and specificity (90%) with fat malabsorption of >10 g/24 hr. Sensitivity drops with stool fat in the range of 6-10 g/24 hr.
D-Xylose test	A test of small intestinal mucosal absorption, used to distinguish mucosal malabsorption from malabsorption due to pancreatic insufficiency. An oral dose of D-xylose (25 g/500 mL water) is administered, and D-xylose excretion is measured in a 5-hr urine collection. Normally, >4 g of D-xylose is excreted in the urine over 5 hr. The test also may be positive in bacterial overgrowth owing to metabolism of D-xylose by bacteria in the intestinal lumen. False-positive test results occur with renal failure, ascites, and an incomplete urine collection. Blood levels at 1 and 3 hr improve sensitivity. May be normal with mild or limited mucosal disease.
Hydrogen breath test	Most useful in the diagnosis of lactase deficiency. An oral dose of lactose (1 g/kg body weight) is administered after measurement of basal breath H_2 levels. The sole source of H_2 in the mammal is bacterial fermentation; unabsorbed lactose makes its way to colonic bacteria, resulting in excess breath H_2. A *late peak* (within 3-6 hr) of >20 ppm of exhaled H_2 after lactose ingestion suggests lactose malabsorption. Absorption of other carbohydrates (e.g., sucrose, glucose, fructose) also can be tested.
SPECIFIC TESTS FOR MALABSORPTION	
Tests for Pancreatic Function	
Secretin stimulation test	The gold standard test of pancreatic function. Requires duodenal test intubation with a double-lumen tube and collection of pancreatic juice in response to IV secretin. Allows measurement of bicarbonate (HCO_3^-) and pancreatic enzymes. A sensitive test of pancreatic function, but labor intensive and invasive.
Fecal elastase-1 test	Stool test for pancreatic function. Equal sensitivity to the secretin stimulation test for the diagnosis of moderate-to-severe pancreatic insufficiency. More specific than the fecal chymotrypsin test. Unreliable with mild insufficiency. False-positive results occur with increased stool volume and intestinal mucosal diseases.
Tests for Bacterial Overgrowth	
Quantitative culture of small intestinal aspirate	Gold standard test for bacterial overgrowth. Greater than 10^5 colony-forming units (CFU)/mL in the jejunum suggests bacterial overgrowth. Requires special anaerobic sample collection, rapid anaerobic and aerobic plating, and care to avoid oropharyngeal contamination. False-negative results occur with focal jejunal diverticula and when overgrowth is distal to the site aspirated.
Hydrogen breath test	The 50-g glucose breath test has a sensitivity of 90% for growth of 10^5 colonic-type bacteria in the small intestine. If bacterial overgrowth is present, increased H_2 is excreted in the breath. A hydrogen level (within 2 hr) of >20 ppm suggests bacterial overgrowth. False-negative results occur with non-hydrogen-producing organisms.
^{14}C-D-xylose breath test	This test uses 1 g of carbon 14–labeled D-xylose. It has a sensitivity and specificity >90% for growth of 10^5 test colonic-type bacteria in the small intestine. Bacteria metabolize D-xylose with release of $^{14}CO_2$, which is absorbed and exhaled. Non-degraded D-xylose is absorbed in the small bowel and does not reach the colon, yielding a greater specificity than the lactulose H_2 breath test. A nonradioactive ^{13}C-D-xylose breath test is suitable for children and pregnant women.
Tests for Mucosal Disease	
Small bowel biopsy	Obtained for a specific diagnosis when there is a high index of suspicion for small intestinal disease. Several biopsy specimens (4-5) must be obtained to maximize the diagnostic yield. Distal duodenal biopsy specimens are usually adequate for diagnosis, but occasionally enteroscopy with jejunal biopsy specimens is necessary. Small intestinal biopsy provides a specific diagnosis in some diseases (e.g., intestinal infection, Whipple's disease, abetalipoproteinemia, agammaglobulinemia, lymphangiectasia, lymphoma, amyloidosis). In other conditions, such as celiac disease and tropical sprue, the biopsy specimens show characteristic findings, but the diagnosis is made on improvement after treatment.
Tests of Ileal Function	
Schilling test	A test of vitamin B_{12} absorption (see Table 167-1 in Chapter 167).
^{75}SeHCAT test	This is a test of bile acid absorption. Seven days after ingestion of radiolabeled synthetic selenium-homocholic acid conjugated with taurine (^{75}SeHCAT), whole body retention is measured by a gamma-counting device. The result is expressed as a fraction of baseline ingestion. Retention values of less than 10% are abnormal and indicate bile acid malabsorption with a sensitivity of 80-90% and specificity of 70-100%. The radiation dose is equivalent to a plain chest x-ray. Liver disease and bacterial overgrowth may give false results. Not approved for use in the United States.

*Not all these tests are readily available. A strong suspicion for any disease may warrant foregoing an extensive work-up and obtaining the test with highest diagnostic yield. In some cases, empirical treatment, such as removing lactose from the diet of an otherwise healthy individual with lactose intolerance, is warranted without any testing.

TREATMENT Ⓡ

Pancreatic enzyme replacement and analgesics are the mainstays of treatment for chronic pancreatitis (Chapter 146). It is difficult to correct fat malabsorption completely with exogenous pancreatic enzymes because of their inactivation by acid and pepsin in the stomach. Normally, 28,000 U of lipase is present in the duodenal lumen with each meal. A high lipase-containing pancreatic enzyme preparation (25,000 to 40,000 U of lipase in the form of uncoated enzymes or enteric-coated, pH-sensitive microspheres) should be prescribed with each meal. Mini-microsphere preparations (e.g., 20,000 U of lipase taken orally with each meal) may be best tolerated owing to their small capsule size. Pancreatic proteases present in enzyme preparations may reduce abdominal pain by inactivating cholecystokinin-releasing factor in the duodenum. Uncoated preparations may be more effective in pain relief because coated preparations release enzymes predominantly distal to the duodenum.

A histamine-2 receptor antagonist (e.g., ranitidine, 150 mg orally taken two times a day) or a proton pump inhibitor (e.g., lansoprazole, 15 to 30 mg orally once a day) should be added to uncoated pancreatic enzyme replacement therapy in patients with a poor response.

In the dumping syndrome, treatment is with a diet that is low in concentrated sugars divided into six small meals. Administration of pectin (15 g with each meal) may slow gastric emptying. In patients who are refractory to dietary measures, a short-acting somatostatin analogue (e.g., octreotide, 25 to 200 µg subcutaneously three times a day) or the better tolerated long-acting octreotide preparation (10 to 20 mg subcutaneously monthly) improves dumping symptoms. In patients with predominant reactive hypoglycemia 1 to 3 hours after a meal (late dumping), an α-glycosidase hydrolase inhibitor (e.g., acarbose, 50 to 100 mg orally three times daily) that blocks carbohydrate absorption in the small bowel may be beneficial. Continuous tube feeding is also effective.

IMPAIRED MICELLE FORMATION

PATHOBIOLOGY

Bile salt concentrations in the intestinal lumen can fall to less than the critical concentration (2 to 3 mmol/L) needed for micelle formation because of decreased bile salt synthesis (severe liver disease), decreased bile salt delivery (cholestasis), or removal of luminal bile salts (bacterial overgrowth, terminal ileal disease or resection, cholestyramine therapy, acid hypersecretion). Fat malabsorption resulting from impaired micelle formation is generally not as severe as malabsorption resulting from pancreatic lipase deficiency, presumably because fatty acids and monoglycerides can form lamellar structures, which to a certain extent can be absorbed. Malabsorption of fat-soluble vitamins (D, A, K, and E) may be marked, however, because micelle formation is required for their absorption.

Decreased Bile Salt Synthesis and Delivery

Malabsorption can occur in individuals with cholestatic liver disease or bile duct obstruction. The clinical consequences of malabsorption are seen most often in women with primary biliary cirrhosis because of the prolonged nature of the illness. Although these individuals can present with steatorrhea, osteoporosis or, less commonly, osteomalacia is the most common presentation. The cause of bone disease in these patients is poorly understood and often is not related to vitamin D deficiency. Bone disease is treated with calcium supplements (and vitamin D if a deficiency is documented), weight-bearing exercise, and a bisphosphonate (e.g., alendronate, 10 mg orally once daily or 70 mg orally once weekly).

Intestinal Bacterial Overgrowth

In health, only small numbers of lactobacilli, enterococci, gram-positive aerobes, or facultative anaerobes can be cultured from the upper small bowel lumen. Motility and acid are the most important factors in keeping the number of bacteria in the upper small bowel low. Any condition that produces local stasis or recirculation of colonic luminal contents allows development of a predominantly "colonic" flora (coliforms and anaerobes, such as *Bacteroides* and *Clostridium*) in the small intestine (see Table 142-4). Anaerobic bacteria cause impaired micelle formation by releasing cholylamidases, which deconjugate bile salts. The unconjugated bile salts, with their higher pK_a, are more likely to be in the protonated form at the normal upper small intestinal pH of 6 to 7 and can be absorbed passively. As a result, the concentration of bile salts decreases in the intestinal lumen and can fall to less than the critical micellar concentration, causing malabsorption of fats and fat-soluble vitamins. Vitamin B_{12} deficiency and carbohydrate malabsorption also can occur with generalized bacterial overgrowth. Anaerobic bacteria ingest vitamin B_{12} and release proteases that degrade brush-border disaccharidases. Although anaerobic bacteria use vitamin B_{12}, they synthesize folate. Individuals with bacterial overgrowth usually have low serum vitamin B_{12} levels but normal or high folate levels; this helps distinguish bacterial overgrowth from tropical sprue, in which vitamin B_{12} and folate levels are usually low because of decreased mucosal uptake.

CLINICAL MANIFESTATIONS

Individuals with bacterial overgrowth can present with diarrhea, abdominal cramps, gas and bloating, weight loss, and signs and symptoms of vitamin B_{12} and fat-soluble vitamin deficiency. Watery diarrhea occurs because of the osmotic load of unabsorbed carbohydrates and stimulation of colonic secretion by unabsorbed fatty acids.

DIAGNOSIS

The diagnosis of bacterial overgrowth should be considered in elderly people and in individuals with predisposing underlying disorders (see Table 142-4). Bacterial overgrowth may be associated with the irritable bowel syndrome (Chapter 139). The identification of greater than 10^5 CFU/mL in a culture of small intestinal aspirate is the "gold standard" in diagnosis but is not readily available. The noninvasive tests with a sensitivity and specificity comparable to intestinal culture are the glucose hydrogen breath test and the ^{14}C- or ^{13}C-D-xylose breath test; in individuals with low vitamin B_{12} levels, a Schilling test before and after antibiotic therapy can be diagnostic (Chapter 167).

TREATMENT

The goals of treatment are to correct the structural or motility defect, if possible; to eradicate offending bacteria; and to provide nutritional support. Acid-reducing agents should be stopped, if possible. Treatment with antibiotics should be based on culture results whenever possible; otherwise, empirical treatment is given. Rifaximin (400 mg orally three times a day) is effective,[6] but less so in individuals with an excluded (blind) intestinal loop. Tetracycline (250 to 500 mg orally four times a day) or a broad-spectrum antibiotic against aerobes and enteric anaerobes (ciprofloxacin, 500 mg orally twice a day; amoxicillin–clavulanic acid, 250 to 500 mg orally three times a day; cephalexin, 250 mg orally four times a day with metronidazole, 250 mg three times a day) should be given for 14 days. Prokinetic agents such as metoclopramide (10 mg orally four times a day) or erythromycin (250 to 500 mg orally four times a day) can be tried to treat small bowel motility disorders, but often they are not efficacious. Octreotide (50 μg subcutaneously every day) may improve motility and reduce bacterial overgrowth in individuals with scleroderma. If the structural abnormality or motility disturbance cannot be corrected, the patient is at risk for malnutrition and deficiencies of vitamin B_{12} and fat-soluble vitamins. Cyclic treatment (1 to 3 weeks out of every 4 to 6 weeks) with rotating antibiotics may be required in these patients to prevent recurrent bouts of bacterial overgrowth. If supplemental calories are needed, medium-chain triglycerides should be given because they are not dependent on micelle formation for their absorption. Monthly treatment with vitamin B_{12} should be considered, along with supplemental vitamins D, A, K, and E and calcium.

ILEAL DISEASE OR RESECTION

Disease of the terminal ileum is most commonly due to Crohn's disease (Chapter 143), which also may lead to ileal resection, but it also can be caused by radiation enteritis, tropical sprue, tuberculosis, *Yersinia* infection, or idiopathic bile salt malabsorption. These diseases cause bile salt wasting in the colon.

The clinical consequences of bile salt malabsorption are related directly to the length of the diseased or resected terminal ileum. In an adult, if less than 100 cm of ileum is diseased or resected, watery diarrhea results because of stimulation of colonic fluid secretion by unabsorbed bile salts. Bile acid diarrhea responds to cholestyramine (2 to 4 g taken at breakfast, lunch, and dinner). If more than 100 cm of ileum is diseased or resected, bile salt losses (>3 g/day) in the colon exceed the capacity for increased bile salt synthesis in the liver, the bile salt pool shrinks, and micelle formation is impaired. As a result, steatorrhea ensues, and fatty acid–induced intestinal secretion synergizes with the bile acid–induced secretion to cause diarrhea. Treatment is with a low-fat diet, vitamin B_{12} (300 to 1000 μg subcutaneously once every month or 2 mg orally once a day), dietary supplements of calcium (500 mg orally two to three times a day, monitor 24-hour urine calcium for adequacy of dose), and a multiple vitamin and mineral supplement. An antimotility agent should be given for diarrhea. Bile salt binders may worsen diarrhea. Screening for fat-soluble vitamin deficiencies (vitamins A and E, 25-OH vitamin D, and prothrombin time) and bone disease (bone densitometry, serum calcium, intact parathyroid hormone, 24-hour urine for calcium) should be done.

Three long-term complications of chronic bile salt wasting and fat malabsorption are renal stones, bone disease (osteoporosis and osteomalacia), and gallstones. Oxalate renal stones occur as a consequence of excess free oxalate absorption in the colon. Free oxalate is generated when unabsorbed fatty acids bind luminal calcium, which is then unavailable for binding oxalate. Renal oxalate stones sometimes can be avoided with a low-fat, low-oxalate diet and calcium supplements. Bone disease is caused by impaired micelle formation with a resulting decrease in absorption of vitamin D; year-round sun exposure reduces this complication. Vitamin D (50,000 U orally one to three times a week) and calcium supplements (500 mg orally two to three times a day) should be given to susceptible individuals, but vitamin D levels and serum and urinary calcium must be monitored for response to treatment because excess vitamin D can be toxic. The mechanism of gallstone formation in these individuals is unclear; pigmented gallstones are most common.

Conditions that Impair Mucosal Absorption

PATHOBIOLOGY

Nutrients are absorbed along the entire length of the small intestine, with the exception of iron and folate, which are absorbed in the duodenum and proximal jejunum, and bile salts and cobalamin, which are absorbed in the distal ileum. The efficiency of nutrient uptake at the mucosa is influenced by the number of villus absorptive cells, the presence of functional hydrolases and specific nutrient transport proteins on the brush-border membrane, and transit time. Transit time determines the contact time of luminal contents with the brush-border membrane and influences the efficiency of nutrient uptake across the mucosa.

Mucosal malabsorption can be caused by specific (usually congenital) brush-border enzyme or nutrient transporter deficiencies or by generalized diseases that damage the small intestinal mucosa or result in surgical resection or bypass of small intestine. The nutrients malabsorbed in these general malabsorptive diseases depend on the site of intestinal injury (proximal, distal, or diffuse) and the severity of damage. The main mechanism of malabsorption in these conditions is a decrease in surface area available for absorption. Some conditions (infection, celiac disease, tropical sprue, food allergies, and graft-versus-host disease) are characterized by intestinal inflammation and villus flattening; others are characterized by ulceration (ulcerative jejunitis, NSAIDs, Crohn's disease), infiltration (amyloidosis), or ischemia (radiation enteritis, mesenteric ischemia).

Long-chain fatty acids are transported across the microvillus membrane of villus epithelial cells by the fatty acid transport protein FATP4. The bile salts from mixed micelles remain in the intestinal lumen and are absorbed in the distal ileum by sodium-dependent cotransport. Oligosaccharides and larger oligopeptides (products of pancreatic enzyme digestion), sucrose, and lactose are hydrolyzed further by enzymes present in the brush-border membrane of villus epithelial cells before they are absorbed. Although only sugar monomers (glucose, galactose, fructose) can be taken up at the apical epithelial cell membrane, dipeptides and tripeptides are readily taken into the cell.

Water-soluble vitamins are readily absorbed throughout the small intestine. Fat-soluble vitamins, minerals, and cobalamin are more difficult to absorb because of the requirement for micelle formation (vitamins D, A, K, and E), a divalent charge (magnesium, calcium, iron), or selected sites of uptake in the intestine (iron, cobalamin). Calcium is absorbed best in the proximal small intestine by a vitamin D–dependent calcium channel. Magnesium is absorbed by the small intestine (throughout its length) by a poorly understood mechanism. Ferrous iron is transported into intestinal epithelial cells by a proton-coupled metal-ion transporter (Nramp2) that has specificity for Fe^{2+} and other divalent cations (Zn^{2+}, Mn^{2+}, Co^{2+}, Cd^{2+}, Cu^{2+}, Ni^{2+}, and Pb^{2+}). The absorption of calcium and nonheme iron is enhanced by solubilization with hydrochloric acid. Intraluminal compounds such as oxalate, phytate, and long-chain fatty acids bind to calcium and magnesium, decreasing their absorption. Individuals with severe mucosal disease or short-bowel syndrome with high fecal fluid outputs lose magnesium and zinc from endogenous secretions.

Folates (Chapters 167 and 225) are both taken in the diet and produced by bacteria in the colon. Dietary folates are absorbed in the proximal small intestine through a reduced folate carrier (RFC1). Deficiency can be caused by poor intake or malabsorption secondary to intestinal disease or drugs. The cobalamins (Chapters 167 and 225) are abundant in foods containing animal proteins (e.g., meat, seafood, eggs, milk). Cobalamin deficiency in industrialized countries is rarely due to poor dietary intake but rather reflects the inability to absorb cobalamin. This inability may be caused by a lack of intrinsic factor, consumption of cobalamin by overgrowth of anaerobic bacteria in the small bowel lumen, ileal disease or resection, or defective transcobalamin II. Large amounts of cobalamin are present in the liver (2 to 5 mg), and cobalamin is reabsorbed from bile through the enterohepatic circulation, thereby limiting daily losses to less than 1 μg. It usually takes 10 to 12 years for cobalamin deficiency to develop after it is eliminated from the diet, but deficiency can occur more rapidly (2 to 5 years) with malabsorptive syndromes. If lack of gastric acid causes food-cobalamin malabsorption, treatment with oral cyanocobalamin supplementation (Chapter 167) is curative.

LACTASE DEFICIENCY

EPIDEMIOLOGY

Acquired lactase deficiency is the most common cause of selective carbohydrate malabsorption. Most individuals, except those of northern European descent, begin to lose lactase activity by the age of 2 years. The prevalence of lactase deficiency is highest (85 to 100%) in persons of Asian, African, and Native-American descent.

PATHOBIOLOGY

The persistence or nonpersistence of lactase activity is associated with a single nucleotide polymorphism C/T_{-13910} that is found upstream of the

lactase gene on chromosome 2q21-22. Hypolactasia is associated with the C/C_{-13910} genotype in diverse ethnic groups. The mechanism by which this variant downregulates the lactase gene is not known, but functional studies suggest genotype-dependent alterations in levels of messenger RNA.

CLINICAL MANIFESTATIONS

Adults with lactase deficiency typically complain of gas, bloating, and diarrhea after the ingestion of milk or dairy products but do not lose weight. Unabsorbed lactose is osmotically active, drawing water followed by ions into the intestinal lumen. On reaching the colon, bacteria metabolize lactose to short-chain fatty acids, carbon dioxide, and hydrogen gas. Short-chain fatty acids are transported with sodium into colonic epithelial cells, facilitating the reabsorption of fluid in the colon. If the colonic capacity for the reabsorption of short-chain fatty acids is exceeded, an osmotic diarrhea results (see later discussion of carbohydrate malabsorption in watery diarrheas).

DIAGNOSIS

The diagnosis of acquired lactase deficiency can be made by empirical treatment with a lactose-free diet, which results in resolution of symptoms; by the hydrogen breath test after oral administration of lactose; or by genetic testing. Many intestinal diseases cause secondary reversible lactase deficiency, including viral gastroenteritis, celiac disease, giardiasis, and bacterial overgrowth.

Congenital Enteropeptidase (Enterokinase) Deficiency

Enteropeptidase is a brush-border protease that cleaves trypsinogen to trypsin, triggering the cascade of pancreatic protease activation in the intestinal lumen. The rare congenital deficiency of enteropeptidase results in inability to activate all pancreatic proteases and leads to severe protein malabsorption. It manifests in infancy as diarrhea, growth retardation, and hypoproteinemic edema.

Abetalipoproteinemia

Formation and exocytosis of chylomicrons at the basolateral membrane of intestinal epithelial cells are necessary for the delivery of lipids to the systemic circulation. One of the proteins required for assembly and secretion of chylomicrons is the microsomal triglyceride transfer protein, which is mutated in individuals with abetalipoproteinemia. Children with this disorder have fat malabsorption and the consequences of vitamin E deficiency (retinopathy and spinocerebellar degeneration). Biochemical tests show low plasma levels of apoprotein B, triglyceride, and cholesterol. Membrane lipid abnormalities result in red blood cell acanthosis (burr cells). Intestinal biopsy is diagnostic; the tissue is characterized by engorgement of epithelial cells with lipid droplets. Calories are provided by treatment with a low-fat diet containing medium-chain triglycerides. Poor absorption of long-chain fatty acids sometimes can result in essential fatty acid deficiency. High doses of fat-soluble vitamins, especially vitamin E, often are needed. Mutations in the apolipoprotein B gene (hypobetalipoproteinemia) and intracellular retention of chylomicrons (Anderson's disease) cause a similar although less severe clinical syndrome.

CELIAC DISEASE

DEFINITION AND EPIDEMIOLOGY

Celiac disease is an inflammatory condition of the small intestine precipitated by the ingestion of wheat, rye, and barley in individuals with certain genetic predispositions. Screening studies for the antiendomysial (EMA) and anti–tissue transglutaminase (anti-tTG) antibodies that are associated with celiac disease suggest a prevalence in white populations of about 1%. High-risk groups for celiac disease include first-degree relatives and individuals with type 1 diabetes mellitus, autoimmune thyroid disease, primary biliary cirrhosis, Turner's syndrome, or Down syndrome. About 20% of patients diagnosed with irritable bowel syndrome or with microscopic (lymphocytic) colitis have celiac disease.

PATHOBIOLOGY

Environmental and genetic factors are important in the development of celiac disease. The alcohol-soluble protein fraction of wheat gluten, the gliadins, and similar prolamins in rye and barley trigger intestinal inflammation in susceptible individuals. Oat grains, which have prolamins rich in glutamine but not proline, are rarely toxic. Gliadins and similar prolamins with high proline content are relatively resistant to digestion by human proteases. A 33-mer peptide that is a natural digestion product of α_2-gliadin may be important in the pathogenesis of celiac disease. This peptide resists terminal digestion by intestinal brush-border proteases and contains three previously identified antigenic epitopes. It also reacts with tissue transglutaminase and stimulates human leukocyte antigen (HLA)-DQ2-restricted intestinal T-cell clones from individuals with celiac disease.

Approximately 15% of first-degree relatives of affected individuals are found to have celiac disease. Predisposition has been mapped to the HLA-D region on chromosome 6. More than 90% of northern Europeans with celiac disease have the DQ2 heterodimer encoded by alleles *DQA1*0501* and *DQB1*0201*, compared with 20 to 30% of controls. A smaller celiac group carries HLA DQ8. The strongest candidate non-HLA alleles identified in genome-wide association studies are 4q27 and 3q28. The DQ2 protein expressed on antigen-presenting cells has positively charged binding pockets; tTG (the autoantigen recognized by EMA) may enhance intestinal inflammation by deamidation of select glutamine residues in gliadin to negatively charged glutamic acid. In the deamidated form, most gliadin peptides have a higher binding affinity for DQ2 and are more potent stimulants of gluten-sensitized T cells. Villous atrophy may be caused by inflammation that is triggered by γ-interferon released from DQ2- or DQ8-restricted CD4 T cells in the lamina propria. Alternatively, intraepithelial lymphocytes may directly kill intestinal epithelial cells under the influence of IL-15 released from stressed enterocytes.

CLINICAL MANIFESTATIONS

Celiac disease usually manifests early in life, at about 2 years of age (after wheat has been introduced into the diet), or later in the second to fourth decades of life, but it can occur at any age. It may first manifest clinically after abdominal surgery or an episode of infectious diarrhea.

Breast-feeding and the time of introduction of wheat in the diet may lessen the risk or delay the onset of celiac disease in children at risk. Adults with celiac disease in the United States often present with anemia or osteoporosis without diarrhea or other gastrointestinal symptoms. These individuals most likely have proximal disease that impairs iron, folate, and calcium absorption but an adequate surface area in the remaining intestine for absorption of other nutrients. Other extraintestinal manifestations of celiac disease include rash (dermatitis herpetiformis), neurologic disorders (peripheral neuropathy, ataxia, epilepsy), psychiatric disorders (depression, paranoia), reproductive disorders (infertility, spontaneous abortion), short stature, dental enamel hypoplasia, chronic hepatitis, or cardiomyopathy.

Individuals with significant mucosal involvement present with watery diarrhea, weight loss or growth retardation, and the clinical manifestations of vitamin and mineral deficiencies. Cobalamin deficiency is more common (10% of patients) than previously thought and usually corrects itself on a gluten-free diet. Symptomatic individuals require supplementation of vitamin B_{12}. Diarrhea is caused by many mechanisms, including a decreased surface area for water and electrolyte absorption, the osmotic effect of unabsorbed luminal nutrients, an increased surface area for chloride secretion (crypt hyperplasia), and the stimulation of intestinal fluid secretion by inflammatory mediators and unabsorbed fatty acids. Some individuals have impaired pancreatic enzyme secretion caused by decreased mucosal cholecystokinin release or bacterial overgrowth that may contribute to diarrhea.

DIAGNOSIS

The diagnosis of celiac disease is made by characteristic changes found on a small intestinal biopsy specimen and improvement when a gluten-free diet is instituted (Figs. 142-6 and 142-7). Mucosal flattening may be observed endoscopically as scalloped or reduced duodenal folds. Characteristic features found on intestinal biopsy include blunted or absent villi, crypt hyperplasia, increased intraepithelial lymphocytes, and infiltration of the lamina propria with plasma cells and lymphocytes. In some individuals, the only abnormal biopsy finding is increased intraepithelial lymphocytes. A hypoplastic mucosa indicates irreversible (end-stage) intestinal disease.

Serologic markers for celiac disease are useful in supporting the diagnosis, in screening first-degree relatives, and in monitoring the response to a gluten-free diet. EMA immunoglobulin A (IgA) antibodies, detected by indirect immunofluorescence, are highly sensitive (90%) and specific (90 to 100%) for active celiac disease in skilled laboratory testing. An enzyme-linked immunosorbent assay (ELISA) test to detect antibodies against tTG has equal sensitivity to the EMA test but is less specific. The newer anti-deamidated gliadin (a biotinylated synthetic γ-gliadin peptide with glutamic acid substituted for glutamine) IgA and IgG antibody immunofluorometric assay has a sensitivity and specificity that approaches that of EMA.

FIGURE 142-6. Intestinal biopsy appearance of flattened villi, hyperplastic crypts, and increased intraepithelial lymphocytes. (Courtesy of John Hart, MD.)

FIGURE 142-7. Regeneration of villi after initiation of a gluten-free diet. (Courtesy of John Hart, MD.)

The anti-tTG IgA antibody test, when obtained with a serum IgA level, is a cost-effective strategy for screening high-risk groups; very high titers of the anti-tTG IgA and EMA antibodies are virtually diagnostic of celiac disease. Patients with mild disease may have negative antibody studies. Anti-tTG, gliadin peptide, and EMA IgA antibodies tests are negative in individuals with selective IgA deficiency (present in up to 2.6% of individuals with celiac disease). In these patients, anti-tTG or gliadin peptide IgG antibodies may be helpful in diagnosis. In equivocal cases (negative serology and equivocal biopsy or positive serology and normal biopsy), HLA genotyping is useful to exclude the diagnosis of celiac disease in persons who lack the DQ2 or DQ8 gene.

TREATMENT   Rx

Treatment consists of a lifelong gluten-free diet. Wheat, rye, and barley grains should be excluded from the diet. Rice and corn grains are tolerated. Oats (if not contaminated by wheat grain) are tolerated by most. Early referral to a reputable celiac support group or website is often helpful in maintaining dietary compliance. Owing to secondary lactase deficiency, a lactose-free diet should be recommended until symptoms improve. Bone densitometry should be performed on all individuals with celiac disease because up to 70% have osteopenia or osteoporosis. Patients with diarrhea and weight loss should be screened for vitamin and mineral deficiencies. Documented deficiencies of vitamins and minerals should be replenished (see Table 142-4), and women of childbearing age should take folic acid supplements. Bone mass often improves on a gluten-free diet alone. Patients with vitamin D or calcium deficiency should receive supplements (Chapter 225), with the dose monitored by 25-OH vitamin D levels and a 24-hour urine test for calcium.

PROGNOSIS

Of patients with celiac disease treated with a gluten-free diet, 90% experience symptomatic improvement within 2 weeks. The most common cause of a poor dietary response is continued ingestion of gluten. Other possibilities include a missed intestinal infection (see later), an alternative diagnosis (e.g., agammaglobulinemia [diagnosed by hypogammaglobulinemia and lack of plasma cells on small bowel biopsy], autoimmune enteritis [diagnosed by a positive antienterocyte antibody and crypt apoptosis or loss of goblet cells on small bowel biopsy]), bacterial overgrowth, pancreatic insufficiency, microscopic colitis, or other food allergies (cow's milk, soy protein).

In a small percentage of patients, symptoms and enteropathy persist despite a strict gluten-free diet. In such patients, repeat intestinal biopsy is indicated. Some patients will have collagen deposition beneath the surface epithelium (collagenous sprue). Others will have ulcerative jejunitis or a monoclonal population of intraepithelial T cells with an aberrant phenotype or clonal T-cell receptor-γ gene rearrangements, which are predictive of enteropathy-associated T-cell lymphoma (Chapter 191) that portends a poor prognosis. Video capsule endoscopy and balloon-assisted enteroscopy may be helpful in establishing these diagnoses. Patients with collagenous sprue, autoimmune enteritis, or refractory sprue with a polyclonal population of intraepithelial T lymphocytes often respond to prednisone (20 to 40 mg orally daily) or budesonide (3 mg orally three times a day).

Individuals with celiac disease are at increased risk for B-cell lymphoma (Chapter 191), gastrointestinal tract carcinomas (esophageal, small bowel, and colonic adenocarcinomas), and increased mortality; a strict gluten-free diet for life may lessen these risks. Intestinal T-cell lymphoma is rare and should be suspected in individuals who have abdominal pain, recurrence of symptoms after initial response to a gluten-free diet, or refractory celiac disease.

TROPICAL SPRUE

Tropical sprue is an inflammatory disease of the small intestine associated with the overgrowth of predominantly coliform bacteria. It occurs in residents or travelers to the tropics, especially India and Southeast Asia. Individuals classically present with diarrhea and megaloblastic anemia secondary to vitamin B_{12} and folate deficiency, but some have anemia only. Intestinal biopsy characteristically shows subtotal and patchy villous atrophy in the proximal and distal small intestine, which may be caused by the effect of bacterial toxins on gut structure or by the secondary effects of vitamin B_{12} deficiency on the gut (megaloblastic gut). Diagnosis is based on history, documentation of vitamin B_{12} or folate deficiency, and the presence of an abnormal small intestinal biopsy report. Treatment is a prolonged course of broad-spectrum antibiotics, oral folate, and vitamin B_{12} injections until symptoms resolve. Relapses occur mainly in natives of the tropics.

Infection

GIARDIA LAMBLIA

Giardia lamblia (Chapter 359) infection, the most common protozoal infection in the United States, can cause malabsorption in individuals infected with many trophozoites, especially the immunocompromised or IgA-deficient hosts. Malabsorption occurs when many organisms cover the epithelium and cause mucosal inflammation, which results in villous flattening and a decrease in absorptive surface area. Stool for ova and parasites at this stage of infection is often negative because of the attachment of organisms in the proximal small intestine. Diagnosis can be made by a stool antigen-capture ELISA test but may require duodenal aspiration and biopsies.

HUMAN IMMUNODEFICIENCY VIRUS

Diarrhea, malabsorption, and wasting are common in individuals with AIDS but are seen less frequently with improved antiretroviral therapy (Chapter 397). In patients who are receiving highly active antiretroviral therapy, diarrhea is more likely to be due to protease inhibitors than to enteric infection.

Malabsorption is usually due to infection with cryptosporidia, *Mycobacterium avium-intracellulare* complex, *I. belli*, or microsporidia. An organism can be identified by stool examination or intestinal biopsy about 50% of the time. *AIDS enteropathy* (a term used if no organism is identified) also can cause malabsorption. Mechanisms of malabsorption and diarrhea include villous atrophy, increased intestinal permeability, rapid small bowel transit (in patients with protozoal infection), and ultrastructural damage of enterocytes (in AIDS enteropathy). Among individuals with AIDS and diarrhea, results of fecal fat and D-xylose absorption are frequently abnormal. Serum albumin, vitamin B_{12}, and zinc levels are often low. Vitamin B_{12} deficiency is caused mainly by ileal disease, but low intrinsic factor and decreased transcobalamin II may be contributing factors. Management of malabsorption should focus on restoring the immune system by treating the underlying HIV infection with antiviral therapy. If possible, the offending organism should be treated with antibiotics. If the organism cannot be eradicated, chronic diarrhea and

malabsorption result; treatment in these cases consists of antimotility agents and a lactose-free, low-fat diet. Pancreatic enzyme replacement therapy can be tried in HIV-infected individuals who are taking highly active antiretroviral therapy or nucleoside analogues and who have fat malabsorption of obscure origin. If supplemental calories are needed, liquid oral supplements that are predigested and high in medium-chain triglycerides (semi-elemental) are tolerated best. Vitamin and mineral deficiencies should be screened for and treated.

WHIPPLE'S DISEASE

Whipple's disease (Chapters 144 and 283), a rare cause of malabsorption, manifests with gastrointestinal complaints in association with systemic symptoms, such as fever, joint pain, or neurologic manifestations. About one third of patients have cardiac involvement, most commonly culture-negative endocarditis. Occasionally, individuals present with ocular or neurologic disease without gastrointestinal symptoms. Men are affected more commonly than women, particularly white men. The organism responsible for causing Whipple's disease is a gram-positive actinomycete, *Tropheryma whippelii*. The epidemiology and pathogenesis of Whipple's disease are poorly understood. The prevalence of the disease is higher in farmers compared with other workers, which suggests that the organism lives in the soil. Using the polymerase chain reaction, *T. whippelii* has been detected in sewage and in duodenal biopsy specimens, gastric juice, saliva, and stool of individuals without clinical disease. Whether the latter represents a carrier state or the presence of non-pathogenic organisms is not known. Immunologic defects and an association with the HLA-B27 gene may be disease factors. Small intestinal biopsy shows villous blunting and infiltration of the lamina propria with large macrophages that stain positive with the periodic acid–Schiff method and are filled with the organism. It is important to distinguish these macrophages from macrophages infected with *M. avium-intracellulare* complex, which stain positive on acid-fast staining and are found in individuals with AIDS. Treatment is with a prolonged course of broad-spectrum antibiotics (e.g., 10 to 14 days of parenteral penicillin G, 1.2 million U every day and streptomycin, 1 g every day; ceftriaxone, 2 g intravenously daily, or meropenem, 1 g intravenously three times daily; then, 160 mg of trimethoprim and 800 mg of sulfamethoxazole orally two times a day for 1 year or 160 mg of trimethoprim and 800 mg of sulfamethoxazole orally two times a day for 1 year). Relapses occur, but initial treatment with parenteral ceftriaxone or meropenem appears to be associated with a low relapse rate.

GRAFT-VERSUS-HOST DISEASE

Diarrhea occurs frequently after allogeneic bone marrow or stem cell transplantation (Chapter 181). Immediately after transplantation, diarrhea is caused by the toxic effects of cytoreductive therapy on the intestinal epithelium. Twenty to 100 days after transplantation, diarrhea is usually due to graft-versus-host disease (GVHD) or infection. Patients with GVHD present clinically with a skin rash, hepatic cholestasis, buccal mucositis, anorexia, nausea, vomiting, abdominal cramps, and diarrhea. The diagnosis of GVHD in the gastrointestinal tract can be made on biopsy of the stomach, small intestine, or colon. In mild cases, the mucosa appears normal on inspection at endoscopy, but apoptosis of gastric gland or crypt cells can be found on biopsy. In severe cases, denudation of the intestinal epithelium results in diarrhea and malabsorption and often requires parenteral nutritional support. Octreotide (50 to 250 µg subcutaneously three times a day) may be helpful in controlling voluminous diarrhea. Treatment of GVHD is with steroids and antithymocyte globulin combined with parenteral nutritional support until intestinal function returns.

SHORT-BOWEL SYNDROME

Malabsorption caused by small bowel resection or surgical bypass is called the short-bowel syndrome. The most common causes in the United States are massive resection due to adhesions, volvulus, ischemia (mesenteric or after intra-abdominal surgery), and gastric bypass surgery. Short-bowel syndrome due to Crohn's disease and radiation enteritis now is less common because of improved medical and radiation therapies. The severity of malabsorption depends on the site and extent of resection; the capacity for hyperplasia, dilation, and elongation; and the function of the residual bowel. Mechanisms of malabsorption after small bowel resection include a decreased absorptive surface area, decreased luminal bile salt concentration, rapid transit, and bacterial overgrowth. Limited jejunal resection usually is tolerated best because bile salt and vitamin B_{12} absorption remain normal. Ileal resection is less well tolerated because of the consequences of bile salt wasting and the limited capacity of the jejunum to undergo adaptive hyperplasia.

When less than 100 cm of jejunum remains, the colon takes on an important role in caloric salvage and fluid reabsorption. Malabsorbed carbohydrates are digested by colonic bacteria to short-chain fatty acids, which are absorbed in the colon.

TREATMENT

Parenteral nutrition may be avoided by a diet rich in complex carbohydrates, oral rehydration solutions, and an antimotility agent. In comparison, individuals with fewer than 100 cm of jejunum and no colon have high jejunostomy outputs and often require intravenous fluids or parenteral nutrition to survive. These individuals waste sodium, chloride, bicarbonate, magnesium, zinc, and water in their ostomy effluent. Dietary modifications should include a high-salt, nutrient-rich diet given in small meals. An oral rehydration solution with a sodium concentration greater than 90 mmol/L is absorbed best. Oral vitamin and mineral doses higher than the usual U.S. recommended daily allowances are required (Table 142-5). Vitamin B₁₂ should be given parenterally (500 to 1000 μg subcutaneously every month). Magnesium deficiencies are often difficult to replenish with oral magnesium because of its osmotic effect in the intestinal lumen. A liquid magnesium preparation added to an oral rehydration solution and sipped throughout the day may minimize magnesium-induced fluid losses. Potent antimotility agents, such as tincture of opium (0.5 to 1 mL orally four times a day), often are needed to slow transit and maximize contact time for nutrient absorption. High-volume jejunostomy outputs can be lessened by inhibiting endogenous secretions with a proton pump inhibitor (e.g., omeprazole, 40 mg orally one to two times a day, or lansoprazole, 30 mg orally one to two times a day) and, in severe cases, octreotide (100 to 250 μg subcutaneously three times a day; if effective, convert to an equivalent long-acting monthly dosage). The benefit of octreotide may be offset by its potential to inhibit intestinal adaptation and impair pancreatic enzyme secretion with doses greater than 300 μg/day.

In the most severe cases, supplemental calories must be provided by nocturnal tube feeding or parenteral nutrition. Treatment with growth hormone (0.1 mg/kg/day subcutaneously) with or without glutamine (30 g once a day orally) for 4 weeks may reduce parenteral nutrition requirements in patients who have had massive intestinal resections.[7] Teduglutide (0.05 mg/kg/day subcutaneously), a glucagon-like peptide-2 analogue that stimulates adaptive hyperplasia in remnant intestine after resection, reduces parenteral nutrition requirements.[8]

PROGNOSIS

Long-term complications include bone disease, renal stones (oxalate stones if the colon is present, urate stones with a jejunostomy), gallstones, bacterial overgrowth, fat-soluble vitamin deficiencies, essential fatty acid deficiency, and D-lactic acidosis. Small bowel transplantation should be considered for individuals who require parenteral nutrition to survive and then develop liver disease or venous access problems.

Conditions That Impair Nutrient Delivery to the Systemic Circulation

Insoluble lipids (present in chylomicrons) are exocytosed across the basolateral membrane of epithelial cells into the intestinal lymphatics. From there, they enter the mesenteric lymphatics and the general circulation through the thoracic duct. Sugar monomers, amino acids, and medium-chain fatty acids are transported across the basolateral membrane of intestinal epithelial cells into capillaries and into the portal circulation. Sugar monomers are transported across the basolateral membrane by the facilitative glucose transporter isoform (GLUT2) and amino acids by facilitative amino acid carriers (see Fig. 142-1A).

IMPAIRED LYMPHATIC DRAINAGE

Diseases that cause intestinal lymphatic obstruction, such as primary congenital lymphangiectasia (malunion of intestinal lymphatics), and diseases that result in secondary lymphangiectasia (lymphoma, tuberculosis, Kaposi's sarcoma, retroperitoneal fibrosis, constrictive pericarditis, severe heart failure) result in fat malabsorption. The increased pressure in the intestinal lymphatics leads to leakage and sometimes rupture of lymph into the intestinal lumen, with the loss of lipids, γ-globulins, albumin, and lymphocytes. The diagnosis of lymphangiectasia can be made by intestinal biopsy, but the specific cause may be more difficult to identify. Individuals with lymphangiectasia malabsorb fat and fat-soluble vitamins and have protein loss into the intestinal lumen. The most common presentation is hypoproteinemic

TABLE 142-5	VITAMIN AND MINERAL DOSES USED IN THE TREATMENT OF MALABSORPTION	
VITAMIN	**ORAL DOSE**	**PARENTERAL DOSE**
Vitamin A*	Water-soluble A, 25,000 U/day†	
Vitamin E	Water-soluble E, 400-800 U/day†	
Vitamin D‡	25,000-50,000 U/day	
Vitamin K	5 mg/day	
Folic acid	1 mg/day	
Calcium§	1500-2000 mg elemental calcium/day Calcium citrate, 500 mg calcium/tablet† Calcium carbonate, 500 mg calcium/tablet†	
Magnesium	Liquid magnesium gluconate† 1-3 tbsp (12-36 mEq magnesium) in 1-2 L of ORS or sports drink sipped throughout the day Magnesium chloride hexahydrate† 100-600 mg elemental magnesium/day	2 mL of a 50% solution (8 mEq) both buttocks IM
Zinc	Zinc gluconate† 20-50 mg elemental zinc/day‖	
Iron	150-300 mg elemental iron/day Polysaccharide-iron complex† Iron sulfate or gluconate	Iron sucrose¶ Sodium ferric gluconate complex¶ Iron dextran (as calculated for anemia) (IV or IM¶; Chapter 162)
B-complex vitamins	1 megadose tablet/day	
Vitamin B₁₂	2 mg/day	1 mg IM or SC/mo**

*Monitor serum vitamin A level to avoid toxicity, especially in patients with hypertriglyceridemia.
†Form best absorbed or with least side effects.
‡Monitor serum calcium and 25-OH vitamin D levels to avoid toxicity.
§Monitor 24-hr urine calcium to assess adequacy of dose.
‖If intestinal output is high, additional zinc should be given. Monitor for copper deficiency with high doses.
¶Parenteral therapy should be given in a supervised outpatient setting because of the risk of fatal reactions. Decreased risk of fatal reactions when compared with iron dextran.
**For vitamin B₁₂ deficiency, 1 mg IM or SC twice a week for 4 wk, then once a month.
ORS = oral rehydration solution.

edema. Nutritional management includes a low-fat diet and supplementation with medium-chain triglycerides, which are absorbed directly into the portal circulation. Fat-soluble vitamins should be given if deficiencies develop.

⬤ WATERY DIARRHEA

Watery diarrhea may be due to osmotic, secretory, inflammatory, or often combined mechanisms (Fig. 142-8).

Ingestion of Nonabsorbable or Poorly Absorbable Solutes

MAGNESIUM AND SODIUM PHOSPHATE AND SULFATE DIARRHEAS

Magnesium, phosphate, and sulfate are poorly absorbed minerals. Individuals who ingest significant amounts of magnesium-based antacids or high-potency multimineral and multivitamin supplements or those who surreptitiously ingest magnesium-containing laxatives or nonabsorbable anion laxatives, such as Na₂PO₄ (neutral phosphate) or Na₂SO₄ (Glauber's or Carlsbad salt) may develop osmotically induced, watery diarrhea that may be high volume.

SORBITOL AND FRUCTOSE DIARRHEA

Dietetic food, chewing gum, candies, and medication elixirs that are sweetened with sorbitol, which is an unabsorbable carbohydrate, can cause diarrhea. Excessive consumption of pears, prunes, peaches, and apple juice, which also contain sorbitol and fructose, a poorly absorbable sugar, can result in diarrhea. Most soft drinks are now sweetened with fructose-containing corn syrup and may be a cause of diarrhea when ingested in high concentrations.

FIGURE 142-8. Approach to the evaluation of watery diarrheas. Many diarrheas have more than one mechanism (i.e., osmotic, secretory, inflammatory). Other causes include medications, postsurgical (vagotomy, Nissan wrap, cholecystectomy), hyperthyroidism, and alcohol. *VIPoma: >3 L output daily "pancreatic cholera," elevated VIP level. Carcinoid: elevated urine 5-hydroxyindole acetic acid, positive OctreoScan. Gastrinoma (Zollinger-Ellison syndrome): elevated gastrin level, positive secretin stimulation test, diarrhea due to high volume of acid secretion. Thyroid medullary cancer: elevated calcitonin level. †May be high or low volume depending on dose ingested, may respond to fast. ‡Carbohydrate malabsorption (CHO) may be due to lactase deficiency, dietary fructose, sorbitol in diabetic candies or liquid medications. §Full-thickness biopsy may be needed for diagnosis. BO = bacterial overgrowth; FGF = fibroblast growth factor; IBS = irritable bowel syndrome; WBCs = white blood cells.

GLUCOSE-GALACTOSE MALABSORPTION AND DISACCHARIDASE DEFICIENCIES

Primary and secondary lactase deficiency is the most common cause of disaccharidase deficiency (see malabsorption). Congenital lactase deficiency causes diarrhea at birth with the first breast feed. Congenital sucrose-isomaltose deficiency presents in infancy when table sugar is introduced into the diet. Glucose-galactose malabsorption is due to mutations in the *SGLT1* gene and causes diarrhea at birth. The mechanism of diarrhea in these disorders is osmotic. Stools are acidic owing to conversion of unabsorbed sugars to short-chain fatty acids in the colon. Treatment is the substitution of fructose for other sugars in the diet. Patients who develop gas, bloating, or diarrhea after the ingestion of mushrooms may have a deficiency in the disaccharidase trehalase.

RAPID INTESTINAL TRANSIT

A small amount of carbohydrate in the diet is unabsorbed by the normal small intestine. Diets that are high in carbohydrate and low in fat may allow rapid gastric emptying and rapid small intestinal motility, thereby leading to carbohydrate malabsorption and osmotic diarrhea. Rapid transit time also occurs in thyrotoxicosis (Chapter 233). Because of the production of H_2 and CO_2 gas by colonic bacteria, abdominal gas and cramping may be the predominant symptoms.

BILE ACID MALABSORPTION

Ileal malabsorption of bile salts results in the stimulation of colonic fluid secretion and watery diarrhea. Three types of bile acid malabsorption induce diarrhea. Type 1 results when severe disease (e.g., Crohn's disease), resection, or bypass of the distal ileum allows bile salts to escape absorption (see earlier). Type 2 may rarely be congenital, owing to a defect in the apical sodium bile acid transporter, or may more commonly be idiopathic. The idiopathic type has been associated with decreased levels of FGF19, an intestinal fibroblast growth factor that normally downregulates bile salt synthesis in the liver. The result is increased bile salt production that overwhelms

reabsorption in the ileum. Type 3 is caused by various conditions, including prior cholecystectomy, celiac disease, pancreatic insufficiency, microscopic colitis, bacterial overgrowth, gastric surgery, or vagotomy. Postulated mechanisms include a bile salt storage problem, increased production, decreased recycling, or saturation of absorption.

> ### TREATMENT Rx
>
> Diarrhea due to types 1 and 2 often responds to cholestyramine, 2 to 4 g given orally two to four times daily, or the more potent and better tolerated bile salt binder, colesevelam, 625 mg tablet orally two to six times daily. Fat-soluble vitamin deficiency is a potential risk with chronic use of bile salt binders.
>
> Although many patients with type 3 respond to cholestyramine, some do not. In these patients, motility-altering drugs such as opiates (e.g., loperamide, 2 to 4 mg orally two to four times daily) and anticholinergics (e.g., hyoscyamine sulfate, 0.125 to 0.250 mg orally two to four times daily) may be of benefit.

Functional Watery Diarrhea (Irritable Bowel Syndrome)

See Chapter 139.

● TRUE SECRETORY DIARRHEAS

Endocrine diseases that can cause secretory diarrheas (see Fig. 142-8) include carcinoid tumors (Chapter 240), gastrinomas (Chapter 201), VIPomas of the pancreas (Chapter 201), and medullary carcinoma of the thyroid (Chapter 254). Diarrhea is also seen in 60 to 80% of patients with systemic mastocytosis (Chapter 263). Diarrhea due to gastrinoma is distinct in that it is caused by high volumes of hydrochloric acid secretion that overwhelm the reabsorptive capacity of the colon and by maldigestion of fat owing to pH inactivation of pancreatic lipase and precipitation of bile salts.

Villous Adenomas

Large (4 to 18 cm) villous adenomas (Chapter 199), particularly in the rectum or occasionally the sigmoid colon, may cause secretory diarrhea of 500 to 3000 mL/24 hours characterized by hypokalemia, chloride-rich stool, and metabolic alkalosis. Increased numbers of goblet cells and increased prostaglandin E_2 are responsible for the diarrhea. Chloride wasting in the stool and metabolic alkalosis are also found in congenital chloridorrhea, which is caused by a defect in the intestinal Cl^-/HCO_3^- transporter. The metabolic alkalosis distinguishes these two diarrheas from most other diarrheas that cause metabolic acidosis. A villous adenoma is usually diagnosed by colonoscopy. The prostaglandin antagonist indomethacin (25 to 100 mg orally daily) reduces the diarrhea in some patients; resection is curative.

Diabetes Mellitus–Related Diarrhea

Constipation is more common than diarrhea in patients with diabetes. High-volume, watery diarrhea, often with nocturnal incontinence, occurs in 20% of poorly controlled type 1 diabetic patients. These patients usually have concomitant neuropathy, nephropathy, and retinopathy. The diarrhea may be due to several causes, including celiac disease, anal incontinence, bacterial overgrowth related to dysmotility, medications (metformin, acarbose), and autonomic neuropathy. If no specific cause is found, clonidine (initial dose 0.1 mg orally twice daily and titrated slowly to a maximal dose of 0.5 to 0.6 mg orally twice daily) may be helpful. Patients with neuropathy frequently have impaired anal sphincter function, and high-dose loperamide (4 mg orally four times a day) may improve the incontinence.

Alcoholic Diarrhea

Diarrhea related to alcohol ingestion (Chapter 32) may be due to rapid intestinal transit, decreased bile and pancreatic secretion, nutritional deficiencies such as folate or vitamin B_{12}, or alcohol-related enteric neuropathy. Diarrhea may be acute with binge drinking, or it may be chronic and watery and persist for days or weeks. The diarrhea slowly resolves with abstinence from alcohol, proper nutrition, and the repletion of vitamin deficiencies.

Factitious Diarrhea

Approximately 30% of patients referred to tertiary centers have chronic diarrhea due to laxative abuse. The diarrhea is usually severe and watery, often with nocturnal symptoms. Some patients may have abdominal pain, weight loss, nausea, vomiting, hypokalemic myopathy, and acidosis. Stool volumes range from 300 to 3000 mL a day depending on the dose of laxative ingested. In the United States, bisacodyl is the most common cause. Other culprits include anthraquinone (senna, cascara, aloe, rhubarb) or osmotic laxatives (neutral phosphate, Epsom salts, and magnesium citrate). Some patients abuse other agents that cause diarrhea, such as the diuretics furosemide and ethacrynic acid.

More than 90% of laxative abusers are women who have underlying eating disorders such as anorexia nervosa or bulimia (Chapter 226) or middle-aged women who have complicated medical histories and who often work in health care. In patients with unexplained diarrhea, laxative screening of stool and urine (see later) should be performed to exclude this syndrome before an extensive medical evaluation is performed for other causes of chronic diarrhea.

Chronic Idiopathic Secretory Diarrhea

In a small subset of patients with secretory diarrhea, no cause is found despite an extensive evaluation. These cases are labeled as chronic idiopathic secretory diarrhea. In most patients, the diarrhea resolves within 6 to 24 months, which suggests a possible postinfectious or Brainerd's diarrhea. If no diagnosis is found after thorough testing and a search for surreptitious laxative abuse, a therapeutic trial with bile salt–binding drugs (e.g., cholestyramine, 4 g orally before meals three times a day, or the more potent colesevelam, 625-mg tablet two to six times daily) or opiates (e.g., loperamide, 2 mg orally four times a day, maximal dose 16 mg a day) is warranted.

⬤ INFLAMMATORY DIARRHEAS

Diarrhea due to inflammation is characterized by watery or bloody stools, fecal leukocytes, and loss of protein in the stool (see Fig. 142-8).

Inflammatory Bowel Disease

See Chapter 143.

Eosinophilic Gastroenteritis

Eosinophilic gastroenteritis is an increasingly recognized condition of unknown etiology characterized by infiltration of eosinophils in the mucosa, muscle, or serosal layers of the gastrointestinal tract. Approximately 50% of patients have atopic histories. Infestation with nematodes (Chapter 365) must be excluded before this diagnosis is made. Diarrhea occurs in 30 to 60% of patients with mucosal disease. Patients with involvement of the muscle layer often present with abdominal pain, nausea, and vomiting indicative of gastric outlet or intestinal obstruction. Peripheral eosinophilia is present in most patients. The disease may involve the entire gastrointestinal tract from esophagus to anus, or it may be isolated to a segment. With diffuse involvement, patients may have steatorrhea, protein-losing enteropathy, and blood loss.

COLLAGENOUS COLITIS AND LYMPHOCYTIC COLITIS

These two conditions, collectively known as *microscopic colitis*, may or may not be the same disease or variants of the same disease. Lymphocytic colitis is equally prevalent in men and women, whereas collagenous colitis occurs ten times more often in middle-aged or elderly women. These conditions may be associated with autoimmune disease or with NSAID use. There is an increased prevalence (15%) of microscopic colitis among individuals with celiac sprue. These diseases may be categorized as either inflammatory or secretory diarrheas. An epidemiologic relationship to medications such as NSAIDs, H_2-receptor blockers, proton pump inhibitors, selective serotonin reuptake inhibitors, and others has been reported, and increased luminal prostaglandin levels may cause the diarrhea. Enteric infections, food hypersensitivity, or intraluminal bile has been proposed as a trigger for prostaglandin release from lymphocytes. The disease disappears with fecal stream diversion. Antidiarrheal agents such as loperamide (2 mg orally four times a day) are the mainstay of therapy. Budesonide (9 mg orally once a day), bismuth subsalicylate therapy (eight chewable 262-mg tablets orally once a day), and 5-aminosalicylates (e.g., mesalamine, 400 to 800 mg orally three times daily) may be useful. Those with refractory disease may require corticosteroids (e.g., prednisone, 40 mg orally once a day).

FOOD ALLERGY

Food allergies or sensitivities, especially to cow's milk and soy protein, are a well established cause of enterocolitis in children, with an estimated frequency of 5%. Symptoms of abdominal cramps, diarrhea, and sometimes vomiting occur shortly after ingestion of the allergen (Chapter 261). The role of food allergy in causing diarrhea in adults is less clear owing to the lack of a reliable diagnostic test. Allergy testing correlates poorly with intestinal allergy. The most common food allergens are milk, soy, eggs, seafood, nuts, and wheat. Sequential elimination diets can be diagnostic and therapeutic.

Protein-Losing Enteropathy

Severe protein loss through the gastrointestinal tract can be caused by mucosal diseases such as lymphangiectasia, lymphatic obstruction, bacterial or parasitic infection, gastritis (Chapter 141), gastric cancer, collagenous colitis, inflammatory bowel disease (Chapter 143), celiac disease, sarcoidosis (Chapter 95), lymphoma (Chapter 191), tuberculosis (Chapter 332), Ménétrier's disease (Chapter 198), eosinophilic gastroenteritis, and food allergies. A variety of extraintestinal diseases, including systemic lupus erythematosus (Chapter 274), heart failure (Chapter 58), and constrictive pericarditis (Chapter 77), also can be causative. Patients with systemic lupus erythematosus (Chapter 274) may present with protein-losing enteropathy as the only manifestation of their disease. Treatment focuses on the underlying disease.

Radiation Enteritis

Patients who receive pelvic radiation for malignancies of the female urogenital tract or the male prostate may develop chronic radiation enterocolitis 6 to 12 months after total doses of radiation greater than 40 to 60 Gy (Chapters 19 and 144). Symptoms can develop 20 years after treatment, however. Early abnormalities include an increase in inflammatory mediators, an increase in cholinergic stimulation of intestinal tissue, and endothelial cell apoptosis that precedes epithelial cell apoptosis. The last finding suggests that vascular injury is the primary event. Vascular endothelial growth factor, basic fibroblast growth factor, and IL-11 protect animal intestine from experimental radiation damage. Diarrhea may be caused by bile acid malabsorption if the ileum is damaged, by bacterial overgrowth if radiation causes small intestinal strictures or bypass, or by radiation-induced chronic inflammation of the small intestine and colon. Rapid transit also may contribute to malabsorption and diarrhea.

Miscellaneous Diseases

Although acute mesenteric arterial or venous thrombosis manifests as an acute bloody diarrhea, chronic mesenteric vascular ischemia (Chapter 145) may manifest as watery diarrhea. Gastrointestinal tuberculosis (Chapter 332) and histoplasmosis (Chapter 340) manifest as diarrhea that may be either bloody or watery, as do certain immunologic diseases, such as Behçet's syndrome or Churg-Strauss syndrome. All of these diseases may be misdiagnosed as inflammatory bowel disease (Chapter 143). Neutropenic enterocolitis, an ileocolitis that occurs in neutropenic leukemic patients, sometimes is caused by *C. difficile* infection.

CLINICAL MANIFESTATIONS OF CHRONIC DIARRHEA

Patients with malabsorption can present with a variety of gastrointestinal or extraintestinal manifestations (Table 142-6). Significant malabsorption of fat and carbohydrate usually causes chronic diarrhea, abdominal cramps, gas, bloating, and weight loss. Steatorrhea (fat in the stool) manifests as oily, foul-smelling stools that are difficult to flush down the toilet. Stools may be large and bulky (e.g., pancreatic insufficiency) or watery (e.g., bacterial overgrowth, mucosal diseases). Individuals with malabsorption also can present with manifestations of vitamin and mineral deficiencies. Dyspnea can be caused by anemia from iron, folate, or vitamin B_{12} deficiency. Manifestations of calcium, magnesium, or vitamin D malabsorption include paresthesias and tetany due to hypocalcemia or hypomagnesemia and bone pain due to osteomalacia or osteoporosis-related fractures. Paresthesias and ataxia are manifestations of cobalamin and vitamin E deficiency. Dermatitis herpetiformis is a blistering, burning, itchy rash on the extensor surfaces and buttocks that is associated with celiac disease.

Inflammatory diarrheas may present with fever and abdominal pain or with edema to suggest chronic protein loss. Patients may have multiple, low-volume, bloody stools with tenesmus to suggest proctitis, or have severe diarrhea due to GVHD or celiac disease. Systemic manifestations of inflammatory bowel disease include polymigratory arthritis, sacroiliitis, erythema nodosum, pyoderma gangrenosum, leukocytoclastic angiitis, uveitis, and oral aphthous ulcers.

DIAGNOSIS OF CHRONIC DIARRHEA

A detailed history, physical examination, and certain screening tests lead to a diagnosis in 75 to 80% of patients with chronic diarrheas (see Table 142-1 and Fig. 142-3). A history of 10 to 20 daily bowel movements that do not respond to fasting suggests secretory diarrhea (see Fig. 142-8). A history of peptic ulcer should suggest gastrinoma (Chapter 201) or systemic mastocytosis (Chapter 263). Physical examination is helpful only if the thyromegaly of medullary carcinoma (Chapter 254), the cutaneous flushing of the neuro-endocrine tumors and systemic mastocytosis, the dermatographism of systemic mastocytosis, or the migratory necrolytic erythema of glucagonoma (Chapter 201) is evident. Autonomic dysfunction (e.g., postural hypotension, impotence, gustatory sweating) is almost invariably present in diabetic diarrhea.

Evaluation for malabsorption begins with a careful elicitation of bowel habits, a description of the stool, weight loss, travel, food or milk tolerance, underlying gastrointestinal or liver diseases, abdominal surgery, radiation or chemotherapy treatments, family history, and drug and alcohol use.

Blood Tests

Blood measurements (see Fig. 142-3) of iron, folate, vitamin B_{12}, vitamin D, or prothrombin time (vitamin K) help evaluate malabsorption. Peripheral blood findings of leukocytosis, eosinophilia, elevated erythrocyte sedimentation rate, hypoalbuminemia, or low total serum protein suggests an inflammatory diarrhea, whose hallmark is the presence of blood, either gross or occult, and leukocytes in the stool. There are no bedside screening tests to establish the diagnosis in watery diarrheas.

Imaging

Malabsorption may be suggested if a flat plate radiograph of the abdomen shows pancreatic calcification (Chapter 135). Some diseases (e.g., previous gastric surgery, gastrocolic fistulas, blind loops from previous intestinal anastomoses, small intestine strictures, multiple jejunal diverticula, abnormal intestinal motility that could lead to bacterial overgrowth) may be shown by computed tomography or magnetic resonance imaging of the abdomen after administration of oral contrast agents or by a traditional upper gastrointestinal radiographic series with small intestine follow-through. A small bowel barium study may show thickening of the intestinal folds (e.g., amyloidosis, lymphoma or Whipple's disease), uniform or patchy abnormalities (e.g., lymphoma or lymphangiectasia), or flocculation of barium and ilealization of jejunum to suggest celiac disease. Routine contrast radiographs of the gastrointestinal tract usually are not helpful in the diagnosis of watery diarrheas, unless they show extensive small bowel resection, the presence of a tumor (carcinoid or villous adenoma), or a bowel filled with fluid (endocrine tumor). Abdominal contrast imaging may show diagnostic evidence of advanced inflammatory bowel disease or changes suggestive of eosinophilic gastroenteritis or radiation enterocolitis. Somatostatin receptor scintigraphy with indium-111-labeled octreotide can be useful in localizing gastrinomas, pancreatic endocrine tumors, and carcinoid tumors.

Endoscopy and Biopsy

Upper endoscopy with distal duodenal biopsy should be undertaken if serologic tests for celiac disease are positive or diagnostic clues suggest small bowel mucosal malabsorption (Chapter 136). Small bowel biopsy is virtually always abnormal when the tTG IgA antibody level is very high (more than five-fold the normal range), and EMA is positive. A biopsy may be avoided in this setting. Some patients may have patchy mucosal disease and require enteroscopy with jejunal biopsies for diagnosis. Wireless video capsule endoscopy (Chapter 136) and balloon-assisted enteroscopy are increasingly used to diagnose diseases that reside deep in the small bowel. Patients with severe watery or elusive diarrhea should have a colonoscopy to assess for villous adenomas, microscopic colitis, mastocytosis, or early inflammatory bowel disease. Colonoscopy may also show brown pigmentation suggestive of melanosis coli due to chronic use of anthracene laxatives. Terminal ileal biopsy may indicate infectious or inflammatory bowel disease.

Other Laboratory Tests
Malabsorption

If chronic diarrhea is the presenting symptom, a stool examination for ova and parasites and a stool antigen-capture ELISA test for *Giardia* should be

TABLE 142-6	CLINICAL CONSEQUENCES OF MALABSORPTION OF NUTRIENTS, WATER, AND ELECTROLYTES

NUTRIENT MALABSORBED	CLINICAL MANIFESTATION
Protein	Wasting, edema
Carbohydrate and fat	Diarrhea, abdominal cramps and bloating, weight loss and growth retardation
Fluid and electrolytes	Diarrhea, dehydration
Iron	Anemia, cheilosis, angular stomatitis
Calcium and vitamin D	Bone pain, fractures, tetany
Magnesium	Paresthesias, tetany
Vitamin B_{12} and folate	Anemia, glossitis, cheilosis, paresthesias, ataxia (vitamin B_{12} only)
Vitamin E	Paresthesias, ataxia, retinopathy
Vitamin A	Night blindness, xerophthalmia, hyperkeratosis, diarrhea
Vitamin K	Ecchymoses
Riboflavin	Angular stomatitis, cheilosis
Zinc	Dermatitis, hypogeusia, diarrhea
Selenium	Cardiomyopathy
Essential fatty acids	Dermatitis

TABLE 142-7   ABNORMALITIES CONDUCIVE TO BACTERIAL OVERGROWTH

STRUCTURAL

Afferent loop syndrome after gastrojejunostomy
Ileocecal valve resection
End-to-side intestinal anastomoses
Duodenal and jejunal diverticula
Strictures (Crohn's disease, radiation enteritis)
Adhesions (postsurgical)
Gastrojejunocolic fistulas

MOTOR

Scleroderma
Diabetes mellitus
Idiopathic pseudo-obstruction

HYPOCHLORHYDRIA

Atrophic gastritis
Proton pump inhibitors
Acquired immunodeficiency syndrome
Acid-reducing surgery for peptic ulcer disease

MISCELLANEOUS

Immunodeficiency states
Pancreatitis
Cirrhosis
Chronic renal failure

obtained. A stool test for fat on a high-fat diet (70 to 100 g/day) is the best available screening test for malabsorption (see Table 142-6). If the fecal fat test result is negative, selective carbohydrate malabsorption or other causes of watery diarrhea should be considered. If the fecal fat test result is positive, further testing should be based on clinical suspicion for particular diseases. If pancreatic insufficiency is suspected, imaging studies of the pancreas should be performed. If proximal mucosal damage is suspected, multiple small intestinal biopsy specimens should be obtained. If there are no clues to the cause of malabsorption, a D-xylose test may help to distinguish mucosal disease from pancreatic insufficiency. However, the D-xylose test result also can be abnormal in individuals with bacterial overgrowth; if this condition is suspected, culture of an intestinal aspirate or a breath test should be obtained (see Table 142-6). Small bowel contrast imaging is useful in detecting ileal disease and structural abnormalities that predispose to bacterial overgrowth (Table 142-7). Some individuals with celiac disease present with selective nutrient deficiencies without diarrhea. In these cases, tTG antibody tests and intestinal biopsy should be performed. In patients hospitalized for severe diarrhea or malnutrition, a more streamlined evaluation usually includes a stool for culture, ova and parasites, and fat; an abdominal imaging study; and a biopsy of the small intestine and colon.

Watery Diarrhea

Breath tests to measure the respiratory excretion of labeled CO_2 after oral administration and metabolism of radioactive carbon-labeled substrates, or of H_2 after administration of carbohydrates, can assess carbohydrate and bile salt malabsorption or bacterial overgrowth (see Table 142-6).

The diagnosis of endocrine tumors, such as carcinoids, gastrinoma, VIPoma, medullary carcinoma of the thyroid, glucagonoma, somatostatinoma, and systemic mastocytosis, is made by showing elevated blood levels of serotonin or urinary 5-hydroxyindoleacetic acid and serum levels for gastrin, vasoactive intestinal peptide, calcitonin, glucagon, somatostatin, histamine, or prostaglandins (Chapter 201). Somatostatin receptor scintigraphy has proved to be sensitive and useful in the diagnosis and evaluation of Zollinger-Ellison syndrome (Chapter 201).

Inflammatory Diarrhea

Stool occult blood, white blood cells, or lactoferrin and calprotectin (components of leukocytes) are helpful tests for bowel inflammation. Video capsule endoscopy (Chapter 136) of the small bowel may detect ulcerations deep in the small bowel not reachable by standard upper or lower endoscopy and not detected with conventional barium contrast radiography. However, the risk of capsule retention in the small bowel is high in patients with Crohn's disease or NSAID use, particularly when there is a history of obstructive symptoms. The most sensitive test for protein-losing enteropathy is measurement of intestinal protein loss by 24-hour stool excretion or clearance of α_1-antitrypsin.

Stool Examination in Elusive Diarrhea

An important adjunct to diagnosing the cause of diarrhea is to examine the stool. The greasy, bulky stool of steatorrhea and the bloody stool of gut inflammation are distinctive. Stool collections (see Table 142-6) can be analyzed for weight, volume, fat, electrolytes ($^+Na^{++}$, K^{++}, Cl^-), osmolality, pH, and a laxative screen (SO_4^{2-}, PO_4^{2-}, Mg^{2+}). Stool or urine can be analyzed for emetine (a component of ipecac), bisacodyl, castor oil, or anthraquinone.

Carbohydrate malabsorption lowers stool pH because of colonic fermentation of carbohydrate to short-chain fatty acids. Stool pH less than 5.3 usually means pure carbohydrate malabsorption, whereas in the generalized malabsorptive diseases, stool pH is greater than 5.6 and usually greater than 6.0.

The normal stool osmotic gap, which is the difference between stool osmolality (or 290 mOsm) and twice the stool Na^{++} and K^{++} concentrations, is 50 to 125. In secretory diarrheas, the colon's capacity for adjusting electrolyte concentrations is overwhelmed, the stool osmotic gap is less than 50, and stool electrolytes more nearly resemble plasma electrolytes ($^+Na^{++}$ concentrations are usually >90 mmol/L, K^+ concentrations usually <10 mmol/L), except for higher HCO_3^- concentrations (usually >50 mmol/L). In osmotic diarrhea, the presence of uncharged solute or unmeasured cation in the colonic lumen draws in water, depresses stool Na^{++} (usually <60 mmol/L) and K^+ concentrations, and results in a stool osmotic gap >125. Stools with Na^{++} concentrations between 60 and 90 mmol/L and calculated osmotic gaps between 50 and 100 can result from either secretory or malabsorptive abnormalities. Patients with Mg^{2+}-induced diarrhea may be diagnosed by fecal Mg^{2+} values of more than 50 mmol/L. Sodium anion–induced diarrheas (Na_2SO_4, Na_2PO_4) mimic secretory diarrhea because the stool Na^{++} content is high (>90 mmol/L), and there is no osmotic gap; this diarrhea may be diagnosed by determining stool Cl^- concentration because these anions displace stool Cl^- resulting in a depressed stool Cl^- value (usually <20 mmol/L).

TREATMENT OF CHRONIC DIARRHEA   Rx

Antidiarrheal Therapy

Antidiarrheal agents are of two types: those used for mild to moderate diarrheas and those used for severe secretory diarrheas. A major shortcoming of opiates, the most commonly prescribed antidiarrheal agents, is that they have no antisecretory effect. Rather, they act by decreasing intestinal motility, thereby allowing longer contact time with the mucosa for improved fluid absorption. The exception is racecadotril, an enkephalinase inhibitor, that blocks intestinal fluid secretion without affecting motility.

Bulk-forming agents (psyllium [7 g in 8 ounces water orally up to five times a day] and methylcellulose [three to six tablets twice a day with 300 mL of water]) act by binding water and increasing the consistency of stool. Pectin has been shown to have proabsorptive activity. These agents may be useful in patients with fecal incontinence. Bismuth subsalicylates (524 mg orally every hour up to eight doses a day) have mild antisecretory and antimotility effects and are effective and safe in mild diarrheas. Agents that bind bile salts (e.g., cholestyramine, 2 to 4 g orally two to four times a day) are effective in the treatment of bile acid diarrheas but may worsen diarrhea in patients with ileal resection or disease of more than 100 cm of ileum.

The opiates may be symptomatically useful in mild to moderate diarrheas. Paregoric, deodorized tincture of opium, codeine, and diphenoxylate with atropine largely have been supplanted by loperamide. Loperamide does not pass the blood-brain barrier and has a high first-pass metabolism in the liver; it has a high therapeutic-to-toxic ratio and is essentially devoid of addiction potential. It is safe in adults, even in total doses of 24 mg/day. The usual dose is 2 to 4 mg two to four times daily. Opiates may be harmful in patients with severe diarrheas because large volumes of fluid may pool in the intestinal lumen (third space), and stool output is no longer a reliable gauge for replacing fluid losses. The antimotility effects are a problem in infectious diarrheas because stasis may enhance bacterial invasion and delay clearance of microorganisms from the bowel. Opiates and anticholinergics also are dangerous in severe inflammatory bowel disease or severe *C. difficile* infection, where they may precipitate megacolon.

Antidiarrhea agents that are used for the treatment of severe secretory and inflammatory diarrheas generally have profiles with more serious side effects. The somatostatin analogue octreotide (initial dose, 100 to 600 µg subcutaneously in two to four divided doses daily; maximal dose, 1500 µg daily) lessens diarrhea in the carcinoid syndrome and in neuroendocrine tumors because it inhibits hormone secretion by the tumor. It is also effective in the treatment of dumping syndrome and chemotherapy-related diarrheas. Long-acting subcutaneous octreotide preparations (20 to 30 mg intramuscularly intragluteally every month) are now available for once-a-month dosing. Octreotide can suppress pancreatic enzyme secretion and make diarrhea worse; it also may be of only limited usefulness in short-bowel syndrome and AIDS diarrhea. Agents such as phenothiazine and calcium-channel blockers have mild antisecretory effects, but side effects limit their use. Clonidine (initial dose, 0.1 mg orally twice daily, titrated slowly to a maximal dose of 0.5 to 0.6 mg twice daily) is most useful in opiate withdrawal diarrhea and is sometimes useful in diabetic diarrhea; postural hypotension may limit its use, particularly in patients with diabetes. Alosetron (0.5 mg orally twice daily for four weeks, maximal dose 1 mg orally twice daily) may be justified for severe diarrhea-predominant irritable bowel syndrome; associations with ischemic colitis and severe constipation have limited its use. Indomethacin (250 to 500 mg orally twice daily), a cyclooxygenase blocker that inhibits prostaglandin production, is useful in the treatment of diarrhea caused by acute radiation, AIDS, or villous adenomas of the rectum or colon; occasionally, it may be useful in neuroendocrine tumors and food allergy. For eosinophilic gastroenteritis, corticosteroids (prednisone, 20 to 40 mg orally once a day for 7 to 10 days) are the mainstay of therapy, but disodium cromoglycate (200 mg orally four times daily) also may be useful; food elimination diets are not usually effective. Treatment of inflammatory bowel disease is described in Chapter 143.

Grade A

1. Lowy I, Molrine DC, Leav BA, et al. Treatment with monoclonal antibodies against *Clostridium difficile* toxins. *N Engl J Med*. 2010;362:197-205.
2. Richardson V, Hernandez-Pichardo J, Quintanar-Solares M, et al. Effect of rotavirus vaccination on death from childhood diarrhea in Mexico. *N Engl J Med*. 2010;362:299-305.
3. Madhi SA, Cunliffe NA, Steele D, et al. Effect of human rotavirus vaccine on severe diarrhea in African infants. *N Engl J Med*. 2010;362:289-298.
4. Sur D, Lopez AL, Kanungo S, et al. Efficacy and safety of modified killed-whole-cell oral cholera vaccine in India: an interim analysis of a cluster-randomised, double-blind, placebo-controlled trial. *Lancet*. 2009;374:1694-1702.
5. Dupont HL, Jiang ZD, Okhuysen PC, et al. A randomized, double-blind, placebo-controlled trial of rifaximin to prevent travelers' diarrhea. *Ann Intern Med*. 2005;142:805-812.
6. Lauritano EC, Gabrielli M, Scarpellini E, et al. Antibiotic therapy in small intestinal bacterial overgrowth: rifaximin versus metronidazole. *Eur Rev Med Pharmacol Sci*. 2009;13:111-116.
7. Byrne TA, Wilmore DW, Iyer K, et al. Growth hormone, glutamine, and an optimal diet reduces parenteral nutrition in patients with short bowel syndrome: a prospective, randomized, placebo-controlled, double-blind clinical trial. *Ann Surg*. 2005;242:655-661.
8. Jeppesen PB, Gilroy R, Pertkiewicz M, et al. Randomized placebo-controlled trial of teduglutide in reducing parenteral nutrition and/or intravenous fluid requirements in patients with short bowel syndrome. *Gut*. 2011. [Epub ahead of print.]
9. Miehlke S, Madisch A, Bethke B, et al. Oral budesonide for maintenance treatment of collagenous colitis: a randomized, double-blind, placebo-controlled trial. *Gastroenterology*. 2008;135:1510-1516.
10. Miehlke S, Madisch A, Karimi D, et al. Budesonide is effective in treating lymphocytic colitis: a randomized double-blind placebo-controlled study. *Gastroenterology*. 2009;136:2092-2100.

SUGGESTED READINGS

Feurle GE, Junga NS, Marth T. Efficacy of ceftriaxone or meropenem as initial therapies in Whipple's disease. *Gastroenterology*. 2010;138:478-486. *Either antibiotic is an effective initial therapy.*

Lopman BA, Hall AJ, Curns AT, et al. Increasing rates of gastroenteritis hospital discharges in U.S. adults and the contribution of norovirus, 1996-2007. *Clin Infect Dis*. 2011;52:466-474. *Norovirus, which causes 10% of cause-unspecified and 7% of all-cause admissions for gastroenteritis, should be routinely considered in hospitalized patients.*

van der Windt DA, Jellema P, Mulder CJ, et al. Diagnostic testing for celiac disease among patients with abdominal symptoms: a systematic review. *JAMA*. 2010;303:1738-1746. *IgA anti-tissue transglutaminase antibodies and IgA antiendomysial antibodies have a high sensitivity and specificity for diagnosing celiac disease among patients with abdominal symptoms.*

Williams JJ, Beck PL, Andrews CN, et al. Microscopic colitis: a common cause of diarrhea in older adults. *Age Aging*. 2010;39:162-168. *About 10 to 30% of older patients with diarrhea and normal colonoscopy have microscopic colitis.*

143

INFLAMMATORY BOWEL DISEASE

GARY R. LICHTENSTEIN

DEFINITION

Inflammatory bowel disease refers to two chronic idiopathic inflammatory disorders, ulcerative colitis and Crohn's disease. These disorders are diagnosed by characteristic clinical, endoscopic, and histologic features, but no single individual finding is absolutely diagnostic for one disease or the other. Ulceration from Crohn's disease may be transmural and may occur anywhere in the gastrointestinal tract, most commonly in the distal ileum and proximal colon. The hallmark of ulcerative colitis is continuous ulceration starting in the rectum and limited to the colon. Approximately 10% of patients with inflammatory bowel disease have indeterminant colitis, a term used when Crohn's colitis cannot be differentiated from ulcerative colitis.

EPIDEMIOLOGY

Inflammatory bowel disease occurs worldwide, but the highest incidence is found in North America, the United Kingdom, and northern Europe. The incidence of Crohn's disease has risen slowly over time, although ulcerative colitis remains slightly more prevalent than Crohn's disease. The incidence of ulcerative colitis in North America is estimated to be 2.2 to 14.3 per 100,000 person years, with a prevalence of 37 to 246 per 100,000. The incidence of Crohn's disease in North America is estimated to be 3.1 to 14.6 per 100,000 person years, with a prevalence of 26 to 199 per 100,000.

Crohn's disease and ulcerative colitis may occur at any age. The peak incidence of Crohn's disease occurs between age 15 and 30 years of age, with a second peak in the seventh decade. There is a 1.2 : 1 female-to-male ratio. Ulcerative colitis also has a bimodal peak age distribution, with an initial peak between 20 and 40 years of age and second smaller peak beyond the seventh decade. There is an equal gender distribution in ulcerative colitis.

Crohn's disease and ulcerative colitis are polygenic disorders, for which family history is a risk factor. Crohn's disease and ulcerative colitis occur in all ethnic groups and races, but their incidence is highest in whites and Jewish people of Eastern European (Ashkenazi Jews) descent. In North America and the United Kingdom, however, the incidence of Crohn's disease in African Americans and African Caribbeans appears to be approaching that of whites. Studies of migrants from underdeveloped countries in South Asia to the United Kingdom suggest an increased prevalence of inflammatory bowel disease in subsequent generations, presumably as a result of environmental influences.

Cigarette smoking is associated with a worse prognosis in patients with Crohn's disease but an improved course in ulcerative colitis. Nonsteroidal anti-inflammatory drugs (NSAIDs) appear to be associated with exacerbations of disease, although evidence for this is less definitive. Appendectomy has been suggested as protective against the development of ulcerative colitis. Diet does not clearly affect the course of inflammatory bowel disease.

PATHOBIOLOGY

Although the trigger for inflammatory bowel disease is not known, three major pathways likely activate the disease: a genetic predisposition, immune dysregulation, and an environmental antigen. A possible explanation is that the inability of the innate immune system to clear microbial antigens, combined with increased intestinal epithelial permeability to antigens, eventually leads to an overactive adaptive immune response.

Genetics

Of patients with inflammatory bowel disease, 5 to 20% have a positive family history. First-degree relatives have a 10- to 15-fold increased risk for developing inflammatory bowel disease. The concordance rate of developing Crohn's disease in identical twins, siblings, and first-degree relatives is 50%, 0 to 3%, and 5 to 10%, respectively. Ulcerative colitis follows similar genetic patterns but with slightly lower risk rates. Twenty percent of patients with a positive family history of inflammatory bowel disease will have discordant disease type: one family member with Crohn's disease and another with ulcerative colitis.

The initial gene associated with Crohn's disease is *NOD2/CARD15*, located on chromosome 16 (16q12), and is expressed in intestinal epithelial Paneth cells, macrophages, and dendritic cells. This gene is involved in the expression of an intracellular receptor that senses muramyl dipeptide, a peptidoglycan component of gram-positive bacteria. Activation of *NOD2* leads to activation of NF-κB, which mediates transcription of numerous proinflammatory cytokines. A mutation in the leucine-rich domain of the NOD2 protein, which interacts with bacterial lipopolysaccharide, leads to failure in activation of NF-κB and is associated with the development of Crohn's disease.

Toll-like receptor-4 gene polymorphisms are associated with both Crohn's disease and ulcerative colitis. Polymorphisms of the interleukin-23 (IL-23) receptor gene are associated with ulcerative colitis and a varied risk of Crohn's disease. Human leukocyte antigen (HLA) class II polymorphisms, especially in HLA-DR molecules, may confer increased risk for ulcerative colitis and possibly Crohn's as well. The *OCTN1* gene, located on chromosome 5, and the *DLG5* gene, located on chromosome 10, have also been associated with

Crohn's disease. *DLG5*, which encodes a scaffolding protein that is important for maintaining epithelial integrity in various organs, may interact with the *NOD2/CARD15* gene to increase susceptibility to Crohn's disease. Gene *OCTN1*, located on chromosome 5q31, codes for an ion channel and also increases the risk of Crohn's disease; mutations in this gene may disrupt ion channels through altered function of cation transporters and cell-to-cell signaling in the intestinal epithelium.

PATHOPHYSIOLOGY

Microbes likely play a part in the development of inflammatory bowel disease. In several animal models of colitis, colitis does not develop in a sterile environment but can be induced after the introduction of commensal bacteria. Diverting the fecal stream away from active mucosal inflammation, such as in an ileostomy, also helps alleviate inflammation in Crohn's disease. Antibiotics, particularly antibiotics with broad-spectrum anaerobic coverage, are helpful in the treatment of Crohn's disease. More recently, several genetic polymorphisms associated with sensing the intestinal microbial environment and triggering an immune response have been linked to inflammatory bowel disease.

Both Crohn's disease and ulcerative colitis are products of a dysregulated innate immune system that triggers T cells and a humoral response. T_H17 cells, which are activated in Crohn's disease and ulcerative colitis, are stimulated by IL-23, which is produced by antigen-presenting cells. Variations in single-nucleotide polymorphisms of the gene encoding the receptor for IL-23 are associated with Crohn's disease.

Pathology
Crohn's Disease
As a result of a dysregulated immune system, patients with Crohn's disease develop aphthous ulcers, which are superficial mucosal ulcers. As the disease progresses, the ulceration becomes deeper, transmural, and discrete; it may form a serpiginous pattern and may occur anywhere from the esophagus to the anus in a noncontinuous pattern. The most common location for ulceration is the ileocecal region. In some patients, chronic disease leads to the formation of fibrotic strictures, and approximately 30% of patients may develop fistulas.

In early Crohn's disease, the histopathology is characterized by an acute inflammatory infiltrate in the lamina propria, with cryptitis, and crypt abscesses. Later in the disease process, the crypt architecture becomes distorted, with a lymphocytic infiltrate and a resulting branching and shortening of the crypts. Noncaseating granulomas, which are present in up to 15% of endoscopic biopsy specimens and as many as 70% of surgical specimens, are not unique to Crohn's disease but help confirm the diagnosis when other classic features are present.

Surgical specimens also may show transmural intestinal wall inflammation and fat creeping on the serosal surface.

Ulcerative Colitis
In mild ulcerative colitis, the mucosa is granular, hyperemic, and edematous in appearance. As the disease becomes more severe, the mucosa ulcerates, and the ulcers may extend into the lamina propria. Ulcerative colitis starts in the rectum and may extend proximally in a continuous pattern, but it affects only the colon. Pseudopolyps may form owing to epithelial regeneration after recurrent acute attacks. With chronic disease, the colonic mucosa may lose the normal fold pattern, the colon may shorten, and the colon may appear narrowed.

In early ulcerative colitis, the histopathology is characterized by epithelial necrosis, an acute inflammatory infiltrate in the lamina propria, cryptitis, and crypt abscesses. In chronic disease, a predominant lymphocytic infiltrate and distortion of crypt architecture are seen.

CLINICAL MANIFESTATIONS

Symptoms of inflammatory bowel disease are varied and may be a consequence of the location of the disease, the duration of disease, and any anatomic complications of the disease, such as strictures and fistulas in Crohn's disease (Table 143-1).

Symptoms
Crohn's Disease
The terminal ileum is affected in about 70% of patients with Crohn's disease. Primary ileal disease occurs in 30% of patients, whereas ileocolonic disease occurs in 40%. Symptoms may include abdominal pain, typically in the right

TABLE 143-1	CLINICAL CHARACTERISTICS OF CROHN'S DISEASE AND ULCERATIVE COLITIS	
	CROHN'S DISEASE	**ULCERATIVE COLITIS**
Peak age of onset (years of age)	15-30, 2nd peak in the 7th decade	20-40, 2nd smaller peak beyond the 7th decade
Sex distribution (F/M)	1.2/1	1/1
Potential sites of gastrointestinal involvement	Esophagus to anus	colon
Skipped areas of involvement	+	–
Transmural inflammation	+	–
Type of ulceration	Usually discrete	Continuous
Fistula	+	–
Stricture	–	–
Perianal disease (fissure, skin tags)	+	–

lower quadrant, diarrhea, hematochezia, and fatigue. With more severe disease, fever and weight loss may be present. Some patients may present with obstructive symptoms, such as abdominal pain, abdominal distention, and nausea.

Only approximately 5% of patients develop Crohn's disease in the upper gastrointestinal tract, and esophageal Crohn's disease occurs in less than 2% of patients. Subjects with upper gastrointestinal Crohn's disease may present with dysphagia, odynophagia, chest pain, or heartburn. Gastroduodenal disease occurs in 0.5 to 4% of patients and commonly occurs along with distal disease. Symptoms may include upper abdominal pain. Isolated jejunal disease is rare; if the jejunum is involved, there is also distal small bowel involvement. Up to 30% of patients have perianal disease (Chapter 147) that may include the development of fistulas, abscesses, fissures, and skin tags. Symptoms of perianal disease include pain and discharge. Fever may be present if there is an abscess.

Fistulas, which are internal tracks that can occur anywhere in the gastrointestinal tract and connect to various sites, occur in 20 to 40% of Crohn's patients. Penetrating Crohn's disease may also cause intra-abdominal and perianal abscesses owing to a fistula with a blind end or intestinal perforation. External fistulas, which present with symptoms of fluid discharge from the cutaneous opening, can be enterocutaneous, or perianal. Internal fistulas can be enteroenteric, rectovaginal, or enterocolonic. Patients may present with persistent abdominal pain and fever with an abscess in this location.

Ulcerative Colitis
As with Crohn's disease, symptoms and signs of ulcerative colitis depend on the extent and severity of disease. At the time of diagnosis, 14 to 37% of patients have pancolitis, 36 to 41% have disease extending beyond the rectum, and 44 to 49% have proctosigmoiditis. Symptoms include hematochezia, diarrhea, tenesmus, passage of mucus, urgency to defecate, and abdominal pain. In the setting of proctitis or proctosigmoiditis, patients may have constipation with difficulty defecating. With more extensive and severe colonic involvement, patients may also have weight loss and fever. Patients may also have nausea and vomiting because of abdominal pain, fatigue because of anemia, and peripheral edema because of hypoalbuminemia.

Physical Examination
Signs on physical examination are representative of the type of disease as well as its location and severity. Oral ulcers may be present in Crohn's disease. The location of abdominal tenderness usually reflects the location of intestinal involvement. In Crohn's disease, abdominal tenderness is classically in the right lower quadrant and may include fullness or a mass depending on the severity of inflammation. Peritoneal signs may occur when penetrating Crohn's disease causes intestinal perforation. Rectal examination may reveal skin tags, hemorrhoids, fissure, and fistulas.

Extraintestinal Manifestations
Arthropathy, the most common extraintestinal manifestation (Table 143-2), affects up to 10 to 20% of subjects. Peripheral arthralgias, arthritis, ankylosing spondylitis (Chapter 273), and sacroiliitis may exacerbate with

TABLE 143-2 EXTRAINTESTINAL COMPLICATIONS OF INFLAMMATORY BOWEL DISEASE

	CROHN'S DISEASE	ULCERATIVE COLITIS
Ocular disorders (uveitis, episcleritis)	+	+
Arthropathy	+	+
Oral ulcers	+	−
Skin disorders (pyoderma gangrenosum, erythema nodosum)	+	+
Nephrolithiasis	+	+
Primary sclerosing cholangitis	+	+
Bone disorders (osteoporosis, osteomalacia)	+	−
Thromboembolic disease	+	+
B$_{12}$ deficiency	+	−

TABLE 143-3 DIFFERENTIAL DIAGNOSIS OF ILEITIS AND COLITIS

INFECTIONS	MEDICATIONS/TOXINS
Bacterial	Nonsteroidal anti-inflammatory drugs
Aeromonas	Pancreatic enzyme supplements—"fibrosing
Campylobacter jejuni	colopathy"
Chlamydia (proctitis)	Phosphosoda bowel preparations
Clostridium difficile	Radiation
Mycobacterium tuberculosis	
Salmonella	
Shigella	
Enterohemorrhagic *Escherichia coli*	
Yersinia	
Viral	
Cytomegalovirus	
Herpes simplex virus (proctitis)	
Human immunodeficiency virus	
Fungal	
Histoplasma capsulatum	
Parasitic	
Entamoeba histolytica	
Helminths	

VASCULAR	INFLAMMATORY
Collagen vascular disease	Appendicitis
Behçet's disease	Diverticular disease
Churg-Strauss syndrome	Eosinophilic gastroenteritis
Henoch-Schönlein purpura	Nongranulomatous ulcerative jejunoileitis
Systemic lupus erythematosus	(celiac disease)
Polyarteritis nodosa	
Ischemia	

NEOPLASIA	MISCELLANEOUS
Carcinoid	Amyloidosis
Carcinoma primary or metastatic	Sarcoidosis
Lymphoma	Endometriosis
Mycosis fungoides	Tubo-ovarian abscesses
Malignant histiocytosis	

Adapted from Aberra FN, Lichtenstein GR. Crohn disease. In Talley NJ, Kane SV, Wallace MD, eds. *Practical Gastroenterology and Hepatology: Small and Large Intestine.* Wiley-Blackwell, 2010:225-235.

gastrointestinal symptoms. Dermatologic disorders, such as erythema nodosum (10 to 15%; see Fig. 448-23 in Chapter 448) and pyoderma gangrenosum (1 to 2%; Chapter 269), develop in up to 15% of patients. Eye disorders, especially uveitis and episcleritis (Chapter 431), may occur in 5 to 15%. Patients with inflammatory bowel disease also have up to a 10% risk of renal calculi, especially calcium oxalate stones (Chapter 128), in the setting of fat malabsorption with Crohn's disease in the small bowel. Uric acid stones can occur in the setting of severe volume depletion. Inflammatory bowel disease patients, especially patients with ulcerative colitis, are at increased risk for primary sclerosing cholangitis (Chapter 158).

Extraintestinal Complications

Patients with inflammatory bowel disease are susceptible to extraintestinal complications from the disease itself or medications used to treat disease. These complications include osteoporosis, osteomalacia, arthritic complications, thromboembolic events, pulmonary disease, and renal, dermatologic, and neurologic complications. Osteoporosis occurs in about 15% of patients, and steroid therapy (Chapter 34) is the major risk factor; avascular necrosis of the hip and septic arthritis are unusual complications of steroids or other immunosuppressive therapies. Cheilitis may be a result of iron deficiency anemia (Chapter 162). Patients with inflammatory bowel disease are at an increased risk for thromboembolic disease, especially in the setting of active intestinal disease, even when compared with other autoimmune diseases such as rheumatoid arthritis and celiac disease. Renal amyloidosis can be a consequence of chronic inflammation. Asthma is the most common pulmonary disorder in Crohn's disease. Patients also are at risk for multiple sclerosis (Chapter 419) and for peripheral neuropathy (Chapter 428) from vitamin B$_{12}$ deficiency, which may occur as a result of poor absorption owing to active small bowel disease or surgical resection.

DIAGNOSIS

When diarrhea (Chapter 142) is the predominant symptom, the initial evaluation should include a thorough medical history, testing for infectious colitis (Chapter 142), and screening for endocrine-metabolic disorders such as hyperthyroidism (Chapter 233) and hypocalcemia (Chapter 253). Infections with organisms such as *Shigella* (Chapter 317), *Amoeba* (Chapter 360), *Giardia* (Chapter 359), *Escherichia coli* O157:H7 (Chapter 312), and *Campylobacter* (Chapter 311) can be accompanied by bloody diarrhea, abdominal cramps, and an endoscopic picture identical to ulcerative colitis. Stool studies are needed to diagnose or exclude these infections. If hematochezia or abdominal pain are the predominant symptom, the differential diagnosis is broad (Table 143-3).

Diagnostic Evaluation
Endoscopic Evaluation

In a patient with symptoms suggestive of inflammatory bowel disease and no evidence for an infection to explain their symptoms, endoscopic evaluation is essential. Colonoscopy is the initial endoscopic test for patients who present with lower gastrointestinal symptoms such as diarrhea and

hematochezia, except in the presence of acute severe peritoneal symptoms. Colonoscopy to the terminal ileum is important if there is a potential diagnosis of inflammatory bowel disease. Small bowel imaging (such as small bowel follow-through or computed tomography [CT] enterography) may also be needed to determine whether there is small bowel disease or to determine the distribution of disease. Capsule endoscopy is useful if all other endoscopic and radiologic testing is nondiagnostic, but Crohn's disease of the small bowel is still suspected. Findings on capsule endoscopy should be followed by endoscopy to obtain biopsies. Capsule endoscopy should not be performed if Crohn's disease is complicated by a known small bowel stricture.

Crohn's Disease

Early endoscopic findings in Crohn's disease include superficial small mucosal ulcers, also called aphthous ulcers. As the severity of Crohn's disease progresses, the ulceration becomes deeper and may become round, linear, or serpiginous. A cobblestone appearance of the mucosa is caused by intersecting longitudinal and transverse ulcers, with "stone" areas representing normal mucosa (Fig. 143-1). Areas of ulceration, which are typically interspersed with normal "skip" areas, may occur anywhere from the esophagus to anus but are most common in the ileocecal region. Isolated colonic disease occurs in 25% of patients, and 60% will have rectal involvement, thereby making it at times difficult to differentiate from ulcerative colitis.

The diagnosis of inflammatory bowel disease is contingent on accurate histopathology, so biopsy of the affected area is key. Findings of an inflammatory infiltrate in the lamina propria and distortion of the crypt architecture support the diagnosis (Fig. 143-2). The diagnosis of Crohn's disease may be made by histopathology alone if noncaseating granulomas are seen, but

FIGURE 143-1. Endoscopic appearance of Crohn's disease with cobblestoning.

FIGURE 143-3. Endoscopic appearance of ulcerative colitis.

FIGURE 143-2. Colonic biopsy histopathology showing features of inflammatory bowel disease with crypt distortion and lymphocytic infiltration in the mucosa. (Adapted from AGA Institute GastroSlides 2010.)

Radiology

Radiologic imaging is vital and should almost always be obtained when inflammatory bowel disease, particularly Crohn's disease, is suspected. Barium studies such as an upper gastrointestinal series, small bowel follow-through, and barium enema are usually necessary to diagnose fistulas and strictures in Crohn's disease. If Crohn's disease is suspected by colonoscopic examination, a small bowel follow-through is generally obtained to assess the extent, severity, and type of disease (strictures and fistulas) in the small intestine. CT enterography and magnetic resonance imaging (MRI) enterography are alternatives to a small bowel follow-through. CT enterography may be preferred for the detection of abdominal abscesses, whereas MRI may be preferred for the detection of perineal abscesses and strictures.

Laboratory Findings

Anemia may result from chronic disease, blood loss or nutritional deficiencies of iron, folate, or vitamin B_{12}. A modestly elevated leukocyte count is indicative of active disease, but a marked elevation suggests an abscess or another suppurative complication. The erythrocyte sedimentation rate and C-reactive protein are nonspecific serum inflammatory markers that are sometimes used to monitor the activity of disease. Hypoalbuminemia is an indication of malnutrition. Ileal disease or resection of more than 100 cm of distal ileum results in a diminished serum vitamin B_{12} level because of malabsorption.

Serologic Markers

Serologic markers are supportive but may not be used independently to diagnose inflammatory bowel disease. Anti–*Saccharomyces cerevisiae* antibodies (ASCA), which are antibodies to yeast, are present in 40 to 70% of patients with Crohn's disease and in less than 15% of patients with ulcerative colitis. The combination of elevated ASCA immunoglobulin A (IgA) and IgG titers is highly specific for Crohn's disease, ranging from 89 to 100%. Perinuclear antineutrophil cytoplasmic antibodies (pANCA) are present in 20% of Crohn's patients, primarily in colon-predominant disease, and in 55% of patients with ulcerative colitis. ASCA-positive and pANCA-negative disease is associated with a sensitivity of 55% and specificity of 93% for Crohn's disease. The antimicrobial antibodies anti-I2 (Crohn's disease–related protein from *Pseudomonas fluorescens*), anti-Cbir1 (flagellin-like antigen), and anti-OmpC (*E. coli* outer membrane porin C) are also associated with Crohn's disease, but the utility of these additional markers has yet to be determined.

granulomas are rarely found on endoscopic biopsies. The diagnosis of Crohn's disease is usually based on a combination of information gleaned from histopathology, colonoscopy, and small bowel imaging. A skipped pattern of ulceration, ulceration in the small bowel or upper gastrointestinal tract or the presence of fistulas supports the diagnosis of Crohn's disease. Colonic and small bowel ulceration occur in several other disorders, including infections that may not be detected by routine stool studies (such as enterohemorrhagic *Escherichia coli*), vascular disorders, immune-related enterocolitis, neoplasia, diverticulitis, radiation, and medications such as NSAIDs (see Table 143-3).

Ulcerative Colitis

The diagnosis of ulcerative colitis is based on endoscopic findings and histopathology. Early in the disease process, patients develop diffuse mucosal erythema with loss of the normal mucosal vascular pattern. In mild disease, the mucosa may have a granular and edematous appearance. As the disease becomes more severe, the mucosa becomes more friable, bleeds easily when the mucosa is touched, and may eventually ulcerate (Fig. 143-3). Endoscopic findings, which start in the rectum and may extend proximally in a continuous pattern, affect only the colon. Pseudopolyps may form owing to epithelial regeneration after recurrent attacks in patients with long-standing disease. With chronic disease, the colonic mucosa may lose its normal fold pattern, and the colon may shorten and appear narrowed.

Features such as crypt distortion, continuous mucosal inflammation starting from the rectum, absence of granulomas, and absence of small bowel disease are all consistent with ulcerative colitis. Early in the disease process, chronic inflammatory findings, such as crypt distortion, may not be present, and the diagnosis may be more difficult to confirm.

TREATMENT **Rx**

The aim of medical therapy is to reduce inflammation and subsequently induce and maintain clinical remission. Medications used to treat inflammatory bowel disease include the categories of 5-aminosalicylate (5-ASA), antibiotics, corticosteroids, immunomodulators, and biologics (infliximab, adalimumab, certolizumab pegol, and natalizumab) (Table 143-4). The specific medical therapy selected is based on the location, extent (nonpenetrating and nonstricturing, stricturing, and penetrating and fistulizing disease), and severity of disease (Fig. 143-4; see Fig. 143-3). Supportive medical therapy, such as antidiarrheal and antispasmodic medications, may also be used.

Categories of Medical Therapy
5-Aminosalicylate

5-ASA, which acts as a topical anti-inflammatory within the lumen of the intestine, is used to treat mild to moderate ulcerative colitis and also has a

TABLE 143-4 MEDICAL THERAPIES FOR INFLAMMATORY BOWEL DISEASE

DRUG	DOSE	RELEASE SITE
5-AMINOSALICYLATES		
Sulfasalazine (Azulfidine)	2-6 g/day	Colon
Mesalamine (Asacol, Lialda, Apriso)	2.4-4.8 g/day	Distal ileum, colon
Olsalazine (Dipentum)	1-3 g/day	Colon
Balsalazide (Colazal)	6.25 g/day	Colon
Mesalamine (Pentasa)	2-4 g/day	Duodenum, jejunum, ileum, colon
Mesalamine (Rowasa), enema, suppository	4 g/day (enema) 1 g/day (suppository)	Rectum/sigmoid Rectum
Mesalamine (Canasa), suppository	1 g/day (suppository)	Rectum
CORTICOSTEROIDS		
Budesonide (Entocort)	Induction: 9 mg PO qd Maintenance: 6 mg PO qd	Small intestine
Prednisone	0.25-0.75 mg/kg PO qd	Systemic
Methylprednisolone	40-60 mg IV qd	Systemic
IMMUNOMODULATORS		
6-Mercaptopurine	1.5 mg/kg/day	Systemic
Azathioprine	2.5 mg/kg/day	Systemic
Methotrexate	Induction: 25 mg SC q wk × 4 mo Maintenance: 15 mg SC q wk	Systemic
Cyclosporine	2-4 mg/kg/day	Systemic
BIOLOGICS		
Infliximab	Induction: 5 mg/kg IV weeks 0, 2, 6 Maintenance: 5 mg/kg IV q 8 wk	Systemic
Adalimumab	Induction: 160 mg SC week 0, 80 mg week 2 Maintenance: 40 mg SC every other week	Systemic
Certolizumab pegol	Induction: 400 mg SC weeks 0, 2, 4 Maintenance: 400 mg SC q 4 wk	Systemic
Natalizumab	300 mg IV q 4 wk	Systemic

IV = intravenously; PO = orally; SC = subcutaneously.

FIGURE 143-4. Ulcerative colitis treatment algorithm.

limited role in Crohn's disease. Sulfasalazine is the combination of a sulfapyridine with 5-ASA; 5-ASA is responsible for the anti-inflammatory property of this drug, whereas sulfapyridine is the carrier that allows 5-ASA to be delivered into the colon. Other oral formulations of 5-ASA allow it to be delivered to the intestine by different mechanisms. Mesalamine is released in the intestine based on a pH delivery model, whereas sulfasalazine, olsalazine, and balsalazide are released in the intestine by bacterial cleavage of a covalent bond between 5-ASA and a prodrug. For rectal and sigmoid disease, 5-ASA suppository and enema preparations are also available. Adverse events associated with 5-ASAs are rare and may include nausea, dyspepsia, hair loss, headache, worsening diarrhea, and hypersensitivity reactions.

Corticosteroids

Corticosteroids are primarily used to treat flares of ulcerative colitis and Crohn's disease. Oral formulations may be used for mild to moderate disease, whereas systemic corticosteroids are used for moderate to severe disease.

Enteric coated budesonide, a pH-dependent ileal release formulation, is an oral corticosteroid with high topical activity and low systemic bioavailability (10%). Enteric coated budesonide is indicated for treatment of active mild to moderate Crohn's disease. Oral corticosteroids such as prednisone and

methylprednisolone are used for moderate to severe disease, starting at doses ranging from 40 to 60 mg once a day. Intravenous methylprednisolone is used for severe disease, with dosing ranging from 40 to 60 mg once a day. Maintenance with systemic corticosteroids is not recommended because of their substantial side effects (Chapter 34).

Immune Modulators

In patients who remain symptomatic despite 5-ASA therapy or who have moderate to severe Crohn's disease or ulcerative colitis, the thiopurine analogues (6-mercaptopurine and azathioprine) may be used; methotrexate also may be used for moderate to severe Crohn's disease. Azathioprine, the prodrug of 6-mercaptopurine, typically is prescribed at a dose of 2 to 3 mg/kg/day; the equivalent dose of 6-mercaptopurine is 1.5 mg/kg/day. A disadvantage of the thiopurine analogs is the slow clinical response that may not be evident for as long as 12 weeks. Their side effects include allergic reactions, pancreatitis, myelosuppression, nausea, infections, hepatotoxicity, and malignancy, especially lymphoma. The white blood cell count and liver chemistries must be monitored routinely. Methotrexate, which is a folic acid antagonist, is given as 25 mg intramuscularly or subcutaneously once per week for 16 weeks for active Crohn's disease and, 15 mg to 25 mg intramuscularly or subcutaneously once per week for maintaining remission.

FIGURE 143-5. Crohn's disease treatment algorithm. NPO = nothing by mouth; TNF-α = tumor necrosis factor-α; TPN = total parenteral nutrition; UGI = upper gastrointestinal.

[1]Proximal colon disease involvement
[2]Abscess should be excluded before initiating medical therapy
[3]Perianal location

Antibiotics

The exact mechanism for the beneficial effect of broad-spectrum antibiotics in the treatment of inflammatory bowel disease is not known. Potential mechanisms include eliminating bacterial overgrowth, eradicating a bacterially mediated antigenic trigger, and potential immunosuppressive properties (e.g., metronidazole). The primary role of antibiotics is in Crohn's disease, where metronidazole (10 to 20 mg/kg daily for 4 to 8 weeks), ciprofloxacin (500 mg orally twice daily for 4 to 8 weeks), or both are primary inductive therapies for perianal fistulas and fissures. Metronidazole may also be a helpful adjunctive treatment for colonic Crohn's disease.

Biologicals

Anti–Tumor Necrosis Factor-α Agents

Antibodies to tumor necrosis factor-α (anti-TNF-α) include infliximab, which is a chimeric mouse-human IgG1 monoclonal antibody that is approved to treat moderate to severe Crohn's disease, fistulizing Crohn's disease, and moderate to severe ulcerative colitis that has failed to respond to conventional therapy. Adalimumab (Humira) and certolizumab pegol (Cimzia) have been approved to treat moderate to severe Crohn's disease that has failed to respond to conventional therapy. Adalimumab is a fully humanized IgG1 antibody that is self-administered subcutaneously. Certolizumab pegol, which is a chimeric pegylated Fab fragment to TNF-α, also is administered subcutaneously.

Antiadhesion molecules

Natalizumab, a humanized IgG4 monoclonal antibody, binds to the α_4 subunit of $\alpha_4\beta_1$ and $\alpha_4\beta_7$ integrins expressed on all leukocytes except neutrophils. Natalizumab inhibits the interactions between α_4 integrins on the surface of leukocytes and adhesion molecules on vascular endothelial cells in the gastrointestinal tract, thereby preventing adhesion and recruitment of leukocytes. Natalizumab is approved for the treatment of moderate to severe Crohn's disease that is refractory to conventional therapy, but there are strict guidelines for prescribing natalizumab because of its associated risk of progressive multifocal leukoencephalopathy (Chapter 378).

Crohn's Disease Medical Therapy

Mild to Moderate Crohn's Disease

Sulfasalazine, 3 to 6 g/day, is superior to placebo for treating active ileocolonic and colonic Crohn's disease, with response rates ranging from 45 to 55% for mild to moderate disease, but is not clearly effective for small bowel disease alone (Fig. 143-5). Mesalamine also has a modest benefit compared with placebo for mild to moderate disease.[1] However, the 5-ASAs are not effective for maintaining remission.

For mild to moderate Crohn's disease involving the distal small intestine or proximal colon budesonide (9 mg by mouth once a day) provides about a 70% response rate after 8 weeks and is significantly more effective than mesalamine, 4 g once a day, for distal ileal and right colonic disease.[2] As a maintenance agent at 3 or 6 mg, the effects of budesonide wane and disappear within 1 year.

Upper gastrointestinal Crohn's disease (jejunal, duodenal, gastric, and esophageal) is uncommon, so few clinical trials are available to assess therapies for this location. Because local therapies such as 5-ASAs and budesonide are not released in these locations, systemic immunosuppressants (azathioprine, mercaptopurine, infliximab, adalimumab, and certolizumab pegol) are the mainstays of therapy.

Moderate to Severe Crohn's Disease

Patients with moderate to severe disease are initially treated with systemic corticosteroids, but corticosteroids should not be used as maintenance therapy. Options to induce a remission or maintain a steroid-induced remission include 6-mercaptopurine, azathioprine, methotrexate, infliximab, adalimumab, and certolizumab.[3-5] After 1 year, approximately 20% more patients treated with combined therapy (corticosteroids, daily azathioprine, and infliximab, 5 mg/kg at weeks 1, 2, and 6) will be in remission compared with conventional treatment (corticosteroids plus azathioprine and then infliximab as needed according to current guidelines).[6] In a randomized trial, infliximab (5 mg/kg at 0, 2, and 6 weeks and then every 8 weeks) alone or infliximab plus azathioprine (2.5 mg/kg/day) was more effective than azathioprine alone.[7] Patients who have not responded to conventional therapy may be considered for natalizumab.

For severe Crohn's disease, patients should be hospitalized, given nothing by mouth, rehydrated with intravenous fluids, and administered parenteral corticosteroids. Patients who respond to parenteral corticosteroids should be switched to high-dose oral corticosteroids (prednisone, 40 to 60 mg/day), with the dose of prednisone gradually reduced. Patients who have severe Crohn's disease and who do not respond to parenteral corticosteroids within a week should be considered for either infliximab or surgery. A course of total parenteral nutrition (Chapter 224) may be useful as adjunctive therapy.

Fistulizing Crohn's disease

Fistulas occur in one third of patients with Crohn's disease, and perianal fistulas represent the most common location. Asymptomatic internal fistulas rarely require therapy. A concomitant abscess, which may occur in the setting of a fistula, must be excluded before initiating immunosuppressive therapy. Surgery may be required. Medical treatment depends on the location and associated complications.

High-output enterocutaneous fistulas in the setting of proximal small bowel involvement can lead to outputs of more than 500 mL/day and can cause severe volume depletion. Initial management requires volume repletion. In the postoperative setting, a fistulous opening is usually in the area of a wound, and it is imperative to protect the healing skin from infection caused by the drainage from either an ostomy bag or a catheter used for a high-output fistula. High-output fistulas will rarely close spontaneously and typically will require surgical closure. Low-output fistulas may be treated initially with azathioprine (or 6-mercaptopurine), methotrexate, or anti-TNF-α therapy (infliximab, adalimumab, or certolizumab).[8]

Perianal fistulas are classified into simple and complex fistulas. A simple fistula is located below most of the anal sphincter and has one track. A complex fistula passes through the intersphincteric (high location), transsphincteric, or suprasphincteric region and may have multiple tracks. Simple fistulas respond well to medical therapy, initially with metronidazole (10 to 20 mg/kg orally daily for 4 to 8 weeks) and ciprofloxacin (500 mg orally twice daily for 4 to 8 weeks) for the fistula and treatment of concurrent mucosal disease. Treatment with immunomodulators or anti-TNF-α agents is also beneficial.[8] Patients with fistulas without rectal mucosal Crohn's disease may respond well to fistulotomy, whereas patients with mucosal involvement may benefit from seton placement rather than fistulotomy. Complex fistulas usually require a combination of surgical and medical therapy. In the setting of intractable disease, colonic or ileal diversion may allow for rectal and perianal healing; in severe cases, proctocolectomy may be necessary.

For Crohn's disease–related rectovaginal fistulas, medical therapy with antimetabolite therapy, or anti-TNF-α agents is usually considered before surgery. Surgical therapy such as fistulotomy and mucosal flap may be considered.

Enterovesicular or colovesicular fistulas may be treated with antimetabolite therapy or anti-TNF-α agents, or both, but recurrent urinary tract infection is an indication for surgery. Surgery usually involves resection of involved bowel and closure of the bladder defect.

Asymptomatic internal fistulas, such as enteroenteric fistulas, do not require surgical intervention, but treatment with an immunomodulator may be considered. Internal fistulas, such as cologastric and coloduodenal, may cause substantial symptoms because of bypass of part of the intestine. If medical management fails or if an abscess forms, surgery is recommended.

Medical Management of Ulcerative Colitis

The anatomic distribution of ulcerative colitis guides therapy. Options include suppositories, retention enemas, topical foam, oral therapy, and parenteral therapy. Suppositories are effective to treat proctitis in the distal 20 cm of the colon. Topical foam and enemas are effective for distal and left-sided colitis. Oral therapy and parenteral therapy are effective for all locations of disease.

Proctitis

For active ulcerative proctitis, topical 5-ASA (enema and suppository) in combination with oral treatment is superior to oral treatment alone.[9] Topical 5-ASA is superior to topical corticosteroids for treatment of active ulcerative proctitis, rectal 5-ASA therapy produces a faster response when given with oral 5-ASA. Corticosteroid enemas, suppositories, or foam can also be used if 5-ASA fails. 5-ASA or corticosteroid retention enemas can be used for active disease up to the splenic flexure (i.e., the rectum, sigmoid colon, and descending colon). Another approach to proctitis or distal colitis is an oral aminosalicylate, although a response may not be evident for 3 to 4 weeks.

Extensive Colitis

In patients with ulcerative colitis of mild to moderate activity and extension of disease proximal to the splenic flexure, the initial drug of choice is an oral 5-ASA; efficacy increases with increasing doses.[10] Even with more extensive disease, supplementation of oral 5-ASA with 5-ASA enemas or suppositories may help reduce the symptoms of urgency that result from rectal involvement. In patients with more than five or six bowel movements per day, in patients in whom a more rapid response is desired, or in patients who have not responded to 3 to 4 weeks of 5-ASA, the treatment of choice is oral prednisone. Patients with severe diarrhea, systemic symptoms, or significant amounts of blood in stool should be started on 40 mg/day; most patients respond to oral corticosteroids within a few days. After the symptoms are controlled, prednisone can be tapered gradually by 5 mg every 1 to 2 weeks. Patients who respond to oral prednisone and can be fully withdrawn from it should be maintained on 5-ASA.

If patients with severe ulcerative colitis do not begin to respond to corticosteroids at the equivalent dose of 60 mg of intravenous methylprednisolone within 5 days or do not completely respond within 7 to 10 days, options include colectomy, infliximab, or cyclosporine. For patients whose disease flares whenever the corticosteroids are withdrawn or their corticosteroid dose is lowered, the continuation of high-dose corticosteroid therapy is the most common management error. If the patient requires a substantial dose (>15 mg/day of prednisone) for more than 6 months, a trial of an immunomodulator, infliximab, or colectomy should be given serious consideration.

The most common indication for hospitalization in patients with ulcerative colitis is intractable diarrhea, although blood loss is also common. Patients with severely active ulcerative colitis should be evaluated for toxic megacolon by abdominal radiography or CT. Antidiarrheal medications and anticholinergic medications are contraindicated in patients with severe ulcerative colitis because of the risk for precipitating toxic megacolon. The mainstays of therapy for severe ulcerative colitis are rehydration with intravenous fluids and intravenous corticosteroids (hydrocortisone, 300 mg/day; prednisolone, 60 to 80 mg/day; or methylprednisolone, 40 to 60 mg/day). Total parenteral nutrition (Chapter 224) may be necessary in patients with malnutrition. Patients with peritoneal signs or signs of systemic infection should be treated with parenteral antibiotics (Chapter 144). Patients who do not improve in 7 to 10 days should be considered for either colectomy, a trial of intravenous cyclosporine,[11] or a trial of infliximab.

Maintenance Therapy

Aminosalicylates reduce recurrent disease in patients with ulcerative colitis, and essentially all patients should receive maintenance therapy[12] with original or newer 5-ASA preparations. Corticosteroids are not effective as maintenance therapy and should not be used. Azathioprine, 6-mercaptopurine, and infliximab are effective for maintenance therapy in patients whose ulcerative colitis has not responded to 5-ASA.

Surgical Therapy

Crohn's Disease

Surgical resection does not cure Crohn's disease, and recurrences are likely after resection, so the approach should be conservative in terms of the amount of tissue removed. Nevertheless, about 40% of patients with Crohn's disease undergo surgery within 10 years of their diagnosis. Failure of medical management is a common cause for resection in patients with Crohn's disease, but complications (e.g., obstruction, fistula, abscess) are often the indications for resection. For Crohn's disease of the small bowel, the most common surgical procedure is segmental resection for obstruction or fistula; the incidence of a recurrence severe enough to require repeat surgery after ileal or ileocolic resection is about 25% after 10 years and 35% after 15 years. For patients with extensive colonic disease that includes the rectum, the procedure of choice is total proctocolectomy with a Brooke (end) ileostomy. Total colectomy with ileal pouch anal anastomosis is not appropriate in Crohn's colitis because recurrence of Crohn's disease in the ileal segment of the new pouch would require a repeat operation and loss of a long segment of ileum.

Ulcerative Colitis

For ulcerative colitis, colectomy is a curative procedure. Approximately 40% of patients with extensive ulcerative colitis eventually undergo colectomy, usually because their disease has not responded adequately to medical therapy. Emergency colectomy may be required in patients with toxic megacolon or a severe fulminant attack without toxic megacolon. The standard operation for ulcerative colitis is proctocolectomy and a Brooke ileostomy. The most popular alternative operation is total proctocolectomy with an ileal pouch anal anastomosis; in this procedure, a pouch is constructed from the terminal 30 cm of ileum, and the distal end of the pouch is pulled through the anal canal. Ileoanal anastomosis is sometimes complicated by inflammation in the ileal pouch (termed *pouchitis*), which can be treated with antibiotics (typically, metronidazole, 500 mg three times daily or 20 mg/kg daily, or ciprofloxacin, 500 mg twice daily for a duration of 2 weeks). The decision for or against colectomy and among types of surgery is influenced by the patient's age, social circumstances, and duration of disease, and this decision requires expert consultation. When other indications are equivocal, the risk of malignancy (see later) may be an indication for colectomy.

Complications

Crohn's Disease

Abscesses

Abscesses, which are common complications in Crohn's disease, result from extension of a mucosal fissure or ulcer through the intestinal wall and into extraintestinal tissue. Leakage of intestinal contents through a fissure into the peritoneal cavity results in an abscess. Abscesses occur in 15 to 20% of patients with Crohn's disease, especially in the terminal ileum. The typical clinical manifestation of an intra-abdominal abscess is fever, abdominal pain, abdominal tenderness, and leukocytosis. Abdominal abscess is most often diagnosed by a CT scan. Broad-spectrum antibiotic therapy, including anaerobic coverage, is indicated. Percutaneous drainage of abscesses in patients with Crohn's disease may improve the clinical picture but does not provide adequate therapy because of persistent communication between the abscess cavity and the intestinal lumen. Resection of the involved intestine is usually required for definitive therapy.

Obstruction

Obstruction is a common complication of Crohn's disease, particularly in the small intestine, and is a leading indication for surgery. Small bowel obstruction in Crohn's disease may be caused by mucosal thickening from acute inflammation, by muscular hyperplasia and scarring as a result of previous inflammation, or by adhesions. Obstruction may also occur because of impaction of a bolus of fibrous food in a stable, long-standing stricture. Obstruction is marked by cramping abdominal pain and diarrhea that worsen after meals and resolve with fasting. Strictures may be evaluated by CT enterography, MRI enterography, oral contrast studies, barium enema, or colonoscopy, depending on the anatomic location. Corticosteroids (e.g., intravenous methylprednisolone, 40 to 60 mg once a day, or intravenous hydrocortisone, 200 to 300 mg once a day, for 5 to 14 days) are useful if acute inflammation is an important component of the obstructive process, but not if the obstruction is caused by fibrosis. A common error in the management of Crohn's disease is inappropriate treatment with long courses of corticosteroids in patients who have obstructive symptoms from fixed anatomic lesions. If the obstruction does not resolve with nasogastric suction and corticosteroids, surgery is necessary.

Perianal Disease

Perianal disease is a potentially disabling complication of Crohn's disease. Ulcerations in the anal canal may coalesce and result in fistula formation. The fistulous openings are most commonly found in the perianal skin but can occur in the groin, the vulva, or the scrotum. Fistulas are accompanied by drainage of serous or purulent material. If the fistula does not drain freely, there is local accumulation of pus (perianal abscess) with redness, pain, and induration. The pain of a perianal abscess is exacerbated by local pressure that may result from defecation, sitting, or walking. The typical physical manifestation of an abscess is redness with tenderness on digital examination; fluctuance also may be present. Adequate evaluation of perianal disease generally requires proctoscopic examination under anesthesia. Cross-sectional CT or MRI can define the presence and extent of perianal abscesses. The goals of therapy for perianal disease are relief of local symptoms and preservation of the sphincter. Limited disease can be approached with sitz baths and metronidazole, but most cases also require adequate external drainage. Azathioprine, infliximab, adalimumab, or certolizumab pegol may be useful in healing perianal disease, but the disease may reactivate when the drug is stopped. Persistent severe perianal Crohn's disease can result in destruction of the anal sphincter and subsequent fecal incontinence.

Ulcerative Colitis

One of the most significant complications of ulcerative colitis is toxic megacolon, which is dilation of the colon to a diameter greater than 6 cm associated with worsening of the patient's clinical condition and the development of fever, tachycardia, and leukocytosis. Physical examination may reveal postural hypotension, abdominal tenderness over the distribution of the colon, and absent or hypoactive bowel sounds. Agents that reduce gastrointestinal motility, such as antispasmodics and antidiarrheal agents, are likely to initiate or exacerbate toxic megacolon. Medical therapy is designed to reduce the likelihood of perforation and return the colon to normal motor activity as rapidly as possible. The patient is given nothing by mouth, and nasogastric suction is begun. Intravenous fluids should be administered to replete water and electrolyte abnormalities, broad-spectrum antibiotics (e.g., ampicillin-sulbactam, given as 1 g ampicillin plus 0.5 g sulbactam, 1.5 to 3 g every 6 hours for 5 to 14 days; levofloxacin, 500 mg intravenously once daily plus metronidazole, 500 mg intravenously or orally twice daily; cefazolin, 500 mg intravenously three times daily plus metronidazole, 500 mg intravenously or orally twice daily; or trimethoprim-sulfamethoxazole, 8 to 10 mg/kg/day intravenously or orally in two to four divided doses plus metronidazole, 500 mg intravenously or orally twice daily for approximately 7 days or until symptomatic improvement) are given in anticipation of possible peritonitis as a result of perforation, and parenteral corticosteroids are administered at a dose equivalent to more than 40 to 60 mg of prednisone per day. Signs of improvement include a decrease in abdominal girth and the return of bowel sounds. Deterioration is marked by the development of rebound tenderness, increasing abdominal girth, and cardiovascular collapse. If the patient does not begin to show signs of clinical improvement during the first 24 to 48 hours of medical therapy, the risk for perforation increases markedly, and surgical intervention colectomy is indicated.

Follow-Up

Colon Cancer, Dysplasia, and Colonoscopic Surveillance

The risk of colorectal cancer is increased beginning after 8 years of disease and continues to increase in subsequent years. Patients with extensive ulcerative colitis have a markedly increased risk for colon cancer, patients with left-sided disease have an intermediate risk, and patients with long-standing ulcerative colitis are at risk for colorectal cancer even if their symptoms have been relatively mild or even quiescent for 10 to 15 years.

Colon cancers are commonly submucosal and may be missed at colonoscopy. Colon cancer in patients with ulcerative colitis is most commonly associated with dysplastic changes in the mucosa, often at multiple sites in the colon. Dysplasia cannot be always be identified by visual inspection, so microscopic examination of biopsy specimens is required.

Current practice guidelines recommend colonoscopy with random biopsies in patients with long-standing ulcerative colitis beginning 8 years after the onset of disease and repeated every 1 to 2 years. If the specimens show dysplasia, colectomy is recommended.

The risk for colon cancer in patients with Crohn's colitis is similar to the risk in patients with a similar extent of ulcerative colitis. Surveillance colonoscopy is also recommended in patients with Crohn's colitis.

Pregnancy

Fertility in women with inflammatory bowel disease usually is normal or only minimally impaired, and the incidence of prematurity, stillbirth, and developmental defects in the offspring of women with inflammatory bowel disease, except fetal complications may be somewhat more likely when the mother's disease is clinically active, regardless of drug therapy. Previous proctocolectomy or the presence of an ileostomy is not an impediment to successful completion of a pregnancy, but women who have had ileal pouch anal anastomosis surgery with a total proctocolectomy have markedly reduced fertility.

If a woman's disease is inactive at the time of conception, it is likely that it will remain inactive during the course of the pregnancy. Ulcerative colitis that is active at the time of conception tends to worsen. In patients with active Crohn's disease at the time of conception, the degree of activity remains the same in two thirds of women; of the other one third, some improve clinically, and others deteriorate.

Sulfasalazine does not harm the fetus, but pregnant women have an increased requirement for folic acid, and sulfasalazine interferes with folate absorption. Therefore, women who are taking sulfasalazine and who are pregnant or considering pregnancy should receive folate supplementation (1 mg twice daily) to ensure that the fetus receives adequate amounts for normal development. The use of corticosteroids by pregnant women with inflammatory bowel disease is associated with an increased rate of premature rupture of the membranes and a higher rate of cleft lip. In general, it appears that the risk to the pregnancy of treatment with sulfasalazine or corticosteroids is less than the risk of allowing disease activity to go untreated.

Most of the data on the teratogenicity of azathioprine and 6-mercaptopurine in pregnancy are derived from the transplant literature and involve higher doses than are commonly used for inflammatory bowel disease. Reported fetal effects in the transplant population include congenital malformations, immunosuppression, prematurity, and growth retardation. The risks of these medications in the inflammatory bowel disease population are not completely known, given that only small a number of such patients have been formally studied.

PROGNOSIS

Ulcerative Colitis

The prognosis of patients with ulcerative colitis is usually characterized by repeated flares and remissions. A rapidly progressive initial attack results in serious complications in about 10% of patients. Complete recovery after a single attack may occur in another 10% of patients, some of whom may actually have had an acute undetected infection rather than true ulcerative colitis. The probability that a patient with clinically inactive disease will remain in remission the following year is 80 to 90%. By comparison, patients with clinically active disease have a 70% probability of relapse during the following year.

Patients who present with ulcerative proctitis have the best overall prognosis, and only about 5% of patients with proctitis will require colectomy over a lifetime. Severe complications are very uncommon, but the disease will spread more proximally in the colon in approximately 10% to 30% of patients. Ulcerative colitis–related mortality has decreased substantially since the introduction of corticosteroids, and recent studies suggest that long-term survival rates for patients with ulcerative colitis are similar to those of the general population.

Crohn's Disease

Crohn's disease classically waxes and wanes. A patient with clinically active Crohn's disease has a 70 to 80% chance of having active disease in the subsequent year, whereas 80% of patients in remission will remain so over the following year. Over the course of a 4-year period, about 25% of patients will have persistently active disease after diagnosis, about 25% will remain in remission, and 50% will have a fluctuating course with years of remission and years with clinically active disease. Approximately 75 to 80% of all patients with luminal and fistulizing Crohn's disease will require surgical intervention for their disease, with approximately 50% of them requiring surgery within 6 months of diagnosis. The rate for a second surgery for luminal Crohn's disease ranges from 25 to 38% within 5 years, and 40 to 70% will need reoperation by 15 years.

Patients with Crohn's disease have an increased mortality rate, about 1.3 to 1.5 times higher than the general population, unrelated to whether they have small intestine or large intestine involvement, or both. This excess mortality, which is most notable in the first few years after diagnosis, is most commonly related to complications of Crohn's disease (e.g., colorectal cancer, shock, volume depletion, protein-calorie malnutrition, and anemia). Whether aggressive use of immunomodulators and biologic therapy will alter the natural course of disease is unknown.

1. Hanauer SB, Stromberg U. Oral Pentasa in the treatment of Crohn's disease: a meta-analysis of double-blind, placebo-controlled trials. *Clin Gastroenterol Hepatol.* 2004;2:379-388.
2. Seow CH, Benchimol EI, Griffiths AM, et al. Budesonide for induction of remission in Crohn's disease. *Cochrane Database Syst Rev.* 2008;16:CD000296.

3. Prefontaine E, Macdonald JK, Sutherland LR. Azathioprine or 6-mercaptopurine for induction of remission in Crohn's disease. *Cochrane Database Syst Rev.* 2009;7:CD000545.
4. Patel V, Macdonald JD, McDonald JW, et al. Methotrexate for maintenance of remission in Crohn's disease. *Cochrane Database Syst Rev.* 2009;7:CD006884.
5. Behm BW, Bickston SJ. Tumor necrosis factor-alpha antibody for maintenance of remission in Crohn's disease. *Cochrane Database Syst Rev.* 2008;23:CD006893.
6. D'Haens G, Baert F, van Assche G, et al. Early combined immunosuppression or conventional management in patients with newly diagnosed Crohn's disease: an open randomised trial. *Lancet.* 2008;371:660-667.
7. Colombel JF, Sandborn WJ, Reinisch W, et al. Infliximab, azathioprine, or combination therapy for Crohn's disease. *N Engl J Med.* 2010;362:1383-1395.
8. Sands BE, Anderson FH, Bernstein CN, et al. Infliximab maintenance therapy for fistulizing Crohn's disease. *N Engl J Med.* 2004;350:876-885.
9. Marshall JK, Thabane M, Steinhart AH, et al. Rectal 5-aminosalicylic acid for induction of remission in ulcerative colitis. *Cochrane Database Syst Rev.* 2010;20:CD004115.
10. Sutherland L, Macdonald JK. Oral 5-aminosalicylic acid for induction of remission in ulcerative colitis. *Cochrane Database Syst Rev.* 2006;19:CD000543.
11. Van Assche G, D'Haens G, Noman M, et al. Randomized double-blind comparison of 4mg/kg versus 2 mg/kg IV cyclosporine in severe ulcerative colitis. *Gastroenterology.* 2003;125:1025-1031.
12. Sutherland L, Macdonald JK. Oral 5-aminosalicylic acid for maintenance of remission in ulcerative colitis. *Cochrane Database Syst Rev.* 2002;4:CD000544.

SUGGESTED READINGS

Abraham C, Cho JH. Inflammatory bowel disease. *N Engl J Med.* 2009;361:2066-2078. *Review.*
Kornbluth A, Sachar DB. Ulcerative colitis practice guidelines in adults: American College of Gastroenterology, Practice Parameters Committee. *Am J Gastroenterol.* 2010;105:501-523. *Comprehensive guidelines.*
Lichtenstein GR, Hanauer SB, Sandborn WJ, for the Practice Parameters Committee of American College of Gastroenterology. Management of Crohn's disease in adults. *Am J Gastroenterol.* 2009; 104:465-483; quiz 464, 484. *Comprehensive review.*
Nielsen OH, Seidelin JB, Munck LK, et al. Use of biological molecules in the treatment of inflammatory bowel disease. *J Intern Med.* 2011. [Epub ahead of print.] *Review.*

144

INFLAMMATORY AND ANATOMIC DISEASES OF THE INTESTINE, PERITONEUM, MESENTERY, AND OMENTUM

CHARLENE PRATHER

APPENDICITIS

DEFINITION AND EPIDEMIOLOGY

Acute appendicitis refers to inflammation of the appendix. Appendicitis is the most common acute surgical emergency involving the abdomen. Although appendicitis occurs most commonly in young adults, it can develop at any age. The lifetime prevalence of acute appendicitis is approximately 7%.

PATHOBIOLOGY

Obstruction of the appendix by a fecalith, which is thought to be the usual inciting event, is found in less than 30% of patients. Other causes of obstruction include ulceration of the appendiceal orifice, lymphoid hyperplasia, tumor (e.g., carcinoid; Chapter 240), inspissation of barium, and ascariasis (Chapter 365). Obstruction blocks the ongoing production of mucus by the appendix, thereby resulting in distention and subsequent mucosal ischemia. This process allows invasion by intraluminal bacteria, infection, and inflammation. Continued obstruction and inflammation can result in perforation, peritonitis, diarrhea, and abscess formation.

CLINICAL MANIFESTATIONS

More than 95% of patients with appendicitis have abdominal pain, but only 50 to 60% have the classic symptoms of appendicitis: an acute onset of periumbilical pain, often with nausea and vomiting and later localizing to the right lower quadrant. The position of the appendix has important implications for the location of pain, with pain from appendicitis occurring in the suprapubic region or the right upper quadrant. Anorexia is nearly universal, nausea is frequent, but vomiting is uncommon. Acute appendicitis occurs with nonspecific abdominal symptoms and signs in elderly patients and in

patients who are immunosuppressed, as from corticosteroid use, organ transplantation, or diabetes mellitus. In elderly patients, the diagnosis is unsuspected 25% of the time.

Adults older than 50 years have a perforation rate of greater than 50%, with an intra-abdominal abscess in one third. Signs of perforation include the presence of peritoneal irritation, fever, and increasing abdominal pain.

DIAGNOSIS

A broad differential diagnosis (Table 144-1) may be narrowed by diagnostic testing, which usually includes a complete blood count, serum electrolytes, and tests of renal function, with the addition of amylase and lipase levels when pancreatitis (Chapter 146) is suspected and liver enzymes (aminotransferase levels and alkaline phosphatase) and a bilirubin level when gallbladder (Chapter 158) or bile duct conditions are suspected. An elevated white blood cell count, usually in the 12,000 to 18,000/mm³ range, is common in acute appendicitis but may not be seen early in the course; the presence and degree of elevation are not helpful in identifying complicated appendicitis.

Computed tomography (CT), which is the preferred test[1] to confirm the diagnosis or suggest other causes (Fig. 144-1), has a sensitivity ranging from 88 to 100%, a specificity of 91 to 99%, a positive predictive value of 92 to 98%, and a negative predictive value of 95 to 100%. With a reported overall diagnostic accuracy of 94 to 98% and the ability to detect abscess formation (Fig. 144-2), CT has become the imaging diagnostic modality of choice. A disadvantage, which is more significant in children and young adults, is the need for ionizing radiation. Intravenous contrast may be used, but CT with rectal contrast is an alternative to avoid the risk of nephrotoxicity.[2] Ultrasound is useful when gynecologic causes, especially an ectopic pregnancy, are also in the differential diagnosis. Plain abdominal radiographs are not useful.

TABLE 144-1	DIFFERENTIAL DIAGNOSIS IN SUSPECTED APPENDICITIS

Crohn's ileitis
Mesenteric adenitis
Right-sided colonic diverticulitis
Yersinia, Campylobacter enterocolitis
Meckel's diverticulitis
Tuberculous colitis
Perforated right colon adenocarcinoma
Nephrolithiasis (right sided)
Foreign body perforation (e.g., toothpick bowel perforation)
Right tubo-ovarian abscess
Tubal pregnancy
Ovarian cyst rupture or torsion

Page: 48 of 97   Compressed 8:1   IM: 48 SE: 2

FIGURE 144-1. **Appendicitis.** A computed tomography scan shows an edematous appendix with a diameter greater than 1 cm *(arrow)*, consistent with acute, uncomplicated appendicitis.

FIGURE 144-2. Appendicitis. A computed tomography scan shows appendicitis complicated by perforation with abscess formation (arrow).

Page: 64 of 95
Compressed 8 :1
IM: 64 SE: 2

TREATMENT Rx

When appendicitis is suspected, emergent surgical consultation is indicated. Treatment of appendicitis is appendectomy, which is increasingly being performed laparoscopically. Two days of intravenous antibiotics followed by 10 days of oral antibiotics is a reasonable short-term alternative in the absence of evidence of perforation when surgery cannot be performed safely in the interim, but about one third of patients will require appendectomy.[3] Laparoscopic appendectomy generally takes longer than the open operation but results in faster recovery and a lower rate of wound infection.[4] Preoperative antibiotics (e.g., cefotetan, 2 g intravenously, or cefoxitin, 2 g intravenously, followed by three postoperative doses, or ticarcillin–clavulanic acid) reduce infectious complications in otherwise uncomplicated appendicitis.

In the presence of a perforated appendix with an appendicular abscess, immediate appendectomy yields similar results to a strategy of percutaneous ultrasound- or CT-guided drainage, intravenous antibiotics, and laparoscopic appendectomy about 10 weeks later.[5] In the setting of perforation, once-daily dosing with ceftriaxone and metronidazole for 7 to 10 days is as good as triple-dose therapy.[6]

PROGNOSIS

The frequency of complications associated with perforated appendicitis is greater than 18%, as opposed to a 10% frequency of complications in non-perforated appendicitis. Overall mortality in patients with perforated appendicitis is 3%, but it can be as high as 15% in elderly patients. Most patients who are operated on for suspected appendicitis, but who do not have it, have benign self-limited disease. In adults, however, appendiceal diverticulitis, granulomatous appendicitis, carcinoid tumors (Chapter 240), and occasionally other tumors may be found.

DIVERTICULITIS OF THE COLON

DEFINITION

Colonic diverticulosis refers to uncomplicated herniations of the colonic mucosa and submucosa through the muscular layer of the colon. Technically, these lesions are actually pseudodiverticula because all layers of the colon are not involved. Diverticular disease encompasses a spectrum of problems occurring in the setting of diverticulosis, including diverticulitis, painful diverticular disease, and complicated diverticular disease (Table 144-2).

EPIDEMIOLOGY

Although colonic diverticulosis is quite common and affects up to 10% of middle-aged adults and 50 to 80% of those older than 80 years, few people are aware that they have them. Diverticulosis is uncommon in individuals younger than 40 years of age. Diverticulosis is predominantly a disorder of industrialized or Western populations, where it correlates with low intake of dietary fiber. Obesity appears to be a risk factor for diverticulosis in young males.

TABLE 144-2	TERMINOLOGY IN DIVERTICULAR DISEASE
Diverticular disease	The entire spectrum of diverticulosis and its complications
Diverticulosis	The presence of one or more diverticula
Diverticulitis	Inflammation or infection of one or more colonic diverticula
Complicated diverticulitis	Diverticulitis with abscess, fistula formation, free perforation, or obstruction
Painful diverticular disease	Abdominal pain and altered bowel habit in the setting of diverticulosis without another explanation (may be a manifestation of irritable bowel syndrome)
Diverticular bleeding	Acute lower gastrointestinal bleeding from a colonic diverticulum

PATHOBIOLOGY

Colonic diverticulosis most commonly occurs at the location where the vasa recta (nutrient artery) penetrates through the muscularis propria. In Western populations, diverticulosis occurs more commonly in the left colon, with the sigmoid colon most frequently involved, perhaps because of the relatively higher pressure present in the lumen of the sigmoid colon. However, in Asian populations, a right-sided distribution is more common.

Diverticulitis, which is infection and inflammation of a diverticulum, develops in 10 to 25% of persons with diverticulosis during their lifetimes. Diverticulitis results from inflammation of a colonic diverticulum with subsequent microperforation, which is thought to occur when particulate debris within the diverticular sac compresses or erodes the blood vessel and thereby leads to perforation. Diverticulitis occurs most commonly in the sigmoid colon. Complications of diverticulitis, which include abscess formation, free perforation, colonic obstruction, and fistula formation, are more common in middle-aged and elderly patients but can also occur in young patients.

CLINICAL MANIFESTATIONS

Patients with diverticulitis most commonly have anorexia, left lower quadrant pain, and fever. The pain in diverticulitis may radiate to the flank, back, or suprapubic region. Patients may report loose stools or constipation. Additional associated symptoms include nausea, vomiting, altered bowel pattern, and urinary symptoms. On physical examination, left lower quadrant tenderness can usually be demonstrated. The examination may also identify localized guarding and, occasionally, a tender painful mass. The presence of peritoneal signs (e.g., rebound) suggests a free perforation.

Diverticular bleeding is manifested as painless rectal bleeding, with massive bleeding occurring in 5% of patients with diverticulosis (Chapter 137). Diverticular bleeding is rare in the setting of acute diverticulitis.

DIAGNOSIS

Leukocytosis is present in 70 to 80% of patients. When the diverticulitis is adjacent to the bladder, pyuria may occur. Conditions with findings similar to those of diverticulitis include gastroenteritis, appendicitis, inflammatory bowel disease (Chapter 143), and a perforating colon cancer (Chapter 199).

CT radiography, which reliably identifies the presence and location of inflammation, may show the colonic diverticula, inflammation involving the pericolic fat, and a colonic wall thicker than 4 mm (Fig. 144-3). Barium radiography, which can demonstrate diverticula (Fig. 144-4), will also identify whether the colon connects with the fluid collection in the setting of perforation and abscess formation; it is not recommended in the acute setting because of a higher risk for colonic perforation from contrast or air insufflation. After the acute syndrome has resolved and the patient has become stable, colonoscopy can also show diverticula (Fig. 144-5) and is essential to exclude malignancy, even in younger patients.

TREATMENT Rx

Uncomplicated diverticulitis may be treated in the outpatient setting with broad-spectrum antibiotics such as ciprofloxacin and metronidazole for 7 to 10 days (Table 144-3). Oral antibiotics are as effective as the intravenous route,[7] and 4 days of treatment are as effective as 7 to 10 days for uncomplicated patients.[8] Patients are started on a clear liquid diet that can be advanced

FIGURE 144-3. **Diverticulitis.** A computed tomography scan shows perforated diverticulitis with abscess formation *(arrow)*. The abscess is identified as the air-filled collection. Residual contrast remains in the diverticulum.

FIGURE 144-4. **Colonic diverticula.** An abdominal flat plate shows residual barium in diverticula scattered throughout the colon.

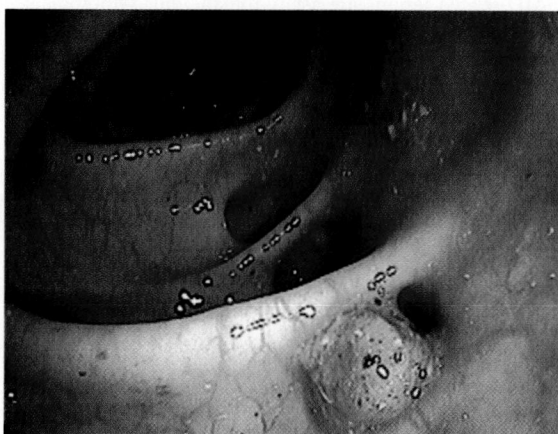

FIGURE 144-5. **Sigmoid diverticula.** A colonoscopic photograph shows sigmoid diverticula.

TABLE 144-3	ANTIBIOTIC OPTIONS FOR ACUTE DIVERTICULITIS*

Ciprofloxacin, 750 mg bid, and metronidazole, 500 mg q6h
Levofloxacin, 750 mg IV q24h, and metronidazole, 500 mg q6h
Trimethoprim-sulfamethoxazole-DS, bid
Piperacillin-tazobactam, 3.375 g q6h
Ampicillin-sulbactam, 3.0 g q6h
Imipenem–cilastatin sodium, 500 mg q6h (reserved for life-threatening infection)

*Four days in uncomplicated patients; 7 to 10 days in others.

as symptoms resolve. Patients unable to maintain oral intake require hospitalization for hydration and intravenous antibiotics.

Elective resection carries a mortality rate of 1 to 4%, and expectant management rather than operative treatment is probably associated with less mortality and fewer colostomies, and it is also less expensive.

However, patients younger than 40 years may experience a more aggressive form of the disease, so surgical resection is sometimes recommended after the first episode of diverticulitis. Patients with conditions resulting in immune system compromise may benefit from earlier (after a first episode) surgery because of their reduced ability to ward off infection and their increased risk for emergency surgery. For sigmoid diverticulitis, laparoscopic resection is preferred over open resection.[9]

Patients with diverticular abscesses are treated by CT-guided drainage and subsequent surgery, usually 6 weeks after successful abscess drainage. Laparoscopic resection, which is increasingly being performed for diverticular disease, results in shorter hospitalization and an early return to full function. Patients with complicated diverticulitis have a mortality of 6.5% and morbidity of 41%; when perforated diverticulitis is excluded, the mortality is less than 2%. Older age, immunosuppressive medications, preexisting medical problems (especially preexisting cardiac and pulmonary disease), and perforated diverticulitis increase postoperative morbidity.

PREVENTION

Randomized trials show that the combination of fiber and rifaximin (400 mg twice daily for 7 days every month), a poorly absorbable antibiotic, decreases symptoms over a 12-month period.[10] Other medications used to reduce recurrent diverticular symptoms included mesalazine and calcium-channel blockers, although the evidence to support their use is inconclusive. The use of nonsteroidal anti-inflammatory drugs (NSAIDs) increases the risk for diverticular perforation.

PROGNOSIS

Most patients with diverticulitis improve quickly over a period of 2 to 3 days, and the risk for a second attack of diverticulitis is less than 25%. After a second attack of diverticulitis, the risk for subsequent episodes of diverticulitis exceeds 50%, and the risk increases with each subsequent episode. Surgical therapy to remove the segment of colon involved with diverticulosis is often recommended after a second episode of diverticulitis. After elective resection, 25% of patients have persistent symptoms, including altered bowel habits and pain that probably reflect a coexistent irritable bowel syndrome (Chapter 139), and 10% have recurrent diverticulitis.

● OTHER INFLAMMATORY CONDITIONS
Neutropenic Enterocolitis

Neutropenic enterocolitis is also referred to as typhlitis. Although originally described in children after induction chemotherapy for acute leukemia, it is an increasingly recognized clinical syndrome in adults as well.

CLINICAL MANIFESTATIONS AND DIAGNOSIS

The syndrome occurs in neutropenic patients (absolute neutrophil count <500/μL) and consists of right lower quadrant abdominal pain, distention, fever, nausea, vomiting, and diarrhea, which may be bloody. Symptoms typically occur 10 to 14 days after high-dose chemotherapy. The clinical findings are nonspecific and overlap with symptoms seen in *Clostridium difficile* colitis (Chapter 304), ischemic colitis (Chapter 145), and colonic pseudo-obstruction (Chapter 138). CT findings include a thickened colonic wall (>4 mm), dilated cecum, and pericecal inflammatory changes (Fig. 144-6).

FIGURE 144-6. Computed tomography scans showing neutropenic colitis. The *left scan* shows a thickened cecal wall *(arrow)*. Eight days latter a follow-up scan showed resolution *(right scan)*.

TREATMENT

Conservative management includes bowel rest, nasogastric suction when bowel dilation is present, and broad-spectrum antibiotics to cover gram-positive and enteric gram-negative organisms, as well as anaerobes. Recombinant granulocyte colony-stimulating factor has been recommended to correct neutropenia. Lower gastrointestinal bleeding resulting from the colitis with a coexisting coagulopathy necessitates correction of the coagulopathy and blood transfusions. Surgery is indicated in the setting of impending or free perforation, when bleeding cannot be stopped, and for otherwise unexplained clinical deterioration. Symptoms improve rapidly as the neutropenia resolves.

Visceral Angioedema

Visceral angioedema is seen with hereditary and acquired C1 esterase inhibitor deficiency (Chapter 260), hypocomplementemia, drugs (especially angiotensin-converting enzyme inhibitors), or foods or may be idiopathic. Acquired C1 esterase inhibitor deficiency may occur as a paraneoplastic syndrome and is occasionally seen in autoimmune disorders. Angioedema of the gastrointestinal tract is commonly manifested as abdominal pain and distention, nausea, vomiting, and diarrhea. The symptoms may be accompanied by swelling of the mucous membrane, hives, wheezing, or dyspnea. CT findings include thickened, fluid-filled loops of small bowel. Ascites may also be present. The symptoms last 1 to 3 days and may recur periodically. The diagnosis is established by identifying suspect drugs, low serum levels of C4, low C1 esterase quantitative levels, or reduced C1 esterase functional activity. Hereditary and acquired C1 esterase inhibitor deficiency can be treated with C1 inhibitor therapy (Chapter 260).

Radiation Enterocolitis

Patients who receive radiation therapy for intra-abdominal and pelvic neoplasms are at risk for radiation-induced injury.

EPIDEMIOLOGY

The risk for injury varies according to the size of the radiation field and the dose received. Chronic radiation enterocolitis occurs approximately a year after completion of radiation therapy but may develop up to 20 years later. Doses greater than 50 Gy increase the risk for chronic changes, such as the development of obliterative arteritis, intestinal wall fibrosis, and serosal thickening. Other risk factors include older age, previous abdominal surgery, and a larger field of radiation. The quantity of small bowel in the radiation field is a strong predictor of subsequent complications.

CLINICAL MANIFESTATIONS AND DIAGNOSIS

Symptoms of acute radiation enterocolitis commonly include diarrhea, intestinal bleeding, and fecal incontinence. These symptoms are typically self-limited and resolve within a few months after the completion of radiation treatment.

Symptoms of chronic radiation enterocolitis commonly include abdominal pain and diarrhea. Gastrointestinal bleeding results from vascular ectasia.

The bleeding is typically chronic and occult, with the development of iron deficiency anemia, but occasionally it is overt. Complete or partial bowel obstruction from adhesions or strictures, fistulas, small bowel bacterial overgrowth, and malabsorption can also occur.

Diagnostic imaging includes CT radiography or colonoscopy. The finding of a stricture necessitates an evaluation to exclude malignancy.

PREVENTION AND TREATMENT

Prevention of radiation enteritis includes minimizing the volume of small bowel and colon in the radiation field. Treatment is predominantly supportive. Management of bleeding includes endoscopic ablation of telangiectatic lesions and chronic iron therapy. Sucralfate enemas (2 g twice daily) may improve symptoms, but the data are not conclusive.

For acute obstruction, bowel rest and nasogastric suction may allow resolution; surgery is reserved for complete bowel obstruction that does not improve or perforation. Poor wound healing, anastomotic leaks, and fistulas may complicate surgical operations. Patients with diarrhea should be evaluated for small bowel bacterial overgrowth. Cholestyramine, loperamide, and diphenoxylate-atropine provide first-line options for treating diarrhea (Chapter 142), but stronger opiates such as codeine, morphine, or tincture of opium are sometimes required. Caution is necessary when using these agents because of the risk for development of bowel dilation and obstipation.

Nonsteroidal Anti-inflammatory Drugs

Small intestinal ulcerations are increasingly being recognized with the advent of small bowel capsule endoscopy (Chapter 136). The most common cause of small intestinal ulcers is the use of NSAIDs (Chapter 36). Small bowel and colonic erosions and ulcerations occur in 60 to 70% of long-term users of NSAIDs. Diaphragm-type strictures of the small bowel and, less frequently, the colon also result from chronic NSAID use.

CLINICAL MANIFESTATIONS AND DIAGNOSIS

Most NSAID-related lesions are asymptomatic, but symptoms suggesting NSAID enteropathy include gastrointestinal bleeding, abdominal pain, iron deficiency anemia, diarrhea, hypoalbuminemia, and obstructive symptoms. Ulceration can be detected by small bowel enteroscopy, small bowel capsule endoscopy, and colonoscopy.

TREATMENT

Treatment consists of discontinuing NSAIDs. When obstruction is present and conservative treatment fails, surgical resection may be required.

Systemic Inflammatory Conditions

Ulcerative jejunitis is an uncommon manifestation of celiac disease (Chapter 142). This diagnosis is suspected in patients with persistent symptoms despite a gluten-free diet.

Mycobacterium tuberculosis (Chapter 332) involvement of the small intestine and occasionally of the colon, especially in the cecum, most commonly manifests as abdominal pain, vomiting, and diarrhea. The disease may be subacute with waxing and waning symptoms or be marked by more fulminant sepsis. The intestinal lesions include nodularity, ulcerations, skip lesions, and strictures, features similar to those found in small bowel Crohn's disease. The diagnosis is made by biopsy, stains, and culture. When the small bowel is not accessible endoscopically, exploratory laparotomy for full-thickness biopsy may be required to make the diagnosis. Treatment with conventional antituberculous therapy results in symptomatic improvement.

Histoplasma capsulatum (Chapter 340) typically involves the gastrointestinal tract in the setting of disseminated disease in immunocompromised patients, predominately in patients with acquired immunodeficiency syndrome. Gastrointestinal involvement is accompanied by bleeding, obstruction, diarrhea, and malabsorption. Small bowel lesions include ulcerations, polypoid lesions, and masses that simulate carcinoma. The granulomatous changes present on biopsy must be differentiated from Crohn's disease, tuberculosis, and less commonly, sarcoidosis. Treatment is directed at the underlying disseminated infection.

Sarcoidosis (Chapter 95) of the gastrointestinal tract is relatively uncommon. Small bowel and colonic involvement has manifestations similar to those of Crohn's disease, with ulceration and non-necrotizing granulomas. Gastrointestinal involvement typically occurs in the setting of other systemic symptoms of sarcoidosis. Patients have abdominal pain, vomiting, diarrhea, or protein-losing enteropathy, or any combination of these findings. Treatment is aimed at the systemic disease.

Systemic lupus erythematosus (Chapter 274) frequently affects the gastrointestinal tract. Abdominal pain may be due to serositis, mesenteric ischemia, vasculitis, intestinal dysmotility, angioedema, or pancreatitis. Clinical manifestations include abdominal pain, nausea, vomiting, abdominal bloating, distention, diarrhea, and malabsorption. Small bowel bacterial overgrowth also occurs, presumably secondary to the underlying dysmotility. Treatment consists of management of the underlying systemic disease.

Ulceration of any part of the gastrointestinal tract may occur in *Behçet's disease* (Chapter 278). Symptoms include abdominal pain, diarrhea, and gastrointestinal bleeding. Most patients with gastrointestinal involvement have ileocecal involvement with a single or few ulcers. In the absence of obvious systemic symptoms, Behçet's disease can be difficult to differentiate from Crohn's disease.

Patients with *polyarteritis nodosa* (Chapter 278) may have intermittent or persistent abdominal complications. Gastrointestinal involvement occurs in half or more of patients with polyarteritis nodosa. Most have abdominal pain, nausea, vomiting, melena, hematochezia, diarrhea, and occasionally, constipation; however, severe abdominal pain can also develop as a result of mesenteric vasculitis with gastrointestinal infarction and perforation. These gastrointestinal complications of polyarteritis nodosa result in considerable morbidity and mortality, with a mortality rate of 23% to greater than 60% when the symptoms include an acute abdomen. The diagnosis is typically made by CT radiography and magnetic resonance or CT angiography; less frequently, angiography is required. Although colonoscopy can identify ischemia, its role is limited in the acute setting because of the risk for perforation. Treatment is directed at the systemic disease (Chapter 278).

Henoch-Schönlein purpura (Chapter 278) is an immunoglobulin A (IgA)-mediated vasculitis with skin, abdominal, and renal manifestations. Abdominal symptoms include pain, nausea, vomiting, diarrhea, and gastrointestinal bleeding. Small bowel thickening and intussusception can be seen on CT radiography. Upper endoscopy and colonoscopy are not usually necessary diagnostically but can show submucosal hemorrhage, erythema, swelling, and ulcerations. Similar changes are also present in the small intestine as imaged by capsule endoscopy. The disease is often self-limited but may require systemic therapy (Chapter 278).

● PERITONEAL DISORDERS
Peritonitis

DEFINITION

The peritoneum is the smooth serous membrane that lines the abdominal and pelvic cavities. The most common clinical disorders of the peritoneum are ascites (Chapter 156) and peritonitis. Peritonitis may be acute or chronic, septic or aseptic, primary or secondary, and localized or diffuse.

EPIDEMIOLOGY AND PATHOBIOLOGY

Acute peritonitis results from acute disruption of the peritoneal cavity with infectious or inflammatory materials. In the setting of perforation of the bowel or an intra-abdominal viscus, the contents themselves may be inflammatory, such as with bile spillage, or may be infectious, such as with contamination from intraluminal contents (e.g., bacteria and fecal material). Aseptic peritonitis results from the introduction of sterile bile, digestive juices, or extrinsic materials (e.g., chemotherapeutic medications) into the peritoneal cavity. Aseptic peritonitis rarely remains that way, with infection typically following in due course. Primary peritonitis refers to spontaneous bacterial peritonitis without an identifiable cause, typically in the setting of chronic liver disease (Chapter 148). Secondary peritonitis results most commonly from a perforated viscus such as the appendix, a diverticulum, peptic ulcer disease, or trauma with secondary spillage of luminal contents into the peritoneum. The most common bacteriology in secondary peritonitis is a mixed flora with *Escherichia coli*, *Streptococcus faecalis*, *Pseudomonas aeruginosa*, *Klebsiella mirabilis*, *Bacteroides fragilis*, *Clostridium* species, and anaerobic streptococci.

CLINICAL MANIFESTATIONS

Clinical manifestations of acute diffuse peritonitis typically include the sudden onset of abdominal pain that is usually constant. The pain may be diffuse or referred to the umbilicus or the portion of the abdomen where the inciting event originated. The peritoneal inflammation may subside or localize, thereby resulting in a reduction in pain and improved localization. Additional symptoms include nausea, vomiting, and fever. The development of progressive tachycardia and a falling temperature are grave signs of impending peritoneal shock from bacterial toxemia and septicemia (Chapter 108) (Fig. 144-7).

Additional physical signs (Chapter 134) include a very still patient. Bowel sounds are typically diminished or absent in the setting of peritonitis. Percussion often reveals tympany from the resultant ileus. On palpation, tenderness and rigidity are present. Rebound tenderness, with increasing pain when the examining hand is lifted from the abdomen, is usually present. Increased pain may also be elicited in the affected area on examination of an uninvolved portion of the abdomen. The abdominal muscles may become boardlike with rigidity, although this sign is frequently absent in elderly patients and in immunosuppressed patients.

DIAGNOSIS

Identifying the cause of the peritonitis depends on the age and sex of the patient. In younger patients, appendicitis and a perforated duodenal ulcer (Chapter 141) are most common. In older patients, perforated diverticula and cancer (Chapter 199) are more common. The use of NSAIDs or aspirin increases the likelihood of a perforated ulcer or diverticula. In young females, tubal pregnancy and a ruptured tubo-ovarian abscess must be considered (Chapters 293 and 308). CT imaging identifies the presence of free air and often is the cause of the intra-abdominal calamity (see Fig. 144-3).

FIGURE 144-7. Computed tomography scan in a patient with peritonitis. Thickening of the duodenal wall *(arrow)* was identified at surgery as a perforated duodenal ulcer.

Treatment focuses on resuscitation, control of infection, and laparoscopy. The presence of suspected acute peritonitis necessitates surgical consultation. Correction of volume depletion and electrolyte disturbances with intravenous fluids is the cornerstone of initial management. Blood should be obtained for culture and broad-spectrum antibiotics administered prophylactically to cover gram-negative and anaerobic bacteria (Table 144-4).

TREATMENT

Treatment of malignant ascites is symptomatic and quite challenging. In general, malignant ascites does not respond to diuretic therapy, except that patients with malignant ascites in the setting of hepatic metastases may respond to spironolactone. Therapeutic paracentesis in the setting of tense ascites improves symptoms, including shortness of breath and abdominal discomfort. Unfortunately, malignant ascites rapidly reaccumulates. The use of intracavitary radioisotopes or chemotherapy has been advocated in some cases for palliation with variable success.

PROGNOSIS

Peritonitis is a life-threatening disorder whose outcome depends on its cause as well as the rapidity of treatment. Mortality rates can be as low as 15% in patients who have correctable causes, such as a perforated appendix, and who do not develop multiorgan failure before treatment, but mortality rates can be as high as 50% for postoperative peritonitis.

Peritoneal Carcinomatosis and Malignant Ascites

Less than 10% of cases of ascites are malignant. Peritoneal carcinomatosis results from the metastatic spread of intra-abdominal malignancy (Table 144-5), usually in the setting of endometrial, colonic, gastric, and pancreatic carcinoma. The manifestation is similar to ascites of other causes (Chapter 148), although the ascites typically occurs rather suddenly in the absence of known portal hypertension, tuberculosis, or right heart failure.

DIAGNOSIS

In the setting of new-onset ascites, diagnostic paracentesis should be performed. Aspirated fluid should be sent for cell count and differential, Gram stain and culture, and measurement of albumin with simultaneous serum albumin measurement. A serum minus ascites albumin value of less than 1.1 g/mL (Chapter 156) supports the diagnosis of malignant ascites but is also seen in pancreatitis, nephrotic syndrome, and peritoneal tuberculosis. In the setting of hepatic metastases, the serum-ascites albumin gradient may be greater than 1.1. Ascitic fluid cytology will identify malignant cells 50 to 60% of the time.

Abnormal ultrasound findings can confirm the presence of ascites, but CT is preferred to help identify the underlying cause (Fig. 144-8). Malignant ascites is frequently loculated, sometimes from previous surgically related adhesions.

PROGNOSIS

The development of malignant ascites is usually a poor prognostic indicator, with few patients surviving beyond 4 months. An exception is the better prognosis with malignant ascites from ovarian (Chapter 205) or breast cancer (Chapter 204).

Peritoneal Tuberculosis

In the United States, tuberculosis (Chapter 332) is relatively uncommon, although it is increasingly being identified in immigrants. Tuberculous ascites also occurs in cirrhosis and in patients with chronic renal disease who are maintained on peritoneal dialysis.

Peritoneal tuberculosis is accompanied by abdominal swelling, fever, anorexia, and weight loss. The diagnosis should be considered in the setting of refractory ascites. Analysis of ascitic fluid reveals an exudative ascites. The fluid protein is typically greater than 2.5 g/100 mL, with a serum-ascites gradient of less than 1.1 g/mL.

TREATMENT AND PROGNOSIS

Treatment involves conventional antituberculous therapy (Chapter 332). Prognosis is dependent on whether tuberculosis is systemic or restricted to the peritoneum. It is important to document clearance of the tuberculosis with repeat paracentesis.

Peritonitis Associated with Continuous Ambulatory Peritoneal Dialysis

Patients in whom peritonitis develops while undergoing continuous ambulatory peritoneal dialysis (Chapter 133) have abdominal pain and cloudy peritoneal fluid. Approximately 50% of patients have fever. Nausea and diarrhea may also occur. On physical examination, abdominal pain is usually present.

Diagnosis is based on the peritoneal fluid cell count and differential. Although Gram stain is rarely positive, any organisms that are seen are predictive of subsequent culture results. Peritoneal cultures are positive 90% of

TABLE 144-4	ANTIBIOTIC OPTIONS FOR INTRA-ABDOMINAL SECONDARY PERITONITIS

Piperacillin-tazobactam, 3.375 g q6h
Ampicillin-sulbactam, 3.0 g q6h
Ciprofloxacin, 400 mg q12h, and metronidazole, 1 g q12h
Levofloxacin, 750 mg q24h
Cefepime, 2 g q12h, and metronidazole, 1 g q12h
Imipenem–cilastatin sodium, 500 mg q6h

TABLE 144-5	CAUSES OF PERITONEAL CARCINOMATOSIS

PRIMARY

Mesothelioma
Sarcoma

SECONDARY INTRA-ABDOMINAL MALIGNANCIES

Gastric adenocarcinoma
Colon adenocarcinoma
Pancreatic adenocarcinoma
Ovarian carcinoma
Neuroendocrine tumors, including carcinoid
Lymphoma

EXTRA-ABDOMINAL MALIGNANCIES

Breast
Melanoma
Lung

FIGURE 144-8. Malignant ascites. A computed tomography scan shows ascites (large arrow) and a gastric mass (small arrow).

the time. Gram-positive organisms predominant, with coagulase-negative staphylococci and *Staphylococcus aureus* most commonly identified. Gram-negative organisms are present about 20% of the time, and 10% of patients have polymicrobial infections. Fungal peritonitis is infrequent and usually due to *Candida* species.

Antibiotic choices for empirical therapy include intraperitoneal cefazolin, cephalothin, and ceftazidime. Aminoglycosides should be used only when residual urine volume is less than 100 mL/day. Once culture results are available, antibiotics are adjusted according to the sensitivity of the organisms.

MISCELLANEOUS DISEASE OF THE MESENTERY AND OMENTUM

Mesenteric disorders are uncommon. Patients with mesenteric cysts complain of abdominal pain, fever, and emesis. Symptomatic cysts are treated surgically.

Mesenteric panniculitis refers to an inflammatory process of the adipose tissue of the mesentery. A variety of other terms are used, including lipodystrophy, sclerosing lipogranulomatosis, lipogranuloma of the mesentery, and mesenteritis. The disease is manifested as thickening or nodularity of the mesentery with fat necrosis. Mesenteric panniculitis is characterized by a variety of nonspecific abdominal symptoms, including fever, abdominal pain, anorexia, weight loss, and altered bowel habits. The diagnosis is made at laparoscopy. Laboratory studies are rarely helpful, although an elevated erythrocyte sedimentation rate may be seen. Surgical resection is required only when obstruction is present.

ANATOMIC AND MECHANICAL DISORDERS
Groin Hernias

In addition to hiatal hernias (Chapter 140), hernias may occur in the groin as inguinal or femoral hernias or as a result of weakness or abnormalities of other abdominal and pelvic muscles.

EPIDEMIOLOGY

About 3 to 4% of men have groin hernias, and the incidence increases with age. Indirect inguinal hernias, caused by a defect in the abdominal wall, account for about two thirds of hernias. Direct inguinal hernias, which protrude through an area bounded by the rectus abdominis muscle, the inferior upper gastric artery, and the inguinal ligament, account for about 30% of hernias in men and about 2% of hernias in women. Femoral hernias, which pass through an opening associated with the femoral artery and vein, represent about 30% of hernias in women and about 2% in men.

CLINICAL MANIFESTATIONS AND DIAGNOSIS

Groin hernias may be asymptomatic or be perceived as a mass that enlarges with standing or with increases in intra-abdominal pressure. If a hernia is not readily reducible (i.e., incarcerated), it may be associated with constant discomfort. With strangulation, ischemia or bowel obstruction may occur. The diagnosis is usually readily apparent by palpation of a soft groin mass that becomes larger with standing or with increases in intra-abdominal pressure.

TREATMENT Rx

Although femoral hernias should be repaired when first diagnosed because of the risk for strangulation, watchful waiting is an acceptable option for men with minimally symptomatic inguinal hernias.[11] Surgical options for both the initial operation and for recurrent hernias include laparoscopic repair and open mesh repair.[12,13]

Other Hernias

Incisional hernias develop after 1 to 4% of laparotomy incisions. These hernias may cause chronic abdominal discomfort, especially with maneuvers that increase intra-abdominal pressure. Repair is usually performed with prosthetic mesh.

Colonic Volvulus

Most cases of colonic volvulus involve the sigmoid colon (>90%), but volvulus can also involve the cecum and transverse colon. Elderly persons are at greatest risk. Volvulus results in colonic obstruction when the colon twists on its mesentery. Patients with volvulus frequently report a history of chronic constipation or laxative use or have previously been noted to have a dilated

colon. A history of psychiatric illness or institutionalization is also associated with an increased risk for the development of volvulus.

CLINICAL MANIFESTATIONS

Symptoms of volvulus include the acute development of abdominal distention, nausea, and vomiting, with abdominal pain present initially in about one third of patients. Progressive or severe pain and tenderness suggest developing colonic ischemia and perforation. Much less commonly, patients have an intermittent history of obstructive symptoms and distention suggesting chronic volvulus.

DIAGNOSIS

The diagnosis of volvulus is made by abdominal radiographs, which show a dilated colon that may lack haustral folds and has a "bent inner tube" appearance, with the apex pointing to the right upper quadrant. Cecal volvulus is suspected radiographically when a dilated cecum is located in the epigastrium or left upper quadrant. Small bowel dilation may also be present. Water-soluble contrast enema will also confirm the presence and site of obstruction with the classic finding of a "bird's beak" configuration at the obstructed site.

TREATMENT Rx

Patients who have suspected colonic volvulus and who exhibit peritoneal signs or have complete obstruction on abdominal radiographs require fluid emergency exploratory laparotomy. In the absence of signs of complete obstruction or impending ischemia and when sigmoid volvulus is suspected, endoscopic sigmoidoscopic examination will document the site of obstruction and endoscopic reduction is the emergent treatment of choice for colonic decompression. Endoscopic procedures are generally avoided in patients with suspected cecal volvulus, however, and surgical resection is required emergently when endoscopic treatment is not appropriate or is unsuccessful or later after endoscopic treatment because of the risk of recurrence.

Intussusception

Intussusception results when a segment of intestine is drawn distally into another segment of intestine, thereby resulting in obstruction. Intussusception may occur in the small intestine itself, or the small intestine may intussuscept into the colon. Intussusception occurs most commonly in children, in whom it is seen in the setting of recent viral enteritis (e.g., rotavirus; Chapter 388), cystic fibrosis (Chapter 89), or Meckel's diverticulum. In adults, intussusception is more likely to occur in the setting of small bowel neoplasia (Chapter 199).

CLINICAL MANIFESTATIONS

Most patients have symptoms of partial small bowel obstruction—crampy abdominal pain, nausea, vomiting, and occasionally, diarrhea. An abdominal mass may be palpable on examination, and patients may have evidence of occult or overt gastrointestinal bleeding (the passage of "currant jelly" mucus-like stool is described in infants and children).

DIAGNOSIS AND MANAGEMENT

The diagnosis is most commonly confirmed by CT radiography, which classically shows a "target" lesion of the small bowel that represents the layers of the small bowel and intussuscepted segment. The finding of intussusception in an adult necessitates abdominal exploration and resection of the intussuscepted segment.

Adhesions

Peritoneal adhesions cause most cases of small bowel obstruction. Adhesions can result from previous laparotomy, with an increased risk for adhesions occurring in patients with intra-abdominal infections, ischemia, and foreign bodies. Symptomatic adhesive bowel obstruction will subsequently develop in 5 to 10% of patients undergoing laparotomy. Adhesive disease may also result in reduced fertility in females. After laparotomy, adhesive-related obstruction can occur at any time from the early postoperative period to many years later.

CLINICAL MANIFESTATIONS

Patients have crampy abdominal pain, nausea, vomiting, and increasing abdominal distention. In the setting of complete bowel obstruction, patients no longer pass stool or flatus.

FIGURE 144-9. Adhesion-related small bowel obstruction. A computed tomography scan shows dilated, fluid-filled small bowel *(white arrow)* and a nondilated colon *(black arrow)*. At laparotomy, an obstruction secondary to adhesions was found in the midileum.

DIAGNOSIS AND TREATMENT ⟨Rx⟩

On an upright abdominal radiograph, findings of adhesive-related bowel obstruction include dilated loops of bowel (>6 cm of small bowel) and air-fluid levels, with reduced air distal to the obstruction. Similar findings are present on CT radiography (Fig. 144-9). Limitations of radiographic examination include subtle findings when the obstruction is very proximal in the bowel or the obstruction is only partial. In these settings, small bowel radiographs with water-soluble or barium contrast may be necessary to make the diagnosis.

Treatment of complete small bowel obstruction is fluid resuscitation and urgent laparotomy. Nasogastric tube decompression reduces nausea, vomiting, and distention. Nonoperative management may be tried in the setting of partial small bowel obstruction, with surgery reserved for patients whose obstruction fails to resolve. Patients with recurrent small bowel obstruction may benefit from a low-roughage diet to reduce the risk for obstruction from nondigestible food residue in a narrowed lumen.

The presence of chronic or recurrent abdominal pain in the absence of bowel obstruction has often been blamed on adhesions. Unless a clearly identified obstruction is present radiographically, surgical intervention for adhesiolysis is not warranted and does not reliably reduce abdominal pain symptoms. The search continues for intraoperative techniques or substances to reduce the development of adhesions.

1. Terasawa T, Blackmore C, Bent S, et al. Systematic review: computed tomography and ultrasonography to detect acute appendicitis in adults and adolescents. *Ann Intern Med.* 2004;141:537-546.
2. Hershko DD, Awad N, Fischer D, et al. Focused helical CT using rectal contrast material only as the preferred technique for the diagnosis of suspected acute appendicitis: a prospective, randomized, controlled study comparing three different techniques. *Dis Colon Rectum.* 2007;50:1223-1229.
3. Varadhan KK, Humes DJ, Neal KR, et al. Antibiotic therapy versus appendectomy for acute appendicitis: a meta-analysis. *World J Surg.* 2010;34:199-209.
4. Sauerland S, Lefering R, Neugebauer EAM. Laparoscopic versus open surgery for suspected appendicitis. *Cochrane Database Syst Rev.* 2004;4:CD001546.
5. St. Peter SD, Aguayo P, Fraser JD, et al. Initial laparoscopic appendectomy versus initial nonoperative management and interval appendectomy for perforated appendicitis with abscess: a prospective, randomized trial. *J Pediatr Surg.* 2010;45:236-240.
6. St. Peter SD, Tsao K, Spilde TL, et al. Single daily dosing ceftriaxone and metronidazole vs standard triple antibiotic regimen for perforated appendix in children: a prospective randomized trial. *J Pediatr Surg.* 2008;43:981-985.
7. Ridgway PF, Latif A, Shabbir J, et al. Randomized controlled trial of oral vs intravenous therapy for the clinically diagnosed acute uncomplicated diverticulitis. *Colorectal Dis.* 2009;11:941-946.
8. Schug-Pass C, Geers P, Hugel O, et al. Prospective randomized trial comparing short-term antibiotic therapy versus standard therapy for acute uncomplicated sigmoid diverticulitis. *Int J Colorectal Dis.* 2010;25:751-759.
9. Klarenbeek BR, Veenhof AA, Bergamaschi R, et al. Laparoscopic sigmoid resection for diverticulitis decreases major morbidity rates: a randomized control trial: short-term results of the Sigma Trial. *Ann Surg.* 2009;249:39-44.
10. Latella G, Pimpo MT, Sottili S, et al. Rifaximin improves symptoms of acquired uncomplicated diverticular disease of the colon. *Int J Colorectal Dis.* 2003;18:55-62.
11. Fitzgibbons RJ Jr, Giobbie-Hurder A, Gibbs JO, et al. Watchful waiting vs repair of inguinal hernia in minimally symptomatic men: a randomized clinical trial. *JAMA.* 2006;295:285-292.
12. Amato B, Moja L, Panico S, et al. Shouldice technique versus other open techniques for inguinal hernia repair. *Cochrane Database Syst Rev.* 2009;4:CD001543.
13. Karthikesalingam A, Markar SR, Holt PJ, et al. Meta-analysis of randomized controlled trials comparing laparoscopic with open mesh repair of recurrent inguinal hernia. *Br J Surg.* 2010;97:4-11.

SUGGESTED READINGS

Eglinton T, Nguyen T, Raniga S, et al. Patterns of recurrence in patients with acute diverticulitis. *Br J Surg.* 2010;97:952-957. *Elective surgery to prevent recurrence and the development of complications should be used sparingly.*
Gupta RK, Agrawal CS, Yadav R, et al. Intussusception in adults: institutional review. *Int J Surg.* 2011;9:91-95. *Review of 38 cases, including causes (about 50% malignant) and rates of successful reduction (58% for ileocolic, 30% for colocolic).*
Merlin MA, Shah CN, Shiroff AM. Evidence-based appendicitis: the initial workup. *Postgrad Med.* 2010;122:189-195. *Review emphasizing CT diagnosis.*
Tan KK, Chong CS, Sim R. Management of acute sigmoid volvulus: an institution's experience over 9 years. *World J Surg.* 2010;34:1943-1948. *Elective definitive surgery is suggested in view of the high recurrence rate (>60%) and the considerable risks of emergency surgery.*
Zielinski MD, Elken PW, Bannon MP, et al. Small bowel obstruction—who needs an operation? A multivariate prediction model. *World J Surg.* 2010;34:910-919. *Intraperitoneal free fluid, mesenteric edema, lack of the "small bowel feces sign," and history of vomiting predict the need for surgery.*

145

VASCULAR DISEASES OF THE GASTROINTESTINAL TRACT

STEPHEN CRANE HAUSER

⬤ INTESTINAL ISCHEMIA

Intestinal ischemia can occur as a result of a variety of conditions that decrease intestinal blood flow. Both diminished arterial blood flow to the gut and compromised venous circulation from the intestine can cause intestinal or mesenteric ischemia. Several conditions, such as adhesions and malignancy (Chapter 199), may predispose to mesenteric ischemia by secondarily diminishing blood flow through extrinsic compression of otherwise normal intestinal arteries or veins (Table 145-1). These disorders and esophageal varices (Chapters 137 and 156) are discussed elsewhere.

EPIDEMIOLOGY

Intestinal ischemia is responsible for about 1 per 1000 hospital admissions. When considering the diagnosis of intestinal ischemia, it is important to distinguish *primary* (occlusive or nonocclusive) from *secondary* (extrinsic to the blood vessel) mesenteric ischemia, *acute* manifestations from *chronic,* *arterial* versus *venous,* and *small bowel* versus *colonic* ischemia. Risk factors for intestinal ischemia include older age (all the disorders discussed) and conditions that predispose to arterial embolism (e.g., cardiac arrhythmias, heart failure, cardiomegaly, dyskinesia, valvular heart disease, recent myocardial infarction, cardiac catheterization, intracardiac thrombus, atheromatous cholesterol embolism), occlusion of arteries (atherosclerosis, fibromuscular dysplasia, abdominal aortic aneurysm, trauma, vasculitis), low-flow states (sepsis, dialysis, reduced cardiac output, vasoconstrictive drugs), and pathologic thromboses (largely venous; hypercoagulable and hyperviscosity states, trauma, malignancy, inflammation).

TABLE 145-1	**CONDITIONS PREDISPOSING TO SECONDARY MESENTERIC ISCHEMIA**

Adhesions
Herniation
Volvulus
Intussusception
Mesenteric fibrosis
Retroperitoneal fibrosis
Carcinoid syndrome
Malignancy (peritoneal, mesenteric, colonic)
Neurofibromatosis
Amyloidosis
Trauma

PATHOBIOLOGY

Arterial or venous disease of the esophagus, stomach, duodenum, and rectum is very unusual for anatomic reasons. The esophagus receives its main blood supply segmentally through multiple small vessels from the aorta, right intercostal artery, bronchial arteries, inferior thyroid artery, left gastric artery, short gastric artery, and left phrenic artery. Likewise, the stomach, duodenum, and rectum have numerous arterial inputs with rich collateralization. Patients who have undergone extensive surgical resection of the esophagus, stomach, or duodenum are at increased risk for ischemia. Vasculitic disorders, which can involve small or large arteries or veins, may affect the esophagus, stomach, duodenum, or rectum.

The arterial supply of blood to the small and large intestine is from the *celiac artery, superior mesenteric artery* (SMA), and *inferior mesenteric artery* (IMA). Collateral vessels, which vary from person to person, may include the meandering mesenteric artery or arc of Riolan at the base of the mesentery (connecting the SMA and IMA), the marginal artery of Drummond along the mesenteric border (connecting the SMA and IMA), the pancreaticoduodenal arcade (connecting the celiac artery and SMA), the arc of Barkow (connecting the celiac artery and SMA), and the arc of Buhler (connecting the celiac artery and SMA). These collaterals can rapidly enlarge in response to localized mesenteric ischemia. During states of low arterial flow, such as in patients with low systemic arterial blood pressure, "watershed" areas such as the splenic flexure, which is farthest away from arterial flow, are more likely to be involved. In contrast, when a major arterial vessel such as the IMA is suddenly occluded, the splenic flexure is less likely to be involved because of collaterals from the SMA circulation.

Intestinal blood flow, which accounts for approximately 10% of cardiac output, increases to as much as 25% of cardiac output after eating a meal. Blood flow to the intestine is regulated by the sympathetic nervous system and a variety of systemic (angiotensin II, vasopressin) and local (prostaglandins, leukotrienes) humoral factors.

Mesenteric ischemia can occur as a result of decreased *arterial* blood flow, which can be *occlusive* (arterial embolus, arterial thrombus, and vasculitis) or *nonocclusive* (low-flow states). *Venous* obstruction (thrombosis, vasculitis) can also result in mesenteric ischemia.

Whatever the cause of mesenteric ischemia, the gut is able to adapt to as much as a 75% reduction in normal blood flow for as long as 12 hours. Increased flow through available and newly opened collateral vessels and increased oxygen extraction help compensate. However, with a more prolonged and more severe reduction in blood flow, generalized mesenteric arterial vasoconstriction often develops and can become irreversible, even with correction of the original underlying condition (i.e., relief of focal arterial obstruction or resolution of a low-flow state). Hypoxia and reperfusion injury by oxygen radicals, reduced endothelial synthesis of nitric oxide, and an enhanced cellular inflammatory response cause microvascular and end-organ damage. Initially, the end-organ damage is primarily mucosal, but damage can rapidly progress to transmural necrosis (gangrene). Some ischemic segments of bowel will heal with fibrosis (strictures).

CLINICAL MANIFESTATIONS

Symptoms of intestinal ischemia at initial evaluation may be acute (sudden, lasting hours), subacute (days), or chronic (intermittent, occurring over a period of weeks to months). With acute and many subacute manifestations, abdominal pain is often the cardinal symptom. Usually the pain is severe, persistent, and poorly localized. Initially, the pain is typically more severe than the findings on abdominal palpation (i.e., pain out of proportion to tenderness). With or without pain, other initial features may include fever, altered mental status, abdominal distention, difficulty eating, nausea, vomiting, and diarrhea. With small bowel ischemia, overt gastrointestinal bleeding (Chapter 137) is a late and ominous finding that often suggests small bowel infarction.

Findings on physical examination can include hypotension, tachycardia, abdominal distention, initially increased and later decreased bowel sounds, and nonspecific diffuse abdominal tenderness, often mild at first. Over time, peritoneal signs with localized to generalized abdominal tenderness, rebound, and rigidity may become manifest. Occult gastrointestinal bleeding can be an early finding.

DIAGNOSIS

Even as the diagnostic evaluation is begun, appropriate attention must be directed to emergency therapy, including fluid resuscitation, antibiotics, and invasive therapy (Fig. 145-1).

Initial Diagnostic Evaluation

The initial laboratory findings in patients with an acute onset of bowel ischemia can be entirely normal. Nonspecific abnormalities such as leukocytosis with a predominance of neutrophils and hemoconcentration may be observed. Elevated serum levels of amylase, lactate, aminotransferases, lactate dehydrogenase, creatine kinase, and phosphate often portend more advanced (necrotic) small bowel ischemia, but these findings lack sensitivity as well as specificity.

Noninvasive Imaging

The presence or absence of radiographic features suggestive of ischemia in patients with acute-onset mesenteric ischemia varies and depends on the duration and extent of ischemia. Plain abdominal radiographs are useful in helping exclude secondary causes of mesenteric ischemia, as well as other causes of acute abdominal pain, nausea, vomiting, or distention, such as obstruction and perforation. Radiographic findings such as "thumbprinting" (caused by submucosal hemorrhage), an ileus pattern, or formless loops of small bowel, or with more advanced disease, pneumatosis intestinalis or portal venous gas (often a sign of transmural necrosis or gangrene) may on occasion be seen. Contrast-enhanced abdominal-pelvic computed tomography (CT) is also helpful to exclude alternative diagnoses. CT may demonstrate entirely normal findings in acute mesenteric ischemia, or findings such as segmental bowel wall thickening, submucosal hemorrhage, mesenteric stranding, mesenteric venous thrombosis, pneumatosis, and portal venous gas may be present (Fig. 145-2). Multidetector CT angiography (MDCTA) has a greater sensitivity and specificity (each up to 95%) than traditional CT (about 65%). Magnetic resonance angiography (MRA) is less sensitive for more peripheral emboli. Subacute manifestations of bowel ischemia may be due to a wide variety of causes, including mesenteric venous thrombosis, which is best diagnosed by CT scan. However, the time needed to obtain a CT scan should not delay resuscitation or arteriography in very ill patients with suspected acute-onset ischemia.

TREATMENT Rx

Acutely ill patients require prompt, definitive diagnosis and treatment, which often requires selective mesenteric angiography (Fig. 145-3). If transmural intestinal necrosis (gangrene) is suspected from peritoneal signs, pneumatosis, or portal venous gas on imaging procedures, emergency laparotomy is indicated. The presence of predisposing conditions (e.g., arrhythmias, systemic hypotension) and their extraintestinal manifestations (e.g., heart failure, sepsis, respiratory insufficiency, acute renal failure, anemia) dictate the initial therapy: volume replacement, optimization of cardiac output, management of respiratory function, avoidance of splanchnic vasoconstrictors such as digoxin, and administration of broad-spectrum antibiotics (e.g., meropenem, imipenem/cilastatin, metronidazole and a third-generation cephalosporin, ciprofloxacin and metronidazole, or piperacillin until symptoms resolve to cover aerobic gram-negative and anaerobic organisms and to prevent sepsis secondary to translocation of bacteria across ischemic gut mucosa.

PROGNOSIS

Acute primary arterial mesenteric ischemia involving the small bowel is an urgent condition, which, if unidentified or untreated, can result in death within hours. Mortality rates may be as high as 70% but are much lower with early diagnosis and prompt therapy. Overall, colonic ischemia has a much better prognosis than does small bowel ischemia. Mesenteric venous thrombosis also has a much better prognosis than acute primary arterial mesenteric ischemia of the small intestine.

Specific Ischemic Bowel Syndromes
SUPERIOR MESENTERIC EMBOLISM

Embolization to the intestine through the SMA (*SMA embolus*) accounts for 5% of peripheral emboli and nearly 50% of cases of primary noncolonic mesenteric ischemia. Emboli originate most commonly from the heart, with an aortic origin being less common (Table 145-2), and tend to obstruct beyond the origin of the SMA.

CLINICAL MANIFESTATIONS AND DIAGNOSIS

Patients who are evaluated early in the course of their illness may have entirely normal CT scans, or the CT findings may be consistent with mesenteric

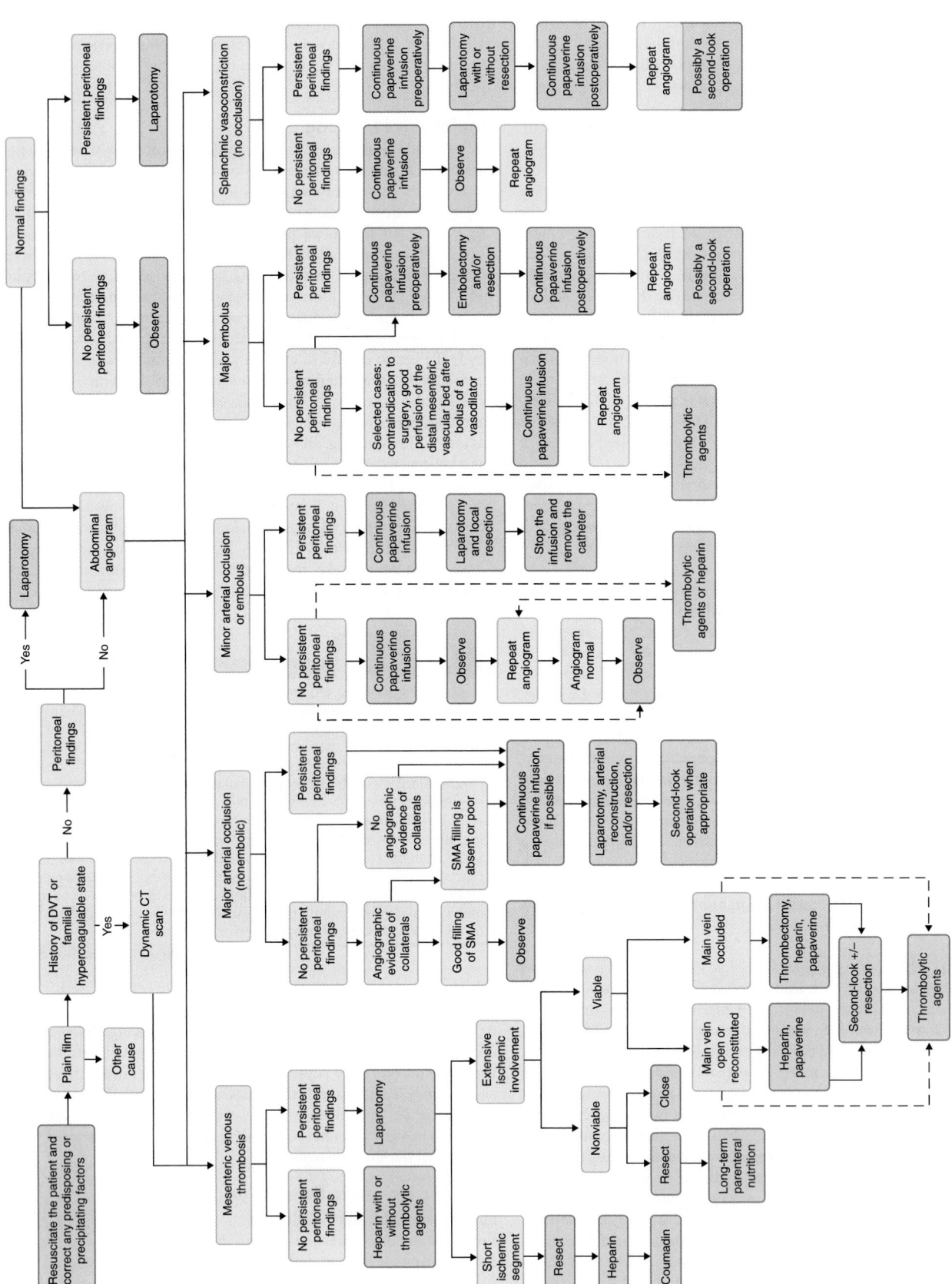

FIGURE 145-1. Algorithm for managing patients with suspected acute mesenteric ischemia: diagnosis and management. *Solid lines* indicate an accepted management plan; *dashed lines* indicate an alternative management plan. CT = computed tomography; DVT = deep venous thrombosis; SMA = superior mesenteric artery. (From American Gastroenterological Association Medical Position Statement: guidelines on intestinal ischemia. *Gastroenterology.* 2000;118:951-953 [corrected algorithm in *Gastroenterology.* 2000;119:281].)

ischemia without features that would suggest alternative diagnoses (e.g., perforation, obstruction). MDCTA is much more likely than standard CT to diagnose embolic disease reliably in the mesenteric arterial vasculature. Selective mesenteric angiography offers the possibility of therapy as well as diagnosis.

TREATMENT Rx

Select patients with acute onset of a partial or small SMA branch occlusion may be candidates for thrombolytic therapy (e.g., streptokinase, urokinase, tissue plasminogen activator) infused through an arterial catheter directly into the vicinity of the embolus; this therapy can lyse the embolus and resolve symptoms such as abdominal pain. Because segmental arterial embolic occlusion of a small portion of the SMA vascular bed results in widespread splanchnic visceral arterial vasoconstriction, which may persist even after the original inciting event (i.e., an embolus) is rectified, infusion of a vasodilator such as papaverine (often given as a 60-mg bolus, followed by a continuous infusion of 30 to 60 mg/hour for 12 to 48 hours) through an arterial catheter reverses this reflex vasoconstriction and improves the outcome, including mortality rates. The same scenario occurs with other arterial occlusive lesions (SMA thrombi), arterial nonocclusive disease (nonocclusive mesenteric ischemia), and disorders associated with mesenteric venous occlusion.

Patients evaluated in the course of their acute embolic illness with peritoneal signs require laparotomy, with or without resection and with or without embolectomy, which is usually performed during surgical exploration. A "second-look" operation 24 hours after embolectomy to make sure that all necrotic tissue has been resected may be necessary.

FIGURE 145-2. Computed tomography of the abdomen in a patient with ischemic colitis as a result of superior mesenteric vein thrombosis. A segmental area of the transverse colon demonstrates a thick wall, as well as considerable fluid and soft tissue stranding in the adjacent mesentery. (From Johnson CL, Schmit GD, eds. *Mayo Clinic Gastrointestinal Imaging Review.* Boca Raton, Fla: Mayo Clinic Scientific Press, Taylor and Francis Group; 2005. By permission of the Mayo Foundation for Medical Education and Research. All rights reserved).

Any patient in whom SMA embolization is diagnosed requires preoperative systemic anticoagulation (e.g., intravenous heparin) to prevent propagation of clot around the embolus and to guard against further embolization to the intestine or other organs (i.e., brain, coronary arteries, kidneys, extremities). Anticoagulation is usually discontinued before surgery and is often resumed 24 to 48 hours postoperatively, depending on the operative findings. Mortality can be as high as 70%.

SUPERIOR MESENTERIC THROMBOSIS

Thrombosis of the SMA (*SMA thrombus*) accounts for nearly 15% of cases of primary noncolonic mesenteric ischemia. Risk factors include older age, atherosclerosis (e.g., hypertension, diabetes mellitus, hyperlipidemia, smoking history), low-flow states, hypercoagulable states, and less often, vasculitis and aortic or mesenteric aneurysms.

CLINICAL MANIFESTATIONS AND DIAGNOSIS

Nearly one third of these patients have a history of symptomatic chronic mesenteric ischemia (see later) antedating their acute manifestation of SMA thrombosis. Proximal mesenteric arterial occlusions are well recognized by MDCTA, MRA, and Doppler ultrasound, but similar abnormalities are common in asymptomatic elderly persons. Similar to acute SMA embolism, the diagnosis is confirmed by selective mesenteric angiography, with intra-arterial infusion of a vasodilator used to reverse reflex-generalized vasoconstriction.

TREATMENT Rx

Although thrombolytic therapy has been helpful in a limited number of case reports, surgical thrombectomy or bypass grafting, with or without bowel resection, is the most common therapeutic approach. Because many thrombi occur near the SMA origin, angioplasty may be therapeutic in very select cases, but the risk for reocclusion is high. Similar to acute SMA embolism, anticoagulation (intravenous heparin) is important preoperatively and at some point postoperatively in the acute state, as is administration of broad-spectrum antibiotics (see earlier).

TABLE 145-2	CONDITIONS ASSOCIATED WITH EMBOLIZATION TO THE GASTROINTESTINAL TRACT

Cardiac arrhythmias
Valvular heart disease
Heart failure
Myocardial infarction
Intracardiac thrombus
Cardiac catheterization
Cardioversion
Atherosclerosis of the aorta

FIGURE 145-3. Selected films from superior mesenteric angiography. **A,** Diffuse vasoconstriction characteristic of nonocclusive mesenteric ischemia. **B,** Intra-arterial infusion of papaverine (30 to 60 mg/hour) resulted in vasodilation.

ACUTE NONOCCLUSIVE, NONCOLONIC PRIMARY ARTERIAL ISCHEMIA

Nonocclusive mesenteric ischemia, which accounts for about 20% of primary noncolonic mesenteric ischemia cases, is caused by low arterial blood flow to the intestine. Risk factors include advanced age, decreased systolic blood pressure (e.g., cardiac arrhythmia, heart failure, myocardial infarction, shock, sepsis, burns, pancreatitis, hemorrhage, multiple organ failure, dialysis, perioperative states), vasospasm (e.g., digoxin, vasopressin, amphetamines, cocaine), and atherosclerotic disease.

CLINICAL MANIFESTATIONS AND DIAGNOSIS

The clinical findings are generally indistinguishable from those of embolic or thrombotic vascular disease, except that symptoms may be less acute. As a result, patients initially may be seen without acute abdominal pain but rather with more nonspecific symptoms such as distention, nausea, fever, altered mental status, and borderline or low systolic blood pressure. Selected mesenteric angiography establishes the diagnosis (lack of embolus or thrombus, alternating areas of vessel spasm and dilation, vascular pruning and spasm).

TREATMENT   Rx

The best specific treatment is prolonged intra-arterial instillation of a vasodilator (e.g., papaverine, often given as a 60-mg bolus, followed by a continuous infusion of 30 to 60 mg/hour) to reverse the vasospasm. Avoidance of vasospastic medications and optimization of cardiac output, blood volume, and blood pressure are crucial. Anticoagulation is generally not necessary, but broad-spectrum antibiotics (similar to those recommended earlier) should be administered to cover aerobic gram-negative and anaerobic organisms. Although many of these patients have serious conditions that predispose them to low-flow states and their ultimate prognosis is dependent on the outcomes of these serious conditions, diagnosis and treatment of acute nonocclusive mesenteric ischemia with therapeutic angiography can be life-saving.

MESENTERIC VENOUS THROMBOSIS

Occlusive disease of the mesenteric venous circulation (*mesenteric venous thrombosis*) usually involves the superior mesenteric vein (SMV) and may be accompanied by symptoms that are acute (hours to days) or subacute (weeks to months) in onset.

EPIDEMIOLOGY AND PATHOBIOLOGY

Thrombosis of the SMV accounts for about 10% of cases of primary noncolonic mesenteric ischemia. Colonic involvement with ischemic colitis is much less common. In contrast to arterial occlusive disease, risk factors and causes for SMV thrombosis are more numerous and diverse. Individuals with a personal or family history of a hypercoagulable state or deep venous thrombosis are at increased risk for SMV thrombosis. Hypercoagulable states, hyperviscosity syndromes, portal hypertension, intra-abdominal infections (e.g., pyelophlebitis, diverticulitis, appendicitis) or inflammation (e.g., Crohn's disease, pancreatitis), malignancy, vasculitis, and trauma may all cause thrombosis of the SMV (Table 145-3).

CLINICAL MANIFESTATIONS

Symptoms in acute-onset cases are similar to those observed in acute occlusive and nonocclusive arterial mesenteric ischemia—abdominal pain, anorexia, nausea, vomiting, abdominal fullness, diarrhea, and constipation— but tend to persist over a longer time period. Some patients may have bacteremia, especially infection with *Bacteroides*. Gastrointestinal hemorrhage, if present, is often indicative of infarction. However, many patients with SMV thrombosis experience more vague symptomatic abdominal pain, nausea, distention, or diarrhea over a period of weeks to months (subacute).

DIAGNOSIS

Abdominal-pelvic contrast-enhanced CT, which is the preferred diagnostic test, usually (>90% sensitivity) demonstrates SMV thrombosis with or without portal vein or splenic vein thrombosis. By definition, chronic mesenteric venous thrombosis is asymptomatic and usually detected as an incidental CT finding in patients with portal hypertension, pancreatitis (acute or chronic), or malignancy. The presence of abundant collateral vessels suggests chronic or sometimes subacute mesenteric venous obstruction.

TABLE 145-3 RISK FACTORS FOR MESENTERIC VENOUS THROMBOSIS

Hypercoagulable and hyperviscosity states
    Protein S deficiency
    Protein C deficiency
    Antithrombin III deficiency
    Factor V Leiden mutation
    Hyperfibrinogenemia
    Antiphospholipid syndrome
    Primary myeloproliferative syndrome
    Sickle cell disease
    Estrogen or progesterone

Intra-abdominal infections and inflammation
    Appendicitis
    Diverticulitis
    Crohn's disease
    Abscess
    Pancreatitis
    Cholecystitis
    Pyelophlebitis
    Neonatal omphalitis

Portal hypertension
    Variceal sclerotherapy

Malignancy

Trauma

Vasculitis

Small bowel radiography may demonstrate segmental bowel wall thickening and separation of bowel loops. Selective mesenteric angiography is not generally necessary.

TREATMENT   Rx

Therapy for acute-onset cases may include laparotomy with or without bowel resection when infarction is suspected, fluid resuscitation, broad-spectrum antibiotics (similar to those recommended earlier to cover aerobic gram-negative and anaerobic organisms), avoidance of vasoconstrictors, and anticoagulation (e.g., intravenous heparin) in the absence of gastrointestinal bleeding. Selected patients may be candidates for thrombolytic therapy (e.g., streptokinase, urokinase, tissue plasminogen activator), followed by anticoagulation. Underlying conditions such as hypercoagulable states, portal hypertension, intra-abdominal infections, intra-abdominal inflammation, and malignancy require concomitant diagnosis and therapy. The indications for anticoagulation in the chronic setting are uncertain, and it is generally avoided in patients who have portal hypertension but do not have symptoms related to their mesenteric venous thrombosis.

CHRONIC MESENTERIC ISCHEMIA

Chronic atherosclerotic stenosis of the visceral arteries is the cause of most cases of chronic mesenteric ischemia, sometimes called *intestinal angina*.

EPIDEMIOLOGY AND PATHOBIOLOGY

Risk factors for chronic mesenteric ischemia are principally older age and the risk factors for atherosclerosis. Rarely, vasculitis or an aortic aneurysm can be manifested as chronic mesenteric ischemia. Atherosclerotic stenoses usually involve the origins of two or all of the three major visceral arteries supplying the intestine. However, many age-matched patients also harbor atherosclerotic lesions and do not have symptoms of chronic mesenteric ischemia.

CLINICAL MANIFESTATIONS

Patients typically complain of episodic ischemic abdominal pain. The pain is usually upper or midabdominal, typically begins 15 to 30 minutes after a meal, lasts 1 to 3 hours, and progresses in severity over time, as well as occurs after smaller meals and more frequently after meals. Patients may lose weight as a result of fear of eating (sitophobia). Nausea, vomiting, bloating, diarrhea, and constipation can also occur. Malabsorption with steatorrhea, otherwise unexplained gastroduodenal ulcerations, and small bowel biopsy findings of villous atrophy, nonspecific surface cell flattening, and chronic inflammation may be seen in some patients. More than one half of patients have a bruit on abdominal examination. In some patients with episodic symptoms, acute thrombotic mesenteric ischemia develops suddenly.

DIAGNOSIS AND TREATMENT Rx

Atherosclerotic lesions usually can be identified by Doppler ultrasound because they are proximal in these vessels and demonstrate increased flow velocity through areas of marked stenosis. MDCTA and MRA are also useful to screen for arterial stenoses consistent with chronic mesenteric ischemia in symptomatic patients, but neither technique is adequately sensitive to exclude the diagnosis of chronic mesenteric ischemia when the pretest probability is high. Thus, selective mesenteric angiography is important to ensure that the anatomic findings are consistent with the diagnosis. Patients must be evaluated thoroughly to exclude other causes of abdominal pain (i.e., gastric cancer, gastroparesis, gastric volvulus, partial small bowel obstruction, small bowel bacterial overgrowth states, pancreatic cancer, biliary disease, paraesophageal hernias). For symptomatic patients with appropriate findings on angiography and no other causes of symptoms, surgical reconstruction provides better long-term outcomes than angioplasty and stenting.

ISCHEMIC COLITIS

EPIDEMIOLOGY AND PATHOBIOLOGY

Ischemic colitis, which is the single most common cause of mesenteric ischemia, accounts for nearly 50% of all cases and for almost 1 in 2000 hospital admissions. Many cases are acute and self-limited and occur in persons older than 60 years without any apparent cause; these cases are probably due to transient nonocclusive hypoperfusion involving a segment of the colon. It is controversial whether subtle hypercoagulable states contribute to the pathogenesis of idiopathic cases. Atherosclerotic or thrombotic occlusion of the IMA or its branches and low-flow states are recognizable causes of ischemic colitis. Less common causes include hypercoagulable states (especially in younger persons), iatrogenic ligation of the IMA (e.g., with aortic surgery), embolism, vasculitis, and any cause of colonic obstruction, including malignancy, stricture, and fecalith, that can produce localized compression of the vasculature with an upstream segment of ischemia. Other unusual associations include long-distance running (dehydration, mechanical trauma to the vasculature, generally involving the cecum), pit viper bite, scuba diving, and intra-abdominal infections or inflammatory disease. A variety of medications, illicit drugs, and chemicals also can result in a chemical picture identical or similar to ischemic colitis (Table 145-4), sometimes probably secondary to vasoconstriction that can affect other parts of the gastrointestinal tract, liver, and other organ systems (e.g., cocaine, amphetamines, pseudoephedrine), sometimes due to constipation (e.g., alosetron), sometimes due to a hypercoagulable effect (e.g., estrogens), and sometimes as a result of a chemical effect (e.g., sodium polystyrene with sorbitol enemas).

CLINICAL MANIFESTATIONS

The clinical presentation of ischemic colitis is acute and, in most patients, includes abdominal pain (mostly left lower quadrant), often with urgency, diarrhea, and passage of bright red blood per rectum. Anorexia, nausea,

TABLE 145-4	MEDICATIONS AND DRUGS ASSOCIATED WITH ISCHEMIC COLITIS

Digitalis
Vasopressin
Pseudoephedrine
Amphetamines
Cocaine
Ergot
Sumatriptan
Gold
Danazol
Estrogens
Progestins
Alosetron
Psychotropics
Nonsteroidal anti-inflammatory drugs
Various enemas
Tegaserod
Interferon/ribavirin

vomiting, abdominal distention, and passage of maroon material per rectum may also occur. Although the blood loss is not usually enough to require transfusion, some patients may be orthostatic because of loss of blood and fluid. Fever, tachycardia, abdominal tenderness over the affected portion of the colon, and distention may be found on physical examination.

DIAGNOSIS

Laboratory findings range from normal to nonspecific findings such as leukocytosis and hemoconcentration to those observed in persons with bowel necrosis (see earlier). Evaluation of patients younger than 50 years should include tests for thrombophilic disorders (Chapter 179).

Plain radiographs of the abdomen may reveal "thumbprinting" or may be normal. Similar to small bowel ischemia, CT scanning can be useful to help exclude other disorders, especially in more symptomatic and ill patients; the findings may be consistent with segmental colonic edema and inflammation, with or without adjacent pericolonic inflammatory stranding. These radiographic features are consistent with ischemic colitis in an appropriate clinical setting but are nonspecific and may be seen in patients with other disorders such as acute diverticulitis (Chapter 144), infectious colitis (Chapter 142), and inflammatory bowel disease (Chapter 143). The diagnosis is best made by colonoscopy, which should provide endoscopic and histologic findings consistent with acute ischemic colitis: segmental patchy ulceration, edema, erythema, single stripe sign, and submucosal bluish purple hemorrhagic nodules (Fig. 145-4).

Typically, visceral angiography is not required because most patients with ischemic colitis have self-limited involvement of the left colon or distal transverse colon–splenic flexure with sparing of the rectum, and findings on urgent angiography in these patients are usually normal. However, about 10% of patients with acute ischemic colitis have predominantly right-sided involvement of the cecum, ascending colon, hepatic flexure, and proximal transverse colon. Because the arterial supply to the right colon is through the ileocolic branch of the SMA, there may be concomitant distal ileal ischemia, often owing to low-flow states (especially hemodialysis patients) or embolization. These patients have more pain, less bleeding, and a much worse outcome and are at risk for small bowel necrosis.

Differential Diagnosis

Gastrointestinal infections, such as with *Escherichia coli* O157:H7, *Clostridium difficile*, *Klebsiella oxytoca*, and cytomegalovirus, can mimic ischemic colitis clinically and even histologically. Acute-onset inflammatory bowel disease involving the colon can also be difficult to distinguish from ischemic colitis. However, patients with subacute or chronic pain, diarrhea, obstructive symptoms, weight loss, or bleeding may be thought to have complicated

FIGURE 145-4. Endoscopy of the splenic flexure of the colon in a patient with ischemic colitis. Note the shallow, irregular, exudative ulceration with interspersed erythema. (From Emory TS, Carpenter HA, Gostout CJ, et al, eds. *Atlas of Gastrointestinal Endoscopy and Endoscopic Biopsies.* Washington, DC: Armed Forces Institute of Pathology, American Registry of Pathology; 2000.)

diverticular disease, Crohn's disease, or malignancy with stricture, and chronic ischemic stricture of the colon may not be correctly diagnosed until after surgery is performed.

Stool culture can exclude infection, especially with *E. coli* O157:H7, *C. difficile*, and parasites. In immunocompromised patients, colonic biopsy can be performed to diagnose cytomegalovirus infection.

TREATMENT   Rx

Patients with right-sided ischemic colitis require visceral angiography not only for diagnosis but also for intra-arterial administration of vasodilators (e.g., papaverine as a 60-mg intravenous bolus followed by an infusion of 30 to 60 mg/hour). Some patients may require urgent surgery. The clinical course in patients with right-sided ischemic colitis may be subacute, with a mortality rate as high as 50% or greater.

By contrast, left-sided acute ischemic colitis, which accounts for most cases, tends to resolve within hours to a few days with supportive therapy, including volume replacement, correction of any low-flow state, broad-spectrum antibiotics (similar to those recommended earlier for patients with small bowel ischemia), avoidance of vasoconstrictive medications, and rarely, blood transfusion; surgery is required only in patients with signs and symptoms of transmural necrosis, perforation, or massive bleeding. Occasional patients with acute-onset left-sided ischemic colitis have persistent or recurrent symptoms of pain, diarrhea, bleeding, sepsis, or stricture formation that develop over a period of weeks to months and may require segmental surgical resection.

VASCULITIS

Many vasculitic syndromes can involve the gastrointestinal tract. Usually, but not always, other organ systems are also involved.

Large and Medium Vessel Vasculitis

Takayasu's arteritis (Chapters 78 and 278) and *giant cell arteritis* (Chapter 279), which affect large to medium-sized muscular arteries, rarely involve the gastrointestinal tract. Takayasu's arteritis has been associated rarely with inflammatory bowel disease.

Medium to Small Vessel Vasculitis

Polyarteritis nodosa (Chapter 278) is characterized by segmental microaneurysms typically involving small and medium-sized arteries. The small bowel is involved more commonly than the large bowel. Many patients will have abdominal pain, fever, hypertension, and multiple organ involvement. Gastrointestinal bleeding or perforation will develop in some patients. The gallbladder, spleen, pancreas, and liver may also be involved. Nearly half of patients with polyarteritis nodosa are infected with hepatitis B virus.

Both *Wegener's granulomatosis* (Chapter 278) and *Churg-Strauss syndrome* (Chapter 278) affect small and medium-sized arteries. Although gastrointestinal involvement is not common in Wegener's granulomatosis with granulomatous inflammation, in up to one third of patients with Churg-Strauss syndrome, abdominal pain or gastrointestinal bleeding may develop as a result of ischemia. Mesenteric venous involvement can also occur with Churg-Strauss syndrome.

Thromboangiitis obliterans (Buerger's disease; Chapter 80) involves small and medium-sized arteries and can cause multiple distal occlusions of the mesenteric arterial circulation. Patients with *Behçet's disease* (Chapter 278) often have lymphocytic inflammation of small and medium-sized arteries, as well as veins. Like Crohn's disease, the ileocecal region is frequently involved with ulceration. Abdominal pain, diarrhea, gastrointestinal bleeding, and perforation may occur.

Small Vessel Vasculitis

Small vessel involvement with immunoglobulin A immune complex deposition in blood vessel walls is typical in *Henoch-Schönlein purpura* (Chapter 278). These patients usually have palpable purpura, arthritis, and abdominal pain, as well as gastrointestinal bleeding. *Hypersensitivity vasculitis* (Chapter 278), which affects small arterioles, venules, and capillaries, is related to a variety of drugs, infections, and chemicals; on occasion there may be gastrointestinal involvement. *Cryoglobulinemia* (Chapter 193) with immune complex involvement of small blood vessels can sometimes involve the gastrointestinal tract. These patients are often infected with hepatitis C virus.

HEMORRHAGIC VASCULAR DISORDERS
Angiodysplasia

DEFINITION AND EPIDEMIOLOGY

Angiodysplasia or vascular ectasia is a thin-walled, dilated, punctate red vascular structure in the mucosa or submucosa of the bowel; it typically involves adjacent venules, capillaries, and arterioles. Angiodysplasia is found in the colon, especially the right colon, in up to 1% of persons and is found also in the stomach and small bowel but rarely in the esophagus. Angiodysplastic lesions may be single or multiple, and they increase in frequency with age. Some data suggest associations with chronic renal failure (Chapter 132), von Willebrand's disease (Chapter 176), and aortic stenosis (Chapter 75); whether correction of these associated disorders diminishes future gastrointestinal hemorrhage (Chapter 137) from angiodysplasia is uncertain.

CLINICAL MANIFESTATIONS

Clinically, these lesions can produce painless bleeding, which may be occult and manifest only by guaiac-positive stools or iron deficiency anemia, or the bleeding may be overt, with hematochezia, maroon stools, melena, and hematemesis.

DIAGNOSIS

Endoscopic procedures most often make the diagnosis of bleeding secondary to angiodysplasia (Fig. 145-5). In some patients, endoscopic procedures may need to be repeated, especially in volume-depleted patients and after the administration of narcotics. Small bowel angiodysplasia, beyond the reach of both a colonoscope from below and an extended-length endoscope from above, may be the cause of major bleeding (Chapter 137) and require video capsule endoscopy (Chapter 136) or small bowel enteroscopy for diagnosis.

TREATMENT   Rx

Electrocoagulation laser therapy or argon plasma coagulation can be accomplished during endoscopy. When very active bleeding makes urgent colonoscopy technically difficult, visceral angiography can be diagnostic and also permit embolization of bleeding lesions or intra-arterial infusion of a vasoconstrictor. Rarely, bowel resection is required.

PROGNOSIS

More than 90% of gastrointestinal angiodysplasias never bleed. If found incidentally in patients without a history of bleeding, they should not be treated.

FIGURE 145-5. Endoscopy of the sigmoid colon in a patient with angiectasia. The lesion is discrete and contains a tight, radiating cluster of ectatic mucosal vessels. (From Emory TS, Carpenter HA, Gostout CJ, et al, eds. *Atlas of Gastrointestinal Endoscopy and Endoscopic Biopsies.* Washington, DC: Armed Forces Institute of Pathology, American Registry of Pathology; 2000.)

Dieulafoy's Lesion

Dieulafoy's lesion is an unusually large submucosal artery typically found in the proximal portion of the stomach within 6 cm of the gastroesophageal junction. Similar lesions may also occur in the rectum, colon, small bowel, and far less often, the esophagus. Dieulafoy's lesion is manifested clinically as sudden, massive bleeding, which may be recurrent.

DIAGNOSIS AND TREATMENT ℞

Urgent endoscopy is required to identify what is usually a very small vascular protuberance (Fig. 145-6) but can rapidly become inapparent once the acute bleeding stops. Ulceration is not seen, and repeat endoscopic procedures during active bleeding may be required to make the diagnosis. Sometimes the diagnosis requires angiography during a bleeding episode. Endoscopic injection and electrocoagulation therapy are generally effective, but endoscopic band therapy and hemoclips may also be used, and surgery is sometimes required.

PROGNOSIS

Endoscopic therapy is successful long-term in nearly 90% of patients.

Other Ectasias

Telangiectases are similar to angiodysplasias but occur in all the layers of the bowel wall, are usually congenital, and often occur in other organ systems. *Hereditary hemorrhagic telangiectasia* (Osler-Weber-Rendu disease; Chapter 176) is an autosomal dominant disorder with telangiectases involving the lips; mucous membranes, especially in the mouth and nose; gastrointestinal tract, especially the stomach and small bowel; liver; lung; retina; and central nervous system. Patients with *Turner's syndrome* (Chapter 243), *scleroderma* (Chapter 275), and the *CREST syndrome* (Chapter 275) (calcinosis, Raynaud's phenomenon, esophageal dysmotility, sclerodactyly, telangiectasia) may also have gastrointestinal tract telangiectases.

Vascular ectasias involving venules and capillaries can also be seen in the small bowel *(congestive enteropathy)*, in the colon *(congestive colopathy)*, and more commonly, in the stomach *(congestive gastropathy)* in patients with portal hypertension (Chapter 156). In contrast to angiodysplasias, these lesions tend to be more diffuse, appear as multiple, fine punctate red spots or as a mosaic pattern similar to the gastritis of *Helicobacter pylori*, and are more often found in the proximal than the distal part of the stomach. Therapies that decrease portal hypertension can reduce or eliminate these lesions and bleeding from them.

FIGURE 145-6. Endoscopy of the stomach in a patient with Dieulafoy's lesion. Note the visible vessel manifested as a pale protuberance surrounded by a clot with adjacent normal-appearing mucosa. (From Emory TS, Carpenter HA, Gostout CJ, et al, eds. *Atlas of Gastrointestinal Endoscopy and Endoscopic Biopsies*. Washington, DC: Armed Forces Institute of Pathology, American Registry of Pathology; 2000.)

Gastric antral vascular ectasia (GAVE), or watermelon stomach, also involves venules and capillaries with thrombosis as well as ectasia. Erythematous streaks similar to the stripes on a watermelon are typically seen in the antrum radiating toward the pylorus. Patients usually have occult bleeding and less often melena. GAVE is associated with connective tissue diseases (e.g., systemic lupus erythematosus [Chapter 274], mixed connective tissue disease [Chapter 275], scleroderma [Chapter 275]), pernicious anemia (Chapter 167), and portal hypertension (Chapter 156). However, unlike congestive gastropathy, treatment of portal hypertension does not eliminate GAVE or bleeding from it. Argon plasma coagulation is the usual therapy if iron replacement alone is not effective. Antrectomy is rarely needed.

Neoplastic Vascular Lesions

Hemangiomas are uncommon, usually benign vascular tumors that can be found throughout the gastrointestinal tract, often in the rectum or colon. They may be single or multiple, bluish purple, and sessile or polypoid. In some persons, these lesions are multiple and associated with skin lesions, such as the *blue rubber bleb nevus syndrome* with purple-blue cutaneous hemangiomas or the *Klippel-Trenaunay* syndrome with port-wine-colored cutaneous hemangiomas, hemihypertrophy, and varicose veins. Rare vascular malignant neoplasms of the gastrointestinal tract include *angiosarcomas* and *hemangioendotheliomas*.

Miscellaneous Vascular Disorders

Aortoenteric fistulas, which most commonly occur after surgery for an aortic aneurysm (Chapter 78), may be related to infection of the graft and can result in torrential gastrointestinal bleeding. Many of these fistulas communicate with the duodenum. Evaluation of bleeding in persons who have previously undergone abdominal aortic surgery should include urgent extended-length upper endoscopy to document a fistula or diagnose another definitive source of the bleeding. Angiography and radiographic tests (CT, magnetic resonance imaging [MRI]) are helpful only if the findings are abnormal (i.e., there is evidence of a fistula) because of their poor sensitivity for the presence of aortoenteric fistulas. If no clear alternative source for the bleeding can readily be found, explorative surgery is indicated.

Celiac artery compression syndrome (median arcuate ligament syndrome) is a very rare pseudo-ischemic syndrome. Patients are often young and healthy and have postprandial upper abdominal pain, most likely caused by extrinsic compression of the celiac axis by the median arcuate ligament of the diaphragm. Sitophobia can result in considerable weight loss, and there may be a loud systolic bruit in the epigastric region on physical examination. Visceral angiography supports the diagnosis, but bruits and celiac axis compression may occur without symptoms. Surgical therapy is indicated after other possible causes of the patient's symptoms have been excluded.

Bowel as well as large vessel rupture can occur as a complication of *Ehlers-Danlos syndrome type IV* (Chapter 268). Similar vascular catastrophes with gastrointestinal or intraperitoneal hemorrhage can occur in patients with *pseudoxanthoma elasticum type I* (Chapter 268) or with *visceral artery aneurysms* (secondary to atherosclerosis, fibrodysplasia, portal hypertension, pregnancy, pancreatitis, vasculitis, or trauma).

● HEPATIC AND SPLENIC VASCULAR DISEASE
Budd-Chiari Syndrome

Budd-Chiari syndrome can occur as a result of any process that interferes with the normal flow of blood out of the liver, including constrictive pericarditis (Chapter 77) and veno-occlusive disease (Chapter 152). Hepatic vein thrombosis, which is the main cause of Budd-Chiari syndrome, may involve one, two, or all three of the major hepatic veins, with or without partial or complete occlusion of the inferior vena cava. Often, Budd-Chiari syndrome is due to a hypercoagulable state (Chapter 179), such as a chronic myeloproliferative disorder (e.g., polycythemia vera [Chapter 169], essential thrombocythemia [Chapter 169], myeloid metaplasia [Chapter 169]), paroxysmal nocturnal hemoglobinuria, or other hypercoagulable conditions (Chapter 179), such as factor V (Leiden) gene mutation, antiphospholipid antibody syndrome, protein C deficiency, protein S deficiency, or antithrombin III deficiency. A high percentage of these patients harbor *JAK2* V617F mutations. Nearly 50% of patients with Budd-Chiari syndrome have more than one risk factor. Malignancies (direct compression or invasion of hepatic veins, hypercoagulable state), infections (liver abscess), pregnancy, inflammatory disorders (e.g., Behçet's syndrome, inflammatory bowel disease, connective tissue disease, sarcoidosis), and membranous

FIGURE 145-7. Budd-Chiari syndrome. A hepatic vein contrast study depicts the "spider web" pattern of venovenous collaterals attempting to bypass a thrombosed hepatic vein. (Courtesy of Patrick Kamath.)

obstruction (webs) of the inferior vena cava are also associated with Budd-Chiari syndrome.

CLINICAL MANIFESTATIONS

The syndrome is usually subacute or chronic, occurs over a period of weeks to months, and is characterized by the insidious onset of upper abdominal pain, hepatomegaly, and ascites. Fulminant or acute presentations, including encephalopathy, jaundice, ascites, and liver failure, are rare.

DIAGNOSIS

Liver function testing usually reveals normal or mild to moderate nonspecific elevations in serum aspartate and alanine aminotransferase levels. Doppler ultrasound of the liver is the initial diagnostic test of choice, but the absence of hepatic venous flow or venous thrombosis (or both) is also readily apparent with contrast-enhanced CT scanning or MRA. Hepatic venography can confirm the diagnosis (Fig. 145-7) and, with imaging of the inferior vena cava, as well as selective venous pressure measurements, can help guide therapy.

TREATMENT   Rx

Therapy includes diagnosis and treatment of underlying conditions, anticoagulation (intravenous heparin; see Table 81-4 in Chapter 81) to prevent the propagation of thrombi, and treatment of the ascites (e.g., diuretics; Chapter 156). To decompress the congested liver, most patients require interventional radiologic procedures, such as angioplasty, stenting, or transjugular intrahepatic portosystemic shunts, to restore hepatic venous flow. Surgical procedures such as surgical shunts to drain the portal or mesenteric venous system into the inferior vena cava can also decompress the liver. Liver transplantation (Chapter 157) should be considered for patients with fulminant liver failure or cirrhosis, or both. Most patients with Budd-Chiari syndrome require lifelong warfarin anticoagulation (Chapter 37), even after liver transplantation. Selective JAK2 inhibitors (Chapter 169) are being tested in preclinical and clinical studies.

PROGNOSIS

Overall, the 5-year survival rate of patients with the Budd-Chiari syndrome is more than 80%. Indices such as levels of serum albumin and bilirubin, the international normalized ratio, ascites, and encephalopathy, as well as the Child-Pugh score (see Table 156-2 in Chapter 156), can be useful in determining prognosis.

Portal Vein Thrombosis

In adults, cirrhosis, hypercoagulable states, intra-abdominal malignancy, inflammatory disorders (e.g., pancreatitis, Crohn's disease), and medical procedures (e.g., splenectomy, cholecystectomy, gastrectomy, liver transplantation, transjugular intrahepatic portosystemic shunt) are most often the cause of acute portal vein thrombosis. Similar to Budd-Chiari syndrome, a substantial number of these patients harbor JAK2 V617F mutations.

CLINICAL MANIFESTATIONS AND DIAGNOSIS

Clinical manifestations include portal hypertension with variceal bleeding and ascites. Abdominal pain and diarrhea may indicate extension of the thrombus into the SMV with intestinal ischemia. The diagnosis of acute portal vein thrombosis is confirmed by Doppler ultrasound, MDCTA, or MRA. CT imaging may reveal multiple small liver abscesses.

TREATMENT   Rx

Anticoagulation (see Table 81-4 in Chapter 81) therapy for at least 3 months is recommended for patients with acute portal vein thrombosis and should be continued long term in those persons with permanent thrombotic risk factors not otherwise correctable, as well as in patients with extension of thrombus into the mesenteric veins.

High fever, chills, a tender liver, and sepsis suggest pylephlebitis, which usually requires treatment with parenteral antibiotics such as piperacillin/tazobactam, ticarcillin/clavulanate, carbapenem, or a third-generation cephalosporin plus metronidazole for at least 6 weeks. Blood cultures can help to guide the choice and course of antibiotics, which should be administered intravenously for at least 2 weeks.

Treatment is less clear in cirrhotic patients with acute or chronic portal vein thrombosis. Endoscopy for the diagnosis and treatment of varices (Chapter 136), with or without pharmacologic treatment of the portal hypertension (e.g., β-blockade with propranolol; Chapter 156), is often beneficial, and surgical shunts are rarely necessary. Antibiotics, such as those recommended previously for pylephlebitis, should be administered in patients with any sign of infection.

Chronic portal vein thrombosis is defined as an obstructed portal vein replaced by collateral veins. Doppler ultrasound, MDCTA, or MRA will confirm the diagnosis. Patients may be asymptomatic but often have hypersplenism and portal hypertension (e.g., subclinical encephalopathy, rare ascites). Some patients may develop jaundice owing to biliary cholangiopathy and will require endoscopic placement of biliary stents. Endoscopic screening and treatment of varices (Chapter 136), with or without pharmacologic treatment of portal hypertension (Chapter 156), is recommended. After treatment of the varices, long-term anticoagulation therapy (see Table 81-4 in Chapter 81) should be considered in noncirrhotic patients whose permanent thrombotic risk factors are not otherwise correctable, unless there is a contraindication.

PROGNOSIS

Mortality rates after treatment of acute portal vein thrombosis are less than 10%, and the prognosis for patients with chronic portal vein thrombosis over 5 years is similar.

Splenic Vein Thrombosis

Splenic vein thrombosis is usually secondary to malignancy (e.g., pancreatic cancer), pancreatitis, or trauma. In many of these patients, isolated gastric varices develop and are difficult to treat by therapeutic endoscopy. Liver function and portal pressure are normal. Most patients with splenic vein thrombosis have splenomegaly (Chapter 171). Doppler ultrasound, MRI, and CT assist in making the diagnosis. Patients with symptomatic isolated splenic vein thrombosis (e.g., gastric variceal bleeding, hypersplenism) are best treated by splenectomy.

Hepatic and Splenic Arterial Disease

Hepatic arterial disease may be nonocclusive or occlusive. Nonocclusive disease, termed *ischemic hepatitis*, occurs when arterial blood flow to the liver is insufficient, usually because of cardiogenic hypotension, volume depletion, or sepsis. Typically, serum aminotransferase rises acutely to levels greater than 1000 U/L. With restoration of adequate hepatic arterial blood flow, serum aminotransferase levels eventually fall back to their baseline by about 40 to 60% per day. Hepatic artery thrombosis is extremely rare except in a post–liver transplantation (Chapter 157) patient, in whom it may be manifested as mild abnormalities in liver function test results, bile duct injury (e.g., biliary stricture, cholangitis, liver abscess), or liver failure. Doppler ultrasound and angiography will confirm the diagnosis, and these patients often require biliary stents, drainage of abscesses, surgical reconstruction of the hepatic artery, or retransplantation of the liver.

The splenic artery or hepatic artery may be predisposed to the development of aneurysmal dilation, usually secondary to atherosclerosis, trauma, portal hypertension, pancreatitis, pregnancy, infection, or vasculitis. Common clinical manifestations include abdominal pain and intra-abdominal hemorrhage. Hemobilia may occur with hepatic artery aneurysms.

Angiography is usually required to make the diagnosis. Symptomatic as well as sizable (variably defined, usually 1 cm or greater for a hepatic aneurysm and 2 cm or greater for a splenic artery aneurysm) aneurysms require surgery. Splenic artery aneurysms discovered during pregnancy are more likely to bleed and should be treated, usually by interventional radiology.

Fistulas from the hepatic artery to the portal vein can occur as a result of trauma, malignancy, or the inherited disorder hereditary hemorrhagic telangiectasia. The resultant portal hypertension may cause abdominal pain, ascites, and gastrointestinal bleeding, and involvement of the hepatic artery may result in biliary strictures and hepatobiliary infection. Radiographic embolization of these fistulas, surgery, or liver transplantation may be required.

SUGGESTED READINGS

Arthurs ZM, Titus J, Bannazadeh M, et al. A comparison of endovascular revascularization with traditional therapy for the treatment of acute mesenteric ischemia. *J Vasc Surg.* 2011;53:687-704. *Endovascular treatment was successful in 87% of patients with thrombotic or embolic arterial occlusions.*

DeLeve LD, Valla DC, Garcia-Tsao G. AASLD practice guidelines: vascular disorders of the liver. *Hepatology.* 2009;47:1729-1764. *Data-supported recommendations for diagnosis and treatment of vascular diseases of the liver.*

Feuerstadt P, Brandt LJ. Colon ischemia: recent insights and advances. *Curr Gastroenterol Rep.* 2010;12:383-390. *Review emphasizing that most patients respond to supportive therapy.*

Reissfelder C, Sweiti H, Antolovic D, et al. Ischemic colitis: who will survive? *Surgery.* 2011;149:585-592. *Nonocclusive ischemic colitis, acute renal failure, extent of bowel ischemia, serum lactate, and duration of catecholamine therapy predict survival.*

146

PANCREATITIS

CHRIS E. FORSMARK

TABLE 146-1 CAUSES OF ACUTE PANCREATITIS

ETIOLOGY	EXAMPLES
Gallstones	Gallstones Microlithiasis
Drugs and toxins	Ethyl and methyl alcohol Tobacco Azathioprine, 6-mercaptopurine, pentamidine, didanosine, sulfonamides, thiazides, aminosalicylates, valproic acid, and others Scorpion venom Insecticides
Metabolic	Hyperlipidemia Hypercalcemia
Trauma	After endoscopic retrograde cholangiopancreatography Blunt or penetrating trauma Postoperative
Obstruction of the pancreatic duct	Benign pancreatic duct stricture Benign ampullary stricture (e.g., celiac disease, diverticulum) Ampullary adenoma or adenocarcinoma Pancreatic ductal adenocarcinoma Intraductal papillary mucinous neoplasm Pancreas divisum Sphincter of Oddi dysfunction
Infections	Cytomegalovirus, mumps, rubella, coxsackie B virus *Candida*, histoplasmosis *Ascaris*
Genetics	*PRSS1* mutations *CFTR* mutation *SPINK1* mutation
Autoimmune pancreatitis	
Idiopathic pancreatitis	

ACUTE PANCREATITIS

DEFINITION

Acute pancreatitis is defined as a discrete episode of cellular injury and inflammation in the pancreas, usually with symptoms of abdominal pain, nausea, and vomiting, and typically accompanied by elevations in serum levels of amylase or lipase and by radiographic evidence of pancreatic inflammation, edema, or necrosis. Although pancreatic morphology and function may appear to recover promptly after the attack, recovery may not be complete if the damage is substantial. With repeated episodes, there is a shift from acute inflammation, necrosis, and apoptosis to the chronic inflammation and fibrosis that is characteristic of chronic pancreatitis. In some patients, it may be difficult to distinguish acute pancreatitis from a flare of chronic pancreatitis.

EPIDEMIOLOGY

The incidence of acute pancreatitis in the United States is estimated to be between 5 and 30 cases per 100,000 population, thereby resulting in about 250,000 hospital admissions annually and making acute pancreatitis the second most common gastrointestinal discharge diagnosis in U.S. hospitals. The cost of caring for these patients is about $4 to $6 billion annually. The incidence of acute pancreatitis is increasing in the United States and many other developed countries, perhaps because of better diagnostic tests but also perhaps owing to an increasing prevalence of gallstones (Chapter 158) in the setting of the obesity epidemic.

PATHOBIOLOGY

Acute pancreatitis is characterized by premature activation of digestive enzymes within the pancreas. In particular, the activation of trypsinogen to trypsin appears to be a critical initial step, with trypsin then activating other proteases within the gland. These activated enzymes produce cellular injury and death, which is a mixture of necrosis, apoptosis, and autophagy. Necrosis may involve not only the pancreas but also the surrounding fat and structures, thereby leading to fluid extravasation into the retroperitoneal spaces ("third space" losses). Although necrosis may be present in many cases, necrosis visible on a contrast-enhanced computed tomography (CT) scan is usually termed *acute necrotizing pancreatitis* and distinguished from the milder interstitial pancreatitis, in which necrosis is not visible on a CT scan. In addition to the local damage, the release of proinflammatory cytokines and activated digestive enzymes into the systemic circulation can produce a systemic inflammatory response syndrome (SIRS; Chapter 108) with hypotension, renal failure, and respiratory failure. Gallstones and alcohol account for about 70 to 80% of all cases of acute pancreatitis, but the cause is unknown in about 10% (Table 146-1).

Gallstones

Passage of a gallstone (Chapter 158) through the ampulla of Vater with transient obstruction of the pancreatic duct is the initiating event for gallstone pancreatitis. Only about 5% of all patients with gallstones develop pancreatitis, and patients with smaller gallstones (≤5 mm), which can pass the cystic duct and reach the ampulla, are at highest risk. Patients with microlithiasis, defined as tiny gallstones or biliary sludge, may account for up to 75% of patients initially labeled as having acute idiopathic pancreatitis.

Alcohol

More than 5 years of alcohol intake averaging more than 5 to 8 drinks daily is usually required before pancreatitis develops, but most people with this level of intake do not develop pancreatitis. A variety of cofactors have been proposed, including a high-fat diet, genetic variability in detoxifying enzymes, and cigarette smoking. By the time patients present with a first episode of acute pancreatitis, most already have evidence of underlying chronic pancreatitis. The mechanism of alcoholic pancreatic injury likely involves a mixture of direct toxicity, oxidative stress, and alterations in pancreatic enzyme secretion.

Drugs, Toxins, and Metabolic Factors

Drug-induced pancreatitis is a rare and generally idiosyncratic event. Implicated drugs include 6-mercaptopurine and azathioprine (up to a 4% attack rate), didanosine, pentamidine, valproic acid, furosemide, sulfonamides, and aminosalicylates. Toxins that may cause acute pancreatitis include methyl alcohol, organophosphate insecticides, and venom from certain scorpions.

Levels of serum triglycerides above 500 mg/dL, and usually more than 1000 mg/dL, can cause acute pancreatitis, but the mechanism is not known. Hyperlipidemic pancreatitis can be caused by the administration of estrogens, which can worsen underlying hypertriglyceridemia. Hypercalcemia is an exceedingly rare cause of acute pancreatitis.

Trauma

Iatrogenic trauma to the pancreas and pancreatic duct during performance of an endoscopic retrograde cholangiopancreatography (ERCP; Chapter 136) is a common cause of pancreatitis, with the risk ranging from less than 5% for those with simple common bile duct stones or malignancy, to as high as 20% for those with suspected sphincter of Oddi dysfunction. The risk of post-ERCP pancreatitis is markedly reduced with the placement of small-caliber temporary pancreatic duct stents.

Penetrating and blunt trauma ranging from a contusion to severe crush injury and even transection of the gland can cause pancreatitis. Acute presentation is the rule, but some patients with milder injury may present in a subacute or chronic fashion. Ischemic injury to the gland can occur after surgical procedures, especially cardiopulmonary bypass, and can be quite severe.

Obstruction of the Pancreatic Duct

In addition to gallstones and microlithiasis, obstruction of the pancreatic duct by a pancreatic ductal adenocarcinoma, ampullary adenoma or carcinoma, or an intraductal papillary mucinous neoplasm can cause acute pancreatitis. The diagnosis is usually established with endoscopic ultrasound (EUS). Benign strictures of the pancreatic duct or ampulla of Vater may be caused by celiac disease and periampullary diverticula. Sphincter of Oddi dysfunction, which is defined by abnormal manometry of the sphincter at the time of ERCP, and pancreas divisum, in which the larger dorsal pancreas drains through the smaller minor papilla, may also cause pancreatitis by obstruction of the pancreatic duct and should be considered in patients with repeated episodes of otherwise unexplained acute pancreatitis.

Infections and Autoimmune Pancreatitis

Ascaris lumbricoides (Chapter 365) may cause pancreatitis by obstructing the pancreatic duct as the worms migrate through the ampulla. Viruses that may infect the pancreatic acinar cells directly include cytomegalovirus (Chapter 384), Coxsackie B virus (Chapter 387), and mumps virus (Chapter 377). Fungal infections of the pancreas are exceedingly rare but may be seen in the setting of immunosuppression. Autoimmune pancreatitis, which can be systemic, affects the salivary glands, retroperitoneum, biliary ducts, and kidneys.

Genetics

Mutations in the cationic trypsinogen gene (*PRSS1*), which have been identified in families with hereditary pancreatitis, are more commonly seen in association with chronic pancreatitis but can be observed rarely in acute pancreatitis. Mutations in the cystic fibrosis conductance regulator (*CFTR*; Chapter 89) and the serine protease inhibitor Kazal type 1 (*SPINK1*) predispose to pancreatitis but do not cause pancreatitis in the absence of other provocations.

Idiopathic Acute Pancreatitis

Of the 25% of patients who do not have an identified cause after a basic initial evaluation, surreptitious alcohol use and microlithiasis are probably the most common underlying explanations. With additional evaluation and testing, only about 10% of patients are ultimately labeled as having idiopathic pancreatitis.

CLINICAL MANIFESTATIONS

Abdominal pain, nausea, and vomiting are the hallmark symptoms of acute pancreatitis. The abdominal pain is usually maximum in the epigastric region and often radiates to the back. The pain is steady, reaches its maximal intensity over 30 to 60 minutes, and persists for days. These characteristic symptoms may be masked in patients who present with delirium, multiple-organ system failure, or coma.

The physical examination usually reveals tachycardia. Hypotension, tachypnea, dyspnea, and fever are seen in more severe cases. Confusion, delirium, and even coma may be present. The abdomen is often distended with diminished bowel sounds. Tenderness to palpation of the abdomen, which may be epigastric or more diffuse, is typical, and rebound and guarding are seen in more severe cases. Dullness to percussion in the lower lung fields may be

noted owing to a pleural effusion. Rare physical findings include ecchymoses of the flank (Grey-Turner sign) or umbilicus (Cullen sign), which occur when fluid and blood tracks into these spaces from the retroperitoneum. Jaundice may be present if there is biliary obstruction by a stone.

The presence of tachycardia, dyspnea, tachypnea, orthostatic hypotension, pleural effusion, oxygen desaturation, or shock signal more substantial third space losses, a higher likelihood of a variety of complications (Table 146-2), and a worse prognosis. More severe pancreatitis is characterized by more substantial pancreatic and peripancreatic necrosis, more peripancreatic fluid collections, and more dysfunction of extrapancreatic organs.

DIAGNOSIS

The diagnosis of acute pancreatitis is suggested by the clinical features and confirmed by laboratory and imaging studies that exclude other serious intra-abdominal conditions, establish the presence of acute pancreatitis, and, hopefully, define the severity and most likely cause of the pancreatitis.

Laboratory Tests

Amylase and Lipase

Most patients with acute pancreatitis have elevations in serum levels of amylase or lipase within a few hours of the onset of symptoms. Lipase tends to remain elevated for longer than amylase, but both decline gradually over several days. Elevations more than three times the upper limit of normal are

---

TABLE 146-2 SCORING SYSTEMS TO ASSESS SEVERITY OF ACUTE PANCREATITIS

SYSTEM	CRITERIA	DEFINITION OF SEVERE PANCREATITIS

Ranson	At admission
	  Age > 55 years
	  WBC > 16,000/μL
	  Glucose > 200 mg/dL
	  LDH > 350 IU/L
	  AST > 250 IU/L
	Within next 48 hours
	  Decrease in hematocrit by > 10%
	  Estimated fluid sequestration of > 6 L
	  Serum calcium < 8.0 mg/dL
	  PaO_2 < 60 mm Hg
	  BUN increase > 5 mg/dL after hydration
	  Base deficit > 4 mmol/L
		Total score ≥ 3

APACHE-II	Multiple clinical and laboratory factors. Calculator available at *www.mdcalc.com/apache-ii-score-for-icu-mortality*	Total score ≥ 8
BISAP	BUN > 25 mg/dL Impaired mental status Presence of SIRS Age > 60 years Pleural effusion	Total score > 2
CT	A: Normal pancreas B: Focal or diffuse enlargement of pancreas C: Grade B plus pancreatic and/or peripancreatic inflammation D: Grade C plus a single fluid collection E: Grade C plus two or more fluid collections or gas in pancreas	Grade > C

CT severity index	CT grade
	  A = 0
	  B = 1
	  C = 2
	  D = 3
	  E = 4
	Plus necrosis grade
	No necrosis = 0
	  <30% necrosis = 2
	  30-50% necrosis = 4
	  >50% necrosis = 6
		Score > 5

AST = aspartate aminotransferase; BUN = blood urea nitrogen; CT = computed tomography; LDH = lactate dehydrogenase; SIRS = systemic inflammatory response syndrome; WBC = white blood count.

most specific for acute pancreatitis. Amylase and lipase levels may be normal in patients with acute pancreatitis, particularly if the measurement is delayed for several days after the onset of symptoms. Marked hypertriglyceridemia also can interfere with their accurate measurement. Both enzymes are cleared by the kidney, and renal failure can falsely raise the level of these enzymes up to five times the upper limit of normal in the absence of pancreatitis. Amylase and lipase also can be elevated in a variety of other conditions that may mimic acute pancreatitis, including intestinal ischemia and infarction (Chapter 145), bowel obstruction (Chapter 144), cholecystitis (Chapter 158), and choledocholithiasis (Chapter 158). In addition, amylase may be elevated from ectopic pregnancy, acute salpingitis, and a variety of extra-abdominal conditions such as parotitis, lung cancer, and head trauma. In some patients, only amylase or lipase may be elevated. Given its improved specificity, equal cost, and equal sensitivity, lipase is preferred over amylase as a single diagnostic test. Serial measurements of amylase or lipase in patients with established acute pancreatitis are not helpful in clinical decision making.

Other Laboratory Tests

In severe pancreatitis, leukocytosis and hemoconcentration may be seen. Failure of the blood urea nitrogen (BUN) level or hematocrit to normalize with fluid resuscitation is associated with a worse prognosis. Hyperglycemia, hypocalcemia, and mild hypertriglyceridemia can develop in more severe cases. Elevations in alanine aminotransferase levels more than three times the upper limit of normal are most suggestive of gallstones, although any significant elevation in liver chemistries should raise the possibility of gallstones (Chapter 158).

Imaging Studies

Imaging studies are used not only in establishing the diagnosis but also in determining etiology and prognosis. In most patients, both ultrasound and CT are used in a complementary fashion.

Abdominal ultrasound can confirm the presence of acute pancreatitis by documenting pancreatic enlargement, edema, or associated peripancreatic fluid collections. Visualization of the pancreas may be limited owing to body habitus or overlying intestinal gas. Importantly, ultrasound is most accurate in identifying gallstones in the gallbladder or a dilated common bile duct.

CT is more accurate than ultrasound in confirming the diagnosis of acute pancreatitis and in documenting the presence of pancreatic necrosis and peripancreatic fluid collections, but it is less accurate in identifying gallstones. CT is also particularly helpful in excluding intra-abdominal conditions that can mimic acute pancreatitis. On contrast-enhanced CT, pancreatic parenchyma that opacifies with intravenous contrast is considered still viable, whereas parenchyma that does not opacify is necrotic (Fig. 146-1). The extent of pancreatic necrosis, which is best seen about 3 days after presentation and may be missed in an early CT, has prognostic importance. CT

FIGURE 146-1. A computed tomographic scan demonstrating a large area of pancreas that does not enhance with intravenous contrast *(arrow)*, consistent with pancreatic necrosis.

scans are not routinely required in patients with acute pancreatitis but should be performed in patients with a first attack, with severe disease, with systemic complications, or when disease is slow to improve or the diagnosis is not clear.

Magnetic resonance imaging (MRI) is equivalent to CT in its ability to document acute pancreatitis, identify necrosis, and diagnose or exclude other diseases that could mimic acute pancreatitis. In addition, MRI with *magnetic resonance cholangiopancreatography* (MRCP) is much better than CT in identifying gallstones. MRI is more difficult than CT to perform in critically ill patients.

ERCP and EUS are important in both diagnosis and therapy of acute pancreatitis. EUS, which is primarily used to establish the cause when the initial evaluation is unrevealing, is particularly accurate in identifying underlying malignancy, premalignant lesions such as ampullary adenoma, and small gallstones or microlithiasis. ERCP is used primarily for therapeutic reasons, but it also may diagnose rare causes of pancreatitis such as pancreas divisum or sphincter of Oddi dysfunction.

Determining Etiology

To identify the cause of acute pancreatitis, the history should focus on alcohol and tobacco use, previous biliary colic, drug history, family history, and recent trauma. Alcohol use may need to be corroborated with family members. Gallstone pancreatitis should be suspected if stones are seen on imaging studies or if liver chemistries are abnormal and then improve over a few days. If these initial studies are unrevealing, EUS can detect small gallstones, microlithiasis, or underlying malignancy, particularly in patients older than 40 years. More specialized investigations like ERCP, sphincter of Oddi manometry, or genetic testing are usually reserved for patients seen in referral centers after multiple attacks of pancreatitis.

Determining Severity

Severe pancreatitis is characterized by organ system failure and by local pancreatic complications such as necrosis, fluid collections, or pseudocysts. Organ failure can be single or multiple, early or late onset, and progressive and persistent or transient. In severe acute pancreatitis, renal failure, pulmonary failure, and circulatory failure most commonly occur as part of the SIRS response. Severe pancreatitis also can be defined by local pancreatic and peripancreatic complications. Necrotizing pancreatitis as defined by CT is associated with a worse outcome, and the degree or amount of necrosis generally correlates with outcome, particularly if infection develops in the devitalized necrotic tissue.

During the acute attack, poorly demarcated fluid collections around the pancreas track into various retroperitoneal and peritoneal spaces. Much of this inflammatory fluid will resolve, but some will form into a more rounded and circumscribed fluid collection, called a *pseudocyst*. This process, which takes weeks, should be distinguished from early areas of pancreatic necrosis that may appear on CT as fluid collections and may be termed *pseudocysts* but in reality are collections of both liquid and solid necrotic material and are better described as *walled-off pancreatic necrosis*. Necrosis on CT, which can be seen in up to 25% of patients with acute pancreatitis and portends a worse outcome and particularly more substantial necrosis, is associated with higher rates of serious pancreatic infections. Organ system failure is quite rare in the absence of pancreatic necrosis.

Clinical features may help identify patients at higher risk, including patients who are older, are obese, or have more serious or more numerous comorbid conditions. In addition, a number of scoring systems can help guide clinicians in gauging prognosis.

The best known multiple-factor scoring systems are the Ranson criteria and Acute Physiology and Chronic Health Evaluation (APACHE) II score (see Table 146-2). Practice guidelines suggest a cutoff of more than 8 APACHE II points or more than 3 Ranson points as the definition of severe disease. Each approach has a high false-positive rate, in that many patients with high scores do not develop organ failure or die. An elevated admission BUN that does not return to normal with fluid therapy is associated with increased mortality, and a C-reactive protein level higher than 150 mg/L at 48 hours may be as accurate as multiple-factor scoring systems at predicting poor outcome. A simpler system is the "BISAP" score (*B*UN > 25 mg/dL, *I*mpaired mental status, *S*IRS, *A*ge > 60, and *P*leural effusion), in which mortality ranges from <1% for patients with none or only one of those risk factors (BISAP score of 0 or 1) to 27% for a BISAP score of 5. Each scoring system should be considered as a guide but not a replacement for clinical judgment.

TREATMENT   Rx

General Supportive Care

Most patients recover within several days, but it is usually not possible to identify these patients at the time of admission. All patients should be made NPO. Pain control usually requires parenteral narcotics, and hydromorphone (in divided doses of 1 to 2 mg given intravenously every 4 to 6 hours initially, with titration as needed, or more commonly as patient-controlled analgesia) is generally preferred. Patients with significant third space loss, often augmented by fluid losses through vomiting, will have evidence of intravascular fluid depletion. Even in mild pancreatitis, fluid losses may be substantial. Appropriate fluid resuscitation, which is one of the few medical interventions that appears to affect outcome, should be accomplished within the first 24 hours of admission to correct the blood pressure and pulse, to reduce the hematocrit and blood urea nitrogen levels to normal, and to ensure a urine output of at least 0.5 mL/kg/hour. Crystalloid, either normal or half-normal saline or lactated Ringer's solution, is preferred. If nausea and vomiting require treatment, promethazine (12.5 to 25 mg intravenously three times daily) is usually successful, although some patients may be more effectively treated with 5-HT3 antagonists (e.g., ondansetron, 8 mg orally or 4 or 8 mg intravenously up to every 8 hours). Nasogastric suction is needed for those with intractable nausea and vomiting. Patients can be fed, preferably with a full solid diet,[1] when bowel sounds and appetite have returned, nausea has resolved, enzyme levels are normalized, and pain is controlled.

In patients with more severe pancreatitis, based on the severity of their comorbid conditions, early organ system failure, or substantial third space fluid losses, admission to an intensive care unit (ICU) is appropriate. Vigorous fluid replacement, as outlined previously, which may reach 5 to 10 L/day, is required. Appropriate fluid resuscitation can be gauged by serial measurements of BUN and hematocrit as well as by urine output. Careful monitoring for progressive organ system failure and metabolic complications is critical in these patients.

Patients who appear to have sufficiently severe disease that they might not be able to eat for 5 to 7 days should be started on nutritional therapy. Trials suggest that enteral nutrition, using an elemental or semi-elemental formula, is associated with fewer complications, including hyperglycemia and line infections, compared with total parenteral nutrition.[2] Nasogastric feeding is easier and may be as good as nasojejunal feeding.[3]

Treatment of Complications

Most patients who develop acute gallstone pancreatitis have already passed the offending stone into the duodenum, but patients with a persistent stone or multiple stones are at higher risk of developing cholangitis and more severe pancreatitis. Data support current practice guidelines that recommend early ERCP in patients who have gallstone pancreatitis and evidence of concomitant cholangitis (e.g., fever, jaundice, right upper quadrant pain) or of a persistent bile duct stone (e.g., visible persistent stone on imaging study, jaundice, persistently dilated bile duct, worsening liver chemistries at 48 hours after admission).[4] Early ERCP is occasionally considered for patients who have severe pancreatitis, as evidenced by early and progressive organ system failure, but who do not have cholangitis or strong evidence of a stone; however, data do not support benefit from this intervention.[5] There is no other role for early endoscopic intervention in patients with acute pancreatitis.

The systemic complications (Table 146-3) that develop from multiple-organ system failure in patients with severe acute pancreatitis include some that are similar to those commonly encountered in other ICU patients as well as specific metabolic complications of severe pancreatitis. Hyperglycemia is commonly a result of the pancreatitis and may be seen with enteral nutrition; hyperglycemia may contribute to higher rates of infections. In severe acute pancreatitis, ionized calcium levels are usually normal, but hypocalcemia is common owing to a diminished serum albumin level; treatment (Chapter 253) is not needed in the absence of signs of hypocalcemia, such as tetany or a Chvostek's sign. Mild hypertriglyceridemia is common, but underlying hypertriglyceridemia is often the cause of acute pancreatitis when levels of triglycerides surpass 1000 mg/dL; triglyceride levels usually drop promptly when the patient is made NPO, but plasmapheresis may be required.

Any hospital-acquired infection dramatically worsens prognosis. Infections in patients with acute pancreatitis include urinary tract infections, pulmonary infections, line infections, and *Clostridium difficile* infection. High-quality nursing care, antibiotic stewardship, and careful attention to catheters and lines can minimize these infections.

For necrotizing pancreatitis, a step-up approach of percutaneous drainage followed, if necessary, by minimally invasive retroperitoneal necrosectomy reduces the risk of multiple-organ failure by more than two thirds and new diabetes by more than 50% with no change in in-hospital mortality compared with routine open necrosectomy.[6] Patients with necrotizing pancreatitis may develop infected pancreatic necrosis, which increases mortality to nearly 30%. Infection of preexisting necrosis typically occurs 2 to 3 weeks into the illness and is heralded by fever, leukocytosis, and worsening abdominal pain. The responsible organisms are usually gram-negative rods and other gut flora, but *Staphylococcus aureus* (Chapter 296) is an important agent as well. If infected necrosis is suspected, a CT scan should be obtained, followed by CT-directed fine-needle aspiration of the necrotic area for culture and Gram stain. If infection is documented, antibiotics tailored to the organism should be promptly initiated. Conservative therapy is continued, often for weeks, to allow the necrotic material to demarcate, begin to liquefy, and become encapsulated. When this walled-off necrosis is sufficiently liquefied to allow less invasive approaches, therapy can include percutaneous, endoscopic, or minimally invasive surgical therapy. Open surgical drainage is reserved for patients with progressive clinical deterioration and sepsis.

Given that infected necrosis has such substantial impact on prognosis, numerous studies have assessed the ability of prophylactic antibiotics to prevent infection in patients with preexisting sterile pancreatic necrosis. Data are unconvincing,[7] and current practice guidelines do not endorse prophylactic antibiotics in sterile pancreatic necrosis.

Fluid collections around the pancreas are common in acute pancreatitis and do not require any specific therapy. Most will resolve spontaneously, whereas some will mature into an encapsulated pseudocyst. It is important to distinguish a pseudocyst (usually outside the confines of the pancreas and filled with fluid) from an area of necrosis (usually inside the confines of the pancreas and a mixture of solid and liquid material). Therapy is not needed for asymptomatic pseudocysts, even if they are large, but therapy is indicated for pseudocysts that cause abdominal pain, obstruct a surrounding hollow viscus, or are associated with infection or bleeding. Bleeding may be limited to within the pseudocyst itself or may reach the intestine through the pancreatic duct if the pseudocyst is in communication with the duct. In some patients, bleeding into the pseudocyst may be caused by a pseudoaneurysm of a nearby visceral artery; this type of bleeding may be massive. Unexplained gastrointestinal bleeding or a sudden, unexplained drop in the hematocrit in a patient with pancreatitis or a pseudocyst should prompt an emergent CT scan, followed by embolization if a pseudoaneurysm is identified. A pseudocyst can be treated successfully using endoscopic, percutaneous or surgical techniques, and the choice among these approaches can be determined by local expertise.

Prevention of Relapse

Preventing relapse requires a clear knowledge of the precipitating causes. Abstinence from alcohol (Chapter 32) and tobacco (Chapter 31) should be strongly encouraged, including referral to appropriate resources. Cholecystectomy (Chapter 158) prevents subsequent attacks of gallstone pancreatitis and should be accomplished within a few weeks of discharge, if not sooner, if gallstones are the cause. In patients who have gallstone pancreatitis but who are not surgical candidates, endoscopic sphincterotomy provides reasonable protection from subsequent attacks. Control of serum lipids (Chapter 213) prevents subsequent attacks of hyperlipidemic pancreatitis. Therapy of lesions that obstruct the pancreatic duct, such as strictures, ampullary adenomas, and possibly sphincter of Oddi dysfunction and pancreas divisum, may also prevent relapse.

TABLE 146-3   COMPLICATIONS OF ACUTE PANCREATITIS

COMPLICATION	EXAMPLES
Systemic complications	Hypotension and shock
	Adult respiratory distress syndrome
	Acute renal failure
	Disseminated intravascular coagulation
	Hypocalcemia
	Hypertriglyceridemia
	Hyperglycemia
	Encephalopathy and coma
Gastrointestinal bleeding	Stress ulceration
	Pseudoaneurysm
Local (pancreatic) complications	Acute fluid collection
	Pseudocyst
	Pancreatic necrosis (infected and sterile)
	Duodenal and biliary obstruction

PROGNOSIS

More than 80% of all patients with acute pancreatitis recover promptly without developing severe pancreatitis. Mortality is usually from progressive multiple-organ system failure, either from the acute pancreatitis itself or from hospital-acquired infections, including infection of pancreatic fluid collections and pancreatic necrosis. The presence of early organ failure (within 24 hours of admission), multiple-organ system failure, and persistent or progressive (present beyond 48 hours after admission) organ failure are associated with prolonged hospitalization, ICU admission, need for surgery, and death. Overall mortality is about 2% but can be as high as 20% in patients referred to tertiary hospitals. Mortality can approach 30% in patients with more severe comorbid conditions and in patients who develop pancreatic necrosis, infection, or organ system failure. Although high-quality ICU care minimizes mortality, no specific therapy is currently available to affect these risks.

CHRONIC PANCREATITIS

DEFINITION

Chronic pancreatitis, which is a complex process rather than an isolated event, implies the presence of irreversible and permanent fibrosis, often with chronic mononuclear cell inflammation, damage to nerves, and loss of ducts, acini, and islets. Chronic pancreatitis evolves after episodes of acute pancreatitis, which may be subclinical, but the transition between acute and chronic pancreatitis may be difficult to identify.

EPIDEMIOLOGY

The prevalence of symptomatic chronic pancreatitis in Western countries is about 25 to 30 per 100,000 population, with an estimated incidence of 3 to 9 cases per 100,000. In the United States, chronic pancreatitis accounts for about 125,000 outpatient visits and 25,000 hospitalizations yearly. Interestingly, the prevalence of histologic evidence of chronic pancreatitis in autopsy studies approaches 5%, indicating that many people apparently develop chronic pancreatic damage as a consequence of normal aging, other diseases, or exposure to toxins, such as consumption of alcohol, but do not develop any symptoms or signs of chronic pancreatitis during life.

PATHOBIOLOGY

Multiple episodes of acute inflammation, whether clinical or subclinical, eventually change the inflammatory milieu of the pancreas, with a shift to chronic inflammation, the activation of pancreatic stellate cells, and the production of fibrosis. This process is self-sustaining and produces the characteristic histologic damage noted previously. Genetic mutations predispose to chronic pancreatitis, but the genetic predisposition is superimposed on exposure to various toxins, which precipitate acute pancreatitis, with cellular necrosis or apoptosis, that progresses in some individuals, particularly those with multiple episodes, to a chronic and fibrotic process. In Western countries, alcohol and tobacco abuse are the dominant causes of chronic pancreatitis.

One important contributor to the pain in chronic pancreatitis is damage to pancreatic nociceptive nerves and the complex neuroimmune interaction driven by the chronic inflammatory state. Chronic pain produces visceral, spinal cord, and central hyperalgesia, and the pain may become self-perpetuating even if therapy on the pancreas is successful. In addition to this neural mechanism, increased pressure within the gland, associated ischemia, obstruction of the pancreatic duct, and a pseudocyst can cause pain.

Alcohol and Tobacco

Alcohol (Chapter 32) causes about 70 to 80% of all cases of chronic pancreatitis in the United States and other major industrial countries. Substantial and prolonged ingestion of alcohol is usually required, on the order of 5 to 8 drinks daily over more than 5 years. Most people who consume this much alcohol do not develop chronic pancreatitis, pointing to important cofactors such as genetic background and cigarette smoking. There is evidence that tobacco alone (Chapter 31) can cause chronic pancreatitis, and the combination of alcohol and tobacco may be synergistic. Most patients will present initially with an episode of acute pancreatitis but will shortly thereafter develop evidence of chronic pancreatitis, but others will have obvious chronic pancreatitis at their first presentation.

Genetic

Hereditary pancreatitis is an autosomal dominant disease characterized by early onset of acute and chronic pancreatitis, the development of exocrine and endocrine pancreatic insufficiency, and a high risk of pancreatic adenocarcinoma. Mutations in the trypsinogen (*PRSS1*) gene in these families appear to cause a gain in function in which the mutant trypsinogen, once activated to trypsin, is difficult to inactivate. This trypsin, if present in an amount that overwhelms normal protective mechanisms, can activate other pancreatic enzymes and lead to pancreatic damage and eventually to chronic

pancreatitis. One of the protective mechanisms is a trypsin inhibitor called *SPINK1*. Loss of function mutations in *SPINK1* may predispose to chronic pancreatitis, but unlike *PRSS1* mutations, are not sufficient to cause chronic pancreatitis. Major mutations in *CFTR* lead to cystic fibrosis (Chapter 89), which is associated with chronic pancreatitis and pancreatic atrophy. Milder mutations in *CFTR*, which predispose to chronic pancreatitis without causing the sinopulmonary features of cystic fibrosis, are encountered in patients with idiopathic chronic pancreatitis.

Other Causes

Autoimmune pancreatitis is a disease that most often presents as a masslike lesion with obstructive jaundice, mimicking cancer, but it also may present as chronic pancreatitis and rarely as acute pancreatitis. Characteristic features of the disease include a diffuse swelling of the pancreas, elevations in serum immunoglobulin G4 (IgG4), and involvement of other organs, especially biliary strictures, salivary gland inflammation, retroperitoneal fibrosis, and renal lesions. Histologically, these organs are infiltrated by chronic inflammatory cells, especially plasma cells bearing IgG4 on their surface.

Tropical pancreatitis is seen primarily in southern India. Characteristic features include childhood onset, exocrine insufficiency, diffuse pancreatic calcifications, and inevitable diabetes. There may be a genetic component (*SPINK1*), but cofactors such as malnutrition and dietary toxins have been suggested. In southern India, this disease is becoming uncommon and is being replaced by alcohol as the most common cause of idiopathic chronic pancreatitis.

Although most chronic pancreatitis evolves from multiple episodes of acute pancreatitis, a single severe acute attack that causes substantial pancreatic necrosis can destroy enough gland to produce exocrine and endocrine insufficiency. In addition, diseases that cause repeated attacks of pancreatitis can lead to chronic pancreatitis. For example, *hypertriglyceridemia* causes acute pancreatitis but commonly leads to chronic pancreatitis.

In about 20% of patients, no clear cause of chronic pancreatitis is found. Some patients may have underlying genetic mutations, and others may be surreptitiously using alcohol or tobacco. Two general forms of idiopathic chronic pancreatitis are seen. In the first, pain is the predominant feature, and the onset of disease is in young adulthood. In the second, the onset is in middle age, and exocrine and endocrine insufficiency, rather than abdominal pain, are the major clinical manifestations.

CLINICAL MANIFESTATIONS

The most common symptom of chronic pancreatitis is abdominal pain. The pain may be episodic or constant, and it is generally felt in the epigastrium with radiation to the back. If pain is episodic, the patient may be labeled as having acute pancreatitis or an acute flare of chronic pancreatitis. When pain is severe, nausea and vomiting may occur. Pain may worsen, improve, or remain stable over time. Up to 5% of patients do not have pain and instead present with exocrine (steatorrhea, weight loss) or endocrine (diabetes) pancreatic insufficiency. The disease tends to be progressive over time, even if the original cause (e.g., alcohol) is removed. The pathophysiology of pain is complex.

DIAGNOSIS

The diagnosis may be suspected based on the clinical features but should be confirmed by tests that identify structural damage to the pancreas or derangements in pancreatic function (Table 146-4). Chronic pancreatitis is a slowly

TABLE 146-4 DIAGNOSTIC TESTS FOR CHRONIC PANCREATITIS

STRUCTURAL	FUNCTIONAL
Biopsy	Hormonal (secretin) test
Endoscopic ultrasound	Fecal elastase
Endoscopic retrograde cholangiopancreatography	Serum trypsin
Magnetic resonance imaging with magnetic resonance cholangiopancreatography	Fecal fat
Computed tomography	Blood glucose
Ultrasonography	
Plain x-ray	

FIGURE 146-2. A computed tomography scan demonstrating diffuse pancreatic calcification in a patient with long-standing chronic pancreatitis (arrows).

FIGURE 146-3. Endoscopic retrograde cholangiopancreatography demonstrating a very irregular pancreatic duct with areas of dilation and structuring in a patient with chronic pancreatitis (arrows).

progressive disease in which visible damage to the gland (e.g., on a CT scan) and functional failure (e.g., steatorrhea or diabetes) may not be apparent for years. All diagnostic tests are most accurate when the disease is far advanced, and all are far less accurate in the early stages of disease.

Tests of Pancreatic Structure

Plain abdominal radiographs may demonstrate diffuse or focal pancreatic calcification in patients with advanced chronic pancreatitis. Although specific for chronic pancreatitis, these findings are quite insensitive.

Abdominal ultrasound is of limited utility because overlying gas often limits the ability to visualize the pancreas. An abnormal pancreatic duct, pancreatic calcifications, gland atrophy, or changes in echotexture are seen in about 60% of patients.

CT is the most widely used diagnostic test for chronic pancreatitis, and high-quality images can be obtained of the pancreas and pancreatic duct. Characteristic findings include a dilated pancreatic duct, ductal or parenchymal calcifications, and atrophy (Fig. 146-2). These structural changes take years to develop, so CT is not as accurate in early or less advanced disease. Like CT, MRI allows detailed images of the pancreas, and the addition of MRCP allows even better assessment of pancreatic duct morphology. At some centers, secretin is administered at the time of MRCP to allow better visualization of the pancreatic duct.

ERCP provides the most detailed images of the pancreatic duct. Changes in the duct, including dilation, irregularity, ductal stones, and strictures, can be appreciated (Fig. 146-3). These findings are not completely specific for chronic pancreatitis and can be seen in other situations, including with pancreatic cancer and in very elderly individuals. ERCP carries risk but has the advantage of providing both diagnostic and therapeutic impact.

EUS allows very detailed images of pancreatic parenchyma and duct (Fig. 146-4). A normal EUS essentially excludes chronic pancreatitis, whereas a very abnormal EUS is highly consistent with chronic pancreatitis.

Tests of Pancreatic Function

Serum trypsinogen (also called *trypsin*) is abnormally low in patients with far advanced chronic pancreatitis but is often normal in patients with less advanced disease. Levels lower than 20 ng/mL are seen in patients with chronic pancreatitis that is sufficient to cause functional failure (e.g., steatorrhea). Serum levels of amylase or lipase are not useful for chronic pancreatitis. Serum glucose levels will be elevated in those with endocrine insufficiency.

Quantification of fat in stool during a 72-hour collection while on a high-fat diet can be used to document steatorrhea (Chapter 142) but is rarely performed. Qualitative analysis of fat with Sudan staining of a stool specimen has poor sensitivity and specificity. Fecal levels of pancreatic elastase are diminished to less than 100 μg/g in patients with advanced chronic pancre-

FIGURE 146-4. Endoscopic ultrasound in a patient with chronic pancreatitis, demonstrating a dilated pancreatic duct (marks on margin of main duct).

atitis and steatorrhea. The test can be performed while patients are taking pancreatic enzyme therapy.

For a pancreatic function test, a tube is passed into the duodenum, where pancreatic secretions are collected over the course of 1 hour in 15-minute aliquots and analyzed for bicarbonate concentration after a supraphysiologic dose of secretin is administered. A normal study is defined by at least one of the samples having a bicarbonate concentration of more than 80 mEq/L. The test becomes abnormal earlier in the disease process than any other test, so it is well suited to diagnose chronic pancreatitis earlier in its clinical course; however, it is not widely available. An alternative, using endoscopy instead of a tube, is possible but somewhat less sensitive.

Diagnostic Approach

As the disease advances over years, structural and functional damage accumulate to the point that essentially all diagnostic tests are positive. In most patients, the diagnosis is established by routine tests such as CT or MRI; EUS and ERCP are rarely needed for diagnostic purposes in patients with long-standing chronic pancreatitis. The diagnostic challenge lies with patients who present with a severe pain syndrome suggestive of chronic pancreatitis but who have a normal CT or MRI. In these patients, EUS is the best choice unless the physician has access to a secretin-based pancreatic function test. ERCP should not be used for purely diagnostic purposes because patients with a normal-appearing pancreas are particularly prone to complications, especially post-ERCP pancreatitis.

TREATMENT Rx

Abdominal Pain

A search for specifically treatable complications should be undertaken before initiating therapy for pain. Causes include a pseudocyst, obstruction of a surrounding hollow organ (e.g., duodenum or bile duct), or superimposed carcinoma. A good-quality CT or MRI image is usually sufficient to exclude these possibilities. These imaging tests also help in choosing appropriate therapy. Patients with a dilated pancreatic duct (generally >5 mm) are candidates for endoscopic and surgical therapy, which involves decompression of the dilated duct. Patients without duct dilation are generally not appropriate for endoscopic and surgical therapy and must rely instead on medical therapy (Table 146-5).

Medical therapy starts with vigorous attempts to assist patients in stopping alcohol and tobacco, if applicable. Most patients will require analgesics. It is appropriate to start with the less potent agents first, such as tramadol (50 mg, usually starting at one dose given every 6 hours). In patients who require more potent narcotics, it may be helpful to add an adjunctive antidepressant (e.g., amitriptyline, starting at 50 mg at night), selective serotonin reuptake inhibitors (see Table 404-5 in Chapter 404), gabapentin (starting at 100 mg at night), or pregabalin (starting at 50 mg three times daily). Antioxidants (mixtures of selenium, vitamins E and C, β-carotene, and methionine) may also have some beneficial effect on pain.[8] Finally, pancreatic enzyme therapy may have some beneficial effect on pain. Non-enteric-coated (tablet) pancreatic enzymes can reduce pancreatic stimulation and reduce pain by digesting a releasing factor present in the duodenum and providing negative feedback on the pancreas; conversely enteric-coated preparations, which are not active in the duodenum, have no proven effect on pain. These nonenteric preparations are not currently approved for clinical use but must be given with an agent to reduce gastric acid because acid will denature the proteases in these tablets. Autoimmune pancreatitis responds promptly to steroid therapy (usually 40 mg of prednisone daily for 4 weeks, with a taper of 5 mg/week over the next 7 weeks), but relapse may occur, particularly in the biliary tree.

Nerve Block and Neurolysis

EUS-guided celiac plexus block, using a local anesthetic and a steroid, or neurolysis, using absolute alcohol, can be performed relatively easily and safely, but substantial relief of pain is achieved for only weeks or months.[9] This therapy generally is considered only as a temporizing measure to provide relief from debilitating pain.

Endoscopic Therapy and Lithotripsy

At the time of ERCP, strictures can be dilated, and stents can be placed across the stricture. Ductal stones, if they are not too large and are not affected, may also be removed. Lithotripsy of larger stones is usually required to reduce the stone to fragments that are manageable. Only a subset of patients with chronic pancreatitis has ductal anatomy that is amenable to this type of therapy. In large case series from expert centers, therapy is technically successful in more than 80% of carefully selected patients, and pain relief may be seen in 70 to 80% of patients who undergo therapy. In patients with large stones, intraductal or extracorporeal lithotripsy is needed.

Surgical Therapy

Surgery for chronic pancreatitis is more effective and more durable than endoscopic therapy.[10],[11] Surgery can involve decompression of the pancreatic duct, resection of the pancreas, or a combination of the two. The most commonly performed procedure, the modified Puestow procedure, involves a longitudinal incision of the pancreatic duct from the body of the pancreas to as close to the duodenum as possible, and this filleted duct is overlaid with a defunctionalized Roux limb. At the time of surgery, ductal strictures can be incised, and ductal stones can be removed. The procedure is relatively simple in patients with a dilated pancreatic duct (>5 mm). Pain relief in the short term is good (>80%), with about 50% obtaining long-term relief of pain. Alternative surgical procedures for pain include some resection of the pancreas, typically the head of the gland, in patients who have an inflammatory mass that causes biliary or duodenal obstruction. These operations, which include the classic pancreaticoduodenectomy (Whipple operation), provide equal short-term pain relief and better long-term pain relief than a modified Puestow, but with a higher morbidity. Total pancreatectomy, usually coupled with autotransplantation of harvested islet cells, is performed at a small number of centers but is generally considered a therapy of last resort, given the fact that diabetes mellitus is common after the procedure and pain relief is inconsistent.

Exocrine Insufficiency

Steatorrhea and maldigestion do not occur until approximately 90% of pancreatic enzyme secretion is lost, usually after 5 to 10 years of disease or even longer. Patients may note weight loss and oily stools, but often do not complain of diarrhea. Patients with chronic pancreatitis and exocrine insufficiency maldigest fat, protein, and carbohydrates, but fat maldigestion is usually most severe. In addition to weight loss, malabsorption of fat-soluble vitamins, particularly vitamin D, may occur. The diagnosis of exocrine insufficiency is usually suggested by symptoms of oily or floating stools and weight loss. A formal 72 stool fat analysis (Chapter 142) is the most accurate method to document steatorrhea and to gauge effectiveness of therapy but is rarely done. Instead, the clinical features and a fecal elastase of less than 100 µg/g stool, coupled with an appropriate response to enzyme replacement therapy, is the best substitute for 72-hour fecal fat testing.

Enzyme therapy (Table 146-6), which significantly reduces fecal fat levels and may reduce weight loss,[12] is divided into enteric-coated capsules and non-enteric-coated tablets. Non-enteric-coated preparations, as noted previously, are not clinically available but theoretically are the agents of choice if the goal is to treat pain. However, the enteric-coated preparations are used more frequently for exocrine insufficiency because they are more potent and require fewer pills. Enzymes are identified by the lipase content of the pill or capsule, although they all contain proteases and amylase as well. The goal of enzyme therapy, which is to administer at least 10% of normal pancreatic output with each meal, translates to approximately 30,000 IU of lipase with each meal. Most current products are measured in U.S. Pharmacopeia (USP) units, which are one third the amount of an international unit (IU) (e.g., up to 90,000 USP units of lipase with each meal). Because most patients are still producing some enzymes (including gastric lipase), it is usually not necessary to use the full dosage of 90,000 USP units with each meal.

Enzymes should be split during the meal (e.g., equally split before, during, and immediately after the meal). Supplementation with vitamin D (400 to 1000 IU daily) and calcium (1.0 to 1.5 g daily) is appropriate because osteoporosis (Chapter 251) and osteopenia are common. Success of enzyme therapy is generally defined as weight gain and reduction or absence of visible oil in the stool. Failure of enzyme therapy is most often due to inadequate dose. Increasing the dose up to the full 90,000 USP units with meals and encouraging compliance are appropriate as a first step. Some enteric-coated preparations may not release sufficient enzymes in the small bowel unless they are used with an agent to reduce gastric acid. Some patients may not respond owing to the presence of a second disease that also causes malabsorption, such as small intestinal bacterial overgrowth.

Endocrine Insufficiency

Like exocrine insufficiency, diabetes mellitus (Chapter 236) is a very late complication of chronic pancreatitis, occurring years or decades after disease onset. Unlike type 1 diabetes mellitus, there is destruction of the entire islet, which reduces secretion of both insulin and glucagon. As a result, overly aggressive therapy may lead to hypoglycemia, which cannot be reversed by

TABLE 146-5	TREATMENT FOR PAIN
TREATMENT	**EXAMPLES**
Medical therapy	Alcohol and tobacco cessation
	Analgesics and adjunctive agents
	Tramadol, 50 mg, one to three times daily
	Amitriptyline, starting at 50 mg at night
	Selective serotonin reuptake inhibitors (citalopram, fluoxetine, sertraline, paroxetine, and others) at recommended starting dose (see Table 404-5 in Chapter 404)
	Gabapentin, starting at 100 mg at night
	Pregabalin, starting at 50 mg three times daily
	Antioxidants
	Typical mixture containing vitamin C (1000 mg), vitamin E (300 IU), selenium (500 µg, methionine 2 g, and β-carotene 10,000 IU) total daily dose
	Non-enteric-coated enzymes (see Table 146-6)
Neurolysis	Endoscopic ultrasound–guided celiac plexus block or neurolysis
	Thoracoscopic splanchnicectomy
Endoscopic therapy	Stent
	Stone removal, lithotripsy
Surgical therapy	Pancreaticojejunostomy (modified Puestow operation)
	Partial pancreatic resection (Whipple operation, duodenum-preserving pancreatic head resection, others)
	Total pancreatectomy with islet cell autotransplantation

TABLE 146-6 ENZYME THERAPY FOR EXOCRINE INSUFFICIENCY*

AGENT†	DOSAGE
Creon 6000	10-15 with meals
Creon 12,000	5-8 with meals
Creon 24,000	3-4 with meals
Zenpep 5,000	12-18 with meals
Zenpep 10,000	6-10 with meals
Zenpep 15,000	4-6 with meals
Zenpep 20,000	3-5 with meals
Pancreaze 4200	15-18 with meals
Pancreaze 10,000	6-10 with meals
Pancreaze 16,800	4-5 with meals
Pancreaze 21,000	3-5 with meals

*Brand names. All contain pancrealipase.
†As more manufacturers receive U.S. Food and Drug Administration approval, this list may change.

FIGURE 146-5. On computed tomography, a large pseudocyst is seen *(black arrows)*. In addition, ascites surrounding the liver *(white arrow)* is due to a leak from the pseudocyst (pancreatic ascites).

the usual natural glucagon surge. In most patients, therefore, insulin treatment is not aimed at exceeding tight glucose control. Unfortunately, these patients are at similar risk for microvascular complications, as are all other patients with diabetes.

Complications

Pancreatic Pseudocyst

Pseudocysts, when they are discovered in patients with chronic pancreatitis, are generally mature and have a visible capsule surrounding them. As in acute pancreatitis, benign pseudocysts in chronic pancreatitis do not require therapy if they are not producing symptoms and are not rapidly enlarging. However, some cystic structures in and around the pancreas are cystic neoplasms, not pseudocysts. Symptomatic pseudocysts require drainage, whereas neoplasms require resection. Features that suggest a cystic neoplasm include a cyst with a thick or nodular wall, a cyst with multiple internal septations, or a cyst occurring in a patient who does not have a history of pancreatitis. Any combination of these features should lead to further investigation, generally with EUS and cyst aspiration.

Symptomatic pseudocysts can be treated with endoscopic, percutaneous, or surgical therapy with equal efficacy. In many centers, EUS-guided drainage is becoming first-line therapy. Both short-term and long-term results are excellent. Complications of pseudocysts include infection, bleeding, and rupture. A visceral artery pseudoaneurysm, which may develop as a consequence of a pseudocyst, can bleed torrentially, sometimes preceded by a brief self-limited bleed that stops when the blood is tamponaded within the pseudocyst. If the pseudocyst is in continuity with the pancreatic duct, blood may traverse the duct and enter the duodenum to cause melena; this release of pressure can produce exsanguinating bleeding. Any evidence of gastrointestinal bleeding or unexplained anemia in a patient with known pseudocyst or pancreatitis should raise the possibility of pseudoaneurysm. Embolization of the pseudoaneurysm is highly effective.

Pseudocysts may leak into the peritoneal compartment (pancreatic ascites) or track into the chest (pancreatic pleural effusion). Patients usually present with abdominal distention or dyspnea, rather than abdominal pain. Amylase level in the fluid is usually higher than 4000 U/L. Endoscopic therapy with stent placement across the connection between pseudocyst and pancreatic duct is highly effective in this situation (Fig. 146-5).

Malignancy

Chronic pancreatitis is a strong risk factor for pancreatic ductal adenocarcinoma (Chapter 200), with a lifetime risk of about 4%. The risk of cancer is much greater in patients with hereditary pancreatitis, in whom the risk may range as high as 40 to 70%. Equally importantly, it may be difficult to distinguish cancer from benign disease, particularly in patients with autoimmune pancreatitis.

PREVENTION

Currently, there are no reliable methods to prevent chronic pancreatitis. Patients at risk for chronic pancreatitis, such as members of families with hereditary pancreatitis and patients with established chronic pancreatitis, should avoid alcohol and tobacco and should probably be placed on a low-fat diet.

PROGNOSIS

With prolonged follow-up of 10 to 20 years, most patients will develop exocrine or endocrine insufficiency. The overall mortality is increased 3.6-fold compared with age-matched controls. Patients who are older, smoke, or have alcohol as the cause are at highest risk of mortality. Overall, 10-year survival approximates 70%, and 20-year survival is about 45%. Death is usually not due to pancreatitis itself, but rather to malignancy, postoperative complications, and complications of alcohol or tobacco.

Grade A

1. Moraes JM, Felga GE, Chebli LA, et al. A full solid diet as the initial meal in mild acute pancreatitis is safe and results in a shorter length of hospitalization: results from a prospective, randomized, controlled, double-blind clinical trial. *J Clin Gastroenterol.* 2010;44:517-522.
2. Petrov MS, van Santvoort HC, Besselink MG, et al. Enteral nutrition and the risk of mortality and infectious complications in patients with severe acute pancreatitis: a meta-analysis of randomized trials. *Arch Surg.* 2008;143:1111-1117.
3. Eatock FC, Chong P, Menezes N, et al. A randomized study of early nasogastric versus nasojejunal feeding in severe acute pancreatitis. *Am J Gastroenterol.* 2005;100:432-439.
4. Ayub K, Slavin J, Imada R. Endoscopic retrograde cholangiopancreatography in gallstone-associated acute pancreatitis. *Cochrane Database Syst Rev.* 2004;4:CD003630.
5. Petrov MS, van Santvoort HC, Besselink MG, et al. Early endoscopic retrograde cholangiopancreatography versus conservative management in acute biliary pancreatitis without cholangitis: a meta-analysis of randomized trials. *Ann Surg.* 2008;247:250-257.
6. van Santvoort HC, Besselink MG, Bakker OJ, et al. A step-up approach or open necrosectomy for necrotizing pancreatitis. *N Engl J Med.* 2010;362:1491-1502.
7. Segarra-Newnham M, Hough A. Antibiotic prophylaxis in acute necrotizing pancreatitis revisited. *Ann Pharmacother.* 2009;43:1486-1495.
8. Bhardwaj P, Garg PK, Maulik SK, et al. A randomized controlled trial of antioxidant supplementation for pain relief in patients with chronic pancreatitis. *Gastroenterology.* 2009;136:149-159.
9. Santosh D, Lakhtakia S, Gupta R, et al. Clinical trial: a randomized trial comparing fluoroscopy guided percutaneous technique vs. endoscopic ultrasound guided technique of celiac plexus block for treatment of pain in chronic pancreatitis. *Aliment Pharmacol Ther.* 2009;29:979-984.
10. Dite P, Ruzicka M, Zboril V, et al. A prospective, randomized trial comparing endoscopic with surgical therapy for chronic pancreatitis. *Endoscopy.* 2003;35:553-558.
11. Cahen DL, Gouma DJ, Nio Y, et al. Endoscopic versus surgical drainage of the pancreatic duct in chronic pancreatitis. *N Engl J Med.* 2007;356:676-684.
12. Shafiq N, Rana S, Bhasin D, et al. Pancreatic enzymes for chronic pancreatitis. *Cochrane Database Syst Rev.* 2009;7:CD006302.

SUGGESTED READINGS

Braganza JM, Lee SH, McCloy RF, et al. Chronic pancreatitis. *Lancet.* 2011;377:1184-1197. *Review.*
Chari ST, Kloeppel G, Zhang L, et al. Histopathologic and clinical subtypes of autoimmune pancreatitis: the Honolulu consensus document. *Pancreatology.* 2011;10:664-672. *Consensus definitions.*
Ksiadzyna D. Drug-induced acute pancreatitis related to medications commonly used in gastroenterology. *Eur J Intern Med.* 2011;22:20-25. *Review emphasizing importance of a high index of suspicion.*

147

DISEASES OF THE RECTUM AND ANUS

ROBERT D. MADOFF

DEFINITIONS

The rectum is best defined anatomically as the level of the large intestine where the taeniae coli splay to form a continuous longitudinal muscle layer. As a practical matter, the rectum begins about 15 cm proximal to the anal margin or verge, where the anus meets the perianal skin. The junction of the colon and rectum bears a variable relationship to the peritoneal reflection, which lies obliquely and at a variable distance from the anal margin.

The anus can be defined both anatomically and histologically. As a practical matter, it is best defined as the distal-most segment of the large bowel that extends from the pelvic floor muscles (levator ani) to the skin. The anorectal junction can be recognized as the point where the rectum angulates posteriorly from the axis of the anal canal. This junction, easily appreciated on digital rectal examination, is caused by the anterior pull of the puborectalis, a U-shaped muscle that loops behind the anorectal junction and pulls it forward. The puborectalis plays an important role in continence, and it is in continuity with the proximal external anal sphincter.

The dentate line lies about 2 cm proximal to the anal margin and roughly corresponds to the level where the distal squamous mucosa meets the more proximal columnar mucosa. Approximately 6 to 12 anal glands located around the perimeter of the dentate line can become infected and become the source of perianal abscesses and fistulas. The anal transition zone, which extends 1 to 2 cm proximal to the dentate line, is the site where many anal cancers develop and marks the proximal boundary for anal cancer surveillance. Hemorrhoids are classified based on their relationship to the dentate line: those proximal are deemed internal, and those distal are external. Anal papillae, the small triangular points of the dentate line, can become hypertrophied and may be mistaken for polyps. Finally, somatic sensation ceases 1 to 2 cm above the dentate line, which explains why hemorrhoid ligation can be performed without anesthesia.

The anal sphincter complex has three major components: the puborectalis, the external anal sphincter, and the internal anal sphincter. The external anal sphincter is composed of skeletal muscle and is under voluntary control. The internal anal sphincter is composed of smooth muscle and represents a continuous though thickened extension of the circular muscle coat of the rectum. The internal anal sphincter is responsible for about 70% of resting anal tone; augmentation of anal sphincter pressure occurs when the individual contracts the external anal sphincter.

SPECIFIC ANORECTAL CONDITIONS
Hemorrhoids

EPIDEMIOLOGY AND PATHOBIOLOGY

The prevalence of hemorrhoids in the United States has been estimated to be 4.4%. However, because many "hemorrhoidal" symptoms are in fact due to other causes, the true incidence and prevalence are unknown.

Despite the commonly held notion that hemorrhoids are always pathologic, hemorrhoids are normal structures, identifiable even in the fetus. Hemorrhoids are vascular cushions that consist of both arterioles and veins. The arteriolar component explains why hemorrhoidal bleeding is typically bright red in color and can be copious in quantity. Hemorrhoids are *not* rectal varices, which are a distinct entity caused by portal hypertension. Many causative factors have been proposed, including constipation, diarrhea, pregnancy, and prolonged straining at stool. Although none of these precipitating factors has been rigorously proved, each can cause either increased abdominal pressure or obstruction of venous return, leading to engorgement and enlargement of the vascular cushions.

CLINICAL MANIFESTATIONS AND DIAGNOSIS

The most common symptom of internal hemorrhoids is bright red rectal bleeding. This bleeding is typically painless and is most often seen on the toilet tissue or in the toilet bowl. The quantity of blood is variable, but some patients complain of blood dripping or squirting into the toilet bowl. Passage of dark blood or blood mixed in the stool suggests a more proximal source. Internal hemorrhoids are classified based on the symptoms they cause. As internal hemorrhoids enlarge, they become associated with redundant rectal mucosa that protrudes from the anus with defecation. Grade 1 hemorrhoids bleed but do not prolapse. Early protrusion reduces spontaneously (grade 2); more advanced protrusion requires digital reduction (grade 3) and, at its most advanced, becomes irreducible (grade 4). Internal hemorrhoids are insensate and are not itchy themselves, but they can cause itching due to associated perianal soiling or mucus deposition caused by mucosal prolapse.

Individuals with anorectal symptoms frequently present complaining of "hemorrhoids." It is always incorrect—and sometimes dangerous—for the physician to apply this diagnosis without completing an adequate evaluation. Fortunately, the initial evaluation is simple, and the correct diagnosis is often suspected based on history alone and confirmed by a limited endoscopic examination. For example, rectal bleeding should never be attributed to hemorrhoids alone, even if hemorrhoids are visible; at a minimum, sigmoidoscopy is required to exclude more proximal pathology. Internal hemorrhoids are best visualized with a slotted anoscope.

External hemorrhoids are usually asymptomatic and should be differentiated from perianal skin tags, which occasionally cause difficulties with hygiene. External hemorrhoids become symptomatic when they thrombose to cause acute-onset pain and swelling (Fig. 147-1). Thrombosed external hemorrhoids are diagnosed by simple inspection.

TREATMENT Rx

Grade 1 hemorrhoids often respond to dietary manipulation: increased dietary fiber, addition of a fiber supplement, and increased water intake (Table 147-1). The goal, which may not be readily achievable, is approximately 25 g of fiber and 8 glasses of water daily. More advanced hemorrhoids require specific therapy, which is almost always office based. The most popular and simplest technique is rubber band ligation, whereby a tiny rubber band (internal diameter approximately 1 mm) is placed around a quantity of redundant rectal mucosa above the prolapsing hemorrhoid. The banded tissue sloughs in 7 to 14 days, an event sometimes heralded by rectal bleeding. Banding can be repeated at 3- to 4-week intervals until bleeding and protrusion are controlled. Bands placed too close to the dentate line cause immediate severe pain and must be removed promptly. Alternative therapies for moderate internal hemorrhoids include injection sclerotherapy and infrared coagulation, which can be performed in the office.

Operative hemorrhoidectomy is needed in only a small minority of patients. Indications for hemorrhoidectomy include irreducible prolapse, a substantial external component, and failure of more conservative therapies. The most common approach is an excisional hemorrhoidectomy, which is generally performed on an outpatient basis. A more recent approach is the stapled hemorrhoidopexy, which entails resecting a ring of rectal mucosa proximal to the internal hemorrhoids using a circular stapling device. This technique is quicker than conventional hemorrhoidectomy and is associated with less postoperative pain and a shorter period of disability; its drawbacks include a higher recurrence rate than conventional surgery and a small but worrisome risk of significant complications. Another alternative approach is Doppler-guided transanal devascularization of internal hemorrhoids, which is directed at obliterating the feeding arterioles. Although early results are promising, the experience to date is limited, and follow-up is short.

External hemorrhoids are usually treated by excision in the office under local anesthesia. However, because the pain associated with thrombosis generally abates within 7 to 10 days, patients who present with resolving symptoms are often best managed conservatively with standard doses of over-the-counter analgesics, sitz baths, and 25 g/day fiber supplementation.

Perianal Abscess

EPIDEMIOLOGY AND PATHOBIOLOGY

Although perianal abscess is a common condition, its exact incidence is not well documented. Most perianal abscesses are caused by infection of the anal glands that track toward the skin. Other causes include simple skin infections, trauma, anorectal surgery, and malignancy.

CLINICAL MANIFESTATIONS AND DIAGNOSIS

Patients most commonly present with complaints of perianal pain and swelling. In most cases, a local area of erythema, tenderness, and fluctuance can be appreciated. However, local swelling, erythema, and fluctuance are often absent in an intersphincteric abscess, which is a small abscess in the plane

FIGURE 147-1. Thrombosed external hemorrhoids.

TABLE 147-1	INTERNAL HEMORRHOIDS: GRADING AND MANAGEMENT	
GRADE	**SYMPTOMS AND SIGNS**	**MANAGEMENT**
1	Bleeding No prolapse	Dietary modifications* Rubber band ligation Infrared coagulation Injection sclerotherapy
2	Prolapse with spontaneous reduction Bleeding, seepage	Rubber band ligation Infrared coagulation Dietary modifications Injection sclerotherapy
3	Prolapse requiring digital reduction Bleeding, seepage	Surgical hemorrhoidectomy Rubber band ligation Dietary modifications
4	Prolapsed, cannot be reduced Strangulated	Surgical hemorrhoidectomy Urgent hemorrhoidectomy

*Dietary modifications include increasing the consumption of fiber, bran, or psyllium and water. Dietary modifications are always appropriate for the management of hemorrhoids and to prevent recurrence after banding or surgery (or both).
Adapted from Nelson H, Dozois RR. Anus. In: Townsend CM, ed. *Sabiston Textbook of Surgery*, 16th ed. Philadelphia: Saunders; 2001:979.

between the internal and external sphincter muscles; these abscesses are suspected based on the history of increasing pain and the physical finding of focal perianal tenderness.

As with all acutely painful anal conditions, digital examination should be avoided. Likewise, office instrumentation with an anoscope or proctoscope is contraindicated because these examinations cause substantial pain and yield little if any diagnostic information. When the cause of the acute pain cannot be determined in the office, prompt examination under anesthesia should be performed.

TREATMENT
Rx

Treatment for perianal abscess is prompt incision and drainage, which can usually be performed in the office. Antibiotics do not adequately penetrate abscess cavities, and extension of a local infection can lead to severe local sepsis and complex long-term problems. Therefore, antibiotic therapy is inadequate and should never be given in an attempt to avoid or delay incision and drainage. Antibiotics usually are not indicated after incision and drainage; exceptions include immunocompromised patients (those with AIDS, transplant recipients, patients undergoing chemotherapy, diabetics) and those at high risk for endovascular infection (e.g., patients with cardiac shunts, prosthetic valves).

Anal Fistula

EPIDEMIOLOGY

An anal fistula represents the chronic form of a perianal abscess. The incidence of anal fistula is about 8.6 per 100,000. Fistulas are two to three times more common in men than in women.

PATHOBIOLOGY

After a perianal abscess is drained, there is about a 50% chance that the internal opening—the site at the dentate line where the infected gland originated—will remain patent, thereby leaving a source for recurrent infection. Multiple or atypical anal fistulas should always raise the diagnostic suspicion of Crohn's disease, which is isolated to the perianal area in approximately 10% of cases.

Anal fistulas are characterized by their relationship to the sphincter complex. The simplest fistula is intersphincteric—located in the plane between the internal and external sphincter muscles. Transsphincteric fistulas, which traverse both the internal and external sphincter muscles, are classified as low fistulas, which traverse only the distal external sphincter, or high fistulas, which traverse the more proximal portions of the external sphincter. Suprasphincteric fistulas loop over the entire sphincter complex. Extrasphincteric fistulas have internal openings remote from the dentate line; most originate from a pelvic abscess caused by a ruptured appendix (Chapter 144), diverticulitis (Chapter 144), or Crohn's disease (Chapter 143). A horseshoe fistula is one with external openings on both sides of the midsagittal plane; these most commonly have a single internal opening in the posterior midline.

CLINICAL MANIFESTATIONS AND DIAGNOSIS

Anal fistulas sometimes present as recurrent abscesses in the same location as the original one, and they sometimes present as persistent purulent drainage from an abscess site that has failed to heal completely. In either case, a persistent track between the external and internal openings remains.

The diagnosis of an anal fistula is established by history and by visualization of an external opening in the perianal skin. A fibrous fistula track can sometimes be palpated along the course of the fistula from the skin toward the anal canal. An internal opening is occasionally visible on anoscopy, but it is not necessary to identify one to make a presumptive diagnosis.

TREATMENT

Treatment of anal fistulas is surgical. Most fistulas are cured by being laid open to eliminate the original source of infection at the internal opening. The fistula track heals by secondary intention. However, this approach divides sphincter muscle and puts the patient at risk for impaired fecal continence in proportion to the quantity of muscle involved. In general, intersphincteric and low transsphincteric fistulas can be safely laid open if the patient has normal baseline continence and no underlying predisposing factors for diarrhea (e.g., colitis) or recurrent fistulas (e.g., Crohn's disease). Because the anterior sphincter mechanism is relatively short and because the anterior sphincter is subject to injury following vaginal delivery, fistulotomy for anterior fistulas in women must be undertaken only after careful consideration.

Treatment of high fistulas is a challenge. When a high fistula is identified, the first step is often placement of a seton, a suture, or other material (now commonly a Silastic vessel loop) that is passed though the fistula track, out the anus, and secured to itself. The seton guarantees that the external fistula opening will not heal over, so a recurrent abscess cannot supervene. Once the track has "matured"—scarred around the seton and become fibrotic—treatment options to eliminate the internal opening include endorectal advancement flap repair and obliteration of the track using fibrin glue or a collagen fistula plug. For individuals with known or suspected Crohn's disease, fistulotomy is avoided, except for the most superficial fistulas. In general, patients with Crohn's disease are best served by placement of long-term draining setons and medical therapy for their underlying disease.

Anal Fissure

EPIDEMIOLOGY

Anal fissures can occur at any age but most frequently affect young adults. Men and women are equally affected.

PATHOBIOLOGY

An anal fissure is a longitudinal tear in the anoderm that occurs just inside the anal margin (Fig. 147-2). The underlying pathophysiology of anal fissures is hypertonia of the internal anal sphincter. Typical anal fissures occur at the midline; most commonly they occur posteriorly, but about 15% are found anteriorly or both anteriorly and posteriorly. "Off-the-midline" fissures should raise the question of other pathology such as anal cancer, Crohn's disease (Chapter 143), syphilis (Chapter 327), HIV, leukemia (Chapter 190), or tuberculosis (Chapter 332). Fissures may occur acutely owing to trauma but are more commonly a subacute condition.

FIGURE 147-2. Anal fissure.

CLINICAL MANIFESTATIONS AND DIAGNOSIS

Patients with anal fissures generally have a typical presentation, and in most cases the correct diagnosis is suspected based on history alone. Following bowel movements, patients describe severe anal pain that may persist for hours or even continue until exacerbation by the next bowel movement. There is sometimes an association with minor red rectal bleeding, most commonly seen in small quantities on the toilet tissue. Anal fissures are frequently associated with a diagnostic triad: the fissure itself, a "sentinel" skin tag (so called because its presence should suggest the presence of an underlying fissure), and a hypertrophied anal papilla located just proximal to the fissure at the dentate line. Well-established fissures may have fibrotic margins and visible internal anal sphincter fibers at their base.

Most fissures can be readily seen on physical examination by applying opposing traction to the buttocks. Once a fissure is identified, no further examination is performed. Digital and endoscopic examination should generally be delayed until the patient has healed to avoid causing pain. However, patients should be advised that they will require subsequent sigmoidoscopy to exclude proximal pathology.

TREATMENT Rx

All therapies are directed at the underlying hypertonia of the internal anal sphincter. Approximately 40% of fissures heal with fiber supplementation and increased fluid intake. Patients are also advised to take warm sitz baths for symptomatic relief, especially following bowel movements.

Two pharmacologic approaches can augment diet and sitz baths: topical sphincter relaxants and botulinum toxin injection. Topical nitroglycerine ointment (0.2 to 0.5%) or diltiazem gel (2%) applied to the anal orifice two to three times daily reduces sphincter tone and usually leads to healing.[3] Both drugs have similar efficacy, but nitroglycerine has the significant disadvantage of causing headaches, lightheadedness, or syncope owing to systemic vasodilation in a substantial minority of patients; commercial 2% nitroglycerine ointment for cardiac use is too potent for perianal use. Botulinum toxin injection is another treatment option, but its usefulness is variable, and the risk of fissure relapse is significant.

For patients who fail medical therapy or who are simply too miserable to pursue it, lateral internal sphincterotomy is an appropriate and generally safe approach.[4] This simple operation is easily performed under monitored local anesthesia in an outpatient setting; recovery is rapid, and fissure healing is expected in more than 90% of cases. Sphincterotomy as first-line therapy provides higher healing rates, fewer relapses, and fewer side effects than topical nitroglycerine,[5] with fewer symptoms, greater satisfaction, and no difference in continence at long-term follow-up.[6] However, a small percentage of patients who undergo sphincterotomy develop minor seepage or actual incontinence, so sphincterotomy should be avoided in individuals who have underlying impaired continence, known sphincter injuries, or diarrheal disorders. When such patients have refractory fissures, a trial of botulinum toxin injection is often a good alternative.

Pruritus Ani

Pruritus ani, or perianal itching, is a very common complaint. It is a symptom and not a disease. The most common cause is inadequate perianal hygiene, often exacerbated by scratching, which leads to excoriation of the skin and further inflammation. Other causes include prolapsing hemorrhoids, anal fistulas, anal incontinence, and specific dermatologic conditions such as contact dermatitis (Chapter 446), psoriasis (Chapter 446), lichen sclerosus (Chapter 448), squamous intra-epithelial neoplasia (Bowen's disease), and perianal Paget's disease (intra-epidermal adenocarcinoma).

TREATMENT Rx

Most cases respond to treatment of the underlying pathology, improved hygiene, avoidance of potential contact allergens, and use of either talc to absorb excess moisture or a barrier cream such as zinc oxide. Some patients benefit from the avoidance of certain foods, including caffeinated beverages, alcohol, milk, chocolate, and tomatoes. Mild topical steroids such as 1% hydrocortisone are sometimes helpful, but stronger steroid preparations are frequently counterproductive and should be avoided when they are not indicated for a specific dermatologic diagnosis. Skin biopsies should be obtained when a primary dermatologic condition is suspected or when the perianal irritation fails to heal with conservative therapy.

Fecal Incontinence

EPIDEMIOLOGY AND PATHOBIOLOGY

Involuntary loss of stool or flatus is a relatively common problem that, when severe, can be socially isolating and debilitating. About 2% of individuals in the United States report incontinence symptoms, but the prevalence is substantially higher in patients visiting primary care providers and gastroenterologists. Almost half of U.S. nursing home patients suffer from fecal incontinence.

CLINICAL MANIFESTATIONS AND DIAGNOSIS

Fecal incontinence can be caused by many disorders. Sphincter disruption related to vaginal delivery is a common cause that often affects young women; many incontinent women who present later in life have an underlying sphincter injury for which they can no longer compensate. Other causes of incontinence include fecal impaction, surgical or traumatic sphincter injury, rectal prolapse, neurologic disorders (e.g., diabetic neuropathy, stroke, multiple sclerosis, brain or spinal cord injury), chronic diarrheal states, dementia, and impaired mobility.

Because incontinence is a symptom and not a disease, the diagnosis is based on history alone. Specific evaluation of the incontinent patient can include anal manometry, anal ultrasound, pudendal nerve testing, and defecography. Anal ultrasound, which is generally the most helpful test, accurately depicts sphincter anatomy and reliably identifies sphincter defects.

TREATMENT Rx

Mild incontinence is often treated successfully with dietary management, addition of a fiber supplement, and use of an antimotility agent such as loperamide 2 to 4 mg up to four times daily (Fig. 147-3). Biofeedback is successful in many patients. For individuals with sphincter disruption, surgical repair leads to substantial improvement in most patients. Sacral nerve stimulation is highly effective for fecal incontinence, although the implantable device has not yet been approved for this indication in the United States. In a randomized trial, transanal submucosal injections of dextranomer in stabilized hyaluronic acid reduced fecal incontinence by at least 50% with minimal adverse effects.[7] For patients with severe refractory incontinence, creation of a colostomy should be strongly considered. Initial reluctance notwithstanding, most patients regain control of their bowel function and report a substantially improved quality of life.

Rectal Prolapse

EPIDEMIOLOGY AND PATHOBIOLOGY

Rectal prolapse is a full-thickness protrusion of the rectum beyond the anal sphincter. The disorder can occur at any age, but prolapse is most frequently seen in older patients, and approximately 90% of adult patients are women. Prolapse is caused by an internal rectal intussusception that, as it becomes more severe, protrudes externally. Uncorrected prolapse frequently leads to

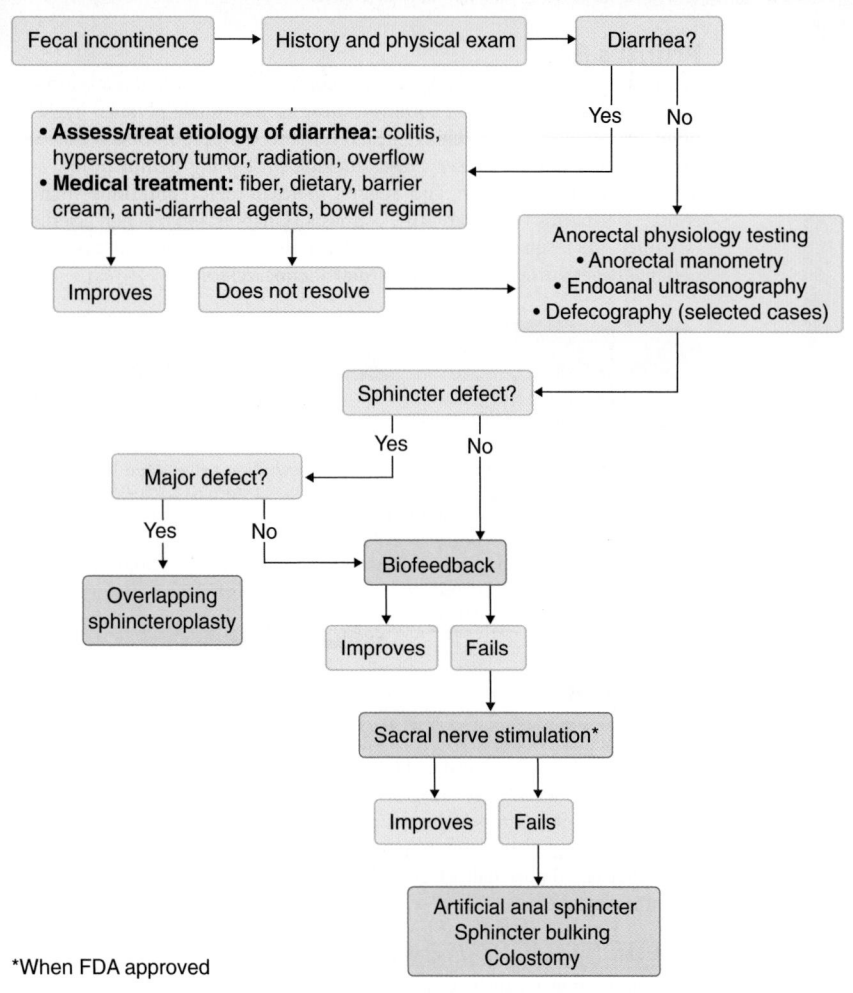

FIGURE 147-3. Algorithm for fecal incontinence. FDA = Food and Drug Administration. (Adapted from Madoff RD, Parker SC, Varma MG, Lowry AC. Faecal incontinence in adults. Lancet. 2004;364:621-632.)

*When FDA approved

fecal incontinence by mechanically stretching the sphincter complex and causing a stretch injury to the pudendal nerves.

CLINICAL MANIFESTATIONS AND DIAGNOSIS

The main clinical manifestation of rectal prolapse is the protruding rectal mass (Fig. 147-4). Most commonly the protrusion occurs with bowel movements, but with time it may occur with coughing or sneezing, and eventually it can occur spontaneously. Some patients present with complaints of fecal incontinence, and many also complain of "constipation," which may be caused by unsuccessful attempts to evacuate the intussuscepting rectum. The protruded rectum may cause minor bleeding and mucus discharge. Occasional patients present with an incarcerated or strangulated prolapse.

The diagnosis of rectal prolapse is confirmed on physical examination. Full-thickness prolapse, which is characterized by concentric mucosal folds, must be differentiated from circumferential mucosal prolapse, which is characterized by radial folds. The prolapse is often best demonstrated by having the patient strain on a commode. Defecography is sometimes helpful to diagnose internal rectal intussusception and associated pelvic floor abnormalities, such as rectocele and enterocele.

TREATMENT Rx

Rectal prolapse is treated by surgical correction. Both transabdominal and transperineal approaches are commonly used.

Human Papillomavirus

EPIDEMIOLOGY AND PATHOBIOLOGY

Human papillomavirus (HPV, Chapter 381), which is the most common sexually transmitted infection, is a cause of anal dysplasia and cancer. The approximately 40 HPV subtypes that can cause anogenital infections are divided into low-risk types (e.g., types 6 and 11) that cause anal warts (condyloma acuminata) and high-risk types (e.g., types 16, 18, and 33) that can

FIGURE 147-4. Rectal mucosal prolapse.

cause anal dysplasia and cancer. HPV infection is associated with cervical, vulvar, vaginal, and penile cancers, and some patients have HPV-related dysplasia or cancer in multiple sites. Approximately 90% of anal cancers are attributable to HPV infection.

The incidence of anal cancer has been steadily increasing, from 0.6 per 100,000 in 1973 to 1.0 per 100,000 in 2001; the female-male ratio decreased from 1.6 : 1 to 1.2 : 1 over the same period. These epidemiologic trends have been attributed to a particularly rapid increase in anal cancers among men who have sex with men, especially men infected with HIV. Anal HPV, including the high-risk types, is highly prevalent in at-risk populations (sex workers, intravenous drug users, transplant recipients, men who have sex with men, and HIV-positive men and women). Furthermore, anal dysplasia is common in at-risk populations; indeed, the prevalence rates of high-grade anal dysplasia are reportedly 40 to 60% among HIV-positive men who have sex with men seen in specialty clinics in New York and San Francisco.

FIGURE 147-5. Perianal condylomata resulting from human papillomavirus infection.

TREATMENT   Rx

Management of the patient with anal dysplasia is controversial. Many authorities advocate a screening and treatment approach based on that used for cervical cancer, another HPV-associated disease. High-risk individuals are screened with anal Papanicolaou smears, and high-definition anal microscopy (analogous to colposcopy of the cervix) is performed when abnormal cytology is detected. Using this technique, dysplastic lesions can be identified and focally ablated or treated with topical imiquimod. More extensive dysplasia requires microscopy-directed targeted ablation in the operating room. Although this overall approach is rational and provides good control of most dysplasia, it is also time-consuming and requires multiple follow-up visits. Cost, recurrence, compliance, and provider manpower all remain significant issues. However, even advocates of less aggressive surveillance report significant rates of anal cancer among patients with dysplasia, especially those who are immunocompromised.

Chemoradiotherapy is now standard first-line treatment for squamous cell cancer of the anal canal. Current radiation protocols most frequently use 45-Gy external beam radiation therapy in 25 fractions, with a boost to the primary tumor and involved inguinal nodes to a total dose of 54 to 59 Gy. Standard chemotherapy utilizes 5-fluorouracil (1000 mg/m^2 per 24 hours continuous infusion for 96 hours, starting on days 1 and 29) in combination with mitomycin C (most commonly 10 mg/m^2 intravenous bolus on days 1 and 29). Abdominoperineal resection with permanent colostomy is reserved for tumors that fail to respond to chemoradiation and those that recur. Similarly, groin dissection is performed only when involved inguinal nodes fail chemoradiation.

Early squamous cell cancers of the anal margin can be locally excised if a satisfactory margin can be obtained without injuring the anal sphincter and if there is no evidence of nodal spread. More advanced anal margin tumors are treated with chemoradiotherapy as described for anal canal tumors.

ANAL WARTS

CLINICAL MANIFESTATION AND DIAGNOSIS

Anal warts can occur in the perianal skin and within the anal canal. The lesions are raised, epithelialized (when external), and narrow based. They can appear as scattered individual warts or as a confluent mass (Fig. 147-5).

TREATMENT   Rx

External warts can be treated with topical podophyllin or imiquimod, but extensive warts usually require surgical excision or fulguration. Untreated warts can rarely progress to form Bushke-Löwenstein tumors—giant, locally invasive condyloma acuminata that frequently contain in situ or invasive cancer.

ANAL CANCER

CLINICAL MANIFESTATIONS AND DIAGNOSIS

The most common symptoms of anal cancer are bleeding, pain, and a palpable mass. The cancer may be seen externally as an ulcerated mass or may be palpated within the anal canal. Anal dysplastic lesions may appear as anal warts or as flat, pigmented lesions, or they may be invisible to the naked eye. They are best visualized using anal microscopy after topical application of 3 to 5% acetic acid (see later). Biopsy is necessary to make the diagnosis.

The terminology of anal cancer is complex, but the great majority of tumors (including epidermoid, cloacogenic, and basaloid carcinomas) are variants of squamous cell carcinoma. The terminology of preinvasive squamous anal lesions is even more confusing because several terms exist for histologically identical pathology. The terms *anal dysplasia, anal intraepithelial neoplasia* (AIN), and *squamous intra-epithelial lesion* (SIL) are used interchangeably. SILs are divided into low-grade and high-grade groups; AIN is similarly divided into AIN 1, 2, and 3, with AIN 2 and 3 being classified as high-grade lesions. Squamous cell carcinoma in situ corresponds to high-grade SIL and AIN 3; these terms are preferable to *Bowen's disease,* which has historically been applied to this lesion. Other significant but less common anal cancers include adenocarcinoma, melanoma, and Paget's disease.

Squamous cell carcinoma of the anus is divided into two groups based on tumor location: cancers of the anal margin (extending from the anal orifice for a distance up to 5 cm) and cancers of the anal canal. Tumors visible externally but extending into the anal canal are considered anal canal lesions.

Other Sexually Transmitted Anorectal Diseases

A number of sexually transmitted diseases (Chapter 293) of the anorectum occur most frequently in individuals who practice anoreceptive intercourse. Common causative agents include *Treponema pallidum* (Chapter 327), *Neisseria gonorrhoeae* (Chapter 307), *Chlamydia trachomatis* (Chapter 326), herpes simplex (Chapter 382), and HIV (Chapter 392). Other sexually transmitted pathogens are *Shigella* (Chapter 317), *Campylobacter jejuni* (Chapter 311), *Haemophilus ducreyi* (Chapter 309), *Calymmatobacterium granulomatis* (Chapter 324), *Entamoeba histolytica* (Chapter 360), *Giardia lamblia* (Chapter 359), and *Isospora belli* (Chapter 361).

The widely variable presentations range from asymptomatic to anal pain, pruritus, discharge, fever, cramps, and bloody diarrhea. Clinical suspicion followed by appropriate and specific testing is necessary to make the correct diagnosis, and clinicians should consider the possibility of simultaneous infections. Treatment addresses the specific infection.

1. Alonso-Coello P, Mills E, Heels-Ansdell D, et al. Fiber for the treatment of hemorrhoids complications: a systematic review and meta-analysis. *Am J Gastroenterol.* 2006;101:181-188.
2. Jayaraman S, Colquhoun PH, Malthaner RA. Stapled versus conventional surgery for hemorrhoids. *Cochrane Database Syst Rev.* 2006.4.CD005393.
3. Nelson R. Nonsurgical therapy for anal fissure. *Cochrane Database Syst Rev.* 2006.4.CD003431.
4. Nelson RL. Operative procedures for fissure in ano. *Cochrane Database Syst Rev.* 2010.20.CD002199.
5. Richard CS, Gregoire R, Plewes EA, et al. Internal sphincterotomy is superior to topical nitroglycerin in the treatment of chronic anal fissure: results of a randomized, controlled trial by the Canadian Colorectal Surgical Trials Group. *Dis Colon Rectum.* 2000;43:1048-1057.
6. Brown CJ, Dubreuil D, Santoro L, et al. Lateral internal sphincterotomy is superior to topical nitroglycerin for healing chronic anal fissure and does not compromise long-term fecal continence: six-year follow-up of a multicenter, randomized, controlled trial. *Dis Colon Rectum.* 2007;50:442-448.
7. Graf W, Mellgren A, Matzel KE, et al. Efficacy of dextranomer in stabilised hyaluronic acid for treatment of faecal incontinence: a randomised, sham-controlled trial. *Lancet.* 2011;377:997-1003.

SUGGESTED READINGS

Balik SH, Gincherman M, Mutch MG, et al. Laparoscopic vs open resection for patients with rectal cancer: comparison of perioperative outcomes at long-term survival. *Dis Colon Rectum.* 2011;54:6-14. *Laparoscopic resection appears to be as good as open resection.*
Herzig DO, Lu KC. Anal fissure. *Surg Clin North Am.* 2010;90:33-44. *Review.*
Rao SS. Advances in diagnostic assessment of fecal incontinence and dyssynergic defecation. *Clin Gastroenterol Hepatol.* 2010;8:910-919. *Review.*

XIII

DISEASES OF THE LIVER, GALLBLADDER, AND BILE DUCTS

148

APPROACH TO THE PATIENT WITH LIVER DISEASE

PAUL MARTIN

The liver has a variety of key functions, including metabolism of the products of ingested food, production of amino acids to form proteins, detoxification of ingested drugs, conversion of nitrogenous substances from the gut into urea for subsequent renal excretion, formation of clotting factors, metabolism of bilirubin, processing of lipids absorbed from the intestine, and excretion of its products as bile. The liver also stores glycogen, which is a source of glucose, and it has a role in containing bacterial infections by removing bacteria from the blood stream. These various functions are achieved by several types of liver cells, including hepatocytes, bile duct cells, and Kupffer cells.

The liver has a dual blood supply: 70% of its blood is delivered by the portal vein, which drains the intestine, and the remainder is from the hepatic artery. After delivery to the liver by the portal vein, nutrient-rich blood passes along the hepatic sinusoids in close contact with the hepatocytes that line them before draining into the hepatic vein. The hepatocytes detoxify, metabolize, and synthesize the products of digestion delivered to them. Bilirubin, the product of the breakdown of red cells and other hemoproteins, is produced by reticuloendothelial cells predominantly in the liver and spleen. Bilirubin is transported to the hepatocytes while bound to albumin; it is then solubilized by the hepatocytes for excretion into the bile ducts.

Clinical consequences of liver disease may reflect the loss of hepatocellular activity, with diminished detoxification, excretory, and synthetic functions. Interruption of bile flow may be caused by ineffective biliary excretion by diseased hepatocytes or by portal hypertension owing to disruption of portal blood flow through a diseased liver. Hepatocyte dysfunction results in diminished production of clotting factors, albumin, and other proteins, as well as the reduced endogenous formation of lipids. Hepatocyte injury from a variety of causes, including viruses, alcohol, autoimmune disorders, and drug hepatotoxicity, is accompanied by leakage of cellular enzymes into the systemic circulation (Chapter 149). Coagulopathy, decreased serum albumin, and hyperbilirubinemia are typical in more profound hepatocellular injury. Portal hypertension occurs because of disruption of the low-pressure intrahepatic blood flow from the portal to the systemic venous circulation, typically owing to fibrosis within the hepatic parenchyma. Consequences of portal hypertension include the accumulation of abdominal ascites and the development of portal-systemic venous collaterals with portal-systemic shunting, thereby resulting in the formation of varices and ultimately in hepatic encephalopathy. Vascular disorders, including portal vein thrombosis, can also result in portal hypertension.

Because of the diverse functions of the liver, its complicated blood supply, and its intimate relationship with the biliary tree, liver disease can present in a variety of ways. The presenting complaint often reflects whether the cause is diffuse, such as when acute viral hepatitis with widespread hepatocyte injury presents as malaise or fatigue, or discrete, such as when biliary obstruction from a gallstone in the common bile duct presents as severe abdominal pain. Patients with liver disease may present with multiple complaints, such as nausea and anorexia owing to hepatocellular disease accompanied by right upper quadrant discomfort due to stretching of the hepatic capsule by parenchymal cell edema and inflammation. Patients with more advanced liver disease, such as decompensated cirrhosis (Chapter 156), may have marked hepatocellular dysfunction with jaundice and coagulopathy in addition to portal hypertension with ascites and bleeding esophageal varices. Many patients who present with hepatic symptoms or signs may have extrahepatic disease; for example, a tender, swollen liver may be caused by a systemic disorder, such as heart failure with hepatic congestion, rather than a primary hepatic disorder. In cirrhotic patients, the initial presentation of previously undiagnosed liver disease may be a major complication such as variceal hemorrhage, which in turn can precipitate hepatic encephalopathy and other features of frank hepatic decompensation.

● HISTORY

Patients with liver disorders come to medical attention for a number of reasons, ranging from the incidental discovery of abnormal liver chemistries to advanced cirrhosis. For patients with possible liver disease, however, a thorough history guides the appropriate diagnostic evaluation. Many complaints related to liver disease, such as fatigue, are nonspecific; unless liver disease is considered in the differential diagnosis, recognition of the hepatic origin of these complaints may be delayed.

In clinical practice, a frequent presentation of liver disease is an asymptomatic patient who is found to have abnormal liver biochemistries (Chapter 149) during a life insurance application, yearly physical examination, or attempt to donate blood. Such patients often have no prior history of liver disease, but it is important to inquire about past occasions when liver biochemistries may have been obtained to determine whether hepatic dysfunction is long-standing or more recent. In a patient with hepatic dysfunction, specific inquiries should be made about the presence of malaise, anorexia, fatigue, and weight change. Jaundice (Chapter 149) is the most typical manifestation of liver disease but is not specific. A patient may first notice lighter-colored stools or dark urine rather than scleral icterus. The absence of these changes suggests that unconjugated hyperbilirubinemia due to hemolysis may be the cause of jaundice rather than intrinsic liver disease. Not infrequently, a patient may be unaware of jaundice until it is noted by a family member or colleague.

Abdominal pain (Chapter 134) related to liver disease can have a variety of causes. Symptomatic gallstones (Chapter 158) can present with the abrupt onset of severe epigastric or right upper quadrant discomfort, often after a large meal and frequently associated with nausea and vomiting. The pain is often steady rather than colicky, and it can radiate widely, including to the chest and back. Patients may not be able to achieve a position that lessens the pain, which may last several hours. More persistent pain, particularly if associated with weight loss and jaundice, raises concern about malignant bile duct obstruction. Pain is also common in parenchymal liver disease in the absence of biliary tract disease. Many patients with chronic hepatocellular disorders, such as chronic hepatitis C (Chapter 151) or nonalcoholic fatty liver disease (Chapter 155), complain of vague right upper quadrant discomfort that has no particular relieving or aggravating factors. Abdominal pain, which can be severe, is also frequent in acute viral hepatitis (Chapter 150), as well as with the hepatic congestion that results from back pressure in heart failure or hepatic vein occlusion, as seen in Budd-Chiari syndrome (Chapter 145).

Fatigue, anorexia, and malaise can be present in both acute and chronic liver disease. In acute liver disorders such as acute viral hepatitis (Chapter 150), drug-induced liver disease (Chapter 152), or an acute presentation of autoimmune hepatitis (Chapter 151), patients may report profound fatigue, nausea, and malaise with decreased appetite and substantial associated weight loss. Distaste for cigarettes is said to be characteristic of acute viral hepatitis. Fatigue is also prominent in chronic liver disease such as chronic hepatitis C (Chapter 151). Pruritus is a prominent feature of cholestatic disorders, such as primary biliary cirrhosis, sclerosing cholangitis, or cholestatic drug reactions, particularly when patients are frankly icteric; however, pruritus also occurs in chronic parenchymal liver disease, most notably chronic hepatitis C, and in acute viral hepatitis. Easy bruisability in those with liver disease reflects coagulopathy and thrombocytopenia.

Fever in a patient with hepatic dysfunction is seen in the prodrome of acute hepatitis A, as well as in alcoholic hepatitis and drug-induced liver disease. In a patient with suspected biliary obstruction, fever suggests complicating bacterial cholangitis or acute cholecystitis.

Ascites is most frequently evidence of cirrhosis and portal hypertension in a patient with liver disease. Patients report increasing abdominal girth, which may be preceded by ankle edema. Weight gain owing to fluid retention may be masked by concomitant loss of muscle mass, and vice versa. The onset of ascites in the absence of a history of liver disease suggests a vascular event, such as hepatic vein occlusion (Chapter 145), or a nonhepatic cause of ascites, such as nephrotic syndrome or heart failure. Accumulation of ascites in a patient with liver disease may be subtle, with a slowly increasing waist circumference, or it may be more rapid, such as in a cirrhotic patient who receives fluid resuscitation following gastrointestinal bleeding. Although ascites in a patient with liver disease implies the presence of cirrhosis, ascites can also complicate severe acute liver disease, including alcoholic hepatitis and viral hepatitis, in which it suggests a poor prognosis.

Hepatic encephalopathy (Chapter 157), which is a neuropsychiatric disorder in patients with liver disease, can range from subtle cognitive impairment to deep coma. Early symptoms include a disturbed sleep pattern with nocturnal insomnia and daytime somnolence. More advanced encephalopathy can result in impairment of memory, confusion, and difficulty completing routine tasks. However, new-onset confusion or coma in a patient with liver disease should not be presumed to reflect hepatic encephalopathy unless other explanations, such as sedative overdose or subdural hematoma, have been ruled out. Important precipitants of hepatic encephalopathy in a cirrhotic patient include gastrointestinal bleeding, bacterial infection, and electrolyte imbalance, all of which need to be excluded during the initial clinical evaluation. In a patient with acute liver failure, coma owing to cerebral edema may be impossible to distinguish from advanced hepatic encephalopathy unless the increased intracranial pressure results in papilledema.

Gastrointestinal hemorrhage due to bleeding varices is usually profuse and often abrupt in onset. It classically presents with hematemesis or melena (Chapter 137), and coexisting postural hypotension and presyncope can reflect profound blood loss. The increased protein load in the gut can cause hepatic encephalopathy. Nonvariceal causes of gastrointestinal bleeding in a patient with liver disease include portal gastropathy (Chapter 137).

RISK FACTORS FOR LIVER DISEASE

An important aspect of the history is the identification of possible risk factors for liver disease. The history should include directed questioning about alcohol consumption, including frequency and pattern (Chapter 32). The age of initial alcohol use and whether its consumption has increased with age should be ascertained. Family members, if present, should also be asked about their perception of the patient's alcohol use and whether it has resulted in difficulties in personal relationships or work performance. Other clues to alcohol abuse are a history of convictions for driving under the influence of alcohol, motor vehicle accidents, and physical symptoms of alcohol dependence (Chapter 32). More circumspect questioning may be required to elicit a history of recreational drug use, especially given societal disapproval of this activity. Not infrequently, a patient with suspected viral hepatitis admits to smoking marijuana or snorting cocaine but does not acknowledge intravenous drug use. With the increasing frequency of nonalcoholic fatty liver disease as a cause of hepatic dysfunction (Chapter 155), the history should assess comorbid conditions such as diabetes mellitus, hyperlipidemia, or weight gain. Ingestion of medications, whether obtained by prescription or over the counter, must be assessed because drug-induced liver disease is an important cause of apparently cryptogenic hepatic dysfunction and is not limited to therapeutic drugs (Chapter 152). Increasingly, herbal and "natural" products (Chapter 38) are ingested for a variety of maladies, and patients may fail to disclose their use because they do not perceive these agents to have side effects or may sense that the physician does not endorse their use. As with alcohol, it is important to quantify the amount of medication ingested and over what period. The social history should also include details about recent travel and contact with individuals with viral hepatitis through intimate, household, or occupational contact. It is also important to ask about vigorous physical activity that can result in elevated aminotransferase levels of nonhepatic origin.

ASSESSING DURATION OF LIVER DISEASE

The differential diagnosis in a patient with liver disease is determined to a large extent by the presenting symptoms, such jaundice or ascites. In many patients, however, the timing of more subtle findings such as elevated aminotransferases is more difficult to determine. Prior blood test results should be retrieved to determine whether hepatic dysfunction is long-standing or more recent. Hepatic dysfunction of less than 6 months' duration is regarded as acute and is frequently self-limited, whereas abnormalities that persist for more than 6 months are chronic and unlikely to resolve spontaneously. If the patient has had a cholecystectomy, it is important to determine the indication; incidental gallstones are sometimes assumed to be the cause of hepatic abnormality in a patient with parenchymal liver disease, leading to unnecessary removal of the gallbladder. Thrombocytopenia owing to portal hypertension in a patient with unrecognized cirrhosis may have been investigated in the past without a firm conclusion being reached.

REVIEW OF OTHER ORGAN SYSTEMS

Despite the appropriate focus on liver-related symptoms, it is important not to overlook other clues, associated disorders, and complications. Sicca symptoms, including dry eyes and mouth, are common in primary biliary cirrhosis (Chapter 158); florid features of scleroderma and the CREST syndrome (Chapter 275) are also seen in association with this liver disease. Dyspnea in

a patient with hepatic dysfunction may reflect cardiac failure with hepatic congestion (Chapter 58). Other explanations include the hepatopulmonary syndrome (Chapter 156), with the characteristic complaint of platypnea–dyspnea (often with chest tightness) that is worse in the upright position owing to aggravation of the ventilation-perfusion mismatch because of intrapulmonary shunting. The hepatopulmonary syndrome can also occur in association with cirrhosis (Chapter 156). A hydrothorax in decompensated cirrhosis can cause dyspnea, as can emphysema in patients with liver disease caused by α_1-antitrypsin deficiency (Chapter 153). A history of premature menopause is common in middle-aged women with cirrhosis, as is decreased libido and sexual potency in male cirrhotic patients. Arthralgias are often reported in viral hepatitis, and hemochromatosis (Chapter 219) may present with involvement of the proximal interphalangeal joints or chondrocalcinosis of the knees; increased skin pigmentation and diabetes mellitus are among other features of this disorder. Accelerated osteopenia occurs in many liver diseases, including primary cirrhosis, primary sclerosing cholangitis, and alcoholic cirrhosis; osteopenia may be aggravated by corticosteroid use in autoimmune chronic active hepatitis. Alcoholic peripheral neuropathy (Chapter 428) can present with pain as well as paresthesia. Tremor and inattentiveness in a younger patient with hepatic dysfunction suggests Wilson disease (Chapter 218). Diarrhea and rectal bleeding in a patient with cholestatic liver disease suggests associated inflammatory bowel disease (Chapter 143).

FAMILY HISTORY

The family history should inquire not only about relatives with liver disease but also about extrahepatic conditions associated with liver disease. Hereditary hepatic conditions, such as Wilson disease and hemochromatosis, may occur in several members of a sibship (Chapter 153). In α_1-antitrypsin deficiency, some family members may experience predominantly emphysema or cirrhosis of unclear cause (Chapter 153). Similarly, renal failure in a family member of a patient with hepatic cysts suggests adult polycystic disease (Chapter 129). A family history of inflammatory bowel disease may be a clue to primary sclerosing cholangitis in a patient with cholestatic liver chemistries. The family history in patients with suspected alcoholic liver disease may reveal other family members with alcoholism.

PHYSICAL EXAMINATION
General Condition

In a patient with suspected liver disease, it is crucial to resist the temptation to palpate the abdomen immediately and ignore other important clues to liver disease as a result. Apart from noting icterus, the initial observation should determine whether muscle wasting, cutaneous stigmata of liver disease, abdominal distention, and peripheral edema are present. The vital signs may reflect the hyperdynamic circulation characteristic of cirrhosis, with a resting tachycardia, wide pulse pressure, and low blood pressure due to peripheral vasodilation. Fetor hepaticus, which is described as a musty smell, may be detected when a cirrhotic patient exhales and must be distinguished from the more frequent halitosis due to poor dental hygiene.

Mucocutaneous Findings

Icterus (Fig. 148-1) is best confirmed by examination of the sclera or, if necessary, under the tongue, where elastin tissue retains bilirubin. Grayish skin discoloration in hemochromatosis may be most evident in the skin folds in

FIGURE 148-1. Scleral icterus.

FIGURE 148-2. Palmar erythema.

FIGURE 148-3. Prurigo nodularis.

FIGURE 148-4. Caput medusae. Photograph shows a caput medusae accentuated by a large amount of ascites in a patient being prepared for liver transplantation. An extensive plexus of veins is seen emanating from the umbilical region and radiating across the anterior abdominal wall. Note the large vein coursing inferiorly along the right flank (arrows). This is the superficial epigastric vein, which drains into the external iliac vein. (From Henseler KP, Pozniak MA, Le FT, et al. Three dimensional CT angiography of spontaneous portosystemic shunts. Radiographics. 2001;21:691-704.)

FIGURE 148-5. Ascites.

the groin or axilla. A Kayser-Fleischer ring (see Fig. 218-1 in Chapter 218), caused by the deposition of copper in Descemet's membrane, is a brownish circle around the periphery of the iris and may require slit lamp examination to detect; it should always be sought in a patient with suspected Wilson disease (Chapter 218). Poor dentition is characteristic in alcoholic or drug-abusing individuals, and excessive dental caries may result from decreased saliva production in the sicca syndrome. Parotid gland swelling is occasionally observed in alcoholic patients. Central cyanosis and clubbing are found in the hepatopulmonary syndrome. Temporal muscle wasting and "paper money" facial skin, owing to atrophy with telangiectasia, are signs of advanced liver disease. Xanthelasma from lipid deposits may be observed on the eyelids and skin around the orbits in patients with cholestatic liver disease. Spider nevi on the face and thorax are not pathognomonic of liver disease, especially in women, but they are suggestive if more than a few are present. Palmar erythema (Fig. 148-2) may be normal in women but suggests liver disease in men. Dupuytren's contracture (see Fig. 155-1 in Chapter 155), the retraction of the palmar fascia with subsequent contracture of the palms and fingers, can be a sign of alcoholic liver disease, although it is also described in persons with epilepsy or diabetes mellitus. Petechiae and ecchymoses reflect impaired production of clotting factors and hypersplenism in advanced liver disease. Patches of white discoloration on the nails may be present in advanced liver disease. Scratch marks from pruritus may be observed on the trunk and extremities of patients with cholestatic liver disease (Fig. 148-3); sparing of the center of the back can lead to a less pigmented butterfly-shaped area, presumably because patients cannot reach that area with their fingernails.

Examination of the Abdomen

Abdominal distention and dilation of collateral veins are the most florid visible signs of advanced liver disease with ascites and portal hypertension. Caput medusae (Fig. 148-4) in the periumbilical area implies recanalization of the umbilical vein due to portal hypertension.

The presence of ascites (Fig. 148-5) can be assessed by percussion of the abdomen and the detection of shifting dullness or a fluid wave. Shifting dullness results from movement of the fluid to the most dependent portion of the abdomen. The subject should be examined in the supine position, and the abdomen should be percussed from the midline toward the right or left flank. A change from a tympanic sound to a dull sound signifies a change from air to fluid, and the location of that change identifies the surface of the fluid pool. Next, the examiner should percuss below the point at which dullness is elicited and ask the subject to turn toward the examiner. With the subject on his or her side, the examiner percusses again at the same point where tympany converted to dullness. If that spot is now tympanic, shifting dullness has been detected as a result of movement of the air-fluid boundary; this finding supports the presence of ascites. This maneuver should be performed sequentially on each side for confirmation. A fluid wave can be felt by placing the medial border of one hand on the abdomen and tapping the right or left lateral abdominal walls; the resulting wave is felt by the first hand. Scrotal edema and abdominal wall hernias are often present in patients with long-standing ascites. Abdominal tenderness in a patient with ascites suggests peritonitis (e.g., spontaneous bacterial peritonitis or due to a perforated viscus). However, it is important to note that abdominal tenderness is frequently absent, even with spontaneous bacterial peritonitis.

The liver is dull to percussion. Percussion of the right upper quadrant can assess the liver span, which is normally 6 to 12 cm in the midclavicular line. The liver span may be diminished in a patient with cirrhosis, whereas hepatomegaly (Fig. 148-6) is detected in hepatic congestion due to heart failure,

FIGURE 148-6. Diagnostic approach to hepatomegaly. *Conditions to be excluded include viral hepatitis, alcohol- and drug-induced liver disease, steatohepatitis, autoimmune liver diseases, and metabolic disorders, including hemochromatosis, Wilson disease, and α_1-antitrypsin deficiency. †Systemic and infiltrative diseases include amyloidosis, lymphoma, sarcoidosis, and infectious processes such as disseminated tuberculosis and fungemia. CT = computed tomography; MRCP = magnetic resonance cholangiopancreatography; MRI = magnetic resonance imaging.

nonalcoholic fatty liver disease, and cholestatic forms of cirrhosis. The liver is best examined with the patient in the supine position, arms parallel to the sides of the body, and knees bent to relax the abdominal muscles. To assess the liver, palpation should begin in the right lower quadrant of the abdomen and move upward toward the rib cage so that the liver edge is felt on the way up. A normal liver edge is smooth and sometimes slightly tender when palpated. In general, a liver edge that is felt up to 2 cm below the right costal margin is considered normal, but a normal-sized liver can be displaced downward by other abnormalities, such as emphysema. In thin subjects, the liver edge may be felt on deep inspiration, even if it is normal in size.

The liver can feel hard and irregular, as in cirrhosis, or slightly tender, enlarged, and smooth, as in acute viral hepatitis or hepatic congestion. The liver can extend across the midline, and the left lobe can be felt in the epigastrium. When the location of the edge of the liver is uncertain, the scratch test may be helpful. It is performed by placing the bell of the stethoscope on the right upper quadrant over the rib cage and scratching the surface of the abdominal wall from the midabdomen toward the liver; the sound of the scratch is amplified in an area under which the liver lies. In the presence of ascites, the liver edge may be detected by exerting quick pressure with the fingertips below the rib cage.

A palpable gallbladder suggests obstruction of the biliary system, whereas tenderness elicited by palpation during inspiration (Murphy's sign) suggests acute cholecystitis. Marked hepatic tenderness with hepatomegaly is observed in patients with a hepatic abscess (Chapter 154).

Splenomegaly may be suggested by dullness to percussion between the 9th and 11th ribs in the left midaxillary line. A palpable spleen tip is highly suggestive of portal hypertension in a patient with chronic liver disease, although an enlarged spleen can also be detected in acute viral hepatitis and infiltrative disorders that involve both the liver and the spleen (see Table 171-7 in Chapter 171). Rectal examination is obligatory if gastrointestinal bleeding is suspected because of melena, anemia, or unexplained hepatic encephalopathy.

Complete Physical Examination

The presence of rales and elevation of the jugular venous pressure suggest heart failure or pericardial disease as a cause of hepatic congestion. Loss of secondary sexual characteristics in liver disease is reflected by a loss of axillary and pubic hair, as well as feminization of body habitus in a male patient. Testicular atrophy may also be present. Peripheral edema is common in decompensated cirrhosis and may occur before ascites is obvious.

Neuropsychiatric alterations can include subtle changes in personality or more overt hepatic encephalopathy. Constructional apraxia (e.g., inability to draw a five-pointed star or to write legibly) in a fully conscious patient is a typical finding of hepatic encephalopathy. Asterixis, which is characterized by a series of extensor and flexor wrist movements, can be elicited by having the patient extend the arms, with dorsiflexion of the wrists, while separating the fingers for at least 15 seconds. Tremors (Chapter 417) are nonspecific but are also common in advanced cirrhosis.

DIAGNOSTIC STUDIES (TABLE 148-1)

Laboratory Studies

The initial evaluation for suspected liver disease involves a battery of blood tests that reflect hepatic necroinflammation (serum aminotransferases), cholestatic biliary tract dysfunction (alkaline phosphatase, γ-glutamyl transpeptidase), excretory function (bilirubin), and synthetic function (coagulation factors, albumin) (Chapter 149). In hepatocellular dysfunction caused by viral hepatitis (Chapter 150), the aminotransferase levels are elevated, with the serum alanine aminotransferase (ALT) level higher than the aspartate aminotransferase (AST) level. In alcoholic hepatitis (Chapter 155), AST elevation exceeds ALT elevation. In patients with biliary obstruction or cholestatic liver diseases (Chapter 158), such as primary biliary cirrhosis or a cholestatic drug reaction, the bilirubin and generally the alkaline phosphatase levels are elevated. Impairment of synthetic function, such as from cirrhosis or severe acute viral hepatitis, can lead to a low serum albumin level over days to weeks. The prothrombin time, expressed as the international normalized ratio (INR), is a more sensitive test of hepatic synthetic function and becomes prolonged within several hours after a major hepatic insult. Portal hypertension owing to advanced hepatic fibrosis or cirrhosis results in a decreased platelet count due to hypersplenism. Although these general patterns of liver dysfunction are helpful in the initial evaluation of liver disease, they are nonspecific. For example, a patient with a predominantly hepatocellular process commonly has elevated bilirubin and alkaline phosphatase levels and a low serum albumin level if the injury is severe. Nevertheless, these blood tests should identify the predominant pattern of abnormality and help focus further diagnostic evaluation with serologies and abdominal imaging.

Abdominal Imaging

Plain abdominal radiographs generally do not have a major role in the evaluation of suspected liver disease. An exception is a patient with severe abdominal pain in whom it is important to exclude a perforated viscus with free air under the diaphragm.

Ultrasonography should be the initial investigation in patients with obstructive jaundice. It can confirm dilated bile ducts in patients with biliary obstruction and can often identify the cause, such as a pancreatic mass or a

TABLE 148-1 APPROACH TO COMMON HEPATIC COMPLAINTS

PRESENTATION	COMMON SYMPTOMS	COMMON PHYSICAL SIGNS	DIAGNOSTIC STUDIES	COMMON DIAGNOSES
Ascites	Abdominal distention and pain, ankle edema	Flank dullness Shifting dullness Fluid wave	Ultrasound with Doppler Diagnostic paracentesis Urinalysis	Cirrhosis Budd-Chiari syndrome Heart failure Nephrotic syndrome
Hepatic encephalopathy	Sleep disorientation, confusion, coma	Asterixis Altered mentation Fetor hepaticus	Serum ammonia Blood cultures Stool Hemoccult Serum creatinine and electrolytes	Decompensated cirrhosis Acute liver failure Other metabolic encephalopathies (renal, respiratory)
Hepatic mass	None or abdominal pain	Hepatic bruit or rub	α-Fetoprotein Ultrasound CT scan MRI Biopsy	Benign lesions: hemangioma, adenoma, focal nodular hyperplasia Malignant lesions: hepatocellular carcinoma, cholangiocarcinoma, metastases
Abdominal pain	Nausea, vomiting, fever	Right upper quadrant tenderness Palpable gallbladder Murphy's sign	Ultrasound HIDA scan Paracentesis for ascites if present	Biliary colic Acute cholecystitis Hepatic congestion Hepatic metastases

CT = computed tomography; HIDA = hepatobiliary iminodiacetic acid; MRI = magnetic resonance imaging.

gallstone lodged in the common bile duct. Ultrasonography can also determine whether the hepatic parenchyma is diffusely abnormal, such as in a patient with acute viral hepatitis; it can identify bright hepatic echo texture in a patient with nonalcoholic fatty liver disease; or it can show a coarsened echo texture in cirrhosis. In addition to confirming the presence of ascites, ultrasonography can identify other signs of portal hypertension, such as splenomegaly or intra-abdominal varices. Blood flow through the portal and hepatic vessels can be assessed by adding a Doppler flow study. An ultrasound study can identify hepatic masses and distinguish a cystic mass from a solid lesion. Computed tomography (CT) and magnetic resonance imaging (MRI) add greater detail to the assessment of the hepatic vasculature, hepatic masses, and hepatic vascular structures. MRI can also obtain a very detailed cholangiogram (see Fig. 202-3 in Chapter 202), thereby avoiding the more invasive endoscopic retrograde cholangiopancreatography in many patients with suspected bile duct obstruction or disease (Chapters 135 and 136).

Liver biopsy remains the definitive test to assess the severity of hepatic inflammation and the extent of fibrosis in diffuse hepatocellular disease. In addition, it can confirm diagnoses suspected by noninvasive testing, such as autoimmune hepatitis, or it can suggest diagnoses, such as drug hepatotoxicity. Because of its potential complications, such as intra-abdominal bleeding, biopsy is recommended only when less invasive testing has not yielded a definitive diagnosis or prognosis or when additional information, such as quantitative determination of hepatic copper in Wilson disease or hepatic iron in hemochromatosis, is necessary for definitive diagnosis.

Transjugular pressure measurements are indicated in patients with atypical presentations of portal hypertension (e.g., when it is unclear whether liver disease is the cause) or to titrate medications to reduce portal pressure. A catheter is advanced under fluoroscopy into the hepatic vein, and the free hepatic venous pressure is measured. The catheter is then advanced farther until it becomes "wedged" in a small hepatic vein venule. The venule is occluded by a small balloon, and the wedged hepatic vein pressure, which reflects hepatic sinusoidal pressure, is obtained. The portal pressure gradient, which is derived by subtracting the free pressure measurement from the wedged pressure measurement, is normally less than 5 mm Hg. Varices form at a gradient above 10 mm Hg, whereas ascites and variceal hemorrhage occur only when the gradient exceeds 12 mm Hg. A transjugular approach also increases the safety of liver biopsy in the presence of ascites, coagulopathy, or thrombocytopenia when standard percutaneous liver biopsy is hazardous. Endoscopy is indicated to screen for varices in any patient suspected of having cirrhosis to determine the need for prophylaxis against hemorrhage.

SUGGESTED READING

Mutter D, Soler L, Marescaux J. Recent advances in liver imaging. *Expert Rev Gastroenterol Hepatol.* 2010;4:613-621. *Review.*

149

APPROACH TO THE PATIENT WITH JAUNDICE OR ABNORMAL LIVER TESTS

PAUL BERK AND KEVIN KORENBLAT

JAUNDICE

DEFINITION

Jaundice, from the French *jaune* (yellow), is the yellow-orange discoloration of the skin, conjunctivae, and mucous membranes that results from elevated concentrations of bilirubin in plasma. Mild hyperbilirubinemia may be clinically undetectable, but jaundice becomes evident at plasma bilirubin concentrations of 3 to 4 mg/dL, depending on the patient's normal pigmentation, the conditions of observation, and the bilirubin fraction that is elevated. Optimal interpretation of an elevated plasma bilirubin concentration is based on an appreciation of its sources and disposition.

Bilirubin Metabolism
Bilirubin Production

Bilirubin is the degradation product of the heme moiety of hemoproteins, a class of proteins involved in the transport or metabolism of oxygen (Fig. 149-1). Normal adults produce about 4 mg of bilirubin per kilogram of body weight per day. Between 70 and 90% of bilirubin is derived from the hemoglobin of erythrocytes, which in turn are sequestered and destroyed by the mononuclear phagocytic cells of the reticuloendothelial system, principally in the spleen, liver, and bone marrow. A minor fraction reflects ineffective erythropoiesis, the premature destruction of newly formed erythrocytes within the bone marrow. The remainder results primarily from the turnover of nonhemoglobin hemoproteins such as myoglobin, the P-450 cytochromes, catalase, and peroxidase. Although this occurs principally in the liver, bilirubin has proved to have antioxidant properties, and recent studies suggest that a limited, regulated production of bilirubin from heme may occur in many cell types and contribute to regulating the intracellular antioxidant environment.

The two-step conversion of heme to bilirubin commences with the opening of the heme molecule at its α bridge carbon by the microsomal enzyme *heme oxygenase*, a process that results in the formation of equimolar quantities of carbon monoxide and the green tetrapyrrole biliverdin, the main excretory product of heme in birds, reptiles, and amphibians. Because biliverdin cannot

FIGURE 149-1. Overview of bilirubin metabolism. Unconjugated bilirubin (UCB) formed from the breakdown of heme from hemoglobin and other hemoproteins is transported in plasma reversibly bound to albumin and is converted in the liver to bilirubin monoglucuronide (BMG) and diglucuronide (BDG), the latter being the predominant form secreted in bile. BMG and BDG together normally account for less than 5% of normal serum bilirubin. In patients with hepatobiliary disease, BMG and BDG accumulate in plasma and appear in urine. Bilirubin glucuronides in plasma also react nonenzymatically with albumin and possibly other serum proteins to form protein conjugates, which do not appear in urine and have a plasma half-life similar to that of albumin. BR = bilirubin.

cross the placenta, its reduction to bilirubin in mammals by a second enzyme, *biliverdin reductase*, allows its transplacental removal from the fetus into the maternal circulation. The unconjugated bilirubin produced in the periphery is transported to the liver in plasma. Because of its insolubility in aqueous media, it is kept in solution by tight but reversible binding to albumin. A number of compounds, including sulfonamides, furosemide, and radiographic contrast agents, competitively displace bilirubin from its binding sites on albumin, a phenomenon of little clinical significance except in neonates, in whom the resulting increased concentration of unbound bilirubin raises the risk of kernicterus.

Disposition of Bilirubin by the Liver

Bilirubin excretion from the body is a major function of the liver (see Fig. 149-1), wherein specialized microanatomy enhances extraction of tightly protein-bound compounds from the circulation. Hepatic translocation of bilirubin from blood to bile involves four distinct steps: (1) uptake of unconjugated bilirubin, by both an incompletely characterized facilitated transport process and by diffusion; (2) intracellular binding, mainly to various cytosolic proteins of the glutathione-*S*-transferase family; (3) conversion of unconjugated bilirubin to bilirubin monoglucuronides and diglucuronides by a specific uridine diphosphate (UDP)-glucuronosyltransferase isoform designated UGT1A1; and (4) transfer of bilirubin monoglucuronides and diglucuronides into bile by a canalicular membrane adenosine triphosphate (ATP)-dependent transporter designated multidrug resistance–associated protein 2 (MRP2) or canalicular multispecific organic anion transporter (cMOAT). MRP2/cMOAT is a member of the *MRP* gene family, other members of which pump certain drug conjugates, as well as unmodified anticancer drugs, out of cells.

Conjugation to bilirubin monoglucuronides and diglucuronides greatly increases the aqueous solubility of bilirubin and thereby enhances its elimination from the body while simultaneously reducing its ability to diffuse across biologic membranes, including the blood-brain barrier. In newborns, a decreased capacity to conjugate bilirubin leads to unconjugated hyperbilirubinemia (physiologic jaundice of the newborn). If severe, this hyperbilirubinemia may lead to irreversible central nervous system toxicity. Phototherapy by exposure to blue light converts bilirubin to water-soluble photoisomers that are readily excreted in bile, protecting the central nervous system from bilirubin toxicity. Gilbert's syndrome and Crigler-Najjar syndrome types 1 and 2, which result from genetic defects in bilirubin conjugation, are characterized by unconjugated hyperbilirubinemia; in contrast, Dubin-Johnson syndrome, which results from inheritable defects in MRP2/cMOAT (see later), is characterized by conjugated or mixed hyperbilirubinemia.

Enterohepatic Circulation and Excretion of Bilirubin
Bilirubin in Bile

Normal bile contains an average of less than 5% unconjugated bilirubin, 7% bilirubin monoconjugates, and 90% bilirubin diconjugates. The proportion of monoconjugates increases with an increased bilirubin load (hemolysis) or defective conjugation (e.g., Gilbert's and Crigler-Najjar type 2 syndromes). After canalicular secretion, conjugated bilirubin passes down the gastrointestinal tract without reabsorption by either the gallbladder or intestinal mucosa.

Urobilinogen and the Enterohepatic Circulation

Although some bilirubin reaches the feces, most is converted to urobilinogen and related compounds by bacteria within the ileum and colon, where the urobilinogen is reabsorbed, returns to the liver through the portal circulation, and is re-excreted into bile in a process of enterohepatic recirculation. Any urobilinogen not taken up by the liver reaches the systemic circulation and is cleared by the kidneys. Normal urine urobilinogen excretion is 4 mg/day or less. With hemolysis, which increases the load of bilirubin entering the gut and therefore the amount of urobilinogen formed and reabsorbed, or with liver disease, which decreases its hepatic extraction, plasma urobilinogen levels rise, and more urobilinogen is excreted in the urine. Severe cholestasis, bile duct obstruction, or broad-spectrum antibiotics that reduce or eliminate bacterial conversion of bilirubin to urobilinogen markedly decrease the formation and urinary excretion of urobilinogen.

Unconjugated bilirubin ordinarily does not reach the gut except in neonates or by ill-defined alternative pathways in the presence of severe unconjugated hyperbilirubinemia (e.g., Crigler-Najjar type 1). In these circumstances, unconjugated bilirubin is reabsorbed from the gut, thereby amplifying the hyperbilirubinemia.

Measurement of Bilirubin in Plasma

The total plasma bilirubin concentration in normal adults is less than 1 to 1.5 mg/dL, depending on the measurement method used. Modern analytic techniques show that normal plasma contains principally unconjugated bilirubin, with only traces of conjugates. Clinical laboratories typically quantify plasma bilirubin by a reaction in which bilirubin is cleaved by a diazo reagent, such as diazotized sulfanilic acid, to azodipyrroles that are quantitated spectrophotometrically. Bilirubin conjugates react rapidly ("prompt" or "direct"-reacting bilirubin). Unconjugated bilirubin reacts slowly because the site of attack by the diazo reagent is protected by internal hydrogen bonding. Accordingly, accurate measurement of the total plasma bilirubin concentration requires addition of an accelerator, such as ethanol or urea, to disrupt this internal bonding and to ensure complete reaction of any unconjugated bilirubin. The "indirect"-reacting bilirubin is calculated by subtracting the direct-reacting bilirubin from the total. Although physicians traditionally equate the direct-reacting fraction of bilirubin in plasma with conjugated bilirubin and the indirect fraction with unconjugated bilirubin, this approach is, at best, a rough approximation, and the unqualified interpretation of direct and indirect fractions as reflecting conjugated and unconjugated bilirubin, respectively, may lead to diagnostic errors, particularly in the diagnosis of hereditary hyperbilirubinemias. In practice, 10 to 20% of bilirubin in normal plasma gives a prompt (direct) diazo reaction even though more than 95% of total bilirubin in normal plasma is unconjugated. Thus, at virtually any total bilirubin concentration, a direct-reacting fraction of less than 15% of the total can be considered as essentially all unconjugated. When the direct-reacting fraction is greater than 15%, a simple dipstick test for bilirubinuria may clarify the situation. Unconjugated bilirubin is not excreted in urine regardless of the height of its plasma concentration because its binding to albumin is too tight for effective glomerular filtration and it is not secreted by the tubules. The canalicular transport mechanism for excretion of bilirubin conjugates is especially sensitive to injury. Accordingly, in parenchymal liver disease or mechanical bile duct obstruction, bilirubin conjugates within the hepatocyte or biliary tract may reflux into the blood stream, resulting in a mixed or, less often, a purely conjugated hyperbilirubinemia. Conjugated bilirubin, which is normally loosely bound to albumin, is readily filtered at the glomerulus; even modest degrees of conjugated hyperbilirubinemia result in bilirubinuria, which is *always* a pathologic finding. With prolonged conjugated hyperbilirubinemia, some of the conjugated bilirubin binds *covalently* to albumin and produces what is designated the delta (δ) bilirubin fraction. Although δ-bilirubin gives a direct diazo reaction, it is not filterable by the glomerulus and does not appear in the urine; it disappears slowly from the plasma, with the 14- to 21-day half-life of the albumin to which it is bound. δ-Bilirubin accounts for the sometimes slow rate at which conjugated (direct) hyperbilirubinemia resolves as hepatitis improves or biliary obstruction is relieved. Although δ-bilirubin is not easily measured, its presence can be inferred when an elevated direct-reacting bilirubin persists after bilirubinuria resolves.

Bilirubin Kinetics

The plasma disappearance kinetics of radiolabeled bilirubin indicate that the plasma unconjugated bilirubin concentration ([UCB]) reflects a balance between the bilirubin production rate (BRP) and hepatic bilirubin clearance (C_{BR}) according to the relationship:

$$[UCB] \approx BRP/C_{BR}$$

C_{BR} is analogous to the creatinine clearance in the test of kidney function; it is a measure of the rate at which bilirubin is extracted from plasma, and is a true quantitative test of liver function. Whereas BRP and C_{BR} are not easily quantified in clinical settings, investigative measurements have yielded useful pathophysiologic insights. This equation indicates that [UCB] increases linearly with an increase in BRP or hyperbolically with a decrease in C_{BR}, thereby providing a basis for classifying unconjugated hyperbilirubinemias according to their pathogenesis.

● APPROACH TO THE PATIENT WITH HYPERBILIRUBINEMIA

Hyperbilirubinemia and jaundice (Fig. 149-2) may result from isolated disorders of bilirubin metabolism, liver disease, or obstruction of the biliary tract. Jaundice represents the most visible sign of hepatobiliary disease of many causes (Table 149-1).

FIGURE 149-2. Severe cholestatic jaundice in a patient with primary biliary cirrhosis. The high level of conjugated bilirubin, maintained over a long period, gives a characteristic dark brown-orange pigmentation to the skin and sclerae. Patients with primary biliary cirrhosis usually develop large xanthelasmas and corneal arcus as a consequence of disordered lipid metabolism. (From Forbes CD, Jackson WF. *Color Atlas and Text of Clinical Medicine*, 3rd ed. London: Mosby; 2003.)

TABLE 149-1 DIFFERENTIAL DIAGNOSIS OF HYPERBILIRUBINEMIA AND JAUNDICE

ISOLATED DISORDERS OF BILIRUBIN METABOLISM

Unconjugated hyperbilirubinemia
  Increased bilirubin production
    Examples: hemolysis, ineffective erythropoiesis, blood transfusion, resorption of hematomas
  Decreased hepatocellular uptake
    Examples: drugs (e.g., rifampin)
  Decreased conjugation
    Examples: Gilbert's and Crigler-Najjar syndromes, physiologic jaundice of the newborn, breast milk jaundice, HIV protease inhibitors
Conjugated or mixed hyperbilirubinemia
  Decreased canalicular transport: Dubin-Johnson syndrome
  Mechanism uncertain: Rotor's syndrome

LIVER DISEASE

Acute or chronic hepatocellular dysfunction
  Acute or subacute hepatocellular injury
    Examples: viral hepatitis A, B, and C, hepatotoxins (e.g., ethanol, acetaminophen, mushroom [*Amanita phalloides*] poisoning), drugs (e.g., isoniazid, α-methyldopa), metabolic diseases (e.g., Wilson's disease, Reye's syndrome), pregnancy-related (e.g., acute fatty liver of pregnancy, preeclampsia), hepatic ischemia (e.g., hypotension, postoperative, hepatic artery thrombosis)
  Chronic hepatocellular disease
    Examples: hepatitis B and C, hepatotoxins (e.g., vinyl chloride, vitamin A), nonalcoholic and alcoholic fatty liver disease, autoimmune hepatitis, metabolic disease (Wilson's disease, hemochromatosis, α$_1$-antitrypsin deficiency)
Hepatic disorders with prominent cholestasis
  Familial cholestatic disorders
  Single-gene disorders
    Examples: benign recurrent intrahepatic cholestasis types 1-3; progressive familial intrahepatic cholestasis types 1-3
  Familial cholestatic disorders of unknown pathogenesis
    Examples: Aagenaes syndrome, Navajo neurohepatopathy, North American Indian cholestasis
  Diffuse infiltrative disorders
    Examples: granulomatous diseases (e.g., mycobacterial and fungal infections, sarcoidosis, lymphoma, drugs, Wegener's granulomatosis), amyloidosis, infiltrative malignancies
  Inflammation of intrahepatic bile ductules and/or portal tracts
    Examples: primary biliary cirrhosis, liver allograft rejection, graft-versus-host disease, drugs (e.g., chlorpromazine, erythromycin)
  Miscellaneous conditions
    Examples: uncommon presentations of viral or alcoholic hepatitis, intrahepatic cholestasis of pregnancy, contraceptive jaundice, estrogens, anabolic steroids, postoperative cholestasis, cholestasis of sepsis, total parenteral nutrition, bacterial infections, drugs

OBSTRUCTION OF THE BILE DUCTS

Choledocholithiasis
  Examples: cholesterol gallstones, pigment gallstones
Diseases of the bile ducts
  Inflammation/infection
    Examples: primary sclerosing cholangitis, AIDS cholangiopathy, hepatic arterial chemotherapy, postsurgical strictures
  Neoplasms (e.g., cholangiocarcinoma)
Extrinsic compression of the biliary tree
  Neoplasms
    Examples: pancreatic carcinoma, metastatic lymphadenopathy, hepatoma
  Pancreatitis with or without pseudocyst formation
  Vascular enlargement (e.g., aneurysm, cavernous transformation of portal vein)

AIDS = acquired immunodeficiency syndrome; HIV = human immunodeficiency syndrome.

DISORDERS OF BILIRUBIN METABOLISM

Hyperbilirubinemia in the absence of hepatocellular dysfunction (pure hyperbilirubinemia) may result from either increased bilirubin production or inherited or acquired defects in specific aspects of hepatic bilirubin disposition.

Increased Bilirubin Production

Increased bilirubin production and consequent unconjugated hyperbilirubinemia can be caused by hemolysis, accelerated destruction of transfused erythrocytes, resorption of hematomas, or ineffective erythropoiesis (e.g., lead poisoning, megaloblastic anemias related to deficiency of either folic acid or vitamin B_{12}, sideroblastic anemia, congenital erythropoietic porphyria, or myeloproliferative or myelodysplastic diseases). In these settings, other liver tests are typically normal and the hyperbilirubinemia is modest, rarely exceeding 4 mg/dL; higher values imply concomitant hepatic dysfunction. However, following brisk blood transfusion or resorption of massive hematomas, the increased bilirubin load may be transiently sufficient to lead to frank jaundice. The causes of hemolysis are numerous (Chapters 163 to 166). Besides specific blood disorders, mild hemolysis accompanies many acquired diseases. In the setting of systemic disease, which may include a degree of hepatic dysfunction, hemolysis may produce a component of conjugated hyperbilirubinemia in addition to an elevated unconjugated bilirubin concentration. Prolonged hemolysis may lead to the formation of bilirubin gallstones, which may cause cholecystitis, obstruction, or any other biliary tract consequence of calculous disease.

Decreased Hepatic Bilirubin Clearance

DECREASED BILIRUBIN UPTAKE

Several drugs (e.g., rifampin, flavaspidic acid, novobiocin, and various cholecystographic contrast agents) competitively inhibit the hepatocellular uptake of bilirubin. The resulting unconjugated hyperbilirubinemia resolves with cessation of the medication. Decreased hepatic bilirubin uptake is also believed to contribute to the unconjugated hyperbilirubinemia of Gilbert's syndrome, although the principal molecular basis for this syndrome is reduction of bilirubin conjugation.

IMPAIRED BILIRUBIN CONJUGATION

The most frequent cause of decreased bilirubin clearance is decreased bilirubin conjugating activity. Bilirubin conjugation with glucuronic acid is catalyzed by a specific UDP-glucuronosyltransferase, designated UGT1A1, encoded by the *UGT1* gene complex. The *UGT1A1* gene is assembled by alternative splicing of a bilirubin-specific variant of exon 1, designated exon A_1, with four common exons (exons 2 to 5) that encode the shared carboxyl terminal end of all *UGT1*-encoded proteins. Its promoter region normally contains an $A(TA)_6TAA$ TATA boxlike construct.

Genetic Disorders of Bilirubin Conjugation

The hereditary hyperbilirubinemias (Table 149-2) are a group of five syndromes in which hyperbilirubinemia occurs as an isolated biochemical abnormality, without evidence of either hepatocellular necrosis or cholestasis. The molecular defects have been identified in all but Rotor's syndrome.

CRIGLER-NAJJAR SYNDROME TYPES 1 AND 2 AND GILBERT'S SYNDROME

These are hereditary unconjugated hyperbilirubinemias that result from mutations in *UGT1A1*. In Crigler-Najjar type 1, essentially no functional enzyme activity is present, whereas patients with Crigler-Najjar type 2 have up to 10% of normal and patients with Gilbert's syndrome have 10 to 33% of normal, leading to bilirubin concentrations of 18 to 45, 6 to 25, and 1.5 to 4 mg/dL, respectively (see Table 149-2). Because total UGT1A1 enzymatic activity must be reduced to less than 50% of normal to produce unconjugated hyperbilirubinemia, phenotypic expression of mutations in this enzyme requires either homozygosity or double heterozygosity. Each of these disorders is inherited as an autosomal recessive trait. Patients with Crigler-Najjar types 1 and 2 are either homozygotes or double heterozygotes for structural mutations within the coding region. In Western countries, patients with Gilbert's syndrome are typically homozygous for an $A(TA)_7TAA$ promoter mutation. Structural mutations in exon 1 of *UGT1A1* causing modest reductions in UGT1A1 enzymatic activity have been reported in some Japanese patients with Gilbert's syndrome.

Crigler-Najjar type 1 is characterized by striking unconjugated hyperbilirubinemia that appears in the neonatal period, persists for life, and is unresponsive to phenobarbital. The majority of patients (type 1A) exhibit defects in the glucuronide conjugation of a spectrum of substrates in addition to bilirubin as the result of mutations in one of the common exons (2 to 5) of the *UGT1* complex. In a smaller subset (type 1B), a mutation in the bilirubin-specific exon A1 limits the defect to bilirubin conjugation. More than 85 structurally diverse *UGT1A1* mutations can cause Crigler-Najjar type 1; their common feature is that they all encode proteins with absent or, at most, traces of enzymatic activity. Before the availability of phototherapy, most patients with Crigler-Najjar type 1 died of bilirubin encephalopathy (kernicterus) in infancy or early childhood. Optimal treatment for a neurologically intact patient includes (1) about 12 hours/day of phototherapy from birth throughout childhood, perhaps supplemented by exchange transfusion in the neonatal period; (2) use of tin-protoporphyrin to blunt transient episodes of increased hyperbilirubinemia; and (3) early liver transplantation, before the onset of brain damage. Transplantation with isolated allogeneic hepatocytes continues to be evaluated as an experimental therapeutic approach.

Bilirubin concentrations are typically lower in Crigler-Najjar type 2, and plasma bilirubin levels can be reduced to 3 to 5 mg/dL by phenobarbital. At least 20 different mutations of *UGT1A1* have been associated with Crigler-Najjar type 2; all encode a bilirubin-UDP-glucuronosyl transferase with markedly reduced but detectable enzymatic activity. Although uncommon in Crigler-Najjar type 2, kernicterus has occurred at all ages, typically associated with factors that temporarily raise the plasma bilirubin concentration above baseline (e.g., fasting, intercurrent illness). For this reason, phenobarbital therapy is often recommended; a single bedtime dose usually maintains clinically safe plasma bilirubin concentrations.

Gilbert's syndrome is the most common hereditary hyperbilirubinemia, with a genotypic prevalence of 12% or less and a phenotypic prevalence of 7% or less. Its high prevalence may explain the frequency of mild unconjugated hyperbilirubinemia in liver transplant recipients. Plasma bilirubin concentrations are most often less than 3 mg/dL, although both higher and lower values are frequent, with increases of two- to three-fold commonly occurring with fasting and intercurrent illness. The phenotypic distinction between mild Gilbert's syndrome and a normal state is often blurred. Phenobarbital normalizes both the bilirubin concentration and C_{BR}. Oxidative drug metabolism and the disposition of most xenobiotics that are metabolized by glucuronidation appear to be normal in Gilbert's syndrome. A critical exception is the antitumor agent irinotecan (CPT-11), whose active metabolite (SN-38) is glucuronidated specifically by UGT1A1. In patients with Gilbert's syndrome, CPT-11 can cause intractable diarrhea, myelosuppression, and other serious toxicities. Life expectancy in Gilbert's syndrome is normal, and the denial of life insurance or employment to these patients is not medically justified.

UNCONJUGATED HYPERBILIRUBINEMIA RELATED TO SELECTIVE INHIBITION OF UGT1A1

This occurs with several human immunodeficiency virus (HIV) protease inhibitors (e.g., indinavir, atazanavir). Abnormal disposition of menthol, estradiol benzoate, acetaminophen, tolbutamide, rifamycin SV, and other agents has not been associated with significant complications, but prudence should be exercised in prescribing agents metabolized by glucuronidation to patients with Gilbert's syndrome.

UNCONJUGATED HYPERBILIRUBIN IN THE NEWBORN PERIOD

Most neonates develop mild unconjugated hyperbilirubinemia between days 2 and 5 after birth because of hepatic immaturity and low levels of UGT1A1. Peak bilirubin levels are typically less than 5 to 10 mg/dL, and levels return to normal within 2 weeks as mechanisms of bilirubin disposition mature. Prematurity, with hemolysis or hepatic immaturity, is associated with higher bilirubin levels that may require phototherapy. The progestational steroid $3\alpha,20\beta$-pregnanediol and certain fatty acids that are found in breast milk (but not serum) of some mothers inhibit bilirubin conjugation and can cause excessive neonatal hyperbilirubinemia (*breast milk jaundice*). By comparison, *transient familial neonatal hyperbilirubinemia* (Lucey-Driscoll syndrome) is caused by a UGT1A1 inhibitor found in maternal serum.

Acquired Conjugation Defects

A modest reduction in bilirubin conjugating capacity occurs in advanced hepatitis or cirrhosis (Chapter 156). However, in this setting, conjugation is better preserved than other aspects of bilirubin disposition, such as

TABLE 149-2   PRINCIPAL FEATURES OF THE HEREDITARY DISORDERS OF BILIRUBIN METABOLISM

FEATURE	Crigler-Najjar Syndrome		GILBERT'S SYNDROME	DUBIN-JOHNSON SYNDROME	ROTOR'S SYNDROME
	TYPE I	**TYPE II**			
Incidence	Very rare	Uncommon	Up to 12% of population	Uncommon	Rare
Total serum bilirubin (mg/dL)	18-45 (usually >20), unconjugated	6-25 (usually ≤20), unconjugated	Typically ≤4 in absence of fasting or hemolysis; mostly unconjugated	Typically 2-5, less often ≤25; about 60% direct reacting	Usually 3-7, occasionally ≤20; about 60% direct reacting
Defect(s) in bilirubin metabolism*	Bilirubin UGT1A1 conjugating activity markedly reduced: trace to absent	Bilirubin UGT1A1 conjugating activity reduced: ≤10% of normal	Bilirubin UGT1A1 conjugating activity typically reduced to 10-33% of normal; reduced bilirubin uptake in some cases; mild hemolysis in up to 50% of patients	Impaired canalicular secretion of conjugated bilirubin due to MRP2/cMOAT mutation	Impaired hepatic secretion or storage of conjugated bilirubin; molecular defect not known
Routine liver tests	Normal	Normal	Normal	Normal	Normal
Serum bile acids	Normal	Normal	Normal	Usually normal	Normal
Plasma sulfobromophthalein removal (% retention of 5 mg/kg dose at 45 min)†	Normal	Normal	Usually normal (<5%); mild 45-min (<15%) retention in some patients	Slow initial decline in plasma concentration (retention ≤20% at 45 min) with secondary rise at 90-120 min	Very slow initial decline in plasma concentration (45-min retention = 30-45%) without secondary rise
Oral cholecystography	Normal	Normal	Normal	Faint or no visualization of gallbladder	Usually normal
Pharmacologic responses/special features	No response to phenobarbital	Phenobarbital reduces bilirubin by ≤75%	Phenobarbital reduces bilirubin, often to normal	Increased bilirubin concentration with estrogens; diagnostic urine coproporphyrin isomer pattern (total is normal, with isomer I increased to ≥80% of total)	Characteristic urine coproporphyrin excretion pattern (total is increased ≥2.5-fold in ~65% of cases, but isomer I always <80% of total)
Major clinical features	Kernicterus in infancy if untreated; may occur later despite therapy	Rare late-onset kernicterus with fasting	None	Occasional hepatosplenomegaly	None
Hepatic morphology/histology	Normal	Normal	Normal; occasionally increased lipofuscin pigment	Liver grossly black; coarse, dark centrilobular pigment	Normal
Bile bilirubin fractions‡	>90% unconjugated	Largest fraction (mean, 57%) monoconjugates	Mainly diconjugates but monoconjugates are increased (mean, 23%)	Mixed conjugates, reported increase in diconjugates	Increased conjugates
Inheritance (all autosomal)	Recessive	Recessive	Promoter mutation is recessive; missense mutation often dominant	Recessive; rare kindred appears dominant	Recessive
Diagnosis	Clinical and laboratory findings: lack of response to phenobarbital	Clinical and laboratory findings: response to phenobarbital	Clinical and laboratory findings: promoter genotyping; liver biopsy rarely necessary	Clinical and laboratory findings: liver biopsy unnecessary if coproporphyrin studies available; BSP disappearance	Clinical and laboratory findings: urine coproporphyrin analysis; BSP disappearance
Treatment	Phototherapy or tin protoporphyrin as short-term therapy; liver transplantation definitive	Consider phenobarbital if baseline bilirubin ≥8 mg/dL	None necessary	Avoid estrogens; no other therapy necessary	No treatment necessary

*UGT1A1 is the bilirubin specific isoform of the UGT1 family of uridine diphosphate glucuronosyl transferases.
†Sulfobromophthalein (BSP) studies: previously used to help distinguish Dubin-Johnson and Rotor's syndromes if coproporphyrin isomer studies not available. However, BSP is no longer approved for clinical use in the United States.
‡Bilirubin in normal bile: <5% unconjugated bilirubin, with an average of 7% bilirubin monoconjugates and 90% bilirubin diconjugates.
BSP = sulfobromophthalein; cMOAT = canalicular multispecific organic anion transporter; MRP2 = multidrug resistance–associated protein 2.

canalicular excretion. Pharmacologic and metabolic perturbations may also lead to acquired reductions in bilirubin conjugation. Various drugs (e.g., pregnanediol, novobiocin, chloramphenicol, gentamicin, and several HIV protease inhibitors) may cause unconjugated hyperbilirubinemia by inhibiting UGT1A1. In all settings in which UGT1A1 inhibitors cause unconjugated hyperbilirubinemia, the hyperbilirubinemia is greater in patients with underlying Gilbert's syndrome.

Conjugated or Mixed Hyperbilirubinemia

Two phenotypically similar but mechanistically distinct inherited disorders, *Dubin-Johnson syndrome* and *Rotor's syndrome*, are characterized by conjugated or mixed hyperbilirubinemia with normal values for other standard liver tests (see Table 149-2). Dubin-Johnson syndrome results from any of several mutations in the gene encoding the ATP-dependent canalicular organic anion transporter MPR2/cMOAT (see Fig. 149-1). The molecular defect in Rotor's syndrome remains unknown. Despite the conjugated hyperbilirubinemia, patients with these syndromes are not cholestatic and can be distinguished noninvasively by analysis of urine coproporphyrins (see Table 149-2), so liver biopsy is not required. Both syndromes carry a benign prognosis without specific therapy.

⬤ LIVER AND BILIARY TRACT DISEASE

Jaundice is a common sign of generalized hepatobiliary dysfunction, both acute and chronic. Icteric hepatobiliary disease is readily distinguished from the isolated disorders of bilirubin metabolism because the increase in plasma bilirubin concentration occurs in association with other markers of hepatobiliary injury. Liver diseases can be categorized as those in which the primary injury results from inflammation and hepatocellular necrosis, inhibition of bile flow (cholestasis), or a combination of the two. The cholestatic disorders can be further subdivided into those due to mechanical obstruction of the bile duct flow (Chapter 158) and those resulting from intrahepatic cholestasis, which may be the consequence of a multitude of conditions that include familial cholestatic syndromes and infiltrative disorders (Chapters 151 to 156), particularly those involving the intrahepatic biliary tree; sepsis (Chapter 108), and certain other inflammatory or neoplastic conditions; and drug reactions (see Table 149-1). It is important to note that chronic cholestasis from any cause may result in the intrahepatic accumulation of compounds such as bile acids, which may themselves be toxic, causing hepatocellular injury.

Familial Cholestasis Syndromes

Benign recurrent intrahepatic cholestasis (BRIC) is a rare disorder characterized by recurrent attacks of cholestatic jaundice beginning either in childhood or in adulthood and varying in duration from weeks to months. Intervals between attacks may vary from months to years. This benign disorder does not progress to chronic liver disease or cirrhosis. There is complete resolution between episodes; treatment during the cholestatic episodes is symptomatic. Three subtypes result from mutations in different canalicular transporters: *BRIC type 1* from a partial deficiency of the familial intrahepatic cholestasis 1 (FIC1) gene product, also designated ATP8B1; *BRIC type 2* from mutations in the bile salt export pump (BSEP, or ABCB11); and *BRIC type 3* from mutations in multidrug resistance–associated protein 3 (MDR3, ABCB4).

Progressive familial intrahepatic cholestasis (PFIC) is a heterogeneous group of cholestatic disorders of childhood that, by contrast, typically lead to hepatic fibrosis and end-stage liver disease before adulthood. The three best-characterized *PFIC* subtypes are type 1 (Byler's disease) and type 2, resulting from functionally more severe mutations in ATP8B1 and BSEP, respectively; and type 3, due to MDR3 deficiency. All forms of *BRIC* and *PFIC* are inherited as autosomal recessive disorders. Diagnostically, γ-glutamyl transpeptidase (GGT) levels are low despite elevations in alkaline phosphatase in types 1 and 2, whereas GGT and alkaline phosphatase are elevated in parallel in PFIC type 3, as in most other forms of cholestatic liver disease. In contrast to the selective bilirubin transport defect in Dubin-Johnson syndrome, the conjugated hyperbilirubinemia in these syndromes reflects generalized bile secretory failure.

Postoperative Jaundice

This multifactorial syndrome can be caused by increased bilirubin production (e.g., breakdown of transfused erythrocytes, resorption of hematomas) or decreased hepatic clearance (e.g., from bacteremia, endotoxemia, parenteral nutrition, perioperative hypoxia). Hyperbilirubinemia, the main biochemical feature, is often accompanied by a several-fold increase in alkaline phosphatase or GGT levels, or both. Aminotransferases are, at most, minimally elevated, and synthetic function is typically normal. The differential diagnosis includes biliary obstruction or hepatocellular injury related to shock, anesthetic injury (Chapter 152), or viral hepatitis (Chapter 150). Postoperative jaundice per se (Chapter 441) is not a threat to the patient, and it usually resolves in parallel with the patient's overall condition.

Jaundice in Pregnancy

Jaundice in pregnancy (Chapter 247) may result from any liver disease that also affects nonpregnant women or from conditions unique to pregnancy. The unique conditions include a generally modest, self-limited elevation of aminotransferase and bilirubin levels during the first trimester, often in patients with hyperemesis gravidarum; intrahepatic cholestasis of pregnancy (ICP), which occurs during the second and third trimesters and usually resolves spontaneously after delivery; or acute fatty liver or the HELLP (*h*emolysis, *e*levated *l*iver enzymes, and *l*ow *p*latelets) syndrome, in association with preeclampsia in the third trimester (Chapters 153, 178, and 247). ICP, as well as cholestasis occurring recurrently in some women taking oral contraceptives, is increasingly being linked to polymorphisms in the same genes responsible for BRIC and PFIC. Acute fatty liver may resemble fulminant hepatic failure, with early delivery a prerequisite to maternal recovery; a defect in the oxidation of long-chain fatty acids is found in some infants born after these pregnancies.

DIAGNOSTIC TOOLS FOR THE EVALUATION OF LIVER DISEASE

Accurate diagnosis and the distinction between acute and chronic disease are often dependent on appropriate selection and interpretation of a spectrum of laboratory and imaging studies.

Tests used in initial evaluation of liver disease fall into two categories: (1) tests that indicate injury, such as release of intracellular enzymes; and (2) tests that measure, or at least reflect, actual function. Tests that reflect injury usually do not measure liver function and should not be called liver function tests.

The important functions of the liver include clearance, biotransformation and detoxification of potentially toxic metabolites and exogenous compounds, synthesis and export of various plasma proteins, and a critical integrative role in the intermediary metabolism of carbohydrates, amino acids, and lipids. In specific diseases, some of these functions may be markedly compromised, whereas others are little affected. Liver tests must be chosen with care and interpreted within the total clinical context. In specific situations, serial determinations are often helpful to assess the course of disease or effects of therapy.

Serum Enzyme Tests

The levels of hepatic enzymes found in plasma are a measure of hepatocyte turnover or injury. Enzymes released during normal hepatocyte turnover are believed to be the principal basis for normal circulating levels. Cell injury and cell death activate phospholipases that create holes in the plasma membrane, thereby increasing the release of intracellular contents.

Aminotransferases

The aminotransferases (formerly called transaminases) catalyze transfer of the α-amino group of aspartate (aspartate aminotransferase, AST) or alanine (alanine aminotransferase, ALT) to the α-keto group of ketoglutarate, with pyridoxal phosphate (vitamin B_6) as a cofactor. Laboratory methods that assay aminotransferase activity require supplementation with vitamin B_6 to avoid falsely decreased activity in vitamin B_6-deficient subjects.

Normal ranges for serum aminotransferases are usually reported to be up to approximately 40 IU/L (see Appendix), but when particular care is taken to exclude obese patients and others with known fatty liver disease from the sampled population, results suggest that less than 30 IU/L is normal for men and less than 19 IU/L for women. Values can exceed 1000 IU/L in acute hepatocyte injury, for example, from viral infection (Chapter 150) or toxins (Chapter 152). ALT is a purely cytosolic enzyme. Distinct isoforms of AST are present in cytosol and mitochondria. Expression of the mitochondrial isoform and its physiologic export from the hepatocyte are upregulated by ethanol. Circulating levels of AST or ALT (or both) are elevated in most hepatic diseases, and the degree of aminotransferase activity found in plasma roughly reflects the current activity of the disease process. There are, however, critical exceptions, and the sensitivity of aminotransferases as markers of hepatocellular injury varies with the disease in question. A subset of patients with proven chronic hepatitis C have normal aminotransferase levels, approximately 25% of morbidly obese patients with biopsy-proven nonalcoholic steatohepatitis may have normal ALT levels, and aminotransferase levels greater than or equal to 200 to 300 IU/L are uncommon in even the most severe cases of alcoholic hepatitis (Chapter 155). By contrast, aminotransferases of 1000 IU/L or greater are often present in even mild acute viral hepatitis (Chapter 150) or shortly after acute biliary obstruction, for example, during passage of a gallstone (Chapter 158). Conversely, aminotransferase levels may decline during the course of massive hepatic necrosis because liver injury is so extensive that little enzyme activity remains (Chapter 157). In rare circumstances, autoantibodies to AST result in autoantibody-enzyme complexes called macroenzymes that have a delayed clearance, detected as an increase in enzyme concentrations in the absence of cellular turnover.

Aminotransferase levels are useful in several distinct ways. First, they provide a relatively specific screening test for hepatobiliary disease. Although AST levels may be increased with disease of other organs (notably myocardial and skeletal muscle), values ten times the upper limit of normal or greater almost invariably indicate hepatobiliary pathology. Moreover, in the total clinical context, the source of increased aminotransferase activity is usually obvious. Aminotransferase levels are also used to monitor the activity of an acute or chronic parenchymal liver disease and its response to therapy. However, levels in a given patient may correlate poorly with the severity of the disease as assessed by liver biopsy, particularly in chronic hepatitis C

(Chapter 151). Aminotransferases are also often normal in advanced cirrhosis (Chapter 156), in which they are of limited prognostic value. Finally, aminotransferase levels may provide diagnostic clues. AST levels 15 or more times normal are unusual in *chronic* bile duct obstruction unless there is concomitant cholangitis, and AST levels 6 or more times normal are uncommon in alcoholic liver disease in the absence of other causes. In most liver diseases, the ratio of AST to ALT is usually less than or equal to 1. However, ratios are typically 2 or higher in alcoholic fatty liver and alcoholic hepatitis (Chapter 155), reflecting increased mitochondrial AST synthesis and secretion into plasma and selective loss of ALT activity because of the pyridoxine deficiency commonly seen in alcoholism. An elevated AST/ALT ratio also occurs in fulminant hepatitis related to Wilson disease (Chapters 153 and 218).

Alkaline Phosphatase

Alkaline phosphatases are widely distributed enzymes (e.g., liver, bile ducts, intestine, bone, kidney, placenta, and leukocytes) that catalyze the release of orthophosphate from ester substrates at an alkaline pH. The normal activity level in adult serum is highly dependent on the measurement method, age, and sex. Two methods in current use have upper limits of normal in adults of 85 and 110 IU/L (see Appendix). Higher levels are normal in children and in pregnancy. Results must always be compared with the appropriate normal range. In bone, alkaline phosphatase participates in the deposition of hydroxyapatite in osteoid. In other sites, including liver, alkaline phosphatase activity may facilitate movement of molecules across cell membranes. Serum alkaline phosphatase activity usually reflects principally the hepatic and bone isozymes; the intestinal form may account for 20 to 60% of the total after a fatty meal. There is a substantial placental contribution to the alkaline phosphatase level late in pregnancy; the *Regan isozyme,* a variant that appears identical to the placental form, is associated with hepatomas (Chapter 202), lung cancer (Chapter 197), and other tumors.

Elevations in serum alkaline phosphatase activity in cholestatic hepatobiliary disease result from two distinct mechanisms: increased synthesis and secretion of the enzyme and solubilization from the apical (canalicular) surface of hepatocytes and the luminal surface of biliary epithelial cells by the increased local concentrations of bile acids that occur with cholestasis. Serum alkaline phosphatase activity may also be increased in bone disorders (e.g., Paget's disease [Chapter 255], osteomalacia [Chapter 252], bone metastases [Chapter 208]), during rapid bone growth in children, in the later stages of pregnancy, with chronic renal failure (Chapter 132), and, occasionally, in the presence of malignancy not involving bones or liver. The source is often obvious, but when it is not, methods such as heat stability and electrophoretic separation can distinguish hepatobiliary alkaline phosphatase from other forms. A simpler alternative is to measure serum levels of GGT or 5′-nucleotidase (5′-NT), which tend to parallel levels of alkaline phosphatase in hepatobiliary disease but are usually not increased in bone disease. With a serum half-life of approximately 1 week, serum alkaline phosphatase may remain elevated for days to weeks after resolution of biliary obstruction. This delay may be especially misleading when it is accompanied by prolonged direct-reacting hyperbilirubinemia owing to delayed clearance of δ-bilirubin.

Modest increases in serum alkaline phosphatase (three times normal or less) occur in many hepatic parenchymal disorders, including hepatitis and cirrhosis. In the absence of bone disease, larger increases (three to ten times normal) usually indicate obstruction of bile flow. Although the highest levels usually reflect obstruction of the common bile duct, elevations can also occur with obstruction of intrahepatic bile ducts from infiltrative conditions that arise from granulomatous processes (sarcoidosis, *Mycobacterium avium-intracellulare, Mycobacterium tuberculosis*), malignancy (lymphoma, cholangiocarcinoma, or metastatic cancer) or amyloidosis.

Other Hepatic Enzymes

5′-NT is a plasma membrane enzyme that cleaves orthophosphate from the 5′ position on the pentose sugar of adenosine or inosine phosphate. *Leucine aminopeptidase (LAP)* is a ubiquitous cellular peptidase. The serum levels of both usually increase in cholestasis. Accordingly, their major use is to confirm whether an elevated serum alkaline phosphatase is hepatic in origin. Both enzymes may be increased in the later stages of a healthy pregnancy.

γ-*Glutamyl transpeptidase (GGT)* is present in many tissues. Its serum activity increases in hepatobiliary disease but also after myocardial infarction; in neuromuscular diseases, pancreatic disease (even in the absence of biliary obstruction), pulmonary disease, and diabetes; and during the ingestion of ethanol and other inducers of microsomal enzymes. Nevertheless, because serum GGT levels are usually normal in bone disease, the enzyme may be

helpful in confirming the hepatic origin of an elevated alkaline phosphatase. Measurement of GGT has been proposed as a sensitive screening test for hepatobiliary disease and for monitoring abstinence from ethanol. Because of its low specificity, many persons who test positive have no identifiable liver disease on further study. GGT offers no clear advantage over LAP or 5′-NT for identifying the source of increased serum alkaline phosphatase activity except in pregnancy. Serum GGT levels may be normal despite elevated hepatobiliary alkaline phosphatase levels in certain rare disorders, including benign recurrent intrahepatic cholestasis and progressive familial intrahepatic cholestasis types 1 and 2 (see earlier and Chapter 158).

Lactate dehydrogenase (LDH) levels are often elevated in hepatic ischemia; otherwise, the enzyme is too ubiquitous in other body tissues to be diagnostically useful.

Tests Based on Clearance of Metabolites and Drugs

A major liver function is to remove various metabolites and toxins from the blood (Chapter 152). In liver disease, clearance of such molecules may be impaired because of loss of parenchymal cells, diminished bile secretion, biliary obstruction, decreased cellular uptake or metabolism, or reduced or heterogeneous hepatic blood flow. When a metabolite is produced at a relatively constant rate (e.g., bilirubin), its serum level can be a sensitive indicator of liver function. The removal rate from plasma of certain exogenous drugs and dyes can be similarly interpreted.

Bilirubin

The differential diagnosis of hyperbilirubinemia (see earlier) includes generalized liver disease, inherited disorders of bilirubin metabolism (e.g., Gilbert's and Crigler-Najjar syndromes), and nonhepatic conditions (e.g., hemolysis). Higher bilirubin levels correlate with a poorer prognosis in acute alcoholic hepatitis (Chapter 155), fulminant hepatic failure (Chapter 157), primary biliary cirrhosis (Chapter 156), and most forms of chronic liver disease.

Ammonia

Ammonia, a byproduct of amino acid metabolism, is removed from blood by the liver, converted to urea in the Krebs-Henseleit cycle, and excreted by the kidneys (Chapter 117). In the setting of portosystemic shunting, severe hepatic dysfunction (e.g., fulminant hepatic failure), or defects in urea cycle metabolism, ammonia levels rise. Measurements of blood ammonia are sometimes used to confirm a diagnosis of hepatic encephalopathy and to monitor the success of therapy, but the correlation of ammonia levels with the degree of encephalopathy is only approximate (Chapter 157). Correlations may be somewhat better if the measurement is made rapidly on an iced arterial blood sample. Elevated ammonia levels also occur when ammonia production is increased by intestinal flora (e.g., after a high-protein meal or gastrointestinal bleeding), by the kidney (in response to metabolic alkalosis or hypokalemia), or in rare genetic diseases that affect the pathway of urea synthesis (Chapter 212).

Drug Clearance

The rate of hepatic clearance of compounds such as sulfobromophthalein, lidocaine, and aminopyrine from the circulation can be measured chemically or with radiolabeled tracers. Although such tests can quantify hepatic function, they are rarely used in clinical practice.

Tests Reflecting Hepatic Synthetic Function
Coagulation Tests

See also Chapters 37 and 174.

Prothrombin Time

The prothrombin time (PT) reflects the plasma concentrations of both extrinsic and common pathway factors, that is, factors VII, X, and V, prothrombin, and fibrinogen. A prolonged PT most often results from vitamin K deficiency, liver disease, or both. Vitamin K, a fat-soluble vitamin found in many foods, is also synthesized by gut bacteria (Chapter 177). Vitamin K deficiency can be caused by poor dietary intake and malabsorptive states, including fat malabsorption resulting from cholestasis, and also occurs with antibiotic suppression of gut flora, particularly in patients receiving inadequate vitamin K replacement.

The half-lives of clotting factors are typically less than 1 day. Factor VII, which has the shortest half-life, is usually the earliest and most severely depressed during periods of defective hepatic synthesis. Because the PT is dependent on the level of factor VII, it responds rapidly with changes in hepatic synthetic function; it is useful for following the course of acute liver diseases, in which a significant or growing prolongation of the PT may indicate a poor prognosis. An abnormal PT that is due solely to vitamin K deficiency usually becomes normal within 24 to 48 hours after parenteral repletion. However, if decreased synthesis of clotting factors reflects hepatocyte dysfunction, there may be little or no response to vitamin K. Finally, prolongation of the PT may also reflect disseminated intravascular coagulation (Chapter 178), which should always be considered in the context of both acute liver failure and end-stage chronic liver disease.

Partial Thromboplastin Time

This test reflects both intrinsic and common pathway factors, that is, all classical clotting factors except factor VII, and is, therefore, complementary to the PT. It is especially useful in detecting circulating anticoagulants (Chapter 178) but adds little to the PT in evaluating hepatic synthetic function.

Albumin

Albumin is produced solely by the liver. Its plasma concentration reflects a balance between its synthetic rate (100 to 200 mg/kg/day) and its plasma half-life of about 21 days. The synthetic rate is affected by the patient's nutritional state, thyroid and glucocorticoid hormone levels, plasma colloid osmotic pressure, exposure to hepatotoxins (e.g., alcohol), and presence of systemic disorders or liver disease. Many conditions increase albumin losses and shorten its plasma half-life, including nephrotic syndrome (Chapter 123), protein-losing enteropathy (Chapter 142), severe burns (Chapter 112), exfoliative dermatitis, and major gastrointestinal bleeding (Chapter 137). In cirrhosis with ascites (Chapters 156 and 157), hypoalbuminemia indicates diminished synthesis or redistribution into ascitic fluid. Thus, a reduced serum albumin concentration can confidently be considered an indicator of decreased hepatic synthetic function only when these other factors are not involved.

Examinations of Urine and Stool

Bilirubinuria always indicates a pathologic increase in plasma conjugated bilirubin levels. It is frequently seen with plasma conjugated bilirubin concentrations of 2 to 3 mg/dL, often appearing before the onset of clinical jaundice and persisting after jaundice has resolved. The quantification of urobilinogen in urine or feces is of limited clinical value. By contrast, stool culture or examination for ova and parasites may provide important information in selected patients. Testing of stool for occult blood may lead to discovery of a gastrointestinal lesion related to hepatobiliary disease (e.g., tumors metastatic to liver, ulcerative colitis associated with sclerosing cholangitis) or may explain the onset or worsening of hepatic encephalopathy.

Hematologic Tests in Liver Disease

In moderate to severe acute liver diseases, varying degrees of cytopenia occur in all three cell lineages. The most common finding is of thrombocytopenia from hypersplenism, which can be a surrogate marker of portal hypertension. Anemia may reflect low-grade hemolysis or marrow depression. Bone marrow suppression may be caused by ethanol or drugs, and aplastic anemia may sometimes complicate acute viral hepatitis (Chapters 150 and 168). Zieve's syndrome (hemolytic anemia and hypertriglyceridemia) is a rare but well-characterized complication of severe alcoholic liver disease (Chapters 155 and 156). Modest leukopenia, often with atypical lymphocytes, may also be present. Coagulopathy frequently complicates both acute and chronic liver failure owing to depressed hepatic synthesis of clotting factors or disseminated intravascular coagulation, or both (Chapters 177 and 178).

A modest increase in erythrocyte mean corpuscular volume occurs with alcohol consumption, hemolysis, or on occasion, liver disease per se. Chronic liver disease, especially if cholestatic, may be accompanied by target cells in the peripheral blood smear. Target cells are erythrocytes with an expanded cell membrane that reflects abnormalities in serum lipids. Spur cells (acanthocytes), most often found in advanced alcoholic cirrhosis, reflect a still greater increase in membrane cholesterol.

Tests for Specific Liver Diseases

Patients who present with a picture of acute or chronic parenchymal liver disease are most likely to fall into one of three categories: viral or toxic hepatitis, including alcoholic and nonalcoholic fatty liver disease; autoimmune liver disease; or an inherited metabolic disorder Specific tests for viral antigens, nucleic acids, and antibodies are available for the conventional hepatitis

viruses (Chapters 150 and 151) as well as Epstein-Barr virus (Chapter 385), cytomegalovirus (Chapter 384), and herpesviruses (Chapters 382 and 383), which are well-established but less common causes of liver disease. The major hepatic autoimmune diseases include primary biliary cirrhosis (Chapter 158), autoimmune hepatitis (Chapter 151), and various overlap syndromes. The starting point for establishing a specific diagnosis within this category is the search for specific serum autoantibodies, including antimitochondrial antibodies against epitopes of the pyruvate dehydrogenase complex, which are virtually diagnostic of primary biliary cirrhosis (Chapter 158), and antinuclear, anti–smooth muscle, and anti–liver microsomal antibodies, which suggest one of the subtypes of autoimmune hepatitis (Chapter 148). The most prevalent of the hereditary metabolic disorders affecting the liver (Chapter 153) include hemochromatosis (Chapter 219), α_1-antitrypsin deficiency (Chapter 153), and Wilson disease (Chapter 218).

Liver Biopsy

Liver biopsy can be of great help in the diagnosis of diffuse or localized parenchymal diseases, including chronic hepatitis, cirrhosis, and primary or metastatic malignancy in the liver. The value of liver biopsy in acute hepatitis or acute cholestatic jaundice may be primarily prognostic because the histologic changes in these settings, although sometimes suggesting a specific diagnosis, are often nonspecific. However, toxic hepatitis (Chapter 152) related to certain medications may display diagnostic features. Liver biopsy for assessment of diffuse disease can be performed percutaneously after localization of the liver by physical examination or ultrasonographic visualization. When specific lesions, such as tumors, must be sampled, the biopsy can be guided by ultrasonographic or radiographic imaging or performed under direct visualization during laparoscopy or laparotomy. Relative or absolute contraindications include coagulopathy, high-grade biliary obstruction, biliary sepsis, ascites, and right pleural disease. Although liver biopsy remains the standard for assessment of hepatic histology in diffuse disease (Chapter 148), its invasiveness and concern for sampling error have generated interest in noninvasive measures of hepatic diseases. Transient elastography uses ultrasound to assess tissue stiffness as a measure of hepatic fibrosis. Commercially available biomarker panels have also been developed to provide a noninvasive assessment of hepatic fibrosis by blood testing alone. These panels typically include standard laboratory measures of hepatic injury (GGT, total bilirubin) and other serum markers (e.g., haptoglobin, hyaluronic acid, apolipoprotein A1). However, the ability of currently available noninvasive markers to assess the extent of hepatic fibrosis across the clinically relevant histologic spectrum remains to be established. Magnetic resonance elastography is another, emerging technique to characterize liver tissue elasticity, and hence fibrosis, noninvasively.

⬤ APPROACH TO THE PATIENT WITH JAUNDICE OR ABNORMAL LIVER TESTS

History, Physical Examination, and Initial Laboratory Studies

Patients with liver disease may present with jaundice or other signs or symptoms, or the disease may be detected in the asymptomatic patient by the finding of abnormal liver tests during a routine evaluation. Regardless of how the patient comes to medical attention, the diagnostic approach (Fig. 149-3) begins with a careful history and physical examination (Chapter 148), as well as screening laboratory studies (complete blood cell count, measurement of plasma bilirubin concentration, assay of ALT, AST, and alkaline phosphatase levels, and PT) to formulate an initial differential diagnosis. The ability to distinguish expeditiously between liver disease and extrahepatic biliary tract obstruction is the major goal of the initial evaluation, in part because the latter may require prompt surgical intervention. Appropriate choice of second-level laboratory tests and imaging studies leads to a definitive diagnosis in most patients. Care in selecting tests, particularly imaging studies, both maximizes the likelihood of making a correct diagnosis and protects the patient from unnecessary discomfort, risk, and expense.

If the patient is asymptomatic and hepatic tests other than bilirubin are normal, hemolysis or an isolated disorder of bilirubin metabolism should be considered. If signs, symptoms, or laboratory abnormalities indicate hepatobiliary disease, certain patterns of findings help to distinguish intrinsic liver disease from biliary obstruction (Table 149-3). Pain in the right upper quadrant accompanied by a predominant increase in serum alkaline phosphatase activity suggests biliary obstruction (Chapter 158), as does a history of prior biliary surgery, right upper quadrant scars, or an abdominal mass. Fever and

FIGURE 149-3. Diagnostic algorithm for the evaluation of hyperbilirubinemia and other liver test abnormalities and/or signs and symptoms suggestive of liver disease. CT = computed tomography; ERCP = endoscopic retrograde cholangiopancreatography; EUS = endoscopic ultrasound; PTC = percutaneous cholangiogram; MRCP = magnetic resonance cholangiopancreatography. (Modified from Lidofsky SD, Scharschmidt BF. Jaundice. In: Feldman M, Scharschmidt BF, Sleisenger MH, eds. *Gastrointestinal and Liver Disease*. 6th ed. Philadelphia: WB Saunders; 1998:227.)

TABLE 149-3   OBSTRUCTIVE JAUNDICE VERSUS CHOLESTATIC LIVER DISEASE

FEATURE	SUGGESTS OBSTRUCTIVE JAUNDICE	SUGGESTS PARENCHYMAL LIVER DISEASE
History	Abdominal pain Fever, rigors Previous biliary surgery Older age Acholic stools	Anorexia, malaise, myalgias, suggestive of a viral prodrome Known infectious exposure Receipt of blood products, use of intravenous drugs Exposure to a known hepatotoxin Family history of jaundice
Physical examination	High fever Abdominal tenderness Palpable abdominal mass Abdominal scar	Ascites Other stigmata of liver disease (e.g., prominent abdominal veins, gynecomastia, spider angiomas, asterixis, encephalopathy, Kayser-Fleischer rings)
Laboratory studies	Predominant elevation of serum bilirubin and alkaline phosphatase Prothrombin time that is normal or normalizes with vitamin K administration Elevated serum amylase	Predominant elevation of serum aminotransferases Prolonged prothrombin time that does not correct with vitamin K administration Blood tests indicative of specific liver disease

rigors, indicative of cholangitis, strengthen this conclusion. The incidences of gallstone disease and malignant neoplasm increase with age, although risk factors such as obesity or recent extensive diet-induced weight loss increase the risk of gallstones. Other risk factors (e.g., hepatitis exposure, transfusions, intravenous drug use, alcohol use, certain medications, and family history of genetic diseases) and a predominant elevation in serum aminotransferase levels favor a diagnosis of parenchymal liver disease. Physical evidence of cirrhosis (e.g., spider angiomas, gynecomastia, ascites, splenomegaly) supports the diagnosis of chronic parenchymal disease.

Despite the general validity of these patterns, many exceptions exist. In particular, parenchymal disorders with prominent cholestasis may mimic biliary obstruction. Both alkaline phosphatase and GGT are usually elevated in patients with cholestasis; the combination of an elevated alkaline phosphatase and normal GGT suggests that the alkaline phosphatase is from bone. Conversely, an isolated elevation of GGT may result from certain drugs (e.g., diphenylhydantoin) or alcohol even in the absence of liver disease. Because of the risk of life-threatening infection in the setting of unrelieved biliary tract obstruction, this possibility must always be considered and excluded if an alternative diagnosis is not definitely established.

Imaging Studies

If extrahepatic obstruction is suspected, it should be possible to determine its site and nature in virtually all patients (see Fig. 149-3). A reasonable initial step is the use of a noninvasive study such as ultrasonography or computed tomography (CT) to determine whether the intrahepatic or extrahepatic biliary system is dilated, implying mechanical obstruction. Because of its

lesser expense, lack of radiation exposure, portability, and convenience, ultrasonography is often the procedure of choice and is substantially better than CT for detecting gallstones. CT may be preferred when better anatomic definition and information about the general level of obstruction are desired. Still more precise resolution may be obtained with magnetic resonance imaging cholangiopancreatography (MRCP). However, all of these techniques can fail to identify dilated ducts, particularly in patients with cirrhosis or primary sclerosing cholangitis. Conversely, a modest degree of ductal dilation is common in a patient with a previous cholecystectomy and does not necessarily signify current obstruction. Ultrasonography has the disadvantage of being highly operator dependent, whereas optimal CT imaging requires the use of intravenous contrast agents that may be nephrotoxic.

If dilated ducts are found, the biliary tree should be examined by endoscopic retrograde cholangiopancreatography (ERCP) or percutaneous transhepatic cholangiography (PTC) (Chapter 136). ERCP involves positioning an endoscope in the duodenum, inserting a catheter through the ampulla of Vater, and injecting contrast medium into the distal common bile duct or pancreatic duct, or both. PTC involves percutaneous passage of a needle through the hepatic parenchyma into a peripheral bile duct, followed by injection of contrast medium into the biliary tree through the peripheral duct. The choice of procedure is based on the suspected site of obstruction (proximal vs. distal); the presence of coagulopathy or a history of prior gastroduodenal surgery that might preclude PTC or ERCP, respectively; the likely need for a therapeutic procedure (e.g., stent placement or endoscopic sphincterotomy); and the skills of available staff. Endoscopic ultrasound (EUS) is a complementary approach that permits internal ultrasonographic analysis of the pancreas, extrahepatic bile ducts, and regional lymph nodes and blood vessels. EUS combined with fine-needle aspiration permits tissue sampling of abnormalities in areas such as the bile ducts and pancreas that typically have been difficult to sample percutaneously.

Selection of Imaging Tests

Liver ultrasound is an ideal screening test to evaluate the liver architecture, assess for surface nodularity and parenchymal mass lesions, and exclude biliary obstruction. Ultrasound is relatively inexpensive in comparison to other imaging modalities, is widely available, and avoids ionizing radiation. The identification of mass lesions on ultrasound commonly prompts further cross-sectional imaging with either CT or magnetic resonance imaging. If there is evidence of biliary obstruction on imaging, or if obstruction is still considered likely despite imaging findings, direct cholangiography by ERCP or PTC, which offer therapeutic as well as diagnostic capabilities, may be an appropriate choice. If obstruction is considered possible but not highly likely, noninvasive imaging with MRCP is a reasonable study. Individual radiology suites have different levels of expertise for these procedures, and the local radiology staff may be quite helpful in recommending the best procedure for a given patient.

● APPROACH TO THE ASYMPTOMATIC PATIENT WITH ABNORMAL LIVER TESTS

The apparently healthy patient with an isolated abnormality of aminotransferase or alkaline phosphatase levels requires careful evaluation to identify any underlying disease while avoiding unneeded testing. Often, no significant disease is found despite extensive evaluation. Common causes of abnormal

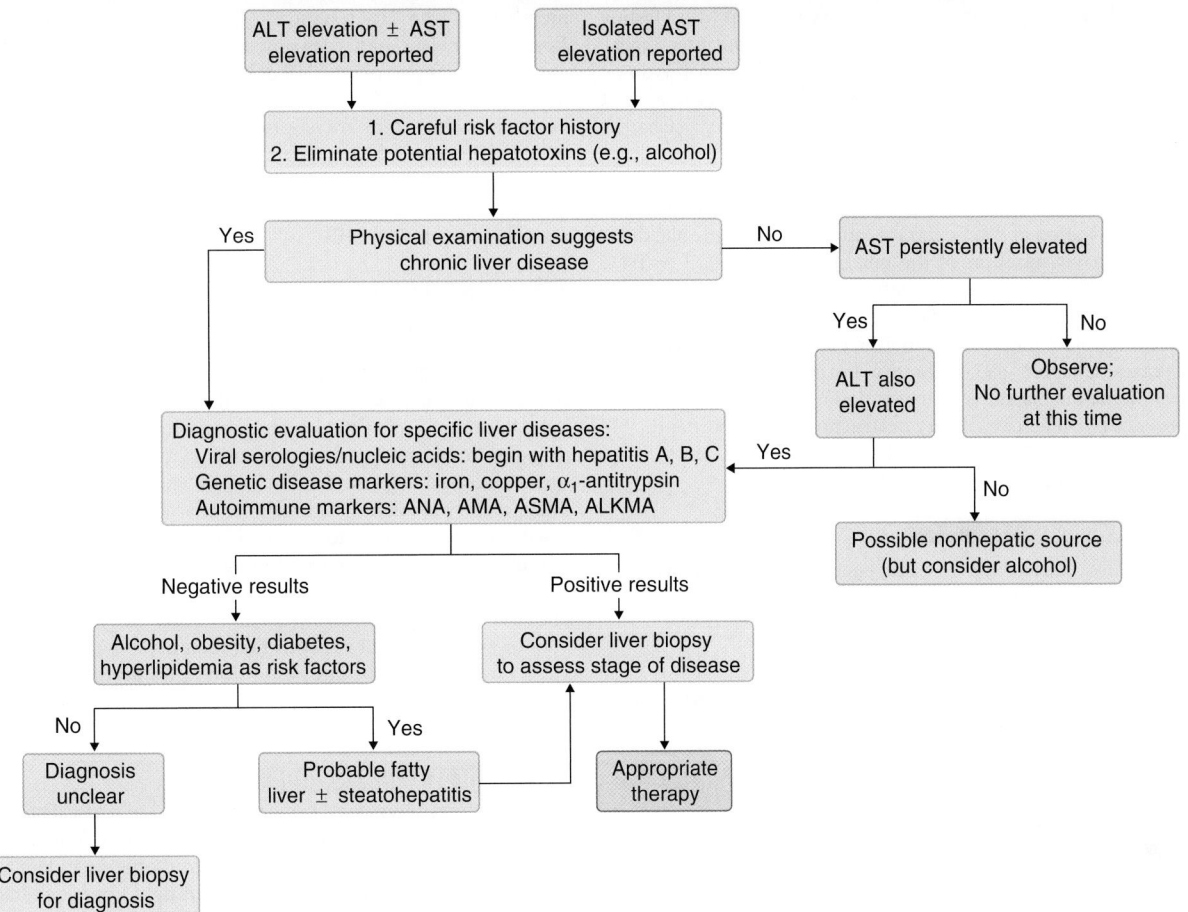

FIGURE 149-4. Approach to the evaluation of isolated elevated levels of serum alanine aminotransferase (ALT) and/or aspartate aminotransferase (AST) in the asymptomatic patient. ALKMA = anti-liver/kidney microsomal antibody; AMA = antimitochondrial antibody; ANA = antinuclear antibody; ASMA = anti–smooth muscle antibody.

enzyme tests include obesity, alcohol consumption, chronic hepatitis C, steatohepatitis, bone disease, and muscle injury.

Asymptomatic Aminotransferase Elevation

Epidemiologic data suggest that up to 25% of asymptomatic adult Americans have a mild to moderate elevation of aminotransferase levels. The incidental discovery of such abnormalities is currently the most frequent means by which liver disease is first recognized. Whereas up to one third of such patients have no elevation on subsequent testing, many others prove to have hepatic steatosis or steatohepatitis (Chapter 155) or chronic hepatitis C (Chapter 151) (Fig. 149-4). Further evaluation is generally indicated only in patients with persistent abnormalities. Initial screening should include a careful history of exposure to hepatotoxins (alcohol, prescription drugs, over-the-counter medications, herbs, chemicals, and occupational exposures). If the abnormal test was an AST, a hepatic origin for the enzyme elevation should be confirmed with an ALT determination. If the ALT is normal, a muscle source is likely, or the elevation may reflect the presence of a macro-enzyme. If the ALT level is abnormal, the patient should be screened serologically for hepatitis B and C; young women in particular should also be screened for markers of autoimmune liver disease. Older persons should be screened for hemochromatosis with an iron and transferrin level (Chapter 219), whereas younger persons should be screened with ceruloplasmin and urine copper for Wilson disease (Chapter 218). If these tests are negative, screening for α_1-antitrypsin deficiency is indicated (Chapter 153). Malaria (Chapter 353), schistosomiasis (Chapter 363), and other parasitic diseases should be considered in appropriate settings. A substantial fraction of patients prove to have fatty liver, with or without nonalcoholic steatohepatitis (NASH; Chapter 155). AST abnormalities caused by alcohol-induced steatosis should become normal with several weeks of abstinence. If the abnormalities persist for 6 to 12 months without an apparent cause, liver biopsy should be considered.

Asymptomatic Alkaline Phosphatase Elevation

Many patients with isolated elevation of the alkaline phosphatase level have nonhepatic causes, such as pregnancy or bone disease (Fig. 149-5). The

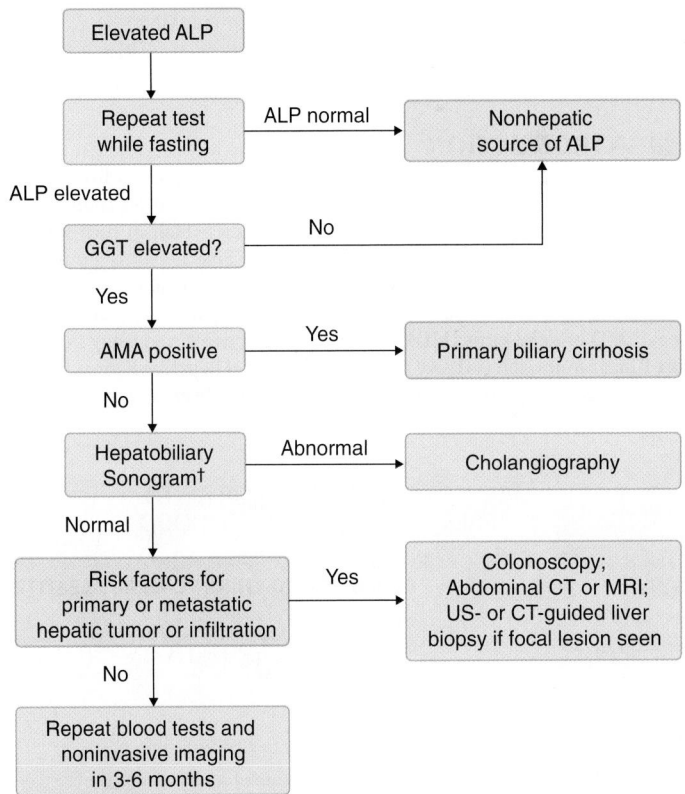

FIGURE 149-5. Approach to the asymptomatic patient with isolated elevated levels of serum alkaline phosphatase (ALP). †In cases with a high index of suspicion of biliary tract disease, such as sclerosing cholangitis, cholangiography may be warranted even in the face of normal ultrasound imaging. AMA = antimitochondrial antibody; CT = computed tomography; GGT = γ-glutamyl transpeptidase; MRI = magnetic resonance imaging; US = ultrasonography.

origin of an elevated alkaline phosphatase should be confirmed with a fasting sample because intestinal alkaline phosphatase may be elevated after a meal. A hepatic source is highly likely if the serum GGT is also abnormal. Women should be screened with an antimitochondrial antibody test; a positive result suggests primary biliary cirrhosis (Chapter 158). A careful history (Chapter 148) identifies patients at risk for intrahepatic cholestasis related to drugs or toxins. Essentially all other patients with persistently abnormal alkaline phosphatase should receive a hepatobiliary sonogram or other noninvasive imaging test. Demonstration of dilated intrahepatic or extrahepatic bile ducts should prompt direct visualization of the biliary tract by ERCP or PTC (Chapters 136 and 158). Evidence of an intrahepatic mass should prompt thorough evaluation for possible malignancy (Chapters 158 and 202). Because colon cancer often metastasizes to liver, colonoscopy may be useful in appropriate cases (Chapter 199). Infiltrative diseases, including schistosomiasis and granulomatous hepatitis (Chapter 154), should also be considered. In the absence of evidence of biliary obstruction or a cause identifiable by noninvasive means, liver biopsy should be strongly considered to complete the evaluation of cholestatic liver test abnormalities.

SUGGESTED READINGS

Castera L, Bedossa P. How to assess liver fibrosis in chronic hepatitis C: serum markers or transient elastography vs. liver biopsy? *Liver Int.* 2011;Suppl 1:13-17. *Discusses the advantages and limitations of liver biopsy and new, noninvasive diagnostic methods in clinical practice.*

Stapelbroek JM, van Erpecum KJ, Klomp LW, et al. Liver disease associated with canalicular transport defects: current and future therapies. *J Hepatol.* 2010;52:258-271. *Review of molecular transporters and their role in inherited and acquired cholestatic disease.*

Strassburg CP. Hyperbilirubinemia syndromes (Gilbert-Meulengracht, Criggler-Najjar, Dubin-Johnson, Rotor syndrome). *Best Pract Res Clin Gastroenterol.* 2010;24:555-571. *Summary of current knowledge.*

150

ACUTE VIRAL HEPATITIS

HEINER WEDEMEYER AND JEAN-MICHEL PAWLOTSKY

INTRODUCTION

Infection with a hepatotropic virus causes an acute episode of liver inflammation, referred to as *acute hepatitis*, which can lead to either spontaneous clearance of the infectious agent or its persistence, which in turn leads to chronic infection for a subset of these viruses. Five hepatitis viruses are responsible for the vast majority of acute hepatitis cases (Table 150-1): hepatitis A virus (HAV); hepatitis B virus (HBV); hepatitis C virus (HCV); hepatitis D or delta virus (HDV), which is a defective viroid using the hepatitis B surface antigen (HBsAg) as its envelope; and hepatitis E virus (HEV). Other viruses may also cause acute inflammatory liver disease, including

members of the Herpesviridae family such as human cytomegalovirus, Epstein-Barr virus, or herpes simplex virus. It is unclear to what extent other viruses, such as parvovirus B19 or human herpesvirus 6, can also cause acute hepatitis. Patients who present with an acute viral hepatitis syndrome but negative virologic tests are referred to as having non A to E hepatitis, perhaps owing to unknown hepatotropic viruses. The worldwide incidence of acute viral hepatitis is decreasing because of global improvement in hygiene and the development and use of efficient vaccines against HAV and HBV, and perhaps in the future, HEV.

GENERAL FEATURES OF ACUTE VIRAL HEPATITIS

PATHOBIOLOGY

Acute viral hepatitis is characterized by acute necroinflammation of the liver. Because none of the hepatotropic viruses is cytopathic, liver injury is thought to be mediated by a strong cytotoxic T-cell-mediated reaction against infected hepatocytes that express viral antigens at their surface. Proinflammatory cytokines, natural killer cells, and antibody-dependent cellular cytotoxicity also appear to play a role in liver necroinflammation. Successful immune elimination may lead to viral clearance, which may or may not be associated with lifelong immunity, depending on the infecting agent. The immune reaction is sometimes so potent that the patient develops subfulminant or even fulminant hepatitis that requires liver transplantation (Chapter 157). In some patients—the proportion varies, according to the virus responsible for acute hepatitis—the immune response fails and chronic infection is established (Chapter 151).

CLINICAL MANIFESTATIONS

After infection, there is an incubation period of a few days to a few weeks, depending on the causative agent (Fig. 150-1). This incubation period is generally characterized by nonspecific symptoms, including fatigue, nausea, loss of appetite, flu-like symptoms, and/or right upper quadrant pain (Table 150-2). The incubation period is often characterized by leukopenia and relative lymphocytosis. Immune-mediated symptoms, including rash, hives, arthralgias, angioneurotic edema, and fever, are observed in 10 to 20% of patients during the preicteric phase.

During the acute stage of the disease, symptoms may vary widely, from asymptomatic to subicteric, icteric or severe, and fulminant. The icteric form, which is not frequent, is characterized by fatigue, anorexia, nausea, dysgeusia, jaundice, dark urine, light colored stool, and weight loss. Physical

TABLE 150-1	VIRUSES RESPONSIBLE FOR ACUTE VIRAL HEPATITIS AND LIKELIHOOD OF CHRONIC EVOLUTION
VIRUS	**EVOLUTION TO CHRONIC VIRAL HEPATITIS**
Hepatitis A	Never
Hepatitis B	>90% (perinatal acquisition) to <1% (adult infection)
Hepatitis C	50-80%
Hepatitis D or delta	2% (coinfection) to 90% (superinfection)
Hepatitis E	Occasionally in immunosuppressed patients

Other viruses
  Human cytomegalovirus
  Epstein-Barr
  Herpes simplex
  Human herpesvirus 6
  Parvovirus B19
	May establish chronic infection, not associated with chronic hepatitis

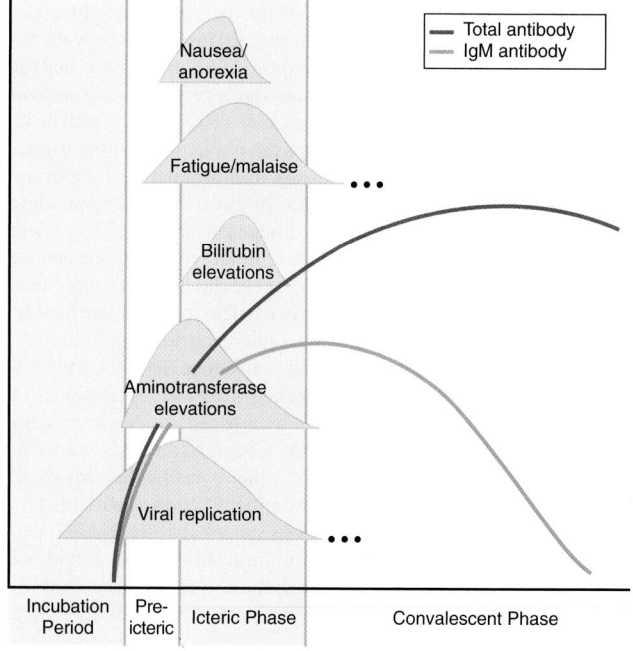

Acute Viral Hepatitis

Nausea/anorexia

Fatigue/malaise

Bilirubin elevations

Aminotransferase elevations

Viral replication

Total antibody — IgM antibody

Incubation Period | Pre-icteric | Icteric Phase | Convalescent Phase

Time After Exposure

FIGURE 150-1. Typical course of acute viral hepatitis.

TABLE 150-2 CLINICAL MANIFESTATIONS OF VIRAL HEPATITIS

PHASES OF INFECTION	DURATION*	MANIFESTATIONS*
Inoculation	2-20 wk	Virus detectable in blood Aminotransferase and bilirubin levels normal No antibody detectable
Preicteric	3-10 days	Nonspecific symptoms: fatigue, anorexia, nausea, vague right upper quadrant pain Viral titers peak Aminotransferase levels begin to rise Serum sickness–like reaction (≈10-20% of cases) with rash, hives, arthralgias, fever
Icteric	1-3 wk	Jaundice appears; dark urine and light stools seen Nonspecific symptoms worsen Weight loss, dysgeusia, pruritus may occur Hepatosplenomegaly may develop Aminotransferase levels typically >10 times normal Antibodies appear Viral titers decline Rare extrahepatic manifestations (aseptic meningitis, encephalitis, seizures, ascending flaccid paralysis, nephrotic syndrome, seronegative arthritis)
Recovery	Up to 6 mo	Symptoms resolve gradually Antibody levels rise Aminotransferase and bilirubin levels normalize
Chronic	After 6 mo	See Chapter 151

*Varies by virus.

TABLE 150-3 LABORATORY TESTING FOR SUSPECTED ACUTE VIRAL HEPATITIS

GENERAL EVALUATION

Alanine aminotransferase
Aspartate aminotransferase
Alkaline phosphatase
International normalized ratio

FIRST-LINE DIAGNOSTIC TESTS

Anti-HAV IgM
HBsAg, anti-HBc IgM
Anti-HCV antibodies
HCV RNA

SECOND-LINE DIAGNOSTIC TESTS

Anti-HAV IgM present: none
HBsAg present: HBeAg, anti-HBeAg, HBV DNA, HDV antigen, anti-HDV antibodies
HCV RNA present with or without anti-HCV antibodies: none
No virologic marker: see Figure 149-4

HAV = hepatitis A virus; HBc = hepatitis B core; HBeAg = hepatitis B e antigen; HBsAg = hepatitis B surface antigen; HBV = hepatitis B virus; HCV = hepatitis C virus; HDV = hepatitis D virus; IgM = immunoglobulin M.

examination reveals jaundice and hepatic tenderness. Hepatomegaly and splenomegaly may be present. On laboratory testing, acute viral hepatitis is characterized by elevated total and direct serum bilirubin levels and aminotransferase levels that are often more than 10 times the upper limit of normal. Cholestatic acute hepatitis is frequently associated with prolonged and fluctuating jaundice and pruritus. After 1 to 3 weeks, on average, both clinical and laboratory signs progressively improve and return to normal. Some patients, however, may experience a relapse before definitive resolution.

Fulminant forms of acute viral hepatitis are characterized by signs of hepatic failure, including changes in personality, aggressive behavior, sleeping disorders, and hepatic encephalopathy (Chapter 157). Coma can supervene rapidly, and widespread hemorrhage may develop.

DIAGNOSIS

The diagnosis of acute hepatitis is suspected based on elevated serum aminotransferase levels, which are generally more than 10 times the upper limit of normal (Table 150-3). Total and direct bilirubin levels are elevated if the acute hepatitis is subicteric or icteric. Alkaline phosphatase levels may be elevated in cases of cholestatic hepatitis.

Serologic and eventually molecular testing identifies the causal agent. Liver biopsy is generally not required. All cases of acute hepatitis should be reported to the local, state, or national health department as soon as possible after diagnosis.

TREATMENT   Rx

In addition to virus-specific therapy for HBV and HCV, patients with acute viral hepatitis should avoid alcohol consumption. Sexual contact should be avoided if the partner is not protected. Patients with subfulminant or fulminant hepatitis should be evaluated for possible liver transplantation and supported in an intensive care unit setting (Chapter 157).

PROGNOSIS

Prognosis depends on the degree of prolongation of the prothrombin time, as well as how high the bilirubin and lactate levels are. A factor V level below 40% or any signs of encephalopathy are indications for hospitalization. Death is extremely rare and occurs only in fulminant cases. Other signs of poor prognosis are persistently worsening jaundice, ascites, and an acute decrease in the size of the liver. Serum aminotransferase levels and viral genome levels have no prognostic value.

HEPATITIS A

The Pathogen

HAV is a member of the Picornaviridae family, genus *Hepatovirus*. The hepatitis A viral particle is a 27-nm nonenveloped icosahedral nucleocapsid that expresses the hepatitis A antigen and contains a positive-stranded RNA genome approximately 7.5 kb long. At least four different HAV genotypes have been described in humans (genotypes I, II, III, and VII), with genotype I predominating worldwide. Other genotypes have been isolated in nonhuman primates. It is currently unclear to what extent different genotypes are associated with distinct clinical courses of infection.

EPIDEMIOLOGY

HAV infection has a worldwide distribution, and infections can be sporadic or occur in epidemic outbreaks. The incidence of acute cases and the seroprevalence vary according to the hygiene, sanitation, housing, and socioeconomic standards of the region, with seroprevalences as low as about 13% in Sweden but up to 100% in many developing countries. In developing countries, infection generally occurs at a young age, and most of the population has been exposed and is protected after age 10 years. In developed countries, however, infection can occur at any age, and the prevalence of exposed, immune subjects slowly increases with age. In the United States, the incidence of acute hepatitis A has declined from 12.0 cases per 100,000 individuals in 1995 to 1.0 case per 100,000 individuals in 2007.

HAV is generally transmitted via the oral-fecal route, most often directly from person to person or through the ingestion of fecally contaminated food or water. Transmission by blood transfusion has been reported, and isolated cases of apparent perinatal transmission have been described. High-risk groups for acute hepatitis A include travelers to developing countries, children in daycare centers and their parents, men who have sex with men, injection drug users, hemophiliacs who receive plasma products, and persons in institutions.

PATHOBIOLOGY

The genome serves as a messenger RNA and contains a single open reading frame that encodes both structural and nonstructural viral proteins. After attachment to a specific receptor at the surface of hepatocytes, the virus penetrates into cells and is uncoated. Subsequent events occurring exclusively in the cytoplasm include translation of the single open reading frame into a polyprotein that is later processed to generate the mature viral proteins; replication in a membrane-bound replication complex that generates new viral genomes, which are subsequently used for viral protein production and viral particle assembly; and packaging of newly formed genomes into new particles that are exported out of the cells. The virus is secreted into bile and, to a lesser extent, serum.

CLINICAL MANIFESTATIONS

Typically, the incubation period is 15 to 45 days (see Table 150-2). In most cases, acute infection takes a mild, often unrecognized course. The incidence of symptomatic, icteric cases increases with the age at infection. Acute hepatitis A in adults may require hospitalization in up to 13% of cases; prolonged courses of 6 to 9 months have been reported in 10% of adult patients with a diagnosis of acute hepatitis A. Hepatitis A is the most common cause of relapsing cholestatic hepatitis.

DIAGNOSIS

The diagnosis of acute hepatitis A is based on the detection of anti-HAV immunoglobulin (Ig) M in serum by enzyme immunoassay. IgM serum levels peak during the second month of infection (Fig. 150-2). HAV RNA can be transiently detected in stool and other body fluids by polymerase chain reaction (PCR) 3 to 10 days before the onset of illness and for 1 to 2 weeks thereafter; however, HAV RNA testing is generally not necessary. When the infection resolves, anti-HAV IgM disappears after 4 to 12 months, but anti-HAV IgG persists for life and confers definitive protection against infection.

TREATMENT   Rx

Because HAV infection is self-limited, no specific antiviral treatment is required. In severe cases, patients may need to be hospitalized. If liver function is deteriorating, patients may need to be assessed for liver transplantation, which is the only therapeutic option for acute liver failure (Chapter 157).

PREVENTION

HAV vaccines consist of inactivated hepatitis A antigen purified from cell culture. Two doses of the vaccine at a 6- to 18-month interval are recommended. All vaccines are highly immunogenic, and virtually all healthy persons who are vaccinated develop protective anti-HAV antibodies. Patients with chronic liver disease also respond to vaccination but may display lower anti-HAV titers. An accelerated vaccine schedule, with vaccination on days 0, 7, and 21, is also effective and may be recommended for those planning to travel to endemic areas. HAV vaccines are well tolerated, and no serious adverse events have been linked with their administration; they can be safely administered with other vaccines or immune globulins without compromising the development of protective antibodies. A combination HAV and HBV vaccine is also available. Seroconversion rates are lower in patients with human immunodeficiency virus (HIV) infection and in other immunocompromised individuals.

HAV vaccination is recommended for nonimmune individuals who plan to travel to endemic countries, medical health professionals, men who have sex with men, persons who are in contact with hepatitis A patients, and individuals with chronic liver diseases. A childhood vaccination program leads to

a significant decline in HAV infection, justifying its use as part of control efforts in endemic countries. Serologic testing for anti-HAV IgG can be performed before vaccination in adults born in endemic countries and in individuals older than 50 years born in industrialized areas; persons with detectable IgG are protected and should not be vaccinated. For postexposure prophylaxis, both HAV vaccination and immune globulin are effective; although immune globulin confers a slightly lower rate of infection, they should be used together.

Long-term follow-up studies after complete HAV vaccination show that anti-HAV titers sharply decline during the first year after vaccination but remain detectable in almost all individuals for at least 10 years. Protective anti-HAV antibody titers persist for at least 27 years after the successful vaccination of children and young adults.

PROGNOSIS

Acute hepatitis A infection generally resolves without complications in 3 to 4 weeks and never evolves to chronic infection. Prolonged elevations of serum aminotransferase levels have been reported. Relapses a few weeks after the acute case have also been observed. Prolonged courses may occur in children and immunosuppressed individuals.

Cholestatic hepatitis A is unusual and has a good prognosis, with full recovery within a few weeks. Fulminant hepatitis A is rare, occurring in less than 0.1% of cases, but its incidence and mortality increase with the patient's age at acquisition. In the United States, 4% of all cases of fulminant hepatitis are caused by HAV infection. Overall, mortality of acute hepatitis A is 1.8% in patients older than 50 years. In patients with chronic hepatitis B, superinfection with HAV is associated with a 6- to 23-fold higher morbidity and mortality.

ACUTE HEPATITIS B

The Pathogen

HBV is a member of the Hepadnaviridae family, genus *Hepadnavirus*. The infectious virion, the Dane particle, is 42 to 47 nm in diameter. It possesses an envelope and a capsid or core that contains the partially double-stranded, circular DNA genome. The HBV genome is the smallest known human virus genome, with approximately 3000 nucleotides.

EPIDEMIOLOGY

Two billion individuals—that is, one third of the human population—have been in contact with HBV, and more than 350 million individuals have chronic infection. In the United States, approximately 0.5% of the population is chronically infected. HBV virions are produced and circulate in very high amounts in HBV-infected individuals, who are highly contagious. Four principal routes of transmission are responsible for acute HBV infections: (1) sexual transmission, which is the principal route in industrialized areas; (2) perinatal mother-to-infant transmission, which is associated with a very high (>90%) rate of chronic infection and is the principal cause of HBV transmission in Asia; (3) horizontal transmission through nonsexual interindividual contact, which is frequent at a young age in Africa and is associated with evolution to chronicity in approximately 15% of cases; and (4) percutaneous transmission by blood and blood products, unsafe medical or surgical materials, or injection drug use.

In industrialized countries, groups at high risk for HBV infection include individuals born in areas where HBV is endemic, including immigrants and adopted children; individuals who were not vaccinated as infants and whose parents were born in regions where HBV is endemic; household and sexual contacts of HBsAg-positive individuals; persons who have ever injected drugs; persons with multiple sexual partners or a history of sexually transmitted disease; men who have sex with men; inmates of correctional facilities; patients infected with HCV or HIV; patients undergoing renal dialysis; recipients of blood or blood products before 1987; and health care workers.

PATHOBIOLOGY

The HBV genome contains at least four overlapping open reading frames that encode a number of structural and nonstructural viral proteins. The pre-S/S gene encodes the three surface proteins—small (S), middle (M), and large (L)—which express HBsAg. The pre-C/C gene encodes the core protein that expresses the hepatitis B core (HBc) antigen and the hepatitis B e (HBe) protein, a nonstructural protein that plays a role in immune tolerance to HBV replication. The P gene encodes the HBV polymerase, whose two motifs—a reverse transcriptase motif and an RNAse H motif—code for two enzymes

Acute Hepatitis A

Jaundice

Symptoms

HAV in stool

— Anti-HAV
--- IgM anti-HAV
•— ALT

0   1   2   3   4   5   6   12

Months after exposure

FIGURE 150-2. Serologic course of acute hepatitis A. ALT = alanine aminotransferase; HAV = hepatitis A virus; IgM = immunoglobulin M.

involved in HBV replication. Finally, the X gene encodes the X protein, which is a transactivator involved in HBV replication that bears oncogenic properties. The blood of infected patients contains not only infectious viruses but also a large excess of empty, noninfectious HBV envelopes.

The complex HBV life cycle involves multiple steps: fixation to an as yet unidentified receptor complex at the surface of hepatocytes; internalization; fusion and release of the nucleocapsid containing the HBV DNA genome and the associated HBV polymerase molecule in the cell cytoplasm; transport into the nucleus, where decapsidation occurs and the DNA genome molecule is released; transformation of the viral genome by the viral polymerase into a covalently closed circular DNA, which is the episomal form responsible for persistence of the HBV genome in the nucleus of infected hepatocytes; generation of messenger RNAs and viral protein synthesis; generation of a pregenomic RNA, which serves as a template for reverse transcription that generates the long DNA strand; degradation of the pregenomic RNA by the RNAse H activity of the viral polymerase; DNA-dependent DNA polymerase activity of the reverse transcriptase motif, which synthesizes the short complementary DNA strand in newly formed nucleocapsids; and, finally, budding into the endoplasmic reticulum, maturation, and export of newly formed virions.

Eight HBV genotypes (A through H), which differ by approximately 8% of their genomic nucleotide sequence, have different geographic distributions and may be associated with different clinical outcomes. Genotype A predominates in northern and western Europe, whereas genotype D is the most frequent genotype in the Mediterranean area and in eastern Europe. In non-Asian populations in the United States, genotype A predominates in men who have sex with men, whereas genotype D is the most frequent in intravenous drug users. In Asia and in Asian immigrants living in industrialized countries, genotypes B and C predominate. Genotype C has been associated with a higher incidence of severe liver disease and hepatocellular carcinoma compared with genotype B in Asia, perhaps because this genotype spread earlier than the others.

CLINICAL MANIFESTATIONS

Typically, the incubation period is 30 to 150 days. Jaundice has been reported in up to one third of adult patients with acute hepatitis B, but most cases are unrecognized. Among symptomatic patients (see Table 150-2), the manifestations are similar to those of other causes of acute viral hepatitis.

DIAGNOSIS

Four markers should be sought for the diagnosis of acute hepatitis B: HBsAg, total anti-HBc antibodies, anti-HBc IgM, and anti-HBs antibodies (Table 150-4). Acute hepatitis B is characterized by the simultaneous presence of both HBsAg and anti-HBc IgM (Fig. 150-3). Total anti-HBc antibodies are also present, whereas anti-HBs antibodies are not. During the convalescence phase, patients lose HBsAg before the appearance of anti-HBs antibodies; they have isolated anti-HBc antibodies, and the diagnosis is based on the presence of anti-HBc IgM. Recovery is characterized by the appearance of anti-HBs antibodies. The presence of both total anti-HBc and anti-HBs antibodies characterizes recovery from acute hepatitis B. Anti-HBc IgG remains at high levels for the patient's lifetime, whereas anti-HBs antibody titers may fluctuate and become undetectable after several years. Quantitative HBsAg assessment may be useful during the course of acute hepatitis B because if the HBsAg level does not rapidly decrease, the patient is at risk for chronic evolution. Patients who remain HBV DNA– and/or HBeAg-positive 6 weeks after the onset of symptoms are likely to develop chronic infection.

FIGURE 150-3. Kinetics of hepatitis B virus (HBV) markers during acute self-resolving hepatitis B. The arrow indicates infection. HBc = hepatitis B core; HBeAg = hepatitis B e antigen; HBs = hepatitis B surface; HBsAg = hepatitis B surface antigen; IgM = immunoglobulin M.

TREATMENT Rx

Acute HBV infection usually does not require antiviral therapy, and most patients spontaneously clear the infection. Antiviral therapy with lamivudine can decrease HBV DNA levels more rapidly but does not result in better clinical or biochemical improvement and may be associated with lower levels of protective anti-HBs at 1 year.[2] However, nonrandomized data in patients with severe acute or fulminant hepatitis B suggest that early antiviral therapy (lamivudine 100 mg daily) is safe and may reduce the need for liver transplantation.

PREVENTION

Because not everyone has been vaccinated, individuals who are aware that they are infected with HBV should take steps to avoid transmitting the infection to others. This is accomplished by ensuring that their sexual contacts and household members are vaccinated; using barrier protection during sexual intercourse; not sharing instruments such as toothbrushes, razors, and combs; cleaning blood spills with detergent or bleach; and not donating blood, organs, or sperm.

Prevention of HBV infection is based on vaccination. Universal infant vaccination programs have been initiated in many countries. High-risk individuals (e.g., health care workers, dialysis patients, family members and sexual partners of HBV carriers, pregnant women, and men who have sex with men) should be screened for HBV infection by HBsAg and anti-HBs antibody testing, and seronegative persons should be vaccinated.

Vaccination consists of the administration of recombinant HBsAg in three injections at 0, 1, and 6 months in adults. A lower dose is given at the same time points in newborns, children, and adolescents. Adults on dialysis require four injections at months 0, 1, 2, and 6. HBV vaccination elicits a potent neutralizing response, characterized by the presence of anti-HBs antibodies at titers greater than 10 U/L (protective titer). The seroconversion rate is higher than 90% in healthy individuals. HBV vaccines are well tolerated. Injection site reactions within 1 to 3 days, as well as mild general reactions, are common and transient. Postvaccination testing for anti-HBs antibodies to document seroconversion is not routinely recommended. However, persons who remain at risk for HBV infection, such as infants of HBsAg-positive mothers, health care workers, dialysis patients, and sexual partners of HBV carriers, should be tested to determine their response to vaccination.

Three percent to 10% of vaccinated subjects respond poorly or do not respond, especially smokers, obese patients, and elderly individuals. Nonresponders should receive another full course of vaccination, often with an increased dose. Other options include intradermal application and the coadministration of adjuvants and cytokines. One to two thirds of vaccinated individuals lose their anti-HBs antibodies after 10 to 15 years. It is unclear whether these subjects are still protected. Thus, persons at risk should receive booster immunization if anti-HBs antibodies have been lost.

TABLE 150-4	SEROLOGIC PROFILES OBSERVED IN DIFFERENT PHASES OF ACUTE, SELF-RESOLVING HEPATITIS B			
PHASE OF INFECTION	**HBsAg**	**ANTI-HBc IgM**	**TOTAL ANTI-HBc ANTIBODIES**	**ANTI-HBs ANTIBODIES**
Incubation	+	+/–	+/–	–
Acute hepatitis	+	+	+	–
Convalescence	–	+	+	–
Recovery	–	–	+	+

HBc = hepatitis B core; HBs = hepatitis B surface; HBsAg = hepatitis B surface antigen; IgM = immunoglobulin M.

When nonimmune persons or vaccinated individuals with an anti-HBs titer below 10 IU/L have contact with HBV-contaminated materials (e.g., needles) or have sexual intercourse with an HBV-infected person, active-passive immunization (i.e., infusion of hepatitis B immune globulin) plus active immunization (vaccination) is recommended within 48 hours after exposure. Vaccination alone is sufficient in persons with anti-HBs antibody titers between 10 and 100 IU/L, and no action is required if the anti-HBs titer is above 100 IU/L.

Infants born to HBsAg-positive mothers must receive hepatitis B immune globulin and be vaccinated within 12 hours of birth; this regimen reduces the rate of vertical HBV transmission from 95% to less than 5%. Mothers with HBV DNA levels above 5×10^7 IU/mL should also be treated during pregnancy with a potent nucleoside/nucleotide analogue with no teratogenic risk; the safest drugs in this setting are lamivudine and tenofovir, with the latter being more potent and having a higher barrier to resistance. Cesarean section is not needed if active-passive immunization is to be performed. Mothers of vaccinated infants can breast-feed, unless oral antiviral medications are present in the breast milk.

PROGNOSIS

Fulminant hepatitis is more frequent in acute HBV infection than in other types of acute viral hepatitis, with an incidence of about 0.1%. Factors associated with adverse outcomes of acute hepatitis B include advanced age, female sex, and perhaps some strains of virus. Whether infection with a precore mutant strain is associated with more severe or fulminant disease is still debated.

Among patients infected at birth, the rate of spontaneous recovery after an acute HBV infection is less than 5%, whereas adult infections spontaneously resolve in 95 to 99% of cases. Spontaneous resolution confers lifelong immunity, which is usually characterized by the presence of anti-HBs antibodies. Anti-HBs antibodies may become undetectable several years after resolution, but patients rapidly produce protective antibodies if they are re-exposed to HBV.

● ACUTE HEPATITIS C

The Pathogen

HCV is a member of the Flaviviridae family, genus *Hepacivirus*. The genome is a single-stranded, positive, linear RNA molecule whose 5′ end contains an internal ribosome entry site involved in polyprotein translation; the genome also includes one single open reading frame and a short 3′ noncoding region involved in replication. The genome is contained in a protein capsid or core, which itself is surrounded by a lipid bilayer envelope into which two inserted viral glycoproteins mediate attachment of the viral particle to receptor molecules at the surface of target cells.

EPIDEMIOLOGY

HCV is present in all continents, and an estimated 120 to 130 million individuals, or 3% of the world population, are chronically infected. In industrialized countries, the incidence of HCV infection has declined considerably owing to blood screening and measures to prevent viral infections in intravenous drug users. However, about 35,000 new cases of acute hepatitis C still occur annually in the United States. In Germany, approximately 8 new infections per 100,000 inhabitants occur each year. HCV prevalence is higher in developing areas of the world, where the main route of HCV infection is unsafe medical or surgical procedures; only about 50% of blood products are screened for anti-HCV antibodies in these countries, and about 40% of all injections are given via reused equipment. Egypt's estimated 9% prevalence is the highest worldwide, owing to unsafe injection campaigns for the treatment of schistosomiasis. Although the incidence of acute hepatitis C has declined in Egypt during the past 15 years, up to 10% of cases of acute hepatitis are still caused by HCV.

HCV is transmitted almost exclusively by infected blood. Preventive screening with highly sensitive enzyme immunoassays and, more recently, nucleic acid testing has virtually eliminated the risk of post-transfusional HCV infection (theoretical risk: 1 in 2 million donations in the United States, 1 in 8 million donations in France). As a result, the principal route of HCV transmission in industrialized countries is now intravenous drug use, which is responsible for 60 to 80% of new cases. The incidence of HCV infection in this high-risk group is as high as 39 per 100 person years. In this context, imprisonment is an important risk factor for acquiring HCV infection in industrialized countries.

Nosocomial transmission through the use of improperly decontaminated materials or the contaminated hands or gloves of health care workers is responsible for a substantial number of new infections worldwide. HCV can also be transmitted by tattooing, piercing, or acupuncture if standard precautions are not implemented. Although HCV can be acquired after accidental needlestick exposure, the risk of infection is low (<1%), and health care workers have only a slightly higher prevalence of HCV than the general population. HCV can be transmitted to household members who share instruments such as scissors, razors, and combs. Sexual transmission is unusual, but outbreaks of acute hepatitis have been reported in HIV-positive communities of men who have sex with men. The risk of mother-to-infant transmission of HCV is less than 5% and is generally related to exposure to the mother's blood in the perinatal period. Cesarean sections are not recommended, and breast-feeding is not contraindicated. The risk of perinatal transmission is higher when the mother is coinfected with HIV. Other factors possibly associated with high transmission rates include the level of HCV viremia and maternal intravenous drug abuse. In 10 to 30% of cases, no apparent risk factor for HCV infection is identifiable, suggesting other potential sources of "community-acquired" hepatitis C.

PATHOBIOLOGY

Entry of HCV into cells is pH dependent through clathrin-mediated endocytosis and is followed by fusion. Decapsidation of viral nucleocapsids liberates free genomic RNAs into the cell cytoplasm, where they serve, together with newly synthesized RNAs, as messenger RNAs for synthesis of the HCV polyprotein. The post-translational processing of the HCV polyprotein results in the generation of at least 10 proteins, including 3 structural proteins (the core protein and the two envelope glycoproteins) and 7 nonstructural proteins. Infection with HCV leads to rearrangements of intracellular membranes, a prerequisite to the formation of the replication complex that associates viral proteins, cellular components, and nascent RNA strands in close proximity. HCV replication is catalyzed by a virally encoded RNA-dependent RNA polymerase within the replication complex. The positive-strand genome RNA serves as a template for the synthesis of a negative-strand intermediate of replication. Then, negative-strand RNA serves as a template to produce numerous strands that have a positive polarity and will subsequently be used for polyprotein translation, synthesis of new intermediates of replication, or packaging into new virus particles. Viral particle formation is initiated by the interaction of the core protein with genomic RNA. Budding of newly formed virions in the endoplasmic reticulum lumen leads to the formation of coated particles. Newly produced virus particles leave the host cell via constitutive secretory pathways.

Phylogenetic analyses of HCV strains isolated in various regions of the world have identified six main HCV genotypes, designated 1 through 6. These HCV types comprise a large number of subtypes, identified by lower-case letters (1a, 1b, etc.). The genotypes' nucleotide sequences differ by between 31 and 34%, and their amino acid sequences differ by approximately 30%; in contrast, the subtypes' nucleotide sequences differ by between 20 and 23%, with marked differences in particular genomic regions. The high prevalence and diversity of HCV genotype 3 and 6 strains in Asia and of genotype 1, 2, and 4 strains in Africa suggest that these types and subtypes emerged and diversified in these regions. In industrialized countries, a small number of HCV genotypes, including 1a, 1b, 2a, 2b, 2c, 3a, and 4a, have been introduced and spread rapidly among exposed populations. Subtypes 1a and 1b predominate all over the world. The most common genotypes in the United States are 1a and 1b (approximately 75%), 2a and 2b (approximately 15%), and 3a (approximately 7%). Genotype 3a is more prevalent in western Europe, where it accounts for up to 35% of cases, especially among intravenous drug users. Genotype 4 is highly prevalent in the Middle East and Africa. Its incidence and prevalence are increasing in intravenous drug users in industrialized countries. Genotype 5 is rare outside South Africa, and genotype 6 is rare outside Southeast Asia. Infections with different genotypes do not differ in terms of the clinical manifestations, progression, or disease severity (although this is debated), but the HCV genotype is a major determinant of the response to interferon-α–based therapies.

CLINICAL MANIFESTATIONS

HCV RNA becomes detectable in the serum 3 to 7 days after exposure. HCV RNA levels rise rapidly during the first weeks, followed by serum aminotransferase levels 2 to 8 weeks after exposure. Anti-HCV antibodies arise late in the course of acute hepatitis C and may not be present at the onset of symptoms and serum aminotransferase elevation.

TABLE 150-5	PATTERNS OF HEPATITIS C VIRUS (HCV) MARKERS AND THEIR SIGNIFICANCE DURING ACUTE HEPATITIS C	
ANTI-HCV ANTIBODIES	**HCV RNA**	**DIAGNOSIS**
–	–	Not acute hepatitis C
–	+	Acute hepatitis C
+	–	Probably not acute hepatitis C (retest in a few weeks)
+	+	Difficult to differentiate acute from chronic hepatitis C

FIGURE 150-5. Kinetics of hepatitis C virus (HCV) markers during acute hepatitis C that evolves toward chronic infection. ALT = alanine aminotransferase; ULN = upper limit of normal.

FIGURE 150-4. Kinetics of hepatitis C virus (HCV) markers during acute self-resolving hepatitis C. ALT = alanine aminotransferase; ULN = upper limit of normal.

After an incubation period that ranges from 15 to 120 days, acute hepatitis C usually remains asymptomatic and is undiagnosed. Nonspecific symptoms such as fatigue, low-grade fever, myalgias, nausea, vomiting, or itching may be present. Jaundice occurs in only 20 to 30% of patients, usually 2 to 12 weeks after infection. Serum aminotransferase levels commonly exceed 10 times the upper limit of normal in the acute stage, even in the absence of symptoms. Fulminant hepatitis C has been reported but appears to be exceptional in the absence of another chronic underlying liver disease.

DIAGNOSIS

When acute hepatitis C is suspected, patients should be tested for both anti-HCV antibodies by enzyme immunoassay and HCV RNA with a sensitive molecular biology technique (i.e., an HCV RNA assay with a lower limit of detection of ≤50 IU/mL). Four marker profiles can be observed, based on the presence or absence of either marker (Table 150-5). The presence of HCV RNA in the absence of anti-HCV antibodies is strongly indicative of acute HCV infection, which will be confirmed by seroconversion (i.e., the appearance of anti-HCV antibodies) a few days to weeks later. Acutely infected patients can have both HCV RNA and anti-HCV antibodies at the time of diagnosis; in this case, it is difficult to distinguish acute hepatitis C from an acute exacerbation of chronic hepatitis C or acute hepatitis of another cause in a patient with chronic hepatitis C.

Acute hepatitis C is very unlikely if both anti-HCV antibodies and HCV RNA are absent or if anti-HCV antibodies are present without HCV RNA (Fig. 150-4). Patients in the latter group should be retested in a few weeks, however, because HCV RNA may be temporarily undetectable owing to transient, partial control of viral replication before the infection becomes chronic (Fig. 150-5). Apart from such cases, the presence of anti-HCV antibodies in the absence of HCV RNA is generally seen in patients who have recovered from a past HCV infection. Nevertheless, this pattern cannot be differentiated from a false-positive enzyme immunoassay result, the exact prevalence of which is unknown.

TREATMENT

Treatment of acute hepatitis C should be considered not only because it prevents chronic HCV infection, which can lead to serious clinical sequelae, but also because HCV viremia, which is associated with a risk of transmitting HCV to other persons, may have social, legal, and economic consequences, especially for infected health care workers. Treatment can be delayed for up to 3 months in patients with symptomatic acute hepatitis C, whereas immediate therapy is recommended if patients are infected with genotype 1 and have asymptomatic disease. Treatment of acute hepatitis C is based on the use of pegylated interferon-α2a or -α2b at doses of 180 μg/week or 1.5 μg/kg/week, respectively. Treatment should be administered for 24 weeks, but a shorter duration may be sufficient in patients with baseline parameters that predict a rapid viral clearance, such as symptomatic disease, high alanine aminotransferase levels, and low HCV RNA levels. Ribavirin should be added in patients who have a delayed or slow HCV RNA decrease with treatment, genotype 1 infection, and/or low or normal baseline alanine aminotransferase levels. With this treatment, 70% to more than 90% of patients have sustained viral clearance.[3] If treatment fails to clear the virus, patients can be retreated with a combination of pegylated interferon-α2a (180 μg/week) or -α2b (1.5 μg/kg/week) and ribavirin (0.8 g/day) for 48 weeks.

After accidental needlestick exposure, neither immune globulin nor preemptive therapy with pegylated interferon-α is recommended. Patients should be monitored with HCV RNA and aminotransferase level testing at baseline, week 2, and 4 and 6 months after exposure. Patients who have documented infection should be treated as above.

PREVENTION

Prevention of HCV transmission is based on standard precautions such as screening of blood and blood products, application of standard medical and surgical hygiene procedures, and safe use of syringes and materials for drug preparation in drug users. Needle exchange programs and education regarding the risks of drug use (including intranasal cocaine) and the risk of transmission from shared injection equipment are important.

No prophylactic vaccine is available against HCV. Phase I vaccine studies using HCV peptides, HCV proteins, or recombinant vectors expressing HCV proteins have induced HCV-specific T-cell responses or antibodies in healthy individuals, but full protection against infection by heterologous strains appears unlikely.

PROGNOSIS

About 50 to 80% of patients are unable to clear HCV spontaneously and develop chronic infection. Spontaneous recovery is more frequent if infection is acquired at birth (approximately 50%) and if acute hepatitis is symptomatic. It is unclear whether the genotype influences recovery rates. Other factors associated with better rates of spontaneous recovery include female sex, early decline of HCV RNA levels, and high aminotransferase or bilirubin levels. Patients who spontaneously recover may retain detectable anti-HCV antibodies for years to decades, but they are not protected against HCV reinfection.

ACUTE HEPATITIS D OR DELTA

The Pathogen

HDV, which is a satellite of HBV, can be transmitted only to patients who are acutely or chronically infected with HBV. Its single, negative-strand, circular RNA genome of approximately 1700 nucleotides folds in native conditions into a nearly complementary rod-like structure that contains a ribozyme. The HDV genome encodes one single structural protein, the hepatitis D (HD) protein, which expresses HDAg. The 36-nm infectious HDV virion comprises the HD protein and the genome, both enclosed within an HBsAg coat derived from empty HBV envelopes.

EPIDEMIOLOGY

Five percent of chronic HBV carriers, or 15 million to 20 million individuals worldwide, are also infected with HDV. The prevalence of HDV infection in HBV-infected patients varies according to the geographic area because it is transmitted primarily through parenteral exposure. As a result, its prevalence is relatively higher in HBsAg-positive intravenous drug users in Western countries, where approximately 8 to 12% of HBsAg-positive patients are infected with HDV. By comparison, the prevalence of HDV has decreased substantially in southern Europe, probably owing to universal HBV vaccination programs, improvement in hygiene and living conditions, and implementation of standard precautions to prevent HIV infection. The incidence of HDV is increasing in Russia, eastern Europe, Japan, and India.

PATHOBIOLOGY

HDV uses host RNA polymerase II for its replication, following the rolling circle model. Within cells, HDV RNA is associated with multiple copies of the HD protein to form a ribonucleoprotein complex. This complex is exported by the HBV envelope, which contains the three HBV envelope proteins, into the Golgi apparatus before being secreted.

HDV has at least eight genotypes, which differ from one another by at least 15% of their nucleotide sequences. Genotype I is the most prevalent HDV worldwide. Additional genotypes have recently been identified in Africa.

CLINICAL MANIFESTATIONS

HDV can be acquired at the same time as HBV (coinfection) or by a chronic HBsAg carrier (superinfection). Coinfection is characterized by one or two episodes of acute hepatitis, depending on the respective amounts of HBV and HDV present in the inoculum; acute hepatitis can range from mild to fulminant. In contrast, when chronic HBV carriers are superinfected by HDV, acute hepatitis D is generally severe, often fulminant, and chronic.

DIAGNOSIS

Three markers of HDV infection are total anti-HD antibodies, anti-HD IgM, and HDV RNA; each can be detected and quantified by real-time PCR. All HBsAg-positive patients should be tested.

In patients with an HBV-HDV coinfection, HDV RNA is only transiently present and is often missed. Anti-HBc IgM indicates concomitant acute HBV infection.

In HDV superinfection of a chronic HBsAg carrier, no anti-HBc IgM is present. HDV RNA is found in serum or plasma before and during the acute episode, whereas both total anti-HD antibodies and anti-HD IgM are present during the acute phase. Both serologic markers remain at high levels if the disease becomes chronic.

TREATMENT Rx

No treatment of acute hepatitis D has been evaluated so far.

PREVENTION

The most effective means of preventing HDV infection is HBV vaccination, because individuals who are protected against HBV cannot be infected with HDV. In chronic HBsAg carriers, standard hygiene and behavioral precautions should be practiced to avoid superinfection with HDV.

PROGNOSIS

In patients who are acutely coinfected with HBV and HDV, only about 2% become chronic HDV carriers. In contrast, when HDV infection is acquired by chronic HBV carriers, about 90% also become chronic carriers of HDV.

ACUTE HEPATITIS E

The Pathogen

HEV is the sole known member of the genus *Hepevirus* in the Hepeviridae family. HEV is a small, nonenveloped virus. Its genome is a positive sense, single-stranded RNA molecule. Five HEV genotypes have been described: genotypes 1 and 2 appear to be strictly human, whereas genotypes 3 and 4 appear to be of swine origin but can also infect humans.

PATHOBIOLOGY AND EPIDEMIOLOGY

HEV transmission is principally oral-fecal. HEV is endemic in most developing areas of the world, where acute infections are sporadic or occur during large epidemics related to the contamination of drinking water. Genotype 1 has been found principally in Asia and North Africa, whereas genotype 2 has been isolated in cases from Central America and western Africa. No animal reservoir is known for these genotypes, and transmission appears to be linked to the contamination of food or drinking water. In industrialized countries, HEV genotypes 1 and 2 are not present. HEV genotypes 3 and 4 are endemic in swine, and zoonotic transmission appears to be the main route of transmission in Europe, the United States, and Asia. Diagnosed cases of acute hepatitis E have increased constantly in western Europe and North America in recent years, and high HEV seroprevalences have been described in special at-risk populations, such as butchers or farmers. Transmission may be favored by the consumption of uncooked meat and direct contact with infected animals.

CLINICAL MANIFESTATIONS

The incubation period is 15 to 60 days. HEV infection causes only mild, nonspecific symptoms in the majority of cases, especially if the infection is acquired early in life. Immunocompetent individuals clear the virus spontaneously. The peak of viremia occurs early during infection, whereas the peak of aminotransferase activity is reached approximately 6 weeks after infection. Severe disease is more frequent in pregnant women and in patients with underlying chronic liver disease, who may rarely progress to fulminant hepatic failure.

DIAGNOSIS

Diagnosis of acute hepatitis E is based on the detection of anti-HEV IgM antibodies, but current assays lack sensitivity and specificity. HEV RNA can also be detected in feces, serum, or plasma, where its presence is transient. Anti-HEV IgG generally persists for life after acute infection.

TREATMENT Rx

Treatment of acute hepatitis E is not recommended because the vast majority of patients recover spontaneously. Severe and fulminant cases should be referred to specialized units.

PREVENTION

Improved public hygiene is the best defense against hepatitis E in developing countries. Travelers to areas of the world where HEV is endemic, particularly pregnant women, should be cautioned about drinking the water and eating uncooked food. An efficient prophylactic vaccine based on recombinant HEV proteins was 100% effective in a phase 3 trial.[4] However, the duration of protection is uncertain, so the vaccine's efficacy in preventing the spread of HEV has yet to be determined.

PROGNOSIS

Acute cases can be severe in elderly patients, and fulminant cases are frequent among pregnant women who are infected during large-scale water-borne epidemics. HEV genotypes 3 and 4 are less virulent than genotypes 1 and 2. Sporadic cases in industrialized areas are generally benign. HEV does not commonly evolve into chronic infection, but immunosuppressed patients and HIV-positive individuals can become chronic carriers.

OTHER TYPES OF ACUTE VIRAL HEPATITIS

Infection by members of the Herpesviridae family, such as cytomegalovirus (Chapter 384), Epstein-Barr virus (Chapter 385), and herpes simplex virus (Chapter 382), should be considered in the differential diagnosis of unclear episodes of elevated liver enzymes in the absence of markers of acute hepatitis virus infection, especially in immunocompromised individuals. For instance, cytomegalovirus infection can be associated with graft loss after liver transplantation (Chapter 157). Parvovirus B19 (Chapter 379) may persist in the liver and worsen liver disease in patients with chronic hepatitis B and perhaps in patients with chronic HCV infection. Human herpesvirus 6 variant A has been linked with syncytial giant-cell hepatitis.

Non A to E Hepatitis

Rare patients develop acute hepatitis of presumed viral cause but have no markers of known hepatitis viruses. Some of these cases may be due to variants of known hepatitis viruses, in particular HBV, that are not detected by the usual serologic and molecular methods. However, the existence of other, unknown hepatotropic viruses cannot be excluded.

1. Victor JC, Monto AS, Surdina TY, et al. Hepatitis A vaccine versus immune globulin for postexposure prophylaxis. *N Engl J Med.* 2007;357:1685-1694.
2. Kumar M, Satapathy S, Monga R, et al. A randomized controlled trial of lamivudine to treat acute hepatitis B. *Hepatology.* 2007;45:97-101.
3. Jeckel E, Cornberg M, Wedemeyer H, et al. Treatment of acute hepatitis C with interferon alfa-2b. *N Engl J Med.* 2001;345:1452-1457.
4. Zhu FC, Zhang J, Zhang XF, et al. Efficacy and safety of a recombinant hepatitis E vaccine in healthy adults: a large-scale, randomised, double-blind placebo-controlled, phase 3 trial. *Lancet.* 2010;376:895-902.

SUGGESTED READINGS

Fitzsimmons D, Hendrickx G, Vorsters A, et al. Hepatitis A and E: update on prevention and epidemiology. *Vaccine.* 2010;28:583-588. *Review.*
Hadziyannis SJ. Milestones and perspectives in viral hepatitis B. *Liver Int.* 2011;1:129-134. *Review.*
Loomba R, Rivera MM, McBurney R, et al. The natural history of acute hepatitis C: clinical presentation, laboratory findings and treatment outcomes. *Aliment Pharmacol Ther.* 2011;33:559-565. *Review.*
Stramer SL, Wend U, Candotti D, et al. Nucleic acid testing to detect HBV infection in blood donors. *N Engl J Med.* 2011;364:236-247. *Triplex nucleic acid testing successfully detected HBV, HIV, and HCV during the window period before seroconversion.*
Wedemeyer H, Manns MP. Epidemiology, pathogenesis and management of hepatitis D: update and challenges ahead. *Nat Rev Gastroenterol Hepatol.* 2010;7:31-40. *Review.*

151

CHRONIC VIRAL AND AUTOIMMUNE HEPATITIS

JEAN-MICHEL PAWLOTSKY AND JOHN MCHUTCHISON

DEFINITION

Chronic hepatitis is defined by chronic necroinflammation of the liver and may be due to various causes, including hepatotropic viruses, autoimmunity, alcohol (Chapter 155), and metabolic disorders (Chapter 153). Chronic infection by hepatitis viruses is by far the main cause of chronic hepatitis worldwide, with more than 500 million individuals chronically infected with hepatitis B virus (HBV) or hepatitis C virus (HCV). Chronic viral hepatitis B and C are the leading cause of cirrhosis (Chapter 156) and hepatocellular carcinoma (Chapter 202) worldwide and account for more than 1 million deaths per year. Chronic HBV infection can be associated with infection by hepatitis D virus (HDV). Hepatitis A virus does not cause chronic hepatitis. Hepatitis E virus (HEV) does not cause chronic hepatitis, except rarely in patients who undergo liver transplantation.

CLINICAL MANIFESTATIONS

The clinical symptoms of chronic viral and autoimmune hepatitis are typically nonspecific, and many patients have no symptoms. Fatigue, sleep disorders, and right upper quadrant pain may be present. Often the diagnosis is made when liver test abnormalities are identified by blood testing during a routine health evaluation or assessment for an unrelated problem or at the time of voluntary blood donation. More advanced symptoms include poor

TABLE 151-1	DIAGNOSIS OF CHRONIC HEPATITIS	
DIAGNOSIS	**SCREENING TESTS**	**CONFIRMATORY TESTS**
Chronic hepatitis B	HBsAg	HBV DNA, HBeAg
Chronic hepatitis C	Anti-HCV antibodies	HCV RNA
Chronic hepatitis D	Anti-HDV antibodies	HDV RNA
Autoimmune hepatitis	ANA (anti-LKM1)	Exclusion of other causes and patterns of clinical disease
Drug-induced liver disease	History	Rechallenge, if necessary, is considered safe
Wilson disease	Ceruloplasmin	Urine copper concentration
Cryptogenic hepatitis	Exclusion of other causes	

ANA = antinuclear antibody; anti-LKM1 = anti–liver-kidney microsomal 1 antibody; HBeAg = hepatitis B e antigen; HBsAg = hepatitis B surface antigen; HBV = hepatitis B virus; HCV = hepatitis C virus; HDV = hepatitis D virus.

appetite, nausea, weight loss, muscle weakness, itching, dark urine, and jaundice. Patients can progress to full-blown cirrhosis (Chapter 156), with its typical clinical manifestations. If cirrhosis is present, weakness, weight loss, abdominal swelling, edema, bruisability, gastrointestinal bleeding, and hepatic encephalopathy with mental confusion may arise. Other findings may include spider angiomas, palmar erythema (see Fig. 148-2 in Chapter 148), ascites (see Fig. 148-5 in Chapter 148), edema, and skin excoriations (see Fig. 148-3 in Chapter 148).

DIAGNOSIS

Levels of alanine aminotransferase (ALT) and aspartate aminotransferase (AST) are usually two to five times the upper limit of normal. The ALT level is generally higher than the AST level, but both can be normal in mild or inactive disease or 10 to 25 times the upper limit of normal during acute exacerbations. Biologic tests can establish the specific diagnosis (Table 151-1).

Alkaline phosphatase and γ-glutamyl transpeptidase levels are usually minimally elevated unless cirrhosis is present. Serum bilirubin and albumin levels and the prothrombin time are normal unless the disease is severe or advanced. Serum immunoglobulin levels are mildly elevated or normal in chronic viral hepatitis but may be very elevated in autoimmune hepatitis. Results that suggest the presence of advanced fibrosis are a platelet count below 160,000, AST levels higher than ALT levels, elevation in serum bilirubin, decrease in serum albumin, prolongation of the prothrombin time, elevation in α-fetoprotein levels, and presence of rheumatoid factor or high globulin levels.

Hepatic ultrasound can determine the texture and size of the liver and spleen, exclude hepatic masses, and assess the gallbladder, intrahepatic bile ducts, and portal venous flow. Computed tomography and magnetic resonance imaging of the liver are helpful if a mass or other abnormality is found by ultrasound. Hepatic elastography can assess liver stiffness as a marker of fibrosis.

Liver biopsy is usually critical for diagnosis and to determine the severity of disease. Hepatocellular necrosis is typically eosinophilic degeneration or ballooning degeneration throughout the parenchyma, greater in the periportal area, spotty, or piecemeal. Fibrosis also typically begins in the periportal regions and can link adjacent portal areas or portal and central areas (bridging fibrosis), distort the hepatic architecture, and lead to cirrhosis and portal hypertension. The histologic grade of chronic hepatitis can be determined by combining scores for periportal necrosis and inflammation, lobular necrosis and inflammation, and portal inflammation. Recently, ultrasound-based methods or serologic markers have proved accurate for the assessment of mild disease and cirrhosis, but they are less accurate for identifying moderate to severe inflammation, except in patients with chronic hepatitis C. Patients with suspected chronic viral or autoimmune hepatitis should be evaluated carefully for fatty liver, alcohol- (Chapter 155) or drug-induced (Chapter 152) liver disease, and metabolic liver diseases (Chapter 153), each of which can coexist with hepatitis. Liver biopsy can exclude other diagnoses that mimic chronic hepatitis, including fatty liver, alcoholic liver disease, steatohepatitis (Chapter 155), drug-induced liver disease (Chapter 152), sclerosing cholangitis (Chapter 158), iron overload (Chapter 219), and veno-occlusive disease (Chapter 145).

TREATMENT AND PROGNOSIS

Chronic HBV infection is not curable, but it can usually be controlled by appropriate antiviral drugs. HCV infection is curable, but less than 50% of patients who have access to therapy are cured. Autoimmune hepatitis responds to immunosuppression with corticosteroids and azathioprine.

CHRONIC HEPATITIS B

EPIDEMIOLOGY

More than 350 million individuals, or 8.5% of the world's population, are chronic HBV carriers. Two billion individuals, or one human being out of three, have been in contact with the virus. In North America, western and northern Europe, and Australia, less than 2% of the population are chronic hepatitis B surface antigen (HBsAg) carriers. In the United States, the prevalence is approximately 0.4%; that is, about 1.25 million Americans are infected. In eastern Europe, South America, the Mediterranean basin, and the Indian subcontinent, the prevalence of chronic HBsAg carriage is between 2 and 8%. Highly endemic areas, with a rate of chronic HBsAg carriage exceeding 8%, include China, Southeast Asia, sub-Saharan Africa, and the native populations of the Far North of America.

HBV is the main cause of primary liver cancer (hepatocellular carcinoma, Chapter 202) worldwide, with about 350,000 new cases attributable to HBV every year. Hepatocellular carcinoma is more likely in the presence of underlying cirrhosis, but HBV has oncogenic properties of its own, and hepatocellular carcinoma can occur in noncirrhotic HBV patients.

PATHOBIOLOGY

HBV is not a cytopathic virus. Rather, liver injury in chronic hepatitis B is a consequence of the local immune response at the immune elimination phase. In particular, liver injury is related to cytotoxic T cells that recognize and kill infected hepatocytes that express HBV antigens at their surface and to the local production of cytokines. Chronic inflammation triggers fibrogenesis through the activation of hepatic stellate cells. The hepatitis B X protein may also directly activate fibrogenesis. As a result, many patients with chronic hepatitis B have progressive fibrosis, which may evolve into cirrhosis.

The rate of chronicity after an acute HBV infection is more than 95% among patients infected at birth. This risk diminishes as the age at acquisition increases, and it is less than 5% in those infected as adults. Chronic HBV infection is defined by HBsAg carriage that persists for more than 6 months after the acute episode. Chronic HBsAg carriage typically evolves through three phases: immune tolerant, immune elimination, and inactive.

The immune tolerant phase is generally short if the infection occurred during adulthood, but it persists for years to decades in patients infected at birth or during early childhood. At the immune tolerant stage, the immune response of the host "tolerates" HBV infection and does not cause liver inflammation or hepatocyte destruction. The immune tolerant phase is characterized by the presence of hepatitis B e antigen (HBeAg), very high levels of HBV DNA in blood, normal serum or plasma aminotransferase levels, and no or minimal inflammatory activity on liver biopsy.

The immune elimination phase is characterized by an active immune response that causes necroinflammatory lesions and triggers hepatic fibrogenesis and progressive fibrosis. ALT and AST levels are increased, but HBV DNA levels are lower than during the immune tolerant phase and frequently

fluctuate. The immune elimination phase has a variable duration, ranging from a few weeks to several decades. HBeAg, when present, defines HBeAg-positive chronic hepatitis B; it can be cleared and replaced by anti-HBe antibodies, defined as HBe seroconversion; or it can be absent while anti-HBe antibodies are present and to define HBeAg-negative chronic hepatitis B. Patients with HBeAg-positive chronic hepatitis B are infected with a wild-type virus and are able to secrete the HBe protein. Patients with HBeAg-negative chronic hepatitis B are infected with so-called precore mutant viruses, which cannot produce the HBe protein because they have a stop codon in the pre-C gene, and/or with core promoter mutant viruses, which produce considerably lower amounts of HBe protein.

The inactive HBsAg carriage phase is the result of successful immune elimination leading to HBe seroconversion. ALT and AST levels are normal, HBV DNA is undetectable or at very low levels, and patients without preexisting cirrhosis have normal liver histology.

CLINICAL MANIFESTATIONS

Chronic hepatitis B is usually asymptomatic. The most common symptom is fatigue, but sleep disorders, difficulty concentrating, and upper right quadrant pain are often observed. Chronic hepatitis B is characterized biologically by elevated aminotransferase levels, and ALT levels can fluctuate substantially during the immune elimination phase. Moderate cholestasis, with mildly elevated alkaline phosphatase and γ-glutamyl transpeptidase levels, can also be present, especially in patients with cirrhosis.

HBeAg-negative chronic hepatitis B is generally more severe than the HBeAg-positive variety. The incidence of spontaneous HBe seroconversion among HBeAg-positive patients is 8 to 12% per year when they are in the immune elimination phase; HBe seroconversion often follows a transient ALT flare. Some of these patients evolve toward inactive HBsAg carriage, whereas others switch into an HBeAg-negative form of chronic hepatitis B, with elevated ALT levels and an HBV DNA level greater than 2000 IU/mL.

The annual incidence of cirrhosis varies from 2 to 10% in patients with chronic HBV infection, with a cumulative incidence of approximately 20% at 5 years. The risk of cirrhosis is two- to four-fold higher in HBeAg-negative patients compared with HBeAg-positive ones, probably because they are older and have more severe disease at the time of diagnosis. The annual incidence of hepatocellular carcinoma in patients with chronic hepatitis B varies from 1% in patients without cirrhosis to 2 to 8% in cirrhotic patients, with the higher rates occurring in older patients. Patients with cirrhosis (Chapter 156) and/or hepatocellular carcinoma (Chapter 202) have the typical signs associated with these conditions. Rarely, chronic HBV infection is associated with extrahepatic manifestations, including glomerulonephritis (Chapter 123), most often in children, and polyarteritis nodosa (Chapter 278), mostly in adults.

DIAGNOSIS

Serologic markers used to diagnose chronic hepatitis B (Table 151-2) include HBsAg, anti-HBs antibodies, total anti–hepatitis B core (HBc) antibodies and anti-HBc immunoglobulin M (IgM), HBeAg, and anti-HBe antibodies. Molecular markers include HBV DNA and HBV resistance substitutions; real-time polymerase chain reaction (PCR)–based assays are the best way to detect and quantify HBV DNA

Chronic HBV infection is defined by the persistence of HBsAg in the serum for more than 6 months after the acute episode. The majority of subjects with isolated anti-HBc antibodies are not viremic. However, some individuals who test positive for anti-HBc antibodies, but not for HBsAg or anti-HBs antibodies, may be viremic; in these cases, the virus's amino acid

					Anti-HBc Ab		
TABLE 151-2 VIROLOGIC MARKER PROFILES IN PATIENTS WITH CHRONIC HEPATITIS B VIRUS (HBV) INFECTION							
	HBsAg	ANTI-HBs Ab	HBeAg	ANTI-HBe Ab	IgM	TOTAL	HBV DNA
Chronic hepatitis							
HBeAg-positive	+	−	+	−	−*	+	>2 × 10⁴ IU/mL
HBeAg-negative	+	−	−	+	−*	+	>2 × 10³ IU/mL
Inactive carrier	+	−	−	+	−	+	<2 × 10³ IU/mL
Reactivation	+	−	+/−	+/−	+/−	+	>2 × 10³ IU/mL

*Anti-HBc IgM can be detected at low titers.
Ab = antibodies; Ag = antigen; HBc = hepatitis B core; HBe = hepatitis B e; HBs = hepatitis B surface; IgM = immunoglobulin M.

FIGURE 151-1. Liver biopsies in patients with chronic hepatitis C. **A,** Lymphoid nodule with germinal center; minimal interface hepatitis (hematein-eosin, magnification ×200). **B,** Mild fibrosis, Metavir score F1 (picrosirius-hemalun, magnification ×100). C, Extensive fibrosis, Metavir score F3 (picrosirius-hemalun, magnification ×20). (Courtesy of Prof. Elie-Serge Zafrani, Department of Pathology, Henri Mondor Hospital, Créteil, France.)

substitutions in the HBsAg sequence make HBsAg undetectable with current enzyme immunoassays. Other individuals may have such low-level HBV replication in their livers that HBV DNA is not detectable in blood ("occult" hepatitis B).

Serum or plasma ALT and HBV DNA levels are important markers of severity and prognosis. The assessment of severity, including the grade of necroinflammation and the stage of fibrosis, is based on the liver biopsy (Fig. 151-1). Noninvasive assessment using serologic markers or transient elastography can discriminate cirrhosis from mild hepatitis and fibrosis; although they are not accurate enough for intermediate stages, these methods will likely replace liver biopsy in the pretreatment assessment of the severity of chronic hepatitis B in many patients in the future.

PREVENTION AND TREATMENT (Rx)

Patients with chronic hepatitis B should be vaccinated against hepatitis A virus, abstain from alcohol, and avoid immunosuppressive therapies unless absolutely necessary. HBV-infected patients who require corticosteroids or chemotherapy for other conditions should receive lamivudine 100 mg daily as prophylaxis against reactivation of hepatitis B. **1**

The goals of therapy are to suppress HBV replication, reduce the histologic activity of chronic hepatitis, and lessen the risk of cirrhosis and hepatocellular carcinoma. HBV infection cannot be completely eradicated because of the persistence of covalently closed circular DNA in the nucleus of infected hepatocytes. As a result, therapy attempts to reduce HBV DNA levels as much as possible—ideally, below the limit of detection of real-time PCR assays (10 to 15 IU/mL)—to ensure a degree of viral suppression that will lead to biochemical remission, histologic improvement, and prevention of complications.

Two different types of drugs for the treatment of chronic hepatitis B are pegylated interferon-α (IFN-α) and nucleoside/nucleotide analogues. Pegylated IFN-α2a, administered subcutaneously at a dose of 180 µg once a week for 48 weeks, improves various markers of HBV infection in both HBeAg-positive (Table 151-3) and HBeAg-negative (Table 151-4) patients. **2** Pegylated IFN-α2b (1.5 µg/kg) is very similar to IFN-α2a and is used by many liver experts, although it is not currently approved for HBV. The most frequent side effects of IFN-α are flu-like symptoms after the injections, fatigue, anorexia, weight loss, and alopecia. The most concerning side effects are neutropenia, thrombocytopenia, anxiety, irritability, depression, and even suicidal ideation.

Nucleoside analogues (lamivudine, telbivudine, and entecavir) require triple phosphorylation to be active, whereas nucleotide analogues (adefovir and tenofovir) need only two phosphorylations to be active. These drugs are given orally once a day at the following dosages: 100 mg for lamivudine, 600 mg for telbivudine, 0.5 mg for entecavir, 10 mg for adefovir (administered

as the pro-drug adefovir dipivoxil), and 300 mg for tenofovir (administered as the pro-drug tenofovir disoproxil fumarate). All have short-term benefits on various markers of HBV infection in HBeAg-positive (see Table 151-3) and HBeAg-negative (see Table 151-4) patients. Entecavir and tenofovir are two of the most potent inhibitors of HBV replication, **3-5** and they are less likely to select for resistant HBV variants. These drugs are generally well tolerated. However, adefovir is nephrotoxic at doses higher than those used for HBV therapy, renal impairment and decreases in mineral bone density are rarely seen with tenofovir, myopathy is a rare complication of telbivudine, and peripheral neuropathy has been observed when telbivudine is combined with pegylated IFN-α.

Patients should be considered for treatment when their HBV DNA levels are greater than 2000 IU/mL and/or their serum ALT levels are abnormal if the liver biopsy shows moderate to severe active necroinflammation and/or fibrosis. Indications for treatment must also take into account the patient's age and health status and the availability of antiviral agents in individual countries. Patients in the immune tolerant phase and those with mild hepatitis on liver biopsy should not be treated, but follow-up ALT levels and HBV DNA assays are mandatory. Patients with compensated cirrhosis and detectable HBV DNA may be considered for treatment even if their ALT levels are normal and/or their HBV DNA levels are below 2000 IU/mL. Patients with decompensated cirrhosis require urgent antiviral treatment.

Two treatment strategies can be considered: a 48-week course of pegylated IFN-α or long-term oral treatment with nucleoside/nucleotide analogues. Whether their combined use improves the rate of sustained virologic response after treatment is currently under study. Pegylated IFN-α can provide a sustained virologic response, defined as a sustained HBe seroconversion (clearance of HBeAg, which is replaced by anti-HBe antibodies) and an HBV DNA level that remains below 2000 IU/mL after a 48-week course of treatment; however, an ALT flare can be observed at the time of HBeAg loss in patients in whom treatment is successful. Pegylated IFN-α treatment should be reserved for patients with the best chance of a sustained virologic response off treatment—HBeAg-positive patients with high baseline ALT levels (more than three times the upper limit of normal) and HBV DNA levels below 2.10^6 IU/mL. Pegylated IFN-α therapy is contraindicated in patients with advanced cirrhosis and in immunosuppressed patients. Patients infected with HBV genotypes A and B generally respond better to IFN-α therapy than do patients infected with genotypes C and D, but the predictive value of the HBV genotype for an individual patient is weak. Patients who fail to achieve a sustained virologic response after a single course of pegylated IFN-α are candidates for nucleoside/nucleotide analogue therapy.

Long-term treatment with nucleoside/nucleotide analogues is indicated in the majority of patients with chronic hepatitis B. Tenofovir or entecavir, which are the most potent drugs with an optimal resistance profile, are recommended as first-line monotherapies. HBV DNA should be suppressed to undetectable levels (<10 to 15 IU/mL) with a sensitive real-time PCR-based assay. If the HBV DNA level is reduced but still detectable in a compliant patient, the other agent may be added; however, the long-term safety of combined tenofovir and entecavir is unknown. When HBeAg-positive patients seroconvert to negative or HBeAg-negative patients lose their HBsAg, treatment should be continued for an additional 6 to 12 months. In all other cases, treatment should be continued for life, and adherence is particularly important.

Virologic breakthroughs—defined by a subsequent increase of the HBV DNA level of 1 log or more above the nadir level—in adherent patients are due to HBV resistance to the administered antiviral drug or drugs. HBV DNA levels most often increase back to baseline levels, and the virologic breakthrough is generally followed a few weeks later by a biochemical breakthrough in which a previously normal ALT level rises above normal. The cumulative rates of resistance in newly treated patients are 70% at 5 years for lamivudine, 17% at 2 years for telbivudine, 1.2% at 6 years for entecavir, 29% at 5 years for adefovir, and 0% at 2 years for tenofovir. These figures illustrate the high genetic barrier against resistance of entecavir and tenofovir. In a patient who develops resistance to any of the available nucleoside/nucleotide analogues, adding a second drug without cross-resistance is the only efficient strategy, although the long-term safety of some of these combinations is not known. In patients with lamivudine, telbivudine, or entecavir resistance, tenofovir should be added. Patients who have resistance to adefovir should be switched to tenofovir and also given lamivudine, telbivudine, or entecavir. In patients with tenofovir resistance, any of these three drugs should be added. The combination of tenofovir and emtricitabine, a nucleoside analogue similar to lamivudine, in a single tablet (approved for HIV but not for HBV therapy) is also a valid option in cases of resistance to any of these drugs.

In patients with cirrhosis, nucleoside/nucleotide analogue therapy is the only option because pegylated IFN-α is contraindicated if cirrhosis is decompensated. Because resistance in this population can be life threatening, some experts recommend de novo treatment with two potent drugs without cross-resistance. In those with decompensated disease, efficient antiviral treatment most often stabilizes the patient's condition and can also delay or obviate the need for liver transplantation. If transplantation is needed, post-transplant administration of anti-HBV immune globulins in combination with a potent nucleoside/nucleotide analogue prevents recurrent HBV in the vast majority of cases.

PROGNOSIS

Every year, approximately 0.5% of inactive HBsAg carriers spontaneously lose HBsAg, and most of them acquire anti-HBs antibodies. Reactivations are possible in inactive HBV carriers, especially if they become immunosuppressed, such as during chemotherapy or corticosteroid administration. HBV reactivations often evolve into a subfulminant or fulminant form.

The risk of cirrhosis in chronic hepatitis B is 2 to 10% per year, and it is significantly associated with a higher HBV DNA level, older age, alcohol consumption, coinfection with other hepatotropic viruses, and coinfection with HIV. The cumulative incidence of liver decompensation is about 15 to 20% at 5 years in patients with compensated cirrhosis. The complications of cirrhosis, including hepatocellular cancer, are among the main causes of mortality in HBV-infected patients, and the annual incidence of death is about 3 to 4%.

The likelihood of developing hepatocellular carcinoma is about 1% per year in patients without cirrhosis and 2 to 8% per year in those with cirrhosis, and it is significantly associated with a higher HBV DNA level, male sex, old age, reversion from anti-HBe-positive to HBeAg-positive, and coinfection with other hepatotropic viruses. HBV carriers at risk for hepatocellular cancer should be screened every 6 to 12 months, ideally with an ultrasound examination and an α-fetoprotein level.

CHRONIC HEPATITIS C

EPIDEMIOLOGY

HCV, which is present on all continents, is estimated to cause chronic infection in approximately 170 million individuals, or 3% of the world's population. The prevalence of chronic HCV infection, which varies geographically, is estimated to be about 1.3% in the United States (affecting 3.2 million individuals), 3.5% in Asia, 1.9% in the Americas overall, 5.2% in Africa, 1.7% in Europe, and 1.8% in Oceania. The highest prevalence is in Egypt (9% overall, but up to 40% in certain rural areas), where infection was initially spread by intramuscular injections for schistosomiasis during treatment campaigns several decades ago.

TABLE 151-3 SHORT-TERM (1-YEAR) RESPONSES TO APPROVED ANTIVIRAL THERAPIES AMONG TREATMENT-NAÏVE PATIENTS WITH HBeAg-POSITIVE CHRONIC HEPATITIS B

	PLACEBO/ CONTROL GROUPS	PEGYLATED IFN-α2A (48 WK)	LAMIVUDINE (48-52 WK)	TELBIVUDINE (52 WK)	ENTECAVIR (48 WK)	ADEFOVIR (48 WK)	TENOFOVIR (48 WK)
Loss of serum HBV DNA (%)*	0-17	25	40-44	60	67	21	76
HBeAg loss (%)	6-12	30/34[†]	17-32	26	22	24	NA
HBe seroconversion (%)	4-6	27/32[†]	16-21	22	21	12	21
HBsAg loss (%)	0-1	3	1	0	2	0	3
ALT normalization (%)	7-24	39	41-75	77	68	48	68
Histologic improvement (%)	NA	38[‡]	49-56	65	72	53	74
Durability of response (%)[§]	NA	NA	50-80	≈80	69	≈90	NA

*HBV DNA levels were assessed with various molecular assays, with different lower limits of detection.
[†]Responses at week 48/week 72 (24 weeks after stopping treatment).
[‡]Post-treatment biopsies at week 72 (24 weeks after stopping treatment).
[§]No or short duration of consolidation treatment for lamivudine and entecavir; most patients had consolidation treatment for adefovir and telbivudine.
Ag = antigen; ALT = alanine aminotransferase; HBe = hepatitis B e; HBs = hepatitis B surface; HBV = hepatitis B virus; IFN = interferon; NA = not available.
Adapted from Lok AS, McMahon BJ. American Association for the Study of Liver Diseases practice guidelines—chronic hepatitis B: update 2009, www.aasld.org.

TABLE 151-4 SHORT-TERM (1-YEAR) RESPONSES TO APPROVED ANTIVIRAL THERAPIES AMONG TREATMENT-NAÏVE PATIENTS WITH HBeAg-NEGATIVE CHRONIC HEPATITIS B

	PLACEBO/ CONTROL GROUPS	PEGYLATED IFN-α2A (48 WK)	LAMIVUDINE (48-52 WK)	TELBIVUDINE (52 WK)	ENTECAVIR (48 WK)	ADEFOVIR (48 WK)	TENOFOVIR (48 WK)
Loss of serum HBV DNA (%)*	0-20	63	60-73	88	90	51	93
ALT normalization (%)	10-29	38	60-79	74	78	72	76
Histologic improvement (%)	33	48	60-66	67	70	64	72
Durability of response (%)	NA	≈20	<10	NA	3	≈5	NA

*HBV DNA levels were assessed with various molecular assays, with different lower limits of detection. ALT = alanine aminotransferase; HBeAg = hepatitis B e antigen; HBV = hepatitis B virus; IFN = interferon; NA = not available.
Adapted from Lok AS, McMahon BJ. American Association for the Study of Liver Diseases practice guidelines—chronic hepatitis B: update 2009, www.aasld.org.

PATHOBIOLOGY

Acute HCV infection evolves into chronic infection in 50 to 80% of cases. Even patients who spontaneously recover and maintain detectable anti-HCV antibodies are not protected against reinfection. Persistence of infection is related to a qualitatively and quantitatively altered CD4$^+$ T-helper cell and cytotoxic T lymphocyte response that fails to eradicate infection. The plasticity of the viral genomes is responsible for the coexistence of closely related but genetically different viral populations in equilibrium in the patient's replicative environment. This genetic diversity allows continuously generated variant viral populations to be selected by timely changes in the replicative environment.

Chronic HCV infection is responsible for necroinflammatory lesions of varying severity, sometimes associated with steatosis, which is the accumulation of triglycerides in hepatocytes. HCV is not a cytopathic virus. Liver injury in chronic hepatitis C is related to the action of immune effectors that recognize and kill infected hepatocytes that express HCV antigens at their surface. Chronic inflammation triggers fibrogenesis through the activation of hepatic stellate cells. Fibrosis progresses at nonlinear rates that are generally faster in older patients, in males, and in the presence of chronic alcohol intake, viral coinfections, or immunosuppression. The severity of chronic hepatitis is independent of the HCV RNA level and of the HCV genotype. This chronic inflammation and progression of fibrosis predispose patients to cirrhosis (Chapter 156) and hepatocellular carcinoma (Chapter 202).

CLINICAL MANIFESTATIONS

Acute hepatitis C (Chapter 150) is most often asymptomatic and therefore undiagnosed. The most common symptom associated with chronic HCV infection is fatigue, but it may remain unapparent for years. ALT levels are usually moderately elevated and fluctuate, but they can remain normal for weeks to months despite active hepatitis on liver biopsy. Moderate cholestasis can be present in patients with cirrhosis. Patients with cirrhosis (Chapter 156) and/or hepatocellular carcinoma (Chapter 202) have the typical signs associated with these conditions.

HCV is the main cause of type II and type III mixed cryoglobulinemia (Chapter 193). Low levels of circulating cryoglobulins, which contain HCV RNA, anti-HCV antibodies, rheumatoid factor, and low levels of complement, can be found in 50 to 70% of cases, whereas elevated rheumatoid factor (Chapter 272) is found in 70% of cases. Less than 1% of HCV-infected patients develop symptoms of cryoglobulinemic vasculitis, including fatigue, myalgias, arthralgias, rash (purpura, hives, and leukocytoclastic vasculitis), neuropathy, and membranoproliferative glomerulonephritis. Cryoglobulinemia can be severe and lead to end-stage renal disease or severe neuropathies, and long-term cryoglobulinemia has been linked to non-Hodgkin's B-cell lymphomas (Chapter 191).

Low titers of antinuclear and anti–smooth muscle antibodies can be found in HCV-infected patients, but they do not have any clinical significance. HCV has been reported to trigger the symptoms of porphyria cutanea tarda (Chapter 217), and an association with lichen planus (Chapter 446) has been suggested.

DIAGNOSIS

Chronic HCV infection is defined by the persistence of HCV RNA for more than 6 months. In patients with clinical and/or biologic signs of chronic liver disease, chronic hepatitis C is diagnosed by the simultaneous presence of anti-HCV antibodies and HCV RNA. Detectable HCV replication in the absence of anti-HCV antibodies is observed almost exclusively in patients who are profoundly immunosuppressed, on hemodialysis, or agammaglobulinemic. The level of HCV replication does not correlate with the severity of liver disease or with the risk of progression to cirrhosis or hepatocellular carcinoma.

The HCV genotype, which has important therapeutic implications, should be determined. Anti-HCV IgM, which is found in about 50% of patients with chronic hepatitis, is of no significance. Laboratory testing often reveals high levels of monoclonal rheumatoid factor and cryoglobulins.

TREATMENT Rx

Chronic HCV infection is curable. The goal of therapy is to achieve a sustained virologic response, defined by undetectable HCV RNA 24 weeks after the end of therapy using a sensitive HCV RNA assay with a lower limit of detection of 50 IU/mL or less.

The decision to treat chronic hepatitis C depends on a precise assessment of the severity of liver disease, the presence of absolute or relative contraindications to therapy, and the patient's willingness to be treated. Treatment typically requires a liver biopsy, but serologic markers of liver fibrosis and/or fibrogenesis and transient elastography have been validated in large series of patients with chronic hepatitis C.

In patients with no indication for therapy or with contraindications to therapy, repeated assessments of aminotransferase levels are recommended on a yearly basis. Assessment of liver inflammation and fibrosis by liver biopsy or noninvasive serologic or ultrasound-based testing is indicated for patients with persistent or intermittently elevated aminotransferase levels.

The current standard treatment for chronic hepatitis C is the combination of ribavirin (0.8 to 1.4 g/day orally) with either pegylated IFN-α2a (180 µg subcutaneously once weekly) or pegylated IFN-α2b (1.5 µg/kg subcutaneously once weekly).[6] The most common side effects of IFN-α are influenza-like symptoms (which can be prevented by acetaminophen), neutropenia, thrombocytopenia, irritability, difficulty concentrating, memory disturbances, thyroiditis, hair loss, sleep disorders, and weight loss. The principal side effect of ribavirin is hemolytic anemia. As a result of these side effects, dose modification is frequently required during therapy. Ribavirin should be decreased in 200-mg increments in patients with severe anemia. For IFN-induced side effects, the pegylated IFN-α dose should be decreased stepwise, from 180 to 135 to 90 µg/week for pegylated IFN-α2a, and from 1.5 to 1.0 to 0.5 µg/kg/week for pegylated IFN-α2b.

The main contraindications to therapy with pegylated IFN-α and ribavirin are decompensated liver disease, renal failure, severe immunosuppression, solid organ transplantation, cytopenias, severe psychiatric disease, and active substance abuse. Ribavirin is also contraindicated in patients with anemia, significant coronary or cerebrovascular disease, or renal insufficiency. Because ribavirin is teratogenic, it is essential that adequate contraception be practiced during therapy and for at least 6 months thereafter in both men and women.

In patients for whom therapy is deemed appropriate, the HCV genotype guides treatment and its duration (Fig. 151-2). Patients infected with HCV genotype 1 require 48 weeks of treatment and a higher, body-weight-based dose of ribavirin (1.0 to 1.4 g/day). Treatment should be tailored to the actual virologic response using a sensitive assay, such as a real-time PCR. The HCV RNA level should be measured before therapy and 4 and 12 weeks after its initiation. The lack of a virologic response (no change or an HCV RNA level that decreases by less than a factor of 100 [2 log$_{10}$]) at 12 weeks indicates that the patient has virtually no chance of achieving a sustained virologic response and should stop treatment. In contrast, treatment must be continued if such a decline in HCV RNA level is observed at week 12. Patients who achieve a rapid virologic response (undetectable HCV RNA at week 4) can stop therapy after 24 weeks if their baseline HCV RNA level is below 400,000 IU/mL. Patients who do not achieve a complete virologic response (i.e., HCV RNA is still detectable) at week 4 but do so at week 12 should be treated for 48 weeks; then they can stop therapy. It is now generally accepted that patients with a slow virologic response (HCV RNA has decreased by more than 2 log$_{10}$ but is still detectable at week 12) should be treated for 72 weeks because prolonged therapy significantly reduces the incidence of post-treatment relapse.

Patients infected with HCV genotypes 2 and 3 require 24 weeks of treatment, but at a lower ribavirin dose of 0.8 g/day. In patients who respond to treatment with an undetectable HCV RNA but relapse after the end of therapy, another 48 weeks of treatment with a higher, weight-based dose of ribavirin (1.0 to 1.4 g/day) is recommended.

Patients infected with HCV genotypes 4, 5, and 6 require 48 weeks of treatment and a higher, body-weight-based dose of ribavirin (1.0 to 1.4 g/day). The same approaches to monitoring and dose adjustment used for genotype 1 probably apply to these genotypes, but they have not been validated in sufficiently large cohorts of patients.

Currently, about 40 to 50% of patients infected with HCV genotypes 1 and 4 and 80% of patients infected with genotypes 2 and 3 achieve a sustained virologic response with the standard combination of pegylated IFN-α and ribavirin; rates for genotypes 5 and 6 are unknown. Predictors of a sustained virologic response include a baseline HCV RNA level less than 800,000 IU/mL, lack of extensive fibrosis or cirrhosis, young age, female sex, nonblack race, and single nucleotide polymorphisms in the host genome. However, none of these negative predictive factors should be used to deny treatment. Long-term maintenance therapy with a low dose of pegylated IFN-α is not beneficial, except perhaps in a small proportion of patients whose HCV RNA levels remain very low or undetectable on treatment.

The results of pegylated IFN-α and ribavirin therapy can be improved by reducing body weight and insulin resistance. Erythropoietin can control ribavirin-induced anemia and minimize ribavirin dose reductions. Granulocyte colony-stimulating factor can be used to reverse severe IFN-induced neutropenia. Careful management of anxiety, sleeping disorders, and depression is also important. Retreatment of patients who do not achieve a sustained virologic response with the same dose of pegylated IFN-α and ribavirin yields sustained virologic response rates of about 10 to 15%; retreatment with higher doses can be tried with careful monitoring and attention to side effects.

FIGURE 151-2. Pegylated interferon-α (IFN-α) and ribavirin treatment algorithm in patients with chronic hepatitis C, according to the hepatitis C virus (HCV) genotype.

New HCV drugs in trials include novel IFNs, alternatives to ribavirin, and direct-acting antiviral drugs that target various functions of the HCV life cycle. Telaprevir 750 mg three times daily or boceprevir 800 mg three times daily, in combination with the standard doses of pegylated IFN-α and ribavirin, has resulted in sustained virologic response rates of 70% in never-treated patients infected with HCV genotype 1 and in about 50% of patients who did not respond to a first course of standard two-drug therapy.[7,8] However, telaprevir frequently causes rashes and pruritus, and boceprevir can aggravate ribavirin-related anemia; furthermore, these drugs have little or no efficacy for genotypes 3 and 4. Similarly, the addition of boceprevir to standard therapy increases viral response in both never-treated[9] and previously treated[10] patients with genotype 1.

In patients with end-stage liver disease, liver transplantation (Chapter 157) is the only option. However, the graft becomes infected in 100% of patients who are viremic at the time of transplantation. Treatment with pegylated IFN-α and ribavirin is difficult in the post-transplant setting and yields disappointing results.

PROGNOSIS

Spontaneous HCV clearance in patients with chronic hepatitis C is exceptional. The HCV RNA level has no prognostic value in chronic hepatitis C.

It is estimated that 20% of patients with chronic hepatitis C develop cirrhosis; this occurs, on average, after 20 years of progression. Cirrhosis remains compensated for many years in the vast majority of patients, but decompensation occurs at an annual rate of 2 to 5% in cirrhotic patients. After a first decompensation, the mortality rate related to portal hypertension, hepatocellular insufficiency, and hepatocellular carcinoma is 10% per year, with a 50% survival rate at 5 years. The risk of death increases with advancing age, male gender, and the severity of cirrhosis.

Hepatocellular carcinoma is rare in patients with chronic hepatitis C without cirrhosis. In patients with cirrhosis, the incidence of hepatocellular carcinoma is 2 to 4% per year, most often in patients with compensated cirrhosis. HCV has become the most common cause of hepatocellular carcinoma in most industrialized countries.

Long-term follow-up shows that HCV does not recur in greater than 99% of patients who achieve a sustained virologic response, even in those who are immunosuppressed or receive chemotherapy. However, the liver disease may continue to evolve even after the infection has been eradicated. In addition, patients with chronic hepatitis C should abstain from alcohol and, unless there are other contraindications, should be vaccinated for hepatitis A and B (Chapter 17).

● CHRONIC HEPATITIS D

EPIDEMIOLOGY

HDV infection occurs only in HBsAg carriers. Only approximately 2% of patients acutely coinfected with HDV and HBV develop chronic hepatitis D. In chronic HBV carriers superinfected by HDV, however, 90% of patients become chronic HDV carriers.

CLINICAL MANIFESTATIONS

Chronic hepatitis D is generally severe, with more than 80% of patients developing cirrhosis. Compared with patients who have chronic hepatitis B alone, patients with chronic infection with both HBV and HDV are three times as likely to develop hepatocellular carcinoma and twice as likely to die.

DIAGNOSIS

Markers of HDV infection should be sought at least once in every chronic HBsAg carrier. Both total anti-HD antibodies and anti-HD IgM remain at high levels in chronic HDV infection, and HDV RNA is present. Although all chronic HDV carriers also are chronic HBsAg carriers, chronic HDV carriers generally have low or undetectable HBV DNA levels because HDV inhibits HBV replication.

TREATMENT

High doses (9 million units three times/week for 1 year) of standard, non-pegylated IFN-α result in sustained normalization of ALT levels 24 weeks after the end of therapy in approximately 50% of cases, sometimes for as long as 20 years. Some patients clear HDV RNA and, eventually, HBsAg.

Pegylated IFN-α2b, 1.5 µg/kg once weekly for 12 months, provides a sustained virologic response in 20 to 40% of cases.[11] Although there is no clear consensus, most experts now recommend 1 year of pegylated IFN-α as first-line treatment of chronic HDV infection.

PREVENTION

Chronic HDV infection is best prevented by preventing primary HBV infection, because individuals who are protected against HBV cannot be infected with HDV. In chronic HBsAg carriers, standard hygiene and behavioral precautions should be practiced to avoid superinfection with HDV. Once acute HDV infection occurs, no secondary prevention strategy is successful.

CHRONIC HEPATITIS E

Although HEV infection was long thought to be self-limited, it can persist and cause liver inflammation in solid organ transplant recipients who harbor HEV RNA in their blood and liver tissues, either from a latent virus reactivated by immunosuppression or from a virus transmitted at the time of transplantation. All cases of chronic infection have been in immunosuppressed patients.

CLINICAL MANIFESTATIONS AND DIAGNOSIS

Chronic hepatitis E occurs after transplantation. Diagnosis is based on the detection of anti-HEV IgM antibodies, but current assays lack sensitivity and specificity. HEV RNA can also be detected in blood or feces, where its presence is transient. Solid organ transplant recipients with chronic hepatitis E harbor repeatedly positive anti-HEV antibodies and HEV RNA in blood.

TREATMENT AND PREVENTION   Rx

There is no validated treatment of chronic HEV infection. Whether candidates for transplantation or immunosuppressive therapies should be vaccinated to prevent chronic HEV infection remains to be determined.

AUTOIMMUNE HEPATITIS

Autoimmune hepatitis is a chronic inflammatory liver disorder characterized by the presence of autoantibodies in serum, high levels of serum immunoglobulins, and a frequent association with other autoimmune diseases.

EPIDEMIOLOGY AND PATHOBIOLOGY

Autoimmune hepatitis typically presents between the ages of 15 and 25 years or between the ages of 45 and 60 years, and it is more common in women. Along with primary biliary cirrhosis (Chapter 158) and primary sclerosing cholangitis (Chapter 158), autoimmune hepatitis is one of the three major autoimmune liver diseases.

Autoimmune hepatitis is believed to be caused by autoimmune reactions against normal hepatocytes in genetically predisposed persons or persons exposed to unidentified triggers of an autoimmune process against liver antigens. Associations are seen with the human leukocyte antigen (HLA) class I B8 and class II DR3 and DR52a loci. In Asians, autoimmune hepatitis is associated with HLA DR4.

CLINICAL MANIFESTATIONS AND DIAGNOSIS

Autoimmune hepatitis tends to be more severe at its onset than chronic hepatitis B or C, and it progresses to end-stage liver disease if not treated with immunosuppression. Although it is occasionally detected by elevated serum aminotransferase levels on a routine health evaluation, most patients present with fatigue and jaundice. Elevations of bilirubin or alkaline phosphatase indicate more severe or advanced disease. Patients typically have marked elevations in serum gamma globulin, specifically immunoglobulin G, as well as autoantibodies directed at non-organ-specific cellular constituents.

Type 1 (classic) autoimmune hepatitis is characterized by the presence of titers of 1:80 or higher (>1:20 in children) of antinuclear, anti-smooth muscle, antiactin, and anti-asialoglycoprotein receptor antibodies. Type 2 autoimmune hepatitis is characterized by similar elevations of anti–liver-kidney microsomal 1 antibodies and anti–liver cytosol 1 antibodies, without antinuclear or anti–smooth muscle antibodies. Liver biopsy shows features that are typical of all chronic types of hepatitis, except plasma cell infiltrates.

TREATMENT   Rx

The clinical symptoms and liver test abnormalities of autoimmune hepatitis generally respond promptly to prednisone, usually at a dose of 20 to 30 mg/day, with a decrease in serum aminotransferase levels to the normal or near-normal range within 1 to 3 months; higher doses may be required in patients with more severe disease. Lack of a biochemical or clinical response should lead to reevaluation of the diagnosis. Azathioprine 50 to 100 mg can be combined with prednisone or added later to reduce long-term steroid side effects.

Maintenance doses, which are typically required indefinitely, are often 5 to 10 mg/day of prednisone combined with 50 to 150 mg/day of azathioprine. Sometimes patients can be maintained on azathioprine (2 mg/kg/day) alone. After 3 years or more of remission, therapy can be carefully withdrawn, but severe and even fatal flares can occur weeks to months later.

PROGNOSIS

The prognosis is generally related to the histologic stage of the disease. Patients who initially respond to therapy may do well for many years. Patients who progress to end-stage liver disease require liver transplantation (Chapter 157).

CRYPTOGENIC CHRONIC LIVER DISEASE

Cryptogenic chronic liver disease refers to chronic hepatitis or cirrhosis of unknown cause after excluding hepatitis B, C, D, and E; autoimmune hepatitis; steatohepatitis (Chapter 155); alcoholic liver disease (Chapter 155); drug-induced hepatitis (Chapter 152); and inherited and metabolic liver diseases (Chapter 153). Tests to exclude these conditions include serum levels of α_1-antitrypsin, iron, and ceruloplasmin and, if necessary, urine and liver copper concentrations. In its later stages, nonalcoholic steatohepatitis may be associated with little or no fat.

1. Loomba R, Rowley A, Wesley R, et al. Systematic review: the effect of preventive lamivudine on hepatitis B reactivation during chemotherapy. *Ann Intern Med.* 2008;148:519-528.
2. Lau GK, Piravisuth T, Luo KX, et al. Peginterferon alfa-2a, lamivudine and the combination for HBeAg-positive chronic hepatitis B. *N Engl J Med.* 2005;352:2682-2695.
3. Chang TT, Gish RG, de Man R, et al. A comparison of entecavir and lamivudine for HBeAg-positive chronic hepatitis B. *N Engl J Med.* 2006;354:1001-1010.
4. Lai CL, Shouval D, Lok AS, et al. Entecavir versus lamivudine for patients with HBeAg-negative chronic hepatitis B. *N Engl J Med.* 2006;354:1011-1020.
5. Heathcote EJ, Marcellin P, Buti M, et al. Three-year efficacy and safety of tenofovir disoproxil fumarate treatment for chronic hepatitis B. *Gastroenterology.* 2011;140:132-143.
6. Fried MW, Shiffman ML, Reddy KR, et al. Peginterferon alfa-2a plus ribavirin for chronic hepatitis C virus infection. *N Engl J Med.* 2002;347:975-982.
7. McHutchison JG, Everson GT, Gordon SC, et al. Telaprevir with peginterferon and ribavirin for chronic HCV genotype 1 infection. *N Engl J Med.* 2009;360:1827-1838.
8. Hézode C, Forestier N, Dusheiko G, et al. Telaprevir and peginterferon with or without ribavirin for chronic HCV infection. *N Engl J Med.* 2009;360:1839-1850.
9. Poordad F, McCone J Jr, Bacon BR, et al. Boceprevir for untreated chronic HCV genotype 1 infection. *N Engl J Med.* 2011;364:1195-1206.
10. Bacon BR, Gordon SC, Lawitz E, et al. Boceprevir for previously treated chronic HCV genotype 1 infection. *N Engl J Med.* 2011;364:1207-1217.
11. Wedemeyer H, Yurdaydin C, Dalekos GN, et al. Peginterferon plus adefovir versus either drug alone for hepatitis delta. *N Engl J Med.* 2011;364:322-331.

SUGGESTED READINGS

Alberti A, Caporaso N. HBV therapy: guidelines and open issues. *Dig Liver Dis.* 2011;43:57-63. *Review of guidelines.*

Ghany MG, Strader DB, Thomas DL. Diagnosis, management and treatment of hepatitis C: an update. *Hepatology.* 2009;49:1335-1374. *Clinical practice guidelines of the American Association for the Study of Liver Diseases.*

Vergani D, Mieli-Vergani G. Pharmacological management of autoimmune hepatitis. *Expert Opin Pharmacother.* 2011;12:607-613. *Most patients respond rapidly to prednisolone and azathioprine.*

Woo G, Tomlinson G, Nishikawa Y, et al. Tenofovir and entecavir are most effective antiviral agents for chronic hepatitis B: a systematic review and Bayesian meta-analyses. *Gastroenterology.* 2010;139:1218-1229. *Conclusions based on meta-analysis.*

152

TOXIN- AND DRUG-INDUCED LIVER DISEASE

WILLIAM M. LEE

DEFINITION

Toxin-induced and drug-induced hepatotoxicity, defined as any degree of liver injury caused by a drug or a toxic substance, is a frequent cause of acute liver injury and accounts for more than 50% of all cases of acute liver failure with hepatic encephalopathy in the United States. Hepatotoxicity has been described with many drugs, although the number of cases is low, given the number of prescriptions written.

EPIDEMIOLOGY

Few data are available on the epidemiology of toxin- and drug-induced liver disease. The precise number of drug-induced liver injuries in the United States is unknown, but European data on adverse drug reactions indicate about 22 cases of drug-induced liver disease per 1 million people per year. In developing parts of the world, drug-induced liver disease is much less common and is related to fewer drugs. It is estimated that less than 10% of actual cases are reported, so the true incidence of toxin- and drug-induced liver disease may be impossible to determine.

PATHOBIOLOGY

The liver is central to the metabolism of exogenous substances. Most drugs and xenobiotics cross the intestinal brush border because they are lipophilic. *Biotransformation* is the process by which lipophilic therapeutic agents are rendered more hydrophilic by the liver, resulting in drug excretion in urine or bile. In most instances, biotransformation changes a nonpolar to a polar compound through several steps. Foremost are oxidative pathways (e.g., hydroxylation) mediated by the cytochromes (CYPs) P-450 (Chapter 28). The next step is typically esterification to form sulfates and glucuronides, a process that results in the addition of highly polar groups to the hydroxyl group. These two enzymatic steps are referred to as *phase I* (CYP oxidation) and *phase II* (esterification). Other important metabolic pathways involve glutathione-*S*-transferase, acetylating enzymes, and alcohol dehydrogenase, but the principal metabolic pathways for most pharmacologic agents involve CYPs and subsequent esterification.

Pathogenesis

The exact details of the pathogenesis of liver injury are unclear for most drugs. A single drug may cause toxic effects in several ways. One overarching approach suggests that high-energy unstable metabolites of the parent drug, the result of CYP activation, bind to cell proteins or DNA and disrupt cell function. Perhaps the best example is acetaminophen. Although used universally for non-narcotic pain relief, acetaminophen, when taken in large quantities, causes profound centrilobular necrosis. The metabolic pathway of acetaminophen involves phase I and phase II reactions, glutathione detoxification, and the formation of reactive intermediates (E-Fig. 152-1). The presence of alcohol, which competes for CYP P-450 2E1, not only inhibits the formation of *N*-aminoparaquinoneamine (NAPQI) but also induces the enzyme so that its half-life is slowed and more enzyme is present. After the cessation of alcohol ingestion, NAPQI formation is enhanced by the presence of the induced enzyme and the lack of competition from alcohol. Toxicity is a dynamic process and may be most pronounced in the 24 hours after the cessation of alcohol. Glucuronidation and sulfation occur as the initial detoxifying step because the parent compound contains a hydroxyl group. Glucuronidation and sulfation capacity greatly exceeds daily needs, so even patients with very advanced liver disease continue to have adequate glucuronidation capacity, which explains why no obvious enhancement of toxicity is observed when cirrhotic patients take acetaminophen.

Genetics
Enzyme Polymorphism

Although acetaminophen is a dose-related toxin, the rarity of idiosyncratic drug toxicity (1 in 10,000 patients) suggests the importance of environmental and host factors (Table 152-1). Genetically variant CYP isoenzymes may partially explain the observed individual variation in response to drugs. An example is debrisoquine, an antihypertensive drug marketed in Europe that is hydroxylated by CYP2D6, an isoform that is totally absent in 5% of normal individuals. Lack of CYP2D6 greatly prolongs the half-life of the parent compound in affected individuals. Another example is the phenomenon of fast versus slow acetylation, which affects different ethnic groups and has been implicated in the differential metabolism of isoniazid. Most of the known genetic variants that occur relatively frequently, however, cannot explain the formation of a toxic intermediate in only a rare individual.

Most drugs are small organic compounds, unlikely to evoke an immune response. Although some toxic drug reactions are associated with an obvious allergic response, most are not. Nevertheless, immune mechanisms not

TABLE 152-1	FACTORS THAT MAY INFLUENCE THE METABOLIC FATE OF DRUGS

AGE

The elderly seem to be affected more often; adults are more susceptible than children to some drugs (acetaminophen, halothane, isoniazid) and less susceptible to others (aspirin, valproic acid)

ALCOHOL, ACUTE AND CHRONIC INGESTION

Induction of CYP2E1 affects drugs metabolized by this pathway, including acetaminophen and isoniazid

GENDER

Females are affected more often, but the reason is unknown

PREGNANCY

Effects of drugs in pregnancy have been poorly studied

PREEXISTING LIVER DISEASE

Hepatic disease may *protect* against idiosyncratic reactions and may *enhance* the toxicity of dose-dependent hepatotoxins (e.g., acetaminophen)

RENAL DISEASE

Slowed disappearance of the parent compound yields higher concentrations and affects P-450 (e.g., enhancement of tetracycline toxicity in renal disease)

CERTAIN FOODS

Grapefruit has an unknown substance that interferes with the metabolism of some drugs

CONCOMITANT DRUGS

Drug-drug interactions are common causes of adverse effects (e.g., valproate and chlorpromazine together lead to enhanced cholestasis)

GENETIC FACTORS

Enzyme polymorphisms (e.g., enhanced phenytoin liver disease in patients with defective epoxide hydrolase activity), HLA phenotypes (e.g., nitrofurantoin susceptibility)

associated with systemic allergic immunoglobulin E (IgE) reactions or skin hypersensitivity might be involved. Studies suggest that the products of CYP P-450 metabolism, the highly reactive intermediates formed within the microsomes, covalently bind to the enzyme itself to form a drug-hapten adduct that disables the enzyme and injures the cell. Haptenization then evokes an immune response directed against the newly formed antigen or neoantigen. P-450s have been shown to traffic to the plasma membrane, thereby allowing the drug–P-450 adduct to become the target of a subsequent cytolytic attack. It is unclear whether the targets are these adducts or the smaller peptides processed and presented by the major histocompatibility complex class I and class II schemes. The association among neoantigens, autoantibodies, and hepatotoxic drugs implicates an immunologic mechanism.

Regardless of whether an individual drug causes significant cell necrosis, the drug–P-450 adducts can evoke an immune response. Any subsequent drug–P-450 adduct present on the hepatocyte surface would evoke a further response. Responses may be antibody mediated or occur as a result of direct cytolytic attack by primed T cells. Specific genetically determined components of the immune response may be important. A specific human leukocyte antigen (HLA) haplotype has been associated with amoxicillin-clavulanate–induced hepatitis, and polymorphisms have been identified for the interleukin-10 promoter and for tumor necrosis factor-α. For every patient with a severe injury caused by drugs, there are often many more individuals with asymptomatic aminotransferase elevations that subsided despite continuing the drug—sometimes referred to as an adaptive response.

Other Mechanisms

In drug-induced cholestasis, disruption of specific transport proteins or processes in hepatocytes or cholangiocytes may be the key event. Estrogen may cause multiple canalicular membrane transport changes that affect, among others, the canalicular bile salt pump. Uncoupling or inhibition of mitochondrial respiration may lead to microvesicular steatosis.

Hepatotoxic Agents

Although there are a few dose-related toxins, most drugs involved in liver disease cause idiosyncratic, unpredictable toxicity.

TABLE 152-2 DRUGS AND TOXINS IN WHICH A DOSE-RESPONSE EFFECT IS OBSERVED

DRUG OR TOXIN	RESPONSE
Acetaminophen	Total dose, single vs. multiple time points
Amiodarone	Total dose over time
Bromfenac	Toxicity occurs only after extended use
Cocaine	Dose-related vascular collapse
Cyclophosphamide	Dose related, worse with previous ALT elevations
Cyclosporine	Cholestasis with toxic blood levels, CYP3A phenotype
Methotrexate	Aminotransferase, fibrosis; single dose/total dose
Niacin	Large doses cause vascular collapse
Oral contraceptives	Prolonged use causes hepatic adenomas
Tetracycline	Total dose, renal dysfunction
Toxins (yellow phosphorus, carbon tetrachloride, *Amanita* toxin, bacterial toxins)	Total dose

ALT = alanine aminotransferase.

TABLE 152-3 TYPES OF TOXIN AND DRUG REACTIONS

REACTION TYPE	IMPLICATED DRUGS OR TOXINS
Autoimmune (attack on cell surface markers)	Lovastatin, methyldopa, nitrofurantoin
Cholestatic (attack on bile ducts)	Anabolic steroids, carbamazepine, chlorpromazine, estrogen, erythromycin
Fibrosis (activation of stellate cells leads to fibrosis)	Methotrexate, vitamin A excess
Granulomatous (macrophage stimulation)	Allopurinol, diltiazem, nitrofurantoin, quinidine, sulfa drugs
Hepatocellular (damage to smooth endoplasmic reticulum and immune cell surface)	Acetaminophen, *Amanita* poisoning, diclofenac, isoniazid, lovastatin, nefazodone, trazodone, venlafaxine
Immunoallergic (cytotoxic cell attack on surface determinants)	Halothane, phenytoin, sulfamethoxazole
Mixed (see above)	Amoxicillin-clavulanate, carbamazepine, cyclosporine, herbs, methimazole
Oncogenic (hepatic adenoma formation)	Oral contraceptives, androgenic agents
Steatohepatitis (mitochondrial dysfunction: β-oxidation and respiratory chain)	Amiodarone, perhexiline maleate, tamoxifen
Vascular collapse (ischemic damage)	Cocaine, ecstasy, nicotinic acid
Veno-occlusive disease (endotheliitis of sinusoidal endothelial cells)	Busulfan, cytoxan

Intrinsic (Dose-Dependent) Agents

Acetaminophen (see later) and a few other agents seem to have a clear dose-response effect, although idiosyncrasy usually plays a role as well (Table 152-2). Some toxins, such as α-amanitine produced by *Amanita* mushrooms, cause dose-related injury. *Amanita* poisoning may occur after ingestion of the mushrooms *Amanita phalloides* (death cap) or *Amanita virosa* (deadly agaric). The dose-dependent toxic effect on the liver is attributed to amatoxin, an ingredient of the mushrooms that enhances the toxic effect by its enterohepatic recirculation characteristics; the toxic effect is exerted on each cycle of the recirculation through the liver.

Idiosyncratic Reactions

Drug reactions occur in 1 in 1000 to 1 in 200,000 patients. Characteristics of these idiosyncratic reactions include their infrequent occurrence, varying time intervals between the initial exposure and the reaction, and varying severity of reactions in affected individuals. There are also similarities such as "class effects" (similar drugs exhibit similar features; see Table 152-3), a consistent pattern for each drug, and the fact that rechallenge with a responsible

agent usually leads to a more severe reaction with a shorter latency than seen after the initial exposure.

Antibiotics, anticonvulsants, and nonsteroidal anti-inflammatory drugs (NSAIDs) are associated more frequently with drug-induced liver disease, whereas hormones, antihypertensive drugs, digoxin, and antiarrhythmic drugs are implicated rarely. In some cases, idiosyncratic reactions are so infrequent that a drug continues to be used if its effectiveness or uniqueness makes the risk acceptable. An example is isoniazid, which is among the few drugs implicated in drug-induced liver injury in developing countries. In individuals receiving isoniazid as a single agent for tuberculosis prophylaxis, increased aminotransferase levels may develop in 15 to 20%, but severe hepatic necrosis develops in only 0.1 to 1% (Chapter 332)—a rate that is high in comparison to idiosyncratic drug reactions, yet low enough for isoniazid, because of its effectiveness, to remain a key drug.

CLINICAL MANIFESTATIONS

Patients may have few or nonspecific complaints despite elevated aminotransferase levels. Clinical features include nausea, fatigue, occasional right upper quadrant pain, and nonspecific symptoms similar to those seen in other forms of acute hepatitis (Chapter 150). Fever or pharyngitis (typically seen in phenytoin reactions) may be present. No specific physical findings to raise suspicion of drug toxicity are noted, except possibly a rash. Any patient in whom jaundice develops is at risk for having a severe or fatal outcome, and patients who continue taking the drug despite jaundice are at highest risk.

DIAGNOSIS

Abnormal aminotransferase levels with the use of a new drug should raise the suspicion of a drug-induced reaction and prompt immediate discontinuation of the drug rather than awaiting diagnostic tests to confirm or exclude the diagnosis. Immediate discontinuation of medication at the first sign of liver disease can prevent most fatal liver injuries.

Evaluation of a patient with a suspected drug reaction is directed toward establishing the timeline for all drugs or herbs the patient may have taken. Responsible drugs have usually been started between 5 and 90 days before the onset of symptoms. Evidence of viral hepatitis (Chapters 150), gallstones (Chapter 158), alcoholic liver disease (Chapter 155), pregnancy (Chapter 247), severe right heart failure (Chapter 58), or a period of hypotension (Chapter 106) points to these specific causes. Less commonly, cytomegalovirus (Chapter 384), Epstein-Barr virus (Chapter 385), or herpesviruses (Chapter 383) can cause hepatic injury, primarily in immunosuppressed individuals. If all these causes can be excluded, the temporal relationship fits, and the patient begins to improve after withdrawal of the drug, the diagnosis is more secure. Liver biopsy is of limited value because the histologic picture in most cases of drug-induced liver injury is no different from that of viral hepatitis (Chapter 150). Nevertheless, an occasional liver biopsy specimen in an enigmatic case might reveal eosinophils or granulomas, consistent with a drug reaction.

Types of Drug Reactions

Although most liver injury involves direct hepatocyte necrosis or apoptosis (hepatocellular injury), some drugs injure primarily the bile ducts or canaliculi and cause cholestasis without significant damage to hepatocytes. Other drugs affect sinusoidal cells or present a particular pattern of liver injury affecting multiple cell types (mixed type). Another approach to drug reactions emphasizes the histologic changes involved and the cell type (Table 152-3 and Fig. 152-1).

Hepatocellular Reactions

Hepatocellular reactions are the most common type of drug-induced liver disease and account for 90% of cases (Table 152-4). They are characterized by a pattern of serum liver test results that reflect hepatocellular injury. Usually, improvement is quick after discontinuation of the drug (1 to 2 months), and fulminant, acute liver failure with hepatic encephalopathy develops in only a few patients.

Histologic findings include necrosis and cellular infiltration. The necrosis may be zonal (e.g., induced by acetaminophen or carbon tetrachloride) or diffuse (e.g., induced by halothane), and the inflammatory response consists of lymphocytes or eosinophils. Massive necrosis may cause acute liver failure and death.

Acetaminophen toxicity is the most common form of acute liver failure in the United States and is the best understood example of direct hepatocyte toxicity. The incidence of acetaminophen poisoning varies widely throughout

FIGURE 152-1. Mechanisms of liver injury. Each form of liver injury targets specific organelles, although multiple organelles may be affected. The hepatocyte in the center may be affected in at least six ways. **A,** Disruption of intracellular calcium leads to actin fibril disassembly at the hepatocyte surface, which results in blebbing of the cell membrane and subsequent rupture and cell lysis. **B,** In cholestatic diseases, disruption of actin filaments may occur with the loss of villous processes. Interference with ion pumps limits the excretion of bilirubin and other organic compounds. **C,** Most hepatocellular reactions involve the cytochrome P-450 system. The high-energy reaction involved may lead to binding of drug to enzyme and create a new adduct. **D,** Enzyme-drug adducts may traffic to the cell surface and serve as target immunogens for cytolytic attack by T cells. **E,** Activation of apoptotic pathways results in cell death. **F,** Inhibition of β-oxidation or respiration in mitochondria results in microvesicular fat accumulation and lactic acidosis, a pattern characteristic of a variety of agents, including nucleoside analogues, tetracycline, and aspirin. ATP = adenosine triphosphate; FAD = flavin adenine dinucleotide; FFA = free fatty acid; NAD = nicotinamide adenine dinucleotide; ROS = reactive oxygen species; TNFR = tumor necrosis factor receptor. (**A,** Adapted from Farrell GC. *Drug-Induced Liver Disease.* Edinburgh: Churchill Livingstone; 1994: 44; **B,** Adapted from Trauner M, Meier PJ, Boyer J. Mechanisms of disease: molecular pathogenesis of cholestasis. *N Engl J Med.* 1998;339:1217-1227; **C,** Adapted from Watkins Zimmerman HJ. *Hepatotoxicity,* 2nd ed. Philadelphia: Lippincott Williams & Wilkins; 2000; **D,** From Robin M-A, Le Roy M, Descatoire V, Pessayre D. Plasma membrane cytochromes P450 as neoantigens and autoimmune targets in drug-induced hepatitis. *J Hepatol.* 1997;26(Suppl 1):23-30; **E,** From Reed JC. Apoptosis-regulating proteins as targets for drug discovery. *Trends Mol Med.* 2001;7:314-319; **F,** Adapted from Pessayre D, personal communication.)

the world, but it is becoming more frequent and widespread. Liver injury occurs predictably after an intentional suicidal overdose (Chapter 110); it also occurs when acetaminophen is used in excessive doses or sometimes even in therapeutic doses for pain relief. Enhanced toxicity occurs when patients are fasting or are chronic alcohol users because of enzyme induction and depletion of glutathione by alcohol and fasting; by comparison, acute alcohol intake may protect against acetaminophen toxicity during the period of alcohol ingestion. Thereafter, a rebound increase in available CYP2E1 results in increased toxicity in the 12 hours after ingestion because of enzyme induction (see E-Fig. 152-1). Patients with an unintentional acetaminophen overdose may fare worse than suicidal patients because the former seek treatment later in their course, even though suicidal patients take larger doses. The better outcome after an acute overdose may be explained by earlier medical attention and the use of N-acetylcysteine, an effective antidote. Nevertheless, one fifth of suicide attempts using acetaminophen are associated with severe liver injury and the potential for a fatal outcome.

The extremely elevated aminotransferase values (often >6000 IU/L, and sometimes as high as 30,000 IU/L) observed in suicidal and unintentional acetaminophen ingestion help distinguish these cases from viral hepatitis or other drug injury. The antidote N-acetylcysteine (Chapter 110) may be given by nasogastric tube on admission and for the next 72 hours to provide glutathione substrate. The standard treatment is intravenous N-acetylcysteine beginning at a dose of 140 mg/kg in 300 mL of 5% dextrose given over 1 hour, followed by a dose of 70 mg/kg in 5% dextrose given over a 1-hour period every 4 hours for 48 hours. A loading dose of 140 mg/kg can be given orally, followed by 70 mg/kg every 4 hours for 17 doses (72 hours). Expected survival rates are greater than 80%, although liver transplantation is occasionally required.

Cholestatic Reactions

Cholestatic reactions have been described for many drugs. Cholestasis is best defined as failure of bile to reach the duodenum, and common symptoms are jaundice and pruritus. *Pure cholestasis,* with no signs of hepatocellular necrosis, is seen almost exclusively in patients taking oral contraceptives, anabolic steroids, or sex hormone antagonists such as tamoxifen. Acute *cholestatic hepatitis* is characterized histologically by cholestasis (dilated canaliculi, brown granules in the cytoplasm of hepatocytes), some degree of liver cell necrosis and bile duct injury, and inflammatory infiltration by polymorphonuclear leukocytes. Drugs that cause this type of reaction include carbamazepine, trimethoprim-sulfamethoxazole, and captopril.

TABLE 152-4	SCORING SYSTEM TO ASSESS CAUSALITY OF HEPATOCELLULAR REACTIONS	
FACTOR		**SCORE***
TEMPORAL RELATIONSHIP OF START OF DRUG TO START OF ILLNESS		
Initial treatment: 5-90 days; subsequent treatment course: 1-15 days		+2
Initial treatment: <5 or >90 days; subsequent treatment course: >15 days		+1
From cessation of drug: ≤15 days†		+1
COURSE		
ALT decreases ≥50% from peak within 8 days		+3
ALT decreases ≥50% from peak within 30 days		+2
If the drug is continued, inconclusive		0
RISK FACTORS		
Alcohol‡		+1
No alcohol‡		0
Age ≥ 55 yr		+1
Age < 55 yr		0
CONCOMITANT DRUG		
Concomitant drug with suggestive time of onset		−1
Concomitant drug known to be a hepatotoxin with suggestive time of onset		−2
Concomitant drug with further evidence of involvement (rechallenge)		−3
NUMBER OF NONDRUG CAUSES		
Hepatitis A, B, or C; biliary obstruction; alcoholism (AST ≥ 2 × ALT); recent hypotension; and CMV, EBV, and HSV infection all excluded		+2
4-5 causes excluded		+1
<4 causes excluded		−2
Nondrug cause highly probable		−3
PREVIOUS INFORMATION ON HEPATOTOXICITY OF DRUG IN QUESTION		
Package insert mentions		+2
Published case reports but not on package label		+1
Reaction unknown		0
RECHALLENGE		
Positive (ALT doubles with drug alone)§		+2
Compatible (ALT doubles, compounding features)§		+1
Negative (increase in ALT but ≤ 2 × ULN)§		−2
Not done		0

*Causality is highly probable (score >8), probable (score 6-8), possible (score 3-5), unlikely (score 1-2), or excluded (score ≤0).
†For cholestatic reactions, ≤30 days.
‡For cholestatic reactions, alcohol, or pregnancy.
§For cholestatic reactions, substitute alkaline phosphatase (or total bilirubin) for ALT.
ALT = alanine aminotransferase; AST = aspartate aminotransferase; CMV = cytomegalovirus; EBV = Epstein-Barr virus; HSV = herpes simplex virus; ULN = upper limit of normal.
Adapted from Danan G, Benichou C. Causality assessment of adverse reactions to drugs. I. A novel method based on the conclusions of international consensus meetings: application to drug-induced liver injuries. *J Clin Epidemiol.* 1993;46:1323-1330; Benichou C, Danan G, Flahault A. Causality assessment of adverse reactions to drugs. II. An original model for validation of drug causality assessment methods: case reports with positive rechallenge. *J Clin Epidemiol.* 1993;46:1331-1336.

Generally, drug-induced cholestasis takes longer to resolve than drug-induced hepatotoxicity. In some cases, segments of the intrahepatic biliary tree may be destroyed progressively, the so-called vanishing bile duct syndrome that occurs after a protracted course (>6 months) of drug-induced cholestasis. The result is a state of chronic cholestasis that resembles primary biliary cirrhosis (Chapter 158). Approximately 30 drugs have been implicated in the vanishing bile duct syndrome, including chlorpromazine and ajmaline. A sclerosing cholangitis–like syndrome with jaundice caused by intrahepatic and extrahepatic strictures in the bile ducts is sometimes observed in patients receiving intra-arterial floxuridine chemotherapy for hepatic metastases of colorectal cancer.

Immunoallergic Reactions

Drugs also may be associated with definite allergic reactions. A combined toxic-immunologic mechanism is involved in liver injury caused by halothane, a fluorinated hydrocarbon anesthetic that causes severe, often fatal liver injury after multiple exposures (Chapter 440). Other fluorinated hydrocarbons, including isoflurane and desflurane, occasionally result in the same response. Although halothane has never been withdrawn, its use has been limited by the advent of safer agents. Hypersensitivity reactions, such as fever, eosinophilia, and rash, are common. Halothane may induce fever, eosinophilia, and antimitochondrial antibodies. Direct cytotoxicity and immune-mediated toxicity are observed, consistent with the clinical observation that severe halothane toxicity occurs with repeated exposure. Although evidence of injury can usually be identified within 1 week of the first exposure, the interval to toxicity is shortened and the damage is more severe with each successive exposure, as befits an immune reaction.

Phenytoin (Chapter 410) induces the simultaneous onset of fever, rash, lymphadenopathy, and eosinophilia. The mechanisms responsible for the combined allergic and hepatotoxic reaction are unknown, but the slow resolution of the illness suggests that the allergen remains on the surface of the hepatocyte for weeks or months. A concurrent mononucleosis-like picture is frequently confused with a viral illness or streptococcal pharyngitis. If phenytoin is not discontinued promptly despite signs of hepatitis, a severe Stevens-Johnson drug eruption (Chapters 447 and 448) and prolonged fever may result. As with any therapeutic agent, rapid recognition of the presence of a toxic drug reaction and immediate discontinuation of the compound are key to limiting hepatic damage. Systemic features of an allergic reaction may not be obvious, even when eosinophilia or granulomas are present on liver biopsy.

Steatohepatitis

Steatosis in the liver (Chapter 155) can be present in a microvesicular or macrovesicular pattern. Macrovesicular steatosis, the most common form, is characterized histologically by a single vacuole of fat filling up the hepatocyte and displacing the nucleus to the cell's periphery. Macrovesicular steatosis is typically caused by alcohol, diabetes, or obesity. Sometimes drugs such as corticosteroids or methotrexate may cause these hepatic changes. Amiodarone (Chapters 64 and 65) has been associated with a picture resembling alcoholic hepatitis, occasionally with progression to cirrhosis. The pathophysiology involves accumulation of phospholipids in the liver, eyes, thyroid, and skin. Treatment is primarily withdrawal of the drug and observation, although the half-life of amiodarone is prolonged. Tamoxifen, which has been used in long-term regimens for the prevention of recurrent breast cancer (Chapter 204), has also been associated with steatohepatitis evolving to cirrhosis.

In microvesicular steatosis, hepatocytes contain numerous small fat vesicles that do not displace the nucleus. Valproic acid, an anticonvulsant (Chapter 410), causes hepatotoxicity, either as a result of microvesicular fat deposition, resembling Reye's syndrome, or in a more chronic, indolent fashion associated with macrovesicular fat accumulation. Toxicity is more severe and frequent in children. These lesions are associated with disruption of mitochondrial DNA, resulting in anaerobic metabolism that leads to lactic acidosis in the most severe cases. Macrovesicular and microvesicular lesions may be observed concomitantly in some patients, and microvesicular lesions are more often associated with a poor prognosis. Hepatocellular necrosis may also be present. Acute fatty liver of pregnancy (Chapter 153) and Reye's syndrome are two examples of severe liver diseases caused by microvesicular steatosis.

Drugs involved in microvesicular steatosis include valproate, tetracycline, and fialuridine. Aspirin use in children has been associated with Reye's syndrome, but the incidence of Reye's syndrome has decreased dramatically since warnings were issued concerning aspirin use in children.

Effects of Sex Steroids

Anabolic steroids, such as methyltestosterone, may cause cholestasis. Androgens may cause peliosis hepatis and benign or malignant tumors. Oral contraceptives (Chapter 246) may cause cholestasis, hepatic adenomas, or Budd-Chiari syndrome (hepatic vein thrombosis). Antiandrogens used to treat prostate cancer (Chapter 207), such as flutamide and nilutamide, and antipituitary drugs, such as cyproterone acetate, have also been associated with severe hepatocellular injury.

Other Drug Reactions

Other less severe drug reactions involving the liver include granulomatous reactions, fibrosis, ischemic injury, and chronic autoimmune liver injury (see Table 152-3). The type of reaction observed can be helpful in determining the probable agent because most drugs have a specific injury profile.

A pattern of veno-occlusive disease with obliteration of small intrahepatic veins, sinusoidal congestion, and necrosis is observed frequently in bone marrow transplant patients (Chapter 181) who receive chemotherapy with cyclophosphamide (Cytoxan) or busulfan. Symptoms, including rapidly accumulating ascites, painful hepatomegaly, and jaundice, develop soon after the chemotherapeutic regimen has begun. Rarely, herbal medicines (Chapter 38) such as pyrrolizidine alkaloids (*Crotalaria* and *Senecio* found in Jamaican bush tea) may cause veno-occlusive disease.

Toxins are associated with direct injury to hepatocytes in a dose-dependent fashion. Organic solvents such as carbon tetrachloride and trichloroethylene (Chapter 110) cause centrilobular injury. Yellow phosphorus, found in firecrackers and rat poisons, is a rare cause of liver injury from either accidental or intentional exposure. Symptoms of poisoning are similar to those of any other type of hepatitis.

Mushroom poisoning (Chapter 110), which follows the ingestion of *A. phalloides* and related species, typically occurs in amateur mushroom fanciers in a dose-related fashion. The associated muscarinic effects, including severe diarrhea, vomiting, and profuse sweating, predominate in the first hours after ingestion. Hepatic failure follows if antidotes (see later) are not given. The overall prognosis for spontaneous recovery is poor; liver transplantation may be life-saving.

Differential Diagnosis

The differential diagnosis of toxin- and drug-induced liver injury includes almost the entire spectrum of liver diseases. Because the clinical picture of drug-induced liver injury ranges from pure hepatocellular to pure cholestatic variants, a high index of suspicion must be maintained, even when toxin- or drug-induced liver injury is not obvious initially.

For dose-dependent hepatotoxins, the diagnosis may be easier to establish than for idiosyncratic drug reactions. Serum levels of acetaminophen, a thorough history, and characteristic biochemical abnormalities (high aminotransferase levels) usually reveal an acetaminophen overdose, whereas a diagnosis of *Amanita* poisoning depends on the history, symptoms of gastroenteritis (muscarinic reaction), and positive mushroom identification.

For idiosyncratic drug reactions, the diagnosis is sometimes more difficult to establish. A standardized reporting form called the RUCAM (Roussel-Uclaf causality assessment method; see Table 152-4), developed by an international panel, provides a worthwhile scoring system. These guidelines outline the steps an experienced clinician might use to assess the likelihood of a drug reaction. Causality assessment factors typically include the temporal relationship, course after cessation of the drug, risk factors, concomitant drugs, a search for nondrug causes (viral hepatitis), previous information concerning the drug, and response to rechallenge, which is typically not required.

TREATMENT   Rx

Prompt discontinuation of a suspected drug is mandatory. Available antidotes should be used for acetaminophen (*N*-acetylcysteine) and *Amanita* poisoning (penicillin 300,000 to 1 million U/kg/day intravenously and thioctic acid 5 to 100 mg every 6 hours intravenously have been recommended, but there are no controlled trials). General supportive therapy ranges from intravenous fluid replacement to intensive monitoring and treatment of patients with hepatic encephalopathy secondary to acute liver failure (Chapter 157). Liver transplantation (Chapter 157) is performed in more than 50% of patients with idiosyncratic drug-induced acute liver failure because the survival rate in this setting without transplantation is less than 20%.

FUTURE DIRECTIONS

Research in pharmacogenomics may allow the patient's own genetic information to guide individualized drug therapy and monitoring of idiosyncratic drug reactions. The genetic information would probably concentrate initially on enzymes with variant alleles associated with poor metabolism, such as CYP1A2 or CYP2C19 for isoniazid, CYP2C9 for piroxicam, or CYP2D6 for nortriptyline. Better postmarketing surveillance of all drugs to identify those with previously unappreciated hepatotoxicity should be a high priority.

PREVENTION

It is reasonable to consider a drug reaction whenever an episode of apparent hepatitis is unexplained, particularly if a new agent has been introduced in the previous 3 months. It is prudent to defer embracing new drugs during their first year of introduction, particularly if they show no unique advantages over accepted formulations. Physicians must strive to instill in their patients a healthy level of alertness with regard to drug-induced liver injury, particularly for agents with known hepatotoxicity. Monitoring of aminotransferase levels on a monthly basis is suggested for known hepatotoxins such as isoniazid or diclofenac, but it is unlikely to be cost-effective when adverse reactions occur less frequently, such as in only 1 in 50,000 patients. Because many drug reactions develop within days, monitoring provides no guarantee. Most fatal drug reactions could have been prevented if the offending agent were withdrawn immediately, at the first sign of illness.

SUGGESTED READINGS

Bjornsson E. Review article: drug-induced liver injury in clinical practice. *Aliment Pharmacol Ther.* 2010;32:3-13. *Practical information for clinicians.*

Chalasani N, Björnsson E. Risk factors for idiosyncratic drug-induced liver injury. *Gastroenterology.* 2010;138:2246-2259. *Review of genetic and non-genetic risk factors.*

Khandelwal N, James LP, Sanders C, et al. Unrecognized acetaminophen toxicity as a cause of indeterminate acute liver failure. *Hepatology.* 2011;53:567-576. *Suggests that many indeterminate cases are unrecognized acetaminophen cases.*

Rockey DC, Seeff LB, Rochon J, et al. Causality assessment in drug-induced liver injury using a structured expert opinion process: comparison to the Roussel-Uclaf causality assessment method. *Hepatology.* 2010;51:2117-2126. *Review of the process of assessing causality.*

153

INHERITED AND METABOLIC DISORDERS OF THE LIVER

BRUCE R. BACON

DEFINITION

Inherited liver diseases (Table 153-1) include hereditary hemochromatosis, (Chapter 219), Wilson disease (Chapter 218), α_1-antitrypsin deficiency (Chapter 88), and cystic fibrosis. Metabolic liver diseases include nonalcoholic fatty liver disease (NAFLD), which is the most common cause of abnormal liver enzymes in Western societies; in addition, 3 to 5% of overweight or obese individuals in the United States may have nonalcoholic steatohepatitis (NASH) (Chapter 155), which has the potential to progress to advanced fibrosis. A variety of systemic metabolic abnormalities are less common causes of liver dysfunction or abnormal liver tests (Chapter 149).

INHERITED LIVER DISEASES
Hereditary Hemochromatosis
EPIDEMIOLOGY AND PATHOBIOLOGY

Hereditary hemochromatosis (Chapter 219) is the most common inherited disorder of the liver. The responsible gene for this inherited disorder of iron metabolism is *HFE*, which encodes for a major histocompatibility complex type 1 protein. Genetic testing is available for the two major mutations (C282Y, H63D) responsible for *HFE*-linked hereditary hemochromatosis. Large-scale population studies demonstrate that C282Y homozygosity is found in about 1 in 250 individuals of northern European descent, about 60% of whom have phenotypic expression of the disease. About 10% of the population are asymptomatic heterozygotes.

CLINICAL MANIFESTATIONS

Most individuals with hereditary hemochromatosis have no symptoms and are identified by screening laboratory tests or family studies. When

TABLE 153-1	INHERITED AND METABOLIC DISORDERS OF THE LIVER

INHERITED LIVER DISEASES

Hereditary hemochromatosis
α_1-Antitrypsin deficiency
Wilson disease
Cystic fibrosis

METABOLIC LIVER DISEASES

Nonalcoholic fatty liver disease
Porphyrias
Lipid storage diseases
Amyloidosis

FIGURE 153-1. Liver biopsy in hemochromatosis (Perls Prussian blue stain for iron). Iron deposition is found in a periportal distribution, predominantly in parenchymal cells (hepatocytes).

symptoms are present, they are frequently nonspecific and include lethargy, fatigue, weight loss, and weakness. More organ-specific symptoms include right upper quadrant abdominal pain or arthralgias of the hands, hips, and knees. Occasionally, patients present with signs of advanced liver disease.

DIAGNOSIS

When symptoms and signs suggestive of hereditary hemochromatosis are present, it is reasonable to consider this diagnosis and order appropriate laboratory studies. Conversely, when abnormal iron studies (Chapter 162) are identified by routine screening or in patients being evaluated for anemia, hereditary hemochromatosis should be considered even in the absence of signs or symptoms.

Definitive diagnosis is relatively straightforward. Transferrin saturation (iron ÷ transferrin or total iron binding capacity × 100%) and ferritin levels are typically elevated in symptomatic patients in both the fasting and nonfasting states. Ferritin, which is an acute phase reactant, can be elevated without increased iron stores in acute illnesses, cancer, inflammatory arthritides, chronic viral hepatitis, and alcoholic and nonalcoholic fatty liver disease.

In patients with elevated transferrin saturation or ferritin levels, genetic testing should be performed. Detection of a C282Y homozygote or a compound heterozygote (C282Y/H63D) confirms the diagnosis of hereditary hemochromatosis. If the ferritin level is greater than 1000 µg/L, the patient should be considered for liver biopsy (Fig. 153-1) to determine whether fibrosis is present. Sensitive magnetic resonance imaging techniques can help determine hepatic iron concentrations when liver biopsy cannot be performed. On liver biopsy, iron deposition is found in periportal hepatocytes, with a periportal to pericentral gradient, and Kupffer cells are spared.

TREATMENT AND PROGNOSIS Rx

Treatment of hereditary hemochromatosis is simple, safe, effective, and inexpensive. It consists of weekly phlebotomy of 1 unit of blood, which contains about 200 to 250 mg of iron, and is designed to reduce total body iron stores with a goal of reducing ferritin levels to 50 to 100 µg/L. Most patients require maintenance phlebotomy of 1 unit of blood every 2 to 3 months. Screening with iron studies and genetic testing should be offered to all first-degree relatives of identified probands. Complications of the disease can be avoided if patients are diagnosed and treated before they develop fibrosis.

α_1-Antitrypsin Deficiency

EPIDEMIOLOGY AND PATHOBIOLOGY

α_1-Antitrypsin deficiency has been identified in all populations, but the disorder is most common in individuals of northern European descent. In North America, about 1 in 1500 to 2000 individuals is affected by the disorder.

α_1-Antitrypsin is a 52-kD glycoprotein produced in hepatocytes, epithelial cells of the lungs, and phagocytes. It inhibits serine proteases, primarily neutrophil elastase. When patients are deficient in α_1-antitrypsin, increased amounts of neutrophil elastase degrade elastin and can lead to progressive lung injury and premature emphysema (Chapter 88). α_1-Antitrypsin deficiency causes liver disease in infancy, early childhood, adolescence, and adulthood.

More than 75 variants have been identified in the proteinase inhibitor (Pi) gene located on chromosome 14. Some alter protein structure, thereby interfering with hepatocellular export. As a result, deformed polymers of α_1-antitrypsin aggregate and accumulate in the endoplasmic reticulum of the hepatocyte. Conventional nomenclature identifies normal variants as PiMM; individuals with these variants have normal blood levels of α_1-antitrypsin. The most common abnormal variants of functional significance are identified as S and Z. Individuals who are homozygous for the Z mutation (PiZZ) have α_1-antitrypsin levels that are only about 15% of normal; these patients are susceptible to liver and/or lung disease, but only about 25% of PiZZ patients develop end-organ disease. Individuals with PiSZ are at risk for developing liver disease and cirrhosis. Null variants have undetectable α_1-antitrypsin and are susceptible to premature lung disease but not liver disease.

CLINICAL MANIFESTATIONS AND DIAGNOSIS

In adults, symptoms of liver disease may be absent, or patients may complain of symptoms ranging from fatigue to complications of chronic decompensated liver disease (Chapter 148). The diagnosis is most frequently considered in patients who present with abnormal liver enzymes (Chapter 149) or as part of an evaluation for the cause of cirrhosis (Chapter 156). Coexistent lung disease at a relatively young age or a family history of liver and/or lung disease can provide clues to the diagnosis. Lung disease is not necessarily present.

The diagnosis is confirmed by a reduced serum level of α_1-antitrypsin, which can be measured specifically or assumed based on a low level of α_1-protein on serum protein electrophoresis, accompanied by Pi determinations. Most patients with liver disease have either the PiZZ or the PiSZ variant; some patients with PiMZ have reduced α_1-antitrypsin levels, but they are usually not low enough to cause disease. Liver biopsy, which is performed to determine the degree of hepatic fibrosis, shows characteristic periodic acid–Schiff–positive, diastase-resistant globules in the periphery of the hepatic lobule (Fig. 153-2).

TREATMENT AND PROGNOSIS Rx

Unfortunately, there is no specific therapy for α_1-antitrypsin deficiency, so treatment is supportive. Other causes of liver injury, such as excessive alcohol ingestion, should be avoided. Evidence of other liver diseases (e.g., viral hepatitis B and C, hemochromatosis, NAFLD) should be sought, and such diseases should be treated if possible. Smoking, which can worsen the progression of lung disease but not liver disease in patients with α_1-antitrypsin deficiency, should be discontinued. In patients with lung disease, weekly infusions of α_1-antitrypsin given indefinitely can halt further lung damage.

The natural history of α_1-antitrypsin deficiency is variable because many individuals with the PiZZ variant never develop disease, whereas others develop cirrhosis in childhood, ultimately leading to liver transplantation. The risk of hepatocellular cancer is increased in patients with cirrhosis. If decompensated liver disease develops, liver transplantation (Chapter 157) should be curative. Following the transplant, patients express the Pi phenotype of the donor.

FIGURE 153-2. Liver biopsy in α₁-antitrypsin deficiency. On a periodic acid–Schiff, diastase-resistant stain, α₁-antitrypsin globules, with a characteristic magenta color, are found at the periphery of the lobule.

Wilson Disease

Wilson disease (Chapter 218), which is an inherited disorder of copper metabolism, leads to a progressive accumulation of copper in the liver and in various other tissues, ultimately causing toxicity and organ damage. The Wilson disease gene (*ATP7B*) encodes for a P-type ATPase that is involved in copper transport and is required for the removal of copper from hepatocytes into hepatic bile.

CLINICAL MANIFESTATIONS AND DIAGNOSIS

Wilson disease usually presents before age 35 years, but it can present in middle age or later. The clinical presentation is quite variable, and hepatic manifestations include chronic hepatitis, hepatic steatosis, and cirrhosis in adolescents and young adults. Patients who present with neurologic manifestations such as dysarthria or choreic or athetoid movement disorders always have concomitant liver disease. On physical examination, patients classically have Kayser-Fleischer rings (see Fig. 218-1 in Chapter 218) owing to copper deposition in Descemet's membrane in the cornea.

Diagnosis includes demonstration of a reduced ceruloplasmin level and an increased 24-hour urine copper excretion. In the presence of neurologic findings and clinical evidence of liver disease, a liver biopsy is not required. If a liver biopsy is obtained, however, the classic findings include an elevated hepatic copper level, hepatic steatosis, chronic hepatitis, and cirrhosis. The genetic diagnosis of Wilson disease is difficult because there are more than 200 mutations in *ATP7B*, with different degrees of frequency and penetration in certain populations.

TREATMENT AND PROGNOSIS   Rx

Treatment consists of copper chelation using medications such as D-penicillamine (1 to 1.5 g/day indefinitely) and trientine. Zinc acetate (75 to 250 mg/day) has been used as maintenance therapy. Medical treatment should be lifelong because discontinuation of therapy has been associated with severe relapses, liver failure, and death. Liver transplantation (Chapter 157), which is indicated for either decompensated cirrhosis or fulminant liver failure, cures the underlying metabolic defect and restores normal copper homeostasis.

Cystic Fibrosis

Cystic fibrosis (Chapter 89) can cause chronic liver disease in adults, although its principal manifestations are chronic lung disease and pancreatic insufficiency. Some adult patients with cystic fibrosis develop biliary cirrhosis with portal hypertension. Combined lung-liver transplantation is recommended for these patients. Ursodeoxycholic acid (13 to 15 mg/kg/day) improves symptoms and liver test abnormalities but is not curative.

● METABOLIC LIVER DISEASES
Nonalcoholic Fatty Liver Disease

NAFLD (Chapter 155), which is seen most commonly in obese, diabetic, and hyperlipidemic nonalcoholic patients, has a prevalence ranging from 15 to 30% in the United States. Not all obese patients have fatty liver disease, but

NASH occurs in about 3 to 5% of the overweight and obese population, and liver fibrosis is increased in up to 40% of these individuals. Most patients with hepatic steatosis have stable, nonprogressive disease, but NASH can progress to cirrhosis. Many patients who were previously described as having cryptogenic cirrhosis are now thought to have NASH, especially because catabolic cirrhosis reduces macrovesicular steatosis, so late biopsy may show just a bland cirrhosis.

Symptoms usually include fatigue and/or vague right upper quadrant discomfort, most likely due to a distended hepatic capsule. However, most patients come to medical attention as a result of incidentally identified elevated liver enzymes or the finding of a fatty liver on imaging studies for other purposes.

Critical to the diagnosis of NAFLD is a careful history to be sure that alcohol ingestion is less than 20 g/day. Routine laboratory testing for other common liver diseases (e.g., hepatitis B and C, hemochromatosis), as well as less common ones (e.g., Wilson disease, α₁-antitrypsin deficiency, autoimmune liver diseases), should be performed. Imaging studies can confirm characteristic features of a fatty liver (e.g., bright liver on ultrasound). These findings are nonspecific, however, and the ultimate diagnosis of NAFLD or NASH requires liver biopsy.

The principal treatments are dietary changes and weight loss, but some medications can also be helpful in selected patients (Chapter 155).

Porphyrias

The porphyrias (Chapter 217) are characterized by defects in the synthesis of heme, which is necessary for incorporation into numerous hemoproteins such as hemoglobin, myoglobin, catalase, and cytochromes. The porphyrias can present both acutely and chronically, with the acute disorders causing recurring bouts of abdominal pain, and the chronic disorders being characterized by skin lesions.

The most commonly encountered porphyria is porphyria cutanea tarda, which is characterized by vesicular-type lesions that appear on sun-exposed areas of the skin, such as the backs of the hands (see Fig. 447-11 in Chapter 447), tips of the ears, or over the cheekbones. About 40% of patients with porphyria cutanea tarda have mutations in *HFE* (Chapter 219), and about 50% have chronic hepatitis C (Chapter 151).

Liver disease associated with the porphyrias typically presents as an asymptomatic elevation of liver enzymes. After appropriate testing to confirm porphyria (Chapter 217), *HFE* mutation analysis, iron studies, and hepatitis C testing should be performed in all patients who present with porphyria cutanea tarda. Excess alcohol use is also associated with porphyria cutanea tarda, so patients should be counseled to decrease or eliminate alcohol use. Iron reduction therapy, using therapeutic phlebotomy, is the cornerstone of treatment for porphyria cutanea tarda, even in the absence of iron overload (Chapter 219). Concomitant chronic hepatitis C should be treated as well (Chapter 151). Skin lesions reverse in the majority of patients. Acute intermittent porphyria (Chapter 217), which is much less common, presents with abdominal pain in the absence of typical findings on physical examination. Intravenous hematin is the treatment of choice.

Lipid Storage Diseases

Lipid storage diseases that involve the liver include Gaucher's disease (Chapter 215) and Niemann-Pick disease (Chapter 215). Other rare disorders include abetalipoproteinemia, Fabry's disease (Chapter 215), Tangier disease (Chapter 213), and types 1 and 5 hyperlipoproteinemia (Chapter 213). On physical examination, the liver is enlarged owing to both fat deposition and increased hepatic glycogen deposition. Liver enzymes may be elevated and diagnosis requires liver biopsy in the appropriate clinical setting. Treatment is supportive, with enzyme infusions as indicated.

Amyloidosis

In patients with systemic amyloidosis (Chapter 194), the liver is commonly involved, but this involvement is sometimes identified only in the premorbid state or documented at autopsy. Characteristic pathologic findings include positive staining with Congo red histochemical stain, where an apple-green birefringence is noted under polarizing light. Liver enzymes may be mildly elevated, but this finding is nonspecific. Treatment is as for the systemic disease.

● LIVER DISEASE IN PREGNANCY

In a pregnant patient with liver enzyme abnormalities, it is important to distinguish between liver diseases that are unique to pregnancy and those

TABLE 153-2 LIVER DISEASES UNIQUE TO PREGNANCY

DISEASE	TRIMESTER OF ONSET	SYMPTOMS	LABORATORY ABNORMALITIES	RECURRENCE WITH FUTURE PREGNANCIES
Hyperemesis gravidarum	1	Nausea, vomiting	Mild to moderate elevation in ALT/AST, occasionally hyperbilirubinemia	
Cholestasis	2, 3	Pruritus, jaundice	Bile acids >8 µM, elevated ALT/AST and bilirubin in more severe cases	Common
Acute fatty liver	3	Nausea, vomiting, abdominal pain	Elevated ALT/AST (100-1000 U/L), bilirubin >5 mg/dL, prolonged prothrombin time*	Rare
HELLP syndrome	2, 3, or postpartum	Abdominal pain, nausea, vomiting	Elevated ALT/AST (60-1500 U/L), platelets <100,000/mm^3, LDH >600 U/L, hemolytic anemia	3-25%

*Useful diagnostic distinction from HELLP syndrome, in which the prothrombin time, partial thromboplastin time, and fibrinogen are usually normal.
ALT = alanine aminotransferase; AST = aspartate aminotransferase; HELLP = hemolysis, elevated liver enzymes, and low platelet count; LDH = lactate dehydrogenase.

that occur commonly in pregnancy (Table 153-2). In normal pregnancy, levels of alkaline phosphatase, bile acids, globulins, fibrinogen, and triglycerides may be increased, whereas levels of albumin, antithrombin 3, protein S, and γ-glutamyltransferase may be reduced.

Hyperemesis Gravidarum

Hyperemesis gravidarum is a syndrome of unknown cause in which patients have fairly intractable nausea and vomiting. It generally occurs in the first trimester, usually before 10 weeks of pregnancy. Risk factors include young age, obesity, and nulliparity. Aminotransferases levels may be increased up to 200 U/L, and bilirubin may be elevated up to 4 mg/dL. No specific abnormalities are found on liver biopsy, but some patients have mild steatosis or mild cholestasis. Treatment is symptomatic with antiemetics.

Intrahepatic Cholestasis of Pregnancy

Intrahepatic cholestasis of pregnancy presents with generalized pruritus. Most cases are associated with a mutation in the multiple drug resistance-3 gene. Ten percent to 25% of patients have visible jaundice, and laboratory abnormalities generally include hyperbilirubinemia less than 6 mg/dL. The alkaline phosphatase level may be elevated, and aminotransferase levels may be 2 to 10 times the upper limit of normal. Serum bile acids are also markedly increased at 2 to 100 times the upper limit of normal. If liver biopsy is performed, a bland cholestasis is identified. Ultrasonography is normal.

Treatment includes ursodeoxycholic acid or cholestyramine to bind bile salts. Phenobarbital has also been used. The syndrome resolves after delivery but is likely to recur with subsequent pregnancies.

Preeclampsia and HELLP Syndrome

Preeclampsia (Chapter 247), seen in as many as 7 to 10% of pregnancies, usually occurs in the third trimester or late in the second trimester. The triad of findings consists of hypertension, proteinuria, and edema. Some patients have severe hypertension, profound proteinuria, and seizures. Liver enzymes can be markedly elevated, and levels of lactate dehydrogenase and bilirubin can be increased by hemolysis. The prothrombin time is usually normal, but some patients may have thrombocytopenia. The *HELLP* syndrome (hemolysis, elevated liver enzymes, and low platelet count) is seen in about 10% of patients with preeclampsia and is considered a severe manifestation of eclampsia. Hepatic infarction is rare, but hepatic rupture can be catastrophic.

The diagnosis is generally made clinically, and a liver biopsy is usually not necessary. Treatment is by delivery.

Acute Fatty Liver Disease in Pregnancy

Acute fatty liver disease occurs in about 1 in 900 to 6000 pregnancies. Abnormalities in mitrochondrial function and adenosine triphosphate (ATP) synthesis have been described, and about 20% of cases have a deficiency in long-chain 3-hydroxyacyl-CoA dehydrogenase, with an abnormality in the beta oxidation of fatty acids. Acute fatty liver is characteristically seen in the third trimester. Patients can have profound hepatic dysfunction, but liver enzymes are usually not markedly elevated and are characteristically less than 10 times the upper limit of normal. The prothrombin time may be prolonged, and the bilirubin level is elevated. Some patients have disseminated intravascular coagulation, and some may have hypoglycemia.

Clinical features are nonspecific, and the clinical course ranges from mild complications to more severe problems. Diagnosis is by ultrasound showing steatosis and liver biopsy showing microvesicular steatosis. Treatment requires urgent delivery.

Other Hepatobiliary Conditions in Pregnancy

Other hepatic conditions that can occur in pregnancy including gallstones (Chapter 158) and Budd-Chiari syndrome (Chapter 145). Acute herpes hepatitis, caused by herpesvirus type 2, occurs in the second and third trimesters and is associated with fever, chills, malaise, and nausea. Liver enzymes may be markedly elevated, and the prothrombin time may be prolonged. Liver biopsy shows typical viral inclusions. Treatment is with antiviral therapy (Chapter 368).

⬤ TOTAL PARENTERAL NUTRITION–INDUCED LIVER DISEASE

As many as 30 to 40% of patients who receive total parenteral nutrition (Chapter 224) develop abnormal liver enzyme levels. These abnormalities range from mild elevations of aminotransferase levels, owing to hepatic steatosis, to cholestatic liver disease with elevated alkaline phosphatase levels. Minor adjustments in the formula usually resolve the abnormalities. Some patients with cholestatic abnormalities may benefit from ursodeoxycholic acid.

SUGGESTED READINGS

Bacon BR, Adams PC, Kowdley KV, et al. AASLD Practice Guidelines. Diagnosis and management of hemochromatosis. *Hepatology.* 2011 (in press). *Practice guidelines.*
Huster D. Wilson disease. *Best Pract Res Clin Gastroenterol.* 2010;24:531-539. *Review.*
Joshi D, James A, Quaglia A, et al. Liver disease in pregnancy. *Lancet.* 2010;375:594-605. *Review.*

154

BACTERIAL, PARASITIC, FUNGAL, AND GRANULOMATOUS LIVER DISEASES ⬤

K. RAJENDER REDDY

⬤ INFECTIONS OF THE LIVER

Infections of the liver can be due to a variety of pathogens, including bacteria, fungi, amebae, protozoa, helminthes, spirochetes, and rickettsial infections. The manifestations of these infections are protean; some are generic to all infections, whereas others are specific to particular infections. The epidemiology can vary and depend on the geographic region of the world. In endemic areas, *Entamoeba histolytica* is a key consideration in the differential diagnosis of a liver abscess (Table 154-1).

TABLE 154-1   FEATURES OF BACTERIAL AND AMEBIC ABSCESSES

	DEMOGRAPHICS	RISK FACTORS	SYMPTOMS	LABORATORY FINDINGS	RADIOGRAPHIC FEATURES	DIAGNOSIS	TREATMENT
Bacterial liver abscess	50-70 years old Male = female	Recent bacterial infection, biliary obstruction, diabetes mellitus	Fevers, chills, malaise, anorexia, diarrhea, cough, pleuritic chest pain, RUQ pain	Leukocytosis, anemia, elevated alkaline phosphatase and bilirubin, low albumin, positive blood cultures (50%)	Multifocal (50%), usually right lobe, irregular margins	Aspirate (70-80% positive)	Percutaneous drainage and antibiotics
Amebic liver abscess	18-50 years old Male > female	Alcohol intake, HLA-DR3, oral and anal sex, contaminated enema apparatus, travel to or living in an endemic area	Fever, RUQ pain, hepatic tenderness, anorexia, weight loss, uncommon to have colitis	Leukocytosis, no eosinophilia, mild anemia, elevated alkaline phosphatase, elevated ESR, positive serology	Single abscess (80%), usually right lobe, wall enhancement seen on CT scan with IV contrast	Aspirate (trophozoites rarely seen) can rule out superimposed bacterial infection, positive serology and risk factors	Metronidazole and iodoquinol

CT = computed tomography; ESR = erythrocyte sedimentation rate; IV = intravenous; RUQ = right upper quadrant.

FIGURE 154-1. A and B, Computed tomographic scans of a pyogenic liver abscess. (Courtesy Dr. Chalermrat Bunchorntavakul, Bangkok, Thailand.)

Pyogenic Liver Abscess

DEFINITION

Pyogenic liver abscess is a focal collection of purulent bacterial material and necroinflammatory debris. It can be solitary or multiple and can be caused by one or more aerobic and anaerobic bacteria (Fig. 154-1).

EPIDEMIOLOGY

Pyogenic liver abscess has an estimated global incidence of approximately 1.1 to 2.3 per 100,000 person-years, whereas in the United States the incidence is reported to be approximately 3.6 per 100,000 and has been rising. Biliary obstruction, caused by a malignancy or benign disease, accounts for 50 to 60% of pyogenic liver abscesses, whereas portal pyemia, owing to appendicitis or other intra-abdominal infections, accounts for about 20% of cases.

PATHOBIOLOGY

Bacteria can enter the liver through the portal system from infections in areas drained by the mesenteric system into the portal system, such as appendicitis (Chapter 144). Other mechanisms for pyogenic liver abscess include bacterial cholangitis owing to benign or malignant obstruction, and infection of the liver from a systemic bacteremia, such as an infection of the oral cavity. Pyogenic liver abscess can also be caused by blunt or penetrating trauma, including such unusual causes as the ingestion of a toothpick or fish bone that can cause an intestinal perforation, fistula to the liver, and subsequent abscess formation. Liver abscesses can occur in a transplanted graft owing to vascular compromise caused by hepatic artery thrombosis and ischemic bile duct strictures.

Multiple organisms can cause pyogenic liver abscess. The most common organism, *Klebsiella pneumoniae*, often is associated with biliary tract disease. Other aerobes include *Escherichia coli*, group D streptococci, β-hemolytic streptococci, and *Staphylococcus aureus*. Anaerobic infection is often seen with colonic disease. Less common causes of liver abscesses include actinomyces, *Nocardia asteroides*, *Yersinia pseudotuberculosis* and *Yersinia enterocolitica*, *Listeria monocytogenes*, *Campylobacter jejuni*, *Legionella pneumophila*, *Mycobacterium tuberculosis*, *Salmonella typhi* or *Salmonella paratyphi*, *Candida albicans*, and *Bartonella henselae*. Most often the organism recovered from an abscess cavity is single, but multiple organisms can be isolated in as many as one third of patients. No bacteria may be isolated from the abscess because of prior antibiotic therapy or the failure to perform proper anaerobic cultures.

CLINICAL MANIFESTATIONS

The signs and symptoms associated with a liver abscess typically include fever, right upper quadrant abdominal pain, chills, nausea, vomiting, weight loss, and jaundice. The presentation can be acute or indolent. An associated bacteremia is seen in approximately 50% of the patients, but frank sepsis is rare.

DIAGNOSIS

Appropriate diagnosis requires a high degree of clinical suspicion, and diagnosis is sometimes delayed. Usually, however, the diagnosis is made promptly with the wide availability of the various radiologic modalities. The two common causes of liver abscesses are pyogenic and amebic abscess, and it is important to make a distinction because the prognosis and management differ. Amebic abscess can become secondarily infected with bacteria.

The diagnosis of an abscess is based on a constellation of clinical, bacteriologic, and radiologic features. Ultrasonography and computed tomography (CT) are the most common radiologic modalities to diagnose an abscess cavity reliably, as either single or multiple lesions, but CT is the preferred test, with sensitivity above 90%. Any concurrent biliary obstruction also can be diagnosed by these imaging studies. Approximately 50% of patients have multiple abscesses. On CT, the lesion is seen as a fluid collection with irregular borders and wall edema. One drawback to this imaging modality is that no specific features differentiate a pyogenic abscess from other infectious causes (i.e., amebic or fungal). Another drawback is that a very early stage abscess may not be well formed and may have characteristics more suggestive of a solid mass. Distinguishing an abscess from a tumor (Chapter 202) or a simple cyst can be difficult on noninvasive imaging if there is bleeding into a cyst, calcification, necrosis, or bleeding into a tumor. The presence of smaller (<2 cm) peripheral lesions that surround a central lesion argues strongly against a hepatic neoplasm. Calcification suggests bleeding into a tumor, but it also can be seen in the wall of an echinococcal cyst. Nonspecific radiologic features, including elevation of the right hemidiaphragm, right lower lung lobe atelectasis, and right pleural effusion, are seen in up to 30% of patients with pyogenic liver abscesses. Magnetic resonance imaging (MRI) and tagged white blood cell scans add little to the diagnosis of a liver abscess.

Microbial cultures are essential. In addition to blood cultures, the abscess cavity should be aspirated percutaneously, with either ultrasound or CT guidance, and the aspirate should be cultured for aerobic and anaerobic organisms as well as for amebae if there is any suspicion of an amebic abscess. Blood cultures are positive in only approximately 50% of cases. In approximately 15 to 20% of cases, multiple organisms are identified in the abscess cavity, but 20 to 30% of cases may have negative cultures despite appropriate culture techniques.

TREATMENT Rx

Immediate broad-spectrum antibiotic coverage, as well as the prompt identification and treatment of the source of the infection, are essential for successful outcomes. Once the etiologic bacteria is identified, the antibiotic regimen can be tailored appropriately based on prevailing bacterial resistance patterns. Monotherapy with a β-lactam or β-lactamase inhibitor such as ampicillin-sulbactam (3 g intravenously every 6 hours), piperacillin-tazobactam (4.5 g intravenously every 6 hours), or ticarcillin-clavulanate (3.1 g intravenously every 6 hours) can be used, or a third-generation cephalosporin such as ceftriaxone (1 to 2 g intravenously daily) plus metronidazole (500 mg intravenously every 8 to 12 hours) can be used. Other potential regimens include a fluoroquinolone (e.g., ciprofloxacin, 400 mg intravenously every 12 hours, or levofloxacin, 500 or 750 mg intravenously daily) plus metronidazole (500 mg intravenously every 8 to 12 hours), or monotherapy with a carbapenem such as imipenem (500 mg intravenously every 6 hours), meropenem (1 g intravenously every 8 hours), or ertapenem (1 g intravenously daily).

The duration of therapy is partly based on the response to therapy. On an average, 4 to 6 weeks of antibiotic therapy appears reasonable, and the last 2 to 4 weeks of the antibiotic regimen can be administered orally. Abscesses that are hard to drain or are slow to demonstrate radiographic resolution require longer courses of therapy. Importantly, radiologic abnormalities resolve more slowly than clinical and biochemical features, so the latter should be used as an indicator for tailoring the therapeutic regimen.

Although antibiotics alone can sometimes successfully resolve small, multiple pyogenic abscesses, it also is critical to address the source of infection. Any underlying biliary source must be resolved, and any biliary obstruction must be relieved. More often, most patients will require drainage of the abscesses. The standard approach is placement of a drain for about 7 days. Alternatively, needle aspiration, repeated as needed when the abscess is large enough to drain percutaneously, provides equivalent results,[1] except in abscesses larger than 10 cm in diameter.[2] Surgical drainage seldom is the first option, except in patients who also have a surgically correctable precipitating lesion, such as appendicitis or biliary obstruction. More often, a biliary obstruction is treated with endoscopic retrograde cholangiopancreatography (ERCP) or transhepatic cholangiography with biliary drainage. For pyogenic abscesses in transplanted livers, management and proper biliary drainage may be difficult to achieve because of the diffuse nature of the biliary strictures.

PROGNOSIS

Abscesses smaller than 10 cm can take up to 16 weeks to resolve, whereas abscesses larger than 10 cm may take, on an average, another 6 weeks to resolve. Mortality from pyogenic liver abscess is associated with older age and with comorbidities such as cirrhosis, diabetes, chronic renal failure, and malignancy. Jaundice is an ominous sign. In developed countries, the mortality rate ranges from 2 to 12%. Patients with bacteremia have a four-fold higher risk for death.

Nonabscess Hepatic Bacterial Infections

Bacterial infections of the liver can also cause more diffuse infections without frank abscess formation. Implicated organisms include *L. monocytogenes* (Chapter 301), *Y. enterocolitica* (Chapter 320), *S. typhi* and *S. paratyphi* (Chapter 316), legionella (Chapter 322), ehrlichia (Chapter 335), and gonococci (Chapter 307). There are no specific features associated with these infections, and these organisms do not necessarily cause abscesses. Patients with chronic liver disease are especially at risk for listerial infection. Patients with active enteric yersinia infection can have secondary liver involvement with or without liver abscesses. Disseminated gonococcal infections (Chapter 307) can cause a perihepatitis (Fitz-Hugh-Curtis syndrome), which can present with right upper quadrant pain and tenderness.

Systemic bacteremia can cause a variety of hepatobiliary abnormalities, which may range from elevated aminotransferase and alkaline phosphatase levels (Chapter 149) to the cholestasis of sepsis with the development of jaundice. Common organisms that can disrupt normal liver function after entering the blood stream include *E. coli*, *Klebsiella* species, *Streptococcus pneumoniae*, and *S. aureus*, especially from pneumonias, urinary tract infections, or soft tissue infections. The hepatic biochemical abnormalities associated with bacteremia may be related to factors such as hemodynamic instability and liver hypoperfusion, as well as to the infection per se. Associated renal failure, a blood transfusion–derived bilirubin load, and drugs may complicate the picture. The course of cholestasis may be prolonged for several days to a few weeks, but it typically resolves with resolution of the systemic infection. There is no specific treatment for the cholestasis related to a systemic infection, but it is important to rule out drug-induced cholestasis that may evolve as a consequence of one or more of the antibiotics.

Fungal Diseases of the Liver

Except for hepatosplenic candidiasis with granuloma formation, clinically significant fungal diseases of the liver are unusual. Other fungal infections also commonly manifest as hepatic granulomas but usually are not accompanied by the high fever that is characteristic of hepatosplenic candidiasis.

HEPATOSPLENIC CANDIDIASIS
EPIDEMIOLOGY AND PATHOBIOLOGY

Hepatosplenic candidiasis typically is caused by *C. albicans*, but other *Candida* species, including *C. tropicalis*, *C. parapsilosis*, *C. glabrata*, and *C. krusei*, have occasionally been reported. It occurs as part of disseminated candidiasis (Chapter 346), almost exclusively in patients with acute leukemia, but rarely in patients with lymphoma, aplastic anemia, and sarcoma. Up to 7% of patients with acute leukemia may develop hepatosplenic candidiasis, and it is more common with acute lymphoblastic leukemia than acute myeloid leukemia. Recently, however, the incidence of hepatosplenic candidiasis has decreased by a factor of four owing to the widespread use of prophylactic antifungal agents early in the disease. Hepatosplenic candidiasis presumably results from translocation of *Candida* species from the gastrointestinal tract into the blood stream as a result of prolonged neutropenia and a breach in mucosal integrity.

CLINICAL MANIFESTATIONS AND DIAGNOSIS

Hepatosplenic candidiasis presents with persistent and high spiking fevers in a patient who was previously neutropenic and has now returned to a normal neutrophil count. The fever may be accompanied by right upper quadrant pain, nausea, vomiting, and anorexia.

Patients typically have elevated levels of alkaline phosphatase and less commonly of aminotransferases, bilirubin, and leukocytes. CT, which is the imaging modality of choice, classically shows multiple areas of lucency representing microabscesses in the liver, spleen, and kidneys. If the CT scan is nondiagnostic but clinical suspicion remains high, an MRI should be performed.

TREATMENT AND PROGNOSIS

The mainstay of therapy is with antifungal therapy for a long duration of treatment. In clinically stable patients, oral fluconazole can be used. In acutely ill patients, a lipid formulation of amphotericin B (3 to 5 mg/kg intravenously daily) is recommended. If the lipid formulation of amphotericin B is not used, other options are caspofungin (70 mg loading dose, then 50 mg intravenously daily), anidulafungin (200 mg loading dose, then 100 mg intravenously daily), or micafungin (100 mg intravenously daily). After 1 to 2 weeks, oral fluconazole (400 mg daily) should be started. Treatment should continue until lesions resolve on follow-up CT scans, typically within 6 months of treatment. In patients who are receiving chemotherapy or stem cell transplantation, however, the high risk for recurrent hepatosplenic candidiasis typically warrants continued prophylactic fluconazole (400 mg orally, daily) to prevent relapse until native immunity is restored.

A definitive diagnosis is usually made on liver biopsy specimens that show multiple granulomas, and, with special stains, yeast and hyphal forms. However, biopsy often will not show evidence of infection, especially in patients who have received prior antifungal therapy. Although biopsy is the only means to establish a definitive diagnosis, it is not often required because other clinical, laboratory, and radiographic manifestations are almost always sufficient for diagnosis.

PROGNOSIS

With prolonged treatment with antifungals, there has been good success at treating hepatosplenic candidiasis.

Other Fungal Diseases

Other fungal infections of the liver are quite rare. Fungal cultures are always necessary to establish a definitive diagnosis.

Coccidioides immitis (Chapter 341) is often asymptomatic but may lead to fungal hepatitis characterized by an increased alkaline phosphatase level and the development of hepatic granulomas. Hepatic *Cryptococcus neoformans* infections (Chapter 344) are rare but are seen in patients with AIDS, who typically develop hepatomegaly. In the much more rare non-HIV-infected patient, disseminated cryptococcosis can result in focal granulomatous hepatitis, which may clinically mimic viral hepatitis, or can present as obstructive jaundice secondary to sclerosing cholangitis. *Histoplasma capsulatum* (Chapter 340) infects individuals who inhale the fungus, but most cases are subclinical. In symptomatic hepatic histoplasmosis, two thirds of patients present with hepatomegaly, with some showing splenic enlargement as well. Histologically, histoplasmosis can cause multiple granulomas diffusely distributed throughout the liver, although a more common finding is portal lymphohistiocytic infiltrate. *Paracoccidioides brasiliensis* (Chapter 343) most commonly infects adult males, and autopsy series have shown hepatic involvement in up to 50% of patients who die from this infection. Some individuals may present with hepatomegaly or jaundice, although the latter is found in less than 6% of patients. Aminotransferase levels are often elevated in the early stages of the disease, with changes in alkaline phosphatase or bilirubin levels tending to occur in the later stages. Biopsy may reveal lesions ranging from small granulomas to diffuse fibrosis and infiltration of yeast forms, often with bile duct involvement.

PARASITIC, PROTOZOAL, AND HELMINTHIC INFECTIONS OF THE LIVER

Amebic Liver Abscess

EPIDEMIOLOGY

Entamoeba histolytica (Chapter 360) is found throughout the world where the barriers between human feces and food and water are inadequate. After malaria, it is the second leading cause of death from parasitic diseases worldwide, accounting for an estimated 40,000 to 100,000 deaths annually. In the United States, most cases of amebiasis arise in immigrants from endemic areas and people living in states that border Mexico. Travelers to endemic areas are also at risk; ingestion of amebic cysts and colonization of the gastrointestinal tract can occur years before the development of a liver abscess. Amebic liver abscesses mainly affect men between the ages of 18 and 50 years but are also more common in postmenopausal women, thereby suggesting a hormonal protective effect. Other risk factors include alcohol intake, HLA-DR3, oral and anal sex, and contaminated enema apparatuses.

TABLE 154-2 PARASITIC INFECTIONS INVOLVING THE LIVER

	CHARACTERISTICS	ENDEMIC AREAS	RISK FACTORS AND ENDEMIC AREAS	MAJOR HEPATIC MANIFESTATIONS
MAJOR PROTOZOA				
Entamoeba histolytica	Ingested cysts develop into invasive trophozoites that colonize the colon and occasionally spread to the liver by the portal blood	Mexico, regions of Central and South America, India, and regions of Africa	Male gender, alcohol intake, HLA-DR3, oral and anal sex, and contaminated enema apparatuses	Amebic liver abscesses develop as a tissue response to trophozoite invasion with acute and chronic manifestations (see text)
OTHER PROTOZOA				
Cryptosporidium species and microsporidia	Ingested cysts develop into trophozoites in intestinal mucosa	Worldwide distribution	AIDS	Biliary tract infection with obstruction and cholangitis
Toxoplasma gondii	Ingestion of oocysts in contaminated soil or water or in infected meat; systemic spread of tachyzoites in the circulation	Worldwide distribution	Consumption of undercooked meat, contact with soil, and travel outside the United States, Europe, or Canada	Immunocompetent: asymptomatic or hepatomegaly and mild LFT elevations Immunocompromised: occasional overt hepatitis
Leishmania species	Sand fly bite transmits promastigotes; proliferation in the reticuloendothelial system	Worldwide distribution	Children <10 yr and immunocompromised adults Contact with sand flies	Hepatosplenomegaly months to years after infection
Plasmodium species	Mosquito (*Anopheles*) bite transmits sporozoites	Multiple regions throughout the world	Exposure to anopheline mosquito bites	Proliferation in hepatocytes causes hepatomegaly, enzyme elevations, and jaundice
Babesia microti	Tick bite transmits the agent, which parasitizes erythrocytes	Europe	Asplenia is a risk for fatal hepatic failure, especially bovine babesiosis	Mild liver enzyme elevations

PATHOBIOLOGY

E. histolytica has a simple life cycle consisting of the cyst (infectious form) and trophozoite (the motile stage associated with disease); it infects only humans and some nonhuman primates. Cysts are ingested and mature into trophozoites in the intestinal lumen. The development of amebic colitis is not essential for liver abscess formation. *E. histolytica* trophozoites penetrate through the mucosa and submucosal tissues and enter the portal circulation. *E. histolytica* blocks intrahepatic portal venules. When the trophozoites reach the liver, they create their unique abscesses, which are well-circumscribed regions of dead hepatocytes, liquefied cells, and cellular debris that are surrounded by a rim of connective tissue, a few inflammatory cells, and amebic trophozoites. The adjacent liver parenchyma is unaffected. Given the small numbers of amebae relative to the size of the abscess, it is suggested that *E. histolytica* can cause hepatocyte death without direct contact.

CLINICAL MANIFESTATIONS

Patients can present with amebic liver abscesses months to years after traveling to an endemic area, so a detailed travel history is essential for the diagnosis. The disease should be suspected in patients with an appropriate travel history, fever, right upper quadrant pain, and substantial hepatic tenderness. Jaundice is extremely uncommon. Symptoms are usually acute (<10 days in duration) but can be chronic, with anorexia and weight loss. Patients with acute disease tend to have multifocal disease, whereas patients with a more indolent course tend to have a solitary lesion. Laboratory data tend to demonstrate a leukocytosis without eosinophilia, mild anemia, an elevated alkaline phosphatase level, and high erythrocyte sedimentation rate.

DIAGNOSIS

Although some individuals with amebic liver abscesses have concurrent amebic colitis, most have no bowel symptoms; hence, stool microscopy for *E. histolytica* trophozoites and cysts are usually negative. The diagnosis relies on identification of a space-occupying lesion in the liver and a positive amebic serology. Both ultrasound and CT scan are very sensitive (Fig. 154-2), but neither provides absolute specificity for amebic liver abscesses. Serologic testing is highly sensitive (>94%) and specific (>95%). False-negative testing can be obtained within the first 7 to 10 days of infection, but repeat testing will usually be positive. Aspiration of the lesion may be necessary to exclude a primary or secondary bacterial infection.

TREATMENT AND PROGNOSIS   Rx

Metronidazole (500 to 750 mg orally three times daily or a 15-mg/kg loading dose followed by 7.5 mg/kg every 6 hours intravenously) usually provides evidence of clinical improvement within 72 to 96 hours but should be continued for 5 to 10 days. Nitroimidazole tinidazole at 2 g daily for 3 days is also effective. Drainage is not necessary,**3** except in patients who do not respond within 5 days. For cysts larger than 10 cm, catheter drainage is preferred over repeated needle aspiration.**2** The abscess usually shrinks by about 50% within a week, but the mean time to complete radiologic resolution is 3 to 9 months. Repeated imaging in a clinically improving patient may lead to unwarranted concern and unnecessary treatment.

Treatment must also address the removal of all of the cysts from the intestinal lumen in patients with evidence of intraluminal infection. A recommended treatment is iodoquinol (650 mg orally three times a day for 20 days) to prevent continued colonization and possible recurrence of the liver abscess. With prompt diagnosis and adequate medical treatment, the mortality rate from amebic abscess is 1 to 3%.

Other Protozoal Liver Diseases

In addition to *E. histolytica*, other protozoal diseases that affect the liver include *Cryptosporidium* species, *Toxoplasma gondii*, *Leishmania* species, *Plasmodium* species, and *Babesia microti* (Table 154-2).

⬤ HELMINTH INFECTIONS
Echinococcosis and Hydatid Cyst Disease

EPIDEMIOLOGY AND PATHOBIOLOGY

Human cystic echinococcosis is a zoonosis caused by the larval cestode *E. granulosus*. It is often referred to as hydatid cyst disease because of the watery cysts that characterize the infection.

SYMPTOMS AND SIGNS	LABORATORY FINDINGS	RADIOGRAPHIC FEATURES	DIAGNOSIS	TREATMENT
Fever, RUQ pain, and substantial hepatic tenderness	Leukocytosis without eosinophilia, mild anemia, elevated serum AP, and high ESR	US, CT, and MRI can detect abscess but cannot always differentiate amebic from pyogenic. On CT or MRI, amebic abscess sometimes appears "cold" with bright rim.	Imaging, serology, stool antigen test (microscopic evaluation of stool has a poor yield)	Metronidazole, 500-750 mg PO tid × 5-10 days, or tinidazole, 2 g daily × 3 days; iodoquinol, 650 mg tid × 20 days, also needed to eradicate intestinal colonization
See Chapter 358	See Chapter 358	See Chapter 358	See Chapter 358	See Chapter 358
See Chapter 357	See Chapter 357	See Chapter 357	See Chapter 357	See Chapter 357
See Chapter 356	See Chapter 356	See Chapter 356	See Chapter 356	See Chapter 356
See Chapter 353	See Chapter 353	See Chapter 353	See Chapter 353	See Chapter 353
See Chapter 361	See Chapter 361	See Chapter 361	See Chapter 361	See Chapter 361

TABLE 154-2 PARASITIC INFECTIONS INVOLVING THE LIVER—cont'd

	CHARACTERISTICS	ENDEMIC AREAS	RISK FACTORS AND ENDEMIC AREAS	MAJOR HEPATIC MANIFESTATIONS
MAJOR HELMINTHS				
Schistosoma species	Cercaria in fresh water penetrate the skin, travel by the circulation to portal vein radicals	*S. mansoni* found in South America, Africa, and Middle East. *S. japonicum* found in Far East (mostly China and Philippines).	Contact with fresh water containing cercaria of schistosomes	Progressive presinusoidal blood flow obstruction, periportal fibrosis, portal hypertension, varices, ascites, splenomegaly
Echinococcus granulosus	Eggs of small (3-7 mm) tapeworms in stool of canid hosts; ingested eggs produce larval oncospheres that migrate to the liver and form cysts in sheep, humans, and other intermediate hosts	Worldwide distribution, found especially in sheep-raising areas (Africa, the Mediterranean region of Europe, the Middle East, Asia, South America, Australia, and New Zealand)	Ingestion of food or water fecally contaminated with eggs and human contact with sheepdogs	Initial infection asymptomatic; liver cysts increase in diameter by 1-5 cm yearly and cause variable abdominal pain, hepatomegaly, and variable eosinophilia; occasional cyst rupture, secondary bacterial infection
Echinococcus multilocularis	Eggs of small tapeworms in stool of foxes; ingested eggs produce oncospheres in the liver of rodents, humans, and other intermediate hosts	Endemic in Northern hemisphere	Human exposure increasing with growing fox populations	Metacestodes colonize the liver as a tumor-like mass of small vesicles
Fasciola species	Leaf-shaped flukes up to 13 × 30 mm derived from ingested cysts; the fluke excysts in the duodenum, migrates directly across the bowel wall into the peritoneal cavity, and burrows directly into the liver (or occasionally out to the skin)	Worldwide distribution	Consumption of freshwater or aquatic plants contaminated by colonized livestock	Adult flukes live in the common and hepatic bile ducts causing obstruction and leading to thickening of the ducts, dilation, and fibrosis of the proximal biliary tree
Opisthorchis species and *Clonorchis sinensis*	Flukes of 8-25 mm derived from ingested cysts; the fluke excysts in the duodenum and migrates into the bile ducts	*Opisthorchis* sp: Southeast Asia, Central and Eastern Europe (particularly Siberia) *C. sinensis*: China, Japan, Vietnam, Korea	Consumption of raw, pickled, dried, smoked, or salted freshwater fish or crayfish originating from East Asia or, in the case of *Opisthorchis felineus*, Russia and Eastern Europe	*Acute:* typically asymptomatic *Chronic:* abdominal pain, fever, anorexia, tender hepatomegaly, sometimes eosinophilia *Late sequelae:* intermittent biliary obstruction, cholelithiasis, cholecystitis, cholangitis, secondary bacterial abscesses, cholangiocarcinoma
Toxocara species	Nematode infection disseminates to cause visceral larva migrans after ingestion of soil contaminated with dog or cat feces	Highest prevalence in southeastern United States	Consumption of food contaminated with soil containing eggs; distributed throughout the United States	Often an asymptomatic cause of eosinophilia (exclude *Trichinella* sp, *Strongyloides* sp, filaria, hookworm, schistosomiasis); hepatomegaly is common, but nonhepatic manifestations dominate the clinical picture
OTHER HELMINTHS				
Ascaris lumbricoides	Ingested eggs develop into larvae that migrate to the lungs and are coughed and swallowed; develop into roundworms 15-30 mm long in the small intestine	Global distribution with higher prevalence in Africa, South America, India, and the Far East; 20% of the world's population is colonized	Consumption of fecally contaminated food or water, particularly in young children	Colonization is typically asymptomatic with eosinophilia; biliary migration of worms can cause symptomatic biliary obstruction, cholangitis, cholecystitis, and secondary bacterial liver abscess
Capillaria hepatica	Ingested eggs develop into larvae in the intestinal mucosa; larvae migrate to the liver by portal blood flow and develop into short-lived roundworms	Human infection is rare	Consumption of food contaminated with rodent feces	Fever, eosinophilia, and hepatomegaly; subsequent foci of liver fibrosis, granulomas, and calcification in involved areas
Strongyloides stercoralis	Ingested eggs develop into 1.5- to 2.5-mm nematodes that invade the hepatic vasculature, lymphatics, and biliary tract	Tropical and subtropical areas, including southeastern United States and Southern and Eastern Europe	Consumption of food contaminated with soil containing eggs, infection with HTLV-1, and immunocompromised individuals	Hepatic disease in the setting of immunosuppression: jaundice, abdominal pain; eosinophilia is uncommon

AP = alkaline phosphatase; CT = computed tomography; ELISA = enzyme-linked immunosorbent assay; ERCP = endoscopic retrograde cholangiopancreatography; ESR = erythrocyte sedimentation rate; HTLV = human T-cell lymphotrophic virus; LFT = liver function test; MRI = magnetic resonance imaging; RUQ = right upper quadrant; US = ultrasonography.

SYMPTOMS AND SIGNS	LABORATORY FINDINGS	RADIOGRAPHIC FEATURES	DIAGNOSIS	TREATMENT
Initial infection presents as itching. Later presentations include fever, diarrhea, chills, headaches, or hives. Hematemesis from ruptured gastroesophageal varices	Eosinophilia and splenomegaly; seroconversion occurs within 4 to 6 weeks	Extensive calcification with typical turtle-back appearance along portal tracts	Rectal biopsy, liver biopsy, microscopic examination of stool	Praziquantel (single dose, 40 mg/kg) with a second dose 6-12 weeks later if necessary
Enlarged hydatid cyst can cause abdominal pain, nausea, hepatomegaly, or a palpable mass. Mild RUQ pain, urticaria, and episodes of pruritus	Positive Weinberg reaction (false negative in 38% of cases) or ELISA analysis; eosinophilia seen in ruptured cysts	On US or CT, cysts appear flaky, sometimes showing daughter cysts or peripheral focal calcification. Fluid is of variable density.	Imaging, Weinberg reaction, or ELISA	Albendazole, 400 mg 2× daily for 3-6 monthly cycles with 10-14 day intervals. Drainage of the cyst is essential. Surgical resection if the cyst communicates with the biliary tree.
See Chapter 362	See Chapter 362	See Chapter 362	See Chapter 362	See Chapter 362
Acute: fever, abdominal pain, eosinophilia *Chronic:* symptomatic biliary obstruction, variable eosinophilia	Serologic tests include hemagglutination, complement fixation, ELISA, and counterimmunoelectrophoresis. Anemia, leukocytosis, eosinophilia, elevated AP, and hypergammaglobulinemia are often seen.	CT is most useful: liver shows hypodense nodules or tortuous tracks; thickening of the liver capsule, subcapsular hematoma, and parenchymal calcification may also be seen	Serology, stool examination	Triclabendazole, 10 mg/kg once or twice
Chronic infection presents as dyspepsia, abdominal pain, diarrhea, nausea, vomiting, anorexia, weight loss, fevers, hepatomegaly, and urticaria. Acute presentation includes serum sickness, intrahepatic pigment stones, and facial edema. Other rare complications are cholangitis, pancreatitis, and obstructive jaundice.	Anemia, leukocytosis, eosinophilia, elevated AP, and hypergammaglobulinemia	US may detect flukes in biliary tree. CT shows small hypodense nodules.	Serology and stool examination	Praziquantel, 25 mg/kg q8h × 3 doses
See Chapter 365	See Chapter 365	See Chapter 365	See Chapter 365	See Chapter 365
Sensitized patients during pulmonary phase present with asthma-like symptoms, hemoptysis, chest pain, and cyanosis. Urticaria and other allergic reactions are sometimes seen. Patients in intestinal phase show cognitive and nutritional impairment with abdominal pain, hepatomegaly, cholangitis, and obstructive jaundice.	Leukocytosis with eosinophilia; hyperbilirubinemia occasionally seen	Movement of the worms within the biliary tree can sometimes be observed. A bull's-eye appearance can be seen on cross-sectional imaging.	Stool examination, imaging, and ERCP	Albendazole, 400 mg once
Persistent fever, eosinophilia, and hepatomegaly are most common. Splenomegaly, anorexia, nausea, vomiting, night sweats, and altered bowel habits are also seen.	Anemia, eosinophilia, moderately elevated liver enzymes, increased ESR, and hypergammaglobulinemia	US shows nonspecific hyperechoic areas in the portal spaces.	Stool and liver biopsy	Mebendazole, 200 mg bid × 20 days
Recurrent urticaria, abdominal pain, diarrhea, and cough; mild jaundice and hepatomegaly in the absence of splenomegaly	Eosinophilia and hypoalbuminemia Patients may have elevated liver enzymes.	Imaging studies not used in diagnosis	Serology and stool examination	Ivermectin, 200 μg/kg/day × 2 days, or albendazole, 400 mg/day × 7 days

FIGURE 154-2. Computed tomographic scan of an amebic liver abscess. (Courtesy Dr. Chalermrat Bunchorntavakul, Bangkok, Thailand.)

The disease remains endemic in sheep-raising areas of the world, including Africa, the Mediterranean region of Europe, the Middle East, Asia, South America, Australia, and New Zealand. Dogs are the definitive hosts for *E. granulosus,* and sheep are the major intermediate hosts, although yaks, goats, and camels are other relevant intermediate hosts. Humans are only accidental hosts when they ingest food or water that is fecally contaminated with eggs. Human contact with sheepdogs that are in frequent contact with livestock is a major risk for infection.

The disease cycle begins when an adult tapeworm infects the intestinal tract of the definitive host (dogs usually). The adult tapeworm then produces eggs, which are expelled in the host's feces. Intermediate hosts become infected by ingesting the eggs of the parasite in fecally contaminated food. Inside the intermediate host, the eggs hatch and release tiny hooked embryos (called oncospheres), which travel in the blood stream and eventually lodge in the liver, lungs, or kidneys, where they develop into hydatid cysts. Inside these cysts grow thousands of tapeworm larvae, the next stage in the life cycle of the parasite.

CLINICAL MANIFESTATIONS

The initial infection is asymptomatic, but an enlarging hydatid liver cyst can cause abdominal pain, nausea, hepatomegaly, or a palpable mass. Patients may describe symptoms of mild upper right quadrant pain, urticarial skin rash, and episodes of pruritus. If the cyst ruptures, serious complications can develop. Cysts that perforate into the peritoneum can lead to the development of extrahepatic cysts and may induce an allergic reaction with eosinophilia, pruritic urticaria, and systemic anaphylaxis. In most cases, however, cysts rupture into bile ducts, where they cause cholestatic jaundice, cholangitis, or biliary pain.

DIAGNOSIS

On ultrasound or CT scans (Fig. 154-3), the hydatid cysts are often large with a flaky appearance that is referred to as *hydatid sand.* CT imaging also may show multiple daughter cysts or a fluid density cyst with peripheral focal areas of calcification. Fluid is of variable density depending on the amount of proteinaceous debris.

Hydatid cysts of liver can be diagnosed by a serologic assay, the Weinberg reaction, but this test can have false-negative results in up to 38% of cases. An enzyme-linked immunosorbent assay (ELISA) may be more sensitive. Eosinophilia is not a feature unless the cyst ruptures; in fact, usually there are no changes in blood chemistries.

TREATMENT AND PROGNOSIS   Rx

Drug therapy includes albendazole, 400 mg twice a day for 3 to 6 monthly cycles separated by 10 to 14 day intervals, but treatment with albendazole alone is not effective, so drainage is essential to the effective treatment of hydatid cysts. In a randomized trial, percutaneous drainage consisting of puncture, aspiration, injection, and reaspiration of scolicidal solutions resulted in a similar rate of cyst disappearance as open surgical drainage but with fewer side effects, provided that patients received preprocedure and postprocedure

FIGURE 154-3. Computed tomographic scan of a hepatic echinococcal cyst.

albendazole therapy.**4** Chlorhexidine, H_2O_2, 80% alcohol, and 0.5% cetrimide are the preferred scolicidal agents. If the cyst communicates with the biliary tree, however, injection of scolicidal agents carries an almost universal risk of secondary sclerosing cholangitis, and so it is contraindicated. In such cases, the cyst must be treated surgically, by either cystectomy or hepatic resection.

The prognosis is generally good, with complete cure expected after successful percutaneous or surgical treatment. However, spillage occurs in 2 to 25% of cases, depending on the location of the cyst and surgeon's experience, and the operative mortality rate varies from 0.5 to 4% for the same reasons.

Schistosomiasis

EPIDEMIOLOGY AND PATHOBIOLOGY

Schistosomiasis is an infection of trematodes. *Schistosoma* species (Chapter 363) cause periportal fibrosis and liver cirrhosis owing to deposition of eggs in the small portal venules. *Schistosoma mansoni* and *Schistosoma japonicum* lead to liver disease. Infection with *S. mansoni* is found in parts of South America, Africa, and the Middle East. Infection with *S. japonicum* is found in the Far East, mostly China and the Philippines. Although primary infection does not occur in the United States, 5% of the world's population may be infected, thereby making it a major international health concern and highly prevalent in immigrants.

Humans become infected after contact with water that contains the infective stage (cercaria) of schistosomes. After penetration of the skin, the larvae migrate to the lungs and then to the venules of the mesentery, urinary bladder, or ureters. They release eggs in the venules of the mesentery, and the eggs enter the liver through the portal vein, where they become lodged in the terminal branches of the portal venules. The lodged eggs cause a granulomatous inflammation, and the lesions heal by periportal fibrosis. *S. japonicum* is more virulent than *S. mansoni* because its infections produce ten times more eggs.

CLINICAL MANIFESTATIONS

Initial infection presents as itching that is caused by skin penetration by larvae. Several weeks later, patients may complain of fever, diarrhea, chills, headaches, or hives. At this time, patients will have eosinophilia. Over the next 5 to 15 years, periportal liver fibrosis develops and leads to presinusoidal portal hypertension, splenomegaly (Chapter 171), and gastroesophageal varices (Chapter 140). With *S. japonicum,* however, the progression can be much more rapid, with little interval between the acute and chronic disease. Hepatic function is generally well preserved, and patients usually present with hematemesis from ruptured gastroesophageal varices.

DIAGNOSIS

Schistosomal eggs typically have lateral or terminal spines and are easy to detect on microscopic examination of feces or on a rectal biopsy. Seroconversion occurs within 4 to 8 weeks of infection but cannot distinguish active infection from a history of exposure. Imaging may show extensive calcification with the typical turtle-back appearance along the portal tracts reflecting the clustered, calcified eggs along the portal triads.

TREATMENT AND PROGNOSIS

Praziquantel (a single dose of 40 mg/kg) is effective in 70 to 100% of cases, but a second dose can be given 6 to 12 weeks later, particularly in patients with eosinophilia, high antibody titers, or persistent symptoms. Treatment of portal hypertension may be necessary (Chapter 156). The mortality rate is 0.05% for severe *S. mansoni* infection and 1.8% for severe *S. japonicum* infection. Bleeding from esophageal varices is the most serious complication. Chronic infection can lead to hepatocellular carcinoma.

GRANULOMATOUS DISEASES OF THE LIVER

Granulomas, which are found in up to 15% of liver biopsies, can be an incidental finding or may represent a wide array of liver diseases (Table 154-3). A granuloma is an accumulation of epithelioid cells, including transformed macrophages, mononuclear cells, and other inflammatory cells. Granulomas may have associated necrosis (caseating) as in tuberculosis (Chapter 332) or may be non-necrotizing (noncaseating) as in sarcoidosis (Chapter 95). In Q fever (Chapter 335), fibrin-ring granulomas are characterized by a vacuole encircled by a ring of fibrinoid necrosis and surrounded by lymphocytes and histiocytes.

An incidental granuloma requires minimal further evaluation. Tuberculosis should be excluded (Chapter 332). Sarcoidosis also should be considered because it is the most common cause of granulomas in the United States. An antimitochondrial antibody should be drawn to rule out primary biliary cirrhosis. The use of potentially causative drugs should be stopped (see Table 154-3).

Sarcoidosis

Sarcoidosis, which is the most frequently identified cause of hepatic granuloma in the United States, affects all racial and ethnic groups and occurs at all ages. In patients with sarcoidosis, the liver is the third most commonly involved organ, after the lymph nodes and lung; about 50 to 80% of patients with sarcoidosis have granulomas in their livers. The classic granuloma is found mainly in the portal triads, with a cluster of large epithelioid cells and often with multinucleated giant cells.

CLINICAL MANIFESTATIONS AND DIAGNOSIS

Hepatic involvement of sarcoidosis is often subclinical, and only a minority of patients present with pruritus, fever, abdominal pain, hepatomegaly, cholestatic jaundice, or portal hypertension. In some patients, the granulomatous injury and destruction of the interlobular bile ducts eventually causes ductopenia and a histologic picture similar to primary biliary cirrhosis (Chapter 158). In other patients, damage to the large bile ducts may lead to a syndrome that mimics primary sclerosing cholangitis (Chapter 158). Other patients may present with focal liver lesions suggestive of malignant neoplasm.

Patients typically have a marked elevation of the serum alkaline phosphatase level. Angiotensin-converting enzyme (ACE) levels also are characteristically elevated but may not be helpful in differentiating sarcoidosis from other chronic liver diseases, such as primary biliary cirrhosis, in which it also may be elevated. The presence of noncaseating granulomas in a patient with clinically suspected sarcoidosis generally establishes the diagnosis. However, granulomas do not correlate with liver function tests or duration of disease.

TREATMENT AND PROGNOSIS

In general, hepatic sarcoidosis does not need to be treated except in patients with other indications for treatment (Chapter 95). Corticosteroids improve liver function tests but do not alleviate portal hypertension, and serial biopsies often show little improvement. Sarcoidosis that leads to portal hypertension and fibrosis may ultimately require liver transplantation (Chapter 157), and sarcoidosis may recur in the new organ.

Other Granulomatous Liver Diseases

In addition to sarcoidosis, another major cause of granulomatous liver disease is tuberculosis (Chapter 332). Military tuberculosis, caused by *Mycobacterium tuberculosis*, commonly results in hepatic granulomas, and patients present with hepatomegaly or abnormal liver function tests, or both. A biopsy revealing caseating granulomas along with a positive purified protein derivative test and active pulmonary tuberculosis can help in establishing a diagnosis. Other mycobacteria known to cause granulomatous liver disease include *M. avium-intracellulare*, *M. gevanese*, and *M. scrofulaceum* (Chapter 333).

Other causes of granulomatous liver disease include zoonotic infections such as cat-scratch disease (Chapter 323), Q fever (Chapter 335), and brucellosis (Chapter 318). Cat-scratch disease is caused by *B. henselae*, with cats serving as the main reservoir for the organism. The disease primarily affects children. Patients typically present with lymphadenopathy associated with persistent pyrexia of unknown origin, abdominal pain, and weight loss. *B. henselae* can be identified by a Warthin-Starry stain, or an imaging study may demonstrate scattered defects in the liver. Q fever is caused by the intracellular gram-negative rickettsial organism *Coxiella burnetii*. Most infections are

TABLE 154-3 CAUSES OF GRANULOMATOUS LIVER DISEASE

DIAGNOSIS	SPECIAL AND UNIQUE FEATURES
Sarcoidosis	Evidence of pulmonary sarcoidosis, granulomas found on biopsy specimens from other organs, elevated ACE level
Bacterial infections	
Mycobacteria tuberculosis	Caseating granulomas on biopsy, + PPD, active pulmonary tuberculosis
Other mycobacteria (*M. avium-intracellulare, M. lepra, M. mucogenicum, M. bovis*)	HIV, exposure history
Other bacteria (brucellosis, listeriosis, melioidosis, tularemia, yersiniosis, bartonellosis, Q fever, syphilis, psittacosis)	Fever, exposure history
Viral infections (cytomegalovirus, Epstein-Barr virus, hepatitis C, hepatitis B, hepatitis A)	Serology for acute or recent exposure
Fungal infections (histoplasmosis, coccidioidomycosis, blastomycosis, nocardiosis, candidiasis)	Fever, immunocompromised
Parasitic infections (schistosomiasis, *Ascaris lumbricoides* infection, toxoplasmosis, visceral leishmaniasis)	Travel to endemic regions, positive serologic testing
Primary biliary cirrhosis	Female sex, positive AMA, elevated IgM
Malignancies (Hodgkin's disease, non-Hodgkin's lymphoma, renal cell carcinoma)	Evidence of malignancy in kidney, lymph node, or bone marrow
Drug reactions (allopurinol, chlorpropamide, phenylbutazone, sulfonamides, carbamazepine, glyburide, quinidine, quinine, diltiazem, hydralazine, rosiglitazone, phenytoin, methyldopa, procainamide, amoxicillin–clavulanic acid, mebendazole, mesalamine, acetaminophen, pyrazinamide, halothane, isoniazid, norfloxacin)	Exposure history
Toxins (beryllium, copper sulfate, Thorotrast)	Previous exposure history
Miscellaneous (talc, Crohn's disease, Wegener's granulomatosis, after jejunoileal bypass, mineral oil lipogranulomas, hepatic allograft rejection, chronic granulomatous disease)	History of IV drug use, history of liver transplantation, diarrhea

ACE = angiotensin-converting enzyme; AMA = antimitochondrial antibody; HIV = human immunodeficiency virus; IV = intravenous; PPD = purified protein derivative.

asymptomatic, but patients may have self-limited influenza-like symptoms, pneumonia, and hepatitis. A liver biopsy may demonstrate fibrin-ring granulomas (doughnut shaped) in the background of nonspecific reactive hepatitis and steatosis. Brucellosis, which is not common in the United States, is caused by at least four species of Brucella: *B. abortus*, *B. suis*, *B. melitensis*, and *B. canis*. The disease presents as recurrent high fevers, drenching sweats, malaise, arthralgia, fatigue, abdominal pain, anorexia, and headaches. Patients often have hepatomegaly and increases in serum levels of aminotransferases and alkaline phosphatase. The granulomas formed by this infection are typically smaller than those caused by sarcoidosis or tuberculosis, and a definitive diagnosis can be established through serologic testing.

It is important to keep in mind that hepatic granulomas are formed naturally as a consequence of the immune response, so they may be seen in many infections with hepatic involvement (see Table 154-3). Examples of infections that can manifest as granulomatous liver disease include listeriosis, yersiniosis, candidiasis, histoplasmosis, coccidioidomycosis, and schistosomiasis. Viral infections (e.g., cytomegalovirus and hepatitis A, B, and C), primary biliary cirrhosis, malignancies, and certain drug reactions have all been etiologically linked to granulomatous liver disease.

1. Yu SC, Ho SS, Lau WY, et al. Treatment of pyogenic liver abscess: prospective randomized comparison of catheter drainage and needle aspiration. *Hepatology.* 2004;39:932-938.
2. Singh O, Gupta S, Moses S, et al. Comparative study of catheter drainage and needle aspiration in management of large liver abscesses. *Indian J Gastroenterol.* 2009;28:88-92.
3. Chavez-Tapia NC, Hernandez Calleros J, Tellez-Avila FL, et al. Image-guided percutaneous procedure plus metronidazole versus metronidazole alone for uncomplicated amoebic liver abscess. *Cochrane Database Syst Rev.* 2009;21:CD004886.
4. Nasseri Moghaddam S, Abrishami A, Malekzade R. Percutaneous needle aspiration, injection, and reaspiration with or without benzimidazole coverage for uncomplicated hepatic hydatid cysts. *Cochrane Database Syst Rev.* 2006;19:CD003623.

SUGGESTED READINGS

Meddings L, Myers RP, Hubbard J, et al. A population-based study of pyogenic liver abscesses in the United States: incidence, mortality, and temporal trends. *Am J Gastroenterol.* 2010;105:117-124. *The most common causes were streptococci (30%) and Escherichia coli (18%).*
O'Farrell N, Collins CG, McEntee GP. Pyogenic liver abscesses: diminished role for operative treatment. *Surgeon.* 2010;8:192-196. *Emphasizes interventional radiology and antimicrobial therapy.*
Reid-Lombardo KM, Khan S, Sclabas G. Hepatic cysts and liver abscesses. *Surg Clin North Am.* 2010;90:679-697. *Review.*

155

ALCOHOLIC AND NONALCOHOLIC STEATOHEPATITIS

NAGA P. CHALASANI

Alcoholic liver disease and nonalcoholic fatty liver disease (NAFLD), which represent two of the most common forms of liver disease, can lead to cirrhosis, liver failure, and death. Although these two conditions have different risk factors and natural histories, in both conditions (Table 155-1) the hepatocytes are characterized by macrovesicular steatosis, which is the accumulation of triglycerides as one large cytoplasmic globule that displaces the nucleus. In microvesicular steatosis, cytoplasmic accumulation of fat occurs as multiple small globules with a central nucleus.

ALCOHOLIC LIVER DISEASE

DEFINITION

Excessive alcoholic consumption (Chapter 32) causes alcoholic liver disease and can significantly worsen other liver disorders such as viral hepatitis (Chapter 151) and hemochromatosis (Chapter 219). Although most individuals who consume alcohol do not consume it excessively and do not develop any physical or social consequences, some alcoholics consume sufficient alcohol and, presumably owing to other predisposing factors, develop alcoholic liver disease. Alcoholic liver disease is a spectrum of chronic liver diseases, ranging from alcoholic fatty liver to alcoholic hepatitis and cirrhosis.

Alcoholic fatty liver disease will develop in nearly 90% of individuals who consume alcohol heavily (on average, >6 drinks per day), and some individuals develop the more severe conditions of alcoholic hepatitis and alcoholic cirrhosis. Nearly 50% of the patients with alcoholic hepatitis have preexisting cirrhosis (Chapter 156), and individuals who do not yet have cirrhosis are at high risk for developing it, especially if they continue to consume alcohol.

EPIDEMIOLOGY

The true prevalence of alcoholic liver disease is not known, but nearly 1% of North American adults are believed to have alcoholic liver disease. Even this figure is considered an underestimation because milder forms of alcoholic liver disease are asymptomatic and often unrecognized. It has been estimated that alcoholic liver disease accounts for 40% of deaths from cirrhosis and 28% of all deaths from liver disease. It is the second most common indication for liver transplantation in the United States once abstinence from alcohol has been established.

PATHOBIOLOGY

The mechanisms underlying alcoholic liver injury can be broadly categorized into those caused by the effects of alcohol directly on hepatocytes and those caused by the effects mediated by Kupffer cells. The hepatocyte mechanisms include the altered redox state induced by alcohol and aldehyde dehydrogenase reactions, the oxidative stress and lipid peroxidation caused by the induction of CYP2E1 enzymes and the mitochondrial electron transfer system, and the effects of alcohol on the nuclear transcription factors (AMP kinase and SREBP-1c), protein adduct formation, and altered methionine and folate metabolism with resulting endoplasmic reticulum stress. Chronic alcohol consumption increases gut permeability, and the resulting portal endotoxemia activates Kupffer cells. Activated Kupffer cells release a number of proinflammatory mediators, including tumor necrosis factor-α (TNF-α), transforming growth factor-β1 (TGF-β1), interleukins 1, 6, 8, and 10, and platelet-derived growth factor (PDGF). TNF-α has plethora of biologic effects and causes hepatocyte apoptosis, whereas TGF-β1 and PDGF play important roles in stellate cell activation, collagen production, and hepatic fibrosis.

Among the known risk factors for developing alcoholic liver disease (Table 155-2), the amount of alcohol consumed is the single most important. For

TABLE 155-1 COMMON CAUSES OF MACROVESICULAR AND MICROVESICULAR STEATOSIS

MACROVESICULAR STEATOSIS	MICROVESICULAR STEATOSIS
Obesity, type 2 diabetes, metabolic syndrome, and dyslipidemia (nonalcoholic fatty liver disease)	Reye's syndrome
	Medications (valproate, antiretroviral medicines, intravenous tetracycline)
Excessive alcohol consumption	Heat stroke
Hepatitis C (genotype 3)	Acute fatty liver of pregnancy
Wilson's disease	HELLP syndrome
Lipodystrophy	Inborn errors of metabolism (lecithin-cholesterol acyltransferase deficiency, cholesterol ester storage disease, Wolman's disease)
Starvation	
Jejunoileal bypass	
Parenteral nutrition	
Abetalipoproteinemia	
Medications (amiodarone, methotrexate, tamoxifen, corticosteroids, antipsychotics)	

HELLP = hemolysis, elevated liver enzymes, and low platelets.

TABLE 155-2 RISK FACTORS FOR ALCOHOLIC LIVER DISEASE AND NONALCOHOLIC FATTY LIVER DISEASE (NAFLD)

ALCOHOLIC LIVER DISEASE	NAFLD
MAJOR	**MAJOR**
Amount and duration of alcohol consumption	Obesity
Female gender	Type 2 diabetes
Genetic factors	Dyslipidemia
Protein-calorie malnutrition	Metabolic syndrome
MINOR	**MINOR**
Type of beverage	Polycystic ovary syndrome
Binge drinking	Hypothyroidism
Obesity	Sleep apnea
African-American and Hispanic ethnicity	Hypopituitarism

FIGURE 155-1. Dupuytren's contracture. (From Gudmundsson KG, Jonsson T, Arngrims-son R. Guillame Dupuytren and finger contractures. Lancet. 2003;362:165-168.)

unclear reasons, only 30 to 35% of individuals with heavy and long-term drinking develop alcoholic hepatitis, and less than 20% develop cirrhosis. Women are at higher risk; for example, the risk of alcoholic cirrhosis increases after 10 years of alcohol consumption at quantities of more than 60 to 80 g/day in men, whereas in women, it can develop at quantities of only more than 20 g/day. Moreover, the peak incidence of alcoholic liver disease in women is approximately a decade earlier than in men. The type of alcoholic beverage consumed may not be as critical, but "spirits" and beer may be more hepatotoxic than wine. African-American and Hispanic ethnic groups may be predisposed to more significant alcoholic liver injury. Both obesity and protein-calorie malnutrition, in which micronutrients and antioxidant capacity are diminished, also are important predispositions.

Polymorphisms in genes associated with alcohol metabolism (alcohol and aldehyde dehydrogenases and cytochrome P-450 enzymes) and dysregulated cytokine production (e.g., TNF-α) may also influence genetic susceptibility. In patients with other forms of chronic liver disease (e.g., viral hepatitis B or C), concomitant alcohol consumption significantly aggravates liver injury.

CLINICAL MANIFESTATIONS

Patients with alcoholic liver disease may have signs and symptoms from underlying alcoholism as well as those caused by liver disease. Stigmata of chronic alcoholism include palmar erythema (see Fig. 148-2 in Chapter 148), spider nevi, bilateral gynecomastia, testicular atrophy, bilateral parotid enlargement, and Dupuytren's contractures (Fig. 155-1). The clinical features of liver disease will depend on the stage of alcoholic liver disease, that is, whether a patient has alcoholic fatty liver or more advanced liver disease such as alcoholic hepatitis and cirrhosis.

Patients with alcoholic fatty liver disease are generally asymptomatic, but some patients may have anorexia, fatigue, right upper quadrant discomfort, and tender hepatomegaly. These patients may also have biochemical evidence of alcoholism and alcoholic liver disease with macrocytosis as well as elevated levels of aspartate aminotransferase (AST) and γ-glutamyl transpeptidase (GGT). Patients with alcoholic fatty liver typically do not have jaundice, ascites, or splenomegaly.

Patients with alcoholic hepatitis may have a more dramatic presentation with severe malaise, fatigue, anorexia, fever, evidence of protein-calorie malnutrition, and features of decompensated liver disease, including jaundice, coagulopathy, ascites, and encephalopathy. Physical examination invariably shows at least some features of chronic alcoholism, and jaundice (see Fig. 148-1 in Chapter 148), ascites (see Fig. 148-5 in Chapter 148), and splenomegaly are common. The laboratory examination is typically abnormal. Common hematologic abnormalities include leukocytosis with neutrophil predominance, macrocytic anemia (Chapter 167), thrombocytopenia (Chapter 175), and a prolonged prothrombin time. Liver biochemistries (Chapter 149) are abnormal with an elevated AST and ratio of AST to alanine transferase (ALT), alkaline phosphatase, GGT, and total bilirubin, but decreased levels of serum albumin. The AST rarely exceeds 300 IU/L. Serum electrolyte abnormalities including hypokalemia (Chapter 119), hypomagnesemia (Chapter 121), hypocalcemia (Chapter 253), and hypophosphatemia (Chapter 121) are frequent. Patients with alcoholic cirrhosis have the same clinical features that are common to other types of cirrhosis (Chapter 156), but also with striking features of underlying chronic alcoholism.

DIAGNOSIS

The diagnosis of alcoholic liver disease strongly depends on the history of excessive alcohol consumption and the presence of liver disease. Although laboratory abnormalities are not specific for alcoholic liver disease, they can be quite suggestive in the context of excessive alcohol consumption. An AST/ALT ratio of more than 2 is typical in alcoholic liver disease, and ALT values greater than 150 to 200 IU/L are very rare in alcoholic liver disease. Serology testing for co-existing chronic viral hepatitis (Chapter 151) is critical. Diagnostic dilemmas arise when a patient denies excessive alcohol consumption in the face of clinical features that are suggestive of alcoholic liver disease. Interviewing family members regarding specific alcohol consumption may be helpful in the accurate ascertainment of alcohol consumption. Elevated blood levels of carbohydrate-deficient transferrin, which is a form of transferrin with fewer than the four sialic acid chains present in normal transferrin, can identify recent heavy alcohol consumption. Hepatic imaging by ultrasound, computed tomography (CT), or magnetic resonance imaging (MRI) will show changes consistent with hepatic steatosis or more advanced forms of liver disease, such as alcoholic hepatitis and cirrhosis. Imaging is also important to exclude other forms of liver disease, including malignancy and biliary obstruction. Imaging findings specific for alcoholic liver disease include an enlarged caudate lobe, greater visualization of the right posterior hepatic notch, and focal fat sparing or geographic fat distribution.

Because specific treatment for alcoholic hepatitis may be harmful in patients with other liver diseases, it is very important to exclude other predominant or coexisting liver diseases, including chronic viral hepatitis (Chapter 151) and drug-induced liver injury, especially from acetaminophen (Chapter 152), by history, blood tests, and biopsy if needed. Hyperferritinemia generally reflects an acute phase reactant, rather than an iron overload disorder, so it usually will return to normal when the acute liver injury resolves.

Liver biopsy is the key to precisely characterizing the nature of alcoholic liver disease and determining whether a patient has fatty liver or more advanced alcoholic hepatitis. Histologic features of alcoholic fatty liver include macrovesicular steatosis that is predominantly zone 3 in nature. In alcoholic hepatitis, the biopsy is more striking and reveals macrovesicular steatosis, lobular neutrophilic infiltration, Mallory's hyaline, balloon degeneration of the hepatocytes, and perivenular fibrosis. In general, patients with alcoholic hepatitis also have histologic evidence of chronic liver injury in the form of more advanced fibrosis (periportal or bridging fibrosis, or cirrhosis).

TREATMENT   Rx

Total abstinence, which is the most important treatment measure, is mandatory for the improvement of the clinical and histologic features of alcoholic liver disease. Its benefits are unequivocal, even in patients with severe decompensation. However, long-term abstinence is difficult to achieve, so a multidisciplinary approach with counseling and medications that promote abstinence should be considered. Disulfiram is not commonly used owing to its poor tolerability and hepatotoxicity. Opioid antagonists, such as naltrexone (50 mg/day for up to 6 months or even longer), nalmefene (20 mg/day as maintenance), and acamprosate (333 mg tablets, 2 tablets three times each day for 1 year) can help promote abstinence when used as part of a multidisciplinary approach (Chapter 32).

Alcoholic fatty liver disease requires no specific treatment other than abstinence. Patients with alcoholic hepatitis, however, have increased short- and long-term mortality and should be considered for therapeutic interventions in addition to mandatory abstinence. If a patient's liver biopsy is consistent with alcoholic hepatitis and there is no evidence of other inflammatory liver diseases, such as hepatitis C (Chapter 151), corticosteroids and pentoxifylline (400 mg three times daily for 28 days) are of some benefit.**[1,2]** Prednisolone (40 mg per day for 4 weeks) should be given to carefully selected patients who have a score of greater than 32 on Maddrey's discriminant function (4.6 × [patient's prothrombin time—control prothrombin time] + total bilirubin level) and encephalopathy, but do not have gastrointestinal bleeding or systemic infection. Recent studies suggested that a Model for End-Stage Liver Disease (MELD) score (see Table 156-2 in Chapter 156) higher than 21 can substitute for Maddrey's score for guiding the use of prednisolone. Two other anti-TNF-α agents, infliximab and etanercept, are not effective and have significant side effects. All patients with alcoholic hepatitis and alcoholic cirrhosis should be assessed and treated for protein-calorie malnutrition and micronutrient deficiency. Hospitalized patients with severe decompensation should be considered for enteral nutrition (Chapter 223).

Complications such as ascites, spontaneous bacterial peritonitis, encephalopathy, variceal bleeding, hepatorenal syndrome, osteoporosis, and hepatopulmonary syndrome may occur in patients with decompensated alcoholic cirrhosis and must be managed carefully (Chapter 156). Liver transplantation is a reasonable option in patients with decompensated alcoholic cirrhosis, but 6 months of abstinence and strong social support are generally required for eligibility (Chapter 157). Patients with alcoholic cirrhosis are at risk for hepatocellular carcinoma (Chapter 202) and should be screened with semiannual liver imaging and serum α-fetoprotein levels. They are also at risk for extrahepatic malignancy, notably head and neck, lung, and esophageal cancer. For Dupuytren's contracture, injection of collagenase clostridium histolyticum can reduce the severity and improve the range of motion significantly.3

PROGNOSIS

Alcoholic fatty liver is generally reversible with total abstinence for a few months. Alcoholic hepatitis carries high mortality, with nearly 40% of patients dying within 6 months after its presentation.

NONALCOHOLIC FATTY LIVER DISEASE

DEFINITIONS

Histologically, NAFLD resembles alcoholic liver disease, but it occurs in individuals without significant alcohol consumption. Average alcohol consumption greater than two drinks per day in men and greater than one drink per day in women generally is not consistent with a diagnosis of NAFLD. In addition, the definition of NAFLD excludes patients with a history of exposure to steatogenic medications such as amiodarone, methotrexate, and tamoxifen.

NAFLD encompasses a spectrum of abnormal liver histology, ranging from simple steatosis to nonalcoholic steatohepatitis (NASH) and cirrhosis. In simple steatosis, liver histology reveals macrovesicular steatosis without ballooning degeneration of hepatocytes or liver fibrosis. NASH, which is a more advanced form of NAFLD, is histologically characterized by macrovesicular steatosis, ballooning degeneration of the hepatocytes, and sinusoidal fibrosis.

EPIDEMIOLOGY

NAFLD is one of the most common causes of elevated liver enzymes and chronic liver disease in the Western world. Its incidence in adults and children is rising rapidly owing to the ongoing epidemics of obesity (Chapter 227), type 2 diabetes mellitus (Chapter 237), and metabolic syndrome. Its prevalence is quite high in certain patient populations; for example, nearly 80% of type 2 diabetic patients and 90% of morbidly obese individuals have imaging evidence of NAFLD. Nearly one third of U.S. adults are estimated to have NAFLD, and up to 5% of U.S. adults may have NASH. These percentages compare reasonably well with other data suggesting that the prevalence of cirrhosis from NAFLD is about 2%. Hispanics and whites are at higher risk for NAFLD, whereas its prevalence is intriguingly quite low in African Americans.

PATHOBIOLOGY

The major risk factors for NAFLD include obesity, type 2 diabetes mellitus, metabolic syndrome, and dyslipidemia (see Table 155-2). Other comorbidities associated with NAFLD include polycystic ovary syndrome (Chapter 243), hypothyroidism (Chapter 233), hypopituitarism (Chapter 231), and sleep apnea (Chapter 100).

Two fundamental defects in NAFLD are insulin resistance/hyperinsulinemia and excessive levels of nonesterified fatty liver within the hepatocytes. An excessive influx of nonesterified fatty acids into the hepatocytes results in macrovesicular steatosis, which is predominantly centrilobular in location.

Additionally, patients with NAFLD have increased de novo intrahepatic lipogenesis. Although patients with NAFLD robustly esterify free fatty acids in neutral triglycerides, free fatty acids within the hepatocytes are considered the primary mediators of cell injury (lipotoxicity). In the background of hepatic steatosis, factors that promote cell injury, inflammation, and fibrosis include oxidative stress, endoplasmic reticulum stress, apoptosis, adipocytokines, and stellate cell activation. The sources of oxidative stress include mitochondria and microsomes. Adipocytokines that play an important role in the pathogenesis of NAFLD include adiponectin and TNF-α. It is unclear why some patients with NAFLD exhibit NASH, whereas other patients with a comparable risk factor profile have only simple steatosis. There is a consistent and significant relationship of PNPLA3 genetic polymorphisms with the severity of steatosis and other histologic features of NAFLD. However, the genetic factors that play a role in NASH and NAFLD have not been fully elucidated.

CLINICAL MANIFESTATIONS

NAFLD is often asymptomatic but may rarely cause fatigue and right upper quadrant pain. Physical examination may reveal hepatomegaly, palmar erythema (see Fig. 148-2 in Chapter 148), and spider nevi. If liver disease is advanced, the features of liver failure, such as ascites, encephalopathy, and abdominal collateral vessels, are present. Simple steatosis is benign with a minimal risk of cirrhosis, whereas NASH is progressive and can lead to cirrhosis (Chapter 156) and liver failure (Chapter 157). In up to 20% of patients with NASH, liver histology will worsen and cirrhosis will develop over a 10- to 15-year period. Severe obesity, advancing age, and diabetes are believed to be risk factors for disease progression. Disease progression during the early phase can be identified only with a repeat liver biopsy, but in later stages, the signs and symptoms of portal hypertension (e.g., abdominal collateral vessels and low platelet count) indicate the development of cirrhosis. Patients with NASH-induced cirrhosis are at risk of developing hepatocellular carcinoma (Chapter 202). Patients with NAFLD have several metabolic risks that predispose them to atherosclerosis, and coronary artery disease is the single most common cause of death in patients with NAFLD.

DIAGNOSIS

NAFLD is generally suspected when aminotransferase levels are asymptomatically elevated in an individual with metabolic risk factors (obesity and diabetes) or when liver imaging (ultrasound, CT, or MRI) obtained for another reason shows fatty infiltration (Fig. 155-2). The diagnosis of NAFLD requires that there is no history of previous or ongoing significant alcohol consumption, no exposure to steatogenic medications, and no evidence of other causes of liver disease, such as viral hepatitis B or C. Elevated levels of aminotransferases, although common, are not required for the diagnosis of NAFLD. In contrast to alcoholic liver disease, ALT levels are higher than AST levels, but they rarely exceed 250 IU/L. In general, AST and ALT levels do not have diagnostic or prognostic significance. Mild hyperferritinemia is common and should not be confused with hereditary hemochromatosis (Chapter 219). Similarly, low-grade autoantibody (antinuclear antibody, anti–smooth muscle antibody) positivity is not uncommon and should not be confused with autoimmune liver disease (Chapter 151). Because steatosis is common in patients with Wilson's disease (Chapter 218), serum ceruloplasmin should be obtained as part of the diagnostic evaluation.

Fatty liver on ultrasonogram has a positive predictive value of only 77% and a negative predictive value of only 67% when compared with liver biopsy. Abdominal MRI is more accurate, but its high cost limits its usefulness in routine practice. Because none of these three tests can differentiate simple steatosis from NASH nor identify cirrhosis until hepatic fibrosis has caused overt portal hypertension, liver biopsy is required to establish the presence of NASH or cirrhosis. Common indications for a percutaneous liver biopsy

FIGURE 155-2. Magnetic resonance image of chronic liver disease due to nonalcoholic fatty liver disease. Out-of-phase T1-weighted images show focal fat infiltration of varying shapes in right lobe (*white arrows*) and left lobe (*black arrow*). (Courtesy of Professor Kumar Sandrasegaran, Indiana University School of Medicine, Indianapolis, Ind.)

FIGURE 155-3. Liver biopsy showing nonalcoholic steatohepatitis, with increased fat and with early cirrhosis. (Courtesy of the NASH Clinical Research Network.)

in patients with NAFLD include persistently high aminotransferase levels, inability to exclude a competing or a coexisting cause (e.g., iron overload or autoimmune liver disease), or clinical suspicion of severe liver disease. In patients with NASH, liver histology shows steatosis, inflammation, ballooning, and fibrosis (Fig. 155-3).

TREATMENT Rx

Lifestyle modification with dietary restriction and regular exercise is the first choice of treatment for NAFLD. It is generally recommended that patients with NAFLD lose 10% of their body weight in a gradual fashion, but this goal is difficult to achieve. If resources are available, a multidisciplinary approach with behavioral therapy, dietary advice, and monitoring by a professional nutritionist and an exercise expert is more successful than a prescriptive approach.[4]

Statins (e.g., atorvastatin 20 mg daily) with or without vitamins C and E can improve liver test results and reduce subsequent NAFLD.[5,6] In a large trial, 800 IU of vitamin E administered daily for 2 years significantly improved liver histology.[7] Thiazolidinedione insulin sensitizers (pioglitazone and rosiglitazone) improve steatosis, inflammation, and ballooning, but may not improve fibrosis.[8] Unfortunately, the weight gain that is common with thiazolidinediones may offset the histologic benefits that they offer. In morbidly obese individuals with NASH and other significant metabolic comorbidities, foregut bariatric surgery can lead to significant improvement in hepatic histology, but the physician must exclude the presence of portal hypertension before offering this type of surgery.[9] Patients with NAFLD often have dyslipidemia that puts them at excessive risk for coronary artery disease; their dyslipidemia (Chapter 213) should be treated aggressively with statins and other lipid-lowering agents, which can be safely administered to patients with NAFLD and NASH. Carefully selected patients with decompensated cirrhosis owing to NASH can be treated with liver transplantation (Chapter 157), but recurrence during the post-transplantation period is common.

PREVENTION

The measures to prevent NAFLD include maintaining optimal body weight, exercising regularly, and treating any associated metabolic comorbidities such as diabetes and dyslipidemia. Avoidance of saturated fat, high fructose intake, and alcohol consumption may reduce the development of NAFLD.

PROGNOSIS

Steatosis alone is generally benign, whereas steatohepatitis is often progressive. Otherwise, however, data are sparse regarding the risk and risk factors for the progression of NAFLD and NASH to cirrhosis and liver failure.

Because NAFLD often coexists with one or more components of the metabolic syndrome, its presence reflects guarded long-term overall prognosis. The long-term complications in patients with simple steatosis generally result from cardiovascular disease and atherosclerosis, not from liver failure.

Patients with NASH also are at risk for liver failure and liver cancer, in addition to their significantly increased risk of cardiovascular disease. For example, among patients with NASH on their initial biopsy, one third or more develop progressive fibrosis over a mean follow-up interval of about 5 years. Older age, diabetes, and ballooning and fibrosis on liver biopsy are important predictors of progression.

Grade A

1. Whitfield K, Rambaldi A, Wetterslev J, et al. Pentoxifylline for alcoholic hepatitis. *Cochrane Database Syst Rev.* 2009;4:CD007339.
2. De BK, Gangopadhyay S, Dutta D, et al. Pentoxifylline versus prednisolone for severe alcoholic hepatitis: a randomized controlled trial. *World J Gastroenterol.* 2009;15:1613-1619.
3. Hurst LC, Badalamente MA, Hentz VR, et al. Injectable collagenase clostridium histolyticum for Dupuytren's contracture. *N Engl J Med.* 2009;361:968-979.
4. Promrat K, Kleiner DE, Niemeier HM, et al. Randomized controlled trial testing the effects of weight loss on nonalcoholic steatohepatitis (NASH). *Hepatology.* 2010;51:121-129.
5. Athyros VG, Tziomalos K, Gossios TD, et al. Safety and efficacy of long-term statin treatment for cardiovascular events in patients with coronary heart disease and abnormal liver tests in the Greek Atorvastatin and Coronary Heart Disease Evaluation (GREACE) study: a post-hoc analysis. *Lancet.* 2010;376:1916-1922.
6. Foster T, Budoff MJ, Saab S, et al. Atorvastatin and antioxidants for the treatment of nonalcoholic fatty liver disease: the St. Francis Heart Study randomized clinical trial. *Am J Gastroenterol.* 2011;106:71-77.
7. Sanyal AJ, Chalasani N, Kowdley KV, et al. Pioglitazone, vitamin E, or placebo for nonalcoholic steatohepatitis. *N Engl J Med.* 2010;362:1675-1685.
8. Musso G, Gambino R, Cassader M, et al. A meta-analysis of randomized trials for the treatment of nonalcoholic fatty liver disease. *Hepatology.* 2010;52:79-104.
9. Mummadi RR, Kasturi KS, Chennareddygari S, et al. Effect of bariatric surgery on nonalcoholic fatty liver disease: systematic review and meta-analysis. *Clin Gastroenterol Hepatol.* 2008;6:1396-1402.

SUGGESTED READINGS

Beier JI, Arteel GE, McClain CJ. Advances in alcoholic liver disease. *Curr Gastroenterol Rep.* 2011;13:56-64. *Review.*
Dowman JK, Tomlinson JW, Newsome PN. Systematic review: the diagnosis and staging of non-alcoholic fatty liver disease and non-alcoholic steatohepatitis. *Aliment Pharmacol Ther.* 2011;33:525-540. *Review.*
Lucey MR, Mathurin P, Morgan TR. Alcoholic hepatitis. *N Engl J Med.* 2009;360:2758-2769. *A state-of-the-art review of pathogenesis, clinical features, and treatment of the alcoholic hepatitis.*
O'Shea RS, Dasarathy S, McCullough AJ, for the Practice Guideline Committee of the American Association for the Study of Liver Diseases and the Practice Parameters Committee of the American College of Gastroenterology. Alcoholic liver disease. *Hepatology.* 2010;51:307-328. *Comprehensive guidelines for the practicing physician.*

156

CIRRHOSIS AND ITS SEQUELAE

GUADALUPE GARCIA-TSAO

DEFINITION

Cirrhosis, which can be the final stage of any chronic liver disease, is a diffuse process characterized by fibrosis and conversion of normal architecture to structurally abnormal nodules (Fig. 156-1). These "regenerative" nodules lack normal lobular organization and are surrounded by fibrous tissue. The process involves the whole liver and is essentially irreversible. Although cirrhosis is histologically an "all or nothing" diagnosis, clinically it can be classified by its status as compensated or decompensated. Decompensated cirrhosis is defined by the presence of ascites, variceal bleeding, encephalopathy, or jaundice, which are complications that result from the main consequences of cirrhosis: portal hypertension and liver insufficiency.

EPIDEMIOLOGY

Because many patients with cirrhosis are asymptomatic until decompensation occurs, it is very difficult to assess the real prevalence and incidence of cirrhosis in the general population. The prevalence of chronic liver disease or cirrhosis worldwide is estimated to be 100 (range, 25 to 400) per 100,000 subjects, but it varies widely by country and by region.

Cirrhosis is an important cause of morbidity and mortality worldwide and in the United States. According to the World Health Organization, about 800,000 people die of cirrhosis annually. In the United States, cirrhosis accounts for about 27,500 deaths each year, or a death rate of 9.3 per 100,000, making it the 12th leading cause of death overall. Importantly, chronic liver disease and cirrhosis are the seventh leading cause of death in the United States in individuals between 25 and 64 years of age. Because chronic liver disease affects people in their most productive years of life, it has a significant impact on the economy as a result of premature death, illness, and disability.

Any chronic liver disease can lead to cirrhosis (Table 156-1). Chronic viral hepatitis C and alcoholic liver disease are the most common causes of

FIGURE 156-1. Gross and microscopic images of a normal and cirrhotic liver. **A,** Gross image of a normal liver with a smooth surface and homogeneous texture. **B,** Microscopically, liver sinusoids are organized, and vascular structures are normally distributed. **C,** Gross image of a cirrhotic liver. The liver has an orange-tawny color with an irregular surface and a nodular texture. **D,** Microscopically, the architecture is disorganized, and there are regenerative nodules surrounded by fibrous tissue.

TABLE 156-1 CAUSES OF CIRRHOSIS

MAIN FACTORS CAUSING CIRRHOSIS

Chronic hepatitis C
Alcoholic liver disease
Nonalcoholic fatty liver disease
Chronic hepatitis B

OTHER CAUSES OF CIRRHOSIS (<2% OF ALL CASES)

Cholestatic and autoimmune liver diseases
    Primary biliary cirrhosis
    Primary sclerosing cholangitis
    Autoimmune hepatitis
Intrahepatic or extrahepatic biliary obstruction
    Mechanical obstruction
    Biliary atresia
    Cystic fibrosis
Metabolic disorders
    Hemochromatosis
    Wilson's disease
    α_1-Antitrypsin deficiency
    Glycogen storage diseases
    Abetalipoproteinemia
    Porphyria
Hepatic venous outflow obstruction
    Budd-Chiari syndrome
    Veno-occlusive disease
    Right-sided heart failure
Drugs and toxins
Intestinal bypass
Indian childhood cirrhosis

cirrhosis, followed by nonalcoholic fatty liver disease and chronic hepatitis B (Chapters 151 and 155). However, the many other causes of cirrhosis include cholestatic and autoimmune liver diseases such as primary biliary cirrhosis, primary sclerosing cholangitis (Chapter 158), autoimmune hepatitis (Chapter 151), and metabolic diseases such as hemochromatosis, Wilson's disease, and α_1-antitrypsin deficiency (Chapter 153). When all the causes have been investigated and excluded, cirrhosis is considered "cryptogenic." Many cases of cryptogenic cirrhosis are now thought to be due to nonalcoholic fatty liver disease (Chapter 155).

It is important to mention that although the entity termed *primary biliary cirrhosis* assumes the presence of cirrhosis, this term is actually misleading. Primary biliary cirrhosis (Chapter 158) is an immune-mediated cholestatic chronic liver disease that is characterized by progressive destruction of intrahepatic bile ducts and progresses over time from an initial stage in which fibrosis is minimal (stage 1) to a final stage in which there is well-established cirrhosis (stage 4).

PATHOBIOLOGY

Liver Fibrosis/Cirrhosis

The key pathogenic feature underlying liver fibrosis and cirrhosis is activation of hepatic stellate cells. Hepatic stellate cells, which are known as *Ito cells* or *perisinusoidal cells*, are located in the space of Disse between hepatocytes and sinusoidal endothelial cells. Normally, hepatic stellate cells are quiescent and serve as the main storage site for retinoids (vitamin A). In response to injury, hepatic stellate cells become activated, as a result of which they lose their vitamin A deposits, proliferate, develop a prominent rough endoplasmic reticulum, and secrete extracellular matrix (collagen types I and III, sulfated proteoglycans, and glycoproteins). Additionally, they become contractile hepatic myofibroblasts.

Unlike other capillaries, normal hepatic sinusoids lack a basement membrane. The sinusoidal endothelial cells themselves contain large fenestrae (100 to 200 nm in diameter) that allow the passage of large molecules with molecular weights up to 250,000. Collagen deposition in the space of Disse,

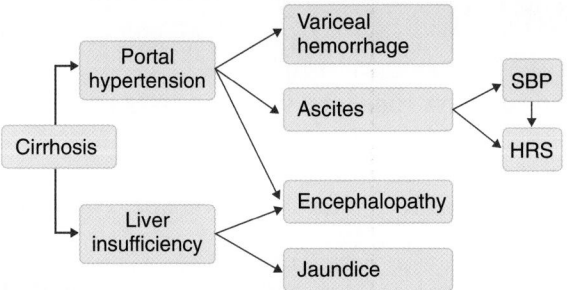

FIGURE 156-2. Complications of cirrhosis result from portal hypertension or liver insufficiency. Varices and variceal hemorrhage are a direct consequence of portal hypertension. Ascites results from sinusoidal portal hypertension and can be complicated by infection (spontaneous bacterial peritonitis [SBP]) or renal dysfunction (hepatorenal syndrome [HRS]). Hepatic encephalopathy results from portosystemic shunting (i.e., portal hypertension) and liver insufficiency. Jaundice results solely from liver insufficiency.

as occurs in cirrhosis, leads to defenestration of the sinusoidal endothelial cells ("capillarization" of the sinusoids), thereby altering exchange between plasma and hepatocytes and resulting in a decreased sinusoidal diameter that is further exacerbated by the contraction of stellate cells.

Complications of Cirrhosis

The two main consequences of cirrhosis are portal hypertension, with the accompanying hyperdynamic circulatory state, and liver insufficiency (Fig. 156-2). The development of varices and ascites is a direct consequence of portal hypertension and the hyperdynamic circulatory state, whereas jaundice occurs as a result of an inability of the liver to excrete bilirubin (i.e., liver insufficiency). Encephalopathy is the result of both portal hypertension and liver insufficiency. Ascites, in turn, can become complicated by infection, which is called *spontaneous bacterial peritonitis,* and by functional renal failure, which is called *hepatorenal syndrome.*

Portal Hypertension and the Hyperdynamic Circulatory State

In cirrhosis, portal hypertension results from both an increase in resistance to portal flow and an increase in portal venous inflow. The initial mechanism is increased sinusoidal vascular resistance secondary to (1) deposition of fibrous tissue and subsequent compression by regenerative nodules (fixed component) and (2) active vasoconstriction (functional component), which is amenable to the action of vasodilators such as nitroprusside and is caused by a deficiency in intrahepatic nitric oxide (NO), as well as enhanced activity of vasoconstrictors.

Early in the portal hypertensive process, the spleen grows and sequesters platelets and other formed blood cells, thereby leading to hypersplenism. In addition, vessels that normally drain into the portal system, such as the coronary vein, reverse their flow and shunt blood away from the portal system to the systemic circulation. These portosystemic collaterals are insufficient to decompress the portal venous system and offer additional resistance to portal flow. As collaterals develop, an increase in portal blood inflow maintains the portal hypertensive state as a result of splanchnic vasodilation, which in turn is secondary to increased production of NO. Thus, the paradox in portal hypertension is that a deficiency of NO in the intrahepatic vasculature leads to vasoconstriction and increased resistance, whereas overproduction of NO in the extrahepatic circulation leads to vasodilation and increased flow.

In addition to splanchnic vasodilation, there is systemic vasodilation, which by causing a decreased *effective* arterial blood volume, leads to activation of neurohumoral systems (renin-angiotensin-aldosterone system), retention of sodium, expansion of plasma volume, and development of a hyperdynamic circulatory state. This hyperdynamic circulatory state maintains portal hypertension, thereby leading to the formation and growth of varices, and plays an important role in the development of all other complications of cirrhosis.

Varices and Variceal Hemorrhage

The complication of cirrhosis that results most directly from portal hypertension is the development of portal-systemic collaterals, the most relevant of which are those that form through dilation of the coronary and gastric veins and constitute gastroesophageal varices. The initial formation of esophageal collaterals depends on a threshold portal pressure, clinically established by a hepatic venous pressure gradient of 10 to 12 mm Hg, below which varices do not develop.

Development of a hyperdynamic circulatory state leads to further dilation and growth of varices and eventually to their rupture and variceal hemorrhage, one of the most dreaded complications of portal hypertension. Tension in a varix determines variceal rupture and is directly proportional to variceal diameter and intravariceal pressure and inversely proportional to variceal wall thickness.

Ascites and Hepatorenal Syndrome

Ascites in cirrhosis is secondary to sinusoidal hypertension and retention of sodium. Cirrhosis leads to sinusoidal hypertension by blocking hepatic venous outflow both anatomically by fibrosis and regenerative nodules and functionally by increased postsinusoidal vascular tone. Similar to the formation of esophageal varices, a threshold hepatic venous pressure gradient of 12 mm Hg is needed for the formation of ascites. In addition, retention of sodium replenishes the intravascular volume and allows the continuous formation of ascites. Retention of sodium results from vasodilation that is mostly due to an increase in NO production because NO inhibition in experimental animals increases urinary sodium excretion, lowers plasma aldosterone levels, and reduces ascites. With progression of cirrhosis and portal hypertension, vasodilation is more pronounced, thereby leading to further activation of the renin-angiotensin-aldosterone and sympathetic nervous systems and resulting in further sodium retention (refractory ascites), water retention (hyponatremia), and renal vasoconstriction (hepatorenal syndrome).

Spontaneous Bacterial Peritonitis

Spontaneous bacterial peritonitis, an infection of ascitic fluid, occurs in the absence of perforation of a hollow viscus or an intra-abdominal inflammatory focus such as an abscess, acute pancreatitis, or cholecystitis. Bacterial translocation, or the migration of bacteria from the intestinal lumen to mesenteric lymph nodes and other extraintestinal sites, is the main mechanism implicated in spontaneous bacterial peritonitis. Impaired local and systemic immune defenses are a major element in promoting bacterial translocation and, together with shunting of blood away from the hepatic Kupffer cells through portosystemic collaterals, allow a transient bacteremia to become more prolonged, thereby colonizing ascitic fluid. Spontaneous bacterial peritonitis occurs in patients with reduced ascites defense mechanisms, such as a low complement level in ascitic fluid. Another factor that promotes bacterial translocation in cirrhosis is bacterial overgrowth attributed to a decrease in small bowel motility and intestinal transit time. Infections, particularly from gram-negative bacteria, can precipitate renal dysfunction through worsening of the hyperdynamic circulatory state.

Encephalopathy

Ammonia, a toxin normally removed by the liver, plays a key role in the pathogenesis of hepatic encephalopathy. In cirrhosis, ammonia accumulates in the systemic circulation because of shunting of blood through portosystemic collaterals and decreased liver metabolism (i.e., liver insufficiency). The presence of large amounts of ammonia in the brain damages supporting brain cells or astrocytes and leads to structural changes characteristic of hepatic encephalopathy (Alzheimer's type II astrocytosis). Ammonia results in upregulation of astrocytic peripheral-type benzodiazepine receptors, the most potent stimulants of neurosteroid production. Neurosteroids are the major modulators of γ-aminobutyric acid, which results in cortical depression and hepatic encephalopathy. Other toxins, such as manganese, also accumulate in the brain, particularly the globus pallidus, where they lead to impaired motor function. Other yet-to-be-elucidated toxins may also be involved in the pathogenesis of encephalopathy.

Jaundice

Jaundice (Chapter 149) in cirrhosis is a reflection of the inability of the liver to excrete bilirubin and is therefore the result of liver insufficiency. However, in cholestatic diseases leading to cirrhosis (e.g., primary biliary cirrhosis, primary sclerosing cholangitis, vanishing bile duct syndrome), jaundice is more likely due to biliary damage than liver insufficiency. Other indicators of liver insufficiency, such as the prothrombin time or the presence of encephalopathy, help determine the most likely contributor to hyperbilirubinemia (Chapter 149).

Cardiopulmonary Complications

The hyperdynamic circulatory state eventually results in high-output heart failure with decreased peripheral utilization of oxygen, a complication that

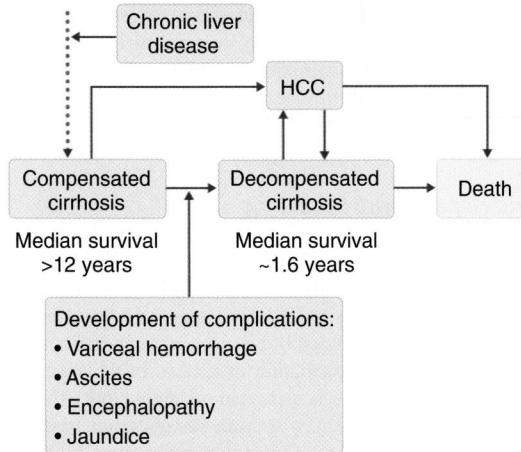

FIGURE 156-3. Natural history of cirrhosis. Any chronic liver disease will lead to cirrhosis. Initially, cirrhosis will be compensated (median survival, >12 years), but once complications (ascites, variceal hemorrhage, encephalopathy, jaundice) develop, it becomes decompensated (median survival, 1.6 years). Hepatocellular carcinoma (HCC) can develop at any stage and precipitate decompensation and death.

TABLE 156-2 THE TWO MOST COMMONLY USED SCORING SYSTEMS IN CIRRHOSIS

1. CHILD-TURCOTTE-PUGH (CTP) SCORE (RANGE, 5-15)

	Points Ascribed		
PARAMETERS	1	2	3
Ascites	None	Grade 1-2 (or easy to treat)	Grade 3-4 (or refractory)
Hepatic encephalopathy	None	Grade 1-2 (or induced by a precipitant)	Grade 3-4 (or spontaneous)
Bilirubin (mg/dL)	<2	2-3	>3
Albumin (g/dL)	>3.5	2.8-3.5	<2.8
Prothrombin time (seconds > control) or INR	<4 <1.7	4-6 1.7-2.3	>6 >2.3

CTP classification: Child A: score of 5-6; Child B: score of 7-9; Child C: score of 10-15

2. MODEL OF END-STAGE LIVER DISEASE (MELD) SCORE (RANGE, 6-40)

$$[0.957 \times LN \text{ (creatinine in mg/dL)} + 0.378 \times LN \text{ (bilirubin in mg/dL)} + 1.12 \times LN \text{ (INR)} + 0.643] \times 10$$

INR = international normalized ratio; LN = natural logarithm.

has been referred to as *cirrhotic cardiomyopathy.* Vasodilation at the level of the pulmonary circulation leads to arterial hypoxemia, the hallmark of hepatopulmonary syndrome. Normal pulmonary capillaries are 8 μm in diameter, and red blood cells (slightly less than 8 μm) pass through them one cell at a time, thereby facilitating oxygenation. In hepatopulmonary syndrome, the pulmonary capillaries are dilated up to 500 μm, so passage of red cells through the pulmonary capillaries may be many cells thick. As a result, a large number of red cells are not oxygenated, which causes the equivalent of a right-to-left shunt.

Conversely, portopulmonary hypertension occurs when the pulmonary bed is exposed to vasoconstrictive substances that may be produced in the splanchnic circulation and bypass metabolism by the liver; the initial result is reversible pulmonary hypertension. However, because these factors result in endothelial proliferation, vasoconstriction, in situ thrombosis, and obliteration of vessels, irreversible pulmonary hypertension ensues.

CLINICAL MANIFESTATIONS

The clinical manifestations of cirrhosis range widely, depending on the stage of cirrhosis, from an asymptomatic patient with no signs of chronic liver disease to a patient who is confused and jaundiced and has severe muscle wasting and ascites. The natural history of cirrhosis is characterized by an initial phase, termed *compensated* cirrhosis, followed by a rapidly progressive phase marked by the development of complications of portal hypertension or liver dysfunction (or both), termed *decompensated* cirrhosis (Fig. 156-3). In the compensated phase, portal pressure may be normal or below the threshold level identified for the development of varices or ascites. As the disease progresses, portal pressure increases and liver function decreases, thereby resulting in the development of ascites, portal hypertensive gastrointestinal (GI) bleeding, encephalopathy, and jaundice. The development of any of these complications marks the transition from a compensated to a decompensated phase. Progression to death may be accelerated by the development of other complications such as recurrent GI bleeding, renal impairment (refractory ascites, hepatorenal syndrome), hepatopulmonary syndrome, and sepsis (spontaneous bacterial peritonitis). The development of hepatocellular carcinoma (Chapter 202) may accelerate the course of the disease at any stage (see Fig. 156-3). Transition from a compensated to a decompensated stage occurs at a rate of approximately 5 to 7% per year. The median time to decompensation, or the time at which half the patients with compensated cirrhosis will become decompensated, is about 6 years.

Compensated Cirrhosis

In this stage, cirrhosis is mostly asymptomatic and is diagnosed either during the evaluation of chronic liver disease or fortuitously during routine physical examination, biochemical testing, imaging for other reasons, endoscopy showing gastroesophageal varices, or abdominal surgery in which a nodular liver is detected. Nonspecific fatigue, decreased libido, or sleep disturbances may be the only complaints. About 40% of patients with compensated cirrhosis have esophageal varices. Nonbleeding gastroesophageal varices are

asymptomatic, and their presence (without bleeding) does not denote decompensation.

Decompensated Cirrhosis

At this stage, there are signs of decompensation: ascites, variceal hemorrhage, jaundice, hepatic encephalopathy, or any combination of these findings. Ascites, which is the most frequent sign of decompensation, is present in 80% of patients with decompensated cirrhosis.

Variceal Hemorrhage

Gastroesophageal varices are present in approximately 50% of patients with newly diagnosed cirrhosis. The prevalence of varices correlates with the severity of liver disease and ranges from 40% in Child A cirrhotic patients (Table 156-2) to 85% in Child C cirrhotic patients.

Both the development of varices and the growth of small varices occur at a rate of 7 to 8% per year. The incidence of a first variceal hemorrhage in patients with small varices is about 5% per year, whereas medium and large varices bleed at a rate of approximately 15% per year. Large varices, severe liver disease, and red wale markings on varices are independent predictors of variceal hemorrhage. Bleeding from gastroesophageal varices can be manifested as overt hematemesis or melena, or both (Chapter 137).

Ascites and Hepatorenal Syndrome

Ascites is the most common cause of decompensation in cirrhosis and occurs at a rate of 7 to 10% per year. The most frequent symptoms associated with ascites are increased abdominal girth, which is often described by the patient as tightness of the belt or garments around the waist, and recent weight gain. When present in small to moderate amounts, ascites can be identified on examination by bulging flanks, flank dullness, and shifting dullness (Chapter 148).

Hepatorenal syndrome is a type of prerenal kidney injury that occurs in patients with cirrhosis and ascites. It is divided into two types based on clinical characteristics and prognosis. Type 1 hepatorenal syndrome is rapidly progressive *acute* kidney injury in which the rise in serum creatinine occurs within a 2-week period. Type 2 hepatorenal syndrome is more slowly progressive and associated with ascites that is refractory to diuretics. Patients with hepatorenal syndrome usually have tense ascites that responds poorly to diuretics, but no specific symptoms or signs typify this entity.

Spontaneous Bacterial Peritonitis

About one third of cirrhotic patients are admitted for or acquire bacterial infections during hospitalization, the most common being spontaneous bacterial peritonitis. The two most important predictors of the development of bacterial infection are the severity of liver disease and admission for GI hemorrhage. The most frequent clinical manifestations of spontaneous bacterial peritonitis are fever, jaundice, and abdominal pain. On physical examination, there is typically abdominal tenderness, with or without rebound tenderness, or ileus (or both). However, patients with spontaneous bacterial peritonitis may have just encephalopathy, acute kidney injury or evidence of shock. Up to one third of patients may be entirely asymptomatic.

Hepatic Encephalopathy

Hepatic encephalopathy, which is the neuropsychiatric manifestation of cirrhosis, occurs at a rate of approximately 2 to 3% per year. Hepatic encephalopathy associated with cirrhosis is of gradual onset and rarely fatal. Clinically, it is characterized by alterations in consciousness and behavior ranging from inversion of the sleep-wake pattern and forgetfulness (stage 1); to confusion, bizarre behavior, and disorientation (stage 2); to lethargy and profound disorientation (stage 3); to coma (stage 4). On physical examination, early stages may demonstrate only a distal tremor, but the hallmark of hepatic encephalopathy is the presence of asterixis (Chapter 157). Additionally, patients with hepatic encephalopathy may have sweet-smelling breath, a characteristic termed *fetor hepaticus*.

Pulmonary Complications

Hepatopulmonary syndrome is associated with exertional dyspnea, which can lead to extreme debilitation. Clubbing of the fingers, cyanosis, and vascular spiders may be seen on physical examination. Hepatopulmonary syndrome is present in approximately 5 to 10% of patients awaiting liver transplantation.

Portopulmonary hypertension is manifested as exertional dyspnea, syncope, and chest pain. On examination, an accentuated second sound and right ventricular heave are prominent (Chapter 68).

DIAGNOSIS

The diagnosis of cirrhosis should be considered in any patient with chronic liver disease. In asymptomatic patients with *compensated cirrhosis*, typical signs of cirrhosis may not be present, and the diagnosis may often require histologic confirmation by liver biopsy, which is the "gold standard" for the diagnosis of cirrhosis. In patients with symptoms or signs of chronic liver disease, however, the presence of cirrhosis can frequently be confirmed noninvasively by imaging studies without the need for liver biopsy.

Physical Examination

On physical examination, stigmata of cirrhosis consist of muscle atrophy, mainly involving the bitemporal muscle regions and the thenar and hypothenar eminences; spider angiomas, mostly on the trunk, face, and upper limbs; and palmar erythema involving the thenar and the hypothenar eminences and the tips of the fingers. Although muscular atrophy is a marker of liver insufficiency, spider angiomas and palmar erythema are markers of vasodilation and a hyperdynamic circulation. Males may have hair loss on the chest and abdomen, gynecomastia, and testicular atrophy. Petechiae and ecchymoses may be present as a result of thrombocytopenia or a prolonged prothrombin time. Dupuytren's contracture, which is a thickening of the palmar fascia, occurs mostly in alcoholic cirrhosis. A pathognomonic feature of cirrhosis is the finding on abdominal examination of a small right liver lobe, with a span of less than 7 cm on percussion, and a palpable left lobe that is nodular with increased consistency. Splenomegaly may also be present and is indicative of portal hypertension. Collateral circulation on the abdominal wall (caput medusae) may also develop as a consequence of portal hypertension. Absence of any of the aforementioned physical findings does not exclude cirrhosis.

Laboratory Tests

Laboratory test results suggestive of cirrhosis include even subtle abnormalities in serum levels of albumin or bilirubin or elevation of the international normalized ratio. The most sensitive and specific laboratory finding suggestive of cirrhosis in the setting of chronic liver disease is a low platelet count ($<150,000/mm^3$), which occurs as a result of portal hypertension and hypersplenism. Other serum markers that are often abnormal include levels of aspartate aminotransferase, γ-glutamyl transpeptidase, hyaluronic acid, α_2-macroglobulin, haptoglobin, tissue metalloproteinase inhibitor I, and apolipoprotein A. Although attempts have been made to use combinations of such markers to predict the presence of cirrhosis, none has sufficient sensitivity and specificity to be useful clinically.

Imaging Studies

Confirmatory imaging tests include computed tomography, ultrasound, and magnetic resonance imaging. Findings consistent with cirrhosis include a

FIGURE 156-4. Computed tomography in a patient with compensated cirrhosis. The liver parenchyma is heterogeneous, there is splenomegaly, and, importantly, there are portosystemic collaterals.

nodular contour of the liver, a small liver with or without hypertrophy of the left or caudate lobe, splenomegaly, and in particular, identification of intra-abdominal collateral vessels indicative of portal hypertension (Fig. 156-4). Transient elastography, a new noninvasive technique based on ultrasound wave propagation, measures liver stiffness and appears to be useful in the diagnosis of cirrhosis. Typical findings on any of these imaging studies, together with a compatible clinical picture, are indicative of the presence of cirrhosis. A liver biopsy then would not be required unless the degree of inflammation or other features require investigation.

In *decompensated cirrhosis*, detection of ascites, variceal bleeding, or encephalopathy in the setting of chronic liver disease essentially establishes the diagnosis of cirrhosis, so a liver biopsy is not necessary to establish the diagnosis. Patients with decompensated cirrhosis often exhibit malnutrition, more severe muscle wasting, more numerous vascular spiders, and hypotension and tachycardia as a result of the hyperdynamic circulatory state.

Portal Pressure Measurements

Direct measurements of portal pressure involve catheterization of the portal vein, are cumbersome, and may be associated with complications. Hepatic vein catheterization with measurement of wedged and free pressure is the simplest, safest, most reproducible, and most widely used method to indirectly measure portal pressure. Portal pressure measurements are expressed as the hepatic venous pressure gradient: the gradient between wedged hepatic venous pressure, which is a measure of sinusoidal pressure, and free hepatic or inferior vena cava pressure, which is used as an internal zero reference point. In a patient with clinical evidence of portal hypertension (e.g., varices), the hepatic venous pressure gradient is useful in the differential diagnosis of the cause of portal hypertension: it will be normal (3 to 5 mm Hg) in prehepatic causes of portal hypertension, such as portal vein thrombosis (Chapter 145), and in intrahepatic but presinusoidal causes, such as schistosomiasis (Chapter 363), but will be abnormal (≥6 mm Hg) in sinusoidal causes of portal hypertension, such as cirrhosis, and in postsinusoidal causes, such as veno-occlusive disease. A hepatic venous pressure gradient of 10 mm Hg or greater ("clinically significant" portal hypertension) predicts the development of complications of portal hypertension, and its reduction on pharmacologic therapy predicts a favorable outcome in patients with cirrhosis.

Complications of Cirrhosis
Varices and Variceal Hemorrhage

Upper GI endoscopy (Chapters 136) remains the main method for diagnosing varices and variceal hemorrhage. Varices are classified as small (straight, minimally elevated veins above the esophageal mucosal surface), medium (tortuous veins occupying less than one third of the esophageal lumen), or large (occupying more than one third of the esophageal lumen). The diagnosis of variceal hemorrhage is made when diagnostic esophagogastroduodenoscopy shows one of the following: active bleeding from a varix, a "white nipple" overlying a varix, clots overlying a varix, or varices with no other potential source of bleeding.

	TABLE 156-3	USING THE SERUM-ASCITES ALBUMIN GRADIENT AND THE ASCITES TOTAL PROTEIN LEVEL TO DIAGNOSE THE CAUSE OF ASCITES

CONDITION	SERUM-ASCITES ALBUMIN GRADIENT*	ASCITES TOTAL PROTEIN LEVEL†
Cirrhosis	High	Low
Malignant ascites	Low	High
Cardiac ascites	High	High

*High is greater than 1.1 g/dL; low is less than 1.1 g/dL.
†High is greater than 2.5 g/dL; low is less than 2.5 g/dL.

Ascites

The most common cause of ascites is cirrhosis, which accounts for 80% of cases. Peritoneal malignancy (e.g., peritoneal metastases from GI tumors or ovarian cancer), heart failure (Chapter 58), and peritoneal tuberculosis (Chapter 332) together account for another 15% of cases. The initial, most cost-effective, and least invasive method to confirm the presence of ascites is abdominal ultrasonography.

Diagnostic paracentesis is a safe procedure that should be performed in every patient with new-onset ascites, even in those with coagulopathy. Ultrasound guidance should be used in patients in whom percussion cannot locate the ascites or in whom a first paracentesis attempt does not yield fluid. The fluid in a patient with new-onset ascites should always be evaluated for albumin (with simultaneous estimation of serum albumin), total protein, polymorphonuclear (PMN) blood cell count, bacteriologic cultures, and cytology. The PMN cell count and bacteriologic culture are useful to exclude infection (either spontaneous or secondary bacterial peritonitis), and cytologic evaluation is needed if peritoneal carcinomatosis is suspected. Depending on the clinical setting, additional tests can be performed on the fluid: glucose and lactate dehydrogenase levels (if secondary bacterial peritonitis is suspected), smear and culture for acid-fast bacilli (if peritoneal tuberculosis is suspected), and an amylase level (if pancreatic ascites is suspected).

The serum-ascites albumin gradient and ascites protein levels are useful in the differential diagnosis of ascites (Table 156-3). The serum-ascites albumin gradient correlates with sinusoidal pressure and will therefore be elevated (>1.1 g/dL) in patients in whom the source of ascites is the hepatic sinusoid (e.g., cirrhosis or cardiac ascites). Protein levels in ascitic fluid are an indirect marker of the integrity of the hepatic sinusoids: normal sinusoids are permeable structures that "leak" protein, whereas sinusoids in cirrhosis are "capillarized" and do not leak as much protein. The three main causes of ascites—cirrhosis, peritoneal malignancy or tuberculosis, and heart failure—can easily be distinguished by combining the results of both the serum-ascites albumin gradient and ascites total protein content. Cirrhotic ascites typically has a high serum-ascites albumin gradient and low protein, cardiac ascites has a high serum-ascites albumin gradient and high protein, and ascites secondary to peritoneal malignancy typically has a low serum-ascites albumin gradient and high protein.

Hepatorenal Syndrome

Hepatorenal syndrome represents the extreme of the spectrum of abnormalities that lead to cirrhotic ascites and is characterized by maximal peripheral vasodilation as well as maximal activation of hormones that cause the retention of sodium and water and intense vasoconstriction of renal arteries. Ascites unresponsive to diuretics is universal, and dilutional hyponatremia is almost always present.

Hepatorenal syndrome, which is a diagnosis of exclusion, should be made only after discontinuing diuretics, expanding intravascular volume with albumin, and excluding or treating any condition that leads to worsening of the hemodynamic status of the cirrhotic patient. The differential diagnosis includes conditions that worsen vasodilation, such as sepsis, the use of vasodilators, and large-volume paracentesis not accompanied by albumin infusion; conditions that decrease effective arterial blood volume, such as gastrointestinal hemorrhage, overdiuresis or diarrhea (often induced by overdoses of lactulose); conditions that induce renal vasoconstriction, such as nonsteroidal anti-inflammatory drugs; and nephrotoxic insults, such as from aminoglycosides.

Spontaneous Bacterial Peritonitis

A high index of suspicion and early diagnosis are key in the management of spontaneous bacterial peritonitis. Diagnostic paracentesis should be performed in any patient with symptoms or signs of spontaneous bacterial peritonitis, including unexplained encephalopathy and renal dysfunction. Because spontaneous bacterial peritonitis is often asymptomatic and frequently community acquired, diagnostic paracentesis should be performed when any cirrhotic patient is admitted to the hospital, regardless of the cause for admission.

The diagnosis of spontaneous bacterial peritonitis is established by an ascitic fluid PMN count greater than 250/mm³. Bacteria can be isolated from ascitic fluid in only 40 to 50% of cases, even with sensitive methods such as inoculation directly into a blood culture bottle. Spontaneous bacterial peritonitis is mostly a monobacterial infection, usually with gram-negative enteric organisms. Anaerobes and fungi very rarely cause spontaneous bacterial peritonitis; their presence, as well as a polymicrobial infection, should raise suspicion of secondary bacterial peritonitis.

Hepatic Encephalopathy

The diagnosis of hepatic encephalopathy is clinical and based on the history and physical examination showing alterations in consciousness and behavior, as well as the presence of asterixis. Ammonia levels are unreliable, and there is poor correlation between the stage of hepatic encephalopathy and ammonia blood levels. Therefore, measurements of ammonia are not useful. Psychometric tests and an electroencephalogram are typically used in research but are not useful for clinical diagnosis. Minimal hepatic encephalopathy, formerly called *subclinical* hepatic encephalopathy, which occurs in about 30 to 70% of patients who have cirrhosis without overt hepatic encephalopathy, is detected by psychometric and neuropsychological testing of attention (e.g., number connection test, digit symbol test) and psychomotor function (e.g., grooved pegboard) alone. However, screening of cirrhotic patients for asymptomatic hepatic encephalopathy is not recommended because diagnostic tests are not standardized and the benefits of treatment are unknown.

Hepatopulmonary Syndrome and Portopulmonary Hypertension

The diagnostic criteria for hepatopulmonary syndrome are arterial hypoxemia with a Pao_2 of less than 80 mm Hg or an alveolar arterial oxygen gradient of greater than 15 mm Hg, along with evidence of pulmonary vascular shunting on contrast echocardiography (Chapter 55) or a ^{99m}Tc-labeled macroaggregated albumin scan demonstrating abnormal shunting of radioactivity to the brain. Portopulmonary hypertension is diagnosed by the presence of mean pulmonary arterial pressure higher than 25 mm Hg on right heart catheterization, provided that pulmonary capillary wedge pressure is less than 15 mm Hg.

TREATMENT

Treatment of cirrhosis should ideally be aimed at interrupting or reversing fibrosis. However, antifibrotic drugs have not been shown to reverse fibrosis consistently or improve outcomes in cirrhotic patients. Treatment of compensated cirrhosis is currently directed at preventing the development of decompensation by (1) treating the underlying liver disease (e.g., antiviral therapy for hepatitis C or B) to reduce fibrosis and prevent decompensation; (2) avoiding factors that could worsen liver disease, such as alcohol and hepatotoxic drugs; and (3) screening for varices (to prevent variceal hemorrhage) and for hepatocellular carcinoma (to treat at an early stage) (Fig. 156-5). Treatment of decompensated cirrhosis focuses on specific decompensating events and the option of liver transplantation.

Varices and Variceal Bleeding

Reducing portal pressure decreases the risk for the development of varices and variceal hemorrhage, as well as the risk for ascites and death. Nonselective β-adrenergic blockers (propranolol, nadolol) reduce portal pressure by producing splanchnic vasoconstriction and decreasing splanchnic venous inflow. In patients with cirrhosis and medium or large varices that have never bled, nonselective β-blockers significantly reduce the risk for first variceal hemorrhage. **1** Propranolol is initiated at a dose of 20 mg orally twice a day, whereas nadolol is initiated at a dose of 20 mg orally every day. The dose should be titrated to produce a resting heart rate of about 50 to 55 beats per minute. Endoscopic variceal ligation (Fig. 136-3 in Chapter 136), a therapy that aims to obliterate varices by placing rubber rings on variceal columns, is as useful as nonselective β-blockers to prevent a first variceal hemorrhage. **2** Because ligation is a local therapy that has no effect on portal pressure and that can lead to hemorrhage from ligation-induced ulcers, a rational approach is to start therapy with β-blockers and to use ligation in patients who cannot tolerate or have contraindications to β-blockers.

In patients with no varices, nonselective β-blockers do not prevent the development of varices and are associated with more side effects. **3** In

FIGURE 156-5. Summary of the management of compensated and decompensated cirrhosis. AFP = α-fetoprotein; BM = bowel movement; d/c = discontinue; EGD = esophagogastroduodenoscopy; GI = gastrointestinal; HCC = hepatocellular carcinoma; INR = international normalized ratio; Na = sodium; NSAIDs = nonsteroidal anti-inflammatory drugs; r/o = rule out; SBP = spontaneous bacterial peritonitis; US = ultrasound.

patients with small varices, data are insufficient to recommend therapy with nonselective β-blockers. Endoscopy should be repeated every 2 to 3 years in patients with no varices, every 1 to 2 years in patients with small varices, and sooner in patients with decompensated disease so that effective therapy can be instituted before the varices grow in size and bleed.

Patients with cirrhosis and variceal hemorrhage require resuscitation in an intensive care unit. However, overtransfusion should be avoided because it can precipitate rebleeding. Hemoglobin values should be maintained at about 7-8 g/dL. Prophylactic antibiotics should be used in this setting not only to prevent bacterial infections but also to decrease rebleeding[4] and death. The recommended antibiotic is oral norfloxacin at a dose of 400 mg twice daily for 5 to 7 days, although intravenous ceftriaxone at a dose of 1 g/day for 5 to 7 days is preferable in patients with advanced liver disease (malnutrition, ascites, encephalopathy, and jaundice) or in those already on norfloxacin prophylaxis.[5]

The most effective specific therapy for the control of active variceal hemorrhage is the combination of a vasoconstrictor with endoscopic therapy.[6] Safe vasoconstrictors include terlipressin, somatostatin, and the somatostatin analogues octreotide and vapreotide; they can be initiated at admission to the hospital and continued for 2 to 5 days. The vasoconstrictor currently available in the United States is octreotide, which is used as a 50-μg intravenous bolus followed by an infusion at 50 μg/hour.

After control of hemorrhage, the 1-year recurrence of hemorrhage without treatment is very high at about 60%. Therefore, therapy to prevent rebleeding should be instituted before the patient is discharged. The lowest rebleeding rates (about 10%) are observed in patients who achieve a significant reduction in the hepatic venous pressure gradient with pharmacologic therapy (β-blockers, with or without isosorbide mononitrate at stepwise dosing starting at 20 mg/day orally and increased as tolerated up to 40 mg twice a day); however, because hepatic venous pressure gradient measurements are not widely used, the next best results (rebleeding rates of about 22%) are obtained with the combination of nonselective β-blockers (propranolol or nadolol), with or without isosorbide mononitrate, and endoscopic variceal ligation.[7] The dose of β-blockers should be the maximal dose tolerated, and endoscopic variceal ligation should be repeated every 2 to 4 weeks until the varices are obliterated.

Shunt therapy, either surgical or through radiologic placement of a transjugular intrahepatic portosystemic shunt (TIPS), should be used in patients whose variceal bleeding has persisted or recurred despite combined pharmacologic and endoscopic therapy. Both types of shunts are equally

effective,[8] and the choice will depend on local expertise. Although uncovered TIPS stents frequently occlude, newer polytetrafluoroethylene-covered stents are associated with lower occlusion rates and lower rates of hepatic encephalopathy.[9]

Ascites

Salt restriction and diuretics constitute the mainstay of management of ascites. Dietary sodium intake should be restricted to 2 g/day. A more restrictive diet is not recommended and may compromise nutritional status. Fluid restriction is not required unless the serum sodium concentration is below 130 mEq/L.

Spironolactone, which is more effective than loop diuretics, should be started at a dose of 100 mg/day (once a day in the morning). The dose should be adjusted every 3 to 4 days to a maximal effective dose of 400 mg/day. Furosemide, at an escalated dose from 40 to 160 mg/day, can be started concurrently with spironolactone if weight loss is inadequate or if hyperkalemia develops on spironolactone alone. The goal is weight loss of 1 kg in the first week and 2 kg/week subsequently. However, diuretics should be reduced if the rate of weight loss is greater than 0.5 kg/day in patients without peripheral edema or more than 1 kg/day in patients with peripheral edema. Side effects of diuretic therapy include electrolyte abnormalities, renal dysfunction, encephalopathy, and painful gynecomastia (with spironolactone).

In the 10 to 20% of patients with ascites who are refractory to diuretics, large-volume paracentesis, aimed at removing all or most of the fluid, plus albumin at a dose of 6 to 8 g intravenously per liter of ascites removed, particularly when more than 5 L is removed at once, is a reasonable approach. The frequency of large-volume paracentesis is dictated by the rapidity at which the ascites reaccumulates. TIPS with uncovered stents is more effective than large-volume paracentesis in preventing recurrent ascites but is associated with a higher rate of encephalopathy without a significant improvement in survival.[10] In patients requiring frequent large-volume paracentesis (more than twice per month), polytetrafluoroethylene-covered TIPS stents should be considered. A peritoneovenous shunt, using a subcutaneously placed silicone tube that transfers ascites from the peritoneal cavity to the systemic circulation, can be used in patients who are not candidates for TIPS or liver transplantation.

Hepatorenal Syndrome

Because hepatorenal syndrome is a functional kidney injury that results from hemodynamic abnormalities secondary to end-stage liver disease and severe portal hypertension, the mainstay of therapy is liver transplantation (Chapter 157). Therapies that have been used to "bridge" a patient to transplantation include vasoconstrictors (terlipressin, noradrenaline, octreotide plus midodrine) plus albumin, TIPS, and extracorporeal albumin dialysis, which is an experimental hemofiltration dialysis method that uses an albumin dialysate. The largest experience is with the use of terlipressin, which at a dose 0.5 to 2.0 mg intravenously every 4 to 6 hours leads to a higher reversal rate of hepatorenal syndrome compared with placebo.[11] Because terlipressin is not yet available in the United States, the most used combination is octreotide (100 to 200 µg subcutaneously three times a day) plus midodrine (7.5 to 12.5 mg orally three times a day), with the dose adjusted to obtain an increase of at least 15 mm Hg in mean arterial pressure. Improvements may become clinically noticeable at day 7.

Spontaneous Bacterial Peritonitis

Empirical antibiotic therapy with an intravenous third-generation cephalosporin (e.g., cefotaxime, 2 g intravenously every 12 hours, or ceftriaxone, 1 to 2 g intravenously every 24 hours) or amoxicillin-clavulanic acid (1 g/0.5 g intravenously every 8 hours) should be initiated as soon as the diagnosis is established and before culture results are available; the minimal duration of therapy should be 5 days. Aminoglycosides should be avoided because of the high incidence of renal toxicity in cirrhotic patients. Repeat diagnostic paracentesis should be performed 2 days after starting antibiotics, by which time the number of PMN neutrophils in ascitic fluid should have decreased by more than 25% from baseline. Lack of response should prompt further investigations to exclude secondary peritonitis. The renal dysfunction associated with spontaneous bacterial peritonitis can be prevented by the intravenous administration of albumin, particularly in patients who have any evidence of renal dysfunction (blood urea nitrogen >30 mg/dL or creatinine >1 mg/dL, or both) or serum bilirubin greater than 4 mg/dL at the time of diagnosis. Albumin has been used at a dose of 1.5 g/kg of body weight at diagnosis, repeated on the third day at an intravenous dose of 1 g/kg of body weight. However, this dosing is empirical and should not exceed 100 g per dose.

The administration of nonabsorbable (or poorly absorbable) antibiotics can prevent the development of spontaneous bacterial peritonitis and other infections in cirrhosis by selectively eliminating gram-negative organisms in the gut. However, the widespread use of prophylactic norfloxacin is associated with a higher rate of infections by antibiotic-resistant organisms. Long-term antibiotic prophylaxis with oral norfloxacin at a dose of 400 mg/day is justified only in two groups: patients who have recovered from a previous episode of spontaneous bacterial peritonitis, and patients who have an ascites protein level of less than 1 g/L with advanced liver and circulatory dysfunction as evidenced by the presence of jaundice, hyponatremia, or renal dysfunction.[12,13]

Hepatic Encephalopathy

Treatment of hepatic encephalopathy involves identifying and treating the precipitating factor and reducing the ammonia level. Precipitating factors include infections, overdiuresis, GI bleeding, a high oral protein load, and constipation. Narcotics and sedatives contribute to hepatic encephalopathy by directly depressing brain function. TIPS is a common precipitant of hepatic encephalopathy, and shunt reduction or occlusion may be required. Agents aimed at decreasing ammonia production in the gut are lactulose (15 to 30 mL orally twice daily adjusted to obtain two to three soft bowel movements per day) or orally administered nonabsorbable antibiotics such as neomycin (500 mg to 1 g three times per day), metronidazole (250 mg two to four times per day), or rifaximin (550 mg two times per day).[14] L-Ornithine, L-aspartate, and benzoate may increase ammonia fixation in the liver. Switching dietary protein from an animal source to a vegetable source may be beneficial, but protein restriction is not necessary and should not be used long term.[15]

Pulmonary Complications

Hepatopulmonary syndrome rarely resolves spontaneously, and medical therapy is disappointing. TIPS is not generally recommended. The only viable treatment is liver transplantation (Chapter 157).

By comparison, portopulmonary hypertension is not an indication for liver transplantation. In fact, a mean pulmonary arterial pressure higher than 50 mm Hg is an absolute contraindication to liver transplantation.

Surgical Therapy

Liver Transplantation

Orthotopic liver transplantation (Chapter 157), which is the definitive therapy for cirrhosis, is indicated when the risk for dying from liver disease is greater than the risk for dying from transplantation, as determined by a Child-Pugh score of 7 or higher (see Table 156-2) or a Model for End-Stage Liver Disease (MELD) score of 15 or higher. MELD (see Table 157-4 in Chapter 157), which is a mathematical model that estimates the risk for 3-month mortality, is used to determine the priority for liver transplantation. The number of available deceased donor organs is lower than the number of patients awaiting liver transplantation; as a result, 15 to 20% of patients awaiting liver transplantation in the United States die before an organ becomes available.

PRIMARY PREVENTION

Treatment of the underlying liver disease, before the development of cirrhosis, is a primary prevention strategy. Because the major causes of cirrhosis are related to lifestyle choices such as injection drug use (Chapter 33), alcohol consumption (Chapter 32), and unprotected sex, primary prevention programs that focus on encouraging alcohol abstinence, reducing high-risk behavior for hepatitis virus infection, and vaccinating for hepatitis B are even better prevention strategies.

PROGNOSIS

The outcome of cirrhosis depends on the patient's stage. Patients with compensated cirrhosis die of liver disease only after transition to a decompensated stage. The 10-year survival rate of patients who remain in a compensated stage is approximately 90%, whereas their likelihood of decompensation is 50% at 10 years. Inception cohort studies of patients with compensated cirrhosis show a median survival of all patients, including those in whom decompensation develops over time, of about 10 years, whereas the median survival after decompensation is about 2 years.

Four clinical stages of cirrhosis have recently been identified, each with a different prognosis. In stage 1 patients without varices or ascites, the mortality rate is about 1% per year. Stage 2 patients, or those with varices but without ascites or bleeding, have a mortality rate of about 4% per year. Stage 3 patients have ascites with or without esophageal varices that have never bled; their mortality rate while remaining in this stage is 20% per year. Stage 4 patients, or those with portal hypertensive GI bleeding with or without ascites, have a 1-year mortality rate of 57%, with nearly half of these deaths occurring within 6 weeks after the initial episode of bleeding. Stages 1 and 2 correspond to compensated cirrhosis, whereas stages 3 and 4 are decompensated cirrhosis. Hepatocellular carcinoma develops at a fairly constant rate of 3% per year and is associated with a worse outcome at whatever stage it develops.

Predictors of survival are different in compensated and decompensated patients, with parameters of portal hypertension (varices, splenomegaly, platelet count, γ-globulin) assuming greater importance in compensated patients, whereas renal dysfunction, hemorrhage, and hepatocellular carcinoma are important predictive factors in patients with decompensated cirrhosis. In clinical practice, the Child-Pugh score is applicable to all cirrhotic patients, and the MELD score is used in decompensated patients to determine priority for liver transplantation.

Grade A

1. D'Amico G, Pagliaro L, Bosch J. Pharmacological treatment of portal hypertension: an evidence-based approach. *Semin Liver Dis.* 1999;19:475-505.
2. Gluud LL, Klingenberg S, Nikolova D, et al. Banding ligation versus beta-blockers as primary prophylaxis in esophageal varices: systematic review of randomized trials. *Am J Gastroenterol.* 2007;102:2842-2848.
3. Groszmann RJ, Garcia-Tsao G, Bosch J, et al. Beta-blockers to prevent gastroesophageal varices in patients with cirrhosis. *N Engl J Med.* 2005;353:2254-2261.
4. Hou MC, Lin HC, Liu TT, et al. Antibiotic prophylaxis after endoscopic therapy prevents rebleeding in acute variceal hemorrhage: a randomized trial. *Hepatology.* 2004;39:746-753.
5. Fernandez J, Ruiz del Arbol L, Gomez C, et al. Norfloxacin vs ceftriaxone in the prophylaxis of infections in patients with advanced cirrhosis and hemorrhage. *Gastroenterology.* 2006;131:1049-1056.
6. Banares R, Albillos A, Rincon D, et al. Endoscopic treatment versus endoscopic plus pharmacologic treatment for acute variceal bleeding: a meta-analysis. *Hepatology.* 2002;35:609-615.
7. Gonzalez R, Zamora J, Gomez-Camarero J, et al. Meta-analysis: combination endoscopic and drug therapy to prevent variceal rebleeding in cirrhosis. *Ann Intern Med.* 2008;149:109-122.
8. Henderson JM, Boyer TD, Kutner MH, et al. Distal splenorenal shunt versus transjugular intrahepatic portal systematic shunt for variceal bleeding: a randomized trial. *Gastroenterology.* 2006;130:1643-1651.
9. Bureau C, Garcia-Pagan JC, Otal P, et al. Improved clinical outcome using polytetrafluoroethylene-coated stents for TIPS: results of a randomized study. *Gastroenterology.* 2004;126:469-475.
10. D'Amico G, Luca A, Morabito A, et al. Uncovered transjugular intrahepatic portosystemic shunt for refractory ascites: a meta-analysis. *Gastroenterology.* 2005;129:1282-1293.
11. Sanyal AJ, Boyer T, Garcia-Tsao G, et al. A randomized, prospective, double-blind, placebo-controlled trial of terlipressin for type 1 hepatorenal syndrome. *Gastroenterology.* 2008;134:1360-1368.
12. Fernandez J, Navasa M, Planas R, et al. Primary prophylaxis of spontaneous bacterial peritonitis delays hepatorenal syndrome and improves survival in cirrhosis. *Gastroenterology.* 2007;133:818-824.
13. Loomba R, Wesley R, Bain A, et al. Role of fluoroquinolones in the primary prophylaxis of spontaneous bacterial peritonitis: meta-analysis. *Clin Gastroenterol Hepatol.* 2009;7:487-493.
14. Bass NM, Mullen KD, Sanyal A, et al. Rifaximin treatment in hepatic encephalopathy. *N Engl J Med.* 2010;362:1071-1081.
15. Cordoba J, Lopez-Hellin J, Planas M, et al. Normal protein diet for episodic hepatic encephalopathy: results of a randomized study. *J Hepatol.* 2004;41:38-43.

SUGGESTED READINGS

Beier JI, Arteel GE, McClain CJ. Advances in alcoholic liver disease. *Curr Gastroenterol Rep.* 2010;13:56-64. *Review of biology and treatment.*

Kremer AE, Oude Elferink RP, Beuers U. Pathophysiology and current management of pruritus in liver disease. *Gastroenterol Clin Biol*. 2011. [Epub ahead of print.] *Review emphasizing potential role of lysophosphatidic acid, a potent neuronal activator.*

Thabut D, Moreau R, Lebrec D. Noninvasive assessment of portal hypertension in patients with cirrhosis. *Hepatology*. 2011;53:683-694. *Noninvasive methods effectively identify severe portal hypertension but not less severe disease.*

Thalheimer U, Triantos C, Goulis J, et al. Management o f varices in cirrhosis. *Expert Opin Pharmacother*. 2011;12:721-735. *Review.*

157

HEPATIC FAILURE AND LIVER TRANSPLANTATION

EMMET B. KEEFFE

Liver transplantation is the treatment of choice for patients with severe liver failure, end-stage liver disease, and certain metabolic liver diseases for which no alternative therapies are available. More than 6000 liver transplantations are performed in the United States annually, with a waiting list that has grown to approximately 16,000 patients. With modern immunosuppressive drug regimens, technical advances, and improved perioperative care, the current 1-year survival rate after liver transplantation is 85 to 90% (Table 157-1). Many studies show that liver transplantation significantly improves the physical, cognitive, and psychological functioning of the recipient. In recent years, the disparity between a limited supply of cadaver donor organs and much greater need for liver transplantation has resulted in an unacceptable number of deaths of patients listed for transplantation and created a mandate to optimize the selection of patients and timing of transplantation.

INDICATIONS AND SELECTION CRITERIA FOR LIVER TRANSPLANTATION

The indications and contraindications for liver transplantation, the most appropriate candidates to receive a transplant, and the organ allocation scheme continue to evolve. The diseases for which liver transplantation is performed in adults include cirrhosis with end-stage liver disease (Chapter 156), acute liver failure, hepatic malignancies (particularly hepatocellular carcinoma; Chapter 202), and metabolic diseases in which the inborn error of metabolism resides in the hepatocytes (e.g., hemochromatosis, α_1-antitrypsin deficiency, Wilson's disease; Chapter 153). The most common indications for liver transplantation are chronic hepatitis C and alcoholic liver disease in adults (together accounting for approximately 50% of transplantations) and biliary atresia and α_1-antitrypsin deficiency in children.

General selection criteria that should be considered in the referral of patients for liver transplantation include the following: (1) the absence of alternative forms of therapy that may reverse liver failure and defer the need

TABLE 157-1 KAPLAN-MEIER PATIENT SURVIVAL RATES FOR LIVER TRANSPLANTATION PERFORMED FROM 1997 TO 2004

DIAGNOSIS	Kaplan-Meier Survival Rate (%)		
	1-YEAR	3-YEAR	5-YEAR
Acute hepatic necrosis	81	72	69
Cholestatic cirrhosis	90	85	80
Noncholestatic cirrhosis	86	77	70
Other liver disease	81	72	63
Metabolic disease	89	84	81
Malignant neoplasm	86	68	54
Benign neoplasm	86	81	68

From The Organ Procurement and Transplantation Network. http://www.unos.org → Data → View data reports → National Data → Survival/Liver/Patient → Survival by recipient diagnosis category. Accessed Nov. 25, 2009.

TABLE 157-2 BIOCHEMICAL AND CLINICAL INDICATIONS FOR LIVER TRANSPLANTATION IN CHRONIC LIVER DISEASE

CHOLESTATIC LIVER DISEASE

Bilirubin >10 mg/dL
Intractable pruritus
Progressive cholestatic bone disease
Recurrent bacterial cholangitis

HEPATOCELLULAR LIVER DISEASE

Serum albumin <3 g/dL
Prothrombin time >3 seconds above control

BOTH CHOLESTATIC AND HEPATOCELLULAR LIVER DISEASES

Recurrent or severe hepatic encephalopathy
Refractory ascites
Spontaneous bacterial peritonitis
Recurrent portal hypertensive bleeding
Severe chronic fatigue and weakness
Progressive malnutrition
Development of hepatorenal syndrome
Detection of small hepatocellular carcinoma

INR = International Normalized Ratio.
From Keeffe EB. Selection of patients for liver transplantation. In Maddrey WC, Sorrell MF, Schiff ER, eds. *Transplantation of the Liver*, 3rd ed. Philadelphia: Lippincott Williams & Wilkins; 2001:5-34.

TABLE 157-3 KING'S COLLEGE CRITERIA FOR LIVER TRANSPLANTATION IN FULMINANT HEPATIC FAILURE

PATIENTS TAKING ACETAMINOPHEN

pH <7.3, or prothrombin time >6.5 (INR) and serum creatinine >3.4 mg/dL

PATIENTS NOT TAKING ACETAMINOPHEN

Prothrombin time >6.5 (INR) *or* any three of the following:
1. Age <10 or >40 yr
2. Etiology: non-A, non-B hepatitis; halothane hepatitis; idiosyncratic drug reaction
3. Duration of jaundice before encephalopathy >7 days
4. Prothrombin time >3.5 (INR)
5. Serum bilirubin >17.6 mg/dL

INR = International Normalized Ratio.
Adapted from O'Grady JG, Alexander GJ, Hayllar KM, et al. Early indicators of prognosis in fulminant hepatic failure. *Gastroenterology*. 1989;97:439-445.

for liver transplantation, (2) the absence of any absolute contraindication to transplantation (discussed later), (3) expected compliance with longitudinal follow-up care, and (4) the ability to provide for the financial costs of liver transplantation and follow-up care, including medications that may be expensive. Insurance coverage for transplantation is typically determined before referral by a financial counselor at the transplantation center.

Referral for Liver Transplantation

Patients with chronic (Table 157-2) or acute (Table 157-3) liver disease should be referred when hepatic decompensation first develops or the presence of hepatocellular carcinoma is first detected. The greatest likelihood of survival and return to an excellent quality of life occurs in patients who undergo liver transplantation before the onset of multiorgan failure. Meticulous attention to medical management of the complications of cirrhosis, such as avoidance of excessive diuretic therapy or aminoglycosides to preserve renal function in patients with ascites or spontaneous bacterial peritonitis, is critical. Blood loss in patients with gastrointestinal bleeding should be replaced judiciously with blood products to avoid fluid overload and pulmonary edema.

For long-term management in patients with chronic liver disease who may ultimately become candidates for transplantation, nonsurgical interventions, such as transjugular intrahepatic portosystemic shunt (TIPS) for refractory portal hypertensive bleeding and endoscopic or radiologic approaches to dominant biliary strictures in patients with primary sclerosing cholangitis, are preferable to abdominal procedures that can cause adhesions. Patients with cirrhosis (Chapter 156) should undergo surveillance for hepatocellular carcinoma with ultrasound or computed tomography and α-fetoprotein testing every 6 months to facilitate early diagnosis of lesions, when they are small and amenable to treatment with modalities such as resection or liver transplantation.

Chronic Liver Disease

Although the survival of patients with compensated cirrhosis is excellent (approximately 90% at 5 years), the development of decompensation with ascites, portal hypertensive bleeding, or encephalopathy implies a lower 5-year survival rate of about 20%. A patient with a Child-Turcotte-Pugh (see Table 156-2 in Chapter 156) score of 5 or 6 (Child's class A cirrhosis) without a history of portal hypertensive bleeding or spontaneous bacterial peritonitis is likely to remain stable for a considerable period of time and does not require listing for transplantation. Suggested criteria for listing should be clinical decompensation or biochemical deterioration of synthetic function that results in a Child's class B or C status, any complication of portal hypertension, or the development of a small hepatocellular carcinoma, although one randomized trial showed no benefit to listing patients with Child's class B alcoholic cirrhosis compared with standard care.■1 Many centers are also using a Model for End-Stage Liver Disease (MELD; see Table 156-2 in Chapter 156) score of 10 to assist in the timing of evaluation for liver transplantation.

Liver transplantation for hepatocellular carcinoma (Chapter 202) is reserved for selected patients who have advanced cirrhosis, who do not have the hepatic reserve to undergo resection, and who have no evidence of extrahepatic tumor after thorough evaluation. Risks for recurrent hepatocellular carcinoma after transplantation include advanced disease (stage 3 or greater) as defined by lymph node involvement, gross vascular invasion by imaging studies, tumor burden (single lesion <5 cm, or two or more lesions >3 cm), or involvement of more than one lobe. In low-risk patients with stage 1 or 2 disease (single lesion of 5 cm, or two or three lesions of ≤3 cm), the actuarial survival rate is about 75% at 4 years, whereas the survival in patients with higher risk is about 50% at 4 years. Evolving data support expanding liver transplantation to patients with early stage 3 hepatocellular carcinoma, but use of these expanded criteria remains experimental.

Acute Liver Failure

Liver transplantation is a major advance in the management of severe acute liver failure. *Fulminant hepatic failure* refers to the presence of acute liver failure with superimposed hepatic encephalopathy developing within 2 to 8 weeks after the onset of illness in a patient without preexisting liver disease. *Subfulminant hepatic failure* (or *late-onset hepatic failure*) is applied to a syndrome that develops more slowly, after 2 to 8 weeks up to 3 to 6 months. The selection of patients with acute liver failure who are likely to die and therefore would benefit from liver transplantation is challenging but can be predicted by certain biochemical and clinical features, the most popular of which was established at King's College Hospital in London (see Table 157-3).

Aggressive supportive care is necessary in patients with fulminant hepatic failure to prevent and treat bleeding, infection, cerebral edema, renal failure, and respiratory failure. These complications are the main reasons that transplantation may not be possible and may also contribute to postoperative morbidity and mortality.

Potential alternative treatment strategies for fulminant hepatic failure include extracorporeal liver assist devices, hepatocyte transplantation, and heterotopic auxiliary liver transplantation, although all of these currently must be viewed as investigational. The goals of these therapies are to prevent irreversible brain damage, provide time for possible hepatic regeneration and recovery of acceptable function, and stabilize patients who do not recover until liver transplantation can be performed. Clinical experience with hepatic support devices, primarily using either porcine or human hepatocytes, is encouraging but limited to ongoing trials. Hepatocyte transplantation and heterotopic liver transplantation have a number of technical problems that limit their application.

Patients with fulminant hepatic failure should be treated in an intensive care unit, with the patient's head elevated at 20 to 30 degrees. Although lactulose is the cornerstone of treatment of chronic hepatic encephalopathy, it is less effective in patients with acute encephalopathy, and the role of antibiotics such as neomycin is unknown. However, a trial of lactulose, 30 mL two to four times daily, adjusted to achieve two to three loose bowel movements daily, is worthwhile, and the drug may need to be administrated by nasogastric tube or by rectal enema. Factors precipitating hepatic encephalopathy, such as gastrointestinal bleeding, hypokalemia, or sepsis, should be identified and treated.

Cerebral edema is manifest frequently by hypertension, bradycardia, and neurologic findings such as decerebrate posturing or abnormal pupillary reflexes. These findings may occur late; therefore, monitoring of intracranial pressure (ICP) with institution of therapy to maintain ICP at less than 20 mm Hg is preferred. ICP may be monitored with either a subdural or an epidural transducer, and the risk for hemorrhage as a complication of placement is outweighed by the benefit of monitoring and early intervention.

Initial treatment of increased ICP is with mannitol (0.5 to 1 g/kg by intravenous infusion over 5 minutes). Repeated doses of mannitol may be required to treat recurrent increases in ICP. Mannitol can be given only if the serum osmolality is less than 320 mOsm/L. Caution is advised in patients with renal failure, and mannitol may need to be administered in combination with hemodialysis or continuous arteriovenous hemofiltration. Other useful therapies include disturbing the patient as little as possible, controlling agitation, and administering moderate hyperventilation to a partial carbon dioxide pressure of 25 to 30 mm Hg. A persistent ICP greater than 40 mm Hg that is refractory to treatment precludes liver transplantation.

Listing for Liver Transplantation

Before final selection and listing for liver transplantation, prospective candidates with acute or chronic liver disease undergo a pretransplantation evaluation to define the current status of systemic diseases and to determine whether any absolute or relative contraindications are present. Routine evaluation includes blood bank and hematologic studies, complete liver and kidney chemistry profiles, viral serology assays (hepatitis A, B, and C viruses; human immunodeficiency virus [HIV]; cytomegalovirus [CMV]), chest radiography, and abdominal computed tomography or Doppler ultrasound studies of the hepatic vasculature. Additional routine tests include skin testing for tuberculosis, creatinine clearance, electrocardiogram, and, in the presence of lung disease, pulmonary function testing. Patients who are at risk for coronary artery disease undergo cardiology consultation and, if indicated, stress testing, cardiac catheterization, or both. Cancer screening, depending on age and gender, includes Papanicolaou smear, mammography, and colonoscopy. Consultations with a social worker, financial counselor, and psychiatrist are routinely performed at the transplantation center.

Patients are generally assigned to one of four categories by the liver transplantation center selection committee: (1) suitable and ready, with listing for transplantation; (2) suitable but too well, with placement on inactive status and continued follow-up with the referring physician; (3) potentially reversible relative contraindication, with treatment and recategorization at a later date; and (4) absolute contraindication, with denial of transplantation. Patients who are approved for liver transplantation are then listed for a donor organ with the United Network for Organ Sharing (UNOS), and final approval by the insurance carrier or third party payer is sought.

Allocation of Donor Organs

In the current UNOS system, patients with fulminant liver failure receive the first priority for available organs. The MELD score (see Table 156-2 in Chapter 156) was adopted by UNOS in 2002 as the severity measure to determine priority for transplantation and allocation of organs to patients with end-stage liver disease (Table 157-4). Recent data indicate that lower serum sodium levels also independently predict higher mortality over and beyond MELD scores alone, but serum sodium has not been included in the formula used to allocate organs.

Contraindications to Liver Transplantation
Absolute Contraindications

The list of absolute contraindications to transplantation is short: advanced cardiopulmonary disease, active untreated sepsis, extrahepatic malignancy, anatomic abnormality precluding transplantation, active alcohol or substance abuse, and documented poor compliance with medical care. In addition, patients should not undergo liver transplantation if they have compensated cirrhosis (Child's class A; Chapter 156) and no history of portal hypertensive bleeding. Patients are not candidates for liver transplantation if they have poor ventricular function or severe valvular heart disease. Coronary artery disease, if anatomically reversible by angioplasty or bypass surgery, is not a contraindication to listing if left ventricular function is adequate.

Nearly 50% of liver transplantation candidates have abnormal arterial oxygenation, but only patients with advanced chronic obstructive pulmonary disease or pulmonary fibrosis are precluded from liver transplantation. Previous tuberculosis is not a contraindication to liver transplantation. The

TABLE 157-4 RELATIONSHIP BETWEEN MELD SCORE AND 3-MONTH MORTALITY IN HOSPITALIZED CIRRHOTIC PATIENTS

MELD SCORE	NO. DEATHS/TOTAL NO. OF PATIENTS	MORTALITY RATE (%)
≤9	6/148	4
10-19	28/103	27
20-29	16/21	76
30-39	5/6	83
≥40	4/4	100

MELD = Model for End-Stage Liver Disease.
Adapted from Wiesner RH, McDiarmid SV, Kamath PS, et al. MELD and PELD: application of survival models to liver allocation. *Liver Transpl.* 2001;7:567-580.

benefits of treating latent tuberculosis before liver transplantation appear to outweigh the risks, providing justification for the strategy of performing a skin test and treating with isoniazid if positive. Active tuberculosis should be treated for at least 2 to 3 weeks and preferably for several months before liver transplantation and for up to 1 year afterward. Hepatopulmonary syndrome (Chapter 156), which is diagnosed on the basis of the triad of chronic liver disease with portal hypertension, intrapulmonary vascular dilation with right-to-left shunting, and arterial hypoxemia, may be reversed by liver transplantation. By contrast, portopulmonary hypertension is associated with high operative mortality; for example, patients with a mean pulmonary artery pressure of 50 mm Hg or greater have a postoperative mortality rate that approaches 100%. Conversely, patients with mean pulmonary artery pressures lower than 35 mm Hg do not have increased perioperative mortality.

Active untreated infection should be controlled before proceeding with liver transplantation. In the setting of spontaneous bacterial peritonitis, most programs defer transplantation until antibiotic treatment has been administered for 48 hours and resolution of infection is documented on repeat paracentesis. Sepsis and pneumonia remain absolute contraindications to liver transplantation. Serious chronic infections such as osteomyelitis, chronic fungal diseases, and abscesses preclude transplantation unless they can be treated effectively. Selected HIV-positive patients are currently undergoing liver transplantation in a few centers in the United States to determine whether the benefits outweigh the risks.

Liver transplantation is not performed in the presence of extrahepatic malignancy, except perhaps for patients with isolated liver metastases from slow-growing neuroendocrine tumors (Chapter 201), such as gastrinoma, insulinomas, glucagonomas, somatostatinomas, and carcinoid tumors. The results of liver transplantation are so poor with cholangiocarcinoma (Chapter 158) that most centers consider this diagnosis to be an absolute contraindication, although a few centers have demonstrated acceptable tumor-free survival rates when liver transplantation is combined with adjuvant chemotherapy and radiation in highly selected patients.

Most programs accept patients with alcoholic liver disease as candidates for liver transplantation only after proven alcohol abstinence for at least 6 months and completion of an inpatient or outpatient rehabilitation program. Isolated portal vein thrombosis, previously considered an absolute contraindication, is only a relative problem in light of novel reconstructive innovations, including thrombectomy or jump grafts.

Relative Contraindications

Patient selection should be based on an assessment of biologic age and absence of major systemic illnesses rather than an arbitrary chronologic age cutoff. Patients undergoing evaluation for liver transplantation may have hepatorenal syndrome, chronic renal failure, or reversible acute renal failure that may be related to intercurrent events such as spontaneous bacterial peritonitis, gastrointestinal bleeding, or excessive diuresis; however, these conditions are not contraindications to transplantation. Chronic renal failure secondary to intrinsic kidney disease is not a contraindication to liver transplantation but necessitates consideration for combined liver and kidney transplantation. Transient deterioration in renal function due to an acute injury usually is not a problem unless it is complicated by the development of hepatorenal syndrome, which is reversible only if urgent liver transplantation can be performed.

THE TRANSPLANTATION PROCEDURE

Donors and recipients are matched according to blood type and body size. In general, organs are transplanted into recipients in keeping with standard ABO compatibility rules. Most surgeons believe that a satisfactory size match exists if the donor's and recipient's body weights are within 20% of one another. The donor organ is harvested according to standard protocols to ensure that the physiologic condition of the donor is close to normal when the organ is removed and to limit warm ischemia time. The cold ischemia time while the organ is in a preservation solution is also kept as short as possible—the usual goal is less than 12 hours—to minimize the risk for delayed graft function or nonfunction.

The recipient undergoes bilateral subcostal incision with upper midline extension. The standard hepatectomy includes removal of both the vena cava and the liver, often with use of a pump-driven venovenous bypass to return the inferior vena cava and portal venous flow to the heart through the axillary vein. A popular alternative method is to preserve the retrohepatic vena cava during hepatectomy. After hepatectomy, the donor liver is put in place, with repair of the inferior vena cava if it was interrupted, portal reperfusion, hepatic arterial reconstruction, and, finally, duct-to-duct reconstruction of the common bile duct. A Roux-en-Y choledochojejunostomy is used when a duct-to-duct anastomosis is not suitable, such as in patients who have primary sclerosing cholangitis, in whom the diseased common bile duct is removed in its entirety.

Evolving Approaches to Liver Transplantation

The growing discrepancy between the number of available organs and the need for transplantation has led to increasing application of novel approaches to liver replacement, including deceased donor split-liver transplantation and adult living donor liver transplantation. Xenotransplantation and hepatocyte transplantation are investigational.

Split-liver transplantation allows two liver transplants from a single deceased donor liver, usually a right lobe implanted into an adult recipient and left lobe or left lateral segment implanted into a pediatric recipient. This technique has the potential to provide grafts to most listed pediatric patients and to decrease substantially the waiting time for adult patients.

Living donor liver transplantation uses the left lateral segment for adult-to-child donation, with a very low risk to the adult donor, who usually is a parent. Good results also have been achieved in recent years with elective adult-to-adult living donor liver transplantation grafting the right lobe (segments 5 to 8), which represents 60 to 65% of the liver, into the recipient. Advantages of living donor liver transplantation include thorough donor screening, optimization of the timing of transplantation, and minimal cold ischemia time. This operation has also been applied to urgent cases with good outcomes. Patients with small hepatocellular carcinomas and those with primary sclerosing cholangitis at risk for cholangiocarcinoma are excellent candidates for a timely living donor liver transplantation. Unfortunately, adult-to-adult living donor liver transplantation is just a partial solution to the donor shortage for adult liver transplantation because only about 15% of potential donors are satisfactory candidates after complete evaluation, and most liver transplantation centers do not routinely pursue this option. The morbidity and mortality rates for the donor average 15 to 30% and 0.3 to 0.5%, respectively, making the operation formidable and necessitating careful informed consent from the donor.

POST-TRANSPLANTATION MANAGEMENT

Allograft dysfunction is the most important complication after liver transplantation. Liver biopsy is critical in differentiating the various causes of dysfunction because many of them share similar but nonspecific clinical and biochemical presentations. Diagnostic evaluations may also include a cholangiogram and duplex ultrasound of the vessels supplying the liver.

Standard Medical Therapies

In general, all patients receive corticosteroids in large intravenous doses during the operation. Steroid doses are rapidly reduced over 5 days and can be discontinued by 3 to 12 months after transplantation in many patients, depending on the underlying disease and the presence or absence of rejection. Either cyclosporine or tacrolimus is initiated at the time of liver transplantation and is used long-term in most patients to prevent acute and chronic allograft rejection. Immunosuppression can be prednisone and a calcineurin agent (cyclosporine or tacrolimus) with early withdrawal of corticosteroids (from 14 days to 3 months after transplantation) followed by use of a calcineurin agent alone. Alternatively, a three-drug regimen (daclizumab, mycophenolate mofetil, and tacrolimus) may reduce rejection and avoid steroid side effects.[2] In patients with renal dysfunction, calcineurin-sparing regimens using mycophenolate mofetil with lower doses of a calcineurin agent or sirolimus alone are used. Calcineurin-sparing regimens reduce the incidence of late renal failure, which approaches 15 to 20% by 20 years after transplantation. Immunosuppressive drugs are typically titrated to therapeutic or slightly subtherapeutic blood levels, but different drug strategies are used in different centers. Other routine medications after liver transplantation include those used for preemptive prevention of viral and fungal infection (see later discussion).

Early Complications after Liver Transplantation

Problems that may occur in the first few days after liver transplantation include hepatic artery thrombosis, portal vein thrombosis, primary graft nonfunction, and hyperacute rejection. Hepatic artery thrombosis, which occurs in about 2 to 8% of adults and in 3 to 20% of children who undergo liver transplantation, is more common among patients who receive sirolimus. Hepatic artery thrombosis typically manifests early after transplantation as fulminant liver failure; occasionally, it occurs 1 to 2 months after transplantation and manifests with stenosis or intimal hyperplasia with eventual rearterialization from collaterals. Early hepatic artery thrombosis is first treated by immediate revascularization through thrombectomy or use of a surgical conduit, but it often requires urgent retransplantation. Hepatic artery stenosis without thrombosis is usually associated with multiple ischemic biliary strictures and manifests somewhat later. Retransplantation is indicated if biliary sepsis or graft failure develops.

Portal vein thrombosis complicates only 1 to 3% of liver transplantation cases. Early acute portal vein thrombosis leads to fulminant liver failure and requires immediate revascularization or urgent retransplantation. Conversely, late portal vein thrombosis manifests as portal hypertension.

Primary graft nonfunction, or delayed ischemia-reperfusion injury, is the most common cause of graft loss within the early postoperative period after a technically successful liver transplantation. The clinical presentation resembles that of fulminant liver failure, with persistent or new hepatic encephalopathy and elevated serum aminotransferase levels (>2500 IU/L).

Initial poor graft function is characteristic of a marginally functioning graft that typically recovers adequate function days to weeks after transplantation. This syndrome has a milder clinical presentation than primary nonfunction, and serum aminotransferases are usually less than 2500 IU/L. Treatment is largely supportive, and most grafts eventually recover.

Acute and Chronic Allograft Rejection

The most common cause of allograft dysfunction after the first postoperative week is acute cellular rejection, which occurs overall in one half to two thirds of cases and is seen within 5 to 30 days of transplantation. The incidence of acute rejection with the use of low-dose prednisone, tacrolimus, and mycophenolate mofetil is 25 to 30%. An acute rejection episode occurring beyond 6 weeks after transplantation should raise suspicion for a subtherapeutic immunosuppressive regimen or for noncompliance with the medical regimen. The patient is usually asymptomatic and presents with increases in serum bilirubin, alkaline phosphatase, and γ-glutamyltransferase in the early post-transplantation course and with predominant elevations in the serum aminotransferases if acute rejection occurs several weeks after transplantation. However, recipients may also present with fever, malaise, abdominal pain, or portal hypertensive changes such as ascites. Histologic examination reveals a mixed portal or periportal inflammatory infiltrate (with neutrophils, eosinophils, plasma cells, and lymphocytes) leading to destructive suppurative cholangitis and endotheliitis. Treatment, which reverses 65 to 85% of episodes, consists of high-dose intravenous corticosteroids, usually 1 g of methylprednisolone, followed by oral prednisone with a rapid taper over 7 days.

Chronic ductopenic rejection now occurs in 2 to 3% of patients, most commonly between 6 weeks and 6 months after transplantation. Cholestatic enzymes, such as alkaline phosphatase and γ-glutamyltransferase, gradually increase for weeks to months before the onset of jaundice that signals the late stage of chronic ductopenic rejection. Histologic evaluation reveals sparse lymphocytic portal inflammation but progressive loss of interlobular and septal bile ducts in at least half of the portal tracts—a condition known as vanishing bile duct syndrome. Approximately 10 to 20% of retransplantations are done because of chronic ductopenic rejection.

Biliary Complications after Liver Transplantation

The biliary tree has very poor regenerative and reparative capacity when damaged and is the most common site for technical complications after transplantation. Biliary complications occur in 10 to 25% of all recipients, with more than two thirds of cases diagnosed within 1 month and 80% within 6 months after transplantation. Causes of biliary complications include technical factors, preservation injury, hepatic artery thrombosis, immunologic factors, and infection, particularly with CMV. Bile leaks and strictures are the most common presentations of biliary complications in the first 3 months after surgery.

Choledochocholedochostomy and choledochojejunostomy are the two methods of primary biliary reconstruction in liver transplantation. The more commonly performed choledochocholedochostomy, or duct-to-duct anastomosis, preserves the sphincter of Oddi and endoscopic access to the biliary tree after transplantation. Choledochojejunostomy, or Roux-en-Y anastomosis, is used for retransplantation, for transplantation of small liver grafts, and in patients with intrinsic disease of the extrahepatic bile ducts, such as primary sclerosing cholangitis.

Bile leakage occurs in up to 25% of all recipients and can be diagnosed by cholangiogram or biliary scintigraphy if the leak is sufficiently large. Patients may present with fever, abdominal pain, peritonitis, hypotension, or sepsis with biloma. For patients who suffer from bile leak after T-tube removal, endoscopic placement of a nasobiliary drain or internal plastic stent allows the leakage to heal as the bile flows preferentially through the ampulla. Surgical creation or revision of choledochojejunostomy should be performed only after failure of endoscopic or radiologic interventions.

Anastomotic biliary stricture, which affects 4 to 10% of all recipients, occurs within the first 6 months after transplantation. Clinical presentation is typical of cholangitis but may be asymptomatic, with only elevation of cholestatic enzymes (predominantly alkaline phosphatase and γ-glutamyltransferase). Balloon dilation or stenting endoscopically or radiologically should be attempted before resorting to surgery. Nonanastomotic biliary strictures, affecting up to 20% of all recipients, occur within the first 4 months after transplantation. The biliary strictures are usually multiple and may be associated with extrahepatic and intrahepatic bile leaks. Management of these strictures depends on their number, location, and severity, as well as liver function. Diffuse strictures in the setting of bile leakage and biloma indicate the need for retransplantation. Focal intrahepatic strictures may benefit from repeated sessions of balloon dilation and stenting performed endoscopically or radiologically.

Infections

Most infections occur within the first 2 months after transplantation, whereas recipients are receiving a high-dose induction immunosuppressive regimen. Bacteria and fungi cause more than 90% of infections during this period. Pneumonia, urinary infection, intra-abdominal and hepatic abscesses, peritonitis, wound infection, and line sepsis are the most common infections. *Candida albicans* is the most common infecting fungal agent in the immediate post-transplantation period. Other frequently seen fungi include *Aspergillus fumigatus* and non-*albicans Candida* species. Despite its nephrotoxicity, amphotericin B is the treatment of choice for invasive fungal infections. Oral fluconazole, 100 mg daily, prevents most fungal infections and is the standard antifungal prophylaxis used for the first 6 weeks after transplantation.

The routine use of trimethoprim-sulfamethoxazole prophylaxis, one single-strength tablet (80/400) daily or one double-strength tablet three times weekly for 3 to 12 months, has made infection with *Pneumocystis jirovecii* (formerly *P. carinii*) rare in liver transplant recipients. Inhalational pentamidine, 300 mg every 4 weeks, and oral dapsone, 50 to 100 mg daily, are alternative prophylactic regimens for patients who are allergic to sulfa. Prophylaxis is administered for 3 months to 1 year after transplantation but should be extended for an extra year if the patient received additional high-dose immunosuppressants (e.g., steroid boluses, muromonab-CD3, increased tacrolimus) during the first year after transplantation.

CMV infection and disease are less common than in the past but remain a risk after liver transplantation. Prophylaxis with acyclovir, ganciclovir, or valganciclovir is effective and reduces mortality[3]; oral valganciclovir (900 mg daily) is most commonly used for the first 3 months after transplantation. Prophylaxis with oral acyclovir (200 mg daily) or valganciclovir is also a useful preventive strategy against the reactivation of oral or genital herpes simplex virus in the first 3 months after transplantation. Reactivation of varicella-zoster virus may manifest as localized dermatomal vesicles or, in patients who were seronegative before transplantation, as cutaneous and visceral dissemination; treatment is with high-dose acyclovir (800 mg four to five times daily for 5 to 7 days).

By 6 months after liver transplantation, recipients who have normal allograft function and are receiving standard doses of immunosuppressive drugs share the same risks as immunocompetent hosts for community-acquired infections and are not at increased risk for opportunistic infections. Conversely, recipients who have been receiving high-dose immunosuppressive drug regimens for antirejection therapy continue to be at high risk for life-threatening opportunistic infections.

Long-Term Follow-up

Long-term management after liver transplantation requires continuing communication and cooperation between the transplantation center and the primary care physician. Patients require careful routine medical management, screening for malignancy, and immunization updates and boosters.

Hypertension

Hypertension (Chapter 67) occurs in two thirds of all liver transplant recipients and is related to cyclosporine and tacrolimus, which cause vasoconstriction in the systemic and renal vasculature, and corticosteroids, which result in sodium retention, increased plasma volume, and weight gain. Management of hypertension in these patients follows a stepwise approach. Dietary sodium restriction, resumption of physical activity, and weight reduction are the first steps. Because of the pathophysiology of vasoconstriction, calcium-channel blockers are the drugs of first choice. The preferred calcium-channel blockers belong to the dihydropyridine class, such as nifedipine. Verapamil, diltiazem, and nicardipine are also effective, but they increase the drug levels of cyclosporine and tacrolimus. Second-line antihypertensive agents include diuretics, β-blockers, and α-adrenergic blockers. Angiotensin-converting enzyme inhibitors should be used with caution because they can aggravate hyperkalemia and, in rare instances, exacerbate leukopenia. Hypertension may improve with time as corticosteroids are discontinued and the dose of cyclosporine or tacrolimus is lowered.

Diabetes Mellitus

Diabetes mellitus (Chapter 237) develops in up to one third of liver recipients after transplantation, with most cases being insulin dependent. The pathogenesis is multifactorial, including genetic predisposition and use of tacrolimus, cyclosporine, and corticosteroids. Steroid tapering is the key to management of early post-transplantation hyperglycemia. Management is otherwise similar to that for the nontransplanted population.

Hyperlipidemia

Hyperlipidemia (Chapter 213) develops in approximately one fourth of all liver transplant recipients. The management of hyperlipidemia includes appropriate dietary restrictions of fat and carbohydrate, weight reduction, regular exercise, and smoking cessation. The preferred medication for patients with resistant hyperlipidemia is 3-hydroxy-3-methylglutaryl coenzyme A (HMG-CoA) reductase inhibitors.

Bone Mineral Density

Bone mineral density decreases during the first few months after transplantation but eventually regains its preoperative level. Fractures most frequently involve trabecular bones such as the vertebrae and the ribs. *Osteonecrosis* or *avascular necrosis* of the hips and, less often, the knees and the humerus bones, may occur. Contributing risk factors to bone disease include preexisting osteopenia, prolonged bed rest, malnutrition, corticosteroids, cyclosporine, tacrolimus, furosemide, and the original diagnosis of primary biliary cirrhosis or primary sclerosing cholangitis with associated metabolic osteodystrophy. Management includes regular exercise and pharmacologic therapies such as calcium supplementation, vitamin D derivatives, and bisphosphonates (Chapter 251).

Cancer

Skin cancer (Chapter 210) is the most common malignancy occurring in the setting of solid-organ transplantation and immunosuppression. Squamous cell carcinoma is more common than basal cell carcinoma or malignant melanoma in this population, and some recipients develop hundreds of squamous cell carcinomas. Patients should seek medical attention if they have a skin growth that bleeds or crusts, increases in size or thickness, or changes in color or texture. Sunscreen with a sun protection factor of at least 15 is recommended. Patients should undergo at least annual skin examinations depending on their previous history of skin cancers.

Colon cancer (Chapter 199) is a common de novo neoplasia after transplantation. Colonoscopic surveillance with multiple biopsies every 6 months for the first 2 years after transplantation, followed by annual examinations, has been recommended for high-risk patients with ulcerative colitis.

If not given before liver transplantation, hepatitis A, hepatitis B, and pneumococcal vaccines (Chapter 17) should be given. Other immunizations include influenza vaccine annually and tetanus toxoid booster every 5 years. Vaccines based on live or attenuated microorganisms should be avoided, including those for measles, mumps, rubella, chickenpox, polio, and bacille Calmette-Guérin (BCG).

 ───○

1. Vanlemmens C, Di Martino V, Milan C, et al. Immediate listing for liver transplantation versus standard care for Child-Pugh stage B alcoholic cirrhosis: a randomized trial. *Ann Intern Med.* 2009;150:153-161.
2. Otero A, Varo E, de Urbina JO, et al. A prospective randomized open study in liver transplant recipients: daclizumab, mycophenolate mofetil, and tacrolimus versus tacrolimus and steroids. *Liver Transpl.* 2009;15:1542-1552.
3. Hodson EM, Jones CA, Webster AC, et al. Antiviral medications to prevent cytomegalovirus disease and early death in recipients of solid-organ transplants: a systematic review of randomised controlled trials. *Lancet.* 2005;365:2105-2115.

SUGGESTED READINGS

Bernal W, Auzinger G, Dhawan A, et al. Acute liver failure. *Lancet.* 2010;376:190-201. *Review.*
Dutkowski P, De Rougemont O, Clavien PA, et al. Current and future trends in liver transplantation in Europe. *Gastroenterology.* 2010;138:802-809. *Overview of liver transplantation in Europe.*
Gali B, Rosen CB, Plevak DJ. Living donor liver transplantation: selection, perioperative care, and outcome. *J Intensive Care Med.* 2011. [Epub ahead of print.] *Review of surgical methods and donor risks.*

158

DISEASES OF THE GALLBLADDER AND BILE DUCTS

NEZAM H. AFDHAL

● THE BILIARY SYSTEM

Definition

The biliary tract consists of the intrahepatic biliary canaliculus; the small, medium, and large intrahepatic bile ducts; the common bile duct; the gallbladder; the cystic duct; and the ampulla of Vater. The primary functions of the biliary system are secretion and storage of bile salts that solubilize intestinal lipids, excretion of cholesterol to maintain cholesterol homeostasis, excretion of excess bilirubin, and excretion of organic ions, including drug metabolites.

● CHOLESTASIS

PATHOBIOLOGY

Cholestasis is the systemic retention of biliary constituents as a result of failure of formation and flow of bile (Table 158-1). In the liver, hepatocytes are organized into cribriform, anastomosing plates along the sinusoids. At the apical pole, between adjacent hepatocytes, is the 1- to 2-μM biliary canaliculus or space. Each hepatocyte can have multiple canaliculi (up to three), which are characterized by microvilli that protrude into the canalicular lumen. Bile consists of water, electrolytes, and organic solutes (Table 158-2). It is continuously modified both by the cholangiocytes that line the bile ducts and by the gallbladder mucosa; therefore, gallbladder bile is markedly different from hepatic bile. The gallbladder mucosa absorbs water and concentrates bile, so the total lipid content of gallbladder bile is much higher than that of hepatic bile (10 vs. 3 g/dL, respectively).

TABLE 158-1 CAUSES OF CHOLESTASIS

EXTRAHEPATIC	INTRAHEPATIC
Choledocholithiasis	Viral hepatitis
Bile duct stricture	Alcoholic hepatitis
Cholangiocarcinoma	Drug induced
Pancreatic carcinoma	Ductopenia syndromes
Chronic pancreatitis	Primary biliary cirrhosis
Papillary stenosis	Benign recurrent intrahepatic cholestasis
Ampullary cancer	Byler's disease
Primary sclerosing cholangitis	Primary sclerosing cholangitis
Choledochal cysts	Alagille's syndrome
Parasites (e.g., *Ascaris, Clonorchis*)	Sarcoid
Acquired immunodeficiency syndrome (AIDS) cholangiopathy	Lymphoma
Biliary atresia	Postoperative
Portal lymphadenopathy	Total parenteral nutrition
Mirrizzi's syndrome	α_1-Antitrypsin deficiency

FIGURE 158-1. Schematic diagram of the metabolism of phospholipid and cholesterol by the hepatocyte. BSEP = bile salt export pump; HDL = high-density lipoprotein; LDL = low-density lipoprotein; MDR2 = multidrug resistant receptor 2 (a phospholipid lipase highly selective for phosphatidylcholine or lecithin); VLDL = very low density lipoprotein.

TABLE 158-2 CONSTITUENTS OF HUMAN CANALICULAR BILE

Bile salts, 12 g/L	Cholates, 35%
Glycine conjugates, 75%	Chenodeoxycholates, 35%
Taurine conjugates, 24.8%	Deoxycholates, 25%
Free bile acids, 0.2%	Lithocholates, 1%
	Miscellaneous, 40%
Phospholipids, 5 g/L	Phosphatidylcholine, 96%
	Phosphatidylethanolamine, 3%
Cholesterol, 1 g/L	Free, unesterified, 99%
Bilirubin, 0.2 g/L	Diglucuronide, 80%
	Monoglucuronide, 18%
	Unconjugated, 2%
Proteins, 2 g/L	Albumin, 50%
	Immunoglobulins, 23%
	Calcium binding protein/anionic peptide fraction, 17%
	Serum proteins, 9%
	Canalicular proteins, 1%
Electrolytes	Sodium, 150 mEq/L
	Magnesium, 2 mEq/L
	Calcium, 3 mEq/L
	Potassium, 5 mEq/L
	Chloride, 110 mEq/L
	Bicarbonate, 30 mEq/L

TABLE 158-3 CANALICULAR ATP-BINDING CASSETTE TRANSPORTERS FOR PRIMARY BILIARY CONSTITUENTS

TRANSPORTER NAME	GENE CODE	SUBSTRATE	ASSOCIATED HEREDITARY DISEASE
FIC1	*ATP8B1*	?	PFIC type 1 (Byler's disease)
BSEP	*ABCB11*	Bile salts	PFIC type 2
MDR3	*ABCB4*	Phosphatidylcholine	PFIC type 3
MDR1	*ABCB1*	Amphipathic drugs	
MRP2 (cMOAT)	*ABCC2*	Anionic neutral drugs	Dubin-Johnson syndrome
ABCG5/ABCG8	*ABCG5/8*	Cholesterol	Sitosterolemia

ATP = adenosine triphosphate; BSEP = bile salt export pump; cMOAT = canalicular multispecific organic anion transporter; MDR = multidrug-resistant receptor; MRP2 = multidrug resistance-associated protein 2; PFIC = progressive familial intrahepatic cholestasis.

1 L/day. The major phospholipid in bile is phosphatidylcholine, also called lecithin. Phosphatidylcholine in bile is derived from newly synthesized hepatic phosphatidylcholine, which is then transported through the hepatocyte by a phosphatidylcholine transfer protein and delivered to the multidrug resistance receptor 3 (MDR3), a phosphatidylcholine-specific transporter for final secretion into bile (see Fig. 158-1). All biliary lipids, including cholesterol, are secreted in a controlled manner by adenosine triphosphate (ATP)–binding cassette transporters (Table 158-3).

CLINICAL MANIFESTATIONS

The clinical manifestations depend on the location and cause of the obstructive process and the degree to which an associated increase in pro-inflammatory cytokines decreases bile salt synthesis and secretion. Intrahepatic cholestasis is usually the result of either hepatocellular dysfunction or injury to the small and medium bile ducts secondary to viruses, alcohol, or drugs.

Bile salt retention can lead to an excess of hydrophobic bile salts, such as deoxycholate, which are hepatotoxic. These retained bile salts can overflow out of the liver and lead to increased levels of bile salts in the serum and skin; the clinical manifestation is pruritus. Excess cholesterol is deposited in all tissues, particularly as tendinous xanthomas and periorbital xanthelasmas, but clinically significant atherosclerosis is uncommon.

In cholestasis, concentrations of intestinal bile salts are inadequate to solubilize dietary lipids; the result is the excretion of excess nonabsorbed fat. Long-chain dietary fats also irritate the colonic mucosa. Steatorrhea is suggested by the presence of stainable fat in stool and confirmed by quantitative analysis of a stool collection.

The major primary bile acids are cholic and chenodeoxycholic acid. The secondary bile acids, lithocholic and deoxycholic acids, which are derived from the intestinal breakdown of primary bile acids, are more hydrophobic, increase in cholestasis, and can be toxic to hepatocytes. Amidation with glycine or taurine results in the formation of bile salts that are preferentially secreted into bile. Bile salts are amphophilic detergent-like molecules synthesized from cholesterol via a pathway dependent on either 7α-hydroxylase or sterol 27-hydroxylase. Bile salt synthesis accounts for approximately 50% of the liver metabolism of cholesterol. Bile salts are secreted into the canalicular space by an energy-dependent bile salt export pump (Fig. 158-1). In the canalicular membrane, bile salts exist as simple (bile salt only) or mixed (with phosphatidylcholine and cholesterol) micelles and are transported into the gallbladder. A fatty meal results in contraction of the gallbladder, with expulsion of bile salts into the duodenum, where they form micelles with intraluminal fat. About 95% of bile acids are absorbed by a sodium-dependent bile acid transporter in the terminal ileum. The total bile acid pool is circulated four to six times per day, and the volume of biliary secretion is approximately

Because malabsorption of the fat-soluble vitamins A, D, E, and K can result in deficiency syndromes, fat-soluble vitamins and essential fatty acids should be given as dietary supplements. The combination of osteomalacia and osteoporosis is a serious consequence of cholestasis and chronic liver disease.

DIAGNOSIS

In pure cholestasis, alkaline phosphatase and γ-glutamyltransferase levels are elevated significantly, whereas aminotransferase levels are normal or only mildly increased (Chapter 149). Bilirubin may be elevated but can be normal even in severe intrahepatic cholestasis until the very late stages of disease. Dilation of the intrahepatic ducts on ultrasonography (US) suggests extrahepatic obstructive cholestasis.

TREATMENT   Rx

Therapy should attempt to remove the cause of cholestasis, such as bypassing an obstructing pancreatic cancer (Chapter 200) with surgery or a stent. In the progressive cholestasis of intrahepatic biliary disease (e.g., primary biliary cirrhosis [PBC]), liver transplantation (Chapter 157) may be the only recourse.

Bile acid binders or sequestrants, such as cholestyramine, can lower the bile acid concentration but are associated with bloating and constipation (Table 158-4). Replacement of hydrophobic bile salts with hydrophilic bile salts, such as ursodeoxycholic acid (UDCA), treats all forms of intrahepatic cholestasis and the associated pruritus. The sensorineural pathway can also be blocked by using opioid antagonists such as naloxone and naltrexone, but care must be taken to avoid the risk for opioid withdrawal syndrome. Hepatic enzyme inducers such as phenobarbital and rifampicin have also been used successfully to treat pruritus. Rifampicin may induce drug-metabolizing transporters, resulting in increased excretion of pruritogens, but with a risk of hepatotoxicity. In some cases of intractable pruritus, marijuana or its synthetic form dronabinol (Marinol) has been useful in controlling symptoms. Finally, for situations such as the intractable pruritus of biliary cirrhosis, liver transplantation is the only option.

Supplementation with calcium, 1500 mg/day, plus vitamin D is essential. If bone density scans show osteopenia, therapy with bisphosphonates should be instituted (Chapter 251).

● BILIARY TRACT DISEASES

Lesions of the intrahepatic and extrahepatic biliary tree, including the ampulla of Vater, are rare.

Biliary Atresia

Biliary atresia is a fibro-obliterative process that affects the perinatal bile ducts from the hilar bifurcation to the duodenum in 1 in every 13,000 live births in the United States. Associated genetic abnormalities in 25% of cases include polysplenia, anomalies of the portal vein and hepatic artery, abdominal situs inversus, intestinal malrotation, and cardiovascular and urinary tract anomalies. The clinical findings consist of jaundice with acholic stools persisting for 2 weeks after birth. The diagnosis can be suspected by endoscopic retrograde cholangiopancreatography (ERCP) or magnetic resonance cholangiopancreatography (MRCP) but is usually confirmed by laparotomy. Surgical correction by portoenterostomy should be performed within the first 60 days of life. About 80% of children grow normally through the first years of life, but subsequent stenosis of the anastomosis, with progressive biliary cirrhosis and liver failure, is common and is an indication for liver transplantation.

TABLE 158-4	CLINICAL FEATURES OF AND THERAPY FOR CHOLESTASIS
CLINICAL SYNDROME	**TREATMENT**
Pruritus	Bile salt binders (e.g., cholestyramine), ursodeoxycholic acid, rifampicin, naltrexone, carbinoids, phenobarbital
Hypercholesterolemia	Bile salt binders (e.g., cholestyramine) Statins—poor effect
Malabsorption	Medium-chain triglycerides, fat-soluble vitamins (A, D, E, K), essential fatty acids
Osteopenia	Calcium, vitamin D, bisphosphonates

Choledochal Cysts

Choledochal cysts are congenital ductal ectasias involving either a segment of the biliary tree or its entirety. The incidence is 1 per 13,000 live births in the United States, but it is 13 times higher in Japan and other parts of Asia. There is a four-fold greater prevalence in females, and choledochal cysts are associated with an abnormal pancreatic ductal junction and congenital hepatic fibrosis. The usual clinical manifestation is a right upper quadrant mass, jaundice, and pain. Acute pancreatitis, cholangitis, variceal hemorrhage, and cyst rupture are alternative findings. The diagnosis is usually made by imaging studies, including US, computed tomography (CT), MRCP, and ERCP. Therapy is generally surgical excision of the cyst with a Roux-en-Y hepaticojejunostomy because of the high (3 to 26%) incidence of malignant transformation of the cysts into cholangiocarcinoma. When there is extensive intrahepatic ductal dilation (Caroli's disease), recurrent cholangitis and intrahepatic stones are common, and liver transplantation is the optimal therapy.

Oriental Cholangiohepatitis

Recurrent cholangitis with hepatolithiasis is endemic in East Asia, especially in Taiwan, where the incidence is as high as 13% in areas where infection with *Ascaris lumbricoides* (Chapter 365) and *Clonorchis sinensis* (Chapter 364) is common. These worms cause local strictures and dilation of the intrahepatic biliary tree. Biliary stasis ensues, and the bile becomes infected with bacteria that are able to deconjugate bilirubin and cause brown stones to form. Recurrent cholangitis is the usual finding, but malignant transformation to cholangiocarcinoma can also occur. The diagnosis is made by US or CT. Treatment includes intravenous fluids and antibiotics. Endoscopic stone removal plus clearance of infected biliary segments is a primary option, but surgical resection of localized segments of the liver may be necessary.

Primary Sclerosing Cholangitis

Primary sclerosing cholangitis is a chronic cholestatic condition characterized by segmental fibrosing inflammation of the intrahepatic and extrahepatic bile ducts.

EPIDEMIOLOGY

The prevalence of primary sclerosing cholangitis is 1 to 6 cases per 100,000 in the U.S. population, with a male-to-female ratio of 2.3 : 1. The mean age at diagnosis is 32 to 40 years, but children can be affected.

PATHOBIOLOGY

The cause remains unknown, but primary sclerosing cholangitis is thought to be a primary autoimmune disease. Genome-wide association studies implicate loci near human leukocyte antigen (HLA)-B on chromosome 6p21 and loci not related to HLA on chromosomes 13q31, 2q35, and 3p21. Even more sophisticated technologies will likely identify specific genes and molecular pathways in the future. The disease is progressive, with the obliteration of small, medium, and large bile ducts leading to three distinct clinical syndromes: (1) cholestasis with eventual biliary cirrhosis, (2) recurrent cholangitis and large duct strictures, and (3) cholangiocarcinoma. The multiple causes of secondary sclerosing cholangitis can be accompanied by symptoms and signs indistinguishable from those of the primary form (Table 158-5).

Primary sclerosing cholangitis is associated with both ulcerative colitis and Crohn's disease of the colon (Chapter 143). Between 70 and 90% of patients with primary sclerosing cholangitis have clinical or microscopic colitis, and between 1.3 and 13% of patients with colitis have primary sclerosing cholangitis. Inflammatory bowel disease usually precedes primary sclerosing cholangitis, but in some cases the colitis is asymptomatic and is discovered by subsequent colonoscopy and biopsy. There is also a crossover syndrome between primary sclerosing cholangitis and primary autoimmune hepatitis (Chapter 151).

CLINICAL MANIFESTATIONS

The most common laboratory finding is an elevated alkaline phosphatase level, which is present in 90% of patients, and mildly elevated aminotransferase levels. The bilirubin level is initially normal in 60% of patients but increases over time and is an important prognostic factor. Autoantibodies, including antinuclear antibodies and anti–smooth muscle antibodies, are seen in 22% of patients, but a positive antimitochondrial antibody (AMA) is rare and suggests PBC. Perinuclear antineutrophilic cytoplasmic antibody (pANCA) is positive in 90% of patients with primary sclerosing cholangitis

TABLE 158-5	DISEASES ASSOCIATED WITH SCLEROSING CHOLANGITIS
PRIMARY SCLEROSING CHOLANGITIS	**SECONDARY SCLEROSING CHOLANGITIS**
Ulcerative colitis	Choledocholithiasis
Crohn's colitis or ileocolitis	Infections in immunocompromised patients (*Cryptosporidium, Trichosporon,* cytomegalovirus, *Cryptococcus,* visceral protothecosis)
Type 1 autoimmune hepatitis	HTLV-1-associated myelopathy
	Ischemic injury to the hepatic artery or arterioles
	Trauma
	Neoplasia
	Toxic injury
	Floxuridine (hepatic artery injection)
	Formalin injection of echinococcal cysts
	Congenital abnormalities
	Celiac sprue

HTLV = human T-lymphotropic virus.

FIGURE 158-2. Endoscopic retrograde cholangiopancreatography for primary sclerosing cholangitis with contrast injected through a balloon catheter (seen in the lower common duct). The intrahepatic ducts are mainly affected and show diminished arborization (pruning); diffuse segmental strictures alternating with normal-caliber or mildly dilated duct segments (cholangiectases) have resulted in a beaded appearance. (From Mahadevan U, Bass NM. Sclerosing cholangitis and recurrent pyogenic cholangitis. In: Feldman M, Friedman LS, Sleisenger MH, eds. *Gastrointestinal and Liver Disease: Pathophysiology/Diagnosis/Management,* 7th ed. Philadelphia: Saunders; 2002:1137.)

and colitis, but pANCA is nonspecific and is also found in ulcerative colitis and in autoimmune hepatitis without primary sclerosing cholangitis.

DIAGNOSIS

The diagnosis is based on pathologic and radiologic findings, and all patients should undergo both liver biopsy and cholangiography. Large duct disease, which is diagnosed most frequently by ERCP or MRCP, includes strictures, beading, and dilation (Fig. 158-2). Liver biopsy shows an obliterative cholangitis with inflammation and characteristic periductular "onion ring" fibrosis (Fig. 158-3). As the disease progresses, ductopenia and secondary biliary cirrhosis predominate. In stage I, inflammation is confined to the portal tracts; in stage II, there is hepatitis and portal fibrosis; in stage III, bridging fibrosis appears; and stage IV is characterized by biliary cirrhosis and regenerative nodules. Associated conditions include pancreatitis (15% of patients), perihepatic lymphadenopathy, and cholangiocarcinoma (27 to 41% of patients at autopsy or transplantation).

TREATMENT ℞

No treatment slows disease progression. Medical therapy includes treatment of cholangitis and endoscopic therapy for large strictures via balloon dilation and stent insertion. Surgery is avoided, if possible, because it increases the risk for recurrent cholangitis. Immunosuppressive therapy is not effective. In randomized trials, UDCA (15 mg/kg/day) improved bilirubin, alkaline phosphatase, and albumin levels, but it provided no definite benefit in terms of survival or time to liver decompensation. Higher doses (>20 mg/kg) have often been used, but a randomized trial suggested that doses of 28 to 30 mg/kg are not beneficial and may actually increase morbidity when compared with placebo.[1]

Liver transplantation (Chapter 157), which is the only potentially curative therapy, provides an actuarial survival rate of 83% at 1 year and 73% at 5 years. All patients with primary sclerosing cholangitis who undergo transplantation should be screened periodically for colon carcinoma because they have chronic colitis (Chapter 143). Recurrent primary sclerosing cholangitis after transplantation is rare and difficult to distinguish from other causes of bile duct injury. If small (<1 cm), incidental cholangiocarcinomas are found at transplantation, survival is not affected, but larger cholangiocarcinomas (>2 cm) detected during the pretransplant evaluation by CT or magnetic resonance imaging are a contraindication to liver transplantation.

Patients with primary sclerosing cholangitis should be screened for possible cholangiocarcinoma by cholangiography of strictures every 6 to 12 months, with brushings and biopsies. If cholangiocarcinoma is detected, patients should be offered surgical resection or radiation therapy (Chapter 202).

FIGURE 158-3. Microscopically, this bile duct in a case of sclerosing cholangitis is surrounded by marked collagenous connective tissue deposition. (Reproduced from http://library.med.utah.edu/WebPath/GUIDE/INTRO.html with permission.)

Primary Biliary Cirrhosis

DEFINITION

PBC is a slowly progressive, obliterative autoimmune cholangiopathy involving the small and medium-sized bile ducts. It leads to ductopenia, progressive fibrosis, cholestasis, and liver failure.

EPIDEMIOLOGY

PBC is predominantly a disease of women (95% of cases) between the ages of 20 and 60 years. The age- and gender-adjusted prevalence has been estimated at 65 and 12 per 100,000 persons, respectively, for women and men. The incidence of the disease may be increasing, and a U.S. study estimated it at 2.7 per 100,000 person years, or 4.5 and 0.7 for women and men, respectively.

PATHOBIOLOGY

PBC is thought to be an autoimmune disorder, but the mechanism of progressive destruction of the small interlobular ducts is unknown. Genome-wide studies show an association with HLA, interleukin (IL) 12A, and IL-12RB2 variants, suggesting that IL-12 signaling might be important. Mouse models have pointed to the potential roles of IL-12Rα and transforming growth factor-βII receptor. The human disease is slowly progressive and can eventually lead to biliary cirrhosis with portal hypertension and liver

PROGNOSIS

The natural history is variable. Some patients have severe recurrent cholangitis, whereas others progress to biliary cirrhosis. The median survival until death or transplantation is approximately 12 years, with a range of up to 21 years. Actuarial survival is greater for asymptomatic patients than for symptomatic ones (10-year survival rate of 80% vs. 50%).

failure. The classic histologic finding is the presence of noncaseating granulomas associated with small bile ducts and an overall paucity of bile ducts in the portal tracts. The presence of significant bridging fibrosis or cirrhosis carries a worse prognosis.

CLINICAL MANIFESTATIONS

Almost 60% of patients with PBC are asymptomatic at diagnosis. The most common symptoms are fatigue (50%) and pruritus (30%). Fatigue is unrelated to the degree of underlying liver injury or cholestasis and can be extremely debilitating. Pruritus is often first noticed in pregnancy but persists after delivery, and many patients are initially referred for dermatologic evaluation.

In addition to the features of cholestasis, multiple clinical syndromes are associated with PBC and are suggestive of an autoimmune origin. Autoimmune thyroid dysfunction (Chapter 233), sicca syndrome (Chapter 276), Raynaud's phenomenon (Chapter 275), and celiac disease (Chapter 142) have all been associated with PBC. Metabolic bone disease can be particularly troublesome because of the long duration of cholestasis; bone density studies are mandatory every 2 years to guide and monitor therapy.

DIAGNOSIS

The most common biochemical abnormality is an elevation in serum alkaline phosphatase, which should be confirmed by an elevated γ-glutamyl transpeptidase and indicates cholestasis. The bilirubin level is not elevated until late in the course of the disease, and most of the elevation usually consists of conjugated bilirubin. US should be performed to image the biliary tree and confirm the absence of extrahepatic disease. AMA, which has a sensitivity and specificity higher than 95% when the titer is greater than 1:40, can be positive before there is any clinical or biochemical evidence of PBC. Total immunoglobulins are generally normal, but the immunoglobulin M fraction can be elevated. Liver biopsy is performed to stage the disease and occasionally to confirm the diagnosis, particularly in AMA-negative patients.

TREATMENT   Rx

UDCA therapy reduces intracellular hydrophobic bile acids and may have a cytoprotective effect on cell membranes. Although initial randomized trials showed a significant increase in survival after up to 4 years of UDCA therapy (12 to 15 mg/kg), as judged by the time to liver transplantation, a more recent meta-analysis of 16 trials showed no benefit in terms of reducing mortality or delaying liver transplantation.[2] Serum bilirubin, alkaline phosphatase, and cholesterol levels improve with UDCA therapy, but treatment does not relieve the fatigue and has a variable effect on pruritus. Side effects are rare, the most common being diarrhea.

There is no definite benefit from steroids, colchicine, or azathioprine. Low-dose methotrexate (2.5 mg three times/week) has been tried, but data are insufficient to support its routine use at this time. PBC is a common indication for liver transplantation (Chapter 157), but there is considerable debate regarding the timing of transplantation.

PROGNOSIS

PBC is a progressive disease, with up to two thirds of asymptomatic patients becoming symptomatic in 2 to 4 years. Median survival is 9.3 years from diagnosis, and the most reliable determinants of prognosis are the serum bilirubin level and the Mayo risk score, a composite score that predicts clinical outcomes and is calculated as follows: $R = 0.871 \log(e)$ (bilirubin in mg/dL) $+ 2.53 \log(e)$ (albumin in g/dL) $+ 0.039$ (age in years) $+ 2.38 \log(e)$ (prothrombin time in seconds) $+ 0.859$ (edema score of 0, 0.5, or 1). Liver failure develops in 26% of patients by 10 years after diagnosis.

Vanishing Bile Duct Syndromes

Vanishing bile duct syndromes are characterized by a paucity of intrahepatic bile ducts and by eventual cholestasis and biliary cirrhosis. Causes include PBC, primary sclerosing cholangitis, autoimmune hepatitis (Chapter 151), graft-versus-host disease, chronic liver allograft rejection (Chapter 157), ischemia, intrahepatic chemotherapy, drug toxicity (e.g., ampicillin, amoxicillin, flucloxacillin, erythromycin, tetracycline, doxycycline, cotrimoxazole), human immunodeficiency virus (HIV) infection (Chapter 397), sarcoidosis (Chapter 95), idiopathic or paraneoplastic bile duct paucity, and histiocytosis. Almost all these conditions are accompanied by chronic cholestasis and

TABLE 158-6	RISK FACTORS FOR GALLSTONE DISEASE

Age
Female gender
Parity
Obesity
Rapid weight loss
Hypertriglyceridemia
Genetic (e.g., Pima Indians, Chileans)
Medications: estrogen, clofibrate, ceftriaxone, octreotide acetate (Sandostatin)
Terminal ileal resection
Gallbladder hypomotility: pregnancy, diabetes, after vagotomy
Somatostatinoma
Total parenteral nutrition
Spinal cord injury

elevated alkaline phosphatase levels. Treatment is for the complications of cholestasis, and UDCA (15 mg/kg) is given to increase bile flow. Most of these conditions are slowly progressive and result in biliary cirrhosis, which ultimately requires liver transplantation.

GALLSTONE DISEASE

DEFINITION

There are three different types of gallstones: cholesterol gallstones, mixed gallstones, and pigment stones, which can be further divided into black and brown stones. Cholesterol and mixed stones account for 80% of gallstone disease in the United States. Cholesterol stones contain more than 70% cholesterol, whereas mixed stones also contain significant amounts of pigments such as bilirubin. Black pigment stones, which are generally associated with hemolytic diseases, contain calcium salts, bilirubin, and proteins. Brown pigment stones are more common in Asia, where they are associated with intrahepatic cholangitis and infection; in the United States, brown stones are seen after cholecystectomy, especially when they manifest as choledocholithiasis.

EPIDEMIOLOGY

Approximately 30 million people in the United States have gallstones, and the estimated annual cost of gallstone disease is $15 billion. In Europe, large ultrasound studies in subjects between 30 and 65 years of age have shown gallstones in 18.8% of women and 9.5% of men. In a study in which 1930 subjects were monitored for 10 years, the cumulative incidence of new stones was 4.6%.

Age is a major risk factor for gallstone disease (Table 158-6); less than 2% of cholecystectomies for gallstones are performed in children, usually because of hemolytic diseases. However, the increased prevalence of obesity in children may result in an earlier incidence of gallstone disease.

The age-adjusted female-to-male ratio for gallstone disease is 2.9:1 between the ages of 30 and 39 years, but it decreases to 1.2:1 between the ages of 50 and 59 years. Women with gallstone disease also appear to be more likely than men to undergo cholecystectomy. Pregnancy appears to be the major risk factor for gallstones in younger women, with a prevalence of 1.3% in nulliparous women versus 13% in multiparous women. Estrogen use is also associated with a higher risk for symptomatic gallstones and cholecystectomy: a relative risk of 2.1 to 3.7 versus no estrogen use. The mechanisms of increased risk include activation of estrogen α-receptor-mediated hepatic cholesterol secretion, a progesterone-induced reduction in gallbladder contraction, and a pregnancy-induced alteration in hydrophobic-hydrophilic bile salt balance.

Obesity increases the risk for gallstones as a result of enhanced cholesterol absorption, synthesis, and secretion. The risk is higher in women and in the morbidly obese, but rapid weight reduction by very low-calorie diets is also associated with gallstones. Diets high in polyunsaturated and monounsaturated fats may reduce the risk for gallstone disease.

PATHOBIOLOGY

Gallstone disease is predominantly an inability to maintain free cholesterol in solution in bile. As canalicular bile passes down the bile duct system, cholangiocytes maintain bile flow and volume by secreting chloride, bicarbonate, and water into bile. In cystic fibrosis (Chapter 89), defects in the cystic fibrosis transmembrane conductance regulator, which in the liver is found only on cholangiocytes, reduces choleresis and results in the formation of mucous plugs, with subsequent focal biliary cirrhosis and gallstone disease.

The gallbladder, which acts as the final storage reservoir for bile, concentrates bile by removing water and thereby increasing the lipid concentration from 3 g/dL in hepatic bile to 10 g/dL in gallbladder bile. Bile salt concentrations can be as high as 300 mM and would digest the biliary epithelium if the gallbladder did not secrete mucin for protection. The gallbladder mucosa also secretes hydrogen ions to prevent calcium salt deposition and maintain a bile pH of about 6.5. A normal gallbladder ejects 10 to 20% of its contents in response to duodenal-gallbladder enteric nervous stimulation. Postprandially, duodenal lipids cause an approximately 70% contraction of the gallbladder, mediated by both the enteric nervous system and cholecystokinin. Impaired contractility is one of the critical steps in the pathogenesis of gallstones.

Genetics

Family history studies have shown that gallstones are twice as common in first-degree relatives of gallstone patients as in age- and sex-matched control subjects. In the United States, descendants of the original Amerindians have a markedly increased prevalence of gallstones, with the highest rates in female Pima Indians older than 25 years, who have a 75% prevalence of cholesterol gallstones. Amerindians in South America and Mexico also have a very high prevalence of gallstones, and these populations have the highest rate of complications of gallstone disease, such as gallbladder cancer, in the world. South Americans of Hispanic origin have much lower rates of gallstone disease.

No specific gallstone genes have been found in humans, but lithogenic genes, including the bile salt export pump gene, have been described in gallstone-susceptible mice. Human gallstone disease is probably a combination of complex multigene susceptibility and environmental factors.

Cholesterol Gallstones

Cholesterol gallstones contain 50 to 90% cholesterol and are the most common form of stones in countries where people consume a Western diet high in protein and fat. Cholesterol is an intensely hydrophobic molecule that can remain soluble in aqueous solution only as saturated micelles and vesicles in conjunction with bile salts and lecithin. Cholesterol in gallbladder bile is found in multiple phases; in the presence of cholesterol supersaturation, unstable cholesterol vesicles nucleate to form cholesterol crystals (Fig. 158-4). Nucleation is promoted by a variety of factors, including proteins and lipids.

Increased biliary secretion of cholesterol results in cholesterol supersaturation of bile. The result is excess secretion of mucus into the gallbladder, formation of a gel layer, and stasis, which causes cholesterol to nucleate and cholesterol crystals to be deposited.

Cholesterol monohydrate crystals are only several hundred micrometers in size and should easily be expelled through the cystic duct. However, the mucous sludge containing calcium salts, bilirubin, mucin, and crystals is not easily expelled by contraction of the gallbladder. Biliary sludge, also known as microlithiasis, can be seen as an echogenic, freely mobile mass in the gallbladder on US. Biliary sludge can cause the symptoms of gallstone disease, including cholecystitis, cholangitis, and pancreatitis.

Biliary sludge can resolve, persist, or progress to stones when its crystals grow to form plates, in part because of an impairment in gallbladder contractility. Cholesterol supersaturation of bile is associated with increased absorption of cholesterol by the gallbladder smooth muscle, a process that impairs smooth muscle contractility and reduces the gallbladder's response to cholecystokinin.

Pigment Gallstones

Black pigment stones contain 10 to 90% calcium bilirubinate in combination with a variety of other calcium salts, such as hydroxyapatite and carbonate. These stones are common in India (40%) but rare in Minnesota (5%). Older age is associated with a higher incidence of pigment stones, as are total parenteral nutrition and hemolytic diseases.

Brown pigment stones represent 30% of gallstones in Japan and up to 90% of gallstones in rural China. They are related to low-calorie, high-vegetable diets; occur in both the biliary tract and the liver; and have a strong association with recurrent pyogenic cholangitis and cholangiohepatitis. In the United States, these stones are seen as postcholecystectomy cholelithiasis, presumably secondary to stasis and infection. Bacterial enzymes deconjugate bilirubin from its glucuronide and hydrolyze phospholipids, leading to precipitation of calcium, bilirubin, and free fatty acids. These stones, which are often soft and easy to crush endoscopically, are commonly treated by endoscopic extraction.

CLINICAL MANIFESTATIONS

The symptoms caused by gallstones are often nonspecific and include nausea, bloating, and right upper quadrant pain. Biliary pain, which is described as an intermittent right upper quadrant or epigastric pain occurring 15 to 30 minutes after a meal, often with radiation to the back, is unpredictable, severe, and usually constant rather than a true colic. The pain persists for 3 to 4 hours and may be associated with nausea and vomiting. In uncomplicated cholecystitis, fever and leukocytosis are absent, the pain can usually be adequately treated with a single dose of narcotic analgesics or nonsteroidal anti-inflammatory drugs (NSAIDs), and the pain generally subsides within 6 hours. Attacks of colic may be separated by days or months.

DIAGNOSIS

Asymptomatic Gallstones

Asymptomatic gallstones, which are frequently diagnosed by US performed for other indications, account for about 85% of gallstones. Patients with asymptomatic stones have a similar incidence of nonspecific symptoms of nausea and bloating as the general population, and complications of gallstone disease rarely develop. Biliary colic, however, is more predictive of gallstones, and it is an indicator of increased risk for cholecystitis or other complications. Because the current standard of care is to treat only symptomatic stones, it is critical to determine whether any symptoms are related to gallbladder stones.

Among patients with asymptomatic stones, biliary colic develops in about 2 to 3% annually. In the absence of antecedent symptoms, complications of gallstone disease (e.g., acute cholecystitis) develop at a rate of less than 1% per year. As a result, the recommendation is to delay cholecystectomy until after biliary colic develops, with prophylactic or incidental cholecystectomy recommended only for Amerindians, transplant recipients, or patients with sickle cell anemia, morbid obesity, an anomalous pancreatic ductal junction, porcelain gallbladder, or gallbladder polyps larger than 1 cm (see Cholecystectomy under Treatment).

Acute Calculous Cholecystitis

Acute cholecystitis, which is the most common serious complication of gallstone disease, can lead to perforation of the gallbladder, peritonitis, fistula into the intestine or duodenum with gallstone ileus or obstruction, and abscesses in the liver or abdominal cavity. Acute cholecystitis is caused by obstruction of the cystic duct, and the ensuing increased intraluminal pressure can lead to vascular compromise of the gallbladder. *Salmonella* and other less common microorganisms such as *Vibrio cholerae*, *Leptospira*, and *Listeria* can cause primary cholecystitis. Clinical differentiation of biliary colic from acute cholecystitis is difficult but can usually be made from clinical and radiologic findings (Table 158-7).

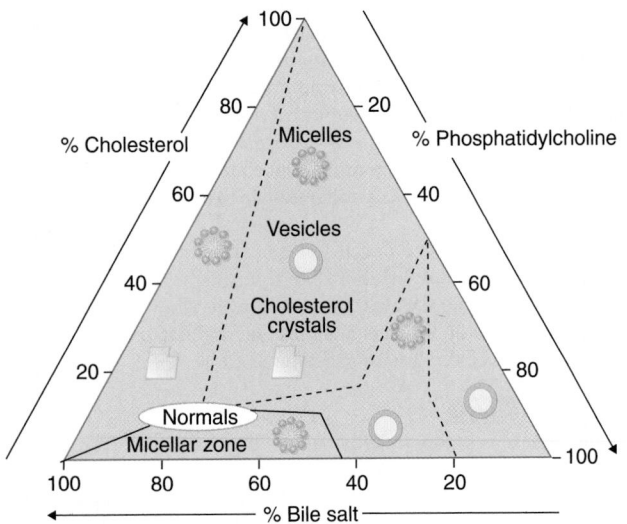

FIGURE 158-4. Equilibrium phase diagram for a lithogenic model bile system with a total lipid content of 10 g/dL.

TABLE 158-7	CLINICAL FEATURES OF BILIARY COLIC COMPARED WITH ACUTE CHOLECYSTITIS	
CLINICAL FINDINGS	**BILIARY COLIC**	**ACUTE CHOLECYSTITIS**
Right upper quadrant pain	Present	Present
Abdominal tenderness	Absent or mild	Moderate to severe, especially over the liver and/or gallbladder (Murphy's sign)
Fever	Absent	Usually present
Leukocytosis	Absent	Usually >11,000/μL
Duration of symptoms	<4 hr	>6 hr
Ultrasound	Gallstones	Gallstones, thickening of gallbladder wall
HIDA scan	Gallbladder visualized within 4 hr	No filling of gallbladder

HIDA = hepatobiliary iminodiacetic acid.

Blood Tests

In uncomplicated acute cholecystitis, laboratory testing usually shows leukocytosis but otherwise is not very helpful. Elevated liver enzyme levels, hyperbilirubinemia, and elevated amylase or lipase levels are not common in cholecystitis and suggest other complications of gallstone disease, such as cholangitis or pancreatitis. When acute cholecystitis is accompanied by an inflammatory mass, the gallbladder can compress the common duct and lead to bile duct obstruction (Mirrizzi's syndrome).

Imaging Studies

Right upper quadrant US noninvasively diagnoses gallstones in 95% of patients with cholecystitis (Fig. 158-5). US can also exclude common bile duct obstruction and may occasionally show bile duct stones. In cholecystitis, the gallbladder wall may be thickened, and free pericholecystic fluid may be present. Murphy's sign is also useful and can be elicited by the ultrasonographer or on physical examination. Gentle pressure is placed by the probe or hand at the border of the rectus sheath in the right upper quadrant, and the patient is asked to inspire. The gallbladder moves down with inspiration onto the examiner's hand or ultrasound probe, and the patient complains of pain when the inflamed gallbladder comes into contact with the examining hand. US can also exclude gangrenous cholecystitis with free air in the gallbladder wall, perforation, and abscess. The most specific test for acute cholecystitis is a technetium-labeled hepatobiliary iminodiacetic acid (HIDA) scan. Intravenously, HIDA is normally taken up by the liver, excreted into the biliary tract, and concentrated in the gallbladder. When a stone obstructs the cystic duct, the gallbladder fails to fill with HIDA; the sensitivity of HIDA scanning is 95%, but the specificity varies markedly and can be as poor as 50% in critically ill or jaundiced patients.

FIGURE 158-5. Ultrasound showing a gallstone.

TREATMENT Rx

Medical Stabilization of Acute Cholecystitis

Treatment of uncomplicated acute cholecystitis is intravenous fluids, antibiotics for 7 to 10 days, and bowel rest. Antibiotic choices include ampicillin (2 g intravenously every 6 hours) and an aminoglycoside (gentamicin 5.1 mg/kg every 24 hours), but cephalosporins (ceftriaxone 1 to 2 g once daily) and ampicillin-sulbactam (1.5 to 3 g every 6 hours) can also be used. Broader coverage should be used in immunosuppressed patients, including the addition of metronidazole (500 mg every 8 hours), piperacillin-tazobactam (3.375 g every 6 hours), and levofloxacin (500 mg to 1 g once daily). Early cholecystectomy during the first hospital admission is generally recommended because it is safe and reduces total hospital stays.[3]

Cholecystectomy

Indications for cholecystectomy include biliary colic, acute and chronic cholecystitis, and acalculous cholecystitis. Diabetic patients may have fewer symptoms because of their neuropathy. As a result, their cholecystitis may be complicated more often by gangrene and perforation; however, prophylactic cholecystectomy is not recommended in patients with diabetes.

Laparoscopic cholecystectomy and small-incision cholecystectomy provide equivalent results for the treatment of gallstones,[4] with some data suggesting that small-incision cholecystectomy reduces operating time and complexity.[5,6] Most patients can be discharged a day after the procedure. A planned laparoscopic approach is changed to open cholecystectomy in only 3% of cases, usually because of difficulty identifying critical anatomic structures such as the cystic or common bile ducts.

Operative cholangiography can be performed during laparoscopic cholecystectomy, and bile duct stones can be removed concurrently or subsequently by ERCP. The incidence of unsuspected, retained common bile duct stones after laparoscopic cholecystectomy is about 2.3%.

The most serious complication of cholecystectomy is bile duct injury, which now occurs in 0.25% of cases. It is more common when the indication for surgery is acute cholecystitis, and it is less common after a surgeon has performed more than 25 laparoscopic surgeries. Bile duct injuries include cystic duct leak, laceration of the duct, complete transection of the duct, and thermal injuries to the duct. Early recognition permits primary open bile duct repair. Leakage from the cystic duct is usually recognized by jaundice, fever, and abdominal pain several days after the procedure; it can be treated successfully by ERCP, with insertion of an endoscopic stent, or by sphincterotomy.

Gallstone Dissolution Therapies

In patients who have relative or absolute contraindications to laparoscopic cholecystectomy, such as concomitant advanced cardiopulmonary or liver disease, a combination of chenodeoxycholic acid (10 mg/kg/day) and UDCA (7 to 15 mg/kg/day) or UDCA alone (15 mg/kg/day) can dissolve multiple small (<5 mm) stones in up to 60% of patients with functioning gallbladders. If CT shows the stones to be calcified, the efficacy is lower, and complete dissolution occurs in only about 10% of patients. Gallstones generally dissolve at a rate of 1 mm/month. After dissolution, gallstones recur at a rate of 10% per year for 5 years, but recurrence is unusual after that time. Continuous therapy may be necessary, thereby making this treatment unattractive except in selected patients in whom cholecystectomy cannot be performed safely.

Extracorporeal shock wave lithotripsy, which uses a focused ultrasound beam, can fragment larger stones. The fragmented stones can then be passed through the cystic duct and expelled into the common bile duct. The fragments that remain behind in the gallbladder should be treated with UDCA for dissolution. Gallstones disappear in more than 50% of patients, but they recur in 50% of successfully treated patients, particularly those with multiple stones and poorly functioning gallbladders.

Topical dissolution therapy involves the insertion of a catheter into the gallbladder under ultrasound guidance; stones are dissolved with methyl ter-butyl ether or ethyl propionate. The technique is still experimental but may soon be ready for widespread testing.

Choledocholithiasis

Common bile duct stones can descend from the gallbladder or arise de novo in a tortuous, dilated common bile duct as a result of infection and biliary stasis (usually cholesterol stones), or they can occur in a postcholecystectomy patient (usually brown stones), in whom they are frequently missed at surgery (2% of cholecystectomies). The clinical findings are cholangitis, pancreatitis, or biliary obstruction; large, obstructing stones can cause jaundice.

Acute bacterial cholangitis, which is most frequently caused by common duct stones that obstruct the common bile duct and raise intrabiliary pressure, is a medical emergency (Fig. 158-6). The bile in these patients is generally infected with *Escherichia coli*, *Bacteroides*, *Klebsiella*, or *Clostridium* species, and the increase in pressure results in transient bacteremia.

FIGURE 158-6. Magnetic resonance cholangiopancreatogram of a dilated biliary tract. The common bile duct (CBD), pancreatic duct (PD), and two large common duct stones (S) are shown.

Clinically, patients are usually very ill with a high temperature, features of systemic sepsis, and obtundation. US may show air in the gallbladder or gallbladder wall; perforation of the gallbladder with peritonitis may then occur. Emergency cholecystectomy is required.

If a fistula develops from the gallbladder to the duodenum, stomach, or colon, a large gallstone can pass through the fistula and into the bowel. If obstruction occurs at the duodenum or the ileocecal valve, gallstone ileus occurs, with symptoms and signs of intestinal obstruction. A plain abdominal radiograph shows bowel obstruction with free air in the gallbladder or biliary tract. Treatment is generally cholecystectomy and removal of the obstructing gallstone.

DIAGNOSIS

Patients with bacterial cholangitis have Charcot's triad of jaundice, abdominal pain, and fever with rigors. Severe renal dysfunction and disseminated intravascular coagulation can complicate severe cholangitis. Aminotransferase, bilirubin, and alkaline phosphatase levels are usually increased. The diagnosis of common bile duct stones can be made with US, which generally shows dilated bile ducts and occasionally identifies a stone. MRCP can identify 95% of stones larger than 1 cm (see Fig. 158-6). ERCP remains the "gold standard" for the diagnosis and treatment of common bile duct stones. If cholangitis is suspected, ERCP should be performed.

TREATMENT   Rx

In patients with concomitant stones in both the gallbladder and the common bile duct, laparoscopic cholecystectomy and bile duct exploration are preferable to a two-stage procedure (ERCP extraction of the common duct stone followed by laparoscopic cholecystectomy).[7][8] For isolated common duct stones, endoscopic therapy includes sphincterotomy and stone extraction with a balloon or basket. Small (<2 cm) stones can be removed easily, whereas larger stones may be crushed with mechanical or ultrasound lithotriptors before removal. Fluids and antibiotics with broad gram-negative coverage (e.g., ceftriaxone 1 to 2 g once daily, ampicillin-sulbactam 1.5 to 3 g every 6 hours, piperacillin-tazobactam 3.375 g every 6 hours, levofloxacin 500 mg to 1 g once daily) are recommended for bacterial cholangitis. In an acutely ill patient, initial decompression of a pus-filled common bile duct with a stent may be the first-line treatment, followed by definitive endoscopic or surgical therapy. After successful endoscopic therapy, laparoscopic cholecystectomy should be performed routinely because of the high risk for recurrent biliary events.[9]

In certain situations, such as after Roux-en-Y choledochojejunostomy, ERCP may not be possible. Alternative approaches include radiologic percutaneous transhepatic cholangiography (PTC) or open exploration of the common bile duct. During PTC, the radiologist can decompress the bile ducts with catheters or stents, and the stones can be removed through the fistula tract by direct cholangiography.

Unusual Complications of Gallstone Disease

Gallstone pancreatitis (Chapter 146) is more common in patients with multiple small stones; it has also been associated with microlithiasis and biliary sludge. Patients have acute epigastric pain radiating into the back, hyperamylasemia, and an imaging study that demonstrates an edematous or necrotic pancreas. Rarely, concomitant cholangitis or jaundice can be seen if the stone is obstructive. Clinical features that suggest gallstone pancreatitis include elevated aspartate aminotransferase and alkaline phosphatase levels. Early ERCP with sphincterotomy plus stone extraction within 24 hours of suspected acute gallstone pancreatitis reduces morbidity and mortality, but in 50% of cases, the stones are not visible or have passed by the time of ERCP. After the successful treatment of common duct stones, any patient who still has a gallbladder should have it removed electively.

Vascular compromise to the gallbladder and the presence of gas-forming bacteria, which are more common in patients who have diabetes or are immunocompromised, can cause gangrenous or emphysematous cholecystitis.

PREVENTION

UDCA, 600 mg at night, markedly reduces gallstone formation in patients on low-fat, low-calorie diets. Primary prevention of cholesterol gallstones is based on dietary alteration to avoid cholesterol supersaturation (i.e., a diet rich in whole grains and roughage and low in cholesterol and saturated fats). Secondary prevention includes using bile acid therapy with UDCA to reduce cholesterol supersaturation, improving gallbladder motility with cholecystokinin analogues, and reducing mucin secretion with aspirin and NSAIDs. All these strategies have been used effectively in high-risk groups, such as patients on low-calorie diets or those maintained on total parenteral nutrition.

PROGNOSIS

Overall, the prognosis of gallstone disease is excellent for younger and otherwise healthy patients. However, with the aging population, there is a higher prevalence of complicated gallstone disease with common duct stones, cholangitis, and pancreatitis, each of which is associated with substantial morbidity and mortality.

ACUTE ACALCULOUS CHOLECYSTITIS

EPIDEMIOLOGY AND PATHOBIOLOGY

Acalculous cholecystitis is inflammation of the gallbladder or the presence of gallbladder-related symptoms in the absence of stones. Acute acalculous cholecystitis accounts for 2 to 17% of all cholecystectomies. Ischemia, infection, chemical injury by biliary contents, and obstruction of the cystic duct have all been implicated as causes (Table 158-8).

TABLE 158-8   RISK FACTORS AND ORGANISMS ASSOCIATED WITH ACALCULOUS CHOLECYSTITIS

RISK FACTORS

Fasting
Total parenteral nutrition
Septicemia, biliary infections
Major trauma
Burns
Major nonbiliary surgery
Childbirth
Multiple blood transfusions
Mechanical ventilation
Opiates
Immunosuppression—chemotherapy, HIV infection, transplantation
Diabetes
Ischemic heart disease
Malignancy

ORGANISMS IMPLICATED AS A PRIMARY CAUSE

Salmonella typhi
Vibrio cholerae
Staphylococcus
Leptospira
Listeria
Pneumocystis carinii
Mycobacterium spp
Cytomegalovirus
Candida
Ascaris
Echinococcus

Primary infection may manifest as acute cholecystitis with unexplained fever, right upper quadrant pain, or clinical deterioration postoperatively or after transplantation, trauma to the abdomen, chemotherapy, or total parenteral nutrition. Pain, fever, leukocytosis, and abnormal liver enzyme test results are common.

DIAGNOSIS

The diagnosis is confirmed by US showing a distended gallbladder, often with a thin wall, pericholecystic fluid, or a positive Murphy's sign (see earlier) in the absence of gallstones. Sludge may be present. Intraluminal gas or bubbles, the so-called champagne sign, indicates emphysematous cholecystitis.

TREATMENT Rx

Treatment includes intravenous fluids, antibiotics as for gallstone disease, and general supportive measures. Because gangrene and perforation are more common in acalculous than calculous cholecystitis, urgent cholecystectomy is recommended. Postcholecystectomy complications such as leak, abscess, and wound infection are also more common and reflect the underlying multisystemic problems. In severely ill patients in whom cholecystectomy is contraindicated, radiologic decompression of the gallbladder via percutaneous cholecystostomy can be performed. The overall mortality associated with acute acalculous cholecystitis is 5 to 20%.

CHRONIC ACALCULOUS CHOLECYSTITIS

Chronic acalculous cholecystitis is a poorly understood clinical syndrome in which patients have symptoms of biliary colic in the absence of gallstones. The gallbladder may be normal or show changes of chronic inflammation. Cholesterolosis may also be present, with deposits of cholesterol in the mucosa and muscle layers of the gallbladder. Affected patients, who are often young and female, have abdominal pain and nonspecific symptoms such as nausea and intolerance of fatty food. Biliary dyskinesia may be diagnosed by food-cholecystokinin-stimulated US or a HIDA scan. In 80 to 90% of patients with abnormal stimulated motility, symptoms are relieved by cholecystectomy.

GALLBLADDER CANCER

Gallbladder cancer constitutes 0.76 to 1.2% of all cancers and is the most common biliary cancer, with about 7200 new cases reported in the United States each year. The highest incidence occurs in Amerindians, particularly in Chile, Mexico, and Colombia. Its incidence is also high in India, perhaps owing to the higher prevalence of pigmented gallstones. Gallbladder cancer is a disease of the elderly and is more common in women than in men. There is a strong association with cholelithiasis, chronic cholecystitis, and inflammation; 90% of patients with gallbladder cancer have concomitant stones. Patients who have a porcelain gallbladder, defined as calcification of the gallbladder wall, have a 25% risk for the development of gallbladder cancer, and patients with an anomalous pancreatic ductal junction in which the pancreatic duct drains into the lower common bile duct instead of the ampulla have an increased risk for gallbladder cancer. Both these lesions are indications for prophylactic cholecystectomy.

About 90% of gallbladder cancers are adenocarcinomas; the remainder are squamous cell or other cancers. Gallbladder cancer spreads locally, with invasion of the liver and to the local lymph nodes and peritoneal cavity. About 90% of patients have symptoms and signs suggestive of cholecystitis. Surgery, which is the only therapeutic option, can be curative when the tumor is confined to the gallbladder. Adjuvant radiation therapy and chemotherapy are not effective. The median survival for all patients with gallbladder cancer is 3 months, with a 1-year survival rate of 14% and a 5-year survival rate of 5%.

DISORDERS OF THE AMPULLA OF VATER

The ampulla of Vater is the final sphincter that controls entry of bile into the duodenum. Hormonal control of the sphincter is mediated by cholecystokinin, which causes the gallbladder to contract and the ampulla to relax. The most common disorder of the ampulla is stenosis or dysfunction after cholecystectomy, the so-called sphincter of Oddi dysfunction.

FIGURE 158-7. Carcinoma of the ampulla of Vater. The carcinoma can be seen toward the bottom of the picture. The bulging swelling above is the grossly dilated common bile duct, which is obstructed by the carcinoma. (From Forbes CD, Jackson WF. *Color Atlas and Text of Clinical Medicine*, 3rd ed. London: Mosby; 2003.)

Sphincter of Oddi Dysfunction or Biliary Dyskinesia

In true sphincter stenosis, the sphincter is narrowed by inflammation and fibrosis secondary to pancreatitis, passage of a gallstone through the papilla, intraoperative trauma, infection, or adenoma. Sphincter stenosis can manifest as abdominal pain and pancreatitis. The common bile duct is often dilated above the stenosis, and treatment is a large sphincterotomy performed at ERCP.

In sphincter of Oddi dyskinesia, a functional disorder of the sphincter leads to intermittent biliary obstruction. Most patients have undergone cholecystectomy and are being evaluated for recurrent biliary pain or, less frequently, pancreatitis. The diagnosis is usually made by ERCP, which can demonstrate delayed excretion of contrast material. In patients who have pain associated with abnormal aminotransferase levels on two or more occasions, a dilated common bile duct, and delayed drainage of contrast material, sphincterotomy is recommended. Patients without all three of these criteria are usually given a trial of relaxants, such as nitrates or calcium-channel blockers.

Ampullary Tumors

Adenocarcinoma of the ampulla has an incidence of 3 per million. Adenomas appear as protruding ampullary lesions, may grow either inside the ampulla or into the duodenum, and can transform into adenocarcinomas (Fig. 158-7). The cancer tends to be locally invasive. Ampullary adenomas are associated with familial adenomatous polyposis (Chapter 199) and the *APC* gene: almost 80% of patients with the *APC* gene have adenomas of the ampulla, and their risk for ampullary cancer is significantly higher than that of the normal population.

The average age at diagnosis is 50 years, with a peak at 70 years; there is no gender predilection. About 80% of patients have jaundice, which is usually progressive and associated with abdominal pain and weight loss. Liver enzymes are generally abnormal, and the diagnosis is suggested by US or CT findings of dilated biliary and pancreatic ducts all the way to the ampulla. Confirmation is by endoscopy, with biopsy and brushings. Staging of the tumor, particularly for lesions growing into the ampulla, is best performed by endoscopic US. Adenomas and small cancers can be removed by endoscopic ampullectomy. The standard, recommended curative operation is pancreaticoduodenectomy (the Whipple procedure), which provides a 25 to 55% 5-year survival rate, depending on the extent of the tumor. Adjuvant chemotherapy and radiation therapy have no proven benefit in the treatment of ampullary lesions.

1. Poropat G, Giljaca V, Stimac D, et al. Bile acids for primary sclerosing cholangitis. *Cochrane Database Syst Rev.* 2011;1:CD003626.
2. Gong Y, Huang ZB, Christensen E, et al. Ursodeoxycholic acid for primary biliary cirrhosis. *Cochrane Database Syst Rev.* 2008;3:CD000551.
3. Gurusamy K, Samraj K, Gluud C, et al. Meta-analysis of randomized controlled trials on the safety and effectiveness of early versus delayed laparoscopic cholecystectomy for acute cholecystitis. *Br J Surg.* 2010;97:141-150.
4. Keus F, Gooszen HG, van Laarhoven CJ. Systematic review: open, small-incision or laparoscopic cholecystectomy for symptomatic cholecystolithiasis. *Aliment Pharmacol Ther.* 2009;29:359-378.
5. Keus F, Werner JE, Gooszen HG, et al. Randomized clinical trial of small-incision and laparoscopic cholecystectomy in patients with symptomatic cholecystolithiasis: primary and clinical outcomes. *Arch Surg.* 2008;143:371-377.

6. Keus F, Gooszen HG, van Laarhoven CJ. Open, small-incision, or laparoscopic cholecystectomy for patients with symptomatic cholecystolithiasis. An overview of Cochrane Hepato-Biliary Group reviews. *Cochrane Database Syst Rev* 2010;1:CD008318.

7. Rogers SJ, Cello JP, Horn JK, et al. Prospective randomized trial of LC+LCBDE vs ERCP/S+LC for common bile duct stone disease. *Arch Surg.* 2010;145:28-33.

8. Bansal VK, Misra MC, Garg P, et al. A prospective randomized trial comparing two-stage versus single-stage management of patients with gallstone disease and common bile duct stones. *Surg Endosc.* 2010;24:1986-1989.

9. Boerma D, Rauws EA, Keulemans YC, et al. Wait-and-see policy or laparoscopic cholecystectomy after endoscopic sphincterotomy for bile-duct stones: a randomised trial. *Lancet.* 2002;360: 761-765.

SUGGESTED READINGS

Barie PS, Eachempati SR. Acute acalculous cholecystitis. *Gastroenterol Clin North Am.* 2010;39:343-357. *Ultrasound of the gallbladder is most accurate for diagnosis.*

Ishibashi H, Komori A, Shimoda S, et al. Risk factors and prediction of long-term outcome in primary biliary cirrhosis. *Intern Med.* 2011;50:1-10. *Review emphasizing sustained serologic presence of anti-gp 210 antibodies as a risk factor.*

Shakespear JS, Shaaban AM, Rezvani M. CT findings of acute cholecystitis and its complications. *AJR Am J Roentgenol.* 2010;194:1523-1529. *Acute cholecystitis is unlikely with a normal CT scan, but an abnormal CT scan requires follow-up with abdominal ultrasound.*

XIV

HEMATOLOGIC DISEASES

159

HEMATOPOIESIS AND HEMATOPOIETIC GROWTH FACTORS

KENNETH KAUSHANSKY

Hematopoiesis is the process by which bone marrow stem cells develop all of the cell types present in the blood (erythrocytes, neutrophils, eosinophils, basophils, monocytes, platelets, T lymphocytes, B lymphocytes, and natural killer cells) (Fig. 159-1). The regulation of the numbers of each cell type is carefully controlled by paracrine and endocrine hematopoietic growth factors, which exert antiapoptotic, proliferative, and differentiating effects on hematopoietic stem, progenitor, and maturing blood cells. Many of these glycoproteins are produced by recombinant DNA technology and have been among the most successful therapeutics in modern medicine.

HEMATOPOIETIC STEM AND PROGENITOR CELLS

Hematopoietic stem cells represent one in 10^5 to 10^6 bone marrow cells, are not morphologically distinguishable from other progenitors or small lymphocytes, but can be purified to homogeneity using physical characteristics and combinations of monoclonal antibodies to cell surface proteins. The two critical characteristics of a hematopoietic stem cell are its abilities to differentiate into all blood cell types and to self-renew. The decision to self-renew or differentiate is a stochastic process, at the stem cell stage and at the subsequent multipotent or unipotent stages of differentiation, that can be influenced by a number of cell extrinsic (growth factors and stromal proteins) and cell intrinsic (transcription factors) molecules.

HEMATOPOIETIC CELL EXPANSION— HEMATOPOIETIC GROWTH FACTORS

A large number of transcription factors regulate stem cell number and differentiation state. Several molecular switches have been identified that determine hematopoietic cell fate.

Equally important to hematopoiesis as the transcription factors is a group of hematopoietic growth factors, which share structural homology and bind to nonredundant type I transmembrane proteins belonging to the cytokine receptor family. Many of these proteins are the physiologic regulators of a specific lineage of blood cells; others appear to represent redundant hematopoietic growth-promoting activities of molecules essential for other biologic functions. Erythropoietin, granulocyte colony-stimulating factor (G-CSF), and thrombopoietin serve as examples of the former; interleukin-3 (IL-3), granulocyte-macrophage colony-stimulating factor (GM-CSF), and IL-11 serve as examples of the latter class of hematopoietic growth factors.

Erythropoietin is produced predominantly by the kidneys, and to a lesser extent in the liver, and acts on marrow erythroid progenitors to enhance their survival, proliferation, and differentiation. Levels of erythropoietin are inversely related to hemoglobin concentrations in the blood, as reflected in renal oxygen tension. In the presence of tissue (renal) hypoxia, the transcription factor hypoxia-induced factor (HIF)1α is stabilized against proteasome-mediated destruction and drives erythropoietin transcription by binding to a critical hypoxia-responsive element located in the 3′ untranslated region of the gene. Genetic elimination of erythropoietin or its receptor results in embryonic lethality, establishing that although other cytokines can influence erythropoiesis, red cell production is absolutely dependent on the hormone.

G-CSF stimulates the production of neutrophils from their marrow progenitors (Fig. 159-2). Levels of the hormone are also inversely related to neutrophil numbers but are regulated primarily by inflammatory stimuli, including tumor necrosis factor-α and IL-1α, acting on endothelial cells, fibroblasts and macrophages. Like the action of erythropoietin on erythroid progenitors, G-CSF acts to enhance the survival, proliferation, and differentiation of neutrophil progenitors. In addition, the cytokine acts to functionally activate the mature cells it helps to produce. Genetic elimination of G-CSF or its receptor in mice reduces neutrophil levels to 25% of normal, the only hormone known to exert this great an impact on granulopoiesis.

Thrombopoietin, the primary regulator of platelet production, is produced in the liver and kidney and by marrow stromal cells and is regulated by both platelet receptor–mediated uptake and destruction and by transcriptional feedback inhibition of the thrombopoietin gene in marrow stromal cells by platelet granule proteins. Like G-CSF, thrombopoietin stimulates the survival, proliferation, and differentiation of its corresponding lineage and megakaryocytes and their precursors, and also prime mature platelets to respond to platelet activation agonists. Genetic elimination of thrombopoietin or its receptor in mice and congenital non-sense or missense mutations in the thrombopoietin receptor in humans result in platelet levels approximately 10% of normal at birth, and in humans leads to aplastic anemia by 1 to 2 years of age.

Other cytokine-receptor systems related to erythropoietin, G-CSF, and thrombopoietin essential for one or more aspects of hematopoiesis include IL-7, critical for all types of lymphocyte production; IL-5, the primary regulator of eosinophil production; IL-4, responsible for immunoglobulin class switching in B lymphocytes; IL-15, essential for normal natural killer cell differentiation; and IL-2, a lymphocyte activation cytokine. They display modest effects on blood cell growth, but their genetic elimination fails to affect basal or stimulated production of those cells.

A second class of cytokines and receptors that influences hematopoiesis is exemplified by the c-kit receptor, a member of the receptor tyrosine kinase family of surface proteins, and its cognate ligand, stem cell factor (also termed *steel* factor or *kit-ligand*). Although the c-kit receptor is structurally distinct from members of the hematopoietic cytokine receptor family, possessing an intrinsic tyrosine kinase motif in its cytoplasmic domain, stem cell factor is structurally related to the cytokines that bind to members of the hematopoietic growth factor family. Genetic elimination of stem cell factor or the c-kit receptor results in the near elimination of hematopoietic stem cells, erythroid precursors, and basophils and mast cells. Two other hematopoietic members of this family of cytokines and receptors are Flt3 ligand and its receptor Flt-3, and monocyte colony-stimulating factor and its receptor, c-Fms. Like stem cell factor, both Flt3 ligand and monocyte colony-stimulating factor play nonredundant roles in hematopoiesis, inducing the formation of dendritic cells and monocytes, respectively.

The molecular mechanisms by which the hematopoietic growth factors affect blood cell survival, proliferation, and differentiation are becoming increasingly well understood. Binding of cognate ligand to each of the hematopoietic cytokine receptors results in activation of one or more tyrosine kinases, either tethered cytoplasmic kinases of the Janus (JAK) family for the hematopoietic cytokine receptor family, or the intrinsic kinase of the cytokines that employ the receptor tyrosine kinase class of receptors (stem cell factor, Flt3 ligand, and monocyte colony-stimulating factor). Once activated, these kinases phosphorylate tyrosine residues within the cytoplasmic domains of each receptor, providing docking sites for cytoplasmic signaling intermediates possessing Src homology (SH)2 domains. Among the best characterized SH2 domain–containing proteins that bind to hematopoietic receptors are nascent transcription factors, such as the signal transducers and activators of transcription (STAT) proteins, adapter proteins, including Grb2, Gab1, tensin2 and SHC, phosphatases (e.g., SHP1 and SHP2), and the regulatory subunit (p85) of phosphoinositol-3-kinase (PI3K). Once bound to one or more of the newly induced phosphotyrosine residues of the cytokine receptor or receptor tyrosine kinase, these secondary molecules are phosphorylated, either by the JAK kinase or by other kinases, making them competent to bind additional molecules (e.g., the adapters that ultimately activate Ras, and p85 PI3K that binds its kinase [p110] subunit) or are activated as transcription factors (e.g., STATs). The downstream effector molecules then activated include a number kinases, transporter molecules, and transcription factors, ultimately leading to hematopoietic cell survival, proliferation, and differentiation.

CLINICAL USES OF HEMATOPOIETIC CELLS AND GROWTH FACTORS

The clinical development of erythropoietin, G-CSF, and thrombopoietin mimetics represents some of the very best examples of harnessing recombinant DNA technology for therapeutic benefit. Patients with renal failure, widespread inflammation, or marrow replacement and those undergoing chemotherapy for cancer all suffer from variable degrees of anemia, often very debilitating. Clinical trials have demonstrated the efficacy of recombinant erythropoietin in patients with renal failure and with cancer and inflammation. Administration of the drug almost invariably results in a rapid reticulocyte response and correction of the anemia. The only patients who regularly demonstrate a poor response are individuals with severe inflammation. Most

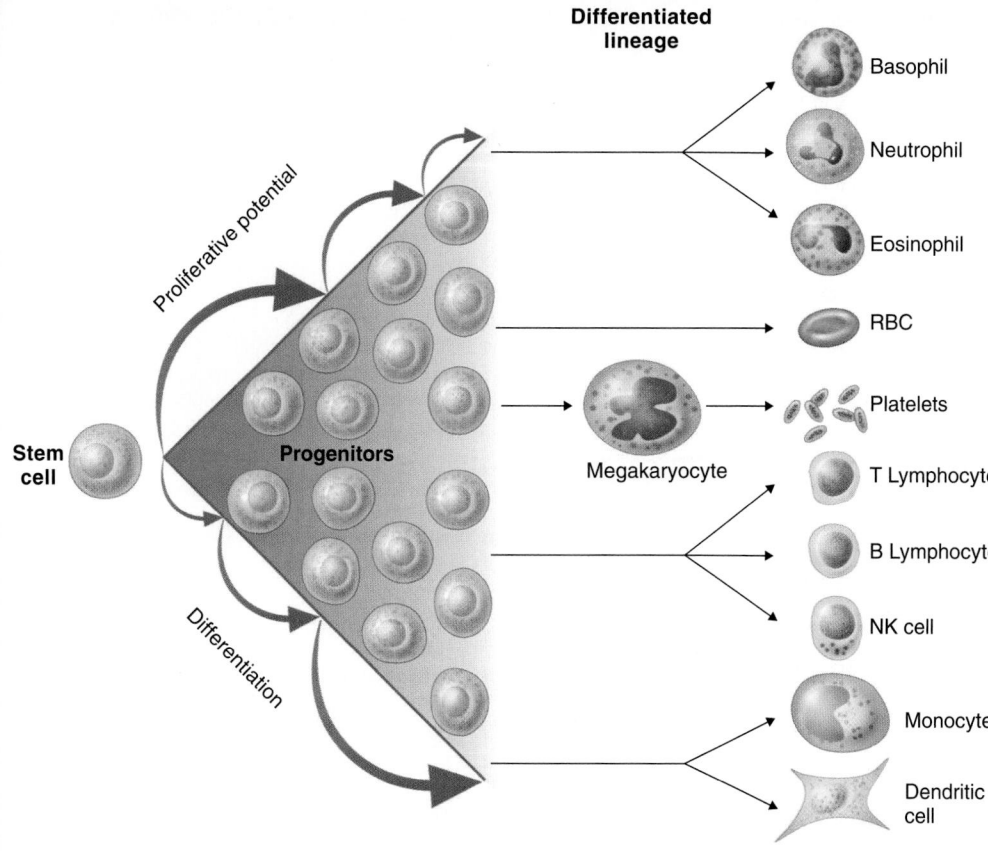

FIGURE 159-1. Hierarchical model of lymphohematopoiesis. NK = natural killer; RBC = red blood cell.

FIGURE 159-2. Neutrophil production system. PMN = polymorphonuclear leukocyte.

patients undergo an enhanced sense of well-being as the blood hemoglobin concentration rises to 10 g/dL. However, quality-of-life studies of doses of erythropoietin higher than those needed to result in a hemoglobin level of 10 g/dL failed to further enhance patient well-being and surprisingly resulted in a number of adverse effects. For example, patients receiving the drug for anemia secondary to kidney failure progressed to requiring dialysis more frequently and experienced greater cardiovascular events, such as myocardial infarction and stroke, than patients on low levels of the hormone sufficient to maintain their blood hemoglobin at 10 g/dL. Patients receiving erythropoietin for cancer also experienced greater relapses of their tumors than individuals not receiving the hormone. Overall, erythropoietin is a safe and effective drug for anemia due to a wide range of conditions, but its use and dose must be carefully considered.

Many patients undergoing cytotoxic therapy for cancer experience severe neutropenia and are thus at substantial risk for life-threatening infection. Clinical trials of recombinant G-CSF in patients undergoing aggressive chemotherapy for leukemia and solid tumors resulted in the U.S. Food and Drug Administration (FDA) approval of the drug for use in patients undergoing chemotherapy of intensity sufficient to produce severe neutropenia. The use of the drug is associated with the more rapid return of neutrophils to safe levels if administered soon after the inciting chemotherapy is completed, but not at the nadir of neutrophil production, and results in lower numbers of severe infections. However, the use of G-CSF has not enhanced survival in patients with any tumor type. Like the use of erythropoietin in patients with cancer, the administration of G-CSF to some patients receiving cytotoxic chemotherapy for cancer (e.g., breast cancer) has been associated with a statistically significant increase in cancer recurrence, although this finding is controversial.

Thrombopoietin was cloned and characterized in 1994 and was quickly advanced to clinical trials following the model of G-CSF use in patients undergoing cancer chemotherapy. Initial results with the intact hormone and a truncated version that included only the receptor-binding domain were mixed, and use of the truncated form of the drug, administration to healthy volunteer donors to improve platelet apheresis yields, resulted in a significant number of subjects developing antidrug antibodies, which cross-reacted with their native thrombopoietin, resulting in severe thrombocytopenia. This experience caused both manufacturers of thrombopoietin to cease clinical trials. Instead, a series of small molecule mimics have been developed that bind to the thrombopoietin receptor and stimulate thrombopoiesis. Two such drugs are approved by the FDA for use in patients with severe immune thrombocytopenia, one a peptibody, which contains four thrombopoietin receptor–binding peptides grafted onto an immunoglobulin scaffold, and one a small organic molecule that is orally bioavailable and binds to a spatially distinct site on the thrombopoietin receptor. The use of each drug results in a high rate of platelet responses into the normal range in patients with severe immune thrombocytopenia (Chapter 175) who were refractory to conventional therapies. However, because thrombopoietin mimics do not affect the underlying immune destruction of platelets and megakaryocytes in patients with this disease, discontinuation of each drug results in rapid relapse to thrombocytopenia. Current clinical trials in other settings of transient myelosuppression are expected to improve platelet recovery but not be associated with rapid relapse.

 Visit expertconsult.com for e-expanded chapter

SUGGESTED READINGS

Kaushansky K. Lineage specific hematopoietic growth factors. *N Engl J Med.* 2006;354:2034-2045. *Overview of the biochemistry, cell biology, clinical use, and potential side effects of these products of recombinant DNA technology.*

Laiosa CV, Stadfeld M, Graf T. Determinants of lymphoid-myeloid lineage diversification. *Ann Rev Immunol.* 2006;24:705-738. *Review of the cell intrinsic (transcription factors) and cell extrinsic (cytokines) factors that determine cell phenotypes.*

Yannaki E, Stamatoyannopoulos G. Hematopoietic stem cell mobilization strategies for gene therapy of beta thalassemia and sickle cell disease. *Ann N Y Acad Sci.* 2010;1202:59-63. *Overview of approaches for gene-engineered stem cell therapy.*

160

THE PERIPHERAL BLOOD SMEAR

BARBARA J. BAIN

With the development of sophisticated automated instruments to count and characterize blood cells, Romanowsky (Wright-Giemsa or May-Grünwald-Giemsa)-stained peripheral blood smears are now performed on only a minority of blood specimens received in a hematology laboratory. Nevertheless, the blood smear remains important for a number of reasons: it can (1) verify the result of an automated instrument, (2) provide an immediate specific diagnosis, or (3) indicate a narrow range of diagnostic possibilities, permitting a focused rather than indiscriminate investigation. A blood film can provide a rapid diagnosis in cases in which speed is crucial, such as in acute promyelocytic leukemia, thrombotic thrombocytopenic purpura, or Burkitt's lymphoma. Sometimes a smear provides unexpected information that is of value in patient management.

Usually, blood smears are initially interpreted by a laboratory scientist. In some countries it is customary for clinicians to examine the blood smears of their own patients because the clinician has the final responsibility for integrating all information and making a diagnosis. However, the interpretation of a blood smear can be difficult, and a trained laboratory hematologist or hematopathologist has a major role in interpreting smears that may have been initially examined by a laboratory scientist. It is crucial that, when requesting a blood count, the clinician provide all the essential information needed to interpret the count and any associated smear. Regardless of whether the clinician examines the blood film, he or she must be able to interpret the written report issued by the laboratory. To do so, the clinician must be familiar with the terms generally used by laboratory staff and the possible significance of the abnormalities described. The most important of these terms are illustrated in Figures 160-1 through 160-20.

REASONS FOR PERFORMING A BLOOD SMEAR

A blood smear may be requested by a clinician or initiated by a laboratory scientist or a laboratory hematologist. Clinical findings that should lead a clinician to request a blood smear are summarized in Table 160-1.

Laboratory scientists and physicians may initiate a blood smear that has not been requested by the clinician if the clinical details indicate the possibility of a significant hematologic abnormality. However, they are

FIGURE 160-1. Normal peripheral blood smear. These normal red cells are described as *normocytic* (i.e., of normal size) and *normochromic* (i.e., their staining characteristics are normal). Normal erythrocytes are biconcave discs, causing them to have an area of central pallor that does not exceed one third the diameter of the cell. There are also scattered normal platelets (×1000).

FIGURE 160-2. Smear showing multiple abnormalities. There is *anisocytosis,* defined as an increased variation in cell size; *poikilocytosis,* defined as an increased variation in cell shape; and *polychromasia,* defined as the presence of erythrocytes with a blue tinge to their cytoplasm—indicating a young cell recently released from the bone marrow in which the polychromasia is due to the presence of RNA. *Polychromatic cells* are erythrocytes with a blue tinge; because polychromatic cells are larger than normal mature erythrocytes, they are known as *polychromatic macrocytes (arrow)*. The film also shows two cells containing bluish purple *Howell-Jolly bodies*; these inclusions are nuclear remnants (×1000).

FIGURE 160-3. Microcytic red cells from a case of thalassemia minor. In a blood smear, a *microcyte* can be defined as a cell with a diameter less than that of the nucleus of a normal small lymphocyte. There are also some cells showing *hypochromia,* an area of central pallor that is larger than one third of the diameter of the red cell. In addition, there are two *target cells,* with a hemoglobinized area in the center of the area of pallor (×1000).

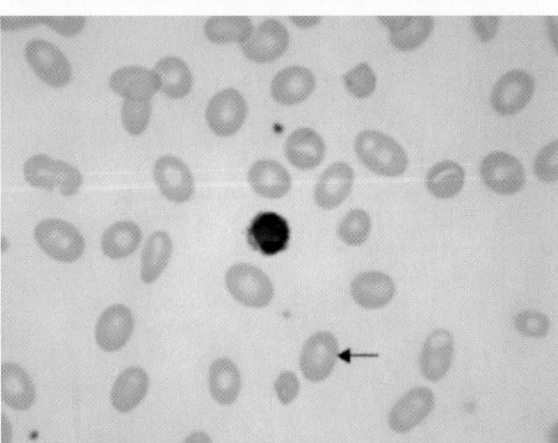

FIGURE 160-4. Macrocytic anemia. A *macrocyte* is recognized on a blood film as a cell with a diameter that is considerably greater than that of the nucleus of a small lymphocyte. In addition, this smear shows *oval macrocytes* (also known as *macro-ovalocytes*), defined as cells that are larger than normal and oval in shape *(arrow)*. They are of considerable diagnostic importance, being characteristic of megaloblastic anemia; they can also be seen in dyserythropoiesis (×1000).

FIGURE 160-7. Sickle cells. A *sickle cell* is a cell with a sickle or crescent shape resulting from the polymerization of hemoglobin S. These cells are seen not only in sickle cell anemia (homozygosity for hemoglobin S) but also in compound heterozygous states such as sickle cell/hemoglobin C disease and sickle cell/β-thalassemia, which also lead to sickle cell disease. This smear also shows target cells and boat-shaped cells with a lesser degree of polymerization of hemoglobin S than in a classic sickle cell (×1000).

FIGURE 160-5. Hereditary spherocytosis. A *spherocyte* is a red cell that lacks central pallor because of its spherical shape. In hereditary spherocytosis, there are usually cells in which the central pallor is reduced rather than absent, and they are intermediate in shape between a spherocyte and a *discocyte*, which is an erythrocyte with the normal shape of a biconcave disc (×1000).

FIGURE 160-8. Red cell fragmentation. *Red cell fragments* or *schistocytes* are defined as fragments of erythrocytes. In addition to small angular fragments, there may be *microspherocytes,* cells of reduced size and spherical in form (also known as *spheroschistocytes*), and *keratocytes,* cells with two horn-like projections. Schistocytes are seen in microangiopathic hemolytic anemias and in mechanical hemolysis (×1000).

FIGURE 160-6. Target cells. A *target cell* is an erythrocyte with a hemoglobinized area in the middle of the normal area of central pallor (×1000).

FIGURE 160-9. Hereditary elliptocytosis. An *elliptocyte* is an elliptical red cell. When seen in the numbers present in this smear, they are indicative of hereditary elliptocytosis; smaller numbers are seen in other conditions such as iron deficiency anemia, in which they are sometimes referred to as *pencil cells* (×1000).

also likely to evaluate a blood smear in response to abnormalities revealed by an automated instrument. These abnormalities may be quantitative or qualitative. Quantitative abnormalities that require evaluation include anemia, polycythemia, macrocytosis, microcytosis, neutrophilia, lymphocytosis, eosinophilia, thrombocytopenia, and thrombocytosis.

Modern automated instruments are able to "flag" the presence of qualitative abnormalities that require a blood film to be examined for confirmation of the abnormality or for further elucidation. "Flags" are generated in response to the electrical impedance or the light scattering characteristics of individual cells. Some instruments are dependent on cytochemical

FIGURE 160-10. Hereditary pyropoikilocytosis. This smear shows striking poikilocytosis, including elliptocytes, microspherocytes and other fragments, and teardrop cells. This congenital condition, which is related to hereditary elliptocytosis, usually results from the inheritance of two different mutated genes from the two parents and is characterized by a severe hemolytic anemia (×1000).

FIGURE 160-13. Numerous Pappenheimer bodies. A *Pappenheimer body* is an iron-containing red cell inclusion *(arrow)*. It is smaller and more angular than a Howell-Jolly body and stains navy blue rather than purple. Pappenheimer bodies are seen following splenectomy and in sideroblastic anemias (×1000).

FIGURE 160-11. Teardrop poikilocytes. *Teardrop poikilocytes*, or *dacrocytes*, are teardrop-shaped red cells; they are characteristic of primary myelofibrosis but are also seen in megaloblastic anemia (×1000).

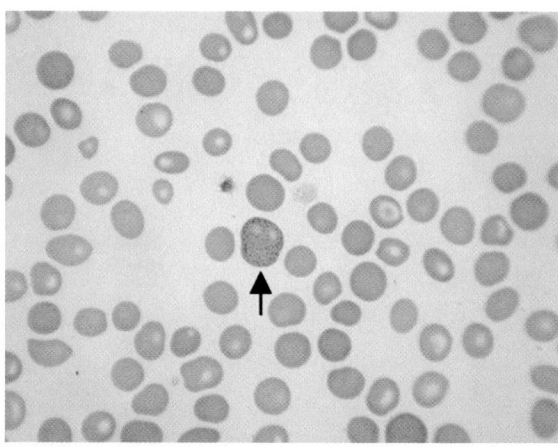

FIGURE 160-14. Basophilic stippling. *Basophilic stippling* means that there are fine (as in this case) or coarse purplish blue dots dispersed through the red cell *(arrow)*. They are a very nonspecific feature occurring in thalassemia trait, lead poisoning, 5′-nucleotidase deficiency, and dyserythropoiesis in general (×1000).

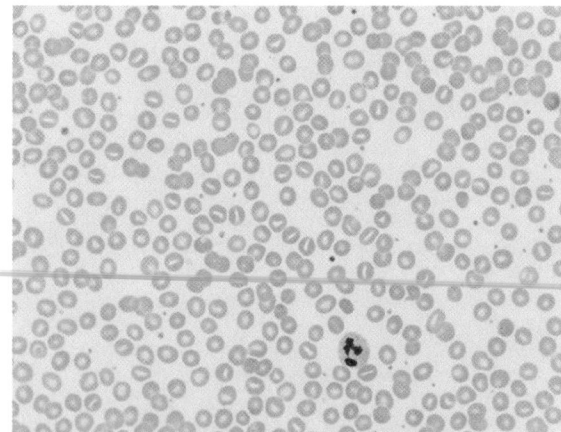

FIGURE 160-12. Stomatocytosis. A *stomatocyte* is a cell that appears to have a central mouth-shaped or slit-like stoma. Among the less common causes is hereditary stomatocytosis. Alcohol and hydroxycarbamide therapy are more common causes (×400).

FIGURE 160-15. Rouleau formation. *Rouleaux* are stacks of red cells, often compared to stacks of coins. They result from an increase of high-molecular-weight globulins in the plasma, either as a reactive change or as a result of secretion of a paraprotein in a plasma cell neoplasm (×1000).

reactions of cells or on the cells' ability to polarize light. Most instruments can indicate the possibility of the presence of blast cells, reactive or other atypical lymphocytes, granulocyte precursors, or nucleated red blood cells. Instruments using a cytochemical reaction for peroxidase to help identify neutrophils, eosinophils, and monocytes may flag the appearance of large, unstained (i.e., peroxidase-negative) cells; such cells may indicate a harmless inherited peroxidase deficiency, but sometimes such cells are lymphoma cells, reactive lymphocytes, or leukemic blast cells. Instruments often flag the possibility of an erroneous platelet count, such as when there is an overlap in size between platelets and red cells or when light scattering characteristics suggest the presence of platelet aggregates (a potential cause of pseudothrombocytopenia).

FIGURE 160-16. Red cell agglutination. *Red cell agglutinates* are irregular aggregates of red cells, as seen in *Mycoplasma pneumoniae* infection. They are also seen in other infections, such as infectious mononucleosis, and in chronic cold hemagglutinin disease (×100). (Courtesy of Jean Schafer.)

FIGURE 160-17. Homozygous hemoglobin C. Three *hemoglobin C crystals* are present, one indicated by an arrow. Hemoglobin C crystals are usually six-sided, with a long axis having parallel edges (×1000).

FIGURE 160-18. Toxic granulation. *Toxic granulation* refers to heavy staining of azurophilic granules of neutrophils. When accompanied by neutrophil vacuolation, it is often indicative of infection, but it can also result from inflammation, tissue damage, and normal pregnancy (×1000).

FIGURE 160-19. Döhle's body. A *Döhle's body* (arrow) is a pale blue-gray amorphous inclusion near the cell membrane of a neutrophil. Döhle's bodies can result from infection and inflammation. Similar but different inclusions (larger and more angular) are seen in the May-Hegglin anomaly (×1000).

FIGURE 160-20. Pelger-Huët anomaly. A *Pelger-Huët anomaly* is a cytologic abnormality of neutrophils in which there is hypolobulation of nuclei and increased chromatin clumping. Nuclei may have a shape resembling a peanut or a pince-nez, as in the examples shown. The Pelger-Huët anomaly is inherited, but similar Pelger neutrophils are seen in myelodysplastic syndromes, in which the neutrophils may also be hypogranular (×1000).

TABLE 160-1 CLINICAL FEATURES SUGGESTING THE NEED FOR A BLOOD SMEAR

CLINICAL FEATURE	REASON TO PERFORM A BLOOD SMEAR
Lymphadenopathy or splenomegaly	May be indicative of infectious mononucleosis or another reactive condition, or of leukemia or lymphoma
Clinically evident anemia	Helps in the differential diagnosis
Bruising or bleeding tendency, including unexplained retinal hemorrhages	May confirm thrombocytopenia or show morphologically abnormal platelets (which may have defective function); sometimes owing to acute leukemia or other condition causing bone marrow failure
Acute renal failure	Hemolytic-uremic syndrome and thrombotic thrombocytopenic purpura should be confirmed or excluded
Jaundice and hypertension in a pregnant woman	May show schistocytes, supporting a diagnosis of HELLP syndrome
Bone pain	May indicate multiple myeloma, bone marrow infiltration, or sickle cell disease
Unexplained chest or abdominal pain or acute splenic enlargement in a child	Possible sickle cell disease
Unexplained hyperbilirubinemia	Assessment of possible hemolysis

HELLP = hemolysis, elevated liver enzymes, low platelets.

International consensus guidelines indicate which automated instrument results require blood smear review. Whether a review is needed is determined in part by whether that specimen is the first one obtained from that patient and whether there has been a significant change from a previously validated result (referred to as a delta check). Laboratory computers can be programmed to indicate when a result meets the criteria for smear review.

Automated red cell measurements can, to some extent, replace examination of the blood film. An increased red cell distribution width indicates the presence of anisocytosis. A decreased mean cell volume is usually a reliable indicator of microcytosis. A reduction in the mean cell hemoglobin concentration indicates hypochromia (for most instruments, however, this measurement is less sensitive than the human eye in the detection of hypochromia). An increased mean cell volume usually indicates macrocytosis, but examination of a smear is necessary both to confirm that the result is not artifactual and to elucidate the cause. Some instruments can measure the hemoglobin concentration in individual cells and thus flag the presence of hyperdense cells; however, a blood film is still necessary to distinguish spherocytes from irregularly contracted cells. Most instruments produce a histogram of the size distribution of red cells, and some do the same for the distribution of hemoglobin concentration; either of these graphic representations may show dimorphic red cells (i.e., two populations of cells).

THE BLOOD SMEAR IN THE DIFFERENTIAL DIAGNOSIS OF ANEMIA

Microcytic Anemias (Chapter 162)

In microcytic anemias, the automated count is of considerable importance and may permit a distinction between iron deficiency and thalassemia heterozygosity. In iron deficiency, there is initially a normocytic normochromic anemia; only when the deficiency becomes more severe is there microcytosis. Conversely, in β-thalassemia heterozygosity, there is usually a normal or near-normal hemoglobin concentration, but the red blood cell count is increased and there is marked microcytosis (low mean cell volume) together with a parallel reduction in mean cell hemoglobin. The blood film provides supplementary information that can favor one diagnosis or the other. Iron deficiency is more likely to be associated with hypochromia and elliptocytes ("pencil cells"), whereas in β-thalassemia heterozygosity there is microcytosis, hypochromia is less marked, and there are more likely to be target cells and basophilic stippling. Individuals with α-thalassemia involving the deletion of two α genes (−α/−α) or (− −/α α) have red cell indices similar to those of β-thalassemia heterozygosity; in this case, the blood film usually does not provide any additional diagnostically useful information, although individuals with nondeletional α-thalassemia due to hemoglobin Constant Spring have prominent basophilic stippling. When there is deletion of a single α gene, the blood count is either less abnormal or normal, and the blood smear does not provide any extra diagnostically useful information. The blood smear is, however, a useful supplement to the blood count in suggesting a diagnosis of hemoglobin H disease (Chapter 165). The count shows anemia, marked microcytosis (low mean cell volume and mean cell hemoglobin), and sometimes a reduction in the mean cell hemoglobin concentration. The smear usually shows marked poikilocytosis in addition to microcytosis, and there may be polychromasia, correlating with an elevated reticulocyte count. Iron deficiency anemia also needs to be distinguished from anemia of chronic disease. The blood counts may be quite similar, but in anemia of chronic disease, the smear often shows features of inflammation, such as increased rouleau formation, background staining (as a result of increased plasma proteins), and sometimes neutrophilia. Other rare microcytic anemias that must be distinguished from iron deficiency include congenital sideroblastic anemia and lead poisoning. In congenital sideroblastic anemia, the film is dimorphic, with one population of hypochromic microcytes and another of normochromic normocytic cells. In lead poisoning, the presence of basophilic stippling and polychromasia in a patient with microcytosis can suggest the diagnosis.

Macrocytic Anemias

A blood film can be important in distinguishing true macrocytosis from factitious macrocytosis as a result of the presence of red cell agglutinates (see Fig. 160-16). Diagnostic features that can suggest the cause of macrocytosis are shown in Table 160-2.

A smear is particularly important in evaluating the possibility of a megaloblastic anemia (Chapter 167) (Figs. 160-4 and 160-21). Sometimes assays of vitamin B$_{12}$ and folate are normal despite a deficiency, and only the blood film features suggest the true diagnosis and indicate the need for further investigation.

Normocytic Normochromic Anemia (Chapter 161)

A blood smear is only occasionally useful in determining the cause of a normocytic normochromic anemia. Signs of inflammation may be present in anemia of chronic disease. Increased rouleau formation and background staining can also indicate multiple myeloma. Polychromasia suggests the

TABLE 160-2 USEFUL FEATURES FOR DETERMINING THE CAUSE OF MACROCYTIC ANEMIA

CAUSE	SMEAR FEATURES
Megaloblastic anemia (vitamin B$_{12}$ or folic acid deficiency)	Oval macrocytes, teardrop poikilocytes, hypersegmented neutrophils; when severe, marked anisocytosis and poikilocytosis, which may include red cell fragments
Ethanol excess	Target cells and stomatocytes; anisocytosis and poikilocytosis less than in megaloblastic anemia
Liver disease	Target cells, stomatocytes
Myelodysplastic syndromes, including sideroblastic anemias	Other dysplastic features such as hypogranular and hypolobulated neutrophils; if erythropoiesis is sideroblastic, a population of hypochromic microcytic cells and Pappenheimer bodies
Chronic hemolytic anemia	Polychromasia; characteristic poikilocytes sometimes present (e.g., irregularly contracted cells if there is an unstable hemoglobin)

TABLE 160-3 BLOOD SMEAR FEATURES SUGGESTING A SPECIFIC CAUSE OF INHERITED OR ACQUIRED HEMOLYTIC ANEMIA

BLOOD SMEAR FEATURES	CONDITIONS SUGGESTED
Spherocytes	Hereditary spherocytosis, autoimmune hemolytic anemia, alloimmune hemolytic anemia (e.g., hemolytic disease of the newborn, delayed hemolytic transfusion reaction), drug-induced immune hemolytic anemia, *Clostridium perfringens* sepsis
Irregularly contracted cells	Glucose-6-phosphate dehydrogenase deficiency, oxidant damage from chemicals or drugs in individuals with normal red cell enzymes (e.g., dapsone administration), liver failure due to Wilson disease (release of copper from liver), unstable hemoglobin, hemoglobin C homozygosity
Sickle cells and boat-shaped cells	Sickle cell disease (e.g., sickle cell anemia or compound heterozygous states such as S/C, S/D-Punjab, S/O-Arab, S/β-thalassemia)
Target cells	Hemoglobin C homozygosity, other hemoglobinopathies, hereditary xerocytosis
Stomatocytes	Hereditary stomatocytosis
Acanthocytes	Liver failure (spur cell hemolytic anemia)
Basophilic stippling	Lead poisoning, pyrimidine 5′-nucleotidase deficiency
Red cell fragments (schistocytes)	Microangiopathic hemolytic anemia (including hemolytic-uremic syndrome, thrombotic thrombocytopenic purpura, HELLP syndrome, and hemolysis associated with disseminated intravascular coagulation), mechanical hemolytic anemia (e.g., defective cardiac prosthetic valve, march hemoglobinuria)

HELLP = hemolysis, elevated liver enzymes, low platelets.

possibility of young red cells as a result of recent blood loss or hemolysis. Small numbers of acanthocytes may indicate hypothyroidism or anorexia nervosa. Dysplastic features, such as in neutrophils, suggest a myelodysplastic syndrome.

Hemolytic Anemias

The possibility of hemolysis is suggested by the presence of polychromasia and macrocytosis. Specific causes of hemolysis are suggested by the presence of various poikilocytes, as shown in Table 160-3.

The distinction between spherocytes and irregularly contracted cells is important; both are dense cells with absent central pallor, but the differential diagnosis is quite different. Recognition of the features of oxidant damage is important in diagnosing glucose-6-phosphate dehydrogenase (G6PD) deficiency, because sometimes an assay for G6PD performed during an acute hemolytic episode is normal (Chapter 164). In addition to irregularly contracted cells, there may be ghost cells, hemi-ghost cells ("blister cells"), and even Heinz bodies protruding from the red cells and confirmed on a Heinz body preparation. The observation of these features is an indication to repeat the assay when the acute hemolytic episode is over.

ASSESSMENT OF THROMBOCYTOPENIA, THROMBOCYTOSIS, AND PLATELET MORPHOLOGY

A blood smear is essential to validate the cell count whenever an automated count shows thrombocytopenia (e.g., a count <60 × 10⁹/l). This should be done quickly before patient management is altered, such as by postponing surgery or initiating further diagnostic work-up. A platelet transfusion should never be given for an unexpected thrombocytopenia without microscopic confirmation of the count. A factitiously low platelet count is often the result of in vitro platelet aggregation and is occasionally the result of platelet satellitism (Chapter 174). To detect aggregates reliably, the edges and the tail of the smear should be examined for aggregates. The presence of fibrin strands also suggests the activation of coagulation and an erroneous count.

If a low platelet count is confirmed, the film may give clues to the cause (Chapter 175). Giant platelets (Figs. 160-22 and 160-23) occur in a number of inherited thrombocytopenias, including Bernard-Soulier syndrome and the May-Hegglin anomaly. Small platelets are less common but are a feature of Wiskott-Aldrich syndrome. Agranular platelets occur in the gray platelet syndrome, and platelets with a reduced number of larger-than-normal granules are seen in Jacobsen/Paris-Trousseau syndrome. The presence of May-Hegglin inclusions (Döhle-like bodies; see Fig. 160-19) in neutrophils indicates that this anomaly is the cause of the thrombocytopenia. In acquired thrombocytopenias, increased platelet turnover is often accompanied by the presence of large platelets, whereas bone marrow failure is associated with platelets of normal size. It is important to look for red cell fragments to confirm or exclude a diagnosis of thrombotic thrombocytopenic purpura in any patient with the apparent recent onset of thrombocytopenia; because platelet transfusions are usually contraindicated in this condition, the smear should be examined before platelet transfusion is contemplated. The smear of any patient with the apparent recent onset of severe thrombocytopenia should be examined carefully for evidence of acute promyelocytic leukemia; the leukemic cells may be infrequent in the circulating blood. Hemorrhagic manifestations and a low platelet count can also be indicative of meningococcal septicemia; in some patients, organisms are seen in the blood smear and the diagnosis is confirmed; in other patients, only marked toxic changes in neutrophils are detected.

Thrombocytosis should also be confirmed on a smear. Factitiously elevated counts may be the result of the presence of red cell fragments (in microangiopathic or mechanical hemolytic anemia, burns, or accidental in vitro heating of the blood sample), white cell fragments (in acute leukemia and, less often, in lymphoma), cryoglobulin precipitates, or microorganisms (particularly *Candida* species). If the count is confirmed, the blood smear may be useful to indicate a likely cause (e.g., features of hyposplenism or the presence of basophilia in a myeloproliferative disorder).

It is sometimes necessary to examine a smear to confirm that an apparently normal platelet count is valid. This should always be done in patients with acute leukemia and an elevated white cell count; the presence of white cell fragments of a similar size to platelets can suggest that the platelet count is at a safe level when it is in fact dangerously low. Counting the ratio of platelets to other particles of similar size permits the count to be corrected. Any unexpectedly normal count should be confirmed; for example, the sudden rise of the automated platelet count in a patient being treated for a hematologic neoplasm may be the result of fungi that have colonized an indwelling intravenous line and are being shed into the blood stream.

LEUKOCYTOSIS AND LEUKOPENIA
(CHAPTER 170)

The finding of leukocytosis is not necessarily an indication for a blood smear. For example, this finding would be expected in a patient with infection or following surgery or trauma, in which case smear confirmation is not required. However, unexpected leukocytosis requires a smear. Artifactual elevation is unusual but can occur as a result of cryoglobulinemia, hyperlipidemia, or the presence of *Candida* species. Distinguishing reactive changes from leukemia on the basis of morphology is usually straightforward. In reactive leukocytosis, there is usually toxic granulation, and Döhle's bodies may be present (see Figs. 160-18 and 160-19). Vacuolation is particularly characteristic of bacterial infection, and there may be some degranulation of neutrophils. The hematologist should be aware of the changes induced by granulocyte colony-stimulating factor so that they are not confused with a response to infection;

FIGURE 160-21. Hypersegmented neutrophils. A *hypersegmented neutrophil* is a neutrophil with more than five nuclear segments or lobes, as in this example from a patient with megaloblastic anemia. Neutrophil hypersegmentation is also said to be present if there are increased numbers of neutrophils with five lobes or if the median lobe count is increased (×1000).

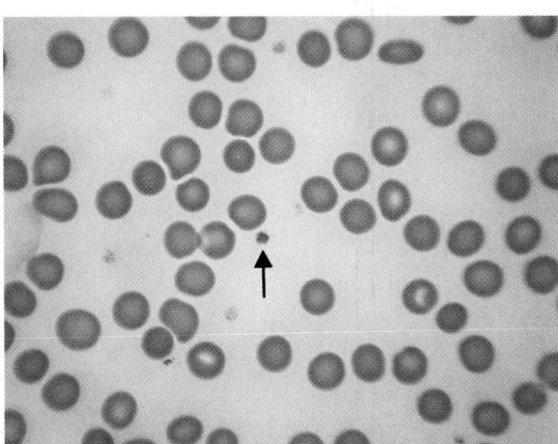

FIGURE 160-22. Normal-sized platelet (arrow). Platelets have central granules, although this is not apparent in this photomicrograph (×1000).

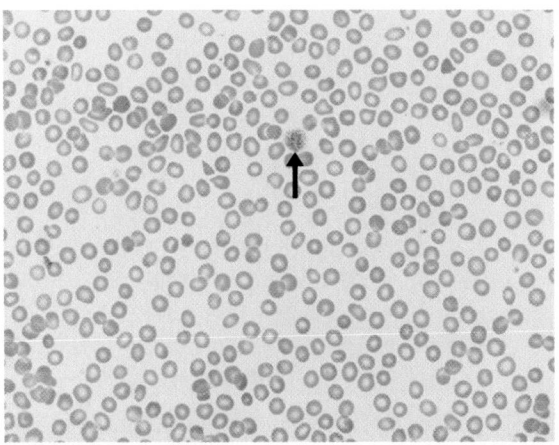

FIGURE 160-23. Giant platelet (arrow). Giant platelets are as large as or larger than normal red cells. Giant platelets can indicate increased platelet turnover or an inherited or acquired defect in thrombopoiesis (×1000).

this cytokine can cause toxic granulation, Döhle's bodies, vacuolation, and the presence of macropolycytes (giant neutrophils) and circulating neutrophil precursors. The changes typical of leukemia are discussed later.

Leukopenia usually requires a film for confirmation and elucidation. The exception is when it is expected in a given clinical context, such as when a patient has had recent chemotherapy. Rarely, an apparent leukopenia is artifactual, owing to the aggregation of neutrophils mediated by an autoantibody or resulting from infection-induced changes in adhesion molecules of the leukocyte surface membrane.

With some automated instruments, it is necessary to confirm that neutropenia is real. If the automated count is based on peroxidase cytochemistry, the presence of an inherited deficiency will lead to an apparent neutropenia associated with an increase of large, unstained (i.e., peroxidase-negative) cells. The scatter plot is characteristic, but because the same features could be due to acute leukemia with neutropenia and circulating blast cells, a smear is needed for confirmation.

LEUKEMIAS AND LYMPHOMAS

The blood smear is critical in the diagnosis of leukemias and lymphomas. The lymphoblasts of acute lymphoblastic leukemia are usually medium-sized agranular cells with relatively scanty cytoplasm (Fig. 160-24), whereas in acute myeloid leukemia, blast cells are generally larger, with more plentiful cytoplasm that may contain granules or Auer rods (Fig. 160-25). Myeloid blast cells vary in appearance according to whether they are myeloblasts or monoblasts. Myeloblasts are usually medium sized and may have plentiful granules, scanty granules, or no visible granules; they may contain Auer rods. Monoblasts are much larger cells with plentiful cytoplasm containing few granules and, very rarely, Auer rods. Megakaryoblasts are present in some

patients and are sometimes cytologically distinctive because of their tendency to form cytoplasmic blebs or develop platelet-type granules.

Chronic myelogenous leukemia has a very characteristic blood smear (Fig. 160-26) in which the most numerous cells are myelocytes and mature neutrophils. Eosinophils and basophils are also present. Dysplastic features are generally absent. In atypical Philadelphia chromosome–negative chronic myeloid leukemia, monocytosis is more frequent and dysplastic features are present. Chronic myelomonocytic leukemia is characterized by increased monocytes, some of them immature, with inconspicuous dysplastic features and infrequent granulocyte precursors.

Chronic lymphocytic leukemia also has a very characteristic blood film, with an increase of small, mature lymphocytes of rather uniform appearance. The chromatin is often irregularly clumped, creating a mosaic effect (Fig. 160-27). Smear cells are almost always increased in number but are not pathognomonic.

Lymphoma in leukemic phase often has cytologic features that aid in the diagnosis. Follicular lymphoma, Burkitt's lymphoma, and splenic marginal zone lymphoma can all be distinctive.

THE INCIDENTAL DETECTION OF CLINICALLY SIGNIFICANT ABNORMALITIES

Sometimes the examination of a blood film reveals unexpected but clinically significant information. Examples are given in Table 160-4. Detection of microorganisms is particularly likely in patients with acquired immunodeficiency syndrome (AIDS), hyposplenic patients, and patients with overwhelming sepsis, but sometimes they are detected in immunologically normal patients with only trivial symptoms. It should be noted that microorganisms in blood smears sometimes represent contaminants, particularly if

FIGURE 160-24. Acute lymphoblastic leukemia. Numerous agranular blast cells with a high nuclear-to-cytoplasmic ratio are present. Platelets are decreased in number (×1000).

FIGURE 160-26. Chronic myelogenous leukemia. In this view there are myeloblasts, a myelocyte, a basophil, and a segmented neutrophil (×1000).

FIGURE 160-25. Auer rod. An Auer rod (arrow) is a rod-shaped inclusion in the cytoplasm of cells of myeloid lineage formed by the crystallization of azurophilic granule constituents. Auer rods are seen only in acute myeloid leukemia and high-grade myelodysplastic syndromes. They are usually seen in blast cells but are occasionally found in maturing cells (×1000).

FIGURE 160-27. Chronic lymphocytic leukemia. There are large numbers of rather monotonous, mature small lymphocytes with chromatin clumping. Smear cells, reflecting the mechanical fragility of the cells, are characteristic but are not seen in this photomicrograph (×1000).

TABLE 160-4	INCIDENTAL BUT CLINICALLY RELEVANT BLOOD SMEAR OBSERVATIONS
OBSERVATION	**POSSIBLE SIGNIFICANCE**
Acanthocytes	Abetalipoproteinemia, neuroacanthocytosis, McLeod phenotype
Howell-Jolly bodies, target cells, and acanthocytes	Hyposplenism (congenital, previous splenectomy, celiac disease, amyloidosis)
Cryoglobulin	Hepatitis C, multiple myeloma
Vacuolated lymphocytes	Inherited metabolic disorders
Parasites (e.g., malaria parasites, *Babesia*, microfilaria, trypanosomes, *Leishmania*)	Parasitic infection
Fungi (*Candida* spp, *Histoplasma capsulatum*, *Penicillium marneffei*, *Cryptococcus neoformans*, *Malassezia furfur*)	Disseminated fungal infection or, in the case of *Candida*, colonization of an indwelling intravenous line
Bacteria (e.g., pneumococcus, meningococcus, *Capnocytophaga canimorsus*, *Borrelia*, *Ehrlichia*, *Anaplasma*, *Yersinia pestis*)	Bacterial infection
Leukoerythroblastic blood film	Bone marrow infiltration (e.g., metastatic malignancy)

TABLE 161-1	NORMAL VALUES FOR RED BLOOD CELL MEASUREMENTS	
MEASUREMENT	**UNIT**	**NORMAL RANGE (APPROXIMATE)***
Hemoglobin	g/dL	Males: 13.5-17.5 Females: 12-16
Hematocrit	%	Males: 40-52 Females: 36-48
Red blood cell (RBC) count	$\times 10^6/\mu L$ of blood	Males: 4.5-6.0 Females: 4.0-5.4
Mean cell volume (MCV)	fL	81-99
Mean cell hemoglobin (MCH)	pg	30-34
Mean cell hemoglobin concentration (MCHC)	g/dL	30-36
RBC size distribution width RDW-CV RDW-SD	% fL	12-14 37-47
Reticulocyte count (absolute number)	No./μL of blood	20,000-100,000
Reticulocyte percentage	% of RBCs	0.5-1.5

*Actual normal ranges for many of these values may vary slightly, depending on factors such as the location and type of laboratory instruments used, altitude above sea level, and patient age.

specimens have been obtained by skin prick or from the umbilical cord and if there has been a delay in making the film.

CONCLUSION

Despite major advances in other diagnostic methods, the blood smear remains very useful in hematologic diagnosis. Sometimes it is critical either because it yields a diagnosis very quickly or because it provides information that is not available in any other way.

SUGGESTED READINGS

Bain BJ. Diagnosis from the blood smear. *N Engl J Med.* 2005;353:498-507. *More examples of how examining a blood smear contributes to diagnosis.*

Barnes PW, McFadden S, Machin SJ, et al. The International Consensus Group for Hematology Review. http://www.islh.org/web/index.php/2009/index.php?page=consensus_preface. Accessed Jan. 1, 2010. *Discussion of how abnormalities in the automated blood count may indicate that a blood film should be examined.*

Froom P, Havis R, Barak M. The rate of manual peripheral blood smear reviews in outpatients. *Clin Chem Lab Med.* 2009;47:1401-1405. *Fewer than 3% of automated peripheral blood smears in outpatients may require manual review.*

Prokocimer M, Potasman I. The added value of peripheral blood cell morphology in the diagnosis and management of infectious diseases—part 1: basic concepts. *Postgrad Med J.* 2008;84:579-585.

Prokocimer M, Potasman I. The added value of peripheral blood cell morphology in the diagnosis and management of infectious diseases—part 2: illustrative cases. *Postgrad Med J.* 2008;84:586-589. *Two articles that show the potential contribution of the blood smear examination to the diagnosis of infectious diseases.*

161

APPROACH TO THE ANEMIAS

H. FRANKLIN BUNN

Anemia is defined as a significant reduction in the mass of circulating red blood cells. As a result, the oxygen binding capacity of the blood is diminished. Because blood volume is normally maintained at a nearly constant level, anemic patients have a decrease in the concentration of red cells or hemoglobin in peripheral blood. As shown in Table 161-1, hemoglobin and hematocrit levels vary with the age of the individual and, in adults, with gender. The values in women of childbearing age are 10% lower than those in men. At altitude, higher values are found, roughly in proportion to the elevation above sea level. Anemic patients' values are more than one standard deviation below the mean values for their gender. However, because of the wide range in normal hemoglobin and hematocrit levels, it is often difficult to document mild anemia.

Sometimes the diagnosis of anemia is confounded by a concomitant change in the plasma volume. For example, if a patient with a low red cell

$$O_2 \text{ Delivery} = \text{Blood Flow} \times \text{Hb Concentration} \times (\text{Asat} - \text{Vsat})$$

In anemia: | ↑ Cardiac output Altered flow distribution | ↑↑ Plasma Erythropoietin | ↓ RBC 2,3-DPG RBC O_2 affinity |

FIGURE 161-1. The Fick equation expresses the three independent variables that determine the transport of oxygen to a given organ or tissue. The impact of anemia on each of these variables is shown beneath the equation. Asat = oxygen saturation of arterial blood (oxyhemoglobin/oxyhemoglobin + deoxyhemoglobin); 2,3-DPG = 2,3-diphosphoglycerate (2,3-bisphosphoglycerate); Hb = hemoglobin; RBC = red blood cell; Vsat = oxygen saturation of venous blood.

mass sustains a loss of plasma volume from dehydration, diarrhea, vomiting, or severe burns, the blood hemoglobin and hematocrit levels will be increased and may even be in the normal range. Another important example, discussed in detail later in this chapter, is acute hemorrhage, in which the loss of both red blood cells and plasma results in a false elevation of hemoglobin and hematocrit. In contrast, hemoglobin and hematocrit values may be falsely low in patients with an expanded plasma volume, such as in pregnancy or congestive heart failure.

PATHOBIOLOGY
Impact of Anemia on Oxygen Transport

In any organ or region of the body, the transport of oxygen is a product of three independent variables expressed in the Fick equation (Fig. 161-1). The middle variable—the oxygen carrying capacity of the blood—is, by definition, low in anemic patients. The two other variables in the Fick equation undergo compensatory changes that, as explained later, greatly enhance oxygen transport.

Blood Flow

Anemia has a marked impact on blood flow, the left-hand variable in the Fick equation. In all anemic individuals, there is enhanced flow to vital organs, including the heart, brain, liver, and kidneys, at the expense of nonvital organs. Anemic patients are pale because blood is diverted away from the skin and mucous membranes to preserve oxygen supply to the critical organs. Resting cardiac output is normal in patients with mild or moderate anemia, but with exercise, it increases more than that of a normal individual. In severe anemia, resting cardiac output is increased, putting patients at risk of developing high-output cardiac failure, particularly those with coronary artery insufficiency or other types of preexisting cardiac disease.

Oxygen Binding to Hemoglobin

The variable on the right side of the Fick equation is the difference in fractional oxygenation between the arterial and venous blood. This difference in

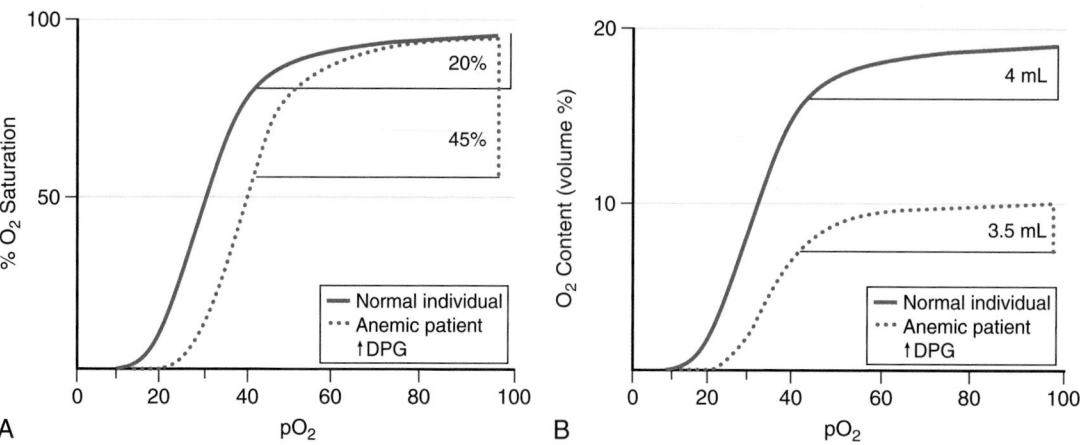

FIGURE 161-2. Oxygen binding curves for hemoglobin of a normal individual and a patient with anemia. **A,** Conventional plot of percent of oxygen (O_2) saturation versus oxygen tension (pO_2). **B,** The Y-axis shows the volume of oxygen in milliliters per 100 mL of blood. DPG = diphosphoglycerate.

oxygen saturation is determined by the hemoglobin oxygen binding curve. A comparison between a normal individual and an anemic patient is shown in Figure 161-2. As shown in part A, the curve is shifted to the right in an anemic patient. At any given oxygen tension (Po_2), the oxygen saturation of hemoglobin is lower. Thus, red cells of anemic patients have decreased oxygen affinity. This change is due entirely to elevated levels of red cell 2,3-diphosphoglycerate (2,3-DPG) in red cells. This glycolytic intermediate is the principal determinant of oxygen affinity in human red cells. The Po_2 in arterial blood is normally approximately 95 mm Hg, resulting in nearly 100% oxygen saturation. During the transit of red cells from an artery through its capillary bed to its vein, oxygen is released to respiring cells. In normal individuals, at a normal venous Po_2 of about 40 mm Hg, the oxygen saturation is approximately 80%. Thus, as shown in Figure 161-2A, 20% of the oxygen in the blood is unloaded. In contrast, in patients with anemia and elevated red cell 2,3-DPG levels, the lower oxygen affinity of their red cells enables a much higher fraction of the oxygen (about 45%) to be unloaded. In Figure 161-2B, the oxygen binding curves are depicted with the volume fraction of oxygen plotted on the Y-axis. One gram of hemoglobin binds up to 1.34 mL of oxygen under standard conditions of temperature and pressure. Thus, in a normal individual having a hemoglobin of 15 g/dL, the oxygen carrying capacity of the blood is 15×1.34, or 20 mL O_2/dL. As mentioned earlier, 20% of this oxygen will be unloaded—that is, 4 mL O_2/100 mL blood during arterial-venous transit. In contrast, an anemic patient with a hemoglobin of 7.5 g/dL has an oxygen binding capacity that is half normal, or 10 mL O_2/dL. If this patient had red cells with normal oxygen affinity, 20%, or only 2 mL of oxygen, would be unloaded per 100 mL of blood. However, because the patient's red cells have a lower affinity for oxygen, 3.5 mL is unloaded, nearly as much as normal. Thus, the decrease in oxygen affinity is an important mechanism by which anemic patients compensate for the deficit in red cell mass.

Methemoglobinemia

In order for hemoglobin to reversibly bind oxygen, the iron atom in the heme must be in the reduced (Fe^{2+}) valence state. As red cells circulate, the heme iron slowly auto-oxidizes to Fe^{3+}, forming methemoglobin, which is incapable of binding oxygen. Normal red cells are endowed with a very efficient enzymatic pathway composed of cytochrome b_5, cytochrome b_5 reductase, and NADH that rapidly reduces the iron in methemoglobin back to its functional Fe^{2+} form. Thus, normal red cells contain less than 0.5% methemoglobin. However, either an inherited deficiency in cytochrome b_5 reductase or exposure to an oxidant drug or toxin can result in methemoglobinemia. Laboratory samples of blood containing methemoglobin are dark brown, whereas patients with greater than 10% methemoglobinemia have cyanosis, a blue discoloration of the skin indistinguishable from that commonly seen in patients having normal hemoglobin but low oxygen saturation owing to pulmonary or cardiac disease. In many hospitals and large clinical laboratories, the instrument that measures oxygen saturation in blood samples also provides an accurate determination of methemoglobin.

Patients with congenital methemoglobinemia inherit an autosomal recessive deficiency in cytochrome b_5 reductase. Heterozygote relatives have low or undetectable methemoglobin levels, whereas affected individuals

(homozygotes and compound heterozygotes) generally have 10 to 35% methemoglobin. These individuals are generally asymptomatic owing to the fact that the methemoglobin is distributed primarily in the older population of red cells. Nevertheless, many affected individuals have cosmetic concerns. Treatment with oral ascorbic acid or riboflavin is effective in lowering the level of methemoglobin below the threshold of detectable cyanosis.

A variety of drugs can cause methemoglobinemia, including acetaminophen (Tylenol), dapsone, nitroprusside, amyl nitrate, and procaine congeners used for local anesthesia. It is not clear why only a very small fraction of those using these drugs develop this complication, but some affected individuals have been shown to be heterozygous for cytochrome b_5 reductase deficiency. When these drugs are taken in prescribed doses, methemoglobinemia seldom reaches levels high enough to cause clinical concern.

In contrast, individuals exposed to industrial toxins such as nitrite, nitrate, or aniline may develop life-threatening levels of methemoglobin. The threshold at which symptoms occur is highly variable. Acute induction of 20% methemoglobin may cause fatigue; at 30%, individuals often develop tachycardia. When methemoglobin exceeds 50%, patients experience weakness, breathlessness, and confusion. At 70 to 80%, coma and death may occur. The toxicity of methemoglobinemia is not just because of the oxidized hemes' inability to bind oxygen; the remaining functional (Fe^{2+}) hemes in the hemoglobin tetramer have increased oxygen affinity and therefore, as suggested in Figure 161-2, are much less effective in releasing oxygen to tissues. Patients with toxic methemoglobinemia can be effectively treated with intravenous infusion of methylene blue (1 to 2 mg/kg).

Regulation of Erythropoiesis by Erythropoietin

Anemia also impacts the middle component of the Fick equation (see Fig. 161-1). As mentioned earlier, hemoglobin levels are, by definition, low in anemic patients. The resultant decrease in the oxygen carrying capacity of the blood causes cellular hypoxia. In all cells of the body, a molecular sensor detects even modest degrees of low oxygen tension and induces a hypoxia-inducible transcription factor called HIF. HIF upregulates expression of the hormone erythropoietin in the kidney and, to a lesser extent, in the liver. Erythropoietin (Chapter 159) binds to a specific receptor abundantly expressed on erythroid progenitor cells in the bone marrow and salvages these cells from apoptosis, thereby enhancing red blood cell production. Normal individuals maintain nearly constant levels of circulating red cells by finely tuned regulation of erythropoietin production. In anemic patients, the hypoxic signal in the kidneys and, to a lesser extent, in the liver results in a robust induction of erythropoietin expression. As the hematocrit falls, the plasma erythropoietin level rises markedly; in severely anemic patients, it may be 1000-fold higher than normal (Fig. 161-3). In patients with anemia due to impaired red cell production, their erythroid progenitors are unresponsive to such high levels of plasma erythropoietin. In contrast, in patients whose anemia is due to hemolysis or blood loss, elevated erythropoietin levels maximize red cell production.

CLINICAL MANIFESTATIONS

Figure 161-4 is a 17th-century painting of a pale young woman clutching her chest, apparently complaining of palpitations. Her physician is feeling her

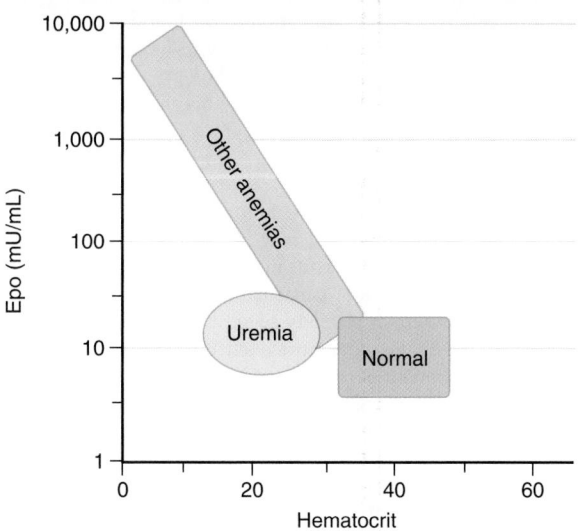

FIGURE 161-3. Plasma erythropoietin (Epo) levels in patients with different degrees of anemia. The subset of anemia patients with chronic renal disease (labeled "Uremia") have much lower plasma erythropoietin levels than those with other types of anemia. Values for normal individuals are also shown.

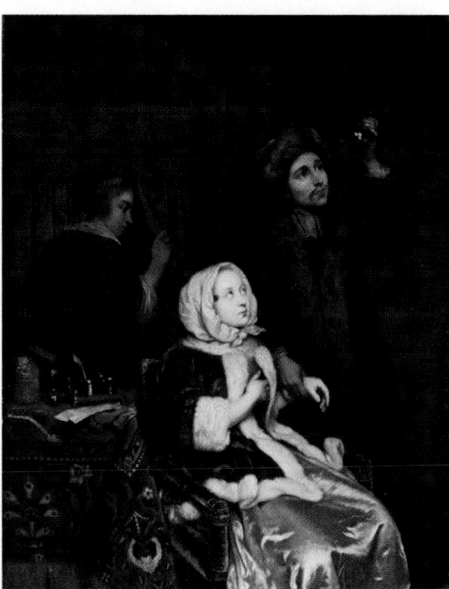

FIGURE 161-4. "The Sick Lady," a 17th-century painting attributed to Caspar Netscher, from the Royal Collection, Buckingham Palace.

pulse, documenting her rapid, forceful heartbeat. These signs and symptoms, common in patients with very low hemoglobin levels, can be readily explained by the cardiovascular adjustments discussed in the preceding section. These clinical findings pertain to anemia per se, irrespective of cause, and are dependent on its severity and chronicity. The history and physical examination may reveal additional findings peculiar to specific causes of anemia or to other comorbid conditions. The degree to which symptoms occur in an anemic patient depends on several contributing factors. If the anemia has developed rapidly, there may not have been adequate time for compensatory adjustments to take place, and the patient may have more marked symptoms than if an anemia of equivalent severity had developed insidiously. Furthermore, the patient's complaints may depend on the presence of local vascular disease. For example, symptoms owing to ischemia in patients with angina pectoris, intermittent claudication, or transient cerebral episodes may be triggered by the development of anemia.

Symptoms
Many individuals with mild anemia have no complaints and are unaware that they have "tired blood." Others may complain of fatigue as well as dyspnea and palpitations, particularly following exercise. Patients with severe anemia are often symptomatic at rest and are unable to tolerate significant exertion.

TABLE 161-2 INITIAL ASSESSMENT OF ANEMIA

Decreased red cell production
   Usually acquired
   Onset is insidious
   Reticulocyte count is inappropriately low
   Red cell indices (MCV, MCHC) are informative
   Bone marrow examination is often required for diagnosis
Increased red cell destruction (hemolysis)
   Often inherited
   Onset may be abrupt or insidious
   Reticulocyte count is increased
   Red cell morphology is usually informative
   Bone marrow examination is usually not indicated
Blood loss—must be ruled out in any patient with anemia

MCHC = mean cell hemoglobin concentration; MCV = mean cell volume.

If the hemoglobin concentration falls below 7.5 g/dL, resting cardiac output is likely to rise, with an increase in both stroke volume and heart rate. The patient may be aware of this hyperdynamic state and complain of a rapid, pounding sensation in the precordium. Patients with compromised myocardial reserve may develop complaints due to cardiac failure.

The symptoms of severe anemia often extend beyond the cardiac or circulatory system. Patients sometimes experience dizziness and headache and, less often, syncope, tinnitus, or vertigo. Many are irritable and have difficulty sleeping or concentrating. Because blood flow is shunted away from the skin, patients may complain of increased sensitivity to cold. In like manner, gastrointestinal symptoms such as indigestion, anorexia, or even nausea are attributable to the shunting of blood away from the splanchnic bed. Females commonly develop abnormal menstruation, either amenorrhea or increased bleeding. Males may experience impotence or loss of libido.

Physical Findings
Pallor is the most commonly encountered physical finding in patients with anemia. As mentioned earlier, this sign is due to the shunting of blood away from the skin and other peripheral tissues, permitting enhanced blood flow to vital organs. The usefulness of pallor as a physical finding is limited by other factors that affect the appearance of the skin. Blood flow to the skin may undergo wide fluctuations. Moreover, the skin's thickness and texture vary widely among individuals. Those with a fair complexion may appear pale even though they are not anemic, while pallor is difficult to detect in deeply pigmented individuals. The amount of melanin in the epidermis is an important determinant of skin color. Pallor may be difficult to detect in patients who have increased melanin pigmentation due to Addison's disease or hemochromatosis. Nevertheless, even in blacks, the presence of anemia may be suspected by the color of the palms or of noncutaneous tissues such as oral mucous membranes, nail beds, and palpebral conjunctivas. When the creases of the palm are as pale as the surrounding skin, the patient usually has a hemoglobin of less than 7 g/dL.

In addition to tachycardia, wide pulse pressure, and hyperdynamic precordium, a systolic ejection murmur is often heard over the precordium, particularly at the pulmonic area. In addition, a venous hum may be detected over the neck vessels. These findings disappear when the anemia is corrected.

DIAGNOSIS
Laboratory Evaluation of the Patient with Anemia
In the clinical assessment of the anemic patient, it is important to proceed in a systematic way so that the diagnosis can be established with a minimum of laboratory tests and procedures. A thorough history and careful physical examination are critical in the initial evaluation of the anemic patient. For example, a family history that reveals a dominant inheritance pattern would reinforce the tentative diagnosis of hereditary spherocytosis. The presence of fever, a new heart murmur, and splenomegaly is an anemic patient suggests subacute bacterial endocarditis.

In evaluating the anemic patient, the clinician must first ask whether the anemia is caused by decreased production of red cells or by loss of blood cells as a result of hemorrhage or hemolysis (Table 161-2). Blood loss may be either the sole cause of the anemia or a significant contributor. Therefore, examination of the stool for occult blood is an indispensable part of the evaluation of all anemic patients.

The laboratory work-up of anemia includes a complete blood count, red cell indices, reticulocyte count, and microscopic examination of the blood smear. In addition, in many cases a bone marrow examination is a critical component of the initial laboratory assessment.

Complete Blood Count

Most hospitals and clinical laboratories use equipment that provides high-throughput analyses of red cell, platelet, and white cell counts and white cell differential, along with measurements of cell size. The mean red cell volume (MCV) is normally 81 to 99 fL. These instruments also provide accurate determinations of hemoglobin concentration. The hematocrit, or fraction of packed red cells over total blood volume, is determined indirectly from the red cell count and the MCV. The mean concentration of hemoglobin within the red cell population (MCHC) is the quotient of hemoglobin divided by hematocrit. The MCV is particularly useful in classifying the anemias caused by decreased red cell production. Microcytic anemias have low MCV values and often low MCHC. Microscopic examination reveals small and often pale red cells. The MCV in the macrocytic anemias is increased, and large, oval cells (macro-ovalocytes) are seen. In contrast to the anemias of underproduction, the hemolytic anemias are either normocytic or slightly macrocytic owing to the preponderance of young red cells that are relatively large. Severe forms of thalassemia (Chapter 165) are an exception; there, microcytic red cells may be accompanied by brisk hemolysis.

Reticulocyte Count

This simple and cost-effective test is extremely useful for distinguishing anemias secondary to decreased red cell production from those caused by hemolysis. With the application of an appropriate supravital stain, the 1- to 2-day-old red cells in the peripheral blood reveal a network of purple strands, which are aggregates of ribosomes. The reticulocyte count in normal individuals is about 1%, consistent with a red cell lifespan of approximately 120 days. An elevated reticulocyte count reflects the release of an increased number of young cells from the bone marrow. The rate of red cell production can be assessed more quantitatively by determining the absolute reticulocyte count, the product of the percentage of reticulocytes and the red cell count. Thus, normal blood contains about 50,000 reticulocytes/mm^3. In interpreting this test, one should consider the distribution of reticulocytes between the bone marrow and the peripheral blood. When erythropoiesis is robust, marrow reticulocytes enter the circulation prematurely. These "shift reticulocytes" appear larger than average on a routine (Wright-stained) blood smear and have a lavender hue, called polychromatophilia. Because the circulation of shift reticulocytes in the peripheral blood is prolonged, the reticulocyte count should be divided by two. This correction should always be made if normoblasts are encountered in the peripheral blood because this finding indicates the premature release of newborn red cells into the circulation.

A failure to produce red cells is reflected in an inappropriately low reticulocyte count. In contrast, a significant elevation of reticulocytes is suggestive of hemolysis. Exceptions include the following:

- The brisk reticulocyte response seen in patients with hemorrhage
- Reticulocytosis encountered in patients recovering from impaired erythropoiesis (e.g., an individual with pernicious anemia who received an injection of cobalamin 1 week earlier)
- Mild to moderate elevations in reticulocytes (3 to 7%) encountered in myelophthisic anemia (Chapter 160), in which the orderly release of cells is affected by alterations of the marrow stroma owing to tumor, fibrosis, or granuloma

These exceptions are generally appreciated in the initial evaluation of the patient.

A number of ancillary laboratory tests described later under Hemolytic Anemias are useful in determining both the extent and the cause of hemolysis.

Examination of the Blood Smear

In the evaluation of any patient with unexplained anemia, the physician should take the time to examine a well-stained peripheral blood film (Chapter 160). Many subtleties escape the attention of the technologist, whose primary aim is to confirm or refine the white cell differential count provided by automated cell counters. The clinician approaches the specimen with a prepared mind and can scrutinize it for specific abnormalities. Examination of the blood film can confirm the size and color of red cells estimated by red blood cell indices. In contrast to the mean statistical values provided by automated cell counters, microscopic examination can reveal variations in red cell size (anisocytosis) or shape (poikilocytosis), abnormalities that are helpful in

diagnosing specific anemias. Examination of the blood smear is particularly important in a patient with hemolysis. Many types of hemolytic anemia have characteristic abnormalities in red cell morphology. The presence of abnormal white cells may be the first clue to a lymphoproliferative or primary bone marrow disorder.

Bone Marrow Examination

A microscopic examination of the bone marrow (aspirate with or without a core biopsy) is often useful and may be critical in the work-up of any *unexplained* anemia. Study of the bone marrow is informative in the diagnosis of anemias of underproduction, particularly those accompanied by abnormalities in white cells and/or platelets, suggesting disordered hematopoiesis. The more severe the anemia, the more likely it is that the procedure will be informative. An assessment of the quantity and quality of red cell precursors may identify a defect in cell production due to either hypoplasia or ineffective erythropoiesis. A marrow biopsy is required for estimating overall cellularity. The ratio of myeloid (M) to erythroid (E) precursors is normally about 2 : 1, but it may be artifactually increased by the inclusion of circulating leukocytes. The ratio is increased in patients with infection, a leukemoid reaction, or neoplastic proliferation of myeloid cells. Rarely, a high M/E ratio is due to selective aplasia of the red cell precursors. A decreased M/E ratio indicates erythroid hyperplasia. Erythroid maturation is normal in hemolysis and hemorrhage, but it is disordered when erythropoiesis is ineffective, such as in megaloblastic and sideroblastic anemias and in β-thalassemia major or intermedia. The bone marrow examination is also important in demonstrating the presence of cellular infiltrates such as those found in leukemia, lymphoma, or multiple myeloma. The demonstration of tumor, fibrosis, or granuloma usually requires a bone marrow biopsy, not just a bone marrow aspiration. A portion of the marrow specimen should be stained with Prussian blue. In addition to providing an assessment of iron stores, this iron stain is required for the identification of erythroid sideroblasts.

● ANEMIA DUE TO BLOOD LOSS

The clinical presentation of anemia resulting from blood loss varies considerably, depending on the site, severity, and rapidity of the hemorrhage. At opposite extremes are acute fulminant bleeding producing hypovolemic shock and chronic occult blood loss leading to iron deficiency anemia.

Acute Blood Loss

Patients who have had a sudden hemorrhage present with clinical findings secondary to hypovolemia and hypoxia. Symptoms and signs depend on the severity of the process. The patient may experience weakness, fatigue, lightheadedness, or stupor and may appear pale, diaphoretic, and irritable. The vital signs reflect cardiovascular compensation for the acute blood loss. The degree of hypotension and tachycardia depends on the extent of the hemorrhage. Elicitation of postural signs is useful in the initial evaluation of a patient with acute blood loss. When a patient is lifted from a supine to a sitting position, an increase in the pulse of 25% or more or a fall in the systolic blood pressure of 20 mm Hg or more signifies significant hypovolemia (blood loss >1000 mL). Acute blood loss in excess of 1500 mL usually leads to cardiovascular collapse.

Following acute hemorrhage, the red cell mass and plasma volume are contracted in parallel; accordingly, there is often not a significant decrease in the hemoglobin or hematocrit level initially. This stress induces a moderate leukocytosis and a "shift to the left" in the white cell differential count. In both acute and chronic blood loss, the platelet count is often increased, particularly if the patient is already iron deficient. During the first few days after acute blood loss, there is usually an increase in reticulocytes. Severe hypoxia may trigger the release of nucleated red cells from the bone marrow into the peripheral blood. Because young red cells are larger than old ones, the MCV generally rises slightly. If significant blood loss continues, reticulocytosis will persist until iron stores have been exhausted. Internal bleeding is often accompanied by an increase in unconjugated bilirubin, reflecting an increase in the catabolism of heme from extravasated red cells. Patients with acute gastrointestinal blood loss sometimes have an elevation of blood urea nitrogen owing to impaired renal blood flow and perhaps to the absorption of digested blood protein.

These patients must be assessed promptly, and treatment must be initiated without delay. Patients with severe acute blood loss require transfusion of packed red cells, with central monitoring of the appropriate amount of volume replacement. The site or sites of bleeding should be emergently identified and controlled. In addition, an emergency coagulation profile should be obtained. The approach to the patient with shock is discussed in detail in Chapter 106.

Chronic Blood Loss

Chronic blood loss is usually due to lesions in the gastrointestinal tract or the uterus. Testing of stool specimens for occult blood is an essential but frequently overlooked part of the evaluation of anemia. It is sometimes necessary to examine serial specimens over a prolonged period because gastrointestinal bleeding may be intermittent. The hematologic manifestations of chronic blood loss are those of iron deficiency anemia, discussed in detail in Chapter 162.

● ANEMIAS DUE TO DECREASED RED CELL PRODUCTION

As shown in Table 161-3, anemias caused by the underproduction of red cells can be conveniently classified according to red cell size: microcytic, macrocytic, and normocytic.

Microcytic Anemias

The presence of small red cells (MCV <77 fL) indicates a defect in the production of hemoglobin. As shown in Figure 161-5, hemoglobin is composed of globin subunits into which heme is inserted. Heme is produced by the insertion of an iron atom into porphyrin (protoporphyrin IX). A defect in any of these three key components can cause microcytic anemia. Most individuals with microcytosis have either iron deficiency anemia (Chapter 162) or thalassemia (Chapter 165). A congenital or, more often, acquired impairment in porphyrin synthesis can lead to a buildup of excess iron in erythroid

cells, resulting in the morphologic entity of ringed sideroblasts, which are identified in red cell precursors in the bone marrow (Chapter 162). Most patients with acquired sideroblastic anemia actually have a normal or somewhat elevated MCV but a broad distribution of red cell size, including a population of microcytes (because of this ambiguity, sideroblastic anemia appears in parentheses in Table 161-3). Iron deficiency anemia, the thalassemias, and sideroblastic anemia all involve some degree of ineffective erythropoiesis.

The anemias of chronic inflammation and malignancy, described in detail later, may be slightly microcytic owing to a defect in the availability of iron. However, these disorders are more often normocytic. Measurement of serum iron and iron binding capacity (Fig. 161-6A) and evaluation of marrow iron stores are particularly useful in distinguishing between iron deficiency and the anemia of chronic inflammation.

Macrocytic Anemias

A modest increase in red cell size is encountered in a variety of conditions, including liver disease, hypothyroidism, acute blood loss, hemolytic anemia, aplastic anemia, and alcoholism. The macrocytes in liver disease and hypothyroidism may be related to an increased deposition of lipid in the red cell membrane. If the MCV exceeds approximately 105 fL, the patient is likely to be deficient in either cobalamin (vitamin B_{12}) or folic acid. The bone marrow reveals megaloblastic morphology, reflecting impaired replication of DNA. Because nuclear maturation lags behind cytoplasmic development, large red cells tend to be produced in the bone marrow. Megaloblastic anemias are discussed in detail in Chapter 167. Like the microcytic anemias, these disorders are maturation defects associated with ineffective erythropoiesis.

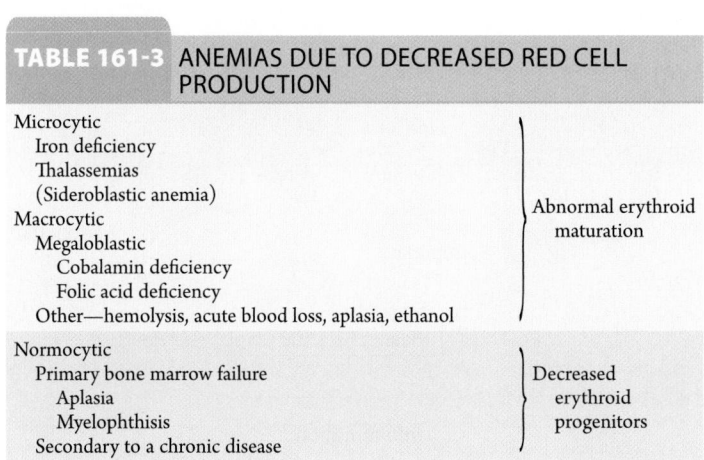

TABLE 161-3	ANEMIAS DUE TO DECREASED RED CELL PRODUCTION

Microcytic
  Iron deficiency
  Thalassemias
  (Sideroblastic anemia)
Macrocytic
  Megaloblastic
    Cobalamin deficiency
    Folic acid deficiency
  Other—hemolysis, acute blood loss, aplasia, ethanol
	Abnormal erythroid maturation

Normocytic
  Primary bone marrow failure
    Aplasia
    Myelophthisis
  Secondary to a chronic disease
	Decreased erythroid progenitors

FIGURE 161-5. Components of hemoglobin that are deficient in the microcytic anemias.

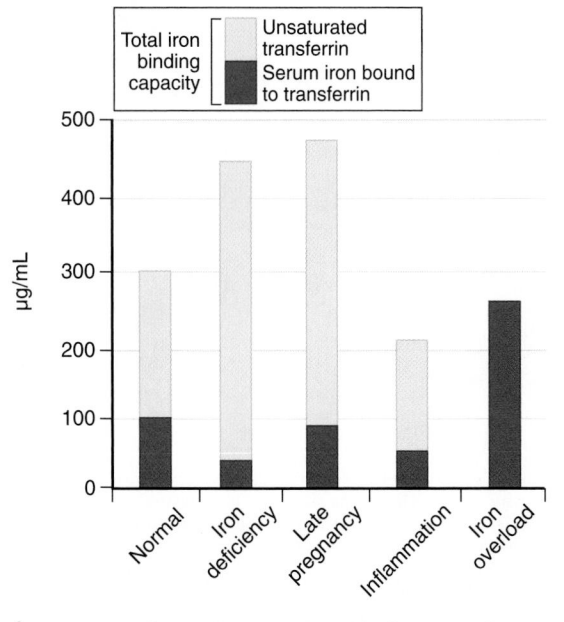

A **Serum iron and iron-binding capacity**

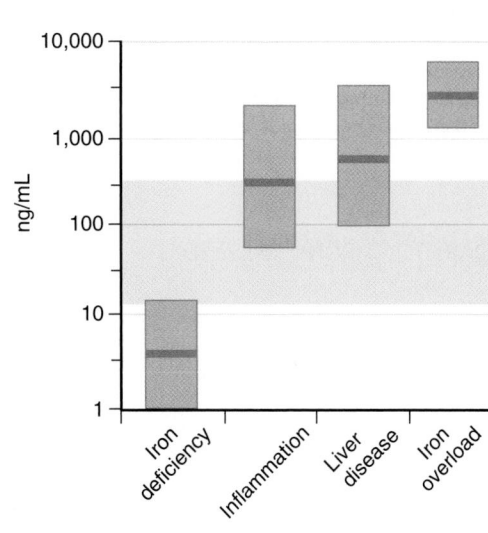

B **Serum ferritin**

FIGURE 161-6. **A,** Serum iron and transferrin saturation in different conditions. **B,** Serum ferritin in different conditions. Note that the Y-axis in this panel is on a log scale. The normal range (10 to 200 ng/mL) is shown by the beige shaded area.

Normocytic Anemias

The normocytic anemias of underproduction are a diverse group of disorders. They can be conveniently divided into two categories: those due to intrinsic pathology within the bone marrow, and those secondary to some other underlying disease.

Primary Bone Marrow Disorders

The primary disorders of the bone marrow, such as the leukemias (Chapters 189 and 190), myelodysplasia (Chapter 188), aplastic anemia (Chapter 168), and myelophthisis, are best approached by microscopic examination of a marrow aspirate and biopsy. This group of anemias is often accompanied by leukopenia and thrombocytopenia. A lesser degree of pancytopenia can also occur in hypersplenism and in the megaloblastic anemias.

Anemias of Chronic Disease

Among the most common anemias and the ones most prevalent in patients hospitalized on a medical service are those secondary to an underlying chronic disease. The diagnosis is usually quite straightforward. However, in some patients the predisposing illness may not be apparent. Thus, the presence of an unexplained normocytic anemia should prompt the search for the disorders listed in Table 161-4. Even if the presence of an underlying illness is established, the physician should investigate whether other factors such as blood loss or a nutritional deficiency are contributing to the patient's anemia. Generally, the anemias due to chronic inflammation, an endocrinopathy, or liver disease are of only moderate severity. In contrast, the anemia of uremia is often severe.

ANEMIA OF CHRONIC INFLAMMATION

If a systemic inflammatory disorder persists for more than a few weeks, it is nearly always accompanied by anemia. As shown in Table 161-4, the most common causes of chronic inflammation are infection, tumor, or a connective tissue disorder. Many chronic infections can be responsible, including tuberculosis, lung abscess, subacute bacterial endocarditis, pyelonephritis, and osteomyelitis. The pathogenesis is more complex in some types of chronic infections. For example, in AIDS, the human immunodeficiency virus can directly attack hematopoietic cells and suppress erythropoiesis. In malaria and babesiosis, the parasite enters circulating red cells and triggers their destruction.

There is considerable variability in tumors' ability to evoke an inflammatory response. Many tumors express inflammatory cytokines as part of their profile of abnormal gene expression. In some cases, impaired supply of oxygen or nutrients to the interior of the tumor mass can lead to necrosis and an inflammatory response. Red cell production may be further compromised by encroachment of the bone marrow with leukemia, lymphoma, or metastatic tumor.

Anemia is also a feature of a broad range of inflammatory conditions that are not associated with either infection or cancer. In some of these disorders, the autoimmune attack on the patient's cells and tissues is met with a robust inflammatory response. Rheumatoid arthritis (Chapter 272) is the most commonly encountered connective tissue disorder and gives rise to the prototypical anemia of chronic inflammation. Even more intense inflammation and, accordingly, more severe anemia are seen in polymyalgia rheumatica and temporal arteritis (Chapter 279). In patients with systemic lupus erythematosus (Chapter 274), the anemia of chronic inflammation is often compounded by either immune hemolysis (Chapter 163) or renal insufficiency (discussed later).

TABLE 161-4 ANEMIAS SECONDARY TO CHRONIC DISEASE
Inflammation
Chronic infections
Cancer
Connective tissue disorders
Renal insufficiency
Endocrine disorders
Hypothyroidism
Hypoadrenalism
Hypopituitarism
Hypogonadism—males
Liver disease
Aging

PATHOBIOLOGY

Recently, the mechanism underlying the anemia of chronic inflammation has been elucidated by the discovery that plasma hepcidin levels are markedly increased as a result of induction by inflammatory cytokines. As shown in Figure 161-7, hepcidin blocks both iron absorption from the gut and the exit of iron from macrophages, thus explaining both reduced levels of serum iron and increased iron stores.

DIAGNOSIS

The anemia of chronic inflammation is associated with disordered iron homeostasis. Increased storage of iron in macrophages within the bone marrow, liver, and spleen results in elevated levels of serum ferritin (Fig. 161-6B). However, because of a block in the transfer of this excess iron into the plasma, serum iron is low (see Fig. 161-6A). The level of total transferrin in the serum is also low for unclear reasons. With the recent development of a reliable assay for hepcidin, elevated serum levels of this "master regulator" of iron homeostasis should become useful in the diagnosis of the anemia of chronic inflammation. Because of the impairment in iron availability, erythropoiesis is somewhat "iron deficient." The amount of cytoplasmic iron is

Normal

Inflammation

Plasma Fe ~25 μg/dL

FIGURE 161-7. Pathogenesis of the block in iron availability in the anemia of chronic inflammation. The primary sources of iron in the plasma are from the breakdown of senescent red blood cells (RBCs) within macrophages and from duodenal absorption. **A,** In the presence of physiologically low levels of hepcidin in the plasma, there is efficient release of iron from the duodenal enterocyte and from macrophages via ferroportin. **B,** In patients with inflammation, the induction of plasma hepcidin by interleukin-6 and other cytokines results in the inactivation of ferroportin and the loss of iron egress from the duodenal enterocyte and from the macrophage.

decreased in erythroid precursors in the bone marrow, and the red cells that enter the circulation are slightly microcytic. This suppression of red cell production is earmarked by a low reticulocyte index. Because this block in iron utilization is subtle, the degree of anemia is seldom severe in patients with inflammatory disorders. If the hemoglobin is less than 8 g/dL, it is necessary to look for additional contributors such as hemolysis or bleeding.

ANEMIA OF RENAL INSUFFICIENCY

A normocytic anemia almost always accompanies uremia (Chapter 132). Although the hemoglobin level is highly variable, the severity of the anemia is roughly proportional to the degree of impaired renal function. The cause of the kidney failure usually has little bearing on the extent of anemia. However, for any level of serum creatinine, patients with polycystic disease tend to be less anemic than those with other types of renal disease. In contrast to the anemias associated with other chronic disorders, the anemia of uremia can be very severe, with hemoglobin levels as low as 4 g/dL.

Examination of the bone marrow seldom reveals any abnormalities. Red cell morphology is usually normal. In a minority of patients, the peripheral blood smear reveals so-called burr cells characterized by an evenly scalloped border. Neither the degree of anemia nor the red blood cell lifespan is influenced by the presence of burr cells. In most patients, the corrected reticulocyte count is low, and the red blood cell survival is only modestly decreased. Thus, the low red blood cell mass is due to decreased red blood cell production.

PATHOBIOLOGY

The primary basis for the anemia is the diseased kidneys' inability to secrete adequate amounts of erythropoietin. Plasma erythropoietin levels are lower than those of nonuremic patients with a comparable degree of anemia (see Fig. 161-3). Erythropoiesis is further impaired but not abolished in patients who have undergone bilateral nephrectomy. In addition, red blood cell production may be suppressed by the accumulation of substances that are normally cleared by the kidneys.

Other factors may aggravate the anemia of renal disease. Uremic patients have a propensity to hemorrhage, owing to a qualitative defect in platelet function. As in other patients, chronic gastrointestinal blood loss leads to iron deficiency. Folic acid deficiency may also occur, owing to the poor nutrition of many patients or to the loss of this vitamin during dialysis. Patients whose renal failure is due to thrombotic thrombocytopenic purpura or hemolytic-uremic syndrome (Chapter 175) have a severe form of microangiopathic hemolytic anemia, with characteristic abnormalities of red blood cell morphology (Chapter 160).

FIGURE 161-8. Response of a uremic patient to recombinant human erythropoietin (rHuEPO) therapy. Before therapy, the patient was severely anemic and transfusion dependent. Treatment with rHuEPO resulted in a reticulocytosis, followed by a progressive increase in hemoglobin. The dose of rHuEPO had to be lowered to prevent the hemoglobin from rising too high. Before rHuEPO therapy the patient was severely iron overloaded. The marked increase in red cell mass following therapy was accompanied by a significant reduction in iron stores. RBC = red blood cell; TIBC = total iron binding capacity. (From Eschbach JW, Egrie JC, Downing MR, et al. Correction of the anemia of end-stage renal disease with recombinant human erythropoietin: results of a combined phase I and II clinical trial. *N Engl J Med.* 1987;316:73-78.)

ANEMIA OF ENDOCRINE HYPOFUNCTION

The in vitro proliferation of erythroid cells is stimulated by a number of hormones, including thyroxine, glucocorticoids, testosterone, and growth hormone. Therefore, it is not surprising that a mild to moderate normocytic anemia generally accompanies endocrine deficiency states, including hypothyroidism, Addison's disease, hypogonadism, and panhypopituitarism.

In the anemia of hypothyroidism, erythropoiesis is suppressed, and the red blood cell lifespan is normal. A minority of patients have macrocytic red blood cells, often owing to cobalamin deficiency. Patients with hypothyroidism have an increased incidence of pernicious anemia. Some patients, particularly females with menorrhagia, develop iron deficiency and a microcytic anemia. The anemia of hypothyroidism may be masked because of a reduction in plasma volume. Because the signs and symptoms of hypothyroidism are sometimes elusive (Chapter 233), this diagnosis should be considered in any patient with unexplained anemia.

The anemia of adrenal insufficiency, including Addison's disease, may also be masked by a decrease in plasma volume. Untreated patients have an average hemoglobin level of about 13 g/dL. Upon hormone replacement, the plasma volume is rapidly reconstituted, and the hemoglobin level falls to 80% of its pretreatment value. With continued therapy, the red blood cell mass returns to normal.

Testosterone influences erythropoiesis in a physiologic manner. In males, the mean hemoglobin level increases from 13 to 15 g/dL during the transition from puberty to adulthood. Eunuchoid males usually have a mild anemia (hemoglobin ≈ 13 g/dL). Pituitary dysfunction or ablation is also associated with a mild anemia.

The anemias secondary to endocrine failure are all readily corrected when adequate hormone replacement is given.

ANEMIA OF CHRONIC LIVER DISEASE

Chronic liver disease, regardless of cause (Chapter 148), is usually accompanied by mild or moderate anemia that is normocytic or slightly macrocytic. An increased plasma volume may artificially lower the hematocrit, making the anemia seem worse than it is. Red cell morphology is normal, except for the presence of target cells and occasional stomatocytes that have a slitlike rather than a circular area of central pallor. These morphologic features reflect an increased red cell membrane surface area due to increased deposits of cholesterol and phospholipid. The bone marrow is usually normal. Erythropoiesis fails to compensate for a modest shortening of the red cell lifespan. The mechanism underlying the anemia of chronic liver disease is not understood. The anemia is usually corrected if the patient regains normal hepatic function.

In patients with alcoholic liver disease (Chapters 155 and 156), the situation is much more complex. Many factors can contribute to the development of anemia. Alcohol in high doses suppresses not only erythropoiesis but also neutrophil and platelet production. In alcoholics who continue to drink up to the time of clinical evaluation, the bone marrow often reveals vacuoles in the cytoplasm of red and white blood cell precursors. In addition, ringed sideroblasts may be observed, especially if there is concurrent malnutrition. Folic acid deficiency is common in alcoholics because of both a suboptimal diet and an impairment of folate utilization. Moreover, the anemia in alcoholics is often compounded by gastrointestinal hemorrhage as a result of gastric erosions, duodenal ulcers, or esophageal varices. The risk of blood loss is further increased by the presence of thrombocytopenia and/or deficiencies in soluble clotting factors. Although alcoholics usually have increased iron stores, they may become iron deficient after prolonged gastrointestinal bleeding. Rarely, patients with alcoholic cirrhosis develop a severe hemolytic anemia accompanied by the appearance of rigid blood cells with irregular borders called acanthocytes or "spur" cells.

ANEMIA OF THE ELDERLY

As individuals age there is a slight and gradual fall in hemoglobin and hematocrit levels. Elderly individuals whose values fall below two standard deviations of normal have significantly enhanced morbidity and mortality. As people age, there is also an increased incidence of cancer, myelodysplasia, renal insufficiency, and chronic inflammatory disorders, all of which can suppress red cell production. Because of the high likelihood of comorbid conditions among the elderly, it is not possible to affirm with any certainty whether aging per se is a cause of anemia. Nevertheless, a fall in hemoglobin in any patient, old or young, should prompt an investigation into the possible presence of one of these underlying disorders.

● HEMOLYTIC ANEMIAS

With the exception of sickle cell disease (Chapter 166), hemolytic anemias are encountered much less frequently than those caused by decreased red cell production. Although they are a diverse group, the hemolytic anemias share a number of clinical and laboratory features. Patients with moderate or severe hemolysis may have icterus owing to an elevation in nonconjugated (indirect) bilirubin. In addition, individuals with various types of hemolytic anemia often have splenomegaly, signifying the primary site of enhanced red cell destruction.

PATHOBIOLOGY

The presence of hemolysis is established by the laboratory tests outlined in Table 161-6. Further evaluation is required to establish the specific diagnosis. The clinician saves both time and money by using the available tests in a rational and orderly manner. Diagnosis of hemolytic anemias is greatly facilitated by the use of a logical and pathophysiologically based classification scheme. Table 161-5 groups these disorders going from the outside of the red cell into the cytoplasm, as well as by whether the defect is inherited or acquired. Hemolytic anemias due to environmental factors such as immune destruction or traumatic rupture (Chapter 163) are acquired. Abnormalities of red cell membrane proteins can also cause hemolysis. Mutations in proteins of the red cell cytoskeleton may cause hemolysis of varying severity. The most commonly encountered is hereditary spherocytosis (Chapter 164). Acquired red cell membrane defects are rare. Paroxysmal nocturnal hemoglobinuria is discussed in Chapter 163, and spur cell anemia was mentioned earlier in the section on anemias secondary to chronic liver disease. The proteins in the cytosol of the red cell include hemoglobin and enzymes. Mutations in these proteins can result in inherited hemolytic anemias. Sickle cell disease (Chapter 166) and the thalassemias (Chapter 165) are the most commonly encountered hemoglobinopathies. Homozygous SS disease and the compound heterozygous states SC disease and S/β-thalassemia are pure hemolytic anemias. In contrast, anemia in the clinically significant forms of β-thalassemia is primarily due to ineffective erythropoiesis. By far the most

TABLE 161-5 CLASSIFICATION OF THE HEMOLYTIC ANEMIAS*

Environmental factors	
Antibody: immunohemolytic anemias	
Mechanical trauma: TTP, HUS, heart valve	
Toxins, infectious agents: malaria, etc.	Acquired
Membrane defects	
Paroxysmal nocturnal hemoglobinuria	
Spur cell anemia	
Hereditary spherocytosis, etc.	
Defects of cell interior	
Hemoglobinopathies: sickle cell, thalassemia	Congenital
Enzymopathies: G6PD deficiency, etc.	

*A more detailed differential diagnosis of the hemolytic anemias is presented in Table 163-2 in Chapter 163.
G6PD = glucose-6-phosphate dehydrogenase; HUS = hemolytic-uremic syndrome; TTP = thrombotic thrombocytopenic purpura.

TABLE 161-6 LABORATORY FEATURES COMMON TO HEMOLYTIC ANEMIAS

Peripheral blood
  Increased reticulocyte count
  Polychromasia
Bone marrow—erythroid hyperplasia
Serum
  Increased nonconjugated (indirect) bilirubin
  Elevated lactate dehydrogenase (isoenzymes 1, 2, and 3)
  Decreased or absent haptoglobin
  Plasma hemoglobin:
    Extravascular hemolysis: moderately increased
    Intravascular hemolysis: markedly increased
Urine
  Hemoglobinuria ⎤
  Hemosiderin in urine sediment ⎦ In intravascular hemolysis

common red cell enzyme defect is glucose-6-phosphate dehydrogenase deficiency (Chapter 164).

DIAGNOSIS

A number of laboratory tests are used to establish the presence of accelerated breakdown of red cells (Table 161-6). As mentioned in the section Laboratory Evaluation of the Patient with Anemia, the reticulocyte count is the simplest and most cost-effective way to distinguish between hemolytic anemias and those due to decreased red cell production. In this test, a supervital stain or a probe for RNA reveals strands of polyribosomes that are present for only 24 to 48 hours after red cells exit the bone marrow. On a routine Wright or Romanowsky stain, these cells often appear relatively large, with a blue-gray hue (so-called polychromasia). The reticulocyte count is nearly always elevated in patients with hemolysis (unless there is concomitant marrow suppression, such as by folic acid or iron deficiency). This test is a reliable index of red cell production. Thus, in patients with hemolytic anemia, the bone marrow nearly always exhibits erythroid hyperplasia. Because this result is predictable, a bone marrow examination is seldom helpful in patients with hemolytic anemia, unless there is suspicion that the hemolysis is due to an underlying lymphoma.

A number of serum and urine tests are available to confirm the presence of hemolysis and assess its magnitude. As mentioned earlier, serum nonconjugated bilirubin is elevated in proportion to the severity of the hemolysis. Lactate dehydrogenase (LDH) isoforms type 1 through 3 are released from red cells during hemolysis, resulting in increased serum LDH. Most kinds of hemolytic anemia are extravascular, with red cell destruction mediated by macrophages in the spleen, liver, and bone marrow. In these patients, a relatively small amount of hemoglobin is released from engulfed red cells into the plasma, where it binds specifically to haptoglobin. The hemoglobin-haptoglobin complex is rapidly cleared from the circulation. Measurement of serum haptoglobin is a useful test of hemolysis. The great majority of patients with clinically significant hemolysis have very low or absent levels. Less often, patients have intravascular hemolysis with much higher levels of free hemoglobin in the plasma, sufficient to traverse renal glomeruli and exceed the tubular reabsorption capacity. These patients have red or brown urine that, after centrifugation, tests positive with a "dipstick" that detects heme protein. Hemoglobinuria can be readily distinguished from myoglobinuria. In the former, both the plasma and the urine are pigmented. In the latter, the plasma remains colorless because the smaller myoglobin molecule rapidly traverses the glomeruli. Hemoglobinuria is often transient. For a week or so after the episode has abated, the urine sediment will contain hemosiderin, which can be readily detected with the Prussian blue iron stain.

Once these general laboratory tests confirm the presence of hemolysis, an array of specific tests is available to establish the specific cause (Chapters 163 through 165).

APPROACH TO THE TREATMENT OF ANEMIA

As in other disorders, the effective treatment of anemia is based on a thorough diagnostic evaluation. Hematinics such as iron, cobalamin, or folic acid should not be administered unless a specific deficiency has been demonstrated or is anticipated. Although indiscriminate treatment with cobalamin is not harmful per se, it lulls both the patient and the physician into a false sense of security. In contrast, the inappropriate use of iron preparations over a prolonged period can be directly harmful, leading to a state of iron overload.

Many kinds of anemias can be corrected if a precipitating cause can be uncovered and reversed. If a drug or toxin is responsible, its withdrawal may allow full recovery. Correction of anemia secondary to a chronic disease usually depends on whether the underlying condition can be reversed. One of the most dramatic dividends of successful renal transplantation is the rapid correction of the anemia of uremia.

Erythropoietin Therapy

The administration of rHuEPO is remarkably effective in certain circumstances. In addition to those with the anemia of chronic renal failure, selected patients with other types of anemia may benefit from rHuEPO. Treatment can lower transfusion requirements in patients with cancer or HIV infection in whom anemia has been aggravated by chemotherapy. In comparison to patients with renal failure, higher doses are required for those with cancer or AIDS to achieve the same increase in red cell mass. Treatment with rHuEPO has also been effective in some patients with primary bone marrow disorders, particularly myelodysplasia (Chapter 188). Transfusion requirements in surgical patients, both perioperatively and postoperatively, may be reduced by prior short-term administration of rHuEPO. Treatment may also benefit rare patients who are unable to receive blood transfusions because of either antigen incompatibility or religious convictions.

A note of caution has emerged from a number of large studies suggesting that high doses of rHuEPO that drive the hemoglobin level above 12 g/dL are associated with a slight but significant increase in the risk of thrombosis and cardiovascular mortality. A meta-analysis of randomized controlled clinical trials of chronic kidney disease patients treated with rHuEPO showed that targeting higher levels of hemoglobin was associated with an increased risk of all-cause mortality and arteriovenous access thrombosis. Administration of the erythropoiesis-stimulating agents erythropoietin and darbepoetin to patients with cancer has been associated with an increased risk of venous thromboembolism and mortality.[2] The possibility of increasing the risk of tumor progression may be mediated by erythropoietin receptors on malignant cells.

Primary bone marrow disorders pose a formidable therapeutic challenge when considering rHuEPO therapy. Aplastic anemia (Chapter 168) can be cured by both immunosuppressive therapy and stem cell transplantation. Long-lasting remissions can be achieved in an increasing fraction of patients with acute leukemias by chemotherapy, often coupled with stem cell transplantation (Chapter 181). Other primary bone marrow disorders that are unresponsive to these interventions are treated with supportive measures such as transfusions of red cells and platelets.

Red Cell Transfusion

The decision whether to transfuse an anemic patient is often challenging. The risks and complications of the administration of blood products are discussed in Chapter 180. Patients with chronic or long-standing anemia are able to compensate in several ways, discussed earlier in this chapter. A considerable reduction in red cell mass can be surprisingly well tolerated, especially if the patient is young or sedentary. Transfusion is seldom indicated in a patient with chronic anemia whose hemoglobin is 9 g/dL or greater. Those who are expected to respond to the administration of a specific agent such as iron,

folic acid, or vitamin B_{12} can usually be spared transfusions. However, if the anemia is severe and accompanied by myocardial or cerebral ischemia or by congestive heart failure, prompt but slow administration of packed red cells is indicated. Whole blood should be given only if the patient is hypovolemic.

Splenectomy

Splenectomy is indicated in the treatment of certain hemolytic anemias. The efficacy of splenectomy correlates with the degree to which the abnormal or defective red cells are destroyed or sequestered in the spleen. Splenectomy is curative in nearly all patients with hereditary spherocytosis (Chapter 164). The operation may be also beneficial in selected patients with immunohemolytic anemia, congestive splenomegaly, spur cell anemia, and certain hemoglobinopathies and enzymopathies. The operative morbidity and mortality from elective splenectomy are very low. The procedure can often be done via mini-laparotomy. Occasional patients develop postoperative left subphrenic abscess. Following splenectomy, young children are at risk of developing overwhelming septicemia. This complication can be partially circumvented by vaccination against pneumococcus and meningococcus. Post-splenectomy sepsis occurs rarely in adults. The risk of sepsis can be circumvented by partial splenectomy. Thrombocytosis generally develops promptly following splenectomy. However, in most cases it is transient. In patients with continued hemolysis or with a myeloproliferative disorder (Chapter 169), the thrombocytosis usually persists and may occasionally be associated with thromboembolic complications.

1. Phrommintikul A, Haas SJ, Elsik M, et al. Mortality and target haemoglobin concentrations in anaemic patients with chronic kidney disease treated with erythropoietin: a meta-analysis. *Lancet.* 2007;369:381-388.
2. Bennett CL, Silver SM, Djulbegovic B, et al. Venous thromboembolism and mortality associated with recombinant erythropoietin and darbepoetin administration for the treatment of cancer-associated anemia. *JAMA.* 2008;299:914-924.

SUGGESTED READINGS

Bunn HF, Aster JA. Pathophysiology of Blood Disorders. New York: McGraw Hill; 2010. *Overview of the anemias, with an emphasis on pathobiology.*
Hussein M, Haddad RY. Approach to anemia. *Dis Mon.* 2010;56:449-455. *Review.*
Price EA, Mehra R, Holmes TH, et al. Anemia in older persons: etiology and evaluation. *Blood Cells Mol Dis.* 2011;46:159-165. *Twelve percent had iron deficiency, 35% had unexplained anemia, and 16% had findings suspicious for myelodysplastic syndrome.*
Theurl I, Aigner E, Theurl M, et al. Regulation of iron homeostasis in anemia of chronic disease and iron deficiency: diagnostic and therapeutic implications. *Blood.* 2009;113:5277-5286. *Thorough and up-to-date review of clinically relevant aspects of iron homeostasis.*

162

MICROCYTIC AND HYPOCHROMIC ANEMIAS

GORDON D. GINDER

The oxygen-carrying hemoglobin molecule executes the principal function of the mature erythrocyte. The hemoglobin content of erythrocytes is determined by the coordinated production of globin protein, the heme porphyrin ring, and the availability of iron. A deficiency in any of these three critical components of hemoglobin results in hypochromic and/or microcytic anemia (see Fig. 161-5 in Chapter 161). Microcytic anemia is typically reported initially by automated red blood cell (RBC) indices. Hypochromic microcytic anemia can be confirmed on the peripheral blood smear (Fig. 162-1). Disorders of globin protein production typically produce microcytosis but not hypochromia and are discussed elsewhere (Chapter 165).

IRON DEFICIENCY ANEMIA

EPIDEMIOLOGY

Iron deficiency is by far the most common cause of anemia worldwide and is among the most frequently encountered medical problems seen by primary

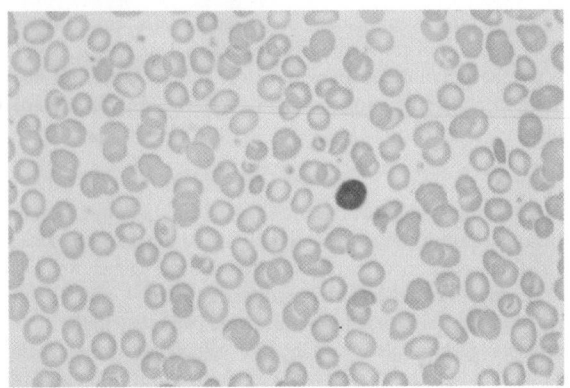

FIGURE 162-1. Iron deficiency anemia. Many of these red blood cells are microcytic (smaller than the nucleus of the normal lymphocyte near the center of the field) and hypochromic (with central areas of pallor that exceed half the diameter of the cells).

Regulation of Body Iron

FIGURE 162-2. Iron homeostasis in normal humans. RBC = red blood cell.

incorporated into porphyrin rings is associated with proteins. Transferrin is the major protein associated with circulating plasma iron, and ferritin is the major protein associated with stored intracellular iron both in the cytoplasm and in mitochondria. Because the normal rate of iron loss is low, only about 1 to 2 mg/day of dietary iron is needed to maintain homeostasis. The average Western diet contains about 20 mg/day, and the efficiency of iron absorption in the duodenum is usually sufficient to maintain the amount of iron required for homeostatic balance.

Control of iron absorption by the duodenal crypt cells is critical because of the lack of any regulated physiologic mechanism for iron excretion. As a result, excessive iron intake can lead to deleterious iron overload, with concomitant organ damage (Chapter 219). Nonheme dietary iron is dissolved in part by the low pH of the stomach effluent. After reduction to the ferrous state by ferroreductase, iron is transferred across the apical crypt cell membrane by divalent metal transporter-1 (DMT-1). Several levels of regulation are involved in iron absorption by the intestine. One of these is modulated by dietary intake; thus, after a large influx of dietary iron, the duodenal absorptive capacity is diminished. A second regulatory mechanism modulates the iron absorption capacity based on total body iron stores. Finally, the so-called erythropoietic regulator modulates the capacity for enterocyte absorption based on the iron needed for erythropoiesis. A paradoxical increase in iron absorption through this mechanism occurs in certain types of anemia characterized by intravascular and intramedullary destruction of erythroid cells: sideroblastic anemia, the thalassemias (Chapter 165), and congenital dyserythropoietic anemias.

Once inside the intestinal absorbing cell, iron is stored in complex with ferritin. Circulating plasma iron is complexed with the iron transport protein transferrin. The transferrin-iron complex is then taken up by erythroid precursors via the transferrin receptor. The high density of transferrin receptors on erythroid precursors ensures the preferential uptake of iron by these cells and explains why erythropoiesis proceeds normally until a critical deficiency of transferrin-bound iron, reflecting a depletion of total body iron, is present. The levels of transferrin, transferrin receptor, ferritin, and other proteins important in iron metabolism are regulated by the iron regulatory proteins IRP-1 and IRP-2.

Hepcidin, a 25–amino acid peptide, is the central regulator of iron homeostasis through its effects on intestinal absorption, macrophage recycling of iron from senescent RBCs, and iron mobilization from hepatic stores. Thus, hepcidin affects all major sites of iron uptake and storage. Hepcidin is produced in the liver and acts as a negative regulator of iron absorption by the intestine and of iron release from storage in the macrophages and hepatocytes (see Fig. 161-7 in Chapter 161). It is believed that hepcidin binds to ferroportin, the major iron transporter in the membranes of the enterocyte, macrophage, and hepatocyte, causing the internalization and degradation of ferroportin. This process blocks the transport of iron across the membrane of the basolateral crypt cell, preventing its incorporation into transferrin-bound plasma iron. Likewise, loss of ferroportin function blocks the major export pathway of iron stores from macrophages and hepatocytes. Hepcidin production is upregulated by iron and downregulated by hypoxia, consistent with its homeostatic role. Because hepcidin is also upregulated by inflammatory cytokines, it is believed to play an important role in the paradoxical lack of transferrin-bound iron available for erythropoiesis in the face of adequate or even excess iron stores found in the anemia of chronic inflammation (see later and Chapter 161).

Blood Loss

Iron deficiency anemia results from an imbalance between available body iron for hemoglobin production and the minimal amount needed to sustain normal hemoglobin production during erythropoiesis (see Fig. 162-2). Because of the combined effectiveness of dietary absorption and retention of iron under normal circumstances, this mismatch is most often due to blood loss, with the gastrointestinal (GI) tract being the most common site (Chapter 137). In developed countries, the blood loss is usually secondary to benign or neoplastic lesions of the GI tract (Chapters 198 and 199) or chronic ingestion of drugs that cause GI mucosal damage (Chapter 141). The most common offending agents are alcohol and salicylates or other nonsteroidal anti-inflammatory agents. In developing countries, helminthic infections, including hookworm (Chapter 365) and schistosomiasis (Chapter 363), are among the most common causes of GI blood loss.

Genitourinary tract blood loss resulting in iron deficiency is most common in menstruating women. Less common are urinary tract malignancies (Chapter 203) and hemoglobinuria due to intravascular hemolysis (Chapter

care physicians in the United States. It is estimated that between 2 and 5% of adolescent females in the United States have iron deficiency sufficient to cause anemia. Elsewhere, the prevalence of iron deficiency–induced anemia is much higher, with estimates that up to 10% of the world population, or more than 500 million people, are affected. The prevalence rates are especially high in developing countries where dietary insufficiency and intestinal parasites are prevalent.

PATHOBIOLOGY

The majority of the approximately 4 g of iron in the adult human body is incorporated into hemoglobin (approximately 2100 mg) in erythrocytes or myoglobin (approximately 300 mg) in muscle. The remainder is chiefly present as storage iron in the liver (1000 mg) and in the reticuloendothelial macrophages of the bone marrow and spleen (600 mg) (Fig. 162-2). Only a small amount of iron (3 to 7 mg) is freely circulating in plasma bound to transferrin, but this pool is kinetically very active, turning over every 3 to 4 hours. Because of the potent conservation mechanisms of iron recycling through the reticuloendothelial macrophage system, only an average of about 1 to 2 mg of iron is normally lost per day, largely through mucosal sloughing, desquamation, and, in females of reproductive age, menstruation.

The ability of iron to donate or accept electrons readily through conversion between the ferrous (Fe^{2+}) and ferric (Fe^{3+}) states makes it a critical component of the hemoglobin and myoglobin porphyrin rings that transport oxygen as well as cytochromes and various other vital enzymes. Free iron is extremely toxic owing to its capacity to catalyze the formation of free radicals, which lead to cellular damage. Therefore, the majority of body iron that is not stably

TABLE 162-1 LABORATORY FINDINGS FOR IRON STUDIES IN MICROCYTIC AND HYPOCHROMIC ANEMIAS							
ANEMIA	SERUM IRON	TIBC	TRANSFERRIN SATURATION (%)	SERUM FERRITIN	SERUM TRANSFERRIN RECEPTOR	MARROW RE IRON	MARROW RINGED SIDEROBLASTS
Iron deficiency anemia	Low	High	0-15	Low (<30 µg/L)	High	Absent	Absent
Anemia of chronic disease	Low	Normal or low	5-15	Normal or high	Normal	Normal or high	Absent
Sideroblastic anemia	High	Normal	60-90	High	Normal or high	High	Present

RE = reticuloendothelial; TIBC = total iron binding capacity.

163). Respiratory tract blood loss is far less common as a cause of iron deficiency.

Reproduction and Growth

In most cases, an increased iron requirement is due to blood loss; other causes include rapid growth in infancy and adolescence and pregnancy and lactation in adulthood. It is estimated that failure to satisfy the increased iron requirements during pregnancy with supplemental iron may result in a deficiency equivalent to a cumulative blood loss of up to 1500 mL.

Inadequate Iron Intake

The other major cause of iron deficiency is inadequate iron intake. Only diets that lack 1 to 2 mg/day fail to provide adequate iron. The average Western meal contains about 6 mg of iron, so dietary insufficiency is not a common cause of iron deficiency. Certain diets that lack iron or contain large quantities of phytates from cereals or tannate from tea, both of which inhibit intestinal iron absorption, may result in iron deficiency. Although iron is usually readily absorbed, primarily in the duodenum, pathologic states that can impair the process include generalized intestinal malabsorption (Chapter 142), atrophic gastritis (Chapter 141) with achlorhydria, and extensive gastric surgery. In contrast, chronic use of H₂-receptor blockers or proton pump inhibitors does not appear to cause iron deficiency. In the United States, celiac disease (Chapter 142) is an increasingly common cause of iron deficiency, with resulting anemia.

CLINICAL MANIFESTATIONS

Because of compensatory physiologic mechanisms, patients with mild iron deficiency anemia may be asymptomatic. Iron deficiency in these patients may be recognized during the evaluation of an underlying disease process or as part of routine laboratory studies. The findings of microcytosis and hypochromia occur only after the hematocrit has fallen to approximately 30%, so neither finding may be present in early stages.

The anemia of iron deficiency, like other anemias, manifests with nonspecific symptoms such as weakness, pallor, dizziness, decreased exercise tolerance, or irritability. Because iron is a critical component of the porphyrin complex in muscle as well as many essential metabolic enzymes, its deficiency affects other organ systems besides the erythron, often resulting in a degree of fatigue, exercise intolerance, and weakness out of proportion to the hemoglobin level. Repletion of iron in iron-deficient individuals may improve cognitive and exercise performance. In addition, intravenous iron treatment in patients with heart failure and coexisting iron deficiency (to which heart failure patients are prone) can improve symptoms, functional capacity, and quality of life, irrespective of the presence or absence of anemia.█

Rare patients, most frequently elderly women, may have dysphagia due to an esophageal stricture or web (Plummer-Vinson syndrome). A clinical manifestation unique to iron deficiency is pica, which is an unusual craving for certain non-nutritional substances. Pica may manifest as a craving for ice (pagophagia) or, less commonly, for clay (geophagia) or starch (amylophagia); pagophagia is believed to be the most specific for iron deficiency.

Physical findings that may be associated with the iron-deficient state include glossitis and angular stomatitis. Other less common but highly specific findings are spooning of the fingernails (koilonychia) and blue-tinged sclerae.

DIAGNOSIS

The diagnosis of iron deficiency anemia is made by laboratory testing. Because microcytic hypochromic RBCs are a sine qua non of this type of anemia, initial screening consists of a determination of hemoglobin levels, mean corpuscular volume, erythrocyte hemoglobin content, and reticulocyte count. In experienced hands, the peripheral blood smear (Chapter 160) is an excellent indicator of iron deficiency anemia. In iron deficiency anemia, most erythrocytes are smaller in diameter than the nucleus of a typical lymphocyte, and the area of central pallor is greater than 50% of the total diameter of the erythrocyte (see Fig. 162-1). Variability of erythrocyte size distinguishes iron deficiency anemia from other conditions that give rise to microcytosis; the calculated variability in RBC volume (the so-called RBC volume distribution width, or RDW) is elevated early in iron deficiency anemia.

The definitive diagnosis of iron deficiency anemia is made by tests that measure total body iron stores: the absence of iron stores that can be mobilized is unique to this microcytic hypochromic anemia. Transferrin and transferrin-bound iron levels may not be reliable indicators of iron deficiency because they are also abnormal in the anemia of chronic disease, despite adequate total body iron stores (see Fig. 161-6 in Chapter 161).

The serum ferritin level is the most reliable, noninvasive, and cost-effective indicator that is routinely available in most clinical laboratories (Table 162-1). In a large study of 259 anemic patients, a serum ferritin level less than 18 µg/L was diagnostic of iron deficiency with greater than 95% specificity and a 55% sensitivity. At a serum ferritin level of 45 µg/L, the sensitivity rose to approximately 70%, and a level higher than 100 µg/L in populations with a less than 40% prevalence of iron deficiency excluded a diagnosis of iron deficiency with more than 90% sensitivity. Although some recent studies have questioned the accuracy of the routine determination of stainable marrow iron, this test is still generally considered to be the "gold standard" for tests of iron deficiency. However, determination of total bone marrow iron stores is rarely necessary to diagnose iron deficiency anemia, except when there is some other complicating process.

One setting in which serum ferritin levels can be spuriously elevated is chronic inflammation or chronic disease. The soluble serum transferrin receptor (StFR) level is an excellent measure of total erythroid precursor mass. The StFR is aberrantly elevated in the presence of iron deficiency, so it is considered a useful test for this condition. A number of studies have demonstrated the utility of the StFR/ferritin ratio in distinguishing iron deficiency from the anemia of chronic disease. However, the lack of reliable standards has prevented this assay from becoming routinely available in clinical practice.

TREATMENT

The treatment of iron deficiency anemia is replenishment of body iron stores. However, the underlying cause should always be investigated before treatment is begun, because in many cases it is a correctable and potentially fatal GI lesion (Chapter 137).

Oral Administration

The preferred route of iron administration is oral. Oral iron is most readily absorbed in the absence of food, especially in the setting of decreased stomach acid production owing to atrophic gastritis, gastric surgery, or chronic suppression of gastric acid with an H₂ antagonist or proton pump inhibitor. The major obstacle to oral iron replacement is unacceptable side effects, chiefly epigastric discomfort or nausea; diarrhea or constipation also occurs in some patients. Reducing the dose often eliminates nausea and epigastric discomfort. Despite the development of a number of orally effective iron-containing compounds, the original salt, ferrous sulfate (325 mg three times daily), remains the most useful. Although some newer oral iron preparations, such as ferrous gluconate (300 mg two or three times daily) or ferrous fumarate (325 mg two or three times daily), may induce fewer GI side effects per milligram of iron, they are also less well absorbed, so there is no net advantage to these costlier formulations except for patients who cannot tolerate ferrous sulfate. Given both the low toxicity and the low cost of oral iron replacement, a therapeutic trial is an alternative means of confirming a diagnosis of iron deficiency anemia.

Parenteral Administration

In situations in which primary blood loss is uncontrollable, iron cannot be absorbed owing to severe malabsorption, or oral iron is not tolerated despite concerted efforts to minimize side effects, parenteral iron is an effective alternative treatment.[1] Intramuscular dosing is limited to 100 mg/injection, so intravenous administration is recommended. Sodium ferric gluconate (given intravenously at a dose of 125 mg over 10 minutes) is the preferred form of parenteral iron owing to the low incidence of adverse reactions. A multi-institutional, double-blind, randomized, placebo-controlled trial of more than 2500 patients showed similar adverse events in patients receiving sodium ferric gluconate versus those receiving placebo, and only one life-threatening complication occurred; in comparison, there were 23 such events among 3768 patients treated with iron dextran in a historical control arm.[2] One limitation of sodium ferric gluconate is that the maximum dose deliverable in a single injection is approximately 125 mg, and a total dose of 500 to 2000 mg is usually required for adequate repletion. Although large doses of iron dextran can be delivered in a single intravenous injection, this is currently reserved for situations in which rapid iron replacement is required because of the life-threatening anaphylactic and delayed adverse reactions that occur in 0.6 and 2.5% of cases, respectively. If iron dextran is to be given intravenously, premedication with diphenhydramine and a slow test-dose injection of 30 to 40 mg diluted in normal saline are recommended.

The response to iron repletion therapy is usually quite rapid, with elimination of symptoms within a few days. Increased reticulocytosis usually begins within 4 to 5 days, and the hemoglobin level often rises within 1 week and reaches a normal level after 6 weeks of therapy if adequate iron replacement is achieved. The goal of therapy, which is to reach a serum ferritin level of greater than 50 mg/L, usually takes 4 to 6 months. Therapy must be continued after adequate replacement is achieved if the underlying cause of iron deficiency is not reversible. Because of the avidity of transferrin receptor–rich erythroid precursors for transferrin-bound iron, the serum ferritin level usually does not rise until hemoglobin levels reach normal.

Failure to Respond to Iron Therapy

An incomplete or lack of response to oral iron therapy, as determined by failure to normalize the hemoglobin level, usually means either that iron replacement has not been adequate (most commonly due to noncompliance with oral iron because of its side effects) or that iron deficiency is not the primary cause of the anemia (e.g., coexisting anemia of chronic disease). Less common causes of failure to respond to oral iron include iron malabsorption (e.g., celiac disease, atrophic gastritis) or blood loss in excess of iron replacement.

TMPRSS6, also called matriptase-2, is a type II transmembrane serine protease that suppresses hepcidin production. Several types of mutations in *TMPRSS6* that are either sporadic or familial (usually autosomal recessive) have recently been described as causes of iron-refractory iron deficiency anemia (IRIDA). Associated with inappropriately increased levels of urinary hepcidin, the defect causes impaired iron absorption and recycling, leading to IRIDA. Characteristically, these patients exhibit no hematologic improvement in response to oral iron intake and are only partially responsive to parenteral iron because of abnormal iron utilization.

PROGNOSIS

In most cases, iron deficiency anemia can be corrected rapidly by either oral or parenteral replacement, but the long-term prognosis ultimately depends on the clinical course of the underlying cause. It is critical that the patient undergo a full evaluation to determine the underlying cause of the iron deficiency, especially because an occult gastrointestinal lesion, often malignant, may be present, particularly in patients older than 50 years (Chapters 198 and 199).

● ANEMIA OF CHRONIC DISEASE AND INFLAMMATION

DEFINITION

Anemia of chronic disease refers to anemia that occurs in the setting of a chronic disease state, usually one associated with elevated levels of inflammatory cytokines. Because of this association, the condition is also referred to as anemia of inflammation. Although anemia of chronic inflammation usually manifests as a normochromic normocytic process (Chapter 161), between 20 and 50% of cases are associated with microcytic RBC indices. The anemia is usually mild to moderate, and it may not be symptomatic.

EPIDEMIOLOGY

Anemia of chronic inflammation is believed to be the second most common cause of anemia, after iron deficiency. It is the most common type of anemia encountered among hospitalized patients. The wide spectrum of underlying diseases includes acute and chronic infections, inflammatory and autoimmune diseases, cancers, and chronic kidney diseases.

PATHOBIOLOGY

There are three major mechanisms of anemia of chronic inflammation, and all are believed to result from the effects of abnormal levels of inflammatory cytokines. The first is dysregulated iron homeostasis, manifested by low serum iron (hypoferremia) in the presence of normal or elevated serum ferritin levels and abundant reticuloendothelial macrophage iron stores. The functional consequence is a limited availability of iron for erythroid progenitor cells and resultant restriction of erythropoiesis. Pro-inflammatory stimuli, including lipopolysaccharides, interferon-γ, and tumor necrosis factor-α (TNF-α), upregulate DMT-1, which increases iron uptake by the reticuloendothelial cells. At the same time, these stimuli cause the downregulation of ferroportin expression; ferroportin is the protein required for the release of ferrous iron from storage cells and for the transport of dietary iron from duodenal enterocytes into the circulation.

Because hepcidin is an iron-regulated, acute phase reactant peptide that blocks both iron uptake in the gut and iron release from hepatocytes and macrophage stores, its upregulation by lipopolysaccharides, interleukin (IL)-6, and possibly IL-1 (indirectly, through induction of IL-6) results in another mechanism of anemia. Also, patients with hepatic adenomas that secrete high levels of hepcidin have iron-refractory anemia in the presence of normal or elevated ferritin and macrophage iron stores, despite the absence of elevated inflammatory cytokine levels. Elevated urinary hepcidin concentrations correlate with ferritin levels in patients with anemia of inflammation, iron overload, and iron deficiency. These relationships are depicted in Figure 161-7 in Chapter 161.

A third pathophysiologic feature of anemia of chronic inflammation is the inhibition of erythroid progenitor expansion. Interferon-γ is the most potent inhibitory factor of erythropoiesis, but similar inhibition is believed to be mediated by IL-1, TNF-α, and interferon-β. These mediators of inflammation act to increase erythroid progenitor apoptosis, downregulate erythropoietin receptors, and antagonize pro-hematopoietic factors. The action of erythropoietin appears to be directly antagonized by these pro-inflammatory cytokines, which would explain why responsiveness to erythropoietin seems to be inversely related to the severity of the underlying chronic inflammation and the levels of interferon-γ and TNF-α. Finally, increased erythrophagocytosis in the presence of inflammation results in a modest shortening of RBC half-life.

CLINICAL MANIFESTATIONS

The clinical manifestations in patients with anemia of chronic inflammation are usually dominated by the underlying disease process. The anemia in this condition is usually mild, with hemoglobin levels in the range of 8 to 10 g/dL. However, supervening blood loss, absolute iron deficiency, or other aggravating factors can produce life-threatening anemia. Even mild to moderate anemia contributes to the debilitating effects of the underlying disease, adversely impacting performance status and quality of life. Moreover, the presence of anemia is associated with a poorer overall prognosis in many of the underlying chronic diseases, although correction of anemia has not been directly demonstrated to improve survival.

DIAGNOSIS

The clinical diagnosis of anemia of chronic disease presenting with microcytic hypochromic RBC indices is one of exclusion, based on low serum iron in the presence of normal or increased total body iron stores (see Table 162-1). Serum ferritin is the best single laboratory marker for assessing iron storage, and it is almost invariably normal or elevated in anemia of chronic disease. If both the serum iron and the transferrin saturation are reduced, reflecting dysregulation of iron homeostasis, the diagnosis of anemia of chronic disease can be made in the appropriate clinical setting after the exclusion of other causes of anemia, such as coexistent blood loss, thalassemia (Chapter 165), and drug-induced suppression of erythropoiesis. In the presence of inflammation, however, up to 30% of patients with true iron deficiency have serum ferritin levels greater than 100 μg/L, potentially obscuring the diagnosis of iron deficiency. Assays for StFR are useful to diagnose iron deficiency in the presence of the inflammation associated with anemia of chronic disease, but problems with standardization have limited this test's availability in clinical practice. Examination of the bone marrow for reticuloendothelial macrophage iron stores (hemosiderin) and erythroblasts containing iron granules (sideroblasts) can provide definitive evidence of absent iron stores in the setting of anemia of chronic inflammation. A low serum erythropoietin level is also useful in supporting a diagnosis of anemia of chronic inflammation, but only when the hemoglobin level is less than 10 g/dL.

TREATMENT Rx

Treatment of the Underlying Disease

The most effective treatment for anemia of chronic disease is successful treatment of the underlying inflammatory disease process, whether it is an acute or chronic infection, treatable cancer, renal failure, or rheumatoid arthritis. Even if definitive treatment is not possible, quality of life and perhaps prognosis can improve if symptomatic anemia is treated directly. Unfortunately, anemia of chronic inflammation remains undertreated, even in developed countries.

Blood Transfusion

Blood transfusion (Chapter 180) offers the immediate resolution of anemia, but it is indicated chiefly when the anemia is life threatening or seriously limits the patient's functioning. These situations almost always involve supervening blood loss or some other acute process that compounds the anemia of chronic disease. Transfusion is not recommended for the long-term treatment of mild or moderate anemia of chronic inflammation because of the secondary risks, which include transfusional iron overload, human leukocyte antigen (HLA) sensitization in the case of potential renal transplantation, and other side effects of transfusion.

Intravenous Iron and Erythropoietin Therapy

If iron replacement is needed for anemia of chronic inflammation, parenteral iron administration is usually required to replenish stores because of the block in intestinal absorption. In hemodialysis patients receiving erythropoietin therapy, intravenous iron therapy improves anemia; however, when intravenous iron replacement raises the transferrin saturation to greater than 20%, there appears to be an increased risk of developing bacteremia, underscoring the complex relationship between iron homeostasis and immunity.

Erythropoietin therapy is currently approved for use in patients with chronic kidney disease, those with HIV infection, and cancer patients who are undergoing myelosuppressive treatment. Patients with demonstrated iron deficiency should receive supplemental iron with intravenous iron gluconate (see the earlier discussion) while being treated with erythropoietin.

In patients undergoing chemotherapy for cancer whose hemoglobin is less than 10 g/dL, erythropoietin therapy improves quality of life and performance status.**3** However, erythropoietin therapy may be associated with cancer progression in some settings. Because of the decreased survival and increased thromboembolic complications that have been reported in cancer patients receiving erythropoiesis-stimulating agents, current recommendations are for cautious use during chemotherapy and against routine use in inpatients not receiving chemotherapy.**3,4**

PROGNOSIS

The overall prognosis of anemia of chronic inflammation is determined almost exclusively by the course of the underlying disease. It is well established that the degree of anemia correlates well with the severity of the underlying disease process and therefore with levels of inflammatory cytokines. In the absence of a supervening process, anemia of chronic inflammation is not life threatening, and treatment of the anemia per se has not been proved to affect overall survival.

SIDEROBLASTIC ANEMIAS

DEFINITION

This heterogeneous group of anemias is distinguished by the characteristic finding of excessive mitochondrial iron in erythroblasts, as manifested by iron-laden, ringed sideroblasts in the bone marrow in the presence of moderate to severe anemia. These disorders result from mitochondrial defects either in the biosynthesis of the heme porphyrin ring or in the metabolism of iron. Both hereditary and acquired types of sideroblastic anemia have been described. Although often characterized by microcytic and sometimes hypochromic anemia, these disorders can manifest with normochromic normocytic RBCs; if the anemia is associated with myelodysplasia (Chapter 188), macrocytic RBC indices may be present.

EPIDEMIOLOGY

Although acquired sideroblastic anemias are relatively rare, they are much more prevalent than hereditary forms. The true incidence of acquired

FIGURE 162-3. The heme synthesis pathway. ALAS-2 = δ-aminolevulinic acid synthase; CoA = coenzyme A.

sideroblastic anemia is not well established, in part owing to the heterogeneity of causes and clinical presentations. Hereditary X-linked sideroblastic anemias usually manifest in childhood or early adulthood.

PATHOBIOLOGY

Genetics

The pathophysiologic mechanisms of hereditary sideroblastic anemias are much better understood than those of the more common idiopathic, acquired variety associated with myelodysplasia. Two main forms of X-linked hereditary sideroblastic anemia have been characterized, and both result from defects in the heme synthesis pathway (Fig. 162-3). The first type is caused by mutations in the gene coding for erythroid-specific δ-aminolevulinic acid synthase, known as ALAS-2, on the X chromosome. These mutations may affect the affinity of the enzyme for pyridoxal phosphate or its structural stability, catalytic site, or susceptibility to mitochondrial proteases. In those cases in which the affinity of ALAS-2 for pyridoxal phosphate is altered, pyridoxine supplementation can ameliorate the associated anemia. The other major group of X-linked sideroblastic anemias results from defects in the adenosine triphosphate binding cassette (ABC) protein known as hABC7. The hABC7 protein is believed to be involved in iron-sulfur [FeS] cluster formation. Because [FeS] cluster–associated proteins include ferrochelatase and the cytosolic IRP-1, defects in hABC7 are believed to result in defective iron metabolism or inadequate incorporation of iron into the heme porphyrin ring by ferrochelatase. This type of X-linked sideroblastic anemia is associated with ataxia.

In addition to the two X-linked causes, both autosomal dominant and recessive forms of hereditary sideroblastic anemia have been described. However, the exact mechanisms involved in these disorders are not known.

Other types of hereditary sideroblastic anemia are believed to result from mutations in the mitochondrial genome rather than in nuclear genes. The inheritance of these disorders is complex, owing to the exclusively maternal inheritance pattern of mitochondria; the ovum is the only source of embryonic mitochondria.

Exposure to Drugs or Toxins

The most common form of acquired sideroblastic anemia results from nutritional deficiency or exposure to exogenous drugs or toxins, especially alcohol. Although sideroblastic anemia is not a common finding in alcoholism, the high incidence of alcohol abuse in Western cultures accounts for its frequency as a cause. Alcohol directly inhibits erythropoiesis, but sideroblastic anemia is usually seen only in the setting of concurrent alcoholism and nutritional deficiencies. Other well-documented drug exposures associated with sideroblastic anemia include isoniazid, chloramphenicol, and cycloserine. Sideroblastic anemia has also been attributed to lead exposure (Chapter 21), but there are limited primary data to support this association. Deficiency of pyridoxine causes sideroblastic anemia in animals and may also occur in the setting of alcoholism in humans, although ethanol is believed to be an antagonist of the interaction of pyridoxal phosphate with 5-aminolevulinic acid as a cofactor in the first step of heme biosynthesis. Copper deficiency, though rare, has also been associated with sideroblastic anemia, usually in the setting of an overdose of bivalent cation chelators such as penicillamine or trientine, used to treat the copper overloading found in Wilson disease (Chapter 218).

Idiopathic Forms

The major cause of acquired sideroblastic anemia is idiopathic, in association with myelodysplastic syndromes (Chapter 188). Refractory anemia with ringed sideroblasts is characterized by abnormalities in all three hematopoietic cell lineages, in addition to the presence of ringed sideroblasts.

A second form, known as pure sideroblastic anemia, is less frequently associated with cytogenetic abnormalities, is characterized by dysplasia only in erythroid progenitors, and lacks cytopenias other than anemia. The prognosis in this type of acquired idiopathic sideroblastic anemia is much better than that in refractory anemia with ringed sideroblasts, in part because of a very low incidence ($\approx$10%) of evolution to acute leukemia.

Because of the important differences in prognosis, it is imperative to evaluate cytogenetics and marrow morphology at the time of diagnosis. Recent evidence suggests that mitochondrial DNA mutations and attendant mitochondrial cytopathies account for many, if not all, cases.

CLINICAL MANIFESTATIONS

Because of the heterogeneous nature of the sideroblastic anemias, many of the clinical manifestations vary according to the underlying pathophysiologic cause. The anemia is usually moderate to severe, with hemoglobin levels in the range of 4 to 10 g/dL. The peripheral blood smear frequently reveals hypochromia, often with basophilic stippling. Microcytosis is often seen in hereditary forms, but normochromic, normocytic, or even macrocytic RBCs may be seen, especially in the setting of myelodysplasia or in a rare X-linked hereditary form known as Pearson's syndrome.

DIAGNOSIS

The most useful diagnostic laboratory test for sideroblastic anemia is bone marrow morphology with Prussian blue iron staining, which reveals abnormally large and numerous bluish green siderosomes within at least 15% of erythroblasts, giving the characteristic appearance of ringed sideroblasts (Fig. 162-4). These ringed sideroblasts distinguish this disorder from iron deficiency anemia and anemia of chronic inflammation. Bone marrow findings in idiopathic acquired sideroblastic anemias include dyspoietic features of erythroid and/or myeloid and megakaryotic cell lineages.

Iron studies usually reveal normal iron stores or evidence of iron overload, which is caused by the ineffective erythropoiesis found in sideroblastic anemia as well as by the transfusion therapy often required for its treatment. Iron deficiency can occur coincident with sideroblastic anemia, complicating the diagnosis owing to the lack of characteristic ringed sideroblasts, particularly in myelodysplastic syndromes in which thrombocytopenia leads to GI blood loss. If coexisting iron deficiency is suspected, a repeat bone marrow examination after iron repletion has failed to correct the anemia reveals the diagnostic ringed sideroblasts.

FIGURE 162-4. Sideroblastic anemia. Prussian blue iron stain of the bone marrow shows ringed sideroblasts, which are nucleated red blood cell precursors with perinuclear rings of iron-laden mitochondria.

TREATMENT

Treatment of Underlying Disease

Most forms of sideroblastic anemia lack a specific therapy aimed at the underlying mechanism. Exceptions are those types caused by alcohol or drugs, for which removal of the offending agent usually results in resolution, or at least improvement, of the anemia. Abstinence from alcohol usually reverses the abnormalities in heme biosynthesis in 1 to 2 weeks, as evidenced by the disappearance of ringed sideroblasts in the marrow.

Pyridoxine markedly improves the relatively rare cases of nutritional deficiency, which are usually associated with alcoholism, and some forms of X-linked hereditary sideroblastic anemias in which the binding of pyridoxine by ALAS-2 is defective. Because of its low toxicity in moderate doses, a trial of pyridoxine, 100 to 200 mg/day orally for up to 3 months, is worthwhile in all patients. In responsive cases, reticulocytosis occurs within 2 to 3 weeks, and the hemoglobin level improves over several months. High-dose pyridoxine has been shown to overcome the defect in ALAS-2 activity in some patients with X-linked sideroblastic anemia, but prolonged high-dose therapy can be associated with peripheral neuropathy.

Transfusion

The mainstay of therapy for most severe sideroblastic anemias remains RBC transfusions. Because of the risks of long-term transfusion therapy, treatment should be aimed at achieving a normal performance status rather than a specific target hemoglobin level. Iron stores should be monitored regularly, and iron chelation therapy should be used in the setting of iron overload.

Erythropoietin

Therapy with erythropoietin, with or without granulocyte colony-stimulating factor (G-CSF), benefits a small percentage of patients with acquired sideroblastic anemia due to myelodysplasia. A meta-analysis of 17 studies in which 205 patients were treated with erythropoietin showed an overall response rate of only 16%. However, patients with a diagnosis other than refractory anemia with ringed sideroblasts who were not transfusion dependent had response rates greater than 50%, whereas none of the patients who had refractory anemia with ringed sideroblasts and a serum erythropoietin level greater than 200 U/L responded. Studies using a combination of erythropoietin and G-CSF showed somewhat higher response rates, although none of these studies were large or randomized. Allogeneic bone marrow transplantation (Chapter 181) benefits eligible patients whose myelodysplasia (Chapter 188) has a high risk of evolving into acute leukemia.

PROGNOSIS

As with the underlying pathophysiology, the prognosis in sideroblastic anemias is highly variable. Secondary acquired forms of the disease due to alcohol or toxins respond well to withdrawal of the offending agent, with rapid and often complete normalization of erythropoiesis. The pure sideroblastic anemia variant of myelodysplasia-associated sideroblastic anemia can usually be managed well for many years with transfusions and, if necessary, concordant iron chelation therapy. Other myelodysplasia-related sideroblastic anemias generally have a poor prognosis because of the frequent coexistence of pancytopenia and the relatively high incidence of progression to acute leukemia.

1. Anker SD, Colet JC, Filippatos G, et al. Ferric carboxymaltose in patients with heart failure and iron deficiency. *N Engl J Med.* 2009;361:2436-2448.
2. Michael B, Coyne DW, Fishbane S, et al. Sodium ferric gluconate complex in hemodialysis patients: adverse reactions compared to placebo and iron dextran. *Kidney Int.* 2002;61:1830-1839.
3. Ludwig H, Crawford J, Osterborg A, et al. Pooled analysis of individual patient-level data from all randomized, double-blind, placebo-controlled trials of darbepoetin alfa in the treatment of patients with chemotherapy-induced anemia. *J Clin Oncol.* 2009;27:2838-2847.
4. Bohlius J, Schmidlin K, Brillant C, et al. Recombinant human erythropoiesis-stimulating agents and mortality in patients with cancer: a meta-analysis of randomised trials. *Lancet.* 2009;373: 1532-1542.

SUGGESTED READINGS

Camaschella C. Hereditary sideroblastic anemias: pathophysiology, diagnosis, and treatment. *Semin Hematol.* 2009;46:371-377. *Basic mechanisms and clinical approach to this heterogeneous group of rare anemias.*

Goodnough LT, Nemeth E, Ganz T. Detection, evaluation, and management of iron restricted erythropoiesis. *Blood.* 2010;116:4754-4761. *Comprehensive review of iron restricted anemias.*

Pietrangelo A. Hepcidin in human iron disorders: therapeutic implications. *J Hepatol.* 2011;54:173-181. *Review emphasizing the potential for therapeutic interventions.*

Zhu A, Kaneshiro M, Kaunitz JD. Evaluation and treatment of iron deficiency anemia: a gastroenterological perspective. *Dig Dis Sci.* 2010;55:548-559. *Approach to the evaluation of iron-deficient patients for a source of GI blood loss, including the frequent problem of nondiagnostic findings on upper and lower endoscopy.*

163

AUTOIMMUNE AND INTRAVASCULAR HEMOLYTIC ANEMIAS

ROBERT S. SCHWARTZ

DEFINITION

The immune-mediated hemolytic anemias are a group of disorders in which antibodies, complement, and macrophages, usually acting in concert, cause the patient's red blood cells to die prematurely. In the most common type, the antibodies bind to native constituents of the membrane of the patient's own red blood cells. For this reason, the antibodies qualify as autoantibodies, and the diseases they cause fall under the rubric of autoimmune hemolytic anemia.

There are also less common types of immune-mediated hemolytic anemia. Some drugs elicit antidrug antibodies that can cause hemolytic anemia if the drug plants itself in the erythrocyte membrane, thereby making the red cell a target of the antibodies. A high titer of immunoglobulin (Ig) M antierythrocyte autoantibodies that bind to red blood cells at cold temperatures is the distinguishing serologic feature of cold agglutinin disease. In paroxysmal cold hemoglobinuria, an IgG antibody binds to the erythrocyte at cold temperatures, setting the stage for complement-mediated hemolysis at warm temperatures. Paroxysmal nocturnal hemoglobinuria (PNH), another disease in which complement mediates hemolysis, arises from a somatic mutation in a hematopoietic stem cell that renders erythrocytes susceptible to complement-mediated lysis in the absence of antibody. The hemolytic transfusion reaction (Chapter 180) is another disorder in which complement-mediated destruction of erythrocytes occurs, but in such cases, the recipient's alloantibodies against the donor's red cell antigens trigger lysis of the transfused cells.

AUTOIMMUNE HEMOLYTIC ANEMIAS
Autoimmune Hemolytic Anemia with IgG Autoantibodies

EPIDEMIOLOGY

Autoimmune hemolytic anemia associated with IgG autoantibodies (generally referred to simply as autoimmune hemolytic anemia) accounts for about 75% of all autoimmune hemolytic anemias. It has also been called warm antibody autoimmune hemolytic anemia because the IgG autoantibodies in this disorder react best with red cells at 37° C. Autoimmune hemolytic anemia can be primary (idiopathic), or it can develop in association with another disease (secondary).

Autoimmune hemolytic anemia is uncommon. The estimated overall (not age-adjusted) annual incidence is about 1 case per 100,000 population; after age 60 years, the annual incidence reaches 10 per 100,000. The disorder can occur at any age, but most patients are older than 40 years. About 65% of patients with primary autoimmune hemolytic anemia are women, and almost all cases that complicate systemic lupus erythematosus (Chapter 274) occur in women.

PATHOBIOLOGY
Red Cell Antibodies

IgG anti–red cell autoantibodies mediate the destruction of red blood cells outside the circulating blood in a process called *extravascular hemolysis*. By contrast, when lytic components of the complement system participate in the process, the destruction of red cells usually occurs directly within the circulation (intravascular hemolysis). The participation of lytic complement components in IgG-mediated autoimmune hemolytic anemia is rare.

Structure of IgG Anti–Red Cell Autoantibodies

Chapter 44 reviews the structure and function of immunoglobulins. To understand how autoantibodies cause the destruction of red cells, recall that IgG antibodies consist of two identical heavy chains and two identical light chains (Fig. 163-1A); each kind of chain contains variable and constant

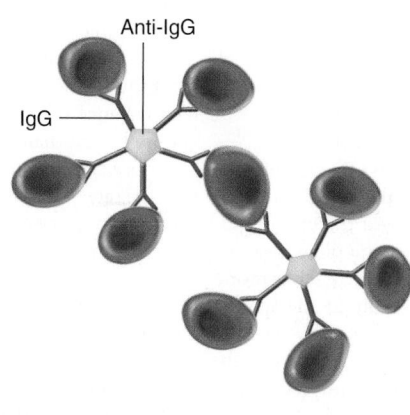

FIGURE 163-1. IgG anti–red cell autoantibodies. **A,** Structure of an IgG molecule demonstrating its variable and constant regions and the heavy and light chains. **B,** Agglutination of red cells by pentameric IgM antibodies, which can join the cells into a lattice. **C,** Coating of red cells by IgG antibodies. The antibodies are unable to agglutinate the cells. **D,** Agglutination of IgG-coated red cells by an anti-IgG antibody.

regions. The four variable regions of IgG form two identical antigen-binding pockets in the molecule. Disulfide bonds hold the constant regions of the heavy and light chains together and give the molecule its characteristic Y shape. An individual B cell produces a monoclonal antibody, a single kind of antibody with a structurally unique antigen-binding pocket, whereas polyclonal antibodies arise from a mixed population of B cells. The constant region (Fc) of the antibody consists of the constant regions of the two heavy chains.

There are two variants of the constant region of light chains: κ and λ. By contrast, the nine heavy chain constant region genes allow nine types of heavy chains: μ (IgM), δ (IgD), γ3 (IgG3), γ1 (IgG1), α1 (IgA1), γ2 (IgG2), γ4 (IgG4), ϵ1 (IgE1), and α2 (IgA2). These various constant regions determine the isotype of the antibody.

During the immune response, B cells produce IgM antibodies at first; later, under the influence of antigen-activated helper T cells (CD4$^+$), they switch to the production of an IgG, IgA, or IgE isotype. In autoimmune hemolytic anemia, the autoantibodies are a mixture of IgG κ and IgG λ molecules. Such a polyclonal population of antibodies marks the participation of activated CD4$^+$ T cells.

Red Cell Destruction
Birth and Death of a Normal Erythrocyte

The blood of a normal adult contains about 2000 mL of erythrocytes, which arise in the bone marrow from hematopoietic precursors with a commitment to the red cell lineage. Under the primary influence of erythropoietin, these precursors differentiate, synthesize hemoglobin, and emerge from the marrow 3 days after they become proerythroblasts (Chapter 159). The earliest red cells in the blood are reticulocytes. They lose the blue-staining remnants of cytoplasmic RNA and ribosomes in a little more than a day to become mature oxygen-transporting erythrocytes. Its biconcave shape, the lack of a nucleus, and the lipid bilayer arrangement of its membrane give the red cell the flexibility it needs for the 100-mile journey it makes through the circulatory system during its lifespan of 4 months.

Normally, production and destruction of erythrocytes are matched. To maintain the steady state, the marrow of a 70-kg adult produces about 25 mL of red blood cells (2×10^{11} erythrocytes) daily. About 1% of the circulating red cells die every day, mainly because worn-out water pumps of the aged erythrocyte can no longer prevent intracellular water overload. The excessive water transforms red cell discs into spheres. These spherocytes constitute 1% of the erythrocytes in blood, a figure equal to the percentage of reticulocytes in blood. In sinusoids of the spleen, lymph nodes, and liver, where blood flow is sluggish, macrophages ingest spherocytes and break down their hemoglobin into bilirubin and amino acids.

In an adult, dead erythrocytes release 6 to 7 g of hemoglobin daily, mostly within macrophages. About 10% of dying spherocytes empty hemoglobin directly into the blood stream, where it binds with high affinity to haptoglobin. The haptoglobin-hemoglobin complexes turn plasma red (whereas in myoglobinuria—the result of massive muscle destruction—the plasma is pale amber because myoglobin does not bind to haptoglobin). Macrophages rapidly engulf the hemoglobin-haptoglobin complexes through the macrophage scavenger receptor (CD163), then catabolize the protein constituents of the complex and deliver the heme iron to transferrin. If massive intravascular hemolysis overwhelms the haptoglobin disposal mechanism, the kidneys excrete unbound (free) hemoglobin into the urine. Renal tubular cells take up and convert urinary hemoglobin into bile pigments and retain most of the heme iron. These tubular cells stain with Prussian blue; the blue cells and the cola-colored urine (hemoglobinuria) are diagnostic of chronic (or massive) intravascular hemolysis. Table 163-1 lists the causes of black or brown urine.

Mechanism of Antibody-Mediated Red Cell Destruction

IgG anti–red cell autoantibodies are opsonins; when bound to autoantigens on red cell membranes, they instigate phagocytosis of the cells by macrophages. Using its Fcγ receptors, the macrophage can ingest the entire IgG-coated erythrocyte or transform it into a spherocyte by nibbling away its surface (Fig. 163-2). Antibody-coated spherocytes cannot resist osmotic forces and ultimately surrender to macrophages, especially in the splenic sinusoids, where blood flows sluggishly.

Macrophages bind to structures in the constant regions of all four subclasses of IgG by means of Fcγ receptors. When IgG or IgM antibodies bind to an antigen, their Fc regions expose a binding site for C1q, the first component of the complement system (Chapter 49). The bound C1q, which

TABLE 163-1	CAUSES OF BLACK OR DARK BROWN URINE

Hemoglobinuria
    Intravascular hemolysis
Myoglobinuria (from rhabdomyolysis, Chapter 115)
    Ischemic muscle damage
    Crush injury
    March myoglobinuria
Drugs
Porphyria cutanea tarda (Chapter 217)
Melanin (metastatic malignant melanoma)
Alkaptonuria
Methemoglobinuria

FIGURE 163-2. Electron micrograph of a macrophage that has ingested two spherocytes (dark circular structures within the cytoplasm) and is pinching off bits of membrane from antibody-coated red cells in contact with the surface of the macrophage. (From Jandl JH. Blood. In: *Textbook of Hematology,* 2nd ed. Boston: Little, Brown; 1996:432.)

resembles a bouquet of polypeptides, initiates activation of the classical complement pathway to its final step—formation of the lytic membrane attack complex. Macrophages display receptors for the later-acting C3b and C4b components of complement (CR1 receptors), and these components cooperate with the corresponding Fcγ receptors to hasten destruction of the red cell by acting as opsonins. In autoimmune hemolytic anemia, the complement system rarely proceeds to the late lytic components because molecules on the red cell surface can block generation of the membrane attack complex. The density and mobility of target antigens on the erythrocyte membrane are important because binding of C1q to the constant region of the anti–red cell antibody requires two closely adjacent Fcγ structures on the red cell membrane.

The Hemolytic Rate

The rate of hemolysis in autoimmune hemolytic anemia depends on the amount of autoantibody on the red cell surface, the affinity and avidity of autoantibodies for the red cell autoantigen, and the number of macrophages in the environment of the antibody-coated erythrocyte. Populations of autoantibodies with high avidity cause a higher rate of red cell destruction than populations with low avidity. Free (monomeric) IgG competes with the interaction of antibody-coated red cells with the Fc receptors of macrophages, but the IgG in plasma has only a minor influence on the hemolytic rate. The importance of the subclasses of IgG is unclear, but IgG3 antibodies seem more potent than IgG1 antibodies in promoting phagocytosis.

The degree of anemia in autoimmune hemolytic anemia depends not only on the rate of red cell destruction but also on the ability of marrow to generate a compensatory increase in erythrocyte production. With an adequate supply of nutrients and growth factors, the marrow can increase red cell production by six to eight times the normal rate. In such cases, there is erythroid hyperplasia in the marrow, and reticulocytes leave the marrow at an accelerated pace and in increased numbers; in some severe cases, even nucleated red cells enter the blood. Anemia does not appear until the half-life of the circulating red cell population drops to about 10 days (the half-life of a population of normal red cells is about 30 days). A half-life of 5 or 6 days is not unusual in autoimmune hemolytic anemia.

Causes of Autoimmune Hemolytic Anemia

The cause of autoimmune hemolytic anemia is unknown. In about a third of cases, the autoantibodies have specificity for an antigen in the Rh system. In another third, the antibodies target proteins in membrane glycoproteins (glycophorins) of the red cell; in other cases, the antibodies have specificity for antigens in the Kell or Duffy blood group system (very rarely for ABO antigens) or for structures in the membrane that are not blood group antigens (e.g., band 3). In all these cases, the patient's own erythrocytes display the relevant antigen.

During fetal life, the thymus deletes lymphocytes with receptors that can bind to autoantigen. This effect, one of the mechanisms of immunologic tolerance of endogenous ("self") antigens, prevents the development of autoantibodies against blood group antigens. The extreme rarity of autoimmune hemolytic anemia secondary to anti-A or anti-B antibodies indicates that the deletion occurs early in ontogeny, because the embryo begins to synthesize A and B substances at 5 weeks of gestation.

A population of CD4$^+$/CD25$^+$ T cells that express the transcription factor Foxp3 restrains immune responses against autoantigens. There is evidence that a deficiency of these regulatory T cells plays a role in the pathogenesis of autoimmune hemolytic anemia, but how this deficiency arises is unknown.

The anti–red cell autoantibodies in autoimmune hemolytic anemia constitute a polyclonal population of IgG antibodies—a typical feature of an antigen-driven immune response. Evidence that cultured T cells from patients with autoimmune hemolytic anemia proliferate in the presence of certain synthetic Rh peptides supports the idea that the patient's own Rh antigens, or exogenous cross-reactive antigens, drive the autoimmune response. These peptides are cryptic—they reside in regions of the Rh protein that are not normally exposed on the red cell surface. By contrast, T cells from Rh-negative persons who were alloimmunized by transfusion of Rh-positive blood respond to peptides in exposed regions of the Rh protein. The weak response of T cells from normal subjects to allogeneic Rh peptides suggests that cross-reactive environmental antigens may prime T cells for an anti-Rh response.

T cells from patients with chronic lymphocytic leukemia (Chapter 190) complicated by autoimmune hemolytic anemia also respond in vitro to self-Rh proteins. Notably, the leukemic B cells are highly effective in presenting Rh protein to T cells. In some cases of chronic lymphocytic leukemia with autoimmune hemolytic anemia, the leukemic cells display surface immunoglobulins with light chain isotypes that differ from those of the patient's anti–red cell autoantibodies, indicating that the source of the autoantibodies in these patients is not the leukemic clone.

Drug-Induced Immune Hemolytic Anemia

Many drugs or drug metabolites have the potential to elicit antidrug antibodies. Drugs that form covalent bonds with proteins in the red cell membrane can bind antidrug antibodies to the red cell surface, causing a positive direct antiglobulin test (see later) and, in some cases, initiating antibody-mediated destruction of red cells. Other drugs, such as the cephalosporins, can bind to red cell membranes and take up IgG nonspecifically from plasma. In these cases, there is no antidrug antibody. The diagnosis of drug-induced immune-mediated hemolytic anemia should be considered if the patient has a history of taking a suspected medication, there is acute complement-mediated hemolysis, only complement components are detectable on the red cell surface, or the patient's serum reacts with red cells in the presence of the suspected drug.

Some drugs can induce true autoantibodies against red cells. Fludarabine, a purine nucleoside analogue used in the treatment of chronic lymphocytic leukemia, and monoclonal antibodies against tumor necrosis factor-α (infliximab and adalimumab), T cells (alemtuzumab), α4 integrin (natalizumab), and interleukin-2 receptor (daclizumab) also have this property, the cause of which is unknown. Notably, there is no sure way of distinguishing drug-induced autoimmune hemolytic anemia from primary autoimmune hemolytic anemia.

CLINICAL MANIFESTATIONS

Autoimmune hemolytic anemia usually unfolds insidiously, but in some cases it begins abruptly with overt symptoms of severe anemia. When the disease is secondary to chronic lymphocytic leukemia (Chapter 190), systemic lupus erythematosus (Chapter 274), or some other disorder, the primary condition generally brings the patient to the physician.

The symptoms are nonspecific and varied. They depend on the age of the patient; the presence of comorbid conditions, especially cardiovascular

disease; whether the autoimmune process is primary or a complication of another disorder; and the degree of anemia. In primary autoimmune hemolytic anemia, symptoms of anemia predominate; asthenia and easy fatigue are typical. Dyspnea suggests coexisting heart disease; angina or myocardial infarction can occur in patients with severe anemia and coronary artery disease.

DIAGNOSIS

History

The history can provide clues that help in the differential diagnosis of hemolytic anemia (Table 163-2). The patient's medical history is the key to the diagnosis of drug-induced hemolytic anemia. It is essential to question the patient about both prescribed and over-the-counter medications, because drug-induced hemolytic anemia can be confused with autoimmune hemolytic anemia, and management of the two conditions differs. It is also important to inquire about comorbid conditions; for example, symptoms of cardiovascular disease will influence management.

Autoimmune hemolytic anemia is a well-known complication of chronic lymphocytic leukemia (Chapter 190) and non-Hodgkin's B-cell lymphomas (Chapter 191). It can also occur occasionally in ulcerative colitis (Chapter 143), rheumatoid arthritis (Chapter 272), and various carcinomas. Autoimmune hemolytic anemia occurs in about 10% of cases of systemic lupus erythematosus (Chapter 274); it may be the initial clinical manifestation of the disease or occur later. It may also complicate the antiphospholipid antibody syndrome; such cases constitute a subset of systemic lupus erythematosus. In most diseases with autoimmune hemolytic anemia as a secondary feature, the primary disorder is at the center of the clinical problem.

Physical Examination

There are no diagnostic findings on physical examination. The combination of pallor, jaundice, and a palpable spleen (Chapter 171) points strongly to hemolytic anemia, but not necessarily to autoimmune hemolytic anemia. Pallor is often difficult to gauge; examination of the palmar creases, buccal mucosa, and subconjunctival membranes, as well as side-by side comparison of the examiner's nail beds with the patient's, can be revealing. More than half of patients have a palpable spleen. The tip of the spleen rarely descends more than 6 cm below the costal margin, except in the presence of lymphoma or chronic lymphocytic leukemia. Hepatomegaly is also frequent; a firm, nontender edge is easily palpable in about 50% of patients.

The examiner should search for an underlying disease because the differences between primary and secondary autoimmune hemolytic anemia influence management and prognosis. The malar rash of systemic lupus erythematosus and the enlarged lymph nodes of lymphoma or chronic lymphocytic leukemia should not be overlooked. A very large spleen also raises the possibility of coexisting lymphoma or chronic lymphocytic leukemia.

Laboratory Findings

The blood smear reflects the marrow's attempt to compensate for accelerated hemolysis and the effects of the interaction between antibody-coated red cells and macrophages. Two populations are evident: large, blue-tinged red cells, which correspond to reticulocytes, and small, dark red spherocytes (microspherocytes) (Fig. 163-3). Such a dimorphic population is characteristic of hemolytic anemia but is not diagnostic of any particular type of hemolytic anemia.

The white blood cell count is often moderately elevated, a reflection of a bone marrow stressed by severe hemolytic anemia. In uncomplicated cases, platelet counts are normal or occasionally increased slightly. Platelet counts may be low in systemic lupus erythematosus or in Evans syndrome, a rare combination of autoimmune hemolytic anemia and immune thrombocytopenia (Chapter 175).

The characteristic finding in bone marrow is erythroid hyperplasia. However, examination of marrow is necessary only if there are unexpected findings or suspicion of lymphoma.

Elevated serum levels of prehepatic (indirect) bilirubin and lactate dehydrogenase (LDH) and a reduced serum haptoglobin concentration are signs of hemolytic anemia. The indirect bilirubin in hemolytic anemia usually does not exceed 4.0 mg/dL unless there is coexisting liver disease. Serum LDH can be useful, especially in cases with intravascular hemolysis, but neither LDH nor the haptoglobin level is specific for hemolytic anemia. Moreover, the presence of inflammation negates the value of measuring haptoglobin, which is an acute phase protein. Oral contraceptives, estrogen replacement therapy, and tamoxifen all increase haptoglobin levels. Laboratory signs of intravascular destruction of red blood cells (hemoglobinemia, hemoglobinuria, and hemosiderinuria; see later) are unusual in autoimmune hemolytic anemia.

The Antiglobulin (Coombs) Test

The antiglobulin test is central to the diagnosis of autoimmune hemolytic anemia and to an understanding of the antibody-mediated mechanism of red blood cell destruction in this disorder (Fig. 163-1B to D).

The terms *complete* and *incomplete antibodies* refer to the ability (or inability) of antibodies to cross-link adjacent red cells, thereby building the lattice needed for the macroscopic clumping of red cells. The strong negative charge of red blood cells suspended in saline keeps them apart, even if they have a coating of antibodies—the average distance between cells is 24 nm. IgM antibodies, being pentamers, are efficient agglutinins; with five antigen-binding sites, they can bridge this distance. In contrast, bivalent IgG antibodies usually cannot cause the clumping of saline-suspended erythrocytes.

The test that reveals antibody-coated red blood cells is the direct Coombs (antiglobulin) test. The indirect Coombs test was devised to seek the presence of incomplete antibodies in the patient's serum. As presently used, the standard antiglobulin reagent contains antibodies against all four classes of IgG and components of complement (usually C3 and C4).

A positive Coombs test requires cautious interpretation when there are no other features of autoimmune hemolytic anemia. False-positive test results are not unusual. The reported incidence of positive antiglobulin tests in normal blood donors and general populations of hospitalized patients varies widely—from 1 in 100 to 1 in 15,000. Differences in the technique used to perform the test account for this variation. The usual reason for a false-positive direct antiglobulin test is nonspecific, low-avidity adherence of IgG to red cells. In rare cases, however, the result is not a false-positive but a harbinger of the development of autoimmune hemolytic anemia. False-negative direct antiglobulin tests are usually due to low-affinity autoantibodies that spontaneously elute from the red cell in vitro or to amounts of erythrocyte-coating antibodies that are below the limit of detection by the antiglobulin test. The distinction between a true-positive and a false-positive direct antiglobulin test can be made by eluting the antibody from the red cells and testing its ability to bind to normal red cells. In a false-positive reaction, the eluted antibody does not bind to normal red cells, whereas binding does occur in a true-positive test.

TREATMENT **Rx**

There are no controlled trials of the treatment of autoimmune hemolytic anemia. A corticosteroid, usually prednisone, is the standard initial treatment. Splenectomy is indicated in patients who fail to attain or sustain a remission. If splenectomy does not result in improvement, one or more immunosuppressive agents can be tried. The physician should not withhold red cell transfusions from symptomatic patients.

TABLE 163-2	DIFFERENTIAL DIAGNOSIS OF HEMOLYTIC ANEMIA

HEREDITARY HEMOLYTIC ANEMIA

The thalassemias
  β-Thalassemia
  α-Thalassemia
  Combined thalassemia and hemoglobinopathy
The hemoglobinopathies
  Sickle cell disease (hemoglobin S)
  Hemoglobin C disease
  Hemoglobin E disease
  Combined hemoglobinopathies (hemoglobin SC disease)
Defects of the red cell membrane
  Hereditary spherocytosis
  Hereditary elliptocytosis
  Acanthocytosis
Deficiencies in red cell enzymes
  Glucose-6-phosphate dehydrogenase deficiency
  Pyruvate kinase deficiency
  Defects of the Embden-Meyerhof pathway

ACQUIRED HEMOLYTIC ANEMIA

Immune-mediated hemolytic anemia
  Autoimmune hemolytic anemia
  Cold agglutinin disease
  Paroxysmal nocturnal hemoglobinuria
  Paroxysmal cold hemoglobinuria
  Drug-induced immune hemolytic anemia
  Hemolytic transfusion reaction
  Hemolytic disease of the newborn secondary to maternal alloantibodies
  Systemic lupus erythematosus
Microangiopathic hemolytic anemia (Fig. 163-4)
  Disseminated intravascular coagulation
  Thrombotic thrombocytopenic purpura
  Hemolytic-uremic syndrome
  Infections (e.g., *Clostridium*, malaria, babesiosis, *Bartonella*)
  Deficiency of factor H
  Giant hemangioma
  Disseminated carcinomatosis
  Chemotherapy (e.g., mitomycin C)
  Solid organ transplantation
  Bone marrow transplantation
  Malignant hypertension
  Scleroderma
  Eclampsia, preeclampsia, HELLP syndrome (hemolysis, elevated liver enzymes, low platelet count)
  Prosthetic materials
    Heart valves
    Ventricular or atrial septal patches
    Left ventricular assist devices
    Vascular grafts
    Transjugular intrahepatic portosystemic shunts
Physical or chemical injuries
Trauma to small vessels (e.g., exercise related)
Burn related
Venoms
Bacterial infection (e.g., *Clostridium*)
Copper
Freshwater near-drowning

FIGURE 163-3. Representative peripheral blood smear in a patient with autoimmune hemolytic anemia. (Courtesy Thomas K. Chacko.)

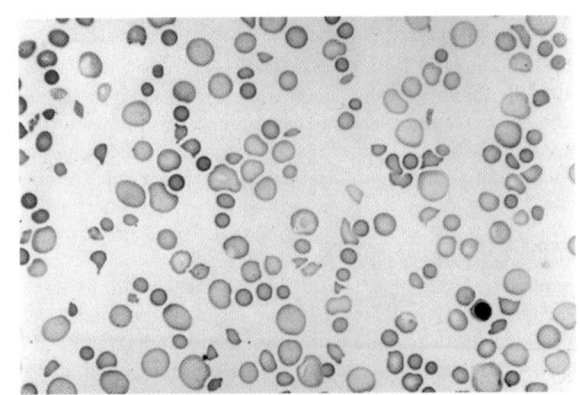

FIGURE 163-4. Microangiopathic hemolytic anemia. A peripheral smear shows fragmental red blood cells or schistocytes in a variety of shapes and sizes.

Initial Therapy
Corticosteroids

In the initial management of the disease, the standard of practice is to administer prednisone at a dose of 1.0 to 1.5 mg/kg/day. The duration of treatment at this dose is an unsettled question, but a response—manifested by a rise in the hematocrit and a fall in the reticulocyte count—is usually evident within 3 to 4 weeks. A patient who fails to improve within this time is unlikely to respond to further treatment with prednisone. In a patient who does respond, slow reduction of the dose of prednisone is essential to avoid a relapse. The usual tapering schedule is a weekly reduction of the initial dose by 10 mg/day to a dose of 30 mg/day, followed by a weekly reduction of 5 mg/day to 15 mg/day. Thereafter, slow, cautious tapering over at least 4 months is the rule. A rise in the reticulocyte count or a fall in the hematocrit should prompt an increase in the dose, usually to the previous level.

About 25% of patients treated with corticosteroids in this manner enter a stable, complete remission; half of patients require continuous, low-dose prednisone; and the remaining 25% respond only transiently or not at all or are unable to tolerate continuous corticosteroid treatment. There is no reliable evidence that alternate-day maintenance treatment is superior to daily treatment, but some patients tolerate this schedule better than daily prednisone. Very high doses of intravenous methylprednisolone have been advocated for stubborn cases, but such treatment is risky and should be considered experimental.

Transfusion

Red blood cell transfusions (Chapter 180) are indicated in patients with disabling symptoms of anemia: marked fatigue, reduced exercise tolerance, or an inability to work. These symptoms often develop when the hemoglobin concentration falls below 10 g/dL, but the decision to administer red cell transfusions should not depend primarily on laboratory tests—the patient's clinical status is the dominant factor. Some patients can tolerate a stable hemoglobin level as low as 8 g/dL; however, symptoms of coronary artery disease or heart failure may force the decision to transfuse before the hemoglobin level falls below 10 g/dL. Regardless of the patient's clinical status, rapid transfusion of large volumes of red cells can have serious adverse consequences. The blood should be administered at a rate that does not exceed 1 mL/kg/hour.

The risk of reactions to blood transfusions (Chapter 180) in patients with autoimmune hemolytic anemia is always present because of the destruction of transfused blood by the patient's autoantibodies. This hazard is increased if the patient also has alloantibodies that were induced by pregnancy or previous transfusions. For these reasons, the blood bank should be alerted to the diagnosis and should be informed if the patient was ever pregnant or has ever had transfusions.

It is important for the managing physician to understand that no patient with symptomatic autoimmune hemolytic anemia should be denied blood transfusions because of an "incompatible crossmatch." The patient's positive antiglobulin test always interferes with compatibility testing. Communication and cooperation between the patient's physician and specialists in transfusion medicine (Chapter 180) are essential in reducing the risks associated with transfusion in patients with autoimmune hemolytic anemia.

Splenectomy

Because the spleen is the major site of red cell destruction in autoimmune hemolytic anemia, splenectomy should be considered for patients who have not responded to corticosteroids or who have maintained a stable but corticosteroid-dependent remission. A complete, durable remission follows splenectomy in one half to two thirds of cases. Attempts to predict responsiveness to splenectomy by measuring the splenic sequestration of ^{51}Cr-labeled erythrocytes have not been reliable. The only way of determining the effectiveness of splenectomy in a given patient is to perform the procedure. Laparoscopic splenectomy, a safe method of removing the organ, is now the preferred surgical technique.

A major risk is post-splenectomy sepsis secondary to encapsulated bacteria, particularly pneumococci and especially in children. Splenectomy also increases susceptibility to babesiosis, ehrlichiosis, and malaria. Preoperative immunization with polyvalent pneumococcal and *Haemophilus influenzae* vaccines reduces the risk of post-splenectomy sepsis. In children, a prophylactic antibiotic, generally penicillin or amoxicillin, is essential after splenectomy. Evidence for the effectiveness of (or need for) prophylactic antibiotics in splenectomized adults is inconclusive. Education of the patient concerning the risk for serious infection after splenectomy is also important.

A rise in the platelet count occurs in almost all patients after splenectomy. The increase rarely exceeds 500,000/mL and usually subsides within 3 to 5 months. The low risk for thromboembolism related to post-splenectomy thrombocytosis argues against the need for routine antithrombotic prophylaxis.

Therapy in Refractory Patients
Rituximab

Rituximab is a chimeric monoclonal antibody with a high affinity for the CD20 antigen on the surface of normal and malignant B lymphocytes (Chapter 35).

The antibody consists of murine variable region sequences and human constant region sequences. The usual dose is 375 mg/m^2 by intravenous infusion once a week for four or eight doses, but it may be continued weekly or biweekly if necessary. Rituximab rapidly depletes the circulation and lymphoid tissue of B cells; it can cause allergic reactions and increase the risk for infection.

Other Monoclonal Antibodies

Monoclonal antibodies against components of the immune system or cytokines have been used in the treatment of autoimmune hemolytic anemia, but most of the literature on this topic consists of small, uncontrolled series. Among the monoclonal antibodies that have been used are alemtuzumab (anti-CD52, a T-cell marker) and natalizumab (α4 integrin). These and similar monoclonal antibodies should be reserved for experimental use in refractory, transfusion-dependent cases.

Immunosuppressive Drugs and Other Modalities

Immunosuppressive drugs other than corticosteroids can be useful in stubborn cases of autoimmune hemolytic anemia, but no head-to-head trials have compared the efficacy of these drugs. The choice usually depends on safety and familiarity with the agent. Azathioprine has the least toxicity; cyclosporine is nephrotoxic; and cyclophosphamide damages the bone marrow, ovaries, and bladder and impairs spermatogenesis. Mycophenolate has also been tried, with some success in refractory cases. In general, these drugs should be administered only by specialists and should be reserved for patients who have failed to respond to splenectomy or who, because of comorbidities, are not suitable candidates for splenectomy.

A variety of other treatments have been used in refractory cases of autoimmune hemolytic anemia, including plasma exchange, vinca alkaloids, danazol (a synthetic androgen), and intravenous IgG. None of these forms of therapy is reliably effective, and none of them has been tested for efficacy in a randomized trial.

Cold Agglutinin Disease

DEFINITION AND EPIDEMIOLOGY

Of the two types of cold agglutinin disease, the acute form is a complication of infection, usually by *Mycoplasma pneumoniae* (Chapter 325) or Epstein-Barr virus (infectious mononucleosis [Chapter 385]). The onset in these cases is abrupt and generally appears during recovery from the infection. The acute disease, which almost always affects young adults, is rare, is self-limited, and seldom requires treatment. The usual type of cold agglutinin disease is a chronic disorder of older patients, many of whom have a B-cell lymphoma (Chapter 191), chronic lymphocytic leukemia (Chapter 190), or Waldenström's macroglobulinemia (Chapter 193). In these cases, the cold agglutinin is a monoclonal IgM antibody, in contrast to the polyclonal IgM cold agglutinins of postinfectious cold agglutinin disease.

PATHOBIOLOGY
Cold Agglutinins

Cold agglutinins are IgM autoantibodies that react with erythrocytes at temperatures below 37° C. Normal serum contains low titers of cold agglutinins, which are usually not detectable in a dilution higher than 1 : 10; in chronic cold agglutinin disease, however, the titer can exceed 1 : 10^5. The temperature at which cold agglutinins react with red cells in vitro—the thermal amplitude of the antibodies—varies considerably, but in almost all cases, red cells agglutinate readily at 4° C and quickly disaggregate at 37° C. The temperature-dependent reversibility of the reaction reflects the weak affinity of cold agglutinins for red cell antigens.

Most cold agglutinins react with polysaccharides on the red cell surface. The principal targets are the i antigen (a straight-chain paragloboside) and the I antigen (a branched paragloboside with the same composition as the i antigen). Less common are the Pr glycoproteins and sialylated polysaccharides. The erythrocytes of almost all adults are I$^+$ and lack the i antigen. The i antigen is characteristic of newborns, because the enzyme that converts i to I becomes active only after birth. Cold agglutinins associated with *M. pneumoniae* infection have anti-I specificity, whereas cold agglutinins related to infectious mononucleosis have anti-i specificity. In chronic cold agglutinin disease, the cold agglutinins are almost always monoclonal IgM, anti-I antibodies with a VH4-34 heavy chain; the shape of the antigen-binding surface of this heavy chain favors attachment to polysaccharides. About 10% of B cells from normal subjects display the VH-34 heavy chain; these cells are probably the source of the cold agglutinins in normal serum. Anti-Pr cold agglutinins tend to have a similar κ light chain variable region; presumably, the binding surface of this light chain promotes attachment of the agglutinins to red cell glycoproteins.

Erythrocyte Destruction in Cold Agglutinin Disease

The basis of red cell destruction in cold agglutinin disease is the ability of IgM antibodies to fix complement. Unlike IgG antibodies, each IgM molecule has two binding sites for C1q. An inhibitor on the red cell surface (the membrane inhibitor of reactive lysis) stops the complement cascade before lytic components can be activated, leaving behind C3b and C4b fragments. This step prepares the erythrocyte for engulfment by phagocytic cells with receptors for C3b and C4b. If such coated cells escape into the circulation, enzymes degrade the C3b and C4b fragments to harmless peptides (C3dg and C4d).

Blood cools sufficiently in the hands and feet to allow cold agglutinins to bind red cells. The adherent IgM attracts C1q, which initiates the generation of C3b and C4b on the erythrocyte's surface. On entering the warmer visceral circulation, the red cell releases the cold agglutinin, but the C3 fragments remain engaged to the CR1 of macrophages, thereby enabling phagocytosis of the red cell. The efficiency of this process depends on the amount of cold agglutinin on the red cell surface and the thermal amplitude of the cold agglutinin. An antibody that binds only at very low temperatures causes little harm, whereas an antibody that binds at a temperature close to 37° C can cause severe hemolytic anemia. These variables account for the widely different degrees of severity of cold agglutinin disease.

CLINICAL MANIFESTATIONS

Most cases of chronic cold agglutinin disease occur between the ages of 50 and 70 years. Anemia causes the main symptoms, which can worsen in cold weather. The degree of anemia, which is usually not severe, can remain static without treatment for many months because of the action of an inhibitor of C3b in serum.

In a patient with high-affinity cold agglutinins, exposure to cold can precipitate an attack of acrocyanosis by inducing massive agglutination of red cells in the capillary circulation of the hands, feet, or both. In such a case, intravascular hemolysis with hemoglobinuria and, rarely, acute renal failure can also occur. The acrocyanosis is neither Raynaud's phenomenon (white, blue, and red digits caused by vasospasm [Chapter 80]) nor the vasculitis of cryoglobulinemia (Chapter 193). Enlargement of the spleen is uncommon unless there is an associated B-cell neoplasm.

DIAGNOSIS

Agglutination of the patient's red cells at room temperature or, more often, on chilling of the blood, followed by disaggregation on warming the blood to 37° C, is typical. Hemagglutination causes red cell clumping in the blood smear and may interfere with automated blood counts. Spherocytosis is not prominent; the reticulocyte count is proportional to the degree of anemia.

The titer of cold agglutinins is often $1:10^5$ or higher, and the direct antiglobulin test is positive if the cold agglutinin has a high thermal amplitude. A monoclonal cold agglutinin indicates the presence of a B-cell lymphoma.

TREATMENT

Cold agglutinin disease, whether postinfectious or chronic, often requires no treatment. Postinfectious cold agglutinin disease is self-limited and generally mild. When chronic cold agglutinin disease is stable, its management requires mainly avoidance of the cold. Safe transfusion is possible; there is no agreement concerning the need for transfusion with warmed blood.

In chronic cold agglutinin disease, prednisone, usually at a dose of 1.0 to 1.5 mg/kg/day for 3 to 6 weeks, can be tried, but it is rarely effective. The use of immunosuppressive drugs such as azathioprine or cyclophosphamide is not recommended. Splenectomy generally fails to induce a remission because the liver is a major site of destruction of C3b-coated red cells. Rituximab (375 mg/m² by intravenous infusion once a week for four or eight doses) has been used successfully in some cases. In patients with chronic cold agglutinin disease and a B-cell neoplasm, treatment should be directed against the tumor.

Paroxysmal Cold Hemoglobinuria

Paroxysmal cold hemoglobinuria is a rare form of immune-mediated hemolytic anemia in which C1q bound to an IgG autoantibody attaches to red cells at low temperatures. The target antigens are globoside and a glycosphingolipid. The antibody dissociates from red cells at 37° C, but C1q remains on the membrane; at the warmer temperature it triggers progression of the complement cascade to its lytic components. The result is intravascular hemolysis.

An unsolved problem is how the lytic components of complement are generated on the red cell surface in paroxysmal cold hemoglobinuria but not in cold agglutinin disease. With the waning of late syphilis in modern times,

the so-called Donath-Landsteiner antibody of paroxysmal cold hemoglobinuria is encountered most often during convalescence from a viral infection, usually a childhood exanthem.

The Donath-Landsteiner autoantibody has no clinical effects unless the patient is exposed to cold temperatures. With cold exposure, even of just an arm or a leg, intravascular hemolysis begins soon after the return to a warm temperature. Chills, fever, back pain, abdominal cramps, and hemoglobinuria are typical. Urticaria is common, acute renal failure is rare, and anemia is an inevitable consequence of severe intravascular hemolysis. The attack is self-limited, lasting only 1 or 2 days.

A positive Donath-Landsteiner test is diagnostic, but the test is relatively insensitive. The procedure should demonstrate hemolysis in the test tube when the patient's blood is chilled and then warmed to 37° C. Addition of normal serum as a source of complement is often necessary to bring out the hemolytic phase of the reaction.

Treatment is generally unnecessary, and spontaneous recovery can be expected within weeks or a few months.

Paroxysmal Nocturnal Hemoglobinuria

DEFINITION

PNH is an acquired form of hemolytic anemia in which a somatic mutation in a hematopoietic stem cell renders erythrocytes susceptible to the lytic components of complement, thereby causing intravascular hemolysis in the absence of an anti–red blood cell antibody.

EPIDEMIOLOGY

PNH can occur at any age but is most common between 10 and 50 years. The median age at diagnosis is about 40 years; median survival after diagnosis is approximately 20 years. It is a rare disorder with an estimated prevalence in the population of 1 in 10^5 to 1 in 10^6. There is no sex preference, and a family history of PNH is unusual.

PATHOBIOLOGY

Genetics

PNH is due to a somatic mutation that causes a defect in the red cell membrane. The disease begins in a single hematopoietic stem cell when the *PIGA* gene on the short arm of the active X chromosome acquires a mutation. The *PIGA* gene encodes PIG-A, an enzyme that is essential for the synthesis of glycosylphosphatidylinositol (GPI). The location of *PIGA* on the X chromosome allows a single mutation in the gene to affect GPI synthesis. This lipid forms a peptide link with the C-terminal amino acid of numerous proteins, anchoring them to the red cell membrane. Molecular genetic studies indicate that the PNH clone upregulates genes that make the PNH clone resistant to apoptosis and immune attack.

The mutation in a hematopoietic stem cell affects PIG-A in blood cells of all lineages. Almost 150 different mutations of *PIGA* have been identified. Most of them inactivate PIG-A and cause total loss of GPI in the descendents of the carrier stem cell. Red cells with complete deficiency of GPI are termed PNH III erythrocytes, and those with partial deficiency are called PNH II erythrocytes. The coexistence of PNH III and PNH II red cells in the same patient indicates the presence of two mutant clones.

A small number of hematopoietic stem cells in normal people bear the *PIGA* mutation; they have no proliferative advantage and persist in small numbers. In normal blood, the frequency of PIG-A–deficient cells is about $1:50,000$ red cells. In contrast to those with PNH, however, the deficient cells in normal subjects arise from committed hematopoietic cells. The presence of PIG-A–deficient cells in normal subjects suggest that PNH involves not only the *PIGA* mutation but also a second step, perhaps a mutation, that allows expansion of the mutated clone.

Functional Consequences of Deficiency of GPI

The membrane inhibitor of reactive hemolysis (CD59, or protectin) and CD55, an inhibitor of C3 convertase, are two of the many proteins that GPI anchors to the red cell. They prevent polymerization of C9, the final step in assembly of the membrane attack complex that begins with cleavage of C5 to C5b. The deficiencies of CD59 and CD55 allow unimpeded assembly of the membrane attack complex on the erythrocyte surface, thereby initiating intravascular hemolysis. A variety of nonspecific factors, such as a reduction in the pH of blood, can activate complement. The morning hemoglobinuria of PNH is probably the result of subtle acidification of blood during sleep.

CLINICAL MANIFESTATIONS

Classically, a patient with PNH arises in the morning and passes urine the color of a cola beverage. During the ensuing hours, the color of the urine gradually returns to yellow. The typical paroxysms of hemoglobinuria occur on a background of chronic, low-grade intravascular hemolysis, the cause of constant hemosiderinuria in PNH. About a third of cases evolve into aplastic anemia (Chapter 168). Transformation to acute myelogenous leukemia is a rare event. Abdominal pain, dysphagia, and erectile dysfunction are additional clinical features. The basis of these symptoms is probably scavenging by free plasma hemoglobin of nitric oxide, a regulator of vasomotor and smooth muscle tone. In about a third of cases, venous thrombosis occurs and can cause Budd-Chiari syndrome (Chapter 145) by obstructing the hepatic veins. Splenomegaly is uncommon; hepatomegaly and ascites point to the complication of hepatic vein thrombosis. Petechiae and susceptibility to infection are indications of bone marrow failure. Hemosiderinuria is the result of chronic intravascular hemolysis. Subtle or overt signs of bone marrow damage (leukopenia and thrombocytopenia) are frequent.

The extent of red cell destruction in PNH depends on the number of PNH red cells in blood, the level of GPI on the red cell membrane (PNH III cells are devoid of GPI), and the activation of complement. The anemia is often aggravated by iron deficiency caused by chronic urinary iron loss in the form of hemosiderinuria. The basis of the tendency to develop venous thrombosis is unclear; hypercoagulability caused by the release of prothrombotic materials in red cell and platelet membranes (which are also abnormal in PNH) and impaired fibrinolysis have been implicated. Nitric oxide scavenging by free plasma hemoglobin may also damage endothelial cells and cause aggregation of platelets.

DIAGNOSIS

Often, the clinical picture is virtually diagnostic. The diagnosis can be established by demonstrating, by flow cytometry, a deficiency of CD59 on erythrocytes. Another reagent with utility in flow cytometry is aerolysin, a bacterial protein that binds to the GPI anchor. Flow cytometry can also measure the proportions of PNH III and PNH II red cells in blood, providing information on the severity of the disease. Laboratory tests that depend on the sensitivity of PNH red cells to complement, such as the Ham acidification test, are insensitive and have largely been abandoned.

TREATMENT   Rx

Eculizumab, a humanized monoclonal antibody against C5, which is essential for formation of the membrane attack complex, can reduce the signs of intravascular hemolysis, the requirement for transfusions, and the tendency to thrombosis. In a randomized trial,[1] the dose of the antibody was 600 mg every week for 4 weeks, followed 1 week later by a 900-mg dose, and then by 900 mg every other week through week 26. A thrombotic event is a strong indication for eculizumab treatment. Warfarin can also be used in patients with a history of a thrombotic event. Oral iron can correct the iron deficiency; treatment with iron does not exacerbate the hemolysis. Transfusions are helpful in supportive care. Aplastic anemia has been treated successfully with immunosuppressive agents (antithymocyte globulin, usually at a dose of 1.5 mg/kg/day for 7 to 14 days) or cyclosporine (3 to 5 mg/kg for at least 3 months). Bone marrow transplantation is risky but can be curative.

Hemolytic Transfusion Reactions

The cause of hemolytic transfusion reactions (Chapter 180) is intravascular lysis of the donor's red cells by antibodies (alloantibodies or isoantibodies) in the recipient that bind to one or more blood group antigens on the transfused cells. The recipient's isoantibodies can be natural anti-A or anti-B antibodies, or they can be induced by previous transfusions or pregnancy. Whether IgM or IgG, the isoantibodies trigger the assembly of lytic complement components on the surface of the donor's red cell. The rapid formation of large amounts of C3a and C5a fragments causes hypotension and bronchial and smooth muscle spasm. Renal failure is a consequence of severe, prolonged hypotension; the main renal lesion is renal cortical ischemia secondary to shunting of blood away from the kidneys. Hemoglobin itself is not nephrotoxic.

The signs and symptoms of a hemolytic transfusion reaction are nonspecific and include fever, back pain, urticaria, dyspnea, hypotension, and

TABLE 163-3 CAUSES OF EXTRAVASCULAR AND INTRAVASCULAR HEMOLYSIS

CONDITION	DIAGNOSTIC FINDING	RED CELL MORPHOLOGY	OTHER FINDINGS	TREATMENT
Autoimmune hemolytic anemia	Positive antiglobulin test	Spherocytosis	Splenomegaly	See text
Drug-induced hemolytic anemia	Drug-dependent antibody	Spherocytosis	History of drug ingestion	See text
Cold agglutinin disease	Cold agglutinins	Normal	Acrocyanosis	See text
Paroxysmal nocturnal hemoglobinuria	Lack of CD59	Normal	Hemoglobinuria, hemosiderinuria	See text
Paroxysmal cold hemoglobinuria	Donath-Landsteiner antibody	Normal	Cold-dependent hemoglobinuria	See text
Prosthetic heart valve	Heart murmur	Schistocytosis	Hemosiderinuria	Iron, folic acid, vitamin B_{12}; valve replacement for severe hemolysis (Chapter 75)
Thrombotic thrombocytopenic purpura	Intravascular hemolysis + thrombocytopenia	Schistocytosis	Renal failure, autoantibody against ADAMTS-13	Chapter 175
Hemolytic-uremic syndrome	Intravascular hemolysis + thrombocytopenia	Schistocytosis	Renal failure, *Shigella* toxin	Chapter 175
HELLP syndrome	Pregnancy	Schistocytosis	Thrombocytopenia, abnormal liver function tests	Chapter 175
Arteriovenous malformations (Kasabach-Merritt syndrome)	Large cavernous hemangioma	Schistocytosis	Thrombocytopenia, DIC	Chapter 175
Postperfusion syndrome	Cardiopulmonary bypass surgery	Ghost erythrocytes	Complement activation	Chapter 74
March hemoglobinuria	History of jogging	No consistent abnormality	Hematuria, hemoglobinuria	Symptomatic
Oxidative hemolysis	Drugs	Heinz bodies	G6PD deficiency	Avoid responsible drug (Chapter 164)
Chemical-induced hemolysis	Strong oxidizing chemicals (e.g., sodium chlorate)	Microspherocytes	Hemoglobinuria, methemoglobinemia, renal failure	Plasma exchange, dialysis
Burns	Severe burn	Spherocytes, schistocytes	Hemoglobinuria	Treatment of burn (Chapter 112)
Malaria	*Plasmodium falciparum* infection	Red cell sporozoites	Hemoglobinuria	Chapter 353
Babesiosis	Tick bite	Intracellular protozoa	Splenectomy scar	Chapter 361
Clostridium perfringens	*C. perfringens* bacteremia	Spherocytosis	Intravascular hemolysis	Chapter 304

DIC = disseminated intravascular coagulation; G6PD = glucose-6-phosphate dehydrogenase; HELLP = hemolysis, elevated liver enzymes, low platelet count.

evidence of disseminated intravascular coagulation. These nonspecific signs appear and worsen during administration of the transfusion. Immediate steps must be taken to stop the transfusion, submit the transfused blood and a sample of the patient's blood to the blood bank, and order tests of plasma and urine for free hemoglobin. Hydration is necessary to ward off renal failure; intravenous fluid, usually normal saline, should be started at once, together with a diuretic (usually furosemide) in amounts to keep urine flow at a rate of at least 100 mL/hour.

● OTHER CAUSES OF INTRAVASCULAR HEMOLYSIS

Conditions in which vascular abnormalities, toxins, infections, or drugs damage red blood cells and cause them to lose pieces of membrane and ultimately fragment into hemoglobin-containing bits should be considered in the differential diagnosis of intravascular hemolysis (Table 163-3; see also Table 163-2). Most of these conditions are readily apparent from the history and physical examination. Treatment focuses on the underlying cause of the hemolysis (see Table 163-3).

1. Brodsky RA, Young NS, Antonioli E, et al. Multicenter phase 3 trial of the complement inhibitor eculizumab for the treatment of paroxysmal hemoglobinuria. *Blood.* 2008;111:1840-1847.

SUGGESTED READINGS

Garratty G. Immune hemolytic anemia associated with drug therapy. *Blood Rev.* 2010;24:143-150. *Of about 125 implicated drugs, the most common are antimicrobials (e.g., cefotetan, ceftriaxone, and piperacillin).*

Gómez-Almaguer D, Solano-Genesta M, Tarin-Arzaga L, et al. Low-dose rituximab and alemtuzumab combination therapy for patients with steroid-refractory autoimmune cytopenias. *Blood.* 2010; 116:4783-4785. *Alemtuzumab 10 mg subcutaneously on days 1 and 3 plus rituximab 100 mg intravenously weekly in 4 doses provided an encouraging response rate.*

Kelly RJ, Hill A, Arnold LM, et al. Long-term treatment with eculizumab in paroxysmal nocturnal hemoglobinuria: sustained efficacy and improved survival. *Blood.* 2011. [Epub ahead of print.] *Survival in treated patients was similar to an age-matched control population and significantly better than historical controls with PNH.*

Rachidi S, Musallam KM, Taher AT. A closer look at paroxysmal nocturnal hemoglobinuria. *Eur J Intern Med.* 2010;21:260-267. *Practical clinical review.*

164

HEMOLYTIC ANEMIAS: RED CELL MEMBRANE AND METABOLIC DEFECTS

PATRICK G. GALLAGHER

The mature erythrocyte differs from all other cells in the body. Lacking a nucleus, DNA, RNA, and ribosomes, it cannot synthesize RNA, DNA, or protein. It does not divide, it has no mitochondria, it cannot perform the Krebs cycle, and it lacks an electron transport system for oxidative phosphorylation. After enucleation, the reticulocyte, the precursor of the mature erythrocyte, leaves the marrow and enters the circulation equipped with a full complement of enzymes, transporters, signaling molecules, and all other proteins necessary to perform the essential functions of the red cell during its life span.

The erythrocyte membrane accounts for only about 1% of the total weight of a red cell, yet it plays a critical role in the maintenance of normal red cell homeostasis through a number of mechanisms. These include retention of vital compounds and removal of metabolic waste, regulation of erythrocyte metabolism and pH, and import of iron required for hemoglobin synthesis during erythropoiesis. The membrane maintains a slippery exterior so that erythrocytes do not aggregate or adhere to endothelial cells. The membrane skeleton, a network of proteins on the inner surface of the red cell, provides the strength and flexibility needed to maintain the normal shape and deformability of the erythrocyte.

The principle functions of erythrocyte metabolism in the mature erythrocyte include maintenance of adequate supplies of adenosine triphosphate (ATP), production of reducing substances to act as antioxidants, and control of oxygen affinity of hemoglobin by production of adequate amounts of 2,3-diphosphoglycerate (2,3-DPG). Because the mature erythrocyte has lost its ability to perform oxidative phosphorylation, its energy is supplied by anaerobic glycolysis though the Embden-Meyerhof pathway, by oxidative glycolysis through the hexose monophosphate (HMP) shunt, and through nucleotide salvage pathways.

● THE ERYTHROCYTE MEMBRANE

Composed of a lipid bilayer and an underlying cortical membrane skeleton (Fig. 164-1), the membrane provides the erythrocyte the deformability and stability required to withstand its travels through the circulation. In one circulatory cycle throughout the body, the erythrocyte is subjected to high sheer stress in the arterial system, dramatic size and shape changes in the microcirculation with capillary diameters as small as 7.5 μm, and marked fluctuations in tonicity, pH, and P_{O_2}.

Membrane Lipids

Red cell membrane lipids are asymmetrically distributed across the bilayer membrane, reflecting a steady state involving a constant exchange of phospholipids between the two bilayer hemileaflets. Glycolipids and cholesterol are intercalated between the phospholipids in the bilayer with their long axes perpendicular to the bilayer plane. Glycolipids, located in the external half of the bilayer with their carbohydrate moieties extending into the aqueous phase, carry several important red cell antigens and serve other important functions. Phospholipids are asymmetrically organized, with the choline phospholipids, phosphatidylcholine and sphingomyelin, primarily in the outer half of the bilayer, and the amino phospholipids, phosphatidylethanolamine and phosphatidylserine (PS), in the inner half of the bilayer. In pathologic states, such as thalassemia, sickle cell disease, and diabetes, loss of phospholipid asymmetry with externalization of PS leads to activation of blood clotting through conversion of prothrombin to thrombin and facilitates macrophage attachment to erythrocytes, marking them for destruction. Mature erythrocytes are unable to synthesize fatty acids, phospholipids, or cholesterol de novo and depend on lipid exchange and fatty acid acylation as mechanisms for phospholipid repair and renewal.

Membrane Proteins

Membrane proteins are classified as *integral*, penetrating or crossing the lipid bilayer and interacting with the hydrophobic lipid core, or *peripheral*, interacting with integral proteins or lipids at the membrane surface but not penetrating into the bilayer core. Integral membrane proteins include the glycophorins, the Rh proteins, Kell and Duffy antigens, and transport proteins such as band 3 (AE1, anion exchanger 1, SLC4A1), Na⁺,K⁺-ATPase, Ca^{2+}-ATPase, and Mg^{2+}-ATPase. Numerous membrane receptors and antigens are present on integral membrane proteins. Peripheral membrane proteins are on the cytoplasmic membrane face and include enzymes such as glyceraldehyde 3-phosphate dehydrogenase and the structural proteins of the spectrin-actin–based membrane skeleton.

Integral Membrane Proteins

Band 3, the major integral protein of the red cell, has two primary functions: ion transport and maintenance of protein-protein interactions. Band 3 mediates chloride-bicarbonate exchange and provides a binding site for glycolytic enzymes, hemoglobin, and the skeletal proteins ankyrin, protein 4.1, and protein 4.2. A single *N*-glycan chain attached to an Asn in the membrane spanning domain of band 3 is composed of *N*-acetyl-D-lactosamine units arranged in an unbranched, linear fashion in fetal erythrocytes (i antigen) and in a branched fashion in adult cells (I antigen).

The glycophorins are the next most abundant family of integral membrane proteins. They provide most of the negative surface charge required by red cells to avoid sticking to each other and to the vascular wall. They are involved in transmembrane signaling and carry receptors for *Plasmodium falciparum*, a number of viruses and bacteria, and several blood group antigens.

Peripheral Membrane Proteins

Spectrin is the major component of the membrane skeleton. It is composed of two subunits, α and β spectrin, that are structurally related but functionally distinct. Spectrin is highly flexible and assumes a variety of conformations, an unusual property that may be critical for normal membrane pliancy. The spectrin-based membrane skeleton is linked to the plasma membrane through the actin-protein 4.1 junctional complex, through spectrin-ankyrin interactions, and through binding of a multiprotein complex containing Rh proteins, Rh-associated glycoproteins, CD47, LW, glycophorin B, and protein 4.2 to ankyrin. Protein 4.1, a protein necessary for normal membrane stability,

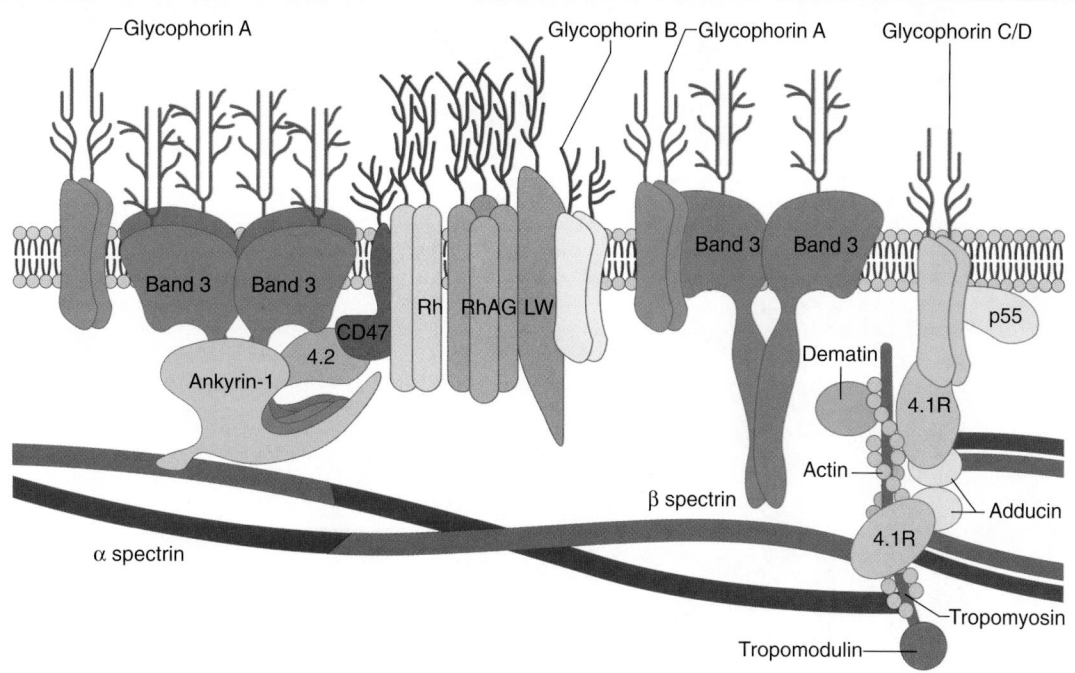

FIGURE 164-1. The erythrocyte membrane. A model of the major proteins of the erythrocyte membrane is shown: α and β spectrin, ankyrin, band 3 (the anion exchanger), 4.1 (protein 4.1) and 4.2 (protein 4.2), actin, and glycophorin. (From Perrotta S, Gallagher PG, Mohandas N. Hereditary spherocytosis. *Lancet.* 2008; 372:1411-1426.)

interacts with spectrin, actin, and other proteins of the red cell membrane. Ankyrin serves as the primary linkage protein for the high-affinity binding of spectrin to the inner membrane through interactions with the cytoplasmic domain of band 3. Protein 4.2 is a peripheral membrane protein that helps link the skeleton to the lipid bilayer through interactions with ankyrin and band 3.

Erythrocyte membrane disorders result from alterations in the quantity or quality (or both) of individual proteins and their dynamic interactions with each other. Disruption of the vertical protein-protein interactions of the membrane, that is, the spectrin-ankyrin–band 3 linkage or the band 3–protein 4.2 interaction, leads to uncoupling of the membrane skeleton from the lipid bilayer. This leads to membrane instability with loss of lipids and some integral membrane proteins, resulting in loss of membrane surface area and the phenotype of spherocytosis. Disruption of the horizontal interactions of membrane skeleton proteins, including perturbation of spectrin self-association or junctional complex protein-protein interactions, leads to membrane instability, altered membrane deformability and mechanical properties, and the phenotype of elliptocytosis.

DISORDERS OF THE ERYTHROCYTE MEMBRANE

Hemolytic anemias due to defects in the erythrocyte membrane comprise an important group of hereditary anemias. Hereditary spherocytosis (HS), hereditary elliptocytosis (HE), and hereditary pyropoikilocytosis (HPP) are the most common disorders among this group. Detailed clinical studies carried out years ago have now been complemented by biochemical and genetic studies, providing both a better understanding of the pathogenesis of these disorders and a better understanding of the normal biology of the erythrocyte membrane.

Hereditary Spherocytosis

DEFINITION

HS refers to a group of disorders characterized by spherical erythrocytes on the peripheral blood smear. Clinical, laboratory, and genetic heterogeneity characterize this group of disorders.

EPIDEMIOLOGY

HS affects approximately 1 in 2000 to 3000 individuals of northern European ancestry. Found worldwide, it is much more common in whites than individuals of African ancestry.

PATHOBIOLOGY

The primary defect in HS is the loss of erythrocyte membrane surface area due to defects in erythrocyte membrane proteins including α spectrin, β spectrin, ankyrin, band 3, and protein 4.2. Qualitative or quantitative defects of one or more of these membrane proteins lead to membrane instability,

which, in turn, leads to membrane loss. In approximately two thirds of HS patients, inheritance is autosomal dominant. In the remaining patients, inheritance is nondominant owing to a de novo mutation or autosomal recessive inheritance. Cases with autosomal recessive inheritance are due to defects in either α spectrin or protein 4.2. Rare cases of homozygous HS have been reported, resulting in fetal death or severe hemolytic anemia. In most cases, HS mutations are "private," that is, each individual has a unique mutation, implying that there is no selective advantage to HS.

The spleen plays a critical, albeit secondary, role in the pathophysiology of HS. Splenic destruction of poorly deformable spherocytes is the primary cause of hemolysis experienced by HS patients. Abnormal erythrocytes are trapped in the splenic microcirculation and ingested by phagocytes. Moreover, the splenic environment is hostile to erythrocytes, with low pH, low glucose, and low ATP concentrations and high local concentrations of toxic free radicals produced by adjacent phagocytes, all contributing to membrane damage.

CLINICAL MANIFESTATIONS

The clinical manifestations of the spherocytosis syndromes vary widely. The classic triad of HS is anemia, jaundice, and splenomegaly. Rarely, patients may suffer from severe hemolytic anemia presenting in utero or shortly after birth, continuing through the first year of life. These patients may require multiple blood transfusions, and in some cases, splenectomy in the first year of life. Many HS patients escape detection throughout childhood. In these patients, the diagnosis of HS may not be made until they are being evaluated for unrelated disorders later in life or when complications related to anemia or chronic hemolysis occur. Although the life span of the erythrocyte in these patients may be shortened to only 20 to 30 days, they adequately compensate for their hemolysis with increased marrow erythropoiesis.

Chronic hemolysis leads to the formation of bilirubinate gallstones, the most frequently reported complication in HS patients. Although gallstones have been observed in early childhood, most appear in adolescents and young adults. Routine interval ultrasonography to detect gallstones should be performed, even if patients are asymptomatic.

Other complications of HS include aplastic, hemolytic, and megaloblastic crises. Aplastic crises occur after virally induced bone marrow suppression and present with anemia, jaundice, fever, and vomiting. The most common etiologic agent in these cases is parvovirus B19 (Chapter 379). Hemolytic crises, usually associated with viral illnesses and occurring before 6 years of age, are generally mild and present with jaundice, increased spleen size, and a decrease in hematocrit. Megaloblastic crises occur in HS patients with increased folate demands, such as the pregnant patient, growing children, or patients recovering from an aplastic crisis.

Uncommon manifestations of HS include skin ulceration, gout, chronic leg dermatitis, cardiomyopathy, spinal cord dysfunction, movement

FIGURE 164-2. Peripheral blood smears in disorders of erythrocyte shape. **A,** Hereditary spherocytosis. Characteristic spherocytes lacking central pallor are seen. **B,** Hereditary elliptocytosis. Smooth, cigar-shaped elliptocytes are seen. **C,** Hereditary pyropoikilocytosis. Pronounced microcytosis, poikilocytosis, fragmentation of erythrocytes and elliptocytes are seen. **D,** Hereditary stomatocytosis.

disorders, and extramedullary erythropoiesis. In patients with untreated severe HS, poor growth and findings attributable to extramedullary hematopoiesis, such as hand and skull deformities, may be found.

DIAGNOSIS

Patients with HS may present at any age, usually with anemia, hyperbilirubinemia, or an abnormal blood smear. In evaluating a patient with suspected HS, particular attention should be paid to the family history, including questions about anemia, jaundice, gallstones, and splenectomy. Initial laboratory investigation should include a complete blood count with a peripheral smear, reticulocyte count, direct antiglobulin test (Coombs' test), and serum bilirubin. When the peripheral smear or family history is suggestive of hereditary spherocytosis, an incubated osmotic fragility test (discussed later) should be obtained. Rarely, additional, specialized testing is required to confirm the diagnosis.

Overall, laboratory findings in HS are heterogeneous. Erythrocyte morphology is distinctive but not diagnostic (Fig. 164-2A). Typical HS patients have blood smears with easily identifiable spherocytes lacking central pallor. Some patients present with only a few spherocytes on peripheral smear, whereas others present with numerous small, dense spherocytes and bizarre erythrocyte morphology. Specific morphologic findings have been identified in patients with certain membrane protein defects such as pincered erythrocytes (band 3) or spherocytic acanthocytes (β spectrin). When examining a smear in a case of suspected spherocytosis, it is important to have a high-quality smear with the erythrocytes well separated and some cells with central pallor in the field of examination because spherocytes are a common artifact on peripheral blood smears. The presence of spherocytosis on peripheral blood smear is not diagnostic of HS. Other disorders with spherocytes on peripheral blood smear are listed in Table 164-1.

The mean corpuscular hemoglobin concentration (MCHC) is increased (between 34.5 and 38) owing to relative cellular dehydration. The mean corpuscular volume (MCV) is usually normal or slightly decreased. Technicon and Advia (Siemens Diagnostics, Deerfield, Ill) blood counters provide a histogram of MCHCs claimed to be accurate enough to identify nearly all HS patients.

In the normal erythrocyte, a redundancy of cell membrane gives the cell its characteristic discoid shape and provides it with abundant surface area. In spherocytes, there is a decrease in surface area relative to cell volume, resulting in their abnormal shape. This change is reflected in the increased osmotic fragility found in these cells. Osmotic fragility is tested by adding increasingly hypotonic concentrations of saline to red cells. Normal erythrocytes are able to increase their volume by swelling, but spherocytes, which are already at maximal volume for surface area, burst at higher saline concentrations than normal. Approximately one fourth of HS individuals will have a normal

TABLE 164-1	DISORDERS WITH SPHEROCYTES ON PERIPHERAL BLOOD FILM

Hereditary spherocytosis
Autoimmune hemolytic anemia
Thermal injuries
Microangiopathic and macroangiopathic hemolytic anemias
Hepatic disease
Clostridial septicemia
Transfusion reactions with hemolysis
Poisoning with certain snake, spider, and Hymenoptera venoms
Severe hypophosphatemia
Heinz body anemias
ABO incompatibility (in neonates)

osmotic fragility on freshly drawn red blood cells, with the osmotic fragility curve approximating the number of spherocytes seen on peripheral smear. However, after incubation at 37° C for 24 hours, HS red cells lose membrane surface area more readily than normal because their membranes have become leaky and unstable. Thus, incubation accentuates the defect in HS erythrocytes and brings out the defect on osmotic fragility, making incubated osmotic fragility the standard test in diagnosing HS. When the spleen is present, a subpopulation of very fragile erythrocytes that have been conditioned by the spleen form the tail of the osmotic fragility curve. This tail disappears after splenectomy. The osmotic fragility test suffers from poor sensitivity, with as many as 20% of mild cases of HS missed after incubation. It is unreliable in patients who have small numbers of spherocytes and in patients who have been recently transfused. It is abnormal in other conditions in which spherocytes are present.

Specialized testing is available for studying difficult cases or cases in which additional information is desired. Useful tests for these purposes include structural and functional studies of erythrocyte membrane proteins, such as protein quantitation, limited tryptic digestion of spectrin, spectrin, and ion transport. Membrane frigidity and fragility may be examined using an ektacytometer. Complementary DNA and genomic DNA analyses are available when a molecular diagnosis is desired.

Other laboratory manifestations in HS are manifestations of ongoing hemolysis. Increased serum bilirubin, increased lactate dehydrogenase, increased urinary and fecal urobilinogen, and decreased serum haptoglobin reflect increased erythrocyte destruction.

After diagnosing a patient with HS, family members should be examined for the presence of HS. This can be of great epidemiologic importance, particularly for very old and very young patients. Prenatal diagnosis of HS has been made in a few cases, but this is rarely necessary.

TREATMENT AND OUTCOME

Splenic sequestration and destruction is the primary determinant of erythrocyte survival in HS patients. Splenectomy cures or alleviates the anemia in most patients, reducing or eliminating the need for transfusions. The risk for cholelithiasis is also decreased to nearly background levels. After splenectomy, spherocytes remain in the peripheral blood, but their life span becomes near normal.

In the past, splenectomy was routinely performed in all HS patients. However, the risk of overwhelming postsplenectomy infection, the emergence of penicillin-resistant pneumococci, and the growing recognition of the increased risk of postsplenectomy cardiovascular disease, particularly thrombosis and pulmonary hypertension, have led to reevaluation of the role of splenectomy in the treatment of HS. In addition, with growing globalization, the important role of the spleen in protection of individuals living in or traveling to geographic regions where parasitic diseases such as malaria or babesiosis occur has re-emerged. When splenectomy is considered, health care providers, the patient, and family members must review and weigh the benefits of splenectomy against the immediate and long-term risks of the procedure. Considering the risks and benefits, a reasonable approach is to splenectomize all patients with severe spherocytosis and all patients suffering from significant signs or symptoms of anemia, including growth failure, skeletal changes, leg ulcers, and extramedullary hematopoietic tumors. Other candidates for splenectomy are older HS patients suffering from vascular compromise of vital organs. Whether patients with moderate HS and compensated, asymptomatic anemia should undergo splenectomy is controversial.

When splenectomy is indicated, laparoscopic splenectomy has become the method of choice. This technique results in less postoperative discomfort, a quicker return to preoperative diet and activities, shorter hospitalization, decreased costs, and smaller scars. Even massive spleens can be removed laparoscopically because the spleen is placed in a large bag, diced intraoperatively, and eliminated through suction catheters. Partial splenectomy, initially advocated for infants and young children with significant anemia associated with erythrocyte membrane disorders to allow for palliation of hemolysis and anemia while maintaining some residual splenic immune function, is now being suggested by some for most HS patients.

Before splenectomy, patients should be immunized with vaccines against pneumococcus, *Haemophilus influenzae* type B, and meningococcus. Postsplenectomy care includes counseling of patients or parents to seek prompt medical care in case of febrile illness. Use of routine antibiotics after splenectomy for prevention of pneumococcal sepsis is controversial. Data are lacking to indicate or refute their prescription. Before splenectomy and, in severe cases, after splenectomy, HS patients should take folic acid (1 mg/day orally) to prevent folate deficiency.

Hereditary Elliptocytosis and Related Disorders

DEFINITION

HE is characterized by the presence of elliptical or oval cigar-shaped erythrocytes on peripheral blood smears of affected individuals (see Fig. 164-2B).

EPIDEMIOLOGY

HE has been estimated to occur in approximately 1 in 2000 to 4000 individuals. The true incidence of HE is unknown because its clinical severity is heterogeneous and many patients are asymptomatic. It is common in African Americans and people of Mediterranean ancestry, presumably because elliptocytes confer some resistance to malaria. In parts of Africa, the incidence of HE approaches 1 in 100.

PATHOBIOLOGY

The principal defect in HE is mechanical weakness or fragility of the erythrocyte membrane skeleton. Qualitative and quantitative defects in a number of red cell membrane proteins have been described in HE, including α spectrin, β spectrin, protein 4.1, and glycophorin C. Most defects occur in spectrin, the principal structural protein of the erythrocyte membrane skeleton. αβ Spectrin heterodimers self-associate into tetramers and higher-order oligomers that are critical for erythrocyte membrane stability as well as erythrocyte shape and function. Most spectrin defects in HE impair the ability of spectrin dimers to self associate into tetramers and oligomers, thereby disrupting the membrane skeleton. Structural and functional defects of protein 4.1 appear to disrupt the spectrin-actin contact in the membrane skeleton. Glycophorin C variants are also deficient in protein 4.1. The precise pathobiology of how elliptocytes are formed in these syndromes is unclear.

Genetically, HE is heterogeneous with multiple genetic loci. A wide variety of mutations have been described in the α spectrin, β spectrin, protein 4.1, and glycophorin C genes, including point mutations, gene deletions and insertions, and messenger RNA processing defects. Several mutations have been identified in a number of individuals on the same genetic background, suggesting a "founder effect" for these mutants, which supports the hypothesis that there has been genetic selection for elliptocytosis because these red cells confer some resistance to malaria. Most cases of HE are inherited in an autosomal dominant pattern, with rare cases of de novo mutations.

CLINICAL MANIFESTATIONS

The clinical presentation of HE is heterogeneous, ranging from asymptomatic carriers to patients with severe, life-threatening anemia. Most HE patients are asymptomatic and are diagnosed incidentally during testing for unrelated conditions. Asymptomatic carriers have been identified who posses the same molecular defect as an affected HE relative but who have normal peripheral blood smears. The erythrocyte life span, normal in most patients, is decreased in only about 10% of patients. It is this subset of HE patients with decreased erythrocyte life span who experience hemolysis, anemia, splenomegaly, and intermittent jaundice. Many of these patients have parents with typical HE and thus are homozygotes or compound heterozygotes for defects inherited from each of the parents. Symptoms may vary among members of the same family, indeed, they may vary in the same individual at different times.

Hereditary Pyropoikilocytosis

HPP is a rare cause of anemia with distinctive erythrocyte morphology on peripheral blood smear (see Fig. 164-2C) and has a picture similar to that seen in patients suffering severe burns. Patients typically present in infancy with severe anemia and peripheral blood smear findings of elliptocytosis, poikilocytosis, pyknocytosis, and fragmentation. Microspherocytosis is common, and the MCV is usually very low (50 to 70 fL). The incubated osmotic fragility is increased. Most patients are of African ancestry, and at least one third of HPP patients have a parent or sibling with typical HE. Patients with HPP tend to experience severe hemolysis and anemia in infancy that gradually improves, evolving toward typical HE later in life.

DIAGNOSIS

Cigar-shaped elliptocytes on peripheral blood smear are the hallmark of HE (see Fig. 164-2B). These normochromic, normocytic elliptocytes vary in number from a few to 100%, with the likelihood of hemolysis not correlating with the number of elliptocytes present. Ovalocytes, spherocytes, stomatocytes, and fragmented cells may also be seen. In some cases, pyknocytes may be prominent. Elliptocytes may be seen in association with other disorders, including megaloblastic anemias, hypochromic microcytic anemias (iron deficiency anemia and thalassemia), myelodysplastic syndromes, and myelofibrosis; however, elliptocytes generally make up less than one third of red cells in these conditions. History and additional laboratory testing usually clarify the diagnosis of these disorders. In typical cases, the incubated osmotic fragility is normal, whereas in severe HE and HPP, osmotic fragility is increased.

Other laboratory findings in HE are similar to those found in other hemolytic anemias and are nonspecific markers of increased erythrocyte production and destruction. The reticulocyte count generally is less than 5% but may be higher when hemolysis is severe.

Like HS, specialized laboratory procedures are available to study the erythrocyte membranes of HE and HPP patients. These studies are not routinely required to make the diagnosis of HE or HPP, but they may be helpful in studying problematic cases and in elucidating the underlying molecular defects.

TREATMENT

Therapy is rarely needed in patients with HE. In rare cases, occasional red blood cell transfusions may be required. In cases of severe HE and HPP, splenectomy has been palliative because the spleen is the site of erythrocyte sequestration and destruction. Many practitioners think that the same indications for splenectomy in HS should be applied to patients with symptomatic HE or HPP. Postsplenectomy patients with HE or HPP experience increased hematocrits, decreased reticulocyte counts, and improvement in clinical symptoms.

Patients should be followed for signs of decompensation during acute illnesses. Interval ultrasonography to detect gallstones should be performed. In patients with significant hemolysis, folate should be administered daily.

Hereditary Stomatocytosis Syndromes

Red cell hydration is primarily determined by the intracellular concentration of monovalent cations. A net increase in sodium and potassium ions causes water to enter, forming *stomatocytes* (see Fig. 164-2D) or *hydrocytes,* whereas a net loss of sodium and potassium produces dehydrated red cells, or *xerocytes.* Numerous descriptions of congenital or familial hemolytic anemias associated with abnormal cation permeability and, in some cases, disturbed red cell hydration have been reported. These span the range from severe hydrocytosis to severe xerocytosis. In most cases, the molecular bases of this group of disorders are unknown. An unusual characteristic of the stomatocytosis syndromes is a predisposition to thrombosis after splenectomy. Acquired stomatocytosis has been associated with acute alcoholism and hepatobiliary disease, vinca alkaloid administration, neoplasms, and cardiovascular disease. Stomatocytosis is also sometimes observed as a processing artifact.

OVERHYDRATED HEREDITARY STOMATOCYTOSIS (HYDROCYTOSIS)

This group of disorders is characterized by stomatocytes, erythrocytes with a mouth-shaped (stoma) area of central pallor on peripheral blood smear (see Fig. 164-2D), severe hemolysis, macrocytosis (110 to 150 fL), elevated erythrocyte sodium concentration, reduced potassium concentration, and increased total Na$^+$ and K$^+$ content. The excess cations elevate cell water, producing large, osmotically fragile cells with a low MCHC (24 to 30%). The clinical severity of overhydrated hereditary stomatocytosis is variable; some patients experience hemolysis and anemia, whereas others are asymptomatic.

DEHYDRATED HEREDITARY STOMATOCYTOSIS (XEROCYTOSIS)

Blood smears from patients with dehydrated hereditary stomatocytosis exhibit contracted and spiculated red cells, dessicytes, a variable number of stomatocytes, and target cells. Most patients have nearly normal erythrocyte morphology, with only a few target cells and an occasional echinocyte or stomatocyte. The MCHC and MCV (95 to 115 fL) are increased, and the osmotic fragility is decreased (i.e., resistance to osmotic lysis). The characteristic biochemical abnormality is a reduced potassium concentration and total monovalent cation content.

INTERMEDIATE SYNDROMES AND HEREDITARY STOMATOCYTOSIS VARIANTS

Hydrocytosis and xerocytosis represent the extremes of a spectrum of red cell permeability defects. A number of families with features of both conditions have been reported. Some patients with severe permeability defects have little or no hemolysis. The proportion of stomatocytes and the degree of sodium influx do not correlate with each other, and neither correlates with the amount of hemolysis or anemia.

● ERYTHROCYTE METABOLISM

The primary functions of the erythrocyte, gas transport and exchange, are maintained without a net change in energy state. However, several critical functions of the erythrocyte depend on the production and expenditure of energy. As erythrocytes age, glucose utilization and ATP levels fall, leading to decreased membrane deformability and, ultimately, shortened life span. Lower potassium levels, higher sodium levels, and decreased membrane lipids are also seen in ATP-deficient, aging erythrocytes.

Erythrocytes do not undergo oxidative phosphorylation and do not store glycogen, thus they must constantly catabolize glucose from the blood stream through the Embden-Meyerhof pathway and the hexose monophosphate shunt as a source of energy (Fig. 164-3). Erythrocytes incorporate glucose from the plasma through facilitated transfer, with erythrocyte glucose levels rapidly equilibrating with changes in blood glucose levels. Glucose is the preferred carbohydrate of the red cell, but fructose and mannose are metabolized almost as readily. Inside the erythrocyte, glucose is converted to glucose-6-phosphate or to fructose by sorbitol. Glucose-6-phosphate follows one of three pathways: (1) most (~90%) enters the Embden-Meyerhof pathway,

FIGURE 164-3. Pathways of energy metabolism in the erythrocyte. Glucose 6-phosphate may be degraded anaerobically to lactate through the Embden-Meyerhof pathway, or oxidatively through the hexose monophosphate shunt. Pentose phosphates (R-5-P) can reenter anaerobic glycolysis as fructose 6-phosphate (F-6-P) and glyceraldehyde 3-phosphate (G-3-P) after conversion by enzymes of the terminal pentose phosphate pathway or as a product of adenosine or inosine degradation. 2,3-Diphosphoglycerate (2,3-DPG) may be generated instead of adenosine triphosphate (ATP) through diversion of triose through the Rapoport-Luebering shunt. Glutathione may be synthesized directly from constituent amino acids; its cycling from oxidized (GSSG) to reduced forms (GSH) depends on reduced pyridine cofactor (NADPH) generation. ADP = adenosine diphosphate; DHAP = dihydroxyacetone phosphate; FDP = fructose 1,6-diphosphate; NAD = nicotinamide adenine dinucleotide; NADP = nicotinamide adenine dinucleotide phosphate; NADPH = nicotinamide adenine dinucleotide phosphate, reduced form; PEP = polyestradiol phosphate.

where it is converted into lactate, pyruvate, and ATP; (2) some (~5 to 10%) enters the hexose monophosphate shunt to produce reduced intermediates and ribulose 5-phosphate, the latter of which eventually enters the Embden-Meyerhof pathway; and (3) a tiny fraction (<1%) is converted to glucose-1-phosphate and then to glycogen.

Embden-Meyerhof Pathway

The Embden-Meyerhof Pathway of glycolysis is the primary source of ATP, 2,3-DPG and nicotinamide adenine dinucleotide, reduced form (NADH) in the erythrocyte (see Fig. 164-3). Most of the energy generated by erythrocytes is through the Embden-Meyerhof pathway, followed by storage as high-energy phosphates such as ATP or as reducing energy in the form of glutathione or pyridine nucleotides (NADH and nicotinamide adenine dinucleotide phosphate, reduced form [NADPH]). This pathway metabolizes about 90% of erythrocyte glucose with the catabolism of 1 mole of glucose yielding 2 moles of ATP and 2 moles of lactate. Two moles of ATP per mole of metabolized glucose seems insignificant compared with the Krebs cycle of intermediary metabolism, in which 1 mole of glucose metabolized produces 38 moles of ATP. However, this ATP production is adequate to renew 150 to 200% of the total red cell ATP every hour.

The Embden-Meyerhof pathway is also the primary source of NADH, a necessary cofactor for NADH methemoglobin reductase, which maintains heme iron in the reduced state. Without this reaction, heme iron would be oxidized to methemoglobin, which is not a functional oxygen transporter.

Finally, the Rapoport-Luebering shunt of the Embden-Meyerhof pathway (see Fig. 164-3) produces 2,3-DPG, a compound found in high concentrations in erythrocytes, but in low concentrations in other cells. Once formed, under physiologic conditions of pH and solute concentrations, 2,3-DPG binds reversibly to tetramers of deoxyhemoglobin with greater affinity than it does to oxyhemoglobin. By binding to deoxyhemoglobin, it allosterically upregulates the release of the remaining oxygen bound to the hemoglobin, enhancing the ability of erythrocytes to release oxygen near tissues that need it most.

Hexose Monophosphate Shunt (Pentose Phosphate Pathway)

In the HMP shunt (see Fig. 164-3), glucose-6-phosphate undergoes oxidation followed by a series of reactions to yield fructose-6-phosphate and glyceraldehyde-3-phosphate, intermediates in the glycolytic pathway. The HMP shunt is the primary source of erythrocyte NADPH, with 2 moles of NADPH produced for each mole of glucose metabolized. NADPH is required for the reduction of oxidized glutathione and some protein sulfhydryl groups.

Mature erythrocytes synthesize large amounts of reduced glutathione (GSH). GSH protects erythrocytes from oxidants, including hydrogen peroxide (H_2O_2), superoxide anions (O_2^-), and hydroxyl radicals (OH), which are produced as byproducts of the oxidation of heme by oxygen. Oxidants are also produced by activated phagocytes (e.g., during infection) and by erythrocytes after exposure to certain agents. When oxidants accumulate, they damage cellular proteins and lipids. Detoxification of H_2O_2 is significantly enhanced by glutathione peroxidase. GSH is converted to oxidized glutathione (GSSG) and to mixed disulfides with protein thiols. GSH levels are restored by glutathione reductase. In this process, NADPH is oxidized to nicotinamide adenine dinucleotide phosphate (NADP), which stimulates the HMP shunt to regenerate NADPH. After oxidant stress, hypoxia, or acidosis, erythrocytes can increase the amount of glucose metabolized through the HMP shunt up to 10- to 20-fold to generate increased amounts of reduced glutathione. The tight coupling of glutathione metabolism with the HMP shunt protects the mature erythrocyte from oxidative stress.

● DISORDERS OF ERYTHROCYTE METABOLISM

Congenital nonspherocytic hemolytic anemia (CNSHA) traditionally includes erythrocyte disorders not due to defects of the red cell membrane or hemoglobin, immune-mediated disease, or other diseases such as paroxysmal nocturnal hemoglobinuria. CNSHA is a heterogeneous group of disorders associated with various metabolic abnormalities of the erythrocyte, including enzymopathies of glucose, glutathione, and nucleotide metabolism. Like the membrane disorders, clinical, biochemical, and genetic heterogeneity are typical within the enzymopathies. Hemolysis may develop as a result of either enzyme or antioxidant deficiency or dysfunction (e.g., abnormal substrate or cofactor binding), altered activation or inhibition characteristics, or decreased stability or specific activity.

Peripheral blood smears in CNSHA, with the exception of pyrimidine 5′-nucleotidase deficiency, are unremarkable. Osmotic fragility of fresh erythrocytes is normal. Response to splenectomy is variable. Inheritance is

heterogeneous. A thorough family history is important and may be of assistance in determining the diagnosis. Manifestations of the metabolic defect are usually confined to the erythrocyte but may occasionally involve nonerythroid cells.

Definitive diagnosis of metabolic abnormalities of the red cell depend on qualitative or quantitative assays of specific enzyme activity or identification of the specific genetic mutation by DNA analysis. Results of enzyme assays should be interpreted with caution because (1) they only sample surviving red cells in the peripheral blood, and the metabolic milieu of these cells is not necessarily comparable to cells already hemolyzed; (2) in vitro enzyme assay conditions may not accurately reflect the in vivo environment; (3) transfusions before the assay may obscure the underlying metabolic defect, and (4) leukocyte contamination may lead to spurious results. Finally, average enzyme activity may not accurately reflect activity in subpopulations of erythrocytes. This is particularly true when there is reticulocytosis, which may yield artificially elevated mean enzyme activity owing to higher enzyme levels found in reticulocytes.

Disorders of the Embden-Meyerhof Pathway

Defects of the Embden-Meyerhof pathway are inherited in an autosomal recessive fashion, and usually hemolysis is seen only in homozygotes or compound heterozygotes. Heterozygotes, whose erythrocytes contain less than normal amounts of mutant enzyme, are clinically normal.

An exception is phosphoglycerate kinase deficiency, an X-linked disorder with hemolysis found only in males. In this group of disorders, hemolysis is chronic, is not typically influenced by drugs or other inciting agents, and is attributed to insufficient levels of erythrocyte ATP. Splenomegaly from trapping of mutant erythrocytes is common. The hostile splenic environment contributes to the shortened erythrocyte life span. When performing specific diagnostic enzyme assays, measurement of glycolytic intermediates may assist in diagnosis because concentrations of intermediates is increased upstream of a defect and decreased downstream of a defect.

PYRUVATE KINASE DEFICIENCY

Pyruvate kinase (PK) deficiency accounts for approximately 90% of inherited defects of the Embden-Meyerhof pathway and is the second most common inherited erythrocyte enzymopathy associated with anemia after glucose-6-phosphate dehydrogenase (G6PD) deficiency (see later). PK deficiency is found worldwide, but it is most common in individuals of northern European descent.

▶ PATHOBIOLOGY

PK catalyzes the conversion of phosphoenolpyruvate (PEP) to pyruvate, generating ATP. Deficient or defective PK leads to decreased levels of erythrocyte ATP, disturbing many cellular processes such as signaling and maintenance of water and ion content, leading to energy failure and dehydration. Upstream catabolites accumulate in the erythrocyte, including 2,3-DPG, which shifts the oxygen dissociation curve to the right, enhancing tissue oxygenation and ameliorating some of the physiologic effects of anemia. Early PK-deficient reticulocytes retain the ability to utilize oxidative phosphorylation to produce ATP, bypassing their defect. This ability is lost as reticulocytes mature and is markedly dampened in the hypoxic environment of the spleen.

PK deficiency is inherited in an autosomal recessive manner. Affected individuals are homozygous or compound heterozygotes for PK defects. Heterozygotes are clinically normal or exhibit very minimal hemolysis.

▶ CLINICAL MANIFESTATIONS

Clinical manifestations in PK deficiency are heterogeneous, ranging from asymptomatic to transfusion-dependent hemolytic anemia. More severely affected patients present in infancy or early childhood with anemia, jaundice, and splenomegaly. Occasionally, patients may escape detection until later in life when complications related to anemia and chronic hemolysis occur such as cholelithiasis or aplastic crisis or when the diagnosis is made during evaluation of the patient for another condition.

▶ DIAGNOSIS

Peripheral blood smear demonstrates normocytic, normochromic erythrocytes, sometimes with spiculations (Fig. 164-4A). Poikilocytes and acanthocytes may also be seen. Reticulocytosis is common. Osmotic fragility of fresh erythrocytes is usually normal. Occasional patients exhibit a population of osmotically fragile cells after incubation.

FIGURE 164-4. Peripheral blood smears in erythrocyte enzymopathies. **A,** Pyruvate kinase deficiency. **B,** Pyrimidine 5′-nucleotidase deficiency; **C,** Glucose-6-phosphate dehydrogenase (G6PD) deficiency. **D,** Heinz bodies in G6PD deficiency. (**B** from Paglia DE. Disorders of erythrocyte glycolysis and nucleotide metabolism. In: Handin RI, Lux SE, Stossel TP, eds. *Blood: Principles and Practice of Hematology.* Philadelphia: JB Lippincott; 1995:1877-1896.)

NADH fluorescence under ultraviolet light is a commonly used screening test for PK deficiency. PEP and NADH are mixed with the patient's blood, incubated, and spotted on filter paper, and fluorescence is measured. Direct enzyme assay, which uses PEP as substrate for PK, can be performed on leukocyte-free hemolysate to confirm abnormal fluorescence tests. Leukocytes must be carefully depleted from the samples because they contain over 300 times the PK activity of erythrocytes.

TREATMENT   Rx

Most patients require only expectant management, with only rare transfusions, such as during an aplastic episode. In severe cases, patients may be transfusion dependent. In these cases, splenectomy typically lessens hemolysis and ameliorates the anemia. After splenectomy, some patients develop marked reticulocytosis, up to 50 to 70%. This paradoxical reticulocytosis is attributed to increased reticulocyte survival after removal of the hostile splenic environment.

OTHER DISORDERS OF THE EMBDEN-MEYERHOF PATHWAY
Other abnormalities of the Embden-Meyerhof pathway have been described. Hexokinase deficiency is quite uncommon, with great phenotypic variability in reported cases. Severely affected patients have suffered from anemia beginning in infancy and may require blood transfusion. Glucose phosphate isomerase (GPI) deficiency is the third most common hemolytic enzymopathy. GPI deficiency usually presents in infancy or early childhood with moderate to severe hemolytic anemia. Phosphofructokinase deficiency may involve erythrocytes, muscle, or both. Presentation is usually in adolescence with exertional myopathy. Hemolytic anemia has been described in isolated cases of 2,3-bisphosphoglycerate mutase deficiency and phosphoglycerate kinase deficiency.

Disorders of Nucleotide Metabolism
Mature erythrocytes lack the ability to synthesize purine and pyrimidine nucleotides de novo. However, they are able to form some nucleotides through salvage pathways.

PYRIMIDINE 5′-NUCLEOTIDASE DEFICIENCY
Pyrimidine 5′-nucleotidase (P5N) degrades the pyrimidine nucleotides of RNA to cytidine and uridine, which can diffuse out of the cell. When P5N is deficient, nondiffusible, partially degraded RNAs accumulate, leading to the marked basophilic stippling characteristic of P5N-deficient erythrocytes

(see Fig. 164-4B). These accumulated pyrimidine nucleotides inhibit the transport of GSSG out of red cells, leading to high levels of erythrocyte glutathione. Clinically, there is mild to moderate hemolytic anemia and splenomegaly. The etiology of the hemolysis remains cryptic. Typically, splenectomy does not ameliorate the hemolysis and anemia.

Disorders of the Hexose Monophosphate Shunt (Pentose Phosphate Pathway) and Associated Pathways
Disorders of the HMP shunt or of the glutathione metabolic pathways (see Fig. 164-3) compromise the ability of the red cell to respond adequately to oxidative stress. In the normal erythrocyte, GSH detoxifies oxidants produced by various agents and infection. In G6PD-deficient erythrocytes, because of the inability to generate NADPH, GSH levels are inadequate, leaving the cell susceptible to oxidant stress. Oxidation of hemoglobin sulfhydryl groups leads to the production of methemoglobin and intracellular hemoglobin precipitates called Heinz bodies. Heinz bodies (see Fig. 164-4D), usually visualized on peripheral blood smears with supravital stains such as methyl violet, attach to and damage the erythrocyte membrane. They induce clustering of immunoglobulins and band 3 protein, marking the erythrocyte for opsonization by phagocytes and eventual removal from the circulation. Heinz bodies are "pitted" from circulating cells by the spleen and are commonly seen on smears of patients after splenectomy. "Bite cells," erythrocytes with localized invaginations, possibly at the site of Heinz body injury or removal, are seen during acute hemolytic episodes. In addition to damage from Heinz body formation, GSH-deficient erythrocytes also undergo peroxidation of membrane phospholipids and oxidative cross-linking of spectrin, decreasing membrane deformability and further promoting splenic trapping.

GLUCOSE-6-PHOSPHATE DEHYDROGENASE DEFICIENCY
G6PD deficiency is the most common inherited disorder of erythrocyte metabolism, affecting more than 400 million people worldwide. The high prevalence of G6PD deficiency is thought to be due to genetic selection because G6PD-deficient erythrocytes have a selective advantage against invasion by the malaria parasite *Plasmodium falciparum*.

EPIDEMIOLOGY AND PATHOBIOLOGY
G6PD is the initial and rate-limiting step in the HMP shunt (see Fig. 164-3), which converts NADP into NADPH. NADPH is required for the generation of glutathione, a critical constituent in the prevention of oxidative damage to

the cell. G6PD-deficient patients may develop acute hemolytic anemia after exposure to oxidative stress. Although G6PD is a ubiquitous enzyme, erythroid cells are particularly susceptible to oxidative stress because the HMP shunt is their only source of NADPH.

Hundreds of G6PD variants have been described, but only a few are common. Variants are classified on the basis of biochemical characteristics, electrophoretic mobility, ability to use substrate analogue, Km for NADP and G6PD, pH activity profile, and thermal stability. The normal enzyme, Gd^B, is present in 99% of white Americans and 70% of African Americans. A normal variant, Gd^{A+}, found in 20% of African Americans, has a faster electrophoretic mobility than Gd^B. Gd^{A-}, the most common variant associated with hemolysis, is found in about 10% of African Americans and in many Africans. Gd^{A-} has decreased catalytic ability compared with Gd^{A+}. Gd^{Med}, the second most common variant associated with hemolysis, is common in the Mediterranean area, in India, and in southeast Asia, with a prevalence of up to 5 to 50%. Gd^{Med} exhibits markedly decreased catalytic activity. Gd^{Canton}, a variant common in Asian populations, produces a clinical syndrome similar to Gd^{A-}.

Gd^B activity decreases as normal cells age, with a half-life of approximately 60 days. Despite very low levels of or no active G6PD, older erythrocytes maintain the ability to produce NADPH and maintain a GSH response to oxidative stress. Gd^{A-} variant has a half-life of only 13 days, so young cells have a normal amount of enzyme activity whereas older red cells are grossly deficient. Because of this heterogeneity in G6PD levels, individuals with the Gd^{A-} variant experience only limited hemolysis after oxidant exposure.

More than 100 mutations in the *G6PD* gene, localized to Xq28, have been described. Most mutations are amino acid substitutions that influence enzyme kinetics, stability, or both, with a few rare deletions and splicing mutations described. Because it is X-linked, G6PD deficiency primarily affects males. Males have only one G6PD allele and express only one G6PD type. Females can express one or two G6PD types. The Lyon hypothesis specifies that only one X chromosome is active in any given cell; thus, any given cell in a heterozygous female is either normal or deficient. In females who are heterozygous for G6PD deficiency, average G6PD activity may be normal or mildly, moderately, or severely reduced, depending on the degree of lyonization. G6PD-deficient erythrocytes in heterozygous females are susceptible to the same oxidant stress as G6PD-deficient cells in males, but, typically, the overall degree of hemolysis is less because there is a smaller population of vulnerable cells.

CLINICAL MANIFESTATIONS

G6PD deficiency is divided into five classes based on clinical severity and degree of enzyme deficiency. Class I is characterized by CNSHA without precipitating cause and severe G6PD deficiency. Class II is characterized by intermittent hemolysis and severe G6PD deficiency. Class III is characterized by hemolysis after oxidant stress and mild G6PD deficiency. Class II and III together represent more than 90% of G6PD variants. Classes IV and V are clinically asymptomatic. The most clinically significant syndromes of G6PD deficiency are acute hemolytic anemia (AHA), neonatal jaundice (NNJ), and rarely, CNSHA.

AHA is the most dramatic clinical presentation of G6PD deficiency with acute intravascular hemolysis after exposure to an oxidative stress. Oxidative stresses include ingestion of certain drugs such as primaquine or sulfa-containing compounds, exposure to naphthalene (mothballs), ingestion of fava beans, or infection, the latter being the most common cause of hemolysis. Table 164-2 lists drugs that should be avoided in G6PD-deficient patients. Presenting symptoms include irritability, fever, nausea, abdominal pain, and diarrhea within 48 hours of oxidant exposure. Hemoglobinuria, jaundice, and anemia ensue. The spleen and liver may be enlarged and tender. Cases with severe anemia may precipitate congestive heart failure. Laboratory findings include a normochromic, normocytic anemia with anisocytosis and reticulocytosis. Poikilocytes and bite cells may be seen. Heinz bodies, a classic finding in G6PD deficiency, may be seen but are an inconsistent finding because these damaged cells are rapidly cleared from the circulation in the spleen. Additional laboratory findings include hemoglobinuria and the presence of free hemoglobin in the blood.

Another clinically significant syndrome of G6PD deficiency is NNJ. Jaundice is seldom present at birth, with the peak incidence of onset between days 2 and 3 of life. The severity of hyperbilirubinemia is variable. It may be severe, resulting in kernicterus or even death. In most cases, however, hyperbilirubinemia is adequately treated with phototherapy. In NNJ, it is important to note that the anemia is very rarely severe. The etiology of NNJ remains controversial. NNJ is increased in G6PD-deficient infants who also carry a

TABLE 164-2 AGENTS TO BE AVOIDED BY GLUCOSE-6-PHOSPHATE DEHYDROGENASE–DEFICIENT PATIENTS*

ANTIMALARIALS

Primaquine (people with the African A⁻ variant may take it at reduced dosage, under surveillance)
Pamaquine
Chloroquine (may be used under surveillance when required for prophylaxis or treatment of malaria)

SULFONAMIDES AND SULFONES

Sulfanilamide
Sulfapyridine
Sulfadimidine
Sulfacetamide (Albucid)
Acetyl sulfisoxazole (Gantrisin)
Salicylazosulfapyridine (Salazopyrin)
Dapsone
Sulfoxone
Glucosulfone sodium (Promin)
Sulfamethoxazole-trimethoprim (Septrin)

OTHER ANTIBACTERIAL COMPOUNDS

Nitrofurans—nitrofurantoin, furazolidone, nitrofurazone
[Nalidixic acid]
Chloramphenicol
p-Aminosalicylic acid

ANALGESICS

Acetylsalicylic acid (aspirin): moderate doses can be used
Acetophenetidin (Phenacetin)
Safe alternative: Paracetamol

ANTHELMINTICS

β-Naphthol
Stibophen
Niridazole

MISCELLANEOUS

Vitamin K analogues (1 mg of menaphthone can be given to babies)
Naphthalene (moth balls)
Probenecid
Dimercaprol (BAL)
Methylene blue
Arsine†
Phenylhydrazine†
Acetylphenylhydrazine†
Toluidine blue
Mepacrine

*Drugs in bold print should be avoided by people with all forms of glucose-6-phosphate dehydrogenase (G6PD) deficiency. Drugs in normal print should be avoided, in addition, by G6PD-deficient people of Mediterranean, Middle Eastern, and Asian origin. Items in normal print and within square brackets apply only to people with the African A⁻ variant.
†These drugs or chemicals may cause hemolysis in normal people if given in large doses. Many other drugs may produce hemolysis in certain individuals.

polymorphism of the uridine diphosphoglucuronyl transferase (*UDPGT1*) gene associated with Gilbert syndrome.

Chronic nonspherocytic hemolytic anemia is associated with uncommon variants of G6PD deficiency, usually mutant enzymes unable to maintain basal NADPH production. Presentation may be in the neonatal period when NNJ is accompanied by anemia in a male. The degree of chronic anemia in CNSHA due to G6PD deficiency has been variable. Some patients have compensated hemolysis, whereas others require intermittent transfusions. Transfusion dependence occurs in the most severe cases.

DIAGNOSIS

The G6PD reaction (glucose-6-phosphate + NADP⁺ → 6-phosphogluconolactone + NADPH + H⁺) reduces NADP⁺ to NADPH. Formation of NADPH and NADH can be observed directly because they fluoresce in the visible spectrum when illuminated with long-wave ultraviolet light. Based on this observation, several simple screening tests performed using inexpensive long-wave ultraviolet light have been devised. These tests are semiquantitative, categorizing a sample as normal or deficient. They are unreliable after an acute hemolytic episode and do not typically detect female heterozygotes. Positive screening tests should be confirmed by spectrophotometric assay or DNA studies.

Definitive assay of the enzyme depends on direct spectrophotometric measurement of NADPH production. Although more sensitive than screening tests, this still requires 20 to 30% G6PD-deficient cells to obtain an abnormal result. Sensitivity can be increased by comparing the level of G6PD deficiency to levels of other age-dependent erythrocyte enzymes, especially when testing is temporally in close proximity to an acute hemolytic episode. The cyanide-ascorbate test measures the ability of erythrocytes to prevent the oxidation of hemoglobin by ascorbate. Employing intact erythrocytes, as few as 10 to 15% deficient cells can be detected, making this test useful for detecting female heterozygotes and males following a hemolytic episode. This test also detects other perturbations of the HMP shunt or glutathione metabolism.

TREATMENT   Rx

The best treatment for the individual with AHA is careful prescription of medications and avoidance of inciting agents (see Table 164-2). Outside of acute hemolytic episodes, these patients do not require any special therapy. AHA episodes are managed with particular attention to hematologic, cardiopulmonary, and renal complications of hemolysis. Management of NNJ does not differ from that recommended for other causes of neonatal hyperbilirubinemia. In CNSHA, management is expectant. Exposure to oxidant stresses should be avoided. Blood transfusions may be necessary during acute hemolytic episodes. In severe cases of CNSHA, splenectomy may ameliorate the anemia.

Disorders of Glutathione Metabolism

Defects of glutathione metabolism may be associated with hemolysis. Erythrocytes from patients lacking glutathione synthetase or γ-glutamylcysteine synthetase, enzymes involved in glutathione synthesis, have very low levels of GSH. Clinically, these disorders resemble G6PD deficiency. There is mild to moderate chronic hemolytic anemia with increased susceptibility to oxidant stress.

 Visit expertconsult.com for e-expanded chapter

SUGGESTED READINGS

Bruce LJ. Hereditary stomatocytosis and cation leaky red cells—recent developments. *Blood Cells Mol Dis.* 2009;42:216-222. *Review of the molecular basis of hereditary stomatocytosis.*

Cappellini MD, Fiorelli G. Glucose-6-phosphate dehydrogenase deficiency. *Lancet.* 2008;371:64-74. *Comprehensive clinical review of the most common human enzyme defect worldwide.*

Iolascon A, Avvisati RA, Piscopo C. Hereditary spherocytosis. *Transfus Clin Biol.* 2010;17:138-142. *Review of the various forms of a condition with a prevalence of about 1 in 2000 among northern Europeans.*

Mohandas N, Gallagher PG. Red cell membrane: past, present and future. *Blood.* 2008;112:3939-3948. *Current concepts of red cell membrane structure and function in health and disease.*

165

THE THALASSEMIAS

MARIA DOMENICA CAPPELLINI

DEFINITION

The thalassemias—or, more comprehensively, the thalassemia syndromes—are a heterogeneous group of inherited hemolytic anemias characterized by deficient or absent production of one of the globin chains of hemoglobin. This leads to imbalanced globin chain synthesis, which is the hallmark of all the thalassemia syndromes.

EPIDEMIOLOGY

Taken together, the thalassemias are the most common single gene disorder in the world population. The estimated number of carriers exceeds 270 million, and more than 300,000 children are born each year with one of the thalassemia syndromes or one of the structural hemoglobin variants. The extremely high frequency of hemoglobin disorders compared with other monogenic diseases reflects natural selection mediated by the relative resistance of carriers against *Plasmodium falciparum* malaria. Other factors that may be involved include the widespread practice of consanguineous marriage

and increased maternal age in poorer countries, and gene drift and founder effects. For these reasons, the thalassemias are most frequent in southeastern and southern Asia, the Middle East, the Mediterranean countries, and northern and central Africa. However, as a result of the mass migration of African populations from high-prevalence areas, thalassemias are now encountered worldwide.

PATHOBIOLOGY

The normal adult red cells contain 97% adult hemoglobin (HbA: $\alpha_2\beta_2$), with approximately 2.5% of the minor component HbA$_2$ ($\alpha_2\delta_2$) and a small amount of fetal hemoglobin (HbF: $\alpha_2\gamma_2$). Because the stable tetramer $\alpha_2\beta_2$ is the major component of hemoglobin after birth, there are two main forms of thalassemia: α-thalassemia and β-thalassemia. Because β-chain synthesis is fully activated only after birth, it follows that the β-thalassemias are not expressed as diseases in intrauterine life; they manifest as γ-chain synthesis declines during the first year of life. In contrast, because α chains are shared by both fetal and adult hemoglobin, α-thalassemias manifest in both fetal and adult life.

As knowledge about their genetic basis and pathophysiologic mechanisms has evolved, the thalassemia syndromes can now be classified at genetic and clinical levels (Table 165-1).

Genetics

Six different types of globin chains (α, β, γ, δ, ε, ζ) are found in normal human hemoglobin at different stages of development. In the very early embryo, hemoglobin synthesis is restricted to the yolk sac and to the production of Hb Gower 1 ($\zeta_2\varepsilon_2$), Gower 2 ($\alpha_2\varepsilon_2$), and Portland ($\zeta_2\gamma_2$). Subsequently, at about 8 weeks of gestation, the fetal liver takes over, synthesizing predominantly HbF ($\alpha_2\gamma_2$) and a small amount (<10%) of HbA. Between about 18 weeks and birth, the liver is progressively replaced by bone marrow as the major site of red cell production. This is accompanied in the later stages of gestation with a reciprocal switch in the production of HbF and HbA; this continues until, by the end of the first year of life, HbF production has dropped to less than 2%. The globin genes are encoded in separate gene clusters. The α cluster (ζ, α_2, α_1) lies at the telomere of chromosome 16, and the β cluster (ε, $^G\gamma$ and $^A\gamma$, δ, β) lies at chromosome 11p15.5. In both clusters the genes are aligned 5′ to 3′ in the order in which they are expressed during development. Both sets of genes are under the regulation of enhancer-like elements (hypersensitive site [HS]-40 for α cluster, and locus control region [LCR] for β cluster) that lie some distance away at the 5′ end of the cluster. Deletion of these enhancer elements results in inactivation of any related globin gene. There are two α genes/alleles (α_2 and α_1) that differ by a few nucleotides in intron 2 and the 3′ untranslated region but produce identical protein products. The output of the α_2 gene exceeds that of the α_1 gene by two- to three-fold. The α cluster also contains pseudo-ζ and pseudo-α genes that are not translated into protein products. The region around a DNase I

TABLE 165-1	GENETIC AND CLINICAL CLASSIFICATIONS OF THE THALASSEMIAS	
	GENETIC	**CLINICAL**
α-Thalassemias	α^0	α-Minor
	α^+	HbH disease
	Deletion (−α)	Hydrops fetalis
	Nondeletion (α^T)	
β-Thalassemias	β^0	β-Minor
	β^+	Thalassemia intermedia
	Variant with high HbA$_2$	Thalassemia major
	Normal HbA$_2$	
	Silent	
	Dominant	
	Unlinked to β-gene cluster	
δβ-Thalassemia	$(\delta\beta)^0$	δβ-Minor
	$(\delta\beta)^+$	Thalassemia intermedia
	$(^A\gamma\delta\beta)^0$	
HPFH	Deletion	Silent increase in HbF
	Nondeletion	
	Unlinked to β-gene cluster	

HbA = adult hemoglobin; HbF = fetal hemoglobin; HbH = hemoglobin H; HPFH = hereditary persistence of fetal hemoglobin.

HS at 40 kb upstream of the ζ-globin gene (HS-40) is the major regulator of α-globin gene expression. The β cluster contains a single pseudo-β gene; the β-cluster "enhancer" consists of five elements marked by erythroid-specific DNase I HSs lying 6 to 20 kb upstream of the ε-globin gene, each of which contains several binding sites for erythroid-specific and other transcription factors. All together, these elements are known as the LCR, and each element contributes to the overall LCR activity. In addition, there is an erythroid-specific HS approximately 20 kb downstream of the β-globin gene; when the cluster is activated, the upstream and downstream HSs are brought into close proximity with the gene promoters to activate their transcription. The individual globin genes share many general features: they consist of three coding sequence exons separated by two introns in identical positions but of variable length, for a total length of approximately 1500 nucleotides. This structure has been highly conserved throughout evolution. The upstream regions flanking the first exon contain a number of sequence motifs that are necessary for specifying correct transcriptional initiation. A TATA box is found at 30 base pairs upstream of the initiation site, together with one or more CCAAT sites at 70 base pairs upstream. The gene promoters also contain a CACCC or CCGCCC box that binds erythroid Krüppel-like factor (EKLF)-1, and some have binding sites for erythroid transcription factor GATA-1. In model systems, mutations introduced into such sequences lead to a reduction in the level of transcription.

All the thalassemias have a similar pattern of inheritance: in most cases, the gene defects are transmitted in a mendelian autosomal fashion. Thus the severe, symptomatic varieties usually result from the interaction of more than one genetic determinant. The inheritance of α-thalassemia is more complicated because it involves the products of the linked pairs of α genes (αα) (see Clinical Manifestations).

Molecular Basis

The α- and β-thalassemias are divided into disorders in which no chains are produced from the affected chromosomes (α^0 and β^0) and those in which the chain output is reduced (α^+ and β^+).

For the α-thalassemias, the most common molecular defects are deletions of one or both α genes, which are designated –α and – –, respectively. The single α gene is believed to have arisen by crossover between two misaligned α genes on the homologous chromosome, which can give rise to chromosomes with either single (–α) or triplicated (ααα) α-globin genes. Depending on the point of crossover, deletions may remove between 2.5 and 5.3 kb of sequence, with the loss of 3.7 ($-\alpha^{3.7}$) or 4.2 ($-\alpha^{4.2}$) kb being most prevalent. Full duplication of the α-globin gene locus, including the upstream regulatory element, has also been reported in subjects of different ancestries, suggesting that this type of homologous genetic recombination occurs relatively frequently in globin loci. To date, more than 20 different deletions that involve both α genes, resulting from illegitimate or nonhomologous recombination, have been reported. The lengths of deletion vary from 5.2 to more than 40 kb, with the most common being those from Southeast Asia, the Mediterranean, and the Philippines, designated $--^{SEA}$, $--^{MED}$, and $--^{FIL}$, respectively. Nondeletion types of α-thalassemia (α^T) are much less common than the deletion forms, and in most cases they result from single oligonucleotide mutations at regions of the α gene sequence that are critical for normal expression. Because expression of the α_2 gene is two to three times greater than that of the α_1 gene, it is not surprising that most of the nondeletion mutants affect predominantly expression of the α_2 gene. The mutations may affect the initiation codon or splicing signals, cause frameshifts, or introduce premature stop codons. At least five single-nucleotide variants affect the natural termination codon (TAA) of the α_2-globin gene. Among these, Hb Constant Spring ($\alpha^{CS}\alpha$) is the most common and extensively studied. Finally, there are several α-globin variants that are so unstable that they undergo very rapid, postsynthetic degradation. In such situations, β chains remain in excess within the red cell, and patient carriers of these α-chain variants, by definition, have α-thalassemia. To date, 17 unstable α variants have been shown to produce the phenotype of α-thalassemia to a greater or lesser extent.

As for the α-thalassemias, the β-thalassemias are classified as β^0 thalassemia (in which no β globin is produced) and β^+ thalassemia (in which some β globin is produced, but less than normal). In some cases the defects in β-chain production are so mild that they are designated β^{++}. So far, more than 200 different thalassemic mutations of the β-globin gene have been reported; the vast majority are point mutations within the gene or its immediate flanking sequence. A few β-thalassemia mutations that segregate independently of the β-globin gene cluster have been described, presumably involving trans-acting regulatory factors. The distribution of alleles is highly variable from one population to another, but within each population, only a few alleles are common. The nondeletion forms of β-thalassemia account for the vast majority of β-thalassemia alleles. An updated list of these mutations is accessible at the Globin Gene Server website: *http://globin.cse.psu.edu.* They include transcriptional mutations, RNA processing mutations, and mutations affecting translation.

Simple deletions of the β-globin gene are rare, ranging in size from 290 base pairs to more than 60 kb. The 619–base pair deletion at the 3′ end of the β gene is relatively common among Sind and Punjabi populations in India and Pakistan. The remaining deletions are restricted to single families and are necessarily β0 thalassemias; interestingly, they are associated with an unusually high level of HbA2 in heterozygotes. Large deletions that affect the entire β-globin gene cluster ($(\epsilon\gamma\gamma\delta\beta)^0$) are rare and restricted to single families. Finally, some highly unstable β-chain variants may manifest as a dominant form of β-thalassemia.

The δβ-thalassemias and the hereditary persistence of fetal hemoglobin (HPFH) are the result of deletions affecting various parts of the β-globin locus. These deletions are partially compensated by an increased expression of the γ genes, which raises the level of HbF. The length of deletion accounts for different forms of δβ-thalassemia, including both $^G\gamma$ and $^A\gamma$ genes or only $^A\gamma$, and this length varies from 9 to 100 kb. Hb Lepore is a hybrid of δ and β chains resulting from a crossover between the two misaligned genes; this hemoglobin is synthesized inefficiently and gives rise to a form of δβ-thalassemia. Deletions of δ and β genes are also the molecular basis for many forms of HPFH that usually have higher levels of compensatory HbF production than the δβ-thalassemias. Other forms of HPFH are due to point mutations in the promoter region upstream from the transcription start site in either the $^G\gamma$ or $^A\gamma$ genes that alter the binding of one or more transcription factors; they are known as nondeletion HPFH. Genetic studies have identified three major quantitative trait loci that account for 20 to 50% of the common variation in HbF levels in patients with β-thalassemia and sickle cell disease, as well as in healthy adults.

CLINICAL MANIFESTATIONS

The clinical manifestations (phenotype expression) of the thalassemia syndromes are extremely variable and depend on the degree of globin chain imbalance.

α-Thalassemias

As previously mentioned, there are two major classes of α-thalassemias: α^0, in which both α genes are inactivated (– –/), and α^+, in which only one of the pair is defective owing to either an α deletion or a mutation (–α or $\alpha\alpha^T$). The clinical spectrum of α-thalassemias correlates well with the number of affected α genes—that is, from normal to the loss of all four genes. The inheritance of a normal allele (αα) with one of the α^+ or α^0 alleles results, most frequently, in α-thalassemia minor (– –/αα, –α/αα, $-\alpha^T/\alpha\alpha$, $\alpha^T\alpha/-\alpha$, –α/–α). In general, carriers of such genotypes have lower levels of total hemoglobin, mean corpuscular volume, and mean cell hemoglobin but a higher than normal red blood cell count. The greatest differences are seen in mean cell hemoglobin, which is usually less than 26 pg. The peripheral blood smear is quite variable, showing different degrees of hypochromia, with some target cells and occasional poikilocytes (Chapter 160). In carriers of α^0-thalassemia (– –/αα), it is possible to generate a few red cell HbH inclusions (β_4). The carriers of nondeletional forms ($\alpha\alpha^T/\alpha\alpha$) show slightly more marked hematologic changes than carriers of deletional forms. The hemoglobin constitution of adults carriers of α^+- or α^0-thalassemia is indistinguishable from normal but has slightly lower levels of HbA2. Traces of Hb Bart's (γ_4) in the neonatal period are detectable in a large proportion of neonates with α-thalassemia, and the levels decline during the first 6 months after birth. The α-thalassemias are common in areas where β-thalassemias are also found at a high frequency. Thus, the coinheritance of α- and β-thalassemia traits may occur and even ameliorate the hematologic parameters. For families in which both α- and β-thalassemias are present, genotype determination is essential to provide genetic counseling. The unstable mutant Hb^{CT} causes a severe reduction in α_2-globin expression from the affected chromosome; therefore, carriers and particularly homozygotes have a more severe phenotype than α-thalassemia minor but not as severe as most cases of HbH disease.

HbH disease most frequently results from the interaction of α^+ and α^0 thalassemia, and not surprisingly, most patients originate from southeastern Asia, the Mediterranean, and the Middle East. HbH disease is a diagnosis attributed to subjects older than 6 months with a sufficient globin imbalance to produce detectable levels of HbH (>1 to 2%) in their peripheral blood, together with inclusion bodies (β_4 tetramers) in their red cells. The clinical phenotypes encompass a wide spectrum, from mild clinical manifestations to thalassemia intermedia. The predominant features are a hypochromic microcytic anemia, with jaundice and hepatosplenomegaly. Because the main mechanism of the anemia is hemolysis rather than dyserythropoiesis, only a few patients have clinical evidence of an expanded erythron. The most common complication is the development of hypersplenism due to severe splenomegaly. Other complications include gallstones, leg ulcers, increased risk of infection, folic acid deficiency, and increased risk of venous thrombosis, mainly following splenectomy. Hemoglobin levels range from 3 to 12 g/dL in different series, and fluctuations may occur after exposure to an oxidant drug, infection, or transient aplasia possibly owing to intercurrent viral infection. Rarely, patients with HbH disease require regular blood transfusions. The anemia is associated with reticulocytosis and typical thalassemic changes of the red cell indices. The relative amount of HbH varies from 1 to 40%. HbA$_2$ values are always reduced. The peripheral blood film shows hypochromia with variable anisopoikilocytosis, target cells, and basophilic stippling. The characteristic feature of HbH disease is that it is always possible to generate multiple inclusions in the red cells after incubation with brilliant cresyl blue. The bone marrow shows marked erythroid hyperplasia.

The most severe form of α-thalassemia is hydrops fetalis, in which all four α-globin genes are deleted (genotype —/—). It is incompatible with life. In fact, because α-globin chains are absent during gestation, Hb Bart's (γ_4) becomes the dominant hemoglobin. Because of its very high oxygen affinity, Hb Bart's is unable to deliver oxygen to tissues, and the intrauterine consequences are progressive severe anemia, severe ineffective erythropoiesis with marked extramedullary erythropoiesis, massive organomegaly, heart failure, severe albuminemia, and edema. Infants with hydrops fetalis syndrome die either in utero (30 to 40 weeks' gestation) or soon after birth. The hemoglobin levels range from 3 to 20 g/dL; the peripheral blood film is characterized by marked anisopoikilocytosis, large hypochromic macrocytes, and many nucleated red cells. The hemoglobin consists almost entirely of Hb Bart's (80 to 90%), with some remaining HbH and Portland. Mothers of these infants often have a history of previous neonatal deaths. Without medical care, women carrying these fetuses may have delivery and postpartum complications (e.g., retained placenta, eclampsia, sepsis).

There are several reports describing α-thalassemia associated with mental retardation (so-called ATR-16 syndrome). These conditions are mainly owing to large deletions (1 to 2 megabases) of the tip of chromosome 16, including the α-globin gene cluster. However, several cases have no deletions or other apparent abnormalities of the α-globin gene cluster. It has been shown that these patients, with a peculiar phenotype characterized by severe mental retardation, dysmorphic facies, genital abnormalities, and α-thalassemia, have a disorder that maps to the X chromosome (ATR-X syndrome).

β-Thalassemias

The β-thalassemias include a heterogeneous group of disorders of hemoglobin synthesis, all of which are characterized by reduced output of the β chains of adult hemoglobin. The clinical classification includes thalassemia major (TM; transfusion dependent), thalassemia intermedia (TI; intermediate severity), and thalassemia minor (asymptomatic) (Fig. 165-1; see Table 165-1). The severity of the clinical manifestations correlates quite well with the degree of imbalance of the globin chains: depending on the β-globin gene defects and their interaction, the production of β-globin chains is quantitatively reduced to different degrees, whereas the synthesis of α-globin continues as normal, resulting in the accumulation of excess unmatched α-globin chains in the erythroid precursors. The free α-globin chains are unable to form stable tetramers; they therefore precipitate in the erythroid precursors, forming inclusion bodies that damage the red cell membrane, thereby causing premature destruction of erythroid precursors in the bone marrow (ineffective erythropoiesis). Ineffective erythropoiesis leads to a sequence of events

• Homozygous disorder • Significant imbalance of αβ globin chains • Severe anemia presenting early in life • Requires lifelong RBC transfusions • If untreated, leads to death usually in first decade	β-Thalassemia major
• Various genetic interactions • Globin chain production moderately impaired • Mild anemia, diagnosed usually in late childhood • Occasional blood transfusions may be required	β-Thalassemia intermedia
• Heterozygous condition • Asymptomatic • May require genetic counseling	β-Thalassemia minor

A

Severity of disease →

	Thalassemia major more likely	Thalassemia intermedia more likely
Clinical		
Presentation (years)	<2	>2
Hb levels (g/dL)	<7	7-10
Liver/spleen enlargement	Severe	Moderate to severe
Hematologic		
HbF (%)	>50	10-50 (may be up to 100%)
HbA$_2$ (%)	>3.5	<4-4.5
Genetic		
Parents	Both carriers of high HbA$_2$ β-thalassemia	One or both carriers: high HbF β-thalassemia, borderline HbA$_2$
Molecular		
Type of β-chain mutation	Severe	Mild/silent
Coinheritance of α-thalassemia	No/rare	Yes
Hereditary persistence of fetal hemoglobin	No	Yes
δβ-thalassemia	No	Yes
Gγ Xmnl polymorphism	No	Yes

B

FIGURE 165-1. A, Clinical classification of β-thalassemias. B, Tentative criteria to differentiate thalassemia major from thalassemia intermedia at presentation. HbA = adult hemoglobin; HbF = fetal hemoglobin; RBC = red blood cell.

FIGURE 165-2. Pathophysiology of β-thalassemias and modifiers of globin chain imbalance. The severity of ineffective erythropoiesis is dependent on the degree of excess free α chains that result primarily from three different mechanisms: (1) inheritance of severe, mild, or silent β-chain mutations; (2) coinheritance of determinants associated with increased γ-chain production; and (3) coinheritance of α-thalassemia. A phenotype of thalassemia intermedia may result from the increased production of α-globin chains by a triplicated (ααα) or quadruplicated (αααα) α genotype associated with β heterozygosity. Inheritance of polymorphisms or mutations of genes involved in bone, iron, and bilirubin metabolism, as well as in infection, may contribute to modify the clinical course of the disease. ESR1 = estrogen receptor 1; HbF = fetal hemoglobin; HFE = hereditary hemochromatosis gene; HLA = human leukocyte antigen; ICAM1 = intercellular adhesion molecule-1; TNF = tumor necrosis factor; UGT1 = UDPglucose: glycoprotein glucosyltransferase 1; VDR = vitamin D receptor.

responsible for bone marrow expansion, anemia, hemolysis, splenomegaly, and increased iron absorption. Any factor that reduces the degree of chain imbalance and the magnitude of α-chain excess, such as coinheritance of α-thalassemia or an innate ability to increase HbF, will ameliorate the clinical expression of the disease (Fig. 165-2).

The major forms of β-thalassemia (still sometimes called Cooley's anemia) are disorders in which life can be sustained only by regular blood transfusions. This condition usually results from the homozygous state or from the compound heterozygous state for severe β gene mutations (β⁰). The typical forms of TM manifest during the first year of life, during which γ chains are switched off but not replaced by β-chain synthesis. These infants, left untreated, are incapable of maintaining a hemoglobin level above 5 g/dL and show marked bone deformities and growth retardation. They develop thalassemic facies due to frontal bossing of the skull and protrusion of the jaws and cheekbones. The magnitude of the increase in erythropoiesis may result in extramedullary masses usually arising from the sternum and ribs. Progressive hepatosplenomegaly is a constant finding, leading to pancytopenia. The early childhood of untreated or inadequately treated TM patients includes various complications, such as recurrent infections, spontaneous fractures, gallstones, and leg ulcers. The mortality rate in such patients was once very high around puberty. Fortunately, this is no longer the case in children with well-treated TM. Children who are transfused to maintain a hemoglobin level above 9 g/dL have relatively normal growth and development, and their future course depends on whether they receive adequate iron chelation (see Treatment). Many children who are adequately transfused and are fully compliant with iron chelation therapy develop normally, enter puberty, and become sexually mature. At present, we are dealing with an adult population of TM patients who may suffer from the side effects of long-term treatment—namely, transfusion-associated infections (particularly hepatitis B and C and, in some populations, HIV) and organ damage (liver, heart, endocrine glands) due to unsatisfactory long-term iron chelation. The main causes of death in adult TM patients is still cardiac complications. Heart failure in these patients is multifactorial, involving chronic anemia, remaining iron overload, myocarditis, pericarditis, and probably many other mechanisms. Furthermore, in addition to the degree of globin chain imbalance, which is dependent on

genetic factors linked to the globin genes (coinheritance of α-thalassemia, innate increased synthesis of HbF), there are many other genetic modifiers that may secondarily impact the outcome of complications. For example, the presence of a polymorphic variant in the UGT1A1 promoter responsible for Gilbert's syndrome (Chapter 149) may increase the predisposition to cholelithiasis, which is already a common complication in thalassemia. Likewise, polymorphisms in genes involved in iron homeostasis or bone metabolism may negatively or positively influence the degree of iron overload or osteopenia and osteoporosis, respectively (see Fig. 165-2). Environmental factors, including social conditions, nutrition, and the availability of medical care, have also been implicated in the variable severity of the clinical manifestations of TM.

TI is a clinical term used to describe patients with anemia and splenomegaly but without the full clinical spectrum of TM. The clinical phenotypes of TI lie between those of thalassemia minor and major, encompassing a wide spectrum. Mildly affected patients are almost completely asymptomatic until adult life, experiencing only mild anemia and spontaneously maintaining hemoglobin levels between 7 and 10 g/dL. Patients with more severe TI generally present between 2 and 6 years of age; although they are able to survive without regular transfusion therapy, growth and development may be retarded. Most TI patients are homozygotes or compound heterozygotes for mild to moderate β gene mutations (β⁺/β⁺, β⁰/β⁺); less commonly, only a single β-globin gene is affected. Because the clinical severity of the disease is dictated by the extent of globin chain imbalance, at least three different mechanisms can promote the mild clinical characteristics of TI versus those of TM: inheritance of mild or silent β gene mutations; coinheritance of determinants associated with increased γ-chain production, which contributes to neutralizing the large proportion of unbound α chains; and coinheritance of α-thalassemia, which reduces the synthesis of α chains, thereby reducing the α/non-α chain imbalance.

Three main factors are responsible for the clinical sequelae in TI patients: ineffective erythropoiesis, chronic anemia, and iron overload. The degree of ineffective erythropoiesis depends primarily on the underlying molecular defects (as already mentioned) and is due to the precipitation of free α chains into erythroid precursors in the bone marrow, causing membrane damage and premature cell death in the marrow. The degree of ineffective erythropoiesis is the primary determinant of the anemia of TI; the peripheral hemolysis of mature, circulating red cells and an overall reduction in hemoglobin synthesis are secondary. Hemolysis per se and damaged red cells that expose negatively charged membrane phosphatidyl-serine residues have been linked to the development of the hypercoagulable state and the increased risk of pulmonary hypertension found in the TI population. Chronic anemia and chronic ineffective erythropoiesis lead to an inappropriate increase in gastrointestinal iron absorption, resulting in iron overload. In contrast, in TM, iron loading results mainly from transfusional iron infusion. It has been shown that chronic anemia and ineffective erythropoiesis, which are characteristic of TI, are associated with the reduced expression of hepcidin, a hepatic peptide that plays a central role in iron homeostasis. Moreover, growth and differentiation factor 15 (GDF15), secreted by erythroid precursors and overexpressed in the presence of ineffective erythropoiesis, may suppress hepcidin synthesis. Taken together, ineffective erythropoiesis (leading to increased GDF15) and chronic anemia and hypoxia result in hepcidin suppression, increased dietary iron absorption from the gut, and increased release of recycled iron from the reticuloendothelial system, leading to an iron overload situation that is very similar to that observed in patients with hereditary hemochromatosis syndromes (which are characterized by impaired hepcidin production; Chapter 219). As a consequence of these pathophysiologic processes, several complications have been identified as unique in TI patients, especially in splenectomized naïve patients. Cholelithiasis is much more common in TI than in TM because of ineffective erythropoiesis and peripheral hemolysis. Extramedullary hematopoiesis, as a compensatory mechanism, leads to the formation of erythropoietic tissue masses that primarily affect the spleen, liver, lymph nodes, and vertebrae. These masses may cause neurologic problems such as spinal cord compression and paraplegia and intrathoracic masses. Leg ulcers are rare in well-transfused TM patients but are quite common in adult TI patients; it remains unclear why, at the same hemoglobin and HbF levels, some patients develop leg ulcers and others do not. Thrombotic risk is definitely increased in TI patients. Several studies have collectively shown that the incidence of thromboembolic events is higher in splenectomized TI patients. Although stroke is rare in TI, asymptomatic brain damage, including ischemia, has been documented by magnetic resonance imaging (MRI) and computed tomography in TI patients. Pulmonary hypertension (Chapter 68) is prevalent in TI patients (approximately 60%) and is thought to be the primary cause of heart failure in this population. Liver disease due to viral infection is less frequent than in TM; however, abnormal liver enzymes are frequently observed in TI patients, primarily owing to hepatocyte damage resulting from iron overload. In some of the oldest patients with TI (>40 years), hepatocellular carcinoma (Chapter 202) has been detected owing to long-term untreated iron accumulation with resultant cirrhosis, as found in genetic hemochromatosis (Chapter 219). Hypogonadism, hypothyroidism, and diabetes mellitus are quite rare. Although patients with TI generally experience puberty late, they have normal sexual development and are usually fertile. Women with TI may have spontaneous successful pregnancies, although complications may occur.

Thalassemia minor is the heterozygous state of β-thalassemia. Subjects with thalassemia minor are "carriers" of a single β-globin gene defect and are usually asymptomatic, except for a mild anemia of pregnancy. The carriers are usually identified as part of a family study, incidentally during an intercurrent illness, or as part of a population survey. The anemia is mild, microcytic, and hypochromic and is associated with an elevated level of HbA$_2$. The blood smear shows characteristic microcytosis and hypochromia, with some variation in size and shape of the red cells. The presence of target cells is very variable. The hematologic features are remarkably similar among different ethnic groups. Carriers of β-thalassemia with normal HbA$_2$ have been observed in settings in which an individual with mild TI was found to have one parent with typical β-thalassemia minor with elevated HbA$_2$ while the other showed either minimal or no hematologic abnormalities and normal HbA$_2$. Subjects with normal HbA$_2$ are usually carriers of silent β mutations (β^{++}).

δβ-Thalassemia and Hereditary Persistence of Fetal Hemoglobin

The clinical manifestations of (δβ)^0-thalassemias are similar to those of TI, whereas the heterozygotes are distinguished from β-thalassemia heterozygotes by normal levels of HbA$_2$ and increased HbF levels of 5 to 20%. Homozygotes for Hb Lepore may have phenotypes similar to either TM or TI. Subjects affected by deletion or nondeletion forms of HPFH are usually asymptomatic.

Any of the β-thalassemia defects may be coinherited with β-chain variants (e.g., HbS, HbC, HbE) and cause a clinically relevant β-thalassemia phenotype of differing severity. These variants illustrate that β-thalassemia syndromes have a wide clinical spectrum and that specific therapeutic approaches may completely change the clinical course and natural history of these disorders.

DIAGNOSIS

The diagnosis of thalassemia may be required in a patient with a suspicious clinical picture or to identify a heterozygote subject as part of a family study or population screening program. The general diagnostic approach is common to any form of thalassemia, regardless of presentation. The primary evaluation is based on hematologic changes: the red cell indices obtained by electronic cell counter and the red cell morphology examined on a well-stained blood film are sufficient to direct further investigations. Individuals with a mean corpuscular volume below 80 fL and mean corpuscular hemoglobin below 27 pg with normal iron parameters need further investigation. The number of red blood cells is usually higher than normal. In the presence of anemia with thalassemic red cell changes, the next step is the evaluation of hemoglobin fractions (HbA, HbA$_2$, HbF, or Hb variants) by electrophoresis on cellulose acetate at alkaline pH or, even better, by high-performance liquid chromatography, which enables the precise measurement of HbA$_2$, HbF, and HbA and the provisional identification of a large number of Hb variants. An HbA$_2$ level greater than 3.5% associated with hypochromic microcytic red cells is diagnostic of β-thalassemia minor. HbA$_2$ values between 3.2 and 3.5% (borderline) should be interpreted with care because they could be due to the interaction of more than one thalassemic defect (α and β), a silent β mutation, or concomitant iron deficiency. If iron deficiency is present, it should be corrected and the HbA$_2$ estimation repeated. The majority of individuals with thalassemic red cell indices and normal or low HbA$_2$ and normal HbF are α^0-thalassemia carriers or α$^+$-thalassemia homozygotes. Carriers of α^0-thalassemia may have a few red cells with HbH inclusions. Microcytosis with low or normal HbA$_2$ levels and elevated HbF (2 to 20%) indicates heterozygosity for δβ-thalassemia. Patients with HPFH usually have normal red blood cell indices but increased levels of HbF with a different intercellular distribution (homogeneous or pancellular, with the exception of

heterocellular HPFH) compared with δβ-thalassemia (uneven or heterocellular). A radioactive method for measuring the α/β-globin synthesis ratio was introduced in the mid to late 1960s and was largely directed at prenatal diagnosis in the pre-DNA era. Although it gives a quantitative assessment of globin production, today its use is limited to difficult cases caused by the interaction of different globin chain defects. Definitive diagnosis of the thalassemia syndromes involves identification of the underlying mutations through DNA analysis. There are several methods available for the diagnosis of any particular mutation, such as polymerase chain reaction (PCR) restriction-enzyme analysis, PCR allele-specific-oligonucleotides, gap PCR, and direct sequencing, which is probably the easiest and most reliable method. For deletion forms of α-thalassemia, multiplex ligation-dependent probe amplification is a useful, recently introduced method.

During their clinical course, patients affected by different forms of thalassemia develop several complications mainly due to iron overload, which must be monitored to direct iron chelation therapy. The principal methods of determining body iron levels (Chapter 219) are measurements of the serum ferritin level and assessment of liver iron concentration from biopsy tissue or, as an alternative noninvasive method, by R2 MRI. High serum ferritin levels (>2500 μg/L) and a high liver iron concentration (>15 g/dry weight) indicate a high risk of significant morbidity and mortality. Cardiac iron can be measured by a recently introduced T2* MRI procedure that allows estimation of the cardiac iron load. MRI T2* less than 10 msec is always associated with severe iron load and a high risk of heart failure within 1 year. MRI T2* greater than 20 msec is considered normal, meaning there is no iron in the heart. Echocardiography may also be useful to evaluate functional changes. For other complications, including endocrinopathies, liver disease, lung disease, thrombophilia, and bone disease, the diagnostic approaches are similar to those used in clinical practice, taking into consideration test cost, performance characteristics, and patient preferences.

TREATMENT   Rx

Conventional Treatment

No specific treatment is required for α- or β-thalassemia heterozygotes (carriers, thalassemia minor), but they should receive appropriate genetic counseling. During pregnancy, particularly during the second and third trimesters, thalassemia-carrying women may become more anemic, so they should be followed carefully and supported with folic acid. When real iron deficiency is associated with thalassemia traits, iron supplementation should be provided, while monitoring transferrin saturation and ferritin. Very few cases of in utero blood transfusions have been reported with Hb Bart's hydrops fetalis syndrome; most of these babies have been delivered prematurely by cesarean section, subsequent development has been abnormal, and survivors required regular blood transfusions after birth. HbH patients in general have rather high hemoglobin levels (8 to 9 g/dL) and do not need regular blood transfusion. Supplementation with folic acid (2 to 5 mg/day) is generally recommended, especially in pediatric patients. The major complications in HbH disease are hemolytic crises that may occur during or after acute infections; in such cases, immediate intervention, including blood transfusions and treatment for infection, should be promptly administered.

The clinical management of TM and TI remains the major issue. The lifespan and quality of life of TM and TI patients have been transformed over the last 10 years, with life expectancy increasing well into the third and fourth decades. Nevertheless, prolongation of life is accompanied by several complications, partly due to the underlying disorder and partly as a consequence of treatment with blood transfusions and iron overload. Moreover, we have to deal with aging-related complications in the context of a multiorgan disease that requires management by a team of clinicians with specific knowledge of thalassemias, working together with different specialists and well-trained nurses. The conventional treatment for TM patients includes regular transfusion therapy and iron chelation. Definition of the optimal transfusion and iron chelation regimen has been the most important advance in the management of TM patients, with the primary objective being to control the ineffective erythropoiesis, its consequences, and the iron burden. The optimal regimen involves regular blood transfusions, usually administered every 2 to 5 weeks, to maintain pretransfusion hemoglobin levels above 9 to 10.5 g/dL. The decision to initiate lifelong transfusion therapy should be based on a definitive diagnosis of severe thalassemia, taking into account the molecular defects, the severity of anemia on repeated measurements, the level of ineffective erythropoiesis, and clinical criteria such as failure to thrive or bone changes. It is advisable for TM patients to receive leukoreduced packed red cells to reduce transfusion reactions and pathogen transmission. Adverse reactions to red blood cell transfusions may occur during or after the transfusion, and they can be hemolytic or nonhemolytic. Transfusion-related acute lung injury (TRALI) is a very rare but severe complication and must be managed immediately

(Chapter 180). Many patients with TM require splenectomy because of hypersplenism. However, with optimal clinical management, the need for splenectomy may be delayed or even obviated. Splenectomy should be considered for patients whose annual blood consumption increases progressively and is responsible for significant increases in iron stores, despite good chelation therapy, and in those experiencing symptoms due to spleen enlargement. Clinical problems related to leukopenia or thrombocytopenia due to hypersplenism are other reasons to consider splenectomy. The major complication of splenectomy is severe and sometimes overwhelming infection. Because removal of the spleen may reduce the primary immune response to encapsulated organisms, it is advisable to delay splenectomy until patients are at least 5 years old. The mortality rate for overwhelming post-splenectomy infection in thalassemia patients is approximately 50%, despite intensive supportive care; therefore, preventive measures are mandatory, including immunoprophylaxis (vaccination against *Streptococcus pneumoniae*, pneumococcus, and meningococcus), chemoprophylaxis, and parent and patient education to recognize and report febrile illnesses.

Iron overload is an inevitable and serious complication of long-term blood transfusion therapy and hyperabsorption of dietary iron, and it requires adequate treatment to prevent early death from iron-induced cardiac disease. Optimal chelation therapy extends complication-free survival (Fig. 165-3). For more than 40 years, the standard chelation therapy has been deferoxamine (DFO), given for 10 to 24 hours a day as a continuous subcutaneous infusion 5 to 7 days per week. The long-term efficacy of DFO has been extensively documented in large cohorts of patients in Italy and elsewhere. Unfortunately, compliance with the rigorous daily regimen is a serious limiting factor, and in noncompliant patients, life expectancy is no different from that in the pre-DFO era. This has been the rationale behind the intensive effort to identify alternative, orally effective iron chelators. At present, two oral iron chelators are in the market: deferiprone (DFP) and deferasirox (DFX). DFP is registered in Europe but is not yet available in the United States. Based on the guidelines of the EMEA countries (Europe, Middle East, and Africa), treatment with DFP at doses of 75 to 100 mg/kg/day is restricted to patients unable to use DFO or those with an unsatisfactory response to DFO as judged by serum ferritin levels and liver iron concentrations. Recent studies indicate that DFP may be more effective than DFO in protecting the heart from the accumulation of iron.[1] A potential benefit of combined DFO/DFP therapy has been observed,[2,3] and according to the Thalassemia International Federation, combination DFO/DFP treatment should be considered for patients with very high levels of heart iron or cardiac dysfunction. The new orally effective iron chelator DFX is safe and effective for removing excess iron from different organs, including the heart. DFX is now available in most countries throughout the world as first-line treatment. Iron chelation therapy must be individualized according age,

compliance history, and other factors. Monitoring and adjusting iron chelation based on repeated measurements of ferritin, calculation of iron intake by transfusions, and, whenever possible, measuring cardiac and liver iron by MRI (at least once) are mandatory.

The management of TI patients is more complicated owing to the wide heterogeneity of TI phenotypes. A number of options are currently available to treat TI patients, including transfusion therapy, splenectomy, modulation of HbF production, and hematopoietic stem cell transplantation. However, increasing evidence is delineating the benefit of transfusion therapy in decreasing the incidence of complications. Thus, although common practice in the past was to initiate transfusion when complications ensued, it may be worthwhile to start transfusion therapy earlier, as a preventive approach and to help alleviate the increased risk of alloimmunization with the delayed initiation of transfusion. The initiation of iron chelation therapy in patients with TI depends not only on the amount of excess iron but also on the rate of iron accumulation, the duration of exposure to excess iron, and various other factors in individual patients.

Bone Marrow Transplantation and Experimental Therapies

Allogeneic hematopoietic stem cell transplantation (HSCT) in thalassemia syndromes has been increasingly successful during the last 2 decades, mainly in β-thalassemia major. Predictors of poor transplant outcome are hepatomegaly, a history of irregular chelation, and hepatic fibrosis. Patients are categorized into three risk classes. Class 1 patients have none of these adverse risk factors, class 2 patients have one or two adverse risk factors, and class 3 patients have all three. In the most recent update of the Pesaro group's experience, the probability of thalassemia-free survival for patients younger than 17 years at the time of HSCT, receiving the allograft from a human leukocyte antigen (HLA)–identical relative, was 87% in class 1 patients, 85% in class 2 patients, and much lower in young class 3 patients. The progressive adjustment of conditioning therapy in class 3 patients and in adults (older than 17 years) has significantly reduced the incidence of transplant-related mortality. Only 25 to 30% of patients with diseases potentially curable by HSCT have suitable HLA-compatible siblings however, and bone marrow transplantation from unrelated donors significantly increases the incidence of acute and chronic graft-versus-host disease, particularly in thalassemia. A study from the Eurocord cooperative group reported the outcome of 33 class 1 and 2 patients with thalassemia who received cord blood HSCT from HLA-identical siblings: no patient died of transplant-related complications, suggesting that this is a safe procedure for thalassemia patients.

An alternative treatment of β-thalassemia consists of the pharmacologic stimulation of HbF synthesis. In humans, the hemoglobin switch from HbF to

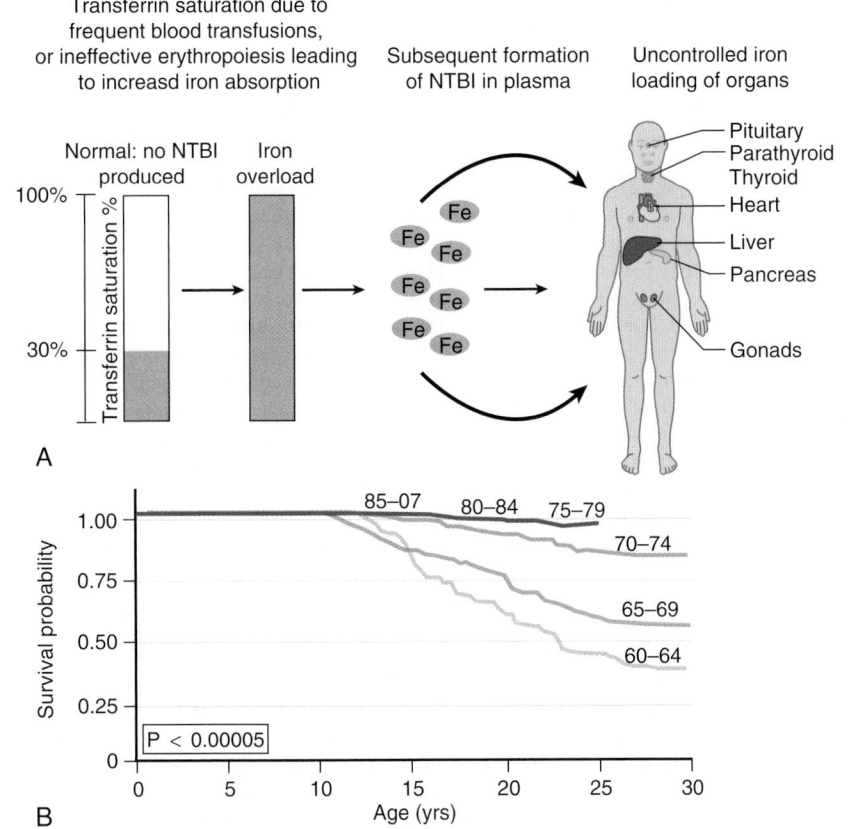

FIGURE 165-3. A, Transfusional iron overload and specific organ iron loading. B, Survival of Italian thalassemia major patients by cohort of birth: 1960 to 1964, 1965 to 1969, 1970 to 1974, 1975 to 1979, 1980 to 1984, and 1985 to 1997. NTBI = non–transferrin-bound iron. (From Borgna-Pignatti C, Rugolotto S, De Stefano P, et al. Survival and complications in patients with thalassemia major treated with transfusion and deferoxamine. *Haematologica.* 2004;89:1187-1193.)

HbA occurs in the period around birth as a result of γ- to β-globin gene switching. A number of pharmacologic agents with the ability to reactivate HbF synthesis have been identified, including hypomethylating agents, histone deacetylase inhibitors, and hydroxyurea. Although the effect of these treatments (particularly hydroxyurea) in sickle cell disease is clear (Chapter 166), their benefit on the clinical course of β-thalassemia is presently limited. This discrepancy in the response to HbF inducers may be related mainly to the higher level of HbF required to achieve clinical results in β-thalassemia compared to sickle cell disease. The limited clinical response to γ-globin inducers observed in the majority of β-thalassemia patients may also be a reflection of the unfavorable effects of these agents on the other globin genes (i.e., increased α-globin synthesis).

Gene therapy is an attractive approach for thalassemia syndromes; however, this strategy poses major challenges in terms of controlling transgene expression, which should be erythroid specific and sustained over time. Treatment of ß-thalassemia, sickle cell disease, and other disorders through lentivirus-mediated gene transfer has been reported in murine and primate models, but few human patients have been treated.

UNSTABLE HEMOGLOBINOPATHIES

More than 80 rare mutant hemoglobins have been reported to cause hemolytic anemia owing to amino acid replacements or deletions that significantly lower solubility. These mutant hemoglobins form intracellular precipitates that can be detected as so-called Heinz bodies when the blood smear is exposed to a supravital stain. Structural abnormalities include mutations that weaken the linkage between heme and globin, disrupt secondary (α-helical) structures, or introduce a charged or polar side group into the hydrophobic interior of the globin subunit.

This disorder, sometimes called congenital Heinz body hemolytic anemia, is inherited in an autosomal dominant manner. Severely affected individuals have jaundice, splenomegaly, and, on occasion, dark brown urine owing to the release of heme and aberrant conversion to dipyroles. The instability of a few of these globin mutants is so extreme that they cannot be detected by routine laboratory methods. This results in a thalassemia phenotype with microcytosis and ineffective erythropoiesis. Like individuals with glucose-6-phosphate dehydrogenase deficiency (Chapter 164), those with unstable hemoglobin mutants often lack clinical symptoms and signs of hemolysis until or unless they develop an infection or are exposed to an oxidant drug.

The diagnosis can be established by the combination of a positive Heinz body preparation and either abnormal hemoglobin electrophoresis or demonstration of a precipitate following exposure of a hemolysate to heat or isopropanol. Some clinics have access to a reference laboratory that can identify the specific mutation by α- and β-globin DNA sequencing.

Most individuals with this disorder do not require treatment. However, some are symptomatic from severe anemia. Splenectomy generally results in a significant increase in red cell mass, but the fraction of Heinz body–positive red cells increases markedly after splenectomy, putting these patients at significant risk of developing pulmonary hypertension and cor pulmonale.

1. Pennell DJ, Berdoukas V, Karagiorga M, et al. Randomized controlled trial of deferiprone or deferoxamine in beta-thalassemia major patients with asymptomatic myocardial siderosis. *Blood.* 2006;107:3738-3744.
2. Tanner MA, Galanello R, Dessi C, et al. A randomized, placebo-controlled, double-blind trial of the effect of combined therapy with deferoxamine and deferiprone on myocardial iron in thalassemia major using cardiovascular magnetic resonance. *Circulation.* 2007;115:1876-1884.
3. Maggio A, Vitrano A, Capra M, et al. Long-term sequential deferiprone-deferoxamine versus deferiprone alone for thalassemia major patients: a randomized clinical trial. *Br J Haematol.* 2009;145:245-254.

SUGGESTED READINGS

Cao A, Galanello R. Beta thalassemia. *Genet Med.* 2010;12:61-74. *Review.*
Pennell DJ, Porter JB, Cappellini MD, et al. Continued improvement in myocardial T2* over two years of deferasirox therapy in β-thalassemia major patients with cardiac iron overload. *Haematologica.* 2011;96:48-54. *Continuous treatment with deferasirox (40 mg/kg/d) continued to remove iron from the heart.*
Pennell DJ, Porter JB, Cappellini MD, et al. Efficacy of deferasirox in reducing and preventing cardiac iron overload in beta-thalassemia. *Blood.* 2010;115:2364-2371. *Deferasirox is effective in removing and preventing myocardial iron accumulation.*
Serjeant GR, Serjeant BE, Fraser RA, et al. Hb S-β-thalassemia: molecular, hematological and clinical comparisons. *Hemoglobin.* 2011;35:1-12. *Clinically, Hb S-β(0)-thal and Hb S-β(+)-thal type I were generally severe.*

Smiers FJ, Krishnamurti L, Lucarelli G. Hematopoietic stem cell transplantation for hemoglobinopathies: current practice and emerging trends. *Pediatr Clin North Am.* 2010;57:181-205. *Improved results are possible with new conditioning regimens and expanded donor pools.*
Taher AT, Musallam KM, Karimi M, et al. Overview on practices in thalassemia intermedia management aiming for lowering complication-rates across a region of endemicity: the OPTIMAL CARE study. *Blood.* 2010;115:1886-1892. *Study of 584 thalassemia intermedia patients, searching for associations among disease characteristics, treatment received, and rate of complications.*
Testa U. Fetal hemoglobin chemical inducers for treatment of hemoglobinopathies. Review. *Ann Hematol.* 2009;88:505-528. *The increase in HbF in response to these drugs varies among patients with thalassemia and sickle cell disease owing to individual genetic determinants.*
Weatherall DJ. The inherited diseases of hemoglobin are an emerging global health burden. *Blood.* 2010;115:4331-4336. *Strong argument for recognition of inherited hemoglobinopathies as a major, growing global health burden.*

166

SICKLE CELL DISEASE AND OTHER HEMOGLOBINOPATHIES

MARTIN H. STEINBERG

SICKLE CELL DISEASE

DEFINITION

Sickle cell disease, caused by a mutation in the β-globin gene (*HBB*), consists of a group of chronic hemolytic anemias, all characterized by vaso-occlusive events, hemolytic anemia, vasculopathy, widespread acute and chronic organ damage, and premature mortality.

EPIDEMIOLOGY

The prevalences of the various forms of sickle cell disease and of the sickle cell trait, which is not truly a form of sickle cell disease, vary in the United States and worldwide (Table 166-1; Fig. 166-1). The sickle hemoglobin mutation became prominent in equatorial Africa, the Middle East, and India several thousand years ago, when deforestation, the rise of agriculture, and stagnant pooling of water permitted *Plasmodium falciparum* infection to become endemic. Carriers of the sickle cell trait were more likely to survive to reproductive age and had a selective advantage where falciparum malaria was present. At least five distinct origins of this identical mutation can be distinguished by the accompanying haplotype of the β-globin gene–like cluster. Slave trading and war spread this mutation to the Americas, throughout the Mediterranean basin, and eastward to the Indian subcontinent. In some sites in Africa, half the population carries the sickle hemoglobin gene.

PATHOBIOLOGY

Globin, the protein portion of hemoglobin, harbors the porphyrin heme ring and permits the molecule to operate efficiently in oxygen transport and its other physiologic functions (Fig. 166-2). Mutations can alter the primary amino acid sequence of the globin polypeptide, sometimes resulting in clinically significant diseases called hemoglobinopathies, including sickle cell disease. Sickle hemoglobin (HbS; $\alpha_2\beta_2^S$) is caused by an adenine (A) to thymidine (T) substitution (GAG → GTG) in codon 6 of the β-globin gene, resulting in replacement of the normal glutamic acid residue by a valine (Glu6Val). HbS polymerizes when it is deoxygenated, a property only of hemoglobin variants that have the *HBB* Glu6Val substitution. Critical amounts of HbS polymer within sickle erythrocytes cause cellular injury and lead to the phenotype of sickle cell disease, which is recognized by hemolytic anemia and vaso-occlusion. Other hemoglobin variants, such as HbE and HbC, are also common. More than 1000 hemoglobin mutations are known, and occasionally they can affect the stability and function of hemoglobin and cause hemolytic anemia (Chapter 161), disordered oxygen transport (Chapter 169), or methemoglobinemia (Chapter 161). However, most globin mutations are clinically insignificant. Thalassemias (Chapter 165) are also caused by mutations in globin genes, but these mutations affect globin gene expression so that synthesis of a globin chain is reduced or absent, although the structure of any globin produced is usually normal.

In sickle cell disease, erythrocytes are heterogeneous as a result of membrane damage and the cellular distribution of fetal hemoglobin (HbF). HbF

TABLE 166-1 GENETIC AND LABORATORY FEATURES OF COMMON SICKLE HEMOGLOBINOPATHIES*

GENOTYPE	GENETICS	PREVALENCE AMONG AFRICAN AMERICANS[†]	HEMATOCRIT (%)	MCV (FL)	HBS (%)	HBA$_2$ (%)	HBF (%)	SEVERITY[‡]
Sickle cell anemia (HbSS)	Homozygous HbS	1:600	18-28	85-95	>85	2-3	2-15	4
HbSS-α-thalassemia	Homozygous HbS α$^+$-thalassemia	30% of HbSS patients	25-33	70-85	>85	4-6	2-15	4
HbSC disease (HbSC)	Compound heterozygous HbS, HbC	1:800	28-40	70-85	50	2-3	1-8	2
HbS-β^0-thalassemia (HbS-β^0-Thal)	Compound heterozygous HbS, β^0-thalassemia	1:1600	20-30	65-75	>85	4-6	5-15	4
HbS-β$^+$-thalassemia (HbS-β$^+$-Thal)	Compound heterozygous HbS, β$^+$-thalassemia	1:1600	30-40	60-70	70-95	4-6	2-10	1-3
HbSE disease (HbSE)	Compound heterozygous HbS, HbE	Rare[§]	30-45	70-80	60	2-3	1	1-2
HbS-HPFH	Compound heterozygous HbS and gene deletion HPFH	Rare	38-45	70-80	70	2	20-30	0
Sickle cell trait (HbAS)[¶]	Heterozygous HbS	1:12	38-50	80-90	35-40	2-3	<1	0
Normal (HbAA)	Homozygous HbA	—	38-50	80-90	0	2-3	<1	—

*Many other abnormal globin genes can be found as compound heterozygotes with the HbS gene. The most common of these are α-thalassemia, HbD, HbO (Arabia), HbG (Philadelphia), HPFH, Hb Hope, and Hb Lepore. Average ranges of laboratory values are shown, but these can vary according to patient age.

[†]These figures differ depending on the prevalence of the involved genes in the population studied. In West and Central Africa, where the disease is most common, approximately 2% of all newborns have sickle cell disease. The prevalence of the HbC trait in African Americans is 3%, and that of the β-thalassemia trait is 1%. About 30% of African Americans carry an α-thalassemia gene, which can alter the phenotype of sickle cell disease by causing microcytosis, reduced cell density, and less hemolysis.

[‡]Severity of disease compared with sickle cell anemia, clinically the most severe genotype. This is a qualitative ranking of the clinical severity of each genotype; within each genotype, there is great clinical heterogeneity.

[§]Although this combination is still a rare genotype, the rising Asian population in the United States (HbE is a Southeastern Asian gene) will make it more frequent with time. With few cases reported compared with the other genotypes, the phenotype of HbSE disease is not totally defined. It may resemble HbS-β$^+$ thalassemia with symptoms appearing mainly in adults.

[¶]Sickle cell trait should not be classified as a form of sickle cell disease. About 8% of African Americans are carriers of HbS. Carriers are hematologically normal with a normal life expectancy. The few abnormalities traceable to the presence of HbS besides the renal lesions (see Table 166-3) include a four-fold increased risk of pulmonary embolism, an increased risk of splenic infarction at high altitude, and a higher risk of dying during the course of exertional heat illness.

Hb = hemoglobin; HPFH = hereditary persistence of HbF; MCV = mean corpuscular volume.

FIGURE 166-1. Worldwide prevalence of the sickle cell trait. Shown are the percentages of individuals with sickle cell trait in regions of the world where the hemoglobin S (HbS) gene is often present. In each geographic area, the prevalence of sickle cell trait can vary markedly according to racial or ethnic group, historical migration patterns, and even from village to village. Not shown is the high concentration of the HbS gene in areas of Europe such as London, Manchester, and Paris, where migrants from Africa or Afro-Caribbean populations have settled.

concentrations vary among patients with sickle cell anemia (homozygosity for HbS) and among erythrocytes of each individual. Because HbF inhibits HbS polymerization (see later discussion), its concentration within each cell and its distribution among all cells influence cell heterogeneity.

Sickle cell anemia is noteworthy for its clinical heterogeneity. Any patient can have almost all known disease complications; some have almost none but die suddenly; some skip one or more phases of the disease but suffer intensely from others. Thus, this prototypical single-gene, mendelian disorder behaves clinically as a multigenic trait with exceptional phenotypic variability. Understanding the vascular and inflammatory components of the disease provides many loci where the disease phenotype can be influenced by modifying

genes. These genes potentially affect the pathogenesis of sickle cell anemia by modulating HbF concentration, inflammation, oxidant injury, nitric oxide (NO) biology, vasoregulation, cell-cell interaction, blood coagulation, and hemostasis. Polymorphisms have been noted in candidate genes that affect these functions, and some may be prognostically useful. The sickle mutation is found on several different haplotypes of the β-globin gene–like cluster, reflecting different origins of the mutation in Africa and the Middle East. The Senegal haplotype is often associated with higher HbF levels than other haplotypes and with a more benign clinical course. Conversely, the Bantu haplotype may be associated with more disease complications; however, there is phenotypic heterogeneity even within a particular haplotype group.

Cation homeostasis is impaired in some sickle cells. A reduced capacity of sickle cells to maintain normal potassium (K$^+$) gradients is mediated by activation of the Gardos and K$^+$/Cl$^-$ cotransport channels. As a result, sickle erythrocytes vary in their density and deformability. Irreversibly sickled cells (ISCs; Fig. 166-3) always appear deformed because of permanent membrane damage, even though they may not contain HbS polymer. In some dense cells, the mean corpuscular hemoglobin concentration reaches 50 g/dL (normal, 27 to 38 g/dL), and HbS polymer is always present. Individuals with the highest numbers of ISCs and dense cells have the most hemolysis and anemia but not necessarily the highest incidence of acute vaso-occlusive events like painful episodes.

Hemolysis is mainly extravascular owing to erythrophagocytosis by reticuloendothelial cells that recognize the damaged sickle erythrocyte. In most patients, intravascular destruction of sickle erythrocytes liberates excessive amounts of hemoglobin into the circulation, thereby depleting haptoglobin and scavenging NO. This process promotes a vasoconstrictive, proinflammatory phenotype (Fig. 166-4). Certain complications of sickle disease, such as pulmonary hypertension, priapism, leg ulcer, and stroke, are epidemiologically linked to the intensity of hemolysis, whereas other complications, such as painful episodes, acute chest syndrome, and osteonecrosis, are linked to high blood viscosity and the interactions among sickle cells, leukocytes, and the endothelium.

Vaso-occlusive events probably depend on features intrinsic to the sickle erythrocyte, such as polymer content and the degree of cellular damage, interacting with factors in the cell's environment, such as endothelial injury, vascular tone, and other blood cells. In the first hours of a painful episode, the number of dense cells falls; it rises again as pain resolves. These observations suggest the possibility that more deformable, more adherent cells might

FIGURE 166-2. Human globin genes. **A,** The β-like globin gene cluster on chromosome 11 is shown above, and the α-like globin gene cluster below. Two β-globin chains and two α-globin chains combine to form the normal hemoglobin A (HbA) tetramer, represented between the globin genes. Each globin chain contains one heme group, and oxygen transport takes place sequentially at the four iron-containing heme groups. Fetal hemoglobin (HbF) is composed of two α- and two γ-globin chains; the minor hemoglobin of adults, HbA₂, contains two α- and two δ-globin chains. Normally present at a level of only 2 to 3%, HbA₂ concentration is increased to 4 to 6% in most carriers of β-thalassemia. The ζ (*HBZ*) and ε (*HBE1*) genes are normally expressed only in the embryo. The 5′ ψα gene has recently been found to be expressed at a very low level and is now called the μ-globin gene (*HBM*). The θ-globin gene (*HBQ1*) is also expressed at low levels. Neither the θ nor the μ gene has been found in a functional hemoglobin. Any of the globin chains participating in hemoglobin formation may have a mutation altering its amino acid sequence. HbS, HbE, and HbC mutations affect the β-globin gene (*HBB*). Other mutations can affect the α- (*HBA1, HBA2*), γ- (*HBG1, HBG2*), and δ-globin (*HBD*) genes. LCR = locus control region. **B,** Expression of globin genes during development. α-Chains are expressed throughout gestation and adult life, fetal γ-globin chains are expressed predominantly in utero, and the β- and δ-globin genes are expressed mainly postnatally. This switching of gene expression patterns accounts for the different hemoglobins present in the embryo, fetus, and adult. It also accounts for the observation that disorders of α-globin can affect both fetus and adult, whereas β-globin chain diseases usually are not clinically apparent in the first months of life, when HbF levels are still high.

initiate vaso-occlusion, whereas dense cells become sequestered or destroyed in the microvasculature. Endothelial cells are responsive to many biologic modifiers that can be generated during sickle vaso-occlusive episodes and infection. Their activation and damage may be provoked by adherent sickle cells and shear stresses that cause release of oxidant radicals, expression of endothelin, and disturbed NO balance. Cellular damage enables adhesive interactions among sickle cells, endothelial cells, and leukocytes. Reperfusion injury can also induce endothelial activation. The association of sickle and endothelial cells by a variety of adhesion molecules and their ligands may sufficiently delay cellular passage so that HbS polymerization, cell sickling, and vaso-occlusion happen before transit through the microvasculature is complete. Reticulocytes that are prematurely released from bone marrow display adhesive ligands that facilitate erythrocyte-endothelial interactions. Individuals with the greatest amount of hemolysis have the highest reticulocyte counts, and these adherent cells provide another link of hemolysis with vaso-occlusion. Neutrophils, which are modulators of inflammation and tissue damage, are increased in patients who have the acute chest syndrome, priapism, or stroke, and their numbers at baseline are a risk factor for survival.

CLINICAL MANIFESTATIONS

The clinical phenotype of sickle cell disease can be a result of many different genotypes, but most patients have either sickle cell anemia, HbSC disease, or HbS-β-thalassemia (see Table 166-1). Although hemolytic anemia and vaso-occlusive events are found in all genotypes, genotypes with higher cellular concentration of HbS are clinically more severe. Within milliseconds to seconds after HbS deoxygenation, depending on the intracellular concentration of HbS, HbS polymer appears in the sickle erythrocyte. In sickle cell trait (i.e., the simple heterozygote carriage of the HbS mutation), each cell contains only 30 to 40% HbS, so polymer is not found under most conditions (see Fig. 166-3). Therefore, carriers have few complications and a normal life expectancy.

The features of sickle cell anemia change as life advances (Table 166-2). The switch from HbF to HbS underlies the clinical shift in life's first decade. This time is typified by acute problems: high risks of severe life-threatening infection, acute chest syndrome, splenic sequestration, and stroke. Chronic organ damage (renal failure, pulmonary hypertension, and late effects of previous cerebrovascular disease) becomes paramount in adults.

Most patients with sickle cell anemia have moderate anemia with a hematocrit between 25 and 30%. Some patients appear to have more severe hemolysis, with hematocrit less than 20%, marked reticulocytosis, and extreme elevation of serum lactic dehydrogenase (LDH). Patients with the most profound hemolysis appear more likely to have stroke, pulmonary

hypertension, priapism, and leg ulcers. Many patients with HbSC disease, especially adult men, have almost normal hematocrits and may have a higher incidence of sickle retinopathy, perhaps owing to their increased blood viscosity. Symptoms of anemia, such as weakness and dyspnea, are not the hallmarks of sickle cell disease, yet hemoglobin concentration can be a prognostic indicator for certain complications (see Table 166-2). Plasma volume in sickle cell anemia may be greatly expanded, making it difficult to predict the red blood cell (RBC) mass based on the hematocrit. Serum erythropoietin levels in sickle cell anemia are inappropriately low for the hematocrit. A consequence of hemolysis is increased turnover of bile pigments, regulated in part by promoter polymorphisms in the uridine diphosphate-glucuronosyltransferase 1A (*UGT1A*) gene, which is also associated with unconjugated hyperbilirubinemia and Gilbert's syndrome (Chapter 149). As a result, more than half of all adults have cholelithiasis (Chapter 158). Hemolytic anemia places patients at risk for acutely developing severe anemia when erythropoiesis is temporarily interrupted by parvovirus B19 infection (Chapter 379), which is the predominant cause of the aplastic crisis. Aplastic crisis is typified by a plummeting hematocrit, reticulocytopenia, and a bone marrow without erythroid precursors. It is a transient process, most common in children, and often requires blood transfusion to maintain circulatory competence until a spontaneous recovery follows. Rarely, if a patient's diet is inadequate, hemolysis-induced accelerated turnover of erythrocytes causes folic acid deficiency and megaloblastic anemia (Chapter 167).

First 20 Years

Although any complication can occur at any age, certain events tend to predominate in different age groups. In life's first decades, the most common sickle cell disease–related clinical events are painful episodes, acute chest syndrome, and stroke. Delayed growth and sexual development, more severe in patients with sickle cell anemia than in those with HbSC disease, become major issues of concern to the adolescent, but sexual maturation is eventually achieved.

Psychosocial problems are common in adolescents with sickle cell disease. Difficulties with medical staff often begin in adolescence and frequently center on issues of pain management and inpatient stay.

The Painful Episode

Pain, presumed to be caused by sickle vaso-occlusion, often starts in young children as the hand-foot syndrome: painful swelling of the hands and feet caused by inflammation of the metacarpal and metatarsal periosteum. Acute painful episodes are the most commonly encountered vaso-occlusive events in patients of all ages, but what triggers an acute painful episode is usually

FIGURE 166-3. Diagnosis of sickle cell disease. **A,** A prototypical family structure in which both parents (I) have sickle cell trait and each offspring (II) has a 25% chance of having sickle cell anemia (SS). Each child of an affected parent (III) will have sickle cell trait (SA) if the other parent has a normal hemoglobin (AA) genotype. The center and right blood films are from patients with sickle cell anemia and HbSC disease, respectively. Note the irreversibly sickled cells (ISCs) in the former and the hemoglobin C (HbC) crystal and target cells in the latter. **B,** High-performance liquid chromatography (HPLC) profiles from patients with sickle cell trait (*left*), sickle cell anemia (*center*), and HbSC disease (*right*). **C,** Amplification refractory mutation system (ARMS)-based separation of the β-globin genes from a normal subject (AA), a carrier of sickle cell trait (AS), and a patient with sickle cell anemia (SS).

unknown. Commonly, painful episodes begin with little warning; some patients, however, may sense one in the offing. These episodes, which last from hours to many days, may wax and wane in intensity and migrate from site to site. No useful laboratory test can tell whether a vaso-occlusive pain episode is occurring, and the history remains the best clue. Sickle cell pain is described as worse than postoperative or traumatic pain. Some women describe the pain of childbirth as paling in comparison with the pain experienced during painful episodes. These agonizing attacks of acute pain must be separated from chronic pain perhaps caused by osteoporosis of the spine, pain associated with osteonecrosis of the hips and shoulders, neuropathic pain, iatrogenic pain, and the milder aches, pains, and soreness that are frequently present between severe episodes.

Patients vary greatly in the number, severity, and frequency of their painful episodes. Painful episodes are often stereotypical, affecting individuals in the same manner from episode to episode. Patients usually know whether the pain they are experiencing is different from their typical painful episode, and the wise physician should heed a patient's advice about the need for hospitalization or the likelihood that the pain has an alternative explanation.

About 40% of patients do not have pain requiring a hospital visit in a given year, whereas 3% have more than six painful episodes per year. Having more

than three pain episodes requiring hospitalization per year is associated with increased mortality among patients 20 years and older. Recent studies suggest that pain is present on about half of all days; most episodes are managed at home and not in a medical setting, so hospital visits underestimate the frequency of pain.

HbF levels are inversely related to the frequency of painful episodes. Concurrent α-thalassemia may increase the pain rate because of its effect on the hematocrit. The day-to-day management of sickle cell disease often equates with the management of acute and chronic pain.

The pain accompanying acute chest syndrome, acute cholecystitis, splenic sequestration crisis, splenic infarction, or right upper quadrant syndrome may sometimes be mistaken for uncomplicated pain episodes. Acute painful episodes often herald the acute chest syndrome, and occasionally pain episodes end with multiorgan failure. Unexplained death can occur during acute painful episodes, perhaps as a result of an arrhythmia secondary to unrecognizable myocardial damage or perhaps as a sequela of pulmonary hypertension. Currently, it is not possible to foretell whether a "usual" pain episode will have an unexpected mortal outcome or presage acute chest syndrome, but the presence of atypically severe pain or an uncommonly high leukocyte count or low hematocrit should be cause for extra scrutiny.

FIGURE 166-4. Pathophysiology of sickle cell disease. An adenine (A) to thymidine (T) transversion (A6T) at codon 6 in the β-hemoglobin gene on chromosome 11 *(HBB)* leads to the substitution of a glutamic acid codon by a valine codon. β⁶ valine endows the hemoglobin S (HbS) molecule ($\alpha_2\beta_2^S$) with the property of polymerization when deoxygenated. HbS polymer injures the erythrocyte and leads to a heterogenous population of sickle cells with damaged membrane cytoskeleton, reduced cation and water content, and altered distribution of membrane lipids. In the vasculature, sickle cells interact with endothelium and other blood cells to cause vaso-occlusion. Some damaged erythrocytes hemolyze intravascularly, thereby releasing heme into the plasma to scavenge nitric oxide (NO) and to reduce hemoglobin to methemoglobin and nitrate. NO, by binding soluble guanylate cyclase, converts cyclic guanosine triphosphate (cGTP) to guanosine monophosphate (GMP), thereby relaxing vascular smooth muscle and causing vasodilation. A state of reduced endothelial NO bioavailability in sickle cell disease impairs the homeostatic vascular functions of NO, such as inhibition of platelet activation and aggregation and transcriptional repression of genes transcribing cell adhesion molecules. Hemoglobin, heme, and heme iron catalyze the production of oxygen radicals and protein nitration, potentially further limiting NO bioavailability and activating endothelium. Lysed erythrocytes also liberate arginase, which destroys L-arginine, the substrate for NO production, providing another mechanism for endothelial NO deficiency. The normal balance of vasoconstriction versus vasodilation is therefore skewed toward vasoconstriction as well as endothelial activation and proliferation. EC = epithelial cell; ISC = irreversibly sickled cell; N = neutrophil; R = reticulocyte; RBC = red blood cell.

TABLE 166-2   FEATURES OF SICKLE CELL ANEMIA

Painful episodes: associated with higher hemoglobin
Acute chest syndrome: associated with higher hemoglobin
Stroke: associated with lower hemoglobin
Osteonecrosis: associated with higher hemoglobin
Priapism: associated with lower hemoglobin
Proliferative retinopathy: associated with higher hemoglobin
Splenic infarction and sequestration
Leg ulcers: associated with lower hemoglobin
Gallstones
Aplastic crisis
Osteopenia—bone marrow hyperplasia
Nutritional deficiencies—folic acid, zinc, calories
Pneumococcal disease and sepsis
Placental insufficiency
Some complications are associated with hemoglobin concentration

Stroke

A major complication of sickle cell anemia in early life is stroke caused by stenosis and occlusion of large vessels (Chapter 414). Sickle erythrocytes and anemia-related high blood flow velocity lead to vascular damage. Hemorrhagic stroke is often caused by rupture of aneurysms. Moyamoya disease, a proliferation of small vessels found in sickle cell patients with stenotic lesions, may also cause hemorrhage in adults (Chapter 414). Hemorrhagic stroke is associated with a mortality rate of more than 20%. Stroke is most common among patients with sickle cell anemia, with much lower rates among those with HbSC disease or HbS-β⁺-thalassemia. Beyond age 1 year, the incidence of stroke in sickle cell anemia is approximately 0.5 events per 100 patient

years until age 40 years. The risk of having a first stroke is 11% by age 20 years, 15% by age 30 years, and 24% by age 45 years. Severe anemia, acute chest syndrome, and elevated systolic blood pressure are associated with ischemic strokes, whereas an elevated leukocyte count is a risk factor for hemorrhagic stroke. α-Thalassemia may protect patients with sickle cell anemia from stroke, perhaps because these patients have less hemolysis and a higher hematocrit. Subclinical neurologic events and silent cerebral infarction are even more common than stroke. The aberrant behavior of some sickle cell patients is most likely a result of otherwise silent cerebral infarction with deteriorating neurocognitive function.

Acute Chest Syndrome

Acute chest syndrome, characterized by fever, chest pain, wheezing, cough, hypoxia, and a new lung infiltrate, is a sometimes lethal complication that affects more than half of all patients with sickle cell anemia. It is the second most common reason for hospitalization and is a frequent cause of death in adults. The syndrome is more frequent in children, in whom its course is often mild, than in adults, in whom it tends to be more severe.

Commonly, acute chest syndrome develops after several days in individuals hospitalized for an acute painful episode (see earlier discussion). Acute chest syndrome also often occurs postoperatively, even when patients are properly prepared with blood transfusion. Other causes include rib infarction with atelectasis and regional hypoxia; fat emboli from the bone marrow (Chapter 98); infection with chlamydia, parvovirus B19, or other viral agents; microvascular or large vessel in situ thrombosis; thromboembolic disease; and vascular injury and inflammation. Fat embolism can be identified by finding lipid within pulmonary macrophages obtained by bronchopulmonary lavage, but this nonstandardized test is not recommended.

In most cases of acute chest syndrome, a cause cannot be found early enough to guide treatment. Elevated concentrations of phospholipase A₂ have been found in patients with sickle cell disease in association with acute chest syndrome and may predict its occurrence, but this test is not used widely.

Acute Anemia

Acute anemia can result from sequestration of blood in the spleen or liver, an aplastic crisis caused by parvovirus B19 infection (Chapter 379), or a severe vaso-occlusive event, such as acute chest syndrome or multiorgan failure. Transfusion may be needed. Megaloblastic arrest of erythropoiesis is uncommon if the diet is adequate in folic acid.

Infection

Because patients with sickle cell anemia are functionally asplenic early in life and hyposplenic later, they are susceptible to infection with encapsulated bacteria. Persistent gross splenomegaly but not normal splenic function is common in patients with sickle cell disease in Africa and is related to endemic malaria. Splenomegaly and splenic function often persist in patients with HbSC disease—hence the reduced incidence of infection but risk of splenic sequestration and infarction in adults. Prevention of mortality from pneumococcal infection is the basis for screening of newborns for sickle cell disease and the use of prophylactic oral penicillin in affected individuals. Pneumococcal vaccines (Chapter 17) are also recommended.

Age 20 to 40 Years
Pregnancy

There is no absolute contraindication to pregnancy for patients with sickle cell anemia, and fertility is probably normal. All approved methods of contraception can be used satisfactorily.

Modern medical management generally achieves good results of pregnancy, but the rates of pyelonephritis, pregnancy-induced hypertension (Chapter 247), and cesarean section are increased, and babies are more likely to have low birthweight. Some obstetricians believe that blood transfusions should be used routinely, but limited data suggest that, with good prenatal care, transfusions do not improve the outcome.

Osteonecrosis and Bone Diseases

Osteonecrosis of the hip and shoulder joints (Chapter 256) affects about half of all patients with sickle cell anemia or HbSC disease. Its onset is insidious but progressive, and most patients with early-stage disease progress to collapse of the femoral head within 2 years. Osteonecrosis of the hip usually manifests with pain in and around the affected joint, or at times with spasm of the surrounding muscles. Patients with higher hematocrits and with sickle cell anemia α-thalassemia have the highest prevalence of osteonecrosis. Osteonecrosis can be detected very early by magnetic resonance imaging, but only more advanced disease is visible on plain radiographs.

Osteomyelitis (Chapter 280) is often difficult to distinguish from bone infarction. Osteomyelitis is usually caused by staphylococcal infection, but salmonella infection is a particular cause of sickle cell osteomyelitis.

Leg Ulcers

About 5 to 10% of patients with sickle cell anemia older than 10 years of age develop leg ulcers, but leg ulcers are rare in HbSC disease or HbS-β$^+$-thalassemia and in children before age 10 years. In the tropics, leg ulcers are more common. Small and superficial leg ulcers heal spontaneously with rest and careful local hygiene. Control of local inflammation and infection remains the mainstay of treatment. Dressing the ulcer with an Unna boot protects the involved area and is a reasonable method of conservative management. Deep, large, painful ulcers may require large doses of narcotic analgesics, prolonged bed rest, and even surgery.

Priapism

Priapism, a prolonged undesirable painful erection, may be seen in 40% of men with sickle cell anemia. Priapism in sickle cell anemia is usually bicorporeal, with only the corpora cavernosa affected. Venous outflow is obstructed rather than arterial flow increased. In bicorporeal priapism, the glans remains soft, and urination is normal. Recurrent, self-limited attacks of priapism can last for several hours with tolerable discomfort. These episodes have been termed stuttering priapism and usually have a nocturnal onset. Erectile function is usually preserved between attacks. Major episodes of priapism often, but not always, follow a history of stuttering attacks, last for days, and can be excruciatingly painful; they often end in impotency. Affected patients have a

higher incidence of stroke, pulmonary hypertension, renal failure, leg ulcers, and premature death than individuals without priapism, perhaps reflecting the severity of vasculopathy.

Digestive Diseases

Sickle hepatopathy, hepatic crisis, and right upper quadrant syndrome are terms applied to sickle cell–associated liver disease. Liver disease may be related to intrahepatic and extrahepatic cholestasis, viral hepatitis (Chapter 150), cirrhosis, hypoxia, infarction, erythrocyte sequestration, iron overload (Chapter 153), or drug reactions (Chapter 152). Differentiation among these potential causes can be difficult. Increased bilirubin levels (Chapter 149) are often the result of unconjugated bilirubinemia and are a manifestation of hemolytic anemia.

Gallstones

Cholelithiasis (Chapter 158), a consequence of the accelerated bile pigment turnover typical of hemolytic anemia, can appear in the first decade of life, and more than half of all adults are affected. Depending on the degree of calcification, pigmented gallstones may be either radiopaque or radiolucent. Ultrasonography is the preferred means of detection, and laparoscopic cholecystectomy is the preferred method of dealing with symptomatic stones. Documented episodes of acute cholecystitis and typical obstructive jaundice are much less frequent than the presence of stones. If stones are asymptomatic or symptoms and laboratory findings suggesting cholecystitis are equivocal, careful observation may be the best course.

Beyond the Fifth Decade
Pulmonary Hypertension

Echocardiographic studies show that 30 to 43% of adults with sickle cell anemia have a tricuspid regurgitant velocity (TRV) of more than 2.5 m/second (Chapter 55), suggestive of pulmonary hypertension (Chapter 68). This is associated with a six- to ten-fold increased risk in mortality. Although it is assumed that many patients with elevated TRV have pulmonary hypertension, pulmonary artery catheterization data in this population are limited, and it is likely that in many instances, an elevated TRV is not synonymous with true pulmonary hypertension. Pulmonary arterial hypertension is present in about half of catheterized patients, but with milder hemodynamics and symptoms compared with idiopathic pulmonary hypertension, particularly early in the course of disease. Increased TRV and the coexistence of relative systemic hypertension, renal disease, and intimal and smooth muscle proliferative changes in conduit vessels suggest the presence of a more widespread vasculopathy, which may be responsible for the observed mortality risk. Increased TRV is also seen in children and in patients with HbSC disease.

Nephropathy

Hyposthenuria is present in almost all patients with sickle cell anemia and even in most carriers of sickle cell trait (Table 166-3). Clinically, the loss of urine concentrating ability is not important unless access to fluid is restricted. Isosthenuria, distal renal tubular acidosis, and impaired potassium excretion are signs of medullary dysfunction.

Glomerular hyperfiltration, increased creatinine secretion, and a very low serum creatinine are characteristic of young patients with sickle cell anemia, so renal dysfunction can be present even with normal serum creatinine values. Glomerulopathy begins very early in life, but an increasing prevalence of renal failure is a hallmark of an aging population of sickle cell anemia patients. About 4% of patients with sickle cell anemia and 2% of those with HbSC develop renal failure, at median ages of 23 and 50 years, respectively. Among sickle cell patients, 60% of those older than 40 years of age have proteinuria, and 30% have renal insufficiency. Nephrotic syndrome is found in 40% of adults with creatinine levels greater than 1.5 mg/dL. Survival time for patients with sickle cell anemia after the diagnosis of sickle renal failure is 4 years, even with dialysis.

Eye Disease

Proliferative sickle retinopathy is present in fewer than 20% of patients with sickle cell anemia but in more than 40% of those with HbSC disease by the third decade of life. Vitreal hemorrhage and retinal detachment can occasionally lead to visual loss, but proliferative lesions may regress spontaneously. Screening for proliferative retinopathy using fluorescence angiography is recommended in patients with HbSC disease to guide possible laser photocoagulation.

TABLE 166-3 RENAL ABNORMALITIES IN SICKLE CELL DISEASE*

DISTAL NEPHRON

Impaired urine concentrating ability
Impaired urine acidification—incomplete renal tubular acidosis
Impaired K+ excretion

HEMATURIA

PAPILLARY NECROSIS

PROXIMAL TUBULE

Increased phosphate reabsorption
Increased β2-microglobulin reabsorption
Increased uric acid secretion
Increased creatinine secretion

HEMODYNAMIC CHANGES

Increased glomerular filtration rate
Increased renal plasma flow
Decreased filtration fraction

GLOMERULAR ABNORMALITIES

Proteinuria
Nephrotic syndrome with focal glomerular sclerosis
Chronic renal failure

*In carriers of sickle cell trait, because of its hypertonicity and oxygen content, HbS can polymerize in the renal medulla and lead to hyposthenuria, a possible increased risk of urinary tract infection during pregnancy, papillary necrosis, and hematuria. A rare tumor, medullary carcinoma, arises from distal nephrons and is associated with sickle cell trait.

Cardiovascular Complications

The heart is usually enlarged, with a hyperactive precordium and systolic ejection murmurs. Myocardial infarction is rare and when present suggests small vessel disease. Sudden unexpected and unexplained death is common in adults and may be due to arrhythmias and pulmonary hypertension.

Patients with sickle cell anemia usually have blood pressures that are in the normal range yet inappropriately high compared with controls who have similar levels of anemia. "Relative" hypertension in sickle cell anemia may reflect endothelial cell damage and NO scavenging. Survival is decreased and the risk of stroke is increased as blood pressure rises. Treatment goals of 120/80 mm Hg or less are generally the same as for other patients (Chapter 67).

DIAGNOSIS

Normocytic, microcytic, or macrocytic hemolytic anemia with reticulocytosis, increased levels of lactate dehydrogenase and aspartate aminotransferase, and a compatible clinical history should suggest the presence of sickle cell disease. Nevertheless, because of the multiple genotypes and considerable clinical heterogeneity of each genotype, milder cases may not be diagnosed for many years.

The Blood

In sickle cell anemia, the erythrocytes are normocytic or macrocytic depending on the reticulocyte count. Microcytosis in a suspected case of sickle cell disease can be seen very early in life, when iron deficiency has developed, or when β-thalassemia or α-thalassemia is present. Sickled cells are usually present in the peripheral blood smear in sickle cell anemia and in HbS-β⁰-thalassemia (see Fig. 166-3A) but are less common in other forms of sickle cell disease. In HbSC disease, target cells are prominent, and HbC crystalizes in some cells (see Fig. 166-3A). ISC numbers remain relatively constant over time, although their percentage may rise early during a painful episode. Finding ISCs has no value for establishing whether a patient is experiencing a vaso-occlusive episode.

Hemoglobin Composition of the Blood

After 1 year of age, hemoglobin fractions are sufficiently stable to be relied on for diagnosis, but the high HbF concentrations of early infancy often make the results of hemoglobin analysis at that time difficult to interpret. In patients with sickle cell anemia, except in infancy, HbS almost always forms more than 80% of the hemolysate. HbS is best detected by high-performance liquid chromatography (HPLC), which is also the method of choice for quantitation of the hemoglobin fractions in newborns and adults (see Fig. 166-3B),

or by isoelectric focusing that provides qualitative information. HPLC provides excellent resolution of hemoglobin fractions, gives quantitative results, and is automated. HbF levels in adults average about 6% but can vary between 1 and 20%. DNA-based methods of detecting HbS are specific but usually are not needed for uncomplicated cases. Nevertheless, they are necessary for antenatal diagnosis and, sometimes, for genetic counseling (see Fig. 166-3C).

Family Studies

The *HBB* gene on chromosome 11 (see Fig. 166-2) is inherited as a codominant trait, implying that both normal and mutant alleles are expressed and are easily detectable. However, the sickle cell phenotype (see Table 166-1) is present only in homozygotes for HbS and in certain compound heterozygotes. Family studies (see Fig. 166-3) can suggest a patient's hemoglobin genotype.

PREVENTION AND TREATMENT   Rx

Primary Prevention

In populations with a high prevalence of the HbS gene, heterozygote detection is simple, but there is little proven benefit of a broad screening effort to detect carriers. A preferred approach consists of educational programs about sickle cell disease and sickle cell trait, followed by counseling for couples who are planning families. These couples are offered the choice of testing, after which the risks of having affected fetuses can be discussed and the availability of antenatal diagnosis by chorionic villus sampling or amniocentesis presented.

General Measures

Sickle cell disease is a chronic disorder, for which good nutrition and timely immunizations are critical. Work should be encouraged.

Older children do not routinely need continued antibiotic prophylaxis. Neonatal screening to detect newborns with sickle cell disease allows early administration of prophylactic penicillin[1] and antipneumococcal immunization. These measures reduce the incidence of and mortality from pneumococcal bacteremia in children younger than 5 years of age who have sickle cell anemia.

Because of increased rates of RBC production and inadequate nutrition, folic acid, 1 mg daily, is generally recommended but may not be necessary with a good dietary intake. There is no evidence that high concentrations of inhaled oxygen are of preventive value.

Hydroxyurea

Hydroxyurea, the sole drug approved by the U.S. Food and Drug Administration for treatment of sickle cell anemia, increases HbF in these patients because its cytotoxicity causes erythroid regeneration and perhaps because its metabolism leads to NO-related increases in soluble guanylate cyclase, with a subsequent increase in cyclic guanosine monophosphate (cGMP) that augments γ-globin gene expression. In a multicenter trial in adults with sickle cell anemia, hydroxyurea reduced the incidence of pain and acute chest syndrome by almost 50%,[2] with little risk during more than 17.5 years of observation.[3,4] In follow-up studies, cumulative mortality was reduced almost 40%, and the favorable result was related to the ability of the drug to increase HbF and reduce painful episodes and the acute chest syndrome. Children have a more robust HbF response to hydroxyurea than adults. Cancer and leukemia have been reported in patients with sickle cell disease treated with hydroxyurea, but whether the incidence is higher than in the general population is not known. Hydroxyurea should be used in nearly all adults with sickle cell anemia and HbS-β⁰ thalassemia (Table 166-4). However, not all patients who might benefit from this treatment receive it. The clinical benefits of hydroxyurea in HbSC disease are just beginning to be studied.

Red Blood Cell Transfusion

Acute transfusions of packed RBCs can be life-saving, and chronic transfusions reduce the incidence and severity of most complications of sickle cell disease. However, repeated transfusions produce iron overload, alloimmunization, loss of venous access, and viral infection. Whether exchange transfusion is preferable to simple transfusion in the acute chest syndrome, stroke, or other acute complications has not been tested in clinical trials. For severe symptomatic anemia or stroke prophylaxis, simple transfusions are preferred.

Treatment of Common Complications
Painful Episodes

A decision as to whether hospitalization is needed can be made after an assessment of the duration and severity of the pain and the response to treatment. Associated factors such as excessive tachycardia, hypotension, body temperature higher than 38.3° C (101° F), marked leukocytosis, a fall in the hematocrit and platelet count, hypoxia, or a new infiltrate on chest radiography should prompt admission.

TABLE 166-4 HYDROXYUREA TREATMENT IN SICKLE CELL ANEMIA*

BASELINE EVALUATION

Blood counts, RBC indices, HbF level, serum chemistries, pregnancy test, willingness to adhere to all recommendations for treatment, not receiving chronic RBC transfusions

INITIATION OF TREATMENT

Hydroxyurea 10-15 mg/kg/day or, for adults, 500 mg every morning for 6-8 wk

CONTINUATION OF TREATMENT

If counts are acceptable by CBC every 2 wk (granulocytes, ≥2000/mm^3; platelets, ≥80,000/mm^3), escalate dose in increments of 200 to 500 mg every 6-8 wk. When a stable nontoxic dose of hydroxyurea is reached, CBC may be done at 4- to 8-wk intervals. Most good responses require 1000 to 2000 mg/day and a final dose more than 30 mg/kg/day should be the top.

GOALS OF TREATMENT

Less pain, increase in HbF (usually measured every 6-8 wk) or MCV, increased hematocrit if severely anemic, acceptable toxicity. Failure of HbF to increase may be due to biologic inability to respond to treatment or, more often, to poor compliance with treatment. If compliance is documented, the dose can be increased cautiously to 2000-2500 mg/day (maximum dose, 30 mg/kg).

*Special caution should be exercised in patients with compromised renal or hepatic function and in those who are habituated to narcotics. Contraception should be practiced by both men and women. Without chronic RBC transfusions or an intercurrent illness suppressing erythropoiesis, a trial period of 6 to 12 months is probably adequate.
CBC = complete blood count; HbF = fetal hemoglobin; MCV = mean corpuscular volume; RBC = red blood cell.

TABLE 166-5 PULMONARY COMPLICATIONS OF SICKLE CELL DISEASE

ACUTE CHEST SYNDROME

Diagnosis: Chest pain, fever, cough wheezing, new infiltrate on chest radiograph, hypoxemia

Management: simple or exchange transfusions, pain relief, oxygen if hypoxemic, bronchodilators, incentive spirometry, antibiotics (broad coverage)

PULMONARY HYPERTENSION

Diagnosis: Tricuspid regurgitant velocity (TRV) ≥ 2.5 m/sec by echocardiography. May also have an elevated N-terminal pro–brain natriuretic peptide (NT-pro-BNP) (≥160 pg/mL) and a reduced 6-min walk distance (≤350 m).

Management: Screen by echocardiography beginning at age 18 yr, repeat echocardiogram periodically according to symptoms. If TRV > 3.0 m/sec, refer for right heart catheterization. Consider anticoagulation, treatment of iron overload and nocturnal hypoxemia. Optimize hydroxyurea, consider chronic transfusions and pulmonary vasodilator therapy.

ASTHMA

ABNORMAL PULMONARY FUNCTION

Physical examination is usually not helpful, but sometimes there is localized swelling and pain over an involved bone. Low-grade fever and a mild increase in leukocytosis can accompany uncomplicated painful episodes, but higher temperature elevations may point to infection or extensive tissue damage.

The cornerstones of pain management (Chapter 29) are fluid replacement and opioid analgesics. Because almost every patient is hyposthenuric, urinary output in patients with sickle cell anemia may exceed 2 L/day, making them susceptible to dehydration. Pain is often accompanied by reduced fluid intake and increased water losses, so increased fluid intake is essential. Administration of 5% dextrose in water and 0.25 to 0.5 normal saline should be used for initial fluid replacement. Although needs vary and hydration should be monitored closely to avoid iatrogenic heart failure or electrolyte imbalance, the daily fluid intake should be approximately 3 to 5 L for adults and 100 to 150 mL/kg for children. Oxygen should be reserved for patients who are hypoxic or have acute respiratory distress. Infection should always be considered and treated early if present, although bacterial infections are uncommon.

Analgesic management presupposes that other treatments, such as hydration, oxygen, and antimicrobial agents, are used if needed. The key to successful pain management is individualized treatment and dosing, taking into account prior pain management and prior use of opioids. Patient-controlled analgesia and a scheduled regimen of drug dosing are preferable, and PRN analgesics should be avoided. Frequent reassessment of the effects of treatment is paramount so that opioid doses can be titrated for pain relief and tapered when relief is obtained. Meperidine should be avoided because its metabolites (e.g., normeperidine) can cause central nervous system excitation. Pain management (Chapter 29) is complicated by the influence of learned pain behavior, pain memories, and pain therapy–induced pain. Management proves extremely difficult in perhaps 10% of all patients, and often enormous doses of opioids are required for relief.

Stroke

For new strokes, after initial stabilization and transfusion, chronic RBC transfusion reduces the chance of recurrent ischemic stroke. However, it is not known how long chronic transfusions should continue. In practice, transfusions are often stopped after children make the transition from pediatric to adult care. Long-term management of hemorrhagic stroke is unclear, and whether transfusion reduces their recurrence is unknown. Increased intracranial flow velocity, measurable only in children, increases the risk of stroke, but its sensitivity is only 10%, with a far from perfect specificity. Children found to be at risk for stroke by transcranial Doppler flow velocities should be started on chronic transfusions,[5] but it is unclear whether or when such transfusions may be discontinued.

Acute Chest Syndrome

Routine treatments for acute chest syndrome initially include bronchodilators (e.g., albuterol nebulizer 0.25 mL in 2.5 mL normal saline; or albuterol metered-dose inhaler during the acute episode), incentive spirometry,

empirical antimicrobial agents as used for community-acquired pneumonia (e.g., ceftriaxone or azithromycin or levofloxacin for 5 to 7 days [Chapter 97]), and supplemental oxygen when hypoxia is noted by continuous or frequent monitoring of blood oxygen saturation. Opioid analgesics (e.g., morphine) are often needed, but their dose should be titrated carefully to avoid respiratory depression and worsening of hypoxia.

Blood transfusion is the cornerstone of treatment when a patient becomes hypoxic, develops respiratory distress, has a clinically significant fall in the hematocrit and platelet count or increase in leukocyte count, or shows any sign of multiorgan failure, such as impaired mentation, rhabdomyolysis, renal failure, or liver failure. Both simple transfusion and exchange transfusions appear to reverse many adverse findings of the acute chest syndrome, but controlled studies have never tested the superiority of either method. Although the death rate in acute chest syndrome is less than 10%, a few patients have a rapidly deteriorating course with sudden development of the acute respiratory distress syndrome (ARDS; Chapter 104), as manifested by increased oxygen requirements, extensive pulmonary opacification, and multiorgan failure. Excessive hydration and fat emboli are potential contributing causes. Successful management of severe acute chest syndrome and ARDS requires close coordination among physicians and nurses. Some patients have repeated episodes of severe acute chest syndrome, and chronic transfusion can reduce the recurrence rate. Hydroxyurea also reduces the rate of acute chest syndrome by about 50%.

Osteonecrosis and Bone Disease

Treatment with reduced weight bearing, nonsteroidal anti-inflammatory drugs (NSAIDs), and physical therapy is the mainstay of conservative management but does not retard progression of osteonecrosis and bone disease. Total hip arthroplasty can be very successful, but about one third of prostheses fail within 4 to 5 years.

Diffuse osteoporosis (Chapter 251) is usually present, and osteomalacia (Chapter 252) due to vitamin D deficiency is common in both children and adults. If vitamin D deficiency is present, treatment with calcium (1000 mg PO daily) and vitamin D (50,000 IU PO every week for 2 months, then 50,000 IU PO every other week) is reasonable.

Priapism

Conservative treatment of priapism includes analgesics, hydration, and transfusions. Aspiration and irrigation of the corporeal bodies should be performed within a 12-hour window from the onset of erection if the episode differs from prior episodes of stuttering priapism. Operative treatment, which should be considered after 24 to 48 hours of priapism, includes the creation of shunts between the corpora cavernosa and spongiosum. For a typical episode of low-flow priapism, a Winter shunt between the glans penis and corpora cavernosa should be performed within 24 to 48 hours. Oral or intra-cavernous administration of α-adrenergic agonists such as pseudoephedrine and sildenafil treatment are being studied.

Pulmonary Hypertension

Patients with sickle cell anemia should be screened by echocardiography for the presence of pulmonary hypertension because of the prognostic importance of an elevated TRV, although management of patients with few symptoms and minimally elevated TRV is ill defined. For symptomatic individuals, optimization of hydroxyurea, transfusions, sildenafil, bosentan, and epoprostenol have all been used, but controlled trials reporting their effectiveness in sickle cell patients have not been (Table 166-5) reported.

Renal Disease

In a small randomized trial, 6 months' treatment with 25 mg/day of captopril caused a 37% reduction in microalbuminuria, compared with a 17% increase in placebo-treated patients; such treatment would be reasonable in patients with known microalbuminuria, but whether screening or long-term treatment is worthwhile is unknown. NSAIDs reduce the glomerular filtration rate in sickle cell anemia and should be avoided in older individuals with creatinine levels of 1.2 mg/dL or higher. Dialysis and renal transplantation are used in end-stage sickle cell nephropathy, but with outcomes less favorable than in other types of renal failure.

Surgery and Anesthesia

Preoperative blood transfusion should be used for all surgeries requiring general anesthesia and selected other surgeries. Simple transfusion to a hematocrit of about 30% before surgery is as effective in preventing postoperative complications as exchange transfusion and causes fewer transfusion-related complications.[6] In some minor surgeries, it is likely that preoperative transfusion is unnecessary.

Implantable infusion ports and catheters have higher risks of complications in sickle cell anemia, including thrombosis of large veins and bacteremia. Low-dose warfarin may retard thrombosis of these devices.

Red Blood Cell Transfusion and Iron Chelation Therapy

The customary level of chronic stable anemia alone is seldom an indication for transfusion. With aging and the onset of renal failure, anemia worsens and can become symptomatic. Transfusion may become necessary, although judicious use of erythropoietin (e.g., darbepoetin, 0.45 μg/kg every 2 weeks, increased as needed) can often restore the hematocrit to prerenal failure levels and should not be higher because of the potential adverse effects of hyperviscosity.

It is advised that patients undergo erythrocyte phenotyping to determine their RBC antigens before embarking on a transfusion program. Otherwise, alloimmunization occurs in about one fourth of frequently transfused patients. In the presence of multiple alloantibodies, it may be difficult to find compatible blood.

With repeated transfusion, iron overload inevitably develops and can result in heart and liver failure and many other complications (Chapter 219). Serum ferritin is an inaccurate means of estimating the iron burden. Liver biopsy might be the most accurate means of determining tissue iron concentration and the response to chelation, but magnetic resonance imaging (FerriScan) correlates very well with this measurement and is noninvasive.

Chelation of excessive iron can be achieved using deferasirox (20 mg/kg orally daily).[7] Increases in serum creatinine and proteinuria occur in about 40% of patients. Desferrioxamine is a parenteral chelator and is usually started with 25 to 30 mg/kg given subcutaneously five times per week in 8- to 12-hour infusions (Chapter 219). Side effects include skin reactions, ototoxicity, retinal toxicity, bone and growth abnormalities, and *Yersinia* infection resulting from the sudden mobilization of iron. Another oral chelator, deferiprone, is less potent than deferasirox or desferrioxamine but is useful instead of or in addition to these drugs; at present, it is approved for use in more than 40 countries but not the United States. Side effects requiring discontinuation of deferiprone, seen in 5 to 10% of patients, include agranulocytosis, neutropenia, arthropathy, and gastrointestinal symptoms.

Stem Cell Transplantation

Successful stem cell transplantation (Chapter 181) can cure sickle cell anemia, but only about 10% of patients have suitable donors. Myeloablative stem cell transplantation carries a 5 to 10% mortality rate and is poorly tolerated in adults. A nonmyeloablative regimen that used total-body irradiation and treatment with alemtuzumab and sirolimus led to stable mixed chimerism in 10 adults transplanted with an HLA-identical family donor, with no graft versus host disease observed. If extended to a larger group of patients and to haploidentical transplants, this approach would be a major advance in treating the most severely ill patients.

FUTURE DIRECTIONS

Experimental treatments to induce higher levels of HbF more consistently and to reduce HbS polymer with drugs that may remodel chromosomal structure (e.g., short-chain fatty acids and their derivatives) or affect hypomethylation of the HbF gene promoters (e.g., decitabine) are undergoing clinical trials. Where malaria is endemic, antimalaria prophylaxis reduces episodes of malaria and increases mean hemoglobin levels. Gene therapy trials are slowly progressing.

PROGNOSIS

Average life expectancy for patients with sickle cell anemia in the United States is between 50 and 60 years; patients with HbSC disease typically live 60 to 70 years. Patients with HbS-β⁰-thalassemia are likely to have a life expectancy similar to those with sickle cell anemia, and the lifespan for patients with the HbS-β⁺ form may resemble that of patients with HbSC disease. Death is often caused by infection, and another 20% of deaths are related to organ failure. However, death in adults often is unexpected, happening in the midst of an acute event such as an acute painful episode, and occurring within the first 24 hours of hospitalization. In areas of the developing world without access to modern medical care, death in childhood is still common.

OTHER HEMOGLOBINOPATHIES

Hemoglobinopathies other than those associated with HbS, HbE, and HbC rarely cause clinically recognizable disorders. HbC (*HBB* Glu6Lys) and HbE (*HBB* Glu26Lys) are common β-globin variants. As with HbS, their high gene frequencies are a result of the positive selective pressure of endemic falciparum malaria. HbC is present in about 2% of African Americans, and HbE is seen in Southeast Asia, where, in some areas, the gene frequency may reach 50%. Heterozygotes with either mutation are asymptomatic, although the blood of HbC trait carriers contains target cells, and HbE carriers may have very mild anemia and microcytosis. Even homozygotes for HbC and HbE have virtually no clinical disease, only mild hematologic abnormalities such as microcytosis, target cells, and mild anemia. Compound heterozygotes for HbE and β-thalassemia usually have the phenotype of transfusion-dependent β-thalassemia, although genotype-phenotype correlations are difficult to make because of the likelihood that other genes affect the expression of disease.

Rare hemoglobinopathies may change the affinity of hemoglobin for oxygen, render it susceptible to oxidation, or cause molecular instability. Amino acid substitutions involving heme-binding residues may lead to irreversible iron oxidation, methemoglobinemia, and cyanosis (Chapter 161). Patients with these conditions have congenital pseudocyanosis but are usually asymptomatic and need no treatment.

Substitutions at contacts between globin subunits may alter the affinity of hemoglobin for oxygen. When hemoglobin-oxygen affinity is increased, less oxygen is available in tissues, erythropoietin production is enhanced, and erythrocytosis results (Chapter 169). Usually, no treatment is required because the erythrocytosis is mild. Hemoglobin-oxygen affinity may also be reduced by some mutations, resulting in anemia or cyanosis. Hemoglobin instability, produced by several molecular mechanisms (including introduction of proline residues into the α-helix, substitutions near the heme ring, and deletion or addition of amino acids) often causes loss of heme from the molecule and hemolytic anemia. Hb Koln is the most common example of this class of hemoglobinopathy, but more than 200 unstable variants have been described. Sometimes, oxidant drugs provoke increased hemolysis. Splenectomy is sometimes effective treatment when the anemia is severe.

1. Gaston MH, Verter J, Woods G, et al. Prophylaxis with oral penicillin in children with sickle cell anemia. *N Engl J Med.* 1986;314:1593-1599.
2. Charache S, Terrin ML, Moore RD, et al. Effect of hydroxyurea on the frequency of painful crises in sickle cell anemia. *N Engl J Med.* 1995;332:1317-1322.
3. Lanzkron S, Strouse JJ, Wilson R, et al. Systematic review: hydroxyurea for the treatment of adults with sickle cell disease. *Ann Intern Med.* 2008;148:939-955.
4. Steinberg MH, McCarthy WF, Castro O, et al. The risks and benefits of long-term use of hydroxyurea in sickle cell anemia: a 17.5 year follow-up. *Am J Hematol.* 2010;85:403-408.
5. Adams RJ, McKie VC, Hsu L, et al. Prevention of a first stroke by transfusions in children with sickle cell anemia and abnormal results on transcranial Doppler ultrasonography [see comments]. *N Engl J Med.* 1998;339:5-11.
6. Vichinsky EP, Haberkern CM, Neumayr L, et al. A comparison of conservative and aggressive transfusion regimens in the perioperative management of sickle cell disease. *N Engl J Med.* 1995;333:206-213.
7. Meerpohl JJ, Antes G, Rücker G, et al. Deferasirox for managing transfusional iron overload in people with sickle cell disease. *Cochrane Database Syst Rev.* 2010;8:CD007477.

SUGGESTED READINGS

Bauer DE, Orkin SH. Update on fetal hemoglobin gene regulation in hemoglobinopathies. *Curr Opin Pediatr.* 2011;23:1-8. *Review.*

Brousseau DC, Owens PL, Mosso AL, et al. Acute care utilization and rehospitalizations for sickle cell disease. *JAMA.* 2010;303:1288-1294. *Acute care encounters and hospitalizations are very common.*

Hsieh MM, Kang EM, Fitzhugh CD, et al. Allogeneic hematopoietic stem-cell transplantation for sickle cell disease. *N Engl J Med.* 2009;361:2309-2317. *Stem cell transplantation with an HLA-identical donor can "cure" sickle cell anemia in adults.*

Rees DC, Williams TN, Gladwin MT. Sickle-cell disease. *Lancet.* 2010;376:2018-2031. *Review.*

Tsaras G, Owusu-Ansah A, Boateng FO, et al. Complications associated with sickle cell trait: a brief narrative review. *Am J Med.* 2009;122:507-512. *Sickle cell trait is "benign" but can be associated with certain complications.*

Wolfson JA, Schrager SM, Coates TD, et al. Sickle-cell disease in California: a population-based description of emergency department utilization. *Pediatr Blood Cancer.* 2011;56:413-419. *Nearly two thirds visited an emergency department each year, and almost 50% were on Medicaid.*

167

MEGALOBLASTIC ANEMIAS

A$OK C. ANTONY

DEFINITION

Megaloblastic anemias, a group of disorders characterized by a distinct morphologic pattern in hematopoietic cells, are commonly due to a deficiency of vitamin B_{12} (cobalamin) or folates. These anemias are globally prevalent and carry a significant burden of morbidity. Folate and cobalamin are both required to sustain one-carbon metabolism, which involves the transfer of one-carbon groups such as methyl-, formyl-, methylene-, methenyl-, and formimino- in enzyme reactions essential for pyrimidine and purine biosynthesis, including the synthesis of three of the four nucleotides of DNA. Thus, a deficiency in cobalamin or folate results in the common biochemical feature of a defect in DNA synthesis, along with lesser alterations in RNA and protein synthesis, leading to a state of unbalanced cell growth and impaired cell division. The majority of megaloblastic cells have DNA values between 2 and 4 N because of delayed cell division. This is morphologically expressed as larger-than-normal "immature" nuclei with finely particulate chromatin, whereas the relatively unimpaired RNA and protein synthesis results in large cells with greater "mature" cytoplasm and cell volume. The microscopic appearance of this nuclear-cytoplasmic asynchrony (or dissociation) is morphologically described as *megaloblastic*. Megaloblastic hematopoiesis commonly presents with anemia, the most easily recognized manifestation of a global defect in DNA synthesis in all proliferating cells (especially of the gastrointestinal and reproductive tracts). Because vitamin replacement is curative, precise identification of the deficient vitamin is essential. In the case of cobalamin, the cause of the deficiency (Table 167-1) dictates the dose and duration of replacement therapy.

EPIDEMIOLOGY
Cobalamin
Nutrition

Cobalamin is a red, water-soluble vitamin with a complex structure that generally resembles the heme molecule, but with cobalt replacing iron in the center of the pyrrole ring. The recommended daily allowance of cobalamin is 2.4 µg for men and nonpregnant women, 2.6 µg for pregnant women, 2.8 µg for lactating women, and between 1.5 and 2 µg for children 9 to 18 years old. Cobalamin is produced in nature only by microorganisms, and humans receive cobalamin solely from the diet. Meat from parenchymal organs is richest in cobalamin (>10 µg/100 g wet weight); fish and animal muscle, milk products, and egg yolks have 1 to 10 µg/100 g wet weight. An average nonvegetarian Western diet with abundant meat, milk and other dairy products, and eggs contains 5 to 7 µg/day of cobalamin, which is adequate to sustain normal cobalamin equilibrium. For vegetarians, the consumption of eggs, milk, and dairy products generally provides less than 0.5 µg/day of cobalamin and cannot sustain cobalamin balance. Other foods, including *nori* (dried seaweed) and *tempeh* (fermented soybean cake), are not reliable sources of cobalamin. Near-vegetarians who consume meat infrequently (usually because of poverty) have a cobalamin status that is only marginally better than that of lacto-ovovegetarians.

Cobalamin is stored exceptionally well in tissues. Of the total body content of 2 to 5 mg in adults, half is in the liver. With a daily loss of 1 µg, dietary cobalamin deficiency can take 5 to 10 years to become apparent. However, it takes about 3 to 4 years to deplete cobalamin stores if dietary cobalamin is abruptly malabsorbed (e.g., ileal resection), thereby interfering with an efficient enterohepatic circulation, which accounts for the turnover of 5 to 10 µg of cobalamin per day and the reabsorption of 75% of cobalamin secreted into bile. Although cobalamin resists high-temperature cooking processes, it is unstable with light exposure and can be converted to inactive analogues.

Folates
Nutrition

Folates are synthesized by microorganisms and plants. Rich food sources include green leafy vegetables (spinach, lettuce, broccoli), beans, fruit (bananas, melons, lemons), yeast, mushrooms, and animal protein (liver, kidney). The recommended daily allowance of folate is 400 µg for adult men and nonpregnant women, 600 µg for pregnant women, 500 µg for lactating women, and 300 to 400 µg for children 9 to 18 years of age. A balanced Western diet can prevent folate deficiency, but the net dietary intake of folate in many developing countries may be insufficient to sustain folate balance and is often less than half of optimum. Folates are susceptible to breakdown during prolonged cooking (>15 minutes), which can destroy 50 to 95% of folate.

PATHOBIOLOGY
Cobalamin
Normal Physiology
Absorption and Transport

Cobalamin in food is usually in coenzyme form (as deoxyadenosylcobalamin and methylcobalamin) and bound to proteins (Fig. 167-1). In the stomach, peptic digestion at low pH is a prerequisite for the release of cobalamin from food protein. Once it is released by proteolysis, cobalamin preferentially binds to a high-affinity cobalamin-binding protein called R protein, which is secreted in salivary and gastric juice. These cobalamin–R protein complexes, along with unbound intrinsic factor, which is produced by gastric parietal cells, pass into the second part of the duodenum, where pancreatic proteases degrade R proteins. This allows the transfer of cobalamin to intrinsic factor.

The stable intrinsic factor–cobalamin complexes then pass through the jejunum to the ileum, where they bind to membrane-associated intrinsic factor–cobalamin receptors (also called *cubam* receptors because they are composed of a complex of two proteins, cubulin and amnionless) on the microvilli of ileal mucosal cells. Within enterocytes, cobalamin is transferred to transcobalamin II, which efficiently binds and delivers cobalamin ultimately to transcobalamin II receptors found on cell surfaces. Another protein, transcobalamin I, which binds approximately 75% of serum cobalamin but does not participate in transport, appears to be a storage protein for cobalamin in blood. A third quantitatively minor protein, transcobalamin III, binds a wide spectrum of cobalamin analogues that are rapidly cleared by the liver into bile for efficient fecal excretion.

Cellular Processing

More than 95% of intracellular cobalamin is bound to two intracellular enzymes: methylmalonyl-coenzyme A (CoA) mutase and methionine synthase. In mitochondria, deoxyadenosylcobalamin is a coenzyme for methylmalonyl-CoA mutase, which converts the product of propionate metabolism, methylmalonyl-CoA, to succinyl-CoA, a form that is easily metabolized. In the cytoplasm, methylcobalamin is a coenzyme for methionine synthase, which catalyzes the transfer of methyl groups from methylcobalamin to homocysteine to form methionine. The methyl group of 5-methyltetrahydrofolate (methyl-THF) is donated to regenerate methylcobalamin, thereby forming the THF that is essential to sustain one-carbon metabolism. The methionine so formed can be adenylated to *S*-adenosylmethionine, which donates its methyl group in a critical series of biologic methylation reactions involving more than 80 proteins, phospholipids, neurotransmitters, RNA, and DNA. An elevation of methylmalonic acid and homocysteine in the blood can point to cobalamin deficiency.

Pathogenesis of Cobalamin Deficiency
Nutritional Cobalamin Deficiency

Vegetarianism and poverty-imposed near-vegetarianism are the most common causes of nutritional cobalamin insufficiency worldwide in all age groups. In such patient populations, low maternal cobalamin status is associated with adverse pregnancy outcomes (preterm birth, intrauterine growth retardation, very early recurrent miscarriage), neural tube defects, reduced neurocognitive performance in children, accelerated bone turnover, and low bone mineral density with fractures.

Inadequate Dissociation of Cobalamin from Food Protein

Failure to release dietary cobalamin from food protein can lead to cobalamin deficiency despite the presence of intrinsic factor. This is a common cause of

TABLE 167-1   ETIOPATHOPHYSIOLOGIC CLASSIFICATION OF COBALAMIN AND FOLATE DEFICIENCIES

I. Cobalamin deficiency
  A. Nutritional cobalamin deficiency (insufficient cobalamin intake)—vegetarians, poverty-imposed near-vegetarians, breast-fed infants of mothers with pernicious anemia
  B. Abnormal intragastric events (inadequate proteolysis of food cobalamin)—atrophic gastritis, hypochlorhydria, proton pump inhibitors, H_2-blockers
  C. Loss/atrophy of gastric oxyntic mucosa (deficient intrinsic factor molecules)—total or partial gastrectomy, adult and juvenile pernicious anemia, caustic destruction (lye)
  D. Abnormal events in the small bowel lumen
    1. Inadequate pancreatic protease (R factor–cobalamin not degraded, cobalamin not transferred to intrinsic factor)
      a. Insufficient pancreatic protease—pancreatic insufficiency
      b. Inactivation of pancreatic protease—Zollinger-Ellison syndrome
    2. Usurping of luminal cobalamin (inadequate binding of cobalamin to intrinsic factor)
      a. By bacteria—stasis syndromes (blind loops, pouches of diverticulosis, strictures, fistulas, anastomosis), impaired bowel motility (scleroderma), hypogammaglobulinemia
      b. By *Diphyllobothrium latum* (fish tapeworm)
  E. Disorders of ileal mucosa/intrinsic factor–cobalamin receptors (intrinsic factor–cobalamin not bound to intrinsic factor–cobalamin receptors [a.k.a. cubam receptors])
    1. Diminished or absent cubam receptors—ileal bypass, resection, fistula
    2. Abnormal mucosal architecture or function—tropical/nontropical sprue, Crohn's disease, tuberculous ileitis, amyloidosis
    3. Cubam receptor defects—Imerslund-Gräsbeck syndrome, hereditary megaloblastic anemia
    4. Drug effects—metformin, cholestyramine, colchicine, neomycin
  F. Disorders of plasma cobalamin transport (TCII-cobalamin not delivered to TCII receptors)—congenital TCII deficiency, defective binding of TCII-cobalamin to TCII receptors (rare)
  G. Metabolic disorders (cobalamin not used by cells)
    1. Inborn enzyme errors (rare)
    2. Acquired disorders (cobalamin functionally inactivated by irreversible oxidation)—nitrous oxide inhalation
II. Folate deficiency
  A. Nutritional causes
    1. Decreased dietary intake—poverty and famine, institutionalization (psychiatric facilities, nursing homes), chronic debilitating disease, prolonged feeding of infants with goat's milk, special slimming diets or fad foods (folate-rich foods not consumed), cultural or ethnic cooking techniques (food folate destroyed)
    2. Decreased dietary intake and increased requirements
      a. Physiologic—pregnancy and lactation, prematurity, hyperemesis gravidarum, infancy
      b. Pathologic
        (1) Intrinsic hematologic diseases involving hemolysis with compensatory erythropoiesis, abnormal hematopoiesis, or bone marrow infiltration by malignant disease
        (2) Dermatologic disease—psoriasis
  B. Folate malabsorption
    1. With normal intestinal mucosa
      a. Drugs—sulfasalazine, pyrimethamine, proton pump inhibitors (via inhibition of proton-coupled folate transporters)
      b. Hereditary folate malabsorption (mutations in proton-coupled folate transporters) (rare)
    2. With mucosal abnormalities—tropical/nontropical sprue, regional enteritis
  C. Defective CSF folate transport—cerebral folate deficiency (autoantibodies to folate receptors) (rare)
  D. Inadequate cellular utilization
    1. Folate antagonists (methotrexate)
    2. Hereditary enzyme deficiencies involving folate
  E. Drugs (multiple effects on folate metabolism)—alcohol, sulfasalazine, triamterene, pyrimethamine, trimethoprim-sulfamethoxazole, phenytoin, barbiturates
III. Miscellaneous megaloblastic anemias not caused by cobalamin or folate deficiency
  A. Congenital disorders of DNA synthesis
    1. Orotic aciduria
    2. Lesch-Nyhan syndrome
    3. Congenital dyserythropoietic anemia
  B. Acquired disorders of DNA synthesis
    1. Deficiency—thiamine-responsive megaloblastic anemia (thiamine transporter 1 mutation)
    2. Erythroleukemia; refractory sideroblastic anemias (pyridoxine responsive?)

CSF = cerebrospinal fluid; HIV = human immunodeficiency virus; TCII = transcobalamin II.

cobalamin deficiency in affluent countries and occurs among 30 to 50% of elderly individuals with low cobalamin status. It is about 10-fold more common than pernicious anemia or loss of functional cubam receptors.

Absent Secretion of Acid and Intrinsic Factor

Deficiency of intrinsic factor as a result of gastric parietal cell atrophy is associated with insufficient hydrochloric acid secretion and can be caused by total or partial gastrectomy; autoimmune destruction (chronic atrophic gastritis), as found in classic pernicious anemia; or destruction of gastric mucosa by caustic (lye) ingestion.

Total gastrectomy invariably leads to cobalamin deficiency in 2 to 10 years, thus warranting prophylactic cobalamin (and iron) replacement. After partial gastrectomy, up to a third of patients may have multifactorial cobalamin deficiency from decreased secretion of intrinsic factor, hypochlorhydria, or intestinal bacterial overgrowth of cobalamin-consuming organisms. Morbidly obese patients following bariatric gastric bypass surgery (Chapter 227) also have food-cobalamin malabsorption, as do those on long-term H_2-blockers or proton pump inhibitors.

In pernicious anemia, the primary event is autoimmune destruction and atrophy of the gastric parietal cell mucosa, leading to the absence of intrinsic factor and hydrochloric acid, which causes severe cobalamin malabsorption and deficiency. The autoimmune gastritis that eventually leads to chronic atrophic gastritis involves the gastric fundus and body. Intrinsic factor antibodies are found in the serum of 60% and in the gastric juice of 75% of patients with pernicious anemia. The incidence of pernicious anemia is approximately 25 new cases per year per 100,000 persons older than 40 years. The average age at onset is about 60 years. Nearly 2% of free-living individuals older than 60 years in Southern California had undiagnosed pernicious anemia, with minimal clinical manifestations of cobalamin deficiency; significantly, in this cohort, 4% of white and African American women had pernicious anemia. Nonetheless, pernicious anemia can be found in persons of all ages, races, and ethnic origins. About 30% of patients have a positive family history, and there is an association with other autoimmune diseases (polyglandular autoimmune syndrome, Graves' disease, Hashimoto's thyroiditis, vitiligo, Addison's disease, idiopathic hypoparathyroidism, primary ovarian failure, myasthenia gravis, type 1 diabetes, adult hypogammaglobulinemia).

FIGURE 167-1. Components and mechanism of cobalamin absorption, with an indication of the locus for malabsorption. Cbl = cobalamin; IF = intrinsic factor; TCII = transcobalamin II. (From Antony AC. Megaloblastic anemias. In: Hoffman R, Benz EJ Jr, Shattil SJ, et al, eds. *Hematology: Basic Principles and Practice*, 4th ed. Philadelphia: Churchill Livingstone; 2005:519-556.)

Abnormal Events Precluding Absorption of Cobalamin

In pancreatic insufficiency (Chapter 142) with a deficiency of pancreatic protease, there is a failure to break down the R proteins to which cobalamin is preferentially bound in the stomach; this precludes the transfer of cobalamin to intrinsic factor. However, with the widespread early use of pancreatic protease replacement, frank cobalamin deficiency is uncommon. Endogenous pancreatic protease can be inactivated by massive gastric hypersecretion arising from a gastrinoma in Zollinger-Ellison syndrome (Chapter 201). Further, if the pH of the luminal contents in the ileum is less than 5.4, the binding of the intrinsic factor–cobalamin complex to cubam receptors will be precluded.

Bacterial overgrowth in the small bowel (arising from stasis, impaired motility, and hypogammaglobulinemia; Chapter 144) favors colonization by bacteria, which can usurp free cobalamin before it can bind to intrinsic factor. This problem can be reversed by a short course of antibiotic therapy. Individuals heavily infested with the fish tapeworm *Diphyllobothrium latum* (acquired by consuming raw or partially cooked freshwater fish from lakes in Russia, Japan, Switzerland, Germany, and the United States) can become cobalamin deficient when these long (10 m) adult worms in the jejunum avidly usurp cobalamin. After the worms have been expelled (with a single oral dose of praziquantel 10 to 20 mg/kg), cobalamin replenishment is curative.

Disorders of the Intrinsic Factor Receptors or Mucosa

Because the distal ileum has the greatest density of cubam receptors, the removal, bypass, or dysfunction of only 1 to 2 feet of terminal ileum can result

in cobalamin malabsorption. Among drugs, the biguanides (e.g., metformin) decrease intrinsic factor and acid secretion and can inhibit the transenterocytic transport of cobalamin in up to a third of patients. This can be avoided by taking calcium (1.2 g/day). Other drugs (extended-release potassium chloride, cholestyramine, colchicine, neomycin) can also impair the transepithelial transport of cobalamin.

Acquired Cobalamin Deficiency

Nitrous oxide (N_2O) irreversibly inactivates cobalamin and results in a state of functional intracellular cobalamin deficiency, which can be bypassed by the administration of 5-formyl-THF (leucovorin). Although N_2O exposure during prolonged surgery can induce megaloblastosis, especially in those with marginal or low cobalamin stores, chronic intermittent (surreptitious, accidental, or occupational) exposure more frequently leads to neuromyelopathic manifestations, in which magnetic resonance imaging shows T2-weighted hyperintensity in affected areas of the spinal cord. Capsules used for making whipped cream are a cheap and easy source of N_2O in the community, and at one college, about 3% of students inhaled it monthly in an on-campus "nitrous club."

Folates
Normal Physiology
Absorption and Transport

In general, only half the folate in food, which is mainly in polyglutamylated form, is nutritionally available (bioavailable), whereas 85% of folic acid added to food or ingested as a supplement is bioavailable. The small intestine can absorb folic acid unchanged, but food folate polyglutamates must be hydrolyzed to monoglutamate by folate polyglutamate hydrolase at the brush border before transport into enterocytes. A luminal surface, proton-coupled, folate transporter protein, which has a low pH optimum in the acid microclimate of the duodenum and jejunum, facilitates the efficient transport of folates into enterocytes, where it is reduced to THF and methylated before being released into plasma as methyl-THF. The normal serum folate level is maintained by dietary folate intake and by an efficient enterohepatic circulation.

From plasma, there is a rapid uptake of folate (methyl-THF and folic acid) into tissues by two physiologic transport processes for cellular entry. Membrane-associated folate receptors bind and take up physiologically relevant methyl-THF, folic acid, and some newer antifolates with high affinity at concentrations found in serum. Following folate receptor–mediated endocytosis, a proton-coupled folate transporter then helps export folate from acidified endosomes into the cytoplasm of cells and also into the cerebrospinal fluid (CSF). Another transporter (reduced folate carrier) is a low-affinity but high-capacity system that can also mediate the uptake of methyl-THF and pharmacologic folates (methotrexate and folinic acid well, but folic acid poorly) into a variety of cells. Passive diffusion also operates to transport folate across biologic membranes at supraphysiologic folate concentrations.

Cellular Retention and Excretion
Polyglutamylation of folate is the major factor in intracellular retention. After glomerular filtration, folate receptors on the brush border membranes of proximal renal tubular cells bind luminal folate and transport it back into blood.

Intracellular Metabolism and Cobalamin-Folate Interactions
After cellular uptake, methyl-THF must first be converted to THF via methionine synthase. Only then can the THF be polyglutamylated by folate polyglutamate synthase, which allows it to play a central role in one-carbon metabolism. THF can be converted to 10-formyl-THF, which can be used for de novo biosynthesis of purines, and to methylene-THF, which can be used for the synthesis of thymidylate.

The central role of methylene-THF is that it can be used either in the thymidylate cycle via thymidylate synthase for the synthesis of thymidine and DNA or in the methylation cycle via methionine synthase, but only after its conversion to methyl-THF by methylene-THF reductase. Inactivation of methionine synthase during cobalamin deficiency results in accumulation of the substrate methyl-THF, which cannot be polyglutamylated and thus leaks out of the cell, resulting in an intracellular THF deficiency and the reduction of one-carbon metabolism. This process explains why cobalamin deficiency responds to replacement with folic acid, which can be converted to THF via dihydrofolate reductase, or to replacement with 5-formyl-THF (folinic acid), which bypasses methionine synthase and can be converted to methylene-THF or 10-formyl-THF via intermediates.

Pathogenesis of Folate Deficiency
Folate deficiency can arise from decreased supply (reduced intake, absorption, transport, or utilization) or increased requirements (from metabolic consumption, destruction, or excretion). One individual may have multiple causes of folate deficiency, but specific tests to define each mechanism are not available clinically. Folate deficiency varies among different populations, and nutritional folate insufficiency is the most common cause worldwide in all age groups, with women and children in developing countries at highest risk. Although food folate fortification has dramatically reduced the prevalence of folate deficiency in the United States, it can still be found among some elderly, infirm, or socially isolated individuals with poor diets.

Nutritional Causes (Decreased Intake or Increased Requirements)
With an abrupt reduction in folate consumption, body stores of folate are adequate for approximately 4 months. However, these stores are depleted faster in individuals who chronically have a negative folate balance and often have multiple nutritional deficiencies (and diseases) that tip them into frank folate deficiency. A seasonal reduction in folate-rich foods, poverty, cultural or ethnic diets that are intrinsically low in folates, cooking techniques that destroy folate, and the anorexia that accompanies chronic illnesses are among the many reasons for folate deficiency, especially in developing countries.

Patients with hematologic diseases involving increased intrinsic cell proliferation or with increased compensatory erythropoiesis in response to chronic peripheral red blood cell destruction are at risk. Folate deficiency in the face of chronic hemolysis can lead to an acute reticulocytopenic (aplastic) crisis, an unexpected increase in transfusion requirements, or a fall in platelets. Exfoliative skin diseases (Chapter 446) also cause folate deficiency when there is an increased demand from excess loss of skin cells.

Pregnancy and Infancy
Poor folate intake during pregnancy is a very common cause of megaloblastic anemia in developing countries because pregnancy and lactation require additional folate for growth of the fetus and maternal tissues. Physiologic transplacental folate transport, which relies on the continued intake of adequate dietary folate by the mother, involves the capture of maternal folate by placental folate receptors, followed by displacement of this pool by dietary folates, a process that leads to transfer to the fetal circulation along a downhill concentration gradient. However, mothers with short intervals between pregnancies, with twin pregnancies, or with hyperemesis gravidarum are unable to maintain adequate folate stores, leading to premature, low-birthweight infants and other predominantly midline developmental abnormalities in the fetus. Low maternal folate status has also been associated with behavioral abnormalities (hyperactivity-inattention and peer problems) in offspring during early childhood. Autoantibodies to folate receptors in mothers have been linked to recurrent neural tube defects among some populations.

Cerebral folate deficiency can be caused by a mutation in folate receptors that perturbs folate transport into the CSF, leading to severe developmental regression in early childhood associated with movement disturbances, epilepsy, and leukodystrophy that is reversed by folinic acid. Alternatively, cerebral folate deficiency can be acquired when autoantibodies to folate receptors (which develop against consumed bovine milk folate-binding proteins that share epitopes with human folate receptors) bind to folate receptors on the choroid plexus and thereby reduce folate transport to the central nervous system. The folate receptor autoantibody titer decreases with the restriction of bovine milk intake but promptly increases upon rechallenge. Cerebral folate deficiency responds to high doses of folinic acid and a bovine milk–free diet. Reduction of folate transport to the central nervous system associated with folate receptor autoantibodies also occurs in two autism spectrum disorders: Rett syndrome and infantile low-functioning autism with neurologic abnormalities. High doses of oral folinic acid can normalize the CSF folate and lead to partial or complete clinical recovery in 12 months.

Hereditary folate malabsorption, an autosomal recessive syndrome, is due to a mutation in the proton-coupled folate transporter that results in the defective transport of folates across the small intestine and across the choroid plexus into the CSF. The proton-coupled folate transporter functions distal to folate receptors in the choroid plexus to facilitate folate transfer to the CSF, and a loss-of-function mutation of the proton-coupled folate transporter can independently interrupt physiologic folate delivery to the brain, despite intact folate receptors. The CSF/blood folate ratio in healthy humans is 3 : 1, but in those with hereditary folate malabsorption, CSF folate is very low or undetectable. Patients present with folate deficiency anemia, hypoimmunoglobulinemia with recurrent infections, chronic diarrhea, and neurologic abnormalities (seizures or mental retardation) that are irreversible if left untreated. High parenteral doses of folinic acid can ensure passive diffusion into the CSF and lead to significant clinical improvement in these children.

Tropical and Nontropical (Celiac) Sprue
With the development of intestinal mucosal abnormalities, patients are at increased risk for folate malabsorption. In tropical sprue (Chapter 142), a dramatic response to a 4- to 6-month course of oral folic acid (5 mg/day) plus tetracycline (250 mg four times a day) can effect a cure in 60% or more of patients. In the short term, malabsorption leads to folate deficiency, but later in the chronic phase of the disease (>3 years), malabsorption of cobalamin also develops. In addition, iron deficiency (Chapter 162), pellagra, and beriberi (Chapter 225) may coexist in these patients.

Drugs
Excess alcohol consumption at the expense of a balanced diet may be the most common cause of folate deficiency in the United States. Inhibition of dihydrofolate reductase by trimethoprim and pyrimethamine or methotrexate can be acutely reversed by the administration of 5-formyl-THF (folinic acid). Sulfasalazine induces megaloblastosis in two thirds of subjects taking full doses (>2 g/day) by decreasing the breakdown of folate polyglutamates to monoglutamates before absorption or by inducing Heinz body hemolytic anemia, which leads to increased requirements. Sulfasalazine, pyrimethamine, and proton pump inhibitors also inhibit the human proton-coupled

folate transporter, reducing folate absorption. Oral contraceptives may increase folate catabolism, whereas anticonvulsants can reduce absorption and induce microsomal liver enzymes. Antineoplastics and antiretroviral antinucleosides (azidothymidine) induce megaloblastosis by perturbing DNA synthesis.

CLINICAL MANIFESTATIONS

The finding of macrocytosis (increased mean corpuscular volume [MCV]) on a routine complete blood count may be the first clinical manifestation. In other patients, the findings may be dominated by the condition causing the deficiency of cobalamin or folate, such as malabsorption, alcoholism, or malnutrition (see Table 167-1).

The clinical manifestations of folate deficiency may include hematologic (pancytopenia with megaloblastic bone marrow), cardiopulmonary (secondary to anemia), gastrointestinal (megaloblastosis with or without malabsorption), dermatologic (hyperpigmentation of the skin, premature graying), genital (megaloblastosis of the cervical epithelium), infertility (sterility), and psychiatric (primarily a flat affect) symptoms. If patients have additional neurologic findings, other diseases that predispose to folate deficiency (e.g., alcoholism with thiamine deficiency) or associated cobalamin deficiency must be considered. Because megaloblastosis secondary to either folate or cobalamin deficiency results in functional folate deficiency, the hematologic manifestations of both deficiencies, including pancytopenia with megaloblastic bone marrow, are indistinguishable (see later). However, only cobalamin deficiency results in a patchy demyelinating process, which is expressed clinically as cerebral abnormalities and subacute combined degeneration of the spinal cord (Chapter 425). This widespread demyelination begins in the dorsal columns in the thoracic segments of the spinal cord and then spreads contiguously to involve the corticospinal tracts and later the spinothalamic and spinocerebellar tracts. Hematologic manifestations, neurologic manifestations, or both may dominate the clinical picture.

With chronic hyperhomocysteinemia associated with cobalamin or folate deficiency (or both), there may be additional clinical manifestations that stem from the fact that homocysteine is a risk factor for occlusive vascular diseases such as coronary artery disease, stroke, and peripheral arterial disease (Chapter 51), as well as arterial and venous thromboembolism (Chapters 81 and 179). Hyperhomocysteinemia is also associated with significant complications of pregnancy (preeclampsia, placental abruption or infarction, recurrent miscarriage) and poor pregnancy outcomes (preterm delivery, neural tube defects, congenital heart defects, intrauterine growth retardation). In addition, there is reduced bone mineral density, with an increased fracture risk, and a greater chance of small-vessel cerebrovascular disease–related stroke. Despite the failure of homocysteine-lowering therapy for the secondary prevention of atherosclerotic disease, this does not negate the risk. Several clinical conditions are benefited by folate supplementation or homocysteine-lowering therapy with combined folic acid, cobalamin, and pyridoxine.[1-7] By inference, patients can present clinically with any of these additional conditions when they have long-standing untreated hyperhomocysteinemia.

DIAGNOSIS

Diagnostic Approach to the Patient

The general approach to a patient with megaloblastic anemia is first to *recognize* that megaloblastic anemia is present; then to *distinguish* whether folate, cobalamin, or combined folate and cobalamin deficiencies have led to the anemia; and finally to diagnose the *underlying disease* and *mechanism* causing the deficiency (see Table 167-1).

Although deficiencies of cobalamin and folate are only two of the causes of macrocytosis, they become increasingly more likely as the MCV increases (see Fig. 167-2). Because perturbed DNA synthesis from any cause (including folate and cobalamin deficiency) results in megaloblastosis of bone marrow precursor cells, the red cells released into the circulation have an MCV that is often greater than 110 fL; on the peripheral blood smear, these large cells appear oval in shape (macro-ovalocytes). When compared with mature red cells, which normally have a central area of pallor that occupies about one third of the cell diameter, the central pallor of macro-ovalocytes is significantly reduced. Assessment of the corrected reticulocyte count is a good starting point to distinguish conditions in which macrocytes are not accompanied by megaloblastosis in the bone marrow (Fig. 167-2). On the hematoxylin-eosin–stained peripheral blood smear, reticulocytes, which are normally 20% larger than mature red cells, are recognized by their polychromatophilic staining; when they are prematurely released from the bone marrow during the stress of acute blood loss or hemolysis, these so-called shift reticulocytes are even larger. In liver disease, an altered lipid composition of the erythrocyte membrane results in an increased cell surface without a proportionate increase in volume; these so-called thin macrocytes are recognized on the peripheral blood smear by their larger area of central pallor (much greater than one third the cell diameter). Thin macrocytes are also found in the post-splenectomy state (because reticulocytes, which normally undergo a form of "remodeling" with a loss of membrane lipids during their maturation in the spleen, escape this process in splenectomized individuals).

Macrocytic Anemia

Complete blood count, peripheral smear, and corrected reticulocyte count

Reticulocyte count >2%
Response to blood loss
Response to hemolysis

- Immune hemolytic anemia (warm antibodies and cold agglutinins)
- Infectious hemolysis (malaria)
- Glucose-6-phosphate dehydrogenase deficiency
- Mechanical destruction of red cells (heart valve, disseminated intravascular coagulation)
- Paroxysmal nocturnal hemoglobinuria

Normal or low reticulocyte count <0.5%

Thin macrocytes

- Post-splenectomy
- Liver disease ± alcoholism
- Aplastic/hypoplastic anemia
- Myelodysplastic (esp. 5q−) syndrome
- Myelophthisic anemia
- Hypothyroidism
- Smoking, chronic lung disease
- Severe hyperglycemia, leukocytosis

Macro-ovalocytes

- Cobalamin or folate deficiency (see Table 167-2)
- Drug-induced disorders of DNA synthesis (antineoplastic or immunosuppressive chemotherapy, antiretrovirals)
- Erythroleukemia (rare)
- Inherited disorders affecting DNA synthesis (rare)

FIGURE 167-2. Algorithm for the evaluation of patients with macrocytosis.

The frequency with which a high MCV is found depends on the patient population studied. Thus, in a U.S. hospital, up to two thirds of cases of macrocytosis (MCV ≥100) can be due to drug therapy (chemotherapy, antiretroviral therapy) or alcoholism and liver disease. But in a developing country where a substantial percentage of the population is vegetarian or near-vegetarian, insufficient intake of cobalamin, folate, or both, with an associated iron deficiency resulting in a dimorphic anemia (with a large red cell distribution width from a mix of macrocytic and microcytic cells), would be common.

The underlying condition predisposing to the development of folate deficiency usually began within the previous 6 months and often dominates the overall clinical picture. Alcoholism can be identified as the basis for folate deficiency from the history and physical examination, but associated thiamine deficiency may result in a more complex manifestation, such as heart failure from cardiovascular disease ("wet beriberi") and peripheral neuropathy ("dry beriberi") with Wernicke-Korsakoff syndrome (Chapters 225 and 425). By contrast, cobalamin deficiency takes several years to manifest clinically. Therefore, the underlying condition is more chronic, symptoms develop more insidiously, and defining the cause is a clinical challenge.

History and Physical Examination

The dietary history may be revealing (food faddism, vegetarianism), whereas the medical or family history may uncover blood diseases, gluten sensitivity, autoimmune diseases, epilepsy treated with an anticonvulsant, use of offending drugs, previous hemolytic anemia, past surgery (e.g., gastrectomy, fistula, bowel resection), inhalation of N_2O, or a travel history predictive for tropical sprue.

Physical examination of cobalamin-deficient vegetarians or those with pernicious anemia may reveal well-nourished individuals. By contrast, patients with folate deficiency are poorly nourished and may have other stigmata of multiple deficiencies from malabsorption (Chapter 142). Associated deficiency of vitamins A, D, and K or protein-calorie malnutrition, or both, may give rise to angular cheilosis, bleeding mucous membranes, dermatitis, osteomalacia, and chronic infections. Varying degrees of pallor with lemon-tint icterus (a combination of pallor and icterus best observed in fair-skinned individuals) are common features of megaloblastosis. The skin may reveal either a diffuse brownish pigmentation or abnormal blotchy tanning. Premature graying is observed in both light- and dark-haired individuals.

Examination of the mouth may reveal glossitis, with a smooth (depapillated), beefy-red tongue and occasional ulceration of the lateral surface. Thyromegaly may be observed with pernicious anemia and associated autoimmune thyroid disease, but it also raises suspicion for (nonmegaloblastic) macrocytosis related to hypothyroidism. The characteristic findings of heart failure from severe anemia may be accompanied by mild splenomegaly and extramedullary hematopoiesis.

In prolonged cobalamin deficiency, neurologic examination reveals evidence of involvement of the posterior columns as well as the pyramidal, spinocerebellar, and spinothalamic tracts. Posterior column dysfunction results in loss of position sense in the index toes (before great toe involvement) (Chapter 425) and loss of the ability to discern vibration of a high-pitched (256 cycles/second) tuning fork. Diminished vibratory sensation and proprioception of the lower extremities are the most common early objective signs. Neuropathic involvement of the legs precedes that of the arms. Upper motor neuron signs may be modulated by the subsequent involvement of peripheral nerves. A positive Romberg's sign and a Lhermitte's sign may be elicited. Loss of sphincter and bowel control or involvement of cranial nerves, such as optic neuritis, may be accompanied by other dysfunction of the cerebral cortex, including dementia, psychoses, and disturbances of mood. Folate deficiency in adults does not give rise to significant neurologic findings. Thus, the coexistence of folate deficiency with neurologic disease should prompt investigations to exclude cobalamin and other nutrient deficiencies arising from dietary insufficiency or malabsorption.

Nutritional cobalamin deficiency in developing countries can manifest as florid pancytopenia, mild hepatosplenomegaly, fever, and thrombocytopenia, with the neuropsychiatric syndrome developing as a later manifestation. However, cobalamin-related neurologic disease has also been found in patients with only mild to moderate anemia secondary to cobalamin deficiency in both developing and developed countries. Between 25 and 50% of patients who have neuropsychiatric abnormalities attributable to cobalamin deficiency may have a normal hematocrit and MCV if they have adequate folate stores to protect them from hematologic abnormalities. In fact, in the United States, there is often an inverse correlation between the hematocrit and neurologic disease in cobalamin deficiency—most subjects have mild neurologic deficits, and 25% have only moderate deficits, with paresthesias or ataxia as the initial symptoms.

Laboratory Tests

Megaloblastosis

To establish the diagnosis of megaloblastosis, the evaluation begins with a complete blood count, MCV (which often reveals a steady increase over a period of several months or years), peripheral smear, and reticulocyte count; a low reticulocyte count with macro-ovalocytes suggests an underlying megaloblastic anemia (see Fig. 167-2). Classic megaloblastosis from cobalamin or folate deficiency may be accompanied by a hemoglobin level of less than 5 g/dL. Neutropenia and thrombocytopenia occur less commonly than anemia and are usually not severe. Occasionally, however, neutrophil counts less than 1000/μL and platelet counts less than 50,000/μL can be seen. Additional abnormalities supporting intramedullary hemolysis include elevated levels of serum lactate dehydrogenase and bilirubin, as well as decreased serum haptoglobin levels.

Peripheral Smear

In peripheral blood, the earliest manifestation of megaloblastosis is an increase in MCV with macro-ovalocytes (up to 14 μm). Nuclear hypersegmentation of neutrophils, diagnosed if more than 5% of polymorphonuclear leukocytes have five lobes or if more than 1% have six lobes on the smear (Fig. 167-3), strongly suggests megaloblastosis, especially when associated with macro-ovalocytosis. However, neutrophil hypersegmentation is not sensitive for the diagnosis of *mild* cobalamin deficiency, and macrocytosis is absent in nearly 50% of cases. There may be associated teardrop-shaped erythrocytes and anisocytosis with mild leukopenia and thrombocytopenia.

Megaloblastic anemia can be masked when there is a coexisting condition that neutralizes the tendency to generate large cells, such as iron deficiency (Chapter 162) or thalassemia (Chapter 165). In these situations, giant myelocytes and metamyelocytes in bone marrow and hypersegmented neutrophils in bone marrow and peripheral blood (see Fig. 167-3) are important clues to a masked megaloblastosis. This problem is clinically relevant because appropriate replacement with cobalamin or folate elicits a maximal hematologic response only when any associated iron deficiency is corrected. Conversely, if a combined iron and cobalamin deficiency (after gastrectomy) or iron and folate deficiency (with pregnancy) is treated with iron alone, megaloblastosis will be unmasked.

Cobalamin and Folate Levels

Laboratory evaluation of suspected cobalamin or folate deficiency begins with measurement of the serum levels of these vitamins and then progresses to confirmatory tests (Table 167-2). Use of clinical information can improve the pretest probability of serum cobalamin and folate levels. Moreover, without detailed clinical information, the combined results of serum cobalamin, folate, and metabolite tests are not sufficiently unambiguous to diagnose and distinguish cobalamin deficiency from combined cobalamin plus folate deficiency.

Serum Cobalamin Levels

A low serum cobalamin level (<200 pg/mL) is a valuable (albeit relatively insensitive) indicator of cobalamin deficiency when compared with metabolite levels. Serum cobalamin is less than 300 pg/mL in 99% of patients with clinical hematologic or neurologic manifestations of cobalamin deficiency,

FIGURE 167-3. Megaloblastic anemia. The peripheral blood has oval macrocytes (large red blood cells) and marked neutrophil hypersegmentation.

TABLE 167-2 STEPWISE APPROACH TO THE DIAGNOSIS OF COBALAMIN AND FOLATE DEFICIENCY

MEGALOBLASTIC ANEMIA OR NEUROLOGIC-PSYCHIATRIC MANIFESTATIONS CONSISTENT WITH COBALAMIN DEFICIENCY PLUS TEST RESULTS ON SERUM COBALAMIN AND SERUM FOLATE

Cobalamin* (pg/mL)	Folate† (ng/mL)	Provisional Diagnosis	Proceed with Metabolites?‡
>300	>4	Cobalamin/folate deficiency unlikely	No
<200	>4	Consistent with cobalamin deficiency	No
200-300	>4	Rule out cobalamin deficiency	Yes
>300	<2	Consistent with folate deficiency	No
<200	<2	Consistent with combined cobalamin plus folate deficiency or with isolated folate deficiency	Yes
>300	2-4	Consistent with folate deficiency or with anemia unrelated to vitamin deficiency	Yes

TEST RESULTS ON METABOLITES: SERUM METHYLMALONIC ACID AND TOTAL HOMOCYSTEINE

Methylmalonic Acid (Normal = 70-270 nM)	Total Homocysteine (Normal = 5-14 μM)	Diagnosis
Increased	Increased	Cobalamin deficiency confirmed; folate deficiency still possible (i.e., combined cobalamin plus folate deficiency possible)
Normal	Increased	Folate deficiency likely; <5% may have cobalamin deficiency
Normal	Normal	Cobalamin and folate deficiencies excluded

*Serum cobalamin levels: abnormally low = <200 pg/mL; clinically relevant low-normal range = 200-300 pg/mL.
†Serum folate levels: abnormally low = <2 ng/mL; clinically relevant low-normal range = 2-4 ng/mL.
‡Any frozen-over sample from the serum folate or cobalamin determination can be subjected to metabolite tests.

whereas a cobalamin level greater than 300 pg/mL suggests folate deficiency or another cause of macrocytosis or neurologic disease.

About 90% of older patients with serum cobalamin levels less than 200 pg/mL show evidence of true tissue cobalamin deficiency, but individuals with neuropsychiatric disorders attributed to cobalamin deficiency may not have anemia and may have normal or only minimally depressed cobalamin levels. The serum cobalamin concentration is falsely low in the absence of true cobalamin deficiency in patients with folate deficiency (one third of patients), pregnancy, multiple myeloma, transcobalamin I deficiency, megadose or vitamin C therapy, or when the serum contains other radioisotopes (e.g., ^{99m}Tc, ^{67}Ga, ^{125}I) from organ scanning.

A falsely raised cobalamin level in the presence of a true cobalamin deficiency leads to clinical manifestations if uncorrected. Examples include an artificial increase in transcobalamin I and II, which can occur with myeloproliferative disorders, hepatomas, and fibrolamellar hepatic tumors; when transcobalamin II–producing macrophages are activated in autoimmune diseases, monoblastic leukemias, and lymphomas; and on the release of cobalamin from hepatocytes during active liver disease in cobalamin-deficient patients. Studies suggest that approximately 10% of the U.S. population, especially the elderly, have true cobalamin deficiency manifested by low or low-normal serum cobalamin levels, as well as elevated levels of serum methylmalonic acid (MMA) and homocysteine that fall to normal with cobalamin therapy.

Serum Folate Levels

When combined with a clinical picture of megaloblastic anemia and the measurement of cobalamin levels, serum folate is the cheapest and best initial biochemical test to diagnose folate deficiency. Although red blood cell folate levels by microbiologic assay correlate well with hepatic folate stores, they are not widely available, and the newer radioisotopic or colorimetric assays are too unreliable for routine clinical use.

The serum folate level is highly sensitive to the intake of a single folate-rich meal. Nutritional folate deficiency first leads to a decline in the serum folate level below normal (<2 ng/mL) in about 3 weeks; thus, it is a sensitive indicator of negative folate balance. Isolated reduction of serum folate in the absence of megaloblastosis (i.e., a false-positive result) occurs in one third of hospitalized patients with anorexia and acute alcohol consumption, in normal pregnancy, and in those using anticonvulsants; because these groups are also at high risk for folate deficiency, additional testing with metabolites or an empirical therapeutic trial may be required. Conversely, in 25 to 50% of alcohol abusers (Chapter 32) with folate deficiency, serum folate levels may be low normal or borderline low.

Metabolite Levels—Homocysteine and Methylmalonic Acid

The serum homocysteine and MMA values rise in proportion to the severity of deficiency (see Table 167-2). Although serum MMA and homocysteine tests are the "gold standard" for confirming the diagnosis of cobalamin deficiency, they are too expensive to use for screening. Serum MMA levels are elevated in more than 95% of patients with clinically confirmed cobalamin deficiency (with median values of 3500 nM). Serum homocysteine concentrations are elevated in both cobalamin deficiency (median values of 70 μM) and folate deficiency (median values of 50 μM). Both homocysteine and MMA rise with dehydration or renal failure. Propionic acid, derived from anaerobic fecal bacterial metabolism, can also contribute to MMA values, which can be lowered by a course of metronidazole. Thus, although these metabolites can help distinguish between isolated cobalamin and folate deficiency, an increase in both metabolites cannot differentiate between isolated cobalamin deficiency and combined cobalamin plus folate deficiency. The abnormally high metabolites return to normal in a week when replaced with the appropriate (deficient) vitamin.

Clinicians can use serum MMA and homocysteine to assist in the diagnosis in patients with (1) borderline cobalamin and folate levels; (2) existing conditions known to perturb folate and cobalamin tests, leading to difficulties in interpreting the results; (3) low levels of both cobalamin and folate, in which case a high MMA level is useful to confirm cobalamin deficiency (rather than attributing the condition to folate deficiency alone); and (4) low serum cobalamin levels when there is an alternative explanation for the syndrome that led to the test (e.g., a diabetic or alcoholic patient with peripheral neuropathy or an alcoholic patient with a high MCV and low cobalamin level without anemia). In the context of diagnosing a subclinical deficiency of cobalamin (or folate) based on increased serum MMA or homocysteine (or both) despite normal serum cobalamin (or folate) levels, a positive diagnosis can be made only after reversal of laboratory values following treatment with cobalamin (and/or folate) has been demonstrated.

Bone Marrow Examination

In florid hematologic disease with or without neurologic disease suggestive of cobalamin or folate deficiency, the identification of nucleated red cells with megaloblastic changes in the peripheral smear—which reflects the morphology in the bone marrow—can clinch the diagnosis of megaloblastosis. If not found, a bone marrow aspirate can be invaluable in making the rapid diagnosis of megaloblastosis. However, in the outpatient setting, when there is less urgency because the anemia is mild to moderate and the patient has a suggestive peripheral smear, or when the manifestation is primarily neuropsychiatric, a good case can be made to initiate the sequence of diagnostic tests without bone marrow aspiration and proceed with the measurement of serum levels of vitamins or metabolites (see Table 167-2 and Fig. 167-2).

In a bone marrow aspirate (Fig. 167-4), which is better than biopsy for observing megaloblastosis, the cells are actually proliferating very slowly despite what looks like exuberant cell proliferation with numerous mitotic figures. In early cobalamin or folate deficiency, normoblasts may dominate the marrow, with only a few megaloblasts seen, but the full spectrum of megaloblastic hematopoiesis is observed in florid deficiency and is accompanied by varying degrees of pancytopenia. In contrast to the normally dense chromatin of comparable normoblasts, megaloblastic erythroid precursors have an open, finely stippled, reticular, sieve-like pattern. The orthochromatic megaloblast, with its hemoglobinized cytoplasm, continues to retain its large, sieve-like immature nucleus, in sharp contrast to the clumped chromatin of orthochromatic normoblasts. The majority of megaloblastic cells (80 to 90%) die in the bone marrow and are scavenged by macrophages in a process called *ineffective erythropoiesis* or *intramedullary hemolysis*. There is an

FIGURE 167-4. Megaloblastic anemia. A bone marrow aspirate shows red blood cell precursors that are giant megaloblasts with nuclear-cytoplasmic dissociation (nuclear maturation lagging behind cytoplasmic maturation). Megaloblastic changes in the leukocyte series are shown by the "giant metamyelocyte."

absolute increase in leukopoiesis, with megaloblastic cells also having a sieve-like chromatin. Giant (20 to 30 μm) metamyelocytes and "band" forms are pathognomonic for megaloblastosis. Hypersegmented polymorphonuclear leukocytes may be seen in the marrow and peripheral blood. Megakaryocytes may be normal or increased in number and can exhibit complex hypersegmentation, with liberation of fragments of cytoplasm and giant platelets into the circulation. The net output of platelets is decreased in severe megaloblastosis.

Determining the Cause of the Vitamin Deficiency

By the time the megaloblastic state is established, the cause of the folate deficiency is usually clear from the history, physical examination, and clinical setting. With rare exceptions, adults with cobalamin deficiency have either cobalamin malabsorption or dietary cobalamin insufficiency. All these conditions can be treated similarly with either monthly parenteral cobalamin or daily oral cobalamin. However, identifying the likely basis for malabsorption can point to the need for additional diagnostic tests (e.g., intestinal biopsy, examination of stool for malabsorption or *D. latum* infestation) and specific therapy (e.g., gluten-free diet, folate, antibiotics, anthelmintics). This evaluation, in turn, indicates whether cobalamin replacement should be lifelong. At this juncture in the diagnostic evaluation, the Schilling test, which was discontinued in 2003, once provided invaluable information on the locus and mechanism of cobalamin malabsorption. Now, only 60% of patients with pernicious anemia can be confidently identified through the measurement of serum anti–intrinsic factor antibodies. However, because most of the conditions predisposing to cobalamin deficiency (see Table 167-1) should be clinically evident by the time cobalamin deficiency is apparent, it is possible to identify several conditions through a detailed dietary history or past medical history that suggests esophagogastroduodenal disease, pancreatic insufficiency, impaired bowel motility, or other autoimmune diseases. The physical examination can provide additional clues and suggest focused testing for rarer conditions (stool for ova, anti–tissue transglutaminase antibodies, lipase, gastrin, intestinal biopsy, or radiographic contrast studies for stasis, strictures, or fistulas). For the younger patient with megaloblastic anemia, juvenile pernicious anemia and congenital intrinsic factor deficiency warrant the measurement of gastric juice for intrinsic factor and achlorhydria and DNA for mutations in cubam receptor (amnionless, cubulin genes) for hereditary megaloblastic anemia and Immerslund-Gräsbeck syndrome.

Measurement of a rise in blood holo-transcobalamin (cobalamin-bound transcobalamin II) levels after the administration of oral cobalamin can indicate the absorption of orally administered doses of cobalamin in otherwise healthy individuals or vegetarians; however, this test must still be clinically validated among various cohorts of patients with cobalamin malabsorption (see Table 167-1).

TREATMENT ℞

First, blood is drawn for a determination of serum folate and cobalamin levels (and enough for the measurement of metabolite levels later, if indicated), and bone marrow aspiration is performed, if necessary, to confirm megaloblastosis. If the patient is decompensated or decompensation is imminent, the patient is then transfused slowly with 1 U of packed red cells; diuretics are administered, if necessary; and both cobalamin and folate are started at full doses. If the patient is moderately symptomatic, transfusions should be avoided because a dramatic improvement in well-being is likely to occur within 2 to 3 days of starting appropriate vitamin replacement, even before hematologic improvement. If the patient is well compensated or is in the ambulatory setting, diagnostic testing should proceed in an orderly sequence (see Fig. 167-2 and Table 167-2) before initiating therapy.

Drug Dosage

Therapy with full doses of parenteral cobalamin (1 mg/day) and oral folate (folic acid 1 to 5 mg) before the type of vitamin deficiency has been established should be reserved for severely ill patients. An aggressive scheme to replace cobalamin rapidly is 1 mg/day of intramuscular or subcutaneous cyanocobalamin (week 1), 1 mg twice weekly (week 2), 1 mg/week for 4 weeks, and then 1 mg/month for life. Because 1 to 2% of an oral dose is absorbed by passive diffusion, even in patients with malabsorption of physiologic cobalamin for any reason, an equally effective alternative to maintenance therapy with monthly cobalamin injections is the daily administration of 2-mg cobalamin tablets orally after rapidly replenishing cobalamin parenterally. In patients with malabsorption of food-bound cobalamin, cobalamin doses of 1 mg/day are required. For patients with nutritional cobalamin deficiency (vegetarians) without absorptive problems, after cobalamin stores are replenished with 2 mg/day of oral cobalamin for at least 3 months, smaller oral cobalamin doses of 5 to 10 μg, using tablets or equivalent cobalamin-fortified foods, taken for life, are sufficient.

Subclinical cobalamin deficiency does not inexorably progress to clinical cobalamin deficiency; indeed, mild or borderline abnormal biochemical results tend to remain unchanged, fluctuate above or below normal values, or even spontaneously resolve. Some physicians follow these patients and treat them with cobalamin only when they exhibit symptoms or signs of frank cobalamin deficiency. Others err on the side of caution, preferring to preemptively replenish depleted cobalamin stores; these patients are treated for 6 months with high-dose daily oral cobalamin (1 mg), and then serum cobalamin levels are followed.

Oral folate (folic acid) at doses of 1 to 5 mg/day results in adequate absorption despite intestinal malabsorption of physiologic food folate. Therapy should be continued until complete hematologic recovery is documented; the subsequent duration of therapy is dictated by the cause. Folinic acid bypasses any block in one-carbon metabolism induced by methotrexate, trimethoprim-sulfamethoxazole, or N₂O.

Prophylaxis with Cobalamin or Folate

Cobalamin must be given to infants of cobalamin-deficient mothers, as well as to patients who have undergone total gastrectomy. For vegetarians, cobalamin-fortified foods (soy or rice beverages, fortified cereals, nutritional yeast) or oral cobalamin tablets 5 to 10 μg/day should suffice. For those with malabsorption of cobalamin from any other mechanism (see Table 167-1), cobalamin replacement is achieved with 1- to 2-mg tablets taken orally each day.

Periconceptional folate supplementation for all normal women (400 μg/day of folic acid) and for women who have previously delivered a baby with a neural tube defect (4 mg/day of folic acid) is now standard and prevents nearly three quarters of neural tube defects. Women of childbearing age who are taking anticonvulsant medications (phenytoin, phenobarbital, carbamazepine) are also at increased risk for delivering babies with neural tube defects and should routinely take 1 mg of folic acid daily. Folate supplementation throughout pregnancy also helps prevent premature delivery of low-birthweight infants and is recommended for premature infants and lactating mothers. Folic acid supplements (1 mg/day orally) are taken by patients with hemolysis or myeloproliferative diseases and to reduce the toxicity of methotrexate in patients with rheumatoid arthritis and psoriasis. Individuals in whom cobalamin deficiency develops while undergoing long-term folate replacement have a pure neurologic syndrome.

The mandatory fortification of food (flour, enriched pasta, cornmeal, cereal foods) with 140 and 150 μg of folic acid per 100 g in the United States and Canada, respectively, has led to several beneficial effects (Table 167-3). Indeed, 94% of U.S. adults who do not consume supplements or consume less than 400 μg/day of folic acid from supplements do not exceed the upper intake limit for folic acid (>1 mg/day), which has potential to mask cobalamin deficiency.

PROGNOSIS

The general response to cobalamin replacement is a dramatic improvement in well-being, with alertness, a good appetite, and resolution of a sore tongue. Megaloblastic hematopoiesis reverts to normal within 12 hours and resolves by 48 hours; the only persistent findings may be giant metamyelocytes in the bone marrow and hypersegmented neutrophils in the blood for up to 14 days. The reticulocyte count peaks by days 5 to 8, followed by a rise in the red cell count, hemoglobin level, and hematocrit. By the end of the first week, the white blood cell count rises, sometimes with a transient left shift, as does the platelet count; both normalize by approximately 2 months.

TABLE 167-3	BENEFICIAL EFFECTS OF HOMOCYSTEINE-LOWERING THERAPY ON NONHEMATOPOIETIC SYSTEMS

FOLIC ACID, COBALAMIN, PYRIDOXINE SUPPLEMENTATION

Reduction in hip fracture[1]
Reduction in progression of carotid intima media thickness (surrogate marker of early subclinical arteriosclerosis)[2]
Reduction in age-related macular degeneration[3]

FOLIC ACID SUPPLEMENTATION

Reduction in stroke[4]
Reduction in rate of cognitive decline among healthy elderly[5]
Reduction in age-related (sensorineural) hearing loss[6]
Reduction in recurrence of neural tube defects[7]

FOLIC ACID FORTIFICATION OF FOOD (POPULATION-BASED STUDIES)

Reduction in neural tube defects (anencephaly, spina bifida, encephalocele, meningocele, iniencephaly)
Reduction in cleft lip with or without cleft palate
Reduction in severe congenital heart disease (endocardial cushion defects, conotruncal defects)
Reduction in congenital pyloric stenosis, stenosis of the pelvicoureteric junction, limb reduction defects, omphalocele
Reduction in stroke mortality
Decreased risk of low-birthweight and small-for-gestational-age babies

With cobalamin replacement, the degree of reversal of neurologic damage is generally inversely related to the extent of disease and the duration of signs and symptoms. Most neurologic abnormalities improve in up to 90% of patients with documented subacute combined degeneration, and most signs and symptoms of less than 3 months' duration are reversible. With signs and symptoms of longer duration, there is invariably some residual neurologic dysfunction. The maximal response often takes up to 6 months, but recovery beyond 12 months is unusual.

Incorrect treatment of cobalamin deficiency with folate does not improve the neuropsychiatric abnormalities, which will continue to progress; hematologic improvements often occur, however. Alternatively, there may be associated iron deficiency or hypothyroidism that needs treatment or another hemoglobinopathy (e.g., sickle cell disease, thalassemia) that limits the normalization of hemoglobin values.

In patients with pernicious anemia, subsequent iron deficiency anemia (Chapter 162), osteoporosis (Chapter 251) with fractures of the proximal end of the femur and vertebrae, gastric cancer (Chapter 198), and cancer of the buccal cavity and pharynx can develop. Some experts recommend periodic endoscopic surveillance.

Grade A

1. Sato Y, Honda Y, Iwamoto J, et al. Effect of folate and mecobalamin on hip fractures in patients with stroke: a randomized controlled trial. *JAMA.* 2005;293:1082-1088.
2. Hodis HN, Mack WJ, Dustin L, et al. High-dose B vitamin supplementation and progression of subclinical atherosclerosis: a randomized controlled trial. *Stroke.* 2009;40:730-736.
3. Christen WG, Glynn RJ, Chew EY, et al. Folic acid, pyridoxine, and cyanocobalamin combination treatment and age-related macular degeneration in women: the Women's Antioxidant and Folic Acid Cardiovascular Study. *Arch Intern Med.* 2009;169:335-341.
4. Wang X, Qin X, Demirtas H, et al. Efficacy of folic acid supplementation in stroke prevention: a meta-analysis. *Lancet.* 2007;369:1876-1882.
5. Durga J, van Boxtel MP, Schouten EG, et al. Effect of 3-year folic acid supplementation on cognitive function in older adults in the FACIT trial: a randomised, double blind, controlled trial. *Lancet.* 2007;369:208-216.
6. Durga J, Verhoef P, Anteunis LJ, et al. Effects of folic acid supplementation on hearing in older adults: a randomized, controlled trial. *Ann Intern Med.* 2007;146:1-9.
7. Grosse SD, Collins JS. Folic acid supplementation and neural tube defect recurrence prevention. *Birth Defects Res A Clin Mol Teratol.* 2007;79:737-742.

SUGGESTED READINGS

Andrès E, Fothergill H, Mecili M. Efficacy of oral cobalamin (vitamin B₁₂) therapy. *Expert Opin Pharmacother.* 2010;11:249-256. *Support for the routine use of oral cobalamin therapy in clinical practice.*
Bukowski R, Malone FD, Porter FT, et al. Preconceptional folate supplementation and the risk of spontaneous preterm birth: a cohort study. *PLoS Med.* 2009;6:e1000061. *This recent paper suggests a role for folate supplements in preventing spontaneous preterm births in developed countries.*
Carmel R. Mandatory fortification of the food supply with cobalamin: an idea whose time has not yet come. *J Inherit Metab Dis.* 2011;34:67-73. *Argues for randomized clinical trials before this potentially beneficial public health intervention is undertaken.*

Clarke R, Halsey J, Lewington S, et al. Effects of lowering homocysteine levels with B vitamins on cardiovascular disease, cancer, and cause-specific mortality: meta-analysis of 8 randomized trials involving 37,485 individuals. *Arch Intern Med.* 2010;170:1622-1631. *No benefit for incident or fatal cancer or cardiovascular disease, or for overall mortality.*
Schlotz W, Jones A, Phillips DI, et al. Lower maternal folate status in early pregnancy is associated with childhood hyperactivity and peer problems in offspring. *J Child Psychol Psychiatry.* 2010;51:594-602. *Maternal nutrition during early pregnancy contributes to an individual's neurodevelopment, with potential consequences for behavior later in life, similar to experimental studies in mice.*

168

APLASTIC ANEMIA AND RELATED BONE MARROW FAILURE STATES

GROVER C. BAGBY

DEFINITION

Aplastic anemia is a life-threatening syndrome characterized by failure of the bone marrow to produce peripheral blood cells and their progenitors. Diverse diseases and environmental factors can cause this syndrome, but its hallmark is bone marrow hypocellularity and hypoplasia of the erythroid, myeloid, and megakaryocyte lines (Fig. 168-1).

EPIDEMIOLOGY

In Europe and North America, the annual incidence is 2 per 1 million persons, and in Asia, 4 to 7 per 1 million. No age group is exempt, and although the syndrome occurs most often in young adults, the age distribution of newly diagnosed patients is bimodal, with peaks at 15 to 25 years and at 60 to 65 years.

PATHOBIOLOGY

Pathology

Peripheral blood pancytopenia is universally present in patients with aplastic anemia, but bone marrow biopsy is required to establish the diagnosis. The diagnosis will be clear-cut if the biopsy specimen is of sufficient size and has been obtained from an anatomic site that has never been exposed to extensive trauma or radiation. As shown in Figure 168-1B, some residual lymphoid cell populations can be found in marrow specimens. Although these lymphoid cells may be of pathophysiologic importance, it is the absence of *nonlymphoid* hematopoietic cells that is important in establishing the diagnosis of this syndrome. However, if the hematopoietic marrow has been suppressed (or "replaced") by the infiltration of neoplastic cells or fibroblasts, the diagnosis of aplastic anemia cannot be made. Therefore, the diagnosis requires not only a dearth of hematopoietic cells in the marrow but also an empty bone marrow.

Some bone marrow failure syndromes affect only one lineage. In those cases, only the marrow precursors of that lineage are missing. In patients with agranulocytosis, for example, there are rare neutrophils and neutrophil precursors present, and the ratio of erythroid to myeloid cells is very high. Likewise, in patients with the disorder known as pure red cell aplasia, few erythroid cells are detectable in the marrow, but the other lineages are well represented and functional. These two disorders are examples of bone marrow failure syndromes but are not examples of aplastic anemia, which involves global suppression of all hematopoietic lineages.

Pathophysiology

Marrow aplasia in a few patients (10%) can be attributed to an inherited bone marrow failure syndrome, but most cases are acquired and caused by factors other than an inherited gene mutation. In all cases, it is clear that the causative factors, genetic or environmental, injure pluripotent hematopoietic stem cells. This is in contrast to the case of the lineage-restricted disorders, wherein the causative agents and factors suppress the growth and development of unipotent progenitor cells committed to that particular lineage. Radiation, viral diseases, cytotoxic drugs, and chemicals are known causes of aplastic anemia, but the most common form of acquired aplastic anemia is immunologically mediated, and evidence is emerging that some marrow failure states attributed to viral infection or to idiosyncratic drug reactions may also result

FIGURE 168-1. Two bone marrow biopsy samples from different patients. **A.** This specimen, from a normal individual, shows an abundance of hematopoietic cells, including myeloid and erythroid precursors and normal-appearing megakaryocytes. **B,** A specimen from a patient with severe aplastic anemia shows few detectable hematopoietic cells, and those that can be seen (one small nest) are largely lymphocytes. Lymphoid cells are often detectable and probably play an important pathophysiologic role in many cases of acquired idiopathic aplastic anemia, a disorder that is most often immunologically mediated. (Courtesy of Dr. Ken Gatter, Oregon Health and Science University.)

TABLE 168-1	MAJOR CAUSES OF APLASTIC ANEMIA AND RELATED BONE MARROW FAILURE STATES

1. Autoimmune aplastic anemia
   a. Acquired
   b. Drug induced
   c. Infections
      i. Hepatitis
      ii. Epstein-Barr virus
2. Autoimmune-mediated failure of single hematopoietic lineages
   a. Agranulocytosis
   b. Pure red cell aplasia
3. Direct stem cell toxicity
   a. Radiation
   b. Chemicals
   c. Drugs
4. Other aplastic states
   a. Pregnancy
   b. Paroxysmal nocturnal hemoglobinuria
   c. Inherited bone marrow failure syndromes

from immune suppression of hematopoiesis. The pathogenesis of the major causes of aplastic anemia and related bone marrow failure states is outlined in Table 168-1.

Pathogenesis
Autoimmune Aplastic Anemia
Acquired Aplastic Anemia
In patients with the most common form of acquired aplastic anemia, autologous lymphocytes suppress the replicative activity and induce the death of hematopoietic stem and progenitor cells. Evidence supporting this model are to be found in studies demonstrating that: (1) removal of T lymphocytes from cultured bone marrow cells enhances hematopoiesis in vitro; (2) patients with aplastic anemia can be effectively treated with immunosuppressive therapy alone; (3) oligoclonal T cells in the marrow and blood of aplastic anemia patients contain high intracellular levels of the myelosuppressive cytokines interferon-γ (IFN-γ) and tumor necrosis factor-α (TNF-α); (4) the IFN-γ/TNF-α-positive T-cell populations are suppressed in patients who respond to immunosuppressive therapy but are not suppressed in patients who do not respond; and (5) the syndrome can be modeled in mice by infusing alloreactive lymphocytes that induce marrow failure.

Drug Induced
Although a wide variety of drugs have been associated with aplastic anemia, the association is loose. Much of the evidence is circumstantial and, apart from drugs that are known to be directly toxic to the marrow (e.g., chemotherapeutic agents; Table 168-2), the cases are not related to total dose of the suspect agent. These "idiosyncratic" reactions are likely autoimmune.

Some agents, chloramphenicol being the classic paradigm, are capable of inducing dose-related myelosuppression in all treated patients (which abates after discontinuation of the drug) and rare idiosyncratic aplastic responses as well (which do not remit after discontinuation of the agent). Drugs that have been repeatedly associated with aplastic anemia are listed in Table 168-2.

Infections
HEPATITIS. About 2 to 5% of patients with severe aplastic anemia have had viral hepatitis (Chapters 150 and 151). Some cases were associated with hepatitis A or B, but most patients with the hepatitis-aplasia syndrome have had hepatitis of unclear type (non-A, -B, -C, -E, or -G). Most patients with this syndrome are younger than 20 years. The natural course is rapid, with a 1-year mortality rate of more than 90%. The immune system is likely involved in the pathophysiology of this syndrome because immunosuppressive therapy has been reported to induce meaningful remissions.

EPSTEIN-BARR VIRUS. In rare patients with aplastic anemia, evidence of active Epstein-Barr virus (EBV) infection has been discovered (Chapter 385). Because the virus does not infect progenitor cells or stem cells, it is most likely that the virus induces an aberrant immune response that generates either immunoglobulin- or T-lymphocyte–mediated hematopoietic suppression. Because only a minority of EBV-infected aplastic patients describe a history of typical infectious mononucleosis, it is equally likely that the aplastic state came first and that EBV was later reactivated.

Autoimmune-Mediated Failure of Single Hematopoietic Lineages
Agranulocytosis
Agranulocytosis is characterized by severe neutropenia and suppression of granulopoiesis. This disorder can be an idiosyncratic reaction to certain drugs and most likely involves immune suppression of granulopoietic progenitor cells. The disease almost always abates when the offending drug is discontinued. Agranulocytosis also occurs in patients with established autoimmune diseases, including systemic lupus erythematosus, Sjögren's syndrome, and rheumatoid arthritis. In some cases, the disorder is caused by myelosuppressive antibodies, and in others, by T lymphocytes that suppress granulopoiesis. Immunosuppressive therapy is often effective in such patients and should be used in patients whose agranulocytosis is severe and associated with recurrent infections.

Pure Red Cell Aplasia
Severe normochromic, normocytic anemia with a marked decrease in reticulocyte number is sometimes associated with selective hypoplasia of the erythroid marrow without loss of megakaryocytes and myeloid precursor cells. In immunocompromised hosts and patients with chronic hemolytic diseases, this disorder, known as pure red cell aplasia, can be caused by parvovirus B19 infection (Chapter 379), an agent that infects erythroid precursor cells and likely generates an erythroid suppressive immune response. This disease can also be mediated by T lymphocytes or natural killer cells that suppress cells of the erythroid lineage and in more uncommon cases by antibody-dependent

TABLE 168-2 DRUGS AND TOXINS ASSOCIATED WITH APLASTIC ANEMIA

DOSE DEPENDENT
Antineoplastic Agents
Antimetabolites: fluorouracil, mercaptopurine, 6-thioguanine, methotrexate, cytosine arabinoside, gemcitabine, fludarabine, cladribine, pentostatin, hydroxyurea
Alkylating and cross-linking agents: busulfan, cyclophosphamide, chlorambucil, nitrogen mustard, melphalan, cisplatin, carboplatin, ifosfamide, nitrosoureas (BCNU and CCNU), mitomycin C
Cytotoxic antibiotics: daunorubicin, doxorubicin, mitoxantrone
Plant alkaloids: vinblastine, paclitaxel
Topoisomerase inhibitors: etoposide

Antimicrobial Agents
Chloramphenicol, dapsone, fluorocytosine

Anti-Inflammatory and Antirheumatic Agents
Colchicine

Insecticides
Chlordane, chlorophenothane (DDT), lindane, parathion

Other Chemicals
Benzene
Benzene-containing chemicals: kerosene, chlorophenols, carbon tetrachloride

DOSE INDEPENDENT
Idiosyncratic, likely immune mediated
(*Note:* Most agents on this list should be considered to be possibly associated with aplastic anemia.)

Antimicrobial Agents
Chloramphenicol, dapsone, sulfonamides, tetracycline, methicillin, amphotericin, quinacrine, chloroquine, pyrimethamine

Anticonvulsants
Hydantoins, carbamazepine, phenacemide, primidone, ethosuximide

Anti-Inflammatory Agents
Phenylbutazone, indomethacin, ibuprofen, oxyphenylbutazone, sulindac, naproxen

Antiarrhythmic Drugs
Quinidine, tocainide, procainamide

Metals
Gold, arsenic, mercury, bismuth

Antihistamines
Cimetidine, ranitidine, chlorpheniramine, pyrilamine, tripelennamine

Diuretics
Acetazolamide, furosemide, chlorothiazide, methazolamide

Hypoglycemic Agents
Chlorpropamide, tolbutamide

Antithyroid Drugs
Propylthiouracil, potassium perchlorate, methylthiouracil, methimazole, carbimazole

Antihypertensive Agents
Methyldopa, enalapril, captopril

Sedatives
Chlordiazepoxide, chlorpromazine, meprobamate, prochlorperazine

suppression of erythropoiesis. Pure red cell aplasia can also develop as a complication of thymoma (Chapters 99 and 430) and in these circumstances is likewise caused by oligoclonal T-cell expansion that specifically suppresses erythroid progenitor cells. This disorder can also be associated with drug exposure (e.g., isoniazid, chlorpropamide, and phenytoin), lymphoid neoplasms (chronic lymphocytic leukemia; Chapter 190), and myelodysplasia (Chapter 188). Rarely, adults with Diamond-Blackfan anemia present with isolated erythroid suppression, but the degree to which the erythroid marrow is suppressed rarely matches the profound suppression seen in acquired cases of immune-mediated pure red cell aplasia.

Direct Stem Cell Toxicity
Radiation
The severity of myelosuppression induced by radiation and the degree to which the marrow can recover from that injury depend on the radiation dose, the timing of exposure, and the fraction of hematopoietic tissues exposed. Low-dose total body radiation causes transient marrow suppression. High doses of total body radiation (700 to 1000 cGy) induce severe injury to the stem cell pool with persistent and life-threatening marrow failure. When limited bone marrow sites are radiated to very high doses (4000 cGy or more), the relatively radioresistant bone marrow stromal cells are eradicated, and thereafter that marrow space can never support hematopoietic activity.

Chemicals
Benzene suppresses the bone marrow in a dose-dependent manner, and chronic exposure to it has been linked with aplastic anemia and myeloid leukemogenesis. Benzene and many of its catabolites are directly toxic to stem cells, damage DNA, suppress the supportive function of the bone marrow microenvironment, and accentuate the responsiveness of hematopoietic progenitor cells to intramedullary apoptotic cues that arise during the inflammatory response. Kerosene, carbon-tetrachloride, and chlorophenols contain benzene, as do many other like products used for paint stripping, refinishing, and degreasing (see Table 168-2).

Drugs
Many agents in use for the treatment of malignant diseases are predictably myelosuppressive and can induce aplastic anemia because they are directly toxic to stem and progenitor cells in the marrow (see Table 168-2). These myelosuppressive responses are completely predictable and dose dependent. In practical terms, unless the patient receives a drug overdose or has an undiagnosed genetic disorder that predisposes the patient to respond to the agent in an exaggerated way (e.g., Fanconi anemia [FA]), most patients treated for neoplastic diseases develop reversible bone marrow aplasia or hypoplasia and recover bone marrow function within a matter of days.

Other Aplastic States
Pregnancy
Aplastic anemia can be diagnosed in pregnancy. In addition, some patients with aplastic anemia have become pregnant after the diagnosis. The prognosis in both instances is poor, and most fatal outcomes are due to bleeding complications. Some women, who have been fortunate enough to recover bone marrow function postpartum, develop aplastic anemia with a subsequent pregnancy. The pathogenesis and causal relationship between pregnancy and aplastic anemia remain unknown but may reflect immunologic activation during pregnancy.

Paroxysmal Nocturnal Hemoglobinuria
Paroxysmal nocturnal hemoglobinuria (PNH) is an acquired disorder that results from the expansion of a clone of hematopoietic stem cells whose progeny are incapable of anchoring essential proteins to their membranes (Chapter 163). The defect is caused by an inactivating somatic mutation of *PIGA*, an X-linked gene that encodes a protein essential for synthesis of the membrane anchor glycosyl phosphatidylinositol (GPI). Some of the GPI-anchored proteins (e.g., CD55 and CD59) are important in normal red cells to protect them from activated complement. Their loss results in chronic intravascular hemolysis. Two less clearly defined features of PNH are thromboembolism, of which there is a very high relative risk in the PNH patient population (Chapter 179), and aplastic anemia. The emergence of "PNH clones" is not uncommon in patients with acquired aplastic anemia, and experimental evidence supports the idea that the evolution of *PIGA*-deficient stem cells is an adaptive response to the immune attack. How the *PIGA*-deficient cells fend off cytotoxic T cells is less clear, but it is likely that their pool expands because they accomplish that task somehow. In effect, in the setting of an immune attack, *PIGA*-deficient stem cells are more fit than normal stem cells, but the complement-sensitive red cells to which they give rise have a short lifespan.

Inherited Bone Marrow Failure Syndromes
Some inherited bone marrow failure syndromes can present in adolescence and adulthood. They include dyskeratosis congenita, Fanconi anemia (FA), and Diamond-Blackfan anemia. The molecular pathogenesis of the bone marrow failure seen in these diseases is unclear. Although the genetic basis of these disorders has been well defined in the past decade, the canonical functions of the proteins encoded by these genes is distinct (Table 168-3) for each disease. For example, in dyskeratosis, the mutations occur in genes that encode proteins and RNAs involved in telomere maintenance. In FA, the mutations involve proteins involved in the DNA-damage response, and in

TABLE 168-3 DISTINGUISHING CLINICAL FEATURES OF THE INHERITED BONE MARROW FAILURE SYNDROMES THAT MAY BE INITIALLY DIAGNOSED IN ADULTHOOD

DISTINGUISHING FEATURES	Diseases		
	FANCONI ANEMIA	**DYSKERATOSIS CONGENITA**	**DIAMOND-BLACKFAN ANEMIA**
History	Skeletal and renal malformations, low birthweight, pancytopenia, family member with bone marrow failure, myelodysplasia (MDS), acute myelogenous leukemia (AML), or squamous cell carcinoma at an early age. Family member with Fanconi anemia	Intrauterine growth retardation, developmental delay, and short stature. Family history of MDS, AML, marrow failure, abnormal fingernails or toenails, leukoplakia, head and neck cancer, or pulmonary fibrosis	Low birthweight, arm and thumb deformities at birth
Physical findings	Thumb and radial malformations, hyperpigmented skin lesions (cafe au lait spots), short stature, MDS, AML, squamous cell carcinoma at young age, renal and cardiac malformations, microcephaly, hypogonadism	Lacy reticular pigmentation of skin, dystrophic fingernails and toenails, premature graying of hair, hair loss, short stature, oral leukoplakia, squamous cell cancer of head and neck, pulmonary fibrosis, osteopenia, hypogonadism	Triphalangeal thumbs, short stature, arm anomalies
Genes inactivated	*FANCA, FANCB, FANCC, FANCD1* (aka *BRCA2*), *FANCD2, FANCE, FANCF, FANCG* (aka *XRCC9*), *FANCI, FANCJ* (aka *BACH1* and *BRIP1*), *FANCL* (aka *PHF9* and *POG*), *FANCM* (aka *Hef*), and *FANCN* (aka *PALB2*) These genes encode proteins known to protect the genome from excessive damage induced by chemical crosslinking agents. These genes account for most cases of Fanconi anemia.	*DKC1, TERC, TERT, TINF2, NOLA2,* and *NOLA3* These genes encode proteins known to participate in maintenance of telomeres. They account for only half of dyskeratosis cases, so there are additional genes to be discovered.	*RPS17, RPS19, RPS24, RPLS, RPL11,* and *RPL35A* These genes encode ribosomal proteins. They account for only half of cases, so there are additional genes to be discovered.
Screening and diagnostic tests	1. Chromosomal breakage test (in response to mitomycin C or diepoxybutane) 2. Complementation analysis (flow cytometric analysis of G₂ arrest in melphalan-exposed cells after transduction with retroviral vectors expressing normal Fanconi anemia genes) 3. Gene sequencing	1. Quantitative analysis of telomere length ("flow FISH") 2. Gene sequencing	*Note:* Isolated erythroid failure is more common than full blown aplastic anemia. 1. There are no screening tests, although serum ADA is often elevated. 2. Gene sequencing

ADA = adenosine deaminase; FISH = fluorescent in situ hybridization.

Diamond-Blackfan anemia, inactivating mutations involve ribosomal proteins known to be involved in ribosome biogenesis. Whether loss of these canonical functions is linked with the pathogenesis of marrow failure is unclear. In fact, studies on hematopoietic cells have revealed noncanonical functions of some of these proteins. Some of the FA proteins, for example, not only function to protect the genome, but also participate directly in survival signaling pathways for hematopoietic cells. Interestingly, some of the pathways disrupted in mutant cells result in hyperactivation of precisely those same cytokine signaling pathways involved in the pathogenesis of acquired autoimmune aplastic anemia.

Genetics

The genetic basis of inherited bone marrow failure syndromes is being rapidly solved. Some of these syndromes (e.g., Shwachman-Diamond syndrome, amegakaryocytic thrombocytopenia, and severe congenital neutropenia) are almost always diagnosed in early life. However, some may be first diagnosed in adulthood (e.g., dyskeratosis congenita, FA, and Diamond-Blackfan anemia). It is critically important to consider these three disorders early in the evaluation of adults with aplastic anemia because the treatment of such patients with conventional stem cell transplantation regimens is associated with high mortality rates (especially in dyskeratosis congenita and FA). Furthermore, immunosuppressive therapy plays no role in these diseases. The clinical and laboratory manifestations of these three diseases and the findings that should prompt genetic testing in such patients are reviewed in Table 168-3. Importantly, adults who present with these diseases were not born with aplastic anemia. Instead, aplasia develops over time and gives rise to symptoms in adulthood. Prospective studies of children and adults who present with bone marrow failure have indicated that nearly 10% will have previously unsuspected FA. ▪ Diagnostic consideration of a hereditary form of aplastic anemia should not be limited to children.

▶ CLINICAL MANIFESTATIONS

The natural course of aplastic anemia is influenced by its severity. Patients with hypoplastic bone marrow have severe aplastic anemia if they meet two

of the following laboratory criteria: (1) absolute neutrophil count less than 0.5×10^9/L, (2) platelet count less than 20×10^9/L, or (3) reticulocytes less than 20×10^9/L. Patients who do not have severe aplastic anemia often progress to severe aplasia, but the pace is slow (about 40% will have progressed in 5 years). Severe aplastic anemia is a life-threatening condition that, untreated, is associated with a mortality rate of 80% in the 24 months after diagnosis. Treatment of any cohort of patients with severe aplastic anemia will prolong life, and many patients, particularly those who have received stem cell transplants, will be cured.

History

Symptoms of this syndrome, cause notwithstanding, are almost always reflective of low blood counts. The most common presenting symptoms are those associated with thrombocytopenia and anemia. Low platelet counts are associated with bleeding, often epistaxis and bleeding gums, bruising with minor or no trauma, and menorrhagia. Anemia accounts for the nearly universal symptoms of fatigue and dyspnea on mild exertion. Some aplastic patients may present with intercurrent bacterial or fungal infection (because of severe neutropenia), but these cases are less common. Family histories that include any of the features listed in Table 168-3 should raise suspicion of an inherited bone marrow failure syndrome.

Physical Examination

Pallor and tachycardia at rest are common signs of anemia but can be absent or unnoticeable in younger patients and in patients whose aplasia is of very recent onset. Often hemorrhagic manifestations classic for thrombocytopenia are found: petechiae (cutaneous or palatal), ecchymoses, and epistaxis. The most common form of aplastic anemia, autoimmune, is rarely associated with lymphadenopathy or hepatosplenomegaly, and when such findings are present, alternative diagnoses should be considered and painstakingly ruled out. Likewise, short stature, endocrinopathies, osteopenia, findings of developmental anomalies of the skin, nails, hands, or arms, or malformations of the heart, liver, or genitourinary tract should trigger concerns of an inherited bone marrow failure disease (see Table 168-3).

Initial Laboratory Findings

Pancytopenia (anemia, leukopenia, and thrombocytopenia) is a universal presenting finding. The morphology of neutrophils, platelets, and red cells on peripheral blood smear is usually normal unless there is concurrent iron deficiency due to bleeding.

Diagnostic Evaluation

The evaluation of pancytopenic patients first requires examination of the peripheral blood smear. If there are morphologic or clinical signs of vitamin B_{12} or folic acid deficiency (e.g., hypersegmented neutrophils and oval macrocytes), those disorders should be ruled out because a bone marrow aspiration and biopsy would not be required in those conditions. In severe aplastic anemia, the peripheral blood smear will not show nucleated red blood cells or other signs that the marrow might be infiltrated with abnormal cells. All patients in whom B_{12} and folate deficiency have been ruled out require a bone marrow aspiration and biopsy. Obtaining both types of samples is important. The biopsy best assesses overall bone marrow cellularity and provides the most sensitive evidence for some infiltrative processes. The aspirated sample can be examined microscopically for the presence of abnormal cells but also provides cells for cytogenetic analyses (which can provide evidence supporting hypoplastic myelodysplasia and acute leukemia). Rarely in the early stages of aplasia, the biopsy can be somewhat cellular. A repeat biopsy in 1 to 2 weeks might be required to establish the diagnosis clearly. As summarized in Figure 168-2, once the diagnosis of aplastic anemia has been made, a series of additional tests must be obtained. In light of the life-threatening nature of this disease, the tests must be obtained simultaneously, but they serve three distinct purposes.

Ruling Out Aplastic Anemia Variants that Are Treated Differently

The best therapeutic option for many different aplastic states is often matched sibling donor stem cell transplantation, but there are some aplastic states that are managed differently. For example, a child with an inherited marrow failure syndrome might have a human leukocyte antigen (HLA)-identical sibling who also has the same genetic defect. If such a diagnosis has been overlooked, the recipient will likely die from complications of the conditioning regimen (e.g., patients with FA are highly intolerant of radiation and crosslinking agents used in conventional conditioning regiments, and patients with dyskeratosis suffer excessive post-transplantation morbidity and mortality) or possibly because the transplanted stem cells (from the undiagnosed affected sibling donor) are equally unfit. Patients with dyskeratosis congenita and children with the Shwachman-Diamond syndrome are also intolerant of conventional transplantation regimens and often suffer severe pulmonary and hepatic toxicity. Although patients with Diamond-Blackfan anemia are more tolerant of standard conditioning regimens, they are more apt to respond to glucocorticosteroid therapy, and if they are transplanted with stem cells from an undiagnosed affected sibling, they too will do poorly. Finally, patients with PNH should be identified using flow cytometric quantification of CD55- and CD59-deficient red cells because more than half of patients with severe aplastic anemia will have PNH clones; when treated with immunosuppressive therapy, the PNH clone often expands and causes clinically significant signs of PNH (hemolysis and thrombosis).

Tests Helpful in Supportive Care

At some point during the course of the disease, red cell and platelet transfusions will be necessary. Radiated and filtered blood products are used to prevent transfusion-associated graft-versus-host disease (GVHD), reduce alloimmunization, and reduce the complication of cytomegalovirus (CMV) infection. ABO and HLA typing are required. Infections can be of bacterial, viral, or fungal origin and must be quickly diagnosed and treated not only because the patients are often neutropenic but also because, once definitive therapy begins, it is likely they will be receiving immunosuppressive therapy (either through primary immunosuppression or through stem cell transplantation). In the acutely infected, severely neutropenic patient, once cultures and biopsies are obtained, empirical antibiotic therapy should be prescribed even before the culture results are available. Post-transplantation CMV infection is best avoided in CMV-seronegative recipients by using CMV-negative blood products (Chapter 180). Many centers routinely infuse radiated and filtered ("CMV-safe") blood products and therefore no longer routinely screen for CMV seronegativity.

Evaluating the Patient as a Candidate for Stem Cell Transplantation

Timing of treatment depends on the severity of the aplastic anemia and the age of the patient (Table 168-4). Patients with mild marrow hypoplasia and mild bone marrow suppression can be followed closely to determine what the pace of hypoplasia might be. In patients up to 40 years of age with either severe acquired aplastic anemia or transfusion dependence, steps should be taken to evaluate them promptly for stem cell transplantation therapy by seeking HLA-identical siblings and, in appropriate cases, searching for matched unrelated donors.

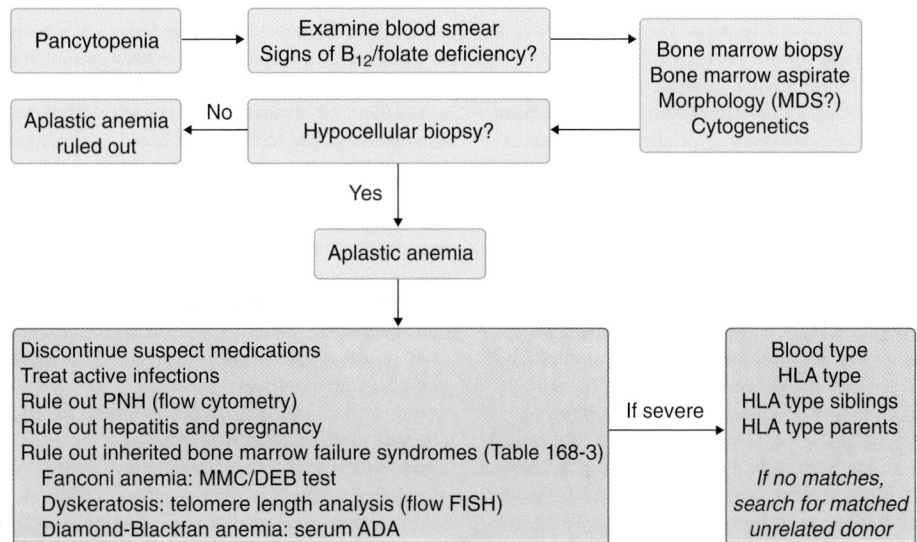

FIGURE 168-2. A pathway for the diagnostic management of patients with aplastic anemia. Patients who present with pancytopenia will require bone marrow biopsy and aspiration unless there are signs of vitamin B_{12} or folate deficiency. If the bone marrow is as cellular as that shown in Fig. 168-1A, the diagnosis of aplastic anemia has been effectively ruled out because the diagnosis requires bone marrow hypocellularity (see Fig. 168-1B). In all patients, regardless of severity, suspect medications should be discontinued, active infections should be treated without delay, and paroxysmal nocturnal hemoglobinuria (PNH) should be excluded, as should pregnancy and hepatitis. For patients with positive family histories or any one of the findings listed in Table 168-3, and all patients younger than 40 years, inherited marrow failure syndromes should be ruled out with screening tests. Patients with severe aplastic anemia are those who have at least two of the following: absolute neutrophil count of less than 0.5×10^9/L, platelet count of less than 20×10^9/L, or reticulocyte count of less than 20×10^9/L. These patients must be treated with definitive therapy and should be evaluated for stem cell transplantation with human leukocyte antigen (HLA) typing (patient and family members) and, if necessary, a search for matched unrelated donors. ADA = adenosine deaminase; DEB = diepoxybutane; FISH = fluorescent in situ hybridization; MDS = myelodysplasia; MMC = mitomycin C.

TABLE 168-4 TREATMENT RECOMMENDATIONS FOR PATIENTS WITH SEVERE ACQUIRED IDIOPATHIC APLASTIC ANEMIA*

	AGE < 20 YR		AGE 20-40 YR		AGE > 40 YR	
HLA-identical sibling?	Yes	No	Yes	No	Yes	No
First-line treatment	MSBMT	IST	MSBMT	IST	IST	IST
Second-line treatment	IST or second MSBMT	IST or MUDT or CBT	IST	IST or MUDT	MSBMT	IST. For failures, consider MUDT.

*This general set of recommendations cannot be applied to patients with inherited bone marrow failure syndromes because they do not respond to immunosuppressive therapy (IST).
CBT = umbilical cord blood transplantation; IST = immunosuppressive therapy; MSBMT = matched sibling bone marrow transplant; MUDT = matched unrelated donor transplant.
Adapted from Bacigalupo A, Passweg J. Diagnosis and treatment of acquired aplastic anemia. *Hematol Oncol Clin North Am.* 2009;23:159-170.

Differential Diagnosis

Most classic aplastic anemia patients have immunologically mediated disease. Notwithstanding strong evidence in support of this mechanism from some research laboratories over the past 30 years, there exists no validated screening tool that can either rule in or rule out immune-mediated disease, a fact that is complicated by the evidence that some cases of drug- and virus-induced disease are also immunologically mediated. Therefore, idiopathic autoimmune aplastic anemia remains a diagnosis of exclusion. For this reason, the obligation of the diagnostician is to consider disease induced by chemical or viral agents and radiation and disease associated with pregnancy. It is also most important to rule out PNH and inherited bone marrow failure syndromes (see Fig. 168-2).

Cytotoxic Drugs, Chemicals, and Radiation

A fastidiously obtained medication history is important. Any drug with the potential of inducing aplastic anemia should be discontinued. It is equally important to ask patients about alternative therapies that they might not consider being "medicines." Some herbal remedies are known to contain molecules (e.g., phenylbutazone) not listed on the label but associated with aplasia (see Table 168-2). A history of exposure to radiation or to chemicals with myelosuppressive capacities (see Table 168-2) should likewise be obtained. Tests for benzene metabolites detect only acute exposure and are not reliable indicators of cumulative exposure in individual patients. Although it is intuitively obvious and prudent to discontinue the use of agents that might have inflicted severe stem cell injury, by the time the injury has progressed to the point of severe aplastic anemia, most of these patients are in need of the same types of therapy prescribed for patients with autoimmune aplastic anemia.

Idiosyncratic Drug Responses

If a medication history unearths an exposure to an agent known to be associated with idiosyncratic (not related to dose) responses, the agent must likewise be discontinued. Because it is likely that these responses are immunologically mediated, the patient should be treated no differently from patients with severe idiopathic aplastic anemia, and the patient should be evaluated as a stem cell transplantation candidate. If, during the diagnostic evaluation of the patient and potential donors, there are signs that the marrow is recovering on its own, a more conservative approach can be taken.

Paroxysmal Nocturnal Hemoglobinuria

PNH can be ruled out by screening for CD55 and CD59 on the surface of granulocytes, monocytes, and red cells using flow cytometry. The proper diagnosis of PNH requires the absence of these or other GPI-anchored proteins on at least two hematopoietic cell types. Other characteristic features of this syndrome can be a high low-density lipoprotein level, high indirect bilirubin, low haptoglobin, and a positive urine hemosiderin test.

Fanconi Anemia

FA should be considered in any adult of any age with a family history of aplastic anemia, acute myelogenous leukemia or myelodysplasia, or a squamous cell carcinoma at an unusually young age. This disease should also be considered in any patient with any physical finding listed in Table 168-3 or in patients with a family member who has any of these findings. Unfortunately, some patients with FA meet none of these standards, so some hematologists advocate testing for it in all patients with aplastic anemia patients who are younger than 40 years. This disease can be ruled out by obtaining a chromosomal breakage test (see Table 168-3). Here, either lymphocytes or skin fibroblasts are exposed to mitomycin C or diepoxybutane for a period of 2 to 3 days, after which metaphase chromosomes are examined for chromosomal breaks and quadriradial forms (in FA cells, these four-armed interchromosomal forms involve at least two chromosomal breaks). If the clinical context is suggestive (see Table 168-3), but results of the lymphocyte chromosomal breakage test are negative or equivocal, testing of skin fibroblasts is required to rule out the diagnosis. Once the diagnosis is made, history, physical examination, blood counts, and chromosomal breakage tests should be performed on all immediate family members.

There are at least 13 different FA genes (see Table 168-3), and sequencing them all using cells from every patient is not practical at this time. Fortunately, the involved gene can be first identified by a variety of more affordable complementation analyses. In this type of test, normal FA genes are introduced into primary cells of the patient in vitro, and the one gene that corrects the defect (i.e. ,reduces hypersensitivity to cross-linking agents [melphalan, mitomycin C, or diepoxybutane]) represents the gene of interest. That gene can then be fully sequenced to identify the precise mutation, information that will be of value to family members for family planning purposes. In rare instances, it can also aid in applying preimplantation genetic diagnosis and in vitro fertilization, a process that has successfully resulted in unaffected offspring and ideal cord-blood stem cell donors for transplantation of an affected sibling.

Dyskeratosis Congenita

Dyskeratosis congenita should be considered in any aplastic adult of any age with a family member who has had aplastic anemia. It should be likewise considered if either the patient or a family member has had acute myelogenous leukemia, myelodysplasia, nail dystrophy, lacy skin pigmentation, pulmonary fibrosis, oral leukoplakia, squamous cell carcinoma at an unusually young age, or any other physical finding listed in Table 168-3. This disease can be frequently ruled out by quantifying the length of telomeres in circulating white cells using a flow cytometric method. Because some of the physical findings overlap, FA should be ruled out in all patients being evaluated for dyskeratosis congenita. The dyskeratosis test quantifies telomere length using fluorescence in situ hybridization. Lymphocytes from dyskeratosis patients have extremely short telomeres (i.e., at or less than the 1st percentile). If two or three leukocyte types from a given patient are above the 1st percentile, the diagnosis of dyskeratosis is unlikely. If telomeres are in the diagnostic range, genetic testing is warranted. It is not yet known whether this test will become a "gold-standard" test as reliable as the chromosomal breakage test is for FA because some investigators report that very short telomeres can be found in patients who have other causes of bone marrow failure. Unlike the genetic strategy employed with FA (at least today), complementation analyses are not routinely performed in dyskeratosis. The molecular diagnosis is based on gene sequencing. Once the diagnosis is made and even before the establishment of a molecular genetic diagnosis (see Table 168-3), all immediate family members of the patient should be seen individually, their history taken, and their physical examination performed along with peripheral blood counts and telomere length analysis.

Diamond-Blackfan Anemia

Diamond-Blackfan anemia is an inherited bone marrow failure syndrome that more often exhibits selective erythroid failure and is an unusual cause of full-blown severe aplastic anemia. Although some patients can present in adulthood, most are discovered within the first year of life and present with anemia but less commonly neutropenia and thrombocytopenia. Phenotypic abnormalities like short stature and skeletal defects are the exception in this disease. There are no screening tests as reliable as those used for FA and dyskeratosis congenita. However, in patients with unexplained erythroid failure, the finding of an elevated adenosine deaminase level in the serum, although unexplained, is strongly suggestive of this disease. Because no helpful screening test exists, there are no reliable or standardized complementation tests.

Consequently, genetic diagnosis requires the application of gene sequencing methods (see Table 168-3).

Other Diagnostic Considerations

Aplastic anemia has been reported in recipients of organ allografts (in which mismatched T cells [either from the donated graft or from blood products that had not been irradiated] induce severe aplasia), patients with myelodysplasia (Chapter 188), patients with congenital and acquired immunodeficiency states (Chapter 258), and patients with established autoimmune diseases including systemic lupus erythematosus (Chapter 274) and eosinophilic fasciitis (Chapter 448), a disease characterized by painful swelling of the skin and subcutaneous tissue.

TREATMENT Rx

For patients with more mild forms of aplastic anemia, aggressive therapy may not be indicated. A passive approach is more problematic in patients with FA and dyskeratosis congenita because transplantation early in life is better tolerated, immunosuppressive therapy is ineffective, and stem cell transplantation provides the only hope for cure of bone marrow failure. If there is evidence of an underlying autoimmune-mediated disease (e.g., isolated granulopoietic or erythroid failure in patients with rheumatic diseases or thymoma), immunosuppressive therapy alone is often highly effective.

Hematopoietic Stem Cell Transplantation: Matched Sibling Donor

For patients with severe aplastic anemia, stem cell transplantation offers the advantages of immunosuppression, an infusion of new "healthy" stem cells, and the expectation that the lymphoid cells that suppressed the marrow in the first place will be replaced by more normal cells that have no myelosuppressive capacity. This expectation is borne out by large retrospective studies indicating the superiority of stem cell transplantation over immunosuppressive therapy alone in the treatment of severe aplastic anemia. Naturally, this approach is relevant to a minority of patients because only 25 to 30% will have an HLA-matched sibling.

Stem cells derived from the bone marrow, not the peripheral blood, should be the source of donor cells. Studies testing the comparative effectiveness of peripheral blood as a source of stem cells demonstrated that the peripheral blood source was associated with excess mortality stemming from an increased incidence of chronic GVHD. The recipient (in whom congenital marrow failure syndromes have been ruled out) initially receives high-dose cyclophosphamide with antithymocyte globulin (ATG) as the preparative regimen. Immunosuppressive therapy begins 2 to 4 days before infusion of stem cells. Common post-transplantation immunosuppression combines cyclosporine and methotrexate. The complication of graft failure with this approach is infrequently seen (<5%), grades II to IV acute GVHD is seen in 30 to 50% of recipients, 25% have chronic GVHD, and short-term (2-year) survival after transplantation is nearly 90%. Ten-year survival rates are highly age dependent: 83%, 73%, and 68% for recipients in the first, second, and third decades of life, respectively. In patients 40 years of age or older, the 10-year survival rate is only 51%. Treatment choices adjusted for patient age are presented in Table 168-4.

Hematopoietic Stem Cell Transplantation: Matched Unrelated Donor

The use of bone marrow from an HLA-matched unrelated donor should be considered for patients who have no HLA-identical siblings, have failed immunosuppressive therapy, and are refractory to transfused platelets. Results have not been as favorable as those associated with the use of marrow from HLA-identical siblings, but this strategy has improved in the past decade in part because of more accurate selection of HLA-matched donors and in part because of adjustments made with pretransplantation conditioning regimens. In fact, in some pediatric populations, some centers are now reporting identical outcomes in children transplanted with marrow cells from HLA-matched related and matched unrelated donors. Conditioning regimens without ATG are associated with inferior outcomes, and less toxic conditioning regimens appear to have improved survival (65% for patients older than 16 years and 75% for those 16 years of age or younger). The improvements have been encouraging enough to recommend strongly that unrelated donor searches be initiated at the time of diagnosis for any patient younger than 30 years. Adults older than 30 years should be considered candidates for alternative donor stem cell transplantation if they have failed two attempts at immunosuppressive therapy because newer fludarabine-based conditioning regimens have improved outcomes of matched unrelated donor transplants remarkably.

Immunosuppressive Therapy

Treatment with ATG alone prolongs survival when compared with supportive care alone, and for patients with mild aplastic anemia (not severe), either no treatment or ATG alone is sufficient. In patients with severe aplastic anemia,

however, the combination of ATG and cyclosporine is superior to treatment with ATG alone. The combination reduces mortality and induces more rapid and higher overall response rates than does ATG as a single agent. Doses vary from center to center, but ATG is given at doses of 12 to 40 mg/kg/day for 4 to 5 days, and cyclosporine doses of 5 to 10 mg/kg/day (targeting blood levels of 150 to 250 ng/mL) are prescribed for 6 months, after which cyclosporine is slowly tapered over a period of 1 year or more. The median time to response is 120 days. Complete responses are defined as the resolution of pancytopenia and the development of normal blood counts. Relapses are uncommon in complete responders (10%). Partial responders are those whose counts do not normalize but who no longer require transfusion support. Forty to 60% of these patients will relapse in 5 years, but most will respond to a repeat course of immunosuppressive therapy. Some will require chronic immunosuppressive therapy with cyclosporine to remain transfusion independent. Those with unresponsive relapses have a poor prognosis.

All age groups can benefit from immunosuppressive therapy. Long-term survival rates do vary with the age of the treated population. In patients younger than 20 years, 10-year survival rates are 80%, but these rates progressively decline to 25% in patients older than 70 years. However, when adjusted for the survival of an age-matched population using the standardized mortality ratio, the corrected risk for death is highest in young patients and declines as age increases. Advanced age is not a contraindication for the prescription of immunosuppressive therapy.

There are some caveats of importance related to the use of immunosuppressive therapy in aplastic anemia patients. First, patients may experience allergic reactions during infusions of ATG. This should not necessarily dissuade one from continuing this agent. Slowing the infusion after premedication with glucocorticosteroids and antihistamines often solves this problem. Fever and rigor can be signs of cytokine release from the targeted T-cell pool, so they likewise should not be used as a reason to stop treatment. Second, if a responsive patient later relapses, a second course of ATG is frequently effective and should be used. Third, it seems clear that a long interval between diagnosis of aplastic anemia and the initiation of immunosuppressive therapy is a negative predictor of response. Treatment should begin as soon as possible; certainly within 3 weeks of initial diagnosis. Fourth, the inclusion of hematopoietic growth factors during immunosuppressive therapy provides no benefit.[2]

Diamond-Blackfan Anemia and Pure Red Cell Aplasia

Although the mechanism by which glucocorticosteroids induce remissions in patients with Diamond-Blackfan anemia is unknown, nearly 80% of patients initially respond. Prednisone treatment is started at 2 mg/kg/day and is tapered after the hemoglobin increases to 10 g/dL. Most patients require a low every-other-day dose, but 15% remain in remission off steroids altogether. In those cases, survival to age 40 years is nearly universal. Of patients who require ongoing steroid support, 75% reach age 40 years. Only half of the patients with steroid-resistant severe anemia survive to age 40 years. Pure red cell aplasia may respond to a synthetic erythropoietin receptor agonist.

Supportive Care

Platelet Transfusions

In the absence of bleeding or infection, platelet transfusions are commonly administered only when the platelet count declines to 10,000/mL or less, but in the presence of active infection or bleeding, transfusion thresholds are often set at 20,000/mL or higher. If bleeding and infection coexist, it is prudent to rule out disseminated intravascular coagulation because fresh-frozen plasma or cryoprecipitate may be required along with platelet transfusions. Drugs (e.g., aspirin) that inhibit platelet function must be avoided, as should activities that might result in trauma. Menstrual activity should be suppressed with oral contraceptives or other agents.

Red Cell Transfusions

Filtered packed red blood cells should be provided to meet the needs of the patient's daily activities. There is no established hemoglobin target number for this purpose, but as a general rule, the number is higher in elderly patients than in young patients. Children with hemoglobin levels of as low as 6 g/dL can compensate reasonably. Adults with underlying cardiopulmonary disease may have symptomatic anemia at 8 g/dL. If chronic transfusion therapy is required, the development of iron overload may require chelation therapy.

Management of Infections

The major infectious challenges result from the immunosuppression used (either as primary therapy or as a component of a stem cell transplantation regimen) more than the neutropenia. For that reason, antibacterial, antiviral, and antifungal prophylaxis is routinely used in transplant recipients. In many centers, patients treated with immunosuppressive therapy alone are treated similarly for a 2- to 3-month period following ATG administration. Importantly, the onset of fever requires prompt clinical evaluation and antibiotic therapy as described in Chapter 289.

PREVENTION

Apart from public health measures controlling exposures to benzene, aromatic hydrocarbons, and radiation, little can be done to prevent acquired aplastic anemia. In the inherited bone marrow failure syndromes, prevention is quite achievable. Once the proband is identified, other affected family members, carriers, and siblings with no mutant allele can be identified, and genetic results can be applied in family planning even to the extent of preimplantation genetic diagnosis followed by in vitro fertilization. Because all somatic cells of children and adults with FA are hypersensitive to alkylating agents and oxidative stress, they must not receive standard doses of radiation or alkylating agents either for transplant conditioning or for treatment of squamous cell carcinoma.

Clonal evolution (e.g., to myelodysplasia and acute leukemia) occurs in 10 to 20% of patients with acquired aplastic anemia survivors and up to 40% of children and adults with dyskeratosis congenita and FA. This complication likely evolves through a process of clonal selection and adaptation and for that reason is seen less commonly in completely responsive patients than in those with less than complete responses (who therefore have ongoing suppression of hematopoiesis). This suggests that more effective strategies of immunosuppressive therapy may better control ongoing marrow damage and decrease the incidence of clonal evolution.

PROGNOSIS

Acquired Idiopathic Aplastic Anemia

The severity of aplastic anemia and age are key determinants of long-term survival. Both these factors influence the choice of therapy (see Table 168-4). Early intervention is associated with a better prognosis, which should inform the pace of diagnostic evaluation. Matched sibling donor transplants are associated with higher response rates, lower relapse rates, long-term survival rates approximating 80%, and a lower incidence of clonal evolution. Immunosuppressive therapy is associated with long-term (10-year) survival rates of 70 to 75% in responders. Infection represents the most common cause of death in patients of any age treated with either immunosuppression alone or stem cell transplantation.

Inherited Bone Marrow Failure Syndromes

Patients with dyskeratosis congenita and FA will not respond to immunosuppressive therapy. Stem cell transplantation with nonmyeloablative approaches has the potential of curing the marrow failure component of these diseases. There are good theoretical reasons for anticipating that successful transplantation will reduce the likelihood of clonal evolution to myelodysplasia and acute leukemia. Unfortunately, the decision to transplant is influenced by other key factors, as described earlier. In light of these complexities, no clearcut when-to-transplant rule can be applied to all patients with these diseases. Taking these difficult issues into account, all patients should be evaluated early in an experienced transplantation center, and family members should be screened by hematologists, geneticists, and genetic counselors using specialty laboratories.

In patients with dyskeratosis, small case series report good outcomes after fludarabine-containing nonmyeloablative conditioning regimens, but studies of sufficient size are not available to permit concrete recommendations except that patients should be referred to an experienced center. In patients with FA, with proper conditioning regimens, matched sibling donor transplant recipients have expected 3-year survival rates of about 85% and matched unrelated recipients (when fludarabine containing nonmyeloablative approaches are used) have 3-year survival rates of 50%. In patients with Diamond-Blackfan anemia, sibling donor transplant recipients have 3-year survival rates of about 80%, but disease-free survival rates after matched unrelated donor transplants have been poor (20 to 30%).

Future Treatments

For patients with acquired aplastic anemia, studies designed to selectively target the T-cell clones responsible for hematopoietic suppression may provide more effective and less toxic strategies for immunosuppressive therapy. For all patients with aplastic anemia, further improvements in matched unrelated transplantation should make this modality more widely available for patients who are not now considered optimal candidates. GVHD control will continue to improve. For children with nonsevere aplastic anemia, the 10-year progression-free survival rate is only about 25%, suggesting that prospective trials of early intervention are warranted. For patients with inherited bone marrow failure syndromes, the genes for which have been largely identified, the possibility of stem cell gene therapy holds enormous theoretical promise.

Grade A

1. Gafter-Gvili A, Ram R, Gurion R, et al. ATG plus cyclosporine reduces all-cause mortality in patients with severe aplastic anemia: systematic review and meta-analysis. *Acta Haematol.* 2008;120:237-243.
2. Gurion R, Gafter-Gvili A, Vial PM, et al. Hematopoietic growth factors in aplastic anemia patients treated with immunosuppressive therapy: systematic review and meta-analysis. *Haematologica.* 2009;94:712-719.

SUGGESTED READINGS

Auerbach AD. Fanconi anemia and its diagnosis. *Mutat Res.* 2009;668:4-10. *A comprehensive, thoughtful up-to-date review of this disease by one of the founders of modern Fanconi anemia research.*

Gafter-Gvili A, Ram R, Raanani P, et al. Management of aplastic anemia: the role of systematic reviews and meta-analyses. *Acta Haematol.* 2011;125:47-54. *Review of hematopoietic cell transplantation, immunosuppressive therapy, hematopoietic growth factors, and supportive care.*

Kwon JH, Kim I, Lee YG, et al. Clinical course of non-severe aplastic anemia in adults. *Int J Hematol.* 2010;91:770-775. *About 20% of patients progress to severe disease, especially those with more severe initial abnormalities.*

Leguit RJ, van den Tweel JG. The pathology of bone marrow failure. *Histopathology.* 2010;57:655-670. *Review.*

Macdougall IC, Rossert J, Casadevall N, et al. A peptide-based erythropoietin-receptor agonist for pure red-cell aplasia. *N Engl J Med.* 2009;361:1848-1855. *A synthetic peptide-based erythropoietin-receptor agonist was effective for the treatment of anemia in pure red-cell aplasia, with 13 of 14 patients no longer requiring regular transfusions.*

Risitano AM. Immunosuppressive therapies in the management of immune-mediated marrow failure in adults: where we stand and where we are going. *Br J Haematol.* 2011;152:127-140. *Review of the pathophysiology and treatment of immune-mediated bone marrow failure states, with a comprehensive list of new immunosuppressive agents in various stages of clinical trial development.*

169

POLYCYTHEMIAS, ESSENTIAL THROMBOCYTHEMIA, AND PRIMARY MYELOFIBROSIS

AYALEW TEFFERI

DEFINITION

Polycythemia vera (PV), essential thrombocythemia (ET), and primary myelofibrosis (PMF) are categorized as myeloproliferative neoplasms (MPNs) in the 2008 World Health Organization (WHO) classification system for hematologic malignancies (Table 169-1). These disorders represent hematopoietic bone marrow stem cell–derived clonal myeloproliferations with a propensity to evolve into acute myeloid leukemia (also called blast-phase MPN). These three clinicopathologic entities, together with

TABLE 169-1   2008 WORLD HEALTH ORGANIZATION CLASSIFICATION OF MYELOID NEOPLASMS

1. Myeloproliferative neoplasms (MPNs)
   1.1. Chronic myelogenous leukemia, *BCR-ABL1* positive (CML)
   1.2. Polycythemia vera (PV)
   1.3. Essential thrombocythemia (ET)
   1.4. Primary myelofibrosis (PMF)
   1.5. Chronic neutrophilic leukemia (CNL)
   1.6. Chronic eosinophilic leukemia, not otherwise specified (CEL-NOS) (Chapter 173)
   1.7. Mast cell disease (MCD) (Chapter 263)
   1.8. MPN, unclassifiable (MPN-U)
2. Myeloid and lymphoid neoplasms with eosinophilia and abnormalities of *PDGFRA*, *PDGFRB*, or *FGFR1* (Chapter 173)
3. Myelodysplastic syndromes (MDS)/MPN
   3.1. Chronic myelomonocytic leukemia (CMML) (Chapter 190)
   3.2. Juvenile myelomonocytic leukemia (JMML)
   3.3. Atypical chronic myeloid leukemia, *BCR-ABL1* negative (aCML) (Chapter 190)
   3.4. MDS/MPN, unclassifiable
4. Myelodysplastic syndromes (MDS) (Chapter 188)
5. Acute myeloid leukemia (AML) and related neoplasms (Chapter 189)

chronic myelogenous leukemia (Chapter 190), used to be referred to as *myeloproliferative disorders*. Because chronic myelogenous leukemia is invariably linked to the Philadelphia translocation (i.e., *BCR-ABL1*), PV, ET, and PMF are operationally labeled *BCR-ABL1–negative MPNs*.

EPIDEMIOLOGY

Incidence figures for *BCR-ABL1*–negative MPNs are estimated at 0.2 to 2.5 per 100,000 for ET, 0.4 to 1.5 per 100,000 for PMF, and 0.8 to 2.6 per 100,000 for PV. The median age at diagnosis for all three MPNs is usually reported as 60 years, but population-based studies report a substantially older age. Family studies suggest a five- to seven-fold increased risk of MPN among first-degree relatives of patients with *BCR-ABL1*–negative MPN; the possibility of there being a hereditary component to disease susceptibility has been further supported by *JAK2* haplotype studies. ET appears to be more common in young women, but this gender imbalance is not as clear in other age groups. PMF has been associated with exposure to ionizing radiation (e.g., in Hiroshima survivors), heavy exposure to petroleum derivatives, and thorium dioxide (Thorotrast) contrast medium, but in the vast majority of cases there is no such exposure history.

PATHOBIOLOGY

The clonal nature of PV, ET, and PMF was established between 1976 and 1981 using glucose-6-phosphate dehydrogenase isoenzyme analysis. These diseases are now believed to derive from a genetically transformed bone marrow stem cell resulting in either monoclonal or oligoclonal myeloproliferation. In 2005, a *JAK2* gain-of-function mutation (*JAK2V617F*) was reported in *BCR-ABL1*–negative MPN, and subsequent studies using sensitive assays have revealed the presence of this mutation in approximately 95% of patients with PV and 60% of those with ET or PMF. Most of the remaining 5% of patients with PV carry another *JAK2* mutation (*JAK2* exon 12), whereas approximately 5 to 15% of *JAK2V617F*-negative patients with ET or PMF carry a *MPLW515* mutation. All these mutations relate to the JAK-STAT intracellular signaling pathway in hematopoietic cells. The JAK-STAT pathway is normally activated by the occupancy of hematopoietic growth factor receptors (the receptor and the thrombopoietin receptor, also known as MPL) by their respective ligands (erythropoietin [Epo], thrombopoietin). Both *JAK2* and *MPL* mutations are also seen, albeit much less frequently, in other myeloid neoplasms. More recently, additional mutations have been described in PV, ET, and PMF and involve *TET2, ASXL1, CBL, IDH, IKZF1,* and *LNK* (Table 169-2). Most of these mutations originate at the progenitor cell level, but they do not necessarily represent the primary clonogenic event, are not mutually exclusive, and do not follow a predictable hierarchy.

The aforementioned molecular alterations in *BCR-ABL1*–negative MPN induce biologic changes that are demonstrated in animal models or ex vivo. For example, *JAK2* or *MPL* mutations induce PV-, ET-, or PMF-like diseases in mice by experimental manipulation of the mutant allele burden. These mutations are also believed to contribute to the growth factor independence or hypersensitivity of erythroid or megakaryocyte colony-forming progenitor cells and the accumulation of anti-apoptotic proteins such as Bcl-X_L. Bone marrow fibrosis, osteosclerosis, and angiogenesis in PMF are currently believed to be reactive and mediated by cytokines; that is, fibroblast proliferation in the bone marrow of patients with PMF is not a primary part of the clonal process.

TABLE 169-2 NOVEL MUTATIONS IN POLYCYTHEMIA VERA, ESSENTIAL THROMBOCYTHEMIA, PRIMARY MYELOFIBROSIS, AND BLAST-PHASE MYELOPROLIFERATIVE NEOPLASM

MUTATION	CHROMOSOME LOCATION	APPROXIMATE MUTATIONAL FREQUENCY (%)	PATHOGENETIC RELEVANCE
JAK2V617F exon 14 (Janus kinase 2)	9p24	PV: 96 ET: 55 PMF: 65 Blast-phase MPN: 50	Believed to contribute to myeloproliferation and progenitor cell growth factor hypersensitivity
JAK2 exon 12	9p24	PV: 3 ET: rare PMF: rare Blast-phase MPN: ?	Believed to contribute to primarily erythroid myeloproliferation
MPL exon 10 (myeloproliferative leukemia virus oncogene; encodes for thrombopoietin receptor)	1p34	PV: rare ET: 3 PMF: 10 Blast-phase MPN: ?	Believed to contribute to primarily megakaryocytic myeloproliferation
TET2 (mutations occur across several of the gene's 12 exons; TET oncogene family member 2)	4q24	PV: 16 ET: 5 PMF: 17 Blast-phase MPN: 17	Might contribute to epigenetic modulation of transcription (TET1 catalyzes conversion of 5-methylcytosine to 5-hydroxymethylcytosine)
ASXL1 exon 12 (Additional Sex Combs-Like 1)	20q11.1	PV: ? ET: ? PMF: ? Blast-phase MPN: 19	Believed to affect regulation of transcription and RAR-mediated signaling
CBL exons 8 and 9 (Casitas B-lineage lymphoma proto-oncogene)	11q23.3	PV: rare ET: rare PMF: 6 Blast-phase MPN: ?	Believed to alter the regulatory function of wild-type CBL against kinase signaling because of defective ubiquitylation of oncoproteins
IDH1/IDH2 exon 4/exon 4 (isocitrate dehydrogenase)	2q33.3/15q26.1	PV: rare ET: rare PMF: 4 Blast-phase MPN: 20	Induces accumulation of 2-hydroxyglutarate, a possible oncoprotein
IKZF1 (mostly deletions, including intragenic; IKAROS family zinc finger 1)	7p12	PV: rare ET: rare PMF: rare Blast-phase MPN: 19	Not clear at this point
LNK exon 2 (encodes a membrane-bound adaptor protein)	12q24.12	PV: rare ET: rare PMF: rare Blast-phase MPN: 10	Wild-type is a negative regulator of JAK2 signaling

ET = essential thrombocythemia; MPN = myeloproliferative neoplasm; PMF = primary myelofibrosis; PV = polycythemia vera; RAR = retinoic acid receptor.

TABLE 169-3	CLINICAL AND LABORATORY FEATURES OF POLYCYTHEMIA VERA

Persistent leukocytosis
Persistent thrombocytosis
Microcytosis secondary to iron deficiency
Increased leukocyte alkaline phosphatase
Splenomegaly
Generalized pruritus (usually after bathing)
Unusual thrombosis (e.g., Budd-Chiari syndrome)
Erythromelalgia (acral dysesthesia and erythema; see Fig. 169-1)

FIGURE 169-1. Erythromelalgia—a painful red discoloration of the hands or toes.

CLINICAL MANIFESTATIONS

Polycythemia Vera

Table 169-3 lists the typical clinical and laboratory features of PV. Increased red cell mass in PV might result in blood hyperviscosity, which leads to a plethora of symptoms and signs. Headaches are frequent, but blurry vision, altered hearing, mucous membrane bleeding, shortness of breath, and malaise are also observed. At least two thirds of PV patients have spleno-megaly. Thrombosis occurs in about 40% of patients, most commonly arterial thrombosis. As in ET, venous thrombosis can occur in unusual sites, such as mesenteric or hepatic vessels, and hepatic vein thrombosis (Budd-Chiari syndrome) or portal vein thrombosis (Chapter 145) may be the presenting manifestation before the full hematologic picture of PV has emerged. Bleed-ing, especially gastrointestinal, is seen in PV, but it is less common than thrombosis. Pruritus is common in PV and may be provoked by warm water ("aquagenic"). Erythromelalgia (described later under Essential Thrombocy-themia) may trouble some patients with PV, as do other vasomotor symp-toms such as paresthesias and headaches.

Essential Thrombocythemia

At presentation, microvascular and vasomotor symptoms are found in 25 to 50% of ET patients. Major thrombosis is seen in 11 to 25% of patients at diagnosis and in 10 to 22% during follow-up; major hemorrhage is observed in 2 to 5% at diagnosis and in 1 to 7% during follow-up. Vasomotor distur-bances (e.g., headaches, lightheadedness, visual symptoms such as blurring and scotomata, palpitations, chest pain, erythromelalgia, distal paresthesias) are not infrequent in ET and might be the result of abnormal platelet-endothelium interactions. Erythromelalgia (Fig. 169-1) is the most dramatic vasomotor symptom, characterized by erythema, warmth, and pain in the distal extremities; this symptom is rare but not entirely specific for ET. Sple-nomegaly is found in about 40% of patients with ET, but it is usually not prominent. Life-threatening complications of ET include large-vessel throm-bosis (both arterial and venous), hemorrhage, and transformation of the disease into either a fibrotic phase resembling PMF or acute myeloid leuke-mia. Venous thrombosis in ET occurs both in sites common to other throm-botic diatheses (e.g., pulmonary embolism, lower extremity deep vein thrombosis) and in more unusual sites (e.g., cerebral sinus thrombosis, retinal vein thrombosis, hepatic and portal vein thrombosis).

Major hemorrhage in ET is most common in the gastrointestinal tract and may be precipitated by aspirin or other nonsteroidal anti-inflammatory drugs. Hemorrhage also occurs in the central nervous system and the retina, but such events are, fortunately, uncommon. Paradoxically, patients with extreme thrombocytosis may be at special risk for bleeding, in part related to the development of an acquired von Willebrand syndrome (Chapter 176) that is thought to be related to the adsorption of large multimers of von Wil-lebrand protein from plasma onto the large number of abnormal circulating platelets. Fibrotic and leukemic transformations of ET are rare events (<5% of patients) during the first 10 years after diagnosis, but the risk increases with time.

Primary Myelofibrosis

Most patients with PMF present with anemia and marked splenomegaly. The anemia of PMF is multifactorial. Contributing factors include ineffective hematopoiesis and hypersplenism. Spleen and liver enlargement in PMF is secondary to extramedullary hematopoiesis (EMH) and may be associated with hypercatabolic symptoms including profound fatigue, weight loss, night sweats, and low-grade fever. Patients also experience peripheral edema, diar-rhea, early satiety, and, occasionally, complications of portal hypertension, including variceal bleeding and ascites.

Splenomegaly in PMF may be complicated by splenic infarction that mani-fests with left upper quadrant abdominal pain and referred left shoulder pain. Computed tomography in such cases may be unremarkable, or it may show wedge-shaped or rounded low-attenuation lesions in the spleen. EMH occurs in many sites throughout the body. Besides the spleen and liver, common sites include the lymph nodes, skin, pleura, peritoneum, lung, and paraspinal and epidural spaces, where lesions may be found incidentally on imaging or may produce mass effects. The latter may result in spinal cord and/or nerve root compression, which is a medical emergency requiring corticosteroids to reduce edema and immediate radiation therapy.

DIAGNOSIS

At present, the 2008 WHO criteria are used for the diagnosis of ET, PV, and PMF (Table 169-4). These criteria are based on morphology and cytoge-netic or molecular studies (Fig. 169-2). Almost all patients with PV carry a *JAK2* mutation (*JAK2V617F* or *JAK2* exon 12 mutation). Therefore, the absence of a *JAK2* mutation makes a diagnosis of PV unlikely. *JAK2V617F* is not specific to PV, however; it is also found in ET (≈55% of cases), PMF (≈65% of cases), and other myeloid neoplasms (usually <5% of cases). *JAK2* exon 12 mutations are relatively specific to *JAK2V617F*-negative PV and occur in approximately 3% of all patients with PV. Thus, the presence of a *JAK2* mutation excludes secondary myeloproliferation (e.g., secondary poly-cythemia or reactive thrombocytosis; see later), and its absence makes a diagnosis of PV very unlikely. The value of *MPL* and other MPN-associated mutations as diagnostic markers is undermined by their low prevalence in ET and PMF.

At present, neither red cell mass measurement nor bone marrow examina-tion is essential for the diagnosis of PV (see Fig. 169-2). However, bone marrow examination with cytogenetic studies is often necessary for the accu-rate diagnosis of ET and PMF and is especially useful in distinguishing ET from prefibrotic PMF. Bone marrow fibrosis associated with *JAK2V617F*, trisomy 9, or del(13q) is highly suggestive of PMF. Figure 169-3 shows the typical peripheral blood smear seen in PMF, and the corresponding bone marrow histology is illustrated in Figure 169-4. Bone marrow morphology in ET also provides additional clues for distinguishing clonal from reactive thrombocytosis (Fig. 169-5).

Erythrocytosis (Polycythemias)

Polycythemia refers to either a real (true polycythemia) or a spurious (appar-ent polycythemia) perception of an increase in red blood cell mass. True polycythemia may represent either a clonal myeloproliferative disorder (PV) or a nonclonal increase in red blood cell mass that is often mediated by Epo (secondary polycythemia). Apparent polycythemia results from a decrease in plasma volume without an actual increase in red cell mass (relative poly-cythemia). Occasionally, a true increase in red blood cell mass may be masked by a normal-appearing hematocrit because of a concomitant increase in plasma volume, often accompanied by marked splenomegaly (inapparent polycythemia).

Most conditions that cause an acute depletion of plasma volume (i.e., rela-tive polycythemia) are clinically obvious (e.g., severe dehydration, diarrhea, vomiting, use of diuretics, capillary leak syndrome, severe burns) and do not require specialized tests to confirm the diagnosis. Conversely, the existence

TABLE 169-4	2008 WORLD HEALTH ORGANIZATION DIAGNOSTIC CRITERIA FOR POLYCYTHEMIA VERA, ESSENTIAL THROMBOCYTHEMIA, AND PRIMARY MYELOFIBROSIS		
CRITERIA	POLYCYTHEMIA VERA*	ESSENTIAL THROMBOCYTHEMIA*	PRIMARY MYELOFIBROSIS*
Major criteria	1 Hb >18.5 g/dL (men), >16.5 g/dL (women) or Hb/Hct >99th percentile of reference range or Hb >17 g/dL (men) or >15 g/dL (women) if associated with sustained increase of ≥2 g/dL from baseline, not otherwise explained or Elevated red cell mass >25% above mean normal predicted value 2 Presence of *JAK*2V617F or similar mutation	1 Platelet count ≥450 × 10⁹/L 2 Megakaryocyte proliferation with large and mature morphology; no or little granulocyte or erythroid proliferation 3 Not meeting WHO criteria for CML, PV, PMF, MDS, or other myeloid neoplasm 4 Demonstration of *JAK*2V617F or other clonal marker or No evidence of reactive thrombocytosis	1 Megakaryocyte proliferation and atypia† accompanied by either reticulin or collagen fibrosis or In the absence of fibrosis, megakaryocyte changes accompanied by increased marrow cellularity and granulocytic proliferation 2 Not meeting WHO criteria for CML, PV, MDS, or other myeloid neoplasm 3 Demonstration of *JAK*2V617F or other clonal marker or No evidence of reactive marrow fibrosis
Minor criteria	1 Bone marrow trilineage myeloproliferation 2 Subnormal serum Epo level 3 EEC growth		1 Leukoerythroblastosis 2 Increased serum LDH 3 Anemia 4 Palpable splenomegaly

*Diagnosis of PV requires meeting either both major criteria and one minor criterion or the first major criterion and two minor criteria. Diagnosis of essential thrombocythemia requires meeting all four major criteria. Diagnosis of PMF requires meeting all three major criteria and two minor criteria.
†Small to large megakaryocytes with an aberrant nuclear-to-cytoplasmic ratio and hyperchromatic and irregularly folded nuclei and dense clustering.
CML = chronic myelogenous leukemia; EEC = endogenous erythroid colony; Epo = erythropoietin; Hct = hematocrit; Hb = hemoglobin; LDH = lactate dehydrogenase; MDS = myelodysplastic syndrome; PMF = primary myelofibrosis; PV = polycythemia vera; WHO = World Health Organization.
From Tefferi A, Vardiman JW. Classification and diagnosis of myeloproliferative neoplasms: the 2008 World Health Organization criteria and point-of-care diagnostic algorithms. *Leukemia.* 2008;22:14-22.

FIGURE 169-2. Diagnostic algorithm for the myeloproliferative neoplasms (MPNs). BM = bone marrow; CML = chronic myelogenous leukemia; Epo = erythropoietin; ET = essential thrombocythemia; MDS = myelodysplastic syndrome; PMF = primary myelofibrosis; PV = polycythemia vera. (From Tefferi A, Skoda R, Vardiman JW. Myeloproliferative neoplasms: contemporary diagnosis using histology and genetics. *Nat Rev Clin Oncol.* 2009;6:627-637.)

of chronic contraction of the plasma volume, such as that postulated to occur in Gaisböck's syndrome or stress polycythemia, is controversial. Accurate reference to the race- and sex-adjusted normal laboratory values should minimize the inappropriate use of the term *apparent polycythemia* in physiologically normal persons with hematocrit values in the upper percentiles of the normal range. In such instances, the performance of costly diagnostic tests, including the measurement of red blood cell mass, is unwarranted.

Table 169-5 provides a comprehensive list of causes of erythrocytosis (polycythemia), including acquired forms (both clonal and secondary) and congenital forms. In each of these, the serum Epo level is helpful in

FIGURE 169-3. Myeloproliferative disorder. A peripheral blood smear from a patient with agnogenic myeloid metaplasia shows a leukoerythroblastic picture. The characteristic findings are teardrop-shaped red blood cells (dacryocytes), nucleated red blood cells (erythroblasts), and immature granulocyte precursors.

FIGURE 169-4. Bone marrow biopsy specimen from a patient with primary myelofibrosis shows reticulin fibrosis, osteosclerosis, and intrasinusoidal hematopoiesis.

FIGURE 169-5. Myeloproliferative disorder. Bone marrow shows megakaryocytic clusters, seen in essential thrombocythemia and other conditions associated with clonal thrombocytosis.

TABLE 169-5	CLASSIFICATION OF ERYTHROCYTOSIS

I. Acquired erythrocytosis
  A. Clonal (polycythemia vera)
  B. Secondary
    1. Hypoxia driven
      a. Chronic lung disease
      b. Right-to-left cardiopulmonary shunts
      c. High-altitude habitat
      d. Tobacco use, carbon monoxide poisoning
      e. Sleep apnea–hypoventilation syndrome
      f. Renal artery stenosis
    2. Hypoxia independent
      a. Use of androgen preparations, erythropoietin injection
      b. Post renal transplant
      c. Cerebellar hemangioblastoma, meningioma
      d. Pheochromocytoma, uterine leiomyoma, renal cysts, parathyroid adenoma
      e. Hepatocellular carcinoma, renal cell carcinoma
II. Congenital erythrocytosis
  A. Associated with reduced p50 (partial pressure of oxygen at which 50% of hemoglobin is saturated with oxygen)
    1. High-oxygen-affinity hemoglobinopathy (usually autosomal dominant)
    2. 2,3-bisphosphoglycerate deficiency (usually autosomal recessive)
    3. Methemoglobinemia (Chapter 161)
  B. Associated with normal p50
    1. *VHL* mutations, including Chuvash polycythemia (usually autosomal recessive)
    2. *PHD2* mutations
    3. *HIF2α* mutations
    4. *EPOR* mutations (usually autosomal dominant)

From Patnaik MM, Tefferi A. The complete evaluation of erythrocytosis: congenital and acquired. *Leukemia.* 2009;23:834-849.

with cardiopulmonary conditions most commonly responsible. Other causes of central hypoxia include high-altitude habitat and carbon monoxide poisoning. Hypoxia in peripheral tissues is exemplified by the acquired polycythemia associated with renal artery stenosis. In both central and peripheral hypoxia-driven secondary polycythemia, the serum Epo level is initially elevated but may fall to within the normal range after the hemoglobin level has stabilized at a higher level. In contrast, in Epo-mediated, hypoxia-independent secondary polycythemia, the serum Epo level often remains elevated despite the rise in hemoglobin. Hypoxia-independent elevation of Epo with an elevated hemoglobin level is associated with malignant or benign tumors of the liver, kidney, uterus, and cerebellum (see Table 169-5). Exogenous administration of drugs such as androgen preparations or Epo itself also causes acquired secondary polycythemia.

Congenital polycythemia can be associated with increased, normal, or decreased serum Epo levels. For example, the serum Epo level is usually increased or normal in the autosomal dominant, high-oxygen-affinity hemoglobinopathies (e.g., 2,3-diphosphoglycerate mutase deficiency) and the autosomal recessive Chuvash polycythemia that is endemic in Russia and is associated with a von Hippel-Lindau (*VHL*) gene mutation. Conversely, the serum Epo level is low in patients with an activating mutation of the Epo receptor gene.

The diagnostic approach to congenital polycythemia should start with measurement of the serum Epo level. The presence of a subnormal serum Epo level in the absence of PV suggests the presence of a germline mutation of the Epo receptor. If the serum Epo level is normal or elevated, the next step is to measure the p50 (the oxygen tension at which hemoglobin is 50% saturated). Decreased p50 suggests the presence of either a high-oxygen-affinity hemoglobinopathy or 2,3-bisphosphoglycerate deficiency. If the p50 is normal, the possibility of *VHL* mutations (usually associated with increased serum Epo levels) should be considered first because they constitute the most frequent mutations in congenital polycythemia.

Thrombocytosis

Table 169-6 outlines the different causes of thrombocytosis, and Figure 169-6 provides an algorithmic approach to the differential diagnosis. By far, the most common cause of thrombocytosis in general medical populations is a reactive or secondary process. Also, the degree of elevation in the platelet count does not clearly differentiate clonal from reactive thrombocytosis. Figure 169-7 illustrates the value of examining the peripheral blood smear

establishing the differential diagnosis. Epo is a 35-kD glycosylated protein synthesized in response to tissue hypoxia, mainly by the peritubular capillary endothelial cells of the renal cortex by means of an intricate oxygen-sensing mechanism. Acquired secondary polycythemia is usually associated with increased Epo production that is either hypoxia driven or hypoxia independent. In the former instance, the hypoxic stimulus is usually central, in cases of thrombocytosis; the finding of Howell-Jolly bodies indicates a post-splenectomy or asplenic state as the cause of secondary (reactive) thrombocytosis.

Bone Marrow Fibrosis (Myelofibrosis)

Other causes of bone marrow fibrosis (myelofibrosis) are outlined in Table 169-7. The diagnosis of post-PV or post-ET myelofibrosis requires full documentation of a previous morphologic diagnosis of PV or ET, respectively.

TREATMENT   Rx

Polycythemia Vera and Essential Thrombocythemia

Drug therapy in PV or ET does not improve survival or prevent disease transformation into post-ET or post-PV myelofibrosis or blast-phase MPN. Instead, the main objective of specific therapy is to prevent thrombosis in high-risk patients (i.e., those older than 60 years or with a history of thrombosis) or to alleviate non-life-threatening symptoms, including microvascular disturbances (e.g., headaches, acral paresthesia, erythromelalgia), pruritus, or symptomatic splenomegaly. Microvascular symptoms are usually effectively treated with low-dose aspirin (81 mg/day). The cause of MPN-associated

TABLE 169-6 CAUSES OF THROMBOCYTOSIS IN UNSELECTED COHORTS OF CONSECUTIVE PATIENTS

CONDITION	Platelet Count (Approximate % of Patients)	
	ADULTS, >500,000/μL	>1 MILLION/μL
Infection	22	31
Rebound thrombocytosis	19	3
Tissue damage (surgery)	18	14
Chronic inflammation	13	9
Malignancy	6	14
Renal disorders	5	<1
Hemolytic anemia	4	<1
Post-splenectomy status	2	19
Blood loss	NS	6
Primary thrombocythemia	3	14

NS = not stated.
From Tefferi A, Gilliland DG. Classification of chronic myeloid disorders: from Dameshek towards a semi-molecular system. *Best Pract Res Clin Haematol.* 2006;19:365-385.

TABLE 169-7 CAUSES OF BONE MARROW FIBROSIS

MYELOID DISORDERS

Primary myelofibrosis
Metastatic cancer
Chronic myeloid leukemia
Myelodysplastic syndrome
Atypical myeloid disorder
Acute megakaryocytic leukemia
Other acute myeloid leukemias
Gray platelet syndrome

LYMPHOID DISORDERS

Hairy cell leukemia
Multiple myeloma
Lymphoma

NONHEMATOLOGIC DISORDERS

Connective tissue disorder
Infections (tuberculosis, kala-azar)
Vitamin D deficiency rickets
Renal osteodystrophy

FIGURE 169-6. Diagnostic evaluation of thrombocytosis in routine clinical practice.

TABLE 169-8   RISK STRATIFICATION AND RISK-ADAPTED THERAPY IN ESSENTIAL THROMBOCYTHEMIA, POLYCYTHEMIA VERA, AND PRIMARY MYELOFIBROSIS

| RISK GROUPS FOR PV AND ET | Management | | | IPSS RISK GROUPS FOR PMF |
	ET	PV	PMF	
Low risk (age <60 yr and no thrombosis history)	Low-dose aspirin	Low-dose aspirin + phlebotomy*	Observation	Low risk (no risk factors[†])
Low risk with extreme thrombocytosis[‡]	Low-dose aspirin[§]	Low-dose aspirin[§] + phlebotomy	Conventional management[∥]	Intermediate-1 risk (1 risk factor[†])
High risk (age ≥60 yr or thrombosis history)	Low-dose aspirin + hydroxyurea[¶]	Low-dose aspirin + phlebotomy + hydroxyurea[¶]	Allo-SCT if age <65 yr, or experimental therapy	Intermediate-1 risk with transfusions or unfavorable karyotype
			Allo-SCT if age <65 yr, or experimental therapy	Intermediate-2 risk (2 risk factors[†])
			Allo-SCT if age <65 yr, or experimental therapy	High-risk (≥3 risk factors[†])

*In the presence of aspirin therapy, the hematocrit target can range between 38 and 50% and is set at a level that maintains best performance status.
[†]The IPSS uses five risk factors for inferior survival: age >65 years, hemoglobin <10 g/dL, leukocyte count >25 × 10⁹/L, circulating blasts ≥1%, and presence of constitutional symptoms.
[‡]Extreme thrombocytosis is defined as a platelet count >1000 × 10⁹/L.
[§]Clinically significant acquired von Willebrand syndrome (ristocetin cofactor activity <30%) should be excluded before using aspirin in patients with extreme thrombocytosis.
[∥]Androgen preparations or thalidomide with prednisone for anemia; hydroxyurea for symptomatic splenomegaly.
[¶]In hydroxyurea-intolerant or -resistant cases, interferon-α (age <60 years) or busulfan or pipobroman (age >60 years) can be used.
Allo-SCT = allogeneic stem cell transplantation; ET = essential thrombocythemia; IPSS = International Prognostic Scoring System; PMF = primary myelofibrosis; PV = polycythemia vera.
From Tefferi A, Vainchenker W. Myeloproliferative neoplasms: molecular pathophysiology, essential clinical understanding, and treatment strategies. *J Clin Oncol.* 2011;29:573-582.

pruritus is poorly understood, but its dramatic response to JAK inhibitor therapy suggests a causal relationship with cytokines that use JAK-STAT signaling. Other therapies for MPN-associated pruritus include antihistamines, selective serotonin re-uptake inhibitors, interferon-α (IFN-α), and phototherapy. Symptomatic splenomegaly is usually managed with hydroxyurea (starting dose 500 mg orally twice a day).

Preventive cytoreductive therapy for thrombosis is indicated only in the presence of high-risk disease (see Prognosis later; Table 169-8). In this regard, randomized studies have demonstrated the value of low-dose aspirin (40 to 100 mg/day) in PV[1,2] and hydroxyurea (starting dose 500 mg orally twice a day) in high-risk ET. Hydroxyurea is a nonalkylating DNA synthesis inhibitor and a myelosuppressive agent. Based on noncontrolled but prospective evidence, most experts agree that low-dose aspirin therapy (81 mg/day) should also be considered for ET and hydroxyurea therapy for high-risk PV (see Table 169-8). In addition, phlebotomy is required for all patients with PV, and the target hematocrit in aspirin-treated individuals should be less than 50%—preferably around 45%. In high-risk patients with ET in whom cytoreductive therapy is indicated, a platelet target of less than 400 × 10⁹/L is reasonable and supported by data from retrospective studies.

High-risk PV or ET patients (see Prognosis) who cannot tolerate or are resistant to hydroxyurea are effectively managed by IFN-α or busulfan. IFN-α is the preferred second-line drug, at least for younger patients. Two recent studies of pegylated IFN-α (≈90 µg by weekly subcutaneous injection) in PV and ET patients reported hematologic remissions of approximately 80%, accompanied by decreases in the *JAK2*V617F allele burden (complete molecular remission rate of 5 to 10%). A controlled study is needed before IFN-α is recommended as first-line therapy in either PV or ET. For older patients, busulfan is started at 4 mg/day; it is withheld in the presence of platelets less than 100 × 10⁹/L or a white blood cell count less than 3 × 10⁹/L, and the dose is reduced to 2 mg/day if the corresponding levels are less than 150 × 10⁹/L and 5 × 10⁹/L.

There is unsubstantiated fear among primary caregivers regarding the leukemogenicity of hydroxyurea and busulfan; no controlled studies in either PV or ET have shown this to be the case. The most recent randomized study in this regard found no difference in leukemia risk among patients receiving either hydroxyurea or anagrelide. Similarly, the two largest noncontrolled studies in ET and PV, as well as long-term studies of patients receiving hydroxyurea for sickle cell disease, do not support the concern that leukemia might be caused by the use of hydroxyurea. The evidence for busulfan's leukemogenicity in the context of treatment for PV or ET is equally weak and inappropriately extrapolated from older patients with advanced disease who were exposed to multiple cytoreductive drugs. Similarly, the safety and efficacy of busulfan treatment in ET were underlined by a more recent long-term study of 36 patients older than 60 years in whom no instances of acute myeloid leukemia or other malignancies were documented after a median follow-up of 72 months.

Anagrelide is a cyclic adenosine monophosphate phosphodiesterase III inhibitor that relatively selectively reduces the platelet count by acting on platelet production in the bone marrow. A large randomized study compared anagrelide with hydroxyurea, both in combination with aspirin, in high-risk patients with ET and demonstrated hydroxyurea's overall superiority.[3] Hydroxyurea was better tolerated and was associated with significantly less risk of arterial thrombosis, major hemorrhage, and fibrotic transformation. In contrast, anagrelide displayed better activity against venous thrombosis. A more recent but smaller randomized study found no difference between hydroxyurea and anagrelide in terms of the incidence of ET-related events, but the treatment discontinuation rate was higher in the anagrelide arm. Other treatment options in PV and ET include pipobroman (not available in the United States) and radiophosphorus. The latter has been associated with a delayed risk of leukemic transformation in patients with PV, and its use is currently limited to patients older than 65 years.

ET is associated with an increased risk (approximately 35% vs. 15% in the control population) of spontaneous abortion in the first trimester of pregnancy. There is no association between the increased risk of spontaneous abortion and the degree of thrombocytosis. Low-risk pregnant patients with ET or PV are managed the same way as their nonpregnant counterparts, and the use of low-dose aspirin has been associated with a decreased prevalence of first trimester miscarriages in retrospective studies. High-risk pregnant women with ET (i.e., those with previous thrombosis) require cytoreductive therapy, just like other high-risk patients. In such patients, there is anecdotal evidence of the safety of using IFN-α and the potential teratogenicity of hydroxyurea.

Major bleeding occurs in less than 10% of ET patients. Extreme thrombocytosis (i.e., platelet count >1 million/µL) appears to be a risk factor for bleeding, in part because of the acquired von Willebrand syndrome (Chapter 176). One approach is to measure ristocetin cofactor activity in patients with extreme thrombocytosis and withhold aspirin therapy if the value is less than 30%.

Primary Myelofibrosis

Drug therapy does not modify the natural history of PMF, although survival has improved in recent years. Patients with PMF who are considered low risk, as determined by the International Prognostic Scoring System (IPSS), can be observed without any therapeutic intervention. IPSS high-risk or intermediate-2-risk patients should be considered for investigational drug therapy or allogeneic stem cell transplantation (Chapter 181). Intermediate-1-risk patients who are transfusion dependent or have an unfavorable karyotype are managed as high-risk patients.

Conventional therapy for PMF is largely palliative and does not improve survival. Anemia and symptomatic splenomegaly are the main indications for treatment. Conventional drugs used to treat PMF-associated anemia include androgen preparations (e.g., oral fluoxymesterone 10 mg twice daily), danazol (400 to 600 mg/day), prednisone (30 to 40 mg/day), and erythropoiesis-stimulating agents. Prostate cancer screening is required in men treated with androgen preparations. Response rates to prednisone, androgen preparations, or danazol are about 20%, and response durations average about 1 to 2 years. Erythropoiesis-stimulating agents may exacerbate PMF-associated splenomegaly and are usually ineffective in transfusion-dependent patients.

Thalidomide and thalidomide-like drugs such as lenalidomide may be effective in the treatment of anemia in PMF. Thalidomide as a single agent (50 to 200 mg/day) is not as effective as its combination with prednisone (30 mg/day), with reported response rates ranging from 20 to 62% for anemia, 25 to 80% for thrombocytopenia, and 7 to 30% for splenomegaly. Response rates with lenalidomide are similar, but the drug works best in the presence of a del(5q) cytogenetic abnormality. The occurrence of peripheral neuropathy with thalidomide and severe pancytopenia with lenalidomide therapy has limited their use in most patients.

The drug of choice for symptomatic splenomegaly in PMF is hydroxyurea (starting dose 500 mg twice daily). Hydroxyurea-refractory cases are often managed by splenectomy because the value of other conventional drugs in this regard is limited. Indications for splenectomy in PMF include mechanical discomfort, symptomatic portal hypertension (i.e., associated with ascites or variceal bleeding), and frequent red blood cell transfusions. The perioperative mortality of splenectomy in PMF is between 5 and 10%. Post-splenectomy complications occur in approximately 50% of patients and include bleeding, thrombosis, hepatomegaly, extreme thrombocytosis, leukocytosis, and an increase in circulating blasts. Prophylactic therapy with hydroxyurea is advised to prevent post-splenectomy thrombocytosis. A transjugular intrahepatic portosystemic shunt might be considered to alleviate symptoms of portal hypertension.

EMH is the main cause of hepatosplenomegaly in PMF and post-PV or post-ET myelofibrosis. Nonhepatosplenic EMH also occurs in PMF and might involve the vertebral column (causing cord compression), lymph nodes, lung (causing pulmonary hypertension), pleura (causing effusion), small bowel, peritoneum (causing ascites), urogenital tract, skin, and heart. Diagnosis is usually tissue based, but imaging studies are sometimes used; myelofibrosis-associated pulmonary hypertension is confirmed by technetium-99m sulfur colloid scintigraphy, which shows diffuse pulmonary uptake.

Radiation therapy is an attractive treatment option in both hepatosplenic and nonhepatosplenic EMH. Splenic irradiation (100 to 500 cGy in 5 to 10 fractions) induces a transient reduction in spleen size but might be associated with life-threatening pancytopenia. More recent studies suggest the relative safety and value of lower-dose treatment (100 cGy total dose in four daily fractions of 25 cGy). Radiation therapy works best for nonhepatosplenic EMH. Single-fraction (100 to 400 cGy) involved-field therapy has also been shown to benefit patients with myelofibrosis-associated pulmonary hypertension or extremity pain.

Symptoms in myelofibrosis that affect quality of life include profound fatigue, night sweats, weight loss, pruritus, bone pain, and nonproductive cough. In an international survey of 1179 patients, standardized fatigue metrics of the Functional Assessment of Cancer Therapy–Anemia (FACT-AN) and Brief Fatigue Inventory (BFI) were used to demonstrate that patients with PV, ET, and PMF suffer from anemia-independent fatigue exceeding that expected in age-matched controls. In a subset analysis of 458 patients with myelofibrosis, more than 50% suffered from moderate to severe fatigue, night sweats, pruritus, and symptomatic splenomegaly, whereas a smaller proportion listed bone pain, weight loss, and fever as additional symptoms. The study also documented the inadequacy of conventional therapy in the management of these symptoms. Recent studies of JAK inhibitor therapy in PMF or post-PV or post-ET myelofibrosis suggest major benefits in terms of constitutional symptoms and cachexia (see later).

Experimental Drug Therapy in Myeloproliferative Neoplasms

Because of the association between MPN and JAK-STAT–relevant mutations (e.g., *JAK2* and *MPL* mutations), several anti-JAK2 small-molecule drugs are currently undergoing clinical trials. One or more of these drugs have demonstrated remarkable activity against splenomegaly and constitutional symptoms, including pruritus, and resolution of leukocytosis and thrombocytosis, as well as reduction in the *JAK2*V617F allele burden. Side effects so far have included gastrointestinal symptoms; anemia; thrombocytopenia; reversible increases in transaminases, amylase, or lipase; and the phenomenon of "cytokine rebound." This phenomenon is seen in some patients receiving JAK2 inhibitors with particularly strong activity in suppressing pro-inflammatory cytokines and consists of the acute and immediate reappearance of symptoms on drug discontinuation.

Allogeneic Stem Cell Transplantation

The largest study of allogeneic stem cell transplantation in PMF was conducted by the Center for International Bone Marrow Transplant Research (CIBMTR) and included 289 subject with a variety of donor types and conditioning regimens. Five-year disease-free survival and treatment-related mortality were 33 and 35% for matched related transplants and 27 and 50% for unrelated transplants, respectively. Outcome was not favorably affected by reduced-intensity conditioning (Chapter 181). In another reduced-intensity conditioning transplant study from the Chronic Leukemia Working Party of the European Group for Blood and Marrow Transplantation, 103 patients (median age, 55 years) with PMF or post-PV or post-ET myelofibrosis were prospectively studied, and 5-year disease-free survival was estimated at 51%.■ Chronic graft-versus-host disease (Chapter 181) occurred in 49% of these patients, and relapse (29%) was predicted by high-risk disease and prior splenectomy. The chronic graft-versus-host disease and relapse rates for matched related transplants in the CIBMTR study were 40 and 32%, respectively, and a history of splenectomy did not affect outcome.

Considering the lack of effective drug therapy for PMF, the risk of transplant-related complications might be justified in patients whose median survival is expected to be less than 5 years and whose leukemia risk is greater than 20%. Using the age-adjusted dynamic prognostic model, this group includes high- or intermediate-2-risk patients, as well as those with either red cell transfusion dependence or an unfavorable karyotype (see Prognosis). In general,

FIGURE 169-7. Peripheral smear showing Howell-Jolly bodies (arrow) in red blood cells. This finding is typical of surgical or functional hyposplenism.

post-transplant outcome is poor in the presence of high-risk disease, advanced age, unrelated donor, or human leukocyte antigen (HLA) mismatch. More studies are needed to clarify the impact of pretransplant *JAK2*V617F presence or allele burden on transplant outcome, but the persistent presence of the mutation after transplantation predicts clinical relapse.

PROGNOSIS

Essential Thrombocythemia and Polycythemia Vera

Neither ET nor PV is presently a curable disease, and current therapy has not been rigorously shown to prolong survival. Fortunately, a normal life expectancy is possible in most patients. Recent studies suggest a median survival that approaches 20 years in both diseases. Fibrotic or leukemic transformation in ET or PV is relatively infrequent (a combined rate of <10% in the first 15 years of disease).

Current risk stratification in PV and ET is designed to estimate the risk of thrombosis (see Table 169-8). Age 60 years or older and history of thrombosis are the two risk factors used to classify patients with PV or ET into low-risk (no risk factors) and high-risk (one or two risk factors) groups. In addition, because of the potential risk for bleeding, low-risk patients with extreme thrombocytosis (platelet count >1000 × 10⁹/L) are considered separately. The presence of cardiovascular risk factors is currently not taken into consideration during formal risk stratification.

Primary Myelofibrosis

The prognosis of PMF is worse than that of ET or PV. Median survival is approximately 6 years and appears to have improved in recent years. The IPSS uses five independent predictors of inferior survival: age older than 65 years, hemoglobin less than 10 g/dL, leukocyte count greater than 25 × 10⁹/L, circulating blasts 1% or higher, and constitutional symptoms. The presence of zero, one, two, or three or more adverse risk factors defines low-, intermediate-1-, intermediate-2-, and high-risk disease, respectively, with corresponding median survivals of approximately 11.3, 7.9, 4, and 2.3 years. A dynamic prognostic model that uses the same variables but can be applied at any time during the disease course was recently published. In addition, red cell transfusion dependency, a platelet count less than 100 × 10⁹/L, and an unfavorable karyotype carry an IPSS-independent prognostic value, and their presence warrants assignment to the high-risk category regardless of IPSS score.

1. Landolfi R, Marchioli R, Kutti J, et al. Efficacy and safety of low-dose aspirin in polycythemia vera. *N Engl J Med.* 2004;350:114-124.

2. Squizzato A, Romualdi E, Middeldorp S. Antiplatelet drugs for polycythaemia vera and essential thrombocythaemia. *Cochrane Database Syst Rev.* 2008;16:CD006503.
3. Harrison CN, Campbell PJ, Buck G, et al. Hydroxyurea compared with anagrelide in high-risk essential thrombocythemia. *N Engl J Med.* 2005;353:33-45.
4. Kroger N, Holler E, Kobbe G, et al. Allogeneic stem cell transplantation after reduced-intensity conditioning in patients with myelofibrosis: a prospective, multicenter study of the Chronic Leukemia Working Party of the European Group for Blood and Marrow Transplantation. *Blood.* 2009;114:5264-5270.

SUGGESTED READINGS

Chen AT, Prchal JT. JAK2 kinase inhibitors and myeloproliferative disorders. *Curr Opin Hematol.* 2010;17:110-116. *Update on the status of early-phase clinical trials of molecularly targeted therapy.*

Harrison CN, Bareford D, Butt N, et al. Guideline for investigation and management of adults and children presenting with a thrombocytosis. *Br J Haematol.* 2010;149:352-375. *Guidelines from U.K. groups on the clinical approach to patients with thrombocytosis.*

Passamonti F, Cervantes F, Vannucchi AM, et al. A dynamic prognostic model to predict survival in primary myelofibrosis: a study by the IWG-MRT (International Working Group for Myeloproliferative Neoplasms Research and Treatment). *Blood.* 2010;115:1703-1708. *A novel model for assessing the prognosis of patients with primary myelofibrosis any time during their clinical course, which is useful for treatment decision making.*

Tefferi A, Vainchenker W. Myeloproliferative neoplasms: molecular pathophysiology, essential clinical understanding, and treatment strategies. *J Clin Oncol.* 2011;29:573-582. *Review.*

Vaidya R, Siragusa S, Huang J, et al. Mature survival data for 176 patients younger than 60 years with primary myelofibrosis diagnosed between 1976 and 2005: evidence for survival gains in recent years. *Mayo Clin Proc.* 2009;84:1114-1119. *Retrospective study of 176 consecutive patients at a single institution showing encouraging survival trends.*

170

LEUKOCYTOSIS AND LEUKOPENIA

NANCY BERLINER

The normal peripheral white blood cell count (WBC) ranges between 4500/μL and 10,000/μL, with a mean of 7500/μL and is composed of neutrophils, lymphocytes, monocytes, basophils, and eosinophils. Because neutrophils usually represent about 60% of the peripheral WBC, derangement in the WBC usually reflects elevation or reduction in the absolute neutrophil count. Leukocytosis, an elevated WBC, and leukopenia, a depressed WBC, may be secondary to an underlying disease or exposure, or they may be manifestations of a primary hematologic disorder. This chapter outlines both the primary and secondary causes of leukocytosis and leukopenia, focusing particularly on neutrophilia and neutropenia.

NORMAL NEUTROPHIL DYNAMICS

To understand the pathogenesis of a high or low WBC, one must understand normal neutrophil dynamics. Neutrophils arise from multipotent progenitor cells in the bone marrow that also give rise to erythrocytes, megakaryocytes, eosinophils, basophils, and monocytes. Neutrophil precursors in the marrow mature over 6 to 10 days to form a storage pool of mature neutrophils

(Fig. 170-1). Together the marrow populations make up about 95% of the body's total granulocyte mass (20% neutrophil precursors, 75% mature bands and neutrophils). The circulating neutrophil pool thus represents only the remaining approximately 5% of the body's total neutrophils, just over half of which at any given time are adherent to the vascular endothelium and the spleen, a phenomenon termed *margination*. These marginated neutrophils are poised for immediate release into the circulation during times of stress. The remaining neutrophils circulate freely in the blood, where they can survive for 6 to 12 hours, or migrate into tissues, where they can survive for 1 to 4 days. In general, then, neutrophilia can occur as the result of increased marrow production, increased release of neutrophils from the storage pool, or mobilization of neutrophils from the marginated pool. Neutropenia, on the other hand, may be due to decreased marrow production, increased margination with or without sequestration by the spleen, or increased destruction of peripheral cells.

NEUTROPHILIA

Most cases of neutrophilia are reactive or secondary to an underlying inflammatory process. This includes neutrophilia due to infection, chronic inflammation, stress, drugs, nonhematologic malignancy, marrow stimulation (as in hemolysis or idiopathic thrombocytopenic purpura), or splenectomy. Primary causes of neutrophilia may be congenital, including hereditary neutrophilia, Down syndrome, and leukocyte adhesion deficiency (LAD), or acquired as in the case of chronic myelogenous leukemia and other myeloproliferative neoplasms (Table 170-1).

Secondary Causes of Neutrophilia
Infection
Many acute bacterial infections can present with a modest leukocytosis with a "left shift," referring to the circulation of more immature myeloid cells. This left shift most commonly is restricted to release of an increased number of band forms; however, in severe stress, one may see circulating metamyelocytes and even earlier cells (see Fig. 170-1) in the peripheral blood. Leukocytosis occurs within hours of infection owing to release of neutrophils from both the marrow and marginated pools. Examination of these neutrophils on peripheral smear may reveal evidence of toxic granulation (see Fig. 160-18 in Chapter 160), Döhle bodies (see Fig. 160-19 in Chapter 160), and cytoplasmic vacuoles. Certain infections (e.g., *Clostridium difficile* or tuberculosis in particular) are known to cause elevations in the WBC to greater than 30,000/μL in about one fourth of infected patients and may result in a *leukemoid reaction*, defined as a WBC of greater than 50,000/μL with a pronounced left shift (Fig. 170-2).

Chronic Inflammation
Leukocytosis due to chronic inflammation results from increased leukocyte (specifically neutrophil and monocyte) production as opposed to altered neutrophil distribution. Mature neutrophil pools become depleted with ongoing inflammation, and the myeloid compartment of the marrow expands to increase neutrophil production. A myriad of cytokines, including tumor necrosis factor-α (TNF-α), granulocyte colony-stimulating factor (G-CSF),

| Myeloblast | Promyelocyte | Myelocyte | Metamyelocyte | Band | Segmented neutrophil |

Nucleolus: should be prominent in myeloblast and much less in promyelocyte, and absent thereafter

Primary Granules: should be present mostly in promyelocytes and myelocytes, and fewer in the later stages.

Secondary Granules: should be present at myelocyte stage and beyond. Lighter pink than primary granules

FIGURE 170-1. Myeloid maturation in the bone marrow. Nucleoli are prominent in myeloblasts, much less frequent in promyelocytes, and absent in more mature forms. Primary granules are present in the cytoplasm of promyelocytes and myelocytes, and secondary granules predominate beyond the myelocyte stage.

TABLE 170-1 DIFFERENTIAL DIAGNOSIS OF NEUTROPHILIA

I. Primary hematologic etiologies
  a. Congenital neutrophilia
    i. Hereditary neutrophilia
    ii. Chronic idiopathic neutrophilia
    iii. Down syndrome
    iv. Leukocyte adhesion deficiency (LAD)
      1. LAD I
      2. LAD II
  b. Acquired hematologic neoplasms
    i. Myeloproliferative disease
      1. Chronic myelogenous leukemia
      2. Polycythemia vera
II. Secondary to other disease entities
  a. Infection
    i. Acute via release from marginated and storage pools
    ii. Chronic via increased myelopoiesis (e.g., tuberculosis, fungal infection, chronic abscess, other chronic infections)
  b. Chronic inflammation
    i. Rheumatic disease: juvenile rheumatoid arthritis, rheumatoid arthritis, Still's disease, and others
    ii. Inflammatory bowel disease
    iii. Granulomatous disease
    iv. Chronic hepatitis
  c. Cigarette smoking
  d. Stress
  e. Drug induced
    i. Corticosteroids
    ii. β-agonists
    iii. Lithium
    iv. Recombinant cytokine administration
  f. Nonhematologic malignancy
    i. Cytokine-secreting tumors (lung, tongue, kidney, urothelial tumors)
    ii. Marrow metastasis (myelophthisis)
  g. Marrow stimulation
    i. Hemolytic anemia, immune thrombocytopenia
    ii. Recovery from marrow suppression
    iii. Recombinant cytokine administration
  h. Postsplenectomy

FIGURE 170-2. Peripheral blood from a patient with leukemoid reaction. From this smear, it would be impossible to distinguish this from chronic-phase chronic myelogenous leukemia (Chapter 190). Distinction would depend on determination of presence or absence of *BCR-ABL* fusion.

granulocyte-macrophage colony-stimulating factor (GM-CSF), macrophage inflammatory protein-1 (MIP-1), interleukin-1 (IL-1), IL-6, and IL-8, have been implicated in this marrow stimulation (Chapter 159). Chronic inflammatory conditions that are particularly associated with leukocytosis and neutrophilia include juvenile rheumatoid arthritis, rheumatoid arthritis, Still's disease, Crohn's disease, ulcerative colitis, granulomatous infection, and chronic hepatitis. The WBC and neutrophil elevation in these cases is typically more modest than that seen in acute infection or inflammation.

FIGURE 170-3. Myelophthisic changes in erythrocyte morphology. Note prominent teardrop forms. (From Rose M, Berliner N. Disorders of red blood cells. In Andreoli TE, Benjamin IJ, Griggs RC, et al, eds. *Andreoli and Carpenter's Cecil Essentials of Medicine,* 8th ed. Philadelphia: Saunders, 2010:522, Fig. 49-2.)

Cigarette Smoking
Cigarette smoking can cause a leukocytosis and neutrophilia in about 25 to 50% of chronic smokers that can persist for even up to 5 years after quitting smoking. The mechanism by which this occurs is unknown.

Stress
Within minutes of exercise, surgery, or stress, one can see an elevation in circulating neutrophils. This is presumed to be due to the effects of catecholamines on marginated neutrophils, with release of neutrophils into the circulation. Some cases of stress-induced neutrophilia can be prevented by pretreatment with β-adrenergic antagonists (e.g., propranolol), supporting the role of catecholamines in the process. Exercise-induced neutrophilia, however, is not blocked by propranolol, suggesting that it may instead be due to flow and mechanical perturbation of neutrophils in the lungs. An elevated WBC has also been noted in the setting of acute myocardial infarction, but whether this is a risk factor for cardiac ischemia or a result of inflammation is unclear.

Drug Induced
Probably the most well-known and widely used drugs associated with leukocytosis are corticosteroids. Other drugs that are associated with elevations in WBC and neutrophil count in particular include β-agonists and lithium. Lithium causes neutrophilia by increasing the production of endogenous colony-stimulating factors (CSFs). G-CSF or GM-CSF treatment likewise may result in neutrophilia, and although this is the desired effect, the neutrophilia can be quite pronounced if not appropriately monitored.

Nonhematologic Malignancy
Leukocytosis can be seen in a number of nonhematologic malignancies. Some tumors (lung, tongue, kidney, bladder) are thought to secrete G-CSF themselves as an ectopic hematopoietic growth factor. Other tumors (lung, stomach, breast), when metastasized to the bone and bone marrow, can cause a *leukoerythroblastic reaction*, characterized by left-shifted leukocytosis, thrombocytosis, and red cell abnormalities including nucleated and teardrop-shaped red blood cells (Fig. 170-3). The presence of nonhematopoietic entities invading the bone marrow (metastatic cancer, fibrosis, granulomatous disease) is termed *myelophthisis*.

Marrow Stimulation
Peripheral destruction of red cells and platelets, as seen with hemolytic anemia and idiopathic thrombocytopenic purpura, can result in stimulation of the bone marrow and a "spillover" leukocytosis. Recovery of cell counts following marrow suppression, as in the case of chemotherapy, can result in a rebound leukocytosis that may last several weeks.

Primary Causes of Neutrophilia
Hereditary Neutrophilia
Hereditary neutrophilia is an autosomal dominant genetic disease that is characterized by an elevated WBC in the 20,000 to 100,000/μL range with

splenomegaly and widened diploe of the skull. The neutrophils in this disorder appear to function normally, and patients have no increased risk for bacterial infection or other sequelae.

Chronic Idiopathic Neutrophilia

Chronic idiopathic neutrophilia is a condition marked by leukocytosis in the 11,000 to 40,000/μL range with a normal bone marrow biopsy. In one series with a 20-year follow-up, patients with this condition had no medical sequelae from this elevated WBC.

Pelger-Huet Anomaly

Patients with the Pelger-Huet anomaly (PHA) are often misdiagnosed as having a left-shifted WBC because many of their mature neutrophils are misinterpreted as band forms. Although these patients do not actually have leukocytosis, the anomaly often raises suspicion for an acute infection or inflammatory process because of this apparent left shift. PHA is due to a mutation in the lamin B receptor gene and manifests with mature neutrophils and condensed, clumped chromatin within a bilobed nucleus (see Fig. 160-20 in Chapter 160). These neutrophils, however, function normally. A number of drugs can reversibly induce pseudo-PHA, including colchicine, sulfonamides, ibuprofen, taxoids, and valproate. Pseudo-PHA is also seen in some patients with myelodysplasia (Chapter 188). Vitamin B_{12} or folate deficiency can cause increased nuclear lobation of neutrophils in patients with PHA, perhaps leading a missed diagnosis. With correction of the vitamin deficiency, however, the aberrant neutrophil nuclear morphology returns.

Down Syndrome

Up to 10% of patients with Down syndrome develop transient myeloproliferative disorder (TMD) related to peripheral blood leukocytosis with blasts in association with an accumulation of megakaryoblasts in the blood, liver, and marrow. Similar reactions have also been reported in patients with trisomy 21 mosaicism who are phenotypically normal. TMD resolves spontaneously in most patients but can progress to acute megakaryoblastic leukemia (AMKL) in 23 to 30% of affected patients. This fascinating disorder is attributable to acquisition of mutations in the *GATA1* gene, which encodes a key transcription factor for hematopoietic regulation, leading to loss of normal GATA-1 expression and expression of a truncated GATA-1 protein. Evidence supports that these mutations are acquired during fetal life, and patients present in early infancy with TMD. The pathogenesis of progression to AMKL presumably requires additional genetic events and is the focus of intense study.

Leukocyte Adhesion Deficiency

Patients with LAD have persistent leukocytosis, defects in stimulus-dependent activation of neutrophils, recurrent infections, and delayed separation of the umbilical cord. LAD is an abnormality of leukocyte adhesion reflecting the loss of surface adhesion molecules. LAD I is due to absence or marked reduction in the common β chain of $β_2$ integrins, resulting in loss of expression of leukocyte function-associated antigen 1 (LFA-1), the C3bi receptor, and GP150;95. This results in a failure to ingest and kill microbes opsonized by C3bi. In LAD II, neutrophils lack sialyl Lewis X, the ligand for L-selectin expressed on endothelial cells. Neutrophils appear morphologically normal but are defective in chemotaxis, adherence, and phagocytosis.

Familial Cold Urticaria

Familial cold urticaria is marked by episodic fevers, leukocytosis, urticaria, rash, conjunctivitis, and muscle and skin tenderness with cold exposure. The rash is composed of infiltrating neutrophils. The syndrome appears to be related to decreased levels of C1-esterase inhibitor and is associated with mutations in the *CIAS1* gene on chromosome 1q.

Chronic Myelogenous Leukemia and Other Myeloproliferative Disorders

Chronic myelogenous leukemia (CML) and the other myeloproliferative neoplasms (namely polycythemia vera [PV] and essential thrombocythemia [ET]) are discussed in detail in Chapters 190 and 169, respectively. They are the principal acquired primary hematologic disorders associated with neutrophilia. They are marked by clonal expansion of myeloid precursors and increased release of both immature and mature myeloid cells into the peripheral blood. CML on presentation often has to be distinguished from a leukemoid reaction. In contrast to a leukemoid reaction, CML is characterized by the presence of abnormalities of other blood cell lines ("panmyelosis") and

by the presence of specific abnormalities. Therefore, the peripheral blood smear in CML (but not leukemoid reaction) demonstrates increased numbers in all cells of the neutrophilic series, classically with a greater proportion of myelocytes to metamyelocytes, and may display concomitant basophilia, eosinophilia, anemia, and thrombocytosis. CML is characterized by the diagnostic presence of the Philadelphia chromosome [t(9;22)], which can be identified in the peripheral blood by the detection of the *BCR-ABL* translocation by fluorescence in situ hybridization (FISH) or reverse transcriptase–polymerase chain reaction (RT-PCR). PV and ET, on the other hand, are notable for a marked increase in red cell mass and a marked thrombocytosis, respectively, which is often accompanied by leukocytosis. Both PV and ET are associated with activating mutations in the *JAK2* gene (95 to 97% and 23 to 75% for PV and ET, respectively).

The leukocyte alkaline phosphatase (LAP) score was historically used in the laboratory evaluation of granulocytosis as a diagnostic marker for myeloproliferative disease. The LAP score is very low (usually 0) in the setting of CML and elevated in PV. The LAP score has a very wide normal range and in practical terms was only definitively helpful in the setting of CML because "high" LAP scores can also be seen in infectious and inflammatory settings. With the availability of direct molecular genetic diagnosis of CML by assay for the *BCR-ABL* fusion gene, it can no longer be recommended as a diagnostic test.

Postsplenectomy

Patients develop leukocytosis following splenectomy, and this may be long-standing, reflecting the loss of a major site of neutrophil margination. This is of no clinical importance, except insofar as it leads to unnecessary evaluation for other pathology.

CLINICAL MANIFESTATIONS AND DIAGNOSIS

As outlined previously, acquired leukocytosis is most commonly the result of acute or chronic infection or inflammation. When it occurs in the absence of fever, aberrations in acute phase reactants, effusions and edema, or other signs and symptoms of inflammation, it still may be secondary to drugs or an underlying nonhematologic malignancy. As such, it should be seen as the sign of a healthy hematopoietic system responding to an outside stress. Bone marrow evaluation is therefore rarely indicated. However, persistence of leukocytosis in the absence of signs and symptoms of inflammation or infection, nonhematologic malignancy, and offending drugs should prompt an evaluation for a primary myeloproliferative disease or clonal hematologic neoplasm, particularly when there is evidence of a leukoerythroblastic reaction. CML and PV can be ruled out by molecular diagnosis on the peripheral blood as described previously. In this setting, bone marrow examination is indicated to evaluate for marrow infiltration by infection, tumor, or fibrosis and should include cultures for tuberculosis and fungal infection as well as cytogenetics and flow cytometry (Fig. 170-4).

Leukocytosis Due to Expansion of Other Cell Lines

Monocytosis and lymphocytosis can also lead to elevations of the WBC. Monocytosis is defined by an absolute monocyte count of greater than 500/μL and usually occurs in the setting of chronic inflammation resulting from infections like tuberculosis, syphilis, or subacute bacterial endocarditis, autoimmune or granulomatous disease, and sarcoidosis. It can also be seen in malignancies, such as preleukemic states, nonlymphocytic leukemia including acute myelomonocytic and monocytic leukemia, histiocytosis, Hodgkin's disease, non-Hodgkin's lymphoma, and various carcinomas. Finally, it can be seen in the setting of chronic neutropenia, after splenectomy, and in the setting of recovery from marrow suppression (Table 170-2).

Lymphocytosis is defined by an absolute lymphocyte count of more than 5000/μL. The most common causes of an elevated lymphocyte count are viral infections such as Epstein-Barr virus and the hepatitis viruses. Although most bacterial infections cause neutrophilia, pertussis and cat-scratch disease due to *Bartonella henselae* can cause an impressive lymphocytosis. Other infections that may cause a secondary lymphocytosis include toxoplasmosis and babesiosis. Hypersensitivity reactions due to drugs or serum sickness may also be associated with lymphocytosis. Primary disorders that cause a lymphocytosis include chronic lymphocytic leukemia (CLL) and monoclonal B-cell lymphocytosis (Table 170-3; see also Table 190-2 and Chapter 190).

Eosinophilia is defined by an absolute eosinophil count of more than 400/μL. Eosinophils proliferate under the influence of IL-5 and play a role in phagocytosis and modulating toxicity due to mast cell degranulation in

FIGURE 170-4. Diagnostic approach to neutrophilia. AID = autoimmune disease; CML = chronic myelogenous leukemia; ddx = differential diagnosis; dx = disease; MPD = myeloproliferative disorder; Ph¹ = Philadelphia chromosome; P. vera = polycythemia vera.

TABLE 170-2 DIFFERENTIAL DIAGNOSIS OF MONOCYTOSIS

 I. Infection
   a. Granulomatous disease (tuberculosis, fungal disease)
   b. Endocarditis
   c. Syphilis
 II. Autoimmune diseases
   a. Lupus, rheumatoid arthritis
   b. Giant cell arteritis
   c. Vasculitis
 III. Inflammatory bowel disease
 IV. Sarcoid
 V. Malignancy
   a. Primary hematologic malignancy
     i. Chronic myelomonocytic leukemia
     ii. Acute myelomonocytic leukemia
     iii. Lymphoma
   b. Solid tumors
 VI. Neutropenia
   a. Associated with chronic neutropenia
   b. Recovery form marrow suppression
 VII. Postsplenectomy

TABLE 170-3 DIFFERENTIAL DIAGNOSIS OF LYMPHOCYTOSIS

 I. Infection
   a. Viral infection
     i. Epstein-Barr virus
     ii. Cytomegalovirus
     iii. Hepatitis
   b. Bacterial infection
     i. Pertussis
     ii. Bartonella
     iii. Tuberculosis
     iv. Syphilis
     v. Rickettsia
     vi. Babesia
 II. Hypersensitivity reactions
   a. Serum sickness
   b. Drug hypersensitivity
 III. Primary hematologic disease
   a. Chronic lymphocytic leukemia
   b. Monoclonal B-cell lymphocytosis
   c. Non-Hodgkin's lymphoma

hypersensitivity reactions. Eosinophilia is therefore most often seen in the setting of drug reactions, allergy, atopy, and asthma. A variety of infections, particularly parasitic infections and, to a lesser degree, fungal infections, can be associated with an increased number of circulating eosinophils. Eosinophilia can also be the result of autoimmune and inflammatory conditions, as in Churg-Strauss vasculitis. Atheroembolic disease and adrenal insufficiency may also cause eosinophilia. There are a number of cancers that have been associated with polytypic expansion of eosinophils, including lymphomas and solid tumors. There are also a number of clonal disorders of eosinophils that occur in the setting of some leukemias. Finally, there is a heterogeneous group of disorders termed *hypereosinophilic syndromes*. A *FIP1L1-PDGFRA* fusion gene has confirmed that some of these are primary clonal disorders of eosinophils; the clonality of other hypereosinophilic syndromes can be difficult to establish (see Table 173-1 in Chapter 173).

NEUTROPENIA

Neutropenia may reflect low numbers of circulating neutrophils with either low or normal neutrophil reserves. The risk for infection in the setting of neutropenia is therefore highly dependent on the size of the neutrophil storage pool. Although neutropenia is defined by an absolute neutrophil count of less than 1500/μL, patients with neutrophil counts below this number may have different risks and rates of infection depending on the cause of neutropenia. For instance, patients who are neutropenic owing to chemotherapy, marrow failure, or marrow exhaustion experience infection at much higher rates than those with chronic neutropenic syndromes and immune-mediated neutropenia. Neutropenia may be congenital or acquired. The following sections first discuss congenital neutropenic disorders, the study of which has provided critical insights into normal myelopoiesis, and then the secondary causes of neutropenia (Table 170-4).

Primary Causes of Neutropenia

Ethnic and Benign Familial (Constitutional) Neutropenia

The normal range of the neutrophil count is genetically determined and can be variable. A number of racial and ethnic groups have been observed to have a relatively large proportion of members who are neutropenic by comparison to the published normal range, usually based on young, largely white individuals. This is termed *constitutional neutropenia* and is seen among a variety of ethnic groups, including African Americans, Yemenite Jews, Falasha Jews, and African Bedouins. Single nucleotide polymorphisms in the gene for the Duffy antigen receptor for chemokine (DARC) have been shown to associate with race and are a postulated candidate to explain racial and ethnic differences in neutrophil counts. There is also an autosomal dominantly inherited

TABLE 170-4 DIFFERENTIAL DIAGNOSIS OF NEUTROPENIA

I. Congenital neutropenia
  a. Ethnic and benign familial (constitutional) neutropenia
  b. Severe congenital neutropenia
    i. Autosomal dominant (*ELANE* mutation)
    ii. Autosomal recessive (Kostmann's syndrome; *HAX2* mutation)
    iii. X-linked (*WASP* mutation)
    iv. Other rare defects (*G-CSFR* mutation, unknown)
  c. Cyclic neutropenia
  d. Shwachman-Diamond syndrome
  e. Fanconi anemia
  f. Dyskeratosis congenita
  g. Glycogen storage disease type Ib
  h. Myelokathexis
  i. Chédiak-Higashi syndrome
  j. Griscelli syndrome type II
  k. Hermansky-Pudlak syndrome II
II. Acquired neutropenia
  a. Infection
  b. Postinfection
  c. Drug induced
  d. Immune neutropenia
    i. Primary immune neutropenia
    ii. Secondary to autoimmune disease
      1. Rheumatoid arthritis
        (a) Felty's syndrome
        (b) Large granular lymphocyte disease
      2. Systemic lupus erythematosus
      3. Wegener's granulomatosis
      4. Hyperthyroidism
    iii. Pure white cell aplasia associated with thymoma
    iv. Large granular lymphocyte disease
  e. Primary bone marrow failure
    i. Aplastic anemia
    ii. Myelodysplastic syndrome
    iii. Acute leukemia
  f. Margination and hypersplenism
  g. Nutritional deficiency
  h. Chronic idiopathic neutropenia in adults (CINA)

ELANE = neutrophil elastase; G-CSFR: granulocyte colony-stimulating factor receptor; WASP = Wiskott-Aldrich syndrome protein.

TABLE 170-5 CONGENITAL NEUTROPENIA SYNDROMES

SYNDROME	INHERITANCE PATTERN	GENE
SCN	Autosomal dominant	ELANE (~60%)
	Autosomal recessive	HAX1 (~5%)
	X-linked	WASP (~5%)
	Autosomal recessive	G6PC3 (~2%)
	Autosomal dominant	Gfi1 (rare)
	Autosomal dominant	G-CSFR (rare)
Cyclic Neutropenia	Autosomal dominant	ELANE
Other Congenital Syndromes		
Shwachman-Diamond syndrome	X-Linked	SBDS
Fanconi anemia	Autosomal recessive	FANCA-FANCO
Dyskeratosis congenita	Variable	Telomerase and related genes
Glycogen storage disease type 1b	Autosomal recessive	G-6-PT
Myelokathexis	Autosomal dominant	CXCR4
Chédiak-Higashi Syndrome	Autosomal recessive	LYST
Griscelli syndrome type 2	Autosomal recessive	RAB27A
Hermansky-Pudlak syndrome type 2	Autosomal recessive	AP3B1

ELANE = neutrophil elastase; G6PC3 = glucose-6-phosphatase catalytic subunit 3; G-6-PT = glucose-6-phosphatase translocase; G-CSFR = granulocyte colony-stimulating factor receptor; LYST = lysosomal trafficking regulatory gene; SBDS = Shwachman-Bodian-Diamond syndrome; SCN = severe congenital neutropenia; WASP = Wiskott-Aldrich syndrome protein.

condition called *benign familial neutropenia* that is characterized by neutrophil counts in the 800 to 1400/μL range. Both ethnic and benign familial neutropenia have been shown to be associated with *no* increased risk for infection.

Severe Congenital Neutropenia
First described by Rolf Kostmann in 1956, severe congenital neutropenia (SCN) is a disorder of severe neutropenia with neutrophil counts of less than 500/μL, presenting in the neonatal period with recurrent bacterial infections. These infections can occur as early as the first months of life and often include omphalitis and perirectal abscesses. There is often an increase in other myeloid cell lines, including monocytes and eosinophils. Bone marrow biopsy in SCN patients reveals a "maturation arrest" with an absence of mature neutrophil elements. SCN can follow autosomal dominant and recessive and X-linked patterns of inheritance and has been shown to be associated with mutations in a variety of genes, as summarized in Table 170-5.

Neutrophil elastase (ELA2, now ELANE) is a serine protease that is synthesized at high levels in the promyelocyte stage of neutrophil maturation and is packaged in primary granules. It was originally hypothesized that mutations in ELANE led to its defective cellular trafficking and cytoplasmic accumulation, subsequently triggering neutrophil apoptosis. Newer evidence, however, supports a mechanism by which accumulation of the mutant neutrophil elastase in the endoplasmic reticulum activates the unfolded protein response, leading to apoptosis. SCN due to these mutations is inherited in an autosomal dominant fashion. Hax-1 is a mitochondrial protein with weak homology to bcl-2, and its absence results in mitochondrial-dependent apoptosis. It is the mutated protein implicated in the original autosomal recessive cases of SCN described by Kostmann. Although all SCN cases were originally referred to as *Kostmann's syndrome*, that term is now reserved for this subgroup of autosomal recessive SCN. Wiskott-Aldrich syndrome protein (WASP) regulates actin polymerization in hematopoietic cells, and

deficiency in this protein results in the Wiskott-Aldrich syndrome, characterized by small platelets in low number, sinopulmonary infections, and eczema. Another phenotype of mutated WASP, however, is X-linked thrombocytopenia and neutropenia. Mutations in glucose-6-phosphatase catalytic subunit 3 (*G6PC3*) are the most recently discovered cause of a subset of SCN patients; homozygous loss of this metabolic enzyme also appears to lead to activation of the unfolded protein response and increased apoptosis of neutrophil precursors.

SCN was formerly a disease of infancy and early childhood because few, if any, patients survived to adulthood. However, the advent of the availability of recombinant G-CSF and the observation that G-CSF is able to raise neutrophil counts and prevent infection in most patients have allowed these children to survive. Some patients require very high doses of G-CSF, but responses are seen in 80 to 90% of individuals. Increased survival led to the emerging realization that SCN predisposes to the development of myelodysplasia and acute leukemia (MDS/AML), with the development of MDS/AML at a rate of approximately 2% per year, and a cumulative risk of about 30% over 10 years. Patients refractory to G-CSF appear to have a higher risk for leukemic transformation. As discussed later, development of MDS/AML is often associated with the acquisition of a mutation in the gene encoding for the G-CSF receptor. Considerable controversy exists concerning the potential contribution of G-CSF administration to the risk for malignant transformation in children with SCN who receive lifelong treatment with G-CSF (see later under Treatment).

Two classes of G-CSF receptor mutations have been associated with SCN and either hyper-responsiveness or hyporesponsiveness of the receptor. Initial studies aimed at demonstrating that SCN was caused by mutation of the G-CSF or G-CSF receptor gene did not implicate such mutations in the pathogenesis of a significant number of patients with SCN. However, a small number of patients have been shown to have mutations in the G-CSF receptor gene that block ligand binding and produce a G-CSF-resistant form of SCN. More important, however, the studies identified an acquired missense mutation that introduces a stop codon and leads to the deletion of the distal intracellular domain of the receptor known to be responsible for differentiation signaling. This has been hypothesized to cause proliferation of hematopoietic progenitors at the expense of maturation and to be associated with hypersensitivity to G-CSF, suggesting that this mutation may play an important role in the development of MDS/AML in the setting of SCN. However, whether this mutation is in fact of pathogenetic importance to the development of MDS/AML and whether G-CSF influences the risk of developing the mutation and influencing leukemic transformation remain subjects of significant controversy.

Cyclic Neutropenia

Cyclic neutropenia is defined as periods of neutropenia (≤200/μL) lasting 3 to 5 days and occurring at approximately 21-day intervals. These periods of neutropenia can be marked by recurrent fevers, mouth sores, and infections of the skin, upper respiratory tract, and ears. The disorder can be dominantly inherited or sporadic. Congenital cyclic neutropenia has also been shown to be associated with mutations in the gene for neutrophil elastase in all cases tested to date. The diagnosis formerly required demonstration of transient neutropenia through blood counts every 2 to 3 weeks over a course of 6 weeks but now can be established by sequencing of the neutrophil elastase gene. It is successfully treated with G-CSF and is not associated with an increased risk for leukemic transformation. Rare cases of cyclic neutropenia acquired in adulthood have been associated with systemic diseases such as large granular lymphocytosis or T-cell lymphoma.

Other Congenital Syndromes with Associated Neutropenia

A number of other congenital syndromes are associated with neutropenia as one of the constellation of disease-associated abnormalities. These include Shwachman-Diamond syndrome, Fanconi anemia, dyskeratosis congenita, glycogen storage disease Ib, myelokathexis, Chédiak-Higashi syndrome, Griscelli syndrome II, and Hermansky-Pudlak syndrome II.

Shwachman-Diamond syndrome usually begins as an isolated neutropenia but progresses to marrow failure and is also associated with pancreatic dysfunction and skeletal abnormalities. The responsible gene has been identified, the Shwachman-Bodian-Diamond syndrome gene (*SBDS*), and is involved in the regulation of ribosomal RNA. These patients carry an increased risk for leukemic transformation.

Fanconi anemia is due to mutations in genes involved in DNA repair, and as such, it takes more time for marrow failure to develop in these patients (median age, 7 years). Patients with Fanconi anemia often have, in addition to marrow failure, short stature with upper limb anomalies and hyperpigmented cafe au lait spots, although about one third have no physical abnormalities. Screening is done by chromosomal fragility testing following exposure to diepoxybutane or mitomycin C as well as direct assessment for known Fanconi gene mutations. Stem cell transplantation is curative but carries a high risk for morbidity and mortality.

Dyskeratosis congenita is a syndrome of nail dystrophy, leukoplakia, and skin pigmentation abnormalities with associated neutropenia or aplastic anemia, or both. It can be inherited in an autosomal dominant or recessive or X-linked fashion and has been shown to be associated with mutations in several genes that are implicated in telomere maintenance. It typically does not present until the second decade of life.

Glycogen storage disease Ib is inherited in an autosomal recessive fashion and characterized by intermittent neutropenia due to defects in the neutrophil respiratory burst with subsequent apoptosis of circulating neutrophils. Hepatomegaly and metabolic crises are also the hallmarks of this disease and are due to mutations in the gene for the glucose-6-phosphatase translocase enzyme.

The neutropenia of *myelokathexis* is due to retention of mature neutrophils in the bone marrow despite a low peripheral neutrophil count. During infection, however, patients with myelokathexis typically have a sudden rise in their neutrophil count, which makes their clinical course relatively more benign. There is an association between this condition and hypogammaglobulinemia and warts, the WHIM syndrome (*w*arts, *h*ypogammaglobulinemia, *i*mmunodeficiency, and *m*yelokathexis). It has been shown to be caused by heterozygous mutations in the gene encoding chemokine receptor CXCR4.

Chédiak-Higashi syndrome, Griscelli syndrome II, and *Hermansky-Pudlak syndrome II* are all syndromes of albinism and neutropenia due to defects in vesicular trafficking. Chédiak-Higashi syndrome is due to mutations in a lysosomal trafficking regulatory gene (*LYST*) and is characterized by oculocutaneous albinism, bleeding, progressive neurologic disease, and increased susceptibility to hemophagocytic syndrome. Patients with Griscelli syndrome II also have an increased susceptibility to hemophagocytic syndrome as well as albinism and periodic neutropenia; Griscelli syndrome II is caused by mutations in the gene encoding the small guanosine triphosphatase RAB27A, which is involved in the release of myeloperoxidase from the primary granules of neutrophils. Finally, Hermansky-Pudlak syndrome II is

due to mutations in the *AP3B1* gene, which encodes a part of a protein transport complex that is involved in vesicular trafficking in many cell types and appears to be involved in the trafficking of neutrophil elastase. It is also marked by albinism, platelet abnormalities, and pulmonary fibrosis.

Secondary Causes of Neutropenia

Infection-Related Neutropenia

Several viral infections have been shown to cause a transient neutropenia that typically resolves as the viremia abates. These include varicella, measles, rubella, hepatitis A and B, Epstein-Barr virus, influenza, parvovirus, and cytomegalovirus. The mechanisms are diverse and can involve redistribution, decreased production, and immune destruction of neutrophils. Human immunodeficiency virus and acquired immunodeficiency syndrome can likewise cause leukopenia and neutropenia, perhaps through splenomegaly with increased sequestration as well as through immune-mediated destruction by antineutrophil antibodies. A myriad of atypical infections like *Mycobacterium tuberculosis*, ehrlichiosis, rickettsia, tularemia, brucellosis, and some staphylococcal infections can cause a moderate neutropenia. Any infection leading to overwhelming sepsis can cause neutropenia, but this is usually through consumption of the marrow neutrophil reserve and is typically seen in newborns and elderly patients and not in individuals with an otherwise healthy and mature marrow. There is also increased margination of neutrophils during sepsis due to systemic activation of complement, exacerbating the neutropenia.

Drug-Induced Neutropenia and Neutropenia Due to Marrow Injury

Drug-induced neutropenia is the most common cause of neutropenia. Multiple drugs have been implicated in neutropenia and agranulocytosis, in both predictable and idiosyncratic patterns. The mechanism of leukopenia is predominantly one that occurs within the marrow compartment, but certain drugs are also associated with increased destruction or clearance of peripheral neutrophils. Within the marrow compartment, many drugs cause direct dose-dependent marrow suppression, whereas others incite immune-mediated destruction. The typical pattern of drug-induced neutropenia is neutropenia that occurs after about 1 to 2 weeks of exposure to the drug with a recovery that begins within days of stopping the drug. However, atypical cases can present long after drug initiation, and others may be associated with a longer interval before recovery of the neutrophil count (Fig. 170-5). Patients with drug-induced agranulocytosis may present with acute sepsis, and it is associated with a significant risk for acute mortality. Recovery is often preceded by the appearance of monocytes and immature neutrophil forms. The more hypercellular the marrow is at diagnosis, the earlier marrow recovery may occur. Some common drugs known to cause neutropenia, in addition to antineoplastic, antiviral, and immunosuppressive agents, include clozapine, the thioamides, and sulfasalazine. Neutrophil recovery is speeded by G-CSF, although there are no definitive data that this improves survival.

Radiation can also result in marrow injury leading to an acute or chronic marrow failure state; in high doses, it is also a risk factor for the development of myelodysplasia and leukemia. These malignant hematopoietic diseases can themselves cause marrow failure because the malignant cells proliferate within the marrow-occupying space and can cause marrow fibrosis, both of which lead to cytopenias. These diseases are discussed in greater detail in Chapters 188 and 189, respectively. Likewise, metastatic carcinoma to the bone can also cause marrow failure because the marrow becomes increasingly occupied by the metastatic cells.

Immune Neutropenia

Infection and drugs cause immune-mediated neutrophil destruction. However, immune neutropenia can also occur as an isolated phenomenon (primary immune neutropenia) or as a manifestation of an underlying systemic autoimmune disease (secondary immune neutropenia). Primary autoimmune neutropenia is a disease of children younger than 4 years; median age of onset is 6 to 12 months. Although infectious risk is increased, treatment is restricted to prophylactic antibiotics, with G-CSF reserved for acute infectious episodes. Ninety-five percent of patients undergo spontaneous remissions within 2 years. Nearly all of these patients have antineutrophil antibodies directed against antigens derived from the FcγIIIb receptor; these antibodies mediate neutrophil destruction by either sequestration in the spleen or complement-mediated neutrophil lysis.

Secondary autoimmune neutropenia is a disease of adults and can be seen in association with hyperthyroidism, Wegener's granulomatosis, rheumatoid

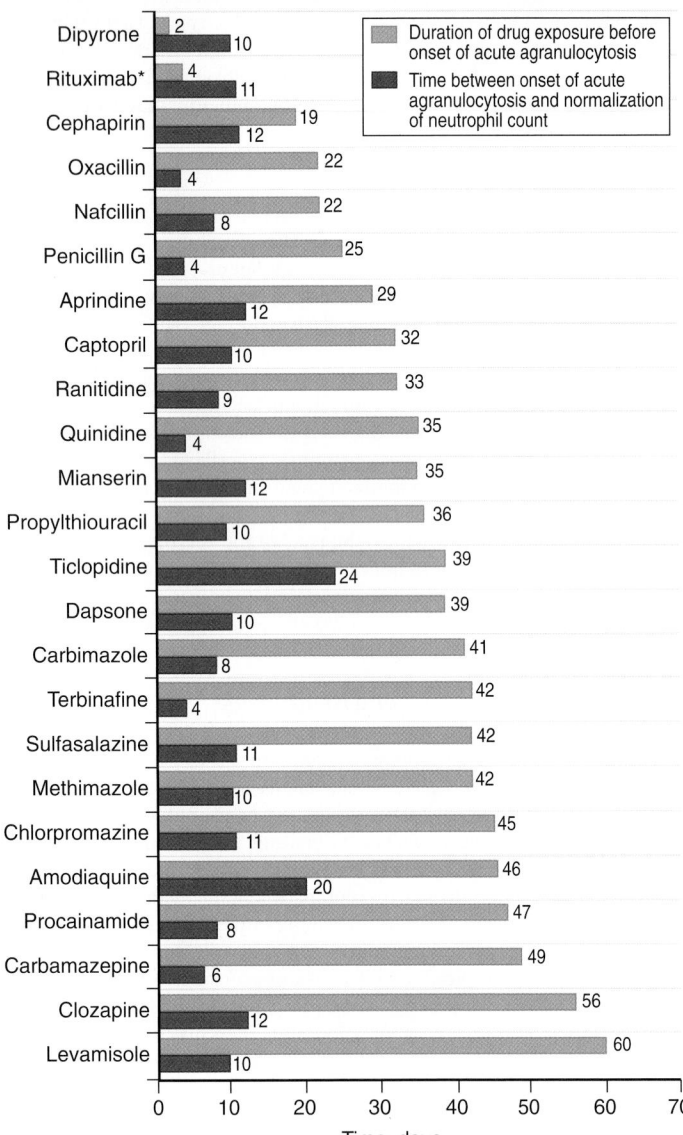

Legend:
- Duration of drug exposure before onset of acute agranulocytosis
- Time between onset of acute agranulocytosis and normalization of neutrophil count

Data (drug: light bar value / dark bar value):
- Dipyrone: 2 / 10
- Rituximab*: 4 / 11
- Cephapirin: 19 / 12
- Oxacillin: 22 / 4
- Nafcillin: 22 / 8
- Penicillin G: 25 / 4
- Aprindine: 29 / 12
- Captopril: 32 / 10
- Ranitidine: 33 / 9
- Quinidine: 35 / 4
- Mianserin: 35 / 12
- Propylthiouracil: 36 / 10
- Ticlopidine: 39 / 24
- Dapsone: 39 / 10
- Carbimazole: 41 / 8
- Terbinafine: 42 / 4
- Sulfasalazine: 42 / 11
- Methimazole: 42 / 10
- Chlorpromazine: 45 / 11
- Amodiaquine: 46 / 20
- Procainamide: 47 / 8
- Carbamazepine: 49 / 6
- Clozapine: 56 / 12
- Levamisole: 60 / 10

Time, days (x-axis: 0 to 70)

FIGURE 170-5. Median duration of treatment and neutropenia. Only drugs with more than three definite or probable reports of the time between onset of acute agranulocytosis and normalization of neutrophil count and the duration of treatment before onset of acute agranulocytosis were considered. (From Andersohn F, Konzen C, Garbe E. Systematic review: agranulocytosis induced by nonchemotherapy drugs. *Ann Intern Med.* 2007;146: 657-665.)

FIGURE 170-6. Peripheral blood with macrocytosis and hypersegmented neutrophils in megaloblastic anemia.

arthritis, and systemic lupus erythematosus (SLE). The role of antineutrophil antibodies in these patients is less clear. More than 50% of patients with SLE, for example, have antineutrophil antibodies, but many have normal neutrophil counts, and there is a poor correlation between the presence of the antibodies and neutrophil number.

Felty's syndrome and *large granular lymphocyte syndrome* deserve separate mention. Felty's syndrome occurs in association with long-standing rheumatoid arthritis (RA) (Chapter 272), and is characterized by splenomegaly and profound neutropenia. Large granular lymphocyte syndrome often occurs in the setting of RA but can also occur as an isolated phenomenon. Both Felty's syndrome and large granular lymphocyte syndrome are associated with a proliferation of large granular lymphocytes, with a characteristic surface phenotype (CD3$^+$, CD8$^+$, CD16$^+$, and CD57$^+$). In the setting of RA, these two syndromes were originally thought to be separate diseases, with Felty's syndrome being polyclonal and large granular lymphocyte syndrome representing a monoclonal proliferation of larger granular lymphocytes, but with increasing sensitivity of detection of monoclonal populations of lymphocytes, this distinction has become blurred. Finally, it has been observed that more than 90% of RA patients with either syndrome are human leukocyte antigen (HLA)-DR4-positive, leading to the postulate that the two entities represent the extremes of a single spectrum of disease. This HLA restriction is not found among non-RA patients with large granular lymphocytes. Both

syndromes cause immune-mediated neutrophil destruction by a wide array of mechanisms, including antineutrophil antibodies and cell-mediated destruction. Some patients may also have G-CSF resistance mediated by inhibitory G-CSF antibodies.

There are other rare forms of immune neutropenia. Isoimmune neonatal neutropenia is a moderate to severe neutropenia of the newborn due to transplacental passage of maternal immunoglobulin G antibodies against alleles inherited from the father, resulting in neutropenia in a manner similar to the development of anemia in Rh hemolytic disease. Pure white cell aplasia is a rare disease associated with severe pyogenic infections, and also with thymoma in more than two thirds of cases. It has also occurred following ibuprofen therapy. There is a complete absence of myeloid precursors on bone marrow examination. It is immune-mediated, but removal of the thymoma in thymoma-associated cases may not be sufficient for remission. Adjuvant therapy with cyclophosphamide, corticosteroids, cyclosporine, and intravenous immunoglobulin may be needed.

Neutropenia Due to Increased Margination and Hypersplenism
Complement activation can result in both acute and chronic neutropenia as a result of increased margination of the circulating neutrophil pool. This is attributed to the fact that C5a renders neutrophils more adherent and thereby prone to aggregation within the pulmonary vasculature. This has been seen in patients suffering from burns and transfusion reactions. Complement activation may also lead to neutrophil destruction, as in paroxysmal nocturnal hemoglobinuria. The circulating neutrophil pool can also be diminished in association with hypersplenism, although this is typically less common and less pronounced than the anemia and thrombocytopenia seen in patients with an enlarged spleen.

Neutropenia Due to Nutritional Deficiency
Several vitamin and mineral deficiencies, particularly B$_{12}$, folate, and copper, are associated with neutropenia. Deficiencies in these vitamins and minerals result in ineffective myelopoiesis, maturation arrest, and megaloblastic changes with nuclear-cytoplasmic dyssynchrony. The characteristic finding in the setting of megaloblastic anemia is hypersegmentation of the neutrophil (Fig. 170-6).

Chronic Idiopathic Neutropenia
Chronic idiopathic neutropenia in adults (CINA) is perhaps the most puzzling form of neutropenia. Patients present with chronic neutropenia that is often an incidental finding on routine blood tests, making it impossible to know how long the neutropenia has been present. They have no evidence of autoimmune disease, nutritional deficiency, or myelodysplasia. The syndrome is heterogeneous, with a wide range of neutrophil counts. A group of these patients from Greece has been studied by Papadaki and colleagues, who reported increased production of transforming growth factor-β (TGF-β) and consequent marrow suppression, leading them to posit an undiagnosed underlying inflammatory disease. These patients, however, tend to have very

mild neutropenia, with an absolute neutrophil count (ANC) that is rarely less than 800. It seems likely that these patients have an ethnic predisposition to neutropenia, and indeed the neutropenia has been demonstrated to be linked to a genetic polymorphism in the TGF-β locus. It seems likely, however, that these patients should be distinguished from other CINA patients, many of whom have an ANC below 200. The etiology of neutropenia in these patients is completely unknown. However, the natural history of CINA, even in the face of very low neutrophil counts, is generally benign. Most patients require no therapy, although those with very low counts must be treated with G-CSF when they develop fever in the setting of infections. Some patients with recurrent infections or troublesome aphthous ulcers require chronic G-CSF treatment. These patients typically respond to fairly low doses of G-CSF, and there is no reported increase in the development of MDS/AML.

CLINICAL MANIFESTATIONS AND DIAGNOSIS

Neutropenia by itself is not associated with many clinical signs and symptoms other than those of the condition that may be causing it. It becomes clinically evident, however, when it results in infection. Although patients with an ANC below 1000/µL do have a slightly increased risk for infection, the risk is substantially increased once the neutrophil count falls below 500/µL. Given the lack of neutrophils, the signs and symptoms of infection may be attenuated; as such, pneumonia may be present with minimal infiltrate on chest radiograph, or a urinary tract infection may yield only a very mild pyuria. Given this, fever in any neutropenic patient must be considered an emergency with prompt acquisition of cultures and administration of empirical antibiotic therapy.

When fever, infection or sepsis, and neutropenia present concomitantly for the first time, it can be difficult to determine whether the neutropenia predated the infection or, rather, is the result of the infection. Examination of the peripheral blood smear can be helpful in this regard because an elevation of band forms and evidence of toxic granulation suggest the latter.

Because drug-induced neutropenia is the most common cause of acquired neutropenia, a careful inventory of all drug and toxin exposures is warranted. Likewise, there should be a careful evaluation for underlying malignant and inflammatory conditions as the precipitant of neutropenia. The time course of the neutropenia and infections can provide clues to the etiology of the

neutropenia (acute versus chronic, persistent versus cyclic, neonatal versus childhood versus adult onset). Attention should be paid to the skin, bones, appendages, and nails because abnormalities in these may point toward one of the congenital neutropenia syndromes. Evaluation of the complete blood count, peripheral blood smear, and vitamin B_{12} and folate levels should also be performed.

When the neutropenia is not severe and is associated with anemia and thrombocytopenia, one should consider the possibility of hypersplenism. In many cases, the diagnosis can be made by the finding of palpable splenomegaly. However, especially in obese patients, abdominal imaging should be used to evaluate spleen size. Abdominal ultrasound allows the assessment of portal venous flow with Doppler studies. If splenic enlargement is confirmed, the etiology of the splenomegaly (Chapter 171) should be determined. It may reflect congestive splenomegaly secondary to portal hypertension (as a result of cirrhosis, fatty liver, or congestive heart failure, among others) or infiltrative splenomegaly due to a benign or malignant process; Felty's syndrome should be considered in the setting of RA.

In patients with chronic neutropenia in the absence of a history of infection or drug or toxin exposure or an evident B_{12} or folate deficiency, bone marrow examination should be performed to rule out myelodysplasia, with assessment of morphology, flow cytometry for large granular lymphocyte syndrome, and cytogenetics. Once a normal marrow has been obtained, further bone marrow examination is not indicated in patients with CINA (Fig. 170-7).

TREATMENT AND MANAGEMENT   **Rx**

The management of neutropenia (Chapter 289) is dependent on the etiology of the depressed neutrophil count as well as its severity and the presence or absence of fever or infection. Neutropenia with fever is a clinical emergency because these patients are at risk for hemodynamic collapse and septic shock. Therefore, these patients should be evaluated thoroughly and cultured promptly, and antibiotics should be administered within 30 to 60 minutes of presentation before obtaining the results of the cultures. The timely empirical administration of a combination of antipseudomonal antibiotics in patients with neutropenia at the onset of fever resulted in significant clinical benefit,

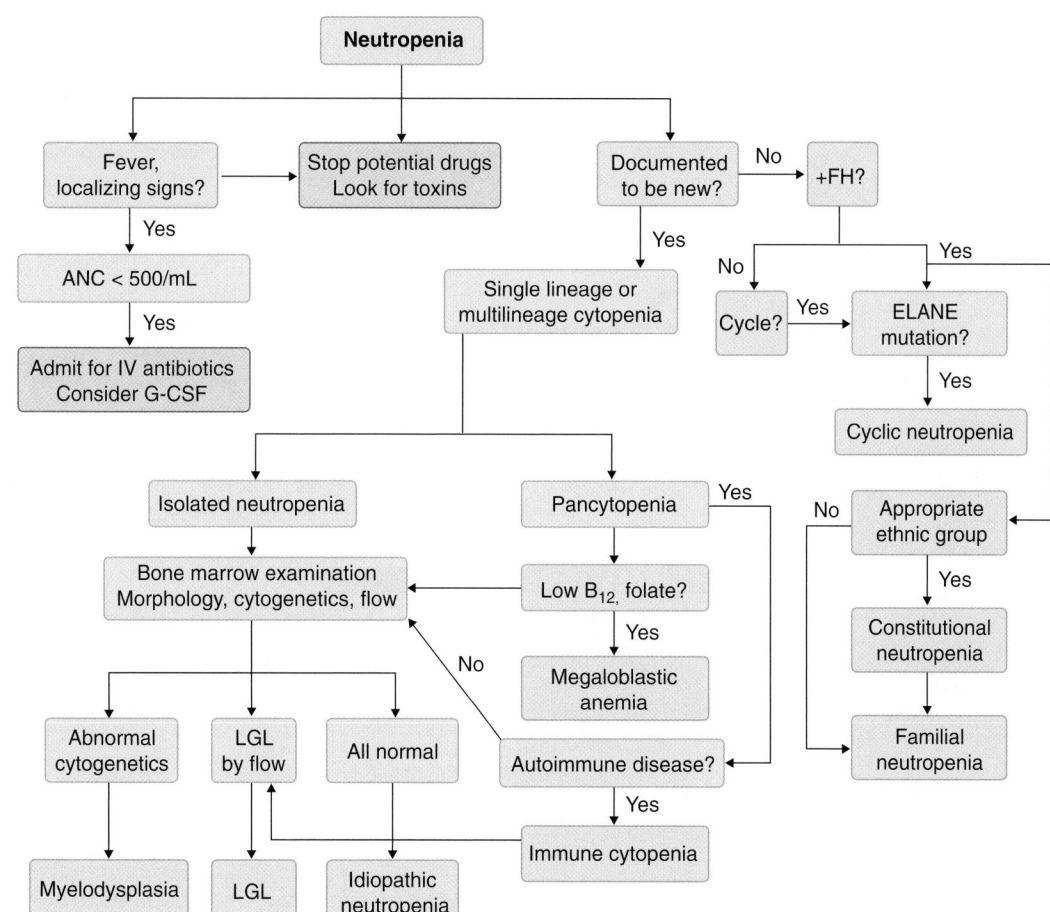

FIGURE 170-7. Diagnostic approach to neutropenia. ANC = absolute neutrophil count; ELANE = neutrophil elastase gene, FH = family history; G-CSF = granulocyte colony-stimulating factor; IV = intravenous; LGL = large granular lymphocyte syndrome.

both with respect to response and survival. With the advent of newer-generation cephalosporins, studies have shown that monotherapy with a third- or fourth-generation cephalosporin at the onset of fever may be sufficient. The addition of a second antipseudomonal agent, vancomycin, or antifungal agent is warranted in patients considered at risk for resistant pseudomonal infection, resistant gram-positive infection, or fungal infections, respectively, or in the face of a failure to defervesce within 3 to 5 days of antibiotic administration. These considerations are discussed in more detail in Chapter 289.

How to manage the uninfected and afebrile neutropenic patient is more nuanced and dependent on the etiology of the neutropenia. Patients with immune-mediated neutropenia are typically treated with immunosuppressive therapy, including steroids, antithymocyte globulin, or cyclosporine, or a combination of these, aimed primarily at treatment of the underlying autoimmune disease. Patients usually respond to G-CSF, although in the setting of RA, this may induce a flare of joint symptoms. Patients with large granular lymphocyte syndrome often respond to therapy with low-dose methotrexate, cyclosporine, or low-dose cyclophosphamide.

Patients with congenital neutropenia, including idiopathic, severe congenital, or cyclic neutropenia, are usually successfully managed with G-CSF for years. Before the use of G-CSF, the mean age of death for these patients was 2 to 3 years. Since the advent of G-CSF, however, life expectancy has been extended by decades into adulthood. Therapy is daily and chronic, with doses varying by the type of neutropenia and the individual responsiveness to therapy. It is usually well tolerated, although accelerated bone loss has been observed. Growth and development do not appear to be affected. Patients with SCN typically require the highest doses, whereas those with idiopathic neutropenia require the lowest, and patients with cyclic neutropenia fall somewhere in between. An increased rate of MDS/AML has been reported with the use of G-CSF in patients with SCN, but this has occurred coincidentally with improved survival. The increased incidence of MDS/AML may then be due to the fact that patients are living longer with a disease whose natural history includes a risk of developing MDS or AML. Certainly, the observation that acquired mutations in the G-CSF receptor are present in 65 to 80% of patients with SCN who develop MDS or AML suggests a potential mutagenic pathway towards leukemogenesis, but whether this is enhanced or accelerated by the administration of G-CSF has yet to be determined. Patients with idiopathic and cyclic neutropenia do not develop MDS or AML, despite therapy with G-CSF. However, recent evidence suggests that the risk for MDS/AML in SCN patients is much higher in those requiring high doses of G-CSF (>10 μg/kg/day), and patients with idiopathic and cyclic neutropenia are usually responsive to much lower G-CSF doses.

In patients with CINA, G-CSF should be reserved for acute febrile episodes unless the patient has recurrent infections. Patients with CINA treated with G-CSF may experience significant side effects, including fever, gastrointestinal symptoms, and splenomegaly. Consequently, in patients with CINA requiring chronic G-CSF administration, the cytokine should be administered at the lowest dose necessary to prevent infections; it is usually sufficient to treat to maintain the ANC higher than 500.

For patients with an inflammatory, infectious, or drug-induced neutropenia, the recommendation is to treat the underlying condition or stop the offending agent. This, however, is not always immediately possible, as in the cases of HIV-infected patients with opportunistic infections or on antiretroviral therapy, solid organ and bone marrow transplant recipients on immunosuppression and antiviral prophylaxis and treatment, and cancer patients undergoing chemotherapy. Prophylactic use of G-CSF in these patients has been shown to be effective in improving the ANC and decreasing rates of infection and febrile neutropenia, but has not been associated with a proven or consistent survival advantage.[1] In light of these findings, many oncologic professional society guidelines recommend the use of prophylactic G-CSF in patients receiving chemotherapy who have a 20% or greater risk of developing febrile neutropenia based on age, comorbid illness, disease characteristics, and myelotoxicity of the chemotherapy regimen. In addition, it is recommended for use during hematopoietic stem cell transplantation, for patients receiving chemotherapy for non-Hodgkin's lymphoma or dose-dense chemotherapy, and for patients with a history of febrile neutropenia receiving further chemotherapy.

The use of prophylactic antibiotics has also been investigated, predominantly in neutropenic patients receiving chemotherapy. Early studies in the 1980s and 1990s demonstrated an improvement in infection-related outcomes but not in infection-related or overall survival. Most recently, several randomized trials of prophylactic quinolones in patients receiving chemotherapy demonstrated an improvement in rates of infection and febrile neutropenia.[2-4] A meta-analysis of studies investigating the use of prophylactic quinolones in patients receiving chemotherapy was the first to document an overall survival benefit as well, although most of these patients had hematologic as opposed to solid tumor malignancies. The current Infectious Diseases Society of America guidelines do not recommend the use of prophylactic antibiotics in cancer patients undergoing myelosuppressive chemotherapy, with the exception of trimethoprim-sulfamethoxazole in patients at risk for *Pneumocystis jirovecii* pneumonia. Antibiotic prophylaxis is not generally used outside of the stem cell transplantation setting. The use of antibiotics to prevent infection in patients with neutropenia due to other causes has not been extensively studied but is typically not recommended and should be based on clinical context.

Stem cell transplantation (Chapter 181) can be curative for a number of the congenital neutropenia and bone marrow failure syndromes. It is, however, not without risk and should therefore be reserved for patients with severe neutropenia complicated by recurrent infection definitively shown to be due to marrow failure.

Leukopenia Due to Deficiency of Other Cell Lines

Lymphocyte production takes place in a variety of anatomic sites, and lymphocyte trafficking from those sites is bidirectional, making it difficult to understand lymphocyte dynamics in the same way that we do for neutrophils. Despite this, the peripheral lymphocyte count seems to be maintained in a narrow range at 2000 to 4000/μL, 20% of which are B cells and 70% of which are T cells. Lymphocytopenia, then, is a total lymphocyte count of less than 1500/μL. It can be the result of decreased production, defective trafficking, or increased loss or destruction. Decreased production can occur as a result of protein and calorie malnutrition; lymphocyte progenitor pool injury secondary to radiation, chemotherapy, or immunosuppressive agents; and congenital immunodeficiency states. Endogenous or exogenous glucocorticoid excess can cause lymphocytopenia by altering lymphocyte trafficking. This can also occur as the result of acute bacterial or fungal infections, certain viral infections, and granulomatous disease. Finally, many viruses can cause direct destruction of lymphocytes, as can antilymphocyte antibodies seen in patients with underlying autoimmune diseases. Lymphocytes can also be lost from intestinal lymphatics in cases of protein-losing enteropathy, primary disease of the gut or intestinal lymphatics, or gut edema secondary to severe heart failure. When lymphocytopenia is discovered, a comprehensive assessment of the immune system should be done, including lymphocyte subtyping, quantitative immunoglobulins, and skin testing to detect deficiencies of cell-mediated immunity. Treatment is typically aimed at the underlying disease, but intravenous immunoglobulin can be administered to patients who are hypogammaglobulinemic, and transplantation can be performed in patients with severe deficiencies of cell-mediated immunity due to impaired lymphocyte production and function.

Monocytopenia, eosinopenia, and basophilopenia can be seen in the setting of bone marrow failure syndromes or as a result of acute infection, malignancy, or severe injury. This is thought to be due to elevations in glucocorticoids, prostaglandins, and epinephrine. A rise in these humoral factors has the greatest impact on eosinophils such that a lack of eosinopenia in any of these settings should prompt suspicion for adrenal insufficiency, a primary myeloproliferative syndrome, parasitic infection, or primary hypereosinophilic syndrome. Monocytopenia is less frequently seen, probably owing to the diverse roles monocytes play in normal human physiology; prolonged and extreme monocytopenia may not be compatible with life.

1. Sung L, Nathan PC, Alibhai SM, et al. Meta-analysis: effect of prophylactic hematopoietic colony-stimulating factors on mortality and outcomes of infection. *Ann Intern Med.* 2007;147:400-411.
2. Bucaneve G, Micozzi A, Menichetti F, et al. Levofloxacin to prevent bacterial infection in patients with cancer and neutropenia. *N Engl J Med.* 2005;353:977-987.
3. Cullen M, Steven N, Billingham L, et al. Antibacterial prophylaxis after chemotherapy for solid tumors and lymphomas. *N Engl J Med.* 2005;353:988-998.
4. Gafter-Gvili A, Fraser A, Paul M, et al. Meta-analysis: antibiotic prophylaxis reduces mortality in neutropenic patients. *Ann Intern Med.* 2005;142:979-995.

SUGGESTED READINGS

Aapro MS, Bohlius J, Cameron DA, et al. 2010 update of EORTC guidelines for the use of granulocyte-colony stimulating factor to reduce the incidence of chemotherapy-induced febrile neutropenia in adult patients with lymphoproliferative disorders and solid tumours. *Eur J Cancer.* 2011;47:8-32. *Consensus guidelines for targeted use.*

Apinantriyo B, Lekhakula A, Rujirojindakul P. Incidence, etiology and bone marrow characteristics of non-chemotherapy-induced agranulocytosis. *Hematology.* 2011;16:50-53. *Antimicrobial agents (63%) and antithyroid agents (14%) are the two most common causes.*

Berliner N. Lessons from congenital neutropenia: 50 years of progress in understanding myelopoiesis. *Blood.* 2008;111:5427-5432. *A review of congenital neutropenia in the context of our understanding of normal myeloid maturation.*

Dale DC, Welte K. Cyclic and chronic neutropenia. *Cancer Treat Res.* 2011;157:97-108. *Review of genetics, clinical manifestations, and the observation that most cyclic neutropenia responds well to G-CSF.*

Wilcox RA. Cancer-associated myeloproliferation: old association, new therapeutic target. *Mayo Clin Proc.* 2010;85:656-663. *New insights into the importance of cancer-associated paraneoplastic leukocytosis, the so-called leukemoid reaction.*

171

APPROACH TO THE PATIENT WITH LYMPHADENOPATHY AND SPLENOMEGALY

JAMES O. ARMITAGE

⬤ LYMPHADENOPATHY

Physiology and Anatomy

Lymph nodes are found throughout the body along the course of the lymphatics, strategically located to allow the filtering of lymphatic fluid and the interdiction of microorganisms and abnormal proteins. Lymphatic fluid enters the node in afferent lymphatic vessels that empty into the subcapsular sinus. The fluid then transverses the node and exits in a single efferent lymphatic vessel. In doing so, the lymph and its contents are exposed to immunologically active cells throughout the node. Lymph nodes are populated predominantly by macrophages, dendritic cells, B lymphocytes, and T lymphocytes. B lymphocytes are located primarily in the follicles and perifollicular areas, whereas T lymphocytes are found principally in the interfollicular or paracortical areas of the lymph node. These cells function together to provide antigen processing, antigen presentation, antigen recognition, and proliferation of effector B and T lymphocytes as part of the normal immune response to microorganisms or foreign proteins.

Because the normal immune response leads to the proliferation and expansion of one or more cellular components of lymph nodes, it often results in significant lymph node enlargement. In young children, who are continuously being exposed to new antigens, palpable lymphadenopathy is the rule. In fact, the absence of palpable lymphadenopathy would be considered abnormal. In adults, lymph nodes larger than 1 to 2 cm in diameter are generally considered abnormal. However, lymph nodes 1 to 2 cm in diameter in the groin are sufficiently common to be considered normal.

Lymphoid proliferation is a normal response to exposure to foreign antigens. The location of the enlarged lymph nodes often reflects the site of invasion. For example, cervical lymphadenopathy would be typical in a patient with pharyngitis. Generalized immune proliferation and lymphadenopathy can occur with a systemic disorder of the immune system, disseminated infection, or disseminated neoplasia. Malignancies of the immune system might manifest as localized or disseminated lymphadenopathy.

Differential Diagnosis

The differential diagnosis of lymphadenopathy (Table 171-1) is vast, and the underlying causes are responsible for either proliferation of immunologically

active cells or infiltration of the lymph node by foreign cells or substances. In practice, the cause of enlarged lymph nodes is often uncertain even in retrospect; in such cases, unrecognized infectious processes are generally blamed.

Infections by bacteria, mycobacteria, fungi, chlamydiae, parasites, and viruses are the major causes of lymph node enlargement. Lymph nodes in the drainage area of essentially all pyogenic infections can enlarge. In certain infections, such as bubonic plague caused by *Yersinia pestis,* dramatic regional lymph node enlargement with fluctuant lymph nodes (i.e., buboes) can be a hallmark of the disease (Chapter 320). Other bacterial infections have lymph node enlargement as a prominent feature (e.g., cat-scratch disease, Chapter 323) and can mimic lymphoproliferative disorders. Mediastinal lymphadenopathy is seen in inhalational anthrax (Chapter 302). In some parts of the world, cervical lymphadenopathy is a sufficiently frequent manifestation of tuberculosis to lead to the institution of antituberculous therapy rather than biopsy. Disseminated lymphadenopathy can be seen in cases of infection by a variety of organisms such as *Toxoplasma,* Epstein-Barr virus (i.e., infectious mononucleosis), cytomegalovirus, and human immunodeficiency virus (HIV).

A variety of nonmalignant disorders of the immune system can lead to localized or disseminated lymphadenopathy. Autoimmune diseases such as rheumatoid arthritis (Chapter 272) and systemic lupus erythematosus (Chapter 274) often have accompanying lymphadenopathy, which can pose a diagnostic challenge because of the increased incidence of lymphoma in patients with these disorders. In the lymphadenopathy that occurs as a reaction to drugs such as phenytoin, lymph node biopsy findings can sometimes be confused with lymphoma. Benign proliferative diseases of the immune system that can also be confused with lymphoma include Castleman's disease (Chapters 191 and 400; angiofollicular lymph node hyperplasia), sinus histiocytosis with massive lymphadenopathy, and disorders seen more frequently in Asia, such as Kawasaki syndrome (Chapter 447) and Kimura's disease.

All the cells in the immune system can become malignant. Several of these malignancies typically manifest as lymphadenopathy, and it can be seen in all of them. Lymphadenopathy as the initial manifestation is the rule for Hodgkin's disease and non-Hodgkin's lymphoma, and it is common in Waldenström's macroglobulinemia and B-cell chronic lymphocytic leukemia; it is seen only occasionally in the myeloid leukemias (Chapters 189 through 192) and is rare in multiple myeloma. Malignancies of all organ systems can metastasize to the lymph nodes and cause lymphadenopathy, which is usually seen in the drainage area of the primary tumor—for example, axillary lymph nodes in patients with breast cancer, hilar and mediastinal lymph nodes in patients with lung cancer, and cervical lymph nodes in patients with head and neck cancer. However, widespread lymphadenopathy can also occur. Other disorders in which lymphadenopathy may be an initial finding include storage diseases such as Gaucher's disease (Chapter 215), endocrinopathies such as hyperthyroidism (Chapter 233), sarcoidosis (Chapter 95), and dermatopathic lymphadenitis. Amyloidosis (Chapter 194) can cause lymphadenopathy in patients with multiple myeloma, hereditary amyloidosis, or amyloidosis associated with chronic inflammatory states.

Among patients with lymphadenopathy actually seen in practices in the United States, diagnoses are not determined in a high proportion (Table 171-2). In such cases, the lymphadenopathy is usually blamed on infection. When the lymphadenopathy is in the drainage site of a known infection (e.g., cervical lymphadenopathy in a patient with pharyngitis) or the patient has a known infection associated with lymphadenopathy (e.g., infectious mononucleosis; Chapter 385), this infectious assumption is usually correct. Alternatively, if a patient has an immunologic disorder that is known to cause lymphadenopathy, such as rheumatoid arthritis, this disorder is usually an acceptable

---

TABLE 171-1 CAUSES OF LYMPHADENOPATHY

Infection
  Bacterial (e.g., all pyogenic bacteria, cat-scratch disease, syphilis, tularemia)
  Mycobacterial (e.g., tuberculosis, leprosy)
  Fungal (e.g., histoplasmosis, coccidioidomycosis)
  Chlamydial (e.g., lymphogranuloma venereum)
  Parasitic (e.g., toxoplasmosis, trypanosomiasis, filariasis)
  Viral (e.g., Epstein-Barr virus, cytomegalovirus, rubella, hepatitis, HIV)
Benign disorders of the immune system (e.g., rheumatoid arthritis, systemic lupus
  erythematosus, serum sickness, drug reactions such as to phenytoin, Castleman's
  disease, sinus histiocytosis with massive lymphadenopathy, Langerhans cell
  histiocytosis, Kawasaki syndrome, Kimura's disease)
Malignant disorders of the immune system (e.g., chronic and acute myeloid and
  lymphoid leukemia, non-Hodgkin's lymphoma, Hodgkin's disease,
  angioimmunoblastic-like T-cell lymphoma, Waldenström's macroglobulinemia,
  multiple myeloma with amyloidosis, malignant histiocytosis)
Other malignancies (e.g., breast carcinoma, lung carcinoma, melanoma, head and
  neck cancer, gastrointestinal malignancies, germ cell tumors, Kaposi's sarcoma)
Storage diseases (e.g., Gaucher's disease, Niemann-Pick disease)
Endocrinopathies (e.g., hyperthyroidism, adrenal insufficiency, thyroiditis)
Miscellaneous (e.g., sarcoidosis, amyloidosis, dermatopathic lymphadenitis)

TABLE 171-2 MOST FREQUENT CAUSES OF LYMPHADENOPATHY IN ADULTS IN THE UNITED STATES

Unexplained
Infection
  In drainage area of infection (e.g., cervical adenopathy with pharyngitis)
  Disseminated (e.g., mononucleosis, HIV infection)
Immune disorders (e.g., rheumatoid arthritis)
Neoplasms
  Immune system malignancies (e.g., leukemias, lymphomas)
  Metastatic carcinoma or sarcoma

TABLE 171-3 FACTORS TO CONSIDER IN THE DIAGNOSIS OF LYMPHADENOPATHY

Associated systemic symptoms
Patient's age
History of infection, trauma, medications, travel experience, previous malignancy
Location: cervical, supraclavicular, epitrochlear, axillary, intrathoracic (hilar vs. mediastinal), intra-abdominal (retroperitoneal vs. mesenteric vs. other), iliac, inguinal, femoral
Localized vs. disseminated
Presence of tenderness or inflammation
Size
Consistency

TABLE 171-4 METHODS OF LYMPH NODE EVALUATION

Physical examination
Imaging
    Chest radiography
    Ultrasonography
    Computed tomography
    Magnetic resonance imaging
    Positron emission tomography
Sampling
    Needle aspiration
    Cutting needle biopsy
    Excisional biopsy

explanation; however, progressive lymphadenopathy in such patients should trigger a biopsy because they are at increased risk for lymphoma. Localized, progressive lymphadenopathy, particularly when associated with fever, sweats, or weight loss, requires biopsy to exclude lymphoma.

Lymph Node Evaluation

Evaluation of a patient with lymphadenopathy includes a careful history, a thorough physical examination, laboratory tests, and sometimes imaging studies to determine the extent and character of the lymphadenopathy. The age of the patient and any associated systemic symptoms might be important clues (Table 171-3). Cervical lymphadenopathy in a child is much less worrisome than equally prominent lymphadenopathy in a 60-year-old adult. The occurrence of fever, sweats, or weight loss raises the possibility of a malignancy of the immune system. The explanation for the lymphadenopathy might become apparent with the identification of a site of infection, a particular medication, a travel history, or a previous malignancy.

Physical examination allows the identification of localized versus widespread lymphadenopathy. The particular sites of involvement can be important hints to the diagnosis because infection and carcinoma are likely to cause lymphadenopathy in the lymphatic drainage of the site of the disorder. In general, tender lymph nodes are more likely to be due to an infectious process, whereas painless adenopathy raises concern for malignancy. Lymph node consistency can also aid in the diagnosis: typically, lymph nodes containing metastatic carcinoma are rock hard, lymph nodes containing lymphoma are firm and rubbery, and lymph nodes enlarged in response to an infectious process are soft.

The larger the lymph node, the more likely it is that a serious underlying cause exists; lymph nodes greater than 3 to 4 cm in diameter in an adult are very worrisome. Physical examination to assess lymph node size is only marginally accurate and reproducible, although it is by far the most widely used method. More precise methods are available with various imaging techniques.

Imaging

Imaging studies, including routine radiographs, computed tomography (CT), ultrasonography, magnetic resonance imaging (MRI), and positron emission tomography (PET), can be used to assess the extent of lymphadenopathy in the chest and abdomen (Table 171-4). Chest radiographs are the most economical and easiest way to assess mediastinal and hilar lymphadenopathy but are not as accurate as CT of the chest. CT and ultrasonography are the most useful modalities for assessing abdominal and retroperitoneal lymphadenopathy. In most patients, CT is probably the most accurate approach, but ultrasonography has the advantage of being less expensive and not requiring radiation exposure. MRI and PET are not first-line studies for the assessment of lymphadenopathy. PET is frequently positive in patients with Hodgkin's disease and aggressive non-Hodgkin's lymphomas and can be used to assess the presence of active lymphoma in patients with lymphadenopathy and a proven diagnosis; it is especially useful for re-evaluating patients after therapy because lymph nodes do not always regress to normal size after treatment, particularly those in the mediastinum and retroperitoneum, even though the malignancy has been eradicated.

Interventional Evaluation

Lymph node aspiration or biopsy is often necessary for an accurate diagnosis of the cause of lymphadenopathy. Fine-needle aspiration is currently popular and is an accurate means of diagnosing infection or carcinoma involving a lymph node. Although lymphomas can occasionally be diagnosed with this

TABLE 171-5 APPROACH TO THE PATIENT WITH LYMPHADENOPATHY

Does the patient have a known illness that causes lymphadenopathy? Treat and monitor for resolution.
Is there an obvious infection to explain the lymphadenopathy (e.g., infectious mononucleosis)? Treat and monitor for resolution.
Are the nodes very large and/or very firm and thus suggestive of malignancy? Perform a biopsy.
Is the patient very concerned about malignancy and unable to be reassured that malignancy is unlikely? Perform a biopsy.
If none of the preceding are true, perform a complete blood cell count and, if unrevealing, monitor for a predetermined period (usually 2 to 8 weeks). If the nodes do not regress or if they increase in size, perform a biopsy.

approach, it is inappropriate as an initial diagnostic maneuver for lymphoma. Cutting needle biopsy occasionally provides sufficient material for an unequivocal diagnosis and subtyping of the lymphoma. However, excisional biopsy, which is most likely to provide the pathologist with adequate material to perform histologic, immunologic, and genetic studies, is also most likely to yield the correct diagnosis.

An Approach to the Patient with Lymphadenopathy

Patients with lymphadenopathy (Table 171-5) come to medical attention in several ways. Perhaps most common is a patient who feels a lymph node in the neck, axilla, or groin and seeks a physician's opinion. Lymphadenopathy might also be an unexpected finding on a routine physical examination or as part of an evaluation for another complaint. Finally, patients might be found to have unexpected lymphadenopathy on imaging studies of the chest or abdomen. When the nodes are multiple or larger than 2 to 3 cm, biopsy via mediastinoscopy, a paramediastinal incision, laparoscopy, or laparotomy is often required for diagnosis.

The approach to a patient complaining of newly discovered lymphadenopathy in the neck, axilla, or groin depends on the size, consistency, and number of enlarged lymph nodes and the patient's general health. In most cases, very large or very firm lymph nodes in the presence of systemic symptoms such as unexplained fever, sweats, or weight loss should lead to lymph node biopsy. Patients who have enlarged lymph nodes in the drainage area of a previously treated malignancy (e.g., neck nodes in a patient with a history of head and neck cancer) might be best approached by lymph node aspiration. Carcinoma can often be diagnosed in this manner, although it is a poor approach for the diagnosis of lymphoid malignancies. For cervical lymph nodes, excisional biopsy should be delayed in a patient in whom head and neck cancer (Chapter 196) is a diagnostic consideration. These patients should initially undergo careful ear, nose, and throat examinations to avoid performing a biopsy that might complicate the patient's subsequent therapy. Some diagnostic possibilities for localized lymphadenopathy are presented in Table 171-6.

In the most common situation—that is, a lymph node is soft and is not larger than 2 to 3 cm and the patient has no obvious systemic illness—observation for a brief period is usually the best approach. Performance of a complete blood cell count and examination of a peripheral smear can be helpful in recognizing a systemic illness (e.g., infectious mononucleosis). These patients are often given antibiotics. If the lymph node does not regress over the course of a few weeks or if it gets bigger, a biopsy should be performed.

TABLE 171-6 SOME DIAGNOSTIC CONSIDERATIONS FOR LOCALIZED LYMPHADENOPATHY

SITE	INFECTIONS	NEOPLASMS	OTHER
Cervical	Pharyngitis, other head and neck infections, mononucleosis, toxoplasmosis, TB	Head and neck cancers, thyroid cancer, lymphoma	
Supraclavicular		Intra-abdominal cancer (particularly left-sided nodes), lung cancer, lymphoma	
Axillary	Cat-scratch disease, distal infections, plague	Breast cancer, melanoma, lymphoma	Silicone implants
Mediastinal	TB, fungal infection, anthrax	Lymphoma, lung cancer, germ cell tumor	Sarcoidosis
Retroperitoneal	TB	Lymphoma, testicular cancer, kidney cancer, upper GI malignancy	Sarcoidosis
Mesenteric	Appendicitis, cholecystitis, diverticulitis, Whipple's disease	Lymphoma, GI cancer	Inflammatory bowel disease, panniculitis
Inguinal	Distal or genital infection, plague, STDs	Lymphoma, melanoma, vulvar cancer	

GI = gastrointestinal; STD = sexually transmitted disease; TB = tuberculosis.

FIGURE 171-1. Howell-Jolly body in an erythrocyte. This is evidence of splenectomy or a nonfunctional spleen.

Part of the care of such patients involves the art of medicine and being responsive to the patient's particular needs. For example, biopsy might be performed more quickly in a patient who is very anxious about malignancy or who needs a definitive diagnosis expeditiously.

SPLENOMEGALY

DEFINITION

The spleen is the largest lymphatic organ in the body and is sometimes approached clinically as though it were a very large lymph node. Although it participates in the primary immune response to invading microorganisms and foreign proteins, the spleen has many other functions. It functions as a filter for the blood and is responsible for removing senescent red blood cells from the circulation, as well as blood cells and other cells coated with immunoglobulins. Blood enters the spleen, filters through the splenic cords, and is exposed to immunologically active cells in the spleen.

The splenic red pulp occupies more than half the volume of the spleen and is the site where senescent red cells are identified and destroyed and red blood cell inclusions are removed by a process known as *pitting*. In the absence of splenic function, basophilic inclusions known as *Howell-Jolly bodies* are seen in circulating red blood cells. The presence of Howell-Jolly bodies (Fig. 171-1) in peripheral blood indicates that the patient has undergone splenectomy or has a process that has rendered the spleen nonfunctional (e.g., sickle cell disease with repeated splenic infarcts, chronic graft-versus-host disease).

The white pulp of the spleen contains macrophages, B lymphocytes, and T lymphocytes; participates in the recognition of microorganisms and foreign proteins; and is involved in the primary immune response. Absence of this splenic function makes individuals particularly susceptible to certain infections, including sepsis with encapsulated organisms such as *Streptococcus pneumoniae*. The risk for overwhelming sepsis is related to the age at the time of splenectomy or other cause of loss of splenic function. Children and young adults are at highest risk. If possible, all patients should undergo vaccination against *S. pneumoniae* and perhaps *Haemophilus influenzae* and *Neisseria meningitidis* before splenectomy. Some physicians have patients take oral penicillin (e.g., phenoxymethyl penicillin 250 mg twice daily) indefinitely if splenectomy has been performed in childhood or adolescence.

TABLE 171-7 CAUSES OF SPLENOMEGALY

Infection
    Bacterial (e.g., endocarditis, brucellosis, syphilis, typhoid, pyogenic abscess)
    Mycobacterial (e.g., tuberculosis)
    Fungal (e.g., histoplasmosis, toxoplasmosis)
    Parasitic (e.g., malaria, leishmaniasis)
    Rickettsial (e.g., Rocky Mountain spotted fever)
    Viral (e.g., Epstein-Barr virus, cytomegalovirus, HIV, hepatitis)
Benign disorders of the immune system (e.g., rheumatoid arthritis with Felty's syndrome, systemic lupus erythematosus, drug reactions such as to phenytoin, Langerhans cell histiocytosis, serum sickness)
Malignant disorders of the immune system (e.g., acute or chronic myeloid or lymphoid leukemia, non-Hodgkin's lymphoma, Hodgkin's disease, Waldenström's macroglobulinemia, malignant histiocytosis)
Other malignancies (e.g., melanoma, sarcoma)
Congestive splenomegaly (e.g., portal hypertension secondary to liver disease, splenic or portal vein thrombosis)
Hematologic disorders (e.g., autoimmune hemolytic anemia, hereditary spherocytosis, thalassemia major, hemoglobinopathies, elliptocytosis, extramedullary hematopoiesis)
Storage diseases (e.g., Gaucher's disease)
Endocrinopathies (e.g., hyperthyroidism)
Miscellaneous (e.g., sarcoidosis, amyloidosis, tropical splenomegaly, cysts)

PATHOBIOLOGY

As with lymphadenopathy, numerous conditions are associated with splenomegaly (Table 171-7). Certain bacterial infections such as endocarditis (Chapter 76), brucellosis (Chapter 318), and typhoid fever (Chapter 316) have splenomegaly as a frequent manifestation. Disseminated tuberculosis (Chapter 332) is often associated with splenomegaly, and splenomegaly can also be seen in cases of disseminated histoplasmosis (Chapter 340) and toxoplasmosis (Chapter 357). Splenomegaly is an almost constant accompaniment of malaria (Chapter 353). Rickettsial disorders such as Rocky Mountain spotted fever are frequently associated with splenomegaly. A wide variety of viral infections typically cause splenomegaly, including infectious mononucleosis associated with Epstein-Barr virus (Chapter 385) and viral hepatitis (Chapters 150 and 151). Splenomegaly can accompany HIV infection. Splenic abscesses, which are usually the result of hematogenous spread of pyogenic organisms, represent an unusual and difficult to diagnose cause of splenomegaly.

Splenomegaly is also seen in a variety of benign disorders of the immune system, including rheumatoid arthritis (Chapter 272); some of these patients have Felty's syndrome and accompanying granulocytopenia. Splenomegaly can be detected in some patients with systemic lupus erythematosus (Chapter 274), certain drug reactions, and serum sickness.

Malignancies of the immune system and nonimmune organs can also lead to splenomegaly. Splenomegaly is usually seen in patients with chronic myeloid leukemia and is frequent in chronic lymphoid leukemia (Chapter 190). It can develop in patients with acute myeloid or lymphoid leukemia, non-Hodgkin's lymphoma, Hodgkin's disease, and Waldenström's macroglobulinemia but is rare in multiple myeloma (Chapter 193). Isolated splenomegaly (i.e., without any enlarged lymph nodes) is characteristic of certain immune system malignancies, including hairy cell leukemia (Chapter 190), the prolymphocytic variant of chronic lymphocytic leukemia (Chapter 190), and splenic marginal zone lymphoma (Chapter 191). Metastasis of carcinomas and sarcomas to the spleen is unusual except for malignant melanoma; even with melanoma, however, palpable splenomegaly is an unusual finding.

Splenomegaly can develop as a result of increased pressure in the splenic circulation, especially in patients with portal hypertension caused by a variety of hepatic disorders, including alcoholic cirrhosis (Chapter 155). However, it also can be due to splenic or portal vein thrombosis.

Hematologic disorders that can lead to palpable splenomegaly include autoimmune hemolytic anemia, hereditary spherocytosis, and a number of other anemias. In cases of idiopathic myelofibrosis, the spleen is frequently a site of extramedullary hematopoiesis (Chapter 169).

A variety of less common conditions can lead to splenomegaly. The storage disorder Gaucher's disease (Chapter 215) usually manifests as splenomegaly. Splenomegaly can be seen in endocrinopathies such as hyperthyroidism (Chapter 233). Sarcoidosis (Chapter 95) and amyloidosis (Chapter 194) can manifest as splenomegaly. *Tropical splenomegaly* is a term used to describe the palpable spleens found in patients who live in tropical areas, for which there may be numerous causes.

DIAGNOSIS

Evaluation of Spleen Size and Function

Physical Examination
The ability to perform an accurate physical examination and determine the presence of an enlarged spleen (Table 171-8) is an important skill, but it is not easily learned. Physical examination of the spleen can be performed with the patient supine or in the right lateral decubitus position. Inspection, percussion, auscultation, and palpation are all important parts of an accurate assessment. It is rare for a spleen to be so large that it is visible and can be seen to move with respiration. However, in patients with such a condition, it is possible to miss splenomegaly by failing to start palpation sufficiently low to find the edge. Occasionally, percussion of the left upper quadrant helps identify an area of dullness that moves with respiration and can lead to the identification of splenomegaly. Spleen size is generally recorded as the number of centimeters the spleen descends below the left costal margin in the midclavicular line on inspiration. Although auscultation is not usually a regular part of splenic examination, the existence of a splenic rub on inspiration can lead to the diagnosis of splenic infarction. The left kidney is sometimes confused with the spleen on physical examination, but its failure to move with respiration in the manner typical for the spleen usually allows its distinction.

Laboratory Evaluation
Laboratory studies are frequently valuable in assessing splenic function. In patients with an absent or nonfunctional spleen, Howell-Jolly bodies will be seen in circulating red blood cells (see Fig. 171-1). Splenic hyperfunction (a condition often referred to as *hypersplenism*) is associated with cytopenias: the spleen is the normal reservoir for a significant proportion of platelets, and this reservoir function can lead to thrombocytopenia in patients with splenomegaly. Patients with autoimmune hemolytic anemia usually have palpable splenomegaly, but patients with idiopathic (immune) thrombocytopenic purpura usually do not.

The spleen can be imaged with ultrasonography, CT, traditional radionuclide scans, and PET (Fig. 171-2). Ultrasonography can provide an accurate determination of spleen size and is easy to repeat. CT frequently gives a better view of the consistency of the spleen and can identify splenic tumors or abscesses that would otherwise be missed. PET can aid in evaluating focal lesions in the spleen. The technetium-labeled liver-spleen scan can be important in identifying liver disease as the cause of splenomegaly; in patients with cryptogenic cirrhosis who are found to have thrombocytopenia, a technetium liver-spleen scan that shows higher activity in the spleen than in the liver might be the first hint of liver disease.

Because of the spleen's location and its propensity to bleed, needle aspiration or cutting needle biopsy of the spleen is rarely performed. In general, splenic "biopsy" involves splenectomy, which can be performed at the time of laparotomy or via laparoscopy. However, performing splenectomy laparoscopically usually leads to maceration of the organ and can reduce the diagnostic information. In very young children, in whom splenectomy leads to a high risk for serious infections such as pneumococcal septicemia, partial splenectomy can sometimes be performed. Patients who undergo splenectomy at the time of splenic trauma and rupture may have seeding of splenic cells to other sites in the abdomen. Some patients have additional small or accessory spleens. Persistent, functional splenic tissue can be the explanation for recurrent immune thrombocytopenia after splenectomy and might be recognized by the absence of Howell-Jolly bodies in circulating red blood cells.

An Approach to the Patient with Splenomegaly
Patients with splenomegaly (Table 171-9) may come to medical attention for a variety of reasons. Patients may complain of left upper quadrant pain or fullness or early satiety. A splenic infarct, which typically manifests as left upper quadrant pain that sometimes radiates to the left shoulder, can be the first clue to the existence of an enlarged spleen. Rarely, splenomegaly initially manifests with the catastrophic symptoms of splenic rupture. Some patients are found to have splenomegaly as a result of evaluation for unexplained cytopenia. Splenomegaly can also be discovered incidentally on physical examination. In recent years, splenomegaly has frequently been discovered on imaging studies of the abdomen performed for other purposes.

The presence of a palpable spleen on physical examination is almost always abnormal. The one exception to this rule is a palpable spleen tip in a slender young woman. In general, the presence of a palpable spleen should be

FIGURE 171-2. Enlarged spleen with metastatic adenocarcinoma.

TABLE 171-8   METHODS FOR EVALUATING THE SPLEEN

Physical examination
Imaging
    Ultrasonography
    Computed tomography
    Liver-spleen scanning
    Positron emission tomography
Biopsy
    Needle aspiration
    Splenectomy
        Laparotomy (total or partial splenectomy)
        Laparoscopy

TABLE 171-9   APPROACH TO THE PATIENT WITH SPLENOMEGALY

Does the patient have a known illness that causes splenomegaly (e.g., infectious mononucleosis)? Treat and monitor for resolution.

Search for an occult infection (e.g., infectious endocarditis), hematologic disorder (e.g., hereditary spherocytosis), occult liver disease (e.g., cryptogenic cirrhosis), autoimmune disease (e.g., systemic lupus erythematosus), or storage disease (e.g., Gaucher's disease). If found, manage appropriately.

If systemic symptoms are present and suggest malignancy, focal replacement of the spleen is seen on imaging studies, and no other site is available for biopsy, splenectomy is indicated.

If none of the above are true, monitor closely and repeat studies until the splenomegaly resolves or a diagnosis becomes apparent.

considered a serious finding, and an explanation should be sought. It is less clear whether the same rules apply to borderline splenomegaly discovered incidentally on routine imaging studies.

The approach to a patient with an enlarged spleen should focus initially on excluding a systemic illness that could explain the splenomegaly. Infectious mononucleosis, leukemia or lymphoma, rheumatoid arthritis, sarcoidosis, cirrhosis of the liver, malaria, and a host of other illnesses would be reasonable explanations for the splenomegaly. The systemic condition should be treated, and then the spleen should be re-evaluated. If the systemic illness can be treated successfully, the spleen should regress to normal size over time.

Patients with no obvious explanation for an enlarged spleen present a difficult diagnostic problem. Careful follow-up of these patients sometimes reveals occult liver disease or an autoimmune process that initially defied diagnosis. Concerns about malignancy, particularly in patients with systemic symptoms such as fever, sweats, or weight loss or in whom imaging studies show a focal abnormality, are sometimes indications for splenectomy. However, in the absence of such findings, it is generally preferable to monitor patients closely with repeated attempts to establish the diagnosis by approaches other than splenectomy. It is particularly important to avoid splenectomy in a patient with occult liver disease and portal hypertension.

Splenectomy was once performed routinely as part of the staging evaluation for Hodgkin's disease or other lymphomas. Today, this procedure is rarely needed to choose the correct therapy, and it should be avoided. Splenectomy can be an effective therapy for immune thrombocytopenic purpura (Chapter 175) and autoimmune hemolytic anemia (Chapter 163), and it is occasionally an appropriate therapy to relieve cytopenias in other conditions such as advanced myelofibrosis (Chapter 169).

SUGGESTED READINGS

Casaccia M, Torelli P, Cavaliere D, et al. Laparoscopic lymph node biopsy in intra-abdominal lymphoma: high diagnostic accuracy achieved with a minimally invasive procedure. *Surg Laparosc Endosc Percutan Tech.* 2007;17:175-178. *Laparoscopic procedures increase the number of patients who can have excisional biopsy.*

Casaccia M, Torelli P, Pasa A, et al. Putative predictive parameters for the outcome of laparoscopic splenectomy: a multicenter analysis performed on the Italian Registry of Laparoscopic Surgery of the Spleen. *Ann Surg.* 2010;251:287-291. *Only 6% of planned laparoscopic splenectomies were converted to open procedures, with an overall perioperative death rate of 0.4%.*

Feng K, Ma K, Liu Q, et al. Randomized clinical trial of splenic radiofrequency ablation versus splenectomy for severe hypersplenism. *Br J Surg.* 2011;98:354-361. *Ablation is an attractive alternative for hypersplenism induced by liver cirrhosis, particularly when more than 50% of the spleen is ablated.*

Harris A, Kamishima T, Hao HY, et al. Splenic volume measurements on computed tomography utilizing automatically contouring software and its relationship with age, gender, and anthropometric parameters. *Eur J Radiol.* 2010;75:e97-e101. *Normal spleen size correlates with age, body weight, body mass index, and body surface area.*

Yong M, Thomsen RW, Schoonen WM, et al. Mortality risk in splenectomised patients: a Danish population-based cohort study. *Eur J Intern Med.* 2010;21:12-16. *Most of the increased risk is due to the underlying indication for splenectomy, not to the splenectomy itself.*

172

DISORDERS OF PHAGOCYTE FUNCTION

MICHAEL GLOGAUER

Neutrophils and monocyte-macrophages are the key phagocytes of the innate immune system. Their principal innate immune role is to recognize and eliminate microorganisms that make their way past primary physical barriers, such as the epithelium and body secretions that protect the external and lining surfaces of the body. Phagocytes identify foreign invaders through a series of pattern recognition receptors, the majority of which belong to the Toll-like receptor family (Chapters 44 and 47). Whereas macrophages carry out sentinel duty looking for microbes in healthy tissue and act as a bridge between the innate and adaptive immune systems, neutrophils appear only in infected or damaged tissue after being recruited by inflammatory mediators released from activated macrophages and endothelial cells or by chemical signals released by invading microorganisms themselves (Table 172-1). After accumulation of these key immune cells at sites of infection, the microbes are eliminated through the process of phagocytosis, which is defined as the engulfment, internalization, and degradation of extracellular material.

● NEUTROPHILS

Neutrophils develop in the bone marrow from myeloid precursors, migrate into the circulation, and, if required, make their way into infected or damaged

TABLE 172-1	PRIMARY IMMUNE ROLES OF MONOCYTE-MACROPHAGES AND NEUTROPHILS

MONONUCLEAR PHAGOCYTE FUNCTIONS

Elimination of invading pathogens
Elimination of cellular debris from sites of tissue damage and the blood stream
Wound healing-remodeling of normal tissue
Amplification of the innate immune response: release of immune regulators
Bridge to the adaptive immune system: presentation of antigens to lymphocytes

NEUTROPHILS

Elimination of invading pathogens

tissue (Fig. 172-1). Their travels are essentially one-way trips because once they leave a compartment, they do not return. After release from the bone marrow compartment, a mature neutrophil has a blood half-life of about 10 hours and may survive up to an additional 48 hours within infected or damaged tissue.

The Bone Marrow Compartment: The Site of Granulopoiesis

Neutrophils are the most abundant white blood cell and account for up to 70% of circulating leukocytes. Neutrophil numbers can increase rapidly by as much as 5- to 10-fold during periods of acute infection. Because these cells have a very short half-life in blood, the bone marrow compartment provides a steady supply of mature neutrophils with the capability to upregulate cell production rapidly during times of infection. Neutrophils originate in the bone marrow from a common population of hematopoietic stem cells through a 10- to 14-day process of proliferation, differentiation, and maturation (Chapter 159).

Steps in Granulopoiesis

The stages of neutrophil granulopoiesis in the bone marrow (Fig. 172-2) are divided and identified by the major transitions from the pluripotent stem cell to the mature neutrophil. The *myeloblast* is the first recognizable progenitor cell committed to granulopoiesis. This proliferating cell is characterized by its large nucleus and agranular cytoplasm. The *promyelocyte* follows and displays the initial development of primary granules. *Myelocytes* occupy the next stage of neutrophil maturation and are characterized by development of the first specific or "secondary" (peroxidase-negative) granules. *Metamyelocytes,* which follow myelocytes, are incapable of further mitosis and are readily identifiable by their now numerous cytoplasmic granules. The functional maturation of metamyelocytes results in the development of *band* cells, which are usually slightly larger than mature neutrophils and have a 15-μm diameter, a horseshoe-shaped nucleus, and a moderate to abundant supply of specific granules. Band cells can be found in the circulation during periods of acute infection. The final mature *neutrophil,* which is released into the circulation, has a diameter of approximately 10 μm with a characteristic nucleus that is segmented and multilobed and occupies about 20% of the cell's volume; the remaining cytoplasm is taken up by granules.

Defects in granulopoiesis are manifested clinically as low circulating levels of neutrophils (neutropenia; Chapter 170). Verification of the stage at which neutrophil developmental arrest occurs can be determined by a bone marrow biopsy to assess the cellularity and characteristics of the neutrophil precursors present in the marrow space.

Regulation of Granulopoiesis

Granulopoiesis is driven by hematopoietic growth factors (Chapter 159). These factors, which are synthesized by a variety of cells, including fibroblasts and endothelial cells, are known to work together with other regulatory molecules, such as cytokines, to regulate hematopoiesis. Hematopoietic growth factors such as *interleukin-3* (IL-3), *granulocyte-macrophage colony-stimulating factor* (GM-CSF), and *granulocyte colony-stimulating factor* (G-CSF) bind to their target cells through specific receptors and are critical for the hematopoietic system to respond rapidly to infection or inflammation by dramatically increasing the production of leukocytes.

G-CSF is a potent cytokine that influences the proliferation, survival, maturation, and functional activation of cells from the neutrophil-granulocyte lineage. In normal individuals, circulating levels of G-CSF are very low (<100 pg/mL). However, in conditions of stress, G-CSF levels can rise to 20 times baseline levels, thereby resulting in a rapid increase in circulating neutrophils. G-CSF may regulate this increased granulopoiesis by increasing the

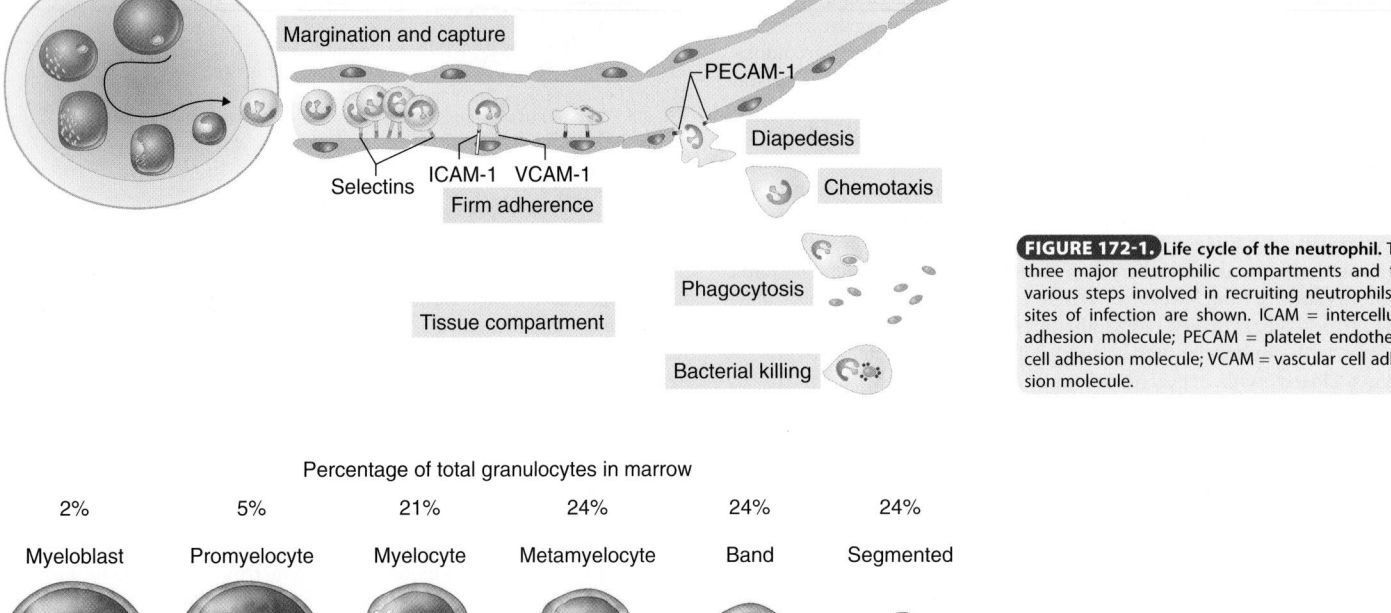

FIGURE 172-1. Life cycle of the neutrophil. The three major neutrophilic compartments and the various steps involved in recruiting neutrophils to sites of infection are shown. ICAM = intercellular adhesion molecule; PECAM = platelet endothelial cell adhesion molecule; VCAM = vascular cell adhesion molecule.

FIGURE 172-2. Cellular stages of granulopoiesis in bone marrow.

TABLE 172-2 MEMBRANE AND MATRIX COMPONENTS OF NEUTROPHILIC GRANULES

COMPONENT	AZUROPHIL GRANULES (PRIMARY; PEROXIDASE POSITIVE)	SPECIFIC GRANULES (SECONDARY; PEROXIDASE NEGATIVE)	GELATINASE GRANULES (TERTIARY; PEROXIDASE NEGATIVE)	SECRETORY VESICLES
Antimicrobial proteins	Defensins Lysozyme Elastase Myeloperoxidase Cathepsin G	Lysozyme Lactoferrin	Lysozyme	
Membrane proteins and receptors	CD63 CD68 Alkaline phosphatase	CD11b fMLP-R Cytochrome b_{558} CR3	CD11b fMLP-R Cytochrome b_{558} CR3 CD45	CD11b fMLP-R Cytochrome b_{558} CR1 CD14 CD16
Matrix proteins	β-Glucuronidase	Collagenase Gelatinase Laminin	Gelatinase	Albumin

Modified from Edwards SW. *Biochemistry and Physiology of the Neutrophil.* Cambridge, UK: Cambridge University Press; 2005:55.

mitotic pool at the promyelocyte and myelocyte stages and shortening neutrophil transit time in bone marrow.

Neutrophil Granules

One of the major mechanisms used by neutrophils to eliminate bacteria is a remarkable arsenal of antimicrobial proteins that are packed into cytoplasmic granules (Table 172-2). These antimicrobial proteins are securely contained within their respective granules and are released only when granules fuse with phagosomes or directly with the plasma membrane. Granulogenesis begins between the myeloblast and promyelocyte stages of neutrophil development and continues throughout the differentiation and maturation process of the cell. *Azurophilic* granules, which make up 30% of granules in a mature neutrophil, are the first to appear at the promyelocyte stage; they contain hydrolytic enzymes, microbicidal peptides, and myeloperoxidase. The *secondary,* or *specific*, granules appear later, beginning at the metamyelocyte stage; they are twice as abundant in the cytoplasm as azurophilic granules and contain

proteins such as collagenase and lactoferrin. The *gelatinase-containing,* or *tertiary,* granules also appear at the metamyelocyte stage. A fourth category of granules, *secretory vesicles,* appear at the very final stages of neutrophil maturation, immediately before release of the cell into the circulation. All the granule types contain membrane proteins such as CR1, CR3, CD45, CD11c, and fMLP (*N*-formyl-methionyl-leucyl-phenylalanine) receptors, which are rapidly transported to the plasma membrane during activation to enhance neutrophil microbicidal activity.

A number of clinical conditions result from specific defects in granule development and formation. Initial assessment for granule defects can be made by microscopic evaluation of a peripheral blood smear (Chapter 160). Examples of obvious clinical diagnoses made with the peripheral smear include specific granule deficiency, which is characterized by bilobed nuclei in more than 80% of the neutrophils, and a significant decrease in cytoplasmic granularity. Abnormally large cytoplasmic granules are seen in individuals with Chédiak-Higashi syndrome.

The Vascular Compartment

Mature neutrophils are released from the postmitotic bone marrow compartment into the circulation, where they have an approximate lifespan of 8 to 12 hours and either circulate within the center of the blood vessel or attach to its endothelial lining, a process termed *margination*. Marginated neutrophils on the vessel walls are able to detach and reenter the circulation when required. For example, corticosteroids and epinephrine induce a rapid increase in circulating neutrophils by releasing neutrophils from the marginated pool. Neutrophils circulate until they are recruited to a site of infection. The initial phase of recruitment involves changes in the endothelial cell surface receptors lining the capillary beds closest to the site of infection or tissue damage. These critical changes in endothelial cells are mediated by immune regulators released by tissue macrophages, which initially detect the tissue damage or bacterial invasion. Emigration of circulating neutrophils from the vasculature to the site of infection or tissue damage requires three steps (see Fig. 172-1): capture and margination, firm adhesion to the endothelial wall, and diapedesis.

Margination and Capture

The marginated pool of neutrophils consists of neutrophils transiently retained against the walls of pulmonary capillaries and postcapillary venules. In the 20-μm diameter of a postcapillary venule, the smaller and faster circulating red blood cells displace the slower-moving and larger neutrophils, which move to the vessel margins, where a low-affinity molecular interaction occurs between surface adhesion molecules of the neutrophil and the endothelial cells. This interaction results in neutrophil rolling and capture along the vessel walls, an event that requires the specific neutrophil receptors *leukocyte selectin* (L-selectin) and the corresponding endothelial ligand, sLe. L-selectin is constitutively expressed in neutrophils, with highest expression in young circulating neutrophils and gradual decline with a cell's age, probably because previous margination events have depleted the receptor. The endothelial ligand for L-selectin, sLe, is a sialylated carbohydrate linked to a mucin-like molecule that can be upregulated by bacterial lipopolysaccharide or other mediators of inflammation. The selectin-ligand interactions are reversible and serve to promote and maintain accumulation of circulating neutrophils on inflamed endothelium.

Adherence to the Endothelial Wall

Low-affinity, selectin-mediated transient interactions must be replaced by high-affinity, adhesive contacts between neutrophils and endothelial cells. During an acute inflammatory event, mediators derived from bacteria, damaged host cells, complement activation, or other immune cells are released from the site of infection and diffuse to the capillary beds, where they induce an immediate and transient vascular response that results in vascular leakage, which further encourages neutrophil margination. Endothelial cells adjacent to the site of inflammation, as well as the activated neutrophils that are bound to them, express integrin receptors that lead to high-affinity attachments between the neutrophils and endothelial cells. These high-affinity connections occur between neutrophil β2 *integrins* and their endothelial counterparts, the intercellular adhesion molecules (ICAMs). Integrins, which are a receptor family of heterodimeric transmembrane glycoproteins made up of an α- and β-subunit, are integral for cell adhesion. Neutrophil β2 integrins consist of three different α-subunits (CD11a, CD11b, and CD11c) that bind to a common β-subunit (CD18). The cytoplasmic tails of these transmembrane receptors possess phosphorylation sites for attachment of signal transduction and cytoskeletal proteins. The neutrophil integrins that mediate this adhesion step are *macrophage antigen-1* (Mac-1; CD11b/CD18) and *lymphocyte-associated function antigen-1* (LFA-1; CD11a/CD18). The receptors are stored in the neutrophil granule compartments to facilitate quick transfer to the plasma membrane during cell stimulation. The integrins bind to endothelial ICAM-1 and ICAM-2 and *vascular cell adhesion molecule-1* (VCAM-1), which are upregulated on the endothelial cell membranes when a cell is exposed to inflammatory cytokines. L-selectin receptors on neutrophils are concentrated on microvillus projections of the cell membrane, whereas the integrins are restricted to the body of the neutrophil. As a result, soon after initial contact during rolling interactions, the projections retract, thereby allowing integrins to interact with their ligands.

Diapedesis

Firm adherence through the L-selectin and integrin receptors facilitates transendothelial migration, or diapedesis, which marks the "point of no return"

in the process of neutrophil recruitment to the site of injury. Unlike rolling and firm adhesion, which require heterophilic interactions between one class of molecules on the neutrophil and another class of molecules on the endothelial cell, diapedesis involves homophilic interactions between the same class of molecules on both cells—the *platelet-endothelial cell adhesion molecule-1* (PECAM-1 or CD31). PECAM-1 is expressed evenly on the surface of neutrophils and concentrated at endothelial cell junctions. Once firmly bound to the endothelial cell surface, neutrophils migrate between the closest tricellular endothelial cell junctions through interactions with PECAM-1 receptors. The neutrophil has now entered the tissue compartment, where it is primed for its final critical role in the elimination of microorganisms and cellular debris.

Laboratory Evaluation of Margination and Firm Adhesion

A defect in neutrophil margination or adhesion to the endothelial lining of the vascular compartment results in neutrophilia (elevated circulating neutrophil levels). This condition is usually associated with leukocyte adhesion deficiency (LAD), which is the result of a lack of CD11/CD18 receptor surface expression in peripheral blood neutrophils. If LAD is suspected, surface expression of these receptors can be measured with a flow cytometer and specific antibodies to CD11, CD18, or CD15 receptors.

The Tissue Compartment
Chemotaxis

Chemotaxis is the directed movement of cells up a chemical concentration gradient of a *chemoattractant*. Chemoattractants are soluble proteins or peptides, including bacterial products, complement factors, and chemokines produced by both inflammatory and noninflammatory cells, that are released from damaged or infected tissue. A concentration difference of 1% at the opposite ends of the neutrophil is sufficient to activate neutrophil chemotaxis. Once a chemoattractant binds to its corresponding neutrophil membrane receptor, a series of cytoplasmic signaling pathways leads to activation of the neutrophil cytoskeleton. This activation results in the neutrophil assuming a polarized state characterized by an actin-rich leading lamella or pseudopod that drives cell motility.

Directional cell crawling, the intrinsic basis of chemotaxis, can be broken down into smaller processes, including extension of the cell membrane, adhesion to the tissue matrix, and contraction of the cell body in an organized and reversible manner. The actin-dependent protrusion of the leading edge, which is a sheetlike structure rich in actin filaments, is critical for normal neutrophil motility. The actin filaments within these lamellar regions are assembled into highly organized structures that push the membrane forward. These structures are formed by different collections of actin-binding proteins under the regulation of specific signal transduction cascades linking chemotactic receptors with cell movement. Defects in actin assembly also result in defects in chemotaxis and recurrent infections.

Actin Assembly Biology

Actin filaments are polar structures, with each end differing in its equilibrium-binding constant for actin monomers (Fig. 172-3). Filaments grow at the high-affinity or barbed end, whereas depolymerization occurs at the low-affinity or pointed end. This difference, generated by the ability of actin to bind and hydrolyze adenosine triphosphate, provides a physical polarity that regulatory proteins use to drive filament dynamics with high temporal and spatial precision. Three classes of proteins regulate the availability of high-affinity actin filament ends: filament-nucleating proteins (e.g., ARP2/3 de novo nucleation), filament-capping proteins (e.g., gelsolin), and filament-severing proteins (e.g., cofilin). Actin-nucleating factors bind actin monomers under conditions otherwise unfavorable for assembly and generate a new filament with a free high-affinity end available for assembly. Actin filament-capping proteins bind to the high-affinity filament end and regulate the addition of monomers by their presence or absence at the end of the filament. Actin-binding proteins are regulated by various second messengers, including calcium. On stimulation, localized changes in the intracellular Ca^{2+} concentration lead to the rapid initiation of actin assembly and disassembly. The changes in actin filament length and the extent of cross-linkage between the filaments may account for the directional extension of actin-rich lamellae and contraction of the tail-like uropod at the other end of the cell. Movement in the neutrophil is therefore the result of lamellar protrusions resulting from the growth of actin filaments. Actin-rich lamellae will continue to be maintained as long as the neutrophil detects the chemoattractant gradient.

Actin Assembly Regulation: Barbed End Regulation

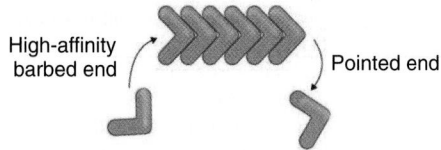

A. ARP 2/3 de novo nucleation

B. Capped barbed end

C. Cofilin-mediated severing

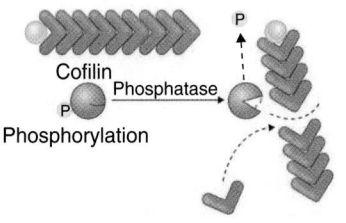

FIGURE 172-3. Regulation of actin assembly through the generation of free barbed ends by actin-binding proteins. **A,** The components below join together to form a nucleation complex (above). **B,** PIP_2 binds the capping protein, leading to its removal from the high-affinity end, allowing for addition and filament growth. **C,** A phosphatase removes the P from cofilin, thereby allowing it to sever the actin filament and leaving a free high affinity end. PIP_2 = phosphatidylinositol 4,5-biphosphate; WASP = Wiskott-Aldrich syndrome protein.

Laboratory Evaluation of Chemotaxis

A defect in neutrophil chemotaxis can be measured in the laboratory with a Boyden chamber, which uses a porous membrane to separate isolated neutrophils from a chemoattractant. A chemical gradient develops across the porous membrane and activates the neutrophils to crawl through the membrane toward the compartment containing the chemoattractant. Defects in chemotaxis can be determined by a lack of neutrophil transmigration through the membrane compared with control neutrophils from a healthy donor.

Phagocytosis

Phagocytosis is the process whereby neutrophils engulf and internalize invading pathogens into membrane compartments called *phagosomes*. Bacterial targets are "highlighted" or opsonized by antibodies (immunoglobulin G) or products from the classical complement pathway that coat the target and serve to mediate phagocytic adhesion. Neutrophilic phagocytosis involves two separate classes of receptors: *Fcγ receptors* (CD32 and CD16) for antibody-coated targets and *complement receptors* (CR1 and CR3) for complement-coated targets. CD32 and CR3 are functional receptors directly involved in neutrophilic phagocytosis, whereas CD16 and CR1 are coreceptors that assist their mate in completing binding and internalization. Activation of Fcγ receptors brings about phosphorylation of their cytoplasmic *immunoreceptor tyrosine-based activation motifs* (ITAMs) through activation of *Src family kinases;* the result is transduction of signals that induce extension of pseudopods, including signaling to the small Rho family of small guanosine triphosphatases (GTPases). These GTPases are responsible for the assembly of actin filaments, thereby leading to remodeling of the plasma membrane and the formation of actin-rich pseudopods, which are essential for the ingestion of particles and formation of phagosomes.

Laboratory Evaluation of Phagocytosis

Neutrophils can be incubated with fluorescently labeled bacteria after opsonization with serum from either the patient or a control. Phagocytosis is assessed by flow cytometry, which measures the increase in neutrophilic fluorescence after uptake of the fluorescently tagged bacteria.

Bacterial Killing

Phagocytes use two potent mechanisms for killing bacteria within the membrane-bound phagosome. The first involves fusion of the previously described storage granules with the phagosome to deliver microbicidal and lytic enzymes into the membrane compartment that contains the ingested microorganisms. The second mechanism uses a multiprotein enzyme complex to generate microbicidal oxidants through partial reduction of oxygen. The multiprotein enzyme complex known as reduced nicotinamide adenine dinucleotide phosphate (NADPH) oxidase generates oxidants by means of oxygen consumption, hence the term *respiratory burst.*

The NADPH enzyme system is made up of four essential polypeptide subunits that are denoted by their molecular weight (kD) and the superscript phox, which denotes phagocyte oxidase. Within the cytoplasmic membrane, the subunits p22^{phox} and gp91^{phox} bind the electron-carrying components of the oxidase (NADPH, a flavin adenine dinucleotide, and two nonidentical hemes) and form the cytochrome b_{558} redox center of the oxidase complex. Cellular activation by inflammatory mediators results in the addition of two cytosolic components, p47^{phox} and p67^{phox}, to the complex along with the Rac small GTPase.

The membrane-bound electron transport chain NADPH oxidase catalyzes the reduction of molecular oxygen to superoxide (O_2^-). The superoxide generated by this process is in turn catalytically converted to hydrogen peroxide and serves as a cosubstrate for myeloperoxidase to oxidize halides and produce hypochlorous acid (HOCl), a very potent antimicrobial agent. These oxidants are able to kill bacteria within the phagosomes by oxidizing their cellular constituents.

Laboratory Evaluation of the Respiratory Burst and Bacterial Killing

Flow cytometry, a rapid and effective method for quantitatively assessing the respiratory burst, measures the fluorescence generated by cytoplasmic fluorescent probes such as dihydrorhodamine, which is converted to rhodamine by H_2O_2. The nitroblue tetrazolium (NBT) test is still used for rapid assessment of the respiratory burst when flow cytometry is not available.

Bacterial killing assays using a patient's neutrophils with either the patient's or control serum and bacteria such as *Staphylococcus aureus* or *Escherichia coli* are a definitive method to determine whether a given patient's neutrophils have an intracellular killing defect. Neutrophils from a healthy control subject phagocytose and kill approximately 95% of the bacteria within 2 hours. In assays in which an intracellular killing defect is present, neutrophils kill less than 10% of bacteria over a 2-hour period. It is necessary to confirm that there is no phagocytic defect before performing the bacterial killing assay to be sure that any defect in bacterial killing is not due to an internalization defect.

Neutrophil Extracellular Traps

It has recently been shown that neutrophils use a newly identified extracellular process to contain and kill bacteria. Neutrophil extracellular traps (NETs) are formed by the release of chromatin and antimicrobial proteins from the neutrophil cytoplasm and granules. The chromatin forms a netlike meshwork that traps the bacteria and brings them in closer proximity to the antimicrobial elements adhered to the chromatin. Activation of NET formation requires simultaneous activation by at least two different receptors and reactive oxygen species are essential to the process. IL-8 has been shown to be a potent activator of NET formation. The importance of NETs was highlighted by work showing that DNase expressing strains of GAS and *Streptococcus pneumoniae* are more virulent than their non-DNase-expressing counterparts because of their ability to escape NETs. The importance of this antibacterial function of neutrophils will become clearer in the years to come.

Clinical Manifestations of Phagocytic Defects

In addition to fever and recurrent infections, the most common findings in patients with phagocytic defects are oral infections resulting in gingival inflammation, periodontal bone loss, mobile or loose teeth, and premature

TABLE 172-3	SYMPTOMS SUGGESTIVE OF A PHAGOCYTIC DISORDER

Recurrent infections that fail to resolve with conventional treatment
Recurrent infections of unusual severity
Recurrent infections in the lung, liver, or bone
Normally nonpathogenic bacteria or fungi identified in cultures from the infection sites
Aphthous ulcers
Severe periodontal diseases, including gingivitis
Lymphadenopathy or hepatosplenomegaly
Severe recurrent cutaneous infections with *Staphylococcus aureus*
Recurrent mycobacterial infections

loss of teeth (Table 172-3). An oral examination should be performed at the initial evaluation, followed by a full dental examination, depending on the findings. The history and laboratory tests can differentiate among the various clinical causes of disordered phagocytosis (Table 172-4).

DEFECTS IN LEUKOCYTE ADHESION

A defect in neutrophil adhesion to the endothelial lining leads to neutrophilia—an accumulation of neutrophils in the circulation, with very few neutrophils at sites of infection. Defects in neutrophil adhesion can be induced by drugs or due to a genetic defect. Drugs such as corticosteroids and epinephrine result in a transient leukocyte adhesive defect that results in an apparent dramatic increase in circulating neutrophils because of release of the marginated neutrophil pool. The major genetic disease that results in an adhesion deficiency is termed *leukocyte adhesion deficiency.*

Leukocyte Adhesion Deficiency
LAD-I
LAD-I is an autosomal recessive inherited disorder in which patients have a mutation in the gene encoding CD18. The result is a deficiency of β2 integrin receptors, which are required for neutrophil migration from the vasculature into the tissues, thereby impairing the binding of neutrophils to C3bi and endothelial ICAM-1 and ICAM-2.

Patients have soft tissue bacterial and fungal infections, delayed wound healing, impaired pus formation, and severe destructive periodontitis with rapid tooth loss. This condition is also characterized by delayed separation of the umbilical cord. Patients usually die during childhood. Flow cytometry is used to measure CD11/CD18 surface expression levels on neutrophils.

Treatment is mainly supportive with prophylactic antibiotics in patients with recurrent infections. In severe cases, bone marrow transplantation is the treatment of choice.

LAD-II AND LAD-III
LAD-II, a variant of LAD-I, is associated with neutrophilia, the Bombay (hh) blood phenotype, dwarfism, and mental retardation. This disorder is due to a mutation in the guanosine diphosphate-fucose transporter gene, which results in impaired expression of CD15s and other selectin ligands. Symptoms are similar to those of LAD-I, and the diagnosis is confirmed by flow cytometry for CD15s. In the most recently described LAD-III, there is a primary activation defect in all three β integrins 1, 2, and 3, and mutations have been found in Kindlin 3, which binds the cytoplasmic tail of integrin.

DEFECTS IN NEUTROPHILIC CHEMOTAXIS

After phagocytes enter the tissue compartment from the vascular pool, they migrate up the concentration gradients of various chemoattractants to the site of focal infection. A number of chemotactic defects result in severe recurrent infections.

Hyperimmunoglobin E Syndrome
Hyperimmunoglobin E syndrome, or hyper-IgE syndrome, also referred to as Job's syndrome, is a group of genetically diverse, multisystem disorders of cytokine signaling. The most common form of the syndrome involves dominant mutations in the gene for signal transducer and activator of transcription 3 (*STAT3*). The neutrophilic disorder is characterized by recurrent skin abscesses, pneumonia, and periodontal diseases. After birth, patients usually have moderate to severe dermatitis, eczematous skin eruptions, nonerythematous abscesses, pneumatoceles, and severe osteoporosis that can result in bone fractures. The organisms most commonly present at infected sites are *S. aureus*, *Haemophilus influenzae*, *E. coli*, and *Candida albicans*. Patients have

elevated IgE levels and eosinophilia. The defect in neutrophilic chemotaxis is less severe than that in Chédiak-Higashi syndrome (see later). Treatment is prophylactic antibiotics and aggressive treatment of infections. In severe cases, bone marrow transplantation may be considered.

Familial Mediterranean Fever
Familial Mediterranean fever (Chapter 269), also known as recurrent polyserositis, is an autosomal recessive inflammatory disease that is widespread among people of Mediterranean descent, including Arabs, Armenians, and Sephardic Jews. The genetic defect is a missense mutation in the *MEFV* gene, which encodes the protein pyrin. Pyrin is believed to be a transcription factor involved in downregulating inflammation, possibly through an effect on chemotaxis in neutrophils and monocytes. The *MEFV* mutation results in a hyperinflammatory response characterized by abundant neutrophilic infiltration into the peritoneal, pleural, and joint spaces.

The most common findings include acute, self-limited attacks of fever accompanied by pleuritis, peritonitis, arthritis, pericarditis, and erythematous skin lesions. Although first attacks may be observed during infancy, clinical disease commonly occurs in childhood or adolescence.

Leukocytosis has been observed during attacks, but the leukocyte count is normal between episodes. Genetic testing is available for the most common mutations. This disease can be fatal if renal failure develops as a result of amyloidosis (Chapter 194), which occurs in up to 25% of those affected.

The hyperinflammatory attacks can be reduced significantly with 0.6 mg of prophylactic colchicine orally two or three times daily. The prognosis is generally good for most affected individuals maintained with colchicine.

DISORDERS OF NEUTROPHILIC DEGRANULATION

Granules supply key membrane proteins, including receptors required for phagocytosis. Granule-related defects result in profound defects in bacterial killing.

Chédiak-Higashi Syndrome
Chédiak-Higashi syndrome is a rare autosomal recessive disorder of the *LYST* gene, which encodes a protein responsible for lysosomal trafficking. Defective targeting of granules to the membrane results in large cytoplasmic granules that are unable to target to the plasma membrane in neutrophils, monocytes, and lymphocytes.

Symptoms are recurrent bacterial infections of the skin, mouth, and respiratory tract; partial albinism; peripheral neuropathy; and mild bleeding disorders as a result of a deficiency in serotonin- and adenosine phosphate–containing granules in platelets. Defects in myelopoiesis result in neutropenia. Death usually occurs by 7 years of age because of infection. Advanced disease is characterized by lymphocytic tissue infiltrates and pancytopenia.

Giant cytoplasmic granules are seen in the peripheral blood smear. Neutrophil function testing shows defects in chemotaxis and bacterial killing. Prophylactic antibiotics should be used to prevent infections. Bone marrow transplantation from an HLA-matched donor may be successful if performed before the disease becomes advanced.

Specific Granule Deficiency
Specific granule deficiency is an autosomal recessive disorder that manifests during infancy as the recurrent appearance of deep and superficial skin infections, respiratory infections, and abscesses. Azurophilic granules in neutrophils lack defensins, gelatinase, cytochrome *b*, and vitamin B_{12}. Neutrophils are morphologically altered and have a bilobed rather than a trilobed nucleus. This disorder is characterized by impaired neutrophil chemotaxis, reduced respiratory burst, and a defect in bacterial killing. Infections are commonly caused by *S. aureus*, *Pseudomonas aeruginosa*, and *C. albicans*. Aggressive treatment of infections is required.

DISORDERS OF OXYGEN-DEPENDENT BACTERIAL KILLING

A genetic defect in any component of the respiratory burst results in delayed or ineffective bacterial killing.

Chronic Granulomatous Disease
PATHOBIOLOGY
Chronic granulomatous disease (CGD) is a genetic disease that occurs in about 1 in 200,000 live births. Neutrophils and macrophages cannot generate

TABLE 172-4 DISORDERS OF PHAGOCYTIC FUNCTION

DISORDER	ETIOLOGY	IMPAIRED FUNCTION	CLINICAL CONSEQUENCE
DEGRANULATION ABNORMALITIES			
Chédiak-Higashi syndrome	Autosomal recessive; disordered coalescence of lysosomal granules Responsible gene found at 1q42-45. The encoded protein (LYST) has structural features homologous to a vacuolar sorting protein	Decreased neutrophilic chemotaxis, degranulation, and bactericidal activity; platelet storage pool defect; impaired NK function; failure to disperse melanosomes	Neutropenia, recurrent pyogenic infections, propensity for the development of marked hepatosplenomegaly in the accelerated phase, partial albinism
Specific granule deficiency	Autosomal recessive; abnormal regulation of various myeloid granule genes by a transacting factor	Impaired chemotaxis and bactericidal activity; bilobed nuclei in neutrophils; reduced content of neutrophil defensins, gelatinase, collagenase, vitamin B_{12}–binding protein, and lactoferrin	Recurrent infections, especially sinopulmonary and skin infections
ADHESION ABNORMALITIES			
Leukocyte adhesion deficiency type 1	Autosomal recessive; absence of CD11/CD18 surface adhesive glycoprotein (β2-integrins) on leukocyte membranes, most commonly arising from failure to express CD18 mRNA	Decreased binding of C3bi to neutrophils and impaired adhesion to ICAM-1 and ICAM-2	Neutrophilia, recurrent bacterial infection associated with lack of pus formation
Leukocyte adhesion deficiency type 2	Autosomal recessive; absence of neutrophil sialyl-Lewis^x	Decreased adhesion to activated endothelium expressing ELAM	Neutrophilia, recurrent bacterial infection without pus
Leukocyte adhesion deficiency type 3	Autosomal recessive; defects in activation of β1, β2, and β3 integrins	Severe leukocyte adhesion dysfunction; abnormal platelet aggregation	Neutrophilia, recurrent bacterial infection without pus, severe bleeding tendency
Neutrophil actin dysfunction	Altered polymerization of neutrophil cytoplasmic actin, perhaps arising from the presence of an inhibitor to F-actin formation	Impaired neutrophil adhesion, chemotaxis, and bacterial killing	Neutrophilia, recurrent bacterial infections without pus
DISORDERS OF CELL CHEMOTAXIS			
Hyperactive Chemotaxis			
Familial Mediterranean fever (FMF)	Autosomal recessive gene responsible for FMF on chromosome 16, which encodes for a protein called pyrin; pyrin may modify neutrophil activation	Excessive accumulation of neutrophils at inflamed sites	Recurrent fever, peritonitis, pleuritis, arthritis, amyloidosis
Depressed Chemotaxis			
Intrinsic defects of the neutrophil, e.g., leukocyte adhesion deficiency, Chédiak-Higashi syndrome, specific granule deficiency, neutrophil actin dysfunction, neonatal neutrophils	In the neonatal neutrophil, there is diminished ability to express β2 integrins and a qualitative impairment in β2 integrin function	Diminished chemotaxis	Propensity for the development of pyogenic infections
Direct inhibition of neutrophil mobility, e.g., drugs	Ethanol, glucocorticoids, cyclic AMP	Impaired locomotion and ingestion, impaired adherence	Possible causes of frequent infections; neutrophilia seen with epinephrine is the result of cyclic AMP release from the endothelium
Immune complexes	Bind to Fc receptors on neutrophils in patients with rheumatoid arthritis, systemic lupus erythematosus, and other inflammatory states	Impaired chemotaxis	Recurrent pyogenic infections
Hyperimmunoglobulin E syndrome	Disorders of cytokine signaling, most commonly due to autosomal dominant mutations in the STAT3 gene	Impaired chemotaxis, impaired IgG opsonization of Staphylococcus aureus	Recurrent skin and sinopulmonary infections
DEFECTS OF MICROBICIDAL ACTIVITY			
Chronic granulomatous disease (CGD)	X-linked and autosomal recessive; failure to express functional gp91^{phox} (in the phagocyte membrane) and p22^{phox} (autosomal recessive). Other autosomal recessive forms of CGD arise from failure to express protein p47^{phox} or p67^{phox}	Failure to activate neutrophil respiratory burst leading to failure to kill catalase-positive microbes	Recurrent pyogenic infections with catalase-positive microorganisms
G6PD deficiency	Less than 5% of normal activity of G6PD	Failure to activate NADPH-dependent oxidase	Infections with catalase-positive microorganisms
Myeloperoxidase deficiency	Autosomal recessive; failure to process modified precursor protein arising from missense mutation	H_2O_2-dependent antimicrobial activity not potentiated by myeloperoxidase	None
Deficiencies of glutathione reductase and glutathione synthetase	Failure to detoxify H_2O_2	Excessive formation of H_2O_2	Minimal problems with recurrent pyogenic infections

TABLE 172-4 DISORDERS OF PHAGOCYTIC FUNCTION—cont'd			
DISORDER	**ETIOLOGY**	**IMPAIRED FUNCTION**	**CLINICAL CONSEQUENCE**
IMPAIRED MACROPHAGE FUNCTION			
Defects in the interferon-γ–IL-12 axis	Interferon-γ receptor ligand-binding chain, interferon-γ receptor signaling chain, IL-12 receptor β1 chain, IL-12 p40 deficiency; the interferon-γ receptor abnormalities may be autosomal dominant or recessive; the IL-12 receptor and IL-12 abnormalities are autosomal recessive	Impaired killing of microorganisms. Fatal BCG infection secondary either to an inability to produce IL-12 by dendritic cells and macrophages or to depressed bactericidal activity of macrophages lacking normal function of the interferon receptor	Infection with atypical mycobacteria, *Salmonella*, and *Listeria*

AMP = adenosine monophosphate; BCG = bacille Calmette-Guérin; ELAM = endothelial leukocyte adhesion molecule; G6PD = glucose-6-phosphate dehydrogenase; ICAM = intracellular adhesion molecule; IL-12 = interleukin-12; NADPH = nicotinamide adenine dinucleotide phosphate; NK = natural killer; phox = phagocyte oxidase.
Modified from Boxer LA. Quantitative abnormalities of granulocytes. In: Beutler E, Lichtman MA, Coller BS, et al, eds. *Williams Hematology*, 6th ed. New York: McGraw-Hill; 2001:836.

superoxide and are therefore unable to kill catalase-positive organisms. This condition results from mutations in one of the four structural genes of the NADPH oxidase complex. The most common genetic defect occurs in the 91-kD component of cytochrome b_{558}, which is coded on the X chromosome. The other mutations are autosomal recessive and have been detected in the 22-, 47-, and 67-kD structural proteins.

CLINICAL MANIFESTATIONS AND DIAGNOSIS

Children are prone to infections or granulomatous lesions in the lungs, skin, and liver. *S. aureus* is the most common organism, but other organisms include *Serratia marcescens*, *Burkholderia cepacia*, *Aspergillus* species, and *Nocardia* species. Staphylococcal liver abscesses are pathognomonic of chronic granulomatous disease. Flow cytometry is used to measure the increase in fluorescence generated when dihydrorhodamine is converted to rhodamine by H_2O_2.

TREATMENT   Rx

Abscesses can be removed by surgery. Trimethoprim-sulfamethoxazole prophylaxis (5 mg/kg/day divided into two equal doses) and antifungal prophylaxis with itraconazole (100 mg/day for <50 kg, 200 mg/day for >50 kg) have been shown to reduce the frequency of infections in these patients. Interferon-γ (50 μg/m² subcutaneously three times per week) prophylaxis is now considered "standard of care" in many centers. Bone marrow transplantation can also be considered for patients with refractory infections. Gene therapy for CGD by gene-modified autologous hematopoietic stem cell transplantation has resulted in transient immune restoration but also genomic instability, monosomy 7, and clonal progression toward myelodysplasia.

Myeloperoxidase Deficiency

Myeloperoxidase deficiency is a relatively common disorder (1 in 4000) in which the enzyme for conversion of neutrophilic hydrogen peroxide to HOCl is absent. This deficiency is not associated with increased susceptibility to infections, probably because of the accumulation of hydrogen peroxide, which is also bactericidal. Myeloperoxidase deficiency is usually asymptomatic, although patients with diabetes mellitus may occasionally experience candidal infections. The diagnosis is made by observation of a negative peroxidase stain of the peripheral blood smear. Symptomatic patients may be treated with prophylactic antibiotics.

Glutathione Synthetase Deficiency

Glutathione, which is a potent antioxidant found in granulocytes, is required for a normal respiratory burst and bacterial killing. Patients with glutathione synthetase deficiency typically have recurrent otitis and hemolytic anemia. The diagnosis is confirmed by verifying low or no glutathione synthetase in red blood cells.

Severe Glucose-6-Phosphate Dehydrogenase Deficiency

Glucose-6-phosphate dehydrogenase (G6PD) deficiency is an X-linked disorder. White individuals with a severe reduction in G6PD activity are subject to recurrent infections, whereas Asians or blacks with similarly reduced G6PD levels are not. G6PD is crucial for regulating the availability of NADPH for the respiratory burst. G6PD deficiency results in recurrent bacterial infections, hemolytic anemia (Chapter 164), and jaundice. The diagnosis can be made with flow cytometry to assess the respiratory burst and to demonstrate the absence of G6PD in all blood cells.

MACROPHAGE-RELATED ABNORMALITIES

Accumulation of monocyte-macrophages at sites of infection occurs after the major influx of neutrophils. Macrophages have a critical role in antigen presentation to lymphocytes, thereby activating the adaptive arm of the immune system. A critical defect in macrophage signaling results in susceptibility to mycobacterial infection.

Interferon-γ Receptor 1 Defects

When macrophages phagocytose mycobacteria, they produce IL-12, which in turn stimulates T cells to produce interferon-γ (IFN-γ). IFN-γ is critical to the killing of mycobacteria and other intracellular bacteria. Patients with recurrent and severe mycobacterial infections who are not infected with human immunodeficiency virus should be assessed for abnormalities in pathways that lead to the generation and utilization of IFN-γ.

Patients with autosomal recessive mutations in the IFN-γ receptors typically have a complete loss of function of the IFN-γ receptors. Autosomal dominant mutations in the IFN-γ receptors result in normal ligand binding but defective intracellular signal transduction because of a cytoplasmically truncated form of the receptor.

Recessive mutations typically manifest as severe disseminated infections and poor formation of granulomas. Multifocal mycobacterial osteomyelitis is pathognomonic of an autosomal dominant mutation in the IFN-γ receptor. Flow cytometry confirms the absence of membrane expression of IFN-γ receptor 1 in the autosomal recessive form and up to ten-fold higher membrane expression levels of the cytoplasmically truncated receptor in the autosomal dominant form.

For patients with autosomal dominant mutations, subcutaneous IFN-γ is effective. For autosomal recessive patients completely lacking IFN-γ receptor function, bone marrow transplantation should be considered. Long-term antibiotic prophylaxis against mycobacterial infections with azithromycin or clarithromycin is recommended.

ASSESSING PHAGOCYTE FUNCTION: MAKING THE DIAGNOSIS

If a phagocyte functional disorder may be the underlying cause of recurrent infections in a patient, a complete blood count (CBC) and peripheral smear guide subsequent definitive testing (Fig. 172-4). Cultures from infected areas allow antimicrobial targeting and also provide critical diagnostic information. If the defect is a result of abnormal neutrophil development and maturation, the CBC will show neutropenia; a bone marrow biopsy might be required. Repeated CBC (twice per week for 6 weeks) is indicated if cyclic neutropenia is suspected because of a periodicity of the infections (Chapter 170).

If the CBC reveals neutrophilia, a defect in the recruitment of neutrophils into tissues is suggested. An assessment of the receptors required for transmigration by flow cytometry and specific antibodies to the surface receptors is indicated.

If circulating levels of phagocytes are normal yet the patient is experiencing recurrent infections, a phagocytic defect within the infected tissue is likely. Laboratory testing to evaluate chemotaxis, phagocytosis, and bacterial killing is indicated.

Finding	Possible diagnosis	Laboratory confirmation testing
Neutrophilia • Rule out chronic infection/inflammation • Rule out myeloproliferative disorders	Leukocyte adhesion deficiency syndrome	FACS for surface receptor expression levels (CD11/CD18) and Slex (CD15) receptor expression levels
Neutropenia	Congenital agranulocytosis, cyclic neutropenia (regular recurrent infections)	Consider bone marrow biopsy; repeat CBC
Abnormal neutrophil morphology	Large cytoplasmic granules—Chédiak-Higashi syndrome Bilobed with decrease in cytoplasmic granules—specific granule deficiency Binucleate neutrophils—myelokethexis MPO deficiency can be diagnosed by the use of appropriate biochemical stains	Special stains to confirm
Normal neutrophil levels and morphology	Chronic granulomatous diseases—(CGD) Abnormal oxidase function Severe deficiency of G6PD or glutathione synthetase—abnormal oxidase function	FACS—DHR reduction or NBT test If CGD ruled out assess G6PD and gluthathione synthetase levels
Normal neutrophil levels, morphology, and oxidase function	Functional phagocyte defect	In order to specifically identify defect consider assays for: Chemotaxis (Boyden Chamber) Phagocytosis (FACS-FL bacteria/beads) Bacterial killing

Obtain cultures (identify pathogens) → Obtain CBC and peripheral smear

FIGURE 172-4. Approach to diagnosing a suspected phagocytic defect. CBC = complete blood count; DHR = dihydrorhodamine; FACS = flow cytometry; FL = fluorescent; G6PD = glucose-6-phosphate dehydrogenase; MPO = myeloperoxidase; NBT = nitroblue tetrazolium.

SUGGESTED READINGS

Bianchi M, Hakkim A, Brinkmann V, et al. Restoration of NET formation by gene therapy in CGD controls aspergillosis. *Blood*. 2009;114:2619-2622. *Positive effects of gene therapy on neutrophils in CGD.*

Bouma G, Ancliff PJ, Thrasher AJ, et al. Recent advances in the understanding of genetic defects of neutrophil number and function. *Br J Haematol*. 2010;151:312-326. *Review.*

Kuhns DB, Alvord WG, Heller T, et al. Residual NADPH oxidase and survival in chronic granulomatous disease. *N Engl J Med*. 2010;363:2600-2610. *Moderate residual production is associated with a significantly better survival.*

Lemos S, Jacob CM, Pastorino AC, et al. Neutropenia in antibody-deficient patients under IVIG replacement therapy. *Pediatr Allergy Immunol*. 2009;20:97-101 *Primary immunodeficient patients, even when treated with IVIg, require monitoring for neutropenia.*

Segal BH, Veys P, Malech H, et al. Chronic granulomatous disease: lessons from a rare disorder. *Biol Blood Marrow Transplant*. 2011;17:S123-S131. *Review.*

EOSINOPHILIC SYNDROMES

MARC E. ROTHENBERG

DEFINITION

Eosinophilic syndromes are a heterogeneous group of disorders that involve eosinophilia, which is defined as the accumulation of eosinophils in peripheral blood and/or tissues. Circulating eosinophils normally account for only 1 to 3% of peripheral blood leukocytes, and the upper limit of the normal range is 350 cells/mm³ of blood. Eosinophilia occurs in a variety of disorders (Table 173-1) and is usually arbitrarily classified according to the degree of blood eosinophilia: mild (351 to 1500 cells/mm³), moderate (>1500 to 5000 cells/mm³), or severe (>5000 cells/mm³). Tissue eosinophilic disorders, such as eosinophil-associated gastrointestinal disorders and eosinophilic fasciitis, are not necessarily associated with blood eosinophilia, so their

TABLE 173-1   CAUSES OF EOSINOPHILIA

REACTIVE EOSINOPHILIA

Allergic diseases—asthma, atopic dermatitis, allergic rhinitis
Drug reactions—including cytokine infusions
Infection—viral (human immunodeficiency virus) or fungal (allergic bronchopulmonary aspergillosis, coccidioidomycosis)
Parasitic infection—mostly helminths

EOSINOPHILIA ASSOCIATED WITH OTHER DISEASES

Eosinophil-associated gastrointestinal disorders—eosinophilic esophagitis, gastroenteritis
Skin—bullous pemphigoid, urticaria, eosinophilic cellulitis, episodic angioedema
Pulmonary—eosinophilic pneumonia, allergic bronchopulmonary aspergillosis
Neurologic—eosinophilic meningitis
Autoimmune—Churg-Strauss syndrome, eosinophilic fasciitis
Primary immunodeficiency—hyperimmunoglobulin E syndrome, Omenn's syndrome
Post-transplantation status—liver (in association with immunosuppression)
Transplant rejection—lung, kidney, liver
Malignancy—Hodgkin's disease, solid tumors
Hypoadrenalism—Addison's disease, adrenal hemorrhage
Renal—drug-induced interstitial nephritis, eosinophilic cystitis, dialysis

PRIMARY CLONAL EOSINOPHILIA

Chronic eosinophilic leukemia
Acute eosinophilic leukemia
Acute myelogenous leukemia with eosinophilia
Acute lymphoblastic leukemia with eosinophilia
Myeloblastic disorders with eosinophilia
Myeloproliferative disorders with eosinophilia
Systemic mastocytosis with eosinophilia
FIP1L1-PDGFRA fusion gene–positive disease

IDIOPATHIC HYPEREOSINOPHILIA

diagnosis is based on the microscopic identification of eosinophil-rich inflammatory infiltrates associated with tissue damage.

Historically, hypereosinophilic syndromes were generally classified as idiopathic and were defined by (1) the presence of eosinophilia (>1500 cells/mm³ for at least 6 months) that remained unexplained despite a comprehensive evaluation for known causes of eosinophilia (such as drug reactions and infections) and (2) evidence of organ dysfunction directly attributable to the eosinophilia. Now, however, it is known that in some patients, a chromosome 4 microdeletion results in the generation of an activated tyrosine kinase (*FIP1L1*-platelet-derived growth factor receptor-α [*PDGFRA*]) that causes a clonal hematologic disorder now better classified as chronic eosinophilic leukemia. Identification of *FIP1L1-PDGFRA*-positive disease has important therapeutic implications because *PDGFRA*-associated disease can be treated with imatinib, a tyrosine kinase inhibitor.

EPIDEMIOLOGY

The most common cause of eosinophilia worldwide is helminth infections, which affect hundreds of millions of people. The most frequent cause in industrialized nations is atopic disease, which affects 10 to 30% of the population. Hypereosinophilic disorders such as *FIP1L1-PDGFRA*-associated disease and Churg-Strauss syndrome (Chapter 278) are very rare. For example, Churg-Strauss syndrome affects 4 to 6 cases per million per year, whereas true idiopathic hypereosinophilic syndromes may affect only 4000 to 5000 people worldwide. Other syndromes such as eosinophil-associated gastrointestinal disorders are more common, with a prevalence of approximately 1 in 10,000 individuals.

PATHOBIOLOGY

Eosinophils are produced in the bone marrow from pluripotential hematopoietic stem cells under regulation of the transcription factor GATA-1 and the cytokines interleukin-3 (IL-3), IL-5, and granulocyte-macrophage colony-stimulating factor (GM-CSF) (Fig. 173-1). Eosinophils are under the regulation of helper type 2 T cells (T_H2) that secrete IL-4, IL-5, and IL-13. Notably, IL-5 is a cytokine that specifically regulates the selective differentiation of eosinophils, their release from bone marrow into the peripheral circulation, and their survival. A humanized anti-IL-5 drug markedly lowers circulating eosinophilia and reduces tissue eosinophilia more modestly. Recent preliminary studies in patients with severe asthma have shown that

anti-IL-5 therapy improves asthma control, including exacerbations, and allows steroid reduction. Similarly, anti-IL-5 has a steroid sparing effect in hypereosinophilic syndromes. Humanized anti-IL-5 therapy is currently in clinical testing for a variety of indications, including eosinophilic esophagitis, asthma, and hypereosinophilic syndromes. IL-4 and IL-13 induce eosinophil recruitment and survival, expression of critical adhesion molecules on the endothelium that bind to the β1 and β2 integrins on eosinophils (such as intercellular adhesion molecule 1 [ICAM-1] and vascular cell adhesion molecule 1 [VCAM-1]), and eosinophil-active chemokines such as the eotaxins. The eotaxins are three structurally related eosinophil chemoattractant and activating proteins that signal exclusively through the eosinophil-selective receptor CCR3. In addition to regulating the baseline homing of eosinophils into various tissues, such as the gastrointestinal tract, wherein most eosinophils reside, the eotaxins are induced by T_H2-associated inflammatory triggers (e.g., IL-13) and thereby promote tissue accumulation of eosinophils. Humanized antibodies against the eotaxins and small-molecule inhibitors against CCR3 are promising new approaches for treating eosinophilic disorders that are in clinical development.

Eosinophil granules contain a crystalloid core composed of major basic protein (MBP-1 and MBP-2), as well as a matrix composed of eosinophil cationic protein (ECP), eosinophil-derived neurotoxin (EDN), and eosinophil peroxidase (EPO). MBP, EPO, and ECP have cytotoxic effects on a variety of tissues in concentrations similar to those found in biologic fluids from patients with eosinophilia. Additionally, ECP and EDN belong to the ribonuclease A superfamily and possess antiviral and ribonuclease activity. ECP can insert voltage-insensitive, ion-nonselective toxic pores into the membranes of target cells, and these pores may facilitate the entry of other toxic molecules. MBP directly increases smooth muscle reactivity by causing dysfunction of vagal muscarinic M₂ receptors, and this process has been postulated to contribute to the airway hyperresponsiveness associated with asthma. MBP also triggers degranulation of mast cells and basophils. Triggering of eosinophils by engagement of receptors for cytokines, immunoglobulins, and complement can lead to the generation of a wide range of inflammatory cytokines, including IL-1, IL-3, IL-4, IL-5, IL-13, GM-CSF, transforming growth factor-α/β, tumor necrosis factor-α, RANTES, macrophage inflammatory protein 1α (MIP-1α), and the eotaxins, thus indicating that eosinophils have the potential to modulate multiple aspects of the immune response. Additionally, eosinophils can directly activate T cells by antigen presentation and help polarize dendritic cells to promote a T_H2 phenotype. Further eosinophil-mediated damage is caused by toxic hydrogen peroxide and halide acids generated by EPO and by superoxide generated by the respiratory burst oxidase enzyme pathway in eosinophils. Eosinophils also generate large amounts of cysteinyl leukotriene C₄ (LTC₄), which is metabolized to LTD₄ and LTE₄. These three lipid mediators increase vascular permeability and mucus secretion and are potent stimulators of smooth muscle contraction. Finally, bipyramidal Charcot-Leyden crystals are derived from a nongranule lysophospholipase in eosinophils and are frequently found in sputum, feces, and tissues infiltrated by eosinophils.

FIGURE 173-1. Schematic representation of eosinophil development, tissue recruitment, and therapeutic intervention. Eosinophil lineage development is specified by the GATA-1 transcription factor and promoted by the cytokines interleukin-3 (IL-3), IL-5, and granulocyte-macrophage colony-stimulating factor (GM-CSF). IL-5 is most selective to the eosinophil lineage and regulates eosinophil movement from the bone marrow into the peripheral blood. Eosinophil adhesion is mediated by β1, β2, and β7 integrins and their interaction with the endothelial adhesion molecules intercellular adhesion molecule 1 (ICAM-1), vascular cell adhesion molecule 1 (VCAM-1), and mucosal address in cell adhesion molecule 1 (MAdCAM-1). Recruitment of eosinophils into tissue is regulated by the eotaxin chemokines that stimulate eosinophilic chemoattraction and activation through their receptor CCR3. Hypereosinophilic syndromes can develop after an 800-kilobase microdeletion on chromosome 4 results in fusion of the *FIP1L1* and *PDGFRA* genes, thereby resulting in activation of an imatinib-sensitive tyrosine kinase. Targeted therapeutic intervention for eosinophilic syndromes includes anti-IL-5 and anti-CCR3/eotaxins, which are currently in clinical development.

CLINICAL MANIFESTATIONS

Hypereosinophilia is often recognized on a routine blood count in a patient who is asymptomatic or being evaluated for unrelated or nonspecific signs or symptoms. On other occasions, the possibility of eosinophilia may be specifically investigated in a patient with gastrointestinal or respiratory symptoms because helminthic disease or allergic causes are suspected. The clinical signs and symptoms of hypereosinophilic syndromes are heterogeneous because of the diversity of the causes and potential organ involvement. Common signs and symptoms include dermatitis, heart failure, neuropathy, and abdominal pain. One of the most serious complications of hypereosinophilia is cardiac disease secondary to endomyocardial thrombus formation and restrictive fibrosis (Chapter 60). Mitral and tricuspid valve regurgitation may result from progressive fibrotic damage to the chordae tendineae, and resultant heart failure can develop from valvular insufficiency and endomyocardial fibrosis. Cardiac involvement can occur in association with eosinophilia from diverse causes, including parasitic infections. Hypereosinophilic syndromes can result in cerebral emboli from cardiac disease, diffuse encephalopathy, and peripheral neuropathy.

DIAGNOSIS

Differential Diagnosis

The differential diagnosis of eosinophilia includes reactive eosinophilia, eosinophilia associated with other primary disorders, and eosinophilia

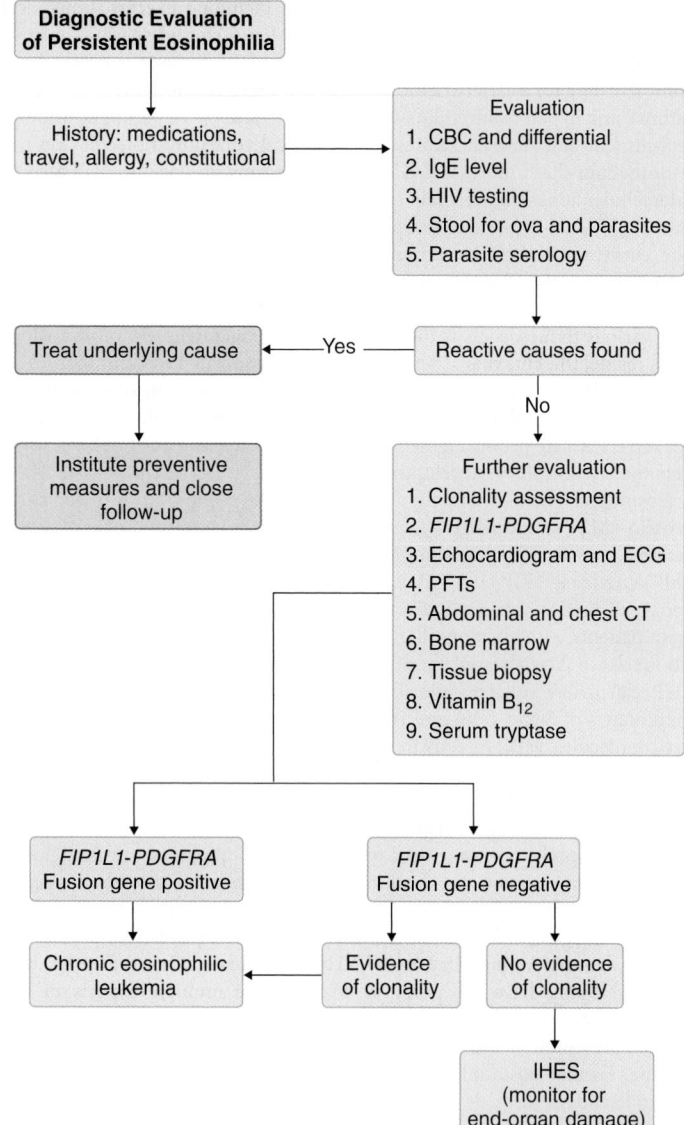

FIGURE 173-2. Diagnostic evaluation of persistent eosinophilia. CBC = complete blood count; CT = computed tomography; ECG = electrocardiogram; IgE = immunoglobulin E; IHES = idiopathic hypereosinophilic syndrome; HIV = human immunodeficiency virus; PDGFRA = platelet-derived growth factor-receptor α; PFTs = pulmonary function tests.

chromosome inactivation patterns in female patients), an elevated level of mast cell tryptase (elevated in myelodysplastic variants of hypereosinophilic syndrome), the presence of aberrant lymphocyte phenotypes (elevated in lymphocytic variants of hypereosinophilic syndrome), abnormal cytogenetics, and the possible presence of specific fusion genes such as *FIP1L1-PDG-FRA* should be investigated.

Other eosinophilic syndromes such as Churg-Strauss syndrome (Chapter 278) should be considered in patients with a history of worsening asthma, sinus disease, neuropathy, or blood eosinophilia and the presence of abnormal laboratory findings associated with autoimmunity, such as an elevated erythrocyte sedimentation rate, C-reactive protein, and antineutrophil cytoplasmic antibodies.

An accumulation of eosinophils that is limited to specific organs is characteristic of particular diseases, such as eosinophilic cellulitis (Wells' syndrome), eosinophilic esophagitis, eosinophilic pneumonias (e.g., Löffler's syndrome [Chapter 92]), and eosinophilic fasciitis (Shulman's syndrome).

Diagnostic Evaluation

Diagnostic studies that should be performed in patients with moderate to severe eosinophilia and considered in patients with persistent mild eosinophilia include morphologic examination of a blood smear, human immunodeficiency virus (HIV) screen, serial stool examinations for ova and parasites, parasite serology, and plasma immunoglobulin E (IgE) level. Parasitic infections that cause eosinophilia are usually limited to helminthic parasites, with the exception of two enteric protozoans, *Isospora belli* (Chapter 361) and *Dientamoeba fragilis* (Chapter 361). *Strongyloides stercoralis* (Chapter 366) infection is important to diagnose because it can cause disseminated fatal disease in immunosuppressed patients; detection of such infection often requires serologic testing. Other infections to consider include trichinosis (Chapter 366), *T. canis* infection (Chapter 365), and HIV infection (Chapter 400).

Patients with sustained hypereosinophilia should be monitored closely for the subsequent development of cardiac disease. A pathologically similar disease, Löffler's endomyocarditis (Chapter 60), has been noted in tropical regions, where antecedent parasite-elicited eosinophilia may be responsible for the cardiac damage.

TREATMENT

Reactive Hypereosinophilia and Hypereosinophilia Associated with Other Diseases

Treatment of reactive hypereosinophilia and hypereosinophilia associated with other diseases centers around identifying the cause and then treating the underlying disease process. For example, reactive eosinophilia typically responds by removal of the inciting triggers (e.g., allergens, parasites, and medications). Eosinophilia associated with other disease processes typically improves after treatment of the underlying disease, such as dietary manipulation in patients with allergic eosinophilic gastroenteritis.

FIP1L1-PDGFRA-Positive Disease

Imatinib should be considered as first-line therapy in patients in whom the *FIP1L1-PDGFRA* fusion gene has been demonstrated and in selected patients with the characteristic clinical and laboratory features of this myeloproliferative subtype of hypereosinophilic syndrome (e.g., male gender, tissue fibrosis, elevated serum vitamin B_{12} and tryptase levels). Clinical responses to imatinib in *FIP1L1-PDGFRA*-positive patients are rapid, with normalization of eosinophil counts generally occurring within 1 week of initiation of treatment and reversal of the signs and symptoms occurring within 1 month. Doses of imatinib as low as 100 mg daily appear to be effective in controlling symptoms and eosinophilia in most patients, but some recommend beginning imatinib treatment at 400 mg daily to achieve molecular remission and then decreasing the dose slowly while monitoring the patient closely for evidence of molecular relapse. In imatinib-resistant patients, sorafenib may be effective. The utility of imatinib therapy in hypereosinophilic patients without a demonstrable *FIP1L1-PDGFRA* mutation remains controversial, although some patients have responded. Nonmyeloablative allogeneic bone marrow transplantation (Chapter 181) has also been used successfully in several patients with hypereosinophilia.

Other Hypereosinophilic Syndromes

Corticosteroids, which have been used for decades in the treatment of idiopathic hypereosinophilic syndromes, remain the first-line treatment for most patients except those with *PDGFRA*-associated hypereosinophilia. The most appropriate initial corticosteroid dose and the duration of steroid therapy have not been subjected to randomized trials, but a general recommendation is to start with a moderate to high dose (≥40 mg prednisone equivalent) and taper very slowly while monitoring the eosinophil count

---

associated with clonal hematopoiesis (see Table 173-1). Evaluation of patients is based on their history and clinical characteristics (Fig. 173-2). The initial goal is to determine whether the eosinophilia is secondary to a reactive cause (i.e., in response to another primary trigger such as allergy, infection, solid tumor, vasculitis). If reactive causes are not identified, further evaluation should determine whether the eosinophilia is secondary to a clonal hematologic disorder. If no evidence of clonality is determined, the patient is considered to have an idiopathic hypereosinophilic syndrome.

The differential diagnosis of eosinophilia requires a review of the patient's history, which may reveal wheezing (Chapter 87), rhinitis (Chapter 259), or eczema (indicating atopic causes); travel to areas where helminth infections (e.g., schistosomiasis [Chapter 363]) are endemic; the presence of a pet dog (indicating possible infection with *Toxocara canis* [Chapter 365]); symptoms of cancer; or drug ingestion (indicating a possible hypersensitivity reaction [Chapter 262]). Eosinophilia caused by drugs (Chapter 262) is usually benign but can sometimes be accompanied by tissue damage, as in hypersensitivity pneumonitis (Chapter 97). In most cases, the eosinophilia resolves when use of the drug ceases, but in some cases, such as eosinophilia-myalgia syndrome secondary to the ingestion of contaminated L-tryptophan, the disease can persist despite withdrawal of the drug.

The presence of abnormal morphologic features of eosinophils, an increase in immature and dysplastic cells in the bone marrow or blood, elevated levels of vitamin B_{12}, and splenomegaly raises suspicion of a clonal hypereosinophilic syndrome. In such cases, evidence of clonality (e.g., by analysis of X closely. With this approach, most patients will respond initially, and some will be able to be maintained on low doses of corticosteroids for prolonged periods.

Monoclonal anti-IL-5 antibody therapy (e.g., mepolizumab or reslizumab) for hypereosinophilia and eosinophil-associated asthma[1,2] has a number of unique advantages related to the specificity of IL-5 for the eosinophil lineage. In patients treated with this agent, eosinophil counts are twice as likely to fall below 600/µL (95% vs. 45%, $P < .001$) with significantly lower prednisone doses.[3] Of the cytotoxic therapies that have been used for steroid-refractory hypereosinophilia, hydroxyurea has been the most extensively studied at doses of 1 to 3 g/day. Vincristine at a dose of 1 to 2 mg intravenously can rapidly lower eosinophilia in patients with extremely high eosinophil counts (>100,000/mm³) and may be useful for the treatment of children whose aggressive disease is unresponsive to other therapies. In patients who have corticosteroid-refractory hypereosinophilic syndromes or who develop intolerable side effects of steroid treatment, immunomodulatory agents that are sometimes helpful include interferon-α, cyclosporine, and alemtuzumab. Responses can often be achieved with relatively low doses of interferon-α (1 to 2×10^6 U/day) and may persist for prolonged periods. Because the effects of interferon-α on eosinophil numbers in peripheral blood may not become evident for several weeks, escalation to an effective dose may require several months. Rarely, patients have remained in remission for extended periods after cessation of interferon-α therapy, suggesting that interferon-α may be curative in a small subset of individuals. Low-dose (500 mg daily) hydroxyurea appears to act synergistically with interferon-α to lower the eosinophil count without increasing side effects.

FUTURE DIRECTIONS

Treatments on the horizon for hypereosinophilic disorders include targeted therapy against the eotaxin chemokines and their receptor CCR3, as well as anti-IL-5 and anti-IL-5 receptor–based antibody therapy.

PROGNOSIS

The prognosis of hypereosinophilic syndromes depends on the primary cause. Whereas *FIP1L1-PDGFRA*-positive disease and other forms of clonal disorders have a poor prognosis (25 to 50% 5-year mortality rate if responsiveness to therapeutic intervention is not achieved), the prognosis of hypereosinophilia from reactive and other causes is usually better.

1. Nair P, Pizzichini MM, Kjarsgaard M, et al. Mepolizumab for prednisone-dependent asthma with sputum eosinophilia. *N Engl J Med.* 2009;360:985-993.
2. Haldar P, Brightling CE, Hargadon B, et al. Mepolizumab and exacerbations of refractory eosinophilic asthma. *N Engl J Med.* 2009;360:973-984.
3. Rothenberg ME, Klion AD, Roufosse FE, et al. Treatment of patients with the hypereosinophilic syndrome with mepolizumab. *N Engl J Med.* 2008;358:1215-1228.

SUGGESTED READINGS

Dulohery MM, Patel RR, Schneider F, et al. Lung involvement in hypereosinophilic syndromes. *Respir Med.* 2011;105:114-121. *About 25% of patients have pulmonary involvement with variable radiologic findings and oftentimes with asthma.*

Ogbogu PU, Bochner BS, Butterfield JH, et al. Hypereosinophilic syndromes: a multicenter, retrospective analysis of clinical characteristics and response to therapy. *J Allergy Clin Immunol.* 2009;124: 1319-1325. *The 11% of patients who were FIP1L1-PDGFRA positive usually responded to imatinib, whereas the 17% with aberrant clonal T-cell populations usually responded to corticosteroids.*

Roufosse F, Weller PF. Practical approach to the patient with hypereosinophilia. *J Allergy Clin Immunol.* 2010;126:39-44.

Sade K, Mysels A, Levo Y, et al. Eosinophilia: a study of 100 hospitalized patients. *Eur J Intern Med.* 2007;18:196-201. *Common causes were asthma or atopic disease (13%), eosinophilic pneumonia (10%), cancer (10%), infections (10%), and drug reactions (6%), but 34% were of unknown cause.*

Schwartz LB, Sheikh J, Singh A. Current strategies in the management of hypereosinophilic syndrome, including mepolizumab. *Curr Med Res Opin.* 2010;26:1933-1946. *Clinical review.*

Sheikh J, Weller PF. Advances in diagnosis and treatment of eosinophilia. *Curr Opin Hematol.* 2009;16:3-8. *Review of the lymphocytic (non-malignant T-cell expansion) and myeloproliferative (abnormal tyrosine kinase activity from a fusion product) variants.*

174

APPROACH TO THE PATIENT WITH BLEEDING AND THROMBOSIS

ANDREW I. SCHAFER

MECHANISMS OF HEMOSTASIS AND THROMBOSIS

The coagulation system is normally quiescent, and blood fluidity is maintained by the actions of a continuous monolayer of endothelial cells that line the intimal surface of the vasculature throughout the circulatory tree. At a site of vascular damage, the antithrombotic properties of endothelium are lost, and thrombogenic constituents of the subendothelial vessel wall become exposed to circulating blood. The result is rapid formation of a hemostatic clot that consists of platelets and fibrin and is localized to the area of vascular injury. Activation of platelets and formation of fibrin occur essentially simultaneously and interdependently to effect hemostasis. Subsequently, vascular repair is accomplished by thrombolysis and recanalization of the occluded site.

Platelet activation at a site of vascular injury begins with the adhesion of platelets to the locally de-endothelialized intimal surface (platelet–vessel wall interaction). Platelet adhesion is mediated by von Willebrand factor, which sticks circulating platelets to the area of damaged vessel wall by binding to its receptors located in platelet membrane glycoprotein Ib. The adherent platelets then undergo a "release reaction," during which they discharge constituents of their storage granules, including adenosine diphosphate (ADP), and simultaneously elaborate thromboxane A_2 from arachidonic acid through the aspirin-inhibitable cyclooxygenase reaction. ADP, thromboxane A_2, and other components of the release reaction act in concert to recruit and activate additional platelets from the circulation to the site of vascular injury. These activated platelets expose binding sites for fibrinogen by forming the surface membrane glycoprotein IIb/IIIa complex. In the process of platelet aggregation (platelet-platelet interactions), fibrinogen (or von Willebrand factor under conditions of high shear stress) mediates the final formation of an occlusive platelet plug.

Fibrin, which anchors the hemostatic platelet plug, is formed from soluble plasma fibrinogen by the action of the potent protease enzyme thrombin (Fig. 174-1). The fibrin mesh is stabilized by covalent cross-linking mediated by factor XIII. Thrombin is formed from its inactive (zymogen) plasma precursor, prothrombin, by the action of activated factor X (Xa) and its cofactor, factor Va. This sequence of reactions has classically been referred to as the *common pathway* of coagulation. Factor X can be activated by either the *tissue factor (extrinsic) pathway* or the *contact activation (intrinsic) pathway* of coagulation. The tissue factor pathway is now considered to be the major physiologic initiator of coagulation activation. It is triggered by the formation of the complex of tissue factor, which is exposed on the surfaces of activated vascular and blood cells, with activated factor VII (VIIa). The contact activation pathway involves a series (or cascade) of zymogen-protease reactions that are initiated by factor XII, high-molecular-weight kininogen, and prekallikrein. Activated factor XII (XIIa) converts factor XI to XIa, which in turn activates factor IX to IXa. Factor IXa is the enzyme that converts factor X to Xa, a reaction that requires factor VIIIa as a cofactor.

Intact, normal endothelium promotes blood fluidity by inhibiting platelet activation. It likewise plays a crucial role in preventing fibrin accumulation. Among the physiologic antithrombotic systems that produce this latter effect are (1) antithrombin III, (2) protein C and protein S, (3) tissue factor pathway inhibitor (TFPI), and (4) the fibrinolytic system. Antithrombin is the major protease inhibitor of the coagulation system: it inactivates thrombin and other activated coagulation factors. Heparin functions as an anticoagulant by binding to antithrombin and greatly accelerating these reactions. Heparin and heparin sulfate proteoglycans are naturally present on endothelial cells, so antithrombin inactivation of thrombin and other coagulation proteases most likely occurs physiologically on vascular surfaces rather than in fluid plasma. Activated protein C, with its cofactor protein S, functions as a natural anticoagulant by destroying factors Va and VIIIa, two essential cofactors of the coagulation cascade. Thrombin itself is the activator of protein C, and this reaction occurs rapidly only on the surfaces of intact vascular endothelial cells, where thrombin binds to the glycosaminoglycan thrombomodulin. TFPI is a plasma protease inhibitor that specifically quenches tissue factor–induced coagulation. Finally, what little fibrin can be produced, despite these potent physiologic antithrombotic mechanisms, is digested rapidly by the endogenous fibrinolytic system. Fibrinolysis is mediated by the protease plasmin, which is generated from plasminogen in plasma by the action of endothelium-derived plasminogen activators.

EVALUATION OF THE PATIENT WITH A POSSIBLE BLEEDING DISORDER

History and Physical Examination

A thorough history is paramount in evaluating a patient for a possible systemic bleeding disorder. In addition to asking the patient about spontaneous bleeding episodes in the past, responses to specific hemostatic challenges should be recorded. A bleeding tendency may be suspected if a patient previously experienced excessive hemorrhage after surgery or trauma, including common events such as circumcision, tonsillectomy, labor and delivery, menses, dental procedures, vaccinations, and injections. Conversely, a history of normal blood clotting after such specific challenges in the recent past is

FIGURE 174-1. **Coagulation cascade.** This scheme emphasizes an understanding of (1) the importance of the tissue factor pathway in initiating clotting in vivo, (2) the interactions among pathways, and (3) the pivotal role of thrombin in sustaining the cascade by feedback activation of coagulation factors. HMWK = high-molecular-weight kininogen; PK = prekallikrein; PL = phospholipid; PT = prothrombin; TF = tissue factor; Th = thrombin. (From Schafer AI. Coagulation cascade: an overview. In: Loscalzo J, Schafer AI, eds. *Thrombosis and Hemorrhage.* Cambridge, MA: Blackwell Scientific Publications; 1994:3-12.)

just as important to note. It may be a better test of the integrity of systemic hemostasis than any laboratory measurement can provide.

In a patient with a history of excessive or unexplained bleeding, the initial goal is to determine whether the cause is a systemic coagulopathy or an anatomic or mechanical problem with a blood vessel. This situation is encountered most frequently in patients with excessive postoperative bleeding, which could be due to either local surgical trauma or a coagulation abnormality. A history of prior bleeding suggests a coagulopathy, as does the finding of bleeding from multiple sites. However, this is not always the case. Even diffuse bleeding may arise from anatomic rather than hemostatic abnormalities. An example of this is recurrent mucosal hemorrhage in patients with hereditary hemorrhagic telangiectasia. Conversely, a single episode of bleeding from an isolated site may be the initial manifestation of a coagulopathy.

The history must include a survey of coexisting systemic diseases and drug ingestions that could affect hemostasis. Renal failure and the myeloproliferative disorders are associated with impaired platelet–vessel wall interactions and qualitative platelet abnormalities, connective tissue diseases and lymphomas are associated with thrombocytopenia, and liver disease causes a complex coagulopathy (Chapter 178). Ingestion of aspirin and other nonsteroidal anti-inflammatory drugs (NSAIDs) that cause nonselective inhibition of cyclooxygenase leads to platelet dysfunction; these drugs are often contained in over-the-counter preparations that patients may neglect to report without specific questioning. Other drugs, such as antibiotics, also may be associated with a bleeding tendency by causing abnormal platelet function or thrombocytopenia. Finally, it is important to elicit a family history of bleeding problems. Although a positive history provides an important clue to a possible inherited coagulopathy, a negative history does not exclude a familial cause; for example, 20% of patients with classic hemophilia have a completely negative family history of bleeding.

Patterns of clinical bleeding, as revealed by the history and physical examination, may be characteristic of certain types of coagulopathy (Table 174-1). In general, patients with thrombocytopenia or qualitative platelet or vascular disorders present with bleeding from superficial sites in the skin and mucous membranes. These may involve petechiae, which are pinpoint cutaneous hemorrhages that appear particularly over dependent extremities (characteristic of severe thrombocytopenia), ecchymoses (common bruises), purpura, gastrointestinal and genitourinary tract bleeding, epistaxis, and hemoptysis. In these types of disorders, bleeding tends to occur spontaneously or immediately after trauma. In contrast, patients with inherited or acquired coagulation factor deficiencies, such as hemophilia, or those on anticoagulant therapy tend to bleed from deeper tissue sites (e.g., hemarthroses, deep hematomas, retroperitoneal hemorrhage) and in a delayed manner after trauma.

Laboratory Testing

Four simple screening tests have traditionally been used in the initial evaluation of patients with a suspected coagulopathy: platelet count, bleeding time, prothrombin time (PT), and activated partial thromboplastin time (aPTT). Thrombocytopenia, reported by electronic particle counting, should be verified by examination of the peripheral smear. Pseudothrombocytopenia, a laboratory artifact of ex vivo platelet clumping, may be caused by the ethylenediaminetetraacetic acid (EDTA) anticoagulant used in tubes for blood cell counts, by other anticoagulants, or by nonphysiologic cold agglutinins acting at room temperature. It should be suspected whenever a very low platelet count is unexpectedly reported in a patient who does not exhibit any clinical bleeding. Pseudothrombocytopenia is indicated by the finding of platelet clumps on the peripheral smear, and the diagnosis is supported by the finding of simultaneously normal platelet counts in blood samples obtained by finger stick, in tubes containing other anticoagulants, or in a tube maintained at 37° C before platelet counting. Examination of the blood smear

	Sites of Bleeding					
TYPE OF DISORDER	**GENERAL**	**SKIN**	**MUCOUS MEMBRANES**	**OTHER**	**ONSET OF BLEEDING**	**CLINICAL EXAMPLES**
Platelet-vascular disorders	Superficial surfaces	Petechiae, ecchymoses	Common: oral, nasal, gastrointestinal, genitourinary	Rare	Spontaneous or immediately after trauma	Thrombocytopenia, functional platelet disorder, vascular fragility, disseminated intravascular coagulation, liver disease
Coagulation factor deficiency	Deep tissues	Hematomas	Rare	Common: joint, muscle, retroperitoneal	Delayed after trauma	Inherited coagulation factor deficiency, acquired inhibitor, anticoagulation, disseminated intravascular coagulation, liver disease

TABLE 174-1 CHARACTERISTIC PATTERNS OF BLEEDING IN SYSTEMIC DISORDERS OF HEMOSTASIS

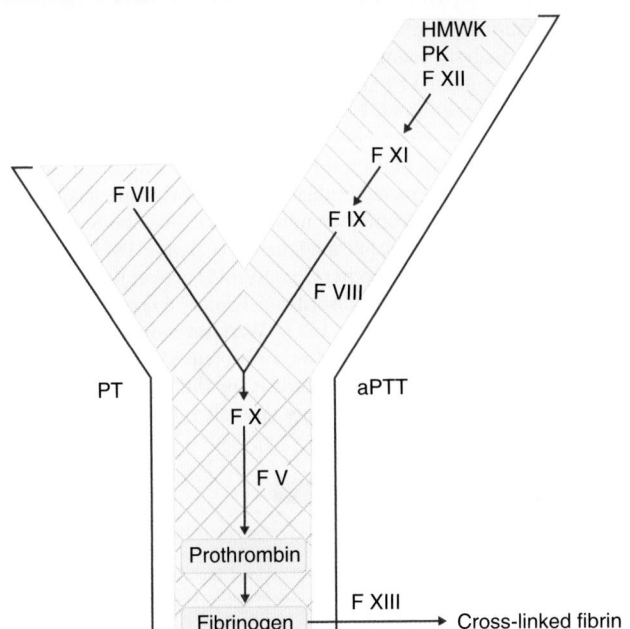

FIGURE 174-2. Classic coagulation cascade. The prothrombin time (PT) measures the integrity of the extrinsic and common pathways, whereas the activated partial thromboplastin time (aPTT) measures the integrity of the intrinsic and common pathways. Factor (F) XIII deficiency is not detected by PT or aPTT. HMWK = high-molecular-weight kininogen; PK = prekallikrein.

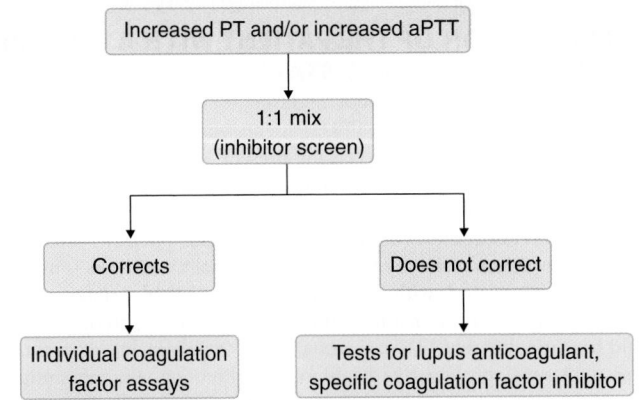

FIGURE 174-3. Approach to evaluating patients with prolonged prothrombin time (PT) or activated partial thromboplastin time (aPTT).

can also reveal clues to the cause of real thrombocytopenia, such as fragmented red blood cells in thrombotic thrombocytopenic purpura.

The bleeding time is a widely used clinical screening test for disorders of platelet–vessel wall interactions. It measures the time to cessation of bleeding after a standardized incision over the volar aspect of the forearm, now most commonly performed by disposable automated devices. The bleeding time is prolonged in thrombocytopenia, qualitative platelet abnormalities, defects in platelet–vessel wall interactions (e.g., von Willebrand disease), and primary vascular disorders. The bleeding time usually is not prolonged in patients with coagulation factor deficiencies. The test is prone to problems related to reproducibility, sensitivity, and specificity, however. Therefore, because von Willebrand disease is the most common genetic cause of abnormal platelet–vessel wall interactions, some experts now recommend replacing the bleeding time with specific tests for von Willebrand disease in the initial evaluation of patients with a suspected coagulopathy (Chapter 176).

The PT measures the integrity of the extrinsic and common pathways of coagulation (factors VII, X, and V; prothrombin; and fibrinogen) (Fig. 174-2). The aPTT measures the integrity of the intrinsic and common pathways of coagulation (high-molecular-weight kininogen; prekallikrein; factors XII, XI, IX, VIII, X, and V; prothrombin; and fibrinogen). The sensitivity of the PT and aPTT in detecting coagulation factor deficiencies may vary with the reagents used to perform these tests, and each laboratory must determine its own reference standards.

With a few notable exceptions, normal results for all these screening tests of hemostasis essentially exclude any clinically significant systemic coagulopathy. However, patients with factor XIII deficiency may have a serious bleeding diathesis but normal screening tests; specific tests for factor XIII deficiency should be performed if this disease is suspected. The PT and aPTT detect only the more severe deficiencies of coagulation factors, usually at levels less than 30% of normal; specific factor levels should be determined if a mild coagulation factor deficiency is suspected. Patients with von Willebrand disease sometimes have normal bleeding times and usually do not have sufficiently reduced levels of factor VIII to affect the aPTT, requiring specific testing for the disease. Rare disorders of fibrinolysis also may be associated with normal screening tests, necessitating more specialized tests when indicated. Abnormalities in the screening tests of hemostasis may be pursued by more specialized tests to establish a specific diagnosis.

The initial approach to a prolonged bleeding time in the absence of thrombocytopenia is to determine whether the patient is taking any drugs that might interfere with platelet function (e.g., aspirin, other NSAIDs) or has a coexisting disease that might explain the finding (e.g., renal failure). If these conditions are absent or if the bleeding time fails to correct after

discontinuation of any potentially offending drugs, further specialized testing may include platelet aggregation studies to identify specific qualitative abnormalities of platelet function and specific assays to exclude one of the types of von Willebrand disease.

The finding of a prolonged PT and/or aPTT indicates either a deficiency of one or more coagulation factors or the presence of an inhibitor, usually an antibody, directed at one or more components of the coagulation system (Fig. 174-3). These two possibilities can be distinguished by performing a simple inhibitor screen, which involves a 1 : 1 mix of the patient's plasma and normal plasma. The premise of the test is that even if the patient's plasma is completely deficient (0% level) in a certain factor, mixing it 1 : 1 with normal plasma (100% level) should bring the concentration of that factor to 50% in the mixture; this is sufficient to correct the prolonged PT or aPTT. If correction occurs with the inhibitor screen, individual coagulation factor levels should be assayed for a specific deficiency state. If the 1 : 1 mix fails to correct the prolonged PT and/or aPTT, an inhibitor is likely to be present, and it is interfering with coagulation in vitro in both the patient's plasma and the normal plasma. Specific assays should then be performed to determine whether there is a true inhibitor against a coagulation factor (e.g., factor VIII antibody) or whether the inhibitor is a lupus anticoagulant.

EVALUATION OF THE ASYMPTOMATIC PATIENT WITH ABNORMAL COAGULATION TESTS

In asymptomatic individuals who are discovered incidentally to have abnormalities in screening laboratory tests of hemostasis, the first critical question is whether the findings are clinically relevant. Patients with inherited deficiencies of one of the contact activation coagulation factors (factor XII, high-molecular-weight kininogen, prekallikrein) characteristically have a markedly prolonged aPTT, yet they do not have a clinical bleeding tendency. Likewise, patients with lupus anticoagulants typically have prolongation of the aPTT and sometimes also the PT; they more often have thrombotic rather than bleeding complications. In patients with heparin-induced thrombocytopenia, a marked decrease in the platelet count is sometimes associated with arterial and venous thrombosis rather than bleeding. It is crucial to view the clinical setting, history, physical examination, and screening laboratory tests as complementary facets of the approach to patients with suspected coagulopathies.

EVALUATION OF THE PREOPERATIVE PATIENT

Routine screening of all preoperative patients with a platelet count, bleeding time, PT, and aPTT not only is uninformative but also may be counterproductive if follow-up testing causes unnecessary expense and delays in surgery (Chapter 439). Preoperative bleeding time, PT, and aPTT do not predict surgical bleeding risk in patients who are not found to be at increased risk on clinical grounds, so a thorough clinical assessment should guide the need for these preoperative screening tests. Laboratory testing and possibly further specialized tests of coagulation are indicated for patients whose bleeding histories are suspicious for a hemostatic abnormality. Preoperative screening tests of coagulation are probably warranted for patients who cannot cooperate with an adequate clinical assessment and for those who will be undergoing procedures in which even minimal postoperative hemorrhage could be hazardous.

EVALUATION OF THE PATIENT WITH A POSSIBLE HYPERCOAGULABLE STATE

Most patients with venous thromboembolism (VTE) have an inherited basis for hypercoagulability (Chapter 179). Patients with inherited hypercoagulable states (or thrombophilia) typically present with an initial episode of VTE in early adulthood, but thrombotic manifestations may begin at any time from early childhood to old age. Patients usually have deep vein thrombosis of the lower extremities or pulmonary embolism, but other uncommon sites of venous thrombosis may be involved. Arterial thrombosis is not characteristically associated with inherited hypercoagulable states. Arterial thrombosis that occurs prematurely or in the absence of apparent risk factors should trigger a different line of investigation, possibly including evaluation for vasculitis, myeloproliferative disorders, hyperhomocysteinemia, antiphospholipid syndrome, and potential sources of systemic embolization.

The primary or hereditary hypercoagulable states (see Table 179-1 in Chapter 179) result from specific mutations or polymorphisms that lead to decreased levels of physiologic antithrombotic proteins or increased levels of procoagulant proteins. In contrast, the secondary or acquired hypercoagulable states (see Fig. 179-2 in Chapter 179) are a heterogeneous group of disorders that predispose to thrombosis by complex mechanisms. VTE is often precipitated by the combination of an underlying hypercoagulable genotype and an acquired prothrombotic, hypercoagulable state such as pregnancy, immobilization, or the postoperative state. Certain clinical characteristics suggest the presence of an inherited hypercoagulable state (Table 174-2). Patients with recurrent thrombosis should be tested for these disorders and, in most cases, committed to lifelong prophylactic anticoagulation. It is not clear whether it is essential to order these tests after a single episode of VTE. Counterintuitively, it has been found that most of the common inherited hypercoagulable states—which, to varying extents, clearly increase the risk of a *first* episode of VTE—are at best only weak predictors of *recurrent* VTE. It has been argued, therefore, that making a specific thrombophilia diagnosis after an initial episode of VTE will not influence the decision about the duration of prophylactic anticoagulation. However, the increased risk of recurrent VTE with the more prothrombotic mutations (e.g., antithrombin III, protein C or S deficiency), combined inherited thrombophilias, or antiphospholipid syndrome may necessitate long-term anticoagulation, and their diagnosis after a first episode of VTE will in fact alter decisions about the duration of anticoagulation. Even if they are not maintained on long-term anticoagulation, patients with diagnosed primary hypercoagulable states should receive prophylactic anticoagulation during situations that pose a high risk for thrombosis, such as the peripartum period. There is no simple screening test for primary hypercoagulable states, and the timing of obtaining these tests is crucial to avoid erroneous diagnoses. Acute thrombosis itself can cause transient decreases in the levels of antithrombin, protein C, and protein S. Heparin therapy can cause a decrease in plasma antithrombin activity. Warfarin therapy lowers the functional levels of protein C and protein S. Inherited deficiency states can be diagnosed spuriously under these conditions.

Patients who present with VTE probably have an increased risk of harboring an occult malignancy (Chapter 187). This association is increased further in patients with recurrent and unprovoked thrombosis. There are conflicting opinions whether an evaluation for occult malignancy in these patients must be exhaustive. Some contend it can be limited to a thorough history, physical examination, routine complete blood cell count and chemistries, test of fecal occult blood, urinalysis, mammogram (in women), and chest radiograph, with further testing guided by any abnormalities found in this initial evaluation. Others argue for routine CT scanning of the chest, abdomen, and pelvis.

In addition to classic deep vein thrombosis and pulmonary embolism, certain characteristic types of thrombosis may provide important clues to the cause and trigger a more directed evaluation. Migratory, superficial thrombophlebitis (Trousseau's syndrome) or nonbacterial thrombotic endocarditis suggests the presence of an occult malignancy (Chapter 187). Hepatic vein thrombosis (Budd-Chiari syndrome; Chapter 145) or portal vein thrombosis may indicate a myeloproliferative disorder (Chapter 169) or paroxysmal nocturnal hemoglobinuria (Chapter 163). Warfarin-induced skin necrosis strongly suggests an underlying protein C or protein S deficiency. Recurrent, spontaneous miscarriages are characteristic of the antiphospholipid syndrome (Chapter 177), although they are also associated with other thrombophilias.

SUGGESTED READINGS

Favaloro EJ, Lippi G. Coagulation udate: what's new in hemostasis testing? *Thromb Res.* 2011;127:S13-S16. *Review of standard and newer tests.*

Favaloro EJ, McDonald D, Lippi G. Laboratory investigation of thrombophilia: the good, the bad, and the ugly. *Semin Thromb Hemostas.* 2009;35:695-710. *Review of the rationale for and current controversies over screening laboratory tests for thrombophilia.*

Kessler CM. The link between cancer and venous thromboembolism: a review. *Am J Clin Oncol.* 2009;32(4 Suppl):S3-S7. *Brief review of the relationship between cancer and venous thromboembolism (VTE) and the value of extensive screening for occult malignancy in patients with a first episode of idiopathic VTE.*

Tsoran I, Saharov G, Brenner B, et al. Prolonged travel and venous thromboembolism findings from the RIETE registry. *Thromb Res.* 2010;126:287-291. *Risk factors include high BMI, previous VTE, hormone use, and, in 16% of patients, a positive thrombophilia test.*

175

THROMBOCYTOPENIA

CHARLES S. ABRAMS

Thrombocytopenia is defined as a platelet count less than the normal range, typically below 150,000/µL. In the absence of qualitative platelet defects (Chapter 176), excessive bleeding does not occur in thrombocytopenic patients following trauma or surgery unless the platelet count is lower than 75,000/µL. In otherwise hemostatically normal patients, spontaneous hemorrhage typically does not occur with platelet counts above 30,000/µL. Patients with platelet counts less than 5000 to 10,000/µL are at high risk for spontaneous, life-threatening hemorrhage. However, there is no absolute threshold for spontaneous bleeding due to thrombocytopenia. It may occur at higher counts when fever, sepsis, severe anemia, and other hemostatic defects are present or when platelet function is impaired by medication. Notably, a prolonged cutaneous bleeding time test does not accurately predict the risk of clinical bleeding. Therefore, it is critical that the physician consider the gamut of possibilities when diagnosing and managing a patient with a low platelet count.

Typically, the first step in diagnosing a patient with a low platelet count is to determine whether the thrombocytopenia is attributable to one of the three broad mechanisms for developing thrombocytopenia: (1) increased destruction, such as that seen in immune-mediated causes; (2) decreased production, usually due to an underlying bone marrow disorder; or (3) sequestration of platelets within the spleen, as occurs in conditions that cause splenomegaly (hypersplenism).

Determining the cause of the patient's thrombocytopenia is essential to select the most appropriate therapy and to avoid unnecessary procedures. Because there is no easy test to differentiate among the three possibilities, clinical evaluation is critical. Therefore, a thorough history and physical examination, with attention to possible alternative explanations for thrombocytopenia, are mandatory. Particular attention should be paid to the duration of symptoms, which helps determine whether the patient has acute or chronic thrombocytopenia. Attention should also focus on the patient's recent exposure to new medications that might induce thrombocytopenia as a side effect.

Preliminary laboratory tests include a complete blood count (CBC) with a differential, along with an examination of the peripheral blood smear.

Venous thromboembolism (>90% of cases)
  Deep vein thrombosis and/or pulmonary embolism most common
  Mesenteric, cerebral vein thrombosis rare but characteristic
Frequent family history of thrombosis
  Typically autosomal dominant
First episode of thrombosis typically in young adulthood (<40 yr)
Often idiopathic (but an acquired thrombosis trigger is not infrequently identified with a careful history)
More common thrombophilias (factor V Leiden, prothrombin 20210G→A) are associated with a lower thrombosis risk; rarer thrombophilias (antithrombin III, protein C, protein S deficiency) are associated with a higher thrombosis risk
Warfarin-induced skin necrosis or neonatal purpura fulminans with protein C or protein S deficiency (very rare)

Abnormalities in the number or morphology of the leukocytes or erythrocytes may indicate a systemic inflammatory disorder or pathology within the bone marrow. Clumping of the platelets on the peripheral blood smear may indicate that the patient has pseudothrombocytopenia (Chapter 174). This anomaly is usually due to an antibody that binds to and thereby agglutinates platelets only in the presence of ethylenediaminetetraacetic acid (EDTA) or when the blood sample is allowed to cool to room temperature. Repeating the platelet count in a blood sample that has been anticoagulated with heparin and kept warm until it is analyzed can help exclude this spurious diagnosis. Any additional testing is based solely on the available clinical information; for example, human immunodeficiency virus (HIV) testing would be prudent in a patient with risk factors. A bone marrow aspirate and biopsy are typically not required for a patient with thrombocytopenia who has an otherwise normal CBC and peripheral blood smear count. However, a bone marrow aspirate and biopsy should be considered in older patients or in patients in whom standard therapy has not been effective.

GENERAL MECHANISMS OF THROMBOCYTOPENIAS

Increased Platelet Destruction

An acute drop in a patient's platelet count implies that a peripheral destructive process is the likely cause. For example, a patient who develops abrupt thrombocytopenia during hospitalization most likely has a low platelet count caused by an infection or a new medication. Both nonimmune and immune processes can lead to a shortened platelet lifespan. Nonimmune reasons for the accelerated destruction of platelets include sepsis, disseminated intravascular coagulation (DIC), thrombotic thrombocytopenic purpura (TTP), hemolytic-uremic syndrome (HUS), preeclampsia or eclampsia, cardiopulmonary bypass, and giant cavernous hemangioma. Thrombocytopenia that occurs in these circumstances usually resolves with treatment of the underlying disorder, and platelet transfusions are rarely necessary. Thrombocytopenia due to TTP, HUS, or heparin-induced thrombocytopenia (HIT) is associated with thrombosis rather than bleeding (Table 175-1), so platelet transfusions are rarely necessary. In addition, controversial reports have noted the clinical deterioration of patients with TTP or HIT following platelet transfusion, suggesting that platelets should not be given to most patients with these disorders.

Immune-mediated platelet destruction can occur owing to drugs, alloimmune sensitization, or autoimmunity. Medications should always be considered as a possible cause of acute thrombocytopenia. The list of potential offending agents is long, but drugs with strong evidence of antibody-mediated platelet destruction include quinine, quinidine, sulfonamides, and gold salts. In addition to stopping the offending medication, platelet transfusions might be required for severe thrombocytopenia.

Platelet Sequestration

Approximately 30% of the circulating platelet mass is normally sequestered within the spleen. Even more platelets may be sequestered when the spleen enlarges owing to portal hypertension or infiltrative diseases. This in turn can result in moderate thrombocytopenia. Because hypersplenism never causes a platelet count less than 40,000 to 50,000/µL, bleeding due to thrombocytopenia from hypersplenism alone is unusual.

Decreased Platelet Production

Decreased platelet production occurs in primary diseases of the bone marrow, such as acute leukemia and aplastic anemia; myelophthisic processes in which marrow is affected by metastatic carcinoma, fibrosis, or other clonal hematopoietic disorders; following chemotherapy and/or radiation therapy; with ethanol toxicity; and during infections with viruses such as HIV, cytomegalovirus (CMV), Epstein-Barr virus (EBV), and varicella. Thrombocytopenia also occurs when normal megakaryocyte proliferation is impaired by myelodysplasia.

PLATELET TRANSFUSIONS

Clinicians usually consider "wet" bleeding to be much more ominous than "dry" bleeding. Signs of wet bleeding include epistaxis, gingival bleeding, gastrointestinal or genitourinary bleeding, or bleeding around intravenous sites. Dry bleeding is defined as ecchymosis or petechiae. Overt wet bleeding that is clearly due to thrombocytopenia is usually treated with platelet transfusion. Prophylactic platelet transfusion for patients who are not bleeding is controversial. When making the decision whether to treat a nonbleeding patient with thrombocytopenia, the practitioner must consider the short lifespan of platelets (10 days), the 5-day shelf life of stored platelets, and the potential for the patient to develop transfusion-induced platelet alloantibodies. In patients undergoing treatment for acute leukemia, the outcome is unchanged when a platelet count as low as 5000 to 10,000/µL is used as the threshold for prophylactic platelet transfusion. In contrast, a higher platelet count is required when patients are bleeding or undergoing an invasive procedure or surgery. For patients experiencing the most extreme hemostatic challenges (e.g., neurosurgery, cardiopulmonary bypass, thyroid surgery, prostatectomy), a platelet count greater than 75,000 to 100,000/µL for the procedure and for the next several days is advisable. For minor invasive procedures, such as colonoscopy with biopsy, a platelet count of 30,000 to 50,000/µL is usually adequate.

A donated unit of blood contains approximately 50 billion platelets. Infusing this number of platelets into a patient should increase his or her platelet count by 20,000/µL divided by the patient's surface area in square meters. Therefore, transfusion into a typical patient should increase the recipient's platelet count by 10,000 to 12,000/µL. Bags of platelets used for transfusions are typically obtained by pooling platelets derived from four to eight blood donors. Therefore, a "unit" at one hospital may be derived from more donors than a "unit" obtained at another hospital.

Large quantities of platelets can be derived from a single donor by using apheresis technology (plateletpheresis). Because there is minimal loss of red blood cells with this technique, plateletpheresis allows one individual to donate very large numbers of platelets (equivalent to the number of platelets obtained from 6 to 10 units of donated blood). As discussed in the following section, the risk of platelet alloimmunization is partially dependent on the number of individuals donating platelets to a patient. Therefore, single-donor plateletpheresis platelets can prevent or at least minimize alloimmunization.

Several trials have addressed how many platelets should be transfused into thrombocytopenic patients to maintain hemostasis and minimize exposure to blood products. The largest of these trials was the multicenter Platelet Dose (PLADO) trial.[1] In this study, patients were randomized to receive transfusions of low-dose (110 billion), medium-dose (220 billion), or high-dose (440 billion) platelets per square meter for thrombocytopenia while recovering from hematopoietic stem cell transplantation. Patients who received the low-dose therapy required more frequent platelet transfusions, but overall, they received fewer transfused platelets over the course of the study. Importantly, bleeding complications were identical with all platelet transfusion strategies. This study demonstrates that low doses of platelets (110 billion/square meter of body surface area) are as safe as larger doses in patients with hypoproliferative thrombocytopenia receiving prophylactic platelet transfusion therapy.

Several complications of platelet transfusion therapy merit mention. First, some patients can become alloimmunized against platelet antigens and can become refractory to future platelet transfusion therapy (discussed in detail later). Second, bacterial contamination of stored platelets is a much more common complication than the infectious risk associated with red blood cell transfusions. Unlike red blood cells, which are stored frozen after being harvested from donated blood, platelets are sensitive to cool temperatures and therefore need to be stored at room temperature. This method of storage results in more bacterial overgrowth in the transfusion bags. Transfusion-associated bacterial sepsis is one of the most frequently reported causes of transfusion-induced mortality in the United States, and platelet transfusions are the most common blood products associated with sepsis. It should also be noted that room temperature storage of platelets contributes to their short shelf life of approximately 5 to 7 days. Consequently, unlike the blood-derived products that can be frozen (such as red blood cells and plasma), there is a constant need for platelet donations year-round. In contrast to the risk of bacterial infection, the risk of viral infection from platelet transfusions is no

TABLE 175-1	DISORDERS THAT CAUSE BOTH THROMBOCYTOPENIA AND THROMBOSIS

Thrombotic thrombocytopenic purpura (TTP)
Hemolytic-uremic syndrome (HUS)
Heparin-induced thrombocytopenia (HIT)
Disseminated intravascular coagulation (DIC)
Paroxysmal nocturnal hemoglobinuria (PNH)
Vasculitis (such as systemic lupus erythematosus)
Antiphospholipid antibody syndrome (APS)

higher than it is for red blood cell transfusions. From a single unit of platelets, the risk of being exposed to HIV is less than 1 in 2.5 million, the risk of exposure to hepatitis B virus is less than 1 in 750,000, and the risk of exposure to hepatitis C virus is less than 1 in 1 million.

Platelet transfusions have been considered contraindicated for thrombocytopenia owing to TTP or HIT. This recommendation is driven entirely by case reports of thrombotic events occurring soon after platelet transfusions in such patients, not by randomized trials addressing this issue. Because thrombotic events are a known complication of both TTP and HIT, it is difficult to determine whether the thrombi were due to the platelet transfusions or merely the intrinsic prothrombotic risk of TTP and HIT. In any case, there is usually no indication for platelet transfusions in patients with TTP and HIT because thrombosis is a much greater risk than hemorrhage in these disorders.

The Transfusion-Refractory Patient

Many patients do not have an optimal increase in the platelet count following transfusion. Although there are various definitions of platelet refractoriness, it is simplest to base this definition on the timing of platelet loss following transfusion. A patient who does not have the predicted rise in platelet count (between 10,000 and 12,000/μL for every unit of donated platelets) should have the platelet count analyzed before the next platelet transfusion, 1 hour after that transfusion, and again 24 hours later. If the platelet count rises appropriately 1 hour after the transfusion but falls substantially 24 hours later, the patient has ongoing platelet consumption. This is often seen in patients with sepsis, DIC, or severe active hemorrhage or as a result of the drug-mediated immune destruction of platelets. In these situations, the best therapy is to treat the underlying cause and to continue to support the patient with platelet transfusions as clinically indicated. Alternatively, some patients fail to have a significant increase in platelets even 1 hour after a transfusion. These patients have (1) hypersplenism, (2) an autoantibody that eliminates not only endogenous platelets but also allogeneic platelets (as in patients with idiopathic thrombocytopenic purpura [ITP]), or (3) alloantibodies that react with antigens on the transfused platelets.

Alloantibodies develop in approximately 20% of patients who are repeatedly exposed to platelet transfusions, and these patients present some of the most challenging management issues in transfusion medicine (Chapter 180). The alloantibodies may be directed against human leukocyte antigen (HLA) class I antigens (HLA-A and HLA-B) or against platelet-specific antigens present on the surface of the platelets. Because it appears that HLA class II antigens present on the surface of leukocytes are essential for the development of antibodies directed against HLA class I antigens, efforts to remove the contamination of leukocytes in platelet transfusion preparations can minimize alloantibody formation. Therefore, the use of filters that trap leukocytes during transfusions are useful to prevent patients from becoming refractory to future platelet transfusions. Once a patient develops alloantibodies against transfused platelets, the clinician and the blood bank should attempt to identify whether the alloantibody is directed against an HLA or against a platelet-specific antigen. If the alloantibody can be identified, platelets derived from donors matched for HLA or the platelet-specific antigen can be used. Corticosteroids, intravenous immunoglobulin, splenectomy, and recombinant factor VIIa are probably of no value in maintaining hemostasis in platelet-refractory patients. Antifibrinolytic agents (e.g., ε-aminocaproic acid) might be helpful for patients with bleeding predominantly in the oral cavity or the genitourinary tract. However, antifibrinolytic agents are contraindicated in patients with DIC (Chapter 178) because these agents can precipitate thrombotic events.

● SPECIFIC CAUSES OF THROMBOCYTOPENIA
Drug-Induced Thrombocytopenia

The abrupt onset of thrombocytopenia implies a high probability of the immune-mediated destruction of platelets. This is particularly likely if the thrombocytopenia is present in the absence of other abnormalities on the CBC. The clinician should first suspect either an infection (viral or bacterial) or a drug. A careful history and physical examination, along with a normal leukocyte count and differential, should help exclude an infectious cause of thrombocytopenia. Drug-induced thrombocytopenia is one of the most frequent causes of cytopenias evaluated by physicians.

The typical drug-induced thrombocytopenia is the result of an immune reaction elicited by either the drug or one of its metabolites. Sometimes the drug is simply deposited on the platelet surface, and antidrug antibodies lead to accelerated platelet clearance, primarily in the spleen. More frequently, the drug binds to a protein on the platelet surface and induces a neoantigen that is ultimately recognized by the immune system. In the absence of the drug or drug metabolites, this platelet neoantigen disappears, and the thrombocytopenia slowly resolves as new platelets are released from the bone marrow. This mechanism explains the vast majority of drug-induced thrombocytopenias, but there are some exceptions. For example, chemotherapy and other bone marrow toxins can decrease platelet production and thereby induce thrombocytopenia by a mechanism independent of the immune system.

Patients with drug-induced thrombocytopenia can have mild, moderate, or even severe forms. Almost all types of drug-induced thrombocytopenia predispose the patient to hemorrhagic but not thrombotic complications. The notable exception to this rule is HIT (discussed separately in the next section). The most difficult diagnostic dilemma is to discern drug-induced thrombocytopenia from ITP. For this distinction, the patient's medical history may be helpful. A gradually progressive thrombocytopenia is more consistent with ITP than with one induced by a medication. Conversely, the rapid onset of thrombocytopenia following the initiation of a new medication indicates that the drug is the most likely culprit. The time between initiation of the offending drug and development of thrombocytopenia has not been well documented for most medications. However, thrombocytopenia typically begins days to a few weeks after the administration of most medications with this type of toxicity. Presumably, this lag represents the period required for the patient to develop an immune response against the drug-platelet complex. Medications that have been taken safely for years before the onset of thrombocytopenia are unlikely to be the offending agents. In addition to an assessment of prescribed medications, a careful evaluation of over-the-counter medications is necessary. Agents that contain quinine lead the list of nonprescribed drugs that can induce life-threatening thrombocytopenia. Quinine is frequently contained in over-the-counter pills for leg cramps. Even the quinine in tonic water can induce severe thrombocytopenia ("gin and tonic purpura") when ingested by certain patients.

Some medications are much more likely to induce thrombocytopenia than others. Table 175-2 contains a partial list of drugs that frequently induce this type of toxicity. One particularly useful online database (*www.ouhsc.edu/platelets/ditp.html*) lists and periodically updates the level of evidence for specific drugs that may induce thrombocytopenia. With the exception of tests for HIT, laboratory tests for drug-induced thrombocytopenia do not have widespread applicability. Usually, drug-induced thrombocytopenia is proved only in retrospect, when the platelet count improves after discontinuation of the suspected medication. Even then, the diagnosis is not conclusive unless thrombocytopenia recurs after rechallenging the patient with the offending drug (a practice that is almost never recommended).

TABLE 175-2 DRUGS THAT ARE STRONGLY ASSOCIATED WITH THROMBOCYTOPENIA

ANTIBIOTICS AND ANTIVIRALS

Quinine/quinidine
Penicillins
Cephalosporins
Vancomycin
Trimethoprim/sulfamethoxazole
Sulfonamides/sulfonylureas
Linezolid
Valacyclovir
Ganciclovir
Indinavir

CARDIOVASCULAR MEDICATIONS

Abciximab
Tirofiban
Eptifibatide
Salicylates
Digoxin
Furosemide

MISCELLANEOUS

Cimetidine
Ranitidine
Famotidine
Valproate
Interferon

The most efficacious method of treating drug-induced thrombocytopenia is to stop all suspected offending medications. Usually, no additional therapy is indicated. The thrombocytopenia typically begins to resolve without further intervention within days to a week of stopping the drug. The notable exceptions involve drugs with particularly long half-lives. Sulfonamides, quinine, and quinidine are particularly notorious for inducing severe or even life-threatening thrombocytopenia. In patients with profound thrombocytopenia (<10,000 to 15,000/μL) or at high risk for bleeding, platelet transfusions are indicated. If ITP cannot be confidently excluded and the thrombocytopenia is life threatening, glucocorticoids can also be initiated (see the discussion of ITP treatment later).

Heparin-Induced Thrombocytopenia

A special case of drug-induced immune-mediated thrombocytopenia associated with arterial and venous thrombosis, rather than bleeding, is HIT. It is seen in 2 to 5% of patients exposed to unfractionated heparin and in 0.7% of patients given low-molecular-weight heparin; it almost never occurs in patients exposed only to fondaparinux. To understand this disease, one must know that platelets can secrete a protein, platelet factor 4 (PF4), that can bind to heparin. HIT is caused by an antibody that binds to this PF4-heparin complex (Fig. 175-1). Large complexes of antibodies directed against heparin-bound PF4 accumulate on the surface of platelets. At times, these anti-PF4 immunoglobulins bind to the Fc receptor that is also present on the platelet surface. The interaction of platelet Fc receptors and anti-PF4 antibodies causes activation of the platelet, release of more PF4, and a cycle of events that leads to the stimulation of even more platelets. Ultimately, it also leads to activation of the coagulation cascade. The activation of platelets and the clotting cascade leads to the formation of thrombi and thrombocytopenia.

When thrombocytopenia is detected in a hospitalized patient, HIT must always be considered. Patients with this syndrome often have multiple potential causes for thrombocytopenia (such as other medications or infections). Therefore, it is important to exclude these other causes. Large retrospective studies of HIT have suggested that the onset of thrombocytopenia relative to the initiation of heparin therapy is useful in establishing or excluding this diagnosis. HIT typically occurs 4 to 14 days after patients are given heparin by any route (even subcutaneously or in extremely low doses by heparin flush). This lag between heparin exposure and the appearance of HIT is due to the time it takes for the immune response to generate the requisite antibodies against the heparin-PF4 complex. Some patients who have been exposed to heparin within the past several months already have preexisting antibodies against the heparin-PF4 complex in their circulation. When these patients are re-exposed to heparin, they may develop an acute onset of HIT within the first day of reinitiating the drug.

The unique timing of acute-onset HIT within hours of heparin re-exposure and the more typical development of HIT within 4 to 14 days of initial heparin exposure emphasize the importance of a careful and critical history in establishing the diagnosis. HIT should be suspected in any patient who develops thrombocytopenia while on heparin therapy. It is important to note that the normal platelet count varies widely (150,000 to 450,000/μL), so some patients may have a substantial decrease in the platelet count but still remain within the normal range. Therefore, a greater than 50% decrease in the platelet count in a patient on heparin should raise suspicion for this syndrome. HIT should also be suspected in any patient who develops a thrombotic event while on heparin therapy.

Several antibody-based laboratory tests are available to confirm this diagnosis (Table 175-3). Although antibodies against the heparin-PF4 complex are almost always present in patients with HIT, these antibodies are also frequently present in heparin-treated patients who do not have this disorder (i.e., those with neither thrombocytopenia nor thrombosis). In addition, several days may elapse before the test results are available. Therefore, in practice, these laboratory assays provide only confirmatory information. Urgent clinical decisions should *not* be deferred until such test results are available. The timing of the thrombocytopenia with respect to the heparin exposure and the degree of platelet drop are the most important pieces of information needed by the physician evaluating a patient suspected of having HIT.

There are two general categories of laboratory assays for the diagnosis of HIT: functional assays and immunologic assays. Functional assays analyze whether the combination of heparin and the patient's plasma can induce normal platelets to aggregate or to secrete serotonin; these assays have very high specificity but relatively low sensitivity. Immunologic assays test the patient's plasma for antibodies that bind to the heparin-PF4 complex; they have very high sensitivity but lack specificity. Consequently, a *negative immunologic assay* is useful in excluding this diagnosis, and a *positive functional assay* is very useful in confirming the diagnosis of HIT.

Because platelets are consumed as they become activated, the clinical presentation of HIT is thrombocytopenia. However, it is unusual for the thrombocytopenia to actually cause bleeding. Instead, HIT is a highly prothrombotic disorder. Both venous and arterial thromboses are common in HIT. Patients with HIT who do not have thrombosis on initial presentation still have a 20 to 30% chance of developing a thrombus within the next month. Nevertheless, the incidence of HIT-related clinical events is greatest immediately after diagnosis. More importantly, clinical studies report that cessation of heparin frequently fails to prevent thromboses or the development of new thrombotic events.

If a patient has HIT, all heparin should be stopped immediately. This includes subcutaneous injections of "minidose" heparin, heparin flushes of intravenous lines, and low-molecular-weight heparin; even heparin-coated intravenous catheters should be withdrawn. Alternative anticoagulation, such as a direct thrombin inhibitor like recombinant hirudin or argatroban (Chapter 37), should be administered, at least until the platelet count normalizes. Warfarin should not be used in cases of acute HIT because of its delayed therapeutic effect and its association with venous limb gangrene. Because patients rarely become profoundly thrombocytopenic as a result of HIT alone, platelet transfusions are typically not required. In fact, some reports suggest that platelet transfusions can actually precipitate thrombotic complications, although this remains controversial.

FIGURE 175-1. Pathophysiology of heparin-induced thrombocytopenia. Platelet factor 4 (PF4) is a protein stored in platelet granules and secreted from platelets upon their activation. Heparin can bind to PF4 and induce a conformational change within PF4 that in some patients produces an antibody-mediated immune response. Large complexes of immunoglobulin (Ig), heparin, and PF4 can accumulate on the platelet surface and stimulate the platelet when the Fc portion of the antibody interacts with the platelet's FcγRII receptor (FcR). Once activated, the platelets contribute to thrombosis. In addition, the activated platelets secrete more PF4, continuing the process.

TABLE 175-3	LABORATORY ASSAYS FOR HEPARIN-INDUCED THROMBOCYTOPENIA			
ASSAY	**SENSITIVITY (%)**	**SPECIFICITY (%)**	**POSITIVE PREDICTIVE VALUE (%)**	**NEGATIVE PREDICTIVE VALUE (%)**
Functional assay (e.g., serotonin release assay)	88	≈100	≈100	81
PF4/heparin enzyme immunoassay (ELISA)	95-98	86	93	95

ELISA = enzyme-linked immunosorbent assay; PF4 = platelet factor 4.

Sepsis

Along with exposure to certain drugs, bacterial and viral infections are the most common cause of acute thrombocytopenia in hospitalized patients. Acute thrombocytopenia can be caused by the deposition of antibody-antigen complexes on the platelet surface via an "innocent bystander" phenomenon. These antibody-coated platelets are then cleared from the circulatory system by Fc receptor–expressing macrophages in the spleen. Thrombocytopenia associated with infections can also be due to DIC. The treatment of sepsis-induced thrombocytopenia is directed at the underlying cause, along with platelet transfusions as clinically indicated.

Idiopathic (Immune) Thrombocytopenic Purpura

DEFINITION

ITP is an autoimmune disorder caused by circulating antiplatelet autoantibodies. An ITP-like picture can also be found in patients with autoimmune diseases such as systemic lupus erythematosus (see later and Chapter 274), low-grade lymphoproliferative disorders such as chronic lymphocytic leukemia (Chapter 190), and HIV infection (Chapter 400).

CLINICAL MANIFESTATIONS

ITP was originally thought to be a disease of young women. Although this description is appropriate for many individuals with this disorder, more recent data indicate that ITP can occur in patients of either sex and at any age. ITP is a chronic, recurring disorder in the vast majority of adults with this disease. This is in stark contrast to pediatric patients, who usually suffer from acute ITP and rarely have the chronic variant of this disorder.

In contrast to patients with coagulation factor deficiencies who present with bleeding deep within tissues, individuals with ITP (or other disorders of platelets) typically have excessive mucocutaneous bleeding. Consequently, the clinician should inquire whether the patient has noticed epistaxis, gingival bleeding, easy bruising, hematuria, melena, or hematochezia. Female patients should also be asked about inappropriate or excessive vaginal bleeding. The physical examination should pay particular attention to signs of mucocutaneous bleeding. Consequently, the patient should be thoroughly examined for petechiae and ecchymosis, as well as for evidence of hemorrhage within the conjunctiva, retina, and central nervous system.

DIAGNOSIS

Except for the thrombocytopenia, the CBC is usually normal, and the peripheral blood smear is remarkable only for a decreased number of platelets, some of which may be larger than normal. Splenomegaly is absent unless the ITP is due to an underlying disorder, such as lymphoma, that is itself associated with splenomegaly. Bone marrow examination is usually not necessary in the absence of findings that suggest a different disease such as myelodysplasia. If performed, the bone marrow aspirate and biopsy typically show normal or increased numbers of megakaryocytes but are otherwise normal, characteristic of other forms of destructive thrombocytopenia.

TREATMENT Rx

Because platelet production is assumed to be increased in patients with ITP, traditional therapy has focused on moderating this immune response that ultimately leads to accelerated platelet destruction. For most of the latter half of the 20th century, splenectomy and corticosteroids were the sole therapies for ITP. Although they remain first-line therapeutic modalities, immunomodulating agents such as intravenous immunoglobulin (IVIG) and anti-D, as well as alternative immunosuppressives, have been introduced for the therapy of ITP. Corticosteroids in the form of high-dose dexamethasone (4-day pulses every 14 to 28 days for four to six cycles) are effective. For selected refractory patients, other immunosuppressives, such as cyclophosphamide, azathioprine, cyclosporine A, mycophenolate mofetil, dapsone, interferon, and etanercept, can be used.

For years, the basic mechanism of and rationale for ITP treatment revolved around altering the immune system through immunosuppressives, splenectomy, or immune modulators such as IVIG or anti-D. A more recent addition to the ITP treatment regimen is rituximab, a "humanized" murine monoclonal antibody against CD20, which is a B-cell antigen. Although rituximab has not been approved by the Food and Drug Administration (FDA) for the treatment of ITP, it is currently widely used in patients who are unresponsive to splenectomy and corticosteroids. Response rates vary significantly between studies, ranging from 28 to 44% in larger trials. The combination of high-dose dexa-

methasone and rituximab was recently shown to be more effective than dexamethasone alone.[2]

Although the vast majority of ITP patients have a compensatory increase in megakaryopoiesis in response to the rapid platelet destruction, plasma derived from some ITP patients was unexpectedly found to inhibit platelet production. This has prompted a re-evaluation of whether impaired megakaryopoiesis contributes to the development of thrombocytopenia in this disease. Thrombopoietin (TPO) is a potent megakaryocyte colony-stimulating factor and, along with other cytokines, increases the size and number of megakaryocytes (Chapter 159). TPO levels are not markedly elevated in ITP, suggesting that supplemental TPO could help increase platelet production and correct the thrombocytopenia.

Early experiments demonstrated that recombinant as well as truncated forms of TPO significantly increased the platelet count in some refractory ITP patients. However, this also induced autoimmune autoantibodies against endogenous TPO, which resulted in profound and persistent thrombocytopenia. Both recombinant TPO and its truncated form were therefore withdrawn from clinical trials. Subsequently, peptides were developed that bear no structural resemblance to TPO but still bind to and activate the TPO receptor; these agents are called *TPO receptor agonists*. Because these recombinant drugs bear little structural similarity to native TPO, they should not trigger autoimmune anti-TPO antibodies. The FDA has approved two of these drugs, and several more are being used in clinical trials. The first of these, called romiplostim, is composed of several copies of the TPO receptor–binding peptide spliced into a recombinant antibody. This peptide agonist competes with TPO for binding to the TPO receptor and activates the receptor in an identical fashion as endogenous TPO. The second FDA-approved TPO receptor agonist is eltrombopag (Promacta). It is an oral drug that activates the TPO receptor by binding to the receptor's transmembrane region.

Both subcutaneously administered romiplostim and orally administered eltrombopag are capable of increasing platelet counts in approximately 70% of patients with ITP. Remarkably, these drugs can also increase the platelet count in patients with ITP that is refractory to other treatment modalities, including splenectomy.[3-7] However, adverse events, including bone marrow fibrosis and thromboembolism, have been reported. It should be noted that the drugs' effects disappear soon after their discontinuation. Therefore, the TPO receptor agonists are not disease modifying and are probably most appropriate for short-term use when a temporary rise in platelet count is required.

General Principles of ITP Therapy

Management of ITP is guided by both symptoms and platelet count.[8] Asymptomatic patients with platelet counts greater than 30,000/µL can be followed without treatment. If the patient is bleeding and/or has a platelet count less than 30,000/µL, treatment with prednisone is recommended (Table 175-4). Refractory patients may require splenectomy, other immunosuppressive medications, or one of the new thrombopoiesis-stimulating agents (Table 175-5). Splenectomy has a long history of success in this disorder; durable complete response rates are approximately 66 to 70%. Approximately half the remaining patients who do not have normal platelet counts following splenectomy achieve a partial response that is clinically meaningful. Unfortunately, 10 to 15% of patients derive no benefit from splenectomy, and there is no test to predict whether a particular patient will respond to this treatment.

ITP patients with severe thrombocytopenia (<5000/µL) and/or internal bleeding should be promptly treated with high doses of pulse corticosteroids and IVIG. Platelet transfusion may be given concurrently with IVIG for critical bleeding. In Rh-positive patients who have not undergone splenectomy, anti-D immune globulin may be substituted for IVIG. However, some patients develop autoimmune hemolysis from this treatment.

TABLE 175-4	THERAPY FOR THE INITIAL MANAGEMENT OF IDIOPATHIC THROMBOCYTOPENIC PURPURA

ORAL PREDNISONE

Effect is dose dependent—approximately 80% of patients respond to 1 mg/kg/day. Toxicity also increases with dose and duration of treatment and includes glucose intolerance, immunosuppression, osteoporosis, and cataracts. Relapse is typical once therapy is discontinued.

INTRAVENOUS IMMUNOGLOBULIN (IVIG)

More rapid than daily prednisone. Administered at a dose of 1 g/kg/day for 2 consecutive days or 0.4 g/kg/day for 5 consecutive days. Response rates are approximately 80%, and effects typically last 2-4 wk. Toxicity includes headache, allergic reactions, and, rarely, thrombosis.

ANTI-D IMMUNOGLOBULIN

Administered at a dose of 50-75 µg/kg IV. Response rates are dose dependent but can approach 75-80%. Hemolysis is a common toxicity. Rarely, hemolysis can be life threatening and can be associated with disseminated intravascular coagulation, renal failure, and end-organ infarction.

Thrombotic Thrombocytopenic Purpura

DEFINITION

TTP is a consumptive thrombocytopenia associated with a mechanical hemolytic anemia. The classic pentad of symptoms—thrombocytopenia, anemia, fever, neurologic problems, and renal abnormalities—is fully present in only a minority of patients. Many patients today have only hemolytic anemia and thrombocytopenia. The poor specificity of the clinical features and laboratory abnormalities makes this disease difficult to diagnose. Historically, untreated TTP had a mortality of 90% within 3 months. With modern therapy, patients with TTP have a mortality of approximately 10 to 20%.

PATHOBIOLOGY

Some patients with recurrent TTP have very large multimers of von Willebrand factor (Chapter 176). Because larger multimers of von Willebrand factor are more efficient at binding and activating platelets than smaller ones, it was speculated that TTP could be due to a deficiency of a protease that cleaves large multimers of von Willebrand factor into smaller, less sticky ones. A genome-wide linkage analysis of patients with inherited recurrent TTP (Upshaw-Schulman syndrome) demonstrated a deficiency of a metalloproteinase that is now called ADAMTS13 (a disintegrin-like and metalloprotease with thrombospondin type 1 repeats). Many patients with adult-onset TTP have an antibody against ADAMTS13 that causes an acquired deficiency

of the enzyme. Inherited or acquired ADAMTS13 deficiency causes the accumulation of ultra-large multimers of von Willebrand factor in plasma, which leads to platelet activation and the microvascular thrombosis characteristic of this disease (Fig. 175-2). Because many patients can have a partial deficiency of ADAMTS13 without having TTP, clinical assays of ADAMTS13 enzymatic activity have not been useful in diagnosing TTP. Levels of ADAMTS13 below 5% of normal are considered highly suggestive of TTP, but levels greater than this are not very helpful. This hypothesis still needs to be validated in large clinical trials. Consequently, analysis of ADAMTS13 enzymatic activity should not be used to diagnose TTP outside of a research setting.

Some patients reportedly developed TTP soon after taking an antiplatelet drug of the thienopyridine class. Approximately 1 of every 2000 patients taking ticlopidine will develop TTP. In several individuals with ticlopidine-induced TTP, an antibody against ADAMTS13 was identified. A few studies have also suggested that clopidogrel can induce TTP at an incidence of 1 in 15,000 to 1 in 250,000. Because the incidence of TTP in the general population is approximately 1 in 100,000, it is difficult to determine whether there is a significant risk of TTP in patients who are prescribed clopidogrel. It should be noted that some patients can also develop TTP after exposure to medications that directly injure the vascular endothelium. The majority of these patients do not have TTP but have the related disorder HUS (discussed later in this chapter).

CLINICAL MANIFESTATIONS AND DIAGNOSIS

Patients often present with symptoms of excessive mucocutaneous bleeding, but they might present with signs of a thrombotic event (including phlebitis, myocardial infarction, or stroke). Many patients complain of abdominal pain that is presumably due to intestinal ischemia. Signs of central nervous system disease, including somnolence and even frank coma, can also be seen on presentation.

The two major hallmarks of this disorder are microangiopathic hemolytic anemia and thrombocytopenia. Microangiopathic hemolytic anemia is a non-immune-mediated hemolytic anemia caused by red cell fragmentation. Patients with this disorder have typical laboratory findings of hemolytic anemia, including a decreasing hemoglobin concentration, high lactate dehydrogenase level, elevated indirect bilirubin, and increased reticulocyte count. Examination of the peripheral blood smear (Chapter 160) shows torn red blood cells (schistocytes) and, frequently, early red blood cell precursor cells (nucleated red blood cells). The thrombocytopenia may be mild if the disease is diagnosed at an early stage, but advanced cases of TTP can have platelet counts less than 10,000/μL. TTP should be considered in any patient who has evidence of hemolysis accompanied by thrombocytopenia.

Unlike most patients with typical thrombocytopenia, who tend to bleed excessively, patients with TTP have few hemorrhagic complications. Instead, they are markedly predisposed to thrombosis. In fact, a thrombotic complication in a thrombocytopenic patient is another clue that TTP might be the cause of the thrombocytopenia (see Table 175-1). Characteristically, the thrombotic occlusions are in the terminal arterioles and capillaries and are composed mainly of platelets within the damaged vascular lumen. In contrast to most blood clots, these occlusions contain very little fibrin and are referred to as hyaline thrombi. Before plasmapheresis was used, TTP typically progressed and caused renal disease, neurologic symptoms, and fever. These symptoms are believed to be due to ischemia and infarction of the affected

TABLE 175-5 THERAPY FOR THE MANAGEMENT OF REFRACTORY IDIOPATHIC THROMBOCYTOPENIC PURPURA

ORAL PREDNISONE

Effect is dose dependent and rapidly dissipates after discontinuation of the medication. Some patients can be maintained on a very low and tolerable daily dose (e.g., 5 mg). Long-term use is associated with infections, diabetes, osteoporosis, avascular necrosis, weight gain, and cataracts.

ORAL DEXAMETHASONE

Administered at a dose of 40 mg/day for 4 consecutive days. Repeated every 2-4 wk for several months. Sustained response rates of 29-42% are possible. Toxicity is similar to that of oral prednisone.

SPLENECTOMY

Durable (often lifelong), significant responses are seen in 65-70% of patients who undergo this procedure. More modest benefits are seen in another 10-15% of patients. There is no useful way to predict who will respond. Splenectomy is associated with surgical morbidity and some mortality (≈1-2%). Produces lifelong immunosuppression to encapsulated and gram-positive organisms.

RITUXIMAB

Given at a dose of 375 mg/m²/wk IV for a total of 4 wk. Significant responses are seen in 28-44% of patients and typically last for months. Toxicity includes reactivation of hepatitis B, immunosuppression, and, rarely, progressive multifocal leukoencephalopathy.

THROMBOPOIETIN RECEPTOR AGONISTS

Administered daily (eltrombopag) or weekly (romiplostim). An effect is typically seen in 2-3 wk and disappears a few weeks after discontinuation of the medication. Toxicity from long-term use is not well known but may include excessive thrombosis and bone marrow fibrosis.

FIGURE 175-2. Pathophysiology of thrombotic thrombocytopenia purpura (TTP). **A,** Von Willebrand factor (vWF) is synthesized in endothelial cells and stored in Weibel-Palade bodies. The vWF is assembled into ultra-large multimers that are cleaved once they are released into the blood stream by the protease ADAMTS13. The resultant smaller multimers of vWF can bind to platelets to participate in normal hemostasis. **B,** Some patients with TTP have a deficiency of ADAMTS13. This results in the accumulation of ultra-large multimers of vWF within the circulation, promoting the excessive adhesion of platelets. This produces large hyaline plugs of vWF and platelets that cause vascular occlusions.

organs. Today, this disease is often diagnosed in its early stages, so patients may have only microangiopathic hemolytic anemia and thrombocytopenia.

TREATMENT[9]

The prompt initiation of plasma exchange (plasmapheresis with plasma replacement) reduces the mortality of TTP from 90% to approximately 15%. The mechanism of this benefit is not entirely known. A randomized trial demonstrated that plasmapheresis is more beneficial than plasma infusion for the treatment of TTP, implying that some of the benefit of plasmapheresis is attributable to the removal of a pathologic substance from the patient's plasma. Assuming that the pathogenesis of most acquired forms of TTP is the antibody-mediated inhibition of ADAMTS13, plasmapheresis might have two benefits. First, it helps remove the pathogenic antibody from the plasma. Second, the normal plasma infused into the patient during plasmapheresis repletes the deficiency of ADAMTS13. Both these benefits probably play a role in the efficacy of plasma exchange in the treatment of this disease.

Because patients with TTP can develop sudden thrombotic events (including stroke and myocardial infarction) without warning and deteriorate quickly, it is prudent to initiate plasma exchange as rapidly as possible. Given the morbidity and mortality of untreated TTP and the relatively low risk of plasmapheresis, this therapy should be initiated even when the diagnosis is not certain. As discussed in the section on HUS, plasmapheresis is not beneficial in children with Shiga toxin–induced microangiopathic hemolytic anemia or in patients who develop HUS following exposure to endothelium-toxic drugs, such as chemotherapy.

Plasma exchange is administered to replace one entire plasma volume and is usually repeated once daily. An average-sized individual requires 20 to 30 units of fresh-frozen plasma for each plasmapheresis session. Therapy is usually administered daily, and the patient is monitored for signs of improvement in thrombocytopenia, hemolysis, neurologic symptoms, fever, and renal disease. Appropriate daily laboratory tests to monitor the patient are CBC, lactate dehydrogenase, reticulocyte count, and creatinine. Once the thrombocytopenia and hemolysis have been corrected for a few days, the daily plasmapheresis can be either discontinued or continued every other day for several more days. A typical duration of therapy is 1 to 2 weeks, although some patients require treatment far beyond this usual time course.

Approximately one third of patients relapse quickly after plasmapheresis is stopped. These patients require a reinitiation of plasma exchange and perhaps the addition of an immunosuppressive drug, such as a glucocorticoid. Some reports indicate that rituximab shows promise in reducing the incidence of relapse. However, given that this drug does not decrease antibody production for weeks to months after its administration, it is likely that if rituximab has any benefit in the treatment of TTP, it is probably only to minimize the incidence of late relapses.

Major complications of plasmapheresis do occur and are often attributable to the use of a central venous catheter. Hypotension, bacteremia, hemorrhage, and thrombosis are among the most common life-threatening complications of plasmapheresis therapy. Two specific complications deserve emphasis. First, patients on angiotensin-converting enzyme (ACE) inhibitor antihypertensives are susceptible to plasmapheresis-induced hypotension owing to these drugs' interference with bradykinin catabolism. Second, a patient who develops recurrent thrombocytopenia and fever several days to a week into treatment may not be having an exacerbation of TTP but may be developing central line–induced sepsis. Consequently, a vigorous investigation for infection should be initiated in patients who appear to be relapsing early.

Hemolytic-Uremic Syndrome

DEFINITION

HUS is another cause of microangiopathic hemolytic anemia, and it may be difficult to distinguish from TTP. When acute renal failure is predominant and there are no neurologic symptoms, many clinicians consider the syndrome to be HUS, not TTP. In contrast to TTP, HUS is not caused by a deficiency of ADAMTS13. However, at this point, it is not clear whether ADAMTS13 levels will be clinically useful to distinguish between HUS and TTP. Because there is such overlap between the signs and symptoms of TTP and those of HUS, the distinction and diagnosis may be impossible in some cases.

PATHOBIOLOGY AND CLINICAL MANIFESTATIONS

A toxin that directly damages endothelial cells can cause HUS. These direct endothelial toxins are either infectious or the result of a drug. Perhaps the best-characterized infectious agent that damages endothelial cells is Shiga toxin–producing enterohemorrhagic *Escherichia coli* (Chapter 312). In Shiga toxin–induced HUS, the renal disease and microangiopathic hemolytic anemia occur after an episode of diarrhea that is often bloody. *E. coli* O157:H7

is the cause of many cases in the United States. The toxin damages endothelial cells within the glomeruli and promotes the adhesion of platelets and the trapping of red blood cells.

Several drugs can induce HUS by directly damaging endothelial cells. These include calcineurin inhibitors such as tacrolimus and cyclosporine; sometimes, lowering the dose of these drugs can reverse the microangiopathic hemolytic anemia. Cytotoxic drugs such as mitomycin C, cisplatin, and bleomycin can also induce HUS by damaging endothelial cells.

Inherited forms of HUS have been described, and they usually involve dysregulation of the complement cascade (Chapter 49). The best-described genetic mutations cause the deficiency of factor H, a complement regulatory protease. HUS-inducing mutations in other components of complement regulation include those found in C3, CD46, and factor I.

TREATMENT AND PREVENTION

Reducing the spread of Shiga toxin–producing *E. coli* is vital, because antibiotics and antimotility drugs do not lower the risk of developing HUS symptoms. In contrast to TTP, there is little evidence that plasma exchange is beneficial.[9] The infusion of plasma or plasmapheresis is reportedly beneficial in the treatment of atypical forms of HUS caused by the dysregulation of complement.

Disseminated Intravascular Coagulation

DIC is a pathologic condition that depletes components of the coagulation system, including platelets. Therefore, in contrast to TTP and HUS, the thrombocytopenia of DIC is associated with the consumption of coagulation factors and increased fibrinolysis, often leading to prolongations of the prothrombin time and activated partial thromboplastin time, as well as increased levels of D-dimers. In its fully manifested state, DIC can be associated with arterial and venous thrombi, hemorrhage, microangiopathic hemolysis, thrombocytopenia, excessive fibrinolysis, and deficiency of coagulation factors such as fibrinogen. For a more complete review of DIC and related disorders, see Chapter 178.

Thrombocytopenia during Pregnancy

Thrombocytopenia occurs in approximately 5% of pregnant women. It may be due to a normal variant of pregnancy (gestational thrombocytopenia), a pregnancy-specific condition (preeclampsia and HELLP syndrome [hemolysis, elevated liver enzymes, and low platelets]), or a condition exacerbated by pregnancy (ITP, vasculitis, TTP). The prognosis and treatment vary tremendously based on the underlying cause.

Gestational thrombocytopenia (incidental thrombocytopenia of pregnancy) is a mild, asymptomatic thrombocytopenia that typically occurs late in pregnancy. There is no association with fetal thrombocytopenia, and this maternal thrombocytopenia resolves spontaneously after delivery. Other than thrombocytopenia during previous pregnancies, women with gestational thrombocytopenia have no prior history of a low platelet count. This lack of previous thrombocytopenia helps distinguish gestational thrombocytopenia from ITP. Additionally, in contrast to other causes of maternal thrombocytopenia, gestational thrombocytopenia does not produce a platelet count lower than 70,000/μL. Consequently, deviation from standard obstetric care is usually not required for a patient with gestational thrombocytopenia.

Preeclampsia is a syndrome that causes the gradual development of proteinuria and hypertension during the later stages of pregnancy (Chapter 247). A minority of women with preeclampsia progress to have seizures; when this occurs, the syndrome is called *eclampsia*. Approximately 15% of women with preeclampsia have thrombocytopenia, and 5% of patients with preeclampsia have platelet counts less than 50,000/μL. Some patients have a more severe form of preeclampsia associated with HELLP syndrome. Preeclampsia and HELLP syndrome are believed to be caused by a factor produced within the placenta, because these syndromes usually resolve rapidly and spontaneously after delivery. They can present post partum, but they still resolve within a few days of delivery. Consequently, immediate delivery of the child is recommended, if possible, because the microangiopathic process stops soon thereafter. If these syndromes do not resolve spontaneously within 3 days, alternative diagnoses such as ITP and TTP should be considered.

Most patients with ITP or vasculitis during pregnancy have a history of thrombocytopenia before pregnancy. The antiplatelet immunoglobulin G antibodies that cause this disease in the mother can cross the placenta and lead to thrombocytopenia in the fetus. However, the platelet count in the unborn child does not correlate well with the platelet count of the mother, and attempts to sample fetal blood to monitor platelet counts are associated with significant risk. Because the vast majority of children born to women with ITP have a platelet count high enough for a successful delivery, the management of ITP focuses on keeping the maternal platelet count acceptable for the mother's safety. In the early stages of pregnancy, a platelet count of 30,000 to 50,000/μL is considered safe. In preparation for delivery, a platelet count of 50,000 to 80,000/μL is more desirable. This can be managed by the use of oral glucocorticoids and, if necessary, by the administration of IVIG. The safety of rituximab and thrombopoiesis-stimulating agents during pregnancy is not known. Splenectomy performed during the first trimester has a risk of inducing miscarriage, and this operation is technically difficult during the later stages of pregnancy because of uterine enlargement. There is no evidence that a cesarean section is safer than vaginal delivery.

The diagnosis of TTP during pregnancy can be difficult because many of the symptoms are identical to those of preeclampsia. If the symptoms develop during the early stages of pregnancy, when preeclampsia is unlikely, the diagnosis of TTP is more certain. The presence of hyperuricemia, hypoproteinemia, elevated liver transaminases, and direct bilirubin is more consistent with preeclampsia. The development of microangiopathic hemolytic anemia and thrombocytopenia in the peripartum period is presumed to be attributable to preeclampsia, and immediate delivery of the fetus is desirable if it is safe to do so. Typically, the thrombocytopenia starts to resolve rapidly after delivery. If no improvement is seen by the third postpartum day, standard management for TTP, including plasma exchange, is recommended.

Post-Transfusion Purpura and Neonatal Alloimmune Thrombocytopenia

Alloimmune thrombocytopenia is due to sensitization to alloantigens such as PI^A1 (HPA-1a). These alloimmune antibodies can cause thrombocytopenia approximately a week after a blood transfusion (post-transfusion purpura, or PTP). A similar alloimmune antibody can cause thrombocytopenia in a fetus when it is produced by the mother (neonatal alloimmune thrombocytopenia, or NAIT). PTP causes profound thrombocytopenia 7 to 10 days after exposure to platelets that contaminate red blood cell transfusions. However, it can be treated with IVIG or plasma exchange. NAIT can cause severe thrombocytopenia and bleeding in neonates and is treated with the transfusion of platelets derived from a PI^A1-negative donor (most conveniently the newborn's mother herself), corticosteroids, and IVIG.

Vasculitis

Autoimmune diseases such as systemic lupus erythematosus, rheumatoid arthritis, and other forms of vasculitis can also involve thrombocytopenia. This can be due to an ITP-like process that occurs in patients with a propensity for the development of autoantibodies. The treatment for these patients is immunosuppression, similar to the treatment for other patients with ITP. Some patients with active vasculitis and endothelial inflammation consume circulating platelets due to this damaged vessel wall, creating a clinical picture that is difficult to distinguish from that of TTP without a tissue diagnosis that documents vasculitis. Owing to the difficulty of discerning TTP from a flare-up of vasculitis, these patients are often treated with both plasma exchange and immunosuppression.

Dilutional Thrombocytopenia

Thrombocytopenia does not typically occur after blood loss, possibly due in part to the release of platelets from the splenic pool. Thrombocytopenia occasionally occurs after massive hemorrhage, but only when the hemorrhage is severe enough to necessitate replacement of 1.5 to 2 times the total blood volume, which usually requires transfusion of at least 15 to 20 units of packed red blood cells over a short period. Even in this circumstance, the thrombocytopenia is only mild to moderate. Therefore, the clinician should remain vigilant for another cause of the thrombocytopenia (such as DIC resulting from hemorrhage-induced hypotension and shock). There is no reason to routinely transfuse platelets in a fixed ratio to packed red blood cells unless thrombocytopenia is present and doing so is otherwise indicated. When indicated, dilutional thrombocytopenia can be corrected with platelet transfusions.

Congenital Thrombocytopenias

Lifelong thrombocytopenia can be due to an inherited defect that affects platelet production or survival. These disorders can be autosomal dominant (May-Hegglin anomaly, Alport's syndrome), autosomal recessive

(Bernard-Soulier disease, Fanconi's anemia, gray platelet syndrome, thrombocytopenia with absent radius syndrome), or X-linked (Wiscott-Aldrich syndrome). Many of these disorders are associated with other abnormalities in addition to thrombocytopenia. A congenital cause of thrombocytopenia should be suspected in a patient who has long-standing moderate thrombocytopenia presumed to be treatment-refractory ITP.

Grade A

1. Slichter SJ, Kaufman RM, Assmann SF, et al. Dose of prophylactic platelet transfusions and prevention of hemorrhage. N Engl J Med. 2010;362:600-613.
2. Zaja F, Baccarani M, Mazza P, et al. Dexamethasone plus rituximab yields higher sustained response rates than dexamethasone monotherapy in adults with primary immune thrombocytopenia. Blood. 2010;115:2755-2762.
3. Kuter DJ, Bussel JB, Lyons RM, et al. Efficacy of romiplostim in patients with chronic immune thrombocytopenic purpura: a double-blind randomised controlled trial. Lancet. 2008;37:395-403.
4. Kuter DJ, Rummel M, Boccia R, et al. Romiplostim or standard of care in patients with immune thrombocytopenia. N Engl J Med. 2010;363:1889-1899.
5. George JN, Mathias SD, Go RS, et al. Improved quality of life for romiplostim-treated patients with chronic immune thrombocytopenic purpura: results from two randomized, placebo-controlled trials. Br J Haematol. 2009;144:409-415.
6. Bussel JB, Provan D, Shamsi T, et al. Effect of eltrombopag on platelet counts and bleeding during treatment of chronic idiopathic thrombocytopenic purpura: a randomised, double-blind, placebo-controlled trial. Lancet. 2009;373:641-648.
7. Cheng G, Saleh MN, Marcher C, et al. Eltrombopag for management of chronic immune thrombocytopenia (RAISE): a 6-month, randomised, phase 3 study. Lancet. 2011;377:393-402.
8. Provan D, Stasi R, Newland AC, et al. International consensus report on the investigation and management of primary immune thrombocytopenia. Blood. 2010;115:168-186.
9. Michael M, Elliott EJ, Ridley GF, et al. Interventions for haemolytic uraemic syndrome and thrombotic thrombocytopenic purpura. Cochrane Database Syst Rev. 2009;1:CD003595.

SUGGESTED READINGS

Arepally GM, Ortel TL. Heparin-induced thrombocytopenia. Annu Rev Med. 2010;61:77-90. Review of current understanding of the pathogenesis, clinical features, diagnostic criteria, and management of this commonly encountered problem in inpatient medicine.

Cines DB, Bussel JB, Liebman HA, et al. The ITP syndrome: pathogenic and clinical diversity. Blood. 2009;113:6511-6521. Focus on the variety of underlying conditions associated with ITP.

George JN, Aster RH. Drug-induced thrombocytopenia: pathogenesis, evaluation, and management. Hematology Am Soc Hematol Program. 2009;153-158. Excellent review of an important consideration in determining the cause of thrombocytopenia.

Kavanagh D, Goodship T. Haemolytic uraemic syndrome. Nephron Clin Pract. 2011;118:c37-c42. Review.

Provan D, Stasi R, Newland AC, et al. International consensus report on the investigation and management of primary immune thrombocytopenia. Blood. 2010;115:168-186. Consensus guidelines.

176

VON WILLEBRAND DISEASE AND HEMORRHAGIC ABNORMALITIES OF PLATELET AND VASCULAR FUNCTION

WILLIAM L. NICHOLS

VON WILLEBRAND DISEASE

DEFINITION AND EPIDEMIOLOGY

Von Willebrand disease (VWD), a usually autosomal dominantly inherited condition affecting both males and females of all ethnicities, is the most common hereditary bleeding disorder worldwide, with prevalence estimates dependent on case definition. It may also occur less frequently as an acquired disorder (acquired von Willebrand syndrome [AVWS]). Von Willebrand factor (VWF) plasma levels are variably decreased (minimally to substantially) in at least 2.5% of humans, whereas approximately 0.1% (1 in 1000) have definite VWD with medically significant bleeding symptoms related to low VWF, and approximately 0.01% (1 in 10,000) have more severe forms of VWD that often result in referral to tertiary care centers including hemophilia centers.

PATHOBIOLOGY

VWD reflects deficiency or dysfunction of VWF, a multimeric plasma glycoprotein that mediates platelet adhesion and aggregation at sites of vascular injury (Chapter 174), and that also carries and stabilizes blood coagulation factor VIII (FVIII) in the circulation. The *VWF* gene is located on chromosome 12, with a partial pseudogene on chromosome 22 that potentially complicates DNA-based mutation detection (which remains primarily a research application, with evolving clinical diagnostic potential). The protein is synthesized by vascular endothelium as ~270-kD subunits (protomers) that are dimerized, then processed and polymerized into very large (up to about 20,000 kD) hemostatically active VWF multimers, and finally secreted into the blood. Vascular endothelial cells additionally provide a storage reservoir of multimerized VWF (in intracellular Weibel-Palade bodies) from which it can be released by stress or drugs such as DDAVP (desmopressin). VWF is also synthesized and multimerized by bone marrow megakaryocytes and stored in circulating blood platelet α granules, from which it is secreted with platelet activation. Platelet-stored VWF represents about 10% of total blood VWF.

Multimerization of VWF is essential for its hemostatic activity that is mainly mediated by the higher-molecular-weight (larger) multimers. Circulating plasma VWF does not interact with platelets, but when VWF binds to injured (de-endothelialized) blood vessel walls, reflecting its collagen-binding activity, multimers can be stretched and unfolded by high intravascular shear forces, such as in the microvasculature, exposing and activating previously cryptic platelet-binding domains to promote platelet adhesion and aggregation to vessel-bound VWF. Simultaneously, activated (stretched) VWF multimers expose protomer cleavage sites for proteolysis by the circulating enzyme, ADAMTS13 (A Disintegrin And Metalloprotease domain with ThromboSpondin type 1 motifs, member 13), ultimately decreasing the size of VWF multimers and thereby downregulating VWF hemostatic function. Severe deficiency of ADAMTS13 is associated with the pathologic microangiopathy of thrombotic thrombocytopenic purpura (TTP) (Chapter 175), in which the microvascular thrombosis is mediated by ultralarge VWF multimers in the circulation.

VWD is classified into three major types that vary in severity and differ in clinical management, such that defining the VWD subtype is important. Type 1 VWD reflects partial quantitative deficiency of normally functioning VWF, of variable severity, and comprises 75 to 80% of individuals with symptomatic VWD. Type 2 VWD reflects qualitative VWF deficiency, with four subtypes (A, B, M, N), and comprises 20 to 25% of persons with VWD. Type 3 VWD reflects the virtual absence of VWF, with secondary near-absence of FVIII, and is rare (<1% of VWD). Inheritance of VWD is usually autosomal dominant, except that type 3 VWD is typically autosomal recessive in inheritance. Table 176-1 summarizes the classification of VWD subtypes and their basic pathophysiology.

The FVIII deficiency that often accompanies different types of VWD (see Table 176-1) is not genetically related to the disease; the gene that encodes FVIII is on the X chromosome, and its primary deficiency causes classic hemophilia (Chapter 177). FVIII deficiency in VWD is due to a primary deficiency or defect in the VWF molecule, which normally carries and stabilizes FVIII in the circulation. Therefore, FVIII is more rapidly cleared from the circulation, leading to its secondary deficiency in VWD.

CLINICAL MANIFESTATIONS

Individuals with VWD usually experience mucocutaneous bleeding symptoms such as easy bruising, prolonged or excessive bleeding from minor cuts or other injuries, nosebleeds or other mucosal bleeding such as gastrointestinal hemorrhage, or heavy menstrual bleeding (in women), and they may be at increased risk for bleeding following surgery or invasive procedures, dental extractions, traumatic injury, or childbirth. Symptoms can range from relatively mild or infrequent bleeding in type 1 VWD to severe, life-threatening bleeding in type 3 VWD. As a group, women with VWD may be more affected by bleeding symptoms than men because of hemostatic challenges of menstruation and childbirth.

DIAGNOSIS

Clinical Assessment

Diagnosis of VWD (or other bleeding disorders) begins with clinical assessment to evaluate for a personal and possible family history of abnormal bleeding, accompanied by focused physical examination to detect signs or symptoms of bleeding (e.g., petechiae, ecchymoses, hematomas, anemia), as well as findings that may suggest other causes of increased bleeding such as liver disease (e.g., hepatosplenomegaly, jaundice), joint or skin laxity (e.g., Ehlers-Danlos syndrome), telangiectasia (e.g., hereditary hemorrhagic telangiectasia), or anatomic lesions on gynecologic examination. Because

TABLE 176-1 CLASSIFICATION OF VON WILLEBRAND DISEASE

TYPE	DESCRIPTION
1	Partial quantitative deficiency of VWF (~75-80% of VWD)
2	Qualitative VWF defect (~20-25% of VWD)
2A	Caused by VWF mutations that decrease the proportion of large functional VWF multimers, leading to decreased VWF-dependent platelet adhesion and aggregation
2B	Caused by VWF mutations that increase platelet-VWF binding, resulting in depletion of large, functional VWF multimers. Circulating platelets are coated with mutant VWF, which may impair platelet adhesion and aggregation at sites of injury. Thrombocytopenia, persistent or intermittent, is observed in most cases. Distinguishing type 2B VWD may require RIPA to detect increased (abnormal) platelet aggregation response to low-dose ristocetin; the latter may also reflect platelet-type (pseudo) VWD caused by rare mutations in the platelet VWF receptor.
2M	Caused by VWF mutations that decrease VWF-dependent platelet adhesion and aggregation, but do not deplete the large VWF multimers. Distinguishing between types 2A and 2M VWD requires VWF multimer gel electrophoretic analysis.
2N	Caused by VWF mutations that impair binding to FVIII, thereby shortening FVIII survival and lowering FVIII levels so that type 2N VWD can masquerade as an autosomal recessive form of hemophilia A. Discrimination from hemophilia A may require assays of VWF-FVIII binding.
3	Virtually complete VWF deficiency, associated with markedly decreased FVIII (<1% of VWD)

FVIII = factor VIII coagulant activity; RIPA = ristocetin-induced platelet aggregation/aggregometry; VWD = von Willebrand disease; VWF = von Willebrand factor.
Adapted and modified from National Heart, Lung, and Blood Institute. *The Diagnosis, Evaluation, and Management of von Willebrand Disease.* Bethesda, MD: National Institutes of Health Publication 08-5832. December 2007 (released Feb 29, 2008). Available at: http://www.nhlbi.nih.gov/guidelines/vwd; and Yawn BP, Nichols WL, Rick ME. Diagnosis and management of von Willebrand disease: guidelines for primary care. *Am Fam Physician.* 2009;80:1261-1268, 1269-1270.

bleeding symptoms are common in apparently normal individuals, with prevalence of certain symptoms as high as 25 to 50%, clinical assessment for VWD or other possible bleeding disorders can be challenging (Chapter 174).

The most important parts of the medical history include (1) family history of a known or suspected bleeding disorder; (2) review of personal surgical or other hemostatic challenges lifelong and recently, including dental extractions and traumatic injuries, and whether abnormal bleeding occurred and its severity; (3) mucocutaneous bleeding symptoms (e.g., bruising, nosebleeds, ecchymoses, gastrointestinal bleeding, menorrhagia), including frequency, severity and spontaneity of events; and (4) assessment for medical conditions that can increase risk for bleeding, such as use of certain drugs that can impede normal hemostasis, including aspirin or other nonsteroidal anti-inflammatory drugs (NSAIDs), clopidogrel, or warfarin or heparin anticoagulants; presence of liver or kidney disease (e.g., cirrhosis, uremia); and history of low or high platelet count and blood or bone marrow disorders.

Bleeding history scoring tools are being developed and applied for studying populations with VWD or other bleeding disorders but are not yet validated for routine clinical use. However, in general, an increasing number of positive or abnormal clinical bleeding history items increases the likelihood that an individual has a bleeding disorder, including VWD, and may merit undergoing appropriate laboratory evaluation (Chapter 174).

Laboratory Evaluation

Because no simple, single laboratory test is available to screen for VWD, the initial laboratory evaluation requires measurements of plasma: (1) VWF antigen (VWF:Ag); (2) ristocetin cofactor activity (VWF:RCo); and (3) factor VIII coagulant activity (FVIII). All three tests are recommended for initial evaluation, and the results may not only establish the diagnosis but also suggest the type and severity of VWD if it is present. These three tests are also used for monitoring therapy. Tests such as the bleeding time (BT) or platelet function analyzer (PFA-100, Siemens) assay lack sufficient sensitivity and specificity and are not recommended for routine screening.

If one or more of the three test results are abnormally low, or if the ratio of VWF:RCo to VWF:Ag is below 0.5 to 0.7, additional laboratory evaluation may include selecting one or more of the following tests, based on the pattern of initial results together with clinical assessment and experience: (1) repeating the three initial VWD tests with timing and procedures optimized for conditions of the patient, the blood sample, and laboratory testing (see later for additional information about these conditions); (2) VWF multimer analysis to help differentiate or exclude types 2A, 2B, or 2M VWD; (3) ristocetin-induced platelet aggregometry (RIPA), including low-dose ristocetin testing to evaluate for type 2B VWD or platelet-type (pseudo) VWD; (4) VWF-FVIII binding assay (or molecular DNA-based VWF testing) to evaluate for type 2N VWD; and (5) other tests such as VWF:CB (collagen-binding activity) to supplement VWF:RCo testing and the overall evaluation. Some of these tests have limited availability and are mainly performed in reference laboratories. Consultation with a hemostasis specialist can help guide test selection.

Multimer analysis visualizes the distribution of plasma VWF multimers, is technically complex, is qualitatively interpreted in conjunction with results of the initial three tests and available clinical information, and is used to help determine the VWD subtype. Therefore, VWF multimer analysis is not recommended for initial VWD screening and should only be performed if initial VWD testing identifies an abnormal result (e.g., abnormally low VWF:RCo or ratio of VWF:RCo to VWF:Ag) or clinical information suggests a high likelihood of abnormal VWF multimer analysis.

Table 176-2 provides prototypical laboratory values for VWD subtypes. Diagnosis, especially for individuals with mildly decreased VWF (30 to 50% or IU/dL), requires correlation of clinical assessment (personal and family history of bleeding) and results of laboratory testing, the latter preferably performed or repeated in the absence of conditions associated with elevation of baseline VWF and with careful attention to blood specimen collection, processing, transportation, and storage.

The laboratory evaluation of a person for possible VWD or AVWS is relatively complex, particularly because results of the laboratory tests can be influenced by certain conditions of the patient and by variables in the blood sample and laboratory testing methodology (Table 176-3). In interpreting test results, therefore, it is important to be aware of these variabilities and the status of the patient at the time of evaluation.

TABLE 176-2 PATTERNS OF LABORATORY TEST RESULTS FOR VON WILLEBRAND DISEASE DIAGNOSIS AND CLASSIFICATION*

CONDITION	VWF:RCo (IU/dL)	VWF:Ag (IU/dL)	FVIII (IU/dL)	VWF:RCo/VWF:Ag RATIO[¶]	RIPA	VWF MULTIMERS
Type 1 VWD	<30[†]	<30[†‡]	↓ or Normal	>0.5-0.7	Often normal	Normal
Type 2A VWD	<30[†]	<30-200[†‡]	↓ or Normal	<0.5-0.7	↓ or Normal	↓ HMW
Type 2B VWD	<30[†]	<30-200[†‡]	↓ or Normal	Usually <0.5-0.7	↑ (Low dose)	↓ HMW
Type 2M VWD	<30[†]	<30-200[†‡]	↓ or Normal	<0.5-0.7	↓ or Normal	No ↓ HMW
Type 2N VWD	30-200	30-200	↓↓	>0.5-0.7	Normal	Normal
Type 3 VWD	<3	<3	↓↓↓ (1-9)	NA	Absent	NA
"Low VWF"[§]	30-50[§]	30-50[§]	Normal	>0.5-0.7	Normal	Normal
Normal	50-200	50-200	Normal	>0.5-0.7	Normal	Normal

*Values in the table represent prototypical cases without additional VWF (or other disease) abnormalities. Exceptions occur, and repeat testing and clinical experience may be necessary for clarification and interpretation of laboratory test results.
[†]VWF values <30 IU/dL (or %) are designated as the level for definite diagnosis of VWD (especially type 1 VWD) because (1) there is a high frequency of blood type O that is associated with "low VWF" levels but not necessarily VWD; (2) bleeding symptoms are reported by a significant proportion of individuals with no disease; and (3) no abnormality in the VWF gene has been identified in many individuals who have only mildly to moderately decreased VWF levels. VWF values of 30-50 IU/dL include both apparently normal persons and those with mild VWD.
[‡]VWF:Ag is <50 IU/dL in most persons with types 2A, 2B, or 2M VWD.
[§]Diagnosis of VWD is not precluded for persons with VWF:RCo of 30-50 IU/dL if there is supporting clinical or family evidence for VWD, nor is the use of agents to increase VWF levels precluded in those who have VWF:RCo of 30-50 IU/dL and who may be at risk for bleeding.
[¶]Until more laboratories clearly define a reference range, the VWF:RCo/VWF:Ag ratio of <0.5-0.7 is recommended to distinguish type 1 vs. type 2 VWD variants (A, B, or M).
FVIII = factor VIII coagulant activity; HMW = high molecular weight VWF multimers; IU/dL = international units per deciliter (e.g., 100 IU/dL = 100% of mean normal level); NA = not applicable; RIPA = ristocetin-induced platelet aggregation/aggregometry; VWD, von Willebrand disease; VWF = von Willebrand factor; VWF:Ag = von Willebrand factor antigen; VWF:RCo = von Willebrand factor ristocetin cofactor activity; ↓, ↓↓, ↓↓↓, ↑, refer to varying degrees of decrease, or an increase, of the test result compared to the laboratory reference range.
Adapted and modified from National Heart, Lung, and Blood Institute. *The Diagnosis, Evaluation, and Management of von Willebrand Disease.* Bethesda, MD: National Institutes of Health Publication 08-5832. December 2007 (released Feb 29, 2008). Available at: http://www.nhlbi.nih.gov/guidelines/vwd; and Yawn BP, Nichols WL, Rick ME. Diagnosis and management of von Willebrand disease: guidelines for primary care. *Am Fam Physician.* 2009;80:1261-1268, 1269-1270.

TABLE 176-3 VARIABLE CONDITIONS OF THE PATIENT, BLOOD SAMPLING, AND LABORATORY TESTING AFFECTING LABORATORY EVALUATION FOR VON WILLEBRAND DISEASE

Phlebotomy conditions—An atraumatic blood draw limits the exposure of tissue factor from the site and the activation of clotting factors, minimizing falsely high or low values. Lipemia should be avoided because it may interfere with photo-optical testing methods, especially some used for VWF:RCo assay.

Patient stress level—Undue stress, such as struggling or crying in children or anxiety in adults, may falsely elevate VWF and FVIII levels. Very recent exercise can also elevate VWF levels.

Additional conditions in the individual—The presence of an acute or chronic inflammatory illness may elevate VWF and FVIII levels, as may pregnancy or administration of estrogen or oral contraceptives. Individuals with blood group O have VWF levels approximately 25% lower than those of other ABO blood groups. African Americans have higher VWF levels than whites.

Sample processing—To prevent cryoprecipitation of VWF and other proteins, blood samples for VWF assays should be transported to the laboratory at room temperature. Plasma should be separated from blood cells promptly at room temperature, and the plasma should be centrifuged thoroughly to remove platelets. If plasma samples will be assayed within 2 hours, they should be kept at room temperature. Frozen plasma samples should be carefully thawed at 37° C and kept at room temperature for <2 hours before assay.

Sample storage—Plasma samples that will be stored or transported to a reference laboratory must be frozen promptly at or below −40° C and remain frozen until assayed. A control sample that is drawn, processed, stored, and transported under the same conditions as the tested person's sample may be helpful in indicating problems in the handling of important test samples. Activity of FVIII typically is 10-20% lower in frozen-thawed plasma than in fresh (nonfrozen) plasma, and can be even lower if blood processing or storage conditions are suboptimal.

Laboratory testing—Calibrators for assays of VWF:Ag, VWF:RCo, and FVIII should be referenced to the World Health Organization (WHO) plasma standard. These three tests have relatively high coefficients of variation (CVs of 10-30%), especially the VWF:RCo assay. The quality of laboratory testing also varies considerably among laboratories (high interlaboratory CV). Test results can be reported as international units per deciliter (IU/dL), rather than as a percentage (%) of mean normal, if WHO-linked calibrators are used. Referencing VWF testing results to the population reference range, rather than to ABO-stratified reference ranges, may be clinically useful.

FVIII = coagulation factor VIII; VWF = von Willebrand factor; VWF:Ag = VWF antigen; VWF:RCo = VWF ristocetin cofactor activity.
Adapted and modified from National Heart, Lung, and Blood Institute. *The Diagnosis, Evaluation, and Management of von Willebrand Disease.* Bethesda, MD: National Institutes of Health Publication 08-5832. December 2007 (released Feb 29, 2008). Available at: http://www.nhlbi.nih.gov/guidelines/vwd; and Nichols WL, Rick ME, Ortel TL, et al. Clinical and laboratory diagnosis of von Willebrand disease: a synopsis of the 2008 NHLBI/NIH guidelines. *Am J Hematol.* 2009; 84: 366-370.

TABLE 176-4   SUGGESTED DURATIONS OF VON WILLEBRAND FACTOR REPLACEMENT FOR DIFFERENT TYPES OF SURGICAL PROCEDURES

MAJOR SURGERY 7-14 DAYS*	MINOR SURGERY 1-5 DAYS*	OTHER PROCEDURES: IF UNCOMPLICATED, SINGLE VWF TREATMENT
Cardiothoracic	Biopsy: breast, cervical	Cardiac catheterization
Cesarean section	Complicated dental extractions	Cataract surgery
Craniotomy	Gingival surgery	Endoscopy (without biopsy)
Hysterectomy	Central line placement	Liver biopsy
Open cholecystectomy	Laparoscopic procedures	Lacerations
Prostatectomy		Simple dental extractions

*Individual cases may need longer or shorter duration depending on the severity of VWD and the type of procedure.

VWF = von Willebrand factor.

Adapted and modified from National Heart, Lung, and Blood Institute. *The Diagnosis, Evaluation, and Management of von Willebrand Disease.* Bethesda, MD: National Institutes of Health Publication 08-5832. December 2007 (released Feb. 29, 2008). http://www.nhlbi.nih.gov/guidelines/vwd.

TABLE 176-5   INITIAL DOSING RECOMMENDATIONS FOR VON WILLEBRAND FACTOR CONCENTRATE REPLACEMENT FOR PREVENTION OR MANAGEMENT OF BLEEDING

MAJOR SURGERY/BLEEDING

Loading dose*: 40-60 U/kg
Maintenance dose†: 20-40 U/kg every 8 to 24 hours
Monitoring: VWF:RCo and FVIII trough and peak, at least daily
Therapeutic goal: trough VWF:RCo and FVIII >50 IU/dL for 7-14 days
Safety parameter: do not exceed VWF:RCo >200 IU/dL or FVIII >250-300 IU/dL
May alternate with desmopressin (DDAVP) for latter part of treatment

MINOR SURGERY/BLEEDING

Loading dose*: 30-60 U/kg
Maintenance dose†: 20-40 U/kg every 12 to 48 hours
Monitoring: VWF:RCo and FVIII trough and peak, at least once
Therapeutic goal: trough VWF:RCo and FVIII >50 IU/dL for 3-5 days
Safety parameter: do not exceed VWF:RCo >200 IU/dL or FVIII >250-300 IU/dL
May alternate with desmopressin (DDAVP) for latter part of treatment

*Loading dose is in VWF:RCo IU/dL.
†Dosing intervals reflect approximately 12-hour average half-lives of plasma VWF and FVIII, without conditions resulting in shortened survival or enhanced clearance such as bleeding or surgery.
FVIII = factor VIII; VWF = von Willebrand factor; VWF:RCo = VWF ristocetin cofactor activity.
Adapted and modified from National Heart, Lung, and Blood Institute. *The Diagnosis, Evaluation, and Management of von Willebrand Disease.* Bethesda, MD: National Institutes of Health Publication 08-5832. December 2007 (released Feb. 29, 2008). http://www.nhlbi.nih.gov/guidelines/vwd.

TREATMENT   Rx

Management of patients with VWD is focused on treatment or prevention of bleeding episodes. There are three main approaches to treatment of VWD that are used individually or in combination: (1) increasing plasma concentration of VWF and FVIII by releasing endogenous VWF stores through stimulation of endothelial cells with DDAVP; (2) replacing or supplementing VWF and FVIII by using human plasma-derived, viral-inactivated concentrates; and (3) promoting hemostasis using hemostatic agents that work by mechanisms other than increasing VWF and FVIII. Regular prophylaxis is seldom required, and treatment is given primarily before and after planned invasive procedures or in response to episodes of bleeding. Table 176-4 outlines usual durations of treatment for a variety of surgical and other invasive procedures.

Desmopressin (DDAVP)

DDAVP (desmopressin: 1-desamino-8-D-arginine vasopressin) is a synthetic derivative of the antidiuretic hormone and causes release of preformed VWF from endothelial cells. It is mainly used in type 1 VWD, is contraindicated for type 2B VWD (because it can cause thrombocytopenia), has limited efficacy for types 2A, 2M, or 2N VWD, and has no efficacy for type 3 VWD. DDAVP is generally administered for short time periods (48 to 72 hours) and usually not more frequently than at 24- to 48-hour intervals, owing to tachyphylaxis and side effects. If it is required for longer periods or more frequently, the patient should be monitored for fluid and electrolyte problems because DDAVP may cause symptomatic hyponatremia. DDAVP therapy is potentially mildly thrombogenic, especially for persons who are at increased risk for atherosclerotic cardiovascular disorders such as stroke or myocardial infarction.

The hemostatic dose of DDAVP is 0.3 μg/kg body weight, infused intravenously over about 30 minutes, or administered subcutaneously; however, a concentrated formulation for the latter is not available in the United States. For outpatients, DDAVP can also be administered nasally, using a concentrated spray (Stimate, CSL Behring) that delivers 150 μg per nostril (300 μg total dose for persons ≥50 kg body weight). Peak increments of plasma VWF and FVIII occur about 1 to 2 hours after DDAVP, typically reaching two- to four-fold higher levels than at baseline, and decline toward baseline during the next 24 hours, reflecting VWF and FVIII plasma half-lives that are about 12 hours on average. However, plasma half-lives depend on the specific VWF subtype and phenotype and also vary considerably among individuals. Because of variability in response, before therapy with DDAVP, it is important to perform a treatment trial with pharmacokinetic monitoring of VWF and FVIII, measuring baseline (pre-DDAVP) and peak (~1 hour post-DDAVP) levels, supplemented with testing about 4 to 6 hours after DDAVP if shortened survival of endogenous VWF is a consideration. A DDAVP treatment trial with extended monitoring can also help diagnose VWD variants with intrinsically heightened VWF clearance. Because of the problem of rapid tachyphylaxis, the trial of DDAVP should be performed at least 1 to 2 weeks before an elective procedure.

Factor Replacement Therapy

Alphanate SD/HT (Grifols), Humate-P (CSL Behring), and Wilate (Octapharma) are U.S. Food and Drug Administration–approved plasma-derived VWF concentrates for treatment of VWD by intravenous infusions. They also contain FVIII but differ in VWF/FVIII ratios and in content of large (high-molecular-weight) VWF multimers. Other VWF-containing concentrates include Koate-DVI (Talecris) and Wilfactin (LFB, France), which lacks FVIII (endogenous levels of which rise secondarily within a few hours after infusion) and is not available in the United States. Cryoprecipitate is no longer recommended for VWF (or for FVIII) replacement, and its use should be limited to urgent situations when VWF concentrates are not available.

Table 176-5 outlines dosing and laboratory monitoring recommendations for treatment or prevention of bleeding in patients with VWD. Whenever possible, and particularly for individuals with more severe forms of VWD, major surgeries or bleeding events should be managed in hospitals with appropriate laboratory capability and clinical staff, including a hematologist and a surgeon skilled in the management of bleeding disorders.

Other Hemostatic Agents

Epsilon-aminocaproic acid and tranexamic acid are oral (or intravenous) antifibrinolytic agents that are useful for mucous membrane bleeding such as dental procedures. Antifibrinolytic therapy is potentially thrombogenic, particularly in patients who have coexisting disseminated intravascular coagulation (DIC) or advanced liver disease (Chapter 178), and caution should be applied for use. Topical agents such as bovine or human thrombin, or fibrin sealants, may be indicated for accessible bleeding sites.

Treatment with combined oral contraceptive pills can ameliorate menorrhagia in women with VWD, mediated partly by hormonal effects on uterine tissues as well as by elevating blood VWF and FVIII. Contraceptive hormonal skin patches have similar effects, and either type of therapy can also increase the risk for thromboembolic events. The levonorgestrel-releasing intrauterine device is an alternative to oral or skin-patch hormonal agents. For pregnancy and delivery in women with VWD, it is important to ensure that VWF and FVIII levels are normalized at the time of delivery, either spontaneously (which often occurs) or by therapy, including before administration of epidural anesthesia and postpartum.

ACQUIRED VON WILLEBRAND SYNDROME

AVWS refers to deficiencies or defects in VWF concentration, structure, or function that are not inherited but are consequences of other medical disorders. AVWS is less common than congenital (hereditary) VWD and is typically etiologically associated with several different mechanisms and medical conditions (Table 176-6).

Laboratory findings in AVWS are similar to those in congenital VWD (types 1, 2A, or 3). Although VWF:RCo values are typically decreased in AVWS (with variably decreased VWF:Ag or FVIII), sometimes only VWF multimer analysis is abnormal, with mild to moderate reduction or loss of the highest-molecular-weight (largest) multimers. This latter situation is more

TABLE 176-6	CAUSES OF ACQUIRED VON WILLEBRAND SYNDROME
PATHOPHYSIOLOGIC CATEGORY*	**DISEASE OR ASSOCIATION**
Antibodies to VWF	Monoclonal gammopathies, lymphoproliferative disorders, or autoimmune diseases such as systemic lupus erythematosus
Shear-induced VWF conformational changes leading to increased proteolysis of VWF	Aortic valvular stenosis, ventricular septal defect, hypertrophic obstructive cardiomyopathy, left ventricular assist device, or primary pulmonary hypertension
Markedly elevated blood platelet count	Essential thrombocythemia, polycythemia vera, myeloid metaplasia with myelofibrosis, or other myeloproliferative disorders
Removal of VWF from circulation by aberrant binding to tumor cells	Wilms' tumor and certain lymphoproliferative or plasma cell proliferative disorders
Decreased VWF synthesis	Hypothyroidism
Drugs associated with AVWS	Ciprofloxacin, valproic acid, hydroxyethyl starch or griseofulvin

*Pathophysiologic categories are listed in descending order of approximate prevalence.
AVWS = acquired von Willebrand syndrome; VWF, von Willebrand factor.
Adapted and modified from Nichols WL, Rick ME, Ortel TL, et al. Clinical and laboratory diagnosis of von Willebrand disease: a synopsis of the 2008 NHLBI/NIH guidelines. *Am J Hematol.* 2009;84:366-370.

likely for AVWS associated with enhanced VWF proteolysis reflecting shear-induced conformational changes in VWF leading to increased proteolysis of VWF by ADAMTS13, such as with severe aortic valvular stenosis and other conditions causing abnormally high shear forces somewhere in the circulation (see Table 176-6). Heyde's syndrome refers to AVWS caused by severe aortic stenosis and accompanied by gastrointestinal bleeding from arteriovenous malformations.

AVWS, and disorders causing it, should be considered in individuals found to have abnormal VWF test results and bleeding symptoms, without a personal or family history consistent with hereditary VWD. Conversely, when bleeding occurs in association with one of the known causative conditions, AVWS should be considered and initial VWD testing performed if indicated.

TREATMENT Rx

Treatment of AVWS should be focused first on elimination or amelioration of the associated causative disorder, if amenable to treatment (e.g., aortic valve replacement or repair for Heyde's syndrome). Survival of both endogenous and infused VWF is often shortened in AVWS, and replacement therapy should be monitored with measurement of plasma VWF (VWF:RCo and VWF:Ag) and FVIII. For AVWS due to immunoglobulin G MGUS (monoclonal gammopathy of undetermined significance), intravenous immunoglobulin infusion may temporarily normalize plasma VWF and FVIII and stop abnormal bleeding by abrogating heightened VWF clearance. However, such treatment reflects an off-label product use.

● BLEEDING DUE TO QUALITATIVE PLATELET DISORDERS
Hereditary Platelet Bleeding Disorders

Hereditary defects in platelet function can occur at all stages of the linked sequence of events involved in hemostatic platelet activation at sites of vascular injury, as described in Chapter 174: (1) platelet adhesion (Bernard-Soulier syndrome [BSS]), (2) platelet release reaction (storage pool disorders), and (3) platelet aggregation (Glanzmann's thrombasthenia [GT]). They lead to varying levels of severity of bleeding.

BERNARD-SOULIER SYNDROME AND GLANZMANN THROMBASTHENIA

These rare, autosomally recessive platelet hypofunctional disorders typically manifest moderately severe (minimally provoked or spontaneous) mucocutaneous bleeding symptoms during childhood and beyond as well as abnormal bleeding with hemostatic challenges such as surgery. BSS results from deficiency or dysfunction of the platelet membrane glycoprotein (GP) Ib-IX-V complex that is the principal receptor for binding VWF, mediating platelet adhesion to injured blood vessels. (In some ways, therefore, BSS is the platelet counterpart of VWD as an adhesion defect, the latter being caused by an abnormality in the VWF rather than the platelets.) GT reflects deficiency or dysfunction of the platelet GPIIb-IIIa complex that is the principal receptor for binding plasma fibrinogen, mediating platelet aggregation. The platelet count and morphology are normal in GT, but BSS demonstrates moderate thrombocytopenia and enlarged (giant) platelets. BT or PFA-100 test results are typically markedly abnormal in both disorders, but nonspecific. Platelet aggregometry findings are usually diagnostic. BSS demonstrates absence of aggregation response to ristocetin, whereas responses to other agonists are relatively normal. GT demonstrates relatively normal response to ristocetin, contrasting with complete absence of aggregation response to other agonists, such as adenosine diphosphate, collagen, arachidonic acid, and epinephrine. Quantitative analysis of platelet membrane GPs by flow cytometry is evolving as a supplemental diagnostic tool for BSS and GT. Mutational DNA-based testing is primarily a research endeavor.

PLATELET STORAGE POOL DISORDERS

Platelet dense (δ) granule storage pool deficiency (DG-SPD) is more common than BSS and GT. Inheritance is typically autosomal recessive, or occasionally dominant, with evolving understanding of different mutational causes. Bleeding symptoms are usually mild but may be clinically significant. Hermansky-Pudlak syndrome (HPS) describes oculocutaneous albinism associated with platelet DG-SPD, with a propensity to develop pulmonary fibrosis or granulomatous colitis. DG-SPD can accompany some other hereditary disorders such as the X-linked Wiskott-Aldrich syndrome, in which it is associated with microthrombocytopenia, or Chédiak-Higashi syndrome with partial albinism and leukocyte inclusions. Isolated DG-SPD, including HPS, demonstrates normal blood platelet count and morphology by peripheral blood smear review. Results of BT, PFA-100, or platelet aggregometry testing may or may not be abnormal. Platelet content and secretion of adenosine triphosphate are decreased in DG-SPD, and platelet electron microscopy can diagnostically confirm absence or marked decrease of dense granules; however, these tests have limited availability.

Platelet α-granule deficiency manifests as the gray platelet syndrome, which is typically autosomal recessive in inheritance and may result in mild bleeding symptoms. Moderate thrombocytopenia is present, and peripheral blood smear review is usually diagnostic, demonstrating enlarged platelets that are "gray" (absence of granulomere staining, reflecting absence of α granules and their contents that include VWF). X-chromosome-linked mutations of GATA1, the gene encoding a transcription factor essential for erythropoiesis and megakaryocytopoiesis, can cause a gray platelet syndrome–like disorder affecting males.

OTHER HEREDITARY PLATELET HYPOFUNCTIONAL DISORDERS

Hereditary platelet secretion disorders (defective release of α- and δ-granule contents without granule deficiency) comprise a variety of abnormalities affecting various platelet receptors or mechanisms of signal transduction and platelet activation, including defective platelet procoagulant activity, with or without thrombocytopenia or other syndromic features, and with variable bleeding propensity and symptoms. Some of these disorders are reviewed in Chapter 175.

TREATMENT

For treating or preventing major bleeding events (e.g., certain surgical challenges), judicious use of platelet transfusion may be indicated for patients with more severe hereditary platelet bleeding disorders such as BSS and GT. To reduce the risk for platelet alloimmunization, single-donor apheresis platelet concentrates are preferred when available, and HLA-matched transfusions may sometimes be indicated. DDAVP administration has been reported to improve hemostasis in DG-SPD, BSS, and some other hereditary platelet disorders. Treatment with recombinant activated coagulation factor VII (NovoSeven, NovoNordisk) has been reported as an alternative or salvage therapy for bleeding in GT and certain other platelet hypofunctional disorders. Antifibrinolytic therapy with epsilon-aminocaproic acid or tranexamic acid can be useful for dental extractions or for surgical procedures involving other tissues with high intrinsic fibrinolytic activity (e.g., nose, mouth and throat, extraocular tissues).

Acquired Platelet Bleeding Disorders
DRUGS

Drugs are a relatively common cause of platelet hypofunction that can result in mild bleeding symptoms, particularly if other bleeding propensities are present, such as thrombocytopenia. Aspirin, thienopyridines (e.g., clopidogrel, prasugrel, ticagrelor), dipyridamole, and inhibitors of platelet GPIIb/IIIa function are used therapeutically or prophylactically for atherosclerotic cardiovascular disorders such as coronary artery or cerebrovascular disease. In addition to aspirin, other NSAIDs can inhibit platelet arachidonic acid metabolism (Chapter 36) and contribute to bleeding. Other agents that may sometimes impair platelet function include certain selective serotonin reuptake inhibitors or antibiotics and some herbal or nutritional supplements. Laboratory testing for platelet hypofunction is not often indicated and may not yield diagnostic findings.

OTHER ACQUIRED PLATELET BLEEDING DISORDERS

Myelodysplastic or myeloproliferative disorders can sometimes manifest intrinsic platelet hypofunction, disproportionate to thrombocytopenia or thrombocytosis when they are present. Cirrhosis or liver failure can cause platelet hypofunction as well as thrombocytopenia. Uremia may induce platelet hypofunction that can be ameliorated by dialysis and erythropoietin therapy. Antibodies causing autoimmune thrombocytopenia (Chapter 175) can sometimes cause acquired platelet hypofunction (e.g., acquired GT or BSS) in addition to the low platelet count.

TREATMENT   Rx

Review of patient medicaments and medical conditions, and modifications of them when feasible and indicated, can often suffice for recognition and management of acquired platelet hypofunctional disorders.

● VASCULAR HEMORRHAGIC DISORDERS
Hereditary Vascular Hemorrhagic Disorders

Hereditary hemorrhagic telangiectasia (HHT), also called Osler-Weber-Rendu syndrome, is an autosomal dominant vascular disorder characterized by development of telangiectases and arteriovenous malformations in the skin, mucous membranes, and certain viscera (especially the central nervous system, lung, and liver), with a propensity for severe recurring nosebleeds and gastrointestinal bleeds resulting in chronic anemia and iron deficiency. Diagnosis primarily relies on physical examination (Fig. 176-1). Several mutations in two genes have been described: endoglin in HHT type 1 and activin receptor-like kinase-1 (ALK1) in HHT type 2. These genes encode proteins that modulate transforming growth factor-β signaling in vascular endothelial cells, and mutations in them in HHT lead to the development of fragile telangiectatic vessels and arteriovenous malformations. Molecular DNA-based testing has limited availability. Supportive treatment includes supplemental iron therapy for iron deficiency anemia. In a small randomized trial, tamoxifen (20 mg per day for 6 months) significantly reduced bleeding in patients with recurrent epistaxis caused by HHT.[1]

Ehlers-Danlos syndrome is caused by mutations in genes encoding fibrillar collagen or related genes and includes at least six subtypes that vary in clinical manifestations, severity, and prognosis. Inheritance is primarily autosomal dominant. Principal manifestations of Ehlers-Danlos syndrome include skin or joint hyperextensibility, with an associated bleeding tendency including easy bruisability (purpura), surgical bleeding, poor wound healing, and menorrhagia in women. Diagnosis depends mainly on physical examination, supplemented with molecular DNA-based testing that currently has limited availability.

Acquired Vascular Hemorrhagic Disorders

Systemic amyloidosis, Waldenström's macroglobulinemia, and cryoglobulinemia are dysproteinemic disorders reflecting monoclonal gammopathies or hyperglobulinemias (Chapters 193 and 194) that can manifest purpuric or other bleeding symptoms caused by either vascular deposition of immunoglobulin fragments (amyloidosis) or inhibition of platelet-vessel hemostatic functions by immunoglobulins. Henoch-Schönlein purpura is primarily a transient disease of children that typically presents with a palpable purpuric rash of the lower extremities, arthralgias, abdominal pain and renal symptoms

FIGURE 176-1. Hereditary hemorrhagic telangiectasia (HHT). Telangiectasias commonly occur on the face, lips, tongue, and fingers as well as in other areas, including nasal and gastrointestinal mucosa, and may develop in certain other internal organs. Skin or mucous membrane lesions typically blanch with pressure, in contrast to petechiae that do not. (**A,** Copyrighted and used with permission of the Mayo Foundation for Medical Education and Research, all rights reserved. **B,** Courtesy of Dr. Andrew Schafer.)

(hematuria, proteinuria) in some cases, manifestations of a systemic vasculitis characterized by deposition of immunoglobulin A–containing immune complexes in the skin, gastrointestinal tract, and kidneys. Palpable purpura can also result from systemic sepsis or DIC. Scurvy is caused by the effects of vitamin C deficiency on collagen structure and often presents with bruising or petechiae, including tiny perifollicular hemorrhages. Senile purpura or purpura simplex is thought to reflect partly the age-related changes of skin vascular structure and is typified by easy bruisability of the dorsa of the hands, forearms, and lower legs. Psychogenic purpuras are controversial entities that include Gardner-Diamond syndrome, which is characterized by recurring focal pain preceding development of ecchymoses, believed to reflect poorly understood psychosomatic mechanisms. It can be difficult to differentiate this rare syndrome from factitious or self-induced purpura and bleeding.

Grade A

1. Yaniv E, Preis M, Hadar T, et al. Antiestrogen therapy for hereditary hemorrhagic telangiectasia: a double-blind placebo-controlled clinical trial. *Laryngoscope.* 2009;119:284-288.

SUGGESTED READINGS

Bowman M, Hopman WM, Rapson D, et al. A prospective evaluation of the prevalence of symptomatic von Willebrand disease (VWD) in a pediatric primary care population. *Pediatr Blood Cancer.* 2010;55:171-173. *Large prospective study using bleeding history scoring tool and laboratory testing, demonstrating about 5% prevalence of bleeding symptoms in children, with VWD prevalence of about 0.1%.*

Eby C. Pathogenesis and management of bleeding and thrombosis in plasma cell dyscrasias. *Br J Haematol.* 2009;145:151-163. *Review includes purpuric dysproteinemic disorders.*

Faughnan ME, Palda VA, Garcia-Tsao G, et al. International guidelines for the diagnosis and management of hereditary haemorrhagic telangiectasia. *J Med Genet.* 2011;48:73-87. *Consensus guidelines.*

Nichols WL, Rick ME, Ortel TL, et al. Clinical and laboratory diagnosis of von Willebrand disease: a synopsis of the 2008 NHLBI/NIH guidelines. *Am J Hematol.* 2009;84:366-370. *Updated synopsis of recommendations for clinical and laboratory diagnosis of VWD and AVWS, including algorithms.*

177

HEMORRHAGIC DISORDERS: COAGULATION FACTOR DEFICIENCIES

MARGARET V. RAGNI

COAGULATION DEFICIENCIES

Severe coagulation deficiencies, or coagulopathies, are typically characterized by spontaneous or traumatic bleeding, such as during surgery or trauma, and may result in life- or limb-threatening complications. By contrast, moderate and mild coagulopathies may remain clinically silent until they are detected coincidentally on routine laboratory screening tests (e.g., prothrombin time [PT], activated partial thromboplastin time [aPTT]) or when these tests are ordered to evaluate the cause of abnormal bleeding or bruising. Much of the morbidity of coagulopathies can be minimized or avoided altogether by prophylactic replacement of the deficient clotting factor proteins. In contrast to the lifelong clinical manifestations of hereditary or congenital coagulopathies, acquired deficiencies usually appear acutely in previously asymptomatic individuals; they may not be suspected and often remit spontaneously or after eradication of an inciting disease state or withdrawal of an offending medication. Acquired coagulation disorders may be associated with more severe bleeding than congenital disorders, in part because of the delay in diagnosis. In general, coagulopathies may result from inadequate synthesis of coagulation factor proteins or from inhibition of activated clotting factor proteins by acquired antibodies or anticoagulant medications. Finally, qualitative defects, either congenital or acquired, may also result in bleeding.

Hereditary Hemophilias

DEFINITION

The hemophilias include hemophilia A and hemophilia B, caused by deficiencies or defects in clotting factor VIII (antihemophilic factor) and factor IX (antihemophilic factor B, or Christmas factor), respectively. A deficiency of either of these intrinsic coagulation pathway proteins results in inadequate formation of thrombin at sites of vascular injury.

EPIDEMIOLOGY

Hemophilia A and B are sex-linked recessive disorders estimated to occur in 1 in 5000 and 1 in 30,000 male births, respectively. The higher incidence of hemophilia A may be due to the greater amount of DNA "at risk" for mutation in the factor VIII gene (186,000 base pairs) compared with the factor IX gene (34,000 base pairs). Hemophilia A and B are observed in all racial and ethnic groups, and in the United States, more than 20,000 individuals are affected. Although carrier testing, genetic counseling, and prenatal diagnosis are widely available in the United States through the network of federally funded hemophilia treatment centers (HTCs), fecundity rates remain high, and few confirmed carriers elect to terminate their pregnancies, even if an affected fetus is detected in utero. These decisions are likely influenced by the wide availability of safe and effective coagulation factor replacement concentrates and by the prospect of an eventual cure for the hemophilias through gene transfer. A substantial proportion (30%) of hemophilia cases arise as new, spontaneous mutations. Overall, the hemophilias are much more common than the autosomal recessive coagulation disorders (see later), which often affect progeny from consanguineous relationships and require the inheritance of two defective alleles for the bleeding manifestations to become evident.

PATHOBIOLOGY
Genetics

As with other sex-linked recessive diseases, the genes for factor VIII and factor IX are located on the long arm of the X chromosome. Males with a defective allele on their single X chromosome transmit this gene to all their daughters, who are obligate carriers, but to none of their sons. Because the offspring of female carriers inherit one affected X chromosome, half of their sons develop the coagulation disorder, and half of their daughters are obligate carriers. Female carriers may manifest hemophilia-like symptoms if the alleles on the X chromosome are unequally inactivated (lyonization); the defective hemophilic allele is expressed in preference to the normal allele, plasma factor VIII levels are below 50%, and phenotypic hemophilia results. Female hemophilia may arise as a result of mating between a hemophilic male and a female carrier (homozygous for the defective factor VIII or IX gene) or in carrier females who have the 45 XO karyotype (Turner's syndrome) and are hemizygous for the defective hemophilia gene.

No single mutation is responsible for the hemophilias. Many missense and nonsense point mutations, deletions, and inversions have been described. Severe molecular defects predominate, with 40 to 50% of all cases of severe hemophilia A evolving from a unique inversion of intron 22 (the largest of the factor VIII introns). This inversion results from the recombination and translocation of DNA within intron 22 of the factor VIII gene, with areas of extragenic but homologous "nonfunctional" DNA located at a distance from intron 22. Other less common severe molecular defects include large gene deletions (5 to 10% of cases) and nonsense mutations (10 to 15% of cases). The encoded proteins resulting from these mutations are defective and do not express any factor VIII activity. Mild or moderate hemophilia A is commonly associated with point mutations and deletions. In contrast, factor IX mutations are more diverse, and severe hemophilia B is more likely caused by large deletions. Mutated clotting factor genes responsible for the hemophilias may also encode for the production of defective nonfunctional proteins that circulate in the plasma and are detected at normal quantitative levels by immunoassays but not by functional assays. A listing of the mutations that cause the hemophilias can be accessed via the Human Gene Mutation Database (*www.hgmd.org*).

CLINICAL MANIFESTATIONS

Hemophilia A and hemophilia B are said to be clinically indistinguishable, with clinical severity corresponding inversely to the circulating levels of plasma coagulant factor VIII or IX activity. Several studies have found a higher bleeding frequency, greater factor use, and more frequent hospitalizations in hemophilia A, suggesting a greater clinical severity than hemophilia B. Individuals with less than 1% of normal factor VIII or IX activity are classified as having "severe" disease, characterized by frequent spontaneous bleeding events in joints (hemarthrosis) and soft tissues and by profuse hemorrhage with trauma or surgery. Although spontaneous bleeding is uncommon in mild deficiencies (>5% normal activity), excess bleeding typically occurs with trauma or surgery. A moderate clinical course is associated with factor VIII or IX levels between 1 and 5%. Approximately 60% of all cases of hemophilia A are clinically severe, whereas only 20 to 45% of cases of hemophilia B are severe.

Severe hemophilia is typically suspected and diagnosed during infancy in the absence of a family history. Among newborns, intracranial hemorrhage is the leading cause of morbidity and mortality, with a cumulative incidence of 3.8%, according to data collected by the Centers for Disease Control and Prevention. Intracranial hemorrhage does not appear to be related to the mode of delivery, although half of such hemorrhages occur in the newborn period; whether prospective computed tomography screening should be instituted at birth remains unknown. Vacuum extraction may increase cephalohematoma formation and is discouraged. Circumcision within days after birth is accompanied by excessive bleeding in less than half of severely affected boys. The first spontaneous hemarthrosis in severely affected hemophiliacs usually occurs between 9 and 18 months of age, when ambulation begins; in moderately affected individuals, it generally does not occur until 2 to 5 years of age. The knees are the most prominent sites of spontaneous bleeds, followed by the elbows, ankles, shoulders, and hips; wrists are less commonly involved.

Acute hemarthroses (Fig. 177-1) originate from the subsynovial venous plexus underlying the joint capsule and produce a tingling or burning sensation, followed by the onset of intense pain and swelling. On physical examination, the joint is swollen, hot, and tender to palpation, with erythema of the overlying skin. Joint mobility is compromised by pain and stiffness, and the joint is usually maintained in a flexed position. Immediate or early replacement of the deficient clotting factor to normal hemostatic levels rapidly reverses the pain. Delayed treatment results in excess pain, morbidity, and joint damage. Optimal management includes rest, ice, (factor) concentrate, and elevation (RICE). Swelling and joint immobility improve as the intra-articular hematoma resolves. Intra-articular needle aspiration of fresh blood is not recommended because of the risk of introducing infection. Short courses of oral corticosteroids may be helpful to reduce the acute joint symptoms in children but are rarely used in adults.

FIGURE 177-1. Acute hemarthrosis of the knee is a common complication of hemophilia. It may be confused with acute infection unless the patient's coagulation disorder is known, because the knee is hot, red, swollen, and painful. (From Forbes CD, Jackson WF. *Color Atlas and Text of Clinical Medicine*, 3rd ed. London: Mosby; 2003.)

FIGURE 177-2. Severe chronic arthritis in hemophilia. The knee is the most commonly affected joint. Both knees are severely deranged in this patient. Note that he is unable to stand with both feet flat on the floor. (From Forbes CD, Jackson WF. *Color Atlas and Text of Clinical Medicine*, 3rd ed. London: Mosby; 2003.)

Recurrent or untreated bleeds result in chronic synovial hypertrophy and, eventually, damage to the underlying cartilage, with subsequent subchondral bone cyst formation, bony erosion, and flexion contractures. Abnormal mechanical forces from weight bearing can produce subluxation, misalignment, loss of mobility, and permanent deformities of the lower extremities (Fig. 177-2). These changes are accompanied by chronic pain, swelling, arthritis, and disability. Plain radiographs and clinical examination of chronic hemarthroses often underestimate the extent of bone and joint damage; serial magnetic resonance imaging is superior to radiography or computed tomography and is the most sensitive and specific means of detecting and monitoring early and progressive disease.

Intramuscular hematomas account for about 30% of hemophilia-related bleeding events and are rarely life threatening. They are usually precipitated by physical or iatrogenic trauma (e.g., after intramuscular injections) and may compromise sensory and motor function or arterial circulation if they entrap and compress vital structures in closed fascial compartments. The latter occurrence, termed *compartment syndrome*, presents with the rapid onset of swelling and severe pain in an extremity, unrelieved by factor infusion and standard analgesics. This is considered a medical emergency and may require fasciotomy to preserve tissue and provide pain relief. Retroperitoneal hematomas may be confused clinically with appendicitis or hip bleeds but should be suspected in a patient who is hunched over and unable to stand erect owing to the pain of muscle extension in the presence of hematoma. Unless these bleeding episodes are treated immediately and aggressively, permanent anatomic deformity, such as flexion contracture, nerve damage, or pseudotumor formation (expanding hematomas that erode and destroy adjacent skeletal structures), may occur. Bleeding from mucous membranes is very common and may be exaggerated by the degradation of fibrin clots by fibrinolytic enzymes contained in secretions. Bleeding involving the tongue or

the retropharyngeal space may rapidly produce life-threatening compromise of the airway. Gastrointestinal hemorrhage typically originates from anatomic lesions proximal to the ligament of Treitz and may be exacerbated by esophageal varices secondary to cirrhosis and portal hypertension or by the use of nonsteroidal anti-inflammatory drugs (NSAIDs) for the treatment of hemarthroses. Spontaneous bleeding in the genitourinary tract secondary to hemophilia is a diagnosis of exclusion after ruling out renal stones and infection. Ureteral blood clots produce renal colic, which may be confused with nephrolithiasis and may be worsened by the use of antifibrinolytic agents. A short course of steroids may be helpful, especially in children, to hasten their resolution. Ninety percent of hemophiliacs experience at least one episode of gross hematuria or hemospermia.

Intracranial bleeds occur in 10% of patients, are usually induced by trauma, and may be fatal in 30% of cases. The risk of developing an intracranial hemorrhage is approximately 2% per year. Neuromuscular defects, seizure disorders, and intellectual deficits may ensue.

Individuals with hemophilia cared for at HTCs have lower mortality and reduced costs of care compared with those receiving treatment elsewhere. The chronic care model practiced at HTCs emphasizes prevention to reduce joint disease and complications, optimization of factor dosing, and counseling regarding safe sports and the avoidance of aspirin and other drugs that inhibit platelet function.

DIAGNOSIS

The diagnosis of hemophilia is suspected on the basis of a family and personal bleeding history and laboratory detection of prolongation of the aPTT (with normal PT). It is confirmed by significantly reduced plasma factor VIII or IX activity. As noted in Chapter 174, the aPTT is not a sufficiently sensitive screening test to be prolonged in mild hemophiliacs, in whom the factor VIII level is sometimes greater than 30% of normal. Severe hemophilia is usually recognized in infancy, with circumcision bleeding; by contrast, moderate or mild disease is recognized later in life after trauma or surgery. Hemophilia can be distinguished from von Willebrand disease (VWD; Chapter 176) by normal ristocetin cofactor and von Willebrand factor antigen levels. In type 2N VWD, factor VIII is significantly lower than ristocetin cofactor and von Willebrand factor antigen levels due to reduced factor VIII binding; this variant of VWD may require genotyping to distinguish it from hemophilia A. Other congenital intrinsic factor deficiencies (e.g., factor XI and XII) can be determined by coagulation factor–specific assays. Vitamin K deficiency (see later and Chapter 178) can be detected by the associated PT prolongation; deficiencies of factors II, VII, IX, and X; and resolution of the coagulation defect with vitamin K. The presence of heparin can be confirmed by correction of the aPTT after running the sample over a heparin absorption column. Failure of the aPTT to correct in a 1:1 mix with normal plasma suggests the presence of an inhibitor; specific inhibitors are associated with a single decreased factor level (usually factor VIII; see Alloantibody Inhibitors to Factors VIII and IX under Treatment), whereas blocking inhibitors cause nonspecific factor level changes associated with a positive hexagonal lipid assay (see Antiphospholipid Syndrome and Lupus Anticoagulant later).

TREATMENT   Rx

Treatment and prevention of acute bleeding events in hemophilia A and B are based on replacement of the missing or deficient clotting factor protein to restore adequate hemostasis (E-Table 177-1). The morbidity, mortality, and overall cost of care for individuals with hemophilia are reduced significantly if care is provided by comprehensive HTCs that have the multispecialty expertise and laboratory capabilities to coordinate and monitor specific patient needs.

The goal of replacement therapy (Table 177-1) is to achieve plasma factor VIII and IX activity levels of 25 to 30% for minor spontaneous or traumatic bleeds (e.g., hemarthroses, persistent hematuria), at least 50% clotting factor activity for the treatment or prevention of severe bleeds (e.g., major dental surgery, maintenance replacement therapy after major surgery or trauma), and 80 to 100% activity for any life-threatening or limb-threatening hemorrhagic event (e.g., major surgery, trauma). After major trauma or if visceral or intracranial bleeding is suspected, replacement therapy adequate to achieve 100% clotting factor activity should be administered *before* diagnostic procedures are initiated. To calculate the initial dose, plasma factor VIII activity generally increases about 2% (0.02 IU/mL) for each unit of factor VIII administered per kilogram of body weight, and factor IX activity increases about 1% (0.01 IU/mL) for each unit of factor IX administered per kilogram of body weight. Therefore, a 70-kg individual with severe hemophilia A or B (factor VIII or IX activity <1% of normal) who requires replacement to 100% activity for major

TABLE 177-1 FDA-APPROVED COAGULATION PROTEINS AND REPLACEMENT THERAPIES AVAILABLE IN THE UNITED STATES

COAGULATION PROTEIN DEFICIENCY	INHERITANCE PATTERN	PREVALENCE	MINIMUM HEMOSTATIC LEVEL	REPLACEMENT SOURCES
Factor I (fibrinogen)			50-100 mg/dL	Cryoprecipitate, FFP, fibrinogen concentrate
Afibrinogenemia	Autosomal recessive	Rare (<300 families)		
Dysfibrogenemia	Autosomal dominant or recessive	Rare (>300 variants)		
Factor II (prothrombin)	Autosomal dominant or recessive	Rare (25 kindreds)	30% of normal	FFP, factor IX complex concentrates
Factor V (labile factor)	Autosomal recessive	1 in 1 million births	25% of normal	FFP
Factor VII	Autosomal recessive	1 in 500,000 births	25% of normal	Recombinant factor VIIa (15-20 μg/kg), FFP, factor IX complex concentrates
Factor VIII (antihemophilic factor)	X-linked recessive	1 in 5000 male births	80-100% for surgery/life-threatening bleeds, 50% for serious bleeds, 25-30% for minor bleeds	Factor VIII concentrates (see E-Table 177-1)
Von Willebrand disease			>50% VWF antigen and ristocetin cofactor activity	DDAVP for mild to moderate disease (except type 2B; variable response to 2A); cryoprecipitate and FFP (not preferred, except in emergencies); factor VIII/VWF concentrates, viral attenuated, intermediate purity (preferred for disease unresponsive to DDAVP and for type 3 (see E-Table 177-1)
Type 1 and 2 variants	Usually autosomal dominant	1% prevalence		
Type 3	Autosomal recessive	1 in 1 million births		
Factor IX (Christmas factor)	X-linked recessive	1 in 30,000 male births	25-50% of normal, depending on extent of bleeding, surgery	Factor IX concentrates; FFP not preferred except in dire emergencies (see E-Table 177-1)
Factor X (Stuart-Prower factor)	Autosomal recessive	1 in 500,000 births	10-25% of normal	FFP or factor IX complex concentrates
Factor XI (hemophilia C)	Autosomal dominant; severe type is recessive	4% of Ashkenazi Jews; 1 in 1 million general population	20-40% of normal	FFP or factor XI concentrate
Factor XII (Hageman factor), prekallikrein, high-molecular-weight kininogen	Autosomal recessive	Not available	No treatment necessary	—
Factor XIII (fibrin stabilizing factor)	Autosomal recessive	1 in 3 million births	5% of normal	FFP, cryoprecipitate, or viral-attenuated factor XIII concentrate

DDAVP = desmopressin; FDA = U.S. Food and Drug Administration; FFP = fresh-frozen plasma; VWF = von Willebrand factor.

surgery should initially receive 3500 IU of factor VIII or 7000 IU of factor IX concentrate. The circulating half-lives of factors VIII and IX require subsequent dosing at half the initial dose every 8 to 12 hours and every 18 to 24 hours, respectively. However, this empirical dosing (based on calculations) should be individualized according to the peak recovery increment within 10 to 15 minutes after bolus infusion, as well as trough activity levels. The frequency of repeat dosing is also determined by the rapidity of pain relief, recovery of joint function, and resolution of active bleeding. Replacement is usually maintained for 10 to 14 days after major surgery to allow proper wound healing. Bolus dosing typically results in wide fluctuations in clotting factor activity levels and requires frequent laboratory monitoring to avoid suboptimal troughs. A continuous infusion regimen, consisting of 1 to 2 IU of factor VIII or IX concentrate per kilogram per hour after a bolus dose, maintains a plateau level without the need for frequent laboratory testing. Continuous infusion also reduces total concentrate consumption by 30 to 75% in surgical settings. Long-acting recombinant factors VIII and IX, linked to the Fc domain of immunoglobulin G (IgG) or to liposomes, are currently in clinical trials. If these preparations prolong the circulation times of factors VIII and IX with similar efficacy and safety as standard recombinant products, they may allow simpler dosing schedules and fewer intravenous factor infusions.

Because of the potential thrombogenicity associated with the repeated administration of prothrombin complex concentrates to replace factor IX deficiency, high-purity, plasma-derived, or genetically engineered factor IX concentrates, which lack activated vitamin K–dependent clotting factors, are preferred in hemophilia B.

Cryoprecipitate (a cold precipitate of fresh-frozen plasma [FFP] after thawing at 4° C) and FFP contain factor VIII, but only FFP contains factor IX. However, neither cryoprecipitate nor FFP is an optimal replacement product for either hemophilia A or hemophilia B because these agents may transmit blood-borne pathogens. All clotting factor concentrates available in the United States (E-Table 177-1), whether plasma derived or genetically engineered, are equally efficacious and are considered extremely safe; none has ever been implicated in the transmission of blood-borne viral pathogens or prions. Newer second- and third-generation recombinant factor VIII and IX concentrates are manufactured free of added human or animal proteins in the culture medium or in the final formulation, eliminating the theoretical risks of transmission of prions or murine viruses.

Hemarthroses

The moderate or severe pain that accompanies acute hemarthroses responds to immediate analgesic relief, temporary immobilization, restraint from weight bearing, and clotting factor replacement. Narcotic analgesics, such as codeine or synthetic derivatives of codeine, should be prescribed alone or combined with doses of acetaminophen that are low enough to avoid hepatic toxicity in patients with chronic hepatitis. Although these medications do not possess significant anti-inflammatory activity, they are preferable to NSAIDs or aspirin, which can exacerbate bleeding complications through their inhibition of platelet aggregation.

Strategies intended to prevent end-stage joint destruction should be initiated at an early age. Although prophylaxis beginning soon after the first bleed is the optimal approach (see later), the majority of adults have not had the benefit of early prophylaxis and thus have advanced arthropathy with reduced motion, disability, and pain, for which surgery may be recommended. Synovectomy through open surgery or arthroscopy removes the inflamed tissue and should result in substantially decreased pain and less recurrent bleeding. Nonsurgical synovectomy (synoviorthosis), which involves the intra-articular administration of a radioisotope, is particularly useful for high-risk patients and for those with alloantibody inhibitors to factor VIII or IX (see later). The occurrence of leukemia in three hemophilic children receiving radioisotopic synoviorthosis has raised concerns about leukemogenesis, especially given the low background rate of cancers in individuals with hemophilia. Neither synovectomy nor synoviorthosis reverses joint damage, but both procedures may delay its progression. Non-weight-bearing exercises, such as swimming and isometrics, are important to periarticular muscle development and maintenance of joint stability for ambulation. Intractable pain and severe joint destruction secondary to repeated hemorrhage require prosthetic replacement. Chronic ankle pain responds best to open surgical or arthroscopic fixation and fusion (arthrodesis).

The ultimate strategy to minimize or eliminate progressive joint destruction by recurrent hemarthroses is predicated on the concept of prophylaxis—the scheduled administration of clotting factor concentrates several times weekly (twice a week for factor IX, three times a week for factor VIII) at doses to maintain trough factor activity levels greater than 1 to 2% of normal. In a prospective, randomized clinical trial, prophylaxis with factor VIII (25 IU/kg every other day) was superior to episodic therapy (on demand) in young children with severe hemophilia in reducing joint bleeding and joint damage as shown by magnetic resonance imaging and radiography.[1,2] Although prophylaxis uses more factor product at greater expense, the benefits of long-term prophylaxis to promote joint health and avert disability have led to the recommendation that it be initiated in young children with severe disease at the time of the first bleed. Compliance with this recommendation is not easy, given the invasiveness of intravenous factor administration, the requirement for central venous access devices, and the complication of access device infection. With the development of long-acting factor VIII and IX preparations, currently in clinical trials, bleeding management may become less invasive and simpler. Some unanswered questions include whether prophylaxis is necessary in adulthood and what the minimal effective dose is for prophylaxis or for acute bleeds. The risk of bleeding is thought to be related to the time spent at nadir factor levels less than 1% (0.01 IU/mL) between dosing. It is generally agreed that spontaneous bleeding may be averted by maintaining factor levels at 1% (0.01 U/mL) or greater, which is supported by animal studies of factor IX gene therapy.

Factor Concentrate–Transmitted Viral Infections

In contrast to other at-risk groups, individuals with hemophilia were exposed at a young age to transmissible agents through clotting factor concentrates. This included hepatitis C virus (HCV), leading to infection in 90% of those transfused from the late 1970s through the mid-1980s, and human immunodeficiency virus (HIV) infection in 80% of those transfused with factor VIII products and 50% of those transfused with factor IX products from 1978 through the mid-1980s. Overall, of those with HCV infection (Chapter 151), 40% have coinfection, and hepatitis C remains the leading cause of death in hemophilia. With the implementation of viral inactivation and recombinant technologies, new HCV and HIV infections have been virtually eliminated in hemophiliacs born since the 1990s. Nevertheless, among those exposed to HCV, a large multicenter biopsy study found that 25% have liver fibrosis, and those with HIV coinfection have a 1.4-fold greater fibrosis rate. Among the latter, those receiving highly active antiretroviral therapy (HAART) experience a significant slowing in the rate of HCV progression, to the rates observed in hemophilic men infected only with HCV.

Hepatitis G, observed in 15 to 25% of hemophiliacs, is susceptible to current viral attenuation procedures. Hepatitis B is now a rare problem for those with hemophilia because vaccination at an early age is the standard of care. Hepatitis A virus was transmitted to a small but significant number of patients through solvent detergent–treated factor VIII and factor IX concentrates in the past; hepatitis A vaccination now eliminates this risk. Parvovirus B19 seroprevalence approaches 80% in older adult hemophiliacs exposed to plasma-derived products. The long-term clinical consequences of hepatitis A and parvovirus B19 are unclear. Cadaver and living-donor liver transplantation (Chapter 157) has improved the survival of hemophilic men with chronic hepatitis-induced liver failure and has also resulted in the phenotypic cure of hemophilia, confirming that the liver is the predominant source of normal synthesis of factors VIII and IX. Liver transplantation can also be performed successfully in men coinfected with HIV and HCV with a good response to HAART therapy.

Ancillary and Other Therapies

Ancillary treatment strategies for the hemophilias include antifibrinolytic agents, such as ε-aminocaproic acid (50 mg/kg 3 to 4 times daily) or tranexamic acid (3 or 4 g PO daily in divided doses), to minimize mucous membrane bleeding and the application of fibrin glue to bleeding sites. Desmopressin (DDAVP) can be administered by nasal insufflation 2 hours before a scheduled surgical procedure (one spray per nostril, to provide a total dose of 300 μg; or, in patients weighing <50 kg, 150 μg administered as a single spray); alternatively, DDAVP can be administered intravenously (dissolved in 50 mL normal saline) over 30 minutes at a dose of 0.3 μg/kg. DDAVP is useful in patients with mild hemophilia A because an adequate incremental rise in factor VIII activity can circumvent the use of clotting factor concentrates. Repeated administration of DDAVP (intravenously or by intranasal spray) may be complicated by facial flushing, tachyphylaxis, hyponatremic seizures (primarily in children), and, rarely, angina.

Alloantibody Inhibitors to Factors VIII and IX

Alloantibodies—that is, antibodies to "foreign" infused factor VIII or, less frequently, factor IX—are usually detected in childhood after a median of 9 to 12 days of exposure to clotting factor. These inhibitors occur preferentially in those with a family history of inhibitors and those with large, multidomain factor VIII and factor IX gene deletions. The incidence of factor VIII alloantibodies among hemophilia A patients is 15 to 25%, with a higher frequency in blacks and Hispanics. Factor IX alloantibodies are observed in 1.5 to 3% of hemophilia B patients and predominate among Scandinavians. Patients with factor IX inhibitors seem to be susceptible to anaphylaxis and the

development of nephrotic syndrome with subsequent exposure to sources of factor IX. Increasing evidence suggests that exposure to high-dose bolus treatment early in life increases the risk of inhibitor development, especially in those with a predisposition, such as a family history and an at-risk mutation (e.g., a large deletion mutation).

The development of an alloantibody inhibitor is suspected when replacement therapy is ineffective in controlling bleeding symptoms. These IgG antibodies, usually of the IgG4 subclass, completely neutralize clotting factor activity and prevent or reduce any increment in factor VIII or IX levels following bolus infusions of concentrate. Characterized as time and temperature dependent, inhibitors are quantitated in Bethesda units (BU): by definition, 1 BU is the amount of inhibitor that neutralizes 50% of the specific clotting factor activity in normal plasma. "High responders," or patients with high-titer inhibitors (>5 BU), mount an anamnestic antibody response to factor VIII clotting factor protein, usually within 5 to 7 days after subsequent exposure. "Low responders," or patients with low-titer inhibitors (≤5 BU), do not manifest anamnesis. Low-titer inhibitors can easily be overwhelmed by large amounts of human factor VIII or factor IX concentrate, usually three to four times the usual dose.

Treatment of patients with high-titer inhibitors against factor VIII or IX is difficult, and no single approach is uniformly successful. There are two components: first, assurance of hemostasis using "bypass therapy," and second, eradication of inhibitor formation. Hemostasis can be provided by "bypass" agents that are used to treat bleeding episodes (see E-Table 177-1); specifically, the activated prothrombin complex concentrate FEIBA VH (75 to 100 IU/kg initially, then 50 to 100 IU/kg every 6 to 8 hours) and recombinant factor VIIa (90 μ/kg every 2 to 3 hours) can be administered until bleeding is controlled. In studies of congenital hemophilia A patients with alloantibody inhibitors, one dose of FEIBA VH or two doses of recombinant factor VIIa controlled hemarthrosis episodes 81 and 79% of the time, respectively. The activated and unactivated prothrombin complex concentrates contain activated vitamin K–dependent clotting factors that "bypass" the intrinsic pathway (factor VIII or IX) inhibitor. As a result, repeated administration over a short time may be complicated by potential thrombogenicity: the aPTT and clotting factor assays are not helpful in monitoring hemostasis. In patients with high-titer inhibitors to factor VIII or IX, recombinant factor VIIa may achieve effective hemostasis, but its use is limited by the need for frequent intravenous dosing, usually every 2 hours to start. Although continuous dosing has been used in some patients, general experience dictates that for surgery or procedures in which significant bleeding is likely, bolus dosing is required to achieve optimal hemostasis—a "thrombin burst." The product has also been effective in patients who experience anaphylactic reactions or nephrotic syndrome after exposure to factor IX–containing replacement products or FFP. Eradication of inhibitor formation is usually attempted with "immune tolerance induction" regimens, which are generally effective if initiated within 12 months of the inhibitor's detection. Tolerance regimens consist of daily doses of factor concentrates to accomplish desensitization to infused factor, a process associated with a 68% success rate. Although factor dose is not critical in achieving tolerance, the higher the inhibitor titer, the greater the time required to achieve tolerance induction. After tolerance is achieved, maintenance prophylaxis with factor VIII or IX concentrate administered two or three times weekly (at 20 to 30 IU/kg) is necessary. Individuals with inhibitors since childhood who have not undergone immune tolerance induction before adulthood are unlikely to respond. An alternative approach involves treatment with single or combination immunosuppressive agents, including rituximab (currently in clinical trials), mycophenolate, or cyclosporine. Because only a minority respond, adults are typically managed with bypass agents alone.

PREVENTION

Carrier Detection and Prenatal Diagnosis

Carrier detection and prenatal diagnosis have become technically feasible, very sensitive, and widely available. The application of these diagnostic tools, however, is influenced by ethical, cultural, religious, economic, educational, and personal considerations. For instance, carrier detection is particularly useful in identifying women who may be at risk for hemorrhagic complications during the delivery process and male offspring who are particularly vulnerable to intracerebral bleeds at birth. Alternatively, these techniques can provide important information used to make difficult reproductive decisions.

PROGNOSIS

The life expectancy of individuals with severe hemophilia is approaching that of the normal population. The age-matched death rate in hemophilia is 2.7-fold greater than that in the general population, although ischemic heart disease mortality is 60% lower than in the general population. Life expectancy is related to the severity of hemophilia: the mortality rate of severely affected patients is 4- to 6-fold greater than that of patients with mild deficiency. Among those with alloantibody inhibitors, mortality rates are significantly higher than in noninhibitor patients. The three leading causes of death are hepatitis C, HIV/AIDS, and central nervous system bleeding. Hepatitis C has become the leading cause of death, accounting for over half; deaths from HIV have declined with the availability of HAART (Chapter 396). Among those with HIV/HCV coinfection, HAART also slows the progression of HCV-related liver disease. Predictors of hepatitis C disease progression in hemophilia include alcohol use, the use of acetaminophen for pain relief of hemophilic arthropathy, hepatitis B surface antigenemia, and HIV coinfection.

The lifetime risk of intracranial hemorrhage is 2 to 8%. It is the leading cause of morbidity and mortality in the newborn period, and prospective monitoring of central nervous system function is a priority as the population ages. Finally, with the essential elimination of disease transmission through blood products in this population, it is anticipated that the normal problems of aging will be increasingly recognized in those with hemophilia, including atherosclerosis, hypertension, hyperlipidemia, obesity, and diabetes. The impact of these conditions on the natural history of hemophilia, given the recognized lower mortality from ischemic heart disease, remains to be seen.

FUTURE DIRECTIONS

Gene Therapy for Hemophilia A and B

The hereditary hemophilias are model diseases for gene therapy because they are caused by specific, well-defined gene mutations; a small, incremental rise in clotting factor synthesis can lead to substantially improved treatment and quality of life; and inadvertent overexpression by successful gene transfer would not be detrimental. Although successful gene transfer techniques have been developed to provide long-term therapeutic benefits in hemophilic mice and dog models, sustained responses have not yet been achieved in patients with hemophilia—a problem at least in part related to immune responses directed against the vector that suppress long-term expression of clotting factor activity. Approaches under study to avert the immune response to vectors include short-term immunosuppression during the first weeks after vector-gene administration; use of modified, less immunogenic vectors; and use of innovative delivery systems, such as platelets.

Novel therapeutic approaches to enhance clotting factor replacement therapy include long-acting factor products pegylated with liposomes or linked to IgG molecules to prolong factor activity half-life, now in clinical trials; oral delivery systems using bioencapsulated proteins; and molecular modifications to enhance the desirable properties of clotting factor, so-called designer molecules.

Acquired Hemophilias

EPIDEMIOLOGY AND PATHOBIOLOGY

Autoantibody inhibitors occur spontaneously in individuals with previously normal hemostasis (nonhemophiliacs). In contrast to alloantibody inhibitors in hemophilic men, which are directed against foreign infused clotting factor, autoantibody inhibitors are directed against a "self" clotting factor, most commonly factor VIII. These autoantibodies typically arise in individuals with no past bleeding history; thus the diagnosis may be missed until a prolonged aPTT and aPTT mix tests are obtained (Chapter 174). Although half of those with autoantibody inhibitors have no obvious underlying cause, autoimmune diseases, lymphoproliferative disorders, idiosyncratic drug reactions, pregnancy, and advanced age are associated in the other half.

CLINICAL MANIFESTATIONS AND DIAGNOSIS

Massive hemorrhagic events, even more severe than in hemophilia patients with alloantibodies, may occur in those with autoantibodies because of a delay in diagnosis and treatment. The laboratory expression of autoantibodies is similar to that of alloantibodies, except that clotting factor activity is not completely neutralized. Residual clotting factor activities between 3 and 20% of normal are frequently observed in patients with autoantibodies.

TREATMENT   Rx

The same principles of replacement therapy for alloantibodies apply to these acquired autoantibody inhibitors. There are two goals of treatment: stop the bleeding and assure hemostasis, and eradicate the inhibitor. For hemostasis, recombinant factor VIIa or factor VIII bypass activity is commonly used, in similar doses used to achieve hemostasis with alloantibody. Porcine factor VIII concentrate is also useful in acquired hemophilia A because little

cross-reactivity usually occurs, even with extremely high titers of anti–human factor VIII antibodies; however, its availability is limited. Clinical studies are under way to assess the utility of long-acting VIIa as well as genetically engineered forms of the porcine factor VIII protein. For eradication of the inhibitor, immunosuppressive therapy is generally more effective than in alloantibody patients; this includes corticosteroids (prednisone 1 mg/kg/day PO), cytotoxic agents (e.g., cyclophosphamide 150 mg/day PO or 500 to 750 mg/m² IV bolus every 3 to 4 weeks), or a combination, with dose titration based on inhibitor levels and complicating cytopenias. Anti-CD20 antibody (rituximab) 375 mg/m² intravenously weekly for 4 weeks is also effective. These agents are continued until the autoantibody inhibitor has disappeared; then they are tapered and discontinued. Whether these agents are also effective for the long-term eradication of autoantibody inhibitors is not known; the question has not been studied in randomized controlled trials. High-dose intravenous gamma globulin may be a useful adjunctive therapy. Immune tolerance induction regimens that combine alkylating agents, the daily administration of clotting factor concentrate, and high-dose corticosteroids have been successful in eradicating autoantibody inhibitors. Rarely, if inhibitor-related hemorrhage is refractory to bypassing agents, extracorporeal plasmapheresis over a staphylococcal protein A column may remove enough neutralizing IgG alloantibody or autoantibody to facilitate successful hemostasis after replacement therapy.

PROGNOSIS

Several large series of patients with acquired hemophilia reveal a substantial mortality rate of 15 to 25%, which is considerably higher than that observed with alloantibody factor VIII inhibitors. A large meta-analysis found that overall survival in acquired hemophilia was influenced primarily by the achievement of a complete remission, age younger than 65 years at diagnosis, and related diseases (malignancy vs. postpartum vs. others). As many as 17% of the deaths were associated with sepsis, and 71% of those arose as a complication of cyclophosphamide-induced neutropenia. Hemorrhagic complications were the primary cause of death, but these could be reduced if the inhibitor could be eradicated. Of note, complete remission was observed in 89% of cyclophosphamide-treated individuals, compared with 70% of those treated with corticosteroids alone and 41% of those who received no treatment.

Von Willebrand Disease

The most common congenital bleeding disorder is VWD. This disorder is inherited in an autosomal dominant fashion and affects both sexes, with a prevalence of 1 to 3% and no ethnic predominance. Homozygous patients are rare and carry a recessive mutant gene. Von Willebrand factor, the protein that is decreased or defective in VWD, is a large, multimeric glycoprotein encoded by the *VWF* gene, located on chromosome 12. Detailed discussion of VWD is provided in Chapter 176.

Factor XI Deficiency

EPIDEMIOLOGY

Factor XI deficiency has a prevalence of 1 in 1 million in the general population and 1 in 500 births in Ashkenazi Jewish families. Factor XI is the only component of the contact phase system (factor XII, prekallikrein, and high-molecular-weight kininogen) of the intrinsic pathway of coagulation that is associated with excessive bleeding complications when a deficiency exists.

PATHOBIOLOGY

Factor XI deficiency is predominantly an autosomal recessive trait, although some mutations may have a dominant transmission pattern. The factor XI gene (*FXI*) is located on chromosome 4, and the protein circulates as a homodimer, with each FXI monomer composed of 4 apple domains encoded by exons 3 through 10 and a protease domain encoded by exons 11 through 15. The Glu117 stop mutation in *FXI* is the most common cause of factor XI deficiency, secondary to poor secretion or stability of the truncated protein or decreased levels of messenger RNA. To date, more than 170 mutations of *FXI* have been identified in factor XI–deficient patients (see *www.factorxi.org*), but close correlation between hemorrhagic phenotype and genotype is lacking. Most are missense or nonsense mutations and are located across all 4 apple domains and the serine protease region. In Ashkenazi Jewish individuals, factor XI deficiency is common, with a heterozygote frequency of 8 to 10%; two predominant gene mutations occur with equal frequency and are designated type II (a stop codon in exon 5) and type III (a single base defect in exon 9). The most severe clinical disease is observed in patients homozygous for type II, who usually have less than 1% factor XI activity.

Homozygous type III individuals also manifest severe symptoms, but typically less severe than those of type II patients; they have slightly higher factor XI levels of about 10 to 20%. Compound heterozygotes, type II/III, make up the bulk of factor XI–deficient patients; they have clinically mild disease, with factor XI levels between 30 and 50%. In non-Jewish individuals, the mutations are more variable, although Cys128 stop has been described in several kindreds, and Cys38Arg has been found in several French Basque families. One third of those who develop inhibitors are homozygous for Glu117 stop, which results in an absent *FXI*. Genotypic identification of affected patients is determined by measuring factor XI levels rather than by defining the specific gene defect.

CLINICAL MANIFESTATIONS

The clinical bleeding tendencies in factor XI deficiency are less severe than those observed in severe hemophilia A or B and, in contrast to the hemophilias, do not correlate with the severity of the deficiency. Most individuals with less than 20% of normal factor XI activity experience excessive bleeding after trauma or surgery; however, a few do not bleed. In contrast, bleeding has been observed in approximately 35 to 50% of mildly affected patients with factor XI levels between 20 and 50% of normal. Spontaneous hemorrhagic episodes, hemarthroses, and intramuscular and intracerebral bleeds are unusual; traumatic and surgical bleeds typically involve the mucous membranes. Patients undergoing tonsillectomy, prostatectomy, or dental extraction are at highest risk for bleeding unless replacement therapy is administered. Women may experience significant menorrhagia, and it has been recommended that women with menorrhagia be screened for both VWD and factor XI deficiency. Patients with mild factor XI deficiency and coincident mild VWD have an increased risk of bleeding.

DIAGNOSIS

Factor XI deficiency is diagnosed in the laboratory by a prolonged aPTT, normal PT, and decreased factor XI activity ascertained in a specific quantitative clotting assay (normal range, 60 to 130%).

TREATMENT   Rx

Not all individuals with factor XI deficiency bleed, so it may be reasonable to monitor with no treatment, especially if there is no family history of bleeding. For surgical or other major bleeding, FFP 15 to 20 mL/kg can be used, although potential complications include fluid overload and infection risk, which can be reduced with the use of pathogen-inactivated FFP, if available. Use of factor XI concentrate, which is available in Europe but not the United States, may be complicated by thrombosis, which occurs in approximately 10% of patients, particularly in older individuals with preexisting cardiovascular disease and malignancy. Replacement dosing levels should not exceed 70% of factor XI activity. Repeat dosing with FFP or factor XI concentrate should take into consideration the long (60- to 80-hour) biologic half-life of factor XI in vivo.

The decision to treat heterozygotes with factor XI at levels greater than 20% is empirical and should be based on the individual's prior history of bleeding after trauma or surgery. Alternatively, a family medical history of bleeding complications can be considered. There is no clear evidence of benefit with the use of DDAVP. Because hemorrhagic complications originate most commonly from mucous membrane surfaces, antifibrinolytic agents such as ε-aminocaproic acid or tranexamic acid are frequently helpful as adjunctive therapy. In women with menorrhagia or postpartum hemorrhage, testing for VWD is recommended because both diseases may be present.

Alloantibody inhibitors, which neutralize the hemostatic effects of exogenously administered factor XI replacement, can develop in patients with severe factor XI deficiency who have been exposed to plasma or factor XI concentrate. Recombinant factor VIIa can prevent bleeding during or after surgery in these patients.

Deficiencies of Contact Activation Factors

Although factor XI plays an important role in the activation of factor IX in the intrinsic pathway generation of thrombin, it is only one of the four components of the contact phase of coagulation. Deficiencies in any of the other three factors (factor XII, prekallikrein, and high-molecular-weight kininogen) produce in vitro laboratory abnormalities. Even among those with severe factor XII deficiency (<1% activity), there is no clinical bleeding; however, up to 8 to 10% with severe factor XII deficiency actually experience venous thromboembolic events, which are occasionally fatal. This finding has led to speculation that factor XII deficiency may lead to hypercoagulability through defective participation of the contact phase proteins in the activation of fibrinolysis.

DIAGNOSIS

Deficiencies of each of these factors prolong the aPTT, often markedly, which may normalize after prolonged incubation of the patient's plasma at 37° C with a negatively charged activator of the aPTT assay (i.e., kaolin or celite). Specific assays are also available to quantitate each of the contact factors.

TREATMENT   Rx

Deficiencies of the contact activation factors, however severe they are and however prolonged the associated aPTT may be, do not cause clinical bleeding problems, even in response to surgery or trauma. Therefore, no therapy is indicated for factor XII deficiency, prekallikrein deficiency, or high-molecular-weight kininogen deficiency. Routine anticoagulation regimens are used to treat thrombogenic events.

Factor XIII (Fibrin-Stabilizing Factor) Deficiency

Factor XIII is a transglutaminase that is activated by thrombin and functions to cross-link fibrin to protect it from lysis by plasmin. It is also involved in wound healing and tissue repair and seems to be crucial for maintaining a viable pregnancy. Homozygous severe deficiency states are rare and are inherited in an autosomal recessive manner, with a prevalence of 1 per 3 million births. Consanguinity is common.

CLINICAL MANIFESTATIONS

Heterozygous carriers are usually asymptomatic, but homozygotes have lifelong bleeding that typically starts shortly after birth with persistent bleeding around the umbilical stump. Intracranial bleeding events, usually precipitated by minimal trauma, occur commonly enough in infants (25%) to justify the initiation of a primary prophylaxis regimen of replacement therapy. Delayed bleeding after surgery and trauma is the hallmark of the disease; however, easy bruising, poor wound healing with defective scar formation and dehiscence, and hemarthroses are characteristic. Spontaneous abortions are increased in severely affected women.

DIAGNOSIS

The diagnosis is usually suspected on clinical grounds, given that factor XIII deficiency is not detected by conventional screening coagulation assays (i.e., aPTT, PT). Most laboratories use a rapid screening assay that assesses the ability of a fibrin clot to remain intact with incubation in 5 mol/L of urea or 1% monochloroacetic acid. With factor XIII levels less than 1% of normal, the clot dissolves within 2 to 3 hours.

TREATMENT   Rx

Replacement therapy for prophylaxis or the treatment of acute bleeds can be accomplished by administering cryoprecipitate, FFP, or, preferably, plasma-derived factor XIII concentrate (Fibrogammin P), which is pasteurized for viral safety. A clinical trial of Fibrogammin P for factor XIII deficiency is under way in the United States, and the product is available under compassionate investigational new drug use through ZLB-Behring Inc., Marburg, Germany, and CSL Behring Inc., King of Prussia, PA. Clinical studies are also in progress to evaluate a placentally derived product. Normal hemostasis is achieved with a factor XIII level of only 5% of normal. The dose of Fibrogammin P is 10 to 20 U/kg intravenously, and because it has a long half-life (10 days), prophylactic replacement can be given every 3 to 4 weeks. Acquired alloantibody inhibitors can develop in severely affected individuals. Autoantibodies also occur, usually in association with systemic lupus erythematosus.

Dysfibrinogenemia and Afibrinogenemia

Approximately 300 abnormal fibrinogens have been described, but few cause hemostatic symptoms. Abnormal fibrinogens are rare, autosomally inherited proteins. Quantitative fibrinogen deficiencies (afibrinogenemia and hypofibrinogenemia) may result from mutations affecting fibrinogen synthesis or processing, whereas qualitative defects (dysfibrinogenemia) are caused by mutations that lead to abnormal polymerization, defective cross-linking, or defective assembly of the fibrinolytic system.

CLINICAL MANIFESTATIONS

More than 50% of the dysfibrinogenemias are asymptomatic, 25% are associated with a mild hemorrhagic tendency (commonly caused by defective release of fibrinopeptide A), and 20% predispose individuals to thrombophilia (usually caused by impaired fibrinolysis) (Chapter 179). Concurrent bleeding and thrombosis also may occur. The prevalence of dysfibrinogenemia in patients with a history of thromboembolic episodes approaches 0.8%. A high prevalence of dysfibrinogenemia has been reported among patients with chronic thromboembolic hypertension, implicating changes in the molecular structure of fibrin in the development of this disorder. Women experience a high incidence of pregnancy-related complications, such as spontaneous abortion and postpartum thromboembolic events. Thrombin times and reptilase times (plasma-based clotting times with the substitution of reptilase snake venom for thrombin) are not helpful in predicting whether an abnormal fibrinogen will be prothrombotic, prohemorrhagic, or asymptomatic. However, clinical history, fibrinopeptide release studies, and fibrin polymerization studies may be useful. Clinically insignificant dysfibrinogenemias may be acquired in association with hepatocellular carcinoma (Chapter 202).

In contrast to the hepatic synthesis of a qualitatively abnormal protein in dysfibrinogenemia, congenital afibrinogenemia, an autosomal recessive disorder, represents the markedly deficient production of a normal protein. Severe life-threatening hemorrhagic complications can occur at any site, beginning at birth with umbilical bleeding. Intracranial hemorrhage is a frequent cause of death. Poor wound healing is characteristic. All coagulation-based assays that depend on the detection of a fibrin clot end point are markedly prolonged. Afibrinogenemia is usually detectable by specific functional or immunologic assays. Platelet dysfunction may accompany afibrinogenemia and exacerbate bleeding.

DIAGNOSIS

Abnormalities are usually detected incidentally when routine coagulation screening assays reveal decreased fibrinogen concentrations and prolonged thrombin clotting times. On further evaluation, discordance between functional and immunologic fibrinogen levels (>50 mg/dL more antigenic than functional) is observed; clotting times using snake venom (reptilase or ancrod) are variably prolonged.

TREATMENT **Rx**

Deficiencies of fibrinogen can be corrected by the administration of FFP or cryoprecipitate; however, viral safety remains an issue. A viral-attenuated (pasteurized), plasma-derived fibrinogen concentrate (Riastap, CSL Behring) was recently approved by the Food and Drug Administration (FDA) for use in congenital fibrinogen deficiency, with a target replacement goal of 100 mg/dL. With a circulating biologic half-life of at least 96 hours, treatment every 3 to 4 days is adequate. Primary prophylaxis regimens may be useful in afibrinogenemia, with on-demand or prophylactic replacement for trauma or surgery. Individuals with thrombophilic manifestations should receive anticoagulation long term, depending on risk-benefit assessment (Chapter 179). Riastap is not recommended for use in dysfibrinogenemia. Solvent detergent- or psoralen-treated FFP (when licensed by the FDA) may provide an alternative therapy.

Factor V Deficiency

Factor V is a component of the prothrombinase complex that assembles factors Va and Xa on the phospholipid membrane of the platelet for prothrombin (factor II) activation to thrombin (Chapter 174).

CONGENITAL FACTOR V DEFICIENCY

Deficiency of factor V is a rare, autosomal recessive disorder (1 in 1 million births). The factor V Leiden protein, which is responsible for resistance to activated protein C and thrombophilia, does not affect factor V coagulant activity (Chapter 179). The severity of plasma factor V deficiency correlates less well with the risk of clinical bleeding than does the factor V content in platelet α-granules. This observation illustrates the critical role of the platelet in promoting adequate hemostasis at bleeding sites and explains why transfusions of normal platelets may be preferred over FFP for the treatment of hemorrhagic episodes secondary to congenital or acquired factor V deficiency. Hemostasis can be maintained without correcting plasma factor V activity (>25% of normal).

COMBINED DEFICIENCIES OF FACTORS V AND VIII

Factors V and VIII are structurally homologous proteins, and combined deficiencies of these factors occur as an autosomal recessive disorder with a prevalence of 1 in 100,000 births among Jews of Sephardic origin. The severity of bleeding is determined by the levels of these factors, which usually range from 5 to 30% of normal. Replacement therapy should be aimed at normalizing both clotting protein activities.

ACQUIRED FACTOR V DEFICIENCY

Acquired factor V deficiency has been described in individuals exposed to bovine factor V, which contaminates the thrombin preparations used topically to control bleeding during cardiovascular surgery. This abnormality probably represents the development of anti–bovine factor V antibodies that cross-react with the human factor V protein. Profuse bleeding accompanies this complication.

Deficiencies of Vitamin K–Dependent Coagulation
DEFICIENCIES OF FACTORS II, VII, AND X

PATHOBIOLOGY AND CLINICAL MANIFESTATIONS

Congenital deficiencies of factors II (prothrombin), VII, and X are rare, autosomally inherited disorders. Heterozygotes (with factor levels approximately 20% of normal) are typically asymptomatic except in the immediate newborn period, when physiologic vitamin K deficiency exacerbates the underlying clotting factor deficiency. Homozygotes with clotting factor levels less than 10% of normal manifest variable symptoms. As with other coagulopathies, these deficiencies are usually suspected after neonatal umbilical stump bleeding. Thereafter, unless replacement or prophylactic therapy is provided, these patients are subject to mucosal bleeding from epistaxis, menorrhagia, and dental extractions; hemarthroses and intramuscular hematomas; and bleeding after surgery or trauma.

Acquired factor VII deficiency has been associated with Dubin-Johnson and Gilbert's syndromes (Chapter 149). Acquired factor IX deficiency has been associated with Gaucher's disease, because factor IX binds to glucocerebroside (Chapter 215). Acquired factor X deficiency and amyloidosis are discussed later.

DIAGNOSIS

In the coagulation laboratory, factor VII deficiency is associated with a prolonged PT and a normal aPTT. This pattern localizes the deficiency to the extrinsic pathway. In contrast, deficiencies of factors II (prothrombin) and X prolong both the PT and the aPTT, with the defects localized to the common pathway of coagulation. A Russell viper venom–based clotting assay can differentiate between these two deficiencies; as a direct activator of factor X, the assay is prolonged with factor X deficiency but not with factor II deficiency. Mixing patient plasma with normal plasma results in a correction of these assays, and specific clotting assays using plasma deficient in the coagulation protein to be studied can confirm the diagnosis.

TREATMENT

Replacement therapy is indicated for acute symptomatic bleeds and for prophylaxis before surgery. In addition to FFP, which has the potential to transmit blood-borne viruses, factor IX complex concentrates can be administered to achieve hemostatic levels of any of these vitamin K–dependent factors (25 to 30% of normal).

Bleeding complications caused by acquired IgG autoantibodies directed against any coagulation factor protein can be reversed rapidly, albeit temporarily, by extracorporeal immunoadsorption over a Sepharose-bound polyclonal antihuman IgG or staphylococcal A column, with concomitant replacement therapy and initiation of immunosuppression. Recombinant factor VIIa is increasingly useful for surgery in those with rare congenital coagulation deficiencies, but typically at lower doses than with hemophilia inhibitors—generally 10 to 15 µg/kg/day or less, for up to several days.

FACTOR DEFICIENCY IN AMYLOIDOSIS

Severe acquired deficiency of factor X, often accompanied by deficiencies of other vitamin K–dependent factors, occasionally occurs in individuals with systemic amyloidosis (Chapter 194). Because amyloid fibrils in the reticuloendothelial system bind endogenous and exogenous sources of factor X, replacement therapy with FFP or factor IX complex concentrates, even in large quantities, may not be sufficient. Recombinant factor VIIa concentrate has been used to reverse acute bleeding. Splenectomy may ameliorate recurrent bleeding complications.

Other Acquired Coagulation Abnormalities
ANTIPHOSPHOLIPID SYNDROME AND LUPUS ANTICOAGULANT

EPIDEMIOLOGY

The antiphospholipid antibody syndrome (APS) is associated with recurrent thrombosis or recurrent pregnancy loss with autoantibodies directed against phospholipids. Antiphospholipid antibodies (APAs) may include lupus anticoagulant (LA), anticardiolipin antibody (CL), or anti-β2-glycoprotein-I (anti-β2-GPI). Thrombocytopenia is also a common finding in this prothrombotic disorder. Rarely, multiorgan failure may arise from widespread thrombosis, termed *catastrophic APS*.

PATHOBIOLOGY

Our understanding of the role of individual antibodies in diagnosing APS continues to be enhanced with clinical studies, which may also contribute to the development of better diagnostic assays. It has been suggested that the prothrombotic effects of APAs may derive from their ability to complex with β2-GPI in vivo (thereby negating their modulatory phospholipid-binding function) or through APA inhibition of protein C activation, interference with antithrombin III activity, and/or disruption of the annexin V "shield," thereby preventing normal clot breakdown (fibrinolysis). Although complement and inflammation play a role in fetal loss in a murine model of APS, the pathogenic mechanism of APS-associated pregnancy loss remains unclear. Although non-β2-GPI antibodies detected by CL enzyme-linked immunosorbent assay (ELISA) may play a role in early obstetric APS, and anti-β2-GPI antibodies with LA activity play a role in late miscarriage, additional studies are needed to better classify, understand, and manage this syndrome.

CLINICAL MANIFESTATIONS

APAs prolong coagulation in in vitro assays but are not generally associated with clinical bleeding. Rarely, clinical bleeding may occur when APA interacts with factor II (prothrombin), producing an acquired prothrombin (factor II) deficiency associated with accelerated clearance of LA-prothrombin complexes from the circulation. Bleeding tendencies also may arise when LA targets platelet membranes and produces quantitative and/or qualitative platelet abnormalities. Other clinical findings in APS include livedo reticularis (Chapter 80), valvular heart lesions, and nephropathy. Clinically, although both arterial and venous thrombosis (Chapter 179) may occur in APS, the most relevant is venous thrombosis and stroke in young adults. A diagnostic work-up in those with arterial thrombosis should include transesophageal echocardiography to exclude a cardiac source for arterial clots. In obstetric patients, other causes of miscarriage should be excluded. Nonpregnant individuals with APS-associated thrombotic manifestations have a 50% risk of experiencing recurrent events over a 5-year period. Typically, recurrent hypercoagulable episodes occur in a pattern consistent with the initial findings (e.g., venous recurrence following an initial deep vein thrombosis).

DIAGNOSIS

By international consensus, a diagnosis of APS is based on both clinical and laboratory criteria. Clinical criteria include (1) arterial, venous, or small-vessel thrombosis in any tissue or organ and (2) pregnancy morbidity. The latter includes one or more pregnancy losses before 10 weeks' gestation; one or more pregnancy losses before 34 weeks due to eclampsia, preeclampsia, or placental insufficiency; or three or more spontaneous abortions before 10 weeks. APS may be suspected in the setting of recurrent spontaneous miscarriages or pregnancy-related thromboembolic events; with the detection of cerebral arterial thromboses in young adults; in those with systemic lupus erythematosus (20 to 40%; Chapter 274) or other autoimmune diseases or lymphoproliferative malignancies; in those receiving psychotropic medications (e.g., chlorpromazine); or when incidental coagulation assays reveal aPTT prolongation.

Laboratory criteria include one or more high-titer APAs (LA, CL, anti-β2-GPI) on at least two occasions at least 12 weeks apart. APAs can be detected by three assays: the LA assay, the CL ELISA assay, and the β2-GPI ELISA assay. The LA assay includes a screening test, based on a prolonged phospholipid-dependent clotting time; a mixing test that distinguishes the inhibitor (fails to correct in a 1:1 mix) from a deficiency state (corrects in a 1:1 mix); and a confirmatory test based on platelet neutralization to demonstrate that the inhibitor is phospholipid dependent (clotting time corrects) or a modified aPTT reagent based on the binding of hexagonal phase phospholipids to LA. The CL ELISA measures antibodies in dilute sera that bind to CL-coated plates, including those that bind to CL alone or bound to bovine β2-GPI and both IgG and IgM, but it may miss CL bound to human β2-GPI. The β2-GPI ELISA detects antibodies that bind to β2-GPI–coated irradiated plates, but it has reduced specificity owing to binding by nonpathogenic antibodies. Positivity in multiple assays is strongly associated with thrombosis and miscarriage. Of the three assays, the β2-GPI ELISA is most strongly associated with thrombosis and early recurrent miscarriage; the LA assay is associated with venous thrombosis, stroke, and late miscarriage. The greatest weight is given to a positive LA test. From a practical standpoint, testing for all three antibodies at diagnosis is recommended to guide follow-up, because oral anticoagulants may interfere with the LA test.

TREATMENT   Rx

Because of the high risk of recurrent thromboembolism, patients with APS should receive antithrombotic therapy. The approach is based on achieving a balance between thrombosis risk and bleeding complications, especially in those with thrombocytopenia. Because of the limited information from randomized clinical trials, the recommendations for APS are similar to those for patients without APS—that is, to use unfractionated heparin or low-molecular-weight heparin (LMWH), with a 4- to 5-day overlap with warfarin, for acute venous thromboembolism (VTE), followed by long-term warfarin to a target international normalized ratio (INR) of 2.0 to 3.0. This recommendation is based on a randomized trial indicating no difference in bleeding rates with high-intensity (INR >3.0) versus low-intensity (INR 2.0 to 3.0) anticoagulation. **3** In individuals with thrombocytopenia, more frequent monitoring of the INR may be warranted to avoid bleeding complications. The duration of anticoagulation in those both with and without APS is based on a balance between VTE recurrence and bleeding.

For women with APS and pregnancy loss but no past thrombosis, the goal is to prevent recurrent pregnancy loss. Based on prospective studies indicating higher birth rates with aspirin plus heparin, recommendations include low-dose aspirin (81 mg) in combination with prophylactic heparin or LMWH in the antepartum period.

Among those with APS-associated thrombocytopenia and a platelet count below 20 to 30 × 10⁹/L, in the setting of bleeding or when bleeding risk exceeds bleeding with VTE treatment, management is similar to that for idiopathic thrombocytopenic purpura (Chapter 175). This includes steroids, intravenous immunoglobulin, and immunosuppressive agents (e.g., cyclophosphamide, azathioprine, off-label rituximab). Case reports indicate that danazol, dapsone, aspirin, or chloroquine may be helpful adjuncts. In pregnant women with APS-associated thrombocytopenia, treatment is advised before epidural anesthesia or cesarean section. In the latter case, early delivery under cover of intravenous immunoglobulin is recommended.

Treatment of APS-associated bleeding is dependent on the site and severity of bleeding. For anticoagulation bleeding, the anticoagulant should be withheld and an antidote (e.g., protamine) given, if available. For thrombocytopenia bleeding, platelet transfusions should be given, along with red blood cell transfusions, if necessary. If both thrombosis and bleeding occur, treatment should be directed at the component that is most life threatening. In those with a high bleeding risk, anticoagulants should be withheld or given at a lower dosage; those with a high thrombotic risk, despite thrombocytopenia, should be anticoagulated and given agents to boost platelet count. For those who receive prolonged heparin, supplemental calcium and vitamin D should be administered to minimize the risks of osteoporosis.

 Visit expertconsult.com for e-expanded chapter

Grade
A

1. Manco-Johnson MJ, Abshire TC, Shapiro AD, et al. Prophylaxis versus episodic treatment to prevent joint disease in boys with severe hemophilia. *N Engl J Med.* 2007;357:535-544.
2. Gringeri A, Lundin B, von Mackensen SV, et al. A randomized clinical trial of prophylaxis in children with hemophilia A (the ESPRIR Study). *J Thromb Haemost.* 2011;9:700-710.
3. Crowther MA, Ginsberg JS, Julian J, et al. A comparison of two intensities of warfarin for the prevention of recurrent thrombosis in patients with the antiphospholipid antibody syndrome. *N Engl J Med.* 2003;349:1133-1138.

SUGGESTED READINGS

Baudo F, Caimi T, de Cataldo F. Diagnosis and treatment of acquired haemophilia. *Haemophilia.* 2010;16:102-106. *The diagnosis is associated with autoimmune diseases, solid tumors, lymphoproliferative diseases, and pregnancy, but 50% of causes are idiopathic.*

Berntorp E, de Moerloose P, Ljung RC. The role of prophylaxis in bleeding disorders. *Haemophilia.* 2010;16:189-193. *Review emphasizing benefits for joint- or life-threatening bleeds, arthropathy, and quality of life.*

Blancette VS. Prophylaxis in the haemophilia population. *Haemophilia.* 2010;16:181-188. *Review.*

Favaloro EJ, Wong RC. Laboratory testing for the antiphospholipid syndrome: making sense of antiphospholipid antibody assays. *Clin Chem Lab Med.* 2011;49:447-461. *Review.*

Giangrande PL, Escobar MA. Management of difficult-to-treat inhibitor patients. *Haemophilia.* 2010;16:52-57. *Case-based review.*

Iorio A, Matino D, D'Amico R, et al. Recombinant Factor VIIa concentrate versus plasma derived concentrates for the treatment of acute bleeding episodes in people with haemophilia and inhibitors. *Cochrane Database Syst Rev.* 2010;8:CD004449. *rFVIIa and aPCC have similar hemostatic effects without increasing thromboembolic risk.*

Kempton CL. Inhibitors in previously treated patients: a review of literature. *Haemophilia.* 2010;16:61-65. *Review.*

Pipe SW. Hemophilia: new protein therapeutics. *Hematology Am Soc Hematol Educ Program.* 2010;2010:203-209. *Review.*

Pengo V. APS—controversies in diagnosis and management, critical overview of current guidelines. *Thromb Res.* 2011;127(suppl 3):S51-S52. *Review.*

178

HEMORRHAGIC DISORDERS: DISSEMINATED INTRAVASCULAR COAGULATION, LIVER FAILURE, AND VITAMIN K DEFICIENCY

ANDREW I. SCHAFER

DISSEMINATED INTRAVASCULAR COAGULATION

DEFINITION

Disseminated intravascular coagulation (DIC), also referred to as *consumptive coagulopathy* or *defibrination,* is caused by a wide variety of serious disorders (Table 178-1). In most patients, the underlying process dominates the clinical picture, but in some cases (e.g., occult malignancy, envenomation),

DIC may be the initial or predominant manifestation of the disorder. DIC never occurs in isolation, without an inciting cause.

PATHOBIOLOGY

DIC is primarily a thrombotic process, although its clinical manifestation may be widespread hemorrhage in acute, fulminant cases. The basic pathophysiology (Fig. 178-1), regardless of cause, is entry into the circulation of procoagulant substances that trigger systemic activation of the coagulation system and platelets with resultant disseminated deposition of fibrin-platelet

TABLE 178-1 MAJOR CAUSES OF DISSEMINATED INTRAVASCULAR COAGULATION

INFECTIONS

Gram-negative bacterial sepsis
Other bacteria, fungi, viruses, Rocky Mountain spotted fever, malaria

IMMUNOLOGIC REACTIONS

Transfusion reactions (ABO incompatibility)
Transplant rejection

OBSTETRIC COMPLICATIONS

Amniotic fluid embolism
Retained dead fetus
Abruptio placentae
Toxemia, preeclampsia
Septic abortion

MALIGNANCIES

Pancreatic carcinoma
Adenocarcinomas
Acute promyelocytic leukemia
Other neoplasms

LIVER FAILURE

ACUTE PANCREATITIS

ENVENOMATION

RESPIRATORY DISTRESS SYNDROME

TRAUMA, SHOCK

Brain injury
Crush injury
Burns
Hypothermia/hyperthermia
Fat embolism
Hypoxia, ischemia
Surgery

VASCULAR DISORDERS

Giant hemangioma (Kasabach-Merritt syndrome)
Aortic aneurysm
Vascular tumors

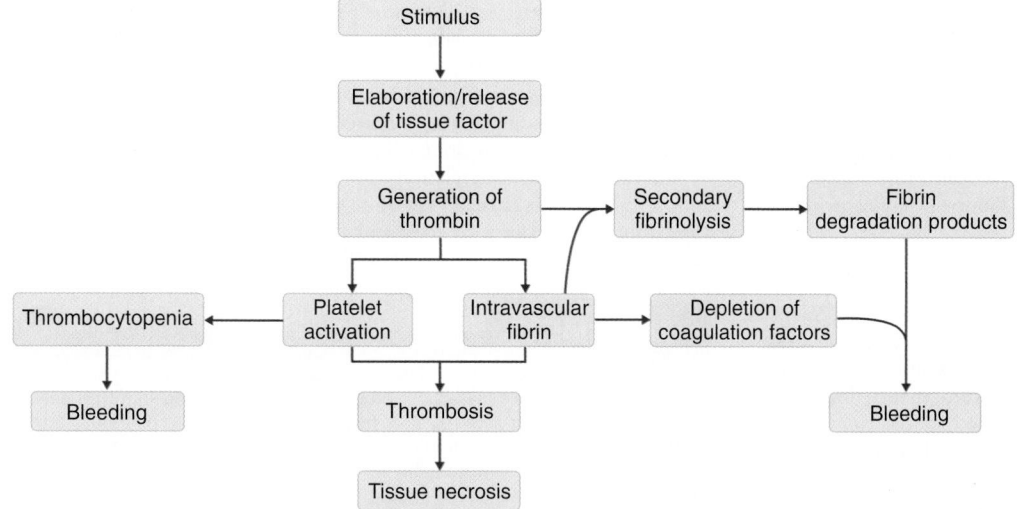

FIGURE 178-1. Pathophysiology of bleeding, thrombosis, and ischemic manifestations in patients with disseminated intravascular coagulation.

thrombi within the microvasculature. In most cases, the procoagulant stimulus is tissue factor, a lipoprotein that is not normally exposed to blood. In DIC, tissue factor gains access to blood by tissue injury, its elaboration by malignant cells, or its expression on the surface of monocytes and endothelial cells by inflammatory mediators. Components of the inflammatory response and the coagulation system are reciprocally activated in some forms of DIC, such as sepsis. Tissue factor triggers generation of the coagulation protease thrombin, which induces fibrin formation and platelet activation. In some specific cases of DIC, procoagulants other than tissue factor (e.g., a cysteine protease or mucin in certain malignancies) and proteases other than thrombin (e.g., trypsin in pancreatitis, exogenous enzymes in envenomation) provide the procoagulant stimulus.

In acute, uncompensated DIC, coagulation factors are consumed at a rate in excess of the capacity of the liver to synthesize them, and platelets are consumed in excess of the capacity of bone marrow megakaryocytes to release them. The resulting laboratory manifestations are a prolonged prothrombin time (PT) and activated partial thromboplastin time (aPTT) and thrombocytopenia. Increased fibrin formation in DIC stimulates the process of secondary fibrinolysis, in which plasminogen activators generate plasmin to digest fibrin (and fibrinogen) into fibrin(ogen) degradation products (FDPs). FDPs are potent circulating anticoagulants that further contribute to the bleeding manifestations of DIC. Intravascular fibrin deposition can cause fragmentation of red blood cells and lead to the appearance of schistocytes in blood smears; however, frank hemolytic anemia is unusual in DIC. Microvascular thrombosis in DIC can compromise the blood supply to some organs and lead to multiorgan failure, particularly when accompanied by systemic hemodynamic and metabolic derangements.

Underlying Causes

DIC always has an underlying cause that generally must be identified and eliminated if the coagulopathy is to be managed successfully. The development of DIC in many of these disorders is associated with an unfavorable outcome. Infection is the most common cause of DIC. The syndrome is particularly associated with gram-negative or gram-positive sepsis (Chapter 108), although it can be triggered by a variety of other bacterial, fungal, viral, rickettsial, and protozoal microorganisms. The placenta and uterine contents are rich sources of tissue factor and other procoagulants that are normally excluded from the maternal circulation; a spectrum of clinical manifestations of DIC may accompany obstetric complications when this barrier is breached, especially in the third trimester. These syndromes range from acute, fulminant, and often fatal DIC in amniotic fluid embolism to chronic or subacute DIC with a retained dead fetus. Other obstetric problems associated with DIC include abruptio placentae, toxemia, and septic abortion. Chronic forms of DIC are caused by a variety of malignancies, particularly pancreatic cancer (Chapter 200) and mucin-secreting adenocarcinomas of the gastrointestinal tract (Chapter 199), in which thrombotic rather than bleeding manifestations predominate. Treatment with all-*trans*-retinoic acid has greatly reduced the incidence of severe DIC in patients with acute promyelocytic leukemia (Chapter 189). It is not known whether liver failure (Chapter 157) can cause DIC or whether its coexistence merely exacerbates intravascular coagulation because of impaired clearance of activated clotting factors, plasmin, and FDPs. Snake venom contains a variety of substances that can affect coagulation and endothelial permeability. Bites from rattlesnakes and other vipers can induce profound DIC by introduction of these exogenous toxins and release of endogenous tissue factor via tissue necrosis. The likelihood and degree of DIC caused by trauma, surgery, and shock (Chapter 106) are related to the extent of tissue damage and the organs involved; the brain is a particularly rich source of tissue factor, so traumatic brain injury (Chapter 406) can precipitate acute DIC. Large aortic aneurysms (Chapter 78), giant hemangiomas, and other vascular malformations can cause subclinical or clinical DIC that is initiated locally within the abnormal vasculature but can "spill" into the systemic circulation.

CLINICAL MANIFESTATIONS

The clinical manifestations of DIC are determined by the nature, intensity, and duration of the underlying stimulus. The coexistence of liver disease exacerbates DIC of any etiology. Low-grade DIC is often asymptomatic and diagnosed only by laboratory abnormalities. Thrombotic complications of DIC occur most often with chronic underlying diseases, as exemplified by Trousseau's syndrome in cancer (Chapter 187). DIC can present as acrocyanosis and gangrene of the digits in critically ill, hemodynamically compromised patients on vasopressors. Hemorrhagic necrosis of the skin

FIGURE 178-2. Disseminated intravascular coagulation resulting from staphylococcal septicemia. Note the characteristic skin hemorrhage ranging from small purpuric lesions to larger ecchymoses. (From Forbes CD, Jackson WF. *Color Atlas and Text of Clinical Medicine*, 3rd ed. London: Mosby; 2003.)

(Fig. 178-2) and purpura fulminans may also be manifestations of DIC. Bleeding is the most common clinical finding in acute, uncompensated DIC. Bleeding can be limited to sites of intervention or anatomic abnormalities, but it tends to be generalized in more severe cases, including widespread ecchymoses and diffuse oozing from mucosal surfaces and orifices.

DIAGNOSIS

The laboratory diagnosis of severe, acute DIC is not usually difficult. Consumption and inhibition of the function of clotting factors cause prolongation of the PT, aPTT, and thrombin time. Consumption of platelets causes thrombocytopenia. Secondary fibrinolysis generates increased titers of FDPs, which can be measured by latex agglutination or D-dimer assays. Some schistocytes may be seen in the peripheral blood smear, but this finding is neither sensitive nor specific for DIC. Chronic or compensated forms of DIC are more difficult to diagnose, with highly variable patterns of abnormalities in "DIC screen" coagulation tests. Increased D-dimers and a prolonged PT are generally more sensitive measures than are abnormalities of the aPTT and platelet count. Overcompensated synthesis of consumed clotting factors and platelets in some chronic forms of DIC may actually cause shortening of the PT and aPTT or thrombocytosis (or both), even though elevated levels of D-dimers indicate secondary fibrinolysis in such cases.

The most difficult differential diagnosis of DIC occurs in patients who have coexisting liver disease. The coagulopathy of liver failure is often indistinguishable from that of DIC, partly because advanced hepatic dysfunction is accompanied by a state of DIC. In liver failure, the combination of decreased synthesis of clotting factors, impaired clearance of activated clotting factors, secondary fibrinolysis, and thrombocytopenia from portal hypertension and hypersplenism may make the coagulopathy practically impossible to differentiate from DIC. In thrombotic microangiopathies, including thrombotic thrombocytopenic purpura and hemolytic-uremic syndrome, platelet consumption and thrombocytopenia are not accompanied by activation of clotting factors or secondary fibrinolysis; therefore the PT, aPTT, thrombin time, and D-dimers are generally normal in these disorders. Schistocytes, often with frank hemolysis, are much more prominent in the peripheral smear in thrombotic thrombocytopenic purpura and hemolytic-uremic syndrome (Chapter 175) than in DIC.

Primary fibrinolysis is disputed as a distinct entity. Some patients with a serious clinical bleeding diathesis, however, have laboratory evidence of predominantly fibrinolysis, including high levels of FDPs (D-dimers) and severe hypofibrinogenemia, with relatively little consumption of coagulation factors and normal or near-normal platelet counts. These unusual findings, which approximate the findings expected with fibrinolytic therapy, are encountered occasionally, particularly in patients with prostate cancer.

TREATMENT   Rx

Successful treatment of DIC (Table 178-2) requires that the underlying cause be identified and eliminated. All other therapies, including hemodynamic support, replacement of coagulation factors and platelets, and pharmacologic inhibitors of coagulation and fibrinolysis, are just temporizing measures. In many patients with asymptomatic, self-limited DIC who have only laboratory manifestations of the coagulopathy, no treatment may be necessary. In

TABLE 178-2	TREATMENT OF DISSEMINATED INTRAVASCULAR COAGULATION

Identify and eliminate the underlying cause
No treatment if mild, asymptomatic, and self-limited
Hemodynamic support, as indicated, in severe cases
Blood component therapy
  Indications: active bleeding or high risk for bleeding
    Fresh-frozen plasma
    Platelets
    In some cases, consider cryoprecipitate, antithrombin III
Drug therapy
  Indications: heparin for DIC manifested by thrombosis or acrocyanosis;
    antifibrinolytic agents generally contraindicated except with life-threatening
    bleeding and failure of blood component therapy

DIC = disseminated intravascular coagulation.

TABLE 178-3	COAGULATION ABNORMALITIES IN LIVER DISEASE

ABNORMALITIES IN COAGULATION

Decreased synthesis of coagulation factors
Impaired vitamin K–dependent γ-carboxylation
Dysfibrinogenemia
Disseminated intravascular coagulation
Increased fibrinolytic activity

ABNORMALITIES IN PLATELETS

Thrombocytopenia (hypersplenism)
Abnormal platelet function

patients with DIC who are actively bleeding or who are at high risk for bleeding, the blood component treatments of choice are transfusions of platelets to improve the thrombocytopenia and fresh-frozen plasma to replace all consumed coagulation factors and correct the prolonged PT and aPTT. Large volumes of plasma (e.g., >6 U/24 hours) may be required to ameliorate bleeding in severe cases. In some patients who have particularly profound hypofibrinogenemia, the additional transfusion of cryoprecipitate, a plasma concentrate that is enriched in fibrinogen, may be useful. The theoretical concern that these blood products could "fuel the fire" and exacerbate the DIC has not been supported by clinical experience.

The use of pharmacologic inhibitors of coagulation and fibrinolysis in DIC is controversial. Heparin is of theoretical benefit because it blocks thrombin activity and quenches intravascular coagulation and the resultant secondary fibrinolysis. In practice, heparin might exacerbate the bleeding tendency in acute DIC. Heparin is usually reserved for special forms of DIC, including those manifested by thrombosis or acrocyanosis and forms that accompany cancer, vascular malformations, retained dead fetus, and possibly acute promyelocytic leukemia. In cases of DIC in which thrombosis or acral ischemia predominates, unfractionated heparin should be used by continuous infusion owing to its short half-life and reversibility in the event of increased bleeding. Monitoring the aPTT in the presence of DIC may be problematic, so heparin infusion in this setting should be followed mainly by clinical response and improvement in other tests of coagulation (e.g., thrombocytopenia). Antifibrinolytic agents, including ε-aminocaproic acid and tranexamic acid, are generally contraindicated in DIC. By blocking the secondary fibrinolytic response to DIC, these drugs cause unopposed fibrin deposition and may precipitate thrombosis. Antifibrinolytic agents may be effective in decreasing life-threatening bleeding in DIC, however, particularly in extreme cases in which aggressive blood component replacement fails to control the hemorrhage; in such situations, simultaneous infusion of low doses of heparin may reduce the risk for thrombosis.

A 96-hour infusion of recombinant human activated protein C (rhAPC; drotrecogin alfa [activated]), which has both anticoagulant and anti-inflammatory properties, significantly reduces mortality in patients with severe sepsis and high risk of death; it should be urgently considered in such specific cases of DIC.[1] However, it does not benefit septic patients with a low risk of death, such as those with only single-organ failure or Acute Physiology and Chronic Health Evaluation (APACHE) II scores of less than 25; in fact, it is associated with increased serious bleeding complications in these patients.[2] Because of the increased risk for intracerebral hemorrhage with severe thrombocytopenia, rhAPC must be used cautiously in patients with DIC and in conjunction with platelet transfusion if the platelet count is less than 30,000/mm³. Although recombinant tissue factor pathway inhibitor and antithrombin III concentrates may have some efficacy in improving laboratory parameters of DIC, the overall survival benefit with these agents in patients with DIC has not been demonstrated.

● LIVER FAILURE

Bleeding complications in patients with advanced liver disease (Chapters 156 and 157) can be severe and even fatal and directly account for about 20% of the deaths associated with hepatic failure. The extent of the bleeding tendency depends on the severity and type of liver disease involved. About one third of deaths in patients undergoing liver transplantation are attributable to perioperative hemorrhage.

PATHOBIOLOGY

The pathophysiology of bleeding in liver failure is complex and multifactorial. Anatomic abnormalities resulting from portal hypertension are frequently the major cause of gastrointestinal bleeding in patients with liver disease.

Upper gastrointestinal bleeding can be caused by esophageal varices or hemorrhagic gastritis (congestive gastropathy), whereas lower gastrointestinal bleeding, although seldom life-threatening, can be due to hemorrhoids.

The complexity of the systemic coagulopathy of liver failure is not surprising inasmuch as the liver is the principal organ site for the synthesis of coagulation and fibrinolytic factors as well as their protein inhibitors (Table 178-3). Hepatocytes produce all of the clotting factors except von Willebrand factor, and advanced parenchymal liver disease results in impaired synthesis of these proteins. Liver disease can also cause impairment in vitamin K–dependent γ-carboxylation of the procoagulant factors II, VII, IX, and X, as well as the anticoagulant proteins C and S. Functional abnormalities of fibrinogen, termed *dysfibrinogenemias*, are frequently found in various forms of liver disease, particularly in hepatocellular carcinoma. Most forms of advanced liver disease are accompanied by some degree of DIC caused by impaired synthesis of inhibitors of blood coagulation and defective hepatocellular clearance of activated coagulation factors. DIC is an especially important potential complication of LeVeen shunts used to treat intractable ascites because this procedure introduces procoagulant-rich ascitic fluid into the systemic circulation. In many of these cases, shunt ligation is required to terminate the DIC. DIC and bleeding risk are exacerbated by the enhanced fibrinolytic activity of liver disease caused by increased levels of tissue plasminogen activator accompanied by decreased synthesis of inhibitors of plasminogen activator and plasmin.

Quantitative and qualitative abnormalities of platelets also contribute to the bleeding diathesis of liver failure. Congestive splenomegaly secondary to portal hypertension causes increased pooling of platelets in the spleen (hypersplenism). The resultant thrombocytopenia, the degree of which generally correlates with spleen size, rarely causes a reduction in the platelet count to less than 50,000/mm³. In alcoholic patients, suppression of bone marrow thrombopoiesis by the acute toxic effects of alcohol or folate deficiency may contribute to the thrombocytopenia. Qualitative platelet abnormalities have also been described in patients with liver disease.

Liver transplantation (Chapter 157) poses special problems to the coagulation system. During the anhepatic stage of surgery, which lasts about 2 hours, the complete cessation of synthesis of coagulation factors causes further prolongation of the PT and aPTT. Release of tissue plasminogen activator from the newly grafted liver leads to increased fibrinolysis and transient exacerbation of bleeding risk in the postoperative period.

CLINICAL MANIFESTATIONS

The most common hemorrhagic complication of liver disease is gastrointestinal bleeding, which is usually caused by anatomic abnormalities and exacerbated by the systemic coagulopathy of liver failure. Bleeding from other mucosal sites, extensive ecchymoses, or more serious hemorrhage into the retroperitoneum or central nervous system generally indicates more significant derangements of the coagulation system.

The severe coagulopathy in patients with liver disease makes liver biopsy a potentially hazardous procedure. The PT and platelet count are the best guides to bleeding risk. In general, liver biopsy can be performed safely if the PT and aPTT do not exceed 1.5 times control values and the platelet count is greater than 50,000/mm³. Fresh-frozen plasma (see Treatment) can be infused to correct the prolonged PT and aPTT. Bleeding time is not a reliable predictor of bleeding risk after biopsy.

DIAGNOSIS

Although the PT and aPTT are often prolonged in patients with advanced liver disease, the former tends to be a more sensitive assay early in the course;

a disproportionate prolongation of the aPTT should raise suspicion of a coexisting coagulation abnormality, such as a lupus anticoagulant or clotting factor inhibitor. A prolonged PT is also a useful prognostic indicator of poor outcome in patients with cirrhosis, acute acetaminophen hepatotoxicity, and acute viral hepatitis; in the latter, it is a better index of prognosis than are serum albumin or transaminases. A disproportionate prolongation of the thrombin time should suggest the presence of dysfibrinogenemia. Hypersplenism (Chapter 171), possibly associated with nutritional folate deficiency or the acute toxic effects of alcohol on bone marrow, often causes mild to moderate thrombocytopenia in patients with liver disease; however, consideration should be given to other coexisting causes of thrombocytopenia if the platelet count is significantly less than $50,000/mm^3$.

The coagulopathy of liver failure is often indistinguishable from that of DIC, in part because some degree of DIC is a necessary accompaniment of advanced liver disease. In general, patients with DIC have more marked decreases in levels of factor VIII and increases in D-dimer than patients with liver failure.

TREATMENT Rx

Therapy for the coagulopathy of liver disease may be directed at preventing the hemorrhagic complications of invasive procedures or treating active bleeding. The most effective treatment is blood component therapy with fresh-frozen plasma (which contains all the coagulation factors) and platelet transfusions (Chapter 180). Some patients require large volumes of fresh-frozen plasma (15 to 20 mL/kg) to lower the prolonged PT; rarely, plasmapheresis with plasma exchange is required to avoid fluid overload in these situations. Because of the short half-lives of some clotting factors, fresh-frozen plasma may have to be administered every 8 to 12 hours to maintain acceptable coagulation test parameters. In some patients, especially those with cholestasis, parenteral administration of vitamin K can at least partially reverse the coagulation abnormalities; however, in patients with advanced hepatocellular failure, vitamin K is largely ineffective. Prothrombin complex concentrates are relatively contraindicated in patients with liver failure, as in those with DIC, because of the risk of thrombotic complications. Because of immediate pooling of transfused platelets in the enlarged spleen of patients with hypersplenism, a higher than calculated dose of platelet concentrates is usually required to increase circulating platelet counts significantly.

A recent randomized, controlled trial failed to demonstrate a beneficial effect of recombinant activated factor VII (rhVIIa) for variceal bleeding in patients with advanced cirrhosis.**3** Routine use of rfVIIa for the coagulopathy of liver disease cannot be recommended at this time. Desmopressin (DDAVP), which can shorten the bleeding time of patients with cirrhosis, may be considered as ancillary therapy in patients undergoing invasive procedures.

● VITAMIN K DEFICIENCY

Vitamin K is required for γ-carboxylation of glutamic acid residues of the procoagulant factors II (prothrombin), VII, IX, and X and the anticoagulant factors protein C and protein S. This post-translational modification normally renders these proteins functionally active in coagulation. The PT is more sensitive than the aPTT in detecting vitamin K deficiency states because factor VII, the only vitamin K–dependent factor that is in the extrinsic pathway of coagulation, is the most labile of these proteins.

The two major sources of vitamin K are dietary intake and synthesis by the bacterial flora of the intestine. In the absence of malabsorption, nutritional deficiency alone rarely causes clinically significant vitamin K deficiency. The condition can arise, however, when eradication of gut flora is combined with inadequate dietary intake. This situation typically occurs in critically ill patients in intensive care units who have no oral intake and are receiving broad-spectrum antibiotics for prolonged periods. Vitamin K deficiency can also develop in patients receiving total parenteral nutrition unless the infusions are supplemented with vitamin K.

Vitamin K is absorbed predominantly in the ileum and requires the presence of bile salts. Clinically significant vitamin K deficiency occurs with malabsorption of fat-soluble vitamins secondary to obstructive jaundice (Chapter 158) or with malabsorption caused by intrinsic small bowel diseases, including celiac sprue, short-bowel syndrome, and inflammatory bowel disease (Chapters 142 and 143).

Warfarin (Chapter 37) acts as an anticoagulant by competitive antagonism of vitamin K. Rare cases of hereditary deficiency of the vitamin K–dependent coagulation factors may cause a lifelong bleeding tendency.

Correction of vitamin K deficiency, when clinically significant, can be achieved with oral supplementation, unless malabsorption is present. In the latter case, parenteral vitamin K (10 mg subcutaneously daily) should be administered. Emergency treatment of bleeding caused by vitamin K deficiency is transfusion of fresh-frozen plasma.

1. Bernard GR, Vincent JL, Laterre PF, et al. Efficacy and safety of recombinant human activated protein C for severe sepsis. *N Engl J Med.* 2001;344:699-709.
2. Abraham E, Laterre PF, Garg R. Drotrecogin alfa (activated) for adults with severe sepsis and a low risk of death. *N Engl J Med.* 2005;353:1332-1341.
3. Bosch J, Thabut D, Albillos A, et al. Recombinant factor VIIa for variceal bleeding in patients with advanced cirrhosis: a randomized, controlled trial. *Hepatology.* 2008;47:1604-1614.

SUGGESTED READINGS

Kitchens CS. Thrombocytopenia and thrombosis in disseminated intravascular coagulation (DIC). *Hematol Am Soc Hematol Educ Progr.* 2009;240-246. *Case-based discussion of contemporary issues in DIC.*
Levi M, Meijers JC. DIC: which laboratory tests are most useful. *Blood Rev.* 2011;25:33-37. *Review including more recently developed dynamic algorithms.*
Montagnana M, Franchi M, Danese E, et al. Disseminated intravascular coagulation in obstetric and gynecologic disorders. *Semin Thromb Hemost.* 2010;36:404-418. *Review.*
Munoz SJ, Stravitz RT, Gabriel DA. Coagulopathy of acute liver failure. *Clin Liver Dis.* 2009;13:95-107. *Review of the epidemiology, pathophysiology, presentation, evaluation, and management of coagulopathy in acute liver failure.*
Takemitsu T, Wada H, Hatada T, et al. Prospective evaluation of three different diagnostic criteria for disseminated intravascular coagulation. *Thromb Haemost.* 2011;115:40-44. *The platelet count, prothrombin time, fibrin and fibrinogen degradation products, and fibrinogen are the key diagnostic criteria.*

179

THROMBOTIC DISORDERS: HYPERCOAGULABLE STATES

ANDREW I. SCHAFER

The *hypercoagulable states,* also referred to as *thrombophilias,* encompass a group of inherited or acquired conditions that cause a risk for thrombosis.

The primary hypercoagulable states are quantitative or qualitative abnormalities in specific coagulation proteins that induce a prothrombotic state. Most of these disorders involve inherited mutations and polymorphisms that lead to either (1) a deficiency of a physiologic antithrombotic factor or (2) an increased level of a prothrombotic factor (Table 179-1). Particularly when they are combined with other inherited prothrombotic mutations (multigene interactions), these primary hypercoagulable states are associated with a lifelong predisposition to thrombosis. The secondary hypercoagulable states, a diverse group of mostly acquired conditions, cause a thrombotic tendency by more complex, often multifactorial mechanisms. The trigger for a discrete, clinical thrombotic event is often the development of one of the acquired, secondary hypercoagulable states superimposed on an inherited state of hypercoagulability.

TABLE 179-1 PRIMARY HYPERCOAGULABLE STATES
DEFICIENCY OF ANTITHROMBOTIC FACTORS
Antithrombin (III) deficiency
Protein C deficiency
Protein S deficiency
INCREASED PROTHROMBOTIC FACTORS
Factor Va (activated protein C resistance; factor V Leiden)
Prothrombin (prothrombin G20210A mutation)
Factor IX Padua (factor IX R338L mutation)
Factors VII, XI, IX, VIII; von Willebrand's factor; fibrinogen (epidemiologic data; molecular mechanisms unknown)

PRIMARY HYPERCOAGULABLE STATES

Antithrombin III Deficiency

EPIDEMIOLOGY AND PATHOBIOLOGY

Inherited quantitative or qualitative deficiency of antithrombin III leads to increased fibrin accumulation and a lifelong propensity to thrombosis (Chapter 174). Antithrombin is the major physiologic inhibitor of thrombin and other activated coagulation factors; therefore, its deficiency leads to unregulated protease activity and fibrin formation.

The frequency of asymptomatic heterozygous antithrombin deficiency in the general population may be 1 in 350. Most of these individuals have clinically silent mutations and never have thrombotic manifestations. The frequency of symptomatic antithrombin deficiency in the general population has been estimated to be between 1 in 2000 and 1 in 5000. Among all patients seen with venous thromboembolism (VTE), antithrombin deficiency is detected in only about 1 to 2%, but it is found in approximately 2.5% of selected patients with recurrent thrombosis or onset of thrombosis at a younger age (<45 years old).

Patients with type I antithrombin deficiency have proportionately reduced plasma levels of antigenic and functional antithrombin that result from a quantitative deficiency of the normal protein. Impaired synthesis, defective secretion, or instability of antithrombin in type I antithrombin-deficient individuals is caused by major gene deletions, single nucleotide changes, or short insertions or deletions in the antithrombin gene. Patients with type II antithrombin deficiency have normal or nearly normal plasma antigen accompanied by low activity levels, characteristics indicative of a functionally defective molecule. Type II deficiency is usually caused by specific point mutations leading to single amino acid substitutions that produce a dysfunctional protein. More than 250 different mutations causing type I or type II antithrombin deficiency have been recognized to date.

The pattern of inheritance of antithrombin deficiency is autosomal dominant. Most affected individuals are heterozygotes whose antithrombin levels are typically about 40 to 60% of normal. These individuals may have the full clinical manifestations of lifelong hypercoagulability. Rare homozygous antithrombin-deficient patients generally have type II deficiency with reduced heparin affinity, a variant that is associated with a low risk for thrombosis in its heterozygous form; other forms of homozygous antithrombin deficiency are probably incompatible with life.

Protein C Deficiency

Protein C deficiency leads to unregulated fibrin generation because of impaired inactivation of factors VIIIa and Va, two essential cofactors in the coagulation cascade.

EPIDEMIOLOGY

The prevalence of heterozygous protein C deficiency in the general population is about 1 per 200 to 500. Protein C deficiency is found in 2 to 5% of all patients with VTE.

PATHOBIOLOGY

AS with antithrombin deficiency, two general forms of protein C deficiency are recognized: type I, in which quantitative deficiency of the protein is associated with a proportionate decrease in protein C antigen and activity, and type II, in which qualitative defects in protein C are associated with disproportionately reduced protein C activity relative to antigen. More than 160 mutations are known to cause protein C deficiency. In the more common type I deficiency, frameshift, nonsense, or missense mutations cause premature termination of synthesis or loss of protein C stability. In type II deficiency, different mutations can cause abnormalities in protein C activation or function. The mode of inheritance of protein C deficiency is autosomal dominant. As in antithrombin deficiency, most affected individuals are heterozygotes.

Protein S Deficiency

Protein S is the principal cofactor of activated protein C (APC), and its deficiency mimics that of protein C in causing loss of regulation of fibrin generation by impaired inactivation of factors VIIIa and Va.

EPIDEMIOLOGY

The exact prevalence of protein S deficiency in the general population is unknown but is estimated to be less than 0.5%. Its frequency in all patients evaluated for VTE (1 to 3%) is comparable to that of protein C deficiency.

PATHOBIOLOGY

Protein S circulates in plasma partly in complex with C4b binding protein; only free protein S, which normally constitutes about 35 to 40% of total protein S, can function as a cofactor of APC. As in antithrombin and protein C deficiencies, quantitative (type I) and qualitative (type II) forms of inherited protein S deficiency are known. In addition, type III protein S deficiency is characterized by normal plasma levels of total protein S but low levels of free protein S.

Relatively few specific mutations of the protein S gene have been described to date. Most involve frameshift, nonsense, or missense point mutations.

Activated Protein C Resistance (Factor V Leiden)

EPIDEMIOLOGY

The factor V Leiden mutation is remarkably frequent (3 to 7%) in healthy white populations but is far less prevalent in certain black and Asian populations. In various studies, APC resistance was found in a wide range of frequencies (10 to 64%) in patients with VTE.

PATHOBIOLOGY

Almost all subjects with functional APC resistance have a single, specific point mutation in the gene for factor V, which is a critical target of the physiologic anticoagulant action of APC. In this mutation, termed *factor V Leiden*, guanine is replaced with adenine at nucleotide 1691 (G1691A), which leads to the amino acid substitution of Arg504 by Gln and renders factor Va incapable of being inactivated by APC. Heterozygosity for the autosomally transmitted factor V Leiden mutation increases the risk for thrombosis by a factor of 5 to 10, whereas homozygosity increases the risk by a factor of 50 to 100.

Prothrombin Gene Mutation

The substitution of G for A at nucleotide 20210 of the prothrombin gene has been associated with elevated plasma levels of prothrombin and an increased risk for venous thrombosis. The allele frequency for this gain-of-function mutation is 1 to 6% in white populations, but it is much less prevalent in other racial groups. The prothrombin G20210A mutation is found in 3 to 8% of all patients with venous thromboembolism.

Other Primary Hypercoagulable States

The first X-linked thrombophilia was recently reported. A family with a gain-of-function mutation in the gene for coagulation factor IX (factor IX-R338L) had juvenile thrombophilia associated with a five- to ten-fold increase in factor IX clotting activity (with normal quantitative protein levels). Elevated levels of factor VIII coagulant activity are a significant risk factor for venous thrombosis, and family studies suggest that high factor VIII levels are often genetically determined. Increased levels of factors VII, IX, and XI, fibrinogen, von Willebrand factor, and thrombin-activatable fibrinolysis inhibitor, as well as very low levels of tissue factor pathway inhibitor, may also confer increased risk. Many other inherited abnormalities of specific physiologic antithrombotic systems may be associated with a thrombotic tendency. Most of these conditions are limited to case reports or family studies, their molecular genetic bases are less well defined, and their prevalence rates are unknown but are probably much lower than those of the disorders described earlier. The other primary hypercoagulable states include heparin cofactor II deficiency, dysfunctional thrombomodulin, and many fibrinolytic disorders that lead to impaired fibrin degradation, including hypoplasminogenemia, dysplasminogenemia, plasminogen activator deficiency, and certain dysfibrinogenemias that cause a thrombotic rather than a bleeding diathesis.

CLINICAL MANIFESTATIONS

The primary hypercoagulable states are associated with predominantly venous thromboembolic complications (see Table 174-2 in Chapter 174). Deep vein thrombosis of the lower extremities and pulmonary embolism are the most frequent clinical manifestations. Venous thromboses occurring in more unusual sites include superficial thrombophlebitis and mesenteric and cerebral venous thrombosis (see Table 174-2 in Chapter 174). Arterial thrombosis involving the coronary, cerebrovascular, and peripheral circulations is not linked to any of the primary hypercoagulable states, although some reports have described its occurrence with protein S deficiency and homozygous antithrombin deficiency. Venous thrombosis can also result in arterial occlusion by paradoxical embolism across a patent foramen ovale.

The initial episode of VTE can occur at any age in patients with primary hypercoagulable states, but it typically takes place in early adulthood. Positive family histories of thrombosis can frequently be elicited. The risk for thrombosis varies among the individual primary hypercoagulable states and is highest in patients with deficiencies of antithrombotic factors (Table 179-2); it is markedly increased with the coexistence of multiple prothrombotic mutations. Patients with homozygous deficiency states tend to have more severe thrombotic complications. A peculiar manifestation of homozygous protein C or protein S deficiency is neonatal purpura fulminans. This serious, sometimes fatal syndrome is caused by ischemic necrosis secondary to widespread thrombosis of small cutaneous and subcutaneous vessels. Fatal purpura fulminans associated with a bleeding diathesis has also been described in a patient with an acquired immunoglobulin G (IgG) inhibitor of protein C. Warfarin-induced skin necrosis (Fig. 179-1) very infrequently complicates the initiation of oral anticoagulant therapy in patients with heterozygous protein C or protein S deficiency. Because both these proteins depend on vitamin K for normal function, their plasma levels in patients with inherited deficiency states may drop to nearly zero within a few days of starting therapy with warfarin, a vitamin K antagonist, and lead to a transient prothrombotic imbalance and skin necrosis caused by dermal vascular thrombosis. Nevertheless, oral anticoagulation provides effective long-term antithrombotic prophylaxis in these individuals.

| TABLE 179-2 | INHERITED HYPERCOAGULABLE STATES (THROMBOPHILIAS): EPIDEMIOLOGY AND RISK OF VENOUS THROMBOEMBOLISM (VTE) |

	Prevalence (%)		Relative Risk	
THROMBOPHILIA	**GENERAL POPULATION***	**UNSELECTED VTE**	**FIRST VTE**	**RECURRENT VTE**
Antithrombin deficiency	0.02-0.3	1-2	5-8	2.5
Protein C deficiency	0.2-0.5	2-5	5-8	2.5
Protein S deficiency	<0.5	1-3	1.7-8	2.5
Factor V Leiden	3-7	10-65	5-10†	1.3
Factor II G20210A	1-6	3-8	1.5-3.8	1.4
FV Leiden + FII G20210A	0.01	—	20-60	2.5

*Data refer to white populations. Prevalence of FV Leiden and FII G20210A is <0.1% in African, African American, and Asian populations.
†Relative risk of first VTE with homozygous FV Leiden is up to ten-fold higher (50-100).
Modified from Coppola A, Tufano A, Cerbone AM, et al. Inherited thrombophilia: implications for prevention and treatment of venous thromboembolism. *Semin Thromb Hemostas.* 2009; 35:683-694.

FIGURE 179-1. Acute skin necrosis in a patient with protein C deficiency who was treated with heparin and warfarin for deep vein thrombosis that occurred after elective hip surgery. Warfarin treatment was withdrawn and anticoagulation continued with heparin. Skin grafting of the affected area was required. (From Forbes CD, Jackson WF. *Color Atlas and Text of Clinical Medicine,* 3rd ed. London: Mosby; 2003.)

In most patients with primary hypercoagulable states, discrete clinical thrombotic complications appear to be precipitated by acquired prothrombotic events (e.g., pregnancy, use of oral contraceptives, surgery, trauma, immobilization), many of which are the secondary hypercoagulable states discussed subsequently. In particular, thrombosis complicates pregnancy, especially during the puerperium, in about 30 to 60% of women with antithrombin deficiency, 10 to 20% with protein C or protein S deficiency, and almost 30% with APC resistance (factor V Leiden), unless prophylactic anticoagulation is administered during this period.

DIAGNOSIS

Laboratory diagnosis (Chapter 174) of the primary hypercoagulable states requires testing for each of the disorders individually because no general screening test is available to determine whether a patient may have such a condition. Factor V Leiden can be diagnosed by a DNA-based assay or by a functional test for APC resistance: the former is required to distinguish between heterozygous and homozygous states. DNA-based assay is required to identify the prothrombin G20210A mutation. In contrast, many different mutations have been found in the genes for antithrombin, protein C, and protein S, so DNA-based tests are not practical for the diagnosis of these inherited deficiency states. Therefore, they are detected by functional and immunologic tests. Because type II ("qualitative") deficiencies of antithrombin, protein C, and protein S exhibit normal immunologic levels, functional assays for these proteins are better screening tests.

A reasonable diagnostic approach at this time is to screen at least all "strongly thrombophilic" patients after an initial episode of VTE: individuals with (1) a documented event before 50 years of age, (2) a positive family history, (3) massive or submassive pulmonary embolism, or (4) spontaneous thrombosis at an unusual site (e.g., intra-abdominal or cerebral). Analysis of results from a recent randomized trial showed that recurrent VTE was not increased in the presence of factor V Leiden, prothrombin G20210A mutation, antithrombin deficiency, or elevated levels of factor VIII, XI, or homocysteine.[1] However, there have been no controlled clinical trials to date that have assessed the benefit of testing for thrombophilia on the risk of recurrent VTE.[2] Although indefinite anticoagulation is recommended for patients who have had two or more VTE events, regardless of whether a primary hypercoagulable state is found, testing these individuals for thrombophilia may also be useful to guide family screening strategies. Individuals with arterial thrombosis generally should not be tested for any of these disorders because primary hypercoagulable states (see Table 179-1) are not clearly associated with an increased risk for arterial thrombosis. In contrast, some of the secondary hypercoagulable states, including hyperhomocysteinemia and the antiphospholipid syndrome (see later), are associated with an increased risk for arterial as well as venous thrombosis.

In general, testing for primary hypercoagulable states is not recommended immediately after a major thrombotic event, but rather in clinically stable patients at least 2 weeks after completing oral anticoagulation following a thrombotic episode. Active thrombosis may transiently consume and deplete some of the proteins in plasma and lead to the erroneous diagnosis of inherited antithrombin, protein C, or protein S deficiency. In addition to acute thrombosis, pregnancy, estrogen use, liver disease, and disseminated intravascular coagulation (DIC) may cause acquired deficiencies of antithrombin, protein C, or protein S. Anticoagulation may also interfere with some of the functional tests for primary hypercoagulable states. Heparin treatment can cause a decline in antithrombin levels to the deficiency range even in normal individuals. In contrast, warfarin can elevate antithrombin levels into the normal range in patients who do have an inherited deficiency state. Warfarin therapy also reduces the functional levels and, less prominently, the immunologic levels of protein C and protein S, thereby potentially leading to a misdiagnosis of inherited deficiency. When testing is indicated in patients in whom interruption of prophylactic oral anticoagulation is considered to be too risky, protein C and protein S levels can be determined after warfarin therapy has been discontinued under heparin coverage for at least 2 weeks.

As noted previously, functional assays are the best screening tests for antithrombin, protein C, and protein S deficiencies because they detect both quantitative and qualitative defects; antigenic (immunologic) assays detect only quantitative deficiencies of these proteins. Functional coagulation assays for protein C and protein S may yield spuriously low values, however, if APC resistance is present. APC resistance can be diagnosed by newer high-sensitivity and high-specificity coagulation assays or by DNA analysis of peripheral blood mononuclear cells for the factor V Leiden mutation.

TREATMENT   Rx

The initial treatment of acute venous thrombosis or pulmonary embolism in patients with primary hypercoagulable states is not different from that in patients without genetic defects (Chapters 37 and 81). As in patients without known thrombophilia, thrombolytic therapy should be considered after massive venous thrombosis or pulmonary embolism. Acute management is initiated with at least 5 days of unfractionated or low-molecular-weight heparin. Oral anticoagulation with warfarin can be started on the first day of heparin use and continued for at least 6 months in patients with VTE in the absence of triggering factors (e.g., postoperative state), with regulation of the dose to maintain an international normalized ratio (INR) of the prothrombin time between 2.0 and 3.0.

Continuing oral anticoagulant prophylaxis beyond the initial 6 to 12 months after an acute episode of VTE must be weighed against continued exposure of the individual patient to the significant risk for bleeding complications. Patients with primary hypercoagulable states who have had two or more thrombotic events should receive indefinite or lifelong prophylactic anticoagulation with warfarin (Chapter 37). Indefinite or lifelong anticoagulation is probably indicated for individuals with recurrent thrombosis even in the absence of identifiable primary hypercoagulable states.

The decision to continue prophylactic oral anticoagulation beyond the initial period after the first episode of thrombosis is more difficult (Table 179-3). After a single episode of thrombosis, patients with inherited hypercoagulable states should probably receive indefinite or lifelong anticoagulation if their initial episodes were life-threatening or occurred in unusual sites (e.g., mesenteric, cerebral venous thrombosis) or if they have more than one prothrombotic genetic abnormality. Some authorities also recommend indefinite or lifelong anticoagulation after an initial venous thromboembolic event in patients whose risk of recurrence likewise appears to be increased: those with isolated heterozygous deficiencies of antithrombin, protein C, or protein S and patients with homozygous factor V Leiden. In the absence of these characteristics, particularly if the initial episode was precipitated by a transient acquired prothrombotic situation (e.g., pregnancy, postoperative state, immobilization), it is reasonable at this time to discontinue warfarin therapy after 6 to 12 months and administer subsequent prophylactic anticoagulation only during high-risk periods.

Asymptomatic individuals with known thrombophilia who have not had previous thrombotic complications do not require prophylactic anticoagulation except during periods of high risk for thrombosis. Because about half of the first-degree relatives of a patient with a primary hypercoagulable state should be affected, these individuals should be counseled about the implications of making a diagnosis.

Management of pregnancy in women with primary hypercoagulable states requires special consideration because of the high risk for thrombosis, particularly during the puerperium. Women with thrombophilia who have previously had thrombosis—and probably also asymptomatic women with thrombophilia—should receive prophylactic anticoagulation throughout pregnancy and for 4 to 6 weeks postpartum, a particularly high-risk period. Coumarin derivatives cross the placenta and have the potential to cause both bleeding and teratogenic effects in the fetus; therefore, oral anticoagulants should not be used during pregnancy. Heparin does not cross the placenta and does not cause these fetal complications. Therefore, either unfractionated heparin or fixed-dose, low-molecular-weight heparin is the anticoagulant of choice during pregnancy. Neither warfarin nor heparin induces an anticoagulant effect in a breast-fed infant when the drug is given to a nursing mother, so either can be given safely when indicated in the postpartum period.

Because warfarin-induced skin necrosis (see Fig. 179-1) is a rare problem, screening of all patients for inherited protein C or protein S deficiency, conditions that are known to predispose to this complication, is not indicated before starting warfarin therapy. Most cases can be avoided by not initiating warfarin therapy with high loading doses and by concomitant coverage with heparin. When the complication does occur, as manifested by painful red and subsequently dark, necrotic skin lesions within a few days of starting warfarin, such therapy must be discontinued immediately, vitamin K administered, and heparin started (Chapter 37). The use of fresh-frozen plasma or purified protein C concentrate to normalize protein C levels rapidly can improve results. Despite this rare complication, warfarin is an effective, long-term prophylactic anticoagulant in patients with inherited protein C or protein S deficiency.

Antithrombin III concentrate purified from normal human plasma may be a useful adjunct to anticoagulation in "heparin-resistant" patients, who represent unusual cases of type II antithrombin deficiency, and in antithrombin-deficient patients with recurrent thrombosis despite adequate anticoagulation. Infusion of antithrombin concentrate can also be considered in some perioperative or obstetric settings in which anticoagulation poses an unacceptable bleeding risk.

TABLE 179-3 LONG-TERM MANAGEMENT OF PATIENTS WITH PRIMARY HYPERCOAGULABLE STATES

RISK CLASSIFICATION	MANAGEMENT
High risk ≥2 spontaneous thromboses 1 spontaneous life-threatening thrombosis 1 spontaneous thrombosis at an unusual site (e.g., mesenteric, cerebral venous) 1 spontaneous thrombosis in the presence of antiphospholipid syndrome, antithrombin deficiency, or more than a single hypercoagulable state	Indefinite anticoagulation or lifelong chronic anticoagulation
Moderate risk 1 thrombosis with an acquired prothrombotic stimulus	Vigorous prophylaxis during high-risk situations
Asymptomatic	

Modified from Bauer K. Approach to thrombosis. In: Loscalzo J, Schafer AI, eds. *Thrombosis and Hemorrhage*, 3rd ed. Philadelphia: Lippincott Williams & Wilkins; 2003:330-342.

● SECONDARY HYPERCOAGULABLE STATES

DEFINITION

The secondary hypercoagulable states (Fig. 179-2) are diverse, mostly acquired disorders that predispose patients to thrombosis by complex, multifactorial pathophysiologic mechanisms. Many of these conditions also represent the acquired precipitating stimuli for clinical thrombotic events in individuals with a genetic predisposition (primary hypercoagulable states). Although each disorder causes thrombosis primarily through abnormalities in blood flow (rheology), the composition of blood (coagulation factors and platelet function), or the vessel wall, multiple overlapping mechanisms are operative in many of them.

Hyperhomocysteinemia

Hyperhomocysteinemia is an elevated blood level of homocysteine, a sulfhydryl amino acid derived from methionine by a transmethylation pathway (E-Fig. 179-1). Homocysteine is remethylated to methionine or catabolized to cystathionine. The major remethylation pathway requires folate and cobalamin (vitamin B_{12}) and involves the action of methylenetetrahydrofolate reductase (MTHFR); a minor remethylation pathway is mediated by betaine-homocysteine methyltransferase. Alternatively, homocysteine is converted to cystathionine in a trans-sulfuration pathway catalyzed by cystathionine β-synthase (CBS), with pyridoxine used as a cofactor.

Homozygous CBS deficiency states that lead to severe hyperhomocysteinemia (homocystinuria) (Chapter 216) cause premature arterial atherosclerotic disease and VTE, as well as mental retardation, neurologic defects, lens ectopy, and skeletal abnormalities. By comparison, adults with heterozygous CBS deficiency, with resultant mild to moderate hyperhomocysteinemia, may have only venous or arterial thrombotic manifestations. Hyperhomocysteinemia resulting from inherited remethylation pathway defects usually involves reduced activity of MTHFR. In homozygous individuals with the autosomal recessive C677T mutation of the *MTHFR* gene, which occurs in 15% of certain populations, moderate hyperhomocysteinemia may occur and is correctable with folic acid, but it does not appear to be related to risk of venous thrombosis. Acquired causes of hyperhomocysteinemia in adults most commonly involve nutritional deficiencies of the cofactors required for homocysteine metabolism, including pyridoxine, cobalamin, and folate.

Acquired and inherited hyperhomocysteinemia is a probable risk factor for both arterial and venous thrombosis. The mechanism of homocysteine-induced thrombosis and atherogenesis involves complex, probably multifactorial effects on the vessel wall. Homocysteine can cause vascular endothelial injury, conversion of the endothelial surface of blood vessels from an antithrombotic to a prothrombotic state, and smooth muscle cell proliferation. These toxic effects of homocysteine on the vessel wall may be mediated by oxidant stress.

Vitamin supplementation with folate, pyridoxine, and cobalamin can normalize elevated blood levels of homocysteine. However, several prospective

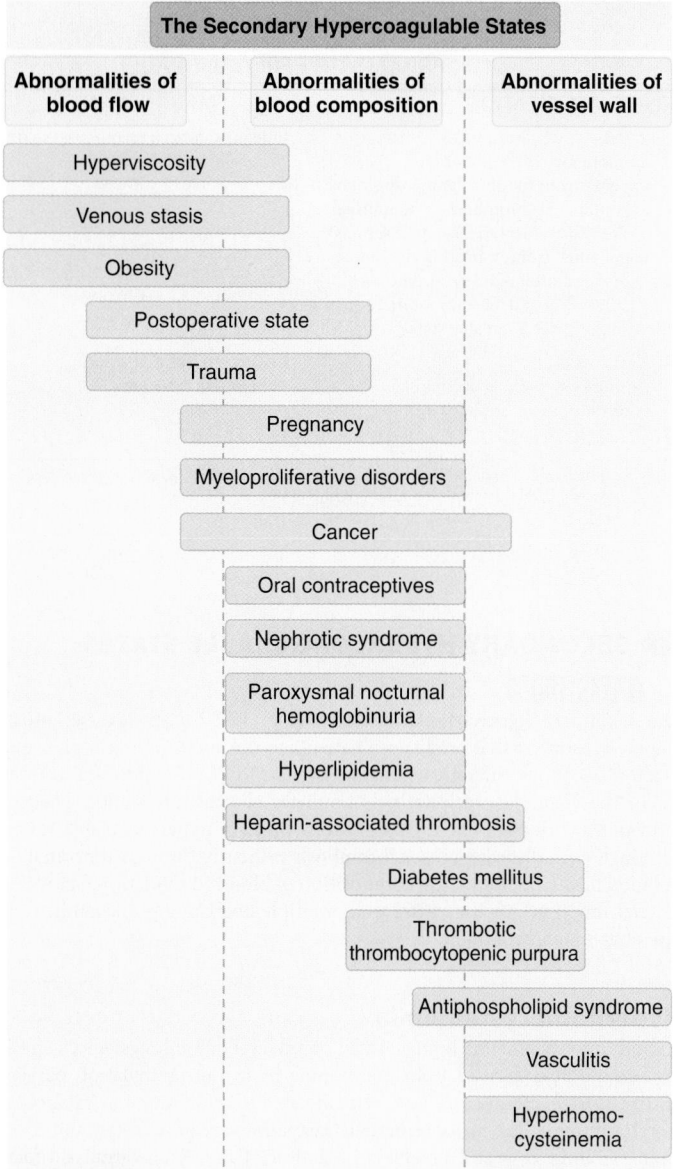

FIGURE 179-2. Secondary hypercoagulable states. The pathophysiologic basis of thrombotic risk in these diverse disorders is complex and multifactorial. Predominant mechanisms of thrombosis for the different secondary hypercoagulable states shown are based on Virchow's triad of thrombogenesis: abnormalities in blood flow, abnormalities in blood composition, and abnormalities of the vessel wall. (Modified from Schafer AI. The primary and secondary hypercoagulable states. In: Schafer AI, ed. *Molecular Mechanisms of Hypercoagulable States.* New York: Chapman & Hall; 1997:16.)

clinical trials of homocysteine-lowering therapy have failed to show reduced rates of vascular events in patients with established vascular disease. It remains to be determined whether this disappointing lack of clinical benefit with homocysteine-lowering vitamin therapy indicates that homocysteine is not a direct atherogenic factor, or that vitamin therapy in this setting might have other, offsetting deleterious effects, or that possibly other mechanisms are operative.

Malignancy

Multiple abnormalities of hemostasis are involved in the hypercoagulable state in cancer patients, many of which initiate a systemic process of chronic DIC (Chapter 178). The thrombotic tendency of patients with cancer may also be related to mechanical factors, such as immobility, indwelling central venous catheters, or a bulky tumor mass compressing vessels, and to comorbid conditions, such as sepsis, surgery, liver dysfunction secondary to metastases, and the prothrombotic effects of certain antineoplastic agents.

The incidence of thrombotic complications in cancer patients depends in part on the type of malignancy. Hypercoagulability is most prominent in patients with pancreatic cancer (Chapter 200), adenocarcinoma of the gastrointestinal tract (Chapters 198 and 199) or lung (Chapter 197), ovarian

cancer (Chapter 205), and hematologic malignancies. The presence of underlying malignancy compounds the independent risk for thrombosis in the postoperative state. Thrombosis most commonly occurs in patients with established or concurrently diagnosed malignancy. In these patients, the risk of venous thrombosis has been found to be highest in the first few months after the diagnosis of malignancy, then decreases progressively over the subsequent 15 years. The same large case-control study showed that the risk of venous thrombosis in cancer patients is approximately 12- to 17-fold increased in those who also have the factor V Leiden or the prothrombin G20210A mutation.

The most frequent thrombotic manifestations in patients with neoplasms are deep vein thrombosis and pulmonary embolism, but more unusual and distinctive thrombotic complications are also found. Trousseau's syndrome, characterized by migratory superficial thrombophlebitis of the upper or lower extremities, is strongly linked to cancer. Nonbacterial thrombotic endocarditis involves fibrin-platelet vegetations on heart valves, which produce clinical manifestations by systemic embolization (Chapter 60). Of patients with nonbacterial thrombotic endocarditis, 75% have underlying malignancies at autopsy. Trousseau's syndrome and nonbacterial thrombotic endocarditis are highly associated with adenocarcinomas. The occurrence of either syndrome in patients without known cancer demands a more vigorous search for occult malignancy than in patients with deep vein thrombosis or pulmonary embolism. Thrombotic microangiopathy (Chapter 175), characterized by hemolysis with red blood cell fragmentation, thrombocytopenia, and microvascular thrombosis with involvement of target organs, occurs in about 5% of patients with metastatic carcinomas, most commonly those with gastric (Chapter 198), lung (Chapter 197), and breast (Chapter 204) primary sites.

TREATMENT   **Rx**

Treatment of acute VTE in cancer patients should be initiated as in other patients, but subsequent prophylactic anticoagulation should be continued while active malignancy is present. Anticoagulation can be difficult in many cancer patients; these patients may be resistant to warfarin prophylaxis. Anticoagulation can also be complicated by bleeding into tumors. Long-term treatment of cancer patients with low-molecular-weight heparin after VTE (Chapter 37) reduces recurrences and possibly decreases bleeding complications when compared with treatment with warfarin.

Myeloproliferative Disorders and Paroxysmal Nocturnal Hemoglobinuria

Thrombosis and, apparently paradoxically, bleeding are major causes of morbidity and mortality in patients with myeloproliferative disorders (Chapter 169) and the related stem cell disorder paroxysmal nocturnal hemoglobinuria (Chapter 163). In uncontrolled polycythemia vera (Chapter 169), increased whole blood viscosity contributes to the thrombotic tendency. Thrombocytosis, abnormal platelet function, and other less well understood factors are also probably involved in the hemostatic defect of the myeloproliferative disorders and paroxysmal nocturnal hemoglobinuria.

In addition to deep vein thrombosis and pulmonary embolism, some distinctive thrombotic manifestations are seen. Hepatic vein thrombosis (Budd-Chiari syndrome) and portal and other intra-abdominal venous thromboses (Chapter 145) are associated with myeloproliferative disorders and paroxysmal nocturnal hemoglobinuria (Chapter 163) and may be the initial manifestations of the disease. Myeloproliferative disorders, particularly polycythemia vera (Chapter 169) and essential thrombocythemia (Chapter 169), may cause erythromelalgia, a syndrome of microvascular thrombosis manifested by intense pain accompanied by warmth, duskiness, and mottled erythema, sometimes resembling livedo reticularis, in a patchy distribution in the extremities, most prominently in the feet; digital microvascular ischemia progressing to vascular insufficiency and gangrene may ensue (Chapter 80). A wide spectrum of neurologic manifestations may be caused by cerebrovascular ischemia, especially in patients with essential thrombocythemia.

TREATMENT   **Rx**

Treatment of VTE in patients with the myeloproliferative disorders and paroxysmal nocturnal hemoglobinuria should be initiated as in patients without these hematologic disorders. In patients with thrombosis associated with polycythemia vera, the hematocrit should be maintained in the normal range with phlebotomies or chemotherapy, or with both (Chapter 169). Low-dose aspirin (100 mg daily) can prevent thrombotic complications without increasing the incidence of major bleeding in patients with polycythemia vera who have no contraindications to such treatment.[5] In patients with essential thrombocythemia, cytoreduction of the elevated platelet count should be achieved with chemotherapy (Chapter 169).

Antiphospholipid Syndrome

Antiphospholipid syndrome (Chapter 177) is characterized by venous and arterial thrombosis, recurrent spontaneous abortions (which may also be due to thrombosis), thrombocytopenia, and a variety of neuropsychiatric manifestations. The syndrome is associated with a heterogeneous group of autoantibodies that bind to anionic phospholipid-protein complexes, a protein cofactor of which is β_2-glycoprotein I. Patients with this syndrome have any combination of positive tests to detect different plasma antiphospholipid-protein antibodies (e.g., anticardiolipin antibodies) and phospholipid-based clotting tests (lupus anticoagulants) (Chapter 265). The predominant prothrombotic effects of these antibodies are probably directed to the vessel wall.

Deep vein thrombosis and pulmonary embolism are the most frequent venous thrombotic events in these patients. Cerebrovascular events are the most common arterial thrombotic complications and are manifested as stroke, transient ischemic attacks (Chapter 414), multi-infarct dementia (Chapter 409), or retinal artery occlusion. Peripheral and intra-abdominal vascular occlusion is encountered more rarely. About one third of these patients have nonbacterial heart valve vegetations (Libman-Sacks endocarditis). The most prominent obstetric complications are recurrent spontaneous abortions and fetal growth retardation, which are probably due to thrombosis of placental vessels. Patients are occasionally seen with "catastrophic" antiphospholipid syndrome involving a series of acute and sometimes fatal vascular occlusive events, or "thrombotic storm." Thrombotic complications are limited largely to patients with primary antiphospholipid syndrome and patients in whom the antibodies are associated with collagen vascular disease, not with drugs or infections.

TREATMENT   **Rx**

Acute management of thrombosis in these patients is essentially the same as in other individuals. Monitoring of heparin anticoagulation is difficult in patients with a lupus anticoagulant because they already have a prolonged activated partial thromboplastin time at baseline; the use of low-molecular-weight heparin, which does not require monitoring, can circumvent this problem. Warfarin is effective in preventing recurrent thrombosis but usually requires prolonged or indefinite therapy with doses to achieve an INR of 2.0 to 3.0.[6] No established treatment of women with antiphospholipid syndrome has been shown to prevent recurrent fetal loss. Treatment with prednisone and aspirin during pregnancy is not effective in promoting live birth and may increase the risk for prematurity.

Pregnancy, Oral Contraceptives, and Hormone Replacement Therapy

The pathophysiology of hypercoagulability associated with pregnancy (Chapter 247) involves a progressive state of DIC throughout the course of pregnancy. Activation of the coagulation system is initiated locally in the uteroplacental circulation, where the placenta is the source of increased thrombin generation. Platelet activation and increased platelet turnover also occur during normal pregnancy, and about 8% of healthy women have mild thrombocytopenia at term. Simultaneously, the fibrinolytic system is progressively blunted throughout pregnancy because of the action of placental plasminogen activator inhibitor type 2. The net effect of these coagulation changes is creation of a state of hypercoagulability that makes pregnant women vulnerable to thrombosis, particularly in the puerperium. These systemic alterations are compounded by prothrombotic mechanical and rheologic factors in pregnancy, including venous stasis in the legs caused by the gravid uterus, pelvic vein injury during labor, and the trauma of cesarean section. Oral contraceptives induce a prothrombotic state by increasing procoagulant effects and decreasing physiologic anticoagulant effects. The use of oral contraceptives is associated with an increased risk for venous thrombosis, myocardial infarction, stroke, and peripheral arterial disease, particularly during the first year of use (Chapter 246). Unexpectedly, third-generation oral contraceptives, which contain less estrogen and a different

progestin, double the risk for venous thromboembolism in comparison to second-generation preparations. Postmenopausal hormone replacement increases the risk for deep venous thromboembolism by a factor of 2 to 3.5, at least during the first year. Hormone replacement therapy has no beneficial and possibly even a detrimental effect on the risk for arterial disease (Chapter 248).

Deep vein thrombosis and pulmonary embolism are the most common thrombotic complications of pregnancy and the use of oral contraceptives or hormone replacement therapy. Coexisting primary hypercoagulable states are an additive risk factor in all these settings. In the absence of a clear family history of venous thromboembolism, there is little justification, however, to screen for prothrombotic mutations with pregnancy or before starting hormone replacement therapy or oral contraceptives. Increasing age, increasing parity, cesarean delivery, prolonged bedrest or immobilization, obesity, and previous thromboembolism are additional prothrombotic risk factors in pregnant women. Most thrombotic events associated with pregnancy occur in the peripartum period, especially after delivery. Special considerations for anticoagulation in the setting of pregnancy are noted in the section on treatment of primary hypercoagulable states.

Postoperative State, Immobilization, and Trauma

Postoperative thrombosis (Chapter 441) is caused by a combination of local mechanical factors, including decreased venous blood flow in the lower extremities, and systemic changes in coagulation (Chapter 81). The level of risk for postoperative thrombosis depends largely on the type of surgery performed. It is probably compounded by coexisting risk factors, such as an underlying inherited primary hypercoagulable state or malignancy, advanced age, and prolonged procedures. Postoperative deep vein thrombosis and pulmonary embolism, the most common thrombotic complications, are often asymptomatic but detectable by noninvasive studies. The incidence of deep vein thrombosis after general surgical procedures is about 20 to 25%, with almost 2% of these patients having clinically significant pulmonary embolism. The risk for deep vein thrombosis after hip surgery and knee reconstruction ranges from 45 to 70% without prophylaxis, and clinically significant pulmonary embolism occurs in 20% of patients undergoing hip surgery. Postoperative thrombosis risk after urologic and gynecologic surgery more closely approximates that found after general surgery. Although the process of thrombosis generally begins intraoperatively or within a few days of surgery, the risk for this complication can be protracted beyond the time of discharge from the hospital, particularly in hip replacement patients.

Patients who are bedridden or experiencing prolonged air travel are at increased risk for VTE. VTE is also one of the most common causes of morbidity and mortality in survivors of major trauma, and asymptomatic deep vein thrombosis of the lower extremities has been detected by venography in more than 50% of hospitalized trauma patients (Chapter 112). The risk for venous thrombosis after trauma is increased by advanced age, need for surgery or transfusions, and the presence of lower extremity fractures or spinal cord injury.

Mechanical methods of prophylaxis against VTE should be considered in high-risk postoperative patients and bedridden patients with medical conditions, either in combination with anticoagulant prophylaxis or instead of it in patients who have an unusually high risk for bleeding with anticoagulation. Such methods include graduated compression stockings, intermittent pneumatic compression devices, and venous foot pumps. For long-distance travelers with thrombophilia, either properly fitted below-knee graduated compression stockings or a single prophylactic dose of low-molecular-weight heparin injected before departure is recommended in addition to general measures such as avoidance of dehydration and frequent stretching of calf muscles.

1. Kearon C, Julian JA, Kovacs MJ, et al. Influence of thrombophilia on risk of recurrent venous thromboembolism while on warfarin: results from a randomized trial. *Blood.* 2008;112:4432-4436.
2. Cohn D, Vansenne F, de Borgie C, et al. Thrombophilia testing for prevention of recurrent venous thromboembolism. *Cochrane Database Syst Rev.* 2009;1:CD007069.
3. Blom JW, Doggen CJ, Osanto S, et al. Malignancies, prothrombotic mutations, and the risk of venous thrombosis. *JAMA.* 2005;293:715-722.
4. Lee AY, Levine MN, Baker RI, et al. Low-molecular-weight heparin versus a coumarin for the prevention of recurrent venous thromboembolism in patients with cancer. *N Engl J Med.* 2003; 349:146-153.
5. Landolfi R, Marchioli R, Kutti J, et al. Efficacy and safety of low-dose aspirin in polycythemia vera. *N Engl J Med.* 2004;350:114-124.

6. Crowther MA, Ginsberg JS, Julian J, et al. A comparison of two intensities of warfarin for the prevention of recurrent thrombosis in patients with the antiphospholipid antibody syndrome. *N Engl J Med.* 2003;349:1133-1138.

SUGGESTED READINGS

Coppola A, Tufano A, Cerbone AM, et al. Inherited thrombophilia: implications for prevention and treatment of venous thromboembolism. *Semin Thromb Hemostas.* 2009;35:683-694. *Review of approaches to prophylaxis and treatment of venous thromboembolism in patients with thrombophilia, based on epidemiology and risk assessment.*

Houbballah R, LaMuraglia GM. Clotting problems: diagnosis and management of underlying coagulopathies. *Semin Vasc Surg.* 2010;23:221-227. *A practical overview of diagnosis and treatment of hypercoagulable states, with a particular focus on patients with arterial thromboembolism seen by the vascular specialist.*

Lim W. Antiphospholipid antibody syndrome. *Hematol Am Soc Hematol Educ Progr.* 2009;233-239. *Concise review of the clinical approach to patients with antiphospholipid syndrome, with an emphasis on management.*

Luxembourg B, Delev D, Geisen C, et al. Molecular basis of antithrombin deficiency. *Thromb Haemost.* 2011;105:635-646. *Review citing nearly 90 different mutations.*

180

TRANSFUSION MEDICINE

LAWRENCE T. GOODNOUGH

DEVELOPMENT OF TRANSFUSION MEDICINE

Issues in blood transfusion and blood conservation include the safety of blood, the formation of guidelines and consensus statements on the use of blood components and products, new strategies in blood conservation, emerging alternatives to blood transfusion, and informed consent for transfusion. The broad-based constituency of transfusion medicine includes blood collection facilities, hospital-based transfusion services, research laboratories, and the commercial sector.

THE TRANSFUSION MEDICINE SPECIALIST

Medical management of the blood bank involves issues related to blood inventory and safety, as well as the oversight of laboratory policies and procedures (Fig. 180-1). Management of the transfusion service includes coordinating blood transfusion and blood conservation activities and serving as a consultant to clinicians whose patients are undergoing massive transfusions, apheresis, or transplantation or who are having difficulty finding compatible blood products. Finally, the transfusion medicine specialist supervises quality assurance to satisfy regulatory and accreditation requirements.

TRANSFUSION

Worldwide, more than 75 million units of whole blood are estimated to be donated every year. In the United States, the yearly transfusion of more than 13 million units corresponds to the transfusion of 1 unit of blood every 0.39 second.

Blood Availability

Blood centers must be able to supply blood in response to acute crises. Sporadic shortages of blood and blood products (e.g., packed red cells, platelet products, albumin, intravenous immunoglobulin, and clotting factor concentrates) are potentially life threatening. Such shortages have been attributed to disruptions in production, increasingly strict criteria for accepting donors, product recalls, increased use (including off-label use), and stockpiling or other market issues.

In the United States, the Department of Health and Human Services monitors sentinel community blood services and hospital transfusion services to track blood collection and transfusion activity. Blood transfusion and collection activities peaked in 1986 and then declined until 1994. However, blood transfusion and collection subsequently increased 8.0% in 1997, 10.2% in 1999, and an estimated 4% to 5% annually thereafter.

Within the American Red Cross, which supplies about half of all blood products in the United States, a 3- to 4-day supply of red blood cell products is typical, but some independent centers have higher reserves. Use of frozen red cells as a hedge against inventory shortages has generally not been practical because the shelf life of thawed units is only 24 hours; however, an automated, functionally closed system for the glycerolization and deglycerolization processes allows a 2-week post-thaw shelf life. With such a system, many blood centers and transfusion services can expand their available red cell

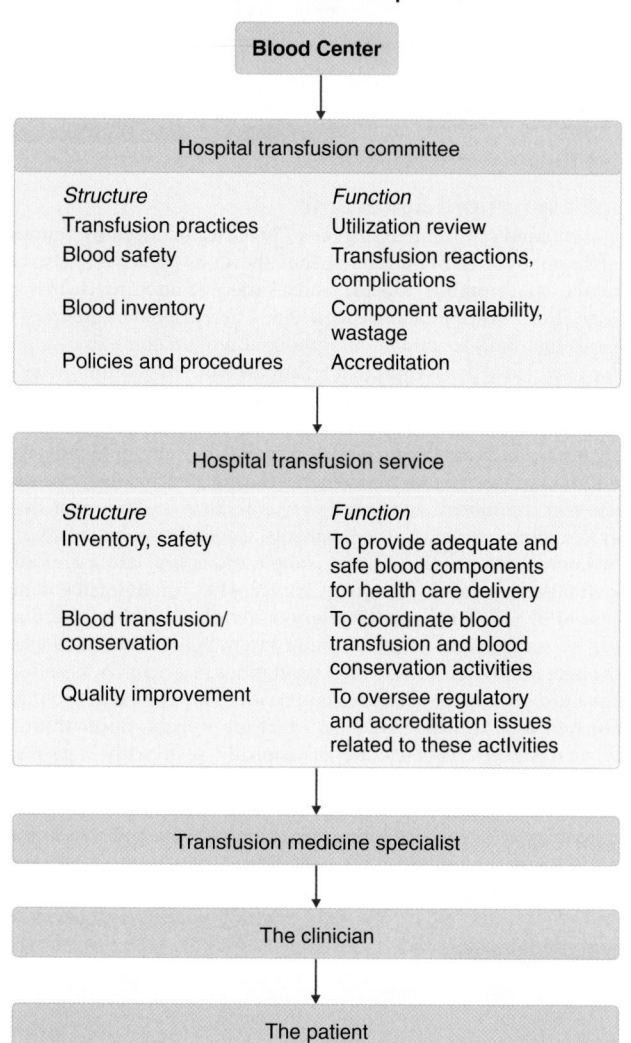

The Flow of Blood Components

FIGURE 180-1. A hospital's transfusion committee and transfusion service can help clinicians manage the availability, safety, and use of blood products. (From Goodnough LT. What is a transfusion medicine specialist? *Transfusion.* 1999;39:1031-1033.)

inventories as reserves. After disasters—human or natural—on-hand blood supplies are adequate in the short term and can be rapidly mobilized over great distances. Because of the need to maintain reserves, blood collection must routinely surpass the anticipated need for blood transfusion.

Red Blood Cell Transfusion
Whole Blood

A unit of blood is collected as a donation of 450 mL ± 10% into a citrate anticoagulant that also contains phosphate and dextrose. The red cell and hemoglobin content is variable and dependent on the donor's hematocrit and the precise volume bled.

Whole blood is stored at 4 ± 2° C to diminish red cells' utilization of adenosine triphosphate and to preserve their viability, which should be at least 70% at the end of a shelf life of 35 days. After 10 days of storage, all predonation 2,3-diphosphoglycerate content in red cells is lost, but up to 50% is regenerated within 8 hours after transfusion.

In Western countries, whole blood is rarely used because within a few hours or days, some coagulation factors (especially factors V and VIII) and platelets decrease in quantity or lose viability. After a 7-day hold at 4° C, factor VIII levels fall to 0.32 ± 0.09 IU/mL, and factor V levels fall to 0.78 ± 0.15 IU/mL. At 4° C, platelets undergo a shape change from discoid to spherical that is irreversible after 8 hours, and their in vivo survival is reduced to 2 days.

Red Cell Components

Red cells are provided in various formats that differ with respect to the presence of additive solutions and the extent to which white cells are removed. Solutions that contain combinations of saline, adenine, phosphate, bicarbonate, glucose, and mannitol provide better red cell viability during storage and allow up to a 42-day shelf life. Red cells and red cells in additive solution can be used interchangeably, with the exception that red cells in additive solution are not recommended for exchange or massive transfusions in neonates.

Red cells should be refrigerated until the time of the transfusion because of the risk for bacterial proliferation within the pack at room temperature. Red cells that have been out of refrigeration for 30 minutes or longer cannot be returned to stock. A unit of red cells should be infused over a maximum period of 4 hours.

Irradiated Cellular Blood Components

Gamma-irradiated cellular blood components are used to prevent the occurrence of transfusion-associated graft-versus-host disease (see later).

Leukocyte-Reduced Blood Components

Blood components are depleted of leukocytes by means of filtration. A leukocyte-reduced component is defined as one with less than 5×10^6 residual white cells per liter, and 100% of tested units should meet this standard. Leukocyte removal should be performed while the cells are still intact by filtering the blood as soon as possible after collection.

Leukocyte reduction reduces the incidence of human leukocyte antigen (HLA) alloimmunization in multitransfused recipients, but immunization rates of 10 to 25% are still seen in women who have already been exposed to HLA alloantigens through previous pregnancy. Leukocyte reduction has less impact on refractoriness to random platelet donations because of the importance of nonimmune factors in the poor response to transfused platelets.

Leukocyte reduction also lowers the risk for nonhemolytic febrile reactions after the transfusion of red cells or platelets. Several, but not all, studies suggest that leukocyte reduction has a beneficial impact on the rate of postoperative infection. The impact of leukocyte reduction on the incidence of transfusion-associated graft-versus-host disease is unknown.

Preventing Transmission of Cytomegalovirus

A small number of studies of prestorage leukocyte reduction have suggested its efficacy in preventing transfusion-transmitted cytomegalovirus (CMV) infection (Chapter 384), which occurs in 4% of cases, even with seronegative components. Prestorage leukocyte depletion reduces the infection rate to less than 1%, suggesting that this technology may be at least equivalent to serologic testing for CMV antibodies for the prevention of CMV transmission; however, CMV testing of leukocyte-reduced components continues to be performed by most transfusion services. Indications for CMV-seronegative components include transfusion in pregnancy, intrauterine transfusion, transfusions to neonates less than 37 weeks' gestation, transfusions to CMV-seronegative patients who are potential or actual recipients of allogeneic bone marrow or peripheral blood progenitor transplants when the donor is also CMV seronegative, and patients infected with human immunodeficiency virus (HIV).

Immunomodulatory Effects

Previous transfusion has an immunomodulatory benefit for the survival of renal allografts, even with the use of potent immunosuppressive drugs, although the exact mechanism of this benefit remains unknown. Retrospective studies suggest an adverse effect of transfusion on the rate of perioperative infections or recurrent cancers.

Typing and Crossmatching

Blood and blood components for transfusion must be compatible with the same blood type as the patient. Obtaining an accurate ABO/Rh grouping for a patient is the most significant serologic test performed before transfusion. When type-specific blood and components are unavailable or emergency circumstances do not allow their identification or use, type O-negative red cells should be used. Group O is the only choice for group O recipients and is the alternative choice for groups A, B, and AB.

Red cell antigens other than ABO and D are not routinely considered when selecting *donor* blood products for transfusion; the exception is when unexpected, clinically significant red cell antibodies are present in the patient, as determined by an antibody screen or previous identification. Red cell alloantibodies are produced by exposure to foreign red cell antigens via previous transfusion, pregnancy, or both. For an antibody to be considered clinically significant, it must be associated with a hemolytic transfusion reaction or decreased survival of transfused incompatible red cells. Most of the clinically significant antibodies are optimally reactive at 37° C or are detected by the antiglobulin test. If an antibody screen is negative in the *recipient*, the probability is greater than 99% that an ABO and Rh crossmatch will also be

compatible. If no unexpected, clinically significant antibodies are detected and there is no record of their previous detection, only serologic testing for ABO incompatibility is required (i.e., antiglobulin testing is not required when the crossmatch is performed).

Red Blood Cell Transfusion

If a transfusion is appropriate, a benefit should occur. In a large study of Jehovah's Witnesses (whose religious beliefs preclude the use of blood transfusion), the risk of death was higher in surgical patients with cardiovascular disease than in those without. A follow-up analysis of a subset of these patients reported that the odds of death in patients with a postoperative hemoglobin level less than 7 g/dL increased 2.5 times for each gram decrease in the hemoglobin level; although no deaths occurred in 98 patients with postoperative levels of 7.1 to 8.0 g/dL, 34.4% of 32 patients with postoperative levels of 4.1 to 5.0 g/dL died. These data suggest that in surgery-induced anemia, survival is improved if blood transfusion is administered to maintain the hemoglobin concentration at greater than 7 g/dL. In a large, retrospective study of elderly patients who underwent surgical repair of hip fractures, the use of perioperative transfusion in those with hemoglobin levels as low as 8 g/dL did not appear to influence 30- or 90-day mortality.

In a multi-institutional study, 418 critical care patients received red cell transfusions when their hemoglobin levels dropped below 7 g/dL and had their levels maintained between 7 and 9 g/dL, whereas another 420 patients received transfusions when their hemoglobin levels dropped below 10 g/dL and had their levels maintained between 10 and 12 g/dL. Thirty-day mortality rates were not significantly different in the two groups, suggesting that a transfusion threshold as low as 7 g/dL may be as safe as a higher threshold of 10 g/dL in critically ill patients.[1] A follow-up analysis found that the more restrictive strategy of red blood cell transfusion also appeared to be safe in most patients with cardiovascular disease.

A retrospective study analyzed the relationships among anemia, blood transfusion, and mortality in nearly 80,000 patients older than 65 years hospitalized for acute myocardial infarction. Anemia, defined as a hematocrit below 39%, was present on hospital admission in 44% of patients and was 33% or less in 10% of patients; blood transfusion in patients with hematocrit levels lower than 33% at admission was associated with a significantly lower 30-day mortality. On the basis of this study, transfusion to maintain hematocrit levels above 33% has been recommended in patients with acute myocardial infarction. In patients with heart failure, transfusion to maintain a hemoglobin level above 10 g/dL appears to improve outcomes. Among patients undergoing cardiac surgery, a restrictive perioperative transfusion strategy is as good as a more liberal strategy.[2]

Guidelines

Guidelines from several professional groups recommend that blood not be transfused prophylactically in patients without risk factors until the hemoglobin level is 6 to 8 g/dL; a threshold of 8 g/dL seems appropriate in surgical patients with no risk factors for ischemia, whereas a threshold of 10 to 11 g/dL can be justified for patients considered to be at risk: those with myocardial ischemia or infarction, heart failure, chronic lung disease, or chronic kidney disease. With substantial improvements in blood safety, now the concern is that some patients may be at risk for undertransfusion.

Platelet Transfusion

The use of intensive chemotherapy regimens and bone marrow or stem cell transplantation has increased the demand for platelet products, particularly in patients with severe thrombocytopenia or bleeding complications. The use of apheresis platelet transfusions (i.e., a platelet unit collected from a dedicated donor via an apheresis procedure) has increased substantially, driven by the need for platelet inventories to support cardiac surgery, oncology, and stem cell transplantation programs. Emerging issues in platelet transfusion therapy include re-evaluation of the platelet threshold for prophylactic transfusion and modification of the dose of platelet transfusions.

Threshold for Platelet Transfusion

The appropriate threshold for platelet transfusion depends on the clinical situation (Fig. 180-2). Prospective, randomized studies indicate that a platelet transfusion threshold of 10,000 cells/μL is as safe and effective as higher thresholds in patients undergoing chemotherapy or stem cell transplantation.[3]

For consumptive thrombocytopenias such as disseminated intravascular coagulation (Chapter 178), platelet therapy is supportive but not effective

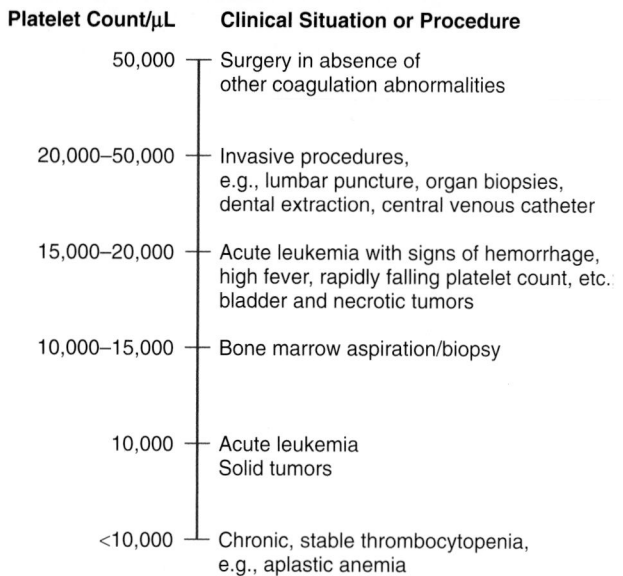

Platelet Count/µL	Clinical Situation or Procedure
50,000	Surgery in absence of other coagulation abnormalities
20,000–50,000	Invasive procedures, e.g., lumbar puncture, organ biopsies, dental extraction, central venous catheter
15,000–20,000	Acute leukemia with signs of hemorrhage, high fever, rapidly falling platelet count, etc. bladder and necrotic tumors
10,000–15,000	Bone marrow aspiration/biopsy
10,000	Acute leukemia Solid tumors
<10,000	Chronic, stable thrombocytopenia, e.g., aplastic anemia

FIGURE 180-2. Threshold for providing platelet transfusions in thrombocytopenic patients.

until the underlying cause is treated. Platelet transfusions are generally not indicated in patients with idiopathic thrombocytopenic purpura or the thrombotic microangiopathies such as thrombotic thrombocytopenic purpura and hemolytic-uremic syndrome (Chapter 175).

Platelet Dose

American Association of Blood Bank (AABB) standards require that 75% of apheresis platelet products contain more than 3×10^{11} platelets; however, no consensus exists for a standardized platelet dose, and clinical trials have used a broad range of doses. In general, higher platelet doses result in greater incremental increases in the platelet count and prolonged time to the next transfusion; however, the estimated platelet half-life is similar, and there are no other differences in outcomes.

Low-dose platelet therapy (i.e., <1 platelet unit) may be more beneficial in thrombocytopenic patients who are receiving prophylactic platelet transfusions. The fixed platelet requirement for hemostasis is estimated to be $7100/\mu L^3/day$, and platelet needs above this threshold are mainly a result of platelet consumption. For patients who become thrombocytopenic as a result of myeloablative therapy, platelet survival decreases with increasing severity of thrombocytopenia. A trial of prophylactic platelet transfusions in patients with hypoproliferative thrombocytopenia found that low doses (1.1×10^{11} per square meter) of platelets led to a decreased number of transfusions but an increased number of platelets transfused (and donor exposures). At doses between 1.1×10^{11} and 4.4×10^4 platelets per square meter, no effect on the incidence of bleeding was demonstrated.

Plasma Transfusion

Plasma therapy provides a source of clotting factors for patients with inherited or acquired coagulation disorders. Patients with inherited disorders such as hemophilia (Chapter 177) or von Willebrand disease (Chapter 176) are now treated primarily with clotting factor concentrates, which are blood derivatives from processed and treated commercial lots from pooled donors. For patients with acquired coagulopathies, there is little systematically derived, evidence-based guidance to inform plasma transfusion decisions. For patients with mild prolongation of coagulation assays such as prothrombin time and partial thromboplastin time (Chapter 174), plasma therapy has little or no value in prophylaxis for invasive procedures. Plasma therapy is indicated in patients undergoing massive hemorrhage (trauma, postpartum hemorrhage, or gastrointestinal bleeding) or for emergent reversal of warfarin-associated coagulopathy (Chapter 37), such as in patients with intracranial hemorrhage. Recommended dosage in these settings is 15 to 30 mL/kg.

● BLOOD SAFETY

Adverse reactions associated with transfusion are listed in Table 180-1.

Errors in Transfusion Medicine

The mistransfusion rate (blood transfused to other than the intended recipient) is about 1 in 14,000 to 28,000 units. About two thirds of the errors occur in the clinical arena (patient misidentification and/or specimen mislabeling

TABLE 180-1	TRANSFUSION-ASSOCIATED ADVERSE REACTIONS	
ADVERSE REACTION	**RISK PER UNIT INFUSED**
ABO-incompatible blood transfusions	1 in 30,000–60,000
Symptoms	40%
Fatalities	1 in 600,000
Delayed serologic reactions	1 in 1600
Delayed hemolytic reactions	1 in 6700
Transfusion-related acute lung injury	1 in 8000
Graft-versus-host disease	Rare
Fluid overload	Underestimated
Febrile, nonhemolytic transfusion reactions	
Red blood cells (non–leukocyte reduced/ leukocyte reduced)	1 in 200/1 in 300
Platelets (non–leukocyte reduced/leukocyte reduced)	1 in 5–20/1 in 25–50
Allergic reactions	1 in 30–100
Anaphylactic reactions	1 in 150,000
Iron overload	After 80–100 U
Post-transfusion purpura	Rare
Immunosuppressive effects	Unknown

Modified from Goodnough LT. Current issues in transfusion medicine. *Clin Adv Hematol Oncol.* 2005;3:614-616.

at time of drawing blood for type and screen/crossmatch, incorrect identification of the recipient of the blood unit, and failure to recognize a transfusion reaction). About half of mistransfusions are ABO incompatible, and about 10% of these are fatal. The frequency of death as a result of ABO error can therefore be estimated at approximately 1 per 600,000 blood units, a risk that is higher than the risk of transmitting HIV or hepatitis C virus.

Transfusion Reactions

Acute Hemolytic Transfusion Reaction

An acute hemolytic transfusion reaction is most commonly defined as hemolysis of donor red cells within 25 hours of transfusion by preformed alloantibodies in the recipient's circulation. Life-threatening acute hemolytic transfusion reactions are most commonly due to ABO-incompatible blood being transfused to a recipient with naturally occurring ABO alloantibodies (anti-A, anti-B, anti-A, B). Clerical errors (mislabeling blood or misidentifying patients) account for 80% of such reactions.

Signs and symptoms of an acute intravascular hemolytic transfusion reaction may develop when as little as 10 to 15 mL of ABO-incompatible blood has been infused. Fever, which is the most common initial manifestation, is frequently accompanied by chills. The patient may complain of a general sense of anxiety or uneasiness or pain at the infusion site or in the back or chest (or both). The most serious sequela is acute renal failure. In an unconscious or anesthetized patient, diffuse bleeding at the surgical site may be the first indication of intravascular hemolysis and may be accompanied by hemoglobinuria and hypotension.

Treatment begins with immediate cessation of the transfusion. The risk for renal failure may be reduced by the administration of crystalloid fluids, including sodium bicarbonate (250 to 500 mg intravenously over a 1- to 4-hour period), to maintain urine pH at 7.0 and by diuresis with 20% mannitol (100 mL/m^2 in 30 to 60 minutes, followed by 30 mL/m^2/hour for 12 hours) or furosemide (40 to 120 mg intravenously).

Febrile Nonhemolytic Transfusion Reactions

Febrile nonhemolytic transfusion reactions are common and are estimated to occur in 0.5% of all red cell transfusions and up to 30% of platelet transfusions. A febrile transfusion reaction is defined as a rise in temperature greater than 1° C, which may be accompanied by chills, rigor, or both.

These reactions are thought to be due to a reaction of HLA or leukocyte-specific antigens (or both) on transfused lymphocytes, granulocytes, or platelets in the donor unit with antibodies in previously alloimmunized recipients. Multiply transfused individuals and multiparous women are most likely to experience this type of transfusion reaction. Febrile nonhemolytic transfusion reactions, especially those associated with platelet transfusions, may be caused by the infusion of biologic response modifiers, such as cytokines, that have accumulated in the platelet concentrate during storage.

Symptoms may occur during the transfusion or may not manifest until 1 to 2 hours after its completion. The diagnosis of a febrile nonhemolytic transfusion reaction is generally made by excluding other causes of fever (e.g., bacterial contamination of blood, acute hemolytic transfusion reaction).

Febrile nonhemolytic transfusion reactions in susceptible populations can often be prevented by administering antipyretics before the transfusion of blood components. Prestorage leukocyte reduction is recommended to prevent reactions resulting from the accumulation of cytokines during storage.

Allergic Reactions

Allergic reactions can be mild, moderate, or life threatening and are associated with the amount of plasma transfused. From 1 to 5% of all blood transfusion recipients experience mild allergic reactions.

Anaphylactic transfusion reactions are sometimes associated with antibodies to immunoglobulin (Ig) A, which are common and have an incidence of approximately 1 in 700 individuals. However, the incidence of anaphylactic transfusion reactions is much lower—1 in 20,000 to 50,000.

Urticarial reactions are not well understood but are believed to be an interaction between antibodies in the recipient's plasma and plasma proteins in the donor blood. There is usually no specific identifiable antigen to which the patient is reacting. Symptoms are generally mild and include localized urticaria, erythema, and itching.

Anaphylactic or anaphylactoid reactions, which can occur after the transfusion of only a few milliliters of blood or plasma, include skin flushing, nausea, abdominal cramps, vomiting, diarrhea, laryngeal edema, hypotension, shock, cardiac arrhythmia, cardiac arrest, and loss of consciousness. Fever is notably absent. In some cases, there may be symptoms indicative of airway involvement, such as hoarseness, wheezing, dyspnea, and substernal pain. Management begins with discontinuation of the transfusion. Treatment is diphenhydramine (25 to 50 mg intravenously), but more severe episodes may require aggressive therapy (Chapters 260 and 261).

Patients who experience recurrent allergic or urticarial reactions can be treated with antihistamines before transfusion. Washed red blood cells may be indicated for patients who experience repeated severe urticarial reactions.

Bacterial Contamination

Bacterial contamination may be introduced into a unit of blood through skin contaminants during venipuncture or from donors with asymptomatic bacteremia. Multiplication of bacteria can occur in blood and blood components stored at refrigerated temperatures but is more likely to occur in platelets stored at room temperature.

Bacterial contamination of red cells is most often due to *Yersinia enterocolitica*, followed by *Serratia liquefaciens*, whereas platelets are most often contaminated with *Staphylococcus* and Enterobacteriaceae. The incidence of bacterial contamination of red cells has been estimated to be 1 in 60,000, with an overall fatality rate of 1 in 1 million. The incidence of bacterial contamination of platelets was estimated to be 1 in 5000 before the initiation of bacterial detection systems in 2004, but it is now estimated to be 50% lower (1 in 10,000).

Recipients of units with low bacterial counts may have relatively mild symptoms such as fever and chills, but those receiving units with high bacterial counts may have severe or fatal reactions. Clinically, the patient may experience high fever, shock, hemoglobinuria, renal failure, and disseminated intravascular coagulation. The blood transfusion must be stopped immediately, the patient's blood and any untransfused blood must be cultured, and broad-spectrum antibiotics (Chapter 108) should be started.

Circulatory Overload

Acute pulmonary edema, caused by the circulatory system's inability to handle an increased fluid volume, can occur in any patient who is transfused too rapidly. Although the true frequency of this type of transfusion reaction is unknown, it is believed to be a common occurrence. Susceptible populations are primarily the very young, the elderly, and patients with a small total blood volume or cardiopulmonary disease. Treatment is the same as for heart failure (Chapter 59).

Delayed Reactions

A delayed hemolytic transfusion reaction generally occurs 3 to 7 days after transfusion of the implicated unit. Hemolysis is usually extravascular, and red cells are destroyed in the recipient's circulation by antibody produced as a result of an immune response to the transfusion. These reactions are most commonly due to an anamnestic response (secondary exposure to a red cell antigen) in a patient with a negative antibody screen despite a low level of antibody as a result of previous exposure to a foreign red cell antigen through either pregnancy or transfusion. Exposure to the same antigen a second time may cause IgG antibody to reappear within hours or days of the transfusion. This subsequent exposure to the antigen produces an anamnestic antibody response, resulting in increased production of IgG antibodies that are capable of reacting with any transfused cells present.

In most cases, anamnestic production of antibody does not result in acute hemolysis, but red cell destruction does occur between 3 days and 2 weeks after the transfusion. Patients are generally asymptomatic, and hemolysis may be noted only by a more rapid decline than usual in the patient's hemoglobin level or by an absence of the expected rise in hemoglobin. Fever, the most common initial symptom, is occasionally noted, along with jaundice; renal failure is rare. Prednisone (1 to 2 mg/kg/day) is indicated for more severe reactions.

Transfusion-Associated Graft-versus-Host Disease

Transfusion-associated graft-versus-host disease results from the transfusion of immunologically competent lymphocytes into an immunologically incompetent host. An individual's risk depends on whether the recipient is immunocompromised (and to what degree), the degree of HLA similarity between the transfusion donor and recipient, and the number of transfused T lymphocytes capable of multiplying and engrafting. The engrafted lymphocytes mount an immunologic response against the recipient's tissue, resulting in pancytopenia with bleeding and infectious complications. Symptoms usually appear within 12 days of transfusion. Transfusion-associated graft-versus-host disease is rare, but it is fatal in approximately 90% of affected patients.

Transfusion-Related Acute Lung Injury

Transfusion-related acute lung injury (TRALI; Chapter 94) is an acute respiratory distress syndrome (Chapter 104) that occurs within 6 hours after transfusion and is characterized by dyspnea and hypoxia secondary to noncardiogenic pulmonary edema. Although the actual incidence is almost certainly underreported, the estimated frequency is approximately 1 in 8000 transfusions. In a prospective nested case control study, 16 of 668 (2.4%) of cardiac surgery patients developed TRALI, suggesting that the incidence of TRALI is particularly high in this population. In approximately 50% of cases, blood donor antibodies with HLA or neutrophil antigenic specificity can be shown to react with the recipient's leukocytes, leading to increased permeability of the pulmonary microcirculation.

Most recently, reactive lipid products from donor blood cell membranes that arise during the storage of blood products have been implicated in the pathophysiology of TRALI. Such substances are capable of neutrophil priming, with subsequent damage to the pulmonary-capillary endothelium of the recipient, particularly in patients who receive massive transfusions during cardiac surgery or for trauma or in patients receiving chemotherapy for malignancy. In each of these settings, the true incidence of TRALI may be underreported because the findings may be blamed on the underlying disease process or the surgical procedure. Similar to other causes of acute respiratory distress syndrome, therapy is supportive, and 90% of patients recover. Ongoing initiatives to reduce TRALI risks include recruiting male plasma donors or female donors with no prior history of pregnancy, and screening female apheresis platelet donors for HLA antibodies and limiting donation to those who are HLA antibody negative.

Transmission of Viral Pathogens

Categories of transfusion-transmitted agents, as well as those currently screened, are listed in Table 180-2. The implementation of nucleic acid testing of multiple minipools (donation samples, test well) from blood donations has markedly reduced the transmission of HIV and hepatitis C virus during the infectious window period. Current estimates of the risk per unit of blood are 1 in 1.4 million to 2.4 million for HIV and 1 in 872,000 to 1.7 million for hepatitis C virus (Fig 180-3).

Only 43% of the World Health Organization's 191 member states test blood for HIV, hepatitis C virus, and hepatitis B virus, so at least 13 million units of blood donated every year are not tested for these transmissible viruses. In the poorest countries, the cost of testing ($40 to $50 per blood donation) is prohibitive. Every year, unsafe transfusions are estimated to account for 8 million to 16 million hepatitis B infections, 2.3 million to 4.7 million hepatitis C infections, and 80,000 to 160,000 HIV infections.

TABLE 180-2   CATEGORIES OF TRANSFUSION-TRANSMITTED AGENTS

AGENTS CAUSING TRANSFUSION-TRANSMITTED DISEASE FOR WHICH DONORS ARE ROUTINELY SCREENED

Hepatitis B virus
Human immunodeficiency virus
Hepatitis C virus
Human T-cell lymphotropic virus
West Nile virus
Bacteria
Trypanosoma cruzi
Cytomegalovirus

AGENTS THAT ARE TRANSFUSION TRANSMISSIBLE BUT HAVE NOT CAUSED ANY KNOWN DISEASE WHEN ACQUIRED THROUGH TRANSFUSION

Agents initially thought to cause hepatitis
Human herpesvirus 8

AGENTS CAUSING TRANSFUSION-TRANSMITTED DISEASE FOR WHICH DONORS ARE NOT ROUTINELY SCREENED

Hepatitis A virus
Parvovirus B19
Dengue fever virus
Babesia spp
Plasmodium spp
Leishmania spp
Brucella spp
Variant Creutzfeldt-Jakob disease prions
Other

Modified from Vamvakes EC, Blajchman MA. Transfusion-related mortality: the on-going risks of allogeneic blood transfusion and the available strategies for their prevention. *Blood.* 2009;113:3406-3417.

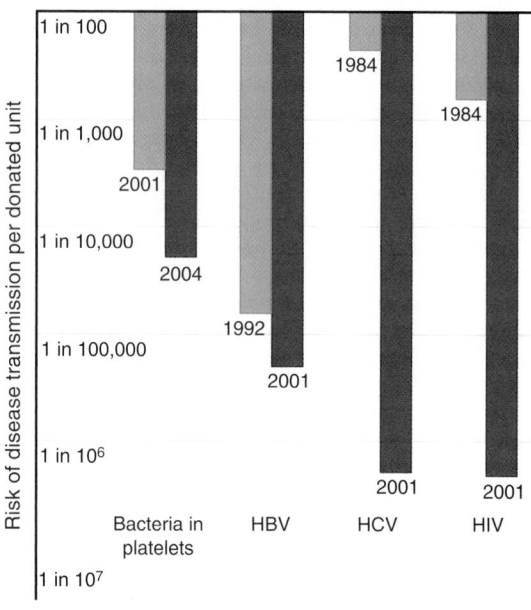

FIGURE 180-3. Risk of transmission of potentially fatal transfusion-acquired infections in the United States. The figures plotted pertain to risk reduction documented between 2001 and 2004 for bacteria in platelets, 1992 and 2001 for hepatitis B virus (HBV), and 1984 and 2001 for hepatitis C virus (HCV) and human immunodeficiency virus (HIV). The risk of bacteria in platelets today is considered to be the same as in 2004, and the risk of HBV, HCV, and HIV is considered to be the same as in 2001, because no further measures to protect the blood supply from these pathogens have been introduced. (From Vamvakas EC, Blajchman MA. Transfusion-related mortality: the on-going risks of allogeneic blood transfusion and the available strategies for their prevention. *Blood.* 2009;113:3406-3417.)

⬤ EMERGING ISSUES AND EVOLVING TECHNOLOGIES

Problems related to blood component storage have long been known, such as depletion of 2,3-diphosphoglycerate in red cell units during storage at 4° C for longer than 35 to 42 days. Recent evidence suggests that in patients undergoing cardiac surgery, transfusion of red cells stored for more than 14 days is associated with a significantly increased risk of postoperative complications, as well as reduced short-term and long-term survival. A prospective, randomized multicenter trial comparing the transfusion of blood less than 10 days old versus blood 21 days or older in adult patients undergoing cardiac surgery is currently under way in the United States. Erythropoiesis-stimulating agents, including recombinant human erythropoietin, modified erythropoietin molecules, and erythropoietin receptor agonists, along with artificial oxygen carriers, can potentially decrease the need for red cell transfusion. It is important that oversight of these biotechnology products and other specialized blood products (e.g., solvent- or detergent-treated plasma, leukoreduced blood products, irradiated blood components, CMV-negative blood components) be placed under the auspices of standing hospital medical committees, such as a transfusion medicine committee. Otherwise, promotion of such products by the commercial sector directly to consumers could undermine both institutional oversight and evidence-based rationales for their use.

Grade Ⓐ ──────────────────────────────── ○

1. Herbert PC, Wells G, Blajchman MA, et al. A multicenter, randomized, controlled clinical trial of transfusion requirements in critical care. *N Engl J Med.* 1999;340:409-417.
2. Hajjar LA, Vincent JL, Galas FR, et al. Transfusion requirements after cardiac surgery: the TRACS randomized controlled trial. *JAMA.* 2010;304:1559-1567.
3. Diedrich B, Remberger M, Shanwell A, et al. A prospective randomized trial of a prophylactic platelet transfusion trigger of 10×10^9 per L versus 30×10^9 per L in allogeneic hematopoietic progenitor cell transplant recipients. *Transfusion.* 2005;45:1064-1072.
4. Slichter SJ, Kaufman RM, Assmann SF, et al. Dose of prophylactic platelet transfusion and prevention of hemorrhage. *N Engl J Med.* 2010;362:600-613.

SUGGESTED READINGS

Goodnough LT, Shander A. How we treat: management of warfarin-associated coagulopathy in patients with intracerebral hemorrhage. *Blood.* 2011, in press. *Review of management with personal perspective.*

Goodnough LT, Viele M, Fontaine MJ, et al. Implementation of a two specimen requirement for verification of ABO/Rh for blood transfusion. *Transfusion.* 2009;49:1321-1328. *The relevance of bedside errors in patient identification and specimen labeling.*

Koch CG, Li L, Sessler DI, et al. Duration of red-cell storage and complications after cardiac surgery. *N Engl J Med.* 2008;358:1229-1239. *Transfusion of red cells that had been stored for more than 2 weeks was associated with a significantly increased risk of postoperative complications and reduced survival.*

McCullough J. Overview of platelet transfusion. *Semin Hematol.* 2010;47:235-242. *Review.*

Shaz BH, Stowell SR, Hillyer CD. Transfusion-related acute lung injury: from bedside to bench and back. *Blood.* 2011;117:1463-1471. *Review.*

Vamakas EC, Blajchman MA. Transfusion-related mortality: the on-going risks of allogeneic blood transfusion and the available strategies for their prevention. *Blood.* 2009;113:3406-3417. *Review of blood risks.*

Vlaar AP, Hofstra JJ, Determann RM, et al. The incidence, risk factors and outcome of transfusion-related acute lung injury in a cohort of cardiac surgery patients: a prospective nested case control study. *Blood.* 2011;117:4218-4225. *Risk factors include age; time on bypass; larger transfusions of blood products, plasma, and RBCs stored for >14 days; and the presence of antibodies in donor blood.*

181

HEMATOPOIETIC STEM CELL TRANSPLANTATION

JULIE M. VOSE

Hematopoietic stem cell transplantation is the process of collecting and infusing hematopoietic stem cells obtained from bone marrow (bone marrow transplantation) or peripheral blood (peripheral blood stem cell transplantation). High-dose chemotherapy followed by bone marrow or peripheral blood stem cell transplantation is increasingly used for the treatment of many hematologic, immunologic, and neoplastic diseases. Hematopoietic stem cells can be obtained directly from bone marrow by multiple aspirations from the pelvic bones while the patient is under general anesthesia. Alternatively, hematopoietic stem cells can be obtained from peripheral blood, after stimulation with hematopoietic growth factors such as granulocyte colony-stimulating factor (G-CSF), followed by leukapheresis, or they can be obtained from cord blood sources. The availability of hematopoietic stem cell transplantation permits the administration of supralethal chemotherapy or combined chemotherapy and radiation therapy to patients with malignancies or, in selected cases, with nonmalignant diseases in an attempt to increase the destruction of the affected cells. Additionally, the healthy transplanted cells may reconstitute the patient's immune system to provide an antitumor effect or, in the case of bone marrow transplantation for congenital diseases, to provide cells that are no longer deficient in certain vital components.

● ALLOGENEIC AND SYNGENEIC TRANSPLANTATION

Allogeneic bone marrow or peripheral blood stem cell transplantation involves the transfer of stem cells from a donor to another person. Syngeneic transplantation, which occurs in only about 1% of transplant procedures, is the special case of a donor and recipient who are genetically identical twins. Myeloablative allogeneic transplants are usually considered only for patients younger than 55 to 60 years; however, older patients are occasionally treated. Results tend to be poorer in older patients because of the increasing incidence of graft-versus-host disease (GVHD) with age. More recently, reduced-intensity nonmyeloablative allogeneic transplants have been used, especially in older patients and others who might not be good candidates for fully myeloablative transplants. In all cases, the decision whether to transplant must take into account all factors, including not only the patient's chronologic age but also his or her physiologic age.

The donor and recipient must be matched for human leukocyte antigens (HLAs); the most important gene pairs include HLA-A, HLA-B, HLA-C, HLA-DR, and HLA-DQ loci, all of which are closely linked on chromosome 6 and inherited in haplotypes. The chance of having an HLA match from a sibling is 25%; however, because of the relatively small size of families in the United States, only about 30% of patients have HLA-matched siblings. For patients who lack HLA-identical sibling donors, other possible solutions include identifying an unrelated but closely HLA-matched person through the National Marrow Donor Program (NMDP), using a partially matched related donor, or identifying one or more cord blood units from a cord blood bank. The genes encoding HLAs are numerous, and the odds that any two unrelated individuals are HLA identical for main loci are less than 1 in 10,000. About 10 million volunteer donors have been HLA-typed through the NMDP registry, however, and a donor can be found for about 50% of patients for whom a search is initiated. It usually takes about 4 months to locate an unrelated donor, which may be too long for some patients with rapidly progressive malignancies.

An allogeneic partially matched sibling or placental or umbilical cord blood is an alternative source of stem cells. Umbilical cord blood stem cells are already stored in cord blood banks, and no additional harvest procedures are needed. Because of the unique immature biology of umbilical cord blood stem cells, these transplants are associated with less GVHD; consequently, the HLA matching requirements are less strict. However, cord blood cells must be partially matched to the recipient, as well as to each other if more than 1 unit is given. The small volume of cord blood stem cells often makes these transplants unsuitable for adult recipients. The time to engraftment and immune reconstitution may also be different for this type of transplant, which sometimes causes late engraftment and an increased rate of post-transplant infection.

When an adequate donor has been identified, the patient is prepared for the allogeneic or syngeneic transplant with high doses of chemotherapy, alone or combined with radiation therapy. This treatment is designed to destroy any remaining malignant cells, provide sufficient immunosuppression to allow engraftment of the new cells, and clear the marrow space for engraftment of the new cells. The preparative agents must have few toxicities at high doses; for this reason, high doses of anthracyclines are often impractical because of their cardiac toxicities. Most regimens consist of total body irradiation combined with alkylating agents, etoposide, or cytarabine. With nonmyeloablative transplants, less intense chemotherapy and/or radiation is used, which is less damaging to the patient. However, acute and chronic GVHD is still a possibility, and in fact, the risk of chronic GVHD may be slightly higher.

An integral component of the regimens for allogeneic transplantation is immunosuppression to prevent GVHD and graft rejection (Chapter 48). Because the recipient's immune system is ablated with high-dose chemotherapy and radiation therapy, graft rejection is a rare event with related donors and a fully ablative transplant. However, reduced-intensity regimens

can have a higher risk of nonengraftment. Drugs commonly used to prevent GVHD include tacrolimus, mycophenolate mofetil, rapamycin, and the combination of cyclosporine and methotrexate. For allogeneic hematopoietic stem cell transplantation, prophylactic immunosuppression is not lifelong; when immunologic tolerance is established, immunosuppressive agents can be slowly withdrawn and discontinued. Another strategy to prevent GVHD is to deplete the donor's T cells from the graft; the disadvantage of this approach is its association with increased rates of disease relapse and infection, and overall survival does not seem to be improved. To accelerate engraftment, hematopoietic growth factors such as G-CSF are administered after transplantation until the neutrophil count recovers. Allogeneic transplantation regimens also include prophylactic antiviral drugs (acyclovir, ganciclovir), antifungal drugs (fluconazole, voriconazole), broad-spectrum antibiotics (cephalosporins, fluoroquinolones), and anti-*Pneumocystis* drugs (trimethoprim-sulfamethoxazole, dapsone, pentamidine).

Leukemias and some indolent lymphomas that relapse after allogeneic stem cell transplantation can sometimes be controlled by further infusions of lymphocytes from the same allogeneic donor. The donor T lymphocytes destroy malignant cells by an immune mechanism called the *graft-versus-tumor effect*. For solid tumors, a graft-versus-tumor effect can sometimes be demonstrated. These observations led to the development of nonmyeloablative transplantation regimens, based on the concept that allogeneic stem cell transplantation is a form of immunotherapy by which the donor lymphocytes eradicate the malignant disease, with high-dose chemotherapy and irradiation not being necessary for success.

● AUTOLOGOUS BONE MARROW TRANSPLANTATION

In autologous bone marrow transplantation, the patient's own hematopoietic cells are infused to reestablish bone marrow function after the administration of high-dose chemotherapy, with or without total body irradiation. These reinfused hematopoietic cells can come from the patient's bone marrow, peripheral blood, or both. Because a major limitation of allogeneic bone marrow transplantation is that only a few patients have HLA-matched sibling donors, the use of autologous hematopoietic cells greatly increases the number of patients eligible for transplantation (Table 181-1). Autologous transplantation can also be used safely in older patients because of the absence of GVHD, which is a major concern in this population. Disadvantages of autologous hematopoietic cell transplantation include the risk of contaminating the graft with viable tumor cells and the lack of graft-versus-tumor effects. Although patients undergoing autologous transplantation have higher relapse rates than those undergoing allogeneic transplantation, the lower rate of other complications seems to translate into similar long-term outcomes. A variety of methods have been developed to decrease the contamination of autologous grafts with tumor cells (graft "purging"), but no prospective data have yet confirmed that these interventions are beneficial because most relapses originate from incompletely eradicated disease in the host.

● INDICATIONS FOR TRANSPLANTATION

For many diseases, hematopoietic stem cell transplantation is now part of standard therapy (Table 181-2). In the United States, more than 17,000 allogeneic and autologous transplants are performed each year for various diseases (Fig. 181-1).

Lymphoproliferative Malignancies
Non-Hodgkin's Lymphoma

As first-line treatment, autologous transplantation results in a higher rate of complete response but not better survival in patients with aggressive

TABLE 181-1	COMPARISON OF ALLOGENEIC AND AUTOLOGOUS TRANSPLANTATION	
FEATURE	**ALLOGENEIC**	**AUTOLOGOUS**
Upper age limits	55–75 yr	Physiologic status limits
Availability	40–60% of patients	Only limitation may be the ability to collect enough stem cells
Main cause of failure	Graft-versus-host disease Infections	Disease relapse

TABLE 181-2	RESULTS OF STANDARD-OF-CARE ALLOGENEIC OR AUTOLOGOUS STEM CELL TRANSPLANTATION IN SPECIFIC DISEASES*	
	Three-Year Survival (%)	
DISEASE	ALLOGENEIC	AUTOLOGOUS
HEMATOLOGIC MALIGNANCIES		
Acute myelogenous leukemia	32–50	43–50
Chronic myelogenous leukemia	28–54	NU
Myelodysplastic syndrome	40–46	NU
Acute lymphocytic leukemia	25–51	NU
Chronic lymphocytic leukemia	35–45	66
Hodgkin's disease	NU	78
Follicular lymphoma	60	76
Diffuse large cell lymphoma	19–30	60
Multiple myeloma	12–40	66
Neuroblastoma	NU	60
NONMALIGNANT CONDITIONS		
Aplastic anemia	33–82	NA
Fanconi's anemia	16–81	NA
Thalassemia major	91 (1 yr)	NA
Sickle cell anemia	91	NA
Severe combined immunodeficiency	59.3	NA

*Information based on the Center for International Bone Marrow Transplant Research report for patients who underwent transplantation between 2000 and 2007. Results are typically better in patients younger than 20 years, patients in earlier stages of the disease, and recipients of HLA-identical sibling transplants.
NA = not applicable; NU = not routinely used.

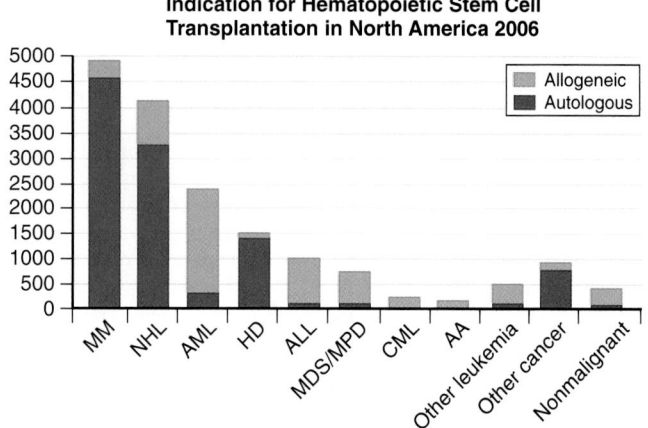

Indication for Hematopoietic Stem Cell Transplantation in North America 2006

FIGURE 181-1. Indications for autologous and allogeneic blood and marrow transplantation in North America. AA = aplastic anemia; ALL = acute lymphocytic leukemia; AML = acute myelogenous leukemia; CML = chronic myelogenous leukemia; HD = Hodgkin's disease; MDS = myelodysplastic syndrome; MM = multiple myeloma; MPD = myeloproliferative disease; NHL = non-Hodgkin's lymphoma. (Information reprinted with permission from the Center for International Bone Marrow Transplant Research [CIBMTR], 2010.)

non-Hodgkin's lymphoma (Chapter 191).∎ Patients with relapsed disease seem to benefit most from this therapy if they undergo transplantation when they still have chemotherapy-sensitive disease. High-risk patients who undergo transplantation early in the course of the disease, during their first partial or complete response, may have a better outcome than similar patients treated with conventional therapy; however, this is considered controversial. The use of high-dose chemotherapy, radiation therapy, and autologous transplantation in patients with indolent disease is associated with a failure-free survival rate of 40 to 60% at a median follow-up of 3 years; because late relapses are common, much longer follow-up is necessary to assess the long-term results of this treatment. Allogeneic stem cell transplantation is typically used for patients who have relapsed after an autologous stem cell transplant or for some lymphomas in which an autologous transplant is not possible owing to circulating lymphoma cells.

Hodgkin's Disease

High-dose chemotherapy followed by autologous hematopoietic stem cell transplantation has been widely accepted for patients with relapsed Hodgkin's disease (Chapter 192). Allogeneic transplantation has not been used as extensively because of increased morbidity and mortality. The outcome is poorer in patients who have received multiple chemotherapy regimens than in those who have undergone less pretreatment. Autologous transplantation during the first remission is being evaluated in patients with "B" symptoms, disseminated disease with bone marrow or pulmonary involvement, and other high-risk features.

Multiple Myeloma

Autologous and allogeneic transplant procedures have been performed successfully in patients with multiple myeloma (Chapter 193). The major concern with conventional myeloablative allogeneic transplantation was its high mortality rate; however, with improvements in supportive care, the transplant-related mortality associated with autografts for multiple myeloma has been reduced to 1%, and randomized trials confirm better progression-free survival but not overall survival after autologous stem cell transplantation compared with conventional chemotherapy.∎ Autologous transplantation for multiple myeloma is more successful in patients who undergo less pretreatment and have a smaller tumor burden. Multiple myeloma is now the most common indication for autologous stem cell transplantation in North America. Studies using autologous tandem transplantation, or an autologous transplant followed by a nonmyeloablative transplant, have shown early promising results.

Lymphoid Leukemias

The results of conventional induction and consolidation chemotherapy for acute lymphoblastic leukemia (ALL) in children are excellent, except for ALL associated with the Philadelphia chromosome (Ph) (Chapter 189). Therefore, in children with ALL, transplantation is generally reserved for these high-risk patients and those who relapse after initial therapy. A much higher percentage of adults fail to respond to initial therapy and have higher-risk disease; therefore, allogeneic stem cell transplantation, which improves overall survival when performed in adults during a first complete remission,∎ should be considered in adult ALL patients, particularly those who are Ph positive.

Selected younger patients with B-cell chronic lymphocytic leukemia (B-CLL) that is refractory or who have relapsed more than once might benefit by transplantation from a related or unrelated donor; durable disease-free survival rates are 40 to 60% (Chapter 190). Because the allogeneic graft-versus-leukemia effect seems to be especially important against B-CLL, this disease is a common indication for nonmyeloablative allogeneic transplantation. Autologous transplantation also yields high rates of remission in pretreated B-CLL patients, but relapse rates are significant.

Myeloproliferative Malignancies
Myeloid Leukemias

Because patients with good-risk or average-risk acute myelogenous leukemia (AML) can be cured with conventional chemotherapy, most centers use transplantation only for relapsed AML in adults or as part of the initial therapy in patients with known poor prognostic characteristics, such as certain high-risk chromosomal abnormalities, including complex abnormalities or deletions (Chapter 189). In these intermediate- and high-risk patients, allogeneic transplantation improves progression-free survival and overall survival when performed during first complete remission.∎

Most patients with chronic myelogenous leukemia (CML) are treated with tyrosine kinase inhibitors rather than allogeneic stem cell transplantation (Chapter 190). If the medications fail, allogeneic transplantation from an HLA-matched sibling donor produces long-term disease-free survival in 55 to 75% of patients with Ph-positive CML. The results seem to be better when younger patients undergo transplantation within the first year of diagnosis. When an HLA-matched related donor is not available, use of alternative donors can yield a cure in about 50% patients with chronic phase CML. However, the development of effective, nontoxic tyrosine kinase inhibitors for the treatment of BCR-ABL–positive CML is tempering enthusiasm for allogeneic transplantation in CML patients, so this procedure is rarely performed.

Myelodysplastic Syndromes

Myelodysplastic syndromes in young, otherwise healthy patients are best treated with an allogeneic transplant (Chapter 188). However, most patients with myelodysplastic syndromes are elderly, which often precludes the use of this therapy.

Solid Tumors

High-dose chemotherapy for the treatment of metastatic breast cancer can result in a higher complete response rate than conventional treatment (Chapter 204). The reported disease-free survival rate in chemotherapy-sensitive stage IV breast cancer is only 10 to 25%, however, and no overall survival benefit has been shown in several randomized trials. As a result, transplantation has lost favor in this condition.

High-dose chemotherapy plus transplantation has had success in the treatment of some chemotherapy-sensitive solid tumors, including testicular cancer (Chapter 206), ovarian carcinoma (Chapter 205), and childhood tumors such as neuroblastoma and Wilms' tumor. Other solid tumors that are refractory to chemotherapy, such as melanoma or many gastrointestinal malignancies, are poor targets for this therapy. Limited reports of a high rate of regression of metastatic renal carcinoma (Chapter 203) after nonmyeloablative allogeneic peripheral blood stem cell transplantation hold promise for its wider use.

Nonmalignant Conditions

Disorders such as Wiskott-Aldrich syndrome or severe combined immunodeficiency syndrome have been treated successfully with HLA-matched sibling transplants or transplants from alternative donors (Chapter 258).

Genetic disorders such as osteopetrosis (Chapter 256), Gaucher's disease (Chapter 215), and Hurler's syndrome (Chapter 268) can be treated successfully with an allogeneic transplant. Other indications for allogeneic transplantation include hemoglobinopathies such as sickle cell anemia (Chapter 166) and thalassemia (Chapter 165) and acquired blood disorders such as paroxysmal nocturnal hemoglobinuria (Chapter 163). The transplant must be performed before the onset of secondary organ failure.

Allogeneic transplantation can lead to long-term disease-free survival in more than 50% of patients with severe aplastic anemia (Chapter 168). When compared with standard immunosuppressive therapy, allogeneic transplantation is more likely to produce a complete and durable reversal of the hematologic abnormalities. Patients with aplastic anemia who are less heavily transfused have better outcomes with allogeneic transplantation. For patients with less severe aplastic anemia, patients older than 40 years, and those without a matched sibling donor, a trial of immunosuppression therapy is usually appropriate before consideration of allogeneic transplantation.

Autologous stem cell transplantation to engraft a tolerant immune system has had promising results in selected patients with systemic lupus erythematosus, rheumatoid arthritis, scleroderma, and multiple sclerosis. Randomized prospective trials comparing conventional treatments are currently under way.

Much attention has focused on the possible use of autologous bone marrow–derived or circulating peripheral blood stem cells to promote the recovery of myocardial function after acute myocardial infarction. To date, the infusion of such cells, usually directly into the relevant coronary artery after successful percutaneous coronary intervention, has shown promising results in improving regional but not necessarily global myocardial function. Further research is required to define the appropriate clinical role for such approaches.

⬤ COMPLICATIONS

Infections

Infections are a major cause of morbidity and mortality after hematopoietic stem cell transplantation, especially allogeneic transplantation, because of prolonged immunosuppression for the prevention or treatment of GVHD. Bacterial infections are frequently related to central venous catheters. Among fungal infections, *Aspergillus* infections typically occur in patients receiving prolonged high-dose steroids for the treatment of GVHD. Viral infections include reactivation cytomegalovirus (Chapter 384), human herpesvirus 6, and Epstein-Barr virus (Chapter 385) infections. These patients are also susceptible to seasonal respiratory viruses. Prophylactic use of G-CSF and granulocyte-macrophage colony-stimulating factor is helpful but does not improve survival.

At 1 year after allogeneic or autologous transplantation, patients should receive the following vaccinations: diphtheria, tetanus, *Haemophilus influenzae* type b, hepatitis A virus, hepatitis B virus, 23-valent pneumococcal polysaccharide, seasonal influenza virus, inactivated poliovirus, and, only in areas of outbreaks, meningococcal vaccine (Chapter 17). Live vaccines against measles, mumps, and rubella should not be administered until 2 years after transplantation, and only in the absence of chronic GVHD and immunosuppressive therapy. Family members can receive routine vaccines, including influenza virus vaccine, but patients should avoid contact with a child who has received oral poliovirus vaccine for about 1 month after vaccination. Despite these recommendations, vaccines may not always induce protective immunity in an immunodeficient patient who has chronic GVHD or is taking immunosuppressive drugs.

Cardiac Toxicity

Most transplant centers screen potential patients for underlying cardiac abnormalities that would place them at increased risk during the procedure. Nevertheless, a few patients experience cardiotoxicity, either acutely during the transplant procedure or later. Pericardial effusion can develop in patients who have disease near the pericardium or are receiving radiation therapy in that area (Chapter 77). An idiosyncratic cardiomyopathy can occur after high doses of cyclophosphamide. Viral cardiomyopathies can also develop.

Pulmonary Toxicity

Pulmonary toxicities include infections from bacterial, fungal, or viral sources during the transplant. In addition, in patients receiving certain chemotherapy agents, such as carmustine, chemotherapy-induced lung damage may develop, but this can usually be treated with steroids. Patients undergoing allogeneic transplantation are at increased risk for pneumonitis caused by cytomegalovirus and fungal infections, for adult respiratory distress syndrome, and for interstitial pneumonia of unknown cause. Chronic GVHD can also manifest in the lung as bronchiolitis obliterans, with or without obstructive pneumonia.

Liver Toxicity and Veno-occlusive Disease

The most frequent liver complication associated with transplantation is veno-occlusive disease of the liver (also called sinusoidal obstruction syndrome). The pathogenesis of this syndrome is damage to hepatic sinusoids, often with occlusion of hepatic venules, associated with chemotherapy drugs and total body irradiation used in conditioning regimens. Symptoms associated with this complication include jaundice, tender hepatomegaly, ascites, and weight gain. Total serum bilirubin is a sensitive but nonspecific test for veno-occlusive disease. Imaging studies may demonstrate hepatomegaly, ascites, periportal edema, and attenuated hepatic venous flow. The diagnosis can be made most definitively by transvenous liver biopsy and hepatic venous pressure measurements. Progressive hepatic failure and multiorgan system failure can develop, but at least 70% of patients recover spontaneously. Predisposing factors seem to be previous hepatic injury, the use of estrogens, and perhaps the use of HLA-mismatched donors.

Renal Toxicity

Acute renal failure requiring dialysis occurs infrequently during the transplant procedure. The judicious use of nephrotoxic agents can decrease the incidence of this complication. Idiopathic or cyclosporine-induced hemolytic-uremic syndrome (Chapter 175) can be a serious complication after allogeneic stem cell transplantation, with a high risk for end-stage renal disease or death.

Graft-versus-Host Disease

In the allogeneic transplant setting, acute GVHD manifests with symptoms in the skin, gastrointestinal tract, and liver within the first 100 days after transplantation. Skin involvement ranges from a maculopapular rash to generalized erythroderma or desquamation. The severity of liver disease is based on bilirubin levels, and the severity of the gastrointestinal disease is graded by the quantity of daily diarrhea. Patients who receive transplants from unrelated donors are at increased risk, and the incidence and severity of GVHD rise with the age of the patient. Other risk factors include a female donor (particularly a multiparous donor), advanced age, and cytomegalovirus seropositivity of the donor or patient. Prophylaxis with cyclosporine or tacrolimus, with or without methotrexate, corticosteroids, or mycophenolate mofetil, reduces the incidence and severity. Treatment of acute GVHD includes high-dose corticosteroids, antithymocyte globulin, or various monoclonal antibodies.

Chronic GVHD occurs more than 100 days after transplantation and is most likely to develop in older patients who also had acute GVHD. Symptoms include the sicca syndrome, chronic sinusitis, rashes, scleroderma-like skin thickening, diarrhea, wasting syndrome, and liver abnormalities. Patients are also at greatly increased risk for infectious complications resulting from either GVHD itself or treatment for it. Adverse prognostic factors for survival include thrombocytopenia, progressive clinical manifestations, involvement of more than 50% of the skin, poor performance status, and elevated bilirubin. Treatment of chronic GVHD includes corticosteroids, cyclosporine, tacrolimus, mycophenolate mofetil, ultraviolet light, and other immunosuppressive agents.

Graft Rejection

Graft rejection occurs when immunologically competent cells of host origin destroy the transplanted cells of donor origin. This complication is rare after fully matched, related donor transplants and occurs more commonly in patients who receive transplants from alternative donors or T-cell–depleted transplants. Graft rejection is less likely in nontransfused patients with aplastic anemia.

Late Complications

As the number of long-term post-transplant survivors increases, complications that develop years later are beginning to be recognized.

Secondary Malignancies

One complication of the chemotherapy or radiation therapy (or both) used to treat malignancy is the development of a secondary malignancy. There have been several reports of the development of secondary AML or myelodysplastic syndrome after autologous transplantation. Some studies have suggested that total body irradiation may increase the risk for these complications. After allogeneic transplantation, the overall incidence of secondary malignancies is 2.2% at 10 years and 6.7% at 15 years after transplantation. Within the first 1 to 2 years, the most common malignancies are Epstein-Barr virus–related lymphoproliferative disorders; solid tumors are more likely to occur more than 3 years after transplantation. Risk factors include the use of antithymocyte globulin to treat GVHD, the use of a T-cell–depleted graft, HLA incompatibility, and perhaps total body irradiation.

Infertility and Hypogonadism

The risk of gonadal failure is likely to be lower with nonmyeloablative preparative regimens. The use of total body irradiation is almost always associated with sterility, but successful pregnancies have occurred in some patients after other regimens. Gynecomastia (sometimes tender) occasionally occurs in males. To address all the complexities of functional castration from high-dose therapy, a reproductive endocrinologist should be consulted before transplantation in patients for whom future fertility is an issue.

Endocrine Dysfunction

Iatrogenic Cushing's syndrome is commonly due to long-term steroid therapy in patients with chronic GVHD (Chapter 34). Particularly disabling are steroid-induced myopathy, avascular necrosis of the hip, and osteoporosis. Because many patients take steroids for many months, tapering can be associated with malaise, nausea, hypotension, and musculoskeletal pains. In these situations, slower tapering over several months or reintroduction of physiologic replacement doses (e.g., 7.5 to 10 mg/day of prednisone) is appropriate. Hypothyroidism (Chapter 233) is typically related to the use of total body irradiation or local irradiation of the head and neck for lymphoma or other cancer. Osteoporosis (Chapter 251) occurs in 50 to 60% of patients after hematopoietic stem cell transplantation. The major contributing causes include hypogonadism, secondary hyperparathyroidism caused by low serum calcium, and post-transplant steroid therapy. Bone mineral density should be evaluated before and after transplantation; osteopenia should be treated as appropriate with bisphosphonates, calcium, vitamin D, estrogen, and testosterone.

Other Complications

The long-term incidence of cataracts is about 20 to 50%; the risk is related to the use of total body irradiation and corticosteroids (Chapter 431). About 50% of patients with cataracts require surgical therapy. Alopecia is typically reversible, but in rare cases it may be irreversible, especially after the use of busulfan-containing preparative regimens.

⬤ FUTURE DIRECTIONS

The safety and efficacy of transplantation may be improved by the use of hematopoietic cytokines to stimulate immunologic reconstitution, ex vivo expansion of progenitors, genetic modulation of cells, improved supportive care for transplant patients, better prophylaxis against GVHD, better HLA typing, and newer anticancer agents. Whether stem cells can be infused to improve the function of adult organs is an area of active investigation.

1. Greb A, Bohlius J, Schiefer D, et al. High-dose chemotherapy with autologous stem cell transplantation in the first line treatment of aggressive non-Hodgkin lymphoma (NHL) in adults. *Cochrane Database Syst Rev.* 2008;1:CD004024.
2. Koreth J, Cutler CS, Djulbegovic B, et al. High-dose therapy with single autologous transplantation versus chemotherapy for newly diagnosed multiple myeloma: a systematic review and meta-analysis of randomized controlled trials. *Biol Blood Marrow Transplant.* 2007;13:183-196.
3. Ram R, Gafter-Gvili A, Vidal L, et al. Management of adult patients with acute lymphoblastic leukemia in first complete remission: systematic review and meta-analysis. *Cancer.* 2010;116:3447-3457.
4. Koreth J, Schlenk R, Kopecky KJ, et al. Allogeneic stem cell transplantation for acute myeloid leukemia in first complete remission: systematic review and meta-analysis of prospective clinical trials. *JAMA.* 2009;301:2349-2361.

SUGGESTED READINGS

Choi SW, Levine JE, Ferrara JL. Pathogenesis and management of graft-versus-host disease. *Immunol Allergy Clin North Am.* 2010;30:75-101. *Review of the immunologic basis of GVHD, risk factors, and management.*

Gooley TA, Chien JW, Pergam SA, et al. Reduced mortality after allogeneic hematopoietic-cell transplantation. *N Engl J Med.* 2010;363:2091-2101. *Mortality from allogeneic hematopoietic stem cell transplantation decreased from 63% in 1993-1997 to 47% in 2003-2007, but the risk of relapse or progression of the underlying disease did not change.*

Wingard JR, Hsu J, Hiemenz JW. Hematopoietic stem cell transplantation: an overview of infection risks and epidemiology. *Hematol Oncol Clin North Am.* 2011;25:101-116. *Review.*

XV

§ONCOLOGY

APPROACH TO THE PATIENT WITH CANCER

MICHAEL C. PERRY

DIAGNOSIS

Few diagnoses produce such emotional responses as *cancer* or *leukemia*, and in the first few moments after those words are uttered, the patient often experiences a storm of feelings that limit useful discussion. When the time is right, however, the physician and the patient must discuss the diagnosis, its implications, and the therapeutic alternatives. It is often best for the patient if family members or close friends are present in the consulting room, both to provide emotional support and to be another "set of ears." It is often useful to ask, "What do you understand about your diagnosis?"

If the physician is not familiar with the latest treatments, consultation in advance with, for example, the National Cancer Institute's Physician Data Query will make the interview more meaningful. Prompt referral to a specialist, whether a surgical oncologist, radiation oncologist, or medical oncologist, is imperative. The generalist should not be a therapeutic nihilist unless he or she is intimately involved in the field and knows about all the current therapies and clinical trials.

The consulting medical oncologist, often advised by a local tumor board comprising medical, surgical, and radiation oncologists, usually outlines the prognosis and the alternatives: standard therapy, possible clinical trials, a second opinion, or no treatment. Many oncologists actively participate in clinical trials and may have investigational drugs available, or they may suggest referral to a tertiary cancer center as appropriate.

Diagnostic Procedures

In most settings, a lesion has been found on physical examination or by abnormal laboratory or radiographic studies, and a biopsy has confirmed the diagnosis. It is critical that the biopsy be representative of the entire tumor and that appropriate investigations (e.g., special stains, flow cytometry, cytogenetics, hormone assays) be performed before treatment is initiated. If there is a question whether the lesion is benign or malignant or about its proper classification, consideration should be given to additional biopsies, and consultation with a reference pathologist may be indicated. There is seldom a need for such rapid therapy that appropriate pretreatment evaluations cannot be performed. For many tumor sites, such as the colon (Chapter 199), there is one predominant histology; in others, such as the lung (Chapter 197), the distinction between small cell lung cancer and non–small cell lung cancer is critical for treatment. For breast cancer (Chapter 204), the treating physician is interested in a variety of factors, such as histology, tumor grade, the presence or absence of estrogen and progesterone receptors, and the presence of ERBB2 (HER2/neu) overexpression.

Staging and Work-up

After a diagnosis has been established, staging is next. The American Joint Committee on Cancer staging system is considered the standard in the United States and is based on the TNM (tumor, node, metastasis) system. The approach to staging depends on the type of cancer, but it commonly includes plain films such as chest radiographs, computed tomography (CT), magnetic resonance imaging (MRI), radionuclide scans, and, increasingly, positron emission tomography (PET). These studies are typically supplemented by routine hematologic and chemistry profiles, tumor markers, and, in some cases, bone marrow aspiration and biopsies.

The keys to the work-up are to identify sites of metastases and to establish an indicator lesion or lesions to monitor therapy. Thus, for most solid tumors, a CT scan and perhaps a bone scan can accomplish both goals, with brain CT or MRI reserved for cases in which central nervous system metastases are most likely (e.g., small cell lung cancer). PET scans supplement CT scans by establishing that a given lesion is likely to be malignant and by clarifying other sites of disease. In patients with known, established advanced disease, they are seldom needed.

TREATMENT Rx

Development of a Treatment Plan

For cancers amenable to surgery, resection is usually the best alternative if the patient is a suitable candidate for anesthesia (Chapter 440) and is otherwise in acceptable condition in terms of concomitant or comorbid illnesses. A joint discussion among the internist, oncologist, surgeon, and anesthesiologist is often very useful in this regard. Determination of the patient's performance score (Table 182-1) is a simple means of assessing functional status. If life expectancy is limited or if the patient is not a good candidate for surgery, radiation therapy is usually considered the next best "local" therapy, with chemotherapy reserved for patients whose disease is extensive or metastatic. The increasing effectiveness of chemotherapy has resulted in its earlier incorporation into therapy, often as part of an "organ-sparing" approach. Ideally, the discussion of treatment with the patient should take a multidisciplinary approach, with clarification of the diagnosis, prognosis, treatment goals, alternatives, side effects, and risks and benefits.

Surgical Therapy

Surgery is used to biopsy a suspected lesion, to remove the primary tumor, to bypass obstructions, and to provide palliation. A preoperative discussion may determine the requirement for placement of a venous access device at the time of surgery, thus eliminating the need for a second anesthesia.

Surgery remains the most common method to cure localized cancers, such as breast cancer (Chapter 204), colorectal cancer (Chapter 199), and lung cancer (Chapter 197), but it is limited by the location of the tumor, its extension, and distant metastases. Even if a tumor cannot be removed, a biopsy provides confirmation of the diagnosis. Occasionally, an obstructing lesion can be bypassed to provide palliation.

Surgical staging also establishes the extent of the disease. For ovarian cancer (Chapter 205), surgical "debulking" aims to remove all visible disease, leaving minimal residual disease, to enhance chemotherapy.

In rare circumstances when the primary tumor is controlled, removal of a single metastasis (metastasectomy) can result in long-term survival; an example is resection of a single liver metastasis found at the time of colectomy for colorectal cancer. A variety of surgical techniques, such as radio frequency ablation or cryoablation, can treat hepatic metastases in carefully selected patients. Adjuvant chemotherapy is often given after surgery in this situation to treat microscopic metastases.

Reconstruction after a disfiguring procedure is critical to long-term physical and emotional functioning. Examples include post-mastectomy breast reconstruction (Chapter 204) and plastic surgery procedures to correct deformities after head and neck surgery (Chapter 196).

Radiation Therapy

Ionizing radiation (Chapter 19) can be delivered using high-energy rays, known as *teletherapy*, via a linear accelerator; by brachytherapy, through the application of radioactive implants, seeds, wires, or plaques; and intravenously by using radioisotopes. Radiation interacts with molecular oxygen, inducing the formation of superoxide, hydrogen peroxide, or hydroxyl radicals that damage DNA, leading to cell death. Like chemotherapy, radiation therapy is most effective against rapidly dividing cells.

As "local" therapies, both surgery and radiation therapy are limited in their effectiveness by the inapparent extension of disease, the location of tumors next to normal structures that must be preserved, and the presence of distant metastases. Normal tissue tolerance, which varies among the different organs and tissues, often prevents the use of radiation doses that could uniformly eradicate cancers. Radiation therapy is also limited by tumor hypoxia: large, bulky tumors are frequently relatively radioresistant, whereas well-oxygenated tumors can be more effectively treated at lower doses.

Radiation therapy can be used as the primary treatment, as part of multimodality therapy, in the adjuvant setting, and for palliation. As a single modality, radiation therapy can be curative for early-stage malignancies such as laryngeal cancer (Chapter 196), cervical cancer (Chapter 205), and prostate cancer (Chapter 207). Breast-conserving surgery (Chapter 204) requires the use of radiation to treat the remaining breast. Partial irradiation techniques using three-dimensional planning with external beam radiation or with a balloon catheter have recently been developed and used in selected patients with appropriately placed and sized breast cancers. For localized prostate cancer (Chapter 207), implanted radioactive seeds of gold or palladium offer an alternative to surgery or external beam radiation therapy, again in carefully selected patients.

It is important to note that the combination of chemotherapy and radiation therapy may result in synergistic toxicities, such as esophagitis (Chapter 140) in the treatment of lung cancer (Chapter 197) or mucositis in the treatment of head and neck cancer (Chapter 196).

Newer techniques, such as intensity-modulated radiation therapy, permit more exact tailoring of the dose to the target, thereby reducing damage to the surrounding normal tissues. Stereotactic radiation therapy or gamma knife techniques allow the treatment of primary or metastatic brain tumors (Chapter 195) measuring up to 3 cm with pinpoint accuracy, minimizing damage to normal brain. Proton therapy has only limited applicability at this time; it is

TABLE 182-1 KARNOFSKY AND ZUBROD PERFORMANCE SCALES

Karnofsky Performance Status Scale

VALUE	LEVEL OF FUNCTIONAL CAPACITY
100	Normal, no complaints, no evidence of disease
90	Able to carry on normal activity, minor signs or symptoms of disease
80	Normal activity with effort, some signs or symptoms of disease
70	Cares for self, unable to carry on normal activity or to do active work
60	Requires occasional assistance but is able to care for most needs
50	Requires considerable assistance and frequent medical care
40	Disabled, requires special care and assistance
30	Severely disabled, hospitalization is indicated although death is not imminent
20	Hospitalization is necessary, very sick, active supportive treatment necessary
10	Moribund, fatal processes progressing rapidly
0	Dead

Eastern Cooperative Oncology Group (Zubrod) Performance Scale

PERFORMANCE STATUS	DEFINITION
0	Asymptomatic
1	Symptomatic; fully ambulatory
2	Symptomatic; in bed <50% of day
3	Symptomatic; in bed >50% of day
4	Bedridden

TABLE 182-2 EXAMPLES OF TIMING OF CHEMOTHERAPY

ADJUVANT THERAPY	NEOADJUVANT THERAPY	ORGAN-SPARING THERAPY	COMBINATION CHEMOTHERAPY
Stage I and II breast cancer	Stage III breast cancer	Anal cancer	Metastatic solid tumors*
Stage III colorectal cancer		Laryngeal cancer	Hematologic malignancies
Stage III melanoma		Esophageal cancer	
Stage I–III lung cancer			

*Usually palliative.

used for some uveal melanomas, skull base tumors, and a few pediatric malignancies.

Low- to moderate-dose palliative radiation is used to ameliorate symptomatic cancer when cure is no longer the goal. For instance, radiation therapy can improve brain metastases (Chapter 195), relieve pain from bone lesions (Chapter 208), relieve obstructing lesions, and sometimes relieve hemoptysis caused by lung cancer (Chapter 197) or bleeding from a gynecologic malignancy (Chapter 205). Bone-seeking radioisotopes such as samarium or strontium may relieve pain from bone metastases in prostate cancer (Chapter 207) or breast cancer (Chapter 204).

Systemic Therapy
Chemotherapy

Pharmacogenomics, the study of inherited interindividual differences in drug disposition and effects, is becoming important in cancer therapy because genetic polymorphisms in drug-metabolizing enzymes are often responsible for the variations in efficacy and toxicity observed with many chemotherapeutic agents. Drugs potentially affected by polymorphisms identified to date include the thiopurines, 5-fluorouracil, irinotecan, and the platinum agents. In patients who are heterozygous or homozygous for deficiencies in metabolizing enzymes, toxicity can be dramatically enhanced.

Currently available tests cannot reliably assess the likelihood of response to therapy, so treatment is largely empirical and based on predictive factors from the tumor itself. Gene expression microarrays currently under development may reliably predict responses in the future. Gene profiles are increasingly used to determine the necessity of therapy, such as the adjuvant therapy of breast or lung cancer.

Assessing Treatment

Assessment of the response to therapy depends largely on tumor size, determined by either direct measurement or diagnostic imaging studies. The categories of response are complete response, with total absence of tumor and correction of tumor-associated changes; partial response, defined as greater than 50% reduction in tumor size; stable disease, defined as greater than 25% but less than 50% reduction in tumor size; and progressive disease, characterized by either tumor growth or the development of new tumors. Leukemias can be assessed by bone marrow aspirates, and multiple myeloma is typically assessed by the measurement of monoclonal proteins, peripheral blood counts, and percentages of malignant plasma cells in bone marrow samples, as well as radiographs of bone lesions.

Chemotherapy is now used in a variety of settings with or without and before, during, or after surgery and radiation therapy (Table 182-2). Considerable experimental evidence suggests that cancers are most sensitive to

chemotherapy during the early stages of growth, as a result of the high growth fraction and shorter cell cycle times. Thus, a given dose of drug exerts a greater therapeutic effect against a rapidly growing tumor than against a larger, quiescent tumor.

Neoadjuvant Chemotherapy

Neoadjuvant therapy, also called *primary* or *induction chemotherapy*, is used before surgery or radiation therapy to decrease the size of locally advanced cancers, thereby permitting better surgical resection, and to eradicate undetectable metastases. It also affords an opportunity to evaluate the effectiveness of treatment by histologic analysis of resected tissue. This approach is most often used for locally advanced breast cancer (Chapter 204), although other primary tumors can be targeted. Disadvantages include the initially incomplete pathologic staging and the possibility that ineffective chemotherapy will permit the tumor to grow beyond the point of resection.

Organ-sparing therapy is the use of chemotherapy, radiation therapy, or both to salvage organs that would have been surgically removed if cure were the intended result. This technique is often effective in patients with cancers of the larynx (Chapter 196), esophagus (Chapter 198), bladder (Chapter 203), and anus (Chapter 199).

Adjuvant Chemotherapy

Adjuvant chemotherapy is used in patients whose primary tumor and all evidence of cancer (e.g., regional lymph nodes) have been surgically removed or treated definitively with radiation but in whom the risk of recurrence is high because of involved lymph nodes or certain morphologic or biologic characteristics of the cancer. Common examples include cancers of the breast (Chapter 204) and colon (Chapter 199). The typical end points of clinical chemotherapy, such as shrinkage of measurable tumor on serial radiographic studies, are not available in this situation; instead, relapse-free survival and overall survival are the principal measures of treatment effect. For an individual patient receiving adjuvant therapy, there is no way to determine whether such therapy is beneficial or necessary, so decisions are generally based on evidence from clinical trials.

Adjuvant therapy has been used in a wide variety of tumors, with variable success. In the case of breast cancer (Chapter 204) and colon cancer (Chapter 199), the number of lives saved by the use of adjuvant therapy is significant because of the large number of affected patients, despite the modest absolute differences between treated and control patients with current treatment programs. Resectable lung cancer (Chapter 197) has recently been added to this list.

Palliative Chemotherapy

Chemotherapy rarely cures cancers that remain after surgical or radiation treatment or that recur after such therapy. Pancreatic cancer (Chapter 200) is perhaps the best example of this scenario, because few patients are deemed eligible for surgery, and most have recurrent cancer after surgery. Most adult patients with recurrent or metastatic disease are considered for palliative therapy if there is no realistic chance of cure but the potential for prolongation of useful life and/or relief of tumor-related symptoms makes such therapy reasonable.

Combination Chemotherapy

Virtually all the curative chemotherapy regimens developed for hematologic malignancies or solid tumors use combinations of active agents. Combination chemotherapy is usually superior to the use of single agents in adjuvant and neoadjuvant therapy as well. The improved results achieved by combination chemotherapy can be explained in several ways. Resistance to any single agent is almost always present at diagnosis, even in clinically responsive tumors. Tumors that are initially "sensitive" to chemotherapy rapidly acquire resistance to single agents, either as a result of selection of a preexisting clone of resistant tumor cells or because of an increased rate of mutation leading to drug resistance. Combination chemotherapy theoretically addresses both phenomena by providing a broader range of coverage against initially resistant clones of cells and preventing or slowing the development of resistant clones.

Combination chemotherapy follows a set of principles. All drugs must be active against the tumor, and all drugs must be given at an optimal dose and on an optimal schedule. The drugs should have different mechanisms of antitumor activity as well as different toxicity profiles, and the drugs should be given at consistent intervals for the shortest possible treatment time.

Hormonal Therapy

Endocrine or hormonal therapy for cancer (Table 182-3), the earliest form of systemic therapy, is almost entirely limited to breast cancer (Chapter 204) and prostate cancer (Chapter 207). Many premenopausal breast cancers are thought to be under the influence of estrogens, and hormonal deprivation (ablation) may produce long-term responses in properly selected patients (those with estrogen and/or progesterone receptor positivity who have predominantly soft tissue or bone disease). This hormonal ablation may take the form of surgical removal of the ovaries, ablative radiation therapy, or the use of luteinizing hormone–releasing hormone antagonists. The antiestrogen tamoxifen is effective against breast cancer, and it may decrease the incidence of contralateral breast cancers in both premenopausal and postmenopausal women with breast cancer. It also has an estrogen-like activity that is responsible for an increased rate of endometrial cancers. Somewhat paradoxically, postmenopausal women who are candidates for hormonal therapy may also respond to tamoxifen.

Aromatase Inhibitors

Patients who have experienced a prolonged objective response or stable disease with hormonal therapy may be candidates for second-, third-, or fourth-line hormonal therapy. However, such responses tend to become less frequent and shorter, and many patients eventually need chemotherapy. Recently, aromatase inhibitors (e.g., anastrozole, letrozole, exemestane), which decrease the conversion of metabolites in fat and muscle into estrogen, have been found to be more effective than tamoxifen as first-line therapy in both the adjuvant and metastatic settings, although the optimal schedule for tamoxifen and the aromatase inhibitors in the adjuvant setting is still under study (Chapter 204).

Prostate cancer (Chapter 207) is androgen dependent, and androgen deprivation through castration or antiandrogens can produce meaningful responses. Estrogen therapy is now used infrequently because of its cardiovascular side effects and the availability of better alternatives. Once prostate cancer becomes androgen independent, second-line hormonal therapy rarely produces useful responses.

Corticosteroids

The corticosteroids (Chapter 34), typically prednisone or dexamethasone, are widely used in the treatment of hematologic and oncologic cancers. In Hodgkin's disease (Chapter 192), the non-Hodgkin's lymphomas (Chapter 191), and multiple myeloma (Chapter 193), corticosteroids have antitumor activity. In solid tumors, they are used as antiemetics and, rarely, for the treatment of hypercalcemia of cancer (Chapter 186), for symptomatic relief of cerebral edema in cases of central nervous system metastases (Chapter 195), or as an adjunct to radiation therapy for spinal cord metastases. Megestrol acetate (Megace) is often used in an attempt to relieve anorexia, which is common among cancer patients.

Immunotherapy

Two cancers characterized by often unpredictable clinical behavior, melanoma (Chapter 210) and renal cell carcinoma (Chapter 203), are treated with interferon, interleukin-2, or both (Table 182-4). Dramatic responses are uncommon, and immunotherapy is only a minor component of cancer therapy.

Molecularly Targeted Agents

Targeted agents (Table 182-5) are drugs directed at a specific molecular point, such as a protein tyrosine kinase, or at the presence of a specific antigen on a tumor cell. The first tyrosine kinase inhibitors were imatinib and erlotinib. The best example of the success of tyrosine kinase inhibitor therapy is the dramatic response of chronic myelogenous leukemia (Chapter 190) to imatinib (Gleevec). Imatinib also has activity against gastrointestinal stromal cell tumors.

Erlotinib, directed against the epidermal growth factor receptor (EGFR), has antitumor effects in patients whose non–small cell lung cancers (Chapter 197) have EGFR mutations. Current research aims to identify the specific types of mutations so that patients can be prospectively selected for therapy, analogous to the measurement of estrogen receptors to select breast cancer patients for hormonal therapy.

The vascular endothelial growth factor receptor (VEGFR) stimulates the formation of new blood vessels that are critical for tumor growth. Anti-VEGFR agents, such as the monoclonal antibody bevacizumab, prevent VEGF from transducing its signal in endothelial cells, thereby preventing their division. Bevacizumab has antitumor effects in metastatic colorectal cancer, non–small cell lung cancer, and breast cancer. Thalidomide inhibits angiogenesis through an unknown mechanism and is used against multiple myeloma (Chapter 193).

Bortezomib (Velcade), a unique drug, is a reversible inhibitor of the proteasome pathway that normally regulates the intracellular concentration of specific proteins, thus controlling homeostasis. It has been effective in the

TABLE 182-3 HORMONAL THERAPY
Corticosteroids
Prednisone
Dexamethasone (Decadron)
Androgens
Fluoxymesterone (Halotestin)
Estrogens
Diethylstilbestrol (DES)
Antiandrogens
Bicalutamide (Casodex)
Flutamide (Eulexin)
Nilutamide (Nilandron)
Antiestrogens
Tamoxifen (Nolvadex)
Toremifene (Fareston)
Progestational agents
Megestrol acetate (Megace)
Luteinizing hormone–releasing hormone analogues
Leuprolide (Lupron)
Goserelin (Zoladex)
Degarelix
Aromatase inhibitors
Anastrozole (Arimidex)
Exemestane (Aromasin)
Letrozole (Femara)
Estrogen receptor antagonist
Fulvestrant (Faslodex)

TABLE 182-4 IMMUNOTHERAPY
Interferon-α (Intron A, Roferon)
Interleukin-2 (Proleukin)

TABLE 182-5 MOLECULARLY TARGETED AGENTS AND MONOCLONAL ANTIBODIES
MOLECULARLY TARGETED AGENTS
Imatinib (Gleevec)
Dasatinib (Sprycel)
Nilotinib (Tasigna)
Erlotinib (Tarceva)—EGFR TKI
Antiangiogenesis agents
Bevacizumab (Avastin)—VEGF inhibitor
Thalidomide (Thalomid)
Lenalidomide (Revlimid)
Multikinase inhibitor
Sorafenib (Nexavar)
Sunitinib (Sutent)
Temsirolimus (Torisel)
Everloimus (Affinitor)
Pazopanib (Votrient)
Lapatinib (Tykerb)
Bortezomib (Velcade)—proteasome inhibitor
MONOCLONAL ANTIBODIES
Trastuzumab (Herceptin)
Rituximab (Rituxan)
Gemtuzumab ozogamicin (Mylotarg)
Alemtuzumab (Campath)
Cetuximab, C-225 (Erbitux)
Tositumomab iodine-131 (Bexxar)
Panitumumab (Vectibex)
Ofatumumab (Arzerra)
Ibritumomab tiuxetan Y 90 (Zevalin)

EGFR = epidermal growth factor receptor; TKI = tyrosine kinase inhibitor; VEGF = vascular endothelial growth factor.

treatment of refractory multiple myeloma (Chapter 193) and non-Hodgkin's lymphomas (Chapter 191).

The development of monoclonal antibodies directed against antigens found on cancer cells represents an additional treatment modality, often complementary to conventional chemotherapy. Examples include alemtuzumab, cetuximab, rituximab, and trastuzumab. Trastuzumab has recently been shown to add significantly to disease-free survival time in patients positive for HER2/neu who receive adjuvant therapy for early-stage breast cancer (Chapter 204). These monoclonal antibodies can be used alone ("naked") or, in some cases, labeled with a radioactive molecule to enhance cell killing. This radioimmuno-conjugate approach has been most effective in the treatment of non-Hodgkin's lymphomas (Chapter 191) and chronic lymphocytic leukemia (Chapter 190). The effectiveness of monoclonal antibodies is limited by changes in the antigenic composition of neoplastic cells, called *antigenic drift*.

Individual Agents

A list of the most commonly used chemotherapeutic agents (Table 182-6) can help in understanding the key issues each one raises. In all cases, the most current information from the manufacturer should be sought before therapy is initiated. The number of new drugs continues to increase, and some older drugs included in previous editions of this textbook have been omitted.

The administration of chemotherapy is best done by specifically trained individuals because of the dual risks of hypersensitivity reactions and extravasation. No doses or schedules are suggested because these agents are often used in combination, and the doses must be reduced in many cases. End-organ function also affects dosing. The administration of chemotherapy during pregnancy is an especially difficult circumstance and requires a particularly high level of expertise.

Unless otherwise specified, all chemotherapeutic agents are capable of producing some degree of nausea and vomiting, myelosuppression, alopecia, mucositis, and/or diarrhea after treatment. Most agents are also teratogenic, mutagenic, and carcinogenic, so these toxicities are not repeated for each agent. Drugs used routinely to offset agent-specific toxicities are also included in Table 182-6.

Bone Marrow or Stem Cell Transplantation

Because the major dose-limiting toxicity of most chemotherapeutic agents is myelosuppression, approaches have been developed to harvest the pluripotent stem cells found in bone marrow, peripheral blood, or, less often, cord blood before marrow-damaging chemotherapy so that the stem cells can be reinfused later (Chapter 181). This technique is most effective for acute leukemias (Chapter 189), relapsed lymphomas (Chapter 191), and germ cell tumors (Chapter 206). The effectiveness of this approach is limited more by the inability to eradicate cancer cells than by the inability to achieve engraftment. Transplants may be syngeneic (from an identical twin), autologous (from oneself), allogeneic (from a matched donor, such as a sibling or parent), or from a matched unrelated donor. Nonablative hematopoietic transplants that do not completely abolish myelopoiesis reduce toxicity and allow the treatment of older and medically infirm patients.

Special Circumstances: Pregnant and Geriatric Patients
Pregnancy

Cancer during pregnancy is not uncommon, with breast, cervical, ovarian, melanoma, thyroid, and hematologic malignancies being most common. This is obviously an emotionally charged time, as the joy of a new birth is contrasted with the possible loss of the mother. Clinical decision making is complicated by ethical, moral, cultural, and religious issues. This is not an area for the inexperienced. If surgery can be safely accomplished, this may be the best course, even if it is only a temporizing measure. Radiation therapy carries the very real risk of radiation exposure to the fetus, and staging is almost always suboptimal and confined to ultrasound examinations. When the disease requires chemotherapy, changes in both the mother and the fetus must be taken into account; for instance, there are major changes is pharmacokinetics during pregnancy, along with changes in renal function and plasma volume, plasma protein levels, hepatic metabolism, gastrointestinal absorption, and placental transfer, not to mention fetal pharmacokinetics and placental excretion. Many of the commonly used chemotherapeutic drugs are classified by the Food and Drug Administration as category D (positive human fetal risk, but the benefits in pregnant women may be acceptable despite the risk) or category X (studies in humans and animal have shown fetal malformations or there is evidence of fetal risk based on human evidence). If the mother's condition permits, it is advisable to defer chemotherapy during the first and perhaps the second trimesters and to treat life-threatening situations during the third trimester after extensive counseling with the parents.

Geriatrics

The aging U.S. population has brought an increasing number of older patients with cancer to the attention of oncologists, and the field of geriatric oncology is a new area of specialization. An increasing proportion of cancers occurs in the older population. The changes that develop with age are covered in another chapter, but they can be briefly summarized here as decreased excretion of drugs and metabolites from the kidneys, decreased volume of distribution of water-soluble drugs, and increased susceptibility to myelosuppression, cardiomyopathy, and neuropathy. Many older adults also have comorbid illnesses that must be taken into account. As a general rule, the suitability of an older patient for therapy can be determined by a comprehensive geriatric assessment (CGA) that evaluates the patient's function, comorbidity, nutrition, medications, and resources. By itself, age is not a barrier to surgery; rather, the patient's performance status and the CGA should determine the likelihood of a good recovery. Tolerance of radiation therapy seems to remain largely intact with increasing age. Chemotherapy

decisions are also based on the performance status and CGA, with the use of growth factors to increase the white blood cell count and to maintain a hemoglobin sufficient to minimize symptoms. Dosage adjustments are also made for individual glomerular filtration rates for patients aged 65 and older. The use of lower chemotherapy doses based on age alone is probably not advisable and may result in ineffective therapy.

Management of Complications
Supportive Care

Nutrition is always a concern for patients newly diagnosed with cancer, even if they have not experienced weight loss. In fact, significant weight loss is an adverse prognostic factor for several cancers, especially lung cancer. Patients are often concerned about whether their diet contributed to development of the cancer and whether diet can influence the results of therapy. In most settings, neither of these scenarios is the case. Malnourished patients should be evaluated by a dietitian to determine whether they are ingesting sufficient calories and whether dietary supplements might be needed. Some patients, such as those with head and neck cancers (Chapter 196) or esophageal cancers (Chapter 198), may require parenteral nutrition through a percutaneous endoscopic gastrostomy tube. Total parenteral nutrition (Chapter 224) is rarely indicated, is not particularly helpful, and is likely to produce an ethical dilemma when therapy fails and the decision to discontinue it must be discussed. Corticosteroids increase appetite but have many undesirable side effects. Megestrol acetate (Megace) at a dose of 800 mg/day improves appetite and allows weight gain in many patients; it is expensive, although the suspension is less costly than the tablets. The synthetic cannabinoid dronabinol (Marinol) stimulates appetite and reduces nausea in some patients, but it can produce dysphoria, particularly in older patients. A multiple vitamin with zinc may help with abnormal taste and provide trace minerals. Larger than recommended doses of vitamins are not helpful and may be toxic. It is always useful to inquire what over-the-counter and alternative medications (Chapter 38) are being contemplated or used by the patient.

Symptom Management

Symptom management is key to successful treatment and the patient's quality of life. Pain control (Chapter 29) can be accomplished with a variety of analgesics, both non-narcotic and narcotic. Oncologists use a 10-point scale for evaluating pain control (Fig. 182-1) and start with nonsteroidal anti-inflammatory drugs (NSAIDs) such as aspirin and acetaminophen, progress through ibuprofen and related drugs, and then through combinations of NSAIDs and narcotics to stronger narcotics.[1] Newer narcotics are available in both short-duration and long-duration forms; some patches last 72 hours, which are ideal for patients who have severe pain and are unable to take oral medications. Oral transmucosal fentanyl is more effective than standard-release morphine in this setting. Oral mucositis, a common complication of intensive therapy for hematologic malignancies, can be treated with local measures or with recombinant human keratinocyte growth factor.[2,3] Oral anti-*Candida* drugs that are absorbed or partially absorbed from the gastrointestinal tract can help prevent oral candidiasis.[4]

Many patients still fear chemotherapy because of the risk of nausea and vomiting. New antiemetics, used in combination, have made this side effect much less common. Chemotherapeutic drugs can be ranked according to their probability of causing nausea and vomiting, with prophylactic treatment given accordingly. The availability of the serotonin 5-hydroxytryptamine type 3 (5-HT$_3$) receptor antagonists (dolasetron, granisetron, ondansetron) has dramatically improved the ability to completely control nausea and vomiting. Although prochlorperazine may be adequate for mildly emetogenic chemotherapy, more emetogenic regimens require combination therapy with a corticosteroid (usually dexamethasone), a 5-HT$_3$ antagonist, and a benzodiazepine (e.g., lorazepam). A newer antiemetic, aprepitant, is particularly useful for the treatment of delayed nausea and vomiting. Treating patients before the development of nausea and vomiting is much more effective and helps patients adhere to their treatment schedules.

Growth factors, such as granulocyte colony-stimulating factor (G-CSF) and granulocyte-macrophage colony-stimulating factor (GM-CSF), permit the more rapid recovery of white blood cell nadirs, thus permitting chemotherapy to be given on schedule, without reducing the dosage in many cases.[5] However, such therapy does not decrease hospitalizations or improve survival. It is possible to determine which individuals are at greatest risk for febrile neutropenia (Chapters 170 and 289) and treat them in advance, based on published guidelines.[6,7] Anemia induced by chemotherapy can be alleviated, the need for transfusions reduced, and quality of life improved by the use of either erythropoietin (Procrit) or darbepoetin (Aranesp).

The bisphosphonates pamidronate (Aredia) and zoledronate (Zometa) are very effective not only to treat tumor-induced hypercalcemia (Chapter 186) but also to reduce pathologic fractures in bones with metastatic lesions, particularly from breast cancer (Chapter 204), prostate cancer (Chapter 207), and myeloma (Chapter 193). They are also used to treat osteoporosis caused by chemotherapy-induced premature menopause in young women with breast cancer. Denosumab (Xgeva) is a human monoclonal antibody that binds to

Text continues on p. 1177

TABLE 182-6 CHEMOTHERAPEUTIC AGENTS

AGENT	CLASS	ACTION	EXCRETION	UNIQUE SIDE EFFECTS	DRUG INTERACTIONS	INDICATIONS
ALKYLATING AGENTS						
Bendamustine (Treanda)	Alkylating agent	Bifunctional with both alkylating and purine-like antimetabolite action	Biotransformation in liver	None	Synergistic with rituximab	CLL, myeloma, Hodgkin's and non-Hodgkin's lymphoma
Carboplatin (Paraplatin)	Platinum coordination compound	Produces interstrand DNA cross-links, similar to those with bifunctional alkylating agents; cell cycle nonspecific	Renal	Nephrotoxicity, ototoxicity, neuropathy, hypomagnesemia, hypersensitivity reactions, hepatotoxicity	Avoid other nephrotoxic or ototoxic drugs	Ovarian cancer, testicular cancer, lung cancer, head and neck cancer, breast cancer
Chlorambucil (Leukeran)	Bifunctional alkylating agent	Formation of interstrand DNA cross-links with resultant inactivation of DNA; cell cycle nonspecific	Hepatic biotransformation, renal excretion	Hepatotoxicity, pulmonary toxicity	None	CLL, Waldenström's macroglobulinemia, Hodgkin's and non-Hodgkin's lymphomas, myeloproliferative disorders, ovarian cancer
Cisplatin (Platinol)	Platinum coordination compound	Produces interstrand DNA cross-links similar to bifunctional alkylating agents; cell cycle nonspecific	Renal	Nephrotoxicity, ototoxicity, neuropathy, hypomagnesemia, hypersensitivity reactions, hemolytic anemia, SIADH	Avoid other nephrotoxic or ototoxic drugs	Testicular cancer, other germ cell tumors, ovarian cancer, bladder cancer, prostate cancer, lung cancer, sarcomas, cervical cancer, endometrial cancer, gastric cancer, breast cancer, adrenal cancer, head and neck cancer
Cyclophosphamide (Cytoxan, Neosar)	Alkylating agent of nitrogen mustard type	Cross-linking of DNA and RNA, inhibits protein synthesis; cell cycle nonspecific	Hepatic biotransformation, renal excretion	Hemorrhagic cystitis, SIADH	Phenobarbital increases rate of metabolism and leukopenia; cyclophosphamide potentiates effects of succinylcholine and may increase oral anticoagulant activity	Breast cancer, ovarian cancer, Hodgkin's and non-Hodgkin's lymphomas, leukemias, neuroblastoma, retinoblastoma, other sarcomas, bladder cancer, lung cancer, cervical cancer, endometrial cancer, prostate cancer, osteogenic sarcoma, Wilms' tumor
Dacarbazine (DTIC-Dome)	Nonclassic alkylating agent	Inhibits DNA and RNA synthesis via formation of carbonium ions; cell cycle nonspecific	Hepatic biotransformation, renal excretion	Pain on injection, flu-like syndrome, hepatic veno-occlusive disease, photosensitivity	Heparin, lidocaine, hydrocortisone, phenytoin, phenobarbital, interleukin-2	Melanoma, Hodgkin's disease, sarcomas
Ifosfamide (Ifex)	Alkylating agent of nitrogen mustard type	Alkylated metabolites interact with DNA; cell cycle nonspecific	Hepatic biotransformation, renal elimination	Hemorrhagic cystitis, nephrotoxicity, CNS toxicity	None	Germ cell tumors, sarcomas, non-Hodgkin's lymphomas, cervical cancer, Ewing's sarcoma, lung cancer
Mechlorethamine, nitrogen mustard (Mustargen)	Bifunctional alkylating agent	Cross-links strands of DNA and RNA, inhibits protein synthesis; cell cycle nonspecific	Rapidly deactivated in body fluids and tissues	Extravasation	None	Hodgkin's disease, intracavitary treatment of effusions; topically for mycosis fungoides
Melphalan (Alkeran)	Alkylating agent of nitrogen mustard type	Forms interstrand, intrastrand, or DNA protein cross-links; cell cycle nonspecific	Deactivated in body fluids and tissues, renal elimination 50%	Pulmonary toxicity	Cimetidine decreases oral bioavailability; cyclosporine enhances risk of renal toxicity	Multiple myeloma, breast cancer, ovarian cancer, rhabdomyosarcoma, bone marrow ablation for stem cell transplantation
Mitomycin (Mutamycin)	Antitumor antibiotic	Acts as bifunctional alkylating agent, inhibiting DNA synthesis; cell cycle nonspecific, but most active in G and S phases	Hepatic biotransformation, renal elimination	Cumulative myelosuppression, extravasation, renal toxicity, pulmonary toxicity, cardiac toxicity, hemolytic-uremic syndrome	Prior treatment with vinca alkaloids may predispose to pulmonary toxicity; if used with doxorubicin, may potentiate cardiotoxicity	Gastric cancer, pancreatic cancer, anal cancer, lung cancer, head and neck cancer, cervical cancer

Drug	Classification	Mechanism of Action	Metabolism/Elimination	Toxicity	Drug Interactions	Clinical Use
Oxaliplatin (Eloxatin)	Platinum coordination compound	Produces interstrand DNA cross-links similar to bifunctional alkylating agents; cell cycle nonspecific	Renal	Nephrotoxicity, neurotoxicity (worse with cold), allergic reactions	Avoid other nephrotoxic drugs, incompatible with 5-fluorouracil	Colorectal cancer
Procarbazine (Matulane)	Nonclassic alkylating agent and MAO inhibitor	Unknown; metabolism produces highly active free radicals that may alkylate and methylate DNA; cell cycle specific, S phase	Renal 70% after hepatic biotransformation	Disulfiram (Antabuse)-like side effects with alcohol ingestion; patients should avoid foods containing tyramine due to the drug's MAO inhibitory effects; central and peripheral neurotoxicity, hepatotoxicity, pulmonary toxicity	>100, including alcohol, antihistamines, anticoagulants, anticonvulsants, hypoglycemics, certain antihypertensives, caffeine-containing preparations, narcotics, methyldopa, metrizamide, sympathomimetics, tyramine or other high pressor amine-containing foods	Hodgkin's disease, brain tumors
Streptozocin (Zanosar)	Nitrosourea	Inhibits DNA synthesis	Renal	Cumulative, dose-related renal toxicity, hepatotoxicity, glucose intolerance	None	Islet cell tumors of pancreas, carcinoid tumors
Temozolomide (Temodar)	Nonclassic alkylating agent	Inhibits DNA and RNA synthesis via formation of carbonium ions; cell cycle nonspecific	Hepatic biotransformation, renal excretion	Photosensitivity	None	Melanoma, brain tumors

DIFFERENTIATING AGENTS

Drug	Classification	Mechanism of Action	Metabolism/Elimination	Toxicity	Drug Interactions	Clinical Use
All-*trans*-retinoic acid (ATRA)	Retinoid	Induces differentiation and/or inhibition of clonogenicity	Conjugation to glucuronic acid with subsequent biliary excretion and enterohepatic circulation	Mucocutaneous toxicity, ocular toxicity, musculoskeletal toxicity, neurologic toxicity, hepatotoxicity, lipid toxicity	None	Acute progranulocytic leukemia
Arsenic trioxide (Trisenox)	Natural product	Induces differentiation of acute progranulocytic leukemia cells	Hepatic metabolism, excreted in urine	Prolonged QT interval, acute progranulocytic leukemia differentiation syndrome, leukocytosis, peripheral neuropathy	Medications that increase QT interval, such as antiarrhythmics and amphotericin	Acute progranulocytic leukemia

ENZYMES

Drug	Classification	Mechanism of Action	Metabolism/Elimination	Toxicity	Drug Interactions	Clinical Use
L-Asparaginase (Elspar)	Enzyme	Hydrolyzes l-asparagine to aspartic acid and ammonia, resulting in cellular deficiency of l-asparagine; sensitive tumor cells lack asparagine synthetase; interferes with protein, DNA, and RNA synthesis; cell cycle specific for G1 phase of cell division	Metabolized in liver	Hypersensitivity reactions, inhibitory effects on protein synthesis with resultant decreases in hepatic synthesis of coagulation factors, pancreatitis, hyperglycemia, CNS depression, hepatotoxicity	Abolishes effects of methotrexate on malignant cells; concurrent vincristine may enhance hyperglycemic effects of asparaginase and increase risk of neuropathy	Acute lymphoblastic leukemia

ANTIMETABOLITES

Drug	Classification	Mechanism of Action	Metabolism/Elimination	Toxicity	Drug Interactions	Clinical Use
5-Azacitidine (Vidaza)	Antimetabolite; pyrimidine nucleoside analogue of cytidine	Causes hypomethylation of DNA and direct cytotoxicity on abnormal hematopoietic cells	Hepatic metabolism, excreted in urine	Renal toxicity, low serum bicarbonate levels	None	Myelodysplasia
Capecitabine (Xeloda)	Antimetabolite of pyrimidine analogue type	Fluoropyrimidine carbamate prodrug form of 5-fluorouracil; given orally; inactive as itself; inhibits DNA and RNA synthesis; cell cycle specific, S phase	Hepatic catabolism	Hand and foot syndrome, angina	Warfarin potentiation, phenytoin, antacids, leucovorin, thymidine	Breast cancer, colorectal cancer

TABLE 182-6 CHEMOTHERAPEUTIC AGENTS—cont'd

AGENT	CLASS	ACTION	EXCRETION	UNIQUE SIDE EFFECTS	DRUG INTERACTIONS	INDICATIONS
Cladribine (Leustatin), 2-chloro-2-deoxy-D-adenosine	Antimetabolite	Purine nucleoside analogue, inhibits both DNA synthesis and repair	Uncertain	Bone marrow suppression, fever, paralysis, and/or acute renal failure when used at very high doses for BMT	None known	Hairy cell leukemia
Clofarabine (Clofar)	Purine nucleoside antimetabolite	Inhibits DNA synthesis and DNA repair	Excreted in urine and other?	Bone marrow suppression, hepatotoxicity	Other renal and hepatotoxic drugs	Relapsed acute lymphoblastic leukemia
Cytarabine (Cytosar-U, Tarabine PFS)	Antimetabolite	Activated to cytarabine triphosphate in tissues, inhibits DNA synthesis; cell cycle specific, S phase	Deaminated in blood and tissues	Pancreatitis; with high doses, cerebral dysfunction, GI damage, hepatotoxicity, pulmonary edema, corneal damage, "Ara-C syndrome"	With high-dose cyclophosphamide, may increase cardiotoxicity	Acute granulocytic leukemia and its variants, non-Hodgkin's lymphoma, myelodysplasia*
Fludarabine phosphate (Fludara)	Antimetabolite of purine type	2-Fluoro-ara-ATP inhibits DNA synthesis by inhibition of ribonucleotide reductase and the DNA polymerases; cell cycle specific, S phase	Renal	Neurologic, pulmonary toxicity	None	CLL
Fluorouracil (5-FU, Adrucil)	Antimetabolite of pyrimidine analogue type	Inhibits DNA and RNA synthesis; cell cycle specific, S phase	Respiratory, small renal elimination	Cerebellar ataxia, myocardial ischemia	None	Breast cancer, GI cancers, head and neck cancer, bladder cancer, ovarian cancer, endometrial cancer, effusions
Floxuridine (FUDR)	Antimetabolite of pyrimidine analogue type	Inhibits DNA and RNA synthesis; cell cycle specific, S phase	Respiratory, small renal elimination	Cerebellar ataxia, myocardial ischemia, hepatotoxicity	Leucovorin enhances activity and toxicity; thymidine rescues toxic effects	Intra-arterial therapy for hepatic malignancies
Hydroxyurea (Hydrea)	Antimetabolite	Inhibits ribonucleotide reductase, causing inhibition of DNA synthesis; cell cycle specific, S phase	Renal after hepatic biotransformation	Megaloblastosis	May enhance effects of anti-HIV drugs	Myeloproliferative neoplasms, ovarian cancer, head and neck cancer, cervical cancer (with radiation therapy)
Mercaptopurine (Purinethol, 6-MP)	Antimetabolite of purine analogue type	Inhibits DNA synthesis; cell cycle specific, S phase	Metabolic alteration by xanthine oxidase, renal excretion	Hepatotoxicity, skin rashes	Dose must be reduced when used with allopurinol; concomitant methotrexate enhances bioavailability of 6-MP; inhibits warfarin (Coumadin) effects	Acute lymphoblastic leukemia
Methotrexate (Folex, Mexate)	Antimetabolite of folic acid analogue type	Inhibits DNA, RNA, thymidylate, and protein synthesis as a result of binding to dihydrofolate reductase; cell cycle specific, S phase	Renal	Hepatotoxicity, lung disease; in high doses, acute renal failure, acute neurologic dysfunction; avoid use with ascites, pleural effusions	Salicylates, NSAIDs, folic acid-containing vitamins, oral nonabsorbable broad-spectrum antibiotics, trimethoprim/sulfamethoxazole, other nephrotoxic drugs	Breast cancer, head and neck cancer, choriocarcinoma, acute lymphoblastic leukemia, non-Hodgkin's lymphomas, osteosarcoma, intrathecal treatment of meningeal leukemia, bladder cancer, lung cancer
Pemetrexed (Alimta)	Antimetabolite of folic acid analogue type	Inhibits thymidylate synthetase, dihydrofolate reductase, and de novo purine synthesis; cell cycle specific, S phase	Renal, after hepatic metabolism	Must be given with folic acid and vitamin B$_{12}$; avoid use with ascites, pleural effusions	Salicylates, NSAIDs	Mesothelioma, breast cancer, lung cancer
Pentostatin (Nipent)	Purine antagonist	Inhibits adenosine deaminase; also inhibits RNA synthesis	Renal	Fever, fatigue, rash, pain, hepatotoxicity, chronic immunosuppression	Enhances effects of vidarabine, a purine nucleoside with antiviral activity; must not be given with fludarabine because of fatal pulmonary toxicity	Hairy cell leukemia, CLL
Pralatrexate (Fotolyn)	Antimetabolite type		Renal	Requires vitamin B$_{12}$ and folate supplementation	Myelosuppression	Relapsed peripheral T-cell lymphomas

NONCOVALENT DNA-BINDING DRUGS

Drug	Classification	Action	Metabolism	Toxicity	Interaction	Indications
Bleomycin (Blenoxane)	Antitumor antibiotic	Inhibition of DNA synthesis; most effective in G2 phase of cell division	Renal	Dose-related pulmonary fibrosis, hypersensitivity reactions, skin and mucocutaneous toxicity, including Raynaud's phenomenon (in combination with other agents), fever, chills; usually considered nonmyelosuppressive	Cisplatin may decrease renal clearance; high oxygen concentrations may enhance pulmonary toxicity, even after therapy	Testicular cancer and other germ cell tumors; Hodgkin's and non-Hodgkin's lymphomas; mycosis fungoides; squamous cell carcinomas of head and neck, cervix, and vulva; pleural effusions
Daunorubicin (Cerubidine)	Antitumor antibiotic	Binds to DNA by intercalation between base pairs and inhibits DNA and RNA synthesis by template disordering and steric obstruction; most active in S phase but not cell cycle phase specific	Hepatic biotransformation with 40% biliary excretion	Dose-related cardiotoxicity, extravasation, red urine	None	Acute granulocytic leukemia and its variants, acute lymphoblastic leukemia
Doxorubicin (Adriamycin, Rubex)	Antitumor antibiotic	Binds to DNA by intercalation between base pairs and inhibits DNA and RNA synthesis by template disordering and steric obstruction; cell cycle specific, S phase	Hepatic biotransformation with 50% biliary excretion	Dose-related cardiotoxicity, extravasation, red urine	None	Acute granulocytic leukemia and its variants, acute lymphoblastic leukemia, breast cancer, bladder cancer, ovarian cancer, thyroid cancer, lung cancer, Hodgkin's and non-Hodgkin's lymphomas, sarcomas, gastric cancer, multiple myeloma, endometrial cancer, bladder cancer, prostate cancer, Wilms' tumor, neuroblastoma
Doxorubicin liposomal (Doxil)	Anthracycline antibiotic	Topoisomerase inhibitor	Liver	Dose-related cardiotoxicity, extravasation, hand-foot syndrome	None	Ovarian cancer, myeloma, Kaposi's sarcoma
Epirubicin (Ellence)	Antitumor antibiotic	Intercalates with DNA	Liver	Dose-related cardiotoxicity	None	Breast cancer adjuvant therapy
Idarubicin (Idamycin)	Anthracycline glycoside	Intercalates DNA and inhibits DNA synthesis, interacts with RNA polymerases, and inhibits topoisomerase II	Hepatic biotransformation, biliary excretion	Dose-related cardiotoxicity, extravasation	None	Acute granulocytic leukemia and its variants
Mitoxantrone (Novantrone)	Antitumor antibiotic	Binds to DNA by intercalation between base pairs and nonintercalative electrostatic interaction, resulting in inhibition of DNA and RNA synthesis; not cell cycle specific, but most active in late S phase	Hepatic biotransformation, biliary/fecal excretion	Dose-related cardiotoxicity, extravasation, blue-green urine	None	Prostate cancer, acute myelogenous leukemia and its variants, breast cancer, non-Hodgkin's lymphomas

INHIBITORS OF CHROMATIN FUNCTION

Drug	Classification	Action	Metabolism	Toxicity	Interaction	Indications
Docetaxel (Taxotere)	Mitotic spindle poison	Unique mitotic spindle inhibitor; cell cycle specific, M phase	Hepatic metabolism, biliary	Hypersensitivity reactions, fluid retention syndrome, nail discoloration, neuropathy, arthralgias	Inhibitors or activators of liver cytochrome P-450 CYP34A enzyme system may affect metabolism	Breast cancer, prostate cancer, lung cancer, ovarian cancer, esophageal cancer, gastric cancer, head and neck cancer, bladder cancer
Etoposide (VP-16, VePesid)	Epipodophyllo toxin	Inhibits DNA synthesis; cell cycle dependent and phase specific, with maximum effect in S and G2 phases	Hepatic biotransformation, renal elimination	Allergic reactions, hepatotoxicity, CNS toxicity, hypotension	None	Testicular cancer, lung cancer, Hodgkin's and non-Hodgkin's lymphomas, choriocarcinoma, Ewing's sarcoma, acute granulocytic leukemia
Irinotecan (Camptosar)	Topoisomerase I inhibitor	Binds to topoisomerase I–DNA complex and prevents relegation of these single-strand breaks	Metabolized in liver	Early and late diarrhea may be severe	None	Colorectal cancer, small cell lung cancer

TABLE 182-6 CHEMOTHERAPEUTIC AGENTS—cont'd

AGENT	CLASS	ACTION	EXCRETION	UNIQUE SIDE EFFECTS	DRUG INTERACTIONS	INDICATIONS
Paclitaxel (Taxol)	Mitotic spindle poison	Unique mitotic spindle inhibitor; cell cycle specific, M phase	Hepatic metabolism, biliary	Hypersensitivity reactions, neuropathy, arthralgias, cardiotoxicity	Enhanced myelosuppression with doxorubicin	Lung cancer, ovarian cancer, breast cancer, esophageal cancer, gastric cancer, head and neck cancer
Paclitaxel protein-bound particles (Abraxane)	Mitotic spindle poison	Unique mitotic spindle inhibitor; cell cycle specific, M phase	Hepatic metabolism, biliary	Hypersensitivity reactions, neuropathy, arthralgias/myalgias, cardiotoxicity	Enhanced myelosuppression with doxorubicin	Metastatic breast cancer
Topotecan (Hycamtin)	Topoisomerase I inhibitor	Binds to topoisomerase I–DNA complex and prevents relegation of these single-strand breaks	Excreted unchanged in urine	—	None	Relapsed ovarian cancer, small cell lung cancer
Vinblastine (Velban)	Vinca alkaloid	Blocks mitosis by arresting cells in metaphase; cell cycle specific, M phase	Biliary/fecal	Extravasation, neurotoxicity	None	Testicular cancer, breast cancer, choriocarcinoma, Hodgkin's and non-Hodgkin's lymphomas, Kaposi's sarcoma, bladder cancer, neuroblastoma, renal carcinoma
Vincristine (Oncovin)	Vinca alkaloid	Blocks mitosis by arresting cells in metaphase; cell cycle specific, M phase	Biliary/fecal	Extravasation, neurotoxicity, constipation, SIADH	Concurrent use with L-asparaginase may increase neurotoxicity	Acute lymphocytic leukemia, neuroblastoma, Wilms' tumor, Hodgkin's and non-Hodgkin's lymphomas, rhabdomyosarcoma, Ewing's sarcoma, breast cancer, small cell lung cancer, multiple myeloma
Vinorelbine (Navelbine)	Vinca alkaloid	Inhibits tubulin polymerization, disrupting formation of microtubule assembly during mitosis; cell cycle specific, M phase	Biliary/fecal	Extravasation, neurotoxicity, constipation, SIADH	Drugs metabolized by liver P-450 system, phenytoin	Non–small cell lung cancer, breast cancer, non-Hodgkin's lymphomas
HORMONAL AGENTS						
Anastrozole (Arimidex)	Nonsteroidal aromatase inhibitor	Inhibits synthesis of estrogens by inhibiting conversion of adrenal androgens to estrogens	Metabolized in liver	Hot flashes, arthralgias	None	Adjuvant and metastatic breast cancer in postmenopausal women
Bicalutamide (Casodex)	Nonsteroidal antiandrogen	Binds to androgen receptors in prostate	Hepatic metabolism	Worsening bone pain, gynecomastia, hot flashes	None	Prostate cancer (usually in conjunction with LHRH antagonist)
Degarelix (Firmagon)	GnRH receptor antagonist	Binds to GnRH receptors in pituitary		Injection site reactions, increased LFTs, QT interval prolongation	None	Prostate cancer
Dexamethasone (Decadron)	Corticosteroid	Multiple	Renal excretion of inactive metabolites	Cushingoid appearance, hyperglycemia, fluid retention, osteoporosis, muscular weakness, peptic ulcer disease, cataracts, psychosis, aseptic necrosis	Efficacy impaired by phenytoin	Acute lymphoblastic leukemia, Hodgkin's and non-Hodgkin's lymphomas, CLL, multiple myeloma, Waldenström's macroglobulinemia, cerebral edema, hypercalcemia, lymphangitic metastases, antiemetic
Diethylstilbestrol (DES)	Estrogen	Stimulation of autocrine growth factors	Renal	Feminization in men, fluid retention, thromboembolic phenomena, induction of endometrial cancer	None	Breast cancer, prostate cancer

Drug	Classification	Mechanism of Action	Clearance/Metabolism	Toxicity	Drug Interactions	Indications
Estradiol	Estrogen	Stimulation of autocrine growth factors	Renal	Feminization in men, fluid retention, thromboembolic phenomena, induction of endometrial cancer	None	Breast cancer, prostate cancer
Estramustine (Emcyt)	Phosphorylated combination of estradiol and nitrogen mustard	Inhibits microtubule structure and function; cell cycle specific, M-phase	Biliary/fecal	Feminization, fluid retention	None	Prostate cancer
Estrogens (conjugated or esterified)	Estrogen	Stimulation of autocrine growth factors, inhibition of pituitary secretion of LH, resulting in decreased serum testosterone concentration	Primarily renal	Feminization in men, fluid retention, thromboembolic phenomena, induction of endometrial cancer	None	Breast cancer, prostate cancer
Exemestane (Aromasin)	Steroidal aromatase inhibitor	Permanently binds to and irreversibly inhibits aromatase, inhibits synthesis of estrogens by inhibiting conversion of adrenal androgens to estrogens	Metabolized in liver	Hot flashes, arthralgias	None	Metastatic breast cancer in postmenopausal women
Fluoxymesterone (Halotestin)	Androgen	Suppresses GnRH, LH, and FSH through negative feedback mechanism involving hypothalamus and anterior pituitary	Renal	Masculinization in women, hepatotoxicity	May increase anticoagulant effects of warfarin (Coumadin); decreased blood glucose, resulting in potential for hypoglycemia in diabetics	Breast cancer
Flutamide (Eulexin)	Antiandrogen	Inhibition of androgen uptake and/or inhibition of nuclear binding of androgen in target tissues; its interference with testosterone at cellular level complements "medical castration" produced by LHRH analogues	Renal	Worsening bone pain, hot flashes, gynecomastia	None	Prostate cancer (usually in conjunction with LHRH antagonist)
Fulvestrant (Faslodex)	Estrogen receptor antagonist	Competitively binds to estrogen receptor and downregulates estrogen receptor protein in breast cancer cells	Cleared by hepatobiliary route	Arthralgias	None	Recurrent breast cancer in postmenopausal women
Goserelin (Zoladex)	Synthetic decapeptide analogue of LHRH	Suppresses pituitary gonadotropins, with fall of serum testosterone into castrate range	Metabolism	Worsening bone pain, hot flashes	None	Breast cancer, prostate cancer
Letrozole (Femara)	Nonsteroidal competitive inhibitor of aromatase	Inhibits synthesis of estrogens by inhibiting conversion of adrenal androgens to estrogens	Metabolized in liver	Hot flashes, arthralgias	None	Adjuvant and metastatic breast cancer in postmenopausal women
Leuprolide (Lupron, Lupron Depot)	Synthetic LHRH analogue	Suppresses secretion of GnRH, with resultant fall in testosterone secretion, producing "medical castration"	Metabolized in liver	Increased bone pain, hot flashes, thromboembolic phenomena	None	Prostate cancer, breast cancer
Medroxyprogesterone (Provera, Depo-Provera)	Progestational drug	Inhibition of pituitary gonadotropin production with resultant decrease in estrogen secretion	Renal	Weight gain, thromboembolic phenomena, fetal hazard	None	Breast cancer, endometrial cancer
Megestrol acetate (Megace)	Progestational drug	Inhibition of pituitary gonadotropin production, with resultant decrease in estrogen secretion	Renal	Weight gain, thromboembolic phenomena, fetal hazard	None	Breast cancer, endometrial cancer

TABLE 182-6   CHEMOTHERAPEUTIC AGENTS—cont'd

AGENT	CLASS	ACTION	EXCRETION	UNIQUE SIDE EFFECTS	DRUG INTERACTIONS	INDICATIONS
Nilutamide (Nilandron)	Nonsteroidal antiandrogen	Binds to androgen receptors in prostate, inhibiting androgen uptake and binding in nucleus	Hepatic metabolism	Worsening bone pain, gynecomastia, hot flashes, visual disturbances, interstitial pneumonitis	Increased warfarin effect; inhibits liver cytochrome P-450 system; increased risk of alcohol intolerance	Prostate cancer (usually in conjunction with LHRH antagonist)
Octreotide (Sandostatin)	Synthetic octapeptide analogue of somatostatin	Suppresses secretion of serotonin and GI peptides; blocks carcinoid flush, decreases serum 5-HIAA, and controls other symptoms associated with carcinoid syndrome	Renal	Hyper/hypoglycemia, hepatic dysfunction	None	Palliative treatment of carcinoid tumors and vasoactive intestinal peptide tumors (VIPomas)
Prednisone (Deltasone)	Corticosteroid	Multiple	Renal excretion of inactive metabolites	Cushingoid appearance, hyperglycemia, fluid retention, osteoporosis, muscular weakness, peptic ulcer disease, cataracts, psychosis, aseptic necrosis	Efficacy impaired by phenytoin	Acute lymphoblastic leukemia, Hodgkin's and non-Hodgkin's lymphomas, CLL, multiple myeloma, Waldenström's macroglobulinemia, cerebral edema, hypercalcemia, lymphangitic metastases, antiemetic
Tamoxifen (Nolvadex)	Nonsteroidal antiestrogen	Competes with estradiol for estrogen receptor protein	In feces, mainly as conjugates	Hot flashes, nausea/vomiting, vaginal bleeding or discharge, hypercalcemia, visual disturbances, thrombocytopenia, endometrial cancer, rare liver dysfunction	When used with coumarin anticoagulants, significant increase in anticoagulant effect may be seen	Adjuvant and metastatic breast cancer

BIOLOGIC RESPONSE MODIFIERS

AGENT	CLASS	ACTION	EXCRETION	UNIQUE SIDE EFFECTS	DRUG INTERACTIONS	INDICATIONS
Aldesleukin (Human Recombinant IL-2, Proleukin)	Lymphokine	Supports T-cell proliferation, augments natural killer cytotoxicity, induces lymphokine-activated killer (LAK) cell development, and participates in activation of monocytes and B cells	Renal	Cardiovascular toxicity, nephrotoxicity, pulmonary toxicity, GI toxicity, endocrine toxicity, dermatologic complications, CNS toxicity, hematologic toxicity, fever and chills, infection, capillary leak syndrome	May potentiate effects of psychotropics, nephrotoxic drugs, and antihypertensive agents; corticosteroids may reduce effectiveness	Renal cancer, melanoma
Erythropoietin (Aranesp, Epogen, Procrit)[†]	Hematopoietic growth factor	Stimulates division and differentiation of committed erythroid progenitors in bone marrow	Metabolized in liver	Headache, hypertension, possible seizures, allergic reactions	None	Correction of anemia in chronic renal failure, azathioprine-treated HIV infection, myelodysplasia, multiple myeloma, chemotherapy-induced anemia
Filgrastim (G-CSF, Neupogen)	Class II hematopoietic growth factor (acts on progenitor cells capable of forming only one differentiated cell type, the neutrophil)	CSFs bind to specific cell surface receptors and stimulate proliferation and differentiation	Metabolized in liver	Pain at site of subcutaneous injection, allergic reactions, arthralgias, bone pain	None	Decreases incidence of infection after myelosuppressive chemotherapy, enhances myeloid engraftment after BMT, enhances peripheral progenitor cell yield
Interferon-α (Intron-A, Roferon)[†]	Interferon	Antiviral, antiproliferative, and immunomodulatory properties	Renal	Fever, flu-like symptoms, cardiotoxicity, neurotoxicity	None	Hairy cell leukemia, Kaposi's sarcoma, renal cancer, non-Hodgkin's lymphoma

Agent	Classification	Mechanism of Action	Metabolism	Toxicity	Drug Interactions	Indications
Sargramostim (GM-CSF, Leukine, Prokine)§	Class I hematopoietic growth factor (stimulates formation of granulocytes and macrophages and is not lineage specific)	CSFs bind to specific cell surface receptors and stimulate proliferation and differentiation	Metabolized in liver	Fever, capillary leak syndrome, pain at site of subcutaneous injection, allergic reactions, arthralgias, bone pain	None	Decreases incidence of infection after myelosuppressive chemotherapy; enhances myeloid engraftment after BMT, enhances peripheral progenitor cell yield
TARGETED AGENTS						
Alemtuzumab (Campath)	Humanized monoclonal antibody	Targets CD52 antigen present on surface of most normal lymphocytes and malignant B and T lymphocytes	Metabolism unclear	Hypersensitivity reactions, immunosuppressive	None	Relapsed B-cell CLL, T-cell prolymphocytic leukemia
Bevacizumab (Avastin)	Recombinant humanized monoclonal antibody to VEGF; inhibits angiogenesis	Binds to all human forms of VEGF, preventing it from binding to its receptors, reducing blood vessel formation	Metabolized	Hemorrhage, hypertension, proteinuria, thrombophlebitis	SN-38 metabolite of irinotecan is higher with concurrent use	Metastatic colorectal cancer, lung cancer, breast cancer
Bortezomib (Velcade)	Targeted agent	Reversible inhibitor of 26S proteasome; inhibits breakdown of ubiquitinated intracellular proteins and disrupts ubiquitin-proteasome pathway, eventually leading to apoptosis	Undergoes oxidative metabolism via cytochrome P-450 enzymes	Myelosuppression, peripheral neuropathy, asthenia, hypotension	Unknown	Relapsed multiple myeloma
Cetuximab (Erbitux)	Chimeric monoclonal antibody targeted against EGFR	Blocks growth factor from binding to EGFR, preventing cell signaling by tyrosine kinase phosphorylation	Metabolized	Hypersensitivity reactions, rash, diarrhea	None	Metastatic colorectal cancer
Dasatinib (Sprycel)	Multitargeted TKI	Inhibits multiple kinases	Metabolized by P-450 microenzyme CYP3A4	Myelosuppression	Multiple	Resistant/refractory CML
Erlotinib (Tarceva)	Targeted agent	Inhibits tyrosine kinase domain of EGFR	Metabolized	Rash, diarrhea, interstitial lung disease	CYP3A4 inducers and inhibitors may alter metabolism	Second- or third-line non–small cell lung cancer
Everolimus (Affinitor)	mTOR inhibitor	Inhibits mTOR	Metabolized by CYP3A4 in liver		CYP3A4 inhibitors/inducers, grapefruit juice	Renal cell carcinoma
Imatinib (Gleevec)	Targeted agent; signal transduction inhibitor	Inhibits BCR-ABL tyrosine kinase	Hepatic metabolism, excreted in feces	Myelosuppression, hypophosphatemia, fluid retention	Drugs inhibiting/stimulating liver microsomal CYP3A4 enzyme	CML, GISTs
Lapatinib (Tykerb)	Tyrosine kinase inhibitor	TKIs of EGFR and HER2/neu inhibitors/inducers	Metabolized by CYP3A4	Diarrhea, hand-foot syndrome	Capecitabine, CYP3A4	HER2/neu+ breast cancer
Lenalidomide§ (Revlimid, CC-5013)	Targeted agent	Induces apoptosis	Renal excretion	Neutropenia, thrombocytopenia, diarrhea, pruritus, rash, fatigue, leg cramps	Other myelosuppressive agents	Myelodysplasia, myeloma
Nexavar (Sorafenib)	Targeted agent	Multikinase inhibitor, inhibits RAF kinase, VEGF, and PDGF receptors	Hepatic	Rash, hand-foot syndrome, fatigue, diarrhea, hair loss	CYP2C9 inducers, UGT1A1 pathway-excreted agents	Renal cell carcinoma
Nilotinib (Tasigna)	Tyrosine kinase inhibitor	Inhibits ATP site of ABL	Metabolized in liver	Prolonged QTc interval	CYP3A 4 inhibitors/inducers (irinotecan)	Resistant/intolerant CML
Ofatumumab (Arzerra)	Monoclonal antibody	Anti-CD20 antibody	Metabolized	Infusion reactions, infections	None	Resistant CLL
Pazopanib (Votrient)	Tyrosine kinase inhibitor	Inhibits multiple TKIs	Metabolized	Hepatotoxicity	CYP3A4 inducers/inhibitors	Renal cell cancer
Rituximab (Rituxan)	Chimeric anti-CD20 antibody	Targets CD20 antigen expressed on lymphocytes	Metabolized	Hypersensitivity reactions, lymphopenia	None	Relapsed low-grade non-Hodgkin's lymphomas

TABLE 182-6 CHEMOTHERAPEUTIC AGENTS—cont'd

AGENT	CLASS	ACTION	EXCRETION	UNIQUE SIDE EFFECTS	DRUG INTERACTIONS	INDICATIONS
Sunitinib (Sutent)	Multitargeted TKI	Inhibits TKIs and angiogenesis	Metabolized by P-450	Bleeding, CHF, prolonged QTc	CYP3A4 inhibitors/inducers	GIST, renal cell cancer
Temsirolimus (Torisel)	mTOR inhibitor	Inhibits mTOR kinase responsible for cell division	Metabolized in liver	Bowel perforation, interstitial lung disease	Affected by CYP3A4 inhibitors/inducers	Renal cell cancer
Thalidomide (Thalomid)	Immunomodulatory agent, antigenic agent	Inhibits TNF-α, may inhibit angiogenesis through inhibition of bFGF and VEGF	Nonenzymatic hydrolysis	Teratogenicity, sedation, constipation, peripheral neuropathy, rash	Sedation enhanced with alcohol, other sedatives	Multiple myeloma
Trastuzumab (Herceptin)	Recombinant humanized monoclonal antibody against HER2/neu	Downregulates expression of ERBB2 pathways	Metabolized	Hypersensitivity reactions	Increased risk of cardiotoxicity when used with anthracyclines or taxanes	Metastatic or adjuvant HER2/neu+ breast cancer

DRUGS TO OFFSET SIDE EFFECTS OF CHEMOTHERAPY

AGENT	CLASS	ACTION	EXCRETION	UNIQUE SIDE EFFECTS	DRUG INTERACTIONS	INDICATIONS
Amifostine (Ethyol)	Cytoprotectant	Free thiol metabolites	Metabolized	Nausea/vomiting, Hypertension	Hypertension	Reduces renal toxicity from cisplatin
Dexrazoxane (Zinecard)	Cardioprotector	Unclear	Excreted in urine	Myelosuppression		Reduces cardiotoxicity
Leucovorin (folinic acid, citrovorum factor, Wellcovorin)	Water-soluble folate vitamin	Increases general body pool of reduced folates	Metabolized in liver	None	In large amounts may counteract action of anticonvulsives	Prophylaxis and treatment of hematopoietic side effects of folic acid antagonists
Kepivance (Palifermin)	Keratinocyte growth factor	Stimulates growth of epithelial cells?		Rash	Heparin, myelotoxic chemotherapy	Decreases mucositis after BMT
Mesna (Mesnex)	Synthetic sulfhydryl compound	Only metabolite, mesna disulfide, reacts chemically with urotoxic ifosfamide metabolites, resulting in their detoxification	Renal	Bad taste, diarrhea	None	Prophylaxis of cyclophosphamide/ifosfamide-induced hemorrhagic cystitis

*An intrathecal formulation, DepoCyt, is used for the treatment of carcinomatous meningitis.

†Dosing differs among agents.

‡Dosages differ among brands.

§An analogue of thalidomide, which is a severe human teratogen; restricted prescribing.

ATP = adenosine triphosphate; bFGF, basic fibroblast growth factor; BMT = bone marrow transplantation; CHF = congestive heart failure; CLL = chronic lymphocytic leukemia; CML = chronic myelogenous leukemia; CNS = central nervous system; CSF = colony-stimulating factor; EGFR = epidermal growth factor receptor; ERBB2 = HER2/neu; FSH = follicle-stimulating hormone; G-CSF = granulocyte colony-stimulating factor; GM-CSF = granulocyte-macrophage colony-stimulating factor; GI = gastrointestinal; GIST = gastrointestinal stromal tumor; GnRH = gonadotropin-releasing hormone; 5-HIAA = 5-hydroxyindolacetic acid; HIV = human immunodeficiency virus; IL = interleukin; LFT = liver function test; LH = luteinizing hormone; LHRH = luteinizing hormone–releasing hormone; MAO = monoamine oxidase; mTOR = mammalian target of rapamycin; NSAID = nonsteroidal anti-inflammatory drug; PDGF = platelet-derived growth factor; SIADH = syndrome of inappropriate secretion of antidiuretic hormone; TKI = tyrosine kinase inhibitor; TNF = tumor necrosis factor; VEGF = vascular endothelial growth factor.

Visual Analogue Pain Scale

What does your pain feel like?

0	1	2	3	4	5	6	7	8	9	10
None		Mild			Moderate			Very bad		Unbearable

FIGURE 182-1. Grading pain in cancer patients.

RANK ligand, a protein found on osteoclasts and involved in bone breakdown. It is administered subcutaneously. Some clinical trials have found denosumab to be superior to zoledronic acid for the prevention of skeletal-related events in cancer patients with bone metastases.[8]

Hematologic malignancies and chemosensitive solid tumors should be treated with prophylactic allopurinol to prevent gout and renal colic from hyperuricemia. The acute tumor lysis syndrome can be defined by laboratory findings—elevated levels of uric acid, potassium, and phosphorus and decreased levels of calcium—or clinically—elevated creatinine, cardiac arrhythmias or sudden death, and seizures. The effects can be minimized by the use of allopurinol, vigorous hydration, and rasburicase and by the careful assessment of serum electrolytes, but anticipating the possibility of its occurrence is the best strategy.

1. Zeppetella G, Ribeiro MD. Opioids for the management of breakthrough (episodic) pain in cancer patients. *Cochrane Database Syst Rev.* 2006;1:CD004311.
2. Worthington HV, Clarkson JE, Bryan G, et al. Interventions for preventing oral mucositis for patients with cancer receiving treatment. *Cochrane Database Syst Rev.* 2010;12:CD000978.
3. Clarkson JE, Worthington HV, Furness S, et al. Interventions for treating oral mucositis for patients with cancer receiving treatment. *Cochrane Database Syst Rev.* 2010;8:CD001973.
4. Worthington HV, Clarkson JE, Khalid T, et al. Interventions for treating oral candidiasis for patients with cancer receiving treatment. *Cochrane Database Syst Rev.* 2010;7:CD001972.
5. Sung L, Nathan PC, Alibhai SM, et al. Meta-analysis: effect of prophylactic hematopoietic colony-stimulating factors on mortality and outcomes of infection. *Ann Intern Med.* 2007;147:400-411.
6. Bucaneve G, Micozzi A, Menichetti F, et al. Levofloxacin to prevent bacterial infection in patients with cancer and neutropenia. *N Engl J Med.* 2005;353:977-987.
7. Cullen M, Steven N, Billingham L, et al. Antibacterial prophylaxis after chemotherapy for solid tumors and lymphomas. *N Engl J Med.* 2005;353:988-998.
8. Fizazi K, Carducci M, Smith M, et al. Denosumab versus zoledronic acid for treatment of bone metastases in men with castration-resistant prostate cancer: a randomized, double-blind study. *Lancet.* 2011;377:785-786.

SUGGESTED READINGS

Aapro MS, Bohlius J, Cameron DA, et al. 2010 update of EORTC guidelines for the use of granulocyte-colony stimulating factor to reduce the incidence of chemotherapy-induced febrile neutropenia in adult patients with lymphoproliferative disorders and solid tumours. *Eur J Cancer.* 2011;47:8-32. *Consensus guidelines recommending their use in patients with ≥20% chance of developing febrile neutropenia.*

Behl D, Hendrickson AW, Moynihan TJ. Oncologic emergencies. *Crit Care Clin.* 2010;26:181-205. *Review including metabolic, cardiac, neurologic, and infectious disorders.*

García Gómez J, Pérez López ME, García Mata J, et al. SEOM clinical guidelines for the treatment of antiemetic prophylaxis in cancer patients receiving chemotherapy. *Clin Transl Oncol.* 2010;12:770-774. *Consensus guidelines.*

Mitera G, Swaminath A, Wong S, et al. Radiotherapy for oncologic emergencies on weekends: examining reasons for treatment and patterns of practice at a Canadian cancer centre. *Curr Oncol.* 2009;16:55-60. *The top reasons for emergency weekend treatment included spinal cord compression (56%), brain metastases (15%), and superior vena cava obstruction (6%).*

National Cancer Institute's Patient Data Query (PDQ). Current version of therapy for cancers and hematologic malignancies, updated every three months. *www.cancer.gov.* Accessed March 9, 2011. *Addresses common management issues.*

Soussain C, Richard D, Fike JR, et al. CNS complications of radiotherapy and chemotherapy. *Lancet.* 2009;374:1639-1651. *Review.*

Swarm R, Abernethy AP, Anghelescu DL, et al. Adult cancer pain. *J Natl Compr Canc Netw.* 2010;8:1046-1086. *Comprehensive review.*

EPIDEMIOLOGY OF CANCER

MICHAEL J. THUN AND AHMEDIN JEMAL

EPIDEMIOLOGY

Overview

All cancers combined account for about 23% of deaths in the United States, placing cancer second only to heart disease as a cause of death. Cancer has also become the second leading cause of death worldwide after heart diseases, owing to increasing longevity, the global dispersion of tobacco use, and Western patterns of diet, physical inactivity, and reproduction. At current rates, nearly one in two men and more than one in three women in the United States will be diagnosed with cancer at some point in life. The National Institutes of Health estimates that the overall costs of cancer in 2008 equaled $228.1 billion.

Research has identified the causes of many types of cancer as well as basic mechanisms that drive carcinogenesis. Various control measures have reduced exposure to tobacco (Chapter 31) and occupational carcinogens (Chapter 18) in most industrialized countries. These advances in prevention, together with progress in early detection and treatment, have achieved a nearly 16% reduction in the death rate from all cancers combined in the United States from 1991 to 2006, and a 6% reduction in the incidence rate from 1999 to 2006.

Measures of Occurrence and Survival
Incidence and Death Rates

Cancer *incidence* and *death rates* are usually expressed per 100,000 people per year and are age-standardized to allow valid comparisons across populations of different sizes and age structures. Age-standardized rates must be standardized to the same age distribution in order for different time periods and geographic areas to be comparable. Conventionally, rates within the United States are standardized to the age distribution of the U.S. population (currently the year 2000 age standard), whereas international comparisons are based on the world population standard in 1960. Data on cancer incidence rates in the United States are collected by population-based tumor registries that now encompass 92% of the population. Temporal trends in cancer incidence have been monitored since 1973 in 10% of the population by the National Cancer Institute (NCI) Surveillance, Epidemiology, and End Results (SEER) program. Deaths from cancer have been tabulated nationally in U.S. vital statistics since 1930. Mortality rates are based on the underlying cause of death as coded from death certificates using systematic nosologic rules. Validation studies have documented that, despite the well-known limitations of death certificates, there is greater than 90% agreement between the clinical diagnosis and the underlying cause of death coded systematically from death certificates for the 17 cancer sites that represent more than two thirds of cancers in the United States.

Relative Survival

Survival in patients with cancer is usually expressed as *relative survival,* which compares the percentage of cancer patients alive after a designated period (often 5 years) with the corresponding percentage in a population without cancer but of similar age, race, and sex. A *relative survival* of 100% signifies that cancer patients have the same survival as people of the same age without cancer. *Relative survival* is different from *absolute survival* in that the latter reflects death from any condition, whether or not it relates to cancer. Trends in *relative survival* have been monitored by the NCI SEER program since 1975. Relative survival has improved substantially for many types of cancer (Table 183-1). Caution is advised, however, in interpreting trends in relative survival for cancer sites detected by screening because of the potential for lead-time bias (see Screening).

Cumulative Incidence

The terms *cumulative incidence* and *cumulative risk* describe the average probability of developing or dying from a specified condition (in this case all cancers or specific cancer sites) over a defined period. Annual incidence and death rates per 100,000 people per year (or alternatively per 1 million

TABLE 183-1 RELATIVE 5-YEAR SURVIVAL RATES* (%) FOR SELECTED CANCER SITES DURING THREE TIME PERIODS, UNITED STATES, SEER

SITE	1975-1977	1984-1986	1999-2005
All sites	50	53	67
Breast (female)	75	79	89
Colon	51	59	67
Leukemia	35	42	54
Lung and bronchus	13	13	16
Melanoma of the skin	82	86	93
Non-Hodgkin lymphoma	48	53	69
Ovary	37	40	46†
Pancreas	2	3	6
Prostate	69	76	100
Rectum	49	57	66
Urinary bladder	73	78	82

*Five-year relative survival rates based on follow-up of patients through 2005.
†Recent changes in the classification of ovarian cancer have affected 1996 to 2005 survival rates.
From Surveillance, Epidemiology and End Results Program (SEER), 1975-2006, Division of Cancer Control and Population Sciences, National Cancer Institute, 2009.

people per year for childhood cancers) correspond to 1-year cumulative risks. The cumulative risk of developing or dying from cancer increases with age. Lifetime cumulative incidence is strongly influenced by life expectancy; improvements in longevity increase the cumulative risk of developing cancer, even if the annual incidence and death rates at every age remain the same.

Geographic Variation

Cancer occurs in all countries of the world, although the predominant types of cancer vary widely (E-Table 183-1). In general, cancers caused by chronic infections (e.g., stomach, liver, cervix) predominate in economically developing countries, whereas those related to Western patterns of tobacco use and diet (lung, breast, prostate, and colon) are most common in high-resource countries. Some of the geographic variation reflects differences in diagnostic capabilities and data quality, yet much of the difference is real, reflecting geographic variation in causal factors. The regional cancer registries that provide these data are maintained by the International Agency for Research on Cancer (IARC), which makes special efforts to improve the completeness of registration. The international variation in cancer occurrence has historically provided important evidence that much of the disease burden from cancer is caused by exposures rather than inherited genetic susceptibility and could, in principle, be prevented.

Lung cancer (Chapter 197) is the most common cancer worldwide in terms of both new cases and deaths. The incidence rate varies from more than 70 per 100,000 among men in Eastern Europe to less than 5 per 100,000 among men in West Africa. The geography of lung cancer principally reflects the progression of populations through the stages of the tobacco epidemic. Within a country, the uptake of smoking manufactured cigarettes typically begins among middle-aged men and then spreads progressively to younger men and women. The resulting increase in lung cancer begins 25 to 30 years later and continues until publicity about the adverse effects of smoking and tobacco control measures cause a downturn in smoking, which is later followed by a downturn in lung cancer.

Breast cancer (Chapter 204) is the most common incident cancer in women worldwide. Incidence rates have increased, even in developing countries, but continue to be about five times higher in North America, Europe, and other Western industrial countries than among women in rural Asia. Increased longevity and the widespread use of screening contribute to the high lifetime risk (12.7%) of breast cancer among women in the United States, as does the prevalence of risk factors such as delayed childrearing, excess body weight, physical inactivity, and hormone use.

Prostate cancer (Chapter 207) is the second most commonly diagnosed cancer in men globally, with nearly three fourths of all cases diagnosed in economically developed countries. Incidence rates are especially high in the United States because of widespread screening with prostate-specific antigen

(PSA), which finds tumors that might otherwise be missed. In contrast, the much higher incidence and death rates among men of African descent in Africa, the Caribbean, and the United States represents a true disparity that is currently unexplained.

Cancers of the colon and rectum (Chapter 199) are more common in economically developed than in developing countries. The incidence rate in the United States is 20 to 30 times higher than in rural India and Southeast Asia. Risk factors thought to contribute to the geographic variation include obesity, physical inactivity, high consumption of red and processed meat, cigarette smoking, and heavy alcohol consumption.

The geographic distribution of several cancers caused by infectious agents or behavioral practices closely parallels the prevalence of the causal agent. For example, the high incidence of liver cancer (Chapter 202) in parts of Asia and sub-Saharan Africa matches the geographic patterns of *hepatitis B virus* (HBV) infection in childhood, just as mortality from stomach (Chapter 198) and cervical (Chapter 205) cancer correlates closely with the prevalence of infection with pathogenic strains of *Helicobacter pylori* and *human papillomavirus* (HPV), respectively. The exceptionally high incidence of oropharyngeal (Chapter 196) cancer throughout much of the Indian subcontinent and Southeast Asia is caused by the practice of chewing betel quid and areca nut, often mixed with tobacco. In contrast, it is not fully understood why squamous cell carcinoma of the esophagus (Chapter 198) was extraordinarily common until the late 20th century in countries surrounding the Caspian Sea. This was attributed to a combination of severe nutritional deficiency corresponding to a seasonal lack of vegetables and the practice of swallowing the charred residue from opium pipes. The incidence of this cancer has decreased rapidly over the past 20 years following improvement of the food supply. Other incompletely understood geographic variations involve why ovarian cancer (Chapter 205) is more common in certain European countries than in others, or how dietary consumption of salted fish may interact with Epstein-Barr virus (EBV) infections and genetic susceptibility to cause nasopharyngeal cancer (Chapter 196) in southern China and in Eskimos in Alaska and Greenland.

Geographic and demographic variations in cancer risk are seen for all cancers combined as well as for individual sites. An extreme example is that the cumulative incidence of being diagnosed with any type of cancer is almost ten times higher among African American men than men of similar age in parts of India. These large variations in overall cancer risk indicate that geographic variability does not simply reflect substitution of one form of cancer for another, but affects disease occurrence overall.

Temporal Variation

Temporal variations in the incidence or death rates from certain cancers further illustrate the importance of potentially modifiable "environmental" factors on the burden of disease. For example, the large changes in mortality from stomach and lung cancer among men and women in the United States (Fig. 183-1A and B) reflect changes in external exposure rather than inherited genetic susceptibility. Cancer of the stomach was one of the most common fatal cancers in the United States in 1930, as was cancer of the uterus (principally uterine cervix) in women. Mortality from these cancers has decreased dramatically over the past 75 years. The global decrease in stomach cancer (Chapter 198) probably reflects an unintended benefit of changes in food preservation and reduced prevalence of *H. pylori* infection. The advent of refrigeration increased the availability of fresh vegetables and fruit and decreased reliance on salted, smoked, and pickled foods, whereas improvements in sanitation and housing and widespread antibiotic use decreased the prevalence of chronic infection with *H. pylori*. Progress in reducing the incidence and death rate from cervical cancer (Chapter 205) is largely attributable to the introduction of Papanicolaou testing and early removal of premalignant and cancerous lesions. The close relationship between global trends in lung cancer (Chapter 197) and cigarette smoking was discussed previously.

Screening

Trends in cancer incidence rates are more difficult to interpret than trends in mortality, especially for sites that are detectable by screening. The introduction of a new screening test can create the appearance of a sudden increase in cancer incidence, especially when the test detects prevalent but undiagnosed tumors that would otherwise be missed. For example, a sudden increase in the incidence rate of prostate cancer (Chapter 207) in the United States in the late 1980s (Fig. 183-2A) coincided with the introduction of PSA screening. The upward trend reversed after 1992 because of saturation of

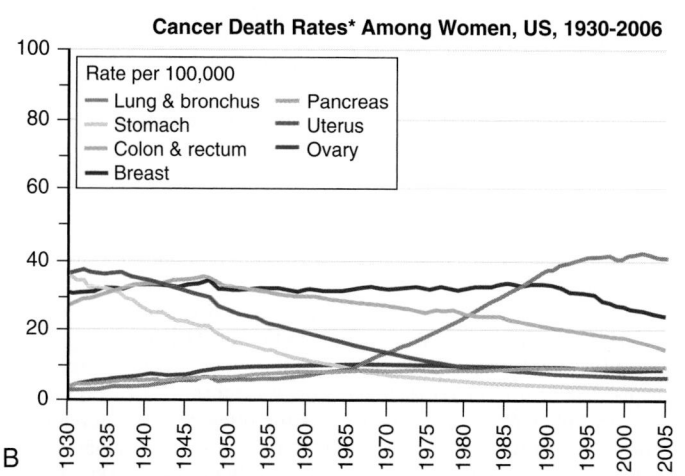

FIGURE 183-1. Cancer mortality rates. **A,** Temporal trends in cancer mortality rates, United States, 1930 to 2006, men. **B,** Temporal trends in cancer mortality rates, United States, 1930 to 2006, women. *Age-adjusted to the 2000 U.S. standard population. (Data from U.S. Mortality Data 1960-2005, U.S. Mortality Volumes 1930-1959, National Center for Health Statistics, Centers for Disease Control and Prevention, 2008.)

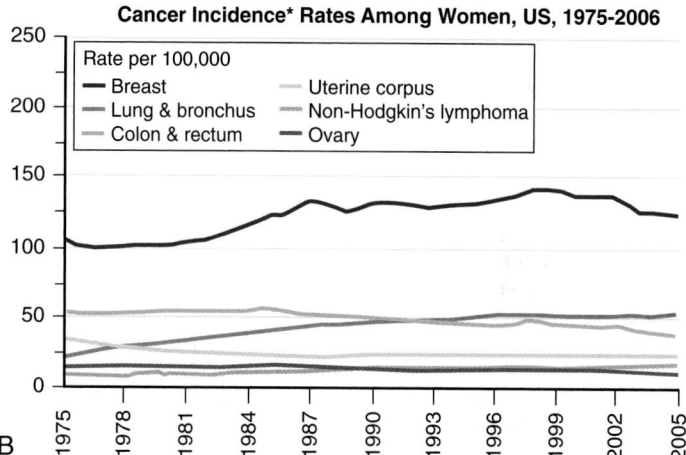

FIGURE 183-2. Cancer incidence rates. **A,** Temporal trends in cancer incidence rates adjusted for delayed reporting, Surveillance, Epidemiology, and End Results (SEER), 1975 to 2006, men. **B,** Temporal trends in cancer incidence rates adjusted for delayed reporting, SEER, 1975 to 2006, women. *Age-adjusted to the 2000 U.S. standard population and adjusted for delays in reporting. (Data from Surveillance, Epidemiology, and End Results Program, Delay-Adjusted Incidence Database: SEER Incidence Delay-Adjusted Rates, 9 Registries, 1975-2005, National Cancer Institute, 2008.)

screening among older men. The upward trend in reported incidence has since returned to the more gradual increase that prevailed before the introduction of PSA testing. Likewise, the introduction of mammography screening during the 1980s contributed to the increase in breast cancer incidence among women (see Fig. 183-2B), although the impact was considerably smaller than that of PSA screening on prostate cancer incidence (see Fig. 183-2A). The introduction of mammography had a much larger impact on the detection of ductal carcinoma in situ (DCIS), which is not included in the incidence rates, than invasive breast cancer.

The introduction of new screening tests also complicates the interpretation of temporal trends in *relative survival* among patients with cancer (see Table 183-1). Screening tests detect cancer earlier, before the tumor would otherwise have been diagnosed, thus creating an apparent lengthening of survival that exaggerates actual progress. This so-called lead-time bias can be difficult to separate completely from improvements in relative survival for sites that are commonly diagnosed by screening, such as breast and prostate cancer, even in analyses that stratify for stage at diagnosis. New screening tests can also alter the mix of cancers being diagnosed by increasing the detection of indolent tumors that may not be life-threatening. Advances in the molecular characterization of tumors may ultimately resolve this problem by providing more homogeneous groupings of tumors in which to measure relative survival.

Demographic Factors

Age

The incidence of most cancers increases exponentially with age from 10 to 84 years (Fig. 183-3). Age is a stronger predictor of cancer risk than any other factor. About three fourths (77%) of all cancers occur in the approximately 19% of the U.S. population 55 years or older. This age-related increase reflects the multistage nature of carcinogenesis and the time required for a single cell line to accumulate all the mutations and epigenetic events needed for malignant transformation (Chapter 185). The apparent decrease in the incidence of cancer after 85 years of age reflects incomplete diagnosis of cancer in elderly people as well as the fact that generations born before 1920 preceded the peak of cigarette smoking.

Age affects the types of cancer that occur as well as their frequency. In the United States, the five most common fatal cancers before age 20 are acute lymphocytic leukemia, cancer of the brain and other nervous system, bones and joints, endocrine system, and soft tissues. In women aged 20 to 59 years, breast cancer is the most common fatal cancer. At age 60 and older, the four most common cancers are lung and bronchus (Chapters 197), breast (Chapter 204), prostate (Chapter 207), and colon and rectum cancer (Chapter 199).

Sex

For most cancers that affect both sexes, the incidence rate is higher in men than women, the exceptions being cancers of the breast, thyroid, gallbladder, and anus. The incidence rate from all cancers combined is higher in men than women except in the age range of 30 to 54 years, when, because of breast cancer, women have higher incidence rates (see Fig. 183-3). The male excess for cancers of the oropharynx, esophagus, larynx, lung, pancreas, and kidney can be attributed to higher tobacco or alcohol use, or both. For other sites, such as brain, hematopoietic, and childhood cancers, however, the reasons for higher risk in men are unclear.

Cancer Incidence Rates* by Age and Sex, US, 1975-2005

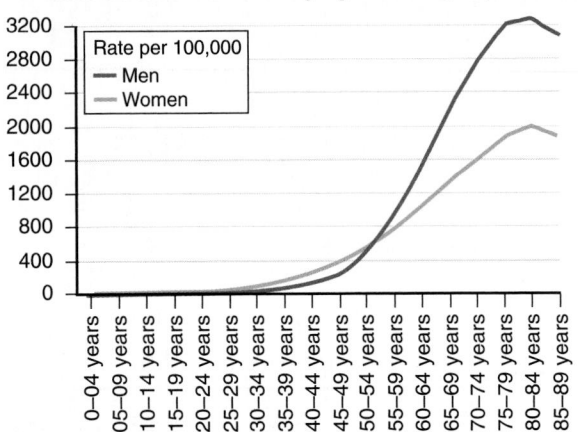

Rate per 100,000
— Men
— Women

FIGURE 183-3. Age- and sex-specific incidence rates for all cancer combined in the nine Surveillance, Epidemiology and End Results (SEER) areas. *Age-adjusted to the 2000 U.S. standard population. (Data from U.S. Mortality Data, National Center for Health Statistics.)

Socioeconomic Status, Race, and Ethnicity

African Americans experience disproportionately high incidence and death rates from most cancers. Racial disparities in death rates are largest for cancers of the prostate, stomach, larynx (men), myeloma, and uterine cervix. Relatively few studies have attempted to separate the impact of biologic differences associated with race from factors related to poverty and its effects on education, risk factors, and access to high-quality care for prevention, early detection, and treatment. Accumulating data suggest that socioeconomic factors account for most of these disparities (Chapter 5). For example, black women have the highest death rate from breast cancer among all racial or ethnic groups in the United States. Although the incidence rate is higher in white than in black women, this paradox likely results from underdiagnosis of breast cancer in black women. Survival among women with breast cancer is lower in black than in white women in the general population, but it is similar in military hospitals where both races have equal access to care. Relative survival is lower in African Americans than in whites for many other cancers, including prostate, uterine cervix and corpus, colon, and rectum cancer.

Other ethnic groups in the United States also have distinctive cancer patterns. Relative to whites, age-adjusted incidence and mortality rates among Hispanics are higher for gallbladder, stomach, and cervical cancer; those among American Indians are higher for cancer of the gallbladder, stomach, and cervix; rates in Japanese Americans are higher for stomach and liver cancer; those in Chinese Americans are higher for nasopharynx, liver, and stomach cancer; Native Hawaiians have higher death rates from breast, esophagus, liver, pancreas, lung, and cervical cancer; and Filipino Americans have a lower risk of most cancers except for cancers of the stomach, liver, oral cavity, and esophagus. Many of these ethnic differences are known to reflect differences in the use of tobacco, dietary habits, infectious exposure, or medical care. Research is needed to identify practical interventions to reduce these disparities.

Causes of Cancer

Whereas infectious diseases are defined by exposure to a specific microorganism, chronic diseases such as cancer may have multiple causes, none of which need be necessary or sufficient for the disease to occur (Table 183-2). For instance, tobacco smoking is the major cause of lung cancer, but it is neither necessary nor sufficient for the disease to occur. Approximately 10 to 15% of lung cancers occur in people who have never smoked actively, and in only about 20% of long-term cigarette smokers does lung cancer develop.

Tobacco

Exposure to tobacco (Chapter 31) is the single largest cause of cancer in the United States. Tobacco smoke contains more than 4000 chemicals, at least 40 of which are known to be carcinogenic in humans or animals, or both. All forms of tobacco can cause cancer. Cigarette smoking causes cancer of the lip, oral cavity, nasal cavity, paranasal sinuses, pharynx (nasal, oral, and hypopharynx), larynx, lung, esophagus (squamous cell and adenocarcinoma),

stomach, colorectum, pancreas, liver, kidney (adenocarcinoma and renal pelvis), urinary bladder, uterine cervix, and myeloid leukemia. Secondhand smoke, or environmental tobacco smoke, contains a similar mix of carcinogens as active smoking at varying concentrations. Each year in the United States, secondhand smoke causes an estimated 3000 deaths from lung cancer and 30,000 to 40,000 deaths from heart disease.

Diet, Obesity, Physical Inactivity

Other important modifiable determinants of cancer risk are dietary patterns, physical inactivity, and obesity. Approximately one third of cancer deaths in the United States are attributed to nutritional factors. Obesity, physical inactivity, and an excess of caloric intake over energy expenditure are known to increase the risk for several types of cancer. Obesity (Chapter 227) is causally related to cancer of the endometrium, kidney, breast (in postmenopausal but not premenopausal women), esophagus, colon (especially in men), and gallbladder (particularly in women). More limited evidence suggests that obesity may also increase the risk for cancer of the liver, pancreas, and stomach as well as some hematopoietic cancers. Excessive alcohol consumption (Chapter 32) is an established cause of cancer of the oropharynx, larynx, esophagus, and liver; even moderate drinking increases the risk for breast cancer. The importance of other specific components of diet to the risk for cancer in Western populations is more controversial. The strongest evidence pertains to increased risk for colon cancer in people who have inadequate intake of folic acid or excessive consumption of red or processed meat.

Infectious Agents

It is estimated that about 17% of cancer cases worldwide are attributable to infectious agents. This percentage is higher in economically developing (26%) than in developed (7.2%) countries. Viruses known to cause cancer in humans include *HPV* (Chapter 381), *hepatitis B virus (HBV)* (Chapter 151), *hepatitis C virus (HCV)* (Chapter 151), *EBV* (Chapter 385), *human immunodeficiency virus (HIV)* (Chapter 400), and *human herpesvirus-8* (Chapter 382). Viruses increase the risk for cancer through a variety of mechanisms, including direct effects on DNA, promotion of tumor development by means of chronic inflammation (*HPV, HBV, HCV*), or suppression of specific elements of the immune system (e.g., *HIV*) (Chapter 185).

H. pylori, which is the only bacterial infection known to cause cancer, is a gram-negative, spiral bacteria that colonizes the mucous layer of the stomach. Chronic inflammation caused by strains of *H. pylori* that express the CagA (a 128-kD cytotoxin-associated gene–A positive) protein promotes the development of gastric ulcers, gastric carcinoma, and mucosa-associated lymphoid tissue (MALT) lymphoma of the stomach (Chapter 198). Parasitic infections known to increase the risk for cancer include *Schistosoma haematobium* (Chapter 363) (bladder cancer) and liver flukes such as *Clonorchis sinensis* (Chapter 364) and *Opisthorchis viverrini* (Chapter 364) (biliary tract cancer, Chapter 202).

Ionizing Radiation

Ionizing radiation (Chapter 19) from x-rays, gamma radiation, and other sources is one of the most extensively studied human carcinogens. Leukemia and cancer of the thyroid and female breast are most strongly associated with radiation, although cancer of the lung, esophagus, stomach, colon, brain, and bladder and myeloma are also causally related. The risk for development of cancer from ionizing radiation depends not only on cumulative exposure but also on the intensity, rate, and nature of the exposure as well as on the age at which it occurs. Childhood exposure from medical treatments or fallout from atomic bombs or nuclear accidents principally increases the risk for leukemia and thyroid cancer. Girls exposed to radiation during adolescence and young adulthood are more susceptible to breast cancer from this exposure than are women exposed later in life. Radioactive isotopes such as iodine-131, radium-224, -226, and -236, and phosphorus-32 concentrate in the thyroid, bone, and bone marrow, respectively, and deliver high localized doses to radiosensitive tissues. Radon-222, a naturally occurring radioactive decay product of uranium-238, was first discovered to cause lung cancer in occupational studies of highly exposed uranium miners. Radon gas is also a common contaminant of household basements and unventilated underground spaces, albeit at much lower concentrations. Exposure to ultraviolet radiation from sunlight and tanning booths is the principal cause of melanoma as well as squamous and basal cell skin cancer. Nonionizing radiation, such as the electromagnetic frequency emissions from cell phones, has not been thought to cause cancer because the energy that is imparted to tissues is too weak to

TABLE 183-2 SELECTED KNOWN CAUSES OF CANCER AND THE ASSOCIATED CANCER SITES*

TOBACCO		RADIATION	
Active and passive smoking	Multiple sites: see text	**Nonionizing Radiation**	
Spit tobacco (snuff, chewing)	Oral cavity, pancreas	Broad-spectrum solar ultraviolet radiation	Skin
NUTRITION, OBESITY, PHYSICAL INACTIVITY, AND FOOD CONTAMINANTS		Sun lamps or sun beds	Skin, eye
Aflatoxins	Liver	**Ionizing Radiation**	
Alcohol	Mouth, pharynx, larynx, esophagus, breast,† liver†	X-radiation and gamma radiation	Leukemia, thyroid, breast, lung
		Radium	Bone sarcoma
Chinese salted fish†	Nasopharynx	Radon	Lung
Obesity	Multiple sites: see text	Thorium dioxide	Liver, leukemia, bone
Physical inactivity	Colon, breast	Neutrons	Leukemia, thyroid, breast, lung
MEDICAL		**OCCUPATION AND ENVIRONMENTAL CHEMICALS**	
Chemotherapy		4-Aminobiphenyl	Bladder
Chlorambucil	Acute nonlymphocytic leukemia	Arsenic compounds, inorganic	Skin, lung, digestive tract, liver, bladder, kidney, lymphatic and hematopoietic systems
Cyclophosphamide	Bladder, leukemia		
Melphalan	Acute nonlymphocytic leukemia		
Methyl-CCNU, Myleran, Thiotepa	Leukemia	Asbestos	Respiratory tract, pleural and peritoneal mesothelioma
Radiotherapy (see Ionizing Radiation)			
Hormones		Benzene	Acute myeloid leukemia
Diethylstilbestrol	Breast, endometrium, cervix, vagina, testicles	Benzidine and dyes	Bladder
		Beryllium and beryllium compounds	Lung
Estrogen, steroidal	Endometrium, breast	1,3-Butadiene	Lymphatic, hematopoietic systems
Tamoxifen	Endometrium (reduces breast cancer risk)	Cadmium and cadmium compounds	Lung, prostate, kidney, bladder
		Bis(chloromethyl) ether and technical-grade chloromethyl methyl ether	Lung
Other Drugs		Chromium hexavalent compounds	Lung, sinonasal cavity
Analgesic mixtures containing phenacetin	Kidney, bladder	Coal tar and coal tar pitch	Skin, scrotum, lung, bladder, kidney, digestive tract, leukemia
Azathioprine	Non-Hodgkin lymphoma, skin, liver, mesenchyma		
Chlornaphazine†	Bladder	Coke oven emissions	Skin, respiratory tract, kidney, bladder
Cyclosporine	Lymphoma, skin		
Methoxsalen with ultraviolet A therapy (PUVA)	Skin	Dioxin	Lung, non-Hodgkin lymphoma
		Erionite	Mesothelioma, lung
INFECTIOUS AGENTS		Ethylene oxide	Leukemia, stomach
Viruses		Formaldehyde†	Nasopharynx
Epstein-Barr virus	Non-Hodgkin lymphoma (Burkitt lymphoma), Hodgkin lymphoma, nasopharynx	Mineral oils (untreated and mildly treated)	Skin, gastrointestinal tract, sinonasal, scrotum, bladder
		Mustard gas	Respiratory tract
Hepatitis B and hepatitis C	Liver	2-Napthylamine	Bladder
Human immunodeficiency virus	Kaposi sarcoma, Hodgkin lymphoma, non-Hodgkin lymphoma	Nickel compounds	Lung, nasal
		Silica, crystalline	Lung
Human papillomavirus	Cervix, vulva, vagina, penis, anus, oral cavity, oropharynx, and tonsil	Soot	Scrotum, skin, lung, prostate, bladder, hematopoietic and lymphatic systems
Human herpesvirus 8	Kaposi sarcoma, lymphoma		
Human T-cell lymphotrophic virus	Leukemia	Strong inorganic acid mists containing sulfuric acid	Larynx, lung
Bacteria			
Helicobacter pylori	Stomach	Vinyl chloride	Liver, brain, lung, lymphatic and hematopoietic systems
Parasites			
Liver flukes (*Clonorchis sinensis* and *Opisthorchis viverrini*)	Bile duct, liver	Wood dust	Nasal cavity, paranasal sinus
Schistosoma haematobium	Bladder		

*Modified from lists compiled by the International Agency for Research on Cancer (IARC) and the National Toxicology Program (NTP).
†Classified as carcinogenic by the IARC but not by the NTP.

damage DNA. Because of the widespread use of cell phones, however, this remains an active area of research.

Iatrogenic Exposures
Many medical diagnostic and therapeutic interventions have been found to increase the risk for cancer, either directly as chemical or physical carcinogens or indirectly through suppression of immune responses. Alkylating drugs and other cytotoxic agents used to treat cancer increase the risk for development of a secondary malignancy, as does radiation therapy. Hormone replacement therapy increases the risk for breast cancer in postmenopausal women. Tamoxifen increases the risk for endometrial cancer, even though this risk is outweighed by the reduction in breast cancer in high-risk women. The

practice of treating pregnant women with diethylstilbestrol was discontinued because of the increased incidence of clear cell vaginal cancer in the daughters of these women during adolescence. Immunosuppressive drugs used to prevent graft rejection in organ transplantation and other autoimmune conditions increase the risk for certain lymphomas (non-Hodgkin B-cell lymphomas), Kaposi sarcoma, malignant melanoma, and liver cancer. Repeated use of diagnostic procedures such as whole body computed tomography results in substantial radiation exposure, although the potential long-term consequences receive surprisingly little attention.

Occupational and Environmental Carcinogens

Occupationally exposed workers (Chapter 18) have unfortunately served as the sentinel for many of the recognized industrial carcinogens, especially in workplaces where prolonged, heavy exposure caused unusual clusters of rare cancers. For example, clusters of scrotal cancer in London chimney sweeps, osteosarcoma of the jaw in watch dial painters exposed to radium, mesothelioma in asbestos workers, and angiosarcoma of the liver in chemical workers exposed to vinyl chloride monomer attest to the carcinogenicity of coal tar, radium, asbestos, and vinyl chloride monomer. In other instances, increases in the risk for common cancers have been sufficiently large to be detected in epidemiologic studies of several thousand workers. Examples include arsenic, asbestos, beryllium, bis(chloromethyl) ether, cadmium, chromium (hexavalent), coal tar, coke oven emissions, nickel, polycyclic aromatic hydrocarbons, and radon.

What Constitutes "Proof" of Causation?

There has been vigorous philosophic and scientific debate over what constitutes "proof" of causation in scientific studies of chronic (i.e., noninfectious) diseases. When policy decisions relate to exposures judged to be harmful, epidemiologic evidence alone is often considered sufficient to justify protective intervention. It is unethical to propose randomized clinical trials to confirm that smoking causes lung cancer, that ionizing radiation causes leukemia, or that HPV causes cervical cancer. Moreover, in these examples, the observational evidence is so strong that the epidemiologic evidence itself is virtually incontrovertible. In other instances, especially when the exposure of interest is difficult to measure and the observed association is weaker, judgments about causality must be based on the weight of the evidence with consideration of all potentially relevant information from observational, clinical, experimental, and basic studies.

The inference that an association is causal is supported when a number of the following apply:

1. The association is strong (higher relative risk being more likely to indicate cause).
2. The risk increases or decreases with exposure in a dose-response gradient.
3. Consistent findings are seen in multiple studies with different investigators, study populations, and designs.
4. The exposure or cause precedes disease onset.
5. It is biologically plausible that the exposure could cause the disease.
6. The association is specific between the exposure and a single disease.
7. The epidemiologic findings fit coherently with information from other types of research and other epidemiologic studies.

Reviews and listings of substances known or suspected to cause cancer in humans are maintained by the National Toxicology Program (NTP) and by the IARC, a branch of the World Health Organization (see Table 183-2). The IARC evaluations classify exposures into one of four categories: (1) "sufficient evidence" of carcinogenicity in humans (in the working group's opinion, chance, bias, and confounding can be excluded with reasonable confidence); (2) "limited evidence" of carcinogenicity (a causal relationship between the agent and risk of cancer in humans is plausible, but chance, bias, and confounding cannot be ruled out with reasonable confidence); (3) "inadequate evidence" of carcinogenicity (available studies are of insufficient quality, consistency, or statistical power to permit a conclusion regarding the carcinogenicity of the agent, or no data on carcinogenicity in humans are available); and (4) "evidence suggesting lack of carcinogenic activity" (several adequate studies of use or exposure are mutually consistent in not showing an increased risk for specified cancer sites, conditions, and levels of exposure). The NTP uses only two categories, "known to be a human carcinogen" and "reasonably anticipated to be a human carcinogen."

⬤ FUTURE DIRECTIONS

An exciting frontier in cancer epidemiology involves efforts to integrate insights from molecular biology and genetics into large-scale population studies to examine how the interaction of inherited genetic susceptibility (nature) with exposure after conception (nurture) influences an individual's risk for the development of cancer. In some cases, information on inherited genetic polymorphisms is now being used clinically to tailor the selection and dose of certain drugs used for chemotherapy or treatment of other conditions. Until now it has been difficult to identify well-established examples of gene-environment interactions that affect cancer risk, mostly because the technology for rapidly genotyping tens of thousands of people has only recently become available and affordable. Advances in proteomics, metabolomics, and epigenetics may soon make it possible to identify early markers and intermediate factors that affect tumor development. These may provide therapeutic targets by which to influence the development or progression of cancer, just as cardiovascular research has identified lipid abnormalities and hypertension as modifiable intermediates of heart disease.

SUGGESTED READINGS

International Agency for Research on Cancer website. http://www.iarc.fr. Accessed Feb. 4, 2011. *Listing of numerous resources on cancer available through the branch of the World Health Organization.*

Jemal A, Siegel R, Ward E, et al. Cancer statistics, 2010. *CA Cancer J Clin.* 2010;60:277-300. *Documents an ongoing decline in cancer-related mortality in 2004, the second consecutive year.*

Garcia M, Jemal A, Ward EM, et al. Global cancer facts and figures 2010. Atlanta, GA: American Cancer Society; http://ntp.niehs.nih.gov. Accessed Feb. 4, 2011. *International cancer statistics.*

National Toxicology Program website. Department of Health and Human Services. http://ntp-server.niehs.nih.gov. Accessed Feb. 4, 2011. *Website lists substances that are known or "reasonably anticipated to be" human carcinogens.*

184

CANCER GENETICS   ⊘

HENRY T. LYNCH AND C. RICHARD BOLAND

⬤ CANCER IS A GENETIC DISEASE

Cancer is caused by alterations in genes. Many genes are involved in the process, and there is a broad range of mechanisms by which the genes may be altered. The genetic alterations are tumor specific, but there are common features to the genes that cause cancer. Also, one must individually consider the differences between somatic mutations (found in the cancers, but not present throughout the rest of the body) and germline mutations (inherited, and present in every cell of the body).

Oncogenes are normal cellular genes that participate in the stimulation of growth pathways and become abnormally activated in cancer. There are several ways for activation to occur. Point mutations may make the protein product unresponsive to downregulating signals, as in the case of mutant *KRAS*. The transcription factor *MYC* is often activated by copy number amplification, or it may be put under the control of an inappropriate promoter, achieving the same result. In the case of the *BCR-ABL* mutation, which is ubiquitous in certain leukemias, a chromosomal translocation relocates a promoter that is active in myeloid cells to a position that drives the unregulated production of a proliferation-promoting tyrosine kinase.

Tumor suppressor genes normally suppress cellular growth or mediate cellular differentiation, and these are inactivated in cancers. Because humans are born with two copies of almost every gene (the X and Y chromosomes in males are the exceptions), it takes two lesions or "hits" to release the cell from the regulatory effects of these genes. Tumor suppressor genes provide the conceptual basis for many of the hereditary forms of predisposition to cancer. The affected person is born with a "germline" mutation in one allele, which is present in every cell of the body. The cancer occurs in a specific cell lineage after the other allele suffers an inactivating "somatic" mutation, which is the second hit. Examples of tumor suppressor genes include the *Rb* gene, *p53*, and *p16*, which are inactivated in some cancers.

DNA repair genes are important in cancer. There are multiple types of DNA repair, each specific to one or more types of DNA damage. When these genes are inactivated, a hypermutability ensues within that cell, and this leads to numerous somatic mutations in the target genes, which will include oncogenes or tumor suppressors, and then leads to cancer. Defective DNA repair states also provide an additional explanation for certain inherited diseases. DNA repair systems inactivated in cancer include the DNA mismatch repair (MMR) system (which is involved in Lynch syndrome [LS]), the base excision repair system (which leads to an autosomal recessive form of familial polyposis called *MYH*-associated polyposis), and nucleotide excision repair (which leads to the autosomal recessive disease xeroderma pigmentosa).

HEREDITARY CANCER SYNDROMES

The tumor suppressor gene concept provides an explanation for how a person could be born with a predisposition to cancer, which occurs when one allele of a gene is mutated in every cell, greatly increasing the likelihood that some cell would eventually lose both copies of the gene—a situation that would be statistically unlikely without the germline mutation. In fact, germline mutations in the previously mentioned tumor suppressors *Rb*, *p53*, and *p16* give rise to familial retinoblastoma, Li-Fraumeni syndrome, and the familial atypical multiple mole melanoma–pancreatic cancer (FAMMM-PC) syndromes, respectively.

Germline mutations in the DNA repair genes create more complex clinical scenarios. In case of hereditary nonpolyposis colon cancer, also known as LS, the most common hereditary CRC syndrome, accounting for approximately 3% of CRC incidence, a germline mutation occurs in one allele of a DNA MMR gene (including *MSH2*, *MLH1*, *MSH6*, or *PMS2*), and the loss of the other allele creates a cell without any DNA MMR activity. The affected cell becomes hypermutable, and mutations accumulate in growth-regulating target genes; this causes the cancer. (There are rare instances in which biallelic mutations in DNA MMR genes create constitutional MMR deficiency and a pediatric cancer diathesis.) More recently it has been discovered that a deletion in the *EPCAM* gene (previously called *TACSTD1*), upstream of *MSH2*, can silence *MSH2*, thereby causing LS without a mutation in the *MSH2* gene itself. Thus, LS is inherited in a classic dominant mendelian fashion, but the cancers occur only after the second hit occurs, meaning that the disease is recessive at the tissue level. Constitutional deficiency of base excision repair occurs when there are biallelic mutations in the *MUTHY* genes (called *MUTHY*-associated polyposis); these patients develop multiple colorectal adenomas and are highly prone to CRC. Similarly, constitutional deficiency of nucleotide excision repair causes xeroderma pigmentosa (Chapter 444), in which patients are unable to tolerate even minimal degrees of sunlight, because the enzyme complex required to repair ultraviolet light–induced DNA changes is defective. These two conditions are classic recessive diseases, and the monoallelic carrier state does not lead to a clinically substantial increase in risk for cancer.

DIAGNOSIS OF FAMILIAL CANCER SYNDROMES

The primary care physician is often the first to apply cancer genetics to clinical care when there is the suspicion of a familial cancer-prone syndrome. It would not be possible to predict which mutations cause what familial cancers based on knowledge of the gene function. The diagnoses depend on pattern recognition and linkage to the known mutations. The recognition of a familial pattern of disease may result in further investigation of potentially affected patients and families. The goal will be effective screening and management recommendations. Examples of the most common familial cancer syndromes include the following:

- Breast and ovarian cancers with *BRCA1/BRCA2* mutations (the hereditary breast and ovarian cancer, or HBOC, syndrome)
- CRC, endometrial, ovarian, stomach, pancreas, and other cancer types with DNA MMR mutations in LS
- Sarcomas, breast cancers, brain tumors, leukemia, lymphoma, and adrenal cortical cancers with *p53* mutations in the Li-Fraumeni syndrome
- Medullary thyroid carcinoma and pheochromocytoma with the *RET* proto-oncogene mutation in the multiple endocrine neoplasia syndromes MEN 2a and 2b
- Malignant melanoma and pancreatic cancer with *CDKN2A* (*p16*) mutation in familial multiple mole melanoma syndrome
- Diffuse gastric cancer and lobular breast cancer with *CDH1* mutation in the hereditary diffuse gastric cancer (HDGC) syndrome
- Multiple adenomatous colonic polyps and CRC with mutations of the *APC* gene in familial adenomatous polyposis (FAP), or biallelic mutations in the *MUTHY* gene in *MUTHY*-associated polyposis

The differential diagnosis is highly complex for common cancers, such as breast and CRC, as shown in Figures 184-1 and 184-2, respectively. Ideally, the family pedigree will cover a minimum of three generations. It must incorporate cancer of all anatomic sites with age of cancer onset and pathology

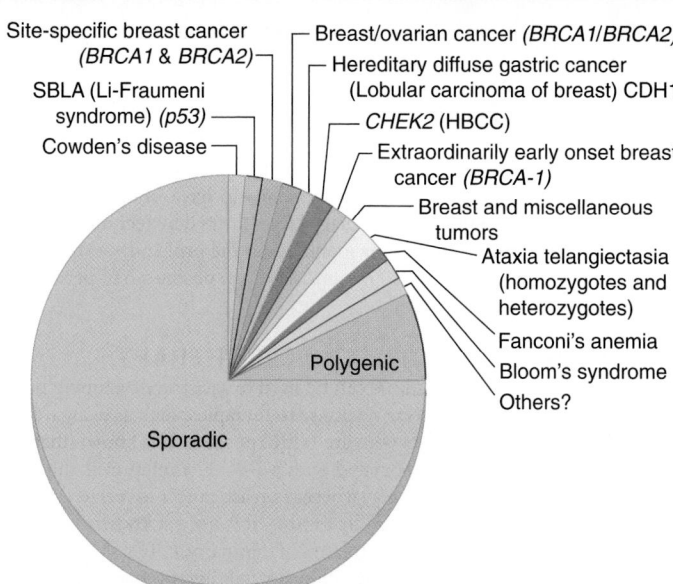

FIGURE 184-1. Schematic depicting heterogeneity in breast cancer. HBCC = hereditary breast and colorectal cancer; SBLA = sarcoma, breast and brain tumors, leukemia, laryngeal and lung cancer, and adrenal cortical carcinoma. (From Lynch HT, Fitzgibbons RJ Jr, Lynch JF. Heterogeneity and natural history of hereditary breast cancer. *Surg Clin North Am.* 1990;70:753.)

FIGURE 184-2. Circle graph depicting the marked genotypic and phenotypic heterogeneity in hereditary colorectal cancer syndromes. AC-1 = Amsterdam Criteria 1; AFAP = attenuated familial adenomatous polyposis; BRRS = Bannayan-Ruvalcaba-Riley syndrome; CD = Cowden's disease; FAP = familial adenomatous polyposis; FJP = familial juvenile polyposis; HBCC = hereditary breast and colorectal cancer; MAP = MUTYH-associated polyposis; MMR = mismatch repair; PJS = Peutz-Jeghers syndrome; TGFBR1 = transforming growth factor-β receptor type 1. (Revised from Lynch HT, Riley BD, Weissman SM, et al. Hereditary nonpolyposis colorectal carcinoma [HNPCC] and HNPCC-like families: problems in diagnosis, surveillance, and management. *Cancer.* 2004;100:53-64.)

documentation. Older individuals will often have passed through the cancer risk age and therefore will be more informative genetically. Pertinent noncancerous phenotypic features, such as perioral pigmentations in Peutz-Jeghers syndrome, multiple colonic adenomas in FAP, multiple atypical moles in the FAMMM syndrome, and the presence of sebaceous adenomas, sebaceous carcinomas, or multiple keratoacanthomas in the Muir-Torre syndrome variant of LS should also be included.

Referral to a medical geneticist or a hereditary cancer center can be made at any time, depending on the physician's individual expertise as well as resources he or she has available. When referral is made, key medical, genetic, and genealogic findings must be made available to the center with the patient's written permission. In every potential hereditary cancer syndrome, it is essential to determine who needs to be tested. Unfortunately, even when a patient has a very strong family history of cancer and would be a candidate for DNA testing for a cancer-causing mutation, rates of referral for such testing are low. Many physicians are intimidated by the profusion of genes linked to cancer and the complexities involved in ordering and interpreting the tests.

Therefore, many patients are not receiving critical information that is available at this time.

The ideal candidate for initial genetic testing will be an individual with an early-onset syndrome cancer who is in the direct line of hereditary descent, and will be the most likely candidate to carry the family's pathogenic mutation. If that mutation can be identified in a likely syndrome carrier, it is then possible for other at-risk members of the family to have "mutation-specific testing." Although the initial genetic diagnosis is limited by technical considerations, once the index mutation is identified in the proband, confirmatory testing is cheaper and is nearly 100% sensitive and specific when performed by the same reference laboratory.

USE OF GENETICS IN CANCER THERAPY

Genetic tests of somatic mutations can be used to assist in developing prognostic estimates and in predicting response to therapies, such as using trastuzumab in breast cancer patients who are *HER2* positive. It is known that the phenotype of breast cancer associated with a *BRCA1* mutation is different from that of sporadic breast cancer, whereas breast cancer associated with a *BRCA2* mutation is similar to sporadic tumors; it is not yet known, however, how these differences should affect treatment. Similarly, CRCs showing MSI do not respond favorably to adjuvant 5-fluorouracil therapy. Imatinib is effective in the treatment of some cancers, including chronic myelogenous leukemia and gastric stromal tumors, which share activating mutations in a tyrosine kinase. Finally, genetic profiling and studies looking for single nucleotide polymorphisms are being investigated as a way to identify incremental forms of cancer predisposition. Genome-wide association studies (Chapter 42) are providing a wealth of new information about risk and are likely to provide clues to developing personalized treatments of cancer.

SUGGESTED READINGS

Boland CR, Goel A. Microsatellite instability in colorectal cancer. *Gastroenterology*. 2010;138:2073-2087. *Scholarly review.*

Leemans CR, Braakhuis BJ, Brakenhoff RH. The molecular biology of head and neck cancer. *Net Rev Cancer*. 2011;11:9-22. *Review of tumor heterogeneity, field cancerization, and molecular pathogenesis.*

McDermott U, Downing JR, Stratton MR. Genomics and the continuum of cancer care. *N Engl J Med*. 2011;364:340-350. *Review.*

Milne RL, Antoniou AC. Genetic modifiers of cancer risk for *BRCA1* and *BRCA2* mutation carriers. *Ann Oncol*. 2011;22:i11-i17. *Review based on GWAS.*

Park YJ, Claus R, Weichenhan D, et al. Genome-wide epigenetic modifications in cancer. *Prog Drug Res*. 2011;67:25-49. *Review of the potential use of DNA methylation for disease detection and prognosis.*

Plon SE, Cooper HP, Parks B, et al. Genetic testing and cancer risk management recommendations by physicians for at-risk relatives. *Genet Med*. 2011;13:148-154. *Review.*

Taylor BS, Ladanyi M. Clinical cancer genomics: how soon is now? *J Pathol*. 2011;223:318-326. *Review of germline and somatic alterations in DNA.*

185

BIOLOGY OF CANCER

JEFFREY A. MOSCOW AND KENNETH H. COWAN

GENETIC CANCER BIOLOGY

Cancer is an acquired genetic disease (Chapter 184). Spontaneous genetic changes overwhelm the mechanisms that maintain normal cellular homeostasis, disrupt the normal tight control of cell division and death, and result in the malignant phenotype.

The genetic damage that results in cancer can occur in several ways: translocations of genes can juxtapose two genes in ways that cause dysregulation of their function; mutations can activate cancer-causing genes or deactivate cancer-preventing genes; and epigenetic modifications of proteins that associate with DNA can alter the expression of critical genes (Chapter 184). Sometimes, the first step is the mutation of genes that normally prevent mutations in other genes—cells then quickly gain additional mutations that,

through a morbid natural selection, ultimately produce the mutant clone that gives rise to a malignancy.

The very processes that generate malignant transformations also present obstacles to their treatment. The genetic plasticity that can manufacture cancer-causing mutations can also generate mutations that result in resistance to anticancer drugs.

Tumor formation after malignant transformation requires changes in cell biology that, in the processes of invasion and metastases, favor propagation of the malignant cells. Because individual cells, like organisms, are programmed to die, cancer cells must learn to evade the intricate systems of apoptosis that ensure cell death. Cancer cells must also enable the formation of new blood vessels to provide nutrition for the growing mass and develop strategies to escape the immune surveillance that suppresses tumor formation. These processes that give rise to malignant tumors can again raise barriers to successful therapies; for example, cells with impaired apoptosis may be resistant to anticancer drugs that kill cells through activation of apoptosis. However, the distinctive biology of malignancies can also provide opportunities for directed therapies.

Specific Mutations, Targeted Therapies

All cancer cells contain some genomic damage. In most cases, several abnormalities must occur, but sometimes even a single mutation appears sufficient to produce malignant transformation. The latter examples demonstrate clearly that cancer is a genetic disease of dysregulated growth, and they demonstrate that identification of a genetic cause can lead to a specific targeted therapy aimed at the product of the damaged gene.

In the case of acute promyelocytic leukemia (APL; Chapter 189), the characteristic t(15;17) translocation is the only identified genetic lesion. This genetic mishap splices the retinoic acid receptor *(RAR)* gene to another gene called *PML*, and the resulting hybrid RAR-PML protein does not function properly. The functional defect of the RAR-PML hybrid protein product can be overcome with pharmacologic doses of a vitamin A analogue, all-*trans*-retinoic acid (ATRA). The addition of ATRA to chemotherapy for APL doubles disease-free survival, from approximately 40% to approximately 80%. Similarly, the accidental genetic recombination that creates the BCR/ABL hybrid protein results in malignant transformation of myeloid cells (Chapter 190), and can be treated with specific inhibitors of the BCR/ABL kinase. Cancers driven by single mutations appear to be restricted to specific tissue types. Thus, genetic alterations that lead to malignant transformation are also dependent on the cellular context in which they occur.

Multistage Evolution of Malignancy

Most cancers do not have a single cause but rather are the products of a progression of genetic lesions that can be years in the making, as evidenced by their multiple and complex genetic alterations. The classical model of two stages of cancer development, initiation and promotion, has been replaced by a more dynamic and multistep model in which accumulated genetic damage leads to dysregulation of cell division and the disarming of the mechanisms of cell death.

Often the first step in the creation of a tumor is the development of genomic instability. During each cell division, some 3 billion nucleotide pairs must be faithfully copied to produce exact replicas in each daughter cell. The process of cancer can begin with alterations in any one of a number of factors that influence the accuracy of this process of genetic replication. Two major mechanisms create this acquired genetic damage: spontaneous mutations can disable the machinery that edits DNA replication and removes damaged genes, or, more frequently, cells are exposed to carcinogens that directly damage DNA, and the imprecise repair of damaged DNA results in an increase in spontaneous mutations.

Heritable conditions that impair the proteins that ensure genomic fidelity cause a predisposition to a variety of types of cancer. Examples of defects in genes that repair DNA damage, leading to increased hereditary cancer risk, are listed in Table 185-1.

Because cancer is a genetic disease, carcinogens are genomic toxins that damage DNA and create mutations. The DNA damage from cigarette smoke (Chapter 31) results from exposure to dangerous hydrocarbon products that bind DNA and disrupt faithful replication. Ultraviolet irradiation causes characteristic DNA damage in the skin that can lead to melanoma and other skin cancers (Chapter 210). Ionizing radiation (Chapter 19) from diagnostic and therapeutic radiation also cause genetic damage and cancer.

One key regulator of genomic integrity is the p53 protein, the product of a tumor suppressor gene that is commonly referred to as the "guardian of the

TABLE 185-1	GENOMIC INSTABILITY GENES ASSOCIATED WITH INCREASED HEREDITARY CANCER RISK	
GENES	**SYNDROME**	**HEREDITARY TUMOR TYPES**
MUTYH	Attenuated polyposis	Colon
ATM	Ataxia-telangiectasia	Leukemias, lymphomas, brain
BLM	Bloom's	Leukemias, lymphomas, skin
BRCA1, BRCA2	Hereditary breast cancer	Breast, ovary
FANCA, FANCC, FANCD2, FANCE, FANCF, FANCG	Fanconi's anemia A, C, D2, E, F, and G	Leukemias
NBS1	Nijmegen breakage	Lymphomas, brain
MSH2, MLH1, MSH6, PMS2	Hereditary nonpolyposis colon cancer (Lynch syndrome)	Colon
XPA, XPC, ERCC2, ERCC3, ERCC4, ERCC5, DDB2	Xeroderma pigmentosum	Skin

TABLE 185-2	TUMOR SUPPRESSOR GENES ASSOCIATED WITH INCREASED HEREDITARY CANCER RISK	
GENES	**SYNDROME**	**HEREDITARY TUMOR TYPES**
p53	Li-Fraumeni	Breast, sarcoma, adrenal, brain
APC	Familial adenomatous polyposis	Colon, thyroid, stomach, intestine
CDH1	Familial gastric carcinoma	Stomach
VHL	von Hippel-Lindau	Kidney
WT1	Familial Wilms' tumor	Wilms'
PTEN	Cowden's	Hamartoma, glioma, uterus
CDKN2A	Familial malignant melanoma	Melanoma, pancreas
CDK4	Familial malignant melanoma	Melanoma
RB1	Hereditary retinoblastoma	Eye
NF1	Neurofibromatosis	Neurofibroma, brain tumors
MEN1	Multiple endocrine neoplasia type 1	Parathyroid, pituitary, islet cell
NF2	Neurofibromatosis	Meningioma, acoustic neuromas

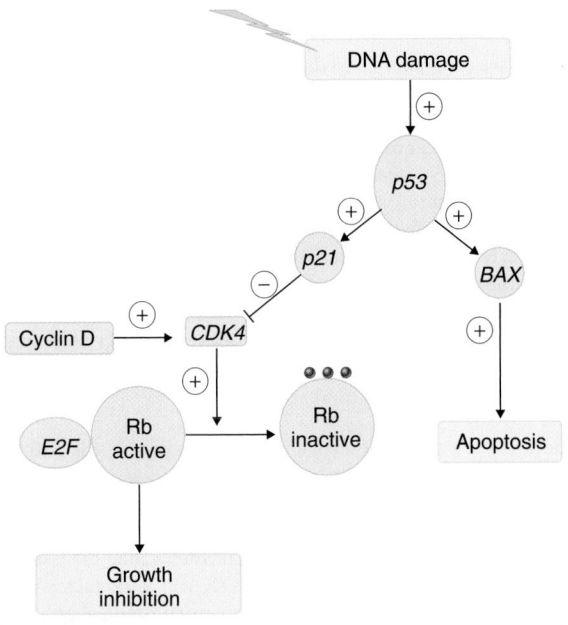

FIGURE 185-1. Response to p53 and DNA damage. After DNA damage, *p53* expression induces the cyclin kinase inhibitor p21, resulting in cell cycle arrest, and *BAX*, which induces apoptosis. Rb = retinoblastoma.

FIGURE 185-2. Protein interactions with *BRCA1* and *BRCA2*. *BRCA1* and *BRCA2* act as molecular scaffolds and promote assembly of protein complexes involved in cell cycle regulation in response to DNA damage as well as DNA repair. Signaling scaffolds, like *BRCA1*, bring together proteins belonging to interlinked pathways and orchestrate specific interactions among signaling proteins. Some of the more than 50 proteins that interact with *BRCA1* are shown.

genome." The p53 protein can sense DNA damage and direct the cell either to cell cycle arrest by increased expression of the cyclin kinase inhibitor p21 (Fig. 185-1), which provides the cell with the opportunity to repair genetic damage before cell division, or down the path of programmed cell death (apoptosis). Inactivating mutations in p53 are among the most common abnormalities observed in cancer, emphasizing the critical role of unrepaired genetic damage in the etiology of cancer. Individuals with inherited mutations of the *p53* gene have the Li-Fraumeni syndrome (Chapter 184), with increased susceptibility to specific types of cancer. The retinoblastoma (*RB*) gene is another tumor suppressor gene whose normal function is to regulate cell growth (see Fig. 185-1). Mutations in a number of other tumor suppressor genes are also associated with specific cancer syndromes (Table 185-2).

Similarly, the heritable breast cancer predisposition genes *BRCA1* and *BRCA2* encode proteins that associate with many intracellular proteins that are involved in DNA repair, including rad50, rad51, ATM, and p53 (Fig. 185-2). Cells defective in *BRCA1* or *BRCA2* display defects both in the response to DNA and in DNA repair. Mutations in the *BRCA1* and *BRCA2* (Chapter 204) are rare, so relatively few women inherit abnormal copies of these gene

alleles from their parents, and only approximately 10% of breast cancers can be attributed to *BRCA1* and *BRCA2* mutations.

DNA damage, whether from heritable conditions, from somatic mutations in the DNA repair mechanisms themselves, or from carcinogen exposure, increases the rate of spontaneous mutations in cells and sets the stage for the natural selection of malignant clones. Although mutations of most of the approximately 25,000 genes in the genome do not result in malignancy, mutations or other disruptions of the right genes in the right cellular context can confer a selective proliferative or survival advantage, and set the stage for malignant progression.

Disease of the Messenger Proteins

In health, cells respond to external stimuli with complex and redundant protein networks that interact with external stimuli and transmit appropriate signals to the nucleus. The proteins involved in signal transduction include cell surface receptors, second messenger systems, and multiple transcription factors that directly regulate gene expression. Each of these elements of the signal transduction network is controlled by multiple proteins that tightly regulate the activation state of each element of the network. Disruption of any of the genes that encode the proteins involved in signal transduction—proteins that relay the external stimulus to the nucleus—occurs frequently in cancer.

Cell surface receptors for external stimuli involve families of receptor tyrosine kinases, proteins that become activated after binding to specific ligands. For example, the epidermal growth factor (ErbB) family receptor kinases are often amplified or found activated by mutations in breast, ovary, gastric, and lung cancers. Identification of such genetic abnormalities in cancer cells has

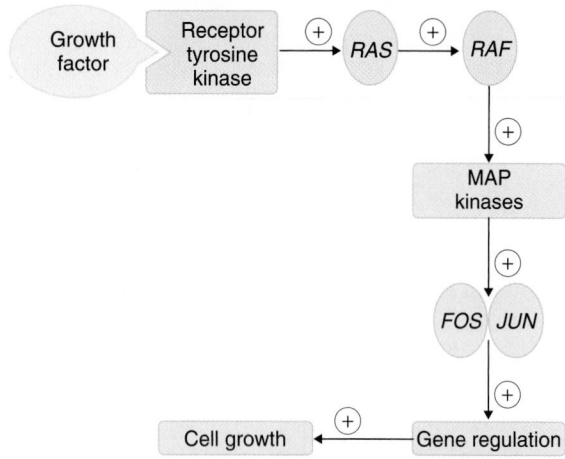

FIGURE 185-3. Growth factor–mediated signal transduction. Upon binding to specific receptor ligands, receptor tyrosine kinases activate downstream signal transduction cascades that result in changes in gene expression and enhanced cell growth. Alterations in various steps in the signal transduction cascade are frequently observed in cancer. MAP = mitogen-activated protein.

provided valuable targets for selective therapies. Thus, trastuzumab, a monoclonal antibody directed against the ErbB2/Her2neu protein, which is amplified and overexpressed in 25% of breast cancers, has been shown to improve disease-free survival and overall survival when given in combination with chemotherapy (Chapter 204). Erlotinib, an inhibitor of ErbB1 (epidermal growth factor [EGF]) receptor, may be effective in treatment of lung cancers that contain mutations in the ErbB1 (EGF) receptor (Chapter 197).

Unregulated growth can also result from mutations that affect downstream signal transduction networks (Fig. 185-3). Receptor tyrosine kinases transmit their signals through biochemical pathways and ultimately drive gene transcription. In some pathways, receptor tyrosine kinases activate Ras proteins, which act as second messengers that amplify and direct signals from receptor tyrosine kinases to other intracellular proteins, which then ultimately generate the cellular response to the stimulus. Ras mutations, which are frequently found in cancer, typically result in the Ras protein being stuck in the "on," or activated, position, which provides a constant, unregulated stimulus to downstream proteins, which in turn creates a cascading effect that stimulates cell growth. Although mutations in other genes are also commonly found in tumors that harbor Ras mutations, mutation of Ras alone has been shown to transform normal cells into malignant cells. Activating mutations of Ras family proteins can frequently be found in melanoma, myeloid leukemias, and cancers of the colon, pancreas, and lung. Genetic abnormalities are also frequently found in the other signaling pathways that transmit signals from receptor tyrosine kinases, including the PIP3/PDK1/Akt pathway, as well as in the nonreceptor tyrosine kinases signaling pathways, including the Jak/STAT and the c-Src pathways.

Disruption of the genes that encode the proteins that regulate gene transcription, which are the downstream targets of signal transduction cascades, can also create malignancy. For example, amplification of the Myc family of transcription factors is frequently observed in neuroblastoma and in cancers of the lung, bladder, breast, stomach, and colon. Certain acute leukemias (Chapter 189) arise when the normal gene recombination process that produces diverse immune responses goes awry and an immunoglobulin or T-cell receptor locus is accidentally spliced onto a gene encoding a transcription factor, resulting in loss of regulation of the transcription factor activity. Several pathognomonic oncogenic chromosomal translocations commonly found in sarcomas also involve genes for transcription factors; for example, the t(11;22) of Ewing's sarcoma (Chapter 209) creates the *EWSR1-FLI1* hybrid transcription factor, and the characteristic t(2;13) of alveolar rhabdomyosarcoma creates the hybrid *PAX3-FOXO1A* DNA binding protein.

Suppression of Tumor Suppressors
Normal cells contain proteins that prevent malignant transformation. Inactivation of the tumor suppressor genes that encode these proteins also leads to cancer. Because a loss of function is required for a malignant effect, both copies of the tumor suppressor gene must be affected. In almost all cases, patients have a physical loss of one copy of a gene and an acquired mutation

of the other. The spontaneous deletion of genetic material, called loss of heterozygosity, is a frequently observed genetic abnormality in tumors.

Some familial cancer predisposition syndromes are based on the inheritance of one damaged copy of a tumor suppressor gene (Chapter 184). Hereditary retinoblastoma, which results from inheritance of a mutated *RB* gene, and the Li-Fraumeni syndrome (Chapter 184), which results from inheritance of a mutant *p53* gene, predispose affected individuals to cancers. Both the Rb and p53 proteins play critical roles in regulating the progression of proliferating cells through the cell cycle, and the loss of this checkpoint regulation can contribute to uncontrolled cell growth and cancer.

The importance of the p53 and Rb signaling pathways in tumor suppression is further revealed by the mechanism by which infection with the human papillomavirus (HPV; Chapter 381) in cervical epithelial cells leads to cervical cancer (Chapter 205). HPV proteins E6 and E7 inactivate p53 and Rb proteins, respectively, thereby creating a virally induced premalignant state in which the machinery that prevents damaged cells from proliferating has been turned off. For this reason, vaccination against certain HPV serotypes holds the promise of preventing most cases of cervical cancer.

DISTINCTIVE CANCER BIOLOGY
Cancer cells do not behave like normal cells. The alterations in the regulation of cell growth, differentiation, and death that give rise to cancer also produce common abnormal biologic characteristics, which are shared by tumors that arise from different cells of origin. These common features conspire to allow the transformed cell to grow into a tumor.

Telomerase
Normal cells are programmed to differentiate and ultimately to die, and this programming is regulated through enzymatic pathways that lead to terminal differentiation, senescence, or apoptosis. Cancer cells evade the mechanisms that are designed to steer cells toward terminal differentiation and senescence by altering the function of telomerase. As primitive cells divide and differentiate, the ends of chromosomes, called telomeres, progressively shorten and ultimately lead to a growth arrest that is termed replicative senescence. An enzyme called telomerase adds length back to the telomeres and reverses the process of replicative senescence. Telomerase is usually expressed at significant levels only in stem cells. However, telomerase is highly expressed in most malignant tissues, demonstrating a common alteration of cell biology that is necessary for creation and maintenance of the malignant phenotype.

Apoptosis
In addition to bypassing senescence, cancer cells disable the pathways that lead to apoptosis. Because apoptosis is literally a life-and-death decision for the cell, it must be tightly controlled by intricate pathways of regulatory proteins. Apoptosis can be triggered through either external or internal pathways that converge to activate a family of enzymes, called caspases, that systematically degrade cellular proteins and DNA in a characteristic pattern resulting in cell death. Cancer cells contain many common aberrations in the machinery that regulates apoptosis, including increased activity of antiapoptotic proteins, such as Bcl-2 and Mcl-1, or increased levels of inhibitors of apoptosis, such as the protein survivin, which inhibits caspase activity.

Cancer Epigenetics
Epigenetic changes in gene expression are also hallmarks of malignancy (Chapter 184). In normal cells, gene expression is controlled by epigenetic processes that limit the physical accessibility of genes to transcription factors. Gene expression can be silenced by processes that methylate specific DNA sequences on chromosomes, called CpG islands. In cancer, tumor suppressor genes are frequently found to be abnormally methylated, leading to a loss of their expression and function. The drugs 5-azacytidine and decitabine reverse methylation and have activity in the myelodysplastic syndrome (Chapter 188) and leukemia. Gene expression is also controlled by histone acetylases, which influence how tightly genomic DNA is spooled around large complex nuclear proteins called histones and alter the interaction of chromatin proteins with DNA. A novel group of drugs called histone deacetylase inhibitors are currently under development as anticancer agents.

Energy Metabolism
Cancer cells also demonstrate characteristic alterations in glucose metabolism, known as the Warburg effect. Malignant cells tend preferentially to shunt glucose into the glycolytic pathway, taking up excessive amounts of glucose and metabolizing glucose into lactate instead of channeling glucose

into the typical aerobic pathway that more efficiently captures energy and creates the end products of carbon dioxide and water. This disruption of normal cellular energy metabolism is thought to be due to dysregulation of a gene that is also involved in the regulation of apoptosis, Akt, and its downstream effectors. This abnormal metabolism of glucose in cancer cells is also the principle behind the use of positron emission tomographic scans to image tumors. Inherited inactivating mutations of the phosphatase and tensin homologue (*PTEN*), which inactivates Akt, are also responsible for Cowden's syndrome, in which the susceptibility to breast and thyroid cancers is increased.

Ubiquitinylation and Proteasomes

Normal cells have tightly regulated mechanisms to degrade and recycle proteins by attaching one or more ubiquitin molecules to a protein. Ubiquitinylation can serve as a signal that a protein should be trafficked to and degraded by lysosomes or the proteasome. Ubiquitinylation plays an important role in the regulation of receptor tyrosine kinases, in cell cycle progression, and in repair of DNA damage. This regulatory mechanism is altered in many types of cancer. The first anticancer drug targeted at this abnormality in cancer cells is bortezomib, which inhibits proteasome activity and is effective in the treatment of multiple myeloma (Chapter 193).

Angiogenesis

Because tumors must find mechanisms to feed themselves as they grow, the malignant transformation must include the ability to stimulate new blood vessel formation, or angiogenesis. Malignant cells have in common the ability to stimulate the formation of endothelial cells and the breakdown of extracellular membranes, often by secreting vasculature endothelial growth factor (VEGF). The resulting tumor vasculature, although functional, does not have the vessel architecture or endothelial wall characteristics of a normal vascular bed. The realization that tumor cells have unique angiogenesis has led to the novel therapeutic approach of targeting tumor vessel formation, and not the malignant cell itself, such as with the monoclonal anti-VEGF antibody bevacizumab in metastatic colorectal cancer (Chapter 199).

Tumor Immune Evasion

Tumors also develop strategies to evade immune surveillance. The T cells and natural killer cells of the immune system play a role in protecting the host against malignancy, just as they also protect against infectious agents. Tumors can grow unimpeded after malignant cells have been selected with properties that disarm the host's immune response to tumors; these mechanisms include downregulation of costimulatory and major histocompatibility complex molecules, as well as secretion of cytokines that inhibit the immune system, such as transforming growth factor-β. The development of therapies designed to harness the immune system for cancer treatment, including tumor antigen vaccines, has been hindered by properties that allow tumors to escape immune destruction.

Drug Resistance

The same genetic plasticity that leads to cancer also gives cancer cells access to the human genome repertoire, with the capability to express and mutate any of its genes—sometimes resulting in resistance to anticancer therapy. Cancer cells can specifically alter the chemotherapy target to become resistant. In the case of imatinib mesylate, the targeted therapy for chronic myeloid leukemia (Chapter 190), cells can become resistant by mutating the binding site of the drug to the already mutant BCR/ABL protein. Cancer cellular resistance to older targeted drugs such as methotrexate, which targets the enzyme dihydrofolate reductase, can be mediated by multiple steps in the folate metabolic pathway. Cancer cells can also reach into their genomes and call on more general mechanisms of protection from stress. Normal cells can upregulate genes to protect against environmental toxins. In cancer, malignant cells use the same proteins to evade chemotherapy, such as adenosine triphosphate–dependent efflux drug pumps MDR1 (for multidrug resistance) and the MRP (for multidrug resistance–related protein) family of transmembrane proteins. Cancer cells also use other detoxification pathways, such as those involving glutathione, for protection against chemotherapy. For every anticancer drug developed, a cancer cell has found a way to circumvent it.

Cancer Stem Cells

Tissues are composed of a vast majority of cells that are irreversibly committed toward terminal differentiation. Hidden within tissues are also a very small minority of primitive, seemingly nondescript cells that are capable of repopulating the tissue with new cells and have the potential for self-renewal, that is, the ability to divide without differentiating; these are called stem cells. The view of cancer as a homogeneous mass of clonally derived malignant cells has been replaced by a view that, in some tumors, cancer cell division is organized more like a tissue in that most of the cells of a tumor do not have unlimited capacity for self-renewal but rather are the progeny of a minute population of cancer-initiating (or stem) cells. In hematopoietic malignancies and other tumors, flow cytometric techniques have demonstrated small, unique populations of cancer cells within tumors that have the ability to re-form the tumor, whereas the vast majority of cells in a malignancy do not have this potential.

This concept of cancer has enormous consequences for the study and treatment of cancer. Most important, all previous studies that have examined the overall expression of genes in a malignancy may not reveal critical and unique characteristics of the cancer-initiating cells from which the tumor has arisen. The pattern of treatment response followed by treatment relapse may be due not only to the acquisition of drug resistance but also to a failure of the therapy to treat the distinctive biology of the cancer stem cell. Isolation and characterization of cancer stem cells may reveal new cancer stem cell–specific targets that distinguish them from both their malignant progeny and normal stem cells. Treatments aimed at cancer stem cells hold the potential for markedly improving cancer therapy.

SUGGESTED READINGS

Frezza C, Pollard PJ, Gottlieb E. Inborn and acquired metabolic defects in cancer. *J Mol Med.* 2011;89: 213-220. *Review of pro-oncogenic signaling.*

Goh AM, Coffill CR, Lane DP. The role of mutant p53 in human cancer. *J Pathol.* 2011;223:116-126. *Review.*

Tsai HC, Baylin SB. Cancer epigenetics: linking basic biology to clinical medicine. *Cell Res.* 2011;21: 502-517. *Review of molecular mechanisms and the possibilities for pharmacological targeting of cancer-specific epigenetic alterations.*

Vander Heiden MG, Cantley LC, Thompson CB. Understanding the Warburg effect: the metabolic requirements of cell proliferation. *Science.* 2009;324:1029-1033. *Review of molecular mechanisms underlying altered glucose metabolism in cancer.*

186

ENDOCRINE MANIFESTATIONS OF TUMORS: "ECTOPIC" HORMONE PRODUCTION

ROBERT F. GAGEL

It is now commonly accepted that genetic abnormalities, either activating or inactivating mutations, cause disordered cell growth leading to cellular transformation. A corollary of this fundamental tenet is that changes in a handful of important cellular genes can result in altered expression of other genes and thereby lead to the production of cellular proteins not normally expressed in the differentiated cell type. Among the more interesting and clinically relevant types of abnormal proteins are those associated with "ectopic" hormone syndromes, a small but clinically important group of disorders.

There are several patterns of "ectopic" hormone production. The most common is the production of small polypeptide hormones by tumors derived from a specific class of neuroendocrine cells. These neuroendocrine cells are widely dispersed throughout the lung, gastrointestinal tract, pancreas, thyroid gland, adrenal medulla, breast, prostate, and skin; they share several common cytologic and biochemical characteristics (amine precursor uptake and decarboxylation), are often derived from the neural crest, and normally produce both biogenic amines and small polypeptide hormones. The list of hormones produced by tumors derived from members of this group of neuroendocrine cells includes adrenocorticotropic hormone (corticotropin, ACTH), calcitonin, vasoactive intestinal peptide, growth hormone–releasing hormone, corticotropin-releasing hormone (CRH), somatostatin, and other small peptides. A second group of tumors, generally derived from squamous epithelium, produces parathyroid hormone–related protein (PTHrP) and vasopressin.

Current evidence suggests that aberrant hormone production is due to reversion to an earlier state of differentiation and an earlier developmental

TABLE 186-1 CLINICAL SYNDROMES OF ECTOPIC HORMONE PRODUCTION

HUMORAL HYPERCALCEMIA

Parathyroid hormone–related protein
  Squamous cell carcinoma
  Breast cancer
  Neuroendocrine tumors
  Renal cell cancer
  Melanoma
  Prostate cancer
Increased calcitriol
  Lymphoma
  Benign conditions: sarcoidosis, berylliosis, tuberculosis, fungal infection

CORTICOTROPIN

Proopiomelanocortin
  Small cell lung cancer
  Pulmonary carcinoid
  Medullary thyroid cancer
  Islet cell tumor
  Pheochromocytoma
  Ganglioneuroma
Corticotropin-releasing hormone
  Medullary thyroid cancer
  Paraganglioma
  Prostate cancer
  Islet cell tumor

HUMAN CHORIONIC GONADOTROPIN

Choriocarcinoma
Testicular embryonal cell carcinoma
Seminoma

HYPOGLYCEMIA

Insulinoma
Sarcomas or large retroperitoneal tumors

INAPPROPRIATE ANTIDIURETIC HORMONE SECRETION

Small cell lung cancer
Squamous cell head and neck cancer

ERYTHROPOIETIN

Renal cell cancer
Hepatoma
Pheochromocytoma
Benign conditions: cerebellar hemangioblastoma, uterine fibroid

---

pattern of transcription factor expression. In hypercalcemia caused by ectopic production of PTHrP, activation of the *ras*–mitogen-activated protein kinase signaling pathway, through mutation, appears to be responsible for PTHrP production by squamous epithelium. For example, normal fibroblasts can be stimulated to express PTHrP by combined expression of an activated *ras* gene and mutated tumor suppressor gene *p53*. In this example, a combinatorial effect of common genetic changes in human cancer results in abnormal expression of this hypercalcemic peptide.

The clinical syndromes associated with ectopic hormone production are important because they are often difficult diagnostic dilemmas, they are a major cause of morbidity and death in cancer patients, and their therapy can be challenging (Table 186-1). Management of these clinical syndromes is often difficult because of the necessity to treat both the cancer and the syndrome caused by excessive hormone production.

● HUMORAL HYPERCALCEMIA OF MALIGNANCY

Hypercalcemia (Chapter 253) is one of the most common hormonal syndromes associated with cancer and is caused by several different pathophysiologic processes. To differentiate among these possibilities and initiate appropriate treatment, each patient must be approached in an organized manner.

PATHOBIOLOGY

Parathyroid Hormone–Related Protein

PTHrP is normally involved in chondrocytic and dermatologic differentiation. Eight of the first 16 amino acids of PTHrP are homologous with parathyroid hormone (PTH), and both peptides exert their various effects through interaction with the PTH receptor. Activation of this receptor in the

osteoblast increases the expression of an osteoblast-specific cell surface protein called receptor activator of nuclear factor-kappa B ligand (RANKL). Interaction of RANKL with the RANK receptor on undifferentiated osteoclasts causes increased osteoclast differentiation and formation, bone resorption, and hypercalcemia. Ectopic production of PTHrP by a wide variety of tumors is one of the most common causes of hypercalcemia associated with malignancy; ectopic production of PTH itself is uncommon.

Increased Production of Calcitriol

Increased production of calcitriol occurs in a high percentage of patients with lymphoma (Chapters 191 and 192). There is compelling evidence for increased expression of 1α-hydroxylase by lymphomatous tissue. Other granulomatous conditions such as sarcoidosis (Chapter 95), berylliosis (Chapter 93), tuberculosis (Chapter 332), or fungal infection can also cause this clinical syndrome. Calcitriol-mediated hypercalcemia is caused by increased calcium absorption and is characterized by a suppression of serum immunoreactive PTH.

Bone Metastasis

Bone metastasis (Chapter 208) should always be considered in the differential diagnosis of hypercalcemia in a cancer patient. Bone metastases are frequently associated with local production of cytokines, PTHrP, or other substances that cause increased bone resorption. Indeed, the distinction between humoral hypercalcemia of malignancy and localized osteolysis has become blurred because of evidence that tumors such as breast cancer (Chapter 204) or myeloma (Chapter 193) cause localized osteolysis by the local production and secretion of PTHrP in addition to RANKL. In breast cancer there is considerable evidence of a local regulatory loop between transforming growth factor-β (TGF-β) and PTHrP production. TGF-β is a normal component of bone matrix. Local PTHrP production by breast cancer cells can stimulate osteoclastic bone resorption and the release of TGF-β. The release of TGF-β in turn stimulates breast cancer growth and greater PTHrP production, accelerating the osteolytic process. Other activators of bone resorption, including tumor necrosis factor, lymphotoxin, endothelin, interleukin (IL)-1, and IL-6, can be produced by other tumors that metastasize to (renal cell carcinoma) or reside in (myeloma) bone.

CLINICAL MANIFESTATIONS

The clinical syndrome associated with elevated levels of PTHrP is nearly identical to that observed with hyperparathyroidism and includes increased osteoclast-mediated bone resorption, as well as an increase in renal tubular calcium resorption and a decrease in renal phosphorus resorption. The only significant clinical difference between PTHrP- and PTH-mediated hypercalcemia is the finding of increased serum calcitriol (1,25-dihydroxycholecalciferol) levels in hyperparathyroidism and low or normal values in PTHrP-mediated hypercalcemia, presumably because of the inhibitory effects of cancer on 1α-hydroxylase, the enzyme that produces calcitriol. PTHrP production is most commonly associated with squamous cell carcinoma (Chapter 197), although production has been observed in other types of cancer as well, including breast (Chapter 204), neuroendocrine (Chapter 201), renal (Chapter 203), skin (Chapter 210), and prostate (Chapter 207) cancer. A notable trend over the past decade has been the reduction of hypercalcemia in patients with breast cancer. Routine bisphosphonate use and more effective therapies for breast cancer, particularly the widespread use of aromatase inhibitors, have led to decreased bone metastasis and hence a substantial reduction in hypercalcemia.

Clinical features that differentiate patients with increased production of calcitriol from those with PTHrP-mediated hypercalcemia include a suppressed intact serum PTH level (Fig. 186-1), an increased or normal serum phosphorus level, hypercalciuria, and no evidence of bone metastasis. An elevated serum calcitriol concentration is found in approximately half of patients with calcitriol-mediated hypercalcemia with a malignancy.

DIAGNOSIS

Measurement of intact PTH provides a useful starting point for diagnosis (see Fig. 186-1). An elevated PTH level in the context of hypercalcemia should prompt further evaluation for parathyroid disease (Chapter 253). However, in the majority of cancer patients with hypercalcemia, the intact PTH value is suppressed, indicating that the malignancy is causing the hypercalcemia. It should be kept in mind that hyperparathyroidism is not an uncommon disease, and a small percentage of patients with hypercalcemia and cancer may have both hyperparathyroidism and cancer-mediated hypercalcemia.

FIGURE 186-1. Strategy for evaluation of hypercalcemia in the context of malignancy based on measurement of intact parathyroid hormone (iPTH). PTHrP = parathyroid hormone–related protein; TNF = tumor necrosis factor.

TREATMENT   Rx

The initial management of hypercalcemia should focus on reversing dehydration and increasing urine calcium excretion by the infusion of normal saline solution at rates of 100 to 300 mL/hour, depending on the patient's cardiac status. A patient with a serum calcium concentration greater than 13 mg/dL (3.25 mM/L), altered mental status, or renal dysfunction should also be treated with a bisphosphonate (intravenous pamidronate 60 to 90 mg over 4 hours, or intravenous zoledronate 4 mg over a 15-minute period), glucocorticoids (prednisone or methylprednisolone 40 to 60 mg/day), gallium nitrate (200 mg/m^2/day, infused for 7 days), or salmon calcitonin (100 to 200 U intravenously or subcutaneously every 6 to 12 hours), alone or in combination. PTHrP-mediated or localized osteolysis is most responsive to bisphosphonates or gallium nitrate; vitamin D–mediated hypercalcemia is most responsive to glucocorticoid therapy (Chapter 253).

Use of high-dose intravenous bisphosphonates for extended periods has been associated with osteonecrosis of the jaw, a condition in which the mandibular or maxillary bone becomes devascularized, leading to loss of the overlying mucosa and exposed bone (Chapter 256). This condition developed in approximately 1 to 2% of patients with breast cancer and 2 to 3% with myeloma who received monthly intravenous pamidronate or zoledronate. Replacement of the devascularized and sclerotic bone occurs slowly—some patients have exposed bone for 3 to 5 years. Because many cases have been associated with dental procedures, such as removal of a tooth or tooth implantation, or with poorly fitting dentures, patients should have any dental issues addressed before the initiation of intravenous bisphosphonate therapy. The benefits of intravenous bisphosphonates in the context of bone metastasis or myeloma are substantial, and their continued use seems appropriate; however, trials are ongoing to determine whether the use of bone turnover markers to monitor suppression of bone resorption will permit use of less intensive bisphosphonate therapy.

Long-term management is focused on treatment of the underlying malignancy. Average survival in a patient with PTHrP-mediated hypercalcemia is less than 3 months, in part related to the underlying malignancy. Long-term therapy for PTHrP-mediated hypercalcemia, like that associated with parathyroid carcinoma, is difficult: patients tend to become less responsive to the effects of bisphosphonate or salmon calcitonin therapy over time and may experience renal toxicity when gallium nitrate therapy is used for extended periods.

Identification of the aforementioned RANKL/RANK receptor system has led to the development of a monoclonal antibody that binds to RANKL, thereby preventing activation of the RANK receptor. This agent, denosumab, is administered subcutaneously and recently approved for treatment of bone metastases; it is comparable to intravenous bisphosphonates in suppressing bone turnover and reducing the risk of skeletal events in patients with cancer-related bone metastases.[1,2]

ECTOPIC ADRENOCORTICOTROPIC HORMONE SECRETION

PATHOBIOLOGY

Inappropriate secretion of ACTH is a rare but important cause of morbidity and mortality in cancer patients. It can be caused by two different mechanisms: expression of the proopiomelanocortin (POMC) gene by a tumor, or ectopic expression of CRH. In cell types that express the POMC gene, posttranslational processing of this gene product can proceed down one of several mutually exclusive pathways and result in the expression of β-lipotropin, γ-lipotropin, and β-endorphin or the expression of big melanocyte-stimulating hormone and ACTH. Although POMC expression by malignant tumors is relatively common, expression of the enzymes necessary to cleave ACTH from the precursor is found less frequently outside the pituitary gland. ACTH production occurs in a broad spectrum of tumors, but it is most commonly associated with small cell carcinoma of the lung (Chapter 197) or classic neuroendocrine tumors such as pulmonary carcinoid (Chapter 240), medullary thyroid carcinoma (Chapter 233), islet cell adenoma or carcinoma (Chapter 238), pheochromocytoma (Chapter 235), and occasional neural tumors such as ganglioneuroma. Ectopic ACTH production causes adrenal cortical hyperplasia and excessive cortisol production (Chapter 234).

CLINICAL MANIFESTATIONS

Ectopic production of CRH causes a clinical syndrome characterized by pituitary corticotrope hyperplasia and laboratory results that mimic those of pituitary Cushing's disease (Chapter 231). Diagnosis requires a high index of suspicion combined with either measurement of CRH in blood or identification of a neoplasm outside the pituitary. Some neoplasms produce both ACTH and CRH. Tumors reported to produce CRH include medullary thyroid carcinoma, paraganglioma, prostate cancer, and islet cell neoplasms.

Hypercorticism associated with ectopic ACTH syndrome may manifest with classic features of Cushing's syndrome, such as easy bruisability, centripetal obesity, muscle wasting, hypertension, diabetes, and metabolic alkalosis. In other patients, particularly those with rapidly growing small cell carcinoma of the lung, the clinical picture may be dominated by profound hypokalemic metabolic alkalosis and hypertension, without the other clinical findings of Cushing's syndrome.

DIAGNOSIS

Evaluation of Cushing's syndrome (Chapter 234) is based on the plasma ACTH measurement in a patient with suggestive clinical and laboratory features (Fig. 186-2). The finding of a marked elevation in the plasma ACTH concentration (>100 pg/mL) should prompt a search for an ectopic source of ACTH. In a patient with a plasma ACTH value greater than 10 pg/mL but

FIGURE 186-2. Evaluation strategy for a patient with Cushing's syndrome and suspected ectopic adrenocorticotropic hormone (ACTH) production. In patients with a plasma ACTH concentration greater than 100 pg/mL, an ectopic ACTH source should be considered, although some patients with pituitary Cushing's disease may have values in this range. In patients with a plasma ACTH concentration between 10 and 100 pg/mL, inferior petrosal sinus sampling for ACTH should be performed after peripheral corticotropin-releasing hormone (CRH) injection (Chapter 234) to separate a pituitary (high central-peripheral ACTH ratio) from an ectopic (low central-peripheral ACTH ratio) ACTH source. In patients with a low basal peripheral ACTH value (<10 pg/mL), a low-dose CRH test (1 µg/kg) should be performed, followed by inferior petrosal sinus sampling in individuals whose plasma ACTH concentration rises to greater than 10 pg/mL.

less than 100 pg/mL, a more detailed evaluation is appropriate. Differentiation between a pituitary and an ectopic source may require stimulation of ACTH secretion by CRH combined with measurement of ACTH in blood from the pituitary venous drainage (inferior petrosal sinus sampling). Lack of an increase in the inferior petrosal sinus ACTH concentration (less than three times the peripheral ACTH concentration) after peripheral CRH stimulation should prompt a search for an ectopic source. In patients with an increased (more than three times the peripheral level) inferior petrosal sinus ACTH level after CRH, a pituitary source is likely. Ectopic CRH can yield confusing results and may not be diagnosed unless the clinician considers the possibility and measures plasma CRH or looks for an ectopic source.

Other approaches have also been applied to the diagnosis of ectopic ACTH syndrome. For example, ACTH production from an ectopic source is not generally suppressed by high-dose dexamethasone. In a patient with an ACTH concentration greater than 10 pg/mL, administration of a single 8-mg oral dose of dexamethasone at 11:00 PM, followed by measurement of the serum cortisol level at 8:00 AM, can differentiate between a pituitary and an ectopic source. The serum cortisol level in pituitary Cushing's disease (caused by a pituitary tumor) is generally suppressed 50% after dexamethasone, whereas levels in ectopic ACTH are usually not suppressed. However, false-positive or false-negative results occur with each of these testing procedures, making the differential diagnosis of Cushing's syndrome one of the most challenging in medicine.

TREATMENT   Rx

Hypercortisolism associated with ectopic ACTH can be managed by removal of the ACTH- or CRH-producing tumor or by inhibition of cortisol synthesis with metyrapone (1 to 4 g/day orally), aminoglutethimide (250 mg orally four times/day with upward titration), or ketoconazole (200 to 400 mg orally twice a day). Parenteral etomidate, used for sedation and induction of anesthesia, rapidly inhibits cortisol synthesis at subhypnotic concentrations. It is titrated from 0.3 to 4 mg/kg/hour to normalize serum cortisol measurements and has been used to rapidly reverse hypercorticism in a small number of patients. Replacement glucocorticoid therapy is needed to prevent adrenal insufficiency in patients receiving inhibitors of cortisol synthesis (Chapter 234). If surgical removal of an ACTH- or CRH-producing tumor is not possible and inhibition of cortisol synthesis is inadequate, bilateral adrenalectomy (with replacement glucocorticoid and mineralocorticoid therapy) may be required. In patients with a rapidly progressive small cell carcinoma of the lung and ectopic ACTH syndrome, the oncologic imperative to initiate immediate cytotoxic therapy must be counterbalanced by the desire to normalize cell-mediated immunity by normalizing cortisol secretion, hypokalemia, and metabolic alkalosis. Cytotoxic chemotherapy should generally be delayed, if possible, until the serum cortisol level is normalized because neutropenic patients with hypercortisolism have a high rate of infection that often causes death. If cancer treatment is initiated, prophylactic therapy for pulmonary *Pneumocystis carinii* (Chapter 349) and fungal infections should be considered.

HUMAN CHORIONIC GONADOTROPIN PRODUCTION

PATHOBIOLOGY

Two different genes encode the α- and β-subunits of human chorionic gonadotropin (HCG). The β-subunit is common to all the pituitary glycoprotein hormones (luteinizing hormone, follicle-stimulating hormone, thyroid-stimulating hormone [TSH], and HCG), whereas each of these hormones has a unique β-subunit gene. Inappropriate production of the α-subunit occurs in a variety of pituitary and nonpituitary tumors and does not cause any discernible clinical syndrome. The β-subunit confers biologic specificity. Production of intact HCG occurs commonly in trophoblastic tumors (choriocarcinoma, testicular embryonal carcinoma, and seminoma; Chapter 206) and less commonly in other tumors such as those of the lung and pancreas.

CLINICAL MANIFESTATIONS AND DIAGNOSIS

Clinical syndromes associated with the production of HCG include precocious puberty, gynecomastia, and hyperthyroidism. Hyperthyroidism results from the low-affinity interaction of HCG with the TSH receptor when β-HCG is present in high concentrations. β-HCG concentrations that are several orders of magnitude higher than normal interact with the TSH receptor and increase the production of thyroid hormone, thereby suppressing endogenous TSH production below normal.

TREATMENT Rx

Therapy for precocious puberty and gynecomastia is directed toward removal or treatment of the underlying tumor. Hyperthyroidism is treated by inhibiting thyroid hormone synthesis, usually with thionamide therapy, followed by therapy for the underlying tumor. Treatment of hyperthyroidism by surgical removal of the thyroid gland or ablation with radioactive iodine is rarely required because the hyperthyroidism resolves rapidly after treatment of the underlying tumor.

HYPOGLYCEMIA ASSOCIATED WITH CANCER

PATHOBIOLOGY

Tumor-associated hypoglycemia is a rare but important cause of morbidity in cancer patients. Three different clinical syndromes cause most cancer-related hypoglycemia. The first is production of insulin by an islet tumor. Although primary insulinomas are rare, dedifferentiation and bulky hepatic metastasis of an islet cell carcinoma may be associated with excessive insulin production (Chapter 238). A second cause of hypoglycemia, insufficient hepatic gluconeogenesis to maintain the plasma glucose concentration in the fasting state, is caused by nearly complete replacement of the liver by metastatic tumor. A third cause of hypoglycemia is increased concentrations of insulin-like growth factor type II (IGF-II), which activates the insulin receptor associated with large abdominal or retroperitoneal tumors such as fibrosarcoma, hemangiopericytoma, or hepatoma. This increased activity appears to be due to the failure to form a normal IGF binding protein 3 (IGFBP-3) and the acid-labile subunit (ALS) complex that normally binds IGF-II; the result is an increase in free IGF-II concentrations. It is usually possible to differentiate among the three causes by measuring serum insulin, C-peptide, proinsulin, IGF-I, IGF-II, and ALS levels during a controlled fast that causes hypoglycemia (Chapter 238).

CLINICAL MANIFESTATIONS, DIAGNOSIS, AND TREATMENT Rx

In all three types of hypoglycemia, the patient is at greatest risk for symptoms during periods of fasting, most commonly while sleeping. Therapy should focus on surgical excision, when possible, or antineoplastic therapy directed at the tumor. Initial therapy for hypoglycemia is focused on frequent meals, and patients occasionally remain symptom free if awakened for one or more snacks during sleeping hours. If the tumor progresses or the patient's caloric intake is inadequate, additional measures may be required. If hepatic replacement by tumor is evident, a continuous infusion of 20% dextrose through a central line may be required, especially during sleep. In patients with insulin-producing or large retroperitoneal tumors, glucagon infusion (0.5 to 2 mg/hour) stimulates hepatic gluconeogenesis and prevents hypoglycemia; however, in rare patients a rash associated with glucagonoma may develop. An increase in glucose concentration after a single injection of glucagon (1 mg) should be documented before initiating therapy. In patients with large retroperitoneal tumors, treatment with growth hormone (3 to 6 μg/kg subcutaneously) or glucocorticoids (20 to 40 mg/day) may reverse the hypoglycemia, possibly by facilitating IGFBP-3/ALS complex formation, thereby reducing free serum IGF-II levels. This condition has also been treated with growth hormone doses as high as 2600 μg/day; long-term treatment with this dose may cause acromegaly. Somatostatin analogues (octreotide or lanreotide) are not generally effective for normalizing the plasma glucose level in patients with islet cell tumors; diazoxide (3 to 8 mg/kg/day in two or three divided doses) may be effective, but problems with fluid retention frequently preclude its long-term use.

SYNDROME OF INAPPROPRIATE ANTIDIURETIC HORMONE SECRETION

PATHOBIOLOGY

Ectopic production of vasopressin by head and neck tumors (3%), small cell carcinoma of the lung (15%), and other lung carcinomas (1%) causes the clinical syndrome of inappropriate antidiuretic hormone (SIADH), which is characterized by hyponatremia, hypo-osmolality, excessive urine sodium excretion, an inappropriately high urine osmolality for the low serum osmolality, and normal function of the kidneys and adrenal and thyroid glands. Other malignant neoplasms (primary brain tumors; hematologic neoplasms; skin tumors; gastrointestinal, gynecologic, breast, and prostate cancers; and sarcomas) are rare causes of this clinical syndrome.

CLINICAL MANIFESTATIONS AND DIAGNOSIS

In most cases the hyponatremia is asymptomatic, although altered mental status and seizures may develop when the serum sodium concentration falls below 120 mEq/L. Hyponatremic women of reproductive age may experience profound cerebral degeneration.

TREATMENT Rx

Fluid restriction may be effective for short-term management, but it is difficult to maintain over long periods. Hypertonic fluids can be given with great caution to symptomatic patients (Chapter 118); the serum sodium concentration should be monitored to prevent an increase of more than 12 mEq/day. Treatment with 150 to 300 mg/day demeclocycline can block the effects of vasopressin on the kidney and is an effective long-term therapy in patients with cancer. Oral tolvaptan☒ and intravenous conivaptan are vasopressin receptor type 2 antagonists that are effective treatments for hyponatremia.

RARE ECTOPIC HORMONE SYNDROMES
Tumor-Induced Osteomalacia

A clinical syndrome characterized by profound hypophosphatemia, muscle weakness, and osteomalacia (Chapter 252) can be produced by mesenchymal tumors (osteoblastoma, giant cell osteosarcoma, hemangiocytoma, and, rarely, prostate and lung carcinoma). Fibroblast growth factor 23 (FGF-23), mutated in autosomal dominant hypophosphatemic rickets (Chapter 252), is overexpressed in neoplasms causing this disorder. Therapy is directed toward correction of hypophosphatemia with either oral or intravenous supplementation and vitamin D treatment. Surgical removal of the tumor is curative. Identification of FGF-23 overexpression as a cause may lead to the development of specific antagonists.

Hematologic Syndromes

The kidney is the primary site of erythropoietin production; therefore, the relatively common erythropoietin production by benign or malignant renal tumors is not an "ectopic" hormone syndrome. Production of erythropoietin by cerebellar hemangioblastomas (Chapter 195), uterine fibroids, pheochromocytomas (Chapter 235), and ovarian (Chapter 205) and hepatic (Chapter 202) tumors is generally considered "ectopic." Patients with excessive erythropoietin production may or may not have polycythemia (Chapter 169). Other ectopic syndromes, less well defined, include production of thrombopoietin or colony-stimulating factor by some tumors. These conditions are treated by removal of the tumor or by appropriate chemotherapy.

Hypertension

Renal (Wilms' tumor, renal cell carcinoma, hemangiopericytoma), lung (small cell carcinoma of the lung, adenocarcinoma), hepatic, pancreatic, and ovarian carcinomas may produce renin. The clinical findings in these patients can include hypertension, hypokalemia, and evidence of increased aldosterone production. Therapy with aldosterone antagonists or angiotensin-converting enzyme inhibitors may be effective.

Growth Hormone and Prolactin Production

Rare examples of growth hormone production have been identified in lung and gastric adenocarcinoma. Ectopic production of growth hormone–releasing hormone has been documented for islet cell tumors (Chapter 238), bronchogenic carcinoids (Chapter 240), and small cell carcinoma of the lung (Chapter 197). Increased prolactin production is a rare phenomenon associated with lymphomas and cancer of the lung, colon, kidney, and oral cavity. Hyperprolactinemia produces galactorrhea and amenorrhea in women and hypogonadism and gynecomastia in men. Treatment with dopamine agonists (bromocriptine, quinagolide, or cabergoline), which is effective in pituitary prolactinoma (Chapter 231), should be tried, but it is most commonly ineffective.

Grade A

1. Lipton A, Steger GG, Figueroa J, et al. Randomized active-controlled phase II study of denosumab efficacy and safety in patients with breast cancer-related bone metastases. *J Clin Oncol.* 2007;25:4431-4437.
2. Body JJ, Lipton A, Gralow J, et al. Effects of denosumab in patients with bone metastases with and without previous bisphosphonate exposure. *J Bone Miner Res.* 2010:25:440-446.
3. Schrier RW, Gross P, Gheorghiade M, et al. SALT Investigators. Tolvaptan, a selective oral vasopressin V2-receptor antagonist, for hyponatremia. *N Engl J Med.* 2007;355:2099-2112.

SUGGESTED READINGS

Alexandraki KI, Grossman AB. The ectopic ACTH syndrome. *Rev Endocr Metab Disord.* 2010;11:117-126. *Review of pathogenesis and diagnosis.*
Kacprowicz RF, Lloyd JD. Electrolyte complications of malignancy. *Hematol Oncol Clin North Am.* 2010;24:553-565. *Concise review of the diagnosis and treatment of life-threatening electrolyte abnormalities in cancer patients, including hyponatremia, hypoglycemia, and hypercalcemia.*
Peri A, Pirozzi N, Parenti G, et al. Hyponatremia and the syndrome of inappropriate secretion of antidiuretic hormone (SIADH). *J Endocrinol Invest.* 2010;33:671-682. *Review.*
Santarpia L, Koch CA, Sarlis NJ. Hypercalcemia in cancer patients: pathobiology and management. *Horm Metab Res.* 2010;42:153-164. *Synthesis of peer-reviewed evidence regarding the pathophysiology and treatment of hypercalcemia in cancer.*
Verbalis JG. Managing hyponatremia in patients with syndrome of inappropriate antidiuretic hormone secretion. *Endocrinol Nutr.* 2010;57:30-40. *Review including the use of tolvaptan.*

187

PARANEOPLASTIC SYNDROMES AND OTHER NON-NEOPLASTIC EFFECTS OF CANCER

HOPE S. RUGO

DEFINITION

The direct clinical manifestations of cancer are usually due to local effects of tumor growth, either in the primary site or at a distant site, or are nonspecific such as anorexia, malaise, weight loss, night sweats, and fever. The term *paraneoplasia,* which means "alongside cancer," has been commonly used to denote remote effects of cancer that cannot be attributed either to direct invasion or to distant metastases.

EPIDEMIOLOGY

These syndromes may be the first sign of a malignancy and affect up to 15% of patients with cancer. However, if patients with cachexia are excluded, the incidence probably drops to only a few percent.

Paraneoplastic syndromes are important clinically for a number of reasons. First, they may be the initial presenting sign or symptom of an underlying malignancy. Up to two thirds of paraneoplastic syndromes arise before an associated malignancy is diagnosed. In some cases, the paraneoplastic syndrome may be associated with relatively small tumors; recognition of these associations may lead to earlier diagnosis and possibly more effective therapy. Second, one of the hallmarks in defining a paraneoplastic syndrome is that the course of the syndrome generally parallels the course of the tumor. Therefore, effective treatment of the underlying malignancy is often accompanied by improvement or resolution of the syndrome. Conversely, recurrence of the cancer may be heralded by return of systemic symptoms. One exception is the neurologic paraneoplastic syndromes, in which damage to structures within the nervous system may not be reversible. Third, the clinical manifestations of the paraneoplastic syndrome (or the toxic effects of electrolyte disturbances) may constitute a more urgent hazard to life or have a greater impact on quality of life than the underlying cancer.

PATHOBIOLOGY

Paraneoplastic syndromes may be caused by a variety of mechanisms; the endocrine (Chapter 186) and neurologic syndromes are the best understood. Possible etiologies include (1) secretion of proteins that are not associated with the normal tissue equivalent of the cancer (e.g., ectopic endocrine syndromes, local destruction of tissues by tumor-secreted cytokines), (2) antibodies that are directed against aberrantly expressed antigens on the tumor cell that cross-react with antigens that are normally expressed on other tissues (e.g., neurologic syndromes), and (3) effects related to unknown mechanisms, such as unidentified tumor products or circulating immune complexes stimulated by the tumor (e.g., osteoarthropathy associated with bronchogenic carcinoma; Chapter 197). Clinical findings may resemble those of primary metabolic, hematologic, dermatologic, or neuromuscular disorders or be specific to a cancer-related syndrome. Even such nonspecific symptoms as fever and weight loss are truly paraneoplastic and are due to the production of specific factors (e.g., tumor necrosis factor) by tumor cells or by normal cells in response to the tumor (see later).

DIAGNOSIS

In a patient who presents with symptoms or signs of a paraneoplastic syndrome, the screening evaluation (Table 187-1) should focus on the most common associated malignancies. If the initial evaluation is unrevealing, a repeated evaluation should be considered after several months. If the relationship between the syndrome and malignancy is less clear or less frequently observed, the evaluation should be focused on the patient's individual risks and symptoms.

The most common cancer associated with paraneoplastic syndromes is small cell cancer of the lung (Chapter 197), probably because of its neuroectodermal origin. Other neoplasms commonly associated with paraneoplastic syndrome include carcinomas of the breast (Chapter 204), ovary (Chapter 205), other adenocarcinomas, lymphoproliferative diseases (especially Hodgkin's disease; Chapter 192), and thymoma (Chapter 99).

NEUROLOGIC PARANEOPLASTIC SYNDROMES

PATHOBIOLOGY

Increasing evidence suggests that the underlying mechanisms of most neurologic syndromes associated with cancer are autoimmune in origin (Table 187-2). Tumors express antigens that are normally isolated to the nervous system and are found on neurons, referred to as onconeuronal antigens. Anti-neuronal antibodies that are produced against the new tumor cell antigen circulate in serum and spinal fluid and, at least in some patients, cause damage at the primary site of normal antigen expression. Pathologically, perivascular and interstitial lymphocytic infiltrates are found in the affected area of the brain. Indirect immunofluorescence of serum detects antibodies reactive with neurons. Disorders mediated by antibodies against neuronal cell surface or synaptic proteins may occur with or without tumor association; both may respond to immunotherapy.

It is unclear what susceptibility factors lead to development of a neurologic paraneoplastic syndrome. In addition to direct antibody-mediated damage, there is evidence that cell-mediated autoimmune mechanisms may

TABLE 187-1   EVALUATION AND DIAGNOSIS OF PARANEOPLASTIC SYNDROMES

Characterize abnormality; obtain laboratory studies and biopsy as necessary.
Carefully elicit any additional symptoms and signs.
Eliminate common causes.
If there is no obvious etiology, consider a paraneoplastic syndrome.
If findings are consistent with a known syndrome, screen for underlying malignancy.
If signs and symptoms are consistent with a known paraneoplastic syndrome, undertake a search for an unknown primary cancer or recurrence or progression of a known primary tumor.
Screening should include a careful physical examination with breast, gynecologic, and prostate evaluations; basic hematology, chemistry, and urine studies; chest radiograph; and mammogram.
Computed tomography (CT) of the abdomen and pelvis or positron emission tomography CT scan is indicated if there are any suspicious symptoms, signs, or laboratory abnormalities. Antibody testing for paraneoplastic neurologic syndromes and/or skin biopsy should be performed as indicated.
Consider treatment of cancer and/or appropriate palliative treatment, including immunosuppressive therapy for paraneoplastic symptoms when possible.

TABLE 187-2 PARANEOPLASTIC NEUROLOGIC SYNDROMES, ASSOCIATED ANTIBODIES, AND MALIGNANCIES

NEUROLOGIC SYNDROME	CLINICAL PRESENTATION	ANTIBODY	ASSOCIATED MALIGNANCY
Lambert-Eaton myasthenic syndrome	See text	Anti-VGCC Anti-SOX1	SCLC (>80%)
Paraneoplastic encephalomyelitis/ subacute sensory neuropathy	See text	Anti-Hu Anti-SOX1 Anti-amphiphysin Anti-Ma Anti-Trk (sensory)	SCLC (75-80%), neuroblastoma SCLC, breast Various carcinomas Lymphoma
	Acute psychosis	Anti-NMDA	Ovarian teratoma
Paraneoplastic cerebellar degeneration	See text	Anti-Yo Anti-SOX1 Anti-Ri Anti-Hu Anti-Tr, Anti-GluR Anti-Ma	Breast, ovarian, and other gynecologic malignancies Breast (50%) SCLC Hodgkin's lymphoma Various carcinomas
Limbic encephalopathy	Subacute amnestic syndrome, affective disorder, seizures DDX: herpes encephalitis Improvement common with treatment of underlying tumor; immunosuppression is of unclear benefit	Anti-Hu, Antiamphiphysin, Anti-SOX1, Anti-VGKC, Anti-AMPA Anti-Ta	SCLC Testicular, breast
Opsoclonus/myoclonus	Saccadic eye movements with ataxia and myoclonus Most occur in children with neuroblastomas Pathology reveals diffuse dropout of Purkinje cells Treatment of underlying tumor may improve symptoms; ACTH, steroids, and IVIG may also benefit	Anti-Ri Anti-Hu Antiamphiphysin Anti-Ta	Breast (70%), ovarian SCLC, neuroblastoma (50%) SCLC Testicular
Stiff-person syndrome	Progressive muscle stiffness and rigidity, with intermittent and painful muscle spasms. EMG: continuous firing of motor unit potentials Treat with muscle relaxants; may improve with cancer therapy	Antiamphiphysin Anti-GAD	Breast, SCLC Breast
Neuromyotonia	Diffuse muscle stiffness and cramps; may be associated with myasthenia gravis Responds to treatment of tumor and immunosuppression	Anti-VGCC	Thymoma
VISUAL SYNDROMES			
CAR	Gradual to acute and progressive visual loss	Antiretinal, antirecoverin	SCLC
MAR	Reports of response to immunosuppressive therapy and plasmapheresis	Antibipolar cell	Melanoma
Bilateral diffuse melanocytic proliferation (BDUMP)		?	Gynecologic malignancy Various adenocarcinomas
SYNDROMES WITH NO ASSOCIATED ANTIBODY IDENTIFIED			
Demyelinating neuropathies (including CDP, mononeuritis multiplex)	Sensory more common than motor or both May improve with treatment of paraprotein, plasmapheresis	IgM paraprotein may cross-react with MAG, cryoglobulins	Plasma cell and lymphoproliferative neoplasms, osteosclerotic myeloma, POEMS, amyloid, SCLC, other carcinomas
Necrotizing myelopathy	Symptoms associated with specific levels of spinal cord dysfunction Rapid deterioration and death		Variety of carcinomas and lymphomas
Motor neuron disease	Similar to ALS with progressive weakness; may improve with plasmapheresis and treatment of paraproteinemia		Plasma cell and lymphoproliferative neoplasms
Polymyositis/dermatomyositis	Unclear relationship to cancer, higher risk with dermatomyositis May improve with treatment of cancer, otherwise treat as idiopathic		Variety of carcinomas

ACTH = adrenocorticotropic hormone; AGNA = antiglial nuclear antibody; ALS = amyotrophic lateral sclerosis; AMPA = α-amino-3-hydroxy-5-methyl-4-isoxazolepropionic acid; amphiphysin = synaptic vesicle–associated protein; CAR = carcinoma-associated retinopathy; CDP = chronic demyelinating polyneuropathy; DDX = differential diagnosis; EMG = electromyogram; GAD = glutamic acid decarboxylase; GluR = glutamate receptor; IgM = immunoglobulin M; IVIG = intravenous immunoglobulin; MAG = myelin-associated glycoprotein; MAR = melanoma-associated retinopathy; NMDA = N-methyl-D-aspartate; POEMS = polyneuropathy, organomegaly, endocrinopathy, monoclonal protein, and skin changes associated with osteosclerotic myeloma; SCLC = small cell lung cancer; VGCC = voltage-gated calcium channel; VGKC = voltage-gated potassium channel.

contribute. The finding of CD8+ T lymphocytes infiltrating neurologic tissue in postmortem studies of patients with neurologic paraneoplastic syndromes, combined with data that patients with antibodies (with or without neurologic paraneoplastic syndromes) may have longer survival rates than otherwise similar patients without circulating antibodies, suggests that CD8+ T lymphocytes play a beneficial role in tumor-directed immune responses. This immune response may be mediated by aberrant expression of native antigens.

CLINICAL MANIFESTATIONS

Neurologic paraneoplastic syndromes may involve the brain, cranial nerves, spinal cord, dorsal root ganglia, peripheral nerves, neuromuscular junction, muscle, or multiple levels of the nervous system. Perhaps because of cross-reactivity of antibodies, it is not uncommon for patients to develop more than one paraneoplastic syndrome, making the diagnosis of a particular syndrome more difficult. Classic paraneoplastic disorders include those whose clinical manifestations are unique and are frequently associated with cancer;

TABLE 187-3 GENETIC SYNDROMES WITH CUTANEOUS MANIFESTATIONS ASSOCIATED WITH AN INCREASED RISK OF SYSTEMIC CANCERS

GENETIC SYNDROME	SKIN LESION	GENETIC MUTATION	ASSOCIATED CANCERS	RISK
Torre's (Muir-Torre)	Multiple sebaceous gland tumors, basal cell cancers	Mutations in DNA mismatch repair genes leading to microsatellite instability (*MSH2*, 2p22-p21)	GI and GU cancers	High
Gardner's	Multiple epidermal and sebaceous cysts of face and scalp, desmoid tumors of skin, osteomas of face and head, GI polyps	Adenomatous polyposis coli tumor suppressor gene (5q21-q22)	GI cancers	High
Cowden's	Multiple hamartomas of skin, mucous membranes (trichilemmomas), lipomas	*PTEN/MMAC1* tumor suppressor gene	Breast, thyroid cancers	High
MEN 2B	Multiple papular mucosal neuromas on lips, oropharynx, conjunctiva	Receptor tyrosine kinase (*RET*) protooncogene	Medullary carcinoma of thyroid, pheochromocytoma	High
Ataxia-telangiectasia	Telangiectasias over face, conjunctiva	*ATM* gene (11q22-23)	Lymphomas	Medium
Neurofibromatosis type 1	Cafe au lait spots, axillary freckles, neurofibromas	*NF1* gene (17q11.2)	Neurofibrosarcoma, pheochromocytoma, acoustic neuromas	Low
Peutz-Jeghers	Pigmented macules on the lips, oral mucosa, hands, feet; hamartomatous GI polyps	*STK11/LKB1* gene (19p13.3)	GI, pancreas, ovary, testes	Low
Basal cell carcinoma nevus (Gorlin's)	Multiple basal cell cancers	*PTCH1* gene (9q22) resulting in activation of hedgehog signaling	Basal cell cancers, medulloblastoma, fibrosarcoma	Low
Bloom's	Telangiectatic redness of skin in photo-exposed areas, stunted growth	DNA helicase gene (*RECQL3*)	Lymphomas, leukemias	Medium

GI = gastrointestinal; GU = genitourinary; MEN = multiple endocrine neoplasia.

nonclassic syndromes frequently occur without cancer and may be difficult to identify. The differential diagnosis of neurologic paraneoplastic syndromes includes idiopathic presentations of the same syndrome, side effects of chemotherapy (Chapter 182) and radiation therapy (Chapter 19; Table 187-2), infections (usually associated with lymphoproliferative diseases), vascular disease (including infarction and hemorrhage), and metabolic and nutritional abnormalities (including hormonal paraneoplastic syndromes). Therapy includes treatment of the underlying tumor as well as immunosuppressive therapy with or without plasmapheresis. Unfortunately, this approach usually results in only modest, if any, improvement of the neurologic deficit.

DIAGNOSIS

A patient presenting with neurologic complaints regardless of a prior diagnosis of malignancy should undergo a standard evaluation for diseases such as a primary central nervous system (CNS) malignancy, a metastatic malignancy, bleeding, vascular events, and infection. Generally, this evaluation includes a careful history regarding onset, associated symptoms, and other general medical conditions, as well as a careful physical and neurologic examination. Studies should include initial contrast-enhanced magnetic resonance imaging (MRI) and examination of the cerebrospinal fluid (CSF) for protein and cells if the MRI is normal or showed leptomeningeal enhancement. If the evaluation does not reveal evidence of primary CNS disease, a body positron emission tomography (PET) or computed tomography (CT) scan along with standard laboratory testing may be useful to screen for undetected malignancies.

If a neurologic paraneoplastic syndrome is suspected, serum and CSF should be tested for antineuronal antibodies targeted to either intracellular or cell surface proteins (see Table 187-2). However, a high degree of specificity of an antibody for a particular syndrome does not prove that the antibody is pathogenic. Finding a circulating antibody is useful but not diagnostic of any particular syndrome; patients can have circulating antibodies without the associated clinical syndrome, and most lung cancers as well as many breast and gynecologic malignancies express neuronal antigens, although the antibody titer is usually much lower than that seen with a neurologic paraneoplastic syndrome. High serum antibody levels and the presence of antibody in the CSF are more specific findings. Diagnosis of a neurologic paraneoplastic syndrome should instigate a reasonable search for the commonly associated malignancy (see Table 187-1). PET and CT scans have been shown to improve the detection of cancers when other screening tests are negative, particularly when patients are found to have antineuronal antibodies.

Lambert-Eaton Myasthenic Syndrome—Anti-VGCC and Anti-SOX1 Antibodies

DEFINITION AND EPIDEMIOLOGY

The Lambert-Eaton myasthenic syndrome (LEMS) is one of the first recognized and most common neurologic paraneoplastic syndromes, and it is one of the only syndromes with direct evidence to support the role of autoantibodies in producing clinical disease. This disorder affects 1 to 2% of patients with small cell cancer of the lung (SCLC), and up to two thirds of the cases are associated with an underlying malignancy.

PATHOBIOLOGY

LEMS is associated with a defect in the release of neurotransmitters (acetylcholine) from the presynaptic neurons at the neuromuscular junction and other sites. Acetylcholine release is mediated by P-type voltage-gated calcium channels (VGCCs); antibodies to VGCC are found in the serum of more than 85% of patients with Lambert-Eaton myasthenic syndrome. Paraneoplastic LEMS and idiopathic LEMS are clinically and immunologically similar, but a recently discovered antibody significantly associates with the presence of SCLC. Antiglial nuclear antibody (AGNA) binds to the SOX1 antigen, found in nuclei of specialized glia cells in the cerebellum. Anti-SOX1 antibodies have been identified in the sera of more than 60% of patients with paraneoplastic LEMS and appear to be a relatively specific marker of an associated underlying malignancy. SOX antibodies, as well as antibodies to the Zic protein, have been found in patients with a number of other paraneoplastic neurologic syndromes associated with SCLC as well as in the serum of patients with SCLC without neurologic symptoms.

CLINICAL MANIFESTATIONS AND DIAGNOSIS

Clinically, patients present with proximal lower limb weakness, with improvement in strength after several seconds of sustained voluntary contraction (Chapter 430). Autonomic symptoms, including dry mouth, ptosis, and impotence, are also common. Patients may also have associated CNS dysfunction, such as encephalomyelitis, cerebellar dysfunction, and peripheral neuropathy resulting from cross-reactivity or the presence of combinations of antibodies. The diagnosis is made by an electromyogram, which shows *increased* muscle action potential with repeated nerve stimulation greater than 10 Hz (the opposite of myasthenia gravis; Chapter 430). As noted previously, the finding of SOX1 antibodies significantly associates with the presence of SCLC.

TREATMENT ℞

Treatment consists of a combination of plasmapheresis, intravenous immunoglobulin (IVIG) to bind circulating antibodies, and immunosuppression (to remove antibodies and suppress their production), as well as treatment of the underlying malignancy. Successful removal of the primary malignancy may result in resolution of symptoms. Pharmacologic facilitation of neuromuscular transmission with pyridostigmine, 3,4-diaminopyridine, and guanidine may be useful.∎

Paraneoplastic Encephalomyelitis and Subacute Sensory Neuropathy—Anti-Hu Antibodies

This heterogeneous group of disorders can affect the cerebral hemispheres, limbic system, cerebellum, brain stem, spinal cord, dorsal root, and autonomic ganglia.

PATHOBIOLOGY

About 75 to 80% of paraneoplastic encephalomyelitis and subacute sensory neuropathy (Chapter 428) is associated with SCLC (Chapter 197), with a variety of other neoplasms representing the remainder. Most patients have circulating antineuronal anti-Hu autoantibodies; a small number have either no antibodies or antibodies to other proteins. One report found evidence of impairment of the Trk-neurotrophin receptor by the serum of a patient with subacute sensory neuropathy, suggesting production of anti-Trk autoantibodies. Although neuronal loss is accompanied by perivascular and leptomeningeal infiltration of lymphocytes, the pathogenesis of this syndrome is unknown.

CLINICAL MANIFESTATIONS

The most common manifestations are related to subacute sensory neuropathy, including patchy or asymmetrical numbness, burning or aching paresthesias, and sensory ataxia with loss of proprioception and vibration sense. Patients may also present primarily with subacute cerebellar degeneration or brain stem encephalitis, and nearly all patients have evidence of multifocal involvement of the CNS and dorsal root ganglia.

DIAGNOSIS

The diagnosis is made on clinical grounds and is aided by finding circulating antibody in serum. MRIs are usually normal, and the CSF can show elevated protein levels with a lymphocytosis. The usual course is deterioration over weeks to months, with stabilization at a level of severe neurologic disability.

TREATMENT ℞

Treatment has been largely unsuccessful, but a small number of patients have improved with immunosuppressive therapy, including prednisone and IVIG.

Paraneoplastic Cerebellar Degeneration— Anti-Yo Antibodies

Paraneoplastic cerebellar degeneration is usually the initial manifestation of cancer. About 90% of patients have breast cancer, ovarian or other gynecologic tumors, SCLC, or Hodgkin's disease.

PATHOBIOLOGY

Patients with paraneoplastic cerebellar degeneration and carcinomas of the breast or ovary or other gynecologic cancers have been found to have high titers of an anti–Purkinje cell antibody, anti-Yo, in the serum and CSF, but other antibodies that react against Purkinje cell antigens can also be found

(see Table 187-2). Autopsy reveals nearly complete loss of cerebellar Purkinje cells, with occasional inflammatory infiltrates.

CLINICAL MANIFESTATIONS AND DIAGNOSIS

Symptoms are often abrupt in onset and include dysarthria, ataxia, and oculomotor dysfunction. Syndromes such as paraneoplastic encephalomyelitis or LEMS may be superimposed. The diagnosis is based on clinical signs and may be aided by the presence of circulating antibody; however, anti-Yo antibodies are also found in patients who have a variety of cerebellar disorders but no evidence of cancer even on follow-up. CSF may reveal a pleocytosis and an elevated protein level or may be normal. MRI may show diffuse cerebellar atrophy but is often normal.

TREATMENT ℞

Treatment of the underlying malignancy occasionally results in significant improvement of cerebellar function. Rarely, responses have been seen to immunosuppressive therapy.

⬤ DERMATOLOGIC PARANEOPLASTIC SYNDROMES

CLINICAL MANIFESTATIONS AND DIAGNOSIS

Recognition of cutaneous manifestations of malignancy can be critical for the early diagnosis and successful treatment of malignancy, but some syndromes are seen only with advanced, incurable disease. Cutaneous manifestations include direct involvement of the skin with tumor as well as the remote effects of cancer.

Benign skin changes may be the only sign of genetic syndromes that predispose to an increased risk for malignancy over a lifetime (see Table 187-3). Recognition of these syndromes is critical for screening, early diagnosis, and genetic counseling of affected family members.

Associations between cutaneous syndromes and underlying malignancies may be difficult to confirm. Generally, and unlike the situation in neurologic paraneoplastic syndromes, the skin condition and cancer should follow a parallel course, and the two diagnoses should be made at about the same time (Table 187-4). Some skin lesions are almost always associated with malignancy. Others, however, are nonspecific and are most commonly seen with nonmalignant conditions, making it difficult or impossible to connect the skin disease with the underlying malignancy. In addition, biopsies of the skin lesion are usually nonspecific, showing features identical to those when the same lesion is seen with a nonmalignant condition. The formation of tumor-related autoantibodies has been rarely associated with dermatologic paraneoplastic syndromes, although inflammatory cell infiltration may be seen.

The finding of a new skin lesion that is almost always associated with an underlying malignancy (e.g., Bazex's syndrome, erythema gyratum repens) should prompt a directed evaluation for that tumor. In contrast, diagnosis of a common problem that is only occasionally associated with cancer (e.g., pruritus, dermatomyositis) should prompt a careful physical examination and routine cancer screening as well as continued awareness of this possible association over time. The etiology of most dermatologic paraneoplastic syndromes is not well understood. The diagnosis of a paraneoplastic dermatologic syndrome is based on characteristic clinical and pathologic findings, including deposition of immunoglobulin G (IgG) and C3 at the basement membrane of affected skin in a variety of syndromes and the finding of an underlying malignancy.

Selected Specific Syndromes
ACANTHOSIS NIGRICANS

One of the most well-known paraneoplastic syndromes is acanthosis nigricans, whose pathogenesis is unclear. The tumor may produce factors that activate insulin-like growth factors or the insulin receptor in skin. Many tumors are known to produce transforming growth factor-α (TGF-α), which might activate epidermal growth factor receptors in skin, causing hyperpigmentation and thickening.

CLINICAL MANIFESTATIONS AND DIAGNOSIS

The skin lesions (Fig. 187-1) arise as velvety, verrucous hyperpigmentation of the neck, axilla, groin, and mucosal membranes, including the lips,

TABLE 187-4 EXAMPLES OF CUTANEOUS AND RHEUMATOLOGIC LESIONS ASSOCIATED WITH MALIGNANT DISEASE

SYNDROME	CLINICAL PRESENTATION	ASSOCIATED MALIGNANCY	ASSOCIATION/RISK
CUTANEOUS			
Acanthosis nigricans	Velvety, verrucous, brown hyperpigmentation involving body folds and mucosal membranes	Gastric cancer (also endocrinopathies)	High
Acquired hypertrichosis lanuginosa (malignant down)	Long, fine, nonpigmented lanugo hairs on face, trunk, limbs, axillae	Carcinomas of the lung, colon, breast, uterus, bladder, and lymphoma (also seen with AIDS, anorexia, thyrotoxicosis, porphyria, medications)	Moderate to high
Acquired tylosis	Hyperkeratosis of palms	Lung cancer, esophageal cancer	Likely low
Bazex's syndrome	Acral hyperkeratotic papulosquamous lesions, onychodystrophy	Squamous cell carcinomas of the oropharynx, larynx, bronchi, esophagus	High
Extramammary Paget's	Nonhealing superficial dermatitis	Genitourinary and rectal cancers	Moderate to high
Sign of Leser-Trélat	Diffuse eruption of seborrheic keratoses	Gastrointestinal cancers (also seen with aging)	Likely moderate
Tripe palms	Thickened, velvety palms	Lung and gastric cancers (almost always seen with acanthosis nigricans)	High
Necrolytic migratory erythema	Circinate erosive erythematous rash, stomatitis	Glucagonoma	Likely moderate
Erythema gyratum repens	Concentric rings on trunk and proximal extremities; may have pruritus	Carcinomas of the lung, esophagus, and breast	High
Erythroderma	Diffuse erythema	Lymphoma	Low to moderate
Paraneoplastic pemphigus	Painful erythematous lesions with blistering; mucous membrane ulcerations	Lymphoma	High
Sweet's syndrome	Red nodules or plaques, fever, dermal neutrophilic infiltrates	Acute myelogenous leukemia (also seen with infection)	Moderate
Pruritus	Excoriations, pruritus occurs on extremities, upper trunk, extensor surfaces	Lymphoma and myeloproliferative neoplasms (especially polycythemia vera)	Low
CUTANEOUS WITH ARTHRITIS OR MYOPATHY			
Amyloidosis	Waxy papules and nodules, occasionally with associated symmetrical arthritis; renal insufficiency	Multiple myeloma	Moderate
Palmar fasciitis-polyarthritis	Thickening of the palmar fascia; inflammatory distal symmetrical arthritis	Ovarian cancer	Low
Panniculitis-arthritis	Erythematous subcutaneous tender nodules; inflammatory monoarticular or polyarticular arthritis	Cancer of the pancreas (also pancreatitis)	Low
Eosinophilic fasciitis	Edema, thickening of the dermis and fascia associated with joint contractures	Breast cancer, myeloproliferative neoplasm, lymphoproliferative disease	Low
Dermatomyositis/polymyositis	Heliotrope rash (erythema in periorbital area); Gottron's papules (erythematous papules over phalangeal joints); proximal myopathy	Various tumors, primarily adenocarcinomas	Low to moderate, more with dermatomyositis
ARTICULAR			
Digital clubbing	Loss of nail bed angle	Lung cancer (also seen with benign cardiopulmonary disorders)	Low
Hypertrophic pulmonary osteoarthropathy	Periostosis of long bones; pain and swelling in distal joints	Lung cancer	High
Carcinoma polyarthropathy	Sudden onset of seronegative arthritis at a late age	Cancers of the breast and lung	Low to moderate
Gout	Classic acute painful gouty arthritis	Acute leukemias, lymphomas associated with rapid tumor cell turnover and tumor lysis	Low
VASCULAR			
Leukocytoclastic vasculitis	Palpable purpura, urticaria, maculopapular rash with or without arthritis	Myeloproliferative and lymphoproliferative neoplasms, myelodysplasia; rarely with adenocarcinoma and melanoma	Low to moderate
Polyarteritis nodosa	Cutaneous and/or mesenteric vasculitis; fever, myalgia; arthritis; mononeuritis multiplex	Hairy cell leukemia	Low
Raynaud's syndrome	Classic Raynaud's with progression to digital necrosis or gangrene common	Lymphoma, leukemia, myeloma, and cancers of the lung, ovary, small bowel, breast, pancreas, kidney	Low to moderate in patients older than 50 years
Erythromelalgia	Painful, erythematous digits, relieved by aspirin	Myeloproliferative neoplasms (especially essential thrombocythemia)	Moderate to high

periocular area, and anus. Although acanthosis nigricans clearly occurs as a benign entity associated with obesity and endocrinopathy, its appearance in older adults, especially when it includes mucosal lesions, has been highly associated with malignancies of the gastrointestinal tract as well as other adenocarcinomas. The lesions often regress with successful treatment of the underlying tumor.

PARANEOPLASTIC PEMPHIGUS

This syndrome is manifested by ulcerative and blistering mucocutaneous lesions with acantholysis; it is primarily associated with lymphoma (Chapters 191 and 192), other lymphoproliferative diseases, and thymic cancers. Patients have high titers of autoantibodies to tumor antigens that cross-react with antigens at the epidermal cell junction, including the plakin family of soles. These lesions can predate the diagnosis of malignancy by as long as 1 year, and they may progress in parallel with the underlying tumor. The main differential diagnosis involves exclusion of benign acral variants of psoriasis.

RHEUMATOLOGIC PARANEOPLASTIC SYNDROMES

DEFINITION AND EPIDEMIOLOGY

A wide variety of rheumatologic paraneoplastic syndromes have been associated with underlying malignancies, but almost all of these syndromes are identical to their benign counterparts (see Table 187-4). The rheumatologic paraneoplastic syndromes can be classified as cutaneous with arthritis, articular, or vasculitic. Paraneoplastic rheumatologic syndromes may either coincide with the diagnosis of malignancy or precede it by several years, although the longer the interval between diagnoses, the less likely the association with cancer. Patients with a variety of rheumatologic diseases are known to have an increased risk of subsequent malignancy. For example, Sjögren's syndrome (Chapter 276) is associated with a slightly increased risk of lymphoproliferative disease, although the cause of this relationship remains unclear.

CLINICAL MANIFESTATIONS

In contrast to the nonparaneoplastic rheumatologic syndromes, rheumatologic paraneoplastic syndromes are associated with rapid onset, late age at onset (>50 years), negative serologies, and effusions characterized by the absence of inflammatory markers. Considerable overlap exists among the rheumatologic, dermatologic, and neurologic paraneoplastic syndromes.

DIAGNOSIS

In general, when a rheumatologic paraneoplastic syndrome is suspected, screening should include a physical examination, laboratory tests, and standard radiographic tests, such as a mammogram.

POEMS Syndrome

Osteosclerotic myeloma (Chapter 193) associated with the POEMS syndrome (*p*olyneuropathy, *o*rganomegaly, *e*ndocrinopathy, *m*onoclonal protein, and *s*kin changes suggestive of *s*cleroderma) is a rare condition that has features of neurologic, rheumatologic, and dermatologic paraneoplastic syndromes owing to the effects of a circulating paraprotein. It is likely that other factors also play a role in the pathogenesis of POEMS syndrome, including production of high levels of vascular endothelial growth factor and inflammatory cytokines.

Hypertrophic Osteoarthropathy

One of the more common and specific rheumatologic paraneoplastic syndromes is hypertrophic osteoarthropathy, which arises as an oligoarthritis or polyarthritis of the distal joints with clubbing, tender periostitis of the distal long bones, and noninflammatory synovial effusions. Hypertrophic osteoarthropathy may affect up to 10% of patients with adenocarcinoma of the lung. It is also seen with a variety of other pulmonary malignancies, including lung metastases from other primary sites. The etiology is unknown. Laboratory studies often reveal an elevation in the erythrocyte sedimentation rate; bone radiographs show linear ossification of the distal long bones separated by a radiolucent zone from the underlying cortex (Fig. 187-2). Treatment is symptomatic with anti-inflammatory agents; successful treatment of the underlying tumor may also improve the signs and symptoms of this syndrome.

Tumor-Induced Osteomalacia

Tumor-induced osteomalacia, a rare paraneoplastic syndrome associated with benign mesenchymal tumors and characterized by inappropriately low levels of serum 1,25-dihydroxyvitamin D and renal phosphate wasting thought to be due to tumor expression of fibroblast growth factor 23, is discussed in detail in Chapter 186.

Dermatomyositis and Polymyositis

Dermatomyositis or polymyositis has been reported to be associated with an underlying malignancy in less than 10% to as high as 60% of cases (Chapter 277). Dermatomyositis is more strongly and frequently associated with malignancy than is polymyositis. Studies of patients with dermatomyositis report a two- to four-fold increased risk of underlying malignancy, including cancer of the lung, ovaries, breast, gastrointestinal tract, and testes. The true incidence of malignancy in patients diagnosed with

FIGURE 187-1. **Acanthosis nigricans. A,** Paraneoplastic acanthosis nigricans with a velvety hyperpigmented rash in the axilla in a patient with gastric cancer. **B,** Acanthosis nigricans of the oral mucosa. This pattern of involvement is almost always associated with cancer. (Courtesy of Dr. Timothy Berger.)

desmosomal proteins and desmogleins; indirect immunofluorescent staining shows IgG and C3 deposition on the surface of keratinocytes and on the basement membrane zone. Antibody titers may correlate with the severity of the skin disease and its response to therapy.

DIAGNOSIS

The diagnosis of paraneoplastic pemphigus should include finding specific major criteria including a polymorphic cutaneous eruption, concurrent internal neoplasia, and a specific immunoprecipitation pattern on testing of serum. Minor criteria include histologic evidence of acantholysis, intercellular and basement membrane staining with antibodies to IgG and C3 on direct immunofluorescence, and staining of rat urothelium with antibodies to desmoplakin on indirect immunofluorescence. The development of paraneoplastic pemphigus in patients with lymphoma (Chapters 191 and 192), chronic lymphocytic leukemia (Chapter 190), Castleman's disease (Chapter 191), and, less commonly, other malignancies is associated with a very poor prognosis and is often associated with pulmonary involvement.

BAZEX'S SYNDROME

Bazex's syndrome is a papulosquamous eruption that is also termed acrokeratosis paraneoplasia owing to the characteristic location of the hyperkeratotic lesions on the palms and soles. It is seen in association with squamous cell carcinoma of the head and neck (Chapter 196) as well as other malignancies involving the oropharynx or larynx. Bazex's syndrome has been postulated to be caused by antibodies that are directed against the tumor but that cross-react with keratinocyte or basement membrane antigens, similar to those in paraneoplastic pemphigus, or a T-cell-mediated immune response to epidermal tumor–like antigens.

CLINICAL MANIFESTATIONS AND DIAGNOSIS

The findings are similar in appearance to psoriatic plaques but are seen in unexpected locations including the ears, nails, nodes, fingers, palms, and

FIGURE 187-2. Hypertrophic pulmonary osteoarthropathy characterized by periosteal elevation of the tibia (*arrow*). (Courtesy of Dr. Lynne S. Steinbach.)

dermatomyositis is probably in the range 10 to 15%. Although the etiology is unknown, autoantibodies to muscle have been described. These autoantibodies are not well characterized and do not appear to be directed to known tumor antigens. The diagnosis of malignancy should be made within 1 year preceding or following the diagnosis of suspected paraneoplastic dermatomyositis; a longer duration of dermatomyositis without the development of cancer substantially decreases the risk of an associated malignancy.

Hematologic Paraneoplastic Syndromes

Routine blood testing may identify a hematologic paraneoplastic syndrome as well as the underlying malignancy. Hematologic paraneoplastic syndromes may involve all three cell lines.

RED CELLS

One of the most prevalent and commonly recognized paraneoplastic syndromes, seen with many cancers, is normochromic, normocytic anemia associated with a low reticulocyte count (Chapter 161). This hypoproductive anemia, generally termed *anemia of chronic disease,* or *anemia of chronic inflammation,* must be differentiated from anemia as a result of side effects of treatment or direct tumor infiltration of the bone marrow. It is associated with inappropriately low serum erythropoietin levels as well as the inability to reuse iron. Cytokines, including interleukin-1 (IL-1), tumor necrosis factor (TNF), and TGF-β, released by the tumor or local inflammatory cells mediate this disorder. Hypoproductive anemia may be effectively treated in patients with advanced malignancies with subcutaneous injections of erythropoietin or darbepoetin, although this treatment may possibly be associated with increased risk of thromboembolism (at high hemoglobin levels) and cancer progression (Chapter 161). Because of the potential risk of tumor stimulation, erythropoietic growth factors are not recommended for use in patients with early-stage or curable cancer. Pure red cell aplasia (Chapter 168) is a rare syndrome associated with cancer of the thymus gland (thymoma; Chapter 99) and is thought to be due to an autoimmune mechanism. Bone marrow examination shows absent red cell precursors.

Paraneoplastic anemia can also be caused by hemolysis (Chapter 163) related to warm- or cold-reacting antibodies in the setting of B-cell malignancies, especially chronic lymphocytic leukemia (Chapter 190) and lymphoma (Chapters 191 and 192). Treatment is directed toward the underlying lymphoproliferative disease but may also include IVIG, steroids, and possibly splenectomy for warm antibody hemolysis; cold-reacting hemolysis may require plasmapheresis. Microangiopathic hemolytic anemia (Chapter 163) with thrombocytopenia may occur with mucinous adenocarcinomas or after specific types of chemotherapy. Erythrocytosis is an uncommon paraneoplastic syndrome that is associated with tumors that produce erythropoietin, including renal cell cancer, hepatocellular carcinoma, and posterior fossa tumors (e.g., cerebellar hemangioblastoma) (Chapters 169 and 195).

WHITE CELLS

Leukocytosis (Chapter 170) is common in advanced cancer. Although infection and myeloproliferative disease must be excluded, the leukocytosis is generally caused by cytokines that are probably produced by the tumor itself, including granulocyte colony-stimulating factor and granulocyte-macrophage colony-stimulating factor. Although paraneoplastic leukocytosis requires no specific treatment, it may represent a poor prognostic sign. Eosinophilia (Chapter 173) can be seen with lymphoproliferative diseases.

PLATELETS

Paraneoplastic thrombocytosis, which is a relatively common laboratory finding, is caused by tumors that produce stimulatory cytokines (IL-6, thrombopoietin); platelet counts usually do not exceed 1 million. This type of secondary or reactive thrombocytosis, in contrast to the myeloproliferative neoplasm essential thrombocythemia (Chapter 169), is generally not associated with complications and does not require specific treatment. However, the underlying neoplasm may cause hypercoagulability by other mechanisms (see later). Iron deficiency, especially caused by gastrointestinal blood loss, should be excluded. Thrombocytopenia is uncommon except when it is associated with microangiopathic hemolytic anemia, disseminated intravascular coagulopathy (DIC), or marrow infiltration.

THROMBOSIS

EPIDEMIOLOGY

The best known and one of the first described hematologic paraneoplastic syndromes is Trousseau's syndrome, or the association of venous or arterial thrombosis with malignancy (Fig. 187-3). Although thrombosis frequently complicates progressive cancer, it may also be the first sign of cancer and predate diagnosis by a year or more. In approximately 10% of patients, deep vein thrombosis may herald an underlying malignancy, particularly in patients who present with an initial episode without other obvious risk factors, in the setting of recurrent thrombosis despite adequate doses of warfarin (warfarin resistance), or when the thrombosis occurs in unusual sites (e.g., subclavian vein, Budd-Chiari syndrome, portal vein thrombosis).

PATHOBIOLOGY

Paraneoplastic thrombosis is most commonly associated with adenocarcinomas, particularly of the stomach, breast, pancreas, and ovary. The etiology of thrombosis in patients with cancer is complex; tumor cells can activate coagulation through a number of mechanisms, including production of procoagulant mediators (e.g., sialic residues of tumor-secreted mucin), release of proangiogenic or inflammatory cytokines, direct interaction with host vasculature (endothelial damage) and blood cells through adhesion molecules, and tumor-mediated endothelial damage . Thrombosis may be associated with low-grade DIC (Chapter 178) and abnormal platelet activation. Risk factors for thrombosis in patients with known malignancy (Chapter 179) include the procoagulant effects of chemotherapy, indwelling catheters, immobility, surgery, older age, infection, obesity, prior thrombosis, and advanced stage of disease.

DIAGNOSIS

The evaluation of patients with a malignancy-associated thrombosis should include laboratory testing for DIC as well as a careful assessment of bleeding risk at sites of tumor, such as metastases to the nervous system, involvement of the gastrointestinal tract, or varices from portal hypertension in patients with liver involvement. It is important to exclude inherited clotting disorders, especially in younger patients who present with deep vein thrombosis without known underlying cause (Chapter 179) and in patients who develop a clot while taking tamoxifen.

FIGURE 187-3. Thrombophlebitis in superficial or deep veins is relatively common in many forms of malignant disease, but it is particularly associated with carcinoma of the pancreas and sometimes is the presenting feature. In this patient, thrombosis in the veins of the upper arm is associated with an extensive collateral circulation in the superficial veins around the shoulder. Recurrent episodes of thrombophlebitis may precede the diagnosis of carcinoma by many months, and their occurrence in an otherwise apparently fit patient should lead to a search for underlying malignancy, especially in the pancreas. (From Forbes CD, Jackson WF. *Color Atlas and Text of Clinical Medicine*, 3rd ed. London: Mosby; 2003.)

TREATMENT   Rx

Treatment for thrombosis without evidence of DIC should include initial standard anticoagulation with heparin. Long-term treatment with low-molecular-weight heparin has been demonstrated to be superior to warfarin for preventing recurrent thromboembolism without increasing the risk of bleeding.[2] Prophylactic low-dose or dose-adjusted subtherapeutic warfarin does not prevent or reduce catheter-related thromboses in patients with cancer.[3] Venous interruption (Chapters 81 and 98) is associated with significant complications and should be reserved for patients without other treatment options; temporary devices may be placed when anticoagulation must be delayed for surgery or other reasons. Successful treatment of the underlying malignancy is the most effective way to reduce the risk of thrombosis.

HEMORRHAGIC PARANEOPLASTIC SYNDROMES

DIC caused by activation of the hemostatic system with consumption of coagulation factors and platelets can result in both thrombosis and hemorrhage (Chapter 178). Acute DIC can be seen with a variety of malignancies. Essentially all patients with acute promyelocytic leukemia (Chapter 189) either present with acute DIC and associated hemorrhage or develop it during treatment. Procoagulant material released from the leukemia cells activates the fibrinolytic pathway; treatment with all-*trans*-retinoic acid and low-dose heparin has significantly reduced the complications of hemorrhage with this leukemia.

Other causes of malignancy-associated bleeding disorders include paraproteins that interfere with fibrin polymerization, amyloid deposits associated with monoclonal gammopathies such as multiple myeloma (Chapters 194), and, rarely, acquired von Willebrand's disease associated with lymphoproliferative and myeloproliferative disorders (Chapter 176). Increased fibrinolysis may be seen in patients with advanced prostate cancer (Chapter 207).

● RENAL PARANEOPLASTIC SYNDROMES

Renal involvement in the setting of malignancy may be due to direct tumor infiltration of the renal parenchyma or, less commonly, to a paraneoplastic syndrome. Paraneoplastic syndromes involving the kidney may be caused by tumor-related hormone production, may directly involve the glomerulus or the microvasculature, may be related to proteins produced by the tumor (e.g., amyloid, paraproteins), or may be caused by electrolyte disorders (hyponatremia, hyperuricemia). Hyponatremia due to the syndrome of inappropriate antidiuretic hormone secretion (SIADH) is commonly associated with both limited and advanced-stage SCLC; some series have suggested a worse outcome in these patients (Chapter 186).

Glomerulonephritis

The renal paraneoplastic syndrome most clearly linked to malignancy is membranous glomerulonephritis, which is characterized by nephrotic range proteinuria, edema, hypoalbuminemia, microscopic hematuria,

hypertension, and increased risk of thrombosis (Chapter 123). Associated cancers include adenocarcinomas of the lung (Chapter 197), breast (Chapter 204), and stomach (Chapter 198), as well as others. The pathology is related to thickening of the glomerular basement membrane from subepithelial deposition of tumor antigen that has reacted with circulating immunoglobulins (IgG) and complement. Other glomerular lesions include minimal change nephropathy complicating lymphoproliferative disorders, in particular Hodgkin's disease (Chapter 192); rapidly progressive glomerulonephritis associated with lymphoplasmacytic diseases; and other glomerulopathies (including nephrotic syndrome and minimal change disease) associated with a variety of malignant diseases.

It may be very difficult to differentiate a renal paraneoplastic syndrome from a benign disorder of the kidney; a biopsy demonstrating immune complex deposition, as well as a parallel course with an underlying malignancy, can help make the diagnosis.

Microvascular Disease

Renal microvascular involvement is uncommon and may be due to vasculitis or microangiopathy. Vasculitis may be caused by cryoglobulinemia in patients with hepatitis C–related hepatocellular carcinoma (Chapter 202) or rarely in patients with IgA monoclonal gammopathy in association with cancer of the lung. Thrombotic microangiopathy (hemolytic-uremic syndrome) or thrombotic thrombocytopenic microangiopathy (Chapter 175) is most commonly a complication of chemotherapy, including mitomycin C, cisplatin, and other drugs, but it may also be seen in association with a variety of advanced-stage adenocarcinomas as well as with promyelocytic leukemia. The etiology is unknown; the underlying malignancy should be treated, if possible, and plasma exchange may be helpful.

● HEPATOPATHY

Paraneoplastic hepatopathy is an uncommon disorder characterized by hepatic dysfunction with elevated liver enzymes and abnormal synthetic function with fever and weight loss. This syndrome has been associated with nonmetastatic renal cell cancer (Chapter 203) and is probably due to either autoimmune effects or direct toxicity from tumor-related products. This unusual syndrome resolves with resection of the tumor.

● FEVER AND CACHEXIA

Fever (Chapters 289), night sweats, and cachexia are nonspecific symptoms that, when seen in the absence of infection or a known disorder, suggest the diagnosis of an underlying malignancy. Cytokines clearly play a pathogenetic role in inducing both fever and cachexia. TNF-α (previously known as cachectin), interleukins (including IL-1 and IL-6), and interferon-γ are produced directly by the tumor or by tumor-associated host inflammatory cells, such as macrophages, which then results in a catabolic state. Cytokines may produce fever directly by acting at the hypothalamic thermoregulatory center (Chapters 289). In addition to the burden of tumor and the production of cytokines, cachexia may be caused or worsened by the side effects of cancer treatment, by intestinal blockage or malabsorption caused by tumor infiltration, and by depression.

Fever is generally cyclic and may be associated with drenching night sweats. Symptoms resolve with treatment of the underlying tumor, and return of fever usually heralds relapse. When treatment of the tumor is not possible or is ineffective, nonsteroidal anti-inflammatory agents or steroids given around the clock significantly improve quality of life. Although fever is most commonly seen in association with lymphoproliferative disease (Chapters 191 and 192), renal cell carcinoma (Chapter 203), and leukemias (Chapters 189 and 190), it may also occur with other cancers.

Cachexia, or the cancer wasting syndrome, is probably the single most common paraneoplastic syndrome, eventually affecting up to 80% of patients with cancer. This syndrome is characterized by anorexia, muscle wasting, loss of subcutaneous fat, and fatigue. It appears to be caused by a combination of protein wasting, malabsorption, immune dysregulation, and increased glucose turnover in the setting of tumor-induced increases in energy expenditure. Successful treatment of the underlying tumor reverses the process; most patients have advanced disease, for which treatment results in modest success at best. Megestrol acetate given in high concentrations in liquid form (400 to 800 mg/day) can significantly improve appetite and result in weight gain, as can dronabinol (Marinol; 2.5 to 5 mg three times a day). Corticosteroids may also help. Although agents that block TNF production are theoretically attractive to treat cancer-related cachexia, there is also concern that such agents may block cytokines that inhibit tumor growth. In addition, preclinical data suggest that antibodies to parathyroid hormone–related protein may block the production of inflammatory cytokines in cancer; whether this effect is of clinical value remains a research question.

1. Wirtz PW, Verschuuren JJ, van Dijk JG, et al. Efficacy of 3,4-diaminopyridine and pyridostigmine in the treatment of Lambert-Eaton myasthenic syndrome: a randomized, double-blind, placebo-controlled, crossover study. *Clin Pharmacol Ther.* 2009;86:44-48.
2. Hull RD, Pineo GF, Brant RF, et al. Long-term low-molecular-weight heparin versus usual care in proximal-vein thrombosis patients with cancer. *Am J Med.* 2006;119:1062-1072.
3. Young AM, Billingham LJ, Begum G, et al. Warfarin thromboprophylaxis in cancer patients with central venous catheters (WARP): an open-label randomised trial. *Lancet.* 2009;373:567-574.

SUGGESTED READINGS

Blum D, Omlin A, Baracos VE, et al. Cancer cachexia: a systematic literature review of items and domains associated with involuntary weight loss in cancer. *Crit Rev Oncol Hematol.* 2011. [Epub ahead of print.] *Review of reduced nutritional intake and catabolic/hypermetabolic changes.*

Giometto B, Grisold W, Vitaliani R, et al. Paraneoplastic neurologic syndrome in the PNS Euronetwork database: a European study from 20 centers. *Arch Neurol.* 2010;67:330-335. *This large study of more than 900 patients suggests that patients with cancer and a PNS have a worse prognosis than those with the underlying malignancy alone.*

Noble S, Pasi J. Epidemiology and pathophysiology of cancer-associated thrombosis. *Br J Cancer.* 2010;102(Suppl 1):S2-S9. *The overall risk of venous thrombosis is increased seven-fold in patients with a malignancy, and thrombosis is associated with significant morbidity and mortality.*

Pelosof LC, Gerber DE. Paraneoplastic syndromes: an approach to diagnosis and treatment. *Mayo Clin Proc.* 2010;85:838-854. *Comprehensive review.*

Rosenfeld MR, Dalmau J. Update on paraneoplastic and autoimmune disorders of the central nervous system. *Semin Neurol.* 2010;30:320-331. *Excellent updated review with a discussion of differential diagnosis, antibodies, and specific syndromes.*

188

MYELODYSPLASTIC SYNDROME

ALAN F. LIST AND RAMI S. KOMROKJI

DEFINITION

Myelodysplastic syndrome (MDS) comprises a heterogeneous group of hematopoietic stem cell malignancies resulting in variable degrees of cytopenias with a tendency to progress to acute myeloid leukemia (AML). Pathologically, the disease is characterized by abnormal morphology and cytologic dysplasia.

EPIDEMIOLOGY

For many years, the incidence of MDS was not well characterized and was underestimated. In 2001, MDS became reportable to the Surveillance, Epidemiology, and End Results (SEER) cancer registry database; from these data, it is estimated that approximately 10,000 MDS cases are diagnosed annually in the United States. The overall incidence of MDS approaches 4 per 100,000, with a male predominance and a clear increase in incidence with age. In populations older than 60 years, the incidence of MDS approaches that for other hematologic malignancies like multiple myeloma and chronic lymphocytic leukemia (CLL), reaching approximately 50 per 100,000. Nonetheless, the complexities in diagnosis, nonspecific symptomatology, and underreporting make accurate estimates of incidence difficult.

Most cases of MDS are sporadic. There are few hereditary syndromes associated with MDS per se, but two ill-defined pediatric conditions, juvenile myelomonocytic leukemia (JMML) and the monosomy 7 syndrome, mimic MDS and show a familial tendency. Heterozygous germline mutations of the runt-related transcription factor 1 (*RUNX1*) gene are associated with an autosomal dominant familial predisposition to platelet abnormalities and MDS, with a median incidence of either MDS or AML among carriers of 35%. In the elderly population, other than senescence, the exact causes of MDS are not well recognized. Risk factors include benzene exposure, chemical or solvent exposure, tobacco smoke, and family history.

Therapy-related MDS (t-MDS) refers to a subset of MDS that is associated with prior exposure to mutagenic antineoplastic drugs or radiation. The increasing success in treatment of solid tumors is accompanied by a challenge

whereby the incidence of t-MDS in survivors is on the rise. The risk of t-MDS varies from less than 1% (adjuvant breast cancer chemotherapy studies) to 15% (heavily treated lymphoma patients), depending on the age of the individual, class of antineoplastics, and duration of cytotoxic therapy.

PATHOBIOLOGY

The pathobiology of MDS is complex and remains under intense investigation. As opposed to other hematologic disorders like chronic myeloid leukemia (CML), there is unlikely to be a sentinel genetic event [i.e., t(9;22)]. The observed morphologic dysplasia is a common pathologic phenotype for the different underlying biology in various subsets of MDS patients. Ineffective erythropoiesis, genetic abnormalities, allelic haploinsufficiency, immune derangements, and microenvironment changes are examples of underlying disease biology.

Accelerated apoptosis is the hallmark of early MDS, which explains the paradoxical findings of normal or hypercellular bone marrow in most patients, accompanied by peripheral cytopenias. The malignant clone has an inherent susceptibility to premature apoptotic cell death. Other factors are recognized that amplify apoptotic sensitivity in MDS and include hematopoietic suppression from stromal production of inhibitory cytokines (e.g., tumor necrosis factor-α) and direct T-cell suppression akin to aplastic anemia. As the disease progresses, additional antiapoptotic signals are acquired, resulting sometimes in clonal evolution and transformation to higher-risk disease and, in some cases, to acute myeloid leukemia.

Cytogenetic Abnormalities

Cytogenetic abnormalities are observed in approximately 50% of MDS patients. The loss of genetic material is highly conserved among MDS and has led to a haploinsufficiency model of tumorigenesis. It is hypothesized that loss of even a single allele in the affected chromosomal regions may decrease the level and activity of critical gene products, presumably tumor suppressor genes. This may lead to dysplastic features, cytopenias, and the propensity to transform to AML. The most common cytogenetic abnormalities in MDS are deletions of the long arm of chromosomes 5, 7, and 20. Chromosome 5q deletion is present in approximately 15% of de novo MDS and 50% of t-MDS; abnormalities of 5q or 7, or both, are present in 70% of t-MDS. A potential validation of the haploinsufficiency model is illustrated in the analysis of a hematologic phenotype resulting from inactivation of genes encoded within the chromosome 5q common deleted region (CDR). Early growth response factor 1 (*EGR1*), a member of the Wilms' tumor 1 (WT1) family of transcription factors, is one such gene located on 5q. It is a direct transcriptional activator of TP53, an important tumor suppressor, and is downstream of many signaling pathways. Ribosomal protein S14 (*RPS14*) is another candidate gene located more distally on 5q, and within the CDR linked to the 5q– syndrome (discussed later). This gene product is required in the 40s subunit of the ribosome and has tumor suppressor properties as well as direct action on erythropoiesis. Haploinsufficiency of the *RPS14* gene alone recapitulates the hematologic features of the 5q– syndrome, resulting in impaired erythroid differentiation and proliferation.

There are some chromosomal abnormalities that are associated with specific MDS subtypes. For example, the *MLL (HRX)* gene localized to chromosome 11q23 has been implicated in the pathogenesis of de novo AML and in t-MDS/AML. It is a translocation t(11;16)(q23;p13), which results in a fusion protein between *MLL* and the promoter of CBP (cyclic adenosine monophosphate response element binding protein [CREB] binding protein). The t(3;21)(q22;q22) translocation is also associated with t-MDS and results in fusion of *RUNX1* (formerly *AML1*) with one of several fusion partners on chromosome 3, including *EAP, EVI1,* and *MDS. RUNX1's* product has been implicated in regulating the expression of important granulocyte elements such as myeloperoxidase and neutrophil elastase. Another translocation, t(5;12)(q33;p13), results in an activating mutation of *PDGFR*-β and is associated with chronic myelomonocytic leukemia (CMML). This is important because the *PDGFR* mutation renders the disease vulnerable to imatinib is some cases.

Epigenetics

Although loss of genetic material is common in MDS, 50% of patients with MDS have a normal karyotype. Therefore, undetectable translocations, point mutations, or epigenetic changes controlling gene expression may be responsible for the hypothesized loss of function. Because of the activity of hypomethylating agents in MDS, the role of epigenetic changes has emerged as a key contributor. DNA methyl transferase (DNMT) is responsible for methylating, and thus inactivating, gene promoters within CpG islands. Aberrant methylation of presumed tumor suppressor genes such as *p15* has been observed in MDS with adverse prognostic connotations, thereby providing an alternate mechanism by which tumor suppressors are inactivated in the pathogenesis of MDS.

Point Mutations

Point mutations represent another mechanism by which tumor suppressor function can be altered. Several activating mutations have been observed in a minority of MDS cases. Activating mutations in the *RAS* gene family occur in 5 to 15% of patients with MDS and are associated with progression to AML. Activating *FLT3* mutations have also been reported and are associated with progression to AML. Recent investigation has described multiple, novel, loss-of-function mutations in a presumed tumor suppressor protein known as TET2. It is hypothesized that these mutations may have a role in MDS progression and AML prognosis, and may be present in up to 15% of MDS cases. Also, previously cryptic mutations have been elucidated using single nucleotide polymorphism technology on c-Cbl, a known regulator of tyrosine kinase. The *c-Cbl* mutation has been seen most in CMML and, in vivo, confers a proliferative advantage.

CLINICAL MANIFESTATIONS

The hallmark clinical manifestation in MDS is persistent or progressive cytopenias. The cytopenia is usually insidious and, in retrospect, may have been present for months before diagnosis. Neutropenia has been reported in 24 to 39% of patients, anemia in 45 to 93%, and thrombocytopenia in 28 to 45%. Symptoms from MDS reflect the magnitude and lineage of cytopenias and their interactions with comorbidities. For example, a patient with coronary artery disease may present with mild anemia associated with an increase in the frequency and duration of angina. A patient on chronic anticoagulation may present with petechiae, bruising, or frank hemorrhage secondary to thrombocytopenia or platelet dysfunction. Or, a diabetic patient may present with signs and symptoms of poor wound healing and infection secondary to neutropenia or neutrophil dysfunction (i.e., impaired chemotaxis and microbial killing in those neutrophils that are produced despite adequate absolute number).

The clinical course of MDS can be subdivided in two broad categories. Approximately 70% of patients with MDS have a clinical course primarily involving progressive cytopenia. The rate of progression of these cytopenias is highly variable, as is their effect on morbidity and mortality. Approximately half of the theses patients die of causes unrelated to MDS, whereas the other half succumb to complications of marrow failure.

The remaining 30% of patients evolve into AML. The clinical course of these patients is grimmer because the transformed AML is notoriously refractory to conventional chemotherapy. If a complete remission is achieved, bone marrow transplantation remains the mainstay of therapy and the only chance for a durable remission.

DIAGNOSIS

The diagnosis of MDS requires the presence of dysplastic hematopoiesis along with the exclusion of disorders that may be a secondary cause of dysplasia. Dysplasia can first be recognized by inspection of the peripheral smear. Neutrophils may show degranulation in the cytoplasm and hyposegmentation of the nucleus (the pseudo-Pelger-Huët anomaly) (Fig. 188-1). The erythrocytes may be mildly macrocytic, a hallmark of MDS, or in cases of refractory anemia with ring sideroblasts, microcytic. The mean corpuscular volume (MCV) ranges between 100 and 110 mm^3, and the erythrocytes are usually hypochromic. Other changes can be seen in the erythrocyte morphology that reflects a hypercellular marrow or even splenomegaly seen in CMML, an MDS variant with myeloproliferative features. Some of these changes include tear drops (dacryocytes), red cell fragments, rouleaux formation, and helmet cells.

Bone marrow aspirate and biopsy are indispensable in the diagnosis of MDS. Dysplastic features may be seen in one or all three hematopoietic lineages. Dysgranulopoiesis, for example, can result in abnormal cytoplasmic granules and pleomorphic nuclear forms. Hyposegmentation of the nucleus and Auer rods (see Fig. 160-25 in Chapter 160) may be seen, with a greater proportion of immature forms including myeloblasts. Dyserythropoiesis is characterized by pleomorphic nuclear forms, ringed sideroblasts, megaloblastic changes, and nuclear-cytoplasmic dyssynchrony. Lastly, dysplasia affecting megakaryocytes can include bizarre nuclear figures, decreased ploidy, separated nuclei (so-called nuclear dispersion), and small micromegakaryocytes. The marrow cellularity is usually increased as a result of ineffective hematopoiesis. Myeloblasts may also be increased, and indeed the percent increase is important in the classification and prognosis of MDS.

FIGURE 188-1. Pseudo-Pelger-Huët phenomenon. Abnormal, acquired, hyposegmented (usually bilobed) nucleus in neutrophil of a patient with MDS, resembling the familial Pelger-Huët anomaly (see Fig. 160-20 in Chapter 160).

TABLE 188-1	DIFFERENTIAL DIAGNOSIS OF MYELODYSPLASTIC SYNDROME

CONGENITAL DISORDERS

Hereditary sideroblastic anemia
Fanconi's anemia
Diamond-Blackfan syndrome
Kostmann's syndrome
Shwachman's syndrome
Down syndrome

VITAMIN DEFICIENCY

B$_{12}$, folate, or iron deficiency

DRUG TOXICITY

Marrow suppression from oral or parenteral medications
Toxins
Chemotherapy and/or radiation therapy
Alcohol

ANEMIA OF CHRONIC DISEASE

Renal failure
Chronic infection, including tuberculosis
Rheumatologic disorders

VIRAL MARROW SUPPRESSION

Including Epstein-Barr virus, parvovirus B19, human immunodeficiency virus, and others

MARROW INFILTRATION

Acute and chronic leukemias
Metastatic solid tumor infiltration

PAROXYSMAL NOCTURNAL HEMOGLOBINURIA

HYPERSPLENISM

Characteristic clonal cytogenetic abnormalities are another helpful clue in the diagnosis of MDS, although normal cytogenetics do not exclude the diagnosis. Most cytogenetic abnormalities in MDS are characterized by loss of genetic material through deletions. Nonrandom chromosomal abnormalities associated with MDS include isolated chromosome 5q deletion (5q–), which occurs in approximately 15% of de novo MDS and 50% of secondary MDS; monosomy 7; trisomy 8; 21q–; 17q–; and 20q–.

Differential Diagnosis

Although MDS should be considered in older adults with an insidious presentation of cytopenia, more common causes should be excluded (Table 188-1). Because this disease predominantly affects elderly people, polypharmacy and vitamin deficiencies (iron, folate, and B$_{12}$ deficiency) should be strongly considered as a cause of cytopenia and corrected before proceeding in the diagnosis of MDS. Infectious causes should be considered to include parvovirus B19, human immunodeficiency virus (HIV), and viral hepatitis. Splenic sequestration should also be considered in the presence of splenomegaly on physical examination, potentially arising from portal hypertension from cirrhosis, myelofibrosis, and infiltrating splenic diseases such as lymphoma. Alcoholism can cause cytopenia secondary to direct myelosuppression, vitamin deficiency, and with intrinsic liver disease, sequestration by the spleen. Autoimmune disorders and hypogonadism in men rarely cause cytopenia. Lastly, a careful history should focus on a personal history of congenital disorders that may causes cytopenias. Once a thorough history and physical examination, review of peripheral smear, and exclusion of the above causes is complete, a bone marrow (BM) biopsy with cytogenetic analysis is warranted. The BM biopsy may then reveal hypercellularity with cytologic dysplasia (MDS), BM aplasia (aplastic anemia), or marrow infiltration with neoplastic cells (metastatic disease, leukemia).

Classification

In 1976, the French-American-British (FAB) classification was first reported and later revised in 1982 to include five MDS subtypes: refractory anemia (RA); refractory anemia with ring sideroblasts (RARS); refractory anemia with excess blasts (RAEB); CMML; and refractory anemia with excess blasts in transformation (RAEB-t). The FAB classification has since been revised by the World Health Organization (WHO) (Table 188-2) and expanded to more accurately classify patients into more homogeneous subgroups. The most important changes include lowering the threshold for AML diagnosis to 20% blasts instead of 30% and thereby omitting FAB RAEB-t subtype; recognizing CMML as a related but stand-alone MDS subtype included in the new category of myelodysplastic myeloproliferative neoplasms (MDS/MPN), and inclusion of the 5q− syndrome, a subtype of MDS that is characterized by this isolated cytogenetic abnormality, clinical distinctness, and unique response to lenalidomide.

TABLE 188-2	WORLD HEALTH ORGANIZATION CLASSIFICATION OF MYELODYSPLASTIC SYNDROME	
CATEGORY	**PERIPHERAL BLOOD**	**BONE MARROW**
1a. RA without dysplasia	Blasts <1%; monocytes <1000/mm³	Blasts <5%; ringed sideroblasts <15%
1b. RA with dysplasia	Same + dysgranulocytes and/or giant platelets	Same + dysgranulocytes and/or dysmegakaryocytes
2a. RARS without dysplasia	Blasts <1%; monocytes <1000/mm³	Blasts <5%; ≥15% ringed sideroblasts
2b. RARS with dysplasia	Same + dysgranulocytes and/or giant platelets	Same + dysgranulocytes and/or dysmegakaryocytes
3a. RAEB-I	Blasts 1-4%; monocytes <1000/mm³	Blasts 5-10%
3b. RAEB-II	Blasts 5-19%; monocytes <1000/mm³	Blasts 11-19%

RA = refractory anemia; RAEB = refractory anemia with excess blasts; RARS = refractory anemia with ringed sideroblasts.

TREATMENT Rx

The International Prognostic Scoring System (IPSS) is currently the most widely used risk stratification tool to tailor treatment options (Table 188-3). In patients in the low and intermediate-1 risk groups, the goals of treatment are improve quality of life and improve cytopenias. In higher-risk MDS patients, (intermediate-2 or high-risk IPSS), the goal of treatment is to alter the natural history of the disease by approaches such as allogeneic stem cell transplantation or hypomethylating agents in order to extend survival and suppress leukemia potential.

Hematopoietic Growth Factors

About 15 to 30% of patients have an erythropoietic response to treatment with a recombinant erythropoietic stimulating agent (ESA), favoring those with low (<200 U/mL) serum endogenous erythropoietin (EPO) levels and low transfusion burden (<2 units/month). Addition of granulocyte-colony stimulating factor (G-CSF) can increase the erythroid response rate in some patients. Responders to ESA may derive a survival benefit with improvement in erythropoiesis.

Epigenetic Therapy

Aberrant hypermethylation of tumor suppressor genes has been implicated in the pathogenesis of MDS. Hypomethylating agents like 5-azacytidine (5-aza) and decitabine aim to reverse this aberrant hypermethylation and restore transcription of tumor suppressor genes. Several trials have explored the use of 5-aza in MDS. A randomized phase III trial compared 5-aza with best supportive care (BSC) in patients with all FAB subtypes and yielded improvements in cytopenias, transfusion dependency, quality of life, and time to AML progression.[1] A more recent phase III trial, Aza-001, compared 5-aza with conventional therapy that included low-dose and intensive chemotherapy in patients with higher risk (intermediate-2, high-risk) MDS. This trial demonstrated a significant improvement in median overall survival (24 months versus 15 months).[2] 5-aza likewise improved overall survival compared with conventional care regimens in the MDS subgroup of elderly patients with low BM blast count AML.[3] Romiplostim, which activates the thrombopoietin receptor, may provide incremental benefit during 5-aza therapy.[4] Decitabine has also been found in a phase III clinical trial to improve time to AML transformation and death compared with BSC; however, no survival advantage was observed compared with BSC.[5,6]

Immunomodulatory Drugs

Lenalidomide, a more potent and less toxic analogue of thalidomide, is approved for the treatment of transfusion-dependent anemia in patients with lower-risk MDS with a chromosomal 5q deletion. In the registration phase II study, 76% experienced a transfusion response, and 67% became transfusion independent that was sustained for a median duration greater than 2 years. Unlike treatment with ESAs, lenalidomide suppresses the del(5q) MDS clone to yield cytogenetic improvement in more 70% of patients. Neutropenia and thrombocytopenia are commonly seen, especially in the initial months of treatment, but are also predictive for hematologic and cytogenetic response. Activity also exists in those without a chromosome 5q deletion, albeit less robust. A multicenter trial in lower-risk patients without del(5q) reported 43% overall transfusion response, with 26% achieving transfusion independence.[7] The mechanism of action of lenalidomide is karyotype specific by clonal suppression in patients with deletion of 5q and erythropoiesis stimulation in non-5q-deletion patients.

TABLE 188-3	INTERNATIONAL PROGNOSTIC SCORING SYSTEM (IPSS)				
	Points				
PROGNOSTIC VARIABLE	**0**	**0.5**	**1.0**	**1.5**	**2.0**
Bone marrow blasts	<5%	6-10%	—	11-20%	21-30%
Karyotype*	Good	Intermediate	Poor	—	—
Cytopenias	0-1	2-3	—	—	—

*Good = normal, -Y, -5q, -20q; intermediate =other abnormal; poor = complex (>3) or monosomy 7. IPSS groups: (1) low = 0 points; (2) intermediate-1 = 0.5-1.0 points; (3) intermediate-2 = 1.5-2.0 points; (4) high = >2.5 points.

Immunosuppressive Therapy

Based on clinical similarities between a subset of hypocellular MDS and aplastic anemia, antithymocyte globulin plus cyclosporine has been used with success in select patients with MDS. A phase III randomized trial has recently demonstrated that immunosuppressive therapy with antithymocyte globulin (15 mg/kg for 5 days) in combination with oral cyclosporine) for 180 days (average daily dose 290 mg) was associated with hematologic response in a subset of patients with MDS, compared with best supportive care, without apparent impact on transformation-free or overall survival.[8]

Hematopoietic Stem Cell Transplantation

Despite novel therapies, allogeneic hematopoietic stem cell transplantation (HSCT) remains the only curative option for MDS (Chapter 181). The overall 5-year survival rate approaches 40%. Based on decision analysis and limited data from randomized trials , the best timing for allogeneic HSCT is on a diagnosis of higher-risk MDS[9]; deferring HSCT until disease progression optimizes survival potential in patients with lower-risk disease with a compatible donor.

Conventional Chemotherapy

Response rates to conventional acute leukemia chemotherapy regimens for MDS patients are low, and mortality and morbidity can be substantial owing to comorbidities and age. Conventional chemotherapies are generally reserved for the setting of hypomethylating agent failure with disease progression.

Signal Transduction Inhibitors

Multiple signal transduction pathways have been implicated in the pathogenesis of MDS. In the rare MDS patient with PDGFR-activating mutations, imatinib is an effective agent. Several other agents are currently in clinical trials targeting different pathways implicated in the pathobiology of MDS.

Iron Chelation

An important consideration in lower-risk patients who are transfusion dependent is iron overload. Iron overload as measured by incremental rise in serum ferritin is an independent prognostic factor in lower-risk MDS, with increased cardiac comorbidity and decrease in survival. In practice, iron chelation therapy is considered in transfusion-dependent lower-risk MDS patients with persistent elevation in ferritin greater than 1000 ng/mL and in patients who have received more than 15 to 20 units of red blood cells. Newer oral iron-chelating agents (e.g., deferasirox) are more appealing and offer a higher expectation for patient compliance.

PROGNOSIS

Unfortunately, most MDS patients will ultimately succumb to complications from the disease or transformation to AML. The IPSS can be applied at the time of diagnosis to estimate the natural history of the disease and therefore guide treatment selection. The cumulative score is based on BM myeloblast percentage, karyotype, and number of cytopenias to risk-stratify patients into four distinct groups: low, intermediate-1, intermediate-2, and high-risk MDS (see Table 188-3). Newer risk models have been proposed to further enhance our ability to predict outcome but more importantly to tailor our therapy according to risk and disease behavior.

FUTURE DIRECTIONS

As our understanding of underlying disease biology improves, one can expect to individualize therapy based on biologic response signatures and enhanced risk stratification.

1. Kornblith AB, Herndon JE 2nd, Silverman LR, et al. Impact of azacitidine on the quality of life of patients with myelodysplastic syndrome treated in a randomized phase III trial: a Cancer and Leukemia Group B study. *J Clin Oncol.* 2002;20:2441-2452.
2. Fenaux P, Mufti GJ, Hellström-Lindberg E, et al. Efficacy of azacitidine compared with that of conventional care regimens in the treatment of higher-risk myelodysplastic syndromes: a randomised, open-label, phase III study. *Lancet Oncol.* 2009;10:223-232.
3. Fenaux P, Mufti GJ, Hellström-Lindberg E, et al. Azacitidine prolongs overall survival compared with conventional care regimens in elderly patients with low bone marrow blast count acute myeloid leukemia. *J Clin Oncol.* 2010;28:562-569.
4. Kantarjian HM, Giles FJ, Greenberg PL, et al. Phase 2 study of romiplostim in patients with low- or intermediate-risk myelodysplastic syndrome receiving azacitidine therapy. *Blood.* 2010;116:3163-3170.
5. Kantarjian H, Issa JP, Rosenfeld CS, et al. Decitabine improves patient outcomes in myelodysplastic syndromes: results of a phase III randomized study. *Cancer.* 2006;106:1794-1803.
6. Wijermans P, Suciu S, Baila L, et al. Low dose decitabine versus best supportive care in elderly patients with intermediate or high risk MDS not eligible for intensive chemotherapy: final results of the randomized phase III study (06011) of the EORTC Leukemia and German MDS Study Groups. *ASH Annual Meeting Abstracts.* 2008;112:226.
7. Raza A, Reeves JA, Feldman EJ, et al. Phase 2 study of lenalidomide in transfusion-dependent, low-risk, and intermediate-1 risk myelodysplastic syndromes with karyotypes other than deletion 5q. *Blood.* 2008;111:86-93.
8. Passweg JR, Glagounidis AA, Simcock M, et al. Immunosuppressive therapy for patients with myelodysplastic syndrome: a prospective randomized multicenter phase III trial comparing antithymocyte globulin plus cyclosporine with best supportive care—SAKK 33/99. *J Clin Oncol.* 2011;29:303-309.
9. de Witte T, Hagemeijer A, Suciu S, et al. Value of allogeneic versus autologous stem cell transplantation and chemotherapy in patients with myelodysplastic syndromes and secondary acute myeloid leukemia: final results of a prospective randomized European Intergroup Trial. *Haematologica.* 2010;95:1754-1761.

SUGGESTED READINGS

Epling-Burnette PK, List AF. Advancements in the molecular pathogenesis of myelodysplastic syndrome. *Curr Opin Hematol.* 2009;16:70-76. *Review of advances in our understanding of the molecular pathogenesis of myelodysplastic syndrome (MDS).*

Greenberg PL, Attar E, Bennett JM, et al. Myelodysplastic syndromes. *J Natl Compr Canc Netw.* 2011;9:30-56. *Review of five subtypes: refractory anemia with or without ringed sideroblasts or excess of blasts, RAEB in transformation, or chronic myelomonocytic leukemia.*

Komrokji RS, Zhang L, Bennett JM. Myelodysplastic syndromes classification and risk stratification. *Hematol Oncol Clin North Am.* 2010;24:443-457. *Comprehensive review of MDS classification and risk stratification.*

Leitch HA. Controversies surrounding iron chelation therapy for MDS. *Blood Rev.* 2011;25:17-31. *Review.*

Loaiza-Bonilla A, Gore SD, Carraway HE. Novel approaches for myelodysplastic syndromes: beyond hypomethylating agents. *Curr Opin Hematol.* 2010;17:104-109. *Review of recent advances in new strategies and targeted therapies for treatment of MDS.*

Tefferi A, Vardiman JW. Myelodysplastic syndromes. *N Engl J Med.* 2009;361:1872-1885. *Review.*

Tehranchi R, Woll PS, Anderson K, et al. Persistent malignant stem cells in del(5q) myelodysplasia in remission. *N Engl J Med.* 2010;363:1025-1037. *Rare treatment-resistant del(5q) myelodysplastic stem cells can be found in patients in remission and can serve as the presumed source of recurrence.*

189

THE ACUTE LEUKEMIAS

FREDERICK R. APPELBAUM

DEFINITION

Normal hematopoiesis (Chapter 159) requires tightly regulated proliferation and differentiation of pluripotent hematopoietic stem cells that become mature peripheral blood cells. Acute leukemia is the result of a malignant event or events occurring in an early hematopoietic precursor. Instead of proliferating and differentiating normally, the affected cell gives rise to progeny that fail to differentiate but continue to proliferate in an uncontrolled fashion. As a result, immature myeloid cells in acute myeloid leukemia (AML) or lymphoid cells in acute lymphoblastic leukemia (ALL)—often called blasts—rapidly accumulate and progressively replace the bone marrow, diminishing the production of normal red cells, white cells, and platelets. This loss of normal marrow function in turn gives rise to the common clinical complications of leukemia: anemia, infection, and bleeding. With time, the leukemic blasts pour out into the blood stream and eventually occupy the lymph nodes, spleen, and other vital organs. If untreated, acute leukemia is rapidly fatal; most patients die within several months after diagnosis. With appropriate therapy, however, the natural history of acute leukemia can be markedly altered, and many patients can be cured.

EPIDEMIOLOGY

Incidence

About 39,000 new cases of leukemia were diagnosed in the United States in 2009, at a rate of about 8.5 cases per 100,000 persons; this rate has remained relatively consistent for the past 3 decades. The leukemias account for about 3% of all cancers in the United States. The impact of leukemia is heightened because of the young age of some patients. For example, with a maximum incidence between ages 2 and 10 years, ALL is the most common cancer and the second leading cause of death in children younger than 15 years. In contrast, the incidence of AML gradually increases with age, without an early peak. The median age at diagnosis of AML is about 60 years.

Determinants

In most cases, acute leukemia develops for no known reason, but sometimes a possible cause can be identified.

Radiation

Ionizing radiation (Chapter 19) is leukemogenic. The incidence of ALL, AML, and chronic myeloid leukemia (CML) is increased in patients given radiation therapy for ankylosing spondylitis and among survivors of the atomic bomb blasts at Hiroshima and Nagasaki. The magnitude of the risk depends on the dose of radiation, its distribution in time, and the age of the individual. Greater risk results from higher doses of radiation delivered over shorter periods to younger patients. In areas of high natural background radiation (often from radon), chromosomal aberrations are reportedly more frequent, but an increase in acute leukemia has not been consistently found. Concern has been raised about the possible leukemogenic effects of extremely low-frequency nonionizing electromagnetic fields emitted by electrical installations. If such an effect exists at all, its magnitude is small.

Oncogenic Viruses

The search for a viral cause of leukemia has been pursued intensely, but only two clear associations have been found. Human T-cell lymphotropic virus type I (HTLV-I), an enveloped, single-stranded RNA virus, is considered the causative agent of adult T-cell leukemia (Chapter 386). This distinct form of leukemia is found within geographic clusters in southwestern Japan, the Caribbean basin, and Africa. Because HTLV-I seropositivity was found with increasing frequency among heavily transfused patients and intravenous drug users, screening of blood products for antibodies to HTLV-I is now routine practice in blood banks in the United States. Epstein-Barr virus (Chapter 385), the DNA virus that causes infectious mononucleosis, is associated with Burkitt's lymphoma (Chapter 191) and its leukemic counterpart, mature B-cell ALL.

Chemicals and Drugs

Heavy occupational exposure to benzene and benzene-containing compounds such as kerosene and carbon tetrachloride may lead to marrow damage, which can take the form of aplastic anemia, myelodysplasia, or AML. A link between leukemia and tobacco use has recently been reported.

With the increasing use of chemotherapy to treat other malignancies, the incidence of AML secondary to prior chemotherapy has increased and may represent 6 to 10% of all cases. Prior exposure to alkylating agents such as melphalan and the nitrosoureas is associated with an increased risk of secondary AML, which often manifests initially as a myelodysplastic syndrome (Chapter 188), frequently with abnormalities of chromosomes 5, 7, and 8 but with no distinct morphologic features. These secondary AMLs typically develop 4 to 6 years after exposure to alkylating agents, and their incidence may be increased with greater intensity and duration of drug exposure. Secondary AML associated with epipodophyllotoxin (teniposide or etoposide) exposure tends to have a shorter latency period (1 to 2 years), lacks a myelodysplastic phase, has a monocytic morphology, and involves abnormalities of the long arm of chromosome 11 (band q23) or chromosome 21 (band q22). Because patients frequently receive combination chemotherapy, it is often difficult to identify a single causative agent.

PATHOBIOLOGY

Genetics

If leukemia develops before 10 years of age in a patient with an identical twin, the unaffected twin has a 20% chance of developing leukemia. Several syndromes with somatic cell chromosome aneuploidy, including trisomy 21 (Down), trisomy 13 (Patau), and XXY (Klinefelter), are associated with an increased incidence of AML. Other inherited mutations, for example, a mutation at 21q22, have been associated with a high incidence of AML in rare families. Several autosomal recessive disorders associated with chromosomal instability are prone to terminate in acute leukemia, including Bloom's syndrome, Fanconi's anemia (Chapter 168), and ataxia-telangiectasia (Chapter 258).

Clonality and Cell of Origin

The acute leukemias are clonal disorders, and all leukemic cells in a given patient are descended from a common progenitor. The clonal nature of acute leukemia suggests that there are leukemic stem cells capable of both self-renewal and proliferation. Recent studies suggest that the leukemic stem cells in AML are rare among the leukemic mass, with a frequency of 0.2 to 10 per 10^6, and are within the primitive $CD34^{++} CD38^-$ fraction. Less is known about the ALL stem cell.

Classification

The World Health Organization (WHO) classification of acute leukemias is based on clinical, morphologic, immunophenotypic, cytogenetic, and molecular features (Table 189-1).

Morphology

Leukemic cells in AML are typically 12 to 20 nm in diameter, with discrete nuclear chromatin, multiple nucleoli, and cytoplasm that usually contains azurophilic granules. Auer rods, which are slender, fusiform cytoplasmic inclusions that stain red with Wright-Giemsa stain, are virtually pathognomonic of AML. The French-American-British (FAB) morphologic system divides AML into eight subtypes: M0, M1, M2, and M3 reflect increasing degrees of differentiation of myeloid leukemic cells; M4 and M5 leukemias have features of the monocytic lineage; M6 has features of the erythroid cell lineage; and M7 is acute megakaryocytic leukemia. The WHO system also recognizes acute basophilic leukemia and acute leukemia with predominant myelofibrosis.

The leukemic cells in ALL tend to be smaller than AML blasts and relatively devoid of granules. ALL can be divided by FAB criteria into L1, L2, and L3 subgroups. L1 blasts are uniform in size, with homogeneous nuclear chromatin, indistinct nucleoli, and scanty cytoplasm with few, if any, granules. L2 blasts are larger and more variable in size and may have nucleoli. L3 blasts are distinct, with prominent nucleoli and deeply basophilic cytoplasm with vacuoles.

Immunophenotyping

Immunophenotyping by multiparameter flow cytometry is used to determine lineage involvement of newly diagnosed acute leukemias and to detect aberrant immunophenotypes, allowing the measurement of minimal residual disease after therapy. Antibodies that react with antigens found on normal immature myeloid cells, including CD13, CD14, CD33, and CD34, also react with blast cells from most patients with AML. Exceptions are the M6 and M7 variants, which have antigens restricted to the red cell and the platelet lineage, respectively. Myeloid leukemia blasts also express human leukocyte antigen (HLA)-DR antigens but usually lack T-cell, B-cell, and other lymphoid antigens. In 10 to 20% of patients, however, otherwise typical AML blasts also express antigens usually restricted to B- or T-cell lineage. Expression of lymphoid antigens by AML cells does not change either the natural history or the therapeutic response of these leukemias.

Approximately 75% of cases of ALL express B-lineage antigens and can be subdivided into four categories. The most immature group, pro-B ALL,

TABLE 189-1　WORLD HEALTH ORGANIZATION CLASSIFICATION OF ACUTE LEUKEMIAS

CLASSIFICATION SUBTYPES (2008)

Acute Myeloid Leukemia (AML) and Related Neoplasms

AML with recurrent genetic abnormalities
    AML with t(8;21)(q22;q22); *RUNX1-RUNX1T1*
    AML with inv(16)(p13.1q22) or t(16;16)(p13.1;q22); *CBFB-MYH11*
    Acute promyelocytic leukemia (APL) with t(15;17)(q22;q12); *PML-RARA*
    AML with t(9;11)(p22;q23); *MLLT3-MLL*
    AML with t(6;9)(p23;q34); *DEK-NUP214*
    AML with inv(3)(q21q26.2) or t(3;3)(q21;q26.2); *RPN1-EVI1*
    AML (megakaryoblastic) with t(1;22)(p13;q13); *RBM15-MKL1*
    Provisional entity: AML with mutated *NPM1*
    Provisional entity: AML with mutated *CEBPA*
AML with myelodysplasia-related changes
Therapy-related myeloid neoplasms
AML, not otherwise specified
    AML with minimal differentiation
    AML without maturation
    AML with maturation
    Acute myelomonocytic leukemia
    Acute monoblastic/monocytic leukemia
    Acute erythroid leukemia
        Pure erythroid leukemia
        Erythroleukemia, erythroid/myeloid
    Acute megakaryoblastic leukemia
    Acute basophilic leukemia
    Acute panmyelosis with myelofibrosis
Myeloid sarcoma
Myeloid proliferations related to Down syndrome
    Transient abnormal myelopoiesis
    Myeloid leukemia associated with Down syndrome
Blastic plasmacytoid dendritic cell neoplasm

B Lymphoblastic Leukemia (ALL)/Lymphoma

B lymphoblastic leukemia/lymphoma, not otherwise specified
B lymphoblastic leukemia/lymphoma with recurrent genetic abnormalities
    B lymphoblastic leukemia/lymphoma with t(9;22)(q34;q11.2); *BCR-ABL1*
    (Philadelphia chromosome–positive ALL)
    B lymphoblastic leukemia/lymphoma with t(v;11q23); *MLL* rearranged
    B lymphoblastic leukemia/lymphoma with t(12;21)(p13;q22); *TEL-AML1*
    (*ETV6-RUNX1*)
    B lymphoblastic leukemia/lymphoma with hyperdiploidy
    B lymphoblastic leukemia/lymphoma with hypodiploidy
    B lymphoblastic leukemia/lymphoma with t(5;14)(q31;q32); *IL3-IGH*
    B lymphoblastic leukemia/lymphoma with t(1;19)(q23;p13.3); *TCF3-PBX1*

T Lymphoblastic Leukemia (ALL)/Lymphoma

ALL = acute lymphoblastic leukemia.

expresses CD19 but not other B-lineage antigens and represents about 10% of cases of ALL. Approximately 50 to 60% of cases of ALL express the common ALL antigen (CALLA, or CD10), a glycoprotein that is also found occasionally on normal early lymphocytes and other nonhematopoietic tissues. CALLA-positive ALL is thought to represent an early pre-B-cell differentiation state. Approximately 10% of cases of ALL have intracytoplasmic immunoglobulin and are termed pre-B-cell ALL. B-cell ALL is signified by the presence of immunoglobulin on the cell surface and accounts for less than 5% of cases of ALL. In general, the best therapeutic outcomes among B-cell ALL types are with early pre-B-cell (CALLA positive) ALL. Among the 25% of cases of ALL that express T-lineage antigens, less than half are so-called pre-T-cell types that express CD3 with either CD4 and CD8 or neither CD4 nor CD8; the majority of cases, termed T-cell ALL, express CD3 and either CD4 or CD8. The prognosis for T-cell ALL is superior to that for pre-T-cell ALL. In about 25% of patients with ALL, the leukemic cells also express myeloid antigens. Historically, the presence of such antigens defined a group of patients with a somewhat worse prognosis; however, with current, more aggressive regimens, the impact of myeloid antigen expression has disappeared.

Acute leukemias of ambiguous lineage are rare cases with no evidence of lineage differentiation (i.e., acute undifferentiated leukemia [AUL]) or those with blasts that express markers of more than one lineage (i.e., mixed phenotype acute leukemia [MPAL]). MPAL can contain either distinct blast populations of different lineages (bilineal) or a single population expressing features of both lineages (biphenotypic). In general, the prognosis of patients with AUL or MPAL is poor when treated with standard chemotherapy.

Cytogenetics and Molecular Biology

In most cases of acute leukemia, an abnormality in chromosome number or structure is found. These abnormalities are clonal, involving all the malignant cells in a given patient; they are acquired and are not found in the normal cells of the patient; and they are referred to as "nonrandom," because specific abnormalities are found in multiple cases and are associated with distinct morphologic or clinical subtypes of the disease. These abnormalities may be simply the gain or loss of whole chromosomes, but more often they include chromosomal translocations, deletions, or inversions. When patients with acute leukemia and a chromosomal abnormality receive treatment and enter into complete remission, the chromosomal abnormality disappears; when relapse occurs, the abnormality reappears. In many cases, these abnormalities have provided clues into the pathobiology of acute leukemia.

The most common cytogenetic abnormalities seen in AML can be categorized according to their underlying biology and prognostic significance. The translocation t(8;21) and the inversion inv(16) result in abnormalities of a transcription factor made up of core binding factor-α (CBF-α) and CBF-β. The t(8;21) results in the fusion of CBF-α on chromosome 21 with the *MTG8* gene on chromosome 8, whereas inv(16) results in the fusion of CBF-β on the q arm of chromosome 16 with the *MYH11* gene on the p arm. Both of these "core binding factor" AMLs are characterized by a high complete response rate and relatively favorable long-term survival. An additional translocation with a favorable prognosis, t(15;17), involves two genes, *PML* and *RAR-α* (a gene encoding the α-retinoic acid receptor), and is invariably associated with acute promyelocytic leukemia (APL), the M3 subtype of AML. Translocations involving the *MLL* gene, located at chromosome band 11q23, carry an intermediate prognosis. *MLL* is perhaps the most promiscuous oncogene partner in oncology, with more than 30 fusion partners identified. Trisomy 8 is among the most common nonrandom cytogenetic abnormalities seen in AML; it accounts for 9% of cases and carries an intermediate prognosis. Trisomies of chromosome 21, chromosome 11, and other chromosomes are sometimes seen as well. Deletions of part or all of chromosome 5 or 7 each account for 6 to 8% of cases of AML. These abnormalities are seen with greater frequency in older patients and in patients with AML secondary to myelodysplasia or prior exposure to alkylating agents, and they are associated with an unfavorable prognosis.

In addition to the abnormalities detectable by routine cytogenetic analysis, other mutations exist in the malignant cells in a substantial proportion of AML cases. Many of these involve signal transduction pathways. Activating mutations in the FLT3 receptor have been found in 20 to 40% of cases of AML. These mutations may be internal tandem repeats (15 to 30%) or point mutations (5 to 10%) and are associated with a poorer overall response to therapy. Mutations in FMS, which, like FLT3, is a receptor tyrosine kinase, are seen in 10 to 20% of cases of AML, and mutations in HRAS, KRAS2, and NRAS1, which are cellular proteins involved with signal transduction, are seen in 15 to 20% of AML cases. Mutations in the nucleophosmin gene (*NPM1*) have been identified in 20 to 30% of AML cases and appear to be associated with a favorable clinical outcome. *CEBPA*, a gene encoding a leucine zipper transcription factor involved in myeloid differentiation, is mutated in 4 to 15% of cases of AML and may be associated with a more favorable outcome. All these mutations are of interest not only for their prognostic importance but also because they may serve as targets for new therapies.

The most common cytogenetic abnormality seen in adults with ALL is the Philadelphia (Ph) chromosome, or t(9;22). This translocation results in fusion of the *BCR* gene on chromosome 22 to the *ABL* tyrosine kinase gene on chromosome 9. This results in the constitutive activation of *ABL*, but the precise mechanism by which this activity leads to leukemia is unclear. The *BCR-ABL* fusion is associated with both ALL and CML (Chapter 190), with a difference in the breakpoint of *BCR* distinguishing the two. A slightly smaller 190-kD fusion protein is usually found in ALL, whereas a larger 210-kD protein is characteristic of CML. The frequency of t(9;22) in ALL increases with age: it is found in approximately 5% of childhood cases, 25% of adults, and 50% of adults older than age 50. Before the development of specific tyrosine kinase inhibitors, ALL with t(9;22) had a poor prognosis; newer regimens combining tyrosine kinase inhibitors with chemotherapy are providing improved outcomes. The most common translocation seen in childhood ALL is t(12;21), which involves the genes *TEL* and *AML1*. Like the AML-associated t(8;21) and inv(16), t(12;21) is thought to result

in abnormal DNA transcription by interfering with the normal function of CBF. Although t(12;21) is difficult to diagnose by routine cytogenetics, by molecular studies it has been shown to account for 25% of childhood ALL and 4% of adult ALL and has a favorable prognosis. Partial deletions in 9p, seen in 5 to 7% of adult ALL, are also associated with a favorable outcome. Other abnormalities sometimes seen in B-cell ALL include t(8;14) and t(8;22), which result in translocation of the *MYC* gene on chromosome 8 and immunoglobulin enhancer response genes on chromosomes 14 or 22; they are associated with a poor therapeutic outcome. T-cell ALLs are frequently associated with abnormalities of chromosome 7 or 14 at the sites of T-cell receptor enhancer genes on these chromosomes. The leukemia cells in about 20% of patients with ALL have a propensity to gain chromosomes, sometimes reaching an average of 50 to 60 chromosomes per cell. Patients with such hyperdiploid leukemias tend to respond well to chemotherapy.

CLINICAL MANIFESTATIONS

The signs and symptoms of acute leukemia are usually rapid in onset, developing over a few weeks to a few months at most; they result from decreased normal marrow function and invasion of normal organs by leukemic blasts. Anemia is present at diagnosis in most patients and causes fatigue, pallor, headache, and, in predisposed patients, angina or heart failure. Thrombocytopenia is usually present, and approximately one third of patients have clinically evident bleeding at diagnosis, usually in the form of petechiae, ecchymoses, bleeding gums, epistaxis, or hemorrhage. Most patients with acute leukemia are significantly granulocytopenic at diagnosis. As a result, approximately one third of patients with AML and slightly fewer patients with ALL have significant or life-threatening infections when initially seen, most of which are bacterial in origin.

In addition to suppressing normal marrow function, leukemic cells can infiltrate normal organs. In general, ALL tends to infiltrate normal organs more often than AML does. Enlargement of lymph nodes, liver, and spleen is common at diagnosis. Bone pain, thought to result from leukemic infiltration of the periosteum or expansion of the medullary cavity, is a common complaint, particularly in children with ALL. Leukemic cells sometimes infiltrate the skin and result in a raised, nonpruritic rash, a condition termed *leukemia cutis*. Leukemic cells may infiltrate the leptomeninges and cause leukemic meningitis, typically manifested by headache and nausea. As the disease progresses, central nervous system (CNS) palsies and seizures may develop. Although less than 5% of patients with ALL have CNS involvement at diagnosis, the CNS is a frequent site of relapse; therefore, CNS prophylaxis is an essential component of ALL therapy. Because the incidence of CNS disease is low in AML, there is no proven benefit to CNS surveillance or prophylaxis. Testicular involvement is seen in ALL, and the testicles are a frequent site of relapse. In AML, collections of leukemic blast cells, often referred to as *chloromas* or *myeloblastomas*, can occur in virtually any soft tissue and appear as rubbery, fast-growing masses.

Certain clinical manifestations are unique to specific subtypes of leukemia. Patients with APL of the M3 type commonly have subclinical or clinically evident disseminated intravascular coagulation (DIC; Chapter 178) caused by tissue thromboplastins released by the leukemic cells. Acute monocytic or myelomonocytic leukemias are the forms of AML most likely to have extramedullary involvement. M6 leukemia often has a long prodromal phase. Patients with T-cell ALL frequently have mediastinal masses.

DIAGNOSIS

Abnormalities in peripheral blood counts are usually the initial laboratory evidence of acute leukemia. Anemia is present in most patients. Most are also at least mildly thrombocytopenic, and up to one fourth have severe thrombocytopenia (platelets <20,000/μL). Although most patients are granulocytopenic at diagnosis, the total peripheral white cell count is more variable; approximately 25% of patients have very high white cell counts (>50,000/μL), approximately 50% have white cell counts between 5000 and 50,000/μL, and about 25% have low white cell counts (<5000/μL). In most cases, blasts are present in the peripheral blood, although in some patients the percentage of blasts is quite low or absent.

The diagnosis of acute leukemia is typically established by marrow aspiration and biopsy, usually from the posterior iliac crest. Marrow aspirates and biopsy specimens are usually hypercellular and contain 20 to 100% blast cells, which largely replace the normal marrow (Figs. 189-1 and 189-2). Occasionally, in addition to the blast cell infiltrate, other findings are present, such as marrow fibrosis (especially with M7 AML) or bone marrow necrosis. Marrow

FIGURE 189-1. Acute leukemia. A, Acute lymphoblastic leukemia (ALL). B, Acute myeloid leukemia (AML). Lymphoblasts in ALL are smaller, with a higher ratio of nuclear to cytoplasmic material and less distinct nucleoli than in the myeloblasts in AML. The nucleoli in the myeloblasts are clear and "punched out."

FIGURE 189-2. Acute myeloid leukemia. The myeloblasts in the smear show Auer rods as cytoplasmic inclusions.

samples should also be evaluated by immunophenotyping and cytogenetics. If AML is suspected, samples should be evaluated for the presence of mutations in *FLT3*, *NPM1*, and *CEBPA*. A diagnostic lumbar puncture is generally recommended in suspected cases of ALL, but not in asymptomatic cases of AML.

The prothrombin and partial thromboplastin times are sometimes elevated. In APL, reduced fibrinogen and evidence of DIC are often seen. Other laboratory abnormalities frequently present are hyperuricemia, especially in ALL, and increased serum lactate dehydrogenase. In cases of high cell turnover and cell death (e.g., L3 ALL), evidence of tumor lysis syndrome may be noted at diagnosis, including hypocalcemia, hyperkalemia, hyperphosphatemia, hyperuricemia, and renal insufficiency. This syndrome, which is more commonly seen shortly after therapy is begun, can be rapidly fatal if untreated.

Differential Diagnosis

The diagnosis of acute leukemia is usually straightforward but can occasionally be difficult. Both leukemia and aplastic anemia (Chapter 168) can manifest with peripheral pancytopenia, but the finding of a hypoplastic marrow without blasts usually distinguishes aplastic anemia. An occasional patient has hypocellular marrow and a clonal cytogenetic abnormality, which establishes the diagnosis of myelodysplasia or hypocellular leukemia. A number of processes other than leukemia can lead to the appearance of immature cells in the peripheral blood. Although other small round cell neoplasms can infiltrate the marrow and mimic leukemia, immunologic markers are effective in differentiating the two. Leukemoid reactions to infections such as tuberculosis can result in the outpouring of large numbers of young myeloid cells, but the proportion of blasts in marrow or peripheral blood almost never reaches 20% in a leukemoid reaction (Chapter 170). Infectious mononucleosis (Chapter 385) and other viral illnesses can sometimes resemble ALL, particularly if large numbers of atypical lymphocytes are present in the peripheral blood and the disease is accompanied by immune thrombocytopenia or hemolytic anemia.

With the development of effective programs of combination chemotherapy and advances in hematopoietic cell transplantation, many patients with acute leukemia can be cured. These therapeutic measures are complex and are best carried out at centers with appropriate support services and experience in treating leukemia. Because leukemia is a rapidly progressive disease, specific antileukemic therapy should be started as soon after diagnosis as possible, usually within 48 hours. The goal of initial chemotherapy is to induce a complete remission (CR) with restoration of normal marrow function. In general, induction chemotherapy is intensive and is accompanied by significant toxicities. Therefore, patients should be stabilized to the extent possible before specific antileukemic therapy is begun.

Preparing the Patient for Therapy

Severe bleeding usually results from thrombocytopenia, which can be reversed with platelet transfusions (Chapter 180). Once thrombocytopenic bleeding is stopped, continued prophylactic transfusions of platelets may be warranted to maintain the platelet count higher than 10,000 to 20,000/μL. Occasionally, patients also have evidence of DIC, usually associated with the diagnosis of M3 AML. If M3 AML is suspected as the cause, all-*trans*-retinoic acid (ATRA) should be started without waiting for molecular confirmation of the diagnosis; the drug can be discontinued if the diagnosis is not M3 AML. If active bleeding is due to DIC (Chapter 178), low doses of heparin (50 U/kg) given intravenously every 6 hours can be of benefit. Platelets and fresh-frozen plasma (or cryoprecipitate) should be transfused to maintain the platelet count higher than 50,000/μL and the fibrinogen level greater than 100 mg/dL until the DIC abates. Whether heparin should be given prophylactically to patients with laboratory evidence of DIC but no active bleeding is an often debated but unsettled question.

Blood cultures should be obtained in patients with fever and granulocytopenia; while awaiting culture results, infection should be assumed and broad-spectrum antibiotics begun empirically (Chapters 170 and 289). It is preferable to bring an infection under control before starting initial chemotherapy if the patient has an adequate granulocyte count. However, patients often have infection but essentially no granulocytes; in this situation, delaying chemotherapy is unlikely to be beneficial.

Patients with very high blast counts (>100,000/μL) may have symptoms attributable to the effect of masses of these immature cells on blood flow. The leukostasis may evolve into vascular injury and local hemorrhage. If this situation occurs in the CNS, the outcome can be fatal. Leukapheresis, immediate whole brain irradiation (600 cGy in one dose), and administration of hydroxyurea (3 g/m²/day orally for 2 or 3 days) can usually prevent this complication.

Before treatment, management in all patients should be aimed at preventing the tumor lysis syndrome. Patients should be hydrated, have their urine alkalinized with acetazolamide 500 mg/day, and be given allopurinol 100 to 200 mg orally three times a day before chemotherapy is initiated. Patients with very high white cell counts may have uremia and anuria secondary to greatly increased serum uric acid levels, with subsequent intratubular crystallization, even before starting therapy. Hyperuricemia usually responds rapidly to rasburicase 0.20 mg/kg/day for up to 5 days intravenously, given over 30 minutes.

The diagnosis of leukemia usually comes as a profound psychological shock to the patient and family. Therefore, in addition to stabilizing the patient hematologically and metabolically, it is worthwhile to have at least one formal conference in which the patient and family are advised about the meaning of the diagnosis of leukemia and the consequences of therapy before treatment is initiated.

Treatment of Acute Lymphoblastic Leukemia

After the patient's condition has been stabilized, antileukemic therapy should be started as soon as possible. Treatment of newly diagnosed ALL can be divided into three phases: remission induction, postremission therapy, and CNS prophylaxis.

Remission Induction

The initial goal of treatment is to induce CR, defined as the reduction of leukemic blasts to undetectable levels and the restoration of normal marrow function. A number of different chemotherapeutic combinations can be used to induce remission; all include vincristine and prednisone, and most add L-asparaginase and daunorubicin, administered over a period of 3 to 4 weeks. With such regimens, CR is achieved in 90% of children and 80 to 90% of adults (Table 189-2). Because vincristine, prednisone, and L-asparaginase are relatively nontoxic to normal marrow precursors, the disease often enters CR after a relatively brief period of myelosuppression. Failure to achieve CR is usually due to either the leukemic cells' resistance to the drugs or progressive infection. These two complications occur with approximately equal frequency.

Postremission Chemotherapy

If no further therapy is given after induction of CR, relapse occurs in almost all cases, usually within several months. Chemotherapy after CR can be given in a variety of combinations, dosages, and schedules. The term *consolidation chemotherapy* refers to short courses of further chemotherapy given at doses

TABLE 189-2 COMMON REGIMENS FOR COMMON FORMS OF ACUTE LEUKEMIA

I. MANAGEMENT OF NEWLY DIAGNOSED ACUTE MYELOID LEUKEMIA

A. Induction—daunorubicin 60-90 mg/m²/day for 3 days (or idarubicin 10-12 mg/m²/day for 3 days) and cytarabine 200 mg/day for 7 days

B. Postremission
  1. Favorable risk—cytarabine 3 g/m² over 3 hr q12h on days 1, 3, and 5 every month for 4 mo
  2. Intermediate risk—as for favorable risk; or, if HLA-matched donor sibling exists, allogeneic hematopoietic cell transplantation
  3. Unfavorable risk—if HLA-matched donor is available, proceed to allogeneic transplantation; if not, treat as for intermediate risk

II. MANAGEMENT OF NEWLY DIAGNOSED ACUTE PROMYELOCYTIC LEUKEMIA

A. Induction—ATRA 45 mg/m²/day until complete remission plus daunomycin 45-60 mg/m²/day for 3 days and cytarabine 200 mg/m²/day for 7 days

B. Consolidation #1—arsenic trioxide 0.15 mg/kg/day 5 days/wk for 5 wk; repeat course after 2-wk rest
  Consolidation #2—ATRA 45 mg/m²/day for 7 days and daunomycin 50 mg/m²/day for 3 days; repeat course 1 mo later

C. Maintenance—ATRA 45 mg/m²/day for 15 days every 3 mo plus 6-MP 100 mg/m²/day and MTX 10 mg/m²/wk for 2 yr

III. MANAGEMENT OF NEWLY DIAGNOSED ADULT Ph-NEGATIVE ACUTE LYMPHOID LEUKEMIA

A. Induction (and courses 3, 5, 7)—cyclophosphamide 300 mg/m² over 3 hr q12h for 6 doses on days 1, 2, 3; doxorubicin 50 mg/m² on day 4; vincristine 2 mg/day on days 4 and 11; and dexamethasone 40 mg/day on days 1-4 and days 11-14

B. Consolidation (courses 2, 4, 6, 8)—MTX 200 mg/m² over 2 hr, followed by 800 mg/m² over 22 hr on day 1; high-dose cytarabine 3 g/m² over 2 hr q12h for 4 doses on days 2 and 3

C. Four intrathecal treatments of MTX 12 mg alternating with cytarabine 100 mg are given during the first four courses of systemic therapy

ATRA = all-*trans*-retinoic acid; HLA = human leukocyte antigen; 6-MP = 6-mercaptopurine; MTX = methotrexate; Ph = Philadelphia chromosome [t(9;22)].

---

similar to those used for initial induction (requiring rehospitalization). Usually, different drugs are selected for consolidation chemotherapy than were used to induce the initial remission. In the case of ALL, such drugs include high-dose methotrexate, cyclophosphamide, and cytarabine, among others. Maintenance involves the administration of low-dose chemotherapy on a daily or weekly outpatient basis for long periods. The most commonly used maintenance regimen in ALL combines daily 6-mercaptopurine and weekly or biweekly methotrexate. The optimal duration of maintenance chemotherapy is unknown, but it is usually given for 2 to 3 years. Optimal chemotherapy for ALL requires both consolidation and maintenance chemotherapy.

Central Nervous System Prophylaxis

Most chemotherapeutic agents that are given intravenously or orally do not penetrate the CNS well, and if no form of CNS prophylaxis is given, at least 35% of adults will develop CNS leukemia. With prophylaxis, relapse in the CNS as an isolated event occurs in less than 10% of patients. Systemic chemotherapy with high-dose methotrexate (e.g., 200 mg/m² intravenously over 2 hours, followed by 800 mg/m² over 22 hours) and cytarabine (e.g., 3 g/m² over 2 hours every 12 hours for 4 doses) can achieve therapeutic drug levels within the CNS. Alternatives are intrathecal methotrexate, intrathecal methotrexate combined with 2400 cGy radiation to the cranium, or 2400 cGy to the craniospinal axis.

Burkitt-Like ALL

Burkitt-like ALL (also called FAB L3 or mature B-cell ALL) is characterized by the presence of monoclonal surface immunoglobulin, cytogenetics showing t(8;14), and the constitutive expression of the *MYC* oncogene. Burkitt-like ALL, which accounts for 3 to 5% of adult cases of ALL, responds well to regimens that incorporate short, intensive courses of high-dose methotrexate (1.5 g/m² over 24 hours with leucovorin), cytarabine (3 g/m² over 2 hours every 12 hours for 4 doses), and cyclophosphamide (200 mg/m²/day for 5 days); this regimen yields high rates of complete response and cures about 50% of patients. Recent results suggest that the addition of rituximab may further improve outcomes.

Philadelphia Chromosome–Positive ALL

Approximately 5% of pediatric cases and 25% of adult cases of ALL have cytogenetics showing t(9;22), the Ph chromosome. Historically, such patients had CR rates slightly lower than those seen in Ph-negative ALL and markedly reduced remission durations, averaging less than a year; few if any such patients were cured with conventional chemotherapy. Therefore, the general recommendation has been that such patients receive an allogeneic transplant from a matched sibling or a matched unrelated donor during the first remission, if possible. With this approach, approximately 50% of patients can be cured. More recently, the addition of the tyrosine kinase inhibitor imatinib mesylate to conventional chemotherapeutic regimens has increased complete response rates, equaling those seen in Ph-negative ALL, but the impact of the addition of imatinib mesylate on the duration of remission is not yet known. The general recommendation remains transplantation during the first remission for this high-risk group of patients.

Prognosis of ALL after Initial Chemotherapy

A number of factors are predictive of outcome in ALL, the most important of which are younger age, a lower white cell count at diagnosis, and favorable cytogenetics. With currently available treatment regimens, 80 to 85% of children and 35 to 40% of adults who initially achieve CR maintain that state for more than 5 years, and these patients are probably cured of their disease.

Treatment of Relapsed ALL

Most relapses occur within 2 years after diagnosis, and most occur in the marrow. Occasionally, relapse is initially found in an extramedullary site such as the CNS or testes. Extramedullary relapse is usually followed shortly by systemic (marrow) relapse and should be considered part of a systemic recurrence. With the use of chemotherapeutic regimens similar to those used for initial induction, 50 to 70% of patients achieve at least a short-lived second remission. A small percentage of patients for whom the initial remission was longer than 2 years may be cured with salvage chemotherapy. If the CNS or testes is the initial site of the relapse, specific therapy at that site is also required, along with systemic retreatment. Because the prognosis of relapsed leukemia treated with chemotherapy is so poor, marrow transplantation is usually recommended in this setting.

Hematopoietic Cell Transplantation

The use of high-dose chemoradiotherapy followed by hematopoietic cell transplantation (Chapter 181) from an HLA-identical sibling can cure 20 to 40% of patients with ALL who fail to achieve an initial remission or who have a relapse after an initial CR; it can cure 50 to 60% of patients who undergo transplantation during a first remission. Although there is still considerable debate, several recent studies have reported improved survival for adults with high-risk or standard-risk ALL who receive a stem cell transplant during a first remission rather than being treated with standard chemotherapy.[1,2] The major limitations of transplantation are graft-versus-host disease, interstitial pneumonia, and recurrence of disease. If an HLA-identical sibling is not available, transplantation from a matched unrelated donor or transplantation of cord blood from a partially matched unrelated donor can be conducted, with results that approach those seen with matched related donors.

Treatment of Acute Myeloid Leukemia
Remission Induction

Treatment with a combination of an anthracycline and cytarabine (100 to 200 mg/m²/day for 7 days) leads to CR in 60 to 80% of patients with AML. Prospective randomized trials have demonstrated that idarubicin (10 to 12 mg/m²/day for 3 days) or a higher dose of daunorubicin (60 to 90 mg/m²/day for 3 days) is superior to the conventional daunorubicin dose of 45 mg/m²/day for 3 days.[3-5] Profound myelosuppression always follows when these agents are used at doses capable of achieving CR. Failure to achieve CR is usually due to either drug resistance or fatal complications of myelosuppression.

Postremission Therapy

Intensive consolidation chemotherapy with repeated courses of daunorubicin and cytarabine at doses similar to those used for induction, high-dose cytarabine (1 to 3 g/m²/day for 3 to 6 days), or other agents prolongs the average remission duration and improves the chances for long-term disease-free survival. The best results reported to date have generally been achieved with repeated cycles of high-dose cytarabine. Unlike the situation with ALL, low-dose maintenance therapy is of limited benefit after intensive consolidation treatment. In AML, leukemic recurrence occurs less often in the CNS (appropximately 10% of cases), most commonly in patients with the M4 or M5 variant. There is no evidence that CNS prophylaxis improves survival in AML.

Prognosis of AML after Initial Chemotherapy

Among patients in whom CR is achieved, 20 to 40% remain alive in continuous CR for more than 5 years, suggesting a probable cure. As with ALL, younger patients and those with a low white cell count at diagnosis have a more favorable outcome. Patients whose disease is characterized by certain chromosomal abnormalities, particularly t(8;21) and inv(16), or those with normal cytogenetics but mutated *CEBPA* and those with normal cytogenetics but mutated *NPM1* and wild-type *FLT3* do somewhat better, whereas those with 5q–, –7, 11q23, inv(3), or t(6;9) do worse. Patients who have a preleukemic phase before their condition evolves into acute leukemia and those whose leukemia is secondary to prior exposure to chemotherapy have a poorer prognosis. Increased expression of the multidrug resistance gene 1 (*MDR1*) is also associated with a worse outcome.

Treatment of Recurrent AML

Patients whose AML recurs after initial chemotherapy can achieve a second remission in about 50% of cases after retreatment with daunorubicin-cytarabine or high-dose cytarabine. The likelihood of achieving a second remission is predicted by the duration of the first remission: 70% in patients whose first remission persisted beyond 2 years, compared with less than 15% in those whose first remission lasted less than 6 months. Older patients may benefit from gemtuzumab ozogamicin (9 mg/m^2 on days 1 and 15), a form of antibody-targeted chemotherapy. Second remissions tend to be short-lived, however, and few patients in whom relapse occurs after first-line chemotherapy are cured by salvage chemotherapy.

Treatment of Acute Promyelocytic Leukemia

CR can be induced in at least 90% of patients with APL by using ATRA (45 mg/m^2/day until CR is achieved) in combination with an anthracycline. Patients treated with ATRA usually have their coagulation disorders corrected within several days. A unique toxicity of ATRA in the treatment of APL is the development of hyperleukocytosis accompanied by respiratory distress and pulmonary infiltrates. The syndrome responds to temporary discontinuation of ATRA and the addition of corticosteroids. By combining ATRA with anthracyclines for induction and consolidation and then using ATRA as maintenance therapy, approximately 70% of patients can be cured. Patients with higher white cell counts at diagnosis do worse. Arsenic trioxide (0.15 mg/kg/day until CR is achieved) is effective in patients with recurrent APL and appears to improve overall survival if used as part of consolidation therapy for patients in their first CR.

Hematopoietic Cell Transplantation

For patients with AML in whom an initial remission cannot be achieved or for those who have a relapse after chemotherapy, hematopoietic cell transplantation (Chapter 181) from an HLA-identical sibling offers the best chance for cure. Fifteen percent of patients with end-stage disease can be saved by this treatment. If the procedure is applied earlier, the outcome is better: approximately 30% of patients who undergo hematopoietic cell transplantation at first relapse or second remission are cured, and 50 to 60% of patients are cured if hematopoietic cell transplantation is performed during the first remission. A large number of studies have prospectively compared the outcome of allogeneic hematopoietic cell transplantation with that of chemotherapy in patients with AML in first remission. The trends in all these studies have been toward higher treatment-related mortality but improved disease-free and overall survival time with allogeneic transplantation. Meta-analyses conclude that survival is improved with allogeneic transplantation from a matched sibling in first remission when compared with continued chemotherapy.[6] This improvement is clearest in patients with high-risk or intermediate-risk cytogenetics and is not seen in those with good-risk cytogenetics. The major limitations of allogeneic hematopoietic cell transplantation are lack of a matched sibling donor, graft-versus-host disease, interstitial pneumonia, and disease recurrence. Because transplant-related toxicities increase with patient age, some centers limit hematopoietic cell transplantation to those 60 years of age or younger. However, recent studies of reduced-intensity or non-myeloablative allogeneic transplantation have shown encouraging results in patients with AML in remission at ages up to 70 years. The results of allogeneic transplantation using matched unrelated donors are not too dissimilar from those using matched siblings, although there is a higher incidence of complications. Autologous hematopoietic cell transplantation offers an alternative for patients without matched siblings to serve as donors. In randomized trials, the use of autologous bone marrow transplantation after consolidation chemotherapy significantly prolonged the duration of disease-free survival for patients with AML in first remission but did not alter overall survival.

Treatment of AML in Older Patients

The benefits of intensive consolidation chemotherapy in younger patients do not translate to patients older than 60 years, in part because older patients are less able to tolerate therapy, but also because AML in older patients is more often associated with unfavorable cytogenetics (particularly abnormalities of chromosomes 5 and 7) and more often overexpresses P-glycoprotein, resulting in the multidrug resistance phenotype. Accordingly, long-term survival rates of only 10 to 15% are seen with chemotherapy in patients older than 60 years. Otherwise healthy older patients can usually tolerate intensive chemotherapy and should be offered this treatment. However, intensive chemotherapy can cause more harm than good in older patients with poor performance status, and such patients may be candidates for supportive care only or for alternative therapies currently under study.

Management of Complications

Treatment of acute leukemia, especially AML, is accompanied by a number of complications, the two most serious and frequent being infection and bleeding. During the granulocytopenic period that follows induction and consolidation chemotherapy, the risk of bacterial infection is high. A Cochrane review examined results of antibiotic prophylaxis compared with placebo in afebrile neutropenic patients. Antibiotic prophylaxis significantly decreased infection-related deaths, with the best results seen with quinolones.[7] Invasive fungal infections are also common following chemotherapy for AML. A review of randomized trials found a significant reduction in death from fungal infection in patients given antifungal prophylaxis. Posaconazole may be more effective than fluconazole or itraconazole. Despite antibiotic and antifungal prophylaxis, many patients are febrile while neutropenic. The most commonly isolated organisms vary somewhat from medical center to medical center, but gram-positive organisms such as *Staphylococcus epidermidis* and gram-negative enteric organisms such as *Pseudomonas aeruginosa*, *Escherichia coli*, and *Klebsiella* (*Aerobacter*) are the most commonly isolated bacteria. Even if no cause for fever is found, bacterial infection should be assumed, and, in general, all patients with fever and neutropenia should begin receiving broad-spectrum antibiotics (Chapters 170 and 289). Commonly used antibiotic approaches include monotherapy with imipenem or a combination of an antipseudomonal penicillin and a third-generation cephalosporin. Once begun, antibiotics should be continued until patients recover their granulocyte counts, even if they become afebrile first. If documented bacterial infection persists despite appropriate antibiotics, the physician should consider removal of indwelling catheters.

In addition to being granulocytopenic, patients undergoing induction chemotherapy for leukemia have deficient cellular and humoral immunity, at least temporarily, and therefore are subject to infections common in other immunodeficiency states, including *Pneumocystis jirovecii* (formerly *Pneumocystis carinii*) infection and a variety of viral infections. *P. jirovecii* infection can be prevented by the prophylactic use of trimethoprim-sulfamethoxazole. Cytomegalovirus (CMV) infection can be prevented in a CMV-seronegative patient by the sole use of CMV-seronegative blood products (Chapter 384). Herpes simplex (Chapter 382) can often complicate existing mucositis and can be prevented with prophylactic acyclovir. Acyclovir is also useful for the treatment of disseminated varicella-zoster virus infection (Chapter 383).

Myeloid growth factors (granulocyte or granulocyte-macrophage colony-stimulating factor; Chapter 159), if given shortly after the completion of chemotherapy, shorten the period of severe myelosuppression by, on average, 4 days. In most studies, this accelerated recovery has resulted in fewer days with fever and less use of antibiotics, but it has not improved the complete response rate or altered survival.

The platelet count that signals a need for platelet transfusion has been the subject of debate. Traditionally, platelet transfusions from random donors were used to maintain platelet counts greater than 20,000/μL, but more recently it has been demonstrated that lowering this threshold to 10,000/μL is safe in patients with no active bleeding. In 30 to 50% of cases, patients eventually become alloimmunized and require the use of HLA-matched platelets (Chapter 180). Transfusion-induced graft-versus-host disease (Chapter 180), manifesting as a rash, low-grade fever, elevated values in liver function tests, and decreasing blood counts, can be prevented by irradiating all blood products before transfusion.

1. Goldstone AH, Richards SM, Lazarus HM, et al. In adults with standard-risk acute lymphoblastic leukemia, the greatest benefit is achieved from a matched sibling allogeneic transplantation in first complete remission, and an autologous transplantation is less effective than conventional consolidation/maintenance chemotherapy in all patients: final results of the International ALL Trial (MRC UKALL XII/ECOG E2993). *Blood.* 2008;111:1827-1833.
2. Ram R, Gafter-Gvili A, Vidal L, et al. Management of adult patients with acute lymphoblastic leukemia in first complete remission: systematic review and meta-analysis. *Cancer.* 2010;116:3447-3457.
3. Mandelli F, Vignetti M, Suciu S, et al. Daunorubicin versus mitoxantrone versus idarubicin as induction and consolidation chemotherapy for adults with acute myeloid leukemia: the EORTC and GIMEMA Groups Study AML-10. *J Clin Oncol.* 2009;27:5397-5403.
4. Fernandez HF, Sun Z, Yao X, et al. Anthracycline dose intensification in acute myeloid leukemia. *N Engl J Med.* 2009;361:1249-1259.
5. Lowenberg B, Ossenkoppele GJ, van Putten W, et al. High-dose daunorubicin in older patients with acute myeloid leukemia. *N Engl J Med.* 2009;361:1235-1248.
6. Koreth J, Schlenk R, Kopecky KJ, et al. Allogeneic stem cell transplantation for acute myeloid leukemia in first complete remission: a systematic review and meta-analysis of prospective clinical trials. *JAMA.* 2009;301:2349-2360.
7. Gafter-Gvili A, Fraser A, Paul M, et al. Meta-analysis: antibiotic prophylaxis reduces mortality in neutropenic patients. *Ann Intern Med.* 2005;142:979-995; erratum in *Ann Intern Med.* 2006;144:704.

SUGGESTED READINGS

Döhner H, Estey EH, Amadori S, et al. Diagnosis and management of acute myeloid leukemia in adults: recommendations from an international expert panel, on behalf of the European LeukemiaNet. *Blood.* 2010;115:453-474. *A comprehensive review of AML from an international group of experts.*

Marcucci G, Haferlach T, Döhner H. Molecular genetics of adult acute myeloid leukemia: prognostic and therapeutic implications. *J Clin Oncol.* 2011;29:475-486. *Review.*

Sanz MA, Lo-Coco F. Modern approaches to treating acute promyelocytic leukemia. *J Clin Oncol.* 2011;29:495-503. *Review including chemotherapy and the use of arsenic trioxide.*

Smith ML, Hills RK, Grimwade D. Independent prognostic variables in acute myeloid leukaemia. *Blood Rev.* 2011;25:39-51. *Review of clinical and molecular risk factors.*

190

THE CHRONIC LEUKEMIAS

HAGOP KANTARJIAN AND SUSAN O'BRIEN

FIGURE 190-1. **The Philadelphia chromosome.** Originally described as a shortened long arm of chromosome 22, the Philadelphia chromosome (Ph) was later found to be the result of a balanced translocation of genetic material between the long arms of chromosomes 9 and 22: t(9;22)(q34;q11.2). This results in the juxtaposition of *ABL* to *BCR*, producing a hybrid *BCR-ABL* oncogene. Depending on the breakpoint on *BCR*, three oncoproteins may be produced: p210$^{BCR-ABL}$, which is associated with 98% or more of the cases of Ph-positive chronic myelogenous leukemia (CML); p190$^{BCR-ABL}$, which is associated with 60 to 80% of cases of Ph-positive acute lymphocytic leukemia (the other 20 to 40% of cases are p210$^{BCR-ABL}$); and p230$^{BCR-ABL}$, which is associated with rare cases of Ph-positive CML. The dysregulated expression of *BCR-ABL*, through phosphorylation of substrate proteins, triggers the abnormal signal transduction of multiple downstream events, some of them thought to cause excessive proliferation, reduced apoptosis, abnormal cytoskeletal regulation and cytoadhesion, and other events contributing to the growth advantage of CML cells.

CHRONIC MYELOGENOUS LEUKEMIA

DEFINITION

Chronic myelogenous leukemia (CML), also called chronic myeloid leukemia, chronic myelocytic leukemia, and chronic granulocytic leukemia, is a clonal myeloproliferative disorder of the primitive hematopoietic stem cell that is characterized by overproduction of cells of the myeloid series, which results in marked splenomegaly and leukocytosis. Basophilia and thrombocytosis are common. A characteristic cytogenetic abnormality, the Philadelphia (Ph) chromosome, is present in the bone marrow cells in more than 90% of cases. Most patients (85 to 90%) present in the chronic phase. Eventually, if poorly controlled, CML evolves into the accelerated and blastic phases.

EPIDEMIOLOGY

CML constitutes one fifth of all cases of leukemia in the United States. It is diagnosed in 1 or 2 persons per 100,000 per year and has a slight male preponderance. This incidence of 5000 to 6000 cases annually has not changed significantly in the past few decades. The incidence of CML increases with age; the median age at diagnosis is 50 to 55 years. Ph-positive CML is uncommon in children and adolescents. No familial association of CML has been noted; for example, the risk is not increased in monozygotic twins or in relatives of patients with CML. Because of the availability of effective therapy, the annual mortality has been reduced from 15 to 20% before 2000 to 1 to 2% at present. Thus, the prevalence of CML is predicted to increase gradually, from 15,000 to 20,000 cases before 2000 up to 250,000 cases by 2040 in the United States.

Often, no etiologic agent is incriminated in CML. Exposure to ionizing radiation (e.g., in survivors of the atomic bomb explosions in Japan in 1945, in those undergoing radiation treatment of ankylosing spondylitis or cervical cancer) increases the risk of CML; the peak incidence occurs 5 to 12 years after exposure and is dose related. No increase in the risk of CML has been demonstrated among individuals working in the nuclear industry. Radiologists working without adequate protection before 1940 were more likely to develop myeloid leukemia, but no such association has been found in recent studies. Benzene exposure increases the risk of acute myelogenous leukemia (AML) but not of CML. CML is not a frequent secondary leukemia after treatment of other cancers with radiation, alkylating agents, or both.

PATHOBIOLOGY

Molecular Pathogenesis

The Ph chromosome abnormality, present in more than 90% of patients with typical CML (Fig. 190-1), results from a balanced translocation of genetic material between the long arms of chromosomes 9 and 22: t(9;22) (q34;q11.2). The breakpoint at band q34 of chromosome 9 results in translocation of the cellular oncogene *ABL1* (previously *c-ABL*) to a region on chromosome 22 coding for the major breakpoint cluster region (BCR). *ABL1* is a homologue of *v-ABL*, the Abelson virus that causes leukemia in mice. This translocation allows juxtaposition of a 5′ portion of a BCR and 3′ position of ABL; the two genetic sequences produce a new hybrid oncogene (*BCR-ABL*), which codes for a novel BCR-ABL oncoprotein with a molecular weight of 210 kD (p210$^{BCR-ABL}$). The p210$^{BCR-ABL}$ oncoprotein results in uncontrolled kinase activity of BCR-ABL, which triggers the excessive proliferation and reduced apoptosis of CML cells, thereby giving CML cells a growth advantage over normal cells and suppressing normal hematopoiesis. Although in most cases 100% of the metaphases on cytogenetic analysis show

BCR-ABL, some normal stem cells emerge on long-term bone marrow culture and after treatment with interferon-α (IFN-α), imatinib, high-dose chemotherapy, and autologous stem cell transplantation.

The constitutive activation of BCR-ABL results in autophosphorylation and activation of multiple downstream pathways that affect gene transcription, apoptosis, cytoskeletal organization, cytoadhesions, and degradation of inhibitory proteins. The signal transduction pathways implicated involve RAS, mitogen-activated-protein (MAP) kinases, signal transducers and activators of transcription (STAT), phosphatidyl inositol 3-kinase (PI3K), MYC, and others. Many of these interactions are mediated through tyrosine phosphorylation and require binding of the BCR-ABL to adapter proteins such as GRB-2, CRK, CRK-like protein (CRKL), and SCR-homology containing proteins (SHC). Although imatinib has been extremely successful at targeting BCR-ABL, understanding of the pathophysiology of the downstream events of BCR-ABL is important for the future development of agents that may target these events.

In Ph-positive acute lymphocytic leukemia (ALL), the breakpoint in BCR is proximal, in the minor BCR, resulting in a smaller *BCR* gene apposing *ABL*; the resulting fusion gene, messenger RNA, and BCR-ABL oncoprotein (p190$^{BCR-ABL}$) are smaller. A third rare, mu (μ) BCR breakpoint distal to the major BCR produces a p230$^{BCR-ABL}$ hybrid oncoprotein, which is associated with a more indolent CML course.

What induces this molecular rearrangement is unknown. Molecular techniques that amplify detection of *BCR-ABL* have demonstrated its presence in the marrow cells of 25 to 30% of healthy volunteers and 5% of infants, but not in cord blood. Because clinical CML develops in only 1 to 2 of 100,000 individuals (i.e., 1 to 2 per 25,000 to 30,000 individuals who express *BCR-ABL* in their bone marrow), immune regulatory processes or additional molecular events presumably contribute to the development of CML.

BCR-ABL is found only in hematopoietic cells and has its origin close to the pluripotent stem cell. For example, the Ph chromosome occurs in erythroid, myeloid, monocytic, and megakaryocytic cells; less commonly in B lymphocytes; rarely in T lymphocytes; and not at all in marrow fibroblasts. The fusion *BCR-ABL* gene and the p210 protein can be found in cases of typical morphologic CML in which no cytogenetic abnormality occurs or in which changes other than the typical t(9;22) (q34;q11.2) are identified. These patients have a survival rate and a response to therapy similar to those of patients with Ph-positive CML. Patients with atypical CML (usually older and more frequently exhibiting anemia, thrombocytopenia, monocytosis, and dysplasia) who are Ph negative and *BCR-ABL* negative have a worse prognosis than those who are either Ph-positive or Ph-negative and *BCR-ABL*–positive; they more closely resemble patients with myelodysplastic syndrome (Chapter 188). Thus, three groups of patients with CML can be identified: (1) those who are positive for Ph and *BCR-ABL,* (2) those who are Ph negative but *BCR-ABL* positive, and (3) those who are negative for Ph and *BCR-ABL. PDGFB* (previously *SIS*), which codes for platelet-derived growth factor (PDGF) and is the homologue of the simian sarcoma virus, is also translocated from chromosome 22 to chromosome 9 in CML, but it is distant from the breakpoint and is not expressed.

CLINICAL MANIFESTATIONS

About 40 to 50% of patients diagnosed with CML are asymptomatic until the disease is found on routine physical examinations or blood tests. In these patients, the white blood cell (WBC) count may be relatively low at diagnosis. The degree of leukocytosis correlates with tumor burden, as defined by spleen size.

The symptoms of CML, when present, are due to anemia and splenomegaly; they include fatigue, weight loss, malaise, easy satiety, and left upper quadrant fullness or pain. Rarely, bleeding (associated with a low platelet count or platelet dysfunction) or thrombosis (associated with thrombocytosis or marked leukocytosis) occurs. Other rare presentations include gouty arthritis (from elevated uric acid levels), priapism (usually with marked leukocytosis or thrombocytosis), retinal hemorrhages, and upper gastrointestinal ulceration and bleeding (from elevated histamine levels due to basophilia). Headaches, bone pain, arthralgias, pain from splenic infarction, and fever are uncommon in the chronic phase but more frequent as CML progresses. Symptoms of leukostasis, such as dyspnea, drowsiness, loss of coordination, or confusion, which are due to leukocyte sludging in the pulmonary or cerebral vessels, are uncommon in the chronic phase despite WBC counts exceeding 50,000 cells/µL, but these symptoms appear more frequently in the accelerated or blastic phases.

Splenomegaly, the most consistent physical sign in CML, occurs in 50 to 60% of cases. Hepatomegaly is less common (10 to 20%) and usually minor (1 to 3 cm below the right costal margin). Lymphadenopathy is uncommon, as is infiltration of skin or other tissues. If present, these findings suggest Ph-negative CML or the accelerated or blastic phase of CML.

DIAGNOSIS

The diagnosis of typical CML is not difficult. Patients with untreated CML usually have leukocytosis ranging from 10,000 to 500,000/µL. The predominant cells are neutrophils, with a left shift extending to blast cells. Basophils and eosinophils are commonly increased. Monocytes may be slightly increased in some cases that overlap with chronic myelomonocytic leukemia (CMML; see later discussion). Thrombocytosis is common, whereas thrombocytopenia is rare and, if present, suggests a worse prognosis. A hemoglobin level of less than 11 g/dL is present in one third of patients. Biochemical abnormalities in CML include a low leukocyte alkaline phosphatase (LAP) score. A low LAP score also occurs in some patients with agnogenic myeloid metaplasia. Serum levels of vitamin B$_{12}$, lactate dehydrogenase, uric acid, and lysozyme are often increased. Some patients demonstrate a cyclic oscillation of the WBC count. The presence of unexplained myeloid leukocytosis (Fig. 190-2) with splenomegaly should lead to a bone marrow examination and cytogenetic analysis.

Bone Marrow

The bone marrow is hypercellular, with marked myeloid hyperplasia and, at times, evidence of increased reticulin or collagen fibrosis. The myeloid-erythroid ratio is 15 : 1 to 20 : 1. About 15% of patients have 5% or more blast cells in the peripheral blood or bone marrow at diagnosis.

Cytogenetics

The presence of the t(9;22)(q34;q11.2) abnormality establishes the diagnosis of CML. If the Ph chromosome is not found in a patient with suspected CML, molecular studies for the presence of the hybrid *BCR-ABL* gene should be performed. About 25 to 30% of patients with a typical morphologic picture of CML who are Ph negative have the *BCR-ABL* rearrangement. The

FIGURE 190-2. Chronic myelogenous leukemia, chronic phase. Peripheral smear shows leukocytosis, with representation by the entire spectrum of leukocyte differentiation, ranging from myeloblasts to mature neutrophils. (Courtesy of Andrew Schafer, MD.)

Ph chromosome is usually present in 100% of metaphases, often as the sole abnormality. Between 10 and 15% of patients have additional chromosomal changes (loss of the Y chromosome, trisomy 8, an additional loss of material from 22q, or double Ph). Some patients have complex chromosomal changes involving chromosome 9 or chromosome 22 (Ph variants, three-way translocations).

Differential Diagnosis

CML must be differentiated from leukemoid reactions (Chapter 170), which usually produce WBC counts lower than 50,000/µL, toxic granulocytic vacuolation, Döhle's bodies in the granulocytes, absence of basophilia, and normal or increased LAP levels; the clinical history and physical examination generally suggest the origin of the leukemoid reaction. Corticosteroids can rarely cause extreme neutrophilia with a left shift, but this abnormality is self-limited and of short duration.

CML may be more difficult to differentiate from other myeloproliferative or myelodysplastic syndromes (Chapters 169 and 188). Patients with agnogenic myeloid metaplasia with or without myelofibrosis frequently have splenomegaly, neutrophilia, and thrombocytosis. Polycythemia vera with associated iron deficiency, which causes normal hemoglobin and hematocrit values, can manifest with leukocytosis and thrombocytosis. Such patients usually have a normal or increased LAP score, a WBC count less than 25,000/µL, and no Ph chromosome.

The greatest diagnostic difficulty lies with patients who have splenomegaly and leukocytosis but do not have the Ph chromosome. In some, the *BCR-ABL* hybrid gene can be demonstrated despite a normal or atypical cytogenetic pattern. Patients who are Ph negative and *BCR-ABL* negative are considered to have Ph-negative CML or CMML (see later discussion). Rarely, patients have myeloid hyperplasia, which involves almost exclusively the neutrophil, eosinophil, or basophil cell lineage. These patients are described as having chronic neutrophilic, eosinophilic, or basophilic leukemia and do not have evidence of the Ph chromosome or the *BCR-ABL* gene. Isolated megakaryocytic hyperplasia can be seen in essential thrombocythemia (Chapter 169), with marked thrombocytosis and splenomegaly. Some patients who present with clinical characteristics of essential thrombocythemia (with marked thrombocytosis but without leukocytosis) have CML; cytogenetic and molecular studies showing the Ph chromosome, the *BCR-ABL* rearrangement, or both lead to the appropriate diagnosis and treatment.

Clinical Course
Evolution to Accelerated and Blastic Phases

More than 90% of patients present with CML in the benign or chronic phase, which becomes asymptomatic once the disease is controlled. Death rarely occurs during the chronic phase of CML.

When poorly controlled, CML evolves into an accelerated phase, usually defined by the presence of 15% or more blasts, 30% or more blasts plus promyelocytes, 20% or more basophils, thrombocytopenia less than 100,000/µL unrelated to therapy, or cytogenetic clonal evolution. The accelerated phase is also characterized by worsening anemia; increasing splenomegaly or hepatomegaly; infiltration of nodes, skin, bones, or other tissues; and fever, malaise, and weight loss. In the accelerated phase, bone marrow studies may

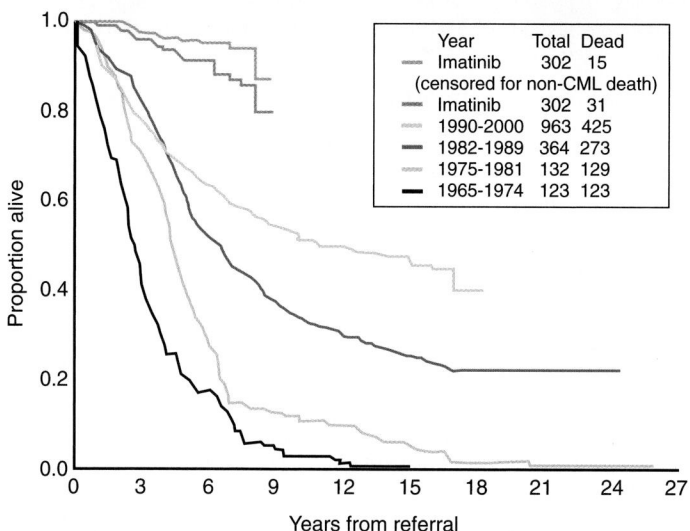

Year	Total	Dead
— Imatinib	302	15
(censored for non-CML death)		
— Imatinib	302	31
— 1990-2000	963	425
— 1982-1989	364	273
— 1975-1981	132	129
— 1965-1974	123	123

FIGURE 190-3. Survival of patients with Ph-positive chronic myelogenous leukemia in chronic phase. (M. D. Anderson data; 1884 patients from 1965 to 2008.)

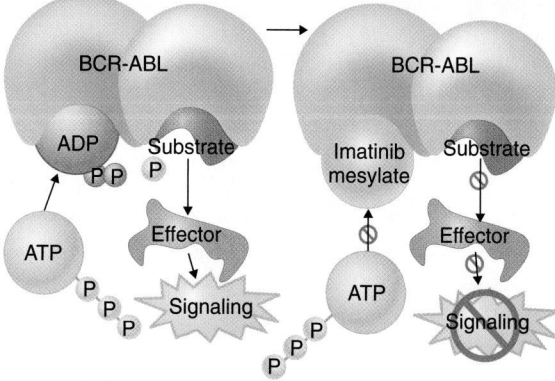

FIGURE 190-4. Mechanism of action of imatinib. By occupying the ATP binding pocket of the ABL kinase domain, imatinib prevents substrate phosphorylation and downstream activation of signals, thus inhibiting the leukemogenic effects of BCR-ABL on cells in chronic myelogenous leukemia. ADP = adenosine diphosphate; ATP = adenosine triphosphate; P = phosphate group.

show dysplastic changes, increased percentages of blasts and basophils, myelofibrosis, and chromosomal abnormalities in addition to the Ph chromosome (clonal evolution). About 5 to 10% of patients present in the accelerated phase.

Before the era of imatinib therapy, the risk of developing accelerated or blastic phase CML was 10% per year in the first 2 years after diagnosis and 15 to 20% per year thereafter, unless therapies such as IFN-α or allogeneic stem cell transplantation were used. With imatinib, the annual incidence of progression of CML from the chronic to the accelerated or blastic phase has been 2% in the first 10 years of observation (Fig. 190-3). Before imatinib therapy, the median survival of accelerated phase CML was 18 months or less, but survival has now increased to 4 years or more.

The blastic phase of CML is diagnosed when 30% or more blast cells are present in the bone marrow and/or peripheral blood or when extramedullary blastic disease is present. Most patients develop features of the accelerated phase before progressing to the blastic phase, but 20% of patients evolve quickly into a blastic phase without warning. Most patients in the accelerated or blastic phase have additional chromosomal abnormalities (clonal evolution) such as duplication of the Ph chromosome, trisomy of chromosome 8, or development of an isochromosome 17. The extramedullary blastic phase of CML can occur in the spleen, lymph nodes, skin, meninges (especially in the lymphoid blastic phase), bones, and other sites; extramedullary transformation is usually followed shortly by evidence of marrow involvement. Blastic phase CML is associated with a very poor median survival time of 5 months. About 25% of patients develop a lymphoid blastic phase; their response rate to anti-ALL–like chemotherapy and imatinib is about 60%, and their median survival time is about 1 year.

Ph-negative and *BCR-ABL*–negative CML often appear to overlap clinically with CMML in terms of behavior, progress, and response to therapy and seem to resemble the myelodysplastic syndromes (Chapter 188) more than Ph-positive CML. A male preponderance and older age are noted; splenomegaly is common (60 to 70%). The WBC count is usually in the range of 25,000 to 100,000/μL. Anemia, thrombocytopenia, and monocytosis are more common than in Ph-positive CML, whereas eosinophilia and basophilia are less common. The median survival time is 18 to 24 months; patients die of infection, bleeding, or transformation to acute leukemia.

TREATMENT

Rx

Choice of Therapy in Chronic Myelogenous Leukemia

Treatment decisions in CML are based on the phase of CML, the patient's age, and the availability of a stem cell donor. For patients presenting in chronic phase CML (>90% of newly diagnosed patients), imatinib mesylate, a selective BCR-ABL tyrosine kinase inhibitor, is first-line therapy in the vast majority of patients. Allogeneic stem cell transplantation is considered effective second-line therapy in chronic phase CML after imatinib failure. Alternative second-line therapies are more potent second-generation tyrosine kinase inhibitors, including dasatinib (dual SRC-ABL kinase inhibitor) and nilotinib (selective and more

potent BCR-ABL kinase inhibitor). Patients with CML in the accelerated or blastic phase should consider allogeneic stem cell transplantation as immediate, definitive therapy; in this situation, the use of tyrosine kinase inhibitors as an interim measure before stem cell transplantation may reduce the CML burden significantly and improve the results of allogeneic stem cell transplantation.

Imatinib Mesylate

Since its discovery in 1999, imatinib mesylate has become standard therapy for CML. Imatinib is a 2-phenylaminopyrimidine derivative that binds to the canonical adenosine triphosphate (ATP) lining the groove between the N and C lobes of the ABL kinase domain, thus blocking the phosphorylation of tyrosine residues on substrate protein. Blocking of ATP binding inactivates the ABL kinase, because it cannot transfer phosphate to its substrate. By inhibiting phosphorylation, imatinib prevents the activation of signal transduction pathways that induce the leukemic transformation processes that cause CML (Fig. 190-4). Imatinib inhibits several tyrosine kinases, including p210$^{BCR-ABL}$, p190$^{BCR-ABL}$, v-ABL, c-ABL, C-kit, and PDGF receptor.

In a randomized trial of 1106 patients with newly diagnosed CML, imatinib 400 mg/day orally provided significantly higher rates of major cytogenetic response (87% vs. 35%) and complete cytogenetic response (76% vs. 14%), as well as lower rates of progression (8% vs. 26%) and transformation (3% vs. 9%) after 12 months of therapy, compared with the prior standard nontransplantation therapy (a combination of IFN-α and cytosine arabinoside).[1][2] The longer-term follow-up results continue to demonstrate outstanding outcomes with imatinib therapy (Table 190-1; see Fig. 190-3): with a median follow-up of 7 years, the complete cytogenetic response rate (occurring at least once on therapy) is 87%, the estimated 5-year durable complete cytogenetic response rate is 65 to 70%, the annual rate of progression to accelerated or blastic phase is only 1 to 2%, and the estimated 7-year survival rate is above 86% (94% if non-CML deaths are censored).[3] Imatinib plus peginterferon alfa-2a is somewhat superior to imatinib alone for providing a persisting molecular response at 12 months,[4] but its precise role in routine treatment remains to be determined.

Most CML experts and physicians now consider imatinib frontline therapy for all patients with newly diagnosed Ph-positive CML in the chronic phase, regardless of age and donor availability. The only possible exceptions are the rare patients who present with p190$^{BCR-ABL}$ CML, who may have a worse prognosis on imatinib.

Imatinib has a 5% or lower rate of serious side effects, which include nausea, vomiting, diarrhea, skin rashes, muscle cramps, bone aches, periorbital or leg edema, weight gain, and, rarely, hepatic, renal, or cardiopulmonary dysfunction; most of these are manageable with dose reductions or treatment interruptions. Drug-related myelosuppression occurs in 10 to 20% of patients with newly diagnosed CML and is manageable with brief treatment interruptions, dose modifications, or both or with the administration of growth factors (erythropoietin for anemia, granulocyte colony-stimulating factor for neutropenia). Hypophosphatemia associated with altered bone metabolism can occur, and the serum phosphate level should be monitored. Chromosomal abnormalities may appear in the Ph-negative diploid cells in 5 to 10% of responding patients, probably due to unmasking of a fragile stem cell prone to the development of CML or to chromosomal instability; such changes disappear spontaneously in 70% of cases and rarely evolve into a myelodysplastic syndrome or acute myeloid leukemia, probably as part of the natural course of CML.

Allogeneic Stem Cell Transplantation

Allogeneic stem cell transplantation, a potentially curative therapy in selected patients with CML, is most effective during the chronic phase, when

TABLE 190-1 EARLY RESULTS OF IMATINIB MESYLATE THERAPY IN CHRONIC MYELOGENOUS LEUKEMIA

| PHASE | % Cytogenetic Response | | ESTIMATED SURVIVAL |
	COMPLETE (Ph 0%)	MAJOR (Ph < 35%)	
Blastic	7	10-20	10-15% at 4 yr
Accelerated	20-40	40-60	40-50% at 4 yr
Chronic, after failure of IFN-α	55-63	60-80	80-85% at 4 yr
Chronic, newly diagnosed	65-85	80-90	86-94% at 7-8 yr

IFN-α = interferon-α; Ph = Philadelphia chromosome.

it is associated with a 20-year survival rate of 40 to 50%. Transplant-related mortality ranges from 5 to 50%, depending on the patient's age, whether the donor is related or unrelated, the degree of matching, and other, less important factors such as positivity for cytomegalovirus, preparative and post-transplantation regimens, and institutional expertise. Disease-free survival rates with related allogeneic stem cell transplantation are 40 to 80% in chronic phase, 15 to 40% in accelerated phase, and 5 to 20% in blastic phase. In chronic phase CML, patients younger than 30 to 40 years have disease-free survival rates of 60 to 80%, compared with only 30 to 40% for patients older than 50 years. A major limitation of allogeneic stem cell transplantation is the availability of related donors. Human leukocyte antigen (HLA)–compatible unrelated donors can be found for 50% of patients; the median time from initiation of the donor search to transplantation is 3 to 6 months.

Nonmyeloablative preparative regimens have expanded the indications for allogeneic stem cell transplantation to older patients and have reduced transplant-related mortality and complications (Chapter 181). Early results show acceptable degrees of engraftment, less mortality and organ damage, more persistent residual disease, and similar degrees of graft-versus-host disease. Patients whose CML recurs after allogeneic stem cell transplantation may respond to donor lymphocyte infusions, imatinib or second-generation tyrosine kinase inhibitors (dasatinib, nilotinib), IFN-α, or a second allogeneic transplant.

The advantage of allogeneic stem cell transplantation is its proven track record, with an estimated cure rate of 40% at 20 years. However, it is associated with a 1-year mortality rate of 5 to 40% and with morbidities such as cataracts, infertility, second cancers (5 to 10%), immune-mediated complications, and chronic graft-versus-host disease. Delaying allogeneic stem cell transplantation beyond 1 to 3 years after diagnosis may be associated with worse results and with occasional sudden blastic transformation, which may not be salvageable. The outcome of allogeneic stem cell transplantation may be even better after imatinib exposure.

Treatment of CML after Imatinib Failure

Imatinib failure is strictly defined as (1) lack of any cytogenetic response after 6 months of imatinib therapy, (2) no major cytogenetic response (Ph ≤35%) after 12 months, (3) no complete cytogenetic response (Ph 0%) beyond the first year of therapy (generally at 18 months or later), or (4) hematologic or cytogenetic relapse or CML transformation at any time. Patients with chronic phase CML on imatinib should be considered for allogeneic stem cell transplantation only if imatinib therapy fails. Alternatively, a more potent tyrosine kinase inhibitor may be tried if imatinib resistance is noted. These include nilotinib (AMN107), which is 20 to 50 times more potent than imatinib, and dasatinib (BMS-354825), which is 300 times more potent than imatinib. Both agents are now approved for the treatment of CML after imatinib failure (dasatinib for all CML phases; nilotinib for chronic and accelerated phases). Dasatinib and nilotinib have been associated with complete hematologic response rates of 70 to 80% and complete cytogenetic response rates of 40 to 50% in chronic phase CML, with estimated 2-year survival rates of 90% (compared with annual mortalities of 10 to 20% after imatinib failure before their availability). They have also shown encouraging results in accelerated or blastic phase CML after imatinib failure. 5,6 An important question is whether these second-generation tyrosine kinase inhibitors can be used as more definitive therapy, thus delaying the consideration of allogeneic stem cell transplantation until the failure of drug therapy. This depends on the patient's age (patients 70 years or older may decide to forgo the risks of allogeneic stem cell transplantation, even though it might be curative), the availability of an ideal donor (e.g., related vs. unrelated; matched vs. mismatched), the initial response to tyrosine kinase inhibitors (major cytogenetic response by 12 months predicts long-term favorable disease control), and the presence and specific type of mutations (e.g., T315I mutations are resistant to all currently approved tyrosine kinase inhibitors; mutations with a high IC_{50} in vitro [drug concentration

that suppresses 50% of clonal growth] to a particular agent are associated with poor long-term disease control).

Treatment of Accelerated and Blastic Phase Chronic Myelogenous Leukemia

Patients with accelerated or blastic phase CML may receive initial imatinib therapy to reduce the CML burden, but they should be considered for early allogeneic stem cell transplantation. Response rates to combination chemotherapy are 20% in nonlymphoid blastic phase CML and 60% in lymphoid blastic phase CML. Median survival times are 3 to 6 months and 9 to 12 months, respectively. The addition of imatinib to chemotherapy has improved the response rates and prolonged the median survival time in blastic phase CML from 3 to 5 months to 6 to 12 months.

At present, allogeneic stem cell transplantation is the only curative therapy for accelerated and blastic phase CML: overall cure rates are in the range of 15 to 40% and 5 to 20%, respectively, and patients with cytogenetic clonal evolution as the only accelerated phase criterion have a long-term event-free survival rate of about 60%. Otherwise, imatinib provides hematologic responses in 80% of patients and an estimated 4-year survival rate of 40 to 55% in accelerated phase CML, but only a 40% response rate and a median survival of 7 months in blastic phase CML. Patients in the accelerated or blastic phase should be encouraged to participate in investigational strategies to improve their prognosis. Combinations of imatinib with chemotherapy may improve results in CML transformation, as may the new tyrosine kinase inhibitors.

Special Therapeutic Considerations

Patients with severe leukocytosis and manifestations of leukostasis may benefit from initial leukapheresis. Severe thrombocytosis uncontrolled with anti-CML measures may respond to anagrelide, thiotepa, IFN-α, 6-mercaptopurine, 6-thioguanine, and platelet pheresis. CML during pregnancy may be controlled with pheresis in the first trimester and then with hydroxyurea until delivery. Use of IFN-α during pregnancy has been reported anecdotally to be safe. There is little experience with the use of imatinib during pregnancy. Splenectomy can be useful as a palliative measure in patients with massive painful splenomegaly, hypersplenism, or thrombocytopenia.

Follow-up
Monitoring Response to Therapy in CML

With improved therapy, the incidences of complete cytogenetic response and minimal residual disease have increased. This has required the development of new techniques to measure these responses more accurately (rather than relying on only 20 metaphases by cytogenetic analysis), less tedious and less painful procedures (peripheral blood rather than marrow studies), and techniques that can measure minimal (molecular) disease below the level of detection by routine cytogenetic studies. Fluorescence in situ hybridization (FISH) studies with improved probes can measure 200 interphase cells using peripheral blood, and they have false-positive rates of less than 2 to 3%. Quantitative polymerase chain reaction (QPCR) studies usually measure the ratio of the abnormal message, BCR-ABL, to a normal message, such as ABL. A BCR-ABL/ABL ratio of 0.1% (International Standard) or less, about a 3-log reduction of disease, has been associated with a very low risk of CML relapse on imatinib therapy. This is now referred to as a major molecular response. A negative QPCR analysis (i.e., undetectable BCR-ABL levels, usually $<10^{-5}$ to 10^{-6}) may be dependent on the technique used and could be referred to as a complete molecular response.

In monitoring the response to imatinib-based therapies, patients require a bone marrow analysis before therapy (to determine the percentages of blasts and basophils and clonal evolution), at 6 and 12 months (to assess cytogenetic response and confirm complete cytogenetic response), and once every 1 to 3 years in those with stable, durable complete cytogenetic responses (to look for chromosomal abnormalities in both Ph-positive and Ph-negative cells). Monitoring in patients with confirmed, durable complete cytogenetic responses can be continued with either FISH or QPCR studies every 6 months (or more often, such as every 3 months, if there are concerns about significant and consistent increases in QPCR levels). The frequency of monitoring depends on the treatment plan; monitoring is more frequent in younger patients, less frequent in very old patients.

"Resistance" to imatinib therapy can be defined as persistent 100% Ph positivity after 6 months of therapy, Ph positivity of more than 35% after 12 months of therapy, or cytogenetic or hematologic relapse. A positive QPCR in a patient with a complete cytogenetic response does not, at present, indicate imatinib resistance or the need to change therapy. The rate of resistance to imatinib in chronic phase CML is less than 4% per year; for those who achieve a complete cytogenetic response, the rate of resistance beyond year 3 of imatinib therapy is 1% or less, suggesting the durable stability of a complete cytogenetic response on imatinib and the predictability of the CML course once such a response is obtained. Several mechanisms of resistance have been identified; the most common are mutations in the BCR-ABL kinase domain. More than 50 different mutations have been reported and can involve any of the important domains in the BCR-ABL structure, including the P-loop (the area where ATP binds), the activation loop, and the catalytic domain, as well as the amino acids where imatinib makes contact with BCR-ABL. The different mutations have considerable variability with respect to resistance to imatinib. Some mutations are overcome by slightly higher concentrations of imatinib than required to inhibit the wild-type form; others are completely insensitive to imatinib. Mutational analysis is useful in patients with imatinib resistance to identify those with the *T315I* mutation, who do not respond to imatinib or the second-generation tyrosine kinase inhibitors (dasatinib, nilotinib, bosutinib) and should be considered for immediate allogeneic stem cell transplantation or therapy with *T315I*-selective inhibitors. In addition, knowledge of the sensitivity of the different mutations, as determined by the IC_{50} for particular agents, can help select the tyrosine kinase inhibitor. Mutational studies may also be helpful in patients who develop cytogenetic or hematologic resistance or relapse on imatinib therapy.

TREATMENT AND PROGNOSIS

Allogeneic stem cell transplantation (Chapter 181), which is the only curative modality, should be considered frontline therapy in candidate patients. Other therapies include hydroxyurea to control leukocytosis, erythropoietin to improve anemia, azacitidine or decitabine (both approved by the U.S. Food and Drug Administration [FDA] for the treatment of CMML), topotecan and cytarabine or other intensive anti-AML (Chapter 189) regimens for CMML transformation, splenectomy for symptomatic splenomegaly and/or hypersplenism, and investigational agents.

Poor prognostic factors include the presence of anemia (hemoglobin <10 g/dL), thrombocytopenia, and more than 5% blasts. Median survival time is 12 to 18 months.

FUTURE DIRECTIONS

Two second-generation tyrosine kinase inhibitors, dasatinib and nilotinib, are now approved for the treatment of CML after imatinib failure. Other tyrosine kinase inhibitors (bosutinib) are under investigation, with promising results. Three randomized studies of the more potent second-generation tyrosine kinase inhibitors nilotinib, dasatinib, and bosutinib against the standard of care, imatinib, are ongoing in patients with newly diagnosed CML. Maturing data suggest that they may significantly improve the complete cytogenetic and major molecular response rates, as well as reduce the transformation rate to the accelerated and blastic phases.[5,6] Equally important are the "third-generation" tyrosine kinase inhibitors such as AP24534, which are also active against CML with the *T315I* mutation. Other active anti-CML agents under development include omacetaxine (previously known as homoharringtonine), decitabine (a hypomethylating agent), and pegylated formulations of interferon. Immunotherapeutic strategies, including vaccines, may improve the eradication of minimal residual disease, potentially obviating the need for indefinite therapy with imatinib. Further understanding of the pathophysiology and events downstream of BCR-ABL may help in the development of new strategies to target these events. Such strategies may include inhibitors of pathways involving Raf, protein farnesylation, mTOR, JAK/STAT, proteasome, MEK/MAPK, PI3K/AKT, or others.

PROGNOSIS

Imatinib therapy has revolutionized the treatment of CML. In cases of newly diagnosed CML, imatinib therapy is associated with an estimated 7-year survival rate of 86% (94% if non-CML deaths are censored). If this favorable trend continues with longer follow-up, the median survival time in CML may exceed 25 years. During the first 7 years of follow-up, the annual mortality has been about 2%. Many well-established poor prognostic factors in CML (e.g., older age, splenomegaly, presence of marrow fibrosis, deletion of derivative 9q) have lost much of their importance since the advent of imatinib therapy. With allogeneic stem cell transplantation, cures can be expected in 40 to 80% of patients with chronic phase CML, 15 to 40% of those with accelerated phase CML, and 5 to 20% of those with blastic phase CML.

CHRONIC MYELOMONOCYTIC LEUKEMIA

DEFINITION AND EPIDEMIOLOGY

Although superficially resembling CML in its clinical and morphologic presentation, CMML should be considered a separate entity because of its particular clinical, therapeutic, and prognostic aspects. CMML is a hybrid entity manifesting as a proliferation of the myeloid monocytic series and dysplasia of the erythroid-megakaryocytic series. Patients with CMML are older (median age, 65 to 70 years) than most patients with CML.

PATHOBIOLOGY

The cytogenetic findings in patients with CMML are normal or involve an additional chromosome 8 or findings other than the Ph chromosome. Patients with CMML have *RAS* mutations in 40 to 60% of cases.

CLINICAL MANIFESTATIONS AND DIAGNOSIS

Patients often present with symptoms related to anemia and thrombocytopenia (fatigue, bleeding). Other typical features include splenomegaly, leukocytosis, and monocytosis. Organ infiltration (lymph nodes, skin, liver) is less common. Basophilia and thrombocytosis are not presenting features.

HAIRY CELL LEUKEMIA

DEFINITION AND EPIDEMIOLOGY

Hairy cell leukemia (HCL) is an uncommon and indolent B-cell leukemia (1 to 2% of all leukemias). The median age at diagnosis is 50 years, and there is a 4 : 1 male preponderance.

PATHOBIOLOGY

The cell of origin of HCL is the B lymphocyte, as documented by the demonstration of heavy and light chain immunoglobulin gene rearrangements. Hairy cells express CD19, CD20, CD11C, CD103, FMC7, and CD22, but not CD21, CD5, CD10, or CD23. The cells demonstrate a κ or γ light chain phenotype excess. The cells also express CD25 (TAC), the low-affinity interleukin-2 (IL-2) receptor, and CD103, a unique hairy cell antigen. High levels of soluble IL-2 receptor (>5 times normal) are present in the sera of almost all patients with HCL, with extremely high levels noted in many cases. A number of different cytogenetic abnormalities have been reported in HCL, but none appears to be consistently present, and all have been described in other hematologic malignancies. Immune dysfunction is wide ranging in HCL. Monocytopenia is universal; B and T lymphocytes are decreased in number; the CD4/CD8 (T helper/T suppressor) ratio is often inverted; and skin test reactivity to recall antigens is impaired, as is antibody-dependent cellular cytotoxicity. Humoral immunity is relatively preserved, with normal immunoglobulin levels. Marrow failure in HCL may be due in part to inhibitory factors (e.g., tumor necrosis factor) produced by the leukemic infiltrate; the pancytopenia is often more marked than would be anticipated from the degree of leukemic infiltration.

CLINICAL MANIFESTATIONS

The majority of patients present with pancytopenia and splenomegaly. Patients may also have fatigue, fever, weight loss, and infection secondary to granulocytopenia or monocytopenia. Leukocytosis is uncommon, and lymphadenopathy is rare. Anemia is present in up to 85% of patients, whereas leukopenia and thrombocytopenia are present in 60 to 75%. The cytopenias are caused by a combination of bone marrow failure due to leukemic infiltration and hypersplenism. Patients may experience repeated infections and, rarely, a systemic vasculitis resembling polyarteritis nodosa. Although bacterial infections occur, as would be expected with neutropenia, patients with HCL have a predilection to develop tuberculosis, atypical mycobacterial infections, and fungal infections, perhaps related to the severe monocytopenia that is characteristic of this disorder.

DIAGNOSIS

In conjunction with the clinical features, careful examination of the peripheral blood smear may demonstrate the occasional typical cells with cytoplasmic projections, giving rise to the name *hairy cell leukemia* (Fig. 190-5). The hairy cells are 10 to 15 mm in diameter, with pale blue cytoplasm, a nucleus with a loose chromatin structure, and one or two indistinct nucleoli. Bone marrow aspiration is often inadequate owing to increased deposition of reticulin, collagen, and fibrin; bone marrow biopsy is usually necessary. Bone marrow involvement is interstitial or patchy, and the infiltrate is characterized by widely spaced nuclei due to the abundant cytoplasm, giving rise to the commonly described "fried egg" appearance.

Hairy cells exhibit a strong acid phosphatase (isoenzyme 5) cytochemical reaction in 95% of cases, a reaction that is resistant to the inhibitory effect of tartaric acid (TRAP). Other lymphoproliferative diseases are rarely TRAP positive. Electron microscopy clearly demonstrates the microvillar

FIGURE 190-5. Hairy cell leukemia. Peripheral smear shows hairy cells with blue-gray cytoplasm; fine, hair-like projections (resembling ruffles); and oval or slightly indented nuclei with loose chromatin and indistinct nucleoli. (Courtesy of Andrew Schafer, MD.)

projections. Often, ribosomal-lamellar complexes, which are characteristic but not diagnostic of HCL, can be identified. The peroxidase stain is negative, and lysozyme activity is absent in hairy cells, thereby differentiating these cells from monocytes.

Differential Diagnosis

The differential diagnosis must distinguish HCL from lymphoma (Chapter 191) or chronic lymphocytic leukemia (CLL), which can manifest with predominant splenomegaly and minimal lymphadenopathy. Some patients with a myelodysplastic syndrome (Chapter 188) or a myeloproliferative syndrome (Chapter 169) have splenomegaly and pancytopenia with only a few atypical cells. Patients with other diseases, such as systemic lupus erythematosus (Chapter 274) and other autoimmune diseases, B-cell and T-cell prolymphocytic leukemias (see later), infiltrative splenomegaly (Chapter 171), or tuberculosis (Chapter 332), may have splenomegaly and cytopenia, but these diagnoses can usually be made by history, physical examination, and appropriate blood and bone marrow tests. Splenomegaly, cytopenia, and nonaspirable marrow in a middle-aged man should create a high index of suspicion for HCL. Splenectomy and lymph node biopsy are sometimes necessary to establish the diagnosis in difficult cases. Cases of HCL variant manifest with higher WBC counts, are TRAP negative, have prominent nucleoli, and are only occasionally positive for antibodies against CD25. HCL variant does not respond as well to the agents that are usually effective in the management of typical HCL.

TREATMENT　　　　　　　　　　　　　　　Rx

A small proportion (<5%) of patients with HCL do not require therapy. These patients have mild cytopenias, are not transfusion dependent, have no history of infections, and have a low level of marrow infiltration by hairy cells.

2-Chlorodeoxyadenosine (cladribine), an adenosine analogue that is resistant to deamination by adenosine deaminase, produces complete remission in more than 80% of HCL patients after a single course of 0.1 mg/kg/day for 7 days given by continuous intravenous infusion, and it is now the recommended first-line therapy. Remissions are durable, and patients who relapse can often attain a second remission after retreatment with cladribine. The drug is well tolerated, with a low infection rate. Despite long-lasting suppression of CD4+ lymphocyte counts, there does not appear to be an increase in late opportunistic infections or second malignancies.

Deoxycoformycin (pentostatin; 4 mg/m² weekly or every 2 weeks for up to 6 months), an adenosine deaminase inhibitor, produces complete remission in 70 to 80% of patients. The response to treatment is rapid, and the drug is active in patients previously treated with IFN. Toxicity includes nausea and vomiting, infection, renal and hepatic dysfunction, conjunctivitis, and photosensitivity, albeit mild in most cases.

Human leukocyte interferon (HuIFN), or r-IFN-α, rapidly improves granulocyte, platelet, and hemoglobin levels (1 to 3 months); reduces spleen size; and decreases marrow infiltration. Peripheral blood cell counts return to normal in 80% of cases, but complete remission is uncommon. In addition, when treatment is discontinued, relapse occurs within 1 to 2 years.

Rituximab, the monoclonal antibody targeting CD20, can also produce responses; 8 weekly infusions appear to be more effective than four.

Two immunotoxins can produce responses in refractory patients. LMB2 is composed of the Fc portion of the anti-TAC antibody linked to a *Pseudomonas* exotoxin. BL22 also contains *Pseudomonas* exotoxin linked to an antibody targeting CD22. Splenectomy is recommended mainly for patients with splenic infarcts or massive splenomegaly.

PROGNOSIS

More than 85 to 90% of patients treated with cladribine or pentostatin are expected to be alive at 10 years.

⬤ CHRONIC LYMPHOCYTIC LEUKEMIA

DEFINITION

CLL is a neoplasm characterized by the accumulation of monoclonal lymphocytes of B-cell origin. The cells accumulate in the bone marrow, lymph nodes, liver, spleen, and occasionally other organs.

EPIDEMIOLOGY

CLL is the most common leukemia (one third of all cases) in the Western world and is twice as common as CML. The disease occurs rarely in those younger than 30 years; most patients with CLL are older than 60 years. CLL increases in incidence exponentially with time; by age 80, the incidence rate is 20 cases per 100,000 persons per year. The male-female ratio is approximately 2 : 1. The incidence of CLL among Asians in Japan and China is only 10% of that in the United States and other Western countries. Intermediate incidence rates are seen in persons of Hispanic origin.

The cause of CLL is unknown. Ionizing radiation and viruses have not been associated with CLL, although hepatitis C infection has recently been associated with splenic lymphoma with villous lymphocytes (another indolent B-cell disorder). Familial clustering in CLL is more common than in other leukemias; first-degree relatives of patients have a two- to four-fold higher risk and develop CLL at a younger age compared with the general population (anticipation). Farmers have a higher incidence of CLL than do those in other occupations, raising the possibility of an etiologic role for herbicides or pesticides. Agent Orange, the defoliating agent used in Vietnam, has been associated with the development of CLL.

PATHOBIOLOGY

Leukemia cells in CLL are homogeneous and have the appearance of normal mature lymphocytes. However, clonality can be documented by the presence of immunoglobulin gene rearrangements and the restriction to either κ or γ light chains on the cell surface. The cells express low-intensity monoclonal surface immunoglobulin (SmIg; usually immunoglobulin [Ig] M ± IgD) and the pan-B-cell antigens CD19, CD20, CD23, and CD24 in almost all cases, as well as CD21 (which includes the receptor for the Epstein-Barr virus and the C3d component of complement) in more than 75% of cases. Almost all cells exhibit Ia antigen and receptors for the Fc fragment of IgG and spontaneously form rosettes with mouse erythrocytes. In addition to B-cell antigens, CLL cells express CD5 (Leu 1, T1, and T101), a pan-T-cell antigen. Other T-cell antigens are absent. CD25 (TAC, IL-2 receptor) antigen is positive in about 25% of cases. T cells are increased in number at diagnosis, and the CD4/CD8 ratio is often inverted, owing to a relatively greater increase in CD8+ cells. The CD4/CD8 ratio declines as the disease progresses and after therapy. The T cells have a blunted response to T-cell mitogens and decreased delayed hypersensitivity reactions to recall antigens. However, these T-cell functions may be impaired by factors produced by the CLL cells, because purified T cells have a normal response to T-cell mitogens.

GENETICS

Standard cytogenetic analysis identifies abnormalities in 40 to 50% of cases of CLL, but CLL cells have low mitotic activity. By FISH, the likelihood of detecting abnormalities increases to 80%. A 13q deletion is the most common abnormality; other abnormalities include 11q deletion (15 to 20%), trisomy 12 (15 to 20%), and 17p deletion (5 to 10%). The 17p deletion increases in frequency as the disease progresses, recurs after therapy, and is associated with a very poor prognosis. The 11q deletion also is associated with a poorer prognosis, whereas the 13q deletion, if present as the sole abnormality, is associated with a favorable prognosis.

CLINICAL MANIFESTATIONS

Most patients with CLL are asymptomatic, and the disease is diagnosed when absolute lymphocytosis is noted in the peripheral blood (see Fig. 190-6) during evaluation for other illnesses or when the patient undergoes a routine physical examination. Symptoms such as fatigue, lethargy, loss of appetite, weight loss, and reduced exercise tolerance are nonspecific. Many patients have enlarged lymph nodes. B symptoms (fever, night sweats, weight loss) are rarely present initially, and their presence in later stages of the disease suggests transformation to large cell lymphoma. The most common infections are sinopulmonary. As the disease progresses, the frequency of neutropenia, T-cell deficiency, and hypogammaglobulinemia increases, resulting in infections with gram-negative bacteria, fungi, and viruses such as herpes zoster and herpes simplex.

The major physical findings relate to infiltration of the reticuloendothelial system. Lymphadenopathy with discrete, rubbery, mobile lymph nodes is present in two thirds of patients at diagnosis. Later, as the lymph nodes enlarge, they can become matted. Enlargement of the liver or spleen is less common at diagnosis (approximately 10% and 40% of cases, respectively) but occurs more frequently with progression. Organ failure resulting from infiltration with CLL is uncommon. Infiltration of the central nervous system in CLL is rare, and central nervous system symptoms are more likely to be caused by opportunistic infections such as cryptococcosis or listeriosis.

DIAGNOSIS

CLL is characterized by absolute lymphocyte counts that typically range from 5000 to 600,000/μL in the peripheral blood. Even with markedly elevated WBC counts, hyperviscosity symptoms rarely occur, probably because of the small size and pliability of the cells. Anemia (hemoglobin <11 g/dL) is present in 15 to 20% of patients at diagnosis, and thrombocytopenia (platelet count <100,000/μL) in 10%. However, bone marrow replacement and hypersplenism, which are seen with progressive disease, increase the frequency of anemia and thrombocytopenia. The anemia is usually normochromic and normocytic, and the reticulocyte count is normal unless the patient has autoimmune hemolytic anemia (Chapter 163), which usually results from the development of a warm-reacting IgG antibody. The diagnosis of autoimmune hemolytic anemia, which occurs in 10% of cases, is confirmed by a positive direct Coombs test (80 to 90% of cases), reticulocytosis, a low serum haptoglobulin concentration, and an elevated unconjugated serum bilirubin level. In such patients, reactive erythroid hyperplasia as a response to the hemolysis may be masked in the bone marrow by the marked lymphocytic infiltration. Cold agglutinin hemolysis occurs rarely in CLL. Autoimmune thrombocytopenia (immune thrombocytopenic purpura; Chapter 175) can be diagnosed in 10 to 15% of cases. The antibodies causing red cell and platelet destruction are not produced by the CLL cells, and the mechanisms for the associated autoimmune diseases are not known. Pure red cell aplasia (Chapter 168) is an additional, underappreciated cause of anemia in CLL.

The lymphocytes in CLL are indistinguishable on light or electron microscopy from normal small B lymphocytes (Fig. 190-6). On bone marrow aspiration, the proportion of lymphocytes is greater than 30% and may be up to 100%. Four patterns of lymphocyte infiltration on bone marrow biopsy

FIGURE 190-6. Chronic lymphocytic leukemia. Peripheral smear shows that the predominant leukocytes are "normal," mature-appearing lymphocytes, with occasional "smudge" cells. (Courtesy of Andrew Schafer, MD.)

occur: nodular (15%), interstitial (30%), mixed nodular and interstitial (30%), and diffuse (35%). Most early-stage cases have one of the first three patterns; diffuse histology is common in advanced-stage disease and becomes more prominent as the disease evolves. A diffuse histologic pattern confers a poor prognosis regardless of the stage of disease.

Differential Diagnosis

There are many diseases that can cause lymphocytosis, including pertussis (Chapter 321), cytomegalovirus (Chapter 384), Epstein-Barr virus mononucleosis (Chapter 385), tuberculosis (Chapter 332), toxoplasmosis (Chapter 357), chronic inflammatory disorders, and autoimmune syndromes. These diseases are seldom confused with B-cell CLL, largely because the lymphocytosis in these conditions is usually less than 15,000/μL and is not sustained. If doubt persists, immunophenotypic or molecular studies can distinguish the monoclonal lymphocytosis in CLL from the T-cell or polyclonal B-cell proliferation in the other disorders.

In individuals 62 to 80 years old, monoclonal CLL-phenotype B cells are found in about 5% of individuals with normal blood counts. In patients with greater than 4000 lymphocytes/mL, about 45% have CLL, about 40% have reactive lymphocytosis, and about 15% have monoclonal CLL-phenotype B cells that confer a 1.1% per year risk of developing CLL. In patients ultimately diagnosed with CLL, B-cell clones were previously present in peripheral blood in 98% of patients, sometimes many years before diagnosis.

Other Chronic Lymphocytic Leukemias

The more difficult differential diagnosis is distinguishing CLL from other lymphoproliferative disorders such as prolymphocytic leukemia (PLL), splenic lymphoma with villous lymphocytes, HCL, the leukemic phase of mantle cell lymphoma, and Waldenström's macroglobulinemia. Although certain clinical features are more common in some of these disorders (e.g., marked splenomegaly with minimal or no lymphadenopathy in PLL, splenic lymphoma, and HCL vs. extensive lymphadenopathy with or without splenomegaly in CLL), none of these clinical features is specific. The differential diagnosis therefore depends largely on histopathologic and, more specifically, immunophenotypic features (Table 190-2).

Prolymphocytic Leukemia

PLL is an uncommon disease (incidence <5% that of CLL), and its characteristics of massive splenomegaly, minimal lymphadenopathy, and markedly elevated WBC count (often >100,000/μL), with 10 to 90% of the cells being prolymphocytes, distinguish this disease from typical B-cell CLL. Prolymphocytes are larger cells that have a distinct nucleolus and express FMC-7. The male-female ratio is 4:1, and the median age at diagnosis is 70 years. Survival is shorter than in CLL (median 3 years), and response to therapies usually applied in CLL is poor. A serum paraprotein, typically IgG or IgA, is present in one third of cases. The immunoglobulin on the surface of the cells is occasionally IgG or IgA, not IgM ± IgD, as in CLL. Several karyotypic abnormalities have been reported in PLL, including t(11;14)(q13;q32). Deletions of 11q3, 23, and 17p are more common in B-cell PLL than in CLL. Abnormalities in the *TP53* oncogene are found in 75% of cases of B-cell PLL. One fifth of PLL cases express a T-cell phenotype.

Small Lymphocytic Lymphoma

Small lymphocytic lymphoma (SLL) shares histopathologic and immunophenotypic features with CLL, differing only in the lack of lymphocytosis in the peripheral blood. The bone marrow in SLL may or may not have more than 30% lymphocytes. LFA-1 adhesion protein is much more commonly expressed on SLL cells than on CLL cells. Other lymphomas, such as follicular and mantle cell lymphomas (Chapter 191), occasionally manifest a leukemic phase on initial presentation. Follicular lymphoma cells are often cleaved on light microscopy, have bright staining for SmIg, and are positive for FMC-7 and CD10. Lymph node biopsy should be performed to identify these cases with greater precision. The presence of lymphoma cells in the blood in follicular lymphoma is more common with advanced disease. Follicular lymphoma can usually be identified by the presence of the translocation t(14;18) and consequent *BCL2* rearrangement, both of which are rare in CLL. The WBC count in Waldenström's macroglobulinemia (Chapter 193) is usually much lower than in CLL (<10,000/μL), and many patients are leukopenic. The cells have a plasmacytoid appearance, CD38 and PCA-1 positivity, and more SmIg and cytoplasmic Ig. A serum monoclonal IgM peak is present in almost all cases of Waldenström's macroglobulinemia but is uncommon in CLL.

TABLE 190-2 DIFFERENTIAL DIAGNOSIS OF INDOLENT LYMPHOPROLIFERATIVE DISORDERS

DISEASE	LYMPHADENOPATHY (%)	SPLENOMEGALY (%)	CELL OF ORIGIN (B/T)	Positive Markers* Smlg	Positive Markers* CD5	Positive Markers* CD19, CD20 (%)	Positive Markers* OTHER
Chronic lymphocytic leukemia (CLL)	75	50	B (20:1)	Weak	>90%	≥90	Mouse red blood cell receptors
Prolymphocytic leukemia (PLL)	33	95	B (4:1)	Bright	T-cell PLL	75	FMC-7
Hairy cell leukemia	<10	80	B (T rare)	Bright	—	>90	CD25, CD11C, CD103
Lymphoma (leukemic phase)	90	90	B (T rare)	Bright	Some	>90	CD10
Splenic lymphoma with villous lymphocytes	10	80	B	Bright	20%	>90	FMC-7, CD22
Waldenström's macroglobulinemia	33	33	All B	Weak	Some	Many	CD38, PCA-1
Large granular lymphocytosis	10	10	All T	Absent	—	—	CD2, CD3, CD8

*CD2 = pan-T cell; CD3 = pan–mature T cell; CD5 = pan-T cell, B-cell CLL; CD8 = T cell (suppressor cytotoxic); CD10 = early B cell; CD11C = hairy cell, activated T cell, NK cell; CD19 = early pan-B cell; CD20 = pan-B cell; CD25 = low-affinity interleukin-2 receptor; CD38 = activated B cell, thymocyte, plasma cell; FMC-7 = PLL, hairy cell leukemia; PCA-1 = plasma cell; SmIg = monoclonal surface immunoglobulin.

TABLE 190-3 RAI AND BINET STAGING SYSTEMS IN CHRONIC LYMPHOCYTIC LEUKEMIA

STAGE	LYMPHOCYTOSIS	LYMPHADENOPATHY	HEPATOMEGALY OR SPLENOMEGALY	HEMOGLOBIN (G/DL)	PLATELETS ×10³/ML
RAI STAGING SYSTEM					
0	+	−	−	≥11	≥100
I	+	+	−	≥11	≥100
II	+	±	+	≥11	≥100
III	+	±	±	<11	≥100
IV	+	±	±	Any	<100
BINET STAGING SYSTEM					
A	+	±	± (<3 lymphatic groups* positive)	≥10	≥100
B	+	±	± (≥3 lymphatic groups* positive)	≥10	≥100
C	+	±	±	<10†	<100†

*The three lymphatic groups are (1) cervical, axillary, and inguinal nodes; (2) liver; and (3) spleen. Each group is considered one group whether unilateral or bilateral.
†The criterion is hemoglobin <10 g/dL and/or platelets <100 × 10³/mL.

T-Cell Leukemias

The predominant clinical manifestation of Sézary's syndrome (a CD4+ T-cell malignant disorder related to mycosis fungoides) is chronic exfoliative erythroderma with a low number of circulating monoclonal T cells. The clinical and laboratory differentiation from CLL is not difficult. Other T-cell malignant disorders with peripheral blood involvement are adult T-cell leukemia-lymphoma and large granular lymphocytosis, also referred to as large granular lymphoproliferative disorder, T-cell lymphocytosis with neutropenia, or T-gamma lymphocytosis syndrome. Adult T-cell leukemia-lymphoma is associated with a retrovirus (human T-lymphotropic virus I) and is common in Japan and the Caribbean. It frequently manifests with lytic bone lesions and hypercalcemia. In T-cell large granular lymphoproliferative disorders, the absolute lymphocyte count is usually low (<5000/μL), with a CD2+, CD3+, CD8+, and CD16+ (T-suppressor) phenotype (T-gamma cells). These patients often have splenomegaly, neutropenia, and rheumatoid arthritis–like symptoms. A subset, called natural killer (NK) cell large granular lymphocytosis, has an NK cell phenotype (CD16−) and no molecular evidence of T-cell receptor rearrangement. The lymphocytes have abundant cytoplasm with azurophilic granules. Most patients have a benign course, although repeated infections can occur.

Staging and Prognostic Factors

The natural history of CLL is heterogeneous, with survival times ranging from 2 to 20 years after diagnosis. Either of two validated clinical staging systems can be used. The Rai staging system (1975) defines five stages and is most frequently used in the United States, whereas the Binet system (1981) defines three stages and is most frequently used in Europe (Table 190-3). Patients with anemia and thrombocytopenia (Rai III and IV, Binet C) have the worst prognosis; patients with lymphocytosis alone (Rai 0, some Binet A patients) have an excellent prognosis. A group of patients with a

lymphocyte count less than 30,000/μL, hemoglobin greater than 13 g/dL, platelet count greater than 100,000/μL, fewer than three involved node areas, and lymphocyte doubling time greater than 12 months has been described as having "smoldering" CLL, with survival equal to that of an age- and sex-matched control population. Patients tend to progress through stages, with many patients developing more sites of involvement over time and eventually experiencing marrow failure; however, anemia and thrombocytopenia can develop abruptly, even without antibody-mediated destruction or markedly increased tumor burden.

Other adverse factors include a diffuse pattern of lymphocytic infiltration observed on bone marrow biopsy; molecular abnormalities, including deletion of 11q or 17p; advanced age; male sex; elevated serum levels of thymidine kinase, β₂-microglobulin, and soluble CD23; rapid lymphocyte doubling time; an increased proportion of large or atypical lymphocytes in the peripheral blood; and lack of somatic mutation of the VH gene within the B-CLL cell or the presence of the ZAP-70 protein or CD38 on the CLL cell surface.

TREATMENT Rx

The major therapeutic questions are when to treat and which therapeutic regimen to use. Patients with CLL are usually older, and the prognosis of the disease is variable (with some early-stage cases being stable for 10 to 20 years). Treatment of early-stage CLL (Rai 0, Binet A) is delayed until the disease progresses. In randomized trials, early treatment with alkylating agents did not prolong survival and was associated with a heightened risk of developing second malignant tumors. Two large clinical trials are currently investigating, in a randomized fashion, whether early treatment benefits asymptomatic patients with high-risk disease. Treatment of Rai stages III and IV (Binet stage C) is recommended at the time of diagnosis because of the morbidities associated with cytopenias and the poor survival time of these patients. Treatment of intermediate-stage disease (Rai I and II, Binet B) is recommended if symptomatic disease (fever, sweats, weight loss, severe fatigue) or massive lymphadenopathy, with or without hepatosplenomegaly, is present.

Medical Therapy

Chemotherapy

Fludarabine monophosphate (25 mg/m^2/day for 5 days every 4 weeks), an adenosine analogue, is approved by the FDA for treatment of relapsed CLL, with overall response rates of 50 to 60%. The dose-limiting toxicity is myelosuppression. When used in conjunction with steroids, the treatment may be complicated by infections with organisms usually associated with immunodeficiency syndromes involving T lymphocytes (e.g., those caused by *Pneumocystis jirovecii* or herpesviruses). In a large randomized trial of initial therapy for CLL, fludarabine resulted in higher overall and complete remission rates, longer duration of remission, and improved response rates on crossover, but there was no survival advantage compared with chlorambucil, the prior standard therapy.[7] However, 10-year follow-up has now shown a survival benefit in the fludarabine arm. Cladribine is used primarily in Europe, where it appears to have efficacy similar to fludarabine; pentostatin has not been as widely studied in CLL as in HCL.

Before the advent of fludarabine, combination regimens were based on alkylating agents and borrowed from regimens used to treat lymphoma. The COP regimen (cyclophosphamide 100 to 300 mg/m^2/day orally on days 1 through 5, vincristine [Oncovin] 2 mg intravenously on day 1, and prednisone 100 mg orally on days 1 through 5) does not have any advantage over chlorambucil alone, usually given at a dose of 0.1 to 0.2 mg/kg/day for 3 to 6 weeks until the desired effect is obtained or until thrombocytopenia or neutropenia develops; the dose is then adjusted for maintenance and is continued for 6 to 12 months. Regimens using cyclophosphamide, doxorubicin, and prednisone with vincristine (CHOP) or without vincristine (CAP) have produced response rates of 50 to 70% in those with Binet stage C disease.

The combination of fludarabine and cyclophosphamide (FC) was a logical attempt to improve on the efficacy of fludarabine alone by combining it with the other most active agent in this disease, an alkylating agent. The FC combination has been compared to fludarabine alone in three randomized trials.[8-10] All these trials consistently showed a higher complete response rate, higher overall response rate, and longer progression-free survival with the FC combination.

After therapy, many patients remain stable for months to years before progressive disease indicates the need for further treatment. The goal of treatment is to achieve complete response (Table 190-4).

Bendamustine is a potent alkylating agent that has some structural similarity to nucleoside analogues, but preclinical data suggest that it does not function as a nucleoside analogue. Bendamustine was recently approved by the FDA for the treatment of CLL based on a randomized trial comparing this agent to chlorambucil as initial therapy for patients with CLL.[11] Complete and overall response rates were higher with bendamustine, and progression-free survival was longer. The main side effect is myelosuppression.

Monoclonal Antibodies

Rituximab, a monoclonal antibody targeting the CD20 antigen, is associated with response rates of about 50% when given at the standard dose (375 mg/m^2/week for 4 weeks) as initial therapy for CLL and significantly lower rates when used in the salvage setting, but complete responses are rare in either setting. The major benefit of this antibody appears to be its use in combination with chemotherapy. Fludarabine combined with rituximab appears to produce better responses than those seen historically with fludarabine alone. In addition, progression-free and overall survival are better than that seen in the historical cohort. A three-drug regimen of fludarabine, cyclophosphamide, and rituximab (FCR) appears to produce the best and most durable complete remission rates when used as first-line therapy. A recent randomized trial compared the activity of FC to that of FCR. More than 800 patients were accrued, and the patient characteristics were balanced between the two arms. FCR produced slightly more neutropenia than FC, but there was no difference in grade 3 or 4 infections. The complete response rate and the overall response rate were significantly higher with FCR, and progression-free and overall survival were significantly longer than with chemotherapy alone.[12] Alemtuzumab (Campath-1H; 30 mg intravenously three times a week for 4 to 12 weeks), a monoclonal antibody that binds to the CD52 antigen, was originally approved for the treatment of fludarabine-refractory CLL. One third of such patients can achieve remission. Recently, alemtuzumab was compared with chlorambucil as initial therapy for symptomatic patients with CLL. Alemtuzumab produced higher complete and overall response rates and longer progression-free survival.[13]

Ofatumumab is a humanized monoclonal antibody that binds to CD20, but to a different epitope than rituximab. This drug was recently approved by the FDA for the treatment of fludarabine- and alemtuzumab-refractory CLL. In the pivotal trial, the drug was given intravenously for 8 weeks and then monthly for 4 months. The overall response rate in this highly refractory population was 58%; the median progression-free survival was 6 months, with a median overall survival of 13.7 months. As with other monoclonal antibodies, the predominant side effects are infusion reactions, which tend to be more common with the initial doses.

Stem Cell Transplantation

Autologous stem cell transplantation has no proven benefit in terms of survival or long-term disease control in CLL. Data on allogeneic stem cell transplantation are limited to young patients with refractory disease, in whom a long-term control rate of 40 to 55% has been reported. Nonmyeloablative stem cell transplantation, which works mainly by its graft-versus-leukemia effect, has been used in older patients with CLL, with some success.

Radiation Therapy

In CLL, radiation therapy is used palliatively to shrink unsightly or painfully enlarged nodal masses or an enlarged spleen.

Autoimmune and Infectious Manifestations

Autoimmune hemolytic anemia and immune-mediated thrombocytopenia do not correlate closely with the activity of CLL. Prednisone (60 to 100 mg/day) is indicated as treatment for autoimmune hemolytic anemia (Chapter 163) and for some cases of immune-mediated thrombocytopenia (Chapter 175) in CLL. If there is no response in 3 to 4 weeks, the treatment has failed, and the dose should be tapered over 1 to 2 weeks. If a response is obtained, the dose is reduced by 25% each week over 4 weeks. Patients for whom corticosteroids fail often respond to low-dose oral cyclosporin 100 mg three times a day. Other therapeutic options include splenectomy, intravenous immunoglobulin, rituximab, and alemtuzumab.

Intravenous immunoglobulin (400 mg/kg every 3 to 4 weeks) significantly decreases the incidence of infections in patients with recurrent infections and hypogammaglobulinemia. However, the cost of this therapy is substantial.

PROGNOSIS

Approximately one third of patients who present with early-stage CLL never require therapy and have the same survival of age-matched controls. Frequent characteristics of such patients include WBC less than 30,000/μL, hemoglobin greater than 13 g/dL, nondiffuse pattern on bone marrow biopsy, and slow lymphocyte doubling time.

A poor response to therapy is an adverse factor in all phases of the disease. As CLL progresses, the development of a prolymphocytic transformation (10% of cases) or transformation to large cell lymphoma portends a median survival time of less than 6 months. Other factors that may suggest transformation are the development of B symptoms, a markedly elevated lactate dehydrogenase level, or fludeoxyglucose-avid disease on positron emission tomography. A high incidence of second malignant tumors (10 to 20% of patients) either precedes or follows the diagnosis of CLL; the roles of therapy versus impaired immune surveillance as causative factors are unclear. Skin

	COMPLETE	

TABLE 190-4 DEFINITION OF REMISSION IN CHRONIC LYMPHOCYTIC LEUKEMIA: THE INTERNATIONAL WORKSHOP IN CHRONIC LYMPHOCYTIC LEUKEMIA–NATIONAL CANCER INSTITUTE WORKING GROUP CRITERIA

CRITERION	COMPLETE REMISSION	PARTIAL REMISSION
Physical examination		
Nodes	None ≥1.5 cm	≥50% decrease
Liver/spleen	Not palpable	≥50% decrease
Symptoms	None	N/A
Peripheral blood		
Neutrophils	≥1500/mL	≥1500/mL or ≥50% increase from baseline
Platelets	>100,000/μL	100,000/μL or ≥50% increase from baseline
Hemoglobin	>11 g/dL	>11 g/dL or >50% increase from baseline
Lymphocytes	≤4000/mL	>50% decrease
Bone marrow	<30%, no B-lymphoid nodules	50% reduction in infiltrate or B-lymphoid nodules

cancer, including melanoma, as well as colorectal and lung cancers are common. CLL tends to develop in older people; in indolent cases, death occurs from other intercurrent illnesses seen in this age group. Almost all patients younger than 60 years and those with progressive disease die as a result of CLL, primarily from infections. Gram-positive organisms usually cause nonfatal infections early in CLL, but most deaths due to infection are associated with gram-negative bacterial or fungal infections. Infection with other opportunistic organisms, such as *Mycobacterium tuberculosis*, herpesvirus, and *P. jiroveci*, may also be fatal.

1. O'Brien SG, Guilhot F, Larson RA, et al. Imatinib compared with interferon and low-dose cytarabine for newly diagnosed chronic-phase chronic myeloid leukemia. *N Engl J Med.* 2003;348: 994-1004.
2. Hughes T, Kaeda J, Branford S, et al. Frequency of major molecular responses to imatinib or interferon alfa plus cytarabine in newly diagnosed chronic myeloid leukemia. *N Engl J Med.* 2003; 349:1423-1432.
3. Druker B, Guilhot F, O'Brien S, et al. Five-year follow-up of patients receiving imatinib for chronic myeloid leukemia. *N Engl J Med.* 2006;355:2408-2417.
4. Preudhomme C, Guilhot J, Nicolini FE, et al. Imatinib plus peginterferon alfa-2a in chronic myeloid leukemia. *N Engl J Med.* 2010;363:2511-2521.
5. Saglio G, Kim DW, Issaragrisil S, et al. Nilotinib versus imatinib for newly diagnosed chronic myeloid leukemia. *N Engl J Med.* 2010;362:2251-2259.
6. Kantarjian H, Shah N, Hochhaus N, et al. Dasatinib versus imatinib in newly diagnosed chronic-phase chronic myeloid leukemia. *N Engl J Med.* 2010;362:2260-2270.
7. Rai KR, Peterson BL, Appelbaum FR, et al. Fludarabine compared with chlorambucil as primary therapy for chronic lymphocytic leukemia. *N Engl J Med.* 2000;343:1750-1757.
8. Eichhorst BF, Busch R, Hopfinger G, et al. Fludarabine plus cyclophosphamide versus fludarabine alone in first-line therapy of younger patients with chronic lymphocytic leukemia. *Blood.* 2006;107:885-891.
9. Flinn IW, Neuberg DS, Grever MR, et al. Phase III trial of fludarabine plus cyclophosphamide compared with fludarabine for patients with previously untreated chronic lymphocytic leukemia: US Intergroup Trial E2997. *J Clin Oncol.* 2007;25:793-798.
10. Catovsky D, Richards S, Matutes E, et al. Assessment of fludarabine plus cyclophosphamide for patients with chronic lymphocytic leukaemia (the LRF CLL4 Trial): a randomized controlled trial. *Lancet.* 2007;370:230-239.
11. Knauf WU, Lissichkov T, Aldaoud A, et al. Phase III randomized study of bendamustine compared with chlorambucil in previously untreated patients with chronic lymphocytic leukemia. *J Clin Oncol.* 2009;27:4378-4384.
12. Hallek M, Fischer K, Fingerle-Rowson G, et al. Addition of rituximab to fludarabine and cyclophosphamide in patients with chronic lymphocytic leukaemia: a randomised, open-label, phase 3 trial. *Lancet.* 2010;376:1164-1174.
13. Hillmen P, Skotnicki AB, Robak T, et al. Alemtuzumab compared with chlorambucil as first-line therapy for chronic lymphocytic leukemia. *J Clin Oncol.* 2007;25:5616-5623.

SUGGESTED READINGS

Bixby D, Talpaz M. Seeking the causes and solutions to imatinib-resistance in chronic myeloid leukemia. *Leukemia.* 2011;25:7-22. Review.
Cramer P, Hallek M. Prognostic factors in chronic lymphocytic leukemia—what do we need to know? *Natl Rev Clin Oncol.* 2011;8:38-47. Review.
Hallek M. Therapy of chronic lymphocytic leukaemia. *Best Pract Res Clin Haematol.* 2010;23:85-96. *Review including fludarabine, bendamustine, alemtuzumab, and rituximab.*
Keating GM. Rituximab: a review of its use in chronic lymphocytic leukaemia, low-grade or follicular lymphoma and diffuse large B-cell lymphoma. *Drugs.* 2010;70:1445-1476. Review.
Okimoto RA, Van Etten RA. Navigating the road toward optimal initial therapy for chronic myeloid leukemia. *Curr Opin Hematol.* 2011;18:89-97. *Review including imatinib, nilotinib, and dasatinib.*

191

NON-HODGKIN'S LYMPHOMAS

PHILIP J. BIERMAN AND JAMES O. ARMITAGE

DEFINITION

Lymphomas are solid tumors of the immune system. Rapidly increasing knowledge of the biology of the immune system has led to a corresponding increase in the understanding of these malignancies. In addition to better systems of classification and clinical evaluation, this new knowledge has led to the development of new therapies. Beneficial treatment is available for essentially every patient with non-Hodgkin's lymphoma, and many patients can be cured.

EPIDEMIOLOGY

In the United States, about 66,000 new cases of non-Hodgkin's lymphoma are diagnosed annually, and about 20,000 people are estimated to die each year of this disease. Non-Hodgkin's lymphomas account for about 4% of new cancers in the United States and result in about 4% of cancer deaths. The U.S. lifetime risk of developing non-Hodgkin's lymphoma is 2.18% (1 in 46) for men and 1.80% (1 in 56) for women. In 2002 the U.S. age-adjusted incidence rate for non-Hodgkin's lymphoma was about 23.2 per 100,000 for men and 16.3 per 100,000 for women. The incidence rate increases dramatically with age and is higher in whites than in other ethnic groups.

Geographic differences in the incidence of non-Hodgkin's lymphomas vary as much as five-fold. The highest rates are seen in the United States, Europe, and Australia, whereas lower rates are seen in Asia. Even more striking are geographic differences in the incidence of certain types of non-Hodgkin's lymphoma, such as Burkitt's lymphoma, follicular lymphoma, extranodal natural killer (NK)/T-cell nasal lymphoma, and adult T-cell leukemia/lymphoma (see later).

Between 1950 and the early 1990s, the incidence rate for non-Hodgkin's lymphomas in the United States increased by about 3 to 4% yearly, but it has declined slightly since the mid-1990s. Increases have occurred among both men and women in all parts of the world. This increase in incidence is partially related to the aging population (Fig. 191-1) and to the acquired immunodeficiency syndrome (AIDS) epidemic (Chapter 400); occupational and environmental exposures (e.g., farm chemicals) may also explain some of the increase. Finally, some of the increase may be explained by improvements in the ability of pathologists to diagnose lymphoma and by improvements in imaging techniques.

PATHOBIOLOGY

For most cases of non-Hodgkin's lymphoma, the cause is unknown, although genetic, environmental, and infectious agents have been implicated (Table 191-1).

Genetic Factors

Familial clusters have been described, and there is a slightly higher risk of non-Hodgkin's lymphoma among siblings and first-degree relatives of patients with lymphoma or other hematologic malignancies. Tumor necrosis factor (308G→A), interleukin (IL)-10 (3575 T→A), and other polymorphisms are associated with the development of diffuse large B-cell lymphoma.

Immune System Abnormalities

Several inherited disorders increase the risk of developing non-Hodgkin's lymphoma as much as 250-fold (see Table 191-1). In some of these conditions, the lymphoma may be related to Epstein-Barr virus (EBV; Chapter 385). For example, patients with X-linked lymphoproliferative disorder have mutations in the *SH2D1A* gene, which encodes proteins that regulate the host immune response against EBV-infected cells; they may develop fatal infectious mononucleosis or non-Hodgkin's lymphoma after primary

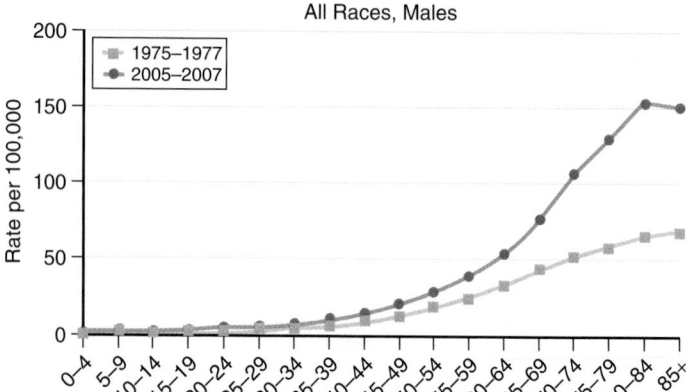

Non-Hodgkin's Lymphoma SEER Incidence by Age
1975-1977 vs. 2005-2007
All Races, Males

FIGURE 191-1. Non-Hodgkin's lymphoma incidence by age in men, 1975-1977 versus 2005-2007. (From the Surveillance, Epidemiology, and End Results [SEER] Program of the National Cancer Institute, http://seer.cancer.gov/csr/1975_2007/.)

exposure to EBV. Acquired immunodeficiency states are also associated with an increased risk of non-Hodgkin's lymphoma. For example, post-transplantation lymphoproliferative disorders occur in as many as 20% of solid organ transplant recipients, related to the proliferation of B lymphocytes that have been transformed during immunosuppressive therapy. The risk of non-Hodgkin's lymphoma is also increased more than 100-fold in patients infected with human immunodeficiency virus (HIV); almost all central nervous system (CNS) lymphomas and approximately 50% of other lymphomas in patients with AIDS are related to EBV. Some studies have shown a two-fold increase in the incidence of non-Hodgkin's lymphomas among patients with rheumatoid arthritis (Chapter 272), and the risk of marginal zone lymphomas is increased approximately 30- to 40-fold in patients with Sjögren's syndrome (Chapter 276). Increases in the incidence of thyroid lymphoma are seen in patients with Hashimoto's thyroiditis (Chapter 233). Enteropathy-type T-cell lymphomas are associated with celiac disease (Chapter 142).

Infectious Agents

EBV is associated with the majority of post-transplantation lymphoproliferative disorders and many AIDS-associated lymphomas. This viral genome is detectable in more than 95% of cases of endemic Burkitt's lymphoma and in approximately 40% of cases of sporadic Burkitt's lymphoma and AIDS-associated lymphomas.

The human T-lymphotropic virus type 1 (HTLV-1; Chapter 386) is detectable in virtually all cases of adult T-cell leukemia/lymphoma. The risk of lymphoma is approximately 3% in patients infected with HTLV-1; in endemic areas, up to 50% of all non-Hodgkin's lymphomas may be related to HTLV-1. Reports of an association between simian virus 40 and non-Hodgkin's lymphoma have not been supported by further research.

Human herpesvirus 8 (HHV-8, Kaposi's sarcoma–associated herpesvirus; Chapter 400), which is associated with expansion of the B-cell population, is also associated with primary effusion lymphoma (see later) in immunocompromised patients and with multicentric Castleman's disease. Patients with primary effusion lymphoma are often coinfected with EBV.

Epidemiologic evidence has linked hepatitis C virus (Chapter 151) to lymphoplasmacytic lymphoma and splenic marginal zone lymphoma. Chronic antigenic stimulation from this virus may lead to the emergence of malignant B-cell clones.

Helicobacter pylori is associated with gastric lymphoma (Chapter 198) of extranodal marginal zone/mucosa-associated lymphoid tissue (MALT). Colonized patients develop gastritis from chronic antigenic stimulation mediated by T cells, which respond to *H. pylori*–specific antigens; malignant B-cell clones emerge. *Borrelia burgdorferi* (Chapter 329) has been associated with marginal zone B-cell lymphoma of the skin. Evidence also links *Chlamydia psittaci* (Chapter 326) with ocular adnexal lymphomas and *Campylobacter jejuni* with immunoproliferative small intestinal disease (Chapter 311).

Environmental and Occupational Exposure

Agricultural chemicals have been associated with an increased risk of developing non-Hodgkin's lymphomas, and the strongest associations involve phenoxy herbicides such as 2,4-dichlorophenoxyacetic acid (2,4-D), which was also a component of Agent Orange (Chapter 18). An increased risk has also been associated with ionizing radiation (Chapter 19), organic solvents, hair dyes, and nitrates in drinking water, although contradictory results have been reported. Some studies have also linked non-Hodgkin's lymphomas to high-fat diets and ultraviolet radiation (Chapter 183). The risk of non-Hodgkin's lymphomas is increased approximately 20-fold after treatment for Hodgkin's disease (Chapter 192). Heavy smokers (Chapter 31) have an increased risk of developing follicular lymphoma.

Pathology

Non-Hodgkin's lymphomas are derived from cells of the immune system at varying stages of differentiation. In some cases, the cell of origin is directly linked to the morphology, immunophenotype, and clinical behavior of the lymphoma (Fig. 191-2 and Table 191-2).

TABLE 191-1	FACTORS ASSOCIATED WITH THE DEVELOPMENT OF NON-HODGKIN'S LYMPHOMA

Inherited immune disorders
   Severe combined immunodeficiency disease
   Common variable immunodeficiency disease
   Wiskott-Aldrich syndrome
   Ataxia-telangiectasia
   X-linked lymphoproliferative disorder
Acquired immune disorders
   Solid organ transplantation
   Acquired immunodeficiency syndrome (AIDS)
   Methotrexate therapy for autoimmune disorders
   Rheumatoid arthritis and systemic lupus erythematosus
   Sjögren's syndrome
   Hashimoto's thyroiditis
Infectious agents
   Epstein-Barr virus
   Human T- lymphotropic virus type 1
   Human herpesvirus 8
   Hepatitis C virus
   Helicobacter pylori
   Borrelia burgdorferi
   Chlamydia psittaci
   Campylobacter jejuni
Occupational and environmental exposure
   Herbicides
   Organic solvents
   Hair dyes
   Ultraviolet light
   Diet
   Smoking

TABLE 191-2	TYPICAL IMMUNOPHENOTYPES OF COMMON NON-HODGKIN'S LYMPHOMAS

LYMPHOMA	CD20	CD3	CD10	CD5	CD23	OTHER
Small lymphocytic	+	−	−	+	+	
Lymphoplasmacytic	+	−	−	−	−	Cytoplasmic Ig+
Extranodal marginal zone MALT	+	−	−	−	−	
Nodal marginal zone	+	−	−	−	−	
Follicular	+	−	+			
Mantle cell	+	−	−	+	−	Cyclin D1+
Diffuse large B cell	+	−				
Mediastinal large B cell	+	−				
Burkitt's	+	−	+			TdT−
Precursor T lymphoblastic	−	+/−				TdT+, CD1a +/−, CD7+
Anaplastic large T cell	−	+/−				CD30+, CD15−, EMA+, ALK+
Peripheral T cell	−	+/−				Other pan-T variable

ALK = anaplastic lymphoma kinase; EMA = epithelial membrane antigen; MALT = mucosa-associated lymphoid tissue; TdT = terminal deoxynucleotidyl transferase.

A

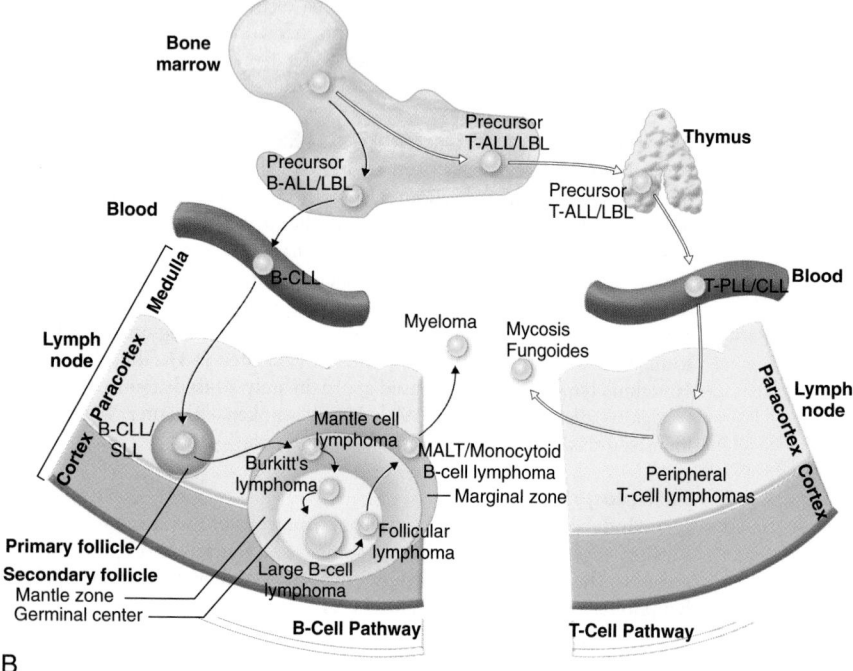

B

FIGURE 191-2. Postulated normal counterparts of currently recognized B- and T-cell malignancies. **A,** Schema of normal B- and T-cell differentiation. Bone marrow–derived lymphoid stem cells differentiate into committed B-cell precursors or into T-cell precursors that undergo further maturation in the thymus. These B- and T-cell precursors mature into naïve B or T cells that circulate to lymph nodes. After antigen exposure, normal B blasts proliferate and undergo further differentiation in the germinal center of the secondary follicle. The germinal center is surrounded by a mantle zone and a marginal zone. Antigen-specific B cells generated in the germinal center leave the follicle and reappear in the marginal zone. Thereafter, immunoglobulin-producing plasma cells accumulate in the lymph node medulla and subsequently exit to the periphery. Antigen-dependent T-cell proliferation occurs in the lymph node paracortex. After antigen exposure, mature T cells become immunoblasts and, subsequently, antigen-specific effector T cells that exit to the periphery. The postulated normal counterparts of many currently recognized T- and B-cell neoplasms are shown. **B,** T- and B-cell malignancies derived from the postulated normal counterparts shown in **A.** ALL = acute lymphoblastic leukemia; CLL = chronic lymphocytic leukemia; LBL = lymphoblastic lymphoma; MALT = mucosa-associated lymphoid tissue; SLL = small lymphocytic lymphoma.

The transformation of cells from the normal immune system into malignant lymphoma reflects the acquisition of specific genetic abnormalities. In many cases, cytogenetic studies can identify chromosomal translocations that underlie the development or progression of the lymphoma. In most cases of non-Hodgkin's lymphoma, the activation of proto-oncogenes is the major abnormality, but occasionally chromosomal translocations can lead to fusion genes that code for chimeric proteins. In addition, some cases are associated with deletion of tumor suppressor genes. Specific genetic abnormalities are associated with some specific subtypes of non-Hodgkin's lymphoma (Table 191-3). It is becoming clear that the tumor microenvironment (i.e., stromal cells associated with the lymphoma cells) is important in tumor cell survival and response to therapy.

Classification

Recognition of the Reed-Sternberg cell approximately 100 years ago made it possible to define Hodgkin's disease (Chapter 192) as a distinct entity, whereas other lymphomas were included under the heading "non-Hodgkin's

lymphomas." In the 1990s a classification system incorporating morphologic, immunologic, genetic, and clinical information (the Revised European-American Lymphoma classification, or REAL) was developed to identify distinct clinicopathologic subgroups representing diseases that can be recognized by clinicians. This system was subsequently adopted as the World Health Organization (WHO) classification of lymphomas in 2008 (Table 191-4).

The WHO classification divides lymphomas on the basis of B-cell or T/NK-cell origin and whether they are derived from primitive precursor cells or from more mature "peripheral" cells. Specific clinical and pathologic entities are recognized within each of these groupings. In the United States and Europe, 85 to 90% of non-Hodgkin's lymphomas are B cell in origin.

The most frequent type is diffuse large B-cell lymphoma, which represents 31% of all non-Hodgkin's lymphomas worldwide. The next most frequent type is follicular lymphoma, which represents 22% of cases; follicular lymphoma is relatively more frequent in North America and western Europe and less frequent in Asia. Less common types, each representing between 5 and

TABLE 191-3 CHROMOSOMAL TRANSLOCATIONS CHARACTERISTIC OF NON-HODGKIN'S LYMPHOMA

LYMPHOMA SUBTYPE	TRANSLOCATION	GENES INVOLVED	FREQUENCY (%)
Diffuse large B cell	t(3q27)	BCL6	35
	t(14;18)(q32;q21)	IgH, BCL2	15-20
	t(18;14)(q24;q32)	MYC (c-Myc), IgH	<5
Burkitt's	t(8;14)(q24;q32)	MYC, IgH	100% have one of these, most commonly t(8;14)
	t(8;22)(q24;q11)	MYC, IgL	
	t(2;8)(p12;q24)	IgK, MYC	
Follicular	t(14;18)(q32;q21)	IgH, BCL2	~90
Mantle cell	t(11;14)(q13;q32)	BCL1, IgH	>90
ALCL	t(2;5)(p23;q35)	ALK, NPM	>80 of ALK+ ALCLs
MALT	t(11;18)(q21;q21)	API2, MALT1	35
	t(14;18)(q21;q32)	IgH, MALT1	20
	t(1;14)(p22;q32)	BCL10, IgH	10

ALCL = anaplastic large cell lymphoma; ALK = anaplastic lymphoma kinase; MALT = mucosa-associated lymphoid tissue.

TABLE 191-4 WORLD HEALTH ORGANIZATION CLASSIFICATION OF NON-HODGKIN'S LYMPHOMA (2008)

PRECURSOR LYMPHOID NEOPLASMS

B-lymphoblastic leukemia/lymphoma
T-lymphoblastic leukemia/lymphoma

MATURE B-CELL NEOPLASMS

Chronic lymphocytic leukemia/small lymphocytic lymphoma
Splenic marginal zone lymphoma
Lymphoplasmacytic lymphoma
Extranodal marginal zone lymphoma of MALT (MALT lymphoma)
Nodal marginal zone lymphoma
Follicular lymphoma
Primary cutaneous follicle center lymphoma
Mantle cell lymphoma
Diffuse large B-cell lymphoma, NOS
Burkitt's lymphoma

MATURE T-CELL NEOPLASMS

Adult T-cell leukemia/lymphoma
Extranodal NK/T-cell lymphoma, nasal type
Enteropathy-associated T-cell lymphoma
Hepatosplenic T-cell lymphoma
Subcutaneous panniculitis-like T-cell lymphoma
Mycosis fungoides
Sézary's syndrome
Primary cutaneous CD30+ T-cell lymphoproliferative disorders
Peripheral T-cell lymphoma, NOS
Angioimmunoblastic T-cell lymphoma
Anaplastic large cell lymphoma, ALK positive
Anaplastic large cell lymphoma, ALK negative

ALK = anaplastic lymphoma kinase; MALT = mucosa-associated lymphoid tissue; NK = natural killer; NOS = not otherwise specified.

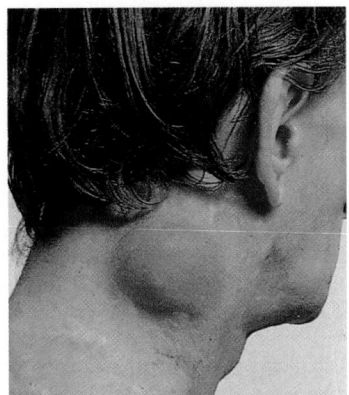

FIGURE 191-3. Non-Hodgkin's lymphoma. Despite the redness of the skin over the enlarged lymph node in this patient, the lesion was completely painless. (From Forbes CD, Jackson WF. *Color Atlas and Text of Clinical Medicine,* 3rd ed. London: Mosby; 2003.)

The use of complementary DNA microarrays has allowed the identification of distinct subsets of patients with diffuse large B-cell lymphoma. Patients with histologically identical lymphomas can be divided into those with tumor gene expression patterns resembling normal germinal center B cells, those whose tumors resemble activated post–germinal center B cells, or those with patterns resembling that seen in Hodgkin's lymphoma; the last pattern is most frequently found in young women who present with large mediastinal masses.

CLINICAL MANIFESTATIONS

The most common presentation of non-Hodgkin's lymphoma is lymphadenopathy (Fig. 191-3; Chapter 171). In many cases, patients notice cervical, axillary, or inguinal adenopathy and seek a physician's advice. In general, lymph nodes containing lymphoma are firm, nontender, and not associated with a regional infection. However, patients are frequently treated with a course of antibiotics before a biopsy is performed to confirm the diagnosis of lymphoma. In other patients, lymphadenopathy occurring in sites such as the mediastinum or retroperitoneum causes symptoms that bring the patient to the physician. Chest pain, cough, superior vena cava syndrome, abdominal pain, back pain, spinal cord compression, and symptoms of renal insufficiency associated with ureteral compression are characteristic.

Non-Hodgkin's lymphomas are often associated with systemic symptoms that may lead to the diagnosis. The most obvious symptoms are fevers, night sweats, and unexplained weight loss. Any of these symptoms without an obvious cause should lead a physician to consider the diagnosis of lymphoma. Other, less characteristic symptoms include fatigue, which is frequently present at the time of diagnosis if the patient is questioned carefully, and pruritus.

Non-Hodgkin's lymphomas can involve essentially any organ in the body, and malfunction of that organ can cause symptoms that lead to the diagnosis.

10% of all non-Hodgkin's lymphomas, are extranodal marginal zone/MALT lymphomas, peripheral T-cell lymphomas, small lymphocytic lymphoma, and mantle cell lymphoma. Other types each represent less than 2% of non-Hodgkin's lymphomas seen in the United States.

The non-Hodgkin's lymphomas recognized in the WHO classification have clinically distinctive characteristics (Table 191-5), such that an experienced hematopathologist can accurately classify 85% or more of patients by WHO criteria when adequate material is available. Some diagnoses, such as follicular lymphoma, can be made with a high degree of accuracy without immunologic or genetic studies. The diagnosis of T-cell lymphomas cannot be made accurately without immunophenotyping. Cytogenetic studies and molecular genetic studies can help resolve difficult differential diagnoses. For example, the presence of a t(8;14) translocation supports the diagnosis of Burkitt's lymphoma, whereas a t(11;14) with cyclin D1 overexpression can confirm the diagnosis of mantle cell lymphoma (see Tables 191-2 and 191-3).

TABLE 191-5 PRESENTING CLINICAL CHARACTERISTICS OF COMMON NON-HODGKIN'S LYMPHOMA SUBTYPES

TYPE OF LYMPHOMA	MEDIAN AGE (YR)	% MALE	Stage (%) I	Stage (%) IV	B SYMPTOMS (%)	BONE MARROW INVOLVED (%)	5-YR SURVIVAL (%)
B-CELL LYMPHOMAS							
Small lymphocytic	65	53	4	83	33	72	51
Lymphoplasmacytic	63	53	7	73	13	73	59
Extranodal marginal zone MALT	60	48	39	31	19	14	74
Nodal marginal zone	58	42	13	40	37	32	57
Follicular	59	42	18	51	28	42	72
Mantle cell	63	74	13	71	28	64	27
Diffuse large B cell	64	55	25	33	33	16	46
Mediastinal large B cell	37	34	10	31	38	3	50
Burkitt's	31	89	37	38	22	33	44
PRECURSOR B/T-CELL LYMPHOMAS							
Precursor T-lymphoblastic	28	64	0	75	21	50	26
T-CELL LYMPHOMAS							
Anaplastic large T cell	34	69	19	39	53	13	77
Peripheral T cell	61	55	8	65	50	36	25

B symptoms = fevers, night sweats, and weight loss; MALT = mucosa-associated lymphoid tissue.
Adapted from Armitage JO, Weisenburger DD, for the Non-Hodgkin's Lymphoma Classification Project. New approach to classifying non-Hodgkin's lymphomas: clinical features of the major histologic subtypes. *J Clin Oncol.* 1998;16:2780-2795.

Examples include neurologic symptoms with primary brain lymphoma (Chapter 195), shortness of breath with MALT lymphomas in the lung, epigastric pain and vomiting with gastric MALT lymphomas or diffuse large B-cell lymphomas (Chapter 198), bowel obstruction with small bowel lymphomas (Chapter 199), testicular masses with diffuse large B-cell lymphoma (Chapter 206), and skin lesions with cutaneous lymphomas (Chapter 448). Many lymphomas involve the bone marrow and occasionally cause extensive myelophthisis (Chapter 168) and bone marrow failure; these patients may present with infections, bleeding, and anemia.

Non-Hodgkin's lymphomas can also manifest with a variety of immunologic abnormalities. For example, autoimmune hemolytic anemia (Chapter 163) and immune thrombocytopenia (Chapter 175) can be the presenting manifestations of non-Hodgkin's lymphoma, especially small lymphocytic lymphoma/chronic lymphocytic leukemia as well as other subtypes, including diffuse large B-cell lymphoma. Peripheral neuropathies (Chapter 428), often associated with overproduction of a monoclonal protein, can be seen in a variety of subtypes but are most characteristic of lymphoplasmacytic lymphoma; sometimes they are also seen with POEMS syndrome (polyneuropathy, organomegaly, endocrinopathy, M protein, skin changes; Chapter 193). Paraneoplastic neurologic complications of non-Hodgkin's lymphoma include demyelinating polyneuropathy, Guillain-Barré syndrome, autonomic dysfunction, and peripheral neuropathy. Paraneoplastic syndromes (Chapter 187) associated with non-Hodgkin's lymphoma can affect the skin (e.g., pemphigus), kidney (e.g., glomerulonephritis), and miscellaneous organ systems (e.g., vasculitis, dermatomyositis, cholestatic jaundice).

The differential diagnosis in patients with non-Hodgkin's lymphoma is broad. Any cause of lymphadenopathy or splenomegaly can potentially be confused with non-Hodgkin's lymphoma (Chapter 171). However, this confusion is resolved by an appropriate biopsy. It is extremely important to recognize that the diagnosis of non-Hodgkin's lymphoma must be considered in patients with compatible clinical presentations and then confirmed by an adequate biopsy read by an experienced hematopathologist. The diagnosis should never be inferred, and patients should not be treated until the diagnosis is confirmed by biopsy. This is also true for patients who achieve a complete remission with initial therapy; they should not be treated for presumed relapse on the basis of symptoms or abnormal images without a biopsy.

DIAGNOSIS

Each new patient with a non-Hodgkin's lymphoma should be thoroughly evaluated in a systematic manner (Table 191-6). Because subtle pathologic distinctions may alter therapy, the most important issue in managing non-Hodgkin's lymphoma is to establish an accurate diagnosis. Core needle

TABLE 191-6 TYPICAL EVALUATION OF A PATIENT NEWLY DIAGNOSED WITH NON-HODGKIN'S LYMPHOMA

1. Biopsy to establish diagnosis
2. Careful history and physical examination
3. Laboratory evaluation
   A. Complete blood count
   B. Chemistry screen, including lactate dehydrogenase
4. Imaging studies
   A. Computed tomography of chest, abdomen, and pelvis
   B. Positron emission tomography
5. Additional biopsies
   A. Bone marrow
   B. Any other suspicious site if results would change therapy

biopsies can occasionally be used for a primary diagnosis if the specimen is handled properly. Fine-needle aspirates should not be used to diagnose lymphoma, and they preclude an accurate diagnosis of the specific subtype of non-Hodgkin's lymphoma. In most cases, an excisional biopsy is necessary (and is always preferred) for the initial diagnosis; another biopsy should be performed if sufficient material is not obtained. Review by an experienced hematopathologist is essential.

Staging and Prognostic Systems

After diagnosis, a meticulous staging evaluation is necessary to estimate prognosis and determine therapy. Staging requires a careful history and physical examination; complete blood count; renal and hepatic function tests; serum lactate dehydrogenase (LDH) level; computed tomography (CT) of the chest, abdomen, and pelvis; and bone marrow biopsy. Positron emission tomography (PET) can be helpful to identify initial sites of involvement and, after treatment, to distinguish persisting lymphoma from residual fibrosis in masses seen on CT. The most common staging system is the Ann Arbor classification, which separates patients into four stages based on anatomic sites of disease (Table 191-7). In addition, each stage is subdivided into A (no defined general symptoms) and B (unexplained weight loss >10% of body weight in the previous 6 months, unexplained temperature >38° C, or night sweats) categories. Known sites of disease can be reexamined later to evaluate the response to therapy.

Although a wide variety of patient factors (e.g., age, symptoms, LDH level) and tumor factors (e.g., bulk, gene expression pattern, proliferation rate) can affect treatment outcomes, two prognostic systems can help in choosing

TABLE 191-7 STAGING OF NON-HODGKIN'S LYMPHOMA

STAGE	DESCRIPTION
I	Involvement of a single lymph node region (I) or a single extralymphatic organ or site (I$_E$)
II	Involvement of ≥2 lymph node regions on the same side of the diaphragm (II) or localized involvement of an extralymphatic organ or site and ≥1 lymph node regions on the same side of the diaphragm (II$_E$)
III	Involvement of lymph node regions on both sides of the diaphragm (III), which may also be accompanied by localized involvement of an extralymphatic organ or site (III$_E$) or by involvement of the spleen (III$_S$) or both (III$_{SE}$)
IV	Diffuse or disseminated involvement of ≥1 extralymphatic organ or tissues with or without associated lymph node enlargement
Subtypes	
A	No B symptoms
B	B symptoms: unexplained weight loss ≥10% of body weight in prior 6 months, unexplained fever >38° C, or night sweats

Adapted from Carbone PP, Kaplan HS, Musshoff K, et al. Report of the Committee on Hodgkin's Disease Staging Classification. *Cancer Res.* 1971;31:1860-1861.

TABLE 191-8 INTERNATIONAL PROGNOSTIC INDEX

CATEGORY	SCORE (NO. OF RISK FACTORS)
ALL PATIENTS*	
Low	0 or 1
Low intermediate	2
High intermediate	3
High	4 or 5
AGE-ADJUSTED INDEX, PATIENTS ≤60 YR†	
Low	0
Low intermediate	1
High intermediate	2
High	3

*Adverse factors for all patients: age >60 yr, ↑LDH, performance status 2–4, >1 extranodal site, Ann Arbor stage III or IV.
†Adverse factors for patients ≤60 yr: ↑LDH, performance status 2–4, Ann Arbor stage III or IV.
LDH = lactate dehydrogenase.
Adapted from Shipp M, Harrington D, Anderson J, et al. A predictive model for aggressive non-Hodgkin's lymphoma. *N Engl J Med.* 1993;329:987-994.

therapy and determining an accurate prognosis. The International Prognostic Index (IPI; Table 191-8) is the most widely used method to predict treatment outcome and survival. The IPI is based on five adverse factors (age older than 60 years, performance status ≤2, elevated serum LDH level, two or more extranodal sites of disease, Ann Arbor stage III or IV), which are summed to give the score. This index was developed for patients with diffuse aggressive lymphoma (predominantly diffuse large B-cell lymphoma), but it can be used to predict treatment outcome with any subtype. For young patients, an abbreviated index that uses only reduced performance status, elevated serum LDH level, and high stage can be applied. Because patients with follicular lymphoma rarely have a reduced performance status or a large number of extranodal sites, an alternative index termed the *Follicular Lymphoma International Prognostic Index* (FLIPI) was developed; it substitutes more than four nodal areas of involvement and a hemoglobin less than 12 g as staging criteria and does a somewhat better job of predicting treatment outcome in follicular lymphoma.

TREATMENT

Lymphomas may behave in an indolent or an aggressive manner. The behavior of many of these neoplasms is distinctive, but within each category, behavior is frequently influenced by disease site, tumor bulk, and performance status of the patient. Some lymphomas can be managed, at least initially, with observation, whereas other situations are medical emergencies, such as spinal cord compression (Chapter 195). It is important to consider three questions before starting therapy: (1) Does treatment have curative potential? (2) Can treatment prolong survival? (3) Will treatment alleviate symptoms?

● SPECIFIC TYPES OF NON-HODGKIN'S LYMPHOMAS
Precursor T-Cell and B-Cell Lymphomas

These tumors are nodal or other solid tissue infiltrates of cells that are morphologically and immunophenotypically identical to the immature cells seen in B-cell or T-cell acute lymphoblastic leukemia (Chapter 189). Patients who have predominantly nodal disease with minimal or no involvement of the bone marrow are frequently classified as having *lymphoblastic lymphoma,* whereas those with more than 25% neoplastic cells in the marrow are classified as having *lymphoblastic leukemia.* These distinctions are arbitrary and reflect the stage of disease rather than different diagnoses. These neoplasms are more common in children than in adults.

B-cell precursor lymphomas frequently manifest as solid tumors with involvement of the skin and bones, whereas T-cell neoplasms typically manifest as a mediastinal mass in a young male. Involvement of the CNS is common. Approximately 90% of patients who present with lymphoblastic

lymphoma have a T-cell phenotype, whereas about 85% of patients who present with acute lymphoblastic leukemia have a B-cell phenotype. Adverse prognostic characteristics include CNS involvement, stage IV disease, and an elevated LDH level.

TREATMENT

Patients with either T-cell lymphoblastic lymphoma or precursor B-cell lymphoblastic lymphoma are typically treated with regimens modeled after those used for acute lymphoblastic leukemia (Chapter 189). These regimens frequently contain cytarabine and high-dose methotrexate, and they often include maintenance therapy. CNS prophylaxis with intrathecal chemotherapy, high-dose methotrexate, or cranial irradiation is also a component of these regimens.

Mature B-Cell Lymphomas
SMALL LYMPHOCYTIC LYMPHOMA/CHRONIC LYMPHOCYTIC LEUKEMIA

Small lymphocytic lymphoma is defined as a lymph node or other tissue infiltrate that is morphologically and immunophenotypically identical to chronic lymphocytic leukemia (Chapter 190). Patients are frequently asymptomatic, and the diagnosis is often made when blood counts are performed for other reasons. Patients frequently have lymphadenopathy or splenomegaly. Fatigue is common. Hypogammaglobulinemia can occur and may lead to an increased susceptibility to infection.

A poor prognosis is associated with advanced stage and systemic symptoms, expression of high levels of CD38 and ZAP-70 on tumor cells, lack of rearranged immunoglobulin heavy chain genes, and genetic abnormalities such as del(17p) and del(11q). Approximately 10% of patients exhibit transformation to diffuse large B-cell lymphoma (Richter's syndrome), which is associated with a poor prognosis.

The median survival time is more than 10 years for patients without adverse characteristics, and these patients can often be managed with observation. Therapy is necessary for patients who have rapidly progressive or symptomatic lymphadenopathy and for those who develop cytopenias.

TREATMENT

Management must be individualized because therapy is not curative, and patients are often elderly. A regimen consisting of fludarabine in combination with cyclophosphamide and rituximab (Table 191-9) is frequently used in the United States for relatively young, fit patients. Single-agent fludarabine plus rituximab is more commonly used in elderly patients. Fludarabine is more effective than chlorambucil, but because chlorambucil is administered orally

TABLE 191-9 COMBINATION CHEMOTHERAPY REGIMENS FOR NON-HODGKIN'S LYMPHOMA

REGIMEN	DOSE	DAYS OF ADMINISTRATION	FREQUENCY
CHOP-R			Every 21 days
Cyclophosphamide	750 mg/m² IV	1	
Doxorubicin	50 mg/m² IV	1	
Vincristine	1.4 mg/m² IV*	1	
Prednisone, fixed dose	100 PO	1-5	
Rituximab	375 mg/m² IV	1	
CVP-R			Every 21 days
Cyclophosphamide	1000 mg/m² IV	1	
Vincristine	1.4 mg/m² IV*	1	
Prednisone, fixed dose	100 mg PO	1-5	
Rituximab	375 mg/m² IV	1	
FCR			Every 28 days
Fludarabine	25 mg/m² IV	1-3	
Cyclophosphamide	250 mg/m² IV	1-3	
Rituximab	375 mg/m²	1	

*Vincristine dose often capped at 2 mg total.

and has few side effects, it is sometimes used in older patients. Bendamustine is an active, newly available drug. Alemtuzumab, a monoclonal antibody directed against the CD52 antigen, is sometimes effective after other treatments have failed. Allogeneic hematopoietic stem cell transplantation may be curative, but few patients are candidates for this approach.

Patients may develop autoimmune thrombocytopenia (Chapter 175), autoimmune neutropenia (Chapter 170), and red blood cell aplasia (Chapter 168). These autoimmune disorders may respond to treatment with corticosteroids, intravenous immune globulin, or splenectomy, as used in patients without underlying lymphoma.

EXTRANODAL MARGINAL ZONE LYMPHOMA OF MUCOSA-ASSOCIATED LYMPHOID TISSUE (MALT LYMPHOMA)

MALT lymphomas are indolent tumors that originate in association with epithelial cells and are seen most commonly in the gastrointestinal tract, salivary glands, breast, thyroid, orbit, conjunctiva, skin, and lung. The majority of cases are stage I or II at diagnosis, although in some series as many as 30% disseminate to bone marrow or other sites. These lymphomas tend to remain localized for extended periods. Local treatment with surgery or radiation therapy cures a high proportion of localized neoplasms. Disseminated disease is treated similarly to follicular lymphoma (see later).

Gastric MALT lymphomas are usually associated with infection by *H. pylori*. Eradication of *H. pylori* with antibiotics leads to complete regression in more than 50% of gastric MALT lymphomas, although polymerase chain reaction analysis demonstrates minimal residual disease in many patients, and the long-term outcome of this approach is unknown. Response to antibiotic therapy is less likely if invasion is deeper, lymph node metastases are found, or the t(11;18) chromosomal translocation is present.

TREATMENT Rx

Patients may have tumors in more than one extranodal site, and these locations can sometimes be successfully treated with local therapy. Asymptomatic patients can be monitored closely without antilymphoma therapy until symptoms progress. Gastric MALT lymphoma that does not respond to antibiotics can be treated with radiation, rituximab as a single agent (similar to its use in follicular lymphoma), or several traditional combination chemotherapy regimens (see Table 191-9).

FOLLICULAR LYMPHOMA

Follicular lymphoma accounts for the majority of indolent or "low-grade" lymphomas in the United States. Follicular lymphoma is divided into three grades based on the proportion of large, transformed cells (centroblasts).

Patients with follicular lymphoma are frequently asymptomatic. The most common presenting complaint is painless lymphadenopathy. Some patients have cough or dyspnea related to pulmonary or mediastinal involvement or pleural effusions. Other patients have symptoms of abdominal pain or fullness related to subdiaphragmatic or splenic disease. A minority of patients have systemic symptoms of fevers, night sweats, or weight loss.

The clinical behavior and treatment of follicular lymphoma grades 1 and 2 are the same and are discussed in this section. Grade 3 follicular lymphoma may have a more aggressive clinical course and is frequently treated similarly to diffuse large B-cell lymphoma (see later).

TREATMENT Rx

Localized Disease

Approximately 5 to 15% of patients have localized disease (stage I or minimal stage II disease) at diagnosis. These lymphomas are usually treated with involved-field radiation, and most series report 10-year disease-free survival rates of approximately 50% and overall survival rates of 60 to 70%. Some retrospective series have reported improved outcomes when chemotherapy is combined with radiation.

Advanced Disease

Most patients with follicular lymphoma have extensive disease at diagnosis. The median survival time of these patients is more than 10 years. Although spontaneous regression has been described, 30 to 50% of patients experience transformation to a more aggressive histology—usually diffuse large B-cell lymphoma. Transformation is frequently associated with new systemic symptoms and rapidly progressive lymphadenopathy, an aggressive clinical course, and a poor prognosis.

Asymptomatic patients, especially elderly patients and those with other medical illnesses, are frequently managed with a "watch and wait" approach. Prospective trials have demonstrated that this approach does not influence overall survival, and patients can sometimes be observed for long periods before treatment is required.

Most patients with follicular lymphoma eventually require treatment because of systemic symptoms, symptomatic or progressive lymphadenopathy, splenomegaly, effusions, or cytopenias. In elderly patients, those who are poor candidates for intensive chemotherapy regimens, and those who want to avoid the side effects (e.g., alopecia) of chemotherapy, single-agent rituximab (375 mg/m² intravenously, given weekly for 4 consecutive weeks) yields an objective response rate of well over 50%. The median duration of response is approximately 1 to 2 years for patients who receive no additional therapy, but the response can be extended with ongoing administration of rituximab once every 2 or 3 months or by repeating the initial four doses every 6 months. When rituximab is combined with standard chemotherapy regimens such as CVP (cyclophosphamide, vincristine, prednisone) or CHOP (cyclophosphamide, doxorubicin, vincristine, prednisone) (see Table 191-9), the response rate, duration of response, and survival are increased compared with the chemotherapy regimen alone, and maintenance rituximab further extends the duration of remission.[1] For aggressive lymphomas, high dose intensity doxorubicin can significantly improve survival.[2] Fludarabine, used alone or in combination with mitoxantrone, is also effective. In one study, ¹³¹I-tositumomab radioimmunotherapy appeared to provide a prolonged benefit. Interferon-α may be beneficial in follicular lymphoma when combined with initial chemotherapy,[3] but it is rarely used as primary therapy in the United States because of its side effects. Some studies have shown an improvement in failure-free survival with the use of autologous bone marrow transplantation in patients who achieve an initial remission, but overall survival is not prolonged.

Salvage Therapy

Most patients respond to initial chemotherapy, and initial responses typically persist for 1 to 3 years. However, follicular lymphoma eventually progresses in most patients with advanced-stage disease. Patients who have a relapse usually respond to additional therapy, often with the same agents, although the duration of response becomes progressively shorter with repeated courses of therapy. Approximately 50 to 60% of patients with relapsed follicular lymphoma respond to rituximab, and maintenance therapy prolongs remission in responding patients; however, less than 10% attain a complete response. Some patients who do not respond to rituximab respond to the radiolabeled antibodies tositumomab or ibritumomab. Radiation therapy may also be useful for patients with a localized site of symptomatic disease.

Prolonged remissions have been observed after autologous hematopoietic stem cell transplantation. Allogeneic hematopoietic stem cell transplantation may cure some patients with relapsed follicular lymphoma.

MANTLE CELL LYMPHOMA

Mantle cell lymphoma is a B-cell neoplasm composed of small lymphoid cells that may resemble small lymphocytic lymphoma or follicular lymphoma. It is most common in elderly patients and is usually at an advanced stage at the time of diagnosis. Males are more frequently affected, and extranodal disease, especially involvement of the bone marrow, Waldeyer's ring, and the gastrointestinal tract, is common. Mantle cell lymphoma is the most common cause of multiple lymphomatous polyposis, and the gastrointestinal tract should be evaluated with endoscopy during the initial evaluation.

Some patients present with involvement of the peripheral blood as well as the bone marrow, a clinical picture that resembles chronic lymphocytic leukemia (Chapter 190). The lymphocytes in both disorders are CD5$^+$, but the t(11;14) and overexpression of cyclin D1 seen in mantle cell lymphoma usually allow an accurate diagnosis.

Mantle cell lymphoma usually has a poor prognosis, with a median survival of 3 to 4 years, although occasional patients may have an indolent course. There is some evidence that prognosis may be improved with aggressive chemotherapy, but mantle cell lymphoma is usually not curable with standard chemotherapy regimens. Autologous hematopoietic stem cell transplantation for patients in their first remission may improve survival, but randomized trials have not been performed. Allogeneic transplantation can be curative but is associated with considerable morbidity and mortality.

DIFFUSE LARGE B-CELL LYMPHOMA

These tumors are the most common type of non-Hodgkin's lymphoma, but their morphology and genetic features are heterogeneous. Signs and symptoms are similar to those of other subtypes, although patients are more likely to have B symptoms or symptoms from the local tumor than are patients with follicular lymphoma.

The WHO classification of non-Hodgkin's lymphomas has identified several variants and subtypes of diffuse large B-cell lymphoma (Table 191-10). Many of these are histologic or genetic subtypes or variants for which treatment is the same as the standard approach for diffuse large B-cell lymphoma. Other subtypes present unusual clinical syndromes or specific therapeutic problems.

TABLE 191-10	DIFFUSE LARGE B-CELL LYMPHOMA, VARIANTS AND SUBTYPES

Diffuse large B-cell lymphoma, not otherwise specified (NOS)
    Common morphologic variants
        Centroblastic
        Immunoblastic
        Anaplastic
    Immunohistochemical subgroups
        CD5$^+$ DLBCL
        Germinal center B-cell–like (GCB)
        Non–germinal center B-cell–like (non-GCB)
Diffuse large B-cell lymphoma, subtypes
    T-cell/histiocyte-rich large B-cell lymphoma
    Primary DLBCL of the CNS
    Primary cutaneous DLBCL, leg type
    EBV-positive DLBCL of the elderly
Other large B-cell lymphomas
    Primary mediastinal (thymic) large B-cell lymphoma
    Intravascular large B-cell lymphoma
    DLBCL associated with chronic inflammation
    Lymphomatoid granulomatosis
    ALK-positive large B-cell lymphoma
    Plasmablastic lymphoma
    Large B-cell lymphoma arising in HHV-8-associated multicentric Castleman's disease
    Primary effusion lymphoma

ALK = anaplastic lymphoma kinase; CNS = central nervous system; DLBCL = diffuse large B-cell lymphoma; EBV = Epstein-Barr virus; HHV = human herpesvirus.

TREATMENT   Rx

Localized Disease

As many as 30% of patients with diffuse large B-cell lymphoma have stage I or minimal stage II disease. These patients are occasionally cured with radiation therapy alone, but initial treatment with chemotherapy is more effective. Although one study in France suggested that a very intensive chemotherapy regimen alone might be better than CHOP plus radiation, most patients in the United States receive CHOP plus rituximab (CHOP-R; see Table 191-9), followed by consolidative radiation therapy.**4** Although the necessity of radiation therapy after CHOP-R has not been tested, this combination is still widely used.

Advanced Disease

CHOP-R is generally considered the "gold standard" treatment for adults of all ages with advanced-stage diffuse large B-cell lymphoma. Among patients older than 60 years, 75% achieve a complete response, with a 5-year event-free survival rate of 47% and a 5-year overall survival rate of 58%. In younger patients the outcome is better.**5**

Salvage Therapy

A variety of chemotherapy regimens have been developed for patients who relapse after attaining a remission with initial chemotherapy. These regimens commonly contain agents such as cisplatin, cytarabine, etoposide, carboplatin, and ifosfamide. Response rates exceeding 50% can be observed with these combinations, although no more than 10% of patients achieve long-term disease-free survival. High-dose therapy followed by autologous hematopoietic stem cell transplantation has become accepted therapy for patients with relapsed diffuse large B-cell lymphoma; approximately 20 to 40% of these patients attain long-term disease-free survival with transplantation if they are still responsive to conventional salvage chemotherapy.

Subtypes of Diffuse Large B-Cell Lymphoma

Primary mediastinal large B-cell lymphoma originates in the thymus and is most common in young women. This entity is distinguished by the presence of a mediastinal mass, which usually causes symptoms of cough, chest pain, or superior vena cava syndrome. A very large mass (>10 cm) or the existence of a malignant pleural effusion is associated with a worse prognosis.

Mediastinal large B-cell lymphoma is treated with the same chemotherapy regimens used for diffuse large B-cell lymphoma, followed, in some cases, by consolidative radiation therapy. The prognosis is similar to that of other diffuse large B-cell lymphomas. Relapses often occur in extranodal sites such as the CNS, lungs, gastrointestinal tract, liver, ovaries, and kidneys.

Intravascular large B-cell lymphoma is an aggressive lymphoma caused by cells that infiltrate the lumens of small blood vessels. Widespread extranodal involvement is common. Focal neurologic deficits and mental status changes are frequent. Cases are often diagnosed at autopsy, although durable responses to combination chemotherapy have been described.

Primary effusion lymphoma is associated with HHV-8 and is seen in HIV-infected and other immunosuppressed patients. Effusions occur in serous body cavities; peripheral lymphadenopathy is not seen. Prognosis is poor despite chemotherapy.

Plasmablastic lymphoma is most often seen in patients with HIV infection and frequently presents with involvement of the head and neck. This tumor does not express CD20 and thus does not benefit from treatment with rituximab.

Primary cutaneous diffuse large B-cell lymphoma of the leg (leg type) is one of two presentations of B-cell lymphoma in the skin. This tumor occurs mostly in older patients and follows an aggressive course. This neoplasm must be distinguished from primary cutaneous follicle center lymphoma, which might also be diagnosed as a cutaneous diffuse large B-cell lymphoma but follows an indolent course and requires only local therapy.

BURKITT'S LYMPHOMA

Burkitt's lymphoma is a highly aggressive B-cell lymphoma that is more common in children and immunosuppressed individuals than in healthy adults (see later). Widespread extranodal involvement is common. The endemic form of Burkitt's lymphoma is seen most frequently in children who reside in equatorial Africa. Involvement of bones of the jaw is common in this form. The sporadic form of Burkitt's lymphoma is seen most commonly in children in the United States. Males are more frequently affected. Both children and adults frequently have bulky abdominal disease, sometimes with involvement of the kidneys, ovaries, and breasts. Bone marrow involvement is seen in about one third of cases.

TREATMENT   Rx

Tumors may progress extremely rapidly, so therapy should be started as soon as possible. Tumor lysis syndrome may occur because of the frequent presence of bulky disease, the high rate of tumor proliferation, and the extreme sensitivity of the tumor to chemotherapy. Patients are usually treated with specialized high-intensity regimens, including rituximab, of relatively short duration. Treatment with the CHOP-R regimen used for diffuse large B-cell lymphoma has a poor outcome. CNS prophylaxis with intrathecal chemotherapy or high-dose methotrexate is required. Cure rates well in excess of 50% are typical with appropriate therapy.

RARE TYPES OF B-CELL LYMPHOMA

Several rare types of lymphoma have distinct clinical features.

Lymphoplasmacytic lymphoma is an indolent lymphoma that frequently involves the bone marrow, peripheral blood, and spleen. Patients frequently have an immunoglobulin M paraprotein (and therefore could be called Waldenström's macroglobulinemia) that may lead to symptoms of hyperviscosity, autoimmune phenomena, or neuropathies (Chapter 193). Plasmapheresis can reduce symptoms of hyperviscosity. Chemotherapy with alkylating agents, combination chemotherapy, or fludarabine may be used. Rituximab is also effective, as are new agents such as the proteosome inhibitor bortezomib.

Splenic marginal zone lymphoma is an indolent lymphoma that usually manifests with splenomegaly and lymphocytosis. A monoclonal gammopathy is frequently seen. Peripheral lymphadenopathy is unusual. Anemia and thrombocytopenia may respond to splenectomy. Chemotherapy with single agents or anthracycline-based combinations may be useful, and when the lymphoma is associated with hepatitis C, antiviral therapy may be effective. Responses to interferon have been described. This lymphoma appears to be particularly responsive to rituximab.

Nodal marginal zone B-cell lymphoma is an indolent disorder that is usually associated with generalized lymphadenopathy. The clinical course and prognosis are similar to those of follicular lymphoma, and it is usually treated in a similar manner.

Small intestinal immunoproliferative disease, a disorder seen most frequently in the Middle East, begins as a polyclonal process and can progress to a large B-cell lymphoma. The process is often associated with *Campylobacter jejuni* infection. Early in the disease, patients may respond to antibiotics, and frank lymphoma may respond to combination chemotherapy regimens.

Mature T-Cell Lymphomas (Peripheral T-Cell Lymphomas)

Peripheral (or mature) T-cell lymphomas are neoplasms of post-thymic T cells. These include relatively indolent disorders such as mycosis fungoides and CD30⁺ cutaneous lymphoproliferative disorders, but most patients diagnosed with peripheral T-cell lymphoma have an aggressive neoplasm. Peripheral T-cell lymphomas represent only 10% of the non-Hodgkin's lymphomas occurring in the United States. Unfortunately, the treatment for these lymphomas has not progressed as rapidly as the treatments for B-cell lymphomas.

MYCOSIS FUNGOIDES

Mycosis fungoides (often referred to as *cutaneous T-cell lymphoma*) is an indolent malignancy that is most common in middle-aged and older adults. The clinical course is usually a slow progression from isolated patches or plaques to thickened, more widespread plaques and then to multiple cutaneous tumors that may ulcerate (Chapter 446). A subset of patients presents with generalized erythroderma and circulating tumor cells, called *Sézary's syndrome.* Lymph node and visceral involvement may occur late in the course of the disease.

TREATMENT Rx

Cutaneous radiation therapy may be curative for patients with limited patch or plaque disease. Patients with early-stage disease (<10% body surface area) are frequently treated with skin-directed therapy that may include ultraviolet radiation, topical steroids, or topical nitrogen mustard.

Patients with more advanced disease frequently benefit from total skin electron beam therapy or extracorporeal photopheresis. Medical treatments include interferon-α, retinoids, monoclonal antibodies, histone deacetylase inhibitors (vorinostat, depsipeptide), the fusion toxin denileukin diftitox, and traditional cytotoxic chemotherapeutic agents; however, these treatments are usually only palliative. Results with autologous hematopoietic stem cell transplantation are usually poor, although allogeneic stem cell transplantation has yielded promising results in some cases.

ADULT T-CELL LYMPHOMA/LEUKEMIA

Adult T-cell lymphoma/leukemia, which is associated with HTLV-1 infection (Chapter 386), is most commonly seen in southern Japan and the Caribbean. Most infected patients are asymptomatic, and the lifetime risk of developing adult T-cell lymphoma/leukemia is approximately 3%.

Patients may have acute leukemia, aggressive lymphoma, or an indolent lymphoproliferative disease. Patients with aggressive disease present with generalized lymphadenopathy, hepatosplenomegaly, cutaneous infiltration, and hypercalcemia. Many patients have characteristic circulating tumor cells with a "flower" or "cloverleaf" nucleus.

TREATMENT

Patients with indolent disease can sometimes be monitored without therapy. Aggressive disease is usually treated with combination chemotherapy, but there is no consensus on the best regimen. Historically, the 5-year survival rate has been less than 10%, although recent trials have reported better outcomes.

CD30⁺ CUTANEOUS LYMPHOPROLIFERATIVE DISORDERS

These disorders represent a spectrum of diseases that may have an identical histologic appearance and overlapping clinical manifestations. Treatment decisions are often based on the clinical behavior of the lesions. These lymphomas express CD30 but do not express the anaplastic lymphoma kinase (ALK) protein (see later).

Lymphomatoid papulosis is a "histologically malignant" clonal disorder consisting of erythematous or skin-colored papules that frequently undergo spontaneous ulceration and necrosis over a period of weeks. The prognosis is excellent, although patients may eventually develop lymphoma.

Primary cutaneous anaplastic large cell lymphoma occurs most commonly in older men and also undergoes frequent spontaneous regression. The 5-year survival rate is greater than 90%. Treatment usually consists of local measures (surgery or radiation), although chemotherapy may be required.

PRIMARY SYSTEMIC ANAPLASTIC LARGE CELL LYMPHOMA

Anaplastic large cell lymphoma (ALCL) is an aggressive, CD30⁺, T-cell non-Hodgkin's lymphoma that is seen most frequently in young males. B-cell lymphomas with similar morphology can occur, but they have clinical features identical to other diffuse large B-cell lymphomas and are not considered part of this disease. A morphologically similar but biologically unrelated and clinically distinct neoplasm, primary cutaneous ALCL, occurs predominantly in older adults and represents part of the spectrum of cutaneous CD30⁺ lymphoproliferative disorders (see earlier). Primary systemic ALCL frequently has a t(2;5) chromosomal translocation that leads to overexpression of ALK, a protein not normally detectable in lymphoid cells.

Patients usually have lymphadenopathy, and involvement of the skin, bone, and gastrointestinal tract may be observed.

TREATMENT Rx

Patients are usually treated with chemotherapy regimens such as CHOP. Patients whose tumors express ALK have an excellent outcome, and 5-year survival rates of 70 to 90% have been observed. ALK-negative ALCL is more common in older patients and is associated with an inferior response rate and shorter survival time. Autologous hematopoietic stem cell transplantation may be curative for patients who relapse.

PERIPHERAL T-CELL LYMPHOMAS, UNSPECIFIED

The largest group of patients with peripheral T-cell lymphomas are defined in the WHO classification as having "peripheral T-cell lymphoma, unspecified." These patients' signs and symptoms are similar to those of patients with aggressive B-cell lymphomas, although systemic symptoms (fevers, night sweats, and weight loss) and extranodal involvement are frequent. The diagnosis of peripheral T-cell lymphoma requires immunophenotyping to demonstrate the T-cell origin.

UNUSUAL SUBTYPES OF T-CELL LYMPHOMA

Angioimmunoblastic T-cell lymphoma is associated with generalized lymphadenopathy, fever, weight loss, skin rash, and polyclonal hypergammaglobulinemia. Results of therapy are similar to those for peripheral T-cell lymphoma, unspecified.

Extranodal NK/T-cell lymphoma usually occurs in extranodal sites, especially the nose, palate, and nasopharynx. Involvement of the nose and face leads to the syndrome that was previously called lethal midline granuloma. This disorder is unusual in the United States, but it is frequent in Southeast Asia and Latin America. The prognosis is extremely poor, although patients with localized disease can sometimes be cured with aggressive combination radiation therapy and chemotherapy.

Hepatosplenic T-cell lymphoma is characterized by sinusoidal infiltration of the spleen, liver, and bone marrow, which leads to hepatosplenomegaly, systemic symptoms, and cytopenias. Lymphadenopathy is unusual. Patients are typically young males, and this disease can occur in allograft recipients and in the setting of immune dysfunction. The prognosis is poor, and remissions are rarely observed with chemotherapy.

Enteropathy-type T-cell lymphoma is usually seen in patients with gluten-sensitive enteropathy (Chapter 142). Patients typically present with abdominal pain and diarrhea and sometimes with bowel perforation. Treatment of celiac disease with a gluten-free diet appears to reduce the risk of lymphoma. The prognosis in these often undernourished patients is poor.

Subcutaneous panniculitis-like T-cell lymphoma manifests with multiple subcutaneous nodules and is often misdiagnosed as panniculitis. Patients with disseminated disease can have a syndrome consisting of fevers, weight loss, hepatosplenomegaly, pancytopenia, and phagocytosis of blood cells (hemophagocytic syndrome). Patients sometimes respond to combination chemotherapy regimens used for diffuse large B-cell lymphoma, interferon, and radiation therapy, but long-term disease-free survival is unusual.

⬤ SPECIAL CLINICAL SITUATIONS

The diagnosis and management of patients with the various types of non-Hodgkin's lymphoma can be profoundly influenced by the site of origin of the lymphoma and by certain clinical characteristics of the patients. Examples of the latter include pregnant patients with lymphoma, elderly patients with lymphoma, and lymphoma in patients who are severely immunosuppressed.

Specific Primary Sites of Diffuse Large B-Cell Lymphoma

Approximately 30% of diffuse large B-cell lymphomas originate in extranodal sites. Presentation in certain extranodal sites is associated with unique clinical behaviors that may necessitate diagnostic studies or additional therapy beyond that used for patients with nodal presentations.

Patients with primary CNS lymphoma (Chapter 195) commonly have ocular involvement, and all patients with this diagnosis should have a slit lamp examination. Surgical resection of primary CNS lymphoma is not beneficial, and the only role for surgery is in diagnosis. Primary lymphomas of the CNS are very sensitive to corticosteroids, but the best results have been observed with chemotherapy regimens that use high-dose methotrexate alone or in combination with other agents such as cytarabine. By comparison, conventional chemotherapy regimens, such as CHOP, are of little benefit. Whole brain irradiation is also effective therapy, although the incidence of leukoencephalopathy is extremely high, especially in elderly patients. Radiation therapy is frequently reserved for relapse rather than being used as adjunctive treatment with primary chemotherapy.

Treatment of primary testicular lymphoma, the most common testicular cancer in men older than 60 years (Chapter 206), usually consists of orchiectomy followed by combination chemotherapy. Relapse in the contralateral testicle is common, and most oncologists recommend adjuvant radiation to the scrotum. CNS involvement is common, and prophylactic intrathecal chemotherapy is usually recommended. Late relapses occur frequently.

Diffuse large B-cell lymphoma of the stomach and gastrointestinal tract is treated differently from gastric MALT lymphoma, even if there is a history of prior MALT lymphoma. Patients can be cured with surgery and adjunctive radiation or chemotherapy, although surgery is rarely performed for gastric lymphomas because of the morbidity associated with gastric resection. Patients should be treated with chemotherapy regimens used for other diffuse large B-cell lymphomas. Radiation therapy is sometimes used after chemotherapy, although the role of combined-modality treatment is not defined.

Lymphoma in AIDS and Post-Transplantation Lymphoproliferative Disorders

Non-Hodgkin's lymphoma is an AIDS-defining illness in HIV-infected individuals (Chapter 400), and the risk of developing a non-Hodgkin's lymphoma is increased more than 150-fold after the diagnosis of another AIDS-defining illness. Most cases are diffuse large B-cell lymphomas or Burkitt's lymphomas. AIDS-associated lymphomas behave aggressively and frequently involve the CNS and other unusual sites, such as the gastrointestinal tract, anus, rectum, skin, and soft tissue (Chapter 400). Factors associated with poor survival include low CD4 counts, poor performance status, older age, and advanced stage. The prognosis of these lymphomas is poor, with median survival times of approximately 6 months in the absence of concomitant aggressive therapy for HIV. If chemotherapy is given in association with highly active antiretroviral agents to patients with a good performance status, the likelihood of controlling the lymphoma is similar to that in patients without HIV infection. Intrathecal prophylaxis is generally recommended because of a higher risk of CNS involvement.

The risk of developing a non-Hodgkin's lymphoma is also markedly increased in patients who have received a solid organ transplant. The histologic appearance of these lymphomas is variable, but they frequently resemble aggressive lymphomas in nonimmunocompromised patients. Similar disorders can be seen in patients who are treated with methotrexate and other drugs for autoimmune disorders and in recipients of allogeneic hematopoietic stem cell transplants, especially if the transplants are T-cell depleted. These post-transplantation lymphoproliferative disorders, which may develop within weeks after surgery, are more common in patients who receive aggressive immunosuppression after transplantation. Involvement of extranodal sites is common, and lymphoma frequently involves the transplanted organ. Post-transplantation lymphoproliferative disorders may respond to reduction or withdrawal of immunosuppression. Some investigators have advocated the use of acyclovir or ganciclovir, because these lymphomas are usually related to EBV, but this practice is controversial. High response rates are also seen with rituximab. Other patients require treatment with combination chemotherapy regimens.

Non-Hodgkin's Lymphoma in Elderly Patients

More than 50% of patients who develop non-Hodgkin's lymphomas are older than 60 years, and the prognosis is generally worse for elderly patients. These poorer outcomes are related to increased toxicity of drug therapy, lower remission rates, increased rates of relapse, and higher death rates from cardiovascular disease and causes other than the lymphoma itself. Older patients are more likely to have other adverse prognostic characteristics (see Table 191-8), which also contribute to poorer outcomes. The practice of arbitrary dose reductions based solely on age should be discouraged if patients have a good performance status and no comorbid illnesses.[6]

Non-Hodgkin's Lymphoma and Pregnancy

Non-Hodgkin's lymphoma in pregnancy involves major clinical and ethical issues, and a multidisciplinary approach is needed (Chapter 247). Although chest radiographs are generally considered safe, ultrasound examination is usually used instead of CT for staging in the abdomen and pelvis.

Treatment can occasionally be delayed until after delivery; however, most women have a tumor that is potentially curable, and treatment delays may decrease the chance for cure. Other patients have conditions such as superior vena cava syndrome that require immediate treatment. After the first trimester, full-dose standard therapy such as CHOP-R may be used; several studies indicate high probabilities of cure without adverse long-term physical or intellectual deficits for the child. Although it is reasonable to offer therapeutic abortion for women in the first trimester, chemotherapy may also be successful in this situation. Regimens using methotrexate must be avoided.

DISEASES SOMETIMES CONFUSED WITH LYMPHOMA

The most common atypical lymphoid proliferations that can be confused with lymphoma are florid reactions to immune stimulation. Follicular hyperplasia with diffuse proliferation of B cells and T cells can be seen in a variety of autoimmune diseases (e.g., Sjögren's syndrome, systemic lupus erythematosus, rheumatoid arthritis) and infectious processes (e.g., EBV, cytomegalovirus, cat-scratch disease) (Chapter 171). If the definitive diagnosis of lymphoma cannot be made even after immunologic and molecular studies, the patient should be closely observed. The clinical course or subsequent biopsies can usually resolve the confusion.

Castleman's disease, or angiofollicular lymph node hyperplasia, usually appears with a hyaline vascular pattern of lymphoid proliferation, but a subset of patients has hyperplastic lymphoid follicles and sheets of plasma cells. Patients with Castleman's disease often present with a localized lymphoid mass, but some patients have a systemic illness with fevers, night sweats, weight loss, and fatigue. Frequently, the systemic symptoms of Castleman's disease are related to excessive production of interleukin-6 (IL-6). Castleman's disease in HIV-infected patients is frequently associated with HHV-8. Patients with disseminated and plasma cell–rich forms of Castleman's disease may occasionally progress to lymphoma. Patients with localized Castleman's disease can be treated with surgical removal or radiation therapy. Patients with systemic disease may respond to treatment with high-dose corticosteroids. Patients with overexpression of IL-6 frequently benefit from treatment with an anti–IL-6 antibody. If other treatments fail, patients sometimes benefit from combination chemotherapy regimens, autologous or allogeneic hematopoietic stem cell transplantation, or both.

Sinus histiocytosis with massive lymphadenopathy, also known as *Rosai-Dorfman disease,* manifests as bulky lymphadenopathy in children and young adults. Extranodal sites such as the skin, upper airways, gastrointestinal tract, and CNS can be involved. The disease is usually self-limited, but it has been associated with autoimmune hemolytic anemia.

Kikuchi's disease (histiocytic necrotizing lymphadenitis) is a disease of unknown origin that most commonly affects young women. Symptoms most commonly consist of painless cervical lymphadenopathy that is often accompanied by fever, flu-like symptoms, and rash. Treatment is symptomatic, and manifestations usually resolve within weeks or months.

1. Salles G, Seymour JF, Offner F, et al. Rituximab maintenance for 2 years in patients with high tumour burden follicular lymphoma responding to rituximab plus chemotherapy (PRIMA): a phase 3, randomised controlled trial. *Lancet.* 2011;377:42-51.
2. Azim HA, Santoro L, Bociek RG, et al. High dose intensity doxorubicin in aggressive non-Hodgkin's lymphoma: a literature-based meta-analysis. *Ann Oncol.* 2010;21:1064-1071.
3. Baldo P, Rupolo M, Compagnoni A, et al. Interferon-alpha for maintenance of follicular lymphoma. *Cochrane Database Syst Rev.* 2010;1:CD004629.
4. Persky DO, Unger JM, Spier CM, et al. Phase II study of rituximab plus three cycles of CHOP and involved-field radiotherapy for patients with limited-stage aggressive B-cell lymphoma: Southwest Oncology Group study 0014. *J Clin Oncol.* 2008;26:2258-2263.
5. Pfreundschuh M, Trumper L, Osterborg A, et al. CHOP-like chemotherapy plus rituximab versus CHOP-like chemotherapy alone in young patients with good-prognosis diffuse large-B-cell lymphoma: a randomized controlled trial by the MabThera International Trial (MInT) Group. *Lancet Oncol.* 2006;7:379-391.
6. Pfreundschuh M, Schubert J, Ziepert M, et al. Six versus eight cycles of bi-weekly CHOP-14 with or without rituximab in elderly patients with aggressive CD20+ B-cell lymphomas: a randomized controlled trial (RICOVER-60). *Lancet Oncol.* 2008;9:105-116.

SUGGESTED READINGS

Chan WC, Armitage JO. Genomic analysis of lymphoma: potential for clinical application. *J Natl Compr Canc Netw.* 2010;8:353-360. *Review of the application of gene expression profiling to the diagnosis and treatment of lymphomas.*

Lenz G, Staudt LM. Aggressive lymphomas. *N Engl J Med.* 2010;362:1417-1429. *Recent progress in the molecular genetics of aggressive lymphomas, focusing on the most common form of this disease: diffuse large B-cell lymphoma.*

Pirani M, Marcheselli R, Marcheselli L, et al. Risk for second malignancies in non-Hodgkin's lymphoma survivors: a meta-analysis. *Ann Oncol.* 2011. [Epub ahead of print.] *Review showing a 1.9-fold increased risk.*

Schultz CJ, Bovi J. Current management of primary central nervous system lymphoma. *Int J Radiat Oncol Biol Phys.* 2010;76:666-678. *Review of most effective whole brain radiation therapy and chemotherapy regimens and the limited role of surgery.*

Tay K, Dunleavy K, Wilson WH. Novel agents for B-cell non-Hodgkin lymphoma: science and the promise. *Blood Rev.* 2010;24:69-82. *Novel agents for lymphoma, including immunotherapy and small molecules.*

192

HODGKIN'S LYMPHOMA

JOSEPH M. CONNORS

DEFINITION

Hodgkin's lymphoma, formerly called Hodgkin's disease, is one of the B-cell lymphomas. It has a characteristic neoplastic cell, the Hodgkin-Reed-Sternberg cell, a distinct natural history, and most important, an excellent response to treatment, with the large majority of patients being cured. Its management, which requires careful multidisciplinary cooperation, serves as a paradigm for the successful application of modern oncologic concepts. Highly effective chemotherapy is the cornerstone of treatment. Carefully selected patients may require the addition of radiation or, if the lymphoma recurs after primary treatment, high-dose chemoradiation therapy and autologous hematologic stem cell transplantation (HDC/HSCT). The current challenge to clinicians managing this neoplasm is to cure the disease while minimizing long-term toxicity.

EPIDEMIOLOGY

The incidence of Hodgkin's lymphoma varies substantially around the world. The highest rates occur in the United States, Canada, Switzerland, and northern Europe. Intermediate rates are seen in southern and eastern Europe and low rates in eastern Asia. No clear explanation for this variation in incidence has been found. Postulated reasons include differences in the age at onset or genotype of any associated Epstein-Barr virus (EBV) infection; crowding during childhood as a result of lower socioeconomic status, predisposing to passage of an as yet undiscovered infectious vector; and intrinsic genetic differences in susceptibility.

Approximately 20,000 new cases are seen annually in North America and Europe. The age-adjusted incidence of Hodgkin's lymphoma declined modestly over the 20 years before 1990 at a rate of approximately 0.9% per year but has leveled off since then and is now approximately 2.7 per 100,000. Age-adjusted annual mortality is 0.5 per 100,000. Hodgkin's lymphoma occurs slightly more often in men and is seen more frequently in whites than African Americans and much less frequently in Asian populations. Much of the difference in incidence between whites and blacks in North America can be attributed to the higher incidence seen in higher socioeconomic classes. The cumulative lifetime risk for development of Hodgkin's lymphoma is approximately 1 in 250 to 1 in 300 in North America.

The incidence of Hodgkin's lymphoma rises from a very low level in childhood to a plateau in early adulthood and then remains stable. In the Western world, only about 5% of cases occur in persons younger than 15 years and 5% in persons older than 70 years. In contrast, however, the age distribution in the Indian subcontinent is strongly shifted into childhood.

PATHOBIOLOGY

The cause of Hodgkin's lymphoma remains unclear. Hodgkin's lymphoma is not associated with exposure to radiation, chemicals, biocidal agents, working in health care–related professions, or previous tonsillectomy. The leading suspect remains EBV, based on much suggestive evidence but no definitive proof.

Epstein-Barr Virus

EBV is a large B-lymphocyte tropic herpesvirus (Chapter 385). Approximately 90% of the general population acquires infection with EBV by early adulthood. In the developing world, this infection usually occurs in childhood, but in developed countries, infection is often delayed into the teens, when it is associated with the syndrome of infectious mononucleosis in up to 30% of new cases. A history of infectious mononucleosis increases the likelihood for subsequent Hodgkin's lymphoma three-fold. Antibodies to the viral capsid antigen reach higher levels in patients with Hodgkin's lymphoma than in controls, and these higher levels appear several years before the neoplasm. In situ hybridization studies have demonstrated that the Hodgkin-Reed-Sternberg cells in approximately 50% of cases of Hodgkin's lymphoma contain EBV-encoded small RNA (EBER), and in these cases, virtually all the Hodgkin-Reed-Sternberg cells are positive for the virus. The EBV genome is amplified 50-fold or more in Hodgkin-Reed-Sternberg cells and is monoclonal in an individual patient's Hodgkin-Reed-Sternberg cells. In some populations, virtually all cases of Hodgkin's lymphoma occur in EBV-positive individuals, but up to 50% of patients in developed countries do not have EBV in their Hodgkin-Reed-Sternberg cells. Thus, although EBV may play an important role in the development of Hodgkin's lymphoma, that role is neither straightforward nor universal.

Genetic Factors

Circumstantial evidence for a genetic contribution to the etiology of Hodgkin's lymphoma comes from studies showing that Hodgkin's lymphoma is almost 100-fold more likely to develop in the monozygotic twin of an affected individual than in a dizygotic twin. First-degree relatives of individuals with the disease have up to a five-fold increased risk for development of the lymphoma. Perhaps genetically predisposed individuals react differently to EBV, thereby increasing the chance that a lymphoid neoplasm will develop.

Polymerase chain reaction–based genotypic analysis has demonstrated the clonal derivation of Hodgkin-Reed-Sternberg cells, including identical $p53$ mutations from multiple Hodgkin-Reed-Sternberg cells extracted from a single biopsy specimen, thereby unequivocally establishing clonality. The presence of clonal immunoglobulin gene rearrangements from multiple cells in the same biopsy specimen also confirms a B-cell origin. Only a few rare cases with a T-cell genotype have been reported, but these are obviously exceptional. The presence of clonal somatic mutations provides proof of the germinal center origin of the neoplastic cells. Finally, identification of cells with identical immunoglobulin gene rearrangements both at diagnosis and at relapse verify that the B-cell clonality of the disease is preserved over time.

Despite their B-cell origin, the neoplastic cells of Hodgkin's lymphoma are incapable of making intact antibodies, perhaps because they lack the ability to make the transcription factors necessary to activate the immunoglobulin promoter. B cells that are incapable of manufacturing antibody should undergo apoptosis, but the Hodgkin-Reed-Sternberg cells avoid this self-destruction. The observation that the antiapoptotic nuclear transcription factor NFκB is constitutively activated in these cells may provide an explanation.

Classic cytogenetics has been unrevealing in Hodgkin's lymphoma. Aneuploidy and hyperploidy consistent with the multinucleated nature of Hodgkin-Reed-Sternberg cells are frequent, but no consistent translocations have been detected.

CLINICAL MANIFESTATIONS

Hodgkin's lymphoma is usually manifested as lymphadenopathy (Chapter 171), typically in the cervical, axillary, or mediastinal areas, and only about 10% of the time as nodal disease below the diaphragm. Although peripherally located nodes seldom reach large size, very large mediastinal masses or, less often, retroperitoneal masses can develop with only modest symptoms. Lymph node involvement in Hodgkin's lymphoma is usually painless, but an occasional patient notes discomfort in involved nodal sites immediately after drinking alcohol.

Approximately 25% of patients with Hodgkin's lymphoma have constitutional symptoms. The classic B symptoms, significant weight loss (>10% of baseline), night sweats, and persistent fever, usually signal widespread or locally extensive disease and imply a need for systemic treatment. Generalized pruritus, occasionally severe, can antedate the diagnosis of Hodgkin's lymphoma by up to several years. Some patients have symptoms suggestive of a growing mass lesion, such as cough or stridor as a result of tracheobronchial compression from mediastinal disease or bone pain secondary to metastatic involvement. Because Hodgkin's lymphoma can involve the bone marrow extensively, an occasional patient has symptomatic anemia or incidentally noted pancytopenia. Paraneoplastic neurologic or endocrine syndromes have been reported with Hodgkin's lymphoma but are rare.

DIAGNOSIS

The diagnosis of Hodgkin's lymphoma is based on recognition of Hodgkin-Reed-Sternberg cells (Fig. 192-1) or Hodgkin's cells (or both) in an appropriate cellular background in tissue sections from a lymph node or extralymphatic organ, such as bone marrow, lung, or bone. Fine-needle aspiration biopsy is not adequate for the diagnosis of Hodgkin's lymphoma. Open biopsy and standard histochemical staining are required to establish the diagnosis unequivocally and to determine the histologic subtype. Immunohistochemical studies can prove helpful in difficult cases or to distinguish special subtypes such as lymphocyte-rich classic Hodgkin's lymphoma and the nodular

FIGURE 192-1. **Nodular sclerosing Hodgkin's lymphoma.** This figure shows a typical case of classic nodular sclerosing Hodgkin's lymphoma with many lacunar cells, occasional diagnostic Hodgkin-Reed-Sternberg cells, and the characteristic background of lymphocytes and eosinophils. (Photomicrograph courtesy of Randy D. Gascoyne, MD, British Columbia Cancer Agency.)

TABLE 192-1 WORLD HEALTH ORGANIZATION CLASSIFICATION OF HODGKIN'S LYMPHOMA SUBTYPES

SUBTYPE NAME	FREQUENCY (%)*
Classic Hodgkin's lymphoma	
Nodular sclerosis	70
Lymphocyte rich	3
Mixed cellularity	10
Lymphocyte depleted	1
Nodular lymphocyte-predominant Hodgkin's lymphoma	7
Hodgkin's lymphoma, not otherwise classifiable	9

*Frequency based on all new cases ($N = 1043$) seen in British Columbia since January 1998 when the category of lymphocyte-rich classic Hodgkin's lymphoma became well established.

lymphocyte-predominant type. In classic Hodgkin's lymphoma, scattered large Hodgkin-Reed-Sternberg cells either are multinucleated or have large polyploid nuclei. Variations include mononuclear cells that are similar to the usual polylobated or multinuclear cells but have only one large nucleus with a prominent nucleolus, as well as lacunar cells, which are Hodgkin-Reed-Sternberg variants with abundant cytoplasm that has retracted as an artifact of formalin fixation. The infrequent Hodgkin-Reed-Sternberg cells are usually present in a background mixture of polyclonal lymphocytes, eosinophils, neutrophils, plasma cells, fibroblasts, and histiocytes. Recently, a high number of associated macrophages have been demonstrated to be a strong predictor of treatment resistance. Occasionally, granulomas form with a prominent histiocytic component.

Hodgkin's lymphoma can typically be classified into one of five well-described subtypes (Table 192-1). Reproducibility of the distinctions among these subtypes has been confirmed in the current widely accepted World Health Organization classification of lymphoid neoplasms. With addition of the new category of lymphocyte-rich classic Hodgkin's lymphoma, this newest classification scheme permits confident identification of nodular lymphocyte-predominant Hodgkin's lymphoma as a separate entity. The most common subtype is nodular sclerosing, which has characteristic course bands of sclerosis surrounding nodules composed of typical Hodgkin-Reed-Sternberg cells in the usual background mixture of reactive and inflammatory cells.

The immunophenotype of the neoplastic cells in Hodgkin's lymphoma can help identify the specific subtype. Typically, the Hodgkin-Reed-Sternberg cells stain positively for CD30 (80 to 100% of cases), CD15 (75 to 85% of cases), and B-cell-specific activating protein (BSAP), which is the product of the *PAX5* gene (>90% of cases). However, often only a minority of the malignant cells stain positively for the CD15 and BSAP markers. CD20, a generally reliable marker of B-cell lineage, is positive in about 40% of cases of classic

Hodgkin's lymphoma, but usually only in a minority of cells, and the staining can be weak. In contrast, nodular lymphocyte-predominant Hodgkin's lymphoma almost always stains strongly positive for CD20 and for the specialized B-cell markers CD79a and CD45, but it is negative for CD30 and CD15. Finally, anaplastic large cell lymphoma (Chapter 191) is reliably negative for CD15, CD20, and CD79a but frequently positive for anaplastic lymphoma kinase (ALK).

Differential Diagnosis

Depending on the site of occurrence and associated symptoms, the differential diagnosis of Hodgkin's lymphoma includes non-Hodgkin's lymphoma (Chapter 191), germ cell tumors (Chapter 206), thymoma (Chapter 430), sarcoidosis (Chapter 95), and tuberculosis (Chapter 332). However, the specific diagnosis is readily determined by obtaining an adequate biopsy specimen for review by an experienced hematopathologist. Proceeding to such a biopsy early in the assessment of patients with lymphadenopathy (Chapter 171), especially of the mediastinum, often saves time and spares the patient needless testing and delay in diagnosis.

With computed tomography (CT) and appropriate biopsy procedures to investigate enlarged central thoracic or intra-abdominal lymph nodes, the diagnosis of Hodgkin's lymphoma seldom presents difficulty. The immunophenotype helps distinguish Hodgkin's lymphoma from other diseases. For example, T-cell-rich B-cell lymphoma (Chapter 191) is distinguished from classic Hodgkin's lymphoma by being CD30 and CD15 negative but positive for CD20 and CD45. However, T-cell-rich B-cell lymphoma (Chapter 191) can be very difficult to distinguish from nodular lymphocyte-predominant Hodgkin's lymphoma because both are negative for CD30 and CD15 but positive for CD45. This distinction is best made by focusing on the histologic pattern of the neoplastic cells. In fact, the combination of appropriate immunohistopathologic evaluation by an expert hematopathologist and clinical assessment has virtually eliminated difficulties with the differential diagnosis. Problems mostly arise when inadequate or improperly processed material is all that is available for diagnosis.

Staging

Physical Examination

Given its tendency to spread in an orderly fashion, usually from initially involved lymph nodes, the stage of Hodgkin's lymphoma can be established by using readily available imaging and laboratory tests (Fig. 192-2 and Table 192-2). The evaluation should start with a careful history to search for the presence of localizing signs, such as bone pain, or the constitutional symptoms of fever, weight loss, or night sweats. The history may also reveal comorbid conditions that may affect the safe delivery of planned treatment. The physical examination may identify lymphadenopathy or organomegaly.

Laboratory Testing

Laboratory testing should include blood cell counts and the erythrocyte sedimentation rate, assessment of liver and renal function, serum albumin level, serum protein electrophoresis, and serologic testing for hepatitis B. Also, the patient should be tested for hepatitis C if liver enzyme abnormalities are detected and human immunodeficiency virus (HIV) antibody if the history indicates an increased risk or if the sites of disease are unusual. Bone marrow aspiration and biopsy are only useful for the minority of patients with constitutional (B) symptoms or those with lower than normal peripheral blood counts at diagnosis.

Imaging

Imaging techniques to evaluate Hodgkin's lymphoma continue to evolve (Fig. 192-3). All patients should undergo contrast-enhanced CT scanning of the thorax, abdomen, and pelvis with slices at intervals of 1 cm or less. Magnetic resonance imaging is occasionally useful when the extent of bone or soft tissue involvement must be determined precisely or for a patient with an absolute contraindication to the use of intravenous contrast agents.

Positron Emission Tomography

Positron emission tomography (PET) is more sensitive and specific than CT or gallium scanning both for staging and for assessment of residual masses after treatment. However, it has not been proved that the addition of PET to standard staging imaging tests for Hodgkin's lymphoma will actually improve outcome, so whether PET could replace other studies is not clear. The greatest usefulness of PET presently appears to be the assessment of residual masses during or after planned treatment so that the minority of patients who

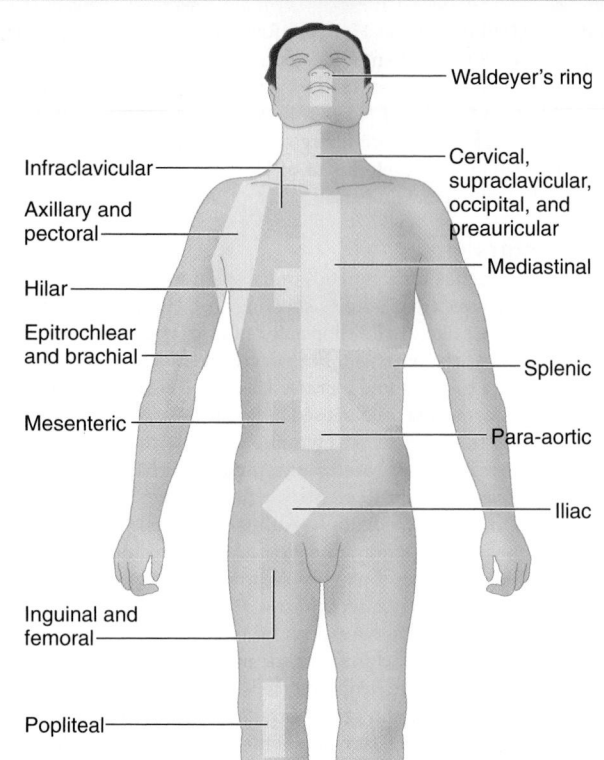

FIGURE 192-2. Anatomic definition of lymph node regions for staging of Hodgkin's disease. (From Kaplan HS, Rosenberg SA. The treatment of Hodgkin's disease. *Med Clin North Am.* 1966;50:1591-1610.)

TABLE 192-2	TESTS REQUIRED FOR STAGING OF HODGKIN'S LYMPHOMA

Complete history to search for B symptoms (fever, weight loss, night sweats) or other symptomatic problems suggesting more advanced disease
Physical examination for lymphadenopathy or organomegaly
Complete blood count
Serum creatinine, alkaline phosphatase, lactate dehydrogenase, bilirubin, and protein electrophoresis (including serum albumin level)
Chest radiograph, posteroanterior and lateral views
Computed tomography scan of the neck, thorax, abdomen, and pelvis
Certain tests are required only for specific manifestations

MANIFESTATION/CONDITION	TEST
B symptoms or WBC count <4.0 × 10⁹/L, Hgb <120 g/L (women) or 130 g/L (men), or platelets <125 × 10⁹/L	Bone marrow biopsy and aspiration
Stage IA or IIA disease with upper cervical lymph node involvement (suprahyoid)	ENT examination

ENT = ear, nose, and throat; Hgb = hemoglobin; WBC = white blood cell.

should receive altered or additional therapy, especially radiotherapy, can be identified.

Staging System

The Ann Arbor staging system with the Cotswold modification (Table 192-3) categorizes patients into four stages. The first three indicate the expanding extent of lymph node disease (see Fig. 192-2): stage I, a single nodal area; stage II, two or more nodal areas but still on one side of the diaphragm; and stage III, nodal disease on both sides of the diaphragm. The spleen and the lymphoid tissue of Waldeyer's ring each count as nodal sites in this system. Stage IV is reserved for extranodal disease, which for all practical purposes is disease in the bone marrow, lung, bone, or liver. Hodgkin's lymphoma at any other extranodal site should prompt questioning of the diagnosis or a search for HIV infection.

Bulky disease is defined as the presence of any tumor mass with the largest diameter greater than 10 cm or a mediastinal mass with a transverse diameter exceeding one third of the largest transverse transthoracic diameter. With CT scanning, use of the mediastinal mass ratio is obsolete, and the term *bulky* is best assigned to tumors exceeding 10 cm in largest single diameter.

FIGURE 192-3. Imaging of Hodgkin's lymphoma. Bulky Hodgkin's disease as seen on chest radiograph (**A**), computed tomography (CT) of the chest (**B**), gallium scan (**C**), and positron emission tomography (PET) (**D**). The *arrows* indicate sites of disease. Note that the PET and CT scans provide more detailed information than the chest radiograph and gallium scan.

TABLE 192-3	MODIFIED ANN ARBOR STAGING SYSTEM FOR HODGKIN'S LYMPHOMA
STAGE	**INVOLVEMENT**
I	Single lymph node region (I) or one extralymphatic site (I$_E$)
II	Two or more lymph node regions, same side of the diaphragm (II), or local extralymphatic extension plus one or more lymph node regions, same side of the diaphragm (II$_E$)
III	Lymph node regions on both sides of the diaphragm (III); may be accompanied by local extralymphatic extension (III$_E$)
IV	Diffuse involvement of one or more extralymphatic organs or sites
A	No "B" symptoms
B	Presence of at least one of the following: Unexplained weight loss >10% of baseline during 6 mo before staging Recurrent unexplained fever >38° C Recurrent night sweats

TABLE 192-4	RATES OF PROGRESSION IN 5 YEARS IN PATIENTS WITH ADVANCED-STAGE HODGKIN'S LYMPHOMA

NO. OF FACTORS*	FREQUENCY (%)	PERCENTAGE WITH PROGRESSION-FREE SURVIVAL AT 5 YEARS
0-3	81	70
4-7	19	47

*Male sex, age older than 45 years, stage IV, hemoglobin level less than 10.5 g/dL, white blood cell count greater than 15,000/mL, lymphocyte count less than 600/mL or less than 8% of the white cell count, or serum albumin less than 4 g/dL.

The E lesion designation identifies patients whose limited extranodal extension of Hodgkin's lymphoma could be included in a reasonable involved field of irradiation. After staging, patients are further subdivided into those with or without fever, night sweats, or weight loss (B symptoms).

TREATMENT ㋡ Rx

Over the past 60 years, Hodgkin's lymphoma has been transformed from a nearly uniformly fatal illness to one that is usually cured. This remarkable success has provided a paradigm on which much of modern oncologic treatment is based. The principles underlying combined-modality treatment and multiagent chemotherapy, the mainstays of today's successful treatment of many malignancies, were first demonstrated to be effective with Hodgkin's lymphoma. The essential involvement of a multidisciplinary team, including pathologists, experts in diagnostic imaging, medical and radiation oncologists, nurses, and support staff, has served as a model for all cancer. The

necessity to balance greater efficacy of initial treatment, which often requires an increase in intensity and therefore toxicity, against troublesome and occasionally fatal late complications has encouraged a long-term perspective.

From a practical therapeutic viewpoint, patients with stage III or IV disease, bulky disease, or B symptoms are defined as having advanced disease, whereas patients without these characteristics have limited-stage disease. In Europe, patients with limited disease are further subdivided into those with favorable and unfavorable outcomes, but cure rates exceed 90 to 95% for all patients with nonbulky stage IA or IIA (limited) disease. However, for patients with advanced-stage disease, independent predictors of progression include gender, age, stage, hemoglobin level, white blood cell count, lymphocyte count, and serum albumin level (Table 192-4). Based on results obtained in the 1980s, the 80% of patients with fewer than four factors had a progression-free survival of 70%, but for the 20% who had four or more factors, the progression-free survival rate fell to less than 50%. However, with better attention to dose delivery, more current results indicate a spread of only 80% to 60% between these two groups. A straightforward plan of treatment for the 90% of patients in whom Hodgkin's lymphoma is diagnosed between the ages of 16 and 70 years can be based on clinical stage, the presence of B symptoms, and bulk of the largest tumor mass (Table 192-5).

Treatment of Limited-Stage Hodgkin's Lymphoma

More than 95% of the one third of patients with Hodgkin's lymphoma initially found to have limited-stage disease can be cured regardless of the site

TABLE 192-5 TREATMENT PLAN FOR ADULT PATIENTS WITH HODGKIN'S LYMPHOMA

STAGE	PROGNOSTIC CATEGORY	TREATMENT
IA or IIA, no bulky disease*		ABVD[†] × 4 if CR after 2 cycles or ABVD × 2 + IRRT
IB, IIB, or any stage III or IV or bulky disease, any stage	≤3 adverse factors[†]	ABVD[†] until 2 cycles past CR (minimum 6, maximum 8)
	≥4 adverse factors[†]	Escalated BEACOPP[‡]

*Bulky refers to disease with the largest diameter of any single mass equal to or greater than 10 cm.
[†]See Table 192-4 note.
[‡]See text for drugs in each regimen. Optimal dosing must be individualized.
CR = complete response; IRRT = involved-region radiation therapy.

of occurrence, the presence of disease above or below the diaphragm, or the histologic subtype. The challenge is to achieve this goal with the least toxicity and cost.

Two cycles of ABVD (Adriamycin [doxorubicin], bleomycin, vinblastine, and dacarbazine) chemotherapy followed by involved-field irradiation cures nearly 95% of patients with limited-stage disease and nearly completely eliminates the risk for infertility, premature menopause, and leukemia and minimizes cardiopulmonary toxicity.[1-3] The chemotherapy in the combined-modality treatment of limited-stage Hodgkin's lymphoma eradicates subclinical disease and allows smaller fields of irradiation to be used. However, a substantial proportion of the excess, long-term mortality in patients with limited-stage Hodgkin's lymphoma is due to cardiovascular disease and second neoplasms that are closely related to the use of irradiation. In a randomized trial that compared four to six cycles of ABVD chemotherapy alone versus irradiation, either alone or augmented with two cycles of ABVD chemotherapy, the strategy of chemotherapy alone proved equivalent to irradiation-based treatment in terms of event-free and overall survival, although the irradiation-based approach did produce a modest improvement in progression-free survival.[4] Longer follow-up will be necessary to see whether the goal of a reduction in cardiovascular events and second neoplasms was accomplished. This trial suggests that more than 90% of patients with limited-stage Hodgkin's lymphoma can be treated with four to six cycles of ABVD alone; for the minority whose lymphoma does not completely regress after two cycles, probably best assessed by PET scanning, the addition of radiation may be optimum.

Treatment of Advanced-Stage Hodgkin's Lymphoma

In advanced-stage Hodgkin's lymphoma (stages IIIA, IIIB, IVA, and IVB), both ABVD and MOPP (mechlorethamine, Oncovin [vincristine], procarbazine, and prednisone)/ABVD are superior to MOPP alone in terms of progression-free survival. Today, ABVD is the most widely used regimen for patients with advanced-stage Hodgkin's lymphoma. The addition of radiation therapy significantly improves progression-free survival at 10 years in patients with advanced-stage Hodgkin's lymphoma, but it does not improve overall survival because it causes significantly more deaths unrelated to lymphoma. Even the addition of radiation therapy for patients in complete remission after chemotherapy for advanced-stage Hodgkin's lymphoma has no significant impact. The adverse long-term effects of radiation therapy and its lack of improvement in overall survival appear to outweigh any benefits for the usual patient with advanced-stage disease. The ability of PET scanning to distinguish between residual fibrosis and persistent lymphoma may provide a mechanism to identify selected patients who might benefit from localized radiation therapy.

Recently devised regimens for patients with advanced Hodgkin's lymphoma are the Stanford V regimen (doxorubicin, vinblastine, mechlorethamine, etoposide, vincristine, bleomycin, and prednisone) and escalated BEACOPP (bleomycin, etoposide, doxorubicin, cyclophosphamide, vincristine, prednisone, and procarbazine) (see Table 192-5). As originally described, both include postchemotherapy irradiation to sites of initial or residual tumor bulk (≥5 cm). Although initial results appeared quite promising, recent results indicate that the Stanford V regimen is no more effective than standard ABVD.[5] BEACOPP plus radiation therapy provides better progression-free and overall survival at a median follow-up of 6.9 years than COPP/ABVD plus radiation therapy despite a higher rate of hematologic toxicity and infertility.[6]

The overall approach to managing advanced-stage Hodgkin's lymphoma must factor in the fact that about 50% of patients who are not cured by primary chemotherapy can be effectively treated with HDC/HSCT (Chapter 181). Thus, for the 80% of patients with zero to three adverse prognostic factors at presentation, who have a 75% chance of cure with primary chemotherapy, the most widely used approach is to start with ABVD. For the 20% of these low-risk patients in whom progressive lymphoma develops despite primary treatment, HDC/HSCT (Chapter 181) should be offered. Such a strategy confines the high cost and toxicity of intensified treatment to the minority of patients whose disease demands it. Conversely, for the 20% of patients with high-risk disease who have four or more adverse factors and only a 60% likelihood of cure with primary chemotherapy, more intense initial treatment with the BEACOPP protocol is reasonable.

Management of Refractory or Relapsed Hodgkin's Lymphoma

HDC/HSCT has become the established treatment for most patients whose Hodgkin's lymphoma persists or recurs despite primary chemotherapy.[7] However, the treatment-related mortality, high levels of toxicity, and cost associated with HDC/HSCT demand that it be reserved for patients in whom it clearly increases the chance of cure over alternative treatments; such patients include those whose disease progresses during or within 3 months of initial multiagent chemotherapy (refractory Hodgkin's lymphoma) and those who relapse more than 3 months after multiagent chemotherapy (relapsed Hodgkin's lymphoma). For relapsed lymphoma, controversy remains, however, for two special subgroups: patients who relapse solely in originally involved but unirradiated lymph nodes and without B symptoms or extranodal disease, who may obtain up to a 40 to 50% cure rate with wide-field irradiation, and patients who relapse without B symptoms more than 1 year after completion of primary chemotherapy, who may achieve up to a 30 to 40% cure rate with additional chemotherapy with or without irradiation. However, even these two subgroups may achieve up to an 80% 10-year disease-free survival rate after HDC/HSCT. Thus, data suggest that standard treatment for patients with progressive Hodgkin's lymphoma after primary chemotherapy for advanced-stage disease should be HDC/HSCT regardless of the characteristics of the relapse.

HDC/HSCT should be reserved for patients who have progressive lymphoma after primary chemotherapy because randomized trials of HDC/HSCT for patients in complete or partial remission after primary chemotherapy for advanced Hodgkin's lymphoma failed to show a difference in outcome.[8]

Management of Complications
Follow-up and Late Complications of Treatment

Most adult patients with Hodgkin's lymphoma are cured and experience minimal long-term toxicity from their treatment. However, the risk for certain predictable and occasional rare and less predictable late effects warrants careful but not intrusive follow-up and selective intervention (Table 192-6). At the conclusion of treatment, a thorough reassessment of the initial sites of lymphoma should be completed to provide post-treatment baseline measurements. Patients should be seen by a specialist knowledgeable in the management of lymphoma, preferably about every 3 months for 2 years, then every 6 months for 3 years, then annually. Patients should be strongly encouraged to refrain from smoking, to perform careful breast and skin examinations on a regular basis, and to undergo regular immunizations for influenza annually, pneumococcus at diagnosis and 5 years after treatment, and diphtheria and tetanus every 10 years (Chapter 17). Patients who have received radiation to the head or neck area should follow a vigorous program of dental prophylaxis in anticipation of the deleterious effect of reduced saliva production and have their thyroid-stimulating hormone (TSH) level checked annually in recognition of the 50% risk for eventual hypothyroidism.

Special Problems in the Management of Hodgkin's Lymphoma
Hodgkin's Lymphoma during Pregnancy

Between 0.5 and 1.0% of cases of Hodgkin's lymphoma occur coincident with pregnancy (Chapter 247). When the lymphoma is discovered during pregnancy, it is almost always possible to keep it under control and allow the pregnancy to go to full term.

Standard staging tests (see Table 192-2) should be completed, except that imaging requiring radiation must be minimized. For example, abdominal ultrasonography can identify bulky retroperitoneal disease, and a single posteroanterior radiograph of the chest, with proper shielding, can identify bulky mediastinal disease.

More than 50% of patients can continue the pregnancy to term without any treatment of the lymphoma. If symptomatic or progressive disease develops, systemic chemotherapy can be given in the second and third trimester with very small risk of injuring the fetus. An attractive alternative is intermittent single-agent vinblastine, given in the lowest dose that can control symptoms until delivery, followed by a full course of six to eight cycles of multiagent chemotherapy after delivery.

Hodgkin's Lymphoma and Acquired Immunodeficiency Syndrome

In patients with HIV infection, the incidence of Hodgkin's lymphoma is increased as much as five- to ten-fold, and the lymphoma manifests differently and pursues a more aggressive natural history (Chapter 400). Hodgkin's lymphoma in HIV-positive individuals is almost always associated with EBV within Hodgkin-Reed-Sternberg cells. The histology is much more likely to be mixed cellularity or lymphocyte depleted. The disease most commonly develops in extranodal sites, especially the bone marrow. More than 80% of patients have advanced-stage disease, and most patients have B symptoms.

TABLE 192-6 MONITORING AFTER SUCCESSFUL PRIMARY TREATMENT OF HODGKIN'S LYMPHOMA

RISK/PROBLEM	INCIDENCE/RESPONSE
Relapse	Ten to 30% of patients experience relapse. Careful attention should be directed to lymph node sites, especially if previously involved with disease and not treated with radiation. New persistent focal symptoms such as bone pain should be investigated with appropriate laboratory and imaging studies.
Dental caries	Neck or oropharyngeal irradiation may cause decreased salivation. Patients should have regular dental care and should make their dentist aware of the previous irradiation.
Hypothyroidism	After external beam thyroid irradiation at doses sufficient to cure Hodgkin's lymphoma, at least 50% of patients eventually become hypothyroid. All patients who have been exposed to neck irradiation should have an annual TSH level determined. Patients whose TSH level becomes elevated should be treated with lifelong thyroxine replacement in doses sufficient to suppress TSH levels to low normal (Chapter 233).
Infertility	ABVD is not known to cause permanent gonadal toxicity, although temporary oligospermia or irregular menses may persist for 1 to 2 years after treatment. Direct or scatter radiation to gonadal tissue may cause infertility, amenorrhea, or premature menopause, but this adverse event seldom occurs with the current fields used for the treatment of Hodgkin's lymphoma. In general, women who continue menstruating are fertile, but men require semen analysis to provide a specific answer.
Secondary neoplasms	Although uncommon, certain secondary neoplasms occur with increased frequency in patients who have been treated for Hodgkin's lymphoma: acute myelogenous leukemia; thyroid, breast, lung, cervical, and upper gastrointestinal carcinoma; and melanoma. It is appropriate to "be vigilant" for these neoplasms for the remainder of the patient's life because they may have a lengthy induction period.

ABVD = doxorubicin (Adriamycin), bleomycin, vinblastine, and dacarbazine; TSH = thyroid-stimulating hormone.

cells, such as those coupling an antibody to the CD30 antigen with a cellular toxin, hold substantial promise to improve treatment outcome.

 Grade A

1. Engert A, Schiller P, Josting A, et al. Involved-field radiotherapy is equally effective and less toxic compared with extended-field radiotherapy after four cycles of chemotherapy in patients with early-stage unfavorable Hodgkin's lymphoma: results of the HD8 trials of the German Hodgkin's Lymphoma Study Group. *J Clin Oncol.* 2003;21:3601-3608.
2. Bonadonna G, Bonfante V, Viviani S, et al. ABVD plus subtotal nodal versus involved-field radiotherapy in early-stage Hodgkin's disease: long-term results. *J Clin Oncol.* 2004;22:2835-2841.
3. Engert A, Plütschow A, Eich HT, et al. Reduced treatment intensity in patients with early-stage Hodgkin's lymphoma. *N Engl J Med.* 2010;363:640-652.
4. Meyer RM, Gospodarowicz MK, Connors JM, et al. Randomized comparison of ABVD chemotherapy with a strategy that includes radiation therapy in patients with limited-stage Hodgkin's lymphoma: National Cancer Institute of Canada Clinical Trials Group and the Eastern Cooperative Oncology Group. *J Clin Oncol.* 2005;23:4634-4642.
5. Hoskin PJ, Lowry L, Horwich A, et al. Randomized comparison of the Stanford V regimen and ABVD in the treatment of advanced Hodgkin's Lymphoma: United Kingdom National Cancer Research Institute Lymphoma Group Study ISRCTN 64141244. *J Clin Oncol.* 2009;27:5390-5396.
6. Engert A, Diehl V, Franklin J, et al. Escalated-dose BEACOPP in the treatment of patients with advanced-stage Hodgkin's lymphoma: 10 years of follow-up of the GHSG HD9 study. *J Clin Oncol.* 2009;27:4548-4554.
7. Schmitz N, Pfistner B, Sextro M, et al. Aggressive conventional chemotherapy compared with high-dose chemotherapy with autologous haemopoietic stem-cell transplantation for relapsed chemosensitive Hodgkin's disease: a randomised trial. *Lancet.* 2002;359:2065-2071.
8. Federico M, Bellei M, Brice P, et al. High-dose therapy and autologous stem-cell transplantation versus conventional therapy for patients with advanced Hodgkin's lymphoma responding to front-line therapy. *J Clin Oncol.* 2003;21:2320-2325.

SUGGESTED READINGS

Armitage JO. Current concepts: early-stage Hodgkin's lymphoma. *N Engl J Med.* 2010;363:653-662. Review.
Farrell K, Jarrett RF. The molecular pathogenesis of Hodgkin lymphoma. *Histopathology.* 2011;58:15-25. Review.
Punnett A, Tsang RW, Hodgson DC. Hodgkin lymphoma across the age spectrum: epidemiology, therapy, and late effects. *Semin Radiat Oncol.* 2010;20:30-44. *Differences in epidemiology, disease biology, and new approaches to prognostic and therapeutic stratification in light of the strong age gradient that exists with respect to patient outcomes in Hodgkin's lymphoma.*
Steidl C, Lee T, Shah SP, et al. Tumor-associated macrophages and survival in classic Hodgkin's lymphoma. *N Engl J Med.* 2010;362:875-885. *Histochemical assessment of tumor-infiltrating macrophages strongly predicts outcome.*

Patients are prone to opportunistic infections, and the interaction of chemotherapeutic agents with other medications may compromise the patient's ability to tolerate treatment. The best approach is a combination of highly active antiretroviral agents (Chapter 396), vigorous supportive care with antiherpetic and antifungal agents and neutrophil-stimulating growth factors, and standard multiagent chemotherapy. With appropriate supportive care, regimens such as ABVD can be delivered. However, more severe than normal toxicity must be anticipated, and cure rates are much lower than in the non-HIV-infected population. Median survival is typically 3 to 4 years.

Hodgkin's Lymphoma in the Elderly Population

Elderly patients with Hodgkin's lymphoma have a worse outcome. For example, the 5-year overall survival rate falls from 80% in patients younger than 65 years to less than 50% in patients older than 65 years. Explanations include more advanced stage at diagnosis, comorbid diseases, delay in diagnosis, incomplete staging, inadequate adherence to treatment protocols, and failure to maintain full dose intensity.

Of note is that elderly patients achieve outcomes equivalent to those of younger patients when they receive similar doses of chemotherapy. The best approach for elderly patients is to attempt to treat them in a manner similar to younger patients, with vigorous supportive care and the addition of neutrophil growth factors if necessary to enable safe delivery of full doses. For patients with preexisting pulmonary or cardiac disease, it might be necessary to reduce or eliminate bleomycin or doxorubicin, respectively.

FUTURE DIRECTIONS

The ability to profile multigene expression patterns and identify genetic polymorphisms associated with specific malignancies may provide better insight into the molecular genesis of Hodgkin's and other lymphomas. Therapeutic agents more specifically targeted at the malignant Hodgkin-Reed-Sternberg

193

PLASMA CELL DISORDERS

S. VINCENT RAJKUMAR

INTRODUCTION

Plasma cell disorders are neoplastic or potentially neoplastic diseases associated with the clonal proliferation of immunoglobulin-secreting plasma cells (Table 193-1). They are characterized by the secretion of electrophoretically and immunologically homogeneous (monoclonal) proteins that represent intact or incomplete immunoglobulin molecules. Monoclonal proteins are commonly referred to as M proteins, myeloma proteins, or paraproteins.

Syndromes associated with plasma cell disorders and monoclonal proteins include monoclonal gammopathy of undetermined significance, multiple myeloma, Waldenström's macroglobulinemia, cryoglobulinemia, and primary amyloidosis (see Table 193-1). Occasionally, free hemoglobin-haptoglobin complexes resulting from hemolysis, large amounts of transferrin in patients with iron deficiency anemia, or increased levels of fibrinogen may simulate the presence of a monoclonal protein in serum.

Serum Immunoglobulins

Intact immunoglobulins consist of two heavy (H) polypeptide chains of the same class and subclass and two light (L) polypeptide chains of the same type (Chapter 44). The heavy polypeptide chains are designated by Greek letters: γ in immunoglobulin G (IgG), α in immunoglobulin A (IgA), μ in immunoglobulin M (IgM), δ in immunoglobulin D (IgD), and ϵ in immunoglobulin E (IgE). The light chain types are kappa (κ) and lambda (λ). Both heavy

TABLE 193-1 PLASMA CELL PROLIFERATIVE DISORDERS

I. Premalignant monoclonal gammopathies
   A. Monoclonal gammopathy of undetermined significance (MGUS)
   B. MGUS in association with chronic lymphocytic leukemia and non-Hodgkin's lymphoma
   C. Biclonal and triclonal gammopathies of undetermined significance
   D. Idiopathic Bence Jones proteinuria and light chain MGUS
   E. Smoldering multiple myeloma
II. Malignant monoclonal gammopathies
   A. Multiple myeloma and related malignancies (IgG, IgA, IgD, IgE, and free light chains)
     1. Symptomatic multiple myeloma
     2. Plasma cell leukemia
     3. Osteosclerotic myeloma (including POEMS syndrome)
     4. Solitary plasmacytoma of bone
     5. Solitary extramedullary plasmacytoma
   B. Waldenström's macroglobulinemia (IgM)
III. Heavy chain diseases (HCDs)
   A. γ-HCD
   B. α-HCD
   C. μ-HCD
IV. Cryoglobulinemia (types I, II, and III)
V. Immunoglobulin light chain amyloidosis

Ig = immunoglobulin; POEMS = polyneuropathy, organomegaly, endocrinopathy, M protein, and skin changes.

chains and light chains have "constant" and "variable" regions with respect to the amino acid sequence. The class specificity of each immunoglobulin is defined by a series of antigenic determinants on the constant regions of the heavy chains (γ, α, μ, δ, and ε) and the two major classes of light chains (κ and λ). The amino acid sequence in the variable regions of the immunoglobulin molecule corresponds to the active antigen-combining site of the antibody.

In the majority of clonal plasma cell disorders, intact immunoglobulin molecules are secreted as monoclonal (M) proteins. In some patients, however, heavy chain expression is completely lost, and only monoclonal light chains (Bence Jones proteins) are secreted. Even less frequently, only heavy chains are secreted, resulting in heavy chain diseases (HCDs). Rare patients with multiple myeloma secrete no identifiable immunoglobulin ("nonsecretory myeloma").

Identification of Monoclonal Proteins

Protein electrophoresis of the serum and urine detects M protein as a narrow peak (like a church spire) on the densitometer tracing or as a dense, discrete band on agarose gel (Fig. 193-1). Electrophoresis also permits quantitation of M proteins. Monoclonal light chains (Bence Jones proteinemia) are rarely seen on serum electrophoresis but are easily detected on urine electrophoresis. Urine electrophoresis requires a 24-hour urine collection.

Immunofixation of the serum and urine is performed when a peak or band is first seen on protein electrophoresis to identify the heavy and light chain type of the M protein. Immunofixation is also a more sensitive test than protein electrophoresis, and it should always be performed in conjunction with electrophoresis when multiple myeloma or related disorders are first suspected in order to detect small, unmeasurable M proteins that may be missed on electrophoresis. This is particularly important in oligosecretory myeloma, primary amyloidosis, and solitary plasmacytoma and after successful treatment of multiple myeloma or macroglobulinemia. In these instances, a small M protein can be concealed in the normal β or γ areas of the electrophoresis gel and may be overlooked. In 5% of patients there is an additional M protein of a different immunoglobulin class; this condition is designated a biclonal gammopathy.

In some patients the M protein has specificity to one of the various antigens. Examples include actin, dextran, antistreptolysin O, antinuclear antibody, riboflavin, von Willebrand's factor, thyroglobulin, insulin, double-stranded DNA, and apolipoprotein. Binding of calcium by an M protein may produce hypercalcemia without symptomatic or pathologic consequences. M proteins have also been found to bind to copper and to phosphate.

Monoclonal proteins must be distinguished from an excess of polyclonal immunoglobulins (one or more heavy chain types and both κ and λ light chains, usually limited to the γ region), which produce a broad-based peak or broad band (Fig. 193-2). This finding is associated with chronic infectious or inflammatory states.

FIGURE 193-1. Serum protein electrophoresis showing a monoclonal (M) protein. **A,** Monoclonal pattern of serum protein as traced by a densitometer after electrophoresis on agarose gel: tall, narrow-based peak of γ mobility. **B,** Monoclonal pattern from electrophoresis of serum on agarose gel (anode on the left): dense, localized band representing monoclonal protein of γ mobility. (From Kyle RA, Katzmann JA. Immunochemical characterization of immunoglobulins. In: Rose NR, Conway de Macario E, Folds JD, et al, eds. *Manual of Clinical Laboratory Immunology*, 5th ed. Washington, DC: ASM Press; 1997:156, with permission of the American Society for Microbiology.)

FIGURE 193-2. Serum protein electrophoresis showing increased polyclonal immunoglobulins. **A,** Polyclonal pattern from a densitometer tracing of agarose gel: broad-based peak of γ mobility. **B,** Polyclonal pattern from electrophoresis of agarose gel (anode on the left). The band at the right is broad and extends throughout the γ area. (From Kyle RA, Katzmann JA. Immunochemical characterization of immunoglobulins. In: Rose NR, Conway de Macario E, Folds JD, et al, eds. *Manual of Clinical Laboratory Immunology*, 5th ed. Washington, DC: ASM Press; 1997:156, with permission of the American Society for Microbiology.)

Detection of Serum Free Light Chains

The serum free light chain assay measures the level of free κ and λ immunoglobulin light chains (i.e., light chains that are not bound to intact immunoglobulin). An abnormal κ/λ free light chain ratio (normal range, 0.26 to 1.65) indicates an excess of one light chain type versus the other and is interpreted as representing a monoclonal elevation of the corresponding light chain type. The serum free light chain assay is more sensitive than electrophoresis or immunofixation in detecting free monoclonal light chains and is useful in the diagnostic evaluation of plasma cell disorders and in risk stratification.

⬤ MONOCLONAL GAMMOPATHY OF UNDETERMINED SIGNIFICANCE

DEFINITION

Monoclonal gammopathy of undetermined significance (MGUS; formerly called *benign monoclonal gammopathy*) is a premalignant clonal plasma cell

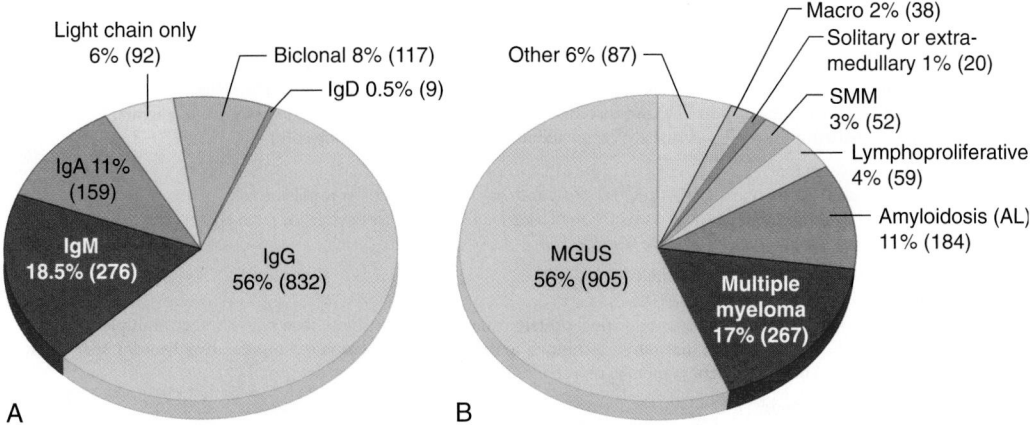

Monoclonal Serum Proteins
Mayo Clinic 2008 n=1485

Light chain only
6% (92)

Biclonal 8% (117)

IgD 0.5% (9)

IgA 11%
(159)

IgM
18.5% (276)

IgG
56% (832)

A

Monoclonal Gammopathies
Mayo Clinic 2008 n=1612

Other 6% (87)

Macro 2% (38)

Solitary or extra-
medullary 1% (20)

SMM
3% (52)

Lymphoproliferative
4% (59)

Amyloidosis (AL)
11% (184)

MGUS
56% (905)

Multiple
myeloma
17% (267)

B

FIGURE 193-3. Monoclonal gammopathy. **A,** Distribution of serum monoclonal proteins in 1485 patients seen at the Mayo Clinic during 2008. **B,** Diagnoses in 1612 cases of monoclonal gammopathy seen at the Mayo Clinic during 2008. Ig = immunoglobulin; Macro = Waldenström's macroglobulinemia; MGUS = monoclonal gammopathy of undetermined significance; SMM = smoldering multiple myeloma.

disorder characterized by the presence of a serum M protein in persons who lack evidence of multiple myeloma, macroglobulinemia, amyloidosis, or other related diseases. MGUS is defined by a serum M protein concentration lower than 3 g/dL, less than 10% clonal plasma cells in the bone marrow, and absence of lytic bone lesions, anemia, hypercalcemia, and renal insufficiency that can be attributed to a plasma cell disorder. The main clinical significance of MGUS is its lifelong risk of transformation to myeloma or related malignancy at a fixed but unrelenting rate of 1% per year.

EPIDEMIOLOGY

More than 50% of patients in whom a serum M protein is detected have MGUS (Fig. 193-3). The prevalence of MGUS in the general population increases with age, from approximately 1% in persons 50 to 60 years old to greater than 5% in those older than 70 years. The age-adjusted prevalence is higher in males than in females and is twice as high in blacks compared with whites.

PATHOBIOLOGY

MGUS represents a limited, nonmalignant expansion of monoclonal plasma cells. The etiology of MGUS is unknown, but age, male gender, family history, immunosuppression, and exposure to certain pesticides are known risk factors. It is hypothesized that infection, inflammation, or other antigenic stimuli, acting in concert with the development of cytogenetic abnormalities in the plasma cells, are the initiating pathogenetic events in most patients. Approximately 50% of MGUS is associated with plasma cell translocations involving the immunoglobulin heavy chain (IgH) locus on chromosome 14q32 (IgH translocated MGUS). These primary IgH translocations commonly involve one of five recurrent partner chromosome loci: 11q13 (CCND1 [cyclin D1 gene]), 4p16.3 (FGFR-3 and MMSET), 6p21 (CCND3 [cyclin D3 gene]), 16q23 (c-maf), and 20q11 (mafB). The remaining 50% lack IgH translocations but are usually associated with hyperdiploidy (hyperdiploid MGUS).

CLINICAL MANIFESTATIONS

MGUS is asymptomatic and is usually diagnosed incidentally on laboratory testing. Patients with MGUS progress to multiple myeloma or related malignancy at a rate of approximately 1% per year. The interval from the time of recognition of the M protein to the diagnosis of serious disease ranges from 1 to 32 years (median, 10.6 years), and the relative risk versus a control population is 25.0 for progression to multiple myeloma, 8.4 for primary amyloidosis, 46.0 for Waldenström's macroglobulinemia, 2.4 for the development of other forms of non-Hodgkin's lymphoma, and 8.5 for plasmacytoma. The relative risk for chronic lymphocytic leukemia (CLL) is not increased. In addition, in a small percentage of patients, the M protein level increases to greater than 3 g/dL and/or the percentage of plasma cells in bone marrow increases to more than 10% without progression to overt myeloma or a related disorder (smoldering multiple myeloma).

DIAGNOSIS

MGUS is differentiated from multiple myeloma and smoldering multiple myeloma by the size of the M protein, the bone marrow plasma cell percentage, and the presence or absence of anemia, renal failure, hypercalcemia, or lytic bone lesions (Table 193-2). Because anemia and renal insufficiency are relatively common in the elderly population with MGUS, the causes of these conditions should be carefully investigated with adequate laboratory studies. For example, in a patient with anemia, tests to exclude iron, vitamin B_{12}, or folate deficiency must be performed. In certain instances, such as unexplained renal failure, a renal biopsy may be needed. Only patients with strong evidence of end-organ damage thought to be directly related to a plasma cell disorder can be considered to have myeloma or a related malignancy.

Levels of the immunoglobulin classes other than M protein (i.e., the normal polyclonal or background immunoglobulins) are generally reduced in multiple myeloma or Waldenström's macroglobulinemia, but a reduction also occurs in almost 40% of patients with MGUS. The presence of osteolytic lesions strongly suggests multiple myeloma, but metastatic carcinoma may produce lytic lesions as well as polyclonal plasmacytosis and must be differentiated from MGUS.

Association of MGUS with Other Diseases

MGUS is associated with numerous diseases. However, because 3% of the general population older than 50 years has MGUS, it is often difficult to determine whether these reported associations are causal or coincidental. Some associations have been verified based on epidemiologic studies; these include peripheral neuropathy (Chapter 428), deep vein thrombosis (Chapter 81), osteoporosis (Chapter 251), and lymphoproliferative disorders (Chapter 191). A secondary form of MGUS also occurs with immunosuppression after organ transplantation (Chapter 48) and autologous or allogeneic stem cell transplantation (Chapter 181). M proteins also occur in the sera of some patients with CLL (Chapter 190) but have no recognizable effect on the clinical course.

Approximately 5% of patients with sensorimotor peripheral neuropathy of unknown cause (Chapter 428) have an associated monoclonal gammopathy (MGUS-associated neuropathy). In half of such patients, the M protein binds to myelin-associated glycoprotein. These patients have a slowly progressive sensory neuropathy more than motor neuropathy, beginning in the distal ends of the extremities and extending proximally. The clinical and electrodiagnostic manifestations of MGUS neuropathy resemble those of a chronic inflammatory demyelinating polyneuropathy. A causal relationship is usually assumed in younger patients and those without other conditions known to cause neuropathy in whom the neuropathy is severe and progressive. Therapeutic approaches include plasmapheresis and, occasionally, chemotherapy (similar to myeloma for IgG or IgA monoclonal proteins, and rituximab or chlorambucil for IgM monoclonal proteins; see the later section on the treatment of multiple myeloma).

TABLE 193-2 CRITERIA FOR THE DIAGNOSIS OF PLASMA CELL DISORDERS

DISORDER	DISEASE DEFINITION
Monoclonal gammopathy of undetermined significance (MGUS)	All 3 criteria must be met: 1. Serum monoclonal protein (IgG, IgA, or IgM) <3 g/dL 2. Clonal bone marrow plasma cells <10% 3. Absence of end-organ damage such as hypercalcemia, renal insufficiency, anemia, and bone lesions that can be attributed to the plasma cell proliferative disorder (or, in the case of IgM MGUS, no evidence of anemia, constitutional symptoms, hyperviscosity, lymphadenopathy, or hepatosplenomegaly)
Smoldering multiple myeloma (also referred to as *asymptomatic multiple myeloma*)	Both criteria must be met: 1. Serum monoclonal protein (IgG or IgA) ≥3 g/dL and/or clonal bone marrow plasma cells ≥10% 2. Absence of end-organ damage such as lytic bone lesions, anemia, hypercalcemia, or renal failure that can be attributed to a plasma cell proliferative disorder
Multiple myeloma	All 3 criteria must be met, except as noted: 1. Clonal bone marrow plasma cells ≥10% 2. Presence of serum and/or urinary monoclonal protein (except in patients with true nonsecretory multiple myeloma) 3. Evidence of end-organ damage that can be attributed to the underlying plasma cell proliferative disorder, specifically hypercalcemia, renal insufficiency, anemia, or bone lesions
Waldenström's macroglobulinemia	Both criteria must be met: 1. IgM monoclonal gammopathy (regardless of the size of the M protein) 2. >10% bone marrow lymphoplasmacytic infiltration (usually intertrabecular) by small lymphocytes that exhibit plasmacytoid or plasma cell differentiation and a typical immunophenotype (surface IgM$^+$, CD5$^{+/-}$, CD10$^-$, CD19$^+$, CD20$^+$, CD23$^-$) that satisfactorily excludes other lymphoproliferative disorders, including chronic lymphocytic leukemia and mantle cell lymphoma
Smoldering Waldenström's macroglobulinemia (also referred to as *indolent* or *asymptomatic Waldenström's macroglobulinemia*)	1. Serum IgM monoclonal protein ≥3 g/dL and/or bone marrow lymphoplasmacytic infiltration ≥10% 2. No evidence of end-organ damage such as anemia, constitutional symptoms, hyperviscosity, lymphadenopathy, or hepatosplenomegaly that can be attributed to a lymphoplasma cell proliferative disorder
Solitary plasmacytoma	All 4 criteria must be met: 1. Biopsy-proven solitary lesion of bone or soft tissue with evidence of clonal plasma cells 2. Normal bone marrow with no evidence of clonal plasma cells 3. Normal skeletal survey and MRI of spine and pelvis (except for the primary solitary lesion) 4. Absence of end-organ damage such as hypercalcemia, renal insufficiency, anemia, or bone lesions that can be attributed to a plasma cell proliferative disorder
POEMS syndrome	All 4 criteria must be met: 1. Presence of a monoclonal plasma cell disorder (almost always *λ*-type) 2. Peripheral neuropathy 3. Any one of the following 3 major features: sclerotic bone lesions, Castleman's disease, elevated levels of vascular endothelial growth factor (VEGF) 4. Any one of the following 6 minor features: organomegaly, edema, endocrinopathy (excluding diabetes mellitus or hypothyroidism), typical skin changes, papilledema, thrombocytosis, polycythemia The features should have a temporal relationship to one another, with no other attributable cause

Modified from Rajkumar SV, Dispenzieri A, Kyle RA. Monoclonal gammopathy of undetermined significance, Waldenstrom macroglobulinemia, AL amyloidosis, and related plasma cell disorders: diagnosis and treatment. *Mayo Clin Proc.* 2006;81:693-703; and Kyle RA, Rajkumar SV. Criteria for diagnosis, staging, risk stratification and response assessment of multiple myeloma. *Leukemia.* 2009;23:3-9.

Certain skin disorders are known to be associated with MGUS. Lichen myxedematosus (papular mucinosis, scleromyxedema) is associated with a cathodal IgG γ protein. Pyoderma gangrenosum and necrobiotic xanthogranuloma are other associated skin disorders.

PREVENTION AND TREATMENT   Rx

No treatment is necessary for MGUS. Low-risk patients (Table 193-3) can be evaluated when symptoms suggestive of myeloma or related disorders occur. In all other patients with MGUS, the M protein level in serum and urine should be measured serially, together with periodic reevaluation of clinical and other laboratory findings, to determine whether multiple myeloma or another related disorder is present. In general, electrophoresis, complete blood count, and creatinine and calcium levels should be repeated at 6 months and, if stable, yearly thereafter.

PROGNOSIS

Differentiating a patient with MGUS in whom the disorder will remain stable for life from one in whom multiple myeloma, macroglobulinemia, or a related disorder will eventually develop is difficult when the M protein is first recognized. The size and type of the M protein at diagnosis of MGUS and an abnormal serum free light chain ratio are prognostic factors for progression (see Table 193-3).

● BICLONAL GAMMOPATHIES

Biclonal gammopathies occur in at least 5% of patients with clonal plasma cell disorders. A biclonal gammopathy of undetermined significance (analogous to MGUS) accounts for about two thirds of such patients. The remainder have multiple myeloma, macroglobulinemia, or other lymphoproliferative diseases. Rarely, triclonal gammopathies may occur.

● LIGHT CHAIN MGUS AND IDIOPATHIC BENCE JONES PROTEINURIA

The diagnosis of typical MGUS requires expression of an intact heavy chain type. In some patients a premalignant clonal plasma cell disorder characterized by the presence of monoclonal immunoglobulin light chains without expression of heavy chains can occur (light chain MGUS). Some patients with light chain MGUS may secrete adequate amounts of monoclonal light chains in the urine, resulting in idiopathic Bence Jones proteinuria. Idiopathic Bence Jones proteinuria is analogous to MGUS, and the urinary excretion of monoclonal light chains can persist for many years without evidence of end-organ damage suggestive of multiple myeloma or related disorders. No therapy is indicated unless progression to malignancy occurs.

● MULTIPLE MYELOMA

DEFINITION

Multiple myeloma is a malignancy of plasma cells characterized by bone marrow infiltration and extensive skeletal destruction resulting in anemia, bone pain, and fractures. Multiple myeloma (commonly referred to as *myeloma*) is defined by the presence of 10% or more clonal plasma cells on bone marrow examination, M protein in serum or urine (except in the case of nonsecretory myeloma), and evidence of hypercalcemia, renal insufficiency, anemia, or bone lesions thought to be related to the plasma cell proliferative disorder. Patients with multiple myeloma must be differentiated from those with MGUS and smoldering multiple myeloma (see Table 193-2).

TABLE 193-3 RISK OF PROGRESSION OF MONOCLONAL GAMMOPATHY OF UNDETERMINED SIGNIFICANCE TO MYELOMA OR RELATED DISORDERS

RISK GROUP	RELATIVE RISK	CUMULATIVE ABSOLUTE RISK OF PROGRESSION AT 20 YEARS (%)*	CUMULATIVE ABSOLUTE RISK OF PROGRESSION AT 20 YEARS ACCOUNTING FOR DEATH AS A COMPETING RISK (%)†
Low risk: serum M protein <1.5 g/dL, IgG subtype, normal free light chain ratio (0.26-1.65)	1	5	2
Low-intermediate risk: any 1 factor abnormal	5.4	21	10
High-intermediate risk: any 2 factors abnormal	10.1	37	18
High risk: all 3 factors abnormal	20.8	58	27

*Estimates in this column represent the risk of progression assuming that patients do not die of other causes during this period.
†Estimates in this column represent the risk of progression calculated by using a model that accounts for the fact that patients can die of unrelated causes during this time.
Ig = immunoglobulin.
Adapted from Rajkumar SV, Kyle RA, Therneau TM, et al. Serum free light chain ratio is an independent risk factor for progression in monoclonal gammopathy of undetermined significance (MGUS). *Blood.* 2005;106:812-817. © The American Society of Hematology.

EPIDEMIOLOGY

Multiple myeloma accounts for 1% of all malignant disease and slightly more than 10% of hematologic malignancies in the United States. The annual incidence of multiple myeloma is 4 per 100,000. Its incidence in blacks is almost twice that in whites. Multiple myeloma is slightly more common in men than in women. The median age of patients at the time of diagnosis is about 65 years; only 2% of patients are younger than 40.

PATHOBIOLOGY

The cause of multiple myeloma is unclear. Exposure to radiation, benzene, and other organic solvents, herbicides, and insecticides may play a role. Multiple myeloma has been reported in familial clusters of two or more first-degree relatives and in identical twins.

Almost all cases of myeloma evolve from a premalignant MGUS phase, although the MGUS is clinically recognized before the diagnosis of myeloma in only a small minority of patients. The progression of MGUS to myeloma suggests a simple, random, two-hit genetic model of malignancy in which the risk of progression is fixed (approximately 1% per year) regardless of the duration of MGUS. Unfortunately, the precise mechanisms of progression are unknown, although several potentially pathogenetic abnormalities have been described in the clonal plasma cells. These include *RAS* and *p53* mutations, p16 methylation, *MYC* abnormalities, and secondary translocations. Changes in the bone marrow microenvironment may also play a role in the pathogenesis, including induction of angiogenesis and abnormal paracrine loops involving cytokines such as interleukin-6 (IL-6), which serves as a major growth factor for plasma cells.

The lytic bone lesions, osteopenia, hypercalcemia, and pathologic fractures in patients with myeloma are a result of abnormal osteoclast activity induced by the neoplastic plasma cells, as well as inhibition of osteoblast differentiation. Osteoclasts are activated by stimulation of the transmembrane receptor RANK (receptor activator of nuclear factor κB), which belongs to the tumor necrosis factor (TNF) receptor superfamily. The ligand for this receptor (RANKL) also has a decoy receptor, osteoprotegerin (OPG). In myeloma, there is an increase in RANKL expression by osteoblasts (and possibly plasma cells), accompanied by a reduction in the level of OPG. The resultant increase in the RANKL/OPG ratio causes osteoclast activation and increased bone resorption and turnover (Chapter 250).

Cytogenetic Abnormalities

As discussed earlier (see Pathobiology of MGUS), primary translocations involving the immunoglobulin heavy chain loci (chromosome 14q32) are seen in up to 50% of patients with multiple myeloma (IgH-translocated or nonhyperdiploid myeloma). The remaining 50% of patients do not have IgH translocations but have evidence of hyperdiploidy (hyperdiploid myeloma). In a small percentage of patients the disease cannot be classified into either of these two types (unclassified). Besides these cytogenetic abnormalities, other secondary cytogenetic abnormalities occur as late events during the course of symptomatic myeloma; these include activating mutations of N- and K-RAS, inactivating mutations of *p53*, and dysregulation of c-MYC. Complete or partial deletions of chromosome 13 are well described in myeloma and have prognostic value, but they also occur at the MGUS stage.

TABLE 193-4 MAJOR CLINICAL MANIFESTATIONS OF MULTIPLE MYELOMA

CLINICAL FINDINGS	APPROXIMATE PERCENTAGE OF PATIENTS WITH ABNORMALITY AT DIAGNOSIS
Skeletal involvement: pain, reduced height, lytic bone lesions, pathologic fractures	80
Anemia (hemoglobin ≤12 g/dL): caused mainly by decreased erythropoiesis; produces weakness and fatigue	75
Renal insufficiency (serum creatinine ≥2 mg/dL): caused mainly by "myeloma kidney" from light chains or hypercalcemia, rarely from amyloidosis	20
Hypercalcemia (≥11 mg/dL)	15
Light chain amyloidosis	10
Evidence of monoclonal protein by immunofixation and serum free light chain assay	97
Evidence of clonal plasma cells ≥10% in bone marrow	96

CLINICAL MANIFESTATIONS

History

Bone pain, particularly in the back or chest and less often in the extremities, is present at the time of diagnosis in more than two thirds of patients (Table 193-4). The patient's height may be reduced by several inches because of vertebral collapse. Weakness and fatigue are common and are often associated with anemia. Fever is rare and, when present, is generally from an infection; in some patients the infection itself is the initial feature. Other symptoms may result from renal insufficiency, hypercalcemia, nephrotic syndrome, radiculopathy, or amyloidosis (Chapter 194).

Physical Examination

Pallor is the most frequent physical finding. The liver is palpable in about 5% of patients, and the spleen in 1%. Tenderness may be noted at sites of bone involvement. Radiculopathy may be caused by spinal compression fractures. Occasionally, extramedullary plasmacytomas are palpable.

DIAGNOSIS

Laboratory Findings

A normocytic, normochromic anemia (Chapter 161) is present initially in approximately 75% of patients, but it eventually occurs in nearly every patient with multiple myeloma. Serum protein electrophoresis shows an M protein in 80% of patients. With serum immunofixation, an M protein can be detected in 93% of patients. When these serum studies are combined with urine electrophoresis plus immunofixation, an M protein can be detected in 97% of patients with myeloma. The serum free light chain assay is more convenient and can be used in place of urine studies in the diagnostic evaluation. The

FIGURE 193-4. Multiple myeloma. A bone marrow aspirate shows a predominance of plasma cells.

FIGURE 193-5. Skull radiograph showing multiple lytic lesions.

type of M protein is IgG in 52%, IgA in 21%, light chain only (Bence Jones proteinemia) in 16%, IgD in 2%, and biclonal gammopathy in 2%; the light chain type is κ in 65% of cases and λ in 35%. In 3% of patients, no secreted M protein can be identified; these patients are considered to have nonsecretory myeloma.

In the bone marrow, plasma cells account for greater than 10% of all nucleated cells in 96% of patients (Fig. 193-4). In 4% of patients, bone marrow examination shows less than 10% plasma cells, even though the patient otherwise meets the criteria for myeloma; because bone marrow involvement in myeloma may be focal rather than diffuse, repeated bone marrow examinations or biopsy of a discrete bone or extramedullary lesion may be required. In most cases, the plasma cells in myeloma are cytoplasmic Ig⁺, CD38⁺, and CD138⁺; only a minority express CD10 and human leukocyte antigen (HLA)-DR, and 20% express CD20. The clonality of the plasma cells is established using the κ/λ ratio, which is abnormal in myeloma (either >4 : 1, indicating a clonal κ population, or <1 : 2, indicating a clonal λ population). This is helpful for differentiating monoclonal plasma cell proliferation in multiple myeloma from reactive plasmacytosis related to connective tissue disease, metastatic carcinoma, liver disease, and infection.

Radiologic Findings

Conventional radiographs reveal abnormalities consisting of punched-out lytic lesions (Fig. 193-5), osteoporosis, or fractures in nearly 80% of patients. The vertebrae, skull, thoracic cage, pelvis, and proximal ends of the humerus and femur are the most frequent sites of involvement. Technetium-99m bone scanning is inferior to conventional radiography and should not be used. Positron emission tomography (PET; Fig. 193-6) and magnetic resonance imaging (MRI) are helpful in patients who have skeletal pain but no abnormality on radiographs and for monitoring the response to therapy.

Organ Involvement

Renal

At diagnosis, the serum creatinine value is increased initially in almost half of patients and is greater than 2 mg/dL in 20%.

The two major causes of renal insufficiency are light chain cast nephropathy (*myeloma kidney*) and hypercalcemia. Light chain cast nephropathy is characterized by the presence of large, waxy, laminated casts in the distal and collecting tubules. The casts are composed mainly of precipitated monoclonal light chains. The extent of cast formation correlates directly with the amount of free urinary light chain and with the severity of renal insufficiency. Dehydration may precipitate acute renal failure.

Hypercalcemia (Chapters 186 and 253), which is present in 15 to 20% of patients initially, is a major and treatable cause of renal insufficiency. It results from destruction of bone. Hyperuricemia may contribute to renal failure. Besides light chain cast nephropathy and hypercalcemia, there are other mechanisms by which renal dysfunction can occur in myeloma. For example, light chain amyloidosis occurs in nearly 10% of patients and may produce nephrotic syndrome, renal insufficiency, or both. Acquired Fanconi's syndrome (Chapter 124), characterized by proximal tubular dysfunction, results in glycosuria, phosphaturia, and aminoaciduria. Deposition of monoclonal light chains in the renal glomerulus (light chain deposition disease) may also produce renal insufficiency and nephrotic syndrome.

Neurologic

Radiculopathy (Chapter 407), the single most frequent neurologic complication, usually occurs in the thoracic or lumbosacral area and results from compression of the nerve by the vertebral lesion or by the collapsed bone

FIGURE 193-6. Positron emission tomography in multiple myeloma. **A,** Extensive bony and extramedullary disease. **B,** Significant improvement after systemic chemotherapy for myeloma.

itself. Compression of the spinal cord occurs in up to 10% of patients. Peripheral neuropathy (Chapter 428) is uncommon in multiple myeloma and, when present, is generally caused by amyloidosis. Rarely, myeloma cells diffusely infiltrate the meninges. Intracranial plasmacytomas almost always represent extensions of myelomatous lesions of the skull.

Other Systemic Involvement

Hepatomegaly from plasma cell infiltration is uncommon. Plasmacytomas of the ribs are common and arise either as expanding bone lesions or as soft tissue masses. The incidence of infections is increased in patients with multiple myeloma. Historically, *Streptococcus pneumoniae* and *Staphylococcus aureus* have been the most frequent pathogens, but gram-negative organisms now account for more than half of all infections. The propensity for infection results from impairment of the antibody response, deficiency of normal immunoglobulins, and neutropenia. Bleeding from coating of the platelets by M protein may occur. Myeloma patients have an increased risk of deep vein thrombosis.

PREVENTION AND TREATMENT   **Rx**

Patients with MGUS or smoldering multiple myeloma should not be treated until evidence of multiple myeloma develops. The approach to treatment of multiple myeloma is illustrated in Figure 193-7.

FIGURE 193-7. Approach to newly diagnosed multiple myeloma.

Initial Therapy of Patients Who Are Candidates for Stem Cell Transplantation

In the approximately 50% of patients with newly diagnosed multiple myeloma who are considered candidates for autologous stem cell transplantation based on good performance status, no or limited comorbid conditions, and younger physiologic age (<65 to 70 years), autologous peripheral blood stem cell transplantation (Chapter 181) with high-dose chemotherapy improves overall survival in comparison to conventional chemotherapy.[1] Currently, it is not possible to eradicate myeloma cells completely with conditioning regimens, and reinfused autologous stem cells are usually contaminated by myeloma cells or their precursors. As a result, autologous transplantation is not curative, but it prolongs event-free and overall survival.

Initial therapy typically consists of low-dose dexamethasone (40 mg once a week) plus lenalidomide (25 mg/day on days 1 to 21, every 28 days) and/or bortezomib (1.3 mg/m² on days 1, 4, 8, and 11, every 21 days) for approximately 4 months to reduce the number of tumor cells in the bone marrow and peripheral blood. As induction before stem cell transplantation in previously untreated myeloma, bortezomib plus dexamethasone has been found to be superior to vincristine plus doxorubicin plus dexamethasone (VAD).[2] Lenalidomide plus high-dose dexamethasone, compared with high-dose dexamethasone only, produced superior 1-year progression-free survival, overall and partial response rates, but not 1-year overall survival.[3] In a randomized trial, lenalidomide plus low-dose dexamethasone (40 mg once a week) was associated with superior overall survival compared with lenalidomide and high-dose dexamethasone (40 mg on days 1 to 4, 9 to 12, and 17 to 20).[4] As a result, high-dose pulse dexamethasone is no longer recommended in the context of initial therapy. Reducing the dose of bortezomib to once a week instead of days 1, 4, 8, and 11 decreases the risk of serious neuropathy and should be considered after the first 1 to 2 months if a bortezomib-based regimen is used.[5] Toxicities of lenalidomide plus dexamethasone include deep vein thrombosis, and all patients must be treated with prophylactic aspirin or an anticoagulant. After induction therapy, peripheral blood stem cells adequate for two stem cell transplants are collected with the use of granulocyte colony-stimulating factor with or without cyclophosphamide to aid in mobilization. Autologous stem cell transplantation (Chapter 181) is performed with

melphalan 200 mg/m² as the conditioning regimen, followed by infusion of the peripheral blood stem cells. Patients who do not achieve a complete or very good partial response with the first autologous transplant are considered for a second autologous transplant.[6]

An alternative approach in patients with newly diagnosed disease is to cryopreserve stem cells for future use after initial therapy. Patients then continue initial therapy, such as lenalidomide plus low-dose dexamethasone, until progression or achievement of a plateau phase, reserving stem cell transplantation for the first relapse. Data from randomized trials comparing early versus delayed transplantation indicate no significant difference in survival between the two strategies. The choice is based on the patient's preferences and other clinical conditions, but early transplantation is often preferred because its mortality is low (<1%) and it avoids the inconvenience, cost, and potential side effects of prolonged chemotherapy.

Role of Allogeneic Bone Marrow Transplantation

Ninety to 95% of patients with multiple myeloma cannot undergo allogeneic bone marrow transplantation because of their age, lack of an HLA-matched sibling donor, or inadequate renal, pulmonary, or cardiac function (Chapter 181). Although a complete response occurs in 40% of patients, most have a relapse; in long-term follow-up there is no apparent survival plateau. The mortality rate from the procedure is approximately 25%, and conventional allogeneic bone marrow transplantation is rarely used in myeloma. An alternative is autologous stem cell transplantation followed by nonmyeloablative ("mini") allogeneic transplantation, but treatment-related mortality is still approximately 20%. Nonmyeloablative allogeneic transplantation for myeloma is best performed only in the context of clinical trials.

Initial Therapy of Patients Who Are Not Candidates for Transplantation

Approximately 50% of newly diagnosed patients are not considered candidates for stem cell transplantation. For decades, the oral administration of melphalan (8 to 10 mg/day for 7 days) and prednisone (20 mg three times a day for the same 7 days) repeated every 6 weeks has been the standard of care. When using melphalan, the leukocyte and platelet levels should be measured every 3 weeks, and the dosage of melphalan must be adjusted until midcycle cytopenia occurs. The addition of thalidomide to the standard regimen of melphalan plus prednisone improves event-free and overall survival compared with melphalan plus prednisone alone in patients with newly diagnosed myeloma who are not candidates for transplantation.[7-9] Similarly, in a randomized trial, the addition of bortezomib to melphalan plus prednisone prolonged event-free and overall survival compared with melphalan plus prednisone alone by 39% among patients not eligible for high-dose chemotherapy and stem cell transplantation.[10] Based on these data, melphalan and prednisone plus either thalidomide (MPT) or bortezomib (VMP) are two recommended treatments for this patient population. Lenalidomide plus low-dose dexamethasone is a third option based on its high efficacy and low toxicity in elderly patients.

MPT is typically administered for 18 months, whereas VMP is given for 9 months. Lenalidomide plus low-dose dexamethasone can be given for 1 year or until progression, based on tolerability. Maintenance therapy is not generally recommended following MPT or VMP. If relapse occurs during the plateau state 6 to 12 or more months after cessation of therapy, the initial chemotherapeutic regimen can be reinstituted. Most patients respond, but the duration and quality of the response are usually inferior to those of the initial response.

Treatment of Relapsed Refractory Myeloma

Almost all patients with multiple myeloma eventually relapse. Single-agent dexamethasone, alkylating agents, thalidomide, lenalidomide, and bortezomib, administered alone or in combination, are all options for the treatment of relapsed refractory myeloma. Methylprednisolone 2 g three times a week intravenously for a minimum of 4 weeks, then reduced to once or twice a week if there is a response, is helpful for patients with pancytopenia and may be associated with fewer side effects than dexamethasone.

Thalidomide (50 to 200 mg/day orally) produces an objective response, with a median duration of about 1 year, in about a third of patients with refractory myeloma. Side effects are sedation, constipation, peripheral neuropathy, rash, bradycardia, and thrombotic events. The addition of dexamethasone to thalidomide increases the response rate to approximately 50%, and combinations of thalidomide, dexamethasone, and alkylating agents produce response rates exceeding 70% in patients with relapsed refractory disease.

The thalidomide analogue lenalidomide is better tolerated and produces objective benefits in approximately 40% of patients with relapsed refractory myeloma as a single agent; in combination with dexamethasone, 60% of patients benefit. Lenalidomide plus dexamethasone significantly prolongs time to progression and overall survival compared with dexamethasone alone.[11,12] The starting dose of lenalidomide is 25 mg orally on days 1 to 21, every 28 days. Lenalidomide has significantly fewer nonhematologic toxicities than thalidomide does; myelosuppression is the most common adverse event.

Bortezomib, an inhibitor of the ubiquitin-proteasome pathway, acts through multiple mechanisms to arrest tumor growth, tumor spread, and angiogenesis. It produces objective responses in about a third of patients with refractory myeloma and is superior to single-agent dexamethasone.[13] Like thalidomide and lenalidomide, bortezomib can also be combined with dexamethasone and other active agents to increase response rates.[10] The starting dose is 1.3 mg/m^2 administered intravenously on days 1, 4, 8, and 11, every 21 days. The most common adverse events are gastrointestinal side effects, fatigue, and neuropathy.

Other novel agents that have shown promise but are not commercially available at this time include pomalidomide (a new analogue of thalidomide) and carfilzomib (a new proteasome inhibitor). Several other novel agents are in clinical trials.

Role of Radiation Therapy

Palliative radiation in a dose of 20 to 30 Gy should be limited to patients who have multiple myeloma with disabling pain and a well-defined focal process that has not responded to chemotherapy and to patients with spinal cord compression from a plasmacytoma. Analgesics in combination with chemotherapy can usually control the pain (Chapter 29).

Management of Complications

Hypercalcemia

Hypercalcemia, present in 15 to 20% of patients at diagnosis, should be suspected in those with anorexia, nausea, vomiting, polyuria, polydipsia, constipation, weakness, confusion, or stupor. If hypercalcemia is untreated, renal insufficiency may develop. Hydration, preferably with isotonic saline plus prednisone (25 mg four times/day), usually relieves the hypercalcemia. Bisphosphonates such as zoledronic acid or pamidronate are recommended and will correct hypercalcemia in almost all patients (Chapter 251).

Renal Insufficiency

The most common cause of acute renal failure is light chain cast nephropathy in patients who have excess excretion of monoclonal protein in urine (myeloma kidney). Aggressive treatment of acute renal failure due to light chain cast nephropathy is critical for long-term overall survival. If the patient is not oliguric, intravenous fluids and furosemide are needed to maintain a high urine flow rate (100 mL/hour). If the underlying cause is thought to be

light chain cast nephropathy based on clinical findings (e.g., serum free light chains >150 mg/dL) or renal biopsy, plasmapheresis is recommended daily for 5 days to reduce the levels of circulating light chains. Hemodialysis is necessary for symptomatic azotemia. The mainstay of therapy is aggressive treatment of myeloma with a regimen such as bortezomib, thalidomide, and dexamethasone (VTD). Allopurinol is necessary if hyperuricemia is present.

Infection

Prompt, appropriate therapy for bacterial infections is necessary. Prophylactic antibiotics such as trimethoprim-sulfamethoxazole should be considered in patients taking high-dose corticosteroids, but trimethoprim-sulfamethoxazole should be avoided in patients receiving thalidomide or lenalidomide to minimize the risk of serious skin reactions. Intravenously administered gamma globulin is reserved for patients with hypogammaglobulinemia and recurrent severe infections. Pneumococcal and influenza immunizations (Chapter 17) should be given to all patients.

Skeletal Lesions

Patients should be encouraged to be as active as possible but to avoid trauma. Pamidronate (90 mg infused intravenously over a 4-hour period every 4 weeks) or zoledronic acid (4 mg intravenously over at least 15 minutes every 4 weeks) reduces the incidence of bone pain, pathologic fractures, and spinal cord compression; such prophylaxis is now routinely recommended for all patients with myeloma bone disease and may improve overall survival.[14] After 1 to 2 years the dosing can be reduced to once every 3 months in patients who are stable, to minimize the risk of osteonecrosis of the jaw, which is a complication of long-term bisphosphonate therapy.

Spinal cord compression from an extramedullary plasmacytoma (Chapter 407) should be suspected in patients who have severe back pain, weakness or paresthesias of the lower extremities, or bladder or bowel dysfunction. Initial treatment is with dexamethasone-based therapy and/or radiation therapy. If the neurologic deficit increases, surgical decompression is necessary.

Miscellaneous Complications

Symptomatic hyperviscosity (see later) is less common than in Waldenström's macroglobulinemia. Anemia that persists despite adequate treatment of underlying myeloma often responds to erythropoietin.

PROGNOSIS

Multiple myeloma is considered incurable at present, but survival has improved significantly in recent years following the arrival of new agents such as lenalidomide and bortezomib. The median survival is approximately 4 years, but it varies widely according to clinical stage and risk stratification factors (Table 193-5). In some patients an acute or aggressive terminal phase is characterized by rapid tumor growth, pancytopenia, soft tissue subcutaneous masses, decreased M protein levels, and fever; survival in this subset is generally only a few months.

FUTURE DIRECTIONS

Future efforts must be directed toward identifying new active agents and developing effective combinations of active drugs. Studies are under way to improve the conditioning regimen used in autologous stem cell transplantation and to better integrate novel therapies with stem cell transplantation.

TABLE 193-5	STAGING AND PROGNOSTIC FACTORS IN MULTIPLE MYELOMA	
STAGE/RISK FACTOR	**MEDIAN SURVIVAL (MO)**
INTERNATIONAL STAGING SYSTEM	
Stage I (serum β_2-microglobulin <3.5 mg/L and serum albumin ≥3.5 g/dL)	62
Stage II (neither stage I nor stage III)	44
Stage III (serum β_2-microglobulin ≥5.5 mg/L)	29
RISK STRATIFICATION	
High-risk myeloma (any one of the following): Fluorescence in situ hybridization: t14;16, t14;20, deletion 17p	24-36
OTHER ADVERSE PROGNOSTIC FACTORS	
Elevated lactate dehydrogenase level	
Poor performance status	
Increased circulating plasma cells	
Plasmablastic morphology	
Increased plasma cell labeling index ≥1%	

● VARIANT FORMS OF MULTIPLE MYELOMA

Smoldering Multiple Myeloma

Smoldering (asymptomatic) multiple myeloma is defined by the presence of an M protein level greater than 3 g/dL in serum or 10% or more plasma cells in bone marrow in the absence of anemia, renal insufficiency, hypercalcemia, or skeletal lesions. Biologically, patients with smoldering multiple myeloma are similar to those with MGUS but carry a much higher risk for progression to myeloma or related malignancy: 10% per year for the first 5 years, 5% per year for the next 5 years, and 1 to 2% per year thereafter. As a result, patients must be observed more closely (every 3 to 4 months), but they should not be treated unless progression to symptomatic multiple myeloma occurs.

Plasma Cell Leukemia

Patients with plasma cell leukemia have more than 20% plasma cells in the peripheral blood and an absolute plasma cell count of 2000/µL or greater. Plasma cell leukemia is classified as primary when it is diagnosed in the leukemic phase (60%) or as secondary when there is leukemic transformation of a previously recognized multiple myeloma (40%). Patients with primary plasma cell leukemia are younger and have a greater incidence of hepatosplenomegaly and lymphadenopathy, a higher platelet count, fewer bone lesions, a smaller serum M protein component, and longer survival (median, 6.8 vs. 1.3 months) than do patients with secondary plasma cell leukemia. Treatment of plasma cell leukemia is unsatisfactory. An aggressive initial treatment regimen that contains bortezomib, dexamethasone, and either thalidomide or lenalidomide for two or three cycles, followed by autologous stem cell transplantation and subsequent maintenance therapy with lenalidomide, is a reasonable strategy if the patient's clinical condition permits such an approach. Secondary plasma cell leukemia rarely responds to chemotherapy because the patients have already received chemotherapy and are resistant.

Nonsecretory Myeloma

Patients with nonsecretory myeloma have no M protein in either serum or urine and account for only 3% of cases of myeloma. To make the diagnosis, the clonal nature of bone marrow plasma cells should be established by immunoperoxidase, immunofluorescence, or flow cytometric methods. Treatment and survival are similar to those in patients with typical myeloma. The serum free light chain assay is abnormal in more than 60% of patients and can be used to monitor the response to therapy.

Osteosclerotic Myeloma (POEMS Syndrome)

This syndrome is characterized by polyneuropathy, organomegaly, endocrinopathy, M protein, and skin changes (POEMS). The diagnosis of POEMS syndrome requires the presence of a monoclonal plasma cell disorder, peripheral neuropathy, plus at least one of the following seven features: osteosclerotic bone lesions, Castleman's disease, organomegaly, endocrinopathy (excluding diabetes mellitus or hypothyroidism), edema, typical skin changes, and papilledema. However, not every patient meeting these criteria has POEMS syndrome; the features should have a temporal relationship to one another, with no other attributable cause. The absence of osteosclerotic lesions makes the diagnosis suspect. Elevations in plasma or serum levels of vascular endothelial growth factor and thrombocytosis are common features of the syndrome and are helpful when the diagnosis is difficult. The major clinical features are a chronic inflammatory-demyelinating polyneuropathy with predominantly motor disability and sclerotic skeletal lesions. The bone marrow usually contains less than 5% plasma cells, and hypercalcemia and renal insufficiency rarely occur. Almost all patients have a λ-type M protein. The diagnosis is confirmed by identification of monoclonal plasma cells obtained at biopsy of an osteosclerotic lesion.

If the lesions are in a limited area, radiation therapy substantially improves the neuropathy in more than 50% of patients. If the patient has widespread osteosclerotic lesions, treatment is with autologous stem cell transplantation or other systemic therapy similar to that used for myeloma.

Solitary Plasmacytoma (Solitary Myeloma) of Bone

The diagnosis of solitary bone plasmacytoma is based on histologic evidence of a solitary tumor consisting of monoclonal plasma cells identical to those in multiple myeloma. In addition, complete skeletal radiographs and MRI of the spine and pelvis must show no other lesions of myeloma, and the bone marrow aspirate must contain no evidence of clonal plasma cells. An M protein may be present in serum or urine at diagnosis, but persistence of the

M protein after radiation therapy is associated with an increased risk for progression to multiple myeloma. Treatment consists of radiation in the range of 40 to 50 Gy. Almost 50% of patients who have a solitary plasmacytoma are alive at 10 years, and disease-free survival rates at 10 years range from 15 to 25%. Progression to myeloma, when it occurs, usually takes place within 3 years, but patients must be monitored indefinitely. There is no convincing evidence that adjuvant chemotherapy decreases the rate of conversion to multiple myeloma.

Extramedullary Plasmacytoma

Extramedullary plasmacytomas outside the bone marrow are most commonly found in the upper respiratory tract (80% of cases), especially in the nasal cavity and sinuses, nasopharynx, and larynx. Extramedullary plasmacytomas may also occur in the gastrointestinal tract, central nervous system, urinary bladder, thyroid, breast, testes, parotid gland, or lymph nodes. Extramedullary plasmacytomas may be solitary, or they may occur in the context of existing myeloma. The diagnosis of solitary extramedullary plasmacytoma is based on detection of a plasma cell tumor in an extramedullary site, absence of clonal plasma cells on bone marrow examination, and absence of other bony or extramedullary lesions on radiographic studies. Treatment of solitary extramedullary plasmacytoma consists of either complete surgical resection or tumoricidal irradiation. The plasmacytoma may recur locally, metastasize to regional nodes, or, rarely, develop into multiple myeloma.

● WALDENSTRÖM'S MACROGLOBULINEMIA (PRIMARY MACROGLOBULINEMIA)

▶ DEFINITION

Waldenström's macroglobulinemia is the result of the uncontrolled proliferation of lymphocytes and plasma cells in which an IgM M protein is produced. The cause is unknown; familial clusters have been reported. The median age of patients at the time of diagnosis is about 65 years, and approximately 60% are male. The diagnostic criteria are IgM monoclonal gammopathy (regardless of the size of the M protein), 10% or greater bone marrow infiltration (usually intertrabecular) by clonal lymphocytes that exhibit plasmacytoid or plasma cell differentiation, and a typical immunophenotype (e.g., surface IgM$^+$, CD5$^{+/-}$, CD10$^-$, CD19$^+$, CD20$^+$, CD23$^-$) that would satisfactorily exclude other lymphoproliferative disorders, including CLL (Chapter 190) and mantle cell lymphoma (Chapter 191).

▶ CLINICAL MANIFESTATIONS

Weakness, fatigue, and bleeding (especially oozing from the oronasal area) are common initial symptoms. Blurred or impaired vision, dyspnea, weight loss, neurologic symptoms, recurrent infections, and heart failure may occur. In contrast to multiple myeloma, lytic bone lesions, renal insufficiency, and amyloidosis are rare. Physical findings include pallor, hepatosplenomegaly, and lymphadenopathy. Retinal hemorrhages, exudates, and venous congestion with vascular segmentation ("sausage" formation) may occur. Sensorimotor peripheral neuropathy is common. Pulmonary involvement is manifested by diffuse pulmonary infiltrates and isolated masses.

Laboratory Evaluation

Almost all patients have moderate to severe normocytic, normochromic anemia. The serum electrophoretic pattern is characterized by a tall, narrow peak or dense band that is of the IgM type on immunofixation. Quantitative IgM levels are high. A monoclonal light chain is detected in the urine of 80% of patients, but the amount of urinary protein is generally modest.

The bone marrow aspirate is often hypocellular, but the biopsy is hypercellular and extensively infiltrated with lymphoid cells and plasma cells. The number of mast cells is frequently increased. Rouleau formation is prominent (Chapter 160), and the sedimentation rate is markedly increased. About 10% of cases may have an associated type I cryoglobulinemia (see later).

▶ DIAGNOSIS

Diagnosis requires the combination of typical symptoms and physical findings, the presence of an IgM M protein, and 10% or greater lymphoplasmacytic infiltration of the bone marrow. The lymphoplasmacytic cells express CD19, CD20, and CD22, whereas expression of CD5 and CD10 occurs in a minority. Asymptomatic patients with 10% or greater lymphoplasmacytic infiltration of the bone marrow are considered to have smoldering Waldenström's macroglobulinemia. Multiple myeloma, CLL, and MGUS of the IgM type must be excluded.

Patients meeting the diagnostic criteria for Waldenström's macroglobulinemia but who have less than 3 g/dL IgM protein at diagnosis have sometimes been classified as having "lymphoplasmacytic lymphoma with an IgM M protein" (Chapter 191). However, except for hyperviscosity, the clinical picture, therapy, and prognosis for these patients do not differ from those of patients with an IgM level of 3 g/dL or greater; thus, these patients are also considered to have Waldenström's macroglobulinemia by the current definition.

PREVENTION AND TREATMENT   Rx

Patients should not be treated unless they have anemia; constitutional symptoms such as weakness, fatigue, night sweats, or weight loss; hyperviscosity; or significant hepatosplenomegaly or lymphadenopathy. Rituximab, a chimeric anti-CD20 monoclonal antibody (Chapter 35), produces a response in at least 50% of untreated patients. Alkylating agents such as cyclophosphamide and chlorambucil with or without corticosteroids are also effective. Another choice for therapy is a purine nucleoside analogue, either fludarabine or 2-chlorodeoxyadenosine. In general, for minimally symptomatic patients, rituximab as a single agent is an excellent choice for initial therapy. For patients with more advanced symptoms, including severe anemia or hyperviscosity, combination approaches are preferred. The combination of rituximab, cyclophosphamide, and dexamethasone is highly active and also preserves the ability to mobilize stem cells for transplantation, if necessary. An alternative is cladribine with or without rituximab.

For relapse, the agents used as initial therapy can be given alone or in combination. Autologous stem cell transplantation can be considered for eligible patients with relapsed disease.

Spuriously low hemoglobin and hematocrit levels may occur because of the increased plasma volume from the large amount of intravascular M protein. Consequently, transfusions should not be given solely on the basis of the hemoglobin or hematocrit value. Symptomatic hyperviscosity should be treated by plasmapheresis. The median survival of patients with macroglobulinemia is 5 years.

HYPERVISCOSITY SYNDROME

Hyperviscosity syndrome occurs in patients with Waldenström's macroglobulinemia who have high levels of serum IgM M protein (>5 g/dL) and occasionally in those with myeloma, especially of the IgA type. Hyperviscosity is disproportionately more common relative to the same serum concentration of IgM and IgA M proteins compared with IgG M proteins, owing to the inherent tendency of IgM and IgA molecules to polymerize. Typically, IgM forms pentamers, whereas IgA forms dimers or sometimes trimers, resulting in high-molecular-weight complexes. Chronic nasal bleeding and oozing from the gums are the most frequent symptoms of hyperviscosity, but postsurgical or gastrointestinal bleeding may also occur. Retinal hemorrhages are common, and venous congestion with sausage-like segmentation and papilledema may be seen (Fig. 193-8). The patient occasionally complains of blurring or loss of vision. Dizziness, headache, vertigo, nystagmus, decreased hearing, ataxia, paresthesias, diplopia, somnolence, and coma may occur. Hyperviscosity can precipitate or exacerbate heart failure. Most patients have symptoms when the relative viscosity is greater than 4 cP, but the relationship between serum viscosity and clinical manifestations is not precise. Patients with symptomatic hyperviscosity should be treated with plasmapheresis and with chemotherapy to treat the underlying malignancy. Plasma exchange of 3 to 4 L with albumin should be performed daily until the patient is asymptomatic. Plasma exchange is rapidly effective (two to three exchanges) in the case of IgM M proteins, which are primarily intravascular; with IgG M proteins, multiple attempts may be needed because a significant amount of IgG can exist in the extravascular space.

HEAVY CHAIN DISEASES

The HCDs are characterized by the presence of an M protein consisting of a portion of the immunoglobulin heavy chain in serum, urine, or both. These heavy chains are devoid of light chains and represent a lymphoplasma cell proliferative process. There are three major types: γ-HCD, α-HCD, and μ-HCD.

γ-HCD

Patients with γ-HCD often initially have a lymphoma-like illness, but the clinical findings are diverse and range from an aggressive lymphoproliferative process (Chapter 191) to an asymptomatic state. Hepatosplenomegaly and lymphadenopathy occur in about 60% of patients. Anemia is found in approximately 80% initially and in nearly all eventually. The electrophoretic pattern

FIGURE 193-8. **Hyperviscosity syndrome.** Right eye retinal image in a patient with Waldenström's macroglobulinemia and hyperviscosity syndrome showing sausaging (focal venular dilations), intraretinal hemorrhages, microaneurysms, and peripapillary cotton-wool spots and disc swelling (papilledema).

often shows a broad-based band more suggestive of a polyclonal increase than an M protein. The diagnosis depends on the identification of an isolated monoclonal γ heavy chain on serum immunofixation, without evidence of either monoclonal κ or λ light chain expression.

Treatment is indicated only for symptomatic patients and consists of chemotherapy with melphalan plus prednisone or regimens used to treat non-Hodgkin's lymphoma (Chapter 191), such as cyclophosphamide, vincristine, and prednisone. The prognosis of γ-HCD is variable and ranges from a rapidly progressive downhill course of a few weeks' duration to the asymptomatic presence of a stable monoclonal heavy chain in serum or urine.

α-HCD

α-HCD is the most common form of HCD and occurs in patients from the Mediterranean region or the Middle East, generally in the second or third decade of life. About 60% are men. Most commonly the gastrointestinal tract is involved, and severe malabsorption with diarrhea, steatorrhea, and weight loss is noted (Chapter 142). Plasma cell infiltration of the jejunal mucosa is the most frequent pathologic feature. Immunoproliferative small intestinal disease is restricted to patients with small intestinal lesions who have the pathologic features of α-HCD but do not synthesize α heavy chains.

The serum protein electrophoretic pattern is normal in half the cases; in the remainder an unimpressive broad band may appear in the α2 or β region. The diagnosis depends on identification of an isolated monoclonal α heavy chain on serum immunofixation, without evidence of either monoclonal κ or λ light chain expression. The amount of α heavy chain in urine is small.

In the absence of therapy, α-HCD is typically progressive and fatal. The usual treatment consists of antibiotics, such as tetracyclines, and the eradication of any concurrent parasitic infection. Patients who do not respond adequately to antibiotics are given chemotherapy similar to that used to treat non-Hodgkin's lymphoma, for example, the cyclophosphamide, hydroxydaunomycin, vincristine (Oncovin), and prednisone (CHOP) regimen (Chapter 191).

μ-HCD

This disease is characterized by the demonstration of an isolated monoclonal μ chain fragment on serum immunofixation, without evidence of either monoclonal κ or λ light chain expression.

The serum protein electrophoretic pattern is usually normal, except for hypogammaglobulinemia. Bence Jones proteinuria has been found in two thirds of cases. Lymphocytes, plasma cells, and lymphoplasmacytoid cells are increased in the bone marrow. Vacuolization of the plasma cells is common and should suggest the possibility of HCD. The course of μ-HCD is variable, and survival ranges from a few months to many years. Treatment is with corticosteroids and alkylating agents.

CRYOGLOBULINEMIA

Cryoglobulins are plasma proteins that precipitate when cooled and dissolve when heated. They are designated as idiopathic or essential when they are not associated with any recognizable disease. Cryoglobulins are classified into

FIGURE 193-9. Skin infarction in cryoglobulinemia. The skin has a reticulated pattern as a result of leakage of red blood cells from damaged skin capillaries. Necrosis and ulceration have occurred in peripheral sites because of vessel blockage. This patient eventually required plastic surgery. (From Forbes CD, Jackson WF. *Color Atlas and Text of Clinical Medicine*, 3rd ed. London: Mosby; 2003.)

three types: type I (monoclonal), type II (mixed monoclonal plus polyclonal), and type III (polyclonal).

Type I Cryoglobulinemia

Type I (monoclonal) cryoglobulinemia is most commonly of the IgM or IgG class, but IgA and Bence Jones cryoglobulins have been reported. Most patients, even with large amounts of type I cryoglobulin, are completely asymptomatic from this source. Others with monoclonal cryoglobulins in the range of 1 to 2 g/dL may have evidence of vasculitis with pain, purpura, Raynaud's phenomenon, cyanosis, and even ulceration and sloughing of skin and subcutaneous tissue (Fig. 193-9) on exposure to cold because their cryoglobulins precipitate at relatively high temperatures. Type I cryoglobulins are associated with macroglobulinemia, multiple myeloma, or MGUS. Therapy for patients with symptomatic type I cryoglobulinemia and significant symptoms is similar to that for Waldenström's macroglobulinemia for the IgM type and multiple myeloma for the non-IgM type.

Type II Cryoglobulinemia

Type II (mixed) cryoglobulinemia typically consists of an immune complex of IgM M protein and polyclonal IgG, although monoclonal IgG or monoclonal IgA may also be seen with polyclonal IgM. Serum protein electrophoresis generally shows a normal pattern or a diffuse, polyclonal hypergammaglobulinemic pattern. The quantity of mixed cryoglobulin is usually less than 0.2 g/dL. Despite the monoclonal component, most patients do not have a clonal plasma cell disorder; rather, they have serologic evidence of infection with hepatitis C virus (Chapter 151). At present, hepatitis C is thought to be the cause of most cases of type II cryoglobulinemia.

Most clinical manifestations are related to the development of vasculitis and include palpable purpura, livedo reticularis, polyarthralgias, and neuropathy. Involvement of the joints is symmetrical, but joint deformities rarely develop. Raynaud's phenomenon, necrosis of the skin, and neurologic involvement may be present. In almost 80% of renal biopsy specimens, glomerular damage can be identified. Nephrotic syndrome may result, but severe renal insufficiency is uncommon.

Early administration of corticosteroids is the most frequent therapy. Treatment should also target underlying hepatitis C infection with interferon-α2 or ribavirin (Chapter 151). Agents to treat the monoclonal component, such as cyclophosphamide, chlorambucil, azathioprine, or rituximab, are used if there is no response. Plasmapheresis (with a warmed circuit) is helpful in the acute management of symptoms by removing circulating immune complexes.

Type III Cryoglobulinemia

Type III (polyclonal) cryoglobulinemia does not have a monoclonal component and is not associated with a clonal plasma cell proliferative disorder. Type III cryoglobulins are found in many patients with chronic infections or inflammatory diseases and are usually of no clinical significance unless associated with hepatitis C infection.

1. Child JA, Morgan GJ, Davies FE, et al. High-dose chemotherapy with hematopoietic stem-cell rescue for multiple myeloma. *N Engl J Med*. 2003;348:1875-1883.

2. Harousseau JL, Attal M, Avet-Loiseau H, et al. Bortezomib plus dexamethasone as induction treatment prior to autologous stem-cell transplantation in newly diagnosed multiple myeloma: results of the IFM 2005-01 phase III trial. *J Clin Oncol*. 2010;28:4621-4629.

3. Zonder JA, Crowley J, Hussein MA, et al. Lenalidomide and high-dose dexamethasone compared with dexamethasone as initial therapy for multiple myeloma: a randomized Southwest Oncology Group Trial (S0232). *Blood*. 2010;116:5838-5841.

4. Rajkumar SV, Jacobus S, Callander NS, et al. Lenalidomide plus high-dose dexamethasone versus lenalidomide plus low-dose dexamethasone as initial therapy for newly diagnosed multiple myeloma: an open-label randomised controlled trial. *Lancet Oncol*. 2010;11:29-37.

5. Mateos MV, Oriol A, Martinez-Lopez J, et al. Bortezomib, melphalan, and prednisone versus bortezomib, thalidomide, and prednisone as induction therapy followed by maintenance treatment with bortezomib and thalidomide versus bortezomib and prednisone in elderly patients with untreated multiple myeloma: a randomised trial. *Lancet Oncol*. 2010;11:934-941.

6. Attal M, Harousseau JL, Facon T, et al. Single versus double autologous stem-cell transplantation for multiple myeloma. *N Engl J Med*. 2003;349:2495-2502.

7. Facon T, Mary JY, Hulin C, et al. Melphalan and prednisone plus thalidomide versus melphalan and prednisone alone or reduced-intensity autologous stem cell transplantation in elderly patients with multiple myeloma (IFM 99-06): a randomised trial. *Lancet*. 2007;370:1209-1218.

8. Palumbo A, Bringhen S, Caravita T, et al. Oral melphalan and prednisone chemotherapy plus thalidomide compared with melphalan and prednisone alone in elderly patients with multiple myeloma: randomised controlled trial. *Lancet*. 2006;367:825-831.

9. Hulin C, Facon T, Rodon P, et al. Efficacy of melphalan and prednisone plus thalidomide in patients older than 75 years with newly diagnosed multiple myeloma: IFM 01/01 Trial. *J Clin Oncol*. 2009;27:3664-3670.

10. San Miguel JF, Schlag R, Khuageva NK, et al. Bortezomib plus melphalan and prednisone for initial treatment of multiple myeloma. *N Engl J Med*. 2008;359:906-917.

11. Dimopoulos M, Spencer A, Attal M, et al. Lenalidomide plus dexamethasone for relapsed or refractory multiple myeloma. *N Engl J Med*. 2007;357:2123-2132.

12. Weber DM, Chen C, Niesvizky R, et al. Lenalidomide plus dexamethasone for relapsed multiple myeloma in North America. *N Engl J Med*. 2007;357:2133-2142.

13. Richardson PG, Sonneveld P, Schuster MW, et al. Bortezomib or high-dose dexamethasone for relapsed multiple myeloma. *N Engl J Med*. 2005;352:2487-2498.

14. Morgan GJ, Davies FE, Gregory WM, et al. First-line treatment with zoledronic acid as compared with clodronic acid in multiple myeloma (MRC Myeloma IX): a randomised controlled trial. *Lancet*. 2010;376:1989-1999.

SUGGESTED READINGS

Landgren O, Waxman AJ. Multiple myeloma precursor disease. *JAMA*. 2010;304:2397-2404. *Review of monoclonal gammopathy of undetermined significance.*
Laubach J, Richardson P, Anderson K. Multiple myeloma. *Annu Rev Med*. 2011;62:249-264. *Review.*
Palumbo A, Anderson K. Multiple myeloma. *N Engl J Med*. 2011;364:1046-1060. *Review.*
Rajkumar SV. Multiple myeloma: 2011 update on diagnosis, risk-stratification and management. *Am J Hematol*. 2011;86:57-65. *Provides a detailed, risk-adapted approach to the treatment of myeloma.*

194

AMYLOIDOSIS

MORIE A. GERTZ

DEFINITION

Immunoglobulin light chain amyloidosis is characterized by a clonal population of bone marrow plasma cells that produces a monoclonal light chain of the κ or λ type, as either an intact molecule or a fragment. The light chain protein, instead of conforming to the α-helical configuration of most proteins, misfolds and forms a β-pleated sheet. This insoluble protein deposits in tissues and interferes with organ function. The β-pleated sheet configuration is responsible for the tinctorial properties; when the protein is stained with Congo red and viewed under polarized light, apple-green birefringence is demonstrated and is required for the diagnosis. Systemic light chain amyloidosis (AL) must be distinguished from the much less common amyloidosis associated with chronic infection and inflammatory arthropathies (secondary or AA) or with inherited amyloid cardiomyopathies and neuropathies (familial or AF).

CLINICAL MANIFESTATIONS

Amyloidosis is particularly difficult to diagnose and is a challenge for internists. The presenting symptoms can be very broad and are mimicked by far more common disorders (Table 194-1). The signs include tongue enlargement with dental indentations and "pinch" or periorbital purpura, a result of vascular fragility. The signs are specific but lack sensitivity, in that they are present in no more than 20% of patients. No single imaging procedure or

TABLE 194-1

TABLE 194-1 SYMPTOMS, SIGNS, AND SYNDROMES IN AMYLOIDOSIS

SYMPTOMS AND SIGNS

Common symptoms: fatigue, edema, dyspnea, anorexia, paresthesias
Rare symptoms: claudication, joint pain and stiffness, sicca syndrome
Common signs: periorbital purpura, glossomegaly, hepatomegaly
Rare signs: waxy infiltration of eyelids, shoulder pad sign

SYNDROMES

Nondiabetic nephrotic syndrome
Nonischemic cardiomyopathy with an echocardiogram showing "hypertrophy"
Hepatomegaly or increased alkaline phosphatase with no imaging abnormality
Peripheral neuropathy with monoclonal gammopathy of undetermined significance or chronic inflammatory demyelinating polyneuropathy with autonomic features
Atypical myeloma with monoclonal light chains and modest marrow plasmacytosis

laboratory study is diagnostic for the disease. The clinician must therefore be aware of the possibility of amyloidosis, or it may be overlooked. The kidney is commonly involved in amyloidosis. The diagnosis should be suspected in any patient who presents with nondiabetic nephrotic-range proteinuria (Chapter 123). One third of patients with amyloidosis have nephrotic syndrome that presents with dramatic increases in the blood cholesterol level (median, 270 mg/dL), and urinalysis for proteinuria should be done in patients with a sudden increase in the serum cholesterol level. A patient with nondiabetic proteinuria may receive an empirical course of corticosteroids for possible minimal-change glomerulopathy. This treatment delays the diagnosis of amyloidosis and allows other organs to become involved. Ten percent of renal biopsy specimens in nondiabetic nephrotic syndrome are subsequently shown to be involved by amyloidosis. The incidence of bleeding after percutaneous renal biopsy is not increased in AL.

The heart is involved in approximately 50% of patients with amyloidosis, and the presentation is subtle because fatigue is often the only manifestation. Because amyloid heart disease (Chapter 60) is a disorder of diastolic failure, the typical findings of cardiomyopathy (enlarged cardiac silhouette on chest radiography, depressed ejection fraction by echocardiography, and pulmonary vascular redistribution) are absent. The effect of amyloidosis on the heart is poor filling during diastole. Patients have low end-diastolic volume and, as a consequence, poor stroke volume despite a completely normal ejection fraction. Electrocardiography frequently shows a pseudoinfarct pattern, which can be interpreted as demonstrating silent ischemic infarction; this finding leads to coronary angiography, which is invariably negative (unless there is coincidental coronary artery disease). Echocardiography, which shows thickening of the heart walls due to amyloid infiltration, is frequently interpreted as showing left ventricular hypertrophy, and the cause of heart failure can be ascribed to silent hypertension or, alternatively, hypertrophic cardiomyopathy. Echocardiography frequently shows valvular insufficiency of the mitral and tricuspid valves. Restrictive cardiomyopathy has been confused with pericardial disease, and patients have undergone unnecessary pericardiectomy, without clinical benefit. The classic granular sparkling appearance of the echocardiogram is not a useful diagnostic finding. Patients with amyloidosis rarely have symptoms of ischemic heart disease. Enhancement on magnetic resonance imaging with gadolinium is delayed in 69% of patients with cardiac amyloidosis. Myocardial enhancement is associated with increased ventricular mass and impaired left ventricular systolic function.

The liver is involved in 13% of patients (Chapter 153). The typical presentation is hepatomegaly and an increased serum alkaline phosphatase value. An increased transaminase value and hyperbilirubinemia are late signs. Imaging is not helpful, and liver uptake is homogeneous. Many patients undergo an evaluation for metastatic malignancy. Liver biopsy is not associated with an increased rate of bleeding and is not contraindicated in the presence of hepatic amyloidosis. Rare patients present with spontaneous splenic rupture. Acquired deficiency of coagulation factor X is specific to AL and can be associated with clinically severe hemorrhage. Levels improve with effective therapy because the cause is binding of the factor to the fibrils of amyloid.

The peripheral neuropathy (Chapter 428) associated with amyloidosis begins in the lower extremities, is symmetrical, and is generally sensory or mixed sensorimotor. When a monoclonal protein is recognized, frequent diagnoses are chronic inflammatory demyelinating polyneuropathy

or neuropathy associated with monoclonal gammopathy of undetermined significance, because amyloidosis has not been considered in the differential diagnosis. Associated autonomic neuropathy occurs in approximately 4% of patients and can be characterized by orthostatic hypotension, which may be misattributed to the cardiac failure. Autonomic dysmotility of the bowel is a common associated finding (Chapter 138). It can be upper intestinal, leading to pseudo-obstruction and recurrent emesis, or lower intestinal, which is characterized by alternating obstipation and fecal incontinence. Diarrhea caused by autonomic failure has been misdiagnosed as collagenous colitis when eosinophilic deposits are found in the bowel mucosa on hematoxylin-eosin staining in the absence of Congo red staining. Carpal tunnel syndrome (Chapter 428) occurs in approximately 13% of patients; it is not clinically distinguishable from the syndrome associated with repetitive stress injury but frequently fails to improve after surgical release. Rarely, interstitial lung disease, pseudoclaudication, periarticular deposits, and unexplained weight loss are presenting symptoms.

Systemic amyloidosis can be confused with early multiple myeloma (Chapter 193). Patients who present with vague symptoms of fatigue and edema are found to have a monoclonal protein in the urine, and a bone marrow biopsy shows a clonal plasmacytosis with a median of 5% plasma cells in the bone marrow; however, a quarter of patients have more than 10% plasma cells in the bone marrow, a finding that qualifies as a diagnosis of multiple myeloma. These patients are often considered to have atypical multiple myeloma when the underlying amyloid syndrome goes undetected. In these patients, a misdiagnosis of myeloma kidney or demyelinating neuropathy is made when an adequate diagnostic evaluation to exclude amyloidosis has not been performed.

DIAGNOSIS

Screening for Amyloidosis

In a patient with nondiabetic proteinuria, cardiomyopathy without ischemic risk factors, unexplained hepatomegaly, peripheral or autonomic neuropathy, or carpal tunnel syndrome, amyloidosis is not the most likely cause. The disorder occurs in only 8 per million persons per year, and routine biopsy is not appropriate whenever consistent symptoms are found. The classic physical finding of periorbital purpura occurs in only 10% of patients, is often limited to petechial eruptions over the eyelids, and is easily overlooked. Enlargement of the tongue occurs in 10 to 15% of patients; therefore, although it is specific, it is not sensitive for the diagnosis. Patients with enlarged tongues may be unrecognized, or they may be evaluated for acromegaly or undergo unnecessary tongue biopsies because of the suspicion of squamous cell cancer. If biopsy is not an appropriate screening technique, what algorithm should be used to recognize light chain amyloidosis?

By definition, amyloidosis is a plasma cell dyscrasia (Chapter 193); therefore, virtually all patients have a detectable immunoglobulin abnormality by immunofixation of the serum or urine, or they have abnormal results on a serum immunoglobulin free light chain assay. When a patient presents with a compatible clinical syndrome, these diagnostic studies should be completed before performing invasive diagnostic studies (Fig. 194-1). Simple electrophoresis without immunofixation is inadequate because the monoclonal proteins are very small in most patients and will not cause a detectable peak on serum protein electrophoresis. When these three diagnostic studies are used in combination, the sensitivity is 100%. If a monoclonal protein is detected, further investigations for amyloid should proceed, as described later. If a monoclonal protein is not found, three possibilities exist: (1) the patient does not have amyloidosis; (2) if the patient is known to have amyloidosis, it may be localized rather than systemic; (3) if the patient is known to have systemic amyloidosis, it may be the senile systemic or familial type rather than the light chain type.

Confirming the Diagnosis of Amyloidosis

In view of the grave prognosis associated with light chain amyloidosis, the diagnosis must be confirmed by biopsy (with Congo red staining) in all cases. Although it is reasonable to biopsy the kidney when proteinuria is the presenting symptom, the heart when cardiomyopathy is recognized, the liver when there is hepatomegaly and increased alkaline phosphatase, or the nerve when there is a sensorimotor functional loss, these invasive and occasionally risky procedures are not required. Subcutaneous fat aspiration is an outpatient procedure that has a 24-hour turnaround time and recognizes amyloid deposits in 70% of patients. Bone marrow is a second convenient biopsy site, and this test is often required to exclude the possibility of associated multiple myeloma. Bone marrow biopsy is positive in 50% of patients. When both

FIGURE 194-1. Algorithm for the cost-effective pursuit of a diagnosis of systemic light chain amyloidosis.

subcutaneous fat aspiration and bone marrow biopsy are done, amyloid is detected in 87% of patients. The remaining patients should have biopsy of the appropriate organ.

Once amyloid deposits are detected in tissues, further diagnostic evaluation is required. The presence of a monoclonal protein in the serum or urine and the presence of congophilic deposits in tissue do not verify that amyloidosis is light chain in origin. Further diagnostic studies are essential to classify the type of amyloid before therapy is initiated. Immunohistochemical studies on the tissue may be useful, but misfolding of the amyloid light chain often prevents epitopes from being recognized by commercial antisera; thus false-negative results are common. Mass spectroscopic analysis of the amyloid deposit can be done on paraffin-embedded tissue and validates the type of amyloid by direct amino acid sequencing, leaving no question about the origin of the amyloid protein as an immunoglobulin light chain. The incidence of monoclonal gammopathies in the elderly ranges from 3 to 5%. Therefore, that fraction of patients with senile systemic, localized, and familial amyloidosis could be expected to have an associated monoclonal gammopathy, which would be misleading. Mass spectroscopic analysis is feasible on subcutaneous fat tissue.

TREATMENT ℞

Previously, amyloidosis was thought to be untreatable and invariably fatal. With current therapy, response rates of about 70% regularly occur, and the median duration of survival is reportedly upward of 5 years. Agents to reverse the misfolding of the protein and render it soluble would be ideal, but they are not available. The source of the immunoglobulin light chain is the clonal plasma cell population in the bone marrow. All known therapies are directed at destruction of the plasma cell clone. The two choices are generally traditional-dose chemotherapy or high-dose chemotherapy with autologous stem cell transplantation. Most patients are not candidates for high-dose therapy because of age, advanced cardiac dysfunction, or renal insufficiency. Current therapies include combinations of melphalan, dexamethasone, bortezomib, and lenalidomide. The role of high-dose therapy with stem cell transplantation in the management of amyloidosis remains controversial.[1][2] Effective therapy has been associated with resolution of nephrotic syndrome, cardiac failure,

and hepatomegaly. Imaging has shown amyloid deposits to regress after the suppression of light chain synthesis.

Assessing the Effect of Therapy

The serum immunoglobulin free light chain assay has been cited as a useful screening test for patients with a compatible clinical syndrome. This assay is also used to measure the therapeutic effect of intervention because the light chain level is quantifiable and reproducible. Based on current hematologic response criteria, successful therapy is characterized by a 50% reduction in the abnormal free light chain level. Because the tissue toxicity associated with amyloid is related to the deposition of small amounts of light chain, it is unclear whether a successful outcome requires complete eradication of the light chain product. Studies have shown that patients achieving complete normalization of the free light chain have a better outcome, but it is uncertain whether patients who do not achieve this level of response should be subjected to more intensive treatment in an effort to remove this pathogenic amyloid serum precursor.

PROGNOSIS

The outcome of patients with light chain amyloidosis depends on the extent of cardiac involvement (Chapter 60). With the advent of routine hemodialysis for this population, death due to renal failure is uncommon. The greater the involvement of the heart, the shorter a patient's survival. Echocardiography provides useful information about the ejection fraction, the thickness of the ventricular septum and left ventricular free wall, and the strain percentage (the rate at which wall shortening occurs). Doppler echocardiography allows quantitative measurements of diastolic function and reflects the slowing of blood flow into the ventricular chamber as the noncompliant left ventricle fills. This "stiffness" measured by the deceleration time provides useful information and correlates well with survival.

Cardiac biomarkers are extremely sensitive measures of myocardial function, are reproducible, and can be used not only for prognosis but also to follow cardiac response after effective therapy. The serum troponin value is a powerful predictor of survival in patients with amyloidosis, and the N-terminal pro-brain natriuretic peptide value predicts survival after a diagnosis of amyloidosis. A staging system has been developed using these two cardiac biomarkers to accurately predict survival. In clinical trials of amyloidosis, half the patients with extreme increases in these markers have been incapable of completing 3 months of therapy.

Other Forms of Amyloidosis

Localized amyloidosis can be confused with systemic amyloidosis, but it has a much better prognosis. Patients with localized amyloidosis generally do not require systemic therapy; management can be supportive or localized to the deposition. The location of the amyloid deposits can be a clue to the localized nature. Typical sites for localized amyloid deposition include the ureter, bladder, urethra, and prostate. Therapy entails cystoscopic resection or intra-vesical instillation of dimethyl sulfoxide. Most forms of cutaneous amyloido-sis are localized, although nodular cutaneous amyloidosis has occurred in systemic light chain AL. Tracheobronchial and laryngeal amyloidosis and nodular pulmonary amyloidosis are localized, are not associated with a plasma cell dyscrasia, and generally require only local therapy. Nodular pul-monary amyloidosis is often diagnosed after thoracotomy for a presumed malignant pulmonary nodule. Most cases of laryngeal amyloidosis are found when the patient presents to an otorhinolaryngologist with hoarseness and amyloid deposits are found on endoscopic biopsy. Patients with localized amyloidosis do not have a demonstrable monoclonal protein in the serum or urine and have a normal free light chain ratio. The localized amyloidosis found in Alzheimer's disease is chemically unrelated to light chain amyloido-sis, and patients with light chain amyloidosis have no increased risk of dementia.

Senile systemic amyloidosis results from the deposition of a normal serum protein, transthyretin, in the myocardium. It has a much better prognosis than cardiac AL and generally necessitates endomyocardial biopsy for diagnosis; most patients are older than 70 years. When a monoclonal protein is present, it is incidental, and confirmation generally requires analy-sis of the amyloid-laden tissues. Therapy is supportive. The clinical presenta-tion of senile systemic amyloidosis is not distinguishable from that of cardiac AL.

Familial amyloidosis is uncommon in the United States and represents only 3% of the cases of systemic amyloidosis. Patients present with the full clinical spectrum associated with amyloidosis, including cardiomyopa-thy, peripheral neuropathy, and proteinuria. Patients do not have a mono-clonal protein because the deposited precursor is a mutant form of transthyretin, fibrinogen, lysozyme, or apolipoprotein A. Selected patients with familial amyloidosis have benefited from liver transplantation. One very important form of familial amyloidosis in the United States is associ-ated with an allele of the normal serum protein transthyretin in which iso-leucine is substituted for valine at position 122 (TTR Val-122-Ile). The prevalence of this mutation in blacks in the United States is as high as 3.9%. Heterozygous inheritance of this mutant TTR is associated with late-onset cardiomyopathy in this population. Wall thickening is found on echocar-diography. The heart failure is often mild at onset. The prognosis is far better than that of cardiac AL, and its recognition has important implications for genetic counseling.

Secondary Amyloidosis

Secondary systemic amyloidosis is the rarest form in Western nations. Previ-ously, it was a consequence of uncontrolled sustained inflammation, usually infectious, and causes included tuberculosis and osteomyelitis. Today it occurs primarily in patients with difficult-to-control inflammatory rheumatic syndromes, including juvenile arthritis and ankylosing spondylitis. These patients present with nephrotic syndrome, diarrhea related to intestinal involvement, and thyromegaly. Suppression of the inflammatory process results in regression of tissue amyloid deposits. There are familial forms of secondary amyloidosis associated with familial periodic fever syndromes, the most common being familial Mediterranean fever (Chapter 269) due to mutations in the tumor necrosis factor receptor.

1. Mhaskar R, Kumar A, Behera M, et al. Role of high-dose chemotherapy and autologous hematopoi-etic cell transplantation in primary systemic amyloidosis: a systematic review. *Biol Blood Marrow Transplant.* 2009;15:893-902.
2. Jaccard A, Moreau P, Leblond V, et al. High-dose melphalan versus melphalan plus dexamethasone for AL amyloidosis. *N Engl J Med.* 2007;357:1083-1093.

SUGGESTED READINGS

Cohen AD, Comenzo RL. Systemic light-chain amyloidosis: advances in diagnosis, prognosis, and therapy. *Hematology Am Soc Hematol Educ Program.* 2010;2010:287-294. *Review.*
Gertz MA. Immunoglobulin light chain amyloidosis: 2011 update on diagnosis, risk-stratification, and management. *Am J Hematol.* 2011;86:180-186. *Review.*
Kumar SK, Gertz MA, Lacy MQ, et al. Recent improvements in survival in primary systemic amyloidosis and the importance of an early mortality risk score. *Mayo Clin Proc.* 2011;86:12-18. *Four-year survival has increased from 21% in 1977-1986 to 42% now.*
Stangou AJ, Banner NR, Hendry BM, et al. Hereditary fibrinogen A alpha-chain amyloidosis: phenotypic characterization of a systemic disease and the role of liver transplantation. *Blood.* 2010;115:2998-3007. *Liver-kidney transplant is curative.*

195

TUMORS OF THE CENTRAL NERVOUS SYSTEM AND INTRACRANIAL HYPERTENSION AND HYPOTENSION

LISA M. DEANGELIS

INTRACRANIAL TUMORS
General Approach to Brain Tumors

EPIDEMIOLOGY

About 17,000 new primary brain tumors and nervous system cancers are diagnosed annually in the United States, making central nervous system (CNS) tumors more than twice as common as Hodgkin's disease and approx-imately one third as common as melanoma. In contrast, intracranial metas-tases are five times more common than primary brain tumors. More than 120 types of primary brain tumors arise from the different cells that make up the CNS (Table 195-1). In addition to classifying tumors by their cell of origin, in clinical practice it is often useful to classify a tumor by its intracranial site as well, such as pineal region tumors or pituitary and suprasellar tumors.

PATHOBIOLOGY

In contrast to tumors arising elsewhere in the body, there is little distinction between benign and malignant tumors when they occur in the brain. The growth of brain tumors is restricted to the CNS; they rarely, if ever, metasta-size to other organs. In the CNS, a malignant tumor is characterized by aggressive pathologic features, including local tissue invasion, neovascularity, regional necrosis, and cytologic atypia. These features confer a growth advan-tage to malignant cells and lead to rapid expansion and, frequently, to early regrowth after treatment. Tumors lacking these aggressive histologic features are preferably classified as low-grade rather than benign. Many low-grade tumors continue to grow within the CNS, causing progressive neurologic disability, and some may acquire a more malignant phenotype over time. The low-grade tumors that transform into high-grade neoplasms are primarily the intra-axial tumors that cannot be cured by resection because of their diffuse infiltration of brain. Almost all truly benign CNS tumors are extra-axial tumors, such as meningiomas and acoustic neuromas that can be cured with complete surgical resection.

CLINICAL MANIFESTATIONS

A patient with a brain tumor can present with one or both of two types of symptoms and signs. *Generalized symptoms,* which typically reflect the increased intracranial pressure (ICP) that often accompanies cerebral tumors, include headache, lethargy, personality change, nausea, and vomiting. *Later-alizing symptoms,* which reflect the specific location of the tumor, include hemiparesis, hemisensory deficits, aphasia, visual field impairment, and sei-zures (Table 195-2).

Most patients have symptoms that progress over a week to a few months. A sudden intensification of symptoms may precipitate the patient's initial visit to the physician; however, a careful history usually reveals symptoms that predated the acute deterioration and slowly worsened over time. Two exceptions are the new appearance of a seizure in a previously asymptomatic individual (Chapter 410) and sudden hemorrhage into a tumor.

TABLE 195-1 WORLD HEALTH ORGANIZATION CLASSIFICATION OF BRAIN TUMORS*

TUMORS OF NEUROEPITHELIAL TISSUE

Astrocytic tumors
  Astrocytoma
  Anaplastic (malignant) astrocytoma
  Glioblastoma multiforme
  Pilocytic astrocytoma
  Pleomorphic xanthoastrocytoma
  Subependymal giant cell astrocytoma
Oligodendroglial tumors
  Oligodendroglioma
  Anaplastic (malignant) oligodendroglioma
Ependymal tumors
  Ependymoma
  Anaplastic (malignant) ependymoma
  Myxopapillary ependymoma (spinal tumor)
  Subependymoma
Mixed gliomas
  Oligoastrocytoma
  Anaplastic (malignant) oligoastrocytoma
Choroid plexus
  Choroid plexus papilloma
  Choroid plexus carcinoma
Neuronal and mixed neuronal-glial tumors
  Gangliocytoma
  Dysembryoplastic neuroepithelial tumor
  Ganglioglioma
  Anaplastic (malignant) ganglioglioma
  Central neurocytoma
Pineal parenchymal tumors
  Pineocytoma
  Pineoblastoma
Embryonal tumors
  Medulloblastoma
  Primitive neuroectodermal tumor

TUMORS OF CRANIAL AND SPINAL NERVES

Schwannoma
Neurofibroma

TUMORS OF MENINGES

Meningioma
Hemangiopericytoma
Hemangioblastoma

PRIMARY CENTRAL NERVOUS SYSTEM LYMPHOMAS
GERM CELL TUMORS

Germinoma
Embryonal carcinoma
Yolk sac tumor (endodermal sinus tumor)
Choriocarcinoma
Teratoma
Mixed germ cell tumors

CYSTS AND TUMOR-LIKE LESIONS

Rathke cleft cyst
Epidermoid cyst
Dermoid cyst
Colloid cyst of the third ventricle

TUMORS OF THE SELLAR REGION

Pituitary adenoma
Pituitary carcinoma
Craniopharyngioma

METASTATIC TUMORS

*Abridged and modified from World Health Organization classification.

TABLE 195-2 FOCAL CLINICAL MANIFESTATIONS OF BRAIN TUMORS

Frontal lobe
  Generalized seizures
  Focal motor seizures (contralateral)
  Expressive aphasia (dominant side)
  Behavioral changes
  Dementia
  Gait disorders, incontinence
  Hemiparesis
Basal ganglia
  Hemiparesis (contralateral)
  Movement disorders (rare)
Parietal lobe
  Receptive aphasia (dominant side)
  Spatial disorientation (nondominant side)
  Cortical sensory dysfunction (contralateral)
  Hemianopia (contralateral)
  Agnosias
Occipital lobe
  Hemianopia (contralateral)
  Visual disturbances (unformed)
Temporal lobe
  Complex partial (psychomotor) seizures
  Generalized seizures
  Behavioral changes
  Olfactory and complex visual auras
  Language disorder (dominant side)
  Visual field defect
Corpus callosum
  Dementia (anterior)
  Memory loss (posterior)
  Behavioral changes
  Asymptomatic (middle)
Thalamus
  Sensory loss (contralateral)
  Behavioral changes
  Language disorder (dominant side)
Midbrain/pineal
  Paresis of vertical eye movement
  Pupillary abnormalities
  Precocious puberty (boys)
Sella/optic nerve/pituitary
  Endocrinopathy
  Bitemporal hemianopia
  Monocular visual defects
  Ophthalmoplegia (cavernous sinus)
Pons/medulla
  Cranial nerve dysfunction
  Ataxia, nystagmus
  Weakness, sensory loss
  Spasticity
Cerebellopontine angle
  Deafness (ipsilateral)
  Loss of facial sensation (ipsilateral)
  Facial weakness (ipsilateral)
  Ataxia
Cerebellum
  Ataxia (ipsilateral)
  Nystagmus

Symptoms of brain tumors can be produced by tumor invading brain parenchyma, tumor and edema compressing brain tissue, cerebrospinal fluid (CSF) obstruction caused directly by the tumor or by a shift of brain tissue, and herniation. Invasion and compression typically produce focal symptoms, many of which can be relieved if the compression is reduced. Obstruction of CSF flow and herniation are frequently a consequence of elevated ICP and typically produce generalized symptoms of headache, nausea, and vomiting, but they can also cause false localizing signs, such as an abducens nerve palsy, as a result of diffuse increased ICP.

Headache (Chapter 405) is a presenting symptom of approximately 35% of brain tumors. It is more common in younger than older patients and more common in patients who have rapidly growing tumors than in those whose tumors have evolved slowly (Fig. 195-1). Mental and cognitive abnormalities may be a reflection of local tumor (e.g., aphasia, alexia, agnosia) or of general impairment (e.g., lethargy, confusion, word finding difficulty, apathy). Seizures affect approximately one third of patients with brain tumors, and they are especially common as the presenting and only symptom of a low-grade tumor. The seizures, which are focal because they originate at the site of the tumor, may remain restricted (e.g., focal motor seizures), or they may generalize secondarily, producing loss of consciousness (Chapter 410), sometimes so quickly that the focal signature is missed by the patient or even an observant witness.

FIGURE 195-1. **Meningioma.** Computed tomography scan with contrast of a meningioma in a patient who presented with mild cognitive deficits, illustrative of the size a slow-growing tumor can attain in the brain. The tumor was completely resected.

FIGURE 195-2. **Glioma.** Magnetic resonance imaging (MRI) view of a low-grade glioma. **Left,** T2-weighted image; **right,** T1-weighted image, gadolinium contrast with minimum enhancement. The images are typical of this tumor, which is being detected with increasing frequency by MRI in seizure patients. Many are invisible on computed tomographic scans.

TABLE 195-3	MAGNETIC RESONANCE IMAGING OF COMMON BRAIN TUMORS		
TUMOR TYPE	**NONCONTRAST T1**	**CONTRAST T1**	**T2**
Malignant glioma	↓ density	+	↑ density
Low-grade glioma	↓ density	−	↑ density
Primary central nervous system lymphoma	↑ density	+	↑ density
Meningioma	Iso to ↑	+	Iso to ↓
Acoustic neuroma	↓ to Iso	+	Iso to ↑
Metastases	↑ to ↓	+	Variable, ↑ to ↓

DIAGNOSIS

Imaging

Magnetic resonance imaging (MRI) is far superior to computed tomography (CT) and should be used in all cases of suspected intracranial tumor. MRI should be performed both without and with intravenous gadolinium. A well-performed MRI scan identifies any intracranial tumor, and normal MRI results effectively exclude a neoplasm. The MRI of some extra-axial tumors (e.g., acoustic neuromas, meningiomas) is so characteristic that histologic confirmation is not required (Table 195-3). A non-contrast-enhancing infiltrative lesion that is visible primarily on T2 or fluid-attenuated inversion recovery (FLAIR) images is most consistent with a low-grade glioma (Fig. 195-2), whereas a contrast-enhancing lesion with an area of central necrosis and surrounding edema is most likely to be a glioblastoma or possibly a brain metastasis. Although these diagnoses must be confirmed histologically, the preoperative diagnostic possibilities affect the choice of surgical procedure and the surgical approach to the lesion.

Perfusion MRI after rapid infusion of gadolinium can measure the relative cerebral blood volume and neovascularity associated with a tumor; high perfusion is associated with higher grade of malignancy. This technique can help estimate the tumor grade preoperatively and guide the planning of treatment.

Magnetic resonance spectroscopy (MRS) noninvasively assesses tissue composition. High-grade primary brain tumors are associated with a decrease in N-acetylaspartate (NAA) and an increase in choline (Cho). More malignant tumors are associated with a greater Cho/NAA ratio and frequently contain areas with elevation of lactate and lipid.

Surgical resection is a major objective in the treatment of almost every kind of brain tumor, but resection must be balanced against possible damage to adjacent normal brain. The development of functional MRI (fMRI), which measures cerebral blood flow when areas of cortex are activated, has greatly enhanced the ability to localize critical neurologic functions and their relationship to the tumor preoperatively. When the fMRI is fused with the anatomic MRI, critical functions can be identified in relationship to the patient's tumor, and a safer and more complete resection may be planned.

On positron emission tomography (PET), high-grade tumors are usually hypermetabolic, whereas low-grade tumors are hypometabolic. New technologies using ^{11}C-methionine PET may differentiate low- from high-grade gliomas much more efficiently than deoxyglucose PET.

CT, without and with intravenous contrast, should be used only for patients who cannot undergo MRI. A CT scan, even with contrast, may miss low-grade tumors and tumors in the posterior fossa.

Currently, angiography has no role in the diagnosis of intracranial tumors. However, angiographic embolization is occasionally useful preoperatively to reduce the vascularity of some meningiomas, thereby making a complete resection safer and more feasible.

Other Tests

Electroencephalography (EEG) is rarely needed in the diagnosis or management of brain tumors. An EEG can occasionally be useful in a patient who has prolonged or unexplained stupor and in whom nonconvulsive status epilepticus is a consideration. Intraoperative monitoring is also frequently used to help guide resection of epileptogenic cortex adjacent to or within brain tumor tissue.

CSF analysis has little role in the diagnosis of most intracranial neoplasms. In primary CNS lymphoma (PCNSL), the diagnosis may be established on CSF cytologic examination in about 15% of patients. Rarely, a lumbar puncture is required to exclude inflammatory conditions or other processes that may be confused with a primary brain tumor. Lumbar puncture must be avoided in patients with cerebellar tumors because the release of pressure through the spinal needle may result in herniation of the cerebellar tonsils through the foramen magnum.

Differential Diagnosis

Patients who present with symptoms of raised ICP or the new onset of central neurologic symptoms such as hemiparesis or seizure should be hospitalized and evaluated rapidly. Prompt neuroimaging discloses a mass, and the radiographic features narrow the differential diagnosis (Table 195-4). Extra-axial tumors, such as a meningioma or acoustic neuroma, can be confused with a dural metastasis. Low-grade intra-axial tumors, which are nonenhancing on MRI, have been confused with infections such as herpes encephalitis when they involve the temporal lobe. Contrast-enhancing intra-axial tumors can be confused with a stroke, brain abscess, or focal plaque of demyelination. Subacute infarction can show brisk contrast enhancement, usually in a gyral pattern, unlike brain tumors, in which enhancement is primarily in the white matter; occasionally, however, the two are indistinguishable radiographically. Brain abscesses typically have a thinner enhancing wall than a malignant tumor, but they sometimes appear similar on MRI. Despite careful evaluation, patients thought to have a malignant glioma occasionally are found at surgery to have a brain abscess. A single large plaque of demyelination can

TABLE 195-4	DIFFERENTIAL DIAGNOSIS OF INTRACRANIAL TUMORS

Infection
    Brain abscess
        Bacterial
        Fungal
        Parasitic (e.g., cysticercosis)
    Herpes encephalitis
Vascular disease
    Stroke
    Intracranial hemorrhage
Inflammatory conditions
    Granuloma (sarcoid)
    Multiple sclerosis: single large lesion
Vascular malformations
    Cavernous angiomas
    Venous angiomas
Congenital abnormalities
    Cortical dysplasia
    Heterotopia

also be confused radiographically with a brain tumor, and sometimes the diagnosis can be established only by biopsy.

When MRI suggests a primary brain tumor, there is no need for an extensive systemic search for a possible source of metastasis. Brain metastases are more common than primary brain tumors, but most occur in patients with known cancer, typically with active systemic disease. If an obvious systemic cancer is not revealed by a thorough general examination, chest radiograph, routine blood tests, and urinalysis, then the patient should proceed to craniotomy. Even if a brain metastasis is found at surgery, resection of a single brain metastasis is the appropriate treatment, and the pathology of the lesion guides the subsequent search for the primary tumor.

TREATMENT   Rx

The treatment for all brain tumors can be divided into two main categories: symptomatic and definitive (Table 195-5). Symptomatic treatment addresses the associated problems, such as cerebral edema, seizures, and thromboembolic disease, which can contribute substantially to clinical symptoms. Definitive treatment addresses the tumor itself.

Symptomatic Treatment

Symptomatic management includes the use of corticosteroids, anticonvulsants, and prophylaxis for deep vein thrombosis (DVT) (Chapter 37). Corticosteroids decrease the vasogenic edema that surrounds primary and metastatic brain tumors. Blood vessels associated with tumor formation are leaky and do not share the normal morphologic and physiologic features that form the blood-brain barrier; corticosteroids effectively reconstitute the blood-brain barrier by decreasing the abnormal permeability of these neovessels. Clinical improvement may begin within minutes, and frequently patients are dramatically improved within 24 to 48 hours.

Dexamethasone is the most commonly used glucocorticoid because it has the least mineralocorticoid activity. The usual starting dose is 12 to 16 mg/day, but this can be adjusted to find the lowest possible dose that alleviates neurologic symptoms. After definitive treatment is instituted, many patients can be tapered off their corticosteroid completely. Chronic high-dose corticosteroid therapy is associated with substantial side effects (Chapter 34). Patients who will be taking glucocorticoids for 6 weeks or longer should receive prophylaxis against *Pneumocystis jiroveci* (formerly *Pneumocystis carinii*; Chapter 349).

Anticonvulsants are administered to any patient who has had a seizure, but prophylactic anticonvulsants should not be prescribed for patients who have never had a seizure, except they may be useful in the perioperative period.[1,2]

DVT, which occurs in about 25% of patients with brain tumors, can occur early in the illness or at any time during treatment. All patients undergoing neurosurgery should have pneumatic compression boots in the postoperative period to reduce the incidence of DVT. Prophylactic anticoagulants have also been used successfully in the immediate postoperative period without increasing postoperative hemorrhage. Appropriately regulated anticoagulation (Chapter 37) is the optimal therapy for DVT and is not associated with an increased risk of intracerebral hemorrhage in patients with intracranial tumors. Inferior vena cava filters can be used for patients who have DVTs or pulmonary emboli and who cannot be fully anticoagulated.

TABLE 195-5	TREATMENT FOR BRAIN TUMORS

SYMPTOMATIC

Glucocorticoids
Anticonvulsants
Deep vein thrombosis prophylaxis and treatment

DEFINITIVE

Surgery
    Goal is gross total excision
Radiotherapy
    Standard external beam
        Fractionated
        Usually focal
    Stereotactic radiosurgery
Chemotherapy
    Limited by intrinsic drug resistance and blood-brain barrier

Definitive Treatment

Surgery

Complete excision is the goal for a primary brain tumor. Surgical excision can often be accomplished for primary extra-axial tumors, such as meningiomas and acoustic neuromas. However, meningiomas often occur in intracranial locations that make resection impossible. Tumors of the skull base are particularly difficult to remove, and partial resection for decompression is often performed to preserve neurologic function. The safe boundaries for resecting cortical lesions while preserving function can often be elucidated by preoperative fMRI and intraoperative cortical mapping. However, lesions involving many critical structures, such as the brain stem or thalamus, cannot be excised safely.

Lesions that cannot be resected are still amenable to biopsy for diagnostic purposes. In particular, the use of stereotactic biopsy has made it feasible to reach lesions in almost any area of the brain with minimal morbidity. The risks of stereotactic biopsy include (1) inadequate tissue sample to make a diagnosis, (2) a tissue sample that does not accurately reflect the most malignant grade of the tumor, and (3) a procedure-related complication, such as hemorrhage. Hemorrhage that causes neurologic impairment occurs in only 2% of stereotactic biopsies, typically in patients with glioblastoma multiforme.

Complete excision can cure extra-axial primary brain tumor and is associated with prolonged survival and better neurologic outcome even in patients with primary intra-axial tumors. Gross total excision, as measured by postoperative neuroimaging, is associated with prolonged survival in patients with malignant gliomas and probably in those with low-grade gliomas as well. However, most low-grade gliomas are not amenable to gross total excision, and usually only partial excision is feasible. Macroscopic tumor can frequently be removed completely in patients with high-grade gliomas, but there is always remaining microscopic disease that infiltrates surrounding brain.

Some tumors, such as brain stem gliomas, are in such critical locations that biopsy is not attempted. Their characteristic radiographic appearance permits diagnosis and initiation of medical treatment.

Radiation Therapy

A course of external beam radiation therapy is delivered in small daily fractions to a total cumulative dose usually between 45 and 60 Gy. Dividing the treatment into small daily fractions permits sublethal repair in normal tissues and markedly reduces neurologic toxicity associated with cerebral radiation. External beam irradiation, which is the most effective nonsurgical treatment for brain tumors, doubles median survival time of patients with malignant primary brain tumors or metastatic lesions. It can also be useful for recurrent meningiomas and acoustic neuromas. However, it only rarely cures any of these lesions, and most patients develop recurrent disease despite maximal radiation therapy.

Stereotactic radiosurgery has been developed to deliver high fractions of focused radiation therapy that spare normal surrounding tissue. The technique is limited to tumors that are 3 cm in diameter or smaller and is less useful for malignant gliomas because of their infiltrative nature.

The neurologic complications of radiation therapy, which are usually observed in patients months to years after completion of treatment, include radionecrosis, dementia, and leukoencephalopathy. The incidence is reported as less than 5%, and most patients die of their brain tumor before the delayed consequences of treatment can be observed. However, in long-term survivors (e.g., patients with low-grade glioma or children with medulloblastoma), the late consequences of radiation therapy are important. Dementia accompanying radiation-induced leukoencephalopathy can progress and result in severe neurologic impairment. Radionecrosis can mimic recurrent tumor with a large contrast-enhancing lesion on MRI. Corticosteroids can reduce the edema and sometimes are sufficient to treat small areas of radionecrosis. However, if the lesion is sufficiently large, resection may be required to decompress the mass and reduce the steroid requirements.

Chemotherapy

Chemotherapy for brain tumors has usually been disappointing because of the intrinsic resistance of these tumors to most conventional agents. Carboplatin and cisplatin are active agents against medulloblastoma, even when the tumor is disseminated in the CSF. Temozolomide (150 to 200 mg/m^2 for 5 days every 4 weeks) is active in all gliomas, and high-dose methotrexate (3 to 8 g/m^2 for 3 to 12 months) is effective for PCNSL. For patients with glioblastoma, polymers impregnated with carmustine (BCNU) and placed in a resection cavity offer modest benefit when compared with no chemotherapy, but they are associated with local tissue injury and edema.

● SPECIFIC TYPES OF BRAIN TUMORS

Primary Extra-axial Tumors

The most common primary extra-axial tumors are meningiomas, pituitary adenomas, and acoustic neuromas. These tumors arise within the intracranial cavity but are not tumors of brain tissue. Almost all are benign; because the brain is rarely invaded, complete excision often enables cure with full recovery of neurologic function. These tumors produce neurologic symptoms and signs by compressing the underlying brain; however, edema of the underlying brain is infrequent, so glucocorticoids have a limited role.

MENINGIOMAS

EPIDEMIOLOGY

Meningiomas are usually benign. Between 5 and 10% of meningiomas are atypical or malignant variants with a more aggressive course. Meningiomas are more common in women, may be multiple in about 10% of patients with sporadic meningioma, and are occasionally part of a familial syndrome. They occur with increased frequency in patients with neurofibromatosis type 2 (Chapter 426).

DIAGNOSIS

Meningiomas grow slowly and produce symptoms that are insidious in onset and typically slowly progressive. Tumors can reach a considerable size, but they grow so slowly that the brain accommodates to the progressive compression. Meningiomas typically occur in specific locations: over the convexity, along the falx and parasagittal area, the olfactory groove, base of the skull near the sphenoid bone, cavernous sinus, cerebellopontine angle, and foramen magnum. Cortical and parasagittal tumors typically manifest with seizures or progressive hemiparesis. Tumors in the anterior cranial fossa can cause slowly progressive changes in personality and cognition. Meningiomas at the base of the skull manifest with cranial neuropathies and gait difficulties when there is brain stem compression. Frequently, tumors are completely asymptomatic and are identified on neuroimaging done for another purpose, such as head trauma.

On MRI, meningiomas have a characteristic appearance consisting of a diffusely enhancing, dural-based lesion that is associated with a thin enhancing dural tail extending from the tumor. Often the radiographic features are so characteristic that surgery is performed for therapeutic purposes only. The radiographic differential diagnosis includes the less common hemangiopericytoma and dural metastasis. Most meningiomas are not accompanied by significant edema, but marked edema is seen with high-grade malignant lesions or the secretory variant.

If small meningiomas are discovered in the absence of clinical symptoms or the symptoms are minor, lesions may be monitored with serial images because growth can be so slow.

TREATMENT   Rx

If treatment is indicated, complete resection is often curative, but even completely resected benign tumors may recur (as many as 20% in some series), so radiologic follow-up is essential. Tumors at the base of the skull often cannot be resected completely and tend to recur despite successive attempts at surgical resection. Radiation therapy can sometimes slow progression and is essential for the treatment of malignant meningiomas. No effective chemotherapy has yet been identified.

Acoustic Neuromas

Acoustic neuromas (Chapter 436), better called vestibular schwannomas, are benign tumors that arise from the eighth cranial nerve. Acoustic neuromas are twice as common in women as in men; the peak age is between 40 and 60 years. Sporadic vestibular schwannomas are unilateral; bilateral acoustic neuromas are pathognomonic of neurofibromatosis type 2 (Chapter 426).

Acoustic neuromas usually arise from the vestibular portion of the nerve and typically manifest with unilateral hearing loss, sometimes preceded or accompanied by tinnitus and a sensation of dizziness or unsteadiness but not true vertigo. The slow, progressive enlargement of the tumor produces ipsilateral facial numbness or weakness by compressing the fifth or seventh cranial nerve, respectively. Tumors originate within the internal auditory meatus but grow out of the acoustic canal and into the cerebellopontine angle, where they can compress the brain stem and cause ataxia and ipsilateral cerebellar signs. Cranial MRI with gadolinium delineates even small acoustic neuromas with ease.

Treatment is often surgical; stereotactic radiosurgery may be an alternative for lesions smaller than 3 cm. It is preferable to treat the tumors when they are small, to preserve facial nerve function and hearing.

Pituitary Adenomas

Pituitary adenomas (Chapter 231) can be classified according to their size as microadenomas (<1 cm in diameter) or macroadenomas; by the presence or absence of endocrine function; and by the endocrinologic syndromes or neurologic syndromes caused by tumor compression. Microadenomas typically manifest with endocrine symptoms as described in Chapter 231. As pituitary tumors enlarge and become macroadenomas, they compress the surrounding neural structures, including the optic chiasm and optic nerves, typically causing bitemporal hemianopia and occasionally causing unilateral visual loss. Macroadenomas are frequently nonsecreting but destroy pituitary tissue, causing panhypopituitarism. Rarely, pituitary tumors manifest with the abrupt onset of headache, ophthalmoplegia, unilateral blindness, and even a depressed level of alertness or coma—a syndrome of *pituitary apoplexy* caused by hemorrhage or infarction.

Cranial MRI, particularly with coronal images and gadolinium administration, can completely outline the pituitary tumor and surrounding neural structures. All macroadenomas and some microadenomas can be treated with transsphenoidal pituitary surgery, which is associated with minimal morbidity. Occasionally, residual or recurrent tumor necessitates radiation therapy. Some hormone-secreting tumors, particularly prolactinomas or growth hormone–secreting tumors, can be treated medically with cabergoline or octreotide, respectively (Chapter 231). These medications not only correct the hormonal excess but also shrink the tumor; they must be taken for life.

Other tumors in the pituitary and suprasellar region include craniopharyngiomas, suprasellar epidermoid cysts, Rathke cleft cysts, germinomas (discussed later), and lymphocytic hypophysitis, which is a benign inflammatory condition that usually manifests with diabetes insipidus (Chapter 232). MRI frequently differentiates these conditions, which are usually suprasellar and erode into the pituitary fossa only secondarily. Some of these lesions also have characteristic radiographic features. These lesions are benign. Except for hypophysitis, which resolves completely with corticosteroid treatment (e.g., methylprednisolone, 120 mg daily for 2 weeks and then tapered for 1 additional week), complete surgical excision is the curative therapy.

Other Extra-axial Tumors

Pineal region tumors all have a characteristic clinical presentation that includes Parinaud's syndrome, which consists of paresis of upward gaze, poor pupillary reaction to light with brisk reaction on accommodation, impairment of convergence, and convergence-retraction nystagmus. Some of these lesions may also cause hydrocephalus and symptoms of increased ICP. Pineal region tumors include pineal parenchymal tumors, such as pineocytomas and the more aggressive pineoblastomas, and germ cell tumors, including germinomas and nongerminomatous germ cell tumors. Germinomas can be completely cured with focal radiation therapy, whereas nongerminomatous germ cell tumors are more aggressive and frequently relapse despite chemotherapy plus cranial irradiation.

Chordomas are rare tumors of residual notochordal tissue. They usually occur at the base of the skull, are locally invasive, and are characterized by multiple recurrences despite surgery and radiation therapy.

Lipomas are benign tumors that can occur in midline structures, particularly near the corpus callosum. They can be cured by complete removal.

Arachnoid cysts are not tumors per se but can manifest with headaches, seizures, or focal neurologic symptoms if they become large enough to compress underlying brain tissue. Many are completely asymptomatic and are found incidentally on neuroimaging. Only symptomatic cysts require removal.

Primary Intra-axial Tumors

Most primary intra-axial brain tumors are gliomas, including the astrocytomas, oligodendrogliomas, and ependymomas. Less common are medulloblastomas, other rare neuroectodermal tumors, and PCNSLs. All of these tumors have a tendency to invade brain tissue, and none can be completely excised surgically.

GLIOMAS

DEFINITION

Astrocytomas, which are the most common glioma, are classified into one of four World Health Organization (WHO) categories: grade I is the pilocytic astrocytoma, grade II is the fibrillary astrocytoma, grade III is the anaplastic astrocytoma, and grade IV is the glioblastoma multiforme. Pilocytic astrocytomas (grade I) are extremely low-grade focal tumors that are more common in children and may be associated with neurofibromatosis type 1; they are often cured by complete surgical excision. Astrocytomas, anaplastic astrocytomas, and glioblastomas are diffuse tumors that tend to infiltrate widely into brain; even grade II tumors progress over time, and most acquire the histologic features and growth patterns of grade III and IV tumors.

EPIDEMIOLOGY

Gliomas occur at any age, but the peak age is 20 to 30 years for an astrocytoma, 40 years for anaplastic astrocytoma, and 55 to 60 years for glioblastoma. Age is the single most important prognostic factor: younger patients live substantially longer than older patients. Histology is also critical: patients with glioblastoma do significantly worse than patients with lower-grade lesions. Performance status, duration of symptoms, and whether a complete resection has been achieved are also strong predictors of improved outcome and prolonged survival. For all grades of glioma, men are more frequently affected than women, and whites significantly more frequently than blacks. Gliomas are typically single lesions, but multifocal disease is seen in approximately 5% of patients with high-grade tumors. A variant of gliomas, called *gliomatosis cerebri*, causes widespread infiltration of the entire brain; most patients have relatively low-grade pathology on biopsy, but focal regions of high-grade transformation can exist.

PATHOBIOLOGY

At least 95% of gliomas are sporadic, and only 5% occur in patients with a family history of brain tumor. Furthermore, patients with a familial history of glioma usually do not fall into a well-recognized hereditary syndrome. However, neurofibromatosis 1 (von Recklinghausen's disease; Chapter 426) is associated with an increased incidence of gliomas, particularly in the optic pathway, hypothalamus, and brain stem. Gliomas also occur with increased frequency in Turcot's syndrome, in which colorectal neoplasms are seen in association with a variety of CNS tumors. Somatic mutations of the isocitrate dehydrogenase 1 and 2 genes (*IDH1* and *IDH2*) have been identified in most low-grade gliomas and secondary glioblastomas: these patients had a better outcome than those with wild-type *IDH* genes.

CLINICAL MANIFESTATIONS AND DIAGNOSIS

Patients with gliomas often present with seizures, headache, and lateralizing signs such as hemiparesis, aphasia, or a visual field deficit. On MRI, low-grade gliomas typically appear as diffuse, nonenhancing lesions with a propensity to occur in the frontal lobe and insular cortex. High-grade gliomas, which typically enhance with contrast, occur in the cortical white matter and are accompanied by significant surrounding edema. Glioblastomas frequently have regions of central necrosis (Fig. 195-3), and hemorrhage can occur in 5 to 8% of patients.

TREATMENT   Rx

For all gliomas, treatment frequently involves surgery, radiation therapy, and chemotherapy. The surgical goal of complete removal of all visible disease is often impossible. The adequacy of resection is best assessed on a postoperative MRI study, without and with gadolinium, performed within 72 to 96 hours after surgery. Surgical removal usually improves neurologic function and reduces dependency on corticosteroids.

FIGURE 195-3. **Temporal lobe glioblastoma.** This T1-weighted gadolinium-enhanced magnetic resonance imaging view shows a typical ring configuration of contrast with central necrosis and marked mass effect.

ANAPLASTIC ASTROCYTOMAS AND GLIOBLASTOMAS

All anaplastic astrocytomas and glioblastomas should be treated with postoperative radiation therapy to a dose of approximately 60 Gy. In a randomized trial of patients with glioblastoma, the alkylating agent temozolomide (75 mg/m² daily), administered concurrently with radiation therapy and followed by adjuvant temozolomide (150 to 200 mg/m² for 5 consecutive days every 4 weeks for 6 cycles), significantly improved survival (median, 14.6 months) compared with radiation therapy alone (median, 12.1 months; *P* < .001), and the 2-year survival rate more than doubled to 26.5%. **3** Patients whose tumors contained a methylated promoter of the O6-methylguanine-DNA methyltransferase *(MGMT)* DNA repair gene benefited most from the addition of temozolomide. Based on these data, combined treatment is the current standard of care for patients with glioblastoma. Chemotherapy is generally well tolerated and associated with minimal toxicity. Elderly patients often do poorly, but a randomized trial showed that radiotherapy (compared with supportive care only) results in a modest improvement in survival, without reducing quality of life or cognition, in elderly patients with glioblastoma.**4** Recurrences can be treated with re-resection, additional chemotherapy, or, occasionally, stereotactic radiosurgery, or a combination of these. Despite aggressive treatment, disease recurs in almost all patients, and the median survival time is 14 to 15 months for glioblastoma. Patients with anaplastic gliomas (including anaplastic oligodendrogliomas) had identical median survivals of about 7 years whether the initial treatment was radiotherapy or chemotherapy.**5** However, some young patients with anaplastic astrocytoma can survive many years before the tumor recurs.

OPTIC AND BRAIN STEM GLIOMAS

Optic gliomas, which can involve the optic nerve or optic chiasm, are usually associated with neurofibromatosis type 1. These gliomas are typically pilocytic tumors that can have an indolent course, including rare spontaneous regression. Often they are not amenable to surgical resection, and they can have a stuttering clinical course, with periods of visual loss punctuated by prolonged periods of visual stability. When necessary, radiation or even chemotherapy may be useful, but often no treatment is required. Brain stem gliomas usually involve the pons, less often the medulla or midbrain. Brain stem gliomas are most commonly seen in children in the first decade of life but can be found even in elderly people; they can have a low-grade or a high-grade histology, but outcome is primarily determined by the location of the tumor. In general, most brain stem gliomas have a dismal outcome with survival of 1 year or less, but relatively benign variants occasionally occur.

LOW-GRADE ASTROCYTOMAS

Low-grade astrocytomas have a variable course. In patients who present with isolated seizures that can be easily controlled with anticonvulsants, treatment with radiation therapy or chemotherapy immediately after surgery does not prolong survival, and patients can be monitored until there is clinical or radiographic evidence of tumor progression.[6] Patients with progressive neurologic symptoms or cognitive impairment require immediate treatment after diagnosis, and focal radiation therapy to a total of about 54 Gy is the optimal choice. An astrocytoma can progress as a low-grade tumor or transform to a higher-grade malignancy, a change that typically is associated with the appearance of contrast enhancement on MRI. Resection or a biopsy may be necessary in these patients, followed by radiation therapy if they have not received it previously; chemotherapy with temozolomide (150 to 200 mg/m^2 for 5 days every 4 weeks for anywhere from 6 to 24 cycles) is also used. Patients with astrocytomas have a median survival of about 5 years.

OLIGODENDROGLIOMAS

Oligodendrogliomas occur as low-grade tumors and, less commonly, as anaplastic lesions. Treatment of these tumors differs from that of their astrocytic counterparts because oligodendrogliomas are uniquely chemosensitive, owing to their characteristic loss of chromosomes 1p and 19q. As with the low-grade astrocytomas, treatment should be withheld in patients with low-grade oligodendrogliomas who have no symptoms other than well-controlled seizures. Patients with progressive neurologic symptoms require treatment, and initial therapy is often chemotherapy, usually with single-agent temozolomide (150 to 200 mg/m^2 for 5 days every 4 weeks for 6 to 24 cycles) or the combination of procarbazine, lomustine, and vincristine. Radiation therapy is withheld until chemotherapy fails.

By comparison, all anaplastic oligodendrogliomas require immediate treatment. The standard approach includes focal radiation therapy. Adjuvant chemotherapy significantly prolongs disease-free survival but not overall survival time.[7] However, there is a growing movement toward treating high-grade tumors with chemotherapy alone and, in some cases, using high-dose chemotherapy with autologous stem cell rescue (Chapter 181). Some success has been reported with this approach, but it should still be considered experimental. Tumor progression should be treated with re-resection, radiation therapy if not previously administered, and additional chemotherapy. Patients with low-grade oligodendrogliomas have a median survival time in excess of 15 years, and those who have anaplastic oligodendrogliomas survive a median of 4 to 5 years.

MEDULLOBLASTOMAS

Medulloblastomas usually occur in the vermis of the cerebellum and principally affect children and young adults. Boys outnumber girls by about 2 : 1, and peak onset is at age 7 years; medulloblastoma in adulthood is rare and usually affects the cerebellar hemisphere.

The most common chromosomal abnormality associated with medulloblastoma is isochromosome 17q, which is found in as many as 60% of tumors. Tumors with an identical histology but different genetics may arise in the cerebral hemispheres and are called *primitive neuroectodermal tumors* (PNETs). PNETs usually have an aggressive course, leading to rapid death despite vigorous treatment.

Medulloblastomas have a characteristic clinical presentation, with ataxia (due to cerebellar and brain stem involvement) and headache, nausea, and vomiting (due to increased ICP from obstructive hydrocephalus). Aggressive surgery with complete excision is strongly associated with improved outcome. Surgery is always followed by neuraxis radiation therapy. Chemotherapy with vincristine, etoposide, carboplatin, and cyclophosphamide significantly improves 5-year event-free survival from 60 to 74% but has not significantly prolonged overall survival, which is about 70 to 80% at 5 years. This vigorous therapy often results in significant delayed complications in survivors, including intellectual deficits, growth impairment, and endocrinologic dysfunction. Late relapses as well as secondary neoplasms compromise long-term outcome.

GANGLIOGLIOMAS

Gangliogliomas, as the name implies, possess both a glial component and a neoplastic neural component (ganglion cell). Some low-grade gangliogliomas are indolent and do not require additional treatment after surgical extirpation. Patients with anaplastic tumors may fare better than patients with malignant gliomas, but recurrence is the rule despite surgery and radiation therapy.

PRIMARY CENTRAL NERVOUS SYSTEM LYMPHOMAS

PCNSLs are associated with immunodeficiency states, particularly acquired immunodeficiency syndrome and organ transplantation, and are seen with increased frequency among the apparently immunocompetent population as well. Men are more frequently affected than women, and the median age at

diagnosis is about 60 years. These tumors are usually large cell, B-cell non-Hodgkin's lymphomas identical to systemic lymphoma (Chapter 191). The tumor can involve the CSF, the eye, and the brain, where it is multifocal in about 40% of patients at presentation. In contrast to all other brain tumors, surgical resection is not associated with improved survival and can cause significant neurologic morbidity; therefore, biopsy, not resection, is the better surgical approach. Chemotherapy is the primary treatment, and high-dose methotrexate (3 to 8 g/m^2 on alternate weeks for 3 to 12 months) is the most important chemotherapeutic agent. In older patients, radiation therapy is avoided because the necessary whole brain irradiation causes significant cognitive impairment when combined with chemotherapy. Furthermore, radiation therapy alone produces a response but is followed by relapse within 1 year. Corticosteroids (e.g., dexamethasone 8 to 16 mg/day), which are frequently used as part of the chemotherapeutic regimen, not only help manage the associated cerebral edema but also can cause tumor regression. With the use of multiagent chemotherapy, with or without cranial irradiation, median survival times are now in the 3- to 5-year range.

OTHER INTRA-AXIAL TUMORS

Rare, intra-axial cerebral tumors include the *ependymoma,* which is optimally treated with surgical excision followed by radiation therapy. *Choroid plexus papillomas* and carcinomas may manifest with hydrocephalus or lateralizing signs. Resection may be sufficient for the benign papilloma, but carcinomas rapidly recur even when postoperative radiation therapy is also used. *Colloid cysts* of the third ventricle are benign tumors that can cause obstructive hydrocephalus; they may be treated with a ventricular peritoneal shunt or with resection using an intraventricular endoscope. *Hemangioblastomas* occur primarily in the cerebellum but can also occur in the spinal cord and the hemispheres. About 15% of patients with a hemangioblastoma have the autosomal dominant disorder, von Hippel-Lindau disease (Chapter 426), which is characterized by hemangioblastomas in the CNS and retina, renal cell carcinoma, pheochromocytoma, endolymphatic sac tumors, and cysts in a variety of visceral organs. Hemangioblastomas are treated by surgical excision and require radiation therapy only for recurrence. Complete removal usually results in cure.

Metastatic Tumors
BRAIN METASTASES

DEFINITION AND EPIDEMIOLOGY

Every systemic cancer is capable of metastasizing to the brain. Melanoma (Chapter 210) has the greatest propensity to spread to the CNS, but the most common causes of CNS metastases are cancers of the breast (Chapter 204) and lung (Chapter 197), followed by cancers of the colon (Chapter 199) and kidney (Chapter 203). CNS metastases are being seen with greater frequency as patients with systemic cancers have prolonged survival with better treatments. In most patients with brain metastases, CNS disease develops late in the course of their illness, but a brain metastasis may be the initial presentation of a systemic cancer. In most of the latter patients, lung cancer is the primary site; in some, however, a primary site is never identified (Chapter 211).

CLINICAL MANIFESTATIONS AND DIAGNOSIS

Patients with brain metastases present with progressive neurologic symptoms and signs that typically include headache, seizures, and lateralizing signs. Metastases are best diagnosed by a cranial MRI with gadolinium enhancement (Fig. 195-4). All lesions can be clearly seen by MRI, which is better than CT for visualizing the posterior fossa. Metastases, which are usually well-circumscribed lesions at the gray matter–white matter junction, are often associated with extensive edema. Hemorrhage into a metastasis occurs most frequently with metastases from melanoma, renal cancer, and thyroid cancer; however, because brain metastases from lung cancer are so common, they are the type most commonly associated with hemorrhage. Sometimes, hemorrhage into a brain metastasis is best visualized by noncontrast head CT.

TREATMENT   Rx

Because brain metastases do not widely infiltrate into brain tissue and tend to have a pseudocapsule around them, they can be completely excised surgically. In randomized controlled studies, complete removal of a single brain metastasis substantially prolonged life and maintained neurologic function for

FIGURE 195-4. Brain metastasis. Multiple metastases from breast carcinoma are seen on this T1-weighted gadolinium-enhanced magnetic resonance imaging view. The multiple smaller tumors were not visible on computed tomography, even after a contrast agent was given.

FIGURE 195-5. Leptomeningeal metastases. Gadolinium-enhanced magnetic resonance imaging of the lumbosacral spine in a patient with leptomeningeal metastases from melanoma. Multiple enhancing nodules are seen on the cauda equina, and the conus medullaris and lower spinal cord are encased by tumor.

a longer period. Postoperative whole brain radiation therapy significantly improves control of CNS disease after resection of a single brain metastasis, but it does not prolong survival[8] because patients die of progressive systemic tumor. Consequently, the use of postoperative whole brain radiation therapy is frequently decided on an individual basis. If multiple lesions can be completely resected, these patients do as well as those with a single lesion that has been removed.

Most patients with multiple brain metastases are best treated with a course of whole brain radiation therapy, most commonly 3 Gy in 10 fractions for a total of 30 Gy. Some patients with single brain metastasis are also treated with whole brain irradiation if they are in poor general condition, have uncontrolled systemic disease, or are not good candidates for surgical treatment.

Stereotactic radiosurgery, using either a gamma knife that delivers gamma radiation from multiple cobalt sources or a linear accelerator that delivers x-rays to a highly focused area involving the tumor, has been quite effective for the treatment of one or a few brain metastases. Most patients tolerate radiosurgery without difficulty, but occasionally the procedure is complicated by seizures or acute swelling that causes more neurologic dysfunction. Approximately 20 to 30% of patients develop radionecrosis, which may be indistinguishable clinically and on MRI from recurrent tumor. One advantage of stereotactic radiosurgery is that most of the normal brain is not exposed to the radiation.

Chemotherapy is used to treat brain metastases from only a few chemosensitive primary cancers such as choriocarcinoma, small cell lung cancer, and, to a lesser extent, breast cancer. Because few patients have a significant response to chemotherapy, it is usually used as a last resort. The oral agent temozolomide (150 to 200 mg/m² for 5 days every 4 weeks) has shown some activity against brain metastases from lung cancer and is very well tolerated.

LEPTOMENINGEAL METASTASES

The brain is the most common intracranial site of metastases, but systemic cancer can spread to the dura and the leptomeninges as well. Dural metastases most commonly arise from breast or prostate cancer, frequently from a metastasis in the overlying calvaria. Metastasis to the leptomeninges often manifests as multifocal neurologic symptoms and signs. These metastases involve the cranial nerves to cause diplopia or bulbar palsy; the cervical and lumbar roots to cause limb pain or weakness; and the intracranial space to cause headache, nausea, vomiting, and elevated ICP. The diagnosis is established by the presence of tumor cells in the CSF or by neuroimaging that definitively outlines tumor in the subarachnoid space (Fig. 195-5). Treatment frequently involves radiation therapy to symptomatic sites; intrathecal chemotherapy, usually through an intraventricular cannula (Ommaya reservoir); or systemic chemotherapy with agents at doses that penetrate into the CSF.

TABLE 195-6	SPINAL TUMORS

Extradural
  Metastasis
  Primary bone tumors arising in the spine
Intradural extramedullary
  Meningiomas
  Neurofibromas
  Schwannomas
  Lipomas
  Arachnoid cysts
  Epidermoid cysts
  Metastasis
Intramedullary
  Ependymoma
  Glioma
  Hemangioblastoma
  Lipoma
  Metastasis

Spinal Tumors

Tumors involving the spine can be classified according to the anatomic area they involve: extradural, intradural extramedullary, and intramedullary tumors (Table 195-6). Extradural tumors typically arise from the bony elements of the spine and cause neurologic symptoms and signs by spinal cord compression. Intradural but extramedullary tumors arise from the pachymeninges or nerve roots (meningiomas or schwannomas) and can cause either radicular symptoms or spinal cord compression. Intramedullary spinal cord tumors arise from the spinal cord parenchyma and have a biology similar to brain tumors. Intramedullary tumors are rare.

EXTRADURAL TUMORS

EPIDEMIOLOGY AND CLINICAL MANIFESTATIONS

Most extradural tumors originate from a metastasis to the bony elements of the spine, typically the vertebral body and occasionally the vertebral lamina or spinous process. Less common are primary tumors of the spine, including chordoma, osteogenic sarcoma, plasmacytoma, and chondrosarcoma. Expansile growth of the bone tumor impinges on the spinal canal and, if untreated, compresses the spinal cord or the nerve roots as they exit the intervertebral foramina. Whereas most of these lesions arise from bony metastases, extradural tumors can also arise from paravertebral metastases that can grow through the intervertebral foramina and into the epidural space; very rarely, a direct metastasis to the epidural space is also seen. The most common primary cancers that cause extradural metastases are prostate (Chapter 207), breast (Chapter 204), and lung cancer (Chapter 197), as well as the lymphomas (Chapter 191). Hematologic malignancies may also be associated with paravertebral disease that grows through the intervertebral foramina.

Whether the mass is a primary bone tumor or a metastasis from a distant source, 98% of patients present with pain that is usually local at the site of the tumor. Because there are more thoracic than cervical or lumbar vertebrae, the tumor and pain are likely to be in the middle or high back, a less common site for benign pain (Chapter 407). Motor impairment and sensory symptoms are present in about 50% of patients, whereas sphincter disturbances are found in only about 25% of patients. Back pain often precedes the development of any other neurologic symptom or sign, frequently by weeks and occasionally by months.

DIAGNOSIS

Severe back pain in a patient with cancer should be evaluated by MRI, which does not require intravenous contrast. Plain films of the spine, bone scans, or even CT scans may show bony disease, but epidural tumor can be seen only on MRI. Furthermore, MRI is the only technique that can reveal paravertebral or direct epidural metastasis. Patients who cannot have an MRI should be imaged by CT myelography.

Differential Diagnosis

The differential diagnosis of extradural tumors includes epidural abscess (Chapter 421), acute or subacute epidural hematomas (Chapter 407), herniated intervertebral discs (Chapter 407), spondylosis (Chapter 407), epidural lipomatosis, and, rarely, extramedullary hematopoiesis. Occasionally, a percutaneous needle biopsy or decompressive laminectomy is required to make a definitive diagnosis.

TREATMENT   Rx

Extradural metastases require immediate treatment because patients can develop acute and unpredictable neurologic deterioration resulting in paraplegia. Patients should be started on high-dose corticosteroids, usually 100 mg IV dexamethasone, which rapidly relieve pain and may contribute to neurologic recovery. Surgery followed by postoperative radiation therapy is superior to radiotherapy alone in preserving the ability to walk[9] and may prolong survival in a wide population of patients with metastatic spinal cord compression. It is much easier to preserve neurologic function than to reverse impairment, so clinically silent areas of extradural tumor that are detected on MRI should be treated before neurologic compromise develops. Patients whose primary tumor arises in the spine, such as an osteogenic sarcoma (Chapter 208), should undergo definitive surgery; the need for postoperative radiation therapy is determined on the basis of the tumor's histology. Patients with extradural metastases can have a good neurologic outcome if treated before the onset of severe neurologic compromise, but their overall survival is usually short because of the presence of widespread metastatic disease.

INTRADURAL EXTRAMEDULLARY TUMORS

Meningiomas

Most intradural extramedullary tumors are benign. Meningiomas are benign, slow-growing tumors that occur primarily in middle-aged women and are predominantly located in the thoracic region. Back pain is a common symptom, but about 25% of patients have no pain and present with slowly progressive neurologic dysfunction, typically a gait disorder that has been slowly progressing, frequently for years. Spinal MRI with gadolinium clearly delineates the lesion. Surgical resection is curative, and a complete resection can usually be accomplished easily.

Nerve Sheath Tumors

Nerve sheath tumors include schwannomas and neurofibromas. Both typically arise from the dorsal root, and the first symptom is often radicular pain that precedes symptoms of spinal cord compression by months or even years. Some patients with spinal neurofibroma or schwannoma have neurofibromatosis type 1 (Chapter 426), but most do not. The diagnosis is clearly established by gadolinium-enhanced MRI of the spine. The treatment is surgical, and complete removal results in cure.

Metastases

Metastasis to the spinal leptomeninges can manifest as an intradural extramedullary lesion. A single large tumor nodule can cause focal symptoms and signs referable to that spinal level, but in most patients, multiple levels of the neuraxis are involved, causing multifocal neurologic symptoms and signs. Cervical and lumbosacral radicular pain, as well as sensory and motor loss, is seen in more than half of patients. The diagnosis is established by gadolinium-enhanced MRI showing multifocal nodules or sometimes a layer of cells coating the spinal cord or nerve roots (see Fig. 195-5). If imaging is negative, the diagnosis can be established by demonstrating tumor cells in the CSF. Treatment is complicated and frequently requires radiation therapy to symptomatic sites of disease, intrathecal chemotherapy best administered through an intraventricular cannula (Ommaya device), and occasionally systemic chemotherapy. Radiation therapy can ameliorate neurologic symptoms, particularly pain, but the disease often has a relentless progressive course, resulting in death in 3 to 6 months despite aggressive therapy. Because of the diffuse nature of the disease, surgery is not an option.

INTRAMEDULLARY TUMORS

Intramedullary spinal cord tumors are similar to neoplasms that arise in brain parenchyma. The most common spinal cord tumors are ependymomas and astrocytomas; hemangioblastomas (particularly in association with von Hippel-Lindau disease; Chapter 426), lipomas, and, rarely, intramedullary metastases are also seen.

CLINICAL MANIFESTATIONS AND DIAGNOSIS

All intramedullary tumors have a similar clinical presentation, and pain is a common initial symptom. Signs of spinal cord dysfunction subsequently ensue and reflect the location of the lesion. In addition, some intramedullary tumors are accompanied by a syrinx (Chapter 426), which can contribute to symptoms. The classic signs of intramedullary spinal cord lesions, such as dissociated sensory loss, sacral sparing, and early sphincter problems, are not sufficiently reliable to distinguish intramedullary from extramedullary lesions on the basis of clinical findings. The diagnosis is established by gadolinium-enhanced MRI.

TREATMENT

Surgery is the first therapeutic intervention, both to obtain a definitive diagnosis and to resect the lesion. Complete resection of spinal cord tumors is possible, particularly in the case of ependymomas and hemangioblastomas. However, spinal cord tumors are rare, and only neurosurgeons experienced in removal of this type of lesion should perform the procedure. High-grade gliomas and residual ependymomas should be treated with postoperative radiation therapy. Low-grade astrocytomas of the spinal cord can be treated with radiation therapy when the patient develops symptomatic neurologic impairment, but presymptomatic treatment does not prevent the development of impairment nor necessarily delay it. Intramedullary metastases do not require surgery because the diagnosis is usually straightforward; radiation therapy provides limited benefit because these patients typically have other CNS metastases.

● INTRACRANIAL HYPERTENSION AND HYPOTENSION

CSF is made, in part, by the choroid plexus in the ventricular system; newly formed fluid circulates out the foramina of Luschka and Magendie, at the bottom of the fourth ventricle, to surround the entire spinal cord and cerebrum. It is reabsorbed back into the circulation through the arachnoid granulations over the convexities. Balance between CSF production and reabsorption keeps the volume relatively constant at about 150 mL in the normal healthy adult. CSF is produced at a rate of roughly 20 mL/hour, implying that the entire volume of CSF is replaced three to four times each day. CSF circulates nutrients to the nervous system and removes waste products from the only organ in the body that lacks a lymphatic system. In addition, CSF performs an important mechanical function by absorbing shock to the brain and spinal cord, cushioning them from the bony surroundings of the skull and spine.

A lumbar puncture provides the opportunity not only for sampling the CSF composition to detect disease processes but also for measuring ICP. CSF

(Chapter 409). Some patients have features of parkinsonism (Chapter 416)

TABLE 195-7	SYMPTOMS AND SIGNS OF INTRACRANIAL HYPERTENSION

COMMON

Headache
Tinnitus
Vomiting (with or without nausea)
Visual obscurations, visual loss, photopsias
Papilledema
Diplopia
Lethargy and increased sleep
Psychomotor retardation
Pain on eye movement

LESS COMMON

Hearing distortion or loss
Vertigo
Facial weakness
Shoulder or arm pain
Neck pain or rigidity
Ataxia
Paresthesias of extremities
Anosmia
Trigeminal neuralgia

TABLE 195-8	CAUSES OF HYDROCEPHALUS

ACUTE

Cerebellar hemorrhage/infarction
Colloid cyst of the third ventricle
Exudative meningitis
Head trauma
Intracranial tumor or hematoma
Spontaneous subarachnoid hemorrhage
Viral encephalitis

CHRONIC

Aqueductal stenosis
Ectasia and elongation of the basilar artery (rare)
Granulomatous meningitis
Head trauma
Hindbrain malformations
Leptomeningeal metastasis
Brain and spinal cord tumors
Spontaneous subarachnoid hemorrhage

pressure is normally maintained between 70 and 195 mm H_2O. ICP is maintained within this narrow window because significant fluctuations, either up or down, can cause marked neurologic dysfunction.

Intracranial Hypertension

Elevated ICP causes symptoms by compressing neural tissue, a process that causes ischemia and sometimes hemorrhage due to associated arterial and venous compression. ICP is partially maintained through the autoregulatory mechanisms of the cerebral blood vessels. Low ICP is caused by diminished CSF volume, and symptoms result from the loss of buoyancy of the brain as it floats within the CSF liquid. Pulling or stretching of the dura and cortical veins, which are the pain-sensitive structures in the cranial vault, causes headache; compensatory vasodilation may also contribute to headache.

The principal symptoms and signs associated with increased ICP are headache, nausea, vomiting, and lethargy; other symptoms are less frequent (Table 195-7). Focal mass lesions that cause a herniation syndrome may produce lateralizing signs such as hemiparesis; by comparison, diffuse elevation of ICP, as in communicating hydrocephalus, rarely does. Three main herniation syndromes are (1) herniation of the medial frontal gyrus under the falx; (2) transtentorial herniation of the uncus, pushing the diencephalon and the brain stem downward and laterally; and (3) herniation of the cerebellar tonsils through the foramen magnum. Generalized increased ICP may be due to obstruction of CSF, which may be caused by blockage of the ventricular system (obstructive or noncommunicating hydrocephalus) or by impairment of CSF reabsorption (nonobstructive or communicating hydrocephalus).

Increased ICP of any cause may produce pressure or plateau waves (episodic increases in ICP), leading to transient symptoms such as headache, vertigo, or diminished consciousness. Plateau waves occur normally and are associated with symptoms only when the baseline ICP is elevated. Plateau waves may be precipitated by a change in body position.

Hydrocephalus

Hydrocephalus refers to ventricular dilation caused by accumulated CSF. Hydrocephalus can be acute, resulting from sudden blockage of CSF outflow, or chronic, developing slowly over many months to years (Table 195-8). Patients with chronic hydrocephalus sometimes have normal CSF pressures, whereas those with acute hydrocephalus always have elevated CSF pressure.

CLINICAL MANIFESTATIONS

Acute hydrocephalus usually manifests with severe headache, lethargy, nausea, vomiting, papilledema, and diplopia from abducens palsy as well as signs from the causative lesion. Diffuse hyperreflexia and bilateral Babinski signs are common. Patients with chronic communicating hydrocephalus often have normal CSF pressure, so-called normal pressure hydrocephalus (NPH), and may present with progressive dementia characterized by memory loss and psychomotor retardation, an unsteady gait, and urgency incontinence (Chapter 409). Some patients have features of parkinsonism (Chapter 416) because of the bradykinesia and psychomotor retardation associated with hydrocephalus, but resting tremor is absent.

DIAGNOSIS

Ventriculomegaly is readily diagnosed by MRI or CT. In older patients, cerebral atrophy and the associated compensating increase in ventricular volume that accompanies normal aging (hydrocephalus ex vacuo) must be considered. Periventricular hyperintensity on T2-weighted or FLAIR MRI may help separate patients with NPH from those with hydrocephalus ex vacuo. MRI is the best test to identify a cause of hydrocephalus.

TREATMENT Rx

If the ICP approaches or exceeds the systolic blood pressure, the cerebral perfusion pressure decreases, and ischemia develops. Marked elevation of ICP is a neurologic emergency that requires immediate intervention (Table 195-9) to reduce the volume of the intracranial contents and to prevent permanent brain damage. Hyperventilation to lower the arterial partial pressure of carbon dioxide ($PaCO_2$) to 25 to 30 mm Hg causes immediate vasoconstriction, which reduces cerebral blood volume. Intravenous mannitol or hypertonic saline can cause a rapid diuresis, which reduces intravascular plasma volume and helps to withdraw water from the extracellular space in the brain. Glucocorticoids, typically as dexamethasone 50 to 100 mg by IV bolus, will require hours to reduce underlying edema; vasogenic edema from brain tumor or brain abscess responds rapidly to corticosteroids, but cytotoxic edema accompanying an acute ischemic stroke or hematoma seldom responds to corticosteroids.

Ultimately, however, definitive treatment of the specific cause is necessary. If such treatment is not immediately feasible, hydrocephalus often responds promptly to ventricular drainage. If temporary drainage is necessary, an external ventricular drain can be placed until the underlying obstruction is relieved. A ventriculoperitoneal shunt is the definitive treatment for chronic hydrocephalus, but it is not reliably effective for "idiopathic" NPH. The clinical response to several days of external lumbar CSF drainage has a high predictive value for determining which patients with NPH are likely to benefit from a shunt. Complications of shunting include subdural hematomas and infection.

Idiopathic Intracranial Hypertension

DEFINITION AND EPIDEMIOLOGY

Idiopathic intracranial hypertension, also called benign intracranial hypertension or pseudotumor cerebri, refers to elevated ICP that develops in an otherwise healthy individual without evidence of a structural CNS

TABLE 195-9 EMERGENCY TREATMENT OF ELEVATED INTRACRANIAL PRESSURE IN ACUTELY DECOMPENSATING PATIENTS

THERAPY	TREATMENT	ONSET (DURATION OF ACTION)	OTHER
Hyperventilation	Lower PaCO$_2$ to 25-30 mm Hg	Seconds (minutes)	Usually requires intubation and mechanical ventilation
Osmotherapy	Mannitol 0.5-2 g/kg IV, repeat as necessary	Minutes (hours)	Brisk diuresis Requires Foley catheter Strict attention to electrolytes
Corticosteroids	Dexamethasone 50-100 mg IV, followed by 50-100 mg/day in divided doses	Hours (days)	Most effective on vasogenic edema (tumors, abscesses) Less effective on cytotoxic edema (stroke)

PaCO$_2$ = arterial partial pressure of carbon dioxide.

TABLE 195-10 SYSTEMIC AND IATROGENIC CONDITIONS ASSOCIATED WITH BENIGN INTRACRANIAL HYPERTENSION

COMMONLY PRESCRIBED DRUGS

Nalidixic acid
Nitrofurantoin
Phenytoin
Sulfonamides
Tetracycline
Vitamin A
Retinoic acid (*cis* or *trans*)

ENDOCRINE AND METABOLIC DISORDERS

Addison's disease
Cushing's syndrome
Hypoparathyroidism
Menarche, pregnancy, oral contraceptives
Obesity (often associated with irregular menses)
Corticosteroid therapy or withdrawal

HEMATOLOGIC DISORDERS

Cryoglobulinemia
Iron deficiency anemia

MISCELLANEOUS DISORDERS

Dural venous sinus obstruction or thrombosis
Head trauma
Internal jugular vein ligation
Systemic lupus erythematosus
Middle ear disease

TABLE 195-11 CAUSES OF INTRACRANIAL HYPOTENSION

Postlumbar puncture
CSF leak following CNS surgery or trauma
CSF fistula
Post-thoracotomy leak into pleural space
Spontaneous/idiopathic dural tear

CNS = central nervous system; CSF = cerebrospinal fluid.

TREATMENT   Rx

The need to treat chronic intractable elevation of ICP is based on the patient's symptoms and serial visual field testing. Headache or new or progressive visual loss on eye examination or perimetry testing should trigger one or more of five treatments: (1) weight reduction (e.g., 20 lb) or correction of underlying endocrinologic or hematologic disorders, or both; (2) repeated lumbar punctures; (3) acute pharmacologic treatments, including corticosteroids, loop diuretics, and acetazolamide, although corticosteroids can contribute to weight gain and their tapering may exacerbate the syndrome; (4) ventriculoperitoneal or lumboperitoneal shunt; and (5) fenestration of the optic nerve sheath, especially for patients with persistently elevated ICP and deteriorating vision.

PROGNOSIS

Outcome is variable: spontaneous remissions may occur; clinical improvement is not always accompanied by a reduction in CSF pressure; and the CSF pressure may remain persistently elevated despite intervention. Furthermore, patients with chronically elevated ICP from idiopathic intracranial hypertension never develop hydrocephalus, so CSF pressure and ventriculomegaly are not linked.

abnormality. Most patients are obese young women, but the disorder can also occur in men, thin patients, older adults, and children. Idiopathic intracranial hypertension can be associated with a variety of systemic disorders and medications (Table 195-10), but the direct cause of ICP elevation is usually unknown. Chronic elevations of ICP can lead to the "empty sella syndrome" (Chapter 231), which refers to enlargement of the sella turcica due to an incompetent diaphragma sellae, leading to CT or MRI evidence of CSF in the sella; the result is a compressed but functioning pituitary gland.

CLINICAL MANIFESTATIONS

Patients usually present with headache that may be accompanied by visual disturbances, including visual loss, nausea, vomiting, diplopia, tinnitus, and vertigo. Examination is notable for bilateral papilledema in an otherwise healthy patient. Loss of vision, which is the most feared complication, is uncommon. Visual fields typically reveal an enlarged blind spot owing to the papilledema, but no other visual impairment. Diplopia can occur from an abducens palsy as a false localizing sign.

DIAGNOSIS

The diagnosis is established by excluding any structural cause of elevated ICP by MRI. Magnetic resonance venography (MRV) also should be performed to exclude dural venous sinus thrombosis or stenosis. Lumbar puncture is performed after neuroimaging and is required to confirm the diagnosis by establishing an elevated opening pressure, frequently greater than 300 mm H$_2$O; however, the composition of the fluid is normal, and the protein concentration is typically in the low-normal range (<20 mg/dL).

Intracranial Hypotension

Intracranial hypotension occurs most commonly after lumbar puncture or after an idiopathic tear of the spinal dura. Evidence suggests that new "atraumatic" needles, as well as smaller-bore needles and few passes of the needle to perform the lumbar puncture, are associated with a lower incidence of postspinal headache.

CLINICAL MANIFESTATIONS AND DIAGNOSIS

Low CSF pressure (Table 195-11) can cause clinical symptoms that are usually mild but occasionally severe and debilitating. Postural headaches occur within 30 seconds after assuming the erect posture and subside completely when the patient lies flat (Chapter 405). The headaches, which are usually bifrontal or occipital, are typically severe, generalized, and throbbing. Headaches may be accompanied by nausea, dizziness, photophobia, neck stiffness, and, rarely, an abducens nerve palsy. All symptoms are relieved when the patient lies down.

TREATMENT AND PROGNOSIS

In most patients, symptoms resolve spontaneously and can be treated with simple analgesics. Some patients develop persistent, symptomatic intracranial hypotension that does not respond to simple measures.

In patients whose symptoms are persistent or disabling, an epidural blood patch is performed by injecting approximately 10 mL of the patient's own blood into the epidural space to seal the presumed dural leak. Occasionally, CSF radioisotope studies must be performed to identify the site of the leak so that surgical repair of the dura can be performed.

1. Forsyth PA, Weaver S, Fulton D, et al. Prophylactic anticonvulsants in patients with brain tumour. *Can J Neurol Sci.* 2003;30:106-112.
2. Mikkelsen T, Paleologos NA, Robinson PD, et al. The role of prophylactic anticonvulsants in the management of brain metastases: a systematic review and evidence-based clinical practice guideline. *J Neurooncol.* 2010;96:97-102.
3. Stupp R, Hegi ME, Mason WP, et al. Effects of radiotherapy with concomitant and adjuvant temozolomide versus radiotherapy alone on survival in glioblastoma in a randomised phase III study: 5-year analysis of the EORTC-NCIC trial. *Lancet Oncol.* 2009;10:459-466.
4. Keime-Guibert F, Chinot O, Taillandier L, et al. Radiotherapy for glioblastoma in the elderly. *N Engl J Med.* 2007;356:1527-1535.
5. Wick W, Hartmann C, Engel C, et al. NOA-04 randomized phase III trial of sequential radiochemotherapy of anaplastic glioma with procarbazine, lomustine, and vincristine or temozolomide. *J Clin Oncol.* 2009;27:5874-5880.
6. Karim AB, Afra D, Cornu P, et al. Randomized trial on the efficacy of radiotherapy for cerebral low grade glioma in the adult. *Int J Radiat Oncol Biol Phys.* 2002;52:316-324.
7. Cairncross G, Berkey B, Shaw E, et al. Phase III trial of chemotherapy plus radiotherapy compared with radiotherapy alone for pure and mixed anaplastic oligodendroglioma: Intergroup Radiation Therapy Oncology Group Trial 9402. *J Clin Oncol.* 2006;24:2707-2714.
8. Aoyama H, Shirato H, Tago M, et al. Stereotactic radiosurgery plus whole-brain radiation therapy vs stereotactic radiosurgery alone for treatment of brain metastases: a randomized controlled trial. *JAMA.* 2006;295:2483-2491.
9. Patchell RA, Tibbs, PA, Regine WF, et al. Direct decompressive surgical resection in the treatment of spinal cord compression caused by metastatic cancer: a randomised trial. *Lancet.* 2005; 366:643-648.

SUGGESTED READING

McPherson CM, Suki D, Feiz-Erfan I, et al. Adjuvant whole-brain radiation therapy after surgical resection of single brain metastases. *Neuro-Oncology.* 2010;12:711-719. *Role of adjuvant whole-brain radiation therapy in reducing local and distal recurrences in subsets of patients following surgical resection of single brain metastases.*

Robertson T, Koszyca B, Gonzales M. Overview and recent advances in neuropathology. Part 1: central nervous system tumours. *Pathology.* 2011;43:88-92. *Review.*

Ryken TC, McDermott M, Robinson PD, et al. The role of steroids in the management of brain metastases: a systematic review and evidence-based clinical practice guideline. *J Neurooncol.* 2010;96:103-114. *Limited data suggest a benefit with a preference toward dexamethasone 16 mg/day tapered slowly over a 2-week time period, or longer in symptomatic patients.*

Suh JH. Stereotactic radiosurgery for the management of brain metastases. *N Engl Med.* 2010;362:1119-1127. *Review.*

196

HEAD AND NECK CANCER

MARSHALL R. POSNER

DEFINITION

The principal cancers of the head and neck include squamous cell cancers arising from the mucosal surfaces of the upper aerodigestive tract and a diverse group of salivary gland neoplasms. Unique cancers of the region include nasopharyngeal carcinoma, thyroid malignancies (Chapter 233), esthesioneuroblastoma, and sinonasal undifferentiated carcinoma. A variety of other cancers arise from structures and tissues in the head and neck, including the more common skin cancers (Chapter 210), lymphomas (Chapters 191 and 192), and sarcomas (Chapter 209).

EPIDEMIOLOGY

Squamous cell carcinomas account for 95% of all malignancies of the head and neck, whereas salivary gland cancers represent nearly all of the remaining 5%. They represent 4% of all malignancies in the United States. Squamous cell cancers of the head and neck can be divided into two distinct groups based on pathogenesis, biology, and prognosis. Environmentally related cancers, caused principally by tobacco and alcohol, have been declining in incidence; however, they remain common. There has been an increasing incidence of human papillomavirus (HPV)-related oropharynx cancer (HPVOC). HPVOC now represents about 65% of oropharynx cancers seen in the United States and Europe. HPVOC affects a younger population (50 to 60 years) than environmental cancers (55 to 65 years). HPVOC patients are also generally healthier.

The mucosal surfaces of the head and neck are divided into six anatomic regions: the oral cavity, oropharynx, hypopharynx, larynx, nasopharynx, and paranasal sinuses. The site of anatomic origin for a squamous cell carcinoma of the head and neck has important, albeit imperfect implications for diagnosis, pathogenesis, spread, prognosis, and treatment because of intrinsic differences in the biology of the mucosal cells and subsequent cancers at the sites of origin, as well as differences in lymphatic drainage patterns and proximity to other structures in this compact region.

Oral Cavity

The oral cavity includes the floor of the mouth, anterior or oral aspect of the tongue, lips, buccal surfaces, hard palate, retromolar trigone, and gums. This region is easily appreciable by physical examination, and thus tumors in this area can frequently be detected early in their course. Tumors of the oral cavity, which are strongly related to the use of smokeless tobacco and other oral tobacco products (Chapter 31), appear on the buccal and gingival surfaces in the sites where tobacco products are held in contact with the mucosa for long periods. Anterior tongue cancers are more common in smokers. Lip cancers are particularly prevalent in transplant recipients and can be caused by DNA damage from solar ultraviolet light.

Oropharynx

The oropharynx consists of the tongue from the circumvallate papillae, posteriorly to the epiglottis, the tonsils, the associated pharyngeal walls, and the soft palate. The oropharynx has become the most common location for head and neck tumors in the United States and is a common site of origin in Europe. This is due to a high rate of HPVOC, which continues to increase in incidence. HPVOC is caused almost exclusively by HPV-16, a high-risk HPV type associated with cervical, anal, and vulvar cancers. HPVOC presents with lower primary T stage (T1 and T2) and higher nodal stage (N2 and N3) than environmental cancers and is frequently a cause of unknown primary cancer because of small and hard to identify primary tumors.

Hypopharynx

The hypopharynx comprises the piriform sinuses, the lateral and posterior pharyngeal walls, and the posterior surfaces of the larynx. These structures surround the larynx posteriorly and laterally. Tumors in this region can be difficult to detect because of the recesses and spaces surrounding the larynx. As a result, primary hypopharyngeal tumors may be asymptomatic and, like oropharyngeal tumors, may initially be recognized in an advanced state or diagnosed as an "unknown primary" (Chapter 211). These tumors are associated with tobacco (Chapter 31) and alcohol (Chapter 32) use.

Larynx

The larynx includes the vocal cords, the subglottis, and the supraglottic larynx, as well as the thyroid, cricoid, and arytenoid cartilages. Tumors arising in the true vocal cords are frequently symptomatic early and rarely spread beyond the confines of the larynx, whereas subglottic and supraglottic cancers can be relatively asymptomatic and have a much higher and earlier risk of spread to the lymphatics and regional sites. Laryngeal cancers are strongly associated with smoking (Chapter 31).

Nasopharynx

The nasopharynx includes the mucosal surfaces and structures of the cavity behind the nasal passages. Nasopharyngeal cancers are common in the Pacific Rim, northern Africa, and the Middle East. In some areas of China and Southeast Asia, nasopharyngeal cancers occur with a frequency that rivals lung cancer. In North America, there are about 2000 cases each year, but numbers are increasing as high-risk ethnic populations settle in North America. Nasopharyngeal cancers are frequently associated with the presence of latent infection of the epithelial tumor cells by Epstein-Barr virus (EBV), the etiologic agent of infectious mononucleosis (Chapter 385). Nasopharyngeal cancers are also associated with both environmental and genetic factors in susceptible populations that have migrated to North America and remain at high risk for this disease. Unlike other squamous cell carcinomas of the head and neck, nasopharyngeal cancers can occur at an early age, with a distinct peak in adolescence and young adulthood. Nasopharyngeal cancers are categorized into three histologic subtypes by the World Health Organization (WHO): the undifferentiated (WHO III) and nonkeratinizing forms (WHO II) are latently infected with EBV in 95% of cases and represent the majority of cases in North America and worldwide; the well-differentiated (WHO I) form is rarer and represents about 5% worldwide but about 15 to 25% of all nasopharyngeal cancers in North America, and it is usually associated with traditional risk factors such as smoking. Nasopharyngeal cancers have a high risk of early regional lymph node involvement, a prolonged natural history, and a very high risk of spread to distant sites.

Paranasal Sinuses

The paranasal sinuses comprise the maxillary, ethmoid, sphenoid, and frontal sinuses as well as the nasal cavity. These are relatively rare locations for tumors of the head and neck in North America, but there is an unexplained higher rate of malignant sinus disease among the Japanese. Squamous maxillary sinus cancers are more common in smokers. Up to 50% of cancers of the sinuses may be of salivary gland origin, often related to exposure to dust from woodworking, tanning, or leather working (Chapter 18). Occasionally, neuroendocrine tumors and the rare sinonasal undifferentiated carcinoma are found. Sinus cancers are frequently diagnosed late in their course at the time of symptomatic invasion of surrounding structures, including the orbit, nasal cavity, base of the skull, and cranial nerves.

Salivary Glands

Salivary glands occur in all the regions described, as well as in the trachea and esophagus. Tumors can develop in all of the major and minor salivary glands with an incidence that is roughly proportional to the quantity of glandular tissue. The most common single site is the parotid. Although tumors can develop at any age, including childhood, the peak incidence is between 55 and 65 years of age. Salivary gland cancers have diverse histologic findings and manifest different behavior based on their histologic classification. A substantial fraction of parotid salivary tumors can be benign. Risk factors for salivary gland cancers are poorly understood, but previous radiation therapy in adjacent areas increases the risk (Chapter 19).

PATHOBIOLOGY

Tobacco products and alcohol are major etiologic and risk factors for squamous cell carcinoma of the head and neck. Both show a clear dose response. Any irritating smoked product increases the risk for local cancer, but nicotine in tobacco, as well as in other tobacco leaf components, directly affects the oral mucosa and increases the risk for squamous cancer (Chapter 31). Alcohol is also a carcinogen, and alcohol consumption (Chapter 32), as well as its direct application in mouthwashes, is associated with an increased risk. Moreover, alcohol affects local and systemic detoxification enzymes and may increase the carcinogenic potential of other environmental carcinogens. Other environmental risk factors include radiation exposure and solar radiation; welding, metal refining, diesel exhaust, wood stove, and asbestos exposure; chronic irritants; vitamin A deficiency; and immunosuppression.

Carcinogenic viruses are responsible for the increasing incidence of head and neck cancer in the United States and Europe. Pathogenic HPV subtypes, specifically HPV-16, independently account for approximately 65% of oropharyngeal cancer cases. HPV is transmitted by epithelial contact, and there is increased risk of HPVOC associated with increasing numbers of individual sexual partners. HPV-16 DNA can be found in the tumor cells, and the oncogenic viral proteins E6 and E7 are responsible and necessary for the growth and survival of the cancer cells by effecting critical signaling pathways. HPVOC patients have a three-fold better prognosis than patients with environmentally related cancers. Nasopharyngeal cancer is predominantly associated with keratinocyte infection with EBV (Chapter 385). The classic nasopharyngeal cancer, which is also called *lymphoepithelioma,* is associated with a brisk lymphoid infiltrate that can be confused with a lymphoma. Careful examination reveals the malignant epithelial cells in the tumor. EBV

is also rarely associated with epithelial tumors of the oropharynx, tonsil, and salivary gland.

Several inherited diseases and genetic abnormalities are associated with the development of head and neck cancer. Fanconi's anemia (Chapter 168), a rare disorder of a family of related gene products, has been linked to the development of tongue cancer, as has Cowden's syndrome (Chapter 184), which is associated with mutation of the *PTEN* gene. Finally, common inherited allelic variants of the alcohol dehydrogenase and P-450 genes may be associated with increased susceptibility to alcohol and other environmental carcinogens.

The development of squamous cell carcinoma of the head and neck is a multistep process in which early genetic changes evolve into frank malignancy. In environmentally related cancers, an abnormal premalignant clone of mucosal cells may be localized to a single site within the head and neck, or clones may occur independently in many sites. The pathogenesis of HPVOC is less well understood. Second cancers are rare with HPVOC in the short term, and long-term risk is unknown. In contrast, about 20% of patients with environmentally caused cancers will develop a second primary cancer, most commonly in the head and neck, lung, and esophagus; 5% of patients are initially seen with a synchronous second primary. In environmentally related cancers, the cell cycle is dysregulated by the early loss of p16, an inhibitor of cyclin D1, or by upregulation of cyclin D1; p53 is disabled through a number of mechanisms preventing programmed cell death; mitogenic signaling is enhanced by upregulation of epidermal growth factor (EGF) receptor function; cyclooxygenase-2 is overexpressed, thereby inhibiting apoptosis and promoting angiogenesis; and chromosomal instability with aneuploidy develops. Many of these early molecular and functional changes occur without obvious alteration in the physical appearance of the oral mucosa, although leukoplakia can occur. In HPVOC, the RB and p53 pathways are inactivated by the HPV oncogenic proteins E6 and E7. As a result, the p16 protein is upregulated as a biomarker of HPV tumor origin. As a consequence of RB and p53 inactivation, these patients have dysregulation of cell growth and DNA damage control/programmed cell death, respectively. The differences between the genetic and molecular determinants of cancer in HPVOC and environmentally related cancers can be differentially targeted for therapy.

In environmentally related cancers, high-risk early lesions can occasionally be identified as leukoplakia and erythroplakia. Leukoplakia (Fig. 196-1A) is diagnosed clinically as a white patch of mucosal tissue in the oral mucosa or larynx. It can unpredictably progresses to cancer over a period of several years in approximately 30% of patients. Erythroplakia (see Fig. 196-1B), a red hyperkeratotic change in the mucosa, is a more advanced premalignant lesion with an approximately 60% rate of progression to oral cancer. Surgical resection of leukoplakia or erythroplakia has no effect on the subsequent development of invasive cancer. There is no proven chemopreventive therapy for persons with oral premalignant lesions. Because continued smoking or alcohol consumption increases the risk for recurrence and second primaries dramatically, patients with prior cancers should stop alcohol and tobacco use.

CLINICAL MANIFESTATIONS

The symptoms and clinical manifestations of tumors in the head and neck can vary broadly and are related to the structures at the site of the primary tumor, as well as regional lymph node drainage. Small tumors of the oral cavity and larynx can be easily appreciated because of physical self-discovery

FIGURE 196-1. High-risk early mouth lesions. **A,** Oral leukoplakia. **B,** Oral erythroplakia.

or early compromise of the function of a critical structure. As a result of the propensity for squamous cell carcinoma of the head and neck to remain a local and regional disease, it is unusual for this cancer to be associated with abnormalities outside the head and neck. Salivary gland malignancies are less constrained and frequently spread distantly; however, because the primary tumors are also frequently accessible to direct physical examination and discovery, it is still uncommon to identify these tumors as a result of metastatic spread outside the region.

Clinical manifestations of *tumors in the oral cavity* include a painless lump, a painful mass or ulcer, or simple thickening of the mucosa. Small lesions in the lateral aspect of the tongue and the floor of the mouth can cause pain referred to the mandible, gums, and ear because of the shared sensory nerves supplying these areas. Antibiotics can relieve symptoms and even reduce the size of a tumor or lymph nodes when superficial infection and inflammation are contributing to the pain; however, recurrent or continued pain in an adult should trigger suspicion about more ominous disease. Speech may be affected late if the tumor causes restricted tongue motion or cranial nerve XII dysfunction. Gingival tumors can loosen teeth and invade the mandible along tooth sockets.

In true vocal cord cancer, hoarseness and other forms of voice change are common and expected early symptoms, but they may be later manifestations of *supraglottic and subglottic laryngeal tumors,* which become relatively large without affecting the voice. Tumors of the piriform sinus can affect the voice when they become large and impair the recurrent laryngeal nerve, or they are associated with deep local invasion; pain in the ear or pain on swallowing referred to the ear is also a common and important feature of these tumors. Adults with ear pain or persistent hoarseness should be referred to an otolaryngologist for evaluation. Because this posterior area is difficult to assess, primary tumors are frequently missed in routine office examinations. *Tumors of the supraglottic region, subglottic cancers, and cancers of the piriform sinus* can also be manifested as acute, emergency airway obstruction. Frequently, patients have a history of wheezing and mild upper airway distress in the period leading up to the emergency situation. Occasionally, such findings are confused with adult-onset asthma.

A middle ear infection or effusion in an adult should also prompt an ear, nose, and throat (ENT) evaluation. Nasopharyngeal cancer may be manifested as an ear infection in young adults. Hemoptysis or epistaxis may be the only clue to a nasopharyngeal cancer or a *paranasal sinus tumor.* Cranial nerve findings from deep invasion of the base of skull are late events and include lateral gaze abnormalities, diplopia, facial pain, or facial nerve paralysis. *Sinus tumors* can also be associated with these later findings, although nasal stuffiness occurs frequently and can be confused with sinusitis. New and persistent symptoms of sinusitis or facial pain should raise suspicion of sinus cancer and prompt an evaluation.

Tumors in the tonsil or base of the tongue can cause local pain and referred ear pain; however, they are frequently asymptomatic and can attain a large size before becoming evident as a result of changes in speech ("hot potato voice"), a sense of globus, or restriction of tongue movement. Manifestation as a painless lump in the neck is increasingly common with the increased incidence of HPVOC. Tumors of the tonsil or base of the tongue may also lose their mucosal component, not be seen or felt on direct inspection, and occur as a solid or cystic neck mass. Isolated neck masses can wax and wane with antibiotics. A mass, especially a cystic mass, in the neck in an adult is cancer and specifically HPVOC until proved otherwise and should prompt an ENT evaluation, before fine-needle aspiration (FNA) or excisional biopsy.

The staging of squamous cell carcinoma of the head and neck is based on the TNM (tumor, node, metastasis) staging system, and prognosis is related primarily to the N and T stages (Table 196-1). The risk of the cancer spreading to lymph nodes is directly related to the location of the primary and secondarily to the size of the primary. Tumors of the oropharynx have a high risk for nodal metastases, followed in risk by the supraglottic larynx and piriform sinus (hypopharynx), oral portion of the tongue, soft palate, oral cavity and floor of the mouth, and larynx. Nasopharyngeal cancer is highly associated with extensive nodal spread, whereas paranasal sinus cancers rarely spread to the lymph nodes. The location of lymph node spread is determined in part by site. Nasopharyngeal cancer spreads to the posterior cervical lymph nodes, as well as the high cervical nodes. Oropharynx, larynx, and piriform sinus tumors spread to the high cervical nodes. Nodal metastases from these locations can be bilateral. Oral cavity tumors spread to the submental nodes and submandibular nodes. Spread tends to be orderly from the submandibular nodes to the midcervical nodes. Oral

cavity cancers can have as high as a 20% risk of clinically unappreciated contralateral spread.

DIAGNOSIS

The relative accessibility of the head and neck to direct inspection makes physical examination critical for diagnosis and staging. Patients with localized symptoms or a sign such as an ulcer or a small mass should have a thorough head and neck office examination performed by their primary physician and by a specialist, including inspection of the visible structures and palpation of the base of the tongue and tonsil areas, as well as the neck. Specialized office examination with fiberoptics should be included in the preliminary assessment. Regardless of whether cancer is suspected, excisional biopsies should be discouraged because margins are frequently violated and inadequate, thereby leading to larger re-excisions. A simple punch biopsy is sufficient for diagnosis, particularly in the oral portion of the tongue where tumors can spread readily though lymphatics.

When cancer is highly suspected and before definitive surgical intervention, a computed tomography (CT) scan from the base of the skull to the clavicles, preferably with the spiral technique, and a chest radiograph should be obtained. Magnetic resonance imaging (MRI) provides added information in evaluating soft tissue involvement, especially in the base of the tongue and the parapharyngeal spaces and for sinus tumors. MRI can distinguish between soft tissue masses and retained secretions, whereas CT is more helpful in assessing nodal spread in the neck and bone invasion. Positron emission tomography (PET) provides an adjunct to CT scanning and can identify occult disease. PET scanning should be performed when cancer is suspected and when the patient has an "unknown primary tumor," before biopsy, in order to guide the evaluation and reduce the risk of inadequate diagnostic and premature therapeutic procedures (Fig. 196-2).

When a biopsy indicates cancer or cancer is highly suspected, an examination under anesthesia with endoscopy should be performed to stage the primary tumor before definitive therapy is undertaken. This procedure, which provides information regarding the extent of disease, the appropriateness of the planned definitive procedure, and the presence of second primaries, is an absolute requirement before definitive therapy can be discussed with a patient. Endoscopy and palpation under anesthesia can identify unexpected local spread or a synchronous second primary (found in about 5% of patients with environmentally related cancers).

Approach to the Patient with an Unknown Primary Site

Patients frequently seek care from their primary physician because of an enlarged lymph node, a cystic mass, or a collection of lymph nodes in the

FIGURE 196-2. Positron emission tomography and computed tomography fused images. A primary human papillomavirus–positive base of tongue cancer and neck adenopathy is shown.

TABLE 196-1 AMERICAN JOINT COMMITTEE ON CANCER STAGING FOR HEAD AND NECK SQUAMOUS CELL CARCINOMA

TUMOR	LARYNX	LIP AND ORAL CAVITY	OROPHARYNX	HYPOPHARYNX
Tis	Carcinoma in situ	Carcinoma in situ	Carcinoma in situ	Carcinoma in situ
T1 T1a T1b	*Supraglottis:* Tumor limited to one subsite of supraglottis with normal vocal cord ability *Glottis:* Tumor limited to the vocal cord(s) (may involve anterior or posterior commissure) with normal mobility Tumor limited to one vocal cord Tumor involves both vocal cords *Subglottis:* Tumor limited to the subglottis	Tumor 2 cm or less in greatest dimension	Tumor 2 cm or less in greatest dimension	Tumor limited to one subsite of hypopharynx and/or 2 cm or less in greatest dimension
T2	*Supraglottis:* Tumor invades mucosa of more than one adjacent subsite of supraglottis or glottis or region outside the supraglottis (e.g., mucosa of base of tongue, vallecula, medial wall of pyriform sinus) without fixation of the larynx *Glottis:* Tumor extends to supraglottis and/or subglottis, and/or with impaired vocal cord mobility *Subglottis:* Tumor extends to vocal cord(s) with normal or impaired mobility	Tumor more than 2 cm but not more than 4 cm in greatest dimension	Tumor more than 2 cm but not more than 4 cm in greatest dimension	Tumor invades more than one subsite of hypopharynx or an adjacent site, or measures more than 2 cm but not more than 4 cm in greatest dimension without fixation of hemilarynx
T3	*Supraglottis:* Tumor limited to larynx with vocal cord fixation and/or invades any of the following: postcricoid area, pre-epiglottic space, paraglottic space, and/or inner cortex of thyroid cartilage *Glottis:* Tumor limited to the larynx with vocal cord fixation and/or invasion of paraglottic space, and/or inner cortex of the thyroid cartilage	Tumor more than 4 cm in greatest dimension	Tumor more than 4 cm in greatest dimension or extension to lingual surface of epiglottis	Tumor more than 4 cm in greatest dimension or with fixation of hemilarynx or extension to esophagus
T4a	Moderately advanced local disease Tumor invades through the thyroid cartilage and/or invades tissues beyond the larynx (e.g., trachea, soft tissues of neck including deep extrinsic muscle of the tongue, strap muscles, thyroid, or esophagus)	Moderately advanced local disease Lip: Tumor invades through cortical bone, inferior alveolar nerve, floor of mouth, or skin of face, i.e., chin or nose Oral cavity: Tumor invades adjacent structures only (e.g., through cortical bone [mandible or maxilla] into deep [extrinsic] muscle of tongue [genioglossus, hyoglossus, palatoglossus, and styloglossus], maxillary sinus, skin of face)	Moderately advanced local disease Tumor invades the larynx, extrinsic muscle of tongue, medial pterygoid, hard palate, or mandible (Note: Mucosal extension to lingual surface of epiglottis from primary tumors of the base of the tongue and vallecula does not constitute invasion of larynx)	Moderately advanced local disease Tumor invades thyroid/cricoid cartilage, hyoid bone, thyroid gland, or central compartment soft tissue (Note: Central compartment soft tissue includes prelaryngeal strap muscles and subcutaneous fat).
T4b	Very advanced local disease Tumor invades prevertebral space, encases carotid artery, or invades mediastinal structures	Very advanced local disease Tumor invades masticator space, pterygoid plates, or skull base and/or encases internal carotid artery	Very advanced local disease Tumor invades lateral pterygoid muscle, pterygoid plates, lateral nasopharynx, or skull base or encases carotid artery	Very advanced local disease Tumor invades prevertebral fascia, encases carotid artery, or involves mediastinal structures

NODE	DEFINITION
NX	Regional lymph nodes cannot be assessed
N0	No regional lymph node metastasis
N1*	Metastasis in a single ipsilateral lymph node, 3 cm or less in greatest dimension
N2*	Metastasis in a single ipsilateral lymph node, more than 3 cm but not more than 6 cm in greatest dimension; or in multiple ipsilateral lymph nodes, none more than 6 cm in greatest dimension; or in bilateral or contralateral lymph nodes, none more than 6 cm in greatest dimension
N2a*	Metastasis in single ipsilateral lymph node more than 3 cm but not more than 6 cm in greatest dimension
N2b*	Metastasis in multiple ipsilateral lymph nodes, none more than 6 cm in greatest dimension
N2c*	Metastasis in bilateral or contralateral lymph nodes, none more than 6 cm in greatest dimension
N3*	Metastasis in lymph node more than 6 cm in greatest dimension

METASTASIS	DEFINITION
M0	No distant metastasis
M1	Distant metastasis present

TABLE 196-1 AMERICAN JOINT COMMITTEE ON CANCER STAGING FOR HEAD AND NECK SQUAMOUS CELL CARCINOMA—cont'd

STAGE	T	N	M
0	Tis	N0	M0
I	T1	N0	M0
II	T2	N0	M0
III	T3	N0	M0
	T1	N1	M0
	T2	N1	M0
	T3	N1	M0
IVa	T4a	N0	M0
	T4a	N1	M0
	T1	N2	M0
	T2	N2	M0
	T3	N2	M0
	T4a	N2	M0
IVb	Any T	N3	M0
	T4b	Any N	M0
IVc	Any T	Any N	M1

*Distribution and prognostic impact of regional lymph node spread from nasopharynx cancer are different from those of other head and neck mucosal cancers and justify the use of a different N classification scheme.
From *AJCC Cancer Staging Manual.* 7th ed. New York: Springer-Verlag; 2010.

upper part of the neck (Fig. 196-3). Such masses in an adult should be considered cancer until proved otherwise. Unless there is an obvious symptom or sign that leads the clinician to the identification of a primary site in the head and neck, such patients are considered to have an unknown primary. Masses in the supraclavicular areas represent primary tumors below the clavicles, and masses in the midneck and cervical regions are almost always from the head and neck. Identification of a primary site is critical to focus therapy, reduce morbidity, and determine prognosis.

The most common primary sites for painless lumps are the oropharynx (base of the tongue and tonsil) and piriform sinus. Oropharynx cancers are frequently due to HPV and a positive HPV-16 polymerase chain reaction test of the biopsy or FNA is presumptive evidence of oropharynx origin. Salivary gland cancers, lymphomas, melanomas, and skin cancers can also be manifested in this manner. Bilateral nodal disease or nodal disease with systemic symptoms may suggest lymphoma. By comparison, pain, warmth, and erythema may suggest an infectious etiology. Intraparotid nodes most likely represent metastases from skin malignancies. Physical examination should include a careful investigation for primary skin cancers. CT, PET, and MRI should be part of the initial evaluation. FNA should be performed and repeated if initially negative. CT-guided biopsy may be indicated if the mass is difficult to approach. If squamous cells are identified, the tumor is most likely a squamous cell carcinoma of the head and neck. Next, endoscopy under anesthesia should be performed with bilateral tonsillectomy and directed biopsies of any abnormalities, areas of firmness, and the base of the tongue, nasopharynx, and ipsilateral piriform sinus, even if they appear normal. Core or excisional (single node <3 cm) biopsy of the lymph node should be performed if the pathology is equivocal and a primary site is not confirmed. Neck dissection can be accomplished if a primary site is not identified and the patient has an N1 or small N2a/b manifestation. Some unknown primaries with squamous histology are never identified. Currently, HPV-16 and EBV are the only molecular markers to distinguish head and neck cancer from skin or salivary gland squamous cancer. EBV positivity indicates a nasopharyngeal cancer, and HPV-16 is an oropharyngeal primary.

In contrast to squamous cell carcinoma of the head and neck, salivary gland cancers are heterogeneous in their natural history and treatment. The three most common histologic types are adenoid cystic carcinoma, mucoepidermoid cancer, and adenocarcinoma. Other histologic types include the aggressive salivary duct cancer and squamous cell cancers, whereas less aggressive histologic varieties include adenocarcinoma ex pleomorphic adenoma and acinic cell carcinoma. Because adenoid cystic carcinoma travels along nerves and can spread hematogenously, careful

assessment of the cranial nerves and the chest by CT is indicated before major surgery is undertaken. Patients should also be evaluated for bone and liver metastases. Formal lymph node dissection is not indicated. Ethmoid and sphenoid sinus adenoid cystic carcinomas are locally and regionally aggressive and require specialized surgery and radiation therapy techniques for local and regional control. The behavior of mucoepidermoid carcinoma is determined by histology. Low- and intermediate-grade lesions rarely metastasize. Isolated high-grade tumors spread to local lymph nodes and by hematogenous routes and carry a high risk for the development of lung metastases. The work-up for high-grade lesions should be similar to that for adenoid cystic carcinoma. Local therapy should be directed at local and regional control with lymph node dissection. Radiation therapy is indicated for close microscopic margins or lymph node involvement. Adenocarcinoma, salivary duct cancers, and squamous cell carcinoma are also poor-prognosis lesions with aggressive local and distant behavior. These tumors should be evaluated in the same fashion as aggressive mucoepidermoid carcinomas. Acinic cell carcinoma and carcinoma ex pleomorphic adenoma are relatively rare. They have a propensity for local and regional recurrence if they are not removed in toto. Metastases are rare and tend to be slow growing.

Other Tumors of the Head and Neck

Lymphomas in the head and neck frequently manifest either as nodal disease in the neck or as tumor involving the lymphoid tissues of Waldeyer's ring (Chapters 191 and 192). A primary head and neck cancer may later develop in patients with lymphoma as a consequence of past exposure to tobacco, radiation therapy, or immunosuppression. The tonsil is a preferred site for mantle cell and undifferentiated lymphomas. Mucosa-associated lymphoid tissue (MALT) lymphomas can affect the salivary glands.

In the context of an isolated neck mass, a systematic evaluation (see Fig. 196-3) should be undertaken, even in young adults without a smoking history. The sinonasal T-cell and natural killer cell lymphomas, also known as *lethal midline granulomas*, represent a unique family of lymphomas of the head and neck. These lymphomas are associated with EBV infection (Chapter 385). Solitary, extramedullary plasmacytoma can also occur in the nasopharynx or paranasal sinuses (Chapter 193).

Sarcomas that arise in the head and neck include osteogenic sarcomas (Chapters 208 and 209) and nerve sheath tumors. Paragangliomas, which are rare malignant tumors of the chief cells of nerve paraganglia, can be extensive, multicentric, and vascular. Rhabdomyosarcomas, which have a predilection for the orbit and sinuses, occur in younger persons; the prognosis tends to be better for tumors of the head and neck than for other locations. Olfactory

Unknown primary neck mass

↓

Assess mass for growth, location, size, and inflammation

↓

High clinical suspicion   Low clinical suspicion

                                 ↓

                                 See Table 171-5

Growth: rapid, slow, fluctuating
High location: cervical, submental, midcervical
Inflammation: may be tender, may become fluctuant
Cystic mass: "cancer until proven otherwise"

↓

ENT referral
Intraoffice oral and oropharyngeal examination with flexible fiberoscopic exam
CT and/or MRI to assess nodes and tongue, respectively
Fine-needle aspiration; repeat if initially negative
HPV testing

↓

Examination under anesthesia with tonsillectomy; biopsy of any abnormalities; and biopsy of nasopharynx, base of tongue, and pyriform sinus, even if normal appearing

No diagnosis   Diagnosis

Core or needle biopsy of large or complex mass (>3 cm); simple neck dissection for simple mass (<3 cm) HPV testing

Therapy based on histology, primary site, and stage

FIGURE 196-3. Evaluation of an unknown primary neck mass. CT = computed tomography; ENT = ear, nose, and throat; HPV = human papillomavirus; MRI = magnetic resonance imaging.

neuroblastomas or esthesioneuroblastomas invade the nasal cavity and base of the skull.

Many skin tumors, including melanoma and squamous cell cancer, can be accompanied by adenopathy of the neck or parotid area (Chapter 210). An unusual skin appendage tumor, Merkel cell cancer, can be confused with other neuroendocrine epithelial tumors.

PREVENTION AND TREATMENT   **Rx**

Selection of a treatment program for an individual patient is based on three factors: the primary site and stage of the tumor, the patient's comorbid conditions and preferences, and the biology of the tumor (Table 196-2). Early-stage lesions, T1N0 and T2N0, are defined by their size, and their prognosis is site specific. For example, early *larynx cancer* involving the true vocal cords has an excellent prognosis and can be treated by local excision. Voice-preserving larynx conservation surgery is effective for selected patients. Radiation therapy is equally effective for early cancer. When there is a risk of lymph node spread, radiation therapy must be given postoperatively, and the primary value of surgery is diminished. Intensity-modulated radiation therapy (IMRT) allows radiation to be delivered in a more conformal manner to the tumor and areas at risk while sparing critical structures such as the spinal cord and noncritical but important structures such as the salivary glands. IMRT is now a standard of care for patients with head and neck cancer.

Oral tongue, piriform sinus, and environmentally related oropharynx tumors have a worse prognosis and are difficult to stage accurately because of submucosal spread or lymphatic involvement. Stage I and II cancers are cured with local and regional surgery or radiation therapy in 70% to 90% of cases. Surgery may be preferred for oral cavity and anterior lesions. In surgically treated patients, those with a positive margin, two or more positive lymph nodes, or extracapsular spread have a poorer survival rate (<30%) at 5 years. Perineural invasion and lymphovascular invasion may also be associated with a poor prognosis. Postoperative cisplatin-based chemoradiotherapy improves local and regional control, as well as survival, and should be given to poor-prognosis patients if their condition permits.[1] At present, aside from HPV status and p16 immunohistochemistry, no molecular or immunohistochemical finding definitively adds to the information gleaned from pathology, staging, and performance status.

When organ preservation and function are issues for stage III or IV cancers or when radiation therapy is required regardless of surgical outcome, primary chemoradiotherapy or sequential therapy should be considered.[2,3] The curative treatment of intermediate (stage III, T1-3N1, T3N0) and locally advanced (stage IV, T1-3N2-3, T4) disease remains controversial. Long-term (3 years) survival rates in patients with stage III disease are generally between 50 and 75%, whereas only 15 to 50% of stage IV patients survive for 3 years. Intermediate-stage tumors are usually resectable, but organ preservation may be an important consideration. In many of these cases, a combined-modality approach that includes chemotherapy is the standard of care.

Patients with anterior lesions may do better with initial surgical treatment. The oral cavity is easy to assess and is relatively forgiving for surgery and reconstruction; postoperative radiation therapy or chemoradiotherapy can be moderated in the absence of bad prognostic features. For intermediate and advanced tumors, radiation therapy or chemoradiotherapy is a necessary adjunct to prevent recurrence. For example, a T3 or N1 lesion of the oropharyngeal tongue or hypopharynx is almost always more extensive than clinically appreciated and may be more suited to a nonsurgical regional and systemic approach. In addition, patients with rapidly growing tumors are more suitable for a combined-modality approach. Patients with extensive N2 or N3 nodal disease (stage IV) should be considered relatively unresectable because of a poor prognosis from regional recurrence and distant metastases. Certain locations such as the nasopharynx and posterior pharynx should also be considered for definitive radiation therapy, sequential therapy, or chemoradiotherapy.

Radiation therapy has been proved by randomized trials to yield better local control and disease-free survival if given in twice-daily fractionated treatments rather than as daily therapy. However, the absolute benefit of hyperfractionated radiation therapy at 5 years is only 3 to 4%, and it is unclear whether a twice-daily schedule is advantageous with chemotherapy.[4]

Induction chemotherapy is the delivery of chemotherapy before definitive local-regional treatment. Sequential therapy adds chemoradiotherapy (see later) to induction chemotherapy. Induction chemotherapy with docetaxel (75 mg/m^2), cisplatin (75 to 100 mg/m^2 by intravenous bolus), plus 5-fluorouracil (750 to 1000 mg/m^2/day for 4 to 5 days by intravenous infusion), repeated every 3 or 4 weeks (TPF) are effective, standard regimens. For patients with advanced oropharynx, larynx, and hypopharynx tumors, sequential chemotherapy using concomitant carboplatin and once-daily radiotherapy improves survival and preserves function compared with radiation, surgery, or cisplatin and 5-fluorouracil chemotherapy (PF).[5,6]

Chemoradiotherapy integrates chemotherapy and radiation therapy together and has led to significant improvements in overall survival in patients with advanced disease compared with radiation therapy alone. For example, patients with unresectable disease who received cisplatin (100 mg/m^2 by intravenous bolus) every 3 weeks during radiation therapy have significantly better survival than do those treated with radiation therapy alone.[7] In a trial of patients with oropharyngeal carcinoma, those treated with carboplatin and 5-fluorouracil plus simultaneous radiation therapy had significantly better survival than did those treated by radiation therapy alone.[8] Cetuximab plus radiotherapy has also proved effective in improving survival in patients with locally advanced head and neck cancer compared with radiotherapy alone.[9]

Patients with locally advanced or unresectable disease (or both) should receive chemotherapy as part of a combined-modality approach. Sequential therapy, induction chemotherapy, and chemoradiotherapy all prolong survival compared with surgery or radiotherapy, or both, and support an organ preservation approach. Organ preservation should be offered to patients who can tolerate the treatment and participate in the post-treatment rehabilitation.

Treatment of *tumors of the paranasal sinuses* is a special case. They rarely metastasize, and treatment should focus on surgical resection with postoperative radiation therapy for resectable stage III and IV disease and on chemoradiotherapy for local and regional control of unresectable disease. Proton beam irradiation may be more suited for tumors in and around the base of the skull and brain.

Follow-up

Patients need lifelong follow-up. A chest radiograph should be performed at least yearly, and surveillance examinations for second primaries and

TABLE 196-2 GENERAL APPROACH TO SQUAMOUS CELL HEAD AND NECK CANCER

STAGE	TNM	DISEASE-SPECIFIC SURVIVAL	TREATMENT APPROACH	SPECIAL CONDITIONS
I	T1N0	85-95%	Surgery or radiation therapy	Consider organ function and long-term toxicity
II	T2N0	75-90%	Surgery, radiation therapy, or chemoradiotherapy	Consider organ function Combined-modality treatment for high-volume tumor Postoperative chemoradiotherapy for poor prognostic findings on pathologic staging
III	T3N0 T1-3N1	50-75%	Combined-modality treatment	Primary chemoradiotherapy or TPF induction therapy or sequential therapy for organ function Postoperative chemoradiotherapy More aggressive approach (sequential therapy) for high-volume disease or hypopharynx tumors
IV	T1-3N2-3 T4N0-3 Any M1	20-60%	Combined-modality treatment	Combined-modality therapy Limited surgery Postoperative chemoradiotherapy Palliative therapy for M1 (curative therapy for isolated lung metastases)

recurrences should be performed monthly to bimonthly in the first year and then less frequently over time. Treatment failure after 3 years is uncommon, but second primaries may continue to be identified in environmentally related cancers. It is important to counsel these patients to avoid tobacco products and any exposure to alcohol.

During therapy and immediately after therapy, patients benefit from pain medications, local anesthetics, mucolytics, and saline mouthwash. Patients must avoid alcohol-containing preparations or irritants. Long-acting agents such as fentanyl or time-release narcotics should be added when needed (Chapter 29). A percutaneous endoscopic gastrostomy feeding tube is effective for maintaining weight, improving healing, and managing nutrition during radiation therapy. Because depression is a major problem, psychiatric support and antidepressants may be very helpful. Salivary function improves over more than 4 years after radiation therapy, but most improvement occurs in the first 2 years. Pilocarpine and cevimeline (Evoxac) are effective stimulants of salivary flow in about 20% of patients.

Long-term sequelae of radiation therapy include dependence on a feeding tube in patients treated with aggressive chemoradiotherapy or radiation therapy alone. Attention should be paid to preserving swallowing function by means of training in speech and swallowing, as well as dilation in selected patients. Hypothyroidism occurs in up to 50% of patients and as early as 3 months after treatment. Patients should be monitored by determining serum thyroid-stimulating hormone levels at regular intervals and then be treated as appropriate (Chapter 233). Dental failure is a common problem. Patients must be counseled to see their dentists regularly for cleanings and to obtain fluoride therapy daily for dental preservation. Patients are at substantial lifelong risk for complications from dental manipulations after radiation therapy. Bone necrosis is painful, can be confused with recurrent tumor, and requires vigorous antibiotic therapy, débridement, and possibly hyperbaric oxygen to promote healing.

Patients with recurrent disease, a second primary, or metastatic disease must be evaluated for potential curability. If patients have a recurrence or second primary, curative treatment options are defined by their current stage, their previous therapy, and the interval from their original therapy. Patients who have previously been treated with surgery but not radiation therapy can undergo surgery, radiation therapy, and chemotherapy as part of a curative treatment plan. Patients with a surgically treatable recurrence in an irradiated field should undergo surgery as appropriate. It is important to recognize that the surgery must encompass the entire recurrence. Symptomatically, persistent pain may be the most important indicator of a recurrence, and repeat biopsy should be considered when a suspicious lesion is observed. Surgical salvage may cure as many as 30% of patients with recurrent oral cavity, larynx, or hypopharyngeal tumors. A repeat course of radiation therapy is also acceptable in selected patients.

Patients who are incurable can be managed effectively with palliative therapy to improve quality of life and survival (e.g., tracheostomy for airway control, laryngectomy for pain and aspiration, percutaneous endoscopic gastrostomy tube for feeding). These maneuvers can improve comfort and care in appropriate patients.

Palliative chemotherapy can provide meaningful benefit to some patients. Response rates with single agents are generally poor, and combination therapy offers higher response rates (30 to 50%). The combination of a platinum (cisplatin or carboplatin) plus 5-fluorouracil with an anti-EGF receptor antibody, cetuximab, significantly improves survival, response rate, and progression-free survival compared with the same chemotherapy without cetuximab.

Salivary Gland Tumors

In contrast to squamous cell carcinoma of the head and neck, salivary gland cancers are heterogeneous in their natural history and treatment; however,

the mainstays of therapy for these tumors are surgery and radiotherapy. Early symptoms of local-regional recurrence include cranial nerve dysfunction and progressive pain. A PET scan may be useful in distinguishing recurrence from the neuropathy that may result from radiation therapy.

There are no highly active agents or combinations for treatment of metastatic salivary gland tumors. Local therapy can include surgical removal of isolated metastases, radio frequency ablation, and radiation therapy. Response rates are generally in the 20 to 35% range, but prolonged responses are occasionally seen.

Future Directions

Antibodies that target the EGF receptor and other molecular targets may improve local and regional control, as well as survival, when delivered with radiation therapy. Vaccines against EBV and HPV may prevent malignancy in high-risk populations.

PROGNOSIS

The prognosis for patients with squamous cell carcinoma of the head and neck (see Table 196-2) is directly related to the presence of HPV, stage, and performance status. The risk for recurrence declines dramatically at 2 years after definitive treatment, and survival and possible cure can be defined after 3 years. HPV status and then N (nodal) stage are the most important prognostic indicators of potential recurrence, with T (tumor) stage and smoking history being next. Stage I patients (T1N0) have a 90% likelihood of tumor control, whereas stage II patients (T2N0) have greater than 70 to 85% tumor control. Tumor control in stage III patients (T1-2N1, T3N0-1) is site dependent and HPV status dependent and varies from 35 to 85%. Patients with stage IVa and IVb environmentally related disease (T1-3, N2-3, or T4NX) have a 20 to 50% tumor-specific 5-year survival rate compared with 60 to 90% 5-year survival for HPVOC. Bad prognostic signs in advanced-stage (IVb) patients are related to N3 nodal disease and invasion of basic structures (carotid artery encasement, base of the skull, pterygoid muscles). Patients with M1 disease are categorized as stage IVc. Isolated patients with single lung metastases can be cured, whether as a second primary or as an isolated recurrence. Patients with recurrent disease and no curative options have a median survival of 6 to 9 months. Death can occur as a result of compromise of local critical structures, including vessels, breathing, and swallowing.

Distant metastases occur in about 15 to 20% of patients, but this rate is increasing as better local and regional control prolongs survival in patients with locally advanced disease. Oropharyngeal, tonsil, and piriform sinus tumors have the highest risk for distant metastases. In approximately 5% of patients, a synchronous lung tumor or metastasis develops. A single lung metastasis in a patient at initial evaluation or at follow-up can be cured in about 20% of cases.

Salivary gland cancers vary in behavior, depending on their histology. Adenocarcinoma, salivary duct cancer, salivary squamous cell cancer, and high-grade mucoepidermoid cancer not only spread to lymph nodes but also spread rapidly hematogenously. The presence of lymph node metastases signals a high risk for distant metastases. Adenoid cystic carcinoma infrequently involves lymph nodes but spreads along nerves. Regional recurrences along cranial nerves are frequent and associated with "skip" lesions. Adenoid cystic carcinoma is also associated with the late development of lung metastases, but these patients can have a prolonged lifespan lasting more than 20 years. Low-grade mucoepidermoid cancer and acinic cell carcinoma have little risk of distant spread and are more notable for local recurrence if not completely removed.

1. Bernier J, Domenge C, Ozsahin M, et al. Postoperative irradiation with or without concomitant chemotherapy for locally advanced head and neck cancer. *N Engl J Med.* 2004;350:1945-1952.
2. Forastiere AA, Goepfert H, Maor M, et al. Concurrent chemotherapy and radiotherapy for organ preservation in advanced larynx cancer. *N Engl J Med.* 2003;349:2091-2098.
3. Pointreau Y, Garaud P, Chapet S, et al. Randomized trial of induction chemotherapy with cisplatin and 5-fluorouracil with or without docetaxel for larynx preservation. *J Natl Cancer Inst.* 2009; 101:498-506.
4. Baujat B, Bourhis J, Blanchard P, et al. Hyperfractionated or accelerated radiotherapy for head and neck cancer. *Cochrane Database Syst Rev.* 2010;12:CD002026.
5. Vermorken JB, Remenar E, van Herpen C, et al. Cisplatin, fluorouracil, and docetaxel in unresectable head and neck cancer. *N Engl J Med.* 2007;357:1695-1704.
6. Lorch JH, Goloubeva O, Haddad RI, et al. Induction chemotherapy with cisplatin and fluorouracil alone or in combination with docetaxel in locally advanced squamous-cell cancer of the head and neck: long-term results of the TAX 324 randomised phase 3 trial. *Lancet Oncol.* 2011;12:153-159.
7. Adelstein D, Li Y, Adams G, et al. An Intergroup Phase III comparison of standard radiation therapy and two schedules of concurrent chemoradiotherapy in patients with unresectable squamous cell head and neck cancer. *J Clin Oncol.* 2003;21:92-98.
8. Denis F, Garaud P, Bardet E, et al. Final results of the 94-01 French Head and Neck Oncology and Radiotherapy Group randomized trial comparing radiotherapy alone with concomitant radiochemotherapy in advanced-stage oropharynx carcinoma. *J Clin Oncol.* 2004;22:69-76.
9. Bonner JA, Harari PM, Giralt J, et al. Radiotherapy plus cetuximab for squamous-cell carcinoma of the head and neck. *N Engl J Med.* 2006;354:567-578.

SUGGESTED READINGS

Ang KK, Harris J, Wheeler R, et al. Human papillomavirus and survival of patients with oropharyngeal cancer. *N Engl J Med.* 2010;363:24-25. *Patients with HPV positive tumors had a significantly better 3-year survival (82% vs 57%).*
Leemans CR, Braakhuis BJ, Brakenhoff RH. The molecular biology of head and neck cancer. *Nat Rev Cancer.* 2011;11:9-22. *Review of tumor heterogeneity and molecular pathogenesis.*
Tham IW, Lu JJ. Controversies and challenges in the current management of nasopharyngeal cancer. *Expert Rev Anticancer Ther.* 2010;10:1439-1450. *Review.*

LUNG CANCER AND OTHER PULMONARY NEOPLASMS

DAVID S. ETTINGER

BRONCHOGENIC LUNG CANCER

DEFINITION

Lung cancer (e.g., bronchogenic carcinoma) arises from the respiratory epithelium. Lung cancer is divided into two major histologic groups: non–small cell lung cancer (NSCLC) and small cell lung cancer (SCLC). NSCLC accounts for approximately 85% of all lung cancer. Other less common pulmonary neoplasms include adenosquamous carcinoma, carcinoid tumors, bronchial gland tumors, soft tissue tumors (e.g., sarcomas), pulmonary blastomas, and lymphoma.

EPIDEMIOLOGY

Worldwide, lung cancer accounts for approximately 13% of all cancer; more than 1.1 million cases of lung cancer are diagnosed annually, and more than 1 million deaths are caused by the disease. In the United States, 28% of all annual cancer deaths (30% in men, 26% in women) are due to lung cancer; lung cancer is the leading cause of cancer death in both men and women.

The incidence and mortality of lung cancer in American men and women reflect their smoking habits (Chapter 31). Lung cancer deaths started rising

TABLE 197-1	LUNG CANCER INCIDENCE AND MORTALITY RATES BY RACE/ETHNICITY AND GENDER					
	Incidence			*Mortality*		
	WHITE	**AFRICAN AMERICAN**	**HISPANIC**	**WHITE**	**AFRICAN AMERICAN**	**HISPANIC**
Male	77.6	104.3	43.2	69.9	90.1	33.9
Female	54.8	54.7	24.7	41.9	40.0	14.4

Incidence and death rates per 100,000 population, 2002 to 2006, from the Surveillance, Epidemiology and End Results (SEER) program in the United States.

in men in the 1950s and in women 10 to 15 years later. Cancer death rates from lung cancer decreased in men by 37% between 1990 and 2005; however, in women, the cancer death rate from lung cancer between 1991 and 2005 increased approximately 8%. Worldwide, increasing lung cancer rates are predicted to continue in less developed countries as a result of increasing endemic use of tobacco.

The U.S. Surveillance, Epidemiology and End Results (SEER) program estimated that 1 in 14 men and women will be at risk for the development of lung cancer during their lifetime. Incidence and mortality rates vary by race/ethnicity (Table 197-1), with African American men having a higher incidence and mortality rate than other racial/ethnic groups. Incidence rates of lung cancer for men and women in the United States from the period 2002 to 2006 are 77.7 and 52.5 per 100,000 people, respectively. The median age at diagnosis in both sexes is 71 years.

Unfortunately, tobacco use in high-school students increased until the mid-1990s, but now it is slowly declining. Despite this decline, 38% of high-school seniors smoke. This smoking at an earlier age may in part explain the occurrence of lung cancer in younger patients.

Risk Factors

Tobacco

It is estimated that cigarette smoking is responsible for approximately 85 to 90% of all cases of lung cancer, including 90% of cases in men and 80% in women. More than 40 carcinogens have been identified in cigarette smoke (Chapter 31). The risk for development of lung cancer correlates with the number of cigarettes smoked per day, lifetime duration of smoking, age at onset of smoking, degree of inhalation, tar and nicotine content of the cigarettes, and use of unfiltered cigarettes. If a lifelong nonsmoker has a relative risk ratio of 1 for the development of lung cancer, cigarette smokers of less than ½ pack/day, ½ to 1 pack/day, 1 to 2 packs/day, and more than 2 packs/day have risk ratios of 15, 17, 42, and 64, respectively. The risk ratio in ex-smokers is dependent on the duration of abstinence of cigarette smoking; to reach a risk ratio of 1.5 to 2.0 requires abstinence of approximately 30 years.

Pipe and cigar smoking are also risk factors for lung cancer, but the risk is thought to be less than that associated with cigarette smoking, possibly because such tobacco products tend to be inhaled less deeply than cigarette smoke. Marijuana and cocaine smoking probably cause an increased risk for lung cancer, but the carcinogenicity of the two drugs is less well studied than that of cigarette smoking.

Environmental Tobacco Smoke

Exposure to environmental tobacco smoke (i.e., passive smoking) by nonsmokers, especially in the workplace, increases the risk for the development of lung cancer. The exposure levels of environmental tobacco smoke depend on the size of the enclosed space and the intensity of smoking.

Other Exposure

The International Agency for Research on Cancer classified the following as group 1 known carcinogens for lung cancer: radon, asbestos, arsenic, beryllium, bis(chloromethyl)ether, cadmium, chromium, nickel, vinyl chloride, and polycyclic aromatic hydrocarbons (PAHs) (Chapters 18 and 93). Group 2A probable carcinogens include acrylonitrile, formaldehyde, and diesel exhaust. Group 2B possible carcinogens include acetaldehyde, silica, and welding fumes. It is estimated that 9% of lung cancers in men and 2% in women are caused by occupational exposure.

Radon, a gaseous decay product of uranium-238 and radium-226, damages lung tissue by emitting alpha particles. Underground mining of uranium

Early	Intermediate	Late	
Normal Epithelium	Hyperplasia	Dysplasia	CIS	Invasive Carcinoma

3p LOH/Small Telomeric Deletions	3p LOH/Contiguous Deletions	~ 80%
Microsatellite Alterations		~ 50%
EGFR (protein)		~ 60%
HER2 (protein)		~ 20%
9p21 LOH		~ 70%
Telomerase Dysregulation	Telomerase Upregulation	~ 80%
MYC Overexpression		~ 60%
8p21-23 LOH		~ 80%
Neoangiogenesis		~ 40%
Loss of Fhit immunostaining		~ 40%
p53 LOH	*TP53* Mutations	~ 70%
Aneuploidy		~ 80%
Methylation		~ 100%
	5q21 *APC-MMC* LOH	~ 30%
	K-ras Mutation	~ 20%

FIGURE 197-1. Sequential changes during the pathogenesis of lung cancer. CIS = carcinoma in situ; LOH = loss of heterozygosity. (From Hirsch FR, Franklin WA, Gazdar AF, et al. Early detection of lung cancer: clinical perspectives of recent advances in biology and radiology. *Clin Cancer Res.* 2001;7:5-22. Updated courtesy of Fred R. Hirsch, MD, PhD, Department of Medical Oncology, University of Colorado Health Sciences Center, and Adi F. Gazdar, MD, Department of Pathology, Southwestern Medical Center.)

exposes miners to radon and its decay products, thus increasing their risk for lung cancer. Radon may appear in homes, especially basements, because it is present in soil rock and ground water and enters the home through defects in pipes or the foundation. The indoor radon level depends on the soil concentration and ventilation rate. Data are conflicting about the risk for lung cancer with exposure to domestic radon, but the consensus is that the risk is increased.

Exposure to asbestos fibers (Chapter 93) occurs in automobile shops, shipyards, mines, and textile and cement plants and in construction and insulation workers. Workers with asbestosis, not just asbestos exposure, have an increased risk for lung cancer. Cigarette smokers with asbestos exposure have a risk of lung cancer that is multiplicative—a 50-fold relative risk compared with unexposed nonsmokers. The latency period for the development of lung cancer in workers exposed to asbestos is 25 to 40 years.

Arsenic, a naturally occurring metal, is a byproduct of copper, lead, zinc, and tin ore smelting. The metal is also present in agricultural pesticides and marine organisms. Exposure to arsenic occurs through air, soil, water, and foods. Cigarette smokers exposed to arsenic are at greater risk for the development of lung cancer than those not exposed to arsenic.

Beryllium, a metal used for alloys, is a pulmonary carcinogen. Exposure occurs in mining and in the manufacture of ceramics and electronic equipment. Bis(chloromethyl)ether is a product of chloromethylation processes used in the manufacture of ion exchange resins, polymers, and plastics. The relative risk for lung cancer in exposed workers is 10, especially for SCLC. Cadmium is a metal used for electroplating metals, batteries, plastics, and pigments. Exposure to cadmium causes an increased risk for lung cancer. Chromium is commonly used for metal alloys, paint pigments, electroplating, cement, rubber, photoengraving, and the composition of floor covering. Exposure to chromium increases the risk for lung cancer two- to three-fold. Nickel is used in electroplating, manufacturing of steel and other alloys, ceramics, storage batteries, electric circuits, and petroleum refining. Nickel exposure increases the risk for lung cancer 1.56-fold. Vinyl chloride is used to make plastics, packaging materials, propellant in cosmetic products, and vinyl floor tiles. Although the risk for development of lung cancer after exposure to vinyl chloride is increased, it is considered small. PAHs are formed from the incomplete combustion of organic material. Exposure to PAHs occurs with cigarette smoke; smelting of nickel-containing ores; aluminum, iron, steel, and coke production; coal tar; and diesel exhaust. PAHs carry a 1.5 to 2.5 relative risk for lung cancer.

Preexisting Lung Disease
Tobacco smoking causes chronic inflammation and destruction of lung tissue, which results in chronic obstructive pulmonary disease (COPD) (Chapter 88). Patients with COPD have an approximately four-fold increased risk for lung cancer. In addition, patients in whom idiopathic pulmonary fibrosis or pulmonary fibrosis from asbestosis or silica develops are at increased risk for the development of lung cancer.

Dietary Factors
Increased consumption of fruits and green and yellow vegetables is associated with a reduced risk for lung cancer, whereas low serum concentrations of antioxidant vitamins such as vitamins A and E are associated with the development of lung cancer. However, β-carotene supplementation increases the incidence of lung cancer.

Increased consumption of dietary fat is also associated with an increased incidence of lung cancer. High blood concentrations of selenium, a mineral involved in the protection of cellular membranes, has been associated with a lower risk for lung cancer.

Gender and Racial Differences
Women who smoke have a 1.2- to 1.7-fold higher risk ratio than men, especially for adenocarcinoma and SCLC. Possible explanations for this difference in lung cancer risk include (1) effects of hormones such as estrogen on the development of lung cancer, (2) gender differences in nicotine metabolism, and (3) gender variations in cytochrome P-450 enzymes involved in the bioactivation of toxic components in cigarette smoke condensate.

The high incidence and mortality of lung cancer in African American males may be due, in part, to (1) increased tobacco use, (2) differences in the metabolism of tobacco smoke, and (3) higher intake of dietary fat.

Human Immunodeficiency Virus Infection
Some studies suggest that the risk for lung cancer is increased in patients infected with human immunodeficiency virus (HIV) (Chapter 398), mostly as a result of cigarette smoking. Most patients are male (10:1) and young, in part reflecting the demographics of HIV infection.

Inheritance
First-degree relatives of patients with lung cancer have a two- to six-fold increase in the risk for lung cancer after adjusting for tobacco use. Second-degree relatives of lung cancer patients have a relative risk of 1.28, and third-degree relatives have a relative risk of 1.14. Nonsmokers with a family history of lung cancer have a two- to four-fold increased risk for lung cancer. The familial risk may be due to shared exposure, such as environmental tobacco smoke, or to shared genetic susceptibility to environmental carcinogens.

PATHOBIOLOGY
The development of lung cancer is the result of a multistep process from a premalignant lesion to frank cancer (Fig. 197-1) after a number of years.

Tobacco smoke or other carcinogens promote sequential genetic and epigenetic changes that result in the loss of normal control mechanisms of cellular growth. These changes affect (1) oncogenes, which are homologues of normal cellular genes and, when mutated, result in activation and gain of function; (2) tumor suppressor genes, which are "cancer" genes, in which loss of function by mutation removes inhibitions to control cell growth; and (3) growth factors (Chapter 185).

Oncogenes

The oncogenes that play a role in the pathogenesis of lung cancer include *ras*, the *myc* family, HER-2/*neu* (ERBB2), and Bcl-2. The *ras* family of oncogenes has three primary members (H-*ras*, K-*ras*, and N-*ras*), one of which, K-*ras*, is activated by point mutations in codon 12 of lung cancer cells. The mutation occurs in 30% of adenocarcinomas of the lung, most often in patients with a history of smoking, but it has not been found in SCLC. Patients who have the K-*ras* mutation have a poorer prognosis, stage for stage.

Amplification and overexpression of the *myc* family oncogenes (a-*myc*, L-*myc*, N-*myc*) are seen in 10 to 40% of SCLC and 10% of NSCLC. The most frequently altered gene, however, is c-*myc*, whose amplification in SCLC tumors that relapse is associated with shorter survival. However, overexpression of the *myc* oncogene is not present in most lung cancers, so its overexpression is probably not a primary event.

The HER-2/*neu* (ERBB2) gene, which encodes growth factor receptor or p185 neu (a tyrosine kinase glycoprotein), is activated in NSCLC but not SCLC. Overexpression of HER-2/*neu* in patients with adenocarcinoma of the lung portends a poor survival. Bcl-2, an oncogene that encodes a protein that inhibits programmed cell death (apoptosis), is also overexpressed in lung cancer, especially in SCLC.

Tumor Suppressor Genes

Tumor suppressor genes include *p53*, *Rb*, and *3p* (Chapter 185). The *p53* mutation correlates with cigarette smoking and has been detected in preneoplastic lesions of the lung. Mutations of *p53* are common in both NSCLC (~50%) and SCLC (~80%).

In SCLC, *Rb* is often mutated or deleted, so the Rb protein is not expressed in 90% of SCLC. In NSCLC, Rb is normally expressed, but when Rb is phosphorylated, uncontrolled cell division can occur in NSCLC.

One of the earliest genetic abnormalities in lung cancer occurs with the deletion of genetic material on the short arm of chromosome 3(3p) (p14-p23). The deletion occurs in approximately 50% of NSCLC and 90% of SCLC. The *FHIT* (fragile histidine triad) gene (3p14.2) is abnormal in many lung cancers and may function as a tumor suppressor gene by suppressing tumor growth and causing apoptosis.

Growth Factors

Growth factors secreted by lung cancer cells may reflect adjacent or regional cells (paracrine stimulation) or cause autonomous proliferation of the cells from which they were secreted (autocrine stimulation). Cells that are affected by this autocrine stimulation secrete a biologically active growth factor. Antibodies that bind to this growth factor will inhibit cell growth.

Autocrine (peptide) growth factors that are important in the growth of lung cancer cells, particularly SCLC, include gastrin-releasing peptide (GRP), insulin-like growth factor type I (IGF-I), and hepatocyte growth factor. GRP occurs in approximately 20 to 60% of SCLC and less frequently in NSCLC. Hepatocyte growth factor is expressed mainly in NSCLC.

The oncogene c-*erB*-1 encodes the epidermal growth factor receptor (EGFR), a 170-kD tyrosine kinase glycoprotein. Activation of EGFR initiates autophosphorylation of the receptor and eventually leads to cell cycle proliferation. Activating mutations in the *EGFR* gene have been found in 10 to 17% of patients with NSCLC; these patients have had an up to 75% response rate to the tyrosine kinase inhibitors, gefitinib or erlotinib.

Epigenetics

Epigenetics refers to a change in gene expression that is heritable but does not involve a change in DNA sequence. One of these epigenetic modifications involves changes in DNA methylation. These changes, which are very common in lung cancer, can include hypomethylation, dysregulation of DNA methyltransferase I, and hypermethylation. Genes that are methylated in NSCLC include *p16*, *RAR-β*, *RASSFIA*, methylguanine-methyltransferase, and death-associated protein kinase (DAP-kinase). This hypermethylation can silence tumor suppressor genes, thereby permitting unregulated cell growth.

CLINICAL MANIFESTATIONS

As many as 15% of patients in whom lung cancer is diagnosed are initially asymptomatic. The diagnosis is usually made incidentally on a chest radiograph obtained for other reasons (e.g., a preoperative study). However, most patients have symptoms and signs that are (1) caused by the pulmonary lesion itself—local tumor growth, invasion, or obstruction; (2) intrathoracic—regional tumor spreading to lymph nodes and adjacent structures; (3) extrathoracic—distant spread of disease; and (4) paraneoplastic syndromes. Nonspecific signs and symptoms of lung cancer include anorexia in about 30% of patients, weight loss, fatigue in third of patients, and anemia and fever in 10 to 20% of patients. More than 80% of patients initially have three or more symptoms or signs as a result of the lung cancer.

Pulmonary Lesion

Symptoms resulting from the primary lung cancer depend on the location and size of the cancer. Such symptoms can be secondary to endobronchial or peripheral growth of the primary tumor. The most common, cough, occurs in approximately 45% of cases, but it is nonspecific and also common in patients who smoke and have COPD. Hemoptysis occurs in more than 30% of patients, but the most common causes of hemoptysis are bronchitis and bronchiectasis. Dyspnea also occurs in 30 to 50% of patients. Wheezing is uncommon as an initial symptom in lung cancer and may signify major airway obstruction, which can cause a postobstructive pneumonia that may not initially be evident on chest radiographs and may be diagnosed only when the pneumonia fails to respond to standard therapy (Chapter 97). Lesions may be cavitary and may be associated with an abscess at the time of diagnosis of the lung cancer.

Peripheral lung tumors may be asymptomatic but are more frequently associated with symptoms of cough and pain from involvement of the pleura or chest wall. Chest pain, which occurs in more than 25% of patients, may be dull in nature, but chest pain that is severe and persists may be due to chest wall involvement.

Intrathoracic Spread

Symptoms associated with intrathoracic spread may be related to direct extension of the tumor or metastasis to regional lymph nodes. Dysphagia may occur secondary to esophageal compression. Although tracheoesophageal or bronchoesophageal fistulas are uncommon, coughing associated with swallowing or the development of aspiration pneumonitis (Chapter 97) should point to this possibility. Hoarseness, which is associated with recurrent laryngeal nerve paralysis, occurs in less than 20% of cases; it is more common with left-sided lung tumors because the nerve on this side has a longer intrathoracic course than the right-sided nerve. Phrenic nerve paralysis with hemidiaphragmatic elevation is associated with dyspnea and hiccups. Apical tumors, such as superior sulcus NSCLC (Pancoast's syndrome), may cause Horner's syndrome (Chapter 427), pain secondary to rib destruction, atrophy of hand muscles, and pain in the distribution of the C8, T1, and T2 nerve roots because of tumor invasion of the brachial plexus.

Blockage of the superior vena cava (SVC) (Chapter 99) as a result of compression or direct invasion by the tumor itself or by enlarged mediastinal lymph nodes may cause dyspnea. Signs of SVC syndrome include facial swelling, plethora, upper extremity swelling, dilated neck veins, and a prominent venous pattern on the anterior surface of the chest. Lung cancer accounts for most cases of SVC syndrome, with most cancer being SCLC and located on the right side.

Other manifestations of intrathoracic spread include pleural effusion (Chapter 99) causing dyspnea; pericardial effusion (Chapter 77) and cardiac extension of the tumor (Chapter 60) causing heart failure, arrhythmia, or tamponade; and lymphangitic spread through the lungs causing dyspnea and hypoxemia.

Extrathoracic Spread

At diagnosis, 30 to 40% of patients with NSCLC and approximately 60% of patients with SCLC have extrathoracic hematogenous spread of their tumor. Bone metastasis occurs in 30 to 40% of patients with lung cancer and commonly involves the vertebrae, ribs, and pelvic bones. Pain is the primary symptom. Liver metastases can produce right upper quadrant abdominal pain as well as nonspecific symptoms of fatigue and weight loss. Adrenal metastases can cause pain but most often cause no symptoms. One gland is usually involved, but bilateral metastases may occur. Brain metastasis, which occurs in 25 to 50% of SCLC and 25% of adenocarcinomas of the lung, may cause no symptoms but is more commonly associated with nausea, vomiting, headaches, seizures, confusion, personality changes, and focal neurologic signs and symptoms, depending on the site of metastatic disease. Epidural, intramedullary spinal cord metastasis and diffuse leptomeningeal involvement are less common than cerebral and cerebellar metastases.

Paraneoplastic Syndromes

Paraneoplastic syndromes (Chapter 187) occur in approximately 10 to 20% of patients with lung cancer. Endocrine syndromes include hypercalcemia, the syndrome of inappropriate antidiuretic hormone secretion, and ectopic adrenocorticotropic hormone secretion (Chapter 186). Other endocrine paraneoplastic syndromes of lesser clinical significance produce hormones such as the β-subunit of human chorionic gonadotropin, prolactin, gastrin, growth hormone, thyroid-stimulating factor, insulin-like substance, and calcitonin.

Neurologic syndromes are relatively rare, are most commonly associated with SCLC, and may have autoimmune mechanisms. Such syndromes include Eaton-Lambert syndrome, limbic encephalopathy, cerebellar degeneration, subacute sensory neuropathy, autonomic neuropathy, and optic neuritis (Chapter 187). Skeletal manifestations include digital clubbing (see Fig. 450-5 in Chapter 450) and hypertrophic pulmonary osteoarthropathy (Chapter 187).

Hematologic and vascular syndromes include hypercoagulable states, migratory thrombophlebitis (Trousseau's syndrome), and nonbacterial thrombotic endocarditis (Chapters 60 and 179). Cutaneous manifestations include dermatomyositis, acanthosis nigricans, erythema gyratum repens, and hyperkeratosis of the palms and soles of the feet (Chapter 187).

DIAGNOSIS

The diagnosis of lung cancer is made by cytologic examination of tissue biopsy specimens, sputum (Fig. 197-2), bronchial washings and brushings of suspicious lesions (Fig. 197-3), bronchoalveolar lavage fluid, and transbronchial and transthoracic needle aspirates (Fig. 197-4). The greater number of viable tumor cells in biopsy specimens from transthoracic, endobronchial, transbronchial, or open biopsy procedures increases the probability of accurate diagnosis. Sputum cytology may be only 20% sensitive for peripheral lung lesions, but it may be 80% sensitive for central lesions. In general, the sensitivity of a single sputum specimen is approximately 50%, whereas examination of three or more specimens increases the sensitivity to nearly 90%. The sensitivity of a single bronchial washing and brushing for detecting lung cancer is approximately 65%. For bronchoalveolar lavage fluid, the sensitivity is 60 to 65%. The sensitivity of fine-needle aspiration biopsy for detecting lung cancer exceeds 85%.

Solitary Pulmonary Nodule

A solitary pulmonary nodule is an asymptomatic lesion less than 3 cm in diameter surrounded by normal lung parenchyma that is incidentally found on a chest radiograph or computed tomography (CT) scan (Fig. 197-5). A solitary pulmonary nodule is found in up to 0.2% of all chest radiographs, and 10 to 70% are malignant. The chance of any solitary pulmonary nodule being cancerous correlates with the size and growth rate of the nodule, the age of the patient, any history of smoking, and a previous history of a malignancy. It is important to compare previous chest radiographs with the one demonstrating the nodule. A nodule that has not changed in size for at least 2 years is probably benign; a high-resolution CT scan with a resolution of 0.3 mm can best assess its size and growth characteristics. Solitary pulmonary nodules smaller than 4 mm have a 1% risk of malignancy, whereas a nodule larger than 8 mm has a 10 to 20% risk. In the latter situation, serial CT scans are indicated; positron emission tomography (PET) and biopsy should be considered. PET is 96.8% sensitive and 77.8% specific for identifying a malignancy, but because both false-negative and false-positive results can occur, tissue is needed for a definitive diagnosis. Transthoracic fine-needle aspiration biopsy, bronchoscopy, thoracotomy, and video-assisted thoracoscopic surgery (VATS) can establish a diagnosis.

Pathology

The histologic classification of lung cancer includes adenocarcinoma (about 40%), squamous cell (epidermoid) carcinoma (~30%), large cell carcinoma (~15%), and small cell carcinoma (~15%). These four histologic types represent more than 95% of all lung cancer.

Squamous cell carcinoma and adenocarcinoma are further classified by their differentiation: well differentiated, moderately differentiated, and

FIGURE 197-2. Adenocarcinoma cells in a sputum smear. (From Forbes CD, Jackson WF. *Color Atlas and Text of Clinical Medicine*, 3rd ed. London, Mosby, 2003.)

FIGURE 197-3. Squamous cell carcinoma. **Left,** Carina between the lingular and upper division bronchus of the left upper lobe. Note the well-defined, sharp features of the carina. **Right,** Carina between the left upper and lower lobes in the same patient. Note the swollen, red, infiltrated appearance of the mucosa and the white exophytic lesion. In addition, there is subepithelial hemorrhage. A biopsy specimen demonstrates squamous cell carcinoma. The patient had increased sputum production, positive sputum cytologic findings, and a nonlocalizing chest radiograph and computed tomography scan.

poorly differentiated. The latter types of cells are more aggressive and may have a worse prognosis than well-differentiated tumors. Adenocarcinoma is the most frequent histologic type in women and nonsmokers. Bronchoalveolar carcinoma, a subtype of adenocarcinoma, is well differentiated, grows along intact alveolar septa, and can be localized, multinodular, multifocal, or diffuse.

From a practical perspective based on biologic differences, clinical features, growth properties, and treatment, bronchogenic lung cancer is divided into two main categories: NSCLC and SCLC. In general, all NSCLCs are generally treated the same way based on the stage of the disease. SCLC is usually characterized by more aggressive biology, and treatment is dependent on whether the SCLC is limited stage (i.e., locally advanced) or extensive stage (i.e., metastatic disease).

Staging

Staging of NSCLC involves classification according to T (tumor size), N (regional lymph node involvement), and M (presence or absence of distant metastases). In October 2009, the TNM staging for NSCLC changed (Table 197-2). For SCLC, TNM staging is not generally used; rather, SCLC is staged as limited disease, defined as disease that can be encompassed by a single radiation portal, or extensive disease, that extending beyond a single radiation portal (usually metastatic).

Staging Procedures

All patients with lung cancer should be clinically staged using a complete history with a focus on performance status and weight loss; physical examination; pathologic review of all biopsy material; complete blood cell and platelet counts; chemistry profile, including renal and liver function tests, electrolytes, glucose, calcium, and phosphorus; and chest radiograph and chest CT (including the upper part of the abdomen and adrenal glands). Magnetic resonance imaging (MRI) of the brain and radionuclide scan of

FIGURE 197-4. Schematic overview for diagnosing, staging, and treating non–small cell and small cell lung cancer. See text for details. (Consult practice guidelines in oncology, non–small cell lung cancer, and small cell lung cancer at www.nccn.org as well for specifics.) *See Tables 197-2 and 197-3. CT = computed tomography; FNA = fine-needle aspiration; MRI = magnetic resonance imaging; PET = positron emission tomography; VATS = video-assisted thoracic surgery.

bones should be performed if metastases to these organs are suspected. Radiographs or MRI should be obtained if bone lesions are suggested by radionuclide scanning. PET is used to assess both regional and metastatic spread of tumor. Pulmonary function tests and arterial blood gas determinations should be obtained only if needed for treatment purposes.

For patients with SCLC, the initial pretreatment staging evaluation is similar to that used for NSCLC patients. For patients with peripheral blood count abnormalities, bone marrow aspiration and biopsy are recommended. Twenty to 30% of patients with SCLC will have tumor in bone marrow at the time of diagnosis.

Imaging
Radiography
A standard posteroanterior and lateral chest radiograph, although inexpensive and easy to perform, has limited value in the staging of lung cancer. Although it can detect pulmonary nodules as small as 3 to 4 mm, it is not reliable in detecting hilar or mediastinal lymphadenopathy.

Computed Tomography
A CT scan is commonly used to evaluate whether lung cancer is present in the hilar and mediastinal lymph nodes, liver, and adrenal glands, but its accuracy in identifying mediastinal lymph node involvement is suboptimal

(sensitivity of 40 to 65% and specificity of 45 to 90% versus either a PET scan or mediastinoscopy). Most importantly, CT will miss small metastatic foci that do not result in mediastinal lymph node enlargement. Mediastinal lymph nodes that are normal in size (≤1 cm) have an 8 to 15% probability of having metastatic disease, whereas mediastinal lymph nodes that are 1 to 1.5 cm, 1.5 to 2 cm, and greater than 2 cm in size will contain metastases 15 to 30%, approximately 50%, and about 90% of the time, respectively.

Positron Emission Tomography
PET, which uses 2-[^{18}F]fluoro-2-deoxy-D-glucose to identify areas of increased glucose metabolism in lung tumors, is more sensitive than CT in staging lung cancer (see Fig. 197-5); it has a sensitivity of 83%, specificity of 96%, and negative predictive value of 96%. However, increased glucose metabolism also occurs with inflammatory processes. Obtaining both PET and CT scans can enhance accuracy in the staging of lung cancer.▮ PET also enhances detection of bone, liver, and adrenal metastases. However, if treatment decisions are to be based on PET scan results, positive PET scan findings require pathologic or other radiologic confirmation.

Evaluation of Mediastinal Tissue
After initial clinical staging, if a patient with NSCLC has potentially surgically resectable disease, the regional lymph nodes (mediastinum) must be sampled

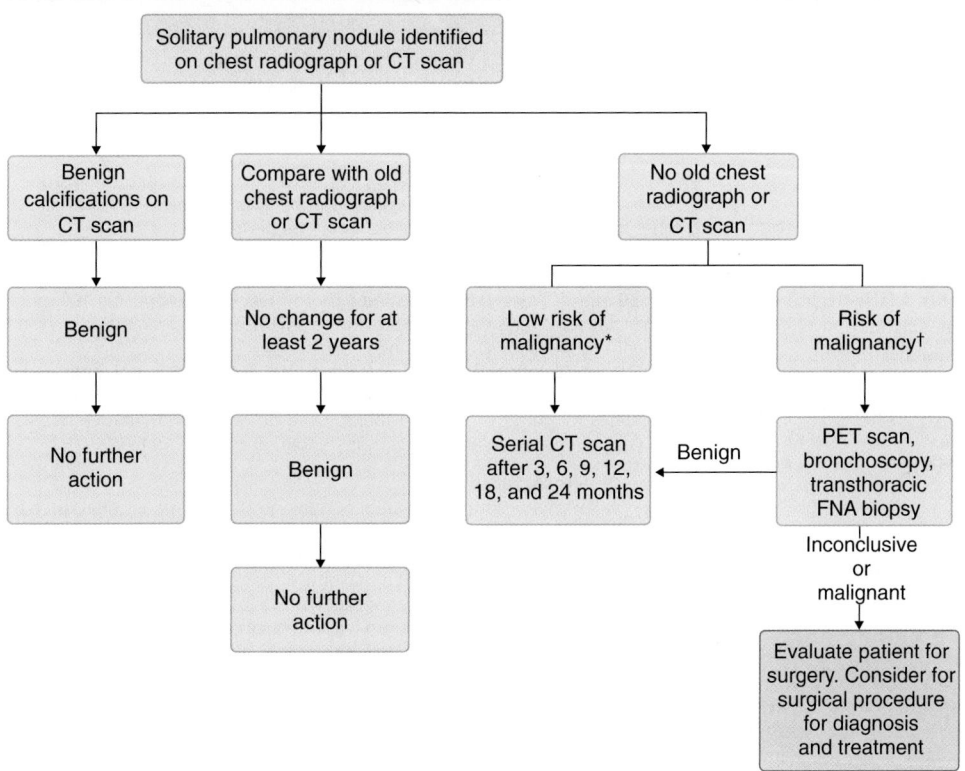

FIGURE 197-5. Evaluation of a patient with a solitary pulmonary nodule. *Patient with a minimal or absent history of smoking and other known risk factors for the development of lung cancer and a nodule 8 mm or smaller in size. †Patient with a history of smoking and other risk factors for the development of lung cancer and a nodule 8 mm or larger in size. CT = computed tomography; FNA = fine-needle aspiration; PET = positron emission tomography.

TABLE 197-2 STAGING OF LUNG CANCER

STAGE	TUMOR	NODE	METASTASIS	GENERAL DESCRIPTION
NON–SMALL CELL LUNG CANCER*				
Local				
IA	T1a,b	N0	M0	T1 tumor: ≤3 cm, surrounded by lung or visceral pleura, not more proximal than the lobar bronchus T1a ≤ 2, T1b > 2 but ≤3 cm
IB	T2a	N0	M0	T2 tumor: >3 cm, but ≤7 cm; or tumor with any of the following: invades visceral pleura; involves main bronchus ≥2 cm distal to the carina; associated with atelectasis/obstructive pneumonia extending to hilum but not involving the entire lung; T2a > 3 but ≤5 cm
IIA	T1a,b T2a T2b	N1 N1 N0	M0	T2b > 5 but ≤ 7 cm N1: involvement of the ipsilateral peribronchial or hilar nodes and intrapulmonary nodes including involvement by direct extension
Locally Advanced				
IIB	T2b T3	N1 N0	M0 M0	T3 tumor: tumor >7 cm or directly invading chest wall, diaphragm, mediastinal pleura, pericardium; or tumor in the main bronchus, <2 cm distal to the carina; or atelectasis or pneumonitis of the entire lung; or separate tumor nodules in the same lobe
IIIA	T1-3 T3 T4	N2 N1 N0,1	M0 M0 M0	N2: involvement of the ipsilateral mediastinal or subcarinal nodes T4 tumor: tumors of any size with invasion of the heart, great vessels, trachea, recurrent laryngeal nerve, esophagus, vertebral body, carina; or separate tumor nodules in a different ipsilateral lobe
Advanced				
IIIB	T4 T1-4	N2 N3	M0 M0	N3: involvement of the contralateral mediastinal or hilar nodes or any supraclavicular nodes
IV	Any T	Any N	M1a,b	M1a: separate tumor nodules in a contralateral lobe; or tumor with pleural nodules or malignant pleural dissemination M1b: distant metastasis
SMALL CELL LUNG CANCER†				
Limited disease				Evidence of tumor confined to the ipsilateral hemithorax; can be encompassed by a single radiation port
Extensive disease				All other diseases, including metastatic disease

The staging classification system was refined by the Union Internationale Contre le Cancer (UICC) and the American Joint Committee on Cancer (AJCC) with help from the International Association for the Study of Lung Cancer (IASLC). T = tumor, N = node, M = metastases. SCLC staging was developed by the Veterans Pulmination Lung Study Group.
*Detterbeck FC, Boffa DJ and Tanoue LT. The new lung cancer staging system. *Chest*. 2009;136:260-271.
†Stahel RA, Ginsberg R, Havermann K, et al. Staging and prognostic factors in small cell lung cancer: a consensus. *Lung Cancer*. 1989;5:119-126.

for possible metastases. Fiberoptic bronchoscopy to assess the bronchi and transbronchial needle aspirates to evaluate for mediastinal lymphadenopathy are recommended. Transbronchial needle aspirates are positive in 35 to 40% of patients when a CT scan demonstrates hilar or mediastinal lymphadenopathy. The larger the size of the lymph node on CT scan, the greater the chance for the aspirate to be positive.

The gold standard for evaluating the mediastinal lymph nodes for metastatic disease during life is transcervical mediastinoscopy. The subaortic and aortopulmonary window lymph nodes are inaccessible by routine mediastinoscopy, and the subcarinal lymph nodes may be difficult to access. The accuracy of the procedure ranges from 80 to 90%, with a false-negative rate of 10 to 12%. Other procedures used to evaluate the mediastinal lymph nodes include extended cervical mediastinoscopy, anterior mediastinotomy, thoracoscopy, and VATS. Endoscopic ultrasound (EUS) and endobronchial ultrasound (EBUS) biopsies of mediastinal lymph nodes can significantly reduce unnecessary thoracotomies when used in the staging of lung cancer.[2]

TREATMENT   Rx

Refer also to Table 197-3 and Figure 197-4.

Non–Small Cell Lung Cancer
Stage I and II Disease

For stage I and II NSCLC, surgery is the initial treatment of choice. Before surgical resection, a comprehensive preoperative medical evaluation is mandatory (Chapter 439). This evaluation must be supplemented by pulmonary function tests (forced expiratory volume at 1 second [FEV_1] and diffusing capacity of the lung for carbon monoxide [$DLCO$]), as well as blood gas analysis (Chapter 85). FEV_1 and $DLCO$ will determine what surgical procedure can be performed safely—pneumonectomy, lobectomy, wedge resection, or segmentectomy. A preoperative FEV_1 less than 40% of predicted and a $DLCO$ less than 40% of normal are associated with an increase in operative mortality. Threshold levels to define resectability include a preoperative FEV_1 greater than 2.0 L and $DLCO$ greater than 60% for pneumonectomy and a preoperative FEV_1 greater than 1.5 L and $DLCO$ greater than 50% for lobectomy. Other factors for determining resectability include exercise tolerance and comorbid disease. The curability of the patient is dependent on the stage of disease and completeness of the resection and not whether lobectomy or pneumonectomy is performed. By comparison, there is a significant risk of local recurrence in patients undergoing wedge resection or segmentectomy rather than more extensive resection of the tumor. Mortality rates for lobectomy and pneumonectomy are 3% and 9%, respectively. For patients older than 70 years, the mortality rate for pneumonectomy rises to 16 to 25%.

For patients with stage I NSCLC who either refuse surgery or have coexisting illnesses that preclude surgery, the use of stereotactic radiotherapy (SRT) shows high local control rates with minimal toxicity. Randomized trials of SRT and surgery for stage I NSCLC are ongoing.

At surgery, a tumor is considered to be unresectable if metastasis is found in the pleura or contralateral mediastinal lymph nodes or if there is tumor invasion of the mediastinum, heart, great vessels, or other structures. In addition to surgical resection of the tumor, sampling or complete removal of all accessible mediastinal lymph nodes should be performed.

Adjuvant cisplatin-based chemotherapy (e.g., cisplatin, 80 mg/m^2 every 3 weeks for four doses or 100 mg/m^2 every 4 weeks for four doses, plus vinorelbine 30 mg/m^2 weekly or vinblastine 4 mg/m^2 weekly or etoposide 100 mg/m^2 per day for 3 days per cycle) provides a small absolute increase in overall survival at 5 years for stage I, II, and III disease.[3]

Adjuvant radiation therapy for stage I and II disease is not indicated. However, in patients with stage I NSCLC who for medical reasons are not candidates for surgery, radiation therapy can be given with curative intent. Five-year survival rates in patients thus treated range from 10 to 30%.

Stage III—Resectable

For patients with stage III resectable disease (ipsilateral mediastinal spread of disease [N2], tumors [T3] involving the chest wall, diaphragm, or pleura; or superior sulcus tumors [Pancoast's]), surgery alone is suboptimal treatment because of the presence of occult metastatic disease. Neoadjuvant (i.e., induction) chemotherapy given in sequence with or concurrent with radiation therapy before surgery improves survival when compared with surgery alone or surgery plus postoperative radiation therapy.[4] However, concurrent chemoradiation therapy causes significant esophagitis when compared with the use of sequential chemotherapy and radiation therapy.

Stage III—Unresectable

Stage IIIA or IIIB disease may be unresectable. Thoracic radiation therapy (total dose, 60 Gy) relieves symptoms in the chest but has little effect on 5-year survival rates unless combined with induction chemotherapy (e.g., vinblastine plus cisplatin for two cycles), which improves median survival from 9.7 months to 13.8 months and the 5-year survival rate from 7 to 19% when compared with radiation therapy alone.

Concurrent chemotherapy and radiation therapy rather than sequential therapy can improve survival in patients with locally advanced NSCLC but increases side effects, particularly esophagitis, by five-fold. To improve the effectiveness of radiation therapy, different fractionation approaches are under evaluation. Three-dimensional treatment planning permits delivery of higher doses of radiation to the primary tumor and regional lymph nodes without increasing toxicity.

Stage IV—Disseminated Disease

For patients with disseminated NSCLC, treatment generally consists of cisplatin or carboplatin combined with paclitaxel, docetaxel, gemcitabine, vinorelbine, pemetrexed, irinotecan, or topotecan. The response rate to such

TABLE 197-3 GENERAL APPROACH TO THE TREATMENT OF LUNG CANCER ACCORDING TO STAGE*

STAGE	PRIMARY TREATMENT	ADJUVANT THERAPY	OUTCOME
NON–SMALL CELL LUNG CANCER			
I	Surgical resection	Chemotherapy (stage 1B)	5-yr survival rate >60-70%
II	Surgical resection	Chemotherapy	5-yr survival rate >40-50%
IIIA (resectable)	Preoperative chemotherapy followed by surgical resection (preferable) or chemotherapy followed by radiation therapy	Chemotherapy with or without radiation therapy	5-yr survival rate 15-30%
IIIA (unresectable) or IIIB (involvement of the contralateral or supraclavicular lymph nodes)	Chemotherapy plus concurrent radiation therapy (preferable) or chemotherapy followed by radiation therapy	None	5-yr survival rate, 10-20%
IV	Chemotherapy with 2 agents for 4-6 cycles Chemotherapy + bevacizumab (selected patients) EGFR-TKI (erlotinib, gefitinib) in patients with positive *EGFR* gene mutation Surgical resection of solitary brain metastasis and surgical resection of primary (T1) lesion	None	Median survival 8-10 mo 1-yr survival rate 30-35% >70% response rate; PFS-HR 0.48; median survival >20 mo 2-yr survival rate 10-15% 5-yr survival rate 10-15%
SMALL CELL LUNG CANCER			
Limited disease†	Chemotherapy plus concurrent radiation therapy	None	5-yr survival rate 15-25%
Extensive disease†	Chemotherapy	None	5-yr survival rate <5%

*All chemotherapy regimens include either cisplatin or carboplatin. The second drug used as part of the regimen may include etoposide, paclitaxel, docetaxel, vinorelbine, gemcitabine, or irinotecan.
†Prophylactic cranial irradiation is recommended for all patients with a complete response to initial therapy.
EGFR = epidermal growth factor receptor; PFS HR = progression-free survival hazard ratio.
Modified from Spira A, Ettinger DS. Multidisciplinary management of lung cancer. *N Engl J Med.* 2004;350:379-392.

therapy is 20 to 50%, with a median survival of 8 to 10 months, 1-year survival rate of 30 to 35%, and 2-year survival rate of 10 to 15%. Data suggest that two-drug combinations are better than single-agent therapy, but three-drug combinations are not more effective than two-drug combinations. The duration of therapy is four to six cycles, and patients older than 70 years who have good performance status respond to and tolerate chemotherapy as well as younger patients.

Over the past several years, the treatment of patients with disseminated NSCLC has changed. The era of "personalized therapy" has arrived, with treatment decisions being made based on histologic subtypes (nonsquamous vs. squamous cell carcinoma) and EGFR mutation analysis. Pemetrexed in combination with cisplatin has been approved for first-line treatment of patients with metastatic nonsquamous NSCLC.[5] The use of bevacizumab (an antiangiogenesis drug) in combination with paclitaxel plus carboplatin demonstrated a significant improvement in overall response rate, progression-free survival, and overall survival compared with chemotherapy alone in patients with non–squamous cell advanced NSCLC.[6] EGFR–tyrosine kinase inhibitors such as erlotinib or gefitinib in patients having tumors with activating mutations in the *EGFR* gene have significant clinical efficacy compared with standard chemotherapy when given as first-line treatment in patients with disseminated NSCLC.[7] Future therapies for patients with NSCLC will be based on genomic, pharmacogenomic, and proteomic strategies.

Patients with a solitary metastasis may occasionally benefit from resection of the isolated metastatic lesion. For example, resection of a solitary brain metastasis followed by whole brain irradiation can potentially be curative, with 5-year survival rates as high as 20%. Patients with metastatic NSCLC can benefit from palliative radiation therapy to specific lesions that cause bronchial obstruction, SVC syndrome, bone pain, brain masses, and spinal cord compression. Early palliative care promotes quality of life and mood as well as survival in patients with metastatic non–small cell lung cancer.[8]

Small Cell Lung Cancer

The mainstay of treatment of SCLC is chemotherapy because the disease is characterized by its propensity for a rapid growth rate and spread to distant sites. Unfortunately, management of SCLC has changed little in the past decade.

Limited Stage

Thirty to 40% of SCLC patients have limited-stage disease. Management usually consists of chemotherapy and radiation therapy, and surgery is indicated only in the approximately 5% of patients who have a solitary peripheral pulmonary nodule without evidence of mediastinal lymph node involvement with clinical staging. After surgical removal of the SCLC nodule, patients with negative mediastinal lymph nodes at surgery require only postoperative chemotherapy with etoposide and cisplatin. The 5-year survival rate in patients with no mediastinal lymph node involvement is 30 to 60%. If the nodes contain metastases, chest irradiation is recommended in addition to chemotherapy.

For most patients with limited-stage SCLC, concurrent chemotherapy and radiation therapy appear to be more effective than sequential therapy. In the United States, etoposide and cisplatin plus concurrent radiation therapy (i.e., twice-a-day irradiation—total dose of 45 Gy) is the treatment of choice and produces a 5-year survival rate of 26% compared with 16% when given with the same dose of radiation once a day.

In patients who achieve a complete response to therapy, prophylactic cranial irradiation (24 to 36 Gy) reduces the risk for brain metastases and provides about a 5% survival advantage, but its higher risk of precipitating cognitive abnormalities must be taken into consideration, especially in elderly patients.

Extensive Stage

For extensive-stage SCLC, chemotherapy is the treatment of choice. In the United States, etoposide plus cisplatin or carboplatin is commonly used. Carboplatin causes significantly less nausea, vomiting, and neurotoxicity. The chemotherapy is administered every 3 weeks for four to six cycles. At this time, there is no evidence that maintenance therapy with either chemotherapy or targeted molecular therapy increases survival rates.

SCREENING AND PREVENTION

Screening

Unfortunately, most patients with lung cancer are initially found to have advanced disease that is not curable. Screening chest radiographs have been unsuccessful in improving outcome. Spiral CT scanning is four- to five-fold more sensitive than chest radiography for detecting malignant nodules in high-risk patients, but spiral CT also detects seven to eight benign nodules for every malignant nodule found. A large trial is currently ongoing to determine whether current or former smokers benefit from screening with spiral CT.

Prevention

Primary prevention of lung cancer focuses on ways to prevent individuals from smoking and promotion of smoking cessation (Chapter 31). Trials of supplemental doses of β-carotene and vitamin E, stimulated by epidemiologic evidence of lower serum levels of these antioxidants in patients with lung cancer, have not only been unsuccessful but actually produced a higher risk of lung cancer in smokers who received either of these supplements. High concentrations of selenium in blood are associated with a lower risk of lung cancer, and an ongoing trial is comparing selenium with placebo in patients who have survived resection for stage I lung cancer.

PROGNOSIS

Most patients in whom lung cancer is diagnosed have incurable disease, with an overall 5-year survival rate of approximately 15%. What determines the chance for survival is the stage of disease in NSCLC and whether the disease is extensive or limited in the case of SCLC (Table 197-4).

OTHER PULMONARY NEOPLASMS

Neuroendocrine Lung Tumors

Neuroendocrine lung tumors are classified into four types: carcinoid tumors, atypical carcinoids, SCLC, and large cell neuroendocrine carcinomas. Carcinoid tumors are low-grade neuroendocrine tumors with a 10-year survival rate of greater than 90%. Atypical carcinoid tumors are intermediate-grade tumors, more aggressive than carcinoid, with survival ranging from 10 months to 3 years. Large cell neuroendocrine carcinoma is an aggressive neuroendocrine tumor that does not meet the criteria for either carcinoid, atypical carcinoid, or SCLC.

Bronchial Carcinoid Tumors

Carcinoid tumors (Chapter 240) of the lung account for 1 to 2% of all lung neoplasms. They are neuroendocrine tumors that trace their origin to the Kulchitsky cell present in bronchial epithelium. Typical and atypical carcinoids differ in the number of mitoses (<2 per 10 high-power fields [HPF] vs. 2 to 10 per 10 HPF, respectively), nuclear pleomorphism (absent vs. present), regional lymph node metastases (5 to 15% vs. 20 to 28%), and distant metastases at initial evaluation (rare vs. 20%). Patients with a typical carcinoid tumors rarely die, whereas patients with atypical carcinoid tumors have a 5-year mortality rate of 27 to 47%. Carcinoid tumors are not associated with cigarette smoking, are twice as common in women as in men, usually occur in patients younger than 40 years, and arise in the perihilar area of the lung. Treatment of bronchial carcinoid tumors is based on the stage of the disease. Usually, mediastinal staging is followed by surgical resection. With mediastinal lymph node involvement, radiation therapy is recommended for typical carcinoid tumors if surgery cannot be performed. For atypical carcinoid or metastatic disease, chemotherapy (etoposide plus cisplatin every 3 weeks for four cycles) plus radiation therapy is commonly used, but there is no evidence for the benefit of one therapy over another.

TABLE 197-4 FIVE-YEAR SURVIVAL RATE FOR NON–SMALL CELL LUNG CANCER BY THE CLINICAL AND SURGICAL TNM (TUMOR, NODE, METASTASIS) INTERNATIONAL STAGING SYSTEM FOR LUNG CANCER

STAGE	TNM SUBGROUPS	5-Year Survival Rate (%)	
		CLINICAL STAGE	SURGICAL STAGE
IA	T1a,b N0 M0	50	73
IB	T2a N0 M0	43	58
IIA	T1a,b N1 M0 T2a N1 M0 T2b N0 M0	36	46
IIB	T2b N1 M0 T3 N0 M0	25	36
IIIA	T3 N1 M0 T1-3 N2 M0 T4 N0 M0	19	24
IIIB	T4 Any N M0 Any T N3 M0	7	9
IV	Any T Any N M1a,b	2	13

Malignant Mesothelioma

Pleural mesotheliomas (Chapter 99) are related to asbestos exposure (Chapter 93), with a peak risk 30 to 35 years after the initial exposure to asbestos. Approximately 50% of patients in whom a mesothelioma develops give no history of direct asbestos exposure. Other possible risk factors for mesothelioma include radiation and SV40 virus. Mesothelioma is generally diagnosed in the fifth to seventh decade of life (median age, 60 years), with the neoplasm developing in men five times more frequently than in women. Common symptoms include shortness of breath (60%) and chest wall pain or discomfort (60%). Chest radiographs usually reveal the presence of a unilateral pleural effusion. When the tumor progresses, it is generally local; symptomatic distant metastases are a late occurrence, if at all. Cytologic evaluation of pleural fluid to establish the diagnosis is difficult and may be inaccurate. The diagnosis is usually made by a biopsy procedure—under CT guidance or thoracoscopically, including VATS if necessary. Several staging systems have been proposed, but none has achieved complete acceptance. Treatment, which depends on the extent of disease, includes surgery (thoracoscopy with sclerosis, pleurectomy, extrapleural pneumonectomy), radiation therapy, and, often, chemotherapy. These three modalities individually have not significantly improved survival rates, and chemotherapy also has not helped control symptoms.[9] Multimodality and molecularly targeted agents are being evaluated. Mesothelioma remains a fatal disease, with a median survival of 9 to 12 months from the time of diagnosis.

Other Lung Tumors

Carcinomas of the salivary gland type include mucoepidermoid carcinoma and adenoid cystic carcinoma. These tumors are slow-growing neoplasms that arise from the bronchial glands. They represent approximately 0.2% of lung cancers and are usually treated surgically.

Primary sarcomas of the lung are very rare and include malignant fibrous histiocytoma, fibrosarcoma, leiomyosarcoma, rhabdomyosarcoma, epithelioid hemangioendothelioma, angiosarcoma, and liposarcoma. Surgery is the primary treatment, but radiation therapy or chemotherapy, or both, may be necessary, depending on the size and grade of the tumor and whether the margins are clear (Chapter 209).

Primary lymphomas of the lung account for approximately 0.3% of all primary cancers of the lung. The most common type is a low-grade small lymphocytic lymphoma. Surgery and chemotherapy (Chapter 191) are the usual treatments.

1. Maziak DE, Darling GE, Inculet RI, et al. Positron emission tomography in staging early lung cancer: a randomized trial. *Ann Intern Med.* 2009;151:221-228.
2. Annema JT, van Meerbeeck JP, Rintoul RC, et al. Mediastinoscopy vs endosonography for mediastinal nodal staging of lung cancer: a randomized trial. *JAMA.* 2010;304:2245-2252.
3. Winton T, Livingston R, Johnson D, et al. Vinorelbine plus cisplatin vs. observation in resected non-small-cell lung cancer. *N Engl J Med.* 2005;352:2589-2597.
4. Albain KS, Swann RS, Rusch VW, et al. Radiotherapy plus chemotherapy with or without surgical resection for stage III non-small cell lung cancer: a phase III randomized control trial. *Lancet.* 2009;374:379-386.
5. Scagliotti GV, Parikh P, von Pawel J, et al. Phase III study comparing cisplatin plus gemcitabine with cisplatin plus pemetrexed in chemotherapy naïve patients with advanced-stage non-small cell lung cancer. *J Clin Oncol.* 2008;26:3543-3551.
6. Sandler A, Gray R, Perry M, et al. Paclitaxel-carboplatin alone or with bevacizumab for non-small-cell lung cancer. *N Engl J Med.* 2006;355:2542-2550.
7. Mok TS, Wu YL, Thongprasert S, et al. Gefitinib or carboplatin-paclitaxel in pulmonary adenocarcinoma. *N Engl J Med.* 2009;361:1-10.
8. Temel JS, Green JA, Muzikansky A, et al. Early palliative care for patients with metastatic non–small-cell lung cancer. *N Engl J Med.* 2010;363:733-742.
9. Muers MF, Stephens RJ, Fisher P, et al. Symptom control with or without chemotherapy in the treatment of patients with malignant pleural mesothelioma (MS01): a multicentre randomized trial. *Lancet.* 2008;371:1685-1694.

SUGGESTED READINGS

Cataldo VD, Gibbons DL, Pérez-Soler R, et al. Treatment of non–small-cell lung cancer with erlotinib or gefitinib. *N Engl J Med.* 2011;364:947-955. *These epidermal growth factor receptor tyrosine kinase inhibitors have a role in advanced disease.*

Clinical Practice Guidelines in Oncology. Non-Small Cell Lung Cancer and Small Cell Lung Cancer. Version 3.2011 (NSCLC), version 1.2011 (SCLC). Available from the National Comprehensive Cancer Network at http://www.nccn.org. *Up-to-date approaches to the treatment of non–small cell and small cell lung cancer.*

NSCLC Meta-analyses Collaborative Group. Adjuvant chemotherapy, with or without postoperative radiotherapy, in operable non–small-cell lung cancer: two meta-analyses of individual patient data. *Lancet.* 2010;375:1267-1277. *In two meta-analyses, adjuvant chemotherapy improved survival of operable non–small-cell lung cancer by 14%.*

Ray M, Kindler HL. Malignant pleural mesothelioma: an update on biomarkers and treatment. *Chest.* 2009;136:888-896. *A concise review of the present and future treatments in pleural mesothelioma.*

Tomaszek SC, Wigle DA. Pretreatment assessment for the optimal management of early-stage lung cancer. *Cancer. J* 2001;17:11-17. *Review.*

Travis WD, Brambilla E, Noguchi M, et al. International association for the study of lung cancer/American Thoracic Society/European Respiratory Society international multidisciplinary classification of lung adenocarcinoma. *J Thorac Oncol.* 2011;6:244-285. *Proposed new classification strategy.*

van Klaveren RJ, Oudkerk M, Prokop M, et al. Management of lung nodules detected by volume CT scanning. *N Engl J Med.* 2009;361:2221-2229. *After one negative screening CT scan, the risk of finding lung cancer on a subsequent screening CT scan was 1/1000 at 1 year and 3/1000 at 2 years.*

NEOPLASMS OF THE ESOPHAGUS AND STOMACH

ANIL K. RUSTGI

NEOPLASMS OF THE ESOPHAGUS

DEFINITION

The esophagus is a hollow tubular organ with primary physiologic functions related to contraction to permit propulsion of solid and liquid food contents into the stomach. Benign disorders of contraction are designated as esophageal motility disorders and discussed in Chapters 138 and 140. The mucosa is a stratified squamous epithelium that covers the submucosa and muscle; the latter is skeletal muscle in the proximal esophagus and smooth muscle in the mid-distal esophagus. Cancers of the esophagus may be classified broadly into epithelial versus nonepithelial. There are benign epithelial tumors referred to as *squamous cell papillomas*. Malignant epithelial tumors are classified into two main subtypes: esophageal squamous cell carcinoma (ESCC) and esophageal adenocarcinoma (EAC) (Table 198-1), which serves as the focus of this chapter's section. Apart from ESCC and EAC, other esophageal epithelially derived tumors include verrucous squamous cell carcinoma, adenosquamous carcinoma, adenoid cystic carcinoma, and mucoepidermoid carcinoma. Benign nonepithelial tumors include leiomyoma, granular cell tumors, fibrovascular polyp, hemangioma, lymphangioma, lipoma, and fibroma. Malignant nonepithelial tumors include leiomyosarcoma and other sarcomas, metastatic carcinoma (originating from breast, lung), and lymphoma.

Esophageal Squamous Cell Carcinoma

EPIDEMIOLOGY

ESCC is the more common type of esophageal cancer worldwide and represents a leading cause of cancer-related mortality in men. ESCC may have rates of up to 100 per 100,000 population in what is often termed the *central Asian belt*, including regions around the Caspian Sea, Iran, India, and China; other areas of high incidence include some Mediterranean countries and South Africa. In the United States, ESCC is more common among African American males than white males, with risks of 15.1 per 100,000 compared with 2.9 per 100,000, respectively. Overall, although the incidence of ESCC

TABLE 198-1	RISK FACTORS FOR ESOPHAGEAL CANCER
Esophageal squamous cell cancer	
Tylosis palmaris et plantaris	
Achalasia	
Plummer-Vinson syndrome	
Cigarette smoking	
Alcohol	
Chronic lye ingestion	
Human papilloma virus infection	
Radiation injury	
Celiac sprue	
Esophageal adenocarcinoma	
Gastroesophageal acid reflux	
Bile reflux	
Obesity	
Barrett's esophagus	

is low in males or females younger than 50 years, it does increase with advancing age.

Risk Factors

Cancers in general are viewed in the context of hereditary or inherited forms versus sporadic or seemingly random diseases that are related to age, environmental exposures, and genetic alterations (see Table 198-1). That being said, the hereditary basis for ESCC is exceedingly rare, consisting of a desquamating condition termed *tylosis palmaris et plantaris*. As implied, the desquamation most dramatically affects the hands and feet, but this extends to the esophagus as well. Another uncommon condition is called *Plummer-Vinson syndrome* or *Paterson-Brown Kelly syndrome*, which entails glossitis, cervical esophageal webs, and iron deficiency anemia. In both conditions, it is likely that chronic inflammation triggers the cascade of events that culminate in ESCC.

The vast preponderance of ESCC cases are attributable to cigarette smoking or alcohol, but especially so in combination because there appear to be synergistic deleterious effects of various chemical carcinogens in both, including *N*-nitroso compounds, polycyclic aromatic hydrocarbons, and aromatic amines. The relative risk for ESCC is 6.2 in those who smoke more than 25 cigarettes on a daily basis. Cessation of cigarette smoking is helpful in attenuating risk after 10 years of abstinence. Cigarette smokers who partake in beer and whiskey have a 10- to 25-fold enhanced risk of developing ESCC. Indeed, it is the type of alcohol and the manner of distillation that are most critical. In endemic areas of the world, deficiencies of vitamins A, B_{12}, C, and E, folic acid, and certain minerals (zinc, selenium, molybdenum) are important risk factors. All these vitamins and minerals exert direct or indirect antioxidant effects, and their deficiencies impair epithelial and tissue homeostasis and regeneration.

Other risk factors for ESCC include achalasia (Chapter 140), a disorder that involves aganglosis of Auerbach's plexus, resulting in dysphagia, chest pain, and weight loss, among other symptoms. The emergence of ESCC may be observed 10 to 20 years after the identification of achalasia in patients. Because head and neck squamous cell carcinoma (HNSCC) (Chapter 196) shares many of the environmental and lifestyle risk factors with ESCC, HNSCC and ESCC may occur synchronously or metachronously. In different parts of the world, ESCC is also associated with chronic esophageal stricture due to lye ingestion, consumption of maté (a hot herb-based beverage), celiac sprue, human papillomavirus infection, and radiation injury.

PATHOBIOLOGY

ESCC involves the transition over time from normal squamous epithelium to squamous dysplasia to cancer. ESCC initiation, progression, and metastasis are associated with a number of genetic alterations. Among the genetic alterations are overexpression of *epidermal growth factor receptor* and *cyclin D1* oncogenes, and inactivation of *TP53*, *p16INK4A*, and *E-cadherin* tumor suppressor genes. The frequency of these changes varies greatly based on the studies, but the oncogenic alterations appear to be generally early onset in dysplasia and early ESCC, whereas the inactivation of the tumor suppressor genes appear to be late events in established primary and metastatic ESCC. From a genomic viewpoint, the SOX-2 transcriptional factor, important in the pluripotent capacity of somatic cells, has been shown to be an important gene involved in ESCC pathogenesis and transformation by virtue of SOX-2 amplification. The ability to model ESCC in vitro and in vivo has witnessed great strides in recent years through the advent and characterization of three-dimensional organotypic culture models, xenograft transplantation mouse models, and genetically engineered mouse models.

CLINICAL MANIFESTATIONS

Symptoms and Signs

Although esophageal squamous dysplasia is typically not associated with symptoms, ESCC, which has a predilection for the proximal to mid esophagus, may be associated with dysphagia, odynophagia, atypical or typical chest pain, gastrointestinal bleeding, nausea, vomiting, weight loss, and malnutrition. ESCC may metastasize to local lymph nodes, lung, liver, and bone. Symptoms attributable to metastatic ESCC may involve bone-related pain, dyspnea, and evidence of jaundice and liver failure, depending on the extent of metastatic disease.

Physical Examination

The patient should be evaluated for changes in hair, skin integrity, and nail beds as a reflection of malnutrition. Weight loss may result in general cachexia and muscle wasting. There may be lymphadenopathy in the anterior cervical and supraclavicular regions. Hepatomegaly and complications of liver disease may be present with metastatic disease to the liver.

Laboratory Studies

There may be progressive iron deficiency anemia due to chronic, indolent upper gastrointestinal bleeding. Additional abnormalities may be reflected in metabolic disturbances, such as metabolic alkalosis due to vomiting and hypernatremia due to dehydration. Liver enzyme abnormalities, both hepatocellular and cholestatic, may reflect metastasis to the liver. There are no specific markers for ESCC, but an elevated carcinoembryonic antigen (CEA) level may be used to aid in diagnosis or to monitor disease recurrence after therapy.

DIAGNOSIS

Barium swallow radiography is useful for the diagnosis of ESCC with depiction of a filling defect due to the mucosal lesion or impaired transit of barium due to luminal growth. However, definitive diagnosis involves direct visualization with upper endoscopy; once the mass is visualized, biopsies are necessary for confirmation by histopathology and possibly immunohistochemistry for cytokeratins associated with proliferation and differentiation. ESCC may involve local lymph nodes, which are best detected by endoscopic ultrasound; as needed, samples can be then analyzed for cytopathology by fine-needle aspiration. Evaluation of metastatic disease involves chest and abdominal/computed tomography (CT) scans. Bone scan might be useful in patients who are symptomatic with bone-related pain. Positron emission tomography (PET) has become increasingly used in some settings, although there are no guidelines for its routine use. In totality, these diagnostic modalities also allow for staging of ESCC (Table 198-2), which is important in guiding therapeutic options.

TREATMENT

Surgical Therapy

Surgery is the cornerstone of therapy for curative intent. Technical advances have led to improvements in both operative mortality and postoperative morbidity. The different surgical techniques include transthoracic, transhiatal, and radical en bloc resections. Depending on the location of the ESCC, either total esophagectomy or subtotal esophagectomy is pursued. For the latter, jejunal or colonic interposition can be done.

Minimally invasive surgery may be done for esophagectomy in selected patients.

Medical Therapy

Depending on the stage, there is some variation in whether to proceed with preoperative (neoadjuvant) chemoradiation therapy or postoperative (adjuvant) chemoradiation therapy.

A study in which patients were randomized to receive surgery alone or surgery plus postoperative chemotherapy with 5-fluorouracil and leucovorin and concurrent radiation therapy revealed that the median survival was 36 months for patients in the adjuvant arm compared with 26 months for those in the surgery-only arm. The 3-year overall survival rates were 50% compared with 40%, respectively.

PROGNOSIS

The 5-year survival for treated ESCC is dependent on stage and types of therapies used as indicated previously. For stages T1 and T2 without lymphadenopathy, surgery alone may be curative in more than 60% of cases. For patients with metastatic disease, therapy is palliative involving endoscopically placed expandable prosthetic stents to open the nearly obstructed lumen for passage of food contents, percutaneous endoscopic gastrotomy tubes for delivery of nutrition to the stomach distal to the mass lesion, total parenteral nutrition, pain control, and systemic chemotherapy.

Esophageal Adenocarcinoma

EPIDEMIOLOGY

EAC affects whites more than African Americans and males much more than females (3 : 1 to 5.5 : 1) and increases in incidence after the age of 40 years. The age-adjusted incidence annually is 1.3 per 100,000. We will deal with EAC as a separate entity from gastroesophageal (GE) adenocarcinomas (so-called GE junctional cancer) and gastric cardia adenocarcinomas, although there has been a tendency by some to think of these in aggregate. That being stated, the incidence of EAC is increasing dramatically in developed

TABLE 198-2 TNM STAGING SYSTEM FOR CANCER OF THE ESOPHAGUS (AMERICAN JOINT COMMITTEE ON CANCER CRITERIA)

PRIMARY TUMOR (T)*

TX	Primary tumor cannot be assessed
T0	No evidence of primary tumor
Tis	High-grade dysplasia†
T1	Tumor invades lamina propria, muscularis mucosae, or submucosa
T1a	Tumor invades lamina propria or muscularis mucosae
T1b	Tumor invades submucosa
T2	Tumor invades muscularis propria
T3	Tumor invades adventitia
T4	Tumor invades adjacent structures
T4a	Resectable tumor invading pleura, pericardium, or diaphragm
T4b	Unresectable tumor invading other adjacent structures, such as aorta, vertebral body, trachea, etc.

*(1) At least maximal dimension of the tumor must be recorded and (2) multiple tumors require the T(m) suffix.
†High-grade dysplasia includes all noninvasive neoplastic epithelia that was formerly called carcinoma in situ.

LYMPH NODE (N)*

NX	Regional lymph nodes cannot be assessed
N0	No regional lymph node metastasis
N1	Metastasis in 1-2 regional lymph nodes
N2	Metastasis in 3-6 regional lymph nodes
N3	Metastasis in 7 or more regional lymph nodes

*Number must be recorded for total number of regional nodes sampled and total number of reported nodes with metastasis.

DISTANT METASTASIS (M)

MX	Metastasis cannot be assessed
M0	No distant metastasis
M1	Distant metastasis

From *AJCC Cancer Staging Manual*, 7th ed. New York: Springer-Verlag; 2010.

countries, especially in the United States (by 4 to 10% annually) and western and northern Europe.

Etiology

Obesity (central) is an important risk factor for EAC. This may be related to either mechanical factors that foster greater gastroesophageal acid reflux disease (GERD) or the release of proinflammatory cytokines and adipokines that track to the esophagus, or both. The major recognized precursor of EAC is Barrett's esophagus (BE). BE is the replacement of the normal stratified squamous epithelium by an incomplete small intestinal type of epithelium (metaplasia) in the distal esophagus projecting from the GE junction in a distal-proximal gradient. In turn, it has been demonstrated that BE is fostered by GERD but also by an admixture of bile acids in the acid refluxate. Patients with scleroderma (Chapter 275) may be at increased risk for BE. A small subset of BE patients may progress to EAC through intermediate stages of low-grade and high-grade dysplasia. In BE, one case of EAC is estimated to arise in 55 to 441 patient years, which corresponds to an approximately 125-fold increased risk for EAC compared with that in the general population.

PATHOBIOLOGY

BE, or incomplete intestinal metaplasia, involves transdifferentiation from normal esophageal epithelium to an epithelium of the small intestine with columnar enterocytes and secretory goblet cells, but without Paneth cells and enteroendocrine cells—hence the designation of incomplete intestinal metaplasia. By itself, BE metaplasia cannot become EAC. However, if and when BE transitions to low-grade and high-grade dysplasia, there is the aforementioned risk for EAC. BE is associated with abnormal DNA ploidy based on flow cytometry analysis, and certain genetic alterations in epidermal growth factor receptor signaling, *TP53* and *p16INK4A*. Microsatellite instability may be noted as well. Whole genome approaches are revealing gains and losses of chromosomal regions that might lead to identification of known and previously unknown genes critical in the pathogenesis of EAC.

CLINICAL MANIFESTATIONS

Symptoms and Signs

It is estimated that 5 to 15% of GERD patients may develop BE, but such population-based studies are difficult to pursue because vast millions of people are affected with GERD, and most GERD patients do not undergo upper endoscopy. Patients with BE may or may not have symptoms related to GERD. Chronic GERD with BE may be associated with distal esophageal strictures. With EAC, patients may suffer from dysphagia, odynophagia, upper gastrointestinal bleeding, chest pain, nausea, vomiting, early satiety, weight loss, and malnutrition.

Physical Examination

Examination of the patient may reveal signs consistent with malnutrition and weight loss. Lymph adenopathy should be explored. There may be hepatomegaly. Paraneoplastic syndromes are unusual with EAC (as well as with ESCC) in contrast to non–small cell lung cancer (NSCLC) or pancreatic adenocarcinoma. Nevertheless, it is important to ensure that EAC is not mistaken for a benign entity such as a primary esophageal motility disorder.

Laboratory Studies

Patients with EAC may suffer from iron deficiency anemia, metabolic derangements, and abnormal liver enzyme tests due to metastatic disease. CEA may be elevated as a tumor serologic marker.

DIAGNOSIS

Barium swallow radiography may lead one to the suspicion of BE and can diagnose luminal mass lesions consistent with EAC in the distal esophagus. However, the mainstay of diagnosis is upper endoscopy. At that time, one will appreciate a salmon-colored mucosa from the GE junction with frondlike projections in a proximal direction. If the extent of BE is less than or equal to 3 cm, it is termed *short-segment BE*; if it is more than 3 cm, it is referred to as *long-segment BE*. This distinction is important in that the risk for EAC in long-segment BE is greater than in short-segment BE. Noting that the normal esophageal mucosa is more pink-white in hue, one can visually distinguish the two different types of epithelia, with the caveat that the gastric cardia mucosa at the GE junction should not be mistaken for BE. With that in mind, endoscopic mucosal biopsies from the BE region (with control biopsies from the normal esophagus and gastric cardia) are required for diagnosis histopathologically. Features of dysplasia are best appreciated in the absence of reflux-related esophagitis that can lead to nuclear architectural distortion; hence, suppression of acid production with proton pump inhibitor therapy for 6 to 8 weeks is needed, with a view to repeat biopsies.

If the patient has BE metaplasia, upper endoscopy should be repeated every 2 to 3 years. However, low-grade dysplasia requires surveillance endoscopy every 6 to 12 months. High-grade dysplasia, if properly evaluated by the pathologist, may require reconfirmation, but then leads to either medical (radiofrequency ablation, endoscopic mucosal resection) or surgical intervention due to the possibility of missed contiguous EAC. Endoscopic ultrasound may be helpful in discriminating between high-grade dysplasia and EAC.

TREATMENT   Rx

The principles are very similar to those applied to ESCC in terms of surgery. Data support adjuvant chemoradiation therapy for EAC, with median survival of 27 months for surgery alone versus 36 months for surgery plus chemoradiation therapy. Overall prognosis for EAC is not too dissimilar from that noted in ESCC. The treatment options of BE, the main precursor of EAC, have witnessed dramatic growth. Initially, photodynamic therapy was viewed with favor. However, for patients who are not surgical candidates because of comorbid illnesses, endoscopic mucosal resection (EMR) and radio frequency ablation are credible options, especially for BE-related high-grade dysplasia or BE associated with intramucosal EAC.

NEOPLASMS OF THE STOMACH

DEFINITION

Gastric neoplasms are predominantly malignant, and nearly 90 to 95% of these tumors are adenocarcinomas. Less frequently observed malignant diseases include lymphomas, especially non-Hodgkin's lymphoma, and sarcomas, such as leiomyosarcoma. Benign gastric neoplasms include leiomyomas, carcinoid tumors, and lipomas.

Adenocarcinoma of the Stomach

EPIDEMIOLOGY

The great geographic variation in the incidence of gastric cancer worldwide strongly indicates that environmental factors influence the pathogenesis of gastric carcinogenesis. Further support for this notion comes from observations that groups emigrating from high-risk to low-risk areas, such as Japanese individuals moving to Hawaii and Brazil, acquire the low risk of the area into which they emigrate, presumably because of adoption of the endogenous lifestyle and exposure to different environmental factors.

Gastric adenocarcinoma was the most frequently observed malignant disease in the world until the mid-1980s, and it remains extremely common among men in certain regions, such as tropical South America, some parts of the Caribbean, and Eastern Europe. Regardless of gender, it remains one of the most common malignancies in Japan and China.

Whereas gastric cancer was the most common cancer in the United States in the 1930s, its annual incidence has steadily decreased. The annual incidence is now fewer than 20,000 new cases per year. However, although the incidence of gastric adenocarcinoma localized to the distal stomach has declined, the incidence of proximal gastric and gastroesophageal adenocarcinomas has been steadily increasing in the United States, a finding that perhaps reflects differences in pathogenic factors. Typically, gastric cancer occurs between the ages of 50 and 70 years and is uncommon before age 30 years. The rates are higher in men than in women by 2 to 1. Five-year survival is less than 20%.

Risk Factors

Risk factors for the development of gastric adenocarcinoma can be divided into environmental and genetic factors as well as precursor conditions (Table 198-3). For example, *Helicobacter pylori* infection is significantly more common in patients with gastric cancer than in matched control groups. Epidemiologic studies of high-risk populations have also suggested that genotoxic agents such as *N*-nitroso compounds may play a role in gastric tumorigenesis. *N*-nitroso compounds can be formed in the human stomach by nitrosation of ingested nitrates, which are common constituents of the diet. High nitrate concentrations in soil and drinking water have been observed in areas with high death rates from gastric cancer. Atrophic gastritis (Chapter 141), with or without intestinal metaplasia, is observed in association with gastric cancer, especially in endemic areas. Pernicious anemia (Chapter 167) is associated with a several-fold increase in gastric cancer. Atrophic gastritis and gastric cancer have certain environmental risk factors in common. It is likely that atrophic gastritis and intestinal metaplasia represent intermediary steps to gastric cancer. The achlorhydria associated with gastritis related to *H. pylori* infection, pernicious anemia, or other causes favors the growth of bacteria capable of converting nitrates to nitrites. The nitrosamine *N*-methyl-*N*′-nitro-*N*-nitrosoguanidine causes a high rate of induction of adenocarcinoma in the glandular stomach of rats. At the same time, most patients with atrophic gastritis do not develop gastric cancer, a finding suggesting that neither atrophic gastritis nor achlorhydria alone is responsible.

Benign gastric ulcers do not appear to predispose patients to gastric cancer. However, patients who have a gastric remnant after subtotal gastrectomy for benign disorders have an increased relative risk for gastric cancer of 1.5 to 3 by 15 to 20 years after surgery.

PATHOBIOLOGY

Gastric adenocarcinomas can be divided into two types based on the Lauren classification: intestinal and diffuse. The intestinal type is typically in the distal stomach with ulcerations, is often preceded by premalignant lesions, and is declining in incidence in the United States. By contrast, the diffuse type involves widespread thickening of the stomach, especially in the cardia, and it often affects younger patients; this form may present as linitis plastica, a nondistensible stomach with the absence of folds and narrowed lumen caused by infiltration of the stomach wall with tumor. Diffuse-type gastric cancers harbor mucin-producing cells. Other conditions may result in linitis plastica, such as lymphoma (Chapter 191), tuberculosis (Chapter 332), syphilis (Chapter 327), and amyloidosis (Chapter 194). The prognosis is generally worse in the diffuse type.

Key histopathologic features of gastric cancer include degree of differentiation, invasion through the gastric wall, lymph node involvement, and the presence or absence of signet ring cells within the tumor itself. Other pathologic manifestations include a polypoid mass, which may be difficult to distinguish from a benign polyp. Early gastric cancer, a condition that is not

TABLE 198-3 CONDITIONS PREDISPOSING TO OR ASSOCIATED WITH GASTRIC CANCER

ENVIRONMENTAL

Helicobacter pylori infection
Dietary: excess of salt (salted pickled foods), nitrates/nitrites, carbohydrates; deficiency of fresh fruit, vegetables, vitamins A and C, refrigeration
Low socioeconomic status
Cigarette smoking

GENETIC

Familial gastric cancer (rare)
Associated with hereditary nonpolyposis colorectal cancer
Blood group A

PREDISPOSING CONDITIONS

Chronic gastritis, especially atrophic gastritis with or without intestinal metaplasia
Pernicious anemia
Intestinal metaplasia
Gastric adenomatous polyps (>2 cm)
Postgastrectomy stumps
Gastric epithelial dysplasia
Ménétrier's disease (hypertrophic gastropathy)
Chronic peptic ulcer

---

uncommon in Japan and that has a relatively favorable prognosis, consists of superficial lesions with or without lymph node involvement.

The leading hypothesis explaining the way in which *H. pylori* predisposes to gastric cancer risk is the induction of an inflammatory response, in which interleukin-1β may be pivotal. Chronic *H. pylori* infection also leads to chronic atrophic gastritis with resulting achlorhydria, which, in turn, favors bacterial growth that can convert nitrates (dietary components) to nitrites. These nitrites, in combination with genetic factors, promote abnormal cellular proliferation, genetic mutations, and eventually cancer. In a mouse model of gastric cancer, *H. pylori* infection may play a role in the recruitment of bone marrow–derived stem cells that facilitate gastric carcinogenesis. Animal models now recapitulate the cardinal features of gastric adenocarcinoma, either through the use of carcinogens or through genetic approaches.

GENETICS

It is clear that genetic factors play a role in gastric cancer. For example, blood group A is associated with a higher incidence rate of gastric cancer, even in nonendemic areas. A three-fold increase in gastric cancer has been reported among first-degree relatives of patients with the disease. Furthermore, albeit rare, germline or inherited mutations in the *E-cadherin* gene have been described in diffuse hereditary gastric cancer, which is seen in young patients. In addition, in hereditary nonpolyposis colorectal cancer type II (Chapter 199), patients have associated extracolonic cancers, including gastric cancer.

It now appears that several genetic mechanisms are important in gastric cancer: oncogene activation, tumor suppressor gene inactivation, and DNA microsatellite instability. For example, loss of heterozygosity of the *APC* (adenomatous polyposis coli) gene has been observed in gastric cancers. The p53 tumor suppressor gene product regulates the cell cycle at the G_1-S phase transition and probably also functions in DNA repair and apoptosis (programmed cell death). The *p53* gene is mutated not only in gastric cancer but also in gastric precancerous lesions, a finding suggesting that mutation of the *p53* gene is an early event in gastric carcinogenesis. Microsatellite DNA alterations or instability in dinucleotide repeats that were originally identified in hereditary nonpolyposis colorectal cancer also occur frequently in sporadic gastric carcinoma. Mutations in genes may accumulate as a result of DNA microsatellite instability.

CLINICAL MANIFESTATIONS

Symptoms and Signs

In its early stages, gastric cancer may often be asymptomatic or may produce only nonspecific symptoms that make early diagnosis difficult. Later symptoms include bloating, dysphagia, epigastric pain, or early satiety. Early satiety or vomiting may suggest partial gastric outlet obstruction, although gastric dysmotility may contribute to the vomiting in patients with nonobstructive cases. Epigastric pain, reminiscent of that associated with peptic ulcer (Chapter 141), occurs in about one fourth of patients, but in most patients with gastric cancer, the pain is not relieved by food or antacids. Pain that radiates to the back may indicate that the tumor has penetrated the pancreas.

When dysphagia is associated with gastric cancer, this symptom suggests a more proximal gastric tumor at the GE junction or in the fundus.

Signs of gastric cancer include bleeding, which can result in anemia that produces the symptoms of weakness, fatigue, and malaise, as well as more serious cardiovascular and cerebral consequences. Perforation related to gastric cancer is unusual. Gastric cancer metastatic to the liver can lead to right upper quadrant pain, jaundice, and fever. Lung metastases can cause cough, hiccups, and hemoptysis. Peritoneal carcinomatosis can lead to malignant ascites unresponsive to diuretics. Gastric cancer can also metastasize to bone.

Physical Examination

In the earliest stages of gastric cancer, the physical examination may be unremarkable. At later stages, patients become cachectic, and an epigastric mass may be palpated. If the tumor has metastasized to the liver, hepatomegaly with jaundice and ascites may be present. Portal or splenic vein invasion can cause splenomegaly. Lymph node involvement in the left supraclavicular area is termed *Virchow's node,* and periumbilical nodal involvement is called *Sister Mary Joseph's node.* The fecal occult blood test may be positive. Metastasis to the ovary is termed *Krukenberg's tumor.*

Paraneoplastic syndromes may precede or occur concurrently with gastric cancer. Examples include the following: Trousseau's syndrome (Chapter 187), which is recurrent migratory superficial thrombophlebitis indicating a possible hypercoagulable state (Chapter 179); acanthosis nigricans (see Fig. 187-1 in Chapter 187), which arises as raised and hyperpigmented skin lesions of flexor areas, neck, axilla, groin, and mucosal membranes; neuromyopathy with involvement of the sensory and motor pathways; and central nervous system syndromes with altered mental status and ataxia (Chapter 187).

Laboratory Studies

Laboratory studies may reveal iron deficiency anemia. Microangiopathic hemolytic anemia has been reported. Abnormalities in liver tests generally indicate metastatic disease. Hypoalbuminemia is a marker of malnutrition. Protein-losing enteropathy is rare but can be seen in Ménétrier's disease, another predisposing condition. Serologic test results, such as those for CEA and CA 72.4, may be abnormal. Although these tests are not recommended for initial diagnosis, they may be useful for monitoring disease after surgical resection.

DIAGNOSIS

The diagnostic accuracy of upper endoscopy with biopsy and cytologic examination approaches 95 to 99% for both types of gastric cancer. Cancer may arise as a small mucosal ulceration, a polyp, or a mass (Fig. 198-1). In some patients, gastric ulceration may first be noted in an upper gastrointestinal barium contrast study. A benign gastric ulcer is suggested by a smooth, regular base, whereas a malignant ulcer is manifested by a surrounding mass, irregular folds, and an irregular base. Although these and other radiographic characteristics historically helped to predict benign versus malignant disease, upper gastrointestinal endoscopy with biopsy and cytologic examination is mandatory whenever a gastric ulcer is found in the radiologic study, even if the ulcer has benign characteristics.

Staging of gastric cancer and, at times, diagnosis have been greatly enhanced by the advent of endoscopic ultrasonography (EUS) (Table 198-4). The extent of tumor, including gastric wall invasion and local lymph node involvement, can be assessed by EUS (Fig. 198-2), which provides information complementary to that obtained from CT scans. EUS can help guide aspiration biopsies of lymph nodes to determine their malignant features, if any.

CT of the chest, abdomen, and pelvis should be performed to document lymphadenopathy and extragastric organ (especially lung and liver) involvement. In some centers, staging of gastric cancer entails bone scans because of the proclivity of gastric cancer to metastasize to bone.

TREATMENT   Rx

Surgical Therapy

The only chance for cure of gastric cancer remains surgical resection, which is possible in only 25 to 30% of cases. If the tumor is confined to the distal stomach, subtotal gastrectomy is performed with resection of lymph nodes in the porta hepatis and in the pancreatic head. By contrast, tumors of the proximal stomach merit total gastrectomy to obtain an adequate margin and to remove lymph nodes; distal pancreatectomy and splenectomy are usually also performed as part of this procedure, which carries with it higher mortality and morbidity rates. The addition of para-aorta nodal dissection does not improve survival. Even if a curative procedure is not possible because of metastasis, limited gastric resection may be necessary for patients with excessive bleeding or obstruction. If cancer recurs in the gastric remnant, limited resection may again be necessary for palliation. Most recurrences in both types of gastric cancer are in the local or regional area of the original tumor.

Medical Therapy

Gastric cancer is one of the few gastrointestinal cancers that is somewhat responsive to chemotherapy.**2** In patients with gastric cancer who undergo gastrectomy and extended lymph node dissection with curative intent, S-1 (an oral fluoropyrimidine, 80 mg daily for 4 weeks followed by 2 weeks off, repeated in 6-week cycles for 1 year starting within 6 weeks after surgery) significantly improves 3-year survival from 70% to 80%.**3** Chemotherapy with the combination of epirubicin, cisplatin, and fluorouracil, given both

TABLE 198-4   TNM STAGING OF STOMACH CANCER

PRIMARY TUMOR (T)

TX	Primary tumor cannot be assessed
T0	No evidence of primary tumor
Tis	Carcinoma in situ: intraepithelial tumor without invasion of the lamina propria
T1	Tumor invades lamina propria, muscularis mucosa, or submucosa
T1a	Tumor invades lamina propria or muscularis mucosa
T1b	Tumor invades submucosa
T2	Tumor invades muscularis propria*
T3	Tumor penetrates subserosal connective tissue without invasion of visceral peritoneum or adjacent structures†,‡
T4	Tumor invades serosa (visceral peritoneum) or adjacent structures†,‡
T4a	Tumor invades serosa (visceral peritoneum)
T4b	Tumor invades adjacent structures

REGIONAL LYMPH NODES (N)

NX	Regional lymph nodes(s) cannot be assessed
N0	No regional lymph nodes metastasis§
N1	Metastasis in 1 to 2 regional lymph nodes
N2	Metastasis in 3 to 6 regional lymph nodes
N3	Metastasis in 7 or more regional lymph nodes
N3a	Metastasis in 7 to 15 regional lymph nodes
N3b	Metastasis in 16 or more regional lymph nodes

DISTANT METASTASIS (M)

M0	No distant metastasis
M1	Distant metastasis

*Note: A tumor may penetrate the muscularis propria with extension into the gastrocolic or gastrohepatic ligaments, or into the greater or lesser omentum, without perforation of the visceral peritoneum covering these structures. In this case, the tumor is classified T3. If there is perforation of the visceral peritoneum covering the gastric ligaments or the omentum, the tumor should be classified T4.
†The adjacent structures of the stomach include the spleen, transverse colon, liver, diaphragm, pancreas, abdominal wall, adrenal gland, kidney, small intestine, and retroperitoneum.
‡Intramural extension to the duodenum or esophagus is classified by the depth of the greatest invasion in any of these sites, including the stomach.
§Note: A designation of pN0 should be used if all examined lymph nodes are negative, regardless of the total number removed and examined.
From *AJCC Cancer Staging Manual,* 7th ed. New York: Springer-Verlag, 2010.

FIGURE 198-1. Benign *(left)* and malignant *(right)* gastric ulcer. Note the shaggy, thickened, and overhanging edges of the cancer. (Courtesy of Pankaj Jay Pasricha, MD.)

FIGURE 198-2. Gastric mass. Endoscopic ultrasonography depicting a large gastric mass that is compressing the liver and gallbladder wall (**A**) and, on a different view, the left lobe of the liver (**B**).

preoperatively and postoperatively, significantly improves 5-year survival from 23% to 36% in patients with resectable gastroesophageal cancer.**4** Similarly, the combination of chemotherapy (fluorouracil and leucovorin) with radiation therapy has been shown to improve median survival from 27 months to 36 months compared with surgery alone in patients with adenocarcinoma of the stomach or gastroesophageal junction.**5**

Single-agent chemotherapy treatment, which provides partial response rates of 20 to 30%, is reserved for patients with a poor performance status. Combination regimens that can yield partial response rates of 35 to 50% include the following: ECF, which is most popular in Europe (epirubicin, 50 mg/m^2 on day 1; cisplatin, 60 mg/m^2 on day 1; 5-fluorouracil, 200 mg/m^2/day as a continuous infusion through a central venous access device [CVAD] given throughout treatment, repeated every 21 days for a maximum of eight cycles); CF (5-fluorouracil infusion, 1000 mg/m^2/day for 4 days; cisplatin, 75 to 100 mg/m^2 on day 1, every 4 weeks); or TCF (docetaxel [Taxotere], 75 mg/m^2 on day 1; cisplatin, 75 mg/m^2 on day 1; and 5-fluorouracil, 750 mg/m^2/day for 5 days, every 3 weeks), or capecitabine plus cisplatin. A randomized trial of triple chemotherapy for advanced esophagogastric cancer showed that oral capecitabine is at least as effective as infused fluorouracil and that oxaliplatin (which does not require hydration) is at least as effective as cisplatin (which does require hydration) with respect to overall survival.**6** Trastuzumab (8 mg/kg intravenously once, then 6 mg/kg every 3 weeks) can increase survival of HER2-positive advanced gastric or gastro-esophageal junction cancer from 11.1 months to 13.8 months.**7** Radiation therapy alone is ineffective and is generally employed only for palliative purposes in the setting of bleeding, obstruction, or pain. Gene therapy and immune-based therapy are currently only investigational in animal models.

General Methods

Implicit in the management of the patient with gastric cancer is meticulous attention to nutrition (jejunal enteral feedings or total parenteral nutrition), correction of metabolic abnormalities that arise from vomiting or diarrhea, and treatment of infection from aspiration or spontaneous bacterial peritonitis. *H. pylori* eradication treatment reduces the risk for metachronous gastric carcinoma by about two thirds.**8** To maintain lumen patency, endoscopic laser treatment or prosthesis placement can be used in a palliative fashion.

PROGNOSIS

Approximately one third of patients who undergo a curative resection are alive after 5 years. In aggregate, the overall 5-year survival rate in patients with gastric cancer is less than 10%. Prognostic factors include anatomic location and nodal status. Distal gastric cancers without lymph node involvement have a better prognosis than proximal gastric cancers with or without lymph node involvement. Other prognostic factors include depth of penetration and tumor cell DNA aneuploidy. Linitis plastica and infiltrating lesions have a much worse prognosis than polypoid disease or exophytic masses. In the subset of mostly Japanese patients with early gastric cancer that is confined to the mucosa and submucosa, surgical resection may be curative and

definitely improves the 5-year survival rate to more than 50%. In fact, when early gastric cancer is confined to the mucosa, endoscopic mucosal resection may be an alternative.

Lymphoma of the Stomach

EPIDEMIOLOGY

Gastric lymphoma represents about 5% of all malignant gastric tumors and is increasing in incidence. Most gastric lymphomas are non-Hodgkin's lymphomas (Chapter 191), and the stomach is the most common extranodal site for non-Hodgkin's lymphomas. Patients with gastric lymphoma are generally younger than those with gastric adenocarcinoma, but the male predominance remains.

CLINICAL MANIFESTATIONS

Patients commonly present with symptoms and signs similar to those of gastric adenocarcinoma. Lymphoma in the stomach can be a primary tumor, or it can be secondary to disseminated lymphoma.

B-cell lymphomas (Chapter 191) of the stomach are most commonly large cell with a high-grade type. Low-grade variants are noted in the setting of chronic gastritis and are termed *mucosa-associated lymphoid tissue* (MALT) lymphomas. MALT lesions are strongly associated with *H. pylori* infection.

DIAGNOSIS

Radiographically, gastric lymphomas usually arise as ulcers or exophytic masses; diffusely infiltrating lymphoma is more suggestive of secondary lymphoma. Thus, upper gastrointestinal barium studies usually show multiple nodules and ulcers for a primary gastric lymphoma and typically have the appearance of linitis plastica with secondary lymphoma. As with gastric adenocarcinoma, however, upper endoscopy with biopsy and cytologic examination are required for diagnosis and have an accuracy of nearly 90%. Apart from conventional histopathologic analysis, immunoperoxidase staining for lymphocyte markers is helpful in diagnosis. As with gastric adenocarcinoma, proper staging of gastric lymphoma involves EUS, chest and abdominal/pelvic CT scans, and bone marrow biopsy as needed.

TREATMENT ℞

Treatment of gastric diffuse large B-cell lymphoma is best pursued with combination chemotherapy with or without radiation therapy (Chapter 191). For MALT lesions, eradication of *H. pylori* infection with antibiotics should be attempted (Chapter 141), but patients with refractory lesions that are confined to the stomach can sometimes be cured with radiotherapy (Chapter 191).

Other Malignant Tumors of the Stomach

Leiomyosarcoma, which constitutes approximately 1% of all gastric cancers, usually occurs as an intramural mass with central ulceration. Symptoms may include bleeding accompanied by a palpable mass. Leiomyosarcomas are often relatively indolent; surgical resection yields a 5-year survival rate of about 50%. Metastasis can occur to lymph nodes and the liver. Other gastric sarcomas include liposarcomas, fibrosarcomas, myosarcomas, and neurogenic sarcomas.

Most gastrointestinal stromal tumors (GISTs) have been associated with activating mutations in the C-*kit* gene; a subset of such tumors are associated with mutations in the platelet-derived growth factor receptor (*PDGFR*) gene. C-*kit* mutations are also found in chronic and acute myelogenous leukemia (Chapters 189 and 190), and approximately 50% of GISTs respond to imatinib mesylate, which is also used in chronic myelogenous leukemia. If imatinib is not successful, sunitinib increases survival.[9] Carcinoid tumors (Chapter 240) may begin in the stomach and are curable by removal if they have not yet spread to the liver.

Primary tumors can also spread to the stomach. In addition to lymphomas, other tumors found in the stomach include primary lung (Chapter 197) and breast (Chapter 204) cancers as well as malignant melanoma (Chapter 210).

LEIOMYOMAS AND BENIGN TUMORS

Leiomyomas, which are smooth muscle tumors of benign origin, occur with equal frequency in men and women and are typically located in the middle and distal stomach. Leiomyomas can grow into the lumen, with secondary ulceration and consequent bleeding. Alternatively, they can expand to the serosa with extrinsic compression. Endoscopy may reveal a mass that has overlying mucosa or mucosa replaced by ulceration. On upper gastrointestinal series, leiomyomas are usually smooth with an intramural filling defect, with or without central ulceration. However, benign leiomyomas can be difficult to distinguish from their malignant counterparts radiographically or endoscopically; tissue diagnosis is imperative. Symptomatic leiomyomas should be removed, but those without associated symptoms do not require therapy.

Other benign gastric tumors include lipoma, neurofibroma, lymphangioma, ganglioneuroma, and hamartoma, the last associated with Peutz-Jeghers syndrome (Chapter 199) or juvenile polyposis (restricted to the stomach).

ADENOMAS

Gastric adenomas and hyperplastic polyps are unusual but may be found in middle-aged and elderly patients. Polyps may be sessile or pedunculated and are also found in nearly 50% of patients with familial adenomatosis polyposis (Chapter 199). Gastric adenocarcinoma arising in the antrum has been described in such patients. Although isolated gastric adenomatous polyps are generally asymptomatic, some patients may have dyspepsia, nausea, or bleeding. Gastric adenomas and hyperplastic polyps are smooth and regular on upper gastrointestinal series, but the diagnosis must be confirmed by upper endoscopy with biopsy. Pedunculated polyps that are larger than 2 cm or that have associated symptoms should be removed by endoscopic snare cautery polypectomy, whereas large sessile gastric adenomatous polyps may merit segmental surgical resection. If polyps progress to an intermediary stage of severe dysplasia or culminate in cancer, treatment is the same as for gastric adenocarcinoma.

1. Shaheen NJ, Sharma P, Overholt BF, et al. Radiofrequency ablation in Barrett's esophagus with dysplasia. *N Engl J Med.* 2009;360:2277-2288.
2. GASTRIC (Global Advanced/Adjuvant Stomach Tumor Reasearch International Collaboration) Group. Benefit of adjuvant chemotherapy for resectable gastric cancer: a meta-analysis. *JAMA.* 2010;303:1729-1737.
3. Sakuramoto S, Sasako M, Yamaguchi T, et al. Adjuvant chemotherapy for gastric cancer with S-1, an oral fluoropyrimidine. *N Engl J Med.* 2007;357:1810-1820.
4. Cunningham D, Allum WH, Stenning SP, et al. Perioperative chemotherapy versus surgery alone for resectable gastro esophageal cancer. *N Engl J Med.* 2006;355:11-20.
5. Macdonald JS, Smalley SR, Benedetti J, et al. Chemoradiotherapy after surgery compared with surgery alone for adenocarcinoma of the stomach or gastroesophageal junction. *N Engl J Med.* 2001;345:725-730.
6. Cunningham D, Starling N, Rao S, et al. Capecitabine and oxaliplatin for advanced esophagogastric cancer. *N Engl J Med.* 2008;358:36-46.
7. Bang YJ, Van Cutsem E, Feyereislova A, et al. Trastuzumab in combination with chemotherapy versus chemotherapy alone for treatment of HER2-positive advanced gastric or gastro-oesophageal junction cancer (ToGA): a phase 3, open-label, randomised controlled trial. *Lancet.* 2010;376:687-697.
8. Fukase K, Kato M, Kikuchi S, et al. Effect of eradication of *Helicobacter pylori* on incidence of metachronous gastric carcinoma after endoscopic resection of early gastric cancer: an open-label, randomised controlled trial. *Lancet.* 2008;372:392-397.
9. Demetri GD, Oosterom AT, Garrett CR, et al. Efficacy and safety of sunitinib in patients with advanced gastrointestinal stromal tumour after failure of imatinib: a randomised controlled trial. *Lancet.* 2006;368:1329-1338.

SUGGESTED READINGS

Ng T, Vezeridis MP. Advances in the surgical treatment of esophageal cancer. *J Surg Oncol.* 2010;101:725-729. *Review of technical improvements in surgical resection of esophageal cancer.*

Paoletti X, Oba K, Burzykowski T, et al, for the GASTRIC (Global Advanced/Adjuvant Stomach Tumor Research International Collaboration) Group. Benefit of adjuvant chemotherapy for resectable gastric cancer: a meta-analysis. *JAMA.* 2010;303:1729-1737. *Meta-analysis showing superiority of fluorouracil-based adjuvant chemotherapy compared with surgery alone in reducing mortality.*

Polk DB, Peek RM Jr. *Helicobacter pylori*: gastric cancer and beyond. *Nat Rev Cancer.* 2010;10:403-414. *Review of mechanisms that regulate the biological interactions of* H. pylori *with its hosts and that promote carcinogenesis.*

Spechler SJ, Fitzgerald RC, Prasad GA, et al. History, molecular mechanisms, and endoscopic treatment of Barrett's esophagus. *Gastroenterology.* 2010;138:854-869. *An excellent review of the diagnosis and management of Barrett's esophagus.*

Wang J, Yu JC, Kang WM, et al. Treatment strategy for early gastric cancer. *Surg Oncol.* 2011. [Epub ahead of print.] *Review.*

199

NEOPLASMS OF THE SMALL AND LARGE INTESTINE

CHARLES D. BLANKE AND DOUGLAS O. FAIGEL

NEOPLASMS OF THE SMALL INTESTINE

EPIDEMIOLOGY

The small intestine accounts for the majority of the length ($\approx$75%) and surface ($\approx$90%) of the gastrointestinal (GI) tract. Nonetheless, it is a rare site for the development of neoplastic disease, as only 1 to 2% of primary GI tumors originate in the duodenum, jejunum, or ileum. In fact, half of all small bowel neoplasms represent metastatic disease from other sites, particularly elsewhere in the GI tract. Small bowel malignancies constitute less than 0.5% of all cancers, although the incidence of small bowel tumors (especially carcinoids) seems to be increasing. Overall, the mean age at diagnosis of a small bowel tumor is about 67 years; neoplasms are more common in males, and they occur more commonly in African Americans than in whites.

PATHOBIOLOGY

Adenocarcinomas, arising from mucosal glands, were formerly the most frequent primary small bowel tumor. They now constitute 25% of small bowel neoplasms, including benign growths, and 40% of all malignant tumors. Adenocarcinomas most commonly arise in the duodenum (65% of all small intestinal adenocarcinomas), even though the duodenum represents only a tiny fraction of the length of the small bowel. They occur less commonly in the jejunum and least commonly in the ileum. The majority are well or moderately differentiated.

Small bowel carcinoids, which derive from enterochromaffin cells in the crypts of Lieberkühn, are now the most common small bowel tumors, accounting for approximately 30 to 40% of malignancies. They tend to be quite well differentiated. In contrast to glandular tumors, small intestinal carcinoids tend to arise in the distal ileum, and up to 30% are multifocal. Other small bowel neuroendocrine tumors are occasionally seen, including biochemically active neoplasms such as gastrinomas and somatostatinomas. Very rarely, high-grade true small cell carcinomas occur.

Malignant connective tissue tumors account for 10% of small bowel neoplasms. Gastrointestinal stromal tumors (GISTs), which derive from the interstitial cells of Cajal or a common precursor, account for approximately 85% of these neoplasms (Fig. 199-1). GISTs, like adenocarcinomas, disproportionately arise in the duodenum, and the small bowel itself is the second most common primary site for these mesenchymal neoplasms (33% derive from small bowel). Morphologically, GISTs often resemble leiomyosarcomas

FIGURE 199-1. Small bowel gastrointestinal stromal tumor with ulceration.

FIGURE 199-2. Histopathology of gastrointestinal stromal tumor.

FIGURE 199-3. Histopathology of small bowel non-Hodgkin's lymphoma. (Courtesy Dr. M. K. Washington.)

(Fig. 199-2), but they can be differentiated by the expression of the Kit protein (CD117). Other small bowel sarcomas such as true leiomyosarcomas are seen more rarely (Chapter 209).

Primary GI lymphomas are the most common extranodal lymphomatous variation, and the small intestine is the second most common GI site for such tumors (Chapter 191). The ileum, rich in submucosal lymphoid follicles, is the most common small bowel site. Tumors may be low or higher grade and can arise from precursor B or T lymphocytes. The overwhelming majority are non-Hodgkin's tumors (Fig. 199-3). Lymphomas involving the small bowel may also be a manifestation of true systemic disease.

Malignant melanoma (Chapter 210) can develop as a primary mucosal small bowel tumor, probably arising from schwannian neuroblasts associated with GI innervation. In addition, the small bowel is the most common GI site for melanoma metastases.

Finally, a variety of common benign tumors may originate in the small bowel, including adenomas, leiomyomas, and lipomas. Desmoids, most often seen in patients with familial adenomatous polyposis (FAP); hamartomas; and hemangiomas are relatively rare. Benign growths are more common in the distal small intestine.

The small intestine can be involved by advanced cancers from other sites through direct invasion, extension of peritoneal metastases, or hematogenous spread. As noted, the small bowel is the most common GI site for melanoma metastases; in addition, involvement is fairly common with ovarian, breast, lung, and other GI neoplasms.

Predisposing Conditions
Inflammatory bowel disease (Chapter 143) predisposes to adenocarcinoma. Additionally, many of the polyposis syndromes are associated with small bowel neoplasms. Most notably, FAP (see later) is associated with adenomas and carcinomas of the duodenum and jejunum, but especially in the ampullary and periampullary region. At least 90% of FAP patients develop duodenal adenomas, and up to 10% develop cancer. The risk of cancer is related to the number of polyps, their size and histologic type, and the presence of high-grade dysplasia. Patients with FAP should undergo regular screening for duodenal neoplasia with both forward- and side-viewing endoscopes beginning around the time of colectomy and repeated at 1- to 5-year intervals, depending on the presence and degree of duodenal polyposis. Patients with MUTYH polyposis likewise develop duodenal neoplasia and should undergo screening. Patients with hereditary nonpolyposis colon cancer (HNPCC) are also at increased risk for small intestine adenocarcinoma, which may be the first manifestation of their disease. HNPCC-associated small bowel cancer may present at a young age (median, 39 years) and occurs with decreasing frequency from the duodenum to the ileum, with about 50% of occurrences in the duodenum. Screening may be considered beginning at age 30. Patients with sprue are at an increased risk for small bowel lymphomas.

CLINICAL MANIFESTATIONS
The most common presenting symptom of small bowel tumors is abdominal pain, especially for those that are true cancers. Less common are symptoms such as weight loss, nausea, GI bleeding, and symptoms related to perforation. Approximately 25% of patients have GI obstruction, and duodenal periampullary tumors can lead to obstructive jaundice. Only a minority of malignancies are asymptomatic, whereas benign tumors may cause no symptoms in up to half of patients. Carcinoid tumors in the small bowel are often asymptomatic, although in the setting of advanced disease they may secrete bioactive amines, leading to flushing, diarrhea, wheezing, and eventually symptoms of right heart failure (related to valvular fibrosis) (Chapter 240). This is more common with tumors originating in the jejunum and ileum. Benign tumors tend to be found incidentally, although intraluminal growth may eventually cause symptoms of obstruction, and some may grow large enough to ulcerate and bleed.

DIAGNOSIS
The physical examination in patients with small bowel tumors is often unremarkable, although there is occasionally a palpable mass and, in more advanced cases, ascites. As discussed earlier, patients with periampullary neoplasms may be jaundiced and/or icteric. Obstructive signs such as hyperperistalsis may be present, and those with lymphoma may also have splenomegaly or other signs of systemic involvement, such as lymphadenopathy. Laboratory findings may include iron deficiency anemia or increased hepatic enzymes (the latter is especially common in those with liver metastases or biliary obstruction). Serum levels of the carcinoembryonic antigen (CEA) tumor marker may be elevated in small bowel adenocarcinoma, especially in advanced cases, but it is neither sensitive nor specific enough for routine diagnostic use. Patients with neuroendocrine tumors may demonstrate elevated levels of serotonin, chromogranin A, tumor-specific bioactive amines (e.g., gastrin), or urinary 5-hydroxyindoleacetic acid. Variants of intestinal lymphomas may show heavy chain immunoglobulin A fragments in serum and urine.

Proper imaging is crucial for both diagnosis and staging of small bowel neoplasms, but no one method is clearly the best. Standard radiographic techniques of value include upper GI with small bowel follow-through (helpful in demonstrating both masses and potential mucosal defects), angiography (which may show a site of bleeding or tumor blush with specific neoplasms), and computed tomography (CT) or magnetic resonance imaging (MRI) enteroclysis (double-contrast studies are both sensitive and specific for small bowel masses). Transabdominal ultrasound and standard CT may indicate a primary mass as well as metastases; MRI appears to be superior to CT in detecting and characterizing liver metastases.

Primary neuroendocrine tumors and their metastases are often apparent on indium-111 octreotide scanning. A wide variety of histologies may have uptake on positron emission tomography (PET) scanning. However, PET does not yet have a well-defined role in the diagnosis of most small bowel malignancies, although PET scans are useful in those with GISTs to monitor response to systemic therapy (see later). Plain films rarely help make the diagnosis, but they may demonstrate intestinal obstruction.

Capsule endoscopy uses a wireless endoscopic device that allows minimally invasive imaging of the small intestine. The system consists of the capsule camera—a swallowable, self-contained battery-operated device that transmits two images per second—a receiver worn on the patient's belt, and a computerized work station for downloading and viewing the images. The primary indications for capsule endoscopy are the evaluation of obscure GI bleeding and Crohn's disease. Tumors are found in about 2 to 3% of patients undergoing capsule endoscopy for obscure GI bleeding, and they may be more common in younger patients. Tumors detected include lymphoma, adenocarcinoma, metastatic disease, carcinoid tumor, and GIST. Capsule endoscopy has also been used to assess the small intestines of patients with FAP and Peutz-Jeghers syndrome (PJS), although its clinical utility for the routine screening of these patients has not been established.

Surveillance

Patients with FAP, MUTYH polyposis, PJS, and probably HNPCC require regular surveillance of the small intestine, with specific recommendations as noted earlier. Patients with sporadic small intestine adenomas and possibly carcinoid tumors should undergo colonoscopy, because they are at increased risk for colonic neoplasia. No specific guidelines exist for following patients with resected small bowel adenocarcinomas.

Staging

The staging systems for small bowel tumors vary by histology. Adenocarcinomas and, more recently, neuroendocrine cancers and GISTs are staged using the American Joint Committee on Cancer's TNM classification of malignant tumors system. Intestinal non-Hodgkin's lymphomas, whether primary or part of a systemic process, are staged in accordance with a modified Ann Arbor system originally used in Hodgkin's disease (Chapter 191).

TREATMENT Rx

In general, surgical excision is the treatment of choice for most localized small bowel tumors. The extent of excision necessary depends on the tumor's location and histology. Adenocarcinomas involving the first and second portions of the duodenum require pancreaticoduodenectomy, whereas those in the more distal small intestine may be treated with segmental or wide local resection, including regional lymph nodes. Low-grade neuroendocrine tumors should be managed with en bloc resection, again including regional nodes. GISTs, which very rarely spread to regional nodes, may be treated with excision without lymphadenectomy (except in cases with gross involvement of nodes). Primary surgery for lymphomas may be offered for low-stage malignancies and may also be required for complications of disease (e.g., intussusception). Local management of benign small bowel tumors varies from observation (incidentally discovered lipomas) to endoscopic polypectomy (small adenomas) to pancreaticoduodenectomy (periampullary villous adenomas).

The need for and types of adjuvant therapy vary as well. Fully resected benign tumors require no additional therapy. Adenocarcinomas are often treated according to the principles developed for colorectal cancer, with some experts advocating fluoropyrimidine-based systemic chemotherapy, at least for patients with nodal involvement. Chemoradiotherapy has also been recommended for those with more locally advanced duodenal adenocarcinomas. So far, no randomized trials have proved either strategy to be superior to surgery alone. Fully excised well- to moderately differentiated neuroendocrine cancers do not require adjuvant therapy. Postoperative imatinib mesylate treatment (see later) clearly postpones the recurrence of intermediate- and high-risk GISTs, but it is not yet known whether the cure rate is improved, and questions remain with regard to dose and duration of therapy. There is no defined role for the postoperative treatment of other mesenchymal tumors. Lymphomas treated with excision alone have high rates of recurrence, and systemic chemotherapy is advocated for high-grade variants; some experts also recommend chemotherapy for low-grade subtypes.

Patients with advanced small bowel adenocarcinomas are often treated with systemic chemotherapy regimens known to be effective against cancers of similar histology originating in the colon. However, the data supporting any specific regimen are scant and are not derived from randomized trials. Approximately 90% of patients with incurable GISTs have durable disease control when treated with the tyrosine kinase inhibitor imatinib mesylate, and the median survival for patients with metastatic disease has recently improved from approximately 18 months to 5 years.

Patients with small bowel lymphomas may be treated with chemotherapy that is effective in tumors of nodal origin.

PROGNOSIS

Patients with small bowel adenocarcinomas generally do worse than those with similarly staged colonic glandular tumors. Also, patients with duodenal primaries may have poorer outcomes than those with more distal small bowel cancers. In general, 5-year survival rates range from 4% for those with metastases to 80% for those with very early disease confined to the small bowel wall. Five-year survival in patients with small bowel carcinoids exceeds 50%. In the pre-imatinib era, patients with surgically resected small bowel GISTs had recurrence rates from 0 to 90% or higher, depending on the tumor's size, precise location, and mitotic rates, and those with more distal tumors had a worse prognosis than those with duodenal primaries. Patients with recurrences almost invariably died within 2 years because salvage surgery and systemic chemotherapy were ineffective. True life expectancy in this era of postoperative imatinib use is unknown, but the median survival of patients with advanced GISTs likely exceeds 5 years. Small intestinal lymphomas have 5-year survival rates surpassing 60%, although this is highly variable and depends on the histologic subtype.

NEOPLASMS OF THE LARGE INTESTINE

Colorectal cancer is the third most common cancer in the United States. Disease that has spread beyond regional lymph nodes is, for the most part, incurable, and colorectal cancer in general remains the second leading cause of neoplastic death. The lifetime risk of developing colorectal cancer for the average patient is about 1 in 18 to 20.

EPIDEMIOLOGY

Almost three quarters of large bowel cancers arise proximally (i.e., are of colonic origin). Although colorectal cancer is primarily a disease of the elderly (median age, ≈73 years), about 10% of cases occur in those 50 years of age or younger. Colorectal cancer incidence and mortality have decreased overall recently, although the incidence has been increasing in the young. Incidence rates for right-sided cancers have also been decreasing, possibly but not solely owing to effective distal large bowel screening with flexible sigmoidoscopy. Colorectal cancer is slightly more common in men than in women and in African Americans than in whites. Men develop colorectal cancer an average of 5 to 10 years earlier than women; similarly, large bowel cancers seem to arise an average of 5 to 10 years earlier in African Americans than in whites. There is much geographic variation in incidence that is probably based more on environmental factors than on genetic ones, as suggested by migration studies.

PATHOBIOLOGY

Between 96 and 98% of colorectal cancers are adenocarcinomas. Rarely seen histologies include neuroendocrine cancers, epidermoid carcinomas, lymphomas, and sarcomas (including GISTs). Additionally, composites, such as adenocarcinomas with neuroendocrine differentiation, are increasingly being described.

Adenocarcinomas derive from colonic columnar glandular epithelium in the colorectal mucosal lining. They are equally common in males and females and are most frequently reported in the sigmoid colon. Adenocarcinomas most commonly present at a localized or regional (nodal) stage. About two thirds are of moderate grade. The majority are nonmucinous, although the mucinous phenotype constitutes up to one fifth of all colorectal cancers. Another variant is the true signet ring carcinoma, identified by large quantities of single tumor cells with nuclear displacement by intracytoplasmic mucin. Mucinous tumors likely have a worse prognosis (data are controversial to date), whereas a signet ring histology almost always indicates a poorly differentiated or undifferentiated tumor and is clearly associated with a worse outcome.

Neuroendocrine cancers can have a variety of histologies, ranging from bland, well-differentiated carcinoids to high-grade small cell carcinomas. True carcinoids are the second most common histologic colorectal subtype. They are more common in nonwhites and make up the vast majority of non-adenocarcinoma epithelial cancers.

Distal bowel carcinoids are hormonally inactive. Noncarcinoid neuroendocrine cancers tend to be high grade and commonly present with hepatic and other distant metastases.

Epidermoid carcinomas are rare overall but still account for up to one fourth of colorectal cancers. Most are squamous cell subtypes. They are more common in women and Hispanics. Epidermoid carcinomas are located in the rectum more than 90% of the time, and they are usually moderately or poorly

TABLE 199-1 GENERAL FEATURES OF THE INHERITED COLORECTAL CANCER SYNDROMES

SYNDROME	POLYP HISTOLOGY	POLYP DISTRIBUTION	AGE OF ONSET	RISK OF COLON CANCER	GENETIC LESION	CLINICAL MANIFESTATIONS	ASSOCIATED LESIONS
Familial adenomatous polyposis	Adenoma	Large intestine, duodenum	16 yr (range, 8-34 yr)	100%	5q (*APC* gene)	Rectal bleeding, abdominal pain, bowel obstruction	Desmoids, CHRPE
Peutz-Jeghers syndrome	Hamartoma	Large and small intestine	First decade	Slightly above average	19p (*STK11*)	Possible rectal bleeding, abdominal pain, intussusception	Orocutaneous melanin pigment spots, other tumors
MUTYH-associated polyposis	Adenoma	Large intestine, duodenum	45-50 yr (range, 13-60 yr)	75% (range, 50-100%)	1p (*MYH* gene)	Rectal bleeding, abdominal pain, bowel obstruction	CHRPE, osteomas
Juvenile polyposis	Hamartoma (rarely adenoma)	Large and small intestine	First decade	≈9%	*PTEN, SMAD4, BMPR1*	Possible rectal bleeding, abdominal pain, intussusception	Pulmonary AVMs
Hereditary nonpolyposis colon cancer	Adenoma	Large intestine	40 yr (range, 18-65 yr)	30%	Mismatch repair genes*	Rectal bleeding, abdominal pain, bowel obstruction	Other tumors (e.g., ovary, uterus, pancreas, stomach)

*Including *hMSH2, hMSH3, hMSH6, hMLH1, hPMS1,* and *hPMS2.*
AVM = arteriovenous malformation; CHRPE = congenital hypertrophy of the retinal pigment epithelium.

differentiated. Interestingly, they commonly present as localized cancers, regardless of their degree of differentiation.

Primary colorectal lymphomas are fairly rare, constituting 10 to 20% of all GI lymphomas but less than 1% of colorectal cancers. They are much more common in males and in the elderly. The cecum is the most common site of origin. Tumors are usually of B-cell origin.

Sarcomas of the large bowel have no gender or racial predilections. More than 50% have been classified as leiomyosarcomas, most commonly found in the rectum. They are usually diagnosed at a localized stage, regardless of grade, although about 40% are actually poorly differentiated. Kaposi's sarcomas and GISTs are other sarcoma histologies found in the large bowel; many of the distal tumors called *leiomyosarcomas* in older registries were likely true GISTs.

Predisposing Conditions

Predisposing conditions for colonic neoplasia include age (discussed previously), gender, race, inflammatory bowel disease, family history, and defined inherited syndromes. Defined genetic cancer syndromes, however, account for only a small percentage of colorectal cancers (see later). Patients with first-degree relatives who also have colon neoplasia (adenomas or carcinomas) are commonly seen. Individuals with a first-degree relative with colorectal cancer face a two- to three-fold increased risk for malignancy, and this risk rises to five- or six-fold if two first-degree relatives are affected. Patients whose relatives have adenomas face a 1.8-fold increased risk for colorectal cancer, and this rises to 2.6 if the relative is younger than 60 years.

Patients with ulcerative colitis and Crohn's disease (Chapter 143) are at increased risk for colorectal cancer in proportion to the amount of bowel involved and the duration of illness. For example, adenocarcinoma of the colon is 10 to 20 times more common in persons with ulcerative colitis than in the general population. Between 2 and 4% of all patients with long-term ulcerative colitis develop this malignancy, and the cumulative incidence over a 25-year period is approximately 12%. Patients with both ulcerative colitis and primary sclerosing cholangitis seem to be at even greater risk. For those with Crohn's colitis, patients with extensive disease involving more than one third of the colon are at increased risk (six- to eight-fold), similar to those with ulcerative colitis. Isolated proctitis is not a risk factor. Patients with ulcerative colitis or extensive Crohn's disease should undergo screening colonoscopy every 1 to 2 years beginning 8 to 10 years after disease onset. At colonoscopy, multiple biopsies (at least 32 for pan-colitis) are obtained, and any suspicious lesions are sampled. The purpose of this is to identify the presence of dysplasia. The presence of high-grade dysplasia, any dysplasia in a mass or lesion that cannot be excised endoscopically, or multifocal low-grade dysplasia should prompt colectomy.

Patients who have had ureterocolostomy and those with acromegaly are also at increased risk. Case-control studies suggest that obesity, low physical activity, smoking, excessive alcohol, high-fat diet, and lack of dietary fiber

FIGURE 199-4. Resected colon lined with hundreds of adenomatous polyps in a patient with familial adenomatous polyposis.

increase the colorectal cancer risk. Patients with *Streptococcus bovis* bacteremia or endocarditis have increased rates of colorectal cancer and should undergo colonoscopy.

Polyposis Syndromes

Several defined dominant and recessive genetic conditions have been identified that convey an increased risk of colorectal cancer (Table 199-1). These include FAP, HNPCC, MUTYH-associated polyposis, PJS, juvenile polyposis, PTEN hamartoma syndrome, and Cronkhite-Canada syndrome.

FAMILIAL ADENOMATOUS POLYPOSIS

FAP is an autosomal dominant condition characterized by the development of hundreds to thousands of adenomatous polyps and colorectal cancer by age 40 (Fig. 199-4). Estimates of disease prevalence are 1 in 8000 to 15,000 births.

PATHOBIOLOGY

FAP is inherited as an autosomal dominant disease with incomplete penetrance. It has been mapped to the adenomatous polyposis coli (*APC*) gene located on the long arm of chromosome 5 (5q21). *APC* is a tumor suppressor gene that is a critical regulator of intestinal epithelial cell growth. Inherited mutations generally result in a truncated gene product. Patients with the familial syndrome inherit one mutant copy of *APC*; when a loss-of-function mutation develops in the other *APC* allele, mucosal epithelial cell growth is no longer controlled normally, and polyps develop. Variable phenotypes can be partly attributed to differences in the location of the *APC* mutation, with attenuated FAP being seen in mutations at the 5′ and 3′ ends of the gene.

CLINICAL MANIFESTATIONS AND DIAGNOSIS

Adenomas begin to appear early in the second decade of life, and GI symptoms begin to appear in the third or fourth decade. Polyps are distributed relatively evenly throughout the colon, although a slight predominance has been noted in the distal colon. Almost all patients with FAP develop frank colorectal carcinoma by age 40 years if the condition is left untreated. Gastric polyps (mostly nonadenomatous) occur in 30 to 100% of patients, and duodenal adenomas are found in 45 to 90%. Periampullary duodenal cancer develops in approximately 10% of cases. Small bowel lesions that are distal to the duodenum rarely progress to malignancy. In attenuated FAP, fewer than 100 colonic adenomas develop, there is a right colon predominance, and cancer develops approximately 10 years later. Genetic testing may identify the mutation in up to 85% of affected individuals and is useful for family screening.

TREATMENT   Rx

The primary treatment option in FAP patients is total proctocolectomy with conventional ileostomy or ileoanal (pouch) anastomosis. Individuals with *APC* mutations and those with no identified mutation but clinical FAP in their families should be screened with annual sigmoidoscopy beginning at age 10 to 12 years. In families with known *APC* mutations, individuals who test negative do not require heightened surveillance but should undergo routine risk screening. FAP patients should be screened for duodenal polyposis with upper endoscopy beginning at age 20 years, with subsequent surveillance depending on polyp burden and histology.

GARDNER'S SYNDROME

Gardner's syndrome is a phenotypic subtype of FAP that is also caused by mutations in the *APC* gene. It is distinguished by the presence of extraintestinal manifestations, including osteomas (particularly mandibular), soft tissue tumors (including lipomas, sebaceous cysts, and fibrosarcomas), supernumerary teeth, desmoid tumors, mesenteric fibromatosis, and congenital hypertrophy of the retinal pigment epithelium. The phenotypic differences between Gardner's syndrome and FAP appear to result from variations in the location of the *APC* mutation, the presence of modifying genes, and environmental factors. Adenomatous polyps in Gardner's syndrome have the same malignant potential as those found in FAP, and colorectal cancer screening and treatment recommendations are the same.

TURCOT'S SYNDROME

A hallmark of Turcot's syndrome is the combination of colorectal polyposis and malignant diseases of the central nervous system. Mutations in the *APC* gene account for two thirds of cases, and the remaining one third result from mutations in the DNA mismatch repair genes that are also mutated in HNPCC. Central nervous system manifestations include medulloblastomas, glioblastomas, and ependymomas.

HEREDITARY NONPOLYPOSIS COLON CANCER

HNPCC, also known as *Lynch syndrome*, is the most common hereditary colorectal cancer syndrome and accounts for approximately 2% of all cases of colorectal cancer (Chapter 184). It is an autosomal dominant trait and is highly penetrant. Clinically, HNPCC has been defined by the presence of all three of the following: (1) three or more relatives with histologically verified HNPCC-associated cancer (colorectal cancer or cancer of the endometrium, small bowel, ureter, or renal pelvis), one of whom is a first-degree relative of the other two, in the absence of FAP; (2) colorectal cancer involving at least two generations; and (3) one or more family members with cancer diagnosed before age 50 years.

PATHOBIOLOGY

HNPCC is caused by loss-of-function germline mutations in a set of genes involved in the repair of DNA base pair mismatches that occur during DNA replication (also known as the *mutation mismatch repair system*). The genetic basis of HNPCC (Lynch syndrome) is described in greater detail in Chapter 184.

CLINICAL MANIFESTATIONS AND DIAGNOSIS

The median age for diagnosis of HNPCC is the mid-40s. Although several adenomas may be present, the diffuse polyposis characteristic of FAP is not found. Colonic neoplasia has a right-sided predominance (proximal to the splenic flexure). Although the cancers tend to be poorly differentiated, they generally have a better prognosis than similar sporadic colorectal cancers. Synchronous and metachronous colorectal cancer is common. Patients with HNPCC are also at high risk for other malignant diseases, especially endometrial carcinoma, as well as cancers of the ovary, stomach, small bowel, hepatobiliary tract, ureter, and pancreas. The Muir-Torre syndrome variant is associated with cutaneous lesions and visceral malignancies. Screening for HNPCC may begin with testing of the tumor for microsatellite instability, performing immunohistochemical staining for products of mismatch repair genes (including *hMSH2, hMSH3, hMSH6, hMLH1, hPMS1,* and *hPMS2*), and/or *BRAF* gene mutation testing. A positive screen does not definitely indicate HNPCC because up to 15% of sporadic tumors may have these features; this should be followed with germline testing.

TREATMENT   Rx

Persons potentially affected with HNPCC should undergo a colonoscopy every 2 years beginning at age 21 years and annually beginning at age 40. Patients with colorectal cancer or large adenomas should undergo subtotal colectomy. Women in HNPCC-affected families should have pelvic examinations every 1 to 3 years beginning at age 18 years; annual pelvic examinations, transvaginal ultrasonography, and endometrial biopsy have been recommended beginning at age 25 years. Prophylactic total abdominal hysterectomy with bilateral salpingo-oophorectomy may also be considered at the time of colectomy.

MUTYH-ASSOCIATED POLYPOSIS

MUTYH-associated polyposis is a recently described autosomal recessive syndrome caused by mutations in the *MYH* gene. It is characterized by colonic polyposis and a high rate of colorectal cancer. In a Finnish colon cancer registry, 0.4% of patients were homozygous for *MYH* mutations.

PATHOBIOLOGY

MUTYH-associated polyposis is caused by a biallelic inherited defect in the *MYH* gene located on chromosome 1p. Inherited as an autosomal recessive trait, this leads to defects in base excision repair and acquired mutations of the *APC* gene and other genes, such as *KRAS*. This results in adenoma formation and the subsequent development of adenocarcinoma.

CLINICAL MANIFESTATIONS AND DIAGNOSIS

Phenotypically, affected patients are similar to those with attenuated FAP. Patients have five to hundreds of adenomas. The onset is later than in classic FAP, with cancers more likely to be right sided and to occur at age 45 to 50 years. Associated extracolonic features include gastroduodenal polyps, duodenal carcinoma, breast and ovarian cancer in female carriers, bladder cancer, skin cancer, congenital hypertrophy of the retinal pigment epithelium, and osteoma. Monoallelic carriers do not appear to have an increased cancer risk.

The diagnosis is suggested by the presence of colonic polyposis in the absence of FAP, or when there appears to be recessive inheritance. In these cases, genetic testing for *MYH* gene mutations should be considered. Whether heterozygote carriers are at increased risk has not been established, but screening similar to that for individuals with first-degree relatives with colorectal cancer may be advisable (i.e., colonoscopy at age 40 and then every 5 years).

TREATMENT   Rx

Patients with numerous polyps should undergo colectomy. Patients with mild disease and a relatively small number of polyps may be considered for colonoscopy with polypectomy and regular surveillance. Colonoscopy should be performed beginning at age 18 to 20 and repeated every 1 to 2 years. Regular endoscopic surveillance for duodenal polyps should also be performed beginning at age 25 to 30.

PEUTZ-JEGHERS SYNDROME

PJS is an intestinal hamartomatous polyposis of the upper and lower GI tract that is associated with characteristic mucocutaneous pigmentation. The

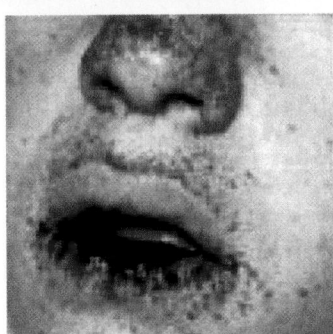

FIGURE 199-5. Mucosal pigmentation in a patient with Peutz-Jeghers syndrome.

average age at diagnosis is in the mid-20s. PHS predisposes to both intestinal and extraintestinal malignancies.

PATHOBIOLOGY

PJS is a rare autosomal dominant syndrome with high penetrance. The prevalence is between 1 in 8300 and 1 in 29,000. The gene responsible for the syndrome is the serine-threonine kinase (*STK11*) gene located on chromosome 19p; a mutation in *STK11* is found in approximately 60% of patients with this syndrome. The hamartomatous polyps in PJS are located predominantly in the small intestine (64 to 96%), stomach (24 to 49%), and colon (60%). Histologically, these polyps are benign; they are unique, in that a layer of muscle that extends into the submucosa or muscularis propria may surround the glandular tissue. Adenomatous and hyperplastic polyps may also be found.

CLINICAL MANIFESTATIONS AND DIAGNOSIS

The most common symptoms are small bowel intussusception, obstruction, and GI bleeding that may require surgery and may be recurrent. PJS is associated with an increased risk of cancer, with an estimated 47% of patients developing a malignancy by age 65. The most common cancers are those of the small intestine, stomach, colon, pancreas, testes, breast, ovary, cervix, and uterus. More than 95% of patients have a characteristic pattern of melanin spots on the lips, buccal mucosa, and skin (Fig. 199-5). Because genetic testing is not widely available, first-degree relatives should be screened beginning at birth with an annual history, physical examination, and evaluation for melanotic spots, precocious puberty, and testicular tumors.

> **TREATMENT**   **Rx**
>
> Standard medical care for patients with PJS involves an annual physical examination that includes evaluation of the breasts, abdomen, pelvis, and testes, as well as a complete blood count. Surveillance for cancer includes small bowel radiography every 2 years, esophagogastroduodenoscopy and colonoscopy every 2 years, and endoscopic ultrasound of the pancreas every 1 to 2 years. For women, annual Pap smear, transvaginal ultrasound, CA125, and mammography are recommended. Polyps larger than 1 cm should be removed endoscopically. Laparotomy and resection are recommended for recurrent or persistent small intestinal intussusception, obstruction, or intestinal bleeding.

JUVENILE POLYPOSIS

Familial juvenile (non-neoplastic, hamartomatous) polyposis is a rare (<1 in 100,000 births) syndrome characterized by 10 or more non-neoplastic, hamartomatous polyps throughout the GI tract or any number of polyps in a patient with a family history of juvenile polyposis. The syndrome is inherited in an autosomal dominant manner with high penetrance and is caused by mutations in the *SMAD4*, *PTEN*, or *BMPR1A* gene. The hamartomas are histologically distinct from the polyps seen in PJS. Patients generally present with rectal bleeding, anemia, abdominal pain, or intestinal obstruction in childhood or early adolescence. Extraintestinal symptoms include pulmonary arteriovenous malformations in some probands. The risk of malignancy in juvenile polyposis is reportedly as high as 20% and occurs in adulthood (median age, 37 years). Affected individuals should undergo regular colonoscopic surveillance. Patients with numerous, large, or high-grade dysplastic polyps may be considered for subtotal colectomy. Family members should

be screened with colonoscopy every 3 to 5 years beginning at age 12 until age 40.

PTEN HAMARTOMA SYNDROME

PTEN hamartoma syndrome is a rare, autosomal dominant syndrome consisting of multiple hamartomatous polyps of the skin and mucous membranes, including GI polyps, facial tricholemmomas, oral papillomas, and keratoses of the hands and feet. It was previously referred to as Cowden's syndrome and Bannayan-Riley-Ruvalcaba syndrome. The causative genetic lesion has been mapped to the *PTEN* tumor suppressor gene. The rate of associated malignancy is high, particularly in the thyroid, breast, and reproductive organs. The polyps in PTEN hamartoma syndrome are benign.

CRONKHITE-CANADA SYNDROME

Cronkhite-Canada syndrome is a rare, sporadic, acquired condition characterized by multiple hamartomatous polyps throughout the GI tract, along with alopecia, dermal pigmentation, and atrophy of the nail beds. Symptoms include diarrhea, protein-losing enteropathy, GI bleeding, intussusception, and rectal prolapse. It carries a poor prognosis, with 5-year mortality rates as high as 55%. Patients are at risk for gastric and colorectal cancer, and endoscopic surveillance has been recommended.

Polyps of the Colon

A *polyp* is defined as a grossly visible mass of epithelial cells that protrudes from the mucosal surface into the lumen of the intestine. A polyp may be sessile, flat, or pedunculated when it is attached by a stalk. Polyps are classified as either non-neoplastic or neoplastic (adenomatous). Polyps may rarely cause symptoms such as bleeding, prolapse, or obstruction. Neoplastic polyps have the potential to become malignant.

NONADENOMATOUS POLYPS

Nonadenomatous polyps, which account for approximately 90% of all mucosal polyps detected in the large bowel, can be found in more than 50% of people older than 60 years. These polyps, which are also termed *non-neoplastic polyps*, can be subcategorized into hyperplastic, inflammatory, lymphoid, and juvenile polyps. Most non-neoplastic polyps are hyperplastic polyps that arise as a result of abnormal maturation of the mucosal epithelial cells; these polyps are usually small in diameter and are found predominantly in the distal sigmoid colon and rectum. Hyperplastic polyps are not malignant and are not thought to be associated with any measurable increase in malignant potential. However, those with multiple, large right-sided hyperplastic polyps may be at increased risk. Patients with inflammatory bowel disease may develop inflammatory pseudopolyps, which may require biopsy or removal to distinguish them from neoplastic polyps. Lymphoid polyps are regions of the mucosa that contain exaggerated intramucosal lymphoid tissue. Juvenile polyps usually develop in the rectum of children younger than 5 years and are termed *hamartomatous* because they are focal malformations that resemble tumors but are caused by abnormal development of the lamina propria; these polyps require no therapy unless they cause symptoms, such as obstruction or severe bleeding, or are part of a genetic syndrome.

ADENOMATOUS POLYPS

DEFINITION

Adenomatous polyps (or adenomas) are neoplastic polyps with malignant potential. They are benign glandular tumors that exhibit either low- or high-grade dysplasia under microscopy. Their anatomic distribution parallels that of colorectal adenocarcinoma. Adenomatous polyps manifest in a range of sizes and may be sessile, flat, or pedunculated in morphology. They are believed to be the precursor lesion to colorectal adenocarcinoma, a process that occurs according to the adenoma-carcinoma sequence. Evidence supporting the adenoma-carcinoma sequence comes from several sources. Patients with genetic conditions that predispose to adenoma formation (e.g., FAP) develop cancer at high rates. Animal studies in which adenomas are induced by either carcinogens or genetic manipulation show carcinoma formation. Correlative evidence includes the observations that the epidemiology is similar for adenomas and carcinomas, that both lesions are more common in the same anatomic locations, and that adenomatous tissue can often be found in small adenocarcinomas. Intervention studies have shown that the removal of adenomatous polyps leads to a significant decrease in the risk for colorectal cancer.

EPIDEMIOLOGY

Adenomatous polyps are relatively common, particularly in elderly populations. Among healthy screening populations older than 50 years, adenomas are found in more than 15% of women and 25% of men. The prevalence of adenomas tends to be high in regions of the world where colorectal cancer is common. The importance of genetic risk factors is clear in the hereditary polyposis syndromes, and sporadic adenomas have a familial component; for example, individuals with a positive first-degree family history have a four-fold greater risk of developing adenomatous polyps. Blacks in the United States have an increased risk for developing adenomas and carcinomas relative to whites; the risk in Asians and Hispanics is similar to that in whites.

PATHOBIOLOGY

The layer of epithelial cells lining the surface of the normal large bowel undergoes continuous self-renewal, with a turnover period of 3 to 8 days. Undifferentiated stem cells located at the base of invaginated crypts give rise to cells that migrate toward the lumen as they differentiate further into specialized enterocytes; these cells are subsequently removed by apoptosis, by extrusion, or by phagocytes underlying the epithelial layer. The development of adenomatous polyps is associated with a sequence-specific accumulation of genetic lesions that cause an imbalance between epithelial cell proliferation and cell death. As a result, cells accumulate at the luminal surface, where they remain undifferentiated and continue to undergo cell division, eventually leading to the abnormal development of a mass of adenomatous tissue.

Adenomas are classified into three main histologic subtypes: tubular adenomas, villous adenomas (Fig. 199-6), and tubulovillous adenomas. Tubular adenomas, which are the most common type, account for 70 to 85% of all adenomas removed at colonoscopy. They are often small and pedunculated, and they consist of dysplastic tubular glands that divide and branch out from the mucosal surface; they rarely contain concomitant high-grade dysplasia or carcinoma. In contrast, villous adenomas are rarer (<5% of all adenomas), are generally large and sessile, and are composed of strands of dysplastic epithelium that project, finger-like, into the lumen of the gut; they have a much higher prevalence of high-grade dysplasia or carcinoma. Tubulovillous adenomas (10 to 25% of all adenomas) have a mixture of tubular and villous architecture. Advanced adenomas are defined as those that measure 1 cm or greater or have any villous histology or high-grade dysplasia. Patients with advanced adenomas or multiple adenomas (three or more) are at much greater risk for synchronous (developing simultaneously) or metachronous (developing after a time interval) colorectal cancer.

CLINICAL MANIFESTATIONS

Patients with adenomatous polyps generally remain asymptomatic, but they may present with an asymptomatic positive stool occult blood test or with evident hematochezia. The lifetime incidence of additional adenomas in a patient with one known adenoma is 30 to 50%. Less than 5% of all adenomas eventually develop into carcinomas. Two critical factors that determine the likelihood of an adenoma developing into an invasive lesion are the size of the polyp and the grade of dysplasia. For polyps less than 1 cm, the risk for carcinoma is 1 to 3%; polyps between 1 and 2 cm have a 10% risk of becoming cancerous; and more than 40% of polyps greater than 2 cm progress to an invasive lesion. All adenomatous polyps contain some degree of dysplasia,

but they can be further categorized as low or high grade to indicate the degree of dysplasia and the corresponding risk for invasive carcinoma. High-grade dysplasia is associated with a 27% rate of eventual transformation into carcinoma.

DIAGNOSIS

Adenomatous polyps in the colon and rectum can be diagnosed by endoscopy, barium radiography, or CT scanning (CT colography or virtual colonoscopy). Colonoscopy is the preferred method for diagnosing adenomas because of its high accuracy and the ability to immediately biopsy and resection most polyps. Barium enema, as assessed in the National Polyp Study, missed 52% of polyps measuring 1 cm or more. CT colography has good sensitivity for detecting large (>1 cm) polyps (>85%) and for detecting cancers (96%), but it is less sensitive and specific for smaller polyps. CT colography requires bowel preparation, exposes the patient to ionizing radiation, and cannot remove polyps. Colonoscopy may miss 6 to 12% of large (≥1 cm) polyps and 5% of cancers. Of note is that nonpolypoid (flat and depressed) colorectal neoplasms are found in about 9% of asymptomatic and symptomatic adults on colonoscopy and are more likely to contain a carcinoma than are polypoid lesions; these lesions may not be visible on barium radiography or CT.

Flexible sigmoidoscopy, which is often used to screen asymptomatic persons at average risk for colorectal adenocarcinoma, detects 50 to 60% of all polyps and cancers. Generally, patients who have polyps detected by barium radiography, CT colography, or flexible sigmoidoscopy should undergo colonoscopy to remove the lesion and search for additional polyps. In one study in which patients with polyps discovered by flexible sigmoidoscopy underwent subsequent colonoscopy, there was an 80% reduction in the incidence of colorectal cancer.

TREATMENT   Rx

The goal of treatment for adenomatous polyps is to remove or destroy the lesion during endoscopy. This recommendation is based on overwhelming evidence that endoscopic polypectomy reduces the subsequent incidence and mortality of colorectal cancer. Pedunculated adenomas are generally removed by snare polypectomy, with subsequent submission of the tissue for pathologic analysis. Piecemeal snare resection may be required to remove sessile polyps. Surgical resection of a polyp is indicated when endoscopic resection of an advanced adenoma is not possible. The biopsied polyp must be evaluated histologically to determine the presence or absence of carcinoma; if a malignant lesion is found, its histologic grade, vascular and lymphatic involvement, and proximity to the margin of resection should be determined. Unfavorable histopathologic factors that should prompt surgical resection include poorly differentiated histology, vascular invasion, lymphatic invasion, and incomplete endoscopic resection. Pedunculated polyps with cancer confined to the submucosa, with no evidence of unfavorable histologic features, can be definitively treated with endoscopic resection, without the need for surgical resection. Whether similar malignant sessile polyps can be managed nonoperatively is controversial. In these cases, the risk of surgery versus the risk of recurrence or lymphatic metastases needs to be balanced.

PROGNOSIS

Patients who have undergone resection of an adenomatous polyp are at increased risk for the subsequent development of adenoma and colorectal adenocarcinoma. This risk is influenced by the size, histology, and number of adenomas, and the surveillance intervals differ (Table 199-2). Low-risk patients—those with only one or two small tubular adenomas—should

FIGURE 199-6. **Villous adenoma.** Large and sessile villous adenomas of the large bowel with finger-like projections into the gut lumen. (Courtesy Dr. M. K. Washington.)

TABLE 199-2 POST–ADENOMA RESECTION SURVEILLANCE INTERVALS

FINDINGS	INTERVAL
1-2 adenomas, <1 cm	5 yr
3-10 adenomas, adenoma with villous features, ≥1 cm, or with high-grade dysplasia	3 yr
>10 adenomas	<3 yr
Sessile adenoma ≥2 cm, piecemeal excision	2-6 mo

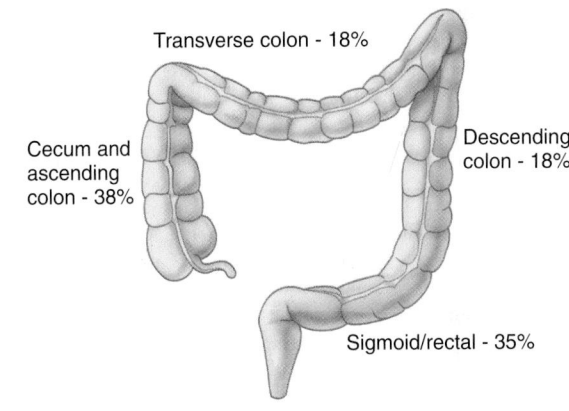

FIGURE 199-7. The molecular basis of colorectal cancer. Sequence-specific genetic lesions result in the transition from normal large bowel mucosa to invasive carcinoma. ACF = aberrant crypt foci; BAX = apoptosis-related protein; CRC = colorectal cancer; HNPCC = hereditary nonpolyposis colorectal cancer; IIR = type II receptor; LOH = loss of heterozygosity; MMR = mutation mismatch repair; MSI = microsatellite instability; TGFβ = transforming growth factor-β.

undergo colonoscopy in 5 years. Patients with multiple (more than two) adenomas, large (≥1 cm) adenomas, or adenomas with villous or high-grade histology should undergo colonoscopy in 3 years. Patients with numerous (>10) adenomas should undergo colonoscopy within 3 years. Patients who have had polypectomy of a large (≥2 cm) adenoma or an adenoma that had to be removed in pieces (piecemeal resection) should undergo colonoscopy within 6 months to evaluate the completeness of the resection.

Adenocarcinoma of the Colon and Rectum

PATHOBIOLOGY

Colorectal cancer is caused by the accumulation of multiple genetic lesions in sequence over time. Both the tissue architecture and the cellular genotype change as the disease progresses (Fig. 199-7). Early in the pathogenesis, mutations occur in either the *APC* gene (approximately 80% of sporadic colon cancers) or one of the mismatch repair genes (15% of sporadic colon cancers). The *APC* gene regulates cell growth and apoptosis, and mutations result in aberrant crypt foci, crypt dysplasia, and adenoma formation; 50% of sporadic adenomas have *APC* mutations. Mismatch repair gene mutations result in the failure to repair DNA transcription errors and the accumulation of additional mutations. Germline mutations in *APC* are the cause of FAP, and germline mutations of mismatch repair genes cause HNPCC (Lynch syndrome). Colorectal cancer pathogenesis requires additional mutations, including *DCC* ("deleted in colon cancer"), a tumor suppressor gene; *p53*, a regulator of the cell cycle; and *KRAS*, involved in the transduction of mitogenic signals across cell membranes. The accumulation of mutations leads to genetic instability and loss of heterozygosity where cells have only one allele of a gene owing to the loss of individual chromosomes during mitosis. DNA methylation can result in inactivation of tumor suppressor genes such as *p14* and *p16*. Other genetic and epigenetic alterations, including the expression of genes capable of cleaving extracellular matrix and a protein tyrosine phosphatase, lead to metastasis.

CLINICAL MANIFESTATIONS

The majority of patients with colorectal cancer present with symptoms that may be emergent. Common symptoms related to primary disease include rectal bleeding with or without manifestations of anemia, abdominal pain, and change in bowel function. Patients with systemic disease may exhibit anorexia, weight loss, and symptoms related to hepatic dysfunction, such as jaundice, icterus, and ascites (the last may also be seen with peritoneal metastases). Symptoms vary, depending on the primary site (Fig. 199-8):

FIGURE 199-8. Sites of development of large bowel adenocarcinoma.

proximal lesions are more likely to present with bleeding and associated symptoms; more distal disease has a higher risk of obstruction and perforation. Rectal cancers can also manifest with tenesmus and changes in stool caliber. They involve sacral nerve plexi, causing significant neuropathic pain. Patients with PJS or Gardner's syndrome may exhibit extraintestinal manifestations.

DIAGNOSIS

The history, physical examination, and judicious use of both laboratory and radiologic tests are important in diagnosing colorectal cancer. The history should include prior colorectal cancer or adenomatous polyps, inflammatory bowel disease, and family history of colonic neoplasia. On physical examination, extraintestinal lesions characteristic of PJS or Gardner's syndrome may be noticed. Metastatic disease is suggested by enlargement, characteristically of the supraclavicular lymph nodes (Virchow's nodes) or the liver, or by the presence of an umbilical mass (Sister Mary Joseph's node) or ascites. The digital rectal examination may reveal a distal rectal cancer or spread of the tumor to the rectal shelf or pelvis (Blumer's shelf). The stool shows evidence of frank or occult blood in 40 to 80% of advanced cases. Iron deficiency anemia or an elevation in liver enzymes may aid in the diagnosis. The CEA level may be elevated, but it cannot be relied on for diagnosis owing to inadequate sensitivity.

FIGURE 199-9. Two manifestations of large bowel adenocarcinoma. **A,** Exophytic growth within the lumen. **B,** Stricturing ("apple core") lesion.

TABLE 199-3	OPTIONS FOR COLORECTAL NEOPLASIA SCREENING*
TEST	**INTERVAL**
TESTS THAT DETECT ADENOMATOUS POLYPS OR CANCER	
Colonoscopy	Every 10 yr
Flexible sigmoidoscopy†	Every 5 yr
CT colography†	Every 5 yr
Double-contrast barium enema†	Every 5 yr
TESTS THAT DETECT PRIMARILY CANCER†	
Fecal occult blood tests	
High-sensitivity guaiac-based fecal occult blood test	Annually
Fecal immunochemical test	Annually
Stool DNA	Interval uncertain

*Beginning at age 50 for average-risk individuals.
†A positive test should prompt full colonoscopy.
CT = computed tomography.

Methods for diagnosing colorectal cancer are similar to those used to detect adenomatous polyps. Colonoscopy is the procedure of choice for all patients who have occult blood in their stools, unexplained iron deficiency anemia, or signs and symptoms suggestive of colorectal cancer (Fig. 199-9). Colonoscopy is more accurate than barium radiographic studies for the detection of colorectal neoplasms of all sizes and has the advantage of enabling the clinician to detect synchronous cancers and to obtain tissue for histologic analysis.

Additionally, accurate *local* staging of rectal cancers is paramount. Endoscopic ultrasound combines high-frequency ultrasonography with videoendoscopy. It is superior to CT and allows an accurate determination of the degree of invasion and detection and sampling of enlarged lymph nodes. Endoscopic ultrasound is also highly sensitive for the detection of rectal cancer recurrence after local resection or low anterior resection. MRI using either endorectal or phased array coils can also provide accurate local staging of rectal cancer. Local staging of nonrectal large bowel cancer is generally not performed preoperatively because this information is not used to guide therapy.

Many expert consensus guidelines now recommend CT scans of the abdomen and pelvis for colorectal cancer patients because liver metastases would preclude resection of an asymptomatic primary. Chest imaging with plain films or CT is recommended as well. PET scans have specific uses in defined cases of colorectal cancer, such as precluding additional systemic disease before resection of a solitary metastatic site. They may also be used to further describe abnormalities seen on CT. However, there is no role for PET in the routine work-up. Plain abdominal films are useful only in diagnosing obstruction.

Screening

The purpose of screening is to reduce colorectal cancer–related mortality by removing the precursor adenomas and detecting prevalent cancers at earlier, more curable stages. The long latency between adenoma development and subsequent cancer, on the order of 10 to 20 years, makes colorectal cancer a preventable disease through colonoscopy with polypectomy. It is an age-associated disease, and most patients should begin screening at age 50. There is a range of options for average-risk individuals (Table 199-3). These can be divided into two categories: stool tests, which include tests for occult blood and abnormal DNA, and structural tests, which include colonoscopy, flexible sigmoidoscopy, CT colography, and double-contrast barium enema. Stool tests are best suited for detecting prevalent cancers (and some advanced adenomas), whereas structural tests detect both cancers and adenomas. These tests may be used alone or in combination. Current multisociety guidelines recognize the multiple screening options but encourage the use of structural tests that have the ability to both detect and prevent colorectal cancer.

Tests for fecal occult blood detect hemoglobin in the stool from bleeding tumors. These tests are either guaiac based or immunochemical based. The guaiac tests detect blood in stool through the pseudoperoxidase activity of heme or hemoglobin. The immunochemical tests react with human globin and are therefore more specific. Guaiac testing consists of collecting two samples from three consecutive stools. To improve test accuracy, individuals undergoing guaiac testing are instructed to avoid aspirin, nonsteroidal anti-inflammatory drugs (NSAIDs), vitamin C, red meat, poultry, fish, and some vegetables. Three large, prospective randomized trials demonstrated that guaiac-based testing decreased colorectal cancer mortality by 15 to 33%, with

one large U.S. study also showing a 20% decrease in colorectal cancer incidence, attributed to the relatively higher rates of colonoscopy in the study group. Guaiac-based tests have sensitivities for cancer from 35 to 80%. Immunochemical-based tests do not rely on a peroxidase reaction and therefore may have fewer false-positives and false-negatives. They do not require the dietary restrictions of guaiac-based tests. Despite these advantages, studies have not demonstrated a clear-cut benefit of immunochemical tests over highly sensitive guaiac-based tests. Fecal occult blood tests are repeated annually, and any positive test should prompt colonoscopy.

Stool DNA tests rely on the observation that both adenomas and carcinomas contain altered DNA, and this DNA is shed in the stool. Tests contain a multiple marker panel designed to detect mutations in *KRAS, APC,* and *p53*; a probe for BAT-26 (a marker of microsatellite instability); and a marker of DNA integrity analysis. Collection kits are designed to facilitate stool collection (at least 30 g) and mailing. In a screening population, stool DNA had better sensitivity for colorectal cancer (52%) than a relatively insensitive guaiac-based test (unrehydrated Hemoccult II; 13% sensitivity). Stool DNA did not have good sensitivity for advanced adenomas (defined as >1 cm, villous, or with high-grade dysplasia), detecting only 15%. Stool DNA testing is more expensive than fecal occult blood testing, and the optimal screening interval has not been defined.

Flexible sigmoidoscopy is capable of examining the distal 60 cm of the colon, or roughly the splenic flexure to the rectum. It can be done with minimal bowel preparation, does not require sedation, and can be performed by primary care providers, nurses, or physician's assistants. Flexible sigmoidoscopy can detect either left-sided cancers or polyps. The detection of an adenoma should prompt referral for full colonoscopy, owing to the high prevalence of synchronous neoplasia in the unexamined proximal colon. In case-control studies, flexible sigmoidoscopy is associated with 60 to 80% reduction in colorectal cancer mortality in the area of the examined colon—an effect that persists for up to 10 years. In one randomized trial, a single flexible sigmoidoscopy performed once between ages 55 to 64 years reduced colorectal cancer incidence by 23% and mortality by 31%.■ Sigmoidoscopy should be repeated every 5 years and may be combined with yearly fecal occult blood testing.

Colonoscopy allows complete examination of the colon, as well as adenoma removal and thus cancer prevention. In the United States it is generally done under sedation, after an oral bowel preparation, and by physicians with specific training in colonoscopy and polypectomy. There are no direct randomized studies assessing the efficacy of colonoscopy for screening, although there is a large amount of indirect evidence. Colonoscopy is generally used as the "gold standard" in assessing other screening methods. In a large, randomized Minnesota study of fecal occult blood testing, a decrease in cancer incidence was observed that could be explained only by the use of colonoscopy and polypectomy at a higher rate in the screened population. Case-control studies of sigmoidoscopy demonstrate a colorectal cancer mortality benefit that should also apply to colonoscopy. The National Polyp Study, which followed patients after polypectomy, found that the incidence of colorectal cancer was reduced 76 to 90% compared to three reference populations. However, recent dietary and chemotherapeutic intervention trials found less of an effect, so the magnitude of the benefit is currently uncertain. If the initial screening colonoscopy is normal, further screening can be deferred for 10 years.

Double-contrast barium enema evaluates the entire colon by coating the mucosal surface with high-density barium and insufflating with air via a rectal tube. Multiple radiographs are obtained while varying the patient's position under fluoroscopy. It requires a colon preparation and exposes the patient to a small amount of ionizing radiation. There are no studies of double-contrast barium enema as a screening test. It is 85 to 97% sensitive for colon cancer, but its sensitivity for detecting large adenomas is only 48 to 73%. It should be repeated every 5 years. The finding of a polyp larger than 5 mm should prompt colonoscopy.

CT colography (also known as *virtual colonoscopy*) uses multidetector CT technology to obtain two- and three-dimensional images of the entire colon. It requires an adequate colon preparation and gaseous distention of the bowel using a rectal tube. Tagging of residual stool with barium or iodinated contrast material is frequently used. CT scanning is performed with the patient in the supine and prone positions. No studies have been done to evaluate the efficacy of CT colography in decreasing colorectal cancer incidence or mortality. CT colography has been compared with standard colonoscopy for the detection of neoplasia in screening populations.**2** The sensitivity of CT colography for large (≥10 mm) polyps is 85 to 93%, with a specificity of 97%. For polyps 6 to 9 mm, CT colography is 70 to 86% sensitive and 86 to 93% specific. Sensitivity for colorectal cancer (96%) is similar to that of colonoscopy. Although the optimal interval for testing has not been established, it is recommended that CT colography screening begin at age 50; if negative, it should be repeated at 5-year intervals. If a polyp greater than 5 mm is found, colonoscopy should be performed.

Staging

Accurate staging of colorectal cancer is of the utmost importance in determining both prognosis and the most relevant and effective therapy. The versions of the TNM classification system for large bowel cancers used by the American Joint Committee on Cancer and the International Union Against Cancer are identical (Table 199-4). Differing from many solid tumors (although not those of other GI origin, except for anal cancer), colorectal cancers are not staged according to size. Stage I cancers penetrate into but not through the bowel wall (T1–2N0M0), while stage II cancers penetrate through the wall without spreading to regional lymph nodes. About 40% of patients present with stage I or II disease in the United States. Stage III cancers involve regional lymph nodes and constitute about 40% of presenting cases. Stage IV colorectal tumors commonly spread to liver, lung, distant nodes, and peritoneum, with about 20% of patients presenting with distant disease. Rectal primaries, because of early access to the systemic circulation, may involve the lungs without liver metastases; this pattern of spread is distinctly unusual in proximal large bowel cancers.

Surveillance

Surveillance should be undertaken in patients fit enough to undergo metastasectomy or systemic therapy for recurrent colorectal cancer. The American Society of Clinical Oncology recommends annual CT of the chest and abdomen for 3 years following resection of high-risk primary tumors, with pelvic CT added in cases of rectal origin. Colonoscopy should also be done at 3 years and then every 5 years, with flexible proctosigmoidoscopy offered to rectal cancer patients who have not received irradiation. Physical examinations should be performed every 3 to 6 months for 3 years, then biannually for at least 2 more years. CEA levels should be checked every 3 months for at least 3 years.

PROGNOSIS

The prognosis for patients with colorectal cancer depends primarily on stage. Five-year survival for patients with proximal (colonic) adenocarcinomas ranges from a low of 6 to 8% for those with metastatic disease to approximately 95% for those with stage I resected tumors. Corresponding rates for rectal cancers are similar to slightly inferior overall, ranging from 4 to 72%. Besides TNM stage, additional factors that are prognostic for poorer outcomes in patients undergoing potentially curative resection include signet ring histologic subtype (see the preceding discussion under Pathobiology), lymphovascular and perineural invasion, absence of host lymphoid response, presence of clinical obstruction preoperatively, high preoperative serum levels of the CEA tumor marker, positive margins, high tumor grade, and microsatellite-stable disease. Differing from many solid tumors originating

STAGE	TUMOR	NODE	METASTASIS
0	Tis	N0	M0
I	T1, T2	N0	M0
IIA	T3	N0	M0
IIB	T4a	N0	M0
IIC	T4b	N0	M0
IIIA	T1, T2	N1	M0
	T1	N2a	M0
IIIB	T3, T4a	N1	M0
	T2, T3	N2a	M0
	T1, T2	N2b	M0
IIIC	T4a	N2a	M0
	T3, T4a	N2b	M0
	T4b	N1, N2	M0
IVA	Any T	Any N	M1a
IVB	Any T	Any N	M1b

TABLE 199-4 STAGING FOR COLORECTAL ADENOCARCINOMAS

Tis = in situ; T1 = submucosa; T2 = muscularis propria; T3 = subserosa, pericolorectal tissues; T4a = visceral peritoneum; T4b = other structures.
N1a = 1 regional node; N1b = 2-3 regional nodes; N1c = satellite(s) without regional nodes; N2a = 4-6 regional nodes; N2b = ≥7 regional nodes.
M1a = 1 organ; M1b = >1 organ, peritoneum.

outside the GI tract, colorectal cancers do not have different prognoses based on size.

Genetic factors are important as well, even in the metastatic setting. Patients with tumors harboring *BRAF* mutations appear to have a worse outcome. *KRAS* mutations were formerly thought to be prognostic but now appear to be only predictive for lack of benefit from certain types of systemic therapy.

TREATMENT

Chemoprevention

NSAIDs, including aspirin, are believed to reduce adenoma formation and inhibit colon cancer development by inhibiting cyclooxygenase and subsequent prostaglandin generation (Chapter 36). Prostaglandins (e.g., E_2) promote cell proliferation and tumor growth. The NSAID sulindac causes regression of existing adenomas and inhibits the formation of new adenomas in patients with FAP. Epidemiologic studies have shown decreased colorectal cancer rates in regular users of NSAIDs. Randomized trials of aspirin have shown 20 to 40% reductions in adenoma recurrence and a 70% reduction in the incidence of colorectal cancer when at least 75 mg of aspirin daily is continual for 5 or more years.**3** The selective cyclooxygenase 2 inhibitor celecoxib has shown similar decreases in adenoma recurrence, but its use is limited by concerns about cardiovascular risk. Calcium supplementation (1200 mg/day) was shown to decrease the rate of metachronous adenomas by 20%. However, the large Women's Health Trial, with 36,000 participants, found that calcium (1000 mg) plus vitamin D (400 IU) had no effect in reducing colorectal cancer incidence.**4** Currently, the routine use of aspirin and calcium for prevention is not recommended, but it may be considered on an individual basis.

Dietary Prevention

Epidemiologic studies have reported correlations between colorectal cancer and obesity, smoking, inactivity, excessive alcohol use, and diets high in fat and low in fruits, vegetables, and fiber. These observations suggest that lifestyle modifications may decrease colorectal cancer risk. Unfortunately, three randomized intervention trials of modest dietary changes (10% less fat, 25 to 75% more fiber, 50% more fruits and vegetables) found no significant reductions in adenomas or colorectal cancer over 3 to 8 years of follow-up.

Surgery

Resection is the primary treatment modality for patients with regionally confined colorectal cancer. Highly selected patients with metastatic disease may also undergo surgery with curative intent. The goal of curative surgery for colonic adenocarcinoma is margin-negative elimination of the tumor, plus en bloc removal of the primary feeding arterial vessel and corresponding lymphatics for that segment of bowel. A minimum of 12 lymph nodes should be retrieved for microscopic examination to assure staging accuracy. Synchronous colon cancers may be removed individually or with subtotal colectomy, and tumors adherent to adjacent structures should be resected en bloc. Prophylactic oophorectomy is no longer recommended, but women with one ovary grossly involved with cancer should undergo bilateral oophorectomy because of the relatively high risk of involvement of the other side. Laparoscopic resection is currently thought to be as effective as open resection and requires a modestly shorter recovery time.[5]

In general, surgical considerations for rectal primaries are similar. Total mesorectal excision (en bloc removal of the lymphovascular and fatty envelope surrounding the rectum) is recommended for distal cancers, whereas tumor-specific mesorectal excision (en bloc removal of the mesorectum 5 cm distal to the tumor) should suffice for upper rectal tumors. Local transanal excision is acceptable for selected low rectal cancers thought to have minimal risk of nodal involvement. Selection criteria include the following: T1 disease, size less than 3 cm, low grade (well differentiated), location within 8 cm of the anal verge, no lymphovascular invasion, and less than one-third circumferential.

Until fairly recently, patients presenting with synchronous colorectal cancer primaries and unresectable metastases underwent resection of the primary tumor, regardless of whether they were symptomatic. This practice pattern could obviously delay systemic treatment in patients who are markedly more likely to die from their metastases before suffering significant complications from the intact large bowel tumor. Recent data suggest that stage IV patients with an asymptomatic primary tumor can safely begin systemic therapy without undergoing surgery, with only a small chance of developing serious complications requiring urgent operative interaction. Patients with rectal primaries may be at slightly higher risk for developing complications than those with tumors originating in the proximal large bowel.

Obstructing tumors that can be fully removed should be resected, with bowel anastomosis usually being acceptable in this setting. Proximal diversion alone, especially in the setting of very locally advanced unresectable cancer, may be necessary; if the primary tumor responds to the point where it can later be removed, resection followed by ostomy closure is reasonable. Endoscopic stenting may be useful to relieve acute obstruction. Perforated bowel is usually resected, with the choice of anastomosis, with or without diversion, depending on a number of factors, including degree of fecal contamination and general health of the patient.

Radiation Therapy

Radiation therapy may be used as curative or palliative treatment of large bowel cancers. In general, it plays a markedly larger role in treating rectal than colonic primaries. Single-institution trials have shown that irradiation improves local control following resection of high-risk proximal large bowel (colonic) cancers, but these findings were not confirmed in a randomized intergroup trial that closed early owing to slow accrual. Current recommendations for adjuvant radiation to the tumor bed following colon cancer resection include positive margins and localized perforation. Some authorities also advocate its use in colon cancers at particularly high risk of local recurrence (T4, T3N1–2 tumors in the ascending or descending colon), but that recommendation is not universally accepted. Irradiation may still play a role in treating colon cancer metastases to bone, brain, liver, and lung, as well as in cases of bleeding, obstruction, and locally advanced unresectable disease.

A major use for radiation in the definitive treatment of large bowel adenocarcinoma involves perioperative therapy for resectable rectal cancer. It is also commonly employed with chemotherapy for locally advanced invasive tumors, which occasionally become resectable after therapy. As with colon primaries, irradiation may be used to palliate bleeding, obstruction, or selected metastases from rectal cancers.

Systemic and Combination Therapies

The backbone of colorectal cancer treatment in both the adjuvant and metastatic settings is a fluorinated pyrimidine. The most commonly used drug is 5-fluorouracil (5-FU), although oral prodrugs are increasingly been utilized. 5FU targets the enzyme thymidylate synthase, inhibiting DNA synthesis and/or repair. It also may be incorporated into RNA, interfering with further processing. Although not particularly effective as a single agent (see later), 5-FU's efficacy can be enhanced by changing its means of administration (prolonging infusion) and by administering it with a variety of biochemical modulators, most commonly leucovorin. Other agents commonly used in treating colorectal cancer include irinotecan, a topoisomerase I inhibitor, and oxaliplatin, a later-generation platin that forms bulky DNA adducts that inhibit replication.

Patients with resected stage I colon cancers have a high cure rate, and this cannot easily be improved on with systemic therapy. Stage II patients have a higher chance of relapse (event-free survival ≈76% at 3 years), and systemic therapy with 5-FU and leucovorin improved that figure by about 3% for an unselected group of node-negative patients. Patients harboring highly microsatellite-unstable tumors have a better prognosis in general but may actually have worse outcomes with 5-FU treatment, although that is controversial. Treatment of stage II patients remains controversial in general: some experts suggest that the proportional benefit of systemic therapy is as great as it is in stage III disease, while others point out the low absolute magnitude of benefit

and do not advocate its use. Some categories of stage II disease are believed to be at particularly high risk for recurrence (e.g., clinical obstruction). These patients usually receive postoperative chemotherapy, often with regimens commonly prescribed for patients with stage III cancer. Radiation has been tested in patients thought to be at higher than average risk of local relapse (T4 tumors), but its use is not standard. Finally, it is likely that gene studies will eventually be used to identify patients at higher risk of relapse or who have a greater chance of benefiting from systemic therapy, and treatment of carefully selected patients with stage II disease may become standard.

Five-year disease-free survival for patients with stage III colon cancer is only in the 40 to 45% range. Barring significant comorbidities or other confounding factors, all patients with node-positive disease receive adjuvant systemic therapy. Combinations of 5-FU and oxaliplatin (usually FOLFOX [fluorouracil, leucovorin, oxaliplatin]) clearly improve long-term survival rates and represent standard care.[6] Regimens containing irinotecan and biologics (bevacizumab, cetuximab) are highly effective in the treatment of advanced disease (see later), but oddly, they do not clearly benefit patients when they are given in the postoperative setting. Patients who are not candidates for combination chemotherapy are sometimes offered capecitabine, an oral prodrug activated to 5-FU in sequential enzymatic steps. Capecitabine has also been combined effectively and relatively safely with oxaliplatin for adjuvant use. Important outstanding questions regarding adjuvant chemotherapy is whether a shorter duration (3 months vs. the standard 6) might be equally effective, and whether elderly patients obtain greater benefit from newer combination regimens versus simple fluoropyrimidine use.

Rectal Adenocarcinoma

Radiation considerations are slightly different for patients with primary rectal adenocarcinomas, owing to the difficulty of achieving negative circumferential (radial) margins. Specifically, the risk of local recurrence is much more significant. In general, rectal cancer patients undergoing standard resection for stage I tumors do not receive additional treatment. However, higher-risk patients (T2 disease, T1 with poorly differentiated histology, perineural or lymphovascular invasion, or close margins) treated with local excision should receive postoperative pelvic irradiation with or without 5-FU chemotherapy, or they should return to the operating room for total mesorectal excision. Irradiation is standard for those with stage II and III rectal adenocarcinomas to decrease local relapse rates, increase the chance of sphincter preservation (when used in selected preoperative settings for low-lying cancers), and possibly improve survival. The major considerations are timing (pre- or postoperative use), course (short or long), and whether to combine it with fluoropyrimidine-based chemotherapy. Short-course (5-day) preoperative irradiation without chemotherapy may be considered and used if tumor downsizing is not necessary. When short-course radiation is used, patients still require postoperative systemic therapy, with either a fluoropyrimidine alone (stage II) or a fluoropyrimidine-oxaliplatin combination regimen (node-positive disease), to minimize the risk of distant metastases. Long-course irradiation (approximately 5.5 weeks) is particularly important when tumor response is necessary to make surgery easier or more feasible. It is usually combined with continuous-infusion 5-FU or capecitabine, and it can be given preoperatively or postoperatively (if the patient did not receive preoperative short-course radiation). Including oxaliplatin preoperatively does not improve results and is not recommended independent of a clinical trial, owing to its higher toxicity profile. Oxaliplatin may be used postoperatively if the pathology specimen demonstrates nodal involvement. With long-course irradiation, preoperative (compared with postoperative) treatment is less toxic and may offer improved local control.[7] However, it requires accurate preoperative staging (to avoid treating patients who might have stage I disease). Highly selected rectal cancer patients thought to be at low risk of local recurrence (T3N0 or T1–2N1) may receive total mesorectal excision plus best systemic therapy without irradiation, usually postoperatively.

Metastatic Colorectal Cancer

Metastatic disease is treated identically, regardless of the site of origin (colon vs. rectum). Patients with incurable metastatic colorectal cancer have a median survival of approximately 6 months with best supportive care alone; however, incremental gains made through the adoption of new systemic therapies have extended that time to almost 2 years. For example, treatment with single-agent fluoropyrimidines leads to median survival in the 10- to 13-month range; adding one more effective chemotherapy drug (either irinotecan or oxaliplatin) affords survival of about 15 to 20 months, and adding both drugs to 5-FU has been reported to extend life to 23 months. Interestingly, long-term results seem to be similar regardless of which drug (oxaliplatin or irinotecan) is added to 5-FU first (although the toxicity pattern varies, depending on which drug is given), or even regardless of whether 5-FU is used first and combination chemotherapy is used subsequently, as long as patients are eventually exposed to all active agents.

Additional improvements have arisen through the development of drugs that are more convenient and/or less toxic than standard agents, although they may not be more effective. Capecitabine, an oral prodrug activated to 5-FU in three sequential enzymatic steps, can be substituted for that agent alone and in combination with oxaliplatin (although patients still need intravenous access for the latter drug).

Recent breakthroughs have all been related to use of biological agents (Chapter 35). Successful drugs to date have all been monoclonal antibodies, whereas small molecule tyrosine kinase inhibitors generally appear to be ineffective. Bevacizumab is a humanized monoclonal antibody directed against vascular endothelial growth factor, an important mediator of angiogenesis. Bevacizumab has little single-agent activity against colorectal cancer, but it improves the interval without progression when added to irinotecan- or oxaliplatin-containing chemotherapy.[8,9] Bevacizumab with FOLFOX or FOLFIRI (fluorouracil, leucovorin, irinotecan) now represents first-line treatment for patients with advanced large bowel cancer in the United States.

The epidermal growth factor receptor (EGFR) is another important target in advanced colorectal cancer. Cetuximab and panitumumab are monoclonal antibodies (chimeric and human, respectively) directed against the EGFR. They have single-agent activity against colorectal cancers,[10] and both may be combined with chemotherapy to improve at least progression-free survival.[11] Although both agents appear effective in front-line or later use, efficacy is restricted to patients whose tumors harbor no mutations in *KRAS*.

Locally Directed Treatment of Metastatic Disease

Complete resection of hepatic or pulmonary metastases may result in long-term survival and is the standard of care for selected patients with colorectal cancer. The majority of data exist for hepatic metastasectomy. Actuarial 5-year survival rates from single-institution series have been in the 25 to 40% range. However, relapse after 5 years still occurs, suggesting that this percentage does not reflect the number actually *cured* with surgery. That figure, calculated from 10-year survival rates, is probably between 17 and 25%, which still compares quite favorably with the survival rate for patients with colorectal cancer metastatic to the liver who do not undergo surgery. The actual role of perioperative systemic therapy in those undergoing metastasectomy is not well defined, but most experts advocate 6 months of fluoropyrimidine-based chemotherapy, with or without oxaliplatin. Importantly, bevacizumab can affect wound healing and should not be used in the immediate perioperative period.

Small liver metastases that are not resectable because of anatomic location or in a frail patient unable to undergo hepatic resection may be treated with radio frequency ablation, which uses alternating electrical current to generate heat, destroying malignant cells through protein coagulation. Although it has never been directly compared with resection in a randomized trial, radio frequency ablation appears to offer inferior local control of disease. Some advocate the placement of a hepatic artery pump to infuse fluoropyrimidine-based chemotherapy to treat unresectable liver-predominant metastases. Other techniques useful in noncolorectal liver-based tumors (e.g., hepatocellular carcinoma), such as chemoembolization, have no proven role for large bowel liver metastases.

CONCLUSION

Colorectal cancer remains a significant problem, despite the fact that most cases can be prevented. Large gains have been made in terms of overall survival, but the vast majority of patients with advanced disease still succumb to their malignancy. Although minimal tailoring can be offered to patients (e.g., selecting a chemotherapeutic agent based on toxicity or not using an anti-EGFR antibody in those with *KRAS*-mutated tumors), the dream of truly individualized therapy remains elusive.

1. Atkin WS, Edwards R, Kralj-Hans I, et al. Once-only flexible sigmoidoscopy screening in prevention of colorectal cancer: a multicentre randomised controlled trial. *Lancet.* 2010;375:1624-1633.
2. Johnson CD, Chen MH, Toledano AY, et al. Accuracy of CT colonography for detection of large adenomas and cancers. *N Engl J Med.* 2008;359:1207-1217.
3. Rothwell PM, Wilson M, Elwin CE, et al. Long-term effect of aspirin on colorectal cancer incidence and mortality: 20-year follow-up of five randomised trials. *Lancet.* 2010;376:1741-1750.
4. Wactawski-Wende J, Kotchen JM, Anderson GL, et al. Calcium plus vitamin D supplementation and the risk of colorectal cancer. *N Engl J Med.* 2006;354:684-696.
5. Fleshman J, Sargent DJ, Green E, et al. Laparoscopic colectomy for cancer is not inferior to open surgery based on 5-year data from the COST study group trial. *Ann Surg.* 2007;246:655-664.
6. Andre T, Boni C, Navarro M, et al. Improved overall survival with oxaliplatin, fluorouracil, and leucovorin as adjuvant treatment in stage II or III colon cancer in the MOSAIC trial. *J Clin Oncol.* 2009;27:3109-3116.
7. Sauer R, Becker H, Hohenberger W, et al. Preoperative versus postoperative chemoradiotherapy for rectal cancer. *N Engl J Med.* 2004;351:1731-1740.
8. Hurwitz H, Fehrenbacher L, Novotny W, et al. Bevacizumab plus irinotecan, fluorouracil, and leucovorin for metastatic colorectal cancer. *N Engl J Med.* 2004;350:2335-2342.
9. Saltz LB, Clarke S, Diaz-Rubio E, et al. Bevacizumab in combination with oxaliplatin-based chemotherapy as first-line therapy in metastatic colorectal cancer: a randomized phase III study. *J Clin Oncol.* 2008;26:2013-2019.
10. Van Cutsem E, Siena S, Humblet Y, et al. An open-label randomized phase 3 clinical trial of panitumumab plus best supportive care versus best supportive care in patients with chemotherapy-refractory metastatic colorectal cancer. *J Clin Oncol.* 2007;25:1658-1664.
11. Van Cutsem E, Köhne C-H, Hitre E, et al. Cetuximab and chemotherapy as initial treatment for metastatic colorectal cancer. *N Engl J Med.* 2009;360:1408-1417.

SUGGESTED READINGS

Cunningham D, Atkin W, Lenz HJ, et al. Colorectal cancer. *Lancet.* 2010;375:1030-1047. *Review.*
Damjanaov N, Weiss J, Haller DG. Resection of the primary colorectal cancer is not necessary in non-obstructed patients with metastatic disease. *Oncologist.* 2009;14:963-969. *Modern literature review with recommendations for treatment (or not) of primary colorectal cancer in patients who also have metastatic disease.*
Gastrointestinal Stromal Tumor Meta-Analysis Group (MetaGIST). Comparison of two doses of imatinib for the treatment of unresectable or metastatic gastrointestinal stromal tumors: a meta-analysis of 1640 patients. *J Clin Oncol.* 2010;28:1247-1253. *Though not limited to intestinal GISTs, this meta-analysis provides results of imatinib therapy for advanced disease, including results for patients with tumors harboring exon 9 mutations (markedly more common in those with small bowel primaries).*
Holden DJ, Jonas DE, Porterfield DS, et al. Systematic review: enhancing the use and quality of colorectal cancer screening. *Ann Intern Med.* 2010;152:668-676. *Review.*
Hyslop T, Weinberg DS, Schulz S, et al. Occult tumor burden predicts disease recurrence in lymph node–negative colorectal cancer. *Clin Cancer Res.* 2011;17:3293-3303. *Molecular tumor burden in lymph nodes is independently associated with time to recurrence and disease-free survival in node-negative colorectal cancer.*

PANCREATIC CANCER

MARGARET TEMPERO AND RANDALL BRAND

DEFINITION

The term *pancreatic cancer* usually refers to ductal adenocarcinomas because more than 90% of pancreatic neoplasms are of ductal epithelial origin. Other pancreatic tumors include endocrine tumors (Chapter 201), carcinoid tumors (Chapter 240), lymphomas, cystic neoplasms, and the rare squamous cell carcinomas, giant cell carcinomas, carcinosarcomas, malignant fibrous histiocytomas, solid pseudopapillary neoplasms, sarcomas, and pancreaticoblastomas.

EPIDEMIOLOGY

Pancreatic cancer is the fourth most common cause of cancer death in the United States despite its low incidence: about 42,500 pancreatic neoplasms are diagnosed and 35,200 will die annually from cancer-related causes. Worldwide, pancreatic cancer accounts for 2% of all malignant diseases. Its incidence is higher in developed than in developing countries, but there is less than a two-fold variation in incidence worldwide. The 5-year survival rate for adenocarcinoma of the pancreas is less than 5%, and most patients die within the first 2 years. The risk for developing a pancreatic carcinoma increases with age, with a mean age of onset in the seventh and eighth decades of life. There is almost an equivalent risk in men and women.

Pancreatic cancer is more common in African Americans, Maori New Zealanders, and Polynesians. Cigarette smoking is the most reproducible environmental risk factor, causing a 1.5- to 5.5-fold increased rate of pancreatic cancer. Other risk factors include increased body mass index, chronic pancreatitis (Chapter 146), high intake of animal fat, and prolonged contact with petroleum products and wood pulp. A modest, less than two-fold increased risk for pancreatic cancer is associated with blood groups A, AB, and B relative to blood group O, and with selected polymorphisms that map to three loci on chromosomes *13q22.1, 1q32.1,* and *5p15.33*.

The association between pancreatic cancer and diabetes is complex. Diabetes or impaired glucose tolerance is observed in up to 80% of patients at the time of diagnosis of their pancreatic cancer, and diabetes is often described as a risk factor. However, the diabetes is usually of recent onset and may improve or resolve after resection of the tumor. A population-based study suggests that about 1% of patients who develop diabetes after age 50 years will have a diagnosis of pancreatic cancer within 3 years before or after the onset of diabetes, and most of these individuals will be diagnosed with diabetes within 6 months of detection of the pancreatic cancer. Thus, diabetes may be a sign of underlying pancreatic cancer.

The greatest risk factor for developing pancreatic cancer is genetic predisposition. It is estimated that up to 10% of patients with pancreatic cancer have one or more first- or second-degree relatives with the disease. Recognized inherited syndromes include hereditary pancreatitis (Chapter 146), mutation of the *BRCA2* gene (Chapter 204), familial atypical multiple mole–melanoma syndrome and a *p16* germline mutation, hereditary nonpolyposis colorectal cancer (Chapter 199), Peutz-Jeghers polyposis (Chapter 199), and ataxia-telangiectasia (Chapter 258). In most families, the genetic factors responsible for the predisposition are unknown.

Pancreatic cysts are increasingly recognized with the widespread use of abdominal imaging and can be categorized as neoplastic or non-neoplastic. Neoplastic cystic lesions consist of those with malignant potential such as intraductal papillary mucinous neoplasms (IPMNs), mucinous cystic neoplasms, and the rare solid pseudopapillary tumors. Those without malignant potential include serous cystadenomas and lymphoepithelial cysts. IPMNs equally affect women and men and are usually located in the head of the pancreas. Other cystic neoplasms most commonly occur in young to middle-aged women and are located in the body or tail of the pancreas.

PATHOBIOLOGY

Three major precursors to invasive pancreatic adenocarcinoma have been identified: pancreatic intraepithelial neoplasia (PanIN), IPMN, and mucinous cystic neoplasm (MCN). The PanIN is the most prevalent type of precursor lesion, arising from the ductal epithelial cells. It is presumed that these lesions follow a pathway of progression from no dysplasia to moderate dysplasia (borderline) to high-grade dysplasia (carcinoma in situ) to invasive carcinoma. As the extent of ductal atypia rises, there is an increasing frequency of associated genetic alterations (Fig. 200-1). Unlike PanIN lesions, the IPMNs and MCNs are detectable by computed tomography (CT) or endoscopic ultrasound (EUS). Although only responsible for a minority of pancreatic cancers (less than 15%), IPMNs and MCNs do offer the opportunity to identify a premalignant lesion in the pancreas, especially with the increasing use of high-resolution noninvasive abdominal imaging procedures.

Ductal adenocarcinoma and its variants are characterized by a dense, desmoplastic reaction surrounding a compact mass of hard pancreatic tissue that can invade surrounding mesenteric vessels and can involve perineuronal tissue and lymphatic channels or nodes. Because approximately 75% of pancreatic carcinomas are located in the head of the pancreas, the usual clinical presentations are related to invasion or compression of the bile or pancreatic ducts. The duodenum, stomach, and colon may be invaded or compressed. Pancreatic cancers other than ductal adenocarcinoma, such as islet cell tumors or lymphomas, tend to be softer and less fibrotic and thus tend to cause distortion rather than encasement or compression of adjacent structures.

Tumor suppressor genes that are most frequently mutated in pancreatic adenocarcinoma are *p16* (95%), *p53* (50 to 75%), and *DPC4* (55%). *K-ras*, which is the most commonly activated oncogene, occurs in about 95% of advanced pancreatic cancers. An extensive genetic analysis of 24 pancreatic cancers, performed using state-of-the-art DNA sequencing of 20,735 genes, as well as both gene expression and gene copy number analysis, revealed on average a total of 63 altered genes per tumor. Although there was marked variability from tumor to tumor in the specific genes that were mutated, 12 cellular signaling pathways and processes that had at least one gene genetically altered in at least 70% of the tumors were identified. The six specific pathways that had alterations of at least one of the genes in all of the 24 pancreatic cancers were *K-ras* signaling, apoptosis, Wnt/Notch signaling, transforming growth factor-β (TGF-β) signaling, hedgehog signaling, and regulation of G_1 to S phase transition.

CLINICAL MANIFESTATIONS

Early symptoms include nonspecific abdominal discomfort, nausea, vomiting, sleeping difficulties, anorexia, and generalized malaise. Despite the historic perception that a mass in the head of the pancreas manifests initially with painless jaundice, the more common presenting symptoms are epigastric pain, obstructive jaundice, and weight loss. Although these symptoms prompt evaluation of the pancreas and biliary tree, they occur late in the disease and are usually associated with advanced tumor at the time of diagnosis. The finding of a palpably distended, nontender gallbladder as a result of obstruction of the distal common bile duct by pancreatic cancer has been called *Courvoisier's sign*. Patients may manifest superficial or deep vein thrombosis (Trousseau's syndrome; Chapter 187).

The most common laboratory abnormalities include anemia and elevation of serum levels of alkaline phosphatase, bilirubin, and aminotransferases. Approximately 80% of patients have jaundice related to biliary obstruction. Diabetes or hyperglycemia is seen in up to 80% of patients, and pancreatic cancer should be considered in the differential diagnosis of the cause of new-onset diabetes in patients who older than 50 years and who do not have a family history of diabetes.

Tumors of other histologic types arising in the pancreas may also cause nonspecific symptoms. Patients with functioning islet cell tumors can present with symptoms related to the overproduction of peptides manufactured in the islets (Chapter 201). Cystic neoplasms generally remain asymptomatic until they become quite large, at which point patients can present with a palpable mass, abdominal pain, nausea, emesis, and weight loss. Obstruction of the common bile duct is less common than with ductal adenocarcinoma. Intraductal papillary mucinous tumors may cause symptoms of acute pancreatitis or pancreatic insufficiency owing to obstruction of the pancreatic duct.

DIAGNOSIS

Differential Diagnosis

The differential diagnosis of pancreatic ductal cancer includes conditions that can manifest as a solid mass in the pancreas or especially acute or, more commonly, chronic pancreatitis (Chapter 146). Ampullary carcinomas and distal cholangiocarcinomas also manifest with biliary obstruction and jaundice (Chapters 158 and 202). It may be difficult to differentiate cystic pancreatic neoplasms from non-neoplastic pancreatic pseudocysts based on noninvasive imaging studies; a cystic neoplasm should always be considered in patients who present with isolated cystic lesions and have no prior history of acute or chronic pancreatitis.

Imaging

For all patients with suspected pancreatic tumors, the preferred imaging study is a multidetector CT scan using dynamic contrast with thin cuts

FIGURE 200-1. Molecular progression model of pancreatic cancer (PanINs). Molecular abnormalities in PanINs can usually be stratified into "early" changes (e.g., expression of *MUC5* and prostate stem antigen, or loss of *p16*), "intermediate" changes (e.g., expression of cyclin D1), and "late" changes (e.g., expression of *p53*, proliferation antigens, *MUC1*, mesothelin, and 14-3-3s, or loss of *SMAD4/DPC4*). (Adapted from Maitra A, Adsay NV, Argani P, et al. Multicomponent analysis of the pancreatic adenocarcinoma progression model using a pancreatic intraepithelial neoplasia tissue microarray. *Mod Pathol.* 2003;16:902-912).

hes1

nestin   Telomere shortening   p16/CDNK2A   TP53
          KRAS2   SMAD4
                                                BRCA2

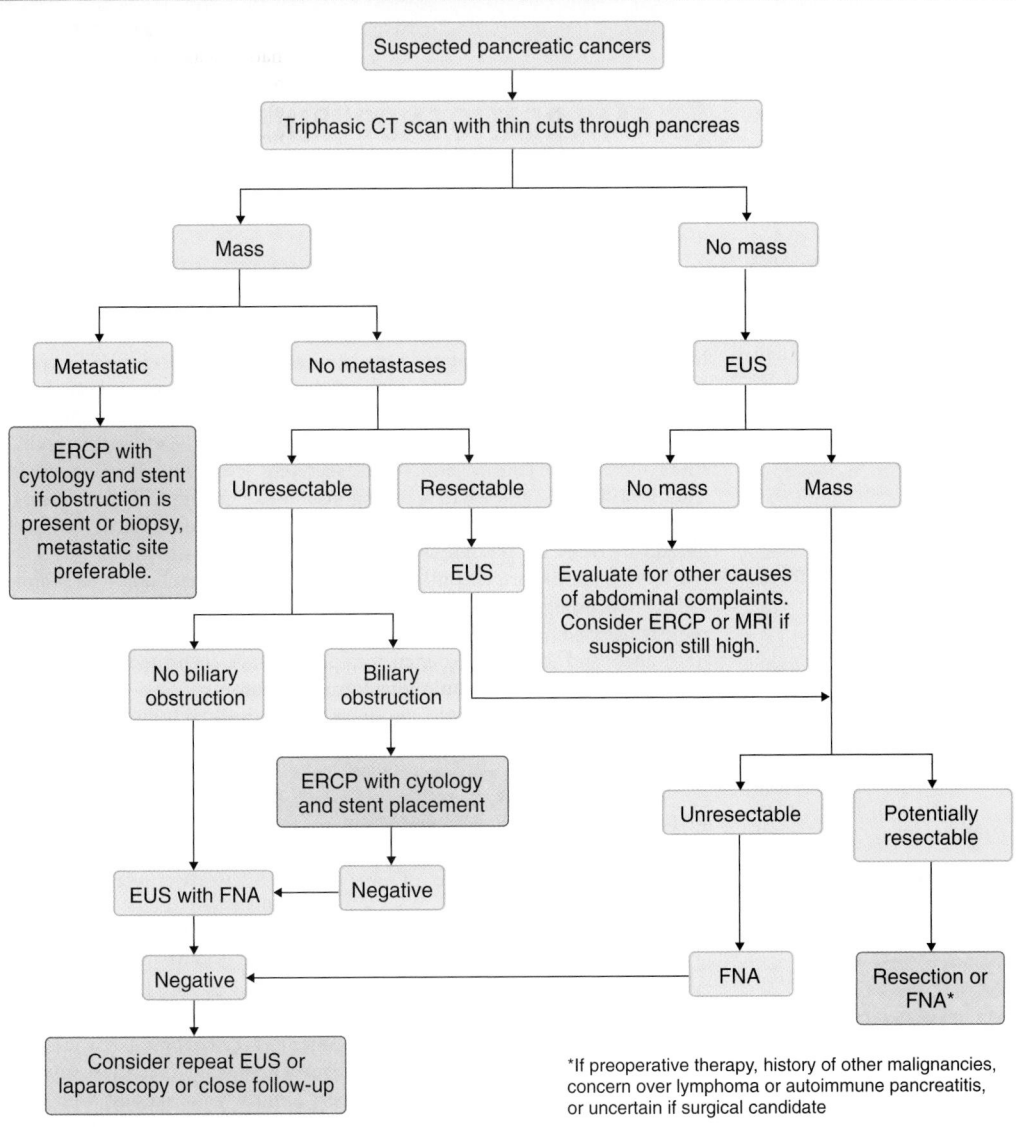

FIGURE 200-2. Diagnostic algorithm for pancreatic cancer. Intraoperative fine-needle aspiration (FNA) is used if the tumor is found to be inoperable during surgery. CT = computed tomography; ERCP = endoscopic retrograde cholangiopancreatography; EUS = endoscopic ultrasonography; MRI = magnetic resonance imaging.

*If preoperative therapy, history of other malignancies, concern over lymphoma or autoimmune pancreatitis, or uncertain if surgical candidate

through the pancreas (Fig. 200-2). The CT scan provides important information about vascular involvement and metastases, and it is approximately 90% accurate in assessing resectability. EUS may be useful in patients with equivocal findings on the CT scan. When a preoperative biopsy is needed, it is preferable to obtain a fine-needle aspiration under endoscopic guidance to minimize the chance of tumor seeding, but patients with potentially resectable disease can proceed directly to surgery. False-negative biopsy findings can result from the desmoplastic reaction characteristic of pancreatic ductal adenocarcinoma. Laparoscopy can identify patients who may have occult metastases in the peritoneum or the surface of the liver. Patients whose CT scans indicate an unresectable tumor based on local extension or the presence of metastases should have a definitive diagnosis established by a fine-needle aspiration biopsy of the primary or metastatic site.

Biomarkers

The clinical role for tumor markers is limited. CA-19-9, a sialylated Lewis[a] antigen associated with circulating mucins, is the most widely used marker for pancreatic disease. At the most commonly used cutoff level of 37 U/mL, its sensitivity ranges from 81 to 85%, and its specificity ranges from 81 to 90%; CA-19-9 levels higher than 1000 U/mL are associated with unresectable disease. Although this test is not a substitute for a histologic diagnosis, it is useful for monitoring the response to treatment.

The aforementioned radiographic studies also apply to other pancreatic tumors. EUS with fine-needle aspiration can be useful in the evaluation of cystic lesions, and it often provides additional detail not seen by CT and permits sampling of the cystic fluid for tumor marker levels, amylase content, viscosity, and cytologic examination. Carcinoembryonic antigen (CEA) levels of 192 mg/mL are approximately 80% accurate for identifying

mucinous as compared with nonmucinous cystic lesions. For obvious reasons, it is important to clarify whether the lesion is a simple cyst, which would suggest a pseudocyst, or a cystic neoplasm.

TREATMENT AND PROGNOSIS

In the absence of metastatic disease, surgical resection is the initial treatment of choice for all patients with pancreatic adenocarcinomas. The procedure should be performed in centers that have a high volume of pancreatectomies because surgical outcomes are improved with more volume and experience. Routine preoperative biliary drainage in patients with obstructive jaundice caused by pancreatic head tumor increases the rate of complications of surgery for the cancer.[1] For periampullary adenocarcinoma, pancreaticoduodenectomy is the standard of care, and distal gastrectomy and extended lymphadenectomy do not improve outcome.[2] Tumors are considered resectable if a clear fat plane is present around the celiac and superior mesenteric arteries and if the mesenteric and portal veins are patent. After successful resection, adjuvant therapy with intravenous 5-fluorouracil (425 mg/m²) and folinic acid (20 mg/m²) daily for 5 days and then monthly for 6 months or gemcitabine (1000 mg/m² over 30 minutes) weekly for 3 weeks out of 4 for 6 months improves survival compared with observation alone,[3,4] but the addition of gemcitabine to fluorouracil plus folinic acid does not provide incremental benefit.[5] Radiation therapy may not confer any added value beyond chemotherapy alone. In general, successful resection followed by adjuvant therapy results in a 5-year survival rate of approximately 20%.

Borderline resectable tumors include those with venous involvement of the superior mesenteric vein (SMV)–portal vein demonstrating tumor abutment with or without impingement and narrowing of the lumen, encasement of the SMV–portal vein but without encasement of the nearby arteries, short-segment venous occlusion secondary to either tumor thrombus, or encasement but with suitable vessel proximal and distal to the area of vessel involvement allowing for safe resection and reconstruction, gastroduodenal artery encasement up to the hepatic artery with either short-segment encasement or direct abutment of the hepatic artery without extension to the celiac axis, and tumor abutment of the superior mesenteric artery (SMA) not to exceed more than 180 degrees of the circumference of the vessel wall. Because there is a higher risk for positive margins with these tumors, some advocate preoperative chemotherapy and radiation, although this is controversial.

Surgery can also have an important palliative role. Patients who undergo surgical exploration but who are found not to have a resectable tumor may benefit from a biliary or gastric bypass procedure, depending on the clinical setting. However, there is now substantial experience in the placement of both biliary and luminal (duodenal) stents, so the more invasive operative procedure can be avoided in most instances. In addition, intraoperative, EUS-guided, or percutaneous chemical splanchnicectomy can provide protracted pain control.

Patients with locally unresectable disease are usually managed with a combination of chemotherapy and radiation therapy, followed by additional chemotherapy. The most commonly used drug is 5-fluorouracil, given by low-dose continuous infusion, combined with radiation therapy, but gemcitabine is also being studied. The median survival time for these patients is 10 to 12 months.

For patients with metastatic disease, single-agent gemcitabine (1000 mg/m^2 intravenously, weekly times 7 for 8 weeks and then weekly times 3 every 4 weeks) remains the standard of care and improves survival. A small improvement in survival has been observed with the addition of erlotinib (orally, 100 mg/day).[6]

For all patients with locally advanced and metastatic disease, optimal management of pain and of local complications is critical. Biliary obstruction can be managed surgically or with placement of a plastic or expandable metal stent. Narcotic analgesics (Chapter 29) and palliative care (Chapter 3) are cornerstones of therapy.

Most patients with a cystic neoplasm should be considered for surgical resection. The long-term survival rate following resection of malignant pancreatic cystic neoplasms exceeds 70%, and adjuvant therapy is currently not recommended.

FUTURE DIRECTIONS

Future research in pancreatic adenocarcinoma will focus on identifying individuals at high risk, developing strategies for early detection, and optimizing treatment. Drugs that interact with tyrosine kinase receptors, downstream signaling events, or tumor-supporting pathways in the microenvironment are under active investigation.

1. van der Gaag NA, Rauws EA, van Eijck CH, et al. Preoperative biliary drainage for cancer of the head of the pancreas. *N Engl J Med.* 2010;362:129-137.
2. Neoptolemos JP, Stocken DD, Friess H, et al. A randomized trial of chemoradiotherapy and chemotherapy after resection of pancreatic cancer. *N Engl J Med.* 2004;351:726.
3. Oettle H, Post S, Neuhaus P, et al. Adjuvant chemotherapy with gemcitabine vs observation in patients undergoing curative-intent resection of pancreatic cancer: a randomized controlled trial. *JAMA.* 2007;297:311-313.
4. Regine WF, Winter KA, Abrams RA, et al. Fluorouracil vs gemcitabine chemotherapy before and after fluorouracil-based chemoradiation following resection of pancreatic adenocarcinoma: a randomized controlled trial. *JAMA.* 2008;299:1019-1026.
5. Neoptolemos JP, Stocken DD, Bassi C, et al. Adjuvant chemotherapy with fluorouracil plus folinic acid vs gemcitabine following pancreatic cancer resection: a randomized controlled trial. *JAMA.* 2010;304:1073-1081.
6. Moore MJ, Goldstein D, Hamm J, et al. Erlotinib plus gemcitabine compared with gemcitabine alone in patients with advanced pancreatic cancer: a phase III trial of the National Cancer Institute of Canada Clinical Trials Group. *J Clin Oncol.* 2007;25:1960-1966.

SUGGESTED READINGS

Brand RE, Nolen BM, Zeh HJ, et al. Serum biomarker panels for the detection of pancreatic cancer. *Clin Cancer Res.* 2011;17:805-816. *Review of promising new approaches.*
Callery MP, Chang KJ, Fishman EK, et al. Pretreatment assessment of resectable and borderline resectable pancreas cancer: expert consensus statement. *Ann Surg Oncol.* 2009;16:1727-1733. *This is the first attempt to define criteria for high-risk resectable tumors.*
Greer JB, Brand RE. New developments in pancreatic cancer. *Curr Gastroenterol Rep.* 2011;13:131-139. *Review of etiology and diagnosis.*
Hidalgo M. Pancreatic cancer. *N Engl J Med.* 2010;362:1605-1617. *Review.*
Petersen GM, Amundadottir L, Fuchs CS, et al. A genome-wide association study identifies pancreatic cancer susceptibility loci on chromosomes 13q122.1, 1q32.1 and 5p15.33. *Nat Genet.* 2010;42:224-228. *Details results of extensive genome-wide association studies on germline DNA and identifies several new susceptibility loci.*
Thomas A, Dajani K, Neoptolemos JP, et al. Adjuvant therapy in pancreatic cancer. *Dig Dis.* 2010;28:684-692. *Review emphasizing 5-fluorouracil and gemcitabine.*

201

PANCREATIC ENDOCRINE TUMORS

ROBERT T. JENSEN

DEFINITION

Pancreatic endocrine tumors (PETs) are also called islet cell tumors; however, because the cell of origin of most is unknown, the general term PET is preferred. This term is also a misnomer because PETs can also occur outside the pancreas. Ten PETs are well established (Table 201-1). Other additional functional PET syndromes have been rarely reported: PETs secreting renin, PETs secreting erythropoietin, PETs secreting luteinizing hormone that causes virilization, and PETs secreting insulin-like growth factor II causing hypoglycemia. In addition, PETs synthesizing neurotensin, calcitonin, and ghrelin are reported, but no distinct syndrome has been described.

PETs frequently are classified as functional or nonfunctional (see Table 201-1) depending on whether a clinical syndrome resulting from the autonomously released hormone is present. Nonfunctional PETs frequently release hormones and peptides (pancreatic polypeptide, neurotensin, α- and β-subunits of human chorionic gonadotropin, neuron-specific enolase, chromogranin A and breakdown products) that cause no distinct clinical syndromes.

EPIDEMIOLOGY

PETs are uncommon, having a prevalence of less than ten cases per 1 million population. Insulinomas, gastrinomas, and nonfunctional PETs are the most common, with an incidence of one to three new cases per 1 million population.

PATHOBIOLOGY

All PETs share certain features. PETs are classified as APUDomas (amine precursor uptake and decarboxylation), which share cytochemical features with carcinoid tumors, melanomas, and other endocrine tumors (pheochromocytomas, medullary thyroid cancer). Except for insulinomas, these tumors are frequently malignant. All PETs appear similar histologically, with few mitotic figures. Ultrastructurally, they have dense granules containing peptides, amines, and products of neuroendocrine differentiation (neuron-specific enolase, chromogranins, synaptophysin). The presence of chromogranin immunoreactivity in the tumor is now widely used to identify these tumors as endocrine tumors.

Molecular studies show that PETs have a different pathogenesis than common gastrointestinal adenocarcinomas because they infrequently demonstrate alterations in common tumor suppressor genes (e.g., retinoblastoma gene, *p53*) or common oncogenes (*ras, c-Jun, c-Fos*). Alterations in p16^{INK4a}, the *MEN1* gene, and the expression of growth factors, as well as chromosomal losses (1q, 3p, 3q, 6p, X) and gains (17p, 17q, 20q), have been associated with a worse prognosis in numerous studies. A number of other factors have prognostic significance, the most important of which is the presence of liver metastases. Recently, a World Health Organization TNM grading and classification system has been proposed for PETs based on tumor size, presence of metastases, invasiveness, and proliferative indices and has been recently shown to have prognostic value in a number of studies.

Four autosomal dominant–inherited disorders are associated with an increased occurrence of PETs: multiple endocrine neoplasia type 1 (MEN 1; 80 to 100% develop PETs), von Hippel-Lindau disease (VHL; 10 to 17% have PETs), von Recklinghausen's disease (neurofibromatosis 1([NF-1]; 12% develop duodenal somatostatinomas), and tuberous sclerosis (<1% develop PETs).

FUNCTIONAL PANCREATIC ENDOCRINE TUMOR SYNDROMES
Zollinger-Ellison Syndrome (Gastrinomas)

DEFINITION AND EPIDEMIOLOGY

Zollinger-Ellison syndrome (ZES) is a clinical syndrome caused by a gastrin-releasing endocrine tumor usually located in the pancreas or duodenum and characterized by clinical symptoms and signs resulting from gastric acid

TABLE 201-1 PANCREATIC ENDOCRINE TUMORS

NAME OF TUMOR	NAME OF SYNDROME	MAIN SIGNS OR SYMPTOMS	LOCATION	MALIGNANCY (%)	HORMONE CAUSING SYNDROME
I. FUNCTIONAL PET					
Gastrinoma	Zollinger-Ellison syndrome	Abdominal pain, diarrhea, esophageal symptoms	Pancreas—30% Duodenum—60% Other—10%	60-90	Gastrin
Insulinoma	Insulinoma	Hypoglycemic symptoms	Pancreas—100%	5-15	Insulin
Glucagonoma	Glucagonoma	Dermatitis, diabetes/glucose intolerance, weight loss	Pancreas—100%	60	Glucagon
VIPoma	Verner-Morrison, pancreatic cholera, WDHA	Severe watery diarrhea, hypokalemia	Pancreas—90% Other—10% (neural, adrenal, periganglionic tissue)	80	Vasoactive intestinal peptide (VIP)
Somatostatinoma	Somatostatinoma	Diabetes mellitus, cholelithiasis, diarrhea	Pancreas—56% Duodenum/jejunum—44%	60	Somatostatin
GRFoma	GRFoma	Acromegaly	Pancreas—30% Lung—54% Jejunum—7% Other—13% (adrenal, foregut, retroperitoneum)	30	Growth hormone–releasing factor (GRF)
ACTHoma	ACTHoma	Cushing's syndrome	Pancreas—4-16% of all ectopic Cushing's cases	>95	Adrenocorticotropic hormone (ACTH)
PET causing carcinoid syndrome	PET causing carcinoid syndrome	Diarrhea, flushing	Pancreas—<1% of all carcinoids	60-90	Serotonin, tachykinins
PET causing hypercalcemia	PET causing hypercalcemia	Signs/symptoms of hypercalcemia	Pancreas (rare cause of hypercalcemia)	>85	PTHrP, other unknown
II. NONFUNCTIONAL PET					
Nonfunctioning PPoma	Nonfunctional PPoma	Weight loss, abdominal mass, hepatomegaly	Pancreas—100%	60-90	None: pancreatic polypeptide chromogranin released but no known symptoms due to hypersecretion

PET = pancreatic endocrine tumor; PP = pancreatic polypeptide; PTHrP = parathormone-related peptide; WDHA = watery diarrhea, hypokalemia, and achlorhydria.

hypersecretion (peptic ulcer disease, diarrhea, esophageal reflux disease). ZES occurs most frequently between the ages of 35 and 65 years and is slightly more common in men (60%).

PATHOBIOLOGY

In recent surgical series, gastrinomas occur two to five times more frequently in the duodenum than in the pancreas. Duodenal gastrinomas are generally small (<1cm), whereas pancreatic gastrinomas are generally larger. Occasionally ZES results from a gastrinoma in the splenic hilum, mesentery, stomach, or only in a lymph node or in the ovary. Extrapancreatic gastrinomas producing ZES have been reported in the heart and as a result of small cell lung cancer. As with other PETs, malignancy can be reliably determined only by demonstrating the presence of metastatic disease, and no light microscopic or ultrastructural finding can clearly establish malignant behavior.

Gastrin stimulates parietal cells to secrete acid and also has a growth effect on cells of the gastric mucosa. Chronic hypergastrinemia thus leads to increased gastric mucosal thickness, prominent gastric folds, and increased numbers of parietal cells and gastric enterochromaffin-like cells. Patients with gastrinomas have increased basal and maximal acid outputs. *Helicobacter pylori* appears not to be important in the pathogenesis of the ulcer disease in ZES, in contrast to that of routine peptic ulcers (Chapter 141). Diarrhea is common because the large-volume gastric acid output leads to structural damage to the small intestine (inflammation, blunted villi, edema), interference with fat transport, inactivation of pancreatic lipase, and precipitation of bile acids. These same mechanisms, if prolonged, can lead to steatorrhea. If acid hypersecretion is controlled, the diarrhea will stop.

CLINICAL MANIFESTATIONS

Abdominal pain resulting from a peptic ulcer is the most common symptom (>80%). Most ulcers occur in the duodenum (>85%), but they occasionally occur in the postbulbar area, jejunum, or stomach, or in multiple locations. Initially, the pain is usually similar to that of patients with typical peptic ulcers

(Chapter 141). With time, the symptoms become persistent and, in general, respond poorly to treatments aimed at eliminating *H. pylori* and to conventional doses of histamine-2 receptor antagonists, as well as to the now rarely used surgical treatments for ulcer disease. By comparison, conventional doses of proton pump inhibitors (PPIs) (e.g., omeprazole, lansoprazole, pantoprazole, esomeprazole, rabeprazole) can mask the symptoms of most patients with ZES and can also cause hypergastrinemia as seen in ZES. The widespread use of PPIs has delayed the diagnosis of ZES.

Heartburn is also common (20%). Diarrhea (60 to 70%) occurs frequently and may be the first symptom (10 to 20%). Twenty to 25% of ZES patients have MEN 1 (Chapter 239). These patients have hyperplasia or tumors of multiple endocrine glands (parathyroid hyperplasia [>90%], pituitary tumors [60%], and PETs [80 to 100%]). In MEN 1, ZES is the most common functional PET syndrome (54%), although patients typically first develop renal stones related to hypercalcemia from hyperparathyroidism or have elevated prolactin levels resulting from pituitary tumors and only later develop ZES. However, studies show that 20 to 40% of patients with MEN and ZES initially present with ZES symptoms.

In ZES patients, almost all the symptoms result from the effects of gastric acid hypersecretion, but late in the disease, patients can have tumor-related symptoms. Approximately one third of patients have metastatic liver disease at presentation, but less than 20% of other patients develop metastatic disease to the liver during a 10-year follow-up period.

Up to 5% of patients with ZES develop Cushing's syndrome (Chapter 234) as a result of adrenocorticotropic hormone (ACTH) secretion by the gastrinoma. These patients usually have a metastatic gastrinoma in the liver, ZES without MEN 1, and a poor prognosis.

DIAGNOSIS

ZES should be suspected in any patient whose peptic ulcer disease is accompanied by diarrhea, is recurrent, does not heal with treatment, is not associated with *H. pylori* infection, is associated with a complication (bleeding, obstruction, esophageal stricture), is multiple or occurs in unusual locations, or is associated with a pancreatic tumor. ZES should also be suspected in patients with chronic secretory diarrhea (Chapter 142), peptic ulcer disease associated with large gastric folds, a family or personal history of renal stones or endocrinopathies, or the laboratory finding of hypercalcemia, hypergastrinemia, or gastric acid hypersecretion.

When suspected, the initial test is a fasting serum gastrin level, which is elevated in 99 to 100% of ZES patients. However, other causes of hypergastrinemia include renal failure, *H. pylori* infections, and a physiologic response to achlorhydria or hypochlorhydria because of pernicious anemia, atrophic gastritis, or the use of PPIs. If the serum gastrin level is elevated, the fasting gastric pH should be determined. If the serum gastrin is more than 1000 pg/mL (normal, <100) and the pH is less than 2.0, the patient almost certainly has ZES; approximately 40% of patients have this combination. If the gastrin is increased more than ten-fold and the pH is less than 2.0, basal acid output and a secretin test should be performed. Basal acid output is increased in patients with ZES, and more than 95% have a value greater than 15 mEq/hour if no previous gastric acid–reducing surgery has been performed. Because of their long duration of action, PPIs must be stopped for at least 1 week, if possible, to ensure that the cause of the hypergastrinemia is not the drug itself.

Differential Diagnosis

A secretin test can exclude *H. pylori* infection, retained gastric-antrum syndrome, antral G-cell hyperfunction or hyperplasia, chronic renal failure, and gastric outlet obstruction that may mimic ZES. Physiologically normal individuals show a less than 120 pg/mL increase in the gastrin level after intravenous secretin, whereas 94% of ZES patients with a fasting gastrin level that is elevated less than ten-fold above normal have a positive test. No false-positive results are reported, except in patients with achlorhydria. In all patients with ZES, evaluation must exclude MEN 1 syndrome by searching for other endocrinopathies and assessing family history.

Imaging and Endoscopy

All patients should have imaging studies to localize the tumor. Somatostatin receptor scintigraphy using single photon emission computed tomography after injection of indium-111–[diethylenetriamine pentaacetic acid-D-phenylalanine-1] octreotide is the localization method of choice; it identifies 60% of primary gastrinomas and more than 90% of patients with metastatic liver disease with a sensitivity equal to all conventional imaging studies (magnetic resonance imaging [MRI], computed tomography [CT], ultrasound, angiography) combined. For pancreatic gastrinomas, endoscopic ultrasound is particularly sensitive. Small duodenal gastrinomas (<1 cm) are frequently not detected by an imaging modality but can be found at surgery if routine duodenotomy is performed. Recent studies show that two new imaging techniques may be useful for small gastrinomas and other PETs: the use of hybrid scanning with CT or MRI and somatostatin receptor scintigraphy (SRS) and the use of positron emission tomographic scanning, especially with gallium-68-labeled somatostatin analogues.

TREATMENT   Rx

Medical Therapy

Patients need medical therapy directed at controlling the gastric acid hypersecretion and, if possible, surgical therapy to remove the gastrinoma. PPIs are now the drugs of choice. Because of their long duration of action, acid hypersecretion can be controlled in all patients with once- or twice-daily doses. The recommended starting dose for omeprazole is 60 mg once a day. In 30% of patients, higher doses are needed, particularly in patients with MEN 1, previous gastric surgery, or a history of severe esophageal reflux. Patients must be treated indefinitely unless surgically cured. Long-term therapy is safe, and patients have been treated for up to 20 years with omeprazole without loss of efficacy, although reduced vitamin B$_{12}$ levels may occur and require vitamin B$_{12}$ supplementation (Chapter 167). Histamine-2 receptor antagonists are also effective, but frequent (every 4 to 6 hours) high doses are needed. Total gastrectomy, the historical treatment, is now performed only for patients who cannot or will not take oral antisecretory medications. Selective vagotomy reduces acid secretion, but many patients continue to require a low dose of drug. Parathyroidectomy should be performed in MEN 1 patients with hyperparathyroidism and ZES because it reduces acid secretion and increases the sensitivity to antisecretory drugs.

Surgical Therapy

Surgical exploration for cure is recommended in all patients without liver metastases, MEN 1, or complicating medical conditions that limit life expectancy. Tumors are found by experienced endocrine surgeons in 95% of patients at surgery. Surgical resection decreases the metastatic rate, increases survival, and results in a 5-year cure rate of 30%. Patients with metastatic gastrinoma in the liver have a poor prognosis, with a 5-year survival rate of 30%.

Metastatic Disease

If the metastatic disease is slowly increasing in size or is symptomatic, treatment with octreotide (100 to 450 µg two to three times daily) alone or in combination with interferon-α (1 to 5 million U 3 to 7 days/week) is effective in inhibiting further tumor growth in 50 to 60% of patients. If this treatment fails or if the tumor is rapidly growing, chemotherapeutic agents (streptozotocin, 5-fluorouracil, doxorubicin) are recommended. For patients with extensive metastatic disease, somatostatin receptor–directed radiation therapy using analogues labeled with yttrium-90, lutetium-177, or indium-111 is increasingly used. Newer treatments targeting PETs using radiolabeled somatostatin analogues or targeting PET growth factors or their receptors, intracellular signaling cascades (mTor), and a DTIC-related compound, temozolomide, show some promise in a small number of gastrinomas and other PET patients. Liver transplantation is occasionally performed in the rare patient with metastases limited to the liver.

PROGNOSIS

Approximately 25% of gastrinomas show aggressive growth. The most important prognostic predictor is the development of liver metastases. The presence of a large primary tumor, a pancreatic tumor, bone metastases, development of ectopic Cushing's syndrome, or a high fasting gastrin level is associated with aggressive growth.

Glucagonomas

DEFINITION

Glucagonomas are endocrine tumors of the pancreas that ectopically secrete glucagons, causing a specific syndrome (see Table 201-1).

PATHOBIOLOGY

Glucagon hypersecretion explains the glucose intolerance. The exact origin of the rash is unclear; some studies report that prolonged glucagon infusions can cause the characteristic skin lesions. A role for possible zinc deficiency has been proposed because of the similarity of the rash to that seen with zinc deficiency (acrodermatitis enteropathica) and because the rash improves in some patients who are given zinc. The hypoaminoacidemia is thought to be secondary to the effect of glucagon on amino acid metabolism by altering gluconeogenesis. The wasting and weight loss are intrinsic parts of the glucagonoma syndrome, and recent studies suggest that a novel anorectic substance distinct from glucagon is responsible.

CLINICAL MANIFESTATIONS

The cardinal clinical features are a distinct dermatitis (necrolytic migratory erythema, seen in 70 to 90%), diabetes mellitus and glucose intolerance (40 to 90%), weight loss (70 to 96%), anemia (30 to 85%), hypoaminoacidemia (80 to 90%) with deficiencies of essential fatty acids, thromboembolism (10 to 25%), diarrhea (15 to 30%), and psychiatric disturbances (0 to 20%). The characteristic skin rash is usually found at intertriginous and periorificial sites, especially in the groin and buttocks (Fig. 201-1). It is initially erythematous, becomes raised, and develops central bullae whose tops detach, with the eroded areas becoming crusty. Healing occurs with hyperpigmentation.

DIAGNOSIS

The diagnosis is established by demonstrating elevated plasma glucagon levels. Normal levels are 150 to 200 pg/mL; in patients with glucagonomas, levels usually (>90%) are higher than 1000 pg/mL. However, in some recent studies, up to 40% of patients had plasma glucagon values of 500 to 1000 pg/mL. Increased plasma glucagon levels also occur in renal insufficiency, acute pancreatitis, hypercorticism, hepatic diseases, celiac disease, severe stress and prolonged fasting, in patients treated with danazol, and in familial hyperglucagonemia. In these conditions, the level is usually less than 500 pg/mL except in patients with hepatic diseases or in those with familial hyperglucagonemia.

FIGURE 201-1. A patient with a glucagonoma with the characteristic rash (necrolytic migratory erythema). The rash is usually at intertriginous areas or periorificial sites and shows various stages of erythema, blistering, and crusting. (From Forbes CD, Jackson WF. *Color Atlas and Text of Clinical Medicine*, 3rd ed. London: Mosby; 2003.)

Glucagonomas are generally large when discovered (mean, 5 to 10 cm), and they most frequently occur in the pancreatic tail (>50%). Liver metastases are commonly present at the time of diagnosis (45 to 80%).

TREATMENT   Rx

Subcutaneous administration of the synthetic long-acting somatostatin analogue, octreotide (100 to 400 micrograms two to three times daily), controls the rash in 80% of patients and improves weight loss, diarrhea, and hypoaminoacidemia, but it usually does not improve the diabetes mellitus. Increasingly, long-acting depot formulations of octreotide (octreotide-LAR) or lanreotide autogel are being given by monthly injection. Zinc supplementation and infusions of amino acids or fatty acids, or both, can diminish the severity of the rash. After tumor localization, surgical resection is preferred; even debulking of metastatic tumor may be of benefit. For advanced disease, chemotherapy (with dacarbazine or streptozotocin and doxorubicin), hepatic embolization, or chemoembolization may control symptoms in refractory cases.

PROGNOSIS

The prognosis is now largely determined by the growth of the tumor per se because the symptoms of glucagon excess can be largely controlled by somatostatin analogues. This is particularly true with glucagonomas because in many series more than 50 to 80% are metastatic at presentation, and patients usually present late with large primary tumors. The mean 5-year survival rate is 50%; however, extended survivals (>15 years) are reported in some patients with treatment with somatostatin analogues and other tumor-directed therapies.

VIPomas

DEFINITION

The VIPoma syndrome, also called the Verner-Morrison syndrome, pancreatic cholera, and the WDHA syndrome (for watery diarrhea, hypokalemia, and achlorhydria), results from an endocrine tumor, usually in the pancreas that ectopically secretes vasoactive intestinal polypeptide (VIP).

EPIDEMIOLOGY AND PATHOBIOLOGY

VIPomas in adults are found in the pancreas in 80 to 90% of cases; rare cases result from intestinal carcinoids, ganglioneuromas, ganglioneuroblastomas, and pheochromocytomas. In children younger than 10 years and rarely in adults (<5%), the VIPoma syndrome is caused by ganglioneuromas or ganglioneuroblastomas at extrapancreatic sites. VIPomas are usually large and solitary; 50 to 75% of these tumors occur in the pancreatic tail, and 40 to 70% have metastasized at diagnosis. VIPomas frequently secrete both VIP and peptide histidine methionine, but VIP is responsible for the symptoms. VIP is a potent stimulant of secretion in the small and large intestine, which causes the cardinal clinical features of the VIPoma syndrome. VIP also causes relaxation of gastrointestinal smooth muscle, and this may contribute to the dilated loops of bowel that are common in this syndrome as well as a dilated, atonic gallbladder that is sometimes seen. Hypochlorhydria is thought to result from the inhibitory effect of VIP on acid secretion, the flushing is related to the vasodilatory effects of VIP, and the hyperglycemia is caused by the glycogenolytic effect of VIP. The mechanism of the hypercalcemia remains unclear.

CLINICAL MANIFESTATIONS

The cardinal clinical feature is severe, large-volume, watery diarrhea (>1 L/day) (100%), which is secretory and occurs during fasting. Hypokalemia (67 to 100%) and dehydration (83%) commonly occur because of the volume of the diarrhea. Achlorhydria is occasionally noted, but hypochlorhydria is usually found (34 to 72% of cases). Flushing occurs in 20% of patients, hyperglycemia in 25 to 50%, and hypercalcemia in 41 to 50%. Steatorrhea is uncommon (16%) despite the volume of diarrhea.

DIAGNOSIS

The diarrhea of VIPomas characteristically persists during fasting and is large in volume (>3 L/day in 70 to 80%); the diagnosis is excluded when fasting stool volume is less than 700 mL/day. To differentiate VIPomas from other causes of large-volume, fasting diarrhea, fasting plasma VIP levels should be determined. The normal value in most laboratories is less than 190 pg/mL, and elevated levels are present in 90 to 100% of patients in various series. The differential diagnosis of large-volume, fasting diarrhea (>700 mL/day) includes ZES, diffuse islet cell hyperplasia, surreptitious use of laxatives, the pseudopancreatic cholera syndrome, and, rarely, human immunodeficiency virus (HIV) infection (Chapter 397). Serum gastrin levels identify patients with ZES, and plasma VIP levels are normal in most patients who abuse laxatives, in 82% of patients with pancreatic islet cell hyperplasias, and in patients with HIV-induced secretory diarrhea.

TREATMENT   Rx

The symptoms caused by the VIP are controlled initially in more than 85% of patients by daily doses of octreotide (50 to 400 µg once to three times daily) or by monthly injections of the depot form, octreotide-LAR or lanreotide autogel, but increased doses may be needed over time. Before the availability of octreotide, small numbers of patients were reported to respond to a variety of agents, including high-dose prednisone (60 to 100 mg/day; 40 to 50%), clonidine, lithium carbonate, indomethacin, loperamide, metoclopramide, and phenothiazines. After tumor localization studies, surgical resection should be attempted if it is possible to remove all visible tumor; however, more than 50% of patients have generalized liver metastases at diagnosis, so complete resection may not be possible. For patients with advanced cases and refractory symptoms, chemotherapy with streptozotocin and doxorubicin, hepatic chemoembolization, and hepatic embolization have been beneficial.

PROGNOSIS

The prognosis is now largely determined by the growth of the tumor per se because the symptoms of VIP excess can be largely controlled by somatostatin analogues. This is particularly true in patients with VIPomas because they frequently (>50%) present with advanced metastatic disease. The mean 5-year survival is 50 to 70%.

Somatostatinomas

DEFINITION AND PATHOBIOLOGY

Somatostatinomas are endocrine tumors that occur in the pancreas or upper small intestine and ectopically secrete somatostatin. In the gastrointestinal tract, somatostatin inhibits basal and stimulated acid secretion, pancreatic secretion, intestinal absorption of amino acids, gallbladder contractility, and release of numerous hormones, including cholecystokinin and gastrin.

CLINICAL MANIFESTATIONS

Most reported somatostatinomas are diagnosed histologically as an endocrine tumor containing somatostatin-like immunoreactivity and are not associated with a distinct clinical syndrome (the somatostatinoma syndrome). The somatostatinoma syndrome includes diabetes mellitus, gallbladder disease, diarrhea, steatorrhea, and weight loss. Sixty percent of somatostatinomas occur in the pancreas, and 40% are found in the duodenum or jejunum. Pancreatic somatostatinomas occur in the pancreatic head in 60 to 80% of cases; 70 to 92% have metastasized at diagnosis, and they are usually large (mean, 5 cm) and solitary. In contrast, duodenal somatostatinomas are smaller (mean, 2.4 cm), frequently associated with psammoma bodies on histologic examination (11%), and less frequently have metastases at diagnosis (30 to 40%).

The somatostatinoma syndrome occurs much more commonly (80 to 95% of all cases) in patients with pancreatic than duodenal or intestinal somatostatinomas. Duodenal somatostatinomas occur in up to 10% of patients with von Recklinghausen's disease and are usually asymptomatic.

DIAGNOSIS

Somatostatinomas are usually found by accident, particularly during exploratory laparotomy for cholecystectomy, during endoscopy, or on imaging studies. The presence of psammoma bodies on histologic examination of a duodenal endocrine tumor or any duodenal lesions in patients with von Recklinghausen's disease should raise the suspicion of a duodenal somatostatinoma. The diagnosis of the somatostatinoma syndrome requires the demonstration of increased concentrations of somatostatin-like immunoreactivity in the plasma and the resected tumor. However, other tumors outside the pancreas or intestine, such as small cell lung cancer, medullary thyroid carcinoma, pheochromocytomas, and paragangliomas, may also have elevated concentrations of somatostatin-like immunoreactivity. Somatostatinomas can be imaged using somatostatin receptor scintigraphy or, if needed, other conventional imaging studies to assess the tumor's location.

TREATMENT Rx

Treatment with octreotide or lanreotide can improve symptoms. Surgery, if possible, or chemotherapy, hepatic chemoembolization, or hepatic embolization may be of value.

PROGNOSIS

Patients with intestinal somatostatinomas, which uncommonly cause the somatostatinoma syndrome and are less malignant, have an excellent prognosis (5-year survival rate, >80%), whereas those with pancreatic somatostatinomas, which frequently cause the somatostatinoma syndrome and present with metastatic disease (>70%), have a much reduced 5-year survival rate (<50%).

GRFomas

DEFINITION

GRFomas are endocrine tumors that frequently originate in the pancreas but also occur in other extrapancreatic locations and ectopically release growth hormone–releasing factor (GRF). The GRF causes acromegaly that is clinically indistinguishable from that caused by a pituitary adenoma.

PATHOBIOLOGY

GRFomas most commonly occur in the lung (54%). Most of the remainder occur in the gastrointestinal tract, including 30% in the pancreas. Pancreatic GRFomas are usually large (mean, 6 cm), 39% are metastatic at diagnosis, 40% occur in combination with ZES, and 33% are in patients with MEN1.

DIAGNOSIS

GRFomas are an uncommon cause of acromegaly. These tumors occurred in none of 177 unselected patients with acromegaly in one study. However, any patient with acromegaly and abdominal complaints, with acromegaly but no pituitary tumor, or with acromegaly and hyperprolactinemia (which occurs in 70% of GRFomas) should be suspected of having a GRFoma. The intraabdominal features of GRFomas result from its metastases and are typical of any malignant PET. The diagnosis is confirmed by performing a plasma assay for GRF and growth hormone.

TREATMENT

The effects of the GRF can be controlled with octreotide or lanreotide in more than 90% of patients. Treatment should be directed at the GRFoma per se, as described for the other more common PETs.

Nonfunctional Pancreatic Endocrine Tumors

DEFINITION

Nonfunctional PETs are endocrine tumors that originate in the pancreas and either secrete no peptides or secrete products that do not cause clinical symptoms.

PATHOBIOLOGY

Frequently secreted, nonfunctional peptides include chromogranin A (100%), pancreatic polypeptide (60%), and the α-subunit (40%) and β-subunit of human chorionic gonadotrophin. Immunocytochemically, even higher percentages contain these peptides as well as insulin (50%), glucagons (30%), and somatostatin (13%).

CLINICAL MANIFESTATIONS

Nonfunctional PETs are frequently diagnosed only late in the course of disease after the patient presents with symptoms or signs of metastatic disease and a liver biopsy reveals metastatic PET. Any symptoms or signs result from the tumor per se and include abdominal pain (36 to 56%), abdominal mass or hepatosplenomegaly (8 to 40%), weight loss or cachexia (8 to 46%), and jaundice (27 to 40%). In 20% of asymptomatic patients, tumors are found incidentally at surgery.

DIAGNOSIS

Any patients with a long survival (>5 years) after a diagnosis of metastatic pancreatic adenocarcinoma should be suspected of having a nonfunctional PET. Most primary tumors are large (70% are >5 cm), and 70% occur in the pancreatic head. Liver metastases are frequent (38 to 62%) at presentation. An elevated plasma chromogranin A or pancreatic polypeptide level or a positive somatostatin receptor scintigraphic scan is strong evidence that a pancreatic mass is a PET. Malignancy correlates with vascular or perineural invasion, a proliferative index of more than 2%, a mitotic rate of 2 or higher, a size of at least 4 cm, capsular penetration, nuclear atypia, lack of progesterone receptors, and the presence of calcitonin immunoreactivity in the tumor.

TREATMENT Rx

Tumor localization, surgical resection, and, for advanced cases, chemotherapy with streptozotocin and doxorubicin, hepatic embolization, or chemoembolization are useful. Survival is better in patients with smaller tumors, patients who are asymptomatic at presentation, patients with no metastases, and patients in whom surgical resection can be performed.

Two novel agents have been recently found to prolong progression-free and probably overall survival in patients with advanced pancreatic neuroendocrine tumors, major proportions of which were nonfunctional. The multitargeted tyrosine kinase inhibitor sunitinib was administered by a daily oral dose of 37.5 mg; the oral inhibitor of mTOR, everolimus, was given at a dose of 10 mg once daily.

PROGNOSIS

The overall 5-year survival rate varies in different series from 30 to 70%, but it is heavily dependent on the extent of the disease at diagnosis, with survival rates of 96% in patients without metastases at presentation, decreasing to 30 to 50% for those with metastatic disease.

ACTHomas and Other Uncommon Tumors

PETs that ectopically secrete ACTH cause 4 to 16% of the cases of ectopic Cushing's syndrome. Cushing's syndrome (Chapter 234) occurs in 5% of all cases of ZES, but in patients with sporadic ZES, it is a late feature, occurring with metastatic liver disease. Its development is associated with a poor prognosis, and the response to chemotherapy is generally poor; however, occasional patients benefit from the use of long-acting somatostatin analogues (octreotide, lanreotide).

Paraneoplastic hypercalcemia (Chapter 186) can result from a PET that releases parathormone-related peptide or an unknown hypercalcemic substance. Tumors are generally large with metastatic liver disease at diagnosis. Somatostatin analogues may help control the hypercalcemia, but surgery, chemotherapy, hepatic embolization, and chemoembolization are the mainstays of treatment.

PETs causing the carcinoid syndrome (Chapter 240) are usually large, and 68 to 88% are malignant. Octreotide may control the symptoms. Surgery, chemotherapy, or hepatic embolization or chemoembolization may be helpful.

A single case of a PET that secreted renin manifested with severe hypertension; the tumor was localized with somatostatin receptor scintigraphy, and the patient's symptoms improved significantly after tumor resection. A single case of an erythropoietin-secreting PET resulting in polycythemia and a single case of a PET secreting insulin-like growth factor II causing hypoglycemia have been described.

Two symptomatic cases of PETs that secreted luteinizing hormone have been described; virilization occurred in the female patient, whereas the male patient had increased acne and a skin rash. In both cases, the tumors were resectable, and symptoms improved postoperatively.

1. Raymond E, Dahan L, Raoul JL, et al. Sunitinib malate for the treatment of pancreatic neuroendocrine tumors. *N Engl J Med.* 2011;364:501-513.
2. Yao JC, Shah MH, Ito T, et al. Everolimus for advanced pancreatic neuroendocrine tumor. *N Engl J Med.* 2011;364:514-523.

SUGGESTED READINGS

Kuiper P, Verspaget HW, Overbeek LI, et al. An overview of the current diagnosis and recent developments in neuroendocrine tumors of the gastroenteropancreatic tract: the diagnostic approach. *Neth J Med.* 2011;69:14-20. *Review of epidemioloty, pathology, and diagnosis.*
Oberg K. Pancreatic endocrine tumors. *Semin Oncol.* 2010;37:594-618. *Review of diagnosis and treatment.*
Wilcox CM, Seay T, Arcury JT, et al. Zollinger-Ellison syndrome: presentation, response to therapy, and outcome. *Dig Liver Dis.* 2011. [Epub ahead of print.] *In a case series, symptoms preceded diagnosis by a median of 9 years and survival was principally related to underlying comorbidity.*

202

LIVER AND BILIARY TRACT TUMORS

LEWIS R. ROBERTS

TABLE 202-1 LIVER AND BILIARY TRACT TUMORS

TUMOR	CHARACTERISTICS ON IMAGING
BENIGN TUMORS USUALLY REQUIRING OBSERVATION ONLY	
Cavernous hemangioma	Peripheral enhancement filling into the center on delayed contrast imaging
Focal nodular hyperplasia	Rapid arterial enhancement with return to isointensity in venous phase; possible central scar with feeding vessel
Simple cyst	Hypoechoic on ultrasound
Focal fatty change	Best characterized by in- and out-of-phase sequences on magnetic resonance imaging
Angiolipoma	Arterial enhancement on contrast imaging
BENIGN TUMORS REQUIRING FURTHER EVALUATION AND TREATMENT	
Hepatic adenoma	Heterogeneous lesion with rapid arterial enhancement
Nodular regenerative hyperplasia	Nonspecific and variable
Cystadenoma	Cystic lesion on ultrasonography with solid components, enhancement of cyst wall; possible septations
Hepatic abscess (Chapter 154)	Cystic lesion on ultrasonography
Inflammatory pseudotumor	Atypical enhancing mass on contrast imaging
Echinococcal cyst (Chapter 154)	Cystic mass with septations, calcified rims, daughter cysts
MALIGNANT TUMORS REQUIRING APPROPRIATE MANAGEMENT	
Hepatocellular carcinoma	Arterial enhancement with portal venous "washout"
Cholangiocarcinoma	Late arterial enhancement that persists in portal phase
Mixed hepatocellular-cholangiocarcinoma	Early to late arterial enhancement
Liver metastases	Peripheral arterial enhancement, usually bilobar, multifocal disease
Cystadenocarcinoma	Solid enhancing mass in cystic lesion
Sarcoma	Solid mass with arterial enhancement
Mixed hepatic tumor	Solid mass with arterial enhancement; possible areas of calcification
Non-Hodgkin's lymphoma (Chapter 191)	Less intense arterial enhancement than hepatocellular carcinoma; possibly diffuse or mimicking hepatocellular carcinoma with venous invasion

Liver and biliary tract tumors are a diverse group of benign and malignant tumors that arise from the different epithelial and stromal tissues of the liver. Various malignant diseases of other tissues metastasize to the liver or extend into or metastasize to the vicinity of the biliary tract, but not all mass lesions of the liver and biliary tract are malignant (Table 202-1).

EVALUATION OF MASS LESIONS OF THE LIVER

Diagnostic Approach

Mass lesions of the liver can be classified as benign lesions usually requiring observation only, benign lesions requiring further evaluation and treatment, or malignant lesions requiring appropriate management (see Table 202-1). The clinical approach to liver mass lesions requires careful history taking, physical examination, appropriate laboratory and imaging studies, judicious use of liver biopsy for histologic confirmation, and optimal management that considers the patient's age and comorbidities (Fig. 202-1).

History and Physical Examination

Because of the increasing use of imaging techniques for the evaluation of abdominal symptoms, many mass lesions of the liver are discovered incidentally as a result of imaging performed to evaluate nonhepatic diseases, such as abdominal pain or discomfort (Chapter 134). Right upper quadrant discomfort is frequently nonspecific and unhelpful in the evaluation of liver masses. Nevertheless, large liver masses may distend the liver capsule and cause pain, which is occasionally referred to the right

shoulder. Patients also may present with episodes of acute, severe pain, which results from bleeding into a hepatic adenoma, a primary hepatocellular carcinoma, or the liver surrounding the lesion. Patients with advanced malignant disease and regional lymph metastases may present with epigastric pain.

Patients with malignant liver disease, whether primary or metastatic, frequently present with constitutional symptoms, which include night sweats, low-grade fever, unintended weight loss, anorexia, and diarrhea. In the United States, the most common malignant lesions in the liver are metastases from other primary cancers, including the esophagus, stomach, colon, pancreas, breast, lung, neuroendocrine, kidney, bladder, and skin cancer. Patients with hepatocellular carcinoma often have symptoms related to their underlying liver disease, such as fatigue from chronic hepatitis or ascites, spontaneous bacterial peritonitis, variceal bleeding, or hepatic encephalopathy resulting from cirrhosis with portal hypertension. Patients with cholangiocarcinoma may present with jaundice from a dominant stricture or with episodes of acute cholangitis in the setting of primary or secondary sclerosing cholangitis (Chapter 158).

When available, previous imaging studies of the liver can be helpful in determining whether a liver lesion is new or enlarging. The patient's characteristics, including age, sex, history of oral contraceptive use (associated with an increased incidence of hepatic adenomas), geographic residence, travel history (relevant in cases of amebic liver abscess and hydatid cysts), alcohol

FIGURE 202-1. Approach to evaluating the patient with a mass lesion in the liver. Flow chart showing an algorithm for evaluating and managing common liver mass lesions. CT = computed tomography; MRI = magnetic resonance imaging.

consumption, and comorbid illnesses (e.g., association between chronic hepatitis or liver cirrhosis and hepatocellular carcinoma; association between ulcerative colitis or primary sclerosing cholangitis and cholangiocarcinoma) can also provide clues to the diagnosis.

On physical examination, patients with chronic liver disease typically have cutaneous stigmata (spider angiomas and palmar erythema), splenomegaly, and bilobar enlargement of the liver or caudate lobe hypertrophy. They may also have an abdominal bruit over a vascular hepatocellular carcinoma. Patients with metastatic disease may have peripheral or intra-abdominal lymphadenopathy or palpable peritoneal carcinomatosis. Jaundice, peripheral edema, and ascites are nonspecific features that may be related to benign or malignant liver disease.

Laboratory Findings

Laboratory studies are often useful in determining the nature of a liver mass or its underlying cause. Laboratory features of chronic liver disease include the following: thrombocytopenia; elevated levels of serum aminotransferase (elevated in active inflammatory liver disease or infiltrative neoplastic diseases), alkaline phosphatase, and bilirubin (markedly elevated in bile duct obstruction from biliary tumor or mass effect; Chapter 149); and low serum albumin levels and an elevated prothrombin time (abnormal in chronic liver disease). Viral markers (e.g., hepatitis B surface antigen and antibody, hepatitis B e antigen and antibody, hepatitis B virus DNA, and hepatitis C antibody and hepatitis C virus RNA), iron studies, and autoimmune markers (e.g., antimitochondrial antibody, antinuclear antibody, and anti–smooth muscle antibody) often help to determine the cause of chronic liver disease. Finally, tumor markers such as α-fetoprotein (AFP; hepatocellular carcinoma), CA-19-9 (cholangiocarcinoma), carcinoembryonic antigen (colorectal metastases or cholangiocarcinoma), and lactate dehydrogenase (lymphoma) have variable sensitivity and utility as screening tests but may be useful in confirming the diagnosis or in predicting prognosis.

COMMON BENIGN TUMORS OF THE LIVER
Cavernous Hemangioma

EPIDEMIOLOGY

Cavernous hemangioma, which is the most common benign tumor of the liver, is present in up to 7% of individuals in autopsy studies. There is a female predominance of 1.5 : 1 to 5 : 1, and hemangiomas are more common in multiparous women. Hemangiomas are multicentric in up to 30% of cases.

CLINICAL MANIFESTATIONS

Cavernous hemangiomas are usually asymptomatic, although large, subcapsular hemangiomas may cause abdominal pain or discomfort. Thrombosis of giant hemangiomas (>10 cm) may cause systemic features of inflammation such as fever, weight loss, and anemia.

Rarely, large hemangiomas are associated with the Kasabach-Merritt syndrome, which is local or disseminated intravascular coagulation with thrombocytopenia, hypofibrinogenemia, and increased fibrin degradation products, usually seen initially in infants (Chapter 178). Most cavernous hemangiomas remain stable over time, and malignant transformation does not occur. Rupture of cavernous hemangiomas is exceedingly rare, considering the high prevalence of hepatic hemangiomas.

DIAGNOSIS
Imaging

Hepatic cavernous hemangiomas have characteristic imaging features. On *ultrasound,* they appear as well-circumscribed, homogeneously hyperechoic lesions with smooth margins. Hemangiomas may also appear hypoechoic in fatty livers. Atypical features include hypoechoic lesions with a thin hyperechoic rim or a thick rind and scalloped borders.

On *dynamic contrast-enhanced multiphasic computed tomography* (CT), hemangiomas are hypoattenuating lesions on nonenhanced scans, with peripheral nodular enhancement during the arterial phase and later filling in toward the center of the lesion. On *contrast magnetic resonance imaging* (MRI) *with gadolinium*, hemangiomas appear as homogeneous, low-intensity lesions on T1-weighted images and as sharply demarcated, hyperintense lesions on T2-weighted images. In the arterial phase, peripheral enhancement occurs and fills in toward the center of the lesion on delayed images.

Technetium-99m-labeled red blood cell scintigraphy is very specific for hemangiomas. It shows low perfusion on early images and a high concentration of isotope that completely fills the lesion on late images. Larger hemangiomas that are complicated by fibrosis, thrombosis, or bleeding may have incomplete filling in on contrast or technetium-99m studies.

Because the imaging features are often characteristic, biopsy is seldom needed to confirm the diagnosis. Biopsy is occasionally useful for small indeterminate lesions and for large lesions with scarring and atypical imaging features. Histologic examination shows a network of vascular spaces lined by endothelial cells and separated by a thin, fibrous stroma. Large hemangiomas may have areas of thrombosis, scarring, and calcification.

TREATMENT   Rx

Observation is the optimal management for most patients with asymptomatic hemangiomas. Surgical enucleation or anatomic resection is recommended for hemangiomas that cause significant pain, enlarge over time, are of uncertain diagnosis, or are associated with the Kasabach-Merritt syndrome. Rarely, liver transplantation has been used for massive unresectable hepatic hemangiomas, particularly in the presence of Kasabach-Merritt syndrome.

Focal Nodular Hyperplasia

DEFINITION

Focal nodular hyperplasia is a benign reaction to a congenital arterial malformation within the liver. The lesion typically consists of a vascular stellate scar with connective tissue, bile ductules surrounded by proliferated hepatocytes, and Kupffer cells separated by fibrous septa.

EPIDEMIOLOGY

Focal nodular hyperplasia occurs predominantly in women of childbearing age. The relationship with oral contraceptive use is controversial; some studies suggest an association of long-term oral contraceptive use with focal nodular hyperplasia and with complications such as hemorrhage or infarction. However, discontinuation of oral contraceptive use usually does not lead to resolution of focal nodular hyperplasia. There is a female predominance of 2 : 1 to 4 : 1, and the lesions are typically diagnosed in women aged 20 to 50 years. Focal nodular hyperplasias are occasionally multiple (10 to 20%) or are associated with cavernous hemangiomas (20%).

CLINICAL MANIFESTATIONS

Most focal nodular hyperplasias are asymptomatic. Patients with large or subcapsular lesions may present with abdominal discomfort or an abdominal mass. In contrast to hepatic adenoma, presentation with acute abdominal pain from tumor bleeding or necrosis is very rare.

DIAGNOSIS

On *ultrasound*, focal nodular hyperplasias are variably hypoechoic, hyperechoic, or isoechoic. The lesions are most commonly hypoechoic except for the central scar. Doppler evaluation frequently shows blood flow within the central stellate scar.

On *dynamic CT*, focal nodular hyperplasias are isoattenuating or slightly hypoattenuating on noncontrast CT. One sees rapid, intense contrast enhancement in the arterial phase and rapid loss of contrast from the lesion, so it becomes isointense in the venous phase. An avascular central scar is often seen, sometimes with a feeding artery coursing into the middle of the lesion.

On *contrast MRI*, the lesions are isointense on T1-weighted images and remain isointense or are slightly hyperintense on T2-weighted images. The central scar is hypointense on T1-weighted images but hyperintense on T2-weighted images. As with contrast CT, rapid, intense contrast enhancement in the arterial phase quickly dissipates. Typically, the central scar has a low signal on T1-weighted images and enhances with contrast.

Technetium-99m-sulfur colloid scintigraphy is occasionally used to characterize focal nodular hyperplasias. Hyperintense or isointense uptake occurs in 50 to 70% of focal nodular hyperplasias because of uptake by Kupffer cells. In contrast, most hepatic adenomas do not have Kupffer cells and so do not take up technetium-99m-sulfur colloid. *Kupffer cell–specific MRI agents* such as ferumoxide are taken up by Kupffer cells and lead to significant signal intensity loss on ferumoxide-enhanced T2-weighted images, which may help to distinguish focal nodular hyperplasia from hepatic adenoma and hepatocellular carcinoma.

Diagnosis is usually made by radiologic studies, and biopsy is rarely needed. When a histologic diagnosis of focal nodular hyperplasia is needed, a core needle biopsy should be performed because fine-needle aspirates may only show benign-appearing hepatocytes in both focal nodular hyperplasia and hepatic adenoma. Histopathologic examination shows a benign hepatic parenchyma with bile ductules in septal fibrosis.

TREATMENT   Rx

The management of asymptomatic focal nodular hyperplasias with characteristic imaging or biopsy features is observation because lesions usually do not enlarge, bleed, or undergo malignant transformation. Patients do not need to discontinue oral contraceptive use because no convincing evidence indicates that discontinuation leads to reduction in size of the lesions. Surgical resection is recommended for indeterminate or symptomatic lesions.

Hepatic Adenoma

EPIDEMIOLOGY

Hepatic adenoma is a benign liver tumor that occurs predominantly in the third and fourth decades of life. There is a female predominance of 2 : 1 to 6 : 1 as well as a strong association with oral contraceptive use. The relative risk of developing a hepatic adenoma is 2.5 after 3 to 5 years of oral contraceptive use and 25 to 40 after 9 years of use, resulting in an incidence of 4 per 100,000 versus 1 per million in the general population.

PATHOBIOLOGY

Hepatic adenomas also occur in users of androgenic steroids, in a familial pattern associated with diabetes mellitus, in the syndrome of maturity-onset diabetes of the young, and in patients with glycogen storage disease types 1A and 3 (Chapter 214), hemochromatosis (Chapter 219), and acromegaly (Chapter 231). Adenomas are multiple in 20% of cases, particularly in patients with glycogen storage disease.

CLINICAL MANIFESTATIONS

Hepatic adenomas are usually asymptomatic and are discovered on imaging studies, but patients may present with intermittent pain or discomfort in the upper abdomen or right upper quadrant of the abdomen. Adenomas also have a propensity to rupture, with intrahepatic hemorrhage and pain or rarely with hemoperitoneum and shock. They may decrease in size after withdrawal of oral contraceptives, but typically they do not, and sometimes they even increase in size.

DIAGNOSIS

On *ultrasound*, hepatic adenomas are variably homogeneous or heterogeneous (because of hemorrhage or necrosis within the tumor). On *dynamic CT*, adenomas, like focal nodular hyperplasias, are isoattenuating on non-enhanced scans; with intravenous contrast, they show early enhancement and then become rapidly isoattenuating in the portal venous phase. Adenomas are often hyperattenuating in a fatty liver. Adenomas typically have well-defined borders and are not lobulated. Approximately 40% of adenomas have intralesional hemorrhage with heterogenous regions of high attenuation. Approximately 5% of adenomas show coarse calcifications within the lesion.

On *contrast MRI*, adenomas are hyperintense or isointense on T1-weighted images and are slightly hyperintense on T2-weighted images. They show early enhancement in the arterial phase and become isointense on delayed imaging.

Technetium-99m-sulfur colloid scintigraphy shows no uptake in 70% of adenomas because of the absence of Kupffer cells. Overall, the relatively nonspecific imaging features make adenomas difficult to differentiate from other lesions.

Biopsy is often required for diagnosis, but a significant risk of misdiagnosis exists in differentiating hepatic adenomas from focal nodular hyperplasias, as well as a potential risk of hemorrhage from core biopsies. Histologic examination shows sheets of well-differentiated hepatocytes without bile ductules, fibrous septa, portal tracts, or central veins. Most adenomas do not contain Kupffer cells.

TREATMENT AND PROGNOSIS   Rx

Management of hepatic adenoma is usually by surgical resection because of the risks of hemorrhage (≤30% for large adenomas) and malignant transformation (the exact risk is unknown). Radiofrequency ablation is used in patients who are high surgical risks. Oral contraceptives should be discontinued, and patients should avoid pregnancy until the adenoma is resected because these lesions often grow during pregnancy. The risk of malignant transformation is small but real.

Benign Liver Cysts

EPIDEMIOLOGY

Benign liver cysts occur in approximately 4% of individuals. There is a female predominance of 4 : 1, and the prevalence increases with age. Liver cysts are often multiple and coexist with other mass lesions in the liver. The inherited autosomal dominant and recessive polycystic kidney diseases (Chapter 129) are both associated with the development of multiple liver cysts. Liver cysts are lined by cuboidal bile duct epithelium and are filled with isotonic fluid. Cysts are typically asymptomatic, but large cysts can cause pressure symptoms or biliary obstruction. Hemorrhage, infection, or rupture of cysts is rare.

DIAGNOSIS

Ultrasound is the best imaging test to confirm the fluid-filled nature of cysts, which are anechoic and show no vascular flow on color flow or duplex Doppler. They demonstrate through-transmission and well-defined posterior walls. Simple cysts may have thin echogenic septa. On *dynamic CT,* cysts appear as water-density lesions. On *contrast MRI,* cysts are hyperintense on T2-weighted images. Small cysts may be difficult to differentiate from a cavernous hemangioma or other small hepatic lesions on CT or MRI because of the volume averaging from adjacent tissue. Biopsy is typically unnecessary because of the classical imaging findings.

Lesions with Focal Fat or Fat Sparing

PATHOBIOLOGY

Fatty infiltration of the liver (Chapter 155) is increasingly common as populations increase in weight across the world. Focal fatty infiltration can look like a mass on imaging studies, as can focal sparing in a liver that is diffusely infiltrated by fat. Associations with fatty change in the liver include obesity, diabetes mellitus, high alcohol consumption, and altered nutritional status as a result of chemotherapy.

CLINICAL MANIFESTATIONS

Patients with focal fatty infiltration are typically asymptomatic. The lesions are usually discovered incidentally and are sometimes mistaken for more sinister masses.

DIAGNOSIS

The characteristic imaging feature of focal fat is that it does not distort the contour of the liver, so normal vessels, especially veins, can be seen coursing through the lesion. Focal fat usually occurs in vascular watersheds such as the region around the falciform ligament. Fat sparing usually occurs adjacent to the gallbladder fossa, in subcapsular areas, and in the posterior aspect of segment IV. On ultrasound, fat is usually hyperechoic. On dynamic CT, fatty liver is hypodense compared with the spleen, but not as low in density as adipose tissue. Venous structures can be seen in the lesion on venous phase studies. On contrast MRI, fatty liver is occasionally hyperintense on T1-weighted and T2-weighted images. The decreased signal intensity on out-of-phase gradient imaging is diagnostic of focal fat.

Biopsy is occasionally useful to rule out other lesions. On histologic examination, areas of fatty infiltration show fat-laden cells.

● PRIMARY MALIGNANT TUMORS OF THE LIVER AND BILIARY TRACT

Hepatocellular Carcinoma

EPIDEMIOLOGY

Hepatocellular carcinoma, the third most common cause of death from cancer worldwide, accounts for approximately 700,000 deaths annually. There is a male preponderance of 2 : 1 to 4 : 1. The major predisposing factor for the development of hepatocellular carcinoma is cirrhosis of the liver (Chapter 156). The risk factors for the development of hepatocellular carcinoma include chronic hepatitis B or C virus infection (Chapter 151), alcoholic cirrhosis, nonalcoholic steatohepatitis (Chapter 155), hereditary hemochromatosis (Chapter 219), α_1-antitrypsin deficiency (Chapter 153), primary biliary cirrhosis (Chapter 158), and autoimmune hepatitis (Chapter 151). The hepatitis B virus almost always integrates into the host genomic DNA and can lead to development of hepatocellular carcinoma in the absence of cirrhosis. The availability of an effective vaccine against hepatitis B has reduced the incidence of hepatitis B–related hepatocellular carcinomas in high-prevalence regions. Long-term exposure to fungal aflatoxins in the diet significantly increases the risk of hepatocellular carcinoma. The fungi are ubiquitous and invade and grow in grains, legumes, and peanuts when they are stored in conditions of high humidity and temperature. The aflatoxin-producing fungal species, *Aspergillus flavus* and *Aspergillus parasiticus,* produce at least 13 different types of aflatoxin, with aflatoxin B1 the most potent. In most parts of the world, the most rapidly increasing groups of patients with hepatocellular carcinoma includes those with chronic hepatitis C virus infection. More than 90% of individuals with hepatitis C virus infection develop chronic infection, and up to 20% of patients with chronic hepatitis C develop cirrhosis. Hepatocellular carcinoma then develops in up to 20% of individuals with cirrhosis from chronic hepatitis C virus, at a rate of 2 to 6% per year. More recently, there has been a progressive increase in obesity-related nonalcoholic fatty liver disease (Chapter 155), which can progress to steatohepatitis, cirrhosis (often previously considered to be of unknown origin or "cryptogenic"), and hepatocellular carcinoma. Diabetes, also obesity related, has recently been shown to be an independent risk factor for the development of hepatocellular carcinoma.

PATHOBIOLOGY

Like most other malignant diseases, hepatocellular carcinoma develops as a result of a combination of the activation of cellular oncogenic pathways and abrogation of tumor suppressor pathways. Chronic hepatic injury resulting from viruses, alcohol, and metabolic or autoimmune mechanisms leads to repeated cycles of liver cell death, regeneration, and repair that ultimately lead to premature senescence of the liver.

Cellular senescence is characterized by a progressive decrease in length of the telomeric regions that protect the ends of chromosomes, with resulting development of chromosomal and genetic instabilities that are recognized by cellular stress response pathways and that trigger the apoptosis of senescent cells in a process known as *telomeric crisis.* In some senescent cells, apoptosis is avoided, and the cells become immortal, either through activation of the cellular telomerase enzyme complex, which maintains telomere ends, or through non-telomerase-dependent mechanisms. These genetically unstable, immortal cells are then prone to the development of additional genetic and epigenetic alterations that result in the cancer phenotype of unconstrained cell proliferation, resistance to apoptosis, enhanced cell migration and invasion, and activation of new vessel formation (angiogenesis).

Many oncogenic pathways normally have intrinsic tumor suppressor activities that limit their growth-promoting procarcinogenic effects; during carcinogenesis, mutations or epigenetic alterations lead to loss of the intrinsic tumor suppressing activity of the oncogenic pathways and result in unconstrained cellular proliferation and the secondary development of the other characteristics of the tumor phenotype. This hypothesis is well illustrated by the phenomenon of aflatoxin-induced mutation of the p53 tumor suppressor. During metabolism of aflatoxin in the liver, an aflatoxin B1-8,9-exo-epoxide intermediate is formed, and it interacts with cellular DNA to mediate formation of specific mutations, most frequently leading to a G-to-T transversion in codon 249 of the *p53* tumor suppressor gene. This mutation leads to loss of the p53 tumor suppressor function. Oncogenic pathways that normally activate p53 and limit proliferation are left without their natural "brake" on proliferation and result in an increased tendency to carcinogenesis. It is well known that aflatoxin B1 has a synergistic effect with the hepatitis B virus in the development of hepatocellular carcinoma.

Another important concept in the pathogenesis of malignant liver diseases is that of the development of malignant diseases within the epithelial stem cell compartment. Progenitor oval cells from the canals of Hering in the liver are capable of differentiating into both the hepatic and biliary lineages during liver regeneration. The development of a neoplastic phenotype within this compartment can result in the formation of cells that subsequently mature partially into more differentiated tumor cells and lead to the formation of a cancer with a "parent" clone of more immature progenitor cells and "daughter" clones of more mature cells. The existence of a tumor stem cell compartment (Chapter 185) has important implications for the development of anticancer therapy because agents that are active against carcinogenic pathways in the daughter cells but not in the parent clones may be capable of suppressing or arresting tumor growth but will not be curative unless they also target the growth pathways within the tumor stem cell compartment.

Integration of hepatitis B virus into host hepatocyte genomic DNA can lead to the development of hepatocellular carcinoma in the absence of cirrhosis. The pathogenic mechanisms include activation of oncogenic pathways through the activity of hepatitis B virus enhancer sequences and mutational inactivation of tumor suppressor genes by insertional mutagenesis. Certain proteins encoded by the hepatitis viruses have been shown to have oncogenic effects; these include the hepatitis B virus X protein, a truncated carboxy terminal variant of the hepatitis B virus S protein, the hepatitis C virus core protein, and NS5A protein.

Specific tumor suppressor and oncogenic molecules and pathways that have been shown to be important in liver carcinogenesis include the p53/p21^{WAF1} pathway, the p16^{INK4a}/CDK4/RB1/E2F pathway, the Wnt/β catenin signaling pathway, transforming growth factor-α, c-myc, the transcription factor NFκB, insulin/insulin-like growth factor I, and the receptor tyrosine kinases (fibroblast growth factor, hepatocyte growth factor, and vascular endothelial growth factor) and their downstream activators.

CLINICAL MANIFESTATIONS

Most patients are asymptomatic except for symptoms of chronic liver disease at cancer diagnosis because ultrasound surveillance in high-risk patients detects cancer in asymptomatic patients. Symptomatic presentation such as abdominal pain often suggests advanced stage cancer. Mild decompensation of cirrhosis can be observed from the replacement of functioning liver tissue with tumor. The sudden onset of severe abdominal pain from hemorrhage within the tumor mass is a rare presentation. Signs on physical examination may include a palpable liver mass and a vascular bruit over the tumor. Hepatocellular carcinomas occasionally cause a variety of paraneoplastic syndromes, including hypoglycemia mediated by insulin-like growth factors, erythrocytosis from erythropoietin generation by the tumor, hypercalcemia related to production of a parathyroid-like hormone, and watery diarrhea from tumor production of vasoactive intestinal peptide and other neuroendocrine hormones (Chapters 186 and 187).

DIAGNOSIS

Approximately 80 to 90% of hepatocellular carcinomas occur in a cirrhotic liver, so the early diagnosis of most hepatocellular carcinomas depends on rigorous efforts of intermittent long-term surveillance for cancer in patients with cirrhosis. Surveillance is usually performed using liver ultrasound every 6 months in patients with any cause of cirrhosis. In patients with chronic hepatitis B who are at increased risk of hepatocellular carcinoma (family history of hepatocellular carcinoma; high viral load or transaminases; Africans older than 20 years; Asian males older than 40 years; Asian females older than 50 years), ultrasound surveillance is indicated even in patients without liver cirrhosis. Any suspicious nodules found by ultrasound are then examined with additional contrast imaging studies.

A serum AFP level is a specific tumor marker for hepatocellular carcinoma. A level greater than 200 ng/mL has a 95 to 100% specificity for hepatocellular carcinoma, and lesions larger than 2 cm with AFP greater than 200 ng/mL is diagnostic for hepatocellular carcinoma; but at the cutoff value of 200 ng/mL, the sensitivity of AFP is only about 20%. Therefore, use of AFP alone for hepatocellular carcinoma surveillance is not recommended.

Contrast imaging studies are diagnostic modalities of choice once suspected nodules are detected during surveillance. On contrast imaging studies, including contrast CT, MRI, ultrasound, and angiography, hepatocellular carcinomas are characterized by bright enhancement in the arterial phase, followed by a loss of enhancement as contrast washes out of the arterial circulation, and a characteristic decreased intensity below that of the surrounding liver during the portal phase, when the surrounding liver is perfused

FIGURE 202-2. Hepatocellular carcinoma. A T1-weighted magnetic resonance image is shown during the arterial (**A**) and portal (**B**) phases after the administration of intravenous gadolinium contrast. The tumor (*arrows*) shows contrast enhancement in the arterial phase and washout in the portal phase.

by contrast to a higher intensity than that of the tumor nodule. This feature, referred to as *washout*, is highly specific for hepatocellular carcinomas occurring in a cirrhotic liver (Fig. 202-2). In patients with cirrhosis, almost all hepatocellular carcinomas 2 cm or larger can be confidently diagnosed using noninvasive imaging criteria. When lesions are between 1 and 2 cm in a cirrhotic liver, characteristic imaging findings should be present in two dynamic imaging studies to diagnose hepatocellular carcinoma.

Lesions smaller than 1 cm should be closely followed at an interval of 3 to 6 months for up to 2 years. Should a lesion not change, the patient can return to routine surveillance.

The diagnosis of small equivocal lesions in a noncirrhotic liver or any lesions in noncirrhotic liver can be established by needle biopsy of the lesion. However, because of the small but real risks of tumor seeding (0.5 to 2%), hemorrhage, and false-negative results from biopsy, many centers avoid biopsy, particularly in patients who may be candidates for liver transplantation and instead rely on imaging characteristics for the diagnosis of hepatocellular carcinoma.

PREVENTION

Universal vaccination against hepatitis B has been shown to reduce the incidence of hepatocellular carcinoma.**1** No vaccine is available against the hepatitis C virus. Individuals who have durable responses to treatment for hepatitis B and C appear to have a reduced risk of developing hepatocellular carcinoma.

TREATMENT Rx

Patients who have early-stage hepatocellular carcinoma and who do not have significant underlying liver dysfunction can be treated by surgical resection. Liver transplantation (Chapter 157) of patients who meet the Milan criteria (one tumor mass lesion ≤5 cm or two to three lesions each ≤3 cm, with no evidence of extrahepatic spread or vascular invasion) provides long-term survival results no different from those of patients receiving liver transplants for nonmalignant indications. In patients who are not candidates for liver transplantation, local ablation of small tumors up to 3 to 4 cm is performed with percutaneous ethanol injection or radiofrequency ablation, which uses probes with small tines that can be deployed through the tumor and energized with high-frequency electrical current to produce coagulation of the tumor and a surrounding rim of benign tissue. Although surgical resection and the local ablative therapies are effective treatments for small hepatocellular carcinomas, patients with cirrhosis still have a residual molecular defect in the remaining liver that makes them susceptible to recurrent tumor, at a rate of approximately 50% by 3 years after surgical resection or local ablation.

Patients with tumors that do not meet the criteria for surgical resection, liver transplantation, or local ablation but that are still limited to the liver are considered to have intermediate-stage disease. Intermediate-stage disease is currently treated using transarterial chemoembolization with chemotherapeutic agents, such as doxorubicin, mitomycin C, and cisplatin, as well as polyvinyl alcohol (Ivalon) or absorbable gelatin (Gelfoam) particles, sometimes combined with iodized poppy-seed oil (Lipiodol or Ethiodol). Randomized trials and meta-analyses have confirmed that transarterial chemoembolization improves survival of patients with intermediate-stage hepatocellular carcinoma.**2** Radioembolization with yttrium-90-impregnated glass microspheres, which is an alternative to transarterial chemoembolization, can be used for patients with portal vein thrombosis because, unlike the Ivalon or Gelfoam particles used for chemoembolization, the 20- to 30-μg glass microspheres used for radioembolization do not occlude the hepatic arterial vascular bed. However, radioembolization has not as yet been subjected to rigorous randomized trials.

Treatment using systemic chemotherapy is complicated by the presence of underlying chronic liver disease and a significantly increased risk of drug toxicity. Current efforts are focused on the use of targeted therapies directed against molecular pathways known to be involved in hepatocarcinogenesis, including receptor tyrosine kinases and the Wnt signaling pathway. Sorafenib, 400 mg twice daily, has been shown to increase median survival significantly in patients with advanced-stage hepatocellular carcinoma, typically by slowing progression but not by inducing remission.**3** Recently, sorafenib, 400 mg twice daily, combined with doxorubicin, 60 mg/m^2 intravenously every 21 days, was shown to be superior to doxorubicin alone in prolonging progression-free survival and overall survival among patients with advanced hepatocellular carcinoma.**4**

PROGNOSIS

Patients with early disease who undergo liver transplantation have an excellent outcome with a 5-year survival rate of 70 to 80% and 5-year recurrence rate of 10% or less. Patients who are ineligible for liver transplantation who undergo surgical resection or local treatment by radiofrequency ablation or percutaneous ethanol injection also have relatively high 5-year survival rates of 50 to 70%; however, because they still have a cirrhotic liver with a predisposition to cancer, these patients have a 3-year recurrence rate of approximately 50%. Patients with intermediate-stage disease who are treated with transarterial chemoembolization have a 1-year survival rate of 50 to 80% and a 2-year survival rate of 25 to 60%. Appropriate selection of individuals with preserved liver function is important for achieving the best outcomes with transarterial chemoembolization because it can decrease survival by inducing liver decompensation. Patients with advanced-stage disease who are currently candidates for treatment trials or symptomatic treatment have a median survival of only 6 to 8 months and a 1-year survival rate of 10 to 30%.

Cholangiocarcinoma

EPIDEMIOLOGY

Although the overall incidence of biliary cancers, or cholangiocarcinomas, is relatively low, these tumors are associated with perhaps the most rapidly rising incidence of any cancer in Western industrial nations. The reason for this trend is unknown. Most cholangiocarcinomas occur incidentally, but the known risk factors for cholangiocarcinoma include primary sclerosing cholangitis (Chapter 158), which is often associated with inflammatory bowel disease (Chapter 143); congenital choledochal cysts or other biliary tract abnormalities; Asian cholangiopathies secondary to liver fluke infections; and secondary chronic bacterial cholangitis, which frequently occurs in individuals who have had intrahepatic biliary stones or a prior biliary-enteric anastomosis. Chronic liver disease from viral or nonviral hepatitis is associated with cholangiocarcinoma, although the strength of association is weaker than with hepatocellular carcinoma.

PATHOBIOLOGY

The pathogenesis of cholangiocarcinoma is not well understood. Current concepts suggest that biliary inflammation results in impairment of DNA repair mechanisms, with the subsequent development of genomic instability and cancer. Genes in pathways shown to be involved in biliary carcinogenesis include *p53, K-ras, c-met, c-erbB2, mcl-1, Bcl-xl, p16^{INK4a}, p14^{ARF}, iNOS,* and *IL-6.*

CLINICAL MANIFESTATIONS

Patients with cholangiocarcinomas typically present with painless jaundice resulting from the presence of hilar or distal biliary strictures or with an intrahepatic mass causing abdominal pain, which may be referred to the shoulder. These patients often have associated pruritus, pale stools, and dark urine. Nonspecific symptoms such as weight loss and low-grade fever may also occur.

DIAGNOSIS

Cholangiocarcinomas are classified as intrahepatic or extrahepatic based on the location of the tumor within the biliary tree. The use of MRI with magnetic resonance cholangiography provides a noninvasive means of imaging the obstructed biliary tract before endoscopic retrograde cholangiopancreatography and allows the endoscopist and surgeon to plan an optimal approach for evaluation and therapy. Patients with unilateral biliary obstruction often have atrophy of the involved liver lobe and compensatory hypertrophy of the other lobe, referred to as the *atrophy-hypertrophy complex* (Fig. 202-3). Because of the presence of a dense fibrous stroma around a relatively sparse number of malignant glandular epithelial elements in many cholangiocarcinomas, cytologic examination from brushings of malignant strictures has a relatively low sensitivity, particularly in early cancers most amenable to successful therapy. However, the examination of biliary brush cytology specimens using advanced cytologic techniques such as DNA flow cytometry, digital image analysis, and fluorescence in situ hybridization with DNA probes for the detection of chromosomal polysomy has improved diagnostic accuracy (Fig. 202-4). These techniques can be applied in patients with primary sclerosing cholangitis who present with a new dominant stricture or clinical deterioration to improve the early detection of malignant transformation. Advanced endoscopic methods such as endoscopic ultrasound, intraductal ultrasound, and choledochoscopy also improve visualization and characterization of biliary strictures and associated metastatic lymphadenopathy.

The CA-19-9 marker is a commonly used tumor marker in cholangiocarcinoma. Although the sensitivity is modest and cholestasis and inflammation of the biliary tract can lead to false positive elevation, CA-19-9 is a tool for determining the effect of treatment or for monitoring recurrence after curative treatment.

TREATMENT Rx

The outcome after development of cholangiocarcinoma is generally poor because the tumor is relatively resistant to chemotherapy and also frequently results in biliary obstruction, which is complicated by episodes of bacterial cholangitis and cholestatic liver dysfunction. The treatment of biliary cancers depends on the extent of involvement of the biliary tree and on the presence of extrahepatic disease.

For disease limited to the liver and biliary tree, with malignant strictures that do not extend beyond the secondary branching of the right or left intrahepatic

FIGURE 202-3. Cholangiocarcinoma. **A,** A T1-weighted magnetic resonance image during the arterial phase after the administration of intravenous gadolinium. The tumor *(arrow)* occludes the left hepatic duct, leading to marked dilation of the left biliary system and atrophy with enhanced contrast enhancement of the left lobe; the right lobe of the liver shows compensatory hypertrophy. This combination of features is called the *atrophy-hypertrophy complex.* **B,** Magnetic resonance cholangiopancreatography from the same patient showing narrowing of the common hepatic duct by the cholangiocarcinoma *(arrow)* and grossly dilated left biliary system. **C,** Endoscopic retrograde cholangiopancreatography showing filling of the right biliary system through the narrowed common hepatic duct *(arrow);* the left biliary system is completely isolated and not filled during injection of contrast.

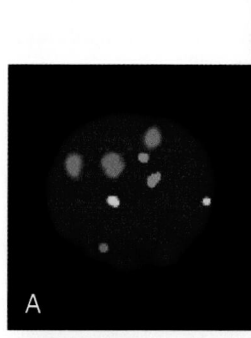

A   **B**

FIGURE 202-4. Fluorescence in situ hybridization for diagnosis of malignancy in biliary strictures. Fluorescent DNA probes for the centromeres of chromosomes 3 (red), 7 (green), 17 (aqua), and the p16 locus at chromosome 9p21 (yellow) are hybridized to brush cytology specimens obtained from biliary strictures at endoscopic retrograde cholangiopancreatography. The normal diploid cell (**A**) has two copies of each of the probes; the malignant polysomic cells (**B**) each have multiple copies of chromosomes 3, 7, and 17.

bile ducts, treatment by surgical resection results in a 5-year survival rate of approximately 20% after successful resection. Patients with distal biliary cancers without distant spread are usually treated by bile duct resection or by Whipple's pancreaticoduodenectomy.

Patients with unresectable disease are generally treated by palliative biliary stenting using plastic or metal stents. Effective stenting of approximately 25% of the total liver volume using the less affected lobe of the liver is usually sufficient to relieve cholestasis and is significantly less likely to result in repeated episodes of cholangitis.

Adjuvant chemotherapy and radiation, with staging laparotomy followed by liver transplantation for selected patients with early hilar cholangiocarcinomas, have resulted in a remarkable 5-year survival rate of 80% in patients who can successfully complete the treatment protocol. Photodynamic therapy with 630-nm laser light treatment administered using a fiber inserted across the biliary stricture after intravenous infusion of a photosensitizing porfimer, which is preferentially taken up by malignant cells, can preserve biliary patency and can improve survival in patients with unresectable malignant biliary strictures.[5]

In patients with locally advanced or metastatic cholangiocarcinoma, gallbladder cancer, or ampullary cancer, combination chemotherapy with cisplatin plus gemcitabine has been found to have survival advantage without the addition of substantial toxicity compared with gemcitabine alone.[6]

PROGNOSIS

Patients eligible for liver transplantation have the best prognosis with a 5-year rate survival of about 80%. Patients with curative resection have 5-year survival rate of about 20 to 40%. In patients with unresectable disease, biliary stenting, photodynamic therapy, and the use of chemotherapy regimens such as gemcitabine and cisplatin generally result in improvements in survival that are measured only in months.

Grade A

1. Chang MH, Shau WY, Chen CJ, et al. Hepatitis B vaccination and hepatocellular carcinoma rates in boys and girls. *JAMA*. 2000;284:3040-3042.
2. Llovet JM, Bruix J. Systematic review of randomized trials for unresectable hepatocellular carcinoma: chemoembolization improves survival. *Hepatology*. 2003;37:429-442.
3. Llovet JM, Ricci S, Mazzaferro V, et al. Sorafenib in advanced hepatocellular carcinoma. *N Engl J Med*. 2008;359:378-390.
4. Abou-Alfa GK, Johnson P, Knox JJ, et al. Doxorubicin plus sorafenib vs doxorubicin alone in patients with advanced hepatocellular carcinoma: a randomized trial. *JAMA*. 2010;304:2154-2160.
5. Ortner ME, Caca K, Berr F, et al. Successful photodynamic therapy for nonresectable cholangiocarcinoma: a randomized prospective study. *Gastroenterology*. 2003;125:1355-1363.
6. Valle J, Wasan H, Palmer DH, et al. Cisplatin plus gemcitabine versus gemcitabine for biliary tract cancer. *N Engl J Med*. 2010;362:1273-1281.

SUGGESTED READINGS

Alves RC, Alves D, Guz B, et al. Advanced hepatocellular carcinoma: review of targeted molecular drugs. *Ann Hepatol*. 2011;10:21-27. *Review emphasizing sorafenib.*
Burak KW, Kneteman NM. An evidence-based multidisciplinary approach to the management of hepatocellular carcinoma (HCC): the Alberta HCC algorithm. *Can J Gastroenterol*. 2010;24:643-650. *Recommendations regarding resection, ablative techniques, liver transplantation, transarterial chemoembolization, transarterial radioembolization, and sorafenib.*

Everhart JE, Ruhl CE. Burden of digestive diseases in the United States. Part III. Liver, biliary tract, and pancreas. *Gastroenterology*. 2009;136:1134-1144. *Documents the increasing incidence of hepatocellular carcinoma and cholangiocarcinoma in the United States over the past 25 years.*
Kim JH, Won HJ, Shin YM, et al. Radiofrequency ablation for the treatment of primary intrahepatic cholangiocarcinoma. *AJR Am J Roentgenol*. 2011;196:W205-W209. *An approach for local tumor control of primary intrahepatic cholangiocarcinomas <5 cm in diameter.*
Marrero JA, Feng Z, Wang Y, et al. Alpha-fetoprotein, des-gamma carboxyprothrombin, and lectin-bound alpha-fetoprotein in early hepatocellular carcinoma. *Gastroenterology*. 2009;137:110-118. *Overview of the diagnostic utility of these assays.*
Rahbari NN, Mehrabi A, Mollberg NM, et al. Hepatocellular carcinoma: current management and perspectives for the future. *Ann Surg*. 2011;253:453-459. *Review.*
Zografos GN, Farfaras A, Zagouri F, et al. Cholangiocarcinoma: principles and current trends. *Hepatobiliary Pancreat Dis Int*. 2011;10:10-20. *Review of surgical and medical treatments.*

203

TUMORS OF THE KIDNEY, BLADDER, URETERS, AND RENAL PELVIS

DEAN F. BAJORIN

RENAL CELL CARCINOMA

DEFINITION

Cancers of the kidney are a heterogeneous group of neoplasms, most of which are of epithelial origin and malignant. Renal cell carcinoma (RCC), classically referred to as clear cell carcinoma or hypernephroma, is not a single malignancy. Rather, RCC comprises a group of distinguishable entities, each with a strong relationship between its morphologic and genetic features. The World Health Organization recognizes these biologic and histologic differences in the classification system of kidney cancers (Table 203-1). The metastatic potential is dependent on the histologic subtype and ranges from the most virulent conventional clear cell carcinomas (75% of total tumors but accounting for 90% of the metastases), to the more indolent papillary and chromophobe carcinomas (20% of the total but only 10% of the metastases), to the benign oncocytomas (5% of all tumors).

EPIDEMIOLOGY

In the year 2009, it is estimated that there will be more than 49,000 new cases and approximately 11,000 deaths from kidney cancer in the United States. Since 1950, there has been a 126% increase in the incidence of renal cancer and a 36.5% increase in annual mortality. The increase in incidence of RCC may be in part related to early detection as a consequence of computed tomography (CT) and magnetic resonance imaging (MRI) of the abdomen for other medical conditions. The male-to-female ratio is approximately 2:1 to 3:1, and the increase in incidence is highest in African Americans and lowest in Asians and Pacific Islanders. The mean age at diagnosis is in the sixth to seventh decade of life. Aside from genetic predisposition, risk factors associated with RCC include cigarette smoking, obesity, hypertension, and the use of diuretics. Increased cigarette smoking has been associated with greater risk in both men and women. The risk may decrease after smoking cessation but requires about 20 years. Obese persons have an increased risk

TABLE 203-1 CLASSIFICATION OF RENAL CELL NEOPLASMS	
BENIGN	**MALIGNANT**
Oncocytoma	Clear cell (conventional) renal cell carcinoma
Papillary (chromophil) adenoma	Papillary (chromophil) renal cell carcinoma
Metanephric adenoma	Chromophobe renal cell carcinoma
Nephrogenic adenofibroma	Collecting duct carcinoma
	Medullary carcinoma
	Mixed tubular and spindle cell carcinoma
	Renal cell carcinoma, unclassified

Modified from Storkel S, Eble JN, Adlakha K, et al. Classification of renal cell carcinoma: Workgroup No. 1. Union Internationale Contre le Cancer (UICC) and the American Joint Committee on Cancer (AJCC). *Cancer*. 1997;80:987-989.

TABLE 203-2 HISTOLOGIC SUBTYPES, GENETICS, AND SYNDROMES

HISTOLOGIC SUBTYPE	%	MAJOR GENETIC/ MOLECULAR DEFECTS	OTHER GENETIC/MOLECULAR DEFECTS	ASSOCIATED SYNDROMES
Conventional (clear cell)	75	LOH* 3p Mutation of 3p25 (VHL)	+5q, −8p, −9p, −14q p53 mutation, c-erB-1 oncogene expression	VHL Hereditary RCC
Papillary 1	5	c-Met gene mutation 7q31	Trisomy 7, 12, 16, and 17; −Y, +7, +17	Hereditary papillary RCC
Papillary 2	10	Fumarate hydratase 1q42	Trisomy 7, 12, 16, 17, 20; −1p, −3p, −9p, −Y, +5q	Hereditary leiomyomatosis RCC
Chromophobe	5	Birt-Hogg-Dubé 17p11	−1p, −2p, −6p, −13q, 21q, −Y p53 mutation	Birt-Hogg-Dubé
Oncocytoma	5	Birt-Hogg-Dubé 17p11	−1, −Y, 11q rearrangement	Familial oncocytoma Birt-Hogg-Dubé
Collecting duct	0.4	−18, −Y	−1q, −6p, −8p, −11, −13q, −21q c-erB-1 oncogene expression	Renal medullary carcinoma

LOH = loss of heterozygosity; RCC = renal cell carcinoma; VHL = von Hippel-Lindau disease.
Modified from Zambrano NR. Histopathology and molecular genetics of renal tumors *J Urol.* 1999;162:1246-1258; and Klatte T, Pantuck AJ, Said JW, et al. Cytogenetic and molecular tumor profiling for type 1 and type 2 papillary renal cell carcinoma. *Clin Cancer Res.* 2009;15:1162-1169.

of RCC, and the risk rises with increasing body mass index. Although there is an elevated risk associated with diuretic use, this association is hard to distinguish from the increased risk associated with hypertension. RCC is more prevalent in patients with preexisting renal conditions such as polycystic kidney disease, horseshoe kidney, and chronic renal failure requiring hemodialysis.

PATHOBIOLOGY

The new classification system for RCC permits a better understanding of the cell of origin for the various subtypes and their chromosomal abnormalities (Table 203-2). The classic clear cell carcinoma constitutes approximately 65% of tumors and is believed to be derived from the proximal convoluted tubule. It is generally solitary and well circumscribed with a golden yellow color because of abundant cytoplasmic lipid. Higher-grade tumors contain less lipid and glycogen. About half of the tumors exhibit either a solid or acinar growth pattern characterized by solid sheets of tumor cells and accompanied by a rich capillary vascular network. Papillary RCCs represent approximately 15% of primary epithelial renal neoplasms. Multifocality, either bilateral or multifocal lesions in the same kidney, is present in about 45% of cases. Most of these tumors exhibit a broad morphologic spectrum, including papillary, papillary-trabecular, and papillary-solid areas; associated necrosis is a common finding. The classic papillary pattern is characterized by discrete papillary fronds lined by neoplastic epithelial cells and containing a central fibrovascular core, easily recognized on low magnification. These tumors are divided into type 1 and type 2 lesions, based on cytologic features and genetic differences. Chromophobe renal cancers make up 5% of renal epithelial tumors. Characteristically, these tumors are solitary and discrete but not encapsulated. The typical histology consists of large round-to-polygonal cells with well-defined cell borders and pale basophilic cytoplasm admixed with a smaller population of polygonal cells with eosinophilic cytoplasm. These tumors may be quite large at diagnosis, with resectable tumors reported as big as 23 cm.

Clear cell carcinoma is characterized by the loss of genetic material of the short arm of chromosome 3 (3p) and mutations in the von Hippel-Lindau (VHL) gene. In patients with von Hippel-Lindau disease, these losses and mutations occur in virtually all cases. The more common sporadic tumors also have somatic mutations or hypermethylation in the same region in approximately 75 to 80% of cases. Conventional clear cell tumors have a mutation in the VHL gene, which is inactivated by a point mutation or by epigenetic gene silencing by promoter methylation. The loss of VHL, responsible for ubiquination and degradation of hypoxia-inducible factor (HIF) genes, leads to upregulation of HIF-responsive genes responsible for angiogenesis and cell growth. Two of these upregulated genes are platelet-derived growth factor (PDGF) and vascular endothelial growth factor (VEGF), which are angiogenic factors thought to induce the neovascularity seen in both primary and metastatic clear cell cancers. Patients with the VHL syndrome more commonly develop tumors at an earlier age and frequently have multiple tumors. Other tumors associated with the syndrome include central nervous system hemangioblastomas (Chapter 195), pancreatic neuroendocrine tumors (Chapter 201), pheochromocytomas, retinal angiomas, and epididymal cystadenomas.

Most sporadic papillary RCCs are characterized by trisomy of chromosomes 7 and 17 as well as loss of chromosome Y. Hereditary papillary renal cancer is a result of germline mutations and activation of the *MET* proto-oncogene, which is located on chromosome 7p. These cells have aberrant hepatocyte growth factor receptors that are unable to deactivate after binding by the growth factor. Somatic *MET* gene amplifications have also been observed in about 10% of sporadic papillary renal cancer. The syndrome of hereditary leiomyomatosis and papillary renal cancers is associated with the gene for fumarate hydratase. Birt-Hogg-Dubé syndrome is a rare disorder predominantly associated with the chromophobe renal cancers but in which clear cell tumors and chromophobe and oncocytic tumors can develop. The gene associated with the Birt-Hogg-Dubé syndrome has been mapped to 17p and expresses a novel protein, folliculin, whose function is not yet characterized. Chromophobe RCCs have genetic loss on chromosomes 1 and Y as well as combined chromosomal losses affecting chromosomes 1, 6, 10, 13, 17, and 21.

CLINICAL MANIFESTATIONS

Although RCC has a high propensity for metastases and has associated paraneoplastic syndromes, most patients are asymptomatic at presentation. Historically, RCC tumor was characterized by the presenting triad of hematuria, a palpable mass, and pain in as many as 10% of patients. However, there has been a migration to the detection of earlier-stage tumors with the increased use of abdominal imaging for unrelated medical conditions in modern series. Up to 48% of tumors may be discovered in this manner, and less than 5% of patients now have a palpable mass at presentation. The more common presenting symptoms are anemia, weight loss, malaise, and anorexia (Table 203-3). The presence of these symptoms has been associated with the disease-free survival after nephrectomy. Patients presenting with RCC frequently have associated paraneoplastic syndromes. Hypercalcemia (Chapter 186) has been observed in approximately 20% of patients and can be due to the secretion of parathyroid hormone, parathyroid hormone–like peptide, and interleukin-6, shown to stimulate osteoclastic bone resorption. Other associated syndromes include hypertension, erythrocytosis (from ectopic erythropoietin production) and the rare Stauffer's syndrome, which is the presence of liver dysfunction without the presence of hepatic metastases; the hepatic dysfunction resolves after surgical resection of the tumor.

DIAGNOSIS

The complete evaluation for patients with suspected RCC should include a complete blood count, chemistry profile, bone scan, and CT scan of the chest, abdomen, and pelvis. CT is the most reliable method for detecting and staging of RCC. The "ideal" CT scan for renal masses can be divided into four phases, including the precontrast images, the arterial phase (about 25 seconds after injection), the nephrographic phase (about 90 seconds into the injection), and the excretory phase. The most important phases for imaging renal tumors are the precontrast and nephrographic images because renal lesions appear low in density in contrast to the uniformly enhanced renal parenchyma. The arterial phase is helpful for identifying renal arteries and small hypervascular masses. The excretory phase aids in assessing the collecting system and the renal pelvis. The CT scan is also helpful in detecting regional

TABLE 203-3 PRESENTING SYMPTOMS AND SIGNS OF RENAL CELL CARCINOMA (BOTH LOCALIZED AND METASTATIC DISEASE)

Anemia	52%
Hepatic dysfunction	32%
Weight loss	23%
Hypoalbuminemia	20%
Malaise	19%
Hypercalcemia	13%
Anorexia	11%
Thrombocytosis	9%
Night sweats	8%
Fever	8%
Erythrocytosis	4%
Hypertension	3%
Chills	3%

Modified from Kim HI, Belldegrun AS, Freitas DG, et al. Paraneoplastic signs and symptoms of renal cell carcinoma: implications for prognosis. *J Urol.* 2003;170:1742-1746.

metastases, and three-dimensional CT imaging is now possible in cases in which "nephron-sparing surgery" or partial nephrectomy is planned. The additional use of ultrasonography and MRI can help distinguish benign from malignant lesions of the kidney and in treatment planning. Ultrasound is used when distinguishing cysts from solid lesions. MRI has the advantage of imaging tumors in patients with poor renal function in which intravenous contrast may be contraindicated. MRI is also helpful for delineating any thrombi that may be extending into the renal vein or inferior vena cava, and magnetic resonance angiography can be used to determine the number and location of renal arteries in patients who are candidates for partial nephrectomy. Once the evaluation is complete, the clinical stage is assessed using the TNM (tumor, node, metastasis) system (Table 203-4).

TREATMENT

Localized Disease

The historical standard of care for patients with an RCC is a radical nephrectomy. Kidney cancers routinely selected for radical nephrectomy include large and centrally localized tumors that have effectively replaced most of the normal renal parenchyma, tumors associated with regional adenopathy (of benign or malignant etiology), those with inferior vena cava or right atrial extension, and even those in which metastatic disease is evident. Nephrectomy can be performed through a flank, transperitoneal, or a transthoracic incision. The ipsilateral adrenal gland is also removed, but a regional lymph node dissection is optional and controversial. The increasing percentage of small tumors has resulted in a corresponding decrease in patients undergoing radical nephrectomy. Partial nephrectomy for tumors of 7 cm or smaller offers rates of local tumor control and survival similar to radical nephrectomy but also reduces the risk of renal insufficiency over time. Partial nephrectomy is further supported by the fact that approximately 35% of renal cortical tumors are the indolent papillary or chromophobe carcinomas. Laparoscopic nephrectomy offers a minimally invasive alternative to the classical radical nephrectomy. Both open and laparoscopic approaches can be used for partial nephrectomy to control disease and preserve renal function.

RCCs are resistant to both radiation therapy and traditional chemotherapy. Neither are used in either the neoadjuvant or adjuvant surgical setting. Immunotherapy with interferon and interleukin-2, used in the treatment of metastatic disease, have shown no benefit in the adjuvant setting after nephrectomy.

Metastatic Disease

About 30% of patients with RCC present with metastatic disease, and an additional 20 to 30% of patients with surgically resected primary tumors relapse with metastases. Complications of metastatic disease include pain from either an unresectable primary tumor or from skeletal metastases. Radiation therapy is frequently used for palliation of bone metastases and in patients with multiple brain metastases. Palliative nephrectomy is sometimes used to provide symptomatic relief of pain. Surgical resection of the primary tumor is considered a mainstay of treatment even in patients with metastatic

TABLE 203-4 TNM STAGING OF RENAL CELL CARCINOMA

TUMOR, NODES, AND METASTASES CLINICAL CLASSIFICATION

PRIMARY TUMOR (T)

TX	Primary tumor cannot be assessed
T0	No evidence of primary tumor
T1	Tumor 7 cm or less in greatest dimension, limited to the kidney
T1a	Tumor 4 cm or less in greatest dimension, limited to the kidney
T1b	Tumor more than 4 cm but not more than 7 cm in greatest dimension, limited to kidney
T2	Tumor more than 7 cm in greatest dimension, limited to kidney
T2a	Tumor more than 7 cm but less than or equal to 10 cm in greatest dimension, limited to the kidney
T2b	Tumor more than 10 cm, limited to the kidney
T3	Tumor extends into major veins or the perinephric tissues but not into the ipsilateral adrenal gland but not beyond Gerota's fascia
T3a	Tumor grossly extends into renal vein or its segmental (muscle-containing) branches, or tumor invades perirenal and/or renal sinus fat but not beyond Gerota's fascia
T3b	Tumor grossly extends into the vena cava below the diaphragm
T3c	Tumor grossly extends into vena cava above the diaphragm or invades the wall of the vena cava
T4	Tumor invades beyond Gerota's fascia (including contiguous extension into the ipsilateral adrenal gland)

Regional Lymph Nodes (N)

NX	Regional lymph nodes cannot be assessed
N0	No regional lymph node metastasis
N1	Metastasis in regional lymph node(s)

Distant Metastasis (M)

MX	Distant metastasis cannot be assessed
M0	No distant metastasis
M1	Distant metastasis

STAGE GROUPING

Stage I	T1, N0, M0
Stage II	T2, N0, M0
Stage III	T1 or T2, N1, M0
	T3, N0 or N1, M0
Stage IV	T4, Any N, M0
	Any T, Any N, M1

From *AJCC Cancer Staging Manual*, 7th ed. New York: Springer-Verlag; 2010.

disease and has been shown to extend survival in these patients.[1] Surgical resection of metastatic sites of disease (i.e., "metastectomy") may also extend survival and even cure a subset of patients. The patients most likely to benefit from surgical resection of metastatic disease are those with a disease-free interval of greater than 1 year, those with a solitary site of metastases, and those with lung metastases. Long-term survival has been observed when the solitary site of resection was the lung (up to 45%) and even the brain (up to 20%). RCC is resistant to most conventional chemotherapy agents, with responses seen in less than 10% of patients.

Immunotherapy with either interleukin-2 or interferon-α (Chapter 35) has been the historical treatment for patients with metastatic disease. High-dose intravenous interleukin-2, a potentially curative treatment, requires a dedicated inpatient setting because of the severe toxicities associated with this therapy, including hypotension, pulmonary edema, renal failure, and central nervous system toxicity. However, most toxicities are reversible, and complete or partial responses are seen in approximately 15 to 20%; approximately 4% of patients achieve long-term, disease-free survival. Interferon-α therapy is given as three to five subcutaneous injections per week, is less toxic than interleukin-2, and has an overall response rate of approximately 15%. However, the number of patients achieving a complete response and long-term survival is substantially less than seen with interleukin-2. Reversible toxicities of interferon-α treatment include influenza-like symptoms such as fever, chills, myalgias, mild myelosuppression, and mild hepatic dysfunction.

RCC has been an ideal candidate for the development of new "targeted" therapies, exploiting the downstream effects of *VHL* mutations. Randomized trials have shown the benefit of tyrosine kinase inhibitors (TKIs), such as sunitinib and sorafenib, that block the actions of *VEGF* and PDGF, and bevacizumab, an antibody that blocks the endothelial growth factor receptor. Sunitinib was found to be superior to interferon as initial therapy and is now a standard of care.**2** Common side effects include fatigue, diarrhea, hypertension, and hand-foot-syndrome, a condition in which blisters appear at areas of contact. The addition of bevacizumab to interferon is superior to interferon alone, and this combination has been approved for first-line treatment as well. Side effects include hypertension and an increased risk of bleeding.**3** Sorafenib was found to be superior to placebo in patients whose disease progressed after cytokine therapy. Side effects are similar to sunitinib. Two new drugs active in RCC target the mammalian target of rapamycin (mTOR) pathway and have also been approved for treatment. Temsirolimus, an intravenous mTOR inhibitor, improves survival of patients with untreated poor-risk disease (those with three or more risk factors; see later).**4** Everolimus, an oral mTOR inhibitor, improves the outcomes of patients who have been previously treated with sunitinib, sorafenib, or bevacizumab.**5** Common side effects include fatigue, skin rashes, and mouth sores.

PROGNOSIS

Survival rates for resected nonmetastatic renal cortical tumors range between 60 and 100% depending on the mode of presentation, tumor histology, tumor size, and pathologic stage (E-Fig. 203-1). The prognosis declines considerably for patients with more advanced disease, with long-term survival seen in only 20% of stage III patients and 5% or less of stage IV patients. Of the more common histologic subtypes of RCC, the prognosis of clear cell carcinoma is less favorable than papillary RCC; chromophobe RCC is the most favorable. For patients with metastatic disease, five clinical features associated with shorter survival are low performance status, high lactate dehydrogenase, low hemoglobin, high calcium, and absence of prior nephrectomy. Three groups have been defined using survival data from patients treated with immunotherapy: favorable (0 zero risk factors), with a median survival of 20 months; intermediate (one or two risk factors), with a median survival of 10 months; and poor (three or more risk factors), with a median survival of 4 months. Immunotherapy treatment of patients and surgical resection of metastases can result in long-term survival of a small percentage of RCC patients. New targeted drugs, a direct result of increased understanding of RCC biology, are now the standard of care for patients with metastatic disease.

BLADDER CANCER

DEFINITION

A spectrum of tumors arise from the urothelial lining of the bladder, renal pelvis, ureters, and urethra, of which transitional cell carcinoma is the most common. Most tumors arise from the bladder, with a minority arising from the upper tracts (renal pelvis and ureters) and even fewer from the proximal urethra. Although transitional cell cancers possess a variable natural history, they have a proclivity for multifocality, high recurrence rates, and progression to higher pathologic stages. These tumors are generally grouped into the three broad categories of superficial, muscle-invasive, and metastatic disease, each of which differs in clinical behavior, prognosis, and primary management. For superficial tumors, the aim is to prevent recurrences and progression to a more advanced stage. In muscle-invasive disease, the medical challenge is to integrate the modalities of surgery, chemotherapy, and radiation to optimize cure and minimize morbidity. For metastatic disease, chemotherapy is used to palliate the symptoms of most patients, but there is a subset of patients in whom combination chemotherapy may result in long-term cure. During the past 30 years, improvements in diagnosis, management, and therapies has resulted in a 5-year survival rate that has increased from 73% in the 1974 to 1976 time period to 82% for those patients diagnosed between 1998 and 2001.

EPIDEMIOLOGY

More than 68,000 estimated new cases of bladder cancer were diagnosed in 2008, of which 14,000 patients are expected to succumb to their disease. The male-to-female ratio of 3:1 is similar in all racial groups, making this disease the fourth most common cancer in men and the ninth in women. The combined bladder cancer incidence for men and women has remained stable from 1986 to 2001 after rising 0.7% per year from 1975 to 1986, whereas the death rate from bladder cancer continues to decline. Bladder cancer is twice as prevalent in whites as in African Americans and is less frequently observed in Asians. The median age at diagnosis is approximately 70 years, and the disease is rarely diagnosed before the age of 40 years.

Carcinogens or their metabolites implicated in the carcinogenesis of bladder cancer are believed to be excreted in the urine, where they can act directly on the urothelial lining. The latency period from initial exposure to the development of cancer is almost 20 years, making it difficult to establish a definitive cause-and-effect relationship between a putative carcinogen and the development of the disease. Cigarette smoking is the leading risk factor for bladder cancer, believed to contribute to 48% of the cancers in men and 28% of the cancers in women. A longer duration of exposure is associated with a higher risk than a more intense exposure (in cigarettes/day) over a shorter time period of time. Overall, smokers have a two- to four-fold higher relative risk of bladder cancer than nonsmokers. Smoking is associated with cellular atypia of the urothelium; individuals who never smoked show atypia in only 4% of cases, in contrast to a 50% incidence of atypia in smokers.

Polycyclic aromatic hydrocarbons such as 2-naphthylamine, 4-aminobiphenyl, and benzidine and benzene or exhausts from combustion gases are associated with an increased risk of bladder cancer. Occupations reported to be at higher risk include aluminum work, dry cleaning, manufacturing of preservatives and polychlorinated biphenyls, and pesticide application. Arylamines, also implicated in carcinogenesis, are metabolically activated to electrophilic compounds by N-hydroxylation in the liver by cytochrome P-450 IA2 and detoxified by N-acetylation; studies suggest that individuals with a fast oxidizer and slow acetylator phenotype are at highest risk. Patients with occupations associated with a higher exposure to arylamines, such as workers in the dye, rubber, or leather manufacturing industries, are believed to be at higher risk of bladder cancer. *Schistosoma haematobium* infection enhances formation of carcinogenic N-nitroso compounds and results in an increased risk of both squamous and transitional cell carcinomas of the bladder. An association has been observed between squamous cell carcinoma (but not transitional cell tumors) and the presence of chronic urinary tract infections seen in paraplegic patients and those with chronic bladder stones and indwelling Foley catheters. The chemotherapy agent cyclophosphamide can increase the risk of bladder cancer nine-fold, and phenacetin-containing compounds have been implicated in the development of renal pelvis and ureteral tumors.

PATHOBIOLOGY

Urothelial tumors can occur anywhere along the urinary tract, including the renal pelvis, ureters, bladder, and urethra. More than 90% of tumors originate in the bladder, 8% in the renal pelvis, and the remaining 2% in the ureter and urethra. Transitional cell carcinomas make up 90 to 95% of urothelial tumors; squamous cell (keratinizing) tumors (3%), adenocarcinomas (2%), and small cell tumors (1%) constitute the remainder. Mixed-histology tumors, consisting of predominantly transitional cell carcinoma with areas of squamous, adenocarcinomatous, or neuroendocrine elements, are frequently observed. Squamous cell tumors are more common in the distal urethra, and adenocarcinomas occur in the embryonal remnant of the urachus on the dome of the bladder and in periurethral tissues. In endemic areas of *S. haematobium* (Chapter 363) infections (such as Egypt), 40% of tumors are squamous cell carcinomas. Rare tumors of the bladder include lymphoma, sarcoma, and melanoma.

Most (70 to 80%) newly detected bladder cancers are classified as superficial tumors and include exophytic papillary tumors confined to the mucosa (Ta), tumors invading the lamina propria (T1), and carcinoma in situ (CIS, also called Tis). Superficial bladder tumors are typically graded according to the World Health Organization/International Society of Urologic Pathology (WHO/ISUP) grading system as low or high grade. If the grading system is not specified, a numerical system can be used: well differentiated (G1), moderately differentiated (G2), poorly differentiated (G3), and undifferentiated (G4). Grading is more important for noninvasive Ta tumors because almost all invasive bladder tumors (T1 or greater) are high grade. Primary CIS (or Tis) without a concurrent Ta or T1 tumor constitutes 1 to 2% of new bladder cancer cases. More frequently, CIS is found in the presence of multiple papillary tumors, either immediately adjacent to another lesion or involving remote mucosa in the bladder. CIS is, by definition, high-grade disease; it is regarded as a precursor to more invasive tumors because 60% of untreated tumors develop more invasive disease within 5 years. A T1 tumor is an aggressive, invasive malignancy. Virtually all T1 tumors are high grade, and 50% have associated CIS. Fifty percent of patients have disease recurrence by 1 year, and 90% within 5 years. A minority of primary tumors at diagnosis are found to invade the muscularis propria (T2), extend to perivesicular fat (T3), or extend into immediately adjacent organs (T4); all primary tumors stage T2 or higher are high grade.

The natural history of a urothelial tumor is to recur either at the same location or at a separate site in the urothelial tract and at the same or a more advanced stage. Several studies support the controversial concept that these recurrences are clonal in origin. Chromosome 9 deletions are the most commonly observed chromosomal changes in bladder cancer. Chromosomal deletions of 17p (the *TP53* locus), 18q (the *DCC* gene locus), and the *RB* gene locus are frequently observed in invasive tumors; deletions of 3p and 11p occur in both superficial and invasive tumors. Associations between specific gene deletions and prognosis have been attempted, particularly for the *TP53* and *RB* genes, but inconsistent findings among studies preclude their routine use in clinical management. The epidermal growth factor receptor is highly expressed (~80%) on bladder cancer tumors, and the Her-2/Neu growth factor receptor is less frequently expressed (~50%). Studies suggest that higher expression of these receptors on bladder cancers is associated with a more advanced and more aggressive phenotype of disease.

CLINICAL MANIFESTATIONS

Hematuria is the presenting symptom in 80 to 90% of bladder cancer cases, but others present with a urinary tract infection. Individuals older than 40 years who develop hematuria should have an evaluation for the presence of urothelial cancer that includes urinary cytology, cystoscopy, and imaging of the urinary tract by either an ultrasound or CT. Screening of asymptomatic subjects for hematuria increases the probability of diagnosing bladder cancer at an earlier stage but does not improve survival; thus, it is not routinely recommended. Urinary frequency and nocturia may be present as a consequence of either irritative symptoms or reduced bladder capacity. Pain, when present, typically reflects the location of the bladder tumor. Lower abdominal pain may occur as a result of a bladder mass, and rectal discomfort and perineal pain can result from tumors invading into the prostate or pelvis. Tumors of the renal pelvis, ureter, or bladder in which the ureteral orifice is obstructed can cause hydronephrosis, reduced renal function, and flank pain. Patients with more advanced disease can present with anorexia, fatigue, weight loss, or pain from a metastatic bone lesion. The physical examination is frequently unremarkable in patients presenting with bladder tumors because most patients have organ-confined tumors.

DIAGNOSIS

The mainstay of bladder cancer diagnosis and staging is the cystoscopic evaluation. The procedure includes the examination under anesthesia to determine whether a palpable mass (either mobile or not) is present. A nonmobile tumor mass is indicative of disease invading the pelvic sidewall, which is unlikely to be resectable. Urine is obtained to evaluate for the presence of malignant cells. A cystoscope is inserted to visually inspect the bladder and detail the size, number, location, and growth pattern (papillary or solid) of all lesions. All visible tumors undergo transurethral resection of the bladder tumor to determine the histologic subtype and depth of invasion. Adequate evaluation, particularly in large tumors that may be invasive, requires that muscle be identified in the pathologic specimen. Repeat biopsy of the resected area is occasionally required to ensure that no muscle invasion is present because invasion into muscle requires consideration of surgical removal of the bladder rather than just endoscopic resection of the tumor. Biopsies from any areas of erythema are performed to assess for CIS. The urethra is inspected during withdrawal of the cystoscope, and specimens are taken if clinically indicated. Patients with a positive cytology but no apparent tumor within the bladder undergo selective retrograde catheterization of the ureters up to the renal pelves to assess for upper tract disease.

The decision whether to image the abdomen and pelvis is based on the cystoscopy results and the pathology of the tumor. An intravenous pyelogram or CT urogram can evaluate the upper urinary tracts, and CT or MRI may distinguish whether a tumor extends to the perivesical fat (T3) or prostate or vagina (T4) and whether regional lymph nodes are involved. In the case of larger, invasive tumors, the presence or absence of distal metastases can be documented with physical examination, CT of the abdomen and pelvis, chest radiograph, and radionuclide bone scan.

All patients with carcinoma of the bladder or of related sites are staged using the TNM system advocated by the American Joint Committee on Cancer (AJCC) (Table 203-5). The TNM system categorizes the depth of invasion of the primary tumor, nodal metastases in the pelvis (or retroperitoneum for upper tract disease) on the basis of the number and size of regional nodes involved, other nonregional lymph node sites, and any visceral sites of disease.

TREATMENT   Rx

Superficial Disease

The standard treatment for superficial tumors is a complete endoscopic resection. Most patients develop new tumors, 30% of which progress to a higher stage, mandating vigilant surveillance at 3-month intervals with cystoscopy, urine cytology, and repeat transurethral resection when indicated. Additional treatment in the form of adjuvant intravesical therapy is dependent on the number of lesions, the size, the depth of invasion, and the number of prior tumors in that individual. Prophylactic or adjuvant intravesical therapy is typically instituted in the setting when a patient has shown either a repeated tendency to develop new lesions in the bladder or is at high risk for recurrence or progression de novo. Intravesical therapy is not warranted for the first Ta tumor that is low grade. Instances of high recurrence and progression warranting intravesical therapy include multifocal or large lesions, high-grade papillary lesions, T1 tumors, CIS, or a combination. It is never advised for muscle-invasive tumors because agents instilled in the bladder do not penetrate beyond a few layers of cells. After allowing sufficient time for healing after the endoscopic resection, intravesical therapy is most frequently initiated with the immunologic agent bacillus Calmette-Guérin (BCG) weekly for 6 weeks.[6] Occasionally, other chemotherapy and cytokines are used when BCG is contraindicated. Treatment outcome is assessed at the 3- and 6-month evaluations following treatment to determine whether the bladder has been rendered tumor free. If disease persists, either a repeat course of BCG treatment or even an immediate cystectomy may be recommended. Bladder toxicity can result from urothelial irritation, including bladder irritability or spasms, hematuria, and pain on urination. A rare complication of BCG is development of a systemic tuberculosis infection requiring treatment with systemic antituberculosis agents. BCG is highly effective in eradicating CIS, with 70% of patients disease free at 1 year and 40% at 10 years. Selected tumors in the ureter or renal pelvis can be managed by ureteroscopic resection, in some cases by instillation of BCG through the renal pelvis, or nephroureterectomy. Tumors of the prostatic urethra are frequently managed by cystoprostatectomy, particularly if a complete resection cannot be accomplished.

Muscle-Invasive Tumors

For patients with tumors infiltrating the muscularis propria, the standard of care in the United States is a radical cystectomy and pelvic lymphadenectomy because of the high incidence of cancer extending into the perivesicular fat or into regional lymph nodes. A prostatectomy is also performed in men; in women, the urethra, uterus, fallopian tubes, ovaries, and anterior vaginal wall are removed. Urinary flow can be directed through either a conduit diversion or a continent reservoir. With a conduit diversion, urine is drained directly from the ureters to a loop of small bowel that is anastomosed to the skin surface with no internal reservoir. Urine is collected in an external appliance. Alternatively, a low-pressure continent reservoir can be created from a detubularized segment of bowel attached to the abdominal wall with a continent stoma that can be self-catheterized at regular intervals. Low-pressure reservoirs can also be anastomosed to the urethra, creating an internal orthotopic neobladder and permitting the patient to void through the normal urethra. The standard pelvic lymphadenectomy includes the distal common iliac, external iliac, obturator, and hypogastric nodes; improved survival and decreased local recurrence are associated with an increased number of lymph nodes removed. Complications of cystectomy include recurrent urinary infections, hyperchloremic acidosis (Chapter 120), oxalate stones (Chapter 128), incontinence, and impotence.

Neoadjuvant chemotherapy before cystectomy for muscle-invasive bladder cancer increases survival.[7] This survival benefit is achieved only with cisplatin-based combinations, which require the patient to have normal renal function and a good performance status. Some physicians prefer immediate cystectomy followed by adjuvant chemotherapy if the pathologic evaluation demonstrates a high risk of recurrence, such as disease extending to either the perivesical fat or the lymph nodes. Radical cystectomy is effective in providing long-term disease control in 75 to 80% of patients with organ-confined disease, approximately 50% of those with tumors extending into the perivesical tissues, and nearly one third of patients with regional lymph node involvement. Some patients prefer a bladder-sparing approach using radiation treatment rather than a cystectomy. The best candidates for this approach are patients with a solitary early-stage lesion and no evidence of hydronephrosis. This trimodality treatment for bladder preservation first requires a successful, near-complete transurethral resection of tumor followed by concurrent chemotherapy and radiation. External beam treatments are delivered in five daily fractions a week, starting with the whole pelvis to a total dose of 40 to 45 Gy followed by 20 to 25 Gy reduced volume to the bladder tumor. Toxicities include inflammation of the skin, impotence, fatigue, and irritative symptoms from the bladder and bowel; persistent proctitis is rare. In this approach, cystectomy is reserved for patients failing to achieve complete response. The 5-year disease-free survival rate with this approach is 50%, with most patients retaining a normally functioning bladder.

TABLE 203-5 TNM DEFINITIONS FOR CANCERS OF THE BLADDER, URETER, AND RENAL PELVIS

PRIMARY TUMORS OF THE BLADDER (T)

TX	Primary tumor cannot be assessed
T0	No evidence of primary tumor
Ta	Noninvasive papillary carcinoma
Tis	Carcinoma in situ ("flat tumor")
T1	Tumor invades subepithelial connective tissue
T2	Tumor invades muscularis propria
pT2a	Tumor invades superficial muscularis propria (inner half)
pT2b	Tumor invades deep muscularis propria (outer half)
T3	Tumor invades perivesical tissue
pT3a	Microscopically
pT3b	Macroscopically (extravesical mass)
T4	Tumor invades any of the following: prostatic stroma, seminal vesicles, uterus, vagina, pelvic wall, abdominal wall
T4a	Tumor invades the prostatic stroma, uterus, vagina
T4b	Tumor invades the pelvic wall, abdominal wall

REGIONAL LYMPH NODES FOR UROTHELIAL TUMORS OF THE BLADDER (N)

Regional lymph nodes include both the primary and secondary drainage regions. All other nodes above the aortic bifurcation are considered distant lymph nodes.

NX	Lymph nodes cannot be assessed
N0	No lymph node metastasis
N1	Single regional lymph node metastasis in the true pelvis (hypogastric, obturator, external iliac, or presacral node)
N2	Multiple regional lymph node metastases in the true pelvis (hypogastric, obturator, external iliac, or presacral node)
N3	Lymph node metastasis to the common iliac lymph nodes

PRIMARY TUMORS OF THE URETER AND RENAL PELVIS (T)

TX	Primary tumor cannot be assessed
T0	No evidence of primary tumor
Ta	Papillary noninvasive carcinoma
Tis	Carcinoma in situ
T1	Tumor invades subepithelial connective tissue
T2	Tumor invades the muscularis
T3	(For renal pelvis only) Tumor invades beyond muscularis into peripelvic fat or the renal parenchyma
T3	(For ureter only) Tumor invades beyond muscularis into periureteric fat
T4	Tumor invades adjacent organs or through the kidney into perinephric fat

REGIONAL LYMPH NODES FOR UROTHELIAL TUMORS (N)* OF URETER AND RENAL PELVIS

NX	Regional lymph nodes cannot be assessed
N0	No regional lymph node metastasis
N1	Metastasis in a single lymph node, 2 cm or less in greatest dimension
N2	Metastasis in a single lymph node, more than 2 cm but not more than 5 cm in greatest dimension; or multiple lymph nodes, none more than 5 cm in greatest dimension
N3	Metastasis in a lymph node, more than 5 cm in greatest dimension

*Note: Laterality does not affect the N classification.

DISTANT METASTASIS FOR ALL UROTHELIAL TUMORS (M)

MX	Distant metastasis cannot be assessed
M0	No distant metastasis
M1	Distant metastasis

AJCC STAGE GROUPINGS FOR BLADDER CANCER

0a	Ta, N0, M0
0is	Tis, N0, M0
I	T1, N0, M0
II	T2a, N0, M0
	T2b, N0, M0
III	T3a, N0, M0
	T3b, N0, M0
	T4a, N0, M0
IV	T4b, N0, M0
	Any T, N1-3, M0
	Any T, Any, N M1

AJCC STAGE GROUPINGS FOR CANCER OF THE RENAL PELVIS AND URETER

0a	Ta, N0, M0
0is	Tis, N0, M0
I	T1, N0, M0
II	T2, N0, M0
III	T3, N0, M0
IV	T4, N0, M0
	Any T, N1, M0
	Any T, N2, M0
	Any T, N3, M0
	Any T, Any, N M1

From *AJCC Cancer Staging Manual*, 7th ed. New York: Springer-Verlag; 2010.

Metastatic Disease

Patients with metastatic disease are treated predominantly with chemotherapy. Cisplatin-based chemotherapy is the standard of care. The two most commonly used regimens are gemcitabine plus cisplatin (GC) and the four-drug regimen of methotrexate, vinblastine, doxorubicin, and cisplatin (MVAC); six cycles of therapy are given are over a 6-month period. The most frequently observed toxicities include anemia, thrombocytopenia, neutropenic fever, mucositis, and fatigue. The GC regimen is better tolerated and has less severe toxicities than MVAC.[8] The median survival of patients treated with both regimens is approximately 14 months, and the 5-year survival rate is 15% or less. Patients with a good performance status and whose metastatic disease is limited to the lymph nodes (i.e., no visceral metastases) have the highest likelihood for response and a 20 to 33% chance of 5-year disease-free survival. Patients with impaired renal function are treated with carboplatin rather than cisplatin owing to less toxicity to the kidney with carboplatin.[9] Carboplatin is administered with either gemcitabine or paclitaxel, and toxicities include myelosuppression and fatigue.

transitional cell CIS requires intravesical immunotherapy therapy with BCG in addition to endoscopic resection. This intravesical treatment can substantially reduce recurrence and progression, with a 5-year disease-free survival rate of 60%. Muscle-invasive disease is most frequently cured with an integrated approach of systemic chemotherapy for micrometastases followed by cystectomy and pelvic lymphadenectomy; cure rates for T2 tumors can be as high as 80% with this multimodality approach. Bladder-sparing approaches associated with an improved quality of life are possible using external beam radiation. Metastatic urinary bladder cancer is a fast growing and often lethal malignancy; despite aggressive chemotherapy, only a small proportion (~15%) of patients are disease free at 5 years.

● CANCERS OF THE RENAL PELVIS AND URETERS

Approximately 10% of transitional cell carcinomas occur in the ureters and the renal pelvis. These tumors can arise either de novo or in the setting of prior tumors. The risk of developing an upper tract tumor in patients with multifocal CIS of the bladder approaches 25% by 10 years. These tumors are morphologically similar to the tumors in the bladder and behave in a similar manner. Hematuria is the most common presenting symptom, although patients with large tumors or ureteral obstruction can present with flank pain. An intravenous pyelogram, CT, or MRI is used to stage the extent of primary disease and to detect regional metastases. Low-grade tumors can be treated endoscopically, but high-grade tumors are most commonly treated

PROGNOSIS

Urinary bladder cancer is a common but heterogeneous disease with a decreasing mortality rate because of improvements in therapy. Superficial Ta G1 lesions, easily treated with endoscopic resection alone, almost never progress. At the other end of the spectrum of superficial disease, aggressive with a nephroureterectomy. In contrast to cystectomy, a regional lymphad-enectomy is not routinely performed. In renal pelvis tumors, the ureter is removed in addition to a nephrectomy because of the high risk of multifocal tumors along the entire upper tract and the inability to monitor the ureteral stump with accuracy. Systemic chemotherapy is used for unresectable primary tumors, patients with regional adenopathy, or recurrent tumors. Upper tract transitional cell carcinomas are staged according to the TNM system (see Table 203-5). Treatment of advanced, nonsurgical disease is with chemotherapy, and these urothelial tumors have the same sensitivity to che-motherapy as bladder cancer, with similar response rates and 5-year survival rates. Cisplatin-based chemotherapy is used in patients with normal renal function. Carboplatin-based chemotherapy is considered if there is renal insufficiency either from obstruction, a prior nephroureterectomy, or medical comorbidity.

1. Flanigan RC, Salmon SE, Blumenstein BA, et al. Nephrectomy followed by interferon alfa-2b com-pared with interferon alfa-2b alone for metastatic renal-cell cancer. *N Engl J Med.* 2001;345: 1655-1659.
2. Motzer RJ, Hutson TE, Tomczak P, et al. Sunitinib versus interferon alfa in metastatic renal-cell carcinoma. *N Engl J Med.* 2007;356:115-124.
3. Escudier B, Pluzanska A, Koralewski, et al, for the AVOREN Trial investigators. Bevacizumab plus interferon alfa-2a for treatment of metastatic renal cell carcinoma: a randomised, double-blind phase III trial. *Lancet.* 2007;370:2103-2111.
4. Hudes G, Carducci M, Tomczak P, et al. Global ARCC Trial. Temsirolimus, interferon alfa, or both for advanced renal-cell cancer. *N Engl J Med.* 2007;356:2271-2281.
5. Motzer RJ, Escudier B, Oudard S, et al, for the RECORD-1 Study Group. Efficacy of everolimus in advanced renal cell carcinoma: a double-blind, randomised, placebo-controlled phase III trial. *Lancet.* 2008;372:449-456.
6. Shelley MD, Mason MD, Kynaston H. Intravesical therapy for superficial bladder cancer: a systematic review of randomised trials and meta-analyses. *Cancer Treat Rev.* 2010;36:195-205.
7. Grossman HB, Natale RB, Tangen CM, et al. Neoadjuvant chemotherapy plus cystectomy compared with cystectomy alone for locally advanced bladder cancer. *N Engl J Med.* 2003;349:859-866.
8. von der Maase H, Hansen SW, Roberts JT, et al. Gemcitabine and cisplatin versus methotrexate, vinblastine, doxorubicin, and cisplatin in advanced or metastatic bladder cancer: results of a large, randomized, multinational, multicenter, phase III study. *J Clin Oncol.* 2000;18:3068-3077.
9. De Santis M, Bellmunt J, Mead G, et al. Randomized phase II/III trial assessing gemcitabine/carbo-platin and methotrexate/carboplatin/vinblastine in patients with advanced urothelial cancer "unfit" for cisplatin-based chemotherapy: phase II—results of EORTC study 30986. *J Clin Oncol.* 2009;27:5634-5639.

SUGGESTED READINGS

Chou R, Dana T. Screening adults for bladder cancer: a review of the evidence for the U.S. preventive services task force. *Ann Intern Med.* 2010;153:461-468. *Clinical guidelines recommending against screening.*

Morgan TM, Keegan KA, Clark PE. Bladder cancer. *Curr Opin Oncol.* 2011;23:275-282. *Comprehensive review of epidemiology, diagnosis, and management.*

Rouprêt M, Zigeuner R, Palou J, et al. European guidelines for the diagnosis and management of upper urinary tract urothelial cell carcinomas: 2011 update. *Eur Urol.* 2011;59:584-594. *Consensus guidelines.*

Singer EA, Gupta GN, Srinivasan R. Update on targeted therapies for clear cell renal cell carcinoma. *Curr Opin Oncol.* 2011;23:283-289. *Review including rapamycin and new biologies.*

204

BREAST CANCER AND BENIGN BREAST DISORDERS

NANCY DAVIDSON

Invasive breast cancer, the most common nonskin cancer in women in the United States, will be diagnosed in about 180,000 women in 2010 and will result in approximately 40,000 deaths. Incidence and mortality from breast cancer appear to be dropping in the United States and parts of western Europe. This decline is believed to reflect early detection by screening mam-mography and widespread use of adjuvant systemic therapy as well as decreased use of hormone replacement therapy.

BREAST CANCER

EPIDEMIOLOGY AND PATHOBIOLOGY

Multiple risk factors for the development of breast cancer have been identi-fied (Table 204-1). The principal risk factor is gender. Breast cancer is largely

TABLE 204-1	RISK FACTORS FOR BREAST CANCER
RISK FACTOR	**RELATIVE RISK**
Any benign breast disease	1.5
Postmenopausal hormone replacement (estrogen with or without progestin)	1.5
Menarche at <12 yr	1.1-1.9
Moderate alcohol intake (two to three drinks/day)	1.1-1.9
Menopause at >55 yr	1.1-1.9
Increased bone density	1.1-1.9
Sedentary lifestyle and lack of exercise	1.1-1.9
Proliferative breast disease without atypia	2
Age at first birth >30 yr or nulliparous	2-4
First-degree relative with breast cancer	2-4
Postmenopausal obesity	2-4
Upper socioeconomic class	2-4
Personal history of endometrial or ovarian cancer	2-4
Significant radiation to chest	2-4
Increased breast density on mammogram	2-4
Older age	>4
Personal history of breast cancer (in situ or invasive)	>4
Proliferative breast disease with atypia	>4
Two first-degree relatives with breast cancer	5
Atypical hyperplasia and first-degree relative with breast cancer	10

a disease of women, although it does occur in men at an incidence of about 1% that seen in women. A second critical risk factor is age. About 75% of breast cancer cases in the United States are diagnosed in women older than 50 years of age.

Family history is a third critical risk factor. About 20% of breast cancer occurs in women with a family history of breast cancer; increased risk is associated with diagnosis of breast cancer in first-degree relatives younger than 50 years. Five to 8% of breast cancer cases occur in high-risk families. Several familial breast cancer syndromes with associated molecular abnor-malities have been identified. Chief among them is the breast ovarian cancer syndrome, which is linked to germline mutations in the breast cancer suscep-tibility genes, *BRCA1* and *BRCA2*. These mutations are inherited in an auto-somal dominant fashion and can therefore be transmitted through the maternal or paternal line. Extensive studies suggest that a germline mutation in either of these genes is associated with a 50 to 85% lifetime risk of develop-ing breast cancer. Testing for *BRCA1* and *BRCA2* mutations is now viewed as a standard option for women with clinical features suggestive of a heredi-tary breast cancer syndrome; these include multiple family members with early-onset breast or ovarian cancer, bilateral breast cancer, or Ashkenazi Jewish heritage. Careful counseling about the implications of a positive or negative test and about the limitations of testing is a prerequisite for testing.

Other hereditary cancer syndromes (Chapter 184) include Li-Fraumeni syndrome, which is linked with germline mutations in the *p53* tumor sup-pressor gene, and Cowden's syndrome, which is associated with inherited mutations in the *PTEN* gene. Finally, in addition to these high-penetrance genetic susceptibility syndromes, recent results from genome-wide associa-tion studies have identified a number of low-penetrance genetic associations, including single nucleotide polymorphisms in a variety of genes. If or how to incorporate these low-penetrance traits into clinical practice remains to be established.

Reproductive risk factors include early menarche, late menopause, nulli-parity, and late first pregnancy. In aggregate, these factors result in prolonged estrogen exposure of the breast. The emerging association between post-menopausal obesity and breast cancer likely reflects estrogen exposure as well. Certain types of breast pathology, including atypical hyperplasia and lobular carcinoma in situ, are also associated with increased risk. The possibil-ity that increased breast density as assessed by mammography is a risk factor has also been raised. Finally, much interest has focused on the possibility that exogenous environmental factors predispose to breast cancer. Among the factors that appear to enhance breast cancer risk are ionizing radiation during adolescence, prolonged use of hormone replacement therapy, ongoing use of oral contraceptives, and alcohol consumption. Large studies have failed to show any convincing association between exposure to estrogenic pesticides or a high-fat diet and breast cancer.

CLINICAL MANIFESTATIONS

Breast cancer usually presents as a mammographic abnormality or a physical change in the breast including a mass or asymmetrical thickening, nipple discharge, or skin or nipple changes. Two unusual clinical presentations include Paget's disease of the nipple and inflammatory breast cancer. The former is a form of adenocarcinoma involving the skin and ducts and is manifested as nipple excoriation. The latter is recognized as a constellation of redness, warmth, and edema that often reflects tumor cell infiltration of dermal lymphatics of the breast; it should not be mistaken for a simple mastitis.

Nipple discharge may be associated with breast malignancy. Although milky discharge is seldom associated with a malignant diagnosis, patients with a clear or bloody nipple discharge require breast examination and mammography and often excisional biopsy of any suspicious area. Ductography and sometimes ductoscopy may be used to identify the inciting lesion. A bloody discharge is frequently caused by an intraductal papilloma.

Breast pain is common, especially as a premenstrual symptom in premenopausal women. But it may also be associated with an underlying malignancy. Patients with localized noncyclic breast pain should undergo breast examination and bilateral mammography. If these are normal, ultrasound or magnetic resonance imaging (MRI) may be used to exclude the small probability of a malignancy.

DIAGNOSIS

Diagnostic evaluation is generally triggered by suspicious findings on screening mammogram or detection of a palpable breast abnormality by the patient or health care provider. For both clinically occult and clinically apparent lesions, pathologic evaluation is mandatory to establish a diagnosis. Today, fine-needle aspiration and core needle biopsy have replaced incisional or excisional biopsy as the standard diagnostic measures. These procedures can be performed in the office in patients with suspicious palpable lesions. For women with nonpalpable lesions, biopsy guided by mammography, ultrasonography, or MRI is now standard. A recently published systematic review showed that stereotactic- or ultrasound-guided core needle biopsies are almost as accurate as and associated with lower complication rates than open surgical biopsy. These technologies permit an accurate diagnosis that can be followed by definitive treatment planning. It is axiomatic, however, that further evaluation must be undertaken for suspicious lesions that give an equivocal diagnosis after needle aspiration or core biopsy. Finally, bilateral breast imaging is always recommended to identify any unsuspected lesions in the contralateral breast that may also require evaluation.

Staging and Prognostic and Predictive Markers

Although staging originally reflected the clinical assessment of tumor size, nodal status, and evidence of metastatic disease, pathologic staging is the most accurate estimate of tumor involvement and prognosis. The staging system for breast cancer was revised in 2002 (Tables 204-2 and 204-3).

Most patients with breast cancer present with stage I or II disease in the absence of symptoms. In these patients, laboratory studies can be limited to blood counts, chemistry panel, and chest radiograph, and more extensive radiologic evaluation is not warranted because of low yield. In contrast, women with clinical evidence of stage III or IV disease should undergo more intensive evaluation of common sites for metastases, including lung, liver, and bone, through computed tomography and radionuclide scanning.

The two most important determinants of prognosis for early-stage breast cancer are pathological lymph node status and tumor size. Other factors that contribute to prognosis are the expression of the estrogen receptor-α (ER), progesterone receptor (PR), and HER2 proteins; these are conventionally measured by immunohistochemistry, although fluorescence in situ hybridization (FISH) for *HER2* gene amplification is also employed. Poor prognosis is associated with high lymph node burden, poor histologic grade, large tumor size, absence of ER and PR expression, and overexpression of HER2.

Recently, the focus has been on the development of predictive markers to guide selection of therapy. There are three established predictive markers for breast cancer—ER, PR, and HER2—and these should be routinely evaluated in every invasive cancer. Most tumors that express ER or PR, or both,

TABLE 204-2 STAGING OF BREAST CANCER: TNM SYSTEM

TUMOR SIZE: T (LARGEST DIAMETER)

TX	Primary tumor cannot be assessed
T0	No evidence of primary tumor
Tis	Carcinoma in situ
Tis (DCIS)	Ductal carcinoma in situ
Tis (LCIS)	Lobular carcinoma in situ
Tis (Paget's)	Paget's disease of the nipple NOT associated with invasive carcinoma and/or carcinoma in situ (DCIS and/or LCIS) in the underlying breast parenchyma. Carcinomas in the breast parenchyma associated with Paget's disease are categorized based on the size and characteristics of the parenchymal disease, although the presence of Paget's disease should still be noted.
T1	Tumor ≤20 mm in greatest dimension
T1mi	Tumor ≤1 mm in greatest dimension
T1a	Tumor >1 mm but ≤5 mm in greatest dimension
T1b	Tumor >5 mm but ≤10 mm in greatest dimension
T1c	Tumor >10 mm but ≤20 mm in greatest dimension
T2	Tumor >20 mm but not ≤50 mm in greatest dimension
T3	Tumor >50 mm in greatest dimension
T4	Tumor of any size with direct extension to chest wall or skin (includes inflammatory carcinoma)

NODAL INVOLVEMENT: N (NODAL STATUS)

NX	Regional lymph nodes cannot be assessed (e.g., previously removed, not removed)
N0	No regional lymph node metastases histologically
N1	Metastases to movable ipsilateral level I, II axillary lymph node(s)
N2	Metastases in ipsilateral level I, II axillary lymph nodes that are clinically fixed or matted; or in clinically detected* ipsilateral internal mammary nodes in the *absence* of clinically evident axillary lymph node metastases.
N3	Metastases in ipsilateral infraclavicular (level III axillary) lymph node(s) with or without level I, II axillary lymph node involvement; or in clinically detected* ipsilateral internal mammary lymph node(s) with clinically evident level I, II axillary lymph node metastases; or metastases in ipsilateral supraclavicular lymph node(s) with or without axillary or internal mammary lymph node involvement
N3a	Metastases in ipsilateral infraclavicular lymph node(s)
N3b	Metastases in ipsilateral internal mammary lymph node(s) and axillary lymph node(s)
N3c	Metastases in ipsilateral supraclavicular lymph node(s)

METASTASES: M

M0	No clinical or radiographic evidence of distant metastases
cM0(i+)	No clinical or radiographic evidence of distant metastases, but deposits of molecularly or microscopically detected tumor cells in circulating blood, bone marrow, or other nonregional nodal tissue that are no larger than 0.2 mm in a patient without symptoms or signs of metastases
M1	Distant detectable metastases as determined by classic clinical and radiographic means and/or histologically proven larger than 0.2 mm

Clinically detected is defined as detected by imaging studies (excluding lymphoscintigraphy) or by clinical examination and having characteristics highly suspicious for malignancy or a presumed pathologic macrometastasis based on fine-needle biopsy with cytologic examination.
From *AJCC Cancer Staging Manual*, 7th ed. New York: Springer-Verlag; 2010.

are responsive to endocrine therapy, whereas those that lack ER and PR expression seldom respond to such therapy. Overexpression of the HER2 protein by immunohistochemistry or *HER2* gene amplification by FISH is associated with response to the HER2-targeted monoclonal antibody, trastuzumab, or the receptor tyrosine kinase inhibitor, lapatinib. Evidence that links expression of ER, PR, or HER2 to chemotherapy efficacy is equivocal.

Modern molecular techniques have provided further insight into molecular classification of breast cancer. Transcriptional profiling has suggested that breast cancers can be divided into at least five molecular subsets—normal mammary, luminal A and B, HER2, and basal. The luminal subtypes frequently express ER, but luminal A appears to be associated with a better

TABLE 204-3 TNM STAGE AND SURVIVAL

STAGE	TNM CATEGORY*	RECURRENCE FREE AT 10 YEARS (NO SYSTEMIC ADJUVANT THERAPY)
0	TisN0M0	98%
I	T1N0M0	80% (all stage I patients)
	T < 1 cm	90%
	T > 1-2 cm	80-90%
IIA	T0N1M0; T2N0M0	60-80%
IIA	T1N1M0	50-60%
IIB	T2 N1M0	5-10% worse than IIA and based on node status
IIB	T3N0M0	30-50%
IIIA	T0 or T1 or T2N2M0; or T3N1 or N2M0	10-40%
IIIB	T4N0 or N1 or N2M0	5-30%
IIIC	Any T, N3M0	15-20%
IV	Any T, any NM1	<5%

*See Table 204-2 for TNM definitions.

TABLE 204-4 CARCINOMA IN SITU: DUCTAL VERSUS LOBULAR

FEATURE	LOBULAR CARCINOMA IN SITU	DUCTAL CARCINOMA IN SITU
Age	Younger	Older
Palpable mass	No	Uncommon
Mammographic appearance	Not detected on mammography	Microcalcifications, mass
Immunophenotype	E-cadherin negative	E-cadherin positive
Usual manifestation	Incidental finding on breast biopsy	Microcalcifications on mammography or breast mass
Bilateral involvement	Common	Uncertain
Risk and site of subsequent breast cancer	25% risk for invasive breast cancer in either breast over remaining lifespan	At site of initial lesion; 0.5% risk/yr of invasive breast cancer in opposite breast
Prevention	Consider tamoxifen or raloxifene	Consider tamoxifen or raloxifene if estrogen receptor positive
Treatment	Yearly mammography and breast examination	Lumpectomy ± radiation; mastectomy for large or multifocal lesions

prognosis and higher likelihood of response to endocrine therapy than luminal B. The basal subtype is dominated by tumors that lack expression of ER, PR, and HER2—the so-called triple-negative breast cancer that lacks a readily identified molecular target. Multigene assays that evaluate these gene expression patterns are under investigation, and several multigene assays are available in clinical practice. One such assay, Oncotype Dx, may assist in the identification of women with early-stage steroid receptor–positive breast cancer who would benefit from the addition of chemotherapy to tamoxifen. A second assay, Mammaprint, may be useful to identify young women with breast cancer with poor prognosis. A number of other assays are under development, and both the Oncotype Dx and Mammaprint assays are the subject of large randomized trials to refine the conditions for their optimal use.

TREATMENT Rx

Local Treatment of Early-Stage Breast Cancer
In Situ Carcinoma
Thanks to heightened breast cancer awareness and use of screening mammography, in situ carcinomas now account for 20 to 25% of newly diagnosed cases of breast cancer (Table 204-4). Most of these are ductal carcinoma in situ (DCIS). These lesions are associated with about a 30% risk for subsequent invasive breast cancer in the same breast. The risk for metastatic breast cancer with a diagnosis of DCIS is extremely small. As a consequence, management decisions are centered on the involved breast, and axillary lymph node evaluation is not routinely performed. Total mastectomy, the traditional therapy, has a high likelihood of cure, but studies suggest that breast conservation is appropriate for many women with DCIS. The major contraindications include poor cosmesis, extensive disease, or patient preference. Several models have suggested that size and grade of lesion and surgical margin status are important determinants of local outcome. Excision to obtain tumor-free margins is critical. Careful mammographic examination of the specimen and postexcision mammography of the breast are crucial to confirm that the DCIS has been adequately excised. A large randomized trial showed that radiotherapy plus lumpectomy decreased the likelihood of in situ or invasive recurrence when compared with lumpectomy alone. Other data sets suggest that some women with favorable histology who are willing to undergo close surveillance are candidates for local excision alone. In addition, the use of tamoxifen for 5 years can reduce ipsilateral breast cancer recurrence and contralateral breast cancer diagnosis by about 50%.

Controversy continues over whether lobular carcinoma in situ (LCIS) is truly a malignant lesion. LCIS is usually an incidental finding on a breast biopsy done for other indications, and it appears to be associated with a 25% risk for development of invasive breast cancer in either breast. Women with LCIS are generally managed expectantly with regular breast examination and mammography. Bilateral total mastectomy is sometimes considered for women with LCIS who have other risk factors or extreme anxiety. Finally, these women are candidates for tamoxifen or raloxifene as a risk-reduction strategy based on the results of several large breast cancer chemoprevention trials.

Invasive Breast Cancer
Surgery
Although radical mastectomy (removal of the breast, axillary contents, and underlying chest musculature) was the mainstay for breast cancer treatment for many years, it is seldom performed today. Multiple randomized trials have consistently shown that breast conservation therapy (BCT) with lumpectomy plus radiotherapy provides identical survival rates to modified radical mastectomy (removal of the breast and lymph nodes) for women with stages I and II breast cancer. Medical contraindications to BCT include multifocal disease, previous radiotherapy, ongoing pregnancy that precludes the timely use of radiotherapy, poor cosmesis, and patient preference. Although the number of patients who receive BCT has increased substantially, there are wide geographic differences within the United States. Patients who undergo mastectomy should be counseled about the availability of a number of autologous tissue and implant options for reconstruction, either at the time of surgery or anytime thereafter.

Because the likelihood of distant micrometastatic spread is highly correlated with the number of pathologically involved axillary lymph nodes, axillary dissection has traditionally been used to provide prognostic information. A drive toward limiting axillary surgery to minimize the incidence of postoperative lymphedema (see later) has led to the development of sentinel node techniques. Here a radioactive tracer or blue dye or both are injected into the area around the primary breast tumor. The injected substance tracks rapidly to the dominant axillary lymph node—the sentinel node—that can be located and removed by the surgeon. If the sentinel node is tumor free, the remaining nodes are likely to be tumor free as well, and no further axillary surgery is required. Currently, women with palpable axillary nodes and those with a histologically involved sentinel node are counseled to undergo axillary dissection. For women with small tumors and a clinically negative axilla, large randomized trials of sentinel node management and traditional axillary dissection suggest similar outcomes.

Adjuvant Radiotherapy
Radiotherapy has been a cornerstone in BCT because women who undergo lumpectomy alone have a breast cancer recurrence rate of up to 40%, whereas the rate of recurrence is less than 10% with whole-breast radiotherapy. Attempts to identify women whose tumors are so favorable that radiotherapy can be withheld are ongoing. One large trial suggested that women older than 70 years with small ER-positive tumors who receive tamoxifen gain little with radiotherapy. Current research is also focused on the possibility that radiotherapy can be delivered safely and effectively to a smaller field (partial breast radiotherapy) or over a shorter period of time.

The role of postmastectomy radiotherapy continues to be a matter of debate. Based on the results of individual randomized trials as well as a meta-analysis suggesting a survival advantage, many radiation oncologists recommend postmastectomy radiation to women with more than three involved nodes and discuss its use for those with involvement of one to three nodes.

Adjuvant Systemic Therapy for Early Breast Cancer
Adjuvant systemic therapy is defined as the use of chemotherapy, endocrine therapy, or biological therapy, or a combination of these, after definitive

local therapy for early breast cancer. Its goal is to suppress or eradicate clinically occult micrometastases. Because current testing does not permit the definitive identification of the patient with micrometastases, recommendations for adjuvant systemic therapy are based on menopausal status, lymph node status, tumor size, and the extent of expression of the ER, PR, and HER2 proteins in breast cancer cells. The treatment algorithms that are currently used are the result of more than 50 years of clinical trials[2]; the results of these trials have been compiled in sequential overview analyses that have evaluated the worldwide experience with use of endocrine therapy and chemotherapy. These analyses have shown that adjuvant therapy results in a proportional reduction in risk of recurrence across all patients regardless of risk of recurrence; this implies that the absolute benefit of adjuvant systemic therapy is greatest for individuals with the greatest risk of recurrence. Tools to assist the clinician and patient to make decisions about the use of adjuvant therapy include guidelines based on evidence and expert consensus such as the National Comprehensive Care Network (NCCN) and St. Gallen conference guidelines, as well as web-based algorithms like Adjuvant Online (Table 204-5).

Adjuvant Endocrine Therapy

Tamoxifen (20 mg/day for 5 years) has been the most widely used endocrine therapy. It improves outcomes in women of all ages with ER- or PR-positive breast cancer. Its side-effect profile includes an increased risk for thromboembolic events and uterine cancer, especially in postmenopausal women, because of its estrogen agonist properties. Potential benefits include promotion of bone density and lowering of cholesterol. The effects of altered activity of the tamoxifen metabolizing enzyme, CYP2D6, by coadministration of pharmacologic inhibitors or single-nucleotide polymorphism variants in the CYP2D6 gene on outcome with tamoxifen is an area of active research.

In recent years, the role of estrogen deprivation has been the subject of intense scrutiny—ovarian suppression or ablation for premenopausal women and aromatase inhibition for postmenopausal women. Ovarian ablation through surgery or radiotherapy is the oldest form of systemic therapy for breast cancer. More recent work has focused on the use of luteinizing hormone-releasing hormone (LHRH) agonists as a means of effecting a temporary and reversible ovarian suppression. Two large meta-analyses have sought to define the role of these approaches. A meta-analysis of trials addressing the efficacy of LHRH agonists in women with early-stage ER-positive breast cancer suggested the following: (1) monotherapy with LHRH agonist has significant activity; (2) the efficacy of LHRH monotherapy is similar to that of certain chemotherapy regimens; and (3) LHRH agonists appear to add benefit to adjuvant chemotherapy, especially in women younger than 40 years, who are less likely than older women to become postmenopausal as a consequence of adjuvant chemotherapy. Unfortunately, these trials did not routinely include tamoxifen because its value in premenopausal breast cancer was recognized only after accrual for these ovarian suppression studies was completed. In sum, however, it appears that ovarian ablation or suppression is a viable strategy for premenopausal women with steroid receptor–positive breast cancer.

In postmenopausal women, the primary source of estrogen is the conversion of androgens synthesized by the adrenal glands to estrogen through the activity of CYP19 or aromatase in peripheral tissues such as the mammary and adipose tissues. The aromatase inhibitors (anastrozole, letrozole, and exemestane) specifically inhibit this conversion, leading to further estrogen deprivation in older women. Randomized trials have shown that efficacy of aromatase inhibitors is similar or superior to that of tamoxifen and that these drugs have an acceptable side-effect profile.[3] Multiple trials have compared monotherapy with tamoxifen or aromatase inhibitor or sequential therapy; in aggregate, they suggest that the use of an aromatase inhibitor at some point should be considered for most postmenopausal women with steroid receptor–positive invasive breast cancer. Side effects include postmenopausal symptoms, osteoporosis and fractures, and arthralgias. Aromatase inhibitors are not useful for receptor-negative breast cancer, nor should they be used as monotherapy in premenopausal women. The simultaneous administration of tamoxifen plus aromatase inhibitor does not improve outcome over aromatase inhibitor alone. In premenopausal women, the combination of LHRH agonist plus aromatase inhibitor is no better than LHRH agonist plus tamoxifen in initial studies.

Duration of endocrine therapy appears to be quite important. Direct evidence suggests that at least 5 years of adjuvant endocrine therapy is associated with better outcomes than shorter periods. Whether longer durations will be more useful remains uncertain.

Adjuvant Anti-HER2 Therapy

Increased understanding of growth and death pathways of breast cancer has led to the identification of critical nonendocrine pathways that are potential targets for therapy. The transmembrane HER2/neu protein is overexpressed in about 20% of breast cancers, generally because of gene amplification. The efficacy and safety of the monoclonal antibody, trastuzumab, in the treatment of women with HER-overexpressing metastatic breast cancer laid the foundation for several adjuvant trials that in aggregate showed that the addition of 1 year of trastuzumab to chemotherapy reduced the risk for recurrence by about 50% in women with high-risk early breast cancer. Thus, use of

TABLE 204-5 ADJUVANT TREATMENT GUIDELINES FOR PATIENTS WITH EARLY-STAGE INVASIVE BREAST CANCER*

PATIENT GROUP*	TREATMENT
FAVORABLE HISTOLOGY (TUBULAR OR COLLOID)	
ER- and/or PR-Positive Breast Cancer	
<1 cm	No adjuvant therapy
1-2.9 cm	Consider adjuvant hormonal therapy[†]
≥3 cm or node-positive	Adjuvant hormonal therapy ± adjuvant chemotherapy[†]
ER- and PR-Negative Breast Cancer	
<1 cm	No adjuvant therapy
1-2.9 cm	Consider adjuvant chemotherapy
≥3 cm or node-positive	Adjuvant chemotherapy
HORMONE RECEPTOR–POSITIVE (ER- AND/OR PR-POSITIVE) BREAST CANCER	
Lymph Nodes Negative	
≤0.5 cm	No adjuvant therapy
0.6-1.0 cm well differentiated and no unfavorable features[‡]	Consider adjuvant hormonal therapy
0.6-1.0 cm moderate or poorly differentiated or unfavorable features	Adjuvant hormonal therapy ± adjuvant chemotherapy
>1 cm	Adjuvant hormonal therapy ± adjuvant chemotherapy
Lymph Nodes Positive	
	Adjuvant hormonal therapy + adjuvant chemotherapy
HORMONE RECEPTOR–NEGATIVE (ER- AND PR-NEGATIVE) BREAST CANCER	
≤0.5 cm	No adjuvant therapy
0.6-1.0 cm	Consider chemotherapy
>1 cm or lymph-node positive	Adjuvant chemotherapy
HER2 POSITIVE	
	Trastuzumab should be added to the suggested treatment above for all node-positive patients; trastuzumab not recommended for tumors ≤1 cm for most node-negative patients; for tumors >1 cm, trastuzumab should be considered for most patients

*Data are insufficient to make chemotherapy recommendations for patients 70 years and older. Treatment should be individualized for these patients based on life expectancy and comorbidity.
[†]In ER-positive or PR-positive patients, decisions regarding the added value of chemotherapy in addition to hormonal therapy alone can be aided by accurately assessing the added value of chemotherapy in individual patients using a web-based model: www.adjuvantonline.com or Oncotype Dx assay.
[‡]Unfavorable characteristics include high-grade tumor, blood vessel or lymphatic invasion by tumor, and high tumor proliferation rate (high S phase by flow cytometry or high Ki-67 value by immunohistochemistry) or HER2-positive status.
ER = estrogen receptor; PR = progesterone receptor.
Modified from National Comprehensive Cancer Network Guidelines. Available at www.nccn.org.

trastuzumab is considered for many women with HER2-positive tumors. Important questions remain regarding long-term risks and benefits, optimal duration of therapy, use of trastuzumab in the absence of chemotherapy, and role of other anti-HER2 agents such as lapatinib in addition to or in place of trastuzumab.

Adjuvant Chemotherapy

Individual trials and the Early Breast Cancer Trialists Collaborative Group meta-analysis have shown the benefit of adjuvant chemotherapy. Benefit varies by age and nodal status such that, in the meta-analysis, the absolute benefit is greatest in women younger than 50 years, in whom 15-year breast cancer mortality decreased from 42% to 32%, whereas it decreased from 50% to 47% for women aged 50 to 69 years.

These trials have established several principles that guide chemotherapy use. Combination therapy appears to be more effective than single-agent chemotherapy. Effective agents include anthracyclines, taxanes, antimetabolites, and cyclophosphamide.[4] Randomized trials have shown that 3 to 6 months of therapy is preferred over longer durations. Dose reduction below the standard level was associated with inferior outcome, but dose escalation through the use of colony-stimulating factors or autologous stem cell support led to excess toxicity without improved outcome. Regimens that use colony-stimulating factors to accelerate schedule of chemotherapy administration have been more successful.

Increased use of adjuvant chemotherapy and longer survival have led to concerns about toxicity. Acute side effects of therapy are nausea and vomiting, bone marrow suppression, and hair loss; all are reversible, and the first may be mitigated by the use of modern antiemetics. Careful use of colony-stimulating agents can minimize complications of neutropenia, but current evidence argues against the use of erythroid-stimulating agents for chemotherapy-induced anemia. Induction of menopause is a common concern for premenopausal women. Its likelihood is related to the type and duration of chemotherapy and the age of the patient; most women older than 40 years will suffer drug-induced menopause. Doxorubicin-related cardiomyopathy is noted in about 1% of women who received doxorubicin-containing adjuvant chemotherapy. Use of standard adjuvant chemotherapy regimens results in a very small incidence of acute leukemia, but there is no evidence of increased incidence of other second tumors. Concerns about cognitive impairment are under evaluation.

Sequencing of Adjuvant Therapy

Women frequently receive several adjuvant interventions, including chemotherapy, radiotherapy, endocrine therapy, or anti-HER2 therapy. A logical question is how best to sequence these therapies. A randomized trial showed no clear difference between the sequence of chemotherapy to radiotherapy and radiotherapy followed by chemotherapy. Concurrent chemoradiotherapy requires that certain drugs be omitted during the radiotherapy to limit toxicity. A common algorithm is surgery followed by chemotherapy followed by radiotherapy. Radiotherapy can be safely administered with endocrine or anti-HER2 therapy.

Because a large randomized trial showed that concurrent chemotherapy plus tamoxifen led to worse outcome than chemotherapy followed by tamoxifen, most practitioners delay the administration of endocrine therapy until after completion of chemotherapy. Conversely, the benefit of trastuzumab appears to be greater when it is coadministered with taxane chemotherapy rather than following completion of taxane.

A number of trials have tested the concept that administration of systemic therapy before primary surgery would improve outcome over the standard sequence of surgery followed by systemic therapy. Together they suggest that, compared with adjuvant therapy, preoperative (also termed neoadjuvant) systemic therapy improves the rate of breast conservation but does not enhance disease-free or overall survival. The possibility that preoperative therapy can provide an in vivo assessment of tumor response to therapy is suggested by the correlation between the finding of a pathologic complete response (absence of invasive cancer in the surgical specimen) and long-term disease-free survival in some studies.

Follow-up of Early Breast Cancer Survivors

A critical question is how longitudinal medical follow-up should be conducted in women who have received appropriate local and systemic therapy for early breast cancer. Randomized trials have addressed the question of the value of serial laboratory and radiology testing as well as the role of primary care versus oncology specialist follow-up. On the basis of these and other studies, the American Society of Clinical Oncology has published evidence-based guidelines for follow-up of asymptomatic survivors of early-stage breast cancer. These guidelines are summarized in Table 204-6.

Stage III Breast Cancer

Locally advanced or inoperable stage III breast cancer accounts for about 10% of breast cancers. It is characterized by large primary tumor or fixed tumor or lymph nodes or neoplastic invasion of the skin or chest wall. Inflammatory breast cancer falls into this category. It has a clinical presentation of breast swelling, warmth, and erythema and may or may not be associated with a mass. Because as many as one third of women with locally advanced breast cancer have distant metastases at the time of diagnosis, many oncologists perform an evaluation for distant disease even in asymptomatic patients. Diagnosis is usually established by fine-needle aspiration or core biopsy, and combined-modality therapy is used to maximize control of local disease and distant micrometastases. Several months of preoperative endocrine therapy or chemotherapy results in tumor regression in most patients, thereby allowing definitive breast surgery of some type to be performed. Postoperative radiotherapy is generally employed to enhance local control, and some studies suggest that administration of further chemotherapy, hormone therapy, anti-HER2 therapy, or a combination thereof (depending on the features of the cancer) is then desirable. Multimodality therapy results in a 5-year disease-free survival rate of about 50%.

Stage IV or Metastatic Breast Cancer

Although seldom curable, advanced breast cancer is a highly treatable illness. Palliation or prevention of symptoms without excess toxicity is the

TABLE 204-6 FOLLOW-UP GUIDELINES FOR PATIENTS WITH EARLY-STAGE BREAST CANCER: AMERICAN SOCIETY OF CLINICAL ONCOLOGY GUIDELINES*

PROCEDURE OR TEST	FREQUENCY
History and physical examination* (eliciting of symptoms of breast cancer)	Every 3-6 mo for first 3 yr, every 6-12 mo for next yr, then yearly
MAMMOGRAPHY	
Mastectomy patients	Yearly
Lumpectomy patients	Yearly
Pelvic examination	Yearly
Breast self-examination	Monthly
Complete blood cell counts and chemistry studies	The literature does not support the use of these tests
Chest radiography, bone scans, PET scans, breast MRI, liver imaging, and tumor marker studies	Not recommended for routine follow-up in asymptomatic patients
Patient education regarding signs and symptoms of recurrence	Each visit

*Limited evaluation: assess for pain, dyspnea, weight loss, and other major changes in function. The limited examination should include an assessment of nodes, axillae, lumpectomy or mastectomy site, chest, and abdomen. Patients should be instructed regarding symptoms of recurrence.
Modified from Khatcheressian JL, Wolff AC, Smith TJ, et al. American Society of Clinical Oncology 2006 update of the breast cancer follow-up and management guidelines in the adjuvant setting. *J Clin Oncol.* 2006;24:5091-5097.

primary goal of treatment. The median survival after diagnosis of metastatic breast cancer is 2 to 3 years, although the range is great, and a small cadre of long-term survivors has been described. Several recent clinical trials have documented small improvements in survival with some of the newer therapies.

Most women with metastatic breast cancer present with symptoms or abnormalities on physical examination. Less than 10% of women present with metastatic disease; rather advanced disease is normally diagnosed in women with a previous diagnosis of early breast cancer for which they received treatment. Common sites for metastases include bone, soft tissues, lung, liver, and brain. If metastatic disease is suspected, relevant hematologic, biochemical, and radiographic evaluation is indicated to assess location and severity of involvement. Because of the import of the diagnosis, pathologic confirmation is preferred. This permits verification of recurrent disease, exclusion of other diagnoses, and reassessment of biologic features such ER, PR, and HER2. Elevation of tumor markers (e.g., CA-2729, carcinoembryonic antigen) or the presence of circulating tumor cells is not diagnostic of recurrent disease, although these markers may be useful adjuncts in the assessment of the effects of therapy.

The role of surgery in metastatic breast cancer is limited. It is useful in certain circumstances such as resection of a chest wall nodule or solitary brain metastasis or orthopedic stabilization to treat or prevent a long-bone fracture. Radiotherapy is a mainstay in the management of advanced disease. It may be used at any time during the patient's course to treat localized disease such as chest wall recurrence, brain metastases, or painful bony metastases. Systemic treatment is the primary mode for management of disseminated disease. Key principles for selection of therapy include maximal palliation of symptoms, minimization of treatment-related toxicity, and prevention of disease complications. An algorithm for treatment of stage IV breast cancer is shown in Figure 204-1.

Endocrine Therapy

Endocrine therapy is preferred as the first intervention for metastatic breast cancer whenever feasible because of its favorable therapeutic index. Factors that support the use of endocrine therapy include the expression of hormone receptors, a long disease-free interval, and absence of symptoms or visceral disease. More than half of the women who meet these criteria respond to an initial course of hormone therapy, with a median response duration of 9 to 12 months. Length of response is a good predictor for the likelihood of response to a second course of endocrine therapy when the first agent fails. A second course of endocrine therapy is less likely to be successful, and the duration of response is shorter; again, duration of response predicts for likelihood of success with third-line therapy. Successful application of this algorithm can result in good disease control with little toxicity for several years in some women.

A number of types of hormone therapy are now available. These include the selective estrogen receptor modulator (SERM) tamoxifen; the selective estrogen receptor–degrading agent, fulvestrant; the aromatase inhibitors; and ovarian suppression by oophorectomy or LHRH agonists. Selection is usually made on the basis of efficacy, toxicity, and menopausal status. Serial

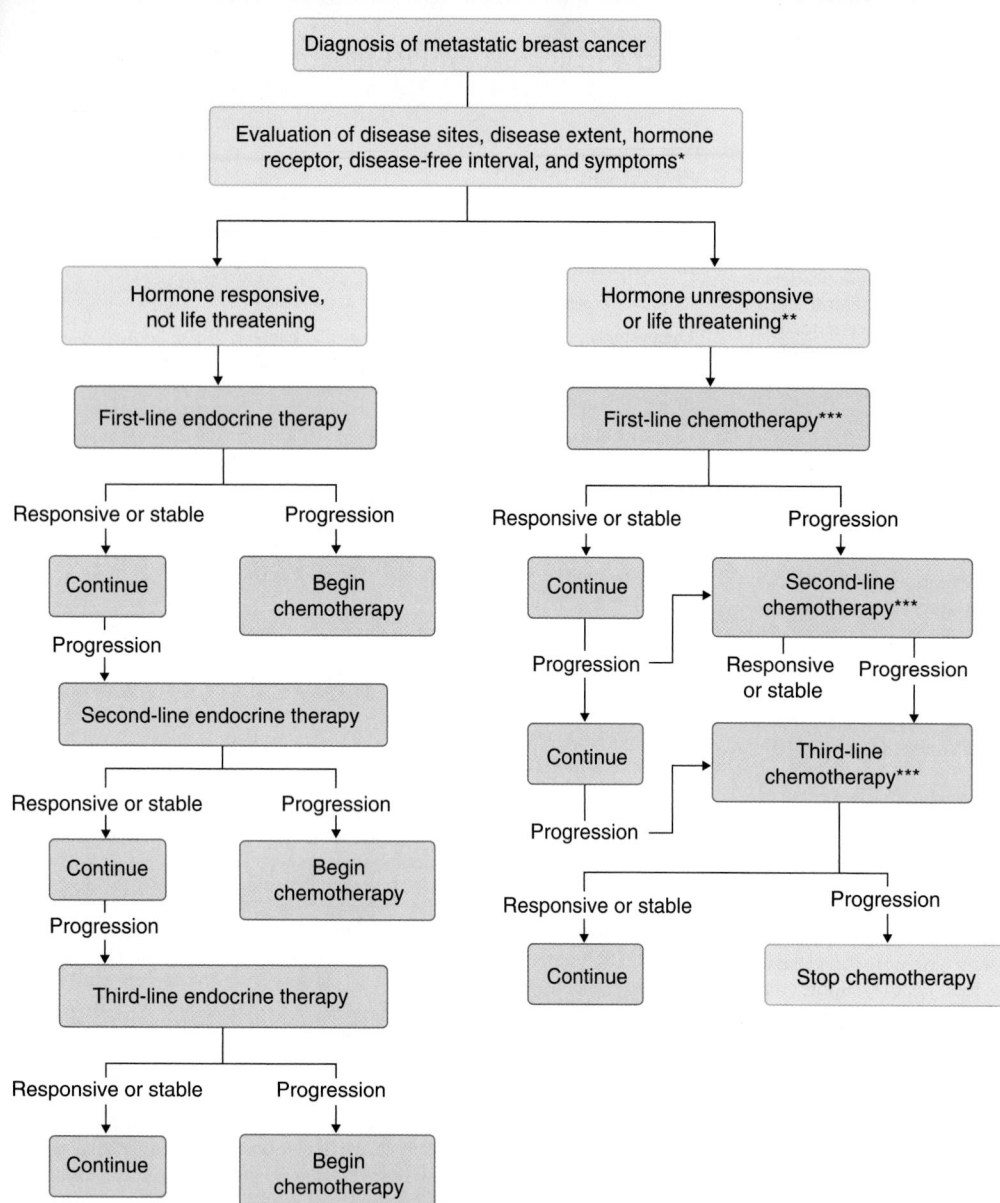

FIGURE 204-1. An algorithm used for the systemic treatment of stage IV breast cancer. *Consider role of bisphosphonate if bone involvement. **Consider integration of anti-HER2 therapy if tumor is HER2 overexpressing. ***Consider using bevacizumab.

administration of agents is the norm; combination therapy (with the possible exception of ovarian suppression plus tamoxifen) does not improve outcomes.

Several months of therapy are needed before the efficacy of a newly introduced endocrine therapy can be assessed. Patients and clinicians should be aware of the possibility of treatment-related tumor flare—a syndrome of worsening symptoms and increased circulating tumor markers—that can occur within the first few weeks of treatment. This response is usually of short duration and should not be confused with disease progression.

Chemotherapy

Most women with advanced breast cancer experience endocrine-unresponsive disease at some point and become candidates for palliative chemotherapy. Serial chemotherapy is the norm. Patients receive two to four cycles of therapy and then are evaluated for disease stabilization or improvement. Duration of therapy is variable for those who are responding to therapy. Several trials compared the approach of continuing therapy until time of disease progression with the approach of administering therapy, followed by a "drug holiday," with resumption of therapy at the time of disease progression. In sum, these studies suggest that survival is the same with these two approaches but that quality of life, as judged by the patients, is often better with continued therapy. Thus, decisions about continuation or cessation of a therapy are driven by perception of side effects and benefits by the patient and clinician.

Many active agents for breast cancer are now available. These include well-established drugs such as cyclophosphamide, doxorubicin, and methotrexate as well as newer agents like paclitaxel, docetaxel, vinorelbine, capecitabine, gemcitabine, carboplatin, ixabepilone, pegylated doxorubicin, and nano-albumin-bound paclitaxel. All these agents are active individually and in combination. There is considerable debate about the value of combination therapy

compared with sequential single-agent therapy for metastatic breast cancer. In addition, much attention has been focused on schedule of administration. For example, weekly paclitaxel regimens appear to be more effective and better tolerated than every-3-week regimens for many women. As with endocrine therapy, response rates and duration diminish with each successive change in therapy. As with early breast cancer, high-dose chemotherapy combined with autologous stem cell or bone marrow support has not shown benefit. A difficult question for patient and doctor is when to stop chemotherapy. No fixed rules exist, but many patients and physicians move to a program of supportive care if two successive chemotherapy regimens fail to produce a tumor response or disease stabilization.

Biological Agents

Enhanced understanding of breast cancer biology has resulted in the identification of new targets for therapy beyond the estrogen receptor pathway. The first agent brought into clinical practice was the monoclonal antibody, trastuzumab (Herceptin), which is active against the transmembrane HER2/neu protein. Administration of trastuzumab monotherapy to women with metastatic HER2-overexpressing breast cancer led to partial or complete tumor regression in about 30% of untreated women. Concurrent trastuzumab with paclitaxel increased response rate and duration and survival compared with paclitaxel alone for women with newly diagnosed metastatic breast cancer. Similar results were seen with concurrent administration of trastuzumab and doxorubicin, but this combination was associated with a 20% incidence of congestive heart failure. This unexpected finding demonstrates the need for careful evaluation of new biological agents as they enter the clinic. Dose and schedule of trastuzumab have been studied, and it appears that every-3-week administration is active with less patient inconvenience. One unanswered question has been how long to continue trastuzumab in advanced breast cancer because discontinuation of a therapy at the time of progression has been the norm. A small provocative study suggests that patients who develop progressive disease while taking paclitaxel and trastuzumab fare better if they are changed to a regimen of trastuzumab and capecitabine rather than capecitabine alone.

Another molecular target of interest is the epidermal growth factor receptor (EGFR, or HER1). Small molecules that target the EGFR tyrosine kinase, gefitinib and erlotinib, or the monoclonal antibody against EGFR, cetuximab, have shown little activity as monotherapy in women with advanced breast cancer. But the dual HER1 and HER2 receptor inhibitor, lapatinib, has been shown to improve outcome for women with advanced HER2-overexpressing breast cancer when added to capecitabine. Further, clinical trials have suggested that addition of lapatinib to trastuzumab at the time of progression on trastuzumab gives superior results to lapatinib alone. Studies of both these agents suggest that their benefit is most marked in women whose tumors overexpress HER2 protein. Other agents that target the HER family members are in clinical testing.

Strategies to block tumor angiogenesis are also employed. One such agent is bevacizumab, a monoclonal antibody that targets the vascular endothelial growth factor. This agent has only modest activity as monotherapy in metastatic breast cancer, but its addition to taxane-based chemotherapy for women with newly diagnosed stage IV breast cancer appears to improve progression-free survival without a major impact on survival. Other studies suggest that it has similar effects when added to subsequent chemotherapy regimens as well. Its use in concert with standard adjuvant chemotherapies is under evaluation.

Multiple other targeted agents are also under development. Of recent interest are the poly-ADP-ribose polymerase (PARP) inhibitors. These small molecule inhibitors of DNA repair show particular activity in women with BRCA mutant breast cancer in early studies. In addition, early information suggests that coadministration of PARP inhibitor with chemotherapy improves outcomes over chemotherapy alone for women with stage IV triple-negative breast cancer. More definitive testing is in progress.

Supportive Care
Bone Health
Because palliation of symptoms and prevention of complications of metastatic disease are the primary goals of treatment for advanced breast cancer, careful attention to supportive care is vital. Bone is the most common site of metastasis in breast cancer, and bone disease can be a source of significant morbidity. Several studies have shown that regular administration of a bisphosphonate such as zoledronate or pamidronate in addition to endocrine therapy or chemotherapy can reduce pain and lower the incidence of skeletal complications of disease. Although such therapy is now the norm, several issues remain unaddressed, including the optimal treatment interval and duration of therapy.

Given the propensity of breast cancer therapy to lead to estrogen deprivation and osteopenia or osteoporosis (Chapter 251), the use of bisphosphonates in the adjuvant setting is under evaluation. Small trials have raised the possibility that bisphosphonates might prevent or delay the development of metastases in women with early-stage breast cancer, and the results of large randomized trials are awaited.

Postmenopausal Symptoms
Postmenopausal symptoms as a consequence of therapy or natural aging are common in breast cancer survivors. In general, hormone replacement therapy should be avoided in women with a history of breast cancer. A short course of treatment can be considered in patients with early-stage breast cancer who have truly disabling symptoms. Topical estrogens are considered for women with vaginal dryness that does not respond to lubricants. Vasomotor symptoms may be reduced with the use of certain antidepressants of the selective serotonin release inhibitor family. Multiple studies have failed to show consistent benefit from many alternative therapies.

Lymphedema
Lymphedema develops in the ipsilateral arm in up to 15% of women after treatment for early breast cancer. Its incidence is lower with sentinel lymph node procedures and meticulous radiotherapy planning. Prevention includes avoidance of trauma and possibly exercises. Early recognition of symptoms is key. Affected patients should be referred to specialists for consideration of treatment such as manual drainage or the use of compression stockings or pumps.

Special Circumstances
The risk for breast cancer is slightly increased during and just after pregnancy. Suspicious breast findings during pregnancy should be investigated vigorously. Surgical therapy for breast cancer can be safely performed after the first trimester of pregnancy, but radiotherapy should be delayed until after delivery. Current data suggest that certain adjuvant chemotherapy regimens can be safely administered in the second and third trimesters of pregnancy, and development is normal in children of mothers who receive this chemotherapy. Administration of antimetabolites should be avoided because of the potential for damage to the placenta. Initiation of endocrine therapy is generally delayed until after delivery. Pregnancy after a diagnosis of early breast cancer does not appear to increase the risk for metastatic disease in limited data sets. The major considerations for women contemplating pregnancy should be its timing with regard to endocrine therapy, which may require 5 or more years to complete, as well as the underlying risk for disease recurrence.

Men account for not more than 1% of breast cancer cases. Failure of the patient or health care provider to diagnose the disease means that it may be diagnosed at a later stage. Most breast cancers in men express ER, and treatment recommendations for these men are generally similar to those for postmenopausal women.

PREVENTION AND SCREENING

There is enormous interest in the development of breast cancer prevention strategies. Currently these include surgical, chemopreventive, and lifestyle modification approaches.

Prophylactic Mastectomy and Oophorectomy
Prophylactic mastectomy appears to reduce the risk of developing breast cancer by about 90% in individuals who are at high risk because of a strong family history or carriage of a germline *BRCA1* or *BRCA2* mutation. Prophylactic oophorectomy in *BRCA* mutation carriers has also been shown to decrease breast cancer incidence by about 50%, presumably because of reduction in ovarian steroids. It is critical that women who opt for prophylactic mastectomy be counseled about the possibility that cancer may develop in remnants of breast tissue that remain after prophylactic mastectomy.

Chemoprevention
The observation that adjuvant endocrine therapy with the SERM tamoxifen also decreased contralateral breast cancer led to evaluation of tamoxifen as a chemopreventive for well women who are at high risk for breast cancer. Meta-analysis of four randomized trials of tamoxifen versus placebo for high-risk women confirmed a 38% reduction in invasive breast cancer with tamoxifen. The largest trial, NSABP P01, randomized 13,388 high-risk women to receive either tamoxifen or placebo for 5 years. Risk factors used to determine eligibility were age ≥60 years, a diagnosis of LCIS, or age 35 to 59 years with a constellation of risk factors that, when combined, resulted in a 1.67% or greater risk for breast cancer within 5 years. This study showed a 50% decrease in the diagnosis of breast cancer across all age groups at a cost of increased risk for endometrial cancer and thromboembolic events in women older than 50 years. These data led to the approval of tamoxifen to reduce incidence of breast cancer in women at high risk as defined by the eligibility criteria for this prevention trial.

Other SERMs have been studied as chemopreventive agents. Two trials have documented the utility of raloxifene as a breast cancer risk-reduction strategy.[5] In one trial, raloxifene administration reduced the incidence of breast cancer in postmenopausal women of average breast cancer risk and elevated cardiovascular risk. A second trial showed that raloxifene was as effective as tamoxifen in preventing invasive breast cancer in postmenopausal women at high risk for breast cancer. Raloxifene use was associated with fewer uterine cancers than tamoxifen but carries the same risk for thromboembolic events. It is approved by the U.S. Food and Drug Administration (FDA) for risk reduction in high-risk postmenopausal women. A vitamin A derivative, fenretinide, showed some impact as a chemopreventive agent for secondary prevention in premenopausal breast cancer survivors but has not found a place in routine practice. Finally, large epidemiologic studies have raised the possibility that aspirin or certain statins might also decrease breast cancer risk, but these agents have not been prospectively tested.

Lifestyle Modification
Prevention strategies that involve lifestyle alterations have been suggested. The Women's Health Initiative did not show a clear role for a low-fat diet as a means of breast cancer prevention. Regular exercise, especially during adolescence, may be associated with reduced breast cancer risk. By extrapolation from the epidemiologic studies mentioned previously, abstinence from alcohol might slightly reduce the risk for breast cancer.

Screening
Screening strategies for breast cancer have traditionally included the triad of breast self-examination (BSE), clinical breast examination (CBE) by a health

TABLE 204-7	BREAST CANCER SCREENING	
TEST	**ACS**	**USPSTF**
Mammography		
40-49 yr	Annual	Insufficient evidence to support
>49 yr	Annual if healthy	Every 2 yr, 50-75 yr
Clinical breast examination	Every 3 yr, 20-39 yr Annually, ≥40 yr	Insufficient evidence to support
Breast self-examination	Optional	Not recommended

ACS = American Cancer Society; USPSTF = U.S. Preventive Services Task Force.

care professional, and screening mammography in well women. Although widely promulgated as an important component of early detection, two large randomized trials of conventional BSE versus observation failed to show any clinical advantage with BSE. As a result, many experts now promote breast awareness rather than regular BSE. The independent value of CBEs has not been rigorously assessed. Rather, it has been studied in conjunction with screening mammography, in which case the two interventions appear to decrease mortality from breast cancer by 25 to 30% in women older than 50 years. Considerable controversy continues over the value of screening mammography in women 40 to 50 years of age and those over 70 years of age as well as the optimal interval between mammograms for women aged 50 to 70 years. Currently, the American Cancer Society and the National Cancer Institute recommend annual screening mammography for women older than 40 years of age who are at standard risk for breast cancer. In contrast, the U.S. Preventive Services Task Force, advising the Department of Health and Human Services, recommended in 2009 that women between 40 and 50 years of age be counseled about the risks and benefits of screening mammography and that screening mammography can be used at 2-year intervals for women aged 50 to 75 years (Table 204-7). A study of digital versus conventional film screen mammography failed to show an overall advantage for digital mammography but suggest that digital mammography may be more useful for women with dense breasts.

The knowledge that screening mammography fails to diagnose about 10 to 15% of breast cancers has led to the evaluation of other imaging modalities. Of these, MRI is the most mature. MRI has been promoted as a useful screening tool for women at high risk by virtue of the *BRCA* mutation; indeed, the American Cancer Society has recommended consideration of screening MRI for women whose predicted risk for breast cancer exceeds 20%. MRI has been shown to detect breast cancer in the contralateral breast in 3% of women with a newly diagnosed breast cancer whose contralateral mammogram showed no abnormality. Use of MRI in the general population is limited by the fact that it is highly sensitive but lacks specificity. Insufficient information exists about other breast imaging modalities such as ultrasound and radionuclide imaging to support their use in screening asymptomatic women.

⬤ BENIGN BREAST LESIONS

Benign breast disease includes *mastalgia* (pain and tenderness), mastitis (including infectious and noninfectious inflammatory conditions), trauma, and benign tumors. In addition, mastalgia can be caused by extramammary conditions, such as myocardial ischemia, pneumonia, pleural irritation, esophageal spasm, costochondritis, rib fracture, and varicella-zoster virus (preceding the skin eruption). After these conditions have been ruled out, mastalgia is considered to be a benign condition that is self-limited. It can be cyclical or noncyclical in timing (where it is thought to be related to hormonal activity), and it may occur in postmenopausal women, even in the absence of hormone replacement therapy.

Mastitis is due to breast inflammation or infection, and it can occur in either nonlactating or lactating women. The typical presentation in nonlactating women is occurrence in their 40s with the acute onset of severe breast pain and tenderness followed by erythema and swelling that tends to be localized in the nipple-areolar area. The cause in most cases is considered to be rupture of dilated subareolar ducts that leads to an inflammatory response to leakage of intraductal contents into periductal tissue. Infection is difficult to rule out, and, in practice, patients are often treated with empirical antibiotics; if symptoms do not resolve within 7 to 10 days on antibiotics, ultrasound is required to rule out abscess. If the latter is found, incision and drainage are required. The most important differential diagnosis with mastitis is inflammatory carcinoma, as noted previously. Therefore, failure to improve with

antibiotics or to find an abscess should lead to evaluation by a breast surgeon. Mastitis in lactating women is often due to infection caused by a break in the skin of the nipple or milk stasis. *Staphylococcal aureus, Staphylococcus albus,* and sometimes *Escherichia coli* or streptococci are the most common pathogens. Treatment requires antibiotics and milk removal.

Nonproliferative and Proliferative Benign Breast Lesions

Nonproliferative benign breast lesions include (1) inflammatory fat necrosis, which follows surgical or blunt trauma, and generally resolves spontaneously; (2) lymphocytic mastitis, which may be seen in diabetic patients; and (3) granulomatous mastitis, associated with foreign body reactions (e.g., silicone and paraffin for breast augmentation and reconstruction after cancer surgery), sarcoid, or certain infections. Other nonproliferative benign breast lesions appear as tumor-like processes, including (4) fibroadenoma, a very common (about 25% of women), usually solitary, sharply demarcated, smooth lesion in younger age groups; (5) phyllodes tumor (previously known as cystosarcoma phyllodes); (6) intraductal papilloma, solitary lesions that may be accompanied by bloody nipple discharge; (7) fibrocystic breast disease, which is now more appropriately called "fibrocystic changes" because it is observed clinically in up to 50% and histologically in 90% of women, composed of varying amounts of fibrosis and cysts sometimes associated with calcifications and inflammation; and (8) simple or complex cysts, which should be aspirated with ultrasound guidance and, when the fluid is not clear, sent for cytologic analysis.

Proliferative benign breast lesions include ductal or lobular hyperplasia; atypical hyperplasias are associated with increased risk for breast cancer.

Breast Cancer Risk

The increasing use of mammography has increased the frequency of breast biopsies, which, in turn, has increased the finding of benign breast lesions, the most common findings on biopsy. The benign breast lesions listed in the previous section encompass the general histologic spectrum of (1) nonproliferative lesions, (2) proliferative lesions without atypia, and (3) atypical hyperplasia, listed in ascending order of risk for breast cancer. A large number of retrospective and prospective studies have shown an overall relative risk for breast cancer of 1.5 to 1.6 for women with biopsy-proven benign breast disease compared with women in the general population. A study of 9087 women with all types of benign histology, followed for a median of 15 years at the Mayo Clinic, found that 707 of them developed breast cancers. Increased risk for cancer persisted for at least 25 years after the original biopsy. Of the three broad histologic categories, the relative risk for cancer development was 4.24 associated with atypia, 1.88 with proliferative changes without atypia, and 1.27 with nonproliferative lesions. It is not known if the finding of a benign breast lesion with atypical histology represents an actual precursor lesion for cancer or if it is only a marker for a general tendency to develop breast cancer. The observations that about half of breast cancers in these patients arise in the contralateral breast suggests the latter hypothesis.

1. Clarke M, Collins R, Darby S, et al, for the Early Breast Cancer Trialists' Collaborative Group (EBCTCG). Effects of radiotherapy and of differences in the extent of surgery for early breast cancer on local recurrence and 15-year survival: an overview of the randomised trials. *Lancet.* 2005; 366:2087-2106.
2. Early Breast Cancer Trialists' Collaborative Group (EBCTCG). Effects of chemotherapy and hormonal therapy for early breast cancer on recurrence and 15-year survival: an overview of the randomised trials. *Lancet.* 2005;365:1687-1717.
3. Dowsett M, Cuzick J, Ingle J, et al. Meta-analysis of breast cancer outcomes in adjuvant trials of aromatase inhibitors versus tamoxifen. *J Clin Oncol.* 2010;28:509-518.
4. Swain SM, Jeong JH, Geyer CE Jr, et al. Longer therapy, iatrogenic amenorrhea, and survival in early breast cancer. *N Engl J Med.* 2010;362:2053-2065.
5. Vogel VG, Costantino JP, Wickerham DL, et al. Update of the National Surgical Adjuvant Breast and Bowel Project Study of Tamoxifen and Raloxifene (STAR) P-2 Trial: preventing breast cancer. *Cancer Prev Res.* 2010;3:696-706.

SUGGESTED READINGS

Bruening W, Fontanarosa J, Tipton K, et al. Systematic review: comparative effectiveness of core-needle and open surgical biopsy to diagnose breast lesions. *Ann Intern Med.* 2010;152:238-246. *Stereotactic and ultrasound-guided breast biopsies are nearly as accurate as open surgical biopsies.*
Burstein HJ, Prestrud AA, Seidenfeld J, et al. American Society of Clinical Oncology clinical practice guideline: update on adjuvant endocrine therapy for women with hormone receptor–positive breast cancer. *J Clin Oncol.* 2010;28:3784-3796. *Consensus guidelines.*

Carlson RW, Allred DC, Anderson BO, et al. Invasive breast cancer. *J Natl Comp Canc Netw.* 2011;9:136-222. *Comprehensive review.*

Henderson TO, Amsterdam A, Bhatia S, et al. Systematic review: surveillance for breast cancer in women treated with chest radiation for childhood, adolescent, or young adult cancer. *Ann Intern Med.* 2010;152:444-455; W144-154. *Women treated with chest radiation for childhood, adolescent, or young adult cancer have a higher risk of breast cancer at a young age and likely benefit from early cancer screening.*

Kabat GC, Jones JG, Olson N, et al. A multi-center prospective cohort study of benign breast disease and risk of subsequent breast cancer. *Cancer Causes Control.* 2010;21:821-882. *Women with proliferative disease without atypia have a modestly increased risk of breast cancer, whereas women with atypical hyperplasia have a substantially increased risk.*

Meissner HI, Klabunde CN, Han PK, et al. Breast cancer screening beliefs, recommendations and practices: primary care physicians in the United States. *Cancer.* 2011. [Epub ahead of print.] *Recommendations of primary care physicians generally followed national guidelines.*

205

GYNECOLOGIC CANCERS

MAURIE MARKMAN

⬤ CERVICAL CANCER

Worldwide there are more than 450,000 cases of invasive cancer of the cervix each year, leading to 250,000 deaths. Overall, this malignancy is the second most common cancer (after breast cancer) in women and the third most common cancer overall.

However, owing to the availability of a highly effective screening strategy (Pap smear), the incidence of invasive cervical cancer and deaths from this illness have decreased substantially in the developed world over the past several decades, with the majority of cases (and deaths) found in the developing world. For example, in the United States it is anticipated that there will be approximately 11,000 new cases accounting for 4000 deaths each year, making cancer of the cervix the 12th most common malignancy in women in this country.

EPIDEMIOLOGY

It is well established that essentially all cases of cervical cancer result from persistent infection (transmitted through sexual exposure) by oncogenic types of human papillomavirus (HPV; Chapter 381). Risk factors for cancer include early age of first sexual encounter; history of other sexually transmitted illnesses (Chapter 293), such as herpes simplex, chlamydia, and human immunodeficiency virus (HIV); multiple sexual partners and pregnancies; extended duration of oral contraceptive use; history of cigarette smoking; and chronic immunosuppression (e.g., renal transplantation, HIV).

Epidemiologic surveys demonstrate that as many as 50% of women will be exposed to HPV within 4 years of their initial sexual encounters. However, the large majority of individuals can spontaneously clear the infection, with subsequent cervical cytologic abnormalities being observed in only 5 to 10% of women experiencing an HPV infection.

The strongest association with cervical cancer involves HPV types 16 and 18, which together are implicated in approximately 70% of cases of the malignancy worldwide. An additional 30 types of HPV have been documented to be oncogenic, and another 70 have been described that are not known to have the potential to lead to cancer of the cervix. Besides types 16 and 18, other relatively common oncogenic HPV types that are responsible for varying percentages of cases in different regions of the world are 45, 31, 33, 52, 58, and 35.

PATHOBIOLOGY

It is important to note that the current level of understanding of the pathogenesis of cervical cancer from the time of viral infection to the development of invasive disease is greater than for any other human malignancy. Evidence suggests that once an oncogenic HPV successfully incorporates into the host genome (becoming a "persistent infection"), viral proteins (E6, E7) are produced that bind to and inactivate essential tumor suppressor proteins (RB1, TP53), leading to a cascade effect that ultimately results in a malignancy.

CLINICAL MANIFESTATIONS

Most cancers of the cervix are of squamous cell histology, although adenocarcinomas currently account for as many as one quarter of all cases of this malignancy. Other less common histologies include neuroendocrine and carcinoid tumors, lymphomas, and sarcomas.

The most common symptoms of invasive cervical cancer are abnormal vaginal or postcoital bleeding and vaginal discharge. These complaints are certainly not specific for cancer, but if they persist or another obvious cause is not evident, the diagnosis of cancer should be considered. A negative Pap test should not preclude further examination of the cervix as a possible site of malignancy in the appropriate clinical setting, because one half of women with documented invasive cervical cancer have a negative test.

With more advanced disease, pelvic pain and difficulty with both defecation and urination may be noted. Finally, with locally advanced cancer or metastatic spread, the patient may complain of back pain, leg swelling (from direct interference with blood flow to the region or development of deep venous thrombosis), or neuropathic pain (from nerve involvement).

DIAGNOSIS

Common diagnostic testing for cervical cancer includes physical examination (which may reveal a mass lesion or friable or necrotic tissue), laboratory testing (revealing possible renal dysfunction due to urethral obstruction), and radiographic imaging. In general, magnetic resonance imaging (MRI) is more sensitive than computed tomography in defining tumor size and extent of disease. Recent data have revealed the superiority of positron emission tomography in determining the presence or absence of nodal involvement in cancer of the cervix.

Screening for Preinvasive Disease

It would not be hyperbole to state that the initial development and subsequent routine use of Pap smears constitute one of the most important public health advances of the past 50 years (Fig. 205-1). It has long been recognized that preinvasive cervical abnormalities precede the development of invasive cancer by many years, permitting highly effective (essentially 100%, if correctly applied) and relatively nonmorbid local interventions.

Liquid-based cytologic testing procedures and HPV testing have improved both the sensitivity and the specificity of screening. However, the basic principle of screening remains the same: early discovery and removal of preinvasive lesions that, if left untreated, would have a substantial risk of developing into invasive cancer. The magnitude of this risk is highlighted by data revealing that as many as one third of documented, untreated carcinoma in situ abnormalities may progress to frank invasive cancer of the cervix over a 10-year period.

Patients with a concerning Pap smear result should be referred to undergo colposcopy and directed biopsies. Subsequent treatment and follow-up are based on the findings from this evaluation.

Recently revised guidelines from the American College of Obstetricians and Gynecologists for routine screening for cervical cancer are as follows:
- Screening should begin at age 21.
- Screening is recommended every 2 years for women aged 21 to 29.
- Either conventional or liquid-based cytology is acceptable.

FIGURE 205-1. Cervical abnormalities on Pap smear. **A,** Low-grade squamous intraepithelial neoplasia. Note the group of mildly dysplastic cells with an increased nuclear-to-cytoplasmic ratio *(single arrow)* contrasted with a normal squamous epithelial cell *(double arrows)* (Papanicolaou stain, × 400). **B,** Cervical adenocarcinoma. Note the three-dimensional cluster of pleomorphic cells with a markedly increased nuclear-to-cytoplasmic ratio, dense nuclear chromatin, and macronucleoli *(single arrow)* contrasted with a normal squamous epithelial cell *(double arrows)* (Papanicolaou stain, × 400).

- Women 30 years of age and older with three consecutive negative results for intra-epithelial lesions can change to an every-3-year screening schedule.
- Women with any of the following risk factors may require more frequent screening: (1) HIV infection; (2) receiving immunosuppressive medication; (3) history of exposure to diethylstilbestrol in utero (see the section on vaginal cancer); (4) prior treatment for cervical intra-epithelial neoplasia (CIN) 2, CIN 3, or cancer.
- Women older than 65 to 70 years with three or more consecutive negative test results over the preceding 10 years can discontinue routine screening.
- Women who have had a total hysterectomy performed for a nonmalignant condition can discontinue routine screening.

TREATMENT Rx

Localized Disease

Following evaluation for the extent of disease involvement, patients with localized cancer of the cervix can be managed with a variety of approaches, including (1) simple hysterectomy (if pretreatment clinical characteristics suggest the risk of lymph node involvement is very low), (2) radical hysterectomy (with removal of pelvic and para-aortic lymph nodes), (3) surgery plus external beam radiation, or (4) external beam radiation plus concurrent chemotherapy (so-called chemo-radiation).

Invasive Disease

Several randomized trials have revealed the superior outcome associated with radiation plus cisplatin-based chemotherapy, compared with radiation alone, in the management of locally advanced, invasive cervical cancer.[1] In patients with nonmetastatic, invasive cervical cancer, long-term disease-free survival is strongly influenced by a number of factors (most prominently, initial tumor stage) and ranges from as high as 95% (early-stage disease without lymphovascular space invasion) to less than 20% for stage IV cancer.

In the presence of metastatic cancer at diagnosis, or if the cancer has recurred following initial management, currently available treatment options provide quite modest palliative benefits. Cisplatin is the single most active antineoplastic agent in cancer of the cervix (20% objective response rate). Patients with an adequate baseline performance status that permits a more intensive approach may be treated with a cisplatin-based combination chemotherapy regimen.[1] Responses in this setting are generally limited in duration (3 to 4 months) and are more likely to occur in areas not previously radiated. In this difficult clinical setting, the limited potential for therapeutic benefit must be weighed against the risk of toxic effects that may negatively impact the quality of a patient's remaining life.

PREVENTION

Two recently licensed vaccines based on HPV types 16 and 18 are highly effective in reducing the risk of developing persistent HPV infection and type-specific cervical dysplasia *if administered before evidence of sexual exposure to the virus.*[2,3] In the large randomized trials conducted to obtain regulatory approval of these preparations, and in extensive post-marketing surveillance evaluations, few serious vaccine-related side effects (e.g., hypersensitivity reactions) have been documented.

There is no convincing evidence of the utility of HPV vaccination in an individual already infected with HPV. These data emphasize the importance of vaccination before an individual's first sexual contact.

Unanswered questions and unresolved issues regarding HPV vaccination include the following: (1) the duration of protective immunity following a single vaccination series (current evidence suggests that sufficient concentrations of antibody persist for more than 5 to 6 years in individuals receiving the complete vaccination regimen); (2) the utility of strategies consisting of fewer than three individual shots (initial vaccination followed by two booster injections) delivered over several months; (3) the benefit of approaches designed to increase the effectiveness of vaccination by adding other oncogenic types (in addition to 16 and 18); (4) the impact on cervical cancer prevention associated with the vaccination of males; and (5) cost, religious, and other societal objections to vaccine use (e.g., mandated vs. voluntary vaccination).

⬤ ENDOMETRIAL CANCER

Endometrial cancer is the most common female pelvic malignancy in the United States; approximately 40,000 new cases are diagnosed each year,

resulting in almost 8000 deaths. Overall, endometrial cancer accounts for almost 50% of all female pelvic malignancies and is the fourth most common cancer type in women. The reported high incidence of endometrial cancer is likely due to several factors, including longer life expectancies, earlier diagnosis, and the reduced incidence of cervical cancer. Worldwide, endometrial cancer trails only cervical cancer as the leading cause of malignant disease in women.

EPIDEMIOLOGY

The major recognized risk factor for the development of endometrial cancer is estrogen exposure, either endogenous or exogenous. Case-control studies conducted more than 20 years ago demonstrated that women exposed to long-term unopposed estrogen have a 4- to 15-fold increased risk of developing this malignancy. In contrast to the impact of unopposed estrogens, the past use of oral contraceptives containing a progestin (either high or low potency) has been shown to reduce the risk for the development of endometrial cancer.

Other risk factors include obesity (an increased mass of fatty tissue is associated with greater aromatization of androstenedione to estrone), nulliparity, eating a "Western-type" (i.e., high-fat) diet, the documented presence of endometrial hyperplasia, a history of hereditary nonpolyposis colorectal cancer, and prior or current treatment with tamoxifen (used to treat or prevent breast cancer, leading to a 3- to 7-fold increased risk for this pelvic malignancy). There is also a documented greater risk of endometrial cancer in women with diabetes (3-fold higher) and in those with hypertension (1.5-fold higher), likely due to these conditions' association with obesity. This is the likely explanation for the "classic triad" frequently used to characterize the endometrial cancer patient: overweight, diabetic, and hypertensive.

For as many as 75% of all patients with endometrial cancer (type 1), it is possible to identify a clinical factor suggesting excessive estrogen exposure (e.g., replacement therapy, obesity). The malignancy in these individuals often begins as endometrial hyperplasia, is well differentiated (grade 1) and of low stage, and has a very favorable prognosis.

Conversely, 25% of patients with this cancer (type 2) have no evidence of excessive estrogen exposure. These women frequently have an atrophic endometrium, the malignancies are of higher grade (grade 3 or undifferentiated) and stage, and their overall survival is poorer.

CLINICAL MANIFESTATIONS

Endometrial cancer is seen predominantly in the postmenopausal population, although in some series as many as one quarter of patients were premenopausal. It is uncommon for endometrial cancer to be diagnosed in a woman younger than 40 years.

The most common presenting symptom is postmenopausal bleeding (80 to 90% of cases), which should lead to a formal gynecologic evaluation (with biopsy). In more advanced cases, pelvic pressure or pain may be noted.

Approximately 90 to 95% of all endometrial cancers are adenocarcinomas. Fortunately, most tumors are low grade and stage I (80%) at diagnosis. However, as previously noted, patients with type 2 endometrial cancer are more likely to present with both a higher-grade and higher-stage malignancy.

Endometrial sarcomas (e.g., uterine leiomyosarcomas) are far less common than adenocarcinomas and have a different natural history. Even in the setting of stage I cancer, as many as half of these patients experience subsequent disease progression.

Uterine carcinosarcomas (mixed müllerian tumors) are another uncommon subtype that frequently demonstrates rapid progression. Despite its name, this tumor is currently considered to be a poorly differentiated epithelial malignancy rather than a true sarcoma.

TREATMENT Rx

Surgical resection is the standard initial treatment for the large majority of women with endometrial cancer, and it is generally considered sufficient therapy for patients with early-stage, low-grade disease. The role of routine postoperative adjuvant therapy is controversial. There is evidence that pelvic radiation decreases the risk of local recurrence, but the impact on overall survival is uncertain.

In patients with disease documented in the upper abdomen (stage III), phase III trial data have revealed the superiority of combination chemotherapy compared with whole abdominal radiotherapy.[4] Despite these data, many oncologists favor a multimodality strategy in the management of high-risk endometrial cancer patients (e.g., those with completely surgically resected disease in the upper abdomen or locally advanced grade 3 cancer), which might include several cycles of systemic chemotherapy followed by pelvic radiotherapy (to reduce the chance of relapse in this region). Unfortunately, phase III trial data are not available to definitively prove the benefits of this approach. Vaginal brachytherapy appears to be as good as external beam radiotherapy.[5]

A number of chemotherapeutic agents have demonstrated biologic activity (objective response rates >20%) in endometrial cancer, including doxorubicin, paclitaxel, cisplatin, and carboplatin. In metastatic disease or in the setting of recurrent cancer, such agents are frequently administered as a combination strategy (e.g., carboplatin plus paclitaxel, cisplatin plus doxorubicin plus paclitaxel), and response rates greater than 50% have been reported. An optimal treatment regimen in this setting has not been defined.[6]

It is also known that patients with low-grade advanced or metastatic endometrial cancer may exhibit clinically meaningful and prolonged responses to high doses of progestational agents (anticipated 15 to 30% response rate). There is no evidence of an added benefit obtained by combining chemotherapy with hormonal therapy in patients with endometrial cancer, and high-grade tumors rarely (if ever) respond to progestational drugs.

Overall 5-year survival in patients with endometrial cancer varies, based on tumor stage. It ranges from greater than 80% for stage I cancer to approximately 25% for individuals who present with metastatic disease. Other factors that influence survival include patient age, evidence of vascular invasion, hormone receptor status (the presence of which suggests a more indolent clinical course), tumor grade, and histologic subtype (papillary, serous, and clear cell morphology being associated with poorer outcomes).

Management of both endometrial sarcoma and carcinosarcoma includes surgical staging and frequently an attempt at maximal surgical cytoreduction. Owing to the substantial risk of recurrence, adjuvant radiation and/or chemotherapy may be employed, but the utility of such treatment is uncertain. Chemotherapy of metastatic disease may prolong survival and favorably impact cancer-related symptoms.

EPITHELIAL OVARIAN CANCER

Epithelial ovarian cancer is the sixth most common cancer in women in the United States, accounting for approximately one quarter of all female pelvic malignancies. However, far more significant than its incidence is the disturbing fact that the majority of women (>70%) initially present with advanced cancer, and overall survival is inferior to that observed in other female pelvic malignancies.

EPIDEMIOLOGY

In rather striking contrast to cancers of the endometrium and cervix, there is no unifying hypothesis or etiologic factor that defines either the epidemiology or the risk of developing this malignancy. Perhaps the most widely accepted theory is that carcinogenesis is initiated during the normal process of damage and repair associated with a woman's monthly ovulatory cycle. This hypothesis is supported by population-based data revealing a lower incidence of ovarian cancer in women with a history of multiple pregnancies, lactation, extended use of oral contraceptives, and late menarche or early menopause. Each of these clinical features is associated with fewer lifetime ovulatory cycles. Conversely, women with a history of infertility, early menarche, or late menopause have a statistically increased risk of experiencing this malignancy.

Overall, an individual woman has a 1 in 70 lifetime risk for the development of ovarian cancer. The single well-established risk factor for ovarian cancer is a family history of either ovarian or early-onset breast cancer, which appears to account for approximately 5 to 15% of all cases of the malignancy. Existing data reveal that the large majority of women with such a family history have either a *BRCA1* or *BRCA2* mutation, which results in a lifetime ovarian cancer risk of 40 to 50% or 10 to 20%, respectively.

CLINICAL MANIFESTATIONS

The large majority of epithelial ovarian cancers are adenocarcinomas. Until recently, the specific ovarian histologic subtypes were not thought to have major prognostic relevance beyond that identified by tumor grade, but it has become evident that both mucinous and clear cell cancers respond poorly to standard ovarian cancer chemotherapy and have a much worse prognosis (when found in an advanced stage) compared with the more common papillary, serous, or endometrioid types.

Unfortunately, symptoms of ovarian cancer are quite nonspecific (abdominal bloating, discomfort, and pain; loss of appetite; early satiety; fatigue) and in the large majority of cases are an indication of advanced disease. Many women present with abdominal fullness and early satiety due to ascites and omental tumor implants. Ascites is commonly observed in patients with advanced disease. There is no evidence that any particular symptom or symptom complex is more suggestive of ovarian cancer in contrast to other equally (or more) common conditions that may be the cause of the reported complaints.

TREATMENT Rx

Standard treatment of suspected or documented epithelial ovarian cancer includes surgical staging and a reasonably aggressive attempt to resect all macroscopic disease (including disease present in the upper abdomen) before the administration of cytotoxic chemotherapy. Extensive published retrospective experience supports the utility of this basic management approach, with superior outcomes anticipated for women who initiate chemotherapy with small-volume macroscopic or only microscopic cancer.

However, it is relevant to note the complete absence of evidence-based data from randomized, controlled trials documenting the superiority of surgery followed by chemotherapy compared with a primary chemotherapy approach (after histologic confirmation of malignant disease) in the treatment of stage III or IV epithelial ovarian cancer. A recently reported international phase III trial demonstrated equivalent survival and reduced morbidity for individuals managed by primary chemotherapy followed by an attempt at surgical resection compared with "standard" cytoreductive surgery followed by chemotherapy.[7] This provides important support for the concept that in certain settings it may be most appropriate for initial treatment to focus on cytotoxic drug delivery.

Ovarian cancer is a highly chemotherapy-sensitive malignancy, with major objective response rates to combination platinum-taxane chemotherapy exceeding 70 to 80%.[8] Prolonged disease-free survival (>5 years) is a realistic possibility for a minority of women who present with advanced (stage III and IV) disease. In women with small-volume residual intraperitoneal disease following surgical cytoreduction, direct delivery of cisplatin into the peritoneal cavity has been shown to improve survival in several randomized trials.

Unfortunately, the majority of responding patients ultimately experience a relapse of the malignancy. Although a number of second-line treatment approaches have been shown to favorably impact symptoms of recurrent disease and improve overall survival, there is no evidence that any such approach can cure the malignancy.

There may also be a role for secondary cytoreductive surgery at the time of documented recurrence of ovarian cancer. In general, patients who have experienced relatively long disease-free intervals (>12 months) following completion of the primary treatment program are the best candidates for surgery designed to remove all visible macroscopic cancer before the initiation of second-line chemotherapy.

It is important to note that carefully considered surgical procedures designed to palliate distressing cancer-related symptoms (e.g., colostomy for large bowel obstruction) may be reasonable therapeutic options, even in the setting of progressive cancer. External beam radiation may also play an important role in the palliation of painful masses in the setting of chemotherapy-resistant disease. Despite encouraging early results, the intraperitoneal administration of chemotherapy has not been incorporated into the mainstream management of advanced ovarian cancer.

PREVENTION

Currently, there is no indication that any screening strategy (e.g., tumor markers such as CA-125, radiographic imaging) can detect recurrent[9] or "early-stage" ovarian cancer, although several such approaches have been proposed. Although it may be tempting to suggest that women at high risk (those with known genetic abnormalities) for the development of ovarian cancer may benefit from some form of routine screening (biomarker or imaging), it must be emphasized that no valid data support the utility of such an approach.

For women with a strong family history of ovarian cancer, particularly those documented to have a *BRCA1* or *BRCA2* genetic abnormality, available data support the conclusion that bilateral oophorectomies can reduce the risk of developing the malignancy by more than 80%. However, the actual extent of the absolute reduction in lifetime risk remains uncertain, because most series have followed individuals for less than 10 years following this cancer prevention surgery. For an individual woman with the appropriate genetic background who is considering undergoing such surgery, it is important to consider the negative aspects of this approach, including infertility, potentially distressing symptoms of early menopause, and the risk of accelerated bone loss.

NONEPITHELIAL OVARIAN MALIGNANCIES

Germ Cell Tumors of the Ovary

Ovarian germ cell cancers are uncommon malignancies observed in adolescent girls and young women. Like their male germ cell counterparts (Chapter 206), these malignances are extremely chemosensitive and have a high cure rate, even if discovered at an advanced stage. Both the diagnosis and the treatment of ovarian germ cell tumors are aided by the presence of two sensitive serum markers (human gonadotropin and α-fetoprotein).

Standard management of ovarian germ cell tumors includes surgical staging and an attempt to remove all gross macroscopic cancer (in the presence of metastatic spread). The majority of ovarian germ cell tumors are unilateral at presentation, permitting the performance of a salpingo-oophorectomy on the involved side and potentially preserving fertility in this young patient population.

Early-stage dysgerminomas can be managed with observation following surgical staging; less than 25% of such patients will experience a relapse. For more advanced disease, chemotherapy is indicated. However, the large majority of nondysgerminous germ cell tumors require chemotherapy because of the high recurrence rate (80% in stage I disease).

Stromal Ovarian Tumors

Granulosa cell and Sertoli-Leydig tumors are uncommon ovarian tumors characterized by being generally localized at presentation and exhibiting long natural histories, even when metastatic spread is documented. In contrast to epithelial ovarian cancer and germ cell tumors, this group of malignancies exhibits modest responsiveness to cytotoxic chemotherapy, which is usually employed only when disease progression has been documented.

VULVAR CANCER

Primary vulvar cancers account for less than 5% of cancers involving the female reproductive tract. As with cervical cancer, HPV has been strongly implicated in the pathogenesis of this malignancy (HPV DNA documented in 70 to 80% of cases).

The majority of patients are symptomatic at presentation (pain, local irritation, pruritus), and these complaints have commonly (>80% of cases) been present for more than 6 months before diagnosis. Most vulvar cancers are of squamous cell histology (Fig. 205-2), but malignant melanoma is also observed in this region.

Standard treatment is surgical excision of the primary tumor and dissection of inguinal lymph nodes. The risk of tumor recurrence is related to the size and extent of tumor involvement, the ability of the surgeon to achieve adequate surgical margins, and the documented presence of metastatic cancer in the inguinal nodes. With advanced local disease, concurrent external beam radiation and chemotherapy are generally employed. There is little evidence for the effectiveness of cytotoxic antineoplastic drugs in the setting of metastatic vulvar cancer.

FIGURE 205-2. Vulvar cancer. Invasive squamous cell carcinoma of the vulva.

VAGINAL CANCER

Vaginal cancers are uncommon malignancies associated with prior persistent HPV infection, and they are generally seen in an elderly population (older than 60 years). The large majority of primary cancers in this region are of squamous cell histology (80 to 90% of cases). Melanomas and sarcomas can also originate at this site.

Women who have undergone successful treatment for cervical cancer have an increased risk for the development of vaginal cancer. Although mainly of historical interest, there is a well-recognized association between in utero exposure to diethylstilbestrol and the development of very rare clear cell vaginal cancer.

The major presenting symptom is vaginal bleeding. Dysuria and vaginal discharge are also noted. In patients with advanced disease, pelvic pain is frequently described.

Depending on the clinical circumstances, standard treatment of vaginal cancers may focus on either radiation or surgical resection. Combined chemo-radiation therapy may be employed in locally advanced disease, but the overall experience with this strategy is limited. In a patient whose performance status is adequate, systemic chemotherapy may provide a modest level of benefit in recurrent or metastatic disease.

UTERINE FIBROIDS

Though not a malignancy, it is appropriate to discuss the management of uterine fibroids in this chapter because this condition is the most common female pelvic tumor (70 to 80% incidence in the female population by age 50). During the reproductive years, the incidence of fibroids may be as high as 40%.

The majority of fibroids are asymptomatic. When present, symptoms can range from mild inconvenience to heavy bleeding and pelvic pressure and pain.

In the past, the most common treatment was surgical removal of the fibroid or of the uterus itself. This procedure can be performed during laparotomy or through less invasive laparoscopic surgery. Over the years, a variety of invasive strategies have been introduced into routine medical practice for the treatment of symptomatic uterine fibroids, including uterine artery embolization, transvaginal temporary uterine artery occlusion, and MRI-guided focused ultrasound.

Noninterventional, hormonally based approaches (e.g., antiprogestins such as mifepristone) have been examined in the management of uterine fibroids. Although they are effective in relieving symptoms, these strategies are potentially limited by long-term drug-related side effects. However, these agents are clinically helpful in reducing the size of fibroids, decreasing dysfunctional uterine bleeding and pain, and improving overall quality of life.

1. Monk BJ, Sill MW, McMeekin DS, et al. Phase III trial of four cisplatin-containing doublet combinations in stage IVB, recurrent, or persistent cervical carcinoma: a Gynecologic Oncology Group study. *J Clin Oncol.* 2009;27:4649-4655.
2. Muñoz N, Manalastas R Jr, Pitisuttithum P, et al. Safety, immunogenicity, and efficacy of quadrivalent human papillomavirus (types 6, 11, 16, 18) recombinant vaccine in women aged 24-45 years: a randomised, double-blind trial. *Lancet.* 2009;373:1949-1957.
3. Paavonen J, Naud P, Salmeron J, et al. Efficacy of human papillomavirus (HPV)-16/18 AS04-adjuvanted vaccine against cervical infection and precancer caused by oncogenic HPV types (PATRICIA): final analysis of a double-blind, randomised study in young women. *Lancet.* 2009;374:301-314.
4. Randall ME, Filiaci VL, Muss H, et al. Randomized phase III trial of whole-abdominal irradiation versus doxorubicin and cisplatin chemotherapy in advanced endometrial carcinoma: a Gynecologic Oncology Group study. *J Clin Oncol.* 2006;24:36-44.
5. Nout RA, Smit VT, Putter H, et al. Vaginal brachytherapy versus pelvic external beam radiotherapy for patients with endometrial cancer of high-intermediate risk (PORTEC-2): an open-label, non-inferiority, randomised trial. *Lancet.* 2010;375:816-823.
6. Humber CE, Tierney JF, Symonds RP, et al. Chemotherapy for advanced, recurrent or metastatic endometrial cancer: a systematic review of Cochrane collaboration. *Ann Oncol.* 2007;18:409-420.
7. Bookman MA, Brady MF, McGuire WP, et al. Evaluation of new platinum-based treatment regimens in advanced-stage ovarian cancer: a Phase III trial of the Gynecologic Cancer Intergroup. *J Clin Oncol.* 2009;27:1419-1425.
8. Vergote I, Tropé CG, Amant F, et al. Neoadjuvant chemotherapy or primary surgery in stage IIIC or IV ovarian cancer. *N Engl J Med.* 2010;363:943-953.
9. Rustin GJ, van der Burg ME, Griffin CL, et al. Early versus delayed treatment of relapsed ovarian cancer (MRC OV05/EORTC 55955): a randomised trial. *Lancet.* 2010;376:1155-1163.

SUGGESTED READINGS

Amant F, Coosemans A, Debiec-Rychter M, et al. Clinical management of uterine sarcomas. *Lancet Oncol.* 2009;10:1188-1198. *A comprehensive review of the management of uterine sarcomas.*

Cragun JM. Screening for ovarian cancer. *Cancer Control.* 2011;18:16-21. *Review concluding that neither CA-125 nor ultrasound has adequate sensitivity or specificity for routine screening.*

Hennessy BT, Coleman RL, Markman M. Ovarian cancer. *Lancet.* 2009;374:1371-1382. *A comprehensive review of the management of ovarian cancer.*

Ramirez I, Chon HS, Apte SM. The role of surgery in the management of epithelial ovarian cancer. *Cancer Control.* 2011;18:22-30. *Review emphasizing that optimal cytoreductive surgery positively impacts survival.*

Wiegand KC, Shah SP, Al-Agha OM, et al. ARID1A mutations in endometriosis-associated ovarian carcinomas. *N Engl J Med.* 2010;363:1532-1543. *ARID1A mutations may predispose to the transformation of endometriosis into cancer.*

Winter-Roach B, Kitchener H, Dickinson H. Adjuvant (post-surgery) chemotherapy for early stage epithelial ovarian cancer. Cochrane Database Syst Rev. 2009;3:CD004706. *Meta-analysis revealing the impact of chemotherapy on high-risk early-stage ovarian cancer.*

206

TESTICULAR CANCER

LAWRENCE H. EINHORN

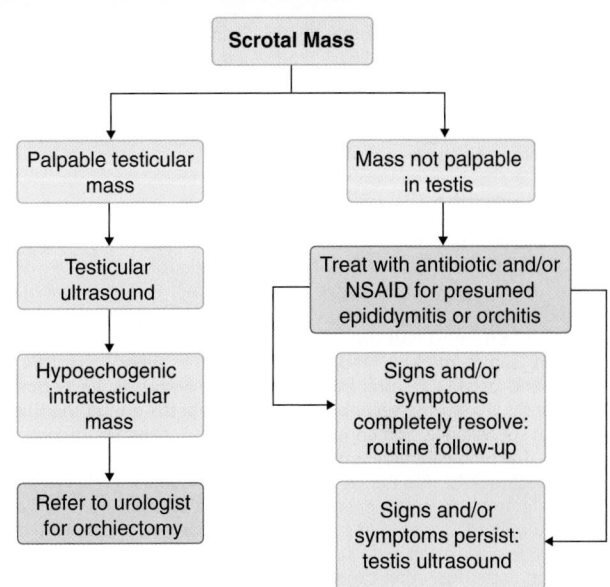

FIGURE 206-1. Management of a scrotal mass. NSAID = nonsteroidal anti-inflammatory drug.

EPIDEMIOLOGY

Testicular tumors are relatively uncommon and account for only 1% of male malignancies in the United States. The highest worldwide incidence occurs in Scandinavian countries; by contrast, testicular cancer is rare in African Americans and Asian Americans. The primary age group is 15 to 35 years for nonseminomatous tumors and a decade older for seminomas.

Male patients with a history of cryptorchidism have a 10- to 40-fold increased risk for the development of testicular cancer. The normally descended testis in these men is also at higher risk, suggesting a dysgenetic abnormality.

PATHOBIOLOGY

More than 95% of tumors of the testis originate from germ cells. Germ cell tumors can be seminomas or nonseminomatous germ cell tumors. Seminomas are more likely to be confined to the testis (stage I) and are exquisitely sensitive to radiation therapy. Pure seminomas never have elevated serum α-fetoprotein (AFP) levels. Nonseminomatous germ cell tumors consist of embryonal cell carcinomas, choriocarcinomas, yolk sac tumors, or teratomas, alone or mixed with other elements. Teratomas do not secrete human chorionic gonadotropin (HCG) or AFP and do not usually metastasize; they grow by local extension and are completely resistant to radiation therapy and chemotherapy.

Most germ cell testicular cancers in adults are associated with the cytogenetic abnormality i12p—an isochromosome of the short arm of chromosome 12—which is a highly specific finding in germ cell tumors. Sertoli cell tumors, Leydig cell tumors, and lymphomas are the most common non–germ cell tumors. In men older than 60 years, most tumors are non-Hodgkin's lymphoma (Chapter 191), with a predilection for bilateral involvement.

CLINICAL MANIFESTATIONS

Most patients with testicular cancer are initially evaluated because of testicular pain or because of a mass in or enlargement of one testis. Others are asymptomatic, and the cancer is first detected during a routine physical examination. Less commonly, the diagnosis is made during an evaluation for infertility, in part because testicular cancer can cause oligospermia.

Metastatic spread is either lymphatic or hematogenous. Lymphatic metastases usually go initially to the ipsilateral retroperitoneal lymph nodes, where they may be associated with flank pain. Lymphatic metastases may continue in a superior direction to the posterior mediastinum and eventually to the left supraclavicular lymph nodes. A large retroperitoneal mass or a supraclavicular lymph node may be palpable on physical examination. Hematogenous spread usually occurs first to the pulmonary parenchyma bilaterally. Pulmonary symptoms such as chest pain, shortness of breath, dyspnea on exertion, coughing, or hemoptysis are seen only with extensive pulmonary metastases. Other sites of hematogenous spread include the liver, bone, or brain. Significant elevation of the serum HCG level may produce gynecomastia.

DIAGNOSIS

Patients with a palpable mass in the testis should be suspected of having testicular cancer, especially if there is a history of cryptorchidism. Other causes of testicular and scrotal abnormalities may be included in the differential diagnosis. Acute pain in the testis suggests torsion. Painful enlargement may be due to a hydrocele, which may be caused by an underlying primary testicular malignancy. Pain and tenderness adjacent to the testis may be due to epididymitis or a varicocele. Tenderness of the testis itself on physical examination may reflect orchitis. However, an underlying neoplasm should always be considered.

Any testicular symptoms, including pain or a suspected mass, require evaluation. Testicular ultrasound is the test of choice in all suspicious cases. A hypoechogenic mass within the testis must be presumed to be testicular cancer and requires referral to a urologist (Fig. 206-1).

When orchiectomy reveals the diagnosis of testicular cancer, a staging evaluation is performed to determine the extent of disease and appropriate therapy. Clinical stage I disease is confined to the testis; stage II disease reflects spread to the retroperitoneal lymph nodes; and stage III is supradiaphragmatic disease, with either nodal metastases to the posterior mediastinum or supraclavicular region or hematogenous spread, especially to the lungs.

In addition to a full history and physical examination, serum HCG and AFP levels should be determined. Because the serum half-life is 1 day for HCG and 5 days for AFP, an AFP level of 1000 may take more than a month to normalize after orchiectomy, even if the tumor has been completely removed. Imaging studies to define the extent of disease include abdominal and pelvic computed tomography (CT) and a chest radiograph. If the chest radiograph does not show pulmonary metastases, a chest CT scan should be performed. Bone scans and head CT scans can be reserved for patients with symptoms suggestive of osseous and central nervous system metastases, respectively.

PREVENTION AND TREATMENT Rx

A careful testicular examination is a mandatory part of the physical examination in men, especially young men (Chapter 14), and is the key means of detecting tumors at an early stage. With the patient lying supine or standing up, the testis is gently palpated with the thumb and second and third fingers; the entire anterior, posterior, and lateral surfaces of the testis should be examined.

Local and Regional Disease
Seminomas
About 70% of seminomas are initially diagnosed at clinical stage I. Although the cure rate with orchiectomy alone is 80 to 95%, treatment can also include 2000 cGy para-aortic irradiation[1] or adjuvant carboplatin.[2]

Twenty percent of patients with seminoma are initially found to have stage II disease (positive abdominal CT scan). For these patients, radiation therapy has a 90% cure rate; in patients who are not cured by radiation therapy, subsequent combination chemotherapy (cisplatin combined with etoposide, with or without bleomycin) is usually curative. If the transverse diameter of the tumor is greater than 3 cm, if there are multiple anatomic levels of nodal metastases, or if stage III disease is present, the preferred initial treatment is cisplatin combination chemotherapy without irradiation; the cure rate is 70 to 100%, depending on the extent of the disease.

Nonseminomatous Germ Cell Tumors

Management of clinical stage I nonseminomatous germ cell tumors begins with orchiectomy, which has a 70% cure rate. This is followed by either retroperitoneal lymph node dissection or close surveillance (which can detect metastases early and guide curative chemotherapy), with or without one course of bleomycin, etoposide, and cisplatin. Most relapses occur in the first year, during which meticulous surveillance should include history and physical examination, serum markers, and chest radiograph every 2 months and abdominal and pelvic CT scans every 4 months. All studies are performed every 4 months during the second year, every 6 months during the third to fifth years of surveillance, and annually thereafter. CT scans are discontinued after 5 years. The physical examination should include palpation of the remaining testis, because these patients have a 1 to 2% chance of developing a contralateral primary tumor. The major complication of retroperitoneal lymph node dissection is inadvertent severing of the sympathetic plexus, with resultant retrograde ejaculation or failure of ejaculation. Nerve-sparing retroperitoneal lymph node dissection can retain antegrade ejaculation in more than 95% of patients. Some centers advocate primary chemotherapy for high-risk clinical stage I disease (embryonal predominant or vascular or lymphatic invasion) with cisplatin combination chemotherapy.**3** However, surveillance is still an option in this patient population.

For clinical stage II disease with persistently elevated serum markers or a transverse tumor diameter greater than 3 cm, chemotherapy is preferred. Other stage II patients are treated with retroperitoneal lymph node dissection, often followed by close surveillance (as described earlier, but without abdominal CT scans) or adjuvant chemotherapy. Testicular cancer has a higher cure rate with surgery alone, despite nodal metastases, than any other cancer.

Chemotherapy for Disseminated or Persistent Disease

The combination of bleomycin, etoposide, and cisplatin repeated every 3 weeks for three to four courses cures 70% of patients with metastatic disease and is the standard chemotherapy for disseminated testicular cancer. Poor-risk disease (Table 206-1) has a 50 to 60% cure rate with standard three-drug therapy, intermediate-risk disease (HCG 5000 to 50,000 IU/mL or AFP 1000 to 10,000 ng/mL) has a 70% cure rate, and all other forms of metastatic disease (good risk) have a 90 to 100% cure rate.

In the 30% of metastatic germ cell tumors that are not cured by initial combination chemotherapy, the use of standard-dose salvage therapy (ifosfamide, cisplatin, and either vinblastine or paclitaxel) or high-dose carboplatin and etoposide therapy, followed by peripheral blood stem cell transplantation, can cure 25 to 70% of refractory cases, depending on patient characteristics.

TABLE 206-1	**DEFINITION OF POOR-RISK DISEASE (ALL NONSEMINOMATOUS TESTICULAR CANCER PATIENTS)**

Presence of any of the following:
Lactate dehydrogenase >10 times the upper limit of normal, human chorionic gonadotropin >50,000 IU/mL, or α-fetoprotein >10,000 ng/mL
Any primary mediastinal nonseminomatous germ cell tumor
Nonpulmonary visceral metastases (e.g., bone, liver, brain)

1. Jones WG, Fossa SD, Mead GM, et al. Randomized trial of 30 versus 20 Gy in the adjuvant treatment of stage I testicular seminoma. *J Clin Oncol.* 2005;23:1200-1208.
2. Oliver RTD, Mason MD, Mead GM, et al. Radiotherapy versus single-dose carboplatin in adjuvant treatment of stage I seminoma: a randomised trial. *Lancet.* 2005;366:293-300.
3. Alberts P, Siener R, Krege S, et al. Randomized phase III trial comparing retroperitoneal lymph node dissection with one course of bleomycin and etoposide plus cisplatin in the adjuvant treatment of clinical stage I non-seminomatous germ cell tumors. *J Clin Oncol.* 2008;26:2966-2972.

SUGGESTED READINGS

Fossà SD, Cvancarova M, Chen L, et al. Adverse prognostic factors for testicular cancer-specific survival: a population-based study of 27,948 patients. *J Clin Oncol.* 2011;29:963-970. *Age over 40 (RR = 2), non-seminomic histology (RR = 2), and metastatic disease (RR = 9) were predictive, but survival has improved significantly in the past 25 years.*

Hotte SJ, Mayhew LA, Jewett M, et al. Management of stage I non-seminomatous testicular cancer: a systematic review and meta-analysis. *Clin Oncol (R Coll Radiol).* 2010;22:17-26. *Review.*
Ilic D, Misso ML. Screening for testicular cancer. *Cochrane Database Syst Rev.* 2011;2:CD007853. *Review emphasizing importance of family history, undescended testis, and testicular atrophy.*
Nakamura T, Miki T. Recent strategy for the management of advanced testicular cancer. *Int J Urol.* 2010;17:148-157. *Comprehensive overview.*
U.S. Preventive Services Task Force. Screening for testicular cancer: U.S. Preventive Services Task Force reaffirmation recommendation statement. *Ann Intern Med.* 2011;154:483-486. *Guidelines recommending against routine screening.*
Winter C, Albers P. Testicular germ cell tumors: pathogenesis, diagnosis and treatment. *Nat Rev Endocrinol.* 2011;7:43-53. *Review.*

PROSTATE CANCER

ERIC J. SMALL

DEFINITION

Prostate cancer is the most common noncutaneous malignant neoplasm in men in the United States, where it results in about 32,000 deaths each year, making it the second most common cause of cancer death in men. Prostate cancer is a single histologic disease with marked clinical heterogeneity ranging from indolent, clinically irrelevant disease to a virulent, rapidly lethal phenotype.

EPIDEMIOLOGY

The incidence of clinically diagnosed prostate cancer reflects the effects of screening by the prostate-specific antigen (PSA) assay. Before PSA testing was available, about 19,000 new cases of prostate cancer were reported each year in the United States; this number reached 84,000 by 1993 and peaked at about 300,000 new cases in 1996. Since 1996, the reported annual incidence of prostate cancer in the United States has declined to about 190,000, a number that may more closely estimate the true incidence of clinically detectable disease. The death rate due to prostate cancer has declined by about 1% per year since 1990. The age-specific decrease in mortality has been greatest in men younger than 75 years. Men older than 75 years still account for two thirds of all prostate cancer deaths. Whether this decline is due to early detection (screening) or to improved therapy has not been proved.

Risk factors for prostate cancer include increasing age, family history, African American race, and dietary factors. Epidemiologic studies have suggested that nutritional factors such as reduced fat intake and increased soy protein may have a protective effect against the development of prostate cancer. The incidence of prostate cancer among African Americans is nearly twice that observed among white Americans. Prostate cancer is diagnosed in African Americans at a more advanced stage, and disease-specific survival is lower in African Americans. The relative contributions of biologic, genetic, and environmental differences, as well as differences in health care access, are not well established. Prior vasectomy and benign prostatic hypertrophy (Chapter 131) do not increase the risk. Prostatic intraepithelial neoplasia, particularly when it is high grade, is recognized as a premalignant lesion, so its presence on biopsy increases the likelihood of subsequent malignancy.

PATHOBIOLOGY

Prostate cancer appears to be common among relatives of men with early-onset prostate cancer. At the molecular level, there appears to be a susceptibility locus for the development of prostate cancer at an early age on chromosome 1, band q24; however, an abnormality at this locus occurs in less than 10% of patients with prostate cancer. Although many genetic abnormalities with both loss and gain of function have been identified, consistent patterns of changes associated with an increased likelihood for the development of prostate cancer have not been identified. Approximately half of prostate cancers demonstrate genetic rearrangements, with fusion of promoters or enhancers of androgen-responsive genes such as *TMPRSS2* (transmembrane protease, serine 2) with oncogenic *ETS* (*E-twenty six*) transcription factors such as *ERG* (*ETS-related gene*). These fusions lead to overexpression of oncogenic transcription factors and appear to define a subset of tumors with more aggressive behavior.

Testosterone is required for maintenance of a normal, healthy prostatic epithelium, but it is also a prerequisite for the development of prostate cancer.

Prostate cancers express robust levels of androgen receptor, and signaling through the androgen receptor results in growth, progression, and invasion of prostate cancer. Inhibition of signaling, typically by the surgical or pharmacologic reduction of testosterone levels, results in prostate cancer apoptosis and involution. Ultimately, however, androgen-deprivation therapy loses clinical efficacy. The biologic events surrounding the clinical development of "androgen deprivation–resistant prostate cancer" are not well delineated, but amplification of the androgen receptor, which is a common event in these patients, presumably makes the cancer sensitive to minute levels of androgen or other ligands of the androgen receptor. The identification of androgen receptor splice variants that are constitutively active and ligand independent raises this as a potential mechanism by which true hormone resistance develops.

CLINICAL MANIFESTATIONS

Most patients with early-stage, organ-confined disease are asymptomatic. Obstructive voiding symptoms (hesitancy, intermittent urinary stream, decreased force of stream) generally reflect locally advanced disease with growth into the urethra or bladder neck, although these symptoms can be indistinguishable from benign prostatic hypertrophy (Chapter 131). Locally advanced tumors can also result in hematuria and hematospermia. Prostate cancer that has spread to the regional pelvic lymph nodes occasionally causes edema of the lower extremities or discomfort in the pelvic and perineal areas. Metastasis occurs most commonly to bone, where it is frequently asymptomatic, but it can also cause severe and unremitting pain. Bone metastasis can result in pathologic fractures or spinal cord compression. Although visceral metastases are rare as presenting features of prostate cancer, patients can have pulmonary, hepatic, pleural, peritoneal, and central nervous system metastases late in the natural history or after androgen-deprivation therapy fails.

DIAGNOSIS

More than 60% of patients with prostate cancer are asymptomatic, and the diagnosis is made solely because of an elevated screening PSA level. A palpable nodule on digital rectal examination, which is the next most common clinical presentation, generally prompts biopsy. Much less commonly, prostate cancer is diagnosed because of advanced disease that causes obstructive voiding symptoms, pelvic or perineal discomfort, lower extremity edema, or symptomatic bone lesions.

Although the digital rectal examination has a low sensitivity and specificity for the diagnosis of prostate cancer, biopsy of a nodule or area of induration reveals cancer 50% of the time, suggesting that prostate biopsy should be undertaken in all men with palpable nodules. The PSA level has a far better sensitivity but a low specificity because conditions such as benign prostatic hypertrophy and prostatitis can cause false-positive PSA elevations (Chapter 131). By use of a PSA threshold of 4 ng/mL, 70 to 80% of tumors are detected. Far greater accuracy is achieved with age-specific PSA thresholds. Thus, for men aged 40 to 49, a PSA greater than 2.5 is considered abnormal; for men 50 to 59, a PSA greater than 3.5 is abnormal; for men 60 to 69, a PSA greater than 4.5 should prompt further evaluation; and patients aged 70 to 79 should have a PSA of 6.5 or less. The positive predictive value for a single PSA level above 10 ng/mL is greater than 60% for cancer, but the positive predictive value for a PSA level between 4 and 10 ng/mL is only about 30%. Assays of the PSA fraction that circulates unbound (percentage of free PSA) may help distinguish prostate cancer from benign processes; in patients with PSA levels of 4 to 10 ng/mL, the percentage of free PSA appears to be an independent predictor of prostate cancer, and a cutoff value of free PSA less than 25% can detect 95% of cancers while avoiding 20% of unnecessary biopsies.

Transrectal ultrasonography with biopsies is indicated when the PSA level is elevated, when the percentage of free PSA is less than 25%, or when an abnormality is noted on digital rectal examination. Extended field specimens (preferably up to six biopsies on each side) are generally obtained. Seminal vesicles are sampled in high-risk patients. A bone scan is warranted only in patients with PSA levels above 10 ng/mL, and abdominal and pelvic computed tomography or magnetic resonance imaging is usually unrevealing in patients with a PSA level below 10 to 20 ng/mL.

The prognosis of prostate cancer correlates with histologic grade and extent (stage) of disease. More than 95% of prostate cancers are adenocarcinomas, and multifocality is common. The histologic (Gleason) grade ranges from 1 to 5, although in the modern era, Gleason grades of 1 and 2 are exceedingly rare; the Gleason score, which refers to the sum of the two most common histologic patterns seen on each tissue specimen, ranges from 4 (2+2) to 10 (5+5). In general, tumors are classified as well differentiated

(Gleason score 2 to 6), of intermediate differentiation (Gleason score 7), or poorly differentiated (Gleason score 8 to 10).

Clinical stage is defined by the extent of disease based on the physical examination, imaging studies, and pathology. Stage T1 is nonpalpable prostate cancer detected only on pathologic examination, noted either incidentally after transurethral resection for benign hypertrophy (T1a and T1b) or on a biopsy specimen obtained because of an elevated PSA level (T1c, the most common clinical stage at diagnosis). Stage T2 is a palpable tumor that appears to be confined to the prostate gland (T2a in one lobe, T2b in two lobes), and stage T3 is tumor with extension through the prostatic capsule (T3a if it is focal, T3b if seminal vesicles are involved). T4 tumors are those with invasion of adjacent structures, such as the bladder neck, external urinary sphincter, rectum, levator muscles, or pelvic sidewall. Nodal metastases can be microscopic and detectable only by biopsy or lymphadenectomy, or they can be visible on imaging studies. Distant metastases are predominantly to bone, but occasional visceral metastases occur.

PREVENTION

The precise role for screening remains controversial. Currently, many organizations recommend screening with PSA, but the U.S. Preventive Services Task Force recommends against screening for men older than 70 years, and it is neither for nor against screening in younger men. Of two large randomized screening trials using PSA levels, one reported a reduction in prostate-cancer–specific mortality,[1] but neither found an overall reduction in mortality.[1,2] At best, an estimated 1410 men would need to be screened to prevent one prostate cancer death over a 10-year period. Randomized trials have shown that vitamins E and C and selenium are not effective at preventing prostate cancer. The use of 5a-reductase inhibitors (both finasteride and dutasteride) reduces the risk for development of prostate cancer.[3,4] However, this approach has not been widely adopted.

TREATMENT   Rx

Localized Prostate Cancer
Principles of Therapy

The principal therapeutic options for men with localized prostate cancer include the following: active surveillance; androgen deprivation; retropubic or perineal radical prostatectomy, with or without postoperative radiation therapy to the prostate margins and pelvis; external beam radiation therapy; and brachytherapy (either permanent or temporary radioactive seed implants), with or without external beam radiation therapy to the prostate margins and pelvis.

Treatment options require individualization, taking into account the patient's comorbidity, life expectancy, likelihood of cure, and personal preferences based on an understanding of the potential morbidity associated with each treatment. A multidisciplinary approach to integrate surgery, radiation therapy, and androgen deprivation is increasingly recommended. For higher-risk patients with a greater likelihood of nodal micrometastases, androgen deprivation is often combined with radiation therapy encompassing both the prostate and the pelvis. In patients at extremely high risk of micrometastatic disease or with comorbidities, systemic therapy alone without concurrent local therapy may be appropriate.

PSA screening has led to the early detection of a large number of nonpalpable tumors, for which conventional clinical means of staging are inadequate. Thus, less emphasis is being placed on clinical stage and more emphasis is being placed on PSA values and other predictors of outcome. Careful risk assessment is required to identify patients who are appropriate candidates for definitive local treatment.

Several studies have confirmed that serum PSA level, clinical stage, and biopsy Gleason score can be used to predict the final pathologic stage after prostatectomy, and that these are independent predictors of survival without PSA elevation after external beam radiation therapy or radical prostatectomy. For example, in a radiation therapy series, clinical stage T3 or higher, PSA level above 10 ng/mL, and biopsy Gleason score of 7 or higher were risk factors for poor outcome (death or PSA elevation); 5-year survival without PSA elevation was 85% for patients with none of these adverse features (good risk), 65% for patients with one adverse feature (intermediate risk), and 35% for patients with two or three adverse features (poor risk). Similar statistics are cited in radical prostatectomy series. The percentage of biopsy specimens that are positive and the rate of increase in the PSA value are each independent predictors of outcome after radical prostatectomy and can be used to counsel patients about their therapeutic options. A number of multivariable prognostic models have been developed and validated and have been used to develop simple nomograms or online risk calculators.

Low- to Intermediate-Risk Disease

In a randomized trial of patients younger than 75 years with clinical stage T1b, T1c, or T2 prostate cancer, radical prostatectomy compared with no therapy significantly reduced the relative risk of death due to prostate cancer by 50% (a 2% absolute risk reduction) and overall mortality by a similar absolute amount at 8.6 years.[5] Reductions in progressive disease and metastases were also significant. The adverse effects on quality of life differed between the two strategies—more sexual dysfunction and urinary leakage after radical prostatectomy, more urinary obstruction with active surveillance—but were of similar magnitude.[6] Nerve-sparing radical prostatectomy was not routinely performed in this study, and many patients already had palpable disease, so the implications for less advanced disease with newer surgical techniques are not known. Nonrandomized data suggest that active surveillance may be judiciously used in patients with low disease volume, Gleason score of 6 or lower, and slow PSA doubling times. Active surveillance is probably not appropriate for young, otherwise healthy men with high-risk features as described earlier (PSA >10 ng/mL, Gleason score of 7 or higher, clinical stage T3 or higher). Whether active surveillance is appropriate for men with intermediate-risk, nonpalpable tumors remains debated. Androgen deprivation has not been carefully studied as primary therapy for localized disease, but it is becoming a more common approach in men who wish to receive some therapy but are not suited for or decline to undergo prostatectomy or radiation therapy.

Men with T1 or T2 prostate cancer who otherwise have a life expectancy of more than 10 years and no significant comorbid illnesses usually should have definitive local therapy with either surgery or radiation therapy. Long-term survival is excellent. Men with T1 or T2 tumors with Gleason scores of 7 or less have 8-year survival rates of 85 to 95%. Patients with T1 or T2 tumors with Gleason scores of 8 to 10 have 8-year survival rates of about 70%.

Nerve-sparing procedures and careful dissection techniques have decreased the risk of postoperative urinary incontinence and impotence. Postoperative urinary incontinence is reported to occur in less than 10% of cases. Postoperative impotence is dependent on a variety of factors, including the patient's age, preoperative erectile function, extent of cancer, and whether a nerve-sparing procedure was performed. In general, impotence rates of 10 to 50% are cited. Robotic-assisted laparoscopic prostatectomies have gained popularity but have not been shown to result in better outcomes. After a radical prostatectomy, the PSA should become undetectable; a detectable PSA implies the presence of cancer cells, either locally or at a metastatic site. Immediate (adjuvant) postoperative radiation therapy improves biochemical progression-free survival and local control in patients with one or more pathologic risk factors (capsule penetration, positive surgical margins, invasion of a seminal vesicle) after radical prostatectomy.[6]

Conventional external beam radiation therapy is being replaced by three-dimensional conformal radiation therapy or intensity-modulated radiation therapy, which permits higher doses to the target tissue with less toxicity. Randomized trials suggest a benefit with higher doses of radiation. Brachytherapy, which is the placement of permanent or temporary radioactive seeds directly into the prostate, is adequate for intracapsular disease with no more than minimal transcapsular extension; otherwise, it should be combined with external beam radiation therapy.

High-Risk Disease

Patients with adverse risk features (Gleason score 8 to 10, PSA >10, stage T3) are at high risk of nodal and micrometastatic disease and are generally treated with aggressive local therapy in combination with androgen deprivation, which is synergistic with radiation therapy.[7] Taken in the aggregate, trials suggest that 4 months of androgen deprivation with radiation therapy can improve local control and prolong progression-free survival in patients with intermediate-risk features, whereas long-term androgen deprivation (up to 3 years) prolongs local control, progression-free survival, and overall survival in patients with high-risk features compared with radiation therapy alone.[8,9] Patients with stage T3 disease and Gleason scores of 7 have intermediate outcomes, with 8-year survival rates of about 70%; patients with stage T3 disease and Gleason scores of 8 to 10 have 8-year survival rates, after radiation therapy, of about 50%. Several randomized controlled trials suggest that patients with high-risk disease who are treated surgically and have capsule penetration, positive margins, or seminal vesicle involvement should receive immediate adjuvant radiation therapy.

Recurrent Disease

Between 30 and 50% of men treated with radiation therapy or prostatectomy have evidence of disease recurrence, as defined by a climbing PSA level. PSA doubling time is predictive of survival, and a short PSA doubling time (<3 to 6 months) is associated with a higher likelihood of systemic disease. For selected patients with clear local recurrences, low PSA levels, and prolonged PSA doubling times (generally), local salvage therapy (surgery for patients previously treated with radiation therapy, radiation therapy for patients previously treated with surgery,[10] and androgen deprivation) can be considered. Although androgen-deprivation therapy readily controls PSA levels, it is unknown whether it prolongs life in patients with PSA-only recurrent disease.

Advanced Disease

In patients whose radical prostatectomy surgery reveals microscopic involvement of lymph nodes, immediate androgen deprivation prolongs survival compared with deferment of androgen deprivation until osseous metastases are detected. Similarly, patients who are at high risk of nodal invasion and who undergo external beam radiation benefit from concurrent short-term hormonal therapy.[9]

In patients with newly diagnosed metastatic prostate cancer, androgen deprivation is the mainstay of treatment and results in symptomatic improvement and disease regression in approximately 80 to 90% of patients. Androgen deprivation can be achieved by orchiectomy or by medical castration with a luteinizing hormone–releasing hormone (LHRH) agonist (leuprolide acetate, goserelin acetate).

Some LHRH agonists cause a transient worsening of signs and symptoms during the first week of therapy as a result of a surge in luteinizing hormone and testosterone, which peaks within 72 hours; an antiandrogen (flutamide, bicalutamide, or nilutamide) should be given with the first LHRH injection to prevent a tumor flare. Medical castration occurs within 4 weeks. The duration of hormone sensitivity is 5 to 10 years for node-positive or high-risk localized (or recurrent) prostate cancer, but it is closer to 24 months in patients with overt metastatic disease. The most common side effects of androgen ablation are loss of libido, impotence, hot flashes, weight gain, fatigue, anemia, and osteoporosis. Bisphosphonates reduce bone mineral loss associated with androgen deprivation.

Castration-Resistant Prostate Cancer

Typically, the first manifestation of resistance to androgen deprivation is a climbing PSA level in the setting of anorchid levels of testosterone. In about 15% of patients, discontinuation of antiandrogen therapy (flutamide, bicalutamide, nilutamide) while continuing treatment with LHRH agonists results in a PSA decline that can be associated with symptomatic improvement and can persist for 4 months or more. If antiandrogen withdrawal fails, treatment with secondary hormonal manipulations, such as ketoconazole or estrogens, is appropriate. Sipuleucel-T is an autologous dendritic cell product that has been shown to prolong life[11] and is appropriate for patients with castration-resistant metastatic prostate cancer who do not have cancer-associated pain, visceral metastases, rapidly progressive disease, or the need for systemic steroids. Thereafter, treatment with chemotherapeutic regimens, such as docetaxel plus corticosteroids or mitoxantrone plus corticosteroids, may be effective. Randomized phase III trials have demonstrated a survival advantage of approximately 25% in patients receiving taxol-based therapy compared with mitoxantrone,[12,13] and docetaxol-prednisone is now considered a standard therapeutic approach in patients with metastatic, androgen deprivation–resistant prostate cancer. Following therapy with docetaxel, patients who remain candidates for further chemotherapy can be treated with cabazitaxel, an agent shown to prolong life in this group of patients. In general, serial PSA levels are the best (albeit imperfect) way to follow up patients, and a decline of 30 to 50% is associated with improved survival. Zoledronic acid or denosumab is indicated in castration-resistant prostate cancer patients with bone metastases, as each reduces the incidence of skeletal-related events.

Palliative Care

Many patients with advanced prostate cancer have bone pain or functional impairments that adversely affect quality of life, and the provision of appropriate palliative care is an integral component of their management. In addition to the usual analgesics, glucocorticoids serve as anti-inflammatory agents and can alleviate bone pain. For patients with widespread bone metastases and pain not easily controlled with analgesics or local irradiation, strontium-89 and samarium-153 can be administered intravenously; they are selectively concentrated in bone metastases and alleviate pain in 70% or more of treated patients.

The approach to the treatment of prostate cancer is detailed in Table 207-1.

PROGNOSIS

In general, the 10-year PSA progression-free survival is 70 to 80% with Gleason scores of 2 to 6, whether treatment is with radiation therapy or surgery; 50 to 70% for Gleason scores of 7; and 15 to 30% for Gleason scores of 8 to 10. For patients with a climbing PSA level after radical prostatectomy, time to detectable PSA, Gleason score at the time of prostatectomy, and PSA doubling time are important prognostic variables. The likelihood of bone metastases at 7 years ranges from 20% for good-prognosis patients to 80% for poor-prognosis patients.

For patients with microscopic nodal disease, 10-year survival approaches 80% in men treated with androgen deprivation. Median survival in men treated with androgen deprivation for established metastatic disease ranges

TABLE 207-1	APPROACH TO THE TREATMENT OF PROSTATE CANCER
EXTENT OF CANCER	**THERAPEUTIC OPTIONS**
Organ confined: low risk (usually T1 or T2, GS <7, PSA <10 ng/mL)	Surveillance Radical prostatectomy External beam radiation therapy to prostate Brachytherapy
Organ confined: intermediate risk (usually T2, GS = 7, PSA = 10-20 ng/mL)	Radical prostatectomy External beam radiation therapy to prostate, possibly to pelvis, with or without AD Brachytherapy
Organ confined: high risk (usually T3, GS >7, PSA >20 ng/mL)	Radical prostatectomy (with adjuvant radiation therapy, if needed) External beam radiation therapy to prostate and pelvis (usually with AD) Brachytherapy plus radiation therapy (usually with AD)
Climbing PSA level after local therapy	AD: antiandrogen monotherapy or combined AD Salvage radiation therapy (for patients with prior prostatectomy) Salvage radical prostatectomy (for patients with prior radiation therapy) Surveillance Investigational therapy
Node positive	Surveillance AD Pelvic or prostate radiation therapy + AD Investigational therapy
Metastatic: untreated hormone-refractory prostate cancer	AD Second-line hormones Sipuleucel-T immunotherapy Chemotherapy Investigational therapy

AD = androgen deprivation; GS = Gleason score; PSA = prostate-specific antigen.

from 3 to 5 years. The median survival for men with androgen deprivation–resistant disease ranges from 20 months if they are minimally symptomatic to 8 to 12 months if they are severely symptomatic.

FUTURE DIRECTIONS

Molecular markers can not only identify patients at risk for the development of progressive disease but also act as therapeutic targets. In addition, the genomic characterization of prostate cancer subtypes will lead to risk-adapted therapy. Enhanced understanding of androgen receptor biology may permit the development of specific hormonal therapies and guide the more rational use of existing agents.

1. Schröder FH, Hugosson J, Roobol MJ, et al. Screening and prostate-cancer mortality in a randomized European study. *N Engl J Med*. 2009;360:1320-1328.
2. Andriole GL, Grubb RL 3rd, Buys SS, et al. Mortality results from a randomized prostate-cancer screening trial. *N Engl J Med*. 2009;360:1310-1319.
3. Thompson IM, Goodman PJ, Tangen CM, et al. The influence of finasteride on the development of prostate cancer. *N Engl J Med*. 2003;349:215-224.
4. Andriole GL, Bostwick DG, Brawley OW, et al. Effect of dutasteride on the risk of prostate cancer. *N Engl J Med*. 2010;362:1192-1202.
5. Bill-Axelson A, Holmberg L, Ruutu M, et al. Radical prostatectomy versus watchful waiting in early prostate cancer. *N Engl J Med*. 2005;352:1977-1984.
6. Steineck G, Helgesen F, Adolfsson J, et al. Quality of life after radical prostatectomy or watchful waiting. *N Engl J Med*. 2002;347:790-796.
7. D'Amico AV, Chen MH, Renshaw AA, et al. Androgen suppression and radiation vs radiation alone for prostate cancer: a randomized trial. *JAMA*. 2008;299:289-295.
8. Bolla M, van Poppel H, Collette L, et al. Postoperative radiotherapy after radical prostatectomy: a randomized controlled trial (EORTC trial 22911). *Lancet*. 2005;366:572-578.
9. Roach M 3rd, DeSilvio M, Lawton C, et al. Phase III trial comparing whole-pelvic versus prostate-only radiotherapy and neoadjuvant versus adjuvant combined androgen suppression: radiation Therapy Oncology Group 9413. *J Clin Oncol*. 2003;21:1904-1911.
10. Stephenson AJ, Shariat SF, Zelefsky MJ, et al. Salvage radiotherapy for recurrent prostate cancer after radical prostatectomy. *JAMA*. 2004;291:1325-1332.
11. Kantoff PW, Higano CS, Shore ND, et al. Sipuleucel-T immunotherapy for castration-resistant prostate cancer. *N Engl J Med*. 2010;363:411-422.
12. Tannock IF, de Wit R, Berry WR, et al. Docetaxel plus prednisone or mitoxantrone plus prednisone for advanced prostate cancer. *N Engl J Med*. 2004;351:1502-1512.
13. de Bono JS, Oudard S, Ozguroglu M, et al. Prednisone plus cabazitaxel or mitoxantrone for metastatic castration-resistant prostate cancer progressing after docetaxel treatment: a randomised open-label trial. *Lancet*. 2010;376:1147-1154.

SUGGESTED READINGS

Berger MF, Lawrence MS, Demichelis F, et al. The genomic complexity of primary human prostate cancer. *Nature*. 2011;470:214-220. *Review of multiple genomic abnormalities.*
Gaster B, Edwards K, Trinidad SB, et al. Patient-centered discussions about prostate cancer screening: a real-world approach. *Ann Intern Med*. 2010;153:661-665. *Practical suggestions for physicians.*
Hayes JH, Ollendorf DA, Pearson SD, et al. Active surveillance compared with initial treatment for men with low-risk prostate cancer: a decision analysis. *JAMA*. 2010;304:2373-2380. *Decision analysis suggests that active surveillance is as effective as initial treatment for men with low-risk prostate cancer.*
Heidenreich A, Bellmunt J, Bolla M, et al. EAU Guidelines on Prostate Cancer. Part I: Screening, Diagnosis, and Treatment of Clinically Localised Disease. *Eur Urol*. 2011;59:61-71. *Consensus guidelines.*
Mottet N, Bellmunt J, Bolla M, et al. EAU Guidelines on Prostate Cancer. Part II: Treatment of Advanced, Relapsing, and Castration-Resistant Prostate Cancer. *Eur Urol*. 2011;59:572-583. *Consensus guidelines.*
Whitson JM, Porten SP, Carroll PR. Prostate cancer: reducing overtreatment: active surveillance in low-risk disease. *Nat Rev Urol*. 2011;8:124-125. *Makes the case for "watchful waiting."*
Wu Y, Rosenberg JE, Taplin ME. Novel agents and new therapeutics in castration-resistant prostate cancer. *Curr Opin Oncol*. 2011;23:290-296. *Review including denosumab, abiraterone, cabazitaxel, and provenge.*

208

PRIMARY AND METASTATIC MALIGNANT BONE LESIONS

ADAM LERNER AND KAREN H. ANTMAN

PRIMARY BONE TUMORS

DEFINITION

Primary bone malignancies are relatively uncommon tumors (0.2% of all neoplasms in the Surveillance, Epidemiology, and End Results [SEER] database, 1.8 new cases/100,000 population/year) that arise from cells that are normal components of bone tissues and that have the potential to metastasize. Malignant tumors are to be distinguished from a variety of more common benign bone lesions, such as osteochondromas and enchondromas, which lack the ability to metastasize.

CLINICAL MANIFESTATIONS AND DIAGNOSIS

Patients with primary malignant and benign bone tumors present with pain, swelling and occasionally pathologic fracture of the involved bone. If radiologic studies suggest a malignant primary bone tumor (see characteristics of each subtype described later), an orthopedic oncologist should be consulted before carrying out a biopsy because improper biopsy technique may compromise subsequent surgical care, particularly limb-sparing surgery. Staging of patients with bone tumors generally requires computed tomography (CT) scans of the chest, abdomen, and pelvis to assess for metastatic disease. Characterization of the primary bone tumor may benefit from magnetic resonance imaging (MRI) assessment of soft tissue extension or CT scan assessment of cortical bone involvement, or both.

MAJOR PRIMARY MALIGNANT BONE TUMORS

Myeloma, the most common primary bone malignancy, is covered in Chapter 193.

Osteosarcoma

Osteosarcoma is the most common malignant sarcoma of bone, representing about 35% of cases. It has a bimodal age distribution, with highest incidence in patients younger than 20 years, most likely related to the normal rapid bone growth that occurs during adolescence. In this age group, most tumors arise in the metaphyseal areas of the long bones of the extremities, particularly around the knee. Males are affected more commonly than females at a ratio of 3:2. A second peak of incidence occurs in adults older than 60 years. The sites of origin in these older patients are somewhat more heterogeneous, with craniofacial and pelvic bones each accounting for 20% of tumors. Radiographically, osteosarcomas usually present as mixed osteoblastic and osteolytic lesions, although pure forms of either appearance can occur. Periosteal elevation (Codman's triangle), cortical destruction, and tumor extension into soft tissue are common on plain films or MRI.

The incidence of osteosarcoma is increased in families that carry germline deletion of retinoblastoma (*Rb*), *p53* (Li-Fraumeni), or *RecQ* DNA helicase (Rothman-Thompson, Werner, or Bloom syndrome) genes. Consistent with these observations, although most younger patients with osteosarcomas have no apparent predisposing factor or family history of bone tumors, alterations in the *p53* and *Rb* genes of such sporadic tumors occur in 40% and 60%, respectively. In older patients, a variety of conditions may predispose patients to osteosarcoma, most convincingly antecedent Paget's disease or prior radiation therapy.

TREATMENT

Osteosarcoma is a highly proliferative neoplasm that metastasizes rapidly. As for most sarcomas, osteosarcoma spreads hematogenously, and the most common site of metastasis is the lung. Despite aggressive surgical resection of the primary bone tumor, the incidence of recurrence with metastatic disease is high in the absence of systemic treatment, consistent with the concept that most patients present with clinically inapparent micrometastatic disease. The development of effective systemic chemotherapy with doxorubicin (Adriamycin) and cisplatin, with or without methotrexate, has had a profoundly positive effect on treatment outcome, with 5-year disease-free survival rates exceeding 65% in patients younger than 40 years with non-metastatic extremity tumors.**1** Most patients are managed with initial neo-adjuvant chemotherapy, delayed resection of the primary tumor, and then further postoperative chemotherapy. Serum alkaline phosphatase levels, often elevated in osteosarcoma patients, can be used to monitor disease status.

Modern surgical techniques have allowed surgical resection of most extremity osteosarcomas without amputation. Although resection of lung metastases can be curative in about 20% of selected patients, detection of radiologically apparent metastatic disease at presentation significantly worsens prognosis. Long-term disease control in older adults with osteosarcoma is substantially lower than in younger patients, with a 5-year overall survival rate of 22% in one series of patients older than 65 years, most likely because of fundamental differences in the underlying molecular pathophysiology of tumors in older adults. Although osteosarcoma is generally considered to be relatively radiation resistant, radiation can play a palliative role in selected patients.

Chondrosarcoma

Chondrosarcoma, a malignant tumor characterized by hyaline cartilage differentiation, is the second most common sarcoma of bone, representing 25% of bone sarcomas. The peak incidence is in the fifth to seventh decades of life. The most common primary sites are in the pelvis, proximal femur, and proximal humerus. Patients present with long-standing complaints of swelling, pain, or both. Radiographically, chondrosarcoma is detected as an area of radiolucency with variable punctate mineralization, with frequent cortical bone erosion or thickening, sometimes with extension into adjacent soft tissue. Distinguishing low-grade chondrosarcomas from benign central enchondromas can be difficult: location in the axial skeleton and size greater than 5 cm favor malignancy.

Up to 15% of chondrosarcomas arise from preexisting peripheral osteochondromas and, like their benign counterparts, harbor mutations in the exostosin *(EXT)* genes. The remaining 85% of chondrosarcomas arise in a central location, some in preexisting enchondromas. Chondrosarcomas are divided into three grades, with higher-grade tumors characterized by greater cellularity and cellular atypia. In one series, 61% of patients had grade 1 tumors; only 4% of such patients developed metastases. In contrast, 36% of patients had grade 2 and 3% grade 3 tumors; among this combined group, 29% developed metastases.

TREATMENT

Unlike osteosarcoma and Ewing's sarcoma, chondrosarcomas generally grow slowly, metastasize less commonly, and have an excellent prognosis after adequate surgical resection. Although chondrosarcomas are considered relatively radiation resistant, radiation therapy may provide palliation for patients with large or recurrent unresectable central chondrosarcomas.

Ewing's Sarcoma

Ewing's sarcoma and primitive neuroectodermal tumor (PNET) are a family of small round cell sarcomas that represent 16% of primary bone sarcomas. As with osteosarcoma, the peak incidence occurs during the second decade of life, but unlike osteosarcoma, the incidence of Ewing's is unimodal, being distinctly unusual in older adults and in nonwhites. Ewing's sarcoma tends to arise in the diaphyseal region of long bones, in the pelvis, or in ribs. Ewing's tumors are characterized radiologically by a permeative or "moth-eaten" appearance of the affected bone, with a multilayered "onion-skin" periosteal reaction. MRI studies frequently document a significant soft tissue mass associated with the bone lesion. Unlike other sarcomas of bone, Ewing's sarcoma may present with symptoms of an inflammatory systemic illness, with intermittent fevers, anemia, leukocytosis, and an increased sedimentation rate.

Eighty-five percent of patients with Ewing's family sarcomas contain a t(11;22)(9q24;q12) chromosomal translocation that juxtaposes the *EWS* gene on chromosome 22 with *FLI1*, an ETS family transcription factor. Another 15% contain a variant in which *EWS* is juxtaposed to *ERG*, another ETS family member on chromosome band 21q22. Because Ewing's sarcoma resembles other small round cell tumors microscopically, reverse transcription–polymerase chain reaction and fluorescent in situ hybridization studies that document such translocations play a critical role in confirming the diagnosis. Ewing's sarcoma/PNET cells characteristically express CD99/MIC2.

TREATMENT

The development of effective systemic chemotherapy regimens has substantially improved long-term control of Ewing's sarcoma. After completion of staging procedures, patients are treated with neoadjuvant chemotherapy. One highly active regimen alternates cycles of vincristine, doxorubicin, and cyclophosphamide with ifosfamide and etoposide. After 3 months of chemotherapy, the primary tumor is resected, radiated, or both, depending on the location and extent of the primary tumor. Chemotherapy is then resumed for a total of up to 1 year of treatment. Using such an approach, the mean 5-year event-free survival rate for patients who present with nonmetastatic disease is 69%.**2** Insulin-like growth factor-1 receptor antagonists have demonstrated clinical activity in recent clinical trials for chemotherapy-refractory disease.

● METASTATIC TUMORS TO BONE

Tumors metastatic to bone are important causes of cancer-related morbidity. Effective prevention and treatment of skeleton-related metastases are an important part of clinical care for many cancer patients. The most common tumors to metastasize to bone are breast in women and prostate in men, followed by lung, kidney, gastrointestinal tract, and thyroid.

Bone metastases typically present as localized or referred pain and less commonly as a fracture. Plain radiographs may demonstrate blastic or lytic lesions. Although prostate cancer is generally blastic and multiple myeloma usually lytic, most other tumors have a mixed appearance. In patients with one documented bone metastasis or in patients with widely metastatic disease and bone pain, a radiologic survey can identify bone metastases that may ultimately place the patient at risk for a pathologic fracture. Technetium diphosphonate bone scans are useful to delineate the extent of bony metastases and in following response to therapy. However, a negative study must be interpreted cautiously for tumors that are potentially purely lytic because these may be undetectable by bone scan. In such tumors (e.g., multiple myeloma), a skeletal survey is therefore preferable. Routine screening for bone metastases is not indicated for cancer patients with no symptoms or signs of bone involvement.

TREATMENT Rx

In the absence of fracture or impending fracture, painful bone metastases are treated with external beam radiation therapy. In patients with numerous bone metastases, systemic chemotherapy or endocrine therapy can play an important palliative role. Pathologic fractures or imminent fractures are generally managed by operative internal fixation.

PREVENTION

In breast cancer, prostate cancer, and multiple myeloma patients, bisphosphonate therapy increases the time to a first skeletal event. Bisphosphonate therapy also appears to prolong survival in patients with metastatic breast cancer. The optimal schedule and duration of administration of bisphosphonates to maximize benefit and minimize potential complications remain to be established.

1. Grier HE, Krailo MD, Tarbell NJ, et al. Addition of ifosfamide and etoposide to standard chemotherapy for Ewing's sarcoma and primitive neuroectodermal tumor of bone. *N Engl J Med.* 2003;348:694-701.
2. Meyers PA, Schwartz CL, Krailo MD, et al. Osteosarcoma: the addition of muramyl tripeptide to chemotherapy improves overall survival—a report from the Children's Oncology Group. *J Clin Oncol.* 2008;26:633-638.

SUGGESTED READINGS

Balamuth NJ, Womer RB. Ewing's sarcoma. *Lancet Oncol.* 2010;11:184-192. *Opportunities for new treatment approaches in a sarcoma of children and adolescents, in which survival has improved from about 10% to about 75% with chemotherapy for localized tumors but patients with metastases still fare badly.*

Geller DS, Gorlick R. Osteosarcoma: a review of diagnosis, management, and treatment strategies. *Clin Adv Hematol Oncol.* 2010;8:705-718. *Review including multiagent chemotherapy.*

Jamil N, Howie S, Salter DM. Therapeutic molecular targets in human chondrosarcoma. *Int J Exp Pathol.* 2010;91:387-393. *Review.*

O'Day K, Gorlick R. Novel therapeutic agents for osteosarcoma. *Expert Rev Anticancer Ther.* 2009;9:511-523. *New therapeutic approaches, including targeted agents, inhibitors of tumor microenvironment, and immunomodulatory agents.*

Riedel RF, Larrier N, Dodd L, et al. The clinical management of chondrosarcoma. *Curr Treat Options Oncol.* 2009;10:94-106. *This review highlights the need for a coordinated multidisciplinary approach to management of these patients.*

209

SARCOMAS OF SOFT TISSUE AND BONE, AND OTHER NEOPLASMS OF CONNECTIVE TISSUES

GEORGE D. DEMETRI

DEFINITION

Sarcomas are a very heterogeneous group of malignant neoplasms of connective tissues, including bone and soft tissue. Sarcomas, as well as other putatively "nonmalignant" neoplasms that affect soft tissue and bone, share a mesenchymal cell of origin with aberrant differentiation and growth potential. Mesenchymal cells (derived from mesoderm), as well as neural crest cells (from ectoderm), are critical for the normal structure and function of humans because they give rise to the connective tissues that hold the organism together and also provide critical functions such as support and nourishment of neural tissues. When the growth, differentiation, or survival of these cells is aberrant, tumors arise, and this is the family of neoplasms to which sarcomas belong. Sarcomas include a vast array of tumor types related to muscle, stromal tissue, adipose tissue, blood and lymphatic vessels, nerves and nerve sheaths, cartilage, bone, and other fibrous tissues.

Sarcomas are tumors with distinct histopathologic abnormalities; other forms of connective tissue neoplasms may also cause significant disease without being classified as sarcomas per se. For example, because of the histopathologically bland appearance of desmoid tumors, pathologists do not classify these myofibroblastic neoplasms as sarcomas, even though they can cause significant morbidity and even death if they are recurrent and unresectable. Similarly, the sarcoma known as gastrointestinal stromal tumor (GIST) was not considered a true sarcoma before 2000, although many GISTs certainly exhibit all the characteristics of aggressive malignancy. In brief, sarcomas represent a broad group of different diseases that can affect any anatomic location, and for this reason, they have puzzled clinicians and intrigued developmental biologists and fundamental researchers.

EPIDEMIOLOGY

True sarcomas represent a very uncommon subset of human malignancies, accounting for less than 1% of cancers in adults but a disproportionately large number of cancers in the pediatric population (approximately 15% of pediatric cancers). The overall incidence of sarcomas of soft tissue and bone is approximately 15,000 cases per year in the United States. Given the fact that there are no sarcoma-specific disease diagnostic codes, however, such numbers must be viewed as rough approximations at best. Nonetheless, it is clear that sarcomas are uncommon compared with carcinomas. The prevalence of sarcomas significantly exceeds the incidence, because sarcomas can be cured with expert multidisciplinary care. This makes it critical that the initial evaluation and management of patients suspected of having sarcomas be performed by an experienced team with relevant expertise and interdisciplinary capabilities (including pathology diagnostic capabilities, surgical specialization, and radiotherapeutic experience and judgment, as well as access to the latest systemic therapy agents and data on their use). Certain patients are at high risk of developing sarcomas, most notably individuals in families with Li-Fraumeni syndrome and those with neurofibromatosis (at risk for malignant peripheral nerve sheath tumors and GISTs) or familial polyposis (at risk for intra-abdominal desmoid tumors). Other risk factors include exposure to radiation (including radiation therapy for other cancers, such as patients with prior irradiated breast cancer or survivors of retinoblastoma). Chemical carcinogens can also increase the risk of sarcoma development, such as the increased risk of sarcomas in Vietnam veterans exposed to Agent Orange or the greatly increased risk of hepatic angiosarcomas associated with occupational exposure to polyvinyl chloride. However, the vast majority of sarcomas appear to be sporadic, with no evident inciting risk factors.

PATHOBIOLOGY

Sarcomas and other connective tissue neoplasms are an overwhelmingly complex and heterogeneous mixture of diseases with a wide range of clinical behaviors and outcomes. Some soft tissue neoplasms, such as localized tenosynovial giant cell tumors, can be cured by expert resection, whereas more advanced tumors of this type (referred to as pigmented villonodular tenosynovitis) often lead to debilitating amputations or even death due to metastatic disease. The bewildering array of polysyllabic names used by pathologists has caused confusion among clinicians and basic science investigators alike. In brief, expert pathologists strive to develop concise, systematic, and reproducible criteria for the diagnosis of specific sarcoma subtypes, but interobserver variability can plague the application of elegant diagnostic categories such as those promulgated by the World Health Organization. Increasing knowledge of the molecular pathways that drive sarcomas has provided more objective diagnostic tools with novel immunohistochemical staining patterns and genetic markers (e.g., pathognomonic chromosomal translocations have defined diseases such as Ewing's sarcoma or synovial sarcoma more objectively than any histopathologic appearance determined by simple light microscopy). In general, sarcomas may exhibit differentiation patterns consistent with defined connective tissues (e.g., well-differentiated liposarcoma may appear as only slightly bizarre fat cells under the microscope), or they may be absolutely unclassifiable. In fact, the terminology used by pathologists for very poorly differentiated sarcomas has also evolved: the current diagnostic category is "unclassifiable pleomorphic sarcoma," whereas 20 years ago most pathologists grouped such poorly differentiated tumors under the misnomer "malignant fibrous histiocytoma." In any case, as diagnostic tools have evolved, it has become possible to place such poorly differentiated tumors more accurately into certain histopathologic categories based on the expression of lineage-related proteins (e.g., smooth muscle actin expression may help categorize tumors as leiomyosarcomas) or on the basis of genomic markers (e.g., overexpression of chromosome 12 material or the *mdm2* gene locus is most consistent with a dedifferentiated liposarcoma).

It may be necessary to refer patient material to expert reference pathologists to accurately define the type of connective tissue neoplasm, and such referral can make an enormous difference in patient care (e.g., differentiating between a benign process that may self-resolve and a truly malignant sarcoma). The complexity of sarcoma and connective tissue tumor diagnosis cannot be overstated, and that is a major reason why all international clinical practice guidelines emphasize the importance of experienced diagnosticians and a low threshold for referral to expert pathology review for patients with connective tissue tumors.

CLINICAL MANIFESTATIONS AND DIAGNOSIS

Given the broad range of sarcomas, it is understandable that the clinical course can range from rapidly evolving and immediately life-threatening cancers (such as most Ewing's sarcomas) to indolent lesions that can take decades to evolve (such as atypical lipomatous tumors, also known as well-differentiated liposarcomas). Most patients with sarcomas present with a mass, often nontender, with a history of abnormal growth over time. For extremity tumors of soft tissues, it is important to note that many benign tumors (e.g., lipomas) cannot be easily distinguished from more worrisome neoplasms or even from frankly malignant sarcomas. Therefore, it is important to include sarcoma in the differential diagnosis of any mass.

The initial biopsy or surgical approach to a sarcomatous lesion is often the most important, and a poorly oriented biopsy or a suboptimal surgical procedure can make the difference between cure with full limb function and disease recurrence with the need for amputation or mutilating surgical re-resection. This lesson was first learned by orthopedic specialists with regard to bone sarcoma (osteosarcoma), but it is true for soft tissue sarcomas as well. The National Comprehensive Cancer Network (NCCN) has developed expert consensus guidelines for clinical practice that emphasize the importance of expert management from the moment a suspected sarcoma presents. The initial diagnosis includes appropriate imaging studies of relevant anatomic areas, including plain radiographs, computed tomography, or magnetic resonance imaging to define the anatomic area of the mass and surrounding tissue, as well as systemic staging because sarcomas can spread in well-defined patterns to distal sites such as the lung or liver. The decision to proceed to diagnostic biopsy, with optimal orientation, is an important one, and for certain lesions, forgoing incisional biopsy and proceeding directly to expertly planned surgical excision may be justified. The most important consideration is to make the correct diagnosis, and there must be sufficient amounts of properly prepared and expertly oriented tissues for optimal diagnostic analysis. In certain tumors with pathognomonic molecular markers (such as the translocation between chromosomes X and 18 that characterizes synovial sarcoma, or the balanced translocation between chromosomes 12 and 16 that defines myxoid and round cell liposarcoma), molecular analyses such as fluorescence in situ hybridization (FISH) may help make the diagnosis. New molecular subtypes of sarcomas enter the pathology literature on an annual basis, and this supports the need for expert pathology review of tumors of soft tissue and bone. These new diagnostic categories may lead to new molecularly targeted therapies. Nowhere has this been more evident than in the rapid evolution of effective therapy against the major pathobiologic cause of GISTs[1] (see later, under Treatment).

The diagnosis of a soft tissue or bone tumor is made by evaluating biopsy material in the clinical context, which includes understanding the tumor's anatomic location and imaging characteristics. Such contextual diagnostics are key to understanding whether a lesion may represent a primary sarcoma or whether it may be the first presentation of metastases from an occult primary tumor located elsewhere. Given the broad spectrum of sarcomas, the diagnostic considerations are quite far-reaching, especially because many benign pathophysiologic conditions can mimic sarcomas. For example, it may be very difficult for an inexperienced pathologist to distinguish among normal fat, inflammatory infiltrates, and liposarcoma. Similarly, certain fibroblastic neoplasms might simulate inflammation or scar. Therefore, a broad differential diagnosis is needed when considering any neoplasm of soft tissue or bone.

TREATMENT   Rx

The most important element of treatment is expert multidisciplinary care. The range of options is too broad to categorize simply, and the specific details of each patient's anatomy, comorbidities, functional status, and personal preferences must be taken into account when defining treatment options and management plans. Therefore, the care of virtually all sarcoma patients should

be managed by an expert multidisciplinary team with expertise in advanced surgical and/or orthopedic oncology techniques, radiation therapy, reconstructive surgery, physical therapy and rehabilitation medicine, systemic therapies such as conventional cytotoxic chemotherapy, hormonal therapy, and modern molecularly targeted therapy with agents such as kinase inhibitors, as well as psychosocial support and specialized nursing care. Sarcomas represent such a complex family of diseases that referral to academic centers makes good sense for patients as well as for the health care system overall. Therefore, appropriate referral to obtain expert opinion and to define the diagnostic and treatment options for patients with suspected sarcomas is exceedingly important.

For most primary localized masses in which sarcoma is in the differential diagnosis, the first step is to obtain the correct diagnosis in a manner that does not compromise patient outcome or function. The need for biopsy must be considered first, because some small, localized sarcomas are best approached through definitive surgical excision following careful staging and expert review of imaging studies. For suspected sarcomas in deeper locations, such as deep within muscle compartments, or for large visceral lesions, biopsy may be necessary to ascertain that the process is in fact a sarcoma, as well as to fully characterize the histopathologic subtype. This may make the difference between initial management with chemotherapy, as might be appropriate for a highly chemosensitive disease such as Ewing's sarcoma, versus surgery, which might be appropriate for a less chemosensitive disease such as dedifferentiated liposarcoma. Expert opinion varies regarding the utility and timing of adjuncts to surgical resection, such as radiation therapy or systemic cytotoxic chemotherapy. This variation can best be appreciated by noting the variety of management options for extremity sarcomas in the NCCN's consensus practice guidelines.

In general, expert surgical resection is first-line therapy for localized sarcomas. Preoperative systemic chemotherapy is standard for most common forms of osteosarcoma, as well as for Ewing's sarcoma and certain rhabdomyosarcomas. Many expert teams favor preoperative radiation therapy for certain sarcomas; irradiation of a large primary tumor can deliver smaller doses to surrounding normal tissues preoperatively compared with postoperatively, but this is a matter of personal preference. A reasonably sized randomized trial of preoperative versus postoperative radiation therapy for large sarcomas of the extremity was performed in Canada, and outcomes were similar, with subtle differences: patients who received preoperative radiation had a higher incidence of serious postoperative wound complications, but the long-term functional outcomes were slightly more favorable.[2] Because of such subtleties in results, sarcoma care is based largely on expert opinion and personal experience, and the vast range of sarcoma diagnoses and clinical presentations adds to this complexity.

Many sarcoma centers disagree about the relative value of cytotoxic chemotherapy, although there is no doubt that chemotherapy has greatly improved disease control rates and cure rates of certain subtypes of aggressive sarcomas such as intermediate- and high-grade osteosarcomas, Ewing's sarcomas, and rhabdomyosarcomas. For other forms of sarcomas originating in bone (e.g., chondrosarcoma) or soft tissue (e.g., leiomyosarcoma, synovial sarcoma), there is no strong evidence that systemic chemotherapy increases cure rates or long-term clinical outcomes, although there may be some improvement in local disease control and recurrence-free survival. This has led to discordant expert opinion: many experts believe that the risks and toxicities of aggressive chemotherapy justify the benefit of longer disease-free survival, whereas others feel that such toxicities are not reasonable without a major improvement in overall survival. Limited series of postoperative adjuvant therapy are often contradictory owing to the relatively small patient groups under study, as well as divergent patient selection factors, such as the inclusion of those with a lower risk of recurrence or death from metastatic disease. Inclusion of a sizable percentage of sarcoma patients with low-risk disease no doubt dilutes the results of even a reasonably effective therapy and runs the risk of making the study result negative; this possibility has remained an irreconcilable point of controversy among sarcoma centers across the United States and around the world.

It is also critical to recognize that treatment may differ radically depending on the histologic diagnosis. The best example of this is GIST, a form of sarcoma that, in more than 95% of cases, is driven by aberrant tyrosine kinase signaling. Routine systemic chemotherapy is completely ineffectual against this disease once it has metastasized or become unresectable owing to extensive local disease. By understanding the pathobiology of the disease and the "short-circuits" of intracellular kinase signaling, it is now possible to use targeted tyrosine kinase inhibitor drugs (e.g., imatinib mesylate, sunitinib malate) to block the abnormally activated tumor cell signaling, leading to dramatic tumor regression and tumor control in more than 85% of patients. Therefore, correctly diagnosing GIST is critical for choosing the proper therapy, and it can have life-or-death consequences for patients. Fortunately, pathologists are increasingly able to recognize this histopathologically and molecularly defined sarcoma. Immunohistochemistry to detect antigens such as CD117 (the Kit receptor tyrosine kinase) and DOG1 (a membrane antigen that is reasonably specific for GIST) and tumor genotyping via molecular genetics have significantly increased the accuracy of GIST diagnosis in the past decade. Tyrosine kinase inhibitor therapy with imatinib has been approved by the Food and

Drug Administration to decrease the risk of disease recurrence following resection of GISTs with significant potential for relapse. It is important to note that patients with a low risk of relapse have not derived substantive benefits from adjuvant imatinib because they have a very good chance of being cured by expert surgery alone.**3** GIST is therefore a paradigmatic example of a sarcoma in which critical therapy decisions must be made in the context of the proper diagnosis and with access to the latest evidence-based medical information.

For soft tissue sarcomas other than GIST, radiation therapy can play a meaningful role in preventing disease recurrence, especially for lesions that arise in the extremities. Radiation therapy can also provide significant palliation of unresectable disease, and it can be surprisingly effective in certain tumors such as desmoid tumor. However, radiation-associated sarcomas are increasingly common after therapeutic radiation therapy (e.g., in patients cured of breast cancer with radiation therapy), and an increasing incidence of poorly differentiated sarcomas or vascular sarcomas has been reported in patients following irradiation for other diseases.

As noted earlier, traditional cytotoxic chemotherapy is dramatically effective at increasing disease control and cure rates for certain sarcomas (especially those most prevalent in pediatric patients, such as osteosarcoma, Ewing's sarcoma, and rhabdomyosarcoma). It appears to be somewhat less effective in improving long-term cure rates for patients with most other forms of soft tissue and bone sarcomas, such as liposarcoma, leiomyosarcoma, synovial sarcoma, and other subtypes. Nonetheless, appropriate use of chemotherapy can lead to objective responses in certain patients and can palliate metastatic disease with disease control and prolongation of progression-free survival. Sarcoma experts often disagree about the relative value and toxicity of combination chemotherapy as opposed to sequential single-agent chemotherapy. In patients with very aggressive and highly symptomatic sarcomas, clinicians may wish to "hedge their bets" and choose a combination chemotherapy regimen, even if there is a greater risk of toxicity, to ensure some measure of rapid disease control or even a greater chance of disease regression. In contrast, in patients with asymptomatic metastatic disease (e.g., a sarcoma patient with indolent pulmonary metastases and no symptoms), the optimal choice might be single-agent chemotherapy to avoid toxicity and to maximize the choice of subsequent chemotherapeutic agents after the benefit of the first agent is fully realized. There is no single "best" choice for all patients, and each clinical situation requires individualization based on the specific details of the case and the patient's preferences. There are no definitive data from rigorously conducted and properly powered randomized trials that any chemotherapy for metastatic sarcoma of soft tissue (other than GIST) improves overall survival, yet there is no room for nihilism. All experts agree that owing to the complexity of the trials, the diseases, and the clinical settings, one must allow for variations in interpretations for individual patients. This explains the greatly discordant practice patterns observed across the country based on referrals, provider experience, and patient characteristics and preferences.

this is being extrapolated to improved understanding of the pathophysiology of other stromal-mediated diseases, such as pathologic conditions of fibrosis (e.g., interstitial pulmonary fibrosis and fibrocystic diseases such as lymphangioleiomatosis). Expert multidisciplinary management of sarcomas is critical to improving outcomes, and ongoing translational and therapeutic research will provide dividends far beyond the relatively low incidence and prevalence of these mesenchymal cell neoplastic disorders.

1. Gastrointestinal Stromal Tumor Meta-Analysis Group (MetaGIST). Comparison of two doses of imatinib for the treatment of unresectable or metastatic gastrointestinal stromal tumors: a meta-analysis of 1640 patients. *J Clin Oncol*. 2010;28:1247-1253.
2. Davis AM, O'Sullivan B, Turcotte R, et al. Canadian Sarcoma Group; NCI Canada Clinical Trial Group Randomized Trial. Late radiation morbidity following randomization to preoperative versus postoperative radiotherapy in extremity soft tissue sarcoma. *Radiother Oncol*. 2005;75:48-53.
3. DeMatteo RP, Ballman KV, Antonescu CR, et al. Placebo-controlled randomized trial of adjuvant imatinib mesylate following the resection of localized, primary gastrointestinal stromal tumor (GIST). *Lancet*. 2009;373:1097-1104.

SUGGESTED READINGS

Bannasch H, Eisenhardt SU, Grosu AL, et al. The diagnosis and treatment of soft tissue sarcomas of the limbs. *Dtsch Arztebl Int*. 2011;108:32-38. *Clinical review with a useful algorithm.*

Casali PG, Blay JY; ESMO/CONTICANET/EUROBONET Consensus Panel of experts. Soft tissue sarcomas: ESMO clinical practice guidelines for diagnosis, treatment and follow-up. *Ann Oncol*. 2010;21:v198-203. *Consensus guidelines.*

Le Cesne A, Ray-Coquard I, Bui BN, et al. Discontinuation of imatinib in patients with advanced gastrointestinal stromal tumours after 3 years of treatment: an open-label multicentre randomised phase 3 trial. *Lancet Oncol*. 2010;11:942-949. *Discontinuation led to high risk of rapid tumor progression.*

National Comprehensive Cancer Network Clinical Practice Guidelines for Soft Tissue Sarcoma and Gastrointestinal Stromal Tumor. http://www.nccn.org/professionals/physician_gls/f_guidelines.asp. *Definitive clinical practice guidelines that cover the complexities of sarcoma management and present algorithms ranging from initial presentation through diagnosis, primary disease management, surveillance, and care of metastatic or recurrent disease.*

Sarcoma on Cancer.Net from the American Society of Clinical Oncology: http://www.cancer.net/patient/Cancer+Types/Sarcoma. *Patient-focused information on sarcomas from the leading professional organization of oncologists.*

Verweij J, Baker LH. Future treatment of soft tissue sarcomas will be driven by histological subtype and molecular aberrations. *Eur J Cancer*. 2010;46:863-868. *Review emphasizing the need for a change in approach to soft tissue sarcomas, a highly heterogeneous group of diseases that have often been studied and treated as if they were all the same.*

PROGNOSIS

As noted earlier, it is relatively meaningless to discuss prognosis for sarcomas overall because they represent such a variety of diseases with widely divergent natural histories. It is estimated that approximately 50% of patients with localized sarcomas can be cured, and the risk of recurrence is related to variables such as tumor grade (low-grade tumors have a lower risk of recurrence or metastasis compared with intermediate- or high-grade tumors), tumor size, and tumor location or depth. For patients with recurrent or metastatic sarcoma, outcome depends on many factors, including the time from initial diagnosis to the first appearance of metastatic disease: a longer disease-free interval is associated with longer survival, probably indicating a slower rate of tumor proliferation. Another factor that may determine outcome is the number of metastatic lesions: it is possible that oligoclonal metastases, with few lesions, can be surgically resected, which itself may be associated with improved survival. Advances in chemotherapy and targeted therapies may also affect survival, as documented by the dramatic improvements in survival and disease control for GIST and other kinase-driven sarcomas, such as dermatofibrosarcoma protuberans, as well as the more recent molecular therapeutic targeting of giant cell tumor of bone, perivascular epithelioid cell–oma (PEComa), and tenosynovial giant cell tumor. The natural history of these diseases will almost certainly be changed by a more complete and mechanistic understanding of the underlying neoplasia-promoting signals that cause the transformation and maintenance of the sarcoma.

The complexities of soft tissue and bone neoplasms and sarcomas are rivaled only by the spectrum of molecular pathways and aberrancies that are at the root of these diseases. Virtually every disease mechanism can be associated with some form of mesenchymal cell neoplasm. Better understanding of sarcoma biology is translating into improvements in sarcoma outcomes, and

210

MELANOMA AND NONMELANOMA SKIN CANCERS

LYNN SCHUCHTER

MELANOMA

EPIDEMIOLOGY

Current estimates are that 1 out of 39 men and 1 of out of 58 women will be diagnosed with melanoma during their lifetime. Each year in the United States, approximately 62,000 new cases of invasive melanoma are detected, and 8400 patients die of melanoma. The explanation for the rising incidence is thought to be increasing sun exposure, especially early in life. Melanoma is the leading cause of death from cutaneous malignant disease, and it accounts for 1 to 2% of all cancer deaths in the United States. Melanoma affects all age groups; the median age at diagnosis is 50 years. Melanoma is largely a disease of whites, with a very low incidence in African Americans, Asians, and Hispanics.

PATHOBIOLOGY

Exposure to sunlight, and especially ultraviolet (UV) radiation (Chapter 19), has been strongly implicated as a causative factor in the development of melanoma. Melanomas originate from melanocytes, which are located predominantly in the basal cell layer of the epidermis and use the enzyme tyrosinase to synthesize melanin pigment, which serves to protect against UV damage (Chapter 443). Worldwide, the incidence of melanoma in whites generally correlates inversely with latitude; that is, rates are generally higher closer to the equator and become progressively lower near the poles.

Risk Factors

Risk factors for melanoma include family history of melanoma, prior melanoma or nonmelanoma skin cancer, inherited genetic susceptibility, and sun exposure. Individuals with fair complexion, blond or red hair, blue eye color, and freckles, who have a tendency to burn rather than tan, have higher rates of melanoma. The pattern of sun exposure may also be important; intermittent intense exposure, rather than long-term exposure, may carry a higher risk of melanoma.

Individuals with an increased number of typical or benign moles or atypical moles or dysplastic nevi (Figs. 210-1 and 210-2) also have an increased risk for melanoma. Atypical moles or dysplastic nevi are important precursor lesions of melanoma and also serve as markers for increasing risk. For example, individuals with dysplastic nevi have a 6% lifetime chance of developing melanoma, and this risk increases to as high as 80% in individuals who have dysplastic nevi and a strong family history of melanoma.

Genetics

Approximately 10% of patients with melanoma have a family history of melanoma. Several chromosomal loci determine susceptibility to melanoma, the most important of which is *p16/CDKN2A*, a gene located on chromosome 9p21. This gene is a member of a class of molecules that play a central role in cell cycle regulation. Of the members of melanoma-prone families, 25 to 40% have mutations in this gene. The risk of developing cutaneous melanoma in an individual who is a CDKN2A carrier is between 30 and 90% by age 80 years and varies by geographic location. Testing for mutations in the *p16/CDKN2A* locus is commercially available, but its clinical utility is unclear at this time. Genetic variability in melancortin-1 receptor (MC1R) plays a key role in pigmentation of skin and hair and more recently has been implicated in melanoma predisposition.

Somatic mutations in primary and metastatic melanoma primarily involve the mitogen activated protein kinase pathway. Activating mutations in *B-RAF* can be found in approximately 40% of melanomas, and 10 to 15% of melanomas are associated with a mutation in *N-RAS*. Recent studies have found that melanoma on mucous membranes, acral skin (soles, palms), and skin with chronic sun damage (i.e., lentigo maligna melanoma) have frequent mutations in *c-kit*. Thus, distinct patterns of genetic alterations are found in primary melanomas based on anatomic location and extent of sun exposure. The discovery of somatic mutations in melanoma and associated aberrant signal transduction pathways has provided leads for the development of molecularly targeted therapy for patients with advanced melanoma.

CLINICAL MANIFESTATIONS

Early detection and recognition of melanoma are key to improving survival. The signs of early melanoma are based on the clinical appearance of the pigmented lesion and a change in the shape, color, or surface of an existing mole. Most patients report a preexisting mole at the site of the melanoma. Itching, burning, or pain in a pigmented lesion should increase suspicion, although melanomas often are not associated with local discomfort. Bleeding and ulceration are signs of a more advanced melanoma. Most melanomas are varying shades of brown, but they may be black, blue, or pink. The ABCDEs for the recognition of melanoma are asymmetry, border irregularity, color variation, diameter greater than 6 mm, and evolution or a change in a skin lesion.

Cutaneous melanoma has been divided into four subtypes. Superficial spreading melanoma, which accounts for 70% of all melanomas, can be located on any anatomic site (Fig. 210-3). Lentigo maligna melanoma, which represents 4 to 10% of all melanomas, tends to occur more commonly in chronically sun-exposed skin in older patients, frequently on the head and neck (Fig. 210-4); clinically, it appears as a macular (flat) lesion, arising in a lentigo maligna. Nodular melanoma (Fig. 210-5) accounts for 15 to 30% of melanomas and manifests as a rapidly enlarging elevated or polypoid lesion, often blue or black. The ABCDE rule does not always apply as well to nodular melanomas. Acral lentiginous melanoma manifests as a darkly pigmented, flat to nodular lesion on the palm, on the sole, and subungually; sunlight is not thought to play a causative role in this form of melanoma. Histologic subtype does not directly correlate with clinical behavior. However, recent data suggest that histologic subtype may correlate with specific genetic abnormalities.

FIGURE 210-1. Nevi. **A,** Common benign nevus. **B,** Dermal nevus.

FIGURE 210-2. Dysplastic nevi. **A** and **B,** Examples of dysplastic nevi.

FIGURE 210-3. Superficial spreading melanoma.

FIGURE 210-4. Lentigo maligna melanoma.

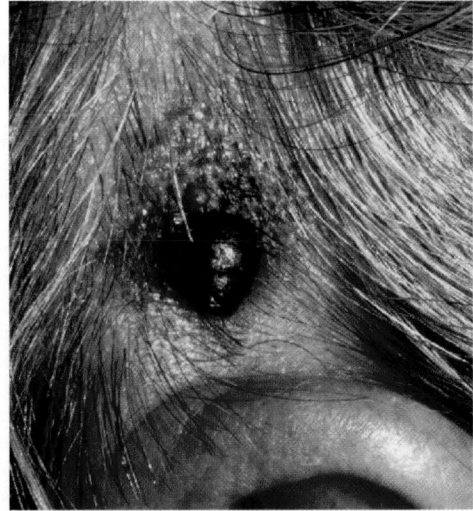

FIGURE 210-5. Nodular melanoma. (From Internal Medicine for Clerkship Students. American College of Physicians, 2006.)

Ocular melanomas arise from the pigmented layer of the eye. Uveal melanoma is the most common intraocular malignancy of adults. Melanomas can also arise from noncutaneous sites, including mucosal epithelium in the gastrointestinal tract, anorectal area, genitourinary tract, and nasal and nasopharyngeal mucosa. Melanomas of the vulva and vagina are relatively rare. In general, mucosal melanomas are diagnosed at a more advanced stage of disease. The mainstay of treatment is surgical.

DIAGNOSIS

Any skin lesion suggestive of melanoma should be sampled using biopsy with complete excision, including a 1- to 2-mm margin of normal skin and

TABLE 210-1	CLINICAL FEATURES OF COMMON NEVI, DSYPLASTIC NEVI, AND MELANOMAS
DISEASE	**CHARACTERISTICS**
Common acquired nevi (moles)	These tend to be small, flat, and round; the border is regular, smooth, and well defined; the color is homogeneous, usually no more than two shades of brown; any site is affected; lesions are usually <6 mm.
Dysplastic nevi (atypical moles)	These occur predominantly on the trunk; they tend to be large, usually >5 mm, with a flat component; the border is characteristically fuzzy and ill defined. The shape can be round, oval, or misshapen. The color is usually brown but can be mottled with dark brown, pink, and tan. Some individuals have only 1 to 5 moles, others more than 100.
Melanoma	The border is more irregular; lesions tend to be larger, often >6 mm; substantial heterogeneity of color is noted, ranging from tan-brown, dark brown, black, pink, red, gray, blue, or white.

some subcutaneous fat. An incisional biopsy may be necessary for lesions too large for complete excision. Shallow shave biopsies, curettage, cryosurgery, laser, and electrodessication are contraindicated in lesions suggestive of melanoma. Other lesions that can be confused with melanoma include blue nevi, pigmented basal cell carcinoma, seborrheic keratosis, and hemangiomas (Table 210-1).

Prognostic Factors

As with most malignancies, the outcome of melanoma is dependent on the stage and extent of disease at presentation. For localized melanoma, the most important prognostic factor is involvement of regional lymph nodes. The most important prognostic factor related to the primary tumor is the depth of invasion (Breslow's thickness) of the melanoma, which is measured in millimeters from the top of the epidermis to the underlying dermis. Increasing thickness is associated with an increased risk for recurrence, regional lymph node involvement, and death from melanoma. Patients whose melanomas are less than 1 mm thick have about an 80 to 90% 10-year survival rate, whereas patients whose melanomas are greater than 4 mm thick have only a 40 to 50% 10-year survival rate. Other poor prognostic factors related to the primary melanoma include the presence of ulceration, an increasing level of invasion (Clark's level), a high mitotic rate, and the presence of microscopic satellites. Regional lymph node involvement (stage III) has a major impact on survival, with 5-year survival rates ranging from 20 to 70%, depending on the number of involved lymph nodes. Melanomas that arise on the extremity tend to have a better prognosis, and women tend to do better than men.

Staging System for Melanoma

Staging and prognosis for melanoma are based on the TNM system, in which T refers to tumor, N to nodes, and M to metastasis, which was updated in 2009 (E-Table 210-1). Stages I and II indicate clinically localized primary melanoma, stage III melanoma indicates regional involvement (lymph nodes or in-transit metastases), and stage IV is metastatic disease beyond the regional lymph nodes (i.e., lung, liver, brain).

Patient Evaluation

The initial evaluation of a patient with melanoma includes a personal history, a family history, a total skin examination, and palpation of regional (draining) lymph nodes. The focus is to identify risk factors, signs or symptoms of metastases, dysplastic nevi, and additional melanomas. A chest radiograph and liver enzyme tests may be performed at the discretion of the physician. Most patients who present with melanoma do not have distant metastatic disease at presentation; therefore, extensive evaluations with computed tomography (CT) to search for distant metastases have an extremely low yield and are not indicated in asymptomatic patients. More extensive staging evaluation with CT or positron emission tomography (PET) can be considered in patients with high-risk disease (primary melanoma >4 mm thick or node-positive disease), in whom the risk of distant metastatic disease is higher.

TREATMENT

Primary Melanoma

Once melanoma is diagnosed, the standard treatment is surgical excision. Several prospective randomized trials have been conducted to define the optimal surgery for primary melanoma.[1] The extent of the surgery depends on the thickness of the primary melanoma. Large surgical excisions are no longer required, and most wide excisions can be performed with primary closure. For melanoma in situ, excision with a 0.5-cm border of clinically normal skin is sufficient. For melanomas less than 1 mm thick, a 1-cm margin is recommended. If the thickness is between 1 and 4 mm, a 1- to 2-cm margin is recommended. For melanomas thicker than 4 mm, at least a 2-cm margin should be taken. In cosmetically sensitive areas (face) or anatomically difficult areas (ear, hands), it may be difficult to achieve the desired margin, but at least a 1-cm margin should be obtained whenever possible.

Management of Regional Lymph Nodes

Clinically Normal Regional Lymph Nodes

In approximately 10 to 20% of patients who do not have clinically apparent lymph node involvement, lymph nodes contain occult micrometastases. The risk for occult lymph node involvement rises with increasing tumor thickness. Results from randomized trials fail to show a survival benefit from elective or prophylactic lymph node dissections in patients with clinically negative lymph nodes.

Sentinel lymph node biopsy (SLNB) is a technique that accurately evaluates whether microscopic melanoma cells involve regional lymph nodes. The technique relies on the concept that specific regions of the skin drain specifically to an initial lymph node within the regional nodal basin through an organized pathway of afferent lymphatic channels. This technique is performed by injecting the primary melanoma site with blue dye (isosulfan blue) or radiolabeled colloid, or both. When both modalities are used in combination, a sentinel node can be identified in 98% of patients; biopsy of the node accurately determines whether melanoma cells have metastasized to that specific lymph node basin. The sentinel node technique also promotes a more comprehensive histologic examination of lymph nodes because limited amounts of pathologic material are submitted.

SLNB allows earlier identification of metastases and earlier lymphadenectomy.[2] The likelihood of detecting melanoma in SLNB increases with thickness of the primary lesion providing the rationale for determining which patients may benefit from the procedure. SLNB is recommended to patients with melanoma 1 mm thick or thicker. The use of this technique for patients with thinner melanomas, that is, less than 1 mm thick, is controversial. The SLNB is generally performed at the same time as the wide excision of the primary tumor. If the SLNB is negative for melanoma, no further lymph node surgery is required. If melanoma is detected by the SLNB, complete lymph node dissection remains the standard of care. SLNB is a useful staging tool; however, its impact on the overall survival of patients is uncertain.

Clinically Apparent Regional Lymph Nodes

Surgical (therapeutic) lymphadenectomy is the preferred treatment of cytologically (fine-needle aspiration) positive or pathologically proven regional lymph node involvement with melanoma. The goal is to provide long-term, disease-free survival and reduce local morbidity of enlarged lymph nodes.

Adjuvant Therapy

Postsurgical adjuvant therapy can be considered for patients at high risk for recurrence (melanomas ≥4 mm thick or node-positive disease). These patients have at least a 25 to 75% chance of dying of melanoma. Adjuvant treatment options include interferon-α (IFN-α), enrollment in a clinical trial, or observation. High-dose IFN-α is the only U.S. Food and Drug Administration (FDA)-approved adjuvant therapy for patients with melanoma. Randomized clinical trials have shown that therapy with IFN-α can prolong disease-free survival but has not improved overall survival.[3] The treatment is given for 1 year and is associated with considerable side effects, which require close monitoring. Intermediate and low doses of IFN-α as well as pegylated IFN-α have also been evaluated in a series of clinical trials. These regimens are not considered standard in the United States but are offered in Europe. Numerous vaccine studies are ongoing but are considered experimental at present.

Treatment and Course of Advanced Melanoma (Stage IV)

The treatment of a patient with metastatic melanoma emphasizes palliation. No evidence indicates that treatment of metastatic melanoma has any impact on survival, which ranges from 5 to 11 months, with a median of 8.5 months. Treatment options include surgery for resection of solitary metastases, single-agent chemotherapy such as dacarbazine, temozolomide (an oral version of dacarbazine), combination chemotherapy, immunotherapy (vaccines, interleukin-2, interferon), or combined immunotherapy. Melanoma can metastasize to virtually any organ, especially the lung, skin, liver, and brain.

The discovery of somatic genetic mutations in melanoma has provided leads for the development of molecularly targeted therapies. The MAP kinase pathway, which is activated in most melanomas due to mutations in BRAF, NRAS, and c-kit, has been the focus of most clinical investigations of signal transduction (kinase) inhibitors. Recent results of a phase I study of PLX4032, a potent and specific BRAF inhibitor in patients with metastatic melanoma whose tumors harbor the V600E BRAF mutation demonstrated a response rate of almost 80% and an estimated median progression free survival of at least 7 months. Recent and preliminary results also show that imatinib can induce regression in patients whose melanoma is driven by KIT mutations.

New immunotherapy approaches are being tested in patients with advanced melanoma. Encouraging results have been reported with ipilimumab, which blocks cytotoxic T-lymphocyte antigen 4 (CTLA-4) in patients with metastatic melanoma.[4]

Surveillance and Follow-up

Patients should be educated on the clinical characteristics of melanoma, the importance of safe sun strategies, and the performance of monthly self-examinations of the skin. Patients should be followed regularly for evidence of local or regional recurrence, distant metastatic disease, and a second primary melanoma. The intensity of the surveillance and the extent of the investigation is influenced by risk for recurrence with more frequent follow-up visits in patients who have thicker tumors or node-positive disease because these patients are at greater risk for recurrence.

For patients with low-risk melanoma (≤1 mm), visits are recommended every 6 months for 2 years and then annually. The surveillance guidelines for patients with high-risk melanoma include evaluation every 3 to 4 months for 2 years, then every 6 months for 3 years. After 5 years, patients are seen once a year. Patients are generally followed for 10 years. However, lifelong dermatologic examination is recommended, particularly for patients with dysplastic nevi or a family history of melanoma. In general, a history and physical examination are performed at each visit. Periodic chest radiographs, laboratory studies, and other imaging studies are performed at the discretion of the treating physician. The physical examination should include a thorough skin examination, because at least 3% of patients develop an additional primary cutaneous melanoma within 3 years. Regional lymph nodes should be thoroughly examined, especially in patients without prior nodal surgery. For the remainder of the examination, one should keep in mind the frequency of metastases to lung, liver, and brain. Follow-up studies may include a complete blood cell count and chemistry studies, including liver enzyme tests. An elevated lactate dehydrogenase level suggests metastatic melanoma.

PREVENTION

The most important measures to prevent melanoma are to reduce excessive sun exposure, particularly to the midday sun, and to avoid sunburns. Sunscreen products with a sun protection factor of 15 or greater and protective clothing are recommended, and one randomized trial found that regular sunscreen use reduced incident melanoma by 50% and invasive melanoma by 75%.[5] Sunscreens block primarily UVB rays, which are considered to be the major causative agent of cutaneous cancers. Newer sunscreen products also block UVA rays, which may contribute to the risk of melanoma.

Screening for skin cancer, whether by self-examination or by a health care provider, is controversial (Chapter 14). Many public health experts do not recommend screening for adults in the general population, but some organizations do. On the basis of the type and number of nevi, family history of melanoma, prior melanoma, and history of severe sunburns, clinicians can identify patients who are at high risk for melanoma and who may benefit from screening programs. In several population studies, screening has detected melanomas at an earlier, curable stage. Physicians, other health care providers, and the public should be educated regarding the early signs of melanoma and the need for prompt biopsy of a suspicious pigmented lesion.

Patients with clinically atypical nevi (see Fig. 210-2), particularly if they have a family history of melanoma, require a regular dermatologic surveillance program. Regular skin examinations should be performed every 6 to 12 months, preferably assisted by the use of serial photography.

Recent studies have focused on the impact of vitamin D levels on the risk for melanoma, and results have been conflicting. The potential health benefits of vitamin D continue to be evaluated, both in terms of melanoma prevention and risk.

BASAL AND SQUAMOUS CELL SKIN CANCER

Nonmelanoma skin cancer (basal cell cancer [BCC] and squamous cell skin cancer [SCC]) is the most common malignant disease in the United States. Although national statistics are imprecise, an estimated 900,000 to 1,200,000 of nonmelanoma skin cancers are diagnosed annually in the United States. SCC accounts for 20%, and most of the remainder are BCC. SCC is associated with a higher absolute mortality rate; most of the 2300 annual deaths from nonmelanoma skin cancer in the United States arise from this tumor.

EPIDEMIOLOGY

Overall, skin cancer incidence rates are rising because of increased recreational sun exposure, longer life expectancy, and depletion of the ozone layer. More than 99% of nonmelanoma skin cancers occur in whites. These skin cancers are most commonly seen in elderly persons, especially those with fair skin and long-standing sun exposure. However, nonmelanoma skin cancers are increasingly being seen in people in their 30s and 40s. The lifetime risk of developing BCC is 30%.

PATHOBIOLOGY

BCC arises from a pluripotential stem cell within the skin. Acquired mutations in the patched gene 1 (*PTCH1*), a tumor suppressor gene in the hedgehog signaling pathway, have been identified in cases of sporadic BCC. Sporadic BCC are also associated with mutations in the genes encoding p53 and ras.

SCC of the skin is a malignant disease of epidermal keratinocytes. Many such carcinomas are derived from actinic keratoses, a precursor that appears as a rough, scaly, often erythematous papule, which often is more apparent on palpation than on visual examination. Estimates of the likelihood of progression of actinic keratoses to squamous cell carcinoma range from 0.025% to as high as 20%. Mutations in the gene encoding the p53 protein and in the *RAS* oncogene have been found in both actinic keratoses and squamous cell carcinomas. Mutations in *p16* have also been reported in squamous cell carcinomas.

Risk Factors

The most important risk factor is exposure to UV radiation from sunlight. The most clearly established association is with UVB radiation, but increasing evidence suggests that UVA is probably carcinogenic as well (Chapter 19). The timing and pattern of sun exposure are associated with different types of skin cancer. In general, SCC is associated with cumulative sun exposure and occurs most frequently in areas maximally exposed to the sun (e.g., the face, back of hands, and forearms). Intermittent, intense exposure to the sun, particularly in childhood, is associated with an increased risk for BCC. Individuals who have fair skin, light-colored eyes, red hair, a tendency to burn rather than tan, and a history of severe sunburns are at increased risk for nonmelanoma skin cancers. Other risk factors, primarily for SCC, include chronic arsenic exposure, therapeutic radiation, chronic inflammatory skin conditions, psoralen plus UVA (PUVA) treatment for psoriasis and other diseases, and immunosuppression. Most cases in African American patients are associated with scarring or burns rather than UV exposure. Human papillomavirus infection (Chapter 381) has also been implicated in some SCCs, particularly in the autosomal dominant disorder epidermodysplasia verruciformis.

BCC can be seen in association with several conditions, including the basal cell nevus syndrome (also called nevoid basal cell carcinoma syndrome or Gorlin's syndrome), albinism, and xeroderma pigmentosum. The basal cell nevus syndrome is a rare autosomal dominant disorder caused by germline mutations in the patched gene (*PTCH*).

CLINICAL MANIFESTATIONS

Basal Cell Carcinoma

Approximately 90% of BCCs occur on sun-exposed areas such as the face, neck, ears, scalp, and arms. The nose is the most common site. Typical BCC appears as slowly growing, shiny, skin-colored to pink translucent papules with telangiectasia and a "pearly" rolled border (Fig. 210-6). As the tumor grows, the center may become ulcerated and bleed, although there is usually no associated pain or tenderness. BCC rarely metastasizes and is usually curable with a variety of treatments. Although the mortality rate is low, these cancers may result in significant morbidity owing to invasive local growth with potential disfigurement and destruction of skin, bone, and cartilage. Clinical trials with inhibitors of the hedgehog pathway for patients with advanced BCC are under way, with very encouraging clinical activity demonstrated.

Squamous Cell Carcinoma

This type of skin cancer usually appears on areas of skin that are heavily damaged by sun exposure. The most common sites include the head or neck, back, forearms, and dorsum of the hand. Clinically, SCC occurs as a discrete

FIGURE 210-6. Basal cell carcinoma.

FIGURE 210-7. Squamous cell carcinoma of the skin.

scaly erythematous papule on an indurated base that can develop on normal-appearing skin or on an actinic keratosis (Fig. 210-7). The lesion may grow over time and may become ulcerated, itchy, painful, or bleeding. Keratoacanthoma is a variant that is characterized by rapid growth and a crateriform appearance with a central plug. Bowen's disease, or squamous cell carcinoma in situ, manifests as an erythematous, scaly, sharply defined plaque.

Untreated SCC may cause significant local destruction. However, unlike BCC, SCC carries a 0.5 to 5% risk for metastasis. Higher-risk lesions are those that are larger than 2 cm, are moderately or poorly differentiated, have perineural involvement, or are located on the ear or the lip, arise in scars, or occur in immunosuppressed patients. Most metastases develop in regional lymph nodes, although metastases may also occur in lung, liver, brain, skin, or bone. For patients with lymph node metastases, the 5-year survival rate is less than 50%.

DIAGNOSIS

The diagnosis of BCC and SCC is frequently suspected by inspection alone, but histologic confirmation is usually indicated. Either a shave or a punch biopsy technique is acceptable (Chapter 444). Care should be taken to include the base of the lesion if a shave biopsy technique is used.

TREATMENT   Rx

Basal Cell Carcinoma

BCCs are classified as low or high risk, based on their clinical features, location, and histology. Treatment options includes cryotherapy (liquid nitrogen), electrosurgery (i.e., curettage and electrodessication), topical treatment (i.e., 5-fluorouracil, photodynamic therapy, or imiquimod), surgical excision, Mohs' surgery, or radiation therapy. Mohs' microsurgery should be considered when treating recurrent cases; microscopically aggressive forms, such as the morpheaform subtype; lesions greater than 2 cm in greatest diameter; and tumors of the ears, eyelids, nose, nasolabial folds, and lips. Cure rates for BCC range between 90 and 99%.

Squamous Cell Carcinoma

As with BCC, SCC can also be cured by traditional surgical excision or Mohs' surgery, cryotherapy, topical therapies, and radiation therapy. Topical 5-fluorouracil, photodynamic therapy, or imiquimod have a role in the management of in situ squamous cell cancers. The optimal approach for a specific patient requires consideration of likelihood of the lesion recurring or metastatic potential, cosmetic factors, and the expertise of the treating physicians.

Mohs' micrographic surgery provides the lowest recurrence rate, with cure rates greater than 90%. Mohs' microsurgery is especially useful for recurrent tumors or lesions that have an increased risk of metastasis.

Follow-up

Patients with BCC and SCC require ongoing follow-up to detect local recurrences and to recognize new skin cancers. The likelihood of developing a second basal cell carcinoma or squamous cell carcinoma has been estimated to be 15% over 3 years. In addition, these patients have an increased risk of developing cutaneous melanoma. Patient education regarding modification of risk factors (i.e., sun exposure) is an important component of follow-up.

PREVENTION

Primary prevention strategies are aimed at reducing long-term sun exposure. Public education and patient education should encourage the regular use of sunscreens with a sun protection factor of 15 or greater, especially in childhood, and sun-protective clothing (e.g., a broad-brimmed hat). Avoidance of tanning parlors and minimizing of total sun exposure, especially to the midday sun, is recommended. The thinning of the ozone layer has been linked to increased UV radiation and increases in the incidence of nonmelanoma skin cancers. Currently, no evidence indicates that total body skin examination is effective at reducing mortality or morbidity from nonmelanoma skin cancer.

1. Thomas JM, Newton-Bishop J, A'Hern R, et al. Excision margins in high-risk malignant melanoma. *N Engl J Med.* 2004;350:757-766.
2. Morton DL, Thompson JF, Cochran AJ, et al. Sentinel-node biopsy or nodal observation in melanoma. *N Engl J Med.* 2006;355:1307-1317.
3. Eggermont AM, Suciu S, Santinami M, et al. Adjuvant therapy with pegylated interferon alfa-2b versus observation alone in resected stage III melanoma: final results of EORTC 18991, a randomised phase III trial. *Lancet.* 2008;372:117-126.
4. Hodi FS, O'Day SJ, McDermott DF, et al. Improved survival with ipilimumab in patients with metastatic melanoma. *N Engl J Med.* 2010;363:711-723.
5. Green AC, Williams GM, Logan V, et al. Reduced melanoma after regular sunscreen use: randomized trial follow-up. *J Clin Oncol.* 2011;29:257-263.

SUGGESTED READINGS

Bower MR, Scoggins CR, Martin RC 2nd, et al. Second primary melanomas: incidence and outcome. *Am Surg.* 2010;76:675-681. *About 2% of patients developed a second primary melanoma during a median follow-up of 5.5 years.*

Lin JS, Eder M, Weinmann S. Behavioral counseling to prevent skin cancer: a systematic review for the U.S. Preventive Services task force. *Ann Intern Med.* 2011;154:190-201. *Consensus guidelines recommending counseling to increase sun-protective behaviors.*

Madan V, Lear JT, Szeimies RM. Non-melanoma skin cancer. *Lancet.* 2010;375:673-685. *Concise review of recent advances.*

211

CANCER OF UNKNOWN PRIMARY ORIGIN

JOHN D. HAINSWORTH AND F. ANTHONY GRECO

DEFINITION

The first signs or symptoms of cancer are frequently the result of metastases to visceral or nodal sites. In most such patients, routine clinical evaluation with a comprehensive history, physical examination, complete blood cell count, screening chemistries, and directed radiologic studies based on specific symptoms or signs identifies the primary tumor. Patients who have no primary tumor located after this routine clinical evaluation are defined as having cancer of unknown primary origin. Further clinical and pathologic evaluation identifies the primary site in only a few patients, and approximately 80% never have a primary site identified during their subsequent clinical course.

EPIDEMIOLOGY

In patients whose primary site of cancer remains undetectable, the primary site has presumably remained small or, less likely, regressed spontaneously. Before the routine use of computed tomography (CT) or magnetic resonance imaging (MRI) for diagnosis, large autopsy series identified small primary sites of cancer in 85% of patients with previously unidentified primary tumors, usually in the pancreas, lung, and various other gastrointestinal sites; with the use of CT and MRI for diagnosis, however, primary sites are identified at autopsy in only 50 to 70% of patients.

Approximately 3% of all patients with cancer have metastatic disease without a known primary site; the annual incidence is approximately 50,000 to 60,000 cases in the United States. Cancer of unknown primary site occurs with approximately equal frequency in men and women, and it increases in incidence with advancing age.

DIAGNOSIS

The initial clinical and pathologic evaluation should focus on identifying a primary site, when possible, and on identifying patients for whom specific treatment is indicated. In most patients with cancer of unknown primary site, the diagnosis of advanced cancer is strongly suspected after the initial history and physical examination. A brief additional evaluation, including complete blood cell counts, chemistry profile, and CT of the chest and abdomen, should be performed. Any specific symptoms or signs should be evaluated with appropriate radiologic and endoscopic studies.

Biopsy

The diagnosis of metastatic cancer should be confirmed by biopsy of the most accessible metastatic lesion. Fine-needle aspiration may or may not provide sufficient material for optimal histologic examination and special pathologic procedures. If tissue is inadequate, a larger biopsy sample should be obtained so that all necessary stains and special studies can be performed.

The initial light microscopic evaluation identifies adenocarcinoma in approximately 60% of patients with cancer of unknown primary site. Other diagnoses obtained by initial light microscopy include poorly differentiated carcinoma (25%), squamous carcinoma (10%), and poorly differentiated neoplasm (inability to distinguish among carcinoma, lymphoma, melanoma, and sarcoma; 5%).

In patients with adenocarcinoma, it is seldom possible for the pathologist to determine a primary site by light microscopic characteristics or with additional pathologic techniques. Specific exceptions include immunoperoxidase staining for prostate-specific antigen (PSA), which is relatively specific for adenocarcinoma of the prostate (Chapter 207); for estrogen and progesterone receptors, which are suggestive of breast cancer (Chapter 204); and for leukocyte common antigen, which can identify non-Hodgkin's lymphoma (Chapter 191) as the primary tumor in up to 50% of patients with poorly differentiated neoplasms. Other diagnoses suggested by immunoperoxidase staining include neuroendocrine carcinomas, melanomas (Chapter 210), and sarcomas (Chapter 209). Electron microscopy should be considered when light microscopy and immunoperoxidase staining fail to identify the tumor, especially in young patients with anaplastic tumors; specific ultrastructural features may suggest neuroendocrine carcinoma (neurosecretory granules), melanoma (premelanosomes), and certain sarcomas.

Occasionally, detection of a tumor-specific chromosomal abnormality can provide a definitive diagnosis. Cancers with recognized specific chromosomal abnormalities include germ cell tumors (i12p; Chapter 206), peripheral neuroepithelioma and Ewing's tumor (t11;22; Chapter 208), and non-Hodgkin's lymphoma (Chapter 191). Chromosomal analysis should therefore be considered, especially in young men who have poorly differentiated mediastinal or retroperitoneal tumors and in whom other pathologic studies have been inconclusive.

Recently, specific gene expression profiles based on the tissue of origin have been identified for many tumor types. Several currently available multigene assays have 80 to 90% accuracy in determining the tissue of origin when performed on metastatic tissue in patients with tumors of known origin. The contribution of molecular profiling to the diagnosis and management of carcinoma of unknown primary site is still being defined; however, it is likely to

TABLE 211-1 RECOMMENDED EVALUATION FOLLOWING INITIAL LIGHT MICROSCOPIC DIAGNOSIS

DIAGNOSIS	CLINICAL EVALUATION*	SPECIAL PATHOLOGIC STUDIES
Adenocarcinoma (or poorly differentiated adenocarcinoma)	PET CT of chest, abdomen Men: serum PSA Women: mammogram Additional directed radiologic or endoscopic studies to evaluate abnormal symptoms, signs, laboratory values	Men: PSA stain Women: estrogen and progesterone receptor stains (if clinical features suggest metastatic breast cancer)
Poorly differentiated carcinoma	PET CT of chest, abdomen Serum hCG, AFP Additional directed radiologic or endoscopic studies to evaluate abnormal symptoms, signs, laboratory values	Immunoperoxidase staining Electron microscopy (if immunoperoxidase stains indeterminate)
Squamous carcinoma, cervical nodes	PET Direct laryngoscopy with visualization; biopsy of nasopharynx, pharynx, hypopharynx, larynx Fiberoptic bronchoscopy (if laryngoscopy is negative)	—
Squamous carcinoma, inguinal nodes	PET Complete examination of perineal area (including pelvic examination) Anoscopy Cystoscopy	—

*In addition to a history, physical examination, complete blood cell counts, chemistry profile, and chest radiograph.
AFP = α-fetoprotein; CT = computed tomography; hCG = human chorionic gonadotropin; PET = positron emission tomography; PSA = prostate-specific antigen.

have an important role in the future both in diagnosing the site of tumor origin and in allowing more site-specific therapy.

Search for the Primary Site

After completion of the brief, directed initial evaluation outlined previously, further diagnostic studies should be limited (Table 211-1). Positron emission tomography (PET) identifies a primary site and guides therapy in about one third of patients, so it should be obtained in all patients with an initially unknown primary tumor. By comparison, other routine radiologic and endoscopic evaluations of asymptomatic areas are not useful in identifying a primary site and therefore are not recommended. Levels of serum tumor markers, including carcinoembryonic antigen, CA-125, CA-19-9, and CA-15-3, are frequently increased in patients with carcinoma of unknown primary site; however, these elevations are nonspecific and should not be used to infer a primary site, even though they can be useful in monitoring response to treatment.

In all men with metastatic adenocarcinoma, serum PSA should be measured. Mammograms and breast MRI should be considered in women with metastatic adenocarcinoma, particularly if clinical features are consistent with metastatic breast cancer (e.g., axillary node involvement, pleural effusion, lytic or blastic bone metastases). In patients younger than 50 years with poorly differentiated carcinoma, serum human chorionic gonadotropin and α-fetoprotein levels should be measured. Patients with metastatic squamous carcinoma involving cervical lymph nodes should have a thorough endoscopic evaluation of the head and neck, including visualization of the structures from the nasopharynx to the larynx and biopsy of any suspicious areas (Chapter 196). Fiberoptic bronchoscopy should also be considered in patients who have low cervical adenopathy and in whom no head or neck primary site is established by endoscopic examination. In patients with metastatic squamous carcinoma involving inguinal lymph nodes, all perineal structures should be carefully inspected, including anoscopy, a urologic evaluation, and a pelvic examination in women.

TREATMENT Rx

Management of Specific Treatable Subsets

Because patients with cancer of unknown primary site have advanced disease, therapeutic nihilism has been common. However, several subsets of patients can benefit from specific treatment, and they can be identified on the basis of clinical and pathologic features (Table 211-2). These patients are important to recognize and treat appropriately, because some individuals in each group have the potential for long-term survival.

Adenocarcinoma
Women with Axillary Lymph Node Metastases

Metastatic breast cancer should be suspected in women who have axillary lymph node involvement with adenocarcinoma, particularly when other metastatic sites are not evident. In these patients, pathologic evaluation of the initial lymph node biopsy should include staining for estrogen and progesterone receptors and for HER-2 expression; elevated levels provide strong evidence for the diagnosis of breast cancer. When no other metastases are identified, these women should be treated as if they had stage II breast cancer, which is potentially curable with appropriate therapy (Chapter 204). Modified radical mastectomy identifies a breast primary site in 44 to 82% of women, even when the breast examination and mammographic findings are normal. Axillary lymph node dissection followed by radiation therapy to the breast appears to give results similar to those of mastectomy, although these two options for primary therapy have not been compared directly. Adjuvant systemic therapy should follow standard guidelines for the treatment of women with stage II breast cancer.

Women with Peritoneal Carcinomatosis

Adenocarcinoma involving the peritoneum in women usually originates from the ovary (Chapter 205), although carcinomas arising in the gastrointestinal tract or breast can occasionally produce this syndrome. However, diffuse peritoneal carcinomatosis occasionally occurs in women who have histologically normal ovaries or who have had previous bilateral oophorectomy. The peritoneum is frequently the only site of tumor involvement, and serum CA-125 levels are usually elevated. When histologic features suggest ovarian cancer, this syndrome has been called *peritoneal papillary serous carcinoma* or *primary extraovarian serous carcinoma*.

Even when the histologic features are not typical, women with adenocarcinoma of unknown primary site involving the peritoneum often have cancers with biologic characteristics similar to those of ovarian cancer (Chapter 205). Treatment of these patients should follow guidelines for stage III ovarian cancer. When feasible, a full laparotomy with maximal surgical cytoreduction should be performed, followed by combination chemotherapy with a taxane/platinum–containing regimen. Measurement of serial serum CA-125 levels provides an accurate assessment of the efficacy of treatment. A few of these patients may have complete responses and long-term survival, particularly when initial surgical cytoreduction leaves minimal residual disease. A similar syndrome of peritoneal carcinomatosis that is responsive to chemotherapy for ovarian cancer has occasionally been reported in men.

Men with Skeletal Metastases and/or Elevated Serum Prostate-Specific Antigen Levels

Metastatic prostate cancer (Chapter 207) should be suspected in men with adenocarcinoma predominantly involving bone, particularly if the metastases are blastic. An elevated serum PSA level or tumor immunostaining for PSA confirms the diagnosis of prostate cancer. Occasionally, men with adenocarcinoma of unknown primary site and patterns of metastasis unusual for prostate cancer (e.g., lung metastases, mediastinal lymph node metastases) are found to have elevated serum PSA levels. These patients should be treated according to guidelines for advanced prostate cancer. Androgen ablation produces excellent responses and substantial palliation in most patients.

Single Metastatic Lesion

Occasionally, a single metastatic lesion containing adenocarcinoma or poorly differentiated carcinoma is identified, and a complete evaluation reveals no other evidence of disease. Such presentations can include a single

TABLE 211-2 SPECIFIC PATIENT SUBSETS AND RECOMMENDED TREATMENT

HISTOLOGIC	Subset-Identifying Features CLINICAL	TREATMENT RECOMMENDATIONS
Adenocarcinoma	Women, isolated axillary adenopathy	Treat as stage II breast cancer
Adenocarcinoma	Women, peritoneal carcinomatosis (Occasionally men?)	Treat as stage III ovarian cancer
Adenocarcinoma	Men, elevated PSA and/or blastic bone metastases	Treat as advanced prostate cancer
Adenocarcinoma, poorly differentiated carcinoma	Single metastatic lesion	Definitive local therapy (resection and/or radiation therapy) with or without chemotherapy
Adenocarcinoma	Colon cancer profile	Treat as metastatic colorectal cancer
Squamous	Cervical adenopathy	Treat as locally advanced head or neck cancer
Squamous	Inguinal adenopathy	Definitive local therapy (node dissection with or without radiation therapy) with or without chemotherapy
Poorly differentiated carcinoma	Young men with midline tumor and/or elevated hCG, AFP	Treat as extragonadal germ cell tumor
Poorly differentiated carcinoma	Diverse clinical features	Empirical chemotherapy with paclitaxel, ,platinum, etoposide
Neuroendocrine carcinoma, poorly differentiated	Diverse clinical presentations	Treat with platinum, etoposide
Neuroendocrine carcinoma, well differentiated	Usually liver metastases	Treat as metastatic carcinoid tumor

AFP = α-fetoprotein; hCG = human chorionic gonadotropin; PSA = prostate-specific antigen.

lymph node or subcutaneous site or single lesions at various visceral sites, including bone, liver, lung, brain, and adrenal gland. The possibility of an unusual primary site mimicking a metastatic lesion should be considered (e.g., a subcutaneous nodule from a primary apocrine or sebaceous carcinoma rather than a metastasis), but this possibility can usually be excluded on the basis of clinical or pathologic features. PET is useful in excluding other metastatic lesions. For patients with only a single identifiable lesion, definitive local therapy is recommended, guided by the site of tumor involvement. Such therapy may include surgical resection, radiation therapy, or a combination of these modalities. Although most of these patients eventually develop other metastatic sites, a significant disease-free interval is often experienced, and local treatment provides substantial palliation. The role of systemic chemotherapy in addition to definitive local therapy is not well defined; younger patients with poorly differentiated carcinoma or poorly differentiated adenocarcinoma are often treated with a short course of a taxane/platinum–based regimen (see Empirical Chemotherapy).

Colon Cancer Profile

The accurate recognition of patients likely to respond to colon cancer regimens has become increasingly important as treatment for this cancer has improved substantially. A "colon cancer profile" has been defined and includes (1) metastases predominantly in the liver and/or peritoneum, (2) adenocarcinoma with histologic features typical of gastrointestinal origin, and (3) typical immunohistochemical staining that is CK20 positive, CK7 negative, and CDX-2 positive. Patients with this profile should be treated according to guidelines for metastatic colorectal cancer (Chapter 199).

Squamous Carcinoma
Cervical Adenopathy

Squamous carcinoma of unknown primary site is relatively uncommon. Most patients with this syndrome have involvement of cervical lymph nodes, usually in the upper or midcervical area. Often, patients with this syndrome are middle-aged or elderly and have a history of substantial tobacco or alcohol use or both. A primary site in the head and neck region should be suspected (Chapter 196); however, complete endoscopic evaluation fails to identify a primary site in approximately 15% of these patients. Even if other tests are negative, PET identifies a primary site in the head and neck region in approximately 25% of such patients and should be part of the initial evaluation.

Even when no primary site is identified, management of these patients should follow standard guidelines for the treatment of locally advanced squamous carcinoma arising in the head and neck. Many reports have documented long-term survival rates of 30 to 60% following definitive local treatment, which should include radiation therapy or combined radiation and cervical lymph node dissection. Outcome of treatment depends on the size and number of involved cervical lymph nodes. Concurrent chemotherapy and radiation therapy are now considered the standard treatment approach for patients with locally advanced head and neck cancers and should be considered in patients with multiple involved lymph nodes or nodes larger than 2 cm in diameter (Chapter 196).

Inguinal Adenopathy

Occasionally, metastatic squamous cancer is found in inguinal lymph nodes. In most of these patients, a primary site can be located in the perineal or anorectal area. For the occasional patient in whom no primary site is identified, long-term survival can result from local therapy with inguinal lymph node dissection, with or without radiation therapy. Recently, combined-modality treatment with concurrent chemotherapy and radiation therapy has improved cure rates in patients with several squamous cancers arising in this region (e.g., cervix, anus, bladder). Although data are incomplete, a reasonable approach is the addition of chemotherapy with a platinum/5-fluorouracil regimen, as described for locally advanced carcinoma of the cervix.

Poorly Differentiated Carcinoma
Extragonadal Germ Cell Cancer Syndrome

Young men with clinical features of extragonadal germ cell tumors, including tumors in the mediastinum or retroperitoneum or those associated with elevated serum levels of human chorionic gonadotropin or α-fetoprotein, should be treated according to guidelines for extragonadal germ cell tumors (Chapter 206). Some of these patients can be proved to have germ cell tumors by identifying an i12p chromosomal abnormality, even when the diagnosis is not possible with other standard pathologic techniques. Approximately 30 to 40% of these patients achieve complete responses and long-term survival following chemotherapy with cisplatin, etoposide, and bleomycin, as used for advanced germ cell tumors.

Anaplastic Lymphoma

An appropriate initial pathologic evaluation should identify most histologically atypical lymphomas. Occasionally, immunoperoxidase staining for leukocyte common antigen is negative or cannot be adequately performed in patients with anaplastic lymphoma. The disease in some of these patients can be recognized using other immunoperoxidase stains (e.g., Ki-1, CD-30) or molecular genetic analysis (detection of immunoglobulin gene rearrangements). All patients with lymphomas identified by special pathologic studies should be treated using standard guidelines for aggressive non-Hodgkin's lymphoma (Chapter 191).

Neuroendocrine Carcinoma

In approximately 10% of poorly differentiated carcinomas, neuroendocrine features are identified by either immunoperoxidase staining or electron microscopy. Treatment of these patients is discussed later (see Neuroendocrine Carcinoma).

Other Poorly Differentiated Carcinomas

In most patients with poorly differentiated carcinoma, there are no clinical or pathologic features that allow their assignment to one of the three preceding subsets. However, this heterogeneous group contains some patients whose carcinomas are highly sensitive to platinum-based chemotherapy. Clinical factors predictive of sensitivity to chemotherapy include site of tumor involvement (lymph nodes as compared with visceral metastases), fewer sites of metastatic disease, and younger age. In selected patients with one or more of these favorable clinical features, treatment with cisplatin-based chemotherapy can produce a greater than 60% response rate, and approximately 15% of patients remain free of disease more than 8 years after completing treatment. Therefore, a brief trial of empirical chemotherapy (see later) is recommended for all patients with poorly differentiated carcinoma, unless they are extremely debilitated at the time of diagnosis. Patients with highly sensitive tumors can be identified within the first 4 to 6 weeks of treatment, and ineffective treatment can be discontinued in the remainder.

Neuroendocrine Carcinoma

Poorly Differentiated Neuroendocrine Carcinoma or Small Cell Anaplastic Carcinoma

These high-grade neuroendocrine tumors are now reliably identified using widely available immunoperoxidase stains. Although the origin of these tumors remains unknown, they are often highly sensitive to combination chemotherapy; with platinum/etoposide chemotherapy, the overall response rate is about 75%, and 25% of patients have complete responses. In patients with locoregional disease, the addition of radiation therapy following chemotherapy is reasonable.

Low-Grade (Carcinoid-Type) Neuroendocrine Tumors

Occasionally, low-grade neuroendocrine tumors are found at a metastatic site. In almost all cases, the liver is the site of involvement, and the histologic features suggest a carcinoid (Chapter 240) or islet cell tumor of gastrointestinal origin (Chapter 201). Various clinical syndromes caused by the secretion of vasoactive peptides (e.g., serotonin, vasoactive intestinal peptide, gastrin) have been described. Like other carcinoid tumors, these tumors often have indolent biologic characteristics, and patients can frequently survive for several years despite multiple liver metastases. Unlike poorly differentiated neuroendocrine tumors, these tumors are relatively resistant to chemotherapy, and intensive combination regimens should usually be avoided. Management of these patients should follow guidelines for metastatic carcinoid tumors (Chapter 240) and may include the use of somatostatin analogues, local ablative procedures (e.g., surgical resection, radiofrequency ablation, chemoembolization), targeted agents (e.g., sunitinib, everolimus), or fluorouracil-based chemotherapy regimens.

Empirical Chemotherapy

Approximately 60 to 70% of patients with carcinoma of unknown primary site do not fit into any of these defined clinical subsets. In these patients, earlier reports of empirical chemotherapy were discouraging, with overall response rates of only 20 to 25% and short median survival times (5 to 7 months). The combination of paclitaxel (200 mg/m^2 IV on day 1) and carboplatin (AUC 6.0 IV on day 1), with or without etoposide (50 mg alternating with 100 mg PO on days 1 to 10), all repeated every 21 days for four courses, produces objective responses in 30 to 45% of patients, with median survival in the 9- to 12-month range. In addition, a few patients obtain a major benefit from treatment; the 2-year survival rate with taxane-containing regimens is 20 to 25%. Regimens containing gemcitabine and cisplatin have produced similar results. The most effective treatment is unknown because randomized comparisons are lacking in this area.

At present, patients with carcinoma of unknown primary site who have a reasonable performance status should be considered for an empirical trial of combination chemotherapy. Patients with responsive tumors can be identified after 4 to 6 weeks of treatment, and they should continue treatment for a standard 4- to 5-month course. Patients who do not respond to initial combination chemotherapy are unlikely to respond to further treatment; palliative care is appropriate in these patients (Chapter 3). For patients who have a poor performance status at the time of diagnosis, palliative care alone is an appropriate approach.

SUGGESTED READINGS

Cerezo L, Raboso E, Ballesteros AI. Unknown primary cancer of the head and neck: a multidisciplinary approach. *Clin Trans Oncol.* 2011;13:88-97. *Review.*

Greco FA, Spigel DR, Yardley DA, et al. Molecular profiling in unknown primary cancer: accuracy of tissue of origin prediction. *Oncologist.* 2010;15:500-506. *Molecular profiling correctly identified the primary site in 15 of 20 cases.*

Morris GJ, Greco FA, Hainsworth JD, et al. Cancer of unknown primary site. *Semin Oncol.* 2010;37:71-79. *Review.*

Pavlidis N, Briasoulis E, Pentheroudakis G; ESMO Guidelines Working Group. Cancers of unknown primary site: ESMO Clinical Practice Guidelines for diagnosis, treatment and follow-up. *Ann Oncol.* 2010;21:v228-v231. *Consensus guidelines.*

XVI

METABOLIC DISEASES

212

APPROACH TO INBORN ERRORS OF METABOLISM

LOUIS J. ELSAS II

DEFINITION

Metabolism is a collective term for integrated biochemical processes that enables homeostasis for the organism by maintaining anabolic and catabolic flow of substrates to products. Inborn errors of metabolism refer to single gene disorders producing loss of function of a single protein that results in altered concentrations of linked metabolites in the reaction sequence.

HISTORY

In the early 20th century, Garrod recognized heritable blocks in normal human metabolic flow that conformed to mendelian mechanisms of inheritance. He first coined the term *inborn error of metabolism,* describing four diseases—alkaptonuria, albinism, cystinuria, and pentosuria. Garrod presumed that a patient expressing the full abnormality was homozygous for mutant alleles affecting a specific metabolic flow whereas the parents were heterozygous for this same inherited block but were clinically normal. The enzyme defect in alkaptonuria was not discovered until 50 years later, when homogentisic acid oxidase was found impaired in the liver and kidneys of patients with this disease. Twenty years ago, the gene for homogentisate 1,2-dioxygenase was cloned, and mutations causing altered function were defined.

Over the past two decades, advances in technology such as fast throughput, genome-wide DNA sequencing, tandem mass spectrometry, and bioinformatics have confirmed Garrod's postulate of chemical individuality and resulted in the discovery of more than 1321 catalogued inborn errors of metabolism, as well as vigorous research exploring normal and abnormal inherited variation in human metabolism for common conditions such as obesity and cancer. The implementation of public health–based newborn screening using these modern technologies defined the clinical power of genetics in presymptomatic prediction and prevention of more than 40 inborn errors.

PATHOBIOLOGY

Protein Diversity

Variations in human proteins do not usually produce disease. Heritable diversity in proteins within normal populations is required for optimal health (e.g., the ability of the immune system to produce γ-globulin in response to a wide range of antigenic epitopes). Nucleotide sequence variations in genes may produce different amino acid changes in the primary protein structure without producing a functional change. When no functional change occurs, the alteration is considered a *polymorphism.* The term *single nucleotide polymorphism* (SNP) is now used to define an individual's diversity after scanning the entire human genome. Continued research is trying to link genomic SNPs to regulatory RNA, messenger RNA, and protein and metabolic variations. Chromatographic separation of physiologic fluids followed by tandem mass spectrometry enables identification of the metabolomic effect of a given SNP on a wide range of molecules, including lipids, amino acids, phospholipids, and glycoproteins.

There are many molecular mechanisms producing normal protein diversity. Normal protein variation can occur through gene rearrangements, as exemplified by the formation of immunoglobins, which give rise to required variations in response to foreign antigens. Post-transcriptional, alternative splicing of RNA is another mechanism for protein variation. There are many examples of alternative splicing that provide organ specificity for protein isoforms. Post-translational modification of proteins produces diversity and is important in directing proteins to subcellular organelles, to the cell surface, or for secretion. Glycosylation of proteins directed to plasma membrane receptors is an example of this post-translational mechanism. As an example of the importance of these mechanisms, consider that humans have more than 250,000 functional proteins but less than 35,000 genes predicted from the human genome sequence. Added to this sequence diversity of proteins

---

TABLE 212-1	CLASSIFICATION OF PROTEIN FUNCTION BY LOCATION IN ORGANISM

Proteins act as follows:
1. Catalyze plasma membrane functions
   a. Substrate transport
   b. Cellular signaling (receptors)
2. Catalyze integrated metabolic pathways in the cytosol, lysosome, peroxisome, mitochondria, nucleus, and endoplasmic reticulum
3. Circulate in blood and provide and maintain various functions (clotting; metal, lipid, and vitamin transport; immunity; oxygen transport; regulation of proteases, hormones, and adhesion proteins)
4. Maintain structural integrity of organs and organelles (collagen, elastin, actin, dystrophin, and fibrillin)

TABLE 212-2	CLASSIC PATHOLOGIC MECHANISMS FOR INBORN ERRORS OF METABOLISM

1. Accumulation of substrates to toxic concentrations in a blocked catabolic reaction. *Examples:* maple syrup urine disease, galactosemia, glucose-galactose malabsorption, Fabry's disease, Gaucher's disease, urea cycle defects
2. Production of toxic byproducts through a normally minor pathway. *Examples:* tyrosinemia type I, adenosine deaminase deficiency
3. Deficiency of an end product in an anabolic pathway. *Examples:* albinism, orotic aciduria, scurvy, plasminogen deficiency
4. Loss of regulation resulting in overproduction of intermediates to toxic levels. *Examples:* congenital adrenal hyperplasia, acute intermittent porphyria, familial hypercholesterolemia

---

are recent biophysical observations that proteins undergo conformational plasticity that can alter their function.

Mutations

The relatively rare circumstance in which a change in a protein impairs function is called a *mutation,* and it may produce an inborn error of metabolism. Naturally occurring mutations that produce pathology also provide insight into the functional role of normal proteins in human metabolism. Inborn errors of metabolism are classified here in accordance with the organ, cell, and subcellular location of normal protein function (Table 212-1) and the abnormal mechanisms that interfere with normal metabolic flow as a result of impaired proteins (Table 212-2).

Current diagnosis and therapy for inborn errors focus on relatively rare mutations in single genes that have major effects on disrupting metabolic flow. Current and future research will provide predictive tools for identifying variations in the genome and metabolome that produce sensitivity to the environment with onset of common illnesses of adults and an opportunity to intervene and prevent them. This concept is called *personalized medicine.*

The correlation of genes that are transcribed and translated approaches only 20% of the genome in any cell or organ. Network perturbation models for essential metabolic pathways are being defined, particularly in the context of drug-induced adverse events, where heritable variations are diagnosed by personalized genomic microarrays before the drug is given and thereby prevent adverse reactions by avoidance. Microarrays for genomic variation in the cytochrome P-450 genes are now commercially available and will assist in predicting some sensitivities to drugs. Similarly, genome microarrays to predict genetic variation producing early-onset heart, liver, eye, lung, and nervous system diseases, including cancers, are in development.

Pathophysiology

One important clinical aspect in defining the genetic component of a metabolic disease is that one can predict, intervene in, and prevent irreversible pathology by a variety of stratagems before irreversible disease is expressed. In general, the severity of an inborn error of metabolism depends on the degree of protein impairment rendered by the genetic mutation and the trauma induced by the environment. A "leaky" mutation may not be expressed until adulthood, whereas a complete block in the same metabolic pathway is lethal in infancy. The age at onset and severity of disease are a result of complex interactions of the gene, environment, or other genes that modify the underlying genetic susceptibility. The pathophysiologic mechanisms outlined in Table 212-2 may occur individually or may combine to produce loss in homeostasis and a disease state. The clinical manifestations are usually *pleiotropic,* which means that one blocked enzyme reaction produces multiple dysfunctions at the organ level. An example is galactosemia, which causes cataracts, ovarian failure, liver disease, and central nervous system dysfunction. The phenotype (clinical outcome) is also affected not only by the specific genetic block but also by alternative metabolic pathways that may remove toxic precursors or supply deficient products of a blocked reaction. Outcome may be adversely affected by an alternative pathway that produces a toxic analyte, and a pathophysiologic mechanism may differ among organs. In galactosemia, the accumulation of galactose can produce excess intracellular galactitol through an alternative pathway catalyzed by aldose reductase and, consequently, cell death of optic lens fibers as a result of the osmotic effect of intracellular galactitol. Accumulation of galactitol causes cataracts, whereas accumulation of galactose 1-phosphate produces hepatic cell death, ovarian failure, and cerebellar dysfunction.

ERRORS IN PROTEINS THAT CAUSE DISEASES

Plasma Membrane Transporter Protein Mutations

Defects of Glucose Transporters

Many disorders are produced by mutant proteins that impair the transport of nutrients into and out of cells (Table 212-3). *Familial glucose-galactose malabsorption syndrome* exemplifies defective transporter proteins and results in the accumulation of nontransported glucose in the intestinal lumen with refractory diarrhea secondary to its osmotic effects. Direct evidence for genetic control of intestinal glucose transport in humans was obtained by in vitro studies of jejunal biopsy material from families in which the affected members expressed refractory diarrhea on ingesting D-galactose or D-glucose but not fructose. Pedigree analysis conformed to autosomal recessive inheritance. These data predicted a gene that coded for a stereospecific, sodium- and energy-dependent transporter protein in human jejunal (and proximal renal tubular) microvilli. Expression cloning of active glucose transport has now confirmed the presence of a family of glucose transporter genes, their

deduced amino acid sequences, and specific codon changes producing the syndromes of familial glucose-galactose malabsorption and renal glycosuria. There are many inherited defects involving the plasma membrane transport of glucose that are caused by mutations of either active or facilitative glucose transport. Glucose transporters are a family of proteins whose definitions of function evolved after their cloning and molecular genetic analysis (Table 212-4). An insulin-responsive, facilitative glucose transporter (GLUT4) is not Na^+ dependent and is expressed primarily in insulin-responsive tissues (fat cells, skeletal muscle). More than one glucose transporter is expressed by most cells. The jejunal epithelial cell uses sodium-glucose cotransporter protein 1 (SGLT1) to concentrate glucose from its luminal surface into the cytosol, then effluxes glucose at its basal-lateral surfaces through GLUT2. GLUT2 is also involved in regulating the amount of glucose transported into β cells of the pancreas, a process that regulates glucose stimulation of insulin release. Indirect evidence suggests that mutations in the *GLUT2* gene are "sensitivity genes" involved in regulating insulin secretion.

Many other facilitative human glucose transporters have been identified by expressed sequence tags (EST) homology searches (GLUT 5, 6, 7, 8, 9, 10, 11, 12, 13). While GLUT5 and GLUT7 have functional assignments as a fructose transporter and as an exporter of glucose from the endoplasmic reticulum, respectively, the functions of these other glucose transporter isoforms are not clearly defined.

Plasma Membrane Receptor Protein Dysfunction

Parathyroid Hormone Resistance

Many diseases characterized by "hormone resistance" are caused by a family of proteins that function as receptors in the plasma membrane and as postreceptor transmitters of signals located in the cytosol and nucleus. The concept of failure to respond to hormone stimulation originated in the early 1940s with a description of *pseudohypoparathyroidism* (Chapter 253). Heritability of resistance to parathormone was suggested before the existence of parathormone receptors, hormone-sensitive adenylate cyclases, or guanine nucleotide-binding proteins was known.

TABLE 212-3 DISEASES CAUSED BY MUTATIONS IN PLASMA MEMBRANE TRANSPORTER PROTEINS

DISEASE	TISSUE AFFECTED	SUBSTRATE	MODE OF INHERITANCE	CLINICAL EXPRESSION
B_{12} malabsorption	Ileum	Vitamin B_{12}	Autosomal recessive	Pernicious anemia
Blue diaper syndrome	Gut	Tryptophan	Autosomal recessive	Hypercalcemia
Primary carnitine deficiency	Kidney + gut	Carnitine	Autosomal recessive	Hypoglycemia, hypotonia
Congenital chloridorrhea	Gut	Chloride	Autosomal recessive	Diarrhea, alkalosis
Cystic fibrosis	Apical epithelia	Chloride	Autosomal recessive	Lung, intestinal obstruction
Cystinuria	Kidney + gut	Cystine + lysine, arginine, ornithine	Autosomal recessive	Renal lithiasis (cystine)
Familial hypophosphatemic rickets	Kidney + gut	Phosphate	X-linked dominant	Rickets
Folate deficiency	Lymphocyte, erythrocyte	Methyltetrahydrofolate	Autosomal recessive	Aplastic anemia
Glucose-galactose malabsorption	Gut + kidney	Glucose and galactose	Autosomal recessive	Refractory diarrhea
Hartnup's syndrome	Gut + kidney	Neutral amino acids	Autosomal recessive (pellagra)	Nicotinic acid deficiency
Hereditary hypophosphatemic rickets	Kidney	Phosphate	Autosomal dominant	Growth restriction, rickets, phosphaturia
Hereditary renal hypouricemia	Kidney	Uric acid	Autosomal recessive	Urolithiasis (uric acid)
Hereditary spherocytosis	Erythrocyte	Sodium	Autosomal dominant or recessive	Hemolytic anemia
Hyperdibasic aminoaciduria (type I)	Kidney	Lysine, arginine, ornithine	Autosomal dominant	Symptoms of growth restriction?
Iminoglycinuria	Kidney + gut	Glycine, proline, hydroxyproline	Autosomal recessive	Benign? Pancreatitis
Isolated lysinuria	Kidney + gut	Lysine	Autosomal recessive	Growth failure, seizures
Lysinuric protein intolerance (type II)	Kidney, fibroblasts, hepatocytes, gut	Lysine	Autosomal recessive	Growth restriction, hyperammonemia, mental retardation
Methionine malabsorption	Gut	Methionine	Autosomal recessive?	Mental retardation, white hair, failure to thrive
Renal glycosuria	Kidney	Glucose	Autosomal recessive	Benign glycosuria
Renal tubular acidosis (type I)	Distal renal tubule	H^+ secretion, citrate, calcium	Autosomal dominant	Hypokalemia, growth restriction, nephrocalcinosis
Renal tubular acidosis (type II)	Proximal renal tubule	Bicarbonate	"Familial"	Hyperchloremic metabolic acidosis

TABLE 212-4 HUMAN GLUCOSE TRANSPORTERS

PROTEIN	kD (AA)	mRNA SIZE (kb)	CHROMOSOMAL LOCALIZATION	EXPRESSION IN TISSUE AND CELLS	FUNCTION	DISORDER
FACILITATIVE GLUCOSE TRANSPORTERS						
GLUT1	55 (492)	2.8	1p35→p31.3	Blood-brain barrier, erythrocyte, fibroblast	Basal glucose transport across most cells, including the blood-brain barrier	Seizures with low cerebrospinal fluid and normal blood glucose
GLUT2	58 (524)	2.8 3.4 5.4	3q26.1→q26.3	Liver, kidney, intestine, β cell of the pancreas	Low-affinity glucose transport	Defective insulin secretion in diabetes
GLUT3	54 (496)	2.7 4.1	12p13.3	Neurons, fibroblasts, placenta, testes	Basal glucose transport, high affinity	?
GLUT4	55 (509)	2.8 3.5	17p13	Fat, skeletal muscle, heart	Insulin-stimulated glucose transport	Defective insulin-stimulated transport, NIDDM?
CONCENTRATIVE GLUCOSE TRANSPORTERS						
SLGT1	75 (664)	2.2 2.6 4.8	22q11→qter	Intestine, kidney (medulla)	Intestinal absorption, renal reabsorption, high affinity (2 Na: 1 glucose)	Glucose-galactose malabsorption
SLGT2	76 (672)	2.4 3.0 3.5 4.5	16p11.2	Kidney (cortex)	Low affinity, high capacity (1 Na: 1 glucose)	Renal glycosuria

AA = amino acids; NIDDM = non-insulin-dependent diabetes mellitus.

In *Albright's hereditary osteodystrophy,* or *pseudohypoparathyroidism* (Chapter 253), a heterogeneous group of mutations affect the gene for the parathormone receptor's guanine nucleotide-binding protein ($G_{s\alpha}$), which links the receptor to adenylate cyclase and stimulates cyclic adenosine monophosphate when the receptor is occupied by parathormone. The gene for $G_{s\alpha}$ is located on chromosome 20q13, and deletions and missense mutations that produce Albright's hereditary osteodystrophy have been defined. Somatic mutations in arginine 201 of the same gene turn the $G_{s\alpha}$ protein constitutively "on" and produce another disease, McCune-Albright-Sternberg syndrome. Cells are mosaic for the mutation, and the syndrome includes nonossifying bone tumors and premature puberty.

Growth Hormone Resistance

Diseases caused by defective transmembrane binding and signaling include *Laron dwarfism,* which results from growth hormone receptor (GHR) defects (Chapter 231). The phenotypic characteristics are *proportionate dwarfism,* hypoglycemia, craniofacial dysmorphology with a doll-like face, balding, frontal bossing, truncal obesity, and wrinkled skin. In this disorder, the growth hormone concentration in blood is elevated, peripheral tissue responses are decreased, and insulin-like growth factor I concentrations in blood are low. An autosomal recessive mode of inheritance has been defined. Dominant or polygenic symmetrical growth restriction may result from mutations in nuclear transproteins, hypothalamic pituitary trophic proteins, growth hormone, GHR, and postreceptor signaling. The *GHR* gene is found on chromosome 5p13-p12, and many different mutations in this gene account for disorders of stature.

Familial Hypercholesterolemia

Familial hypercholesterolemia defines a phenotype of autosomal dominant hypercholesterolemia and early-onset heart disease (Chapter 213). This disorder affects an estimated 1 in 500 individuals in the general population. An autosomal dominant mode of inheritance for early-onset adult heart disease is caused by many different mutations in the trafficking and function of low-density lipoprotein (LDL) cholesterol receptors. Dysfunction of LDL receptors results in a loss of the cell's ability to downregulate endogenous cholesterol synthesis and incorporate LDL cholesterol into cells. Increased intravascular accumulation of LDL cholesterol results in atherosclerosis and heart disease before the sixth decade of life (see Table 212-2).

Errors of Insulin Resistance
Leprechaunism

Leprechaunism has become a prototypical inborn error of severe insulin resistance and loss of cellular signal transduction through the insulin receptor. Affected infants have low birthweight, acanthosis nigricans, cystic changes in organs, and loss of glucose homeostasis. Affected patients have remarkably elevated plasma insulin concentrations greater than 500 mIU/mL. Specific impairment in iodine-125-labeled insulin binding is evident in cells cultured from patients, and a spectrum of mutations produces a variety of severe insulin-resistant syndromes (leprechaunism, Rabson-Mendenhall syndrome, and type A diabetes with acanthosis nigricans). Obligate heterozygotes (parents) of patients with leprechaunism have partially impaired insulin binding and glucose tolerance curves suggesting type 2 diabetes mellitus. The insulin receptor transduces its signal by phosphotransfer to the insulin receptor signal protein 1 (IRS-1), and a cascade of downstream phosphorylations occurs, leading to stimulation of glucose transport.

Impaired Cytosolic Enzymes

Inborn errors affecting proteins of the cytosolic compartment within a cell are the more "traditional" inborn errors of metabolism (Table 212-5). They impair the catalytic reactions of anabolic or catabolic pathways and are usually classified by the class of biochemical involved, such as impairment of glucose, lipid, fatty acid, amino acid, purine, organic acid, vitamin, or drug metabolism.

Phenylketonuria

Phenylalanine is essential for growth, and its anabolic products include tyrosine, thyroid hormone, adrenergic neurotransmitters, and melanin. *Phenylketonuria* (PKU) is caused by mutations in the gene encoding phenylalanine hydroxylase, the first enzyme in this anabolic flow that catalyzes tyrosine production. PKU may also occur if coenzymes are deficient in this reaction, such as dihydropteridine reductase or enzymes involved in biopterin biosynthesis.

Albinism

Albinism is an example of an inborn error in an anabolic pathway in which the pathophysiologic mechanism is related directly to the lack of an end product (see mechanism 3, Table 212-2). Tyrosine is converted by the action of a cytosolic tyrosinase first to dopa and then to dopamine. Dopamine can be converted either to the red-yellow pigment pheomelanin or to the black-brown pigment eumelanin. These reactions occur in the melanosomes produced in melanocytes and exported to keratinocytes. Color of skin is an inherited factor that depends on many genes (polygenic) and is a function of the intensity of the pigment in the skin and not the number of melanocytes, which is constant for all humans. Although skin color is a polygenic trait, single genes can have a profound effect on this color, as evidenced by the albino phenotype. In humans, *oculocutaneous albinism* (OCA) is inherited as an autosomal recessive trait. X-linked forms of *ocular albinism* also exist. Individuals with OCA are classified as tyrosinase negative or positive for tyrosinase activity in hair bulbs. Tyrosinase-negative individuals form no pigment. The gene for tyrosinase has been localized to chromosome 11q14, and many mutations have been defined. A tyrosine-positive OCA has been associated

TABLE 212-5 SOME DISEASES CAUSED BY IMPAIRED CYTOSOLIC ENZYMES

DISORDER	ENZYME DEFECT	PHENOTYPE	INHERITANCE
CARBOHYDRATES			
Fructosuria	Fructokinase	Benign	Autosomal recessive
Hereditary fructose intolerance	Fructose 1-phosphate aldolase	Liver dysfunction, early death	Autosomal recessive
Galactosemia	Galactose 1-phosphate uridyltransferase	Liver dysfunction, cataracts, sepsis, mental retardation, death	Autosomal recessive
Hereditary fructose-1,6-*bis*-phosphate deficiency	Fructose-1,6-*bis*-phosphatase	Apnea, ketosis, lactic acidosis	Autosomal recessive
AMINO ACIDS			
Phenylketonuria	*p*-Hydroxyphenylalanine hydroxylase	Mental retardation (teratogenic)	Autosomal recessive
Tyrosinemia			
Type II	Tyrosine aminotransferase	Palmar bullae, corneal lesions	Autosomal recessive
Type I	Fumarylacetoacetate hydrolase	Succinyl acetone accumulation	Autosomal recessive
Homocystinuria	Cystathionine β-synthase	Marfanoid habitus, arterial thrombosis, lens dislocation, mental retardation	Autosomal recessive
Hyperornithinemia	Ornithine aminotransferase	Gyrate atrophy of the retina	Autosomal recessive
Lesch-Nyhan syndrome	Hypoxanthine phosphoribosyltransferase	Neurologic dysfunction with self-destructive tendency	X-linked

with an autosomal recessive gene located on chromosome 15q11-13 (the P gene), and X-linked ocular albinism is caused by *OCA1* gene mutations. Wide variation in the phenotypic expression of albinism, ranging from severe neurologic deficiency with ocular and sarcomatous skin cancers to mild cosmetic problems, has been reported. Therapy requires total body skin protection and eye avoidance of ultraviolet light.

Errors of the Urea Cycle (Cytosol and Mitochondrial Interaction)

Inborn errors of the urea cycle are represented by defects in the integration of anabolic and catabolic pathways and the distribution of catalytic proteins between mitochondria and cytosol. The role of the urea cycle is to convert ammonia, a byproduct of protein breakdown, to urea and to synthesize arginine and ornithine. Reactions to complete this anabolic cycle require mitochondrial enzymes, cytosolic enzymes, and mitochondrial transporter proteins. Inherited disorders affecting the function of these proteins are known. Individuals with defects in any of the enzymes have varying degrees of hyperammonemia caused by protein ingestion or a nutritional state in which muscle is catabolized. With the exception of the gene for ornithine transcarbamylase found on the short arm of chromosome X, the other proteins are encoded on autosomes, and defects are inherited as autosomal recessive traits. Many principles of diagnosis and therapy for inborn errors of metabolism are exemplified by disorders of the urea cycle.

Errors in Mitochondrial Proteins

A group of inborn errors of metabolism are caused by mutations in both mitochondrial and nuclear genes that encode mitochondrial proteins. Collectively, they are considered disorders of organic acid metabolism (Table 212-6). Branched-chain α-ketoacid dehydrogenase is a multienzyme complex located on the matrix side of the mitochondrial inner membrane in all tissues. When any of these proteins is impaired, the autosomal recessive disorder *maple syrup urine disease* may result. In addition to nuclear-encoded genes, 13 proteins of mitochondrial complexes involved in oxidative phosphorylation are encoded in the mitochondrial DNA genome. Only complex II is encoded entirely by the nuclear genome. A wide range of disorders affecting the eye, brain, and muscle are caused by mutations in mitochondrial DNA that impair oxidative phosphorylation. The inheritance pattern of disorders encoded by the mitochondrial genome is distinguished from disorders caused by mutations in nuclear DNA by being transmitted through an affected mother to all of her offspring. Males do not transmit mitochondrial mutations to their offspring, hence the term *maternal inheritance*. Because there are about 10,000 mitochondrial genomes per cell, variation in disease expression is caused by differences in the ratio of mutant to normal mitochondrial genomes (*heteroplasmy*) and the environment.

Lysosomal Disorders

Another group of inborn errors of metabolism are collectively categorized as *lysosomal disorders* (Chapter 215) to indicate the subcellular localization of

TABLE 212-6 ORGANIC ACIDEMIAS: DISORDERS OF METABOLISM BY MITOCHONDRIAL PROTEINS

DISORDER	ENZYME DEFECT	INHERITANCE
Isovaleric acidemia	Isovaleryl-CoA dehydrogenase	Autosomal recessive
Methylcrotonic aciduria	3-Methylcrotonyl-CoA carboxylase	Autosomal recessive
Glutaconic aciduria	3-Methylglutaconyl-CoA hydratase	Autosomal recessive
Glutaric aciduria (1)	3-Hydroxy-3-methylglutaryl-CoA lyase	Autosomal recessive
Mevalonic aciduria	Mevalonate kinase	Autosomal recessive
Thiolase deficiency	2-Methylacetoacetyl-CoA thiolase	Autosomal recessive
Isobutyric aciduria	3-Hydroxyisobutyryl-CoA deacylase	Autosomal recessive
Propionic aciduria	Propionyl-CoA carboxylase	Autosomal recessive
Methylmalonic aciduria	Methylmalonyl-CoA mutase	Autosomal recessive
Lactic acidosis	Pyruvate carboxylase Pyruvate dehydrogenase	Autosomal recessive
Acyl-CoA dehydrogenase deficiencies	Short-, medium-, and long-chain fatty acyl-CoA dehydrogenase	Autosomal recessive
Branched-chain α-ketoacidemia	Branched-chain α-ketoacid dehydrogenase	Autosomal recessive
Glutaric acidemia type II	Electron transfer factor deficiency	Autosomal recessive
Leber's optic atrophy	Mitochondrial oxidative phosphorylation complexes	Maternal
Myoclonic epilepsy and ragged red fibers	Mitochondrial oxidative phosphorylation complexes	Maternal
Leigh's disease	Mitochondrial oxidative phosphorylation complexes	Maternal

these enzymes that function in this acidic environment. Most of these enzymes are involved in the breakdown of endocytosed membrane components, and when defective, their nondegraded substrates accumulate in the lysosomes and macrophages of affected organs. Enzyme replacement therapy and substrate deprivation therapy are available interventions for some of these disorders.

I-Cell Disease

I-cell disease is an inborn error of post-translational processing of proteins directed to the lysosome. Clarification of this pathophysiology led to an understanding of the mechanisms by which lysosomal enzymes are trafficked and polarized through phosphorylation to remain in the acidic lysosomes. Patients with I-cell disease have inherited defects in the recognition markers required to direct enzymes to the endocytic receptor of the plasma membrane and to their capture in the acidic milieu of the lysosome. Patients lack all cellular lysosomal enzymes. Instead, empty lysosomes look like inclusion bodies ("I cell"). The misdirected lysosomal enzymes are secreted and are present in excess in plasma but are missing from cells. These extracellular enzymes were found to lack mannose 6-phosphate residues, and this observation led to an understanding of the post-translational mechanisms by which enzymes are directed to the lysosome and recaptured into endosomes by adding phosphorylated mannose to their protein structure. Individuals with I-cell disease lack this phosphotransferase activity.

Disorders of Mucopolysaccharides and Gangliosides

Inborn errors affecting single enzymes in the degradative pathway for mucopolysaccharides and gangliosides helped define the steps required for the breakdown of these complex macromolecules. Disorders of mucopolysaccharide metabolism include Hurler's syndrome; Scheie's syndrome; Hunter's syndrome; Sanfilippo's syndrome types A, B, C, and D; Morquio's syndrome types A and B; and Sly's syndrome (Chapter 268). Disorders of ganglioside metabolism include Fabry's disease, Gaucher's disease, Niemann-Pick disease (Chapter 215), Tay-Sachs disease, I-cell disease, fucosidosis, mannosidosis, sialidosis, and aspartylglycosaminuria.

Peroxisomal Diseases

Another group of inborn errors of metabolism defined by altered organelle function are *peroxisomal diseases* (Table 212-7). Peroxisomes are radiodense organelles, 0.5 to 1 nm in diameter, bounded by a single trilaminar membrane. Anabolic and catabolic reactions occur in this organelle. Primary pathways synthesize plasmalogens (unique fatty acids containing vinyl ethers), cholesterol, and bile acids. Other biosynthetic reactions include gluconeogenesis from amino acids and the formation of oxalic acid by the action of alanine-glyoxylate aminotransferase. Catabolic reactions include breakdown of hydrogen peroxide by peroxisomal catalase, a traditional protein of the peroxisome; polyamine oxidation; purine breakdown; ethanol oxidation; hydroxylation of phytanic acid; and degradation of pipecolic acid. A major function of the peroxisome is β-oxidation of very-long-chain fatty acids (>24 carbons). Diagnosis of these disorders entails finding an excess of very-long-chain fatty acids but reduced plasmalogen in blood.

An understanding of the importance of many reactions that occur in the peroxisome has come from identifying patients with either defects in individual biochemical pathways or lack of peroxisomes. The targeting signal for peroxisomal proteins may lie in their carboxyl-terminal end, and mutations in alanine-glyoxylate aminotransferase have resulted in mistargeting of this enzyme to mitochondria with consequent *familial hyperoxaluria*.

Errors In Nuclear Proteins

Several inborn errors are caused by abnormalities in proteins that function in the nucleus and are involved in gene expression or DNA repair (see class 2, Table 212-1). Patients expressing these inherited disorders carry a high risk for the development of cancer. Among these inborn errors of DNA repair are rare disorders, such as *xeroderma pigmentosum, Bloom's syndrome, ataxia-telangiectasia*, and *Fanconi's anemia*; diseases associated with early aging, such as *progeria, Cockayne's syndrome*, and *Werner's syndrome*; and more common adult-onset *nonpolyposis colon cancer*. Collectively, the disorders show increased sensitivity and delayed repair of DNA damaged as a result of ultraviolet, x-ray, or alkylating cross-link mechanisms. Disorders of nucleotide expansion of repeating elements such as -CGG- in the promoter region of the fragile-X protein (FMR1) result in cytosine methylation that turns off FMR1 protein expression with consequent dysregulation of the RNAs to which FMR1 binds.

Errors in Blood-Circulating Proteins

Many inborn errors involve proteins that circulate in blood (see class 3, Table 212-1). Stable circulating proteins in blood perform a variety of functions, including immunologic, hemostatic, regulatory, hormonal, and interorgan transport of trace metals, lipids, and other nutrients. Some inherited disorders affecting circulating proteins are tabulated in Table 212-8. Proteins involved in oxygen transport, coagulation, and immunity are detailed in other chapters, but the pathophysiologic mechanisms and genetic approaches of screening, diagnosis, and intervention to restore homeostasis and prevent an expected disease state make them appropriate to consider here as inborn errors of metabolism.

Abnormal Matrix Proteins

Abnormal matrix proteins produce inborn errors, such as Marfan syndrome (fibrillin), osteogenesis imperfecta (collagen type I) (Chapter 268), spondyloepiphyseal dysplasia (collagen type II), and Sachs' disease (collagen type III). These disorders exemplify class 4 of inborn errors of metabolism (see Table 212-1). The enzymes involved in post-translational processing of these proteins can also cause these syndromes. An example is Ehlers-Danlos syndrome (Chapter 268) type VI, in which procollagen lysyl hydroxylase

TABLE 212-7 INBORN ERRORS OF PEROXISOMES

NAME	GENE DEFECT	ABNORMAL ANALYTES
DISORDERS OF BIOGENESIS		
Zellweger's spectrum	PEX 1, 2, 3, 5, 6, 10, 12, 13, 14, 16, 19, 26 DLP1	Increased plasma very-long-chain fatty acids; bile acids intermediates, phytanic and pipecolic acids Decreased erythrocyte plasmalogen
Rhizomelic chondrodysplasia punctata, type I	PEX 7	Increased plasma phytanic acid Decreased erythrocyte plasmalogen
DISORDERS OF β-OXIDATION		
X-linked adrenoleukodystrophy	ABCD1	Increased plasma very-long-chain fatty acids
Acyl CoA oxidase deficiency	ACOX1	
Methylacyl CoA racemase deficiency	AMACR	Increased plasma very-long-chain fatty acids Increased plasma bile acid intermediates phytanic and pristanic acids
DISORDER OF PLASMALOGEN BIOSYNTHESIS		
Dihydroxyacetone phosphate acyltransferase deficiency	GNPAT	Decreased erythrocyte plasmalogen
DISORDER OF α-OXIDATION		
Refsum's disease	PHYH	Increased plasma phytanic acid only
DISORDER OF GLYOXALATE METABOLISM		
Hyperoxaluria, type I (alanine glyoxylate aminotransferase misplacement)	AGXT	Oxaluria

TABLE 212-8 SOME INBORN ERRORS OF PROTEINS THAT CIRCULATE IN BLOOD

FUNCTIONAL CLASS	PROTEIN	PHENOTYPE
Transport	Ceruloplasmin	Wilson's disease
	Albumin	Analbuminemia
	Hemoglobin	Hemoglobinopathies
	α-Lipoprotein	Analphalipoproteinemia
	β-Lipoprotein	Abetalipoproteinemia
	Transcobalamin II	Megaloblastic anemia
Hormones	Growth hormone	Pituitary dwarfism
	Insulin	Diabetes mellitus (insulin dependent)
	Somatomedin	Pituitary dwarfism
Coagulation	Factors I-XIII	Coagulopathies
	Kininogen	Kininogen deficiency
	Prekallikrein	Prekallikrein deficiency
Immune system	Complement components	Hypocomplementemias
	Immunoglobulins	Hypogammaglobulinemias
Inhibitors	α$_1$-Antitrypsin	Pulmonary emphysema and/or cirrhosis
	C1 esterase inhibitor	Angioneurotic edema
Drugs	Pseudocholinesterase	Prolonged paralysis after succinylcholine (Anectine) exposure

TABLE 212-9 APPROACHES TO TREATING INBORN ERRORS OF METABOLISM

Genetic counseling: prospective therapy
Diagnosis, recurrence risk assessment, informational transfer, support for resource allocation, identification of and intervention for "at-risk" relatives

Reproductive alternatives
Contraception, abstinence, artificial insemination, in vitro fertilization, risk taking with or without prenatal monitoring

Environmental engineering
Avoiding the offending agent
Supplemental physical, speech, occupational therapy

Metabolic management
Promote anabolism
Limit precursor of toxic substrate
Detoxify through alternative metabolic route
Provide feedback inhibitor
Provide supraphysiologic amounts of vitamin precursor

Molecular management
Provide gene expression and protein production
Provide stop codon read-through
Provide chaperone for misfolded protein

Protein and enzyme replacement
Infuse engineered enzyme
Provide clotting factors and peptide hormones
Transplantation
    Organ transplantation
    Bone marrow transplantation
    Stem cell transplantation (adult, hematopoietic, embryonic, nuclear transfer)

Genetic engineering
Somatic gene therapy
    Random insertion
    Homologous recombination (site specific)
Germline therapy

deficiency produces poorly hydroxylated lysyl residues in collagen. Inborn errors of matrix proteins are exemplified by disorders of collagen metabolism. More than 20 different genes dispersed on nine chromosomes are currently known to code for more than 13 different types of collagen. Abnormal proteins of matrix such as fibrillin 1 in the aorta may cause aberrant transforming growth factor-β signaling, inflammation, and consequent cystic medial necrosis with aortic dissection.

TREATMENT   (Rx)

Because the metabolic diseases considered in this chapter have in common causation by genes of large effect that disrupt normal homeostasis, we can consider a general approach to their treatment, as outlined in Table 212-9. The level at which therapy is rendered depends on the level of understanding of the pathophysiologic mechanisms producing disease and the interventional methods available.

Genetic Counseling

Genetic counseling is a unique and fundamental aspect of the management of inherited metabolic diseases and is used for all inherited diseases, even those whose mechanisms are not yet understood and for which no other treatment is available. Patients, their parents, and relatives usually ask questions such as the following: Why did this disease occur? Will this disease happen to me or my children? Can it be cured or prevented? Genetic counseling tries to answer these questions through processes involving probabilities derived from pedigree analysis. One cannot overemphasize the importance of an accurate family history, clinical diagnosis, and prognosis. A genetic discriminant is necessary for other family members before entering into formal genetic counseling. The genetic discriminant can be at the clinical, histologic, biochemical, or molecular level and must define whether an individual family member has or has not inherited the mutant allele or alleles. Transferring information about the burden of the phenotype, variation of clinical outcome including genotype-phenotype associations, and recurrence risks are important components of genetic counseling.

Environmental Engineering

Environmental engineering is the most commonly used approach to preventing disease in patients affected by inherited metabolic disease. Environmental factors (nutritional intake, exposure to toxins, sun, stress, climatic variation, and drug therapy) may produce a disease state in individuals who have inherited single genes or polygenic susceptibility to specific environmental stress. Newborn screening for galactose 1-phosphate uridyltransferase deficiency identifies infants susceptible to accumulation of galactose 1-phosphate, if they ingest human or cow milk. Restriction and replacement of lactose with sucrose save the lives of infants with galactosemia. Pharmacogenetic disorders exemplify the simple treatment of *avoidance* when the genetic susceptibility is identified. Health can be viewed as a continual adaptation between the genes and the environment. Environmental engineering is a form of genetic therapy in which individual genetic susceptibility is identified and the environment is altered to provide optimal health for the individual's unique genetic constitution. The frequency of diseases caused by genetic susceptibility to the environment varies from rare to 100%. *Scurvy* develops in all humans unless ascorbate is provided in the diet because we are unable to convert glucuronic acid to glucuronolactone and ascorbate. Humans and primates lost this anabolic pathway during evolution. By contrast, humans can usually synthesize tetrahydrobiopterin, a cofactor in many hydroxylase reactions, including phenylalanine hydroxylase. In some rare diseases (about 1 in 500,000) of increased blood phenylalanine and severe neurodegeneration, biopterin is not synthesized. Tetrahydrobiopterin can be provided to ameliorate this decreased product from the metabolic block.

Medical Therapy

Nutritional management and chemoprevention involve correction of the metabolic imbalance and return of the patient to homeostasis through diet manipulation and drug therapy. Many of the diseases mentioned in this chapter are amenable to several concurrent therapeutic approaches listed in Table 212-9.

For example, in disorders of the urea cycle, protein intake is limited, and anabolism is encouraged to reduce accumulation of ammonia from either protein intake or catabolism of lean body mass. Arginine is supplemented to provide deficient product of the blocked reaction, and alternative pathways are induced for nitrogen excretion. The latter therapy is made possible by a ubiquitous enzyme, *N*-glycine-acylase, that forms adducts with benzoic acid and glycine to produce hippuric acid, which is excreted, thereby eliminating one nitrogen molecule. Phenylacetylglutamine transferase is also used by giving phenylacetate to produce and excrete two nitrogen molecules as phenylacetylglutamine. Orotic aciduria is caused by mutations in the bifunctional enzyme orotate phosphoribosyltransferase-orotidine-5'-monophosphate decarboxylase. The disease process, which includes severe anemia and immune deficiency, is caused by a deficient end product, uridine, and is treated by replacing 100 to 200 mg/kg/day of uridine, up to 1 g three times daily (orally). Feedback inhibition of pituitary adrenocorticotropic hormone production is important in treating congenital adrenal hypertrophy with replacement doses of hydrocortisone to prevent virilization from overproduction of testosterone.

Vitamin dependency disorders require supraphysiologic amounts of a specific vitamin as the precursor for an active cofactor required for holoenzyme function. Many vitamin-dependent metabolic disorders are known and include pyridoxine (vitamin B$_6$)–dependent homocystinuria (Chapter 216) and vitamin C–dependent Ehlers-Danlos syndrome type VI (Chapter 268). In vitamin B$_6$–dependent homocystinuria, mutant cystathionine β-synthase is stabilized to biologic degradation when saturated with pyridoxal phosphate. Others include vitamin B$_{12}$–dependent methylmalonic aciduria, thiamine-dependent maple syrup urine disease, biotin-dependent multiple carboxylase deficiency, and biopterin-dependent hyperphenylalaninemia. Some blocked metabolic reactions can be augmented by inducing transcription of their gene. Phenobarbital and several other drugs induce hepatic uridine diphosphate glucuronyl transferase gene expression and reduce the accumulation of unconjugated bilirubin in Gilbert's syndrome (Chapter 149). In tyrosinemia type I, the drug NTBC blocks the catabolic pathway by which tyrosine produces the toxin, succinylacetone, when fumarylacetoacetate hydrolase is defective, and successfully prevents hepatic and renal dysfunction.

If the specific protein or enzyme has been purified and engineered to function in its specified organ or subcellular organelle, it can be used to treat an inherited metabolic disease. One good example is glucocerebrosidase, the enzyme that is impaired in Gaucher's disease (Chapter 215). This enzyme has been purified in large quantities from the placenta and from recombinant mammalian cells. The secreted enzyme is biochemically engineered to contain the mannose recognition site for cellular uptake by macrophages into lysosomal compartments. It has been used successfully to prevent and reverse the hypersplenism, pancytopenia, and bone disease of type I Gaucher's disease (Chapter 215). Many proteins are now made through recombinant techniques to treat metabolic disease. Enzymes now include glucocerebrosidase, factor VIII for hemophilia type A, growth hormone for growth hormone deficiency, α-galactosidase to treat Fabry's disease, iduronidase for Hurler-Scheie syndrome, and acid maltase for Pompe's disease. Several other engineered proteins used to treat inherited metabolic disease include 1-deamino-8-D-arginine vasopressin to treat X-linked recessive diabetes insipidus and recombinant α$_1$-antitrypsin made stable by inactivating methionine-385 for the treatment of α$_1$-antitrypsin deficiency. Some enzymes, such as adenosine deaminase, have been modified with polyethylene glycol to reduce immunogenicity and prolong their biologic half-life in blood. It is used to treat severe combined immunodeficiency. Chemoprevention is being developed for heritable cancers. Cyclooxygenase-2 inhibitors may prevent progression of colon polyps to adenocarcinoma, and estrogen receptor inhibitors may ameliorate some forms of breast cancer.

Treatment using chaperones and substrate reduction therapy represent novel approaches for lysosomal disorders in which substrate accumulation in brain cannot be reduced by intravenous therapy of bulky enzymes that do not cross the blood-brain barrier. Small molecules that inhibit ceramide glucosyl-transferase reduce the rate of glucosylceramide accumulation in Gaucher's disease types II and III as well as glycosphingolipids that accumulate in the brain of patients with Niemann-Pick disease type C (Chapter 215). Rhodamine B inhibits glucosamine-glycans accumulation in mucopolysaccharidosis. Chaperones are used to protect misfolded enzymes that will otherwise be destroyed before reaching their lysosomal compartment. Structural analogues of substrates for genetically misfolded α-galactosidase (Fabry's disease) (Chapter 215) are in trial as chaperones for missense mutations. Future use of "read-through molecules" for mutations producing stop codons are in trial. For example, gentamicin will read through stop codons in *CFTR* (cystic fibrosis) and dystrophin (Duchenne muscular dystrophy) genes.

Surgical Therapy

Surgical intervention may be a useful adjunct for treating heritable disorders. Stabilization of hypoplastic cervical vertebrae may prevent quadriparesis or death in a variety of chondrodysplasias and mucopolysaccharidoses accompanied by hypoplasia of the odontoid process or atlantoaxial instability. In Marfan syndrome (Chapter 268), careful monitoring of aortic root diameter with surgical removal of the aorta and prosthesis may prevent lethal aortic dissection. Losartan therapy may prevent the inflammatory response to mutant fibrillin and mitigate the need for this surgery. Evaluation of polyps and early colectomy may prevent disseminated adenocarcinoma in families with the autosomal dominant forms of familial polyposis coli. Molecular diagnosis of mutations in the *APC* gene helps identify at-risk family members and reassure members who did not inherit the mutant allele. Preventing heritable cancer by surveillance and early surgical excision is therapeutic for medullary thyroid carcinoma, Wilms' tumors, and the neurofibromas of von Recklinghausen's disease. Other examples of the benefit of preventive surgery for inborn errors include splenectomy for hemolytic anemias associated with spherocytosis, pyloroplasty for pyloric stenosis, and mastectomy and oophorectomy for patients with *BRCA1* or *BRCA2* mutations.

Transplantation

Organ transplantation (Chapter 48) for metabolic disorders that are lethal and have no other available therapy may be life-saving. Liver transplantation is an option in the long-term treatment of patients with urea cycle defects. Stem cells from cord blood (Chapter 181) are being used to treat neurodegenerative disorders in early childhood. Cloned embryonic cells or stem cells that are still naïve to adult antigens and adult bone marrow are promising therapeutic agents in research. Adult stem cells from differentiated organs are proving useful in improving myocardial function after heart failure from infarction.

Several principles are required for successful treatment of an inherited metabolic disorder by organ transplantation: (1) the normal enzyme, protein, or function must be provided by the transplanted organ or adult stem cell; (2) the pathogenesis must be understood to decide whether the affected organ should be removed; and (3) the host must be immunologically tolerant to the gene product being introduced, in addition to the transplanted organ itself. These principles are particularly relevant when displacement bone marrow transplantation is used. In the latter, normal donor stem cells differentiate and provide their enzymes to the recipient's reticuloendothelial system. Diseases associated with accumulation of products in the central nervous system are not yet ameliorated by bone marrow transplantation, although accumulation in bone, liver, and spleen is reduced. In one group of metabolic diseases, stem cell bone marrow transplantation is performed to prevent leukemia caused by inherited syndromes that are associated with defective DNA repair, such as Fanconi's anemia, Bloom's syndrome, and ataxia-telangiectasia. Liver or kidney transplantation can reverse growth and developmental delay in type I glycogen storage disease, cystinosis, acute intermittent porphyria, type I tyrosinemia, Fabry's disease, oxalosis, and non-neuronotropic lysosomal storage diseases. Lung transplantation has been successful for cystic fibrosis and α$_1$-antitrypsin deficiency, and prophylactic aortic transplantation has prevented aortic dissection in patients with Marfan syndrome.

Somatic Gene Therapy

Somatic cell gene therapy (Chapter 43) to treat patients with genetic disease continues in the arena of clinical research. Numerous laboratories throughout the world are actively designing strategies by which exogenous DNA can be incorporated into the genomic DNA of specific organs to provide a missing gene function and its protein product. Somatic gene therapy for many inherited metabolic diseases continues to be a goal of the future and awaits a nontoxic, stable vector with which to transfer normally transcribed genes.

SUGGESTED READINGS

Blau N, van Spronsen FJ, Levy HL. Phenylketonuria. *Lancet.* 2010;376:1417-1427. *Review of diet, tetra-hydrobiopterin therapy, and possible future treatments.*

GeneTests and GeneClinics. http://www.genetests.org/cgi-bin. Accessed Nov. 30, 2010. *This newly merged website offers updated information for physicians and investigators on the availability of diagnostic tests and reviews of diagnosis and intervention for many inherited metabolic disorders.*

National Center for Biotechnology. http://www3.ncbi.nlm.nih.gov/Omim. *The database can be searched by disease name and contains updated information on the history, biochemistry, and molecular biology of all inherited disorders caused by mutations in single genes.*

Society for Inherited Metabolic Disorders. http://www.simd.org. Accessed Nov. 30, 2010. *This website has links to an international collection of websites dealing with diagnosis and treatment guidelines for inherited metabolic disorders. Includes patient support groups.*

213

DISORDERS OF LIPID METABOLISM

CLAY F. SEMENKOVICH

Despite considerable progress, morbidity and mortality from vascular diseases are substantial and are likely to increase, given the epidemic of lipid-associated diseases such as obesity and diabetes, as well as the export of Western habits to the developing world. Recently discovered mediators of lipid metabolism continue to provide new insight into the mechanisms causing abnormal levels of cholesterol and triglycerides, among the most common problems encountered by practicing physicians.

COMPONENTS OF LIPID TRANSPORT

Cholesterol and Triglycerides

Cholesterol is a critical constituent of eukaryotic cell membranes and the precursor for the synthesis of steroid hormones such as cortisol, vitamin D, progestins, estradiol, and testosterone. Triglycerides carry fatty acids, nutrients that are used preferentially by muscle tissue and are especially important as an energy source in the fasting state. Because both cholesterol and triglycerides are essentially insoluble in water, the lipid transport system evolved to transport fats from one site to another through an aqueous environment.

Lipoproteins

Cholesterol and triglycerides are transported in lipoproteins (Table 213-1), spherical particles that differ in size and composition, depending on their site of origin. Each particle is composed of a central core consisting of cholesteryl esters (the product of an esterification reaction between the polar cholesterol molecule and a fatty acid) and triglycerides, both nonpolar compounds. Free cholesterol, phospholipids, and apolipoproteins are found on the particle surface.

Chylomicrons and their remnants are the largest lipoproteins. Produced by the intestine, these particles carry fats that are absorbed from the diet. Their residence time in the circulation after a meal is short, on the order of minutes in healthy people. Chylomicrons are large and light; that is, their density is low. Because fat floats on water, particles with high fat and low protein content have lower density. Very low density lipoprotein (VLDL) is a triglyceride-rich particle produced by the liver. The removal of triglycerides from VLDL converts this particle to intermediate-density lipoprotein (IDL), which is subsequently metabolized to yield low-density lipoprotein (LDL, popularly known as "bad cholesterol"). A covalent modification of the apolipoprotein (apo) in LDL, apo B100, results in the formation of lipoprotein (a). High-density lipoprotein (HDL, or "good cholesterol") is formed in the blood as a byproduct of the metabolism of triglyceride-rich lipoproteins and the acquisition of esterified cholesterol from peripheral tissues.

Apolipoproteins

Apolipoproteins are amphipathic molecules capable of interacting with both the lipids of the lipoprotein core and the aqueous environment of the plasma. They function as biochemical keys, allowing lipoprotein particles access to specific sites for the delivery, acceptance, or modification of lipids. Major apolipoproteins, their chromosomal locations with sequence accession numbers, and functions are shown in Table 213-2. Serum measurements of apolipoproteins may have clinical utility. For example, increased levels of apo B and decreased levels of apo AI are associated with vascular disease. Apo B48, specific for gut-derived particles, derives its name from the fact that it

TABLE 213-1 LIPOPROTEIN CHARACTERISTICS

LIPOPROTEIN	APOLIPOPROTEIN CONTENT	MAJOR LIPIDS	SIZE (NM DIAMETER)	DENSITY (G/ML)
Chylomicrons, chylomicron remnants	Apo B48, apo E, apo AI, apo AII, apo AIV, apo CII, apo CIII	Triglycerides from diet	80-500	<<1.006
VLDL	Apo B100, apo E, apo CII, apo CIII	Triglycerides from liver	30-80	<1.006
IDL	Apo B100, apo E	Cholesteryl esters, triglycerides	25-35	1.006-1.019
LDL	Apo B100	Cholesteryl esters	18-25	1.019-1.063
HDL	Apo AI, apo AII, apo AV	Cholesteryl esters, phospholipids	5-12	1.063-1.210
Lp(a)	Apo B100, apo(a)	Cholesteryl esters	~30	1.055-1.085

Apo = apolipoprotein; HDL = high-density lipoprotein; IDL = intermediate-density lipoprotein; LDL = low-density lipoprotein; Lp(a) = lipoprotein (a); VLDL = very low density lipoprotein.

TABLE 213-2 MAJOR APOLIPOPROTEINS

APOLIPOPROTEIN	CHROMOSOMAL LOCATION, GENBANK SEQUENCE IDENTIFICATION	FUNCTIONS
Apo B100	2p24-p23, M14162	Structural component of atherogenic lipoproteins (VLDL, IDL, LDL), VLDL secretion, ligand for LDL receptor, elevated levels associated with vascular disease
Apo B48	Same as apo B100	Chylomicron secretion from intestine
Apo E	19q13.31, K00396	Ligand for binding of triglyceride-rich particles to LDL receptor and LRP, potential roles in Alzheimer's disease and neuronal injury
Apo AI	11q23-q24, X02162	Structural component of HDL, activates LCAT, elevated levels associated with protection from vascular disease
Apo AII	1q21-Q23, NM_001643	Genetically and biochemically associated with familial combined hyperlipidemia
Apo AIV	11q23-qter, NM_000482	Potential role in regulating food intake
Apo AV	11q23, AF202889	Required for normal lipolysis of triglyceride-rich lipoproteins
Apo CII	19q13.2, X00568	Activator of LPL
Apo CIII	11q23-qter, X01388	Inhibitor of LPL
Apo (a)	6q26-q27, X06290	Covalent bond with apo B100 forms Lp(a) and renders particle resistant to uptake by LDL receptor

Apo = apolipoprotein; HDL = high-density lipoprotein; IDL = intermediate-density lipoprotein; LCAT = lecithin-cholesterol acyltransferase; LDL = low-density lipoprotein; Lp(a) = lipoprotein (a); LPL = lipoprotein lipase; LRP = LDL receptor–related protein; VLDL = very low density lipoprotein.

TABLE 213-3 IMPORTANT RECEPTORS AND PROTEINS IN LIPID TRANSPORT

PROTEIN	CHROMOSOMAL LOCATION, GENBANK SEQUENCE IDENTIFICATION	FUNCTIONS
LDL receptor	19p13.3, AY114155	Clearance of apo B100 and apo E–containing lipoproteins, activity increased by statin drugs, deficiency causes familial hypercholesterolemia
LDL receptor–related protein (LRP)	12Q13-Q14, NM_000014	Clearance of apo E–containing lipoproteins
Scavenger receptor B1 (SR-B1)	12q24.32, Z22555	HDL receptor
Lipoprotein lipase (LPL)	8p22, NM_000237	Rate limiting for triglyceride metabolism, deficiency causes chylomicronemia syndrome
Lecithin-cholesterol acyltransferase (LCAT)	16q22.1, NM_000229	Esterifies cholesterol in HDL to increase HDL cholesterol levels, deficiency decreases HDL levels
Cholesteryl ester transfer protein (CETP)	16q13, NM_000078	Exchanges cholesteryl ester in HDL for triglycerides in apo B–containing lipoproteins, deficiency increases HDL levels
ABCA1	9q31, AJ12376	Transfers cholesterol in tissues to nascent HDL particles, deficiency causes Tangier disease
PCSK9	1p32.3, NC_000001.10	Degrades LDL receptor, deficiency decreases LDL levels

ABCA1 = ATP binding cassette A1; apo = apolipoprotein; HDL = high-density lipoprotein; IDL = intermediate-density lipoprotein; LDL = low-density lipoprotein; PCSK9 = proprotein convertase subtilisin-like/kexin type 9.

is about 48% of the size of apo B100. Apo B100 and apo B48 are products of the same gene, with B48 resulting from the post-transcriptional introduction of a premature stop codon in the apo B messenger RNA by apobec1, a cytidine deaminase. Genetic variants in apolipoproteins can be associated with well-defined clinical syndromes.

Receptors and Proteins

Several receptors and proteins required for normal lipid transport are listed in Table 213-3.

Low-Density Lipoprotein Receptor

The LDL receptor mediates the removal of LDL as well as some VLDL and IDL particles by binding to apo B100 and apo E. The most important site of

LDL receptor expression is the liver, where its regulation is mediated by sterol regulatory element-binding proteins (SREBPs). SREBPs are found in inactive forms in the endoplasmic reticulum (ER). When cellular cholesterol levels rise after the delivery of cholesterol by the LDL receptor, increased ER sterol content causes cholesterol to bind to Scap, a protein that promotes the migration of SREBPs from the ER to the Golgi. In the Golgi, SREBPs undergo proteolytic conversion to active forms that move to the nucleus and stimulate the expression of genes involved in cholesterol synthesis. The binding of cholesterol to Scap induces a conformational change that causes it to bind to Insigs, ER anchor proteins. However, when intracellular cholesterol levels are high, the Scap/SREBP complex does not move to the Golgi, SREBPs are not processed, and cholesterol synthesis stops. When cholesterol levels are low, Scap is released from Insigs, the Scap/SREBP complex moves to the Golgi,

SREBPs are converted to active forms, and genes important for cholesterol synthesis and acquisition (such as the LDL receptor) are transcribed. Statin drugs effectively lower cholesterol. They inhibit 3-hydroxy-3-methylglutaryl coenzyme A (HMG-CoA) reductase, the rate-limiting enzyme in cholesterol synthesis. Cholesterol levels fall, Scap is free to shepherd SREBPs to the Golgi for activation, an active SREBP stimulates transcription of the LDL receptor gene, and increased levels of the LDL receptor protein on the surface of the hepatocyte bind and remove LDL particles from the circulation.

Low-Density Lipoprotein Receptor–Related Protein

The LDL receptor–related protein (LRP), also called the chylomicron remnant receptor, participates in the removal of intestine-derived lipoproteins by interacting with apo E. Chylomicron remnants carry apo B48, which is missing the LDL receptor binding domain, but these particles are also cleared by the LDL receptor through apo E binding.

Scavenger Receptor B1

Scavenger receptor B1 (SR-B1) is a protein expressed in liver that binds HDL. Unlike the LDL receptor that endocytoses LDL particles, SR-B1 does not appear to internalize HDL particles but instead facilitates the transfer of cholesteryl ester from HDL to the liver. Its genetic manipulation in mice has raised clinically relevant questions regarding the significance of elevated HDL levels. Inactivation of SR-B1 elevates HDL cholesterol levels but promotes atherosclerosis, presumably because of disruption of the transport of cholesterol from peripheral cells, where it can cause disease, to the liver, where it is excreted. These results suggest that it is not the level of HDL per se but the flux of cholesterol through HDL that affords protection from vascular disease.

Lipoprotein Lipase

Lipoprotein lipase (LPL) is rate limiting for the metabolism of triglyceride-rich lipoproteins and is required for the generation of HDL particles because HDL is absent from LPL-deficient mice. Deficient LPL activity thus provides a physiologic explanation for the common association between high triglyceride levels and low HDL cholesterol.

Lecithin-Cholesterol Acyltransferase

Another protein important in HDL metabolism is lecithin-cholesterol acyltransferase (LCAT). LCAT is associated with HDL in the circulation, where it esterifies free cholesterol to form cholesteryl esters that are easily stored in the nonpolar core of the lipoprotein. LCAT deficiency, a rare disorder, is characterized by low HDL as well as anemia and renal failure, clinical features probably related to disruption of the normal membrane function by the accumulation of excessive amounts of unesterified cholesterol.

Cholesteryl Ester Transfer Protein

Cholesteryl ester transfer protein (CETP) exchanges one molecule of cholesteryl ester in HDL for one molecule of triglyceride in apo B–containing particles such as VLDL. The resulting HDL particle is triglyceride enriched, enhancing its clearance (especially by an enzyme related to LPL, hepatic lipase) and lowering HDL. Inhibition of CETP activity increases HDL levels.

ATP Binding Cassette A1

ATP binding cassette A1 (ABCA1) is a cell membrane protein that mediates the transfer of cholesterol and phospholipids from cells to lipid-poor apo AI, a process that promotes HDL formation. ABCA1 in the liver contributes to the genesis of HDL, and overexpression of ABCA1 in macrophages may diminish atherosclerosis. Heterozygous ABCA1 deficiency is responsible for isolated low HDL cholesterol levels that occur in some kindreds (also known as familial hypoalphalipoproteinemia, based on an older term for HDL). Rare homozygotes for ABCA1 mutations have Tangier disease, characterized by the accumulation of cholesteryl esters in macrophages and resulting in distinctive features, including orange-yellow tonsils, neuropathy, and hepatosplenomegaly. HDL is very low to absent. Atherosclerosis is probably increased in these patients, but its extent may be moderated by concomitant low LDL levels.

Proprotein Convertase Subtilisin–Like/Kexin Type 9

Proprotein convertase subtilisin–like/kexin type 9 (PCSK9) is a secreted enzyme that promotes the degradation of the LDL receptor. Its overexpression decreases the LDL receptor, resulting in hyperlipidemia. PCSK9 deficiency in humans is associated with low LDL levels and less atherosclerosis.

Pharmacologic inhibition of PCSK9 would be predicted to have similar effects.

● EXOGENOUS LIPID METABOLISM

Animal products containing cholesterol and triglycerides are eaten regularly by most people. Dietary fats are broken down in the gut to free cholesterol and fatty acids, which are then transported across cell membranes into the enterocyte. There, they are re-esterified into cholesteryl ester and triglycerides and then packaged onto apo B48. These particles gain access to the plasma through the thoracic duct and acquire other apolipoproteins in part by transfer from HDL. These mature chylomicrons circulate to peripheral tissues. LPL, bound to the capillary endothelium in tissues such as adipose tissue and muscle, is activated by apo CII on chylomicrons, and fatty acids hydrolyzed from triglycerides by LPL are released and transported into adipose tissue for storage or into muscle for energy. This process also requires apo AV, an apolipoprotein transported in HDL that appears to facilitate the interaction between LPL and triglyceride-rich lipoproteins, as well as glycosylphosphatidylinositol-anchored high-density lipoprotein–binding protein 1 (GPIHBP1), a recently discovered protein that forms a platform for triglyceride metabolism at the endothelium.

Progressive hydrolysis of triglyceride converts chylomicrons into chylomicron remnants, which are relatively enriched in cholesteryl esters. Chylomicron remnants are removed in the liver by species that bind apo E: LRP, the LDL receptor, and cell surface glycosaminoglycans. Chylomicrons are large, and it is unlikely that they contribute to atherosclerosis. Chylomicron remnants are enriched in cholesteryl esters, the major lipid component of the atherosclerotic lesion, and small enough to enter the subendothelial space, where they are taken up by macrophages. Remnants are atherogenic, consistent with the idea that the progression of atherosclerotic lesions can occur in the postprandial state, a potential contributor to morbidity that is not assessed by current practices, which focus on the measurement of fasting lipoproteins.

Chylomicrons are not soluble. Their presence causes the "tomato soup" appearance of blood drawn after a fatty meal. Because they are mostly triglycerides, they float to the top of serum that is refrigerated overnight, leaving a layer of "cream" on top of the sample. The detection of chylomicrons in fasting serum has clinical relevance because it indicates a risk for pancreatitis and other elements of the chylomicronemia syndrome.

● ENDOGENOUS LIPID METABOLISM

Fats deposited in the liver are further metabolized into component lipid species, re-esterified as cholesteryl ester and triglycerides, and either stored in hepatocytes or exported as lipoproteins (Fig. 213-1). The liver produces the triglyceride-rich VLDL. Its rate of production appears to depend on the availability of triglycerides. Apo B100 is the major apolipoprotein of VLDL, but under normal conditions, regulation of the apo B gene does not appear to play an appreciable role in the control of VLDL synthesis. Production of the apo B100 protein depends on its cotranslational stabilization. As the message is translated into protein, the presence of triglyceride stabilizes the peptide and allows the continued addition of amino acids. In the absence of triglycerides, the apo B molecule is degraded. The transfer of triglycerides to the growing apo B peptide is mediated by microsomal transfer protein (MTP). Mutations in MTP cause abetalipoproteinemia, a rare disease characterized by the absence of circulating apo B. In the absence of apo B, the metabolism of fat-soluble vitamins (normally carried in lipoproteins) is disrupted, and patients with abetalipoproteinemia suffer from multisystem defects, including severe neurologic dysfunction and retinopathy that are presumably caused by deficiency of vitamins E and A. Drugs that interfere with MTP function lower lipids but, not surprisingly, cause the accumulation of triglyceride in the liver. The apo B gene is normal in patients with abetalipoproteinemia. Mutations in the apo B gene cause another condition known as hypobetalipoproteinemia, caused by shortened forms of the apo B protein. Subjects with hypobetalipoproteinemia have very low, but not absent, levels of circulating lipids and appear to be healthy.

Nascent VLDL containing one apo B100 molecule per particle is secreted into the plasma, where it acquires apo E, apo CII, and apo CIII. In a process analogous to that occurring with chylomicrons, apo CII on VLDL activates LPL, and fatty acids hydrolyzed from triglycerides by LPL are released in capillary beds and transported into tissues. With continued hydrolysis and the loss of both phospholipids and apolipoproteins to HDL, VLDL is converted to IDL, a cholesteryl ester–rich particle with an apolipoprotein

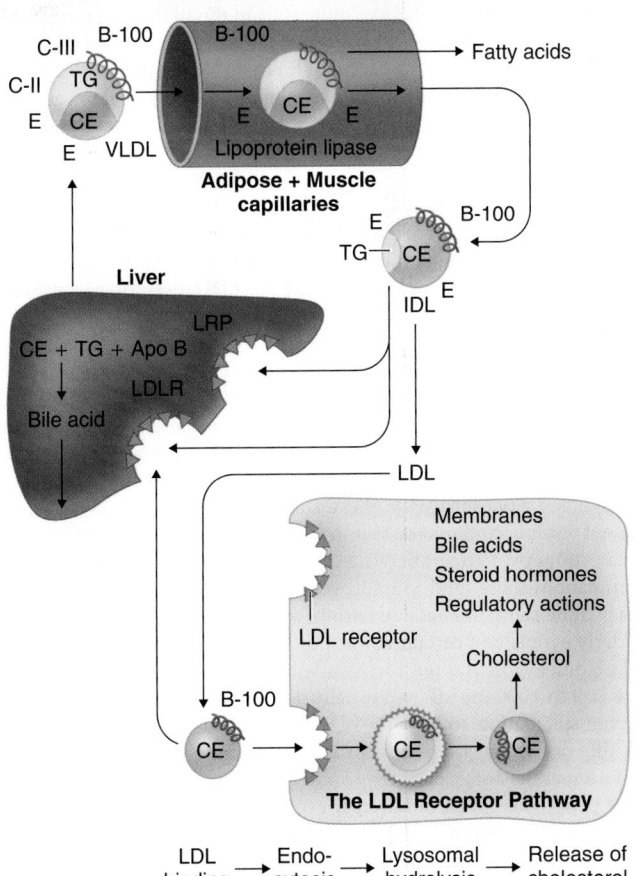

FIGURE 213-1. Endogenous lipid metabolism. In the liver, triglycerides (TG), cholesteryl esters (CE), and apolipoprotein B100 are packaged as very low density lipoprotein (VLDL) particles. TG is hydrolyzed by lipoprotein lipase to generate intermediate-density lipoprotein (IDL), which is further metabolized to generate low-density lipoprotein (LDL). This particle can be removed by the liver or by peripheral cells. Cholesterol derived from LDL regulates several processes and can be used for the synthesis of bile acids, steroid hormones, and cell membranes. LDLR = low-density lipoprotein receptor.

FIGURE 213-2. Reverse cholesterol transport and high-density lipoprotein (HDL) metabolism. Unesterified cholesterol (UC) in peripheral cells can be transferred to HDL and esterified by lecithin-cholesterol acyltransferase (LCAT). This cholesterol ester (CE) in HDL can be transferred to the liver directly through scavenger receptor B1 (SR-B1). Alternatively, it can be transferred to apolipoprotein B100–containing lipoproteins in exchange for triglycerides (TG) through the action of cholesteryl ester transfer protein (CETP). IDL = intermediate-density lipoprotein; LDL = low-density lipoprotein; LDLR = low-density lipoprotein receptor; VLDL = very low density lipoprotein.

beyond the determination of total cholesterol, triglycerides, LDL cholesterol, and HDL cholesterol.

REVERSE CHOLESTEROL TRANSPORT AND HIGH-DENSITY LIPOPROTEIN METABOLISM

Lipid metabolism is dynamic. At the same time lipoproteins are being processed to modify their nonpolar lipids, particles are interacting with one another, exchanging surface materials, apolipoproteins, and nonpolar lipids. HDL is an important reservoir for components cast off during the metabolism of other lipoproteins as well as lipids discarded by cells. Nascent HDL is generated by the liver and intestine as a phospholipid disc containing apo AI and apo AII. It accepts unesterified (free) cholesterol (UC in Fig. 213-2) and phospholipids shed from cells. This unesterified cholesterol is converted to cholesteryl ester by the action of LCAT and stored in the center of the disc, allowing it to become a spherical particle. The particle is further modified as a consequence of the action of LPL on triglycerides in apo B–containing lipoproteins. As the core triglycerides of VLDL are metabolized, the particle collapses, leaving redundant surface lipids (phospholipid in the form of lecithin and unesterified cholesterol) and excess apolipoproteins such as apo CII, apo CIII, and apo E, which are transferred to HDL. LCAT again esterifies the cholesterol to increase the content of cholesteryl ester in the HDL.

Reverse cholesterol transport is the beneficial process by which cholesterol present in peripheral cells, such as foam cells in a growing atherosclerotic lesion, is transported back to the liver for excretion. There are at least two well-defined pathways mediating this transfer. First, after accepting cholesterol from peripheral cells and esterifying it through the action of LCAT, HDL can interact directly with the liver by binding to SR-B1 and transferring cholesteryl ester to the hepatocyte. Second, HDL can transfer cholesteryl ester to apo B100–containing lipoproteins such as VLDL (see bottom of Fig. 213-2) through the action of CETP. This cholesteryl ester can ultimately be transported to the liver after conversion of VLDL to IDL to LDL and uptake by the LDL receptor (LDLR in Fig. 213-2). This pathway is not direct because the transfer of cholesteryl ester to apo B–containing lipoproteins results in cholesterol-enriched particles that may be taken up by foam cells in atherosclerotic plaques before being cleared by the liver. Humans with genetic defects in CETP have high HDL levels and appear to be healthy. An inhibitor of CETP, torcetrapib, increases HDL cholesterol but also increases adverse events, perhaps in part related to its adverse effects on blood pressure. The benefits of raising HDL with medications are uncertain; a meta-analysis of more than 100 randomized trials showed no reduction in coronary heart disease events by simply increasing HDL.∎

complement of only apo B and apo E. These particles, like chylomicron remnants, are thought to have high atherogenic potential. Unlike chylomicron remnants, IDLs are included in current management schemes because reporting of LDL cholesterol levels by most clinical laboratories includes IDL. IDL can be taken up by either the LRP or the LDL receptor in the liver. In the presence of a normal apo E molecule, IDLs are converted to LDL, consisting of one molecule of apo B100 per particle and a cholesteryl ester with essentially no triglycerides. About 75% of LDL is removed from the plasma by the LDL receptor pathway, and most of this takes place in the liver. The uptake of LDL results in the migration of LDL particles to lysosomes, where cholesterol is released for (depending on the cell type) plasma membrane localization, bile acid synthesis, steroid hormone synthesis, and interaction with Scap for the control of SREBP activation. A minority of LDL enters the subendothelial space of the vascular wall, where its modification by oxidation or other processes promotes its uptake by macrophages in atherosclerotic lesions.

Most VLDL particles are large and are not thought to promote vascular disease. However, some small VLDL particles as well as IDL and LDL are atherogenic. Because the majority of VLDL is triglyceride, most patients with elevated levels of fasting triglyceride have either increased numbers of VLDL particles or an increased triglyceride content in each VLDL. LDL has a plasma half-life of 2 to 5 days. The detection of elevated levels of fasting cholesterol usually reflects the presence of either increased numbers of LDL particles or increased cholesteryl ester in each LDL. LDL also exists in a range of sizes. Small, dense LDL tends to occur in the setting of concomitant hypertriglyceridemia. This type of lipoprotein is thought to have greater atherogenic potential than larger LDL species, perhaps because of easy access to the vascular wall and greater susceptibility to oxidative modification. Lipoprotein particle size and number can be quantified by nuclear magnetic resonance techniques, but it is not clear that these data provide diagnostic advantages

● LIPID-ACTIVATED NUCLEAR RECEPTORS AND LIPID METABOLISM

Nuclear receptors are transcription factors that are activated by ligand binding to increase the expression of specific sets of genes. Several nuclear receptors are activated by lipids, play important roles in systemic lipid metabolism, and are current or potential targets of medications for altering lipids in patients.

Peroxisome proliferator-activated receptors (PPARs, so named because their activation increases peroxisomes in rodents) are thought to be activated by fatty acids or their derivatives, such as phospholipids. There are at least three types: PPARα, PPARγ, and PPARδ. PPARα appears to be particularly important in liver and muscle. It stimulates the expression of genes mediating fatty acid oxidation as well as those promoting the formation of HDL. Fibrate drugs such as gemfibrozil and fenofibrate work by activating PPARα. They lower triglycerides by accelerating the oxidation of fatty acids in the liver, so that less lipid is available for stabilizing apo B100 in VLDL secretion, and they elevate HDL by increasing the expression of apo AI, LPL, and other genes. PPARγ is expressed mostly in adipose tissue and macrophages, but it also has measurable effects in other tissues, such as muscle. It increases the expression of genes promoting the development of fat tissue and appears to suppress chronic inflammation. Thiazolidinedione drugs such as pioglitazone and rosiglitazone work by activating PPARγ. They lower blood glucose in people with diabetes by decreasing insulin resistance, a complex process that also results in multiple lipid effects, including lower triglycerides and higher HDL (expected to be beneficial) and higher LDL (expected to be detrimental). Their use is complicated by volume expansion and an increased risk of heart failure. Combined PPARα-PPARγ agonists are in development. PPARδ is expressed widely; has multiple potential effects, including increased fatty acid oxidation; and is the subject of intense pharmacologic investigation.

Two other nuclear receptors are activated by lipids and modulate lipid physiology. Liver X receptors (LXRα and LXRβ) are activated by oxidized derivatives of cholesterol. In the liver, they promote the synthesis of fatty acids and triglycerides in addition to stimulating both the conversion of cholesterol into bile acids and the excretion of bile acids into the gut. In the intestine, they suppress the absorption of cholesterol. The farnesoid X receptor (FXR) is activated by bile acids. FXR stimulates the secretion of bile acids into bile as well as the reabsorption of bile acids from the intestine.

Together, these receptors help orchestrate two important, futile cycles in lipid metabolism. In one, fatty acids exported from the liver (in the form of triglycerides within VLDL) and from the intestine (in chylomicron triglycerides) are released to peripheral tissues by the action of LPL. Some are taken up by muscle, where their activation of PPARα accelerates their oxidation in mitochondria, yielding adenosine triphosphate. Others enter adipose tissue, where they are re-esterified into triglycerides. From there, fatty acids are released in a process stimulated by catecholamines and glucagon. This process is complicated, involving hormone-sensitive lipase, a recently discovered enzyme known as adipose triglyceride lipase, and the remodeling of proteins that coat lipid droplets to alter their accessibility to lipases. Following lipolysis, fatty acids bind to albumin and return to the liver, where they can fuel the production of more VLDL particles. Nicotinic acid improves lipids in part by blocking the release of fatty acids from adipose tissue. A G protein–coupled receptor for nicotinic acid has been identified.

In another futile cycle, bile acids (formed from cholesterol and constituting the major pathway for the excretion of cholesterol from the body) are secreted into the intestine through events stimulated by LXR and FXR. Bile acids are reabsorbed in the terminal ileum. Treatment with bile acid sequestrants such as colesevelam interrupts this enterohepatic circulation, and the increased excretion of cholesterol (in the form of bile acids) depletes cholesterol content in the liver, leading to the induction of LDL receptors and thereby lowering circulating levels of LDL. This treatment also tends to elevate triglyceride levels, the result of de-repression of several processes mediated by FXR that decrease fatty acids and triglycerides. Through effects likely involving both LXR and FXR, colesevelam lowers blood glucose in people with type 2 diabetes.

● IMPORTANT CLINICAL DISORDERS OF LIPID METABOLISM
Familial Hypercholesterolemia

EPIDEMIOLOGY

Familial hypercholesterolemia (FH) is an autosomal dominant form of hypercholesterolemia caused by defects in LDL receptor activity. The vast majority of affected patients have mutations in the LDL receptor gene. Heterozygotes for LDL receptor mutations occur at a frequency of perhaps 1 in 500 in the population, but they account for up to 5% of premature myocardial infarctions (those occurring in males younger than 55 and females younger than 65).

PATHOBIOLOGY

In addition to defects in the LDL receptor gene, other mutations can cause autosomal dominant hypercholesterolemia that is clinically indistinguishable from FH. These include familial defective apo B, caused by mutations that interfere with the ability of LDL to bind the LDL receptor, and variants in PCSK9.

CLINICAL MANIFESTATIONS

Total cholesterol levels are usually greater than 300 mg/dL, with LDL cholesterol levels greater than 200 mg/dL. Triglycerides are generally normal. Clinical features include thickening of the Achilles tendon as well as xanthomas at the extensor tendons of the knees and hands, reflecting the infiltration of lipid-laden macrophages at these sites. There is evidence that clinically apparent tendon xanthomas occur in a minority of patients with FH. Arthralgias are common, perhaps because of the presence of macrophage-mediated inflammation; these tend to improve with cholesterol lowering. Other features include xanthelasmas and corneal arcus, although the latter is also seen in elderly people and certain ethnic populations independent of cholesterol levels. Homozygotes (about 1 in 1 million) have total cholesterol levels in the range 800 to 1000 mg/dL and usually do not survive to adulthood without liver transplantation to provide LDL receptors. Children and adolescents with this disease may develop aortic valve disease because of macrophage infiltration at the aortic origin.

The penetrance of cardiovascular events in heterozygous FH is variable, with some subjects presenting with sudden death or accelerated disease in their 20s and others (generally women without other risk factors) surviving beyond menopause without clinically evident disease.

TREATMENT Rx

Treatment should address any associated risk factors for vascular disease, such as smoking, hypertension, and diabetes. Patients should be instructed in maintaining a diet low in saturated fat and cholesterol, and most require more than one cholesterol-lowering medication to achieve goals. The National Cholesterol Education Program provides periodic updates on the approach to screening and treating hyperlipidemia (Fig. 213-3). It is not uncommon for FH patients to be treated with a statin drug, a bile acid sequestrant such as colesevelam, and nicotinic acid. Some with aggressive disease require LDL apheresis, which involves perfusing blood through a column that extracts apo B–containing lipoproteins.

Familial Combined Hyperlipidemia

EPIDEMIOLOGY

Familial combined hyperlipidemia is an autosomal dominant form of hyperlipidemia that is present in up to 2% of the general population. It accounts for as many as 20% of cases of premature coronary artery disease.

PATHOBIOLOGY

The specific molecular defect is uncertain. Familial combined hyperlipidemia also appears to be associated with the metabolic syndrome (Chapter 237). The disorder is characterized by the primary overproduction of apo B. VLDLs secreted by the liver are small. Small, dense LDLs, thought to be particularly atherogenic, accumulate. For a given concentration of LDL cholesterol, patients with familial combined hyperlipidemia have greater numbers of LDL particles and an increased apo B concentration.

DIAGNOSIS

The diagnosis is made in the setting of a family history of premature coronary disease with different lipid phenotypes combined in the same family. Affected family members may have elevated triglycerides, elevated LDL cholesterol, or both, or they may have hypertriglyceridemia with low HDL cholesterol. Lipid phenotypes commonly change over time.

FIGURE 213-3. Approach to lipid screening and treatment. BP = blood pressure; CHD = coronary heart disease; HDL = high-density lipoprotein; LDL = low-density lipoprotein; PVD = peripheral vascular disease; TG = triglycerides. * >20% 10-year risk of cardiovascular events. (Based on recommendations from Executive summary of the third report of the National Cholesterol Education Program [NCEP] expert panel on detection, evaluation, and treatment of high blood cholesterol in adults [Adult Treatment Panel III]. *JAMA.* 2001;285:2486-2497.)

Familial Hypertriglyceridemia

Familial hypertriglyceridemia is also a common autosomal dominant disorder, occurring in 1 to 2% of the general population. Affected family members have isolated elevated triglycerides. A unifying molecular mechanism is lacking. The phenotype is stable, with affected family members consistently showing isolated hypertriglyceridemia on repeated analyses. The disorder is characterized by primary overproduction of triglyceride. Lipoprotein particles tend to be large, consisting of increased amounts of triglyceride relative to apo B. For a given level of cholesterol, these patients have lower numbers of lipoprotein particles and a decreased apo B concentration. The relationship between this disorder and cardiovascular risk is uncertain. Affected kindreds do not appear to have a propensity for premature vascular disease, but these individuals are at risk for the chylomicronemia syndrome when an additional stimulus for hypertriglyceridemia, such as uncontrolled diabetes, is present.

Chylomicronemia Syndrome

PATHOBIOLOGY

This syndrome occurs when triglycerides are extremely elevated, usually greater than 2000 mg/dL. Individuals with homozygous defects in the LPL gene can present with the syndrome in infancy, although the penetrance of clinical sequelae is extremely variable. Some individuals suffer repeated episodes of the syndrome throughout life, whereas others with triglycerides consistently above 2000 mg/dL remain completely asymptomatic. The basis for the wide spectrum of symptoms despite similar degrees of severe hypertriglyceridemia is unknown. Other molecular defects responsible for the syndrome include mutations in apo CII and apo AV.

Although defects in LPL, apo CII, and apo AV can cause the syndrome, the disorder is most likely to occur when patients with a common predisposition to hypertriglyceridemia (familial combined hyperlipidemia or familial hypertriglyceridemia) develop another defect associated with elevated triglycerides (such as uncontrolled diabetes, obesity, and treatment with glucocorticoids, estrogens, or other drugs).

CLINICAL MANIFESTATIONS

Clinical features include eruptive xanthomas on the back, buttocks, knees, and elbows; lipemia retinalis (a white appearance of retinal blood vessels, usually seen with triglycerides >4000 mg/dL); severe abdominal pain and pancreatitis (which can be life threatening); hepatosplenomegaly; dyspnea; lymphadenopathy; and neurologic dysfunction, such as memory loss and peripheral neuropathy.

DIAGNOSIS

Evaluation can be complicated by the presence of extreme hypertriglyceridemia, which interferes with the determination of amylase (pancreatic lipase should be measured when pancreatitis is suspected) and artifactually lowers serum glucose, sodium, and other analytes.

TREATMENT

Treatment consist of intravenous hydration and other supportive care for pancreatitis, complete elimination of dietary fat (which usually causes striking decreases in lipids within 24 to 48 hours), and appropriate blood glucose control with insulin in the setting of diabetes.

Dysbetalipoproteinemia

This rare disorder is caused by a mutation in apo E. There are three common variants of the apo E protein: E2, E3 (considered normal), and E4. Subjects with one or more E4 alleles are at risk for Alzheimer's disease. Subjects with two E2 alleles are at risk for dysbetalipoproteinemia. The frequency of this genotype is about 1% in the general population, but dysbetalipoproteinemia is rare, requiring an additional poorly defined factor. Hypothyroidism is known to precipitate the disorder. Subjects classically present with equal elevations of triglycerides and cholesterol in the range of about 300 to

600 mg/dL and xanthomas, especially in the palmar creases of the hands. They are at substantial risk for coronary artery disease. Unlike patients with FH, patients with dysbetalipoproteinemia are also at risk for severe peripheral vascular disease. Atherosclerosis occurs in part because of the presence of elevated concentrations of chylomicron remnants, which are not removed normally because of the presence of apo E2, and IDL particles, which are not converted normally to LDL in the presence of apo E2. It is unknown why the remnants that accumulate in dysbetalipoproteinemia cause both peripheral vascular disease and coronary disease, whereas the LDL particles that accumulate in FH tend to cause only coronary disease.

Diabetic Dyslipidemia

PATHOBIOLOGY

Insulin is a critical regulator of lipid metabolism, and because diabetes represents impaired insulin signaling, lipid disorders are common in both type 1 and type 2 diabetes (Chapters 236 and 237). Hypertriglyceridemia is the hallmark of diabetic dyslipidemia. This is driven by two mechanisms. First, LPL is insulin dependent. In the absence of insulin or in the presence of insulin resistance, LPL enzyme activity is deficient, and triglyceride-rich lipoproteins cannot be metabolized appropriately. Second, insulin suppresses the release of free fatty acids from adipose tissue stores. Insulin deficiency or resistance results in unabated release of free fatty acids, and these return to the liver, where they stabilize apo B synthesis and increase VLDL production.

TREATMENT Rx

The lack of insulin in patients with type 1 diabetes causes diabetic ketoacidosis, in which elevated triglycerides can be severe and are corrected by reinstitution of insulin therapy (Chapter 236). Intensive insulin therapy in type 1 diabetes decreases triglycerides, LDL, and often lipoprotein (a). Patients gain weight with intensive insulin therapy, and increased adiposity tends to lower HDL levels, which may explain why HDL does not always increase in intensively treated type 1 patients. Patients with type 2 diabetes usually have increased triglycerides and decreased HDL. These abnormalities improve but seldom normalize with better glycemic control. Most of the improvement occurs with initial pharmacologic glucose-lowering therapy, regardless of its mechanism of action.

Diabetes is frequently classified as a secondary cause of lipid disorders. However, lipid abnormalities are intrinsic to diabetes, and people with diabetes who lack clinical evidence of vascular disease have the same risk for cardiovascular events as those with established coronary disease. Therefore, every person with diabetes should be evaluated for lipid disorders, and adequate control of lipid levels often requires treatment with a statin drug. In patients with diabetes, cholesterol-lowering therapy reduces vascular mortality.[2] This intervention should not be delayed while glycemic control is optimized.

EVALUATION AND THERAPY OF LIPID DISORDERS

Diagnosis

The initial evaluation should include a complete history and physical examination, with careful attention to potential secondary causes of lipid disorders (Table 213-4). Diabetes, hypothyroidism, and excess alcohol intake are probably the most common secondary contributors to abnormal lipid metabolism.

Among prescription medications, β-adrenergic blocking agents are frequent contributors to abnormal lipid profiles. These agents have proven beneficial effects after myocardial infarction but also tend to promote weight gain, elevate triglycerides, and decrease HDL. Many clinicians are using lower doses of these agents and relying on more lipid-neutral drugs (angiotensin-converting enzyme inhibitors and angiotensin receptor blockers) for blood pressure control.

It is now common for internists to encounter patients with human immunodeficiency virus (HIV) infection with hyperlipidemia. Some series estimate that more than half of HIV patients treated with protease inhibitors for 2 years develop dyslipidemia, frequently with a redistribution of fat resembling that in genetic lipodystrophy syndromes (Chapter 396). Newer protease inhibitors appear to have fewer metabolic sequelae than older agents such

TABLE 213-4 SECONDARY CAUSES OF LIPID DISORDERS

CONDITION/MEDICATION	COMMENTS
Diabetes	Common contributor to dyslipidemia; abnormal lipids are seldom normalized by glycemic control alone
Hypothyroidism	Thyroid hormone regulates multiple steps in lipid metabolism, including LDL receptor expression and LPL activity
Alcohol	Can cause hypertriglyceridemia in susceptible patients, but mild intake linked to decreased risk of vascular disease
Renal disease	Increased LDL in nephrotic syndrome, hypertriglyceridemia in end-stage renal disease
Obstructive liver disease	Can be associated with very high cholesterol levels; some evidence that diseases such as primary biliary cirrhosis are not associated with increased vascular events despite dyslipidemia
Diuretics	Increased LDL with high doses; current practice of using low doses of thiazides decreases vascular events and has minimal effect on lipids
β-Adrenergic receptor blockers	Increased triglycerides and decreased HDL, probably by inhibiting LPL
Anabolic steroids	Can result in very low HDL (<10 mg/dL)
Estrogens	Exacerbate hypertriglyceridemia when given orally; this effect is not seen with topical estrogen therapy
Protease inhibitors	Increased triglycerides and decreased HDL especially in the setting of HIV-associated lipodystrophy
Glucocorticoid excess	Increased triglycerides and decreased HDL, probably related to exacerbation of insulin resistance
Antipsychotics	Increased triglycerides and decreased HDL, probably related to increased adiposity and insulin resistance
Retinoids	Increased triglycerides
Systemic lupus erythematosus	Chronic inflammation may increase risk of vascular disease independent of effects on lipid metabolism
Acute intermittent porphyria	Many agents used to treat lipid disorders reported to provoke episodes of abdominal pain

HDL = high-density lipoprotein; HIV = human immunodeficiency virus; LDL = low-density lipoprotein; LPL = lipoprotein lipase.

as ritonavir. In addition to appropriate management of other risk factors, lipid-lowering therapy should be tailored to the ongoing HIV drug regimen. Pravastatin is least likely to interact with protease inhibitors but is less effective at lowering LDL cholesterol. Agents such as simvastatin that are substantially metabolized by the cytochrome P-450 3A4 system should not be used in patients treated with protease inhibitors because of delayed clearance of the statin. PPARα agonists such as fenofibrate can be used to lower triglycerides, but the effects are limited because their clearance is accelerated by protease inhibitor treatment.

Antipsychotics have complex effects on metabolism. Some of the newer agents used to treat schizophrenia promote hyperlipidemia, obesity, and insulin resistance. Although therapeutic decisions should be based on psychiatric responses, substituting for agents with prominent metabolic side effects, such as olanzapine, can improve lipid profiles.

Laboratory Evaluation

After an 8- to 12-hour fast (subjects should be told that it is acceptable to drink water and other calorie-free beverages during this period), total triglycerides, total cholesterol, HDL cholesterol, and LDL cholesterol should be measured. In most clinical laboratories, LDL cholesterol is still calculated using this formula: LDL = total cholesterol − HDL cholesterol − (triglycerides/5). This formula is not valid when triglycerides are greater than 400 mg/dL, however. It is also possible to measure LDL directly, which is sometimes useful for monitoring the therapeutic effects on LDL alone, and this determination does not require patients to fast. Excessive lipid determinations may not be helpful. Biologic and random variability in cholesterol levels is considerable, and for patients with levels that are 19 mg/dL or more below their goal, serial monitoring is more likely to detect false-positive than true-positive increases over a period of 3 years.

What constitutes "normal" lipid levels is unknown. For triglycerides, the Adult Treatment Panel III of the National Cholesterol Education Program identified a normal triglyceride level as less than 150 mg/dL. Values from 150 to 199 are borderline high, 200 to 499 is considered high, and above 500 is very high. In patients with fasting triglycerides greater than 500 mg/dL, triglycerides are a primary target of therapy in order to decrease the risk of pancreatitis and chylomicronemia syndrome. These individuals are treated with a very low fat diet (usually 15% of calories from fat), an exercise program, a weight-loss regimen in the setting of obesity, glycemic control in the setting of diabetes, and either nicotinic acid or a fibrate drug alone or in combination with fish oils.

Risk Assessment

In 2001 the Adult Treatment Panel III identified therapeutic goals for LDL cholesterol levels based on the 10-year risk of coronary heart disease, and it updated these goals in 2004. High risk, with a greater than 20% probability of a vascular event in 10 years, includes those with coronary heart disease (myocardial infarction, angina of any type, previous coronary artery procedure, known myocardial ischemia) or a coronary heart disease equivalent (diabetes, carotid artery disease, abdominal aortic aneurysm, peripheral vascular disease, multiple risk factors indicating a 10-year risk >20%). For these high-risk patients, the LDL goal is less than 100 mg/dL; less than 70 mg/dL is an optional goal.

Risk factors for coronary heart disease include smoking, hypertension (or treatment for hypertension), family history of premature coronary heart disease (younger than 55 years in males, 65 in females), low HDL (<40), and age (older than 45 in men, 55 in women). For those with two or more risk factors and a calculated 10-year risk for coronary heart disease less than 20%, the LDL goal is less than 130 mg/dL. For those with one or no risk factors, the LDL goal is less than 160 mg/dL.

These recommendations are likely to be modified as new data are incorporated into practice. The most recent updates, as well as 10-year risk calculators that are useful for customizing recommendations for individuals patients, are available at http://www.nhlbi.nih.gov/guidelines/cholesterol.

TREATMENT Rx

General Measures
Intensive Lowering of Low-Density Lipoproteins

Randomized clinical trials support the concept that intensive LDL lowering is appropriate for patients with coronary heart disease and its equivalents. In the Heart Protection Study, those who entered the study with LDL less than 100 mg/dL benefited from further lowering of LDL with simvastatin.[3] In the Pravastatin or Atorvastatin Evaluation and Infection Therapy trial, patients with acute coronary syndrome derived greater benefit with an LDL of 62 mg/dL achieved with atorvastatin than with an LDL of 95 mg/dL achieved with pravastatin.[4] In the Treating to New Targets study, patients with stable coronary heart disease had fewer clinical events with an LDL of 77 mg/dL achieved with 80 mg of atorvastatin than with an LDL of 101 mg/dL achieved with 10 mg of the same drug.[5] Those with metabolic syndrome also accrued benefits in the Treating to New Targets study.[6] In the Incremental Decrease in End Points through Aggressive Lipid-Lowering study, there were fewer secondary end points among patients with stable coronary heart disease with an LDL of 81 mg/dL achieved with 80 mg of atorvastatin compared with an LDL of 104 mg/dL achieved with 20 mg of simvastatin.[7] In healthy individuals with LDL less than 130 mg/dL and C-reactive protein greater than 2 mg/dL, rosuvastatin (20 mg/day) reduced major cardiovascular events by 44% and all-cause mortality by 20%.[8]

Lifestyle Changes

Therapeutic lifestyle changes should be recommended as part of the treatment regimen. These include smoking cessation, weight reduction, exercise on most days of the week, reduced intake of dietary cholesterol to less than 200 mg/day, reduction of saturated fat to less than 7% of total calories, increased soluble fiber intake (to at least 10 g/day), and consumption of plant stanols or sterols (2 g/day).

Medical Therapy

Medications commonly used to treat lipid disorders are listed in Table 213-5.

Statins

Statins are by far the most effective. An analysis of results from 90,000 participants in statin trials suggested that the 5-year incidence of cardiovascular events decreases by about 1% for each 2 mg/dL decrease in LDL. The benefit appears to be independent of a patient's baseline lipid values. Patients at sufficient risk should be treated so that LDL is lowered by 30 to 40%, regardless of initial levels.

Statins are well tolerated. Up to 5% of patients have mildly elevated serum transaminases with therapy, which is usually asymptomatic and resolves

TABLE 213-5 MEDICATIONS USED TO TREAT LIPID DISORDERS

CLASS	SIDE EFFECTS	LIPID EFFECTS	SPECIFIC AGENTS (DOSE)
Statins (HMG-CoA reductase inhibitors)	Mildly increased liver enzymes, myalgias without evidence of muscle disease, constipation, insomnia, rhabdomyolysis (rare)	↓↓LDL, 18-55% ↑HDL, 5-15% ↓TG, 7-30%	Simvastatin (20-80 mg/day) Atorvastatin (10-80 mg/day) Pravastatin (20-80 mg/day) Fluvastatin (20-80 mg/day) Lovastatin (20-80 mg/day) Rosuvastatin (10-40 mg/day)
Nicotinic acid	Flushing, nausea, diarrhea, hyperglycemia, hyperuricemia, hepatotoxicity (rare)	↑↑HDL, 15-35% ↓↓TG, 20-50% ↓LDL, 5-25% ↓Lp(a), variable	Extended-release or crystalline niacin (1-2 g/day)
Fibrates	Mildly increased liver enzymes, dyspepsia, gallstones, hepatotoxicity (rare), rhabdomyolysis (rare)	↓↓TG, 20-90% ↑HDL, 10-20%	Gemfibrozil (1.2 g/day) Fenofibrate (34-200 mg/day)
Cholesterol absorption inhibitor	Hepatitis, abdominal pain, back pain, arthralgias	↓LDL, 18%	Ezetimibe (10 mg/day)
Bile acid sequestrants	Constipation, decreased absorption of some drugs	↓LDL, 15-30% ↑TG, variable ↑HDL, 3-5%	Colesevelam (2.5-3.75 g/day); this agent also approved for lowering glucose in type 2 diabetes Cholestyramine (4-16 g/day) Colestipol (2-16 g/day)
Fish oils	Eructation, dyspepsia	↓TG, variable ↑ LDL, variable	Omega-3-acid ethyl esters (variable)

HDL = high-density lipoprotein; HMG-CoA = 3-hydroxy-3-methylglutaryl coenzyme A; LDL = low-density lipoprotein; Lp(a) = lipoprotein (a); TG = triglyceride.

spontaneously. Therapy should be discontinued if elevations exceed three times the upper limit of normal or if patients have symptoms of liver dysfunction (especially fatigue and weight loss). Rhabdomyolysis is rare and more likely in the setting of concurrent treatment with azole antifungals, erythromycin, cyclosporine, and several other agents. Common side effects include constipation, abdominal pain, and difficulty sleeping. A substantial minority of patients treated with statins develop myalgias without physical findings or laboratory evidence of muscle dysfunction. The cause of this side effect is unknown. Patients with this complaint should be evaluated for hypothyroidism, vitamin D deficiency, rheumatologic disorders, and depression. The problem may be resolved by changing to a different statin or by stopping the medication, allowing symptoms to resolve, and restarting at a much lower dose with gradual increases over weeks.

Given the success of statins, it is not surprising that they are also formulated with other agents. Pravastatin with aspirin, atorvastatin with amlodipine, simvastatin or lovastatin with extended-release niacin, and simvastatin with ezetimibe are available as single pills. Outcome data for these combinations are not available. If both agents are indicated, these combinations can enhance compliance and decrease patients' copayment costs.

Nicotinic Acid

Nicotinic acid is a B complex vitamin required to prevent pellagra. When administered in high doses, it has potent triglyceride-lowering and HDL-elevating effects and a modest LDL-lowering effect. A once-daily extended-release form appears to be safe and effective. The most common side effect is flushing, which frequently diminishes over time. The intensity of flushing can be diminished with aspirin, by taking the medication with a small snack, and by avoiding hot beverages at that time. Nicotinic acid has been used safely with simvastatin in patients with vascular disease to induce atherosclerotic regression.

Fibrates

Fibrates are effective for lowering triglycerides in patients with very high levels who are at risk for pancreatitis, especially those who cannot tolerate niacin. These drugs increase HDL (although not as effectively as niacin) but also tend to increase LDL in patients with high triglycerides. The effects of fibrates in clinical trials have been mixed.[9] Many clinicians use fibrates with statins in high-risk patients with mixed hyperlipidemia, which should be done cautiously because of the increased risk of rhabdomyolysis with this combination. The combination of fenofibrate and simvastatin did not reduce nonfatal myocardial infarction, nonfatal stroke, or fatal cardiovascular events compared with simvastatin alone in patients with type 2 diabetes.[10]

Other Agents

Ezetimibe lowers both LDL and triglycerides, with minimal effects on HDL. It is effective at achieving additional LDL lowering when used in combination with a statin. However, there is currently no evidence that LDL lowering with ezetimibe provides a corresponding reduction in clinical events. In those with coronary disease or a coronary risk equivalent, combining extended-release niacin with statin therapy was superior to combining ezetimibe with statin therapy in terms of decreasing carotid intima-media thickness.[11] There were fewer cardiovascular events in the niacin-statin group.

Bile acid sequestrants have been shown to lower LDL and decrease cardiovascular event rates. They are especially effective when combined with statins. Acceptance by patients is limited because of gastrointestinal side effects. These agents also tend to elevate triglycerides and decrease the absorption of some drugs, an effect that is less of an issue with colesevelam.

Fish oils may be used as an adjunct in the therapy of patients with very high triglycerides. These omega-3 fatty acids, which occur naturally in cold-water fish, may work by activating PPARα. They tend to elevate LDL but may also have beneficial anti-inflammatory properties.

● PRIMARY PREVENTION

The results of clinical trials (see Treatment) strongly support lipid lowering for secondary prevention, that is, preventing events in those with known disease. Data are less compelling for primary prevention, that is, preventing events in those without known disease. There is evidence that the use of a statin to lower lipids is effective for primary prevention in at least three groups: patients with multiple risk factors, individuals with type 2 diabetes, and middle-aged and older people with relatively low LDL levels in the setting of elevated C-reactive protein. In the Anglo-Scandinavian Cardiac Outcomes Trial—Lipid-Lowering Arm, subjects with hypertension and at least three other risk factors had fewer events with an LDL of 90 mg/dL achieved with atorvastatin than with an LDL of about 130 mg/dL in control subjects.[12] In the Collaborative Atorvastatin Diabetes Study, people with type 2 diabetes had fewer events with an LDL of about 75 mg/dL achieved with atorvastatin compared with placebo-treated subjects with an LDL of about 119 mg/dL.[13] In the Justification for the Use of Statins in Prevention:

An Intervention Trial Evaluating Rosuvastatin, men over the age of 50 and women over the age of 60 had fewer events and were less likely to die with an LDL of about 55 mg/dL achieved with rosuvastatin compared with placebo-treated subjects with an LDL of about 108 mg/dL.[8]

In short, there does not appear to be a threshold effect of LDL on atherogenesis. In people with established coronary heart disease and those with diabetes, reaching very low LDL cholesterol levels is desirable. The absolute value at which maximal benefit is reached is unknown, and higher doses of statins are associated with more side effects (especially increased serum transaminases), but some analyses assume that an LDL of 40 mg/dL represents no increased risk of vascular disease.

1. Briel M, Ferreira-Gonzalez I, You JJ, et al. Association between change in high density lipoprotein cholesterol and cardiovascular disease morbidity and mortality: systemic review and meta-regression analysis. *BMJ.* 2009;338:b92.
2. Cholesterol Treatment Trialists' (CTT) Collaborators, Kearney PM, Blackwell L, et al. Efficacy of cholesterol-lowering therapy in 18,686 people with diabetes in 14 randomised trials of statins: a meta-analysis. *Lancet.* 2008;371:117-125.
3. Heart Protection Study Collaborative Group. MRC/BHF Heart Protection Study of cholesterol lowering with simvastatin in 20,536 high-risk individuals: a randomised placebo-controlled trial. *Lancet.* 2002;360:7-22.
4. Cannon CP, Braunwald E, McCabe CH, et al. Intensive versus moderate lipid lowering with statins after acute coronary syndromes. *N Engl J Med.* 2004;350:1495-1504.
5. LaRosa JC, Grundy SM, Waters DD, et al. Intensive lipid lowering with atorvastatin in patients with stable coronary disease. *N Engl J Med.* 2005;352:1425-1435.
6. Deedwania P, Barter P, Carmena R, et al. Reduction of low-density lipoprotein cholesterol in patients with coronary heart disease and metabolic syndrome: analysis of the Treating to New Targets study. *Lancet.* 2006;368:919-928.
7. Pedersen TR, Faergeman O, Kastelein JJ, et al. High-dose atorvastatin vs usual-dose simvastatin for secondary prevention after myocardial infarction: the IDEAL study: a randomized controlled trial. *JAMA.* 2005;294:2437-2445.
8. Ridker PM, Danielson E, Fonseca FA, et al. Rosuvastatin to prevent vascular events in men and women with elevated C-reactive protein. *N Engl J Med.* 2008;359:2195-2207.
9. Keech A, Simes RJ, Barter P, et al. Effects of long-term fenofibrate therapy on cardiovascular events in 9795 people with type 2 diabetes mellitus (the FIELD study): randomised controlled trial. *Lancet.* 2005;366:1849-1861.
10. The ACCORD Study Group: Effects of combination lipid therapy in type 2 diabetes mellitus. *N Engl J Med.* 2010;362:1563-1574.
11. Taylor AJ, Villines TC, Stanek EJ, et al. Extended-release niacin or ezetimibe and carotid intima-media thickness. *N Engl J Med.* 2009; 361:2113-2122.
12. Sever PS, Dahlof B, Poulter NR, et al. Prevention of coronary and stroke events with atorvastatin in hypertensive patients who have average or lower-than-average cholesterol concentrations, in the Anglo-Scandinavian Cardiac Outcomes Trial—Lipid Lowering Arm (ASCOT-LLA): a multicentre randomised controlled trial. *Lancet.* 2003;361:1149-1158.
13. Colhoun HM, Betteridge DJ, Durrington PN, et al. Primary prevention of cardiovascular disease with atorvastatin in type 2 diabetes in the Collaborative Atorvastatin Diabetes Study (CARDS): Multicentre randomised placebo-controlled trial. *Lancet.* 2004;364:685-696.

SUGGESTED READINGS

Joy TR, Hegele RA. Narrative review: Statin myopathy. *Ann Intern Med.* 2009;150:858-868. *A review of how to approach a poorly understood but common problem in clinical practice.*

Jun M, Foote C, Lv J, et al. Effects of fibrates on cardiovascular outcomes: a systematic review and meta-analysis. *Lancet.* 2010;375:1875-1884. *Fibrates can decrease major cardiovascular events by about 10 to 13%.*

Kuklina EV, Yoon PW, Keenan NL. Trends in high levels of low-density lipoprotein cholesterol in the United States, 1999-2006. *JAMA.* 2009;302:2104-2110. *The prevalence of high LDL-C levels in the U.S. decreased from about 32% to about 21% from 1999 to 2006.*

National Heart, Lung, and Blood Institute. National Cholesterol Education Program. www.nhlbi.nih.gov/about/ncep/index.htm. *Website with information for health professionals and patients.*

Nichols GA, Arondekar B, Carrison LP Jr. Patient characteristics and medical care costs associated with hypertriglyceridemia. *Am J Cardiol.* 2011;107:225-229. *Severe hypertriglyceridemia with levels ≥500 mg/dL was independently associated with increased medical care costs, but less severe elevations were not.*

Stein EA. Other therapies for reducing low-density lipoprotein cholesterol: medications in development. *Endocrinol Metab Clin North Am.* 2009;38:99-119. *Assessment of novel approaches for lowering atherogenic lipoproteins.*

GLYCOGEN STORAGE DISEASES

JOSEPH I. WOLFSDORF AND DAVID A. WEINSTEIN

▶ DEFINITION

Glycogen, a highly branched polymer of glucose, is the storage form of glucose in mammals. The major sites of glycogen deposition are skeletal muscle and liver. Several other tissues and organs, including cardiac and smooth muscle, kidney, brain, and intestine, are sites of glycogen synthesis, which can be impaired in the glycogen storage diseases (GSDs).

EPIDEMIOLOGY

The overall frequency of the GSDs is approximately 1 per 20,000 to 25,000 births. Fifteen distinct types have been identified, and they are referred to by either the deficient enzyme or a numbering system that reflects the historical sequence of their description. All are uncommon, and some are extremely rare. Six types account for approximately 97% of GSD cases: GSD I (25%), GSD II (15%), GSD III (24%), GSD IV (3%), and GSD VI and IX (30%).

PHYSIOLOGY

Glucose transporter type 2 (GLUT2) predominates in the liver (and pancreatic beta cells) and has a high K_m ($\approx$15 to 20 mmol/L); consequently, the free glucose concentration in hepatocytes increases in direct proportion to the increase in plasma glucose concentration. Glucose is rapidly phosphorylated by glucokinase to form glucose-6-phosphate, which is converted to glucose-1-phosphate, the starting point for glycogen synthesis (Fig. 214-1). Hepatic glycogen synthase catalyzes the formation of α-1,4-linkages, which elongate the chains of glucose molecules. A branching enzyme leads to the formation of α-1,6-linkages at branch points along the chain. The concentration of GLUT4 in the plasma membrane of skeletal muscle increases markedly after exposure to insulin and in response to exercise, resulting in increased glucose transport into skeletal muscle, where it is either oxidized to provide energy for contracting muscle or converted to glycogen.

In the intervals between meals and during the overnight fast, a cascade of enzymatic reactions (including adenylyl cyclase, phosphorylase b kinase, and cyclic adenosine monophosphate–dependent protein kinase) activates hepatic glycogen phosphorylase, the rate-limiting enzyme in glycogenolysis, leading to the formation of glucose-6-phosphate. Glucose-6-phosphatase catalyzes the terminal reaction of both glycogenolysis and gluconeogenesis, the hydrolysis of glucose-6-phosphate, thereby allowing glucose to be released from the liver into the systemic circulation. This process is critical for the maintenance of glucose homeostasis. Because muscle lacks glucose-6-phosphatase, it cannot release glucose for systemic use. Muscle glycogen is used to meet the energy requirements of contracting muscle and is a source of lactate, pyruvate, and alanine for gluconeogenesis early in starvation. The rate of glycogenolysis in muscle is most rapid during the first 5 to 10 minutes of exercise. As exercise continues and blood flow to muscle increases, blood-borne substrates (glucose and free fatty acids) become increasingly important sources of energy.

PATHOBIOLOGY

The glycogen storage diseases (GSDs) or glycogenoses comprise several inherited disorders of glycogen synthesis or degradation. All are autosomal recessive with the exception of a subtype of GSD IX that is X-linked. They are caused by mutations in the genes that code for enzymes involved in the synthesis or degradation of glycogen and may involve the liver, skeletal muscle, and the kidney. They are all characterized by an abnormal tissue concentration or structure (or both) of the glycogen molecule. Molecular genetic testing performed on DNA extracted from blood or saliva is used to diagnose all the common forms of GSD.

CLINICAL MANIFESTATIONS

Hepatomegaly and hypoglycemia are the principal clinical manifestations of the hepatic glycogenoses, whereas muscle cramps, exercise intolerance, easy fatigability, and progressive weakness are the major manifestations of the muscle glycogenoses. Features of the most common GSDs are shown in Table 214-1.

TREATMENT   Rx

The goal of treatment of the hepatic forms of GSD is to prevent hypoglycemia and glucose counter-regulation. The specific details of therapy depend primarily on whether normal gluconeogenesis can occur. In GSD I, abnormal glucose-6-phosphatase activity impairs both glycogenolysis and gluconeogenesis. In contrast, gluconeogenesis is intact in the other liver forms of GSD, allowing protein to be used as a substrate for endogenous glucose production.

Treatment of GSD I consists of providing a continuous dietary source of glucose to maintain blood glucose levels at 75 to 90 mg/dL before meals and overnight. Glucose concentrations must be maintained above 70 mg/dL to prevent counter-regulation, which causes the shunting of glucose-6-phosphate into alternative pathways, resulting in hyperlactacidemia, hyperuricemia, and hypertriglyceridemia. In infants, continuous glucose can be provided by frequent feeds during the day and continuous intragastric feeds at night via a nasogastric or gastrostomy tube. Beginning at 6 to 12 months of age, uncooked cornstarch (UCS), which is slowly digested and absorbed into

---

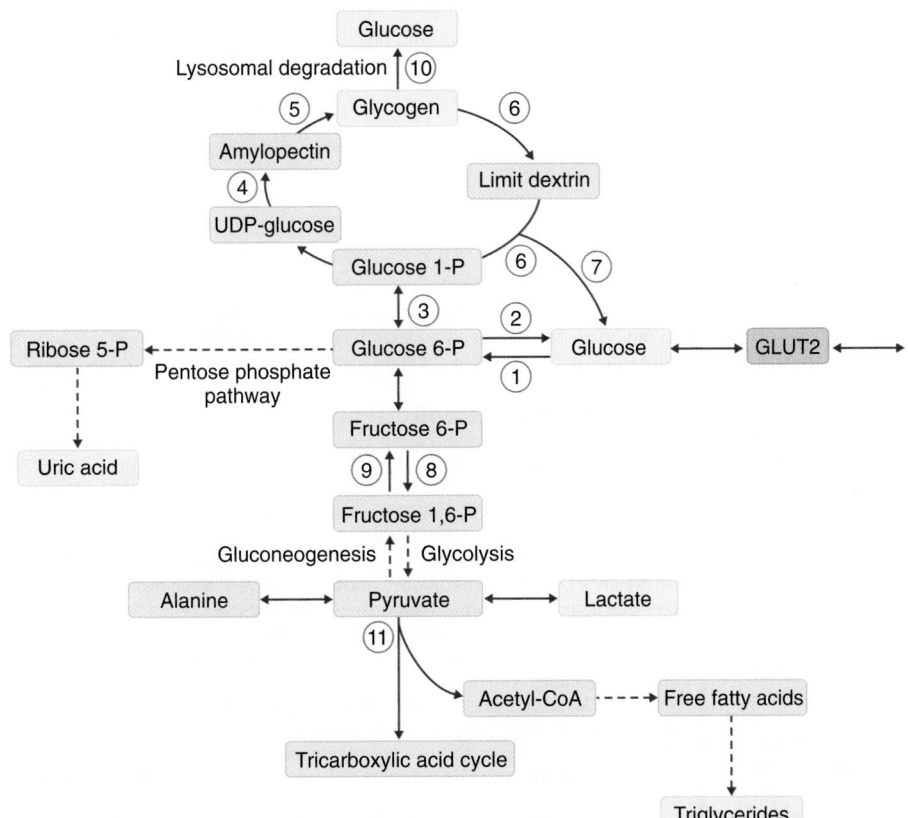

FIGURE 214-1. Simplified scheme of glycogen synthesis and degradation in the liver. Note that in skeletal muscle, GLUT4 transports glucose across the cell membrane, and glucose-6-phosphatase is absent. UDP-glucose = uridine diphosphoglucose. 1, hexokinase/glucokinase; 2, glucose-6-phosphatase; 3, phosphoglucomutase; 4, glycogen synthase; 5, branching enzyme; 6, glycogen phosphorylase; 7, debranching enzyme; 8, phosphofructokinase; 9, fructose 1,6-bisphosphatase; 10, acid maltase; 11, pyruvate dehydrogenase.

TABLE 214-1 PRINCIPAL FEATURES OF THE COMMON GLYCOGEN STORAGE DISEASES

TYPE*	DEFECTIVE ENZYME	CHARACTERISTIC CLINICAL FEATURES	HIGH-RISK POPULATIONS	THERAPY
0	Hepatic glycogen synthase	Liver small or normal in size, fasting ketotic hypoglycemia, postprandial hyperglycemia and hyperlactatemia	French Canadian Italian	UCS, especially at bedtime, with high-protein diet
Ia (Von Gierke's disease)	Glucose-6-phosphatase	Hepatomegaly, failure to thrive, growth retardation, severe hypoglycemia, lactic acidosis, hyperuricemia, hyperlipidemia	Ashkenazi Jew Mexican Chinese Japanese	UCS during the day and at night or continuous overnight intragastric feeding
Ib	Glucose-6-phosphate transporter	Same as type Ia; also neutropenia, recurrent bacterial infections, inflammatory bowel disease	Native American Iranian Jew	UCS as for type Ia; granulocyte colony-stimulating factor
II (Pompe's disease)[1]	Lysosomal acid maltase (α-glucosidase)	Infantile form: severe generalized hypotonia, muscle weakness, hypertrophic cardiomyopathy leading to cardiorespiratory failure usually by age 1 yr; Juvenile and adult forms: skeletal myopathy with slowly progressive muscle weakness; markedly increased serum creatine kinase	None	Intravenous enzyme replacement with recombinant human α-glucosidase
III (Cori's or Forbes' disease)	Debranching enzyme	Hepatomegaly, moderate to severe ketotic hypoglycemia, muscle weakness and wasting, hypertrophic cardiomyopathy (IIIa); increased transaminases without muscle involvement (IIIb)	Faroe Islander First Nation (Canada) Inhabitants of Indian subcontinent	High-protein diet with low-dose UCS supplementation
IV (Andersen's disease)	Glycogen branching enzyme	Clinically heterogeneous; typical presentation is liver disease in early childhood progressing to lethal cirrhosis; less common neuromuscular presentation is divided into four groups by age at onset: perinatal, congenital, childhood, adult	None	No specific treatment; liver transplantation has resulted in decreased glycogen storage in heart and skeletal muscle
V (McArdle's disease)	Muscle glycogen phosphorylase	Symptoms usually begin in adolescence or early adulthood with exercise intolerance, fatigue, myalgia, muscle cramps, muscle swelling; transient myoglobinuria due to rhabdomyolysis may occur after exercise; severe myoglobinuria may lead to acute renal failure; later in adult life, persistent and progressive muscle weakness and atrophy with fatty replacement occurs; increased serum creatine kinase	None	High-protein diet (50% carbohydrate, 25-30% protein); oral sucrose before sustained aerobic exercise may be beneficial[2]
VI (Hers' disease)	Hepatic glycogen phosphorylase	Hepatomegaly; growth retardation; moderate ketotic hypoglycemia; increased serum transaminases, cholesterol, and triglycerides	Mennonite	UCS dosed to prevent hypoglycemia and ketosis
VII (Tarui's disease)	Muscle phosphofructokinase	Presents in childhood with fatigue, muscle cramps, exercise intolerance; rhabdomyolysis and myoglobinuria with strenuous exertion; increased serum creatine kinase; may have mild hemolytic anemia and mild hyperbilirubinemia; hyperuricemia	None	No specific treatment; avoid strenuous exercise
IX	Phosphorylase *b* kinase	Hepatomegaly, mild ketotic hypoglycemia, growth retardation, increased serum transaminases, hypercholesterolemia, hypertriglyceridemia; may be X-linked or autosomal recessive	Mayan	UCS dosed to prevent hypoglycemia and ketosis

*GSD types X-XIV are very rare disorders and are not presented here due to limited cases and lack of formal recommendations.
UCS = uncooked cornstarch.

the circulation as glucose, can be used as an alternative method of providing glucose. Initially, UCS is given every 3 hours. As children age, and guided by the results of periodic blood glucose and lactate monitoring, the interval between feeds is eventually increased to 4 to 6 hours. Galactose and fructose must be restricted because they cannot be converted to glucose, and large quantities may exacerbate the biochemical derangements. Optimal care usually ameliorates the biochemical abnormalities; however, if optimal dietary management does not lower serum uric acid and triglycerides to acceptable levels, treatment with allopurinol and gemfibrozil, respectively, is indicated. Neutropenia (Chapter 170) in GSD Ib responds well to low-dose granulocyte colony-stimulating factor therapy; however, untoward effects of therapy are common. The recommended starting dose (2.5 µg/kg/day) is therefore lower than in other conditions, and the lowest possible dose that prevents infection is used. An enterocolitis that resembles Crohn's disease (Chapter 143) occurs almost universally in GSD Ib, and mesalamine (Pentasa) is first-line therapy because small intestinal disease predominates.

Patients with the other forms of GSD utilize a high-protein diet (2 to 3 g/kg) supplemented with complex carbohydrates and UCS, which is typically administered every 6 to 8 hours to maintain glucose concentrations above 75 mg/dL. Because β-oxidation of fatty acids can occur in these forms of GSD, ketosis can develop rapidly, and UCS doses are titrated to maintain normal blood ketone concentrations (<0.3 mmol/L). Strict avoidance of fructose and sucrose is unnecessary; however, consumption of concentrated sweets is discouraged to avoid excessive storage of glycogen. This is particularly important in GSD III, because excessive glycogen storage has been associated with worsening of the associated hypertrophic cardiomyopathy.

Treatment of the muscle glycogenoses is shown in Table 214-1.

Management of Complications

Despite improvements in care, long-term complications are common in GSD I and III. Hepatic adenomas develop in the majority of patients with GSD I during adolescence or early adulthood; the tumors may gradually enlarge, undergo malignant transformation, or hemorrhage into the peritoneal cavity. Nephrocalcinosis and nephrolithiasis, caused by hypocitraturia, are also common and can be prevented by the use of oral citrate supplementation. Maintenance of optimal metabolic control can prevent renal tubular dysfunction, focal segmental glomerulosclerosis, gout, and osteoporosis.

In GSD III, hypertrophic cardiomyopathy develops in the majority of patients during mid-childhood. Hepatic adenomas develop in 25% of patients; cirrhosis and hepatocellular cancer are rare. Most patients with GSD III do not have myopathic symptoms during childhood or early adulthood. Progressive myopathy develops in most people in the third or fourth decade of life.

Short stature and osteoporosis are the only common complications in GSD 0, VI, and IX, but these can be prevented by maintenance of optimal metabolic control.

1. van der Ploeg AT, Clemens PR, Corzo D, et al. A randomized study of alglucosidase alfa in late-onset Pompe's disease. *N Engl J Med.* 2010;362:1396-1406.
2. Quinlivan R, Martinuzzi A, Schoser B. Pharmacological and nutritional treatment for McArdle disease (glycogen storage disease type V). *Cochrane Database Syst Rev.* 2010;12:CD003458.

SUGGESTED READINGS

Association for Glycogen Storage Disease website. http://www.agsdus.org. *Provides basic information about GSDs for people affected by the diseases, their families, and other interested parties.*

Dagli AI, Weinstein DA. Glycogen storage disease type VI. *GeneReviews* at GeneTests: Medical Genetics Information Resource, 2009. *Online database sponsored by the National Institutes of Health.*

Kishnani PS, Austin SL, Am P, et al. Glycogen storage disease type III diagnosis and management guidelines. *Genet Med.* 2010;12:446-463. *Consensus guidelines.*

Quinlivan R, Buckley J, James M, et al. McArdle disease: a clinical review. *J Neurol Neurosurg Psychiatry.* 2010;81:1181-1188. *Review of 45 cases, most of whom had symptoms from early childhood but whose diagnosis frequently was delayed until after 30 years of age.*

215

THE LYSOSOMAL STORAGE DISEASES

DONNA M. KRASNEWICH AND ELLEN SIDRANSKY

The lysosomal storage diseases encompass a group of more than 45 different inherited disorders, all sharing a defect in lysosomal function. Lysosomes are acidic, membrane-bound organelles present in the cytoplasm that contain enzymes that degrade macromolecules. These disorders ensue when one or more of the hydrolytic enzymes are deficient or when essential lysosomal transporters, receptors, cofactors, or protective proteins are defective or lacking. Typically, complex macromolecules, including glycolipids, mucopolysaccharides, and glycoproteins, are delivered to the lysosome, where they undergo sequential modification by a series of hydrolases. An enzymatic deficiency becomes clinically important when macromolecules accumulate owing to inadequate degradation. Different categories of defects resulting in lysosomal dysfunction are encountered in the lysosomal storage disorders, and examples of each type are listed in Table 215-1.

Although most lysosomal storage disorders are quite rare, as a group their frequency is estimated to be 1 per 7000 to 8000 live births. This is an underestimate, because milder or attenuated forms of these disorders are often not identified. All the disorders have an autosomal recessive pattern of inheritance, with the exception of Fabry's disease and Hunter's disease (mucopolysaccharidosis [MPS] II), which are X-linked. As a whole, these disorders are characterized by a vast spectrum of manifestations, often causing them to evade diagnosis. Many were traditionally classified into infantile, juvenile, and adult types, based on the patient's age at the onset of manifestations, but atypical presentations complicate these distinctions. Among the factors contributing to this phenotypic diversity are the amount of residual enzyme activity, cellular localization of the enzyme, genotype, and the genetic background of the affected individual, as well as other genetic, environmental, or epigenetic influences.

With the advent of new therapies for some of the lysosomal storage disorders, establishing the diagnosis early is paramount. Suggestive clinical findings include coarse facial features; organomegaly; progressive loss of developmental skills; specific eye findings, including corneal clouding or a cherry red spot (of the macula); and skeletal abnormalities, notably dysostosis multiplex. Disorders associated with each of these findings are listed in Table 215-2. There should be a greater index of suspicion whenever these features occur in concert, the findings are progressive, or the patient appears dissimilar to other family members.

The diagnostic work-up includes a careful history, with analysis of the family pedigree and assessment of developmental milestones in childhood and adolescence. A family history of consanguinity, other affected siblings, or early deaths can aid in making the diagnosis. Ethnicity can be a helpful clue because some of the lysosomal disorders occur with increased incidence in specific populations, such as Ashkenazi Jews (Gaucher's disease type 1, Tay-Sachs disease, mucolipidosis type IV) and Scandinavians (mannosidosis, aspartylglucosaminuria, Salla's disease, Gaucher's disease type 3). On physical examination, special attention should be paid to head circumference,

TABLE 215-1 CLASSIFICATION OF LYSOSOMAL STORAGE DISORDERS BASED ON THE TYPE OF DEFECT*

SPHINGOLIPIDOSES

Fabry's disease (α-galactosidase)
Farber's disease (ceramidase)
GM₁ gangliosidosis/Landing's disease (β-galactosidase)
GM₂ gangliosidosis/Tay-Sachs disease (β-hexosaminidase A)
Sandhoff's disease (α-hexosaminidases A and B)
Gaucher's disease (glucocerebrosidase)
Niemann-Pick disease types A and B (sphingomyelinase)
Metachromatic leukodystrophy (arylsulfatase A)
Krabbe's disease (β-galactocerebrosidase)

LIPID STORAGE DISORDERS

Wolman's disease (acid lipase)
Neuronal ceroid-lipofuscinosis (adult)/Kufs' disease/Parry's disease (CLN4, heterogeneous)

MUCOPOLYSACCHARIDOSES

Type I/Hurler's disease (α-L-iduronidase)
Type II/Hunter's disease (iduronate-2-sulfatase)
Type III/Sanfilippo's disease (four different enzymes in the degradation of heparan sulfate defining types A-D)
Type VI/Maroteaux-Lamy disease (N-acetylgalactosamine-4-sulfatase)
Type VII/Sly's disease (α-glucuronidase)

OLIGOSACCHARIDOSES

Aspartylglucosaminuria (aspartylglucosaminase)
Fucosidosis (α-fucosidase)
α-Mannosidosis (α-mannosidase)
Schindler's disease (α-N-acetylgalactosaminidase)
Sialidosis I (sialidase)
Sialidosis II/mucolipidosis I (sialidase)

MUCOLIPIDOSES

Mucolipidosis II/I-cell disease (N-acetylglucosaminylphosphotransferase)
Mucolipidosis III/pseudo-Hurler (N-acetylglucosaminylphosphotransferase)
Mucolipidosis IV (MCOLN1 mutation)

LYSOSOMAL GLYCOGEN STORAGE DISORDER

Glycogenosis type II/Pompe's disease (α-1,4-glucosidase)

LYSOSOMAL TRANSPORT DISORDERS

Sialic acid storage disease/Salla's disease (sialin/SLC17A5)
Cystinosis (cystine transporter)
Niemann-Pick disease type C (intracellular cholesterol transport)

MULTIPLE ENZYME DEFICIENCIES

Galactosialidosis (β-galactosidase and sialidase)
Multiple sulfatase deficiency/Austin's disease (sulfatases)

*Full chapters describing each of these disorders are available in Scriver CR, Sly WS, Childs B, Beaudet AL. *The Metabolic and Molecular Bases of Inherited Disease*, 8th ed. New York: McGraw-Hill Professional; 2001.

facial appearance, enlargement of the tongue, hepatosplenomegaly, skeletal manifestations (including kyphosis), broadening of the long bones, and stiffness of the joints. Skin evaluation may reveal angiokeratoma, especially around the umbilicus and in skin creases. The eye evaluation should include a funduscopic and slit lamp examination, as well as an assessment for atypical eye movements, which may be pathognomonic for disorders such as neuronopathic Gaucher's disease and Niemann-Pick type C. A careful neurologic and cognitive evaluation can be quite fruitful because some of the later presentations include dementia or psychiatric manifestations. Moreover, regression of milestones can provide an early diagnostic clue. Preliminary diagnostic studies include urine for thin-layer chromatography, a blood smear for vacuolated white blood cells, skeletal x-rays, and an ophthalmologic examination.

For the most part, the diagnosis of a specific lysosomal storage disorder is made by assaying enzymatic activity in a blood sample or fibroblast cell line. A lysosomal panel, evaluating the activity of multiple lysosomal enzymes from the same sample, should be the first-tier test. If a lysosomal storage disorder is still suspected, a tissue biopsy, most often of the bone marrow or liver, can be considered, although this is rarely indicated. Most of the genes encoding for the lysosomal enzymes have been identified, and mutation analysis is available. However, in most cases there is vast genotypic

TABLE 215-2 MANIFESTATIONS OF LYSOSOMAL STORAGE DISORDERS

FINDING	DISORDERS
Hepatosplenomegaly	GM$_1$ gangliosidosis, Niemann-Pick disease, Gaucher's disease, Wolman's disease, fucosidosis, Pompe's disease, mannosidosis, multiple sulfatase deficiency, sialidosis, galactosialidosis, several mucopolysaccharidoses, cystinosis
Coarse facies	GM$_1$ gangliosidosis, fucosidosis, Pompe's disease, mannosidosis, multiple sulfatase deficiency, I-cell disease, several mucopolysaccharidoses, mucolipidosis II, sialic acid storage disease, aspartylglucosaminuria
Skeletal findings	GM$_1$ gangliosidosis, Gaucher's disease, fucosidosis, mannosidosis, sialidosis, galactosialidosis, several mucopolysaccharidoses, I-cell disease, mucolipidosis III
Cherry red spot	Infantile forms of GM$_1$ gangliosidosis, Sandoff's disease, Tay-Sachs disease, Niemann-Pick disease, sialidosis, galactosialidosis, I-cell disease
Corneal clouding	GM$_1$ gangliosidosis, several mucopolysaccharidoses, mannosidosis, I-cell disease, mucolipidosis III and IV, multiple sulfatase deficiency, galactosialidosis
Cognitive impairment	GM$_1$ gangliosidosis, Sandoff's disease, Tay-Sachs disease, Niemann-Pick disease, Gaucher's disease type 2, Wolman's disease, fucosidosis, mannosidosis, multiple sulfatase deficiency, sialidosis, galactosialidosis, several mucopolysaccharidoses, sialic acid storage disease, aspartylglucosaminuria, I-cell disease, mucolipidosis III and IV, Krabbe's disease, metachromatic leukodystrophy, neuronal ceroid-lipofuscinosis
Hematologic: Foam cells	GM$_1$ gangliosidosis, Niemann-Pick disease, Gaucher's disease, acid lipase deficiency, fucosidosis
Granulated/ vacuolated WBCs	Several mucopolysaccharidoses, sialidosis, galactosialidosis, neuronal ceroid-lipofuscinosis, Niemann-Pick disease, Wolman's disease, fucosidosis, mannosidosis, aspartylglucosaminuria, I-cell disease, mucolipidosis III, multiple sulfatase deficiency
Psychiatric or behavioral manifestations	Several mucopolysaccharidoses (especially Sanfilippo), sialidosis, galactosialidosis, Fabry's disease, mannosidosis, neuronal ceroid-lipofuscinosis, metachromatic leukodystrophy, Tay-Sachs disease, Niemann-Pick disease type C
Newborn presentations	Gaucher's disease type 2; GM$_1$ gangliosidosis; Krabbe's disease; Niemann-Pick disease types A and C; mucopolysaccharidosis I, IVA, and VII; Pompe's disease; sialidosis types I and II; mucolipidosis I and II; Schindler's disease; Wolman's disease; infantile sialic acid storage disease; sialuria; Salla's disease; galactosialidosis; multiple sulfatase deficiency; prosaposin deficiency

WBC = white blood cell.

heterogeneity, and mutation screening is useful only when a mutation has already been identified in a specific family.

Improved care and new therapeutic modalities have transformed the natural history of several of these disorders. With patients' increased longevity, diseases that were once encountered only by pediatricians have now made their way to the offices of internists. Moreover, many of the classic complications are now avoided by early therapeutic interventions such as enzyme replacement therapy. However, in some instances, prolonged longevity has unmasked unanticipated clinical manifestations. Physicians' increased awareness of the range of manifestations and presentations of lysosomal disorders may lessen the long delays in diagnosis that patients frequently describe. Lysosomal disorders encountered in adult patients are discussed here, with a focus on Gaucher's disease and Fabry's disease. A brief discussion of specific disorders frequently diagnosed during adulthood, as well as childhood-onset lysosomal disorders that persist through adulthood, is included.

GAUCHER'S DISEASE

Gaucher's disease, the autosomal recessively inherited deficiency of the lysosomal enzyme glucocerebrosidase, is a disorder primarily of the reticuloendothelial system. Lysosomes within macrophages become engorged with the substrate glucocerebroside, giving rise to the characteristic Gaucher cells, with a wrinkled-paper appearance resulting from intracytoplasmic substrate deposition. The accumulated glycolipid glucosylceramide derives from the degradation of senescent leukocytes or erythrocyte membranes. Clinically, Gaucher's disease has been divided into three types, based on the absence or presence and the rate of progression of neurologic involvement. Type 1, the non-neuronopathic form, is the most common type and can manifest at any age. Type 2, the acute neuronopathic form, presents before or shortly after birth and has a rapid and progressive course. Type 3 is the subacute neuronopathic form. The spectrum of manifestations encountered in this disorder ranges from asymptomatic octogenarians to infants that succumb in utero, and some patients defy classification into one of the three types. It is a panethnic disorder, although type 1 Gaucher's disease is more frequent among Ashkenazi Jews, where the carrier frequency is about 1 in 16; in contrast, the approximate carrier frequency in the general population is 1 in 100.

The gene encoding glucocerebrosidase (GBA) is located on chromosome 1q21, and more than 300 different mutations have been found in patients. Several mutations are encountered with increased frequency in type 1 Gaucher's disease; for example, among Ashkenazi Jews, mutation N370S is the most common allele. However, the mutations identified do not adequately account for the range of manifestations encountered.

In recent years, an association between Gaucher's disease and parkinsonism (Chapter 416) has been reported. Both patients with Gaucher's disease and carriers of mutations in GBA have a higher incidence of Parkinson's disease and Lewy body disorders. Studies in cohorts of patients with Parkinson's disease around the world demonstrate that they have a greater than five-fold increased frequency of GBA mutations, rendering this the most common genetic risk factor for parkinsonism identified to date.

CLINICAL MANIFESTATIONS

Commonly encountered symptoms in all types of Gaucher's disease include easy bruisability, hepatomegaly, splenomegaly, chronic fatigue, and bone pain or pathologic fractures. Laboratory findings include anemia, thrombocytopenia, and elevations of ferritin, acid phosphatase, angiotensin-converting enzyme, and, at times, liver enzymes. Painless splenomegaly is the most common presentation in patients with type 1 Gaucher's disease, and the spleen can be massively enlarged. Occasional patients have pulmonary involvement or pulmonary hypertension. Bone involvement is a significant cause of morbidity and can manifest with extreme bone pain or pathologic fractures. Most patients have radiologic evidence of skeletal involvement, including the classic Erlenmeyer flask deformity of the distal end of the femur and osteopenia (Fig. 215-1A). Pathologic fractures, especially of the hip or spine; lytic bone lesions; and osteoporosis may occur. Painful bone crises, episodes of bony infarcts, can last for weeks and may require aggressive pain management.

Type 2 disease, which is rare, is characterized by a rapid neurodegenerative course with extensive visceral involvement; death usually occurs within the first 2 years of life. The disease is diagnosed prenatally or in infancy and is associated with increased tone, strabismus, and organomegaly. Failure to thrive and stridor from laryngospasm are typical. Progressive psychomotor degeneration leads to death, usually secondary to an intercurrent respiratory infection and respiratory compromise.

Type 3 disease is clinically variable and is often noted in infancy or childhood. In addition to organomegaly and bone involvement, patients have abnormal horizontal eye movements, and some develop myoclonic epilepsy or neurodegenerative manifestations. A subgroup of patients has cardiac calcifications, hydrocephalus, and other atypical manifestations, and all carry the mutation D409H in the GBA gene.

DIAGNOSIS

Gaucher's disease should be considered in the differential diagnosis of patients of all ages with unexplained organomegaly, easy bruisability, or bone pain. The diagnosis can be made by demonstration of deficient glucocerebrosidase activity in leukocytes or cultured cells. In some populations, particularly Ashkenazi Jews, mutation analysis can be diagnostic, and mutation N370S accounts for about 70% of mutant alleles. However, the presence of a highly homologous pseudogene sequence nearby can complicate molecular analyses. Bone marrow and liver biopsies show pathologic changes

FIGURE 215-1. **A,** Radiographic image showing the Erlenmeyer flask deformity seen in Gaucher's disease. There is cortical thinning and widening of the medullary cavity of the metaphysis and adjacent diaphysis. **B,** Gaucher cells—reticuloendothelial cells storing abnormal amounts of lipid. **C,** Angiokeratomas, the nonblanching punctuate skin lesion seen in Fabry's disease.

(Fig. 215-1B) but are not indicated for diagnosis. Carrier identification is best achieved by DNA testing when the mutant allele is known. Prenatal diagnosis is possible by determining the enzymatic activity or specific mutations in chorionic villi or cultured amniotic fluid cells.

TREATMENT Rx

Enzyme replacement with recombinant glucocerebrosidase is available for the treatment of symptomatic patients with type 1 disease. Studies show that anemia, thrombocytopenia, and organomegaly are reversed within 12 to 36 months using enzyme doses between 30 and 120 IU/kg given monthly. The treatment is ongoing, administered intravenously, and extremely expensive. Several companies are now testing different forms of recombinantly produced enzyme. The enzyme does not cross the blood-brain barrier and does not alter the neurologic progression of patients with neuronopathic forms of Gaucher's disease, but it can still be useful in alleviating visceral manifestations. Efforts are also under way to develop alternative therapies, including substrate reduction therapy, chemical chaperones, and gene therapy. One oral form of substrate reduction therapy, an iminosugar derivative, has been approved and is efficacious for some of the systemic manifestations of type 1 Gaucher's disease. Useful supportive therapies include bisphosphonates for osteoporosis, orthopedic surgery for bone fractures, and palliative therapy and hydration for bone crises. Total or partial splenectomy, once commonly performed in patients with Gaucher's disease, is now rarely indicated. Bone marrow transplantation (Chapter 181) has improved systemic but not neurologic manifestations.

● FABRY'S DISEASE

Fabry's disease, an X-linked inherited deficiency of the lysosomal enzyme α-galactosidase A, has intermediate penetrance in females and is considered a systemic vascular disorder. This defect in the hydrolytic cleavage of the terminal molecule of galactose from glycolipids causes lysosomal accumulation of globotriaosylceramide and galabiosylceramide in many cell types. Lysosomal inclusions or lipid deposits can be seen in vascular cells, including both endothelial and smooth muscle cells; cardiac cells, including endocardial cells, cardiomyocytes, and cardiac valves; kidney epithelial cells, including tubular and glomerular cells and podocytes; and nerve cells, including dorsal root ganglia and some central nervous system neurons. Clinically, angiokeratomas—nonblanching, punctate, blue-black skin lesions—debilitating pain, and corneal opacities can occur in early childhood and may lead to the diagnosis. If the diagnosis is missed, the disease can result in progressive renal and cardiac deterioration. Patients have a propensity to develop ischemic stroke, sometimes in their 20s but more commonly in the fourth and fifth decades of life. As with many metabolic disorders, there is a

spectrum of presentations that can mimic more common disorders, and many patients are undiagnosed. The disease incidence is about 1 in 117,000 live male births. Evidence suggests that 50% of females with Fabry's disease are asymptomatic or are not identified.

The gene encoding α-galactosidase A, *GLA*, is located on Xq22.1. More than 431 mutations have been described, including missense/nonsense mutations, small deletions, large deletions, splice defects, and complex rearrangements. Most affected individuals may have 2 to 25% residual activity, but the most severe form of Fabry's disease has been correlated with complete absence of α-galactosidase A activity.

CLINICAL MANIFESTATIONS

Fabry's disease typically presents in childhood with episodes of extremity pain. Angiokeratomas develop in adolescence, followed by progressive renal and cardiac deterioration. Adults may experience ischemic strokes, initially occurring between their 20s and 50s. Acroparesthesia, or a "Fabry crisis," occurs in the majority of patients and is characterized by excruciating, burning pain that may be either continuous or episodic. The pain typically affects the feet first, followed by the hands, and may be triggered by exercise, stress, and extremes in environmental temperatures. Abdominal or flank pain, simulating renal colic, may occur.

Angiokeratomas (Fig. 215-1C) are often the first sign of Fabry's disease and are accompanied by hypohidrosis. These classic skin lesions increase in number and size over time and are typically most dense between the umbilicus and the knees; however, they may occur anywhere, including the buccal mucosa. Ophthalmologic findings include conjunctival and retinal tortuosity and corneal opacities (cornea verticillata). Characteristic lenticular lesions are observed during slit lamp examination and are present in affected males and 70% of female heterozygotes. Progressive hearing loss is also common.

Renal involvement manifests as progressive proteinuria with birefringent "Maltese crosses" in the urinary sediment. Declining glomerular filtration rates lead to end-stage renal disease in the second to fourth decades. Hyperfiltration precedes the decline in renal function. Cardiovascular findings may include decreased exercise capacity, hypertension, progressive hypertrophic cardiomyopathy, conduction defects and arrhythmias, and valvular disease (insufficiency or stenosis). Abnormal electrocardiograms and echocardiography are common. Affected individuals have an estimated twenty-fold increased risk of ischemic stroke and transient ischemic attacks compared with the general population. Asymptomatic lesions of the brain, typically in white matter, are often seen on magnetic resonance imaging.

The intermediate penetrance of this X-linked disorder is reflected in the fact that 70% of females carrying the mutation have symptoms. Affected or carrier females have more variable and less severe symptoms with a later onset, but they may develop progressive renal disease, cardiac symptoms, and stroke.

DIAGNOSIS

Fabry's disease should be considered in individuals with angiokeratoma, acroparesthesia, and corneal lesions, as well as in patients with cryptogenic strokes, idiopathic cardiomyopathy, or renal disease. However, the identical corneal abnormalities can result from the use of chloroquine or amiodarone, and exposure to silicone dust can result in similar renal findings. Angiokeratoma should be differentiated from Fordyce's disease, benign angiokeratomas of the scrotum, and angiokeratoma circumscriptum. Angiokeratomas are also seen in mannosidosis, fucosidosis, sialidosis, and β-galactosidase and β-hexosaminidase deficiency. A presumed diagnosis can be confirmed by low α-galactosidase activity in peripheral white blood cells or cultured skin fibroblasts. Levels below 20% of normal should be considered diagnostic, and levels 35% of normal should be considered suspicious. *GLA* mutation analysis is available and is critical for confirmation in heterozygote females because random X chromosome inactivation may lead to only slightly reduced or normal enzyme activity.

TREATMENT Rx

Symptomatic treatment of the clinical manifestations of Fabry's disease should follow standard medical care. Antiplatelet agents such as clopidogrel and aspirin or long-acting dipyridamole should be used for the prevention of strokes in individuals with Fabry's disease. The use of angiotensin-converting enzyme inhibitors and angiotensin receptor blockers is appropriate to manage hypertension and preserve renal function. Renal transplantation is effective in individuals with end-stage renal disease. Neuropathic pain can be treated with relatively low doses of antiepileptic medications, antidepressants, topical anesthetics, or pain relievers.

Enzyme replacement therapy has been available since 2001, and evidence continues to be gathered about its efficacy in modifying the natural course of the disease. Enzyme replacement therapy appears to slow the decline in renal function, but there is no evidence thus far that it can change the progression of cardiac disease; nor has a reduction of stroke risk been demonstrated. Treatments targeted at chaperoning the enzyme to the lysosome to enhance enzymatic degradation are in development.

OTHER LYSOSOMAL DISORDERS FREQUENTLY ENCOUNTERED IN ADULTS

Metachromatic leukodystrophy, the deficiency of arylsulfatase A, results in the accumulation of sulfatides in the central and peripheral nervous systems, leading to demyelination of axons and peripheral nerves. It presents with a spectrum of manifestations, divided into childhood and adult variants. In both, gait disturbance and cognitive regression are seen. The adult form is associated with behavioral disturbances and dementia, often mistakenly resulting in a diagnosis of psychosis. Metachromatic leukodystrophy is a recognized underlying cause of psychiatric illness in adults, and prominent features include auditory hallucinations, bizarre delusions, behavioral changes, personality changes, disinhibition and disorganization in daily life, and catatonic posturing. The diagnosis can be especially difficult in these individuals. Other neurologic signs such as dysarthria and spasticity present later as the disease progresses. The diagnosis is made initially by demonstrating low arylsulfatase A activity. However, because there can be a pseudodeficiency, it must be confirmed by molecular diagnosis or the demonstration of the excretion of sulfatides in urine.

Tay-Sachs disease, caused by β-hexosaminidase A deficiency, is characterized by an excessive accumulation of the fatty acid derivative ganglioside GM$_2$ in neurons. There are three clinical variants, based on the age of onset: type 1—infantile acute, type 2—subacute (2 to 18 years), and type 3—late onset. The main features of the disease are neurologic and cognitive deterioration, as well as blindness, the macular "cherry red spot," and deafness. In patients with late-onset GM$_2$ gangliosidosis, psychiatric signs can manifest years before the appearance of motor signs. The most common psychiatric signs include acute psychosis, mania, and depression without psychosis. Either recurrent progressive psychosis, consistent with schizophrenia-hebephrenia, or major depression followed by psychotic features may occur. Dysarthria and progressive speech loss are also common. The disorder is diagnosed by measuring β-hexosaminidase A activity in the serum or white blood cells in the presence of normal or elevated activity of the β-hexosaminidase B (HEX B) isoenzyme. In pregnant women or those taking oral contraceptives, the test should be performed only in leukocytes.

Niemann-Pick disease type C has a spectrum of features, ranging from a rapidly progressive, fatal neonatal phenotype to an adult-onset chronic, neurodegenerative course. Progressive ataxia, vertical supranuclear ophthalmoplegia, dystonia, and dementia are variable. Hepatosplenomegaly is frequently encountered. The disorder results from an error in cellular trafficking of exogenous cholesterol, leading to lysosomal accumulation of unesterified cholesterol. The diagnosis is made by demonstrating impaired cholesterol esterification in cultured fibroblasts or by molecular genetic testing for mutations. Glycosphingolipids and cholesterol accumulate in different tissues such as the liver, spleen, bone marrow, and brain. In adults, psychiatric manifestations consistent with acute psychosis, paranoid delusions or schizophrenia with delusions, hallucinations, disorganized behavior, and aggressiveness are observed.

Aspartylglucosaminuria, a disorder more common in Finland than elsewhere in the world, is an autosomal recessive defect in glycoprotein degradation characterized by a slow or progressive delay in psychomotor development. Delayed speech and motor defects are often accompanied by repeated upper respiratory infections. Patients typically achieve the developmental competency of a 5- to 6-year-old child at around puberty; subsequently, they may experience progressive deterioration, resulting in the severe cognitive impairment seen in adulthood. The characteristic coarse facial features, thick calvaria, and osteoporosis result from mild connective tissue transformation. About 20% of patients experience seizures during the later stages of the disease, resulting primarily from abnormalities in the differentiation between gray and white matter and delayed myelination. The diagnosis is made by the detection of elevated urine oligosaccharides and deficient aspartylglucosaminidase activity in leukocytes.

The neuronal ceroid-lipofuscinoses are divided into four major groups—infantile, classic late infantile, juvenile, and adult—reflecting the age of symptom onset and the appearance of storage material on electron microscopy. Although generally inherited in an autosomal recessive fashion, the adult type can be inherited as a dominant allele. These diseases are characterized clinically by visual impairment leading to blindness, gait abnormalities, seizures, dementia, and early death. They are a genetically heterogeneous group of progressive, hereditary neurodegenerative diseases with a variable onset. To date, approximately 160 mutations causing neuronal ceroid-lipofuscinoses have been found in eight human genes, complicating genetic analysis. Symptoms result from deficiencies in palmitoyl-protein thioesterase 1 and tripeptidyl-peptidase 1. The diagnosis is based on diminished enzyme activity and molecular genetic testing and, in some cases, on clinical findings and electron microscopy of biopsied tissues. Accumulation of autofluorescent ceroid lipopigments is seen in the brain and other tissues. Adult patients may exhibit behavioral disturbances and cognitive decline, and parkinsonian features may be prominent.

Pompe's disease is discussed in Chapters 214 and 429.

The mucopolysaccharidoses are a group of disorders resulting from defective lysosomal degradation of glycosaminoglycans. These chronic, progressive storage disorders show clinical manifestations that vary by type. Findings include coarse facial features, dysostosis multiplex, organomegaly, and neurologic manifestations with regression. All types are inherited in an autosomal recessive pattern except for MPS II/Hunter, which is X-linked. The mucopolysaccharidoses were once typically thought of as pediatric disorders, but with the advent of enzyme replacement therapy and the recognition of milder forms, more patients are reaching adulthood. Classically, patients with MPS type IS/Scheie, II/Hunter, III/Sanfilippo, IV/Morquio, and VI/Maroteaux-Lamy may have life expectancies beyond the pediatric years. Patients with MPS IS may present with normal to short stature, normal intelligence, degenerative joint disease, corneal opacities, and cardiac valve lesions. Patients with MPS II/Hunter share the symptoms of MPS I/Hurler, except that airway involvement may be more significant in individuals with Hunter's syndrome, and the corneas are clear. Patients with MPS III/Sanfilippo have primarily central nervous system manifestations, with mild somatic involvement. They have progressive speech impairment, with the development of severe behavioral and sleep disturbances. Later they have unrelenting loss of skills and deterioration into a vegetative state, with death in the third decade. Individuals with MPS IV have severe skeletal dysplasia, with normal intelligence in type A and a degenerative course in type B. Trials exploring enzyme replacement therapy are ongoing for MPS IS, MPS II, and MPS IV. Medical management is type specific. Generally, attention should focus on airway involvement resulting from progressive storage in the soft tissue of the upper airway and the need to optimize joint mobility and function by physical therapy. Patients with MPS I, II, and VI should be monitored for the development of cervical myelopathy due to dural thickening, which may lead to loss of endurance before ascending paralysis becomes apparent.

Cystinosis is a lysosomal storage disorder with three clinical phenotypes: the most common infantile or nephropathic form, an intermediate or juvenile-onset form, and a benign form typically seen in adults and affecting primarily the eyes. Lysosomal cystine accumulation results from mutations in the gene CTNS, which codes for cystinosin, a lysosomal carrier protein. Individuals with the nephropathic form have lysosomal cystine accumulation leading to multiorgan system involvement, including progressive renal disease, corneal crystals, and effects on the thyroid, gonads, pancreas, muscle, and central nervous system. The adult form has only corneal crystals. Treatment is supportive and should include cysteamine, which is an oral medication that decreases cystine accumulation.

SUGGESTED READINGS

Balwani M, Fuerstman L, Kornreich R, et al. Type I Gaucher disease: significant disease manifestations in "asymptomatic" homozygotes. Arch Intern Med. 2010;170:1463-1469. Almost all asymptomatic homozygotes had disease manifestations and may become candidates for appropriate medical treatment.

Beck M. Therapy for lysosomal storage disorders. IUMBMBLife. 2010;62:33-40. Overview of therapies for lysosomal storage disorders.

Deegan PB, Pavlova E, Tindall J, et al. Osseous manifestations of adult Gaucher disease in the era of enzyme replacement therapy. Medicine (Baltimore). 2011;90:52-60. Review.

Grabowski GA, Kacena K, Cole JA, et al. Dose-response relationships for enzyme replacement therapy with imiglucerase/alglucerase in patients with Gaucher disease type 1. Genet Med. 2009;11:92-100. Demonstrates dose-dependent improvement.

Mehta A, Beck M, Elliott P, et al. Enzyme replacement therapy with agalsidase alfa in patients with Fabry's disease: an analysis of registry data. Lancet. 2009;374:1986-1996. Agalsidase alfa treatment has substantial and sustained benefit for improving quality of life and clinical symptoms in patients with Fabry's disease.

Sidransky E, Nalls MA, Aasly JO, et al. Multicenter analysis of glucocerebrosidase mutations in Parkinson's disease. *N Engl J Med.* 2009;361:1651-1661. *Results of a multicenter study of more than 5000 patients with Parkinson's disease demonstrating that the frequency of Gaucher's mutations is five-fold higher than in matched controls.*

Staretz-Chacham O, Choi J, Wakabayashi K, et al. Psychiatric and behavioral manifestations of lysosomal storage disorders. *Am J Med Genet B Neuropsychiatr Genet.* 2010;153B:1253-1265. *Overview of psychiatric and behavioral features encountered among patients with different lysosomal storage disorders.*

216

HOMOCYSTINURIA AND HYPERHOMOCYSTEINEMIA

BRUCE A. BARSHOP

DEFINITION

Homocysteine is a nonprotein amino acid and an intermediate in methionine metabolism that arises when methionine (through *S*-adenosylmethionine) acts as a donor in methylation reactions (Fig. 216-1). The fate of homocysteine is either remethylation to methionine or transsulfuration of serine (through cystathionine) to cysteine. Homocystinuria results from the accumulation of homocysteine because of a defect in either transsulfuration or remethylation. The classic finding of the disulfide homocystine in urine gives this class of disorders its common name. The free sulfhydryl form, homocysteine, is present in lower amounts in blood. The term *total homocyst(e)ine* is used to describe the mix of homocysteine and homocystine present as sulfhydryl and disulfide, although here the term *total homocysteine* is considered equivalent. The defining finding in blood is hyperhomocysteinemia, which is distributed about 10% as free homocysteine and 90% as protein-bound and soluble disulfides (e.g., homocystine or cysteine-SS-homocysteine).

EPIDEMIOLOGY

Incidence and Prevalence

Minimum estimates of the incidence of cystathionine β-synthase deficiency by newborn screening programs have ranged from 1 in 60,000 to 1 in 300,000 live births, varying with the population and the screening method. Estimates of its incidence in Europe have been in the area of 1 in 40,000, which corresponds to a carrier (heterozygote) frequency of about 1%, but studies screening for known mutations suggest that the prevalence may be more than twice that rate. The incidence of severe homocysteine remethylation defects

appears to be less than 1 in 500,000. In contrast, partial remethylation deficiencies seem to have a much greater incidence, which may be clinically relevant in the predisposition to thrombotic disorders, because evidence of deficiency has been reported in 15 to 30% in some series of patients with vaso-occlusive disease. The methylenetetrahydrofolate reductase (MTHFR) C677T polymorphic allele is homozygous (T/T) in approximately 10% of Western populations.

PATHOBIOLOGY

The classic form of homocystinuria is cystathionine β-synthase deficiency, which results in decreased transsulfuration and hypermethioninemic hyperhomocysteinemia. Homocystinuria may also result from defective remethylation, as in a deficiency of MTHFR, or from a disorder in the delivery, generation, or utilization of the methylcobalamin cofactor of methionine synthase. Defects of remethylation give rise to hyperhomocysteinemia with normal or low methionine. All these disorders are inherited in an autosomal recessive manner (Table 216-1).

Homocysteine has effects on vascular endothelium, platelets, and coagulation factors that predispose to thrombosis. Endothelial dysfunction can be elicited in normal individuals when hyperhomocysteinemia is induced transiently. There is evidence of inflammatory mediator activation in experimental systems related to the pro-oxidant effects of homocysteine, but there remains some controversy about the relevance of these factors in humans. Modification of connective tissue proteins may cause the skeletal and ocular manifestations associated with homocystinuria. These effects are probably related to fibrillin, which is a component of the matrix of periosteum and perichondrium, the major component of the zonular fibers of the ocular lens, and a protein singularly rich in cysteine. Fibrillin structure is affected by the linking of homocysteine to cysteine; as a result, some features of homocystinuria are also associated with fibrillin mutations (Marfan syndrome; Chapter 268). The neurologic effects of homocysteine may be due predominantly to agonism of the *N*-methyl-D-aspartate receptor by homocysteic acid, although cerebral vascular effects may contribute as well.

CLINICAL MANIFESTATIONS

Cystathionine β-synthase deficiency is pleiotropic, with effects in the eye, skeleton, and central nervous and vascular systems (Table 216-2). The eye and skeletal system changes resemble those in Marfan syndrome. Nontraumatic dislocation of the ocular lens can be an initial finding. Some abnormality of the skeletal system develops in almost all untreated patients. Between one third and three fourths of untreated patients have mild or moderate mental retardation, and cerebrovascular thrombosis may play a role in the neurologic picture. Affected patients are at lifelong risk of thromboembolic phenomena, which are the major cause of mortality in those with untreated disease. Arterial and venous occlusion, in small or large vessels, may occur at

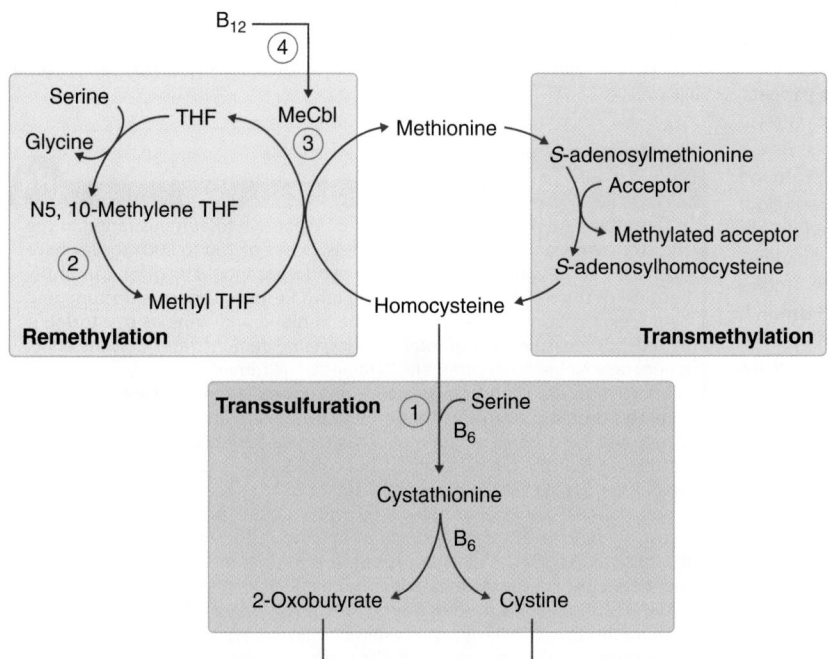

FIGURE 216-1. Pathways of homocysteine metabolism. The systems of remethylation, transmethylation, and transsulfuration are marked. Steps discussed are numbered: (1) cystathionine β-synthase; (2) methylenetetrahydrofolate reductase; (3) methionine synthase and methyltransferase reductase; (4) systems of cobalamin absorption, distribution, and reduction. B_6 = pyridoxine; B_{12} = cyanocobalamin/hydroxocobalamin; MeCbl = methylcobalamin; THF = tetrahydrofolate.

TABLE 216-1 GENETIC DEFECTS ASSOCIATED WITH HOMOCYSTINURIA

FUNCTIONAL DEFECT	COMMON NAME	ENZYME DEFECT	GENE	CHROMOSOME LOCUS
Transsulfuration	"Classic" homocystinuria	Cystathionine β-synthase	CBS	21q22.3
Remethylation	Folate-dependent homocystinuria	Methylenetetrahydrofolate reductase	MTHFR	1p36.3
	Cbl E	Methyltransferase reductase	MTRR	5p15.2-p15.3
	Cbl G	Methionine synthase (methyltransferase)	MTR	1q43
Cobalamin transport	TC-II	Transcobalamin II	TCN2	22q11.2-qter
	Cbl F	Lysosomal B$_{12}$ translocase	LMBRD1	6q13
Cobalamin processing	Cbl C	Intracellular cobalamin chaperone?	MMACHC	1p34.1
	Cbl D	Cobalamin reductase?	MMADHC	2q23.2

TABLE 216-2 CLINICAL FEATURES OF HOMOCYSTINURIA

CLASS	Biochemical Features			Clinical Features	
	HCYS	MET	MMA	SYSTEM	SIGNS
Cystathionine β-synthase deficiency	↑	↑	–	Ocular	Ectopia lentis, myopia, glaucoma, optic atrophy, retinal detachment
				Skeletal	Elongated and thinned bones, arachnodactyly, genu valgum, pectus malformation, scoliosis
				Vascular	Thromboembolic events (arterial or venous)
				Neurologic	Mental retardation in untreated cases, cerebrovascular thromboses, seizures
					Psychiatric disorders, personality disorder
Methylenetetrahydrofolate reductase deficiency	↑	↓	–	Ocular	Ectopia lentis
				Vascular	Thromboses
				Neurologic	Variable—psychiatric to severe neurologic
Transcobalamin II deficiency	–/↑	–/↓	+/–	Hematologic	Pancytopenia, macrocytosis
				Pansystemic	MMA, ketoacidosis, stomatitis
Cbl F	–/↑	?	+/–	Pansystemic	MMA, macrocytosis, stomatitis
Cbl C, Cbl D	–/↑	–/↓	+	Hematologic	Pancytopenia
				Neurologic	Mental retardation
Cbl E, Cbl G	↑	–/↓	–	Vascular	Vaso-occlusive phenomena
				Neurologic	Spasticity, dystonia

Cbl = cobalamin; Hcys = homocystinemia/homocystinuria; Met = plasma methionine; MMA = methylmalonic acidemia.

any time in life, including infancy. Treatment with pyridoxine, the cofactor of the enzyme, may be effective in nearly half these patients, particularly those with relatively high residual activity and spared amounts of immunologically detectable enzyme. Blood total homocysteine concentrations may be intermediately elevated in heterozygotes, especially after a methionine load, and heterozygotes are at some increased risk for vaso-occlusive events. Although increased vascular complications have not been formally demonstrated in outcome studies of obligate heterozygotes, a considerable number of studies show a highly disproportionate fraction of patients with various vaso-occlusive complications who manifest either total blood homocysteine concentrations or fibroblast cystathionine β-synthase activities that fall in the range observed for heterozygotes.

MTHFR deficiency has been described in a limited number of patients, and the spectrum of manifestations includes neurologic symptoms, thrombosis, and lens dislocation, but without conspicuous skeletal changes. Severe deficiencies may present in infancy with cerebral hypoplasia and profound developmental delay. Partial deficiencies and thermolabile variants (including homozygosity for the 677T polymorphism) have been observed in otherwise normal subjects who have premature vaso-occlusive disorders. Relative risks are not well established. Meta-analysis of incidence studies have predicted that lowering total homocysteine concentrations by 3 μmol/L could reduce the risk of heart disease by 11 to 16% and stroke by 19 to 24%, but recent secondary intervention studies did not confirm a benefit, perhaps because of an insufficient statistical power. Polymorphisms in MTHFR have also been associated with spinal closure defects, a class of disease known to be influenced by folate. Cobalamin metabolic disorders generally occur in early childhood and are characterized by neurologic symptoms, megaloblastic anemia, and, in some cases, methylmalonic acidemia.

DIAGNOSIS

Qualitative detection using sodium nitroprusside led to the recognition of homocystinuria early in the history of biochemical genetics, but it is neither specific nor sensitive. Assay of plasma amino acids by routine methods may not reveal homocysteine as a result of the high degree of protein binding.

Because of lower protein concentrations, routine amino acid analysis of urine is more successful, hence the common name *homocystinuria*. The preferred diagnostic method is total homocysteine, which is measured in plasma treated with a reducing agent to release bound homocysteine before deproteinization. Plasma amino acids indicate a transsulfuration or remethylation defect, depending on the presence or absence of hypermethioninemia (see Table 216-2). The clinical diagnosis of remethylation defects is facilitated by the detection of urine methylmalonate and blood vitamin B$_{12}$ and folate. The normal range of total homocysteine in blood extends up to about 15 μmol/L, and it may be more than 50% higher 2 to 4 hours after an oral methionine load. A standard methionine load (100 mg/kg) may identify individuals with partial defects, which could increase their susceptibility to vascular disease.

TREATMENT Rx

Cystathionine β-synthase deficiency is responsive to administration of the cofactor pyridoxine in about 50% of cases. Doses of 100 to 500 mg/day have been used successfully. Higher doses of pyridoxine should be given cautiously because of the risk of peripheral neuropathy. Responsiveness is documented by the elimination of free homocysteine in blood and urine as pyridoxine is added, but measurement of total homocysteine demonstrates that the effect is generally far less than complete. Betaine (*N,N,N*-trimethylglycine, Cystadane) is effective in reducing homocysteine through an alternative remethylation step. This drug is particularly important in pyridoxine-unresponsive cases, but it may also be used as an adjunct in responsive patients. Betaine 6 g/day in divided doses is the typical regimen, but considerably higher doses have been used. The dose in children is generally 100 to 250 mg/kg. There have been two reports of cerebral edema associated with betaine, presumably caused by unusually high levels of methionine or betaine. In the absence of pyridoxine responsiveness, special diets are adopted to restrict methionine and supplement cysteine. Folic (or folinic) acid may be effective in remethylation defects, and it is also generally used as a supplement (10 to 20 mg/day) in all forms of homocystinuria. Vitamin B$_{12}$ preparations may be life-saving in disorders of cobalamin metabolism, although their effectiveness in the most common forms of cobalamin C or D defects is far from complete. Initial doses are usually 1000 µg/day, and hydroxocobalamin may be more effective than cyanocobalamin. It is prudent to adopt measures to decrease thrombosis, such as using low-dose aspirin or dipyridamole and avoiding smoking and oral contraceptives. Nitrous oxide may also be relatively contraindicated because it can inhibit methionine synthase. Surgery poses serious risks but can be performed safely as long as attention is paid to the patient's hydration and coagulation status.

PROGNOSIS

In cases of cystathionine β-synthase deficiency, pyridoxine responsiveness generally correlates with higher residual enzyme activity, and the prognosis is significantly better than that for unresponsive cases, with or without treatment. Skeletal, ocular, vascular, and neurologic risks are all reduced with successful treatment. Without the early institution of treatment, the median IQ in a large outcome study was 57 for unresponsive patients and 78 for responsive patients. With early treatment, pyridoxine-unresponsive patients have a nearly normal median IQ. For patients who are responsive to treatment, the prognosis for intellectual development is very good, but significant elevations in total homocysteine generally persist, and some increased risk for vascular complications probably remains.

SUGGESTED READINGS

Clarke R, Halsey J, Lewington S, et al. Effects of lowering homocysteine levels with B vitamins on cardiovascular disease, cancer, and cause-specific mortality: meta-analysis of 8 randomized trials involving 37,485 individuals. *Arch Intern Med.* 2010;170:1622-1631. *Lowering homocysteine levels does not reduce cardiovascular events or overall or cancer mortality.*

Joseph J, Handy DE, Loscalzo J. Quo vadis: whither homocysteine research? *Cardiovasc Toxicol.* 2009;9:53-63. *Review of recent population intervention studies that is particularly interesting for its discussion of why, despite clear evidence that elevated homocysteine is associated with cardiovascular disease, there have been numerous studies aimed at lowering homocysteine with negative and/or inconclusive outcomes.*

Urreizti R, Moya-Garcia AA, Pino-Ángeles A, et al. Molecular characterization of five patients with homocystinuria due to severe methylenetetrahydrofolate reductase deficiency. *Clin Genet.* 2010;78:441-448. *Missense mutations may cause a less severe phenotype than do mutations that cause severe alterations of the MTHFR protein.*

Zacho J, Yazdanyar S, Bojesen SE, et al. Hyperhomocysteinemia, methylenetetrahydrofolate reductase c.677C>T polymorphism and risk of cancer: cross-sectional and prospective studies and meta-analyses of 75,000 cases and 93,000 controls. *Int J Cancer.* 2011;128:644-652. *Increased plasma homocysteine levels are not associated with an increased age-adjusted risk of any cancer.*

THE PORPHYRIAS

KARL E. ANDERSON

DEFINITION

Porphyrias are due to altered activity of specific enzymes of the heme biosynthetic pathway and, when clinically expressed, are associated with striking accumulations of heme pathway intermediates. Porphyria cutanea tarda (PCT), the most common of these disorders, is primarily an acquired, iron-related disorder. The others occur only with mutations of an enzyme in the heme biosynthetic pathway. Porphyrias are more prevalent and more often manifested in adults than are most metabolic diseases and are likely to be encountered by physicians in many disciplines. The three most common porphyrias differ considerably from each other and are managed differently.

The Heme Biosynthetic Pathway and the Porphyrias
The genes encoding all eight enzymes of this important pathway (Fig. 217-1) have been sequenced and their chromosome locations identified (Table 217-1). Loss-of-function mutations for each enzyme have been associated with specific types of porphyrias, with the exception of δ-aminolevulinic acid (ALA) synthase. Loss-of-function mutations of the erythroid-specific form of this enzyme (ALAS2), the first in the pathway, are found in X-linked sideroblastic anemia. Interestingly, however, gain-of-function mutations of this enzyme were recently identified in a variant, X-linked form of erythropoietic protoporphyria (EPP) (standard abbreviations for these diseases are shown

in Table 217-1). Because all porphyrias are heterogeneous at the molecular level, different mutations are to be expected in unrelated families.

Heme is synthesized in the largest amounts in bone marrow and liver, where it is used primarily to make hemoglobin and cytochrome P-450 enzymes, respectively. Hepatic heme biosynthesis is regulated primarily by the ubiquitous form of ALA synthase (ALAS1), which is rate limiting and under sensitive feedback control by a regulatory pool of cellular heme. Hepatic ALAS1 is induced by many of the same drugs and steroids that induce P-450 enzymes. Additional pathway enzymes and cellular uptake of iron are important in regulating heme synthesis in erythroid cells.

Intermediates in the pathway (see Fig. 217-1) are normally conserved during heme synthesis and excreted only in small amounts. The porphyrin precursors ALA and porphobilinogen (PBG) are normally excreted in much larger amounts than porphyrins. Porphyrinogens undergo auto-oxidation outside cells and are excreted primarily as porphyrins. ALA, PBG, and porphyrinogens are colorless and nonfluorescent. Porphyrins are reddish and fluoresce on exposure to long-wave ultraviolet light. ALA, PBG, uroporphyrin, and the heptacarboxyl, hexacarboxyl, and pentacarboxyl porphyrins are excreted mostly in urine; coproporphyrin (a tetracarboxyl porphyrin), in urine and bile; and harderoporphyrin and protoporphyrin, in bile and feces.

CLASSIFICATION

Porphyrias are classified as erythropoietic or hepatic types, depending on whether overproduction of heme pathway intermediates occurs primarily in bone marrow or liver, and also on the basis of clinical features. The acute porphyrias are characterized by neurologic effects. In the cutaneous porphyrias, photosensitivity results from activation of porphyrins by long-wave ultraviolet light (UVA) with generation of oxygen radicals that damage the skin.

THE MOST COMMON PORPHYRIAS

The three most common types of porphyrias differ markedly from each other with regard to major clinical manifestations, exacerbating factors, tests important for diagnosis, and effective therapies (Table 217-2). Because their features are so distinct, a feature learned about one of these porphyrias will not apply to the others. On the other hand, acute intermittent porphyria (AIP) and PCT (see Table 217-2) share some important features with certain less common porphyrias.

Acute Intermittent Porphyria
AIP, an autosomal dominant disorder, results from an approximately 50% deficiency of PBG deaminase. Penetrance is low, that is, most subjects with PBG deaminase deficiency remain asymptomatic.

EPIDEMIOLOGY
AIP occurs in all races. Its prevalence in most countries has not been precisely estimated, but it may be most common (perhaps 5 per 100,000) in northern European populations.

PATHOBIOLOGY
More than 300 different mutations of the gene encoding PBG deaminase have been identified. Most mutations decrease enzyme activity in all tissues. However, there are two isoenzymes of PBG deaminase, an erythroid-specific and a ubiquitous or "housekeeping" form, both of which are transcribed by alternative messenger RNA (mRNA) splicing from the same gene. The erythroid-specific isoenzyme is encoded by exons 2 to 15, and the erythroid promoter, which functions only in erythroid cells, is found immediately upstream from exon 2. The ubiquitous enzyme is encoded by exons 1 and 3 to 15, and the ubiquitous promoter is immediately upstream from exon 1. For some mutations—in or near exons 1 or 3—only the ubiquitous isoenzyme is deficient. Therefore, in individuals with this type of mutation, the enzyme activity is deficient in nonerythroid tissues but normal in erythrocytes.

The fact that most heterozygotes are asymptomatic and have normal levels of ALA and PBG indicates that the partial deficiency of PBG deaminase does not of itself greatly impair hepatic heme synthesis or induce ALAS1. However, when certain drugs, hormones, or nutritional factors induce hepatic ALAS1, which can occur directly or by inducing cytochrome P-450 enzymes and increasing the demand for heme synthesis, the deficient enzyme becomes limiting for heme synthesis. ALA and PBG accumulate in the liver and increase in the plasma and urine. Excess porphyrins originate nonenzymatically from PBG or enzymatically from ALA transported to tissues other than the liver.

FIGURE 217-1. Intermediates and enzymes of the heme biosynthetic pathway and the major diseases of porphyrin metabolism that have been associated with altered activity of specific enzymes. The initial and last three enzymes (in *pink*) are mitochondrial, and the other four (in *brown*) are cytosolic. Heme is synthesized from glycine and succinyl coenzyme A (CoA). Intermediates in the pathway include δ-aminolevulinic acid (an amino acid used exclusively for heme synthesis), porphobilinogen (a pyrrole), and hydroxymethylbilane (a linear tetrapyrrole). Uroporphyrinogen III cosynthase catalyzes closure of hydroxymethylbilane, with inversion of one of the pyrroles, to form a porphyrin macrocycle, uroporphyrinogen III (nonenzymatic closure occurs without inversion of this pyrrole, forming uroporphyrinogen I, which is not metabolized beyond coproporphyrinogen I). The next two enzymes result in decarboxylation of six of the eight side chains of uroporphyrinogen III, with sequential formation of heptacarboxyl porphyrinogen, hexacarboxyl porphyrinogen, pentacarboxyl porphyrinogen, tetracarboxyl porphyrinogen (coproporphyrinogen III), tricarboxyl porphyrinogen (harderoporphyrinogen), and dicarboxyl porphyrinogen (protoporphyrinogen IX). The final two enzymes catalyze oxidation of protoporphyrinogen IX to protoporphyrin IX and insertion of ferrous iron into the porphyrin macrocycle to form heme (iron protoporphyrin IX). With the exception of protoporphyrinogen IX, all porphyrin intermediates are in their reduced forms (hexahydroporphyrins or porphyrinogens). Chemical structures of two intermediates are shown. ALAD = δ-aminolevulinic acid dehydratase.

FIGURE 217-2. Treatment of porphyria cutanea tarda by repeated phlebotomy. The patient was a 37-year-old woman with a history of excess alcohol intake and chronic hepatitis C. Each *arrow* indicates removal of 450 mL of whole blood. Phlebotomies are stopped when serum ferritin is near the lower limit of normal. Further iron depletion is of no additional benefit and may cause anemia and associated symptoms. Plasma porphyrins become normal, and appearance of new skin lesions ceases within several months. After remission, ferritin can return to normal without recurrence, in most cases. In some cases, relapses occur and respond to another course of phlebotomies. (Modified from Anderson KE. The porphyrias. In Boyer T, Wright T, Manns M, eds. *Zakim and Boyer's Hepatology*. Philadelphia: WB Saunders; 2006:1391-1432.)

Most drugs that are harmful in AIP induce hepatic ALAS1 and cytochrome P-450 enzymes. Some, such as sulfonamide antibiotics, are harmful for reasons not understood. Reduced calorie and carbohydrate intakes enhance induction of ALAS1 in animals and can increase ALA and PBG in AIP and precipitate symptoms. The peroxisome proliferator-activated receptor-γ coactivator 1α (PGC-1α) mediates induction of ALAS1 by fasting and is an important link between nutritional status and acute porphyrias.

Porphyrias and related disorders associated with increased ALA have similar neurologic manifestations, but the mechanism of neural damage is not established. It seems most likely that ALA or another product of the heme pathway is neurotoxic. ALA is structurally analogous to γ-aminobutyric acid (GABA) and can interact with GABA receptors. Alternatively, heme deficiency in nervous tissue may lead to neurologic dysfunction.

CLINICAL MANIFESTATIONS

Symptoms occur intermittently as acute attacks in some heterozygotes lasting for several days or longer, usually followed by complete recovery. There is often no family history of porphyria. Attacks are rare before puberty. Abdominal pain, the most common symptom, is usually steady and poorly localized, but it may be cramping. Tachycardia, hypertension, restlessness, fine tremors, and excess sweating may be due to sympathetic overactivity. Other manifestations include nausea and vomiting; constipation; pain in the limbs, head, neck, or chest; muscle weakness; and sensory loss. Ileus, with distention and decreased bowel sounds, is common. However, increased bowel sounds and diarrhea may be seen. Because the abdominal symptoms are neurologic rather than inflammatory, tenderness, fever, and leukocytosis are generally absent or mild. Dysuria and bladder dysfunction may occur. Recurrent attacks tend to be similar in a given patient.

Peripheral neuropathy in AIP is primarily motor and results from axonal degeneration. This does not develop in all patients with acute attacks, even when abdominal symptoms are severe. Rarely, motor neuropathy develops apart from abdominal symptoms. Weakness most commonly begins in proximal muscles (often requiring a careful examination to be detected) and more often in the arms than in the legs. It can be asymmetrical and focal. Tendon reflexes may be little affected or hyperactive in early stages but are usually decreased or absent with advanced neuropathy. Cranial and sensory nerves can be affected. Progression to respiratory and bulbar paralysis and death is unlikely if porphyria is promptly recognized, harmful drugs are discontinued, and appropriate treatment is instituted. Sudden death, presumably from cardiac arrhythmia, sometimes occurs.

TABLE 217-1 ENZYMES OF THE HEME BIOSYNTHETIC PATHWAY AND CLASSIFICATION AND INHERITANCE OF DISEASES ASSOCIATED WITH THEIR ALTERED ACTIVITIES*

ENZYME	CHROMOSOME LOCATION	DISEASE	INHERITANCE	Classifications of Porphyrias			
				HEPATIC	ERYTHROPOIETIC	ACUTE	CUTANEOUS
ALA synthase							
Erythroid	Xp11.21	Sideroblastic anemia	X-linked recessive				
		X-linked protoporphyria	X-linked recessive		X		X
Housekeeping	3p21	None known					
ALA dehydratase	9q34	ALA dehydratase-deficient porphyria (ADP)	Autosomal recessive	X (?)		X	
Porphobilinogen deaminase†	11q24.1→ q24.2	Acute intermittent porphyria (AIP)	Autosomal dominant	X		X	
Uroporphyrinogen III cosynthase	10q25.2→q26.3	Congenital erythropoietic porphyria (CEP)	Autosomal recessive		X		X
Uroporphyrinogen decarboxylase	1p34	Porphyria cutanea tarda (PCT)‡	Autosomal dominant	X			X
		Hepatoerythropoietic porphyria (HEP)	Autosomal recessive	X	X		X
Coproporphyrinogen oxidase	3q12	Hereditary coproporphyria (HCP)	Autosomal dominant	X		X	X
Protoporphyrinogen oxidase	1q23	Variegate porphyria (VP)	Autosomal dominant	X		X	X
Ferrochelatase	18q21.3	Erythropoietic protoporphyria (EPP)	Autosomal recessive§		X		X

*The most precise classification is according to the specific enzyme deficiencies. Other classifications based on the major tissue site of overproduction of heme pathway intermediates (hepatic vs. erythropoietic) or the type of major symptoms (acute neurovisceral vs. cutaneous) are useful but not precise or mutually exclusive.
†This enzyme is also known as *hydroxymethylbilane synthase* and formerly as *uroporphyrinogen I synthase*.
‡Inherited deficiency of uroporphyrinogen decarboxylase is partially responsible for familial (type 2) porphyria cutanea tarda.
§EPP was previously classified as autosomal dominant with variable penetrance but is now recognized as recessive at the molecular level, with inherited mutations affecting both *FECH* alleles. Most patients have a null mutation trans to a hypomorphic mutation, IVS3-48T>C, that is common in the population but does not itself cause disease.
ALA = δ-aminolevulinic acid.

TABLE 217-2 THE THREE MOST COMMON HUMAN PORPHYRIAS AND THE MAJOR FEATURES OF THESE DISORDERS THAT ARE DISTINCTLY DIFFERENT FROM EACH OTHER

	PRESENTING SYMPTOMS; TREATMENT	EXACERBATING FACTORS	MOST IMPORTANT SCREENING TESTS
Acute intermittent porphyria	Neurovisceral (acute); heme, glucose	Drugs (mostly P-450 inducers), progesterone, dietary restriction	Urinary porphobilinogen
Porphyria cutanea tarda	Blistering skin lesions (chronic); phlebotomy, low-dose hydroxychloroquine	Iron, alcohol, estrogens, hepatitis C virus, halogenated hydrocarbons	Plasma (or urine) porphyrins
Erythropoietic protoporphyria	Painful skin and swelling (mostly acute); β-carotene		Total erythrocyte protoporphyrin

The central nervous system can be involved. Anxiety, insomnia, depression, disorientation, hallucinations, and paranoia, which can be especially severe during acute attacks, may suggest a primary mental disorder or hysteria. Seizures may occur as an acute neurologic manifestation of AIP, as a result of hyponatremia, or secondary to causes unrelated to porphyria. Hyponatremia may be due to hypothalamic involvement and inappropriate antidiuretic hormone secretion, vomiting, diarrhea and poor intake, or excess renal sodium loss.

An attack may resolve rapidly after several days. Attacks during the luteal phase of the menstrual cycle usually resolve with onset of menses. Even advanced neuropathy seen with a prolonged attack is potentially reversible. Frequently recurring attacks and chronic symptoms including pain and depression sometimes occur.

Chronic hepatic abnormalities are common in AIP. Risk for hepatocellular carcinoma (not associated with hepatitis B or C) is also increased. AIP may predispose to chronic hypertension and be associated with impaired renal function.

Homozygous AIP is extremely rare. It presents in early childhood primarily with delayed development and neurologic dysfunction, but not with acute attacks.

Precipitating Factors

Certain drugs, steroid hormones, and nutritional alterations are commonly implicated in causing attacks. Features such as onset after puberty and more frequent clinical expression in women suggest that endogenous hormones are important. Recurrent cyclic attacks are troublesome in some women and occur when progesterone levels are highest. Progesterone and its metabolites are potent inducers of hepatic ALAS1, whereas estrogens are not.

Exacerbations may be seen after administration of progestin-containing steroid combinations. Although pregnancy is usually well tolerated (despite high progesterone levels), attacks may become more frequent, and hyperemesis gravidarum, reduced calorie intake, and harmful drugs (e.g., metoclopramide) may contribute.

Drugs remain important as causes of AIP attacks. Barbiturates and sulfonamides are most notorious, whereas benzodiazepines, which have largely replaced barbiturates in clinical practice, are less hazardous. The major drugs known to be harmful or safe in the acute porphyrias are listed in Table 217-3. Many drugs are not easily classified. Advice can be sought from interactive websites maintained by the European Porphyria Initiative (www.porphyria-europe.com) or from the American Porphyria Foundation (www.porphyriafoundation.com). Some drugs and other factors that contribute in porphyria cutanea tarda are seldom implicated in acute porphyrias (see later).

Attacks may be provoked by reduced calorie intake (usually instituted in an effort to lose weight), infections, and major surgery. Cigarette smoke contains chemicals that can induce hepatic heme synthesis and may predispose to attacks. Attacks are almost always due to two or more factors acting in an additive fashion. Probably for this reason, (1) drugs may produce attacks in adults but rarely in children, (2) anticonvulsants do not produce attacks in all PBG deaminase-deficient subjects, and (3) barbiturate anesthetics more frequently exacerbate porphyria if symptoms are present before anesthetic exposure.

DIAGNOSIS

A high index of suspicion is necessary for diagnosis of AIP and other acute porphyrias because they are uncommon, their symptoms are nonspecific,

TABLE 217-3 SELECTED DRUGS CONSIDERED UNSAFE AND SAFE IN ACUTE INTERMITTENT PORPHYRIA, HEREDITARY COPROPORPHYRIA, AND VARIEGATE PORPHYRIA

UNSAFE	SAFE
Alcohol	Acetaminophen
Barbiturates*	Acetazolamide
Calcium-channel blockers	Allopurinol
Carbamazepine*	Amiloride
Carisoprodol*	Angiotensin-converting enzyme inhibitors[†]
Clonazepam	Angiotensin receptor antagonists[†]
Danazol*	Aspirin
Diclofenac and possibly other nonsteroidal anti-inflammatory drugs*	Atropine
Ergots	β-Adrenergic antagonists[†]
Ethchlorvynol*	Bromides
Glutethimide*	Cimetidine
Griseofulvin*	Erythropoietin*[,‡]
Mephenytoin	Estrogens*[,§] (?)
Meprobamate* (also mebutamate,* tybutamate*)	Gabapentin
Methyprylon	Gentamicin
Metoclopramide*	Glucocorticoids
Phenytoin*	Insulin
Primidone*	Narcotic analgesics
Progesterone and synthetic progestins*	Ofloxacin
Pyrazinamide*	Penicillin and derivatives
Pyrazolones (aminopyrine, antipyrine)	Phenothiazines
Rifampin*	Ranitidine*[,‡]
Succinimides (ethosuximide, methsuximide)	Streptomycin
Sulfonamide antibiotics*	Tetracycline
Valproic acid*	

*Porphyria is listed as a contraindication, warning, precaution, or adverse effect in U.S. labeling for these drugs. For drugs listed here as unsafe, absence of such cautionary statements in U.S. labeling does not imply lower risk.

[†]Some drugs in these classes may be safer than others: see websites of the American Porphyria Foundation (*www.porphyriafoundation.com*) and the European Porphyria Initiative (*www.porphyria-europe.com*).

[‡]Although porphyria is listed as a precaution in U.S. labeling, these drugs are regarded as safe by other sources.

[§]There is little evidence that estrogens alone are harmful in acute porphyrias. They have been implicated as harmful mostly on the basis of experience with estrogen-progestin combinations and because they can exacerbate porphyria cutanea tarda.

and physical findings are minimal. In some European countries, almost all families with acute porphyrias have been identified and studied, but in the United States, many cases still present without a known family history. The diagnosis of acute porphyria is established initially by demonstrating a marked increase in urinary PBG. Urinary PBG excretion in excess of approximately 6 mg/day is virtually diagnostic of AIP, variegate porphyria (VP), or hereditary coproporphyria (HCP). Excretion is generally in the range of 50 to 200 mg/day for PBG (reference range, 0 to 4 mg/day) and 20 to 100 mg/day for ALA (reference range, 0 to 7 mg/day) during attacks of AIP, but increases are less in HCP and VP, and these levels generally decrease with clinical improvement. PBG levels become normal after hemin therapy (usually transiently) and sometimes with prolonged clinical latency. Urinary ALA and PBG decrease to normal levels more readily in HCP and VP than in AIP. Fecal porphyrins are usually normal or minimally increased, which distinguishes AIP from HCP and VP. Urinary uroporphyrin and coproporphyrin are often considerably increased and erythrocyte protoporphyrin may be slightly increased in AIP, but these findings are not specific.

PBG levels often remain variably elevated between attacks of AIP. Diagnosis of a recurrent attack is based on clinical findings, rather than by a particular level of increased PBG, and exclusion of other potential causes of the presenting symptoms.

Laboratory testing for acute porphyrias becomes less sensitive with time after symptoms have subsided. However, in many cases, these disorders may still be recognized and differentiated by more extensive testing to include urinary ALA and PBG, porphyrins in urine and in plasma and feces, and erythrocyte PBG deaminase. An attempt to provoke increases in ALA and PBG for diagnostic purposes by glycine loading or administration of phenobarbital may be dangerous and is not definitive.

Decreased PBG deaminase (most conveniently measured in erythrocytes) helps confirm a diagnosis of AIP. However, erythrocyte PBG deaminase activity is normal in some AIP patients because (1) some PBG deaminase mutations only reduce the nonerythroid enzyme (as noted earlier), (2) erythrocyte PBG deaminase has a wide normal range (up to three-fold) that overlaps the AIP range, and (3) the erythrocyte enzyme is increased by inapparent concurrent conditions that stimulate erythropoiesis. Furthermore, this measurement is not useful in acutely ill patients because it does not distinguish between active and latent stages of AIP, and is normal in other acute porphyrias. The assay is useful for analysis of pedigrees of known AIP patients if it is established that an index case has a low value. However, because DNA studies are more dependable, it is now recommended that the specific PBG deaminase mutation be determined, and then relatives can be tested reliably for latent AIP. Diagnosis in utero is possible but seldom indicated in view of the favorable outlook for most PBG deaminase-deficient subjects.

TREATMENT

Acute attacks usually require hospitalization for treatment of severe pain, nausea, and vomiting and for the intravenous administration of glucose and hemin. Patients should be observed for neurologic complications, respiratory impairment, electrolyte imbalances, and nutritional status. Precipitating factors—usually multiple—should be identified and removed whenever possible. Symptomatic therapy includes narcotic analgesics, which are usually required for severe pain, and small to moderate doses of a phenothiazine for nausea, vomiting, anxiety, and restlessness. Short-acting benzodiazepines in low doses may be safe for insomnia if a minor tranquilizer is required. Bladder distention may require catheterization. After recovery, continued treatment with a phenothiazine is seldom indicated.

Hemin therapy and carbohydrate loading are both specific therapies because they repress hepatic ALAS1 and overproduction of ALA and PBG. Hemin is more effective and should be initiated early, but only after the initial diagnosis of acute porphyria is confirmed by a marked increase in urinary PBG (spot samples of urine, plasma, and feces are saved for later differentiation of AIP, HCP, and VP). Diagnosis is more difficult after hemin is started, which at least transiently lowers ALA and PBG, often to normal levels. Recurrent attacks in patients with persistently high levels of PBG are diagnosed primarily on clinical grounds, and a spot urine sample may be obtained for PBG measurement and treatment with hemin started before the result is available.

The standard regimen for hemin treatment is 3 to 4 mg of hemin per kilogram of body weight infused intravenously once daily for 4 days. A longer course of treatment is seldom necessary if treatment is started early. Efficacy is reduced and recovery less rapid when treatment is delayed and neuronal damage is more advanced. It is not effective for chronic symptoms of AIP. Hemin is available in the United States as a lyophilized hematin (hydroxyheme) preparation. The product is unstable when it is reconstituted with sterile water, and degradation products adhere to endothelial cells, platelets, and coagulation factors, causing a transient anticoagulant effect and frequently a phlebitis at the site of infusion. Reconstitution with human albumin enhances the stability of hematin and prevents these side effects. Heme arginate (available in Europe and South Africa) is more stable and has fewer side effects.

Carbohydrate loading may suffice for mild attacks (e.g., pain not requiring narcotics, and without paresis, seizures, or hyponatremia) and can be given orally as sucrose, glucose polymers, or carbohydrate-rich foods. If oral intake is poorly tolerated or contraindicated by distention and ileus, intravenous administration of glucose (at least 300 g daily) is usually indicated, although larger amounts may be more effective. However, this may entail administration of a large volume of fluids and increase the risk for hyponatremia. A central venous line facilitates more complete parenteral nutrition support and avoids excess fluid volumes. The effect of glucose is mediated in part by elevation of insulin, which reduces expression of PGC-1α in the liver.

Treatment of seizures is problematic because almost all antiseizure drugs can exacerbate AIP. Bromides, gabapentin, and probably vigabatrin can be given safely. β-Adrenergic blocking agents may control tachycardia and hypertension in acute attacks of porphyria, but they may be hazardous in patients with hypovolemia, in whom increased catecholamine secretion may be an important compensatory mechanism. Cimetidine has been reported to be beneficial, but controlled studies are lacking, and it should not be used in place of hemin. Numerous other therapies have been tried in this disease but have not been consistently useful.

Liver transplantation can be curative for patients with repeated disabling attacks that are refractory to hemin therapy and prophylaxis, but without advanced motor neuropathy. This experience, albeit limited to date, strongly indicates that the liver is central to the neurologic manifestations of this disease.

PREVENTION

Some specific measures are helpful in preventing clinical expression of AIP. Family members should be screened, preferably by DNA methods, to detect latent cases. Potentially harmful drugs should be avoided. "Crash diets" for weight reduction and even brief periods of starvation (e.g., during postoperative periods or intercurrent illnesses) should be avoided; diet regimens for obesity should provide for gradual weight loss during periods of clinical remission of porphyria. Gonadotropin-releasing hormone analogues can prevent frequent cyclic attacks in women; oophorectomy is not an acceptable option for preventing cyclic attacks. Single hemin infusions once or twice weekly sometimes prevent frequently recurring attacks. Because suicide is a risk in AIP, a preventive approach is appropriate, especially in patients with chronic symptoms and depression.

PROGNOSIS

If acute attacks are treated promptly, inciting factors removed, and precautions taken to prevent further attacks, the outlook for patients with AIP is usually very good. Recurrent attacks occur in some patients and can be disabling, but they do not occur throughout adult life. Chronic pain, depression, and other symptoms can increase the risk for suicide but may improve in the long term.

Most relatives with PBG deaminase deficiency never develop symptoms, especially if they have normal urinary porphyrin precursors. Such individuals with latent AIP may be less sensitive to inducing drugs or other factors that exacerbate AIP than are patients with prior porphyric symptoms, but they should follow the same precautions as those who have had symptoms.

Porphyria Cutanea Tarda

DEFINITION

Porphyria cutanea tarda (PCT), the most common and readily treated form of porphyria, is an iron-related disorder caused by inhibition of uroporphyrinogen decarboxylase (UROD) in the liver. It presents with blistering cutaneous lesions on sun-exposed areas.

PATHOBIOLOGY

PCT is mostly an acquired disorder in which hepatic UROD activity is reduced to less than about 20% of normal. (The hepatic UROD protein remains at its genetically determined level, as measured immunochemically.) A UROD inhibitor has been isolated as a uroporphomethene (derived from uroporphyrinogen by oxidation of one of its four methane bridges, or possibly from hydroxymethylbilane); iron, along with one or more cytochrome P-450 enzymes, and oxidative stress are believed to be involved in its formation. A normal or increased amount of hepatic iron is essential for development of PCT, although iron does not directly inhibit UROD. Multiple genetic, viral, and chemical susceptibility factors are known, and at least several are combined in individual patients.

Most patients with manifest PCT (~80%) do not have *UROD* mutations and are classified as sporadic (type 1). Those with *UROD* mutations are said to have familial (type 2) disease but usually present sporadically (without a family history of PCT) because penetrance of familial PCT is low. Heterozygous carriers of *UROD* mutations are more susceptible because their genetically determined levels of UROD are half-normal from birth. Type 2 cases can be distinguished by finding half-normal UROD activity in erythrocytes, but DNA studies are more reliable. Clustering of related individuals with features of type 1 PCT, including absence of *UROD* mutations, has been referred to as type 3, but the genetic basis is not known. Types 1 to 3 are clinically similar, although age at disease onset may on average be earlier in type 2.

Halogenated polyaromatic hydrocarbons are rarely associated with PCT in humans. Most notably, an extensive outbreak of porphyria occurred in eastern Turkey in 1955 to 1958 after seed wheat containing the fungicide hexachlorobenzene was consumed during a famine. 2,3,7,8-Tetrachlorodibenzo-*p*-dioxin (TCDD, dioxin) has been implicated in smaller outbreaks. Such exposures are seldom evident in sporadic cases of PCT.

Most of the following susceptibility factors are readily identified clinically in patients with PCT. Several are found in almost all patients, although none is essential.

- **Alcohol** abuse has long been recognized as an important contributor and may increase hepatic iron by downregulation of hepcidin, induce cytochrome P-450 enzymes, and cause oxidative stress in hepatocytes.
- **Smoking** (Chapter 31) has been considered a potential contributor more recently. Constituents of cigarette smoke can induce hepatic cytochrome P-450 enzymes that may be involved in generation of a UROD inhibitor (especially CYP1A2).
- **Estrogen** use is strongly associated with PCT in women and may also lead to the production of reactive oxygen species in hepatocytes.
- **Hepatitis C**, which downregulates hepcidin and causes hepatic oxidative stress and steatosis, is highly prevalent in PCT in most geographic areas (e.g., 70% or greater in the United States and southern Europe).
- **Human immunodeficiency virus infection** is less commonly associated but is probably an additional risk factor for PCT.
- **Hemochromatosis gene (*HFE*) mutations** (Chapter 219) favor increased iron absorption by downregulation of hepcidin. About 10% of PCT patients of northern European origin are homozygous for the *C282Y* mutation, and a corresponding number are *C282Y/H63D* compound heterozygotes.
- **UROD mutations,** which identify patients with type 2 disease, are most reliably found by DNA studies; most will have half-normal erythrocyte UROD activity.

Other factors undoubtedly are important. Reduced levels of antioxidants, such as vitamin C and carotenoids, have been reported. A *CYP1A2* polymorphism that favors induction of this enzyme was more common in PCT than in controls in several case series. Drugs are sometimes associated with PCT and may play an additive role. Those so indicated in U.S. labeling are several nonsteroidal anti-inflammatory drugs, sulfonylureas, and busulfan. Associations with systemic lupus erythematosus, bone marrow disorders, and end-stage renal disease have been described. Because porphyrins are poorly dialyzed, porphyrin levels are often much higher in patients with advanced renal disease, and skin lesions are more severe.

PCT is a chronic disease, and massive amounts of porphyrins accumulate in the liver, probably over many months, before excess porphyrins appear in plasma and urine. Hepatic ALAS1 may be little increased because the amount of excess porphyrins produced in PCT is small relative to the rate of hepatic heme formation. This contrasts with the acute porphyrias, in which much larger amounts of intermediates are excreted as porphyrin precursors, particularly during attacks, and ALA synthase is substantially induced.

The pattern of porphyrins that accumulate in PCT is complex and characteristic. Decarboxylation of uroporphyrinogen occurs in four sequential steps. Therefore, when UROD is markedly deficient, uroporphyrin and the heptacarboxyl, hexacarboxyl, and pentacarboxyl porphyrins (type I and III isomers derived from the corresponding porphyrinogens) accumulate. In addition, pentacarboxyl porphyrinogen can be metabolized by coproporphyrinogen oxidase to a series of tetracarboxyl porphyrinogens termed *isocoproporphyrinogens*. The corresponding isocoproporphyrins are excreted primarily in bile and feces and are diagnostic of UROD deficiency.

CLINICAL MANIFESTATIONS

Cutaneous photosensitivity is the major clinical feature. Vesicles and bullae develop most commonly on the dorsum of the hands as well as on the face, forearms, legs, and feet. Sun-exposed skin becomes friable, and minor trauma may precede the formation of bullae or cause denudation of the skin. Small white plaques (milia) may precede or follow vesicle formation. Involved skin tends to heal slowly. Hypertrichosis and hyperpigmentation sometimes occur even in the absence of vesicles. Thickening, scarring, and calcification of affected skin (pseudoscleroderma) may be striking. Neurologic effects are not observed.

Abnormal liver test results—especially transaminases—are common in PCT and can occur in the absence of hepatitis C. Liver histopathology is nonspecific, other than the finding of fluorescence due to porphyrins, which appear as inclusions in fixed tissue. Liver iron is often increased. Risk for cirrhosis and hepatocellular carcinoma increases with disease duration. Rarely, hepatic tumors themselves contain and presumably produce excess porphyrins. Some of these cases have resembled PCT.

DIAGNOSIS

Skin lesions in PCT, VP, and HCP are indistinguishable clinically and histologically. It is important to differentiate these conditions by laboratory testing before therapy is started. A predominance of uroporphyrin and heptacarboxyl porphyrin in urine is diagnostic of PCT, and increased isocoproporphyrin in feces provides further confirmation. In PCT, urinary ALA may be slightly increased, whereas PBG is normal. Total fecal porphyrins are usually less increased in PCT than in HCP and VP. Plasma porphyrins are virtually always increased in patients with porphyrias causing blistering skin lesions; the fluorescence spectrum of plasma can distinguish VP and erythropoietic protoporphyria from PCT (see later).

TREATMENT   Rx

All three types of PCT respond to treatment; with remission, hepatic UROD activity returns to its genetically determined level (which for type 2 is half-normal). A course of phlebotomies is the preferred treatment. Patients are also advised to discontinue alcohol, estrogens, iron supplements, or other contributing factors. Because iron stores in PCT are seldom markedly increased, removal of only 5 to 8 units of blood at 2-week intervals is usually sufficient. Many more phlebotomies are needed in the minority of patients with very high ferritin levels. Plasma (or serum) ferritin and porphyrin levels should be followed (Fig. 217-2). Deferoxamine, an iron chelator, may be effective but is much less efficient.

A course of low-dose hydroxychloroquine (100 mg) or chloroquine (125 mg) twice weekly for several months is usually effective when repeated phlebotomies are contraindicated. The mechanism of their effects in PCT, which involves release of porphyrins from hepatocytes, has not been established. If usual doses of these drugs are given to patients with PCT, marked increases in photosensitivity and porphyrin levels in plasma and urine are seen and may be accompanied by nausea, malaise, fever, and hepatocellular damage. Although these adverse effects are generally transient and are followed by complete remission, it is prudent to avoid them by use of a low-dose regimen. These may not be effective in patients with marked iron overload.

Therapy is more difficult when PCT occurs with advanced renal disease. However, treatment with recombinant erythropoietin can mobilize excess iron, support phlebotomy, and lead to remission of PCT in these patients.

Erythropoietic Protoporphyria

DEFINITION

EPP, which is the third most common porphyria in adults and the most common in children, causes nonblistering photosensitivity of the skin. EPP is usually due to a deficiency of ferrochelatase (FECH), with increased protoporphyrin in erythrocytes, plasma, bile, and feces. Urine porphyrins are not increased. Rarely, the EPP phenotype results from gain of function mutations of ALAS2.

PATHOBIOLOGY

Several different underlying molecular abnormalities can cause this disease. In more than 90% of affected families, EPP is due in part to 1 of about 110 reported severe mutations of the ferrochelatase gene (FECH). FECH activities, however, are as low as 15 to 25% of normal in patients with EPP, which is accounted for by inheritance of a severe FECH mutation from one parent and a common hypomorphic FECH mutation from the other. The latter is an intronic single nucleotide alteration, IVS3-48T>C, that results in expression of an aberrantly spliced mRNA that is degraded by a nonsense-mediated decay mechanism, which decreases the steady-state level of FECH mRNA. The IVS3-48T>C mutation by itself does not cause disease, even when it is homozygous. Because both FECH alleles are altered in affected individuals, inheritance of the disease is described as recessive at the molecular level. In a few families, two severe FECH mutations (and not the IVS3-48T>C mutation) are found, with at least one allele producing some enzyme protein. Late-onset cases of EPP may be associated with a myeloproliferative disorder and expansion of a clone of erythroid cells carrying a somatic or inherited FECH mutation.

Examination of lineages in a recently described variant form of EPP, in which FECH activity is normal and there are no FECH mutations, suggested X-linked inheritance. Because the ALAS2 gene, which encodes the erythroid-specific form of ALAS, had been localized to the X chromosome, this observation led to the discovery of gain of function C-terminal deletions of this gene in these families. X-linked EPP is also termed X-linked protoporphyria.

Erythrocyte protoporphyrin is increased in many red cell disorders, such as iron deficiency, anemia of chronic disease, and lead poisoning, and is mostly complexed with zinc. FECH activity accounts for formation of zinc protoporphyrin as well as heme. In EPP, the large amounts of protoporphyrin in erythrocytes is mostly free, and only 0 to 15% is complexed with zinc. In X-linked EPP, in which FECH is normal, free protoporphyrin is increased, but zinc protoporphyrin may account for 15 to 50% of the total. Free protoporphyrin diffuses more readily into plasma than does zinc protoporphyrin, especially after light exposure.

Protoporphyrin is markedly increased in bone marrow, erythrocytes, and bile, and less increased in plasma and feces in EPP. Bone marrow reticulocytes that are actively synthesizing heme and hemoglobin are the primary source of the excess protoporphyrin entering the plasma in EPP. Circulating erythrocytes and perhaps the liver contribute smaller amounts. Protoporphyrin is increased in plasma and undergoes hepatic uptake, biliary excretion, and perhaps enterohepatic circulation. Protoporphyrin in large amounts is cholestatic and can cause liver disease that may progress rapidly.

CLINICAL MANIFESTATIONS

Photosensitivity substantially affects lifestyle and quality of life, typically begins early in childhood, and is distinctly different from other cutaneous porphyrias. Burning, itching, erythema, and swelling can occur within minutes of sun exposure. Diffuse edema of sun-exposed areas may resemble angioedema (Chapter 260). Characteristic chronic changes include skin lichenification, leathery pseudovesicles, labial grooving, and nail changes. Scarring is rarely severe or deforming. Vesicles, pigment changes, friability, and hirsutism are unusual. No fluorescence of the teeth and (except with severe hepatic failure) no neuropathic manifestations are present. Drugs that exacerbate hepatic porphyrias are not known to worsen EPP but are generally avoided as a precaution.

Mild microcytic anemia is common, and erythropoiesis and iron absorption may be decreased. These effects may be mediated by excess protoporphyrin, but the mechanism is unclear. Hemolysis is uncommon or mild in uncomplicated cases. Gallstones containing protoporphyrin may require cholecystectomy if they are symptomatic.

Liver function is usually normal in this condition. However, less than 5% of patients with EPP develop *protoporphyric hepatopathy*, which results from the cholestatic effects of protoporphyrin, and can progress rapidly to death from liver failure. Intercurrent factors such as viral hepatitis, alcohol, iron deficiency, fasting, and oral contraceptive steroids have played a role in some patients. Because protoporphyric hepatopathy progressively impairs hepatobiliary excretion of protoporphyrin, plasma and erythrocyte porphyrins increase further, photosensitivity worsens, often with skin blistering, and even a severe motor neuropathy may develop.

DIAGNOSIS

Delay in diagnosis of this porphyria is longer on average than with any other. An increase in erythrocyte protoporphyrin that is primarily free (not complexed with zinc) is diagnostic of EPP. Both free and zinc protoporphyrin are increased in the X-linked form of the disease. Because laboratory methods and terminology are inconsistent, measurement of total erythrocyte protoporphyrin is preferred for initial screening, followed, if elevated, by fractionation of free and zinc protoporphyrin. Plasma porphyrins are more light sensitive and often less elevated than in other cutaneous porphyrias, especially with mild disease. Urinary porphyrins and porphyrin precursors are normal. Hepatic complications of EPP are heralded by abnormal liver tests and increasing levels of erythrocyte and plasma protoporphyrin. Some patients with undiagnosed photosensitivity since childhood are first recognized to have EPP with onset of hepatopathy in adult life.

TREATMENT

β-Carotene (Lumitene) was originally developed primarily for treatment of EPP and found to be beneficial in large series of patients. Its mechanism of action may involve quenching of singlet oxygen or free radicals. Carotenemia with mild, dose-related skin discoloration is expected. Iron supplements are warranted in patients with marginal levels of serum ferritin. Vitamin D and calcium supplements, hepatitis A and B immunizations, and avoidance of alcohol and other hepatotoxins are recommended. Calorie restriction and drugs or hormone preparations that impair hepatic excretory function should be avoided.

Protoporphyric hepatopathy may improve at least partially when treated with transfusions to correct anemia, hemin, cholestyramine, ursodeoxycholic acid, and vitamin E. Liver transplantation is sometimes required. Filters for operating room lights are available to prevent severe skin and peritoneal burns. Hematopoietic stem cell transplantation (Chapter 181) corrects protoporphyrin overproduction and is increasingly considered to prevent damage to the transplanted liver.

● LESS COMMON PORPHYRIAS
ALA Dehydratase-Deficient Porphyria

In this rare autosomal recessive disorder, ALA dehydratase is markedly reduced (usually 1 to 2% of normal). Only six cases (all males) with a total of 11 mutant alleles have been documented, but it is likely that cases are commonly undiagnosed. Three cases were in adolescents, with symptoms resembling AIP. Severe neurologic impairment beginning in childhood was observed in one case. An adult-onset case was associated with a myeloproliferative disorder. Urinary ALA and coproporphyrin III and erythrocyte zinc protoporphyrin are increased. In this and other disorders in which ALA accumulates, coproporphyrin III may originate from excess ALA by metabolism in tissues other than its tissue of origin.

Lead poisoning (Chapter 21) and hereditary tyrosinemia type 1 are also associated with ALA dehydratase deficiency and can present with symptoms (abdominal pain, ileus, and motor neuropathy) that are strikingly similar to those of the acute porphyrias. Lead concentrates in erythroid cells and reversibly inhibits erythrocyte ALA dehydratase by displacing zinc from the enzyme. In lead poisoning, as in ALA dehydratase-deficient porphyria, erythrocyte protoporphyrin and urinary coproporphyrin are increased. In hereditary tyrosinemia type 1, a deficiency of fumarylacetoacetase leads to accumulation of succinylacetone (2,3-dioxoheptanoic acid). This structural analogue of ALA is a potent inhibitor of ALA dehydratase. Other heavy metals or styrene exposure can also inhibit ALA dehydratase.

Congenital Erythropoietic Porphyria
DEFINITION

Congenital erythropoietic porphyria (CEP) is an autosomal recessive disorder that is due to a deficiency of uroporphyrinogen III cosynthase (UROS, also known as *uroporphyrinogen III synthase*). Fewer than 250 cases have been reported.

PATHOBIOLOGY

Many different *UROS* mutations have been identified in CEP. Most patients have unrelated parents and have inherited a different mutation from each parent. The severity of the disease is variable and relates to the degree of enzyme deficiency caused by the particular mutations. Hydroxymethylbilane (the substrate of the deficient enzyme) accumulates and is converted nonenzymatically to uroporphyrinogen I, which is metabolized to coproporphyrinogen I. These porphyrinogens and the corresponding porphyrins accumulate in bone marrow erythroid cells that are actively synthesizing hemoglobin and lead to intramedullary and intravascular hemolysis. Even in the most severe cases, some residual UROS activity is present, and heme production is actually increased in response to hemolysis. Splenomegaly can contribute to anemia and cause leukopenia and thrombocytopenia. The liver is not affected, and drugs and other factors that are harmful in the hepatic porphyrias do not affect this erythropoietic disease.

CLINICAL MANIFESTATIONS

In most cases, reddish urine and severe cutaneous photosensitivity are noted in early infancy. In a few very severe cases, CEP was manifested as nonimmune hydrops, and intrauterine transfusions were administered. Neonatal hyperbilirubinemia may be present at birth, but phototherapy may cause marked blistering and scarring and should be avoided. Late-onset cases are likely to be associated with myeloproliferative disorders and expansion of a clone of cells carrying a *UROS* mutation.

Lesions on sun-exposed skin resemble those in porphyria cutanea tarda but are usually more severe. Bullae and vesicles are likely to rupture and become infected, which contributes to loss of digits and facial features and corneal scarring. Other features include areas of hypopigmentation and hyperpigmentation and hypertrichosis. Porphyrins are deposited in the teeth (producing a red-brown color termed *erythrodontia*) and in bone. Bone demineralization can be substantial and due in part to marrow hyperplasia

and possibly vitamin D deficiency. Hemolysis and splenomegaly are almost always present, but there are no neurologic manifestations. Life expectancy is often shortened by infections or hematologic complications.

DIAGNOSIS

Porphyrin levels and excretion are generally much greater in CEP than in other forms of porphyria. Porphyrins are primarily uroporphyrin I and coproporphyrin I in urine and mostly coproporphyrin I in feces. ALA and PBG are normal. In most cases, uroporphyrin I predominates in erythrocytes. A predominance of protoporphyrin in red cells has been described in some cases with milder disease. Cutaneous features of CEP are readily distinguished from erythropoietic protoporphyria but may resemble hepatoerythropoietic porphyria (see later) and homozygous cases of VP and HCP. These conditions are distinguishable by patterns of porphyrins and porphyrin precursors and should be confirmed by molecular studies.

TREATMENT ℞

Protection of the skin from sunlight and minor trauma and prompt treatment of secondary bacterial infections help prevent scarring and mutilation. Improvement may occur after splenectomy. Oral charcoal may be helpful by increasing fecal excretion of porphyrins. Blood transfusions, sometimes combined with hydroxyurea, may suppress erythropoiesis sufficiently to reduce porphyrin overproduction. Vitamin D and calcium supplementation is recommended. Hematopoietic stem cell transplantation (Chapter 181) may be the most effective current therapy. Gene therapy may eventually be possible.

PREVENTION

In affected families, heterozygotes can be detected by molecular studies, and CEP can be diagnosed in utero. Therefore, options are available to prevent genetic transmission.

Hepatoerythropoietic Porphyria

This rare autosomal recessive disease is clinically similar to CEP but is the homozygous form of familial (type 2) porphyria cutanea tarda, with porphyrin patterns in urine and feces resembling that disease. In addition, erythrocyte UROD activity is markedly decreased, and erythrocyte zinc protoporphyrin is substantially increased. At least one of the *UROD* mutations in a patient with hepatoerythropoietic porphyria (HEP) expresses some enzyme activity because two null mutations would be lethal. Increased erythrocyte protoporphyrin probably reflects an earlier accumulation of uroporphyrinogen III in erythroblasts, which after completion of hemoglobin synthesis, is metabolized to protoporphyrin. A similar explanation can account for increased erythrocyte protoporphyrin in other homozygous forms of porphyria.

Hereditary Coproporphyria and Variegate Porphyria
EPIDEMIOLOGY

These autosomal dominant acute hepatic porphyrias are clinically similar to AIP but are less common in most countries. Unlike AIP, these disorders can cause blistering cutaneous photosensitivity. Variegate porphyria is prevalent in South Africa, where most cases have been traced to a couple who emigrated from Holland in the late 1600s, one of whom carried a disease-causing mutation.

Pathobiology

Hereditary coproporphyria (HCP) and variegate porphyria (VP) are due to approximately 50% deficiencies of coproporphyrinogen oxidase (CPO) and protoporphyrinogen oxidase (PPO), respectively. Many different mutations in the genes for these enzymes have been described. A specific mutation of the *PPO* gene (R59W) is common in South Africa. ALA and PBG are increased during acute attacks, although the degree and duration of increases are usually less than in AIP. Increases in ALA and PBG occur when hepatic ALA synthase (ALAS1) is induced by factors such as endogenous steroids, drugs, and nutritional alterations and because PBG deaminase activity is almost as low as ALAS1 activity even in the normal liver. Coproporphyrinogen III may accumulate in VP because of a functional association between CPO and the deficient PPO in mitochondria. Furthermore, coproporphyrinogen is more readily lost from the liver than are other porphyrinogens, and

TABLE 217-4 FIRST-LINE LABORATORY TESTS FOR SCREENING FOR PORPHYRIAS AND SECOND-LINE TESTS FOR FURTHER EVALUATION WHEN THE INITIAL TEST RESULT IS POSITIVE*

		Symptoms Suggesting Porphyria	
		CUTANEOUS PHOTOSENSITIVITY	
TESTING	**ACUTE NEUROVISCERAL SYMPTOMS**	*Blistering*	*Nonblistering*
First line	Urinary ALA, PBG, and total porphyrins (quantitative; random urine)[‡]	Total plasma porphyrins[†]	Total erythrocyte protoporphyrin
Second line	Urinary ALA, PBG, and total porphyrins[§] (quantitative) Total fecal porphyrins[§] Erythrocyte PBG deaminase Total plasma porphyrins[†]	Erythrocyte porphyrins Urinary ALA, PBG, and total porphyrins[§] (quantitative) Total fecal porphyrins[§]	Fractionate free and zinc protoporphyrin

*All tests are quantitative, except for a rapid method for urinary PBG using a kit. DNA studies are indicated after a diagnosis has been established biochemically.
[†]The preferred method is by direct fluorescent spectrophotometry.
[‡]Semiquantitative testing for PBG using a kit is preferred in acutely ill patients (see text).
[§]Random urine with measured creatinine or a 24-hour collection. Fractionation of urinary and fecal porphyrins is useful only if the total is increased.
ALA = δ-aminolevulinic acid; PBG = porphobilinogen.

its loss increases further when heme synthesis is stimulated. In one form of HCP, termed *harderoporphyria*, a structurally altered CPO with reduced substrate affinity results in accumulation of harderoporphyrin (tricarboxyl porphyrinogen) as well as coproporphyrinogen. The excess porphyrinogens are auto-oxidized to the corresponding porphyrins. Rare homozygous cases of HCP and VP have severe photosensitivity and developmental abnormalities but few acute attacks.

Clinical Manifestations

Drugs, steroids, and nutritional factors that are detrimental in AIP provoke exacerbations of HCP and VP. Neurologic manifestations are identical to those in AIP. Blistering skin lesions, which are much more common in VP than in HCP, are identical to those in PCT and may occur apart from the neurovisceral symptoms. Impaired biliary excretion by concurrent liver diseases or drugs such as contraceptive steroids can cause porphyrin retention and worsen photosensitivity.

Diagnosis

Urinary ALA and PBG are commonly increased during acute attacks. With resolution of symptoms, ALA and PBG normalize more readily than in AIP. Increases in urinary porphyrins are more persistent. A marked, isolated increase in fecal coproporphyrin III is distinctive for HCP. Fecal coproporphyrin and protoporphyrin are about equally increased in VP. The fluorescence spectrum of plasma porphyrins (at neutral pH) is characteristic and useful for rapidly distinguishing VP from the other porphyrias and is the most sensitive porphyrin test, in adults, for detection of VP, including latent cases. However, identification of specific CPO and PPO mutations is recommended and facilitates screening of relatives.

TREATMENT   **Rx**

Acute attacks of both HCP and VP are treated as in AIP. The striking decreases in attacks and deaths from VP in South Africa have been attributed to identification of latent cases, avoidance of potentially harmful drugs, and better treatment during acute attacks. Avoiding sunlight and wearing clothing material designed to protect the skin from sunlight are helpful to prevent photosensitivity. Phlebotomies and hydroxychloroquine are not effective.

Dual Porphyria

Dual porphyria refers to patients with porphyria and deficiencies of more than one enzyme of the heme biosynthetic pathway. Examples include deficiencies of both PBG deaminase and UROD (with symptoms of AIP, PCT, or both), UROS and CPO, and ALA dehydratase and CPO. Dual enzyme deficiencies may be suspected from patterns of porphyrin precursors and porphyrins, but molecular diagnosis is essential.

● LABORATORY DIAGNOSIS OF PORPHYRIAS

Porphyrias in patients with symptoms are readily detected and misdiagnoses avoided by relying on a few first-line tests that are both specific and sensitive,

and on further testing when an initial result is abnormal. This avoids overuse of tests that are expensive and commonly misinterpreted. The preferred tests for screening, as outlined in Table 217-4, are the following:

1. Urinary porphyrin precursors (ALA and PBG) and total porphyrins for patients with concurrent or recent neurovisceral symptoms—for initial diagnosis of AIP, HCP, VP, and very rarely, ADP. Increases are expected to be so striking during an attack of acute porphyria that quantitation in a random urine sample is highly informative. A substantial increase in PBG is highly specific for AIP, HCP, or VP, and is not found in other medical conditions. Assays for PBG employ Ehrlich's aldehyde (*p*-dimethylaminobenzaldehyde), which forms red-purple chromogens with PBG, urobilinogen, and other substances in urine. Qualitative methods for increased PBG (e.g., the Watson-Schwartz and Hoesch tests) are obsolete. A kit that is reliable for screening for increased PBG in urine includes color standards to aid interpretation (Trace PBG kit, Thermo Fisher Scientific).

2. Plasma total porphyrins in patients with blistering skin lesions—to detect PCT, HCP, VP, CEP, and HEP. Total plasma porphyrins are virtually always increased in patients with active, blistering skin lesions due to these conditions. Measurement of urinary porphyrins is an alternative, but elevations are less specific. Fractionation of urine or plasma porphyrins during screening is not helpful because slight elevations in individual porphyrins are not diagnostically important if the total is normal. Measurement of plasma porphyrins is best carried out by a simple and direct fluorometric method. Plasma porphyrins in VP are mostly covalently bound to plasma proteins and may not be detected by other methods.

3. Total erythrocyte protoporphyrin for patients with nonblistering photosensitivity—to detect EPP.

More extensive biochemical testing is required if an initial screening test provides a positive result or may also be necessary initially if subclinical porphyria is suspected. This should include not only urinary ALA, PBG, and total porphyrins, total plasma porphyrins, and erythrocyte protoporphyrin, but also fractionation of urinary porphyrins and fecal total porphyrins (and fractionation if elevated). If plasma total porphyrins are elevated, fluorometric scanning (particularly to differentiate VP) should be done. Elevation in urinary porphyrins (especially coproporphyrin) in the absence of increases in plasma, erythrocyte, or fecal porphyrins is nonspecific, is common in liver and bone marrow disorders and other medical conditions, and is unlikely to indicate a type of porphyria. Erythrocyte protoporphyrin is increased in many red cell disorders, such as iron deficiency and lead poisoning, but in these conditions, it is complexed with zinc rather than metal free, as in EPP. Fecal porphyrin determinations are semiquantitative and subject to interference by diet and other factors. Once a biochemical diagnosis of a specific type of porphyria is established, molecular studies are important to identify the inherited mutation. In most cases of PCT, there is no underlying *UROD* mutation, but a thorough evaluation for all major susceptibility factors is clinically important.

Laboratory testing of asymptomatic relatives is usually not appropriate until test results have firmly established a diagnosis of porphyria in an index case. Results of testing of the index case guide the choice of tests for relatives. Consultation with a physician and laboratory with experience in testing for porphyrias is helpful in these situations. Cytosolic heme biosynthetic pathway enzymes (ALA dehydratase, PBG deaminase, UROS, and UROD) can be measured in erythrocytes. This is not recommended for initial screening of patients with symptoms suggestive of porphyria. The other heme pathway enzymes are mitochondrial and are measured in cells such as lymphocytes; these assays are not widely available. Demonstration of a specific mutation in a family greatly facilitates detection of relatives who carry the same mutation.

Laboratory data that were the basis for an original diagnosis of porphyria should remain available for future reference. Incorrect diagnoses of porphyria are not uncommon when in fact symptoms are due to other diseases. There is little evidence for the suggestion that porphyria is common in disorders such as multiple chemical sensitivity syndrome.

SUGGESTED READINGS

Anderson KE, Bloomer JR, Bonkovsky HL, et al. Recommendations for the diagnosis and treatment of the acute porphyrias. *Ann Intern Med.* 2005;142:439-450. *Detailed recommendations on diagnostic methods and treatment for acute porphyrias.*

Frank J, Poblete-Gutiérrez P. Delayed diagnosis and diminished quality of life in erythropoietic protoporphyria: results of a cross-sectional study in Sweden. *J Intern Med.* 2011;269:270-274. *Review emphasizing the potential adverse effects of delay.*

Jalil S, Grady JJ, Lee C, et al. Associations among behavior-related susceptibility factors in porphyria cutanea tarda. *Clin Gastroenterol Hepatol.* 2010;8:297-302. *A large case series of patients with porphyria cutanea tarda with emphasis on the multiplicity of susceptibility factors and their associations.*

Puy H, Goulya L, Deybach JC. Porphyrias. *Lancet.* 2010;375:924-937. *Comprehensive review and approach to diagnosis of the porphyrias.*

Siegesmund M, van Tuyll van Serooskerken AM, Poblete-Gutiérrez P, et al. The acute hepatic porphyrias: current status and future challenges. *Best Pract Res Clin Gastroenterol.* 2010;24:593-605. *Review of diagnosis and treatment.*

Whatley SD, Mason NG, Holme SA, et al. Molecular epidemiology of erythropoietic protoporphyria in the United Kingdom. *Br J Dermatol.* 2010;162:642-646. *Prevalence of each type of EPP in the United Kingdom and the importance of molecular studies for genetic counseling.*

218

WILSON'S DISEASE

STEPHEN G. KALER

DEFINITION

Wilson's disease is an autosomal recessive disorder of copper transport. Affected individuals accumulate abnormal levels of copper in the liver and later in the brain as a consequence of mutations in both alleles of the Wilson's disease gene *(ATP7B)*. The gene was identified in 1993 and encodes a copper-transporting ATPase expressed primarily in the liver, where its major function is excretion of hepatic copper into the biliary tract.

The clinical condition was first described in 1912 by S. A. K. Wilson, an American neurologist working in England. Thirty-six years later, pathologist J. N. Cummings proposed an etiologic connection with copper overload. Therapy with copper chelation by penicillamine was introduced in 1956 by J. M. Walshe, a British physician working at Boston City Hospital in Massachusetts.

EPIDEMIOLOGY

The incidence of Wilson's disease, defined as the occurrence of new cases, is approximately 1 in 30,000 to 40,000 live births. For special populations in which consanguineous mating is common, the risk of autosomal recessive traits such as Wilson's disease is higher.

In the general population, the prevalence of heterozygous gene carriers (defined as the ratio of all individuals with one mutant *ATP7B* allele to the population at risk of harboring one) is estimated to be 1 in 90. These individuals may represent a group susceptible to liver disease related to environmental copper exposure.

PATHOBIOLOGY

Individuals consume 1 to 3 mg of dietary copper daily, of which approximately 50% is absorbed through the gastrointestinal tract. Most diets contain adequate amounts of copper, and certain foods (e.g., shellfish, liver, mushrooms, chocolate, nuts) contain particularly high quantities. In normal homeostasis, copper is absorbed from the stomach and duodenum, where absorption is mediated by specific copper uptake genes (e.g., *hCTR1*). The Menkes disease gene *(ATP7A)*, which encodes a copper-transporting ATPase with high homology to *ATP7B*, transports copper from intestinal epithelial cells into the blood stream, where it is bound by albumin or amino acids and carried to the liver and other organs and tissues.

Within the liver, copper may be (1) incorporated into ceruloplasmin, a multifunctional 132-kD α_2-glycoprotein enzyme containing six or seven copper atoms per molecule; (2) used in the synthesis of other copper-requiring enzymes; (3) bound by metallothionein, a low-molecular-weight, cysteine-rich protein that provides a storage and detoxification depot for copper and other trace metal elements; or (4) excreted into the bile.

In Wilson's disease, metallation of ceruloplasmin is usually impaired, reflecting impaired transport of copper into the trans-Golgi compartment, where processing of ceruloplasmin occurs. This results in low circulating levels of the ceruloplasmin holoenzyme. Copper excretion into bile is invariably impaired, producing massive hepatic copper overload if the disease is unrecognized. These findings indicate that copper incorporation into ceruloplasmin and biliary excretion of copper are both mediated by the Wilson's disease gene product in the normal state.

Circulating levels of ceruloplasmin and total serum copper are low in many patients with Wilson's disease. However, these biochemical abnormalities are not necessarily associated with liver disease, as illustrated by the inherited disorders aceruloplasminemia, Menkes disease, and occipital horn syndrome. A feature that distinguishes Wilson's disease from these conditions is the amount of non-ceruloplasmin-bound serum copper, which is about five times normal in Wilson's disease patients.

Thus, the major pathophysiologic component of Wilson's disease is hepatic copper overload resulting from defective biliary excretion of the metal. If this diagnosis goes unrecognized, copper overload subsequently involves other tissues, including the brain, which is particularly sensitive to perturbations in trace metal homeostasis.

CLINICAL MANIFESTATIONS

Presenting clinical features of Wilson's disease include nonspecific liver disease, neurologic abnormalities, psychiatric illness, hemolytic anemia, renal tubular Fanconi's syndrome, and various skeletal abnormalities.

Age influences the specific presentation in Wilson's disease. Nearly all individuals who present with liver disease are younger than 30 years, whereas those presenting with neurologic or psychiatric signs may range in age from the first to the fifth decade. This reflects the sequence of events in the pathogenesis of this disease (see earlier discussion). However, regardless of clinical presentation, some degree of liver disease is invariably present. In one series of 400 adult patients with Wilson's disease, approximately 50% presented with neurologic and psychiatric symptoms, 20% with neurologic and hepatic symptoms, and 20% with purely hepatic symptoms.

In patients with neurologic presentations, abnormalities include speech difficulty (dysarthria), dystonia, rigidity, tremor or choreiform movements, abnormal gait, uncoordinated handwriting, and (rarely) a combined motor and sensory peripheral neuropathy. Wilson's disease may properly be classified as a movement disorder. The neurologic signs and symptoms reflect a predilection for involvement of the basal ganglia (e.g., caudate, putamen) in the brains of these individuals. Parkinson's disease or other movement disorders may be mistakenly diagnosed.

In psychiatric presentations, changes in personality (irritability, anger, poor self-control), depression, and anxiety are common symptoms. Patients presenting in this fashion are typically in their late teens or early 20s, a period during which substance abuse is also a diagnostic consideration. Wilson's disease should be formally excluded in all teenagers and young adults with new-onset psychiatric signs.

In hepatic presentations, signs and symptoms include jaundice, hepatomegaly, edema, and ascites. Secondary endocrine effects of liver disease may include delayed puberty or amenorrhea. Viral hepatitis and cirrhosis are often initial diagnostic considerations in individuals with Wilson's disease.

In addition to the brain and liver, the eye is a primary site of copper deposition in Wilson's disease, producing a pathognomonic sign—the Kayser-Fleischer ring (Fig. 218-1). The Kayser-Fleischer ring is a golden to green-brown annular deposition of copper in the periphery of the cornea. This important diagnostic sign first appears as a superior crescent, then develops inferiorly and ultimately becomes circumferential. Slit lamp examinations are required to detect rings in their early stage of formation. Copper can also accumulate in the lens and produce "sunflower" cataracts.

FIGURE 218-1. Kayser-Fleischer ring in a newly diagnosed patient with Wilson's disease.

Approximately 95% of patients with neurologic signs manifest the Kayser-Fleischer ring, compared with approximately 65% of those with hepatic presentations. Copper chelation therapy causes fading and even disappearance of corneal copper over time.

Hemolytic anemia resulting from the direct toxic effects of copper on red blood cell membranes has been observed in Wilson's disease. This is usually associated with the release of massive quantities of hepatic copper into the circulation, a phenomenon that can be sudden and catastrophic.

Renal dysfunction in Wilson's disease is tubular in nature and leads to abnormal losses of amino acids, electrolytes, calcium, phosphorus, and glucose. This effect is presumably related to copper toxicity. High copper levels have been noted previously in the kidneys of patients with Wilson's disease. Treatment with copper chelation often improves the renal disturbances.

There can be skeletal effects of Wilson's disease, including osteoporosis and rickets; these may be attributable to renal losses of calcium and phosphorus. Osteoarthritis primarily affecting the knees and wrists also occurs in Wilson's disease patients and may involve excess copper deposition in the bone and cartilage.

DIAGNOSIS

The presence of the clinical abnormalities described earlier is valuable in the clinical diagnosis of Wilson's disease. Laboratory findings that support the diagnosis include low levels of serum copper and serum ceruloplasmin, elevated hepatic transaminase levels, aminoaciduria, and hemolytic anemia. Incorporation of radiolabeled ^{64}Cu into serum ceruloplasmin, measured as the appearance of copper in the serum after an oral load, is a highly specific diagnostic test; patients with Wilson's disease incorporate very little ^{64}Cu into ceruloplasmin.

Increased urinary excretion of copper (>100 mg/24 hours) is another easily performed and important diagnostic test for this disorder. Acid-washed (copper-free) collection containers should be used. A variation involving serial urine copper measurements is the penicillamine "challenge," in which 500 mg of penicillamine is administered orally after collection of a baseline 24-hour urine specimen. The penicillamine dose is repeated after 12 hours, the midpoint of the second 24-hour urine collection. A several-fold increase in copper excretion in the second collection is highly suggestive of the diagnosis. Some workers believe the challenge does not add enormously to the diagnostic evaluation compared with the baseline measurement alone.

Although it is an invasive technique, percutaneous needle liver biopsy for quantitative measurement of hepatic copper remains the "gold standard" for diagnosis. Hepatic copper values greater than 200 mg/g of dry weight (normal, 20 to 50 mg/g dry weight) are characteristic of Wilson's disease. Atomic absorption spectrometry is the preferred method; histochemical staining for copper in a liver biopsy specimen is unreliable.

A Wilson's disease mutation database (http://www.wilsondisease.med .ualberta.ca/database.asp) contains nearly 300 different mutations reported at the *ATP7B* locus. For families in which the mutant alleles have been determined, molecular diagnosis is highly reliable.

In summary, in the absence of formal molecular evidence, the diagnosis of Wilson's disease can be reliably rendered by the presence of at least two of the following: a positive family history, Kayser-Fleischer rings, Coombs-negative hemolytic anemia, low serum copper and ceruloplasmin, elevated hepatic copper, increased 24-hour urine copper, and a positive penicillamine challenge result.

TREATMENT   Rx

Penicillamine, a free thiol that binds (chelates) copper, does not formally correct the basic defect of impaired copper excretion in the bile; however, it greatly enhances urinary excretion of copper and thereby prevents copper overload and its effects. Faithful compliance with oral penicillamine treatment has enabled the good health of thousands of Wilson's disease patients worldwide over the past 50 years. Pyridoxine (vitamin B_6) should be prescribed concomitantly to counter the vitamin B_6 deficiency that tends to develop with long-term penicillamine administration.

Certain individuals are intolerant of penicillamine. Significant side effects include nephrotoxicity; hematologic abnormalities; and a distinctive rash, elastosis perforans serpiginosa, which often involves the neck and axilla. Furthermore, in some Wilson's disease patients with neurologic presentations, penicillamine treatment induces paradoxical worsening of the clinical phenotype.

Even though penicillamine is the therapy with the longest experience, other pharmaceutical agents are available that may eventually supplant it as a first-line drug. For example, triethylene tetramine dihydrochloride (trien) is a suitable alternative chelating agent with a somewhat less significant side effect profile.

Oral zinc acetate also has proved highly effective in Wilson's disease. The mechanism involves induction of metallothionein synthesis in intestinal epithelial cells; increased metallothionein synthesis results in greater binding of dietary copper and thus decreased absorption. Zinc monotherapy has particular value in young, presymptomatic patients; in patients who are pregnant, given the possible fetal teratogenic effects of other compounds; and as maintenance therapy for patients after their initial "de-coppering" is accomplished. Zinc acetate has minimal side effects. The only drawback to its use is the relatively long time (4 to 6 months) needed to restore the proper copper balance if zinc is used alone in the initial stages of treatment.

Tetrathiomolybdate is a molecule that forms stable tripartite complexes with protein and copper. This drug both decreases copper absorption and reduces circulating free copper. It is fast acting and can restore normal copper balance within several weeks, compared with the several months required with other copper chelators or with zinc. Tetrathiomolybdate is especially appropriate for the initial treatment of patients with neurologic presentations, based on a completed clinical trial.[1]

Regardless of the specific regimen chosen, treatment of Wilson's disease is lifelong, because noncompliance eventually leads to fulminant liver failure.

Liver transplantation is a rare consideration in Wilson's disease because the condition is typically responsive to medical therapy. It is generally necessary only when delayed diagnosis or poor compliance results in irreversible hepatic damage.

Apart from pharmacologic treatment, there are several other important considerations in the treatment of Wilson's disease. These include dietary restriction of shellfish and liver, both copper-rich foods. The major sources of patients' drinking water should be tested for copper concentration and avoided if levels approach 1.3 mg/L, which is the current maximum contaminant level goal (MCLG) established by the U.S. Environmental Protection Agency. The MCLG for copper in drinking water is set at a concentration at which no known or expected adverse health effects occur and for which there is an adequate margin of safety.

In newly diagnosed patients, there is frequently a need for speech therapy and physical or occupational therapy, as well as psychological and genetic counseling.

Wilson's Disease Heterozygotes

There is some debate about the risk of copper overload among individuals who are heterozygous for Wilson's disease. Even though Wilson's disease is a classic autosomal recessive trait—that is, requiring two mutant alleles at the *ATP7B* locus for expression of the disease—a report from the National Academy of Sciences suggested that heterozygous Wilson's disease carriers may be a relatively sensitive population in terms of copper overload, particularly when dietary or drinking water copper exposure is higher than usual. Abnormally increased urinary copper excretion has been documented among some siblings of Wilson's disease patients, although genetic confirmation of the carrier or noncarrier status of these individuals was not available. Further patient and family studies are needed to formally address these questions.

PROGNOSIS

The prognosis in Wilson's disease is generally favorable. Current therapeutic approaches can prevent or reverse most of the significant clinical signs and symptoms, including Kayser-Fleischer rings. However, if treatment is stopped, potentially fatal liver damage inevitably occurs.

FUTURE DIRECTIONS

Gene therapy for Wilson's disease is a possibility. Because the Wilson's copper transporter is expressed most prominently and functions most critically in the liver, this organ could be specifically targeted by the use of adenoviral or adeno-associated viral vectors (e.g., AAV8). Hepatocyte transfer, an alternative to gene therapy, may also be applicable to the treatment of liver-specific metabolic disorders through therapeutic liver repopulation.

Grade A

1. Brewer GJ, Askari F, Lorincz MT, et al. Treatment of Wilson disease with ammonium tetrathiomolybdate: IV, comparison of tetrathiomolybdate and trientine in a double-blind study of treatment of the neurologic presentation of Wilson disease. *Arch Neurol.* 2006;63:521-527.

SUGGESTED READINGS

Bruha R, Marecek Z, Pospisilova L, et al. Long-term follow-up of Wilson disease: natural history, treatment, mutations analysis and phenotypic correlation. *Liver Int.* 2011;31:83-91. *Comprehensive follow-up data on 117 Wilson disease patients.*

Lorincz MT. Neurologic Wilson's disease. *Ann N Y Acad Sci.* 2010;1184:173-187. *Review.*

Lowette KF, Desmet K, Witters P, et al. Wilson's disease: long-term follow-up of a cohort of 24 patients treated with D-penicillamine. *Eur J Gastroenterol Hepatol.* 2010;22:564-571. *All but one patient had beneficial results with very long-term treatment.*

Schilsky ML, Ala A. Genetic testing for Wilson disease: availability and utility. *Curr Gastroenterol Rep.* 2010;12:57-61. *Useful summary of molecular diagnostics.*

Weiss KH, Gotthardt DN, Klemm D, et al. Zinc monotherapy is not as effective as chelating agents in treatment of Wilson disease. *Gastroenterology.* 2011. [Epub ahead of print.] *Case series suggesting that chelator therapy is better than zinc therapy.*

Wiggelinkhuizen M, Tilanus ME, Bollen CW, et al. Systematic review: clinical efficacy of chelator agents and zinc in the initial treatment of Wilson disease. *Aliment Pharmacol Ther.* 2009;29:947-958.

219

IRON OVERLOAD (HEMOCHROMATOSIS)

BRUCE R. BACON

DEFINITION AND EPIDEMIOLOGY

Hereditary hemochromatosis (HH) is a common inherited disorder of iron metabolism. The genetic abnormality responsible in most patients with typical HH is found in homozygous form in about 1 in 250 persons of northern European descent. It is characterized by an increase in iron absorption from the upper gastrointestinal tract, with subsequent tissue iron deposition in parenchymal cells of the liver, heart, pancreas, joints, and endocrine organs. The autosomal recessive inheritance pattern of HH was clearly shown in the 1970s, and the gene responsible for most cases of HH was identified in 1996 by investigators using a positional cloning technique. The gene is called *HFE* and encodes for a novel major histocompatibility complex (MHC) class 1–like molecule that binds with transferrin receptor (TfR) and affects hepcidin homeostasis (Fig. 219-1). Recent prospective population studies have demonstrated that only about 50% of patients who are homozygous for the major mutation found in *HFE* (called C282Y) have evidence of phenotypic expression of iron overload, and only a small percentage (<10%) go on to develop tissue damage from excess iron deposition. These studies have changed modern thinking about HH and must be considered when evaluating patients for this disease in a physician's office and when developing national health policy regarding screening for this genetic disorder.

The discovery of *HFE* has had a tremendous impact in a number of areas. The ability to accurately diagnose disorders of iron overload has been strengthened, family screening is improved, and the evaluation of patients with other forms of liver disease complicated by moderate to severe iron overload is possible. Furthermore, with the discovery of *HFE*, a considerable new body of knowledge regarding the mechanisms of iron absorption has been identified, both in the normal situation and in the pathologic condition seen when *HFE* mutations are present.

PATHOBIOLOGY
Classification of Iron Overload Syndromes

The term *hereditary hemochromatosis* should be reserved for inherited disorders of iron metabolism (see Fig. 219-1) that lead to tissue iron loading (Table 219-1). The most common form of this disease, *HFE*-related HH, is caused primarily by homozygosity for the C282Y mutation in the *HFE* gene. Other heritable forms of iron overload have also been recognized (non-*HFE*-related HH). These include (1) autosomal recessive forms of HH characterized by rapid iron accumulation and caused by mutations in the genes for hemojuvelin and hepcidin (also called juvenile hemochromatosis), (2) an autosomal dominant form of HH caused by mutations in the ferroportin gene, (3) an autosomal recessive form of HH resulting from mutations in the gene for *TfR-2*, and (4) rare forms of HH resulting from mutations in the *DMT-1* gene or in the regulatory region of ferritin messenger RNA. Some other types of iron overload may have a familial or inherited component, but the genes involved have not yet been identified. For example, African iron overload is a familial disorder of iron loading prevalent in sub-Saharan Africa that is exacerbated by the ingestion of iron-rich home-brewed beer. Many of these patients have mutations in ferroportin. The degree of iron loading can be similar to that seen in *HFE*-related HH, but the cellular and lobular distribution of iron is different. In addition, a rare disorder termed neonatal iron overload is characterized by a modest increase in hepatic iron accompanied by severe liver injury present at birth.

It has been recognized over the last several years that many patients who have *HFE*-linked hemochromatosis have no evidence of iron overload. With this in mind, four stages of HH have been described:
1. Genetic predisposition with no phenotypic abnormality
2. Iron overload (approximately 2 to 5 g total body iron) without symptoms
3. Iron overload with mild or early symptoms
4. Iron overload with organ damage, such as cirrhosis

The ability to establish a genetic diagnosis has led to a much greater understanding of genotype-phenotype correlations.

Genetics and Pathophysiology of Hemochromatosis

Since the classic linkage studies of Simon and colleagues in the mid-1970s, it has been known that the gene for hemochromatosis is located in the human leukocyte antigen (HLA) region on chromosome 6. In 1996 a team of molecular geneticists using a positional cloning technique identified a candidate gene for HH, which is now called *HFE*. *HFE* codes for a novel MHC class 1–like molecule, which, like all MHC proteins, requires interaction with β_2-microglobulin for normal presentation on the cell surface. Three principal missense mutations have been identified in *HFE*: one results in a change of cysteine at position 282 to tyrosine (Cys282 → Tyr, C282Y), the second results in a change of histidine at position 63 to aspartate (His63 → Asp, H63D), and the third results in a change of serine at position 65 to cysteine (Ser65 → Cys, S65C). A few other mutations have been identified in *HFE*, but their frequency is low and their clinical impact is limited. In the original study by Feder and associates, 83% of typical phenotypic HH patients were found to be homozygous for the C282Y mutation. Several other studies from around the world in predominantly white populations demonstrated that, among patients with typical hemochromatosis, about 85 to 90% were homozygous for C282Y. Thus, about 10 to 15% of patients with typical HH have some reason other than C282Y homozygosity for their iron overload.

Nearly all absorption of dietary iron occurs in the duodenum, where iron may be taken up either as ionic iron or as heme. Ionic iron requires reduction to the ferrous state, which is accomplished by the ferric reductases (e.g., duodenal ferric reductase), expressed on the luminal surface of the duodenal enterocytes (see Fig. 219-1). This ferrous iron crosses the apical membrane via divalent metal transporter 1, and iron taken up by the enterocyte is either stored as ferritin or transferred across the basolateral membrane to the plasma. This latter process occurs via the iron transporter ferroportin and requires oxidation of iron to the ferric state by the ferroxidase hephaestin.

Hepcidin is a 25–amino acid peptide that influences systemic iron status such that it is now considered to be the principal iron regulatory hormone (see Fig. 219-1). Dysregulation of hepcidin expression is thought to play a role in the pathogenesis of HH. Patients with *HFE*-related HH have low hepatic expression of hepcidin, as do *HFE* knockout mice, despite excess hepatic iron stores. Conversely, overexpression of hepcidin in *HFE* knockout mice prevents the HH phenotype. Studies have revealed that iron-induced regulation of hepcidin expression involves a bone morphogenetic protein

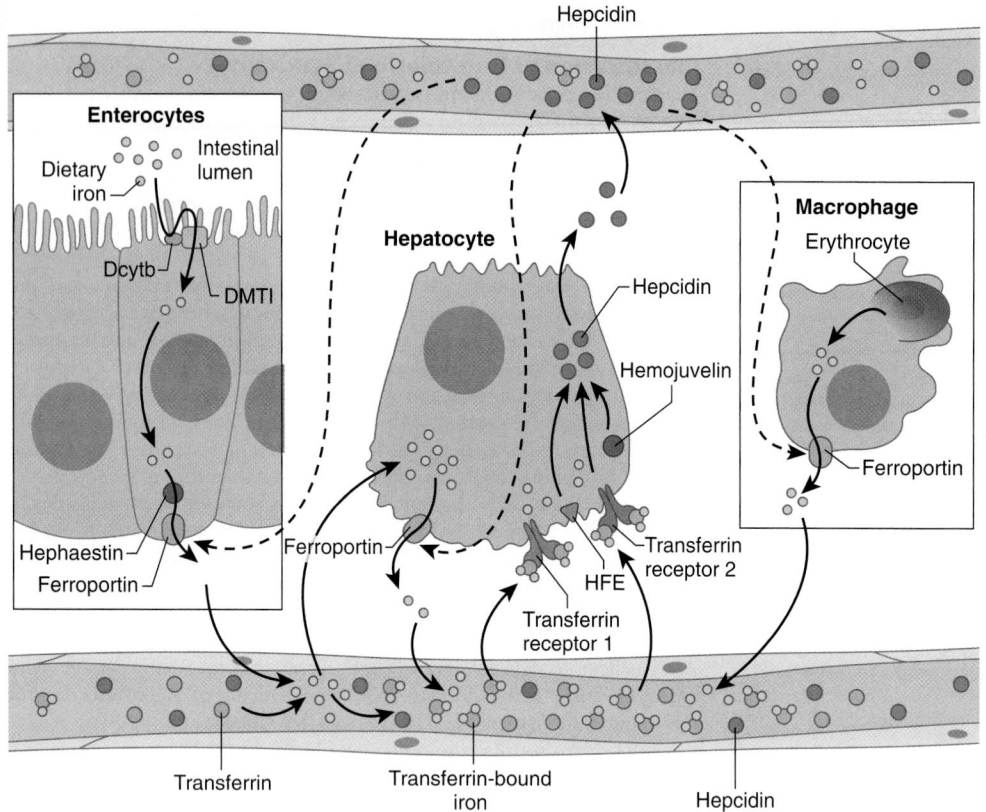

FIGURE 219-1. Orchestration of iron homeostasis. In the duodenal enterocyte, dietary iron is reduced to the ferrous state by duodenal ferric reductase (Dcytb), transported into the cell by divalent metal transporter 1 (DMT1), and released by way of ferroportin into the circulation. Hephaestin facilitates enterocyte iron release. Hepatocytes take up iron from the circulation either as free iron or as transferrin-bound iron (through transferrin receptors 1 and 2). Transferrin receptor 2 may serve as a sensor of circulating transferrin-bound iron, thereby influencing expression of the iron regulatory hormone hepcidin. The hepcidin response is also modulated by HFE and hemojuvelin. Hepcidin is secreted into the circulation, where it downregulates the ferroportin-mediated release of iron from enterocytes, macrophages, and hepatocytes (dashed lines). (From Fleming RE, Bacon BR. Orchestration of iron homeostasis. *N Engl J Med.* 2005;352:1741-1744.)

TABLE 219-1 CLASSIFICATION OF IRON OVERLOAD SYNDROMES

HEREDITARY HEMOCHROMATOSIS

HFE Related

C282Y/C282Y
C282Y/H63D
C282Y/S65C
Other mutations

Non–*HFE* Related

Hemojuvelin (*HJV*) mutations (autosomal recessive)
Hepcidin (*HAMP*) mutations (autosomal recessive)
Ferroportin (*SLC40A1*) mutations (autosomal dominant)
Transferrin receptor 2 (*TfR-2*) mutations (autosomal recessive)
Divalent metal transporter 1 (*SLC11A2*) mutations (rare)
Ferritin regulatory mutations (rare)

Miscellaneous

African iron overload
Neonatal iron overload (rare)

SECONDARY IRON OVERLOAD

Anemia Caused by Ineffective Erythropoiesis

Thalassemia major
Sideroblastic anemias
Congenital dyserythropoietic anemias
Congenital atransferrinemia

Liver Disease

Alcoholic liver disease
Chronic viral hepatitis B and C
Porphyria cutanea tarda
Nonalcoholic steatohepatitis
After portacaval shunt

Miscellaneous

Transfusional iron overload
Excessive parenteral iron administration

(BMP)–dependent signaling pathway. BMPs bind to specific receptors on hepatocytes, thereby triggering SMAD protein–dependent activation of hepcidin expression. Selective inhibition of BMP signaling abrogates iron-induced upregulation of hepcidin. Hemojuvelin is a BMP coreceptor and facilitates the binding of BMP to its receptor; knockout of the hemojuvelin gene markedly decreases BMP signaling and hepcidin expression and causes iron overload. It has been hypothesized that *TfR-2* in hepatocytes may act as an iron sensor. Mutations in *TfR-2* cause a rare form of HH in humans, and *TfR-2* mutant mice have an HH phenotype. In HH, excess iron (both transferrin bound and non–transferrin bound) is avidly taken up by hepatocytes and stored. Iron stores increase to the point at which iron-induced oxidative damage occurs, resulting in cell injury and cell necrosis with phagocytosis by Kupffer cells. Iron-laden Kupffer cells become activated and produce profibrogenic cytokines (transforming growth factor-β, platelet-derived growth factor), which stimulate hepatic stellate cells to synthesize excess collagen and other matrix proteins. Increased fibrosis and then cirrhosis result.

CLINICAL MANIFESTATIONS

Several symptoms and clinical findings have been identified in patients with fully established HH, and all physicians should be aware of these symptoms and findings, which are summarized in Tables 219-2 and 219-3. Table 219-4 summarizes the typical laboratory findings in symptomatic and asymptomatic patients with HH. Recent series have revealed that many asymptomatic patients who are C282Y homozygotes are now coming to medical attention because they are identified by family screening studies or population surveys or after abnormal iron studies are discovered on routine blood chemistry testing. It is ideal to identify patients who have some phenotypic expression with abnormal iron studies but no evidence of organ damage. Several large population screening studies have shown evidence of phenotypic expression with abnormal iron studies in about 40 to 50% of C282Y homozygotes, but less than 10% of these individuals actually have signs and symptoms of the disease.

DIAGNOSIS

Because patients with genetic abnormalities can be identified before there is evidence of phenotypic expression, the method of diagnosing HH has undergone a change. The role of liver biopsy has lessened considerably with the advent of genetic testing. Nonetheless, some general principles should be acknowledged. If the diagnosis of HH is being considered, blood tests,

TABLE 219-2 SYMPTOMS IN PATIENTS WITH HEREDITARY HEMOCHROMATOSIS

ASYMPTOMATIC

Abnormal serum iron studies on routine screening chemistry panel
Abnormal liver tests
Identified by family screening
Identified by population screening

NONSPECIFIC SYSTEMIC SYMPTOMS

Weakness
Fatigue
Lethargy
Apathy
Weight loss

SPECIFIC ORGAN-RELATED SYMPTOMS

Abdominal pain (hepatomegaly)
Arthralgias (arthritis)
Diabetes (pancreas)
Amenorrhea (cirrhosis)
Loss of libido, impotence (pituitary, cirrhosis)
Congestive heart failure (heart)
Arrhythmias (heart)

TABLE 219-3 PHYSICAL FINDINGS IN PATIENTS WITH HEREDITARY HEMOCHROMATOSIS

ASYMPTOMATIC

No physical findings
Hepatomegaly

SYMPTOMATIC

Liver

Hepatomegaly
Cutaneous stigmata of chronic liver disease
Splenomegaly
Liver failure: ascites, encephalopathy

Joints

Arthritis
Joint swelling

Heart

Dilated cardiomyopathy
Congestive heart failure

Skin

Increased pigmentation

Endocrine

Testicular atrophy
Hypogonadism
Hypothyroidism

TABLE 219-4 LABORATORY FINDINGS IN PATIENTS WITH HEREDITARY HEMOCHROMATOSIS

MEASUREMENTS	NORMAL SUBJECTS	Patients with Hereditary Hemochromatosis ASYMPTOMATIC	SYMPTOMATIC
BLOOD (FASTING)			
Serum iron level (μg/dL)	60-180	150-280	180-300
Serum transferrin level (mg/dL)	220-410	200-280	200-300
Transferrin saturation (%)	20-45	45-100	80-100
Serum ferritin level (ng/mL)			
Men	20-200	150-1000	500-6000
Women	15-150	120-1000	500-6000
GENETIC (*HFE* MUTATION ANALYSIS)			
C282Y/C282Y	wt/wt[‡]	C282Y/C282Y	C282Y/C282Y
C282Y/H63D*	wt/wt	C282Y/H63D	C282Y/H63D
LIVER			
Hepatic iron concentration			
μg/g dry weight	300-1500	2000-10,000	8000-30,000
μmol/g dry weight	5-27	36-179	140-550
Hepatic iron index[†]	<1	1 to >1.9	>1.9
Liver histology			
Perls' Prussian blue stain	0, 1+	2+ to 4+	3+, 4+

*Compound heterozygote.
[†]Calculated by dividing the hepatic iron concentration (in μmol/g dry weight) by the age of the patient (in years). With the increased use of genetic testing in patients with iron overload, the specificity of the hepatic iron index has diminished.
[‡]wt/wt: wild type (normal).

concentration with calculation of the hepatic iron index (HII). The HII is the patient's hepatic iron concentration (in μmol/g dry weight) divided by the patient's age in years. Previously, when the HII was greater than 1.9, the diagnosis of HH was established. Recent studies with genetic testing have shown that many (>50%) HH patients may have an HII less than 1.9. Thus, the HII is no longer important in the diagnosis of HH.

Currently, when abnormal iron studies are identified, it is reasonable to proceed to genetic testing. Among individuals who are C282Y homozygotes or compound heterozygotes (C282Y/H63D), liver biopsy is reserved for those with elevated liver enzymes or ferritin levels greater than 1000 ng/mL (Fig. 219-2). Several studies have shown that advanced fibrosis or cirrhosis is not seen in HH patients when ferritin levels are less than 1000 ng/mL or when liver enzymes are normal. Accordingly, as genetic testing has become more widely available, liver biopsy is less necessary.

When liver biopsy is performed, iron deposition is found preferentially in a periportal (acinar zone 1) region of the hepatic lobule, with a decrease in gradient in acinar zones 2 and 3. With significant iron loading, sinusoidal lining cell (Kupffer cell) iron deposition can be identified, and iron can be found in bile duct cells and in fibrous tissue in portal tracts or septa. In patients with secondary iron overload related to alcoholic liver disease or chronic viral hepatitis, iron deposition is typically in Kupffer cells as well as in hepatocytes, and it occurs in a panlobular (as opposed to a periportal) distribution. Histologic evaluation of iron-staining patterns provides information complementary to that obtained by traditional biochemical testing for iron overload along with genetic testing.

TREATMENT Rx

Even though there have been advances in the molecular and cellular biologic understanding of HH, and although the impact of *HFE* mutation analysis on diagnosis has been significant, the treatment of HH remains simple, inexpensive, and safe. Patients should have therapeutic phlebotomy of 500 mL of whole blood (approximately 200 to 250 mg of iron, depending on the hemoglobin concentration) on a weekly basis, if tolerated. Therapeutic phlebotomy should be performed until iron-limited erythropoiesis develops, identified by failure of the hemoglobin level and hematocrit to recover before the next phlebotomy. It is reasonable to monitor transferrin saturation and ferritin levels periodically (every 3 months) to predict iron stores' return to normal and

including transferrin saturation (serum iron ÷ transferrin or total iron binding capacity × 100%) and ferritin levels, should be obtained. A recent study from the HEIRS trial showed that transferrin saturation does not need to be measured in the fasting state to obtain reliable results. In patients with symptoms (see Table 219-2), both these values are elevated; however, transferrin saturation is typically the earliest phenotypic marker of HH and may be elevated in young C282Y homozygotes with normal ferritin levels. Serum ferritin is sometimes elevated in other conditions, such as certain cancers and chronic inflammatory disorders, in which there is no evidence of iron overload. Furthermore, in patients with other types of liver disease, such as chronic hepatitis C, nonalcoholic steatohepatitis, and alcoholic liver disease, ferritin levels can be elevated in as many as half the patients studied. Thus, ferritin is relatively sensitive but not specific for iron overload in the presence of these other disorders. The development of a widely available genetic test has contributed to better characterization of patients with underlying liver disease and abnormal serum iron studies.

In the past, if an elevated transferrin saturation or ferritin level was identified, a liver biopsy would be performed to establish a diagnosis using histochemical iron stains and biochemical determination of the hepatic iron

FIGURE 219-2. Algorithm for evaluation of possible hereditary hemochromatosis in a person with a negative family history. ALT = alanine transaminase; AST = aspartate transaminase.

to provide encouragement to patients who are undergoing phlebotomy. Therapeutic phlebotomy should be continued until the transferrin saturation is less than 50% and the ferritin level is less than 50 ng/mL. It is not necessary for patients to become anemic or iron deficient—just depleted of excess iron stores. Some patients may require weekly phlebotomy for 1 year or longer. Once the initial therapeutic phlebotomy has been completed, most patients require maintenance phlebotomy, with 1 unit of blood removed every 2 to 3 months. This requirement is derived empirically, with the intent being to maintain transferrin saturation at less than 50% and ferritin at less than 50 ng/mL.

With successful iron depletion, patients have an improved sense of well-being, right upper quadrant abdominal pain dissipates, liver test results improve, and diabetes may be easier to manage. Established cirrhosis, arthropathy, and testicular atrophy generally do not improve.

Iron chelation therapy may be necessary for patients who are anemic and cannot tolerate phlebotomy. Parenteral infusions (administered either subcutaneously using an infusion pump or intravenously overnight via a port) of deferoxamine are used. Ototoxicity and ocular toxicity are possible with deferoxamine, and appropriate monitoring should be performed. An orally administered iron chelator, deferasirox, is approved and available for treating secondary iron overload in patients with iron-loading anemias. This therapy is not yet approved for HH in the United States and is quite expensive.

PREVENTION

Family Screening
Once an HH proband is recognized, all first-degree relatives should be offered testing. In the past, HLA haplotyping was performed, but now *HFE* mutation analysis is recommended, along with the determination of transferrin saturation and ferritin levels. In probands with children, *HFE* mutation analysis is performed in the spouse to accurately predict the genotype in the child. If the spouse has either mutation, testing of the child is necessary, although the value and availability of genetic testing in children are debated. If an adult relative of a C282Y homozygote is identified and is either a C282Y homozygote or a compound heterozygote, and if blood iron studies are abnormal, a presumptive diagnosis can be made, and therapeutic phlebotomy can be initiated using the guidelines already discussed.

Population Screening
Because HH is a common disorder with a well-described treatment and a long latent period (i.e., time before disease occurs), some have suggested that

it is an ideal candidate for population screening by genetic testing. However, recent studies have showed a less than expected phenotypic expression and a decreased number of patients with clinical manifestations of iron-mediated disease, raising questions about this recommendation. Initial results from a large National Institutes of Health–sponsored screening study in North America demonstrated a prevalence of C282Y homozygosity of 1 in 227. The C282Y homozygotes had higher ferritin levels than the general population, but 25% had normal ferritin levels. When screening for iron overload as opposed to screening for *HFE*-linked HH, transferrin saturation should be measured. In this situation, when abnormal iron studies are identified and the patient does not have a mutation in *HFE*, liver biopsy should be considered to clarify the situation relative to iron stores.

PROGNOSIS

If patients are identified, diagnosed, and treated before the development of cirrhosis, their life expectancy is the same as for an age- and sex-matched control population. If patients are not identified and treated before the development of cirrhosis, they are at risk for premature death from either complications of chronic liver disease or hepatocellular cancer. Treated cirrhotic patients are still at risk for hepatocellular cancer and should undergo surveillance abdominal imaging every 6 to 12 months.

Mutation Analysis in Patients with Liver Disease
Many patients with liver disease have abnormalities in serum parameters of iron metabolism. These abnormalities are more commonly seen in patients with hepatocellular liver diseases than in those with cholestatic liver diseases. Several clinical studies have shown that approximately 50% of patients with alcoholic liver disease, chronic viral hepatitis C, and nonalcoholic steatohepatitis (NASH) have abnormalities in serum iron studies. Usually this abnormality is an elevation in serum ferritin, but elevated transferrin saturation is occasionally seen as well. When liver biopsy is performed, increased iron deposits can be seen, usually in a panlobular distribution, with iron in both hepatocytes and sinusoidal lining cells (Kupffer cells). Hepatic iron concentrations may be slightly increased or normal. When *HFE* mutations have been evaluated in patients with alcoholic liver disease, there has been no increased incidence of either C282Y or H63D (either heterozygote or homozygote) compared with control populations. Furthermore, there was no increase in *HFE* mutations in patients with alcoholic liver disease who had an increased amount of fibrosis. Thus, the abnormal iron studies frequently seen in patients

with alcoholic liver disease are most likely due to mechanisms other than mutations in *HFE*.

In chronic hepatitis C, the relationship of abnormal iron studies and elevated hepatic iron concentration with a response to interferon monotherapy has been known for several years. Numerous studies have shown that patients who fail to respond to interferon monotherapy have a higher hepatic iron concentration than those who do respond. A corollary to this observation involves therapeutic phlebotomy to deplete iron stores in the hope of improving response to therapy. Reduction in iron stores by therapeutic phlebotomy does reduce liver enzymes and has had some marginal beneficial effect on liver histology, but it does not have any virologic effects. When *HFE* mutation analysis has been investigated in patients with chronic hepatitis C, the frequency of C282Y and H63D has been equivalent to that in control populations. Most studies have shown that when *HFE* mutations are present, they correlate with increased iron stores seen histologically. Some studies have shown a synergistic effect with the development of fibrosis. At present, it is recommended that *HFE* mutation analysis be done when abnormal iron studies are seen in patients with chronic hepatitis C. Also, iron stains are typically performed on liver biopsy samples when biopsies are done to grade and stage chronic hepatitis C. If iron stores are increased, it is reasonable to perform therapeutic phlebotomy to deplete excess iron stores before initiating antiviral therapy.

In patients with NASH, several studies have provided conflicting results. Some have shown an increase in *HFE* mutations in patients with NASH, and others have shown no difference from control populations. When there has been an increased prevalence of *HFE* mutations in NASH, there has been good correlation between abnormal serum parameters of iron and a correlation with hepatic iron concentration. Furthermore, some studies have shown an increase

in fibrosis in NASH patients with *HFE* mutations. Finally, one study showed a reduction in elevated liver enzymes and improvement in parameters of insulin resistance in patients with NASH treated by phlebotomy to produce near iron deficiency. These observations suggest an interaction between the expression of fatty liver disease and iron metabolism. Finally, in porphyria cutanea tarda (PCT), the relationship between abnormalities of iron metabolism and the role of therapeutic phlebotomy has been known for many years. Also, it has recently been shown that as many as 70% of patients with PCT are infected with hepatitis C virus, and many patients with PCT drink excessive amounts of alcohol. An increased prevalence of *HFE* mutations has been shown in both European and American studies of PCT patients, and the use of phlebotomy to deplete excess iron stores is still recommended.

Thus, *HFE* mutation analysis is of value in patients with PCT and may be of value in patients with chronic hepatitis C and NASH. It is probably not of value in patients with alcoholic liver disease.

SUGGESTED READINGS

Brittenham GM. Iron-chelating therapy for transfusional iron overload. *N Engl J Med.* 2011;364:146-156. *Case-based review.*

Carroll GJ, Breidahl WH, Bulsara MK, et al. Hereditary hemochromatosis is characterized by a clinically definable arthropathy that correlates with iron load. *Arthritis Rheum.* 2011;63:286-294. *An arthropathy was found in 24% of patients with hereditary hemochromatosis.*

Gurrin LC, Bertalli NA, Dalton GW, et al. HealthIron Study Investigators. HFE C282Y/H63D compound heterozygotes are at low risk of hemochromatosis-related morbidity. *Hepatology.* 2009;50: 94-101. *Estimation of the prevalence of elevated iron indices and morbidity in HFE compound heterozygotes.*

Pietrangelo A. Hereditary hemochromatosis: pathogenesis, diagnosis, and treatment. *Gastroenterology.* 2010;139:393-408. *Comprehensive review.*

Rochette J, Le Gac G, Lassoued K, et al. Factors influencing disease phenotype and penetrance in HFE haemochromatosis. *Hum Genet.* 2010;128:233-249. *Review.*

XVII

NUTRITIONAL DISEASES

NUTRITION'S INTERFACE WITH HEALTH AND DISEASE

DOUGLAS C. HEIMBURGER

OLD AND NEW PARADIGMS IN THE SCIENCE OF NUTRITION

Nutrition science was characterized by two major phases in the 20th century. During the first phase, nutrition scientists discovered, characterized, and synthesized the essential nutrients and described their deficiency syndromes in detail. The dietary requirements for these nutrients were estimated and periodically updated as recommended dietary allowances (RDAs). Beginning in 1997, the RDAs were reformulated in a series of volumes containing dietary reference intakes (DRIs); in addition to the recommended intakes judged to be sufficient to meet the nutrient requirements of nearly all healthy individuals, the DRIs include estimates of tolerable upper intake levels—that is, the highest intake levels likely not to pose any adverse health risks.

More fundamentally, the DRIs focus on accumulating evidence related to the relationships of diet and nutritional status to the diseases that plague Western societies, such as coronary heart disease, cancer, diabetes, and the other leading causes of death. DRIs recommend intake levels that not only prevent deficiencies but also may promote long-term health and disease prevention.

NUTRITION'S INFLUENCE ON MORTALITY AND MORBIDITY

Evidence of a Connection between Diet and Disease

It has been estimated that between 300,000 and 800,000 deaths per year could be prevented in the United States if Americans followed evidence-based dietary recommendations. Substantial additional benefits from reduced morbidity and enhanced functional status would also accrue. However, the causal connections between diet and chronic diseases are difficult to tease out of the complex network of other risk factors, including social and behavioral variables, so a wide variety of studies must be relied on to establish these connections with reasonable certainty.

Epidemiologic studies are unable to infer causal relationships and may be confounded by variables that have not been examined. They are also challenged by the difficulty of accurately assessing the diets of free-living individuals.

Animal and in vitro studies can overcome some of these drawbacks but may be confounded by experimental conditions that differ from those encountered by humans. A large number of prospective, randomized human intervention trials have been undertaken to test the effects of dietary change on risk for disease. However, even these trials are not always conclusive because of pitfalls associated with selecting study populations and isolating individual dietary factors.

Taken together, epidemiologic, animal, in vitro, and intervention studies are proving that human dietary habits contribute importantly to the pathogenesis of most of the major causes of death in developed countries.

Diseases Influenced by Nutrition

Table 220-1 lists 8 of the top 15 causes of death in the United States that are influenced by nutrition. Five are strongly linked to dietary habits, and three are associated with alcohol abuse. The table also outlines dietary contributions to obesity, atherosclerosis, osteoporosis, diverticular disease, and neural tube defects. A meta-analysis indicates that vitamin D supplementation reduces mortality in adults.[1] Table 220-2 summarizes the 2005 Dietary Guidelines for Americans, and Table 220-3 compares dietary recommendations promulgated by professional societies for risk reduction and/or management of the major chronic diseases. The close agreement among these recommendations enhances their credibility.

Coronary Heart Disease

Nutritional influences on the leading cause of death in the United States, coronary heart disease (CHD), have been the subject of a great deal of research. The overall U.S. mortality rate from CHD peaked in the 1960s and, in a trend that has surprised medical science, has declined steadily since then. Changes in lifestyle, including diet, are responsible for a substantial proportion of this decline. Elevated plasma low-density lipoprotein (LDL) cholesterol levels are a major risk factor for CHD and peripheral atherosclerosis, and they correlate strongly with dietary saturated fat intake and less strongly with cholesterol intake. Intake of both these substances in the United States is derived largely from foods of animal origin, such as meats, dairy products, and eggs. Attempts to produce less atherogenic substitutes for some of these foods have not always proved beneficial. For instance, hydrogenation of vegetable oils to create margarine and shortening results in the formation of *trans*-fatty acids, which affect serum cholesterol levels in a manner similar to—and are perhaps even worse than—the saturated fatty acids found in butter and lard. LDL cholesterol levels can be lowered modestly by increasing the intake of soluble fiber from legumes, fruits, vegetables, and flax seed, as well as by consuming proteins and isoflavones from soy foods. LDL must be oxidized before it induces injury to the arterial wall. Although adequate dietary levels of the antioxidant vitamins C and E and β-carotene have been shown to inhibit LDL oxidation, pharmacologic doses of these vitamins have not reduced CHD events when tested in randomized trials. In fact, pharmacologic doses of vitamin E (>400 IU/day) and other antioxidants have no benefit and may increase all-cause mortality.[2]

Epidemiologic evidence suggests that fish consumption may reduce CHD risk, perhaps through the action of omega-3 fatty acids. Evidence also indicates that moderate consumption of alcohol, especially wine, is associated with a decreased risk for CHD, possibly by increasing high-density lipoprotein (HDL) cholesterol levels, preventing the oxidation of LDL, or both. The polyphenols in red wine are also apparently beneficial. Traditional Mediterranean lifestyle patterns—with diets high in vegetables, fruits, olive oil, fish, nuts, complex grains and carbohydrates, and red wine, along with physical activity—are associated with reduced risks of cardiovascular disease.[3] A conservative estimate suggests that moderate dietary modification by the U.S. population, consisting mainly of replacing saturated fats with complex carbohydrates, fiber, monounsaturated fats, and fish, could easily lead to a 10% reduction in serum cholesterol levels and a 20% or greater reduction in CHD. The actual risk reduction could be much greater.

Cancer

Nutrients, non-nutritive dietary constituents, and nutritional status can influence the risk for cancer in a variety of ways. Nutrition interacts with each step of carcinogenesis (carcinogen activation and tumor initiation, promotion, and progression). Excess energy intake may favor the generation of free radicals and reduce the body's ability to detoxify carcinogens. By contrast, antioxidant nutrients scavenge free radicals and other (pre)carcinogens and may thereby inhibit their activation, their ability to initiate mutations, or both. Folic acid may improve a cell's ability to preserve, repair, and methylate its DNA, either preventing or reversing the tendency toward mutation. Folic acid supplementation, however, may increase the cancer risk in some individuals, so supplementation beyond the levels present in multivitamins is not advised.[4] Obesity has emerged as a major risk factor for many cancers, perhaps by inducing insulin resistance and elevating serum levels of insulin, insulin-like growth factor, and related hormones. Excessive alcohol intake promotes tumor growth.

Lung Cancer

Evidence indicates that the number-one cancer killer, lung cancer (Chapter 197), is influenced by diet. Although the most important causal factor is cigarette smoking, consumption of fruits and vegetables is inversely associated with lung cancer risk in both smokers and nonsmokers. It is probable that both nutrients and the non-nutritive phytochemicals in fruits and vegetables are responsible for the protective effects. However, in view of the disappointing results of randomized trials of supplementation with β-carotene, which increased mortality from lung cancer and other causes, antioxidant supplements should not be relied on to reduce disease risk.

Breast Cancer

The number-two cause of cancer deaths in women, breast cancer (Chapter 204), is positively associated with obesity, especially when excess adiposity is located predominantly in the abdomen, and with physical inactivity. The positive association between obesity and postmenopausal breast cancer has been attributed in part to the synthesis of estrogen (a risk factor for breast

TABLE 220-1 DIETARY INFLUENCES ON MAJOR CAUSES OF DEATH AND MORBIDITY IN THE UNITED STATES

CAUSE OF DEATH OR MORBIDITY	FACTORS ASSOCIATED WITH DECREASED RISK	FACTORS ASSOCIATED WITH INCREASED RISK
DEATH		
Heart disease	Intake of complex carbohydrates, particular fatty acids (e.g., monounsaturated, polyunsaturated, and omega-3 fatty acids from fish), soluble fiber, polyphenols, soy proteins, antioxidants (vitamins E and C, β-carotene, selenium), folic acid, moderate alcohol	Intake of saturated fat, cholesterol, excess calories, sodium; abdominal distribution of body fat
Cancer	Intake of fruits and vegetables (for β-carotene; vitamins A, C, D, and E; folic acid; calcium; selenium; phytochemicals), fiber	Intake of excess calories, fat, alcohol, red meat, salt- and nitrite-preserved meats, possibly grilled meats; abdominal distribution of body fat
Cerebrovascular disease	Intake of potassium, calcium, omega-3 fatty acids	Intake of sodium, alcohol (as with hypertension)
Accidents		Excess alcohol consumption
Diabetes mellitus	Intake of fiber	Intake of excess calories, fat, alcohol; abdominal distribution of body fat
Suicide		Excess alcohol consumption
Chronic liver disease and cirrhosis		Excess alcohol consumption
Hypertension and hypertensive renal disease	Intake of fruits and vegetables, potassium, calcium, magnesium, omega-3 fatty acids	Intake of sodium, alcohol, excess calories, total and saturated fat; abdominal distribution of body fat
MORBIDITY		
Obesity		Intake of excess calories and fat
Osteoporosis	Intake of calcium, vitamin D, vitamin K	Intake of excess vitamin A, sodium, protein
Diverticular disease, constipation	Intake of fiber	
Neural tube defects	Intake of folic acid	

cancer) in adipose tissue. Epidemiologic evidence suggests that alcohol intake may also be a risk factor for this disease, particularly in women with lower intakes of folic acid.

Colorectal Cancer
Colorectal cancer (Chapter 199) is the third leading cause of cancer mortality in men and women. The risk for colorectal cancer correlates positively with the intake of red meat (especially when it is overcooked) and dietary fat and with obesity, and the risk correlates inversely with the intake of calcium and folic acid. Evidence regarding the effect of dietary fiber is somewhat equivocal, but the preponderance of evidence points to a protective effect; there is no evidence of harm. Higher physical activity is associated with a 30 to 50% lower risk for colon cancer.

Summary
The interaction of all these influences is powerful enough to suggest that diet and physical inactivity contribute to well over 35% of cancer deaths in Western countries. Even though the independent influences of potentially protective nutrients such as carotenoids, vitamins C and E,[5,6] folic acid, selenium,[7] and fiber are not known with certainty, because they are all present in vegetables and fruits, a liberal intake of fruits and vegetables is strongly recommended. A very large randomized trial indicated that lowering dietary fat intake did not reduce rates of breast cancer[8] or colon cancer,[9] but it is very likely that maintaining an appropriate body weight and being physically active can reduce cancer risks.

Hypertension
Elevated blood pressure (Chapter 67) is a major risk factor for stroke, CHD, heart failure, peripheral vascular disease, and renal disease. It is often associated with obesity, especially abdominal obesity, and weight reduction in obese hypertensives generally leads to an improvement in blood pressure. Sodium restriction also usually reduces blood pressure levels. The Dietary Approaches to Stop Hypertension (DASH) diet, which is rich in fruits, vegetables, and low-fat dairy products and advocates a reduced saturated and total fat content, can also decrease blood pressure levels; reducing one's sodium intake provides an additional benefit when included as part of the DASH diet.[10] Because alcohol intake elevates blood pressure, its use should be limited in hypertensive patients.

Diabetes Mellitus
Type 2 diabetes mellitus (Chapter 237) is strongly associated with obesity, especially abdominal obesity. Sugar consumption does not lead to diabetes, except to the extent that it may promote weight gain. The previous recommendation to restrict total carbohydrate intake in diabetics has been abandoned for lack of evidence; 55 to 60% of a diabetic's energy intake should come from carbohydrates, preferably unrefined carbohydrates that include fiber. Because higher-fat diets tend to promote both obesity and CHD, for which diabetics are at high risk, dietary fat intake should be kept low. Alcohol can cause hypoglycemia, hyperglycemia, and increased triglyceride levels in diabetics, and its use should be limited. In both diabetics and nondiabetics, excess alcohol intake is responsible for many deaths, particularly from accidents and liver disease, and it is a factor in some suicides.

Osteoporosis
Osteoporosis (Chapter 251) is influenced by several dietary factors. Inadequate calcium intake during adolescence can result in suboptimal peak bone mass in early adulthood, and during later life it can lead to accelerated bone loss, thereby increasing the risk for osteoporosis. Sodium and protein, which are consumed by Americans in greater quantities than required, may promote excess bone loss. Excessive supplementation with vitamin A reduces bone mass and increases fracture risk. Vitamin D, vitamin K, and magnesium assist in maintaining optimal bone mass.

Other Conditions
Obesity
The causes and health effects of obesity, the most prevalent nutritional disorder in the United States, are reviewed in Chapter 227. The metabolic syndrome, a constellation that includes obesity with an enlarged waist circumference; increased serum glucose, triglycerides, and blood pressure; and reduced HDL cholesterol, is strikingly prevalent in the United States and is a major risk factor for CHD, cancer, type 2 diabetes, and hypertension (Chapter 67).

Intestinal Diverticular Disease
Low dietary fiber intake causes constipation, and it is thought to be a cause of intestinal diverticular disease.

TABLE 220-2 DIETARY GUIDELINES FOR AMERICANS: KEY RECOMMENDATIONS FOR THE GENERAL POPULATION

ADEQUATE NUTRIENTS WITHIN CALORIE NEEDS

Consume a variety of nutrient-dense foods and beverages within and among the basic food groups while choosing foods that limit the intake of saturated and *trans*-fats, cholesterol, added sugar, salt, and alcohol.

Meet recommended intakes for energy needs by adopting a balanced eating pattern, such as the U.S. Department of Agriculture (USDA) Food Guide or the Dietary Approaches to Stop Hypertension (DASH) eating plan.

WEIGHT MANAGEMENT

To maintain body weight in a healthy range, balance calories consumed from foods and beverages with calories expended.

To prevent gradual weight gain over time, make small decreases in food and beverage calories and increase physical activity.

PHYSICAL ACTIVITY

Engage in regular physical activity and reduce sedentary activities to promote health, psychological well-being, and a healthy body weight.

To reduce the risk for chronic disease in adulthood, engage in at least 30 minutes of moderate-intensity physical activity, above usual activity levels, at work or at home on most days of the week.

For most people, greater health benefits can be obtained by engaging in physical activity of more vigorous intensity or longer duration.

To help manage body weight and prevent gradual, unhealthy body weight gain in adulthood, engage in approximately 60 minutes of moderate- to vigorous-intensity activity on most days of the week while not exceeding caloric intake requirements.

To sustain weight loss in adulthood, participate in at least 60-90 minutes of daily moderate-intensity physical activity while not exceeding caloric intake requirements. Some people may need to consult a health care provider before engaging in this level of activity.

Achieve physical fitness by including cardiovascular conditioning, stretching exercises for flexibility, and resistance exercises or calisthenics for muscle strength and endurance.

FOOD GROUPS TO ENCOURAGE

Consume a sufficient amount of fruits and vegetables without exceeding energy needs: 2 cups of fruit and 2½ cups of vegetables per day are recommended for a reference 2000-calorie intake, with higher or lower amounts depending on the calorie level.

Choose a variety of fruits and vegetables each day. In particular, select from all five vegetable subgroups (dark green, orange, legumes, starchy vegetables, and other vegetables) several times a week.

Consume ≥3 ounce-equivalents of whole-grain products/day, with the rest of the recommended grains coming from enriched or whole-grain products. In general, at least half the grains should come from whole grains.

Consume 3 cups/day of fat-free or low-fat milk or equivalent milk products.

FATS

Consume <10% of calories from saturated fatty acids and <300 mg/day of cholesterol, and keep *trans*-fatty acid consumption as low as possible.

Keep total fat intake between 20 and 35% of total calories, with most fats coming from sources of polyunsaturated and monounsaturated fatty acids such as fish, nuts, and vegetable oils.

When selecting and preparing meat, poultry, dry beans, and milk or milk products, choose those that are lean, low fat, or fat free.

Limit intake of fats and oils high in saturated and/or *trans*-fatty acids, and choose products low in such fats and oils.

CARBOHYDRATES

Choose fiber-rich fruits, vegetables, and whole grains often.

Choose and prepare foods and beverages with little added sugar or caloric sweeteners, such as amounts suggested by the USDA Food Guide and the DASH eating plan.

Reduce the incidence of dental caries by practicing good oral hygiene and consuming sugar- and starch-containing foods and beverages less frequently.

SODIUM AND POTASSIUM

Consume <2300 mg sodium/day (approximately 1 teaspoon of salt).

Choose and prepare foods with little salt. At the same time, consume potassium-rich foods such as fruits and vegetables.

ALCOHOLIC BEVERAGES

Those who choose to drink alcoholic beverages should do so sensibly and in moderation—defined as the consumption of up to 1 drink/day for women and up to 2 drinks/day for men.

Alcoholic beverages should not be consumed by some individuals, including those who cannot restrict their alcohol intake, women of childbearing age who may become pregnant, pregnant and lactating women, children and adolescents, individuals taking medications that can interact with alcohol, and those with specific medical conditions.

Alcoholic beverages should be avoided by individuals engaging in activities that require attention, skill, or coordination, such as driving or operating machinery.

FOOD SAFETY

To avoid microbial food-borne illnesses, do the following:

Clean hands, food contact surfaces, and fruits and vegetables. Meat and poultry should not be washed or rinsed.

Separate raw, cooked, and ready-to-eat foods while shopping, preparing, or storing foods.

Cook foods to a safe temperature to kill microorganisms.

Chill (refrigerate) perishable food promptly, and defrost foods properly.

Avoid raw (unpasteurized) milk or any products made from unpasteurized milk, raw or partially cooked eggs or foods containing raw eggs, raw or undercooked meat and poultry, unpasteurized juices, and raw sprouts.

Congenital Neural Tube Defects

Inadequate maternal folic acid intake has been definitively proved to be a major risk factor for congenital neural tube defects such as spina bifida and myelomeningocele. For this reason, cereal and grain products have been fortified in the United States with folic acid since 1998.

⬤ TRANSLATING EVIDENCE INTO DIETARY CHANGE

Thus, the evidence is strong that dietary habits can influence the incidence and severity of many incapacitating or lethal diseases in the United States. No justification exists for the belief that modification of the "usual" American diet is unnecessary or futile. The only questions are whether change is feasible and what is required to effect it. Various health agencies and the U.S. government have used public education, particularly the publication of dietary goals, as their primary means (see Table 220-3). The Department of Agriculture and the Department of Health and Human Services have developed and periodically revised the Dietary Guidelines for Americans (see Table 220-2) and a food guidance system, now called MyPyramid (Fig. 220-1). Although some have commented that MyPyramid, released in 2005, is complex and overly ambitious, both it and the Dietary Guidelines for Americans are more evidence based than previous versions, and MyPyramid provides detailed recommendations tailored to individual characteristics entered online by the user.

Physicians can influence their patients' health by encouraging them to optimize their dietary habits and providing them with instructional materials

TABLE 220-3 DIETARY GUIDELINES PROMULGATED BY NATIONAL ORGANIZATIONS*

	Organization				
	U.S. DEPARTMENT OF AGRICULTURE AND DEPARTMENT OF HEALTH AND HUMAN SERVICES: DIETARY GUIDELINES FOR AMERICANS 2005	**NATIONAL CHOLESTEROL EDUCATION PROGRAM ADULT TREATMENT PANEL III: THERAPEUTIC LIFESTYLE CHANGE DIET (2002)**	**NATIONAL HIGH BLOOD PRESSURE EDUCATION PROGRAM/JOINT NATIONAL COMMITTEE: 7 DIETARY APPROACHES TO STOP HYPERTENSION (DASH, 2006)**	**AMERICAN DIABETES ASSOCIATION (2004)**	**AMERICAN CANCER SOCIETY (2006)**
Indication or objective	General health promotion and disease prevention	Elevated cholesterol, heart disease prevention	Prehypertension and hypertension	Diabetes	Cancer prevention
NUTRIENT/FOOD GROUP					
Total energy	Adequate energy intake to maintain a healthy weight		Reduce energy intake to lose weight if overweight	Reduced energy intake and modest weight loss can improve glycemia and insulin resistance	Balance calorie intake with physical activity; choose foods and drinks that help achieve and maintain a healthy weight
Fruits/vegetables	2 cups of fruit and 2.5 cups of vegetables/2000 calories/day		8-10 servings/day		≥5 servings/day
Meat			≤6 servings/day		Limit consumption of processed and red meats
Dairy	2-3 servings/day of low-fat dairy		2-3 servings/day of low-fat dairy		
Grains	≥3 ounce-equivalents of whole-grain products		6-8 servings of whole grains and whole-grain products		Choose whole grains over processed (refined) grains
Fat	20-35% of daily energy intake	25-35% of daily energy intake	<27% of daily energy intake		
Saturated fats	<10% of daily energy intake	<7% of daily energy intake	6% of daily energy intake	<10% of daily energy intake; those with LDL cholesterol ≥100 may benefit from lowering saturated fat to <7%	
Polyunsaturated fats	Up to 10% of daily energy intake	Up to 10% of daily energy intake		Up to 10% of daily energy intake	
Monounsaturated fats	10-20% of daily energy intake	Up to 20% of daily energy intake		15-20% of daily energy intake; combination of MUFA and carbohydrates should equal 60-70% of total energy intake	
Trans-fats	<1% of daily energy intake	Intake should be kept low		Intake should be minimized	
Cholesterol	<300 mg/day	<200 mg/day	150 mg/day	<300 mg/day; those with LDL cholesterol ≥100 may benefit from lowering cholesterol intake to 200 mg/day	
Carbohydrates	45-65% of daily energy intake	50-60% of daily energy intake	55% of daily energy intake	Total amount of carbohydrate is more important than the source or type	
Sugar	Limit added sugars			Sucrose and sucrose-containing foods do not need to be restricted	
Protein		Approximately 15% of daily energy intake	18% of daily energy intake	10-20% of daily energy intake if renal function is normal	
Alcohol	Up to 2 drinks/day for men and up to 1 drink/day for women; persons in special circumstances (e.g., pregnancy, history of alcoholism) should abstain		<2 drinks/day for men and <1 drink/day for women	If individuals choose to drink, limit to 2 drinks/day for men and 1 drink/day for women	No more than 1 drink/day for women and 2 drinks/day for men
Sodium	Up to 2300 mg/day		<2400 mg/day	<2400 mg/day	
Potassium			4700 mg/day		
Calcium			1250 mg/day	1000-1500 mg/day	
Magnesium			500 mg/day		

*For further details, see the websites listed in this chapter.
LDL = low-density lipoprotein; MUFA = monounsaturated fatty acid.
Adapted from Heimburger DC, Ard JD, eds. _Handbook of Clinical Nutrition_, 4th ed. Philadelphia: Elsevier; 2006.

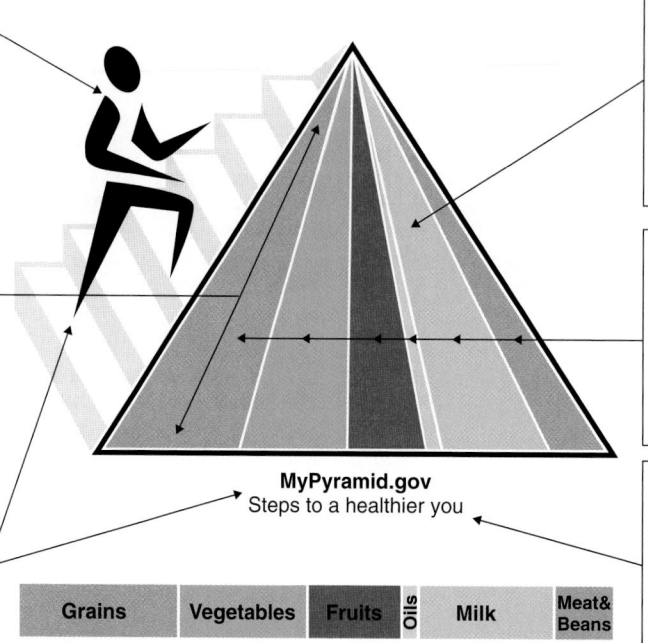

Activity

Activity is represented by the steps and the person climbing them, as a reminder of the importance of daily physical activity.

Moderation

Moderation is represented by the narrowing of each food group from bottom to top. The wider base stands for foods with little or no solid fats or added sugars. These should be selected more often. The narrower top area stands for foods containing more added sugars and solid fats. The more active you are, the more of these foods can fit into your diet.

Personalization

Personalization is shown by the person on the steps, the slogan, and the URL. Find the kinds and amounts of food to eat each day at *www.MyPyramid.gov.*

Proportionality

Proportionality is shown by the different widths of the food group bands. The widths suggest how much food a person should choose from each group. The widths are just a general guide, not exact proportions. Check the web site for how much is right for you.

Variety

Variety is symbolized by the 6 color bands representing the 5 food groups of the Pyramid and oils. This illustrates that foods from all groups are needed each day for good health.

Gradual Improvement

Gradual improvement is encouraged by the slogan. It suggests that individuals can benefit from taking small steps to improve their diet and lifestyle each day.

MyPyramid.gov
Steps to a healthier you

FIGURE 220-1. U.S. Department of Agriculture's MyPyramid. One size doesn't fit all. The new MyPyramid symbolizes a personalized approach to healthy eating and physical activity. It has been developed to remind consumers to make healthy food choices and to be active every day. An interactive version of MyPyramid, with individually tailored nutritional information, is available at www.MyPyramid.gov.

and assistance from dietitians in making needed changes. A significant barrier to practical nutritional interventions could be removed if health insurers would reimburse dietitians' services.

1. Autier P, Gandini S. Vitamin D supplementation and total mortality: a meta-analysis of randomized controlled trials. *Arch Intern Med.* 2007;167:1730-1737.
2. Bjelakovic G, Nikolova D, Gluud LL, et al. Mortality in randomized trials of antioxidant supplements for primary and secondary prevention: systematic review and meta-analysis. *JAMA.* 2007; 297:842-857.
3. Sofi F, Abbate R, Gensini GF, et al. Accruing evidence about benefits of adherence to the Mediterranean diet on health: an updated systematic review and meta-analysis. *Am J Clin Nutr.* 2010;92: 1189-1196.
4. Ebbing M, Bønaa KH, Nygård O, et al. Cancer incidence and mortality after treatment with folic acid and vitamin B12. *JAMA.* 2009; 302:2119-2126.
5. Lin J, Cook NR, Albert C, et al. Vitamins C and E and beta carotene supplementation and cancer risk: a randomized controlled trial. *J Natl Cancer Inst.* 2009; 101:14-23.
6. Gaziano JM, Glynn RJ, Christen WG, et al. Vitamins E and C in the prevention of prostate and total cancer in men: the Physicians' Health Study II Randomized Controlled Trial. *JAMA.* 2009;301:52-62.
7. Lippman SM, Klein EA, Goodman PJ, et al. Effect of selenium and vitamin E on risk of prostate cancer and other cancers: the Selenium and Vitamin E Cancer Prevention Trial (SELECT). *JAMA.* 2009;301:39-51.
8. Prentice RL, Caan B, Chlebowski RT, et al. Low-fat dietary pattern and risk of invasive breast cancer. *JAMA.* 2006; 295:629-642.
9. Beresford SA, Johnson KC, Ritenbaugh C, et al. Low-fat dietary pattern and risk of colorectal cancer. *JAMA.* 2006; 295:643-654.
10. Champagne CM. Dietary interventions on blood pressure: the Dietary Approaches to Stop Hypertension (DASH) trials. *Nutr Rev.* 2006;64:S53-S56.

SUGGESTED READINGS

Food and Nutrition Board, Institute of Medicine: *Dietary Reference Intakes.* http://www.nal.usda.gov/fnic/etext/000105.html. *Review.*

Kaiser M, Bandinelli S, Lunenfeld B. Frailty and the role of nutrition in older people: a review of the current literature. *Acta Biomed.* 2010;81(Suppl 1):37-45. *Summary of the contribution of poor nutrition to frailty.*

Martinez-Gonzalez MA, Bes-Rastrollo M, Serra-Majem L, et al. Mediterranean food pattern and the primary prevention of chronic disease: recent developments. *Nutr Rev.* 2009;67(Suppl 1): S111-S116. *Review.*

U.S. DHSS, USDA. Dietary Guidelines for Americans, 2005. Washington, DC: Government Printing Office; 2005. Available at US DHHS/USDA Center for Nutrition Policy and Promotion Publications, http://www.cnpp.usda.gov/Publications.htm. *A detailed expansion of the recommended dietary habits covered in this chapter to promote health and prevent disease.*

SUGGESTED WEBSITES

American Cancer Society: www.cancer.org.
American Diabetes Association: www.diabetes.org.
American Heart Association: www.americanheart.org.
National Cholesterol Education Program: www.nhlbi.nih.gov/about/ncep/index.htm.
National High Blood Pressure Education Program: www.nhlbi.nih.gov/guidelines/hypertension.
Nutrition Data.com: www.nutritiondata.com.
USDA MyPyramid: www.MyPyramid.gov.

221

NUTRITIONAL ASSESSMENT

BRUCE R. BISTRIAN

GOALS AND IMPORTANCE OF NUTRITIONAL ASSESSMENT

Nutritional assessment in clinical medicine has three primary goals: to identify the presence and type of malnutrition, to define health-threatening obesity, and to devise suitable diets as prophylaxis against disease later in life. The focus of this chapter is on the diagnosis of protein-energy malnutrition because of its wide prevalence and major impact on disease outcome. Other deficiency diseases are of much less relevance in that most occur in conjunction with protein-energy malnutrition or in specific disease states, such as thiamine deficiency in alcoholic liver disease and fat-soluble vitamin deficiency in malabsorptive states. The classic deficiency diseases, whether primary or secondary, are considered elsewhere in those chapters specifically dealing with the diseases mentioned here. The widespread availability of parenteral and enteral therapeutic measures since the mid-1980s that can provide adequate feeding regimens for virtually any disease condition makes a rudimentary knowledge of the pathophysiology of protein-energy malnutrition and its nutritional assessment essential for all primary care practitioners (Chapter 220).

CLINICAL NUTRITIONAL ASSESSMENT

Clinical assessment of protein nutritional status is based principally on the clinical history, physical examination including simple anthropometry, and measurement of the levels of several secretory proteins.

Clinical History

Although detailed dietary assessment can at times be helpful, in most circumstances physicians can safely limit their diet questions to whether patients have been following a prescribed diet, how much alcohol they drink, and whether they habitually take dietary supplements, including vitamins, minerals, and herbs. In ambulatory patients, the ability to maintain usual and adequate weight generally indicates that serious micronutrient deficiency is probably not the result of dietary inadequacy. Isolated vitamin deficiencies in the absence of weight loss or symptoms are rare, except perhaps for folate and vitamin B_{12} (Chapter 167). Although nutritional anemias do exist, the role of dietary deficiency in folic acid–related or vitamin B_{12}–related anemias is minimal in the absence of underlying disease or weight loss. Only iron deficiency is a reasonable cause of dietary anemia (Chapter 162). By contrast, full dietary assessment and diet prescriptions are likely to help patients with conditions such as fat malabsorption accompanied by weight loss, cramps, or diarrhea. Such evaluations are most effectively carried out by dietitians. Thus, detailed nutritional assessment of protein-energy malnutrition with secondary assessment of vitamin and mineral deficiencies is usually needed only when protein-energy malnutrition or a specific disorder known to interfere with nutrient metabolism coexists, such as celiac disease, pernicious anemia, or nutrient-drug interactions. Even then, the assessment should emphasize the likely deficiencies. For fat malabsorption (Chapter 142), one should check levels of the fat-soluble vitamins A, D, E, and K, important divalent and trivalent cations (calcium $[Ca^{2+}]$, zinc $[Zn^{2+}]$, magnesium $[Mg^{2+}]$, and iron $[Fe^{3+}]$), and phosphorus and alkaline phosphatase. When ileal resection has occurred, serum vitamin B_{12} levels should be measured, and the potential for bile salt depletion should be considered. Weight loss resulting from short-gut syndrome should prompt assessment of the fat-soluble vitamins, folic acid, vitamin B_{12}, calcium, magnesium, phosphorus, zinc, and iron. At least initially, levels of the water-soluble vitamins likely to have clinical impact such as thiamine and ascorbic acid should be checked, but provision of the full complement of vitamins should be routine in the management of this condition. Measurements of body water status (weight, blood urea nitrogen, serum creatinine, serum sodium) and acid-base balance (serum carbon dioxide combining power, chloride and potassium, and urine and arterial pH) should be obtained if the diarrhea is profuse (Chapter 142).

Clinically obvious marasmus, cachexia syndromes, and hypoalbuminemic malnutrition (protein-energy undernutrition), the three common types of protein-energy malnutrition, affect 25 to 50% of patients hospitalized for acute care and are secondary to the underlying disease in most instances. Many of these patients can benefit from nutritional support and require a thorough clinical nutritional assessment, including a dietary history, physical examination, and laboratory tests that serve to confirm clinical impressions. The history should list information about the timing and amount of weight loss, medical illnesses, medications, gastrointestinal symptoms (abdominal pain, diarrhea, dysphagia), diet habits (eating fewer than two meals per day, alcohol consumption, dietary supplement intake, dental status), social habits (eating alone, needing assistance in self-care), economic status (having enough money for food), and mental status, particularly the presence of depressive symptoms. A special focus should be reserved for elderly people, in whom protein-energy malnutrition secondary to these last factors is more common (Chapter 23).

Nutritional Support

Four factors principally determine the timing, need, and appropriateness of nutritional support: (1) the presence and severity of protein-energy malnutrition, defined primarily by degree of weight loss and weight-to-height ratio as a percentage of standard or body mass index (BMI); (2) the presence and severity of the systemic inflammatory response, defined principally by the serum albumin level but also by the presence of fever, leukocytosis, and increased band forms; (3) the actual or expected duration of inadequate nutritional intake; and (4) the prognosis of the underlying condition. Well-nourished individuals have a 7- to 10-day reserve of energy and protein to withstand a moderate systemic inflammatory response without adverse nutritional consequences. Greater degrees of systemic inflammatory response and preexisting protein-energy malnutrition dramatically shorten the period that

semistarvation, defined as consuming less than 50% of the energy and protein needs, can be tolerated.

Weight Loss

A recent unintended weight loss of 10 lb, or more than 5% of usual weight, should prompt efforts to diagnose the underlying disorder or social circumstance. Weight loss alone does not distinguish the composition of tissue loss, which can range from 25 to 30% lean tissue in semistarvation alone to 50% lean tissue loss following semistarvation plus injury and as much as 75% of the weight loss with the severest forms of injury, severe sepsis, major body burns, severe closed head injury, and multiple trauma. Therefore, unintentional weight loss of more than 10 lb indicates a need for thorough nutritional assessment. Weight loss in excess of 10% of usual weight should be considered to represent protein-energy malnutrition that will impair physiologic function, particularly muscle strength and endurance. Weight loss in excess of 20% should be considered severe protein-energy malnutrition that will substantially impair most organ systems. If major elective surgery is planned (Chapter 439), such individuals would benefit from adequate feeding preoperatively or at least early nutritional intervention postoperatively. If palliative or curative radiation therapy or systemic chemotherapy is planned, adequate feeding during therapy with the use of supplemental formulas, tube feeding, or parenteral nutrition (in that order) is indicated. However, if the weight loss represents end-stage systemic illness, commonly seen as a cachexia syndrome of loss of weight and muscle mass with symptoms of weakness (e.g., cancer; end-stage liver, renal, or lung disease; acquired immunodeficiency syndrome) for which no primary therapy is planned or is effective, invasive nutritional support is rarely indicated.

Physical Examination

Although the patient's external appearance and a check of the skin, eyes, mouth, hair, and nails often provide clues to the presence of nutritional abnormalities (Table 221-1), the physical findings of deficiency syndromes of vitamins, essential fatty acids, and trace metals are relatively insensitive and nonspecific. With respect to protein-energy malnutrition, only the marasmic form of semistarvation resulting from semistarvation alone and cachexia syndromes resulting from semistarvation and a mild systemic inflammatory response are evident at examination. Loss of subcutaneous fat and skeletal muscle is manifested by sunken temples, thin extremities, wasting of the muscles of the hand, and, rarely, edema. Although kwashiorkor in children is characterized by severe edema and a potbelly appearance from hepatomegaly and ascites, one rarely encounters these clinical signs in cases of hypoalbuminemic malnutrition that develops in the setting of systemic inflammation resulting from disease in industrialized societies.

Body Weight

The most useful element in the physical examination is body weight, which is expressed as a relative value to evaluate the patient in relation to the healthy population. Weight and height are easily obtained, and standards for comparison have been established (Table 221-2). Although newer standards are available, they reflect the increasing prevalence of obesity in the U.S. population. Use of the 1959 standards allows the same tables to be used to diagnose significant protein-energy malnutrition (<85% of desirable weight, which approximates the fifth percentile) and significant obesity, defined as obesity predisposing to excessive mortality risk (>130% of desirable weight or BMI of ≥30). Although severe protein-energy malnutrition often occurs at levels greater than 85% of desirable weight because of the greater likelihood of preexisting obesity, this condition is generally detected by percentage of weight loss or by upper arm anthropometry. Height can be measured in a reclining patient with a tape measure, and in certain situations the clinician may rely on the patient's history. The major confounding variable that limits the value of weight and height as an index of protein-energy malnutrition is the tendency for water retention with disease, and thus weight gain may not reflect an increase in lean body mass or protein content. Fluid retention is particularly a problem in patients with hypoalbuminemic malnutrition because of the effects of aldosterone, antidiuretic hormone, and insulin stimulated by the stress response, which causes sodium and fluid retention. Fluid retention, however, does not usually confound weight assessment in patients who are first seen at the physician's office, except in those patients with diseases such as cardiac failure, end-stage liver disease, and severe renal disease in whom the disturbance in water metabolism results from the underlying disease and not principally from the hormonal response to systemic inflammation.

TABLE 221-1 CLINICAL SIGNS AND SYMPTOMS OF NUTRITIONAL INADEQUACY IN ADULT PATIENTS

	CLINICAL SIGN OR SYMPTOM	NUTRIENT
General	Wasted, skinny appearance	Calorie
	Loss of appetite	Protein-energy, zinc
Skin	Psoriasiform rash, eczematous scaling	Zinc, vitamin A, essential fatty acids
	Pallor	Folate, iron, vitamin B_{12}, copper
	Follicular hyperkeratosis	Vitamin A, vitamin C
	Perifollicular petechiae	Vitamin C
	Flaking dermatitis	Protein-energy, niacin, riboflavin, zinc
	Bruising	Vitamin C, vitamin K
	Pigmentation changes	Niacin, protein-energy
	Scrotal dermatosis	Riboflavin
	Thickening and dryness of skin	Linoleic acid
Head	Temporal muscle wasting	Protein-energy
Hair	Sparse and thin, dyspigmented	Protein
	Easy to pull out	Protein
	Corkscrew hairs	Vitamin C
Eyes	History of night blindness (also impaired visual recovery after glare)	Vitamin A, zinc
	Photophobia, blurring, conjunctival inflammation	Riboflavin, vitamin A
	Corneal vascularization	Riboflavin
	Xerosis, Bitot's spots, keratomalacia	Vitamin A
Mouth	Glossitis	Riboflavin, niacin, folic acid, vitamin B_{12}, pyridoxine
	Bleeding gums	Vitamin C, riboflavin
	Cheilosis	Riboflavin, pyridoxine, niacin
	Angular stomatitis	Riboflavin, pyridoxine, niacin
	Hypogeusia	Zinc
	Tongue fissuring	Niacin
	Tongue atrophy	Riboflavin, niacin, iron
	Nasolabial seborrhea	Pyridoxine
Neck	Goiter	Iodine
	Parotid enlargement	Protein
Thorax	Thoracic rosary	Vitamin D
Abdomen	Diarrhea	Niacin, folate, vitamin B_{12}
	Distention	Protein-energy
	Hepatomegaly	Protein-energy
Extremities	Edema	Protein, thiamine
	Softening of bone	Vitamin D, calcium, phosphorus
	Bone tenderness	Vitamin D
	Bone ache, joint pain	Vitamin C
	Muscle wasting and weakness	Protein, calorie, vitamin D, selenium, sodium chloride
	Muscle tenderness, muscle pain	Thiamine
Nails	Spooning	Iron
	Transverse lines	Protein
Neurologic	Tetany	Calcium, magnesium
	Paresthesias	Thiamine, vitamin B_{12}
	Loss of reflexes, wristdrop, footdrop	Thiamine
	Loss of vibratory and position sense	Vitamin B_{12}
	Ataxia	Vitamin B_{12}
	Dementia, disorientation	Niacin
Blood	Anemia	Vitamin B_{12}, folate, iron, pyridoxine
	Hemolysis	Phosphorus, vitamin E

TABLE 221-2 DESIRABLE WEIGHT IN POUNDS IN RELATION TO HEIGHT FOR MEN AND WOMEN 25 YEARS OR OLDER*

Men, Medium Frame				Women, Medium Frame			
HEIGHT		WEIGHT (LB)		HEIGHT		WEIGHT (LB)	
Ft	In	Range	Midpoint	Ft	In	Range	Midpoint
				4	8	93-104	98.5
				4	9	95-107	101
				4	10	98-110	104
				4	11	101-113	107
				5	0	104-116	110
5	1	113-124	118.5	5	1	107-119	113
5	2	116-128	122	5	2	110-123	116.5
5	3	119-131	125	5	3	113-127	120
5	4	122-134	128	5	4	117-132	124.5
5	5	125-138	131.5	5	5	121-136	128.5
5	6	129-142	135.5	5	6	125-140	132.5
5	7	133-147	140	5	7	129-144	136.5
5	8	137-151	144	5	8	133-148	140.5
5	9	141-155	148	5	9	137-152	144.5
5	10	145-160	153	5	10	141-156	148.5
5	11	149-165	157				
6	0	153-170	161.5				
6	1	157-175	166				
6	2	162-180	171				
6	3	167-185	176				

*Corrected to nude weights and heights by assuming 1-inch heel for men, 2-inch heel for women, and indoor clothing weight of 5 and 3 lb for men and women, respectively.
Adapted from the Metropolitan Life Insurance Company Statistical Bulletin 1959;4:1.

30 or greater, with morbid obesity defined as a BMI of 40 and greater. Evidence from developing countries suggests that the BMI is better correlated with outcome than are weight and height.

Upper Arm Anthropometry

Approximately 50% of body fat is subcutaneous. The use of skinfold calipers to define the triceps skinfold (TSF) is the most practical technique to estimate body fat. Standards for skinfold measurement are available from the National Health and Nutrition Examination Surveys I and II and were derived from a probability sample of the U.S. population. Generally, a value lower than the fifth percentile is used to define abnormality (Table 221-3). The principal value of the TSF measurement is to determine the arm muscle circumference (AMC) or arm muscle area.

$$AMC\,(cm) = arm\ circumference - (\pi)(TSF\,[mm])/10$$

The AMC is a specific measure of protein-energy malnutrition if the fifth or tenth percentile is chosen as the cutoff point, and it is particularly valuable in patients in edematous states and in amputees, in whom weights are inaccurate or insensitive. The TSF and AMC measurements are most useful in initially defining marasmic-type malnutrition or the mixed disorder. Many dietitians are skilled in upper arm anthropometry.

Serum Proteins

Despite many concerns, the serum albumin level remains the traditional standard for nutritional assessment by virtue of its extensive history and its continued use to separate the two principal forms of protein-energy malnutrition. Hypoalbuminemia is a strong predictor of risk for morbidity and mortality in both hospitalized and ambulatory patients. In almost all cases, except perhaps for hereditary analbuminemia, excessive loss secondary to nephrotic syndrome (Chapter 123) and, occasionally, protein-losing enteropathy, hypoalbuminemia identifies the recent or ongoing presence of a systemic inflammatory response. A value for serum albumin of less than 3.5 g/dL is considered to indicate a mild systemic inflammatory response, whereas a value of less than 2.4 g/dL represents a severe systemic inflammatory response, reflecting systemic inflammation that produces anorexia (limiting

Body Mass Index

The BMI, which is the weight in kilograms divided by the height in meters squared, has gained favor as a nutritional measure because of two valuable attributes. The measure is relatively independent of height, and the same standards apply to male and female patients. The following BMI values are used: normal nutrition, BMI of 20 to less than 25; significant protein-energy malnutrition, less than 18.5; overweight, from 25 to less than 30; and obesity,

| TABLE 221-3 | FIFTH, TENTH, AND FIFTIETH PERCENTILES FOR TRICEPS SKINFOLD AND MID-UPPER ARM MUSCLE CIRCUMFERENCE OF U.S. MEN AND WOMEN FROM THE FIRST NATIONAL HEALTH AND NUTRITION EXAMINATION SURVEY | | | | | |

AGE GROUP	MUAMC (cm) PERCENTILE			TSF (mm) PERCENTILE		
	5TH	10TH	50TH	5TH	10TH	50TH
MEN						
18-74	23.8	24.8	27.9	4.5	6	11
18-24	23.5	24.4	27.2	4	5	9.5
25-34	24.2	25.3	28	4.5	5.5	12
35-44	25	25.6	28.7	5	6	12
45-54	24	24.9	28.1	5	6	11
55-64	22.8	24.4	27.9	5	6	11
65-74	22.5	23.7	26.9	4.5	5.5	11
WOMEN						
18-74	18.4	19	21.8	11	13	22
18-24	17.7	18.5	20.6	9.4	11	18
25-34	18.3	18.9	21.4	10.5	12	21
35-44	18.5	19.2	22	12	14	23
45-54	18.8	19.5	22.2	13	15	25
55-64	18.6	19.5	22.6	11	14	25
65-74	18.6	19.5	22.5	11.5	14	23

MUAMC = mid-upper arm muscle circumference; TSF = triceps skinfold.
From Bishop CW, Bowen PE, Ritchey SJ. Norms for nutritional assessment of American adults by upper arm anthropometry. *Am J Clin Nutr.* 1981;34:2530-2539.

food intake) and increases protein catabolism and thus accelerates the development of protein-calorie malnutrition. With a half-life for albumin of 18 to 20 days and the fractional replacement rate of about 10% per day, the return of serum albumin to normal takes about 2 weeks of feeding when the stress response remits. Adequate feeding in the presence of systemic inflammation will not increase the serum albumin concentration, even though substantial nutritional benefit will occur in terms of wound healing and immune function. Levels of other proteins, such as transferrin, prealbumin, and retinol-binding protein with respective half-lives of 7 days, 2 days, and half a day, also fall acutely with injury and respond more quickly when systemic inflammation remits. Serum transferrin also varies with iron status, however, and prealbumin and retinol-binding protein vary with dietary carbohydrate and renal function. As a result, these proteins do not reliably identify the presence and severity of the systemic inflammatory response any better than does albumin, but they reflect the nutritional response more quickly when inflammation lessens.

Composite Screening Tools

Investigators have made numerous attempts to combine the various components of nutritional assessment, including clinical history, physical examination, anthropometry, and serum proteins, into a single score. Some of the more widely used tools include the following: the Subjective Global Assessment, which classifies patients as A, B, or C or as having normal, mild, or moderate malnutrition; the Nutritional Risk Index, which is based on weight loss and serum albumin only; and the more extensive evaluations with the Mini-Nutritional Assessment and Malnutrition Universal Screening Tool. A clear advantage of one technique over another has not been established.

● NUTRITIONAL THERAPY AND ITS ASSESSMENT

The same indices that are used in the baseline nutritional assessment can be used to assess response to therapy, provided certain points are kept in mind.

Assessing Lean Body Mass and Total Body Water

In a stressed, hospitalized patient receiving nutritional support, day-to-day weight changes generally reflect changes in fluid balance rather than energy balance. In an ambulatory setting, weight increases or decreases are most likely to reflect changes in protein nutritional status and body fat because the underlying illness is usually less severe. Even the most sensitive research

methods for assessing changes in lean body mass, however, do not offer major improvements in diagnosis in the more seriously ill patients. Techniques that measure total body water, such as isotope dilution and underwater weighing, from which lean tissue is extrapolated, fail to account for the distortion in hydration of lean tissue with illness. Surrogate measures of total body protein to estimate lean tissues such as total body potassium measurement and dual x-ray absorptiometry do not adjust for differing body composition with disease. A newer method, single-frequency or multifrequency body impedance analysis, does show promise as a simple, accurate, noninvasive method that may allow distinction between intracellular and extracellular water, with the former used to estimate lean tissue for an initial assessment. However, the inherent difficulties resulting from the greater disturbance of total body water in critically ill patients have not been overcome with this technique. Magnetic resonance imaging and total body nitrogen analysis are the most reliable tools for assessing the amount of lean tissue but are primarily useful for research purposes.

Restoration of Lean Tissue

In an unstressed patient with marasmus, appropriate protein and calorie intake should cause a positive nitrogen balance of 2 to 6 g/day (60 to 180 g lean tissue) and slow weight gain, depending on the positive energy balance. For instance, a 300-kcal excess of intake over expenditure would provide approximately 120 g of lean tissue (100-kcal equivalent) in addition to 200 kcal (22 g) as fat, for a total of approximately 140 g, or approximately one third of a pound of weight per day. Weight gains in excess of this number usually reflect sodium and thus water retention from the insulin stimulated by dietary carbohydrate. Such overhydration can be improved by reducing salt and limiting fluid intake. In patients with hypoalbuminemic malnutrition who are no longer stressed, a similar nutritional regimen will lead to a comparable gain of tissue, but weight change is often less as edema becomes mobilized, with normalization of serum albumin in 2 to 4 weeks and of retinol-binding protein, prealbumin, and transferrin more quickly. In stressed patients with hypoalbuminemic malnutrition, appropriate nutritional support often does not restore lean tissue but does improve other important functions, such as wound healing and immunocompetence. These are important treatment goals, and they improve the ultimate clinical outcome. Both the systemic inflammatory response and the limited activity level reduce the efficiency of skeletal muscle repletion, which represents 30% of body weight and 75% of actively metabolizing lean tissue. Functional testing of muscle strength and endurance, such as hand dynamometry, can be useful as a means of assessing this response but has not found wide clinical acceptance. Similarly, any reduction in other physiologic functions or impairment in the patient's ability to perform the usual activities of daily living will accentuate the consequences of protein-energy malnutrition. Cachexia syndromes reflect the loss of lean tissue with mild to moderate persistent inflammation due to an underlying chronic disease. Response to nutritional therapy is generally poor unless there is improvement or correction of the basic disease process.

Measures of Energy Expenditure and Caloric Need

Although caloric expenditure can now be reliably and easily measured with portable indirect calorimeters, estimated energy expenditure is sufficient in most clinical situations. The three components of total energy expenditure are basal energy expenditure (~55 to 65% of total energy expenditure), thermal effect of feeding (~10% of total energy expenditure), and activity energy expenditure (25 to 33%). An energy intake of 30 to 35 kcal/kg of body weight will maintain weight in most sedentary ambulatory patients, with adjustments upward or downward in 200- to 300-kcal increments as prompted by biweekly changes in weight. Although young, severely burned, or traumatized patients may require 35 to 40 kcal/kg in the acute phase to meet total energy expenditure, providing energy intakes principally as carbohydrates that exceed 35 kcal/kg substantially increases the likelihood of hyperglycemia. Evidence strongly implicates hyperglycemia in excess of 180 mg/dL as a major risk factor for nosocomial infection, thus emphasizing the importance of better glycemic control by the use of insulin infusions or by reducing the level of energy intake, or both. Most postoperative patients who require invasive nutritional support for mechanical or infectious complications usually require approximately 25 kcal/kg to meet energy needs and not more than 30 kcal/kg because of their older age and reduced activity and energy expenditure. Overfeeding should be avoided in such patients, and modest underfeeding for the first several weeks of acute illness may actually improve outcome in seriously ill patients.

SUGGESTED READINGS

Dorner B, Friedrich EK, Posthauer ME. Position of the American Dietetic Association: individualized nutrition approaches for older adults in health care communities. *J Am Diet Assoc.* 2010;110:1549-1553. *Consensus recommendations.*

Formiga F, Ferrer A, Chivite D, et al. Predictors of long-term survival in nonagenarians: the NonaSantfeliu study. *Age Ageing.* 2011;40:111-116. *Emphasizes the high risk of malnutrition and its adverse effects in the elderly.*

Jensen GL, Bistrian BR, Roubenoff R, et al. Malnutrition syndromes: a conundrum vs continuum. *JPEN J Parenter Enteral Nutr.* 2009;33:710-716. *A commentary regarding the proposed roles of semistarvation and the systemic inflammatory response in producing the continuum of protein-energy malnutrition from marasmus through cachexia to protein-energy undernutrition.*

Jensen GL, Mirtallo J, Compher C, et al. Adult starvation and disease-related malnutrition: a proposal for etiology-based diagnosis in the clinical practice setting from the International Consensus Guideline Committee. *JPEN J Parenter Enteral Nutr.* 2010;43:156-159. *An update on the proposed mechanisms for the development of malnutrition syndromes.*

Serón-Arbeloa C, Puzo-Foncillas J, Garcés-Gimenez T, et al. A retrospective study about the influence of early nutritional support on mortality and nosocomial infection in the critical care setting. *Clin Nutr.* 2011. [Epub ahead of print.] *Data suggesting that early nutritional support reduces ICU mortality in critically ill patients.*

222

PROTEIN-ENERGY MALNUTRITION

SAMUEL KLEIN

DEFINITION

Normal nutritional status represents a healthy relationship between nutrient intake and nutrient requirements. An imbalance between intake and requirements over time can lead to malnutrition, manifested by alterations in intermediary metabolism, organ function, and body composition. The term *protein-energy malnutrition* has been used to describe macronutrient deficiency syndromes, which include kwashiorkor, marasmus, and nutritional dwarfism in children and wasting associated with illness or injury in children and adults.

PATHOBIOLOGY

Primary protein-energy malnutrition is caused by lack of access to adequate nutrient intake and usually affects children and elderly persons. The functional and structural abnormalities associated with primary protein-energy malnutrition are often reversible with nutritional therapy. However, prolonged primary protein-energy malnutrition can cause irreversible changes in organ function and growth.

Secondary protein-energy malnutrition is caused by illnesses that alter appetite, digestion, absorption, or nutrient metabolism and can be divided into three general, but often overlapping, categories: (1) diseases that affect gastrointestinal tract function, (2) wasting disorders, and (3) critical illness. Gastrointestinal disease can cause protein-energy malnutrition by premucosal (maldigestion), mucosal (malabsorption), or postmucosal (lymphatic obstruction) defects (Table 222-1). The nutritional status of patients with protein-energy malnutrition caused by gastrointestinal tract dysfunction can often be restored to normal if adequate nutritional support can be provided by dietary manipulations, enteral tube feeding, or parenteral nutrition. Wasting disorders, such as cancer, acquired immunodeficiency syndrome (AIDS), and rheumatologic diseases, are characterized by involuntary loss of body weight and muscle mass in the setting of a chronic illness. These patients often experience wasting because of (1) inadequate nutrient intake related to anorexia and possibly gastrointestinal tract dysfunction and (2) metabolic abnormalities caused by alterations in regulatory hormones, cytokines, and systemic inflammation. The alterations in metabolism are responsible for the greater loss of muscle tissue observed in these patients than in those with pure starvation or semistarvation. Restoration of muscle mass is unlikely with nutritional support unless the underlying inflammatory disease is corrected. Weight gain that occurs after nutritional support is started is usually caused by increases in fat mass and body water, without significant increases in muscle tissue. Patients with critical illness exhibit marked metabolic alterations, manifested by increased energy expenditure, altered endogenous glucose production and lipolytic rates, and protein breakdown. Therefore, protein and energy requirements are increased in critically ill patients. However, providing aggressive nutritional support may ameliorate but does not prevent net lean tissue losses without correction of the underlying illness or injury.

TABLE 222-1 CLASSIFICATION OF MALDIGESTIVE AND MALABSORPTIVE DISORDERS

PRIMARY ABNORMALITY	PATHOPHYSIOLOGY	REPRESENTATIVE DISORDERS
Premucosal defect	Pancreatic insufficiency	Chronic pancreatitis Cystic fibrosis Pancreatic duct obstruction
	Bacterial overgrowth	Motility diseases Blind loop syndromes Small intestine diverticula
	Rapid gastric emptying and intestinal transit	Post–gastric surgery syndrome
Mucosal defect	Inadequate bowel syndrome	Intestinal resection Gluten-sensitive enteropathy Immunoproliferative small bowel disease Radiation enteritis Intestinal ischemia Crohn's disease AIDS enteropathy
Postmucosal defect	Lymphatic obstruction	Congenital intestinal lymphangiectasia Milroy's disease Secondary intestinal lymphangiectasia Retroperitoneal carcinoma Lymphoma Retroperitoneal fibrosis Chronic pancreatitis Tuberculosis Sarcoidosis Whipple's disease Constrictive pericarditis Chronic congestive heart failure

AIDS = acquired immunodeficiency syndrome.

METABOLIC RESPONSE TO STARVATION

The adaptive response to starvation involves a series of metabolic alterations that enhance the chance for survival by increasing the use of body fat as a fuel, sparing the use of glucose, minimizing body nitrogen losses, and decreasing energy expenditure. A marked shift in fuel use occurs during the first day of starvation. By 24 hours of fasting, the use of glucose as a fuel has decreased; only 15% of liver glycogen stores remain, and the rates of hepatic glucose production and whole body glucose oxidation have decreased. Conversely, endogenous fat stores become the body's major fuel, and the rates of adipose tissue lipolysis, hepatic ketone body production, and fat oxidation are increased. After 3 days of fasting, the rate of glucose production is reduced by one half, and the rate of lipolysis is more than double the value found at 12 hours of fasting. The increase in fatty acid delivery to the liver, in conjunction with an increase in the ratio of plasma glucagon to insulin concentration, enhances hepatic ketone body production. Ketone bodies provide a water-soluble fuel, derived from water-insoluble adipose tissue triglycerides, which can be safely transported through the circulation and which readily cross the blood-brain barrier. By 7 days of fasting, plasma ketone body concentrations have increased 75-fold, and ketone bodies provide 70% of the brain's energy needs. In addition, body energy requirements are substantially decreased by 7 days of fasting because of fatigue-induced decrease in physical activity and a 15% reduction in resting metabolic rate.

The use of ketone bodies by the brain greatly diminishes glucose requirements and thereby reduces the need for muscle protein degradation to provide glucose precursors. Furthermore, thyroid hormone inactivation and plasma ketones inhibit muscle protein breakdown and prevent rapid protein losses. If postabsorptive protein breakdown rates were to continue throughout starvation, a potentially lethal amount of muscle protein would be catabolized in less than 3 weeks. As fasting continues, the kidney becomes an important site for glucose production; glutamine, released from muscle, is converted to glucose in the kidney and accounts for almost half of total glucose production.

Adaptation is maximum during more prolonged starvation (>14 days of fasting). At this time, adipose tissue provides more than 90% of daily energy requirements. Total glucose production has decreased to about 75 g/day, providing fuel for glycolytic tissues (40 g/day) and the brain (35 g/day). Muscle protein breakdown has decreased to less than 30 g/day, which causes a marked decrease in urea nitrogen production and excretion. The diminished urea load to the kidneys decreases urine volume to 200 mL/day, thereby minimizing fluid requirements. Resting energy expenditures decrease by approximately 25%. Prolonged starvation causes a marked decrease in body fat mass, muscle protein, and the sizes of most organs, whereas the weight and protein content of the brain remains relatively stable.

UNDERNUTRITION-INDUCED ALTERATIONS IN TISSUE MASS AND FUNCTION

BODY COMPOSITION. All body tissue masses are affected by undernutrition, but fat mass and muscle mass are the most severely affected. In lean adults, these two tissues account for almost two thirds of body weight. Therefore, the loss of weight that occurs in malnourished patients is principally the result of a loss in muscle and fat mass. Body adipose tissue can be almost completely depleted and up to half of muscle mass can be consumed before death from starvation occurs.

BODY WATER. Many patients who are malnourished have intravascular volume depletion because of inadequate water and sodium intake. However, the percentage of body weight that is composed of water may be increased. Decreased plasma proteins, leaky capillaries, leaky cells, and increased interstitial ion content may cause intravascular volume depletion and expansion of the interstitial space. Therefore, malnourished patients may have diminished intravascular volume in the presence of whole body fluid overload.

SKIN. The skin is a large organ that regenerates rapidly: a basal cell of the dermis reaches the cornified layer and dies in 10 to 14 days. Frequently, undernutrition causes the skin to be dry, thin, and wrinkled, with atrophy of the basal layers of the epidermis and hyperkeratosis. Severe malnutrition may cause considerable depletion of skin protein and collagen. Patients with kwashiorkor experience sequential skin changes in different locations. Hyperpigmentation occurs first, followed by cracking and stripping of superficial layers, leaving behind hypopigmented, thin, and atrophic epidermis that is friable and easily macerated.

HAIR. Scalp hair becomes thin and sparse and is pulled out easily. In contrast, the eyelashes become long and luxuriant, and there may be excessive lanugo hair in children. Children with kwashiorkor experience hypopigmentation with reddish brown, gray, or blond discoloration. Adults may lose axillary and pubic hair.

GASTROINTESTINAL TRACT. Starvation and malnutrition cause structural and functional deterioration of the intestinal tract, pancreas, and liver. The total mass and protein content of the intestinal mucosa and pancreas are markedly reduced. Mucosal epithelial cell proliferation rates decrease, and intestinal mucosa becomes atrophic with flattened villi. The synthesis of mucosal and pancreatic digestive enzymes is reduced. Intestinal transport and absorption of free amino acids are impaired, whereas hydrolysis and absorption of peptides are maintained. Gastric and biliary secretions are diminished. The abdomen may become protuberant because of hypomotility and gas distention. Hepatomegaly is common in severe malnutrition because of excessive fat accumulation caused by decreased very low density lipoprotein synthesis and triglyceride export. Synthesis of most hepatic proteins is decreased.

HEART. Chronic undernutrition affects cardiac mass and function. Cardiac muscle mass decreases, and the decrease is accompanied by fragmentation of myofibrils. Bradycardia (heart rate can decrease to less than 40 beats/minute) and decreased stroke volume can cause a marked decrease in cardiac output and low blood pressure. For example, a hypocaloric diet in physiologically normal volunteers that caused a 24% decrease in body weight was associated with a 38% decrease in cardiac index.

LUNGS. Respiratory function is altered because of decreased thoracic muscle mass and electrolyte imbalances, which cause a decrease in vital capacity, tidal volume, minute ventilation, and ventilatory response to hypoxia.

KIDNEYS. Renal mass and function are relatively well preserved during undernutrition, provided adequate water is consumed to prevent a severe decrease in renal perfusion and acute renal failure. However, when malnutrition is severe, decreases are noted in kidney weight, glomerular filtration rate, the ability to excrete acid, the ability to excrete sodium, and the ability to concentrate urine. Mild proteinuria may also occur.

BONE MARROW. Severe undernutrition suppresses bone marrow red blood cell and white blood cell production and leads to anemia, leukopenia, and lymphocytopenia.

MUSCLE. Muscle function is impaired by malnutrition because of both a loss of muscle mass and impaired metabolism. Decreased sodium pump activity causes an increase in intracellular sodium and a decrease in intracellular potassium, which affects myocyte electrical potential, contributing to fatigue.

BRAIN. The weight and protein content of the brain remain relatively stable during long-term starvation. Therefore, the integrity of the brain is preserved at the expense of other organs and tissues. However, data from one study found that cerebral atrophy was associated with protein-energy malnutrition in children, a finding suggesting that the brain is not completely protected from malnutrition during childhood.

IMMUNE SYSTEM. Severe undernutrition causes atrophy of all lymphoid tissues, including thymus, tonsils, and lymph nodes. Cell-mediated immunity is diminished more than antibody production. Alterations in cell-mediated immunity cause impaired delayed cutaneous hypersensitivity and anergy. The ability to kill bacteria is diminished because of decreased complement and impaired neutrophil function. Gastrointestinal immunoglobulin A secretion is also decreased. Malnourished patients are at increased risk for opportunistic infections and should be considered immunocompromised.

ENDOCRINE SYSTEM. Decreased plasma insulin concentrations and glucose intolerance are common in severe malnutrition. Growth hormone is usually increased and is much greater in the kwashiorkor type than the marasmic type of protein-energy malnutrition. Serum thyroxine levels are low, and the conversion of thyroxine to triiodothyronine is decreased, with increased conversion to reverse triiodothyronine. Plasma cortisol concentration is usually greater than normal. The decrease in plasma leptin concentration that occurs early during energy restriction may be an important initiator of the neuroendocrine response to fasting.

ENERGY METABOLISM. Starvation and undernutrition decrease basal energy expenditure because of diminished organ size and function, increased conversion of active thyroid hormone to its inactive form, decreased sodium pump activity, decreased protein turnover, decreased body core temperature, absence of shivering and nonshivering thermogenesis, and suppression of sympathetic nervous system activity. Energy is also conserved by the onset of fatigue, which leads to decreased physical activity.

DEATH FROM STARVATION

At the terminal phase of starvation, body fat mass, skeletal muscle mass, and the size of most organs are markedly decreased. During this final phase of starvation, body fat stores are nearly depleted, energy derived from body fat decreases, and muscle protein catabolism is accelerated. The mechanism responsible for death from starvation in humans is not well understood, but many patients ultimately succumb to infection. It has been suggested that there are lethal levels of body weight loss (loss of 40% of body weight), of protein depletion (loss of 30 to 50% of body protein), of fat depletion (loss of 70 to 95% of body fat stores), or of body size (body mass index of 13 kg/m² for men and 11 kg/m² for women) in humans. The duration of survival depends on the amount of available endogenous fuels and the amount of lean tissue. Data from Irish Republican Army hunger strikers demonstrate that death occurs in lean men after approximately 2 months of starvation when more than 35% (~25 kg) of body weight is lost. Obese persons can survive much longer periods of starvation because of their increased fat stores and lean tissue mass. The longest reported fast is that of a severely obese (207 kg) man who safely lost 61% (126 kg) of his initial weight after completing a 382-day fast in which he ingested only acaloric fluids, vitamins, and minerals.

CLINICAL MANIFESTATIONS

Protein-Energy Malnutrition in Children

Undernutrition in children differs from that in adults because it affects growth and development. Much of our understanding of undernutrition in children comes from observations and studies in developing nations where poverty, inadequate food supply, and unsanitary conditions lead to a high prevalence of protein-energy malnutrition. The Waterlow classification of malnutrition and subsequent modification by the World Health Organization (WHO) are used widely and take into account that undernutrition affects childhood growth. Therefore, nutritional status is assessed by comparing a child's weight for height (wasting) and height for age (stunting) with normal standards (Table 222-2). The characteristics of the three major clinical

TABLE 222-2   WATERLOW AND WHO CLASSIFICATIONS OF PROTEIN-ENERGY MALNUTRITION IN CHILDREN

MEASURE	NORMAL	MILD	MODERATE	SEVERE
WEIGHT FOR HEIGHT (WASTING)				
Percentage of median NCHS standard	90-110	80-89	70-79	<70
Standard deviation from the NCHS median	+Z to −Z	−1.1 to −2 Z	−2.1 to −3 Z	≤−3 Z
HEIGHT FOR AGE (STUNTING)				
Percentage of median NCHS standard	95-105	90-94	85-89	<85
Standard deviation from the NCHS median	+Z to −Z	−1.1 to −2 Z	−2.1 to −3 Z	≤−3 Z

NCHS = National Center for Health Statistics; WHO = World Health Organization; Z = 1 standard deviation.

TABLE 222-3   FEATURES OF PROTEIN-ENERGY MALNUTRITION SYNDROMES IN CHILDREN

CHARACTERISTIC	KWASHIORKOR	MARASMUS	NUTRITIONAL DWARFISM
Weight for age (% expected)	60-80	<60	<60
Weight for height	Normal or decreased	Markedly decreased	Normal
Edema	Present	Absent	Absent
Mood	Irritable when picked up Apathetic when alone	Alert	Alert
Appetite	Poor	Good	Good

TABLE 222-4   CLASSIFICATION OF PROTEIN-ENERGY MALNUTRITION IN ADULTS BY BODY MASS INDEX

BODY MASS INDEX (KG/M²)	NUTRITIONAL STATUS
18.5-24.9	Normal
17.0-18.4	Mildly malnourished
15.0-16.9	Moderately malnourished
<15.0	Severely malnourished

FIGURE 222-1. Kwashiorkor and marasmus in brothers. The younger brother, on the left, has kwashiorkor with generalized edema, skin changes, pale reddish yellow hair, and an unhappy expression. The older child, on the right, has marasmus, with generalized wasting, spindly arms and legs, and an apathetic expression. (From Peters W, Pasvol G, eds. *Tropical Medicine and Parasitology*, 5th ed. London: Mosby; 2002, Fig. 986.)

syndromes of protein-energy malnutrition in children are outlined in Table 222-3. Although these three syndromes are classified separately, they may coexist in the same patient. The use of mid-upper arm circumference has been proposed as a useful screening tool in underserved areas because height is difficult to measure accurately in ill children and accurate assessment of weight depends on access to functioning scales. Mid-upper arm circumference of up to 11.5 cm in children 1 to 5 years old can predict subsequent inpatient mortality as reliably as the Waterlow and WHO classifications.

MARASMUS. Weight loss and marked depletion of subcutaneous fat and muscle mass are the characteristic features in children with marasmus. Loss of fat and muscle makes ribs, joints, and facial bones prominent. The skin is thin, loose, and lying in folds. These children are typically weak and lethargic.

KWASHIORKOR. The word *kwashiorkor* comes from the Ga language of West Africa and can be translated as "disease of the displaced child" because it was commonly seen after weaning. The presence of peripheral edema distinguishes children with kwashiorkor from those with marasmus and nutritional dwarfism (Fig. 222-1). Children with kwashiorkor also have typical skin and hair changes (see earlier sections on hair and skin changes). The abdomen is protuberant because of weakened abdominal muscles, intestinal distention, and hepatomegaly, but these children do not have ascites. In fact, the presence of ascites should prompt the clinician to search for liver disease or peritonitis. Children with kwashiorkor are typically lethargic and apathetic when left alone but become quite irritable when they are picked up or held. Kwashiorkor is not caused by a relative deficiency in protein intake, as was previously believed; in fact, protein and energy intakes are similar in children with kwashiorkor and marasmus. The pathogenesis of kwashiorkor is not clear, but it is likely related to the physiologic stress of an infection that induces a deleterious metabolic cascade in an already malnourished child. This explains why kwashiorkor is an acute illness compared with the chronicity of undernutrition alone and why marasmus and kwashiorkor overlap.

Kwashiorkor is characterized by leaky cell membranes that permit the movement of potassium and other intracellular ions to the extracellular space. The increased osmotic load in the interstitium causes water movement and edema.

NUTRITIONAL DWARFISM. The child with failure to thrive may be of normal weight for height but has short stature and delayed sexual development. Providing appropriate feeding can stimulate catch-up growth and sexual maturation.

Protein-Energy Malnutrition in Adults

The diagnosis of protein-energy malnutrition in adults is different from that in children because adults are no longer growing in height. Therefore, undernutrition in adults causes wasting rather than stunting and can be assessed by determining body mass index, defined as the patient's weight (in kilograms) divided by the patient's height (in meters squared) (Table 222-4). In addition, although kwashiorkor and marasmus can occur in adults, most studies of adult protein-energy malnutrition have evaluated hospitalized patients with secondary protein-energy malnutrition and coexisting illness or injury. The current methods that are used clinically to evaluate protein-energy malnutrition in hospitalized adult patients shift nutritional assessment from a diagnostic to a prognostic instrument in an attempt to identify patients who can benefit from nutritional therapy. Therefore, common nutritional assessment parameters are affected by non-nutritional factors that make it difficult to separate the influence of the disease itself from the contribution of inadequate nutrient intake. At present, no "gold standard" exists for determining protein-energy malnutrition in ill patients. The most commonly used methods include a careful history, physical examination, and selected laboratory tests.

TREATMENT

Initial Evaluation

A careful clinical examination is needed to identify life-threatening complications of protein-energy malnutrition that require immediate treatment. The presence of fluid, plasma glucose, electrolyte, and acid-base abnormalities should be determined. A search for infections (e.g., obtaining a white blood cell count, urine analysis and culture, blood cultures, and chest radiograph) should be considered even in the absence of physical findings because many patients are not able to mount a normal inflammatory response. The evaluation must also include a careful analysis of the possible route for nutritional support and whether the gastrointestinal tract can be used or parenteral nutrition is needed for refeeding.

Initial Supportive Care: Resuscitate and Stabilize

Judicious resuscitation with fluids and electrolytes may be necessary before beginning feedings, with frequent evaluations to prevent congestive heart failure from fluid overload. Vitamin supplementation should be given routinely. Severely malnourished patients are poikilothermic, and a warm ambient temperature and warming blankets may be necessary to raise their core temperature slowly. However, if warming blankets are used, patients must be carefully monitored to avoid hyperthermia.

Refeeding: Nutritional Rehabilitation

The goal of feeding the severely malnourished patient can be divided into three phases: (1) to prevent further deterioration and correct life-threatening abnormalities, (2) to restore normal organ function and metabolism, and finally (3) to replete deficient nutrient stores. Oral or enteral tube feedings are preferred to parenteral feeding because of fewer serious complications and enhanced gastrointestinal tract recovery. Feedings should be given in small amounts at frequent intervals to avoid overwhelming the body's limited capacity for nutrient processing and to prevent hypoglycemia, which can occur during brief nonfeeding intervals. Therefore, small amounts of oral feeding should be given frequently (every 1 to 4 hours), enteral tube feeding by continuous drip, or parenteral nutrition by continuous infusion. Sodium intake should be limited during early refeeding, but liberal amounts of phosphorus, potassium, and magnesium should be given to patients who have normal renal function. Daily monitoring of body weight, fluid intake, urine output, and plasma glucose and electrolyte values is critical during the first few days of refeeding so that nutritional therapy can be appropriately adjusted when necessary. Appetite will have usually improved during the second phase. Protein and energy intake should be marginally higher than estimated requirements to provide for adequate maintenance and repair. Additional protein and energy should be provided during phase 3 for repletion and synthesis of new tissue.

The use of nutrient-rich, ready-to-use therapeutic foods is an easy and effective approach for treating malnutrition at home, particularly in developing nations where access to appropriate foods is limited. The manufacturing and processing of ready-to-use-therapeutic foods make it possible to add functional ingredients in an attempt to improve clinical outcome. However, adding probiotics and prebiotics to standard nutritional therapy does not have additional therapeutic effects.

Refeeding Complications

Refeeding can be harmful and may even cause death because of impaired organ function and depleted nutrient stores resulting from previous starvation. The adverse consequences caused by initiating feeding too aggressively are known as the *refeeding syndrome* and usually occur within the first 5 days. (Refeeding syndrome as a complication of parenteral nutrition is briefly discussed in Chapter 224.) Refeeding syndrome complications include fluid overload, electrolyte imbalances, glucose intolerance, cardiac arrhythmias, and diarrhea.

Fluid Overload

Severely malnourished patients are at increased risk for fluid retention and congestive heart failure after nutritional therapy because of compromised cardiac and renal function. Because the ability to excrete sodium is impaired, even normal amounts of dietary sodium intake can be excessive. In addition, carbohydrates increase the concentration of circulating insulin, which stimulates sodium and water reabsorption by the renal tubule. The presence of heart failure requires discontinuation of feeding until cardiac status is stabilized.

Mineral Depletion

Carbohydrate refeeding stimulates insulin release and intracellular uptake of phosphate, which is used for protein synthesis and glucose metabolism. Therefore, plasma phosphorus concentrations can sometimes fall precipitously to less than 1 mg/dL after initiating nutritional therapy if adequate phosphate is not given. Severe hypophosphatemia, associated with muscle weakness, paresthesias, seizures, coma, cardiopulmonary decompensation, and death, has occurred in severely malnourished patients after they received enteral or parenteral nutritional therapy.

Decreased body cell mass and decreased sodium, potassium–adenosine triphosphatase activity, or leaky cell membranes in the malnourished patient lead to depletion of the major intracellular cations, potassium and magnesium. Nonetheless, serum potassium and magnesium concentrations may remain normal or near normal during starvation because of their release from tissue and bone stores. During refeeding, increases in protein synthesis, body cell mass, and glycogen stores require generous intakes of potassium and magnesium. In addition, hyperinsulinemia during refeeding increases cellular uptake of potassium and can cause a rapid decline in its extracellular concentrations.

Glucose Intolerance

Malnourished patients are predisposed to hypoglycemia because of decreased hepatic glucose production. However, starvation and malnutrition impair insulin's ability to suppress endogenous glucose production and stimulate glucose uptake and oxidation. Therefore, providing enteral or parenteral carbohydrates can cause hyperglycemia, glucosuria, dehydration, and hyperosmolar coma. Furthermore, because of the importance of thiamine in glucose metabolism, carbohydrate refeeding in patients who are thiamine deficient can precipitate Wernicke's encephalopathy (Chapter 425).

Cardiac Arrhythmias

Sudden death from ventricular arrhythmias can occur during the first week of refeeding in severely malnourished patients and has been reported in conjunction with severe hypophosphatemia. A prolonged QT interval may be a contributing cause of the rhythm disturbances.

Gastrointestinal Dysfunction

Alterations in gastrointestinal tract function limit the ability of the gastrointestinal tract to digest and absorb food. Mild diarrhea after initiating oral-enteral feeding usually resolves and is not clinically important if fluid and electrolyte homeostasis can be maintained. However, in some severely malnourished patients, oral feeding is associated with severe diarrhea and death. Therefore, aggressive fluid and electrolyte replacement and a search for enteric pathogens should be considered in patients with prolonged or severe diarrhea.

SUGGESTED READINGS

Johansson L, Sidenvall B, Malmberg B, et al. Who will become malnourished? A prospective study of factors associated with malnutrition in older persons living at home. *J Nutr Health Aging.* 2009;13:855-861. *This longitudinal study identified the factors that increase older adult risk for malnutrition.*

Matilsky DK, Maleta K, Castleman T, et al. Supplementary feeding with fortified spreads results in higher recovery rates than with a corn/soy blend in moderately wasted children. *J Nutr.* 2009;139:773-778. *Randomized controlled trial, conducted in moderately wasted Malawian children, which demonstrates ready-to-use therapeutic foods are superior than standard fortified corn and soy blended flour in treating malnutrition.*

Morley JE. Nutrition and the brain. *Clin Geriatr Med.* 2010;26:89-98. *Review.*

Oshikoya KA, Sammons HM, Choonara I. A systematic review of pharmacokinetics studies in children with protein-energy malnutrition. *Eur J Clin Pharmacol.* 2010;66:1025-1035. *Review of common drugs.*

Scrimshaw NS, Viteri FE. INCAP studies of kwashiorkor and marasmus. *Food Nutr Bull.* 2010;31:34-41. *Review.*

Panteli JV, Crook MA. Refeeding syndrome still needs to be recognized and managed appropriately. *Nutrition.* 2009;25:130-131. *Reviews the pathophysiology, clinical manifestations, and management of refeeding syndrome.*

223

ENTERAL NUTRITION

STEPHEN A. MCCLAVE

The provision of early enteral nutrition (EN) to the critically ill patient in the intensive care unit (ICU) exerts a beneficial physiologic effect that down-regulates inflammation and improves patient outcome. Because the gut is the largest immune organ in the body, the timing, volume, and content of nutrient that is infused into the lumen of the gut have a major impact on the level of oxidative stress, the tone of systemic immune responses, and the likelihood for complications. A window of opportunity exists shortly after admission to the ICU, during which placement of enteral access and initiation of feeding will improve patient outcome, by reducing rates of infection, overall complications, organ failure, length of hospital stay, and in some disease processes, even mortality. Failure to utilize the gut in critical illness results in a different physiologic response, whereby the gut becomes a proinflammatory organ and outcome is worsened. Depending on the patient population, the window of opportunity for such modulation may be very narrow. Burns are considered to be "nutritional emergencies," in which the window of opportunity may be as short as 3 to 6 hours before increased permeability occurs. In other disease processes, such as pancreatitis or major elective operations, the window may be longer (i.e., 48 to 72 hours). At some point, the ability to modulate the immune system and contain gut barrier function begins to diminish. Preventing increases in permeability of the gut is easier than containment once barrier function is compromised. The main purpose of early EN in the hospitalized critically ill patient then is to maintain gut integrity and modulate systemic immunity. With time, provision of nutrients to prevent the deterioration of nutritional status and the development of malnutrition becomes increasingly important. Therefore, EN is indicated in any critically ill patient who is unable to eat, and should be initiated as soon as the patient receives full volume resuscitation. If the patient is not critically ill, EN is indicated if the patient is anticipated to be unable to eat for more than 7 days. The only true contraindications to feeding are bowel ischemia, mechanical obstruction of the gut, and peritonitis. It is important for the clinician to realize that although ileus, pancreatitis, nausea, vomiting, and other such factors may make enteral feeding difficult, none is an absolute contraindication to providing EN.

PHYSIOLOGIC BENEFIT OF ENTERAL NUTRITION

The provision of EN maintains both the functional and structural integrity of the intestinal epithelium. Early EN stimulates intestinal contractility and causes release of trophic substances such as bile salts, gastrin, bombesin, and motilin. Good contractility controls the overall number of bacteria within the lumen of the gut by peristaltic movement of organisms downstream. EN stimulates the release of secretory immunoglobulin A (IgA), which helps coat luminal bacteria and prevents their adherence to the epithelial wall (Table 223-1). EN stimulates blood flow to the gut and supports the mass of gut-associated lymphoid tissue (GALT). EN stimulates the production of T_H2 anti-inflammatory CD_4 helper lymphocytes, which enter the systemic circulation and support immune function. Secretory IgA-producing immunocytes form mucosal-associated lymphoid tissue (MALT), which generates further production of secretory IgA. EN promotes the role of commensal bacteria, which provide *direct protection* by degrading bacterial toxins and *indirect protection* by preventing colonization of pathogenic organisms (such as *Pseudomonas aeruginosa*). By fermenting prebiotic fiber to short-chain fatty acids, commensal bacteria stimulate butyrate receptors in the colon, which further downregulates inflammation. EN also simulates the immune process of oral

tolerance, which further supports the anti-inflammatory functions of T_H1 and T_H3 lymphocytes and the production of the anti-inflammatory agent transforming growth factor-β (TGF-β). The T_H2 cytokines that are produced in this process suppress the adhesion molecule E-selectin, which functions to trap neutrophils within the vasculature. T_H2 cytokines also stimulate the release of mucosal addressin cell adhesion molecule-1 (MAdCAM), which allows GALT cells to extirpate from the splanchnic circulation and return to the lamina propria of the gut.

The addition of certain pharmaconutrient agents to an enteral formula exerts a synergistic effect to the benefit already induced by standard enteral formula alone. The effect of the additional pharmaconutrients is most evident in cancer patients undergoing major elective operations and, to a lesser extent, in patients sustaining burns, trauma, sepsis, or respiratory failure requiring mechanical ventilation. The addition of arginine has a direct stimulant effect on immune function and thus may further support the T_H2 response, proliferation of lymphocytes and secretory IgA-producing immunocytes created by the delivery of enteral feeding. The addition of antioxidants, particularly selenium, serves to decrease oxidative stress. Providing fat in the form of fish oil reduces stimulation of the inflammatory ligand toll-Like receptor-4 (TLR-4) on macrophages, neutrophils, and adipocytes, reducing the production and generation of NFκ-B and tumor necrosis factor-β. Provision of fish oil generates alternative prostaglandins (PGE_3, PGE_1), leukotrienes (LTB_5), and thromboxane (TxA_3), which have a downregulatory effect on inflammatory mediators compared with similar products produced from omega-6 fatty acids (PGE_2, LTB_4, TxA_2). Glutamine added to an enteral formula serves as an antioxidant and helps maintain gut integrity. Zinc has a direct effect on the zona occludens, maintaining tight junctions between the gut epithelial cells.

CONSEQUENCES OF NOT PROVIDING ENTERAL NUTRITION

For the critically ill patient, failure to provide enteral feeding generates a different physiologic response that is proinflammatory and is associated with worsened outcome. Increases in gut permeability allow activation of macrophages and neutrophils and upregulation of the innate immune responses. Engagement of the luminal bacteria by adherence to the gut epithelium with loss of barrier function adversely affects the acquired immune response, with stimulation and proliferation of T_H1 lymphocytes. Reduced contractility of the gut promotes bacterial overgrowth. Bacteria express virulent genes, which allow them to adhere to the epithelium. A contact-dependent activation of the epithelial cells results in the release of cytokines into the lymphatic channels. A gut-lung axis of inflammation is initiated, in which cytokines pass through the lymphatic channels and the thoracic duct to the systemic circulation and the capillary system of the lungs, promoting acute respiratory distress syndrome (ARDS) and pneumonia. The production of T_H1 cytokines stimulates the adhesion molecule E-selectin, which allows extravasation of activated neutrophils out of the vascular space and into the pulmonary alveoli. The same cytokines suppress the release of MAdCAM, which effectively traps GALT cells in the vascular space, preventing their return to the intestinal lamina propria. With the increases in gut permeability and the upregulation of immune responses, the gut becomes a proinflammatory organ and contributes its own component to the systemic inflammatory response syndrome (SIRS).

INITIATING ENTERAL FEEDING

In most cases, enteral access may be achieved quickly and easily by placing a nasogastric tube and initiating EN immediately after full volume resuscitation and attainment of hemodynamic stability. Although oral gastric feeding may reduce the incidence of sinusitis compared with nasogastric feeding, it may be more difficult to secure a tube adequately that is protruding from the patient's mouth. Surprisingly, more than 95% of critically ill patients will tolerate gastric feeding despite risk for ileus and aspiration. Compared with small bowel feeding, gastric feeding tends to be initiated almost 1 full day sooner. Small bowel feeding quickly "catches up" such that the overall mean provision of calories and time to advancement to goal calories is the same between the two levels of feeding. Small bowel feeding does reduce the risk for aspiration but may not significantly reduce the incidence of pneumonia. Small bowel feeds are perceived to be tolerated better because residual volumes are lower compared with gastric feeding. Percutaneous access is required only in those patients anticipated to require tube feeding for longer than 4 weeks.

TABLE 223-1 COMPARISON OF PHYSIOLOGIC EFFECTS OF FEEDING VERSUS STARVATION		
	ENTERAL FEEDING	**STARVATION**
Intestinal contractility	Increased	Decreased
Release of secretory IgA from gut	Increased	Decreased
Release of trophic agents (bile salts, gastrin)	Increased	Decreased
Splanchnic intestinal blood flow	Increased	Decreased
Luminal microbiota Organisms Population	Commensal Normal	Pathogenic Overgrowth
Gut integrity and epithelial cell tight junctions	Intact	Permeable
Mass of GALT	Maintained	Diminished
Support of MALT at distant sites	Maintained	Diminished
Population of CD_4 helper lymphocytes emerging from gut into systemic circulation	T_H2 (Anti-Inflam)	T_H1 (Pro-Inflam)
Expression of adhesion molecules	MAdCAM	E-Selectin
Cell line affected (pass out of vascular space)	GALT cells	Neutrophils

GALT = gut-associated lymphoid tissue; IgA = Immunoglobulin A; MALT = mucosal-associated lymphoid tissue; MAdCAM = mucosal addressin adhesion molecule.

With initiation of feeding, it is important to advance to goal as quickly as possible (within 24 to 36 hours). Accurate determination of caloric requirements helps avoid the danger of overfeeding. The caloric goal can be determined by weight-based equations, such as 25 kcal/kg/day, or by measuring requirements with indirect calorimetry. Protein requirements are best estimated again by weight-based equations, such as 1.2 to 1.5 g/kg/day, or by calculating nitrogen balance with a 24-hour urine-urea nitrogen (protein requirement = 1 g urine urea nitrogen × 6.25 g protein/1 g N).

Formula selection has been simplified with the advent of pharmaconutrient formulas. The initial decision in any critically ill patient is whether they are a candidate for an immune-modulating formula. Patients expected to benefit from a pharmaconutrient formula (compared with a standard formula) are those who require major elective gastrointestinal surgery (esophagectomy, gastrectomy, or pancreatectomy), patients who have experienced major trauma (with an Abdominal Trauma Index score >20, especially with head injury), burn patients (total body surface area >30%), patients with head and neck cancer, or critically ill patients on mechanical ventilation. If patients do not meet these criteria, a standard enteral formula providing 1.0 to 1.5 kcal/mL should be selected. The only other type of clinical scenario in which a specialty formula is required is when the patient demonstrates evidence of malassimilation (either maldigestion from pancreatic disease or malabsorption from compromise of small bowel absorption). In these patients, a formula composed of small peptides and medium-chain triglyceride oil or a fiber-containing formula should be initiated. Specialty formulas designed for specific organ failure are rarely indicated, owing to their increased expense and the fact that their use has not been shown to alter patient outcome.

Once feeds are initiated, the clinician must assess tolerance of EN (Table 223-2). Patients should be assessed to make sure they have achieved adequate volume resuscitation before initiation. Evaluating gut motility is important in selecting the proper tube, the level of feeding within the gastrointestinal tract, and whether there is need for simultaneous gastric decompression while feeding into the small bowel. Adequate gastric contractility is indicated by a nasogastric output of less than 1200 mL/day. Small bowel contractility may be assessed by bowel distention, bowel sounds on physical examination, and air-fluid levels on abdominal radiograph. Colonic contractility is evaluated by passage of stool and flatus. In the absence of risk for ischemia (such as a patient who is hypotensive on pressor agents), ileus is not a contraindication to feeding. In fact, feeding will stimulate promotility agents such as

bombesin and motilin. Clinicians should be encouraged to "feed an ileus." Rapid ramp-up in the rate of feeding is tolerated better than slow ramp-up, and enteral feeding protocols should be in place to prevent inappropriate cessation of feeding. The head of the patient's bed should be elevated 35 to 45 degrees, and oral hygiene with chlorhexidine mouthwash twice a day should be used to decrease the bacterial count in oropharyngeal secretions. Physicians should have a low threshold for initiating prokinetic agents, should monitor laboratory tests to avoid the adverse effect of electrolyte abnormalities on motility, and may use the narcotic antagonist naloxone infused through the feeding tube to reverse the effects of any opioid narcotic in order to promote intestinal contractility.

Gastric residual volume (GRV) is a poor marker of gastric emptying and risk for aspiration. Raising the GRV cut-off level for cessation of feeds does not lead to increased aspiration, and lowering the number does not protect the patient from aspiration or pneumonia. Enteral feeding protocols should set the cut-off value for GRV somewhere between 400 and 500 mL, and feeds should not be stopped for the first GRV above this set point. After the first elevated GRV, the head of the bed should be elevated, the patient should be rolled over if possible into the right lateral decubitus position to promote gastric emptying, promotility agents should be considered, and the EN may be continued. In the absence of other signs of intolerance, the feedings should not be stopped for a single GRV above this cut-off point alone. Only after a second GRV is obtained above the cut-off level 4 hours later should feeds be stopped and the patient assessed further for evidence of intolerance.

● COMPLICATIONS OF ENTERAL FEEDING

Aspiration is the most feared complication arising from provision of EN, but the ability of the clinician to monitor such events is limited. Studies using a very specific and very sensitive laboratory marker for aspiration (tracheal pepsin levels) have shown that most critically ill patients (>75%) show signs of aspiration, occurring at a frequency of 22 to 36% of bedside assessments done every 4 hours. These aspiration events are unwitnessed and unmeasurable by clinical parameters, but an increase in their frequency does correlate with increased risk for pneumonia. Ironically, aspiration of bacteria-laden oropharyngeal secretions is more likely to cause pneumonia than aspiration of bacteria-laden gastric contents. Likelihood for developing pneumonia may be reduced in the high-risk patient by elevating the head of the bed, switching from bolus to continuous infusion, displacing the levels of feeds lower in the gastrointestinal tract below the ligament of Treitz, adding a prokinetic agent, initiating oral hygiene twice daily with chlorhexidine mouthwash, and adding simultaneous gastric decompression.

Tube occlusion occurs when acid from the stomach comes in contact with the formula in the tube and forms a clot. The best declogging agent is a Viokase pancreatic enzyme preparation combined with sodium bicarbonate tablets mixed in warm water. This combination is more than twice as effective as soft drinks or papain meat tenderizer. Failure to declog the tube with these agents may necessitate mechanical declogging with some kind of cytology brush, stylette, or commercial corkscrew device.

Although diarrhea is a frequent complaint in the ICU for patients on tube feeding, most cases represent low-volume incontinence. Although diarrhea in the ICU represents a nursing problem, feeding does not need to be stopped. The most frequent cause of diarrhea in the ICU is the addition of sorbitol as a mixing agent for drugs infused through the feeding tube. Pseudomembranous colitis from *Clostridium difficile* occurs in less than 20% of patients (Chapter 304). Rarely, diarrhea is related to the osmolarity of the formula. Switching to a small peptide formula with medium-chain triglyceride oil or adding fiber to a formula often corrects the problem.

Bowel ischemia (Chapter 145) is a rare and unpredictable complication of enteral feeding. This complication is more often described in patients undergoing surgical placement of a small bowel feeding tube, but cases nonetheless have been shown to occur with nasoenteric feeding tubes. In the patient on EN who becomes hypotensive, feeds should be held if pressor therapy is being initiated, the dose of pressors are being increased, or a second or third agent is being added to the first. Feeds may be restarted in the hypotensive patient on pressor agents if they have been stable for 24 to 36 hours or the doses have already been reduced, or both. It is important to confirm adequate volume resuscitation, fiber should be avoided in these situations, and it may be safer to feed into the stomach than into the small bowel. Enteral feeding in the patient on pressor agents should be held for any sign of intolerance, such as increases in nasogastric output, sudden abdominal distention, new abdominal pain, or cessation of flatus and stool, because these may be the first signs of intestinal ischemia.

TABLE 223-2 ENTERAL NUTRITION (EN) PROTOCOL FOR NASOGASTRIC FEEDING

1. Elevate head of bed 30-45 degrees at all times.
2. Scrutinize and correct electrolyte abnormalities (esp. K^+, Ca^{2+}, Mg^{2+}, and phosphorus)
3. Initiate proton pump inhibitor intravenously q8h
4. Place nasal bridle
   Place 12-French nasogastric tube into stomach
   Secure tube to bridle
   Confirm position by abdominal radiograph
5. Initiate EN feeds with small peptide/medium-chain triglycerides (MCT) oil formula full strength at 25 mL/hr
   Advance by 25 mL/hr q12h as tolerated to goal
   State Goal Feeds: _____ kcal/day, infused at final rate _____ mL/hr
6. Chlorhexidine mouthwash with good oral hygiene nursing care bid
7. Check Gastric Residual Volume (GRV) q4h
   Return all contents < 500 mL to the patient
8. If GRV > 400 mL, initiate the following:
   Continue EN at the current rate
   Turn patient to right lateral decubitus position if possible for 30 minutes
   Begin metoclopramide 10 mg IV q6h (if patient is receiving opioid narcotics)
   Begin naloxone 8 mg in 10 mL saline per tube q 6 hrs
   Recheck GRV in 4 hr
9. Only if second GRV 4 hr later is >400 mL, hold EN
   Recheck GRV q2h and restart EN when GRV is <400 mL
   If no other signs of intolerance, restart at same rate
   If other evidence of intolerance is present, consider reducing rate by 25 mL/hr when GRV <400 mL (or to baseline 25 mL/hr)
10. If tube in small bowel and GRV > 50 mL, recheck position of tube by abdominal radiograph. Consider switching to Aspirate/Feed nasojejunal tube.

One other complication that is seen even today in modern urban university-based hospitals is the refeeding syndrome, a syndrome of sudden death associated with abrupt refeeding. Potential candidates for refeeding syndrome are patients who are severely malnourished, those who require mechanical ventilation and are prone to hypercapnia, and those with congestive heart failure. The mechanism of the refeeding syndrome is related to underlying cardiomyopathy and congestive heart failure, electrolyte shifts when the patient becomes anabolic, or volume overload from the feeding itself. Refeeding syndrome may be prevented by closely monitoring fluid volume, electrolytes, and caloric requirements, starting at a low rate of infusion with a mixed fuel substrate and advancing to goal slowly over 3 to 4 days.

CONCLUSION

The provision of early enteral feeding is one of the most important proactive therapeutic strategies that can favorably alter the outcome of critically ill patients through their course of hospitalization. A fairly narrow window of opportunity in time exists during which to initiate feeds in order to achieve attenuation of oxidative stress and modulate systemic immune responses. The timing, dose, and aspects of delivery of EN determine whether the patient receives the full benefit. The physiologic response seen from enteral feeding cannot be duplicated with parenteral nutrition or starvation. Instituting infusion protocols, improving clinician education (regarding issues such as ileus, GRVs, and perceived tolerance), and having the skills for deep jejunal placement of feeding tubes are all factors that promote the delivery of early EN in the ICU setting.

SUGGESTED READINGS

Blackburn GL, Wollner S, Bistrian BR. Nutrition support in the intensive care unit: an evolving science. *Arch Surg.* 2010;145:533-538. *Review.*

Cangelosi MJ, Auerbach HR, Cohen JT. A clinical and economic evaluation of enteral nutrition. *Curr Med Res Opin.* 2011;27:413-422. *Analysis demonstrating the potential cost savings of shifting from parenteral to enteral nutrition for hospitalized patients.*

Montejo JC, Minambres E, Bordeje L, et al. Gastric residual volume during enteral nutrition in ICU patients. The REGANE study. *Intens Care Med.* 2010;36:1386-1393. *This multicenter study from Spain shows the effect of raising the GRV cut-off value to promote delivery of enteral nutrition.*

224

PARENTERAL NUTRITION

ALEXANDER WILMER AND GREET VAN DEN BERGHE

Malnutrition is a pathologic state resulting from unmet metabolic needs. It is associated with reduced body mass, reduced organ function, abnormalities in blood chemistries, and increased morbidity and mortality. On admission to the hospital, 30 to 60% of patients have some degree of malnutrition, and it may be severe in 10 to 25%. Many patients, especially elderly patients, those with prolonged hospitalization, and those with severe disease, are at increased risk for development of malnutrition in the hospital. Frequent reasons for malnutrition include increased catabolism, decreased calorie intake, or impaired anabolism.

Parenteral provision of nutritional support can modulate the catabolic response and correct or prevent nutritional deficits associated with disease. A state of malnutrition induced by starvation can usually be reversed by parenteral nutrition. However, in disease states associated with hypercatabolism, such as in critically ill patients, the provision of parenteral nutrients can at best be supportive. The use of parenteral nutrition is costly and associated with risks. It has grown into a standard of care despite a lack of objective evidence for a beneficial effect on outcome.

NUTRITIONAL SCREENING AND INDICATIONS

All patients who are malnourished or at risk for malnutrition should receive specialized nutritional care on the basis of the premise that this will improve outcome. A nutritional screening process should always precede the provision of artificial nutrition. This assessment should determine whether parenteral nutrition is truly necessary and whether nutritional treatment is likely to influence outcome. In the most recent practice guidelines of 2002, the

---

TABLE 224-1　NUTRITIONAL RISK SCREENING (NRS 2002): INITIAL SCREENING

	YES	NO
1. Is BMI <20.5?		
2. Has the patient lost weight within the last 3 months?		
3. Has the patient had a reduced dietary intake in the last week?		
4. Is the patient severely ill (e.g., in intensive therapy)?		

Yes: If the answer is yes to any question, the screening in Table 224-2 is performed.
No: If the answer is no to all questions, the patient is rescreened at weekly intervals. If the patient is scheduled for a major operation, a preventive nutritional care plan is considered to avoid the associated risk status.
From Kondrup J, Allison SP, Elia M, et al. ESPEN guidelines for nutritional screening 2002. *Clin Nutr.* 2003;22:415-421.

American Society for Parenteral and Enteral Nutrition suggests that nutritional screening should incorporate data such as height, weight, weight change, primary diagnosis, and comorbidities for all patients in an ambulatory, hospital, home, or alternative site care setting. If nutritional screening identifies a patient to be at risk, a formal assessment should be performed, including a combination of clinical (history and physical examination) and biochemical parameters. However, there is no single method with sufficient sensitivity and specificity to screen for nutritional risk or to assess malnutrition, and none of the existing screening systems has been validated with respect to outcome. The Nutritional Risk Screening 2002 is a scoring system developed to detect the presence of malnutrition and the risk for development of malnutrition in the hospital (Tables 224-1 and 224-2). This system has good reliability, high practicability, and reasonably good predictive validity to identify patients who will benefit from nutritional support (likelihood ratio, 1.4 [1.9-1.0]).

There is no evidence that previously healthy patients without risk factors for malnutrition will benefit from enteral or parenteral feeding if the expected duration of insufficient provision of nutrients is less than 7 to 10 days. In those patients in whom nutritional assessment has revealed need for specialized nutritional support, parenteral nutrition should be initiated only in the presence of contraindications to the use of the gastrointestinal tract, such as perforation, proximal high-output fistulas, small-bowel necrosis, severe diarrhea or emesis, important abdominal distention, severe gastrointestinal bleeding, complete bowel obstruction, or severe hemodynamic instability. An indication for initiation of parenteral nutrition within 24 to 48 hours is commonly accepted if one or more of these conditions are likely to persist for more than 3 to 7 days.

Enteral nutrition frequently results in hypocaloric feeding. Even though the evidence for or against it is controversial, it seems reasonable to supplement enteral with parenteral nutrition as a safe and effective means to achieve earlier optimal caloric intake when the enteral approach does not deliver the targeted calories. It is recommended that in critically ill patients receiving less than their targeted enteral calories, supplemental parenteral nutrition should be initiated after 2 days (one guideline) or after 7 days (another guideline).

Frequently cited contraindications for parenteral nutrition include important risk for volume overloading, severe electrolyte disturbances, and major risks for catheter placement.

ORDERING PARENTERAL NUTRITION

Estimation of Fluid and Calorie Needs

Before parenteral nutrition is ordered, the fluid requirements of the patient should be evaluated. These will vary according to the age of the patient, the disease, and the impact of the disease on organ function. Fluid requirements will generally be met with 30 to 40 mL/kg per day or at 1 to 1.5 mL/kcal expended. A more accurate formula for patients with a body weight of 20 kg or more is 1500 mL + 20 mL/kg for each kilogram above 20 kg.

A second step in ordering parenteral nutrition is to estimate the calorie needs of a patient, which remains a difficult task. The total calorie intake should be determined in relation to the energy expenditure. Age, gender, body size, physical activity, fever, and severity of the disease are factors that modulate energy expenditure. Total energy expenditure is the amount of calories burned during 24 hours and can be measured directly by heat loss (direct calorimetry) or indirectly by the relation between oxygen consumption and carbon dioxide production (indirect calorimetry). Calorimetry is

TABLE 224-2 NUTRITIONAL RISK SCREENING (NRS 2002): FINAL SCREENING

IMPAIRED NUTRITIONAL STATUS		SEVERITY OF DISEASE (= INCREASE IN REQUIREMENTS)	
Absent **Score 0**	Normal nutritional status	Absent **Score 0**	Normal nutritional requirements
Mild **Score 1**	Weight loss >5% in 3 mo *or* Food intake below 50-75% of normal requirement in preceding week	Mild **Score 1**	Hip fracture* Chronic patients, in particular with acute complications: cirrhosis,* COPD* *Chronic hemodialysis, diabetes, oncology*
Moderate **Score 2**	Weight loss > 5% in 2 mo or BMI 18.5-20.5 + impaired general condition *or* Food intake 25-60% of normal requirement in preceding week	Moderate **Score 2**	Major abdominal surgery* Stroke* *Severe pneumonia, hematologic malignancy*
Severe **Score 3**	Weight loss >5% in 1 mo (>15% in 3 mo) or BMI <18.5 + impaired general condition *or* Food intake 0-25% of normal requirement in preceding week	Severe **Score 3**	Head injury* Bone marrow transplantation* *Intensive care patients (APACHE >10)*
		Sum of both scores	**= Total score**
Age	If ≥70 years: add 1 to total score above	**= age adjusted total score**	

Score ≥ 3: the patient is nutritionally at risk and a nutritional care plan is initiated.
Score < 3: weekly rescreening of the patient. If the patient is scheduled for a major operation, a preventive nutritional care plan is considered to avoid the associated risk status.
NRS 2002 is based on an interpretation of available randomized clinical trials.
*Indicates that a trial directly supports the categorization of patients with that diagnosis.
Nutritional risk is defined by the present **nutritional status** and risk for impairment of present status due to **increased requirements** caused by stress metabolism of the clinical condition.
A **nutritional care plan** is indicated in all patients who are (1) severely undernourished (score = 3), or (2) severely ill (score = 3), or (3) moderately undernourished + mildly ill (score 2 + 1), or (4) mildly undernourished + moderately ill (score 1 + 2).
Diagnoses shown in *italics* are based on the following prototypes:
Prototypes for severity of disease
Score = 1: a patient with chronic disease admitted to the hospital because of complications. The patient is weak but out of bed regularly. Protein requirement is increased but can be covered by oral diet or supplement in most cases.
Score = 2: a patient confined to bed because of illness (e.g., after major abdominal surgery). Protein requirement is substantially increased but can be covered, although artificial feeding is required in many cases.
Score = 3: a patient in intensive care with assisted ventilation, for example. Protein requirement is increased and cannot be covered even by artificial feeding. Protein breakdown and nitrogen loss can be significantly attenuated.
Modified from Kondrup J, Allison SP, Elia M, et al. ESPEN guidelines for nutritional screening 2002. *Clin Nutr.* 2003;22:415-421.

TABLE 224-3 MACRONUTRIENTS IN PARENTERAL NUTRITION

MACRONUTRIENT	MINIMUM NEED	MAXIMUM NOT TO BE EXCEEDED	TOTAL CALORIES
Carbohydrate	100-150 g/day	4-5 g/kg/day	40-70%
Protein	0.8 g/kg body weight	2 g/kg/day	15-20%
Lipids	2-4% of total calories	2.5 g/kg/day	15-40%

Females: $655 + (9.6 \times \text{weight in kg}) + (1.8 \times \text{height in cm}) - (4.7 \times \text{age in yr})$

Males: $66.5 + (13.8 \times \text{weight in kg}) + (5.0 \times \text{height in cm}) - (6.8 \times \text{age in yr})$

Stress and activity factors are added to this calculation. The predicted amount usually falls between 20 and 35 kcal/kg per day. A more practical method, for unstressed subjects, is to calculate calorie needs on the basis of an average value of 1 kcal/kg per hour for men; in women, subtract 5 to 10%. Yet another simple method is given by the following formulas (calculated for ideal body weight):

$$\text{Women} >60 \text{ yr} = 20 \text{ kcal/kg/day}$$

$$\text{Women} <60 \text{ yr} = 25 \text{ kcal/kg/day}$$

$$\text{Men} >60 \text{ yr} = 25 \text{ kcal/kg/day}$$

$$\text{Men} <60 \text{ yr} = 30 \text{ kcal/kg/day}$$

Forty percent to 50% of Americans are obese, and obesity makes accurate prediction of calorie needs even more difficult. Based on empirical data, a possible approach is to calculate the ideal body weight and to add a percentage (25 to 45%) of the excess body weight to the ideal weight. A formula to calculate ideal body weight is

$$\text{Women} = 45.5 + 0.91 \times (\text{length in cm} - 152.4)$$
$$\text{Men} = 50 + 0.91 \times (\text{length in cm} - 152.4)$$

Formulations

Total parenteral nutrition is the term used to describe a means of feeding whereby all or almost all of the estimated calorie needs are met solely by intravenous administration of nutrients. Supplementary parenteral nutrition refers to a patient who is receiving part of his or her nutritional needs through the gastrointestinal tract and the rest by parenteral infusion. Parenteral nutrition administered through a central vein is referred to as central parenteral nutrition (often also called total parenteral nutrition); when it is given through a peripheral vein, it is referred to as peripheral parenteral nutrition. The main difference is that formulations for peripheral parenteral nutrition need to be isotonic with blood to avoid phlebitis. Hypertonic parenteral formulas are given through a central vein, in which the high flow rapidly dilutes the contents. The main limitation of peripheral parenteral nutrition is that larger volumes are necessary for the nutritional needs of the patient to be met.

The products found in parenteral nutrition formulations typically include macronutrients (protein, carbohydrates, fat emulsions) and micronutrients (vitamins, minerals, and trace elements) (Table 224-3).

Carbohydrates

Carbohydrates are the main source of calories in almost all parenteral nutrition formulations. In the body, glucose is the main metabolic fuel. In the food industry, the natural form of glucose (D-glucose) is also frequently referred to as dextrose. Provision of parenteral glucose has a protein-sparing effect because it decreases the need for skeletal muscle breakdown to provide amino acid precursors for gluconeogenesis. Glucose also stimulates insulin release, thus decreasing lipolysis. The oxidation of 1 g of glucose yields 4 kcal. To meet the needs of the brain, the minimum daily amount of glucose is estimated to be 100 to 150 g. Parenteral nutrition formulations classically contain glucose concentrations ranging from 5 to 70%; the selection depends on the estimated calorie needs and the total volume requirement. In the stressed patient, the maximal oxidation rate of glucose is 4 to 7 mg/kg/minute (for a 70-kg patient, 400 to 700 g/day). To decrease the risk for

viewed as the "gold standard" in measuring energy expenditure. Unfortunately, time limitations and financial constraints preclude this method for everyday clinical practice. Total energy expenditure is the sum of cold- and diet-induced thermogenesis, energy consumed by physical activity, and resting energy expenditure. In hospitalized patients, resting energy expenditure is the most variable component and is highly influenced by body composition and degree of inflammation. The variability for the same disease can be as much as 100%, depending very much on the severity of the disease and the time course. This is why all of the frequently cited equations to predict energy expenditure are often inaccurate in patients with more acute and severe disease and can be associated with a substantial risk for overfeeding or underfeeding.

The Harris-Benedict equation, which was developed in normal individuals and calculates resting energy expenditure, is the most popular of these equations:

metabolic alterations, the maximal rate of glucose infusion should not exceed 5 mg/kg/minute.

Protein

In parenteral nutrition, nitrogen is administered as amino acids containing all essential and almost all nonessential amino acids. Amino acids are a source of calories and precursors for the biosynthesis of proteins involved in almost every body function. Protein can be oxidized and yields 4 kcal/g. In steady-state conditions, protein oxidation equals protein intake, and under such conditions, exogenous protein serves as an energy supply. However, in Europe, it is generally assumed that in critically ill patients, the structural or biosynthetic function of amino acids outweighs their function as a metabolic fuel. Therefore, parenteral protein in that part of the world is usually not included in the calculation of calorie needs. The dietary reference intake for healthy adults is 0.8 g per kilogram of body weight per day, assuming that total calorie intake is adequate. In patients with more severe disease, such as critically ill patients, 1.2 to 1.5 g/kg may seem more appropriate. Burn patients and patients with important gastrointestinal losses presumably fare better with high-protein regimens (>1.5 g/kg).

The standard formulations for amino acids include solutions containing amino acids only or combinations of amino acids with glucose. Standard amino acid solutions are also available with or without electrolytes. Within the amino acid solutions, different formulations have been tailored to specific disease states. For example, patients with hepatic encephalopathy may benefit from solutions with increased amounts of branched-chain amino acids (valine, leucine, and isoleucine) and reduced amounts of aromatic amino acids. Branched-chain amino acids are oxidized in muscle tissue and therefore may decrease the metabolic burden on the liver. Standard amino acid solutions do not contain glutamine because crystalline L-glutamine is poorly soluble and degrades during heat stabilization. However, glutamine participates intimately in many metabolic processes, including protein synthesis and acid-base balance. Under normal conditions, glutamine is not an essential amino acid, but in critically ill patients, plasma levels fall because endogenous production does not meet increased demand. In critically ill patients, supplemental glutamine in the form of intravenous alanyl-glutamine dipeptide has been shown to improve morbidity and to reduce mortality. However, the interpretation of the available evidence differs, with one guideline recommending the routine use of supplemental glutamine in all patients receiving parenteral nutrition (independent of the concomitant use of enteral nutrition) and another guideline recommending the use only for patients who are exclusively fed with parenteral nutrition.

There is no convincing evidence for specific amino acid compositions in patients with acute renal failure, who may need as much as 1.5 g/kg/day of protein when undergoing renal replacement therapies. This is in contrast to stable patients and those with chronic renal failure, for whom a moderate protein restriction (0.7 to 1.0 g/kg/day) is recommended.

Lipids

Lipids are fat emulsions used for provision of energy and to supply linoleic acid and linolenic acid, which are essential, polyunsaturated fatty acids. Linoleic acid is the basic substance of the long-chain ω-6 fatty acids, and linolenic acid is the equivalent of the ω-3 fatty acid family. Lipid emulsions are iso-osmolar and contain a core made essentially of triglycerides stabilized by a layer of phospholipids. Phospholipids serve as an emulsifying agent; glycerol is used to make the emulsion isotonic. Fat emulsions are available in concentrations of 10%, 20%, and 30%. Conventional lipid emulsions use soybean oil or safflower oil or a mixture of both containing only long-chain triglycerides. More recent emulsions contain a mixture of both medium- and long-chain triglycerides. Medium-chain triglycerides are derived from coconut oil and contain mainly saturated fatty acids. They have a number of advantages, such as faster clearance from the blood stream, faster oxidation for energy production, no accumulation in liver tissue, and no storage in adipose tissue. However, hepatic metabolism results in ketogenesis and may lead to acidosis. Olive oil has recently been introduced into fat emulsions. Olive oil is rich in monounsaturated oleic acid and, compared with safflower or soybean oil, may have beneficial influences on inflammatory and immunologic mechanisms. Research on the importance of ω-6 and ω-3 fatty acids in the standard Western diet has led to the development of lipid emulsions based on fish oil. Deep-sea fish oil is an important source of the very long chain, polyunsaturated ω-3 fatty acids eicosapentaenoic acid and docosahexaenoic acid. An increased incorporation of ω-3 fatty acids into plasma membranes derived from fish oil, compared with ω-6 fatty acids derived from vegetable oils and animal fats, increases the release of eicosapentaenoic acid rather than arachidonic acid. The lipid mediators derived from these substances differ markedly. Those derived from eicosapentaenoic acid are mainly anti-inflammatory; those derived from arachidonic acid are more pro-inflammatory. The ratio of ω-6 to ω-3 fatty acids in soybean emulsions and in mixtures of long- and medium-chain triglycerides is 7 : 1; in olive oil emulsions, it is 9 : 1. Outside the United States, manufacturers are marketing lipid emulsions with a ratio of ω-6 to ω-3 fatty acids of less than 4 : 1 with the hope of improved nutritional immunomodulation.

Use of lipids as an energy source can have important benefits. Oxidation of 1 g of intravenous fat supplies 9 kcal. It allows a reduced prescription of parenteral glucose and can thereby reduce the risk or severity of hyperglycemia, especially in stressed patients with insulin resistance. Because of a lower respiratory quotient of 0.7, less carbon dioxide is produced during oxidation of 1 g of lipids compared with 1 g of glucose, although substrate oxidation of glucose is probably not decreased. Only 10% of parenteral nutrition is needed as fat to meet essential fatty acid needs. However, most parenteral nutrition formulations now contain 15 to 40% as lipids. Adults usually receive 0.5 to 1.5 g/kg/day. In patients with hypertriglyceridemia (more than 4 to 5 mmol/L or 350 to 400 mg/dL), lipid emulsions should not be started or should be temporarily interrupted.

Micronutrients

Vitamins are essential organic micronutrients, and most of them are used as necessary precursors of coenzymes. Thirteen different vitamins are required in the diet of human beings; nine of these are water soluble, and four are fat soluble. The essential trace elements include iron, iodine, copper, manganese, zinc, cobalt, molybdenum, selenium, vanadium, and nickel. These trace elements are needed as enzyme cofactors or prosthetic groups.

Vitamins and trace elements are usually administered as combination products; some are also commercially available as single-item injection. The ideal amount of micronutrients remains poorly defined. It is commonly recommended and accepted that all patients should receive daily micronutrient supplementation in standard doses routinely with parenteral nutrition. In critically ill patients, it may be advantageous to increase the dose of vitamins C and E and of selenium because of their role as nonenzymatic reactive oxygen species scavengers. Unless there is clear clinical suggestion of potential deficiency, routine monitoring of serum levels of vitamins or trace elements is not recommended.

● PARENTERAL NUTRITION DELIVERY

Total parenteral nutrition can be given in different ways: as separate solutions for carbohydrates, amino acids, and lipids; as a primary amino acid and glucose solution (two-in-one) with the lipid component as piggyback; or as a three-in-one admixture (all-in-one infusion). Several manufacturers now make all-in-one infusions of varying volumes and varying but predefined contents of lipids, glucose, and protein. These have become popular in many institutions because pharmacy and handling costs are decreased and potential breaks in sterility are avoided. However, compared with prescriptions tailored specifically to an individual patient, these all-in-one infusions are less precise in meeting individual nutritional needs.

Because faster infusion rates are associated with a higher incidence of acute adverse effects, during the first days, lipid emulsions should not be infused at a rate faster than 0.1 g/kg/hour with long-chain triglycerides and 1.5 g/kg/hour with mixed medium- and long-chain triglycerides.

Vascular Access

Solutions for peripheral parenteral nutrition are hypertonic to blood, and their osmolality should not exceed 900 mOsm/L. When solution osmolality exceeds 900 mOsm/L, the incidence of phlebitis, inflammation, and pain is clearly increased. Adding 5000 units of heparin to a peripheral parenteral nutrition solution may prolong the duration of the peripheral line.

In most cases, parenteral nutrition is delivered through a central venous access. The selection of the site for catheter insertion and the type of catheter needs to be individualized. If the aim of the intervention is to provide an access for parenteral nutrition only, a single-lumen catheter is preferred. In general, the favored site for insertion is the subclavian vein. Placement in the internal jugular vein, compared with the subclavian vein, appears to be associated with a slightly higher risk of infection and a clearly higher risk of thrombosis. It is also less comfortable for mobile patients. Placement in the subclavian vein is associated with a small risk of pneumothorax and a slightly higher risk of stenosis. The femoral vein should be used only when placement in the jugular or subclavian vein is contraindicated or not possible. A femoral vein access is associated with the highest risk of infection or thrombosis. Most catheters are introduced by skin puncture; catheters intended for long-term use are placed surgically. Peripherally inserted catheters are inserted through a peripheral, usually antecubital, vein and then advanced into a central vein. They can be placed if the intended duration of parenteral nutrition is more than 2 weeks, and they can be used for up to 6 months in stable patients. The main advantage of these catheters is the avoidance of the risks associated with the puncture of a central vein, but they may lead to a higher rate of phlebitis.

Before placement of a vascular access, patients should be well hydrated and the coagulation status checked. Strict aseptic technique is necessary, and correct positioning of the catheter should be controlled by a chest radiograph before central parenteral nutrition is initiated. Proper catheter care includes regular inspection of the insertion site and dressing with gauze or transparent, semipermeable dressings.

Mechanical complications during placement include arterial puncture, pneumothorax, and hematoma. Infectious complications related to a central venous access occur in 4 to 20% of hospitalized patients, especially in immunocompromised patients and in critically ill patients. In patients with central parenteral nutrition, any sign of fever or sepsis should prompt the thought of catheter-related septicemia or catheter infection. Thrombosis detected by ultrasound examination is frequent, but its clinical relevance remains unclear.

METABOLIC COMPLICATIONS AND MONITORING OF PARENTERAL NUTRITION

The metabolic complications related to parenteral nutrition are numerous. Acute metabolic complications include electrolyte deficiencies, particularly potassium, magnesium, phosphorus, and calcium. These deficiencies are common but can be prevented by adequate monitoring of plasma levels and treated. The same is true for trace elements and vitamin deficiencies, particularly thiamine.

Glucose infused by parenteral nutrition can aggravate illness-induced *hyperglycemia*. Hyperglycemia is common during critical illness and associated with adverse outcome. Large observational studies have revealed a J-curved relationship between blood glucose level and the risk for mortality, with the lowest risk roughly at the "normal for age" blood glucose level. The first randomized controlled trial of "intensive insulin therapy" (IIT) using aggressive parenteral nutrition and central venous continuous insulin infusion targeted a "strictly normal level for fasting blood glucose," compared with tolerating hyperglycemia as an adaptive response and thus starting insulin only when blood glucose levels exceeded the renal threshold (12 mmol/L or 215 mg/dL). This study of cardiac and high-risk noncardiac surgery patients in a Surgical Intensive Care Unit (SICU) setting showed reduced mortality with the use of IIT. A number of other trials have demonstrated no effect of IIT on mortality in different ICU settings and other hospitalized patients, and a meta-analysis of 21 trials found no benefit associated with IIT on short-term hospital or ICU mortality.[2] The recently reported, multicenter NICE-SUGAR (Normoglycemia in Intensive Care Evaluation—Survival Using Glucose Algorithm Regulation) study showed an actual increase in mortality with target glucose levels of 80 to 108 mg/dL, compared with a target of <180 mg/dL.[3] Recent American College of Physicians (ACP) clinical practice guidelines regarding the use of intensive insulin therapy for the management of glycemic control in hospitalized patients have recommended not using IIT to strictly control blood glucose in either non-SICU/medical ICU (MICU) patients or in SICU/MICU patients, with or without diabetes mellitus.

Hypertriglyceridemia is another complication of parenteral nutrition that can increase the risk for liver steatosis. Infusion of lipids over a period of 4 to 8 hours can result in pulmonary hypertension (Chapter 68). Serum triglyceride levels should be determined before starting parenteral nutrition and once a week thereafter. When instituting parenteral nutrition, patients with renal failure are more susceptible to uremia and those with volume depletion to metabolic acidosis. Prevention of hyperglycemia with insulin in intensive care unit patients has been shown to reduce the risk and the severity of hypertriglyceridemia.

Liver steatosis is usually caused by overfeeding and may give rise to elevated aminotransferases and parenchymal abnormalities on ultrasound. *Cholestatic liver disease* may be serious and should be suspected in the setting of elevated γ-glutamyl transferase and alkaline phosphatase, often also in combination with hyperbilirubinemia. The etiology remains unclear, and early reinstitution of enteral feeding and the insulin-titrated prevention of hyperglycemia have been shown to reduce its occurrence. Other complications of the hepatobiliary tract associated with parenteral nutrition are *gallbladder stasis*, which leads to increased risk for gallbladder sludge, gallstones, and acalculous cholecystitis.

Finally, the *refeeding syndrome* is a potentially life-threatening complication of parenteral nutrition. This syndrome comprises a series of metabolic and physiologic derangements resulting from reinstitution of nutrition, possibly because the provision of full specialized nutritional support is initiated too rapidly. Patients who have lost a large amount of weight or who are chronically malnourished are at greatest risk for this syndrome. Usually, this syndrome manifests within the first 2 weeks after start of parenteral nutrition with malaise, edema, weakness, and cardiac arrhythmias. Typical metabolic features are hypophosphatemia, hypokalemia, hypomagnesemia, thiamine deficiency, and fluid overload. Refeeding syndrome is further discussed in Chapter 222.

Grade A

1. Van Den Berghe G, Wouters P, Weekers F, et al. Intensive insulin therapy in the critically ill patients. *N Engl J Med.* 2001;345:1359-1367.
2. Kanasagara D, Fu R, Freeman M, et al. Intensive insulin therapy in hospitalized patients: a systemic review. *Am Intern Med.* 2011;154:268-282.
3. NICE-SUGAR Study Investigators, Finfer S, Chittock DR, Su SY, et al. Intensive versus conventional glucose control in critically ill patients. *N Engl J Med.* 2009;360:1283-1297.

SUGGESTED READINGS

Heyland DK, Dhaliwal R, Drover JW, et al, for the Canadian Critical Care Clinical Practice Guidelines Committee. Canadian clinical practise guidelines for nutritional support in mechanically ventilated, critically ill adult patients. *JPEN.* 2003;27:355-373 (update January 2009, available at http://www.criticalcarenutrition.com). *Summarizes the most recent Canadian guidelines on parenteral nutrition in ICU patients.*

Kumar PR, Crotty P, Raman M. Hyperglycemia in hospitalized patients receiving parenteral nutrition is associated with increased morbidity and mortality: a review. *Gastroenterol Res Pract.* 2011;2011. pii: 760720. *Data showing a consistent association between hyperglycemia and mortality in patients receiving parenteral nutrition.*

Matheson PJ. Parenteral nutrition: future directions. *Arch Surg.* 2010;145:538-539. *Review.*

McClave SA, Martindale RG, Vanek VW, et al. Guidelines for the provision and assessment of nutrition support in the critically ill patient: Society of Critical Care Medicine (SCCM) and American Society for Parenteral and Enteral Nutrition (ASPEN). *JPEN.* 2009;33:277-316. *Summarizes the most recent American guidelines on parenteral nutrition in ICU patients.*

Mueller C, Compher C, Ellen DM; American Society for Parenteral and Enteral Nutrition (A.S.P.E.N.) Board of Directors. A.S.P.E.N. clinical guidelines: nutrition screening, assessment, and intervertion in adults. *JPEN J Parenter Enteral Nutr.* 2011;35:16-24. *Consensus guidelines.*

Qaseem A, Humphrey LL, Chou R, et al. Use of intensive insulin therapy for the management of glycemic control in hospitalized patients: a clinical practice guideline from the American College of Physicians. *Ann Intern Med.* 2011;154:260-267. *ACP guidelines based on evidence for the link between intensive insulin therapy and outcomes in hospitalized patients.*

Singer P, Berger MM, Van den Berghe G, et al. ESPEN guidelines on parenteral nutrition: intensive care. *Clin Nutr.* 2009;28:387-400. *Summarizes the most recent European guidelines on parenteral nutrition in ICU patients.*

Smith PJ, Marks DJ, Forbes A. Parenteral nutrition. *Br J Hosp Med (Lond).* 2010;71:185-189. *Review.*

Thibault R, Pichard C. Parenteral nutrition in critical illness: can it safely improve outcomes? *Crit Care Clin.* 2010;26:467-480. *Review suggesting supplemental parenteral nutrition only when enteral nutrition is insufficient in meeting energy requirements.*

225

VITAMINS, TRACE MINERALS, AND OTHER MICRONUTRIENTS

JOEL B. MASON

MICRONUTRIENTS IN NUTRITIONAL SCIENCE

Dietary Requirements

Micronutrients are a diverse array of dietary components necessary to sustain health. The physiologic roles of micronutrients are as varied as their

TABLE 225-1	FACTORS THAT DETERMINE DIETARY REQUIREMENT OF A MICRONUTRIENT

PHYSIOLOGIC FACTORS

Bioavailability: the proportion of a micronutrient that is ingested and is capable of being assimilated and used for physiologic purposes

Quantity required to fulfill physiologic roles

Extent to which the body can reuse the micronutrient

Distribution of nutrient in the body: storage compartments

Gender

Stage of life cycle: intrauterine development, childhood, adulthood, elder adulthood, pregnancy, lactation

PATHOPHYSIOLOGIC AND PHARMACOLOGIC FACTORS

Inborn errors of metabolism: variously affect assimilation, utilization, or excretion of micronutrients

Acquired disease states that alter the amounts required to sustain homeostasis (e.g., malabsorption, maldigestion, states that increase use)

Lifestyle habits: smoking, ethanol consumption

Drugs: may alter bioavailability and/or utilization

composition; some micronutrients are used in enzymes as either coenzymes or prosthetic groups, others as biochemical substrates or hormones; in some instances, the functions are not well defined. Under normal circumstances, the average daily dietary intake for each micronutrient that is required to sustain normal physiologic functions is measured in milligrams or smaller quantities. In this manner, micronutrients are distinguished from macronutrients, which encompass carbohydrates, fats, and proteins, as well as the macrominerals calcium, magnesium, and phosphorus.

Optimal Intake

For orderly homeostasis to proceed, most dietary nutrients must be ingested in quantities that are neither too small nor too great. Disorders may arise, therefore, when intake regularly falls outside of this physiologic window. The size of this physiologic window varies for each micronutrient and should be kept in mind, particularly in this era when the administration of large quantities of certain micronutrients is increasingly explored for possible therapeutic implications. The dietary requirement for a particular micronutrient is determined by many factors, only one of which is the amount needed to sustain those physiologic functions for which it is used (Table 225-1). The U.S. Institute of Medicine Food and Nutrition Board regularly updates dietary guidelines that define the quantity of each micronutrient that is "adequate to meet the known nutrient needs of practically all healthy persons." These *recommended dietary allowances* (RDAs) were most recently revised between 1998 and 2001, and the values for adults appear in Tables 225-2 and 225-3. Also established for the first time for each micronutrient were *tolerable upper limits* (TULs), which are the "maximal daily levels of oral intake likely to pose no adverse health risks" (see Tables 225-2 and 237-3). *Adequate intake,* the amount necessary to prevent a deficiency state, is not necessarily synonymous with *optimal intake.*

TYPES AND FUNCTION OF MICRONUTRIENTS

Vitamins

Vitamins are categorized as either fat soluble (A, D, E, K) or water soluble (all the others), as shown in Table 225-2. This categorization remains physiologically meaningful. None of the fat-soluble vitamins appears to serve as coenzymes. Intestinal absorption of the fat-soluble vitamins is primarily through a micellar phase, and pathophysiologic conditions associated with fat malabsorption frequently are associated with selective deficiencies of the fat-soluble vitamins. Most of the functions of the water-soluble vitamins are as coenzymes, and they are not absorbed through the lipophilic phase in the intestine.

Trace Elements

Fifteen trace elements have been identified as essential for health: iron, zinc, copper, chromium, selenium, iodine, fluorine, manganese, molybdenum, cobalt, nickel, tin, silicon, vanadium, and arsenic (see Table 225-3), but only for the first 10 of these has compelling evidence indicated that they are essential nutrients in humans. Cobalt appears to be essential solely as a component of vitamin B_{12}, but an isolated deficiency state has never been described.

Deficiency syndromes for several of the essential trace elements were not recognized until recently because of their exceedingly small requirements and because of the ubiquitous nature of these elements in foodstuffs. Only under exceptional circumstances, such as long-term reliance on total parenteral nutrition lacking these elements, have some of the deficiency syndromes been observed.

The biochemical functions of trace elements appear to be as components of prosthetic groups or as cofactors for enzymes. Determination of essential trace element status is problematic with the exception of iron. The low concentrations of these elements in bodily fluids and tissues, the finding that blood levels frequently do not correlate well with levels in the target tissues, and the fact that functional tests cannot be devised until their biochemical functions are better understood preclude an accurate laboratory method of assessing the adequacy of most trace elements.

Additional Compounds with Nutritional Relevance

Evidence indicates that humans also have an absolute requirement for the dietary component choline, which is a necessary precursor for acetylcholine and phospholipids and is needed to sustain normal levels of biologic methylation. To date, the most significant adverse effect of dietary inadequacy has been hepatic inflammation. Deficiency is nevertheless thought to be extremely rare, although pregnancy, and particularly lactation, increases the apparent requirement. Individuals whose long-term nutritional requirements are solely derived from total parenteral nutrition appear to be susceptible to choline deficiency. Both an RDA (425 mg, women; 550 mg, men) and a TUL (3.5 g) have now been established.

L-Carnitine is a dietary component that participates in fatty acid metabolism in mitochondria. Although no evidence exists for a dietary requirement in children or adults, premature infants have very low stores of skeletal muscle carnitine. Therefore, preterm infants receiving parenteral nutrition without carnitine supplements appear to be the group at high risk for deficiency. Parenteral supplementation of carnitine in such infants may increase serum carnitine concentration and improve lipid tolerance, weight gain, and nitrogen retention.

CONDITIONS THAT INCREASE REQUIRED DIETARY INTAKE

Many physiologic, pathophysiologic, and pharmacologic factors increase the dietary requirements for micronutrients (see Table 225-1), thereby enhancing the risk of developing a deficiency state.

Physiologic Factors

Stages of the life cycle frequently have a significant impact on the requirements of nutrients. Phases of rapid growth and development, such as in utero development, infancy, adolescence, and pregnancy, are associated with increases in the utilization of certain micronutrients on a per-kilogram basis.

Pregnancy

Requirements for most micronutrients are increased in pregnancy, but, proportionately, the observed increases in the maternal requirements for iron and folate are particularly great and are related to the rapid proliferation of the placental and fetal tissues. Periods of lactation are similarly associated with remarkable increases in requirements; a lactating woman experiences disproportionately large increases in her requirements for zinc and vitamins A, E, and C to meet the metabolic demands incurred by milk production in addition to the aforementioned needs observed in pregnancy.

Aside from its general role in supporting the rapid proliferation of placental and fetal tissues, folate plays a specific role in the prevention of particular birth defects. A 20 to 85% reduction in births complicated by neural tube defects (NTDs, i.e., spina bifida and anencephaly) has been realized by providing women with a daily supplement of folic acid in the form of supplements or fortified foods. The optimal dose is not well defined, but 200 to 400 μg/day clearly affords a substantial degree of protection. Populations with a high background rate of NTD births attain the largest reductions in NTDs from supplemental folate. However, because the nascent neural tube closes about day 20 after conception, the additional folate must be provided before this time in order to be effective.

Text continues on p. 1405

TABLE 225-2 VITAMINS AND THEIR FUNCTIONS

	BIOCHEMISTRY AND PHYSIOLOGY	DEFICIENCY [RDA*]	TOXICITY [TUL†]	ASSESSMENT OF STATUS
FAT-SOLUBLE VITAMINS				
Vitamin A	A family of the retinoid compounds, each member having biologic activity qualitatively similar to retinol. Carotenoids are structurally related to retinoids. Some carotenoids, most notably β-carotene, are metabolized into compounds with vitamin A activity and are therefore considered to be provitamin A compounds. Vitamin A is an integral component of rhodopsin and iodopsins, light-sensitive proteins in rod and cone cells in the retina. *Additional functions:* induction and maintenance of cellular differentiation in certain tissues; signal for appropriate morphogenesis in the developing embryo; maintenance of cell-mediated immunity. One microgram of retinol = 3.33 IU of vitamin A.	Follicular hyperkeratosis and night blindness are early indicators. Conjunctival xerosis, degeneration of the cornea (keratomalacia), and de-differentiation of rapidly proliferating epithelia are later indications of deficiency. *Bitot spots* (focal areas of the conjunctiva or cornea with foamy appearance) are an indication of xerosis. Blindness, due to corneal destruction and retinal dysfunction, ensues if left uncorrected. Increased susceptibility to infection is also a consequence. [F: 700 µg; M: 900 µg]	In adults, >150,000 µg may cause *acute* toxicity: fatal intracranial hypertension, skin exfoliation, and hepatocellular necrosis. *Chronic* toxicity may occur with habitual daily intake of >10,000 µg: alopecia, ataxia, bone and muscle pain, dermatitis, cheilitis, conjunctivitis, pseudotumor cerebri, hepatocellular necrosis, hyperlipidemia, and hyperostosis are common. Single, large doses of vitamin A (30,000 µg), or habitual intake of >4500 µg/day in early pregnancy can be teratogenic. Excessive intake of carotenoids causes a benign condition characterized by yellowish discoloration of the skin. Habitually large doses of canthaxanthin, a carotenoid, have the additional capability of inducing a retinopathy. [3000 µg]	Retinol concentration in the plasma and vitamin A concentrations in the milk and tears are reasonably accurate measures of adequate status. Toxicity is best assessed by elevated levels of retinyl esters in plasma. A quantitative measure of dark adaptation for night vision or an electroretinogram are useful functional tests.
Vitamin D	A group of sterol compounds whose parent structure is cholecalciferol (vitamin D₃). Cholecalciferol is formed in the skin from 7-dehydrocholesterol (provitamin D₃) by exposure to UVB radiation. A plant sterol, ergocalciferol (provitamin D₂) can be similarly converted into vitamin D₂ and has similar vitamin D activity. The vitamin undergoes sequential hydroxylations in the liver and kidney at the 25 and 1 positions, respectively, producing the most bioactive form of the vitamin, 1,25-dihydroxy vitamin D. Maintains intracellular and extracellular concentrations of calcium and phosphate by enhancing intestinal absorption of the two ions and, in conjunction with PTH, promoting their mobilization from bone mineral. Retards proliferation and promotes differentiation in certain epithelia. One microgram is = 40 IU.	Deficiency results in disordered bone modeling called *rickets* in childhood and *osteomalacia* in adults. Expansion of the epiphyseal growth plates and replacement of normal bone with unmineralized bone matrix are the cardinal features of rickets; the latter feature also characterizes osteomalacia. Deformity of bone and pathologic fractures occur. Decreased serum concentrations of calcium and phosphate may occur. [15 µg, ages 19-70 yr; 20 µg, age >70 yr]	Excess amounts result in abnormally high concentrations of calcium and phosphate in the serum: metastatic calcifications, renal damage, and altered mentation may occur. [50 µg]	The serum concentration of the major circulating metabolite, 25-hydroxyvitamin D, is an excellent indicator of systemic status except in chronic renal failure, in which the impairment of renal L-hydroxylation results in disassociation of the mono- and dihydroxyvitamin concentrations. Measuring the serum concentration of 1,25-dihydroxyvitamin D is then necessary.
Vitamin E	A group of at least 8 naturally occurring compounds, some of which are tocopherols and some of which are tocotrienols. At present, the only dietary form that is thought to be biologically active in humans is α-tocopherol. Acts as an antioxidant and free radical scavenger in lipophilic environments, most notably in cell membranes. Acts in conjunction with other antioxidants such as selenium.	Deficiency due to dietary inadequacy rare. Usually seen in (1) premature infants, (2) individuals with fat malabsorption, and (3) individuals with abetalipoproteinemia. Red blood cell fragility occurs and can produce a hemolytic anemia. Neuronal degeneration produces peripheral neuropathies, ophthalmoplegia, and destruction of posterior columns of spinal cord. Neurologic disease is frequently irreversible if deficiency is not corrected early enough. May contribute to the hemolytic anemia and retrolental fibroplasia seen in premature infants. Reported to suppress cell-mediated immunity. [15 mg]	Depressed levels of vitamin K-dependent procoagulants and potentiation of oral anticoagulants has been reported, as has impaired WBC function. Doses of 800 mg/day have been reported to increase slightly the incidence of hemorrhagic stroke. [1000 mg]	Plasma or serum concentration of α-tocopherol is most commonly used. Additional accuracy is obtained by expressing this value per mg of total plasma lipid. RBC peroxide hemolysis test is not entirely specific but is a useful functional measure of the antioxidant potential of cell membranes.

TABLE 225-2   VITAMINS AND THEIR FUNCTIONS—cont'd

	BIOCHEMISTRY AND PHYSIOLOGY	DEFICIENCY [RDA*]	TOXICITY [TUL†]	ASSESSMENT OF STATUS
Vitamin K	A family of naphthoquinone compounds with similar biologic activity. Phylloquinone (vitamin K_1) is derived from plants; a variety of menaquinones (vitamin K_2) is derived from bacterial sources. Serves as an essential cofactor in the post-translational γ-carboxylation of glutamic acid residues in many proteins. These proteins include several circulating procoagulants and anticoagulants as well as proteins in a variety of tissues.	Deficiency syndrome, uncommon except in (1) breast-fed newborns, in whom it may cause "hemorrhagic disease of the newborn," (2) adults with fat malabsorption or who are taking drugs that interfere with vitamin K metabolism (e.g., coumarin, phenytoin, broad-spectrum antibiotics), and (3) individuals taking large doses of vitamin E and anticoagulant drugs. Excessive hemorrhage is the usual manifestation. [F: 90 μg; M: 120 μg]	Rapid intravenous infusion of K_1 has been associated with dyspnea, flushing, and cardiovascular collapse; this is likely related to the dispersing agents in the solution. Supplementation may interfere with coumarin-based anticoagulation. Pregnant women taking large amounts of the provitamin menadione may deliver infants with hemolytic anemia, hyperbilirubinemia, and kernicterus. [no TUL established]	Prothrombin time is typically used as a measure of functional K status; it is neither sensitive nor specific for vitamin K deficiency. Determination of undercarboxylated prothrombin in the plasma is more accurate but less widely available.

WATER-SOLUBLE VITAMINS

	BIOCHEMISTRY AND PHYSIOLOGY	DEFICIENCY [RDA*]	TOXICITY [TUL†]	ASSESSMENT OF STATUS
Thiamin (vitamin B_1)	A water-soluble compound containing substituted pyrimidine and thiazole rings and a hydroxyethyl side chain. The coenzyme form is thiamin pyrophosphate (TPP). Serves as a coenzyme in many α-ketoacid decarboxylation and transketolation reactions. Inadequate thiamin availability leads to impairments of above reactions, resulting in inadequate adenosine triphosphate synthesis and abnormal carbohydrate metabolism, respectively. May have an additional role in neuronal conduction independent of aforementioned actions.	Classic deficiency syndrome ("beriberi") described in Asian populations consuming polished rice diet. Alcoholism and chronic renal dialysis are also common precipitants. High carbohydrate intake increases need for B_1. *Mild deficiency*: irritability, fatigue, and headaches. *More severe deficiency*: combinations of peripheral neuropathy, cardiovascular dysfunction, and cerebral dysfunction. Cardiovascular involvement ("wet beriberi"): congestive heart failure and low peripheral vascular resistance. Cerebral disease: nystagmus, ophthalmoplegia, and ataxia (Wernicke's encephalopathy); hallucinations, impaired short-term memory, and confabulation ("Korsakoff's psychosis"). Deficiency syndrome responds within 24 hr to parenteral thiamin but is partially or wholly irreversible after a certain stage. [F: 1.1 mg; M: 1.2 mg]	Excess intake is largely excreted in the urine, although parenteral doses of > 400 mg/day are reported to cause lethargy, ataxia, and reduced tone of the gastrointestinal tract. [TUL not established]	The most effective measure of B_1 status is the erythrocyte transketolase activity coefficient, which measures enzyme activity before and after addition of exogenous TPP: RBCs from a deficient individual express a substantial increase in enzyme activity with addition of TPP. Thiamin concentrations in blood or urine are also used.
Riboflavin (vitamin B_2)	Consists of a substituted isoalloxazine ring with a ribitol side chain. Serves as a coenzyme for a diverse array of biochemical reactions. The primary coenzymatic forms are flavin mononucleotide (FMN) and flavin adenine dinucleotide (FAD). Riboflavin holoenzymes participate in oxidation-reduction reactions in a myriad of metabolic pathways.	Deficiency is usually seen in conjunction with deficiencies of other B vitamins. Isolated deficiency of riboflavin produces hyperemia and edema of nasopharyngeal mucosa, cheilosis, angular stomatitis, glossitis, seborrheic dermatitis, and a normochromic, normocytic anemia. [F: 1.1; M: 1.3]	Toxicity not reported in humans. [TUL not established]	The most common method of assessment is determining the activity coefficient of glutathione reductase in RBCs (the test is invalid for individuals with glucose-6-phosphate dehydrogenase [G6PD] deficiency). Measurements of blood and urine concentrations are less desirable methods.
Niacin (vitamin B_3)	Refers to nicotinic acid and the corresponding amide, nicotinamide. The active coenzymatic forms are composed of nicotinamide affixed to adenine dinucleotide, forming NAD or NADP. More than 200 apoenzymes use these compounds as electron acceptors or hydrogen donors, either as a coenzyme or as a co-substrate. The essential amino acid tryptophan is a precursor of niacin; 60 mg of dietary tryptophan yields approximately 1 mg of niacin. Dietary requirements thus depend partly on tryptophan intake. Requirement is often determined on basis of caloric intake (i.e., niacin equivalents/1000 kcal). Large doses of nicotinic acid (1.5-3 g/day) effectively lower low-density lipoprotein cholesterol and elevate high-density lipoprotein cholesterol.	*Pellagra* is the classic deficiency syndrome and is often seen in populations in which corn is the major source of energy. Still endemic in parts of China, Africa, and India. Diarrhea, dementia (or associated symptoms of anxiety or insomnia), and a pigmented dermatitis that develops in sun-exposed areas are typical features. Glossitis, stomatitis, vaginitis, vertigo, and burning dysesthesias are early signs. Reported to occasionally occur in carcinoid syndrome because tryptophan is diverted to other synthetic pathways. [F: 14 mg; M: 16 mg]	Human toxicity known largely through studies examining hypolipidemic effects. Includes vasomotor phenomenon (flushing), hyperglycemia, parenchymal liver damage, and hyperuricemia. [35 mg]	Assessment of status is problematic: blood levels of vitamin not reliable. Measurement of urinary excretion of the niacin metabolites, N-methylnicotinamide and 2-pyridone, is thought to be the most effective means of assessment at present.

TABLE 225-2 VITAMINS AND THEIR FUNCTIONS—cont'd

	BIOCHEMISTRY AND PHYSIOLOGY	DEFICIENCY [RDA*]	TOXICITY [TUL†]	ASSESSMENT OF STATUS
Vitamin B$_6$	Refers to several derivatives of pyridine, including pyridoxine (PN), pyridoxal (PL), and pyridoxamine (PM), which are interconvertible in the body. The coenzymatic forms are pyridoxal-5-phosphate (PLP) and pyridoxamine-5-phosphate (PMP). As a coenzyme, B$_6$ is involved in many transamination reactions (and thereby in gluconeogenesis), in the synthesis of niacin from tryptophan, in the synthesis of several neurotransmitters, and in the synthesis of δ-aminolevulinic acid (and therefore in heme synthesis). It also has functions unrelated to coenzymatic activity: PL and PLP bind to hemoglobin and alter O$_2$ affinity; PLP also binds to steroid receptors, inhibiting receptor affinity to DNA and thereby modulating steroid activity.	Deficiency usually seen in conjunction with other water-soluble vitamin deficiencies. Stomatitis, angular cheilosis, glossitis, irritability, depression, and confusion occur in moderate to severe depletion; normochromic, normocytic anemia has been reported in severe deficiency. Abnormal electroencephalograms and, in infants, convulsions have also been observed. Some sideroblastic anemias respond to B$_6$ administration. Isoniazid, cycloserine, penicillamine, ethanol, and theophylline can inhibit B$_6$ metabolism. [Ages 19-50 yr: 1.3 mg; >50 yr: 1.5 mg for women, 1.7 mg for men]	Long-term use with doses exceeding 200 mg/day (in adults) may cause peripheral neuropathies and photosensitivity. [100 mg]	Many useful laboratory methods of assessment exist. The plasma or erythrocyte PLP levels are most common. Urinary excretion of xanthurenic acid after an oral tryptophan load or activity indices of RBC alanine or aspartic acid transaminases (ALT and AST, respectively) are all functional measures of B$_6$-dependent enzyme activity.
Folate	A group of related pterin compounds. More than 35 forms of the vitamin are found naturally. The fully oxidized form, folic acid, is not found in nature but is the pharmacologic form of the vitamin. All folate functions relate to its ability to transfer one-carbon groups. It is essential in the de novo synthesis of nucleotides and in the metabolism of several amino acids, and is an integral component for the regeneration of the "universal" methyl donor, S-adenosylmethionine. Inhibition of bacterial and cancer cell folate metabolism is the basis for the sulfonamide antibiotics and chemotherapeutic agents such as methotrexate and 5-fluorouracil, respectively.	Women of childbearing age are most likely to be deficient. *Classic deficiency syndrome*: megaloblastic anemia, diarrhea. The hematopoietic cells in bone marrow become enlarged and have immature nuclei, reflecting ineffective DNA synthesis. The peripheral blood smear demonstrates macro-ovalocytes and polymorphonuclear leukocytes with an average of more than 3.5 nuclear lobes. Megaloblastic changes also occur in other epithelia that proliferate rapidly (e.g., oral mucosa, gastrointestinal tract), producing glossitis and diarrhea, respectively. Sulfasalazine and diphenytoin inhibit absorption and predispose to deficiency. [400 µg of dietary folate equivalents (DFE); 1 DFE = 1 µg food folate = 0.6 µg folic acid]	Doses >1000 µg/day may partially correct the anemia of B$_{12}$ deficiency and may therefore mask (and perhaps exacerbate) the associated neuropathy. Large doses also reported to lower seizure threshold in individuals prone to seizures. Parenteral administration is rarely reported to cause allergic phenomena, which is probably due to dispersion agents. [1000 µg]	Serum folate measures short-term folate balance, whereas RBC folate is a better reflection of tissue status. Serum homocysteine rises early in deficiency but is nonspecific because B$_{12}$ or B$_6$ deficiency, renal insufficiency, and older age may also cause elevations.
Vitamin C (ascorbic and dehydroascorbic acid)	Ascorbic acid readily oxidizes to dehydroascorbic acid in aqueous solution. The latter can be reduced in vivo, so it possesses vitamin C activity. Total vitamin C is therefore the sum of ascorbic and dehydroascorbic acid content. It serves primarily as a biologic antioxidant in aqueous environments. Biosyntheses of collagen, carnitine, bile acids, and norepinephrine, as well as proper functioning of the hepatic mixed-function oxygenase system, depend on this property. Vitamin C in foodstuffs increases the intestinal absorption of nonheme iron.	Overt deficiency is uncommon in developed countries. The classic deficiency syndrome is *scurvy*: fatigue, depression, and widespread abnormalities in connective tissues, such as inflamed gingivae, petechiae, perifollicular hemorrhages, impaired wound healing, coiled hairs, hyperkeratosis, bleeding into body cavities. In infants, defects in ossification and bone growth may occur. Tobacco smoking lowers plasma and leukocyte vitamin C levels. [F: 75 mg; M: 90 mg; increase requirement for cigarette smokers by 35 mg/day]	≥500 mg/day (in adults) may cause nausea and diarrhea. >1 g/day modestly increases risk for oxalate kidney stones. Supplementation may interfere with laboratory tests based on redox potential (e.g., fecal occult blood testing, serum cholesterol, and glucose). Withdrawal from chronic ingestion of high doses of vitamin C supplements should be done gradually because accommodation appears to occur, raising a concern of "rebound scurvy." [2 g]	Plasma ascorbic acid concentration reflects recent dietary intake, whereas WBC levels more closely reflect tissue stores. Women's plasma levels are approximately 20% higher than men's for any given dietary intake.

TABLE 225-2   VITAMINS AND THEIR FUNCTIONS—cont'd

	BIOCHEMISTRY AND PHYSIOLOGY	DEFICIENCY [RDA*]	TOXICITY [TUL†]	ASSESSMENT OF STATUS
Vitamin B_{12}	A group of closely related cobalamin compounds composed of a corrin ring (with a cobalt atom in its center) connected to a ribonucleotide through an aminopropanol bridge. Microorganisms are the ultimate source of all naturally occurring B_{12}. The two active coenzyme forms are deoxyadenosylcobalamin and methylcobalamin. These coenzymes are needed for the synthesis of succinyl coenzyme A (CoA), which is essential in lipid and carbohydrate metabolism, and for the synthesis of methionine. The latter reaction is essential for amino acid metabolism, for purine and pyrimidine synthesis, for many methylation reactions, and for the intracellular retention of folates.	Dietary inadequacy is a rare cause of deficiency except in strict vegetarians. Most deficiencies arise from loss of intestinal absorption, which may occur with pernicious anemia, pancreatic insufficiency, atrophic gastritis, small bowel bacterial overgrowth, or ileal disease. Megaloblastic anemia and megaloblastic changes in other epithelia (see "Folate") are the result of sustained depletion. Demyelination of peripheral nerves, posterior and lateral columns of spinal cord, and nerves within the brain may occur. Altered mentation, depression, and psychoses occur. Hematologic and neurologic complications may occur independently. Folate supplementation, in doses of 1000 μg/day, may partly correct the anemia, thereby masking (or perhaps exacerbating) the neuropathic complication. [2.4 μg]	A few allergic reactions have been reported to crystalline B_{12} preparations and are probably due to impurities, not the vitamin. [TUL not established]	Serum, or plasma, concentrations are generally accurate. Subtle deficiency with neurologic complications, as described in the "Deficiency" column, can best be established by concurrently measuring the concentration of plasma B_{12} and serum methylmalonic acid because the latter is a sensitive indicator of cellular deficiency.
Biotin	A bi-cyclic compound consisting of a ureido ring fused to a substituted tetrahydrothiophene ring. Endogenous synthesis by intestinal flora may contribute significantly to biotin nutriture. Most dietary biotin is linked to lysine, a compound called biotinyl lysine, or biocytin. The lysine must be hydrolyzed by an intestinal enzyme called biotinidase before intestinal absorption occurs. Acts primarily as a coenzyme for several carboxylases; each holoenzyme catalyzes an ATP-dependent CO_2 transfer. The carboxylases are critical enzymes in carbohydrate and lipid metabolism.	Isolated deficiency is rare. Deficiency in humans has been produced by prolonged total parenteral nutrition lacking the vitamin and by ingestion of large quantities of raw egg white, which contains avidin, a protein that binds biotin with such high affinity that it renders it biounavailable. Alterations in mental status, myalgias, hyperesthesias, and anorexia occur. Later, a seborrheic dermatitis and alopecia develop. Deficiency is usually accompanied by lactic acidosis and organic aciduria. [30 μg]	Toxicity has not been reported in humans with doses as high as 60 mg/day in children. [TUL not established]	Plasma and urine concentrations of biotin are diminished in the deficient state. Elevated urine concentrations of methyl citrate, 3-methylcrotonylglycine, and 3-hydroxyisovalerate are also observed in deficiency.
Pantothenic acid	Consists of pantoic acid linked to β-alanine through an amide bond. An essential component of CoA and phosphopantetheine, which are essential for synthesis and β-oxidation of fatty acids, as well as synthesis of cholesterol, steroid hormones, vitamins A and D, and other isoprenoid derivatives. CoA is also involved in the synthesis of several amino acids and δ-aminolevulinic acid, a precursor for the corrin ring of vitamin B_{12}, the porphyrin ring of heme, and of cytochromes. CoA is also necessary for the acetylation and fatty acid acylation of a variety of proteins.	Deficiency rare: only reported as a result of feeding semisynthetic diets or an antagonist to the vitamin. Experimental, isolated deficiency in humans produces fatigue, abdominal pain, vomiting, insomnia, and paresthesias of the extremities. [5 mg]	In doses of 10 g/day, diarrhea is reported to occur. [TUL not established]	Whole blood and urine concentrations of pantothenate are indicators of status; serum levels are not thought to be accurate.

*Recommended daily allowance (RDA) established for female (F) and male (M) adults by the U.S. Food and Nutrition Board, 1999-2001. In some instances, insufficient data exist to establish an RDA, in which case the adequate intake (AI) established by the board is listed.
†Tolerated upper intake (TUL) established for adults by the U.S. Food and Nutrition Board, 1999-2001.
PTH = parathyroid hormone; UVB = ultraviolet B.

TABLE 225-3 NUTRITIONAL TRACE ELEMENTS AND THEIR CLINICAL IMPLICATIONS

	BIOCHEMISTRY AND PHYSIOLOGY	DEFICIENCY [RDA*]	TOXICITY [TUL†]	ASSESSMENT OF STATUS
Chromium	Dietary chromium consists of both inorganic and organic forms. Its primary function in humans is to potentiate insulin action. It accomplishes this function as a circulating complex called *glucose tolerance factor*, thereby affecting carbohydrate, fat, and protein metabolism.	Deficiency in humans only described in long-term total parenteral nutrition (TPN) patients receiving insufficient chromium. Hyperglycemia or impaired glucose tolerance occurs. Elevated plasma free fatty acid concentrations, neuropathy, encephalopathy, and abnormalities in nitrogen metabolism are also reported. Whether supplemental chromium may improve glucose tolerance in glucose-intolerant individuals remains controversial. [F: 25 μg; M: 35 μg]	Toxicity after oral ingestion is uncommon and seems confined to gastric irritation. Airborne exposure may cause contact dermatitis, eczema, skin ulcers, and bronchogenic carcinoma. [no TUL established]	Plasma or serum concentration of chromium is a crude indicator of chromium status; it appears to be meaningful when the value is markedly above or below the normal range.
Copper	Copper is absorbed by a specific intestinal transport mechanism. It is carried to the liver where it is bound to ceruloplasmin, which circulates systemically and delivers copper to target tissues in the body. Excretion of copper is largely through bile, and then into the feces. Absorptive and excretory processes vary with the levels of dietary copper, providing a means of copper homeostasis. Copper serves as a component of many enzymes, including amine oxidases, ferroxidases, cytochrome c oxidase, dopamine β-hydroxylase, superoxide dismutase, and tyrosinase.	Dietary deficiency is rare; it has been observed in premature and low-birthweight infants fed exclusively a cow's milk diet and in individuals on long-term TPN without copper. Clinical manifestations include depigmentation of skin and hair, neurologic disturbances, leukopenia, hypochromic microcytic anemia, and skeletal abnormalities. Anemia arises from impaired utilization of iron and is therefore a conditioned form of iron deficiency anemia. The deficiency syndrome, except the anemia and leukopenia, is also observed in Menkes' disease, a rare inherited condition associated with impaired copper utilization. [900 μg]	Acute copper toxicity has been described after excessive oral intake and with absorption of copper salts applied to burned skin. Milder manifestations include nausea, vomiting, epigastric pain, and diarrhea; coma and hepatic necrosis may ensue in severe cases. Toxicity may be seen with doses as low as 70 μg/kg/day. Chronic toxicity is also described. Wilson's disease is a rare, inherited disease associated with abnormally low ceruloplasmin levels and accumulation of copper in the liver and brain, eventually leading to damage to these two organs. [10 mg]	Practical methods for detecting marginal deficiency are not available. Marked deficiency is reliably detected by diminished serum copper and ceruloplasmin concentrations as well as low red blood cell (RBC) superoxide dismutase activity.
Fluorine	Known more commonly by its ionic form, fluoride. It is incorporated into the crystalline structure of bone, thereby altering its physical characteristics.	Intake of <0.1 mg/day in infants and <0.5 mg/day in children is associated with an increased incidence of dental caries. Optimal intake in adults is between 1.5 and 4 mg/day. [F: 3 mg; M: 4 mg]	Acute ingestion of >30 mg/kg body weight is likely to cause death. Excessive chronic intake (0.1 mg/kg/day) leads to mottling of teeth (dental fluorosis), calcification of tendons and ligaments, and exostoses and may increase the brittleness of bones. [10 mg]	Estimates of intake or clinical assessment are used because no good laboratory test exists.
Iodine	Readily absorbed from the diet, concentrated in the thyroid, and integrated into the thyroid hormones, thyroxine (T₄) and triiodothyronine (T₃). These hormones circulate largely bound to thyroxine-binding globulin. They modulate resting energy expenditure and, in the developing human, growth and development.	In the absence of supplementation, populations relying primarily on food from soils with low iodine content have endemic iodine deficiency. Maternal iodine deficiency leads to fetal deficiency, which produces spontaneous abortions, stillbirths, hypothyroidism, cretinism, and dwarfism. Permanent cognitive deficits may result from iodine deficiency during first 2 years of life. In the adult, compensatory hypertrophy of the thyroid goiter occurs along with varying degrees of hypothyroidism. [150 μg]	Large doses (>2 mg/day in adults) may induce hypothyroidism by blocking thyroid hormone synthesis. Supplementation with >100 mg/day to an individual who was formerly deficient occasionally induces hyperthyroidism. [1.1 mg]	Iodine status of a population can be estimated by the prevalence of goiter. Urinary excretion of iodine is an effective laboratory means of assessment. Thyroid-stimulating hormone (TSH) blood level is an indirect, and therefore not entirely specific, means of assessment.
Iron	Conveys the capacity to participate in redox reactions to a number of metalloproteins such as hemoglobin, myoglobin, cytochrome enzymes, and many oxidases and oxygenases. Primary storage form is ferritin and, to a lesser degree, hemosiderin. Intestinal absorption is 15-20% for "heme" iron and 1-8% for iron contained in vegetables. Absorption of the latter form is enhanced by the ascorbic acid in foodstuffs; by poultry, fish, or beef; and by an iron-deficient state. It is decreased by phytate and tannins.	The most common micronutrient deficiency in the world. Women of childbearing age are the highest-risk group because of menstrual blood losses, pregnancy, and lactation. The classic deficiency syndrome is hypochromic, microcytic anemia. Glossitis and koilonychia ("spoon" nails) are also observed. Easy fatigability often is an early symptom, before anemia appears. In children, mild deficiency of insufficient severity to cause anemia is associated with behavioral disturbances and poor school performance. [postmenopausal F and M: 8 mg; premenopausal F: 18 mg]	Iron overload typically occurs when habitual dietary intake is extremely high, intestinal absorption is excessive, repeated parenteral administration occurs, or a combination of these factors exists. Excessive iron stores usually accumulate in the reticuloendothelial tissues and cause little damage ("hemosiderosis"). If overload continues, iron eventually begins to accumulate in tissues such as the hepatic parenchyma, pancreas, heart, and synovium, causing hemochromatosis (Chapter 219). Hereditary hemochromatosis results from homozygosity of a common recessive trait. Excessive intestinal absorption of iron is seen in homozygotes. [45 mg]	Negative iron balance initially leads to depletion of iron stores in the bone marrow: a bone marrow biopsy and the concentration of serum ferritin are accurate indicators of early depletion. As the severity of deficiency proceeds, serum iron (SI) decreases and total iron-binding capacity (TIBC) increases: an iron saturation (SI/TIBC) of <16% suggests iron deficiency. Microcytosis, hypochromia, and anemia ensue. Elevated levels of serum ferritin or an iron saturation of >60% suggest iron overload, although systemic inflammation elevates serum ferritin regardless of iron status.

TABLE 225-3 NUTRITIONAL TRACE ELEMENTS AND THEIR CLINICAL IMPLICATIONS—cont'd

	BIOCHEMISTRY AND PHYSIOLOGY	DEFICIENCY [RDA*]	TOXICITY [TUL†]	ASSESSMENT OF STATUS
Manganese	A component of several metalloenzymes. Most manganese is in mitochondria, where it is a component of manganese superoxide dismutase.	Manganese deficiency in the human has not been conclusively demonstrated. It is said to cause hypocholesterolemia, weight loss, hair and nail changes, dermatitis, and impaired synthesis of vitamin K–dependent proteins. [F: 1.8 mg; M: 2.3 mg]	Toxicity by oral ingestion is unknown in humans. Toxic inhalation causes hallucinations, other alterations in mentation, and extrapyramidal movement disorders. [11 mg]	Until the deficiency syndrome is better defined, an appropriate measure of status will be difficult to develop.
Molybdenum	A cofactor in several enzymes, most prominently xanthine oxidase and sulfite oxidase.	A probable case of human deficiency is described as being secondary to parenteral administration of sulfite and resulted in hyperoxypurinemia, hypouricemia, and low sulfate excretion. [45 µg]	Toxicity not well described in humans, although it may interfere with copper metabolism at high doses. [2 mg]	Laboratory means of assessment not meaningful until deficiency syndrome is better described.
Selenium	Most dietary selenium is in the form of an amino acid complex. Nearly complete absorption of such forms occurs. Homeostasis is largely performed by the kidney, which regulates urinary excretion as a function of selenium status. Selenium is a component of several enzymes, most notably glutathione peroxidase and superoxide dismutase. These enzymes protect against oxidative and free radical damage of various cell structures. The antioxidant protection conveyed by selenium apparently operates in conjunction with vitamin E because deficiency of one seems to potentiate damage induced by a deficiency of the other. Selenium also participates in the enzymatic conversion of thyroxine to its more active metabolite, triiodothyronine.	Deficiency is rare in North America but has been observed in individuals on long-term TPN lacking selenium. Such individuals have myalgias and/or cardiomyopathies. Populations in some regions of the world, most notably some parts of China, have marginal intake of selenium. In these regions *Keshan's disease*, a condition characterized by cardiomyopathy, is endemic; it can be prevented (but not treated) by selenium supplementation. [55 µg]	Toxicity is associated with nausea, diarrhea, alterations in mental status, peripheral neuropathy, loss of hair and nails: such symptoms were observed in adults who inadvertently consumed 27-2400 mg. [400 µg]	Erythrocyte glutathione peroxidase activity and plasma, or whole blood, selenium concentrations are the most commonly used methods of assessment. They are moderately accurate indicators of status.
Zinc	Intestinal absorption occurs by a specific process that is enhanced by pregnancy and corticosteroids and diminished by coingestion of phytates, phosphates, iron, copper, lead, or calcium. Diminished intake of zinc leads to an increased efficiency of absorption and decreased fecal excretion, providing a means of zinc homeostasis. Zinc is a component of more than 100 enzymes, among which are DNA polymerase, RNA polymerase, and transfer RNA synthetase.	Zinc deficiency has its most profound effect on rapidly proliferating tissues. *Mild deficiency:* growth retardation in children. *More severe deficiency:* growth arrest, teratogenicity, hypogonadism and infertility, dysgeusia, poor wound healing, diarrhea, dermatitis on the extremities and around orifices, glossitis, alopecia, corneal clouding, loss of dark adaptation, and behavioral changes. Impaired cellular immunity is observed. Excessive loss of gastrointestinal secretions through chronic diarrhea and fistulas may precipitate deficiency. *Acrodermatitis enteropathica* is a rare, recessively inherited disease in which intestinal absorption of zinc is impaired. [F: 8 mg; M: 11 mg]	Acute zinc toxicity can usually be induced by ingestion of >200 mg of zinc in a single day (in adults). It is manifested by epigastric pain, nausea, vomiting, and diarrhea. Hyperpnea, diaphoresis, and weakness may follow inhalation of zinc fumes. Copper and zinc compete for intestinal absorption: long-term ingestion of >25 mg/day of zinc may lead to copper deficiency. Long-term ingestion of >150 mg/day has been reported to cause gastric erosions, low high-density lipoprotein cholesterol levels, and impaired cellular immunity. [40 mg]	No accurate indicators of zinc status exist for routine clinical use. Plasma, RBC, and hair zinc concentrations are often misleading. Acute illness, in particular, is known to diminish plasma zinc levels, in part by inducing a shift of zinc out of the plasma compartment and into the liver. Functional tests that determine dark adaptation, taste acuity, and rate of wound healing lack specificity.

*Recommended daily allowance (RDA) established for female (F) and male (M) adults by the U.S. Food and Nutrition Board, 1999-2001. In some instances, insufficient data exist to establish an RDA, in which case the adequate intake (AI) established by the board is listed.

†Tolerated upper limit (TUL) established for adults by the U.S. Food and Nutrition Board, 1999-2001.

Infancy

Infancy carries particular vulnerabilities to specific micronutrient inadequacies. Healthy infants in the United States are typically supplemented with vitamin K at birth and with iron and vitamin D during the course of the first year because of their particular susceptibility to deficiencies of these nutrients.

Women of Childbearing Age

The ability to maintain adequate iron status from menarche through menopause is compromised in women by the additional losses incurred by menstruation, pregnancy, and lactation. Therefore, it is not surprising that the population subset that almost invariably displays the highest rate of iron deficiency is women of childbearing age.

Elderly Persons

Specific dietary recommendations for elderly people have been formally incorporated into the RDAs because aging has an impact on the need for certain micronutrients. Vitamin B_{12} status declines significantly with aging, in large part because of the high prevalence of atrophic gastritis and its associated impairment in protein-bound vitamin B_{12} absorption. Estimates suggest that 10 to 20% of the elderly population is at risk for clinically significant vitamin B_{12} deficiency. Consequently, elderly persons should consume some of their vitamin B_{12} requirement in the crystalline form rather than solely from the naturally occurring protein-bound forms found in food because absorption of the former is not impaired by atrophic gastritis. Elderly people also require greater quantities of vitamins B_6 and D to maintain health compared with younger adults, as reflected in the new RDAs (see Table 225-3). For instance, the RDA of vitamin D in persons over the age of 70 is now set at 20 μg/day (800 international units), as opposed to adults who are 70 or younger, whose RDA is 15 μg/day. This increase appears to result from diminished cutaneous synthesis of vitamin D by senile skin and from decreased sun exposure, which is particularly important in elderly patients in institutional facilities. The need for crystalline vitamin B_{12} and for a quantity of vitamin D that is difficult to achieve without resorting to a supplement suggests that universal use of a daily supplement pill containing these nutrients would benefit elderly people. Widespread use among elders of a multivitamin that contains a wide spectrum of micronutrients is more controversial, in part because of concerns regarding subtle toxicity. For example, elders with chronic renal failure appear to have a vulnerability to vitamin A toxicity, suggesting that use of supplements containing this vitamin is contraindicated.

● PATHOPHYSIOLOGIC AND PHARMACOLOGIC FACTORS

Diseases of the Gastrointestinal Tract

Intestinal malabsorptive and maldigestive states predispose to multiple micronutrient deficiencies. Both fat-soluble and water-soluble micronutrients (except vitamin B_{12}) are absorbed predominantly in the proximal small intestine. Therefore, diffuse mucosal diseases affecting the proximal portion of the gastrointestinal tract are likely to result in deficiencies. Even in the absence of mucosal disease of the proximal small intestine, extensive ileal disease, small bowel bacterial overgrowth, and chronic cholestasis can each interfere with the maintenance of adequate intraluminal conjugated bile acid concentrations and can thereby impair absorption of fat-soluble vitamins. Maldigestion is usually the result of chronic pancreatitis. Untreated, it frequently causes malabsorption and deficiencies of fat-soluble vitamins. Vitamin B_{12} malabsorption can often be demonstrated in this setting, a result of inadequate R-protein digestion, but clinical vitamin B_{12} deficiency is rarely reported.

Inborn Errors of Metabolism

Myriad rare inborn errors of metabolism have been described for vitamins and minerals that impair an individual's ability to assimilate, utilize, or retain a particular micronutrient (Chapter 212). Such defects are usually partial and can often be overcome, to a certain extent, by administering doses of the nutrient that are several degrees of magnitude greater than usually required. Suspicion for such defects should be entertained if (1) a known defect exists in the family, (2) a deficiency syndrome arises at birth or during infancy, or (3) the deficiency syndrome is present despite adequate dietary intake and the absence of any disease that would impair the ability to assimilate the nutrient.

TABLE 225-4	DRUG-MEDIATED EFFECTS ON MICRONUTRIENT STATUS: EXAMPLES	
DRUG	**NUTRIENT**	**MECHANISM OF INTERACTION**
Dextroamphetamine, fenfluramine, levodopa	Potentially all micronutrients	Induces anorexia
Cholestyramine	Vitamin D, folate	Adsorbs nutrient, decreases absorption
Omeprazole	Vitamin B_{12}	Modest bacterial overgrowth, decreases gastric acid, impairs absorption
Sulfasalazine	Folate	Impairs absorption and inhibits folate-dependent enzymes
Isoniazid	Pyridoxine	Impairs utilization of B_6
Nonsteroidal anti-inflammatory drugs	Iron	Gastrointestinal blood loss
Penicillamine	Zinc	Increases renal excretion

Medications

Long-term administration of many drugs may adversely affect micronutrient status. The manner in which drug-nutrient interactions occur varies; some of the more common mechanisms are outlined in Table 225-4. Some drugs exert their therapeutic effects by specifically inhibiting the actions of a micronutrient. Examples include coumarin, which inhibits γ-carboxylation reactions mediated by vitamin K, and methotrexate, which binds tightly to dihydrofolate reductase, thereby inhibiting folate metabolism.

Toxins

Tobacco smoking alters the metabolism of several vitamins, including folate and vitamins C and E. In large surveys, diminished plasma levels of folate and ascorbic acid have been observed in chronic smokers. Smoking is also associated with diminished levels of folate in cells of the oral mucosa, diminished ascorbic acid levels in leukocytes, and decreased concentrations of vitamin E in the alveolar fluid, findings providing evidence that many tissues can be affected by smoking and that the effect does not simply represent a shift of these micronutrients out of the plasma compartment.

● ADVANCES IN NUTRITIONAL SCIENCE

New Frontiers in Marginal Deficiency States of Micronutrients

Does Optimal Intake of Micronutrients Optimize Health?

Updating the definition of a micronutrient deficiency and establishing recommended daily intakes that are consistent with the most recent evidence has proved difficult for several reasons. In some instances, a novel biochemical or physiologic role for a nutrient has been identified, but an appropriate question that arises is whether optimization of such functions translates into optimization of health. For example, providing supplemental vitamin E to elderly individuals who are vitamin E replete enhances T-lymphocyte responsiveness; nevertheless, it is unclear whether this translates into diminished infection rates. Another difficult problem pertains to the use of micronutrients in supraphysiologic quantities that exceed all conventional concepts of what is necessary for health. Some micronutrients, when taken in such large quantities, have effects on physiologic functions that impart apparent health benefits. The ingestion of gram quantities of niacin to reduce low-density lipoprotein (LDL) cholesterol is an example. Such physiologic effects are not observed at more conventional levels of intake and are therefore usually considered pharmacologic effects of the nutrient. Thus, the determination of optimal nutrient intake is highly dependent on which physiologic effect is sought. Furthermore, if only a segment of the population will benefit from supraphysiologic quantities of a nutrient, should dietary guidelines for the remainder of the population be established according to this effect?

Determining an adequate level of intake implies the existence of a means of measuring nutrient status. In seeking an appropriate measure of nutrient status, the diversity of function often makes it difficult to decide which measurement is the most germane. Tobacco smoking, for example, diminishes vitamin E levels in alveolar fluid but not in the serum. Thus, the concepts of localized nutrient deficiencies and tissue-specific requirements add an additional level of complexity to the determination of nutrient status.

Redefinition of Nutritional Requirements

Folate

An example of the complexities that have arisen in redefining the criteria for vitamin deficiencies and vitamin requirements is the water-soluble vitamin, folate. In the past, guidelines regarding its necessary intake were straightforward because they were based solely on the prevention of megaloblastic anemia. Measuring serum and erythrocyte folate concentrations were the most common means of assessing status, and maintaining these levels within accepted normative ranges provided assurance that folate status was adequate to prevent anemia. However, degrees of deficiency that are insufficient to cause anemia may still disturb normal biochemical and physiologic homeostasis and, in some instances, cause clinical disease. Clinical trials have demonstrated that women taking folic acid supplements at the time of conception have a markedly lower chance of delivering a baby with an NTD compared with women who are not folate supplemented but whose folate status falls within a conventionally accepted range. This observation compelled the U.S. government to mandate the fortification of flour, beginning in 1998. Present recommendations are that women of childbearing age consume 400 µg/day of folic acid in the form of supplements or fortified foods, although the dose-response curve of this effect is ill defined.

Less than optimal intake of folate is also evidenced by an increase in serum homocysteine, an amino acid that is normally metabolized by a folate-dependent pathway. Before the federally mandated fortification of flour, the median intake of folate among adults was one half of the present RDA, and a substantial minority of Americans had significantly elevated serum homocysteine levels. Elevated homocysteine has been associated with the development of occlusive vascular disease and accelerated cognitive decline. In randomized clinical trials, however, supplementation with folate, vitamin B_{12}, and vitamin B_6 has shown no benefit against cardiovascular disease despite its ability to lower homocysteine levels.[1] Such supplementation also has no clear benefit for cognitive function, except perhaps in patients with low baseline folate levels.[2]

A compelling body of observations in both humans and animals has demonstrated that habitually low consumption of folate is also associated with a substantial increase in the risk for colorectal cancer, and perhaps cancers of other organs such as those of the breast and pancreas. This inverse relationship is observed even when folate status (or dietary intake) falls within the range of conventionally accepted normative values. This relationship has further complicated the determination of what constitutes an optimal intake of folate. The issue is further confounded by newer observations suggesting that an exceptionally high intake of folate among those who unknowingly harbor precancerous or cancerous lesions may paradoxically enhance the progression of these neoplasms, thereby underscoring the potential for harm produced by taking a nutrient outside of its physiologic window.

The most recent update of the U.S. RDA for folate, which occurred in 1998, raised the value from 200 to 400 µg/day, citing both the prevention of anemia and optimization of serum homocysteine as criteria, and recommended that women capable of becoming pregnant consume an additional 400 µg/day in the form of supplements or fortified food. The issues surrounding the prevention of cardiovascular disease, cancer, and cognitive decline were not incorporated into the 1998 determination because the existing data at the time were thought to be inconclusive. However, it may prove appropriate to integrate some of the knowledge surrounding these issues in future revisions of the RDAs. The potential for toxicity, the criterion for which was primarily linked to its ability to mask vitamin B_{12} deficiency, was dealt with by setting the TUL at 1000 µg/day of folic acid obtained from supplements and fortified foods in addition to that obtained from natural food sources (see Table 225-2).

The electronic version of this chapter describes two other instances that exemplify how our expanding understanding of the biologic effects of micronutrients has complicated the process of determining guidelines for optimal intake.[3-5]

Table 225-5 lists several examples of biochemical functions of vitamins that have only recently been identified. As the clinical significance of each of these new roles is defined and as quantities of each vitamin needed to optimize such functions are determined, redefinition of the desirable range of vitamin status is likely to occur. Future efforts to refine appropriate dietary goals further for each micronutrient will, however, need to take into consideration an important theme that is underscored by the previous discussion: that the level of consumption of a particular micronutrient that conveys health benefits to one segment of the population is not necessarily beneficial, or even appropriate, for all segments of society.

TABLE 225-5	NEWLY IDENTIFIED ROLES FOR VITAMINS	
VITAMIN OR PROVITAMIN	**CLASSIC ROLE**	**NEW ROLE**
β-Carotene	Pro-vitamin A	Antioxidant, free radical
Niacin	NAD/NADP coenzyme	Reduction of LDL, elevation of HDL and cholesterol
Folate	Hemopoietic factor	Diminishes homocysteinemia
Vitamin A	Transduction of visual input in retina	Induction and maintenance of epithelial differentiation, signal in embryogenesis
Vitamin D	Regulator of calcium	Retards epithelial proliferation; promotes differentiation
Vitamin B_6	Coenzyme for transamination	Modulation of steroid activity

HDL = high-density lipoprotein; LDL = low-density lipoprotein; NAD = nicotinamide adenine dinucleotide; NADP = nicotinamide-adenine dinucleotide phosphate.

⊗ Visit expertconsult.com for e-expanded chapter

Grade A

1. SEARCH Collaborative Group. Effects of homocysteine-lowering with folic acid plus vitamin B_{12} vs placebo on mortality and major morbidity in myocardial infarction survivors: a randomized trial. *JAMA.* 2010;303:2486-2494.
2. Balk EM, Raman G, Tatsioni A, et al. Vitamin B_6, B_{12}, and folic acid supplementation and cognitive function: a systematic review of randomized trials. *Arch Intern Med.* 2007;167:21-30.
3. Bjelakovic G, Nikolova D, Gluud LL, et al. Mortality in randomized trials of antioxidant supplements for primary and secondary prevention: systematic review and meta-analysis. *JAMA.* 2007;297:842-857.
4. Sanyal AJ, Chalasani N, Kowdley KV, et al, for the NASH CRN. Pioglitazone, vitamin E, or placebo for nonalcoholic steatohepatitis. *N Engl J Med.* 2010;362:1675-1685.
5. Age-Related Eye Disease Study Research Group. A randomized, placebo-controlled, clinical trial of high-dose supplementation with vitamins C and E, beta carotene and zinc for age-related macular degeneration and vision loss: AREDS report no. 8 [erratum in *Arch Ophthalmol.* 2008;126:1251]. *Arch Ophthalmol.* 2001;119:1417-1436.

SUGGESTED READINGS

Larsson SC, Orsini N, Wolk A. Vitamin B_6 and risk of colorectal cancer: a meta-analysis of prospective studies. *JAMA.* 2010;303:1077-1083. *Systemic review with meta-analysis concluding that vitamin B_6 intake and blood levels of the active form of vitamin B_6 are inversely associated with the risk for colorectal cancer.*

Ross AC, Manson JE, Abrams SA, et al. The 2011 report on dietary reference intakes for calcium and vitamin D from the Institute of Medicine: what clinicians need to know. *J Clin Endocrinol Metab.* 2011;96:53-58. *Review concluding that the prevalence of vitamin D inadequacy in North America has been overestimated.*

Swanson AM, Hughey LC. Acute inpatient presentation of scurvy. *Cutis.* 2010;86:205-207. *An unusual case report.*

226

EATING DISORDERS

MARSHA D. MARCUS AND JENNIFER E. WILDES

DEFINITION

The eating disorders are psychiatric syndromes characterized by abnormal eating behaviors and maladaptive thoughts or beliefs about eating, shape, or weight. The American Psychiatric Association's *Diagnostic and Statistical Manual of Mental Disorders* (DSM-IV-TR) describes two primary eating disorders, anorexia nervosa (AN) and bulimia nervosa (BN). A third disorder, binge-eating disorder (BED), also is included as a diagnosis requiring further study. All other presentations of clinically significant eating problems are represented by the residual diagnosis, eating disorder not otherwise specified (EDNOS).

⬤ ANOREXIA NERVOSA

The hallmark features of AN are persistent unwillingness or inability to maintain a minimally adequate body weight, which is defined in DSM-IV-TR as less than 85% of that expected, coupled with an intense fear of gaining weight

TABLE 226-1	DSM-IV-TR* DIAGNOSTIC CRITERIA FOR ANOREXIA NERVOSA

A. Refusal to maintain body weight at or above a minimally normal weight for age and height (e.g., weight loss leading to maintenance of body weight less than 85% of that expected; or failure to make expected weight gain during period of growth, leading to body weight less than 85% of that expected).

B. Intense fear of gaining weight or becoming fat, even though underweight.

C. Disturbance in the way in which one's body weight or shape is experienced, undue influence of body weight or shape on self-evaluation, or denial of the seriousness of the current low body weight.

D. In postmenarchal females, amenorrhea, that is, the absence of at least three consecutive menstrual cycles (a woman is considered to have amenorrhea if her periods occur following only hormone, e.g., estrogen, administration).

Specify type:

Restricting type: During the current episode of anorexia nervosa, the person has not regularly engaged in binge eating or purging behavior (i.e., self-induced vomiting or the misuse of laxatives, diuretics, or enemas).

Binge-eating/purging type: During the current episode of anorexia nervosa, the person has regularly engaged in binge eating or purging behavior (i.e., self-induced vomiting or the misuse of laxatives, diuretics, or enemas).

*Diagnostic and Statistical Manual of Mental Disorders. 4th ed., text revision. Copyright 2000 American Psychiatric Association.

TABLE 226-2	DSM-IV-TR* DIAGNOSTIC CRITERIA FOR BULIMIA NERVOSA

A. Recurrent episodes of binge eating. An episode of binge eating is characterized by both of the following:

  1. Eating, in a discrete period of time (e.g., within any 2-hour period), an amount of food that is definitely larger than most people would eat during a similar period of time and under similar circumstances.

  2. A sense of lack of control over eating during the episodes (e.g., a feeling that one cannot stop eating or control what or how much one is eating).

B. Recurrent inappropriate compensatory behavior in order to prevent weight gain, such as self-induced vomiting; misuse of laxatives, diuretics, enemas, or other medications; fasting; or excessive exercise.

C. The binge eating and inappropriate compensatory behaviors both occur, on average, at least twice a week for 3 months.

D. Self-evaluation is unduly influenced by body shape and weight.

E. The disturbance does not occur exclusively during episodes of anorexia nervosa.

Specify type:

Purging type: During the current episode of bulimia nervosa, the person has regularly engaged in self-induced vomiting or the misuse of laxatives, diuretics, or enemas.

Nonpurging type: During the current episode of bulimia nervosa, the person has used other inappropriate compensatory behaviors, such as fasting or excessive exercise, but has not regularly engaged in self-induced vomiting or the misuse of laxatives, diuretics, or enemas.

*Diagnostic and Statistical Manual of Mental Disorders. 4th ed., text revision. Copyright 2000 American Psychiatric Association.

or becoming fat. There is no clear definition for the 85% weight cutoff in AN. In the United States, this criterion often is applied with respect to the Metropolitan Life Insurance Tables, while guidelines specified by the International Classification of Diseases (ICD-10) suggest a body mass index (BMI) of less than or equal to 17.5 as a threshold for AN diagnosis. AN has two subtypes, binge-eating/purging and restricting. DSM-IV-TR criteria for AN are presented in Table 226-1.

● BULIMIA NERVOSA

BN is characterized by recurrent episodes of binge eating (i.e., the intake of an exceptionally large amount of food given the context accompanied by a sense of loss of control over eating) that are coupled with compensatory behaviors (e.g., self-induced vomiting, fasting) intended to undo the effects of binge episodes. BN also has two subtypes, purging and nonpurging. Diagnostic criteria are detailed in Table 226-2.

● BINGE-EATING DISORDER

BED is characterized by recurrent binge eating in the absence of regular, inappropriate compensatory behaviors. Although classified in DSM-IV-TR as an example of EDNOS, BED is likely to be included as an official diagnosis in the next version of the DSM because there now is substantial evidence documenting the disorder's conceptual validity and clinical utility.

● EATING DISORDER NOT OTHERWISE SPECIFIED

A complete discussion of the residual category of eating disorders, EDNOS, is beyond the scope of this chapter. However, it is important to note that EDNOS is the most common diagnosis at many eating disorders programs, reflecting considerable fluidity in the presentation of disordered eating over time and the limitations of current diagnostic criteria. For example, there is little evidence to support the frequency criteria for binge eating or purging in the diagnosis of BN or the utility of the amenorrhea criterion for a diagnosis of AN. Consequently, many cases of EDNOS are subsyndromal variants of AN or BN, but there also are other patterns of disordered eating. For example, purging disorder, or recurrent purging behaviors in the absence of binge eating, has been described.

EPIDEMIOLOGY

Epidemiologic data on the incidence and prevalence of eating disorders are limited. Available evidence indicates that AN is relatively uncommon, with lifetime prevalence estimates ranging from 0.3% to 2.2% in women. Lifetime prevalence estimates for BN range from 1% to 4.6%, whereas estimates for BED range from 0.6 to 3.5% in community samples and are higher among overweight individuals, especially those seeking weight-loss treatment.

AN and BN are more common among women than men, with ratios of approximately 10:1. In contrast, differences between the sexes in rates of BED are less pronounced, with the female to male ratio estimated at 3:1. Available data suggest that AN and BN are equally common in white, Hispanic, and Native American women and less common in African American

and Asian women. However, BED appears to occur with equal frequency in white, African American, and Hispanic women.

PATHOBIOLOGY

The etiology of eating disorders is complex, likely involving the interaction of genetic, constitutional, psychological, family, and sociocultural factors. Family history and twin studies provide strong support for the role of genetics in the pathogenesis of disordered eating. The results are particularly compelling in the case of restricting AN. However, evidence also suggests that BN and binge eating run in families and that much of the variance in observed cases is explained by genetic factors. Genetic linkage and association studies have implicated several susceptibility loci for AN and BN. Research also has suggested a relation between neonatal complications and subsequent onset of AN that may be mediated by maternal genetic variables.

Multiple psychological traits, including neuroticism and perfectionism, have been identified as putative risk factors for disordered eating. Familial overweight or obesity and parental concerns about eating, shape, and weight also have been implicated as potential contributors to the vulnerability for disordered eating. Finally, in industrialized nations, a sociocultural emphasis on shape and weight and a marked preference for a thin body type have been implicated in the complex pathogenesis of eating disorders. Thus, a given case of eating disorder likely reflects some combination of risk or vulnerability factors whose expression may be promoted by a cultural milieu in which thinness is overvalued.

CLINICAL MANIFESTATIONS

Symptoms and Signs

Patients with eating disorders often present with depression, anxiety, and social withdrawal, as well as the specific symptoms of disordered eating. In AN, psychiatric symptoms such as irritability, obsessionality, and preoccupation with food may be secondary to semistarvation and may remit with refeeding. Physical symptoms of semistarvation or malnutrition affect virtually all systems and may include osteopenia or osteoporosis, dehydration, hypothermia, cardiovascular or renal irregularities, gastrointestinal and endocrine disturbances, and changes in neuropsychological functioning. Laboratory results may be normal, especially in restricting AN, but patients still may be at risk for cardiac events resulting from malnutrition.

Signs and symptoms of BN are most commonly associated with purging behavior and include dental enamel erosion secondary to vomiting, gastrointestinal symptoms, salivary gland hypertrophy, and electrolyte disturbances. Misuse of stimulant laxatives can cause hypomagnesia or hypophosphatemia and ultimately disrupt normal bowel functioning. Binge eating is associated with gastric distention and, in rare cases, gastric rupture.

Natural History

Age at onset of AN typically is during adolescence, but prepubertal onset does occur. New-onset AN is not common in adult women; these cases often appear to be triggered by life crisis. The onset of BN typically is during later adolescence or early adulthood, whereas onset of BED can occur well into adulthood.

Information about the natural course of eating disorders is limited. The few studies that have examined the course of AN in community samples have documented recovery rates of about 50 to 60% over 5 to 10 years of follow-up, although significant psychiatric morbidity still was present in about half of individuals. With respect to BN, spontaneous recovery rates range from 49 to 91% in community samples, but most individuals continue to report symptoms, and about 40% experience relapse. Finally, data regarding the natural course of BED and EDNOS are mixed, with some studies reporting high rates of spontaneous and sustained recovery and others suggesting that individuals with BED and EDNOS exhibit a course similar to AN and BN.

DIAGNOSIS

As is the case in all psychiatric disorders, eating disorder diagnoses are documented by review of the patient's history, symptoms, and behaviors in the course of a collaborative interview. Evaluation of comorbid psychiatric problems, particularly mood, anxiety, and substance use disorders, is critical. Assessment for the presence of suicidal ideation or behavior also is warranted. Involvement of the family is crucial for all children and adolescents who present for assessment of disordered eating. A complete physical examination is recommended for all patients, with particular attention to body mass index (weight in kilograms divided by height in meters squared), vital signs, cardiovascular function, hematologic assessment, and blood chemistries.

Patients with eating disorders frequently are examined for gastrointestinal problems or amenorrhea; however, these symptoms often remit with successful treatment of the eating disorder. Marked weight loss in young women in the absence of substance dependence, severe depression, or other documented illness suggests the need for an eating disorder evaluation.

TREATMENT   Rx

Anorexia Nervosa

Research evidence to guide the treatment of AN is limited. For emaciated patients, the cornerstone of treatment is medical monitoring and supervised nutrition rehabilitation to restore body weight and normalize eating behavior. Markedly underweight individuals may require a hospital-based program to achieve weight restoration, which usually is accomplished with supervised meals and snacks provided in a supportive environment. When patients refuse to eat, nasogastric feeding may be used; continuous feeding is better tolerated than bolus feeding. "Refeeding syndrome," which is characterized by fluid and electrolyte abnormalities, most notably hypophosphatemia, as well as cardiac, neurologic, and hematologic complications, is a rare but serious adverse effect associated with behavioral management of AN (see Chapter 224 for additional information about refeeding syndrome). To prevent refeeding syndrome in AN, nutrition rehabilitation should be initiated gradually and include close medical monitoring.

With regard to psychotherapy, which is the mainstay of AN treatment when adequate nutrition is restored, several small clinical trials have documented the benefit of family therapy in the treatment of adolescent AN of short duration. The Maudsley model, in which families are helped to play a central role in the management of AN, has shown promise, but replication of the positive results in larger samples is required. The evidence base for psychotherapeutic interventions in adults with AN is meager. Preliminary reports have suggested the utility of cognitive behavior therapy (CBT), but there is no compelling evidence for the efficacy of any form of psychotherapy for adults with AN.

Similarly, there is no strong evidence favoring the use of any particular medication in treating AN. Although some research has suggested the potential utility of selective serotonin reuptake inhibitors in preventing relapse, a well-controlled clinical trial failed to show any benefit of fluoxetine for weight-restored individuals with AN.[1] Several reports have suggested that second-generation antipsychotic agents, particularly olanzapine, may be helpful in the management of AN, but additional research is needed. Hormone treatment and vitamin supplements are not considered useful, although supplemental calcium and vitamin D often are recommended.

Bulimia Nervosa

The evidence base for treatment of BN is stronger than that for AN, but the quality of extant studies is variable. Several forms of psychotherapy have been studied; available evidence provides the best support for CBT, conducted individually or in a group format, as a means of decreasing aberrant eating and reducing the psychological symptoms of BN. Nevertheless, CBT has a significant nonresponse rate, with up to one third of patients failing to benefit.[2] Almost all studied antidepressant agents have a moderate impact on the symptoms of BN, but as is the case with psychotherapy, there is a significant nonresponse rate. Fluoxetine at 60 mg/day is the best studied agent, and there is a U.S. Food and Drug Administration–approved indication for its use at that dose in the treatment of BN. There is no strong evidence in support of medications other than antidepressants in the treatment of BN. In clinical practice, antidepressant medication often is provided in addition to some form of psychotherapy, but there is no compelling support for the benefits of combined treatment.

BED and EDNOS

Numerous trials have examined the use of CBT, interpersonal therapy, behavioral weight management, and medications in the treatment of BED. Available evidence indicates that most overweight patients can be helped with either a behavioral weight control program or an eating disorders treatment, although the results of a recently published randomized controlled trial suggest that psychotherapy is superior to behavioral weight control in the sustained amelioration of binge eating.[3] Pharmacotherapy with antidepressant, anticonvulsant, or anti-obesity agents also may reduce binge eating, but generally does not add to the effectiveness of psychosocial treatment. Cases of EDNOS that reflect subsyndromal variants of AN and BN usually are treated with methods appropriate for management of threshold-level eating disorders.

PREVENTION

Prevention programs for eating disorders typically focus on reducing risk factors for disordered eating and preventing the onset of broadly defined eating pathology. Meta-analytic reviews have identified several characteristics of effective eating disorder prevention programs, including a focus on at-risk individuals, the use of an interactive (versus a didactic) session format, and program content that focuses on reducing eating disorder risk factors as opposed to providing information about the development of eating problems. Numerous trials have documented that a dissonance intervention, in which young women critique the thin ideal endorsed in Western culture, is superior to various control conditions in reducing risk factors for disordered eating and the onset of symptoms. However, little is known about the utility of prevention programs for reducing the incidence of threshold-level eating disorders.

PROGNOSIS

Anorexia Nervosa

Numerous studies have described the outcome of AN in cohorts of treated patients, but the interventions have varied, and many studies have significant methodologic limitations. A meta-analysis of this literature documented that about half of individuals did not meet criteria for AN at follow-up, but most had eating disorder symptoms, and about 20% developed a chronic course of illness. Approximately 50% of patients with AN develop bulimic symptoms over time, but information relating to the temporal onset of binge eating or purging is limited. Studies consistently indicate better outcomes for adolescent patients, but time to recovery nevertheless may be protracted (5 to 6 years). Mortality rates for AN are as high as those for any psychiatric disorder; the primary causes of death are suicide and complications related to chronic starvation.

Bulimia Nervosa

The outcome of BN appears to be better than that for AN, but on average, problematic eating behaviors persist for several years in treated patients. Studies that have followed patient cohorts over time have documented that most individuals with BN achieve full recovery at some point, but rates of relapse are high (i.e., 35%), and approximately one third of patients continue to exhibit some symptoms. There are no consistent predictors of outcome in BN, although depression has been associated with a poorer response to treatment in several studies. Unlike AN, BN does not appear to be associated with an increased risk for premature death.

BED and EDNOS

Few studies have documented long-term outcomes in patients with BED. One report found that 36% of individuals who received inpatient treatment for BED continued to have an eating disorder at 12-year follow-up, which was comparable to the proportion of individuals with BN exhibiting a chronic course of illness (28%). Virtually nothing is known about the prognosis of individuals with EDNOS.

1. Walsh BT, Kaplan AS, Attia E, et al. Fluoxetine after weight restoration in anorexia nervosa: a randomized controlled trial. *JAMA*. 2006;295:2605-2612.
2. Agras WS, Walsh BT, Fairburn CG, et al. A multicenter comparison of cognitive behavioral therapy and interpersonal psychotherapy for bulimia nervosa. *Arch Gen Psychiatry*. 2000;57:459-466.
3. Wilson GT, Wilfley DE, Agras WS, et al. Psychological treatments of binge eating disorder. *Arch Gen Psychiatry*. 2010;67:94-101.

SUGGESTED READINGS

Attia E, Walsh BT. Behavioral management for anorexia nervosa. *N Engl J Med*. 2009;360:500-506. *Provides guidance on the evaluation and treatment of individuals with anorexia nervosa.*

Huas C, Caille A, Godart N, et al. Factors predictive of ten-year mortality in severe anorexia nervosa patients. *Acta Psychiatr Scand*. 2011;123:62-70. *The ten-year mortality rate of 11% was associated with older age, longer duration, history of suicide attempt, diuretic use, intensity of symptoms, and desired body mass index.*

Konstantakopoulos G, Tchanturia K, Surguladze SA, et al. Insight in eating disorders: clinical and cognitive correlates. *Psychol Med*. 2011;7:1-11. *Substantially impaired insight is a significant feature of about 25% of patients.*

Treasure J, Claudino AM, Zucker N. Eating disorders. *Lancet*. 2010;375:583-593. *Provides a comprehensive overview of eating disorder phenomenology, course, and treatment with an emphasis on biological mechanisms and interventions.*

227

OBESITY

MICHAEL D. JENSEN

Obesity is the most common nutritional disorder in the United States and directly or indirectly accounts for a significant portion of health-related expenses. The safest and most effective treatment approaches (lifestyle change and behavior modification) are not those commonly employed by physicians and require considerable time to implement. Recently, progress has been made in understanding the pathophysiology and treatment of obesity.

DEFINITION

The National Institutes of Health and National Heart, Lung and Blood Institute (NHLBI) report entitled "Clinical Guidelines on the Identification, Evaluation and Treatment of Overweight and Obesity" provides clear, scientifically based definitions of overweight and obesity. Body mass index (BMI) is now the recommended means to categorize weight relative to height for adults. BMI is calculated as weight (in kilograms) divided by height squared (in meters). To calculate BMI using pounds and inches, the formula is modified as follows: weight (lb)/[height (inches)]$^2 \times 703$. The weight classifications according to BMI are summarized in Table 227-1. Individuals who are overweight (BMI of 25.0 to 29.9) may or may not be overfat. Some men may be overweight because of increased muscle mass, which is a straightforward clinical judgment. Although in general the risk of developing weight-related health problems increases with a BMI of greater than 25, the guidelines point

out that intervention or discussion of weight issues with the patient may not be necessary for overweight adults who are entirely healthy or are not overfat. On the other hand, some individuals with a BMI of 27 to 29.9 develop serious metabolic complications that improve with weight loss and are candidates for more aggressive treatment, including pharmacotherapy if needed. Some populations develop the typical metabolic complications of obesity at an even lower BMI and waist circumference. The guidelines for at-risk BMI in Asian populations is 23-24, much lower than whites, Hispanics, blacks, and Polynesians.

The prevalence of comorbidities increases considerably at a BMI of greater than 30, the definition of obesity. Obesity is divided into three classes, also depending on BMI (see Table 227-1). Treatment approaches may differ for those who are overweight and for different classes of obesity. For example, current U.S. Food and Drug Administration guidelines indicate that pharmacotherapy can be adjunct treatment for any class of obesity, even if medical complications are not present. Familiarity with the guidelines is important. Supervisory agencies and third-party payers use them to determine who is eligible for treatment benefits. Extreme obesity (BMI > 40) is one of the key features that would prompt consideration of a patient for bariatric surgery when medical treatments have failed. Patients with class II obesity (BMI of 35.0 to 39.9) may be considered for bariatric surgery if medical treatments have failed and if severe, life-threatening complications are present.

In addition to using BMI, the NHLBI Guidelines recommend using the waist circumferences as another office assessment tool that can help with the treatment decision-making process. A waist circumference of more than 102 cm or 40 inches for men and more than 88 cm or 35 inches for women is an additional indication of risk for overweight and obesity. This measure is primarily relevant to disease risk in overweight and class I obesity categories, however. In overweight individuals, a large waist circumference changes the relative from "increased" (relative to someone with a normal BMI) to "high." In class I obesity, a large waist circumference increases the risk of disease from "high" to "very high." A large waist circumference does not affect disease risk in those with class II or class III obesity. These definitions of overweight and obesity and of high-risk waist circumference are generally applicable to those of European and African descent, but lower values are recommended for those of Asian descent. The risks of metabolic abnormalities occur at lower BMI and lower waist circumference in these populations.

EPIDEMIOLOGY

Prevalence of Obesity

The number of overweight and obese adults in the United States has increased dramatically over the past 30 years, but the rate of increase has slowed in the last 5 years. Approximately 60% of U.S. men and 51% of U.S. women are overweight or obese, although a greater percentage of women are obese than men. There are substantial differences in the prevalence of obesity by age, race, and socioeconomic status. The prevalence of obesity in adults tends to rise steadily from ages 20 to 60 years, decreasing in later years. It has been estimated that almost 75% of men aged 60 to 69 years in the United States have a BMI of more than 25. The increase in mean BMI with age is not as much of a threat to population health as a similar increase in the BMI of younger populations. The lowest mortality rates for young adults are for a BMI in the lower part of the normal range (18.5 to 24.9), whereas the BMI associated with the lowest mortality rates is somewhat above 25 kg/m^2 for those in the 60s and 70s age groups. Physicians who provide care for individual patients will want to base their weight recommendations based upon whether adverse health consequences associated with obesity are present.

The differences in overweight and obesity among African Americans, Mexican Americans, and European Americans are not subtle. African-American women and Mexican Americans of both sexes have the highest rates of overweight and obesity in the United States. When interpreting these data, however, it is important to keep in mind that there is an inverse relationship between socioeconomic status and obesity, especially among women (Chapter 5). Women in lower socioeconomic classes are much more likely to be obese than those in higher socioeconomic classes. This association reduces but does not eliminate the racial differences in the prevalence of obesity. Whether the remaining racial differences in the prevalence of obesity are due to genetic, constitutional, or social factors is not yet known.

PATHOBIOLOGY

Etiology

There are significant genetic and constitutional susceptibility aspects to obesity that are heavily affected by environmental factors. Evidence from

	OBESITY CLASS	BMI KG/M^2
TABLE 227-1 CLASSIFICATION OF OVERWEIGHT AND OBESITY BY BODY MASS INDEX		
Underweight		<18.5
Normal		18.5-24.9
Overweight		25.0-29.9
Obesity	I	30.0-34.9
Obesity	II	35.0-39.9
Extreme obesity	III	≥40

Data from Clinical Guidelines on the Identification, Evaluation, and Treatment of Overweight and Obesity in Adults: The Evidence Report. National Institutes of Health; National Heart, Lung, and Blood Institute Publication 1998:98-4083.

adoption studies and studies of twins strongly support the concept that within a given environment, a significant portion of the variation in weight is genetic. That said, however, the tremendous increase in the prevalence of obesity in the United States over the past several decades can hardly be ascribed to mass changes in the genetic makeup of Americans.

Genetic Aspects of Human Obesity

There is strong evidence for a hereditary tendency toward the regulation of body weight. The single gene defects resulting in obesity include a number of classic genetic syndromes, such as Prader-Willi and Laurence-Moon-Biedl. More recently, extremely rare monogenic forms of human obesity due to mutations in the leptin gene and leptin receptor gene have been described. The result is an actual or functional leptin deficiency, much like that seen in *ob/ob* or *db/db* mice, the animal models that stimulated the discovery of leptin. There have also been reports of inherited forms of human obesity due to mutations of genes that regulate appetite neuropeptide synthesis. Genome-wide association studies have reported a number of genes associated with higher BMI. Those that appear to predict the greatest amount of variance in BMI include the fat mass and obesity-associated *(FTO)* gene and the melanocortin-4 receptor *(MC4R)* gene. Other genes that have been reliably associated with obesity include *TMEM18, KCTD15, GNPDA2, SH2B1, MTCH2,* and *NEGR1*. Together, however, the combined effects of all the identified genetic contributions account for less than 1% of the variance in BMI. This emphasizes both the huge environmental effects and the polygenic nature of susceptibility to obesity.

Constitutional Influences on Obesity

A number of environmental influences can result in long-term, gene-like affects on body weight regulation and the tendency to be susceptible to obesity-related health problems. These modifications of gene expression without modification of the underlying DNA are termed *epigenetic effects* and are ascribed to processes such as DNA methylation and chromatin remodeling. The effect of the intrauterine environment and the perinatal period on subsequent weight and health is best studied. Undernutrition in the last trimester of pregnancy and in the early postnatal period results in a decreased risk of adult obesity, however, the low birth weight associated with undernutrition (or smoking) in late pregnancy also increases the risk of adulthood hypertension, abnormal glucose tolerance, and cardiovascular disease. In contrast, undernutrition limited to the first two trimesters of pregnancy is associated with an increased probability of adult obesity. The infants of diabetic mothers tend to be fatter than those of nondiabetic mothers, and children of diabetic mothers have a greater prevalence of obesity when they are 5 to 19 years old, independent of their mother's obesity status. Finally, intrauterine exposure to the diabetic environment results in an increased risk of diabetes mellitus and obesity in the offspring. Thus, the issue of the genes versus the environment in regard to obesity and metabolic complications of obesity is blurred in the intrauterine and perinatal time intervals. One of the striking and worrisome aspects of these metabolic effects is not only the long-term effects on the individual's weight regulation and health, but also the suggestion that these traits can be passed on to future generations.

Environmental Contributors to Human Obesity

Few would argue that there have been dramatic changes in the environment over the past 50 years. These changes allowed reduced physical activity for most Americans. In addition, alterations in the food supply have either increased or failed to allow the expected decrease in energy intake that would be needed to match the reduced energy expenditure.

Food

A number of environmental factors can influence food intake (Table 227-2). Consuming energy-dense foods results in greater energy intake because many adults respond to the volume of food taken in rather than the energy content of food. This factor likely accounts for the association between high-fat diets and excess body weight; many high-fat foods are also energy dense. When humans consume diets that are high in fat, but low in energy density, energy intake in not greater than would be expected based on the energy density of the foods. Larger food portion size has also been shown to increase food intake. Given the trend in the United States to serve larger portions of food and beverage, this could be a contributing variable toward obesity. Food variety can also affect energy intake. An increased variety of entrees, sweets, snacks, and carbohydrates in the diet is associated with an increase in body fatness and food intake. In contrast, an increase in variety of vegetables

TABLE 227-2	ENVIRONMENTAL FACTORS PROMOTING OBESITY
DIETARY	**ACTIVITY**
↑ Energy density of foods	↑ Sedentary behavior
↑ Portion size	↓ Activities of daily living
↑ Variety*	↓ Employment physical activity
↑ Palatability	
↑ Availability	
↓ Cost	
↑ Caloric beverages (soft drinks, juices)	

*Variety of sweets, snacks, and entrees.

available does not result in an increased energy intake and is not associated with increased body fatness. Other factors that may have broad population effects in the United States include the reduced costs of food, increased availability, and palatability. Finally, there is evidence that consumption of beverages such as soft drinks and fruit juices is not accompanied by a decrease in food intake to offset the extra energy intake. The implication is that some types of beverages will add to the energy intake during the day and promote weight gain. The evidence that is available to date suggests that dairy products do not share this property and that consumption of low-fat dairy products in the context of a weight loss program may be beneficial under some circumstances.

Several individual factors may also influence how the properties of food affect energy intake. Individuals vary with respect to their dietary restraint (the tendency to consciously limit food intake to control weight), their feelings of hunger, or their disinhibition (the tendency to overeat opportunistically). It has been proposed that interindividual differences in these factors may modify how food variety, portion size, and so forth affect the eating profile. There are also effects of the social context under which food is consumed and the emotional state of the individual.

Physical Activity

Physical activity can be divided into three categories: (1) exercise (fitness- and sports-related activities); (2) work-related physical activity; and (3) non-exercise, nonemployment (spontaneous) activity. Tables are widely available that allow one to calculate energy expenditure based on an individual's weight as well as the type and duration of exercise. Only a fraction of Americans engage in exercise at the recommended frequency, intensity, or duration that could be expected to have a protective effect on the development of obesity and other health problems. The portion of Americans who exercise regularly is about 30%, and this does not appear to be changing; therefore, it seems unlikely that a change in exercise habits over the past several decades is causing the increase in obesity. Recent data suggest that the amount of time spent in sedentary activities (e.g., watching television, computer) is an independent predictor of metabolic abnormalities associated with obesity over and above the effects of exercise per se. Thus, to the extent reduced physical activity is contributing to the epidemic of obesity, it is likely that it is reduced employment-related and spontaneous physical activity that is changing.

It is difficult to measure the energy expended in nonexercise activity. Although it seems obvious that employment physical activity has decreased with the advent of more automated systems in the workplace, there are few data in this regard. One estimate suggests that between 1982 and 1992, energy expenditure at work decreased by about 50 kcal/day. The additional changes in the workplace since that time have likely further reduced employment physical activity.

The other component of nonexercise physical activity, the activities of daily living, is equally difficult to measure. A plethora of labor-saving conveniences (e.g., drive-through food and banking, escalators, remote controls, e-mail, online shopping) have been introduced into the modern environment. Each of these further reduces the energy humans must expend to get through the day. Again, there are few hard data to assess how much of a change has actually occurred, although a reduction in daily walking trips and an increase in daily automobile trips has been documented.

Perhaps because it is easier to assess, information on how differences in sedentary activity (television watching, video games, and computer use) relate to obesity is more readily available. There is compelling evidence that more time spent in sedentary pursuits is associated with an increased risk of overweight and obesity. The striking aspect to these studies is that the adverse effect of sedentary activities is independent of participation in traditional exercise activities.

Understanding the contributions of decreased work-related physical activity, decreases in activity of daily living, and increases in sedentary behavior can help the physician working with the patient to uncover patterns that may relate to weight gain. Physicians who are aware of these environmental factors are in a better position to help their obese patients identify which of these environmental factors are contributing to the problem and develop plans for intervention.

Regulation of Body Weight and Energy Balance

The regulation of adult body weight must be a well-balanced process. For example, the typical U.S. adult will take in and expend approximately 2000 to 3000 kcal/day. If there were a consistent error of even 1% in overconsumption of food, this would result in the gain of approximately 25 to 30 pounds of fat every 10 years if there were no change in energy expenditure. It follows that most adults regulate the average energy balance with greater than 1% precision. There appears to be regulation both of energy intake and energy expenditure through conscious and unconscious processes.

The excess energy consumed by adults is generally stored as triglycerides in adipocytes. Humans continuously recruit new adipocytes from a large preadipocyte pool, to replace dying adipocytes. Although the primary means by which adipose tissue mass expands is through increased fat cell size (adipocyte hypertrophy), this process can only store a limited amount of fat. If sufficient fat is deposited, eventually there will be a net increase in adipocyte number as more new adipocytes are created than needed to replace dying cells. Some adults recruit new adipocytes more readily than others and thus gain weight more so from adipocyte hyperplasia than from hypertrophy. Those who gain fat with large adipocytes, especially if associated with an adipose tissue inflammatory response (greater numbers of macrophages and other immune cells), are more likely to be insulin resistant and have signs of low-grade systemic inflammation (increased C-reactive protein, mildly elevated interleukin-6 and tumor necrosis factor-α).

The discovery of leptin, a protein from the cytokine family that is secreted almost exclusively by adipocytes, was the first confirmation that adipose tissue can secrete hormones that have central nervous system effects on food intake. Leptin also has other hypothalamic-pituitary functions and is proposed to have diverse peripheral physiologic actions. The leptin-deficient animal model of obesity, the *ob/ob* mouse, is severely obese, hyperphagic, hypometabolic, and sexually immature and has low levels of spontaneous activity. Administering leptin to this animal corrects all of these defects. A few humans have been found to have leptin deficiency due to mutations in the leptin gene. These children had very low plasma leptin concentrations and were hyperphagic and severely obese. They responded to exogenous leptin administration with dramatic weight loss, reduced food intake, and accelerated maturation of the pituitary-gonadal axis. With the exception of these rare mutations, however, obese humans are not leptin deficient. In fact, because plasma leptin concentrations increase logarithmically with percentage of body fat, obese humans typically have very high plasma leptin concentrations. Likewise, because women normally have more body fat than men, they also have higher plasma leptin concentrations. From what is currently known, screening for leptin deficiency is not warranted except in severe, hyperphagic obesity that begins in early childhood, is accompanied by sexual immaturity, and exists in the absence of other known causes (e.g., Prader-Willi syndrome).

Some animal models of genetic obesity (the *db/db* mouse and *fa/fa* rat) have defective leptin receptors, making them unresponsive to leptin. Although rare cases of obese humans with defective leptin receptor genes have been reported, again it appears that leptin resistance due to leptin receptor defects (or genetic post-receptor signaling abnormalities) is extremely uncommon. Clinical screening for leptin receptor mutations is not warranted given that no treatment exists.

Leptin secretion can increase 30 to 40% with brief periods of overfeeding (before changes in body composition) and is reduced by 50% in response to brief periods of underfeeding. Clinical studies indicate that low or absent leptin results in extreme hunger. Attempts to treat overweight patients with recombinant leptin have not been successful. Clinical studies suggest that falling leptin plays a role in modulating the hypothalamic-pituitary response to undernutrition, thereby serving the endocrine adaptation to starvation (reduced thyroid-stimulating hormone and gonadotrophins). In summary, the discovery of leptin has been an important advance in understanding the biology of obesity. Defects in leptin secretion or inherited defects in leptin action are very rare.

Energy Intake

Much of what has been learned about the biologic regulation of food intake has been from the study of animal models. These signals may affect different aspects of eating behavior. They can affect hunger—the compelling need or desire for food; satiation—the state of being satisfactorily full and unable to take on more; or satiety—the sense of no longer being hungry, a complex set of postprandial events that affect the interval to the next meal or the amount consumed at the next meal. Some of the signals that alter eating behavior affect one aspect, and others affect multiple aspects. For example, ghrelin, a peptide produced by the stomach, increases hunger but does not appear to affect satiation or satiety. Cholecystokinin causes satiation, but has no effect on satiety. Leptin appears to act on multiple pathways—leptin deficiency is associated with increased hunger and reduced satiation and satiety.

Peripheral satiety signals act to inhibit further food intake at some point during meal consumption. Some of the signals reach the brain through the vagus nerve and some through the systemic circulation. Examples of the proposed factors modulating appetite are listed in Table 227-3. The compounds range from gut-derived (ghrelin, cholecystokinin, glucagon-like peptide 1) and pancreas-derived (insulin) hormones to peptides such as apolipoprotein A-IV, which is secreted with chylomicrons. The signals are thought to be triggered both by mechanical stimuli (e.g., the fullness of the stomach) and the presence of nutrients in the jejunum and ileum.

The central nervous system regulation of food intake is becoming better understood. A number of neuropeptides, lipid derivatives, and monoamines have either anabolic (increased food intake with or without decreased energy expenditure) or catabolic (decreased food intake with or without increased energy expenditure) properties. A list of these molecules is provided in Table 227-4. Many of these compounds serve more than one function, such as regulation of hormone secretion (thyrotropin-releasing hormone and corticotropin-releasing hormone), wakefulness (norepinephrine), or behavior-reinforcing systems (endocannabinoids).

Energy Expenditure

There is a wide range of daily energy expenditure in adults, from less than 1400 kcal/day to more than 5000 kcal/day, with larger, more physically active individuals having the greatest energy needs. Typically, daily energy expenditure is divided into resting (or basal) metabolic rate, the thermic effect of food, and physical activity energy expenditure.

Basal Metabolic Rate

The basal metabolic rate (BMR) is the energy expenditure of laying still at rest, awake, in the overnight postabsorptive state. The resting metabolic rate (RMR) is similarly defined but is not necessarily measured before arising from bed. For most sedentary adult Americans, the RMR represents the major portion of energy expended during the day, and may range from less than 1200 to more than 3000 kcal/day. Most (~80%) of the BMR can be explained by the amount of lean tissue an individual has.

TABLE 227-3	SUGGESTED BIOLOGIC MODULATORS OF FOOD INTAKE
PERIPHERAL SIGNAL	**PROPOSED EFFECT ON FOOD INTAKE**
Vagal	–
Cholecystokinin (CCK)	–
Apolipoprotein A-IV	–
Insulin	–
PYY_{3-36}	–
Glucagon-like peptide 1 (GLP-1)	–
Other glucagon-related peptides	–
Leptin	+ when leptin ↓↓
Ghrelin	+
Tumor necrosis factor-α	–
Obestatin	–

TABLE 227-4 CENTRAL NERVOUS SYSTEM MODULATORS OF ENERGY BALANCE

CENTRAL ANABOLIC (↑ INTAKE)	CENTRAL CATABOLIC (↓ INTAKE)
Neuropeptide Y	α-Melanocyte-stimulating hormone
Agouti-related protein	Corticotropin-releasing hormone
Melanin-concentrating hormone	Thyrotropin-releasing hormone
Hypocretins and orexins	Cocaine- and amphetamine-regulated transcript (CART)
Galanin	Interleukin-1β
Norepinephrine	Urocortin
Endogenous endocannabinoids (anandamide and 2-arachidonoylglycerol)	Oxytocin
	Neurotensin
	Serotonin

Not all components of lean tissue consume oxygen at the same relative rates. Visceral or splanchnic bed tissues account for about 25% of resting metabolic rate but a much smaller proportion of body weight. The brain, which is only a few percent of body weight, accounts for almost 15% of RMR. Likewise, the heart (~7%) and kidneys (~5 to 10%) account for greater portions of resting energy needs than their relative contribution to body mass. In contrast, resting muscle makes up 40 to 50% of lean tissue mass but accounts for only 25% of RMR. This contribution changes dramatically with exercise, however, at which time muscle can account for 80 to 90% of energy expenditure. Adipose tissue is a minor contributor to daily energy expenditure, consuming only approximately 3 kcal/kg of body fat per day. Brown fat is adipose tissue that expresses large amounts of uncoupling protein-1, a protein that allows a mitochondrial membrane proton leak, resulting in heat release as opposed to chemical work from adenosine triphosphate— "uncoupling" of substrate oxidation from chemical or mechanical work. This thermogenic tissue was thought to be present only in human infants but has recently been shown to exist in adults, albeit in amounts insufficient to have measurable thermogenic properties.

Although most of the RMR can be accounted for by the mass of lean tissue, there are also other, more subtle influences on RMR. Age, sex (women have slightly lower BMR even corrected for fat-free mass), and fat mass affect RMR. Small changes in BMR occur during the menstrual cycle (luteal phase > follicular phase). There is also evidence that heritable or family factors influence BMR, accounting for as much as 10% of the interindividual differences.

There are both obligatory and facultative components to resting metabolic rate. With an energy-restricted diet, significant reductions in BMR relative to the amount of fat-free mass occur. Reductions in the production of triiodothyronine from thyroxine and the sympathetic nervous system drive are thought to contribute to this phenomenon. Likewise, during brief periods of overfeeding, resting metabolic rate increases above that which would be expected for the amount of lean tissue present.

It has been proposed that individuals with basal metabolic rates lower than predicted are at increased risk of future weight gain. Published data suggest that the relative risk is small, and clinical effort to identify such patients is not warranted. Measurement of BMR is sometimes helpful in the evaluation of patients who insist they are unable to lose weight while following diets containing less than 1000 kcal/day. Almost without fail, their BMR is substantially greater than their reported food intake. This underscores the fact that most adults are unreliable in assessing their own food intake.

The Thermic Effect of Food

Approximately 10% of the energy content of food is expended in the process of digestion, absorption, and metabolism of nutrients. There is a significant interindividual variability in this value, however, ranging from a low of about 5% to a high of about 15% of meal calories that are "wasted" in the postprandial interval. The thermic effect of a meal is related to its carbohydrate and protein caloric content; the fat content has little stimulatory effect. Both obligatory (60 to 70%) and facultative (30 to 40%) components of the thermic effect of food have been identified. The obligatory components no doubt reflect the energy costs of digestion, absorption, and storage of nutrients. The two factors thought to play a role in the facultative component of the thermic effect of food are the postprandial insulin response and activation of the sympathetic nervous system. The thermic effect of food is somewhat lower in insulin-resistant and obese humans, but this has not been linked to future obesity.

Physical Activity Energy Expenditure

The energy expenditure of physical activity is a product of the amount of work done and the work efficiency of the individual. Although tracking the total amount of physical activity humans perform throughout the day is not easy, when it is possible to do so, it is also possible to calculate the energy expended because the published values for estimating the energy costs of work performed are generally quite accurate. Work units are expressed as metabolic equivalents (METs), a multiple of the resting metabolic rate. If an individual's resting metabolic rate is 1 kcal/minute (1440 kcal/day), a workload of 5 METs would be 5 kcal/minute. Highly trained athletes can work at extremely high METs (>16) for extended periods of time, but most sedentary individuals can only work for a limited amount of time at much lower workloads. This is because athletes have both a greater peak work capacity (or maximal amount of calories or oxygen that can be consumed) and a higher lactate threshold. The lactate threshold can be thought of as the level at which exercise begins to become so uncomfortable that it cannot be maintained much longer. The biochemical definition of lactate threshold describes the progressive rise in blood lactate concentrations observed during sufficiently high-intensity exercise. The lactate threshold may range from 50 to 90% of an individual's peak work capacity. Training raises the lactate threshold closer to the maximal workload and thus allows individuals to work at higher rates for longer periods. Thus, highly fit individuals can expend much greater amounts of energy per minute of exercise with less sense of discomfort than can obese, sedentary individuals who typically have low aerobic fitness and low lactate thresholds (sometimes on the order of 4 to 5 METs). The lactate threshold can be even lower in obese patients with type 2 diabetes, such that walking a mere 3 miles per hour can exceed their lactate threshold. Appreciating the physical limitations of patients, which can usually be overcome with a carefully designed training program, is necessary to provide realistic activity recommendations.

Exercise (fitness and sports-related activities) is commonly considered the main component of physical activity thermogenesis. Because most adults do not exercise at high levels or for a sufficient duration to expend a large amount of energy, focusing solely on "exercise" as the main component of physical activity will miss significant opportunities for improving energy balance. The benefits and energy costs of nonexercise activity can be far greater than the usual amount of exercise in which most patients can engage.

Nonexercise activity thermogenesis (NEAT) is the caloric expense of performing all activities other than exercise—employment-related and spontaneous activity. The range of observed NEAT under controlled (metabolic chamber) conditions has been from less than 100 to up to about 800 kcal/day. The energy expended from a physically demanding job or volitional exercise may or may not be offset by reductions in spontaneous (nonemployment) activity. For example, when young adult men and women take in extra exercise for more than 1 year, they respond differently: men lose weight and women do not, despite the absence of detectable change in food intake. This suggests either that woman reduce spontaneous activity in response to exercise and men do not or that subtle increases in food intake occur in women and not men. It has also been shown that unconscious increases in NEAT can serve to offset the tendency to gain weight in response to overeating. Low levels of NEAT have been reported to predict future weight gain in some populations, and there may be differences between lean and obese persons in the daily amount of NEAT, which could relate to differential tendencies to regulate weight.

Secondary Causes of Obesity

Medications

A growing number of medications cause weight gain in some or most of those patients for whom they are prescribed. Awareness of the medications that have this potential can facilitate weight loss treatment in some patients. Table 227-5 lists a number of medications that are associated with weight gain as well as alternative treatment approaches, if any, for the underlying condition.

Diseases

Less than 1% of obese patients have an underlying disease that can explain the development of their obesity. Endocrinopathies are the most common

TABLE 227-5 PHARMACOLOGIC INFLUENCES IN WEIGHT GAIN AND ALTERNATIVE THERAPIES

DRUGS THAT MAY PROMOTE WEIGHT GAIN	ALTERNATIVE TREATMENTS—WEIGHT NEUTRAL OR WEIGHT LOSS
PSYCHIATRIC AND NEUROLOGIC MEDICATIONS	**ALTERNATIVE PSYCHIATRIC AND NEUROLOGIC MEDICATIONS**
Antipsychotics: olanzapine, clozapine, respiridone, quetiapine, aripiprazole	Ziprasidone
Antidepressants	Nortriptyline, bupropion, nefazodone, fluvoxamine, sertraline, duloxetine
Tricyclics: imipramine, amitriptyline	Topiramate, zonisamide (weight loss), lamotrigine (less weight gain)
Triazolopyridines: trazodone	
Serotonin reuptake inhibitors: paroxetine, fluoxetine, citalopram	
Tetracyclics: mirtazapine	
Monamine oxidase inhibitors	
Antiepileptic drugs: gabapentin (higher doses), valproic acid, carbamazepine, divalproex	
Mood stabilizers: lithium, carbamazepine, lamotrigine, gabapentin (higher doses)	
STEROID HORMONES	**ALTERNATIVES TO STEROID HORMONES**
Progestational steroids	Barrier methods, IUD
Corticosteroids	Nonsteroidal anti-inflammatory drugs
Hormonal contraceptives	
ANTIDIABETES AGENTS	**ALTERNATIVE ANTIDIABETES AGENTS**
Insulin (most forms)	Metformin
Sulfonylureas	Acarbose, miglitol
Thiazolidinediones	Exenatide
	DPP-4 inhibitors
ANTIHISTAMINES	**DECONGESTANTS, MAST CELL STABILIZERS, ANTAGONISTS OF ENDOGENOUS MEDIATORS OF INFLAMMATION**
Commonly reported with older agents; also oxatomide, loratadine and azelastine	
ANTIHYPERTENSIVE AGENTS	**ALTERNATIVE ANTIHYPERTENSIVE AGENTS**
α-Adrenergic and β-adrenergic receptor blockers	Angiotensin-converting enzyme inhibitors,
Calcium channel blockers: nisoldipine	Calcium channel blockers—most other agents
	Angiotensin receptor blockers
	Diuretics
HIGHLY ACTIVE ANTIRETROVIRAL THERAPY	

secondary cause of obesity. These include Cushing's syndrome (Chapter 234), hypothalamic damage resulting in overeating (most commonly after pituitary surgery), insulinoma (Chapter 238), and hypothyroidism (Chapter 233). A Cushing's syndrome–like fat distribution is common; therefore, other physical or laboratory findings are the best clues to whether to test for this condition. These include the classic purple striae, thinning skin, easy bruising, proximal muscle weakness, and electrolyte abnormalities. Correction of Cushing's syndrome commonly results in substantial loss of excess body fat. Insulinoma is a rare tumor, and a small portion of patients with insulinoma develop obesity; only some patients consciously prevent spells by eating more often, and thus become obese. The weight gain associated with hypothyroidism is largely due to fluid retention and resolves dramatically with thyroid hormone replacement. Unfortunately, successful treatment is not available for hyperphagia due to hypothalamic damage. Occasionally, adult patients with growth hormone deficiency, most commonly following hypophysectomy, lose excess body fat with growth hormone replacement therapy.

Psychosocial Aspects of Obesity

Sexual, physical, and emotional abuse, especially in women, can result in long-term adverse consequences that include obesity. The effects of the abuse tend to be most profound if it occurs in childhood and adolescence. These women may be severely obese, suffer from chronic depression, and experience a number of psychosomatic symptoms, particularly chronic gastrointestinal distress. Identifying these issues before initiation of weight loss programs is important because successful weight loss may actually aggravate the distress experienced by these women. In addition, appropriate referral for psychiatric help may be needed before initiation of treatment for obesity.

PATHOPHYSIOLOGY

Metabolic Complications of Obesity

A central or upper body fat distribution, more so than total fat mass, is predictive of the metabolic complications of obesity. Adipose tissue release of free fatty acids (FFAs) and glycerol into the circulation through lipolysis provides 50 to 100% of daily energy needs. Adipose tissue lipolysis is regulated primarily by insulin (inhibition) and catecholamines (stimulation), although growth hormone and cortisol also stimulate lipolysis. Upper body obesity is associated with several abnormalities of adipose tissue lipolysis, most remarkably with higher FFA concentrations due to excess release postprandially. Abnormally high FFA concentrations can contribute to a number of the metabolic complications of obesity.

Insulin Resistance

The term *insulin resistance* is typically used when referring to the ability of insulin to promote glucose uptake, oxidation, and storage as well as to inhibit the release of glucose into the circulation. The primary site of insulin-stimulated glucose uptake, oxidation, and storage is skeletal muscle. The principal site of glucose production is the liver. Insulin resistance initially leads to hyperinsulinemia and may eventually lead to the development of type 2 diabetes mellitus (Chapter 237).

The ability of insulin to promote glucose uptake, oxidation, and storage in muscle and to suppress plasma FFA concentrations is reduced in upper body obesity. High plasma FFA concentrations can induce a state of insulin resistance both in the muscle (glucose uptake) and in the liver (glucose release), independent of obesity. Thus, abnormal regulation of adipose tissue FFA export is a major component of the development of insulin resistance.

Dysregulated production of a number of adipose-derived hormones, also called adipokines, is hypothesized to contribute to insulin resistance and the metabolic complications of obesity. For example, reduced secretion of adiponectin, an adipocyte-derived hormone that improves insulin action, is seen in obesity and diabetes. Increased production of resistin, interleukin-6, tumor necrosis factor-α, and retinol-binding protein-4 by adipose tissue has been linked to insulin resistance in animal models. Visfatin is another adipocyte hormone that is secreted preferentially by omental and mesenteric adipocytes and appears to function to increase insulin action, albeit through a different mechanism than adiponectin. To date, there is insufficient experimental evidence from human studies to know what role adipokines play in the metabolic complications of obesity.

Islet Cell Failure and Type 2 Diabetes Mellitus

Type 2 diabetes is generally the result of defects in both insulin secretion and insulin action (Chapter 237). Many obese individuals are insulin resistant, yet only a subset will develop diabetes mellitus. It follows that those who develop type 2 diabetes develop pancreatic β-cell decompensation with subsequent hyperglycemia. Animal (rodent) studies have suggested that a process referred to as lipotoxicity is involved in pancreatic β-cell failure. In this model, increased FFAs are proposed to contribute to the insulin secretory abnormalities seen in obesity and ultimately lead to β-cell failure. A small number of studies have suggested that FFAs have adverse effects on islet β-cell function in humans. Another explanation for the development of β-cell failure in obesity is the overproduction of islet amyloid polypeptide. This protein is co-secreted with insulin and, because of its tertiary structure, can form toxic amyloid deposits in β cells. Amyloid deposits have been found in the pancreatic islets obtained at autopsy from patients with type 2 diabetes mellitus.

Hypertension

Blood pressure can be increased by a number of mechanisms (Chapter 67). Increased circulating blood volume, abnormal vasoconstriction, decreased vascular relaxation, and increased cardiac output may all contribute to hypertension in obesity. The effect of hyperinsulinemia to increase renal sodium absorption may contribute to hypertension through increased circulating blood volume. Abnormalities of vascular resistance also contribute to the pathophysiology of obesity-related hypertension. Under some experimental conditions, elevated FFAs have been found to cause increased vasoconstriction and reduced nitric oxide–mediated vasorelaxation, similar to that seen in the metabolic syndrome. Some obese adults have increased sympathetic nervous system activity, which could contribute to obesity-associated hypertension. Finally, angiotensinogen (also produced by adipocytes) is a precursor of the vasoconstrictor angiotensin II and is proposed to contribute to elevated blood pressure.

Dyslipidemia

Upper body obesity and type 2 diabetes mellitus are associated with increased triglycerides, decreased high-density lipoprotein (HDL) cholesterol, and a high proportion of small, dense low-density lipoprotein (LDL) particles (Chapter 213). This dyslipidemia contributes to the increased cardiovascular risk observed in the metabolic syndrome. Fasting hypertriglyceridemia is caused by increased hepatic very low density lipoprotein (VLDL) secretion, which may be driven by increased delivery of FFAs to the liver coming from both visceral fat and upper body subcutaneous fat. The reduced HDL cholesterol concentrations and the increased small, dense LDL particle concentrations associated with upper body obesity are likely an indirect consequence of elevated triglyceride-rich VLDL. Increased cholesterol ester transfer protein activity and hepatic lipase activity can theoretically account for the atherogenic shifts in triglycerides and cholesterol between lipoproteins. Genetic influences play a significant role in the expression of these lipid abnormalities. Polymorphisms in the genes for apolipoprotein E, lipoprotein lipase, apolipoprotein B-100, and apolipoprotein A-II are correlated with increased triglycerides and decreased HDL.

Endocrine Manifestations of Obesity

Obesity is associated with abnormalities of the endocrine system. One of the most common abnormalities is polycystic ovarian syndrome (PCOS). This syndrome is characterized by mild hirsutism and irregular menses or amenorrhea with anovulatory cycles. It is most commonly linked with obesity and often improves with weight loss and other treatments that improve insulin resistance. Thus, it is thought that the insulin resistance associated with obesity may trigger the development of PCOS in susceptible individuals. Whereas mild to moderate androgen overproduction is a feature of upper body obesity in women, obese men may suffer from mild to severe hypothalamic hypogonadism. This androgen deficiency improves with weight loss and does not appear to benefit substantially from testosterone replacement. There has been some concern that testosterone treatment of obese men may increase the risk of obstructive sleep apnea. Although estrogens are not elevated in obese premenopausal women, they remain somewhat above postmenopausal levels in obese postmenopausal women. Serum growth hormone concentrations are commonly low in obese adults, but insulin-like growth factor-I concentrations are often normal, and growth hormone concentrations increase with weight loss. Treatment of these patients with growth hormone has been reported to worsen insulin resistance and glucose intolerance and cannot be justified considering the costs and poor risk-to-benefit ratio.

Mechanical Complications of Obesity

The excess body weight associated with obesity is thought to be responsible for the increased prevalence of lower extremity degenerative joint disease. Extreme obesity can result in premature degenerative joint disease, and this may be especially difficult to treat surgically given the greater stress on joint replacements. Severely obese individuals may also have problems with venous stasis, which is occasionally aggravated by right heart failure (see later).

Obstructive Sleep Apnea

Sleep apnea (Chapter 100) is common in severely obese patients, tending to be more prevalent in men and in women with an upper body obese phenotype. Sleep apnea is most likely explained by enlargement of upper airways

soft tissue, resulting in collapse of the upper airways with inspiration during sleep. The obstruction leads to apneas, with hypoxemia, hypercarbia, and high catecholamine and endothelin levels. The frequent arousals to restore breathing result in poor sleep quality. Sleep apnea is associated with an increased risk of hypertension, and if sleep apnea is severe, it can lead to right heart failure and sudden death. A history of daytime hypersomnolence, loud snoring, restless sleep, or morning headaches is suggestive of obstructive sleep apnea. Treatment of sleep apnea is important to improve cardiovascular risk, and the failure to recognize and treat this complication may make weight loss intervention strategies much less successful.

Cancer

The risk of breast cancer and endometrial cancer is increased in obese women (Chapter 183). It is thought that this may be due to the increased estrogen levels associated with obesity in the postmenopausal women. Obese men also have a higher mortality of cancers of the prostate and colon. The reasons for this association are unknown.

Gastrointestinal Disorders

Gastroesophageal reflux disease and gallstones are more prevalent in obese patients. Likewise, fatty liver and nonalcoholic steatohepatitis (Chapter 155) is more common in obesity. Nonalcoholic steatohepatitis can eventually progress to life-threatening hepatic cirrhosis. Weight loss and interventions that improve insulin sensitivity have been shown to improve fatty liver and nonalcoholic steatohepatitis.

DIAGNOSIS

Evaluation of Obesity

In the office practice, obtaining an accurate height and weight allows calculation of BMI, and under some circumstances, measurement of the patient's waist circumference can be useful in assessing risk (see earlier). Accurate measure of blood pressure, which may require a large blood pressure cuff, is important. The presence or absence of dyslipidemia (HDL cholesterol < 45 mg/dL for women, HDL cholesterol < 35 mg/dL for men, or triglycerides > 150 mg/dL), hypertension, glucose intolerance and diabetes, and hyperuricemia should be documented. A history suggestive of sleep apnea should prompt a referral for overnight oximetry or a sleep disorder evaluation.

A review of the patient's lifestyle, including an assessment of physical activity level and eating habits, may help provide information about why the patient is obese. A family history of obesity, or long-standing obesity, provides evidence against a secondary cause of obesity. A careful medication history and social history may help the clinician identify precipitating factors that can be modified.

Before entering a weight management program, it is important to ensure the patient is interested and ready to make lifestyle changes and has realistic goals and expectations. Often patients expect to lose large amounts of weight in short periods of time. Medical treatment programs, even if they include pharmacotherapy, seldom result in greater than 10% weight loss. This degree of weight loss is sufficient to reduce markedly the medical complications of obesity, but disappointment with "only" 10% weight loss may cause patients to quit a medically successful program. Helping the patient to realize and accept that 10% weight loss is a reasonable, initial goal can be one of the more challenging aspects for a physician.

It is sometimes necessary to delay entry into treatment programs if a patient is not ready to make lifestyle changes. In this case, a reasonable strategy is to remind the patient periodically of the potential health benefits of improved activity and eating habits. Once a willingness to make changes is apparent, treatment is more likely to succeed.

TREATMENT   Rx

Obesity represents an individual's response to the environment based on genetics and learned behavior and is best viewed as a chronic disease. Therefore, treatment must be considered a long-term issue, much like diabetes, hypertension, or dyslipidemia. Substantial weight loss can be induced through severe caloric restriction, but without approaches to ensure behavioral changes, body fat is invariably regained. To the extent that environmental factors contribute to a patient's overweight status, and to the extent that the macroenvironment is unlikely to change, patients must learn how to make permanent lifestyle changes (eating and activity behavior) in order to hope for permanent weight loss. Behavior modification approaches often seek to help patients recognize and circumvent environmental cues for sedentary behavior and overeating as a means to accomplish these lifestyle changes.

Reducing energy intake is the most efficient and effective means to lose weight. For example, creating a 500 kcal/day deficit by reduced food intake can allow the loss of 1 pound of fat per week. Although possible, it is much more difficult to increase energy expenditure by 500 kcal/week through exercise. Higher levels of physical activity can prevent weight gain (or weight regain after weight loss). Some patients are able to change eating and activity habits on their own given the proper information, whereas others require formal or informal behavior modification interventions (see later) to help make these changes. In some instances, pharmacotherapy or surgery may be needed for treatment of obesity. A flow diagram on how to evaluate and manage patients with overweight and obesity is presented in Figure 227-1.

Diet

Changes in eating habits must be permanent if weight loss is to be maintained. An experienced registered dietitian can be helpful in the evaluation of a patient's eating habits and will be able to provide the needed education. The diet history may identify eating behaviors that result in excess energy intake. Although it is important to address specific adverse eating behaviors, patients need to understand some general principles regarding diet. Reducing the energy density of food (most commonly accomplished by reducing dietary fat) can allow patients to feel satiated while consuming fewer calories. A common mistake, however, is for patients to consume large quantities of easy-to-eat "nonfat" foods, thereby offsetting the expected benefits of the diet. In addition to reducing the intake of high-fat foods, patients should understand that increasing the consumption of foods high in water and fiber (fruits, vegetables, legumes, and soups) can provide satiety without excess calories. It is also important to avoid the excess intake of beverages containing substantial calories with little or no satiety. Finally, a regular pattern of eating should be encouraged.

New, fad diets are continuously being promoted with the promise of easy weight loss. A common feature of these diets is the claim that special properties of certain foods help people lose weight or are the cause of obesity. If followed, most of these diets result in weight loss because of a reduced energy intake. The reduced intake can be related to the monotony of the diet, and there have been no diets identified that cause persons to lose weight not in accordance with physiologic principles. No published data exist to support the use of fad diets in the long-term treatment of obesity. Recent studies have shown that many types of diets are able to help patients achieve long-term, medically significant weight loss.[1] Thus, it may be less important what specific type of diet (DASH diet, Mediterranean diet, high-carbohydrate/low-fat or high-fat/low-carbohydrate diet) is recommended than for the patient to find it relatively easy to adhere to the diet.

Very low calorie diets (<800 calories per day) have been used for years to achieve accelerated weight loss. The rationale for this approach is now in question, given that the long-term results of these diets is no better and sometimes worse than the results from the standard low-calorie diet combined with behavior modification. The expensive laboratory monitoring required for very low calorie diets without an improved long-term outcome raises questions about the costs versus benefits of this approach.

Physical Activity

A long-term increase in physical activity, either through the activities of daily living or through regular exercise, is key to preventing weight regain, thereby increasing the amount of successful, long-term weight loss.[2] Unfortunately, many overweight and obese patients are quite unfit, being unable to walk even 1 mile continuously. It is not possible for most adults to burn large numbers of calories. For example, only about 100 kcal is expended by a 70-kg adult walking 1 mile. Losing weight solely by increasing exercise is impractical for most patients. However, increasing physical activity as a means of maintaining weight loss is an attainable goal for most patients.

Successful maintenance of weight loss requires that daily energy expenditure be an average of 80 to 90% above RMR. This is a considerable increase for most patients. For example, someone with an RMR of 1500 kcal/day would need to expend about 1000 kcal/day in physical activity to meet this target. Activities other than "exercise" are important means to achieve this goal. The most commonly applicable approach is by increasing the amount of walking done throughout the day.

There are important health benefits from regular physical activity over and above the effects on weight. These include lower cardiovascular and all-cause mortality, independent of weight. The options for increasing physical activity include exercise (sports or fitness pursuits) or using lifestyle approaches. Both methods can improve fitness and allow weight stability; however, persuading obese patients to become more active is not easy. Physicians can begin by asking patients about their current and past activity habits as well as what barriers they see to increasing physical activity. This accomplishes the goal of stimulating patients to think about the issue in a tactful manner. It can help to ask the patient what personal benefits they envision as a result of increasing their level of activity. If patients agree to begin an exercise or physical activity program, they will need to monitor their activity and set realistic goals for the amount of exercise they are going to achieve. The ready availability of step counters offers a practical means for patients to track physical activity throughout the day and to assess the effects of changes in lifestyle on their activity level. There are a variety of step counters available, and the accuracy of many is questionable. Before advising a specific type, it is important to examine the literature or look for data regarding accuracy. Self-monitoring of how many steps are taken each day for 1 to 2 weeks can give the patient a good sense of their level of activity. Many Americans take as few as 4000 to 5000 steps per day, whereas it may take as many as 15,000 to 17,000 steps per day to help those who have lost significant amounts of weight to maintain that lower weight. Gradually increasing the number of steps regularly taken during the day through a series of changes in habits (e.g., parking further away, walking during work breaks) is more likely to result in long-term success for most persons than setting aside 2 hours or more for continuous walking.

Behavior Modification

Patients who are unable to make changes in eating activity habits on their own or with informal office counseling may benefit from referral to a behavior

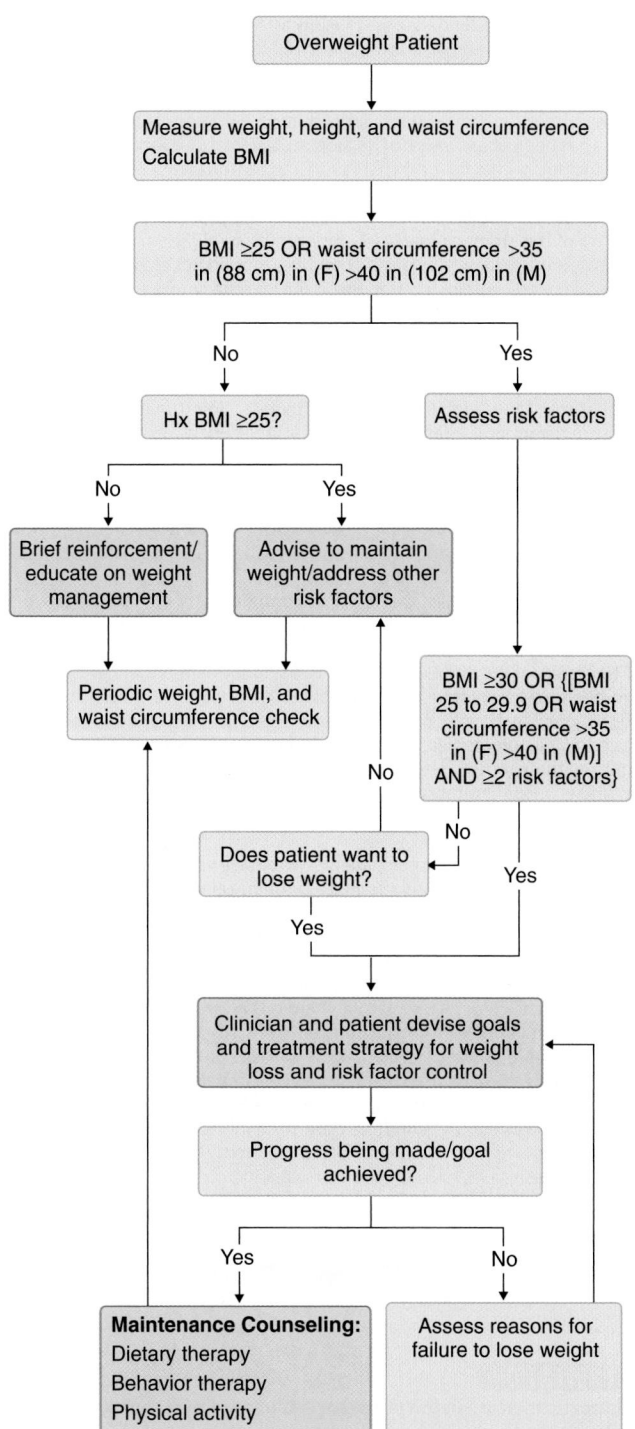

FIGURE 227-1. Flow diagram for the evaluation and management of overweight and obesity. BMI = body mass index. (Adapted from NIH/NHLBI. Clinical guidelines on the identification, evaluation and treatment of obesity in adults: the evidence report. *Obes Res.* 1998;6:51S-209S.)

therapist. The goals are to help patients modify their eating, activity, and thinking habits that predispose to obesity and to focus on specific pathways to achieve the goals. These pathways may include identifying and removing barriers to developing better eating or activity habits. Small, incremental, and consistent changes in behavior are encouraged. Self-monitoring of food and activity is considered a key feature to success because most obese patients underestimate food intake and overestimate exercise. Cognitive restructuring has been introduced as a way to help overcome the thought processes that can lead to failure of a weight management program. Patients are taught to identify, challenge, and correct self-defeating thoughts.

Pharmacotherapy

A limited number of drugs are currently available to help patients with weight loss. The limited amounts of weight loss that most patients experience seems to have dampened the enthusiasm of many physicians to prescribe weight loss drugs, even under circumstances that justify their use. In addition, not all overweight or obese patients are candidates for pharmacologic treatment of obesity. Table 227-6 provides criteria that should help select patients for pharmacologic treatment. Because pharmacologic treatment of obesity exposes patients to some risks and expense, it is reasonable to require an objective benefit. A rational argument can be made that prioritization should be given to those with one or more medical complications or conditions that are likely to improve with weight loss. Numerous studies have shown that medications used alone are much less effective than when they are used as a part of a comprehensive program that includes diet, exercise, and behavior modification.▨ When prescribing antiobesity medications, it is important to set clear goals with respect to both weight loss and health benefits.

Currently Available Medications

The medications currently available for long-term use act either through appetite reduction (phentermine) or through inhibition of pancreatic lipase (orlistat), which results in fat malabsorption. Phentermine is currently approved for short-term (3 months) use. Because weight that is lost with pharmacotherapy (especially when used without a comprehensive program) is quickly regained once the medication is discontinued, agents that are approved for long-term use (orlistat) are more rational therapeutic choices.

Orlistat at the typical dose of 120 mg three times daily with meals causes about 30% of dietary fat to be malabsorbed. As expected, adverse gastrointestinal side effects, such as oily spotting, abdominal pain, excess flatus, fecal urgency, and fatty or oily stools, are not uncommon. These side effects decrease over time, and the concomitant use of bulk-forming laxatives (e.g., psyllium, methylcellulose) can reduce these symptoms. A daily multivitamin is recommended for those on long-term orlistat therapy. It is not necessary to take orlistat if a nonfat meal is being consumed.

Orlistat is now available as an over-the-counter medication. Orlistat improves the results of medical treatment programs that include diet, exercise, and behavior modification, resulting in almost twice as many patients achieving goal weight loss (10% of body weight.)

Success of Medical Therapy

It has been estimated that more than 95% of those embarking on self-diets or fad diets fail to maintain a significant weight loss for a period of time that would have meaningful health benefits. The published results of commercial programs are not impressively better, mostly because of high dropout rates. In contrast, organized, scientifically based weight management programs that employ behavior modification in addition to dietary instruction, physical activity, and medications (when indicated) can achieve impressive results. Although these programs tend to be more selective (accepting only motivated patients), the dropout rates can be acceptable (<30%), and of those remaining in the program, weight loss of more than 10% can be achieved and maintained for more than 1 to 2 years in 40 to 60% of patients. These results are more impressive than those reported with older, less comprehensive programs, wherein almost all patients regained all weight in less than 6 months.

Bariatric Surgery

Surgical treatment may be indicated for severely obese patients with severe medical complications that could be expected to improve with successful weight loss. Patients with a BMI of 35 to 40 with life-threatening complications can be considered, but more typically patients with a BMI of greater than 40 and several complications are candidates for surgery, assuming past attempts at medical treatment have failed. Because the risks and costs of surgical treatment are greater than for medical treatment, it is reasonable practice to select patients who stand to obtain more potential benefit from surgery. Contraindications to surgery include active substance abuse, defined noncompliance or inability to comply with medical care, and certain psychiatric disorders (schizophrenia, borderline personality disorder, uncontrolled depression).

A multidisciplinary team, including a physician, dietitian, psychologist or psychiatrist with expertise in this area, and surgeon experienced in bariatric procedures, is important for optimal outcome. Defining realistic expectations is an important part of the evaluation process. Patients undergoing bariatric surgery are not likely to be reduced to their ideal body weight. Successful weight loss is typically defined as losing an average of 50 to 60% of excess body weight. For example, if someone is 100 kg *overweight,* a reasonable definition of success is to lose 50 kg. Follow-up to support the necessary changes in long-term behavior is recommended to optimize weight loss outcomes.

A variety of bariatric surgical procedures have been used. The jejunoileal bypass has been abandoned for decades because of delayed, severe complications, including liver failure, renal failure, and arthropathy. If these complications are identified before end-stage organ failure, reversal of the procedure can improve or stabilize organ function. Several procedures that modify the capacity of the stomach (gastroplasty, vertical stapling, vertical banded gastroplasty, gastric sleeve and gastric banding), but do not create malabsorption of nutrients, are employed, but these are generally less effective than the Roux-en-Y gastric bypass in terms of long-term weight loss and outright surgical failure. The partial pancreaticobiliary bypass, the very long limb Roux-en-Y gastric bypass, and the duodenal switch procedures have become popular because they create a degree of malabsorption that results in greater weight loss that the standard Roux-en-Y gastric bypass. Unfortunately, the incidence of severe, even fatal vitamin and mineral deficiencies is much higher with these procedures. The laparoscopic approach has allowed the time of hospitalization to be reduced considerably and with lesser rates of incisional hernias compared with open procedures.

Following surgery, almost all of the weight loss that occurs will happen during the first 1 to 2 years. Long-term (>5 year) success rates are outstanding in good programs. Virtually all patients with successful weight loss will have a dramatic improvement in the medical complications of obesity. For these reasons, bariatric surgery has become an important tool in the treatment of severe, medically complicated obesity.

The results of the Roux-en-Y gastric bypass for treatment of morbid obesity have been very favorable. Approximately 70% of patients achieve success as defined previously with this procedure. The mortality and morbidity (e.g., infection, anastomotic leak, wound dehiscence) of this procedure are low in centers with expertise, despite the high-risk population. Laparoscopic gastric banding is becoming more popular. Following any of the malabsorptive procedures, the patients deserve permanent follow-up specifically for adverse nutritional consequences.

The long-term follow-up of patients who have undergone gastric bypass surgery is needed to ensure adequate protein, calorie, vitamin, and mineral nutrition. Supplemental vitamin B_{12}, iron, and calcium are routinely added to standard multivitamins. The most common nutritional consequences of malabsorptive procedures are disorders of calcium and vitamin D metabolism (Chapter 252). An increase in bone alkaline phosphatase may signal calcium or vitamin D deficiency. Low plasma vitamin D levels and low urinary calcium excretion should prompt aggressive replacement therapy. Iron deficiency, other fat-soluble vitamin deficiencies, and cases of copper deficiency occurring more than 5 to 10 years after surgery have been described. There have also been cases of pancreatogenous hypoglycemia that develop after bariatric surgical procedures. The symptoms are primarily postprandial and may be severe enough to warrant partial pancreatectomy. Findings at the time of surgery in these cases have ranged from islet hyperplasia and hypertrophy to multiple small insulinomas. Thus, it is important not to dismiss symptoms of postprandial cognitive dysfunction in patients who have undergone gastric bypass surgery.

TABLE 227-6	INDICATIONS FOR PHARMACOLOGIC TREATMENT OF OBESITY

Body mass index > 27 kg/m²
One or more complications or conditions that are likely to improve with weight loss
Previous failure of conservative treatment with diet and exercise
Agree to 2- to 4-wk trial of making initial changes in diet and exercise before starting pharmacotherapy
Agree to continued treatment with diet, exercise, and behavioral modification while on pharmacologic treatment
Agree to periodic follow-up
Premenopausal women (able to have children) must use some form of contraception
Consider a pregnancy test when initiating treatment if any possibility of pregnancy
No contraindications to the specific drug used for pharmacologic treatment

PREVENTION

The dramatic increase in the prevalence of obesity over the past few decades strongly suggests that preventive strategies are needed. Public health approaches that emphasize education have been almost uniformly unsuccessful at preventing weight gain or producing weight loss. Public health strategies that virtually impose behavior change are more successful in this regard. Unless widespread efforts are made to address the problem of obesity, it is likely that its prevalence and complications will become an ever-increasing health burden.

1. Sacks FM, Bray GA, Carey VJ, et al. Comparison of weight-loss diets with different compositions of fat, protein, and carbohydrates. *N Engl J Med.* 2009;360:859-873.
2. Shaw K, Gennat H, O'Rourke P, et al. Exercise for overweight or obesity. *Cochrane Database Syst Rev.* 2006;2:CD003817.
3. Wadden TA, Berkowitz RI, Womble LG, et al. Randomized trial of lifestyle modification and pharmacotherapy for obesity. *N Engl J Med.* 2005;353:2111-2120.

SUGGESTED READINGS

Bessonova L, Marshall SF, Ziogas A, et al. The association of body mass index with mortality in the California Teachers Study. *Int J Cancer.* Jan 4, 2011. [Epub ahead of print.] *All-cause mortality was increased for BMI < 18.5 and BMI ≥ 30 relative to a BMI of 18.5 to 24.9.*

Birkmeyer NJ, Dimick JB, Share D, et al. Hospital complication rates with bariatric surgery in Michigan. *JAMA.* 2010;304:435-442. *Serious complications occurred in 0.9% of gastric banding procedures and were inversely associated with procedure volume.*

Knowler WC, Barrett-Connor E, Fowler SE, et al, for the Diabetes Prevention Program Research Group. Ten-year follow-up of diabetes incidence and weight loss in the Diabetes Prevention Program Outcomes Study. *Lancet.* 2009;374:1677-1686. *Continued health benefit of lifestyle intervention 10 years after starting the DPP.*

XVIII

ENDOCRINE DISEASES

228

APPROACH TO THE PATIENT WITH ENDOCRINE DISEASE

DAVID R. CLEMMONS

Most endocrine disorders are due to either an excess or a deficiency of a hormone that is transported in the systemic circulation and therefore result in multiorgan manifestations. It is unusual for patients to present with a single isolated set of symptoms that are referable to only one organ system. Additionally, generalized nonspecific symptoms such as weakness, difficulty concentrating, lack of energy, and change in appetite occur commonly in patients with endocrine disorders. Often, a constellation of symptoms is required to point the clinician in the direction of the correct diagnosis, and single symptoms evaluated in isolation are rarely helpful even if one considers an exhaustive differential diagnosis (Table 228-1). Another important feature of the evaluation of patients presenting with endocrinologic disease is obtaining a good longitudinal history. The duration of exposure to a hormone excess or deficiency often dictates the severity of symptoms, and characterizing the symptomatic changes that occur over time can be very helpful in both selecting the tests to confirm the diagnosis and either substantiating the need for treatment or selecting the correct mode of treatment. Physical examination is helpful for confirming the likelihood of a diagnosis; for example, the presence of a symmetrically enlarged thyroid gland indicates that Graves' disease is the most likely cause of hyperthyroidism. However, because of the accuracy and precision of modern endocrinologic testing, endocrine disorders sometimes are diagnosed in the absence of symptoms or signs of overt disease (e.g., hyperparathyroidism). In such instances, a thorough history and physical examination are still important because they establish that the patient is truly in the asymptomatic phase of the disease, and this is often helpful in determining whether therapy or observation is required. A careful temporal history of a symptomatic change may also be helpful in the differential diagnosis, for example, in ascertaining whether a thyroid mass is likely due to a hemorrhagic cyst (i.e., occurring suddenly) or is a thyroid adenoma that might have evolved over an extended period. A thorough general history and physical examination may help to establish the diagnosis of diseases that are associated with endocrinologic abnormalities, such as cancers that ectopically secrete hormones, or may help to exclude the likelihood of an endocrinologic etiology of a specific disease manifestation.

Precise genetic testing to establish the etiology of endocrinologic syndromes is becoming more prevalent; therefore, an accurate family history can be useful in determining the need for genetic testing and familial screening. A thorough evaluation of medication use is also mandatory. Some medications can clearly mask the symptoms of overt endocrine disease, such as β-blockers in hyperthyroidism, and others can exacerbate the findings, such as hydrochlorothiazide use in hyperparathyroidism. Often, specific medications will confound laboratory evaluation, such as diuretics in patients with hyperaldosteronism or antihypertensive drugs in patients being screened for pheochromocytoma. Appropriate withdrawal of the medication may be required to establish a firm diagnosis. Medications may also directly alter a laboratory test, such as use of oral contraceptives in attempting to diagnose hyperthyroidism or hypothyroidism. Finally, an accurate history of the specific complaint may be challenging. For example, in evaluating male sexual dysfunction, a corroborating history from the patient's partner is often necessary for verification.

COMMON SYMPTOMS OF ENDOCRINOLOGIC DISEASE

Generalized symptoms such as weakness and fatigue are prominent features of adrenal insufficiency, hyperthyroidism and hypothyroidism, hypopituitarism, and poorly controlled diabetes mellitus. Pain is an uncommon complaint in endocrinologic disorders and is usually only seen with acute endocrinologic emergencies, such as diabetic ketoacidosis or acute adrenal insufficiency (abdominal pain). Chronic pain seen in primary or secondary hyperparathyroidism due to bone reabsorption and in osteomalacia (Chapter 252) can occur in the shafts of the long bones. Symptoms of

menstrual dysfunction are common in women with adrenal insufficiency, hypopituitarism, Cushing's syndrome, hyperprolactinemia, hyperthyroidism or hypothyroidism, and polycystic ovarian disease and primary ovarian failure. Weakness and easy fatigability can be secondary to anemia, which is common in adrenal insufficiency, androgen deficiency, hypothyroidism, hyperparathyroidism, and panhypopituitarism.

The most common endocrine-related symptom of intestinal dysfunction is constipation. This occurs frequently in patients with diabetic autonomic neuropathy and in hypercalcemia, hypothyroidism, or pheochromocytoma. Diarrhea can be an early and prominent symptom in hyperthyroidism and metastatic carcinoid tumors. Fever, like abdominal pain, usually only occurs in endocrine emergencies, typically in severe adrenal insufficiency and very severe hyperthyroidism. Generalized hair loss not related to androgen excess occurs in hypothyroidism, hypopituitarism, and thyrotoxicosis. Typical male-pattern baldness can be a feature of hirsutism in women as well as Cushing's syndrome and acromegaly. Persistent recurrent headaches are a feature of expanding pituitary tumors, whereas episodic headaches occur frequently in patients with pheochromocytoma and hypoglycemia. Changes in libido are often present in patients with hyperthyroidism, hypopituitarism, hypogonadism, Cushing's syndrome, and poorly controlled diabetes mellitus. Polyuria and nocturia are features of both diabetes insipidus and diabetes mellitus and can also occur in severe hypercalcemia.

Weight gain is an early symptom of Cushing's syndrome and hypothyroidism. Weight loss accompanied by anorexia is common in adrenal insufficiency in metastatic hormone-producing tumors such as ectopic adrenocorticotropic (ACTH) hormone syndrome, type 1 diabetes mellitus, and panhypopituitarism. Weight loss with no change or an increase in appetite is common in hyperthyroidism (see Table 228-1). An important differential diagnostic issue in patients with weight loss is depression. Depression can occur concomitantly in patients with adrenal insufficiency, Cushing's syndrome, hypercalcemia, and hypothyroidism.

An important neuropsychiatric symptom is widening of mood swings, that is, an exaggeration of normal cyclothymic changes. This occurs in hyperthyroidism and Cushing's syndrome. A history of skin changes occurs with several endocrine disorders. Acanthosis nigricans occurs with severe obesity, polycystic ovarian disease, severe insulin resistance syndromes, Cushing's syndrome, and acromegaly. Acne is a symptom of androgen excess and occurs with androgen-producing tumors, polycystic ovarian disease, and Cushing's syndrome. Generalized hyperpigmentation occurs in Addison's disease and Nelson's syndrome. Dry skin is present in almost all patients with hypothyroidism. It also occurs in panhypopituitarism. In Cushing's syndrome, skin changes such as striae, plethora, and easy bruisability are common. Vitiligo occurs in association with several endocrine autoimmune diseases, most prominently with autoimmune thyroid disease and Addison's disease.

Assessment of any of these symptoms in isolation is unlikely to lead a clinician to the correct diagnosis. However, assessment of combinations of these symptoms (e.g., the combination of weight gain, constipation, cold intolerance, and dry skin in hypothyroidism) is likely to lead to the correct set of diagnostic decisions.

PHYSICAL EXAMINATION

Physical examination of a patient with a suspected endocrine disorder is extremely helpful in terms of confirming the significance of findings that were ascertained by a careful medical history (Table 228-2). Examination of the skin is important because endocrinopathies lead to skin changes that progress over time. These often occur early in the course of the illness and can be a major aid in making the correct diagnosis. Primary adrenal failure is usually accompanied by increased skin pigmentation, particularly over the creases of the palms and extensor surfaces. The oral mucosa is often hyperpigmented, which can be helpful in African Americans. Patients with Cushing's syndrome present with persistent facial plethora, acne, and characteristic striae, which are generally larger than 1 cm and exhibit a dark red to purplish hue. These are most common over the abdomen. The presence of axillary purpura is also suggestive of Cushing's syndrome and results from increased capillary fragility. Patients with acromegaly often present with excessive skin tags that increase in number over time and multiple types of benign skin tumors such as dermatofibromas and lipomas. The skin is also much thicker over the dorsum of the hand, and the amount of subcutaneous tissue in the palms is prominent. Patients with Cushing's syndrome have thinning of the skin over the forehead and around the eyes. Patients with hypothyroidism often present with evidence of hyperkeratosis, particularly over the extensor surfaces. Severe long-standing thyroid disease is also accompanied by myxedema of

TABLE 228-1 SYMPTOM CONSTELLATIONS SUGGESTING SPECIFIC ENDOCRINE DISORDERS

SYMPTOM CONSTELLATION	DIAGNOSIS
Weakness, fatigue, anorexia, loss of appetite, postural blood pressure changes	Adrenal insufficiency
Cold intolerance, dry skin, constipation, weight gain	Hypothyroidism
Fatigue, easy bruising, striae, proximal muscle weakness, central obesity, hypertension, acne	Cushing's syndrome
Weight loss, increased appetite, palpitations, tremor, emotional lability, diffuse hair thinning	Hyperthyroidism
Galactorrhea, amenorrhea, headaches	Prolactin-producing pituitary tumor
Weight loss, anorexia, loss of pubic and axillary hair	Hypopituitarism
Episodic palpitations, tremor, anxiety, headaches, sweating, weight loss	Pheochromocytoma
Episodic flushing, palpitations, abdominal cramping, and diarrhea	Carcinoid syndrome

TABLE 228-2 PHYSICAL SIGNS THAT SUGGEST SPECIFIC ENDOCRINE DISORDERS

1. Hyperpigmentation of palms, extensor surfaces, and buccal mucosa	Adrenal insufficiency
2. Facial plethora, moon facies, striae, purpura	Cushing's syndrome
3. Skin tags, acral enlargement, prognathism, orthodontia	Acromegaly
4. Proptosis, lid lag, symmetrically diffuse thyroid enlargement, hyperreflexia	Graves' disease
5. Retinal microaneurysms, macular edema	Diabetic retinopathy
6. Short stature, web neck, loss of tears	Turner's syndrome
7. Shield-like chest, short fourth vertebra	Primary ovarian failure

the extremities, a specific skin finding of thickening of both the dermis and epidermis due to mucopolysaccharide accumulation. In contrast, patients with Graves' disease present with thinning of the skin, but more prominently with skin that is moist and warm. Both adrenal insufficiency and hyperthyroidism or hypothyroidism can be associated with vitiligo. The nails in hyperthyroidism reveal onycholysis in cases of longer duration. Hair changes occur commonly with several endocrinopathies. In hypothyroidism, the hair becomes coarse, whereas in hyperthyroidism, diffuse thinning occurs. Longstanding hypothyroidism can be accompanied by loss of the lateral third of the eyebrow hair. Hirsutism with hair growth over the areolae and along the linea alba is present in patients with gonadal dysfunction or with hyperandrogenism due to polycystic ovarian disease or androgen-producing tumors. In contrast, patients with hypopituitarism or hypogonadism often present with loss of pubic and axillary hair.

The eye examination can be helpful in establishing the diagnosis of hyperthyroidism. Graves' ophthalmopathy occurs in 40% of patients and presents with exophthalmos that can be unilateral. Extraocular movement assessment is important in patients with pituitary tumors because local expansion of these tumors can lead to third, fourth, or sixth nerve palsies, whereas compression of the optic tracts can cause the distinctive visual field defect of bitemporal hemianopsia. On neck examination, ascertainment of whether a goiter is smooth, symmetrical, and multinodular or a single nodule can be helpful in guiding further work-up in the evaluation of hyperthyroidism.

Cardiovascular evaluation is helpful for evaluating the severity and duration of endocrine illness. Patients with hyperthyroidism have evidence of increased sympathomimetic activity, including tachycardia, a widened pulse pressure, and prominent precordial activity. Flow murmurs may be heard as a result of increased cardiac output, and occasionally a bruit is easily heard on auscultation of the thyroid. In patients with hypothyroidism and Addison's disease, these findings are reversed. Specific cardiac abnormalities, such as coarctation of the aorta, may be present in patients with primary ovarian failure due to Turner's syndrome. Patients with pheochromocytoma often have a postural blood pressure change of greater than 20 mm Hg. Cardiomyopathy can be a feature of acromegaly. Hypertension is common in many

endocrine disorders, including hypercalcemia, hyperparathyroidism, acromegaly, diabetes mellitus, obesity, Cushing's syndrome, primary aldosteronism, and pheochromocytoma.

Nearly all patients with acromegaly demonstrate evidence of hand and foot enlargement, a very unusual occurrence in adulthood. This often manifests as a history of changing ring size or shoe size and is easily demonstrable on physical examination. Patients with hyperthyroidism often have a significant hand tremor and evidence of peripheral bruits on auscultation. Evaluation of the extremities is also helpful in the differential diagnosis of metabolic bone disease. The presence of bowing of the legs can be found in either dietary or X-linked hypophosphatemic rickets. The presence of edema is usually an early sign of disorders of hormone-producing tumors that result in salt retention, including Cushing's syndrome and hyperaldosteronism. Measurement of upper to lower segment ratios and span is helpful in establishing the timing and onset of puberty in primary gonadal disorders.

Pelvic examination is a major aid to the differential diagnosis of ovarian disorders. The presence of polycystic ovaries can sometimes be determined by palpation as well as the absence of ovarian tissue. The absence of a uterus is important in the differential diagnosis of pseudohermaphroditism, and the evaluation of external genitalia can be important in establishing the presence of congenital adrenal hyperplasia. Vaginal dryness is a sign of severe estrogen deficiency, as is breast atrophy. Hyperprolactinemia often first manifests as the presence of expressible galactorrhea.

Neurologic changes can occur in a variety of diseases. Evaluation of the ability to detect monofilament or vibratory sensation is an important tool for evaluating the presence of diabetic neuropathy. The presence of peripheral motor nerve defects in diabetes is also an important presenting sign, as is the presence of a cranial nerve palsy, such as third nerve palsy. Funduscopic examination can reveal microaneurysms, even in patients with undiagnosed type 2 diabetes, and this can be helpful for estimating antecedent duration of illness. Hyporeflexia with a delayed relaxation phase is one of the earliest physical changes in hypothyroidism and is prominent in most patients with clinically significant disease; hyperreflexia occurs in hyperthyroidism. Patients with Cushing's syndrome often have extreme proximal muscle weakness, and this occurs in severe long-standing hyperthyroidism. Midgut carcinoids frequently present with severe flushing and diarrhea. The skin characteristically has an unusual purplish hue, and this change typically lasts for the duration of the episode, about 20 to 30 minutes. Mental status changes occur frequently in patients with Cushing's syndrome, hyperthyroidism, and extreme hypercalcemia.

LABORATORY EVALUATION

Patients with endocrinologic diseases are frequently diagnosed in an asymptomatic state as a result of abnormal radiologic evaluation or hormonal testing abnormalities.

The most common radiologic conundrums occur in patients who are noted incidentally to have small pituitary, thyroid, or adrenal masses. Although most of these patients generally do not have a hormonal dysfunction syndrome, proper evaluation to exclude the presence of a functionally active tumor is usually necessary. For pituitary tumors, the minimal evaluation would include measurements of a baseline serum prolactin level and, in cases with suggestive symptoms, of 24-hour urine free cortisol and of growth hormone after glucose suppression. In patients with incidentally found adrenal masses ("incidentalomas"), important findings are a large tumor mass (i.e., >4 cm), the hypertension or hypokalemia, and symptoms and signs of Cushing's syndrome. If any of these are present, appropriate evaluation to exclude hyperaldosteronism, Cushing's syndrome, and pheochromocytoma should be undertaken.

The sensitivity and specificity of hormonal testing have reached levels that have significantly changed the initial evaluation of patients for endocrine disorders. For example, screening of asymptomatic patients for thyroid disease, disorders of lipoprotein metabolism, and disorders of gonadal dysfunction are common and widespread.

Hormones are often measured using immunologic detection methods. Most measurements use blood or urine samples to detect the active hormone. Occasionally, measurement of a metabolite of the active hormone, such as 25-hydroxycholecalciferol (a vitamin D metabolite), is more reliable than that of the parent hormone. Some hormones (e.g., thyroxine) have a very long half-life in plasma, and therefore a measurement at any time of day reflects the ability of the gland to produce that hormone. However, other hormones (e.g., growth hormone) are secreted episodically, and therefore a static measurement may or may not be indicative of hormone excess or deficiency. In these cases, suppression or stimulation testing is used to confirm the diagnosis. Usually, an exogenous substance (e.g., ACTH) is administered either orally or intravenously, and the production of the hormone (e.g., cortisol) by the gland is either stimulated or suppressed.

Many hormones are present in the circulation bound to binding proteins. With the exception of peptide hormones that circulate in the free (unbound) form, this can cause problems in interpretation: medications or concomitant illnesses can result in a major change in the concentration of the binding protein, which, in turn, alters the total hormone concentration. This problem can be obviated either by measuring the binding protein itself or by direct measurement of the free hormone, such as measurement of free thyroxine. Free hormone measurements, however, can be less reliable than total hormone measurements; therefore, a decision sometimes needs to be made wherein the reliability of the assay is compared with the quality of the information that will be provided.

Often, static hormone measurements are used for screening, for example, morning cortisol in screening for the presence of hypoadrenalism. Subsequently, stimulation or suppression testing is used for confirmation of the diagnosis. In some cases, plasma measurements are much less reliable than urinary testing (e.g., in ruling in or out the presence of pheochromocytoma). In these cases, 24-hour urinary measurement of hormone is often required to document overproduction or deficiency. Urinary assays have the advantage of providing integrative assessment over 24 hours and thus are less likely to be susceptible to errors due to episodic hormonal secretion over time. Occasionally, measurements of other substances, such as electrolytes or metabolites, are also informative for confirming the diagnosis. For example measurement of 24-hour urinary calcium can be important in the differential diagnosis of hypercalcemia. Metabolites in the urine may be extremely important in the evaluation of adrenal disorders and in documentation of pheochromocytoma and carcinoid syndrome. Simultaneous measurements of two substances is extremely helpful in the diagnosis of some disorders. Measurement of simultaneous serum calcium and parathyroid hormone (PTH) is important for confirming the presence of hyperparathyroidism. Likewise, simultaneous measurement of blood glucose and insulin can be important in screening for the presence of an insulin-producing tumor. Indirect measurement of hormonal status can also be important; for example, measurement of insulin-like growth factor-I, which is inducible by growth hormone (GH), provides an integrative measure of GH secretion. Similarly, measurement of hemoglobin A_{1c} provides an integrative measurement of long-term blood sugar control in diabetes.

Imaging studies are commonly used in endocrine diagnosis. Magnetic resonance imaging and computed tomography are helpful in evaluating pituitary and adrenal masses. Scanning of the thyroid gland using radioactive iodine is useful for evaluation of the functional status of thyroid nodules and the functional activity of the thyroid gland as a whole. Bone mineral density testing is now commonplace in screening of patients for osteoporosis and in the evaluation of patients with established fracture syndromes. Imaging can also be combined with hormonal measurements. Specifically, cannulation of the adrenal veins can be helpful in confirming the presence of functioning adrenal tumors such as aldosteronomas and pheochromocytomas. Likewise, determining the location of ectopically located tumors such as those producing ACTH can often be confirmed by venous sampling procedures. Similarly, intraoperative measurements of hormones that change rapidly, such as intraoperative PTH, can help determine whether surgical removal of the hormone-secreting tumor has been adequate. The primary use of biopsy in endocrinologic diagnosis is fine-needle aspiration of the thyroid gland. This procedure can be done safely in the outpatient setting, often aided by ultrasound guidance. It is a highly accurate method for determining whether further diagnostic evaluation or therapeutic intervention is necessary.

GENETIC EVALUATION

Use of genetic testing in endocrinologic diagnosis has become much more commonplace. Polymerase chain reaction amplification of DNA obtained from peripheral blood cells is often used to determine the presence of a specific disorder. This has been extremely useful in differential diagnosis, for determining prognosis, and for deciding whether family screening is required (e.g., in the presence of multiple endocrine neoplasia). Whether genetic testing is required is often dictated by whether this information is necessary to solve a differential diagnostic problem (e.g., disorders of vitamin D metabolism) or to decide whether more extensive surgery should be required (e.g., in pheochromocytoma) or whether family screening is necessary (e.g., in multiple endocrine neoplasia 2 syndrome).

EVALUATION OF THE RESPONSE OF AN ENDOCRINE DISEASE TO TREATMENT

Most hormone excess syndromes are treated surgically by removal of the particular endocrine gland that is oversecreting the hormone. However, follow-up of these patients mandates that (1) it be established that the disease has truly been cured by gland resection or (2) if residual disease is present, and (3) determining whether repeat operation is likely to be of benefit to the patient or some other means of treating the patient should be undertaken. These decisions generally need to be made in consultation with surgeons and radiotherapists. If an endocrine deficiency is present, hormone replacement therapy is most often used to correct the disorder. In some cases, the efficacy of substitution therapy can be measured directly by laboratory testing, such as measurement of thyroid-stimulating hormone during thyroxine replacement. In other cases (e.g., measurement of ACTH suppression during substitution therapy for adrenal insufficiency), testing could lead to misleading information and overtreatment of patients; therefore, a combination of return of symptoms and signs to normal, laboratory testing, and indirect tests (e.g., potassium, blood urea nitrogen, and creatinine in the case of adrenal insufficiency) is required to determine the adequacy of replacement therapy. Understanding the pharmacology of the particular synthetic hormone used is important for proper replacement therapy. For example, synthetic glucocorticoids vary greatly in their half-life, and therefore dosage and timing of administration are important issues for patients receiving these hormones. Some patients, such as those with hypopituitarism, require substitution with multiple hormones, and often these need to be coordinated (e.g., glucocorticoid dosage in a patient with panhypopituitarism is dependent on the dosage of thyroid hormone that is administered). Because monitoring thyroid-stimulating hormone is not useful in such patients, empirical substitution with both hormones is required to establish that the therapeutic regimen results in return of functional activity to normal. At times, hormone excesses may have to be treated with ancillary medications; for example, β-blockade may be useful in patients with hyperthyroidism, and both α- and β-blockade are often necessary in patients with pheochromocytoma. The etiology of osteoporosis is often unknown. In most cases, this disease is generally treated by administration of agents that inhibit bone reabsorption by a variety of mechanisms, including the bisphosphonates, estrogen replacement therapy, and calcitonin.

Hormones are also used throughout medicine for treatment of other disorders, and sometimes these treatments result in a hormone excess syndrome. The most common example is administration of high-dose glucocorticoid therapy for immune suppression resulting in Cushing's syndrome. Similarly, growth hormone may be administered to children with short stature who do not have GH deficiency. PTH is the only agent available for stimulation of an anabolic effect in bone; therefore, it is administered to patients with osteoporosis even though they do not have hypoparathyroidism. Octreotide acetate, a long-acting derivative of somatostatin, can be useful for controlling gastrointestinal symptoms in patients with neuroendocrine tumors. Supraphysiologic doses of progesterone are commonly used as contraceptives. Hormone antagonists are also used in both endocrine and nonendocrine disorders. Estrogen receptor antagonists are commonly used in breast cancer therapy, as are androgen receptor antagonists in prostate cancer therapy. Similarly, gonadotropin-releasing hormone agonists have been found to be useful in patients with prostate cancer that is metastatic to bone. Prostaglandin antagonists are commonly used in acute and chronic inflammatory disorders, and angiotensin receptor antagonists as well as renin antagonists are used in the treatment of hypertension, whether it is due to an endocrine or nonendocrine etiology. A comprehensive knowledge of the actions of these hormones can intelligently guide the proper use of these agents in treating nonendocrine disorders.

SUGGESTED READINGS

Nieman LK. Approach to the patient with an adrenal incidentaloma. *J Clin Endocrinol Metab.* 2010;95:4106-4113. *Review emphasizing precontrast Hounsfield units and contrast washout on computed tomography.*

Petersenn S, Quabbe JH, Schöfl C, et al. The rational use of pituitary stimulation tests. *Dtsch Arztebl Int.* 2010;107:437-443. *An algorithmic approach to the diagnostic evaluation of possible pituitary insufficiency.*

Shivaraj G, Prakash BD, Sonal V, et al. Thyroid function tests: a review. *Eur Rev Med Pharmacol Sci.* 2009;13:341-349. *A practical approach to ordering and interpreting the variety of available tests.*

Vazquez BJ, Richards ML. Imaging of the thyroid and parathyroid glands. *Surg Clin North Am.* 2011;91:15-32. *Review including ultrasonography, nuclear scintigraphy, computed tomography, and magnetic resonance imaging.*

229

PRINCIPLES OF ENDOCRINOLOGY

DAVID R. CLEMMONS

REGULATION OF THE ENDOCRINE SYSTEM

Following their synthesis and secretion, hormones either act locally on neighboring cells (termed *paracrine actions*) or, after secretion into the general circulation, are transported to a distant site and function to stimulate target tissues. They also act on a cell of origin (termed an *autocrine action*). The endocrine system is under finely tuned control, most importantly through the process of negative feedback regulation, which functions to maintain homeostasis. Negative feedback regulation occurs when the hormone or metabolite level in blood reaches a concentration to which the system is set to respond in terms of altering hormone biosynthesis or secretion. For example, the pituitary gland, which secretes thyroid-stimulating hormone (TSH) to stimulate the thyroid gland to produce triiodothyronine (T_3) and thyroxine (T_4), is highly sensitive to feedback regulation (Fig. 229-1). The T_3 and T_4 from the circulation are transported to the pituitary, where they bind to the thyroid hormone receptor. When T_3 or T_4 reaches a threshold concentration, the receptor transmits a signal to stop the synthesis of TSH. In some cases, such as parathyroid hormone feedback, regulation occurs through the concentration of the primary metabolite (e.g., calcium), which feeds back directly onto the calcium-sensing receptor in the parathyroid glands. This receptor then transmits a signal to the nucleus to shut down parathyroid hormone (PTH) synthesis. In this way, each hormonal feedback loop maintains homeostasis. Sometimes, this can occur through a physical stimulus rather than a biochemical action. In the case of blood pressure regulation, when the renin and aldosterone concentrations have reached a certain level, changes in arterial blood pressure and renal blood flow feed back through the juxtaglomerular apparatus in the kidney to suppress renin production. This results in less conversion of angiotensinogen to angiotensin I and maintenance of blood pressure regulation. The result of hormone excess syndromes is disruption of this equilibrium, leading to an unrestrained excess of the hormone, which disrupts negative feedback regulation. Although under these conditions negative feedback regulation may still exist, either the set point is changed, or the tumor produces the hormone in such an episodic fashion that negative feedback regulation becomes irrelevant. The latter example would apply to Cushing's syndrome caused by an adrenal adenoma, whereas if the primary problem is an adrenocorticotropic hormone (ACTH)-producing pituitary tumor, the set point of the tumor is altered, resulting in production of ACTH that is subject to altered feedback regulation. Under certain circumstances, loss of negative feedback regulation results in significant hormonal abnormalities but no pathophysiologic changes. For example, in patients with ACTH-producing pituitary tumors, after removal of the adrenal glands, there is excess secretion of ACTH, but no effect will ensue other than hyperpigmentation.

A hormone may be produced by an endocrine gland (e.g., cortisol by the adrenal gland), or it may be produced by several cell types scattered throughout the body (e.g., prostaglandins). A hormone may be produced by a single cell type that occurs in multiple locations, such as adiponectin production by adipose tissue. The chemical structures of many hormones are similar. Steroid hormones are derived from cholesterol, as is vitamin D. Retinoids are derived from carotenoids in the diet and the eicosanoids from fatty acids. Some peptide hormones require not only synthesis and secretion by their gland of origin but also proteolytic processing following their release into the circulation. For example, angiotensinogen is secreted by the liver as an inactive prohormone that is proteolytically cleaved twice. The first cleavage occurs in the kidney by renin and results in angiotensin I, which is still inactive, and the second is in the lung by converting enzyme to form angiotensin II, a potent vasoconstrictor. Thyroid hormone contains the amino acid tyrosine, which is modified by iodination. Thus, ambient iodine intake and factors that control iodine uptake by the thyroid gland are important determinants of thyroid hormone production. Neurotransmitters can also function as hormones. Catecholamines are secreted not only by nerve endings but also by the adrenal medulla into the general circulation and are necessary for maintenance of normal blood pressure and cardiac function.

Several processes are involved in the synthesis of hormones. Peptide hormone synthesis is initiated with transcription of the encoding gene under the direct regulation of transcription factors. The nascent RNA is processed and translated into the peptide hormone. The peptide hormone is then modified by glycosylation or proteolytic cleavage and stored in storage granules until it is released. Some hormones are stored for extended periods and then released abruptly in response to stimuli. For example, insulin is stored in granules in the islet cells of the pancreas and released in response to fluctuations in blood glucose. This allows for rapid minute-to-minute regulation of plasma glucose concentrations based on carbohydrate intake or demands by tissues. Chronic exposure to the appropriate stimulus can also lead to increased cell number within the target endocrine gland. Thus, chronic exposure to hypoglycemia will increase islet cell size and number, leading to increased insulin secretion. Long-term exposure to hypocalcemia will result in the same change within the parathyroid glands. Excess TSH or ACTH will result in hypertrophy and hyperplasia of thyroid or adrenal cortical tissue, respectively.

Steroid hormones are derived from cholesterol by actions of several enzymes on the cytochrome P-450 class of oxidases. The first step in steroid hormone synthesis is rate limiting and involves cleavage of the cholesterol side-chain residues to pregnenolone. Trophic hormones such as ATCH stimulate the transcription of an enzyme termed *steroidogenic acute regulator*, or *STAR*, which acts within the mitochondria to activate the transport of cholesterol and its cleavage to pregnenolone. Steroid synthesis is then regulated by the specific enzymes that are induced by the specific trophic hormone; for example, if glucocorticoid production is required, 17- and 21-hydroxylases are activated, whereas if mineralocorticoid synthesis is required, 18-hydroxylase, a distinct enzyme, is activated.

HORMONE TRANSPORT IN THE GENERAL CIRCULATION

Because so many important hormones have to be transported through the circulation to their distal sites of action to achieve target cell effects, the capacity to bind and transport hormones can be an important determinant not only of the ambient plasma concentration but also of the amount that is bioavailable to cells and tissues. Steroid hormones and thyroxine are transported almost solely in protein-bound form. The globulins that bind these hormones are synthesized in the liver, and their synthesis is influenced by a variety of factors, including estrogens and androgens, genetic defects, and a variety of medications. These binding globulins can be measured directly, and sometimes this is necessary to determine whether a suspected deficiency or excess is in fact really due to a major change in the binding protein. Occasionally, peptides such as vasopressin or insulin-like growth factor-I also bind to binding proteins, and therefore binding proteins can be determinants of their plasma concentrations. At times, measurement of free hormone is required to ascertain whether a hormone excess or deficiency is present because of the severity of the binding protein abnormality (Chapter 228).

Hormone Action

Both peptide and steroid hormones bind specifically to receptors, which are complex, multifunctional proteins located on the surface of the cells (peptide hormone receptors) or in the cytoplasm (steroid hormone receptors). The

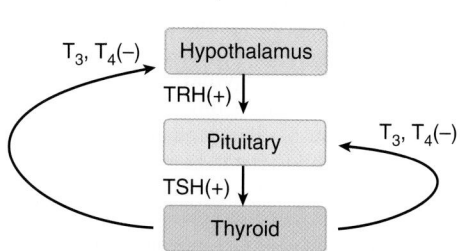

Thyroid Axis

FIGURE 229-1. Hypothalamic-pituitary-thyroid axis illustrating negative feedback regulation. Following thyroid-stimulating hormone (TSH) secretion by the pituitary, the thyroid gland secretes T_3 and T_4, which feed back on the hypothalamus and pituitary to suppress further increases in thyrotropin-releasing hormone (TRH) and TSH secretion.

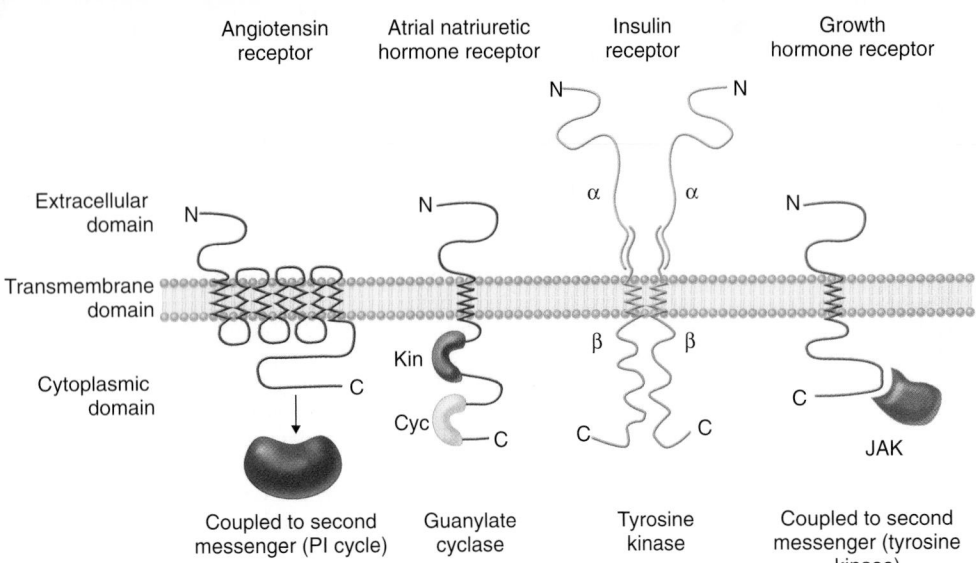

FIGURE 229-2. Structures of different types of peptide hormone receptors.

peptide hormone receptors have a ligand recognition domain, a domain that spans the plasma membrane, and a cytoplasmic domain. The extracellular domain contains the hormone recognition sequence, and the cytoplasmic domain contains the signal transduction apparatus.

Based on this general structure, peptide hormone receptors have been classified into four types (Fig. 229-2). The most common form is the 7-transmembrane domain receptor. These receptors contain the amino-terminal domain, which contains the hormone-binding unit, seven regions that cross the plasma membrane, and a cytoplasmic domain that is coupled to guanylate nucleotide–binding proteins or G proteins. Binding of the ligand to the receptor activates the G protein by a series of conformational changes resulting in a change in the shape of the cytoplasmic domain that allows it to interact directly with the G protein. The G proteins then function through a subunit signaling mechanism resulting in coordinate activation of enzymes such as adenylate cyclase or phospholipase C. These enzymes initiate a series of intracellular signaling events that trigger specific enzymatic reactions or downstream signaling events that initiate the biochemical changes that mediate the hormone's actions. Examples include calcium mobilization in cells by PTH, thyroxine biosynthesis in response to TSH, or steroidogenesis in response to ACTH or luteinizing hormone (LH).

A second group of receptors, the tyrosine kinase receptors, also contain an extracellular domain that is involved in ligand recognition. Ligand-binding sites within this group are highly specific, and this is a major determinant of activation of this class of receptors. Following hormone binding, these receptors undergo a conformational change that causes autocatalytic activation of intrinsic enzymatic activity contained within the sequence of the cytoplasmic domain (see Fig. 229-2). The prototype of this group is the insulin receptor, wherein the cytoplasmic domain contains an enzyme with protein kinase enzymatic activity. Once the enzyme is autocatalytically activated, it autophosphorylates intrinsically located tyrosines, which then form docking sites for signal transduction proteins that contain specific sequences that can bind to phosphorylated tyrosines, called SH2 or PTB domains. These sequences recognize a particular amino acid sequence surrounding the phosphotyrosine, which provides another level of specificity of activation. Activation of the insulin receptor then triggers binding of a transducer protein, termed *insulin receptor substrate-1* (IRS-1), that binds to these SH2 or PTB domains. IRS-1 undergoes further tyrosine phosphorylation by the intrinsic kinase activity of the insulin receptor. The phosphotyrosines act as docking sites for other important catalytic enzymes. The most important for glucose transport is the PI-3 kinase enzyme. This enzyme binds to specific phosphorylated tyrosines that are surrounded by specific flanking amino acids within the IRS-1 sequence. Its binding results in PI-3 kinase activation, which further activates a series of downstream signal transduction events leading to stimulation of glucose transport. Tyrosine kinase receptors can also activate a series of signaling events that lead to an increase in the transcription of specific genes. For example, activation of the IGF-I receptor leads to stimulation of an enzyme called MAP kinase. Its activation leads to its translocation to the nucleus, wherein it specifically activates gene transcription. Thus, tyrosine kinases represent an extremely diverse and functionally significant class of

enzymes that are able to regulate multiple pleiotropic events within cells and greatly influence hormone action.

A third class of receptors is the cytokine receptors. The peptide hormones, growth hormone and leptin, both activate cytokine receptors to initiate signaling (see Fig. 229-2). Unlike receptors with intrinsic tyrosine kinase activity, once these receptors undergo a conformational change, they recruit tyrosine kinases to their cytoplasmic domain. These kinases then phosphorylate the receptor directly. The phosphorylated tyrosines on the receptor mediate the binding of a specific class of transcription factors termed *signal transducers of activators of transcription* (STATS). The STATS are then further phosphorylated by the same tyrosine kinase that phosphorylates the receptor, resulting in their activation and transport to the nucleus where they initiate gene transcription. A fourth class of membrane proteins that interact with hormones is termed *ligand regulated transporters*. These bind to a diverse set of ligands such as low-density lipoprotein, transferrin, and atrial natriuretic peptide. The cytoplasmic domain is not involved in signaling; instead, after transport of the active substance such as low-density lipoprotein across the cell membrane, the substance is endocytosed and further processed. This is also the model for the receptors for atrial natriuretic hormone and transferrin, with the latter being internalized together with its bound iron molecule.

Nuclear Receptors
Nuclear receptors, present in the cytoplasm of target cells, are important for mediating the actions of steroid hormones, thyroid, retinoids, vitamin D, fatty acids, and prostaglandins (Fig. 229-3). After ligand binding, the receptor-hormone complex is translocated to the nucleus. Each receptor contains a DNA-binding domain that contains zinc fingers or regions of a protein that are linked to a zinc atom that allows the receptor to assume a conformation that fits in a groove in the DNA. The complex binds to specific regions of DNA (called promoters) that control the gene transcription. In general, these receptors dimerize before binding. At times, heterodimers form instead of homodimers. An example of this is steroid hormone receptors that bind with the retinoid X receptor to form a heterodimer. Specific DNA sequence domains that are arranged in repetitive sequences form the nuclear receptor–binding site. Small variations in these sequences provide specificity. Although specificity for binding to this sequence is relatively high, there is some overlap. For example, high concentrations of ligand-activated progesterone receptor can bind to glucocorticoid receptor–regulated genes. In some cases, the activated hormone receptor, such as the thyroid hormone receptor, interacts with a specific protein in the nucleus, in this case CREB-binding protein, to activate transcription. These binding proteins are capable of interacting with more than one transcription factor. In many cases, the ligand-hormone complex interacts with the DNA in a *cis* manner and enhances transcription of target genes. Hormone-activated receptors can also repress transcription. Several major negative feedback loops operate through this process. For example, the activated cortisol receptor will suppress ACTH secretion, and activated thyroid hormone receptors will suppress TSH α- and β-subunit transcription. Other cytoplasmic signaling molecules can modify these responses through DNA-binding proteins. An example is cyclic adenosine

FIGURE 229-3. How steroid hormone receptors function. *Left,* Glucocorticoid receptor family members bind as homodimers to palindromic DNA sites. Thyroid hormone receptor family members bind primarily as heterodimers with retinoid X receptor to direct repeat DNA sites separated by varying numbers of base pairs. *Right,* As a result of hormone binding, repressor complexes dissociate and activator complexes bind to nuclear receptors. Repressor complexes contain histone deacetylase (HDAC), and activator complexes contain histone acetylase (CAF).

monophosphate binding, which regulates CREB activation. CREB then binds to DNA to control gene transcription by peptide hormones.

SUGGESTED READINGS

Migliarini B, Piccinetti CC, Martella A, et al. Perspectives on endocrine disruptor effects on metabolic sensors. *Gen Comp Endocrinol.* 2011;170:416-423. *Review of how endocrine-disrupting chemicals increase or block metabolism of peptide and steroid hormones by activating or antagonizing nuclear receptors.*

Visser WE, Friesema EC, Visser TJ. Minireview: thyroid hormone transporters: the knowns and the unknowns. *Mol Endocrinol.* 2011;25:1-14. *Review of TH transporter proteins and how they facilitate movement across the plasma membrane to regulate intracellular effects.*

Wang C, Tian L, Popov VM, et al. Acetylation and nuclear receptor action. *J Steroid Biochem Mol Biol.* 2011;123:91-100. *Review emphasizing how acetylation of transcription factors can regulate cellular growth.*

230

NEUROENDOCRINOLOGY AND THE NEUROENDOCRINE SYSTEM

MARK E. MOLITCH

NEUROENDOCRINE REGULATION

Neuroendocrinology refers to the area of endocrinology in which the nervous system interacts with the endocrine system to link neural activity with metabolic and hormonal homeostatic activity. The *neurohypophysial* neurons originate from the paraventricular and supraoptic nuclei, traverse the hypothalamic-pituitary stalk, and release vasopressin and oxytocin from nerve endings in the posterior pituitary. The *hypophysiotropic* neurons, localized in specific hypothalamic nuclei, project their axons to the median eminence to secrete their peptide and bioamine releasing and inhibiting hormones into the proximal end of the hypothalamic-pituitary portal vessels (Fig. 230-1). The median eminence receives its blood supply from the superior hypophysial artery, which arborizes into a rich capillary bed. The capillary loops extend into the median eminence and coalesce to form the long portal veins that traverse the pituitary stalk and end in the pituitary. The neuroendocrine system operates through a series of feedback loops that regulate pituitary and target organ hormone levels. Target organ hormones can feed back at both the hypothalamic and the pituitary levels to complete the loop. The feedback loops can be perturbed, resulting in alterations of set points by such factors as length of day (circadian periodicity), stress, nutritional status, and systemic illness.

Hypophysiotropic Hormones

Regulation of pituitary hormones by the hypophysiotropic hormones is quite complex, in part because of the multiplicity of substances present in the hypothalamus that can affect pituitary hormone secretion and in part because of the redundancy and overlapping nature of the feedback loops alluded to earlier. In addition, some hypophysiotropic hormones exert effects on more than one pituitary hormone.

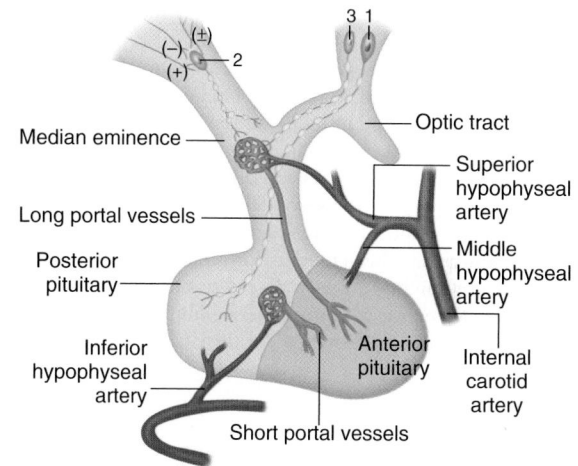

FIGURE 230-1. Neuroendocrine organization of the hypothalamus and pituitary gland. The posterior pituitary is fed by the inferior hypophyseal artery and the hypothalamus by the superior hypophyseal artery, both branches of the internal carotid artery. Most of the blood supply to the anterior pituitary is venous by way of the long portal vessels, which connect the portal capillary beds in the median eminence to the venous sinusoids in the anterior pituitary. Hypophysiotropic neuron 3 in the parvocellular division of the paraventricular nucleus and neuron 2 in the arcuate nucleus are shown to terminate in the median eminence on portal capillaries. These neurons of the tuberoinfundibular system secrete hypothalamic releasing and inhibiting hormones into the portal veins for conveyance to the anterior pituitary gland. Neuron 2 is innervated by monoaminergic neurons. Note that the multiple inputs to such neurons, using neuron 2 as an example, can be stimulatory, inhibitory, or neuromodulatory, in which another neuron may affect neurotransmitter release. Neuron 1 represents a peptidergic neuron originating in the magnocellular division of the paraventricular nucleus or supraoptic nucleus and projecting directly to the posterior pituitary by way of the hypothalamic-neurohypophyseal tract. (From Gay VL. The hypothalamus: physiology and clinical use of releasing factors. *Fertil Steril.* 1972;23:50-63, with permission of the American Society for Reproductive Medicine.)

Thyrotropin-Releasing Hormone

The primary neuroendocrine functions of thyrotropin-releasing hormone (TRH) are to stimulate the synthesis and release of thyroid-stimulating hormone (TSH) and prolactin. In cases of hypothyroidism, the increased TRH synthesis and binding to the pituitary results in increased TSH and prolactin levels. Correction of the hypothyroidism with thyroid hormones decreases the elevated TSH and prolactin levels. Conversely, in cases of hyperthyroidism, TSH levels are markedly suppressed. Although TRH is the major regulator of TSH synthesis and secretion, the role of TRH as a physiologic prolactin-releasing factor (PRF) is undefined.

Gonadotropin-Releasing Hormone

Gonadotropin-releasing hormone (GnRH) is a 10–amino acid peptide; its neurons originate in the epithelium of the medial part of the olfactory placode. This origin of GnRH-producing neurons from olfactory epithelium is of clinical interest with respect to the entity of Kallmann's syndrome, in which GnRH deficiency is associated with agenesis of the olfactory bulbs.

One form of Kallmann's syndrome is caused by loss of function of a protein (anosmin) that facilitates the embryologic migration of these GnRH-producing neurons. The primary function of GnRH is to stimulate the secretion of luteinizing hormone (LH) and follicle-stimulating hormone (FSH). Only one GnRH has been identified, and the differential secretion of LH and FSH is due to variations in sensitivity of the feedback effects of steroid and peptide hormones and variations in sensitivity to GnRH. GnRH pulsatile secretion directly increases its own receptor number whereas continuous administration of GnRH is associated with a decrease. In women, positive and negative steroid hormone feedback regulation of the hypothalamic-pituitary-gonadal axis occurs at both the pituitary and the hypothalamic levels, the hypothalamic effects being alteration of GnRH pulse amplitude and frequency and the pituitary effects being modulation of the gonadotropin response to GnRH. In males, testosterone decreases GnRH pulsatile secretion, with a resultant decrease in gonadotropin pulse amplitude and frequency as well as a decreased gonadotropin response to exogenous GnRH.

The negative feedback effects of inhibin, a peptide produced by testicular Sertoli cells and ovarian granulosa cells, are predominantly on FSH at the pituitary, where inhibin causes a decrease in the sensitivity of gonadotrophs to GnRH. The related ovarian protein activin stimulates basal and GnRH-stimulated FSH synthesis and release from the pituitary, but its primary action is to facilitate the response of ovarian granulosa cells to FSH. Another gonadal peptide, follistatin, also inhibits the oophorectomy- and GnRH-induced rise in FSH selectively, primarily by binding to activin. These ovarian peptides are also found in the pituitary and may therefore have additional local effects on gonadotropin secretion.

GnRH has been administered in pulsatile fashion to individuals with hypogonadotropic hypogonadism secondary to GnRH deficiency with great success, that is, restoration of normal sexual function and fertility. Long-acting GnRH agonists have been used to downregulate GnRH receptors and gonadotropin secretion in a variety of conditions, including precocious puberty, prostate cancer, breast cancer, uterine fibroids, and endometriosis. Direct GnRH antagonists that compete for the GnRH receptor are used for similar conditions.

Somatostatin

Somatostatin (also known as *somatotropin release-inhibiting factor*) inhibits GH secretion. The interaction of somatostatin and growth hormone–releasing hormone (GHRH) on GH secretion is complex. GH secretory episodes are associated with increased GHRH secretion, often accompanied by low somatostatin levels; the basal or trough GH levels are associated with low GHRH levels and more elevated somatostatin levels. Somatostatin also inhibits basal and stimulated TSH secretion. However, GH is about 10-fold more sensitive to inhibition by somatostatin than is TSH, thus suggesting that the physiologic role of somatostatin in inhibiting TSH secretion is limited.

Somatostatin is also present in D cells of the pancreatic islets, the gut mucosa, and the myenteric neural plexus. Through paracrine and endocrine actions, it suppresses the secretion of insulin, glucagon, cholecystokinin, gastrin, secretin, vasoactive intestinal polypeptide (VIP), and other gastrointestinal hormones, as well as such functions as gastric acid secretion, gastric emptying, gallbladder contraction, and splanchnic blood flow. Analogues of somatostatin have been developed for the treatment of acromegaly, carcinoid tumors, VIP-secreting tumors, TSH-secreting pituitary tumors, and islet cell tumors.

Corticotropin-Releasing Hormone

Corticotropin-releasing hormone (CRH) releases adrenocorticotropic hormone (ACTH), β-endorphin, β-lipotropin, melanocyte-stimulating hormone (MSH), and other peptides generated from pro-opiomelanocortin (POMC) in equimolar amounts. CRH mediates 75% of the ACTH response to stress. The remaining 25% is due to vasopressin. CRH and vasopressin have synergistic effects on ACTH release. CRH and vasopressin are not always released coordinately, however, and stress selectively activates the vasopressin-containing subset of CRH neurons. Cortisol feeds back to decrease ACTH secretion at both the hypothalamic and the pituitary levels. ACTH and β-endorphin also feed back negatively to decrease CRH release by the hypothalamus. Central bioamines, opioids, and peptides influence CRH secretion. Monokines released by inflammatory tissue, such as interleukin-1, interleukin-6, and tumor necrosis factor-α, stimulate the synthesis and release of CRH and vasopressin from the hypothalamus. The consequent increase in cortisol then reduces the intensity of the inflammatory response and release of these monokines, thus completing the feedback loop. CRH receptors are widely distributed in the brain, and increases in CRH are associated with activation of the sympathetic nervous system, suppression of the parasympathetic nervous system, stimulation of arousal, and increased learning performance. CRH may also be involved in the regulation of body weight; with overfeeding, increased leptin stimulates CRH, which causes decreased food intake and increased energy expenditure.

Biosynthetic human CRH has become available for clinical use. Its major utility is in the differential diagnosis of Cushing's disease versus ectopic ACTH syndrome, with the finding that patients with Cushing's disease respond with a greater than 35% increment, whereas those with ectopic ACTH secretion have a lesser response. If the results are equivocal, CRH testing during bilateral inferior petrosal sinus sampling for ACTH often provides additional discriminatory information.

Growth Hormone–Releasing Hormone

GHRH dose-dependently stimulates GH secretion. With repetitive administration, GHRH can cause the release of sufficient GH in children with GHRH deficiency to result in an increase in IGF-I levels and an acceleration of growth. Both IGF-I and GH feed back negatively on GH secretion. This negative feedback results in both a decrease in GHRH and an increase in somatostatin. The feedback effect of IGF-I is clinically relevant, as documented by the high circulating GH levels that occur in IGF-I-deficient states, such as renal insufficiency and cirrhosis. In children with mutations of the GH receptor resulting in their not being responsive to GH (GH insensitivity syndrome, also known as Laron-type dwarfism), IGF-I levels are very low, and GH levels are correspondingly elevated. A separate GH-stimulating system for GH secretion involves a distinct receptor, termed the *GH secretagogue* (GHS) receptor, that interacts with a 28–amino acid peptide called Ghrelin that was initially isolated from the stomach. GHS receptor and Ghrelin messenger RNA are both present in the pituitary and hypothalamus of humans. The interaction of Ghrelin physiologically with GHRH and somatostatin is complex but appears to be of minor importance. However, Ghrelin may play a more important role in the regulation of appetite and food intake.

Prolactin Inhibitory Factor

The inhibitory component of hypothalamic regulation of prolactin secretion predominates over the stimulatory component. Dopamine is the major physiologic prolactin inhibitory factor. It is likely that in most physiologic circumstances that cause a rise in prolactin, such as lactation, a simultaneous fall in dopamine occurs along with a rise in a PRF such as VIP. Blockade of endogenous dopamine receptors by a variety of drugs, such as the neuroleptics, causes a rise in prolactin. Lesions that interrupt the basal hypothalamic neuronal pathways carrying dopamine to the median eminence or that interrupt portal blood flow, such as craniopharyngiomas or other large mass lesion, result in decreased dopamine reaching the pituitary and hyperprolactinemia.

Prolactin-Releasing Factor

A number of hypothalamic peptides other than TRH have also been shown to have PRF activity. VIP stimulates prolactin synthesis and release at concentrations found in hypothalamic-pituitary portal blood. Within the VIP precursor is another similarly sized peptide known as peptide histidine methionine, which also has PRF activity. The precise roles of VIP versus peptide histidine methionine are not clear. It appears to be of negligible physiologic importance in humans.

Endogenous Opioid Peptides

Most data now suggest a modest role for endogenous opioid peptides in neuroendocrine regulation. The endogenous opioid peptides have a common 5–amino acid sequence at their amino termini (Tyr-Gly-Gly-Phe-Met [or Leu]) that is important for their binding to endogenous opioid receptors and bioactivity. Three major opioid peptide receptors and three major groups of opioid peptides are recognized. The μ-receptor mediates most of the endocrine effects and analgesia. The primary peptide ligand for the μ-receptor is β-endorphin, which is derived from POMC. The δ-receptor mediates behavioral, analgesic, and some endocrine effects and has as its primary peptide ligands met- and leu-enkephalins, which are derived from proenkephalin A. It is much less well blocked by naloxone than is the μ-receptor. The κ-receptor mediates sedation and ataxia and binds primarily dynorphin and the neo-endorphins. A fourth receptor has recently been described that has considerable sequence homology with the δ-receptor and binds to an endogenous 17–amino acid peptide called nociceptin (also known as orphanin FQ).

POMC is a 31-kD precursor peptide that harbors within it ACTH, β-lipotropin, and β-endorphin. POMC undergoes tissue-specific post-translational processing. In the anterior pituitary, its major cleavage products are β-lipotropin and ACTH, with a significant proportion of β-lipotropin being further processed to β-endorphin. In the pituitary intermediate lobe, the major products are α-MSH, corticotropin-like intermediate peptide, β-endorphin, and γ-lipotropin. Brain POMC, however, is processed primarily to β-endorphin, γ-lipotropin, and ACTH, with most of the ACTH being further processed to corticotropin-like intermediate peptide and α-MSH. The pentapeptide enkephalins are derived from the 28-kD precursor proenkephalin A. Neuronal perikarya containing the enkephalins are widely distributed throughout the brain. Dynorphin is a 17–amino acid peptide derived from a 28-kD precursor called proenkephalin B or prodynorphin. Shorter peptides called α- and β-neoendorphin, which have 10 and 9 amino acids, respectively, have also been isolated. These peptides react almost exclusively with the κ-receptor. Nociceptin is a 17–amino acid peptide derived from a κ precursor called pronociceptin. High concentrations of nociceptin and its receptor are present in the hypothalamus as well as in other areas of the brain that serve as the sources of monoamine neurotransmitters. In general, nociceptin appears to have an anti-opioid or antinociceptive effect. The hypothalamus contains abundant opioid receptors. The effects of opioid peptides on anterior pituitary hormone secretion are produced through modulation of hypothalamic bioamines and hypophysiotropic factors.

The specific functions of the various opioid peptides and the opioid receptors are still not completely understood, although evidence links them to a number of body functions, including stress, mental illness, narcotic tolerance and dependence, eating, drinking, gastrointestinal function, learning, memory, reward, cardiovascular responses, respiration, thermoregulation, seizures, brain electrical activity, locomotor activity, pregnancy, and neuroimmune activity. Endogenous opioids have an inhibitory influence on gonadotropin secretion through action on GnRH secretion. Exogenous β-endorphin and enkephalin analogues increase serum GH and prolactin levels, but blockade of endogenous opioid pathways with naloxone does not alter basal or stimulated GH or prolactin levels. Opioids feed back negatively on ACTH and β-endorphin secretion, and naloxone can increase basal and stimulated ACTH levels. Overall, the effects of the endogenous opioids on normal physiologic regulation of the various pituitary hormones in humans is minimal.

Central Nervous System Rhythms and Neuroendocrine Function

Pituitary hormones are secreted in a pulsatile fashion with a number of rhythms superimposed. The pulse amplitude of a pituitary hormone reflects the amount of releasing hormone and factors that alter sensitivity to that releasing hormone. Thus, the amplitude can be altered by the presence of inhibitory factors (e.g., GHRH versus somatostatin), nutritional factors, feedback effects of target organ hormones, and prior stimulation that depletes the releasable hormone pool. Pulse frequency is governed by the frequency of release of the hypophysiotropic factor, which is regulated by the hypothalamic pulse generator system.

The pituitary has an intrinsic rhythm of small amplitude with a frequency of every 2 to 10 minutes. Superimposed on this intrinsic rhythm is a rhythm caused by the pulsatile release of hypophysiotropic releasing factors, with or without the withdrawal of a corresponding inhibitory factor. Rhythms that are shorter than 1 day are referred to as *ultradian* rhythms. The next layer of rhythmicity is the *circadian* rhythm, that is, a rhythm with approximately 24-hour periodicity. These rhythms are usually synchronized with the 24-hour period by a periodic environmental cue such as the dark-light cycle. The suprachiasmatic nucleus functions as a circadian pacemaker and receives light-induced electrical impulses from the retina transmitting those impulses to the pineal gland, where they are converted to hormonal signals. Signals for a rhythm with a periodicity longer than 24 hours, an *infradian* rhythm, include the gravitational influence of the moon, which gives rise to the menstrual cycle.

A number of factors may influence circadian and infradian rhythms. One of the most important is the sleep-wake cycle. GH, TSH, prolactin, ACTH, and pubertal LH secretion are all entrained more to the sleep-wake cycle than to the dark-light cycle. Each has an increase and maximal level that occur following sleep onset. The profound diurnal variation in cortisol and ACTH is often used as an index of "normality" of the system. Loss of this diurnal rhythm occurs with disordered regulation by CRH, which may be due to endogenous depression or excessive alcohol intake, or autonomous secretion of ACTH in Cushing's disease. Loss of the diurnal rhythm of cortisol has been used as a diagnostic test for Cushing's syndrome.

Interesting changes occur in gonadotropin secretion as a child passes through puberty into adulthood. Early in puberty, the amplitude of the pulses increases during sleep at night, especially for LH, but in adulthood, this nocturnal rise is lost. In patients with anorexia nervosa, the pattern of gonadotropin secretion often reverts to this pubertal pattern. This phenomenon suggests that body composition may in some way affect regulation of the pulsatile secretion of gonadotropins. The percentage of body fat has been proposed as being important in the timing of the onset of puberty. Recent studies implicate leptin as the signal indicating this change in body composition.

● NEUROENDOCRINE DISEASE
Diseases of the Hypothalamus

Diseases may affect the hypothalamus by discrete localization in the hypothalamus, being part of a generalized central nervous system (CNS) disease such as neurosarcoidosis, or indirectly by a process such as hydrocephalus (Table 230-1). Furthermore, hormonal changes mediated by functional alterations in hypothalamic regulation may occur in systemic illnesses.

The axons projecting to the median eminence that contain the various hypophysiotropic factors are concentrated in the basal portion of the

---

TABLE 230-1 ETIOLOGY OF HYPOTHALAMIC DISEASE

NEONATES

Congenital embryopathic disorders: agenesis of the corpus callosum, cleft palate (*HESX1*)
Congenital disorders: isolated hormone and receptor mutations, combined pituitary hormone deficiency (*PIT1, PROP1*), Laurence-Moon-Bardet-Biedl syndrome, Prader-Labhart-Willi syndrome
Tumors: glioma, hemangioma
Trauma
Hydrocephalus, hydranencephaly, kernicterus

1 MONTH TO 2 YEARS

Tumors: glioma, especially optic glioma, hemangiomas
Infiltrative disease: Langerhans cell histiocytosis, meningitis
Hydrocephalus

2-10 YEARS

Tumors: craniopharyngioma, glioma, dysgerminoma, hamartoma, leukemia, ganglioneuroma, ependymoma, medulloblastoma
Infiltrative disease: Langerhans cell histiocytosis, meningitis, tuberculosis, encephalitis
Irradiation: for nasopharyngeal tumors, intracranial tumors, leukemia
Functional: psychosocial deprivation

10-25 YEARS

Congenital disorders: Kallmann's syndrome, gonadotropin-releasing hormone receptor defects
Tumors: craniopharyngioma, pituitary tumors, glioma, hamartoma, dysgerminoma, dermoid, lipoma, neuroblastoma
Trauma: subarachnoid hemorrhage, vascular aneurysm, arteriovenous malformation
Infiltrative diseases: Langerhans cell histiocytosis, sarcoidosis, tuberculosis, meningitis, encephalitis, leukemia
Chronic hydrocephalus or increased intracranial pressure
Functional: hypogonadotropic hypogonadism associated with weight loss, exercise

25-50 YEARS

Tumors: pituitary tumors, meningioma, craniopharyngioma, Rathke's cleft cyst, glioma, lymphoma, angioma, colloid cysts, ependymoma
Infiltrative diseases: sarcoidosis, Langerhans cell histiocytosis, tuberculosis, viral encephalitis
Subarachnoid hemorrhage, vascular aneurysms, arteriovenous malformation
Irradiation: for pituitary adenoma, nasopharyngeal tumors, intracranial tumors
Nutritional: Wernicke's disease
Functional: hypogonadotropic hypogonadism associated with weight loss, exercise

50 YEARS AND OLDER

Tumors: pituitary tumors, meningioma, craniopharyngioma, sarcoma, glioblastoma, lymphoma, colloid cysts, ependymoma
Vascular: infarct, subarachnoid hemorrhage, pituitary apoplexy, aneurysm
Irradiation: for pituitary adenoma, nasopharyngeal tumors, intracranial tumors
Infiltrative diseases: encephalitis, sarcoidosis, meningitis
Nutritional: Wernicke's disease

Modified from Plum F, Van Uitert R. Non-endocrine diseases of the hypothalamus. In: Reichlin S, Baldessarini RJ, Martin JB, eds. *The Hypothalamus.* New York: Raven Press; 1978:415.

hypothalamus. Thus, lesions located within this final common pathway might be expected to cause significant decreases in secretion of some or all of the pituitary hormones except prolactin, which may increase because of the elimination of tonic inhibition by dopamine. Diabetes insipidus (Chapter 232) may also occur. Symptoms resulting from hypothalamic dysfunction are related to the size of the lesion and consequently to the area of the hypothalamus involved, as well as to the rapidity of the increase in lesion size. Slowly growing lesions tend to cause problems of hormone dysregulation rather than dramatic symptoms. Large, slowly growing lesions may cause more acute problems, such as when a slight increment in growth eliminates the remaining vestiges of vasopressin or ACTH secretion. The best way of discerning lesions affecting the hypothalamus is by magnetic resonance imaging (MRI) with gadolinium enhancement, although computed tomographic scanning with intravenous contrast is also effective. Formal visual field testing may discern impingement of the optic nerves and chiasm by hypothalamic lesions. Detailed testing of hypothalamic-pituitary function may reveal evidence of functional hypothalamic disruption with great sensitivity.

CONGENITAL EMBRYOPATHIC DISORDERS

The most common embryopathic disorders to affect the hypothalamus are the midline cleft syndromes, which cause varying degrees of defects of midline structures, especially the optic and olfactory tracts, the septum pellucidum, the corpus callosum, the anterior commissure, the hypothalamus, and the pituitary. The clinical features of patients with midline cleft defects varies in severity from cyclopia to cleft lip and from isolated hypothalamic hormone defects to panhypopituitarism. The combination of absent septum pellucidum associated with optic nerve hypoplasia is referred to as septo-optic dysplasia and is associated with abnormalities of hypothalamic and other diencephalic structures. Some patients with septo-optic dysplasia and hypothalamic hypopituitarism have sexual precocity, presumably caused by a lack of inhibitory influences from other parts of the hypothalamus and intact GnRH-producing structures. Children with very mild midline cleft defects consisting of cleft lip, cleft palate, or both have an increased risk of GH and other pituitary hormone deficiencies. MRI studies of patients with "idiopathic" GH deficiency show absence of the infundibulum in nearly 50%.

Mutations responsible for these developmental defects are the subject of active investigation. Mutations in the human HESX1 gene cause agenesis of the corpus callosum and panhypopituitarism. Case reports of mutations in other transcription factors, such as Pitx2 (Rieger's syndrome) and GLI2, describe patients with varying brain and skull developmental abnormalities along with varying degrees of hypopituitarism. Kallmann's syndrome is a condition characterized by anosmia or hyposmia and hypogonadotropic hypogonadism. The diagnosis is made by finding anosmia and low gonadotropin levels, and MRI will show absence or hypoplasia of the olfactory bulbs. The X-linked form of Kallmann's syndrome, representing about 85% of cases, is due to a gene defect (KAL1) resulting in loss of function of a protein called anosmin that facilitates the embryologic migration of GnRH-producing neurons from the olfactory placode to the hypothalamus and the olfactory nerves to the olfactory bulbs. The pituitary is usually intact in this condition, and treatment with pulsatile GnRH therapy or gonadotropins results in spermatogenesis and normal gonadal function. In some patients, other neurologic abnormalities may be present, including cerebellar ataxia, nerve deafness, color blindness, cleft lip and palate, mental retardation, and disordered thirst.

TUMORS

The most common tumors affecting the hypothalamus are pituitary adenomas that have significant suprasellar extension. These tumors can cause varying degrees of hypopituitarism and hyperprolactinemia, either by compressing the normal pituitary or, more commonly, by affecting the pituitary stalk and mediobasal hypothalamus. Surprisingly, diabetes insipidus (Chapter 232) is a rare finding in patients with pituitary adenomas. In patients with normal or elevated prolactin levels, pituitary function often returns following therapy.

Craniopharyngiomas are the next most common tumors affecting the hypothalamus. Microscopically, craniopharyngiomas consist of cysts alternating with stratified squamous epithelium. The cyst fluid is usually thick and dark, and the material is often calcified. They arise from remnants of Rathke's pouch. A closely related lesion is Rathke's cleft cyst, which develops from the space between the anterior and rudimentary intermediate lobes. Rathke's cleft cysts are lined with cuboidal as opposed to squamous epithelium, and

the cyst fluid is usually a white, mucoid fluid. Craniopharyngiomas may be difficult to remove in their entirety, and postoperative radiation reduces recurrences. Rathke's cleft cysts less commonly recur. Craniopharyngiomas most commonly arise during childhood, but they may also occur in adults and even elderly people. These tumors come to attention because of mass effects, including headache, vomiting, visual disturbance, seizures, hypopituitarism, and polyuria. Some patients have galactorrhea, amenorrhea, and hyperprolactinemia, features suggestive of a prolactinoma. Careful endocrine testing reveals varying degrees of hypopituitarism in 50 to 75%, modest hyperprolactinemia in 25 to 50%, and often diabetes insipidus. Surgical extirpation of craniopharyngiomas commonly causes a worsening of pituitary function, often resulting in complete panhypopituitarism and diabetes insipidus because of stalk section, and may cause damage to the hypothalamic centers that regulate thirst, body temperature, and food intake. Irradiation may also be helpful, especially in children.

Suprasellar dysgerminomas arise from primitive germ cells that have migrated to the CNS during fetal life and are structurally identical to germ cell tumors of the gonads. They most commonly occur in children, in whom they cause decreased growth because of hypopituitarism, as well as diabetes insipidus and visual problems. Hyperprolactinemia occurs in more than 50% of affected children, and 10% have precocious puberty from the production of human chorionic gonadotropin by the tumor. The finding of an elevated human chorionic gonadotropin level in the spinal fluid may be diagnostic. As opposed to craniopharyngiomas, these tumors are very radiosensitive, and radiation therapy combined with chemotherapy is the preferred treatment.

A hypothalamic hamartoma is a nodule of growth of hypothalamic neurons attached by a pedicle to the hypothalamus between the tuber cinereum and the mammillary bodies and extending into the basal cistern. Asymptomatic hamartomas may be present in up to 20% of random autopsies; rarely, these lesions may enlarge and disrupt hypothalamic function because of compression of adjacent tissue. A variant of hamartoma consisting of similar tissue present within the anterior pituitary but without a neural attachment to the hypothalamus is called a choristoma or gangliocytoma. These neuronal tumors are of particular endocrine interest because they can produce hypophysiotropic hormones. A number of cases associated with precocious puberty have been reported in which the hamartomas produced GnRH. Successful treatment has been reported with surgery and with the administration of a long-acting GnRH analogue, which suppresses gonadotropin secretion but does not affect the tumor itself. If the hamartoma does not cause other problems from mass effects, medical therapy with the GnRH analogue may be the best choice because surgery can be noncurative or even fatal. Some gangliocytomas have been reported that produce GHRH and acromegaly or CRH and Cushing's syndrome.

Other tumors and space-occupying lesions occurring in the suprasellar area include arachnoid cysts, meningiomas, gliomas, astrocytomas, chordomas, infundibulomas, cholesteatomas, neurofibromas, lipomas, and metastatic cancer (particularly from the breast and lung). Any such lesion may manifest as varying degrees of hypopituitarism, diabetes insipidus, and hyperprolactinemia, and surgical therapy often worsens the hormonal deficit and may cause other hypothalamic damage.

INFLAMMATORY AND INFILTRATIVE DISORDERS

CNS involvement in cases of sarcoidosis occurs (Chapter 95) in 1 to 5% of patients, as determined on clinical grounds, and in up to 16% of cases at autopsy. Isolated CNS sarcoidosis is uncommon. When sarcoidosis does involve the CNS, the hypothalamus is involved in 10 to 20% of cases. Sarcoid granulomas can involve the hypothalamus, stalk, or pituitary and may be infiltrative or occur as a mass lesion. The most common endocrine findings are varying degrees of hypopituitarism, diabetes insipidus, and hyperprolactinemia. Obesity secondary to hypothalamic involvement by sarcoidosis has also been reported. In patients with isolated CNS sarcoidosis, the diagnosis may be extremely difficult. Examination of cerebrospinal fluid usually shows elevated protein levels, low glucose levels, pleocytosis, and variable elevations of angiotensin-converting enzyme. However, biopsy is often necessary. Although corticosteroid therapy has been reported to at least partially reverse the thirst disorders, anterior pituitary hormone deficits usually do not respond.

Langerhans cell histiocytosis infiltration of the hypothalamus may cause diabetes insipidus, varying degrees of hypopituitarism, and hyperprolactinemia. It is the most common cause of diabetes insipidus in children. Usually, this infiltration appears as a thickening of the pituitary stalk, but it may also appear as a mass lesion of the hypothalamus or the pituitary. Osteolytic lesions may be present in the jaw or mastoid, so radiographs of the jaw are a worthwhile part of the diagnostic evaluation of an unknown suprasellar mass or diabetes insipidus. Therapy consists of local surgery, focal irradiation, or chemotherapy with alkylating agents and high-dose corticosteroids.

VASCULAR DISEASE

An enlarging aneurysm may manifest as a mass lesion of the hypothalamic-pituitary area and may cause hypopituitarism and visual field defects. Obviously, the distinction must be made before surgery. Tumors and aneurysms may also coexist, and careful radiologic evaluation with MRI is necessary to discern such association. Hypothalamic disease caused by vascular infarction is extremely rare. In the past several years, it has been found that subarachnoid hemorrhage may be associated with varying degrees of hypopituitarism in almost half of cases. On the other hand, diabetes insipidus is uncommon.

TRAUMA

Traumatic brain injury (TBI) can cause defects ranging from isolated ACTH deficiency to panhypopituitarism with diabetes insipidus. Within the first 72 hours of trauma, GH, LH, ACTH, TSH, and prolactin levels may actually be elevated in blood, perhaps because of acute release. These levels subsequently fall, and either pituitary function returns to normal or hypopituitarism develops. Overall, the frequency of hypopituitarism in TBI is less than in subarachnoid hemorrhage, occurring in about one fourth of surviving patients. In patients dying of head injury, anterior pituitary infarction has been found in 16% of cases, posterior pituitary hemorrhage in 34%, and hypothalamic hemorrhage or infarction in 42% of cases. The paraventricular and supraoptic nuclei and median eminence are particularly involved with microhemorrhages, hence the high frequency of panhypopituitarism with diabetes insipidus. With frontal injuries, the brain travels backward, but the pituitary cannot move; consequently, the pituitary stalk becomes avulsed, with interruption of the portal vessels. Most patients with head injury are hyperprolactinemic, which clinically confirms that the hypothalamus or stalk is the primary site of injury. In the past, pituitary function in patients with TBI and subarachnoid hemorrhage has not been assessed, and the role of untreated hypopituitarism in the long-term disability of such patients is unknown.

Irradiation

Whole-brain irradiation for intracranial neoplasms frequently results in hypothalamic dysfunction, as evidenced by endocrine abnormalities and behavioral changes. The most common endocrine abnormality is hyperprolactinemia, but hypopituitarism also occurs. When the radiotherapy is targeted to the hypothalamic area, hypopituitarism occurs even more frequently. The frequency of loss of pituitary function is so high that all patients who have had their pituitary and hypothalamic areas irradiated must be monitored periodically for the purpose of detecting these deficits. However, the development of such deficiencies may take many years, so that yearly testing is warranted for up to 20 years. It appears that stereotactic irradiation using the gamma knife apparatus or a linear accelerator for pituitary and other parasellar tumors causes a risk of hypopituitarism similar to that of conventional irradiation.

Effects of Hypothalamic Disease on Pituitary Function

Hypothalamic disease can cause both pituitary hyperfunction and hypofunction in varying degrees of severity. Although severe disease can cause absolute deficiencies of the various hormones, milder disease may cause a subtle alteration in feedback loops and timing such that, for example, the integration of signals necessary for menstrual cycling is lost, with subsequent "hypothalamic" amenorrhea. Furthermore, the hypothalamic defects may be interrelated. The rather common finding of hyperprolactinemia occurring with hypothalamic dysfunction causes a hypogonadotropic hypogonadism that is reversible when the elevated prolactin levels are brought down to normal. In many cases, no structural lesion can be found on MRI, and a functional defect caused by altered neurotransmitter regulation is invoked.

Growth Hormone

Loss of normal GH secretion is the most common hormonal defect occurring with structural hypothalamic disease. About three fourths of cases with congenital, idiopathic GH deficiency have a normal GH response to exogenous GHRH, which implies that the defect is probably disordered hypothalamic regulation. Defects in the gene for GHRH have not been found, but a rare form of GH deficiency has been found to be caused by a mutation in the GHRH receptor. A reversible form of idiopathic GH deficiency caused by inadequate parental care and affection is referred to as the emotional deprivation syndrome or psychosocial dwarfism. Restoration of a proper social environment for such a child results in prompt normalization of GH secretion and growth. It has been hypothesized that the disordered GH regulation is due to psychogenic alteration of the neurotransmitter balance necessary for normal GHRH and somatostatin secretion. Other systemic illnesses such as inflammatory bowel disease, often occult, may also cause decreased GH secretion and growth; treatment of the systemic illness will correct the growth abnormality. Treatment of children and adults with GH deficiency is discussed in Chapter 231.

Gonadotropins

Hypothalamic Hypogonadism

The primary defect in this group of disorders is thought to involve the secretion of GnRH, with resultant impairment in pituitary gonadotropin secretion and gonadal function. The disorders causing these conditions may be primary, that is, congenital defects, or acquired. Depending on the time of onset, they are manifested as either delayed puberty, interruption of pubertal progression, or loss of adult gonadal function. The lesions causing these disorders may cause loss of other hormones or may be isolated to GnRH. Loss of gonadotropin secretion as the result of hypothalamic structural damage is the second most common defect after GH deficiency. However, a substantial portion of these defects are due to hyperprolactinemia and are reversible with correction of the hyperprolactinemia. In some cases, the defect is idiopathic. Defects in the gene for GnRH have not been found, but mutations in the GnRH receptor do occur.

In children, if the disorder is limited to GnRH and the gonadotropins, prior growth and development are normal, but the growth spurt occurring at puberty is lost. Undescended testes are present in 50% of patients with GnRH deficiency, probably secondary to the absence of gonadotropins during fetal development. The most common congenital lesion causing prepubertal GnRH deficiency is Kallmann's syndrome, which affects 50% of males and 37% of females seen with isolated gonadotropin deficiency (see earlier). In patients with GnRH deficiency, replacement of GnRH through subcutaneous administration every 2 hours with a portable pump causes a rapid rise in LH and FSH, a rise in testosterone to normal, and the development of normal spermatogenesis. Similar approaches in women result in ovulatory cycles in 80%. The success of such therapy confirms the original hypothesis of a primary defect of GnRH secretion. In men, comparable results can be obtained with exogenous gonadotropins given three times per week and is much more practical. GnRH therapy is not successful in those with GnRH receptor mutations. Replacement with testosterone alone causes adequate androgenization but does not result in an increase in testicular size or in spermatogenesis.

Loss of formerly normal GnRH secretion in adults may be due to structural hypothalamic damage such as a tumor, a functional change unassociated with a detectable lesion, or hyperprolactinemia. Structural disease must be excluded in such patients by computed tomography or MRI. Most cases of functional hypogonadotropic hypogonadism occur in women, the most common causes being weight loss, excessive exercise, psychogenic stress, or systemic illness, but idiopathic forms occur as well. In some patients, the exercise results in a loss of body fat not detected with total body weight measures, and it is unclear whether the hypogonadism is directly due to the loss of body fat or to the exercise per se. Studies of pulsatile gonadotropin secretion in such patients reveal absent pulses. Usually, the gonadotropin response to injected GnRH is normal. Regain of weight and stopping of the exercise result in resumption of normal gonadal function. Furthermore, the administration of leptin to such women results in a resumption of normal gonadotropin pulsatile secretion and ovulation, confirming the key role that leptin has in mediating the influence of body energy stores on reproductive function. Hyperprolactinemia occurring postpubertally can also decrease GnRH and the pulsatile secretion of LH and FSH and thereby result in anovulation with oligomenorrhea and amenorrhea in women and impotence and infertility in men.

Two goals in the treatment of idiopathic, functional hypogonadotropic amenorrhea are (1) restoration of a normal estrogen status to promote well-being and to prevent osteoporosis and (2) facilitation of ovulation for fertility. The former can generally be achieved with cyclic estrogen and progesterone, whereas the latter may require clomiphene or GnRH or gonadotropin therapy. In men, similar goals may be achieved with testosterone or GnRH or gonadotropins.

Hypothalamic Hypergonadism (Precocious Puberty)

Precocious puberty is defined as the onset of puberty before the age of 8 years in girls or 9 years in boys. Pseudoprecocious puberty is that resulting from peripheral (gonadal or adrenal) causes. Central, "true," or GnRH-dependent precocious puberty is characterized by hormonal changes similar to those that occur at the time of normal puberty, that is, an increase in the pulsatile release of LH, an increase in the gonadotropin response to GnRH, and an increase in gonadal steroid secretion. GnRH-dependent precocious puberty therefore represents premature activation of the GnRH pulse generator by a variety of lesions, or it may also be idiopathic. Fewer than one fourth of cases of central precocious puberty occur in boys, but they tend to have more serious underlying disease. In boys with central, GnRH-dependent precocious puberty, hypothalamic hamartomas account for 38% of cases, other CNS lesions represent 31%, familial disease accounts for 23%, and idiopathic disease accounts for only 8%. The picture is quite different in girls, however: hypothalamic hamartomas account for only 15% of cases, other CNS lesions represent 14%, the McCune-Albright syndrome (polyostotic fibrous dysplasia) accounts for 6%, and fully 65% are idiopathic. Dysgerminomas in the suprasellar or pineal region can produce chorionic gonadotropin, which acts like LH in its stimulation of gonadal function. Usually, such tumors cause increased sex steroid formation but fail to cause ovulation.

Therapy for central GnRH-dependent precocious puberty consists of surgical removal of the tumor or medical therapy with a long-acting GnRH analogue. The latter can suppress gonadotropin and sex steroid hormone levels and cause a stabilization or even regression of secondary sex characteristics and a slowing of growth and bone maturation in most cases. When therapy is discontinued at the normal time of puberty, sex steroid levels increase, secondary sexual characteristics again develop, growth increases, and regular menses develop spontaneously.

Prolactin

Hypothalamic Hyperprolactinemia

Structural or infiltrative lesions of the hypothalamus, such as those discussed earlier, can decrease the amount of dopamine reaching the lactotrophs and thus cause modest hyperprolactinemia (usually <100 ng/mL). Because their therapy is quite different, it is very important to differentiate nonsecreting pituitary adenomas with extensive suprasellar extension causing prolactin elevations in this range from prolactin-secreting adenomas, which usually cause prolactin elevations 5 to 50 times higher. A peculiarity of some two-site immunoassays, referred to as the "hook effect," can sometimes cause a very high prolactin level to read falsely normal or just mildly elevated; a 1:100 dilution of the serum sample with saline will show the true level when the specimen is rerun. If there is any question about an assay being susceptible to the hook affect, in patients with very large tumors, prolactin should be measured undiluted and at 1:100 dilution to avoid this important spurious finding. A number of medications, antipsychotics in particular, can cause hyperprolactinemia, primarily by interfering with central catecholamines (Table 230-2).

Therapy is generally directed at the underlying cause. The hyperprolactinemia itself may impair gonadal function, so efforts may also be made to lower prolactin levels with dopamine agonists. Prolactin levels usually fall quite readily in such patients. Restoration of gonadal function is not automatic, however, because the primary hypothalamic lesion may also directly impair release of GnRH. In that circumstance, both dopamine agonists and sex steroid replacement may be necessary. When administration of psychotropic medications that cause the hyperprolactinemia cannot be stopped, dopamine agonists may be used but very rarely have been reported to exacerbate the psychosis. In such cases and in others in which fertility is not an issue, treatment with cyclic estrogen and progesterone replacement can be carried out safely.

Idiopathic Hyperprolactinemia

Idiopathic hyperprolactinemia is a diagnosis of exclusion. Prolactin levels in this condition are usually less than 100 ng/mL. In such cases, small pituitary or hypothalamic tumors could exist that are beyond the resolution of current imaging techniques, but when such patients are monitored for many years, it is very uncommon for tumors to later be visualized. Idiopathic hyperprolactinemia can cause amenorrhea, galactorrhea, impotence, infertility, and loss of libido, just as occurs with hyperprolactinemia of other causes, so the idiopathic hyperprolactinemia may need to be treated. Premature osteoporosis related to the estrogen deficiency may also occur. The only possible treatment

TABLE 230-2	ETIOLOGIES OF HYPERPROLACTINEMIA

PITUITARY DISEASE

Prolactinomas
Acromegaly
Empty sella syndrome
Lymphocytic hypophysitis
Cushing's disease
Pituitary stalk section

HYPOTHALAMIC DISEASE

Craniopharyngiomas
Meningiomas
Dysgerminomas
Nonsecreting pituitary adenomas
Other tumors
Sarcoidosis
Langerhans cell histiocytosis
Neuraxis irradiation
Vascular

NEUROGENIC

Chest wall lesions
Spinal cord lesions
Breast stimulation

OTHER

Pregnancy
Hypothyroidism
Chronic renal failure
Cirrhosis
Pseudocyesis
Adrenal insufficiency
Idiopathic

MEDICATIONS

Antipsychotics
Atypical antipsychotics
Monoamine oxidase inhibitors
Tricyclic antidepressants
Reserpine
Methyldopa
Metoclopramide
Domperidone
Cocaine
Verapamil
Serotonin reuptake inhibitors

Modified from Molitch ME. Medication-induced hyperprolactinemia. *Mayo Clin Proc.* 2005;80:1050-1057.

is dopamine agonists, and these agents are successful in more than 90% of cases. Alternatively, cyclic estrogen and progesterone replacement may be given, but fertility will not be restored.

Thyroid-Stimulating Hormone

Hypothalamic hypothyroidism is due to a central lesion that impairs the secretion of TRH, usually along with the loss of other hormones. It occurs considerably less commonly than hypothalamic GH and gonadotropin deficiency. Defects in the gene for TRH have not been detected, but a case has been reported of a TRH receptor mutation causing hypothyroidism. TSH levels in this syndrome are generally normal or even slightly elevated. TSH in these patients is biologically less active than normal and binds to the TSH receptor less well because of altered glycosylation as a result of the TRH deficiency. Treatment is with L-thyroxine, and monitoring of therapy is done solely by measurement of free thyroxine (T_4) levels and not TSH levels.

Adrenocorticotropic Hormone

ACTH deficiency caused by hypothalamic lesions is uncommon. It may occur with the loss of other hormones but may also appear as an isolated deficiency. In the absence of CNS lesions or a history of trauma, most cases of isolated ACTH deficiency appear to be a pituitary autoimmune disorder. However, in patients with hypothalamic disease as the cause, basal ACTH levels are low, and the ACTH response to injected CRH may be prolonged and exaggerated, much as is the TSH response to TRH. Treatment is with glucocorticoids; mineralocorticoids are not needed.

Vasopressin

Diabetes insipidus can develop as a result of destructive lesions in the supraoptic and paraventricular nuclei or in the mediobasal hypothalamus in the path of the neural fibers containing vasopressin (Chapter 232) that are passing on to the posterior pituitary. Irritative lesions can trigger the release of vasopressin in an unregulated fashion and thereby result in the syndrome of inappropriate antidiuretic hormone (vasopressin) secretion.

Effects of Hypothalamic Disease on Other Neurometabolic Functions

A number of functions that affect the internal milieu, in addition to anterior and posterior pituitary function, are regulated, at least in part, by the hypothalamus and include temperature control, behavior, consciousness, memory, sleep, food intake, and carbohydrate metabolism.

Alterations in Food Intake

Hypothalamic Obesity

Destruction of the mediobasal hypothalamus will sometimes inhibit satiety and may result in hyperphagia and hypothalamic obesity. The hyperphagia is due to destruction of noradrenergic fibers originating in the paraventricular nucleus and passing through the mediobasal hypothalamus. Because of their location, such lesions also usually produce hypopituitarism and diabetes insipidus. In a number of rare syndromes (Prader-Willi, Laurence-Moon-Biedl-Bardet) with obesity as a major characteristic, hypothalamic causes have been postulated but not proved. Prader-Willi is the most common of these syndromes and occurs in 1 in 25,000 births. It is characterized by hypotonia, obesity, short stature, mental deficiency, hypogonadism, and small hands and feet. About 70% of patients with Prader-Willi syndrome have a chromosome 15 deletion (15q11-q13) on the paternally derived chromosome. In the few cases studied at autopsy, no discernible hypothalamic lesions were detected.

Hypothalamic Anorexia

Lesions of the lateral hypothalamus, which destroy nigrostriatal dopaminergic fibers that pass through this area, produce hypophagia along with an increase in peripheral norepinephrine turnover and metabolic rate. This syndrome is very rare, probably owing to the requirement for bilateral lesions. The hormonal changes that occur in anorexia nervosa appear to all be secondary to the weight loss, and no evidence has been found for a primary hypothalamic disorder in this syndrome.

Hyperglycemia

Hypothalamic activation as part of the generalized response to stress can cause release of GH, prolactin, and ACTH, which serve as counter-regulatory hormones with respect to insulin. These hormones promote lipolysis, gluconeogenesis, and insulin resistance, resulting in glucose elevation. Of more importance in the acute response to stress, this hypothalamic response results in sympathetic activation with release of catecholamines that inhibit insulin secretion and stimulate glycogenolysis.

Temperature Regulation

The anterior hypothalamus and preoptic area contain temperature-sensitive neurons that respond to internal temperature changes by initiating certain thermoregulatory responses necessary to restore a constant temperature. Measures that dissipate heat include cutaneous vasodilation, sweating, and panting, and measures that increase body heat include increasing metabolic heat production, shivering, and cutaneous vasoconstriction.

Rare patients have been reported with anterior hypothalamic lesions that cause paroxysmal or sustained hypothermia or hyperthermia from failure of these thermoregulatory activities. Some cases of paroxysmal hypothermia and hyperthermia respond to anticonvulsant medications, which suggests that the neuronal discharge effecting the temperature changes is seizure-like.

Poikilothermy results from an inability to dissipate or generate heat to keep the body temperature constant in the face of varying ambient temperatures. This condition results from bilateral lesions in the posterior hypothalamus and rostral mesencephalon, which are the areas responsible for the final integration of thermoregulatory neural efferents. Patients with this condition do not feel discomfort with temperature changes and are unaware of having a problem. Depending on the ambient temperature, they may experience life-threatening hypothermia or hyperthermia.

SUGGESTED READINGS

Caronia LM, Martin C, Welt CK, et al. A genetic basis for functional hypothalamic amenorrhea. *N Engl J Med.* 2011;364:215-225. *Review of genes associated with idiopathic hypogonadotropic hypogonadism.*

Chung S, Parks GS, Lee C, et al. Recent updates on the melanin-concentrating hormone (MCH) and its receptor system: lessons from MCH1R antagonists. *J Mol Neurosci.* 2011;43:115-121. *Review of the endogenous system and its regulation of food intake, anxiety, depression, reward, and sleep.*

Donato J Jr, Cravo RM, Frazão R, et al. Hypothalamic sites of leptin action linking metabolism and reproduction. *Neuroendocrinology.* 2011;93:9-18. *Review including how leptin acts indirectly on gonadotropin-releasing hormone–secreting cells.*

Morrison SF, Nakamura K. Central neural pathways for thermoregulation. *Front Biosci.* 2011;16:74-104. *Review of homeostatic mechanisms that maintain body temperature during environmental challenges.*

Pandit R, de Jong JW, Vanderschuren LJ, et al. Neurobiology of overeating and obesity: the role of melanocortins and beyond. *Eur J Pharmacol.* 2011;660:28-42. *Overview of the hypothalamus and its neural interactions.*

Papadimitriou A, Priftis KN. Regulation of the hypothalamic-pituitary-adrenal axis. *Neuroimmunomodulation.* 2009;16:265-271. *Overview of the axis and the factors that regulate its function.*

231

ANTERIOR PITUITARY

MARK E. MOLITCH

ANATOMY AND EMBRYOLOGY

The pituitary is divided into anterior (adenohypophysis) and posterior (neurohypophysis) lobes. The optic chiasm, formed by the decussation of the optic nerves, is positioned directly above the pituitary gland. Specialized vascular structures located in the median eminence of the hypothalamus drain into portal veins that course down the pituitary stalk to join the sinusoidal capillaries of the anterior lobe. Hypothalamic hormones enter these capillaries and flow to the anterior pituitary. Venous drainage from the anterior lobe is into the cavernous sinuses, which drain into the petrosal sinuses. The six major pituitary cell types include somatotrophs (growth hormone [GH] producing), lactotrophs (prolactin [PRL] producing), corticotrophs (ACTH producing), thyrotrophs (thyroid-stimulating hormone [TSH] producing), and gonadotrophs (follicle-stimulating hormone [FSH] and luteinizing hormone [LH] producing).

The pituitary is formed from the fusion of Rathke's pouch (which gives rise to the anterior pituitary) and a portion of the ventral diencephalon (which gives rise to the posterior pituitary). Several transcription factors are important in the development of the various types of pituitary cells. Lhx3 is present in somatotrophs, lactotrophs, and thyrotrophs, and mutations in this gene result in complete deficits of GH, PRL, TSH, and the gonadotropins. Mutations in *HESX1* usually are associated with dysplasia of the septum pellucidum and optic tracts in addition to multiple pituitary hormone deficits. The transcription factor Pit-1 is produced in somatotrophs, lactotrophs, and thyrotrophs. Mutations in the *PIT1* gene prevent the development of these cells and cause deficiencies of GH, PRL, and TSH. This lineage relationship explains why some GH-producing tumors also secrete PRL and some TSH-producing tumors co-secrete GH. Prop-1, another transcription factor, is critical for the development of somatotrophs, lactotrophs, and thyrotrophs. Mutations in the *PROP1* gene result in deficiencies of GH, PRL, and TSH and in some affected individuals there is delayed puberty. Combined pituitary hormone deficiency (GH, PRL, TSH) has an incidence of about 1 in 8000 births, and 10% have an affected relative. More than half of these cases are due to *PIT1* or *PROP1* mutations. Pitx1 and Pitx2 activate the expression of genes coding for the development of all five types of pituitary cells, and mutations of the *PITX2* gene have been found to cause combined GH-TSH and GH-ACTH deficiencies. Tpit is specific to corticotroph cells, and *TPIT* gene mutations cause isolated ACTH deficiency.

Somatotrophs constitute 40 to 50% of anterior pituitary cells; lactotrophs, 15 to 25%; corticotrophs, 10 to 20%; and gonadotrophs 10%. Only 5% of pituitary cells are thyrotrophs.

RADIOLOGY OF THE PITUITARY

Magnetic resonance imaging (MRI) provides excellent resolution of the pituitary and surrounding cerebrospinal fluid (CSF) and vascular and central nervous system structures. There is less radiation exposure with MRI than with computed tomography (CT), allowing repeated imaging. However, bone structures are not as well defined by MRI compared with CT. On MRI, the normal anterior pituitary appears isointense with brain white matter, whereas the posterior pituitary exhibits high signal intensity ("bright spot"). The optic chiasm is readily identified because it is surrounded by hypodense areas. Pituitary adenomas typically appear hypointense on T1-weighted images and show less enhancement with gadolinium than surrounding normal tissue. Focal hypodense areas are also seen in about one fourth of normal individuals, which may correspond to cysts or nonfunctioning small adenomas, emphasizing the importance of endocrine evaluation.

● REGULATION OF THE PITUITARY AXIS

The pituitary gland integrates the influences of an array of positive and negative signals to modulate hormone secretion. PRL is the only major pituitary hormone that is not subject to feedback inhibition by hormones produced in target tissues. It is controlled by positive and negative input from the hypothalamus, the latter being dominant.

The principles of feedback regulation are illustrated by the hypothalamic-pituitary-thyroid axis. Hypothalamic thyrotropin-releasing hormone (TRH) stimulates TSH secretion from the pituitary. TSH increases thyroid hormone secretion, which in turn suppresses hypothalamic TRH as well as pituitary TSH. A typical regulatory loop therefore has both positive (TRH, TSH) and negative (thyroxine [T_4], triiodothyronine [T_3]) components, allowing a high degree of control of hormone levels. The pituitary gland integrates positive TRH signals and the negative effects of thyroid hormone. The concept of feedback regulation is important not only for understanding pituitary physiology but also because it provides the basis for analyzing pituitary gland function using stimulation and suppression tests.

The feedback regulatory systems just described are superimposed on hormonal rhythms that are used for adaptation to the environment. Seasonal changes, the daily occurrence of the light-dark cycles, and stress have major impacts on the secretion of pituitary hormones (Chapter 230). Because many hormones are released in a pulsatile manner and in a rhythmic fashion, these characteristics of secretion should be considered when attempting to relate serum measurements to normal values. Although it is possible to characterize pulsatile patterns of hormone secretion using frequent blood sampling (every 10 minutes), this is not practical in a clinical setting. Alternative approaches include stimulation and suppression tests or the use of "integrated" measurements of hormone production, such as 24-hour urine free cortisol as an index of ACTH secretion or insulin-like growth factor-I (IGF-I) as a biologic marker of GH action.

● HYPOPITUITARISM

Pituitary hormone deficiencies can be caused by loss of hypothalamic stimulation or by direct loss of pituitary function. When hypopituitarism is accompanied by diabetes insipidus or hyperprolactinemia, one should consider hypothalamic etiologies.

▶ PATHOBIOLOGY

A variety of congenital and acquired causes of hypopituitarism have been described (Table 231-1). Congenital deficiencies of multiple pituitary hormones are often caused by mutations in the genes for the transcription factors mentioned previously (*HESX1, LHX3, PIT1, PROP1*). Gene mutations have been found at several steps leading to pituitary hormone secretion, including those for the hypophysiotropic releasing factor receptors for gonadotropin-releasing hormone (GnRH), growth hormone–releasing hormone (GHRH), and TRH; those for the pituitary hormone structures for GH, ACTH, and the β-subunits of FSH, TSH, and LH; and those for the target organ receptors for GH, ACTH, TSH, and LH. Mutations of the GH gene have been shown to be heterogeneous. Some are large deletions that are inherited in an autosomal recessive manner and involve genetic recombination between related DNA sequences in the duplicated GH gene cluster. Point mutations have also been described, and some of these can be inherited in an autosomal dominant manner. Mutations of the other types described earlier generally cause autosomal recessive forms of selective hormone deficiencies. The congenital embryopathic disorders causing hypopituitarism are discussed in Chapter 230.

Neoplastic lesions, particularly pituitary macroadenomas, are the most common cause of acquired hypopituitarism. Pituitary adenomas cause hypopituitarism in several different ways. In some cases, there is direct destruction or compression of the normal pituitary. Compression of the pituitary stalk

TABLE 231-1 CAUSES OF HYPOPITUITARISM

GENETIC DEFECTS

Hypophysiotropic hormone gene defects
Hypophysiotropic hormone receptor gene defects
   GHRH receptor defect
   GnRH receptor defect
   TRH receptor defect
Pituitary hormone gene defects
   Gonadotropins: LH β- and FSH β-subunit gene defects
   Growth hormone: defects in GH gene
   Thyrotropin: defects in TSH β-subunit gene
   Multiple hormone (GH, PRL, TSH) defects: due to mutation in *PIT1* gene and *PROP1* gene
Pituitary hormone receptor genetic defects
   Growth hormone receptor defects: GH insensitivity syndrome (Laron-type dwarfism)
   ACTH receptor defects: congenital insensitivity to ACTH
   LH receptor defects
   FSH receptor defects
   TSH receptor defects

CONGENITAL EMBRYOPATHIC DEFECTS

Anencephaly
Midline cleft defects: septo-optic dysplasia, basal encephalocele, cleft lip and palate
Pituitary aplasia
Kallmann's syndrome (GnRH defect with anosmia)

ACQUIRED DEFECTS

Tumors: pituitary adenomas, craniopharyngiomas, dysgerminomas, meningiomas, gliomas, metastatic tumors, hamartomas, Rathke's cleft cysts
Irradiation
Trauma: surgery, external blunt trauma
Empty sella syndrome
Vascular
   Pituitary apoplexy
   Sheehan's syndrome
   Internal carotid aneurysm
   Vasculitis
   Subarachnoid hemorrhage
Inflammatory and infiltrative diseases
   Sarcoidosis
   Langerhans' cell histiocytosis (histiocytosis X, eosinophilic granuloma)
   Tuberculosis, syphilis
   Meningitis
   Lymphocytic hypophysitis, infundibulohypophysitis
Metabolic
   Hemochromatosis
   Amyloidosis
   Critical illness
   Malnutrition
   Anorexia nervosa
   Psychosocial deprivation
Idiopathic

ACTH = adrenocorticotropic hormone; FSH = follicle-stimulating hormone; GH = growth hormone; GHRH = growth hormone releasing hormone; GnRH = gonadotropin-releasing hormone; LH = luteinizing hormone; PRL = prolactin; TRH = thyrotropin-releasing hormone; TSH = thyroid-stimulating hormone.

can impair blood supply to the pituitary as well as decrease input from hypothalamic hormones. Hemorrhage into tumors can lead to pituitary infarction. A mild degree of hyperprolactinemia (usually <200 ng/mL) is characteristic of disorders that cause stalk compression, and hyperprolactinemia further impairs gonadotropin secretion. A variety of other neoplasms that occur near the sella, such as craniopharyngiomas, can also cause hypopituitarism (see Table 231-1).

Radiation causes hypopituitarism primarily because of its effects on hypothalamic function, although high-dose radiation (e.g., proton beam) can also cause direct pituitary damage. The sellar region is subjected to radiation in the treatment of pituitary adenomas, craniopharyngiomas, optic gliomas, meningiomas, dysgerminomas, and neoplasms of the oropharynx. The effects of radiation can be delayed several years, and patients at high risk should be evaluated yearly. Although GH and gonadotropin deficiencies develop first in most patients, ACTH or TSH deficiencies occasionally occur first, emphasizing the need to evaluate each of the major axes.

Empty sella syndrome can occur as a primary or as an acquired condition. It is caused by defects in the diaphragma sella that allow herniation of the arachnoid membrane into the hypophyseal fossa. In long-standing cases, sellar enlargement occurs, probably because of persistent transmission of intracranial pressure. Imaging studies reveal the pituitary gland as a flattened rim of tissue along the floor of the sella. Primary empty sella occurs most commonly in women and may be associated with features of benign intracranial hypertension. Pituitary function is usually normal, but 10% have mild hyperprolactinemia, probably because of stretching of the pituitary stalk. Acquired forms may occur as a result of surgery, radiation, or pituitary infarction (usually of an adenoma).

Pituitary apoplexy is a syndrome caused by hemorrhage into a tumor with associated infarction and leakage of the blood into the arachnoid space, with resultant fever and stiff neck. When the hemorrhage is large, there can be mass effects with headache and cranial nerve compression within the cavernous sinus. Asymptomatic infarctions are found in about 10 to 15% of pituitary adenomas. In the absence of a tumor, predispositions to apoplexy include trauma, pregnancy, anticoagulation, sickle cell anemia, and diabetes mellitus. Pituitary infarction in the peripartum period (*Sheehan's syndrome*) is usually associated with significant obstetric hemorrhage and hypovolemia. Although Sheehan's syndrome can manifest acutely with vascular collapse, it more commonly has a subacute manifestation consisting of postpartum inability to lactate, amenorrhea, and symptoms of adrenal insufficiency.

Infiltrative diseases such as sarcoidosis, histiocytosis, and tuberculosis cause hypopituitarism by infiltrating the hypothalamus and stalk rather than the pituitary. In lymphocytic hypophysitis, there is massive infiltration of the pituitary by lymphocytes and plasma cells with destruction of the parenchyma; it is believed to have an autoimmune basis. The lesion is usually large, and patients present with either symptoms or signs of hypopituitarism or those of a mass lesion (i.e., visual field defects and headaches). Some patients may have mild hyperprolactinemia and diabetes insipidus. Almost all cases have been reported in women, and most present during or after pregnancy. Because of the presentation as a mass lesion during pregnancy, such lesions may be confused with prolactinomas. Mild PRL elevation points to a nonsecretory lesion rather than a prolactinoma. MRI cannot reliably differentiate pituitary adenoma from hypophysitis, although hypophysitis usually manifests with a diffuse enlargement of the pituitary that enhances, rather than as a focal lesion. Diagnosis is usually made by biopsy, but the lesion may be suspected clinically if it manifests during or just after pregnancy. Careful pituitary function testing is mandatory because many patients have died of adrenocortical insufficiency. Although the prognosis is not clear, a number of cases have resolved spontaneously. An entity with similar histologic findings involving the stalk and posterior pituitary, referred to as *infundibuloneurohypophysitis*, can cause diabetes insipidus. A third variant, *panhypophysitis*, involves both lobes of the pituitary. These last two forms occur in both sexes and are generally not associated with pregnancy. The causes and interrelationships between these entities remain unknown.

The pituitary may undergo damage because of iron deposition in patients with hemochromatosis (Chapter 219) and amyloid fibrils in patients with systemic amyloidosis (Chapter 194). Functional, reversible hypopituitarism of varying degrees occurs in patients with severe systemic illness, severe psychosocial and emotional deprivation, and severe weight loss—particularly in those with anorexia nervosa.

DIAGNOSIS AND TREATMENT

The diagnosis of hypopituitarism rests on the stimulation tests that are summarized in Table 231-2. Therapy depends on the nature and severity of the hormone deficiencies as well as on the desired clinical end points. The goals are to replace hormones in a physiologic manner and to avoid the consequences of over-replacement. Examples of hormonal replacement paradigms are provided in Table 231-3. Adjustment of hormone doses is done primarily based on clinical findings; TSH levels are not helpful for adjusting thyroxine doses in patients with central hypothyroidism. Even when conventional hormone replacement (adrenal, thyroid, gonadal) is carried out appropriately, there is a twofold excess risk for death. Although untreated GH deficiency has been hypothesized to be the cause of this excess risk, this has not been proved. The benefits of GH therapy are less clear than those of the other pituitary hormones and include improvements in body composition, bone, lipids, and quality of life; although there are few adverse effects, treatment involves daily injections.

PITUITARY TUMORS

PATHOBIOLOGY

Pituitary tumors are classified according to the hormones that they produce and their size: microadenomas, less than 10 mm in diameter; macroadenomas, more than 10 mm in diameter; and macroadenomas with extrasellar extension. In general, the levels of hormones produced by the tumors parallel the size of the tumors. The prevalence of the different types of pituitary adenomas, based on surgical data, is summarized in Table 231-4. Immunohistochemical studies, using antibodies specific for each of the major pituitary hormones, have been used to define tumor phenotype. Pituitary adenomas are rarely malignant but can be locally invasive.

Most pituitary tumors are monoclonal. This finding does not exclude a role for hormonal stimulation as a predisposing factor for somatic mutations, and the hormonal environment may also affect the rate of tumor growth (e.g., Nelson's syndrome). Supporting the concept that somatic mutations lead to pituitary tumorigenesis, a subset (35 to 40%) of somatotroph adenomas have activating mutations in the gene for the Gsα-subunit, resulting in two different amino acid (Arg201 and Glu227) substitutions. Either mutation causes the Gsα-subunit to stimulate adenylyl cyclase in a constitutive manner. The elevated intracellular cyclic adenosine monophosphate levels lead to increased cell growth as well as GH production. Mutations in other oncogenes, such as *ras, Rb,* and *p53* are uncommon in pituitary tumors. Thus, the nature of the somatic mutations causing most pituitary tumors remains unknown.

Three types of inherited predispositions to pituitary tumors are recognized. Patients with McCune-Albright syndrome (Chapter 239) occasionally develop pituitary adenomas as well as characteristic abnormalities in other tissues, particularly the ovary, bone, and thyroid. Interestingly, the McCune-Albright syndrome is also caused by mutations in the gene for the Gsα-subunit. However, the somatic mutations in McCune-Albright occur early during development, so that multiple tissues are affected. In multiple endocrine neoplasia type 1 (MEN 1) (Chapter 239), the predisposition to pituitary tumors is inherited in an autosomal dominant manner and occurs in conjunction with tumors of the parathyroid and pancreas. Familial isolated pituitary adenoma (FIPA) syndrome is autosomal dominant and has low or variable penetrance. Germline mutations have been found in the gene for the aryl hydrocarbon receptor–interacting protein (*AIP*), which functions as a tumor suppressor. Such mutations have been found in about one third of FIPA families, most commonly in those with GH- and PRL-producing tumors.

CLINICAL MANIFESTATIONS

Mass Effects of Pituitary Adenomas

Many of the clinical manifestations of pituitary adenomas are related to the hypersecretion of hormones. However, the mass effects of the enlarging tumor can also lead to specific signs and symptoms (Chapter 195). Particularly in the case of nonfunctioning tumors or in those that produce gonadotropins, the primary clinical manifestations are related to effects of the tumor on surrounding structures.

Headaches are common in patients with macroadenomas and appear to be caused by expansion of the diaphragma sellae or by invasion of bone. The sudden onset of severe headache associated with nausea, vomiting, and altered consciousness can also be caused by hemorrhagic infarction with sudden enlargement of a pituitary adenoma. Severe cases require glucocorticoid treatment and possible surgical decompression.

Pituitary tumors that extend superiorly can affect visual fields. Expansion into the suprasellar region exerts pressure on the optic chiasm, usually in the central region where nerves emanating from the inferior and medial part of the retina (superior and temporal visual fields) cross, leading to bitemporal hemianopsia. Visual field loss is variable, however, and is affected by the location and flexibility of the chiasm as well as by the direction and extent of tumor growth. Large tumors may invade the cavernous sinus or surround an optic nerve, leading to other patterns of visual field changes or loss of visual acuity. The tumor size and the direction and degree of extrasellar extension are best evaluated with MRI with gadolinium. If the tumor abuts the chiasm on MRI, formal visual field testing should be performed. Even long-standing visual loss may be reversible.

The normal pituitary is often compressed into a thin rim of tissue by large pituitary adenomas. Hypopituitarism probably results more from compression of the hypothalamic-pituitary stalk than from direct pressure on the normal pituitary. GH deficiency and hypogonadotropic hypogonadism are

TABLE 231-2 TESTS OF PITUITARY INSUFFICIENCY

HORMONE	TEST	INTERPRETATION
Growth hormone (GH)	*Insulin tolerance test:* Regular insulin (0.05-0.15 U/kg) is given IV and blood is drawn at −30, 0, 30, 45, 60, and 90 min for measurement of glucose and GH.	If hypoglycemia occurs (glucose < 40 mg/dL), GH should increase to >5 µg/L.*
	Arginine-GHRH test: GHRH 1 µg/kg IV bolus followed by 30 min infusion of L-arginine (30 g)	Normal response is GH > 4.1 µg/L.
	Glucagon test: 1 mg IM with GH measurements at 0, 60, 90,120, 150 and 180 min	Normal response is GH >3 µg/L.
Adrenocorticotropic hormone (ACTH)	*Insulin tolerance test:* Regular insulin (0.05-0.15 U/kg) is given IV and blood is drawn at −30, 0, 30, 45, 60, and 90 min for measurement of glucose and cortisol.	If hypoglycemia occurs (glucose < 40 mg/dL), cortisol should increase by >7 µg/dL or to >20 µg/dL.
	CRH test: 1 µg/kg ovine CRH IV at 8 AM with blood samples drawn at 0, 15, 30, 60, 90, 120 min for measurement of ACTH and cortisol	In most normal individuals, the basal ACTH increases twofold to fourfold and reaches a peak (20-100 pg/mL). ACTH responses may be delayed in cases of hypothalamic dysfunction. Cortisol levels usually reach 20-25 µg/dL.
	Metyrapone test: Metyrapone (30 mg/kg to max. 2 g) at midnight with measurements of plasma 11-deoxycortisol and cortisol at 8 AM. ACTH can also be measured. A 3-day test is also available. Basal cortisol should be >5-6 µg/dL before test.	A normal response is 11-deoxycortisol > 7.5 µg/dL or ACTH > 75 pg/mL. Plasma cortisol should fall below 4 µg/dL to ensure an adequate response.
	ACTH stimulation test: ACTH 1-24 (Cosyntropin), 0.25 mg IM or IV. Cortisol is measured at 0, 30, and 60 min.	A normal response is cortisol >18 µg/dL. In suspected hypothalamic-pituitary deficiency, a low-dose (1-µg) test may be more sensitive.
Thyroid-stimulating hormone (TSH)	*Basal thyroid function tests:* free T₄, free T₃, TSH	Low free thyroid hormone levels in the setting of TSH levels that are not appropriately increased.
Luteinizing hormone (LH), follicle-stimulating hormone (FSH)	*Basal levels of LH, FSH, testosterone, estrogen*	Basal LH and FSH should be increased in postmenopausal women. Low testosterone levels in conjunction with low or low-normal LH and FSH are consistent with gonadotropin deficiency.
	GnRH test: GnRH (100 µg) IV with measurements of serum LH and FSH at 0, 30, and 60 min	In most normal persons, LH should increase by 10 IU/L and FSH by 2 IU/L. Normal responses are variable, and repeated stimulation may be required.
	Clomiphene test: clomiphene citrate (100 mg) is given orally for 5 days. Serum LH and FSH are measured on days 0, 5, 7, 10, and 13.	A 50% increase should occur in LH and FSH, usually by day 5.
Multiple hormones	*Combined anterior pituitary test:* GHRH (1 µg/kg), CRH (1 µg/kg), GnRH (100 µg) are given sequentially IV. Blood samples are drawn at −30, 15, 30, 60, 90, and 120 min for measurements of GH, ACTH, LH, and FSH.	Combined or individual releasing hormone responses must be evaluated in the context of basal hormone values and may not be diagnostic (see text).

*Values are with polyclonal assays.
CRH = corticotrophin-releasing hormone; GHRH = growth hormone-releasing hormone; GnRH = gonadotropin-releasing hormone; IM = intramuscularly; IV = intravenously; T₃ = triiodothyronine; T₄ = thyroxine; TRH = thyrotropin-releasing hormone.

TABLE 231-3 HORMONAL REPLACEMENT THERAPY IN HYPOPITUITARISM*

PITUITARY AXIS	HORMONAL REPLACEMENTS
Growth hormone (GH)	In children, GH (0.25 mg/kg) SC daily. In adults, GH (0.3-1.2 mg) SC daily. Titrate dose to achieve IGF-1 levels in middle to upper part of normal range. Women receiving oral estrogens require higher doses.
Prolactin	None
Adrenocorticotropic hormone–cortisol	Hydrocortisone (10-15 mg PO q AM; 5-10 mg PO q PM) or prednisone (2.5 mg PO q AM; 2.5 mg PO q PM). Dose adjusted on clinical basis. Stress dosing: 50-75 mg hydrocortisone IV q8hr
Thyroid-stimulating hormone–thyroid	L-Thyroxine (0.075-0.15 mg) PO qd
Gonadotropins-gonads	FSH and LH (or hCG) can be used to induce ovulation in women. hCG alone or with FSH can be used to induce spermatogenesis in men. Pulsatile GnRH (via pump) is less commonly used for GnRH-deficient subjects.
	In men, testosterone enanthate (100-300 mg) IM q1-3wk or testosterone cyclopentylpropionate (100-300 mg) IM q1-3wk. Testosterone transdermal patches can also be used (5 mg qd). Testosterone gel (1%) 1-2 packets (5-10 g) daily
	In women, conjugated estrogens (0.625-1.25 mg) or mestranol (35 mg) PO days 1-25 each month cycled with medroxyprogesterone acetate (5-10 mg) PO days 15-25 each month. Low-dose contraceptive pills may also be used.
	Estrogen-containing transdermal patches are also available.
Posterior pituitary	Desmopressin, 0.05-0.2 mL (5-20 µg) intranasally once or twice daily, or tablets (0.1-0.4 mg q8-12hr) or 0.5 mL (2 µg) SC.

*Replacement therapy is dictated by the types of hormone deficiencies and by the clinical circumstances. In each case, the recommended preparations and doses are representative but need to be adjusted for individual patients. Other hormonal preparations are also available.
FSH = follicle-stimulating hormone; GnRH = gonadotropin-releasing hormone; hCG = human chorionic gonadotropin; IGF-I = insulin-like growth factor-I; IM = intramuscularly; LH = luteinizing hormone; PO, orally; SC = subcutaneously.

particularly common. Slightly elevated PRL levels (generally <200 ng/mL) occur in cases of stalk compression because of diminished inhibition by dopamine. It is important not to mistake such tumors for prolactinomas because they will not decrease in size in response to medical therapy with dopamine agonists. A peculiarity of some two-site immunoassays, referred to as the "hook effect," can sometimes cause a very high prolactin level to read falsely normal or just mildly elevated; a 1:100 dilution of the serum sample with saline will show the true prolactin level. Preoperative hypopituitarism caused by a large pituitary mass is reversible in up to half of patients after surgical decompression. Diabetes insipidus (vasopressin deficiency) is rarely caused by pituitary tumors and should raise the suspicion of a craniopharyngioma or other hypothalamic disorders.

TABLE 231-4	PREVALENCE OF DIFFERENT TYPES OF PITUITARY ADENOMAS		
TYPE OF PITUITARY ADENOMA	**DISORDER**	**HORMONE PRODUCED**	**PREVALENCE (%)***
Somatotroph	Acromegaly and gigantism	Growth hormone	10-15
Lactotroph (prolactinoma)	Hypogonadism, galactorrhea	Prolactin	25-40
Corticotroph	Cushing's disease	Adrenocorticotropic hormone	10-15
Gonadotroph	Mass effects, hypopituitarism	Follicle-stimulating hormone and luteinizing hormone	15-20
Thyrotroph	Hyperthyroidism	Thyroid-stimulating hormone	<3
Nonfunctioning/ null cell	Mass effects, hypopituitarism	None	10-25

*The prevalence rates represent ranges described in several different large surgical series. Mixed tumors (e.g., growth hormone and prolactin) and plurihormonal adenomas are not shown. Rates vary depending on methods used to establish the diagnosis. Prolactinomas were underestimated in most recent pathologic series because they are largely managed medically. Most glycoprotein hormone–producing pituitary tumors were classified as nonfunctioning adenomas until the application of immunohistochemical studies.

TREATMENT Rx

Surgery

Except for prolactinomas, surgery is the primary mode of therapy for pituitary tumors that warrant intervention. Indications for surgery include reduction in hormone levels and decompression to relieve mass effects or to prevent further tumor expansion. Currently, the transsphenoidal route, usually with an endoscopic, endonasal approach, is used almost exclusively for decompression or extirpation of pituitary tumors. Because of substantially greater morbidity, subfrontal craniotomy is reserved for patients with tumors that require extensive exploration of the suprasellar region and surrounding structures. In experienced hands, transsphenoidal surgery is effective, and complications are uncommon (<5% complication rate) but include CSF leak, hemorrhage, optic nerve injury, hypopituitarism, and sinusitis. Transient diabetes insipidus occurs in about 5% of patients after surgery but rarely persists long term. Mortality rates are less than 1%. Complication rates increase with increasing size of the tumor and when a craniotomy is performed.

Surgical cure rates are largely a function of the size and location of the pituitary mass. When stringent hormonal criteria are used to assess surgical success rates, less than 30% of macroadenomas are cured by transsphenoidal surgery, although considerable improvements in hormone levels or mass effects can be achieved. On the other hand, hormone hypersecretion by microadenomas can be corrected completely in 80 to 90% of patients, although the cure rates vary considerably at different institutions. Even with apparent surgical cure, 10 to 20% of tumors may recur over several years, resulting in a redevelopment of the hormone oversecretion syndrome.

Radiation Therapy

Irradiation is usually used as adjunctive therapy after surgery or in combination with medical therapy. Radiation has typically been administered over 5 weeks at a dose of 45 Gy using cobalt-60 or a linear accelerator. Proton beam therapy delivers very high doses of radiation within a localized region, but it is limited to intrasellar lesions and is not widely available. More recently, a radiation therapy technique referred to as stereotactic radiotherapy has been employed for many patients with pituitary tumors. With this technique, approximately the same dosage of radiation is administered as a single dose through multiple ports using a computerized matching of irradiation to tumor geometry. Response rates are slow (several years, but somewhat more rapid with stereotactic therapy). Complete remission is rarely achieved with any of these types of irradiation. Stereotactic radiotherapy appears to be particularly useful for residual tumor in the cavernous sinus because the normal structures that course through that area (carotid artery, cranial nerves III, IV, V_1, V_2, VI) are relatively radioresistant. Because the time to recurrence for most nonfunctioning macroadenomas is 5 to 10 years, and not all tumors recur, it is often reasonable to follow patients with imaging techniques, reserving irradiation for those with evidence of residual tumor or recurrence if no tumor was visible postoperatively.

Complications of irradiation are dose related but can also be idiosyncratic. Partial or complete hypopituitarism occurs in 50 to 70% of patients and is primarily due to hypothalamic injury. Conventional irradiation is associated with an increased risk for stroke. Second tumors occur in the radiation field in about 2% of patients over a 20-year period. Less common complications include optic nerve damage, brain necrosis, and cognitive dysfunction. Whether stereotactic radiotherapy will have similar rates of complications is at present unknown. Early studies show that hypopituitarism is developing at a rate similar to that seen with conventional therapy.

Medical Therapy

The emergence of medical therapies for pituitary tumors has dramatically affected patient management. Dopamine agonists, bromocriptine and cabergoline, have a primary role in the management of prolactinomas. They induce a rapid fall in PRL levels and, importantly, decrease tumor size. Dopamine agonists are also used in the management of acromegaly, although the GH responses and effects on tumor size are much less pronounced than in prolactinomas. Somatostatin analogues, such as octreotide and lanreotide, act to suppress the secretion of a number of hormones, including GH and TSH, and have been used to treat acromegaly and TSH-producing tumors. Medical therapy for Cushing's disease is primarily directed toward inhibition of steroid biosynthesis. These drugs include ketoconazole, metyrapone, etomidate, and mitotane. Because of substantial side effects and because patients with Cushing's disease tend to escape from the cortisol-suppressing effects of these drugs, medical therapy is used primarily as an adjunctive treatment or to reduce cortisol levels preoperatively. Another new category of drugs to treat pituitary tumors includes the receptor blockers. Pegvisomant is a GH analogue with altered binding to the GH receptor that competitively inhibits GH binding to its receptor and is used in the treatment of acromegaly. Mifepristone can block the action of cortisol at its receptor and is being evaluated for the treatment of Cushing's syndrome.

● GROWTH HORMONE

The most important regulators of GH are the hypothalamic hormones: GHRH, which is stimulatory, and somatostatin, which is inhibitory. GH increases the production of IGF-I (formerly known as somatomedin C). The Gsα-subunit, which is coupled to the GHRH receptor, is one of the targets for activating mutations that lead to somatotroph adenomas.

IGF-I inhibits GH secretion, and it acts at both the pituitary and hypothalamic levels. In addition to reflecting GH action (primarily at the liver), serum IGF-I is also sensitive to nutritional and metabolic changes. In cases of starvation, anorexia nervosa, and poorly controlled diabetes, IGF-I levels are low, resulting in increased levels of GH. In cases of obesity, GH levels are low, and GHRH responses are blunted, but IGF-I levels are generally normal and actually increase with increasing body mass index. Stress, exercise, and a variety of neurogenic stimuli also increase GH secretion. Estrogens stimulate GH secretion, but their effects are less pronounced than for PRL, and they inhibit the stimulatory effect of GH on IGF-I production.

Large bursts of GH secretion characteristically occur at night in association with slow-wave sleep. GH levels increase during puberty and decline gradually in adulthood. The amplitude of GH pulses is greater in women than in men, likely reflecting the effects of estrogens. Spontaneous GH pulses can reach 50 ng/mL; consequently, random GH levels can be quite variable. GH responses to GHRH are also variable even within an individual, owing to changes in endogenous somatostatin tone.

GH acts through a single transmembrane receptor that is structurally related to PRL and cytokine receptors. The GH molecule has two distinguishable receptor binding domains that allow it to contact two separate receptor molecules to induce receptor dimerization. Mutations in the gene for the GH receptor cause GH resistance and severe growth retardation, a condition referred to as the GH insensitivity syndrome (Laron-type dwarfism). GH levels are elevated and IGF-I levels are low, reflecting the inability of the mutant receptor to transduce the GH signal. Mutations have also been found in signaling intermediates (such as the signal transducers of activators of transcription *STAT5b* gene) that mediate GH actions.

Many of the growth and metabolic effects of GH are transmitted indirectly through the actions of IGF-I. GH stimulates IGF-I production in most tissues, where it then exerts autocrine or paracrine effects. Circulating IGF-I is derived predominantly from the liver and is a useful marker of GH action because it has a longer half-life and integrates the effects of GH pulses. Although IGF-I levels are used in the diagnosis of acromegaly and to assess the integrity of the GH axis, factors other than GH (e.g., malnutrition) can alter IGF-I levels. IGF-I acts through widely distributed receptors that are structurally related to insulin receptors. In addition to its growth-promoting and anabolic effects, IGF-I also stimulates mitogenesis in many tissues. The bioactivity of IGF-I is itself modulated by six IGF-binding proteins (IGFBPs). These IGFBPs can inhibit or enhance IGF actions. IGFBP-3 is the major IGFBP in plasma; it is regulated by GH, and its levels generally parallel those of IGF-I.

GH has its major effects on linear growth but also influences a variety of metabolic pathways. Some of these effects are mediated by GH directly, whereas others are conferred by IGF-I. Although the relative roles of GH and IGF-I are debated, their actions are cooperative in many cases. The effects of GH on linear growth appear to be mediated largely by IGF-I, which has been used to stimulate growth in patients with the GH insensitivity syndrome. Linear growth in the fetus and neonate is not GH dependent, as illustrated by the fact that GH-deficient infants have normal birth lengths, although intrauterine IGF-I and IGF-II may be important for fetal growth independent of GH. In contrast, normal postnatal linear growth requires GH, as illustrated by the clinical manifestations of GH deficiency. GH and IGF-I act together to accelerate linear growth markedly, particularly at the time of puberty when sex steroids enhance GH and IGF-I levels.

Growth hormone also induces lipolysis and stimulates anabolic activity, including amino acid uptake and protein synthesis. As a result, it reduces body fat, increases lean body mass, and leads to positive nitrogen balance. These properties of GH are most strikingly seen in GH-deficient children who have undergone replacement. GH opposes many of the actions of insulin and can be considered diabetogenic. In diabetic individuals, nocturnal GH secretion accounts in large part for the dawn phenomenon, in which there is a decrease in glucose utilization, causing a tendency toward hyperglycemia.

GROWTH HORMONE DEFICIENCY

Causes of GH deficiency include hypothalamic-pituitary disorders, GHRH receptor mutations, GH gene mutations, combined pituitary hormone deficiencies, GH receptor mutations, IGF-I receptor mutations, radiation, and psychosocial deprivation (Chapter 230). The clinical manifestations of GH deficiency depend on the time of onset and the severity of hormone deficiency. Children with complete GH deficiency have slow linear growth rates (approximately 3 cm/year), and they rapidly fall below normal on standardized growth charts. GH-deficient children have normal skeletal proportions, and many have a pudgy, youthful appearance because of decreased lipolysis. Particularly in the setting of cortisol deficiency, there is a predisposition to hypoglycemia.

Basal GH does not provide a reliable measure of GH reserve, whereas low IGF-I is consistent with GH deficiency. However, not all patients documented to have GH deficiency by stimulation testing have IGF-I levels that are below the normal range. GH deficiency is assessed using insulin-induced hypoglycemia, which activates central nervous system pathways, leading to stimulation of both GH and ACTH secretion (see Table 231-2). The insulin tolerance test requires careful monitoring for symptoms of severe hypoglycemia, such as confusion or depressed consciousness. This test should be avoided in patients with seizure disorders or coronary artery disease. Insulin doses (0.1 to 0.15 U/kg) may need to be decreased if glucocorticoid deficiency is suspected or increased in conditions of insulin resistance (e.g., obesity). Alternatives to the insulin tolerance test for evaluation of GH are a combination of arginine and GHRH given intravenously or glucagon given intramuscularly.

TREATMENT   Rx

In children with well-documented GH deficiency, GH replacement is effective and is essential to increase final adult height. In a typical regimen, recombinant GH (0.025 mg/kg) is given daily as subcutaneous injections. The efficacy of GH treatment depends on when it is initiated as well as replacement of other hormone deficiencies, if they coexist. In the setting of multiple hormone deficiencies, replacement of thyroid hormone and cortisol is necessary for effective GH action. On the other hand, sex steroids lead to epiphyseal closure and limit linear growth. Consequently, GH is more effective before puberty; if exogenous sex steroids are given, low doses should be used. GH has also been shown to increase the final height of girls with Turner's syndrome (chromosomal XO state) and children with end-stage renal disease.

Only about one third of children with isolated, idiopathic GH deficiency are found to be GH deficient when retested as adults. Thus, all such patients should be retested before GH therapy is continued or restarted unless they have proven molecular defects as the cause of their GH deficiency. Studies show that GH treatment can increase lean body mass, decrease fat mass, and improve the sense of well-being in adults with documented GH deficiency. In most studies, safety data for long-term GH administration show negligible adverse effects. Whether GH treatment in adults will affect the increased mortality rate associated with hypopituitarism remains to be seen. Adverse effects occur at lower doses in adults compared with children; a starting dose of 0.2 to 0.3 mg/day has been recommended, with gradual titration guided by clinical benefits, adverse effects, and IGF-I levels.

GROWTH HORMONE EXCESS: ACROMEGALY AND GIGANTISM

PATHOBIOLOGY

GH-producing pituitary tumors account for 10 to 15% of pituitary tumors (see Table 231-4). GH-producing tumors are frequently mixed tumors that secrete more than one hormone. PRL is produced in about 40% of somatotroph adenomas, and some patients may present because of symptoms due to the hyperprolactinemia (i.e., amenorrhea, galactorrhea, or both). Ectopic production of GHRH (usually carcinoid or pancreatic islets) is a well-documented but rare (<1%) cause of acromegaly that can result in somatotroph hyperplasia. Activating Gsα-subunit mutations occur in 35 to 40% of somatotroph adenomas. Molecular defects in the remaining 60 to 65% of somatotroph adenomas remain unidentified.

CLINICAL MANIFESTATIONS

Tumors that secrete GH cause acromegaly in adults and gigantism in children in whom GH excess occurs before epiphyseal closure. Acromegaly affects men and women with equal frequency and is most often recognized when patients are in their 30s or 40s, usually after a decade of GH excess. The most striking features of acromegaly usually involve the face, hands, and feet. The diagnosis is often suspected because of changes in facial appearance that include enlargement of the lower jaw (prognathism), the nose and lips, and the sinuses (causing frontal bossing) (Fig. 231-1). Oral cavity changes include malocclusion, increased spacing between the teeth, and enlargement of the tongue. A hollow, resonant voice is caused by changes in the vocal cords and the soft tissues of the hypopharynx. Sleep apnea may occur in patients with soft tissue obstruction of the pharynx but may also occur because of a central disorder. In addition to bony enlargement, there is a marked increase in the soft tissue of the hands and feet, leading to progressive increases in ring, glove, and shoe size. A moist, doughy, enveloping handshake is characteristic

1977   1981

1983   1988

FIGURE 231-1. Clinical features of acromegaly. Serial photographs of a 64-year-old woman with acromegaly. Over an 11-year period, there is a progressive coarsening of facial features, including enlargement of the nose and lips and development of prognathism. She also experienced hypertension, arthropathy, and enlargement of the hands (not shown). (From Molitch ME. Clinical manifestations of acromegaly. *Endocrinol Metab Clin North Am.* 1992;21:597-614.)

of acromegaly. Arthritis (hands, feet, hips, knees) is common (75%) and is caused by cartilage and synovial overgrowth. Some degree of carpal tunnel syndrome is seen in about half of patients. Skin changes include increased skinfolds, particularly over the brow and forehead. The skin is usually oily, owing to increased sebaceous activity and sweating. Skin tags are common, and their presence correlates with the presence of colonic polyps. Galactorrhea may be seen in women, and reproductive dysfunction occurs in both women and men when PRL levels are elevated. Headaches, visual field defects, and other neurologic symptoms depend on the location and extent of tumor growth.

Acromegaly causes a two- to three-fold increase in mortality rate. Most of the increased mortality can be attributed to cardiovascular and cerebrovascular diseases and may be related to the increased prevalence of hypertension (25 to 35%) and diabetes mellitus (10 to 25%) in patients with acromegaly. There is evidence for cardiac hypertrophy in most patients, and symptomatic heart disease, consisting of coronary ischemia or congestive heart failure or both, occurs in 15 to 20% of patients. Sleep apnea may predispose patients to cardiac dysrhythmias. Some analyses have found an increased risk of premalignant polyps and colon cancer, and screening with colonoscopy is generally recommended. The disfigurement, metabolic complications, and increased mortality associated with acromegaly emphasize the importance of early diagnosis and implementation of appropriate therapy to lower the GH levels into the normal range.

DIAGNOSIS

Because GH is secreted in a pulsatile manner, and because the amplitude of normal GH pulses can be large (>50 ng/mL), random GH level measurements are not very useful in making the diagnosis of acromegaly. IGF-I levels provide an integrated index of GH production and provide a better screening test for acromegaly. IGF-I levels decrease with age, so normal ranges must be age adjusted. IGF-I levels correlate well with 24-hour GH production rates and with disease activity. The most standardized test for acromegaly is the glucose tolerance test (Table 231-5). In acromegaly, increased glucose levels fail to suppress GH levels to below 1 ng/mL with polyclonal antibody immunoassays and to levels below 0.4 ng/mL using newer monoclonal antibody two-site assays. Co-secretion of PRL should be evaluated. After the diagnosis of acromegaly is made, radiologic studies, preferably using MRI, should be used to evaluate the extent of tumor growth. Unlike in Cushing's disease and prolactinomas, most patients with acromegaly have macroadenomas.

TABLE 231-5 SELECTED TESTS OF EXCESS PITUITARY FUNCTION

HORMONE	TEST	INTERPRETATION
Growth hormone (GH)	Basal IGF-1	Elevated IGF-1 levels are consistent with acromegaly when interpreted in the context of age and nutritional status.
	Oral glucose suppression test: after 75-g glucose load, GH is measured at −30, 0, 30, 60, 90, 120 min	GH should be suppressed to <1 μg/L in normal persons with polyclonal radioimmunoassays; <0.4 μg/L with two-site monoclonal assays. GH may paradoxically increase in acromegaly.
Prolactin	Basal prolactin levels	Elevated prolactin (>200 μg/L) is consistent with a prolactinoma. When prolactin levels are between 20 and 200 μg/L, other causes of hyperprolactinemia should be considered.
Adrenocorticotropic hormone (ACTH)	Measurement of 24-hr urine free cortisol	Elevated level is suggestive of Cushing's syndrome, but it has several other causes as well.
	Midnight salivary cortisol: special tubes with cotton pledgets available to collect saliva at 11 PM to midnight	In normal persons, the midnight salivary cortisol is very low because of the normal diurnal variation. In patients with Cushing's syndrome, the salivary cortisol is elevated.
	Overnight dexamethasone suppression test: dexamethasone (1 mg) PO at midnight followed by 8 AM plasma cortisol	In normal persons, AM cortisol should be suppressed to <5 μg/dL. Normal test excludes Cushing's syndrome. Other disorders can cause failure to suppress normally.
	Low-dose dexamethasone suppression test: dexamethasone (0.5 mg) q6hr for eight doses with basal and end of treatment measurements that may include 24-hr urine collections for free cortisol or 17-hydroxysteroids and AM plasma cortisol and ACTH.	Urine free cortisol should be <20 μg/24 hr; serum cortisol should be suppressed to <6 μg/dL. Failure to suppress cortisol production is consistent with the diagnosis of Cushing's syndrome.
	High-dose dexamethasone suppression test: dexamethasone (2 mg) q6hr for eight doses with basal and end-of-treatment measurements that may include 24-hr urine collections for free cortisol or 17-hydroxysteroids and AM plasma cortisol and ACTH.	The high-dose test is intended to distinguish Cushing's disease (pituitary adenoma), ectopic ACTH production, and adrenal adenoma. The 90% suppression of urine free cortisol production is suggestive of Cushing's disease. Less than 50% suppression suggests ectopic ACTH or adrenal adenoma. Low ACTH levels are consistent with adrenal adenoma.
	CRH test: ovine CRH (1 μg/kg) is administered IV, and ACTH and cortisol are drawn at −15, 0, 15, 30, 60, 90, and 120 min	In Cushing's disease, there is usually a 50% increase in ACTH and a 20% increase in cortisol. Adrenal adenoma is associated with suppressed ACTH. Ectopic ACTH is associated with high basal ACTH and cortisol levels that are not affected by CRH.
	Petrosal sinus ACTH sampling: the inferior petrosal sinus is catheterized, ideally bilaterally, and plasma ACTH is compared with simultaneous peripheral samples. The sampling can be done in conjunction with CRH stimulation.	In Cushing's disease, the ratio of ACTH in the petrosal sinus to the periphery is at least 2 basally and at least 3 after CRH. In ectopic ACTH, the ratio of petrosal sinus to peripheral level is <1.5.
Thyroid-stimulating hormone (TSH)	Basal thyroid function tests	An inappropriate normal or elevated TSH in the setting of increased free thyroid hormone levels is consistent with a TSH-producing tumor or other causes of inappropriate TSH secretion.
	Free α-subunit level	Elevated levels associated with inappropriately elevated TSH are suggestive of a TSH-producing tumor.
Follicle-stimulating hormone (FSH), luteinizing hormone (LH)	Basal FSH, LH, testosterone	Increased LH and testosterone levels in males are consistent with LH-secreting tumors. Elevated FSH and low-normal testosterone are suggestive of an FSH-producing tumor if primary gonadal failure is not present. In females, assessment of excess hormone secretion is difficult because of changes during the menstrual cycle and at menopause.
	TRH test: TRH (200 μg) is given IV with measurements of serum FSH, LH, FSH β-, and LH β-subunits at 0, 20, 60 min.	Stimulation of LH, FSH, or their free β-subunits is suggestive of a gonadotropin-producing adenoma. TRH is not available in the United States.

CRH = corticotropin-releasing hormone; IGF = insulin-like growth factor; TRH = thyrotropin-releasing hormone.

TREATMENT

The goals of therapy are to reverse or prevent tumor mass effects and to reduce the long-term morbidity and mortality that result from excess GH production. Correction of the disorder prevents further physical disfigurement and can result in substantial resolution of soft tissue changes and improvements in metabolic derangements. Although reductions in GH levels are associated with improvements in symptoms, the ultimate goal is to achieve normal GH and IGF-I levels and to prevent tumor recurrence without incurring hypopituitarism.

Transsphenoidal surgery results in GH levels below 2.5 ng/mL in 80% of patients with microadenomas when performed by experienced neurosurgeons. This level, along with GH suppression below 1 ng/mL during an oral glucose tolerance test, and a normal IGF-I level have been associated with a normalization of the increased mortality of acromegaly. Patients with macroadenomas are less often cured by surgery (<30%) but usually have reductions in GH levels.

Medical therapies for acromegaly include dopamine agonists, such as cabergoline; somatostatin analogues, such as octreotide and lanreotide; and a GH receptor antagonist, pegvisomant. Although cabergoline can reduce GH and IGF-I levels in many patients, normal levels are achieved in only about 10 to 20%. Long-acting preparations of octreotide and lanreotide that can be given by intramuscular injection every 4 weeks reduce GH and IGF-I levels in almost all patients, with normal levels of IGF-I being achieved in about 50 to 60% of cases. Tumor size is reduced modestly in about one half of cases. Of those achieving normal levels of GH and IGF-I, about 10 to 20% can eventually be successfully withdrawn from treatment after several years. Somatostatin analogues are useful as adjunctive therapy in patients who are not cured by surgery or radiation and in some cases are used primarily when a surgical cure is not possible, such as in those with cavernous sinus invasion. Side effects of somatostatin analogues include diarrhea and increased risk of cholelithiasis, although cholecystitis and need for cholecystectomy are rare. Some patients experience additive beneficial effects from combining these two classes of medications while keeping the dose of each drug low enough to avoid adverse effects. Pegvisomant is a biosynthetic GH analogue that prevents binding of GH to its receptor. It is capable of normalizing IGF-I levels in more than 90% of patients with corresponding clinical benefits, but it has no effects on the tumor itself. Pegvisomant is given by daily subcutaneous injection; although it generally has been held in reserve for patients not responding optimally to other treatment modalities, there is increasing use now as initial medical therapy when tumors are not large because of its high biochemical and clinical efficacy.

Radiation is not recommended as primary therapy for acromegaly because of the long time (5 to 10 years) required for reductions in GH levels and the high incidence of hypopituitarism and other complications. Adjunctive radiation therapy may be required for patients with macroadenomas when GH levels or mass effects persist after transsphenoidal surgery and medical therapy. Recent data suggest that stereotactic radiotherapy may be the most efficacious form of radiotherapy for acromegaly.

⬤ PROLACTIN

Prolactin and GH appear to be derived from a common ancestral gene, which accounts for the similarities in their structures and some overlap in their functional properties. Although large molecular weight forms of PRL due to binding to immunoglobulin G (IgG), termed *macroprolactin*, react in radioimmunoassays, they have diminished biologic potency. Estrogen stimulates lactotroph proliferation, and their number is consequently greater in females than in males and during pregnancy (~70% of pituitary cells).

Secretion of PRL is controlled by tonic inhibition by dopamine, which acts through D_2-type receptors on lactotrophs. PRL biosynthesis and secretion are stimulated by the hypothalamic peptides TRH and vasoactive intestinal peptide (VIP). Hypothyroidism causes increased TRH output and increased sensitivity of the lactotrophs to TRH and can result in hyperprolactinemia. Dopamine inhibition is the dominant influence for PRL secretion; therefore, PRL is the one pituitary hormone that increases after pituitary stalk section. Secretion of PRL is pulsatile and increases with sleep, stress, chest wall stimulation, and pregnancy. PRL levels are usually less than 15 to 20 ng/mL in women and 10 to 15 ng/mL in men. The primary function of PRL is to induce and sustain lactation. During pregnancy, PRL levels increase, and, in conjunction with other hormones (estrogens, progesterone, thyroid hormone, cortisol, and insulin), breast epithelium is stimulated to proliferate, and milk synthesis is induced. High levels of estrogen and progesterone inhibit lactation during pregnancy, and their decline post partum permits lactation to occur. Neural pathways leading to the secretion of oxytocin provide the "let-down" reflex that induces lactation in response to suckling. Early in the postpartum period, PRL secretion is stimulated by suckling, but this response becomes damped with time as the frequency of suckling episodes decreases. PRL also suppresses gonadotropins, probably by a direct action on GnRH-secreting neurons. As a result, breast-feeding can suppress ovulation.

⬤ PROLACTIN DEFICIENCY

Prolactin deficiency is rare and occurs primarily in the setting of combined hormone deficiencies. The only recognized consequence of PRL deficiency is the absence of postpartum lactation, and this scenario may be found with pituitary infarction occurring as a result of obstetric hemorrhage (Sheehan's syndrome). No effects on breast development or other tissues have been described in PRL deficiency.

⬤ HYPERPROLACTINEMIA

PATHOBIOLOGY

Hyperprolactinemia can occur as a consequence of pharmacologic alterations in the pathways that control PRL secretion or of physiologic or metabolic effects on PRL production and clearance or as a neoplastic condition. Prolactinomas are neoplastic growths of lactotroph cells and are the most common type of pituitary adenoma (25 to 40%). Estrogen is a potent stimulus for lactotroph proliferation; however, there is no clear association between estrogens (e.g., oral contraceptive use) and the incidence of prolactinomas. However, the very high estrogen levels present during pregnancy may cause about 30% of large prolactinomas to increase in size. Diminished dopamine tone, such as may occur with prolonged treatment with antipsychotic agents, results in increased PRL but has not been shown to cause prolactinomas.

Microprolactinomas constitute the great majority of tumors in premenopausal women. In contrast, macroadenomas are more commonly seen in men and postmenopausal women. The predominance of smaller tumors in premenopausal women may be accounted for by an ascertainment bias because elevated PRL levels in this group lead to clinical manifestations (amenorrhea, galactorrhea, or infertility). Subclinical prolactinomas exist in men and many older women, and about 5% of apparently normal individuals have PRL-positive microadenomas in autopsy series.

CLINICAL MANIFESTATIONS

Hyperprolactinemia causes galactorrhea and oligomenorrhea or amenorrhea in premenopausal women. Estrogen facilitates PRL-induced galactorrhea, which explains why it is less common in postmenopausal women and in women with prolonged hypogonadism. Amenorrhea is primarily a consequence of PRL suppression of GnRH, although PRL may also have inhibitory effects at the level of the pituitary and the gonad. Amenorrhea is associated with infertility, and PRL levels should be a routine part of the hormonal evaluation of infertility. Estrogen deficiency can cause decreased libido, vaginal dryness, and dyspareunia. Long-standing estrogen deficiency also leads to osteopenia in many women. Oral contraceptives may mask PRL-induced oligomenorrhea or amenorrhea that becomes apparent on their discontinuation. In postmenopausal women, prolactinomas are often identified because of mass effects rather than because of their hormonal effects.

In men, hyperprolactinemia causes hypogonadism with suppressed LH and FSH levels and low testosterone levels. Hypogonadism causes diminished libido, impotence, infertility, and, rarely, gynecomastia or galactorrhea. Diminished libido may also reflect suppression of GnRH because testosterone replacement is not as effective as suppression of hyperprolactinemia. Hyperprolactinemia is found in 1 to 2% of men being evaluated for sexual dysfunction.

DIAGNOSIS

There are four primary categories of causes of hyperprolactinemia that must be distinguished if the correct therapy is to be instituted: (1) physiologic or metabolic hyperprolactinemia; (2) pharmacologic hyperprolactinemia; (3) hypothalamic or pituitary stalk compression; and (4) prolactinoma (see Table 231-4). With the exception of pregnancy and renal failure, physiologic causes of increased PRL result in minor elevations in PRL, usually less than 50 ng/mL. Primary hypothyroidism should be excluded as a cause of mild hyperprolactinemia. A careful drug history should be obtained in all patients with hyperprolactinemia because of the large number of agents that can stimulate PRL secretion. Psychotropic medications, in particular, can increase PRL either by reducing dopamine production or by blocking its action. In most cases, the degree of hyperprolactinemia caused by drugs is less than 150 ng/mL. A variety of suprasellar and parasellar mass lesions cause hyperprolactinemia (generally between 20 and 100 ng/mL) because of compression of the hypothalamus or pituitary stalk. Unless there is very good evidence for physiologic or drug-induced hyperprolactinemia, even patients with mild hyperprolactinemia should be evaluated with CT or MRI to distinguish among idiopathic hyperprolactinemia, microprolactinomas, and other large mass lesions that cause stalk compression, resulting in decreased dopamine reaching the lactotrophs. However, a specific caution is needed when some two-site assays are used because patients with very high PRL levels may appear to have PRL levels that are normal or only modestly elevated, owing to the "hook effect," in which the very high PRL levels saturate the antibodies in the assay. To avoid this problem, PRL levels should be remeasured at 1:100 dilution in patients with macroadenomas and normal to modestly elevated PRL levels because PRL levels in samples with the hook effect will then increase dramatically. When no pituitary lesions are seen by radiographic studies and physiologic and pharmacologic causes of hyperprolactinemia cannot be identified, the diagnosis of idiopathic hyperprolactinemia is made. Idiopathic hyperprolactinemia may represent microprolactinomas too small to be detected accurately by imaging or altered hypothalamic regulation of PRL secretion. Whether such patients should be treated depends on the clinical effects of hyperprolactinemia. When followed for several years, few of these patients develop large tumors, only 10 to 15% show MRI evidence of microadenomas, and in one third of cases, the hyperprolactinemia resolves.

TREATMENT   Rx

The natural history of prolactinomas has been evaluated in several series. Although large prolactinomas evolve from smaller lesions, it is uncommon (~7%) for microprolactinomas to progress to macroadenomas. Because of the slow rate of growth, it is reasonable to monitor patients with microprolactinomas without treatment by periodic measurement of PRL levels unless the hyperprolactinemia is causing symptoms that warrant therapy.

When hyperprolactinemia causes hypogonadism, osteopenia, or infertility, a dopamine agonist such as cabergoline or bromocriptine is the therapy of choice. Dopamine agonists normalize PRL levels and correct amenorrhea-galactorrhea in 80 to 90% of patients. Cabergoline is more effective, has fewer adverse side effects than bromocriptine, and has the additional advantage in only having to be taken once or twice weekly. Bromocriptine must be started in low doses with gradual increases to avoid side effects (nausea, dizziness, somnolence, and nasal stuffiness).

Cabergoline may cause a considerable reduction in tumor size in patients with macroprolactinomas, about 80 to 90% having a greater than 50% reduction in tumor size, but such size reduction is seen in only about two thirds of patients treated with bromocriptine. Visual field defects are a very sensitive index of tumor size, and improvements can be seen in about 90% of patients with defects. Thus, it is reasonable to use cabergoline as first-line therapy even in patients with visual field defects as long as visual acuity is not threatened by rapid progression or recent tumor hemorrhage. Many patients treated with cabergoline whose tumors shrink to the point of nonvisualization on MRI and whose PRL levels are normal can maintain normal PRL levels and not experience tumor re-expansion after therapy has been discontinued. In some cases, prolactinomas appear to be resistant to a dopamine agonist, but it is important to ensure compliance and to be certain that the underlying lesion is a prolactinoma and not some other cause of hyperprolactinemia. In these cases, switching from bromocriptine to cabergoline may be successful. Larger than standard doses (>2 mg/week) of cabergoline may be effective in normalizing PRL levels. The very high doses of cabergoline used in patients with Parkinson's disease have been associated with cardiac valvular abnormalities; such abnormalities have not been found with conventional doses of cabergoline used in patients with prolactinomas, but monitoring with echocardiography may be prudent in patients taking larger than standard doses. Alternatively, transsphenoidal surgery may be used. Although initial remission rates (80 to 90%) for transsphenoidal surgery of microprolactinomas are good, there is long-term recurrence in about 20% of patients. For macroprolactinomas, the initial remission rates with surgery are closer to 30%, with a similar recurrence rate. Radiation therapy, usually stereotactic, is reserved for patients with macroadenomas not responding to either medical or surgical treatment.

Dopamine agonist therapy for infertility, or when there is a possibility of pregnancy, deserves special consideration. These medications can induce ovulation in 80 to 90% of patients with hyperprolactinemia. Although neither bromocriptine nor cabergoline has been associated with congenital malformations, most physicians and patients prefer to avoid their use once pregnancy has been achieved. A form of barrier contraception is usually recommended until two to three regular menstrual cycles have occurred. Subsequently, pregnancy can be confirmed if a menstrual period is missed, allowing discontinuation of medication with exposure of the fetus to the drug for

only 3 to 5 weeks. At present, the safety data for pregnancy outcome are much more limited for cabergoline; therefore, some clinicians prefer bromocriptine when fertility is desired. Less than 2% of patients with microadenomas, but 31% of patients with macroadenomas, develop symptoms of tumor enlargement (headaches, visual field defects) during pregnancy. If symptoms develop, MRI and formal visual field testing should be performed. If there is evidence of visual field compromise or tumor growth, dopamine agonist therapy should be restarted to shrink the tumor. PRL levels are not very useful because they are normally increased in pregnancy and an enlarging tumor may not cause PRL production to increase substantially. Because problems of tumor growth occur most often in patients with macroadenomas, consideration can also be given to the option of transsphenoidal decompression before pregnancy in women with large tumors, as long as fertility can be preserved. If the patient is far advanced in her gestation at the time tumor growth occurs, consideration could also be given to delivering the baby.

⬤ ADRENOCORTICOTROPIC HORMONE

Adrenocorticotropic hormone is a 39–amino acid peptide that is derived from a precursor polypeptide pro-opiomelanocortin (POMC; 241 amino acids), which encodes several peptides, including ACTH and β-lipotropin (Chapter 230). The biologically active portion of ACTH resides within the first 18 of its 39 amino acids. However, because a synthetic peptide (cosyntropin) that includes the first 24 amino acids has a longer half-life, it is used clinically to assess adrenocortical function. In cases with neoplastic ectopic production of ACTH, the levels of precursor peptides or their processed products may be elevated.

The primary effect of ACTH is to stimulate the adrenal gland to produce cortisol. It also stimulates secretion of adrenal androgens and mineralocorticoids, although production of mineralocorticoids is controlled primarily through non–ACTH-dependent mechanisms (i.e., the renin-angiotensin system) (Chapter 234). Consequently, mineralocorticoid function is preserved in ACTH deficiency, in contrast to primary adrenal insufficiency, which is characterized by loss of glucocorticoid and mineralocorticoid function. Long-term stimulation by ACTH causes adrenal hyperplasia and enlargement. On the other hand, ACTH deficiency leads to adrenal atrophy.

Hypothalamic CRH is the most important stimulator of ACTH secretion. Chronic stimulation by CRH causes corticotroph cell hyperplasia, which can be seen in cases of ectopic CRH production. Cortisol inhibits ACTH secretion, blunts the ACTH response to CRH, and inhibits CRH production. After prolonged glucocorticoid suppression of the hypothalamic-pituitary-adrenal axis, the amount of endogenous CRH secretion appears to be rate limiting and can require several months to recover.

Plasma ACTH is secreted in discrete pulses (10 to 80 pg/mL), so random measurements are of little value. Most clinical tests are therefore based on levels of cortisol or its metabolites, which tend to integrate the effects of ACTH. ACTH and cortisol secretion exhibit marked diurnal rhythms, being greatest at night several hours after the initiation of sleep. Cortisol levels are greatest in the early morning and reach a nadir in the late afternoon and evening. Patients with Cushing's disease lose or exhibit a blunted diurnal rhythm of ACTH and cortisol secretion. ACTH secretion can be stimulated by a variety of different forms of stress, including psychological stimuli such as fright, anticipation of athletic competition, or surgery. Depression is associated with activation of the hypothalamic-pituitary-adrenal axis and impaired dexamethasone suppressibility. Hypoglycemia induces ACTH secretion through a central mechanism. The resulting increase in cortisol secretion represents one of several counter-regulatory mechanisms that increase glucose production. Insulin-induced hypoglycemia provides a mechanism for testing the integrity of the hypothalamic-pituitary-adrenal axis (see Table 231-2). Serious trauma and infection activate an array of cytokines that stimulate CRH and ACTH secretion. Because cortisol levels are often increased up to 10-fold in these circumstances, similar adjustments in cortisol replacement doses may be required in seriously ill patients with adrenal insufficiency.

⬤ ADRENOCORTICOTROPIC HORMONE DEFICIENCY: SECONDARY HYPOCORTISOLISM

Secondary hypocortisolism causes symptoms of glucocorticoid deficiency, including nausea, vomiting, weakness, fatigue, fever, and hypotension. In addition to reduced levels of cortisol, abnormal laboratory test findings can include hyponatremia, hypoglycemia, and eosinophilia. Depending on its cause, the severity of cortisol deficiency in cases of secondary adrenal insufficiency is often not as marked as in primary adrenal insufficiency

(Chapter 234). In addition, mineralocorticoid function is preserved in secondary adrenal deficiency. Consequently, the clinical manifestations of volume depletion are less pronounced, and hyperkalemia is not a feature of ACTH deficiency. Because ACTH levels are low, hyperpigmentation is not seen as in primary adrenal insufficiency. In women, reduced adrenal androgens can decrease libido and cause loss of axillary and pubic hair.

The most common cause of ACTH deficiency is treatment with exogenous glucocorticoids, which causes suppression of the hypothalamic-pituitary-adrenal axis. Sudden withdrawal of glucocorticoids or an increased requirement induced by the superimposition of severe illness can elicit symptoms of glucocorticoid deficiency. Congenital forms of ACTH deficiency are rare. When present, ACTH deficiency usually occurs in combination with the loss of other pituitary hormones, although acquired, isolated ACTH deficiency does occur, particularly in women with lymphocytic hypophysitis.

ACTH reserve is most often evaluated using the insulin tolerance test. Caution should be exercised before inducing hypoglycemia in patients with suspected adrenal insufficiency. Insulin-induced hypoglycemia stimulates central responses to neuroglycopenia and mimics some stresses that activate ACTH secretion. The metyrapone test provides an alternative to the insulin tolerance test. By blocking the 11-hydroxylation step, metyrapone inhibits cortisol production, resulting in stimulation of ACTH secretion and an increase in precursor adrenal steroids (e.g., 11-deoxycortisol). Patients should be monitored closely for evidence of adrenal insufficiency, and metyrapone should be used only in patients with at least some evidence of adrenocortical function. ACTH stimulation tests using $ACTH_{1-24}$ (cosyntropin) can accurately evaluate primary adrenocortical insufficiency but may less accurately assess secondary adrenal insufficiency. A variation of the ACTH stimulation test using the low dose of 1 μg has been found to be useful for diagnosing secondary adrenal insufficiency in some studies.

Deficiency of ACTH is treated by replacement with glucocorticoids. Doses need to be individualized and are based largely on clinical criteria in which symptoms of glucocorticoid deficiency are balanced against features of glucocorticoid excess. Typical amounts of hydrocortisone are in the range of 15 to 20 mg/day in divided doses. Such doses are usually doubled in the event of mild-to-moderate illness. Patients should wear MedicAlert tags and be instructed in the warning signs of cortisol deficiency, including nausea, vomiting, abdominal pain, low-grade fever, fatigue, and postural dizziness. Emergency injection kits of hydrocortisone are frequently provided for home use in the event that vomiting precludes taking oral steroids or for severe, sudden stress (e.g., a fracture). Stress doses of steroids should be used during times of illness. Current recommendations call for doses in the range of 50 to 75 mg every 8 hours for severe stress. Mineralocorticoid replacement is not required in patients with ACTH deficiency.

CUSHING'S DISEASE

PATHOBIOLOGY

Cushing's disease results from a pituitary adenoma that causes excess production of ACTH. It should be distinguished from a variety of other causes of *Cushing's syndrome* (glucocorticoid excess), which include adrenal causes of cortisol excess, ectopic production of ACTH and CRH, and physiologic states that result in overproduction of cortisol. Cushing's disease accounts for 60 to 70% of cases of Cushing's syndrome. Ten to 15% of pituitary tumors secrete ACTH. Cushing's disease occurs about eight times more often in women than in men.

Most ACTH-producing pituitary neoplasms, like other pituitary tumors, are monoclonal, implying a primary defect in corticotroph cells. In addition, there are rare cases of corticotroph hyperplasia causing Cushing's syndrome that are secondary to CRH production by either adjacent CRH-producing intrasellar gangliocytomas or ectopic CRH-producing cancers. Most (80 to 90%) of the ACTH-secreting tumors are microadenomas at the time of diagnosis. The clinical features of cortisol excess may allow detection of corticotroph adenomas before they have grown to a larger size. High levels of cortisol may also restrain tumor growth. ACTH-secreting macroadenomas may be locally invasive.

CLINICAL MANIFESTATIONS

The clinical features of Cushing's disease are caused by the effects of excess glucocorticoids and by the hypersecretion of ACTH and other POMC peptide products. The severity of the features of Cushing's disease varies greatly and appears to reflect not only the level of free cortisol but also the duration of the disease and perhaps the sensitivity to glucocorticoid action.

FIGURE 231-2. Clinical features of Cushing's disease. A 25-year-old woman presented with severe Cushing's disease. **A,** Facial features of Cushing's syndrome, including plethora, moon facies, and hirsutism, are evident. **B,** Dramatic resolution of the manifestations of cortisol excess after successful transsphenoidal surgery. (Photographs courtesy of Dr. Beverly M. K. Biller.)

TABLE 231-6 CLINICAL FEATURES OF CUSHING'S DISEASE

GENERAL
Obesity (centripetal distribution)
"Moon facies" and mild proptosis
Increased supraclavicular fat and "buffalo hump"
Hypertension

SKIN
Hyperpigmentation
Facial plethora
Hirsutism
Violaceous striae and thin skin
Capillary fragility and easy bruising
Acne
Edema

MUSCULOSKELETAL
Muscle weakness (proximal)
Osteoporosis and back pain

REPRODUCTIVE
Decreased libido
Oligomenorrhea and amenorrhea

NEUROPSYCHIATRIC
Depression
Irritability and emotional lability
Psychosis

METABOLIC
Hypokalemia and alkalosis
Hypercalciuria and renal stones
Glucose intolerance or diabetes mellitus
Impaired wound healing
Impaired resistance to infection
Granulocytosis and lymphopenia

TUMOR MASS EFFECTS
Headache
Visual field loss
Hypopituitarism

In florid cases of Cushing's disease (Fig. 231-2), the constellation of symptoms and physical features is readily recognized. Early in the disease or in mild cases, it can be challenging to distinguish the clinical features of Cushing's disease from similar traits that are seen in the normal population. Clinical suspicion is of paramount importance. On the other hand, one must be discriminating and not formally evaluate everyone with obesity, hypertension, and glucose intolerance. Of the many features listed in Table 231-6, some are relatively specific for Cushing's disease. For example, the centripetal distribution of fat with the characteristic "buffalo hump," "moon facies," and deposition of fat in the supraclavicular area but not in the extremities, is much more specific than generalized obesity. Striae that are wide (>1 cm) and purple reflect steroid-induced thinning of the dermis and can be distinguished from the more common "stretch marks." Numerous spontaneous ecchymoses also occur because of thinning of the skin and capillary fragility. Proximal muscle weakness represents another manifestation of glucocorticoid excess. Osteopenia and hypokalemia, when present, provide objective evidence consistent with ACTH excess. Hypokalemia results from the effects of ACTH on mineralocorticoid production but also from the ability of high levels of cortisol to saturate 11β-dehydrogenase, an enzyme in the kidney that inactivates cortisol. As a result, cortisol can "spill over" and act on mineralocorticoid receptors in the distal tubule. The hyperpigmentation associated with Cushing's disease is not as striking as one encounters with Addison's disease or in ectopic ACTH syndrome; but in association with other findings, it should raise the suspicion of Cushing's disease and help to distinguish it from adrenal causes of hypercortisolemia. Hirsutism and acne are caused by the increased production of adrenal androgens and are more prominent in patients with Cushing's disease than in those with adrenal adenomas, in whom glucocorticoids tend to be the predominant product. Oligomenorrhea and amenorrhea probably have several causes, including androgen effects on the reproductive axis and glucocorticoid inhibition of GnRH, which may also account for diminished libido. Hypertension and glucose intolerance are caused by glucocorticoid excess. Immunosuppression, opportunistic infections, and impaired wound healing can lead to considerable morbidity. Neuropsychiatric symptoms, including depression, can be prominent effects of Cushing's disease. Suicide occurs with increased frequency in patients who receive no treatment for Cushing's disease.

DIAGNOSIS

The screening tests and differential diagnosis of Cushing's syndrome represent one of the greatest diagnostic challenges in endocrinology (Chapter 234). The first step is to determine whether a patient truly has cortisol excess. After confirmation of Cushing's syndrome, one must distinguish among (1) adrenal causes of cortisol excess; (2) pituitary causes of ACTH excess (Cushing's disease); (3) ectopic sources of ACTH; and (4) ectopic CRH (Table 231-7).

In screening for hypercortisolism, random cortisol levels are not useful because of diurnal variation of the hormone. The overnight dexamethasone test is the most widely used screening test (see Table 231-5). A normal result of the dexamethasone test excludes Cushing's syndrome. It should be noted, however, that abnormal overnight dexamethasone suppression can be seen in up to 30% of hospitalized patients and in many patients with depression or during alcohol withdrawal. An elevated 24-hour urine free cortisol value provides an alternative, or additional, screening test for hypercortisolism. Often, two sequential specimens are collected because of day-to-day variations in hormone production. The sensitivity and specificity of urinary free cortisol measurements are greater than those of the overnight dexamethasone suppression test, particularly in hospitalized patients. A third test takes advantage of the observation that there is a loss of diurnal variation of cortisol levels in all forms of Cushing's syndrome. This test consists of finding elevation of a midnight cortisol level in the serum or saliva. Kits are available for patients to obtain a late-night salivary cortisol sample.

After demonstrating that cortisol excess is present, the next step is to determine the source of excess ACTH or cortisol. The classic approach is to perform a low-dose, followed by a high-dose, dexamethasone suppression test (see Tables 231-5 and 231-7). The low-dose dexamethasone test excludes or confirms the presence of Cushing's syndrome. On the second day of the test, normal individuals suppress plasma cortisol to less than 5 μg/dL and reduce the urinary free cortisol to less than 20 μg per 24 hours. All forms of Cushing's syndrome fail to suppress according to these criteria.

The high-dose dexamethasone test is one of several means to distinguish ACTH-independent and ACTH-dependent causes of Cushing's syndrome and to discriminate between pituitary and ectopic causes of ACTH-dependent Cushing's syndrome (see Table 231-7). Because adrenal sources of cortisol excess are autonomous and ACTH independent, plasma and urinary cortisol levels are not affected by dexamethasone suppression, even at high doses. In addition, plasma ACTH levels are low in adrenal causes of Cushing's syndrome because the hypothalamic-pituitary axis is suppressed. Pituitary and ectopic causes of Cushing's disease are both ACTH dependent but respond differently to high-dose dexamethasone. Pituitary adenomas have an altered set point for glucocorticoid inhibition but retain a partial ability to respond to high-dose dexamethasone. The exact criteria for dexamethasone suppression in the high-dose test are debated. In most cases of ACTH-producing pituitary adenomas, urinary free cortisol is suppressed below 90% of baseline during the high-dose dexamethasone test.

The ectopic ACTH syndrome (Chapter 186) should be suspected in patients with known malignancies, particularly small cell carcinoma of the lung; bronchial, thymic, or gastrointestinal carcinoids; islet cell tumors; and medullary carcinoma of the thyroid, among others. Plasma ACTH levels are often very high (>200 pg/mL) and can be associated with hyperpigmentation. Clinical features of Cushing's syndrome may be altered by the rapid onset of extreme hypercortisolemia coincident with elements of tumor cachexia. Pronounced weakness, fluid retention, glucose intolerance, hypokalemia, and poor skin integrity are often seen. Ectopic ACTH syndrome is readily recognized in its classic form. However, a subset of tumors, particularly carcinoids (Chapter 240), exhibit dexamethasone suppression that is similar to that seen with pituitary adenomas. When suspected, carcinoids can sometimes be detected by CT or MRI, but many are too small to be seen even with these techniques. Because of these exceptions to the high-dose dexamethasone test, a variety of procedures have been devised in an attempt to further distinguish ectopic and pituitary dependent sources of ACTH. CRH testing may also prove useful, with pituitary tumors exhibiting an increase in ACTH and tumors making ACTH ectopically having little or no response.

In recent years, inferior petrosal sinus sampling has been used to distinguish pituitary and ectopic sources of ACTH when the source of ACTH is not obvious based on the clinical circumstances, biochemical evaluation, and imaging studies. This test requires an experienced radiologist for safe and effective catheterization of the petrosal sinuses. Blood samples are taken simultaneously from the left and right petrosal sinuses and from the periphery before and after CRH stimulation. In the case of ACTH-producing pituitary adenomas, there is a gradient in ACTH levels between the central and peripheral blood specimens. When clinical and biochemical studies suggest the presence of a pituitary adenoma, pituitary imaging should be performed using CT or MRI. Most ACTH-secreting pituitary adenomas are small and scans are normal in more than half of patients.

TREATMENT   Rx

The efficacy of transsphenoidal surgery for Cushing's disease is greatly aided by making the correct diagnosis preoperatively. In experienced hands, surgical cures of ACTH-producing microadenomas occur in 75 to 90% of patients undergoing a first operation. As in other pituitary tumors, complete remissions with macroadenomas are much less common. In the event of surgical remission or cure, postoperative hypocortisolism is to be expected because of suppression of the hypothalamic-pituitary axis. After coverage for steroid withdrawal in the postoperative period, cortisol replacement should gradually be decreased to allow recovery of the hypothalamic-pituitary-adrenal axis; recovery may take up to 1 year.

TABLE 231-7 TESTS USED IN THE DIFFERENTIAL DIAGNOSIS OF CUSHING'S SYNDROME*						
ETIOLOGY	OVERNIGHT DEXAMETHASONE SUPPRESSION TEST	PLASMA ACTH	LOW-DOSE DEXAMETHASONE	HIGH-DOSE DEXAMETHASONE	CORTICOTROPIN-RELEASING HORMONE STIMULATION OF ACTH	PETROSAL-TO-PERIPHERAL ACTH RATIO
Normal	Suppression	Normal	Suppression		Normal	
Pituitary	No suppression	Normal or high	No suppression	Suppression	Normal or increased	>2
Ectopic	No suppression	High or normal	No suppression	No suppression	No response	<1.5
Adrenal	No suppression	Low	No suppression	No suppression	No response	

*Classic responses are indicated. Certain cases of ectopic adrenocorticotropic hormone (ACTH) production are suppressed by high-dose dexamethasone or are stimulated by corticotropin-releasing hormone. In these cases, petrosal sinus sampling is the most reliable method for distinguishing pituitary and ectopic sources of ACTH.

If transsphenoidal surgery is unsuccessful, reoperation may be indicated and can result in remission in up to 50% of patients; in this circumstance, consideration should be given to performing a total hypophysectomy at reoperation. If transsphenoidal surgery cannot be performed or has failed, alternative forms of therapy should be used to prevent the long-term consequences of hypercortisolism. Pituitary irradiation is usually the second line of treatment for Cushing's disease. It is more efficacious in children and in younger patients, but even in older adults, remissions can be achieved in 50 to 60% within 2 years. To prevent the continued ravages of hypercortisolism during this period, however, concomitant medical therapy is usually given. Bilateral adrenalectomy represents another alternative for patients with severe hypercortisolism after transsphenoidal surgery. It rapidly and effectively lowers cortisol levels but is associated with relatively high morbidity and mortality rates (as high as 5%) because of the associated metabolic and immune system alterations caused by hypercortisolism. The morbidity has been reduced in recent years by introduction of the laparoscopic approach. After adrenalectomy, patients must be maintained on glucocorticoids and mineralocorticoids and are at risk for the development of Nelson's syndrome (see later).

Medical therapy for Cushing's disease has its primary role in preparation for surgery or control of hypercortisolism during the interval when radiation therapy is taking effect. Because most pituitary adenomas are responsive to changes in cortisol levels, they have a tendency to "escape" from adrenal blockade caused by some therapies by producing higher levels of ACTH. The antifungal agent ketoconazole is highly effective in decreasing glucocorticoid biosynthesis and also inhibits ACTH secretion so that it has become the medical therapy of choice. Alternative medications include metyrapone, mifepristone, etomidate, and mitotane.

● NELSON'S SYNDROME

Nelson's syndrome was initially described as the appearance of a pituitary adenoma after bilateral adrenalectomy. In addition to an enlarging pituitary mass, the syndrome is characterized by very high ACTH levels and hyperpigmentation. It is caused by a preexisting ACTH-producing tumor that grows in the absence of feedback inhibition by high levels of glucocorticoids. The incidence of clinically significant Nelson's syndrome after adrenalectomy for Cushing's disease varies from 10 to 50% in different series. Patients with Cushing's disease who have undergone adrenalectomy should be followed with imaging studies and plasma ACTH levels because tumors that cause Nelson's syndrome can be very aggressive. When there is evidence of mass effects or rapid growth, transsphenoidal surgery should be performed. Postoperative irradiation may provide additional benefit, although it appears to be less efficacious than in other ACTH-producing adenomas.

● GONADOTROPINS (FOLLICLE-STIMULATING HORMONE AND LUTEINIZING HORMONE)

The pituitary glycoprotein hormones include FSH, LH, and TSH. Chorionic gonadotropin, which is structurally very similar to LH, is made in the placenta. Each of the glycoprotein hormones has a specific β-subunit that forms a noncovalently bound dimer with the common α-subunit. The α- and β-subunits each undergo glycosylation, which is important for correct hormone folding, intracellular transport, and secretion. Glycosylation is also required for biologic activity, presumably because of effects on the tertiary structure of the hormones. The gonadotropins are involved in sexual differentiation, sex steroid production, and gametogenesis. The regulation and physiologic roles of gonadotropins are quite different in males and females.

In males, receptors for FSH are located on Sertoli cells and seminiferous tubules, whereas LH receptors are located on Leydig cells in the testis. LH stimulates androgen production by the Leydig cells. FSH is involved primarily in sperm maturation in the seminiferous tubules. Thus, FSH and LH act together to induce spermatogenesis (Chapter 242).

In females, ovarian FSH receptors are located on granulosa cells, where they induce enzymes involved in estrogen biosynthesis. LH receptors are located predominantly on thecal cells in the ovary and stimulate the production of ovarian androgens and steroid precursors that are transported to granulosa cells for aromatization to estrogens. The pattern of FSH and LH secretion during the menstrual cycle results in follicular recruitment and maturation (largely FSH-mediated), followed by ovulation (largely LH-mediated) and steroid production by the corpus luteum (Chapter 243).

Gonadotropin secretion is regulated primarily by the hypothalamic decapeptide GnRH. The gonadotroph cell is exquisitely sensitive to the pattern of GnRH stimulation. Continuous, rather than pulsatile, exposure to GnRH causes gonadotroph desensitization and suppression of LH and FSH. Gonadotroph sensitivity to GnRH is modulated by sex steroids and probably other hypothalamic peptides, such as neuropeptide Y. Increased GnRH secretion, in combination with a higher density of GnRH receptors and rising estradiol concentrations, accounts in part for the dramatic release of gonadotropins that induces ovulation.

In women, the pattern of GnRH pulse frequency varies across the menstrual cycle (Chapter 243). The combination of GnRH stimulation, in conjunction with ovarian feedback regulation, results in a complex orchestration of positive and negative hormonal signals that converge at the gonadotroph to regulate LH and FSH secretion. The typical 28-day menstrual cycle is divided into follicular and luteal phases that are separated by ovulation on day 14. Unlike chronic exposure to low concentrations of estrogens, which exert negative feedback regulation and inhibit GnRH, the increasing concentration of estrogen before the LH surge exerts positive feedback regulation that results in increased GnRH pulse frequency. Increased GnRH, in combination with increased gonadotroph sensitivity to GnRH, results in the LH-FSH surge. During the luteal phase, the gonadotropin pulse frequency is reduced. In addition to feedback regulation by steroids, ovarian peptides such as inhibin also play a role in control of the reproductive axis. Inhibin causes selective suppression of FSH, without affecting LH secretion. A homodimer of inhibin β-subunits, referred to as *activin*, has opposite actions and selectively stimulates FSH, but its predominant physiologic action is to increase ovarian granulosa cell responsivity to FSH. Circulating inhibin provides one of the negative feedback inputs that leads to FSH suppression as the follicle develops. The perimenopause is characterized by a gradual cessation of ovarian function. After several years of menstrual cycles that are sometimes anovulatory or irregular, menses cease, thereby defining the menopause (Chapter 248). At menopause, the decline in estrogen and progesterone causes loss of feedback inhibition and a marked increase in LH and FSH levels.

In males, the regulation of the hypothalamic-pituitary-gonadal axis is relatively constant. Testosterone inhibits the hypothalamic-pituitary axis, although its actions are mediated, in part, by aromatization to estrogens. Most of the inhibition by gonadal steroids occurs at the hypothalamic level. In contrast to menopause in women, there is no analogous abrupt change in hormone levels in men. There is, however, a gradual decline in testosterone levels associated with an increase in LH and FSH with aging.

● HYPOGONADOTROPIC HYPOGONADISM

Clinical features of hypogonadotropic hypogonadism in women are primarily due to estrogen deficiency and include breast atrophy, vaginal dryness, and diminished libido. Hot flashes are uncommon, in contrast to postmenopausal estrogen deficiency. In premenopausal women, normal menstrual cycles provide evidence for an intact hypothalamic-pituitary-gonadal axis. LH and FSH levels should be increased in postmenopausal women, and normal levels may indicate deficiency. Hypogonadism in men causes decreased libido and sexual function. In men, low testosterone without elevation of LH and FSH is consistent with impaired hypothalamic-pituitary reserve. GnRH stimulation can distinguish hypothalamic and pituitary deficiency but may require multiple injections to prime the pituitary.

TREATMENT

In premenopausal women, preparations of estrogen and progestins should be used for hormonal replacement and to allow cyclical growth of the endometrium. Pulsatile GnRH (for GnRH-deficient subjects) has been given to induce ovulation and fertility but is not commonly used at present. Gonadotropin injections are more commonly used. Testosterone can be replaced in men using intramuscular injections that are given at 2- to 4-week intervals. Doses and the intervals between injections should be adjusted on an individual basis using libido and testosterone levels before the next injection as a guide. Oral preparations of androgens should be avoided because of hepatotoxicity. Transdermal patch and gel preparations are also available and maintain more stable testosterone levels but are more expensive. Induction of spermatogenesis requires pulsatile GnRH (for GnRH-deficient subjects) or, more commonly, injections of gonadotropins.

A congenital form of hypogonadotropic hypogonadism is caused by deficiency of GnRH, which in turn causes deficiencies of LH and FSH. When associated with anosmia (absent sense of smell), the condition is referred to as Kallmann's syndrome (Chapter 230). Pulsatile GnRH has been used to induce puberty and fertility in both males and females with Kallmann's syndrome and other forms of GnRH deficiency, but more commonly, injections of gonadotropins are used.

Secondary hypogonadotropic hypogonadism is relatively common. In most cases, it is reversible and is caused by weight loss, anorexia nervosa, stress, heavy exercise, or severe illness. Reversible forms of secondary hypogonadotropic hypogonadism are caused by GnRH deficiency and are more common in women than men. The condition is ideally treated by correcting the underlying cause. Many women have a discrete threshold for weight or exercise level that will cause loss of menstrual periods. When it is not possible to correct the underlying abnormality, hormonal replacement can be used in women for protection against osteopenia and to cycle the endometrium. Permanent, idiopathic hypogonadotropic hypogonadism can also occur in both sexes and will require hormone replacement.

A variety of pathologic conditions can cause secondary hypogonadotropic hypogonadism, often in association with deficiencies of other pituitary hormones (see Table 231-1). These include hypothalamic lesions and central nervous system irradiation. Pituitary tumors can suppress gonadotropins because of stalk compression and disruption of pulsatile GnRH input as well as by direct destruction of normal pituitary tissue. Hyperprolactinemia can suppress GnRH and lead to reduced gonadotropin levels.

In contrast to the aforementioned causes of hypogonadotropic hypogonadism, which result from GnRH deficiency, primary deficiencies of LH and FSH are uncommon. An acquired form of isolated gonadotropin deficiency is rarely encountered and may have an autoimmune basis. Mutations in the *LHβ* or *FSHβ* genes have been described in case reports and cause selective loss of individual gonadotropins. Inactivating mutations in the GnRH receptor and the LH and FSH receptors causing hypogonadotropic hypogonadism have also been reported.

FOLLICLE-STIMULATING HORMONE– AND LUTEINIZING HORMONE–PRODUCING TUMORS

PATHOBIOLOGY

The majority (70 to 80%) of pituitary tumors classified previously as nonfunctioning adenomas can be shown to produce low levels of intact glycoprotein hormones or their uncombined α- or β-subunits. Biosynthetic defects in the tumor cells account for relatively inefficient hormone secretion as well as the propensity to produce uncombined subunits. FSH is produced more commonly than LH. Elevated levels of free α-subunits are noted more often than increased free β-subunits.

CLINICAL MANIFESTATIONS

Gonadotropin-producing tumors are somewhat more common in men than women and increase in prevalence with age. FSH- and LH-producing tumors do not usually cause a characteristic hormone excess syndrome. The tumors, typically large macroadenomas, present as clinically nonfunctioning tumors with symptoms and signs related to local mass effects. Visual field loss is found in more than 70% of patients. Many are detected incidentally by CT and MRI performed for unrelated indications. Symptoms of hypogonadism with loss of libido are also common. Men with predominantly FSH-secreting tumors may present with testicular enlargement from hypertrophy of the seminiferous tubules but may also be hypogonadal due to low levels of testosterone. These patients must be distinguished from those with primary hypogonadism due to testicular dysfunction. Tumors that primarily secrete LH are rare but can cause increased testosterone levels. Premenopausal women with gonadotropin-producing tumors may experience menstrual irregularity or secondary hypogonadism. Postmenopausal women often show reduced gonadotropin levels because the mass effects of the gonadotropin-producing tumors cause stalk compression, impairing GnRH stimulation of gonadotropins from normal pituitary cells.

DIAGNOSIS

Because of the absence of a clinical syndrome in most patients, almost all gonadotropin-producing pituitary tumors are diagnosed by postoperative immunohistochemistry because they had presented with mass effects. There is no particular clinical benefit to distinguish whether a nonfunctioning adenoma is truly a gonadotroph adenoma. Some patients can have moderately elevated PRL levels that are caused by tumor mass effects. It is important to distinguish this group from patients with true prolactinomas. As noted earlier, many women, including those in the postmenopausal group,

have paradoxically low gonadotropin levels. Thus, the absence of elevated gonadotropins does not exclude the diagnosis of a gonadotropin-producing tumor.

TREATMENT   Rx

Because the major symptoms of the gonadotropin-producing tumors are due to extrasellar extension and local mass effects, the main aim of treatment is reduction in the size of the tumor. Complete or partial reversal of visual field defects and hypopituitarism can be accomplished by surgery, unless these conditions have been of long standing. Transsphenoidal surgery is rarely curative, however. Patients with significant residual tumor may benefit from radiation therapy. Because most tumors are slow growing, when no tumor is visible postoperatively by MRI, the patient may be followed with yearly monitoring for tumor recurrence using visual fields and CT or MRI. If tumor markers such as free α- or β-subunit levels are available, they can also be used to monitor tumor function. When follow-up studies show tumor regrowth, repeat surgery, radiation therapy, or both are indicated. Medical therapy with dopamine agonists and somatostatin analogues has been successful in only a minority of patients.

THYROID-STIMULATING HORMONE

Like the other glycoprotein hormones, TSH is a heterodimer composed of the common α-subunit and the unique TSH β-subunit. Normal levels of TSH range from 0.4 to 4.0 µU/mL. The detection limit for current TSH assays is less than 0.01 µU/mL, allowing measurement of suppressed TSH levels in patients with hyperthyroidism. Thyroid-stimulating hormone controls thyroid hormone (T_4 and T_3) synthesis and secretion from the thyroid gland. Hypothalamic TRH stimulates TSH synthesis and secretion. Somatostatin and dopamine can inhibit TSH secretion, but their roles in normal physiology have not been clearly elucidated. Thyroid hormones have an inhibitory effect on the production of TRH and TSH and constitute a powerful negative feedback loop acting at both the hypothalamic and pituitary levels. Secretion of TSH is pulsatile, but the amplitude of the pulses is relatively small and does not create the difficulties in measurement of TSH that are encountered with measurements of other pituitary hormones. Because of the integrated nature of the hypothalamic-pituitary-thyroid axis, thyroid function tests are best interpreted when concentrations of TSH, free T_4, and free T_3 levels are known. Except in conditions of secondary hypothyroidism or TSH-secreting pituitary tumors (see later), TSH levels provide an excellent screening test for thyroid dysfunction.

CENTRAL HYPOTHYROIDISM

Central forms of hypothyroidism are due to loss of either TSH or TRH. Three different types of congenital TSH deficiency are caused by genetic mutations. One type involves mutations in the *TSHβ* gene. A second involves mutations in *PIT1*, which causes combined deficiencies of GH, PRL, and TSH (see earlier). A third involves a mutation in the gene for TRH. Acquired, central forms of hypothyroidism are often associated with other pituitary hormone deficiencies, and usually there is no goiter because of low TSH levels.

Tests for TSH deficiency are best performed by analyzing free T_4 levels in combination with TSH. Low free T_4 without elevated TSH is consistent with central hypothyroidism. In some patients with hypothalamic disease, the TSH level is partially elevated in the presence of low levels of free T_4, but the bioactivity of the TSH is reduced. Central forms of hypothyroidism must be distinguished from the sick-euthyroid condition (Chapter 233). Laboratory tests in the sick-euthyroid syndrome progress through several phases but can include prolonged periods when both TSH and free thyroid hormone levels are low. It can be very difficult in these patients to exclude central hypothyroidism unequivocally. In addition to the clinical setting in which thyroid function tests are measured, the presence of normal thyroid function tests before the illness and the absence of known hypothalamic or pituitary disease make true central hypothyroidism unlikely. Increased levels of reverse T_3 are suggestive of sick-euthyroidism, and free T_4 and T_3 may be in the normal or low-normal range in sick-euthyroid patients. When TSH deficiency is documented, thyroid hormone is replaced using daily doses of L-thyroxine (0.05 to 0.15 mg/day). Because TSH cannot be used as an end point, one monitors the patient clinically and with serum levels of free T_4 and T_3.

THYROID-STIMULATING HORMONE–SECRETING TUMORS

TSH-secreting tumors are rare and account for between 1 and 3% of pituitary tumors. As many as 30% of TSH-producing tumors are plurihormonal. GH and PRL are co-secreted most often, perhaps reflecting the common cellular lineage for thyrotrophs, somatotrophs, and lactotrophs. Long-standing severe hypothyroidism can cause thyrotroph hyperplasia and pituitary enlargement. These hyperplastic masses regress with thyroid hormone replacement therapy, however. Most true TSH-producing tumors are relatively autonomous and respond weakly, if at all, to TRH stimulation or thyroid hormone suppression.

TSH-secreting tumors are usually macroadenomas by the time a diagnosis has been made. Consequently, many patients exhibit mass effects of the tumor as well as hyperthyroidism. The clinical features of TSH-secreting tumors resemble those of Graves' disease, except that features of autoimmunity such as ophthalmopathy are absent. Circulating levels of T_4 and T_3 range widely but can be elevated as much as two- to three-fold. Diffuse goiter is present in most patients with TSH-producing tumors, and the 24-hour uptake of radioiodine is elevated.

Because feedback inhibition of TSH is impaired in TSH-producing tumors, TSH levels are inappropriately elevated in the presence of high levels of T_4 and T_3. TSH levels produced by tumors range from the low-normal range to as high as 500 μU/mL, but most levels are minimally elevated. Most TSH-producing tumors (>80%) secrete excess free α-subunit, and its assessment can be very useful in confirming the diagnosis. Thus, the diagnosis can usually be made by demonstrating that a hyperthyroid patient has a detectable serum TSH level associated with excess secretion of the free α-subunit. The finding of a mass lesion on CT or MRI confirms the diagnosis. Several other causes of inappropriate TSH secretion should be considered, including resistance to thyroid hormone and familial dysalbuminemic hyperthyroxinemia and other disorders that alter serum thyroid hormone binding proteins.

TREATMENT   Rx

The goals of therapy are to treat the underlying TSH-secreting tumor and to correct the hyperthyroidism. Transsphenoidal surgery alone is rarely curative because of the large size of most tumors, but it can alleviate mass effects and lower TSH levels. As in other large pituitary tumors, adjunctive irradiation may be required to control tumor growth. Somatostatin analogues have been used as adjunctive medical therapy, and they decrease TSH and α-subunit levels in about 80% of patients with TSH-secreting tumors, but consistent effects on tumor growth have not been demonstrated. Hyperthyroidism caused by TSH-secreting tumors can also be treated using antithyroid drugs or radioiodine.

CLINICALLY NONFUNCTIONING PITUITARY TUMORS

Most clinically nonfunctioning adenomas can be shown to produce low levels of the free α-subunit, free β-subunits of FSH and LH, and intact FSH and LH when analyzed by immunocytochemistry or messenger RNA expression. A smaller fraction can be shown to produce low levels of other pituitary hormones, particularly ACTH or GH, that escaped detection based on routine endocrine testing. Even with detailed analyses of hormone production, a subset (10 to 20%) of nonfunctioning adenomas does not appear to produce any of the known pituitary hormones.

The clinical features and management of nonfunctioning tumors are similar to those for gonadotropin-producing tumors. The major signs and symptoms result from tumor mass effects that cause visual field defects, headache and other neurologic symptoms, and hypopituitarism. Transsphenoidal surgery is the primary mode of treatment, with a goal of debulking the tumor to relieve mass effects. Because there are no serum tumor markers, patients must be followed by CT or MRI in conjunction with visual field tests.

Some pituitary tumors are discovered as incidental findings on CT or MRI scans that were done for other reasons. Such tumors should be screened for hormone oversecretion with measurement of PRL, IGF-1, and a midnight salivary cortisol or an overnight dexamethasone suppression test, but most will be found to be nonfunctioning. If the tumor abuts the optic chiasm, a formal visual field examination should be performed. Over several years, about 10% of incidental microadenomas and 20% of macroadenomas enlarge. Indications for surgery include compression of the optic chiasm with or without visual field defects and significant tumor enlargement. Hypopituitarism is also a relative indication for surgery.

SUGGESTED READINGS

Buyukbayrak EE, Karageyim Karsidag AY, Kars B, et al. Effectiveness of short-term maintenance treatment with cabergoline in microadenoma-related and idiopathic hyperprolactinemia. *Arch Gynecol Obstet.* 2010;282:561-566. *Cabergoline at a dose as low as 0.125 mg orally twice weekly can maintain remission.*

Clemmons DR. Clinical laboratory indices in the treatment of acromegaly. *Clin Chim Acta.* 2011;412:403-409. *Review of the value of growth hormone and insulin-like growth factor 1 levels.*

Clemmons DR. The diagnosis and treatment of growth hormone deficiency in adults. *Curr Opin Endocrinol Diabetes Obes.* 2010;17:377-383. *Practical guidelines for selecting patients who are candidates for long-term replacement therapy and those in whom such therapy should be reassessed.*

Klibanski A. Clinical practice: prolactinomas. *N Engl J Med.* 2010;362:1219-1226. *Case-based review.*

Lleva RR, Inzucchi SE. Diagnosis and management of pituitary adenomas. *Curr Opin Oncol.* 2011; 23:53-60. *Overview, including medical and surgical management.*

Mann WA. Treatment for prolactinomas and hyperprolactinaemia: a lifetime approach. *Eur J Clin Invest.* 2011;41:334-342. *Review suggesting that lifetime treatment is usually required.*

Tritos NA, Biller BM, Swearingen B; Medscape. Management of Cushing disease. *Nat Rev Endocrinol.* 2011;7:279-289. *Review reporting remission in 70-90% of cases after a first transsphenoidal surgery and a 50-70% rate after a second surgery.*

232

POSTERIOR PITUITARY

JOSEPH G. VERBALIS

ANATOMY AND HORMONE SYNTHESIS

The hormones of the posterior pituitary, vasopressin and oxytocin, are synthesized in specialized neurons in the hypothalamus, the neurohypophysial neurons. These neurons, notable for their large size, are termed magnocellular neurons. In the hypothalamus, magnocellular neurons are clustered in the paired paraventricular and supraoptic nuclei (Fig. 232-1). Vasopressin and oxytocin are synthesized in parvicellular (i.e., small cell) neurons of the paraventricular nuclei, and vasopressin (but not oxytocin) is also synthesized in the suprachiasmatic nucleus.

Transcription of vasopressin and oxytocin messenger RNA and translation of the vasopressin and oxytocin prohormones occur entirely in the cell bodies of the neurohypophysial neurons. The prohormones provasopressin and pro-oxytocin are packaged along with processing enzymes into neurosecretory granules that are transported out of the perikaryon of the neurohypophysial neurons through microtubules and down the long axons that form the supraopticohypophysial tract and terminate in the posterior pituitary. During

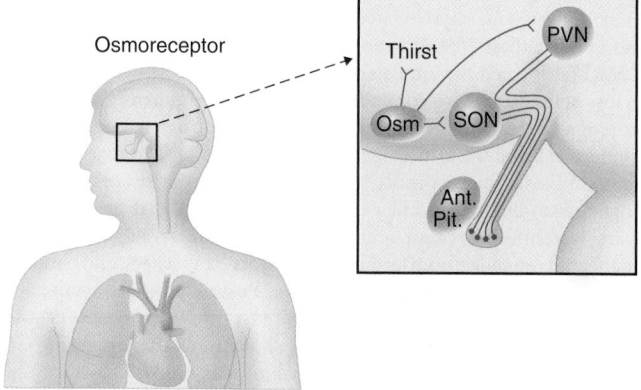

FIGURE 232-1. Sagittal view of the head demonstrating the position of the neurohypophysis. The magnocellular neurons are clustered in two paraventricular nuclei (PVN) and two supraoptic nuclei (SON). Only one nucleus of each pair is illustrated. The supraoptic nuclei are lateral to the edge of the optic chiasm, whereas the paraventricular nuclei are central along the wall of the third ventricle. The axons of the four nuclei combine to form the supraopticohypophysial tract as they course through the pituitary stalk to their storage terminals in the posterior pituitary. The osmostat (Osm) is in the hypothalamus anterior to the third ventricle; the thirst center (Thirst) is distributed across different brain areas. Ant. Pit. = anterior pituitary. (From Buonocore CM, Robinson AG. Diagnosis and management of diabetes insipidus during medical emergencies. *Endocrinol Metab Clin North Am.* 1993; 22:411-423.)

transport, the processing enzymes cleave provasopressin into vasopressin (9 amino acids), vasopressin-neurophysin (95 amino acids), and vasopressin glycopeptide, or copeptin (39 amino acids). Pro-oxytocin is similarly cleaved to oxytocin (which differs from vasopressin by only two of nine amino acids) and oxytocin-neurophysin. The neurophysins form neurophysin-hormone complexes that stabilize the hormones. The hormone within the granules is always bound. Stimulatory (e.g., glutamatergic, cholinergic, and angiotensin) neurotransmitter terminals and inhibitory (e.g., γ-aminobutyric acid and noradrenergic) neurotransmitter terminals control the release of vasopressin by the activity of synaptic contacts on the cell bodies. Physiologic release of vasopressin or oxytocin into the general circulation occurs at the level of the posterior pituitary, where, in response to an action potential, intracellular calcium is increased and causes the neurosecretory granules to fuse with the axon membrane, thereby releasing each hormone in the free form in the general circulation. The mature vasopressin and oxytocin are the only biologically active components of the prohormones. Factors that stimulate the release of neurohypophysial hormones also stimulate their synthesis. Because synthesis is delayed, maintenance of a large store of hormone in the posterior pituitary is essential for the instantaneous and massive release of each hormone that is necessary with acute hemorrhage (vasopressin) or during parturition (oxytocin). In most species, sufficient vasopressin is stored in the posterior pituitary to support maximal antidiuresis for several days and to maintain baseline levels of antidiuresis for weeks.

Vasopressin

Vasopressin and Regulation of Osmolality

The primary physiologic action of vasopressin is its function as a water-retaining hormone. The central sensing system (osmostat) for controlling the release of vasopressin is anatomically discrete, located in a small area of the hypothalamus just anterior to the third ventricle (see Fig. 232-1). The osmostat controls the release of vasopressin to cause water retention and also stimulates thirst to cause water repletion.

Osmotic regulation of vasopressin release and osmotic regulation of thirst are usually tightly coupled, but they can be dissociated under pathologic conditions. The primary extracellular osmolyte to which the osmoreceptor responds is sodium. Under normal physiologic conditions, glucose and urea readily traverse neuron cell membranes and do not stimulate the release of vasopressin. Although basal osmolality in normal subjects is between 280 and 295 mOsm/kg H_2O, extracellular fluid osmolality for each individual is maintained within narrow ranges. Increases in plasma osmolality as small as 1 to 2% stimulate vasopressin release. Basal plasma levels of vasopressin are generally 0.5 to 2 pg/mL, which is sufficient to maintain urine osmolality above plasma osmolality and urine volume in the range of 2 to 3 L/day. When vasopressin levels are suppressed below 0.5 pg/mL, maximal urine osmolality decreases to less than 100 mOsm/kg H_2O, and a free water diuresis (or "aquaresis") ensues at levels approaching 800 to 1000 mL/hour (18 to 24 L/day). Increases in plasma osmolality cause a linear increase in plasma vasopressin and a corresponding linear increase in urine osmolality. At a plasma osmolality of approximately 295 mOsm/kg H_2O, urine osmolality is maximally concentrated to 1000 to 1200 mOsm/kg H_2O. Thus, the entire physiologic range of urine osmolality is accomplished by relatively small changes in plasma vasopressin of 0 to 5 pg/mL (Fig. 232-2).

To maintain fluid balance, water must be not only conserved but also consumed to replace insensible water losses and obligate urine output. Thirst is not stimulated until a somewhat higher plasma osmolality (5 to 10 mOsm/kg H_2O) than the threshold for release of vasopressin. Most humans derive sufficient water from habitual fluid intake and catabolism of food to maintain plasma osmolality below the threshold that activates thirst. Therefore, under normal physiologic conditions, water balance (and hence plasma osmolality) is regulated more by secretion of vasopressin than by thirst. However, with severe degrees of dehydration, thirst is essential to restore body water deficits.

Vasopressin acts on V_2 or antidiuretic receptors in the collecting duct cells of the kidney to cause water retention, or antidiuresis. Vasopressin V_2 receptors are G protein–coupled receptors that activate adenylate cyclase, with subsequent increased intracellular cyclic adenosine monophosphate (cAMP) levels upon ligand activation of the receptor. The increased cAMP initiates the movement of aquaporin-2 water channels to the apical (luminal) membrane of the collecting duct cells. These channels allow facilitated, rapid transport of water from the collecting duct lumen into the cell along osmotic gradients. The water then exits the cell through the basolateral membrane, into the kidney medullary circulation through aquaporin-3 and aquaporin-4

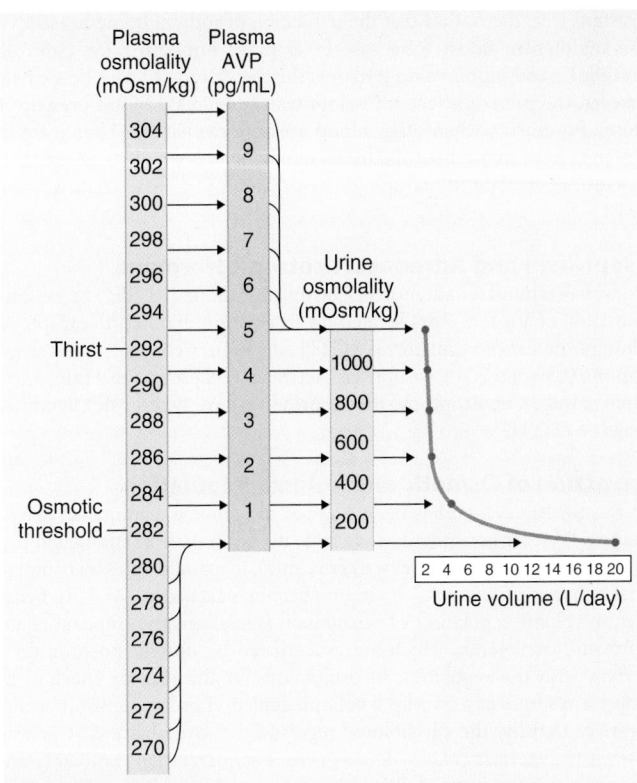

FIGURE 232-2. Idealized schematic of the normal physiologic relationships among plasma osmolality, plasma vasopressin (AVP), urine osmolality, and urine volume. The entire physiologic range of urine osmolality occurs with plasma vasopressin levels from 0 to 5 pg/mL. Increases in plasma osmolality above approximately 290 to 295 mOsm/kg H_2O result in increases in plasma vasopressin but no further concentration of the urine, which is limited by the maximal osmolality in the inner medulla. The relation of volume (calculated on the basis of a constant osmolar load) is inversely exponential to the other parameters. Because of this relationship, urine volume does not change substantially until there is nearly absent vasopressin secretion, after which urine volume increases dramatically. (Calculated from formulas presented in Robertson GL, Shelton RL, Athar S. The osmoregulation of vasopressin. *Kidney Int.* 1976;10:25-37. Figure drawn by J. G. Verbalis, Georgetown University, Washington, DC.)

water channels. This entire process is termed *antidiuresis*. In the absence of vasopressin, the aquaporin-2 channels are re-internalized from the apical membrane into subapical vesicles. This prevents active reabsorption of water from the collecting duct lumen, resulting in diuresis. In addition to this rapid "shuttling" of the aquaporin-2 channels to regulate water reabsorption on a minute-to-minute basis, vasopressin acts through V_2 receptors to regulate long-term stores of aquaporin-2; that is, increased vasopressin stimulates aquaporin-2 synthesis, and the absence of vasopressin results in decreased aquaporin-2 synthesis. The hypertonic medullary interstitium determines the maximal concentration of the urine, which is isotonic with the inner medulla of the kidney under conditions of maximal antidiuresis (Chapter 117).

Vasopressin and Pressure and Volume Regulation

High-pressure baroreceptors are located in the aorta and carotid sinus, and low-pressure baroreceptors are located in the right and left atria. Decreases in blood pressure or intravascular volume stimulate vasopressin release, whereas situations that increase blood volume or left atrial pressure (e.g., negative-pressure breathing) decrease the secretion of vasopressin. The release of vasopressin in response to changes in volume or pressure is less sensitive than the release in response to osmoreceptors, and generally a 10 to 15% reduction in blood volume or pressure is needed to stimulate the release of vasopressin. However, once arterial pressure falls below this threshold, the stimulated response is exponential, and plasma levels of vasopressin are markedly greater than those from osmotic stimulation.

The pressor effects of vasopressin are mediated through a separate receptor subtype, the V_{1a} receptors, located on vascular smooth muscle. The relatively insensitive regulation of vasopressin secretion by changes in volume and pressure and the modest role of vasopressin to regulate blood pressure are consistent with the notion that the regulation of sodium homeostasis by the renin-angiotensin-aldosterone system is more important for controlling extracellular and blood volume than is the regulation of water homeostasis. However, the pressor effects of vasopressin to increase blood pressure can become prominent when other blood pressure regulatory systems are deficient (e.g., autonomic neuropathy or renin-angiotensin-aldosterone system blockade) or in states of pathologic vasodilation (e.g., liver cirrhosis, septic shock).

Vasopressin and Adrenocorticotropic Hormone

Vasopressin stimulates adrenocorticotropic hormone (ACTH) secretion via stimulation of V_{1b} receptors located on anterior pituitary corticotroph cells. Although the major regulator of ACTH secretion is corticotropin-releasing hormone (Chapter 231), vasopressin activates a different signal transduction system in the corticotrophs, so these hormones have synergistic effects in the release of ACTH.

Interaction of Osmotic and Volume Regulation

The vasopressin system has been adapted to optimize mammalian drinking behavior. Water is consumed as available in the absence of stimulated thirst, and then vasopressin regulates water excretion to maintain plasma osmolality. Thirst serves as a backup if dehydration becomes excessive. Similarly, because pressure-volume regulation of vasopressin is less sensitive, modest changes in pressure or volume, which are exacerbated by upright posture, do not interfere with the regulation of osmolality. Yet the pressor effect of high vasopressin serves as a backup if volume depletion or hypotension becomes excessive. Usually, the physiologic regulation of osmolality and pressure-volume are synergistic. Dehydration causes an increase in osmolality and a decrease in volume, both of which stimulate the release of vasopressin. Excess administration of fluid causes a decrease in osmolality and an expansion of volume, both of which inhibit vasopressin secretion.

In addition, other factors can modulate the osmotic release and action of vasopressin. With volume expansion, natriuretic factors such as atrial natriuretic peptide and brain natriuretic peptide are released from atrial myocytes and act at the kidney to induce natriuresis. Atrial natriuretic peptide is also synthesized in the hypothalamus, where it may act to decrease vasopressin secretion. During pregnancy, there is a decrease of plasma osmolality by approximately 10 mOsm/kg H_2O as a result of a resetting of the osmostat, and the osmostat for thirst is reset in parallel. This effect may be mediated by the placental hormone relaxin.

Abnormalities in water and electrolyte balance are common in the elderly. This is due in part to age-related changes in body volume (as much as a 50% decrease in total body water in those older than 75 years) and renal function. The elderly also have a decreased appreciation for thirst. Although there is a normal or even increased ability to secrete vasopressin with age, there is a decreased ability to achieve either maximal urine concentration to retain water or maximal dilution of urine to excrete water. Consequently, the elderly are particularly prone to hypernatremia or hyponatremia with diseases that affect water balance or from the drugs used to treat various diseases.

Oxytocin

Prolactin is the main hormone necessary for milk production, but oxytocin is essential for milk secretion. Suckling stimulates tactile receptors, producing an afferent signal to the hypothalamus that causes the release of oxytocin from the posterior pituitary. Oxytocin binds to oxytocin receptors in the breast and induces contraction of myoepithelial cells around the alveoli and ductules to eject milk. In addition, upregulation of the uterine receptors for oxytocin dramatically increases the response to oxytocin at the end of pregnancy. The greatest release of oxytocin occurs with, not before, delivery of the infant, probably secondary to stretching of the vaginal wall. Oxytocin release may be more important to induce uterine contraction to inhibit blood loss after delivery than to initiate parturition. No pathologic syndromes of either increased or decreased secretion of oxytocin have been defined. However, because of the structural similarity between vasopressin and oxytocin, at high plasma levels oxytocin can activate vasopressin receptors, and vasopressin can activate oxytocin receptors.

⬤ SYNDROME OF INAPPROPRIATE ANTIDIURETIC HORMONE SECRETION

Excess secretion of vasopressin can be caused by abnormal secretion from the posterior pituitary or by ectopic synthesis and secretion of vasopressin by a tumor. The inappropriate secretion of vasopressin causes renal water retention and volume expansion of body fluids, with a secondary natriuresis and consequent hyponatremia. This disorder is called the syndrome of inappropriate antidiuretic hormone secretion and is discussed in Chapter 118.

⬤ DIABETES INSIPIDUS

▬ DEFINITION

Diabetes insipidus is the excretion of a large volume of hypotonic, insipid (tasteless) urine, usually manifested by polyuria (increased urination) and polydipsia (increased thirst). The large volume, usually in excess of 50 to 60 mL/kg/day, must be distinguished from increased frequency of small volumes and from large volumes of isotonic or hypertonic urine, both of which have other clinical significance.

▬ PATHOBIOLOGY

Four pathophysiologic mechanisms must be considered in the differential diagnosis of diabetes insipidus.

1. Central diabetes insipidus is caused by the inability to secrete (and usually to synthesize) vasopressin in response to increased osmolality. No concentration of the dilute glomerular filtrate takes place in the renal collecting duct, and consequently, a large volume of hypotonic (i.e., dilute) urine is excreted. This produces an increase in serum osmolality, with stimulation of thirst and secondary polydipsia. Levels of vasopressin in plasma are unmeasurable or inappropriately low for plasma osmolality.

2. Nephrogenic diabetes insipidus is caused by the inability of an otherwise normal kidney to respond to vasopressin. As in hypothalamic diabetes insipidus, the dilute glomerular filtrate entering the collecting duct is excreted as a large volume of hypotonic urine. The rise in plasma osmolality that occurs stimulates thirst and produces polydipsia. Unlike central diabetes insipidus, however, measured levels of vasopressin in plasma are high or appropriate for plasma osmolality.

3. Gestational diabetes insipidus is a rare condition produced by elevated levels or activity of placental cystine aminopeptidase (oxytocinase or vasopressinase) during pregnancy. The rapid destruction of vasopressin produces diabetes insipidus with polyuria and secondary stimulation of thirst with polydipsia. Because of the circulating vasopressinase, plasma vasopressin levels usually cannot be measured.

4. Primary polydipsia is a disorder of excess fluid ingestion rather than of vasopressin secretion or activity. Excessive ingested water produces a mild decrease in plasma osmolality that shuts off the secretion of vasopressin. In the absence of vasopressin action on the kidney, urine does not become concentrated, and a large volume of hypotonic urine is excreted. The amount of vasopressin in plasma is unmeasurable or low but is appropriate for the low plasma osmolality.

Although the pathophysiologic mechanisms for each of these four disorders are distinct, patients in each category usually manifest polyuria and polydipsia. The serum sodium level is normal because the normal thirst mechanism is sufficiently sensitive to maintain water homeostasis in the first three disorders, and the normal kidney has sufficient capacity to excrete the excess water load in the fourth.

▬ CLINICAL MANIFESTATIONS

Central Diabetes Insipidus

The sudden appearance of hypotonic polyuria after transcranial surgery in the area of the hypothalamus or after head trauma with basal skull fracture and hypothalamic damage obviously suggests the diagnosis of central diabetes insipidus. In these situations, if the patient is unconscious and unable to recognize thirst, hypernatremia is a common accompaniment. However, even in patients with more insidious progression of a specific disease or in patients with idiopathic central diabetes insipidus, the onset of polyuria is often relatively abrupt and occurs over several days or weeks. The initial problem is the volume of urine and polydipsia, not the decrease in urine osmolality. Most patients do not report polyuria until urine volume exceeds 4 L/day, and as illustrated in Figure 232-2, urine volume does not exceed 4 L/day until the ability to concentrate the urine is severely limited and plasma vasopressin is nearly absent. As few as 10% of the normal number of vasopressinergic neurons in the hypothalamus can maintain asymptomatic urine volume, but the further loss of these few neurons produces a rapid increase in urine volume and symptomatic polyuria. Urine volume seldom exceeds the amount of dilute fluid delivered to the collecting duct (about 18 to 24 L in humans), and in many cases, urine volume is less because patients voluntarily restrict fluid intake, which causes some mild volume contraction and increased proximal tubular reabsorption of fluid. Patients often express a preference for cold liquids, which are more effective in assuaging thirst. Both thirst and increased urine output persist through the night. Patients with partial central diabetes insipidus have some ability to secrete vasopressin, but this secretion is markedly attenuated at normal levels of plasma osmolality. Therefore, these patients have symptoms and urine volume similar to those of patients with complete central diabetes insipidus. Because most patients with central diabetes insipidus have sufficient thirst to drink fluid to match urine output, few laboratory abnormalities are present at the time of initial evaluation. The serum sodium level may be in the high-normal range, whereas the blood urea nitrogen level may be low secondary to the large urine volume. Uric acid is relatively high due to the modest volume contraction and the lack of action of vasopressin on V_{1a} receptors in the kidney, which stimulate the clearance of uric acid. Uric acid levels greater than 5 mg/dL can distinguish diabetes insipidus from primary polydipsia.

A variant of central diabetes insipidus is the syndrome of osmoreceptor dysfunction. This syndrome has been referred to as essential hypernatremia and adipsic hypernatremia because such patients have a chronically increased serum sodium concentration and an absence of thirst. Physiologic maneuvers demonstrate that when patients are euvolemic, an increase in plasma osmolality produces neither secretion of vasopressin nor a sensation of thirst. However, vasopressin is still synthesized by the hypothalamus and stored in the posterior pituitary because stimulation of baroreceptors by hypovolemia or hypotension results in the prompt secretion of vasopressin; the kidney is responsive because vasopressin release by volume receptor stimulation causes urinary concentration. Because patients lack thirst, they are chronically dehydrated, with increased serum sodium levels. However, it is the dehydration-induced volume depletion, not the increased osmolality, that eventually stimulates the secretion of vasopressin. The volume of urine output depends on the degree of dehydration-induced secretion of vasopressin. If sufficient fluid replacement is given to return extracellular fluid volume to normal, these patients are unable to regulate vasopressin by osmolality and become polyuric, thereby manifesting their underlying diabetes insipidus.

Central diabetes insipidus can be inherited as an autosomal dominant disease that is typically characterized by an asymptomatic infancy and an onset later in childhood. Most genetic defects are either in the signal peptide of the pre-prohormone or in the neurophysin portion of the prohormone. Mutations involving the vasopressin sequence itself are few. Most cases are believed to result from disruption of cleavage from the signal peptide or abnormal folding of the neurophysin, which slows trafficking of the mutant prohormone through the endoplasmic reticulum, leading to neuronal cell dysfunction and death. Because this is a cumulative process, this explains the later onset of central diabetes insipidus with these types of mutations.

Myxedema and adrenal insufficiency both impair the ability to excrete free water by renal mechanisms. The simultaneous occurrence of either of these diseases with central diabetes insipidus (as can occur with a tumor of the hypothalamus or pituitary) may decrease an otherwise large urine output, masking the symptoms of diabetes insipidus. Replacement treatment for the anterior pituitary deficiency, especially glucocorticoids, can then cause a sudden and massive excretion of dilute urine. Similarly, the onset of either hypothyroidism or adrenal insufficiency during the course of diabetes insipidus can decrease the need for vasopressin replacement and in some cases can even cause hyponatremia. Central diabetes insipidus is extremely common in patients with severe brain ischemia and is usually indicative of brain death. Treatment of the diabetes insipidus along with any coexistent anterior pituitary hormone deficiencies has been advocated to preserve donor organs in such cases.

Nephrogenic Diabetes Insipidus

Nephrogenic diabetes insipidus is caused by mutations of the vasopressin V_2 receptor or the vasopressin-induced water channel aquaporin-2 or by impairments in the signal transduction system linking the V_2 receptor and aquaporin-2. Familial nephrogenic diabetes insipidus is a rare disease, most cases of which (>90%) are due to mutations of the V_2 receptor. More than 100 different V_2 receptor mutations have been described, which can be classified into several different general categories based on differences in transport of the mutant receptor to the cell surface and vasopressin binding or stimulation of adenylate cyclase. Because the gene for the V_2 receptor is located on the X chromosome, this is an X-linked recessive disease. Symptoms are noted only in affected males, who present with vomiting,

constipation, failure to thrive, fever, and polyuria during the first week of life. Hypernatremia is found with a hypotonic urine. The phenotype is similar in the less than 10% of patients with mutations of the aquaporin-2 water channel, but because the aquaporin-2 gene is located on chromosome 12, mutations cause autosomal recessive disease; consequently, consanguinity and a family history of the disease in men and women is common, and this disorder should be suspected when the proband is female.

Nephrogenic diabetes insipidus can also be acquired during treatment with certain drugs, such as demeclocycline (which is used to treat inappropriate secretion of vasopressin), lithium carbonate (used to treat bipolar disorders), and fluoride (previously used in fluorocarbon anesthetics), and from electrolyte abnormalities such as hypokalemia and hypercalcemia. All causes of acquired nephrogenic diabetes insipidus have in common the decreased synthesis and function of aquaporin-2 due to impaired vasopressin signaling from V_2 receptor binding and activation. Other diseases of the kidney produce polyuria and inability to concentrate the urine secondary to altered renal medullary blood flow or to other disorders that inhibit maintenance of the hyperosmolar concentrating gradient in the inner medulla. Renal manifestations of such disorders (e.g., sickle cell disease, sarcoidosis, pyelonephritis, multiple myeloma, analgesic nephropathy) are discussed in Chapter 123.

Gestational Diabetes Insipidus

In pregnancy, there is an increased metabolism of vasopressin due to cystine aminopeptidase (oxytocinase or vasopressinase), an enzyme that normally degrades oxytocin and prevents premature uterine contractions. Normally, this is compensated for by increased synthesis of vasopressin. Rarely, women with normal regulation of vasopressin develop diabetes insipidus because of markedly elevated levels of vasopressinase. Some of these patients have accompanying preeclampsia, acute fatty liver, and coagulopathies, but causal relations between diabetes insipidus and these abnormalities have not been identified. In general, diabetes insipidus is not found after the pregnancy ends or in subsequent normal pregnancies.

Polyuria can also manifest in patients who have limited vasopressin reserve (partial central diabetes insipidus) or who respond poorly to vasopressin action (compensated nephrogenic diabetes insipidus). Treatment may be required only during the pregnancy, and the patient often returns to her previous baseline function without the need for therapy when the pregnancy ends. Less commonly, central diabetes insipidus of another cause first becomes symptomatic during pregnancy and then persists, following the usual course of diabetes insipidus.

Primary Polydipsia

Excessive fluid intake also causes hypotonic polyuria and, by definition, polydipsia. This disorder must be differentiated from the various causes of diabetes insipidus. Despite normal pituitary and kidney function, patients with this disorder share many characteristics of both central diabetes insipidus (vasopressin secretion is suppressed as a result of decreased plasma osmolality) and nephrogenic diabetes insipidus (kidney aquaporin-2 expression is decreased as a result of suppressed plasma vasopressin levels). Many different names have been used for this excessive fluid intake, but primary polydipsia is the best descriptor.

Primary polydipsia is sometimes due to a severe mental illness such as schizophrenia, mania, or obsessive-compulsive disorder, in which case it is called psychogenic polydipsia. These patients usually deny true thirst and attribute their polydipsia to bizarre motives, such as a need to cleanse the body of poisons. The incidence in psychiatric hospitals can be as high as 42%, and there is no obvious explanation for the polydipsia. Primary polydipsia can also be caused by an abnormality in the osmoregulatory control of thirst, in which case it is termed dipsogenic diabetes insipidus. These patients have no overt psychiatric illness and invariably attribute their polydipsia to a nearly constant thirst. Dipsogenic diabetes insipidus is usually idiopathic, but it can also be secondary to organic structural lesions in the hypothalamus identical to those causing central diabetes insipidus, such as neurosarcoidosis of the hypothalamus, tuberculous meningitis, multiple sclerosis, or trauma. Consequently, all polydipsic patients should be evaluated with magnetic resonance imaging (MRI) of the brain before it is concluded that excessive water intake is due to an idiopathic or psychiatric cause. Primary polydipsia can also be produced by drugs that cause a dry mouth or by any peripheral disorder causing marked elevations of renin or angiotensin.

Finally, primary polydipsia is sometimes caused by physicians, nurses, lay practitioners, or health writers who recommend a high fluid intake for valid (e.g., recurrent nephrolithiasis) or unsubstantiated health reasons. These patients lack overt signs of mental illness, but they also deny thirst and usually attribute their polydipsia to habits acquired from years of adherence to a drinking regimen. Laboratory studies in these patients are generally normal, although the serum sodium concentration is sometimes at the low end of the normal range, and the level of uric acid is lower than in patients with other forms of diabetes insipidus.

DIAGNOSIS

Physiologic Diagnosis

Diabetes insipidus should be considered in all patients presenting with significant polyuria (i.e., urine output >50 mL/kg/day). Although osmotic diuresis secondary to hyperglycemia, intravenous contrast agents, or renal injury is a more common clinical cause of polyuria, the medical history, an isotonic urine osmolality, and routine clinical laboratory tests generally distinguish these disorders from diabetes insipidus. A diagnosis of diabetes insipidus can be made when urine osmolality is inappropriately low in the presence of an elevated plasma osmolality as a result of increased serum sodium concentration. These criteria are sometimes met at the initial examination, especially in cases of acute diabetes insipidus occurring after trauma or after surgery with inadequate fluid replacement. In such patients with hypernatremia and hypotonic urine osmolality with normal renal function, one need only administer a vasopressin agonist to differentiate central diabetes insipidus, in which a renal response with decreased urine volume and increased urine osmolality occurs, from nephrogenic diabetes insipidus, in which a subnormal renal response is seen. Sometimes in the postoperative state, a water diuresis occurs as a result of water retention during the surgical procedure. Vasopressin is normally secreted in response to surgical stress, causing fluid administered intravenously during the procedure to be retained. During recovery, vasopressin levels fall, and a diuresis of the retained fluid occurs. In this case, however, the serum sodium level is almost always normal; however, if additional fluid is administered to match the urine output, persistent polyuria might be mistaken for diabetes insipidus. In this situation, the physician should decrease the rate of fluid administered and follow the urine output and serum sodium level. If the urine output decreases and the serum sodium level remains normal, no treatment is necessary; if serum sodium rises above the normal range and the urine remains hypotonic, diabetes insipidus is likely, and the response to a vasopressin agonist can ascertain the type.

Most outpatients with diabetes insipidus are not hypernatremic because the polydipsia produced by a normal thirst response is generally sufficient to maintain water homeostasis. Instead, they present with polyuria, polydipsia, and a normal sodium level. In these patients, further testing is necessary to increase serum osmolality and then measure the plasma vasopressin level or the urinary response to an administered vasopressin agonist. The best described test is the water deprivation test (Fig. 232-3), which should be

carried out under controlled observation in the hospital or an appropriately equipped outpatient area. The timing of the test depends on the patient's symptoms. If the patient has marked polyuria during the night, it is best to begin the test during the day because the patient may become dehydrated overnight. However, if the patient has only two or three episodes of nocturia per night, it is best to begin the test in the evening so that the major part of the dehydration takes place when the patient is asleep. In either case, the patient is weighed at the beginning of the test, and all subsequent fluids are withheld. The volume and osmolality of all excreted urine are measured, and the patient is reweighed after each liter of urine output. When three consecutive urine samples have an osmolality differing by no more than 10% and the patient has lost at least 2% of body weight, a blood sample is obtained for the measurement of serum osmolality, sodium, and plasma vasopressin. The patient is then given 2 μg of desmopressin intravenously or intramuscularly and observed for an additional 2 hours.

Adults with normal vasopressin secretion can concentrate their urine to greater than 800 mOsm/kg H$_2$O and have less than a 10% increase in urine osmolality in response to administered desmopressin. Patients with complete central diabetes insipidus have minimal concentration of the urine with dehydration, and a marked increase in urine osmolality (usually >50%) in response to administered desmopressin. Patients with nephrogenic diabetes insipidus usually have no increase in urine concentration in response to administered desmopressin, although in some cases of acquired nephrogenic diabetes insipidus, some increased urinary concentration (generally <10%) can occur. Nephrogenic diabetes insipidus is best distinguished from central diabetes insipidus by the measurement of vasopressin in plasma; plasma vasopressin levels are normally elevated in cases of nephrogenic diabetes insipidus, especially after dehydration.

In patients with partial central diabetes insipidus and patients with primary polydipsia, the urine is often somewhat concentrated in response to dehydration, but not to the maximum of a normal person. The chronically reduced level of vasopressin downregulates the synthesis of aquaporin-2 water channels, and the large urine volume, regardless of cause, washes out the medullary osmotic gradient that determines the maximal urine concentration. When desmopressin is administered, patients with partial central diabetes insipidus have a further increase (usually >10% but <50%) in urine osmolality, whereas most patients with primary polydipsia have no further increase (i.e., <10%). However, the reliability of distinguishing between these two disorders by the water deprivation test is suboptimal. Some patients with primary polydipsia may not become sufficiently dehydrated to secrete maximal vasopressin and hence have an increase in urine osmolality in response to administered desmopressin. Alternatively, some patients with partial central diabetes insipidus can become sufficiently dehydrated that their maximal concentration of urine is reached during the test, and no further concentration is seen with administered desmopressin. Plasma vasopressin levels at the end of dehydration are better at discriminating between these two disorders, but only at high serum sodium concentrations (>145 mmol/L). Consequently, some investigators advise a limited infusion of hypertonic (3%) sodium chloride solution to achieve these levels if they are not achieved by the water deprivation itself. It is important to maintain adequate follow-up of patients with suspected partial central diabetes insipidus to ensure that, during treatment with vasopressin, a good therapeutic response is obtained. In some difficult cases, the response to treatment with a vasopressin agonist can be an adjunct to the diagnosis. If a decrease in polyuria and thirst with maintenance of normal serum sodium concentration occurs, a diagnosis of partial central diabetes insipidus is confirmed; however, if polydipsia persists and hyponatremia develops, a diagnosis of primary polydipsia is confirmed.

Etiologic Diagnosis

If the water deprivation test confirms that inadequate vasopressin secretion or function is responsible for the polyuria, the underlying cause must be determined. MRI of the hypothalamic-pituitary area is the most important diagnostic tool in these cases. The three areas of interest are the immediate suprasellar region of the hypothalamus, the pituitary stalk, and the posterior pituitary within the sella turcica (see the earlier discussion of anatomy). Most slow-growing tumors confined to the sella do not cause diabetes insipidus. To cause central diabetes insipidus, tumors in the hypothalamic area immediately above the sella must be either sufficiently large to destroy 80 to 90% of the vasopressin cells or located where the paths of the four nuclear groups converge at the origin of the pituitary stalk, just above the diaphragma sellae. Primary tumors, especially craniopharyngioma and suprasellar germinoma;

FIGURE 232-3. Responses to the water deprivation test to differentiate various types of diabetes insipidus (DI) and primary polydipsia (as described by Miller M, Dalakos T, Moses AM, et al. Recognition of partial defects in antidiuretic hormone secretion. *Ann Intern Med.* 1970;73:721-729). The response to dehydration reaches a plateau, and the subsequent change in urine osmolality in response to administered desmopressin is illustrated. See the discussion in the text.

metastatic tumors; and infiltrative diseases can also cause diabetes insipidus by infiltration of the pituitary stalk, which is then thickened on MRI. In addition, on T1-weighted MRI, the vasopressin and oxytocin stored in neurosecretory granules in the posterior pituitary are visualized as a "bright spot" in the sella turcica. Most but not all normal subjects have this bright spot; in most but not all patients with central diabetes insipidus, the bright spot is lost. Thickening of the stalk and absence of the bright spot are therefore especially suggestive of a hypothalamic disease process.

Tumors that cause central diabetes insipidus are most often benign primary intracranial tumors such as craniopharyngioma, ependymoma (suprasellar germinoma), and pinealoma, which arise in the third ventricle. Primary tumors of the anterior pituitary (Chapter 231) cause diabetes insipidus only when substantial suprasellar extension is present. However, rapidly growing intrasellar lesions, such as metastases from carcinomas of the lung, breast, and melanoma or hemorrhage into pituitary adenomas, can cause diabetes insipidus because there is insufficient time for the vasopressin axons to adapt. Metastasis to the hypothalamus can also destroy the supraopticohypophysial tract and produce diabetes insipidus. Granulomatous diseases, such as Langerhans cell histiocytosis, sarcoidosis, tuberculosis, and leukemic infiltrates and lymphomas of the hypothalamus, can cause diabetes insipidus by destroying vasopressin cells. In such patients, the diagnosis is usually suspected on the basis of peripheral manifestations of the respective diseases. Lymphocytic infundibuloneurohypophysitis is an autoimmune disease similar to lymphocytic hypophysitis of the anterior pituitary (Chapter 231) in which lymphocytes infiltrate the neurohypophysis to produce diabetes insipidus. The hallmarks of this process are a thickened pituitary stalk and an absence of the pituitary bright spot in a patient with the abrupt onset of polyuria and polydipsia, particularly a postpartum female. The diagnosis was originally demonstrated by pituitary biopsy but is now generally made by regression of the thickened stalk with continued follow-up. When no cause is found, the diagnosis of exclusion is idiopathic diabetes insipidus, but most such cases are probably caused by an autoimmune disease, and other autoimmune diseases are often recognized in affected patients. When central nervous system disease is suspected but not diagnosed by MRI or general physical examination, cerebrospinal fluid obtained by lumbar puncture may be helpful in identifying tumor cells or markers of tumors or inflammatory processes (e.g., elevated angiotensin-converting enzyme levels in neurosarcoidosis).

TREATMENT Rx

Because excess diuresis of water is the primary manifestation of diabetes insipidus, water replacement in adequate quantities avoids the metabolic complications of this disease. However, oral or intravenous administration of the volume of fluid required to replace urinary losses in diabetes insipidus is difficult and inconvenient. The goal of therapy is to reduce the amount of polyuria and polydipsia to a tolerable level while avoiding overtreatment, which can produce water retention and hyponatremia. The best therapeutic agent for the treatment of hypothalamic diabetes insipidus is the vasopressin agonist desmopressin. Desmopressin is different from vasopressin, in that the amino group of the N-terminal cystine residue has been removed to prolong the duration of action, and D-arginine has been substituted for L-arginine in position 8 to decrease the vasopressor effects. At therapeutic dosages, this agent acts on V_2 or antidiuretic receptors, with minimal activity at V_{1a} or pressor receptors. Desmopressin is available in tablets of 0.1 or 0.2 mg for oral administration and in either a spray bottle that delivers a fixed dose of 10 μg in 100 μL or a bottle with a rhinal catheter that can deliver 50 to 200 μL (5 to 20 μg) for intranasal administration. When therapy is initiated, it is generally best to begin with a low dose (e.g., half of a 0.1-mg tablet, 5 μg by the rhinal tube, or a single 100 μL spray of 10 μg) at bedtime to allow the patient to sleep through the night, and then determine the duration of action by quantifying the polyuria the next day. The duration of action of a single dose varies from 6 to 24 hours, but in most patients, a good therapeutic response can be achieved on an every-12-hour schedule for the nasal spray or an 8- or 12-hour schedule for the tablets. Desmopressin is also available for parenteral use in 1-mL vials of 4 μg/mL. Parenteral administration is especially useful postoperatively or when a patient is unable to take the nasal preparation. In hospitalized patients, some physicians add vasopressin directly to a crystalloid solution to infuse doses in the range of 0.25 to 2.7 mIU/kg/hour to cause modest but persistent urinary concentration as a treatment of diabetes insipidus. With any parenteral administration, serum sodium levels should be monitored frequently to prevent the development of hyponatremia.

Some orally administered pharmacologic agents are also useful in treating diabetes insipidus. Chlorpropamide in doses of 100 to 500 mg/day enhances the effect of vasopressin at the renal tubule and is especially useful in patients with partial central diabetes insipidus. An antidiuretic effect is noted in 1 to 2 days, but maximal antidiuresis may not be achieved until after several days of administration. Thiazide diuretics cause sodium depletion and volume contraction and decrease urine volume by increasing proximal tubular reabsorption of glomerular filtrate. Prostaglandin synthase inhibitors (e.g., indomethacin) block the action of prostaglandin E to inhibit the action of vasopressin on the kidney. Chlorothiazide, amiloride, and prostaglandin synthase inhibitors are useful to reduce polyuria in nephrogenic diabetes insipidus. However, none of these agents has been approved by the Food and Drug Administration for the treatment of diabetes insipidus; therefore, the prescribing physician should be aware of potential toxicities and side effects. In cases of drug-induced nephrogenic diabetes insipidus, the most direct therapy is discontinuation of the offending agent, if possible. Symptomatic nephrogenic diabetes insipidus is usually treated with a thiazide diuretic, which is enhanced by the coadministration of the potassium-sparing diuretic amiloride. Amiloride can be especially beneficial in cases of nephrogenic diabetes insipidus induced by lithium because the drug decreases the entrance of lithium into cells in the distal tubule. When diuretics are used to treat nephrogenic diabetes insipidus, special attention should be paid to the possibility that the induced dehydration may increase the concentration of other drugs.

Some situations require special attention during therapy. Rarely, if patients with diabetes insipidus are unable to drink or are given a hypertonic solution, severe hypernatremia can develop acutely. Osmotic equilibrium with the intracellular water of neurons and glia produces shrinking of the brain. The brain is in a closed vault (i.e., the skull), and when the brain shrinks, traction on the vasculature of the central nervous system can cause the rupture of blood vessels and subarachnoid or intracerebral hemorrhage. If the hypernatremia persists for a longer time, the neurons accommodate by producing organic osmoles (previously called idiogenic osmoles), which limit the amount of brain shrinkage. Once this adaptation has occurred, a too rapid lowering of osmolality in the extracellular fluid will produce a shift of water into the brain and cause cerebral edema. In this situation, desmopressin can be administered to produce constant antidiuresis, and the amount of water given can be regulated to decrease osmolality by no more than approximately 1 mEq every 2 hours. Postoperatively or after head trauma, diabetes insipidus can be transient (see Prognosis), and the need for long-term maintenance therapy cannot be immediately established. During pregnancy, vasopressinase increases the metabolism of vasopressin but not of desmopressin, so desmopressin is the drug of choice. The vasopressinase activity subsides by a few weeks after delivery, and patients with the onset of partial diabetes insipidus during pregnancy may become asymptomatic after delivery. An additional advantage of desmopressin is that it has little action on the oxytocin receptors of the uterus. During pregnancy, normal plasma osmolality decreases by approximately 10 mOsm/kg H_2O because of changes in serum sodium, so pregnant patients with diabetes insipidus require only enough desmopressin to maintain the serum sodium at this lower level.

PROGNOSIS

The prognosis of properly treated diabetes insipidus is excellent. If nephrogenic diabetes insipidus is diagnosed and treated early, intracranial calcification and mental retardation do not occur. When the diabetes insipidus is secondary to a recognized disease process, that disease generally determines the ultimate prognosis. In some specific clinical situations, the course is different and characteristic. The development of diabetes insipidus after surgical or traumatic injury to the neurohypophysis can follow any of several well-defined patterns (Fig. 232-4). In some patients, polyuria develops 1 to 4 days after injury and resolves spontaneously. Less often, the diabetes insipidus is permanent and continues indefinitely. Most interestingly, one can see a "triphasic" response that has been well described after pituitary stalk transection. The first phase of diabetes insipidus is due to axon shock and lack of function of the damaged neurons. This phase lasts several hours to several days and is followed by a second, antidiuretic phase that is due to the uncontrolled release of vasopressin from the disconnected and degenerating posterior pituitary or from the remaining severed neurons. Overly aggressive administration of fluids during this second phase does not suppress the uncontrolled vasopressin release from the damaged neurohypophysis and can lead to hyponatremia. The antidiuresis can last 2 to 14 days, after which diabetes insipidus recurs after depletion of the vasopressin from the degenerating posterior pituitary gland (third phase). Transient hyponatremia without preceding or subsequent diabetes insipidus has been reported after transsphenoidal surgery for pituitary microadenomas.

Once a deficiency of vasopressin secretion has been present for more than a few days or weeks, it rarely improves, even if the underlying cause of the neurohypophysial destruction is eliminated. The major exception to this is postoperative diabetes insipidus, in which spontaneous resolution is the rule. Although recovery from diabetes insipidus that persists more than several weeks postoperatively is less common and is distinctly uncommon after 1

Transient DI

A

Permanent DI

B

Triphasic Response

C

FIGURE 232-4. A to C, Diagrammatic summary of the major patterns of postoperative and post-traumatic diabetes insipidus (DI). The abscissa represents time (T) after the initial injury *(arrow)*; the ordinate represents urinary volume (U_v) relative to a hypothetical "normal" urine output of 2 to 3 L/24 hours *(solid line)*. See the discussion in the text. During the triphasic response **(C)**, uncontrolled release of vasopressin from the disconnected or damaged posterior pituitary gland causes an antidiuresis that can lead to water retention and a dilutional hyponatremia. Diabetes insipidus returns as the third phase after the stored hormone in the posterior pituitary has been depleted. (From Verbalis JG, Robinson AG, Moses AM. Postoperative and post-traumatic diabetes insipidus. In: Czernichow AP, Robinson A, eds. *Diabetes Insipidus in Man: Frontiers of Hormone Research.* Basel: S Karger; 1985:247.)

year of continued diabetes insipidus, well-documented cases of recovery as long as 10 years after the initiating event have been reported. Potential return of function is another reason for occasionally withholding therapy during long-term treatment. Diabetes insipidus should not be considered idiopathic until at least 4 years of follow-up. During this interval, annual computed tomography or MRI is indicated to search for a tumor or infiltrative process that may not have been detected at the initial examination.

SUGGESTED READINGS

Ananthakrishnan S. Diabetes insipidus in pregnancy: etiology, evaluation, and management. *Endocr Pract.* 2009;15:377-382. *Review of diabetes insipidus in pregnancy, emphasizing the need for increased awareness of the syndrome to permit early diagnosis and appropriate treatment to reduce maternal and fetal morbidity.*

Los EL, Deen PM, Robben JH. Potential of nonpeptide (ant)agonists to rescue vasopressin V2 receptor mutants for the treatment of X-linked nephrogenic diabetes insipidus. *J Neuroendocrinol.* 2010;22:393-399. *V2R-specific cell-permeable agonists are promising therapeutics.*

Noda Y, Sohara E, Ohta E, et al. Aquaporins in kidney pathophysiology. *Nat Rev Nephrol.* 2010;6:168-178. *Recent advances in understanding the pathophysiology of the multiple kidney aquaporin water channels, including their role in nephrogenic diabetes insipidus.*

Ross HE, Young LJ. Oxytocin and the neural mechanisms regulating social cognition and affiliative behavior. *Front Neuroendocrinol.* 2009;30:534-547. *Brain oxytocin is an important modulator of social behaviors.*

Viero C, Shibuya I, Kitamura N, et al. Oxytocin: crossing the bridge between basic science and pharmacotherapy. *CNS Neurosci Ther.* 2010;16:e138-e156. *Review of oxytocin's diverse effects on male and female reproductive function and social behavior.*

233

THYROID

MATTHEW KIM AND PAUL LADENSON

The adult thyroid gland contains two lobes that wrap along the right and left anterolateral aspects of the trachea midway between the thyroid cartilage and

the suprasternal notch. Each lobe is demarcated into upper, middle, and lower poles. The right and left lobes are connected by an isthmus on the anterior aspect of the trachea just below the cricoid cartilage. The normal terminus of the thyroglossal duct can persist as a pyramidal lobe. A pyramidal lobe is often palpably enlarged in diffuse thyroid disorders such as autoimmune thyroiditis and Graves' disease.

After thyroid enlargement, the attachment of the sternothyroid muscle to the trachea limits upward expansion of the superior aspect of each lobe. Lateral and posterior growth may cause inferior expansion that may extend into the superior mediastinum, compressing the trachea and veins at the thoracic outlet. The parathyroid glands usually lie beneath the posterior aspects of each thyroid lobe. The recurrent laryngeal nerves course upward along the tracheoesophageal groove, from which branches pass behind each thyroid lobe to innervate the larynx.

Thyroid tissue is composed of clustered spherical follicles, each containing a single layer of follicular epithelial cells known as *thyrocytes* that surround a lumen containing colloid. The principal component of colloid is thyroglobulin, a thyrocyte-specific protein. Parafollicular C cells, which are derived from neural crest tissue and produce calcitonin, are widely dispersed between follicles.

● PHYSIOLOGY

Thyroid Hormone Synthesis and Secretion

Dietary iodine in the form of iodide (I^-) or iodate (IO_3^-) is absorbed from the gastrointestinal tract and distributed in the extracellular fluid. The average daily intake of iodine in the United States equals the recommended daily intake of 150 μg because of the widespread use of iodized salt. Circulating iodide is actively transported into the thyrocyte by the sodium-iodide symporter. Within the thyrocyte, iodide is rapidly oxidized by H_2O_2 in a reaction catalyzed by thyroid peroxidase. The reactive intermediate formed is covalently bound to tyrosyl residues present in thyroglobulin to generate monoiodotyrosine and diiodotyrosine residues through a process known as *organification*. Thyroid peroxidase also catalyzes the coupling of the monoiodotyrosine and diiodotyrosine residues to generate thyroxine (T_4) and triiodothyronine (T_3). T_4 and T_3 are secreted after proteolysis of thyroglobulin. This hydrolytic process may be inhibited by exposure to excessive amounts of iodide or lithium. In the normal state, approximately 100 μg of T_4 and 5 μg of T_3 are directly released into the circulation each day.

Thyroid Hormone Transport and Metabolism

Circulating thyroid hormones are more than 99% bound to three classes of plasma proteins. Thyroxine-binding globulin (TBG) functions as the principal transport protein. Thyroxine-binding prealbumin and albumin make lesser contributions to T_4 and T_3 transport in blood. Pregnancy and exposure to pharmacologic doses of estrogens can increase TBG levels, as can hepatitis, familial TBG excess, and certain medications, including 5-fluorouracil, tamoxifen, and methadone. Conversely, decreased TBG levels may occur with systemic illness, severe hepatic disease, nephrotic syndrome, and treatment with androgens, glucocorticoids, and slow-release nicotinic acid. Whereas total T_4 and T_3 levels rise and fall with changes in TBG, free T_4 and T_3 levels remain constant. Familial dysalbuminemic hyperthyroxinemia is an autosomal dominant disorder characterized by the production of albumin that binds T_4 with a high affinity. Affected individuals may present with high total T_4 levels and normal free T_4 levels. The receptor binding and biologic activity of T_3 is eight-fold greater than that of T_4. More than 80% of the T_3 present in target tissues is derived from T_4 through the action of deiodinase enzymes that convert T_4 to both T_3, which contributes to the pool of T_3 in the circulation, and biologically inactive reverse T_3. The activity of deiodinase may be inhibited by systemic illness; iodide-containing compounds, including amiodarone and radiocontrast agents; glucocorticoid therapy; and selenium deficiency. Type 2 deiodinase is present in the pituitary gland and brain. Type 3 deiodinase is present in the glial cells of the central nervous system. It deactivates thyroid hormone by inner ring monodeiodination, a process that converts T_4 to inactive reverse T_3 (rT_3) and T_3 to inactive diiodothyronine (T_2). Type 3 deiodinase is also expressed in placenta, accounting for the increased thyroxine dose requirement in pregnant women.

Control of Thyroid Function

The growth of thyroid tissue and the synthesis and secretion of thyroid hormones are controlled by the hypothalamus and the pituitary gland.

Thyrotropin-releasing hormone (TRH) is synthesized by the hypothalamus and is transported to the pituitary gland, where it binds to receptors on thyrotrophic cells, stimulating the synthesis and secretion of thyroid-stimulating hormone (TSH). TSH is a heterodimeric glycoprotein composed of a unique β-subunit coupled to an α-subunit, identical to that present in follicle-stimulating hormone, luteinizing hormone, and human chorionic gonadotropin (HCG). It is transported in the circulation to the thyroid gland, where it binds to the TSH receptor on thyrocytes. The binding of TSH to the TSH receptor stimulates iodide transport, hydrolysis of thyroglobulin, and secretion of thyroid hormone. Circulating T_4 and T_3 exert negative feedback at the levels of both the hypothalamus and the pituitary gland, inhibiting the synthesis and secretion of TRH and TSH, respectively.

Thyroid Hormone Action

Thyroid hormone binds receptors that are members of the nuclear receptor superfamily, regulating expression of thyroid hormone–responsive genes. Isoforms of the thyroid hormone receptors (α_1, β_1, and β_2) bind to a specific hexameric oligonucleotide sequence in the transcriptional regulatory region of thyroid hormone–responsive genes. For example, T_3 increases expression of the low-density lipoprotein (LDL) receptor, resulting in accelerated LDL cholesterol degradation. In myocardium, T_3 increases myocyte contractility and relaxation by altering myosin heavy chain and sarcoplasmic reticulum adenosine triphosphatase (ATPase), respectively. In the cardiac conducting system, T_3 increases the heart rate by altering sinoatrial node depolarization and repolarization. Other physiologic effects of thyroid hormone include increased mental alertness, ventilatory drive, gastrointestinal motility, and bone turnover. During fetal development, thyroid hormone plays critical roles in brain development and skeletal maturation.

DIAGNOSIS

Physical Examination

Examination of the thyroid begins with inspection of the lower anterior portion of the neck to check for diffuse or asymmetrical gland enlargement, tracheal deviation, lymphadenopathy, and jugular venous distention. Palpation can be performed by an anterior or posterior approach. Anterior palpation can be performed by using the thumb of one hand to locate the isthmus of the gland beneath the cricoid cartilage. The right lobe of the thyroid gland can be palpated by placing the left thumb along the left side of the trachea to brace the contralateral lobe, using the tips of the fingers of the right hand to laterally retract the right sternocleidomastoid muscle at the level of the isthmus, and using the pads of the fingers of the right hand to explore and define the tissue composing the lobe. The mass of tissue that moves beneath the fingertips when the patient swallows represents the lobe. This maneuver can be reversed to examine the left lobe.

Laboratory Findings
TSH and Thyroid Hormone Levels

TSH is a sensitive indicator of primary thyroid gland dysfunction. Current TSH immunoassays permit the accurate detection of all common causes of thyroid hormone deficiency and excess. Indeed, TSH levels become abnormal when patients' thyroid hormone levels remain within broad reference ranges, conditions termed *subclinical hypothyroidism* and *subclinical thyrotoxicosis*. In most patients with primary thyroid gland dysfunction, measurement of a single TSH level permits an accurate classification of the thyroid status. Limitations of TSH testing occur when there is TSH-mediated secondary thyroid dysfunction, reduced biologic activity of T_3 or TSH itself, temporary disequilibrium of the hypothalamic-pituitary-thyroid axis, or analytic problems affecting the TSH immunoassay.

Measurements of T_4 and T_3 levels confirm the significance of an abnormal TSH level, define the severity of thyroid dysfunction, and provide a clue to the underlying cause. Whereas assays that measure total T_4 and T_3 levels are accurate, their results do not distinguish between large plasma protein–bound and free fractions of each hormone. Consequently, congenital and acquired derangements of TBG (and, less commonly, transthyretin and albumin) can alter total but not free T_4 and T_3 levels. These conditions can be misdiagnosed as abnormal thyroid function unless a discordance in TSH is noted or one of these underlying conditions is suspected (Tables 233-1 and 233-2). There are several methods of estimating unbound T_4 and T_3 levels. Free T_4 and free T_3 immunoassays are widely employed for this purpose and yield reliable results in common conditions that alter plasma protein levels, such as estrogen-induced TBG excess. Free T_4 measurement after

TABLE 233-1 CAUSES OF EUTHYROID HYPERTHYROXINEMIA (INCREASED TOTAL T_4, NORMAL TSH, NORMAL FREE T_4)

Increased synthesis of thyroxine-binding globulin
   Pregnancy
   Hepatitis
   Acute intermittent porphyria
   Drugs
      Estrogens
      Tamoxifen
      Raloxifene
      Methadone
      5-Fluorouracil
Increased binding of thyroid hormone to albumin
   Familial dysalbuminemic hyperthyroxinemia
Increased binding of thyroid hormone to transthyretin
   Hereditary variants
   Pancreatic neuroendocrine tumors

TABLE 233-2 CAUSES OF EUTHYROID HYPOTHYROXINEMIA (DECREASED TOTAL T_4, NORMAL TSH, NORMAL FREE T_4

Increased metabolism of thyroid hormone
   Drugs
      Phenytoin
      Phenobarbital
      Carbamazepine
      Rifampin
Decreased synthesis of thyroxine-binding globulin
   Severe liver disease
   Malnutrition
   Drugs
      Androgens
      Danazol
      L-Asparaginase
Increased clearance of thyroxine-binding globulin
   Nephrotic syndrome
   Protein-losing enteropathy
Decreased binding of thyroid hormone to thyroxine-binding globulin
   Drugs
      Salicylates (high dose)
      Phenytoin (high dose)
      Furosemide (intravenous)

equilibrium dialysis of serum is the most accurate approach, but it is technically demanding and not readily available in most settings.

Other Laboratory Tests

Measurement of thyroid autoantibody titers can be useful in the evaluation of thyroid dysfunction. Antithyroid peroxidase and antithyroglobulin antibody titers can confirm a diagnosis of autoimmune thyroiditis. Thyroid-stimulating immunoglobulin activity levels can be measured to evaluate Graves' disease. The erythrocyte sedimentation rate can be helpful in the diagnosis of subacute thyroiditis. Serum thyroglobulin and calcitonin levels are used as tumor markers when observing patients treated for differentiated and medullary thyroid cancers, respectively.

Imaging
Anatomic Imaging

Ultrasonography provides detailed views that help measure the size of the thyroid gland, characterize its texture, and identify structural abnormalities, including solid nodules and simple or partially cystic nodules. Diffuse heterogeneity may suggest autoimmune thyroiditis. Certain characteristics of nodules—including the appearance of capsules, vascularity, and patterns of calcification—can alter the probability of malignancy but do not confirm or exclude thyroid cancer with certainty. Imaging of surrounding structures may identify cervical lymphadenopathy not detectable on physical examination.

The value of computed tomography (CT) and magnetic resonance imaging (MRI) is their ability to delineate tracheal deviation, narrowing, and substernal extension of the thyroid into the mediastinum. Cervical CT scanning can also help define and localize regional lymphadenopathy. Positron emission tomography (PET) plays a role in the localization of residual thyroid cancer.

Functional Imaging

Radionuclide scanning takes advantage of the fact that gamma ray–emitting tracers transported into thyrocytes by the sodium-iodide symporter can generate images that reflect the regional activity of thyroid tissue. Technetium -99m (^{99m}Tc) and iodine-123 (^{123}I) are commonly used. ^{99m}Tc-pertechnetate is rapidly trapped by thyrocytes, and ^{99m}Tc scans can be acquired 20 to 30 minutes after injection. ^{123}I and ^{131}I thyroid scans generate images that provide a more accurate representation of regional thyroid tissue function and can indicate whether a nodule is hypofunctioning (cold), hyperfunctioning (hot), or equivalent in function to extranodular tissue (warm). Radionuclide imaging no longer plays a central role in the differential diagnosis of most thyroid nodules. When it is necessary, ^{123}I is the preferred tracer because of its lower thyroidal and whole body radiation dose.

Thyroid Uptake

The fraction of an administered radioactive iodine or technetium dose taken up and retained by the thyroid gland during a defined period represents an index of the gland's activity. Typically, technetium pertechnetate uptake ranges from 0.5 to 3%; radioiodine uptake usually ranges from 8 to 28%. These fractional thyroid uptakes can be useful in the differential diagnosis of thyrotoxicosis. Radioiodine uptake values are also used to calculate effective ^{131}I doses for the treatment of hyperthyroidism and thyroid cancer.

⬤ HYPOTHYROIDISM

DEFINITION

Primary hypothyroidism (termed *myxedema* when it is severe) refers to hormone deficiency caused by intrinsic dysfunction of the thyroid gland that disrupts the synthesis and secretion of T_4 and T_3 (Table 233-3). Overt hypothyroidism is characterized by an elevated TSH level, usually greater than 10 mIU/L, in conjunction with a free T_4 level below the lower limit of the reference range. In subclinical hypothyroidism, the TSH level is only modestly elevated; the free T_4 level remains in the low-normal to normal range.

Secondary or central hypothyroidism refers to deficient thyroid gland function that is the result of inadequate stimulation by TSH. This is due, in turn, to production of either insufficient or ineffective TSH from a number of congenital or acquired pituitary and hypothalamic disorders (Chapter 231).

EPIDEMIOLOGY

Primary hypothyroidism is common—present in 5% of individuals. Mild hypothyroidism is present in as many as 15% of older adults. Hypothyroidism is more commonly diagnosed in women. It is more prevalent among whites and Latinos. Secondary hypothyroidism is rare, representing less than 1% of cases.

PATHOBIOLOGY

Dietary iodine deficiency is an important cause of primary hypothyroidism in children in certain underdeveloped countries. The most common cause of primary hypothyroidism in developed countries is autoimmune (or Hashimoto's) thyroiditis, a condition in which altered T-cell-mediated immunity causes destruction of thyroid tissue and impaired gland function. The condition is characterized by a lymphocytic infiltrate and fibrosis. Circulating antithyroid antibodies directed against thyroid peroxidase and thyroglobulin are markers of the disease, but glandular inflammation is principally the result of altered T-cell-mediated function. There is a genetic predisposition to the condition. Linkage studies suggest a polygenic basis. Patients with autoimmune thyroiditis may have other endocrine and nonendocrine autoimmune disorders. It may be a component of the type 2 polyglandular autoimmune syndrome associated with autoimmune adrenal insufficiency and type 1 diabetes mellitus. It is less commonly a component of the type 1 syndrome, which includes adrenal insufficiency, hypoparathyroidism, and chronic mucocutaneous candidiasis (Chapter 239). Other nonendocrine autoimmune conditions associated with autoimmune thyroiditis include atrophic gastritis, pernicious anemia, systemic sclerosis, Sjögren's syndrome, celiac disease, and vitiligo. Individuals treated with interferon-α may develop autoimmune thyroiditis with transient or permanent hypothyroidism.

Surgical resection of thyroid tissue predictably leads to hypothyroidism. Radioactive iodine therapy for treatment of hyperthyroidism commonly destroys sufficient thyroid tissue to cause postablative hypothyroidism. External beam radiation therapy for head and neck cancer can cause thyroid gland failure. Exposure to certain pharmacologic and radiocontrast agents that contain large amounts of iodine, such as amiodarone, radiocontrast dyes, some expectorants, and topical disinfectants, can disrupt thyroid hormone production. Lithium inhibits secretion of T_4 and T_3, leading to hypothyroidism in 10% of treated patients. Other pharmacologic agents reported to cause hypothyroidism include stavudine, thalidomide, sunitinib, and aminoglutethimide.

There are a number of other rare causes of primary hypothyroidism (see Table 233-3). Congenital hypothyroidism can be due to agenesis or dysgenesis of the thyroid gland, or to mutations in genes encoding the enzymes catalyzing thyroid hormone synthesis. Infiltrative disorders can disrupt thyroid function, including hemochromatosis, amyloidosis, systemic sclerosis, and invasive fibrous thyroiditis (also known as *Riedel's thyroiditis*). The thyroid gland inflammation that occurs with subacute thyroiditis and painless (postpartum) thyroiditis causes transient hypothyroidism, from which most patients recover.

Secondary or central hypothyroidism may be caused by a number of disorders that impair normal hypothalamic or pituitary control of the thyroid gland (Chapter 231). Infiltrative disorders affecting the hypothalamus that can interfere with TRH secretion include sarcoidosis, hemochromatosis, and histiocytosis. Masses that impinge on the pituitary stalk can impede TRH delivery through the hypophysial portal system. Compression of thyrotrophic cells by pituitary adenomas and other masses in the sella turcica can inhibit synthesis and secretion of TSH. Surgery and radiation therapy to treat pituitary adenomas can destroy thyrotrophic cells, leading to secondary hypothyroidism that develops as a component of pan-hypopituitarism. Other disorders that may be associated with secondary hypothyroidism include lymphocytic hypophysitis, pituitary metastases from primary malignant neoplasms, apoplexy, infarction caused by hemorrhage at the time of delivery in women (also known as *Sheehan's syndrome*), and head trauma.

TABLE 233-3 ETIOLOGIES OF HYPOTHYROIDISM

PRIMARY HYPOTHYROIDISM

Insufficient functioning thyroid tissue
  Congenital absence of thyroid tissue
  Autoimmune destruction of thyroid tissue
    Autoimmune thyroiditis (Hashimoto's thyroiditis)
  Surgical removal of thyroid tissue
  Radioablation of thyroid tissue by radioactive iodine or external beam radiation
  Infiltrative destruction of thyroid tissue
    Hemochromatosis
    Scleroderma
    Amyloidosis
Impaired thyroid hormone synthesis
  Iodine deficiency
  Congenital enzymatic defects that disrupt thyroid hormone synthesis
  Drug-mediated inhibition of thyroid hormone production and release
    Thionamides
    Amiodarone
    Lithium
    Aminoglutethimide

SECONDARY HYPOTHYROIDISM

Insufficient secretion of TRH or TSH
  Hypothalamic disorders
    Tumor (lymphoma, germinoma, glioma)
    Irradiation
    Inflammation (sarcoidosis, vasculitis)
  Hypopituitarism
    Mass lesions
    Pituitary surgery
    Pituitary radiation
    Hemorrhagic apoplexy (Sheehan's syndrome)
    Infiltration (hemochromatosis, tuberculosis, fungal infection)
    Lymphocytic hypophysitis
  Thyroid hormone resistance syndrome

CLINICAL MANIFESTATIONS

Symptoms and Signs

Symptoms of hypothyroidism include fatigue, lethargy, weight gain despite poor appetite, cold intolerance, hoarseness, constipation, weakness, myalgias, arthralgias, paresthesias, dry skin, and hair loss. Females may develop precocious puberty, menorrhagia, amenorrhea, and galactorrhea. Affected individuals may experience depressed mood with limited initiative and sociability. Cognitive deficits can range from mild lapses in memory to delirium, dementia, seizures, and coma. The nonspecific nature of most of these symptoms makes it difficult to determine which patients presenting with them have hypothyroidism rather than other causes. In most cases, hypothyroidism is insidious in onset, making its recognition difficult. Symptoms that are new, progressive, or present in combination are more likely to be due to hypothyroidism.

The physical findings associated with hypothyroidism vary according to the age at onset and disease severity. Children may present with delayed linear growth despite weight gain, precocious or delayed puberty, and pseudohypertrophy of muscle. Adults can present with bradycardia, diastolic hypertension, and mild hypothermia. The skin may be coarse, dry, yellow, and cool to the touch as a result of peripheral vasoconstriction. Diffuse thinning of scalp hair accompanied by thinning of the lateral eyebrows may occur. The nails may be brittle. Examination of the chest may reveal distant heart sounds. The extremities may reveal diffuse nonpitting edema caused by the deposition of glycosaminoglycans. Neurologic examination may reveal slow, dysarthric speech and diffuse slowing of deep tendon reflexes with a marked delay in the terminal relaxation phase.

Examination of the neck may reveal a range of findings. Healed cervical incisional scars in this region indicate a history of surgical resection of thyroid tissue. The thyroid gland may be normal in size, diffusely enlarged, or atrophic to the point where it may be difficult to palpate with any degree of certainty. It may be soft and smooth with a lobular texture or firm and irregular with a variegated nodular texture.

Other Routine Test Abnormalities

Blood tests may reveal anemia, hyponatremia, hypoglycemia, and elevated creatine phosphokinase, prolactin, homocysteine, triglyceride, and total and LDL cholesterol levels. Electrocardiography may show sinus bradycardia with low voltage in the limb leads. Chest radiography may show a widened cardiac silhouette, and echocardiography may confirm a pericardial effusion.

DIAGNOSIS

Suspected primary hypothyroidism is confirmed by an elevated TSH level (Fig. 233-1). Established reference ranges for TSH levels typically extend from 0.5 to 4.5 mIU/L. However, the distribution of values within this range is skewed toward the lower half, such that the mean TSH level is estimated to be 1.5 mIU/L. Measurement of the free T_4 level confirms the diagnosis of primary hypothyroidism and characterizes its severity. A low free T_4 level in conjunction with a persistently elevated TSH level represents overt primary hypothyroidism, whereas a low-normal free T_4 level with an elevated TSH level is termed *mild primary hypothyroidism*. Other uncommon causes of isolated TSH elevation should be considered in appropriate settings, including recovery from severe systemic illness, renal failure, and adrenal insufficiency.

Testing to determine the underlying cause of primary hypothyroidism is usually unnecessary. When confirmation is required (e.g., to convince a patient that the condition is permanent), serum antithyroid antibodies may be assessed. Measurement of antithyroid peroxidase antibody is a more sensitive test than antithyroglobulin antibody for this purpose. However, 10% of patients with histologically documented autoimmune thyroiditis have no circulating antithyroid antibodies.

When clinical findings such as the presence of a sellar mass, previous pituitary surgery or irradiation, or other pituitary axis hormone deficiencies suggest the possibility of secondary hypothyroidism, the TSH level cannot be relied on to provide an accurate index of thyroid function. In these settings, the serum free T_4 level must be assessed, and a low or even low-normal free T_4 level can confirm the diagnosis. The TSH level in patients with secondary hypothyroidism can be low, normal, or even modestly elevated.

TREATMENT   Rx

The goals of thyroid hormone replacement therapy are straightforward: to replace endogenous thyroid hormone production, to avoid iatrogenic thyrotoxicosis, and, rarely, to treat systemic complications of severe hypothyroidism. Levothyroxine sodium (hereafter thyroxine) is the hormonal preparation of choice. Thyroxine has a number of favorable pharmacokinetic characteristics. It is well absorbed, and its plasma protein binding gives it a 7-day half-life, permitting daily dosing. Thyroxine is physiologically deiodinated to the more biologically active T_3 in peripheral tissues. However, thyroxine is a narrow therapeutic index drug, and doses differing by as little as 12% can have clinical consequences. Tablets of multiple dose strengths ranging from 25 to 300 µg are available. Regulatory standards ensure pharmaceutical equivalence in terms of mass of thyroxine, but bioavailability may differ by as much as 12% among different preparations. Consequently, adherence to a single thyroxine formulation is advisable.

The optimal dose of thyroxine for replacement therapy is related to lean body weight, with most adults requiring a daily dose of 1.8 µg/kg. The dose requirement for elderly adults is typically lower (e.g., 1.0 µg/kg/day) because of reduced metabolic clearance. Patients with postsurgical or postablative hypothyroidism usually require a higher daily dose than patients with autoimmune thyroiditis, who may have some residual gland function. Patients with coexisting malabsorptive disorders may require higher and variable doses. Certain medications, mineral supplements, and foods can interfere with thyroxine absorption, including ferrous sulfate, calcium carbonate, aluminum hydroxide, sucralfate, cholestyramine, and soy-containing foods (Table 233-4). Thyroxine doses should be separated from these substances by 4 hours or longer.

Thyroxine dose requirements may increase as a result of accelerated metabolic clearance in several circumstances. Patients with nephrotic syndrome and other systemic illnesses that lead to rapid clearance of thyroid hormone require higher daily doses. Dose requirements increase by an average of 75% in most pregnant women, probably as a result of placental metabolism of thyroxine. Simultaneous treatment with phenytoin, phenobarbital, carbamazepine, or rifampin also typically accelerates thyroxine metabolism. One third of postmenopausal women beginning estrogen replacement therapy have increased dose requirements.

FIGURE 233-1. Laboratory assessment of suspected hypothyroidism.

TABLE 233-4 INTERFERENCE WITH THYROXINE REPLACEMENT THERAPY

FACTORS CONTRIBUTING TO UNDERREPLACEMENT

Inadequate prescribed dose
Limited compliance
Decreased absorption due to ingestion of agents that bind thyroxine
   Ferrous sulfate
   Calcium carbonate
   Aluminum hydroxide
   Sucralfate
   Cholestyramine
   Soy protein
Increased metabolism of thyroxine
   Pregnancy
   Drugs
      Phenytoin
      Phenobarbital
      Carbamazepine
      Rifampin
Diminishing residual thyroid function
Changing formulations

FACTORS CONTRIBUTING TO OVERREPLACEMENT

Excessive prescribed dose
Factitious ingestion of additional doses
Decreased metabolism of thyroxine due to aging
Increasing residual thyroid function
Changing formulations

TABLE 233-5 ETIOLOGIES OF THYROTOXICOSIS

HYPERTHYROIDISM

Antibody-mediated stimulation of thyroid tissue
   Graves' disease
Autonomously functioning thyroid tissue
   Toxic multinodular goiter
   Toxic adenoma
   Iodine exposure
Autonomously functioning heterotopic thyroid tissue
   Struma ovarii
   Metastatic differentiated thyroid cancer
Excessive secretion of TSH
   TSH-secreting pituitary adenoma

NONHYPERTHYROID THYROTOXICOSIS

Ingestion of exogenous thyroid hormone
   Pharmacologic
      Levothyroxine
      Liothyronine
      Combination preparations
   Nonpharmacologic
      Dietary supplements
   Improperly processed meat products
Inflammation causing release of endogenous thyroid hormone
   Subacute thyroiditis
   Autoimmune thyroiditis

Most adults without known or suspected coronary artery disease can be started on a full replacement dose of thyroxine. The initial dose can be calculated on the basis of the patient's weight and age, rounding down to the nearest available dose strength. For patients with primary hypothyroidism, adequacy of thyroxine therapy can be assessed by TSH measurement 4 to 6 weeks after therapy is started. The target TSH level for most individuals should be the lower half of the reference range (i.e., 1.0 to 2.0 mIU/L). Once an adequate dose has been established, the TSH level should be checked annually. In patients with secondary hypothyroidism, the serum free T_4 level should be monitored 2 to 4 weeks after the thyroxine dose is started or adjusted, with a target free T_4 level in the upper half of the reference range.

Management of Complications

Complications of thyroxine therapy are limited to iatrogenic thyrotoxicosis and, rarely, adverse effects of restoring euthyroidism. Typical symptoms and signs of thyrotoxicosis accompany overtreatment. Even a modestly excessive thyroxine dose can induce bone mineral loss, especially in postmenopausal women, and it can increase the risk of atrial fibrillation in older individuals. In patients with underlying coronary artery disease, the positive chronotropic and inotropic effects of thyroxine may exacerbate myocardial ischemia. Adults with known or suspected ischemic heart disease should be started on a low dose that is titrated upward in small increments once tolerance is ensured (e.g., starting with 25 μg daily, then increasing the dose by 12.5 to 25 μg every 4 to 6 weeks). In some cases, β-blocker therapy may need to be intensified to counter the induction of myocardial ischemia. Deliberate suboptimal dosing of thyroxine should be avoided. If necessary, coronary revascularization may be required before euthyroidism can be fully restored. Coexisting adrenal insufficiency associated with hypopituitarism or the type 2 polyglandular autoimmune syndrome may be unmasked when cortisol clearance is accelerated by a return to the euthyroid state. Other adverse effects that infrequently occur with thyroxine therapy include transient hair loss, acute sympathomimetic symptoms that resolve with dose reduction and slow advancement, and pseudotumor cerebri in children.

A minority of patients with thyroxine-treated hypothyroidism continue to report bothersome symptoms despite biochemical evidence of adequate thyroid hormone replacement. Some of these patients improve with a higher thyroxine dose that restores the serum free T_4 level to the upper limit of normal. Eight trials have now shown that combined T_3 and T_4 therapy—whether as desiccated thyroid or combined synthetic hormones—is not superior to T_4 alone.

Subclinical and Mild Hypothyroidism

Whether individuals diagnosed with subclinical hypothyroidism (i.e., an elevated or high-normal TSH level with a free T_4 level within the reference range) benefit from thyroxine therapy is controversial. In practice, many providers opt for a trial of therapy in mildly hypothyroid patients who are symptomatic, have underlying hypercholesterolemia, or demonstrate a high likelihood of progressing to overt hypothyroidism. Predictors of progressive thyroid failure include age older than 65 years, TSH level higher than 10 mIU/L, and the presence of circulating antithyroid antibodies, indicating underlying autoimmune thyroiditis.

Myxedema Coma

Severe hypothyroidism can culminate in myxedema coma, a life-threatening condition characterized by hypothermia, bradycardia, hypotension, altered mental status, and multisystem organ failure. Risk factors include advanced age, poor access to health care, and other underlying major organ system diseases. Most patients have long-standing thyroid hormone deficiency. Treatment should include thyroxine (1.8 μg/kg/day, with or without a 500-μg loading dose). Some experts advocate coadministration of triiodothyronine in divided doses to compensate for impaired conversion of T_4 to T_3. No controlled trials have been performed to evaluate the relative benefits and risks of these different approaches. Glucocorticoids should be administered in stress doses after a cosyntropin stimulation test has been performed to check for evidence of concomitant adrenal insufficiency (Chapter 234). Care should be taken to avoid exposure to potent sedative or analgesic agents that may exacerbate altered mental status. Hypothermia should be treated with external warming to reduce the risk of circulatory collapse.

Nonthyroidal Illness

In patients with severe nonthyroidal illness, a characteristic constellation of thyroid function test changes occurs that often appears to be consistent with hypothyroidism (see Fig. 233-1). The T_3 level usually declines as a result of decreased extrathyroidal T_4-to-T_3 conversion. With increasingly severe disease, total T_4 and free T_4 levels also decline. TSH levels are usually low to low-normal. During the course of recovery, the TSH level can rise above the upper limit of the normal range, producing a profile that can be mistaken for primary hypothyroidism. Clinical correlation is essential to assess thyroid function in severely ill patients (e.g., a history of preexisting thyroid or pituitary disease, the presence of a goiter, or features suggesting other elements of hypopituitarism). Because no benefit of thyroid hormone treatment has been shown for these patients, observation with retesting 6 to 8 weeks after recovery is the preferred approach.

THYROTOXICOSIS

DEFINITION AND EPIDEMIOLOGY

Thyrotoxicosis is a systemic syndrome caused by exposure to excessive thyroid hormone (Table 233-5). Its prevalence is 1 in 2000 adults, affecting 1% of all individuals during the course of their lifetime.

PATHOBIOLOGY

Hyperthyroidism develops when there is excessive synthesis and secretion of thyroid hormone caused by thyrotropic stimulus or autonomous function of thyroid tissue. Strictly speaking, *hyperthyroidism* refers to those forms of *thyrotoxicosis* that are caused by excessive production of thyroid hormone by the thyroid gland (see Table 233-5). The two terms are often used interchangeably. In Graves' disease, the most common cause of hyperthyroidism, the thyroid gland is stimulated by autoantibodies that bind to and activate the TSH receptor. Excessive secretion of TSH causes hyperthyroidism in patients with rare TSH-secreting pituitary adenomas (Chapter 231). HCG, a glycoprotein with high TSH homology, can cause transient gestational hyperthyroidism during pregnancy when a choriocarcinoma or a germ cell tumor produces variant forms of HCG that are more active, or when mutant TSH receptors bind HCG more avidly, as occurs in familial gestational thyrotoxicosis.

Autonomous production of thyroid hormone occurs when thyrocytes function independently of TSH receptor activation. This can occur as a result of growth of a benign functioning thyroid adenoma or growth of multiple autonomously functioning nodules forming a toxic multinodular goiter; in rare cases, it can occur when patients with well-differentiated thyroid cancer present with functioning metastases. In some toxic adenomas, somatic mutations in the TSH receptor gene lead to constitutive activation. In patients whose thyroid glands have the potential for autonomous function, exposure to excessive amounts of iodine in the form of amiodarone or iodinated contrast agents can provoke hyperthyroidism.

Transient thyrotoxicosis can also be caused by inflammatory conditions that release an excessive amount of thyroid hormone stored in the gland (see the section on thyroiditis). These include subacute thyroiditis, which is believed to be caused by a viral infection; acute or suppurative thyroiditis, caused by bacterial infection; radiation-induced thyroiditis; and pharmacologic thyroiditis, precipitated by exposure to amiodarone. Autoimmunity can also provoke an inflammatory thyroiditis that causes transient thyrotoxicosis. This commonly occurs in the setting of *lymphocytic thyroiditis* (also known as *silent*, *painless*, or *postpartum thyroiditis*). It rarely occurs in the setting of autoimmune thyroiditis (also known as *Hashimoto's thyroiditis*).

In rare cases, excess thyroid hormone can be secreted by ectopic thyroid tissue located anywhere from the base of the tongue to the mediastinum, or by heterotopic thyroid tissue that develops as part of an ovarian teratoma (a condition known as *struma ovarii*).

Thyrotoxicosis can also be caused by ingestion of excessive amounts of thyroid hormone. This is most often the result of the prescription of excessive doses of pharmacologic preparations of thyroid hormone, but it can rarely be due to surreptitious or accidental ingestion.

CLINICAL MANIFESTATIONS

Symptoms and Signs

The classic symptoms of thyrotoxicosis include weight loss despite a hearty appetite, heat intolerance, palpitations, tremor, and hyperdefecation (increased frequency of formed bowel movements). Thyrotoxicosis can escape early detection because of its presentation with common nonspecific symptoms such as fatigue, insomnia, anxiety, irritability, weakness, atypical chest pain, or dyspnea on exertion. Delayed recognition may also occur when atypical symptoms such as headache, weight loss, periodic paralysis, or nausea and vomiting dominate the clinical picture. Elderly patients may present with apathetic thyrotoxicosis typified by weight loss and the absence of sympathomimetic symptoms and signs.

Signs of thyrotoxicosis include resting tachycardia; systolic hypertension with a widened pulse pressure; warm, moist skin with a velvety texture; onycholysis; and a staring gaze with lid lag (noted to be present when a rim of sclera is visible between the upper eyelid and the superior margin of the iris on downward gaze). Cardiac examination may reveal a prominent apical impulse and a systolic flow murmur. Neurologic findings may include a restless, impatient demeanor; pressured speech; proximal muscle weakness; distal hand tremor; and brisk deep-tendon reflexes.

Clinical findings often provide a strong indication of the underlying cause. In Graves' disease, the gland is diffusely enlarged, with a smooth or slightly lobulated contour, and may manifest an audible bruit. Ophthalmopathy and dermopathy are also unique to Graves' disease. In patients with toxic nodular goiter, one or more discrete nodules may be appreciated. In subacute thyroiditis, the gland is modestly enlarged, extremely tender, and firm. A history of

recent pregnancy suggests possible painless thyroiditis. Recent exposure to amiodarone, other iodine-containing compounds, interferon-α, or pharmacologic preparations of thyroid hormone may suggest the characteristic forms of thyrotoxicosis associated with these agents.

Graves' Disease

DEFINITION

Graves' disease is an autoimmune disorder characterized by a variable combination of hyperthyroidism, ophthalmopathy (also known as *thyroid eye disease*), and dermopathy.

EPIDEMIOLOGY

Graves' disease is more common among women, but it also affects men. It can develop at any time during life, but the onset most often occurs between 30 and 60 years of age.

PATHOBIOLOGY

The proximate cause of hyperthyroidism in Graves' disease is the production of thyroid-stimulating immunoglobulins (autoantibodies) that bind to and activate the TSH receptor, promoting thyroid hormone secretion and growth of the thyroid gland. Thyrotropin (TSH) receptor antibodies of the stimulating variety are the hallmark of hyperthyroidism in Graves' disease. Other thyroid autoantibodies commonly identified in the setting of Graves' disease include antithyroid peroxidase antibodies, antithyroglobulin antibodies, and anti-TSH receptor antibodies that block TSH binding. The fundamental pathogenesis of Graves' disease remains unknown. A genetic predisposition is implicated by a higher incidence in monozygotic twins and first-degree relatives of affected individuals. Environmental factors implicated in triggering the onset of Graves' disease include exposure to cigarette smoke, high dietary iodine intake, stressful life events, and certain antecedent infections.

CLINICAL MANIFESTATIONS

Affected individuals usually present with thyrotoxicosis and a thyroid gland that is diffusely enlarged with a rubbery consistency, smooth contour, definable pyramidal lobe, and audible bruit or palpable thrill due to increased blood flow. When it is clinically evident, thyroid eye disease usually presents within a few months of onset. In rare cases, it may develop long before, long after, or without any biochemical confirmation of hyperthyroidism.

PROGNOSIS

The hyperthyroidism associated with this condition often follows a persistent and progressive course, but one fourth of patients with Graves' disease demonstrate spontaneous disease remission.

OPHTHALMOPATHY

DEFINITION

Thyroid eye disease is a distinctive disorder characterized by inflammation and swelling of the extraocular muscles and orbital fat, eyelid retraction, periorbital edema, episcleral vascular injection, conjunctival swelling (chemosis), and proptosis (also called *exophthalmos*). Swelling of soft tissues within the confines of the orbits precipitated by fibroblast growth and inflammatory cell infiltrate can cause proptosis, entrapment of extraocular muscles, and compression of the optic nerve.

CLINICAL MANIFESTATIONS

Affected individuals typically complain of a change in eye appearance, ocular irritation, foreign body sensation, dryness, and, ironically, excessive tearing. More severe involvement may cause exposure keratitis with corneal ulceration, diplopia, and blurred vision. On examination, patients may have a staring gaze; a rim of sclera visible between the upper eyelid and the superior margin of the iris during downward gaze (lid lag); signs of conjunctival inflammation; periorbital edema; and abnormalities of conjugate gaze, color vision, and visual acuity (Fig. 233-2). The precise degree of proptosis can be measured by an exophthalmometer. Orbital imaging with CT scanning or ultrasonography can confirm the diagnosis, which must sometimes be distinguished from other causes of bilateral and unilateral proptosis.

TREATMENT   Rx

Treatment of mild thyroid-related eye disease focuses on protecting the cornea from exposure and desiccation with moisturizing drops and ointment, glasses, and sometimes taping the eyelids closed at bedtime. High-dose systemic glucocorticoid therapy can attenuate orbital inflammation. Orbital irradiation may be helpful in controlling inflammatory symptoms in some patients. Persistent corneal exposure, diplopia, altered vision due to optic nerve compression, and cosmetic issues may require surgery to decompress the orbits and readjust the extraocular muscles. Immunosuppressive agents and plasmapheresis have been used in severely affected patients, with anecdotal success.

DERMOPATHY

Infiltrative dermopathy, the least common complication of Graves' disease, is precipitated by the deposition of glycosaminoglycans in the dermis of the skin. Affected individuals usually present with mildly pruritic, orange peel–like thickening of the skin along the anterior aspects of the shins, commonly known as *pretibial myxedema*. The dorsal aspects of the feet and fingers, the extensor surface of the elbows, and the face are more rarely affected.

The diagnosis can be confirmed by skin biopsy. Treatment of early infiltrative dermopathy with topical glucocorticoids under an occlusive wrap may

FIGURE 233-2. Graves' ophthalmopathy. **A,** A 59-year-old woman with excess proptosis, moderate eyelid edema, and erythema with moderate eyelid retraction affecting all four eyelids. Conjunctival chemosis (edema) and erythema with bilateral edema of the caruncles, with prolapse of the right caruncle, are evident. **B,** A 40-year-old woman with excess proptosis, minimal bilateral injection, and chemosis with slight erythema of the eyelids. She also had evidence, on slit lamp examination, of moderate superior limbic keratoconjunctivitis. (From Bahn RS. Graves' ophthalmopathy. *N Engl J Med.* 2010;362:726-738. Copyright 2010, Massachusetts Medical Society. All rights reserved.)

limit its progression. Treatments involving the use of intradermal or systemic glucocorticoids, long-acting somatostatin analogues, and even surgical resection of soft tissue have shown limited success.

Toxic Adenoma

A toxic adenoma is a solitary, autonomously functioning thyroid neoplasm that synthesizes and secretes excessive amounts of thyroid hormone independent of TSH stimulation. These neoplasms are almost always benign. Most grow large enough to be palpated by the time they present with thyrotoxicosis. Somatic gene mutations causing constitutive activation of the TSH receptor and the stimulatory subunit of the guanine nucleotide ($G_s\alpha$) have been identified in a subset of toxic adenomas. Hyperthyroidism caused by a toxic adenoma does not remit spontaneously, except in unusual cases complicated by hemorrhagic infarction of the neoplasm.

Toxic Multinodular Goiter

A toxic multinodular goiter is composed of multiple autonomously functioning thyroid nodules that synthesize and secrete excessive amounts of thyroid hormone. In some patients with nontoxic multinodular goiters, hyperthyroidism can be precipitated by exposure to excessive amounts of iodine. Most affected individuals have a goiter with multiple palpable thyroid nodules. Progressive enlargement may go undetected when there is substernal extension of nodular tissue. Toxic multinodular goiter is more common among older individuals.

TSH-Secreting Pituitary Adenoma

TSH-secreting pituitary adenomas represent less than 1% of all functioning pituitary tumors (Chapter 231). Patients may present with typical clinical manifestations of thyrotoxicosis, a diffuse goiter, symptoms and signs precipitated by an expanding sellar mass, syndromes associated with co-secretion of other anterior pituitary hormones (growth hormone, prolactin, or adrenocorticotropic hormone), or symptoms and signs of hypopituitarism. The key to suspecting the condition is usually recognition of an inappropriately nonsuppressed TSH level in a patient with thyrotoxicosis. The diagnosis is confirmed in most cases when laboratory testing reveals an elevated circulating level of the pituitary glycoprotein α-subunit in conjunction with a radiographically definable sellar mass.

DIAGNOSIS

Laboratory Findings

Abnormalities detected in routinely ordered laboratory tests are often the first clues to the presence of thyrotoxicosis. Thyrotoxic patients may have hypercalcemia or hypercalciuria, increased alkaline phosphatase levels, modestly elevated transaminase levels, and low or declining total and LDL cholesterol levels. When they are measured, ferritin and angiotensin-converting enzyme levels are often increased. Electrocardiography typically reveals resting sinus tachycardia or atrial tachyarrhythmias, particularly atrial fibrillation with a rapid ventricular response. In severe cases, chest radiography may reveal cardiomegaly.

In most patients with suspected thyrotoxicosis, the diagnosis can be determined by measurement of TSH (Fig. 233-3). Sensitive TSH immunoassays

FIGURE 233-3. Laboratory assessment of suspected thyrotoxicosis.

with a detection limit of less than 0.02 mIU/L can accurately discriminate between clearly suppressed TSH levels, characteristic of all common forms of thyrotoxicosis, and mildly suppressed levels that fall just beneath the reference range, as may occur in otherwise sick and elderly euthyroid individuals. Only the rare conditions associated with TSH-mediated hyperthyroidism (TSH-secreting pituitary tumors and isolated pituitary resistance to thyroid hormone) yield false-negative TSH results in screening for thyrotoxicosis. In these conditions, serum free T_4 and T_3 levels are not elevated on subsequent testing.

Measurement of serum free T_4 and total or free T_3 levels confirms a diagnosis of thyrotoxicosis, defines its severity, and occasionally provides a clue to its underlying cause. Overt thyrotoxicosis is characterized by free T_4 or T_3 levels above the upper limit of the reference range, whereas mild or subclinical thyrotoxicosis is characterized by a suppressed TSH level with free T_4 and T_3 levels within the normal reference range. When only the free T_4 or T_3 concentrations are elevated, the terms T_4 *toxicosis* and T_3 *toxicosis* are applied, respectively.

Differential Diagnosis

Once thyrotoxicosis is confirmed, it is important to define its underlying cause to determine the most appropriate treatment. The relative degrees of T_4 and T_3 elevation sometimes can be helpful. Predominantly T_3 toxicosis is typical of Graves' disease and can also occur with toxic nodular goiter. In contrast, predominantly T_4 toxicosis is more typical of subacute or painless thyroiditis. T_4 toxicosis is also more common in patients with iodine-induced hyperthyroidism.

Other laboratory tests are sometimes helpful in differential diagnosis. Antithyrotropin-receptor antibodies are pathognomonic of Graves' disease. Levels of antithyrotropin-receptor antibodies are especially high in thyroid dermopathy and correlate positively with the clinical features and prognosis of Graves' ophthalmopathy. An elevated erythrocyte sedimentation rate is typically seen in subacute thyroiditis.

Imaging studies can be helpful for the differential diagnosis. The fractional thyroidal uptake of radiotracer within the thyroid gland on scintigraphic scanning often helps establish a definitive diagnosis (Table 233-6). Thyroid ultrasonography can confirm the presence of solitary or multiple thyroid nodules. Chest radiography and CT scanning may help delineate a substernal goiter.

TABLE 233-6	RADIOGRAPHIC EVALUATION OF SUSPECTED THYROTOXICOSIS	
ETIOLOGY	**FRACTIONAL 24-HOUR RADIOIODINE UPTAKE (%)**	**THYROID SCAN APPEARANCE**
Graves' disease	35-95	Diffuse increased homogeneous uptake; visible pyramidal lobe extending from isthmus
Toxic adenoma	20-60	Solitary focus of intense uptake; suppression of uptake in remainder of thyroid
Toxic multinodular goiter	20-60	Patchy heterogeneous foci of increased uptake interspersed with regions of diminished uptake
Subacute thyroiditis	0-2	Minimal to absent uptake
Autoimmune thyroiditis	0-2	Minimal to absent uptake; patchy heterogeneous uptake during recovery
Iodine-induced hyperthyroidism	0-2	Minimal to absent uptake
Exogenous thyroid hormone intoxication	0-2	Minimal to absent uptake
Metastatic differentiated thyroid cancer	0-5	Focal uptake in metastases
TSH-secreting pituitary adenoma	30-80	Diffuse increased homogeneous uptake

TREATMENT Rx

Selection of the most effective treatment for a specific condition causing thyrotoxicosis requires an understanding of the underlying pathophysiologic process and natural history. For example, toxic multinodular goiter does not remit and requires radioiodine treatment or surgery; subacute thyroiditis subsides spontaneously and requires only temporizing symptomatic therapy.

β-Blockers

β-Blockers help alleviate the sympathomimetic manifestations of thyrotoxicosis, regardless of the underlying cause. Palpitations, tremor, and anxiety can often be promptly controlled. However, other clinical features of thyrotoxicosis, including weight loss, heat intolerance, and fatigue, are not ameliorated by these agents. In thyrotoxic patients with marked sinus tachycardia or atrial fibrillation with a rapid ventricular response rate, β-blockers can be used as rate-controlling agents. Propranolol also partially inhibits extrathyroidal conversion of T_4 to T_3, which may be of added benefit in patients with severe thyrotoxicosis.

Propranolol can be started at a dose of 20 to 40 mg every 8 hours and titrated upward to a maximal daily dose of 240 mg on the basis of symptom control. Sustained-release propranolol or longer-acting β-blockers, such as metoprolol and atenolol, can also be used. Esmolol can be used when a short-acting parenteral agent is required. β-Blockers should be used with caution in thyrotoxic patients with a history of heart failure, obstructive pulmonary disease, or Raynaud's phenomenon.

For patients with transient forms of thyrotoxicosis (subacute thyroiditis, autoimmune thyroiditis, or exogenous thyroid hormone intoxication), a β-blocker may be the only treatment required. In patients with more sustained conditions, such as Graves' disease or toxic nodular goiter, β-blockers provide prompt initial relief of symptoms while definitive treatment with antithyroid drugs, radioiodine, or surgery is implemented.

Antithyroid Drugs

The thionamides inhibit thyroid hormone biosynthesis by competitively inhibiting iodine organification and iodotyrosine coupling. These agents are used for the treatment of thyrotoxicosis caused by the overproduction of thyroid hormones. Because the thionamides block only new thyroid hormone synthesis, glandular stores of preexisting thyroid hormone must be exhausted before they are fully effective. This may require 3 to 8 weeks in patients with Graves' disease or toxic multinodular goiter. Although antithyroid drugs can provide long-term control of hyperthyroidism, they are most appropriately used when there is a possibility that the underlying condition will remit, as in Graves' disease, or when thyrotoxicosis must be attenuated before radioiodine treatment or surgery.

Two thionamide agents are currently available: methimazole and propylthiouracil. Methimazole can be taken as a single daily dose because of its longer half-life and higher effective intrathyroidal concentration. This can bolster patients' adherence and drug effectiveness. Propylthiouracil also inhibits extrathyroidal conversion of T_4 to T_3, an effect that may be beneficial in patients with severe complicated thyrotoxicosis. Propylthiouracil is preferred for pregnant women with thyrotoxicosis because it crosses the placental barrier less readily than methimazole does. However, the shorter half-life of propylthiouracil necessitates the administration of three or four daily doses. Concerns about the potential risk of severe hepatotoxicity associated with the use of propylthiouracil have prompted the recommendation that it not be used as a first-line agent to treat hyperthyroidism in children or adults. It is still recommended for the treatment of thyrotoxicosis that develops during the first trimester of pregnancy, however.

For patients with mild to moderate hyperthyroidism, methimazole is usually started at a dose of 10 to 30 mg once daily and increased to as much as 90 mg/day. For patients with more severe hyperthyroidism, thyrotoxicosis complicated by cardiac disease, or concomitant pregnancy, propylthiouracil can be started at a dose of 50 to 200 mg every 6 to 8 hours. Methimazole can be given rectally if necessary. The anticipated duration of treatment depends on the underlying cause. In patients with toxic multinodular goiter, antithyroid drugs are generally used only to restore euthyroidism in anticipation of definitive therapy. An effective dose can be continued for 6 to 24 months in a patient with Graves' disease before it is tapered off to determine whether there has been a remission of the patient's autoimmune thyroid disease. Patients most likely to respond are those who present with mild clinical and biochemical hyperthyroidism, a small thyroid gland, and no active ophthalmopathy.

Patients treated with antithyroid drugs should have thyroid function tests every 3 to 12 weeks during dose titration to monitor for iatrogenic hypothyroidism. Common side effects include rash, pruritus, fever, and arthralgias, which affect 5% of thionamide-treated patients. Agranulocytosis and hepatitis are rare but potentially fatal adverse reactions to thionamide medications. Their presentations are relatively sudden in onset and unpredictable. Monitoring of leukocyte counts and liver function test results is not useful as a preventive measure. Patients who are prescribed antithyroid drugs should be cautioned about manifestations of these adverse reactions and should be instructed to discontinue treatment and seek medical attention if they develop a high fever, pharyngitis, jaundice, or abdominal pain.

Radioactive Iodine

The selective uptake and concentration of iodide in thyrocytes permits the use of radioactive iodine to treat hyperthyroidism. Once it is concentrated in the gland after oral administration, ^{131}I destroys thyroid tissue, effectively controlling hyperthyroidism. The dose of ^{131}I can be calculated on the basis of the fractional uptake of radioiodine, but the outcome of dosimetry is not superior to that achieved with the administration of 10 mCi. Patients can be treated on an outpatient basis, with precautions taken to prevent the exposure of others. Approximately three quarters of patients are cured with a single dose of radioiodine.

The principal side effect of radioactive iodine therapy is postablative hypothyroidism, which develops in most individuals receiving treatment for Graves' disease and a lesser proportion of patients treated for toxic nodular goiter. Lifelong monitoring of thyroid function is required because patients develop postablative hypothyroidism at a rate of 3% per year. Another less common complication is a transient exacerbation of thyrotoxicosis, which occurs in one quarter of patients during the first month after treatment as a result of radiation thyroiditis. Long-term follow-up studies have shown that radioiodine-treated patients with Graves' disease do not have any greater risk of thyroid cancer or other malignant neoplasms. However, hyperthyroid children and adolescents treated with radioactive iodine are more likely to develop benign nodules. Among hyperthyroid women treated with radioiodine, the incidences of infertility, spontaneous abortion, and children with birth defects are not increased. Diagnostic or therapeutic radioactive iodine is contraindicated in women during pregnancy, and treated women should avoid pregnancy until euthyroidism has been confirmed 3 to 6 months after administration of a dose.

Other Drugs

A saturated solution of potassium iodide (SSKI) or Lugol's solution transiently inhibits the synthesis and release of thyroid hormone from the gland. It may be used to accelerate recovery after radioactive iodine treatment, to prepare patients for thyroidectomy, and to augment other treatments used to control severe thyrotoxicosis (see later). Iodinated radiocontrast agents inhibit the release of thyroid hormone while blocking peripheral conversion of T_4 to T_3. Lithium carbonate also inhibits the release of thyroid hormone. Rarely, these agents are used in combination with thionamides to treat patients with severe thyrotoxicosis. They may also help provide temporary control of hyperthyroidism when severe allergies preclude the continued use of thionamides. Cholestyramine can be used to bind thyroid hormone in the gut to interrupt enterohepatic circulation in cases of suspected exogenous thyroid hormone intoxication.

Surgery

Surgery has a limited role because of its potential to injure the adjacent recurrent laryngeal nerves and parathyroid glands. Resection of a toxic adenoma by lobectomy is curative and often preserves sufficient normal thyroid tissue for euthyroidism to be maintained. Consequently, it is often recommended in younger individuals. Toxic multinodular goiters causing compressive symptoms or cosmetic disfigurement may be appropriately managed with surgical resection. Although surgery is seldom recommended for the treatment of hyperthyroid Graves' disease, it may be appropriate when other modalities are contraindicated, such as when there has been an adverse reaction to an antithyroid drug in pregnancy, when a thyroid nodule is thought to be malignant, or when hyperparathyroidism also requires surgical intervention.

Specific Treatment Scenarios
Pregnancy

Pregnant patients with hyperthyroidism present special challenges. Diagnosis requires a careful assessment of symptoms, especially heat intolerance, palpitations, and vomiting, which also occur during normal pregnancy. The serum total T_4 level is elevated because of increased TBG, and the TSH level can be suppressed in the first trimester as a result of HCG-mediated thyroid stimulation. Diagnostic radioiodine studies are contraindicated. After diagnostic confirmation, hyperthyroidism must be treated because it is associated with an increased risk of spontaneous abortion, premature labor, low birthweight, and toxemia. β-Blockers should be used only transiently to treat severe symptoms. Propylthiouracil is the preferred thionamide for treatment of Graves' disease during the first trimester of pregnancy because it crosses the placenta less readily than methimazole and because methimazole has been rarely linked to congenital malformations (i.e., choanal atresia and cutis aplasia). However, owing to the risk of very rare but potentially fatal propylthiouracil-related hepatitis, methimazole is preferred after the first trimester. Because Graves' disease often remits later in pregnancy, antithyroid drug dose requirements often decline as gestation progresses. Measurement of maternal thyroid-stimulating immunoglobulin levels can help predict the risk of an infant's developing neonatal Graves' disease.

Subclinical and Mild Hyperthyroidism

Patients with mild hyperthyroidism (i.e., a suppressed serum TSH with normal free T_4 and T_3 levels) may have symptoms that justify treatment. In patients with a serum TSH level suppressed to less than 0.1 mIU/L, bone mineral loss can lead to osteoporosis, particularly in postmenopausal women. Atrial fibrillation occurs more commonly in mildly hyperthyroid patients aged 60 years and older with TSH suppression below normal. It is less clear, however, whether younger, asymptomatic patients with modestly suppressed TSH levels (e.g., 0.1 to 0.5 mIU/L) require anything more than periodic monitoring.

Thyrotoxic Crisis

Thyrotoxic crisis, also known as *thyroid storm*, is a potentially life-threatening syndrome that is usually the end result of severe and sustained thyrotoxicosis. It can affect patients with other medical conditions that render them vulnerable to the cardiovascular, neuropsychiatric, and gastrointestinal effects of exposure to excessive amounts of thyroid hormone. Thyrotoxic crisis typically develops in the setting of inadequately treated Graves' disease and may be precipitated by intercurrent illness, surgery, or treatment with radioactive iodine. Affected individuals present with fever, atrial tachyarrhythmias, congestive heart failure, nausea and vomiting, diarrhea, and seizures. Mental status changes can include agitation, delirium, psychosis, and coma. Prompt recognition and treatment in a monitored setting are crucial. A multifaceted treatment regimen should incorporate antipyretics, β-blockers, thionamides, iodinated contrast agents, and glucocorticoids, as well as aggressive evaluation and management of underlying medical problems.

● THYROIDITIS
Subacute (de Quervain's) Thyroiditis

PATHOBIOLOGY

Transient thyrotoxicosis results from the uncontrolled release of thyroid hormone from the inflamed gland. After 2 to 8 weeks, when the supply of stored hormone is exhausted, thyrotoxicosis resolves spontaneously. Hypothyroidism ensues because the gland's biosynthetic capabilities remain impaired. This is also transient (lasting approximately 1 month), with subsequent restoration of normal thyroid function in most patients.

CLINICAL MANIFESTATIONS

Subacute thyroiditis is characterized by painful enlargement of the thyroid, systemic inflammatory symptoms, and transient thyrotoxicosis that is often followed by transient hypothyroidism. The histologic pattern shows inflammatory cell infiltrates that are believed to be the result of a viral infection. Many patients with subacute thyroiditis report antecedent upper respiratory infections.

Patients usually present with pain localized to the thyroid or radiating to the throat, ears, or jaw. Constitutional symptoms, including fever, chills, sweats, and malaise, are generally present. On occasion, these features may dominate the presentation. Examination of the thyroid typically reveals an exquisitely tender, modestly enlarged, and woody, hard gland.

DIAGNOSIS
Differential Diagnosis

The differential diagnosis of thyroid pain must be considered in the evaluation of patients presenting with pain and tenderness localized to the lower anterior neck. In addition to subacute thyroiditis, potential causes of thyroid pain include acute (suppurative) thyroiditis; hemorrhage into an existing thyroid nodule; and rapid growth of anaplastic thyroid cancer, diffusely infiltrating thyroid cancer, or thyroid lymphoma.

Laboratory Findings

Laboratory testing in patients with subacute thyroiditis reveals a profile of overt thyrotoxicosis. Elevated T_4 levels are usually proportionately higher than T_3 levels. Patients typically have an elevated erythrocyte sedimentation rate during the acute phase. The fractional uptake of radioiodine is typically less than 2% at 24 hours (see Table 233-6).

TREATMENT

High-dose aspirin or naproxen sodium can be used to treat thyroid pain and systemic inflammatory symptoms. Patients who fail to respond may require glucocorticoid therapy, but it must be tapered over several weeks to prevent a relapse, prolonging the overall course of the illness. Symptoms ascribed to transient thyrotoxicosis may respond to treatment with a β-blocker continued for a limited course of 1 to 3 weeks. Patients who progress to symptomatic hypothyroidism may then need short-term thyroxine replacement therapy, but most do not require long-term thyroid hormone replacement.

Lymphocytic (Postpartum, Painless, Silent) Thyroiditis

EPIDEMIOLOGY

Lymphocytic thyroiditis occurs most commonly in postpartum women, affecting as many as 6% of women 2 to 12 months after delivery or termination. Rarely, this condition occurs in non-postpartum women or in men. Predisposing factors include a history of previous episodes of postpartum thyroiditis, type 1 diabetes mellitus, and circulating antithyroid autoantibodies.

PATHOBIOLOGY

This painless inflammation of the thyroid gland can cause transient thyrotoxicosis followed by transient or persistent hypothyroidism. Each of these phases of thyroid dysfunction typically lasts 2 to 8 weeks. This condition is believed to reflect transient autoimmunity.

DIAGNOSIS

The diagnosis of lymphocytic thyroiditis is often overlooked when nonspecific symptoms of thyrotoxicosis (e.g., weight loss, insomnia, anxiety) or hypothyroidism (e.g., fatigue, depression) are misinterpreted as common postpartum complaints. The thyroid gland is nontender and either normal in size or modestly enlarged. Once it is considered, a diagnosis of lymphocytic thyroiditis can be readily confirmed or excluded by laboratory testing, which reveals a suppressed TSH level during phases of thyrotoxicosis and an elevated TSH level during phases of hypothyroidism. This condition must be distinguished from Graves' disease, which can also present in the same time frame after delivery. Relative degrees of T_4 and T_3 elevation can sometimes provide a clue to which condition is present; lymphocytic thyroiditis is typically characterized by predominant increases in T_4 levels. Fractional uptake of radioiodine is either absent or very low in the setting of lymphocytic thyroiditis but increased in active Graves' disease, thus providing a useful diagnostic test (see Table 233-6).

TREATMENT Rx

Lymphocytic thyroiditis can often be managed with reassurance and observation alone. Symptomatic thyrotoxicosis can be treated with a limited course of β-blocker therapy. Overt hypothyroidism may require transient thyroxine replacement.

PROGNOSIS

Whereas most affected patients eventually return to a euthyroid state, 25% develop persistent hypothyroidism due to classic autoimmune thyroiditis.

Acute (Suppurative) Thyroiditis

Infection of the thyroid gland is a rare condition that typically presents with severe thyroid pain, fever, and other systemic manifestations of infection. Bacterial infection of thyroid tissue can be the result of direct spread of gram-positive or gram-negative pathogens through fistulas communicating with the piriform sinus or the skin. Hematogenous spread of bacterial, mycobacterial, fungal, or parasitic organisms, especially *Pneumocystis carinii*, can occur in immunocompromised individuals. On examination, affected patients are typically febrile, with asymmetrical swelling of a thyroid that is tender, warm, and fluctuant to firm in consistency beneath erythematous skin. Ultrasonography may reveal an abscess that can be aspirated to identify a pathogen. Patients with suppurative thyroiditis require prompt treatment with appropriate antibiotics. Surgical drainage of abscesses may be required.

Other Forms of Thyroiditis

Certain drugs can cause thyroid gland inflammation. Amiodarone can produce a painless thyroiditis associated with thyrotoxicosis. Whenever possible, this should be distinguished from the iodine-induced form of thyrotoxicosis that can also be associated with amiodarone therapy. The former is

optimally treated with glucocorticoid therapy, whereas the latter is managed with antithyroid drugs. Interferon-α can provoke a painless thyroiditis associated with transient thyrotoxicosis. This must be differentiated from interferon-α–induced Graves' disease because the former is managed with β-blockers and the latter with antithyroid drugs.

Riedel's thyroiditis or struma is characterized by fibrotic replacement of the thyroid, with adherence and infiltration of adjacent structures that causes local compressive symptoms. In this idiopathic condition, the thyroid is substantially enlarged, hardened, and fixed. Affected patients may also develop mediastinal and retroperitoneal fibrosis, sclerosing cholangitis, or orbital pseudotumor. Diagnosis requires open biopsy. Surgical excision is difficult or impossible. Glucocorticoid therapy and tamoxifen therapy have been anecdotally reported to be effective.

GOITER

DEFINITION

Goiters can be classified as diffuse or nodular, nontoxic or toxic (i.e., associated with thyroid hormone overproduction), and benign or malignant. Thyroid enlargement can be the result of thyrocyte proliferation stimulated by circulating factors (e.g., TSH and thyroid-stimulating autoantibodies), infiltration of the gland by inflammatory or malignant cells, or benign or malignant neoplastic changes within the gland itself. In a patient with a goiter, three clinical issues must be considered: local compressive or cosmetic problems, gland hyperfunction or hypofunction, and potential malignancy.

EPIDEMIOLOGY

Dietary iodine deficiency represents the most common cause of goiter worldwide. It is encountered in the United States only among immigrants from iodine-deficient regions. Younger patients present with diffuse or simple goiters that shrink in response to adequate iodine supplementation. In older individuals, iodine-deficient goiters become multinodular and do not decrease in size with iodine repletion. Excessive iodine exposure can provoke thyrotoxicosis in these patients.

PATHOBIOLOGY

Benign multinodular goiter or adenoma can be the result of genetic defects that lead to dyshormonogenesis, including mutations in the thyroglobulin, thyroid peroxidase, dual oxidase, and pendrin genes. Similarly, exposure to goitrogenic substances in foodstuffs, water, or drugs (e.g., lithium carbonate) that inhibit the normal steps in thyroid hormone synthesis can lead to goiter. In most patients the underlying cause is unknown.

Autoimmune thyroiditis typically produces a modest goiter as a result of glandular infiltration with lymphocytes, inflammatory changes in thyrocytes, and fibrosis. The hypothyroid state caused by autoimmune thyroiditis results in increased TSH, which further stimulates thyroid enlargement. Graves' disease is also characterized by diffuse thyroid enlargement due to the action of thyroid-stimulating immunoglobulins. Other forms of thyroiditis can present with goitrous enlargement of the thyroid gland, including subacute, lymphocytic, and acute (suppurative) thyroiditis (see earlier sections).

Malignant neoplasms that involve the gland diffusely, including thyroid lymphoma and infiltrative papillary, medullary, and anaplastic thyroid cancers, may present as rapidly enlarging goiters (see later sections). Affected patients often experience local pain and symptoms related to tumor expansion.

DIAGNOSIS
Clinical Examination

The first step in evaluating a suspected goiter is to confirm whether swelling represents enlargement of the thyroid. Redundant skin and subcutaneous fat in the lower anterior neck can be mistaken for an enlarged thyroid. These findings can usually be distinguished from true thyroid enlargement by palpating a normal thyroid beneath the misleading soft tissue and by observing that the fullness does not rise and fall with deglutition. Ultrasonography may help resolve uncertainty.

A patient's history can provide important clues to the underlying cause. A childhood history may confirm previous iodine deficiency. Symptoms of hypothyroidism may suggest autoimmune thyroiditis, whereas clinical evidence of thyrotoxicosis may suggest Graves' disease or toxic multinodular goiter. Clinical findings may lead to recognition of one of the various forms of thyroiditis (e.g., pain in subacute thyroiditis or postpartum status in lymphocytic thyroiditis). Symptoms suggesting the invasion of adjacent structures may raise concerns about malignant disease or Riedel's thyroiditis.

Careful examination of the thyroid is informative. Diffuse enlargement favors one of the forms of thyroiditis, Graves' disease, or a diffusely infiltrating malignant neoplasm. Nodular enlargement is more likely to reflect a benign multinodular goiter or malignant neoplasm. The precise size of the gland should be documented. Dysphonia, tracheal deviation, cervical lymphadenopathy, and venous engorgement in the neck should be noted. Subtotal obstruction of the thoracic outlet may be revealed by having the patient touch his or her hands together above the head (Pemberton's maneuver) while checking for signs of facial plethora and cervical venous distention.

Laboratory Findings

A TSH level determines whether there is primary hypothyroidism or thyrotoxicosis. Elevated antithyroid peroxidase antibody titers can confirm suspected autoimmune thyroiditis. In asymptomatic patients with a modest diffuse goiter, no further evaluation may be indicated. Other blood tests (e.g., erythrocyte sedimentation rate for subacute thyroiditis or calcitonin for medullary thyroid cancer) can be useful when clinical clues suggest specific diagnoses.

Imaging

Cervical ultrasonography is usually the best imaging technique to define the character and extent of a goiter limited to the neck. It can help determine whether a goiter is diffuse or nodular, whether the thyroid is impinging on other cervical structures, and whether lymphadenopathy is present. When a goiter extends posteriorly or beneath the sternal notch into the thorax, CT or MRI may be required. The administration of iodine-containing radiocontrast dye should be avoided in the evaluation of patients with goiters because the stable iodide load may interfere with subsequent radioiodine imaging or therapy. Thyroid uptake studies may help define whether quantitative tracer uptake is subnormal or supranormal. Radioiodine scanning can help determine whether a superior mediastinal mass is thyroid tissue. Barium swallow radiographs with fixed-diameter markers and pulmonary function testing with flow-volume loops can help determine whether symptoms are directly related to compression of the esophagus or trachea, respectively. Laryngoscopy is useful to evaluate vocal cord function in patients with potential recurrent laryngeal nerve involvement.

TREATMENT   Rx

Once thyroid dysfunction and malignant disease have been excluded, asymptomatic patients with goiters can be observed, with periodic clinical assessment. Ultrasonography can be relied on as a reproducible technique for monitoring the size of an enlarged thyroid gland. Thyroxine therapy to suppress TSH levels is effective in shrinking goiters in only a minority of patients. Furthermore, chronic thyroid hormone treatment carries the risks of symptomatic thyrotoxicosis, atrial fibrillation, and bone mineral loss.

Patients with benign multinodular goiters causing local compressive symptoms or cosmetic concerns can be treated with surgery or radioactive iodine therapy. Surgery is often preferred when a patient has substantial gland enlargement causing compressive complications, especially when there is substernal extension of the goiter or acute obstructive symptoms. When surgery is contraindicated by the patient's health status, radioactive iodine therapy has been shown to reduce goiter size by an average of 50% over 12 to 24 months.

⬤ THYROID NODULES

EPIDEMIOLOGY

Thyroid nodules are common, being detected by palpation in 6% of women and 2% of men. Contemporary high-resolution ultrasonography identifies thyroid nodules in as many as 50% of all adults. Although the majority of these represent small, benign adenomatoid nodules or cysts, 5 to 10% of thyroid nodules are malignant. Less commonly, thyroid nodules are clinical problems by virtue of being hyperfunctioning or causing local compressive symptoms or cosmetic dissatisfaction.

DIAGNOSIS

Thyroid nodules are usually noted by the patient or the physician in the absence of any other complaints. It is also common for thyroid nodules to be detected incidentally on imaging procedures, such as carotid ultrasonography and cervical spine CT or MRI. Symptoms of compression or invasion of adjacent tissues suggest that a nodule may be malignant. These include pain in the lower anterior neck, cough or dyspnea due to tracheal compression, hemoptysis due to tracheal invasion, dysphonia due to recurrent laryngeal nerve encasement, and dysphagia or odynophagia due to esophageal compression. Certain other symptoms and signs lead to the consideration of specific underlying conditions. A toxic adenoma should be suspected in a patient with a thyroid nodule and the classic clinical manifestations of thyrotoxicosis. Hypothyroid symptoms and signs suggest autoimmune thyroiditis with asymmetrical thyroid enlargement. Hypercalcitoninemia associated with the metastatic spread of medullary thyroid cancer can cause pruritus, flushing, and diarrhea. The clinical assessment should also include symptoms and signs related to common sites of thyroid cancer metastasis, such as chest pain, dyspnea, bone pain, and neurologic findings. Thyroid nodules rarely can be due to metastasis from other primary malignant neoplasms, including kidney, colon, and breast cancer.

History

A special predisposition to thyroid cancer is suggested by a personal history of therapeutic neck irradiation in childhood. Family history can be informative if relatives have had medullary or papillary thyroid cancers, which are familial in 50% and 10% of cases, respectively. The possibility of medullary thyroid cancer should also be considered when there is a personal or family history of clinical problems associated with multiple endocrine neoplasia type 2 (MEN 2) syndrome, including hyperparathyroidism and pheochromocytoma (Chapter 239).

Physical Examination

Physical examination of the thyroid nodule should seek to define its size, consistency, surface texture, mobility, and tenderness. The presence of malignant disease is suggested by fixation and ipsilateral regional adenopathy or vocal cord paresis. Multinodularity of the gland may reflect benign nodular goiter, but it is not sufficiently reassuring to dispense with further diagnostic testing. This is particularly true for a so-called dominant nodule, which is larger, enlarging faster, or more symptomatic than others present in the thyroid.

Laboratory Findings

Routine laboratory testing includes measurement of TSH levels to identify patients with hyperthyroidism or hypothyroidism. When the TSH level is low or undetectable, the possibility of a benign autonomously functioning toxic adenoma can be pursued with radionuclide thyroid scanning (see Table 233-6). If an elevated TSH level indicates primary hypothyroidism, antithyroid peroxidase antibody titers can confirm whether the patient has autoimmune thyroiditis. Ultrasonography can distinguish asymmetrical enlargement caused by autoimmune thyroiditis from a discrete nodule. Calcitonin levels should be measured in patients with a known or suspected family history of MEN 2 or familial medullary thyroid cancer. Serum thyroglobulin measurement is not helpful in distinguishing benign from malignant thyroid abnormalities.

Imaging

Cervical ultrasonography is not required before biopsy, but it can help confirm that a mass is within the thyroid, accurately define its size, classify it as cystic or solid, and determine whether additional nodules are present. Ultrasonography occasionally reveals other suspicious findings, such as fine calcifications, irregular nodule borders, and cervical adenopathy.

Radionuclide scanning with radioiodine or technetium pertechnetate is helpful only in selected cases. In patients with a thyroid nodule and a suppressed TSH level, scanning can confirm that the nodule is hyperfunctioning or "hot," in which case biopsy is usually not required.

Invasive Evaluation
Fine-Needle Aspiration Biopsy

Fine-needle aspiration biopsy is the most accurate test to exclude or confirm malignant disease in patients with a nodule and a normal TSH level (Fig. 233-4). Most solid nodules and complex cysts larger than 1.0 to 1.5 cm in diameter should be sampled. Although aspiration can be directed by palpation alone when a nodule is readily definable, ultrasonography provides more certain guidance for the sampling of poorly localized lesions, often revealing additional nodules that should be assessed.

FIGURE 233-4. Evaluation of a thyroid nodule.

The cytologic assessment of aspirated material must first confirm that there is adequate material for assessment (e.g., six clumps of 10 cells on two slides). Biopsies with inadequate specimens, which are more common in cystic lesions, must be repeated. Ultrasonographic guidance and on-site preliminary cytologic assessment can improve the yield of biopsy. In accordance with the recently developed Bethesda System for Reporting Thyroid Cytopathology, a sampled nodule can be categorized as benign, malignant, or indeterminate (suspicious).

Benign nodules typically yield samples containing clusters of normal-appearing follicular epithelial cells with colloid. Pure colloid cysts may have scant epithelium. This classification is highly accurate, with a false-negative rate of less than 1% in sonographically directed biopsy specimens, and surgical resection is not required. In most cases, conservative observation based on yearly clinical or sonographic reassessment can be recommended. Further enlargement during observation should prompt repeated biopsy. Surgical resection should be considered if a cytologically benign nodule continues to grow, causing compressive symptoms or cosmetic disfigurement.

Cytologic material classified as malignant typically contains abundant epithelial cells with atypical nuclear features and scant or absent colloid. This is also a highly reliable finding, with 97 to 99% of such lesions found to be thyroid cancers on subsequent resection. Consequently, bilateral thyroidectomy is indicated in patients without contraindications to operation. Samples that contain sparser quantities of epithelial cells with similar atypical nuclear features may be classified as suspicious for malignancy. More than 60 to 75% of nodules falling into this category represent thyroid cancers.

One in five biopsies yields adequate but diagnostically indeterminate cytologic material. Specific findings that classify an indeterminate nodule as suspicious for a follicular neoplasm include abundant follicular or Hürthle cells in microfollicles, with little or no colloid and minor degrees of nuclear atypia, potentially indicative of papillary cancer. Although the majority of such indeterminate nodules are benign follicular adenomas, 15 to 30% are thyroid carcinomas. Consequently, surgery is advisable in most otherwise healthy patients with nodules that fall within this diagnostic category. Unilateral thyroid lobectomy has the advantage of a lower incidence of surgical complications and postoperative hypothyroidism when the lesion is benign, but it necessitates a subsequent completion thyroidectomy for most patients who prove to have cancer. For patients with no clinical features of malignancy, particularly middle-aged or older women with multinodular glands, in whom the prevalence of malignancy is 5% or less, vigilant observation with serial sonography is an alternative.

Biopsy samples that reveal nuclear or architectural features considered to be abnormal but not clearly suspicious for malignancy or a follicular neoplasm are classified as demonstrating atypia of undetermined significance. Nodules that initially fall into this category have been estimated to harbor malignancy at rates ranging from 5 to 15%. Repeat sampling may provide a more definitive diagnosis to guide further management in 75 to 85% of cases.

THYROID CANCER

Cancers of the thyroid gland have a spectrum of behavior that ranges from incidentally detected and clinically inconsequential microcarcinomas to aggressive and virtually untreatable anaplastic malignant neoplasms. When thyroid cancer is diagnosed early, treatment is effective for most types. Most thyroid cancers present as thyroid nodules that are either asymptomatic or associated with local cervical symptoms or adenopathy. Less often, thyroid cancers first present with manifestations of metastatic disease, such as a pulmonary mass or bone pain.

Papillary and Follicular (Epithelial) Thyroid Carcinomas

Papillary and follicular thyroid cancers arise from follicular epithelium and often retain responsiveness to TSH, produce thyroglobulin, and concentrate iodide. They are distinguished by their histopathologic appearances and characteristic patterns of progression. Hürthle cell carcinoma of the thyroid is composed of thyrocytes with abundant cytoplasm and behaves like a follicular thyroid cancer, although it typically does not retain iodine-concentrating ability.

EPIDEMIOLOGY

Approximately 34,000 new cases of thyroid cancer are diagnosed annually in the United States. Thyroid cancer is three times more common in women, in whom its incidence is currently rising fasting than that of any other malignancy. There are estimated to be 350,000 U.S. thyroid cancer survivors, who require lifelong follow-up for recurrence. Papillary thyroid carcinoma is the most common form of thyroid cancer, representing 90% of cases. The mean age at diagnosis is 45 years, but papillary thyroid carcinoma does occur in children and increases in incidence with age.

PATHOBIOLOGY

Irradiation of the thyroid gland in childhood is a risk factor, as evidenced by the epidemics of thyroid cancer that follow both external beam radiation therapy for benign childhood conditions and radioiodine exposure after nuclear incidents. A substantial body of evidence now implicates *RET/PTC* and *B-Raf kinase* gene mutations that activate the MAP kinase signaling pathway in the pathogenesis of papillary thyroid cancer. Most papillary thyroid carcinomas are slow growing and either remain confined to the gland or metastasize to cervical lymph nodes. Papillary microcarcinomas are a common incidental pathologic finding in 5% of thyroid glands excised for other reasons. Some papillary thyroid carcinomas are more aggressive, with extension into adjacent tissues, extensive nodal involvement, and distant metastatic spread, most commonly to the lungs. This is more common in older patients.

Follicular and Hürthle cell thyroid carcinomas account for 10% of all thyroid cancers. When these tumors show histologic evidence of invading only the tumor capsule, they are termed *minimally invasive* and generally behave like papillary thyroid carcinomas. However, follicular and Hürthle cell carcinomas with vascular invasion are more likely to be associated with distant metastatic disease, which most commonly involves the lungs and skeleton.

TREATMENT   Rx

Treatment of epithelial thyroid cancer entails surgery, often followed by radioiodine ablation of remnant thyroid tissue. Total or near-total thyroidectomy with selective central compartment lymph node resection is usually the appropriate initial surgical procedure. Thyroid surgery can be complicated by hypoparathyroidism or recurrent laryngeal nerve injury, which causes hoarseness if it is unilateral and airway obstruction if it is bilateral. The rationale for bilateral surgery is the frequent presence of bilateral disease in papillary thyroid cancer and the lower risk of recurrence. In addition, there is greater accuracy in detecting residual disease after the eradication of all remaining normal thyroid tissue.

Follow-up

Postoperatively, ^{131}I administration can ablate the small amount of normal thyroid tissue that usually remains. This tissue, if it is not destroyed, leaves patients with circulating thyroglobulin and iodine-concentrating tissue, thus decreasing the utility of TBG measurements to detect recurrence. In nonrandomized trials, radioiodine has been associated with a lower rate of tumor recurrence in patients with advanced disease at presentation (see later), but there is no clear clinical benefit for patients with lower stages of disease. TSH stimulation of residual thyroid tissue is essential for effective radioiodine therapy. This can be accomplished either by the administration of recombinant thyrotropin or by the temporary withdrawal of thyroid hormone therapy to promote endogenous TSH production.

Thyroxine therapy is appropriate for all patients with treated thyroid cancer, regardless of the extent of surgery and whether they received radioiodine ablative therapy. Thyroid hormone therapy is intended to suppress the patient's circulating TSH level to reduce the likelihood of thyroid tumor recurrence. In determining the extent to which the TSH level should be suppressed, the patient's risk of cancer recurrence must be balanced against potential complications such as bone mineral loss in postmenopausal women and atrial fibrillation in older patients.

Long-term monitoring of patients entails periodic clinical assessment, measurement of thyroglobulin levels, radioiodine imaging in the early postoperative phase, and occasional use of ultrasonography. Clinically, patients should be assessed for local neck symptoms or recurrent cervical masses, as well as for optimization of thyroid hormone therapy. For patients with treated epithelial thyroid cancers, thyroglobulin is a more specific tumor marker if all remaining normal thyroid tissue has been ablated. For patients with undetectable thyroglobulin levels on TSH-suppressive thyroid hormone therapy, thyroglobulin measurement after recombinant TSH stimulation can sometimes reveal residual disease. Radioiodine scanning after TSH stimulation can be helpful in patients who have previously undergone radioiodine ablation, but once iodine imaging is normal, it offers little or no advantage over measurement of stimulated thyroglobulin levels. This is particularly true in recurrent papillary thyroid cancers, which often lose the ability to concentrate iodine. Unfortunately, thyroglobulin testing is impossible in the 20% of patients who have circulating thyroglobulin autoantibodies that interfere with thyroglobulin immunoassays. Because most epithelial thyroid cancer recurrences are in cervical nodes or soft tissues, ultrasonography is useful for postoperative monitoring, particularly in patients who presented with extensive cervical disease or who have persistent detectable serum thyroglobulin. CT scanning of the chest should be employed to detect intrathoracic disease in patients whose findings suggest recurrence outside the neck. In patients with substantial detectable thyroglobulin levels (>10 ng/dL) and normal findings on standard imaging studies, PET scanning can identify sites of residual disease in more than 50% of patients.

Localization of recurrent cervical disease is usually an indication for comprehensive compartmental neck dissection. Distant and nonresectable metastases that are iodine avid, which occur more commonly in patients with invasive follicular thyroid cancer, can be treated with repeated doses of [131]I. Symptomatic hilar node and bone metastases can be treated palliatively with external beam radiation therapy. Surgery can be employed for isolated metastatic disease sites. Conventional chemotherapy has limited efficacy in the treatment of differentiated thyroid cancer, but newer biologic agents targeting the molecular pathogenesis of these tumors hold promise. For example, in a phase II study of patients with progressive disease, treatment with the multikinase inhibitor motesanib produced stable disease in 67% of patients, and stability was sustained for 24 weeks or longer in 35% of cases.

PROGNOSIS

The TNM (tumor, node, metastasis) staging system is commonly used to stage epithelial thyroid cancers. In addition to tumor size, extent of node involvement, and presence of distant metastatic disease, the age of the patient at presentation is an important predictor of outcome. Patients younger than 45 years have a better prognosis than older individuals. The overall age-adjusted 10-year survival rates for patients with papillary and follicular thyroid cancer are 98% and 92%, respectively. However, disease recurrence is relatively common, (e.g., one third of patients with papillary thyroid cancer). Consequently, patients with treated thyroid cancer must be monitored for recurrent disease.

Medullary Thyroid Carcinoma

Patients with medullary thyroid cancer (Chapter 254) typically present with a thyroid nodule, cervical adenopathy, distant disease, or clinical manifestations of markedly elevated circulating calcitonin levels that may include flushing, diarrhea, and pruritus. Features of the other elements of MEN 2a (e.g., hypertension) or MEN 2b (e.g., marfanoid habitus, submucosal neuromas) should be sought.

Anaplastic Thyroid Carcinoma

Anaplastic thyroid carcinoma is a rare, histologically undifferentiated and clinically aggressive malignant neoplasm that typically arises in older patients, one fourth of whom present with evidence of a preceding differentiated thyroid cancer. Affected patients present with a rapidly enlarging mass in the anterior or lateral neck associated with pain, tenderness, and compressive symptoms including dysphagia, dysphonia, and stridorous dyspnea. Fine-needle aspiration biopsy of the mass usually yields large, pleomorphic, undifferentiated cells, but open surgical biopsy is sometimes required to confirm the diagnosis.

Most cases are unresectable at presentation because of invasion of cervical structures. Surgery is not curative and should aim to secure the patient's airway. A percutaneous gastrostomy tube is often placed to ensure adequate nutrition in the face of esophageal impingement. Conventional therapy consisting of combined external beam radiation therapy and chemotherapy with doxorubicin with or without cisplatin produces an initial response in 25% of patients. Those with disease limited to the neck may have extended survival, but almost all patients relapse within a few months and succumb to their disease, with median survival ranging from 3 to 7 months. Current research is focused on the use of targeted antiangiogenic agents to treat unresponsive disease.

Thyroid Lymphoma

Lymphoma rarely arises in the thyroid gland, typically presenting in older persons as a rapidly enlarging and painful diffuse goiter. Patients often have a preceding history of autoimmune thyroiditis. The diagnosis is further suspected when fine-needle aspiration biopsy yields abundant lymphocytes without other cellular features of autoimmune thyroiditis. Immunohistochemical staining and flow cytometry of sampled material can characterize a monoclonal lymphocyte population. Surgical biopsy is sometimes required to establish the diagnosis. In 50% of cases, lymphoma is primary to the thyroid gland, and it is usually an intermediate-grade non-Hodgkin's–type lymphoma (Chapter 191).

Surgical resection of the thyroid is not indicated, but elective tracheostomy should be considered as a prophylactic measure when tracheal compression is imminent. Most patients respond to treatment with combined external beam radiation therapy and chemotherapy. Disease-free survival rates vary with the disease stage at diagnosis and the initial response to combination therapy.

 Visit expertconsult.com for e-expanded chapter

SUGGESTED READINGS

Bahn RS. Graves' ophthalmopathy. *N Engl J Med.* 2010;362:726-738. *Review of Graves' ophthalmopathy, hyperthyroidism, and thyroid dermopathy.*

Cooper DS, Doherty GM, Haugen BR, et al. Revised American Thyroid Association management guidelines for patients with thyroid nodules and differentiated thyroid cancer. *Thyroid.* 2009;19:1167-1214. *Guidelines for the management of thyroid nodules and thyroid cancer.*

Gerdes AM, Iervasi G. Thyroid replacement therapy and heart failure. *Circulation.* 2010;122:385-393. *Review.*

Gharib H, Papini E, Paschke R, et al. American Association of Clinical Endocrinologists. Associazione Medici Endocrinologi, and European Thyroid Association medical guidelines for clinical practice for the diagnosis and management of thyroid nodules: executive summary of recommendations. *J Endocrinol Invest.* 2010;33:51-56. *Consensus guidelines.*

Parle J, Roberts L, Wilson S, et al. A randomized controlled trial of the effect of thyroxine replacement on cognitive function in community-living elderly subjects with subclinical hypothyroidism: the Birmingham Elderly Thyroid study. *J Clin Endocrinol Metab.* 2010;95:3623-3632. *No evidence of improved cognitive function from treating elderly subjects with SCH with T4 replacement therapy.*

Ross DS. Radioiodine therapy for hyperthyroidism. *N Engl J Med.* 2011;364:542-550. *Review.*

FIGURE 234-1. Magnetic resonance images of the abdomen showing the position and relative size of the normal adrenal glands.

Capsule
Zona glomerulosa
Zona fasciculata
Zona reticularis
Medulla

FIGURE 234-2. Histologic section through a normal adult adrenal gland showing the progression (from outside to inside) of the zona glomerulosa, zona fasciculata, zona reticularis, and medulla.

234

ADRENAL CORTEX

LYNNETTE K. NIEMAN

The adrenal glands weigh 6 to 8 g in adults (Fig. 234-1). Each contains a cortex, which makes steroid hormones, and a medulla, which produces catecholamines. Diseases of the adrenal medulla are discussed in Chapter 235. In the adrenal cortex, production of the three major classes of steroids occurs in specific zones: the outermost layer, the glomerulosa, produces mineralocorticoids, primarily aldosterone; the middle layer, the fasciculata, produces glucocorticoids, primarily cortisol; the innermost layer, the reticularis, produces adrenal "androgens," primarily dehydroepiandrosterone (DHEA) and its sulfated conjugate (DHEA-S) (Fig. 234-2). This division reflects the fact that certain critical enzymes are restricted to specific zones, resulting in the ability or inability to synthesize specific end products.

FUNCTION

The actions and regulation of these steroid classes differ. Mineralocorticoids act through the renal mineralocorticoid receptor to promote the reabsorption of sodium and the secretion of potassium. Aldosterone secretion is stimulated primarily by hyperkalemia and angiotensin II (which itself is stimulated by hypovolemia and excess renin). These agents increase the production of aldosterone synthase to restore homeostasis through this feedback loop. Aldosterone production is stimulated to a much smaller degree by adrenocorticotropic hormone (ACTH).

Cortisol and other glucocorticoids act through the glucocorticoid receptor type 2 and its isoforms. The actions of this class of steroids are much broader, including effects on carbohydrate handling, lipid and calcium metabolism, and the immune and nervous systems. Cortisol production is regulated primarily by ACTH, which is secreted in a circadian rhythm in response to corticotropin-releasing hormone (CRH) so that cortisol levels are highest in the morning and fall to a nadir around midnight. Cortisol coordinates ACTH production through negative feedback at the pituitary (ACTH) and hypothalamus (CRH). Vasopressin secretion also plays a role in stimulating ACTH release.

DHEA and DHEA-S are the most abundant products of the adrenal gland. They exert their estrogenic and androgenic effects as prohormones, being converted to estrogens and testosterone in the peripheral tissues and activating the androgen and estrogen receptors. There is no known regulator of DHEA synthesis, but its production declines with age.

DISORDERS OF ADRENAL FUNCTION

Most disorders of the adrenal cortex reflect overproduction or underproduction of the products of a single synthetic zone—cortisol, aldosterone, or testosterone or estrogen (Fig. 234-3). The congenital adrenal hyperplasias are an exception and present with both overproduction and underproduction. Abnormal secretion is suggested by clinical features of each disorder and is reflected in plasma or urine levels of the relevant hormones or by the consequent increases or decreases in feedback systems, which form the basis of the biochemical diagnostic tests.

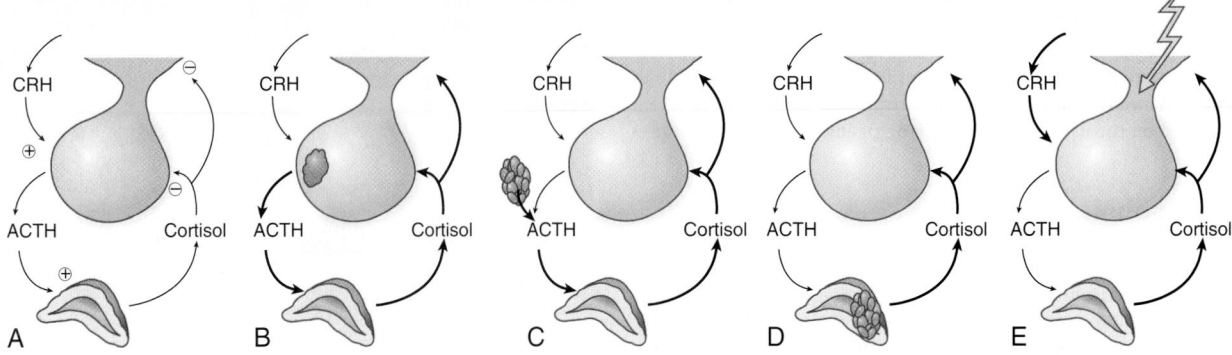

FIGURE 234-3. Physiology of the adrenal axis in health, Cushing's syndrome, and pseudo-Cushing states. **A,** In healthy individuals, cortisol production is stimulated by the increased hypothalamic release of corticotropin-releasing hormone (CRH), which then travels down the pituitary stalk to stimulate adrenocorticotropic hormone (ACTH) secretion and release by corticotropes. Circulating ACTH stimulates adrenal gland production and secretion of cortisol. Cortisol then functions in a negative feedback mechanism to inhibit both CRH and ACTH. **B,** In Cushing's disease, a pituitary tumor releases excessive amounts of ACTH, which results in increased cortisol secretion by the adrenal glands. **C,** In ectopic ACTH secretion, a nonpituitary ACTH-secreting tumor releases excessive amounts of ACTH, which results in increased cortisol secretion by the adrenal glands. **D,** In ACTH-independent adrenal forms of Cushing's syndrome, the adrenal tumor autonomously releases excess amounts of cortisol. In all forms of Cushing's syndrome, the negative feedback effects of excessive cortisol inhibit endogenous CRH and ACTH secretion, so that circulating ACTH levels reflect the underlying tumor (levels are normal or increased) or independent cortisol production (levels are suppressed). **E,** In pseudo-Cushing states, central stimulation increases CRH secretion, which in turn increases ACTH and hence cortisol production. In this setting, the negative feedback effects of excessive cortisol inhibit endogenous CRH and ACTH secretion, so that cortisol levels are ultimately constrained, albeit at an increased level.

Glucocorticoid Excess: Cushing's Syndrome

CLINICAL MANIFESTATIONS

Cushing's syndrome is a symptom complex that reflects excessive tissue exposure to cortisol. Classic features of Cushing's syndrome include weight gain, plethora, hypertension, and striae (Table 234-1). Not all patients have all features; the number and severity of features correlate roughly with the duration and severity of hypercortisolism. Because many of the signs and symptoms are nonspecific, the diagnosis may be confused with psychiatric disorders, polycystic ovary syndrome, the metabolic syndrome, simple obesity, fibromyalgia, or acute illness. However, because worsening hypercortisolism may precipitate hypertension, glucose intolerance, infections, psychiatric disturbances, impaired cognition, and hypercoagulability, it is important to identify this treatable disorder to prevent its associated morbidity and mortality.

Changes in mood and cognition are useful markers of hypercortisolism. These include irritability, crying, and restlessness; depressed mood; decreased libido; insomnia; anxiety; and decreased concentration and impaired memory.

DIAGNOSIS

Clinical Examination

Cushing's syndrome screening is most likely to be positive in the presence of signs that are typical of glucocorticoid excess, such as abnormal fat distribution in the supraclavicular and temporal fossae, proximal muscle weakness, wide (>1 cm) purple striae, and new irritability, decreased cognition, and decreased short-term memory. Testing is indicated when clinical features have progressed over time. For example, oligomenorrhea is more suggestive of Cushing's syndrome if a woman previously had regular menses. Serial seven subtractions and recall of three cities (or objects) are useful bedside strategies to identify deficits in cognition and memory.

Laboratory Findings

Exogenous administration of glucocorticoid should be excluded before screening for endogenous Cushing's syndrome. Two different screening tests should be abnormal to establish the diagnosis.

Urine, Saliva, and Serum Cortisol Measurements

Urine free cortisol (UFC) excretion during 24 hours is a good screening test. Specific, structurally based assay techniques, such as high-performance liquid chromatography and tandem mass spectrometry, are the "gold standard." The upper-normal limit of these tests is much lower and more specific than that of antibody-based assays, in which other steroids may cross-react.

UFC excretion also may be increased in the so-called pseudo-Cushing states, including psychiatric disorders (depression, anxiety disorder, obsessive-compulsive disorder), chronic pain, severe exercise, alcoholism,

SIGN OR SYMPTOM	PERCENTAGE
Decreased libido in men and women	100
Obesity or weight gain	97
Plethora	94
Round face	88
Menstrual changes	84
Hirsutism	81
Hypertension	74
Ecchymoses	62
Lethargy, depression	62
Striae	56
Weakness	56
Electrocardiographic changes or atherosclerosis	55
Dorsal fat pad	54
Edema	50
Abnormal glucose tolerance	50
Osteopenia or fracture	50
Headache	47
Backache	43
Recurrent infections	25
Abdominal pain	21
Acne	21
Female balding	13

TABLE 234-1 THE FREQUENCY OF CLINICAL SIGNS AND SYMPTOMS OF CUSHING'S SYNDROME

uncontrolled diabetes, and morbid obesity. Here, it is hypothesized that higher brain pathways stimulate CRH release and activation of the entire hypothalamic-pituitary-adrenal axis. Cortisol negative feedback inhibition on CRH and pituitary ACTH release restrains the resulting hypercortisoluria to less than four-fold greater than normal. Thus, Cushing's syndrome cannot be diagnosed with certainty unless values reach this threshold. Conversely, patients with Cushing's syndrome may have normal UFC excretion because of intermittent hypercortisolism or altered renal metabolism of cortisol. If UFC is only mildly elevated and clinical features are minimal, it is best to treat any pseudo-Cushing state and to remeasure UFC excretion with the expectation that it will normalize. Alternatively, if UFC values are normal but clinical suspicion is high, repeated measurement might disclose intermittent hypercortisolism.

Measurement of plasma cortisol at midnight distinguishes pseudo-Cushing states from Cushing's syndrome with 95% diagnostic accuracy; a level greater than 7.5 μg/dL is required for the diagnosis of Cushing's syndrome. Measurement of salivary cortisol at bedtime or at midnight works just as well and is more convenient. However, the criteria for its interpretation differ, so each assay must be validated before it is used for this purpose.

Dexamethasone Suppression Tests

The dexamethasone suppression test is a simple screening test that takes advantage of the negative feedback effect of glucocorticoids to reduce ACTH (and hence serum cortisol). Dexamethasone 1 mg is given orally between 11:00 PM and midnight, and plasma cortisol is measured between 8:00 and 9:00 the next morning. The test has an 8% false-negative rate in patients with Cushing's disease and a 30% false-positive rate in chronic illness, obesity, psychiatric disorders, and normal individuals. As a result, Cushing's syndrome cannot be diagnosed by this test alone unless the result is extremely abnormal.

The 2-day, 2-mg dexamethasone suppression test discriminates patients with a pseudo-Cushing state if plasma cortisol end points of less than 1.4 or 2.2 μg/dL are used. Dexamethasone 500 μg is given orally every 6 hours for eight doses, and plasma cortisol is measured 2 hours after the last dose. The test has excellent sensitivity (90 to 100%) and specificity (97 to 100%) for discriminating Cushing's syndrome, but it is costly and requires excellent patient compliance. The immediate subsequent administration of CRH (1 μg/kg body weight intravenously) and the measurement of cortisol 15 minutes later increased the sensitivity and specificity to 100% in a small study of 58 patients, with values above 1.4 μg/dL indicating Cushing's syndrome. Although this combined dexamethasone-CRH test has high diagnostic accuracy, it has the same disadvantages as the 2-day dexamethasone suppression test and the added cost of CRH testing. Because of these drawbacks, these tests are usually reserved for patients with ambiguous or confusing results on other screening tests. CRH is available commercially (Acthrel), with Food and Drug Administration–approved labeling for the differential diagnosis of Cushing's syndrome. Its use in the dexamethasone-CRH test is an off-label use.

Any dexamethasone test may give false results in patients with abnormal metabolic clearance of the drug. Agents that induce the cytochrome P-450 CYP3A4 enzymes (alcohol, rifampin, phenytoin, phenobarbital) increase dexamethasone clearance, whereas renal or hepatic failure decreases it. Measurement of a dexamethasone level can determine whether its clearance has been altered.

Differential Diagnosis

The causes of endogenous Cushing's syndrome can be divided broadly into ACTH-dependent (80%) and ACTH-independent (20%) forms (Table 234-2). Hypercortisolism from autonomously functioning adrenal tumors suppresses ACTH, whereas in primary disorders of ACTH excess, the adrenal glands respond to ACTH. Plasma ACTH concentration distinguishes between these causes. ACTH is usually less than 10 pg/mL in primary adrenal disorders but is also suppressed by exogenous steroids, whether they are prescribed intentionally (iatrogenic Cushing's syndrome) or taken factitiously. Patients in the latter group often have had multiple surgical procedures and do not reveal that they are self-administering steroids. As a result, patients must be queried closely about exogenous steroid administration, recognizing that parenteral, inhaled, and topical steroids can all cause glucocorticoid excess. Patients with endogenous Cushing's syndrome and low ACTH concentrations undergo adrenal imaging to identify the site of adrenal abnormality. Nonautonomous adrenal tissue atrophies when ACTH support is subnormal. Because of this, the common ACTH-independent forms of Cushing's syndrome—adrenal adenoma and carcinoma—present as a unilateral adrenal mass, with atrophy of the adjacent and contralateral tissue on magnetic resonance imaging or computed tomography.

Bilateral forms of primary adrenal disease are rare and may present with small or large adrenal nodules. Primary pigmented nodular adrenal disease occurs primarily in children and young adults and is characterized by small to normal-sized adrenal glands containing small (<5 mm) black-brown cortical nodules. About half these patients have additional features, termed Carney's complex, which are often inherited in an autosomal dominant fashion. The clinical features of Carney's complex include myxomas of the skin, breast, and heart; spotty pigmentation, such as lentigines and blue nevi; and other endocrine overactivity, such as acromegaly and testicular tumors. Some of these patients have mutations leading to a truncated form of protein kinase A regulatory 1α subunit. The resultant increase in protein kinase A activation by cyclic adenosine monophosphate presumably allows tumor formation. Bilateral nodular hyperplasia with Cushing's syndrome can occur in the setting of McCune-Albright syndrome, mostly in infants. Massive macronodular adrenal disease generally presents after age 40 years with huge adrenal glands and aberrant expression of "illicit" receptors for various ligands (gastric inhibitory polypeptide, β-adrenergic, vasopressin), which presumably mediates autonomous cortisol production.

A normal or elevated plasma ACTH level (>15 pg/mL; 3.3 pmol/L) is consistent with an ACTH-producing tumor. Intermediate ACTH concentrations between 5 and 15 pg/mL (1.1 to 3.3 pmol/L) are not diagnostic. In these patients, suboptimal cortisol responses to CRH stimulation may identify the minority of cases of ACTH-independent Cushing's syndrome with borderline basal ACTH values. In addition, a suppressed plasma DHEA-S value supports the diagnosis of an ACTH-independent disorder.

Cushing's disease, an ACTH-secreting pituitary adenoma, is the most common cause of Cushing's syndrome. It is more common in women than in men (6:1 ratio), with a mean age at onset in the fourth decade. ACTH also may be secreted ectopically by a variety of neuroendocrine tumors, as shown in Table 234-3 (see also Chapter 186).

Pituitary magnetic resonance imaging shows a tumor in only about 40 to 50% of patients with Cushing's disease, but it is obtained routinely in patients with ACTH-dependent disease to exclude a macroadenoma or abnormal anatomy before petrosal sinus sampling or surgery. Biochemical tests must be used to distinguish among the ACTH-dependent causes of Cushing's syndrome, and they must be performed after a 6- to 8-week period of sustained hypercortisolism sufficient to suppress normal corticotrope function.

TABLE 234-2 ETIOLOGY OF CUSHING'S SYNDROME

EXOGENOUS	ENDOGENOUS
Most common cause of Cushing's syndrome	ACTH independent—autonomous adrenal activation (20% of all cases)
Glucocorticoid or ACTH driven	Adrenal adenoma (40-50%)
May be factitious or iatrogenic	Adrenal carcinoma (40-50%)
	Primary pigmented nodular adrenal disease
	McCune-Albright syndrome
	Massive macronodular adrenal disease
	Gastric inhibitory polypeptide or food induced
	ACTH dependent—adrenal activation by excessive ACTH (80% of all cases)
	Corticotrope adenoma (80%)
	Ectopic ACTH secretion (20%)
	Ectopic CRH secretion (rare)

ACTH = adrenocorticotropic hormone; CRH = corticotropin-releasing hormone.

TABLE 234-3 THE INCIDENCE AND TYPES OF TUMORS CAUSING THE SYNDROME OF ECTOPIC ACTH SECRETION

TUMOR TYPE	PERCENTAGE
Carcinoma of lung (small cell or oat cell)	19-50
Carcinoid of bronchus	2-37
Carcinoid of thymus	8-12
Pancreatic tumors, carcinoid and islet cell	4-12
Pheochromocytoma, neuroblastoma, ganglioma, paraganglioma	5-12
Medullary carcinoma of the thyroid	0-5
Miscellaneous*	<1

*Miscellaneous tumors reported to secrete ACTH in 1 to 10 cases include carcinoma of the ovary, prostate, breast, thyroid, kidney, salivary glands, testes, gallbladder, esophagus, and appendix; gastric carcinoid and renal carcinoid; acute myeloblastic leukemia; melanoma; and cloacogenic carcinoma of the anal canal.

ACTH = adrenocorticotropic hormone.

Inferior petrosal sinus sampling is the best test to distinguish between a pituitary and an ectopic source of excess ACTH; worldwide, the overall sensitivity and specificity are about 94%. The test involves catheterization of a peripheral vein and the petrosal sinuses draining the pituitary gland, simultaneous measurement of ACTH levels at each site before and after administration of CRH, and calculation of the central-to-peripheral ACTH ratio at each time point. Ratios of more than 2 before CRH administration or more than 3 after CRH administration are consistent with Cushing's disease.

Although it is accurate in experienced hands, inferior petrosal sinus sampling carries a small risk of stroke, is expensive, and is not widely available. Other tests, such as the CRH test and the 8-mg dexamethasone suppression test, may be useful if both responses indicate Cushing's disease. In this setting, the likelihood of ectopic ACTH secretion is low. However, the diagnosis is not clear if both responses are negative or if they are mixed.

If endocrine tests suggest ectopic ACTH secretion, imaging is obtained to localize the tumor (see also Chapter 186). Computed tomography and magnetic resonance imaging of the chest are the best initial screens because these tumors are most often in the thoracic cavity. Octreotide scintigraphy is a useful adjunctive test. Measurement of serum calcitonin and gastrin and measurement of plasma or urine catecholamines may identify medullary carcinoma of the thyroid, gastrinoma, and pheochromocytoma. The process can be repeated every 6 to 12 months; tumors that make ACTH ectopically have a spectrum of malignant potential, and annual screening should continue, regardless of treatment for hypercortisolism.

TREATMENT   Rx

Surgical Therapy

The optimal treatment of Cushing's syndrome is surgical resection of the lesion that is producing excessive ACTH or cortisol. In ACTH-dependent Cushing's syndrome, if this is unsuccessful or cannot be done, bilateral adrenalectomy is an option. Medical therapy can also be used for patients with occult ectopic ACTH-secreting tumors and in combination with pituitary irradiation to treat Cushing's disease.

Transsphenoidal resection of a microadenoma is the optimal therapy for a patient with Cushing's disease, with up to a 90% chance of cure in the hands of an experienced neurosurgeon. A successful outcome is less likely if the initial surgery is not curative, in cases of recurrence, and for macroadenomas. Controversy exists about the criteria for remission; although a low postoperative cortisol level is encouraging, it does not preclude later recurrence. If recurrence develops, additional resection or alternative therapy should be considered.

Radiation Therapy

Radiation therapy to the pituitary gland, with adjunctive medical therapy to normalize cortisol levels, is a good option for Cushing's disease patients who cannot undergo surgery, for those in whom the risk of Nelson's syndrome is deemed great, and for those with recurrent disease. This is usually delivered in 200-rad daily increments to a total dose of 4500 cGy. The disadvantage of radiotherapy is the length of time needed for a full response—up to 10 years—and the possibility of hypopituitarism. There is less experience with high-energy radiosurgery, such as the gamma knife, which has the advantage of requiring only one or two treatments. Adrenalectomy is preferable if rapid normalization of hypercortisolism is needed, and this option may be chosen by patients who have concerns about radiation-induced hypopituitarism and loss of reproductive function.

Medical Therapy
Combination Surgical and Medical Therapy

Medical therapy alone is rarely appropriate for Cushing's disease because it requires close monitoring and adjustment of dose and has low long-term efficacy.

Patients with ectopic ACTH secretion can be cured if the tumor can be removed and is not metastatic. Otherwise, adrenalectomy or medical therapy is chosen. Adrenalectomy is appropriate when the patient cannot tolerate the cost, medical toxicity, or adverse psychological effects of long-term medical therapy and monitoring; if the patient requires rapid correction of hypercortisolism; or if maximal daily doses of ketoconazole (1600 mg) and metyrapone (2 g) given in combination do not render the patient eucortisolemic.

Nonmalignant primary adrenal causes of Cushing's syndrome are cured by resection of the abnormal tissue. Laparoscopy is the preferred approach. Surgery is the mainstay in the treatment of adrenal cancer; multiple operations may be needed to resect primary lesions, local recurrences, and hepatic, thoracic, and intracranial metastases. Adjuvant adrenolytic therapy with mitotane may provide a chemotherapeutic benefit.

Mineralocorticoid Excess

DIAGNOSIS

Patients with mineralocorticoid excess often have few clinical symptoms apart from fatigue and muscle weakness or cramps related to hypokalemia. Most often the condition is suspected because of hypertension, especially if it occurs at an early age in association with spontaneous hypokalemia or is difficult to control. Mineralocorticoid excess can result from primary adrenal disease, in which aldosterone (or another mineralocorticoid) is produced autonomously (and renin levels are low), or it may be due to nonadrenal causes as a result of elevated renin values, which stimulate aldosterone secretion. The latter situations include states of contracted arterial volume, such as congestive heart failure or cirrhosis with ascites, decreased renal arterial blood flow, and tumor production of renin (Table 234-4).

RENIN-INDEPENDENT MINERALOCORTICOID EXCESS

DIAGNOSIS

Although most of these conditions result from excessive aldosterone production by one or both adrenal glands, excessive production of other mineralocorticoids or constitutive activation of the renal sodium channel must be excluded. In these latter conditions, both aldosterone and renin values are low, resulting in the so-called syndrome of apparent mineralocorticoid excess. In this setting, diagnostic information is obtained by history (licorice ingestion) or measurement of other mineralocorticoids (see Table 234-4).

The diagnosis of primary hyperaldosteronism rests on the demonstration of an increased plasma aldosterone value greater than 15 pg/mL with an increased ratio (>20) of aldosterone to plasma renin activity. Salt loading, by one of four possible tests, is used to confirm primary hyperaldosteronism by demonstrating a lack of aldosterone suppression. The plasma aldosterone concentration should decrease to less than 5 ng/dL in normal individuals.

TABLE 234-4   CAUSES OF MINERALOCORTICOID EXCESS

PRIMARY HYPERALDOSTERONISM: HIGH ALDOSTERONE, LOW RENIN

Aldosterone-producing adenomas (30-50%)
Bilateral zona glomerulosa hyperplasia
Familial hyperaldosteronism
    Type 1: glucocorticoid-remediable hyperaldosteronism—this results from formation of a chimeric gene containing the regulator portion of 11β-hydroxylase (normally regulated by ACTH) and the synthetic region of aldosterone synthase; as a result, ACTH stimulates aldosterone synthase and hence aldosterone production
    Type 2: adrenal adenomas or hyperplasia expressed in a familial pattern
Aldosterone-producing adrenal carcinoma
Ectopic aldosterone secretion (rare): kidney, ovary

SECONDARY HYPERALDOSTERONISM: HIGH ALDOSTERONE, HIGH RENIN

Renovascular hypertension and aortic stenosis
Diuretic use
Renin-secreting tumors
Severe cardiac failure

APPARENT MINERALOCORTICOID EXCESS: LOW ALDOSTERONE, LOW RENIN

Licorice ingestion: licorice (candy or flavored tobacco) containing glycyrrhetinic acid (or similar compounds such as carbenoxolone) inhibits renal 11β-hydroxysteroid dehydrogenase type 2, reducing cortisol conversion to cortisone and enabling cortisol to act as an endogenous mineralocorticoid
Severe hypercortisolism: similar in mechanism to licorice ingestion; very high cortisol levels are thought to overwhelm the ability of 11β-hydroxysteroid dehydrogenase type 2 to convert cortisol to cortisone in the kidney; cortisol itself then acts as a potent mineralocorticoid
Liddle's syndrome: mutation of the β or γ subunit of the collecting tubule sodium channel leads to a constitutive increase in sodium reabsorption and potassium excretion
11β-Hydroxylase deficiency form of congenital adrenal hyperplasia: 11-deoxycortisol accumulates because of an inability to convert it to cortisol
17-Hydroxylase deficiency form of congenital adrenal hyperplasia: deoxycorticosterone and corticosterone are increased

Differential Diagnosis

Having made the diagnosis of aldosterone-dependent mineralocorticoid excess, one must differentiate between the two most common adrenal causes—hyperplasia and adenoma—after excluding potential rare causes of hyperaldosteronism. Glucocorticoid-suppressible hyperaldosteronism is a rare cause of aldosterone excess caused by a genetic swap of the promoter for *CYP11B1* (11β-hydroxylase) with that of *CYP11B2* (aldosterone synthase), forming a chimeric gene in which ACTH stimulates aldosterone synthase. Glucocorticoid-suppressible hyperaldosteronism should be suspected in the setting of familial hyperaldosteronism, particularly if there is a history of cardiovascular accidents at an early age. Serum 18-hydroxycortisol and 18-oxocortisol concentrations are elevated in glucocorticoid-suppressible hyperaldosteronism, and gene testing confirms the diagnosis (see *http://www.brighamandwomens.org/gra*).

For the more common conditions, adrenal computed tomography scans may show nonfunctioning nodules and falsely suggest an adenoma. The responses to physiologic maneuvers, such as upright posture, and salt loading with oral or intravenous sodium tend to be preserved in patients with hyperplasia, but there is significant overlap among groups of patients. The best diagnostic test involves the measurement of cortisol and aldosterone in bilateral adrenal venous effluent and a peripheral vein before and during an ACTH infusion. Cortisol is used to evaluate catheter placement in the adrenal veins, as levels from the two sides should be similar. When an adenoma is present, the aldosterone-to-cortisol ratio on one side is usually at least five-fold greater than the other, which may be similar to the periphery, indicating suppression. Bilateral hyperplasia tends to produce similar values on each side.

TREATMENT   Rx

Treatment of primary hyperaldosteronism includes laparoscopic resection for adenomas. Afterward, hypokalemia generally resolves, but hypertension persists in up to 65% of patients. The mineralocorticoid antagonist spironolactone or amiloride is used to treat patients unable to undergo surgery or those with hyperplasia. Antihypertensive agents are continued. Eplerenone is a newer, more selective mineralocorticoid antagonist (with fewer side effects of sexual dysfunction and gynecomastia compared with spironolactone). It is currently approved by the Food and Drug Administration for the treatment of hypertension and congestive heart failure.

Androgen Excess

DEFINITION

Women with excess circulating androgens or increased sensitivity to androgens present with complaints of hirsutism, acne, and anovulation or infertility. When testosterone is secreted in great excess, women may virilize and exhibit a deepened voice, clitorimegaly, masculinized body habitus, and alopecia.

DIAGNOSIS

The adrenal causes of hyperandrogenism—congenital adrenal hyperplasia, Cushing's disease, adrenal cancer, and androgen-producing adrenal adenoma—are uncommon. Most women have no clear-cut cause (idiopathic hirsutism) or polycystic ovary syndrome. Rarely, androgen-secreting ovarian tumors, hyperprolactinemia, glucocorticoid resistance, or exogenous drugs cause hyperandrogenism. Patients with an adrenal source of hyperandrogenism usually have increased serum levels of DHEA-S or androstenedione, in contrast to the testosterone excess that is more typical of an ovarian source. DHEA and DHEA-S are weak androgens that can be converted locally to testosterone in the hair follicles. Because DHEA and DHEA-S levels decline throughout adult life, these values must be interpreted within age-specific normal ranges. Although a tumor is more likely if DHEA-S is greater than 500 μg/dL or testosterone is greater than 200 ng/mL, it is not excluded at lower levels.

Imaging identifies nearly all adrenal tumors but may miss a small intraovarian one. UFC may be elevated in patients with virilizing adrenal carcinoma or Cushing's disease (see earlier) and in those with glucocorticoid resistance. By contrast, androgen-secreting adrenal adenomas do not have glucocorticoid excess. In women suspected of having nonclassic forms of congenital adrenal hyperplasia, precursor and product hormones should be measured before and after ACTH to confirm the diagnosis.

TREATMENT

Treatment of adrenal causes of hyperandrogenism varies according to the disorder. Tumors are resected. Late-onset congenital adrenal hyperplasia is treated by glucocorticoids to normalize ACTH and hence androgen levels (typically, dexamethasone 0.125 to 0.375 mg at bedtime).

Mixed Mineralocorticoid and Glucocorticoid Deficiency: Adrenal Insufficiency

PATHOBIOLOGY

Primary Adrenal Insufficiency
Autoimmune Destruction

Autoimmune destruction is the most common cause of primary adrenal insufficiency in industrialized countries and may occur alone or, rarely, in association with autoimmune polyglandular syndromes. These syndromes tend to present either in childhood (type 1), in association with hypoparathyroidism and mucocutaneous candidiasis, or in adulthood (type 2), in association with insulin-dependent diabetes mellitus, autoimmune thyroid disease, alopecia areata, and vitiligo. The glands are small on imaging.

Adrenoleukodystrophy

Adrenoleukodystrophy, a rare (1 in 25,000) X-linked condition, is characterized by a deficiency of peroxisomal membrane adrenoleukodystrophy protein, which transports activated acyl-coenzyme A derivates into the peroxisomes, where they are shortened by β-oxidation. This deficiency results in the accumulation of very long chain fatty acids in the central nervous system and other tissues and increased plasma $C_{26:0}$ fatty acids. Incomplete penetrance of the genetic defect and variable accumulation of very long chain fatty acids in the adrenal gland, brain, testis, and liver account for the clinical phenotypes, which differ by age and presentation.

Infection

Infections cause about 15% of primary adrenal insufficiency. Typical infections include tuberculosis and systemic fungal diseases (histoplasmosis, coccidioidomycosis, blastomycosis), in which the adrenal tissue is replaced by caseating granulomas. End-stage AIDS-associated opportunistic infections, such as cytomegalovirus or *Mycobacterium avium-intracellulare,* may reduce adrenal function. Adrenal tissue may be replaced by bilateral metastases (most commonly primary carcinoma of the lung, breast, kidney, or gut) or primary lymphoma, although adrenal insufficiency is uncommon. Intraadrenal hemorrhage may also lead to insufficient steroidogenesis. Hemorrhage typically occurs in a stressed, hospitalized patient receiving long-term prophylactic anticoagulation and is often accompanied by back pain. The adrenal glands tend to be large on imaging.

Congenital Adrenal Hyperplasias

The congenital adrenal hyperplasias are a disparate group of diseases caused by a genetic deficiency of one of the enzymes needed for adrenal steroidogenesis. Patients with nearly complete deficiency of an enzyme required for cortisol synthesis present in infancy with adrenal insufficiency and salt-wasting crisis. This is most problematic in patients with mutation of the 21-hydroxylase (*CYP21*) or 11β-hydroxylase (*CYP11B1*) gene. The increase in ACTH levels caused by cortisol deficiency drives the intact steroidogenic pathways so that there is excessive production of the steroids just proximal to the enzymatic block—17-hydroxyprogesterone and 11-deoxycortisol, respectively, in 21-hydroxylase and 11β-hydroxylase deficiency. The increased levels of precursor steroids enable increased adrenal androgen synthesis, so that severely affected girls may be virilized in utero. Girls and women with nonclassic congenital adrenal hyperplasia present later. They have greater enzyme activity, so that cortisol production is adequate, but increased ACTH levels cause hyperandrogenism.

Rare Causes

Other rare causes of primary adrenal insufficiency include ACTH resistance, congenital adrenal hypoplasia, Smith-Lemli-Opitz syndrome, and amyloidosis. Patients with primary adrenal insufficiency should undergo further evaluation to determine its cause (Table 234-5). Detection of antibodies to 21-hydroxylase identifies nearly all patients with idiopathic disease. In a male

TABLE 234-5 CAUSES OF ADRENAL INSUFFICIENCY AND ANCILLARY TESTS

SPECIFIC CAUSES	SUGGESTIVE CLINICAL FEATURES	USEFUL ANCILLARY TESTS
Primary adrenal insufficiency	Hyperpigmentation, orthostatic hypotension	Hyperkalemia, elevated ACTH
Idiopathic autoimmune destruction	Most common cause (80%) in developed countries; with or without other endocrinopathies, as below	Antibodies to 21-hydroxylase are present; on imaging, adrenal glands are small
Polyglandular failure type 1	Hypoparathyroidism, mucocutaneous candidiasis, vitiligo; age <20 yr	
Polyglandular failure type 2	Insulin-dependent diabetes, autoimmune thyroid disease, alopecia areata, vitiligo; age >40 yr	On imaging, adrenal glands are small
Infections: tuberculosis, systemic fungal diseases, AIDS-associated opportunistic infections (e.g., cytomegalovirus)	15% of patients in U.S. series	Adrenal glands tend to be large on CT and may be calcified
Space-occupying adrenal lesions	Metastases from carcinoma of lung, breast, kidney, gut; lymphoma or hemorrhage (heparin use)	Abnormal shape of adrenal glands on CT; evidence of hemorrhage
Bilateral adrenalectomy or treatment with steroidogenesis inhibitors		Ketoconazole, mitotane, aminoglutethimide, trilostane, and metyrapone reduce cortisol levels
Adrenoleukodystrophy	X-linked—screen males; in childhood, cognitive and gait disturbances; in adults, spastic paraparesis	Deficiency of peroxisomal very long chain acyl-coenzyme A synthetase leads to elevated plasma $C_{26:0}$ fatty acid levels
Secondary adrenal insufficiency		
Suppression of the adrenal axis by exogenous or endogenous glucocorticoids	Medication history; history of Cushing's syndrome	Adrenal glands are small on imaging
Structural lesions of the hypothalamus or pituitary gland (tumors, destruction by infiltrating disorders, x-irradiation, and lymphocytic hypophysitis)	Other pituitary deficiencies	Adrenal glands are normal or small on imaging; MRI or CT may show pituitary or hypothalamic lesion
Isolated ACTH deficiency		
Head trauma		

ACTH = adrenocorticotropic hormone; AIDS = acquired immunodeficiency syndrome; CT = computed tomography; MRI = magnetic resonance imaging.

with negative results, measurement of very long chain fatty acids will detect adrenoleukodystrophy. Taken together, this strategy identifies the cause in nearly all adult patients with idiopathic adrenal insufficiency. Patients with autoimmune disease should be tested for other endocrine deficiencies, and those with adrenoleukodystrophy require neurologic evaluation.

Secondary Adrenal Insufficiency
Suppression of the Pituitary Axis
Suppression of the hypothalamic-pituitary-adrenal axis by exogenous or endogenous glucocorticoids is the most common cause of secondary adrenal insufficiency. This phenomenon depends on the dose, duration, and schedule of glucocorticoid administration. Thus, adrenal suppression is unusual with "replacement" doses of glucocorticoid that are roughly equivalent to daily production (e.g., total daily doses of 20 mg hydrocortisone, 5 mg prednisone, or 0.3 to 0.5 mg dexamethasone). At higher doses, adrenal suppression is usually not seen until after 3 weeks of administration, and a single morning administration is less suppressive than are divided doses given during the day. When potentially suppressive doses of glucocorticoids are stopped, symptoms of adrenal insufficiency may occur within 48 hours, and the entire axis may not recover for up to 18 months. During this time, the patient should receive replacement glucocorticoid treatment and/or supplemental steroids at times of physiologic stress, depending on the degree of impairment (see later).

Lesions of the Hypothalamus or Pituitary
Secondary adrenal insufficiency also may result from structural lesions of the hypothalamus or pituitary gland that interfere with CRH production or transport or with corticotrope function. These causes include tumors, trauma, destruction by infiltrating disorders, x-irradiation, and lymphocytic hypophysitis. In general, these are not reversible conditions. Patients with secondary adrenal insufficiency not ascribed to glucocorticoid use should undergo imaging of the pituitary and hypothalamus to exclude a structural or infiltrating lesion, as well as tests of other pituitary function to exclude additional deficiencies.

CLINICAL MANIFESTATIONS
The clinical presentation of adrenal insufficiency reflects the cause and duration of this uncommon condition. Primary adrenal insufficiency eventually destroys the entire adrenal cortex, with loss of both glucocorticoid and mineralocorticoid activity. By contrast, secondary adrenal insufficiency reflects an inability of the hypothalamic-pituitary unit to deliver CRH or ACTH, thus reducing trophic support to otherwise normal glands. As a result, only cortisol production decreases, because mineralocorticoid production is not very ACTH dependent.

The characteristic clinical presentation of acute primary adrenal insufficiency includes orthostatic hypotension, agitation, confusion, circulatory collapse, abdominal pain, and fever. These features are most likely to be caused by hemorrhage, metastasis, or acute infection and can lead to death if not treated. In contrast, the typical history and clinical findings of chronic primary adrenal insufficiency include a longer history of malaise, fatigue, anorexia, weight loss, joint and back pain, and darkening of the skin (especially in the creases of the hands, extensor surfaces, recent scars, buccal and vaginal mucosa, and nipples). Patients may crave salt and may develop unusual food preferences, such as drinking the brine from pickles. Associated biochemical features for both presentations include hyponatremia, hypoglycemia, hyperkalemia, unexplained eosinophilia, and mild prerenal azotemia.

Chronic secondary adrenal insufficiency presents in a similar way, but without hyperpigmentation or mineralocorticoid abnormalities.

DIAGNOSIS
Biochemical testing confirms the diagnosis of adrenal insufficiency. A morning serum cortisol measurement is an inexpensive but relatively insensitive screening test for adrenal insufficiency in patients who are not acutely ill. Adrenal insufficiency is virtually excluded by values greater than 19 μg/dL (524 nmol/L) and is likely if the value is less than 3 μg/dL (83 nmol/L). However, because of the pulsatile nature of cortisol secretion, both healthy individuals and patients with adrenal insufficiency may have results in the intermediate range of 3 to 19 μg/dL, requiring additional evaluation.

Patients with acute adrenal insufficiency should be evaluated for sepsis or for hemorrhage or metastasis in the adrenal glands. Imaging of the glands and other testing may reveal an infectious cause. Individuals thought to have congenital adrenal hyperplasia should undergo additional measurement of ACTH-stimulated precursor and product hormones to delineate the site of enzymatic deficiency. In acute adrenal insufficiency, a serum cortisol value is generally inappropriately normal or subnormal in the setting of hypotension (in which cortisol values are usually well above 18 μg/dL). There is controversy about the best test for the diagnosis of chronic adrenal insufficiency. Many use the cortisol response to exogenous ACTH as a "gold standard" test of adrenal steroidogenic ability. In the classic test, 250 μg of ACTH (1-24, cosyntropin) is given intravenously or intramuscularly at any time of day. This supraphysiologic dose of ACTH is a maximal stimulus to the adrenal gland, so that the serum cortisol level measured 30 to 60 minutes later is greater than 18 μg/dL. Lower values indicate adrenal insufficiency. Insulin-induced hypoglycemia, metyrapone stimulation, and lower doses of ACTH stimulation have been proposed as better tests for patients with mild or recent secondary adrenal insufficiency, who may respond to pharmacologic doses of ACTH. None of these is an ideal test. Also, because there is no commercial formulation of ACTH for lower-dose tests, the product must be diluted and delivered on site, leading to concerns about the accuracy of the administered dose and the validity of results. Metyrapone has limited availability in the United States.

Cerebral adrenoleukodystrophy, presenting in childhood, is characterized by cognitive and gait disturbances; the adult form, adrenomyeloneuropathy, is characterized by spinal cord and peripheral nerve demyelination. In both forms, the accumulation of very long chain fatty acids in the adrenal cortex alters membrane function and inhibits signal transduction by ACTH. Because a substantial minority of patients in both groups present first with adrenal insufficiency, boys and young men with adrenal insufficiency should be screened for adrenoleukodystrophy.

Differential Diagnosis

Primary and secondary adrenal insufficiency can be distinguished by measuring plasma ACTH. In primary adrenal insufficiency, ACTH levels are generally above the normal range and may exceed the normal range before the cortisol response to exogenous ACTH stimulation is subnormal. In addition, hyperkalemia and elevated renin values are characteristic of primary but not of secondary adrenal insufficiency.

TREATMENT   **Rx**

Acute Adrenal Insufficiency

In suspected acute adrenal insufficiency, hydrocortisone is the treatment of choice because it has both glucocorticoid and mineralocorticoid activity. Treatment with intravenous saline for volume expansion, glucose for hypoglycemia, and intravenous hydrocortisone (100 mg) is started immediately after placement of an intravenous line and withdrawal of blood for documentation of the cortisol value.

Chronic Adrenal Insufficiency

Therapy for chronic adrenal insufficiency aims to provide the physiologic replacement of steroids. Glucocorticoid replacement is achieved by administering 10 to 12 mg/m^2 of hydrocortisone daily in one or two oral doses, attempting to mimic the physiologic diurnal variation of cortisol concentrations. Hydrocortisone offers the advantage of multiple-dose tablets, which allows fine adjustment and splitting of the daily dose. Ideally, the morning dose is given as soon after waking as possible; for individuals who feel extremely fatigued in the morning before the agent is absorbed, a strategy of taking the medication 30 minutes before arising may be helpful. Although many patients do well with a single dose, others complain of pronounced fatigue in the afternoon and evening. For them, a split-dose regimen, in which about one third of the daily dose is given around 4:00 PM, may be useful.

Other glucocorticoids may be used for daily replacement therapy. Prednisone, 5 to 7.5 mg daily, has the advantage of a long half-life and may be particularly helpful in patients with afternoon or evening fatigue. Dexamethasone may be used, but because of variable interindividual metabolism, it is difficult to recommend a specific replacement dose; in addition, few options for fixed doses are available, so it is difficult to adjust the dose.

Patients with primary adrenal insufficiency should be encouraged to salt their food and not to limit salt intake. Nearly all patients also require a mineralocorticoid, such as fludrocortisone 50 to 300 µg/day. The dose is adjusted until plasma renin activity is normal. If a mineralocorticoid is not given, the dose of hydrocortisone or other steroid with mineralocorticoid activity is often mistakenly increased to reduce hyperkalemia or salt craving. The problem with this approach is that the amount of glucocorticoid increases beyond physiologic replacement, and the patient becomes cushingoid.

Patients with primary adrenal insufficiency also have decreased serum DHEA levels. Controversy exists regarding its replacement. A recent meta-analysis concluded that there is insufficient evidence to support its routine use in these patients.

Ensuring Proper Dosing
Education of the Patient

All patients receiving chronic glucocorticoid replacement therapy should be instructed that they must take the glucocorticoids as prescribed and that failure to take or absorb the medication will lead to adrenal crisis and possibly death. They should wear medical information bracelets or necklaces that identify this requirement. It is important to educate patients and their families about glucocorticoid adjustment during physiologic stress conditions, including the emergency administration of intramuscular glucocorticoid by means of a kit containing prefilled syringes with injectable steroid.

Dosing for Stress

The daily oral glucocorticoid dose is usually doubled for "stressful" physiologic conditions such as fever, nausea, and diarrhea, although there are few data to support this strategy. In addition, this practice may lead to chronic overmedication by the patient because of a liberal interpretation of what constitutes physical stress. Thus, education regarding when and how to change the dose of steroid should be reinforced periodically, preferably with written material, and the dangers of excessive steroid use should be emphasized. If the patient is vomiting, has severe diarrhea, or has collapsed, intramuscular glucocorticoids should be given before transport to a medical facility.

The glucocorticoid dose is increased in proportion to the amount of stress. Thus, during maximally stressful situations (e.g., adrenal crisis, major surgery, trauma, labor and delivery), the daily hydrocortisone dose is 100 to 300 mg (few data support the need for this pharmacologic rather than physiologic replacement dose, but the safety of not following this practice has not been established). The dose is usually tapered by 50% per day as long as the patient is clinically stable. For more moderate stress, such as that of cholecystectomy, 75 to 100 mg hydrocortisone is given on the day of surgery, and the dose is tapered more rapidly. Patients undergoing minimal stress, such as tooth extraction or short operative orthopedic procedures, may not require any additional supplementation.

Clinical Assessment to Ensure Proper Dosing

Clinical assessment is the best way to judge whether the glucocorticoid dose is correct. Symptoms of adrenal insufficiency improve with adequate therapy. The development of cushingoid features or osteopenia suggests frank or subtle overreplacement, respectively, and the presence of adrenal insufficiency symptoms (fatigue, anorexia, weight loss) suggests underreplacement. In women, DHEA replacement increases testosterone levels, so that hirsutism, acne, or other signs of androgen excess may suggest overreplacement. In primary adrenal insufficiency, adequate hormone replacement results in plasma ACTH levels that decrease but remain elevated, in the range of 100 to 200 pg/mL. Renin values, however, normalize completely and may be used to judge the adequacy of mineralocorticoid replacement. Although hydrocortisone is metabolized to cortisol, plasma cortisol values should not be used to monitor therapy because clearance from the blood stream is rapid, and circulating values are low for most of the day. UFC does not reflect adequate replacement; the increase in plasma cortisol levels after a single daily dose may exceed corticosteroid-binding globulin capacity, resulting in excessive urine levels and overestimation of integrated cortisol levels.

Mineralocorticoid Deficiency

DEFINITION

Hypoaldosteronism may be classified as a low-normal or a high renin state on the basis of plasma renin activity after 4 hours of upright posture. Renin deficiency is the most common cause of hypoaldosteronism, occurring most often in older patients with mild, nonoliguric renal disease who often have insulin-dependent diabetes and potentially diabetic nephropathy. Indomethacin and other prostaglandin synthesis inhibitors, as well as autonomic dysfunction associated with prolonged bedrest, can also result in hyporeninemic hypoaldosteronism.

CLINICAL MANIFESTATIONS

There are few clinical features associated with mineralocorticoid deficiency; as a result, it is usually suspected when laboratory results reveal hyperkalemia, hyponatremia, and a mild metabolic alkalosis. If glucocorticoid deficiency is excluded, isolated hypoaldosteronism is established if the circulating level of aldosterone is inappropriately low.

High renin states of hypoaldosteronism include congenital adrenal hyperplasias with mineralocorticoid deficiency and primary adrenal insufficiency when it is treated with pure glucocorticoid replacement.

Treatment of these conditions involves sodium replacement with at least 10 mEq/kg/day, roughly equivalent to the 4 g of sodium chloride found in a typical diet in the United States. For individuals who do not maintain such a diet (often the elderly or the young), fludrocortisone can be given at the same doses used in primary adrenal insufficiency.

SUGGESTED READINGS

Alkatib AA, Cosma M, Elamin MB, et al. A systematic review and meta-analysis of randomized placebo-controlled trials of DHEA treatment effects on quality of life in women with adrenal insufficiency. *J Clin Endocrinol Metab.* 2009;94:3676-3681. *Comprehensive meta-analysis of DHEA replacement.*
Bornstein SR. Predisposing factors for adrenal insufficiency. *N Engl J Med.* 2009;360:2328-2339. *Review.*
Fassnacht M, Allolio B. Clinical management of adrenocortical carcinoma. *Best Pract Res Clin Endocrinol Metab.* 2009;23:273-289. *Overview of the medical and surgical treatments for these tumors.*

Guignat L, Bertherat J. The diagnosis of Cushing's syndrome: an Endocrine Society clinical practice guideline: commentary from a European perspective. *Eur J Endocrinol.* 2010;163:9-13. *An update on the 2008 Endocrine Society guidelines.*

Husebye ES, Perheentupa J, Rautemaa R, et al. Clinical manifestations and management of patients with autoimmune polyendocrine syndrome type I. *J Intern Med.* 2009;265:514-529. *Excellent clinical review, including unusual features of this rare condition.*

Kempers MJ, Lenders JW, van Outheusden L, et al. Systematic review: diagnostic procedures to differentiate unilateral from bilateral adrenal abnormality in primary aldosteronism. *Ann Intern Med.* 2009;15:329-337. *CT/MRI will misdiagnose the cause of primary aldosteronism in nearly 40% of cases, so adrenal vein sampling is needed for accurate diagnosis.*

Loriaux DL, Fleseriu M. Relative adrenal insufficiency. *Curr Opin Endocrinol Diabetes Obes.* 2009;16:392-400. *Up-to-date review of the literature regarding the use of corticosteroids in critical illness.*

Reisch N, Arlt W. Fine tuning for quality of life: 21st century approach to treatment of Addison's disease. *Endocrinol Metab Clin North Am.* 2009;38:407-418. *Comprehensive review of the treatment of adrenal insufficiency.*

Song JH, Mayo-Smith WW. Incidentally discovered adrenal mass. *Radiol Clin North Am.* 2011;49:361-368. *Review of imaging and evaluation.*

Speiser PW, Azziz R, Baskin LS, et al. Cogenital adrenal hyperplasia due to steroid 21-hydroxylase deficiency: an Endocrine Society clinical practice guideline. *J Clin Endocrinol Metab.* 2010;95:4133-4160. *Consensus guidelines for diagnosis and treatment.*

Terzolo M, Bovio S, Pia A, et al. Management of adrenal incidentaloma. *Best Pract Res Clin Endocrinol Metab.* 2009;23:233-243. *Comprehensive review of the work-up for adrenal masses.*

Tritos NA, Biller BM, Swearingen B. Management of Cushing disease. *Nat Rev Endocrinol.* 2011;7:279-289. *Comprehensive review of surgical, radiation, and medical treatments.*

Westerdahl C, Bergenfelz A, Isaksson A, et al. Primary aldosteronism among newly diagnosed and untreated hypertensive patients in a Swedish primary care area. *Scand J Prim Health Care.* 2011;29:57-62. *Eleven (5.5%) of 200 patients had adrenal adenomas (3 patients) or bilateral adrenal hyperplasia (8 patients).*

235

ADRENAL MEDULLA, CATECHOLAMINES, AND PHEOCHROMOCYTOMA

WILLIAM F. YOUNG JR.

ADRENAL MEDULLA AND CATECHOLAMINES

The adrenal medulla occupies the central portion of the adrenal gland. Adrenomedullary cells are called chromaffin cells (they stain brown with chromium salts). Chromaffin cells differentiate in the center of the adrenal gland in response to cortisol; some chromaffin cells also migrate to form paraganglia. The largest cluster of chromaffin cells outside the adrenal medulla is near the level of the inferior mesenteric artery and is referred to as the organ of Zuckerkandl.

The term *catecholamine* refers to substances that contain catechol (*o*-dihydroxybenzene) and a side chain with an amino group—the catechol nucleus (Fig. 235-1). Epinephrine is synthesized and stored in the adrenal medulla and released into the systemic circulation. Norepinephrine is synthesized and stored not only in the adrenal medulla but also in the peripheral sympathetic nerves. Dopamine, the precursor of norepinephrine, is found in the adrenal medulla and peripheral sympathetic nerves.

Catecholamines affect many cardiovascular and metabolic processes, including increasing the heart rate, blood pressure, myocardial contractility, and cardiac conduction velocity. Specific receptors mediate the biologic actions. The three types of adrenergic receptors are α, β, and DA; their receptor subtypes are α_1, α_2, β_1, β_2, β_3, DA_1, and DA_2. The α_1 subtype is a postsynaptic receptor that mediates vascular and smooth muscle contraction; stimulation causes vasoconstriction and increased blood pressure. The α_2 receptors are located on presynaptic sympathetic nerve endings and, when activated, inhibit the release of norepinephrine; stimulation causes suppression in central sympathetic outflow and decreased blood pressure. Stimulation of the β_1 receptor causes positive inotropic and chronotropic effects on the heart, increased renin secretion in the kidney, and lipolysis in adipocytes as well as bronchodilation, vasodilation in skeletal muscle, glycogenolysis, and increased release of norepinephrine from sympathetic nerve terminals. The β_3 receptor regulates energy expenditure and lipolysis. DA_1 receptors are localized to the cerebral, renal, mesenteric, and coronary vasculature; stimulation causes vasodilation in these vascular beds. DA_2 receptors are presynaptic and localized to sympathetic nerve endings, sympathetic ganglia, and brain; stimulation inhibits the release of norepinephrine, inhibits ganglionic transmission, and inhibits prolactin release.

Catecholamines are synthesized from tyrosine by a process of hydroxylation and decarboxylation (see Fig. 235-1). Tyrosine is derived from ingested food or synthesized from phenylalanine in the liver, and it enters neurons and chromaffin cells by active transport. Tyrosine is converted to 3,4-dihydroxyphenylalanine (dopa) by tyrosine hydroxylase, the rate-limiting step in catecholamine synthesis. α-Methyl-*p*-tyrosine (metyrosine) is a tyrosine hydroxylase inhibitor that may be used therapeutically in patients with catecholamine-secreting tumors. Aromatic L-amino acid decarboxylase catalyzes the decarboxylation of dopa to dopamine. Dopamine is actively transported into granulated vesicles to be hydroxylated to norepinephrine by the dopamine β-hydroxylase. These reactions occur in the synaptic vesicle of adrenergic neurons and the chromaffin cells of the adrenal medulla. In the adrenal medulla, norepinephrine is released from the granule into the cytoplasm, where phenylethanolamine *N*-methyltransferase converts it to epinephrine. Expression of phenylethanolamine *N*-methyltransferase is regulated by glucocorticoids. Thus, catecholamine-secreting tumors that secrete primarily epinephrine are localized to the adrenal medulla. In normal adrenal medullary tissue, approximately 80% of the catecholamine released is epinephrine.

The biologic half-life of circulating catecholamines is between 10 and 100 seconds. Thus, plasma concentrations of catecholamines fluctuate widely. Catecholamines are removed from the circulation by either reuptake by sympathetic nerve terminals or metabolism through two enzyme pathways (see Fig. 235-1), followed by sulfate conjugation and renal excretion. Almost 90% of catecholamines released at sympathetic synapses are taken up locally by the nerve endings (uptake 1). Uptake 1 can be blocked by cocaine, tricyclic antidepressants, and phenothiazine. Extraneuronal tissues also take up catecholamines (uptake 2). Most of these catecholamines are metabolized by catechol-*O*-methyltransferase. Metanephrine and normetanephrine are oxidized by monoamine oxidase to vanillylmandelic acid by oxidative deamination. Monoamine oxidase may also oxidize epinephrine and norepinephrine to 3,4-dihydroxymandelic acid, which is then converted by catechol-*O*-methyltransferase to vanillylmandelic acid. In the storage vesicle, norepinephrine is protected from metabolism by monoamine oxidase. Monoamine oxidase and catechol-*O*-methyltransferase metabolize dopamine to homovanillic acid (see Fig. 235-1).

PHEOCHROMOCYTOMA AND PARAGANGLIOMA

DEFINITION

Catecholamine-secreting tumors that arise from chromaffin cells of the adrenal medulla and the sympathetic ganglia are referred to as pheochromocytomas and extra-adrenal catecholamine-secreting paragangliomas, respectively. Because the tumors have similar clinical presentations and are treated with similar approaches, many clinicians use the term *pheochromocytoma* to refer to both entities. However, the distinction between pheochromocytoma and paraganglioma is an important one because there are differences in the risk for associated neoplasms, risk for malignant transformation, and type of genetic testing that should be considered.

EPIDEMIOLOGY

Catecholamine-secreting tumors are rare; the annual incidence is 2 to 8 cases per million people. Nevertheless, it is important to suspect, confirm, localize, and resect these tumors. The associated hypertension is curable with surgical removal of the tumor, a risk of lethal paroxysm exists, and at least 10% of the tumors are malignant. Fifteen percent to 20% of cases are familial, so detection of this tumor in the proband may result in early diagnosis in other family members.

PATHOBIOLOGY

Genetics

Approximately 15 to 20% of patients with catecholamine-secreting tumors have germline mutations (inherited mutations present in all cells of the body) in genes associated with genetic disease. Hereditary catecholamine-secreting tumors typically present at a younger age than sporadic neoplasms do. Sporadic pheochromocytoma is typically diagnosed on the basis of symptoms or incidental discovery on computed imaging, whereas syndromic pheochromocytoma is frequently diagnosed earlier in the course of disease because of biochemical surveillance or genetic testing.

Multiple Endocrine Neoplasia

Multiple endocrine neoplasia (MEN) type 2a is an autosomal dominant disorder (Chapters 239 and 254). The phenotype includes adrenal pheochromocytoma in 50% (usually bilateral and may be asynchronous), medullary

FIGURE 235-1. Biosynthetic and metabolic pathways for catecholamines. The term *catecholamine* comes from the catechol (*o*-dihydroxybenzene) structure and a side chain with an amino group—the catechol nucleus *(top left)*. Tyrosine is converted to 3,4-dihydroxyphenylalanine (dopa) in the rate-limiting step by tyrosine hydroxylase (TH). Aromatic L-amino acid decarboxylase (AADC) converts dopa to dopamine. Dopamine is hydroxylated to norepinephrine by dopamine β-hydroxylase (DBH). Norepinephrine is converted to epinephrine by phenylethanolamine *N*-methyltransferase (PNMT); cortisol serves as a cofactor for phenylethanolamine *N*-methyltransferase, and this is why epinephrine-secreting pheochromocytomas are almost exclusively localized to the adrenal medulla. Metabolism of catecholamines occurs through two enzymatic pathways. Catechol-*O*-methyltransferase (COMT) converts epinephrine to metanephrine and norepinephrine to normetanephrine by meta-*O*-methylation. Metanephrine and normetanephrine are oxidized by monoamine oxidase (MAO) to vanillylmandelic acid by oxidative deamination. Monoamine oxidase also may oxidize epinephrine and norepinephrine to dihydroxymandelic acid, which is then converted by catechol-*O*-methyltransferase to vanillylmandelic acid. Dopamine is also metabolized by monoamine oxidase and catechol-*O*-methyltransferase, with the final metabolite homovanillic acid.

carcinoma of the thyroid in 100%, hyperparathyroidism in 20 to 30%, and cutaneous lichen amyloidosis in 5%. Medullary carcinoma of the thyroid is usually detected before pheochromocytoma. Numerous activating mutations in the *RET* proto-oncogene have been documented in persons with MEN type 2a (these are described in detail in Chapter 254).

MEN type 2b is also an autosomal dominant disorder, and it represents approximately 5% of all MEN type 2 cases. The phenotype includes pheochromocytoma in 50% (usually bilateral), medullary carcinoma of the thyroid in 100%, mucosal neuromas (typically involving the tongue, lips, and eyelids) in most patients, thickened corneal nerves, intestinal ganglioneuromatosis, and marfanoid body habitus. MEN 2b–associated tumors are caused by mutations in the RET protein's intracellular domain, as described in detail in Chapter 254.

Von Hippel-Lindau Disease

Von Hippel-Lindau (VHL) disease is an autosomal dominant disorder characterized by pheochromocytoma (frequently bilateral), paraganglioma (mediastinal, abdominal, pelvic), hemangioblastoma (involving the cerebellum, spinal cord, or brain stem), retinal angioma, clear cell renal cell carcinoma, pancreatic neuroendocrine tumor, endolymphatic sac tumor of the middle ear, serous cystadenoma of the pancreas, and papillary cystadenoma of the epididymis and broad ligament. Pheochromocytoma is reported to occur in about 10 to 20% of patients with VHL disease. Nearly 100% of patients have an identifiable gene mutation (VHL tumor suppressor gene). Certain missense mutations appear to be associated with a "pheochromocytoma only" presentation of VHL disease.

Neurofibromatosis

Neurofibromatosis type 1 (NF1) is an autosomal dominant disorder characterized by neurofibromas, multiple café au lait spots, axillary and inguinal freckling, iris hamartomas (Lisch nodules), bony abnormalities, central nervous system gliomas, pheochromocytoma and paraganglioma, macrocephaly, and cognitive deficits. The expression of these features is variable. Approximately 2% of patients with NF1 develop catecholamine-secreting tumors; in these patients, the tumor is usually a solitary benign adrenal pheochromocytoma, occasionally bilateral adrenal pheochromocytomas, and rarely an abdominal paraganglioma. Inactivating *NF1* mutations cause the disorder (NF1 tumor suppressor gene).

Familial Paraganglioma

Familial paraganglioma is an autosomal dominant disorder characterized by paragangliomas that are located in the head and neck, thorax, abdomen, and pelvis. Most cases of familial paraganglioma are caused by mutations in the succinate dehydrogenase (SDH; succinate:ubiquinone oxidoreductase) subunit genes (*SDHB, SDHC, SDHD, SDHAF2, SDHA*), which compose portions of mitochondrial complex II. Inactivating germline mutations in *SDHD* have been identified in multigenerational families with head and neck parasympathetic paragangliomas that are usually nonfunctional, and occasionally in those with adrenal pheochromocytoma. In patients with *SDHD* mutations, penetrance depends on the mutation's parent of origin. Hence, the disease does not manifest when the mutation is inherited from the mother but is highly penetrant when it is inherited from the father. This phenomenon is known as maternal imprinting. Missense mutations in *SDHC*, located on chromosome 1q21, have been reported in families with head and neck parasympathetic paragangliomas that are usually nonfunctional. Multiple cofactors are required for normal activity of the SDH complex, including flavin-adenine dinucleotide (FAD) in the SDH1subunit. FAD is covalently attached to Sdh1, and deletion of *SDHAF2* causes a complete loss of FAD cofactor attachment (flavination) of Sdh1. Germline loss-of-function mutations in the *SDHAF2* gene, located on chromosome 11q13.1, have been associated with disease in a family with hereditary paraganglioma. Like families with mutations in *SDHD*, those with mutations in *SDHAF2* also exhibit maternal imprinting and parasympathetic paragangliomas that typically occur in the head and neck. Inactivating mutations in the tumor suppressor gene *SDHB*, located on chromosome 1p35-36, are associated with paragangliomas in the abdomen, pelvis, and mediastinum. Adrenal pheochromocytomas may also be found in patients with *SDHB* mutations. Patients with *SDHB* mutations have an increased risk for malignant paraganglioma.

Genetic Testing

Genetic testing should be considered if a patient has one or more of the following: paraganglioma, bilateral adrenal pheochromocytomas, unilateral adrenal pheochromocytoma and a family history of pheochromocytoma or paraganglioma, onset of unilateral adrenal pheochromocytoma at a young age (before 30 years), or other clinical findings suggestive of one of the previously discussed syndromic disorders. Genetic testing can be complex; testing of one family member has implications for related individuals. Genetic counseling is recommended to help families understand the implications of genetic test results; to coordinate the testing of at-risk individuals; and to help families work through the psychosocial issues that may arise before, during, or after the testing process. A list of clinically approved molecular genetic diagnostic laboratories is available at *www.genetests.org*.

CLINICAL MANIFESTATIONS

Catecholamine-secreting tumors occur with equal frequency in men and women, primarily in the third, fourth, and fifth decades of life. These tumors are rare in children; when discovered, they may be multifocal and associated with a hereditary syndrome. When symptoms are present, they are due to the pharmacologic effects of excess concentrations of circulating catecholamines (Table 235-1). The resulting hypertension may be sustained (in approximately half of patients) or paroxysmal (in approximately a third of patients). The remaining patients have normal blood pressure. Episodic symptoms may occur in spells, or paroxysms, that can be extremely variable in presentation but typically include forceful heartbeat, pallor, tremor, headache, and diaphoresis. The spell may start with the sensation of a "rush" in the chest and a sense of shortness of breath, followed by a "pounding" heartbeat in the chest that typically progresses to a throbbing headache. Peripheral vasoconstriction with a spell results in cool or cold hands and feet and facial

TABLE 235-1	SIGNS AND SYMPTOMS ASSOCIATED WITH CATECHOLAMINE-SECRETING TUMORS

SPELL RELATED

Anxiety and fear of impending death
Diaphoresis
Dyspnea
Epigastric and chest pain
Headache
Hypertension
Nausea and vomiting
Pallor
Palpitation (forceful heartbeat)
Tremor

CHRONIC

Anxiety and fear of impending death
Cold hands and feet
Congestive heart failure—dilated or hypertrophic cardiomyopathy
Constipation
Diaphoresis
Dyspnea
Ectopic hormone secretion–dependent symptoms (e.g., CRH/ACTH, GHRH, PTH-RP, VIP)
Epigastric and chest pain
Fatigue
Fever
General increase in sweating
Grade II to IV retinopathy
Headache
Hyperglycemia
Hypertension
Nausea and vomiting
Orthostatic hypotension
Painless hematuria (associated with urinary bladder paraganglioma)
Pallor
Palpitation (forceful heartbeat)
Tremor
Weight loss

NOT TYPICAL OF PHEOCHROMOCYTOMA

Flushing

ACTH = adrenocorticotropic hormone; CRH = corticotropin-releasing hormone; GHRH = growth hormone–releasing hormone; PTH-RP = parathyroid hormone–related peptide; VIP = vasoactive intestinal polypeptide.
Modified from Young WF Jr. Pheochromocytoma: 1926-1993. *Trends Endocrinol Metab.* 1993;4:122-127.

pallor. Increased sense of body heat and sweating are common symptoms that occur toward the end of the spell. Spells may be spontaneous or precipitated by postural change, anxiety, medications (e.g., metoclopramide, anesthetic agents), exercise, or maneuvers that increase intra-abdominal pressure (e.g., change in position, lifting, defecation, exercise, colonoscopy, pregnancy, trauma). Although the types of spells experienced by patients are highly variable, spells tend to be stereotypical for each patient. Spells may occur multiple times a day or as infrequently as once a month. The typical duration of a pheochromocytoma spell is 15 to 20 minutes, but it may be much shorter or last several hours. The clinician must recognize that most patients with spells do not have a pheochromocytoma.

Additional clinical signs of catecholamine-secreting tumors include hypertensive retinopathy, orthostatic hypotension, angina, nausea, constipation (megacolon may be the presenting symptom), hyperglycemia, diabetes mellitus, hypercalcemia, Raynaud's phenomenon, livedo reticularis, erythrocytosis, and mass effects from the tumor. Fasting hyperglycemia and diabetes mellitus are caused in part by the α-adrenergic inhibition of insulin release. Painless hematuria and paroxysmal attacks induced by micturition and defecation are associated with urinary bladder paragangliomas. Some of the co-secreted hormones that may dominate the clinical presentation include corticotropin (Cushing's syndrome), parathyroid hormone–related peptide (hypercalcemia), vasopressin (syndrome of inappropriate antidiuretic hormone secretion), vasoactive intestinal peptide (watery diarrhea), and growth hormone–releasing hormone (acromegaly) (see Table 235-1). Cardiomyopathy and congestive heart failure are the symptomatic presentations of pheochromocytoma that are most frequently unrecognized by clinicians. Cardiomyopathy, whether dilated or hypertrophic, may be totally reversible with tumor resection. Some patients with pheochromocytoma may be

FIGURE 235-2. Contrast-enhanced computed tomography of the abdomen in a 32-year-old second-year medical student with the peripartum discovery of a pheochromocytoma. The plasma fractionated metanephrines were abnormal: metanephrine, 0.19 nmol/L (normal, <0.5 nmol/L); normetanephrine, 28.6 nmol/L (normal, <0.9 nmol/L). The 24-hour urine studies were abnormal: norepinephrine, 781 µg (normal, <170 µg); epinephrine, 2.4 µg (normal, <35 µg); dopamine, 197 µg (normal, <700 µg); metanephrine, 117 µg (normal, <400 µg); normetanephrine, 8760 µg (normal, <900 µg). The axial image shows a typical 5-cm heterogeneously enhancing right adrenal mass, consistent with pheochromocytoma (*arrow*). After α- and β-adrenergic blockade, a 5.3- × 5.0- × 2.0-cm, 40-g pheochromocytoma was removed laparoscopically.

TABLE 235-2	MEDICATIONS THAT MAY INCREASE MEASURED LEVELS OF CATECHOLAMINES AND METANEPHRINES

Tricyclic antidepressants (including cyclobenzaprine)

Levodopa

Drugs containing adrenergic receptor agonists (e.g., decongestants)

Amphetamines

Buspirone and antipsychotic agents

Prochlorperazine

Reserpine

Withdrawal from clonidine and other drugs

Ethanol

Acetaminophen (may increase measured levels of plasma fractionated metanephrines in some assays)

asymptomatic despite high circulating levels of catecholamines, probably reflecting adrenergic receptor desensitization related to chronic stimulation.

Pheochromocytomas are localized to the adrenal glands, with an average diameter of 4.5 cm (Fig. 235-2). Paragangliomas are found where there is chromaffin tissue: along the para-aortic sympathetic chain, within the organs of Zuckerkandl (at the origin of the inferior mesenteric artery), in the wall of the urinary bladder, and along the sympathetic chain in the neck or mediastinum. Paragangliomas in the head and neck region (e.g., carotid body tumors, glomus tumors, chemodectomas) usually arise from parasympathetic tissue and typically do not hypersecrete catecholamines and metanephrines, whereas paragangliomas in the mediastinum, abdomen, and pelvis usually arise from sympathetic chromaffin tissue and usually do hypersecrete catecholamines and metanephrines.

DIAGNOSIS

Differential Diagnosis
Numerous disorders can cause signs and symptoms that may lead the clinician to test for pheochromocytoma. These disorders span much of medicine and include endocrine disorders (e.g., primary hypogonadism), cardiovascular disorders (e.g., idiopathic orthostatic hypotension), psychological disorders (e.g., panic disorder), pharmacologic causes (e.g., withdrawal from an adrenergic inhibitor), neurologic disorders (e.g., postural orthostatic tachycardia syndrome), and miscellaneous disorders (e.g., mast cell disease). Indeed, most patients tested for pheochromocytoma do not have it. In addition, fractionated catecholamines and metanephrines may be elevated in several clinical scenarios: withdrawal from medications or drugs (e.g., clonidine, alcohol), any acute illness (e.g., subarachnoid hemorrhage, migraine headache, preeclampsia), and administration of many drugs and medications (e.g., tricyclic antidepressants, cocaine, phencyclidine, lysergic acid diethylamide, amphetamines, ephedrine, pseudoephedrine, phenylpropanolamine, isoproterenol) (Table 235-2).

Pheochromocytoma should be suspected in patients who have one or more of the following: hyperadrenergic spells (e.g., self-limited episodes of nonexertional palpitations, diaphoresis, headache, tremor, or pallor); resistant hypertension; a familial syndrome that predisposes to catecholamine-secreting tumors (e.g., MEN type 2, NF1, VHL disease); a family history of pheochromocytoma or a history of a resected pheochromocytoma and a present history of recurrent hypertension or spells; an incidentally discovered adrenal mass; hypertension and diabetes; pressor response during anesthesia, surgery, or angiography; onset of hypertension at a young age (before 20 years); and idiopathic dilated cardiomyopathy.

Laboratory Findings
The diagnosis must be confirmed biochemically by increased concentrations of fractionated catecholamines and fractionated metanephrines in the urine

or plasma (Fig. 235-3). Most laboratories now measure fractionated catecholamines (dopamine, norepinephrine, and epinephrine) and metanephrines (metanephrine and normetanephrine) by high-performance liquid chromatography with electrochemical detection or tandem mass spectroscopy. These techniques have overcome the problems with fluorometric analysis (e.g., false-positive results caused by α-methyldopa, labetalol, sotalol, and imaging contrast agents). One of the most reliable methods of identifying catecholamine-secreting tumors is measurement of metanephrines and catecholamines in a 24-hour urine collection (sensitivity, 98%; specificity, 98%). If clinical suspicion is high, plasma fractionated metanephrines should also be measured. Some groups have advocated the measurement of plasma fractionated metanephrines as a first-line test for pheochromocytoma; the predictive value of a negative test result is extremely high, and the finding of normal plasma fractionated metanephrines excludes pheochromocytoma, except in patients with early preclinical disease and those with strictly dopamine-secreting neoplasms. A plasma test is also attractive because of its simplicity. Although measurement of plasma fractionated metanephrines has a sensitivity of 96 to 100%, the specificity is poor at only 85 to 89%; the specificity falls to 77% in patients older than 60 years. It has been estimated that 97% of patients with hypertension seen in a tertiary care clinic who have abnormal plasma fractionated metanephrine measurements do not have pheochromocytoma. This high false-positive rate results in excessive health care expenditures because of subsequent imaging and potentially inappropriate surgery. Thus, plasma fractionated metanephrines lack the necessary specificity to be recommended as a first-line test; this measurement is reserved for cases in which the index of suspicion is high. In addition, measurement of plasma fractionated metanephrines is a good first-line test for children because it is difficult to obtain a complete 24-hour urine collection.

The index of suspicion for pheochromocytoma should be high (see Fig. 235-3) in patients with the clinical scenarios described earlier and in those with an incidentally discovered adrenal mass that has imaging characteristics consistent with pheochromocytoma. These include marked enhancement with intravenous contrast medium on computed tomography (CT), high signal intensity on T2-weighted magnetic resonance imaging (MRI), cystic and hemorrhagic changes, bilaterality, and large size (>4 cm) (see later).

Although it is preferable for patients not to receive any medications during the diagnostic evaluation, treatment with most medications can be continued. Tricyclic antidepressants interfere most frequently with the interpretation of 24-hour urinary fractionated catecholamines and metanephrines. For the effective detection of catecholamine-secreting tumors, treatment with tricyclic antidepressants and other psychoactive agents listed in Table 235-2 should be tapered and discontinued at least 2 weeks before any hormonal assessments. Furthermore, catecholamine secretion may be appropriately increased in situations of physical stress or illness (e.g., stroke, myocardial infarction, congestive heart failure, obstructive sleep apnea). Therefore, the clinical circumstances under which catecholamines and metanephrines are measured must be assessed in each case.

Imaging
Localization studies should not be initiated until biochemical studies have confirmed the diagnosis of a catecholamine-secreting tumor (see Fig. 235-3). Computer-assisted imaging of the adrenal glands and abdomen with CT or

FIGURE 235-3. Evaluation and treatment of catecholamine-secreting tumors. Clinical suspicion is triggered by the following: paroxysmal symptoms (especially hypertension); hypertension that is intermittent, unusually labile, or resistant to treatment; family history of pheochromocytoma or associated conditions; or incidentally discovered adrenal mass. The details are discussed in the text. CT = computed tomography; ^{123}I-MIBG = ^{123}I-metaiodobenzylguanidine; Met = metanephrine; MRI = magnetic resonance imaging; nl = normal; Nmet = normetanephrine; PET = positron emission tomography. (Modified from Young WF Jr. Pheochromocytoma: 1926-1993. *Trends Endocrinol Metab.* 1993;4:122.)

MRI should be the first localization test (sensitivity, >95%; specificity, >65%). Approximately 85% of these tumors are found in the adrenal glands, and 95% are found in the abdomen. If the results of abdominal imaging are normal, scintigraphic localization with ^{123}I-labeled metaiodobenzylguanidine (^{123}I-MIBG) is indicated (see Fig. 235-3). This radiopharmaceutical agent accumulates preferentially in catecholamine-producing tumors (sensitivity, 88%; specificity, 84%). If a typical (<10 cm) unilateral adrenal pheochromocytoma is found on CT or MRI, ^{123}I-MIBG scintigraphy is superfluous, and the results may even cause confusion. If the adrenal pheochromocytoma is larger than 10 cm in diameter or if a paraganglioma is identified on CT or MRI, ^{123}I-MIBG scintigraphy is indicated because the patient has an increased risk of malignant disease and additional paragangliomas.

Other localizing procedures that can be used but are rarely required include computer-assisted imaging of the chest, neck, and head; somatostatin receptor imaging with [^{111}In]pentetreotide; and positron emission tomography scanning with [^{18}F]fluorodeoxyglucose, [^{11}C]hydroxyephedrine, or 6-[^{18}F]fluorodopamine (see Fig. 235-3). Because of marked gradients between the adrenal glands in non–pheochromocyotma patients, adrenal venous sampling for catecholamines is not helpful in the investigation of adrenal pheochromocytoma.

TREATMENT Rx

Medical Therapy

Some form of preoperative pharmacologic preparation is indicated for all patients with catecholamine-secreting neoplasms. However, no randomized controlled trials have compared the different approaches. Combined α- and β-adrenergic blockade is one approach to control blood pressure and to prevent intraoperative hypertensive crises. α-Adrenergic blockade should be started 7 to 10 days preoperatively to normalize blood pressure and to expand the contracted blood volume. A longer duration of preoperative α-adrenergic

blockade is indicated in patients with recent myocardial infarction, catecholamine cardiomyopathy, and catecholamine-induced vasculitis. Blood pressure should be monitored with the patient in the seated and standing positions twice daily. Target blood pressure is less than 120/80 mm Hg (seated), with systolic blood pressure greater than 90 mm Hg (standing); both targets should be modified on the basis of the patient's age and comorbid disease. On the second or third day of α-adrenergic blockade, patients are encouraged to start a diet high in sodium content (≥5000 mg daily) because of the catecholamine-induced volume contraction and the orthostasis associated with α-adrenergic blockade. This degree of volume expansion may be contraindicated in patients with congestive heart failure or renal insufficiency. After adequate α-adrenergic blockade has been achieved, β-adrenergic blockade is initiated, which typically occurs 2 or 3 days preoperatively.

Phenoxybenzamine is the preferred drug to control blood pressure and arrhythmia preoperatively. It is an irreversible, long-acting, nonspecific α-adrenergic blocking agent. The initial dosage is 10 mg once or twice daily, and the dose is increased by 10 to 20 mg in divided doses every 2 or 3 days as needed to control blood pressure and spells. The final dosage of phenoxybenzamine is typically between 20 and 100 mg daily.

The β-adrenergic antagonist should be administered only after α-adrenergic blockade is effective; with β-adrenergic blockade alone, hypertension may be more severe from the unopposed α-adrenergic stimulation. Preoperative β-adrenergic blockade is indicated to control the tachycardia associated with both the high concentrations of circulating catecholamines and the α-adrenergic blockade. The clinician should exercise caution if the patient is asthmatic or has congestive heart failure. Chronic catecholamine excess can produce a cardiomyopathy that may become evident with the initiation of β-adrenergic blockade, resulting in acute pulmonary edema. Therefore, the β-adrenergic blocker should be administered cautiously and at a low dose. Other agents that may be used to prepare the patient with pheochromocytoma for surgery include α-methyl-*p*-tyrosine (metyrosine) and calcium-channel blockers. Acute hypertensive crises may occur before or during an operation, and they should be treated with intravenous sodium nitroprusside, phentolamine, or nicardipine.

Surgical Therapy

The treatment of choice for pheochromocytoma is complete surgical resection. Surgical survival rates are 98 to 100% and are highly dependent on the skill of the endocrinologist–endocrine surgeon–anesthesiologist team. Careful preoperative pharmacologic preparation is crucial for successful treatment. Most catecholamine-secreting tumors are benign and can be totally excised. Tumor excision usually cures hypertension.

In the past, an anterior midline abdominal surgical approach was generally used to resect adrenal pheochromocytoma. However, the laparoscopic approach to the adrenal gland is currently the procedure of choice for a solitary intra-adrenal pheochromocytoma smaller than 8 cm in diameter. Laparoscopic adrenalectomy for pheochromocytoma should be converted to open adrenalectomy in cases of difficult dissection, invasion, adhesions, or an inexperienced surgeon. An anterior midline abdominal surgical approach is indicated for abdominal paragangliomas. The midline abdomen should be inspected carefully. Paragangliomas of the neck, chest, and urinary bladder require specialized approaches.

Management of Complications

Hypotension may occur during and after surgical resection of the pheochromocytoma, and it should be treated with fluids and colloids and then intravenous pressor agents if necessary. Postoperative hypotension is less frequent in patients who have had adequate preoperative α-adrenergic blockade and volume expansion. If both adrenal glands were manipulated during surgery, adrenocortical insufficiency should be considered a potential cause of postoperative hypotension. Because hypoglycemia can occur in the immediate postoperative period, blood glucose levels should be monitored, and intravenous fluids should contain 5% dextrose.

Approximately 1 to 2 weeks after surgery, fractionated catecholamines and metanephrines should be measured by collection of a 24-hour urine specimen. If the levels are normal, resection of the pheochromocytoma should be considered complete. Increased levels of fractionated catecholamines and metanephrines detected postoperatively are consistent with residual tumor due to either a second primary lesion or occult metastases. Common sites of metastasis include lymph nodes, liver, and bone.

Follow-up

The 24-hour urinary excretion of fractionated catecholamines and metanephrines or plasma fractionated metanephrines should be checked annually for life. Annual biochemical testing assesses for metastatic disease, tumor recurrence in the adrenal bed, or delayed appearance of multiple primary tumors. Follow-up CT or MRI is not needed unless the metanephrine or catecholamine levels become elevated or the original tumor was associated with minimal or no catecholamine or metanephrine excess.

MALIGNANT PHEOCHROMOCYTOMA AND PARAGANGLIOMA

Distinguishing between benign and malignant catecholamine-secreting tumors is difficult on the basis of clinical, biochemical, or histopathologic characteristics. Malignant disease is rare in patients with an adrenal familial syndrome but common in those with familial paraganglioma caused by mutations in *SDHB*. Although the 5-year survival rate for patients with malignant pheochromocytoma is less than 50%, the prognosis is variable; approximately 50% of patients have an indolent form of the disease, with a life expectancy of more than 20 years, and the other 50% have rapidly progressive disease, with death occurring 1 to 5 years after diagnosis. The clinician should assess the pace of the malignant disease and base the level of therapy on the aggressiveness of the tumor's behavior. A multimodality, multidisciplinary individualized approach is indicated to control catecholamine-dependent symptoms, local mass effects, and overall tumor burden.

PHEOCHROMOCYTOMA IN PREGNANCY

Pheochromocytoma in pregnancy can cause the death of both the fetus and the mother. The approach to the biochemical diagnosis is the same as for nonpregnant patients. MRI without gadolinium enhancement is the preferred imaging modality, and ^{123}I-MIBG scintigraphy is contraindicated. The treatment of hypertensive crises is the same as for nonpregnant patients, except that nitroprusside should be avoided. Although the most appropriate management is debated, adrenal pheochromocytomas should be removed promptly after α- and β-adrenergic blockade if the diagnosis is made during the first two trimesters of pregnancy. The preoperative preparation is the same as for nonpregnant patients. If the pregnancy is in the third trimester, one operation is recommended for cesarean delivery and removal of the adrenal pheochromocytoma at the same time. Spontaneous labor and delivery should be avoided.

The management of catecholamine-secreting paragangliomas in pregnancy may require modification of these guidelines, depending on tumor location.

SUGGESTED READINGS

Ayala-Ramirez M, Feng L, Johnson MM, et al. Clinical risk factors for malignancy and overall survival in patients with pheochromocytomas and sympathetic paragangliomas: primary tumor size and primary tumor location as prognostic indicators. *J Clin Endocrinol Metab.* 2011;96:717-725. *Size and location (mediastinum or infradiaphragmatic para-aortic area) were significant risk factors for metastasis and decreased survival.*

Chen H, Sippel RS, O'Dorisio MS, et al. The North American Neuroendocrine Tumor Society consensus guideline for the diagnosis and management of neuroendocrine tumors: pheochromocytoma, paraganglioma, and medullary thyroid cancer. *Pancreas.* 2010;39:775-783. *Consensus guidelines.*

Opocher G, Schiavi F. Genetics of pheochromocytomas and paragangliomas. *Best Pract Res Clin Endocrinol Metab.* 2010;24:943-956. *Review of genetics and genetic and family testing.*

Wiseman GA, Pacak K, O'Dorisio MS, et al. Usefulness of ^{123}I-MIBG scintigraphy in the evaluation of patients with known or suspected primary or metastatic pheochromocytoma or paraganglioma: results from a prospective multicenter trial. *J Nucl Med.* 2009;50:1448-1454. *A large prospective study found 88% sensitivity and 84% specificity for ^{123}I-MIBG imaging used in the diagnostic assessment of primary or metastatic pheochromocytoma or paraganglioma.*

236

TYPE 1 DIABETES MELLITUS

SILVIO E. INZUCCHI AND ROBERT S. SHERWIN

TYPE 1 DIABETES MELLITUS

DEFINITION

Diabetes mellitus is a chronic disorder characterized by hyperglycemia and the late development of vascular and neuropathic complications. Regardless of its cause, the disease is associated with a common hormonal defect—namely, insulin deficiency—that may be absolute or relative in the context of coexisting insulin resistance. The effect of insufficient insulin plays a primary role in the metabolic derangements linked to diabetes; hyperglycemia, in turn, plays an important role in disease-related complications.

CLASSIFICATION

The American Diabetes Association classification scheme for diabetes mellitus is summarized in Table 236-1. Clinical diabetes is divided into four general subclasses: type 1, primarily caused by autoimmune pancreatic β-cell destruction and characterized by absolute insulin deficiency; type 2, characterized by insulin resistance and relative insulin deficiency; other specific types of diabetes (associated with identifiable clinical conditions or syndromes); and gestational diabetes mellitus. In addition to these clinical categories, impaired glucose tolerance, impaired fasting glucose, and a high glycohemoglobin (hemoglobin A_{1c} [HbA_{1c}] 5.7 to 6.4%), sometimes referred to as *pre-diabetes*, describe intermediate metabolic states between normal glucose homeostasis and overt diabetes. Both impaired glucose tolerance and impaired fasting glucose significantly increase the risk for the future development of diabetes mellitus and in many cases are part of the disease's natural history. Patients with any form of diabetes may require insulin therapy; for this reason, the previously used terms *insulin-dependent diabetes* (type 1) and *non-insulin-dependent diabetes* (type 2) have been eliminated.

EPIDEMIOLOGY

In 2008 the Centers for Disease Control and Prevention estimated that nearly 24 million Americans (or nearly 8% of the U.S. population) fulfilled the diagnostic criteria for diabetes mellitus. Most (90 to 95%) have type 2 diabetes, and approximately one in four of these individuals is unaware of the diagnosis (Chapter 237). In those older than 60 years, the prevalence is now estimated at almost 25%. An additional 57 million Americans have prediabetes. Since 1980, the prevalence of diabetes in the United States has more than quadrupled. The number of affected patients continues to rise, with current estimates exceeding 1.6 million new cases per year in those older than 20 years. The most recent estimates of diabetes in youth reveal that approximately 15,000 are diagnosed with type 1 diabetes and nearly 4000 with type 2 diabetes each year. It is estimated that one of every three Americans born in the past decade will develop diabetes in their lifetime. Diabetes is the fourth most common reason for contact with a physician, accounting for

TABLE 236-1   CLASSIFICATION OF DIABETES MELLITUS

ESTABLISHED DIABETES MELLITUS

Type 1 diabetes, formerly known as insulin-dependent diabetes mellitus or
  juvenile-onset diabetes (primarily due to β-cell destruction, usually leading to
  absolute insulin deficiency)
  Immune mediated
  Idiopathic
Type 2 diabetes, formerly known as non-insulin-dependent diabetes or adult-onset
  diabetes (may range from predominantly insulin resistance with relative insulin
  deficiency to predominantly secretory defect with insulin resistance)
Other specific types ("secondary diabetes")
  Genetic defects of β-cell function (e.g., maturity-onset diabetes of the young,
    types 1 to 9; point mutations in mitochondrial DNA)
  Genetic defects in insulin action (e.g., type A insulin resistance, leprechaunism,
    Rabson-Mendenhall syndrome, lipoatrophic diabetes)
  Disease of the exocrine pancreas (e.g., pancreatitis, trauma, pancreatectomy,
    neoplasia, cystic fibrosis, hemochromatosis, fibrocalculous pancreatopathy)
  Endocrinopathies (e.g., acromegaly, Cushing's syndrome, hyperthyroidism,
    pheochromocytoma, glucagonoma, somatostatinoma, aldosteronoma)
  Drug or chemical induced (e.g., vacor, pentamidine, nicotinic acid,
    glucocorticoids, thyroid hormone, diazoxide, β-adrenergic agonists, thiazides,
    phenytoin, interferon-α)
  Infections (e.g., congenital rubella, cytomegalovirus)
  Uncommon forms of immune-mediated diabetes (e.g., "stiff-man" syndrome,
    anti-insulin receptor antibodies)
  Other genetic syndromes (e.g., Down syndrome, Klinefelter's syndrome, Turner's
    syndrome, Wolfram's syndrome, Friedreich's ataxia, Huntington's disease,
    Laurence-Moon-Biedl syndrome, myotonic dystrophy, porphyria, Prader-Willi
    syndrome)
Gestational diabetes mellitus

RISK CATEGORIES FOR DIABETES MELLITUS

Impaired fasting glucose
Impaired glucose tolerance
Increased glycohemoglobin

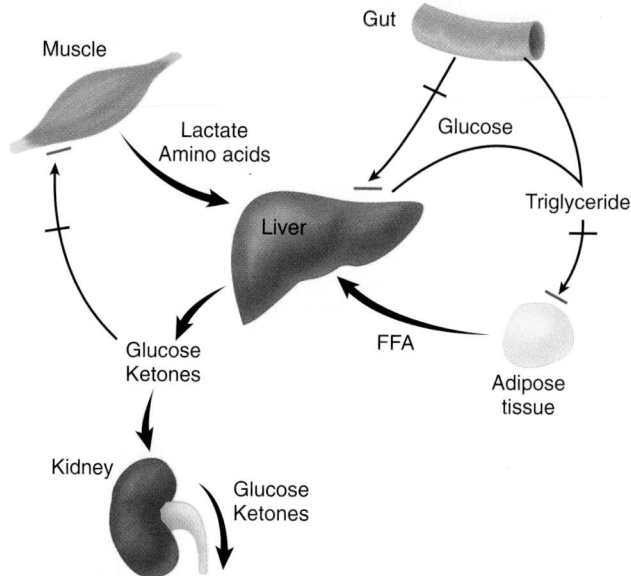

FIGURE 236-1. Effects of severe insulin deficiency on body fuel metabolism. Lack of insulin leads to mobilization of substrates for gluconeogenesis and ketogenesis from muscle and adipose tissue, accelerated production of glucose and ketones by the liver, and impaired removal of endogenous and exogenous fuels by insulin-responsive tissues. The net results are severe hyperglycemia and hyperketonemia that overwhelm renal removal mechanisms. FFA = free fatty acids.

approximately 14% of U.S. health care dollars and total annual costs exceeding $174 billion in 2007—$116 billion in direct medical costs, and another $58 billion in indirect costs due to losses in productivity. Worldwide, diabetes affects more than 220 million people; this figure is projected to double by the year 2030. The rate of increase in diabetes is greatest in developing nations as a result of urbanization and Westernization of lifestyle habits where barriers still exist to proper diagnosis and treatment.

Diabetes is a leading cause of both mortality and early disability; in the United States, it is the leading cause of blindness among working-age adults, end-stage renal disease, and nontraumatic limb amputation. Diabetes increases the risk of cardiac, cerebral, and peripheral vascular disease two- to seven-fold and is a major contributor to neonatal morbidity and mortality. A growing body of evidence, however, suggests that most if not all of the debilitating complications of diabetes can be prevented or delayed by the prospective treatment of hyperglycemia and other cardiovascular risk factors. In treating diabetes, the timing of therapy is crucial; clinical outcomes depend on early recognition and treatment of the disease.

Incidence and Prevalence

Prevalence rates for type 1 diabetes are relatively accurate because these patients invariably become symptomatic. In the United States, this rate is approximately 0.3%, with an annual incidence in youths of approximately 19 per 100,000. Type 1 diabetes is more prevalent in Finland, Scandinavia, and the United Kingdom; less prevalent in most of southern Europe and the Middle East; and relatively uncommon in Asian nations. The annual incidence appears to have risen in the last half century, which could imply the introduction of unidentified environmental factors. Prevalence rates are strikingly different among ethnic groups living in the same geographic region, probably because of genetic differences in susceptibility to the disease.

The recognition that type 1 diabetes has a protracted preclinical phase has shed new light on some epidemiologic characteristics of the disease. Type 1 diabetes has an increased incidence in the winter months and may be associated with specific viral epidemics. These observations may be explained in part by the superimposition of illness-provoked insulin resistance in patients with marginal β-cell function. Similarly, the common appearance of type 1

diabetes during puberty may be attributed to insulin resistance; even under normal circumstances, puberty is accompanied by impaired insulin-stimulated glucose metabolism. New methods for tracking islet-directed autoimmunity have led to a reappraisal of the age at which type 1 diabetes first appears. Although the age-specific incidence rises progressively from infancy to puberty and then declines, incidence rates persist at low levels for many decades; in fact, nearly 30% of patients are diagnosed after the age of 20 years. In patients with a later onset, the clinical syndrome tends to evolve more slowly; in addition, islet-directed antibody titers may be lower, and human leukocyte antigen (HLA) types may be different from those of younger patients. As a result, type 1 diabetes is initially misdiagnosed as type 2 in many of these patients.

PATHOBIOLOGY

Detailed discussion of the normal physiology of insulin secretion and action, the roles of other secretagogues and incretins, and the pathobiology of metabolic defects in diabetes is provided in the Web version of this chapter. Figure 236-1 summarizes the effects of insulin deficiency on body fuel metabolism.

Pathogenesis

Type 1 diabetes produces profound β-cell failure with secondary insulin resistance, whereas type 2 diabetes is associated with less severe insulin deficiency but greater impairment of insulin action. Given their similarities overall, it is not surprising that the two major forms of diabetes share many pathophysiologic features. However, despite the apparent phenotypic similarity, the underlying pathogenetic mechanisms leading to type 1 and type 2 diabetes are strikingly different (see Chapter 237 for the pathogenesis of type 2 diabetes). Type 1 diabetes most likely results from an interplay of genetic, environmental, and autoimmune factors that selectively destroy insulin-producing β cells (Fig. 236-2).

Genetic Factors

The role of genetic factors in type 1 diabetes is underscored by data in identical twins showing concordance rates of 30 to 40%. It has been assumed that because concordance rates are not 100%, environmental factors must be important for disease expression. Although the presence of an environmental trigger is highly likely, even identical twins do not express identical T-cell receptor and immunoglobulin genes; as a result, total concordance might not be expected.

Although many of the genes linked to type 1 diabetes have not been identified, some are known. HLA genes, located on the short arm of chromosome

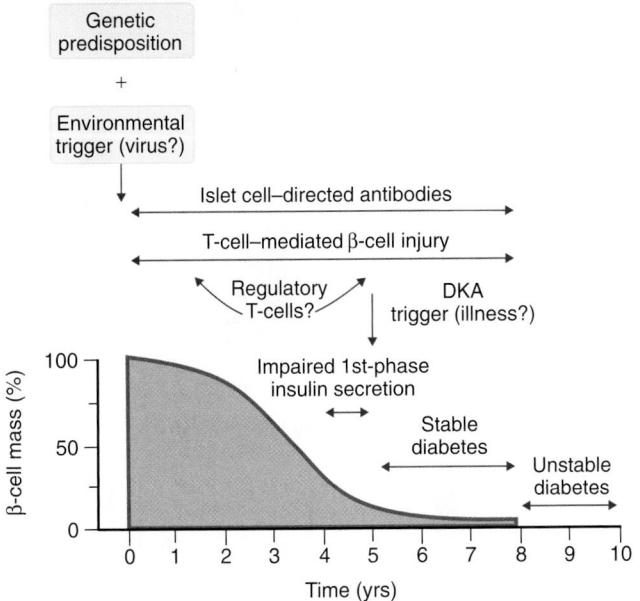

FIGURE 236-2. Summary of the sequence of events that lead to pancreatic β-cell loss and ultimately to the clinical evolution of type 1 diabetes. DKA = diabetic ketoacidosis.

6, clearly play a dominant role; in nonaffected siblings, the risk of developing diabetes is 15 to 20% if they are HLA identical, approximately 5% if they share one HLA gene, and less than 1% if no HLA genes are shared. Specific HLA haplotypes have been linked to type 1 diabetes; 90 to 95% of type 1 patients express DR3 or DR4 class II HLA molecules (compared with 50 to 60% of the general population), whereas 60% express both alleles, a rate more than 10-fold that of the general population. Another class II allele, DQB1*0602, has a negative association with the disease. Specific class II DQ haplotypes (e.g., DQ8 and DQ2) correlate even more strongly with disease susceptibility in white individuals; this susceptibility is associated with polymorphisms of the allele encoding the β chain of the DQ class II HLA molecule. The presence of aspartic acid at position 57 protects against disease, whereas substitution of a neutral amino acid at this position is associated with higher disease frequency. Other polymorphisms, such as the substitution of arginine at position 52 of the DQ α chain, may confer additional risk. Overall, it seems clear that significant genetic heterogeneity exists and that no single class II HLA gene accounts for all HLA-associated susceptibility to disease. Association of the disease with specific class II HLA genes implies the involvement of CD4+ T cells in the autoimmune process because these molecules are critical for both the presentation of antigenic peptides to CD4+ T cells and the selection of the CD4+ T-cell repertoire in the thymus.

Other genes likely contribute to the genetic susceptibility to type 1 diabetes. *IDDM2* (chromosome 11p), a noncoding promoter region of the insulin gene, may influence insulin gene expression in the thymus and may therefore affect thymic selection of insulin-reactive T cells. *CTLA4* (chromosome 2q) plays a role in T-cell action and regulation. Protein tyrosine phosphatase N22 (*PTPN22*) on chromosome 1 is also a regulator of T-cell activation. Many other genes have also been implicated, underscoring the polygenic nature of this disease.

Environmental Factors

Although environmental factors such as diet and toxins have been proposed as triggers of diabetes, most of the scientific attention has focused on putative viruses. Epidemics of mumps, congenital rubella, and coxsackievirus infection have been associated with an increased frequency of type 1 diabetes. Moreover, specific and convincing examples of virus-induced diabetes have been reported. However, it is likely that acute, lytic viral infections are responsible for only an occasional case of diabetes. Instead, if viruses are involved, it is far more likely that they trigger an autoimmune response. If a virus contains an epitope resembling a β-cell protein, viral infection could theoretically abrogate self-tolerance and trigger autoimmunity. It has recently been suggested, based on rodent models of type 1 diabetes, that disease expression may also be influenced by the microorganisms present in the gastrointestinal tract, the greatest surface area for interaction with the environment.

Autoimmune Factors

About 80% of patients with new-onset type 1 diabetes have islet cell antibodies. Antibodies to a variety of β-cell constituents have been identified, including insulin, isoforms of glutamic acid decarboxylase (GAD 65 and GAD 67), and the secretory granule protein islet cell antigen (ICA) 512 or IA-2, which contains a tyrosine phosphatase–like domain. The concept that type 1 diabetes is a chronic autoimmune disease with acute clinical manifestations is supported by the fact that islet antigen-directed antibodies may be present in asymptomatic first-degree relatives of patients. Such antibody-positive individuals are at risk for the development of type 1 diabetes, although the clinical onset may be delayed by many years. The likelihood of developing type 1 diabetes is greater than 50% if autoantibodies are present to more than one β-cell antigen (i.e., insulin, GAD 65, ICA 512); diabetes rarely develops in antibody-negative relatives. If antibodies appear at a young age, the risk for clinical diabetes is particularly high.

The listed antibodies appear to be markers for, rather than the cause of, β-cell injury. β-cell destruction (by apoptotic and cytotoxic mechanisms) is mediated by a variety of cytokines or by direct T-lymphocyte activity. Supporting this notion, type 1 diabetes has been transferred through bone marrow cells from a diabetic patient to a nondiabetic recipient. In addition, autopsies performed on patients who died soon after disease onset have shown islet-restricted monocytic cellular infiltrates (termed *insulitis*) that are composed of CD8+ and CD4+ T cells, macrophages, and B cells. Usually, as the disease progresses, the islets become completely devoid of β cells and inflammatory infiltrates; α, δ, and pancreatic polypeptide cells are left intact, thus illustrating the exquisite specificity of the autoimmune attack. At the time of clinical diagnosis, about 10 to 20% of the original β-cell mass typically remains (see Fig. 236-2). In most patients, there is gradual loss of these remaining β cells; some patients continue to exhibit residual insulin production for many years. These patients are generally easier to control with insulin and have fewer complications.

A critical role for T cells is supported by studies involving pancreatic transplantation in identical twins. Monozygotic twins with diabetes who received kidney and pancreas grafts from their nondiabetic, genetically identical siblings required little or no immunosuppression for graft acceptance. Nevertheless, the islets were soon selectively invaded by mononuclear cells, predominantly CD8+ T cells, with the subsequent recurrence of diabetes. Thus, decades after the original onset of the disease, the immune system retains the ability to selectively destroy β cells. Evidence implicating T cells also derives from clinical trials using immunosuppressive drugs. Drugs such as cyclosporine or antibodies directed against a component of the T-cell receptor (anti-CD3) or that alter antigen presentation by B cells (anti-CD20) slow the progression of recent-onset diabetes, but this effect is not sustained if immunosuppression is withdrawn. Further supporting data for T cells' primary role derive from NOD mice, in which insulitis and islet autoantibodies develop at about 4 weeks of age, and diabetes ultimately develops after 12 to 24 weeks; in these mice, a variety of treatments designed to deplete T cells can prevent diabetes. Most important, adoptive transfer of T cells isolated from diabetic mouse donors into immune-incompetent NOD mice rapidly produces diabetes. Both CD4+ and CD8+ T cells are generally required for the transfer of disease, which suggests that both are necessary for disease expression. These diabetogenic T cells target specific β-cell antigens, including insulin and GAD. A likely role for GAD or insulin is also suggested by data showing that if NOD mice are made tolerant to GAD or insulin (or to peptides derived from these molecules) early in life, insulitis and diabetes fail to develop. In keeping with the concept of immunomodulation, administration of a GAD vaccine reportedly slows the loss of β-cell function in patients with recent-onset diabetes. Finally, the chronic, smoldering nature of type 1 diabetes suggests the presence of regulatory or protective influences. In keeping with this observation, T cells that release immunoregulatory cytokines and, in turn, protect the islet from immune attack have been isolated from the islets of NOD mice. Such findings suggest that the rate of appearance and clinical expression of disease may be modulated by the balance between diabetogenic and protective populations of T cells. "Tipping the scales" in favor of protective T-cell proliferation is the goal of protective immunization.

CLINICAL MANIFESTATIONS

Patients with type 1 diabetes mellitus have little or no insulin secretory capacity and depend on exogenous insulin to prevent metabolic decompensation and death. Classically, symptoms appear relatively abruptly (i.e., over days or weeks) in previously healthy, nonobese children or young adults who may have close relatives with the disease but more commonly do not. Older patients often present more gradually. At the time of initial evaluation, most type 1 diabetic patients are ill and symptomatic, most commonly presenting with polyuria, polydipsia, polyphagia, blurred vision, fatigue, and weight loss; such patients may also present with ketoacidosis. Type 1 diabetes is believed to have a prolonged asymptomatic preclinical phase (often lasting years), during which pancreatic β cells are gradually destroyed by an autoimmune attack influenced by HLA and other genetic factors, as well as by the environment (see Fig. 236-2). In some patients, an acute illness and the development of secondary insulin resistance may speed the transition from the preclinical phase to clinical disease.

Initially, most type 1 patients require high-dose insulin therapy to restore a disordered metabolism. However, a so-called honeymoon period may follow (lasting weeks or months), during which smaller doses of insulin are needed because of partial recovery of β-cell function and reversal of the insulin resistance caused by acute illness. Thereafter, insulin secretory capacity is gradually lost; in some patients, particularly older individuals, this process commonly takes several years, sometimes referred to as latent autoimmune diabetes of adulthood. The rate of decline is slowed by intensive insulin therapy targeting near normoglycemia.

DIAGNOSIS

Because diagnosis and screening are more germane to the evaluation of patients with type 2 diabetes or other forms of diabetes, this topic is reviewed in Chapter 237.

TREATMENT   Rx

In type 1 diabetes, the primary focus of treatment is to replace the insulin secretion that has been lost. A healthy lifestyle is also required to facilitate insulin therapy and to optimize health. In the short term, the goals of diabetes treatment are to optimize metabolic control, improve the patient's sense of clinical well-being, and prevent long-term complications.

Management of Complications
Relation between Diabetes Control and Its Complications

Whether the vascular and neuropathic complications of diabetes mellitus can be prevented or delayed by improved glycemic control was debated for more than half a century. The definitive answer was provided by the Diabetes Control and Complications Trial (DCCT), a 9-year multicenter study involving 1441 type 1 patients aged 13 to 39 years who were randomly assigned to either intensive insulin therapy or conventional care.[1] The intensive therapy group used multiple insulin injections or an insulin pump to maintain premeal blood glucose levels of 70 to 120 mg/dL, postprandial blood levels of less than 180 mg/dL, and glycohemoglobin (HbA1c) values as close as possible to normal. In the conventional care group, the primary goal was simply to maintain clinical well-being, usually with two injections per day. The DCCT achieved a clear separation of glucose levels between the two groups during the study period. HbA1c and mean glucose levels in the intensive therapy group were 1.5 to 2.0% and 60 to 80 mg/dL lower, respectively, than in those receiving conventional care. Intensive therapy reduced the development of retinopathy by 76% in the primary prevention group and the progression of retinopathy by 54% in the secondary intervention group (Fig. 236-3); the latter effect became apparent after only 4 years. In addition, intensive therapy reduced the risk of microalbuminuria by 39%, frank proteinuria by 54%, and clinical neuropathy by 60%. The incidence of major cardiovascular events also tended to be lower, but the number of events was insufficient for statistical proof; at the very least, intensive therapy did not pose a risk for macrovascular complications. An exponential relationship over time between the average blood glucose level (as reflected by HbA1c) and the progression of retinopathy in the intensive care group suggests that there may be no threshold level at which complications occur. These findings imply that any degree of improvement in glycemic control has benefit and that normalization of glucose levels is not required to slow the progression of diabetic complications.

However, the benefits achieved by intensive control in the DCCT were not without risk. Weight gain was more common in the intensive care group. Most important, the frequency of severe hypoglycemia (including multiple episodes in some patients) was three-fold higher in the intensive care group. It is reasonable to conclude that in some patients, the risks of intensive therapy may outweigh the benefits; possibly included are patients with recurrent severe hypoglycemia and decreased perception of hypoglycemia, patients with advanced complications that are less likely to benefit from glucose lowering, young children, and patients who are unable or unwilling to participate in their management (e.g., self-monitoring of blood glucose level). Such individuals are likely to benefit from less aggressive therapy designed to lower glucose levels moderately without the risk of hypoglycemia. Despite the higher rate of

FIGURE 236-3. Summary of the results of the Diabetes Control and Complications Trial (DCCT).

hypoglycemia, intensive therapy in the DCCT had no detectable long-term effects on cognitive function.

Translating these results into clinical practice remains a challenge because patients require significant motivation to comply with the intensive monitoring and insulin administration regimens necessary. Significant expertise is also required on the part of practitioners to manage these individuals properly on an ongoing basis. An important lesson from these studies is that successful treatment of diabetes is largely accomplished through the efforts of the patients themselves, as well as by nurse educators, dietitians, and diabetes counselors.

In an update involving the original DCCT cohort, the Epidemiology of Diabetes Interventions and Complications (EDIC) study, the beneficial effect of intensive glycemic control on microvascular complications persisted.[2] Even more important, the intensively treated group had long-lived cardiovascular benefits. Among the 1375 volunteers who agreed to participate in this observational extension of the DCCT, the intensively treated patients had less than half the number of cardiovascular events (myocardial infarction, coronary revascularization, stroke) of the conventionally treated group (46 vs. 98 events) during a total of 17 years of follow-up. These results were all the more impressive because the mean HbA1c in the intensively treated group had actually risen to about 8% from about 7% during the EDIC study, whereas the conventionally treated group improved their mean HbA1c from about 9% to about 8%. Therefore, despite nearly equal glycemic control during most of the EDIC study, a persistent benefit in terms of macrovascular end points was observed after intensive treatment. Some have referred to this process as "metabolic memory" or the "legacy effect" of tight glucose control.

Medical Therapy
Insulin Preparations and Pharmacokinetics

A variety of highly purified insulin preparations are commercially available (Table 236-2). Premixed insulin preparations are also available and offer added convenience for selected patients with residual endogenous insulin secretion. Nearly all insulin preparations contain 100 U/mL (U-100), although a more concentrated preparation of 500 U/mL (U-500) of regular insulin can be obtained for severely resistant patients.

Short- and Rapid-Acting Insulin Preparations

After subcutaneous injection, regular (R) insulin begins to act in about 30 minutes and should therefore be administered 20 to 30 minutes before a meal. Because it acts relatively quickly and has a relatively short duration of action (5 to 8 hours), it is effective for blunting postprandial glucose excursions and

TABLE 236-2 INSULIN PREPARATIONS: ONSET OF EFFECT, PEAK EFFECT, AND DURATION OF ACTION AFTER SUBCUTANEOUS ADMINISTRATION

CLASS	PREPARATION	ONSET OF EFFECT	PEAK EFFECT (HR)	DURATION OF ACTION (HR)
Rapid acting	Lispro, aspart, glulisine	10-15 min	1-2	3-4
Short acting	Regular (R)	30 min	2-4	5-8
Intermediate acting	NPH (N)	2-4 hr	6-12	16-24
Long acting	Glargine	2-4 hr	No peak	>24
	Detemir	1 hr	No peak	Up to 24

for facilitating rapid dose adjustments based on measured blood glucose values. The properties of regular insulin are especially helpful in managing glucose elevations that occur during illness or after the consumption of large meals. Given by intravenous infusion, regular insulin is also effective in the perioperative period and in the management of severely ill hospitalized patients and acute hyperglycemic complications.

In regular insulin preparations, insulin molecules exist predominantly in hexameric form. Before being absorbed, insulin hexamers must first be diluted in subcutaneous interstitial fluid, then dissociate into single molecules; this property accounts for the slightly delayed absorption of regular insulin from subcutaneous injection sites. Advances in recombinant DNA technology led to the development of several insulin analogues intended to limit this property, allowing more rapid absorption in an effort to more closely mimic the normal brisk increase in endogenously secreted insulin in response to meals. Insulin lispro was the first analogue approved by the Food and Drug Administration (FDA), with amino acids in positions B28 (lysine) and B29 (proline) reversed. Lispro thereby has a reduced capacity for hexameric self-association and is more rapidly absorbed. Its effects begin within 10 to 15 minutes of administration and generally wane within 3 to 4 hours. In insulin aspart, a neutral proline residue at position B28 is replaced by negatively charged aspartic acid, resulting in a reduced capacity for self-association and faster absorption. The pharmacokinetic properties of insulin aspart are similar to those of insulin lispro; insulin aspart may have a slightly longer duration of effect. In a third rapid-acting insulin, insulin glulisine, lysine in position B29 is replaced by glutamic acid, and asparagine at position B3 is replaced by lysine, with changes in polarity similar to those seen with lispro and aspart. Because of their quick onset of action, these analogues can be administered a shorter time (<30 minutes) before eating, which greatly simplifies the planning and consumption of meals; also, because the effects wane more rapidly, there is a reduced risk of "late" hypoglycemia if the next meal is delayed. With their use, postprandial glucose and HbA$_{1c}$ reductions are equal to or better than those achieved with regular insulin, and there is a reduced incidence of delayed hypoglycemia. For these reasons, and because of their greater convenience and flexibility, rapid-acting analogues have become the standard in intensive treatment regimens. However, these differences in response are relatively modest, and these formulations are significantly more expensive than older insulins.

Intermediate- and Long-Acting Insulin Preparations

The longer-acting insulin preparations have been modified to delay their absorption from injection sites, resulting in a longer duration of insulin activity. The addition of protamine and zinc yields intermediate-acting neutral protamine Hagedorn (NPH) insulin. Ideally, NPH is given twice per day, offering a compromise between some degree of meal coverage (coinciding with peak activity) and the provision of basal insulin levels. It is likely the most cost-effective insulin product.

Insulin glargine, the first long-acting basal insulin analogue, differs from human insulin both at position A21, where asparagine is replaced by glycine, and at the carboxyl terminus of the B chain, where two arginine residues have been added. Insulin glargine is soluble at acidic pH and less so in physiologic conditions; injected at a pH of 4, it is neutralized in subcutaneous tissue and forms microprecipitates, delaying its absorption and prolonging its duration of activity. The primary advantages of glargine insulin are its longer than 24-hour activity (allowing once-daily dosing) and the near absence of peak concentrations; both characteristics are desirable for the provision of consistent basal insulin levels. Disadvantages include a higher cost, a higher incidence of mild injection site discomfort (compared with NPH, 6.0% vs. 0.3%), and the inability to mix glargine with other insulins. Insulin detemir is another basal insulin analogue. It has been engineered with a unique fatty acid side chain that facilitates self-association at the injection site and, once absorbed, binding to circulating serum albumin. Both these features allow a smooth basal profile when insulin detemir is taken once or twice daily. Although it has a shorter duration of action compared with glargine, it appears to have less intraindividual variation in activity.

Insulin Regimens

Although it is a simple concept, the clinical use of insulin to treat diabetes mellitus, especially absolutely insulin-deficient type 1 diabetes, can be extraordinarily complex. There are many important interpatient (and intrapatient) variables, so a predictable algorithm cannot be uniformly applied to all patients or to a single patient at all times. In general, subcutaneous insulin regimens for type 1 diabetes can be classified as conservative or intensive. Continuous subcutaneous insulin infusion with insulin pumps is becoming increasingly popular, mainly in patients with type 1 diabetes, and this mode of therapy provides the most flexible and refined insulin replacement regimen to date.

Conservative Insulin Therapy

Through the early stages of type 1 diabetes, some degree of β-cell function is usually preserved, allowing many patients to achieve near-normal glycemic control with less intensive effort. Because intermediate-acting insulins are not generally sustained during a 24-hour period, and because insulin requirements tend to increase early in the morning, many of these patients can start with two daily injections consisting of a mixture of intermediate-acting and short- or rapid-acting human insulins administered before breakfast and before dinner. Regardless of the initiation method used, insulin dose adjustments are inevitably required. Initially, doses of the intermediate-acting insulin should be adjusted to optimize predinner and fasting (morning) glucose levels. Once these goals are accomplished, short- or rapid-acting insulin doses should be adjusted to optimize postprandial, prelunch, and bedtime glucose values. Some patients may experience a brief "honeymoon" period, during which β-cell function partially recovers and insulin needs are temporarily reduced.

Premixed combinations of intermediate insulins and short- or rapid-acting insulins are also available (NPH/regular 70/30, neutral protamine lispro/lispro 75/25, and neutral protamine aspart/aspart 70/30). The fixed proportions in these insulin products make their titration more challenging.

Intensive Therapy: Multiple Subcutaneous Injections

Within several years after the onset of type 1 diabetes, residual insulin secretion typically ceases. When this occurs, twice-daily insulin injections are no longer acceptable, even if they continue to control marked hyperglycemia and diabetic symptoms. For optimal glycemic control, insulin delivery should more closely simulate the "normal" pattern of insulin secretion; continuous or "basal" insulin levels are required throughout the day, whereas brief increases in insulin levels ("boluses") should coincide with the ingestion of meals. Successful management of diabetes begins with fasting glucose control. Failure to control the morning glucose level often results in the stubborn perpetuation of hyperglycemia throughout the day. The key factors responsible for fasting hyperglycemia are inadequate overnight delivery of insulin and sleep-associated growth hormone release. The "dawn phenomenon" is most pronounced in patients with type 1 diabetes because of their inability to compensate by raising endogenous insulin secretion. The magnitude of the dawn phenomenon can be attenuated by designing insulin regimens to ensure that the effects of exogenous insulin do not peak in the middle of the night and dissipate by morning. Several approaches to insulin therapy can reduce this problem; some of the more common regimens are displayed in Figure 236-4. For patients seeking the tightest control, multidose insulin regimens have gained in popularity. These incorporate rapid-acting insulin analogue injections before each meal with one or two daily doses of a long-acting basal insulin. Ideally, the rapid insulin dose is calculated based on carbohydrate intake, typically using a fixed ratio such as 1 U for every 15 g consumed. Many intensive programs adjust this calculated dose based on the preprandial blood glucose reading and/or any anticipated exercise after the meal. Such regimens require a motivated patient and intensive education and monitoring. Pen-style insulin injectors are also available; these may make multidose regimens more convenient for patients.

Pramlintide

Amylin is a natural peptide that is normally secreted by the pancreatic β cell with insulin in response to meals. It has several beneficial effects on glucose homeostasis, including the suppression of glucagon secretion, the retardation of gastric emptying, and the promotion of satiety. Pramlintide, a synthetic amylin analogue, is currently approved for use in patients with type 1 diabetes (as well as those with insulin-requiring type 2 diabetes) who are inadequately controlled with their current regimens. It is given before meals, usually in conjunction with prandial insulin, but in a separate subcutaneous injection. Its major role is to decrease postprandial glucose excursions, stabilizing glycemic control. In clinical trials, the absolute reduction in HbA$_{1c}$ is modest (−0.3 to 0.5%), although it is associated with mild weight loss, which distinguishes it from insulin therapy. Side effects include nausea and vomiting, especially at higher doses. At this time, its niche appears to be for poorly controlled type 1 (and type 2) diabetes in patients already on intensive insulin regimens but whose glucose profile shows postprandial hyperglycemia not adequately addressed by increasing the dose of pre-meal rapid-acting insulin.

Continuous Subcutaneous Insulin Infusion

In continuous subcutaneous insulin infusion, rapid-acting insulin is administered around the clock by an externally worn, battery-powered,

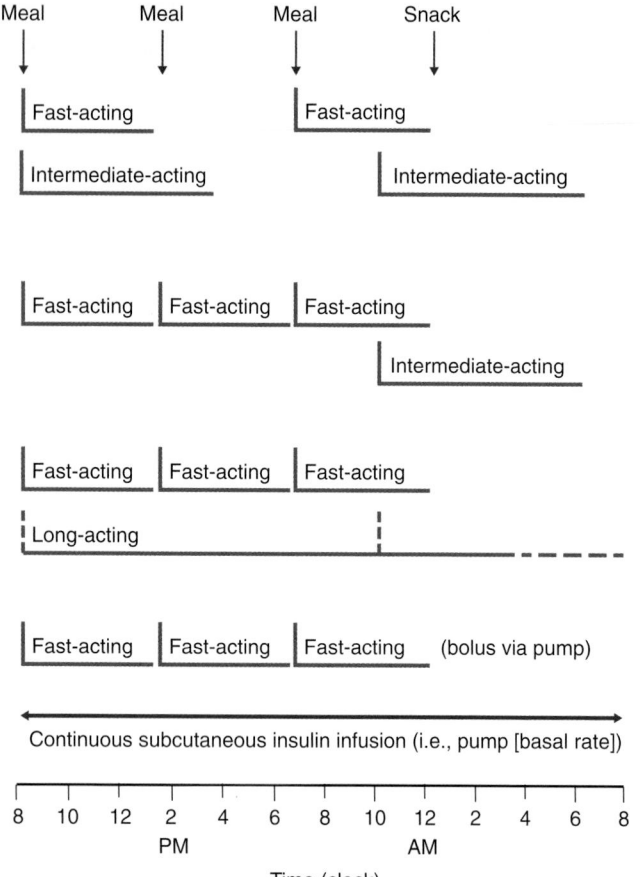

FIGURE 236-4. Several intensive insulin regimens commonly used in the treatment of type 1 diabetes. Each is designed to provide a continuous supply of insulin around the clock and to make extra insulin available at the time of meals, thereby simulating more closely the normal physiologic pattern of insulin secretion. The *dashed lines* for long-acting insulin indicate that it can be given either in the morning or at bedtime.

computer-controlled infusion pump (see Fig. 236-4). **3** The pump delivers a continuous basal rate and can be programmed to vary the flow rate automatically for set periods, such as reducing the rate after bedtime and increasing the flow to compensate for increased insulin requirements in the predawn hours. Boluses, determined by self-monitoring of blood glucose concentration and expected mealtime carbohydrate intake, are given by manual or remote electronic pump activation. Most insulin pumps contain an insulin reservoir (typically containing up to 300 U) attached to a subcutaneous catheter (the catheter is inserted subcutaneously by an introducer needle, which is then removed). Catheters are generally best placed in the abdomen to standardize absorption and to maximize visibility. Overall, continuous subcutaneous insulin infusion provides diabetic patients with the highest degrees of lifestyle flexibility and glucose control. Certain units now communicate by radio frequency to separate capillary blood glucose–monitoring meters, even offering supplemental insulin dosing suggestions. Subcutaneous interstitial sensors that provide continuous glucose monitoring are also electronically linked to modern pumps. At present, the glucose data are displayed by the pump, but there is no automatic feedback control of insulin delivery. There is an active research program aimed at developing an "artificial pancreas," whereby the infusion pump will be largely regulated by the glucose sensor data. Several obvious hurdles in terms of precision, accuracy, and safe, reliable interfaces need to be passed before such closed-loop devices will be ready for commercial use.

The continuous subcutaneous insulin infusion approach has several limitations. One obvious disadvantage of pump therapy is the need to wear the pump itself; the device can be removed only for very brief periods during such activities as intense exercise, contact sports, submersion in water, or personal intimacy. Furthermore, because continuous subcutaneous insulin infusion uses only rapid-acting insulin, any interruption in flow (most commonly because of occlusions within or at the terminus of the catheter) can lead to the rapid deterioration of metabolic control. Local infections at the catheter site occasionally occur, necessitating a site change every 2 or 3 days.

The intensive treatment regimens described are not for everyone. In appropriate patients, however, intensive insulin therapy should be strongly encouraged to reduce the risk of late diabetic complications. Pregnancy is an absolute indication for intensive therapy, and reduction of the excess neonatal morbidity and mortality associated with diabetic pregnancies requires tight glycemic

TABLE 236-3 LIFESTYLE MODIFICATIONS FOR PATIENTS WITH DIABETES

DIETARY PRESCRIPTION

Weight loss to achieve or maintain ideal body weight

Restriction of saturated fat to <10% of total calories, to be replaced in the diet by carbohydrates and monounsaturated fats; if low-density lipoprotein cholesterol (LDL-C) reduction is also desired, saturated fats should be further restricted to <7% of daily calorie intake

Decreased cholesterol intake to <300 mg/day; if LDL-C reduction is also desired, cholesterol intake should be further restricted to <200 mg/day

Sodium restriction (< 2.4 g/day) in patients with hypertension; with overt nephropathy, sodium intake should be further restricted to < 2.0 g/day

Protein restriction to <20% of total calories; with nephropathy, protein intake should be further restricted to <0.8 mg/kg/day or to about 10% of daily calorie intake

EXERCISE PRESCRIPTION*

A combination of aerobic exercise and resistance training is preferred; avoid extreme heavy lifting, straining, and Valsalva maneuvers, which can raise blood pressure and may aggravate proliferative diabetic retinopathy

Intensity: increase heart rate "moderately" to at least 55% of "maximal" heart rate (220 minus age in years), with adjustments based on the patient's cardiovascular fitness; patients with improved cardiovascular fitness can proceed to "harder" activities, achieving heart rates >70% of maximum

Duration: 30 min, preceded and followed by stretching and flexibility exercises for a minimum of 5-10 min

Frequency: at least 3 days/wk; results are best if exercise occurs nearly every day and, to have a consistent effect on blood glucose, at the same time each day

Avoid strenuous exercise if fasting glucose levels are ≥250 mg/dL; avoid any exercise if glucose levels are ≥300 mg/dL or ketosis is present

Monitor blood glucose level before, during, and after exercise to learn responses to different exercise conditions and to identify when changes in insulin or food intake might be necessary

Consume additional foods as needed to avoid hypoglycemia; a rapidly absorbed carbohydrate source should be readily available during exercise and for up to 8 hr after exercise is completed

*Exercise limitations are imposed by preexisting coronary or peripheral vascular disease, proliferative retinopathy, peripheral or autonomic neuropathy, and poor glycemic control.

control. Ideally, intensive insulin therapy should be instituted in type 1 patients before conception to minimize the risk of fetal anomalies. After conception, blood glucose targets are more stringently applied than at other times, with the specific aim of maintaining glucose levels in the normal range.

General Measures
Lifestyle Changes
Diet and exercise contribute importantly to the care of patients with type 1 diabetes. Patients should be educated about balancing calorie intake (diet) with energy expenditure (exercise), and they should understand the basic concepts of insulin therapy as it relates to stress and physical activity. If they are properly managed and sufficiently motivated, diabetic patients should be able to consume the foods they enjoy and participate fully in exercise and sports.

Diet
The introduction of intensive insulin regimens has increased meal flexibility by allowing more latitude in varying the size, content, and timing of meals. New approaches offer the opportunity for a more normal lifestyle, thus reducing compliance problems and optimizing acceptance by and satisfaction of patients. Meals should be nutritionally sound, carbohydrate controlled, and designed to reduce cardiovascular risk, and they should provide sufficient calories to meet the energy needs of growing children, active young adults, and pregnant women; the 1800-kcal diet classically prescribed for overweight type 2 diabetic patients is grossly insufficient in these and other individuals. Furthermore, diabetic diets should specifically aim to minimize long-term cardiovascular risk by minimizing the ingestion of sodium, cholesterol, and saturated fats (Table 236-3).

Because type 1 patients depend on exogenous insulin, proper management is facilitated by a meal plan designed to match the time course of the selected insulin regimen. Patients should learn to compensate for departures from the meal plan by adjusting their insulin doses and for periods of altered activity by adjusting their consumption of food. Even in patients on basal-bolus regimens or those receiving continuous subcutaneous insulin infusion, an effort should be made to avoid long delays between meals, and small snacks may be helpful at times of peak insulin action to avoid hypoglycemia. The potential for insulin-induced weight gain requires special emphasis on portion control; to control hypoglycemia, patients should master the determination of appropriate carbohydrate intake and avoid overcompensation.

Exercise

Regular exercise is important to promote overall health and to reduce cardiovascular complications. Through accelerated insulin absorption (due to increased local blood flow at the injection site) and increased muscle glucose consumption, exercise can rapidly reduce blood glucose levels, particularly when it coincides with the peak action of an insulin injection. In nondiabetic individuals, blood glucose levels remain stable during exercise, as decreased endogenous insulin secretion promotes increased hepatic glucose production to match the increased rate of glucose consumption. In diabetic patients receiving exogenous insulin, however, this finely tuned homeostatic mechanism is perturbed. The continued presence of exogenous insulin during exercise further accelerates glucose uptake and, more important, blocks the compensatory increase in glucose production; as a result, circulating glucose levels can fall precipitously during exercise. Because the magnitude of this fall is not easily titrated, hypoglycemia may occur if the patient is unable to adjust diet and insulin appropriately before, during, and after physical activity. Some general guidelines useful in regulating the glycemic response to exercise are summarized in Table 236-3.

Monitoring

Self-Monitoring of Blood Glucose Concentration

Self-monitoring of blood glucose concentration has revolutionized the management of diabetes. It actively involves patients in the treatment process, allows more rapid treatment adjustments, and reinforces dietary changes. Self-monitoring provides patients with the tools necessary to assist in management of the disease; it is especially useful during periods of stress and for patients who are susceptible to hypoglycemia. Urine glucose testing provides only a gross approximation of recent glucose status and should be used only in patients who cannot or refuse to test their blood.

Newer glucose meters are small, portable, and reliable; they provide a digital readout and have a computerized memory to facilitate record keeping. Blood sampling is facilitated (and made less painful) by automated, spring-operated lancet devices and the option of testing at sites other than the finger (e.g., the arm), which are less painful. Self-monitoring of blood glucose concentration is of maximal value if patients perform tests on a regular basis, can accurately measure glucose levels, and can make use of the results. Patients must become familiar with what a normal glucose value is, what the glucose targets are, and how levels can vary with changes in diet, activity, and insulin absorption. At a minimum, patients should be able to adjust to repetitive patterns of hypoglycemia or hyperglycemia, as well as to periods of stress and illness ("sick days").

Continuous Glucose Monitoring

Traditional self-monitoring of blood glucose concentration is often inadequate to optimize metabolic control. Continuous glucose monitoring of interstitial fluid has revealed that tight glycemic control is often achieved at the expense of unacceptably high rates of nocturnal hypoglycemia, and postprandial glucose excursions are often larger than expected. To minimize these highs and lows, continuous glucose monitoring systems have been approved for clinical use, despite some limitations in accuracy. Data from the first generation of "real-time" glucose sensors were evaluated post hoc, similar to a cardiac Holter monitor, to alert clinicians to previously undetected nocturnal hypoglycemia and postprandial glucose elevations. Current models are needle-like percutaneous glucose sensors inserted under the skin by the patient; the sensors use an enzyme (glucose oxidase) coupled to electrochemical detectors to measure glucose levels for several days to 1 week before they must be replaced. Mechanical continuous glucose sensors give patients (and parents of young children) the ability to view real-time glucose levels (every 5 minutes), review trends and fluctuations in recent blood glucose levels, and receive alerts when blood glucose levels become too high or too low. Recent clinical trials suggest that continuous glucose monitoring, if used daily, helps patients improve glycemic control without increasing the near-term risk of hypoglycemia.[4]

Glycohemoglobin

Glycohemoglobin (glycosylated hemoglobin) assays have emerged as the "gold standard" for long-term glycemic control. The test does not rely on a patient's ability to self-monitor blood glucose levels and is not influenced by acute glycemic changes or by recent meals. Glycohemoglobin is formed when glucose reacts nonenzymatically with the hemoglobin A molecule; it is composed of several fractions, the largest being HbA$_{1c}$. HbA$_{1c}$ (expressed as the percentage of total hemoglobin) varies in proportion to the average level of glucose during the lifespan of the red blood cell, thereby providing an index of glycemic control during the preceding 8 to 12 weeks. Several assay methods have been developed, but all are now standardized to the DCCT assay, as approved by the National Glycohemoglobin Standardization Program.

Although ambient glucose levels are the dominant influence on glycohemoglobin levels, other factors can confound the interpretation of the test result. For example, any condition that increases red blood cell turnover (e.g., pregnancy, hemolytic anemia) spuriously lowers glycohemoglobin levels, regardless of the assay used. Some assays yield spuriously low values in patients with hemoglobinopathies (e.g., sickle cell disease or trait, hemoglobin C or D) or high values when either hemoglobin F is increased (e.g., thalassemia,

myeloproliferative disorders) or large doses of aspirin are consumed. HbA$_{1c}$ can also be affected in uremia and iron deficiency anemia. In addition, poorly understood genetic factors may affect the results of this test, and although estimated average glucose ranges have been proposed for each percentage HbA$_{1c}$, there remains a fair degree of variability from patient to patient (the so-called glycation gap).

Treatment Planning

A management plan should take into consideration the life patterns, age, work and school schedules, psychosocial needs, educational level, and motivation of each individual patient. The plan should include lifestyle changes, a meal plan, medications, monitoring instructions (including sick-day management), and education about the prevention and treatment of hypoglycemia. Importantly, all components of the plan must be both understood and accepted by the patient. The patient's active participation in problem solving, as well as ongoing support from the health care team, is critical for the successful management of diabetes.

At each visit, the management plan should be reviewed and the patient's progress in achieving glucose targets should be assessed. If goals are not being met, causes need to be identified, and the plan should be modified accordingly. Regular clinical evaluation should focus on early signs and symptoms of retinal, cardiovascular, neurologic, and podiatric complications and on reinforcement of the diet and exercise prescription. A complete ophthalmologic examination, assessment of cardiovascular risk factors, and measurement of urinary albumin excretion (through either a timed collection or the more convenient spot urine albumin-to-creatinine ratio) should be performed annually. Specialized podiatric care is also recommended for all patients with evidence of peripheral neuropathy, foot deformities, history of ulcerations, or evidence of peripheral vascular disease. Table 236-4 presents target glycemic guidelines for nonpregnant diabetic patients as well as targets for other clinical factors (e.g., blood pressure, lipids) related to the development of diabetic complications.

Surgical Therapy

Pancreas or Islet Transplantation

Intensive insulin therapy rarely if ever restores glucose homeostasis to levels achieved in nondiabetic individuals. As a result, a more effective method of treatment remains a crucial long-term goal of diabetes research. Pancreas transplantation is conceptually promising in this regard; with growing experience in recent years, there have been substantial improvements in the outcome of pancreas transplantation surgery. Unfortunately, because of the need for long-term immunosuppression, pancreas transplantation is currently an option for only a select group of patients, mainly type 1 diabetic patients who already require immunosuppression for a renal allograft. In such individuals, successful pancreas transplantation may also be effective in preventing nephropathy in the grafted kidney. In the absence of indications for kidney transplantation, pancreas transplantation alone should generally be considered only in rare diabetic patients with a history of frequent, severe metabolic complications (e.g., life-threatening hypoglycemia with or without recurrent ketoacidosis) in whom insulin therapy consistently fails to achieve metabolic control.

TABLE 236-4	THERAPEUTIC TARGETS FOR NONPREGNANT DIABETIC PATIENTS	
PARAMETER	**NORMAL**	**TARGET***
Preprandial plasma glucose (mg/dL)	<100	90-130
2-hr postprandial glucose (mg/dL)	<140	<160-180
Bedtime plasma glucose (mg/dL)	<120	110-150
Hemoglobin A$_{1c}$ (%)[†]	<6	<7
LDL cholesterol (mg/dL)	<130	<100[‡]
HDL cholesterol (mg/dL)	>40 (m), >50 (w)	>45 (m), >55 (w)
Fasting triglycerides (mg/dL)	<150	<150
Blood pressure (mm Hg)	<140/90	<130/80[§]

*Clinical targets vary for individual patients, depending on an assessment of overall health and the risk-benefit ratio.
[†]Whereas the hemoglobin A$_{1c}$ goal in general is <7%, a goal as close as possible to normal (<6%) without significant hypoglycemia is advisable. Also, less stringent goals may be appropriate for some patients (those with a history of severe hypoglycemia, limited life expectancy, or significant comorbidities, and very young children or older adults).
[‡]<70 mg/dL is an optional target in very high risk patients, such as those with overt cardiovascular disease.
[§]<125/75 is the target in patients with overt nephropathy or proteinuria.
HDL = high-density lipoprotein; LDL = low-density lipoprotein; m = men; w = women.

Pancreatic islet cell transplantation holds many potential advantages over whole gland transplantation because it is simpler to perform and less costly. Initially, this still largely experimental procedure involves the intraportal injection of isolated islets from cadaveric sources. Although initial reports appeared encouraging, subsequent follow-up of patients beyond 1 to 2 years reveals that most must resume insulin therapy and many have little or no β-cell function. The critical issue of an adequate source of islets remains a major challenge, and extensive research efforts are being directed at the bioengineering of islets from noncadaveric sources ("islet farming").

ACUTE METABOLIC COMPLICATIONS

Hyperglycemic States

Metabolic decompensation in diabetes is generally classified into one of two broad clinical syndromes: diabetic ketoacidosis (DKA) or hyperosmolar hyperglycemic syndrome (HHS). Although DKA is generally seen in type 1 patients, whereas HHS affects patients with type 2 diabetes (Chapter 237), lines of classification are commonly blurred. For example, HHS can present with variable degrees of ketosis and acidosis, and DKA is seen with increasing frequency in obese type 2 patients. Criteria for both conditions can be met by some patients who experience an overlap syndrome. Despite aggressive treatment, mortality rates remain high for both conditions, approaching 5% for DKA and 15% for HHS. Mortality is associated with advanced age and comorbidity and is usually due to an associated catastrophic illness (e.g., myocardial infarction, cerebrovascular accident, sepsis) or acute complications, including aspiration, cardiac arrhythmias, and cerebral edema. Treatment of hyperglycemic states therefore involves far more than the administration of insulin to reverse hyperglycemia; it also depends on prompt attention to the accompanying fluid and electrolyte disturbances, as well as the detection and treatment of any precipitating illness.

Diabetic Ketoacidosis

PATHOBIOLOGY

DKA may herald the onset of type 1 diabetes, but it most often occurs in established diabetic patients as a result of intercurrent illness (e.g., infection), inappropriate reduction in insulin dosage, or missed insulin injections (especially in adolescents). A common scenario is a patient who fails to adjust insulin therapy or to maintain adequate volume status during an illness, typically a viral gastroenteritis or an influenza-like syndrome. A list of common precipitants appears in Table 236-5.

The three cardinal biochemical features of DKA—hyperglycemia, ketosis, and acidosis—result from the combined effects of deficient circulating insulin activity and the excessive secretion of counter-regulatory hormones. These hormonal imbalances mobilize the delivery of substrates from muscle (amino acids, lactate, pyruvate) and adipose tissue (free fatty acids, glycerol) to the liver, where they are actively converted to glucose or to ketone bodies (β-hydroxybutyrate, acetoacetate, acetone). Both are ultimately released into the circulation at rates that greatly exceed the capacity of tissues to use them. The end results are hyperglycemia (>250 mg/dL), ketoacidosis

---

TABLE 236-5 PRECIPITANTS OF DIABETIC KETOACIDOSIS AND HYPEROSMOLAR HYPERGLYCEMIC STATE

MOST COMMON PRECIPITANTS

Infections (30-50%): pneumonia, urinary tract infections, sepsis, gastroenteritis
Inadequate insulin treatment (20-40%): includes noncompliance, insulin pump failure
Myocardial ischemia or infarction (3-6%): often clinically "silent" in diabetic patients

OTHER PRECIPITANTS

Cerebrovascular accident
Intracranial bleeding (e.g., subdural hematoma)
Acute pulmonary embolism
Intestinal or mesenteric thrombosis
Intestinal obstruction
Acute pancreatitis
Alcohol intoxication or abuse
Severe burns; hyperthermia or hypothermia
Endocrine disorders: Cushing's syndrome, thyrotoxicosis, acromegaly
Total parenteral nutrition
Drugs: corticosteroids, pentamidine, sympathomimetics, thiazides

---

(arterial pH <7.30), and an osmotic diuresis that promotes dehydration and electrolyte loss.

CLINICAL MANIFESTATIONS

The clinical history of DKA typically involves deterioration over several days, with advancing polyuria, polydipsia, and other symptoms of progressive hyperglycemia. Other common clinical features are weakness, lethargy, nausea, and anorexia. Abdominal pain in the setting of DKA is classically periumbilical and can mimic an acute abdomen. Reduced motility of the gastrointestinal tract or, in severe cases, paralytic ileus may further contribute to diagnostic confusion. Nausea and vomiting are ominous symptoms because they preclude oral replacement of fluid losses; severe volume depletion may follow quickly. Physical findings in DKA are mainly secondary to dehydration and acidosis; these include dry skin and mucous membranes, reduced jugular venous pressure, tachycardia, orthostatic hypotension, depressed mental function, and Kussmaul (deep, rapid) respirations. Ketosis may be recognizable by a sweet, sickly smell on the patient's breath.

DIAGNOSIS

The diagnosis of DKA is usually straightforward and needs to be made promptly. The clinical picture and the presence of hyperglycemia should alert the clinician to test for ketones, assess the acid-base status, and measure arterial pH. Initial laboratory tests to be performed include routine serum chemistries (including divalent cations), complete blood count with differential, and urinalysis. Cardiac enzymes and liver and pancreatic function tests should also be checked. An electrocardiogram and a chest x-ray are routinely obtained, and culture specimens should be taken from blood, urine, and other potential sources as clinically indicated. In DKA, glucose levels may vary from 250 to more than 1000 mg/dL, serum bicarbonate concentration drops below 18 mEq/L, and there is an excess anion gap that is generally proportional to the decrease in serum bicarbonate. Hyperchloremia may be superimposed if the patient maintains an adequate glomerular filtration rate and is able to exchange ketoacid anions for chloride in the kidney. The degree of depression of arterial pH depends largely on respiratory compensation. In mild cases the pH may range from 7.20 to 7.30; in severe cases it can fall below 7.00. In general, the clinical severity of DKA depends more on the magnitude of acidosis than on hyperglycemia; as a result, arterial pH is widely used as a reference indicator of DKA severity (Table 236-6). On occasion, a degree of superimposed metabolic alkalosis (e.g., caused by vomiting or diuretic use) may obscure the true severity of the ketoacidosis. An anion gap out of proportion to the fall of bicarbonate should suggest this possibility. Other laboratory abnormalities commonly seen in DKA include a reduced measured serum sodium concentration (due to hyperosmolarity and the resulting osmotic shift of intracellular water into the intravascular space),

---

TABLE 236-6 DIAGNOSTIC CRITERIA FOR DIABETIC KETOACIDOSIS AND HYPEROSMOLAR HYPERGLYCEMIC SYNDROME

CRITERION	MILD DKA	MODERATE DKA	SEVERE DKA	HHS
Plasma glucose (mg/dL)	>250	>250	>250	>600
Effective serum osmolality (mOsm/kg)*	Variable	Variable	Variable	>320
Urine or serum ketones (NP reaction)	Positive	Positive	Positive	Negative to small
Arterial pH	7.25-7.30	7.00-7.24	<7.00	>7.30
Serum bicarbonate (mEq/L)	15-18	10-15	<10	>15
Anion gap (mEq/L)	>10	>12	>12	Variable, usually <12
Typical mental status	Alert	Drowsy	Stupor or coma	Stupor or coma

*Effective serum osmolality (mOsm/kg) = 2 [measured serum sodium (mEq/L)] + [serum glucose (mg/dL)/18]. Normal range = 285 ± 5 mOsm/kg. Urea nitrogen is an "ineffective osmole" (i.e., it diffuses freely across compartments) and is therefore purposely excluded from this equation.
DKA = diabetic ketoacidosis; HHS = hyperosmolar hyperglycemic syndrome; NP = nitroprusside.
Modified from Kitabchi AE, Umpierrez G, Miles JM, et al. Management of hyperglycemic crises in patients with diabetes. *Diabetes Care.* 2009;32:1335-1343.

prerenal azotemia, and hyperamylasemia. The last is usually of nonpancreatic origin and can lead to an erroneous diagnosis of pancreatitis. Normal, elevated, or reduced concentrations of potassium, phosphate, and magnesium may exist when DKA is diagnosed; however, large deficits of these electrolytes invariably accompany the osmotic diuresis and become readily apparent during the course of treatment. The serum triglyceride concentration is frequently elevated, a reflection of deranged lipid metabolism in the setting of insulin deficiency. The white blood cell count is typically elevated; the hemoglobin and hematocrit may be elevated, reflecting volume contraction.

Special care should be taken in interpreting serum or urine ketone results. Because quantitative measurements of β-hydroxybutyrate and acetoacetate are not readily available, rapid diagnosis usually requires qualitative assessment of serum ketones by the use of serum dilutions and reagent strips (e.g., Ketostix) or tablets (e.g., Acetest), which depend on a nitroprusside reaction with acetoacetate. However, acetone reacts weakly with nitroprusside, and β-hydroxybutyrate does not react at all; thus, the results of qualitative testing for ketones can be misleadingly low. Furthermore, because of the presence of intracellular acidosis, β-hydroxybutyrate levels are often much higher than acetoacetate levels, which may further conceal the true degree of ketoacidosis. Conversely, after insulin therapy begins, the nitroprusside reaction may give the "false" impression of sustained ketoacidosis for hours or even days. This results because nonacidic acetone is slowly cleared from the circulation and also because, as acidosis improves, β-hydroxybutyrate is converted to acetoacetate, giving the illusion of worsening ketonemia.

HHS is discussed in Chapter 237.

TREATMENT ℞

The initial goals of therapy for both hyperglycemic states are to replace fluid and electrolyte deficits and to slowly correct hyperglycemia. Unless it is severe, ketoacidosis is generally corrected with these measures and requires no specific therapy. Current management guidelines of the American Diabetes Association are presented in Figure 236-5 and summarized here. In the treatment of hyperglycemic states, special attention must be paid to both the precipitating illness and potential complications that may arise during (or as a result of) medical therapy.

Conventional Medical Therapy

In the early hours of treatment, the primary considerations are to restore intravascular volume, correct tissue hypoperfusion, and restore insulin sensitivity. With DKA, large total body deficits of water (5 to 10 L), sodium (5 to 10 mEq/kg), and other electrolytes (see later) may exist (these losses are even more profound in HHS, which typically develops over a longer time). Although water loss usually exceeds the loss of sodium, it is almost always preferable to begin fluid replacement with isotonic normal saline (0.9% NaCl solution) for efficient intravascular volume restoration. Fluid replacement regimens vary, but it is common to administer 1 L of normal saline within the first hour, followed by a continuous infusion with either 0.45% NaCl or 0.9% NaCl, depending on the corrected serum sodium concentration, the patient's hemodynamic status, and the clinical assessment of tissue perfusion. Likewise, the rate of infusion (commonly 250 to 500 mL/hour) should be adjusted according to both biochemical responses and the age and clinical status of the patient (e.g., oliguria or underlying cardiovascular disease). In pediatric patients with DKA, isotonic solutions are generally preferred because they are less likely than hypotonic solutions to accelerate water shifts into the intracellular space and contribute to cerebral edema. During the course of treatment, once the blood glucose concentration falls below 250 mg/dL, dextrose should be added to intravenous fluids to avoid eventual hypoglycemia because continued insulin delivery will be required to correct the often persistent acidosis.

Although insulin resistance is present in both DKA and HHS, supraphysiologic doses of insulin are unnecessary and are more likely to provoke hypokalemia, hypophosphatemia, and delayed hypoglycemia. A typical insulin replacement regimen uses an intravenous bolus of 0.15 U/kg of rapid-acting (e.g., regular) insulin, followed by 0.1 U/kg/hour thereafter. Intravenous administration is the most predictable way to deliver insulin to target tissues, particularly in severely hypovolemic patients with reduced peripheral blood flow. If intravenous administration is not possible, intramuscular or subcutaneous routes of administration can be used. It is ideal if blood glucose levels fall at a steady and predictable rate (50 to 75 mg/dL/hour), so it is important to monitor blood glucose levels hourly during insulin therapy to ensure an appropriate rate of decline. Blood glucose levels should not fall too rapidly, especially in young children, in whom accelerated correction of plasma glucose concentrations has been associated with cerebral edema.

After a stable blood glucose level below 250 mg/dL is achieved, with resolution of the anion gap acidosis, subcutaneous administration of insulin can be started, and the intravenous insulin infusion may be discontinued. With DKA, it is important to overlap the intravenous and subcutaneous routes by 1 to 2 hours to avoid the return of ketoacidosis. After the return of normoglycemia, long-term medical management should be initiated (or resumed), with both long-acting and short-acting insulins, to approximate the discharge regimen. A temporary "regular insulin sliding scale" is not advisable because such therapy will likely allow the glucose levels to rise into the hyperglycemic range before insulin is administered. More proactive insulin replacement regimens are preferred. The eventual dosage and frequency of insulin depend on multiple factors, including body habitus, comorbidity, insulin sensitivity, and effectiveness of prior therapeutic regimens.

Potassium replacement in DKA (and HHS) is vital. Hypokalemia can result in muscle weakness, cramps, and nausea; both hyperkalemia and hypokalemia are associated with cardiac arrhythmias. At the time of initial evaluation, patients have a severe total body potassium deficit (about 3 to 7 mEq/kg), yet measured serum potassium levels may be normal or high, especially if acidosis or renal failure is present. Once intravenous fluids and insulin are started, serum potassium levels fall quickly because of an insulin-mediated shift of potassium into the intracellular space. In addition, fluid replacement causes extracellular dilution of potassium, leading to improved renal perfusion and increased urinary potassium excretion. This rapid decline can be countered by potassium replacement based on measured serum levels. A low potassium level (<3.5 mEq/kg) requires prompt treatment with up to 40 mEq/hour, whereas "normal" serum levels (3.5 to 5.0 mEq/kg) call for less aggressive repletion (10 to 30 mEq/hour), assuming adequate urine output. In patients who may have lost potassium for additional reasons, such as diuretic use or gastrointestinal loss, one should anticipate the need for greater potassium supplementation.

In the majority of patients with mild to moderate DKA, ketoacids clear spontaneously with standard therapeutic measures, and artificial correction with alkali (bicarbonate) is unnecessary. Suppression of lipolysis by insulin reduces free fatty acid flux to the liver and blocks ketogenesis. The remaining ketoacids are then cleared or oxidized, with subsequent regeneration of bicarbonate and restoration of arterial pH. In cases of severe acidosis (pH <6.9 to 7.0), however, bicarbonate administration may be indicated; the hyperventilatory drive of severe acidosis is uncomfortable, and severe acidosis also impairs cardiac function and peripheral vasodilation. Bicarbonate therapy should be used with caution, however, and only at the minimal doses required to stabilize the patient, because it can further provoke hypokalemia. In addition, by causing a sudden left shift of the dissociation curve for oxyhemoglobin, bicarbonate may impair oxygen delivery to the tissues. Therefore, if alkali therapy is given, small amounts should be administered slowly: 50 mEq (one ampoule) of NaHCO₃ over 1 hour for arterial pH 6.9 to 7.0, and 100 mEq (two ampoules) over 2 hours for pH below 6.9. After bicarbonate administration, arterial pH (and serum potassium levels) should be rechecked every 2 hours, and alkaline therapy should be discontinued when the pH rises above 7.0.

In the setting of DKA, phosphate losses average 3 to 7 mmol/kg; magnesium losses reach 1 to 2 mEq/kg. (Magnitudes of depletion for both ions may be greater for HHS because of a more prolonged osmotic diuresis.) Phosphate is shifted extracellularly during hyperosmolar states, so initial serum levels may be falsely elevated and may drop rapidly during therapy. Complications of hypophosphatemia generally occur at serum levels below 1.0 mg/dL and include respiratory and skeletal muscle weakness, impaired cardiac systolic performance, and hemolytic anemia. Phosphate repletion should be used in patients with serum phosphate levels below 1.0 mg/dL and in patients with evidence of cardiac or respiratory compromise, hypoxia, or hemolytic anemia. An effective means of replacing phosphate is to replace one third to one half of the potassium losses (discussed previously) as potassium phosphate. In severe hypophosphatemia, cautious intravenous administration of additional small amounts of potassium phosphate may be necessary. Because of calcium binding, hypocalcemic tetany may complicate phosphate therapy unless magnesium supplements are also provided; for this reason, serum calcium, phosphate, and magnesium levels should be monitored during any phosphate infusion.

Management of Complications

The most common complications of therapy for hyperglycemic states are hypoglycemia, hypokalemia, hypophosphatemia, and fluid overload; precautions to avoid these complications are described earlier. Cerebral edema, which occurs primarily in pediatric patients, is associated with overaggressive correction of hyperglycemia and with hypotonic fluid replacement. It is likely the result of the osmotically driven movement of water into the central nervous system when plasma osmolarity declines too rapidly. Clinically, cerebral edema is characterized by lethargy and headache, with progressive decline in mental status and neurologic deterioration. The acute respiratory distress syndrome is also attributed to rapid reductions in colloid osmotic pressure, causing increased lung water content, decreased lung compliance, and noncardiogenic pulmonary edema.

PREVENTION

Prevention of DKA requires extensive education in sick-day insulin and fluid management, as well as home-based assessment of urine ketones whenever severe hyperglycemia or physical illness is noted.

Adult patient with DKA or HHS

Complete initial evaluation, including (but not limited to):

Medical history and physical examination

Complete blood count with differential

Fingerstick blood glucose

Serum chemistries ("Chem-10" plus serum ketones)

Urine for urinalysis and ketones

Cultures as indicated (wound, blood, urine, etc.)

Chest ± abdominal x-ray

12-lead ECG

Concurrently, begin empirical fluid resuscitation with 0.9% NaCl at 1000 mL/hr

Consider volume expanders if hypovolemic shock is present

Continue fluid resuscitation until volume status and cardiovascular parameters (pulse, BP) have been restored

IV Fluids

Based on corrected serum sodium*

If high/normal, use 0.45% NaCl

If low/normal, use 0.9% NaCl

Continue IV fluids at 250–1000 mL/hr, depending on volume status, cardiovascular history, and cardiovascular status (pulse, BP)

Insulin Therapy

Regular insulin bolus, 0.15 U/kg

IV infusion, 0.10 U/kg/hr

Check serum glucose hourly—should fall by 50–80 mg/dL/hr

If serum glucose falling too rapidly, back off on insulin infusion

If serum glucose rising or falling too slowly, increase insulin infusion rate by 50–100%

Continuing Management:

Follow and replete serum electrolytes (including divalent cations) q2–4h until stable

After resolution of hyperglycemic state, follow blood glucose q4h and initiate sliding scale regular insulin coverage

Convert IV insulin to subcutaneous injections (or resumption of prior therapy), ensuring adequate overlap

Begin clear liquid diet and advance as tolerated. Encourage resumption of ambulation and activity

Review and update diabetes education, with special attention to prevention of further hyperglycemic crises

When Serum Glucose Reaches 250–300 mg/dL:

For DKA, add dextrose to IV fluids and reduce insulin infusion, adjusted to maintain serum glucose ~200 mg/dL until anion gap has closed

For HHS, continue IV fluids but may reduce insulin infusion until plasma osmolality drops below 310 mOsm/kg

Begin more exhaustive search for precipitant of metabolic decompensation

Potassium (K⁺) Repletion

Obtain baseline serum potassium

Obtain 12-lead ECG

[K⁺] ≥ 5.5 mEq/L

Hold K⁺ therapy

Treat hyperkalemia if ECG changes present

Recheck [K⁺] in 2 hr

[K⁺] < 5.5 mEq/L and adequate urine output

Add K⁺ to IV fluids (Use KCl and/or KPhos)

[K⁺] = 4.5–5.4: add 20 mEq/L IV fluids
[K⁺] = 3.5–4.4: add 30 mEq/L IV fluids
[K⁺] < 3.5: add 40 mEq/L IV fluids

Follow serum [K⁺] every 2–4 hours until stable: anticipate rapid drop of serum [K⁺] during therapy, due to dilution and intracellular shifting

Ensure adequate urine output to avoid over-repletion and hyperkalemia

Continue K⁺ repletion until serum [K⁺] is stable at 4–5 mEq/L

If refractory hypokalemia, ensure concurrent magnesium repletion

Repletion may need to be continued for several days, as total body losses may reach up to 500 mEq

Bicarbonate Therapy

Obtain ABG

Obtain baseline serum bicarbonate

pH < 6.9

100 mEq (2 amps) NaHCO₃ over 2 hr

6.9 ≤ pH < 7.0

50 mEq (1 amp) NaHCO₃ over 1 hr

pH ≥ 7.0

Bicarbonate therapy usually not necessary

Repeat ABG after bicarbonate administration

Repeat NaHCO₃ therapy until pH ≥ 7.0, then discontinue therapy

Follow serum bicarbonate q4h until stable

*Sodium correction: Serum sodium should be corrected for hyperglycemia. For every 100 mg/dL of glucose elevation above 100 mg/dL, add 1.6 mEq/L to the measured sodium value; this will yield the corrected serum sodium concentration.

FIGURE 236-5. Management of diabetic ketoacidosis (DKA) and hyperosmolar hyperglycemic syndrome (HHS). ABG = arterial blood gases; BP = blood pressure; ECG = electrocardiogram; IV = intravenous.

Hypoglycemia

DEFINITION

Hypoglycemia is the most frequent complication of insulin therapy for type 1 diabetes. Nearly all patients are symptomatically affected at least once per year, and a significant percentage have severe hypoglycemia requiring medical assistance. Studies using continuous glucose monitoring of type 1 diabetics have shown alarmingly high rates of hypoglycemia, especially at night, when sleeping patients are unaware of its existence.

PATHOBIOLOGY

Symptoms of low blood glucose concentration result from changes in autonomic activity and brain function. Autonomic symptoms, including sweating, tremor, and palpitations, are often the earliest subjective warning signs of hypoglycemia. Central nervous system symptoms and signs of glucose deficiency, termed *neuroglycopenia*, may be nonspecific (e.g., fatigue, weakness) or more clearly neurologic (e.g., double vision, oral paresthesias, slurring of speech, apraxia, personality change, behavioral disturbances). Hypoglycemia affects type 2 patients as well; most cases occur during treatment with insulin or insulin secretagogues, especially the longer acting sulfonylureas. Because of the long-acting nature of some oral insulin secretagogues, low blood glucose concentration can recur up to 24 to 48 hours after drug withdrawal, and a more extended course of therapy is often required.

It is well known that prolonged, severe hypoglycemia can cause irreversible brain damage. What is less clear, however, is whether significant neurologic damage results from shorter, milder episodes of low blood glucose concentration over time. Nevertheless, hypoglycemia may provoke seizures, accidental injury, and a catecholamine response that can induce cardiac ischemia or arrhythmias in patients with underlying cardiac disease. Overall, hypoglycemia is thought to account for 3 to 4% of deaths in insulin-treated diabetic patients. Hypoglycemia also has far-reaching social implications. On a personal level, it can induce great fear, preclude comfortable engagement in routine activities (e.g., driving), and lead both patient and clinician to aim deliberately for less than optimal glycemic control.

In nondiabetic persons, hypoglycemia provokes a rapid, multitiered metabolic response intended to restore normal blood glucose levels. The brain cannot store more than a few minutes' supply of energy; in the short term, its function is exclusively dependent on a constant supply of glucose for fuel. To preserve central nervous system function, spontaneous recovery from hypoglycemia involves both the activation of endogenous glucose production and reduced peripheral glucose use. Three fundamental mechanisms are responsible for this process: dissipation of endogenous insulin; counter-regulatory hormone activity; and subjective awareness of hypoglycemia, resulting in hunger and subsequent carbohydrate ingestion. Early hormonal changes are triggered when the plasma glucose concentration approaches the hypoglycemic range (65 to 70 mg/dL). A rise in glucose production, attributable mainly to stimulation of hepatic glycogenolysis, is initiated by the release of glucagon from pancreatic α cells in conjunction with falling levels of endogenous insulin. Catecholamines are also released, producing "alarm" symptoms of hypoglycemia (e.g., hunger, tremor, palpitations) and further promoting the synthesis of glucose through the stimulation of hepatic glycogenolysis, mobilization of substrates for gluconeogenesis, and further suppression of insulin production. When hypoglycemia is sustained, additional counter-regulatory hormones such as growth hormone and corticosteroids are released; through a variety of complementary mechanisms, these hormones also help promote continued glucose availability. For a more in-depth discussion of metabolic responses to hypoglycemia, refer to Chapter 238.

Patients with type 1 diabetes are more likely to have hypoglycemia, for several reasons. First, injected insulin enters the circulation from a nonphysiologic source (e.g., a subcutaneous depot) and therefore cannot be curtailed by any counter-regulatory response to falling glucose levels, as may occur in type 2 patients who have residual endogenous insulin secretion. In addition, patients with type 1 diabetes, as a rule, are insulin sensitive, as opposed to their type 2 counterparts. Type 1 patients also lose their glucagon response to hypoglycemia; this appears to be a stimulus-specific phenomenon because their glucagon response to other stimuli may be unaffected. Defective glucagon responses develop in most type 1 patients 2 to 5 years after diagnosis, at about the same time they become completely insulin deficient, implying that the loss of endogenous insulin regulation is a contributory factor. Once this occurs, glucose counter-regulation must rely predominantly on epinephrine release. Unfortunately, half of patients with long-standing type 1 diabetes exhibit diminished epinephrine responses to hypoglycemia as well, further predisposing them to severe episodes. In addition, patients may lose the ability to recognize hypoglycemia and take corrective action. In some cases the irritability and confusion that occur during hypoglycemia may prevent the patient's awareness of its cause. In other cases, patients may lose the autonomic warning symptoms of hypoglycemia and may recognize the condition (or even fail to recognize it) only when somatic neurologic function becomes impaired. This so-called hypoglycemic unawareness syndrome has been associated with a number of factors, including duration of diabetes and autonomic neuropathy.

Hypoglycemia unawareness may also occur when patients are switched to intensive insulin regimens. The introduction of intensified treatment regimens can lower the glucose level that triggers epinephrine release and adrenergic symptoms, which at least partly explains the increased frequency of severe hypoglycemia reported in the DCCT. This leads to an increased incidence of iatrogenic hypoglycemia during intensified insulin therapy. It has been shown that even brief periods of antecedent hypoglycemia can suppress counter-regulatory responses during subsequent hypoglycemic episodes.

CHRONIC DIABETIC COMPLICATIONS

The pathogenesis of the microvascular and neuropathic complications of diabetes is complex and poorly understood. However, these complications are undoubtedly mediated in large part by the metabolic derangements associated with diabetes, especially hyperglycemia. It has been suggested that glucose-induced cell injury is particularly pronounced in those cell types that are unable to regulate their intracellular glucose concentration (e.g., endothelial cells and neurons) and that this leads to increased production of reactive oxygen species (superoxide) as well as advanced glycation end products (AGEs), accelerated polyol and hexosamine pathways, and protein kinase C activation.

Studies suggest that hyperglycemia-mediated intracellular overproduction of reactive oxygen species may be the common mechanism triggering a variety of pathways thought to contribute to cell injury in diabetes. In addition, a variety of proteins are nonenzymatically glycosylated in vivo (including hemoglobin, collagen, laminin, low-density lipoprotein particles, and peripheral nerve proteins) in direct proportion to prevailing levels of glucose. AGE cross-linking capabilities render them resistant to natural degradation. The consequent AGEs accumulate in a variety of tissues (including the kidneys and blood vessels), where they bind to a receptor for AGE (RAGE). Of particular interest, the binding of AGEs to RAGE is thought to contribute to cell injury through a variety of mechanisms, including stimulation of oxidative reactions as well as pro-inflammatory cytokines, complement, and growth factors. In the polyol pathway, increased activity of intracellular aldose reductase leads to accumulation of sorbitol and fructose, resulting in decreased glutathione antioxidant activity (through decreased NAD^+), and enhanced formation of diacylglycerol. Diacylglycerol formation, in turn, can activate specific isoforms of protein kinase C, which stimulate transforming growth factor-β release and play an important role in cell proliferation and vascular permeability. In experimental diabetic animals, prevention of superoxide accumulation, inhibition of AGE formation, and specific protein kinase C inhibitors reduce diabetic complications.

Hemodynamic changes in the microcirculation may also contribute to microangiopathy. In the diabetic kidney, glomerular filtration rate is increased out of proportion to renal plasma flow owing to an elevation in the transglomerular pressure gradient. It is assumed that raised glomerular pressures promote the passage of proteins and AGEs; with time, their accumulation in the mesangium is likely to trigger the proliferation of mesangial cells and matrix production, eventually leading to glomerulosclerosis. Compensatory hyperfiltration and a decreasing number of functional glomeruli would exacerbate matters, increasing intraglomerular pressure and resulting in progressive glomerular damage.

Although microvascular complications can affect patients with either type 1 or type 2 diabetes, they are discussed in this chapter. The macrovascular complications, which are particularly common in type 2 diabetes, are discussed in Chapter 237.

Diabetic Retinopathy

DEFINITION

Diabetic retinopathy refers to progressive pathologic alterations in the retinal microvasculature, leading to areas of retinal nonperfusion, increased vascular permeability, and the pathologic proliferation of retinal vessels.

CLINICAL MANIFESTATIONS
Nonproliferative Diabetic Retinopathy

E-Table 236-1 details the revised international classification (disease severity scales) for this complication. The earliest pathologic changes associated with retinopathy are termed mild nonproliferative diabetic retinopathy. In type 1 patients, these changes generally begin no sooner than 5 years after diagnosis. The first signs of mild nonproliferative diabetic retinopathy are microaneurysms, which arise most often in areas of capillary occlusion. Subsequently, increasing vascular permeability leads to retinal blot hemorrhages (round, with blurred edges) and "hard" exudates (sharply defined and yellow). Infarctions of the nerve fiber layer, known as soft exudates or cotton-wool spots, appear as white or gray, rounded swellings. At this early stage of retinopathy, visual acuity is generally unaffected, and the risk of progression to high-risk proliferative diabetic retinopathy (see later) is about 15% at 5 years.

Moderate nonproliferative diabetic retinopathy is characterized by intraretinal microvascular abnormalities, including venous caliber changes, beading, and increased capillary dilation and permeability. Later changes, termed severe or very severe nonproliferative diabetic retinopathy, include progressive retinal capillary loss and ischemia, with further development of extensive hemorrhages, exudates, and microaneurysms. After 5 years, moderate and severe nonproliferative diabetic retinopathy are associated with a 30% and 60% risk of progression to high-risk proliferative diabetic retinopathy, respectively.

Proliferative Diabetic Retinopathy

Proliferative diabetic retinopathy involves neovascularization—the growth of fine tufts of new blood vessels and fibrous tissue from the inner retinal surface or the optic head. Early proliferative changes are confined to the retina, but later invasion of the vitreous body constitutes high-risk proliferative diabetic retinopathy; during this end stage, fibrosis and contracture of the neovasculature result in retinal detachment and hemorrhage, the most important determinants of blindness. On occasion, new vessels can invade the iris and anterior chamber, leading to sight-threatening closed-angle glaucoma.

Clinically Significant Macular Edema

Clinically significant macular edema results from vascular leakage at the macula and can occur either with or without the stages of retinopathy described earlier. Clinically significant macular edema is suggested by hard macular exudates on funduscopic examination and can be confirmed with slit lamp biomicroscopy. In general, maculopathy is more common in type 2 patients, in whom it is an important contributor to the loss of visual acuity. As discussed later, the treatment of clinically significant macular edema runs parallel to the treatment of other forms of diabetic retinopathy.

TREATMENT   Rx

Medical Therapy

At present, medical management of diabetic retinopathy is aimed at controlling risk factors for progression. The value of tight glycemic control was proved by the DCCT,[1] whose primary prevention arm demonstrated an impressive 76% risk reduction for the onset of retinopathy with intensive therapy. In the secondary prevention arm, patients with early nonproliferative diabetic retinopathy undergoing intensive therapy demonstrated a 47% risk reduction in the development of severe nonproliferative diabetic retinopathy or proliferative diabetic retinopathy, a 51% risk reduction in the need for laser treatment, and a 26% risk reduction in the development of clinically significant macular edema. Other targets for medical management, all associated with accelerated retinal damage, include control of hypertension and hyperlipidemia, treatment of nephropathy, and careful follow-up during pregnancy, when accelerated retinal disease has been linked to preexisting diabetes (but not gestational disease). Fenofibrate can reduce the progression of retinopathy and the need for laser treatment by about one third, with the benefit not clearly related to a reduction in lipid levels.[5] In the Diabetic Retinopathy Candesartan Trials (DIRECT) involving 3326 adults with type 1 diabetes, the angiotensin II receptor blocker candesartan modestly reduced the incidence of diabetic retinopathy, a finding of borderline significance, but it could not prevent its progression in those with established disease.[6]

Surgical Therapy

Surgical management of retinopathy is aimed at slowing disease progression, because baseline visual acuity is difficult to recover. In the 1980s large-scale prospective clinical trials such as the Diabetic Retinopathy Study and the Early Treatment Diabetic Retinopathy Study established photocoagulation as the treatment of choice when retinopathy threatens vision. Most patients with proliferative diabetic retinopathy, and selected patients with severe nonproliferative diabetic retinopathy, are now treated primarily with scatter (panretinal) photocoagulation; cryotherapy or vitrectomy may be required if laser treatment is unfeasible for technical reasons or because of extensive disease. Clinically significant macular edema is treated with focal photocoagulation, with the possible exception of patients exhibiting no or minimal nonproliferative diabetic retinopathy. In such patients, close follow-up at 2- to 4-month intervals is an acceptable option. The decision to treat depends not only on stage of retinopathy and extent of clinically significant macular edema but also on the type of diabetes, the patient's general medical status, compliance with follow-up, and the status of the contralateral eye.

These considerations make it imperative for physicians to prospectively identify diabetic patients at risk for retinopathy and visual loss. Nonspecialists

may have difficulty diagnosing the stages of retinopathy. Accordingly, patients should be referred to an experienced eye specialist for a complete examination, including a dilated funduscopic examination, tonometry, and slit lamp biomicroscopy. The most recent guidelines of the American Diabetes Association recommend an initial eye examination within 5 years of diagnosis of type 1 diabetes and at the time of diagnosis in type 2 patients.

Follow-up

Follow-up of all patients should occur at least annually, with the possible exception of those with retinopathy-free type 2 diabetes. Even in the latter cases, the American Diabetes Association recommends yearly examinations to avoid lost follow-up and to identify patients with more aggressive ocular disease. Of special note, because retinopathy rarely develops in children before puberty, patients with early-onset type 1 diabetes generally do not require screening before 10 years of age. Also, the acceleration of retinopathy during pregnancy demands that all patients with preexisting diabetes be examined during the first trimester. Recently, the availability of high-quality retinal photography with remote interpretation by specialists has become available. This is now thought to be a reasonable substitute when an in-person evaluation is not possible (e.g., in remote areas).

Diabetic Nephropathy

RISK FACTORS

There are several known risk factors for the development of diabetic nephropathy: duration of disease; elevated glycohemoglobin levels; and concurrent hypertension, hyperlipidemia, and tobacco use. Race is known to play a major role as well, as demonstrated by a higher prevalence of nephropathy in African American, Hispanic, and Native American patients. There is also a high concordance rate in families; studies in both type 1 and type 2 diabetic families revealed a three- to four-fold increase in the prevalence of nephropathy among those with affected siblings. Strong associations have been noted with several other factors as well, including a deletion polymorphism of the angiotensin-converting enzyme (ACE) gene, increased sodium-lithium countertransport, and degree of insulin resistance.

CLINICAL MANIFESTATIONS

Natural History

Details are less clear in type 2 diabetes, but the natural history of diabetic nephropathy in type 1 diabetes is well described (Fig. 236-6). The period immediately after diagnosis is best characterized by glomerular hyperfiltration. During this time there is renal hypertrophy, increased renal blood flow, increased glomerular volume, and increased transglomerular pressure gradient, all contributing to a rise in glomerular filtration rate. Importantly, these changes depend at least in part on hyperglycemia, as they are diminished by intensive diabetes treatment. Three to 5 years after diagnosis, early glomerular lesions appear, characterized by thickening of glomerular basement membranes, mesangial matrix expansion, and arteriolosclerosis. Albumin excretion remains low during early glomerular changes; however, as pathologic changes mount, the glomeruli lose their functional integrity, resulting in glomerular filtration defects and increased glomerular permeability. Although the results of routine tests of renal function (creatinine concentration and urinalysis) remain normal, microalbuminuria (30 to 300 mg/day) appears. Systemic hypertension is also present at this time in more than 50% of cases.

Without intervention, approximately 80% of patients with type 1 diabetes who develop sustained microalbuminuria experience an increase in albuminuria on the order of 10 to 20% per year, with overt nephropathy (≥300 mg/24 hours) appearing over 10 to 15 years. Once overt nephropathy occurs, the glomerular filtration rate begins a relentless decline (10 mL/minute/year or more), which is eventually reflected by an increase in serum creatinine concentration. The appearance of massive proteinuria and the nephrotic syndrome is common in this context and often heralds progression to end-stage renal disease (ESRD). Once the serum creatinine concentration rises (reflecting an approximately 50% decline in glomerular filtration rate), ESRD develops in most patients within 10 years. This course is highly variable, however, particularly in type 2 diabetics, who may exhibit moderate proteinuria for several years without a substantial deterioration of renal function. A simple but useful method of monitoring progression to renal failure is to plot the reciprocal of the serum creatinine concentration as a function of time. This technique allows better assessment of both therapeutic interventions and the time at which renal replacement therapy will become necessary. Notably, in

Diagnosis	3 Years	5 Years	15 Years	25 Years
				ESRD

| Renal hypertrophy (gross)
Normal microarchitecture
Normal microvasculature | Thickened GBM
Mesangial matrix expansion
Early arteriolosclerosis | Early GS
K-W nodules
Advanced arteriolosclerosis | Progressive GS (End-stage fibrosis)
Vessel obliteration |
| Increased GFR
Normal serum CR
Normoalbuminuria
Normotensive | Increased GFR
Normal serum CR
Reversible albuminuria
Mostly normotensive | "Pseudonormalization" of GFR
Normal serum CR
Microalbuminuria
~50% hypertensive | Declining GFR
Rising serum CR
Albuminuria
~100% hypertensive |

FIGURE 236-6. Pathogenesis of diabetic nephropathy. CR = creatinine; ESRD = end-stage renal disease; GBM = glomerular basement membrane; GFR = glomerular filtration rate; GS = glomerulosclerosis; K-W = Kimmelstiel-Wilson.

patients with diabetes who have no sustained microalbuminuria after 20 years of disease, the development of significant nephropathy is rare.

Most diabetic patients with nephropathy exhibit diffuse glomerulosclerosis; only a minority have pathognomonic Kimmelstiel-Wilson nodular lesions. Although pathologic changes continue to mount throughout the disease, glomerulosclerosis extensive enough to cause ESRD develops in a minority of patients.

TREATMENT Rx

Early-Stage Treatment

Treatment of nephropathy has become an important focus of recent research and depends heavily on the stage of disease. Early in the course of diabetes (before the onset of microalbuminuria), strict glycemic control is of the utmost importance. The DCCT demonstrated that intensive therapy reduced microalbuminuria by 39% and overt albuminuria by 54% in type 1 diabetics, with a mean follow-up of 6.5 years. A similar result was demonstrated in the United Kingdom Prospective Diabetes Study (UKPDS) of patients with type 2 diabetes (Chapter 237), in which a less dramatic improvement in glycemic control reduced microalbuminuria and overt albuminuria by 24% and 33%, respectively, with a mean follow-up of 9 years. In normotensive, normoalbuminuric type 2 diabetics, treatment with ACE inhibitors retards microalbumin production, but studies achieving similar results with β-blockers and calcium-channel blockers suggest that blood pressure lowering may be responsible for this effect. Studies using ACE inhibitors and angiotensin II receptor blockers have consistently shown that both drug classes can delay the progression of both proteinuria and declining glomerular filtration rate.[7] These drugs are therefore widely favored in diabetic patients, whose blood pressure should be maintained at 130/80 mm Hg or less if possible. Lower targets (<125/75) are endorsed for those with overt nephropathy.

Later Stage Treatment

Once clinical nephropathy becomes evident, aggressive efforts at strict glycemic control have marginal value in slowing the progression of nephropathy. As noted before, efforts aimed at reducing hypertension and glomerular pressure have become the mainstay of therapy. Dietary protein restriction (i.e., 0.8 g/kg body weight) may add limited benefit, and adherence is difficult. Aggressive lipid management is useful in preventing both renal and extrarenal vascular complications. As ESRD approaches, long-term treatment plans should proceed much as they would in nondiabetic uremic patients, but therapy should usually be initiated sooner. It is well known that diabetic patients have a poorer tolerance for uremia than their nondiabetic counterparts do. Protein wasting is accelerated, hypertension becomes more difficult to control, and there is acceleration of generalized atherosclerosis, with extensive cardiovascular morbidity. Current options for ESRD patients include hemodialysis, peritoneal dialysis, kidney transplantation, and combined kidney-pancreas transplantation (Chapter 133). Choosing among these options is complex, and decisions must be made on an individual basis. Careful attention to and treatment of coexisting anemia (due to erythropoietin deficiency; Chapter 161) and optimization of calcium–vitamin D homeostasis are also very important in any patient with advancing renal disease, but especially in those with diabetes. Finally, mortality associated with both dialysis and organ transplantation is higher in diabetic than in nondiabetic patients, usually because of cardiovascular comorbidity and the more rapid development of complications such as vascular insufficiency.

Management of Complications

Glomerular nephropathy is not the only entity that commonly affects the genitourinary system in diabetic patients. Asymptomatic bacteriuria and pyelonephritis are twice as common in diabetic women because of several factors, including autonomic bladder dysfunction, impaired organ perfusion, and glycosuria. Papillary necrosis is also associated with diabetes, and renal artery stenosis is more common as well. Hyperkalemia, another frequent complication of diabetes, is due to a variety of factors, including insulin deficiency, metabolic acidosis, reduced glomerular filtration rate, use of pharmacologic modulators of the renin-angiotensin axis, and the syndrome of hyporeninemic hypoaldosteronism commonly seen in elderly patients with impaired renal function. Finally, diabetic patients are at notable risk for azotemic complications after the injection of contrast dye for radiologic studies. For this reason, aggressive hydration with intravenous fluids, especially those containing sodium bicarbonate, before and after the study or the prophylactic use of N-acetylcysteine is critical in these cases.

Diabetic Neuropathy

PATHOBIOLOGY

The term *diabetic neuropathy* describes a wide variety of clinical syndromes representing a complex interplay of pathogenic factors. Chronic, more insidious neuropathies may be mediated by metabolic factors, whereas the more acute, self-limited neuropathies most likely have a vascular cause. Also, nerve growth factor is diminished in the neurons of patients with neuropathy, perhaps limiting regenerative capacity. Autoimmune mechanisms may also be involved; in affected type 1 diabetics, autonomic nerve bundles may show monocytic infiltration, and the sera may contain complement-fixing antibodies to sympathetic ganglia. Because of the multifactorial nature of diabetic neuropathy, current classification schemes are based largely on clinical presentation. Current taxonomy includes focal, diffuse, and autonomic neuropathies. Our suboptimal understanding of the underlying causes of diabetic neuropathy has slowed the development of appropriate medical therapies.

CLINICAL MANIFESTATIONS

Focal Diabetic Neuropathies

Focal diabetic neuropathies (mononeuropathies) typically present with pain, but motor losses and abnormal deep tendon reflexes can be present. They usually begin suddenly, suggesting a vascular cause. Although any cranial or peripheral nerve can be involved, the most common sites include the oculomotor, median, radial, and lateral popliteal nerves. Painful radiculopathy may also occur in the distribution of one or more spinal roots and can easily be confused clinically with internal organ disease or postherpetic neuralgia. Because of the self-limited nature of focal neuropathy, treatment is generally aimed at pain control, with physical therapy as needed to maintain function of the affected muscle groups. Focal neuropathies are generally self-limited, with an average duration of 6 to 8 weeks; chronicity can occur but is less common.

Distal Symmetrical Polyneuropathy

Distal symmetrical (sensorimotor) polyneuropathy (Chapter 428) is the most common neurologic syndrome seen in diabetes. This process involves all somatic nerves but has a strong predilection for distal sensorimotor nerves of the feet and, to a lesser extent, the hands. Sensory fibers are generally preferentially affected; disease affects both small, unmyelinated C fibers (transmitting pain and temperature) and larger, myelinated Aδ/Aβ fibers, which carry touch, vibration, and proprioception. Early on, most patients with distal neuropathy are asymptomatic, with subtle abnormalities on examination, including the loss of vibration sense, light touch, two-point discrimination, and thermal sensitivity. Once they become symptomatic, patients typically report numbness and tingling of the distal extremities, often in the classic "stocking-glove" distribution. Pain is also common, involving either C fibers (burning, dysesthesia, and allodynia) or the large fibers, usually described as gnawing or like a toothache. Severe, spontaneous, short-lived lancinating pains may also occur. Left unchecked, all types of pain may gradually gain in intensity, with a tendency to worsen at night, and there may be progressive loss of sensorimotor function as well. Later stages of disease can involve severe sensory loss, small muscle wasting of the hands and feet, sensory ataxia, and neuropathic arthropathy (Charcot joints).

Proximal Motor Neuropathy

Proximal motor neuropathy (diabetic amyotrophy), although classified as a polyneuropathy, is a unique condition that deserves special mention. This syndrome primarily affects elderly type 2 patients and is more common in men. It classically begins with pain in the bilateral thighs, hips, and buttocks, followed by weakness and atrophy of the proximal pelvic muscle groups. Iliopsoas, obturator, and adductor muscles of the pelvis are preferentially affected, with relative preservation of the hamstrings and gluteal muscles. Weight loss may also occur.

Autonomic Neuropathy

Symptomatic autonomic diabetic neuropathy (Chapter 427) carries a poor prognosis and is thankfully now less common than it once was. Autonomic neuropathy typically accompanies other chronic complications of diabetes and may play a pathogenetic role through disturbed regulation of local blood flow.

Cardiac

Common cardiovascular abnormalities seen with autonomic neuropathy include resting tachycardia (due to preferential dysfunction of parasympathetic fibers), diminished heart rate variability, prolonged QTc, and silent myocardial ischemia. Diabetic patients often have defective heart rate and blood pressure responses to exercise, and their lack of autonomic regulation places them at high risk for myocardial infarction, congestive heart failure, and sudden cardiac death.

Vascular

Postural hypotension is probably caused by an impaired sympathetic vasoconstrictor response and impaired cardiac reflexes. Non-neurogenic causes of orthostasis, such as volume depletion, impaired cardiac function, and infectious causes, should be ruled out before the diagnosis is made. Tilt-table testing can be useful to confirm the diagnosis (Chapter 62). Nonpharmacologic measures, such as a raised head position at night, reduction of rapid positional changes, and supportive elastic stockings, can be useful in mild cases. Disabling disease may require pharmacologic intervention; first-line agents include mineralocorticoids (9-α-fluorohydrocortisone) and α-agonists (midodrine).

Gastrointestinal

Altered gastrointestinal function is commonly seen in diabetes. Constipation is the most common clinical syndrome. Diarrhea is another frequent complaint and can be caused by a variety of conditions, including hypermotility (impaired sympathetic inhibition), hypomotility with bacterial overgrowth, pancreatic insufficiency, and bile salt irritation. Treatment is generally aimed at the underlying condition and may include antidiarrheals, intermittent use of broad-spectrum antibiotics, pancreatic enzymes, and bile acid sequestrants (cholestyramine).

Gastroparesis is a particularly disabling condition, often presenting with bloating, early satiety, nausea, and vomiting. Labile glycemic control can result from delayed delivery of nutrients to the small bowel. Treatment of gastroparesis begins with small, frequent meals and the use of metoclopramide, a central dopaminergic agonist with gastric cholinergic activity. Early treatment is useful, but the drug's effect may diminish over time. In selected cases, erythromycin, which acts on the motilin receptor to promote gastric motility, may also be considered. Recently, gastric pacemakers have been used as experimental therapy in selected cases.

Genitourinary

Impaired parasympathetic innervation leads to bladder hypotonia, incomplete bladder emptying, dribbling, and overflow incontinence. Bethanechol, a parasympathomimetic agent, can be helpful to reverse these symptoms, but its use is often limited by side effects, including salivation, lacrimation, diarrhea, and bronchoconstriction. α-Blockers help by relaxing the urinary sphincter, but these agents potentiate postural hypotension, which is already prevalent in diabetic patients. Advanced cases of bladder dysfunction often require intermittent straight catheterization or, if absolutely necessary, the placement of an indwelling catheter. Chronic bacterial colonization and actual infections may result, however.

Erectile dysfunction is commonly seen in male diabetic patients. Selective oral inhibitors of phosphodiesterase type 5 (sildenafil, tadalafil, vardenafil) inhibit the local breakdown of cyclic guanosine monophosphate, which, in the presence of nitric oxide, leads to selective engorgement of the corpus callosum. Caution should be used in patients with suspected coronary disease, and such drugs are contraindicated in combination with nitrate therapy. In men who do not respond to these drugs, intrapenile injections of locally acting vasomotor agents, such as alprostadil and papaverine, have been used with moderate success but carry the risk of priapism, infection, and local fibrosis with repeated use. In refractory cases, urologic referral for a penile prosthetic implant should be considered.

TREATMENT   Rx

Early treatment of diabetic sensory neuropathy should include tight glycemic control. In the DCCT, intensive therapy slowed the onset of neuropathy by 70% and the progression of early neuropathy by 57%; in the UKPDS, glucose control in type 2 diabetes was associated with improved vibratory sensation.

The use of several therapies for neuropathic pain (Chapters 29 and 428) has been supported by randomized controlled trials. Tricyclic antidepressants, including amitriptyline, desipramine, and nortriptyline, are moderately effective and well tolerated at low doses, but dose escalation can result in drowsiness, anticholinergic effects, potentiation of cardiac arrhythmias, and worsening of glaucoma. Anticonvulsants, such as carbamazepine and gabapentin, are also effective, but carbamazepine can cause hematologic abnormalities, and patients taking gabapentin may report dizziness, fatigue, headaches, or diarrhea. Two drugs have been specifically approved by the FDA for use in diabetic neuropathy. The first, duloxetine, is a selective serotonin and norepinephrine reuptake inhibitor (related to venlafaxine) that is also approved as an antidepressant. The second, pregabalin, an analogue of γ-aminobutyric acid (GABA; related to gabapentin), modulates calcium channels and GABAergic neurotransmission. Both are modestly effective in decreasing neuropathic pain. Topical therapies, such as capsaicin cream (which depletes stores of axonal substance P) and lidocaine gels, can be moderately effective.

The Diabetic Foot

DEFINITION

The diabetic foot is characterized by slowly healing plantar ulcers that result from apparently insignificant trauma. Left untreated, superficial ulcers may penetrate to underlying tissues, leading to complications including cellulitis, abscess formation, joint sepsis, and osteomyelitis. Gangrene may occur, and amputation may be required.

CLINICAL MANIFESTATIONS

To varying degrees, the diabetic foot is characterized by the combination of chronic sensorimotor neuropathy, vascular disease, autonomic neuropathy, and impaired immune function. Sensory neuropathy prevents the detection of minor traumatic events, so that ill-fitting shoes (or sharp objects in the shoe) may erode the skin surface without signaling pain. Pedal neuropathy also produces abnormalities in both proprioception and intrinsic muscle motor function, pathologically altering weight distribution on the metatarsal heads and leading to "clawing" of the metatarsophalangeal joints. In advanced cases, abnormal loading of the foot can result in repeated painless fractures and the displacement of normal joint surfaces, producing the so-called Charcot foot or Charcot joint. Aortic and peripheral vascular disease often coexist. Diminished cardiac output or disturbed autoregulatory mechanisms of the microcirculation may further contribute to impaired blood flow and delay ulcer healing. Finally, abnormal immune function (secondary to hyperglycemia) can predispose to prolonged inflammation and infection,

TABLE 236-7	FOOT CARE PRESCRIPTION FOR DIABETIC PATIENTS WITH LOWER EXTREMITY SENSORY NEUROPATHY

Avoid walking barefoot
Do not apply very hot water or heating pads to the feet
Inspect the feet daily, using a mirror for plantar surfaces
Wash the feet daily, drying thoroughly between the toes
Lubricate dry skin to avoid cracking
Wear clean, soft, cotton socks
Wear properly fitting, well-cushioned shoes (insoles)
Break in new shoes slowly
Consider a second pair of shoes for evenings (larger size to account for any dependent edema)
Cut toenails straight across
Schedule regular visits to a diabetic foot care specialist, especially if there are any signs or symptoms of neuropathy, vascular disease, or bony deformity

TABLE 236-8	KEY ELEMENTS OF A COMPREHENSIVE MANAGEMENT PLAN FOR PATIENTS WITH DIABETES MELLITUS

LIFESTYLE CHANGES

Healthy diet
Aerobic exercise
Weight control
Smoking cessation
Stress reduction

CONTROL OF MODIFIABLE METABOLIC FACTORS

Glucose
Lipids
Blood pressure
Aspirin prophylaxis in higher risk patients

PREVENTIVE CARE

Regular medical screening examinations
Regular screening for albuminuria
Regular ophthalmologic examinations
Regular podiatric examinations (and self-examinations)
Regular dental check-ups
Yearly influenza vaccinations
Pneumococcus vaccination

further slowing wound closure and increasing the likelihood of ulcer complications.

PREVENTION

Prevention of the diabetic foot parallels general diabetes care, with an emphasis on proper nutrition, tight glycemic control, and medical risk factor modification, including smoking cessation. A general foot care prescription (Table 236-7) is valuable, and office visits should routinely include careful examination of the feet. In affected patients, examination by a specialist is recommended at least once per year. In cases of deformed feet, pressure relief (offloading) is essential and may include the use of orthotics, specialty shoes, assistive devices, or a total-contact cast to direct pressure away from a high-risk area.

TREATMENT   Rx

Once an ulcer has formed, it should be treated aggressively with antibiotics, appropriate local wound care, and débridement of necrotic tissue. In selected cases, local application of recombinant human platelet-derived growth factor can moderately accelerate wound healing. Bioengineered tissue therapies, containing human dermal-epidermal components, are also effective in refractory cases. These products act as biologic dressings and contain live human fibroblasts that deliver growth factors and extracellular matrix components directly to damaged skin. For extensive cases of gangrene or deep tissue infections, surgical amputation may be required. A compromised peripheral circulation makes such an outcome more likely. If poor circulation is a dominant clinical feature, a vascular surgeon should be consulted for consideration of revascularization.

Key elements of a comprehensive management plan for the care of diabetic patients are summarized in Table 236-8.

 Visit expertconsult.com for e-expanded chapter

Grade **A**

1. Diabetes Control and Complications Trial Research Group. The effect of intensive treatment of diabetes on the development and progression of long-term complications of insulin-dependent diabetes mellitus. *N Engl J Med.* 1993;329:927.
2. Diabetes Control and Complications Trial/Epidemiology of Diabetes Intervention and Complications (DCCT/EDIC) Study Research Group. Intensive diabetes treatment and cardiovascular disease in patients with type 1 diabetes. *N Engl J Med.* 2005;353:2643-2653.
3. Misso ML, Egberts KJ, Page M, et al. Continuous subcutaneous insulin infusion (CSII) versus multiple insulin injections for type 1 diabetes mellitus. *Cochrane Database Syst Rev.* 2010;1:CD005103.
4. Juvenile Diabetes Research Foundation Continuous Glucose Monitoring Study Group, Tamborlane WV, Beck RW, et al. Continuous glucose monitoring and intensive treatment of type 1 diabetes. *N Engl J Med.* 2008;359:1464-1476.
5. Keech AC, Mitchell P, Summanen PA, et al. Effect of fenofibrate on the need for laser treatment for diabetic retinopathy (FIELD study): a randomised controlled trial. *Lancet.* 2007;370:1687-1697.
6. Chatuervedi N, Porta M, Klein R, et al. Effect of candesartan on prevention (DIRECT-Prevent 1) and progression (DIRECT-Protect 1) of retinopathy in type 1 diabetes: randomised, placebo-controlled trials. *Lancet.* 2008;372:1394-1401.
7. Strippoli GF, Bonifati C, Craig M, et al. Angiotensin converting enzyme inhibitors and angiotensin III receptor antagonists for preventing the progression of diabetic kidney disease. *Cochrane Database Syst Rev.* 2006;4:CD006257.

SUGGESTED READING

American Diabetes Association. Standards of medical care in diabetes—2011. *Diabetes Care.* 2011;34:S11-61. *An up-to-date summary of the current classification of diabetes and clinical practice recommendations for the management of diabetic patients, including goals of treatment.*
Cheung N, Mitchell P, Wong TY. Diabetic retinopathy. *Lancet.* 2010;376;124-136. *Review.*
Diabetes Control and Complications Trial/Epidemiology of Diabetes Interventions and Complications (DCCT/EDIC) Research Group, Nathan DM, Zinman B, et al. Modern-day clinical course of type 1 diabetes mellitus after 30 years' duration: the diabetes control and complications trial/epidemiology of diabetes interventions and complications and Pittsburgh epidemiology of diabetes complications experience (1983-2005). *Arch Intern Med.* 2009;169:1307-1316. *A good overview of the epidemiology of the complications of type 1 diabetes, based on a large clinical trial and an observational study.*
Dib SA, Gomes MB. Etiopathogenesis of type 1 diabetes mellitus: prognostic factors for the evolution of residual beta cell function. *Diabetol Metab Syndr.* 2009;1:25-32. *A brief review of the autoimmune underpinnings of type 1 diabetes, with mention of ongoing prevention studies in this area.*
Dronavalli S, Duka I, Bakris GL. The pathogenesis of diabetic nephropathy. *Nat Rev Endocrinol.* 2008;4:444-452. *Excellent summary of our current understanding of the etiology of diabetic kidney disease.*
Kitabchi AE, Umpierrez GE, Miles JM, et al. Hyperglycemic crises in adult patients with diabetes. *Diabetes Care.* 2009;32:1335-1343. *An excellent summary of the recognition and evidence-based therapy of diabetic ketoacidosis and hyperosmolar hyperglycemic syndrome.*
Simó R, Hernández C. Advances in the medical treatment of diabetic retinopathy. *Diabetes Care.* 2009;32:1556-1562. *Update on medical interventions demonstrated to prevent or delay retinopathy in diabetes.*
Tesfaye S, Boulton AJ, Dyck PJ, et al. Diabetic neuropathies: update on definitions, diagnostic criteria, estimation of severity, and treatment. *Diabetes Care.* 2010;33:2285-2293. *Consensus review of peripheral neuropathies and autonomic neuropathy.*
Tridgell DM, Tridgell AH, Hirsch IB. Inpatient management of adults and children with type 1 diabetes. *Endocrinol Metab Clin North Am.* 2010;39:595-608. *Review of ketoacidosis, uncontrolled hyperglycemia, and hypoglycemia including perioperative insulin management.*

237

TYPE 2 DIABETES MELLITUS

SILVIO E. INZUCCHI AND ROBERT S. SHERWIN

DEFINITION

In this chapter, we discuss the pathogenesis and treatment of type 2 diabetes and other forms of the disease. See Chapter 236 for a general overview of normal carbohydrate metabolism and the complex physiology of insulin secretion and action. Although type 2 diabetes has many similarities to type 1 diabetes, there are many important differences from the vantage point of both biology and therapeutics.

Type 2 diabetes accounts for most cases of diabetes encountered in clinical practice. Patients retain some endogenous insulin secretory capacity; however, their insulin levels are low relative to their ambient glucose concentrations and magnitude of insulin resistance. Type 2 patients are not dependent on insulin for immediate survival, and ketosis rarely develops, except under conditions of great physical stress. Nevertheless, many of these patients will require insulin therapy for optimal glycemic control over time. Although type 2 diabetes has recently been found with increasing frequency in children, adolescents, and young adults, it is usually associated with advancing

TABLE 237-1   DIAGNOSTIC CATEGORIES*: DIABETES MELLITUS AND AT-RISK STATES

FASTING PLASMA GLUCOSE LEVEL	2-Hour (75-g) OGTT Result		
	<140 MG/DL	140-199 MG/DL	≥200 MG/DL
<100 mg/dL	Normal	IGT[†]	DM
100-125 mg/dL	IFG[†]	IGT[†] and IFG[†]	DM
≥126 mg/dL	DM	DM	DM
HbA₁c LEVEL	<5.7%	5.7-6.4%	≥6.5%
	Normal	High-risk[†]	DM

*These diagnostic categories are based on the combined fasting plasma glucose level and a 2-hour, 75-g oral glucose tolerance test (OGTT) result. Note that a confirmed random plasma glucose level of 200 mg/dL or higher in the appropriate clinical setting is diagnostic of diabetes and precludes the need for further testing.
[†]May be referred to as prediabetes.
DM = diabetes mellitus; IFG = impaired fasting glucose; IGT = impaired glucose tolerance.

age; most cases are diagnosed after the age of 45 years. Type 2 diabetes has a high rate of genetic penetrance unrelated to HLA genes and is associated with obesity and a lack of physical activity. The clinical features of type 2 diabetes can be insidious; classic symptoms may be quite mild. Fatigue, weakness, dizziness, blurred vision, and other nonspecific complaints often dominate the clinical picture, but these may be tolerated for many years before the patient seeks medical attention. Moreover, if the degree of hyperglycemia is insufficient to produce any symptoms at all, the diagnosis can be made only after the development of vascular or neuropathic complications.

The general classification scheme for diabetes mellitus is summarized in Table 237-1.

Other Specific Types of Diabetes

This category encompasses a wide variety of diabetic syndromes attributed to a specific disease, drug, or condition. Categories include genetic defects of β-cell function or insulin action, diseases of the exocrine pancreas (e.g., chronic pancreatitis), other endocrinopathies (e.g., Cushing's syndrome, acromegaly), drug- or chemical-induced diabetes (e.g., due to glucocorticoids), infections, and other immune-mediated and genetic syndromes associated with diabetes mellitus.

Maturity-onset diabetes of the young (MODY), formerly classified as a subtype of type 2 diabetes, has now been more accurately described as a consequence of genetic research. Clinically, patients with MODY generally present in adolescence or young adulthood; unlike patients with classic type 2 diabetes, they are usually nonobese, normotensive, and normolipidemic at the time of diagnosis. MODY is a heterogeneous disorder encompassing several monogenic defects of β-cell function; it has an autosomal dominant inheritance and a penetrance exceeding 80%. Mutations of at least nine genetic loci have been identified. The most common form, MODY type 3, is associated with a mutation of *HNF1α* (hepatocyte nuclear factor-1α), a gene transcription factor encoded on chromosome 12. A subgroup of MODY type 2 patients has a mutation in the gene encoding glucokinase, the key enzyme responsible for the phosphorylation of glucose within the β cell and the liver. A variety of glucokinase mutations, each capable of interfering with the transduction of the glucose signal in the β cell, have been identified in different families. These forms of diabetes may respond to insulin secretagogues, such as sulfonylureas or, if needed, to insulin injections.

Severe illness (e.g., burns, trauma, sepsis) can provoke stress hyperglycemia as a result of the hypersecretion of insulin antagonistic hormones (e.g., catecholamines, cortisol). Although this may represent the unmasking of underlying diabetes, the metabolic disturbance may be self-limited and should therefore not be formally classified as diabetes until the precipitating illness has resolved (unless there is evidence of more chronic hyperglycemia, as reflected by a hemoglobin A₁c [HbA₁c] of 6.5% or greater). Whereas most patients can be readily classified on clinical grounds, a small subgroup of patients is difficult to categorize because they display features common to both type 1 and type 2 diabetes. Such patients are classically nonobese, with reduced insulin secretory capacity but little tendency for ketosis. Many of these patients initially respond to oral agents; however, nearly all of them will eventually require insulin therapy. Many of these patients appear to have a slowly evolving form of type 1 diabetes, with measurable titers of autoimmune markers, referred to as *latent autoimmune diabetes of adulthood* (LADA).

Gestational Diabetes Mellitus

The term *gestational diabetes mellitus* (Chapter 236) describes women with abnormal glucose tolerance that appears or is first detected during pregnancy. Women with known diabetes before conception are not classified as having gestational diabetes. Gestational diabetes mellitus usually appears in the second or third trimester, when pregnancy-associated insulin antagonistic factors (many placentally derived) reach their peak. After delivery, glucose tolerance generally (but not always) reverts to normal. However, within 10 years, type 2 diabetes develops in most women with prior gestational diabetes; on occasion, pregnancy can precipitate type 1 diabetes as well. As a whole; gestational diabetes occurs in approximately 7% of U.S. pregnancies, accounting for approximately 200,000 cases per year; local prevalence rates may rise as high as 14% in high-risk populations. Although patients with gestational diabetes generally present with mild, asymptomatic hyperglycemia, rigorous treatment is indicated to protect against hyperglycemia-associated fetal morbidity. Most respond to diet, but pharmacotherapy is often required, with insulin remaining the standard treatment approach in these individuals.

EPIDEMIOLOGY

Systematic screening for asymptomatic type 2 diabetes mellitus is generally limited to high-risk populations, rendering broader prevalence estimates imprecise. Total U.S. prevalence is now estimated at 8%, but probably exceeds 25% in persons older than 65 years. Type 2 diabetes is more common in Native Americans, Hispanic Americans, and African Americans, in whom the prevalence exceeds 12 to 13%, than in whites,; these patients also typically present at an earlier age. Prevalence rates vary worldwide; type 2 diabetes has a propensity for Asiatic Indians, Polynesians-Micronesians, and Latin Americans. Interestingly, African blacks, Australian Aborigines, Asians, and Pacific Islanders all have an increased risk for diabetes after emigration to the United States; this may be attributable to a genetically determined inability to adapt metabolically to "Western" behavior patterns (i.e., reduced physical activity and a high-fat, high-calorie diet).

Although relatively little is known about the specific genetic abnormalities associated with type 2 diabetes, the personal factors promoting disease expression are well established. Increased age, reduced physical activity, and obesity are risk factors for the disease, especially in genetically susceptible persons. The severity and duration of obesity contribute significantly to diabetes risk; patients with high waist-to-hip ratios (i.e., central or upper body obesity) are also more prone to the disease. Family history is also important because type 2 diabetes occurs more frequently in persons with diabetic parents or siblings. Identical twin concordance rates approach 100%; in these cases, affected twins will even often develop diabetes at a similar age.

Impaired Fasting Glucose and Impaired Glucose Tolerance

In 2008, the Centers for Disease Control and Prevention estimated that 57 million adults had prediabetes in the United States. There is only partial overlap between the impaired fasting glucose (IFG) and impaired glucose tolerance (IGT) groups, as demonstrated by the fact that approximately 37% of patients with IFG also have IGT, whereas approximately 24% of patients with IGT also have IFG. Because of the insidious nature of both conditions, precise rates of progression to overt diabetes are difficult to establish; current estimates approach 5 to 10% per year for each condition, with even higher rates if both conditions are present. In general, IGT appears to have a greater sensitivity for predicting the future development of diabetes; it is also an independent risk factor for cardiovascular complications. Recently, high HbA₁c levels (5.7 to 6.4%) have been added to the laboratory criteria that define prediabetes. As with IFG and IGT, there is imperfect concordance between individuals with HbA₁c levels in this range and those with the glucose-based abnormalities that define prediabetes. Nonetheless, each identifies a group of patients at increased risk for developing diabetes and for which preventive strategies should be considered.

PATHOBIOLOGY

Whereas the pathogenesis of hyperglycemia in patients with type 1 diabetes is reasonably straightforward (lack of insulin due to β-cell destruction), the metabolic underpinnings of type 2 diabetes are comparatively more varied, and to a large degree enigmatic, involving defects in both insulin action and secretion. Hyperglycemia in type 2 diabetes probably results from complex genetic interactions, the expression of which is modified by environmental factors such as body weight and exercise. With type 2 diabetes, identical twin

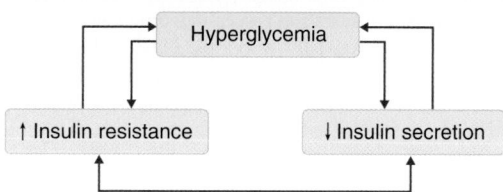

FIGURE 237-1. Elevations of circulating glucose initiate a vicious circle in which hyperglycemia begets more severe hyperglycemia.

concordance rates approach 100%, although disease onset and course can vary greatly on the basis of environmental factors. Hyperglycemia itself is known to impair insulin secretion and action; elevated free fatty acid levels also play an important pathogenic role. By the time that hyperglycemia is detected, nearly all type 2 patients exhibit both defective insulin secretion and insulin sensitivity; this makes it somewhat of a challenge to determine which of the two factors is primarily responsible for the vicious cycle leading to disease (Fig. 237-1). Nonetheless, it is difficult to develop diabetes if β-cell function remains adequate for the peripheral demands for insulin action.

Genetics

Although monogenic forms of diabetes have been identified (e.g., MODY types), most cases are likely to be polygenic in nature. Type 2 diabetes shows clear familial aggregation but does not segregate in classic mendelian fashion; this implies that the disease results either from a combination of genetic defects or from the simultaneous presence of multiple susceptibility genes and predisposing environmental factors. Candidate gene mutations for polygenic forms of type 2 diabetes include mutations of the transcription factor-7–like 2 (*TCF7L2*), the coding region of the insulin gene, peroxisome proliferator-activated receptor-γ (PPAR-γ), β-cell adenosine triphosphate-sensitive potassium channel, intestinal fatty acid–binding protein 2, calpain 10, and β$_3$-adrenergic receptor. These and other mutations have been associated with isolated clusters of patients with type 2 diabetes. *TCF7L2* has received substantial attention recently because single nucleotide polymorphisms in this gene have been strongly associated with type 2 diabetes risk and impaired insulin secretion.

Pathogenesis
Insulin Secretion

It is now quite apparent that the driving force in the progression from normal glucose tolerance to IGT to frank type 2 diabetes is the progressive loss of insulin secretory capacity. Once type 2 diabetes becomes manifested, fasting insulin levels in type 2 diabetes generally appear normal or elevated, yet they are *relatively* low given the degree of coexisting hyperglycemia. As the disease progresses and hyperglycemia becomes more severe, basal insulin levels eventually fail to keep up and may even decline. Indeed, autopsy studies demonstrate that β-cell mass is reduced by 50% in such patients. The insulin secretory defect usually correlates with the severity of fasting hyperglycemia and is more evident after carbohydrate ingestion. In its mildest form, the β-cell defect is subtle, involving the loss of the "first-phase" insulin response and the normal oscillatory pattern of insulin secretion. Although the overall insulin response may appear to be fairly intact, this "normal" response is actually totally inadequate to maintain glucose tolerance when it is viewed in the context of simultaneous insulin resistance. During this early stage, the β-cell defect is usually specific for glucose; other secretagogues (e.g., amino acids) maintain their potency, and insulin deficiency is thus less pronounced during the ingestion of mixed meals. Patients with more severe fasting hyperglycemia lose this capacity to respond to the other insulin secretagogues; thus, their secretory defect worsens as their disease progresses. The underlying cause of the secretory defect remains uncertain and is probably multifactorial, involving both functional and anatomic defects, and to large degree genetically determined.

Studies in rodents suggest that the loss of glucose-stimulated insulin secretion is associated with a decreased expression of GLUT 2, the primary glucose transport protein of the pancreatic β cell. Pathologic studies of islets from patients with long-standing type 2 diabetes have demonstrated amyloid-like deposits composed of islet amyloid polypeptide, or amylin, a peptide synthesized in the β cell and co-secreted with insulin. Chronic hypersecretion of amylin may lead to intra-islet precipitation of the peptide, which over time might also contribute to impaired β-cell function. Experiments in gene knockout mice suggest a potential role for impaired insulin receptor signaling in the development of impaired β-cell function. A link between insulin resistance and secretion is also suggested by the accumulation of fat within the β cell, which may interfere with normal insulin secretion. Finally, studies in patients with type 2 diabetes demonstrate reduced circulating glucagon-like peptide 1 (GLP-1) concentrations, particularly in response to meals. Whether this phenomenon is a causative factor or occurs secondarily in patients with preexisting hyperglycemia is uncertain.

Insulin Resistance

With few exceptions (e.g., a subgroup of African American patients), type 2 diabetes is characterized by impaired insulin action. The insulin dose-response curve for augmenting glucose uptake in peripheral tissues is shifted to the right, representing decreased insulin sensitivity, and maximal response is reduced, particularly in the setting of severe hyperglycemia. Other insulin-dependent processes, such as inhibition of hepatic glucose production and lipolysis, also show reduced sensitivity to insulin. The mechanisms responsible for insulin resistance remain poorly understood. Studies suggest that an important contributory factor is impaired mitochondrial function and the resulting accumulation of free fatty acids and their metabolites in insulin-responsive tissues ("ectopic fat theory").

Early studies of insulin resistance focused on defects of the insulin receptor. Mutation of the insulin receptor gene can produce leprechaunism (Chapter 212), characterized by severe growth retardation, extreme insulin resistance, and early infant death. Other syndromes related to mutated insulin receptors include the Rabson-Mendenhall syndrome, also associated with tooth and nail abnormalities and pineal gland hyperplasia, and "type A insulin resistance," most often affecting young females with acanthosis nigricans, polycystic ovaries, and hirsutism. Another example of extreme insulin resistance involves the presence of anti-insulin receptor antibodies; it is associated clinically with acanthosis nigricans and a number of autoimmune phenomena. These disorders are not involved in most patients with or at risk for type 2 diabetes.

Although insulin receptors may be abnormal in a few type 2 patients, defects in more distal "postreceptor" pathways play a far greater role in insulin resistance. One important aspect of insulin resistance is a reduced capacity for translocation of GLUT 4 to the cell surface in muscle cells. A separate defect in glycogen synthesis also is likely to be present. Whether the defects uncovered are primary or secondary to the disturbance in glucose metabolism is not entirely known, but the bulk of the experimental data would suggest that insulin resistance is a primary defect in this disease. Potentially, a variety of genetic abnormalities in cellular transduction of the insulin signal may individually or in concert produce an identical clinical phenotype. It is uncertain whether mechanisms of insulin resistance in nonobese patients are identical to those of their obese counterparts; however, the coexistence of obesity clearly accentuates the severity of the resistant state. In particular, upper body or abdominal (compared with lower body or peripheral) obesity is associated with insulin resistance and diabetes. Intra-abdominal visceral fat deposits, detected by computed tomography or magnetic resonance imaging, have a higher lipolytic rate than peripheral fat and are more resistant to insulin. The resulting increase in circulating free fatty acid levels promotes fat deposits within the liver and muscle, worsening insulin resistance. Intracellular free fatty acid metabolites appear to promote insulin resistance through complex mechanisms involving serine (rather than tyrosine) phosphorylation of insulin signaling molecules. Disordered cortisol secretion or enhanced local cortisol generation from relatively inactive cortisone in the adipocyte or hereditary factors may also influence the distribution of body fat, the latter contributing an additional genetic influence on the expression of disease.

Adipocyte-Derived Hormones and Cytokines

Adipocytes, once thought of as inert fat storage cells, are now known to produce a number of metabolically active hormones that may affect insulin sensitivity (Chapter 227). Leptin, for example, acts on the hypothalamus to promote satiety and energy expenditure and may accelerate glucose metabolism. Adiponectin, another fat-derived hormone, circulates at levels that correlate inversely with both adiposity and degree of insulin resistance. The administration of adiponectin to obese mice causes a transient, dose-dependent, insulin-independent decrease in circulating glucose levels; adiponectin also improves insulin sensitivity by decreasing triglycerides in the liver and muscle, probably by increasing the expression of molecules (e.g., adenosine monophosphate kinase) involved in fatty acid combustion and energy dissipation. Weight loss paradoxically increases adiponectin, as does pharmacologic therapy that improves insulin sensitivity. Interestingly, adiponectin may have some beneficial effects on atherosclerosis, which may explain at least to some degree the increased prevalence of cardiovascular disease in obesity and type 2 diabetes. Finally, adipose tissue is an abundant source of the cytokine tumor necrosis factor-α, which is known to inhibit muscle glucose metabolism by inducing serine phosphorylation of insulin-signaling molecules. The precise impact that these and other adipocyte-derived factors (resistin, angiotensinogen, interleukin-6, transforming growth factor-β, and plasminogen activator inhibitor 1) exert on insulin resistance and on diabetes and its vascular complications is an active area of scientific research but has yet to be firmly established.

Glucotoxicity and Lipotoxicity

Hyperglycemia per se impairs the β-cell response to glucose and promotes insulin resistance. Reversal of this "glucotoxicity" can disrupt the vicious circle that perpetuates hyperglycemia (see Fig. 237-1). Similarly, circulating lipids can also adversely affect glucose metabolism; increased free fatty acid levels accelerate hepatic gluconeogenesis, inhibit muscle glucose metabolism, and impair pancreatic β-cell function. As is the case with glucotoxicity, the reversal of lipotoxicity can rapidly improve metabolic control and facilitate favorable therapeutic outcomes.

What Is the Primary Defect?

It remains uncertain whether insulin resistance or defective insulin secretion is the primary defect in type 2 diabetes (Fig. 237-2). This issue is difficult to resolve once diabetes has developed; therefore, research attention has focused primarily on high-risk nondiabetic subjects. Studies in high-risk populations (e.g., Pima Indians, Mexican Americans) have suggested that insulin resistance is the initial defect; similar findings have been reported in first-degree relatives of type 2 diabetic patients and in healthy prediabetic offspring of two diabetic parents. Interestingly, hyperinsulinemia has been detected in prediabetic subjects as early as one to two decades before clinical onset, suggesting that the development of diabetes can be exceedingly slow. Although these studies support the view that insulin resistance generally antedates insulin deficiency, the presence of insulin resistance alone is generally insufficient to generate hyperglycemia; this implies that for diabetes to occur, impaired insulin secretion is required (see Fig. 237-2). It is possible that the appearance of a secretory defect is a secondary phenomenon resulting from "β-cell exhaustion," excess fatty acid delivery, amylin accumulation, or factors associated with β-cell growth. Perhaps more likely, diminished insulin secretion may result from an independent defect that becomes evident only on chronic β-cell stimulation, such as a subtle genetic defect in insulin signaling or β-cell replication.

The sequence of events described—underlying insulin resistance followed by a secretory defect—is common but clearly does not describe all type 2 diabetic patients. For example, a subgroup of African American patients exhibits little or no insulin resistance. (An insulin deficiency–predominant phenotype is also encountered not infrequently in clinical practice in other racial groups, although, admittedly, many of these individuals may potentially have a slowly progressive form of type 1 diabetes.) In addition, diminished

glucose-stimulated insulin secretion is seen in women with gestational diabetes in whom type 2 diabetes later develops. Finally, the demonstration of functional β-cell-associated gene mutations in patients with MODY indicates that primary β-cell defects are capable of producing a similar phenotype. Taken together, these lines of evidence strongly suggest that type 2 diabetes cannot be explained by insulin resistance alone or indeed by any single pathogenic mechanism.

DIAGNOSIS

The diagnosis of diabetes mellitus is straightforward when classic symptoms of polyuria, polydipsia, and unexplained weight loss are present. In these cases, a random (or "casual") plasma glucose measurement of 200 mg/dL or more is sufficient to confirm the diagnosis. Although glycosuria is strongly suggestive of diabetes, urine test results should never be used exclusively to diagnose diabetes because an altered renal threshold for glucose excretion can produce similar findings. If suspected diabetes is not confirmed through random glucose determination, additional diagnostic testing should be performed.

An 8-hour (overnight) fasting plasma glucose measurement is most convenient; diabetes is established if fasting glucose levels are 126 mg/dL or higher on two separate occasions. Alternatively, a 75-g oral glucose tolerance test may be employed. The oral glucose tolerance test should be performed after an overnight fast, with use of a glucose load containing 75 g of anhydrous glucose dissolved in water; 2-hour postload glucose levels of 200 mg/dL or higher confirm the presence of diabetes. An important note about the oral glucose tolerance test: although it is able to detect diabetes in its earliest stage, this test should be performed under controlled conditions to ensure its accuracy. Common factors that can nonspecifically interfere with the oral glucose tolerance test result include antecedent dietary carbohydrate restriction, bedrest or severe inactivity, medical or surgical stress, drugs (e.g., thiazides, β-blockers, glucocorticoids, phenytoin), smoking, and anxiety from repeated phlebotomies. As a result, the oral glucose tolerance test should not be performed in acutely ill patients, and patients undergoing the oral glucose tolerance test should ideally stop smoking and consume a liberal carbohydrate diet for at least 3 days before testing. More recently, with global standardization of HbA$_{1c}$ assays, this test is now widely endorsed as an acceptable, and more convenient, screening test for diabetes, with the diagnostic cutoff point set at 6.5%. This threshold was chosen because it correlates with the presence of retinopathy, similar to the diagnostic thresholds for fasting and 2-hour plasma glucose.

The current (2010) American Diabetes Association (ADA) criteria (see Table 237-1) for the diagnosis of diabetes mellitus are as follows. In the absence of unequivocal hyperglycemia with acute metabolic decompensation, each criterion should be confirmed by repeated testing on a separate occasion:

1. Classic symptoms of diabetes (polyuria, polydipsia, and unexplained weight loss) *plus* random plasma glucose concentration ≥200 mg/dL (≥11.1 mmol/L); *or*
2. Fasting (≥8-hour) plasma glucose concentration ≥126 mg/dL (≥7.0 mmol/L); *or*
3. A 2-hour postload plasma glucose concentration ≥200 mg/dL (≥11.1 mmol/L) during a 75-g oral glucose tolerance test; *or*
4. An HbA$_{1c}$ ≥6.5% (nonfasting).

In certain scenarios, clinicians may have available to them results from easily obtained tests, namely fasting plasma glucose and HbA$_{1c}$. Not uncommonly, the results of these tests may be discordant. That is, a patient may have an HbA$_{1c}$ of 6.5% or greater but a "subdiabetic" fasting plasma glucose, or vice versa. In this circumstance, it is recommended that the diagnosis default to the most abnormal test because both measures correlate with retinopathy risk.

The two traditional risk categories for diabetes, IFG and IGT, are associated with an increased risk for development of diabetes as well as subsequent cardiovascular events, with IGT being a much stronger predictor for both sequelae. Diabetes mellitus is established if fasting glucose levels are 126 mg/dL or higher; however, a fasting glucose concentration of 99 mg/dL is now designated the upper limit of normal. Patients with fasting glucose levels between 100 and 125 mg/dL are classified as having IFG (see Table 237-1). Because individuals with IFG may exhibit significant postprandial hyperglycemia, a 75-g oral glucose tolerance test may be considered to rule out diabetes, although the need for this will be less, now that HbA$_{1c}$, which captures both fasting and postprandial hyperglycemia, is recommended as a diagnostic test. During the 75-g oral glucose tolerance test, 2-hour postload glucose

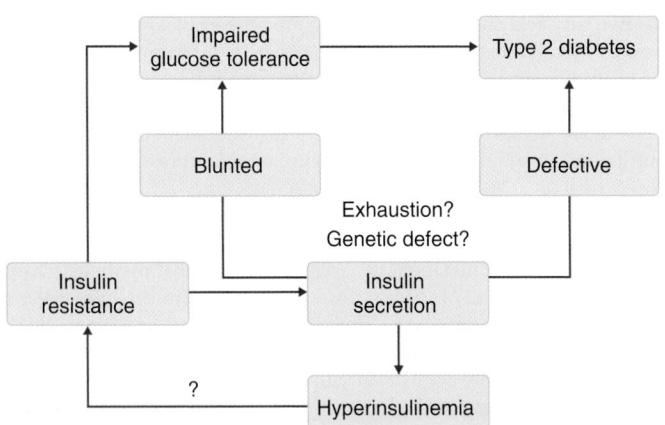

FIGURE 237-2. A proposed sequence of events leading to the development of type 2 diabetes. Insulin resistance resulting from genetic influences, central obesity, inactivity, or a combination of these factors leads over time to a progressive loss of the β cell's capacity to compensate for this defect.

concentrations of 200 mg/dL or higher are diagnostic of diabetes; patients with levels between 140 and 199 mg/dL are defined as having IGT. Patients displaying IFG and IGT simultaneously have a greater risk for development of diabetes. It should be noted that the thresholds that define these "states" are somewhat arbitrary because the risk for diabetes actually runs along a continuum. In fact, the World Health Organization, which is in accord with the other diagnostic thresholds, has kept the lower bound of the IFG range at 110 mg/dL because individuals with levels above this range appear to be at increased cardiovascular risk, similar to those with IGT. As noted previously, the ADA has also recently endorsed the use of the HbA$_{1c}$ for diabetes screening, based on the recommendations of the International Expert Committee, with a diagnostic threshold of 6.5% or higher. In so doing, it considered elevated but not frankly diabetic levels to represent high risk, defining this range as 5.7 to 6.4%. Table 237-1 summarizes the diagnosis of IFG, IGT, and overt diabetes mellitus. Patients with IFG or IGT or increased glycohemoglobin, each of which may be referred to as prediabetes, should be advised about healthy lifestyle changes, including diet and exercise, and should be screened annually for progression to diabetes. In very high risk individuals, such as those with both IFG and IGT, a Consensus Statement from the ADA and the European Association for the Study of Diabetes (EASD) has proposed that, in addition to lifestyle change, metformin be considered as adjunctive therapy (see Prevention).

The clinical utility and cost-effectiveness of screening for diabetes mellitus have never been directly demonstrated. However, because patients with diabetes may harbor the disease for many years before symptoms are appreciated, the ADA has endorsed the screening at 3-year intervals beginning at 45 years of age (Table 237-2). More frequent screening is advised for high-risk individuals, such as those with a personal history of IFG, IGT, gestational diabetes mellitus, obesity, hypertension, or dyslipidemia, patients in high-risk ethnic groups, and patients with first-degree relatives with diabetes. In most cases, a fasting plasma glucose level has been the screening test of choice; however, the oral glucose tolerance test has the advantage of detecting patients with IGT and early diabetes. The more convenient HbA$_{1c}$ test will likely be used more often now that it is endorsed as a screening test by the ADA, but there is little information about its predictive value across various groups of patients.

Gestational Diabetes Mellitus

Because even mild glucose elevations can have serious adverse effects on a developing fetus, an aggressive screening approach is recommended during pregnancy (Chapter 247). Women with a high clinical risk of gestational diabetes (personal history of gestational diabetes mellitus, obesity, glycosuria, or a strong family history of diabetes) should undergo screening as soon as possible after conception; in these patients, screening *before* pregnancy is preferred if possible. At 24 to 28 weeks of gestation, screening is recommended for *all* pregnant women, except those in the lowest risk category who meet *all* of the following clinical characteristics:

- Age younger than 25 years
- Weight normal before pregnancy
- Member of an ethnic group with a low risk for gestational diabetes (e.g., whites)
- No known diabetes in first-degree relatives
- No history of abnormal glucose tolerance
- No history of poor obstetric outcome

In pregnant women, a casual plasma glucose level of 200 mg/dL or higher or a confirmed fasting plasma glucose level of 126 mg/dL or higher establishes the diagnosis of gestational diabetes mellitus and precludes the need for a glucose challenge. In the absence of overt hyperglycemia, a screening 1-hour 50-g glucose challenge test should be performed between 24 and 28 weeks of gestation. If the fasting glucose level is 105 mg/dL or higher or the 1-hour postload value is 140 mg/dL or higher, a diagnostic 3-hour 100-g oral glucose tolerance test is indicated. Gestational diabetes is then diagnosed if two or more values equal or exceed the upper limits of normal: fasting, 95 mg/dL; 1 hour, 180 mg/dL; 2 hour, 155 mg/dL; and 3 hour, 140 mg/dL. To save time and effort, proceeding directly to the 100-g diagnostic oral glucose tolerance test is an acceptable alternative, particularly in those deemed at higher risk. The Hyperglycemia and Adverse Pregnancy Outcomes (HAPO) study included more than 25,000 pregnancies, examining adverse clinical outcomes associated with mild elevations in plasma glucose during oral glucose tolerance testing. The investigators found that increases in plasma glucose above 75 mg/dL fasting, 105 mg/dL at 1 hour, and 90 mg/dL at 2 hours were associated with a higher risk for several adverse fetal and maternal outcomes (e.g., increased birthweight, primary cesarean delivery, and neonatal hypoglycemia). Importantly, no specific glucose thresholds could be identified, suggesting that adverse outcomes occur over a continuum of blood glucose elevations during pregnancy. These data will likely lead to a reevaluation of the current screening guidelines and diagnostic categories for gestational diabetes.

TREATMENT

Complications

As discussed in Chapter 236, the Diabetes Control and Complications Trial (DCCT), involving solely patients with type 1 diabetes, conclusively determined that improved glucose control reduces the risk for microvascular complications. It was assumed but not entirely known if the same relationship would apply to patients with type 2 diabetes. Ultimate evidence for such a benefit came from the United Kingdom Prospective Diabetes Study (UKPDS).[1] The UKPDS initially recruited 5102 patients with newly diagnosed type 2 diabetes; after 3 months of diet therapy, the 3867 patients with fasting glucose levels between 6.1 and 15.0 mmol/L (110 and 270 mg/dL) were randomized to a more intensive regimen, consisting of sulfonylurea or insulin, or maintained on the conventional dietary regimen, focused primarily on symptom reduction. Subjects were monitored for an average of 10 years. Although glycemic control gradually deteriorated in all groups, the intensified treatment group had lower overall mean HbA$_{1c}$ levels than their conventionally treated counterparts (7.0% vs. 7.9%). This modest improvement was associated with 25% and 12% reductions in all microvascular complications ($P < .001$) and any diabetes-related event ($P = .03$), respectively. The intensified treatment group also experienced a 16% reduction in a combined end point—nonfatal or fatal myocardial infarction or sudden death—that did not quite reach statistical significance ($P = .052$). Epidemiologically, a continuous relationship was again noted between glycemic control and diabetic complications. Also similar to the DCCT, no glycemic threshold for microvascular complications was observed. In a smaller substudy within the UKPDS, 753 overweight patients were randomized to metformin versus diet. Metformin-treated subjects experienced relative risk reductions of 32% for any diabetes related point ($P = .002$), 39% for myocardial infarction ($P = .01$), 42% for diabetes-related death ($P = .02$), and 36% for all-cause mortality ($P = .01$). Moreover, among patients allocated to intensive control, metformin had a greater effect than sulfonylureas or insulin on any diabetes-related end point, stroke, and overall mortality. These data suggested a cardiovascular benefit to metformin in overweight diabetic patients compared with either sulfonylureas or insulin.

In the more recent 10-year follow-up study of 3277 patients from the original UKPDS cohort, clinical outcomes were assessed using the original treatment assignment.[2] Differences in HbA$_{1c}$ were lost between groups after the first year of follow-up, as occurred in the DCCT long-term follow-up study. Despite this, however, relative risk reductions for any diabetes-related end point (9%, $P = .04$) and microvascular disease events (24%, $P = .001$) persisted

---

<table>
<tr><td colspan="2">TABLE 237-2   CRITERIA FOR DIABETES SCREENING IN ASYMPTOMATIC INDIVIDUALS</td></tr>
</table>

1. Testing should be considered in all adults who are overweight (BMI > 25 kg/m^{2*}) and have additional risk factors:
   - Physical inactivity
   - A first-degree relative with diabetes
   - High-risk ethnic population (e.g., African American, Hispanic American, Native American, Asian American, Pacific Islander)
   - Delivered a baby weighing more than 9 pounds or diagnosed with gestational diabetes mellitus
   - Systemic hypertension (blood pressure > 140/90 mm Hg or on antihypertensive therapy)
   - High-density lipoprotein cholesterol level < 35 mg/dL or triglyceride level > 250 mg/dL
   - Polycystic ovary syndrome
   - Hemoglobin A$_{1c}$ ≥ 5.7%, impaired glucose tolerance or impaired fasting glucose on prior testing
   - Other clinical conditions associated with insulin resistance (e.g., severe obesity, acanthosis nigricans)
   - History of cardiovascular disease
2. If none of the above criteria are present, screening for diabetes should begin at age 45 years.
3. If the results are normal, screening should be repeated at least every 3 years. Depending on initial results and risk status, more frequent testing may need to be considered.

*In some ethnic groups, such as Asians, at-risk body mass index (BMI) may be lower.
Modified from American Diabetes Association. Diagnosis and classification of diabetes mellitus. *Diabetes Care.* 2010;33(Suppl. 1):S14.

in the sulfonylurea-insulin cohort. In addition, as more events occurred over time, significant relative risk reductions for myocardial infarction (15%, $P = .001$) and all-cause mortality (13%, $P = .007$) emerged. In the metformin-assigned subjects, risk reductions of 21% ($P = .01$) were maintained throughout the follow-up period for any diabetes-related event; 33% ($P = .005$) for myocardial infarction, and 27% ($P = -.002$) for all-cause mortality. By comparison, more aggressive treatment to lower HbA$_{1c}$ below 6.0% in the Action to Control Cardiovascular Risk in Diabetes (ACCORD) trial increased 5-year mortality despite reducing the risk of nonfatal myocardial infarction.**3**

What conclusions can be drawn from these various studies? The primary message is that "glucose matters"—particularly when treated early in the course of the disease and especially for microvascular complications. In both type 1 and type 2 diabetes patients who are willing and able to participate actively in their management, the goal should be to achieve the best possible level of glycemic control as rapidly as possible without undue risk. These studies also demonstrate that most patients benefit from lower glucose levels, even if normalization is not achieved. For most type 2 patients, effective glucose reductions can be achieved by diet, oral agents, or less complicated insulin regimens than are required in type 1 diabetes. Although a statistically significant benefit on macrovascular outcomes could not be detected in the sulfonylurea-insulin tight control arm of the UKPDS, this may have been limited by the HbA$_{1c}$ convergence during follow-up study of the initially randomized groups. Metformin had a more convincing beneficial effect in this regard. It is also noteworthy that extensive epidemiologic data have shown a linear relationship between glycemia and cardiovascular events—even into the "normal" range for glucose. Accordingly, it was theorized by some that in order to achieve substantive cardiovascular risk reduction by glycemic control, euglycemia needed to be achieved. This was the hypothesis tested by an important trio of clinical cardiovascular trials recently reported in patients with type 2 diabetes (see later). Finally, a central conclusion from the UKPDS was that β-cell function continues to decline after the diagnosis of diabetes is made, mandating more aggressive treatment regimens.

Glycemic Control and Cardiovascular Disease Outcomes

Although there is a strong and irrefutable epidemiologic association between glycemic control and cardiovascular events and mortality, clinical trial data to support an effect of glucose control to reduce macrovascular events has been generally elusive. Some had proposed that this phenomenon might reflect a failure of earlier trials to normalize glycemia, which might actually be required to influence the atherosclerotic process once it been initiated. As a result, several large randomized clinical trials (ACCORD,**4** Action in Diabetes and Vascular Disease: Preterax and Diamicron Modified Release Controlled Evaluation [ADVANCE],**5** and the Veterans Affairs Diabetes Trial [VADT]**6**) were initiated in an attempt to answer this question. Each trial examined the potential cardiovascular benefit of more intensive glucose control (HbA$_{1c}$ target, 6 to 6.5%) compared with standard therapy over a period of 3 to 5 years in patients with long-standing type 2 diabetes, most of whom had evidence of cardiovascular disease (CVD) (Table 237-3). In each circumstance, the study failed to reduce CVD outcomes. In ADVANCE, the primary end point,

a composite of both microvascular and macrovascular events, was modestly reduced in the intensive control arm, but this was driven solely by a reduction in renal outcomes. On the other hand, in ACCORD, all-cause mortality was actually *increased* by 22% in the intensive control cohort, mainly driven by increased cardiovascular mortality.**3** The explanation for this finding remains controversial, however. Hypoglycemia was definitely more common in patients who died in both intensive and standard control groups, but subsequent analyses have not been able to demonstrate a precise cause-and-effect relationship. Whether the results may have reflected significant weight gain or the use of complex polypharmaceutical regimens (most participants in ACCORD's intensive arm were receiving at least three oral agents simultaneously with or without aggressive insulin strategies) is also not known.

Importantly, the results of ACCORD, ADVANCE, and VADT do not invalidate the earlier findings from the DCCT and UKPDS. Those studies were quite different insofar as they enrolled different types of patients—those with type 1 diabetes in the DCCT and newly diagnosed type 2 patients without underlying CVD in the UKPDS. Additionally, the patients in the UKPDS were randomized to "intensive control" strategies that were not nearly as stringent as those pursued in the more recent trials, and in the DCCT, the comparator "conventional control" group essentially had poorly controlled type 1 diabetes. So, a rational synthesis of the data would appear to be that the target of lowering HbA$_{1c}$ to approximately 7% will result in major reductions in microvascular disease risk and, over time, a modest benefit on cardiovascular end points in patients in the early stages of the disease without preexisting cardiovascular complications. However, more intensive control in an attempt to near-normalize glucose levels, especially if applied to older patients with significant risk for or preestablished cardiovascular disease, leads to no further benefit and to apparent adverse effects**3,4** over a treatment duration of 3 to 5 years. Given that these trials examined patients at a later stage of diabetes, they cannot answer the question of whether near-normalization of blood glucose control may have a cardiovascular benefit when initiated at the time of diagnosis and maintained for a longer duration, before vascular complications can become established.

General Measures

As in individuals with type 1 diabetes, the primary long-term goals in type 2 patients are to minimize complications and to preserve the patient's sense of clinical well-being. Glucose control should not be addressed in a vacuum. Lifestyle modification should be the primary focus of the patient's care. Also, aggressive lowering of lipids and blood pressure should be routinely incorporated into the treatment program.

In many type 2 diabetic patients, diet**7** and exercise**8** are the only therapeutic interventions required to restore metabolic control. As a result, drug therapy is not required in all patients and may be avoided in motivated individuals who have embraced the important concepts of a healthy lifestyle and can achieve their glycemic targets nonpharmacologically. However, it should also be realized that diabetes tends to be progressive, and the early use of antihyperglycemic medications is usually a wise maneuver. Indeed, a

---

TABLE 237-3 MAJOR CLINICAL TRIALS TO TEST THE ASSOCIATION BETWEEN GLYCEMIC CONTROL AND CARDIOVASCULAR DISEASE OUTCOMES

STUDY PARAMETER	ACCORD	ADVANCE	VADT
No. of subjects	10,251	11,140	1791
Mean age (yr)	62	66	60
Body mass index (kg/m^2)	32	28	31
Mean follow-up (yr)	3.5	5	5.6
Hemoglobin A$_{1c}$ targets	<6.0% vs. 7.0-7.9%	≤6.5% vs. standard	<6% vs. 8-9%
Mean baseline A$_{1c}$	8.3%	7.5%	9.4%
Mean end point A$_{1c}$	INT: 6.4% vs. STD: 7.5%	INT: 6.3% vs. STD: 7.0%	INT: 6.9% vs. STD: 8.4%
Major macro- or microvascular event	—	0.9 (0.82-0.98), $P = .01$	0.88 (0.74-1.05), $P = .14$
Nonfatal myocardial infarction/ stroke, cardiovascular death	HR 0.9 (0.78-1.04), $P = .16$	HR 0.94 (0.84-1.06), $P = .32$	—
All-cause mortality	HR 1.22 (1.01-1.46), $P = .04$	0.93 (0.83-1.06), $P = .28$	1.07 (0.81-1.42), $P = .62$
Nonfatal myocardial infarction	HR 0.76 (0.62-0.92), $P = .004$	0.98 (0.77-1.22), $P = $ NS	0.82 (0.59-1.14), $P = .24$
Hypoglycemic events	INT: 10.5% vs. STD: 3.5%, $P < .001$	INT: 2.7% vs. STD: 1.5%, $P < .001$	INT: 8.5% vs. STD: 3.1%, $P = .000$
Weight change	> +10 kg, INT: 27.8% vs. STD: 14.1%, $P < .001$	INT: −0.1 kg vs. STD: −1.0 kg, $P = $ NS	INT: +8.1% vs. STD: 4.1%, $P = .01$

HR = hazard radio; INT = intensive control group; NS = not significant; STD = standard control group.
Data from the Action to Control Cardiovascular Risk in Diabetes (ACCORD) study group. Effects of intensive glucose lowering in type 2 diabetes. *N Engl J Med.* 2008;358:2545-2559; The ADVANCE Collaborative Group. Intensive blood glucose control and vascular outcomes in patients with type. 2 diabetes. *N Engl J Med.* 2008;358:2560-2572; and Duckworth W, Abraira C, Moritz T, et al, for the VADT Investigators. Glucose control and vascular complications in veterans with type 2 diabetes. *N Engl J Med.* 2009;360:129-139.

consensus statement, sponsored by the ADA and EASD on the treatment of hyperglycemia in type 2 diabetes, has advised using metformin (barring any contraindications) along with lifestyle change at diagnosis.

Diet

Irrespective of initial weight, modest weight reduction (on the order of 5 kg) in obese diabetic patients leads to improved glycemic control. The dramatic impact of weight loss is mediated by changes in insulin-responsive tissues as well as by enhanced β-cell activity; insulin resistance diminishes, glucose production declines, and lower glucose levels improve glucose-stimulated insulin secretion. The beneficial effects of weight loss are not restricted to glucose; dietary therapy also yields improved lipoprotein profiles and systemic blood pressure. In general, it matters little how weight loss is achieved, provided good health is preserved and adequate nutrition is maintained. Successful weight loss (Chapter 227) is best achieved by the combination of a supportive environment that emphasizes the gradual achievement of goals, regular exercise to increase energy expenditure, and long-term behavior modification. Please see Table 236-3 in Chapter 236 for lifestyle changes advised for patients with diabetes.

A popular alternative to diet is bariatric surgery; both Roux-en-Y gastric bypass and gastric banding procedures are being performed with increased frequency in obese patients both with and without diabetes. Without question, these techniques result in greater degrees of weight loss than are usually achieved through diet or medications. Both short-term and long-term safety considerations persist, although several longitudinal studies have suggested an overall health benefit. Importantly, in patients with type 2 diabetes, very often glucose levels normalize postoperatively, and antihyperglycemic therapy can be stopped or at least markedly curtailed. The rapidity of the improvement in glucose levels, which occurs before substantial weight loss has occurred, suggests a direct metabolic benefit, perhaps owing to rapid onset of severe calorie deprivation or altered transit of nutrients through the bowel, or both, which might be promoting the actions of incretins on glucose metabolism.

Exercise

Regular exercise is a powerful (and often forgotten) adjunct in the treatment of type 2 diabetes. Long-term studies demonstrate consistent beneficial effects of regular exercise on carbohydrate metabolism and insulin sensitivity that can be maintained for several years. Exercise also facilitates weight loss and its maintenance, which further improves glycemic control and also has beneficial effects on cardiovascular risk and general well-being. Regular exercise lowers triglyceride-rich very low density lipoprotein (VLDL) levels, raises high-density lipoprotein (HDL) levels, and improves fibrinolytic activity. In general, "moderate" levels of exercise should be prescribed most days of the week (see Table 236-3 in Chapter 236). Limitations may be imposed by preexisting coronary or peripheral vascular disease, proliferative retinopathy, peripheral or autonomic neuropathy, and poor glycemic control.

Medical Therapy

Oral Glucose-Lowering Agents

Sulfonylureas were the only oral agents available in the United States for more than four decades. Over the decade and a half since the 1995 approval of metformin by the U.S. Food and Drug Administration (FDA), many new classes of oral agents have become available for the treatment of type 2 diabetes (Table 237-4 and Fig. 237-3). Indeed, at present there are as many classes to treat glucose in type 2 diabetes as there are antihypertensive medication categories. Currently available noninsulin classes include the sulfonylureas, nonsulfonylurea insulin secretagogues (glinides), thiazolidinediones, α-glucosidase inhibitors, glucagon-like peptide (GLP)-1 agonists, amylin mimetics, dipeptidyl peptidase (DPP)-4 inhibitors, bile acid sequestrants, and dopamine-2 agonists. Oral agents are indicated in patients in whom diet and exercise fail to achieve treatment goals and may be favored over insulin in older patients with relatively mild degrees of hyperglycemia. Patients with more severe hyperglycemia may require insulin during the initial phases of treatment; once glucose levels have stabilized and the "toxic" effects of severe hyperglycemia on β-cell function and insulin action have been minimized, many of these patients may then be converted to oral agents. Of these agents, rosiglitazone must be used cautiously because of its increased risk of heart failure and myocardial infarction compared with other agents.[9,10] By comparison, pioglitazone appears to be protective.[11]

For a detailed review of the oral antihyperglycemic agents, refer to the online version of this chapter. Table 237-4 summarizes the key aspects of each drug class.

Insulin Therapy in Type 2 Diabetes

The principles of insulin therapy and details of insulin preparations, regimens, and monitoring are discussed in the previous chapter on type 1 diabetes (Chapter 236). Insulin is commonly used as first-line therapy for nonobese, younger, or severely hyperglycemic type 2 diabetic patients and is often temporarily required during times of severe stress (e.g., injury, infection, surgery) or during pregnancy. Insulin should not be used as first-line therapy for patients who are poorly compliant, unwilling to self-monitor glucose levels, or at high risk for hypoglycemia (e.g., very elderly patients). In obese patients, profound insulin resistance often necessitates the use of large doses of insulin,

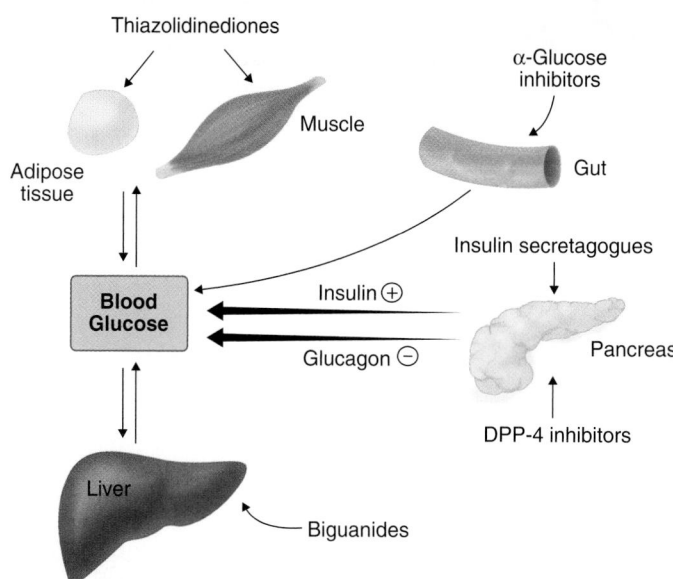

FIGURE 237-3. Sites of action of the most widely used oral antihyperglycemic agents.

which can interfere with efforts to restrict calorie intake and achieve weight loss. In leaner patients and in patients with relatively mild fasting hyperglycemia (who continue to maintain endogenous insulin secretory capacity), relatively small doses of basal insulin (e.g., 0.3 to 0.4 U per kilogram of body weight per day) given once or twice per day may be sufficient to achieve glucose targets. Many of these patients retain some degree of meal-stimulated endogenous insulin secretion and may therefore require no or less rapid-acting insulin as well.

Although a common practice has been to administer a single dose of NPH insulin in the morning, the glucose-lowering effect of this regimen does not usually extend during a full 24-hour period. Because a key element of successful insulin treatment is to counteract accelerated rates of endogenous glucose production in the morning, it is generally more effective to split the dose and to administer sufficient amounts of intermediate-acting insulin in the evening (preferably at bedtime) to optimize control. Alternatively, premixed insulins containing 70 to 75% NPH and 25 to 30% of a short- or rapid-acting insulin (e.g., regular human insulin, lispro, or aspart) can be given twice daily. Although somewhat inflexible because of their combined contents in fixed ratios, these insulins provide a level of convenience for some patients who are not able or willing to mix insulins or use strategies involving three or four injections per day. With the availability of long-acting, basal insulins over the past decade, such as glargine and detemir, one injection per day is an increasingly favored approach in many patients. This may be combined with oral glucose-lowering agents to facilitate endogenous insulin release and action. Typically these agents are offered at bedtime, but they can actually be administered at any time of day. In patients taking large doses or in whom it is suspected that the hypoglycemic effect is waning before 24 hours (as is more commonly seen with detemir), twice-daily dosing can be used.

With regard to the initiation of even more advanced insulin replacement regimens, which are required in certain insulin-deficient type 2 patients (and are similar to the optimal regimens in type 1 patients), there are several acceptable approaches. The optimal insulin strategy in type 2 diabetes is not clear. In general, the more insulin injections, the tighter the control, but this must be balanced against convenience and the commitment on the patient's part to injections and the requisite monitoring. The total daily dose of insulin should first be estimated from body weight; total insulin requirements range between 0.5 and 1.0 U/kg/day, typically higher than those used in type 1 diabetes. One classic method for starting insulin is to divide the total daily dose unevenly, with two thirds given before breakfast and the remaining third before dinner. Each of the two doses is then further subdivided: at breakfast, two thirds of the dose is given as intermediate-acting insulin and the other third as a short- or rapid-acting preparation; at dinner, the dose is divided into two equal parts. As an example, for a 90-kg man with estimated requirements of 0.67 U/kg/day, 60 U of insulin may be required. By use of this method, the patient might receive 27 units of NPH with 13 units of regular insulin or a rapid-acting insulin analogue (e.g., lispro, aspart, or glulisine) before breakfast, then 10 units of NPH with 10 units of analogue before dinner. More refined "basal-bolus" regimens using more modern insulins offer more physiologic insulin replacement. The regimen in the most motivated and capable patients is ideally adjusted on the basis of the anticipated carbohydrate intake ("carbohydrate counting") as well as the before-meal blood glucose level. These regimens are more complex and require frequent dosage adjustments and more intensive glucose monitoring. In the absence of hyperglycemic complications,

TABLE 237-4   ORAL AGENTS AVAILABLE FOR TREATMENT OF DIABETES MELLITUS

AGENT	EXAMPLES	MECHANISM	ACTION	↓ IN HEMOGLOBIN A_{1c}	ADVANTAGES	DISADVANTAGES	COST
Sulfonylureas	*First generation:* Chlorpropamide Tolazamide Tolbutamide *Second generation:* Glyburide Glipizide Glimepiride	Closes K_{ATP} channels	↑ Pancreatic insulin secretion	1-2%	↓ Microvascular risk Convenience	Hypoglycemia Weight gain May blunt myocardial ischemic preconditioning ? β-cell "exhaustion"	$
Glinides	Repaglinide Nateglinide	Closes K_{ATP} channels	↑ Pancreatic insulin secretion	1-1.5%	More physiologic ↓ Postprandial glucose	Hypoglycemia, weight gain, May blunt myocardial ischemic preconditioning ? β-cell "exhaustion" Dosing frequency	$$$
Biguanides	Metformin	Activates AMPK	↓ Hepatic glucose production	1-2%	Weight loss/weight neutrality No hypoglycemia ↓ CVD	Diarrhea, abdominal cramping Lactic acidosis risk (rare) Vitamin B_{12} deficiency Multiple contraindications to consider (e.g., CKD)	$
Thiazolidinediones	Rosiglitazone Pioglitazone	Activates PPAR-γ	↑ Peripheral insulin sensitivity	0.5-1.5%	No hypoglycemia β-cell preservation ↑ HDL-C ↓ Triglycerides ? ↓CVD (pioglitazone)	Weight gain Edema/heart failure ↑ Bone fractures (women) ↑ LDL-C ? ↑CVD (rosiglitazone)	$$$
α-Glucosidase inhibitors	Acarbose Miglitol	Blocks SB α-glucosidase	↓ Intestinal carbohydrate absorption	0.5-1%	? ↓ CVD Nonsystemic medication ↓ Postprandial glucose	Gas, abdominal bloating Dosing frequency	$$
GLP-1 receptor agonists	Exenatide Liraglutide	Activates GLP-1 receptors	↑ Insulin secretion ↓ Glucagon secretion Slows gastric emptying ↑ Satiety	1%	Weight loss ? β-cell preservation ? Cardiovascular benefits	Nausea/vomiting ? Pancreatitis ? C-cell hyperplasia/ tumors Injectable	$$$
Amylin mimetics	Pramlintide	Activates amylin receptors	↓ Glucagon secretion Slows gastric emptying ↑ Satiety	0.5%	Weight loss ↓ Postprandial glucose	Nausea/vomiting Dosing frequency Injectable	$$$
DPP-4 inhibitors	Sitagliptin Saxagliptin	Inhibits DPP-4, ↑ endogenous incretins	↑ Insulin secretion ↓ Glucagon secretion	0.5-0.8%	No hypoglycemia	? Urticaria/angioedema ? Pancreatitis	$$$
Bile acid sequestrants	Colesevelam	Binds bile acid cholesterol	Unknown	0.5%	No hypoglycemia ↓LDL-C	Constipation ↑ Triglycerides	$$$
D2 agonists	Bromocriptine	Activates dopaminergic receptors	Alters hypothalamic regulation of metabolism ↑Insulin sensitivity	0.5%	No hypoglycemia	Dizziness/syncope Nausea Fatigue Rhinitis	?

AMPK = adenosine monophosphate–activated protein kinase; ATP = adenosine triphosphate; CKD = chronic kidney disease; CVD = cardiovascular disease; GLP = glucagon-like peptide; D2 = dopamine-2; DPP = dipeptidyl peptidase; HDL-C = high-density lipoprotein cholesterol; LDL-C = low-density lipoprotein cholesterol; PPAR = peroxisome proliferator–activated receptor; SB = small bowel.

clinicians should generally begin with more conservative doses of insulin to minimize hypoglycemia and to smooth the patient's transition to multiple-dose subcutaneous insulin therapy. In short, the complexity of the regimen should be individualized according to the clinical context, the patient's abilities and capacities to perform self-care, and most important, the patient's level of education and motivation.

The Treating-To-Target in Type 2 Diabetes (4-T) trial compared glycemic outcomes from various insulin regimens in more than 700 patients whose diabetes was inadequately controlled despite therapy with metformin and sulfonylurea.[12] The participants were randomized to (1) premixed insulin analogue injections twice a day (aspart 70/30 before breakfast and supper), (2) prandial rapid-acting insulin analogue (insulin aspart) three times daily, or (3) a basal insulin analogue (insulin detemir) once (or twice) daily, with the goal of achieving an HbA_{1c} level of 6.5% or less. After 1 year, if the HbA_{1c} was not at target, the sulfonylurea was discontinued and a second type of insulin initiated. For those on the premixed regimen, once-daily aspart was added before lunch; for those on the prandial-only strategy, once-daily basal analogue was added; and for those using basal insulin alone, the regimen was advanced to incorporate three times per day prandial rapid insulin. At 3 years, the median HbA_{1c} across groups was 6.9% (premixed, 7.1%; prandial, 6.8%; basal, 6.9%); however, almost three in four patients required two types of insulin in combination. More patients who had started therapy with a basal insulin only

(43.2%) or a prandial insulin only (44.8%) achieved target than those initially randomized to the premixed (31.9%). Weight gain amounted to 3.6 kg, 5.7 kg, and 6.4 kg in the basal, premixed, and prandial groups, respectively. Less hypoglycemia occurred in those randomized to the basal insulin approach (1.7 per patient year) than the premixed (3.0 per patient year) or prandial (5.7 per patient year) insulin regimens. These findings provide support for treatment to begin with basal insulin once a day, and then add mealtime insulin if glycemic targets are not met. However, in patients not able to handle more complex regimens, premixed insulin twice daily is a reasonable option as well.

Experience with the use of intensified insulin treatment, including continuous subcutaneous insulin infusion pumps and multiple subcutaneous injection regimens, is growing in patients with type 2 diabetes. Preliminary results suggest that intensified treatment may be successfully applied to selected patients.

In many cases, the combination of intensive insulin therapy with oral hypoglycemic agents (e.g., TZDs or metformin) may reduce insulin dose requirements and improve glycemic control. Although this is growing in acceptance, the potential benefit of reducing circulating insulin levels (by combination therapy) on the development of atherogenesis remains to be established. As in patients with type 1 diabetes, weight gain and hypoglycemia are potential side effects of insulin therapy. It is noteworthy, however, that the incidence of severe hypoglycemia is markedly lower (<5%) than that seen in patients with type 1 diabetes.

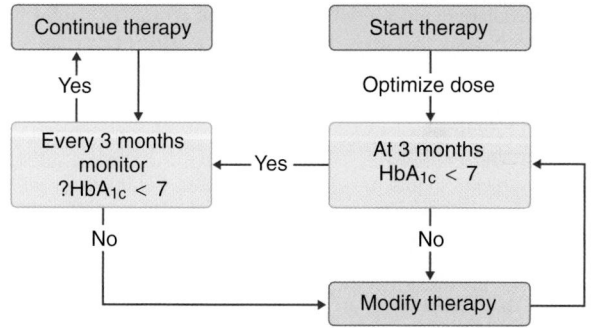

FIGURE 237-4. Overall strategy for the treatment of type 2 diabetes.

Treatment Strategies for Type 2 Diabetes

In contrast to type 1 diabetes, in which insulin therapy is required, many pharmacologic options exist for the management of type 2 diabetes. The pros and cons of the various oral hypoglycemic agents have been discussed; often, it is difficult to justify the use of one oral agent over another, although the general consensus of endocrinologists is to recommend metformin as first-line therapy in the absence of contraindications, given its effectiveness, the lack of hypoglycemia associated with its use as monotherapy, its low cost, and weight neutrality. It is now believed that in most cases metformin therapy should be initiated early, is concurrent with lifestyle intervention, and is gradually increased to the maximally effective dose over 1 to 2 months. In the event these interventions fail to achieve the glycemic goals set for the patient within about 3 months, another drug should be added to the regimen (Fig. 237-4). What the next step should be is much more controversial and remains uncertain. Most studies comparing oral drugs have focused on glycemic end points, and most show modest differences, with few exceptions. Few studies, however, have compared drugs for more relevant clinical outcomes such as mortality or microvascular and macrovascular complications. To date, the largest study to address such outcomes in type 2 diabetes was the UKPDS.[1] In the UKPDS, the long-term follow-up of the study participants assigned to more intensified therapy demonstrated improved outcomes for microvascular complications and myocardial infarction and reduced mortality for patients given insulin and sulfonylureas (as well as metformin). The ability of the study to detect differences among the different treatments was limited because of drug crossovers and the frequent need for drug combinations as the study progressed. On the other hand, the long-term benefits of newer antidiabetic agents have not been established.

The choice of second-line pharmacologic therapy for type 2 diabetes should be influenced in part by the severity of fasting hyperglycemia, the presence and magnitude of hyperglycemic symptoms, and the degree of obesity. Other factors such as age, comorbid conditions, propensity to certain side effects, drug cost, and convenience should also be considered. Published clinical trials comparing drug combinations with monotherapy have generally shown additive reductions in HbA$_{1c}$; with few exceptions, the magnitude of HbA$_{1c}$ reduction approximates that achieved when the added agent is used as monotherapy. As is the case with monotherapy, there is no convincing evidence favoring one combination regimen over another, and most combinations have been approved by the FDA. Triple therapy, or combining three agents to achieve glucose targets, is also used in clinical practice (although not formally with FDA approval) and appears to be effective. Ultimately, if glucose targets cannot be met by combining oral agents, insulin remains an effective treatment option.

Two published algorithms include one from a consensus group representing the ADA and the EASD (see Nathan in Suggested Readings) and one from the American Association of Clinical Endocrinologists/American College of Endocrinology (Rodbard in Suggested Readings).

Monitoring

See Chapter 236 for details. Patients with type 2 diabetes generally require less frequent self-monitoring of blood glucose concentration, particularly those managed with oral agents or less intensive insulin regimens. Glucose and HbA$_{1c}$ targets should be the same as in type 1 diabetes (see Table 237-4), with the recently appreciated caveat that older patients (>65 to 70 years) may not benefit from more stringent goals, especially in the setting of long disease duration (>12 years) or significant underlying risk for or overt cardiovascular disease. Importantly, each patient's desirable glucose range must be an individual decision between the practitioner and the patient. Elements of this decision must take into account the motivation and capacities of the patient, propensity for hypoglycemia and its unawareness, presence or absence of complications, and, of course, other established comorbidities.

Inpatient Management of Diabetes

Much attention has been paid recently to the inpatient management of hyperglycemia, both in patients with an established diagnosis of diabetes and in those whose glucose elevations are a response to illness. Observational studies previously have correlated the degree of hyperglycemia and outcomes in a variety of settings, including after cardiac surgery, in the critically ill, and in patients with acute myocardial infarction and stroke. Acutely, hyperglycemia has a notable detrimental effect on the immune system, wound healing, endothelial function, and cardiac metabolism. When glucose elevations are severe, dangerous fluid shifts and electrolyte fluxes may occur. However, multiple studies have failed to confirm a benefit from aggressive control of inpatient glucose levels and studies have actually raised the probability of a mortality risk with intensive intravenous insulin therapy targeting a blood glucose level lower than 108 mg/dL.[13] This was in the setting of (but not clearly the result of) a several-fold increase in the risk for severe hypoglycemia. Importantly, the conventional therapy groups in most of these studies were targeted to a lower blood glucose value than the initial investigations. This raised the concern that the randomized groups were no longer as distinct from a glycemic standpoint, which might attenuate or even eliminate the benefits of glucose control. Whether there is any short-term benefit of tight glucose control in noncritically ill hospitalized patients is unknown because adequate clinical trials have not been conducted in this setting.

Reasonable approaches to both these patient groups have been proposed by the ADA, the American Association of Clinical Endocrinologists (AACE), and the American College of Physicians,[14] with current targets set at 140 to 180 mg/dL using intravenous insulin in the intensive care setting, and maintaining preprandial blood glucose levels lower than 140 mg/dL in other patients. As in the outpatient arena, individualization is important; patients with severe comorbidities or with short life expectancy can be reasonably kept at a more conservative range. Multidisciplinary inpatient diabetes management teams have been shown to be useful in assisting hospitals to improve the quality of their diabetes care and in reducing the length of stay of diabetic patients.

PREVENTION

With our increasing understanding of the pathogenesis of type 2 diabetes and our appreciation of the often lengthy period between impaired glucose metabolism and overt diabetes, there has been significant attention directed to the possibility of preventing this disease in at-risk individuals.

In the Diabetes Prevention Program, more than 3000 overweight subjects with IGT were randomized into four treatment arms: (1) intensive lifestyle changes aimed at reducing body weight by 7% through a low-fat diet and 150 minutes of weekly exercise; (2) treatment with metformin, 850 mg twice per day; and (3) treatment with placebo pills, twice per day.[15] The last three groups also received standard information about diet and exercise. The trial was stopped a year early because of definitive results. In the placebo group, 29% of patients developed diabetes during the average follow-up period of 3 years, compared with 22% of patients taking metformin and only 14% of patients undergoing intensive diet and exercise. The relative risk reduction for patients taking metformin was 31% versus standard care, whereas patients undergoing intensive lifestyle interventions reduced their risk by an impressive 58%. This risk reduction was identical to that measured by Finnish investigators in the Diabetes Prevention Study, involving a similar study design but focusing on lifestyle change alone. This suggests that patients with IGT can sharply lower their immediate risk for diabetes with intensive lifestyle changes (or in some cases with metformin).

Whether screening, identifying, and then treating patients with IGT in routine clinical practice is cost-effective or even doable remains somewhat controversial. Certainly, if recommendations regarding healthy lifestyle changes were followed by high-risk patients, the incidence of type 2 diabetes would decrease. If such therapy is durable, this would necessarily translate to fewer microvascular complications over time. Whether such interventions will mitigate the risk for macrovascular disease is less clear, although Diabetes Prevention Program participants on diet and exercise did experience some amelioration in cardiovascular risk factors.

How drug therapy fits into this equation is similarly a point of controversy. Notably, after metformin therapy was washed out in Diabetes Prevention Program participants for 2 weeks, 25% of those whose diabetes was apparently prevented developed the disease. Similarly, in the STOP-NIDDM diabetes prevention trial involving the α-glucosidase inhibitor acarbose, a 25% decrease in the appearance of type 2 diabetes during a 3-year period was demonstrated. In two studies involving TZDs, larger risk reductions have been observed. In DREAM, rosiglitazone therapy reduced the progression to diabetes in high-risk patients by 62%, and in the ACT NOW trial, pioglitazone was associated with an 81% risk reduction. Moreover, pioglitazone has recently been reported to diminish carotid intimal thickening by 38% in patients with IGT in a multicenter clinical trial. Importantly, no drug is currently approved by the FDA for diabetes prevention, although metformin is used not uncommonly in such efforts.

A consensus statement from the ADA and the EASD has endorsed lifestyle change in anyone identified with a prediabetic state. It also advised the consideration of metformin therapy in those at especially high risk, such as individuals with both IFG and IGT, combined with other high-risk features such as family history and characteristics that predict an effective response to metformin, based on the DPP. The latter include age younger than 60 years, body mass index greater than 35 kg/m², and fasting plasma glucose level of 110 mg/dL or higher. An approach that emphasizes healthy lifestyle changes is likely more cost-effective and accompanied by other health benefits than one focused on pharmacotherapy. With now more than 50 million individuals in the United States considered to be at high risk for developing diabetes, the economic implications of any broad recommendations will need careful consideration.

ACUTE METABOLIC COMPLICATIONS
Diabetic Ketoacidosis
See Chapter 236 for a discussion of diabetic ketoacidosis.

Hyperosmolar Hyperglycemic Syndrome
CLINICAL MANIFESTATIONS
The metabolic state formerly known as the hyperglycemic hyperosmolar nonketotic state or coma has been renamed the *hyperosmolar hyperglycemic syndrome* (HHS) to highlight two important points: (1) ketosis (and acidosis) may be present to varying degrees in HHS, and (2) alterations in sensorium most commonly occur in the absence of coma. In fact, only 10% of HHS patients present with frank coma, and an equal percentage show no signs whatsoever of mental status change.

As shown in Table 236-6 in Chapter 236, the hallmarks of the HHS are severe hyperosmolarity (>320 mOsm/L) and hyperglycemia (>600 mg/dL). Severe hyperglycemia occurs because patients cannot consume enough liquid to keep pace with a vigorous osmotic diuresis. The resulting impairment in renal function eventually further reduces glucose excretion through the kidney, leading to remarkable blood glucose elevations, sometimes exceeding 1000 mg/dL. In contrast to diabetic ketoacidosis, even though glucose concentrations are generally higher, severe acidosis and ketosis are generally absent in the HHS. This is probably explained by the residual insulin secretory capacity retained by patients with even several decades of type 2 diabetes. That is, their insulin levels remain sufficient to suppress lipolysis and to avoid significant keto acid production. However, some type 2 patients with depressed endogenous insulin secretion may be unable to suppress ketone production fully in the face of elevated counter-regulatory hormones produced by physical illness. Because HHS patients have higher portal vein insulin concentrations than do patients with diabetic ketoacidosis, keto acid production by the liver is relatively mild, yielding only mild acidosis. In the HHS, in the absence of concurrent acid-base disturbances, arterial pH rarely drops below 7.30, and serum bicarbonate levels typically do not fall below 18 mEq/L.

In the hyperosmolar hyperglycemic state, clinical severity and levels of consciousness generally correlate with the severity and duration of hyperosmolarity. Clinical signs indicate profound dehydration; gastrointestinal symptoms are seen less frequently than in diabetic ketoacidosis. A variety of often reversible neurologic abnormalities may exist, including grand mal or focal seizures, extensor plantar reflexes, aphasia, hemisensory or motor deficits, and worsening of a preexisting organic mental syndrome. The laboratory picture is dominated by the effects of uncontrolled diabetes and dehydration; renal function is impaired, hemoglobin and hematocrit are elevated, and liver function test results may be abnormal because of baseline hepatic steatosis. Although severe hyperglycemia would be expected to lower measured serum sodium concentration, it is not uncommon to see normal or even elevated sodium levels because of the severity of dehydration. The serum osmolality can be measured directly or estimated by the following formula, which excludes urea because it is freely diffusible throughout the body and therefore has little influence on the osmotic pressure gradient:

$$\text{Effective osmolarity (mOsm/L)} = 2\,[\text{measured serum Na}^{+}\,(\text{mEq/L})] + [\text{glucose (mg/dL)}/18]$$

TREATMENT

Patients with HHS should be treated as aggressively as are those with diabetic ketoacidosis, although those with the former tend to have more dramatic volume contraction (Chapter 236). By definition, acidosis is not present or is minimal in degree. Accordingly, patients may not require the coadministration of dextrose along with insulin, as is recommended in patients with diabetic ketoacidosis to allow ketones to clear and the acidosis to resolve. Also, it is important to volume-resuscitate the patient adequately before insulin is administered for fear that intracellular fluid shifts that occur as glucose levels are reduced may worsen systemic tissue perfusion. Because, by definition, there is no significant acidosis to clear in HHS, patients may be transitioned directly from insulin infusion to subcutaneous injections, without need for any coadministration of dextrose as is necessary in diabetic ketoacidosis to allow further clearance of ketone bodies. Some patients with HHS may ultimately be able to be managed with oral agents alone. However, the development of HHS signifies a significant degree of insulin deficiency. As a result, it is always best to prescribe insulin injections before the patient is discharged and to reserve judgment about the appropriateness of oral agents until the patient's progress can be monitored and reassessed in the outpatient setting.

HYPOGLYCEMIA
See Chapter 236 for a full discussion of this complication of diabetes therapy. As previously mentioned, hypoglycemia is encountered less frequently in individual patients with type 2 diabetes because of biologic as well as practical reasons. Because the typical type 2 patient retains some residual endogenous insulin secretion, the development of mild hypoglycemia will lead to its abrupt reduction. Accordingly, type 2 diabetic patients can autoregulate portal insulin levels to a degree not possible in the absolutely insulin deficient type 1 patients. Also, patients with type 2 diabetes are, almost by definition, insulin resistant and therefore less likely to develop abnormally low blood glucose levels even when taking insulin injections. Perhaps more important, type 2 patients are more commonly treated with oral agents than with insulin. Many of these drugs reduce glucose levels through nonpancreatic mechanisms and therefore do not predispose to hypoglycemia when they are used as monotherapy or in combination with each other. On the other hand, severe hypoglycemia may be less well tolerated by the aging brain, and therefore it needs to be scrupulously avoided, particularly in elderly patients and especially given the recent clinical trial evidence of an association between hypoglycemia and increased cardiovascular mortality in those at high cardiovascular risk.

CHRONIC DIABETIC COMPLICATIONS
The pathogenesis of the microvascular and neuropathic complications of diabetes is discussed in Chapter 236. Patients with both forms of diabetes are at risk for retinopathy, nephropathy, and nerve dysfunction.

Atherosclerosis
Atherosclerosis (Chapter 70) involving the coronary, cerebral, and peripheral (lower extremity) arteries is the predominant cause of diabetes-related mortality, responsible for up to 70% of all deaths in patients with this disease. The atherosclerotic process in diabetes is essentially indistinguishable from that of the nondiabetic population, but it begins earlier and is often more extensive and more severe. A predilection to cardiovascular disease is observed over the entire spectrum of diabetes, from poorly controlled insulin-dependent patients to those with mild, diet-controlled hyperglycemia. For unclear reasons, the disparity between diabetic and nondiabetic persons is more pronounced in women. When it is accompanied by other major cardiovascular risk factors such as hypertension, dyslipidemia, and smoking, diabetes markedly augments the incidence of macrovascular complications. For example, the observed 2- to 3-fold greater risk for myocardial infarction with diabetes rises to 8-fold in the presence of hypertension and to nearly 20-fold if both hypertension and dyslipidemia are present; smoking increases these risks even further. As a result, the diagnosis of diabetes mellitus should lead to a careful review of coexisting and compounding cardiovascular risk factors and the initiation of aggressive preventive measures.

Diabetes is an *independent* risk factor for accelerated atherosclerosis. Its association with vascular disease is not solely attributable to an increased

FIGURE 237-5. Theoretical construct of the link between insulin resistance (as occurs in patients with metabolic syndrome) and cardiovascular disease.

prevalence of other recognized vascular risk factors, such as hypertension and dyslipidemia. Many abnormalities induced by the diabetic state may contribute to atherosclerosis, including lipid abnormalities (e.g., increased total VLDL and LDL, increased small dense [atherogenic] LDL, decreased HDL, increased lipoprotein oxidation, increased lipoprotein glycosylation, decreased lipoprotein lipase activity), accentuated platelet aggregation and adhesion, endothelial cell dysfunction, and induced procoagulant state (e.g., increased clotting factors and fibrinogen; decreased levels of antithrombin III, protein C, and protein S; and decreased fibrinolytic activity). It has been suggested that hyperinsulinemia per se may contribute to macrovascular disease; proposed pathogenetic mechanisms include insulin-induced stimulation of vascular endothelial and smooth muscle cells, enhanced insulin-like growth factor-I expression, and augmented synthesis of atherogenic factors such as endothelin and plasminogen activator inhibitor. Moreover, insulin resistance appears to be an independent risk factor for vascular events and may exert its effect through many of these disease intermediaries.

The prevention of cardiovascular disease in type 2 diabetes requires a comprehensive and multifactorial approach. Such an approach has been shown to reduce cardiovascular events by almost 50% (Steno-2 study[16]). Two cardinal areas for prevention concern the management of hypertension and dyslipidemia. Figure 237-5 shows a theoretical scheme that links insulin resistance and the metabolic syndrome with cardiovascular disease. The reader is referred to the online version of this chapter and to Chapters 67 and 213 in this text for a more detailed discussion of these topics.

🔵 **Visit expertconsult.com for e-expanded chapter**

1. United Kingdom Prospective Diabetes Study (UKPDS) Group. Intensive blood-glucose control with sulphonylureas or insulin compared with conventional treatment and risk of complications in patients with type 2 diabetes (UKPDS 33). *Lancet.* 1998;352:837-853.
2. Holman RR, Paul SK, Bethel A, et al. 10-Year follow-up of intensive glucose control in type 2 diabetes. *N Engl J Med.* 2008;359:1577-1589.
3. ACCORD Study Group, Gerstein HC, Miller ME, et al. Long-term effects of intensive glucose lowering on cardiovascular outcomes. *N Engl J Med.* 2011;364:818-828.
4. The Action to Control Cardiovascular Risk in Diabetes Study Group. Effects of intensive glucose lowering in type 2 diabetes. *N Engl J Med.* 2008;358:2545-2559.
5. The ADVANCE Collaborative Group. Intensive blood glucose control and vascular outcomes in patients with type 2 diabetes. *N Engl J Med.* 2008;358:2560-2572.
6. Duckworth W, Abraira C, Moritz T, et al, for the VADT Investigators. Glucose control and vascular complications in veterans with type 2 diabetes. *N Engl J Med.* 2009;360:129-139.
7. Diabetes Prevention Program Research Group, Knowler WC, Fowler SE, et al. 10-year follow-up of diabetes incidence and weight loss in the Diabetes Prevention Program Outcomes Study. *Lancet.* 2009;S74:1677-1686.
8. Church TS, Blair SN, Cocreham S, et al. Effects of aerobic and resistance training on hemoglobin A1c levels in patients with type 2 diabetes: a randomized controlled trial. *JAMA.* 2010; 304:2253-2262.
9. Nissen S, Wolski K. Effect of rosiglitazone on the risk of myocardial infarction and death from cardiovascular causes. *N Engl J Med.* 2007;356:2457-2471.
10. Home PD, Pocock SJ, Beck-Nielsen H, et al. Rosiglitazone evaluated for cardiovascular outcomes in oral agent combination therapy for type 2 diabetes (RECORD): a multicentre, randomised, open-label trial. *Lancet.* 2009;373:2125-2135.
11. Dormandy JA, Charbonnel B, Eckland DJ, et al, for the PROactive investigators. Secondary prevention of macrovascular events in patients with type 2 diabetes in the PROactive Study (PROspective pioglitAzone Clinical Trial In macroVascular Events): a randomised controlled trial. *Lancet.* 2005;366:1279-1289.
12. Holman RR, Farmer AJ, Davies MJ, et al. Three-year efficacy of complex insulin regimens in type 2 diabetes. *N Engl J Med.* 2009;361:1736-1747.
13. The NICE-SUGAR Study Investigators. Intensive versus conventional glucose control in critically ill patients. *N Engl J Med.* 2009;360:1283-1297.
14. Kansagara D, Fu R, Freeman M, et al. Intensive insulin therapy in hospitalized patients: a systematic review. *Ann Intern Med.* 2011;151:268-282.
15. Knowler WC, Barrett-Connor E, Fowler SE, et al, for the Diabetes Prevention Program Research Group. Reduction in the incidence of type 2 diabetes with lifestyle intervention or metformin. *N Engl J Med.* 2002;346:393-403.
16. Gaede P, Lund-Andersen H, Parving H-H, et al. Effect of a multifactorial intervention on mortality in type 2 diabetes. *N Engl J Med.* 2008;358:580-591.

SUGGESTED READINGS

American Diabetes Association. Standards of medical care in diabetes—2011. *Diabetes Care.* 2011; 34(Suppl 1):S11-S61. *Updated guidelines from the leading professional organization in diabetes.*
American Diabetes Association. Diagnosis and classification of diabetes mellitus. *Diabetes Care.* 2011;33(Suppl 1):S62-S69. *Includes new guidelines for use of the HbA$_{1c}$ to diagnose diabetes.*
Blonde L. Current antihyperglycemic treatment guidelines and algorithms for patients with type 2 diabetes mellitus. *Am J Med.* 2010;123;s12-s18. *Review.*
Bonora E, Kiechl S, Mayr A, et al. High-normal HbA1c is a strong predictor of type 2 diabetes in the general population. *Diabetes Care.* 2011;34;1038-1040. *Risks of type 2 diabetes were increased 3.8-fold for an HbA$_{1c}$ level of 5.50-5.99% and 12-fold for a level of 6-6.49%.*
Brown A, Reynolds LR, Bruemmer D. Intensive glycemic control and cardiovascular disease: an update. *Nat Rev Cardiol.* 2010;7:369-375. *This review discusses the effects of intensive glycemic control on cardiovascular disease and examines key differences in several major trials that might have contributed to their disparate findings.*
Lebovitz HE. Type 2 diabetes melitus—current therapies and the emergence of surgical options. *Nat Rev Endocrinol.* 2011. [Epub ahead of print.] *Review including control of glucose, blood pressure, and lipids as well as the possible role of gastric bypass surgery in morbidly obese individuals.*
Zoungas S, Patel A, Chalmers J, et al. Severe hypoglycemia and risks of vascular events and death. *N Engl J Med.* 2010;363:1410-1418. *Type 2 diabetes patients who have episodes of severe hypoglycemia have a nearly 3-fold increased risk for vascular events and death compared with other type 2 diabetics, but the reason for this association is not clear.*

238

HYPOGLYCEMIA AND PANCREATIC ISLET CELL DISORDERS

ADRIAN VELLA, ROBERT A. RIZZA, AND F. JOHN SERVICE

⬤ HYPOGLYCEMIA

DEFINITION

Hypoglycemia is a clinical syndrome of diverse causes in which low levels of serum glucose can eventually lead to neuroglycopenia.

PATHOBIOLOGY

Regulation of Carbohydrate Metabolism
Interactions Between Insulin and Counter-Insulin Hormones
Under normal circumstances, serum glucose concentration averages 70 to 100 mg/dL before meals and rarely exceeds 140 to 150 mg/dL after meals. The brain is almost totally dependent on glucose for energy, although over the long term it can adapt to substrates other than glucose (e.g., ketone bodies). Because severe hypoglycemia can impair mental function and, if prolonged, can cause permanent brain damage, a series of well-developed, and at times redundant, homeostatic processes defend against hypoglycemia. Insulin suppresses glucose production by inhibiting both glycogenolysis and

gluconeogenesis. Insulin also stimulates glucose uptake in muscle, liver, and fat. Glucagon, epinephrine, cortisol, and growth hormone, collectively referred to as the counter-regulatory or counter-insulin hormones, oppose the effects of insulin.

In healthy nondiabetic subjects, insulin concentration increases as glucose concentration increases and falls as glucose concentration falls. In contrast, counter-regulatory hormone concentrations change (in general) in the opposite direction of insulin, by falling as glucose rises and rising as glucose falls. By doing so, insulin and the counter-insulin hormones act in concert to ensure that the amount of glucose entering and leaving the blood stream is closely matched in both the fed and the fasted state. Excess amounts of insulin or insulin-like material (e.g., insulin-like growth factor [IGF]-I or IGF-II), inadequate secretion of counter-insulin hormones, insufficient substrate, or defects in the gluconeogenic or glycogenolytic pathways alone or in combination can disrupt this balance and can cause hypoglycemia.

Regulation of Glucose Concentration in the Fed State

After an overnight fast (e.g., 8 to 10 hours), rates of glucose production and utilization average about 2 mg/kg/minute. At this time, most of the glucose is released from the liver, and a small amount is produced by the kidney. Carbohydrate ingestion increases glucose concentration, which stimulates secretion of insulin from the pancreatic β cells and suppresses secretion of glucagon from the pancreatic α cells. The resultant rise in the insulin-to-glucagon ratio increases hepatic glycogen synthesis and inhibits both glycogenolysis and gluconeogenesis, thereby increasing hepatic glycogen content. Glucose concentrations continue to rise until the rate of glucose uptake by peripheral tissues exceeds the net amount of glucose (meal-derived and endogenously produced) released from the splanchnic bed. Glucose concentration then begins to fall toward preprandial levels. This results in a progressive fall in insulin and a progressive rise in glucagon concentration, which, in turn permit a gradual increase in endogenous glucose production and a gradual fall in glucose utilization to basal rates. Depending on the amount and type of food ingested, both glucose concentration and turnover return to basal levels between 4 and 6 hours after the start of a meal.

Thus, the rate of carbohydrate absorption, the timing as well as the amount of insulin and glucagon secreted, the ability of the liver to store and subsequently release glucose, and the response of the liver, muscle, and fat to insulin and counter-insulin hormones all interact to minimize the rise in glucose concentration after a meal as well as to ensure a smooth return of glucose concentrations to preprandial levels during the transition from the fed to the postabsorptive state.

Regulation of Glucose Concentrations in the Fasted State

The contribution of gluconeogenesis becomes progressively more important as the duration of fast is extended and hepatic glycogen stores are depleted. The rate of glycogen depletion depends on a variety of factors, including antecedent diet and exercise, but the process is nearly complete after 24 to 48 hours of fasting. Anything that lowers the demand for glucose lessens the need to break down protein stores. This is accomplished by changing from a primarily carbohydrate-based metabolism in the fed state to a primarily fat-based metabolism in the fasted state.

As hepatic glycogen is depleted, the glucose concentration falls, and insulin decreases. Concentrations of glucagon, growth hormone, and cortisol all increase. This change in the hormonal milieu stimulates lipolysis and ketogenesis, which result in an increase in plasma glycerol, free fatty acid, and ketone body concentrations. Glycerol serves as a gluconeogenic substrate, thereby sparing amino acids. Free fatty acids are metabolized by muscle, liver, and other tissues in place of glucose. Free fatty acids also are converted by means of ketogenesis to acetoacetate and β-hydroxybutyrate, which can substitute for glucose as a fuel for the brain. These metabolic adaptations normally permit glucose to decrease gradually to 40 to 50 mg/dL during a fast without provoking symptoms of hypoglycemia. Inadequate glycogen stores or breakdown, insufficient gluconeogenesis resulting from defects in enzyme activity, lack of substrate availability, and persistent elevations of insulin or of insulin-like activity, alone or in combination, can cause or exacerbate hypoglycemia.

Recovery from Hypoglycemia

If counter-regulation is intact, hypoglycemia (regardless of the cause) will result in a decrease in insulin secretion and an increase in glucagon, epinephrine, cortisol, and growth hormone secretion. Glucagon provides the major defense against acute hypoglycemia. Epinephrine appears to become progressively more important when hypoglycemia is prolonged or severe. Permissive amounts of cortisol and growth hormone are required for a normal hepatic response to glucagon and epinephrine. Drugs or diseases that inhibit counter-regulatory secretion or action predispose patients to hypoglycemia.

CLINICAL MANIFESTATIONS

Symptoms of hypoglycemia have been classified into two major groups: those arising from activation of the autonomic nervous system (autonomic) and those related to insufficient glucose supply to the brain (neuroglycopenic). During acute insulin-induced hypoglycemia in healthy persons, autonomic symptoms are recognized at a threshold of approximately 60 mg/dL (3 mM), and impairment of brain function manifested by neuroglycopenic symptoms occurs at a threshold of approximately 50 mg/dL (2.8 mM) in arterialized venous blood (Fig. 238-1). Comparable venous levels would be about 3 mg/dL (0.16 mM) less. The rate of glucose descent has little if any influence on the occurrence of symptoms and signs of hypoglycemia in nondiabetic persons.

Variations among reports regarding allocation of symptoms to the autonomic and neuroglycopenic types may be ascribed to the specific groups of patients examined. These include patients with diabetes versus those without it, patients with type 1 versus type 2 diabetes, clinical versus experimental conditions, and, most important, differences among persons regarding their perception of symptoms. During experimentally induced hypoglycemia in 20 persons with and 25 persons without diabetes, a principal component analysis allocated sweating, trembling, feeling of warmth, anxiety, and nausea to the autonomic group and dizziness, confusion, tiredness, difficulty with speaking, headache, and inability to concentrate to the neuroglycopenic group. Hunger, blurred vision, drowsiness, and weakness could not be allocated to either group with any confidence. In another study of 10 nondiabetic persons, partitioning of symptoms during insulin-induced hypoglycemia allocated the categories of shaky/tremulous, heart pounding, nervous/anxious, sweaty, hungry, and tingling to the autonomic group and warm, weak, difficulty thinking/confused, and tired/drowsy to the neuroglycopenic group.

In a retrospective analysis of 60 patients with insulinoma, 85% had various combinations of diplopia, blurred vision, sweating, palpitations, and weakness; 80% had confusion or abnormal behavior; 50% were amnesic for the episode or had coma; and 12% had generalized seizures. None of the symptoms noted earlier, regardless of type, is specific for hypoglycemia. It is

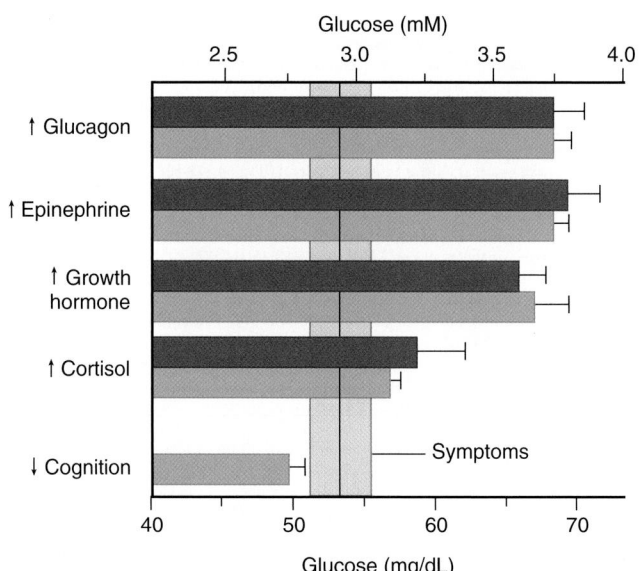

FIGURE 238-1. Arterialized (*blue*) and venous (*green*) glycemic (mean ± standard error) thresholds for increments in plasma glucagon, epinephrine, growth hormone, and cortisol for symptoms of hypoglycemia and for impairment of cognitive function during decrements in serum glucose in normal humans from two independent studies. (From Cryer PE. Glucose counterregulation: the physiological mechanisms that prevent or correct hypoglycemia. In: Frier B, Fisher BM, eds. *Hypoglycaemia and Diabetes: Clinical and Physiological Aspects.* London: Edward Arnold; 1993:34-55.)

unlikely that autonomic symptoms alone, in the absence of at least one event of neuroglycopenia, are indicative of a hypoglycemic disorder.

DIAGNOSIS

Classification

A useful approach for the clinician is a classification based on clinical characteristics (Table 238-1). Persons who appear healthy are likely to have hypoglycemic disorders that are different from those of persons who are ill. Hospitalized patients are at additional risk for hypoglycemia, often from iatrogenic factors.

TABLE 238-1 CLINICAL CLASSIFICATION OF HYPOGLYCEMIC DISORDERS

I. PATIENT APPEARS HEALTHY*

A. No coexistent disease
   1. Drugs
      a. Ethanol
      b. Salicylates
      c. Quinine
      d. Haloperidol
   2. Insulinoma
   3. Islet hypertrophy/nesidioblastosis
   4. Noninsulinoma pancreatogenous hypoglycemia syndrome
   5. Post–gastric bypass hypoglycemia
   6. Factitial hypoglycemia from insulin or sulfonylurea use
   7. Exercise
   8. Autoimmune insulin syndrome
B. Compensated coexistent disease
   1. Drugs
      a. Dispensing error

II. PATIENT APPEARS ILL

A. Drugs
   1. Pentamidine and *Pneumocystis* pneumonia
   2. Sulfamethoxazole-trimethoprim and renal failure
   3. Propoxyphene and renal failure
   4. Quinine and cerebral malaria
   5. Quinine and malaria
   6. Topical salicylates and renal failure
   7. Unripe ackee fruit and undernutrition
B. Predisposing illness
   1. Infant small for gestational age
   2. Beckwith-Wiedemann syndrome
   3. Erythroblastosis fetalis
   4. Infant of diabetic mother
   5. Glycogen storage disease
   6. Defects in amino acid and fatty acid metabolism
   7. Reye's syndrome
   8. Cyanotic congenital heart disease
   9. Hypopituitarism
   10. Isolated growth hormone deficiency
   11. Isolated adrenocorticotropic hormone deficiency
   12. Addison's disease
   13. Hereditary fructose intolerance
   14. Carnitine deficiency
   15. Defective type 1 glucose transporter in the brain
   16. Acquired severe liver disease
   17. Non–islet cell tumor hypoglycemia
   18. Sepsis
   19. Renal failure
   20. Congestive heart failure
   21. Lactic acidosis
   22. Starvation
   23. Anorexia nervosa
   24. Postoperative removal of pheochromocytoma
   25. Insulin receptor antibody hypoglycemia
   26. Spinal muscular atrophy
C. Hospitalized patient
   1. Diseases predisposing to hypoglycemia
   2. Total parenteral nutrition and insulin therapy
   3. Questran interference with glucocorticoid absorption
   4. Shock

*Mutations in the β-cell sulfonylurea receptor gene, glutamate dehydrogenase gene, and glucokinase gene are rare causes of hyperinsulinemic hypoglycemia, usually manifested in infancy or childhood.

Evaluation

The direction and extent of evaluation depend on the clinical presentation. The healthy-appearing patient with no coexistent disease who has a history of episodic symptoms suggestive of hypoglycemia requires an approach quite different from the hospitalized patient with acute hypoglycemia.

The Healthy-Appearing Patient

Serum Glucose

Because symptoms of hypoglycemia are not specific, it is essential to document a low serum glucose concentration at the time of the occurrence of spontaneous symptoms and relief of symptoms through correction of the low serum glucose concentration before concluding that a patient has a hypoglycemic disorder. Furthermore, reliance solely on a low blood glucose value to diagnose a hypoglycemic disorder fails to take into consideration the possibility of laboratory error, artifactual hypoglycemia, and, indeed, the finding that physiologically normal persons may have serum glucose levels much lower than 50 mg/dL (2.8 mM) during prolonged fasting. A normal serum glucose concentration (when measured reliably) obtained during the occurrence of spontaneous symptoms absolutely eliminates the possibility of a hypoglycemic disorder; no further evaluation is required. Although hypoglycemic disorders are uncommon, symptoms suggestive of hypoglycemia are quite common.

Recently published evidence-based guidelines recommend evaluation and management of hypoglycemia only in patients in whom Whipple's triad is documented. Often, however, measurement of serum glucose is not feasible while spontaneous symptoms are occurring during ordinary life activities. Under such circumstances, judging whether to proceed with further evaluation depends on a detailed history. Elicitation of a history of neuroglycopenic symptoms or evidence of a confirmed low serum glucose concentration warrants further testing. If a venipuncture sample cannot be obtained during the spontaneous occurrence of suspected hypoglycemia, the circumstances observed to provoke hypoglycemia should be reproduced: a 72-hour fast for persons with hypoglycemia in the food-deprived state and a mixed-meal test for persons with postprandial hypoglycemia.

Seventy-Two-Hour Fast

The prolonged supervised (72-hour) fast is an important diagnostic test. It should be conducted in a standardized fashion. A suggested protocol is shown in Table 238-2. For patients who experience signs or symptoms of hypoglycemia and who have simultaneously measured serum glucose in the hypoglycemic range, the fast should be terminated at that point. Studies in patients who have neither should not be extended beyond 72 hours.

The decision to end the fast may not be easy. Some patients have slightly depressed glycemic levels without symptoms or signs of hypoglycemia. Other patients may experience the symptoms they have had in ordinary life but have serum glucose levels higher than the hypoglycemic range. Young, lean, healthy women and, to a lesser degree, men may have serum glucose levels in the range of 40 mg/dL during prolonged fasting. Careful examination and testing for subtle signs of symptoms of neuroglycopenia should be conducted repeatedly when the patient's serum glucose level is near or in the hypoglycemic range. The 72-hour fast may be ended when the serum glucose concentration is

---

TABLE 238-2 PROTOCOL FOR 72-HOUR FAST

1. Date the onset of the fast as of the last ingestion of calories; discontinue all nonessential medications.
2. The patient may drink calorie-free and caffeine-free beverages.
3. The patient must be active during waking hours.
4. Measure plasma glucose, insulin, C-peptide, and β-hydroxybutyrate (on the same venipuncture specimen) every 6 hours until plasma glucose reaches ≤60 mg/dL (3.3 mM), when frequency should be every 1 to 2 hours.
5. End the fast when the plasma glucose is ≤45 mg/dL (2.5 mM) and the patient has symptoms or signs of hypoglycemia, or plasma glucose is ≤55 mg/dL if Whipple's triad* had been demonstrated previously.
6. At the end of the fast, measure plasma glucose, insulin, C-peptide, β-hydroxybutyrate, and sulfonylurea (on the same venipuncture specimen); then inject glucagon, 1 mg intravenously, and measure plasma glucose every 10 minutes three times. After this, feed the patient.

*Whipple's triad is: (a) symptoms or signs consistent with hypoglycemia, (b) a low plasma glucose concentration, and (c) resolution of those symptoms or signs after the plasma glucose concentration is raised.

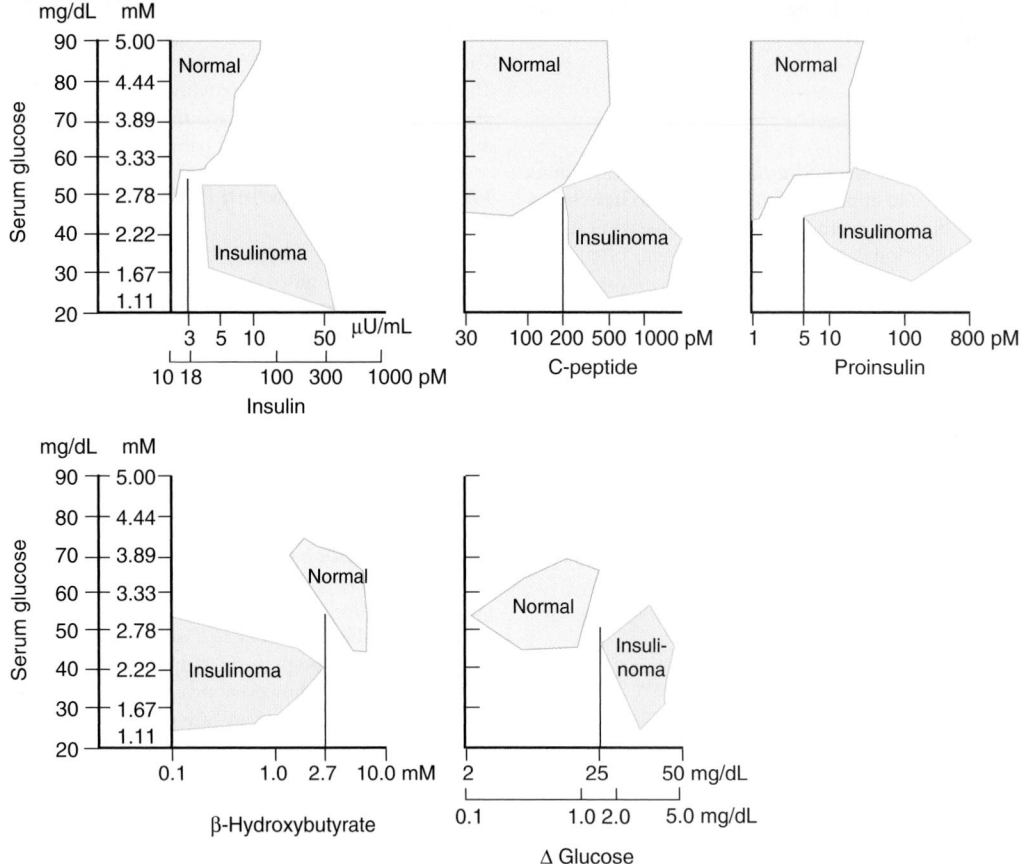

FIGURE 238-2. Distributions of plasma insulin, C-peptide, proinsulin, β-hydroxybutyrate, and serum glucose (Δ glucose) response to intravenous glucagon versus serum glucose at the end of the prolonged fast (72 hours in normal persons [*n* = 25] or at Whipple's triad for patients with histologically confirmed insulinoma [*n* = 40]). The *shaded area* represents serum glucose level less than or equal to 50 mg/dL (2.8 mM). The *vertical line* represents the diagnostic level for insulinoma. Criteria for insulinoma are insulin level greater than or equal to 3 μU/mL (18 pM), C-peptide level greater than or equal to 200 pM, proinsulin level greater than or equal to 5 pM, β-hydroxybutyrate level less than or equal to 2.7 mM, and Δ glucose level greater than or equal to 25 mg/dL (1.4 mM).

55 mg/dL or less if Whipple's triad (see Table 238-2) had previously been demonstrated. β-Cell polypeptides are suppressed in healthy persons when serum glucose is 55 mg/dL or less. Although most patients with insulinoma become hypoglycemic before 72 hours (33% in 12 hours, 65% in 24 hours, 84% in 36 hours, 93% in 48 hours, and 99% in 72 hours in a group of 170 patients with insulinoma), continuation of the fast to 72 hours is necessary to rule out the likelihood of organic hypoglycemia. Although the 72-hour fast has usually been considered to be an inpatient procedure, it may be initiated in an endocrine testing center after an overnight fast. Forty percent of patients have had positive results of the fast in the outpatient setting. Those patients whose fast result is not positive by the end of the outpatient evaluation period are admitted to the hospital to complete the 72-hour fast.

The interpretation of concentrations of β-cell polypeptides (insulin, C-peptide, and proinsulin) during the 72-hour fast is predicated on the concomitant serum glucose concentration. The normal overnight fasting ranges for these polypeptides do not apply when the serum glucose level is less than 55 mg/dL.

Insulin-mediated hypoglycemic disorders are characterized by plasma insulin concentrations greater than or equal to 3 μU/mL (immunochemiluminometric assay) (Fig. 238-2). Persons with insulinomas have insulin concentrations that rarely exceed 100 μU/mL. Values of 1000 μU/mL or greater suggest recent insulin administration or the presence of insulin antibodies. Ratios of glucose to insulin, and vice versa, including the "amended ratio," have been used in an effort to identify relative hyperinsulinemia when the insulin concentration is in the normal overnight fasting range. Unfortunately, these ratios have very poor diagnostic utility (see Fig. 238-2).

Criteria for hyperinsulinemia using C-peptide and proinsulin (each measured by immunochemiluminometric assays) are 200 pmol/L or more and 5 pmol/L or more, respectively (see Fig. 238-2). The molar ratio of insulin to C-peptide is the same for patients with insulinomas as it is for healthy individuals (~0.2). Although the molar ratio of proinsulin to insulin is increased in patients with insulinoma, it appears to have no diagnostic utility.

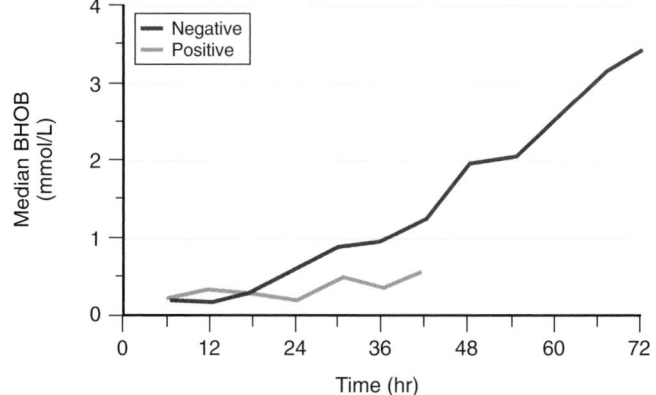

FIGURE 238-3. Median concentrations of β-hydroxybutyrate (BHOB) during 72-hour fasts are shown for patients with insulinoma, all of whom had positive fasts, and for persons with negative fasts. (From Service F. Increasing serum B-hydroxybutyrate. *J Clin Endocrinol Metab.* 2005;90:4555-4558. Copyright 2005, The Endocrine Society.)

Because of the antiketogenic effect of insulin, plasma β-hydroxybutyrate measurement at the end of the fast (72 hours in healthy individuals and when Whipple's triad is fulfilled in patients during a diagnostic fast) is useful. This parameter is considered to be an insulin surrogate. Patients with insulin-mediated hypoglycemia have concentrations of less than 2.7 mmol/L, whereas others (healthy individuals and those with non–insulin-mediated hypoglycemia) have higher levels (see Fig. 238-2). The progressive rise of β-hydroxybutyrate concentration early in the 72-hour fast in persons destined to have a negative test, in contrast to the sustained suppressed level in patients with insulinoma (Fig. 238-3), provides the opportunity to end the fast before the 72-hour point either by attaining a level of 2.7 mmol/L or higher or by having two successive concentrations measured at 6-hour intervals that exceed the concentration at the 18-hour time point. Another insulin surrogate is the response of serum glucose to 1 mg of glucagon injected intravenously at the end of the fast. The rationale for this procedure is that insulin is glycogenic and antiglycogenolytic. Patients with insulin-mediated hypoglycemia have a maximal increment at least 25 mg/dL greater than the terminal fasting serum glucose, whereas others (healthy individuals and those with non–insulin-mediated hypoglycemia) have lower increments (see Fig. 238-2). When the serum glucose concentration exceeds 60 mg/dL at the end of the fast, measurement of the β-cell polypeptides and insulin surrogates is uninformative and unnecessary.

Measurement of sulfonylureas and meglitinides in the plasma when a patient develops hypoglycemia is an essential component of the prolonged supervised fast. The pattern of serum glucose and β-cell polypeptides in sulfonylurea-induced hypoglycemia is identical to that observed in persons with insulinoma. A liquid chromatographic tandem mass spectrography method provides a sensitive measurement of first- and second-generation sulfonylureas and meglitinides (Table 238-3 provides diagnostic interpretation).

Mixed-Meal Test

For persons with a history of neuroglycopenic symptoms within 5 hours of food ingestion, a mixed-meal test may be conducted. The patient should eat a meal similar to that leading to symptoms during ordinary life activities. The test result is positive when the patient experiences neuroglycopenic symptoms and a concomitant serum glucose level is low (e.g., ≤50 mg/dL). No standards exist for the interpretation of levels of β-cell polypeptides measured during this test. However, one can expect insulin levels to be suppressed during postprandial hypoglycemia, provided five half-lives (~30 minutes) have elapsed from peak insulinemia. A positive mixed-meal test in and of itself does not provide a diagnosis, only biochemical confirmation of the history. A surprisingly high percentage of patients (~10%) with insulinoma report neuroglycopenic symptoms after meals, and in some instances only after meals. Patients with a positive mixed-meal test may require a 72-hour fast to document both fasting and postprandial hypoglycemia. For those patients with a positive mixed-meal test result and a negative 72-hour fast result, glucagon levels during the mixed-meal test should be determined to ensure a counter-regulatory response to the low serum glucose concentration. Gastric emptying studies may be performed to look for accelerated transit as

a cause of postprandial hypoglycemia. If this is found, measurement of prokinetic gastrointestinal hormones may be indicated. The combination of a positive mixed-meal test and a negative 72-hour fast may occur in a patient with insulinoma or with noninsulinoma pancreatogenous hypoglycemia syndrome. The 5-hour oral glucose tolerance test should not be used as a diagnostic test for hypoglycemia because a substantial percentage of healthy persons may have a serum glucose nadir less than or equal to 50 mg/dL. Similarly, in patients who are experiencing hypoglycemia-like symptoms after Roux-en-Y gastric bypass, it is important to ensure that the test meal avoids simple carbohydrates and liquid calories, which can provoke symptoms in most patients who have had such surgery.

C-Peptide Suppression Test

The C-peptide suppression test is based on the observation that β-cell secretion (as measured by levels of C-peptide) is suppressed during hypoglycemia to a lesser degree in persons with an insulinoma than in physiologically normal persons. It is rarely used because interpretation requires normative data adjusted for the patient's body mass index and age.

Insulin Antibodies

The detection of insulin antibodies was once considered to be firm evidence of factitious hypoglycemia resulting from inappropriate self-administration of insulin, especially when animal insulin was the only commercially available type. Because of the use of human insulin, which is less antigenic than that derived from animals, such patients usually have no detectable insulin antibodies. Hypoglycemia that can be directly attributed to the spontaneous generation of antibodies to native insulin has been reported to occur primarily in Asians and rarely in whites. In patients with insulin autoimmune hypoglycemia from the spontaneous generation of insulin antibodies, such antibodies may be monoclonal or polyclonal and are present in very high titers, in contrast to the much lower titers in insulin-treated diabetes. It is important to test for the presence of insulin antibodies because even low titers, which may have no diagnostic significance, may cause spurious results of the assay for insulin. Hypoglycemia in such instances may have a variable association with fasting or meal ingestion.

Glycated Hemoglobin

Although glycated hemoglobin concentrations are statistically significantly lower in patients with insulinomas than in physiologically normal subjects, too much overlap exists to provide a diagnostic criterion.

TABLE 238-3 DIAGNOSTIC INTERPRETATION OF THE RESULTS OF A 72-HOUR FAST*

	SIGNS AND SYMPTOMS	GLUCOSE[†] (MG/DL)	INSULIN[‡‡] (μU/ML)	C-PEPTIDE[‡§] (PMOL/L)	PROINSULIN[‡‖] (PMOL/L)	β-HYDROXYBUTYRATE (MMOL/L)	GLUCOSE[¶] (MG/DL)	SULFONYLUREA IN PLASMA
Normal	No	≥40	<3	<200	<5	>2.7	<25	No
Insulinoma	Yes	≤45	≥3[ǀ]	≥200	≥5	≤2.7	≤25	No
Factitious hypoglycemia from insulin	Yes	≤45	≥3**	<200	<5	≤2.7	≥25	No
Sulfonylurea-induced hypoglycemia	Yes	≤45	≥3	≥200	≥5	≤2.7	≥25	Yes[††]
Hypoglycemia mediated by insulin-like growth factor	Yes	≤45	≤3	<200	<5	≤2.7	≥25	No
Non–insulin-mediated hypoglycemia	Yes	≤45	<3	<200	<5	>2.7	<25	No
Inadvertent feeding during the fast	No	≤45	<3	<200	<5	≤2.7	≥25	No
Nonhypoglycemic disorder	Yes	≥40	<3	<200	<5	>2.7	<25	No

*Measurements are made at the point the decision is made to end the fast.
[†]Sequential plasma glucose measurements in the hypoglycemic range fluctuate. Plasma glucose levels ≤45 mg/dL at the time a decision is made to end the fast may rise to as much as 56 mg/dL when the fast is actually ended approximately 1 hour later. Plasma glucose levels may be as low as 40 mg/dL during prolonged fasting in normal women.
[‡]In normal subjects, plasma insulin, C-peptide, and proinsulin levels may be higher if the plasma glucose level is >60 mg/dL.
[§]Measured by the immunochemiluminometric technique (lower limit of detection, 33 pmol/L).
[‖]Measured by the immunochemiluminometric technique (lower limit of detection, 0.2 pmol/L).
[¶]In response to intravenous glucagon (peak value minus value at end of fast).
[ǀ]Ratios of insulin to glucose are of no diagnostic value in patients with insulinomas.
**Plasma insulin levels may be very high (>100 μU/mL or even = 1000 μU/mL) in factitious hypoglycemia produced by insulin.
[††]Unlike the first generation of sulfonylurea drugs, which were easily measured, second-generation drugs are difficult to measure.
[‡‡]Measured by immunochemiluminometric assay, lower limit of detection is 0.1 μU/mL.

Insulin Response to Selective Arterial Calcium Injection

The diagnosis of a hypoglycemic disorder is made entirely from biochemical evidence. Should the data document hyperinsulinemic hypoglycemia, localization procedures are undertaken. Standard radiologic tests are conducted solely in an effort to localize a lesion, rather than for diagnostic purposes. With the availability of the selective arterial calcium stimulation test, which is predicated on hyper-responsive β cells for a positive result, the purposes of regionalization and diagnosis of β-cell hyperfunction may both be served. This test requires access to various intra-abdominal vessels, including the right hepatic vein, splenic artery, gastroduodenal artery, and superior mesenteric artery. A two- to three-fold increase in insulin concentration in the right hepatic vein in response to calcium injection into one or more of the arteries supplying the pancreas suggests that the region served by that artery harbors abnormally functioning β cells, whether from insulinoma or islet hypertrophy or nesidioblastosis.

The Ill-Appearing Patient

Hypoglycemia in persons with coexistent disease sometimes occurs as a discrete episode, which may be asymptomatic if the patient has preexisting blunting of consciousness. Recognition of the underlying disease and its propensity for hypoglycemia and action taken to minimize recurrence may be sufficient. Confirmation of the suspected mechanism for the hypoglycemia may be pursued. Mechanisms may include low insulin and C-peptide levels in cases of non–insulin-mediated hypoglycemia (e.g., ethanol hypoglycemia), elevated IGF-II in cases of non–β-cell tumor-related hypoglycemia, low levels of cortisol in cases of adrenal insufficiency, and blunted serum glucose responses to intravenous glucagon in cases of hypoglycemia resulting from abnormal liver function, glycogen storage disease, sepsis, or congestive heart failure.

Patients who are in hospitals today generally are severely ill and have multisystem disease. These patients are at risk for iatrogenic hypoglycemia in addition to the potential risk generated from the underlying disease. In one tertiary medical center, 1.2% of all patients admitted over a 6-month period experienced hypoglycemia (serum glucose ≤49 mg/dL). The primary causes among persons without diabetes were renal insufficiency, malnutrition, liver disease, infection, and shock. Several patients had more than one risk factor. Not infrequently, nondiabetic patients become hyperglycemic because of treatment with enteral or parenteral nutrition or glucocorticoids. Use of insulin to control hyperglycemia puts patients at risk for hypoglycemia, especially if feedings are interrupted, the dose of glucocorticoid is abruptly reduced or stopped, or glucocorticoid availability is diminished through simultaneous administration of a bile acid sequestrant. In ferreting out the cause of hypoglycemia in the seriously ill hospitalized patient, diligent examination of the record is profitable.

TREATMENT   Rx

The treatment of hypoglycemic disorders encompasses two distinct components: (1) relief of neuroglycopenic systems by restoration of the low serum glucose level to the normal range, and (2) correction of the underlying cause of the hypoglycemia. Unlike diabetes, in which restoration of euglycemia is the ideal goal, overtreatment of hypoglycemia in a nondiabetic person has no sequelae. For the patient with an as-yet undiagnosed disorder, blood by venipuncture should be obtained for measurement of glucose, β-cell polypeptides, and β-hydroxybutyrate before treatment. Both diagnosis and treatment can be achieved by intravenous injection of glucagon with monitoring of the serum glucose response. Depending on the response, the patient may require intravenous glucose administration as a bolus of 50% or a continuous infusion of 5 or 10% or may recover sufficiently to take oral nutrition.

Treatment of the underlying cause of the hypoglycemia depends on the specific cause. Once a biochemical diagnosis of insulinoma has been made, preoperative localization should be attempted. Because of the rarity of insulinoma, only a few referral centers have generated sufficient experience to assess the effectiveness of various localization procedures: computed tomography, magnetic resonance imaging, endoscopic and transabdominal ultrasonography, octreotide scan, celiac axis angiography, and selective arterial calcium stimulation and transhepatic portal venous sampling. Experts differ in their preferred approaches because of differences in experience and skill level. Ultrasonography has the advantage of precise localization, especially in relation to the pancreatic duct. Magnetic resonance imaging and octreotide scanning are not useful. Transhepatic portal venous sampling has been abandoned in centers that once used this technique. There is general agreement that intraoperative ultrasonography combined with careful palpation of the pancreas by an experienced surgeon provides the highest success rate in localization.

Specific Causes

Insulinoma

Insulinoma is a rare tumor. The incidence is estimated to be 4 cases per 1 million person years, similar to that of pheochromocytoma. Insulinoma occurs at any age, is slightly more common in women (59%), and is associated with low rates of malignancy (6%), multiplicity (9%), multiple endocrine neoplasia syndrome (Chapter 239) (8%), and recurrence (8%). After successful removal of an insulinoma, the patient can look forward to a normal life expectancy. Medical therapy for the patient whose insulinoma is missed at pancreatic exploration, or for the patient unsuitable for surgery, or for the patient with metastatic insulinoma may include diazoxide, verapamil, phenytoin, propranolol, or octreotide. Insulinoma is occasionally suspected in patients with labile diabetes, especially when insulin therapy has apparently been suspended. One case of documented insulinoma in a person with type 1 diabetes and a few cases in persons with type 2 diabetes have been reported. Optimal treatment is surgical resection.

Noninsulinoma Pancreatogenous Hypoglycemia

Adults with episodes of hyperinsulinemic hypoglycemia resulting in neuroglycopenia may harbor islet hypertrophy/nesidioblastosis but no insulinoma (noninsulinoma pancreatogenous hypoglycemia syndrome). The clinical features are uniquely different from those of insulinoma: predominance of male patients, postprandial neuroglycopenia, negative 72-hour fast result, negative radiologic localization studies, positive selective arterial calcium stimulation test, and relief of symptoms with gradient-guided partial pancreatectomy. A subgroup of these patients has been identified who have the unique characteristic of a history of Roux-en-Y gastric bypass surgery.

Insulin Factitial Hypoglycemia

Insulin factitial hypoglycemia usually is manifested by neuroglycopenic symptoms that occur erratically. This disorder is observed more often in women, usually those in a health-related occupation. Once confronted with the diagnosis, about half of the patients admit to self-abuse, and most cease this activity. Insulin autoimmune hypoglycemia may be very difficult to distinguish from insulin factitial hypoglycemia because of similar biochemical features. However, some patients with the former have evidence of another autoimmune disease, and the insulin antibody titers are very high.

Other Causes

Mutations in the β-cell sulfonylurea receptor gene, glutamate dehydrogenase gene, and glucokinase gene have been reported to cause hyperinsulinemic hypoglycemia (i.e., inappropriately elevated insulin and C-peptide concentrations). Patients usually present at an early age, and often a familial pattern is detected. Physical exercise–induced hypoglycemia also has been described in some families. Insulin-like material can be secreted by some malignant tumors (e.g., hemangiopericytomas, fibromas, fibrosarcomas, hepatomas). In such instances, plasma insulin and C-peptide concentrations are low at the time of hypoglycemia, whereas pro-IGF-II concentrations are elevated.

● ISLET CELL TUMORS

DEFINITION

Tumors of the endocrine pancreas generally are malignant. Insulin-producing tumors are the exception because they are usually benign. Islet cell tumors are commonly referred to as either functioning or nonfunctioning. Functioning tumors release one or more hormones in amounts sufficient to raise plasma concentrations. Nonfunctioning tumors may contain one or more hormones but, by definition, do not release substantial amounts into the systemic circulation.

Functioning tumors generally manifest with symptoms relating to the hormones secreted, whereas nonfunctioning tumors generally manifest as a pancreatic mass or as a metastasis. Nonfunctioning tumors tend to be larger and more advanced at the time of diagnosis because their presence is not heralded by symptoms generated by hormone excess.

PATHOBIOLOGY

Functioning islet cell tumors are commonly associated with one of five widely recognized syndromes (Table 238-4). The insulinoma, Zollinger-Ellison, glucagonoma, VIPoma, and somatostatinoma syndromes are believed to result (at least in part) from excess secretion of insulin, gastrin, glucagon, vasoactive intestinal polypeptide (VIP), and somatostatin, respectively.

TABLE 238-4 CHARACTERISTICS OF FUNCTIONING ISLET CELL CARCINOMAS

SYNDROME	CLINICAL PRESENTATION	BIOCHEMICAL DIAGNOSIS	RATE OF MALIGNANCY (%)	METASTASES AT DIAGNOSIS (%)	LOCALIZATION (RADIOGRAPHIC)	ECTOPIC SITES (NONPANCREATIC)
Insulinoma	Neuroglycopenia Adrenergic response	Blood glucose ≤45 mg/dL Insulin >3 μU/mL Absence of insulin antibodies Elevated C-peptide	<10	<10	Ultrasonography Spiral CT Selective calcium stimulation test	Rare
Zollinger-Ellison syndrome	Dyspepsia/ulcer Diarrhea	Elevated basal gastrin Elevated basal acid output Positive secretin test	50-60	50-80	Ultrasonography, CT, angiography, PVS	Duodenum, rarely other
WDHA (VIPoma)	Profuse, secretory diarrhea Hypokalemia Hypochlorhydria/achlorhydria Hypercalcemia Hyperglycemia	Elevated VIP	50	50	CT, PVS, angiography	Retroperitoneum, occasionally lung
Glucagonoma	Dermatitis Diabetes Weight loss Anemia	Elevated glucagon	75	60-70	CT	Rare
Somatostatinoma	Diabetes Cholelithiasis Diarrhea Steatorrhea	Elevated somatostatin	90-100	50-75	CT	Duodenum

CT = computed tomography; PVS = portal venous sampling; VIP = vasoactive intestinal peptide; WDHA = watery diarrhea, hypokalemia, achlorhydria.
Adapted from Grant CS. Surgical management of malignant islet cell tumors. *World J Surg.* 1993;17:498-503.

However, additional symptoms also can occur because these tumors frequently secrete more than one hormone (e.g., pancreatic polypeptide, adrenocorticotropin, calcitonin, neurotensin, human chorionic gonadotropin, growth hormone–releasing factor, prostaglandins, and parathyroid hormone), and the amount and type of the hormone secreted can change over time. Islet cell tumors either are sporadic or can occur in association with other known genetic syndromes, such as multiple endocrine neoplasia type 1. Sporadic tumors occur at any age but most commonly are detected between 40 and 60 years of age. The diagnosis can be confirmed by obtaining tissue during surgical resection or by needle biopsy.

TREATMENT Rx

With the exception perhaps of insulinomas, the optimal treatment of islet cell tumors is currently not known because their rarity has made the conduct of randomized therapeutic trials extremely difficult. Furthermore, in the absence of metastases, no reliable histologic criteria distinguish benign from malignant lesions. Islet cell tumors most commonly metastasize to the liver and adjacent lymph nodes. Metastases to lung, bone, adrenal gland, kidney, and ovary may also occur. Fortunately, the rate of growth of malignant islet cell tumors is generally slow. Therefore, many clinicians recommend surgery if the pancreatic tumor is resectable and if the extent of metastatic disease (if present) is limited. "Debulking" of metastases, whether by surgery or by hepatic embolization, may improve symptoms by lowering circulating hormone concentrations. Treatment with chemotherapeutic agents such as streptozotocin (alone or in combination with 5-fluorouracil), doxorubicin, dacarbazine, or interferon-β also may improve symptoms and, in some instances, perhaps improve survival. Somatostatin is a potent inhibitor of hormone secretion. Treatment with long-acting analogues of somatostatin can result in a dramatic, albeit at times temporary, decrease in symptoms, particularly those associated with glucagonomas and VIPomas.

SUGGESTED READINGS

Cryer PE, Axelrod L, Grossman AB, et al. Evaluation and management of adult hypoglycemic disorders: an Endocrine Society Clinical Practice Guideline. *J Clin Endocrinol Metab.* 2009;94:709-728. *Consensus guidelines on diagnosis and treatment.*

Druce MR, Muthuppalaniappan VM, O'Leary B, et al. Diagnosis and localization of insulinoma: the value of modern magnetic resonance imaging in conjunction with calcium stimulation catheterization. *Eur J Endocrinol.* 2010;162:971-978. *Of 36 patients, 16 were localized by CT and 21 by MRI.*

Ekeblad S. Islet cell tumours. *Adv Exp Med Biol.* 2010;654:771-789. *Overview of pancreatic endocrine tumors that can cause hormonal symptoms by over-secretion.*

Placzkowski KA, Vella A, Thompson GB, et al. Secular trends in the presentation and management of functioning insulinoma at the Mayo Clinic, 1987-2007. *J Clin Endocrinol Metab.* 2009;94:1069-1073. *Review of changes in the presentation, diagnosis, and radiological evaluation of patients with surgically confirmed insulinoma at the Mayo Clinic over two decades.*

Watts AG, Donovan CM. Sweet talk in the brain: glucosensing, neural networks, and hypoglycemic counterregulation. *Front Neuroendocrinol.* 2010;31:32-43. *Review of the organization of the neural systems that are engaged by glucosensing mechanisms when blood glucose concentrations fall to levels that pose a physiological threat.*

239

POLYGLANDULAR DISORDERS

HENRY M. KRONENBERG

Internists need to recognize diseases that involve independent abnormalities of more than one endocrine gland, for several reasons. First, the known patterns of multiglandular disease can alert the clinician to look for a second disorder when one is diagnosed. Second, the treatment of many of the individual diseases that occur in polyglandular disorders may differ from the appropriate treatment for the same diseases when they manifest in isolation. Third, because many of these diseases appear in characteristic familial patterns, recognition of the syndromes can lead to useful family screening. Fourth, an understanding of the pathogenesis of these unusual disorders is likely to clarify the pathogenesis of more common single-gland disorders as well. This chapter discusses the best-characterized polyglandular disorders, with these four considerations as the primary focus. Other chapters should be consulted for more detailed discussion of the diseases of individual glands.

NEOPLASTIC SYNDROMES

Three mechanistically distinct neoplastic syndromes involve more than one endocrine gland. Although known by a variety of different names in the past, they are now most frequently called multiple endocrine neoplasia type 1, multiple endocrine neoplasia types 2a and 2b, and McCune-Albright syndrome.

Multiple Endocrine Neoplasia Type 1

DEFINITION

Multiple endocrine neoplasia type 1 (MEN 1) is an autosomal dominant disorder characteristically involving the parathyroid glands, the pancreatic islets, and the anterior pituitary. Less commonly, adrenal cortical neoplasia and foregut carcinoids (primarily of thymus and lung) occur. Nonendocrine manifestations include lipomas, facial angiofibromas, and collagenomas.

PATHOGENESIS

The gene for MEN 1 is located at chromosome 11, band 11q13, and it encodes a 610–amino acid protein called menin. Menin is a widely expressed nuclear protein that forms complexes with proteins that methylate histones in chromatin and also binds many transcription factors. Menin increases gene transcription by poorly understood mechanisms. Although the normal physiologic roles of menin are poorly understood, the abnormalities in MEN 1 suggest that the menin gene is a tumor suppressor gene. The inherited mutations in the menin gene vary widely, are located throughout the gene, and often generate truncated, presumably nonfunctional, menin peptides. In addition to this genetic abnormality, which is present in all cells in the body, MEN 1 tumors usually harbor deletions of the normal allele of the menin gene. Presumably, loss of both copies of the tumor suppressor gene, one by inherited mutation and one by mutation in one particular cell, confers a selective advantage to the cell that proliferates to become a clonal tumor. Such clonal deletions have been found in 100% of parathyroid tumors removed at surgery from patients with MEN 1. Other acquired genetic abnormalities accumulate in these tumors; thus, the tumors in MEN 1 follow the pattern of multistep tumorigenesis found in malignant tumors. The two-hit tumor suppressor model has been confirmed by the generation of mice missing one or both copies of the menin gene in specific target cell types.

The two-hit tumor suppressor model can explain many of the clinical features of MEN 1. Clinical presentation of an inherited disorder in adulthood can be explained by the requirement for a second mutation before clonal expansion. The asymmetrical but relentless nature of the parathyroid disease may be explained by asynchronous but inevitable somatic mutations in each of the parathyroid glands. Multiple islet tumors may result from the same process. What remains completely unexplained is the particular vulnerability of parathyroid, pancreatic islet, and pituitary cells, given the widespread expression of the menin gene.

The menin gene is mutated in about 20% of sporadic parathyroid adenomas, a fraction of sporadic malignant endocrine tumors of the pancreas, and some sporadic carcinoid tumors of the lung as well. Because these mutations occur only in the tumor and not in the patient's normal cells, no familial clustering occurs in these sporadic tumors.

DIAGNOSIS

Screening

Genetic screening for menin gene mutations is now available in reference laboratories. Because inactivating mutations can occur anywhere within the gene, standard surveys of the borders of exons and introns detect only 70% of the genetic abnormalities in families affected by MEN 1. Occasional families inherit mutations in the gene encoding the cyclin-dependent kinase inhibitor p27, but the abnormal genes in a small fraction of MEN 1 patients remain unknown. Thus, the specific mutation in menin in an index case should be ascertained before family members are screened. Because no safe and effective therapies are available for asymptomatic MEN 1 tumors, the precise role for genetic screening has not been established.

To detect active disease, the most useful test to complement a thorough history and physical examination is measurement of blood calcium, particularly ionized calcium, at intervals after age 15 years. Prolactin, gastrin, and fasting blood glucose measurements can also be useful.

PARATHYROID DISEASE. Hyperparathyroidism (Chapter 253), the most common abnormality in MEN 1, is found in more than 90% of patients. Elevated blood calcium levels usually first appear between age 20 and 40 years, considerably earlier than in sporadic primary hyperparathyroidism; however, the disease usually does not present during childhood. At first, the disease is asymptomatic, but it subsequently leads to all the expected consequences of primary hyperparathyroidism. Unlike sporadic hyperparathyroidism, the disease is relentlessly progressive and, with prolonged follow-up, always involves all four parathyroid glands. The involvement is characteristically asymmetrical and asynchronous. This pattern can lead to inappropriately limited parathyroid surgery. If fewer than three parathyroid glands are removed, hypercalcemia always recurs, although not necessarily immediately. Surgical results in patients with MEN 1 are generally less satisfactory than in patients with sporadic four-gland parathyroid disease. At some centers, all four glands are removed, and a portion of one gland is reimplanted in the easily accessible forearm in an attempt to avoid the hazards of too much or too little surgery. The difficulty in attaining long-term normocalcemia has led many clinicians to postpone surgery when the disease is asymptomatic. This strategy may need to be modified if the patient develops Zollinger-Ellison

syndrome (see later), because hypercalcemia can dramatically increase the gastrin levels in such patients.

PANCREATIC ISLET DISEASE. As many as 80% of patients have pancreatic abnormalities at autopsy; many correspondingly have increased blood levels of gastrin, insulin, pancreatic polypeptide, somatostatin, vasoactive intestinal polypeptide, or glucagon during stimulation or suppression tests. The pancreas is often diffusely involved with microadenomas and macroadenomas and apparently hyperplastic lesions. Endoscopic ultrasound can now detect very small tumors of the head or body of the pancreas; the precise role of such early detection is an area of great research interest. Characteristically, more than one islet hormone is secreted from the multiple tumors often present in MEN 1. Despite this underlying pattern of multiple cellular involvement, patients characteristically present with symptoms of only one hormonal disorder. The most common disease is Zollinger-Ellison syndrome (Chapter 201), a peptic ulcer disease associated with gastrin-producing tumors. Identification of disease-causing tumors has proved difficult. The gastrinomas in MEN 1 are often multiple, are very small, and are found in the duodenal wall considerably more often than in the pancreas. Macroadenomas observed in the pancreas by computed tomography (CT) or intraoperative ultrasonography in patients with MEN 1 who have Zollinger-Ellison syndrome may well synthesize hormones other than gastrin.

Although some centers continue to experiment with aggressive attempts at surgical cure, the high recurrence rate after surgery limits its role in this disease. Medical therapy with histamine (H$_2$)-receptor antagonists and hydrogen, potassium–adenosine triphosphatase inhibitors can usually adequately control the secretion of stomach acid. The tumors are slow growing but frequently metastasize locally and to the liver. Chemotherapy is only partially effective and does not cure the disease.

Insulinomas are the second most common, clinically important islet tumor in patients with MEN 1. These tumors are often small and multiple and are much less frequently malignant than are gastrinomas. Despite the frequently diffuse nature of the disease, dominant insulin-producing tumors can often be identified by selective portal venous sampling. Removal of the dominant tissue or, if necessary, subtotal (80%) pancreatectomy is the primary therapeutic strategy.

PITUITARY DISEASE. As in sporadic disease, pituitary disease (Chapter 231) can manifest with a hypersecretion syndrome or with symptoms resulting from a sellar mass or from hypopituitarism. Pituitary tumors occur in about one third of patients with MEN 1. Prolactinomas are the most common tumors. Adrenocortical hyperfunction can result from a pituitary adenoma or from production of adrenocorticotropic hormone or corticotropin-releasing hormone by a foregut carcinoid. Although nonfunctioning adrenal neoplasms are common in patients with MEN 1, primary adrenal neoplasms causing glucocorticoid excess are rare. Acromegaly can result from a pituitary neoplasm or as a consequence of the production of growth hormone–releasing hormone by pancreatic islet tumors. After consideration of ectopic hormone and releasing hormone production by nonpituitary tumors, the course and treatment of pituitary disease in MEN 1 resemble those of sporadic pituitary disease.

PROGNOSIS

The most life-limiting disorders in MEN 1 are the malignant tumors of the pancreatic islets. Whereas sporadic gastrinomas causing Zollinger-Ellison syndrome can sometimes be cured surgically, the gastrinomas in MEN 1 have not been cured by any surgical approach reported thus far. Although vigorous acid control is possible and has dramatically increased life expectancy, these tumors metastasize to the liver and have been poorly responsive to chemotherapy. Other functioning and nonfunctioning pancreatic islet tumors can metastasize and cause death as well. Thus, periodic CT and/or magnetic resonance imaging (MRI) of the abdomen to detect, monitor, and remove growing islet tumors is common practice. The parathyroid tumors are almost always benign, but they recur with a relentlessness much greater than in sporadic multiple-gland parathyroid disease. Thus, even after resection of three and a half glands, recurrence of hyperparathyroidism is common. The course of pituitary tumors, in contrast, resembles the course of sporadic pituitary tumors of an analogous hormonal type.

Multiple Endocrine Neoplasia Types 2a and 2b

DEFINITION

Multiple endocrine neoplasia type 2a (MEN 2a) is an autosomal dominant disease that manifests with medullary carcinoma of the thyroid (MCT;

Chapter 254), pheochromocytoma (Chapter 235), and, less commonly, hyperparathyroidism (Chapter 253). MEN 2b is closely related to MEN 2a because it also manifests with MCT and pheochromocytoma and because both diseases involve mutations in the *RET* proto-oncogene (see later). Patients with MEN 2b present with certain abnormalities not found in patients with MEN 2a, however. These include mucosal neuromas of the tongue, lips, eyelids, and gastrointestinal tract and a marfanoid habitus. Hyperparathyroidism rarely occurs in patients with MEN 2b. MEN 2b is less common than MEN 2a.

PATHOGENESIS

In MEN 2a and 2b, the MCTs and pheochromocytomas often appear bilaterally. Careful prospective analysis of families with MEN 2a has demonstrated that diffuse C-cell hyperplasia precedes a clinically obvious appearance of MCT. C-cell hyperplasia can be detected during the first decade of life by measuring calcitonin after the administration of gastrin, although this test has been supplanted clinically by genetic screening (see later). Virtually all patients with MEN 2a eventually develop C-cell disease. Complete thyroidectomy of patients with C-cell hyperplasia has dramatically decreased the incidence of MCT, which has been the major cause of death in patients with MEN 2a.

Almost all patients with MEN 2a harbor point mutations in the *RET* proto-oncogene, found in the pericentromeric region of chromosome 10. *RET* encodes a member of the tyrosine protein kinase family of cell surface receptors. The gene is expressed in spinal cord, in certain cultured blood cell lines, and in all tested MCT and pheochromocytoma cell lines (both from patients with MEN 2 and from those with sporadic tumors). *RET* interacts with other transmembrane receptors, which in turn bind ligands of the glial cell line–derived neurotrophic factor (GCNF) family. This complicated system of ligands and receptors controls the migration, proliferation, and survival of neural crest cells that populate the thyroid gland, the adrenal gland, and the intrinsic nervous system of the gut. Mutations in *RET* have been found in five different cysteines located in the portion of the receptor that forms the extracellular, ligand-binding domain. The mutant *RET* gene signals in a ligand-independent manner, thereby acting as an oncogene. The mutant *RET* genes can transform cultured cells and cause MCT in transgenic mice.

The transition from diffuse hyperplasia of thyroidal C cells or adrenal medullary cells to clonal neoplasms of the thyroid or adrenal gland probably requires subsequent somatic mutations. Such mutations include the loss of genetic markers on chromosomes 1p, 3p, 3q, and 22q, which frequently occur in these tumors.

Patients with MEN 2b harbor point mutations in the substrate binding pocket of the *RET* kinase, most commonly a change of methionine-918 to threonine. These mutations activate the kinase and change its substrate specificity.

Familial MCT, without tumors of the adrenal or parathyroid gland, is also caused by mutations of the *RET* gene. These mutations include the same mutations that cause MEN 2a, as well as unique mutations in the *RET* gene's kinase domain. Systematic analysis of the *RET* gene has demonstrated that inheritable *RET* gene abnormalities can occur in patients with apparently sporadic MCT as well. Inherited *RET* gene abnormalities are sometimes found in patients with apparently isolated pheochromocytomas, but not in those with sporadic parathyroid adenomas. Remarkably, some patients with familial Hirschsprung's disease (Chapter 138), associated with the absence of neurons in the enteric sympathetic nervous system, have inactive *RET* genes.

DIAGNOSIS

Screening

Direct genetic testing has replaced calcitonin testing as a screening tool in families with MEN 2. These genetic studies have shown that calcitonin testing and even histologic analysis of thyroid tissue can lead to false-positive and false-negative assignment of disease within families. The limited number of sites in the *RET* gene that cause inherited disease makes genetic testing routinely feasible.

Half the patients with MEN 2a develop pheochromocytomas. Family screening allows the detection of pheochromocytoma before the development of hypertension. Plasma metanephrine levels are consistently elevated in patients with MEN 2a pheochromocytomas, as they are in patients with sporadic pheochromocytomas. The tumors are usually found in the adrenal glands and can be documented preoperatively by CT, MRI, and iodine-131-metaiodobenzylguanidine scanning.

TREATMENT

Surgery to prevent MCT is now generally performed before age 5 years in patients with MEN 2a (with some variation, depending on the specific *RET* mutation) and before 6 months of age in patients with the more severe MEN 2b disease.

PROGNOSIS

Because of early detection and curative surgery, MCT can be prevented or cured in virtually all children with MEN 2a or 2b after appropriate genetic testing at a young age. When tumors are seen clinically, however, because such testing was not performed or because the patient represents an index case in a family, the prognosis resembles that of sporadic tumors, except for the high frequency of multiple primary tumors. Similarly, the pheochromocytomas and parathyroid tumors are multiple but otherwise resemble their sporadic counterparts in terms of prognosis.

McCune-Albright Syndrome

DEFINITION

McCune-Albright syndrome is a noninherited disorder consisting of the triad of polyostotic fibrous dysplasia, light brown pigmented skin lesions (café au lait spots), and an endocrinopathy, usually precocious puberty. Multiple endocrine abnormalities can occur.

PATHOGENESIS

Precocious puberty, seen more often in girls than in boys, is gonadotropin independent. Hyperthyroidism is caused by autonomous thyroid nodules. Acromegaly is caused by pituitary adenomas that produce growth hormone and, usually, prolactin. Adrenocortical hyperfunction is caused by adrenocorticotropic hormone–independent adrenal adenomas. Hypophosphatemic rickets, with normal blood calcium levels, phosphate wasting, and low or inappropriately normal levels of 1,25-dihydroxyvitamin D, results from the release of fibroblast growth factor 23 from the dysplastic fibrous tissue.

This somewhat bewildering array of endocrine abnormalities has been rationalized by the observation that cells in the involved tissues harbor mutations in the α-subunit of the G_s protein. The G_s protein links cell surface receptors to the activation of adenylate cyclase. The mutations in McCune-Albright syndrome are point mutations at arginine-201 in the G_s subunit; these mutations lead to prolonged activity of G_s and inappropriate activation of adenylate cyclase. Increased levels of cyclic adenosine monophosphate (cyclic AMP) lead to cellular proliferation and hormone secretion. Patients with McCune-Albright are genetic mosaics. Presumably, at an early stage in embryonic development, a point mutation occurs in the G_s gene of a cell that then proliferates, differentiates, and variably populates normal bone, skin, and endocrine tissues. In cell types in which elevations in cyclic AMP lead to proliferation, abnormal cells become predominant and lead to disease. Because the disease is never inherited, the mutation is presumably lethal when it is present in all cells of the embryo. In contrast, the same mutations at arginine-201 have been found in cases of isolated acromegaly and autonomous thyroid nodules. One can therefore speculate that McCune-Albright syndrome is the most dramatic example of a spectrum of disorders that vary in severity and presentation, depending on the stage of development of the original mutant cell.

TREATMENT

The treatment of the individual hormonal disorders is identical to that of the corresponding sporadic tumor. The polyostotic bone lesions require orthopedic correction when functional disability occurs, and bisphosphonate therapy may slow their growth.

PROGNOSIS

The prognosis of each hormonal component of the syndrome is similar to that of the corresponding sporadically occurring disorder.

AUTOIMMUNE SYNDROMES

Organ-specific autoimmune disease, characterized by lymphocytic infiltration and organ-specific autoantibodies, commonly results in endocrine hypofunction or hyperfunction. Clinical manifestations of disease are usually limited to one gland. Not uncommonly, however, disorders of more than one

TABLE 239-1   CLINICAL FEATURES OF AUTOIMMUNE POLYGLANDULAR SYNDROMES

FEATURE	TYPE 1	TYPE 2
Mucocutaneous candidiasis	Very common	Not seen
Hypoparathyroidism	Common	Rare
Addison's disease	Common	Common
Primary hypogonadism	Common	Occurs
Autoimmune thyroid disease	Rare	Common
Autoimmune diabetes	Occurs	Common
Hypophysitis	Occurs	Occurs
Autoimmune hepatitis	Occurs	Not seen
Pernicious anemia	Occurs	Occurs
Vitiligo	Occurs	Occurs
Malabsorption syndrome	Occurs	Occurs in celiac disease
Alopecia	Common	Occurs
Myasthenia gravis	Not seen	Occurs
Keratopathy	Common	Not seen
Tympanic membrane calcification	Common	Not seen
Inheritance	Autosomal recessive	HLA association
Age at onset	Usually childhood	Usually adulthood

HLA = human leukocyte antigen.

endocrine gland appear in families or in individual patients. Characteristic patterns of disease presentation and genetic inheritance allow the definition of two syndromes with overlapping manifestations (Table 239-1).

Autoimmune Polyglandular Syndrome Type 1

DEFINITION

Autoimmune polyglandular syndrome type 1 is a rare disease that is also known as autoimmune polyendocrinopathy, candidiasis, and ectodermal dystrophy syndrome. It typically manifests in early childhood.

PATHOGENESIS

Autoimmune polyglandular syndrome type 1 is an autosomal recessive disorder caused by a variety of inactivating mutations in the gene encoding autoimmune regulator-1 (AIRE-1), a nuclear protein that influences gene transcription, perhaps by acting as an enzyme—an E3 ubiquitin ligase—that ligates the protein ubiquitin to other nuclear proteins. AIRE-1 is expressed in epithelial cells of the thymus, cells that normally express a wide variety of genes usually expressed only in peripheral tissues. The synthesis of these "peripheral" proteins by thymic epithelial cells may be important for the normal ablation of lymphocytes reactive to these "self-proteins." In an animal model of AIRE-1 gene ablation, the thymic epithelial cells fail to express many of these "peripheral" proteins, perhaps leading to the persistence of lymphocytes responsible for autoimmune attack. The appearance of organ-specific autoantibodies precedes disease presentation and predicts the development of specific end-organ damage. The role of these antibodies is unknown, however.

CLINICAL MANIFESTATIONS

Mucocutaneous candidiasis (Chapter 346) occurs in virtually all patients and is usually the first manifestation of disease. Hypoparathyroidism and Addison's disease are the most common endocrine manifestations; each of these diseases occurs in 70 to 80% of patients. Hypoparathyroidism usually precedes Addison's disease; both diseases typically manifest before age 15 years. Premature ovarian failure (in 60% of affected women) usually presents as secondary amenorrhea; testicular failure occurs less frequently. Insulin-dependent diabetes mellitus occurs in 12% of patients, usually in adulthood; hypothyroidism is uncommon.

Nonendocrine components of this syndrome, in addition to the mucocutaneous candidiasis, include alopecia, vitiligo, corneal opacities, autoimmune hepatitis, enamel hypoplasia of teeth, tympanic membrane calcification, nail dystrophy that correlates only loosely with obvious candidiasis, parietal cell atrophy and vitamin B_{12} malabsorption, and more general intestinal malabsorption with steatorrhea. Asplenism, with Howell-Jolly bodies on peripheral

blood smears (Chapter 160), has been noted in several patients. Each of the disease components should be sought when any patient presents with hypoparathyroidism, primary adrenal insufficiency, or mucocutaneous candidiasis.

TREATMENT

The hypoparathyroidism is treated like the sporadic disease with oral calcium and 1,25-dihydroxyvitamin D, although variable intestinal malabsorption can present a particular therapeutic challenge. The candidiasis can be satisfactorily controlled with ketoconazole.

PROGNOSIS

The prognosis of the variably expressed hormonal disorders is similar to that of their sporadic counterparts. When the diagnosis of autoimmune polyglandular syndrome type 1 is made, surveys for other components of the syndrome can allow earlier treatment than would otherwise occur.

Autoimmune Polyglandular Syndrome Type 2

PATHOGENESIS

Autoimmune polyglandular syndrome type 2 is usually inherited in families with characteristic (normal) variants of genes that regulate the presentation of antigens to T cells and subsequent T-cell function. The most common genetic locus associated with this syndrome is the human leukocyte antigen (HLA) locus. The HLA associations do not predict disease absolutely, even in identical twins, so environmental factors must contribute to disease presentation. Abnormal expression of the gene encoding cytotoxic T-lymphocyte antigen-4 (CTLA-4) can also predispose to autoimmune polyglandular syndrome type 2. The protein tyrosine phosphatase nonreceptor type 22 gene that encodes the lymphoid tyrosine phosphatase opposes signaling from the activated T-cell receptor. A variant of this gene is enriched in families with both type 1 diabetes mellitus and autoimmune thyroid disease. Genome-wide association studies have identified a large number of genes associated with type 1 diabetes. Although this approach has not yet been used for autoimmune polyglandular syndrome type 2, it seems likely that many of the genes identified in these studies will prove relevant because a large fraction of them appear to influence immune responsiveness.

CLINICAL MANIFESTATIONS

Autoimmune polyglandular syndrome type 2 is considerably more common than type 1 and typically manifests in adulthood. Insulin-dependent diabetes mellitus and thyroid dysfunction, either autoimmune hypothyroidism or Graves' disease, are the most frequent manifestations. Addison's disease (Chapter 234) is the third major endocrine component of this disorder. Although most patients who present with autoimmune diabetes or thyroid disease have clinical involvement of only one gland, many patients with autoimmune Addison's disease develop clinically evident disease in other endocrine glands. Less common components of the type 2 polyglandular syndrome include primary hypogonadism and hypophysitis. Pernicious anemia, vitiligo, celiac disease, alopecia, and myasthenia gravis are also associated with this syndrome.

Organ-specific antibodies appear before clinical disease and predict subsequent disease. The role of these antibodies in organ hypofunction has not been established, however.

TREATMENT

The treatment of each component of this syndrome is identical to the treatment of each disorder in isolation, although possible clustering of diseases must be kept in mind during the evaluation and follow-up of all patients with each individual component disorder. Thyroid hormone therapy can precipitate symptoms of adrenal insufficiency in patients with both disorders. Consequently, a careful history, including family history; physical examination; and a low threshold for specific laboratory testing for adrenal insufficiency should be part of the evaluation of every patient with autoimmune hypothyroidism. Further, combinations of hypothyroidism, adrenal insufficiency, and hypogonadism can mimic hypopituitarism, although specific hormonal testing can easily distinguish these disorders. Because multiple components of the syndrome can appear asynchronously, periodic evaluation for the early appearance of additional disease components is indicated.

The prognosis of the individual components of autoimmune polyglandular syndrome type 2 is the same as for the sporadic versions of each component.

SUGGESTED READINGS

Husebye ES, Perheentupa J, Rautemaa R, et al. Clinical manifestations and management of patients with autoimmune polyendocrine syndrome type I. *J Intern Med.* 2009;265:514-529. *Review focusing on clinical presentation and therapy.*

Thakker RV. Multiple endocrine neoplasia type 1 (MEN 1). *Best Pract Res Clin Endocrinol Metab.* 2010;24:355-370. *Review of regulation and proliferation and how they disrupt the interactions of menin with other proteins and alter cell cycle regulation and proliferation.*

Wiebolt J, Koeleman BP, van Haeften TW. Endocrine autoimmune disease: genetics become complex. *Eur J Clin Invest.* 2010;40:1144-1155. *Review.*

240

CARCINOID SYNDROME

KENNETH R. HANDE

The term *carcinoid syndrome* refers to the systemic signs and symptoms resulting from the release of neuroendocrine mediators by some carcinoid tumors. Cutaneous flushing, diarrhea, and cardiac valvular lesions are the most common manifestations of the carcinoid syndrome.

THE NEOPLASMS

Carcinoids are neuroendocrine tumors that arise from enterochromaffin cells. These cells are located throughout the body; however, carcinoid tumors occur most often in the lung (15% of all carcinoid tumors), stomach (5%), small intestine (25%), appendix (25%), and rectum (15%). Carcinoid tumors demonstrate a histologic pattern of dense nests of cells of uniform size and nuclear appearance that contain secretory granules. The neurosecretory granules may contain various amines, such as 5-hydroxytryptamine (serotonin), peptides, tachykinins, and prostaglandins. Only 8 to 10% of all carcinoid tumors are associated with the carcinoid syndrome, usually ileal carcinoids with hepatic metastasis. Carcinoid tumors arising from organs of the embryonic foregut (e.g., bronchus, stomach, pancreas, thyroid) are infrequently associated with the carcinoid syndrome; carcinoids from the distal large intestine may metastasize but do not exhibit endocrine effects. The incidence of carcinoid tumors (2 to 5 per 100,000 population) has been increasing over the past 20 years. Because carcinoid tumors are relatively slow growing, their prevalence is actually greater than that of esophageal, gastric, or pancreatic cancers.

PATHOBIOLOGY

Endocrine Function of Carcinoid Tumors

SEROTONIN. Most carcinoid tumors contain the enzyme tryptophan hydroxylase, which catalyzes the formation of 5-hydroxytryptophan (5-HTP) from tryptophan (Fig. 240-1). The typical ileal carcinoid tumor also contains aromatic L-amino acid decarboxylase, which catalyzes the conversion of 5-HTP to 5-hydroxytryptamine (5-HT or serotonin). Gastric carcinoids are frequently deficient in this decarboxylase and release 5-HTP from the tumor. Following its release from carcinoid tumors, serotonin is oxidized to 5-hydroxyindoleacetaldehyde, which is rapidly converted to 5-hydroxyindoleacetic acid (5-HIAA) by aldehyde dehydrogenase (see Fig. 240-1). This acid is excreted into the urine, and almost all circulating serotonin can be accounted for as urinary 5-HIAA.

TACHYKININS. Peptides of the tachykinin family are stored in carcinoid tumors and are released during flushing. Several tachykinins are derived from a common precursor, β-preprotachykinin; of these, neuropeptide K, neurokinins A and B, and substance P have been identified in tumors and blood from patients with the carcinoid syndrome.

OTHER BIOLOGICALLY ACTIVE SUBSTANCES. Some carcinoid tumors, particularly those of gastric origin, release excessive amounts of histamine. This can be detected by an increased urinary excretion of histamine

Tryptophan

Tryptophan hydroxylase

5-Hydroxytryptophan

Aromatic L-amino acid decarboxylase

5-Hydroxytryptamine (serotonin)

Monoamine oxidase

5-Hydroxyindoleacetaldehyde

Aldehyde dehydrogenase

5-Hydroxyindoleacetic acid (5-HIAA)

FIGURE 240-1. Synthesis and degradation of serotonin.

or its metabolite, *N*-methylhistamine. Carcinoid tumors have been associated with a number of ectopic endocrine syndromes, including hyperadrenocorticism, which results from the ectopic production of adrenocorticotropic hormone, and acromegaly in response to the secretion of growth hormone–releasing hormone by the tumor. Secretion of a variety of prostaglandins by carcinoids has also been demonstrated.

PATHOPHYSIOLOGY OF SEROTONIN OVERPRODUCTION. Serotonin contributes to the intestinal hypermotility and diarrhea associated with the carcinoid syndrome. A secondary effect of serotonin overproduction occurs when a large fraction of dietary tryptophan is shunted into the hydroxylation pathway, leaving less tryptophan available for the formation of nicotinic acid and protein. When urinary excretion of 5-HIAA exceeds 100 mg/day, low levels of plasma tryptophan and evidence of nicotinic acid deficiency (pellagra) can be seen. The interaction of serotonin with platelets and the cardiac endothelium is considered the cause of carcinoid heart disease. This hypothesis is supported by the finding of valvular heart disease in patients taking appetite suppressants, such as fenfluramine, that release serotonin. The risk of valvular heart disease in patients with the carcinoid syndrome is correlated with the amount of 5-HIAA excreted in the urine.

MECHANISM OF THE FLUSH. Most evidence points to the tachykinins as mediators of the carcinoid flush. Tachykinins, particularly neuropeptide K, can be identified in plasma during flushing. Tachykinin levels have been shown to be increased during pentagastrin-induced flushing; when pentagastrin-induced flushing is inhibited by somatostatin, the rise in tachykinin levels is also blocked. Tachykinins are known vasodilators. Serotonin does not appear to be the mediator of flushing. Flushing attacks can be attributed to histamine in certain gastric carcinoids.

Flushing can be triggered by catecholamines, and this probably accounts for the association of flushing with exercise and emotional stimuli. Injection of isoproterenol or pentagastrin can also trigger flushing, an action that may explain the provocation of flushes by eating in some patients. Because the hemodynamic changes associated with such pharmacologically induced attacks can be severe, epinephrine and other β-adrenergic amines, as well as pentagastrin, should be administered with great caution. Flushing episodes can be blocked by somatostatin.

CLINICAL MANIFESTATIONS

Carcinoid tumors typically have a slow rate of growth, and many patients with the carcinoid syndrome survive for years after the disease is recognized. The carcinoid syndrome occurs when mediators produced by the tumor and normally metabolized by the liver escape into the systemic circulation. Thus, most patients with the carcinoid syndrome have hepatic metastasis. For much of the duration of the illness, morbidity results largely from the endocrine functions of the tumor. Death is usually caused by cardiac or hepatic failure and by complications associated with tumor growth.

VASODILATOR PAROXYSMS. Cutaneous flushing, which occurs in 80% of patients with the carcinoid syndrome, is the most common clinical feature. The typical flush is dark red to violaceous and involves the head, neck, and upper trunk (blush area). The flush usually lasts for 30 seconds to 3 minutes. Carcinoid tumors of the foregut produce a slightly different flush, characteristically bright salmon pink to red. Prolonged flushing attacks may be associated with lacrimation and periorbital edema. The flush may be accompanied by tachycardia. The blood pressure usually falls or does not change. A rise in blood pressure during flushing is rare, and the carcinoid syndrome is not a cause of sustained hypertension. Flushing may be provoked by excitement, exertion, eating, and ethanol ingestion. In patients with the bronchial carcinoid variant, flushing may last for hours.

TELANGIECTASIA. In addition to paroxysms of cutaneous vasodilation, some patients develop telangiectasia, primarily on the face and neck, which is most marked in the malar area. These patients may have the characteristic features of rosacea.

PELLAGRA. Tryptophan is normally used to form nicotinic acid. In patients with the carcinoid syndrome, up to 60% of dietary tryptophan may be used to form 5-HTP and 5-HT. Nicotinic acid levels are occasionally depleted, resulting in symptoms of pellagra (dermatitis, diarrhea, and dementia) (Chapter 225).

GASTROINTESTINAL SYMPTOMS. Intestinal hypermotility with borborygmi and cramping occurs in 50 to 70% of patients with the carcinoid syndrome. Explosive secretory diarrhea may occur, although chronic diarrhea with a secretory component is more common (Chapter 142). When diarrhea is severe, malabsorption may occur. Gastrointestinal transit times through the small and large bowel are two- to six-fold faster than in physiologically normal patients.

CARDIAC MANIFESTATIONS. Symptomatic valvular heart disease is present in 15 to 20% of patients with the carcinoid syndrome. Up to 50% of patients have echocardiographic evidence of heart disease (Chapter 60). Plaque-like thickening of the endocardium of the valvular cusps and cardiac chambers occurs primarily on the right side of the heart but may rarely involve the left side (<10%). The endocardial thickening is composed of smooth muscle cells embedded in a stroma rich in mucopolysaccharides. The thickening and deformation of the valve cusps, chordae tendineae, and papillary muscles interfere with valvular function and may lead to regurgitation, stenosis, or combined functional lesions. Lesions of the tricuspid valve (usually regurgitation) are present in 65% of patients with carcinoid heart disease, and pulmonic valvular disease (again, usually regurgitation) is seen in 20% of those with heart disease. Cardiac function may be further compromised by impaired atrial and ventricular compliance and by the occasional occurrence of a high cardiac output that probably results from continuing release of a vasodilator.

PULMONARY SYMPTOMS. Bronchoconstriction, usually most pronounced during flushing attacks, is a less common feature of the syndrome, but it may be severe.

GENERAL FEATURES. Intestinal obstruction may result from the primary tumor or from the desmoplastic reaction in the surrounding mesentery. The desmoplastic reaction is believed to develop in response to the secretion of growth factors, such as platelet-derived growth factor, insulin-like growth factor, epidermal growth factor, and transforming growth factor-β, or by interstitial cells in response to 5-HT. Infrequently, the primary tumors cause gastrointestinal bleeding. Necrosis of hepatic tumor masses may produce an acute syndrome of abdominal pain, tenderness, fever, and leukocytosis. Hepatomegaly from the metastatic disease is often present. Generalized fatigue and debilitation are underappreciated features of the carcinoid syndrome. Attacks of severe and sustained flushing with life-threatening hemodynamic compromise and bronchoconstriction may occur and are referred to as *carcinoid crisis*. Precipitating factors include anesthesia, surgery, tumor necrosis, and catecholamine infusion.

DIAGNOSIS

When all its clinical features are present, the carcinoid syndrome is easily recognized. The diagnosis also must be considered when any one of its clinical manifestations is present.

The diagnostic hallmark consists of overproduction of 5-hydroxyindoles accompanied by increased excretion of urinary 5-HIAA in a patient with a biopsy-proven carcinoid tumor. Normally, excretion of 5-HIAA does not exceed 9 mg/day. Ingestion of foods containing serotonin may complicate the biochemical diagnosis of the carcinoid syndrome; bananas, walnuts, and certain other foods contain enough serotonin to produce abnormally elevated urinary excretion of 5-HIAA after their ingestion. Selected drugs (e.g., guaifenesin, acetaminophen) may also falsely elevate urinary 5-HIAA measurements. Instructing the patient to avoid these foods and medications during the collection of urine for analysis of 5-HIAA can prevent falsely elevated levels. When dietary 5-hydroxyindoles are excluded, urinary excretion of 25 mg/day of 5-HIAA is diagnostic of the carcinoid syndrome. Elevation in the range of 9 to 25 mg/day may be seen with the carcinoid syndrome, nontropical sprue, vomiting, or acute intestinal obstruction. Measurement of serotonin in blood or platelets is of interest but has less diagnostic value than assay of the major metabolite of serotonin in the urine.

Plasma chromogranin A concentrations are often elevated in carcinoid patients, including those who do not have the carcinoid syndrome, and may serve as a marker of tumor mass. The diagnostic value of plasma chromogranin A is relatively low, however, because this substance may be elevated in a variety of neuroendocrine tumors and is increased in patients with renal failure, those with atrophic gastritis, and patients taking proton pump inhibitors. Assessment of the extent and localization of both primary and metastatic tumor is aided by computed tomography of the abdomen and chest and by imaging with radionuclide-labeled somatostatin receptor ligands.

Differential Diagnosis

Attacks of flushing in a patient with normal urinary excretion of 5-HIAA raise other diagnostic possibilities. Systemic mastocyte activation disorders, including systemic mastocytosis and idiopathic anaphylaxis, produce flushing and diarrhea and should be considered when 5-HIAA excretion is not elevated. Flushing also occurs in genetically predisposed individuals following ethanol ingestion, in the postmenopausal state, and in conjunction with other neuroendocrine tumors such as VIPomas (tumors that produce excessive vasoactive intestinal peptide) and medullary carcinomas of the thyroid.

Variants of the Carcinoid Syndrome

The origin of the tumor influences the biologically active substances produced and their storage and release. The typical carcinoid syndrome usually results from tumors of midgut origin, which almost invariably secrete serotonin. In contrast, tumors arising from the embryonic foregut have a lower serotonin content and may secrete 5-HTP. Patients with gastric carcinoids may exhibit unique flushing, which begins as bright, patchy erythema with sharply delineated serpentine borders; these patches tend to coalesce as the blush heightens. Food ingestion is especially likely to produce flushes. Ectopic hormone production (e.g., Cushing's syndrome, acromegaly) and multiple endocrine adenomas are more likely to be associated with tumors of embryonic foregut. Roughly 10% of patients with multiple endocrine neoplasia type 1 (MEN 1) develop a carcinoid tumor. With carcinoid tumors arising from the bronchus, attacks of flushing tend to be prolonged and severe and may be associated with periorbital edema, excessive lacrimation and salivation, hypotension, tachycardia and tachyarrhythmias, anxiety, and tremulousness. Nausea, vomiting, explosive diarrhea, and bronchoconstriction may progress and become severe. This group is therapeutically unique, in that severe flushes can often be prevented by corticosteroids.

TREATMENT

Treatment of the carcinoid syndrome is directed toward pharmacologic therapy for humorally mediated symptoms and reduction of the tumor mass.

Somatostatin Analogues

More than 80% of carcinoid tumors have somatostatin receptors on the cell surface. Somatostatin can bind to these receptors and prevent the flushing and other endocrine symptoms of the carcinoid syndrome. However, the half-life of somatostatin is short. The development of analogues of somatostatin with longer biologic half-lives than the native hormone has made subcutaneous administration feasible and has been a major advance in the treatment of these patients.

Octreotide

One of the somatostatin analogues, octreotide, improves the flushing and other endocrine manifestations in most patients with the carcinoid syndrome. This therapy is frequently associated with a reduction in urinary 5-HIAA excretion and in tachykinin levels in blood. With the improvement of these endocrine symptoms, including fatigue, a considerable improvement in quality of life may be achieved. Long-acting somatostatin analogues (octreotide LAR and lanreotide) have been developed, permitting once-monthly dosing. Two to 4 weeks may be required to achieve steady-state levels of octreotide following the administration of octreotide LAR, during which time supplementation with subcutaneous octreotide may be needed. An uncommon but severe adverse effect of octreotide is hypoglycemia, probably as a result of the inhibition of glucagon and growth hormone secretion. The suppression of pancreatic exocrine function by octreotide can cause steatorrhea, and inhibition of the release of cholecystokinin can cause cholelithiasis. Octreotide should be used to prevent or treat carcinoid crises that accompany the massive release of mediators that may occur during operative procedures and tumor necrosis. In patients with histamine-secreting gastric carcinoids, blockade of both H_1 and H_2 receptors markedly ameliorates flushing. In patients receiving octreotide, about 5% achieve a regression in tumor mass. Octreotide has recently been demonstrated to slow the growth rate of carcinoid tumors. ▣

Surgery

Early diagnosis of the carcinoid syndrome has led to complete surgical cure in a few patients with tumors arising in ovarian or testicular teratomas or in the bronchus. By releasing their humoral mediators directly into the systemic circulation, these tumors can produce the syndrome before metastatic disease occurs. In contrast, tumors that release humoral substances into the portal circulation, to be largely metabolized by the liver, usually produce the syndrome only after liver metastases occur. Given the slow progression of this neoplasm, effective reduction in tumor mass can ameliorate morbidity and improve quality of life even after metastases have occurred. In selected patients, this goal can be achieved by surgical debulking of tumor, including partial hepatectomy for unilobar metastases, excision of large superficial hepatic metastases, and removal of the primary tumor together with regional lymph nodes containing metastases. Elective cholecystectomy during the surgical intervention prevents the cholelithiasis that may result from octreotide treatment. Because the blood supply of hepatic metastases is largely arterial, percutaneous embolization of the hepatic arterial supply to the most involved hepatic lobe can sometimes reduce inoperable hepatic metastases; the procedure carries a risk of serious complications.

Chemotherapy

Chemotherapy with single or combination cytotoxic agents given on a short-term basis has produced little benefit. For patients who exhibit tumor progression or whose clinical syndrome has failed to improve following cytoreduction and octreotide, interferon-α and antiangiogenic agents (bevacizumab and sunitinib) have been considered as palliative therapy.

PROGNOSIS

A concerted strategy consisting of removal of the primary tumor, reduction in tumor bulk, and administration of octreotide can lead to considerable amelioration of symptoms, improvement in the quality of life, reduction in the release of the humoral substances that engender cardiac lesions, and prolongation of survival. The median survival of patients with metastatic carcinoid tumor and the carcinoid syndrome now exceeds 5 years in carefully managed patients.

1. Rinke A, Muller HH, Schade-Brittinger G, et al. Placebo-controlled, double-blind, prospective randomized study on the effect of octreotide LAR in the control of tumor growth in patients with metastatic neuroendocrine midgut tumors: a report from the PROMID Study Group. *J Clin Oncol.* 2009;27:4656-4663.

SUGGESTED READINGS

Dumoulein M, Verslype C, van Cutsem E, et al. Carcinoid heart disease: case and literature review. *Acta Cardiol.* 2010;65:261-264. *Review including surgical valve replacement.*

Klibanski A, Melmed S, Clemmons DR, et al. The endocrine tumor summit 2008: appraising therapeutic approaches for acromegaly and carcinoid syndrome. *Pituitary.* 2010;13:266-286. *Consensus guidelines.*

Landerholm K, Falkmer S, Järhult J. Epidemiology of small bowel carcinoids in a defined population. *World J Surg.* 2010;34:1500-1505. *The annual age-adjusted incidence was 1.12 per 100,000 persons with a median age at diagnosis of 69 years; 50% of patients presented with abdominal pain.*

Pasieka JL. Carcinoid tumors. *Surg Clin North Am.* 2009;89:1123-1137. *Review, with a focus on surgical approaches.*

Yao JC, Hassan M, Phan A, et al. One hundred years after "carcinoid": epidemiology of and prognostic factors for neuroendocrine tumors in 35,825 cases in the United States. *J Clin Oncol.* 2008;26:3063-3072. *Analysis of the incidence and prevalence of carcinoid tumors.*

DISORDERS OF SEXUAL DEVELOPMENT

PERRIN C. WHITE

DEFINITION

This chapter reviews the concepts underlying the initial evaluation and management of patients with disorders of sexual development (DSD). By definition, such an individual has lack of concordance of various aspects of gender. These include chromosomal sex (46,XX, 46,XY, or other), gonadal or reproductive sex (ovaries, fallopian tubes, and uterus versus testes, seminal vesicles, prostate gland, and ejaculatory ducts), genital sex (vagina and clitoris versus scrotum and penis), and gender-specific behavior. Depending on chromosomal sex, most patients can be classified as incompletely masculinized 46,XY males, virilized 46,XX females, and patients with abnormalities of sex chromosomes, such as those with mixed gonadal dysgenesis. (In the past, 46,XY and 46,XX DSD patients were referred to as male and female pseudohermaphrodites, respectively, but these terms are no longer preferred.) Many conditions can cause DSD (Table 241-1).

Normal Sexual Differentiation
Gonadal Differentiation

At 5 to 6 weeks' gestation, the gonadal primordia (gonadal ridges) develop from the coelomic epithelium overlying the medial surface of the mesonephros (primitive kidneys; Fig. 241-1). These primitive gonads are identical in both sexes. Germ cells form at 3 to 4 weeks' gestation and migrate through the gut mesentery into the gonads at this early bipotential stage. Whether germ cells are directed toward male or female gametogenesis depends largely on the environment generated by surrounding somatic cells rather than on factors intrinsic to the germ cells.

During the seventh week, XY male gonads begin to differentiate under the influence of testis-determining genes. The first to be expressed is *SRY*, the key gene on the Y chromosome controlling male differentiation, which initiates the development of Sertoli cells. Sertoli cells surround germ cells to form testis cords, which nourish primordial germ cells and direct them into the pathway for male gametogenesis. Recruitment of endothelial cells leads to development of a testis-specific vasculature that is required for normal organization of the testis.

Steroidogenic cells develop from the mesonephros and migrate into the developing adrenal cortex and testis at 8 weeks. In the testis, they become Leydig cells, which secrete the testosterone required for subsequent male reproductive development. In the first trimester, testosterone secretion is mainly under the control of human chorionic gonadotropin (HCG); it subsequently requires luteinizing hormone (LH) secreted by the fetal anterior pituitary.

Ovaries are recognizable at about 10 weeks. The signaling molecule WNT4 plays an active role in ovarian development, repressing expression of testis-specific genes and vascular development. Germ cells in the ovary continue into the first meiotic prophase beginning at 12 weeks' gestation and continuing until 7 months' gestation.

Development of Male and Female Internal Reproductive Tracts

The reproductive tracts are derived from intermediate mesoderm. The male reproductive tract develops from the mesonephric (wolffian) ducts, whereas the female reproductive tract develops from the paramesonephric (müllerian) ducts (Fig. 241-2). Both sets of ducts are present in normal embryos.

Development of wolffian or müllerian structures depends on the presence or absence of normally functioning testes. The Sertoli cells secrete antimüllerian hormone (AMH, also termed müllerian inhibiting substance) starting when the testes differentiate. Expression of AMH is controlled by several

TABLE 241-1	DISORDERS OF SEXUAL DEVELOPMENT*

VIRILIZATION OR SEX REVERSAL IN XX FEMALES

Virilizing forms of congenital adrenal hyperplasia
  21-Hydroxylase deficiency (1 : 15,000 births) [CYP21]: salt-wasting or simple
    virilizing forms
  11β-Hydroxylase deficiency [CYP11B1]
  3β-Hydroxysteroid dehydrogenase deficiency [HSD3B2]
  Cytochrome P-450 oxidoreductase deficiency (also has a maternal effect) [POR]
Maternal or exogenous androgens
  Drugs (danazol, progestins)
  Luteoma
  Aromatase deficiency [CYP19]
  Transcription factor mutations
Mutations in genes affecting gonadal differentiation
  SRY (translocation to X)
  SOX9 (duplication)
  WT1 (Denys-Drash syndrome)
Structural/idiopathic

UNDERVIRILIZATION OR SEX REVERSAL IN XY MALES

Biosynthetic defects
  Lipoid adrenal hyperplasia [STAR]
  17α-Hydroxylase/17,20 lyase [CYP17]
  3β-Hydroxysteroid dehydrogenase [HSD3B2]
  17-Ketosteroid reductase [HSD17B3]
  5α-Reductase [SRD5A2]
  Cytochrome P-450 oxidoreductase deficiency [POR]
  Smith-Lemli-Opitz syndrome (1 : 20,000) [DHCR7]
Androgen insensitivity (1 : 20,000) [AR]: complete or partial
Luteinizing hormone insensitivity [LHR]
Mutations in genes affecting gonadal differentiation
  SRY
  SOX9 (camptomelic dysplasia)
  SF1 (sometimes associated with adrenal hypoplasia)
  WT1 (WAGR and Denys-Drash syndromes)
  DAX1 or WNT4 duplications
  DHH (associated with peripheral neuropathy)
  ATRX (X-linked α-thalassemia and mental retardation)
Exposure to 5α-reductase inhibitors, other endocrine disruptors

MICROPENIS

Panhypopituitarism [including PROP1 mutations]
Septo-optic dysplasia [including HESX mutations]
Hypogonadotropic hypogonadism
  Kallmann's syndrome [KAL1]
  Prader-Willi syndrome [paternal chromosome 15q11 deletion]
  Adrenal hypoplasia congenita [DAX1]
Vanishing testes (may also cause ambiguous genitalia)

OTHER SYNDROMES AFFECTING REPRODUCTIVE SYSTEMS

Chromosomal aneuploidy
  Turner's syndrome (1 : 2500): 45,X; 45,X/46,XX mosaics; 46,XXr; 46,XXq–
  Klinefelter's syndrome (1 : 1000): 47,XXY
  Mixed gonadal dysgenesis: 45,X/46,XY; 45,X/47,XXY
  Other: trisomy 13, trisomy 18, triploidy, 4p–, 13q–
Persistent müllerian duct syndrome in XY males
  Type 1 [AMH]
  Type 2 [AMHR2]
Mayer-Rokitansky-Küster-Hauser syndrome (vaginal atresia) [WNT4]

*Frequencies of relatively common (at least 1 : 20,000) diseases are noted in parentheses. When causative genetic mutations have been identified, the affected locus is noted in square brackets. WAGR = Wilms' tumor, aniridia, genitourinary abnormalities or gonadoblastoma, and mental retardation.

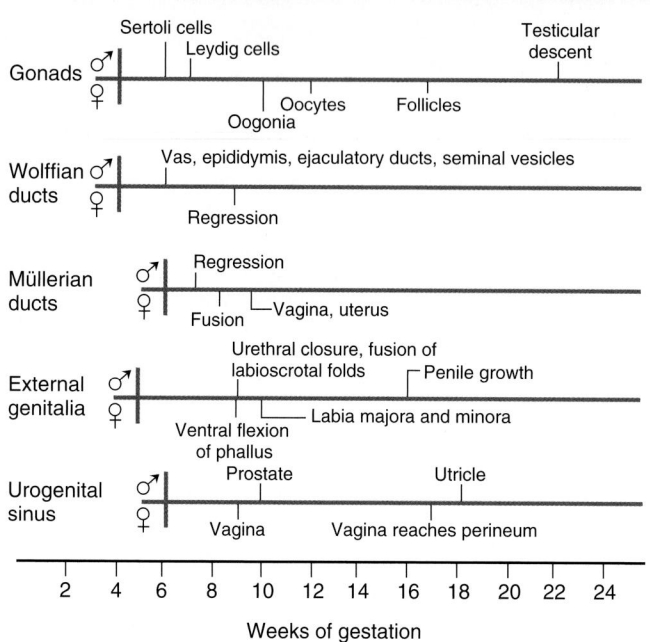

FIGURE 241-1. Time course of prenatal sexual differentiation in male and female fetuses. (Adapted from Barthold JS, Gonzalez R. Intersex states. In: Gonzales ET, Bauer SB, eds. *Pediatric Urology Practice*. Philadelphia: Lippincott Williams & Wilkins; 1999.)

insufficient to develop wolffian structures. Thus, in conditions in which the gonads develop asymmetrically (e.g., true hermaphroditism or mixed gonadal dysgenesis; see later), wolffian structures develop asymmetrically as well. Development of wolffian structures requires an intact androgen receptor.

Development of the External Genitalia
External genital structures are also bipotential in early gestation and consist of the genital tubercle, genital folds (later, urethral-labial folds), and genital swelling (later, labioscrotal folds) (see Fig. 241-2). Differentiation to male genitalia occurs from about 8 to 14 weeks' gestation under the influence of dihydrotestosterone, which must interact with an intact androgen receptor. The genital tubercle becomes the glans penis; the genital folds fuse to become the shaft of the penis and penile urethra, and the labioscrotal folds (derived from the genital swelling) fuse to become the scrotum. Without androgens, these structures become the clitoris, labia minora, and labia majora, respectively.

Normal Gonadal and Adrenal Steroidogenesis
Many forms of genital ambiguity result from defects in steroid biosynthesis in the testes or adrenal cortex or from defective steroid metabolism in the placenta or in target tissues (Fig. 241-3 and E-Fig. 241-1).

Steroid biosynthesis in the testes and adrenals begins with the importation of cholesterol into mitochondria, a highly regulated process controlled largely by the steroidogenic acute regulatory (StAR) protein; levels of StAR are controlled within the adrenals by adrenocorticotropic hormone (ACTH) and within the testis by HCG during the first trimester and by LH later in pregnancy.

Within mitochondria, the side chain of cholesterol is cleaved between carbons 20 and 22 by the cholesterol side-chain cleavage enzyme (cholesterol desmolase, CYP11A), a cytochrome P-450 enzyme. The product is pregnenolone, which is transported to the endoplasmic reticulum. Some pregnenolone is converted by 17α-hydroxylase (CYP17) to 17-hydroxypregnenolone. Both 17-hydroxypregnenolone and the remaining pregnenolone are converted by 3ß-hydroxysteroid dehydrogenase (HSD3B2) to 17-hydroxyprogesterone and progesterone, respectively. The side chain of 17-hydroxypregnenolone is cleaved by the 17,20-lyase activity of CYP17 to dehydroepiandrosterone (DHEA). DHEA may also be converted to androstenedione by HSD3B2.

All the preceding steps can occur in the adrenal cortex, in Leydig cells of the testis, and (after puberty) in theca cells of ovarian follicles. Subsequent biosynthetic steps are specific to different glands. In the adrenal cortex, 17-hydroxyprogesterone is converted by 21-hydroxylase (CYP21, a

transcription factors: SF1 and WT1 (Wilms' tumor locus) synergize to promote transcription, whereas DAX1 antagonizes it. The overall effect of AMH is to induce regression of müllerian structures between 8 and 12 weeks' gestation. In its absence, development of the müllerian ducts proceeds, and the female internal structures (fallopian tubes, uterus, cervix, and upper vagina) are formed.

Development of the structures derived from the wolffian ducts, including the epididymis, ductus deferens, ejaculatory ducts, and seminiferous tubules, requires high local concentrations of testosterone secreted from Leydig cells of the testis beginning at about 7 weeks' gestation. In the absence of testosterone, wolffian ducts regress. Levels of testosterone in the circulation are

Internal Genitalia

FIGURE 241-2. Differentiation of the internal and external genitalia of the human fetus. (Adapted from Griffen JE, Ojeda SR, eds. *Textbook of Endocrine Physiology.* New York: Oxford University Press; 1996.)

microsomal P-450) to 11-deoxycortisol, which is then converted in mitochondria to cortisol by 11ß-hydroxylase (CYP11B1). Additionally, progesterone is converted to deoxycorticosterone by CYP21, which is then converted to aldosterone by aldosterone synthase (CYP11B2).

In Leydig cells of the testis, androstenedione is converted to testosterone by 17-ketosteroid reductase (17ß-hydroxysteroid dehydrogenase type 3 [HSD17B3]); the same reaction occurs in theca cells of the ovary, catalyzed by 17ß-hydroxysteroid dehydrogenase type 1 (HSD17B1). In granulosa cells of the ovary (after puberty), androstenedione and testosterone are converted by aromatase (CYP19) to estrone and estradiol, respectively. In skin of the developing male external genitalia, steroid 5α-reductase (SRD5A2) converts testosterone to a more potent androgen, dihydrotestosterone.

The placenta is a steroid-synthesizing and -metabolizing tissue as well; it has high steroid sulfatase activity that converts DHEA sulfate from the fetal adrenal gland back to DHEA. This is then successively converted by 3ß-hydroxysteroid dehydrogenase type 1 (HSD3B1) and aromatase (CYP19) to androstenedione and estrone, respectively, which are then converted to estradiol by HSD17B1.

DEFECTS OF SEX DIFFERENTIATION
Defects of Steroidogenesis

PATHOBIOLOGY

Genital ambiguity in genetic females is usually the result of exposure to excessive levels of androgens. Virilizing congenital adrenal hyperplasia (CAH), the most common cause of genital ambiguity in female infants, occurs in 1 in 15,000 births.

Conversely, severe deficiencies of androgens, if present early in gestation, cause ambiguous or female-appearing external genitalia in male infants. Usually, müllerian structures such as the uterus, cervix, and upper vagina are not present because the testes are able to secrete müllerian inhibitory substance. Thus, individuals with these conditions have a short vagina ending in a blind pouch.

CONGENITAL ADRENAL HYPERPLASIA

The fundamental defect among patients with any form of CAH is inadequate synthesis of cortisol (see Fig. 241-3 and E-Fig. 241-1). Inefficient cortisol synthesis signals the hypothalamus and pituitary to increase corticotropin-releasing hormone and ACTH, respectively (Chapter 230). Consequently, the adrenal glands become hyperplastic, and steroid precursors accumulate proximal to the block in biosynthesis. In some conditions, these precursors can be converted to androgens.

LIPOID HYPERPLASIA. Lipoid hyperplasia results from mutations in the *STAR* gene. Cholesterol is not imported efficiently into mitochondria and thus accumulates in cells. Steroid biosynthesis is drastically reduced because of the lack of substrate, and the lipid accumulation quickly kills steroid-synthesizing cells in both the adrenals and the testes. Thus, affected male patients are born as phenotypically female because they cannot synthesize testosterone. Affected female patients may undergo transient spontaneous puberty because human ovarian granulosa cells do not synthesize steroid hormones (and thus do not accumulate cholesterol) until puberty. Both sexes have adrenal insufficiency and are unable to synthesize either cortisol or aldosterone.

17α-HYDROXYLASE/17,20 LYASE DEFICIENCY. Severe mutations in the *CYP17* gene prevent the synthesis of any sex hormones. Affected male patients have female-appearing external genitalia but have no müllerian structures because the testes synthesize AMH. Affected female patients remain sexually infantile without hormone replacement. Milder mutations result in ambiguous genitalia in male patients. Although cortisol synthesis is also abolished, even severely affected individuals are able to synthesize corticosterone, an active glucocorticoid, as well as aldosterone. Thus, they do not develop adrenal insufficiency. On the contrary, they secrete excessive levels of deoxycorticosterone, which has mineralocorticoid activity, and are therefore prone to develop hypertension.

3β-HYDROXYSTEROID DEHYDROGENASE DEFICIENCY. Severe mutations in the *HSD3B2* gene prevent the synthesis of aldosterone, cortisol, testosterone, and estrogens. Because DHEA, a weak androgen, is synthesized and secreted at high levels, some degree of phallic growth is present. Thus, affected male patients have severely ambiguous genitalia, but affected female patients may have clitorimegaly. Both sexes develop adrenal insufficiency if they are untreated.

Because many children with premature adrenarche (early development of axillary and pubic hair), as well as many women with polycystic ovary syndrome, have elevated levels of DHEA, it was once thought that such individuals could have a mild form of HSD3B2 deficiency. However, mutations in *HSD3B2* are rarely if ever found in such individuals, who have an imbalance in the relative levels of HSD3B2 and CYP17 activity within the adrenal cortex.

21-HYDROXYLASE DEFICIENCY. More than 90% of cases of CAH are caused by 21-hydroxylase deficiency resulting from mutations in the *CYP21* (or *CYP21A2*) gene. The relatively high incidence of this condition is a consequence of the proximity of a highly homologous pseudogene, *CYP21P* (or *CYP21A1P*), which contains approximately 10 mutations that are deleterious to expression, messenger RNA processing, or enzymatic activity. *CYP21* and *CYP21P* are located within the major histocompatibility complex on chromosome 6p21.3, a genomic region noteworthy for a high rate of recombination. More than 90% of all mutations are the result of intergenic recombination between *CYP21* and *CYP21P*. Most are transfers of deleterious mutations from *CYP21P* to *CYP21*, whereas 20% are net deletions of *CYP21* resulting from unequal meiotic crossover.

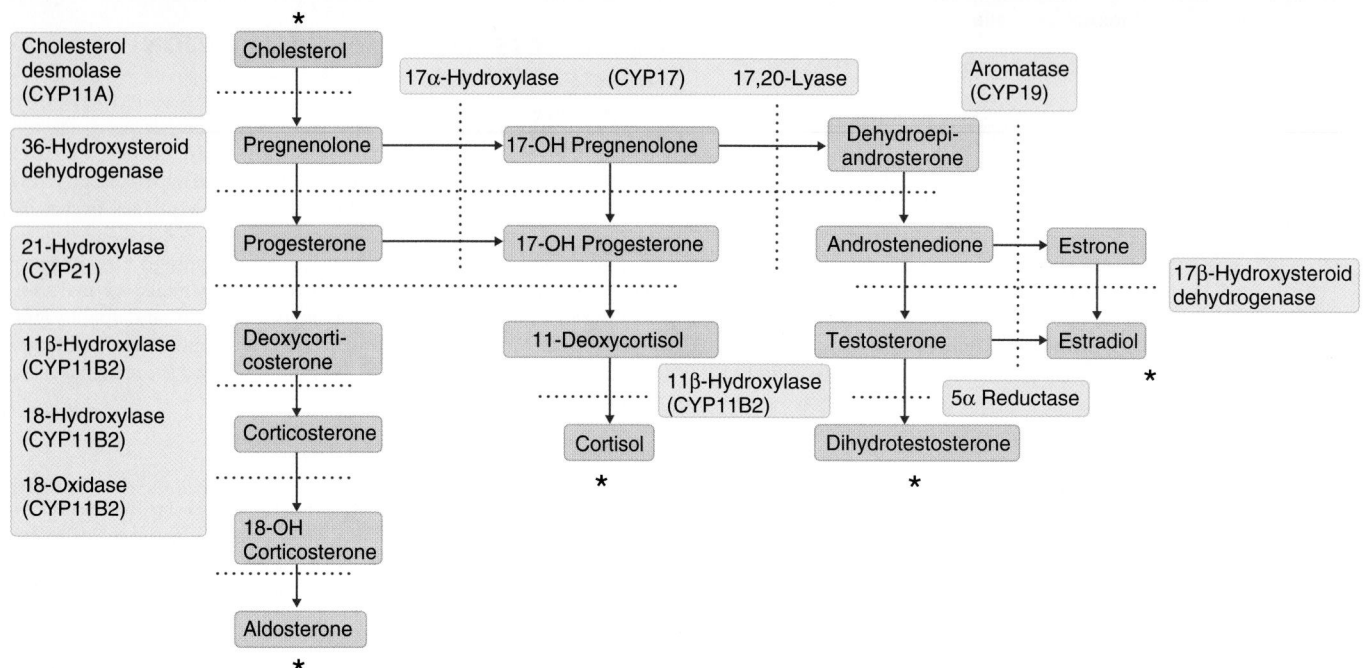

FIGURE 241-3. Steroidogenesis. Pathways for the synthesis of progesterone and mineralocorticoids (aldosterone), glucocorticoids (cortisol), androgens (testosterone and dihydrotestosterone), and estrogens (estradiol) are arranged from left to right. The enzymatic activities catalyzing each bioconversion are written in boxes. For those activities mediated by specific cytochrome P-450 subsets, the systematic name of the enzyme (CYP followed by a number) is listed in parentheses. CYP11B2 and CYP17 have multiple activities. *For an expanded version of this image, including planar structures for cholesterol and the end products of each pathway, see E-Figure 241-1.

In patients with 21-hydroxylase deficiency, the adrenals produce excess 17-hydroxyprogesterone, 17-hydroxypregnenolone, and progesterone, which are further metabolized to DHEA and androstenedione. Once secreted, these substances are further metabolized to active androgens (testosterone and dihydrotestosterone) and, to a lesser extent, to estrogens (estrone and estradiol).

Adrenal secretion of excess androgen precursors does not significantly affect male sexual differentiation. In affected female patients, the urogenital sinus is in the process of septation when the fetal adrenal begins to produce excess androgens, which function to prevent the formation of separate vaginal and urethral canals. Further adrenal-derived androgens interact with androgen receptors in genital skin and induce clitoral enlargement, promote fusion of the labial folds, and cause rostral migration of the urethral/vaginal perineal orifice. However, internal wolffian structures such as the prostate gland and spermatic ducts are usually not virilized, presumably because development of the wolffian ducts requires markedly higher local concentrations of testosterone than the external genitalia. Nevertheless, severely affected female patients occasionally have some development of typically male internal genital structures.

Thus, the typical result in severely affected girls is ambiguous or male-appearing external genitalia with perineal hypospadias and chordee, but without palpable testes (Fig. 241-4). The severity of virilization is often quantitated using a five-point scale developed by Prader (Fig. 241-5). Not all female patients with classic CAH develop the same degree of genital ambiguity. One could speculate that the physical signs of androgen excess depend not only on direct adrenal secretion of androgen precursors but also on the efficiency with which such hormones are converted to more potent products, such as dihydrotestosterone, by peripheral enzymes such as 5α-reductase. Additionally, the concentration and transcriptional activity of androgen receptors may play a role in determining genital phenotype.

Most patients (75%) cannot synthesize sufficient aldosterone to maintain sodium balance and are termed *salt wasters.* These patients are predisposed to episodic and potentially life-threatening hyponatremic dehydration. Patients with sufficient aldosterone production to prevent salt wasting and who have signs of prenatal virilization and/or markedly increased production of hormonal substrates of 21-hydroxylase (e.g., 17-hydroxyprogesterone) are termed *simple virilizers.*

11β-HYDROXYLASE DEFICIENCY. Patients with 11β-hydroxylase deficiency have mutations in the *CYP11B1* gene. They have elevated levels of deoxycorticosterone and 11-deoxycortisol, as well as earlier cortisol precursors such as 17-hydroxyprogesterone. These patients secrete excess adrenal

FIGURE 241-4. Virilized external genitalia in a female infant with congenital adrenal hyperplasia caused by 21-hydroxylase deficiency. No gonads are present in the scrotum.

androgens, with consequences similar to those seen in 21-hydroxylase deficiency. However, patients with 11β-hydroxylase deficiency synthesize aldosterone normally and do not have problems with salt wasting. Instead, they are likely to become hypertensive as a result of elevated levels of deoxycorticosterone and its metabolites.

DEFECTS OF ANDROGEN BIOSYNTHESIS

Lipoid hyperplasia, 17-hydroxylase/17,20 lyase deficiency, and HSD3B2 deficiency affect the biosynthesis of both corticosteroids and sex hormones. In contrast, two enzymatic defects affect only androgen biosynthesis. They have similar phenotypes. Affected male patients are born with ambiguous genitalia, but they virilize at puberty and often reassign themselves to a male gender if they were raised as females. They have absent müllerian structures as a result of the secretion of AMH by the testes.

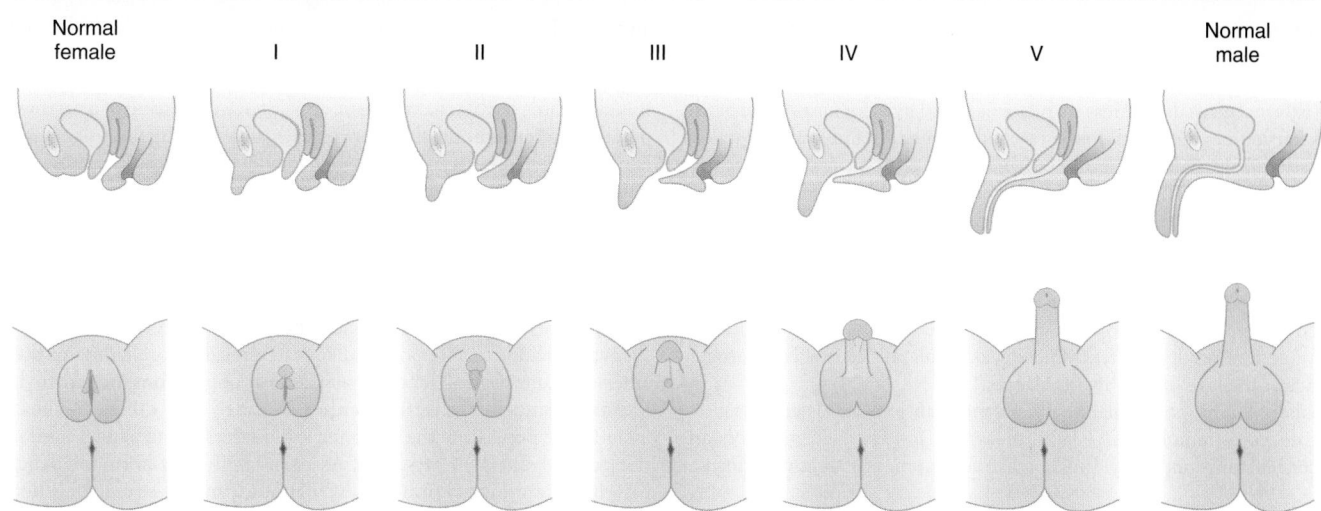

FIGURE 241-5. Abnormal differentiation of the urogenital sinus and external genitalia. Schematic representations of normal female and male anatomy flank a series of schematics illustrating different degrees of virilization of females, graded using the scale developed by Prader. The uterus (shaded) persists in virilized females even when the external genitalia have a completely masculine appearance (Prader grade V). (Adapted from Prader A. Der Genitalbefund beim Pseudohermaphroditismus femininus der kengenitalen adrenogenitalen Syndroms. *Helv Paediatr Acta.* 1954;9:231-248.)

17-KETOSTEROID REDUCTASE (17-HYDROXYSTEROID DEHYDRO-GENASE 3) DEFICIENCY. This disorder is caused by mutations in the *HSD17B3* gene. Although testosterone is not synthesized well, androstenedione, an active androgen, is synthesized. Because several other isozymes have 17-ketosteroid reductase activity in other tissues, some testosterone is invariably synthesized, especially at puberty, when circulating levels of androstenedione increase.

5α-REDUCTASE DEFICIENCY. Patients with 5α-reductase deficiency resulting from mutations in the *SRD5A2* gene synthesize entirely normal amounts of testosterone, but they cannot synthesize adequate amounts of dihydrotestosterone, the most potent naturally occurring androgen. This enzyme is not expressed at high levels in the testes (circulating levels of dihydrotestosterone are relatively low); instead, it is expressed in genital skin. Internal wolffian structures do not require this enzyme and are intact; high testosterone levels at puberty induce significant phallic growth without 5α-reductase activity.

OTHER DEFECTS OF STEROIDOGENESIS

AROMATASE DEFICIENCY. Mutations in *CYP19* cause aromatase deficiency in both the fetus and the placenta. The placenta can convert DHEA sulfate to androstenedione and testosterone normally, but it cannot convert these androgens to estrone and estradiol. These androgens accumulate in both the fetal and the maternal circulations and virilize both the mother and the affected fetus if it is female. Affected male infants are phenotypically normal. Affected female patients virilize further at puberty if they are untreated. The lack of aromatase activity within bone leads to tall stature in both sexes (because estrogens are required to close the growth plates) and later to osteoporosis.

CYTOCHROME P-450 OXIDOREDUCTASE DEFICIENCY. This deficiency is one form of Antley-Bixler syndrome, which is characterized by skeletal anomalies and craniosynostosis; most patients also have ambiguous genitalia associated with mutations in the *POR* gene. Antley-Bixler syndrome without genital abnormalities is caused by mutations in the FGF receptor (*FGFR2*) gene.

Because this disorder affects the activity of all microsomal cytochrome P-450 subsets, complete deficiency of cytochrome P-450 oxidoreductase (POR) is lethal, and identified mutations in humans yield POR with partial activity. *POR* mutations may cause skeletal anomalies by interfering with cholesterol synthesis. Genital ambiguity is caused by several mechanisms. Decreased activity of 17α-hydroxylase/17,20 lyase (CYP17) affects androgen synthesis and leads to undervirilization in males. Conversely, decreased activity of 21-hydroxylase (CYP21) can virilize affected females. These two deficiencies can also cause adrenal insufficiency. Finally, decreased activity of placental aromatase (CYP19) virilizes both the mother and the affected fetus (if female).

SMITH-LEMLI-OPITZ SYNDROME. This relatively frequent (1 in 20,000 northern Europeans) disorder of the final step of cholesterol biosynthesis (conversion from 7-dehydrocholesterol) is caused by mutations in the *DHCR7* gene encoding 7-dehydrocholesterol reductase. The syndrome is characterized by multiple congenital anomalies, including short stature, microcephaly, mental retardation, aggressive behavior, seizures, hypotonia, polydactyly, cleft palate, cardiac defects, lung hypoplasia, and renal anomalies. Male patients have ambiguous genitalia. The range of clinical severity is wide and depends on the nature of the mutations. Pathogenetic mechanisms for the ambiguous genitalia may include insufficient provision of cholesterol for steroid hormone biosynthesis or toxic effects of the precursor, 7-dehydrocholesterol, on steroidogenic cells.

MATERNAL CONDITIONS AFFECTING THE FETUS
Luteoma of Pregnancy

Luteomas are the most common causes of maternal virilization during pregnancy. They often occur bilaterally. Although many luteomas are discovered incidentally during cesarean sections or postpartum tubal ligations, one fourth of mothers virilize during the latter half of pregnancy, and half of female infants born to these mothers also exhibit signs of virilization, most typically clitorimegaly and labial fusion. Spontaneous regression of the luteoma generally begins within days after delivery.

Drug Exposure

Depending on the agent, maternal drug exposure may affect either male or female fetuses. Females may be virilized by androgens such as 19-nortestosterone or progestins administered to prevent spontaneous abortion. Undervirilized males can be born to women exposed to 5α-reductase inhibitors such as finasteride. The antifungal agent fluconazole can inhibit many cytochrome P-450 enzymes and can lead to a condition closely resembling Antley-Bixler syndrome.

The synthetic estrogen diethylstilbestrol was used several decades ago to prevent spontaneous abortion (it was actually ineffective for this purpose). Males exposed to this agent in utero were born with testicular hypoplasia, cryptorchidism, hypospadias, and/or microphallus. Females had uterine, cervical, and vaginal abnormalities and an increased risk of clear cell adenocarcinoma of the vagina. Considering that many cases of genital ambiguity are idiopathic, it is likely that additional endocrine disruptors in the environment have not yet been identified.

HORMONE INSENSITIVITY SYNDROMES AND OTHER HORMONE DEFICIENCIES
Androgen Insensitivity

Males normally carry a single copy of the X-linked androgen receptor gene. Thus, a single mutation can completely inactivate the receptor in males and lead to complete androgen insensitivity (formerly termed *testicular feminization syndrome*). This is one of the most frequent forms of 46,XY DSD, occurring in approximately 1 in 20,000 male births.

Patients with the complete form of androgen insensitivity have normal female external genitalia. Unless suspicion is raised by prior knowledge of the infant's karyotype, the condition is rarely discovered before puberty unless the testes are palpated in the groin or labia on routine examination. Because the testes secrete AMH, müllerian structures are absent, including the uterus, fallopian tubes, and cervix. Thus, the vagina is usually shallow and ends blindly. Wolffian structures are also absent. The testes may be located in the abdomen or in the labia majora and do not undergo spermatogenesis. AMH levels are elevated during the first year and (if the testes have not been removed) after puberty. Testosterone and LH levels in infancy and at puberty are elevated as a result of defective feedback regulation caused by androgen resistance at the level of the hypothalamus.

At puberty, pubic and axillary hair is scant or absent. Testosterone can be aromatized to estradiol by CYP19 in breast fat, and estrogen receptors are unaffected in this condition. Thus, breast development is that of a normal female.

Partial androgen insensitivity (Reifenstein's syndrome) is characterized by a variable degree of genital ambiguity, and both virilization and breast development occur at puberty. Mild androgen insensitivity can also occur with a male phenotype, with gynecomastia and infertility as the sole manifestations. Mutations in the androgen receptor are not detected in many mild cases, which may result from defects in other factors affecting actions of the receptor.

Leydig Cell Agenesis

Leydig cell agenesis or hypoplasia is a rare autosomal recessive syndrome caused by mutations in the *LHGCR* gene encoding the LH receptor. Without stimulation by LH (or by HCG early in gestation), Leydig cells do not differentiate normally and do not secrete testosterone. Thus, affected male infants are born with female-appearing or ambiguous external genitalia. Müllerian structures are absent because of unaffected secretion of AMH by Sertoli cells. LH levels are high in infancy and at puberty, and they respond normally to gonadotropin-releasing hormone, whereas testosterone levels are low and do not respond to stimulation by HCG. Affected females are phenotypically normal but may have oligomenorrhea resulting from primary ovarian dysfunction.

Persistent Müllerian Duct Syndrome

Persistent müllerian duct syndrome (PMDS) is a rare autosomal recessive condition that results from mutations in the genes for either AMH (PMDS type I) or the AMH receptor (*AMHR2* gene, PMDS type II). The two are distinguished clinically by low or absent AMH levels in patients with AMH mutations and by AMH levels in the high-normal range in those with AMH receptor mutations.

Affected male patients have unimpaired testosterone secretion and thus have normal external genitalia and wolffian structures. However, the lack of AMH action prevents regression of müllerian structures, so these patients also retain a uterus and fallopian tubes. These structures are often closely approximated to the vas deferens. The müllerian structures are usually dragged into the inguinal canal by the descending testes. However, these structures typically prevent the testes from descending into the scrotum and thus cause bilateral inguinal hernias (with the uterus on one side) and bilateral or occasionally unilateral cryptorchidism. The condition is usually discovered only at surgery. Fertility in affected patients may be normal or impaired, with an increased risk of malignant disease in undescended testes left in the abdomen.

Hypogonadotropic Hypogonadism

Milder or later-appearing deficiencies of androgen biosynthesis (after 13 to 14 weeks) may allow complete fusion of the labioscrotal folds and normal positioning of the urethral meatus, but subsequent growth of the phallus is suboptimal. Such individuals have a micropenis. The most common cause is lack of gonadotropin (specifically, LH) secretion; even when LH is lacking, early male development is normal because testosterone secretion is controlled mostly by HCG during the first trimester.

Defective LH and follicle-stimulating hormone secretion can result when the neurons that normally secrete gonadotropin-releasing hormone fail to migrate into the hypothalamus. This condition, Kallmann's syndrome, is most often X-linked, resulting from mutations in the *KAL1* gene. It is often associated with anosmia. Other conditions that affect hypothalamic development

and cause hypogonadotropic hypogonadism include Prader-Willi syndrome, which is a result of paternal deletions, methylation defects, and maternal uniparental disomy of imprinted loci on chromosome 15q12. Children with this syndrome have a characteristic appearance consisting of a narrow bitemporal diameter, almond-shaped eyes with an antimongoloid slant, and small hands and feet. They typically have marked hypotonia as infants, with subsequent moderate developmental delay and slow somatic growth. Hypothalamic obesity develops during childhood. Patients with adrenal hypoplasia congenita resulting from mutations in the DAX1 transcription factor have defective development of the ventromedial hypothalamus and consequent hypogonadotropic hypogonadism, associated with adrenal insufficiency that typically presents with aldosterone deficiency and salt wasting.

Hypogonadotropic hypogonadism often results from failure of the entire anterior pituitary gland, or particular cellular populations therein, to develop. Pituitary gland abnormalities can be associated with other midline defects, including hypoplasia of the optic nerves and the septum pellucidum, a condition termed *septo-optic dysplasia*. Associated pituitary hormone deficiencies may include growth hormone, ACTH, and thyroid-stimulating hormone. These deficiencies may present in the neonatal period as hypoglycemia or hypothyroidism (detected by newborn screening programs). Optic nerve dysfunction is difficult to detect by routine examination in the neonatal period, but it causes a characteristic wandering nystagmus after a few months of age.

Although panhypopituitarism is most often sporadic, mutations in transcription factors controlling pituitary development have been documented (Chapter 231), particularly PROP1, and septo-optic dysplasia has been associated with mutations in the *HESX* gene. Rarely, mutations in the gene encoding the β-subunit of LH may yield a phenotype similar to hypogonadotropic hypogonadism.

● OTHER GENETIC CONDITIONS
Aneuploidy of Sex Chromosomes

TURNER'S SYNDROME. Patients with Turner's syndrome have normal female external genitalia and a normal uterus and fallopian tubes, but they have dysgenetic streak ovaries. Most fetuses with Turner's syndrome spontaneously abort, but the incidence in live births is approximately 1 in 2500. Classically, the karyotype is 45,X, but many patients retain an abnormal second X chromosome or even a fragment of a Y chromosome lacking *SRY*. Other patients are mosaic for 46,XX and 45,X cells and may have relatively mild phenotypes.

Untreated patients are short. Many have typical dysmorphic features, including lymphedema of the neck at birth, webbed neck, low posterior hairline, increased carrying angle of the arms, shield chest with widely spaced nipples, low-set ears, and micrognathia. Patients typically have primary amenorrhea and are infertile, but they occasionally have menarche followed by premature ovarian failure.

KLINEFELTER'S SYNDROME. In this condition, male patients have normal development of the penis and scrotum, but the testes are small and firm. Patients tend to be tall. At adolescence, gynecomastia is frequent. Signs of testosterone deficiency occur in most affected adults, and most have azoospermia. The usual karyotype is 47,XXY. Hormonal findings include elevated gonadotropin levels and a decreased serum testosterone concentration. Klinefelter's syndrome is a common disorder that occurs in 1 in 500 to 1000 men.

Mixed Gonadal Dysgenesis

Mixed gonadal dysgenesis, a frequent cause of sexual ambiguity, occurs in approximately 1 in 20,000 births. The karyotype is usually mosaic 45,X/46,XY. Gonadal pathologic features can vary from fibrous streaks indistinguishable from those in Turner's syndrome to normally developed testes and a normal male phenotype. Typically, patients have a testis on one side and a fibrous streak on the other. Some patients may have a Turner-like phenotype. A fallopian tube is usually present on the side of the streak gonad. Leydig cell function, evaluated by testosterone response to HCG, and Sertoli cell function, evaluated by serum AMH levels, vary from poor to normal.

XX Male Syndrome

Males with a 46,XX karyotype have normal external and internal male genitalia; however, they resemble patients with Klinefelter's syndrome in that they have small testes, azoospermia, and infertility. Translocation of the *SRY* gene to the X chromosome is detected in 75 to 90% of sporadic cases; this can occur because the gene is located very near the pseudoautosomal region, where the short arms of the X and Y chromosomes are homologous and meiotic recombination is possible. Duplication of the SOX9 transcription factor may be responsible for some familial cases of XX sex reversal.

XY Female Syndromes

Patients with pure XY gonadal dysgenesis (Swyer's syndrome) have a normal female phenotype, including a uterus and fallopian tubes, but they have streak gonads. These patients are free of Turner-like malformations and attain normal height. Mutations of the *SRY* gene have been identified in 15% of cases. Unlike 45,X patients with Turner's syndrome, these patients have an increased risk of gonadoblastoma.

Similar phenotypes result from duplication of the region of the X chromosome containing the *DAX1* gene, from duplication of the *WNT4* gene, or from haploinsufficiency of the SF1 transcription factor (associated in some cases with adrenal hypoplasia). XY sex reversal can also result from mutations in the SOX9 transcription factor that are associated with camptomelic dysplasia, a form of dwarfism. Mutations of *DHH* cause XY gonadal dysgenesis, associated with peripheral neuropathy.

Other 46,XY patients with absent gonads have various degrees of sexual ambiguity and no müllerian derivatives. The implication that some testicular tissue was functional at least up to 10 weeks' gestation and subsequently regressed led to the name *fetal testicular regression syndrome*. Testicular regression may occur in late pregnancy or even postnatally; these fully virilized male patients have isolated anorchia.

Vaginal Atresia

Mutation of *WNT4* affects the development of müllerian structures but permits normal ovarian development, thus causing vaginal atresia and uterine abnormalities. This disorder is termed *Mayer-Rokitansky-Küster-Hauser syndrome*.

True Hermaphroditism

True hermaphroditism, a rare and usually sporadic disorder, is defined as the coexistence of seminiferous tubules and ovarian follicles. Most patients have an ovotestis with either an ovary or a testis on the opposite side; a gonad in the scrotum is usually a testis but may be an ovotestis.

The genitalia are usually ambiguous, but they may appear completely masculine or feminine. The anatomy of the internal reproductive tract depends on the nature of the gonads, particularly whether they secrete AMH. A uterus or uterine horn is present in 90% of cases. Testosterone response to HCG is variable, and AMH levels are usually low. Most patients experience breast development, ovulation, and even menstruation at puberty; pregnancy and successful childbirth are possible if selective removal of testicular tissue is feasible. Unless sex of rearing has already been chosen, male gender assignment should be restricted to patients with no uterus and descended testicular tissue because the latter is usually dysgenetic and prone to malignant degeneration. Most true hermaphrodites have a 46,XX karyotype. Despite the presence of testicular tissue, true hermaphrodites usually lack *SRY*; this suggests that the condition is the result of constitutive activation of a gene normally triggered by *SRY*.

● MANAGEMENT OF INDIVIDUALS WITH DISORDERS OF SEXUAL DEVELOPMENT: GENDER ROLE AND IDENTITY

The influence of prenatal sex steroid exposure on personality is controversial. In considering this question, it is important to distinguish among gender role, sexual orientation, and gender identity.

Gender Role

Gender role refers to gender-stereotyped behaviors, such as the choice of toys by young children. For example, parents of young girls with CAH often report that their daughters prefer to play with trucks rather than dolls and tend to be tomboyish later in childhood. Decreased interest in maternal behavior, beginning with infrequent doll play in early childhood and extending to lack of interest in child rearing in older girls and women, occurs frequently.

Sexual Orientation

Sexual orientation refers to homosexual versus heterosexual preferences. In many studies, a significant minority of women with CAH are actively

homosexual or bisexual or have an increased tendency toward homoerotic fantasies. These characteristics occur more frequently in women with the salt-wasting form of 21-hydroxylase deficiency.

Gender Identity

Gender identity refers to self-identification as male or female. Gender self-reassignment back to male has been reported in cases of male patients with penile trauma or exstrophy of the bladder who were raised as girls. This may also occur in 46,XY DSD patients raised as girls, especially in cases of 5α-reductase or 17-ketosteroid reductase deficiencies, in which the brain may be exposed to high circulating levels of androgens. Conversely, female-to-male transsexuals may have relatively high levels of androgens and a high incidence of polycystic ovary syndrome. Self-reassignment to the male gender is unusual in women with CAH. When it occurs, it may be related to delays in gender assignment or genital surgery or to inadequate suppression of adrenal androgens with glucocorticoid therapy. Severely virilized girls are more likely to be raised as boys in cultures that value boys more highly or in developing countries owing to a delay in diagnosis. Few studies have directly compared psychosexual functioning in severely virilized genetic female patients with CAH who were raised as girls versus boys, but those raised as boys are not psychologically better adjusted than those raised as girls. The role of external genital anatomy before and after genital surgery in causing gender identity problems is unclear compared with the roles of prenatal hormone exposure, rearing by the family, and community attitudes.

⬤ DIAGNOSIS

Management of a child born with ambiguous genitalia presents a difficult challenge to medical personnel. It is important to refrain from assigning sex until diagnostic information can be gathered. Usually, test results can be obtained within 24 to 48 hours, and parents can be advised about the child's chromosomal and gonadal sex and the anatomy of internal sexual structures.

In addition, the physician must keep in mind that DSD may be associated with life-threatening biochemical or anatomic abnormalities. In particular, the most common cause of severely masculinized external genitalia in females, the salt-wasting form of CAH resulting from steroid 21-hydroxylase deficiency, may cause hyponatremia, hyperkalemia, hypovolemia, and shock. In contrast, male patients with ambiguous genitalia may have lipoid adrenal hyperplasia or a salt-wasting form of HSD3B2 deficiency. Males with micropenis may have panhypopituitarism, in which case they are at risk for significant hypoglycemia resulting from low cortisol (because of low ACTH) and low growth hormone levels, or they may have adrenal hypoplasia congenita, in which case they could have adrenal insufficiency. Finally, patients with ambiguous genitalia are at increased risk for renal anomalies, or they may have chromosomal syndromes with other associated anomalies.

History

The gestational history should concentrate on potential exposure to agents that could interfere with normal sexual differentiation. For a female infant with virilized genitalia, these include progestational agents, whereas the mother of a male with incompletely masculinized genitalia may have been exposed to a 5α-reductase inhibitor through her husband's use of such an agent for male pattern baldness or prostate enlargement. It should be determined whether amniocentesis and karyotyping have been performed. A family history should elicit similar cases of genital ambiguity or cases of sudden death, which could raise suspicion of undiagnosed salt-wasting CAH.

Physical Examination

The physical examination should document the size of the phallus (clitoris or penis), the degree of chordee (ventral bowing of the phallus), and the extent of fusion of the labioscrotal folds. The urethral meatus should be identified, and there must be careful palpation for gonads in the inguinal canals and labia or scrotum. Bilateral cryptorchidism, even if an isolated finding in a phenotypic male patient, should always lead to evaluation for a possible DSD.

Biochemical Evaluation of the Virilized Female

The minimal diagnostic tests should include measurement of basal serum 17-hydroxyprogesterone, androstenedione, and testosterone. Preferably, a complete profile of adrenocortical hormones is obtained before and 1 hour after stimulation of the adrenal cortex with 125 to 250 µg of cosyntropin (ACTH$_{1-24}$). These assays should be deferred until after the first 24 hours of life. They will identify potential defects in adrenal steroidogenesis (i.e., CAH); 21-hydroxylase deficiency is identified by elevations in 17-hydroxyprogesterone, whereas 11-deoxycortisol and 11-deoxycorticosterone are high in 11β-hydroxylase deficiency.

Biochemical Evaluation of the Undervirilized Male

In 46,XY DSD patients, it is necessary to test adrenal and gonadal function as well as extragonadal androgen metabolism. With regard to adrenal defects, 11-deoxycorticosterone and the ratio of pregnenolone to 17-hydroxypregnenolone are high in 17α-hydroxylase deficiency, 17-hydroxypregnenolone and DHEA are high in HSD3B2 deficiency, and all steroids are low in lipoid hyperplasia.

Defects in gonadal steroidogenesis are best evaluated after stimulation with HCG (1500 IU intramuscularly on days 1, 3, and 5, with blood drawn on day 6). However, 17-hydroxylase and HSD3B2 deficiencies affect both the gonads and the adrenal cortex and thus are often diagnosed by cosyntropin stimulation testing. Low levels of all androgen precursors suggest lipoid hyperplasia, 17α-hydroxylase/17,20 lyase deficiency, or a generalized defect in testicular function, such as the vanishing testis syndrome or gonadotropin insensitivity. A high ratio of androstenedione to testosterone is indicative of 17-ketosteroid reductase (HSD17B3) deficiency, and a high ratio of testosterone to dihydrotestosterone is diagnostic of 5α-reductase deficiency. The diagnosis of androgen insensitivity syndrome is suspected when a 46,XY patient has ambiguous or female-appearing external genitalia despite normal or high circulating levels of testosterone and dihydrotestosterone.

Gonadal Biopsies

Patients with mixed gonadal dysgenesis, true hermaphroditism, or unclear diagnoses should undergo bilateral gonadal biopsies (histology of the two gonads is often not identical). Dysgenetic gonads have a high potential for malignant transformation and usually need to be removed in childhood.

TREATMENT

Initial Medical Management

Patients with CAH resulting from 21-hydroxylase or HSD3B2 deficiencies or those with lipoid hyperplasia require replacement of both glucocorticoids and mineralocorticoids, usually with hydrocortisone (15 to 20 mg/m²/day in divided doses) and fludrocortisone (usually 0.1 mg/day, but as much as 0.4 mg/day in neonates with salt-wasting crises), respectively. Neonates with severe salt losses may require sodium chloride supplementation (≤8 mEq/kg/day). Patients with 11ß-hydroxylase or 17α-hydroxylase deficiencies have normal aldosterone biosynthesis and usually require only glucocorticoids. Patients with panhypopituitarism usually require treatment with hydrocortisone, thyroxine, and growth hormone.

All male infants with ambiguous genitalia or micropenis in whom rearing as a boy is contemplated should have a 3-month therapeutic trial of monthly depot testosterone injections (25 mg) to attempt to increase the size of the phallus during infancy. This treatment may improve social acceptability of the genitalia later in childhood and adolescence and may make reconstructive surgery easier. In cases of suspected partial androgen insensitivity, this treatment also documents the degree to which the patient is androgen responsive and thus may provide useful information about whether rearing as a boy is feasible. Higher doses of testosterone (75 mg every 4 weeks) may be used under these circumstances.

Considerations Related to Sex Assignment

In large medical centers, a team consisting of a neonatologist, a pediatric endocrinologist, a urologist, and preferably an experienced social worker and/or child psychiatrist should promptly review the early diagnostic data and make a recommendation to the family as to the sex of rearing and any medical or surgical treatments. These recommendations should be based on both current knowledge of psychosexual development in DSD individuals and the feasibility of surgical correction (see later).

In general, the recommended sex assignment should be that of the genetic/gonadal sex, if for no other reason than to retain the possibility of reproductive function. This is especially true for female infants with CAH who have normal internal genital structures and the potential for childbearing. An exception may be considered in a genetically female infant with completely male-appearing genitalia, especially if the child has been raised as a boy for more than a few months. Such children need to be castrated at puberty to avoid feminization.

Conversely, genetic male infants with completely female-appearing external genitalia (usually resulting from complete androgen insensitivity syndrome, but also seen with severe testosterone biosynthetic defects) should be raised as female because the potential for reconstruction of male genitalia is poor. They, too, need to be castrated by early adulthood to avoid malignant

transformation of the testes. However, male infants with 17-ketosteroid reductase or 5α-reductase deficiency should usually be reared as boys because they have normal levels of androstenedione or testosterone, respectively, and often virilize significantly at puberty. Indeed, many of these patients reassign themselves to the male gender when they are made aware of the diagnosis. The same considerations pertain to male patients with normal testosterone biosynthesis who have penile trauma or anatomic abnormalities such as bladder exstrophy.

Recommendations for sex assignment are to some extent culture specific. In cultures that value boys over girls, parents may strongly resist rearing a female infant with ambiguous genitalia as a girl, and many girls with severely virilized external genitalia will be raised as boys.

Corrective Surgery

Surgery for Ambiguous Genitalia

Whether, how, and when to intervene surgically in the correction of genital anomalies are the subject of continuing debate. Some adult patients with DSD conditions are unhappy with their gender assignments or surgical outcomes. Some physicians advocate postponing cosmetic genital surgery until the affected individual is able to provide informed consent, thus keeping all the options open if the adult patient wishes to function sexually with abnormal genitalia that nevertheless have sensation undiminished by surgery or chooses to reassign his or her gender. Declining or postponing surgery should not be confused with raising the child with an indeterminate gender, a concept currently well outside the mainstream. The option of deferring surgery should always be presented as part of the informed consent process. Nevertheless, most parents want their child to look as "normal" as possible, and they often resist suggestions to postpone corrective surgery.

In addressing this question, it is best to consider the various general types of genital surgery separately. The greatest change in practice over the past few decades probably pertains to male infants with ambiguous (but not completely female) external genitalia. Physicians are far less likely to recommend that such patients be reared as female because it is now recognized that many of these patients reassign themselves as male at puberty. Thus, the ambiguous genitalia in such patients should rarely be "corrected" to female. On the contrary, surgical techniques for hypospadias repair have advanced significantly, and reconstruction of male genitalia is attempted more often, particularly if the infant responds to a course of testosterone with significant phallic growth.

Surgery for female infants with ambiguous genitalia may need to address an enlarged clitoris, the lack of a vaginal introitus, and the presence of a urogenital sinus. The clitoris is normally prominent in many infant girls. Even when enlarged in a girl with virilizing CAH, the clitoris can be prevented from growing larger with adequate suppression of adrenal androgens by glucocorticoids, and it will become less prominent as the patient grows. Thus, mild to moderate clitorimegaly is often best managed without surgery. When clitoroplasty is attempted, one must keep in mind the important role of clitoral sensation in the female sexual response. Such surgery must be performed only by experienced operators with scrupulous attention to the preservation of clitoral innervation.

Consensus is still lacking regarding the best age for vaginoplasty. Although many surgeons advocate a first procedure in infancy, it is difficult to maintain a functionally adequate introitus in the absence of estrogen exposure and mechanical dilation (with dilators or through sexual intercourse), and many patients require reoperation as young adults.

There is a dearth of large longitudinal studies comparing outcomes in patients who have had early genital surgery versus those who have had no surgery or surgery in adolescence. According to self-assessment surveys among sexually active women with CAH who have had genital surgery, most are able to have satisfactory sexual intercourse. As surgical and medical treatment regimens have improved in recent years, more women with CAH have successfully conceived spontaneously, completed pregnancies, and given birth. Most often, delivery is by cesarean section because of an inadequate introitus, but vaginal delivery is possible in some cases.

Hypospadias repair is usually begun in the first year of life, after testosterone treatment (if necessary to increase phallic size). Depending on the degree of hypospadias, more than one surgical procedure may be required.

Removal of Intra-abdominal Testes in 46,XY DSD Patients

Intra-abdominal testes are at increasing risk for malignant transformation over time. In a boy with cryptorchidism who is being reared as male, orchiopexy should be performed as quickly as possible; this also maximizes the possibility of fertility when the underlying condition does not preclude it. Dysgenetic gonads that cannot be brought into the scrotum should be removed soon after diagnosis because the risk of malignant transformation in childhood is relatively high.

There is a lack of consensus regarding nondysgenetic testes in severely undervirilized genetic male infants in whom rearing as female is planned. In patients with complete androgen insensitivity or complete defects in testosterone biosynthesis, no possibility of fertility exists, and so there seems to be no reason to retain the testes. Conversely, the risk of malignant transformation in such gonads is low before puberty, and patients with complete androgen insensitivity can undergo spontaneous breast development at puberty. At that time, patients themselves can assent or consent to gonadectomy, which can usually be accomplished laparoscopically. This is of particular importance in genetic male patients with partial androgen insensitivity or incomplete defects of testosterone biosynthesis, because such patients may eventually desire a male gender role.

Patients with persistent müllerian duct syndrome have a reduced but still appreciable potential for fertility, and virilization is unaffected. Thus, the testes should be removed only if they cannot be brought into the scrotum. Because the müllerian and wolffian structures are closely approximated in these patients, surgical excision of the uterus and fallopian tubes may result in ischemic and/or traumatic damage to the vas deferens and testes; thus, salpingectomy and hysterectomy are indicated only in patients whose müllerian structures limit intrascrotal placement of the testes.

Prenatal Diagnosis and Treatment

Many conditions causing ambiguous genitalia can be detected by karyotyping of chorionic villus samples (for chromosomal abnormalities) or by direct molecular genetic testing. In most cases, this information is useful only for counseling purposes. In the case of virilizing forms of CAH (particularly 21-hydroxylase deficiency), the mother of an affected female fetus can take dexamethasone (20 µg/kg/day), which can cross the placenta and suppress the fetal adrenal gland, thus reducing the secretion of androgens and ameliorating virilization of the external genitalia. To be most effective, this treatment should be started by the sixth week of gestation, before the sex or genotype of the fetus is known. Thus, seven unaffected or male fetuses must be treated with dexamethasone to avoid genital ambiguity in one affected female, until chorionic villus sampling can be performed. Although effective in reducing prenatal virilization, this dose of dexamethasone can cause Cushing's syndrome in the mother, and the long-term sequelae in the fetus are not known. Therefore, many endocrinologists believe that this treatment should be used only under approved research protocols that allow for case registries and long-term follow-up.

Psychosocial Support

Families of DSD patients should be assessed for emotional health, initially by the pediatrician and/or pediatric endocrinologist. Parents should be offered psychological counseling soon after the diagnosis is made. Intermittent assessment of family functioning may be a useful tool in predicting future problems. As children mature, they should repeatedly be informed about their condition by parents and physicians in a sensitive and age-appropriate manner. When psychotherapy is undertaken, medical and psychiatric caregivers should communicate with each other so both are aware of the patient's and family's status. Unfortunately, many locales lack mental health professionals with experience in counseling patients with DSD and their families.

Although the psychosexual development of individuals with DSD cannot be predicted with confidence, patients' families should receive anticipatory counseling. For example, counseling of parents of girls affected with CAH should address the high likelihood that such girls will exhibit tomboyish behavior, masculine play preferences, and perhaps, when older, a preference for a career over domestic activities. In the contemporary United States, these preferences usually have a high degree of social acceptance. Parents should also be told that most (but not all) girls with CAH function heterosexually, although they may require repeated genital surgical procedures to have satisfactory sexual intercourse. The endocrinologist and/or mental health professional (depending on inclination and experience) caring for the adolescent girl with CAH should address sexual orientation, both fantasized and actual. Health care professionals should accept that some women with CAH may be most comfortable as homosexuals and that such individuals should be helped to come to terms with their situation. Adult patients should also be made aware of relevant patient advocacy groups.

SUGGESTED READINGS

Auchus RJ. Congenital adrenal hyperplasia in adults. *Curr Opin Endocrinol Diabetes Obes.* 2010;17:210-216. *Review of approaches to infertility, neoplasia, and consequences of chronic glucocorticoid therapy.*

Caronia LM, Martin C, Welt CK, et al. A genetic basis for functional hypothalamic amenorrhea. *N Engl J Med.* 2011;364:215-225. *Rare genetic variants associated with idiopathic hypogonadotrophic hypogonadism are found in women with hypothalamic amenorrhea.*

Dauber A, Kellogg M, Majzoub JA. Monitoring of therapy in congenital adrenal hyperplasia. *Clin Chem.* 2010;56:1245-1251. *Practical review.*

Davenport ML. Approach to the patient with Turner syndrome. *J Clin Endocrinol Metab.* 2010;95:1487-1495. *Review of growth failure, cardiovascular disease, gonadal failure, and learning disabilities, with an emphasis on the importance of growth hormone, estrogen therapy, and screening for cardiovascular abnormalities.*

Lambert SM, Vilain EJ, Kolon TF. A practical approach to ambiguous genitalia in the newborn period. *Urol Clin North Am.* 2010;37:195-205. *Recommendations regarding use of karyotyping and sex hormone testing.*

Radicioni AF, Ferlin A, Balercia G, et al. Consensus statement on diagnosis and clinical management of Klinefelter syndrome. *J Endocrinol Invest.* 2010;33:839-850. *Emphasizes the benefits of making the diagnosis and initiating therapy among men who typically have hypogonadism and/or infertility.*

Speiser PW, Azziz R, Baskin LS, et al. Congenital adrenal hyperplasia due to steroid 21-hydroxylase deficiency: an Endocrine Society clinical practice guideline. *J Clin Endocrinol Metab.* 2010;95:4133-4160. *Consensus guidelines.*

242

THE TESTIS AND MALE SEXUAL FUNCTION

RONALD S. SWERDLOFF AND CHRISTINA WANG

PHYSIOLOGY

The testis is a bifunctional organ serving as the site of sex steroid (i.e., testosterone) synthesis and sperm production in the male. Androgens and their metabolites (including estrogens) also act on nonreproductive organs and serve essential roles in muscles, adipose tissues, bones, metabolism, and brain functions.

The male reproductive axis consists of six main components: (1) extrahypothalamic central nervous system (CNS), (2) hypothalamus, (3) pituitary, (4) testes, (5) sex steroid–sensitive end organs, and (6) sites of androgen transport and metabolism (Fig. 242-1). The components of this system function in an integrative fashion to control the concentrations of circulating gonadal steroids required for normal male sexual development and function and for androgen- and estrogen-mediated metabolic effects on critical end organs. The reproductive axis is also responsible for normal germ cell development and maturation and sperm transport function necessary to ensure male fertility.

Hypothalamic-Pituitary Function

The hypothalamus is responsible for the normal pulsatile secretion of gonadotropin-releasing hormone (GnRH) (Chapter 231). The pulsatile release of GnRH provides the signals for the timing of the release of luteinizing hormone (LH) and follicle-stimulating hormone (FSH), which occurs every 60 to 90 minutes in men. The secretion of GnRH is regulated by neuronal input from higher cognitive and sensory centers and by circulating levels of sex steroids and peptide hormones such as prolactin and leptin (Chapter 230). Testosterone or its metabolic products (i.e., estradiol and dihydrotestosterone) inhibit the secretion and release of GnRH, LH, and FSH. Prolactin is also a potent inhibitor of GnRH secretion.

Both LH and FSH consist of two subunits (α and β). Both subunits are required for biologic activity; the subunits can be detected in serum and may

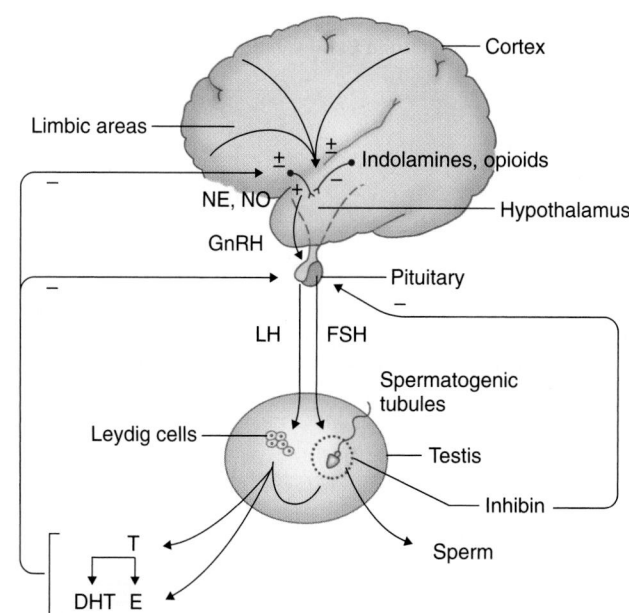

FIGURE 242-1. The hypothalamic-pituitary-gonadal axis in the male. DHT = dihydrotestosterone; E = estrogen; FSH = follicle-stimulating hormone; GnRH = gonadotropin-releasing hormone; LH = luteinizing hormone; NE = norepinephrine; NO = nitric oxide; T = testosterone.

be increased in certain pathologic conditions (e.g., α-subunit elevations in gonadotropin-secreting pituitary adenomas). LH has a shorter half-life than FSH. Feedback regulation of LH and FSH secretion also occurs at the pituitary, with testosterone, dihydrotestosterone (DHT), and estrogens inhibiting the synthesis or release of both gonadotropins. The circulating testicular peptide inhibin, produced by Sertoli cells, also selectively inhibits FSH. LH and FSH act predominantly through specific cell surface receptors on the Leydig and Sertoli cells of the testes, respectively.

Testosterone

The testis is a complex organ consisting of (1) seminiferous tubules containing Sertoli cells and germ cells and (2) the interstitium, which contains the steroid-secreting (Leydig) cells. Leydig cells synthesize steroid hormones under the regulation of LH. The LH receptors on the cell surface of the Leydig cells lead to G protein–, adenyl cyclase–, and cyclic adenosine monophosphate–mediated activation of steroid biosynthesis.

Testosterone is the principal male hormone secreted by the testes; about 5 to 10 mg/day is produced in adult men. Testosterone synthesis occurs in the human testes through either the Δ^4 or the predominant Δ^5 pathway. The enzymatic rate-limiting steps in the process are the LH-inducible steroid acute regulatory (StAR) protein and the conversion of cholesterol to pregnenolone by the cholesterol side-chain cleavage enzyme P450SCC (Fig. 242-2).

Testosterone circulates mainly bound to two plasma proteins: sex hormone–binding globulin (SHBG) and albumin. In young adult men, about 54% of testosterone is bound to albumin, 44% is bound to SHBG, and 2 to 3% is unbound. Bioavailable testosterone refers to the sum of albumin-bound and free testosterone and is measured by separating SHBG-bound testosterone from total testosterone. Serum SHBG levels are increased in hyperestrogenemic states, hyperthyroidism, aging, phenytoin treatment, anorexia nervosa, and prolonged stress. SHBG levels are lowered with androgen treatment, obesity, acromegaly, and hypothyroidism. In most instances, measurement of serum total testosterone provides biochemical support for the diagnosis of androgen deficiency. In conditions with abnormal SHBG levels, however, the total testosterone measurement may be misleading, and direct measurement of free testosterone, measurement of bioavailable testosterone, or calculation of the free testosterone by a formula requiring the serum testosterone and SHBG concentrations may be necessary to separate true testosterone deficiency from binding protein problems.

Testosterone exerts its effects either through direct action or after conversion to DHT by two separate 5α-reductase isozymes (1 and 2) or to estradiol by the aromatase enzyme (Fig. 242-3). Thus, testosterone can act directly on the androgen receptor or as a precursor for DHT which also binds to the androgen receptor. Different tissues have coactivators or coinhibitors that modify the action of the androgen-receptor complex, providing tissue selectivity and amplification. Testosterone can also serve as a precursor for estradiol in some tissues, and after conversion, estrogen binds the estrogen receptors (α or β) to induce its effects. Various end organs differ in their 5α-reductase isoenzyme concentrations and aromatase activity. Congenital and acquired defects in these two enzymes, as well as in the estrogen and androgen receptors, result in distinct syndromes with characteristic phenotypes (Chapter 241).

Spermatogenesis

The spermatogenic compartment of the testis consists of the Sertoli and germ cells that are intimately interactive with the interstitial compartment. The Sertoli cells bridge the entire space between the basement membrane and the lumen of the tubules. They are the target of androgenic and FSH stimulation of spermatogenesis and also the source of a multitude of paracrine regulators of spermatogenesis (e.g., inhibin, activin, growth factors, cytokines).

Germ cell development and maturation are dependent on the proper hormonal (FSH) and paracrine (testosterone) milieu. Not all germ cells reach maturity. Considerable data indicate that a major effect of both testosterone and FSH is to limit the amount of germ cell death (apoptosis).

After spermatogenesis is completed, mature spermatozoa are released into the excretory system and travel through the rete testes and epididymis, where they become functionally mature and acquire fertilizing capacity before traversing the vas deferens. The seminal fluid gains constituents from the seminal vesicles, prostate, and bulbourethral glands before ejaculation.

Normal Sexual Function and Erectile Physiology

Normal sexual function in men requires normal sexual desire (libido) and erectile, ejaculatory, and orgasmic capacity. The process is complex, involving cognitive, sensory, hormonal, autonomic neuronal, and penile vascular integrative actions for normal function. Defects can occur at multiple levels.

The brain is the integrative center of the sexual response system. It processes sensory input and hormonal signals to create the hypothalamic neuronal message that traverses the spinal cord to the T9–12 sympathetic and sacral parasympathetic outflow tracts. The nonadrenergic, noncholinergic autonomic plexus nerves initiate vasodilation of the cavernosal arterial and corpora cavernosal sinusoids of the penis through the release of local vasodilators such as nitric oxide and vasoactive intestinal peptide from the vascular endothelium and the smooth muscle cells of the sinusoids (Fig. 242-4). Nitric oxide produces smooth muscle dilation through the generation of cyclic guanosine monophosphate (cGMP) and the modification of calcium flux. The neurogenic mechanisms leading to vasodilation of the cavernosal arterioles and sinusoids lead to a rapid increase in penile blood flow and expansion of the vascular channels; this, in turn, inhibits venous return through compression of the venous channels against the tunica albuginea and limits venous drainage.

Testosterone Synthesis in the Testis

FIGURE 242-2. The steroid acute regulatory (StAR) protein mobilizes cholesterol from cellular stores to the mitochondria. Intratesticular steroidogenic pathways for the synthesis of testosterone. Although both the Δ^5 (left) and Δ^4 (right) pathways exist, the Δ^5 pathway predominates in the testis. DHEA = dehydroepiandrosterone; HSD = hydroxysteroid dehydrogenase.

FIGURE 242-3. Testosterone action is mediated directly (androgen receptor), after conversion to estradiol (estrogen receptor α or β), or after conversion to dihydrotestosterone (DHT; androgen receptor). (From Kuiper GCJM, Carlquist M, Gustafsson JA. Estrogen is a male and female hormone. Sci Med. 1998;5:36-45.)

FIGURE 242-4. The interaction among cholinergic, adrenergic, and nonadrenergic, noncholinergic (NANC) neuronal pathways and their contribution to penile smooth muscle contraction and dilation (arrows). NO = nitric oxide; VIP = vasoactive intestinal polypeptide. (From Lue TF. Physiology of penile erection and pathophysiology of erectile dysfunction and priapism. In: Walsh P, Retick A, Vaughn E, Wein A, eds. *Campbell's Urology,* 7th ed. Philadelphia: WB Saunders; 1998:1164.)

FIGURE 242-5. Diagram of the timing of the various components of puberty. The range of ages at which each parameter begins and is completed is shown for each bar. These data were obtained from European children 40 years ago. Since then, there may be a slight trend for an earlier onset of puberty. (From Marshall WA, Tanner JM. Variations in the pattern of pubertal changes in boys. *Arch Dis Child.* 1970;45:13-23.)

TABLE 242-1 PUBERTAL STAGES IN BOYS

STAGE	PUBIC HAIR	GENITAL
1	Absence of pubic hair	Child-like penis, testes, and scrotum (testes 2 mL)
2	Sparse, lightly pigmented hair mainly at base of penis	Scrotum enlarged with early rugation and pigmentation; testes begin to enlarge (3-5 mL)
3	Hair becomes coarse, darker, more curled, and more extensive	Penis has grown in length and diameter; testes now 8-10 mL; scrotum more rugated
4	Hair adult in quality, but distribution does not include medial aspect of thighs	Penis further enlarged, with development of glans; scrotum and testes (10-13 mL) further enlarged
5	Hair is adult and extends to thighs	Penis and scrotum fully adult; testes ≥15 mL

Modified from Marshall WA, Tanner JM. Variation in pattern of pubertal changes in boys. *Arch Dis Child.* 1970;45:13-23.

Testosterone's primary effect on erectile function is to enhance libido, with secondary effects on nitric oxide synthase activity. Sexual desire and fantasy are highly sensitive to testosterone, explaining the preservation of erectile capacity in many men with partial androgen deficiency. Erectile dysfunction (see later) is common in older men despite normal serum testosterone levels; this effect appears to be the result of impaired penile vasodilatory capacity probably due to atherosclerosis. Men presenting with erectile dysfunction may also have increased risk for the metabolic syndrome and cardiovascular disease. Erectile dysfunction can be treated by the oral administration of penile-selective phosphodiesterase-5 inhibitors (sildenafil, vardenafil, tadalafil) or through local (intracavernosal or transurethral) administration of potent vasodilators (prostaglandins, papaverine, phentolamine). Combined androgen deficiency with decreased libido and decreased penile responsiveness due to impaired nitric oxide synthase activity may be common in elderly men. With the availability of effective penile vasodilatory medications to ensure erectile capacity, complaints of diminished libido can be effectively treated with androgen supplementation.

Physiology in Development and Aging
Reproductive Axis Development during Childhood and Puberty
Adrenarche and Puberty

Adrenarche occurs at about 7 or 8 years of age when the zona reticularis of the adrenal gland undergoes maturation, leading to increased secretion of androstenedione, dehydroepiandrosterone (DHEA), and DHEA sulfate (DHEA-S). The process is under the control of adrenocorticotropic hormone, not LH or FSH. Androstenedione and DHEA are technically androgenic prehormones, and the prepubertal growth spurt as well as the early development of pubic and axillary hair are mediated by the conversion of these precursors to testosterone and DHT in peripheral tissues.

Initiation of puberty is determined by an increase in the pulsatile pattern of hypothalamic GnRH secretion. This is marked by nocturnal bursts of LH secretion. As puberty progresses, feedback sensitivity of the hypothalamus and pituitary to circulating steroids lessens, thus increasing the secretion of gonadotropins. The increasing concentrations of intratesticular testosterone and circulating FSH stimulate the Sertoli cell to produce factors leading to the maturation of spermatogenesis. The majority of the extratesticular end-organ events of puberty are secondary to the increased testosterone and its metabolic products (DHT and estradiol) (Table 242-1). The penis and scrotum grow and become pigmented. As spermatogenesis advances, the testes increase in size from 1 to 2 mL at the outset of puberty to 15 to 35 mL in adulthood. There is a progressive increase in facial, axillary, chest, abdominal, thigh, and pubic hair; frontal scalp hair regresses, and the voice deepens (Fig. 242-5). Genital and sexual hair development and temporal scalp hair regression require DHT. The increased levels of sex steroids result in closure of the epiphysis and achievement of adult height.

Aberrations of Timing of Puberty

Delayed puberty, more common in boys than in girls, is usually defined as a temporary form of hypothalamic hypogonadotropic hypogonadism in which sexual development has not begun by age 13.5 years. Height age (the age representative of 50% of normal children at the patient's height) is delayed with respect to chronologic age, but it is concordant with bone age. Once initiated, puberty is completed within 4.5 years. The majority of boys with delayed development eventually attain full sexual adulthood. There is often a family history of a parent or sibling being a "late bloomer." The *GPR54* gene encodes a kisspeptin-responsive G protein–coupled receptor whose absence results in hypogonadotropic hypogonadism due to impaired secretion of GnRH. Careful documentation of changing physical findings and measurement of serum LH, FSH, and testosterone concentrations may provide valuable clues to the beginning of puberty. An increase in testicular size to more than 3 mL usually heralds other signs of pubertal onset. Inquiring and testing for hyposmia or anosmia and other midline defects may indicate a common variant of congenital hypogonadotropic hypogonadism (Kallmann's syndrome). The decision to institute early treatment depends on the perceived degree of psychological stress associated with the maturational delay. The major concern is early fusion of the epiphyses induced by treatment with testosterone, which compromises optimal height; however, with proper dosing and monitoring of bone age, this is unusual. In adolescent boys with delayed puberty and low levels of gonadotropins, periodic withdrawal of treatment is used to determine whether spontaneous puberty has occurred. Many adult men diagnosed with and treated for hypogonadotropic hypogonadism achieve normal reproductive function when they discontinue therapy.

Precocious puberty in boys is defined as the onset of pubertal (genital and secondary sexual) development before 9 years of age. Sexual precocity can be subcategorized as true (complete and incomplete) isosexual precocious puberty and pseudo–precocious puberty. The distinction is that true precocious puberty is associated with increases in GnRH-stimulated LH and FSH secretion (hypothalamic-pituitary origin), whereas pseudo–precocious puberty is independent of GnRH stimulation of LH and FSH secretion. True precocious puberty in boys is often associated with CNS disease (two thirds of boys), including hypothalamic tumors, cysts, inflammatory conditions, and seizure disorders. Diagnostic findings include sexual precocity, inappropriately elevated serum LH levels, and associated elevations of testosterone. Magnetic resonance imaging (MRI) can localize most lesions. Another cause of central precocious puberty is human chorionic gonadotropin secretory germinomas (testicular, hepatic, hypothalamic, or pineal tumors). Pseudo–precocious puberty is characterized by increased testosterone with suppressed LH. Causes of pseudo–precocious puberty include congenital virilizing adrenal hyperplasia, testicular testosterone-secreting neoplasms, and constitutively active LH receptor mutations, resulting in uncontrolled testosterone secretion (testotoxicosis). Treatment of true precocious puberty is removal or correction (with surgery or radiation therapy) of the CNS lesion, if possible, and treatment with GnRH analogues to completely suppress LH and FSH secretion. Treatment of pseudo–precocious puberty depends on the cause but includes glucocorticoids for congenital virilizing adrenal hyperplasia and ketoconazole (to suppress steroidogenesis), with or without antiandrogens (e.g., spironolactone, flutamide).

Male Senescence: Decreased Testosterone and Other Anabolic Hormones
Testosterone Deficiency in the Elderly
Blood concentrations of testosterone, other anabolic hormones (e.g., growth hormone), and prehormones (e.g., DHEA, DHEA-S) are significantly lower in older men than in young adult men. There is a gradual decline in the serum testosterone concentration beginning in young adulthood. Both total and bioavailable or free serum testosterone levels progressively decrease with aging (Fig. 242-6). The percentage decline in serum testosterone has been estimated at between 0.8 and 1.6% per year. Many men with low serum testosterone do not have the typical symptoms of hypogonadism seen in younger androgen-deficient men. Serum SHBG levels also rise with age in men, resulting in a higher percentage of circulating testosterone that is tightly bound and less bioavailable. Between 40 and 80% of men older than 70 years have blood levels of bioavailable or free testosterone below the normal range for young adults (Fig. 242-7). Many older men with serum testosterone below the young adult reference range do not complain of symptoms attributable to low testosterone.

The effects of low testosterone levels in aging men are similar to those observed in younger hypogonadal men. These include decreases in muscle mass, muscle strength, bone mass, libido, and erectile function and impaired mood and sense of well-being. Older men have increased body fat, particularly visceral fat. The benefits of testosterone treatment for symptomatic older men with low serum testosterone levels remain controversial because large-scale randomized, controlled international trials have not been performed. Beneficial effects of testosterone replacement have been demonstrated in elderly men with relatively low serum testosterone levels. Testosterone replacement therapy (up to 3 years) decreases fat mass, increases lean body mass, improves strength, and increases bone mineral density.[1-4] In larger, more recent studies of elderly men with borderline low serum testosterone levels, treatment with testosterone did not change functional status in symptomatic individuals in one study,[3] but it improved muscle strength and physical function in another study in frail elderly men.[4] Because erectile dysfunction in the older man is multifactorial (see later), with impaired vasodilatory function in the penis predominating in many cases, testosterone replacement therapy in older men may enhance libido but often does not improve erectile dysfunction. At present, testosterone treatment is not recommended for men known to have or suspected of having prostate cancer, severe and uncorrected sleep apnea, and high red blood cell mass.

A digital rectal examination should be performed, prostate-specific antigen level determined, and symptoms of severe urinary tract obstruction evaluated to ensure that there are no findings suggestive of severe benign prostatic hypertrophy or prostate cancer (nodules, irregularities).

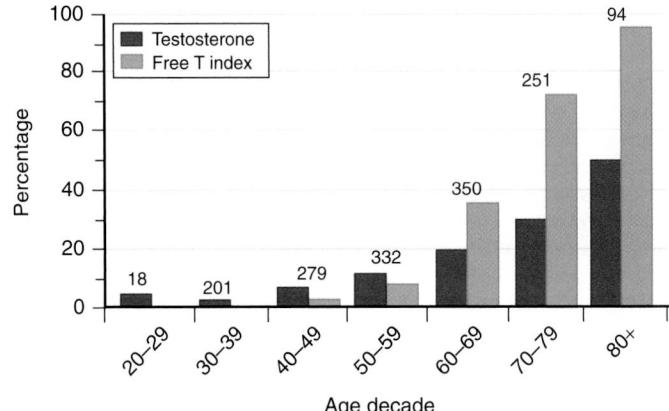

FIGURE 242-7. Hypogonadism in aging men. Bar height indicates the percentage of men in each 10-year interval, from the third to the ninth decades, with at least one testosterone value in the hypogonadal range. The criteria used for these determinations are total testosterone less than 11.3 nmol/L (325 ng/dL) and testosterone and sex hormone–binding globulin (free T index) less than 0.153 nmol/nmol. The numbers above each pair of bars indicate the number of men studied in the corresponding decade. The fraction of men who are hypogonadal increases progressively after age 50 years by either criterion. More men are hypogonadal by free T index than by total testosterone after 50 years, and there seems to be a progressively greater difference, with increasing age, between the two criteria.

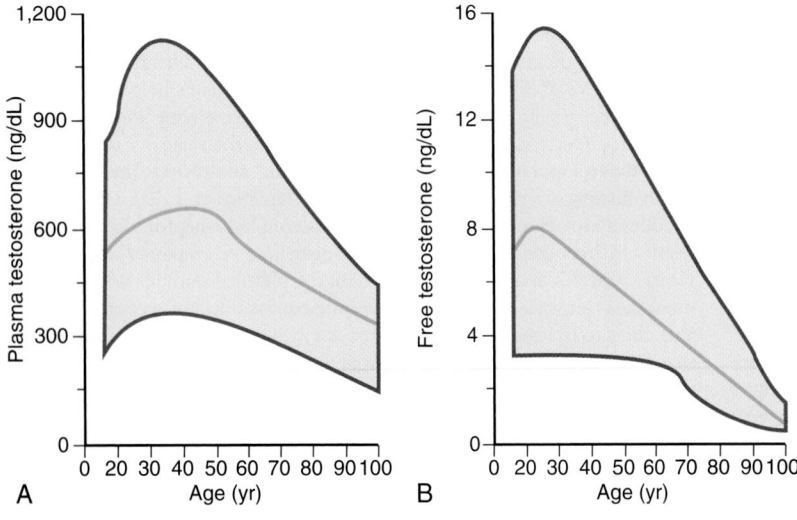

FIGURE 242-6. Relationship between plasma testosterone (A) and free testosterone (B) levels and age in normal males. (From Baker HWG, Berger HG, DeKretser DM, et al. Changes in the pituitary-testicular system with age. *Clin Endocrinol.* 1996; 5:349-372.)

Deficiency of Adrenal Androgen in Older Men

In recent years, a marked decline in the circulating levels of adrenal androgens, especially DHEA and DHEA-S, has been recognized in elderly men and women (Chapter 242). Serum levels of DHEA and DHEA-S peak at about the third decade of life and then decline at about 2% per year, resulting in levels 10 to 20% of baseline by 80 years of age. DHEA is a precursor to androgens such as testosterone and DHT. Studies have shown that the oral administration of 50 mg of DHEA to older men raises serum DHEA and DHEA-S concentrations to the levels found in young men without changing serum levels of testosterone, with no beneficial effects on quality of life, sexual function, mood, body composition, or exercise capacity.[5,6] In the United States, DHEA is available without prescription as a health supplement and is widely used, making large-scale multicenter, prospective, placebo-controlled trials difficult to perform.

● MALE HYPOGONADISM

DEFINITION

Hypogonadism refers to low circulating levels of testosterone. Most androgen-deficient men are infertile. Primary hypogonadism indicates that the abnormality originates in the testis; secondary hypogonadism indicates a defect at the hypothalamus or pituitary, resulting in decreased gonadotropins (LH, FSH, or both). Combined primary and secondary hypogonadism occurs in aging and in a number of systemic diseases, such as alcoholism, liver disease, diabetes mellitus, human immunodeficiency virus (HIV) infection, hemochromatosis, and sickle cell disease. Obesity leads to low total and free testosterone levels. Greater decreases are seen in the total testosterone level because obesity not only decreases testosterone secretion but also lowers SHBG levels. Decreased androgen action with normal or elevated testosterone levels, mimicking androgen deficiency, may occur in patients with androgen receptor defects (androgen resistance), postreceptor signaling abnormalities, and inability to convert testosterone to the active metabolite DHT (5α-reductase abnormalities).

Many of the causes of primary and secondary hypogonadism are listed in Tables 242-2 and 242-3 (see also Chapter 241).

CLINICAL MANIFESTATIONS

History

The medical history should focus on testicular descent, pubertal development, shaving frequency, changes in body hair, and present and past systemic illnesses. A complete sexual history includes changes in libido, erectile and ejaculatory functions, frequency of masturbation, coital activity, and fertility (including that of present and previous partners). Information should be obtained on previous orchitis, sinopulmonary complaints, sexually transmitted diseases, HIV status, genitourinary infections, and previous surgical procedures that might affect the reproductive tract (e.g., vasectomy, hernia repair, prostatectomy, varicocele ligation). Social history includes tobacco and alcohol intake. Medication and drug history includes recreational drugs; opioids; anabolic steroids; psychiatric, antihypertensive, antiandrogenic, cytotoxic, and alternative medicine therapies; environmental toxins; and exposure to heat (including saunas and Jacuzzis) and irradiation.

Physical Examination

The general physical examination is supplemented by height and span measurements; assessment of muscle mass and adiposity; characterization of facial, pubic, and body hair distribution; presence of acne and facial wrinkling; breast examination for gynecomastia; measurement of penile length and urethral integrity; digital rectal prostate examination; and visual field assessment. The scrotal examination should include an assessment of midline fusion (e.g., bifid scrotum, hypospadias); testicular size and consistency; presence of intratesticular masses; abnormalities of the epididymis; bilateral presence of vas deferens; and presence of varicoceles, hydroceles, or hernias. Normal testicular size ranges from 3.6 to 5.5 cm in length, 2.1 to 3.2 cm in width, and 15 to 35 mL in volume in white and black men. Asian men have a slightly smaller mean testicular size. A decrease in testicular volume usually implies decreased spermatogenic cells because the seminiferous tubules account for more than 80% of testicular volume.

Laboratory Studies

Because there is a strong diurnal rhythm in testosterone secretion in young men (highest in the morning), testosterone, LH, and FSH are routinely determined from morning blood samples. There is a broad range of reference values due in part to measurement variability. Most laboratories used immunoassay methods to measure serum testosterone, which may lack precision at low serum testosterone levels. Recent studies suggest that methods using

---

TABLE 242-2	CAUSES OF PRIMARY TESTICULAR FAILURE AND END-ORGAN RESISTANCE

Congenital disorders
  Chromosome disorders
  Klinefelter's and related syndromes (e.g., XXY, XXY/XY, XYY, XX males)
  Testosterone biosynthetic enzyme defects
  Myotonic dystrophy
Developmental disorders
  Prenatal diethylstilbestrol syndrome
  Cryptorchidism
Acquired defects
  Orchitis
  Mumps and other viruses
  Granulomatous disease (e.g., tuberculosis, leprosy)
  Human immunodeficiency virus infection
  Infiltrative disease (e.g., hemochromatosis, amyloidosis)
  Surgical, traumatic injuries, torsion of testis
  Irradiation
Toxins (e.g., alcohol, fungicides, insecticides, heavy metals, cottonseed oil, DDT, other environmental "endocrine disruptors")
Drugs
  Cytotoxic agents
  Inhibitors of testosterone synthesis and antiandrogens (e.g., ketoconazole, cimetidine, flutamide, cyproterone, spironolactone)
  Ethanol, opioids, other recreational drugs
Autoimmune testicular failure
  Isolated
  Associated with other organ-specific disorders (e.g., Addison's disease, Hashimoto's thyroiditis, insulin-dependent diabetes)
Systemic diseases (e.g., cirrhosis, chronic renal failure, sickle cell disease, acquired immunodeficiency syndrome, amyloidosis)
Aging*
Androgen resistance syndromes
5α-Reductase deficiency

*Aging produces a mixed pattern of testicular and hypothalamic-pituitary dysfunction.

TABLE 242-3	CAUSES OF HYPOGONADOTROPIC HYPOGONADISM

IDIOPATHIC OR CONGENITAL

Isolated deficiency of gonadotropin-releasing hormone
  With anosmia (Kallmann's syndrome)
  With other abnormalities (Prader-Willi syndrome, Laurence-Moon-Biedl syndrome, basal encephalocele)
Partial deficiency of gonadotropin-releasing hormone (fertile eunuch syndrome)
Multiple hypothalamic and pituitary hormone deficiency
Pituitary hypoplasia or aplasia

ACQUIRED

Trauma, post surgery, post irradiation
Neoplastic
Pituitary adenoma (prolactinoma, other functional and nonfunctional tumors)
Craniopharyngioma, germinoma, glioma, leukemia, lymphoma
Pituitary infarction, carotid aneurysm
Infiltrative and infectious diseases of hypothalamus and pituitary (sarcoidosis, tuberculosis, coccidioidomycosis, histoplasmosis, syphilis, abscess, histiocytosis X, hemochromatosis)
Autoimmune hypophysitis
Aging*
Obesity
Malnutrition and systemic disease
Anorexia nervosa, starvation, renal failure, liver failure
Exogenous hormones and drugs
Antiandrogens, estrogens and antiestrogens, progestogens, glucocorticoids, cimetidine, spironolactone, digoxin, drug-induced hyperprolactinemia (metoclopramide, tranquilizers, antihypertensives)

*Aging produces a mixed pattern of central and testicular dysfunction.

liquid or gas chromatography and mass spectrometry may give more accurate results even at low serum testosterone levels. Elevated LH and FSH levels distinguish primary from secondary hypogonadism (both have low serum testosterone levels), but many older men with low serum testosterone levels have normal LH concentrations. Serum prolactin levels should be measured in all cases of hypogonadotropic hypogonadism, pituitary mass lesions, and galactorrhea. DHT is measured in cases of abnormal differentiation of the genitalia and when DHT deficiency is suspected. Serum estradiol should be measured in cases of gynecomastia. Assessment of other testosterone precursors and products may be required in special circumstances, including suspected congenital enzyme defects. The semen analysis is the "cornerstone" of the laboratory examination for male infertility.

Hypogonadism and Androgen Resistance
PRIMARY TESTICULAR HYPOGONADISM

Primary hypogonadism refers to a condition of androgen deficiency with or without infertility in which the pathologic process lies at the testis level. A list of common causes is given in Table 242-2. Congenital defects are described in Chapter 241.

PATHOBIOLOGY
Acquired Defects
Mumps, Orchitis, Leprosy, HIV Infection, and Hemochromatosis
After puberty, mumps (Chapter 377) is associated with clinical orchitis in 25% of cases, and 60% of those affected become infertile. During acute orchitis, the testes are inflamed, painful, and swollen. This is followed by a gradual decrease in size. The testes may return to normal size and function, or they may atrophy. Spermatogenic defects occur more often and earlier than Leydig cell dysfunction. Thus, patients with postorchitic infertility may have normal testosterone and LH levels with increased serum FSH levels. Over time, elevations in LH and lower serum testosterone levels may appear. Leprosy (Chapter 334) may also cause orchitis and gonadal insufficiency. HIV infection is often associated with hypogonadism, which can be either hypogonadotropic or hypergonadotropic. Hemochromatosis (Chapter 219) may affect the hypothalamus-pituitary as well as act directly on the testis.

Trauma
The exposed position of the testes in the scrotum makes them particularly susceptible to injury. Surgical injury during scrotal surgery for hernia, varicocele, and vasectomy can result in permanent testicular damage.

Irradiation
Accidental exposure of the testes to irradiation for the treatment of an associated malignant disease produces testicular damage.

Drugs and Toxins
Chemotherapy, in particular alkylating agents such as busulfan, frequently leads to irreversible germ cell damage. Heavy metals (lead, cadmium) and cottonseed oil (gossypol) cause damage to the germ cells. Leydig cells are relatively less susceptible to most chemotherapeutic drugs than are Sertoli and germ cells. Some medications may interfere with testosterone biosynthesis (e.g., ketoconazole, spironolactone) or action (e.g., cyproterone, flutamide). Ethanol, independent of its role in causing liver disease, inhibits testosterone biosynthesis. Marijuana, heroin, methadone, medroxyprogesterone acetate, other progestins, and estrogens lower testosterone, mainly by decreasing LH. Medical treatment with androgens such as testosterone, DHT, and synthetic anabolic steroids or their illicit use (e.g., in athletes, bodybuilders) lowers serum LH and FSH and sperm counts. Serum testosterone levels are low after the use of DHT and synthetic anabolic agents. Environmental toxins such as fungicides and insecticides (e.g., DBCP, metabolites of DDT, vinclozolin) and byproducts of the plastics industry (e.g., phthalates, bisphenol A) are called "endocrine disruptors" because these chemicals may have either weak estrogenic or antiandrogenic effects and have been shown to cause testicular dysgenesis in male offspring when administered in large doses to pregnant female rodents.

Autoimmune Testicular Failure
Antibodies against the microsomal fraction of the Leydig cells may occur either as an isolated disorder or as part of a multiglandular disorder (Chapter 239) involving, to variable degrees, the thyroid, pituitary, adrenals, pancreas, and other organs.

Hypogonadism Associated with Systemic Diseases
Abnormalities of the hypothalamic-pituitary-testicular axis occur in a number of systemic diseases, including liver failure, renal failure, severe malnutrition, sickle cell anemia, advanced malignant disease, severe obesity, diabetes, cystic fibrosis, and amyloidosis, as well as in those on chronic hemodialysis. The effects of cirrhosis of the liver on testicular function are complex and may be either independent of or associated with the direct toxic effects of the continued use of alcohol. Gynecomastia, testicular atrophy, and impotence are concomitant signs of cirrhosis. Decreased spermatogenesis with peritubular fibrosis occurs in 50% of cases. Estradiol levels are usually elevated. This results in an increased ratio of serum estradiol to testosterone, often associated with gynecomastia. Boys with sickle cell anemia may have impaired sexual maturation, and men are often infertile. Diabetes and obesity are two major factors in hypogonadism. Emerging data show that type 2 diabetes is associated with low blood testosterone levels mainly due to hypothalamic-pituitary dysfunction; the decrease in serum testosterone correlates with the degree of hyperglycemia.

SECONDARY GONADAL INSUFFICIENCY (HYPOGONADOTROPIC HYPOGONADISM)
Hypogonadotropic hypogonadism represents a deficiency in the secretion of gonadotropins (LH and FSH) due to an intrinsic or functional abnormality in the hypothalamus or pituitary glands (see earlier and Chapter 241). Such disorders result in secondary Leydig cell dysfunction (see Table 242-3). The clinical manifestations depend on the age of the patient at the onset of the disorder.

Acquired Hypogonadotropic Disorders and Functional Disorders
Anorexia Nervosa and Weight Loss
Anorexia nervosa (Chapter 226) and weight loss are examples of functional defects resulting in low serum testosterone levels. Men and women with anorexia nervosa present with manifestations of hypogonadotropic hypogonadism. Starvation may also reduce gonadotropic secretion. Strenuous exercise has minimal effects on testicular function in men.

Stress and Illness
Severe stress (e.g., surgery, trauma) and systemic illness also lower gonadotropin and testosterone levels. Organic hypothalamic-pituitary disorders include neoplastic, granulomatous, infiltrative, and post-traumatic lesions in the region of the hypothalamus and pituitary.

Pituitary Tumors
Prolactinomas present differently in men and women (Chapter 231). In men these tumors are usually large (>1 cm in diameter; macroadenomas) by the time they are detected. Male patients with prolactin-secreting macroadenomas usually present with hypogonadism, erectile dysfunction, and visual manifestations from suprasellar extension. In small tumors, hypogonadotropic hypogonadism may be due to suppressive effects on GnRH described earlier, but in large tumors, it may also be due to a mass effect damaging the non-neoplastic gonadotrophs.

Large non-prolactin-secreting pituitary tumors (growth hormone, adrenocorticotropic hormone, glycopeptide, and null cell) may also produce gonadotropin insufficiency from damage to the adjacent normal pituitary gland (Chapter 231), resulting in decreased serum LH and testosterone levels.

ANDROGEN RESISTANCE (ANDROGEN-SENSITIVE END-ORGAN DEFICIENCY)
Certain conditions have clinical phenotypes mimicking testosterone deficiency in the absence of lowered testosterone levels. These are either drug-induced (antiandrogens) or congenital defects in the androgen receptor, postreceptor defects, or 5α-reductase deficiency (Chapter 241).

DIAGNOSIS
The diagnosis is based on clinical symptoms and signs and a reduced serum testosterone level. The normal range of serum total testosterone in a young adult male population varies for different laboratories but should be in the general range of 300 to 1000 ng/dL (10 to 38 nmol/L). Accurate measurements of testosterone in the severely hypogonadal range are best done by gas

or liquid chromatography followed by tandem mass spectrometry. Total testosterone measurements may be misleading indicators of Leydig cell status in conditions in which SHBG levels are abnormal (see earlier section). In these circumstances, a measurement of free testosterone (by an equilibrium dialysis method), bioavailable testosterone (consisting of free plus albumin bound), or calculated free testosterone (by total testosterone and SHBG measurements) may be useful.

The following rules apply to most young and middle-aged men thought to have hypogonadism. If a morning serum total testosterone level is repeatedly below 250 ng/dL (8.5 nmol/L), the patient is probably hypogonadal, and testosterone replacement is indicated. If the serum testosterone level is between 250 and 300 ng/dL with normal serum LH levels, the patient may not be hypogonadal, and androgen replacement may not improve the symptoms (e.g., sexual dysfunction). Thus, when serum total testosterone is borderline and LH is not increased, one of the measurements of bioactive testosterone is indicated. The guidelines for men older than 60 years are less certain. Because SHBG levels are increased, total testosterone levels may overestimate the biologically active forms. A serum total testosterone level above 400 ng/dL argues strongly against hypogonadism, a serum level below 250 ng/dL is almost always clinically significant, and total testosterone concentrations between 250 and 400 ng/dL deserve further testing with one of the tests of bioactive testosterone.

TREATMENT [Rx]

The main medical indication for androgen replacement therapy is male hypogonadism (Table 242-4). In about 10% of men with idiopathic hypogonadism reversed by testosterone therapy, the reversal is sustained after therapy is stopped. This suggests that some patients with low serum testosterone may have a transient cause of the defect. Administration of testosterone to elderly men with low-normal testosterone concentrations increases lean body mass and decreases fat mass but may not improve functional status or cognition.[1-4] Carefully designed studies of the efficacy of testosterone treatment in older men are ongoing.

Absolute contraindications to androgen replacement therapy include carcinoma of the prostate and the male breast. Androgens should be used with caution in older men with enlarged prostates and urinary symptoms, elevated hematocrits, and sleep-related breathing disorders.

Testosterone esters, such as testosterone enanthate (or cypionate) injections, are widely used in the United States and throughout the world (Table 242-5). The recommended dose is 150 to 200 mg administered intramuscularly once every 2 to 3 weeks. Testosterone undecenoate injections administered every 10 to 12 weeks are available in many parts of the world but not yet in the United States.

Modified 17α-alkylated androgens (methyltestosterone and many anabolic steroids), which are available in oral preparations, are not recommended as androgen replacement. These agents may lead to abnormalities in liver function, marked decreases in high-density lipoprotein cholesterol, and increases in total cholesterol levels compared with the testosterone esters. Transbuccal delivery of testosterone by mucoadhesive tablets (30 mg applied twice daily) results in physiologic-range testosterone levels through direct absorption into the systemic circulation, thus avoiding first-pass effects on the liver.

Implants consist of pellets of crystalline testosterone. Serum testosterone levels are maintained in the physiologic range for 4 to 6 months. Implants are not very popular in the United States but are widely used in Australia and the United Kingdom.

Transdermal testosterone delivery through skin patches and hydroalcoholic gels is available. The nonscrotal patches deliver 5 mg/day of testosterone, which is the physiologic production rate. These patches deliver levels of testosterone within the normal range but have a high incidence of skin irritability (redness, swelling, and blisters). Hydroalcoholic testosterone gels have been developed for transdermal application and have become the most widely used testosterone formulations in the United States. The usual dosage is 5 to 10 g of 1% testosterone gel applied daily. This results in a reasonably constant serum concentration and causes little skin irritation. Transfer from the user to others is possible during routine use and may be a concern if there is close skin contact with women and children. Protective clothing or a shower is necessary to avoid transferring testosterone through skin-to-skin contact.

Table 242-6 shows the benefits and potential side effects of androgen treatment. In hypogonadal men, androgen replacement leads to the development and maintenance of secondary sexual characteristics. Testosterone has important anabolic effects on muscle and bone and improves libido and sexual dysfunction. It has less effect on erectile dysfunction. It has no major short-term effects on prostate tissue[7] but appears to increase the risk of cardiovascular events, at least in elderly men.[8]

TABLE 242-4 INDICATIONS FOR ANDROGEN THERAPY

Androgen deficiency (hypogonadism)
Microphallus (neonatal)
Delayed puberty in boys
Elderly men with low total or bioavailable or free testosterone levels
Angioneurotic edema
Other possible uses or under investigation
    Hormonal male contraception
    Wasting disease associated with cancer, human immunodeficiency virus infection, chronic infection
    Postmenopausal women

TABLE 242-5 ANDROGEN PREPARATIONS

ROUTE	PREPARATION	DOSE AND FREQUENCY OF ADMINISTRATION
Oral*	Testosterone undecenoate (not available in United States; available in Canada, Mexico, Europe, Asia)	40-80 mg orally two or three times/day
Buccal	Transbuccal testosterone, mucoadhesive tablets (Striant)	30 mg two times/day
Injection	Testosterone enanthate and cypionate	100 mg/wk intramuscularly or 150-200 mg intramuscularly every 2-3 wk
	Testosterone undecanoate (not available in United States)	750-1000 mg intramuscularly every 10-12 wk
Implant	Testosterone implants	75-mg pellets (in United States), 6-10 inserted once every 4-6 mo
Transdermal	Scrotal patch	One patch delivering 4 or 6 mg testosterone per day
	Nonscrotal patch, Androderm	Two patches, each delivering 2.5 mg testosterone per day; or one patch delivering 5 mg testosterone per day
	Testoderm TTS	One patch delivering 5 mg testosterone per day
Transdermal hydroalcoholic gel	AndroGel or Testogel; Testim	5-10 g containing 50-100 mg testosterone applied once daily

*Oral modified 17α-alkylated androgens such as methyltestosterone, fluoxymesterone, oxymetholone, stanozolol, and oxandrolone are not recommended for the treatment of androgen-deficient states because of potential hepatotoxicity and adverse effects on serum lipids.

TABLE 242-6 ANDROGEN THERAPY: RISKS VERSUS BENEFITS

BENEFITS	RISKS
Development or maintenance of secondary sex characteristics	Fluid retention
	Gynecomastia
Improved libido and sexual function	Acne, oily skin
Increased muscle mass and strength	Increased hematocrit
Increased bone mineral density	Decreased high-density lipoprotein cholesterol (oral 17α-alkylated agents produce the greatest effect)
Decreased body and visceral fat	
Improved mood	Sleep apnea
Effect on cognition (?)	Aggressive behavior (?)
Effect on vitality and quality of life (?)	Prostate disease
	Benign prostatic hyperplasia (?)
	Carcinoma of prostate (aggravate existing cancer)

● MALE INFERTILITY

DEFINITION

Infertility is defined as the failure of a couple to achieve pregnancy after at least 1 year of frequent unprotected intercourse. If a pregnancy has not occurred after 3 years, infertility will most likely persist without medical treatment.

FIGURE 242-8. Algorithmic approach to the diagnosis and treatment of male infertility. ART = assisted reproductive technology; FSH = follicle-stimulating hormone; GnRH = gonadotropin-releasing hormone; ICSI = intracytoplasmic sperm injection; LH = serum luteinizing hormone; T = serum testosterone.

EPIDEMIOLOGY

Studies in the United States and Europe showed a 1-year prevalence of infertility in 15% of couples. The prevalence in developing countries is likely to be higher because of the higher prevalence of genital tract infection. Thirty percent to 35% of subfertility can be attributed to predominantly female factors, 25 to 30% to male factors, and 25 to 30% to problems in both partners.

PATHOBIOLOGY

Hypothalamic-pituitary disorders are infrequent causes of male infertility and are discussed in the section on hypogonadism and androgen deficiency. Testicular disorders are the most frequent identifiable cause of infertility (see Table 242-2). Y chromosome microdeletions are increasingly recognized as a genetic cause of azoospermia and severe oligozoospermia. Up to 20% of infertile men have microdeletions in the long arm of the Y chromosome, many of which map to the Yq11 region of the chromosome, which is called the azoospermic factor (AZF).

DIAGNOSIS

The approach to the diagnosis of an infertile couple includes management of both the male and the female partner (Figs. 242-8 and 242-9).

Examination of the ejaculate is the cornerstone for the investigation of an infertile man (Table 242-7). Semen samples are collected at the physician's office or at home, preferably after 2 to 7 days of abstinence from sexual intercourse. The generally accepted reference values for a semen analysis are given in Table 242-8. A normal sperm concentration is greater than 15 million/mL, with a total sperm number greater than 39 million per ejaculate; however, men with lower sperm counts can be fertile. More than 40% of the spermatozoa should be motile, and more than 32% should demonstrate a progressive motility pattern. Using a strict criterion to assess sperm morphology, the percentage of morphologically normal forms should be above 4%. There is considerable overlap in the semen quality of fertile and subfertile men. There is no definite threshold below which a man is infertile, except when azoospermia is present.

In patients with abnormal semen analyses, measurements of serum FSH, LH, and testosterone are indicated (see Fig. 242-7). Elevated FSH levels usually indicate severe germinal epithelium damage. A decreased serum inhibin β level also reflects poor Sertoli cell function and may indicate spermatogenic dysfunction. Elevated serum LH and FSH concentrations together with a low serum testosterone level indicate pantesticular failure. Low serum FSH, LH, and testosterone concentrations suggest hypothalamic-pituitary dysfunction; serum prolactin should be measured, and additional investigations may be required. A low sperm concentration and suppressed

FIGURE 242-9. Algorithmic approach to the diagnosis and treatment of male infertility in patients with normal serum hormone concentrations. ART = assisted reproductive technology; FSH = follicle-stimulating hormone; ICSI = intracytoplasmic sperm injection; LH = serum luteinizing hormone; T = serum testosterone.

TABLE 242-7	MALE INFERTILITY: BASIC LABORATORY TESTS
SEMEN ANALYSES	**HORMONE ANALYSES (IN PATIENTS WITH ABNORMAL SEMEN ANALYSES)**
Volume, pH	Serum luteinizing hormone and follicle-stimulating hormone
Microscopy: agglutination, debris	Serum testosterone
Sperm: concentration, motility, morphology, vitality	If luteinizing hormone and testosterone levels are low, serum prolactin
Leukocytes	
Immature germ cells	
Sperm autoantibodies (sperm and semen biochemistry, sperm function tests)	

TABLE 242-8	SEMEN ANALYSIS: REFERENCE RANGE FROM FERTILE MEN*
PARAMETER	**REFERENCE RANGE**
Semen volume	>1.5 mL
Sperm	
Concentration	>15 million/mL
Total count	>39 million/ejaculate
Motility	>40% motile
	>32% progressively motile
Morphology	>4% normal†
Vitality (live)	>58%
Leukocytes	<1 million/mL

*Men whose partners had a time-to-pregnancy of ≤12 months were chosen to provide reference distributions for semen parameters.
†This value is based on the strict criteria for assessing sperm morphology in studies using in vitro fertilization as an end point. This value will likely be adjusted to a lower level based on recent studies in fertile men.

LH level with an increased, normal, or low serum testosterone level (without clinical manifestations of androgen deficiency) may suggest exogenous androgen use. The hormonal pattern in androgen insensitivity (an uncommon cause of male infertility) is elevated LH, normal FSH, and high-normal to increased serum testosterone levels. Normal hormonal parameters in azoospermic (no sperm in the ejaculate) men with normal-sized testes may suggest congenital or acquired obstruction in the epididymis or vas deferens.

TREATMENT   Rx

An algorithmic approach to the treatment of male infertility is illustrated in Figures 242-8 and 242-9. The principles of managing male infertility can be summarized as follows: (1) Men with mild to moderate oligozoospermia, with or without decreased sperm motility and some impairment of motility, are subfertile rather than infertile. Spontaneous pregnancies can occur in this group. (2) Reliable medical treatment is limited to the 1 to 2% of infertile men with gonadotropin insufficiency. (3) Assisted reproductive technologies, including in vitro fertilization and intracytoplasmic sperm injection, have dramatically improved pregnancy rates. (4) Azoospermia (absence of sperm in the ejaculate) may occur in men with obstruction of the ejaculatory system. In these patients, in vitro fertilization and intracytoplasmic sperm injection after either percutaneous epididymal sperm extraction or microsurgical epididymal sperm extraction are highly successful. (5) Azoospermia due to impaired spermatogenesis may not be a sterile state, because sperm may be present within the testes. These sperm can be extracted, and intracytoplasmic sperm injection can be performed with good success, even in patients with Klinefelter's syndrome.

⬤ SEXUAL DYSFUNCTION

Sexual dysfunction can be divided into four main categories: (1) loss of desire (libido), (2) erectile dysfunction, (3) ejaculatory insufficiency, and (4) anorgasmic states.

Decreased Libido

Loss of libido refers to a reduction in sexual interest, initiative, and frequency and intensity of responses to internal or external erotic stimuli. Causal factors include psychogenic factors, CNS disease, androgen deficiency and resistance, and side effects from medications (e.g., antihypertensives, psychotropics, alcohol, narcotics, dopamine blockers, antiandrogens). Treatment is directed toward the causal mechanism.

Ejaculatory Failure and Impaired Orgasm

Ejaculatory insufficiency refers to absent or reduced seminal emission or impaired ejaculatory contraction. It is usually associated with neurologic conditions and medication therapy. An anorgasmic state is a distressing but relatively uncommon condition in men in which the normal process of erection and ejaculation occurs in the absence of the subjective sensation of pleasure initiated at the time of emission and ejaculation. Premature ejaculation is the most common form of male sexual dysfunction. Estimates of prevalence vary, but 25 to 30% seems to be a reasonable estimate. The fourth edition of the *Diagnostic and Statistical Manual of Mental Disorders* defines the diagnostic criteria for premature ejaculation as follows: persistent or recurrent ejaculation with minimal sexual stimulation that (1) occurs before, upon, or shortly after penetration and before the person wishes, (2) is associated with marked distress or interpersonal difficulty, and (3) is not a direct effect of substance abuse such as opiate withdrawal.

Erectile Dysfunction

Erectile dysfunction can be defined as a man's inability to obtain rigidity sufficient to permit coitus of adequate duration to satisfy himself and his partner.

Current estimates suggest that 10 to 15% of all American men suffer from erectile dysfunction, with the incidence progressively increased as men become older. Data from the Massachusetts Aging Study report that 52% of men 40 to 70 years of age experience some degree of erectile dysfunction.

The causes of erectile dysfunction are many, but they can generally be categorized as follows: psychological, endocrine, systemic illness, neurologic, iatrogenic, drug related, and aging.

TREATMENT   Rx

Medical Therapy
Oral Medications

Oral and selective inhibitors of cGMP phosphodiesterase-5 (the primary phosphodiesterase in the penile cavernosal tissue) are effective for at least 50% of men. Inhibition of phosphodiesterase-5 causes persistence of normally (sexually) stimulated cGMP in the corpora cavernosa, resulting in protracted cavernosal tumescence and rigidity. Patients with diabetes mellitus, spinal cord injuries, prostatic surgery, and pelvic irradiation also benefit, but with a somewhat lower response rate. The usual starting dose of sildenafil is 50 mg, increasing in 25-mg increments up to 100 mg. The most serious side effect is cardiovascular collapse, particularly in patients taking long-acting nitrate or nitroglycerin preparations. Because of its mechanism of action, sildenafil is used on demand; it is administered 20 to 60 minutes before intercourse. Two additional phosphodiesterase-5 inhibitors (vardenafil and tadalafil) are widely used for the treatment of erectile dysfunction and appear to be equally effective. Vardenafil has a relatively longer duration of action (4 to 6 hours), and tadalafil has a much longer duration of action (17.5 hours). Hypogonadal men with erectile dysfunction and low libido may benefit from combined treatment with testosterone and phosphodiesterase-5 inhibitors.

Apomorphine is a selective dopamine receptor agonist that stimulates the CNS, generating an arousal response that includes a penile erection. Apomorphine has not been approved by the Food and Drug Administration and appears to be inferior to phosphodiesterase-5 inhibitors. Yohimbine is an indolalquinolonic alkaloid with central-acting effects, including α_2-adrenergic blockade and cholinergic and dopaminergic stimulation. Despite its widespread use, placebo-controlled studies have shown variable degrees of success, and yohimbine seems to be most useful in conditions in which there is organic disease. Trazodone, an antidepressant, possesses both serotonin and α_2-adrenergic antagonistic properties. It appears to be moderately effective in one third of patients; the main side effect is sedation.

Intracavernosal Injection

The intraurethral prostaglandin E_1 suppository alprostadil is believed to work locally on the corpora cavernosa as a vasodilatory agent. The suppository is apparently successful in improving erectile function in one third to two thirds of cases. Until the recent availability of oral phosphodiesterase-5 inhibitors, intracavernosal injection with prostaglandin E_1 and other vasodilators (papaverine, phentolamine) was the mainstay of pharmacologic therapy for erectile dysfunction. The medications are injected with a 27- to 30-gauge needle and may be useful in men who are refractory to oral agents.

Grade A

1. Page ST, Amory JK, Bowman FD, et al. Exogenous testosterone (T) alone or with finasteride increases physical performance, grip strength, and lean body mass in older men with low serum T. *J Clin Endocrinol Metab*. 2005;90:1502-1510.
2. Amory JK, Watts NB, Easley KA, et al. Exogenous testosterone or testosterone with finasteride increases bone mineral density in older men with low serum testosterone. *J Clin Endocrinol Metab*. 2004;89:503-510.
3. Emmelot-Vonk MH, Verhaar HJ, Nakhai Pour HR, et al. Effect of testosterone supplementation on functional mobility, cognition, and other parameters in older men: a randomized controlled trial. *JAMA*. 2008;299:39-52.
4. Srinivas-Shankar U, Roberts SA, Connolly MJ, et al. Effects of testosterone on muscle strength, physical function, body composition, and quality of life in intermediate-frail and frail elderly men: a randomized, double-blind, placebo-controlled study. *J Clin Endocrinol Metab*. 2010;95:639-650.
5. Baulieu EE, Thomas G, Legrain S, et al. Dehydroepiandrosterone (DHEA), DHEA sulfate, and aging: contribution of the DHEAge Study to a sociobiomedical issue. *Proc Natl Acad Sci USA*. 2000;97:4279-4284.
6. Nair KS, Rizza RA, O'Brien P, et al. DHEA in elderly women and DHEA or testosterone in elderly men. *N Engl J Med*. 2006;355:1647-1659.
7. Marks LS, Mazer NA, Mostaghel E, et al. Effect of testosterone replacement therapy on prostate tissue in men with late-onset hypogonadism: a randomized controlled trial. *JAMA*. 2006;296:2351-2361.
8. Basaria S, Coviello AD, Travison TG, et al. Adverse events associated with testosterone administration. *N Engl J Med*. 2010;363:109-122.

SUGGESTED READINGS

Bhasin S, Cunningham GR, Hayes FJ, et al. Testosterone therapy in adult men with androgen deficiency syndromes: an Endocrine Society clinical practice guideline. *J Clin Endocrinol Metab.* 2006;91:1995-2010. *Recommended approaches to diagnose and treat androgen deficiency.*

Cooper TG, Noonan E, Von ES, et al. World Health Organization reference values for human semen characteristics. *Hum Reprod Update.* 2009. http://humupd.oxfordjournals.org/cgi/content/full/dmp048v2. *Defines the reference ranges of sperm parameters in men.*

Hatzimouratidis K, Amar E, Eardley I, et al. Guidelines on male sexual dysfunction: erectile dysfunction and premature ejaculation. *Eur Urol.* 2010;57:804-814. *Consensus guidelines.*

243

OVARIES AND DEVELOPMENT

ROBERT W. REBAR AND GREGORY F. ERICKSON

DEFINITION

The ovaries or female gonads episodically release female gametes (oocytes or eggs) and secrete sex steroid hormones, principally androstenedione, estradiol, and progesterone. Oocytes are released only during the adult reproductive years, when sex steroid secretion is also greatest, but the ovaries are physiologically active throughout life.

Sex steroids affect the growth, differentiation, and function of a variety of tissues and organs throughout the body; therefore, abnormalities of the ovaries and of sex steroid secretion should be recognized by all physicians. A rational approach to the diagnosis and treatment of reproductive disorders in women requires an understanding of the functions of the ovaries and of their most important unit, the follicle, throughout life.

PHYSIOLOGY

Embryology

Embryogenesis and Differentiation

Organogenesis of the ovaries occurs during fetal life. Ovarian cells are derived from two different sources: (1) primordial germ cells (PGCs) originate at a site outside the prospective gonads, and (2) somatic cells differentiate from the coelomic epithelium and gonadal mesenchyme. In females, PGCs become oocytes, whereas somatic cells differentiate into a variety of cell types, including granulosa, theca, and vascular cells.

PGCs in the human embryo can be distinguished at the gastrula stage (Fig. 243-1). Shortly after formation, PGCs migrate through the dorsal mesentery to the genital ridges. Chemotaxis plays a role in directing PGCs to the gonads. During migration, PGCs proliferate in response to growth factors, most notably Kit ligand. The importance of Kit is demonstrated by the finding that loss-of-function mutations result in a paucity of PGCs, which in turn results in premature ovarian failure.

The genital ridges are characterized by a thickening of the coelomic epithelium and underlying primary mesenchyme. Initially, the gonads are sexually indifferent. Male gonadal differentiation is triggered by the Y chromosome–encoded testis-determining factor SRY. SRY expression results

in the differentiation of Sertoli cells and the secretion of müllerian-inhibiting substance, which induces regression of the müllerian ducts. Testicular interstitial cells differentiate into Leydig cells, which secrete testosterone, which in turn stimulates wolffian duct development. In the female, the absence of müllerian-inhibiting substance and testosterone leads to the degeneration of the wolffian ducts and the development of the müllerian ducts. Thus, the development of the ovaries and female reproductive system is considered a "default" pathway.

When PGCs enter the genital ridges, they begin gametogenesis (see Fig. 243-1). In females, this process is termed *oogenesis* and involves the differentiation of PGCs into oogonia and oocytes. When sex-specific differentiation of the ovary commences, the inactive X chromosome in the PGCs becomes active. This denotes the formation of mitotically active oogonia. The importance of two functional X chromosomes during oogenesis is emphasized by the fact that 45,X females lack oocytes and undergo premature menopause.

After repeated mitosis, oogonia initiate meiosis and become oocytes (see Fig. 243-1). At approximately the same time, granulosa cells differentiate within the gonadal mesenchyme and establish intimate associations with oocytes. Oocytes that become surrounded by granulosa cells stop meiosis after diplotene, and the bivalents enter an interphase state known as dictyotene. If an oocyte is not surrounded by granulosa cells, meiosis continues to diakinesis, and the oocyte dies by apoptosis. Granulosa cells, therefore, are critical for oocyte survival. The majority of oocytes die during fetal ovary development (Fig. 243-2), apparently from a lack of contact with granulosa cells.

With further development, the oocyte–granulosa cell complex becomes a primordial follicle. This occurs between the sixth and ninth months of gestation (Fig. 243-3). A primordial follicle consists of a single layer of squamous granulosa cells, a small (about 15 μm in diameter) dictyotene oocyte, and a thin basal lamina (see Fig. 243-3). In the human female, all potential future eggs have entered diplotene of meiosis at the time of birth, and no reserve oogonia remain.

Anatomy
The Adult Ovary

The ovaries, which normally measure 2.5 to 5.0 cm long, 1.5 to 3.0 cm wide, and 0.6 to 1.5 cm thick in adults, are organized into two principal parts. A central zone, the medulla, is surrounded by a prominent peripheral zone, the cortex (Fig. 243-4). Growing follicles at different stages of development are

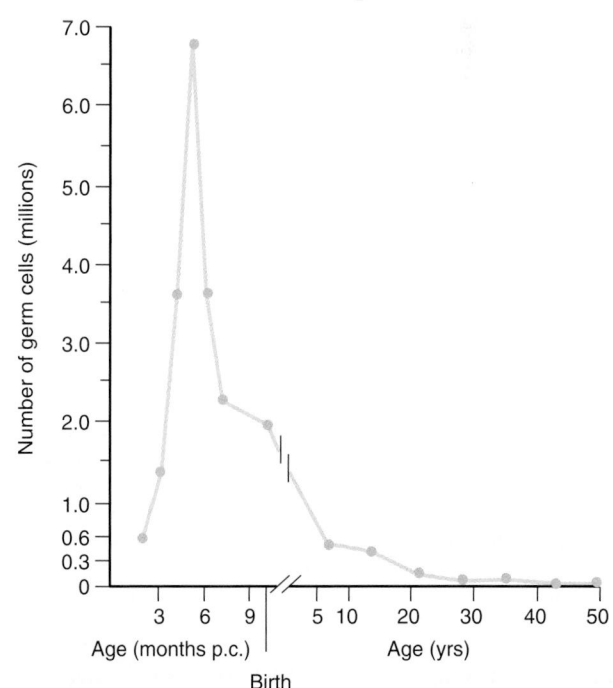

FIGURE 243-2. Changes in the total number of germ cells in the human ovaries during aging. At early to mid-gestation, the number of germ cells increases to almost 7 million; shortly thereafter, the number declines rapidly to about 2 million at birth. The number continues to decline until no oocytes are detected at 50 years of age. p.c. = post conception. (From Baker TG. Radiosensitivity of mammalian oocytes with particular reference to the human female. *Am J Obstet Gynecol.* 1971;110:746-761.)

FIGURE 243-1. Diagram illustrating the developmental timetable of the major events that ultimately lead to the formation of primordial follicles during the process of human ovary organogenesis. PGC = primordial germ cell.

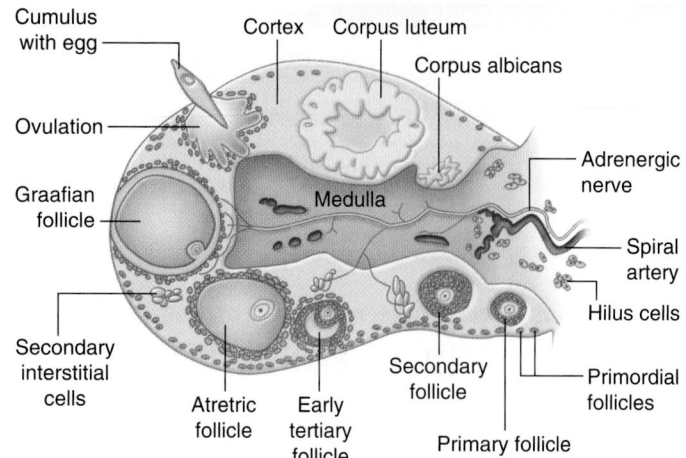

FIGURE 243-4. Diagram showing the anatomy of the human ovary during the reproductive years. Developing follicles and the corpus luteum are located in the cortex; the hilus cells, autonomic nerves, and spiral arteries are present in the medulla. (From Erickson GF. The ovary: basic principles and concepts. In: Felig P, Baxter JD, Broadus AE, et al, eds. *Endocrinology and Metabolism*, 3rd ed. New York: McGraw-Hill; 1995.)

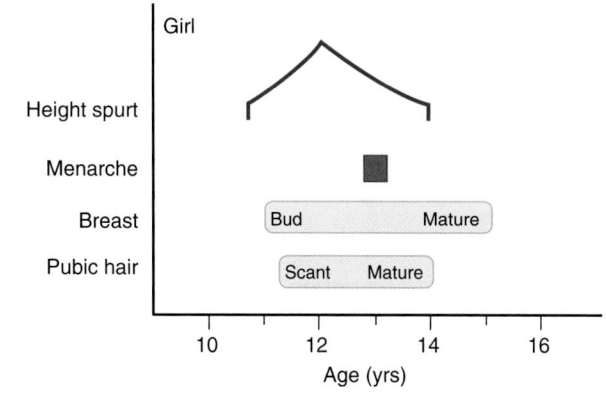

FIGURE 243-5. Temporal sequence of events for the "average" girl during puberty. (From Rebar RW. Practical evaluation of hormonal status. In: Yen SSC, Jaffe RB, Barbieri RL, eds. *Reproductive Endocrinology: Physiology, Pathophysiology, and Clinical Management*, 4th ed. Philadelphia: WB Saunders; 1999:710.)

FIGURE 243-3. A, Drawing showing gametogenesis in the human fetal ovary leading to the formation of primordial follicles. At 3 months (1), oogonia divide mitotically. At 4 months (2), some oogonia deep within the cortical cords enter meiosis (arrowheads). At 7 months (3), the cords are no longer distinct, and all germ cells are in meiotic prophase I. At 9 months (4), some oocytes become associated with granulosa cells and appear as primordial follicles (asterisks). B, Electron micrograph of human primordial follicle. Granulosa cells (arrowheads), oocyte nucleus (N), and Balbiani's body (asterisk) are shown. (From Erickson GF. The ovary: basic principles and concepts. In: Felig P, Baxter JD, Broadus AE, et al, eds. *Endocrinology and Metabolism*, 3rd ed. New York: McGraw-Hill; 1995.)

present in the cortex. Typically, one follicle per cycle reaches maturity and ovulates its ovum. After ovulation, the follicle transforms into a corpus luteum. The corpus luteum of the cycle lasts for about 14 days, after which it dies and becomes a nodule of dense connective tissue, the corpus albicans (see Fig. 243-4).

The medulla is composed of loose connective tissue with numerous blood vessels and associated nerves. The arterial supply to the ovary originates from two principal sources: the ovarian artery and the uterine artery. These two vessels, which enter the medulla from opposite directions, form an anastomotic trunk and become a common vessel called the ramus ovaricus artery. This artery gives rise to a series of primary branches (spiral arteries) that enter the hilum. In the hilum, numerous secondary and tertiary branches are given off to supply the medulla and the follicles and luteal tissue in the cortex (see Fig. 243-4). The hilum also contains the hilus cells (see Fig. 243-4), which, like the testicular Leydig cells, contain Reinke crystals and secrete testosterone. The physiologic role of the hilus cells is still unknown.

Ovarian Function in Childhood and Puberty
Physical Changes at Puberty

Puberty extends from the earliest signs of sexual maturation until the attainment of physical, mental, and emotional maturity. Pubertal changes in girls

result directly or indirectly from maturation of the hypothalamic-pituitary-ovarian unit. Human puberty is characterized hormonally by a resetting of the negative gonadal steroid feedback loop, the establishment of new circadian and ultradian (frequent) gonadotropin rhythms, and the acquisition in the female of a positive estrogen feedback loop controlling the menstrual cycle as interdependent expressions of the gonadotropins and ovarian steroids. In girls, pubertal development generally occurs between 7 and 14 years of age. The age at onset and the rate of progress through puberty are variable and depend on genetic, socioeconomic, nutritional, physical, and psychological factors. It appears that there are racial differences in the onset of pubertal development. In the United States, development begins earlier in African American than in white girls.

Physical changes occur in an orderly sequence during a definite time frame in puberty (Fig. 243-5). Breast budding in girls is usually the first pubertal change, followed shortly by the appearance of pubic hair, with menarche occurring late in pubertal development. The time from breast budding (mean age of 10.0 years in white girls and 8.9 years in African Americans) to menarche is 2 years. Breast development results from increasing ovarian estrogen production, and pubic and axillary hair results from increasing ovarian androgen production. Estrogens are required for the growth of pubic hair as well.

The ovarian sex steroids join with growth hormone and adrenal androgens to produce the adolescent growth spurt. Peak growth velocity is achieved relatively early, with little growth observed after menarche. It has been estimated that more than 50 genes play roles in determining final adult height. It is now clear that estrogen, and not testosterone, is the primary hormone mediating pubertal bone growth in both males and females. Lean body mass, skeletal mass, and body fat are equal in prepubertal boys and girls, but by maturity, women have twice as much body fat as men and less lean body mass and skeletal mass as a result of differences in sex steroid secretion. Estrogens are necessary for the normal formation, mineralization, and maturation of bones. Well-established standards exist for determining whether bone age is appropriate for chronologic age, typically by examining radiographs of the bones of the wrist. Estrogen deficiencies retard, and excesses advance, bone age in relation to chronologic age.

Hormonal Changes

The ovaries function even in early childhood. Low levels of luteinizing hormone (LH) and follicle-stimulating hormone (FSH) are normally present, and these levels increase if the ovaries are removed before puberty, just as they do later in life, indicating the exquisite sensitivity of the hypothalamic-pituitary unit to extremely low circulating sex steroid levels. As puberty nears, there is a progressive decrease in sensitivity of the hypothalamic-pituitary unit to sex steroids, leading to the increased secretion of pituitary gonadotropins, stimulation of sex steroid output, and development of secondary sex characteristics. Increased secretion of both LH and FSH initially occurs at night with sleep and is associated with increased estradiol secretion the next morning (Fig. 243-6). As is true for most hormones, LH and FSH are secreted in an episodic or pulsatile rather than a continuous fashion. Later in puberty, secretion of LH and FSH is increased throughout the 24-hour period, except during the early follicular phase, when nighttime increases still occur. Basal levels of estradiol, the major estrogen secreted by the ovaries, increase throughout puberty. A "critical body mass" may be required for positive estrogen feedback and ovulation. During the first 2 years after menarche, up to 90% of menstrual cycles may be anovulatory because of a delay in synchronization of the hypothalamic-pituitary-ovarian axis.

⬤ ABERRATIONS IN PUBERTAL DEVELOPMENT

Abnormalities of pubertal development can be divided into four major categories (Table 243-1):

1. *Precocious puberty* represents any pubertal changes before age 9 years in white girls and before age 8 years in African-American girls. This remains controversial. Some clinicians believe evaluation is warranted only if pubertal development begins before age 7 years in white girls and 6 years in African-American girls. A compromise may involve careful screening by history and physical examination of girls with early-onset puberty, looking for central nervous system (CNS) symptoms, behavioral concerns, and any other abnormal findings that might warrant further evaluation. The nearer pubertal development begins to the mean age of puberty

FIGURE 243-6. The changing patterns of luteinizing hormone (LH), follicle-stimulating hormone (FSH), and estradiol (E₂) concentrations in peripheral blood throughout the life of a woman. Not shown is the fact that both LH and FSH are secreted in a pulsatile fashion. The pubertal period has been expanded to illustrate the sleep-associated increases in LH and FSH followed by morning increases in E₂ that are observed during puberty. (Reprinted with permission from Endocrine and Metabolism Continuing Education Quality Control Program, 1982. Copyright American Association for Clinical Chemistry Inc.)

onset, the less likely it is to have a pathologic basis. Precocious development is *isosexual* when it is common to the phenotypic sex of the individual and *heterosexual* when the development is characteristic of the opposite sex. *True* or *central precocious puberty* is due to premature maturation of the hypothalamic-pituitary axis. In the absence of increased hypothalamic-pituitary activity, *precocious pseudopuberty* exists.

2. *Delayed* (or *interrupted*) *puberty* is defined as the absence of any secondary sex characteristics by age 13 years, the absence of menarche by age 16 years, or the passage of 5 years or more from breast budding to menarche.

3. *Asynchronous pubertal development* occurs when there is deviation from the normal pattern of pubertal development.

4. *Heterosexual pubertal development* occurs at the appropriate time but has some features characteristic of the opposite sex.

Precocious Puberty

> **DIAGNOSIS**

The overall incidence of precocious puberty has been estimated at 1 in 5000 to 10,000 children. About 10 times as many girls as boys are affected.

Differential Diagnosis

The temporal sequence in which the signs and symptoms of sex steroid hormone excess appear is most important. *Incomplete isosexual precocious puberty* indicates premature development of only a single pubertal feature. If breast budding occurs before age 8 years in the absence of any other development, the diagnosis may be *premature thelarche*. Premature thelarche is believed to be due to transient increases in estrogen secretion or increased breast sensitivity to the small quantities of circulating estrogens present before puberty. Simple ovarian cysts may be present in some girls with this disorder and may be due in some cases to the same genetic abnormality found in girls with McCune-Albright syndrome (Chapters 239 and 256). If pubic or axillary hair develops alone and persists, *premature pubarche* and *adrenarche* must be considered. These abnormalities are associated with slight increases in adrenal androgen secretion but not with clitorimegaly or other signs of virilization. These syndromes require no treatment, and affected girls typically begin true puberty at the usual age. Careful follow-up is required to distinguish these disorders from true precocious puberty.

When precocious development is isosexual, the purpose of the evaluation is to determine whether the cause is central (true precocious puberty) or peripheral, in which case it is considered gonadotropin-releasing hormone (GnRH)–independent precocious puberty or precocious pseudopuberty. Careful questioning of the patient and her parents may indicate the inadvertent ingestion or absorption of sex steroids (iatrogenic or factitious). As many as 20% of individuals with true precocious puberty have one of several organic brain diseases, including any of several neoplasms, tuberous sclerosis, neurofibromatosis, encephalitis, meningitis, vascular malformations, and hydrocephalus. Because of the seriousness of intracranial lesions, girls with precocious puberty must have radiographic evaluation of the CNS, most effectively by magnetic resonance imaging (MRI). In at least 75% of girls with true precocious puberty, however, no cause is identified (idiopathic or constitutional).

The physical examination may also provide critical information about the cause of the precocious development. Cutaneous café au lait spots, facial asymmetry, polyostotic fibrous dysplasia and other skeletal abnormalities, cranial nerve deficits, and multiple ovarian follicular cysts suggest McCune-Albright syndrome (Chapters 239 and 256) in a girl with precocious development. It is now known that various clones of cells in the endocrine glands of girls with this disorder function autonomously with respect to cyclic adenosine monophosphate production as a consequence of a mutation within exon 8 of the G protein α–subunit. This same mutation probably accounts for the bone lesions and café au lait hyperpigmentation. Other endocrine cells may be similarly affected and lead to pituitary adenomas (usually secreting growth hormone), hyperthyroidism, and, rarely, adrenal hyperplasia.

Precocious development associated with short stature, congenital body asymmetry, triangular facies, and clinodactyly suggests Silver-Russell syndrome. Characteristic signs and symptoms may suggest the coexistence of primary hypothyroidism and precocious puberty, especially if galactorrhea is also present. In these patients, thyroid hormone replacement therapy halts the progression of pubertal development until the expected age of puberty (enigmatically, primary hyperthyroidism may also lead to delayed pubertal development).

TABLE 243-1 ABERRATIONS OF PUBERTAL DEVELOPMENT

PRECOCIOUS DEVELOPMENT	Hypogonadotropic or normogonadotropic hypogonadism (LH and FSH <10 mIU/ mL, or LH and FSH 6-25 mIU/mL with at least one being >10 mIU/mL)
Isosexual precocity	Isolated gonadotropin deficiency
Incomplete sexual precocity	In association with midline defects (Kallmann's syndrome)
Premature thelarche	Independent of associated disorders
Premature pubarche	Neoplasms of the hypothalamic-pituitary axis
Premature adrenarche	Craniopharyngiomas
True (central) precocious puberty	Pituitary tumors
Idiopathic (constitutional)	Others
Due to central nervous system lesions	Infiltrative processes (Langerhans-type histiocytosis)
Primary hypothyroidism	Idiopathic hypopituitarism
Silver-Russell syndrome	"Hypothalamic" forms of amenorrhea
Precocious pseudopuberty (of peripheral origin)	Psychogenic
Ovarian neoplasms	Exercise associated
Adrenal neoplasms	Associated with malnutrition
Iatrogenic (estrogen-containing preparations)	Anorexia nervosa
Human chorionic gonadotropin–secreting neoplasms distinct from central nervous system and ovarian tumors	Miscellaneous disorders
McCune-Albright syndrome	Prader-Labhart-Willi syndrome
Heterosexual precocity	Laurence-Moon-Bardet-Biedl syndrome
Ovarian neoplasms	Primary hypothyroidism
Adrenal neoplasms	Constitutional delayed puberty
Congenital adrenal hyperplasia	**ASYNCHRONOUS PUBERTAL DEVELOPMENT**
Other rare disorders of sexual differentiation	Incomplete forms of androgen insensitivity
DELAYED PUBERTAL DEVELOPMENT*	Complete forms of androgen insensitivity
Anatomic abnormalities	**HETEROSEXUAL PUBERTAL DEVELOPMENT**
Müllerian agenesis or dysgenesis (Rokitansky-Küster-Hauser syndrome)	Polycystic ovary syndrome
Distal genital tract obstruction	Congenital adrenal hyperplasia (female pseudohermaphroditism)
Transverse vaginal septum	21-Hydroxylase deficiency
Imperforate hymen	11β-Hydroxylase deficiency
Vaginal agenesis	3β-ol-Hydroxysteroid dehydrogenase deficiency
Hypergonadotropic hypogonadism (FSH >30-40 mIU/mL)	Male pseudohermaphroditism due to 5α-reductase deficiency
Gonadal dysgenesis	Male pseudohermaphroditism due to partial androgen insensitivity
With stigmata of Turner's syndrome	Mixed gonadal dysgenesis
Pure (46,XX or 46,XY)	Androgen-producing neoplasms
Mixed	Ovarian
Ovarian failure with normal ovarian development	Adrenal
Genetic disorders	Cushing's syndrome
Autoimmune disorders	
Gonadotropin receptor or postreceptor defects (resistant ovary or Savage's syndrome?)	
Enzymatic defects (17α-hydroxylase deficiency, galactosemia)	
Physical causes	
Irradiation	
Chemotherapeutic agents	
Viral agents	
Idiopathic	

*No development by age 13 yr, absence of menarche by age 15 yr, or passage of ≥5 yr from breast budding without menarche.
FSH = follicle-stimulating hormone; LH = luteinizing hormone.

Abdominal and rectal examination may reveal a mass, suggesting an adrenal or ovarian tumor. Because palpable ovarian cysts may rarely develop before ovulation in true precocious puberty, the presence of a mass does not confirm the diagnosis of precocious pseudopuberty.

When vaginal bleeding is the only sign of development, the diagnosis of sexual precocity should be suspect. Common causes of bleeding in this age group include irritation from a vaginal infection or foreign body, sexual assault, prolapse of the urethral meatus, and ingestion of estrogen-containing medications (most commonly, oral contraceptive preparations). A vaginal or cervical neoplasm is also a rare possibility. Thus, vaginal bleeding requires a vaginal examination, which is often best performed with the patient under anesthesia, before further evaluation is undertaken.

Heterosexual precocity in an apparent prepubertal female is almost always due to congenital adrenal hyperplasia or to an androgen-secreting adrenal or ovarian neoplasm. Only rarely must another disorder of sexual differentiation be considered (Chapter 241). It is important to examine the external genitalia carefully, because congenital adrenal hyperplasia is usually associated with some degree of sexual ambiguity.

Excessive androgens produced endogenously by abnormal fetal adrenal glands in utero or diffusing across the placenta to the fetus from the mother can virilize the external genitalia and result in female pseudohermaphroditism. The extent of virilization varies from only an enlarged clitoris to sexual ambiguity sufficient to make gender assignment difficult.

Excessive maternal androgen secretion, typically from an ovarian or adrenal neoplasm, can lead to virilization of a female fetus. This occurs very rarely because of the great capacity of the placenta to aromatize naturally occurring androgens to estrogens. Virilization of a female fetus is much more likely to occur if a pregnant woman has ingested a synthetic steroid preparation with androgenic properties, because synthetic compounds generally cannot be aromatized.

Excessive androgen secretion beginning in utero is usually associated with defective cortisol synthesis. As a consequence, pituitary corticotropin secretion is increased, resulting in congenital adrenal hyperplasia and excessive androgen secretion. The three different enzyme defects in the steroidogenic pathway that can lead to virilization of the female fetus are described in Chapter 241. The most common form of congenital adrenal hyperplasia is 21-hydroxylase deficiency, accounting for the disorder in more than 90% of affected individuals. The defect may vary from partial to complete deficiency of the enzyme.

Diagnostic Tests
Measurement of Peptide and Steroid Hormones
Increased levels of immunoreactive human chorionic gonadotropin (HCG) may suggest an HCG-secreting neoplasm, most commonly an ovarian teratoma or dysgerminoma. In such cases, the HCG, which is antigenically and

biologically similar to LH, stimulates ovarian steroid secretion and pseudo-pubertal development. Because even specific LH immunoassays show some cross-reactivity with HCG, values for serum LH may be elevated in individuals with HCG-secreting tumors. Immunoreactive HCG is always elevated in the presence of such tumors. Levels and ratios of FSH and LH typical of pubertal as opposed to prepubertal girls help in the diagnosis of true precocious puberty. Timed urine collections rather than blood samples can be used to measure gonadotropin secretion if necessary. The use of exogenous GnRH to stimulate endogenous LH and FSH secretion can help differentiate gonadotropin-dependent from gonadotropin-independent precocious puberty and is regarded as the "gold standard" in the diagnosis of central precocious puberty. If GnRH is not available, a GnRH analogue can be substituted. Excessively high circulating levels of estrogen (>100 pg estradiol) suggest an estrogen-producing neoplasm or a functioning ovarian cyst. High levels of serum testosterone suggest an ovarian source of excess androgen in girls with heterosexual development, whereas increased levels of dehydroepiandrosterone or its sulfate (the principal precursors of 17-ketosteroids) suggest an adrenal source. High levels of serum l7-hydroxyprogesterone imply congenital adrenal hyperplasia secondary to 21-hydroxylase deficiency, whereas high levels of serum 11-deoxycortisol imply an 11β-hydroxylase deficiency (Chapter 241). In congenital adrenal hyperplasia, these hormone levels should decrease promptly after the oral administration of suppressive doses of dexamethasone. Suppression in response to exogenous corticoids occurs much less consistently in individuals with adrenal cortical adenomas and carcinomas (Chapter 234) and rarely in those with ovarian androgen-secreting neoplasms.

Additional Studies

Imaging of the CNS is the most important test if true precocious puberty is present or if there are any neurologic deficits. Ultrasonography of the adrenals and ovaries or computed tomography (CT) of the adrenals may be indicated to confirm clinical suspicions. In girls with ovarian or adrenal neoplasms, the tumor can almost always be localized radiographically. Catheterization of the ovarian and adrenal veins and measurements of the effluent steroids from each gland should be pursued only when CT, ultrasonography, or MRI fails to identify a suspected neoplasm. Radiographic estimation of bone age is also indicated and serves as a useful tool to follow the results of treatment.

TREATMENT   Rx

Treatment of precocious puberty should be initiated promptly so that the patient's ultimate height is not compromised as a result of sex steroid–induced premature epiphyseal closure and to prevent or attenuate emotional disturbances in the patient and her parents.

GnRH analogues are now the preferred therapy for suppressing gonadotropin secretion, and they also may prevent early bone maturation. No randomized trials have been conducted, but there is universal acknowledgment that GnRH analogues increase ultimate adult height in girls presenting before 6 years of age. Two unresolved issues are whether to initiate treatment with GnRH analogues in girls between 6 and 8 years of age and at what age to stop treatment. The analogues are not effective in children with McCune-Albright syndrome, and ketoconazole and testolactone have been only marginally successful. Aqueous depot medroxyprogesterone acetate (100 to 200 mg intramuscularly every 2 to 4 weeks) also may be used to suppress gonadotropin secretion; however, it does not always prevent premature epiphyseal closure and the resultant short stature.

Individuals with CNS or steroid-secreting neoplasms must undergo therapy appropriate for the particular lesion. Girls with congenital adrenal hyperplasia are appropriately managed with glucocorticoids (plus mineralocorticoids when indicated), as outlined in Chapter 241.

Delayed Puberty

Girls who have no evidence of thelarche by age 13 or who fail to undergo menarche by age 15 have delayed puberty and should be evaluated. Ovarian failure, congenital absence of the uterus and vagina, and constitutional delay constitute about two thirds of cases in large series. Because of the anxiety generated by delayed puberty, some evaluation is always indicated regardless of the age of the patient.

When pubertal development progresses normally but menstruation does not begin, an abnormality in the genital tract should be considered. Congenital malformations of the müllerian ducts are uncommon, occurring in 0.02% of all women. Most do not cause amenorrhea, and many do not impair reproduction. The anomalies associated with amenorrhea vary in severity from an imperforate hymen to complete aplasia of all müllerian duct derivatives, with vaginal atresia. Although aplasia generally involves all the müllerian duct derivatives, defects may involve only a single part of the distal genital tract. Family aggregates of the most common disorders of müllerian differentiation in females—müllerian aplasia and incomplete müllerian fusion—do occur and are best explained by polygenic or multifactorial inheritance. It is clear that the HOX genes, a family of regulatory genes that encode transcription factors, are essential for proper development of the müllerian tract.

A müllerian duct anomaly is suggested by (1) normal levels of serum gonadotropins and steroids, (2) an abnormal outflow tract, (3) a history of cyclic abdominal pain with or without a palpable mass, and (4) normal development of secondary sex characteristics. Normal ovarian function still induces endometrial growth and shedding after menarche if the uterus is normal. In the absence of a normal outflow tract, however, the menstrual effluent is retained and may or may not be able to escape into the abdominal cavity. Free in the abdominal cavity, the effluent may cause endometriosis. Constrained to the uterine cavity, the effluent causes hematometra and a large abdominal mass. In the absence of a mass or cyclic pain, karyotyping is indicated in girls with evidence of an abnormal genital tract to rule out disorders of sexual differentiation (Chapter 241). Such disorders, however, almost never occur together with completely normal pubertal development. In girls with a normal karyotype and a genital tract anomaly, examination under anesthesia and diagnostic laparoscopy should be undertaken to delineate the extent of the defect. When the abnormality consists of an imperforate hymen or transverse vaginal septum only, surgical restoration can be accomplished relatively simply. Attempts to provide an outflow tract for the uterus should not be undertaken if there is no cervix because of the high risk of recurrent pelvic infection. Even with a functional cervix, the construction of an outflow tract that permits successful pregnancy is unlikely. A functional vagina can be constructed surgically or by the daily use of ever-larger dilators. To prevent shrinkage and scarring, surgery should be deferred until the patient is willing to use dilators on a daily basis or she is about to become sexually active.

Other causes of delayed puberty and primary amenorrhea are the same as those that cause amenorrhea in older women (Chapter 244). When no apparent cause of delayed development is found, constitutional delayed puberty must be entertained as a diagnosis of exclusion. A strong family history of delayed maturation supports this presumption. Small doses of estrogen can be administered to induce some pubertal development, but this may obscure a pathologic cause of the delay and may compromise linear growth and ultimate height.

Asynchronous Pubertal Development

Asynchronous pubertal development is characteristic of male pseudohermaphroditism due to androgen insensitivity, especially complete testicular feminization. This syndrome of androgen insensitivity is inherited as either an X-linked recessive trait or a sex-limited autosomal dominant trait. Despite the presence of intra-abdominal or inguinal testes, there is complete failure of virilization. Affected individuals develop breasts (but only to Tanner stage 3) and a typical female habitus with unambiguous female external genitalia, but with the absence of internal female structures and generally only a foreshortened, blind-ending vagina. Little or no pubic and axillary hair develops. The karyotype is 46,XY in these individuals. Circulating testosterone levels are equivalent to or higher than those found in normal men, LH levels are elevated, and FSH levels are normal compared with those in menstruating women. For a more detailed description, see Chapter 241.

Heterosexual Pubertal Development
POLYCYSTIC OVARY SYNDROME

Polycystic ovary syndrome (PCOS), by far the most common cause of heterosexual pubertal development, is associated with the development of some secondary sex features characteristic of males at the normal age of puberty. Feminization occurs in affected girls, and they develop normal breasts and a typical female habitus, but masculinization also occurs (in contrast, girls with congenital adrenal hyperplasia generally show little if any female development at puberty). A heterogeneous syndrome, PCOS typically begins at or near puberty with hirsutism and irregular menses from the time of menarche. Many girls who develop PCOS are overweight in childhood, and obesity is clearly a risk factor. It now appears that many girls who develop PCOS were growth restricted in utero. Menarche may be delayed in a few cases, so young women may present with primary amenorrhea. Basal LH levels tend to be somewhat elevated in perhaps two thirds of cases, and circulating levels of all androgens are moderately elevated. Some degree of insulin resistance is almost invariably present as well, and hypercholesterolemia may predispose to cardiovascular disease later in life. This is discussed more completely in Chapter 244.

CONGENITAL ADRENAL HYPERPLASIA

Congenital adrenal hyperplasia is generally diagnosed before puberty, and heterosexual precocious pseudopuberty is typical. However, if the defect is mild and changes to the external genitalia are minimal, masculinization may occur at the expected age of puberty. This attenuated or nonclassic form of 21-hydroxylase deficiency seems to occur in families with a strong history of hirsutism. Affected girls generally have some defemination, with flattening of the breasts, severe hirsutism, relatively short stature, and obesity. For a more detailed description, see Chapter 241.

MIXED GONADAL DYSGENESIS

Mixed gonadal dysgenesis designates asymmetrical gonadal development, with a germ cell tumor or a testis on one side and an undifferentiated streak, rudimentary gonad, or no gonad on the other. The extent of genital virilization before puberty is variable in this rare disorder. Most individuals are reared as girls, in whom virilization occurs at puberty; some may note breast development as well. Affected individuals generally have a mosaic karyotype, with 45,X/46,XY being most common. Short stature and other stigmata associated with a 45,X karyotype in Turner's syndrome are less common in patients with tumors than in patients with testes. Gonadectomy is indicated in all individuals with a Y chromosome to eliminate the increased neoplastic potential of such dysgenetic gonads and in all patients in whom virilization occurs at puberty to remove the source of androgen. Estrogen replacement therapy is warranted after gonadectomy. Other causes of male pseudohermaphroditism associated with heterosexual pubertal development are described in Chapter 241.

OTHER CAUSES

An androgen-producing adrenal neoplasm or Cushing's syndrome may occur rarely during the pubertal years and lead to heterosexual development (Chapter 234).

SUGGESTED READINGS

Bhangoo A, Jacobson-Dickman E. The genetics of idiopathic hypogonadotropic hypogonadism: unraveling the biology of human sexual development. *Pediatr Endocrinol Rev.* 2009;6:395-404. *Review of what is known about the genetics of isolated hypogonadotropic hypogonadism.*

Carel JC, Eugster EA, Rogol A, et al. Consensus statement on the use of gonadotropin-releasing hormone analogs in children. *Pediatrics.* 2009;123:e752-e762. *Guidelines for the use of GnRH analogues for the treatment of precocious puberty.*

Caronia LM, Martin C, Welt CK, et al. A genetic basis for functional hypothalamic amenorrhea. *N Engl J Med.* 2011;364:215-225. *Variants of hypogonadotrophic hypogonadism genes may increase the risk of hypothalamic amenorrhea.*

Mogensen SS, Aksglaede L, Mouritsen A, et al. Diagnostic work-up of 449 consecutive girls who were referred to be evaluated for precocious puberty. *J Clin Endocrinol Metab.* 2011;96:1393-1401. *Review of 449 consecutive cases, including 88 with central precocious puberty, 68 with premature thelarche, 49 with premature adrenarche, and 129 with early-normal variant.*

Richards JS, Pangas SA. The ovary: basic biology and clinical implications. *J Clin Invest.* 2010;120:963-972. *Review.*

244

REPRODUCTIVE ENDOCRINOLOGY AND INFERTILITY

ROBERT W. REBAR AND GREGORY F. ERICKSON

THE NORMAL MENSTRUAL CYCLE

Between menarche and menopause, the reproductive organs of normal women undergo a series of closely coordinated changes at monthly intervals that constitute the normal menstrual cycle. The menstrual cycle is the expression of the coordinated interactions of the hypothalamic-pituitary-ovarian

axis, with associated changes in the target tissues (endometrium, cervix, vagina) of the reproductive tract.

A menstrual cycle begins with the first day of genital bleeding (day 1; menses) and ends just before the next menstrual period. The median menstrual cycle length is 28 days but ranges from 21 to 35 days. Menstrual cycles vary most in the years immediately after menarche and preceding menopause, partly because of an increase in anovulatory cycles. Irregularities in menstrual cycle length may be caused by changes in diet, exercise, emotional disturbances, parturition, or abortion. The menstrual cycle has three distinct phases: follicular, ovulatory, and luteal.

Follicular (Preovulatory) Phase

The follicular phase begins with the first day of bleeding and extends to the day before the preovulatory luteinizing hormone (LH) surge. A rise in serum follicle-stimulating hormone (FSH) begins in the late luteal phase of the previous menstrual cycle and continues into the early follicular phase. This initiates development of a group of follicles (Fig. 244-1). The preovulatory follicle destined for ovulation is selected from this cohort. After the early follicular phase, FSH levels fall, and LH levels rise slowly. About 7 days before the preovulatory LH surge, estradiol and estrone increase until the day before the LH surge. The divergence in LH and FSH levels may be related to secretion of inhibin B, which inhibits the release of FSH. Several days before the LH surge, plasma androgens and some progestins begin to increase. They peak on the day of the LH surge. Progesterone does not increase until just before the LH surge onset.

Ovulatory Phase

During this phase, the ovum is released from the mature graafian follicle about 32 to 34 hours after the preovulatory LH surge. The ovulatory phase extends from 1 day before the LH surge to 1 day after the LH surge (see Fig. 244-1). Some women experience unilateral pelvic pain near the time of

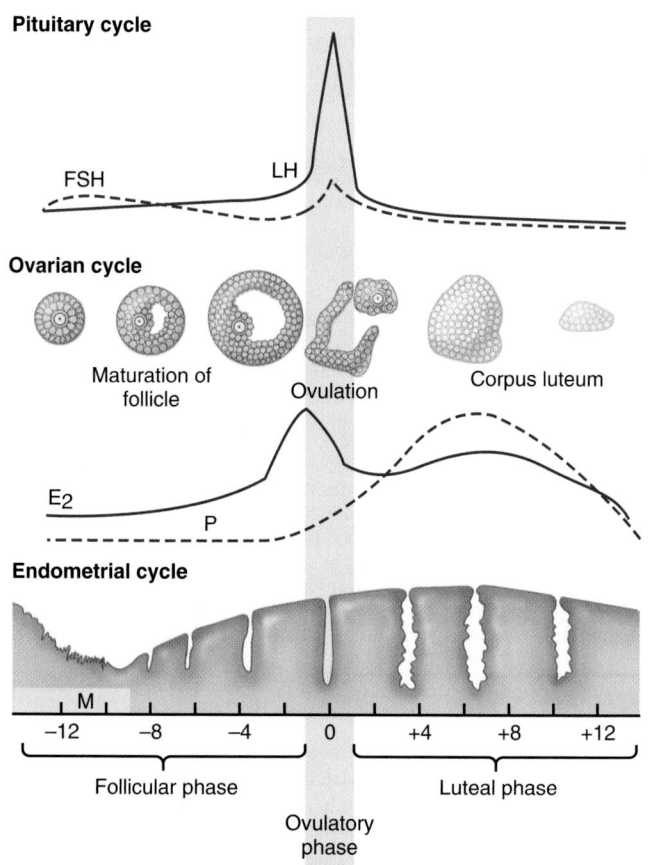

FIGURE 244-1. The idealized cyclic changes observed in gonadotropins, estradiol (E₂), progesterone (P), and uterine endometrium during the normal menstrual cycle. The data are centered on the day of the luteinizing hormone (LH) surge (day 0). Days of menstrual bleeding are indicated by M. FSH = follicle-stimulating hormone; LH = luteinizing hormone. (From Endocrine and Metabolism Continuing Education Quality Control Program, 1982. Copyright American Association for Clinical Chemistry, Inc.)

ovulation, termed *mittelschmerz,* which occurs before or after ovulation. During the ovulatory phase, a rapid rise in plasma LH in response to positive estrogen feedback leads to ovulation. As peak LH levels are reached, estradiol levels drop, but progesterone levels increase.

Luteal (Postovulatory) Phase

The luteal phase is about 14 days in length and ends with the onset of menses (see Fig. 244-1). This phase includes the functional lifespan of the corpus luteum, which supports the released ovum by secreting progesterone. Progesterone secretion increases up to 8 days after the LH surge. Smaller increases in 17α-hydroxyprogesterone, estradiol, and estrone occur. Progesterone decreases before menses unless the ovum is fertilized and pregnancy results. A serum progesterone level higher than 10 ng/mL 1 week before menses is probably diagnostic of normal ovulation.

● CYCLIC CHANGES IN TARGET ORGANS

Endometrium

The endometrium undergoes histologic and cytologic changes that culminate with menstrual bleeding when the corpus luteum ceases to secrete progesterone (see Fig. 244-1). The basal layer of the endometrium then regenerates the superficial layer of compact epithelial cells lining the uterine cavity and an intermediate layer of spongiosa. Both layers are shed at menstruation. Endometrial glands proliferate under the influence of estrogen, and the mucosa thickens. In the luteal phase, the glands become coiled and secretory, with increased vascularity and edema of the stroma. When estradiol and progesterone decline, the stroma becomes edematous, endometrial and blood vessel necrosis occurs, and bleeding ensues. Local release of prostaglandins may initiate vasospasm with ischemic necrosis and uterine contractions that accompany menstrual flow. Prostaglandin synthetase inhibitors can relieve menstrual cramping. The histologic changes are characteristic; therefore, endometrial biopsies can be used to characterize the stage of the cycle and to assess the tissue response to gonadal steroids.

Cervix and Cervical Mucus

During the follicular phase, cervical vascularity, congestion, and edema increase as a result of estrogen. Cervical mucus increases in quantity (10- to 30-fold) and in elasticity. So-called ferning becomes prominent. Progesterone stimulates cervical mucus thickening and loss of elasticity and ability to fern. These characteristics are useful in evaluating the stage of the cycle and the amount of estrogen present.

Vagina

Low estrogen is associated with pale, thin vaginal epithelium. As estrogens rise, the number of cornified epithelial cells increases. Subsequently, progesterone decreases the percentage of cornified cells and increases the number of precornified intermediate cells. There is also increased cellular debris and clumping of shed desquamated cells. Histologic changes in the vaginal epithelium are sensitive indicators of estrogen status.

Ovary

The ovaries produce a single dominant graafian follicle that grows and develops to the preovulatory stage during the follicular phase. This process is brought about by combined action of FSH and LH on the follicle wall to increase estradiol biosynthesis. The LH surge acts on the preovulatory follicle to cause the secretion of the mature fertilizable oocyte. After ovulation, the follicle wall transforms into the corpus luteum, which produces progesterone and estradiol. If implantation does not occur, the corpus luteum undergoes luteolysis and stops hormone production. In the late luteal phase, another dominant follicle develops, and a new menstrual cycle begins.

Chronology of Folliculogenesis

The preovulatory follicle begins its development when a primordial follicle is recruited into the pool of growing follicles. There are two major phases of folliculogenesis: the preantral (gonadotropin-independent) and the antral (gonadotropin-dependent) periods. The first phase is characterized by growth of the oocyte and granulosa proliferation. Preantral folliculogenesis proceeds slowly, requiring at least 300 days. During the second phase, granulosa and theca cells proliferate, and the antrum enlarges. The graafian follicle increases relatively rapidly as it develops. The mature graafian follicle that will ovulate requires 40 to 50 days to complete the antral phase.

Selection

The dominant follicle is selected from a cohort at the end of the luteal phase of the previous menstrual cycle. The selected follicle requires 20 days to develop to the ovulatory stage.

Shortly after the midluteal phase of the cycle, the granulosa cells show a sharp increase in the rate of mitosis. The first indication of selection is that the granulosa cells continue dividing at a high rate. As a consequence of the high sustained mitotic rate and the progressive accumulation of follicular fluid, the dominant follicle undergoes remarkable growth. The increase in plasma FSH levels that begins at the end of luteal phase and continues through the early follicular phase evokes follicle selection. The concentration of FSH in the follicular fluid of the healthy (dominant) follicle increases but does not increase in the nondominant atretic follicles. The manner in which this selective increase in FSH is controlled is unknown. More than 99.9% of all follicles are not selected and undergo atresia.

Mechanism of Follicle-Stimulating Hormone Action

FSH exerts its influence on follicle growth and development by stimulating granulosa cell mitosis and cytodifferentiation. FSH activates high-affinity receptors on the granulosa cell. The binding event is transduced into an intracellular signal through the cyclic adenosine monophosphate (cAMP)-dependent protein kinase A signal transduction pathway (E-Fig. 244-1). This leads to an increase in cell number and cytodifferentiation.

The granulosa cells in the chosen follicle continue to divide at a relatively rapid rate throughout the follicular phase of the cycle, increasing from 1×10^6 cells to 50×10^6 cells at ovulation. FSH induces granulosa cytodifferentiation in the dominant follicle. Expression of cytochrome P-450 aromatase (P450arom) is induced by FSH (see E-Fig. 244-1). The temporal pattern of expression of P450arom determines when and how much estradiol is produced. FSH also induces the expression of LH receptors. This is delayed until the dominant follicle is fully differentiated at day 12. The large number of LH receptors in the granulosa cells is essential for the LH surge to trigger ovulation. The terminal differentiation of the granulosa cells is characterized by the accumulation of other FSH-regulated gene products, including inhibin B, activin, and follistatin.

Mechanism of Luteinizing Hormone Action

The primary function of LH in follicle development is to stimulate androgen production by the theca interstitial cells (see E-Fig. 244-1). LH binds to LH human chorionic gonadotropin (hCG) receptors located on theca cells, which interact with G proteins and activate adenylate cyclase, leading to the synthesis of cAMP, which stimulates gene expression through protein kinase A. This leads to increased conversion of cholesterol to androstenedione. Theca cells express insulin receptors, and insulin stimulates theca androgen production. The crosstalk between the insulin and LH receptor signaling is clinically relevant because of the relationship between hyperinsulinemia and hyperandrogenism in women.

One of the most important consequences of FSH and LH action on the dominant follicle is the production of estradiol. This physiologically important process is called the *two-gonadotropin, two-cell concept* of follicular estrogen production (see E-Fig. 244-1).

Ovulation

At midpoint in the menstrual cycle, the preovulatory surges of LH and FSH act on the preovulatory follicle to initiate the events leading to ovulation (E-Fig. 244-2). The LH surge induces meiotic maturation, a process that converts the oocyte into a fertilizable egg arrested at the second meiotic metaphase. During meiotic maturation, the granulosa cells next to the oocyte are stimulated by FSH to undergo cumulus expansion. This is a prerequisite for the egg's pickup and transport by the oviduct. The LH surge also stimulates production of proteolytic enzymes in the vicinity of the presumptive stigma. This process requires the LH stimulation of progesterone and prostaglandins, which are obligatory for stigma formation. After 36 hours, the fertilizable egg and surrounding cumulus cells are secreted through the stigma (see E-Fig. 244-2).

Luteogenesis

Ovulation leads to changes in the granulosa and theca cells of the ovulated follicle that result in increased production of progesterone and estradiol during the first week of the luteal phase. This event, termed *luteinization,* is important for the formation and development of a secretory endometrium.

Three major physiologic mechanisms are responsible for luteinization: removal of luteinization inhibitors; secretion of LH by the pituitary; and delivery of high levels of cholesterol. The induction of StAR, P450c22, and 3β-hydroxysteroid dehydrogenase in the granulosa lutein cells leads to progesterone production by the corpus luteum. The two-cell, two-gonadotropin mechanism is responsible for estradiol production. If implantation does not occur, the corpus luteum initiates luteolysis, leading to decreases in progesterone, estradiol, and apoptosis. When luteolysis occurs, another dominant follicle is selected, and a new menstrual cycle begins.

Neuroendocrine Regulation of the Ovaries

Neurons containing various peptide hormones that can release or inhibit secretion of the gonadotropins are found in the hypothalamus (Chapter 230). Cells containing gonadotropin-releasing hormone (GnRH) occur in the arcuate nucleus, median eminence, and preoptic area. Axons from these neurons run in the tuberoinfundibular tract and terminate on capillaries within the median eminence, allowing delivery of their products to the anterior pituitary gland. Neurotransmitters, including norepinephrine, dopamine, and serotonin, as well as neuromodulators, such as endogenous opiates and prostaglandins, influence secretion of GnRH. Estrogens and androgens bind to cells in the hypothalamus and the anterior pituitary, and progestins bind to cells in the hypothalamus, to influence hypothalamic-pituitary regulation of ovarian function.

GnRH is secreted in a pulsatile fashion and is responsible for pulsatile release of gonadotropins. Pulsatile gonadotropin release accounts for the pulsatile secretion of sex steroids from the ovaries. The ovarian sex steroids feed back on the hypothalamic-pituitary unit to modulate both the frequency and amplitude of the gonadotropin pulse (Fig. 244-2). Gonadotropin pulses vary throughout the menstrual cycle. Pulses occur at approximately 60- to 90-minute intervals in the follicular phase and at intervals of 180 minutes in the luteal phase.

Gonadal steroids can exert both negative and positive feedback effects on gonadotropin secretion. 17β-Estradiol is the most potent inhibitor of gonadotropin secretion. For women to ovulate, estradiol must also elicit a positive feedback effect on gonadotropin release. The feedback effects are both time and dose dependent. In the normal menstrual cycle, the positive feedback action of estradiol leading to the LH surge is preceded by a period when lower estradiol levels are present.

It appears that the ovary is the "clock" for the timing of ovulation, with the hypothalamus stimulating pulsatile release of the gonadotropins. The follicle complex and corpus luteum develop in response to gonadotropin stimulation. For appropriate ovarian regulation of reproductive function in women, three biologic characteristics are necessary: an appropriate balance and sequence of negative and positive feedback actions; differential feedback effects on the release of LH and FSH; and local intraovarian controls on follicular growth and maturation.

ABNORMALITIES OF THE REPRODUCTIVE YEARS
Dysmenorrhea and Endometriosis

DEFINITION

Dysmenorrhea, defined as painful menstruation, affects about 50% of postpubertal women and can be classified as primary or secondary. *Endometriosis*, which may result in dysmenorrhea, infertility, and dyspareunia (i.e., painful intercourse), is the ectopic occurrence of endometrial tissue, most commonly within the abdominal cavity but sometimes in surgical scars, on the vulva, in the umbilicus, and elsewhere.

PATHOBIOLOGY

Primary dysmenorrhea occurs only in ovulatory cycles. Prostaglandins produce dysmenorrhea by initiating painful, exaggerated uterine contractions and myometrial ischemia. Associated systemic symptoms include nausea, diarrhea, headache, and emotional changes. In secondary dysmenorrhea, there is a pathologic cause, with endometriosis being the most common. Other causes include pelvic inflammatory disease; congenital abnormalities, such as atresia of a portion of the distal genital tract and cystic duplication of the paramesonephric ducts; and cervical stenosis. Recent studies suggest the possibility that the pain of endometriosis is caused by the presence of nerve fibers within ectopic endometrium.

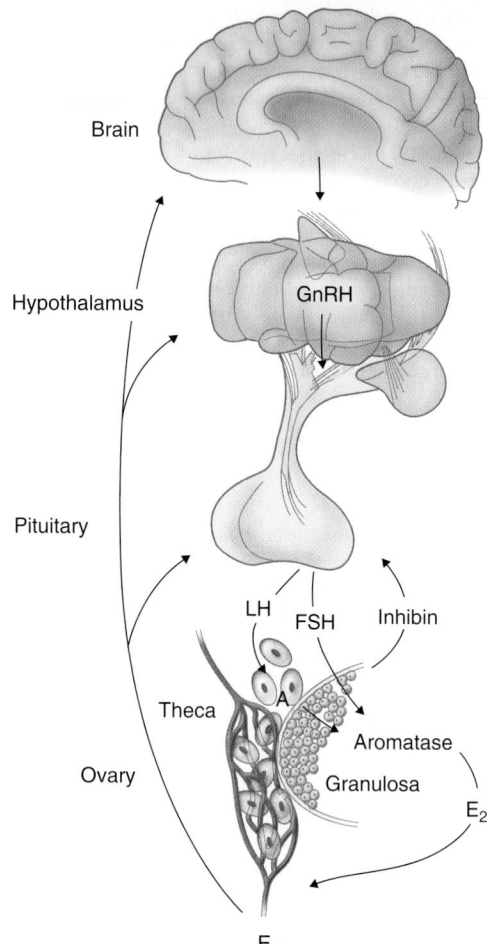

FIGURE 244-2. The hypothalamic-pituitary-ovarian axis in the regulation of follicular maturation and steroidogenesis. A = androgens; E_2 = estradiol; FSH = follicle-stimulating hormone; GnRH = gonadotropin-releasing hormone; LH = luteinizing hormone. (Modified from Endocrine and Metabolism Continuing Education Quality Control Program, 1982. Copyright American Association for Clinical Chemistry, Inc.)

TREATMENT   Rx

Prostaglandin synthetase inhibitors (Chapter 36), such as naproxen, ibuprofen, mefenamic acid, and indomethacin, are used to treat primary dysmenorrhea. If the dysmenorrhea persists, addition of an oral contraceptive to inhibit ovulation and limit prostaglandin release is generally effective. In cases in which the pelvic pain remains intractable, additional evaluation is warranted. If thorough evaluation of the gastrointestinal and urinary tracts fails to reveal a definitive cause, examination under anesthesia and diagnostic laparoscopy may be indicated.

If endometriosis is diagnosed at laparoscopy, treatment varies according to the severity of the disease and the goals of the patient regarding fertility. It may be possible to fulgurate implants or to lyse adhesions. Available data support ablation at the time of initial diagnosis as the preferred approach to controlling symptoms. From this point onward, efforts should be directed toward treating endometriosis medically, with additional surgery deferred until infertility (if present) becomes manifest. Medical therapy can consist of continuous suppression with oral contraceptives, progestins (oral, injectable, or implantable), or GnRH analogues or danazol for 3 to 6 months. GnRH analogues are currently the most frequently used form of medical suppressive therapy. After a course of treatment, use of oral contraceptive agents should probably be continued until fertility is desired. Conservative surgical resection of endometriotic tissue should almost always be deferred until it is established as the cause of infertility. Surgery may be required, however, for continuing severe pain, severe endometriosis, or large ovarian cysts containing endometriosis (endometriomas). If symptoms continue despite adequate treatment or if psychological overlay is suspected, psychiatric evaluation may be indicated. Medical causes of dysmenorrhea, however, should be eliminated first.

Premenstrual Syndrome

DEFINITION

Premenstrual syndrome (PMS), also known as *premenstrual tension*, is a complex of physical and emotional symptoms that occur repetitively in a cyclic fashion before menstruation and that diminish or disappear with menstruation.

DIAGNOSIS

The cyclic symptoms typically are sufficiently severe to interfere with some aspects of life. More than 150 different symptoms are now thought to vary with the menstrual cycle (Table 244-1). Estimates of the prevalence of PMS range from 25 to 100%. The *Diagnostic and Statistical Manual of Mental Disorders* classifies severe PMS as premenstrual dysphoric disorder (PMDD). For most women, PMS is merely annoying; severe PMS (or PMDD) causes serious difficulties for 3 to 5% of women of reproductive age. The diagnosis of both PMS and PMDD is best established by requiring patients to keep prospective daily records of symptoms during a 2- to 3-month period. Less than 50% of women complaining of PMS are found to have the syndrome when such records are examined.

Most women seek help for PMS in their 30s after 10 or more years of symptoms. Many report that their symptoms began at menarche; approximately half state that symptoms followed childbirth. Severity and duration of symptoms are often reported to increase after each successive pregnancy and to become more severe with advancing age. Women with severe long-standing PMS almost always describe associated psychological reactions, including social difficulties, such as marital discord, difficulty relating to their children, difficulty maintaining friendships, and withdrawal from social activities.

TABLE 244-1 COMMON SYMPTOMS OF CYCLIC PREMENSTRUAL SYNDROME

SOMATIC SYMPTOMS	
Abdominal bloating	Constipation or diarrhea
Acne	Headache
Alcohol intolerance	Peripheral edema
Breast engorgement and tenderness	Weight gain
Clumsiness	

EMOTIONAL AND MENTAL SYMPTOMS	
Anxiety	Insomnia
Change in libido	Irritability
Depression	Lethargy
Fatigue	Mood swings
Food cravings (especially salt and sugar)	Panic attacks
Hostility	Paranoia
Inability to concentrate	Violence toward self and others
Increased appetite	Withdrawal from others

TREATMENT Rx

General Measures

The cause of PMS is unknown, and patients should be informed that no one therapy has been effective in all women. Women with mild premenstrual symptoms often benefit from simple changes in lifestyle, including daily mild aerobic exercise; reduction in intake of xanthine-containing beverages, salt, and refined sugar, particularly in the luteal phase; stress reduction; and adequate rest.

Medical Therapy

Women with more severe PMS may benefit from symptomatic treatment. Bromocriptine (generally 2.5 mg twice a day) or danazol (100 to 400 mg/day in two divided doses) may be given continuously for relief of mastalgia (breast pain), although this use is not listed in the manufacturer's directive or approved by the U.S. Food and Drug Administration (FDA). Prostaglandin synthetase inhibitors may help reduce dysmenorrhea and may alleviate headaches. Mild sedatives and tranquilizers may help reduce insomnia and anxiety. Low doses of fluoxetine (20 mg) and other selective serotonin reuptake inhibitors, administered either daily or for the last 2 weeks of each menstrual cycle, are highly effective in reducing the emotional symptoms associated with PMS. Mild diuretics (especially spironolactone at doses up to 100 mg each morning) may benefit cyclic edema.

Natural progesterone, given in the form of vaginal suppositories, has been used, but results of double-blind placebo-controlled trials show no efficacy. Likewise, the value of large quantities of multiple vitamins or of oil of evening primrose, containing the essential fatty acid γ-linolenic acid, a precursor of prostaglandins, is unsubstantiated.

Surgical Therapy

Because PMS requires the occurrence of cyclic ovulation, oophorectomy is occasionally considered for patients with particularly intractable symptoms. However, oophorectomy may create new problems related to estrogen deficiency for women with PMS treated in this permanent fashion. Several trials employing a GnRH agonist together with exogenous steroids have been described as reducing PMS. Whether such therapy can be used in the long term remains to be determined.

Abnormal Uterine Bleeding

DIAGNOSIS

Differential Diagnosis

Because there is considerable confusion about terminology of abnormal uterine bleeding, it is important to determine just what is being included in any term used other than *abnormal uterine bleeding*. Postmenarchal bleeding in adolescents secondary to immaturity of the hypothalamic-pituitary-ovarian axis (resulting in anovulation) accounts for about 20% of cases, and perimenopausal bleeding consequent to incipient ovarian failure constitutes more than half.

The causes of abnormal uterine bleeding in the reproductive years include complications from the use of oral contraceptives; complications of pregnancy, especially threatened, incomplete, or missed miscarriages and ectopic pregnancy; coagulation disorders, most commonly idiopathic thrombocytopenic purpura and von Willebrand's disease; and pelvic disease, such as intrauterine polyps, leiomyomas, and tumors of the vagina and cervix. Clear cell adenocarcinoma of the vagina or cervix may occur in women exposed to diethylstilbestrol during fetal life. Affected women may also have congenital abnormalities of the upper vagina, cervix, and uterus. Women with a history of diethylstilbestrol exposure should be reassured that the incidence of malignant change is extremely low. Trauma (coital or otherwise), foreign bodies, systemic illnesses including various endocrinopathies (such as diabetes mellitus, hypothyroidism and hyperthyroidism, Cushing's syndrome, and Addison's disease), leukemia, and renal disease may also be associated with abnormal bleeding as the presenting manifestation.

Abnormal uterine bleeding with no demonstrable organic genital or extragenital cause (75% of cases) is most frequently associated with anovulation and is appropriately termed *anovulatory* (sometimes termed *dysfunctional*) *bleeding*. Most anovulatory bleeding is due to either estrogen withdrawal or estrogen breakthrough bleeding. In anovulatory women, estrogen stimulates the endometrium unopposed by progesterone. The endometrium proliferates, becomes thicker, and may shed irregularly. Anovulatory bleeding tends to occur at less frequent intervals, and organic lesions tend to cause bleeding more frequently than cyclic menses.

CLINICAL EVALUATION

All cases of abnormal bleeding should be evaluated, beginning with a thorough history emphasizing the amount and duration of blood loss. Prospective charting of the days on which bleeding occurs may be required to evaluate the bleeding pattern. Complications of pregnancy or a bleeding diathesis must always be ruled out.

The findings on physical examination (including the Papanicolaou smear) are normal in anovulatory bleeding except for signs of anemia in the more severe cases. Laboratory tests should include a complete blood count, platelet count, coagulation studies, thyroid function tests, and fasting blood glucose concentration. Anovulatory bleeding must be a diagnosis of exclusion, with management depending on the age of the patient and the extent of the bleeding. A sample of the endometrium should be obtained by biopsy or by dilation and curettage from all women older than 35 years and from those at increased risk for endometrial carcinoma because of prolonged anovulatory bleeding.

TREATMENT

Even profuse bleeding in anovulatory women can almost always be successfully treated by the administration of one combination oral contraceptive pill every 6 hours for 5 to 7 days, although this use is not listed in the manufacturer's directive or approved by the FDA. Bleeding should cease within 24 hours, but patients should be warned to expect heavy bleeding 2 to 4 days after therapy is stopped. If anemia is profound, blood transfusion may be necessary. If the bleeding continues despite therapy, curettage can be carried out. Recurrence can be prevented by giving the patient combination oral contraceptive agents cyclically. If spontaneous cyclic menses do not resume and pregnancy is not desired, the patient can be treated with cyclic progestin (medroxyprogesterone acetate, 5 to 10 mg for 10 to 14 days each month) or oral contraceptive agents. If pregnancy is desired, ovulation can be induced.

Acute episodes of anovulatory bleeding can also be treated with conjugated estrogens administered intravenously (25 mg every 4 hours for up to three doses) until bleeding ceases, although this use is not listed in the manufacturer's directive or approved by the FDA. Progestin therapy (medroxyprogesterone acetate, 5 to 10 mg orally for 10 days) should be started simultaneously. Withdrawal bleeding occurs after cessation of therapy, and the patient can then be treated with oral contraceptive agents for at least three cycles.

For individuals with anovulatory bleeding without an episode of profuse bleeding, treatment with cyclic oral contraceptive agents or progestin can be provided unless pregnancy is desired, in which case ovulation must be induced.

Endometrial ablation by any of several methods is being used increasingly to treat persistent bleeding. However, ablation is not 100% effective, and medical management remains the first line of therapy for most women. Hysterectomy may be an appropriate choice for a small number of women.

Amenorrhea

DEFINITION

Amenorrhea is the absence of menstruation for 3 months or more in women with past menses (secondary amenorrhea) or the absence of menarche by the age of 15 years regardless of the absence or presence of secondary sex characteristics (primary amenorrhea).

PATHOBIOLOGY

If an intact genital outflow tract exists and there is no primary disease of the uterus, amenorrhea is a sign of failure of the hypothalamic-pituitary-ovarian axis to produce cyclically the hormones necessary for menses. Amenorrhea is physiologic in the prepubertal girl, during pregnancy and early in lactation, and after menopause. At any other time, it is pathologic and demands evaluation. Use of the term *postpill amenorrhea* to refer to failure to resume menses within 3 months of discontinuation of oral contraceptives is inappropriate. Women so affected should be evaluated in the same manner as any woman with amenorrhea. Similarly, individuals with menses occurring at infrequent intervals of more than 40 days or having fewer than nine menses per year, termed *oligomenorrhea*, should be evaluated identically to women with amenorrhea.

DIAGNOSIS

Clinical Evaluation

In patients with amenorrhea, even subtle hormonal abnormalities may lead to signs and symptoms. Breast development indicates exposure to estrogens, and the presence of pubic and axillary hair indicates androgenic stimulation.

Patients should be questioned especially closely for evidence of psychological disturbances, dietary and exercise habits, lifestyle, environmental stresses, family history of genetic anomalies, abnormal growth and development, and signs of hyperandrogenism, including hirsutism, temporal balding, deepening of the voice, increased muscle mass, clitorimegaly, and increased libido, and signs of defeminization, including decreasing breast size and vaginal atrophy. Any history of galactorrhea should be determined. A history of symptoms related to thyroid and adrenal dysfunction should also be sought (Chapters 231, 233, and 234).

The physical examination should focus on the evaluation of body dimensions and habitus, extent and distribution of body hair, breast development and secretions, and genitalia. In normal adult women, the arm span is similar to the height; in hypogonadal women, the span is generally more than 5 cm greater than the height. The distribution and quantity of body hair should be considered in view of the family history. The extent of any hirsutism should be recorded, preferably by photographs. Other signs of virilization should be sought carefully. Breast development should be graded according to the method of Tanner (Table 244-2). Breast secretion should be sought by applying pressure to the breasts while the patient is seated. Any secretion should be examined microscopically for the presence of perfectly round fat globules of varying size, which indicate galactorrhea. Finally, the female genitalia should be examined carefully because they are such sensitive indicators of the hormonal milieu. The Tanner stage of pubic hair development should be noted (see Table 244-2).

Because the sensitivity of the genitalia to androgens decreases onward from early in fetal development, the extent of any virilization is important. Fusion of the labia and enlargement of the clitoris with or without formation of a penile urethra are observed in women exposed to androgens during the first 3 months of fetal development (Chapter 241). Significant clitorimegaly in the absence of other signs of sexual ambiguity and in the presence of other signs of virilization requires marked androgenic stimulation and strongly implicates an androgen-secreting neoplasm. The development of the labia minora in postpubertal women indicates the influence of estrogens. Overt anomalies of the distal genital tract and any evidence of obstruction to the escape of menstrual blood should be sought. Under the influence of estrogen, the vaginal mucosa changes during sexual maturation from a tissue with a shiny, bright red appearance with sparse, thin secretions to a dull, gray-pink rugated surface with copious, thick secretions.

The history and physical examination quickly differentiate among several causes of amenorrhea (Table 244-3). The various disorders of sexual differentiation and the other anatomic causes are often apparent on inspection. Distal genital tract obstruction should be identified at the time of pelvic examination even if the specific abnormality is not obvious. The physical stigmata of Turner's syndrome, discussed subsequently, generally make the diagnosis simple. Any sexual ambiguity indicates the need for chromosomal

---

TABLE 244-2 CRITERIA FOR DISTINGUISHING TANNER STAGES 1 TO 5 DURING PUBERTAL MATURATION

TANNER STAGE	BREAST	PUBIC HAIR
1 (Prepubertal)	No palpable glandular tissue or pigmentation of areola; elevation of areola only	No pubic hair; short, fine vellus hair only
2	Glandular tissue palpable with elevation of breast and areola together as a small mound; areolar diameter increased	Sparse, long, pigmented terminal hair chiefly along the labia majora
3	Further enlargement without separation of breast and areola; although more darkly pigmented, areola still pale and immature; nipple generally at or above midplane of breast tissue when individual is seated upright	Dark, coarse, curly hair, extending sparsely over mons
4	Secondary mound of areola and papilla above breast	Adult-type hair, abundant but limited to mons and labia
5 (Adult)	Recession of areola to contour of breast; development of Montgomery's glands and ducts on areola; further pigmentation of areola; nipple generally below midplane of breast tissue when individual is seated upright; maturation independent of breast size	Adult-type hair in quantity and distribution; spread to inner aspects of the thighs in most racial groups

Data from Ross GT. Disorders of the ovary and female reproductive tract. In: Wilson JD, Foster DW, eds. *Textbook of Endocrinology*, 7th ed. Philadelphia: WB Saunders; 1985:206; Speroff L, Glass RH, Kase N. *Clinical Gynecologic Endocrinology and Infertility*, 3rd ed. Baltimore: Williams & Wilkins; 1983:377; and Kustin J, Rebar RW. Menstrual disorders in the adolescent age group. *Primary Care.* 1987;14:139-166.

analysis and the measurement of 17α-hydroxyprogesterone to rule out congenital adrenal hyperplasia. Pregnancy and gestational trophoblastic disease may be confirmed by measurement of hCG. The possibility of intrauterine synechiae or adhesions (Asherman's syndrome) must be considered in individuals in whom amenorrhea develops after curettage or endometritis. Tuberculous endometritis, especially in younger women, may also lead to this disorder. Without hormonal measurements, it may be impossible to distinguish between individuals with chronic anovulation, in whom hypothalamic-pituitary-ovarian function is insufficiently coordinated to produce cyclic ovulation, and those with ovarian failure. However, it is generally possible to form a clinical impression about the cause of the amenorrhea. It can be noted whether the patient has absence of, incomplete, or complete development of secondary sex characteristics. The presence of excess body hair or galactorrhea may provide clinical evidence of the pathogenesis of the amenorrhea.

TABLE 244-3 CAUSES OF AMENORRHEA

ANATOMIC CAUSES

Pregnancy
Various disorders of sexual differentiation
    Distal genital tract obstruction (müllerian agenesis or dysgenesis)
    Gonadal dysgenesis*
    Ambiguity of external genitalia (male and female pseudohermaphroditism)
Intrauterine adhesions (Asherman's syndrome)
Gestational trophoblastic disease

CHRONIC ANOVULATION

Due to CNS-hypothalamic-pituitary dysfunction
With inappropriate steroid feedback (e.g., polycystic ovary syndrome)
Due to thyroid or adrenal disorders

OVARIAN "FAILURE"

Menopause
Genetic abnormalities
Physical and environmental causes (e.g., chemotherapeutic agents, irradiation)
Autoimmune disorders
Idiopathic

*Gonadal dysgenesis may be viewed as both a disorder of sexual differentiation and a form of gonadal "failure."
CNS = central nervous system.

Signs and symptoms of adrenal or thyroid dysfunction may be important as well. Administration of a progestin (typically medroxyprogesterone acetate, 5 to 10 mg given orally for 5 to 10 days, or progesterone in oil, 100 mg given intramuscularly) has been advocated to assess the level of endogenous estrogen. This test is of limited value, however, because almost half the young women with premature ovarian failure experience withdrawal bleeding in response to progestin.

To ascertain whether the outflow tract is intact, an orally active estrogen, such as 2.5 mg of conjugated estrogen daily for 21 days, with 5 to 10 mg of oral medroxyprogesterone acetate for the last 5 to 10 days, is administered. Withdrawal bleeding should occur if the endometrium is normal. Still, hysterosalpingography and hysteroscopy may be required for the diagnosis of Asherman's syndrome because some patients continue to have some withdrawal bleeding.

Laboratory Findings

Basal levels of FSH, prolactin, and thyroid-stimulating hormone (TSH) should be measured in all amenorrheic and oligomenorrheic women to confirm the clinical impression (Fig. 244-3).

Increased TSH levels with or without increased levels of prolactin imply primary hypothyroidism, and further evaluation for this disorder is indicated (Chapter 233). Although hypothyroidism commonly results in anovulation, amenorrhea occurs in only some hypothyroid women. Menorrhagia and oligomenorrhea may occur as well. The sensitive immunoassays for TSH permit identification of women with hyperthyroidism as well because TSH levels are suppressed in those individuals.

If the prolactin concentration is minimally increased and the TSH level is normal, measurement of the prolactin concentration should be repeated before more extensive evaluation is undertaken because prolactin levels are increased by nonspecific stressful stimuli, sleep, and food ingestion. Prolactin levels may be elevated in as many as one third of women with amenorrhea.

Increased FSH levels (generally above 30 mIU/mL) imply ovarian failure and require further evaluation. Incipient ovarian failure should be considered in any woman with basal FSH levels of 15 mIU/mL or higher other than during the midcycle LH surge. Many clinicians believe that chromosomal evaluation is indicated in all individuals with elevated FSH levels before age 40 years, and it is certainly indicated if hypergonadotropic amenorrhea begins before age 30 years.

If FSH levels are low or normal, the measurement of total testosterone levels may be helpful whether or not there is any evidence of hirsutism or

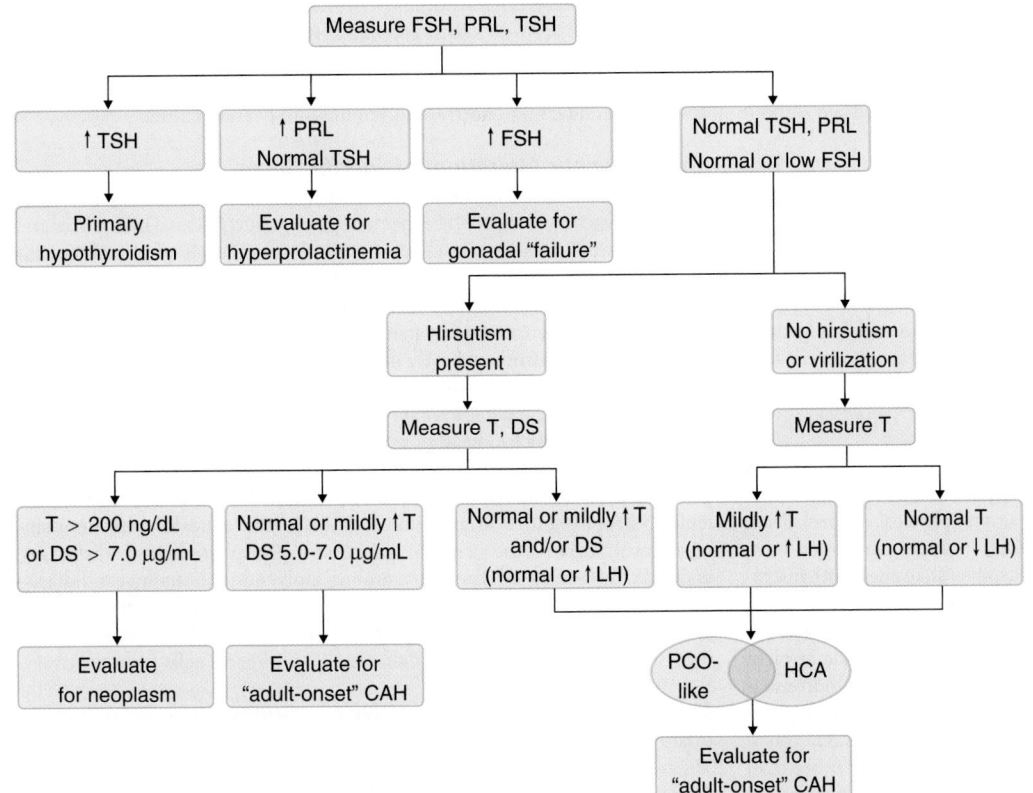

FIGURE 244-3. Biochemical evaluation of amenorrhea. This schema must be considered an adjunct to the clinical evaluation of the patient. See text for details. CAH = congenital adrenal hyperplasia; DS = dehydroepiandrosterone sulfate; FSH = follicle-stimulating hormone; HCA = hypothalamic chronic anovulation; LH = luteinizing hormone; PCO-like = polycystic ovarian syndrome–like; PRL = prolactin; T = testosterone; TSH = thyroid-stimulating hormone.

virilization. Hyperandrogenic women need not be hirsute because some have relative insensitivity of the hair follicles to androgens. Mildly increased levels of testosterone (and perhaps dehydroepiandrosterone sulfate as well) suggest polycystic ovary syndrome (PCOS). However, total circulating androgen levels need not be elevated because of the alterations in metabolic clearance rate and sex hormone–binding globulin that are present in PCOS. Consequently, some clinicians prefer to measure circulating free testosterone levels.

Circulating levels of LH and FSH may aid in differentiation of PCOS from hypothalamic-pituitary dysfunction. LH levels are often elevated in PCOS so that the ratio of LH to FSH is increased; however, LH levels may be identical to those observed in normal women in the follicular phase. In contrast, levels of LH and FSH are normal or slightly reduced in hypothalamic-pituitary dysfunction. There is some overlap between women with "polycystic ovarian–like" disorders and those with hypothalamic-pituitary dysfunction. Radiographic assessment of the sella turcica is indicated in all amenorrheic women in whom both LH and FSH levels are consistently low (both below 10 mIU/mL) to exclude a pituitary or parapituitary neoplasm (Chapter 231). Other pituitary functions should be evaluated in any individual with significantly impaired LH and FSH secretion. Both total testosterone and dehydroepiandrosterone sulfate levels should be measured in hirsute or virilized women. Testosterone levels greater than 200 ng/dL should lead to investigation for an androgen-producing neoplasm, most likely of ovarian origin. Dehydroepiandrosterone sulfate levels greater than 7.0 μg/mL should lead to evaluation for an adrenal neoplasm, and levels between 5.0 and 7.0 μg/mL should lead to evaluation for adult-onset congenital adrenal hyperplasia (Chapter 241).

HYPERGONADOTROPIC AMENORRHEA (PRESUMPTIVE OVARIAN FAILURE, PRIMARY HYPOGONADISM, PRIMARY OVARIAN INSUFFICIENCY)

DIAGNOSIS
Differential Diagnosis
Gonadal failure may begin at any time during embryonic or postnatal development and may result from many causes. Normally, the ovaries fail at menopause, when virtually no functioning follicles remain. However, premature loss of oocytes before the age of 40 years may occur and lead to premature ovarian failure. Most causes of premature ovarian failure involve FSH secretion or action. Circulating gonadotropin levels increase whenever ovarian failure occurs because of decreased negative estrogen feedback to the hypothalamic-pituitary unit.

PATHOBIOLOGY
There are several causes for premature ovarian failure, including genetic causes (a growing list that includes karyotypic abnormalities, single gene mutations, and complex multifactorial polygenic inheritance), physical and environmental causes, and autoimmune disturbances. In addition, there may be families in which menopause begins earlier than the expected age without any further pathologic cause.

Genetic Abnormalities
Several pathologic conditions with dysgenetic gonads involve elevated gonadotropin levels and amenorrhea as well as abnormalities of the X chromosome. The term gonadal dysgenesis refers to individuals with undifferentiated streak gonads without any association with either extragonadal stigmata or sex chromosome aberrations. Because individuals with gonadal dysgenesis have the normal complement of oocytes at 20 weeks of fetal age but virtually none by birth, this disorder is a form of premature ovarian failure.

Turner's Syndrome
Turner's syndrome (also see Chapter 241) describes patients with streak gonads composed of fibrous stroma and four cardinal features: a female phenotype; sexual infantilism; short stature; and several physical abnormalities, sometimes including webbed neck, low-set ears, multiple pigmented nevi, double eyelashes, micrognathia, epicanthal folds, shieldlike chest with microthelia, short fourth metacarpals, increased carrying angle of the arms, and certain renal and cardiovascular defects (most commonly coarctation of the aorta and aortic stenosis). The diagnosis can sometimes be made at birth because of unexplained lymphedema of the hands and feet. The syndrome is associated with an abnormality of sex chromosome number, morphology, or both. Most commonly, the second sex chromosome is absent (45,X). This is the single most common chromosome disorder in humans, but more than 95% of such fetuses are aborted, and the incidence in newborns is

approximately 1 in 3000 to 5000. Chromosome breakage and mosaicism occur as well. In mosaic individuals with a normal 46,XX cell line, sufficient follicles may persist postnatally to initiate pubertal changes and to cause ovulation so that pregnancy is possible. Deletions of the X-chromosome-linked SHOX gene explain many of the dysmorphic skeletal features that are present, including the short stature. It is believed that the number of phenotypic findings may be related to the percentage of cells that are 45,X. There may be an effect of imprinting with the variation in phenotype partly explained by the parental origin of the one remaining X chromosome.

Pure Gonadal Dysgenesis
Pure gonadal dysgenesis is the term given to phenotypically female individuals with streak gonads who are of normal stature and have none of the physical stigmata associated with Turner's syndrome. Such individuals have either a 46,XX or 46,XY karyotype. The 46,XX defect may be inherited as an autosomal recessive, with 10% having associated nerve deafness. The 46,XY defect may be inherited as an X-linked recessive, with clitorimegaly occurring in 10 to 15% and gonadal tumors developing in 25% if the gonads are not removed.

Mutations in the X Chromosome Associated with Premature Ovarian Failure
Several regions of the X chromosome are now recognized to contain mutations in genes that may result in premature ovarian failure. Of particular note is the fragile X mental retardation (FMR1) gene. More than 5% of women with 46,XX spontaneous premature ovarian failure have mutations of the FMR1 gene. This risk is increased if there is a family history of premature ovarian failure. A family history of fragile X syndrome, unexplained mental retardation, dementia, developmental delay of a child, or tremor-ataxia syndrome is reason for genetic counseling. Mutations in the FMR1 gene are known to be associated with a neurodegenerative disorder. Women with mutations in the FMR1 gene are at risk of having a child with mental retardation, should they be one of the 6 to 8% of women with premature ovarian failure who conceive spontaneously. For FMR1, a CGG repeat sequence occurs, with up to 60 repeats being normal. Expansion to more than 200 repeats leads to the fragile X syndrome, with the high level of repeats causing hypermethylation of the gene promoter and silencing of the gene. Female carriers of the permutation have an unstable intermediate number of repeats (i.e., 60 to 199) and the predisposition for premature ovarian failure.

Trisomy X
Trisomy X (46,XXX karyotype) is also associated with premature menopause, although many such individuals have normal reproductive lives. Premature menopause can also occur in mosaic individuals with cell lines with excess X chromosomes. When gonadal abnormalities occur in women with excess X chromosomes, they seem to occur after ovarian differentiation so that some ovarian function is possible. Only later in life do such women develop secondary amenorrhea and premature ovarian failure.

Known Genetic Alterations of Specific Genes
In girls with the rare syndrome of 17α-hydroxylase deficiency involving p450c17 who survive until the expected age of puberty, sexual infantilism and primary amenorrhea occur together with elevated levels of gonadotropins (also see Chapter 241). Defects in the 20,22-lyase (p450scc) or aromatase (p450arom) enzymes may also lead to ovarian failure. Women with galactosemia also experience ovarian failure early in life, even when a galactose-restricted diet is introduced early in infancy.

Mutations of several autosomal genes result in premature ovarian failure. Included in this growing list are mutations involving FSHR (the FSH receptor gene), FOXL2 (a forkhead transcription factor associated with the blepharophimosis-ptosis-epicanthus inversus syndrome), INHA (the inhibin-α gene), E1F2B (a family of genes associated with central nervous system leukodystrophy and ovarian failure), PMM2 (the gene for phosphomannomutase), GALT (the gene for galactose-1-phosphate uridyltransferase), and AIRE (leading to the autoimmune polyendocrinopathy-candidiasis-ectodermal dystrophy syndrome). Myotonic dystrophy (Chapter 429) is caused by an autosomal triple repeat mutation, like the fragile X syndrome, that is similarly associated with premature loss of germ cells from the ovary.

Mutations Involving Reproductive Hormones, Their Receptors, and Action
The resistant ovary (Savage's) syndrome occurs in young amenorrheic women who have elevated peripheral gonadotropin concentrations, normal

(although immature) follicles present on ovarian biopsy, 46,XX karyotype with no evidence of mosaicism, fully developed secondary sex characteristics, and ovarian resistance to stimulation with human menopausal or pituitary gonadotropins.

At least one form of premature ovarian failure is caused by mutations in the FSH receptor. Affected individuals present with primary or secondary amenorrhea and elevated levels of FSH and may still have ovarian follicles detectable on transvaginal ultrasonography.

Other Causes
Physical and Environmental
Irradiation and chemotherapeutic agents used to treat various malignant diseases may also cause premature ovarian failure. Ovulation and cyclic menses return in some of these patients even after prolonged intervals of hypergonadotropic amenorrhea associated with signs and symptoms of profound hypoestrogenism. Rarely, mumps affects the ovaries and causes ovarian failure.

Autoimmune Disorders
Premature ovarian failure may occur in conjunction with a variety of autoimmune disorders. The most well known syndrome (autoimmune polyglandular syndrome type 1) involves hypoadrenalism, hypoparathyroidism, and mucocutaneous candidiasis together with ovarian failure (Chapter 239). Testing for adrenal antibodies by indirect immunofluorescence will identify the 4% of women with spontaneous premature ovarian failure who have steroidogenic cell autoimmunity and are at risk for adrenal insufficiency. Thyroiditis is the most commonly associated abnormality. Antibodies to the FSH receptor have been identified in a few cases. These associations make it mandatory to rule out other potentially life-threatening endocrinopathies in young women with hypergonadotropic amenorrhea.

TREATMENT   Rx

Women with hypergonadotropic amenorrhea and ovarian failure should be treated identically whether or not they have signs of hypoestrogenism or desire pregnancy. Counseling and psychological support are indicated in women in whom the diagnosis of premature ovarian failure is made. Ovarian biopsy is not indicated to document the existence of follicles because only a small portion of each ovary can be sampled and because pregnancies have resulted in patients who had biopsy samples devoid of follicles. Estrogen replacement is warranted to prevent the accelerated bone loss known to occur in affected women (Chapter 251). The estrogen should be given sequentially with a progestin to prevent endometrial hyperplasia. Young women with ovarian failure may require twice as much estrogen as postmenopausal women for relief of signs and symptoms of hypoestrogenism. Inexplicably, women with premature ovarian failure may conceive while taking exogenous estrogen, even in the form of oral contraceptive agents, at the same rate as those not taking estrogen, so barrier contraception should be discussed if pregnancy is not desired.

Women with hypergonadotropic amenorrhea are rarely able to become pregnant. It is not clear why pregnancy may rarely occur in such women, but the spontaneous pregnancy rate is 6 to 8%. Infertility treatment of young women with hypergonadotropic amenorrhea involves hormone replacement to mimic the normal menstrual cycle and embryo transfer by use of donor oocytes. Pregnancy rates are higher than in other women undergoing in vitro fertilization and exceed 30% per cycle. Whether women with gonadal dysgenesis should be offered pregnancy by use of donor oocytes is now the subject of debate because a markedly increased incidence of aortic rupture during pregnancy secondary to medial necrosis has been documented. Women with Turner's syndrome contemplating pregnancy should be counseled regarding the risks.

CHRONIC ANOVULATION

Chronic anovulation, the most frequent form of amenorrhea encountered in women of reproductive age, implies that functional ovarian follicles remain and that cyclic ovulation can be induced with appropriate therapy (Table 244-4). The cause of the anovulation should be determined. The pathophysiologic bases for several forms of anovulation are unknown, but the anovulation can be interrupted transiently by nonspecific induction of ovulation in most affected women. Anovulation can result in either amenorrhea or irregular (generally less frequent) menses.

TABLE 244-4   CAUSES OF CHRONIC ANOVULATION

Chronic anovulation of hypothalamic-pituitary origin
  Hypothalamic chronic anovulation
    Psychogenic
    Exercise associated
    Associated with diet, weight loss, or malnutrition
    Anorexia nervosa and bulimia
    Pseudocyesis
  Forms of isolated (idiopathic) hypogonadotropic hypogonadism
    (including Kallmann's syndrome)
  Due to hypothalamic-pituitary damage
    Pituitary and parapituitary tumors
    Empty sella syndrome
    Following surgery
    Following irradiation
    Following trauma
    Following infection
    Following infarction
  Idiopathic hypopituitarism
  Hypothalamic-pituitary dysfunction or failure with hyperprolactinemia
    (multiple causes)
  Due to systemic diseases
Chronic anovulation due to inappropriate feedback (i.e., polycystic ovary syndrome)
  Excessive extraglandular estrogen production (i.e., obesity)
  Abnormal buffering involving sex hormone–binding globulin (including liver
    disease)
  Functional androgen excess (adrenal or ovarian)
  Neoplasms producing androgens or estrogens
  Neoplasms producing chorionic gonadotropin
Chronic anovulation due to other endocrine and metabolic disorders
  Adrenal hyperfunction
    Cushing's syndrome
    Congenital adrenal hyperplasia (female pseudohermaphroditism)
  Thyroid dysfunction
    Hyperthyroidism
    Hypothyroidism
  Prolactin or growth hormone excess
    Hypothalamic dysfunction
    Pituitary dysfunction (microadenomas and macroadenomas)
    Drug induced
  Malnutrition

Hypothalamic Chronic Anovulation

DEFINITION
Hypothalamic chronic anovulation (HCA) represents a heterogeneous group of disorders with similar manifestations. Emotional and physical stress, excessive exercise, nutritional deficiencies, weight loss, reduced body fat, and other unrecognized factors may contribute in varying proportions to the anovulation. Women with HCA have normal neuroanatomic findings.

Anorexia Nervosa
Individuals with amenorrhea and significant weight loss should be examined for the possibility of anorexia nervosa (Chapter 226).

Isolated Hypogonadotropic Hypogonadism
Affected individuals have absence of spontaneous pubertal development. Most have functional GnRH deficiency, but some have abnormalities of gonadotropin deficiency localized to the pituitary gland.

Kallmann's syndrome is a familial disorder consisting of gonadotropin deficiency, anosmia or hyposmia, and color blindness in men or, more rarely, in women (Chapter 230). Partial or complete agenesis of the olfactory bulb is present on autopsy, accounting for use of the term *olfactogenital dysplasia*. Isolated gonadotropin deficiency in the absence of anosmia occurs as well. Sexual infantilism with a eunuchoid habitus is the clinical hallmark of this disorder, but moderate breast development may occur. Circulating LH and FSH levels are low but almost always detectable. Ovulation induction requires use of exogenous gonadotropins and hCG or pulsatile GnRH. Estrogen replacement therapy is indicated in these women until pregnancy is desired. It may not be possible to distinguish between partial isolated gonadotropin deficiency and functional HCA in all cases.

Hypopituitarism
Hypopituitarism may be obvious on cursory inspection or sufficiently subtle to require endocrine testing (Chapter 231). The clinical presentation depends

on the age at onset, the cause, and the nutritional status of the individual. Failure of development of secondary sex characteristics must always raise the question of hypopituitarism. Ovulation can be induced successfully with exogenous gonadotropins when pregnancy is desired and after the hypopituitarism is treated appropriately. Replacement therapy with estrogen is indicated.

Hyperprolactinemia

Galactorrhea associated with hyperprolactinemia, whatever the cause, almost always occurs together with amenorrhea caused by hypothalamic-pituitary dysfunction or failure. Many conditions can cause excess prolactin secretion (Chapter 231). A prolactinoma must be excluded. Hirsutism may be observed occasionally in association with amenorrhea-galactorrhea and hyperprolactinemia. Elevated levels of the adrenal androgens dehydroepiandrosterone and dehydroepiandrosterone sulfate may be observed and may account for the polycystic-type ovaries present in some hyperprolactinemic women.

Failure of the Hypothalamic-Pituitary Unit

The hypothalamic-pituitary unit may also fail to function normally in a number of stressful, debilitating, systemic illnesses that interfere with somatic growth and development. Chronic renal failure, liver disease, and diabetes mellitus are the most prominent examples.

DIAGNOSIS

Abrupt cessation of menses in women younger than 30 years who have no anatomic abnormalities of the hypothalamic-pituitary-ovarian axis and no other endocrine disturbances suggests a diagnosis of HCA. Affected individuals tend to be bright, educated, and engaged in intellectual occupations and may well give a history of psychosexual problems and socioenvironmental trauma. HCA is characterized by low to normal levels of gonadotropins and relative hypoestrogenism. Rarely, however, do affected women present with signs and symptoms of estrogen deficiency. It is important to rule out a central lesion as the cause of the hypogonadotropic hypogonadism in women who appear to have HCA.

TREATMENT   Rx

Psychological counseling or a change in lifestyle, especially for women engaged in strenuous exercise programs, may be effective in inducing cyclic ovulation and menses in women with functional HCA. Cognitive behavior therapy is effective in a proportion of women with functional HCA. For women desiring pregnancy, ovulation can also be induced with clomiphene citrate (50 to 100 mg/day for 5 days beginning on the third to fifth day of withdrawal bleeding). Treatment with exogenous gonadotropins to induce follicular maturation followed by hCG to induce follicular rupture may be effective in women who do not ovulate in response to clomiphene. Because women with HCA have low circulating levels of leptin, investigators have given recombinant leptin and documented that ovulation may resume in some affected women. Given the heterogeneous nature of the disorder, it is not surprising that exogenous leptin is not effective in all women.

Most physicians advocate the use of exogenous gonadal steroids to prevent osteoporosis. A regimen can consist of daily oral conjugated or esterified estrogens (0.625 to 1.25 mg), ethinyl estradiol (20 μg), or micronized estradiol-17β (1 to 2 mg) or transdermal estradiol-17β (0.05 to 0.10 mg) daily, with oral medroxyprogesterone acetate (5 to 10 mg) added for the first 12 to 14 days of each month. Sexually active women can be given oral contraceptive agents as an alternative. If steroid therapy is administered, patients must be informed that the amenorrhea will probably be present when therapy is discontinued. Other physicians believe that only periodic observation is indicated, with barrier methods of contraception recommended for fertility control. Adequate ingestion of calcium should be ensured regardless of therapy. Contraception is needed for sexually active women with HCA because the functional defect is mild in these disorders and may resolve spontaneously at any time, with ovulation occurring before any episode of menstruation.

Chronic Anovulation Related to Inappropriate Feedback

DEFINITION

PCOS is a heterogeneous disorder in which there is considerable clinical and biochemical variability among affected individuals. PCOS is currently considered to exist in women with any two of the following: (1) oligo-ovulation

or anovulation, (2) hyperandrogenism, or (3) polycystic ovaries on ultrasound, and in whom other etiologies have been eliminated.

PATHOBIOLOGY

Current evidence suggests that the hypothalamic-pituitary unit is intact and that a functional derangement, perhaps involving insulin-like growth factors such as IGF-I within the ovary, results in abnormal gonadotropin secretion. PCOS is characterized by insulin resistance and compensatory hyperinsulinemia. The insulin resistance has been found in affected women of many racial and ethnic groups, implying that it is a universal characteristic and that a common defect may be present. There is increasing evidence of specific genetic abnormalities in some women with PCOS.

CLINICAL MANIFESTATIONS

Although patients usually present with amenorrhea, hirsutism, and obesity, affected women may instead complain of irregular and profuse uterine bleeding, may not have hirsutism, and may be of normal weight. Excess androgen from any source or increased extraglandular conversion of androgens to estrogens can lead to the typical findings of PCOS. Included are such diverse disorders as Cushing's syndrome, mild congenital adrenal hyperplasia, virilizing tumors of adrenal or ovarian origin, hyperthyroidism and hypothyroidism, obesity, and primary PCOS with no other recognizable cause.

In the primary syndrome, the irregular menses, mild obesity, and hirsutism begin during puberty and typically become more severe with time. Obesity alone can lead to a polycystic ovarian–like syndrome, with the degree of obesity required to cause anovulation varying widely. The increase in the prevalence of obesity is leading to an increased prevalence of PCOS. All such patients are well estrogenized regardless of whether they present with primary or secondary amenorrhea or dysfunctional bleeding. LH concentrations tend to be elevated, with relatively low and constant FSH levels, but both may be in the normal range for the follicular phase of the menstrual cycle. Levels of most circulating androgens, especially testosterone, tend to be mildly elevated.

DIAGNOSIS

A consensus conference in Rotterdam in 2003 concluded that after exclusion of other etiologies, two of the following three are required for diagnosis of PCOS: (1) hyperandrogenism (clinical or biochemical); (2) oligo-ovulation or anovulation; (3) polycystic ovaries on ultrasound examination or at surgery.

This definition is confusing to clinicians because it implies that hirsute women with polycystic ovaries on ultrasound examination who ovulate regularly should be considered to have PCOS. Moreover, it is clear that polycystic ovaries may be identified on ultrasound examination in normal women. In any case, the aim of the diagnostic evaluation is to rule out any causes (such as neoplasms) that require definitive therapy. Hirsutism should be evaluated as detailed in Chapter 444.

A particularly severely affected subset of women present with marked obesity, anovulation, mild glucose intolerance with high levels of circulating insulin, acanthosis nigricans, hyperuricemia, severe hirsutism, and elevated circulating androgen levels. These women have hyperthecosis of the ovaries, in which the androgen-producing cells in the stromal, hilar, and thecal regions are increased greatly in number. Hyperthecosis should probably be viewed as a part of the spectrum of disorders constituting PCOS.

TREATMENT   Rx

Patients generally require therapy for hirsutism, for induction of ovulation if pregnancy is desired, and for prevention of estrogen-induced endometrial hyperplasia and cancer. No ideal therapy exists; the therapeutic approach must be individualized. The risks for metabolic syndrome, cardiovascular disease, and diabetes mellitus are increased in women with PCOS, presumably at least in part because of the increased androgens and insulin resistance. Moreover, many women have elevated cholesterol levels.

Medical Therapy

In the anovulatory woman not desiring pregnancy who is not hirsute, therapy with intermittent progestin administration (such as medroxyprogesterone acetate, 5 to 10 mg orally for 10 to 14 days each month) or oral contraceptives can be provided to reduce the increased risk for endometrial carcinoma that is present in such a woman with unopposed estrogen. All women using intermittent progestin administration should be cautioned about the need for effective contraception if they are sexually active because these agents do not inhibit ovulation when they are administered intermittently.

Improvements in insulin sensitivity in women with polycystic ovaries, either through lifestyle changes (i.e., exercise and diet) or through pharmacologic intervention, consistently result in improvements in the reproductive and metabolic abnormalities. Resumption of ovulation may occur in up to 60 to 70% of affected women.

The longest and largest published experiences with any agent that improves insulin sensitivity in PCOS is with metformin, a biguanide that functions primarily by suppressing hepatic gluconeogenesis and also improves insulin sensitivity. Its use in PCOS leads to reductions in insulin and androgen levels and resumption of menses in some women. Divided doses of 1500 to 2000 mg/day have proved effective.

Some clinicians advocate giving metformin to all women with polycystic ovaries, whereas others would administer such an agent only to those with documented insulin resistance. Some clinicians also advocate giving metformin first to women who desire pregnancy and then adding an agent to induce ovulation if the metformin proves ineffective. These agents are not approved for use in pregnant women or for the induction of ovulation.

Treatment Considering Pregnancy

Oral contraceptive agents are the first line of therapy for hirsute anovulatory woman not desiring pregnancy and offer protection from endometrial hyperplasia. In women with PCOS desiring pregnancy, clomiphene citrate can be used to induce ovulation. About 75 to 80% conceive with such therapy. In addition to insulin-sensitizing agents, other possible methods of inducing ovulation include use of exogenous gonadotropins and hCG, and laparoscopic ovarian surgery with multiple punctures of the ovary by diathermy or laser. A large clinical trial documented that clomiphene citrate is more effective than metformin in inducing ovulation and resulting in pregnancy; there was no further improvement when the two agents were used concurrently.∎

Surgical Treatment

Laparoscopic ovarian surgery can achieve unifollicular ovulation or make it easier for medical ovulation induction, but increases the risk for development of ovarian adhesions (themselves leading to infertility). Its use should be restricted to women desiring fertility who do not have funds for ovulation induction or who are unable to undergo the extensive monitoring required for medical ovulation.

Chronic Anovulation Related to Other Endocrine and Metabolic Disorders

Adrenal hyperfunction appears to cause chronic anovulation by inducing a polycystic ovarian-like syndrome secondary to increased adrenal androgen secretion. Both hyperthyroidism and hypothyroidism are associated with a variety of menstrual disturbances, including dysfunctional uterine bleeding and amenorrhea as a result of alterations in the metabolism of androgens and estrogens. These metabolic changes in turn result in inappropriate steroid feedback and chronic anovulation.

LUTEINIZED UNRUPTURED FOLLICLE SYNDROME

The luteinized unruptured follicle syndrome refers to the development of a dominant follicle without its subsequent disruption and release of the ovum. The abnormality can be diagnosed by ultrasonography or by the absence of evidence of ovulation when the ovary is viewed at laparoscopy. The disorder occurs infrequently and is not a significant cause of infertility. Menstrual cycles in which no ovum is released are characterized by presumptive evidence of ovulation, including biphasic basal body temperatures, secretory endometrium, normal LH surge, and normal progesterone production in the luteal phase.

LUTEAL PHASE DYSFUNCTION

PATHOBIOLOGY

Progesterone secretion in the luteal phase may be reduced in duration (termed *luteal phase insufficiency*) or in amount (termed *luteal phase inadequacy*). More rarely, the endometrium may be unable to respond to secreted progesterone because of the absence of progesterone receptors. These disorders represent causes of infertility (because of inability of fertilized ova to implant) in less than 5% of infertile couples. Abnormalities of the follicular phase, especially in the frequency of gonadotropin pulses, may account for most luteal phase defects. Luteal phase defects may also occur sporadically in normally ovulating women.

DIAGNOSIS

Luteal phase dysfunction may be associated with several clinical entities, including mild or intermittent hyperprolactinemia, strenuous physical exercise, inadequately treated 21-hydroxylase deficiency, and habitual abortion. Luteal dysfunction occurs more commonly at the extremes of reproductive life and in the first menstrual cycles after full-term delivery, abortion, or discontinuation of oral contraceptives. It may also occur during ovulatory cycles induced with clomiphene citrate or exogenous gonadotropins and hCG.

TREATMENT Rx

Treatment of luteal dysfunction is controversial. Any underlying defect should be treated. If subsequent luteal function depends on prior follicular development, modification of follicular development with either clomiphene citrate (25 to 100 mg daily by mouth for 5 days beginning on cycle day 3 to 5) or FSH (75 to 300 IU intramuscularly for 3 to 5 days beginning on cycle day 3 to 5) can be used; hCG (2500 to 5000 IU intramuscularly at 2- to 3-day intervals beginning with the shift in basal body temperature), or progesterone (12.5 mg intramuscularly in oil daily or 25 mg twice a day as rectal or vaginal suppositories) can be used as well. Bromocriptine may correct the abnormality in individuals with hyperprolactinemia. Synthetic progestational agents should not be used to treat luteal phase defects because of their possible association with congenital anomalies. Furthermore, the synthetic progestins produce an abnormal endometrium. None of these agents has been shown to increase the pregnancy rate.

Infertility

DEFINITION

The World Health Organization (WHO) has defined *infertility* as "a disease of the reproductive system defined by the failure to achieve a clinical pregnancy after 12 months or more of regular unprotected sexual intercourse." *Sterility* is total inability to reproduce. More than 10% of couples in the United States seek medical assistance for infertility.

The requirements for pregnancy to occur are several:
- The male must produce adequate numbers of normal, motile spermatozoa.
- The male must be capable of ejaculating the sperm through a patent ductal system.
- The sperm must be able to traverse an unobstructed female reproductive tract.
- The female must ovulate and release an ovum.
- The sperm must be able to fertilize the ovum.
- The fertilized ovum must be capable of developing and implanting in appropriately prepared endometrium.

In approximately 40% of cases, infertility is caused by the male (Table 244-5). In one third of couples, more than one cause contributes to the infertility.

Peak age for fertility in the female is 25 years. For nulliparous women of this age, the average time during which unprotected intercourse occurs until conception is 5.3 months. For parous women, the average duration of intercourse until conception is 2.7 months. The reproductive performance of couples is influenced by the ages of the female and male partners, the frequency of intercourse, and the length of time the couple has been attempting to conceive. There is a decline in both female and male reproductive performance after the age of 25 years.

DIAGNOSIS

Couples who complain of infertility merit evaluation regardless of the length of infertility. Evaluation is warranted in all women after 12 months and in women 35 years of age or older after 6 months of regular unprotected intercourse.

The evaluation begins with a detailed history obtained from both partners and physical examinations of both individuals. If possible, the couple should be seen together. Each couple should be questioned together and separately because separate interviews may uncover information that would not be imparted in the presence of the partner.

Initial evaluation for infertility includes assessment of semen; documentation of ovulation by basal body temperature, serum progesterone

TABLE 244-5 CAUSES OF INFERTILITY AND THEIR APPROXIMATE INCIDENCE

Male factors (40%)
  Decreased production of spermatozoa
    Varicocele
    Testicular failure
    Endocrine disorders
    Cryptorchidism
    Stress, smoking, caffeine, nicotine, recreational drugs
  Ductal obstruction
    Epididymal (after infection)
    Congenital absence of vas deferens
    Ejaculatory duct (after infection)
    After vasectomy
  Inability to deliver sperm into vagina
    Ejaculatory disturbances
    Hypospadias
    Sexual problems (i.e., impotence), medical or psychological
  Abnormal semen
    Infection
    Abnormal volume
    Abnormal viscosity
  Immunologic factors
    Sperm-immobilizing antibodies
    Sperm-agglutinating antibodies
Female factors
  Fallopian tube disease (20-30%)
    Pelvic inflammatory disease or puerperal infection
    Congenital anomalies
    Endometriosis
    Secondary to past peritonitis of nongenital origin
  Amenorrhea and anovulation (15%)
  Minor ovulatory disturbances (<5%?)
  Cervical and uterine factors (10%)
    Leiomyomas and polyps
    Uterine anomalies
    Intrauterine synechiae (Asherman's syndrome)
    Destroyed endocervical glands (after surgery or after infection)
  Vaginal factors (<5%)
    Congenital absence of vagina
    Imperforate hymen
    Vaginismus
    Vaginitis
  Immunologic factors (<5%)
    Sperm-immobilizing antibodies
    Sperm-agglutinating antibodies
  Nutritional and metabolic factors (5%)
    Thyroid disorders
    Diabetes mellitus
    Severe nutritional disturbances
Idiopathic or unexplained (<10%)

determination 6 to 8 days before menses, serum thyroid hormone, or (rarely) endometrial biopsy less than 3 days before onset of menses; and evaluation of the female genital tract by hysterosalpingography or sonohysterography. Diagnostic laparoscopy with tubal dye instillation may be performed if results of all previous tests are normal because 30 to 50% of women are found to have endometriosis or tubal disease on surgical evaluation; alternatively, patients with initial normal findings may be merely treated as having idiopathic infertility.

TREATMENT   Rx

Treatment must be predicated on the findings of the infertility evaluation. Abnormalities of sperm are difficult disorders to treat. Low sperm count or poor motility is best treated either by donor insemination or in vitro fertilization with intracytoplasmic injection of a single viable sperm into each oocyte. Obstruction of the fallopian tubes may be amenable to surgical intervention, but success rates are often greater with in vitro fertilization. Endometriosis causing infertility may be treated by surgery or various suppressive drugs as indicated; however, here, too, in vitro fertilization may prove indicated.

Induction of ovulation is one of the most successful therapies when used in anovulatory women.

Induction of Ovulation in Anovulatory Women and "Controlled Ovarian Hyperstimulation" in Unexplained Infertility

Induction of ovulation should never be attempted until serious disorders precluding pregnancy are ruled out or treated. Furthermore, ovulation induction should not be used in women with ovarian failure because they are unresponsive to any form of ovulation induction.

Clomiphene citrate is the agent that usually induces ovulation most easily. Clomiphene should be used in individuals without hyperprolactinemia who have the ability to release LH and FSH. A typical course of clomiphene therapy is begun on the third to fifth days after either spontaneous or induced uterine bleeding. The initial dosage is 50 mg daily for 5 days. Clomiphene appears to act as an antiestrogen and stimulates gonadotropin secretion by the pituitary gland to initiate follicular development. If ovulation is not achieved in the first cycle of treatment, the daily dosage is increased to 100 mg. If ovulation is still not achieved, dosage is increased in a stepwise fashion in 50-mg increments to a maximum of 200 to 250 mg daily for 5 days. The highest dose should be continued for 3 to 6 months before the patient is regarded as unresponsive to clomiphene. The quantity of drug and the length of time that it can be used, as suggested here, are greater than those recommended by the manufacturers and the FDA but conform to published series.

The ovulatory surge of LH may occur 5 to 12 days (average, 7 days) after the completion of the last day of clomiphene treatment. Couples are advised to have intercourse every other day during this interval. Ovulation can be documented by monitoring changes in basal body temperature or preferably by measuring serum progesterone 14 days after the last clomiphene dose. Menses should occur after 3 weeks. Withdrawal bleeding with progestin can be induced if the patient fails to bleed within 4 weeks of therapy and if a serum hCG level documents that the patient is not pregnant. Testing the urine for an LH surge may also be useful in timing ovulation.

Some clinicians give 5000 to 10,000 IU of hCG intramuscularly 7 days after the last day of clomiphene therapy to trigger ovulation, but this approach has not been established to increase effectiveness. The administration of hCG, however, does serve to time ovulation and may be helpful in selected couples. Ovulation can be expected to occur approximately 36 hours after hCG administration.

Of appropriately selected patients, 75 to 80% ovulate, and 40 to 50% can be expected to become pregnant. About 15% of pregnancies can be expected with each ovulatory cycle. The multiple pregnancy rate is about 8%, with almost all being twins. The incidence of congenital anomalies is not increased.

Side effects of clomiphene are uncommon and rarely serious. The most serious ones include vasomotor flushes (10%), abdominal discomfort (5%), breast tenderness (2%), nausea and vomiting (2%), visual symptoms (1.5%), and headache (1%). Ovarian enlargement may occur but is rare (5%). Concern has been raised about the potential for clomiphene to increase the risk for epithelial ovarian cancer. The bulk of the evidence now indicates that clomiphene does not increase this risk.

The addition of dexamethasone, 0.5 mg orally at bedtime, to blunt the nighttime secretion of adrenocorticotropic hormone may be useful in hyperandrogenic women who fail to ovulate in response to clomiphene. Other individuals who do not respond to clomiphene typically require exogenous gonadotropins and hCG or perhaps pulsatile GnRH to induce ovulation.

Both bromocriptine and cabergoline are effective in inducing ovulation in hyperprolactinemic women. The drug should be stopped when pregnancy is confirmed. Ovulatory menses and pregnancy are achieved in about 80% of patients with galactorrhea and hyperprolactinemia. Most women with prolactin-secreting pituitary tumors remain asymptomatic during pregnancy. It is rare for a patient with either a microadenoma or a macroadenoma to develop a problem related to the tumor that affects either the mother or the fetus during pregnancy. Monitoring during pregnancy need consist only of questioning the patient about the development of visual symptoms and headaches. Formal assessment of visual fields and computed tomography or magnetic resonance imaging should be carried out in any patient experiencing suggestive symptoms. Symptoms generally abate with institution of therapy with a dopamine agonist. No adverse effects of dopamine agonists on fetuses or pregnancies have been reported. Concerns have been raised that ergot-derived dopamine agonists, in the large doses used in the treatment of Parkinson's disease, may increase the risk for cardiac valve regurgitation. Although there is no evidence of risk in women treated with much lower doses for hyperprolactinemia, they should be counseled about this potential side effect.

Several preparations of purified and synthetic biochemically engineered gonadotropins for use for induction of ovulation now exist. Synthetic preparations consist entirely of FSH, whereas most purified preparations contain some LH as well. Each vial typically contains 75 IU of gonadotropin. Individuals with gonadotropin deficiency require a preparation containing some LH. Exogenous gonadotropins are typically administered at doses of two to four vials (intramuscularly or subcutaneously, depending on the preparation) for 5 to 12 days to achieve follicular development as monitored by ultrasonography and serum or urinary estradiol concentrations; hCG, 5000 to 10,000 IU, is administered as a single intramuscular dose when follicular maturation is apparent.

The hCG should be withheld if more than three follicles mature together. GnRH analogues are now being used to suppress endogenous follicular activity before initiation of therapy with exogenous gonadotropins and continued until hCG is given in older women and those with poor responses to exogenous gonadotropins. Use of the analogues necessitates administration of larger doses of exogenous gonadotropins. Success rates, however, appear to be somewhat improved with this combined therapy. Because of the expense and the complication rate, thorough evaluation should be carried out to exclude other causes of infertility before exogenous gonadotropins and hCG are used. Ovulation can be induced in almost 100% of patients, but pregnancy occurs in only 50 to 70%. There is no increased risk for congenital anomalies with exogenous gonadotropins and hCG. The rate of multiple pregnancies with exogenous gonadotropins and hCG may approach 30%, with 5% being triplets or more.

Ovarian hyperstimulation (*ovarian hyperstimulation syndrome*, or OHSS) is the major side effect and may be life-threatening. The ovaries enlarge remarkably, and multiple follicle cysts, stromal edema, and multiple corpora lutea are present. There is a shift of fluid from the intravascular space into the abdominal cavity with resultant hypovolemia and hemoconcentration. The cause of the ascites is unknown. The most serious complications of OHSS may include thromboembolism, renal failure, adult respiratory distress syndrome, and hemorrhage from ovarian rupture. Treatment is conservative, with monitoring of fluid and electrolyte status. Pelvic examinations should not be performed for fear of rupturing the ovaries. The hyperstimulation generally resolves slowly during about 7 days but lasts longer if the cycle results in pregnancy.

Use of clomiphene citrate or exogenous gonadotropins together with intrauterine insemination of spermatozoa is increasing in women with unexplained infertility as so-called controlled ovarian hyperstimulation (COH). The intent is to stimulate several oocytes to be ovulated, but multiple (sometimes high-order) gestations are a significant risk. A randomized trial has noted that the risk for multiple gestation and the costs are reduced if COH with gonadotropins is not used and patients are advanced immediately to treatment by in vitro fertilization.[2]

Assisted Reproductive Technologies

The assisted reproductive technologies, in which by definition both eggs and sperm are handled outside of the body, are being used with increasing frequency to treat infertile couples with tubal disease, endometriosis, oligospermia and azoospermia, sperm antibodies, and unexplained infertility. The procedure consists of in vitro fertilization and several variants. In vitro fertilization involves ovarian hyperstimulation, oocyte retrieval, fertilization, embryo culture, and embryo transfer. Ovarian hyperstimulation with clomiphene citrate and exogenous gonadotropins, gonadotropins alone, or a GnRH agonist or antagonist plus gonadotropins typically causes 1 to 20 oocytes to mature, depending on the patient's age and ovarian "reserve." After follicular growth is judged sufficient by ultrasound examination, hCG is given to induce final follicular maturation. About 34 hours after hCG administration, the oocytes are retrieved by direct needle puncture of each follicle, usually transvaginally with ultrasound guidance. The oocytes are then inseminated in vitro with washed sperm, or a single sperm is injected directly into a single egg (so-called intracytoplasmic sperm injection). The embryos are cultured for about 40 to 120 hours, after which one or more embryos are transferred to the uterine cavity. Embryos may be cultured to the blastocyst stage (at 120 hours) before transfer. Additional embryos can be frozen in liquid nitrogen for transfer in a subsequent natural cycle. The success rate is most dependent on the age of the woman. In the United States, the percentage of cycles resulting in live births ranges from 40% in women younger than 35 years to 11.5% in women aged 41 to 42 years. Approximately 30% are twins and 3% are triplets or higher-order multiples. Thus, the greatest current problem with in vitro fertilization involves the number of high-order (three or more) multiples resulting.

It is now possible to test the early embryo for genetic abnormalities by removal of either a single cell (i.e., blastomere) or a polar body from the embryo in vitro and testing it with probes by fluorescent in situ hybridization, with the assistance of polymerase chain reaction, or most recently by comparative genomic hybridization. Identification of normal and abnormal embryos allows only normal embryos to be transferred in families with recognized and testable genetic abnormalities.

● SEXUAL FUNCTION AND DYSFUNCTION
Sexual Function

DEFINITION

Sexual responses historically have been divided into four phases: excitement, plateau, orgasm, and resolution. With sexual arousal and excitement, vasocongestion and muscle tension increase progressively, primarily in the genital region, manifested by vaginal lubrication in the female. The lubrication is due to formation of a transudate in the vagina. Sexual excitement is initiated by any of a variety of psychogenic or somatogenic sexual stimuli and must be

reinforced to result in orgasm. With continued stimulation, the excitement phase increases in intensity into a plateau phase during which a high state of sexual interest is maintained. The plateau phase may be short or long, and it is from this phase that an individual can shift to orgasm. The orgasmic phase tends to be brief and is characterized by rapid release from the developed vasocongestion and muscle tension. The orgasmic release is also known as the climax because peak psychological and physical intensity is achieved and there is an attendant feeling of satisfaction. Copious secretions and transudate may flow during orgasm in women. Characteristic genital and extragenital responses occur during these phases. Estrogens magnify the sexual responses, but responses may occur in estrogen-deficient women. For women, these changes occur in the breasts and in the pudendal region and are variable from one response cycle to another. For some women, excitement proceeds quickly through plateau to orgasm, and orgasm is explosive and accompanied by vocalization and involuntary contractions of the pelvic skeletal muscles. For other women, the responses are slow in building, controlled in amplitude, and long lasting. For a few women, orgasm never occurs; for many, it is intermittently absent.

The somatic sensate focus enabling orgasmic release is variable and may include stimulation of the breasts, vagina, or clitoris. The psychological aspect of coitus may involve concentration on the current partner or act or fantasies about other times and persons. Although orgasms may vary in physiologic intensity, what is important is psychological satisfaction. Satisfaction for both men and women may be had without orgasm.

Many clinicians have noted several limitations of this traditional human sex response cycle. More and more clinicians and researchers see the cycle as circular with stimuli of different types leading to arousal. Clinicians in this field now have extended this theory to include desire and arousal. Women seek sexual experiences for intimacy as well as for sexual gratification. Women may be receptive to or seek out sexual stimuli to enhance intimacy. Biologic and psychological factors contribute to the processing of these stimuli and can enhance arousal and desire simultaneously.

Sexual Dysfunction

Women may seek consultation because of disturbances in normal sexual arousal or orgasm. Such sexual dysfunction may be due to either organic or functional disturbances.

A variety of diseases affecting neurologic function, including diabetes mellitus and multiple sclerosis, may prevent sexual arousal. So, too, may local pelvic disorders, such as endometriosis and vaginitis, which cause dyspareunia and lead to sexual avoidance. Estrogen deficiency causing vaginal atrophy and dyspareunia is a relatively common cause of sexual dysfunction. Debilitating systemic diseases such as malignant disease may also affect sexual function indirectly.

In most cases, the cause of sexual dysfunction is psychological. For instance, vaginismus involves involuntary contractions of the muscles surrounding the introitus and leads to dyspareunia. It is a conditioned response engendered by a previous imagined or real traumatic sexual experience. Feelings of guilt (caused by incest or rape, as examples), of inadequacy (caused by hysterectomy or mastectomy), or of depression or anxiety may lead to failure to be aroused. Failure to achieve orgasm may be viewed as a dysfunction if the woman is frustrated or dissatisfied.

TREATMENT   **Rx**

Treatment of sexual dysfunction should eliminate functional causes and provide the patient, often together with her partner, with appropriate psychological counseling. Behavioral modification is effective in treating many women with psychological sexual dysfunction. In one randomized trial, self-reported sexual satisfaction was increased in women treated with testosterone. However, dosing guidelines are not clear, and the therapy cannot be considered standard care based on current evidence.

 Visit expertconsult.com for e-expanded chapter

Grade **A**

1. Legro RS, Barnhart HX, Schlaff WD, et al. Clomiphene, metformin, or both for infertility in the polycystic ovary syndrome. *N Engl J Med.* 2007;356:551-566.
2. Reindollar RH, Regan MM, Neumann PJ, et al. A randomized clinical trial to evaluate optimal treatment for unexplained infertility: the fast track and standardized (FASSTT) trial. *Fertil Steril.* 2009;94:888-899.

SUGGESTED READINGS

Bulun SE. Endometriosis. *N Engl J Med*. 2009;360:268-279. *Review of endometriosis with focus on steroid-related mechanisms.*

De Vos M, Devroey P, Fauser BC, Primary ovarian insufficiency. *Lancet*. 2010;376:911-921. *Review.*

Dey SK. How we are born. *J Clin Invest*. 2010;120:952-955. *Introduction to a series of review articles in the same issue, providing updates on the current understanding of various reproductive processes.*

Gordon CM. Clinical practice: functional hypothalamic amenorrhea. *N Engl J Med*. 2010;363:365-371. *Clinical review.*

Rebar RW. Premature ovarian failure. *Obstet Gynecol*. 2009;113:1355-1363. *Clinical review.*

Richards JS, Pangas SA. The ovary: basic biology and clinical implications. *J Clin Invest*. 2010;120:963-972. *Review.*

XIX

WOMEN'S HEALTH

245

APPROACH TO WOMEN'S HEALTH

KAREN FREUND

An approach to the care of women must go beyond an understanding of differences in the incidence of disease between men and women. Providers need to consider the impact of sex differences (those based on genetic and hormonal differences) and gender differences (those attributable to the roles men and women are ascribed in society). Therapeutic decisions should take into account both genetic and environmental differences in the presentation of disease and the effectiveness of therapeutic options, the patient's reproductive life stage, comorbidities, and social and cultural contexts of care. Empirical evidence about care for women has expanded since 1994, when the National Institutes of Health required the inclusion of women as research subjects. The increased number of women participating in clinical research, coupled with initiatives through the Office on Research and Women's Health, has led to a broad expansion of knowledge and a greater recognition of the need for gender-specific data when evaluating the impact of any therapeutic intervention.

LIFESPAN GROUPS

Many important women's health issues are linked to the social, psychological, and biologic context at certain ages and stages of life. When considering both preventive care and common causes of mortality and morbidity, these lifespan stages provide a context for organizing care (Table 245-1).

For the majority of women, young adulthood (15 to 44 years) is marked by social transitions in family structure, such as forming one's own family and parenting, and entering the work force. Mortality rates are low, and health visits can focus on behavioral decisions that will influence the risk for future disease, such as those pertaining to sexual behavior, smoking, alcohol and drug use, diet, and exercise. Major sources of morbidity include intentional and unintentional injury, including interpersonal violence (Chapter 249) and motor vehicle accidents. HIV is a leading cause of morbidity and mortality in this age group. Depression and anxiety are common in this and all life stages. Reproductive issues are considered in most therapeutic decisions.

The middle years (ages 45 to 65 years) continue to be influenced by behavioral decisions, especially diet, exercise, and alcohol and substance use. The social context includes role changes as children reach adulthood and caregiving responsibilities for children and possibly grandchildren, as well as aging parents. The menopausal transition may be accompanied by new symptomatic concerns. Common causes of morbidity, including diabetes and obesity, now reflect earlier behavioral decisions. Cancer is the leading cause of mortality.

Health issues in older women (65+ years) may occur in the context of loss of function and independence, and because women commonly survive their male partners, they are more likely at this stage of life to be single and possibly more isolated. Cardiovascular disease is the major cause of mortality, followed by cancer, cerebrovascular disease, chronic obstructive lung disease, and pneumonia. Loss of independence is related to cognitive decline, osteoarthritis, osteoporotic fractures, and incontinence.

HEALTH DISPARITIES AMONG WOMEN

It is critical to consider the racial and ethnic differences in outcomes for most common causes of mortality and morbidity when addressing the health status of women. American women with a minority racial or ethnic affiliation, including those of African descent (whether born in the United States or abroad), women from many Asian and Pacific Island nations, Native Americans, and women of Latino background, share poorer outcomes for a wide variety of conditions. This broad finding of poorer outcomes across many diverse ethnic and racial groups points away from specific genetic differences in these populations and toward social determinants of health. Minority racial and ethnic affiliation is correlated with lower educational attainment, lower income, residence in neighborhoods with higher crime and more environmental health hazards, and less access to comprehensive health insurance. Common recommendations for health promotion, including a diet low in fats and processed sugars and high in whole grains, fruits, and vegetables along with regular exercise, such as walking, may be difficult to follow in high-crime neighborhoods or in those without markets offering a variety of affordable, nutritious food options. Barriers to health care access and poor adherence to medical therapy are more common in low-income women. For instance, they may have difficulty scheduling appointments that do not interfere with their work schedules or unpaid time off from clerical or service jobs. The need to care for dependent children or elders may interfere with women's ability to address their own health care needs. Lack of health literacy and cultural barriers can create additional barriers (Chapter 5).

COMMON CAUSES OF MORTALITY IN WOMEN

Cardiovascular Disease

Cardiovascular disease (CVD; Chapter 51) is the overall leading cause of death in women. However because CVD-related death occurs most often in women older than 65 years, its impact is often underrecognized or underestimated. Racial ethnicity plays a large role in the risk for CVD; African American women have much higher rates of CVD and death from CVD than any other racial or ethnic group.

The incidence rate of CVD in women lags 10 years behind that of men from ages 40 through 70; that is, a 65-year-old woman has the same risk as a 55-year-old man. There is no abrupt increase in CVD risk at menopause in women, suggesting that menopause and changes in estrogen or progesterone status do not account for this sex difference. Furthermore, randomized clinical trials have confirmed that hormone therapy in women does not prevent CVD and is not indicated for CVD prevention.[1] Re-analysis of the Women's Health Initiative confirmed the increased risk of CVD *with* hormone therapy, even when treatment is initiated within 10 years of menopause.[2] Other risk factors for CVD in women are the same as those in men: elevated lipids, lack of physical activity, obesity, smoking, hypertension, and diabetes. Women with diabetes have the same risk of CVD as men of the same age with diabetes. Because smoking rates in current cohorts of young women are equal to or exceed those of men of the same age, it is becoming one of the more important behavioral risk factors of CVD in women. The incidence of many known risk factors, including obesity, hypertension, and hypercholesterolemia, is greater in African American women than in white women.

The presentation of coronary disease in women differs from that in men. Although chest pain is the most common presentation in women, atypical and noncardiac pain is a more common presentation in women than in men, and fewer women have typical chest tightness or pressure as their presenting complaint. For this and other reasons, women present for emergency care at a later time than men, which may limit some therapeutic options and increase the severity of disease complications, including congestive heart failure.

Guidelines for the management of lipid disorders in the prevention of CVD are the same for men and women (Chapter 213). The decision to begin pharmacotherapy is based on both the absolute low-density lipoprotein (LDL) level and risk factors for CVD events. Elevated high-density lipoprotein (HDL) levels confer protection and are therefore considered to reduce one's risk. This factor requires particular attention before beginning therapy in many women. Aggressive LDL management to levels below 100 mg/dL (some suggest <80 mg/dL) is recommended for women with diabetes or known vascular disease, including cerebrovascular disease.

Medical management is similar for men and women with acute coronary syndromes, including unstable angina and acute myocardial infarction (Chapter 72). The use of aspirin, β-blockers, angiotensin-converting enzyme (ACE) inhibitors, heparin, and thrombolytic therapy and recommendations for noninvasive testing are the same for women and men. Randomized controlled trial data show that low-risk women with unstable angina or non–ST segment elevation myocardial infarction do not benefit from early revascularization and that medical management is indicated.[3]

Type 2 Diabetes

The rates of type 2 diabetes (Chapter 237) continue to rise, with a greater risk in women who are overweight or obese and physically inactive. Rates are higher in many racial and ethnic groups than among white women, including African Americans, Asians, Native Americans, and Latinas. Although most guidelines do not currently recommend universal screening, given the high rates of undiagnosed diabetes, screening women for known risk factors (e.g., obesity, family history) seems prudent. For women who develop gestational diabetes (Chapter 247), the risk of developing type 2 diabetes later in life increases five-fold; therefore, screening with fasting glucose testing at least biennially is indicated.

TABLE 245-1 IMPORTANT HEALTH ISSUES FOR WOMEN THROUGH THE LIFESPAN

ISSUE	Ages		
	15-44 YEARS	45-65 YEARS	65+ YEARS
Behavioral issues	Risk behaviors Sexual behavior Smoking Alcohol and drug use Exercise Diet	Risk behaviors Smoking Alcohol and drug use Exercise Diet	Risk behaviors Smoking Exercise
Social roles	Entering work force Relationship transitions Parenting	Caregiving to several generations Transitions in family and work environments	Losses and social isolation
Reproductive issues	Reproductive health issues	Menopause transition	
Injury	Intentional and unintentional interpersonal violence Motor vehicle accidents		Falls
Common causes of mortality and morbidity	Depression Anxiety HIV/AIDS	Cancer Obesity Diabetes Depression Anxiety	Cardiovascular disease Cancer Cognitive decline Osteoporosis Osteoarthritis Incontinence Depression Anxiety

The incidence of diabetes is rising in women at younger ages, with significant perinatal implications. Ongoing discussion of fertility control and family planning is critical in diabetic women with childbearing potential. Tight glycemic control before conception and through the first trimester is critical to reduce the risk of birth anomalies, and it is important later in pregnancy to reduce the risk of adverse fetal events, including macrosomia (large for gestational age) and preterm birth (Chapter 247). Ideally, women planning a pregnancy should switch from oral agents to insulin, with home glucose monitoring for tight control (Table 245-2).

Cancer

Cancer is the leading cause of death in women 40 through 65 years, and it is the leading cause of years of life lost in women younger than 65. Breast cancer (Chapter 204) is the most common type of cancer and the second leading cause of cancer death in women, although most women who develop breast cancer do survive. Studies indicate that many women significantly overestimate their personal risk of the disease. The lack of understanding of the cause of most breast cancers and the limitations and uncertainties of the imaging modalities used as screening tests have limited efforts at breast cancer control. After decades of an increasing incidence of breast cancer in the United States, incidence rates have fallen in the past 3 to 5 years. The cause of this decline is not understood; reduced use of postmenopausal hormone therapy and recent declines in screening rates have both been implicated.

Lung cancer (Chapter 197) is the leading cause of cancer death in women, and rates continue to rise, commensurate with the number of women who took up smoking in the 1940s and 1950s and the lower rates of smoking cessation in women compared with men. Most lung cancers are smoking related, although women are more likely than men to have lung cancers that are not tobacco related. There is no effective screening modality for lung cancer.

Colorectal cancer (Chapter 199) has a similar incidence in both women and men. Testing for occult blood in the stool, sigmoidoscopy, and colonoscopy are effective at detecting precancerous lesions and thereby reducing rates of both new cancers and later-stage disease.

Ovarian cancer (Chapter 205) is relatively rare, with 21,500 cases in the United States annually, but mortality is high owing to its presentation at late stages in most cases. Lower abdominal or pelvic pain, urinary symptoms, and changes in bowel habits are nonspecific and common in many women,

limiting the ability to detect this cancer at an early stage. There is no effective screening test for women at average risk. CA-125 has both low sensitivity and low specificity, with normal levels in early-stage disease and elevations with nonmalignant ovarian pathology. Recent studies suggest that serial CA-125 levels in postmenopausal women may have increased predictive value.

The greatest recent advance in cancer prevention is the development of vaccines against the most carcinogenic subtypes of human papillomavirus (HPV) associated with cervical cancer (Chapters 205 and 381) and anal cancer. The vaccine has the potential to reduce significant morbidity caused by the management of premalignant lesions, including the risk of cervical incompetence and preterm labor. New guidelines advocate delaying Pap test screening in women until age 21 years and increasing the screening interval to every 2 years in women aged 20 to 29 years and every 3 years in women 30 years and older if previous screening has demonstrated no high-risk subtypes of the HPV.

Osteoporosis

Hip fracture due to osteoporosis (Chapter 251) is one of the major causes of disability, loss of independence, and mortality in older women. Osteoporosis prevention through calcium and vitamin D intake and weight-bearing exercise begins at puberty and extends throughout adulthood. Women require a calcium intake of 1000 mg/day, increasing to 1300 mg in puberty and breast-feeding and 1200 mg after menopause, in order to maintain the structural strength of bone. Vitamin D is a necessary element for the absorption of calcium, and it is available through direct sun exposure or vitamin D supplementation of milk (not other dairy products) and some juices. Epidemiologic data suggest widespread vitamin D deficiency in women in the United States. This is attributed to low levels of dietary replacement, decreased sun exposure with the use of sunscreens, and lack of vitamin D production in the skin (even with sun exposure) in northern climates during the winter months. Screening for a single baseline serum 25-hydroxyvitamin D level can provide women with useful information about the adequacy of their diets, with levels above 30 ng/mL considered sufficient or ideal. Short-term, high-dose therapy consisting of 50,000 IU/week for 12 weeks is recommended in women with serum 25-hydroxyvitamin D levels less than 20 ng/mL, followed by daily replacement with 600 to 800 IU. Daily replacement of vitamin D of 600 IU is recommended for women, with 800 IU recommended after age 70.

Although no long-term outcome data exist on the benefits of dual-energy x-ray absorptiometry (DXA) screening (DEXA bone densitometry), many advocate a single screen within 2 years of menopause and a follow-up 2 to 5 years later to determine both absolute bone density and rate of loss. An algorithm to assess risk of bone fracture based on DXA and individual risk factors is available through the World Health Organization and can guide decision making on preventive therapy. Long-term estrogen therapy is not recommended for osteoporosis prevention. Initial enthusiasm for bisphosphonate therapy has been tempered by reports of rare but debilitating jaw osteonecrosis (Chapter 256). This complication has been seen in women with and without risk factors, such as dental disease. Raloxifene, a selective estrogen receptor modulator, has the benefits of preventing osteoporosis while reducing breast cancer risk without increasing the risk of CVD; it has been underutilized as a preventive agent.

● COMMON CAUSES OF MORBIDITY IN WOMEN

Obesity

Obesity rates continue to rise, and the prevalence of obesity is higher in women than men, especially among minority and low-income women (Chapter 227). Dietary reduction in calories and increased caloric output with aerobic exercise are the short- and long-term strategies for care. Studies suggest that no single diet is superior to others, and many common diet strategies can reduce weight. Increasing activity during the course of one's daily routine is as effective as shorter intervals of more strenuous activity. The most effective programs include a combination of behavioral therapy, either individually or in groups, to address behavioral patterns in food intake, along with diet and exercise. Weight loss targets of 1 to 2 lb/week and a total loss of up to 5 to 10% of body weight are realistic goals. Even modest changes in weight and modest increases in physical activity reduce morbidity and mortality on a population basis.

Exercise and diet changes are difficult for many people to achieve, for a wide variety of reasons. The physical environment may not be conducive to

TABLE 245-2 PREFERRED MEDICATIONS FOR WOMEN OF REPRODUCTIVE POTENTIAL

COMMON CONDITIONS IN WOMEN OF REPRODUCTIVE POTENTIAL	ISSUES TO BE AWARE OF	PREFERRED MEDICATIONS OR GROUPS OF MEDICATIONS
Depression	Must consider effects of untreated depression on mother and infant Paroxetine may cause congenital heart defects	Avoid newer medications when older drugs with more information are available SSRIs are generally considered safe; fluoxetine is preferred, with most safety data
Anxiety	Commonly associated with depression in women	Benzodiazepines are not associated with cleft lip and have no known harmful effects; choose those with shorter half-life
GERD	No data on harmful effects of either H$_2$-blockers or PPIs Misoprostol is contraindicated; can cause miscarriage, fetal death, congenital anomalies	Calcium-containing antacids are first-line therapy H$_2$-blockers preferred over PPIs
Acne	Oral isotretinoin and topical tazarotene are contraindicated owing to congenital defects	Most other topical agents are considered classes B and C
Asthma	Extensive data on safety of common drug categories: benefit ratios far exceed risk in treating women	Cortisone inhalers Systemic prednisone for flares Short- and long-acting bronchodilators
Seizure disorders	Difficult to separate effects of medication from effects of seizure on fetal development All agents associated with some increased risk of fetal abnormality (4-8%, compared with 1-2% in general population)	Monotherapy at lowest doses recommended Avoid medication changes in first trimester Folate supplementation in preconception period
Hypertension (not preeclampsia)	ACE inhibitors and ARBs are contraindicated in pregnancy; possibly associated with cardiovascular and neurologic anomalies in first trimester; may cause abnormalities in renal hemodynamics in third trimester Most data suggest thiazide diuretics are safe if stable use before pregnancy	β-blockers, especially labetalol, and methyldopa are first-lines choices Calcium-channel blockers are also considered safe
Lipid disorders	Circulating lipid levels are elevated with pregnancy and breast-feeding.	No medications during pregnancy; ideally, stop statins before conception
Analgesics for fever and pain management	Controversy about whether NSAIDs slightly increase risk of miscarriage in first trimester	Acetaminophen preferred; aspirin also considered safe
Headache	Controversy about whether NSAIDs slightly increase risk of miscarriage in first trimester	Acetaminophen preferred; aspirin also considered safe
Diabetes	First-generation sulfonylureas contraindicated in pregnancy; may cause fetal hyperinsulinemia and birth defects	Conversion to insulin during planned preconception period Insulin, metformin, and glyburide preferred in women of childbearing potential
Autoimmune conditions	Must weigh benefits of immunosuppressive use against potential risks to both mother and infant Methotrexate is contraindicated in pregnancy, as it induces miscarriage No data on safety or risk of TNF and IL-1 inhibitors	Prednisone generally considered safe in pregnancy Azathioprine, sulfasalazine, cyclosporine, and hydroxychloroquine generally preferred if required
Tobacco control	Cigarette smoking has known harmful effects on fetus In one small randomized controlled trial, nicotine replacement was associated with reduced levels of nicotine and improved birth outcomes Bupropion is linked with reports of some fetal anomalies	Try nonpharmacologic approaches to cessation first Short course of nicotine replacement likely better for fetus than smoking
Polycystic ovarian disease	Metformin can restore ovulatory cycles; use with contraception	
Bacterial infections	Tetracyclines accumulate in fetal bone and teeth Sulfa drugs may increase risk of neural tube defects with use in first trimester and kernicterus with use in third trimester Trimethoprim interferes with folic acid metabolism Streptomycin and kanamycin associated with bilateral deafness	Penicillins, cephalosporins, erythromycin, azithromycin

ACE = angiotensin-converting enzyme; ARB = angiotensin receptor blocker; GERD = gastroesophageal reflux disease; IL-1 = interleukin-1; NSAID = nonsteroidal anti-inflammatory drug; PPI = proton pump inhibitor; SSRI = selective serotonin re-uptake inhibitor; TNF = tumor necrosis factor.

physical activity owing to the sedentary nature of most workplaces, the lack of safe areas to exercise, and architectural design features, such as the lack of easy access to stairs instead of elevators. The use of prepared foods and the consumption of fast foods, high in fat and calories and low in nutritional content, increase the risk obesity.

There are currently no evidence-based interventions to support weight reduction in the setting of a brief office visit. Most guidelines focus on assessing body mass index (BMI) in all women and recommending weight reduction with diet restriction and exercise, including behavioral therapy to support these behavioral changes. For obese women with a BMI greater than 40, or those with a BMI greater than 35 and major comorbidities such as diabetes, sleep apnea, or osteoarthritis, bariatric surgery (Chapter 227) is indicated once other weight loss methods have failed. Bariatric surgery leads to short- and long-term benefits in multiple comorbidities and reduced mortality due to improvements in comorbidities. Critical to the success of this intervention is a team approach, with psychological assessment and diet and exercise programs beginning before and continuing after surgery.

Depression

Major depression and other related disorders, including dysthymia, predominate in women (Chapter 404). Multiple short screening tools have been developed to identify depression. Women with depression are highly likely to come to the attention of the health care system, for two reasons. First, chronic medical conditions are associated with higher rates of depression and are treated by both generalists and specialists. Depression is a significant comorbidity in many chronic medical conditions affecting both younger and older women. Screening for depression should be considered for women with chronic medical conditions, and management of depression is necessary to prevent adverse outcomes from these conditions. Second, somatic complaints are a common presentation of depressive disorders and are more common in women than in men. All specialties are likely to see patients with unexplained symptoms, such as chest pain, headache, abdominal pain, and other complaints. It is critical to include depression as either a primary or a secondary diagnosis and to treat depression as part of the overall management plan.

Anxiety Disorders

Anxiety disorders also predominate in women. They commonly coexist with depressive disorders. Anxiety disorders, including post-traumatic stress disorder, may be a consequence of violence against women, which often remains unidentified (Chapter 249). Benzodiazepines have been demonstrated to be safe and effective in trials for short-term use. Selective serotonin re-uptake inhibitors (SSRIs) and behavioral therapies are effective for the long-term management of anxiety disorders.

Osteoarthritis

Osteoarthritis (Chapter 270) is one of the most common causes of morbidity and functional status limitation, especially as women age. Assessment of pain and functional status is at the core of management. Physical and occupational therapy to restore functional status is a critical component of care. Joint replacement (Chapter 285) should be considered and recommended when functional status interferes with activities of daily living and supportive care and other symptom management strategies are ineffective.

Smoking

Tobacco use, most commonly cigarette smoking, continues to be one of the major preventable causes of morbidity and mortality in women (Chapter 31). Although there has been much progress in smoking cessation efforts, lower-income women and younger women continue to start smoking and fail to quit smoking at high rates. In the 1990s more teenage girls than teenage boys started to smoke, and more than 25% of teenage girls became smokers owing to increased marketing to teens generally and to girls specifically. With community- and school-based efforts to promote tobacco control and the increased cost of cigarettes through taxes, smoking rates for girls and boys are now the same, with about 18% of teens smoking. Public health efforts and resources to promote smoking cessation are highly effective. Health care providers can achieve 1 to 2% smoking cessation rates by asking all patients about their smoking status and making a simple statement encouraging smokers to quit. Further gains in smoking cessation are possible with targeted counseling, which involves assessing the patient's stage of readiness to change and providing counseling relevant to that stage.

Nicotine replacement is equally effective in women and men. Smokers with a physiologic addiction to nicotine (those who smoke more than one pack daily or smoke within 20 minutes of awakening) benefit the most from nicotine replacement. Many women report weight gain as a major barrier to smoking cessation. Chapter 31 describes approaches to smoking cessation.

Incontinence

Urinary incontinence (Chapter 25) is a frequently overlooked cause of major functional status limitations in middle-aged and older women. As many as half of affected women underreport this problem to their physicians and alter their lifestyles to adapt to the problem, including reducing fluid intake, avoiding activities that exacerbate the problem, or restricting travel where access to facilities is uncertain. There are two broad categories of incontinence—stress incontinence and urge incontinence—although women commonly have aspects of both types. Stress incontinence is defined as leaking with increases in intra-abdominal pressure, such as occurs with sneezing or coughing as well as running or walking. The most common reasons are pelvic floor laxity, often from childbirth. Kegel exercises are frequently recommended but are of limited value. A number of surgical procedures are available to address this condition. Less invasive procedures may be tried first, include the fitting of a vaginal pessary or periurethral injections with biodegradable materials such as collagen or with nonbiodegradable materials. Urge incontinence, described as detrusor muscle instability, results in the urge to void with low volumes. Anticholinergic medications and bladder training are both effective. Urodynamic evaluation should be considered if the history does not clearly identify a cause.

HIV Disease

The risk factors for HIV disease in women are heterosexual contact in 80% of new cases and injection drug use in 20%. HIV continues to affect minority women disproportionately, with 61% of incident cases affecting African American women. Incidence rates remain lower in women than in men, with only 27% of incident cases affecting women; in large part, this is due to the fact that male-to-male sexual contact continues to account for 72% of new cases in men. However, the absolute number of new infections from heterosexual contact is twice as high in women as it is in men. Women with HIV/AIDS continue to have poorer survival than men, despite the availability of antiretroviral therapies. Some data suggest that women are less likely than men to adhere to an antiretroviral therapy regimen. The gender difference in therapy adherence was associated with caring for dependent children in one study, suggesting that women's caregiving roles may be a barrier to their own care. Cervical and anal dysplasia and cancer are more common among women with HIV than those without. Therefore, annual Pap tests are recommended for all women with HIV infection, even in the absence of positive HPV testing. There is insufficient evidence to support anal screening for dysplasia, but providers should be aware of the increased risk and perform an external examination for evidence of lesions.

REPRODUCTIVE HEALTH ISSUES

All providers caring for women with reproductive potential should consider the reproductive implications of preventive and therapeutic decisions. With half of all pregnancies in the United States unplanned, providers should routinely inquire about contraceptive practices and consider these in their care plans.

All primary care providers should be comfortable counseling patients about contraceptive choices and prescribing oral contraceptives. The absolute contraindications to oral contraceptives are a personal history of CVD, thromboembolic disease, or gynecologic or breast cancer. A family history of cancer is not considered a contraindication; in fact, data suggest that the use of oral contraceptives decreases the risk of both endometrial and ovarian cancer. Smoking while using oral contraceptives increases the risk of thromboembolic events in all women, but especially in those older than 30 years. Oral contraceptive use is considered safe in nonsmoking women until menopause. Although factor Leiden V has been associated with an increased risk of deep vein thrombosis in those taking oral contraceptives, the absolute risk to any woman is still very low; therefore, screening for this and other genetic thrombophilias is not indicated. Preexisting hypertension is a relative contraindication to oral contraceptive use. Some women develop elevated blood pressures on oral contraceptives; therefore, blood pressure should be monitored at 3 months after starting the drug and then annually.

Providers should consider the reproductive implications of all chronic medications in women of reproductive potential (Chapter 247). Given that the teratogenic effects of medications may occur during the first trimester and before an initial obstetric assessment, the principle when choosing chronic medications for women during their reproductive years is to select those with the greatest safety profile during the first trimester of pregnancy. Table 245-2 outlines common drug categories and recommendation for use in pregnancy.

Antidepressant medications deserve particular attention because of the conflicting data regarding their use in pregnancy. Some initial reports suggested that antidepressants, especially paroxetine, were associated with congenital defects; however, further study suggests that other medications are safe, with fluoxetine having the most data. For women who wish to take no medication during pregnancy, the recommendation is to gradually reduce the dosage over the course of several weeks and not to abruptly stop taking the medication. The risk of untreated depression during pregnancy and the risk of postpartum depression to the woman and her infant are substantial. Therefore, treatment goals should be to provide adequate dosing to prevent the worsening of depression during this period.

1. Rossouw JE, Anderson GL, Prentice RL, et al. Risks and benefits of estrogen plus progestin in healthy postmenopausal women: principal results from the Women's Health Initiative randomized controlled trial. *JAMA.* 2002;288:321-333.
2. Toh S, Hernández-Díaz S, Logan R, et al. Coronary heart disease in postmenopausal recipients of estrogen plus progestin therapy: does the increased risk ever disappear? A randomized trial. *Ann Intern Med.* 2010;152:211-217.
3. Lagerqvist B, Safstrom K, Stahle E, et al. Is early invasive treatment of unstable coronary artery disease equally effective for both women and men? FRISC II Study Group Investigators. *J Am Coll Cardiol.* 2001;38:41-48.

SUGGESTED READINGS

FRAX WHO Risk Assessment Tool. http://www.shef.ac.uk/FRAX/. *Algorithm to assess the risk of osteoporotic fracture in women with osteopenia and to guide preventive therapy.*

Gupta K, Hooton TM, Naber KG, et al. Executive summary: international clinical practice guidelines for the treatment of acute uncomplicated cystitis and pyelonephritis in women: a 2010 update by the Infectious Diseases Society of America and the European Society for Microbiology and Infectious Diseases. *Clin Infect Dis.* 2011;52:561-564. *Consensus guidelines, including antimicrobial resistance.*

Mosca L, Benjamin EJ, Berra K, et al. Effectiveness-based guidelines for the prevention of cardiovascular disease in women—2011 update: a guideline from the American Heart Association. *Circulation.* 2011;123:1243-1262. *Consensus guidelines.*

Partridge EE, Abu-Rustum NR, Campos SM, et al. Cervical cancer screening. *J Natl Compr Canc Netw.* 2010;8:1358-1386. *Overview of screening techniques, including HPV testing.*

Santen RJ, Allred DC, Ardoin SP, et al. Postmenopausal hormone therapy: an Endocrine Society scientific statement. *J Clin Endocrinol Metab.* 2010;95:s1-s66. *Consensus guidelines.*

Schwarz EB, McNamara M, Miller RG, et al. Update in women's health for the general internist. *J Gen Intern Med.* 2011;26:207-213. *Review.*

246

CONTRACEPTION

DANIEL R. MISHELL JR.

● CONTRACEPTIVE USE AND EFFECTIVENESS

Contraceptive Use

Reversible contraception, the temporary prevention of fertility, includes all contraceptive methods except sterilization. Sterilization should be considered permanent despite the possibility of surgical reversal. There are advantages and disadvantages of each contraceptive method. During contraceptive counseling, these advantages and disadvantages should be thoroughly explained so that the individual will choose the most acceptable method and not discontinue use prematurely and have an unwanted pregnancy.

In the United States in 2006-2008 (the latest years for which data are available), there were about 61.8 million women in the reproductive age group (15 to 44 years), and 38 million (62%) were using a method of contraception. Of the remainder, about 2% were sterile (prior hysterectomy), 9% were pregnant or trying to conceive, and 19% were never sexually active or had no recent sexual activity. About 7.3% of women who were sexually active were not using a method of contraception, an increase from the 5.2% incidence of this group in 1995.

In the United States in 2006-2008, the most common methods of fertility prevention were oral contraceptives (OCs) and female sterilization, used by 17.3% and 16.7% of women aged 15 to 44 years, respectively. Next in frequency of use was the male condom (10.0%), followed by male sterilization (6.1%). The injectable progestin was used by 2.0%, but the intrauterine device (IUD), the most effective method of reversible contraception, was used by only 3.4%. Between 1982 and 2006-2008, there was a marked decrease in diaphragm use and an increase in condom use. Between 2002 and 2006-2008, diaphragm use virtually disappeared, IUD use tripled, and condom use stabilized. About 80% of reproductive-age women who have had intercourse have used OCs at some time.

Contraceptive Effectiveness

Despite an increased use of contraceptive methods by U.S. women since 1982, more than half the pregnancies that occur are unintended. Of the 6.4 million pregnancies that occurred in the United States in 2002 (the most recent data available), about half were unintended, and 42% of these pregnancies were terminated by elective abortion. Of the women with an unintended pregnancy, 50% stated they were using a method of contraception in the month they conceived.

Typical Use versus Perfect Use

The terms *method effectiveness* and *use effectiveness* (or *method failure* and *patient failure*) were previously used to describe the frequency of conceptions that occurred while the method was being used correctly or incorrectly. These terms have been replaced by the terms *typical use* and *perfect use*. Methods used at the time of coitus have higher failure rates than OCs, implants, injections, IUDs, and sterilization. Cumulative failure rates for use of long-acting methods are low. The cumulative pregnancy rate for 5 years' use of the levonorgestrel-releasing IUD is 0.5% and for 10 years' use of the copper T380 IUD is 1.7%. The cumulative failure rate of all types of tubal sterilization is 1.31% during the first 5 years after the procedure and 1.85% after 10 years, being highest for tubal fulguration and lowest for segmental resection. When women conceive while using these long-acting methods, the ectopic pregnancy rates are high: about 30% with tubal sterilization failure and 5% with copper IUD failure.

● TYPES OF CONTRACEPTIVES

Spermicides and Barriers

All spermicidal agents contain a surfactant, usually nonoxynol 9, that immobilizes or kills sperm on contact. They also provide a mechanical barrier and need to be placed into the vagina before each coital act. There is no increased risk for birth defects in the offspring of women who conceive while using spermicides.

Diaphragm

A diaphragm must be carefully fitted by the health care provider. The largest size that does not cause discomfort or undue pressure on the vagina should be used. The diaphragm should not be left in place for more than 24 hours because it may cause ulceration of the vaginal epithelium. Diaphragm users have an increased risk for urinary tract infection.

Male Condom

Use of the latex male condom by individuals with multiple sex partners should be encouraged because it is the most effective way to prevent sexually transmitted infections (Chapter 293). The natural membrane condoms do not prevent sexually transmitted infections, but polyurethane condoms do.

Female Condom

The female condom consists of a soft, loose-fitting prelubricated sheath and two flexible polyurethane rings. The female condom can be inserted before beginning sexual activity and left in place for a longer time than the male condom after ejaculation occurs. Because the female condom covers the external genitalia, it may prevent transmission of genital herpes. Because polyurethane is stronger than the latex used in most male condoms, the female condom is less likely to rupture. Both polyurethane and latex prevent virus transmission and should reduce the risk for acquiring human immunodeficiency virus infection.

Oral Steroid Contraceptives

There are three major types of OC formulations: fixed-dose combination, combination phasic, and daily progestin. The combination formulations are the most widely used and most effective. They consist of tablets containing both an estrogen and a progestin, usually given continuously for 3 weeks. No steroids are given for the next 7 days (except for one formulation in which estrogen alone is given for an additional 5 days), after which time the active combination is given for an additional 3 weeks. Three formulations provide active tablets for 24 days with 4 days of inactive tablets. Other formulations provide active tablets for 84 days followed by 7 days without active tablets or a low dose of estrogen to allow withdrawal bleeding. The endometrium usually begins to slough 1 to 3 days after steroid ingestion is stopped, causing withdrawal bleeding, which usually lasts 3 to 4 days. The uterine blood loss with OC use averages about 25 mL per cycle, less than the 35 mL average for ovulatory cycles.

Constituents and Action

All formulations are made from synthetic steroids. There are two major types of synthetic progestins: derivatives of 19-nortestosterone (which are used in OCs) and derivatives of 17α-acetoxyprogesterone (pregnanes). Pregnanes are structurally related to progesterone and are used in injectable contraceptives but are not used in OCs.

The 19-nortestosterone progestins used in OCs are of two major types, estranes and gonanes, and both have androgenic activity. The estranes currently used in several OCs are norethindrone and its acetates, norethindrone acetate and ethynodiol diacetate. Gonanes have greater progestational activity per unit weight than estranes, and thus a smaller amount of these progestins is used in OC formulations. One other progestin that is structurally related to spironolactone has been formulated in an OC. This progestin is called drospirenone and has antimineralocorticoid and antiandrogenic activity as well as progestational activity without androgenic activity.

With the exception of a daily progestin-only formulation, the progestins are combined with varying dosages of three estrogens, ethinyl estradiol and its 3-methyl ether, mestranol, as well as one agent with estradiol valerate. The estrogen-progestin combination is the most effective type of OC formulation because these preparations consistently inhibit the midcycle gonadotropin surge and thus prevent ovulation. The progestin-only formulation has a lower dose of progestin than the combined agents and does not consistently inhibit ovulation, even though it is ingested every day. Both types of formulations also act on the cervical mucus and tubal motility to interfere with sperm transport. Progestins also alter the endometrium so that if fertilization occurs, implantation may be prevented. For contraceptive effectiveness to be maintained with the combination formulations, it is important that the pill-free interval be limited to no more than 7 days. This is best accomplished by ingestion of either a placebo or an iron tablet daily during the steroid-free interval.

Metabolic Effects

The synthetic steroids in OC formulations have many metabolic effects in addition to their contraceptive actions. These effects can cause the more common, less serious side effects as well as the rare, serious complications. The magnitude of these effects is directly related to the dosage and potency of the steroids in the formulations.

Symptoms Due to Estrogen and Progestin

The most frequent symptoms produced by the estrogen component include nausea, breast tenderness, and fluid retention (bloating). The progestins can produce certain androgenic effects, such as weight gain, acne, and nervousness. Because estrogens decrease sebum production, women who have acne should be given a formulation with a low progestin-to-estrogen ratio. Unscheduled (breakthrough) bleeding is usually produced by insufficient estrogen, too much progestin, or a combination of both. This problem is more common with formulations containing 20 µg of estrogen than with those containing 30 to 35 µg and is increased in women who also smoke cigarettes. Shortening the pill-free interval to 3 or 4 days should prevent ovarian follicular development and may decrease the incidence of unscheduled bleeding with low-estrogen formulations.

The synthetic estrogens used in OCs cause an increase in the hepatic production of several proteins. The progestins do not affect protein synthesis except to reduce levels of sex hormone–binding globulin. Some of the proteins that are increased by ethinyl estradiol, such as factors V, VIII, and X and fibrinogen, have the potential to enhance thrombosis, whereas an increase in angiotensinogen levels may elevate blood pressure in some users. Blood pressure should be monitored in all users of OCs and the agent discontinued if there is a clinically significant increase. The incidence of both venous and arterial thrombosis in OC users is higher with 50-µg estrogen formulations than with those with 20 to 35 µg of estrogen.

Glucose and Lipid Metabolism

The effect of OCs on glucose metabolism is directly related to the dose, potency, and type of progestin. Although high-progestin formulations caused peripheral insulin resistance, the low-progestin formulations in current use do not significantly alter levels of glucose, insulin, or glucagon after a glucose load. High-progestin formulations have an adverse effect on the lipid profile; because of the direct beneficial effect of estrogen on the arterial wall and serum lipids, however, users of these agents do not have an increased risk for cardiovascular disease. The newer combination formulations with less androgenic progestins have a more favorable effect on the lipid profile.

Complications and Risk Factors
Thrombosis

The cause of the increased incidence of both venous and arterial cardiovascular disease in users of OCs is thrombosis, not atherosclerosis. The background rate of venous thrombosis and embolism in women of reproductive age is about 0.8 per 10,000 woman years. Among users of OCs with 30 or 35 µg of ethinyl estradiol, it is 3 per 10,000 woman years, about four times the background rate but half the rate of 6 per 10,000 woman years that occurs in association with pregnancy. The risk for venous thrombosis and embolism is higher among women ingesting OCs with 50 µg of ethinyl estradiol than those with 30 to 35 µg. In the presence of an inherited coagulopathy disorder (Chapter 179), the risk for venous thrombosis is increased several-fold. It is not recommended that screening for coagulation deficiencies be undertaken before women are started on OC use unless the individual has a personal or family history of thrombotic events. Women with known inherited or acquired thrombophilic conditions should not use estrogen-containing steroid contraceptives in pills, rings, or patches because each of these agents has thrombophilic effects. Some epidemiologic studies have found that the risk for venous thromboembolism is greater in individuals ingesting OCs with the newer less androgenic progestins than those containing levonorgestrel with the same amount of estrogen. However, other studies have reported that the risk is similar with formulations containing these two types of progestins. These studies are all observational and thus subject to bias.

Myocardial Infarction

The use of high-dose OCs by women who smoke cigarettes significantly increases the risk for myocardial infarction. Therefore, combination OCs should not be prescribed to women older than 35 years who smoke cigarettes or use alternate forms of nicotine. Epidemiologic studies indicate that use of low-dose OCs by nonsmoking women without hypertension is not associated with a significantly increased incidence of either myocardial infarction or hemorrhagic or thrombotic stroke.

Delayed Fertility

For about 2 years after the discontinuation of contraceptives, the rate of return of fertility is slightly lower for users of OCs than for users of barrier methods. OCs do not cause permanent infertility or adversely affect pregnancies that occur after their discontinuation. OCs are not teratogenic if they are accidentally ingested during pregnancy.

Breast Cancer

An analysis of worldwide epidemiologic data in 1988 showed that the risk for breast cancer diagnosis was increased by about 25% in young women who were currently using OCs, but this increased risk was no longer present 10 years or more after they stopped using OCs. Several studies have reported that use of OCs by women with a family history of breast cancer does not increase their risk of developing breast cancer (Chapter 204). A large study of women aged 35 to 64 years in the United States reported that there was no significantly increased risk for breast cancer among current and former OC users compared with women who had not used OCs. A very large cohort study in Great Britain of OC users and aged-matched nonusers was initiated in 1968. Data accumulated until 2004 showed a similar incidence of breast cancer in both groups.

Cervical Cancer

The epidemiologic data regarding the risk for invasive cervical cancer as well as cervical intraepithelial neoplasia and OC use are conflicting. Most well-controlled studies indicate that there is no change in risk for cervical intraepithelial neoplasia with OC use. However, it is likely that a causal relationship exists between OC use and a reported increased risk for cervical adenocarcinoma. OC users need annual cervical cytologic screening (Chapter 205).

Endometrial Cancer

Several studies have shown that the use of OCs has a protective effect against endometrial cancer. Moreover, the decrease in risk persists for many years after OCs are stopped. Women who use OCs for at least 1 year have a 50% reduced risk for endometrial cancer development between the ages of 40 and 65 years compared with nonusers. This protective effect is related to duration of use, increasing from a 20% reduction with 1 year of use to a 60% reduction with 4 years of use.

Epithelial Ovarian Cancer

In addition, OCs reduce the risk for development of epithelial ovarian cancer as well as cancers with low malignant potential. The magnitude of the decrease in risk is directly related to the duration of OC use, increasing from about a 40% reduction with 4 years of use to a 60% reduction with 12 years of use. The protective effect continues for at least 20 years after the use of OCs ends. As with endometrial cancer, the protective effect occurs only in women of low parity (fewer than four), who are at greatest risk for this type of cancer. Studies have reported that OCs significantly reduce the risk for development of colorectal cancer by about 20%.

Benign Hepatocellular Adenoma

The development of a benign hepatocellular adenoma was a rare occurrence in long-term users of high-dose OCs containing mestranol, but it is not increased by use of ethinyl estradiol OCs. There is no increased risk for liver cancer associated with OC use.

Contraindications

The OCs can be prescribed for most women of reproductive age. An absolute contraindication is a history of vascular disease, including systemic diseases that affect the vascular system, such as lupus erythematosus and diabetes with retinopathy or nephropathy. Cigarette smoking by a woman older than 35 years and uncontrolled hypertension are also contraindications, as are a personal history of cancer of the breast or endometrium and cholestatic jaundice of pregnancy. Pregnancy and any undiagnosed cause of uterine bleeding are also contraindications. Women with functional heart diseases should not use OCs because the fluid retention could result in congestive heart failure. There is no evidence, however, that individuals with asymptomatic mitral valve prolapse should not use OCs. Women with active liver disease should not take OCs. However, women who have recovered from liver disease, such as viral hepatitis, and whose liver function test results have returned to normal can safely take OCs. The presence of migraine headaches without aura is not a contraindication to OC use, but if auras are present, combination OCs should not be prescribed because of a possible increased risk for stroke. Relative contraindications to OC use include undiagnosed causes of amenorrhea and depression. OC use does not increase the risk for development of malignant melanoma or prolactin-secreting pituitary adenomas. In 2004, the World Health Organization established eligibility criteria for women with various medical problems for use of all types of contraception except female and male sterilization. Medical eligibility for each contraceptive was classified into four categories: (1) no restriction for use of the method, (2) advantages of use outweigh risks, (3) risks outweigh the benefits, (4) the method represents an unacceptable health risk. These criteria were updated in 2008 and are available on the Internet (see Suggested Readings). In 2010, the United States Centers for Disease Control and Prevention created the United States Medical Eligibility Criteria for Contraceptive Use, an adaptation of the WHO criteria. These criteria are also available on the Internet.

Initiation of Therapy and Surveillance

If a healthy woman has no contraindications to OC use, it is unnecessary to perform any laboratory tests, including cervical cytology, before use unless these are necessary for routine health maintenance. Routine use of laboratory tests is not indicated unless the woman has a family history of diabetes or arterial vascular disease at a young age, in which case a fasting glucose or lipid panel should be obtained. After the first three cycles of OC use, a nondirected history should be obtained and blood pressure measured. After this visit, the woman should be seen annually; at each visit, a nondirected history should again be taken, blood pressure and body weight measured, and a physical examination (including breast, abdominal, and pelvic examination with cervical cytology) performed. It is not necessary to measure lipids, other than the routine cholesterol screening every 5 years, in women with no cardiovascular risk factors, even if they are older than 35 years. There is no reason to discontinue OC use unless pregnancy is desired. Intermittent discontinuation is unnecessary and may result in an unwanted pregnancy.

Although synthetic sex steroids can retard the biotransformation of certain drugs (e.g., phenazone and meperidine) as a result of substrate competition, such interference is usually not important clinically. However, some drugs can interfere clinically with the action of OCs by inducing liver enzymes that convert the steroids to more polar and less biologically active metabolites. These drugs include barbiturates, sulfonamides, cyclophosphamide, griseofulvin, and rifampin. There is a high incidence of OC failure in women ingesting rifampin, and these two agents, as well as systemic griseofulvin, should not be given concurrently. Products containing St. John's wort reduce contraceptive effectiveness and cause breakthrough bleeding. Women taking certain medications for epilepsy should be treated with 50-μg estrogen formulations because many antiepileptic medications lower ethinyl estradiol levels and cause breakthrough bleeding, which may cause premature discontinuation of use. Because of their many health benefits, including reduction in risk for endometrial and ovarian cancer and induction of regular cyclic uterine bleeding, OC use can be continued until menopause in normotensive nonsmoking women without contraindications.

Transdermal and Intravaginal Steroid Contraceptives

Transdermal Patch

Two novel long-acting methods of delivering contraceptive steroids other than the oral route are marketed in the United States. One of these is a transdermal patch with an area of 20 cm^2, which delivers 150 μg of the progestin norelgestromin, the active metabolite of norgestimate, and 20 μg of ethinyl estradiol daily into the systemic circulation for 7 days. After this time span, the patch is removed and another is attached to a different area of the skin. The steroids are absorbed into the circulation at a constant rate, yielding fairly constant circulatory levels of each steroid while the patch is attached. This pharmacodynamic pattern differs from the peaks and valleys of steroid levels that occur after ingestion of an OC. After three patches are applied, no patch is used for the fourth week to allow withdrawal bleeding. Contraceptive efficacy, bleeding patterns, and side effects are similar to those associated with OCs, but in one comparative study, compliance was better with the patch than with the OC.

Intravaginal Ring

Another method of administering contraceptive steroids at a constant rate is by use of a flexible vaginal ring, which is 58 mm in outside diameter and 4 mm thick. The ring is composed of ethinyl vinyl acetate and contains the progestin etonogestrel and ethinyl estradiol. The rings are all the same size and do not have to be fitted. The ring is inserted and removed by the woman herself and is left in place for 3 weeks, after which time it is removed for 1 week to allow withdrawal bleeding. Each day, 120 μg of etonogestrel and 15 μg of ethinyl estradiol is released from the ring, and bleeding with the ring in place is uncommon. Contraceptive efficacy and side effects are similar to those of OCs.

Injectable Steroid Contraceptives

Constituents and Use

Several types of injectable steroid formulations are in use for contraception throughout the world. The one most widely used in the United States is depot medroxyprogesterone acetate (DMPA). The initial formulation of this contraceptive was administered as an intramuscular injection of 1 mL of an aqueous suspension containing 150 mg of crystalline medroxyprogesterone acetate once every 3 months. A recently developed formulation that is administered subcutaneously (DMPA-SC) contains 105 mg of DMPA in 0.15 mL of solution. This lower dose formulation has a lower peak medroxyprogesterone acetate concentration than DMPA and a long duration of action that suppresses ovulation for at least 13 weeks and is not affected by body mass. Other injectable contraceptives include norethindrone enanthate, given in a dose of 200 mg every 2 months, and several once-a-month injections of combinations of different progestins and estrogens. DMPA has a low failure rate, 0.1% at 1 year and 0.4% at 2 years. The major contraceptive action of both formulations is inhibition of ovulation, and they also impede sperm transport. With DMPA and DMPA-SC, serum medroxyprogesterone levels rapidly increase to contraceptively effective blood levels (>0.5 ng/mL) within 24 hours after the injection. With DMPA, medroxyprogesterone levels plateau for about 3 months, after which there is a gradual decline until levels become undetectable 7 to 9 months after the injection. With DMPA-SC, medroxyprogesterone levels steadily decline after the initial peak and reach 0.2 ng/mL 3 to 4 months after the injection.

Side Effects

With both formulations, mean endogenous estradiol levels remain above the postmenopausal range (40 to 60 pg/mL), and symptoms of estrogen deficiency do not occur. Although DMPA may decrease bone mineral density during use, it is unnecessary to measure bone mineral density or to administer bone antiresorptive agents in DMPA users because the bone loss is temporary and reversible after stopping DMPA.

Because of the lag time it takes to clear DMPA from the circulation, resumption of ovulation is delayed for a variable time after the last injection. It may take as long as 1 year for ovulatory cycles to return. After this initial delay, fecundity resumes at a rate similar to that found after discontinuation of a barrier contraceptive.

Disruption of the Menstrual Cycle

The major side effect of DMPA is complete disruption of the menstrual cycle. Because this formulation contains only a progestin, without an estrogen, endometrial integrity is not maintained, and usually light uterine bleeding occurs at irregular and unpredictable intervals. As duration of therapy increases, the incidence of frequent bleeding steadily declines and the incidence of amenorrhea steadily increases, so that at the end of 2 years, about 70% of users are amenorrheic. Women who use this method of contraception should be counseled about this. Most DMPA users gain between 1.5 and 4 kg in their first year of use and continue to gain weight thereafter. If weight gain occurs, calorie intake should be decreased. Because there is no estrogen in DMPA, its use does not cause hypertension or thromboembolism.

In cycling women, the initial injection should be given no later than day 5 of the cycle to be certain to inhibit ovulation in the initial treatment cycle. The first injection should be given within 5 days after delivery in nonlactating women but not until after 6 weeks in lactating women. Because the major reason for discontinuance of all progestin-injectable contraceptives is menstrual irregularity, several combined progestin-estrogen injectables that are given once monthly and produce regular withdrawal bleeding have been developed.

Subdermal Implants
Constituents and Use
Several types of subdermal implants containing only progestins are effective long-acting methods of contraception. The initial formulation that was marketed consisted of six 3.4-cm polydimethylsiloxane (Silastic) capsules, each containing 36 mg of levonorgestrel, and was very effective.

A formulation containing levonorgestrel in two 4-cm Silastic rods has a pharmacologic pattern similar to that of the six capsules with similar effectiveness and side effects. The two rods are easier to insert and to remove than the six capsules and are effective for 5 years. A single 4-cm by 2-mm ethylene vinyl acetate rod containing 68 µg of etonogestrel, the active metabolite of desogestrel, provides effective contraception for 3 years. This rod is packaged in a disposable metal trocar inserter and does not require a skin incision for insertion, only for removal. Ovulation is inhibited by the circulating etonogestrel levels, and no pregnancies were reported in three large clinical trials. As with other progestin-only implants, irregular bleeding is the most common clinical complaint. This implant has recently become available in the United States and is the only implant currently marketed in the United States.

Emergency Contraception
For a woman not using contraception, if emergency contraception is given within 72 hours after a single coitus, about 75 to 85% of pregnancies will be prevented. If more than one episode of coitus has occurred, or if treatment was initiated later than 72 hours after coitus, the method is less effective. Previously, the most commonly used regimen was ingestion of four tablets of the OC containing 50 µg of ethinyl estradiol and 0.5 mg DL-norgestrel, in doses of two tablets 12 hours apart. The pregnancy rate with this regimen is 2%, about one fourth that of the 8% expected rate. Another formulation consisting of a 750-µg single tablet of levonorgestrel given once every 12 hours is more effective than the two tablets of the combination steroid formulation without the estrogenic side effects. This formulation prevents about 85% of the expected pregnancies, for a pregnancy rate of 1 to 3%. A single dose of 1500 µg of levonorgestrel is as effective as two doses of 750 µg and both formulations are now marketed. Another recently approved effective agent for emergency contraception is the selective progesterone receptor modulator ulipristal acetate given as a single 30-mg dose. This agent is as affective as levonorgestrel and is effective for 5 days after intercourse.

Intrauterine Devices
Constituents and Use
The main benefits of IUDs are a high level of effectiveness, a lack of systemic metabolic effects for copper IUDs, and the need for only a single act of motivation for long-term use. Despite these advantages, only about 3% of reproductive-age women use the IUD in the United States, compared with 15 to 30% in most European countries and Canada. The copper T380A IUD is approved for use in the United States for 10 years and maintains its high levels of effectiveness for at least 12 years. A levonorgestrel-releasing IUD is also marketed in the United States and elsewhere. A dose of 20 µg of levonorgestrel diffuses from the device into the endometrial cavity each day. Because of the progestational effect on the endometrium, the amount of uterine bleeding is markedly reduced with use of this device, and it is approved to treat menorrhagia. This device has a high level of effectiveness for 5 years, which is the approved duration of use.

The main mechanism of contraceptive action of copper-bearing IUDs is spermicidal. This effect is caused by a local sterile leukocytic response produced by the copper as well as the plastic IUD. The levonorgestrel-releasing IUD acts mainly by preventing transport of spermatozoa through the cervical mucus and thus preventing fertilization of the ovum. After removal of each type of IUD, the inflammatory reaction rapidly disappears and resumption of fertility is prompt.

Pregnancy Rate
In the first year of use, IUDs have less than a 1% pregnancy rate, a 10% expulsion rate, and a 15% rate of removal for medical reasons, mainly bleeding and pain. The incidence of each of these events, especially expulsion, diminishes steadily in subsequent years. Mefenamic acid ingested in a dosage of 500 mg three times a day during the days of menstruation has been shown to reduce significantly the amount of uterine bleeding in IUD users.

Side Effects
Development of acute salpingitis more than a month after insertion of the IUD is due to infection with a sexually transmitted pathogen and is unrelated to the presence of the device. All IUD-related upper genital tract infections occur only during the insertion process. If there is clinical suspicion that cervicitis is present, the endocervix should be cultured and the insertion delayed until the results reveal that no pathogenic organisms are present. It is not cost-effective to administer antibiotics routinely with IUD insertion.

The IUD is not associated with an increased incidence of either endometrial or cervical carcinoma. The IUD is a particularly useful method of contraception for women who have completed their families, and its effectiveness is similar to that of tubal sterilization. It was calculated that after 5 years of use, the IUD is the most cost-effective of all methods of contraception, including sterilization.

SUGGESTED READINGS

American College of Obstetricians and Gynecologists. ACOG Practice Bulletin No. 112: emergency contraception. *Obstet Gynecol.* 2010;115:1100-1109. *Practice guidelines.*

Centers for Disease Control and Prevention (CDC). U.S. medical eligibility criteria for contraceptive use, 2010. *MMWR Recomm Rep.* 2010;59:1-86. *Consensus guidelines including for women with a variety of medical conditions.*

Espey E, Ogburn T. Long-acting reversible contraceptives: intrauterine devices and the contraceptive implant. *Obstet Gynecol.* 2011;117:705-719. *Overview with evidence suggesting potential benefits of shifting from short-acting methods to long-acting reversible methods to reduce unintended pregnancy rates.*

247

COMMON MEDICAL PROBLEMS IN PREGNANCY

KAREN ROSENE-MONTELLA

INTRODUCTION

There are 62 million women of childbearing age in the United States, 85% of whom will give birth by age 44 years. The majority of these women will not have obtained preventive health services in any given year, and more than half the pregnancies will be unplanned or unintended. At least 25% will enter pregnancy with a chronic medical illness, and more than half will be overweight or obese, making the role of the internist paramount in maternal health. In the most recent confidential inquiry into maternal mortality in the United Kingdom, more than half of all women who died from direct or indirect causes were overweight or obese, and more than 15% of all deaths were in morbidly obese women. Sixteen percent of pregnant women have depression in the perinatal period, and depression rates are even higher in those with chronic illnesses such as diabetes or asthma.

By the time pregnant patients are seen by their obstetricians, most major teratogenic abnormalities have already occurred (Fig. 247-1), and the window of opportunity to enter pregnancy in a quiescent disease state, on the safest possible medication profile, may have passed. For this reason, internists

FIGURE 247-1. The developing fetus. CNS = central nervous system. (From Moore K. *The Developing Human: Clinically Oriented Embryology*. Philadelphia: WB Saunders; 1982; with permission from Annals of Internal Medicine; Rosene-Montella K, et al. *Medical Care of the Pregnant Patient*, 2nd ed. Copyright 2008 by American College of Physicians, with permission.)

caring for women of childbearing age have a unique responsibility to provide preconception care at a time when interventions will be of maximum benefit to both the fetus and the mother. Table 247-1 describes preconception interventions for women with chronic medical illnesses.

The basic principles involved in the care of pregnant patients with medical disorders are reviewed here, followed by a more detailed discussion of certain medical conditions, selected because of their contribution to maternal mortality or because of the frequency with which they occur.

BASIC PRINCIPLES

Pregnancy is associated with significant but normal physiologic changes that impact the diagnosis and management of disease states and the pharmacokinetics of most drugs (Table 247-2). The physiologic changes required during pregnancy may stress the woman's ability to adapt, particularly in the presence of an underlying disease. The mother's response to pregnancy often unmasks diseases or predicts future risk, so pregnancy is an opportunity to identify women at risk for other non-pregnancy-related illnesses. For example, gestational diabetes is predictive of an increased risk for type 2 diabetes; preeclampsia is predictive of increased risk for ischemic heart disease and stroke; and thrombosis, late fetal loss, or preeclampsia may unmask an underlying thrombophilia.

Fetal well-being depends on maternal well-being. Although there is often thought to be a dichotomy between maternal and fetal needs, they are usually one and the same. The fetus is dependent on maternal perfusion, oxygenation, and nutrition. Thus, more harm may be done by withholding necessary treatments and investigations from pregnant women than by providing them. Uninvestigated symptoms lead to the progression of untreated disease, and untreated maternal disease compromises fetal safety, growth, and development. The major cause of asthma exacerbations and seizures during pregnancy is abrupt discontinuation of medications, exposing the fetus to hypoxemia and acidosis in an effort to save the fetus from drug exposure. In the U.K. Confidential Enquiry, in more than half the cases of maternal death from pulmonary embolism, failure to make the diagnosis was due to the unfounded fear that diagnostic testing would be harmful to the fetus.

Most diagnostic imaging can be used safely in pregnancy. The effects of radiation in utero depend on both the gestational age at exposure and the level of exposure. Recommendations on fetal exposure from the National Commission on Radiation Protection (NCRP) are summarized in Table 247-3. Radiation exposure from specific diagnostic tests is provided in Table 247-4.

The effect of contrast agents is related to the bioavailability of iodine, and there is concern about the impact on the fetal thyroid. Iodine availability is extremely low, and single-dose exposures, even if they are high, are unlikely to be harmful. Therefore, contrast agents may be used when necessary. There are limited data on gadolinium, so the current recommendation is to avoid gadolinium exposure if possible.

The use of medications to treat pregnant women requires a rational risk-benefit analysis and a good understanding of the maternal indications. It is helpful to view treatment as justifiable or not justifiable, rather than as safe or not safe. It is important to consider (1) whether the condition is self-limited or harmless, (2) what the maternal and fetal consequences of discontinuing a medication will be, and (3) the safety data for the drug. U.S. Food and Drug Administration categories may be misleading and often do not include adequate data for a proper risk-benefit analysis. Resources such as the Teratology Information Service, TERIS, found at *http://departments.washington.edu/-terisweb/teris*, offer more complete information.

The list of known human teratogens is small and includes warfarin, cyclophosphamide, diethylstilbestrol, lithium, thalidomide, penicillamine, isotretinoin, methotrexate, acetazolamide, and the antiepileptic drugs phenytoin, carbamazepine, phenobarbital, and valproic acid. Of these, valproate has the most significant data, and it is the only antiepileptic drug for which discontinuation during pregnancy is recommended, if there is an effective alternative. Angiotensin-converting enzyme (ACE) inhibitors and angiotensin II receptor blockers (ARBs) should be added to this list, based on new data confirming that first trimester exposure is associated with fetal renal agenesis and renal failure. Tetracyclines should be avoided owing to later effects on fetal teeth and bone. Resources for prescribing drugs during pregnancy are listed in Suggested Readings.

TABLE 247-1	PRECONCEPTION INTERVENTIONS FOR WOMEN WITH MEDICAL ILLNESSES

TYPE 1 AND TYPE 2 DIABETES

Discuss importance of a normal hemoglobin A_{1C} before conception and importance of contraception until that is achieved

Evaluate for microvascular complications
    Obtain remission for proliferative retinopathy
    Emphasize need to discontinue ACE inhibitor after first missed period

Discontinue thiazolidinediones and statins

Consider change to insulin therapy for type 2 diabetic patients on oral agents unless using metformin for ovulation induction in PCOS

Discuss probable need to reduce insulin dose in first trimester

THYROID DISEASE

Screen for hypothyroidism in women at risk

Normalize TSH and free T_4 before pregnancy

Counsel women taking levothyroxine on probable need to increase dose soon after conception

Diagnose cause of hyperthyroidism and consider ablative therapy for women with Graves' disease requiring high doses of PTU

CHRONIC HYPERTENSION/RENAL DISEASE

Rule out secondary causes of hypertension if appropriate

Evaluate extent of end-organ disease

Quantify GFR and proteinuria

Discuss drugs of choice for hypertension and replace ACE inhibitor

Discuss risk of superimposed preeclampsia and use of low-dose aspirin for women at significant risk of preeclampsia

THROMBOEMBOLIC DISEASE

Consider evaluation for congenital or acquired thrombophilias in women with previous VTE, previous poor obstetric outcome, or family history

Discuss risks of warfarin in pregnancy, need to discontinue warfarin by 4-6 weeks' gestation, and conversion to unfractionated or low-molecular-weight heparin

Discuss options to combined oral contraceptives

EPILEPSY

Determine whether patient is a candidate for withdrawal of antiepileptic drugs

Consider monotherapy with most effective agent at lowest dose possible

Prescribe folate at 1 to 4 mg/day

Discuss possible ineffectiveness of low-dose contraceptives with phenobarbital, phenytoin, and carbamazepine

Consider discontinuing valproate

CARDIAC DISEASE

Obtain baseline echocardiography if congenital disease, stenotic lesion, or pulmonary hypertension suspected

Evaluate for coronary artery disease in women with multiple risk factors

ASTHMA

Verify patient's asthma action plan and peak flowmeter use

Discuss relative safety of all asthma medications except leukotriene modifiers

SYSTEMIC LUPUS ERYTHEMATOSUS AND AUTOIMMUNE DISEASE

Evaluate for renal and cardiopulmonary disease and antiphospholipid, anti-Ro, anti-La antibodies

Avoid pregnancy if disease is active

Discuss relative safety of most immunosuppressants

ACE = angiotensin-converting enzyme; GFR = glomerular filtration rate; PCOS = polycystic ovary syndrome; PTU = propylthiouracil; T_4 = thyroxine; TSH = thyroid-stimulating hormone; VTE = venous thromboembolism.
From Rosene-Montella K, et al. Chapter 2 of *Medical Care of the Pregnant Patient*, 2nd ed. Table 2-3. Copyright 2008 by American College of Physicians, with permission.

TABLE 247-2	NORMAL PHYSIOLOGIC CHANGES IN PREGNANCY

CARDIAC

Cardiac output increased 40%

Blood volume increased 30-50%

Heart rate increased 10-20 beats/min

Blood pressure decreased 10-15 mm Hg

ECG changes related to widened thorax, dextrorotation of heart, elevation of diaphragm

PULMONARY

Upper airway hyperemia and glandular hyperactivity leading to increased edema and friability

Nasal congestion, gestational rhinitis, snoring

Difficult airway management and failed intubation

Minute ventilation increased (owing to an increase in tidal volume, *not* respiratory rate, which remains unchanged), which leads to relative respiratory alkalosis (pH 7.4-7.45)
    Normal Pao_2 100-105 mm Hg
    Normal $Paco_2$ 28-32 mm Hg

RENAL

Increased GFR to 150-180 mL/min/1.73m^2

Normal serum creatinine <0.8 mg/dL

Increased renal excretion of bicarbonate, limiting buffering capacity in patients who become acidotic

Decreased oncotic pressure

ALTERED PHARMACOKINETICS

Increased renal and hepatic clearance of drugs

Altered absorption

Altered protein binding

Increased volume of distribution

ECG = electrocardiogram; GFR = glomerular filtration rate.

TABLE 247-3	NATIONAL COMMISSION ON RADIATION PROTECTION (NCRP) RECOMMENDED PREGNANCY EXPOSURES

TOTAL EXPOSURE DURING PREGNANCY (RADS)	NCRP RECOMMENDATIONS
≤5	Acceptable; low likelihood of problems
5-10	Low risk for problems
10-15 (at ≤8 wk gestation)	Higher risk; consideration of termination
>15	Termination of pregnancy recommended

From Rosene-Montella K, et al. Chapter 8 of *Medical Care of the Pregnant Patient*, 2nd ed. Table 8-3. Copyright 2008 by American College of Physicians, with permission.

TABLE 247-4	RADIATION EXPOSURE

STUDY	RADIATION EXPOSURE (RADS)
Chest x-ray	<0.001
Lung scan	0.01-0.02 ventilation 0.01-0.03 perfusion
Pulmonary angiogram	<0.050 via brachial route 0.2-0.3 via femoral route
CT angiogram	0.2-0.3
Ultrasound	None
MRI/MRA/MRV	None
Upper GI series	0.1
Lumbar spine series	0.9
Barium enema	1
Complete IVP	0.5
Head CT	<0.01
CT of abdomen	2.0-3.0

CT = computed tomography; GI = gastrointestinal; IVP = intravenous pyelogram; MRA = magnetic resonance angiography; MRI = magnetic resonance imaging; MRV = magnetic resonance venography.

HYPERTENSIVE DISORDERS OF PREGNANCY

DEFINITION

Hypertension in pregnancy is defined as a blood pressure (BP) of 140/90 mm Hg or higher. It is defined as chronic hypertension when it predates pregnancy, is diagnosed before 20 weeks' gestation, or persists post partum. Transient late or gestational hypertension occurs toward term and resolves post partum in the absence of any other signs or symptoms of preeclampsia.

EPIDEMIOLOGY

Chronic hypertension is the most common medical condition encountered in women of childbearing age. The incidence is increasing parallel to the increase in obesity, insulin resistance, and pregnancies in women older than 30 years. Hypertension complicates 5 to 8% of pregnancies and is associated with a 20% risk for the development of preeclampsia.

PATHOBIOLOGY

Systemic arterial BP decreases by 10 to 15 mm Hg during normal pregnancy, with a greater fall in diastolic than systolic pressures, likely owing to the decreased sensitivity to angiotensin II that has been demonstrated in pregnant women. BP begins to fall in the first trimester, reaching a nadir toward the end of the second trimester and returning toward baseline at term. This decrease may be exaggerated in women with chronic hypertension, making the diagnosis of chronic hypertension very difficult during pregnancy and affecting both diagnostic and therapeutic considerations.

DIAGNOSIS

The diagnosis of hypertension relies simply on a BP measurement, in the sitting position at the level of the heart, of 140/90 or greater on two occasions 6 hours apart. Later in pregnancy, inferior vena cava compression by the gravid uterus may lower BP substantially in the supine position, so it is critical to measure maternal BP in the sitting position. The initial evaluation should also document target organ damage, such as left ventricular hypertrophy, renal disease (creatinine, urinalysis, and potassium), and retinopathy, so that a baseline is established. Consideration of secondary causes is necessary in this young population (Chapter 67), but the diagnosis of secondary causes of hypertension is complicated by normal pregnancy-related changes. The diagnosis of Cushing's syndrome is complicated by increased levels of cortisol and the placental production of adrenocorticotropic hormone and corticotropin-releasing hormone, so the best test is a 24-hour urine free cortisol using higher pregnancy-specific reference ranges. Primary hyperaldosteronism (Chapter 234) may also be difficult to diagnose in the face of normal pregnancy-related elevations in plasma renin activity and aldosterone, because progesterone ameliorates both the hypertensive and the kaliuretic effects of aldosterone. Primary hyperaldosteronism should be strongly considered in any patient with chronic hypertension in whom there is a marked increase in BP toward term or post partum. Pheochromocytoma (Chapter 235) is associated with a very high maternal and fetal mortality rate, in large part owing to a delay in diagnosis. Both magnetic resonance imaging and magnetic resonance angiography (which do not require gadolinium) can be used safely in pregnancy to evaluate the adrenal glands and renal arteries.

TREATMENT   Rx

Patients previously on drug therapy can often discontinue antihypertensives and restart them when BP gradually rises to prepregnant values toward term. It is very difficult to determine whether rising BP represents a normal physiologic return to earlier pressure or the development of preeclampsia. Baseline preeclampsia laboratory tests (see later), very close follow-up, and comanagement with the patient's obstetrician are required. Patients with good BP control may prefer to continue safe medications or switch to another regimen. The drugs for which there is grade A evidence of efficacy and safety are methyldopa and labetalol (Table 67-5). Nifedipine, hydralazine and other β-blockers, especially those with intrinsic sympathomimetic activity, have also been studied and are acceptable second- and third-line agents.

Dosing should take into consideration the increase in renal and hepatic clearance and the increased volume of distribution, which may require narrowed dosing intervals during pregnancy. ACE inhibitors and ARBs should be discontinued at the diagnosis of pregnancy because of their teratogenicity and their association with fetal and neonatal renal agenesis and renal failure when used later in gestation.

The goal of antihypertensive therapy in pregnancy is not clear. Most consensus recommendations, which address fetal concerns and short-term maternal safety only, recommend keeping BP less than 160/100. Given the long-term data, most centers prefer to keep maternal BP, particularly in patients with diabetes or renal disease, below 140/90. Consensus recommendations agree that maintaining BP above 120/80 is necessary to preserve placental perfusion. There is no evidence that salt restriction or dietary changes improve BP control in pregnancy, and weight loss is not recommended. Likewise, there is no evidence that BP control decreases the risk of preeclampsia. It is important to obtain baseline preeclampsia laboratory tests (complete blood count, platelet count, creatinine, uric acid, aspartate transaminase, urinalysis) in all patients with hypertension, given the 20% risk of preeclampsia, and low-dose aspirin and calcium supplementation should be considered to prevent preeclampsia (see later). Fetal monitoring with serial ultrasound for growth and amniotic fluid volume, non-stress testing (fetal heart rate acceleration in response to

movement) once or twice a week after 32 weeks, and consideration of Doppler flow velocimetry are recommended.

Most antihypertensives are safe for breast-feeding, which should be encouraged. Hydrochlorothiazides, α-methyldopa, nifedipine, acebutolol, and metoprolol are all approved by the American Academy of Pediatricians. There is no evidence that hydrochlorothiazides affect milk volume. There is evidence that propranolol and atenolol are concentrated in breast milk, so they should be avoided. Enalapril and captopril are the preferred ACE inhibitors in breast-feeding women, but it may be prudent to delay ACE inhibitors for the first few weeks of the baby's life and for mothers of premature babies, given the adverse pregnancy data.

PROGNOSIS

Hypertension may increase the risk of abruption, intrauterine growth restriction (IUGR), and low-birthweight babies. The major risk, however, is its contribution to the risk for preeclampsia and the associated increase in perinatal morbidity and mortality. Women who develop hypertension during pregnancy are at increased lifetime risk for the development of chronic hypertension, even if the BP normalizes post partum.

● PREECLAMPSIA

DEFINITION

Preeclampsia is a multisystem disorder defined as BP 140/90 or greater, accompanied by proteinuria greater than 300 mg/24 hours after the 20th week of gestation in a previously normotensive patient. When it is diagnosed in a patient with preexisting chronic hypertension, it is referred to as chronic hypertension with superimposed preeclampsia.

A urine protein-creatinine ratio of at least 0.3 may become a criterion for proteinuria, but the American College of Obstetricians and Gynecologists has not yet added this to the definition. Edema and hyperreflexia are no longer considered diagnostic criteria, and the 30 mm Hg increase in systolic pressure and/or 15 mm Hg increase in diastolic pressure have been dropped from the criteria for hypertension. Severe preeclampsia is defined as the presence of one of the following symptoms or signs in the presence of preeclampsia: (1) systolic BP 160 mm Hg or greater, or diastolic BP 110 mm Hg or greater, on two occasions at least 6 hours apart; (2) proteinuria greater than 5 g in a 24-hour period; (3) pulmonary edema; (4) oliguria (<400 mL in 24 hours); (5) persistent headaches; (6) epigastric pain and/or impaired liver function; (7) thrombocytopenia; and (8) IUGR.

EPIDEMIOLOGY

Preeclampsia complicates 6 to 8% of pregnancies worldwide. Preeclampsia/eclampsia is a leading cause of maternal mortality in the developing world and continues to contribute to maternal mortality in the United States, despite the availability of antihypertensives and antiseizure medications. In the United States, preeclampsia is believed to be responsible for 15% of premature deliveries and 17.6% of maternal deaths. Worldwide, preeclampsia and eclampsia are estimated to be responsible for approximately 14% of maternal deaths per year (50,000 to 75,000).

Primigravida and multigravida women with new partners are at increased risk, suggesting a role for paternal antigens. Additional risk factors include prior history of preeclampsia, black race, diabetes or insulin resistance, systemic lupus erythematosus (SLE), renal disease, hypertension, thrombophilia, obesity, molar pregnancy, multiple gestation, and extremes of age (younger than 20 or older than 40).

PATHOBIOLOGY

Preeclampsia is a disorder of abnormal placentation that begins very early in gestation, well before its manifestations are clinically apparent. In normal pregnancy, uterine spiral arteries undergo remodeling when they are invaded by fetal cytotrophoblastic cells, resulting in an adhesion receptor switch from cells with characteristics of epithelial cells to cells with the phenotype of endothelial cells. This leads to the transformation of previously narrow, high-resistance maternal uterine blood vessels into dilated, high-capacitance blood vessels. The proximal portions of the spiral arteries are further dilated by the hormonal effects of estrogen and progesterone, resulting in an overall increase in uterine blood flow from 45 mL/minute during menstruation to 750 mL/minute at term. In preeclampsia, this cell switching does not occur, and the fetal cells' only superficial invasion into maternal vasculature results in limited

FIGURE 247-2. Model for the pathogenesis of preeclampsia. CNS = central nervous system; PIGF = placental growth factor; sFlt-1= soluble film-like tyrosine kinase; VEGF = vascular endothelial growth factor. (From Rosene-Montella K, et al. *Medical Care of the Pregnant Patient*, 2nd ed. Copyright 2008 by American College of Physicians, with permission.)

placental perfusion. As the pregnancy progresses, abnormal placentation produces relative hypoxia and ischemia as this compromised uterine blood flow cannot keep up with the growing demands of the fetus and the placenta. The result is diffuse endothelial dysfunction that manifests as the clinical syndrome of preeclampsia (Fig. 247-2).

Recent work on the potential mechanism of the endothelial dysfunction that underlies this disease state has focused on the imbalance between pro- and anti-angiogenic factors, arising from studies showing elevated concentrations of placental soluble film-like tyrosine kinase 1 in the plasma of women with preeclampsia. This protein prevents the interaction of placental growth factor and vascular endothelial growth factor with endothelial receptors, inducing endothelial dysfunction. A placenta-derived soluble transforming growth factor-β coreceptor, soluble endoglin, is elevated in the sera of patients with preeclampsia, inducing vascular permeability and hypertension; the degree of elevation correlates with disease severity, and levels fall after delivery. Current studies to address both the cause of and the mechanism linking preeclampsia and the risk of cardiovascular disease are ongoing and focus on endothelial dysfunction.

DIAGNOSIS

The diagnosis of preeclampsia depends on a BP of 140/90 or greater and proteinuria greater than 300 mg/24 hours after 20 weeks' gestation. Eclampsia is diagnosed when a patient with preeclampsia has a seizure. Additional abnormalities that contribute to the diagnosis include hyperuricemia, hemoconcentration, elevated creatinine or liver function tests, and thrombocytopenia. The HELLP syndrome (hemolysis, elevated liver function tests, and low platelets) is likely a more severe form of preeclampsia. The diagnosis of severe preeclampsia depends on the criteria previously listed.

Diagnostic evaluation should include a careful history, asking about headache, visual complaints, epigastric pain, weight gain, and edema and reviewing the presence of risk factors. The physical examination should include a careful neurologic examination, looking for funduscopic changes (retinal vasospasm, edema, or hemorrhage) or hyperreflexia, and any focal findings suggestive of mass effect, hepatic tenderness, and edema. Laboratory testing for preeclampsia includes a complete blood count, platelet count, urine protein-creatinine ratio or 24-hour urine protein, liver function tests, creatinine, and uric acid. Additional evaluation includes fetal testing and close maternal monitoring for life-threatening consequences such as severe hypertension, seizures, pulmonary edema, cerebral hemorrhage, hepatic infarction or rupture, disseminated intravascular coagulation, and renal failure.

Currently, diagnosis depends on development of the full clinical syndrome, but earlier diagnosis may be possible based on biomarkers. It is likely that a combined model that looks at soluble endoglin, soluble film-like tyrosine kinase 1, and placental growth factor concentrations will be a better prediction instrument before 20 weeks' gestation than any individual marker.

The differential diagnosis of each individual manifestation of preeclampsia is broad, so the diagnosis centers on the constellation of signs and symptoms that suggest preeclampsia. The clinical conditions that can mimic preeclampsia include SLE with nephritis, thrombotic thrombocytopenic purpura, and hemolytic-uremic syndrome. Differentiating preeclampsia from a flare of SLE with nephritis (Chapter 274) is very difficult because both can cause hypertension, proteinuria, thrombocytopenia, and rises in serum creatinine. The differential diagnostic features that favor SLE include falling serum complement levels, rising anti-DNA antibodies, and extrarenal manifestations of SLE such as rash and arthralgias. The proteinuria and hypertension in preeclampsia are more likely to be of sudden onset.

TREATMENT   Rx

Once it occurs, the only known treatment of preeclampsia is delivery as soon as obstetrically feasible.[1] Nevertheless, it is important to note that preeclampsia can present post partum, and both preeclampsia and eclampsia have been reported up to 21 days after delivery. Management of preeclampsia includes treatment of hypertension, seizure prophylaxis, and limitation of fluids due to the risk of pulmonary edema. Treatment of severe hypertension in preeclampsia is reviewed in Table 247-5. Magnesium sulfate ($MgSO_4$) is recommended as first-line treatment for eclampsia as well as prophylaxis against eclampsia in women with severe and nonsevere preeclampsia.[2] Phenytoin and benzodiazepines should not be used for eclampsia prophylaxis or treatment, unless there is a contraindication to $MgSO_4$ or it is ineffective. There is evidence from two randomized controlled trials that magnesium is superior to phenytoin for the prevention of both primary seizures and recurrent seizures in eclampsia.

Treatment of acute seizures in eclampsia includes airway protection, fetal monitoring, magnesium, BP control, and benzodiazepines as needed to stop seizures acutely. Treatment of severe hypertension is as outlined in Table 247-5.

Severe maternal manifestations of preeclampsia that may warrant early delivery include seizure, renal failure, severe hypertension, severe thrombocytopenia or hemolysis, aspartate transaminase or alanine transaminase elevation greater than two to three times normal, pulmonary edema, retinal hemorrhage, or other symptoms suggestive of end-organ damage (headache, visual disturbance, epigastric or right upper quadrant pain). Fetal indications for delivery may include significant IUGR, oligohydramnios, or nonreassuring fetal testing. Women with preeclampsia before 34 weeks' gestation should receive a corticosteroid that crosses the placenta, such as betamethasone or dexamethasone, to accelerate fetal lung maturation.

PREVENTION

Multiple trials of antihypertensives, antioxidant supplementation with vitamins C and E,[3] magnesium, protein or salt restriction, fish oil, and other dietary changes have failed to prevent preeclampsia. Low-dose aspirin in high-risk populations is the only intervention with data to support a positive effect. Initial trials showed limited effects, but a subsequent meta-analysis found that low-dose aspirin (<100 mg/day) decreases both the risk of preeclampsia and fetal and neonatal deaths.[4] We recommend aspirin 81 mg/day in all patients with risk factors for preeclampsia. Trials of calcium supplementation have shown conflicting results, but given the inverse relationship between dietary calcium intake and BP in the general population, calcium supplementation of at least 1 g/day is recommended for women with a low dietary intake of calcium (<600 mg/day). An alternative to supplementation may be to increase dietary calcium by eating three to four servings per day of dairy products (assuming 250 to 300 mg calcium per serving).

PROGNOSIS

Women who have had preeclampsia are at increased risk of heart disease, stroke, and cardiovascular death. Preeclampsia is also a marker for increased risk of end-stage renal disease. One year after delivery, preeclampsia patients had evidence of increased insulin resistance, BP, cholesterol, and triglycerides, which may be the first manifestations of the metabolic syndrome. It is unclear whether there is a shared pathogenesis, an unmasking of already established disease, or a contribution to the development of disease. It is possible that preexisting abnormal endothelial function predisposes to renal

and vascular disease later in life and is, in fact, the same abnormality that disturbs implantation, resulting in preeclampsia and fetal loss. It is also possible that preeclampsia itself contributes to the later development of disease.

Continuing care beyond 6 weeks post partum is strongly recommended. Women with a history of severe preeclampsia should be screened for preexisting hypertension, underlying renal disease, thrombophilia, and possibly secondary causes of hypertension. They should also be informed of the risk for preeclampsia in subsequent pregnancies, particularly if the birth interval is less than 2 years or greater than 10 years. Women who are overweight should be advised to normalize their body mass index before another pregnancy and to reduce long-term risk. Both women with preexisting hypertension and those whose BP normalizes are likely to benefit from an overall assessment of cardiovascular risk that includes a lipid profile, smoking cessation, and early interventions to reduce risk.

⬤ DEEP VEIN THROMBOSIS, PULMONARY EMBOLISM, AND THROMBOPHILIA (CHAPTERS 81, 98, AND 179)

Pulmonary embolism (PE) is the leading medical cause of maternal mortality in the developed world. It was responsible for 30% of direct maternal deaths in the most recent U.K. Confidential Enquiry. Despite our best efforts, mortality rates from PE in pregnancy have not changed in more than 2 decades, and the incidence of PE in the United States is rising, likely owing to the increase in obesity and cesarean deliveries. Current strategies to reduce risk from PE must address the widespread use of appropriate prophylaxis, early detection of venous thromboembolism (VTE), and prompt, safe, and effective therapy.

EPIDEMIOLOGY

More than half the VTE events in women younger than 40 years occur in association with pregnancy. VTE is 10 times more common in pregnant versus nonpregnant women of comparable age. It occurs in 5 to 12 of 10,000 pregnancies ante partum and 3 to 7 of 10,000 post partum. The risk of VTE with pregnancy is increased by the presence of additional risk factors, including prolonged bedrest, cesarean section, preeclampsia, three or more children, smoking, obesity, previous superficial thrombophlebitis, previous VTE, thrombophilia, and family history of VTE.

PATHOBIOLOGY

Pregnancy is a hypercoagulable state (Chapter 179) characterized by venous stasis, increased clotting factors and decreased fibrinolysis, and endothelial disruption. Venous stasis occurs as a result of progesterone-induced venodilation early in pregnancy and is later increased by the compressive effects of the gravid uterus. Compression of the left iliac vein by the right iliac artery further increases venous stasis on the left, which may explain the finding that more than 90% of cases of deep vein thrombosis (DVT) in pregnancy occur in the left leg. Endothelial damage occurs with preeclampsia and with both vaginal and operative delivery, further contributing to VTE risk.

Genetic and Acquired Thrombophilias

A positive family history for VTE (possibly a marker for thrombophilia) or a known thrombophilia significantly increases the risk for VTE in pregnancy. The best-described genetic thrombophilias include deficiencies in protein C, protein S, and antithrombin III, all of which appear to have autosomal dominant inheritance with variable penetrance and the presence of the single gene mutations, factor V Leiden, or prothrombin G202010. Of these, antithrombin-deficient homozygotes and compound heterozygotes have the highest risk of VTE in pregnancy. The thrombophilias have also been associated with obstetric complications, including IUGR, abruption, both early and late pregnancy loss, and early, severe, or recurrent preeclampsia. The antiphospholipid antibody syndrome is the major acquired thrombophilia for which there are compelling pregnancy data supporting a link with both thrombosis risk and obstetric complications, as well as the use of thromboprophylaxis to prevent poor obstetric outcome. A large international, multicenter trial—the Thrombophilia in Pregnancy Prophylaxis Study (TIPPS)—is currently under way, randomizing patients with thrombophilias and adverse pregnancy outcomes to surveillance versus thromboprophylaxis.

DIAGNOSIS

The diagnosis of VTE during pregnancy is complicated by both normal pregnancy-related physiologic changes and the reluctance to use diagnostic

TABLE 247-5	TREATMENT OF SEVERE HYPERTENSION IN PREECLAMPTIC PATIENTS		
MEDICATION	**ONSET AND DURATION OF ACTION**	**ACUTE DOSING FOR SEVERE HYPERTENSION**	**MAINTENANCE DOSE**
Labetalol	Begins to work in 5-10 min Lasts 3-6 hr	Given as a series of boluses until BP reaches the desired level: 10 mg IV push; then in 10 min, 20 mg IV push; then in 10 min, 40 mg IV push; then in 10 min, 80 mg IV push; then in 10 min, 80 mg IV push, up to a total dose of no more than 300 mg Follow with PO labetalol or labetalol drip	100-200 mg PO bid-tid (100-600 mg bid–tid; maximum 2400 mg/day) IV infusion 0.5-2.0 mg/min (labetalol comes in vials of 100 mg/20 mL Put 5 vials (100 mL) labetalol into 150 mL IV fluid (D_5W, LR, or NS) to get a solution of 2 mg/mL Start at 15 mL/hr (0.5 mg/min) Titrate up to as high as 60 mL/hr (2 mg/min)
Nifedipine	Begins to work in <30 min Lasts 4-5 hr	10-20 mg PO q30min to a maximum of 50 mg	10-20 mg PO tid of short-acting nifedipine, or 30-120 mg once daily of long-acting formulation
Hydralazine	Begins to work in 10-20 min Lasts for 3-6 hr	2.5-10 mg IV q30min	Start at 10 mg PO qid; can be gradually increased to 50 mg PO qid

BP = blood pressure; D_5W= dextrose 5% in water (solution); LR = lactated Ringer's (solution); NS = normal saline.
From Rosene-Montella K, et al. Chapter 16 of *Medical Care of the Pregnant Patient*, 2nd ed. Table 16-7. Copyright 2008 by American College of Physicians, with permission.

imaging in pregnancy. Clinical signs are unreliable, and leg swelling and complaints of dyspnea are common during pregnancy, making it very difficult to decide when to investigate for VTE. The finding that 90% of DVT occurs in the left leg led to the observation that the combination of symptoms in the left leg, calf circumference difference of 2 cm or greater, and first trimester presentation (when leg swelling is less likely) is highly predictive of DVT. Most DVTs occur ante partum, and events are evenly distributed throughout gestation. The majority of fatal PEs in most studies occurred in the postpartum period, so vigilance is required for a prolonged period following delivery. Diagnosis of DVT requires compression ultrasonography that includes the iliac veins and the inferior vena cava at the level of the liver. It also requires repeat compression ultrasonography if there is a negative scan but high pretest probability and continuing symptoms. In patients with suspected iliac or pelvic vein thrombosis and negative ultrasound studies, magnetic resonance imaging or magnetic resonance venography is recommended.

The diagnosis of PE is even more problematic, given the frequency of dyspnea, the likelihood of normal oxygenation in young patients with no underlying cardiopulmonary disease, and the more invasive nature of diagnostic testing. Arterial blood gases are not helpful; the A-a gradient was normal in 60% of pregnant patients with documented PE in a retrospective review done at two centers.

The radiation exposure from imaging required for the diagnosis of PE is well below that allowed by the NCRP (see Table 247-3), so testing should never be withheld out of concern for fetal exposure. Ventilation-perfusion (V/Q) scanning is still the diagnostic test of choice in most centers outside the United States. It is better validated in pregnancy, involves no contrast administration, and has good negative predictive value in normal scans and in low-probability scans when paired with leg studies. If V/Q is used, it must be understood that there is still a significant risk of PE in patients with "intermediate" and "indeterminate" scans, so additional testing is required in those cases. Computed tomography (CT) angiography has replaced V/Q scanning in most U.S. centers, based on its use in the nonpregnant population. The technique is dependent on cardiac output and plasma volume, both of which are increased during pregnancy. This may lead to poor opacification of the vessels, causing artifacts to be read as filling defects or the failure to visualize clots, so the technique must be adjusted for pregnancy. It is a sensitive, cost-effective test that offers an alternative diagnosis in 25 to 40% of cases, and it is preferred if there is an abnormal chest x-ray. It is well tolerated and has a shorter breath-holding time than V/Q scans, so it is also preferred in unstable patients, especially if an alternative diagnosis is suspected. It is important to note that CT angiography exposes the maternal breast to 2 to 3.5 rads, and exposure of the breast to 1 rad increases the lifetime risk of breast cancer by 13%. The use of breast shields decreases this exposure by about 50% without compromising the integrity of the test, so breast shields are strongly recommended.

The role of D-dimer testing in pregnancy has not yet been elucidated because D-dimer is elevated during normal pregnancy. It may have some use for its negative predictive value, but studies are inadequate to recommend its use at this time.

TREATMENT   Rx

The safety of unfractionated heparin (UFH) and low-molecular-weight heparin (LMWH) (Chapter 37) for the fetus is well established, so they are the drugs of choice for both the treatment and the prevention of VTE. Warfarin is a teratogen that crosses the placenta and has been associated with fetal bleeding and central nervous system abnormalities later in gestation, so it is not used for this indication in pregnancy. Initial treatment is either intravenous UFH followed by subcutaneous UFH or LMWH, or an initial adjusted dose of LMWH that is then continued; both are acceptable.

LMWH causes less thrombocytopenia and osteoporosis, so, given the prolonged exposure during pregnancy, it is the preferred agent. LMWH has increased bioavailability, but the ease of administration in pregnancy is mitigated by the need for twice daily dosing and frequent monitoring. Dosing requirements increase with increasing gestation, so it is necessary to follow anti-Xa levels. Because LMWH has limited reversibility with protamine, and because it has been associated with epidural hematomas in nonpregnant patients given spinal or epidural anesthesia, most centers recommend a switch to UFH by 34 to 36 weeks. This allows patients the option of epidural anesthesia for delivery, and in the event of an emergent delivery prior to holding anticoagulation, UFH can be reversed with protamine. Specific treatment recommendations are outlined in Table 247-6.

TABLE 247-6   TREATMENT OF VENOUS THROMBOEMBOLISM IN PREGNANCY: ANTEPARTUM ANTICOAGULATION

| DRUG | Prophylaxis | | Aggressive Prophylaxis | | |
	FIRST 20 WEEKS	20-37 WEEKS	FIRST 20 WEEKS	20 WEEKS TO TERM	FULL TREATMENT
Dalteparin	5000 U/day	5000 U q12h	100 U/kg/day	100 U/kg/day	100 U/kg q12h with anti-Xa monitoring
Enoxaparin	30 mg/day	30 mg q12h	1 mg/kg/day	1 mg/kg/day	1 mg/kg q12h with anti-Xa monitoring
Tinzaparin	4500 U/day	4500 U q12h	88 U/kg/day	88 U/kg/day	88 U/kg q12h with anti-Xa monitoring
Heparin	Alternative if LMWH unaffordable: 750 U bid first 20 wk; 10,000 U bid wk 20-37		Alternative if LMWH unaffordable: 10,000 U bid to achieve anti-Xa level of 0.1-0.3 U/mL		Adjusted to mid-interval anti-Xa of 0.35-0.67 with q12h SC injections

LMWH = low-molecular-weight heparin.
Adapted from Bourjeily G, Rosene-Montella K, eds. Venous thromboembolism in pregnancy In: *Pulmonary Problems in Pregnancy, Respiratory Medicine.* New York: Humana Press; 2009: table 18.3.

PREVENTION

The overall recurrence risk of VTE during pregnancy ranges from 5 to 20%, depending in part on the circumstances of the index clot. Patients with a previous idiopathic VTE (while not pregnant) or a secondary VTE that occurred during a previous pregnancy or while on oral contraceptives, and patients with a positive family history or identified thrombophilia, are at the highest risk. The thrombophilias with the highest recurrence risk are the antiphospholipid antibody syndrome and homozygosity or compound heterozygosity with more than one mutation and antithrombin deficiency. Thromboprophylaxis is required in all these groups, and its intensity is related to the severity of the risk (see Table 247-6). The lowest risk of recurrence, based on retrospective data, appears to be in patients without a family history or thrombophilia in whom the previous VTE occurred in association with a transient risk factor other than pregnancy or oral contraceptive use. The American College of Chest Physicians consensus guidelines allow surveillance in this group, but most U.S. centers would also offer antepartum thromboprophylaxis. Prophylaxis should be continued for at least 6 to 8 weeks post partum, when the hemostatic changes of pregnancy return to prepregnant values. Additional groups that should be considered for thromboprophylaxis are patients who have undergone cesarean section, particularly if they have an additional risk factor for VTE, and patients on prolonged bedrest. Patients on continued prophylactic or treatment doses post partum have the option of switching to warfarin, which is safe in breast-feeding women.

PROGNOSIS

VTE during pregnancy may be the first manifestation of a hypercoagulable state, as pregnancy acts as a stress test for thrombophilia. Fifty percent of initial episodes of VTE in women younger than 40 present in association with pregnancy. A thrombophilia evaluation is indicated in all patients who present with VTE during pregnancy to assess long-term maternal and family risk and to guide future secondary prophylaxis recommendations. Patients with an identified thrombophilia and an adverse pregnancy outcome are at risk for a similar outcome in a subsequent pregnancy and should be counseled about this risk and considered for thromboprophylaxis.

Patients who have had a DVT during pregnancy have a very high risk of postphlebitic syndrome and venous insufficiency. Two randomized controlled trials demonstrated a 50% risk reduction in symptoms of post-thrombotic syndrome when compression stockings were used within 1 month of diagnosis and continued for a minimum of 1 year after diagnosis.

● ASTHMA (CHAPTER 87)

Maintaining adequate control of asthma during pregnancy is important for both maternal and fetal outcome. Asthma may be associated with increased perinatal mortality, preterm birth, IUGR, and preeclampsia. Well-controlled asthma reduces the likelihood of these adverse outcomes back to baseline, so it is safer for both mother and fetus to treat maternal asthma than to allow exacerbations to occur.

EPIDEMIOLOGY

Asthma is the most common respiratory disease in pregnancy. It affects 3.7 to 8.4% of pregnancies in the United States and 12 to 13% of pregnancies in Australia and the United Kingdom.

Effect of Pregnancy on Asthma

The course of asthma in pregnancy is unpredictable, and most studies have found that a third of patients improve, a third worsen, and a third stay the same. The most likely predictor in any individual patient is her course during a previous pregnancy. In most studies, the majority of exacerbations occurred between 17 and 32 weeks, with some improvement reported by 36 weeks' gestation. Patients with mild asthma do well during labor and delivery, but almost 50% of patients with severe asthma worsen during labor and delivery. Risk factors for exacerbations include severe asthma; poor compliance with medications, especially inhaled corticosteroids; obesity; viral infections; rhinitis; and poor prenatal care. The highest morbidity and mortality are reported in African American patients.

Effect of Asthma on Pregnancy

Pregnancy and perinatal outcome are unchanged when asthma is well controlled. Poorly controlled asthma increases the risk of spontaneous abortion, low birthweight, IUGR, and cesarean section. Preterm delivery and preeclampsia have also been associated with poorly controlled asthma, but it is unclear how systemic steroids contribute to these complications. Systemic steroids have been associated with an increased risk of premature rupture of membranes, preeclampsia, prematurity and low birthweight, and gestational diabetes.

PATHOBIOLOGY

The normal physiologic changes of pregnancy may contribute to variations in asthma severity. Factors contributing to the worsening of asthma include gastroesophageal reflux disease (GERD) and rhinitis or sinusitis—triggers for asthma that are common during pregnancy. GERD may present initially during pregnancy or worsen in patients with preexisting reflux owing to both hormonal and mechanical effects. Progesterone acts as a smooth muscle dilator that reduces lower esophageal sphincter pressure and contributes to delayed gastric emptying. Later in gestation, uterine enlargement further contributes to gastric displacement and increased reflux. Rhinitis and sinusitis clearly contribute to asthma exacerbations in nonpregnant patients. Gestational rhinitis related to hormonal effects is present in most pregnant women, and its behavior seems to parallel that of asthma. Bacterial sinusitis is five to six times more common in pregnancy and should be treated aggressively.

Hormonal effects on the airway may also contribute to asthma status. There is a progressive increase in serum cortisol and estradiol, which impacts the quality of mucus production, and in progesterone, which decreases smooth muscle contractility and thereby causes airway dilation and improves minute ventilation. Immunologic factors during normal pregnancy may also contribute to the course of asthma. There is a suppression of cell-mediated immunity, with a predominant T_H2 environment and high interleukin-5 and tumor necrosis factor messenger RNA. In pregnant women with asthma (not receiving inhaled corticosteroid therapy), the T_H2/T_H1 ratio is even higher, possibly contributing to exacerbations.

The mechanism by which asthma exacerbations affect perinatal outcome is likely related to chronic maternal hypoxia, with consequent placental dysfunction and decreased uteroplacental flow, which contributes to decreased fetal growth. Poorly controlled asthma increases low birthweight 2.5-fold. Relative placental ischemia in asthma, particularly in disease that was poorly controlled before conception, is likely the link to an increased risk for preeclampsia. Placentas from women with asthma show a change in response to vasodilators and constrictors in vitro, similar to that seen in preeclampsia.

DIAGNOSIS

The diagnosis of asthma during pregnancy is the same as in the nonpregnant state: normal forced expiratory volume in 1 second (FEV_1)/forced vital capacity on baseline pulmonary function tests with an obstructive physiology during exacerbations that is reversible either spontaneously or with

medications. Airway hyperresponsiveness, as demonstrated by a methacholine challenge causing a 20% drop in FEV_1 from baseline, is also useful for diagnosis in pregnancy. The classification of asthma severity in pregnancy is the same as in nonpregnant patients and uses the new classification of asthma severity that incorporates short-acting β-agonist use. The new classification includes both level of impairment (daytime and nighttime frequency, quality of life and interference with normal activities, lung function) and adds the risk of exacerbations based on frequency and severity of prior exacerbations.

Differential Diagnosis

Dyspnea of pregnancy is a benign condition that often occurs later in pregnancy and is characterized by an increased awareness of the work of breathing that is disturbing for many patients. It is not likely to be acute, occurs less with rest, and should not interfere with normal daily activities. Dyspnea of pregnancy should not be accompanied by an increase in respiratory rate, wheezing, or hypoxia. It is important to consider pulmonary edema in any pregnant patient complaining of shortness of breath. Pregnancy-related causes of pulmonary edema and acute respiratory distress syndrome include tocolytics (drugs that slow contractions), preeclampsia, gastric aspiration, amniotic fluid embolism, sepsis (related to pyelonephritis, chorioamnionitis, endometritis, septic abortion), abruption, and obstetric hemorrhage. Cardiac causes should be suspected when pulmonary edema presents at the peak of blood volume (28 to 32 weeks), when occult valvular disease is most likely to be unmasked. Additional cardiac considerations are peripartum cardiomyopathy, preeclampsia, and ischemic heart disease, which in pregnancy may also be caused by coronary dissection.

TREATMENT

Management of asthma during pregnancy does not differ greatly from that of the nonpregnant patient. However, normal arterial carbon dioxide pressure ($PaCO_2$) in pregnancy is 28 to 32 mm Hg, so a tachypneic pregnant patient with a $PaCO_2$ above this range may be in impending respiratory failure. Minute ventilation in pregnancy increases via an increase in tidal volume, but respiratory rate is unchanged by pregnancy, so tachypnea is always an abnormal finding.

The goal of asthma therapy during pregnancy is to maintain adequate control to ensure maternal and fetal health. It is always safer for pregnant women with asthma to be treated with asthma medications than to experience symptoms and exacerbations. Careful monitoring during all prenatal visits, preferably with spirometry, and stepped-up therapy are required both for maternal asthma control and to ensure appropriate oxygenation of the fetus. Maternal arterial oxygen saturation should be maintained at 95% or greater, or the arterial oxygen pressure (PaO_2) should be maintained at 80 mm Hg or greater, to maintain fetal oxygenation. E-Figure 247-1 outlines the classification of asthma and care for pregnant patients with asthma. More detailed recommendations for the home management of exacerbations and for hospitalization and emergency care for pregnant patients can be found in the *National Asthma Education and Prevention Program Working Group Report for Managing Asthma during Pregnancy*.

Albuterol is the preferred short-acting β-agonist because it has an excellent safety profile and the most data related to safety during human pregnancy. Inhaled corticosteroids are the preferred medication for long-term control. Budesonide is the preferred inhaled corticosteroid solely because of the amount of reassuring data on its use in pregnant patients. There are, however, no adverse data on the other inhaled corticosteroids. Data on the effectiveness and safety of long-acting β-agonists during pregnancy are limited, although it is reasonable to assume that they have a similar safety profile to that of albuterol. Salmeterol is the preferred agent, based only on its longer availability and no reports of adverse outcomes in exposed pregnancies. Cromolyn has an excellent safety profile but has limited effectiveness compared with inhaled corticosteroids.

Minimal published reports are available on the use of leukotriene receptor antagonists during pregnancy; however, animal safety data are reassuring. Current guidelines do not recommend leukotriene receptor antagonists owing to the limited data, unless a patient's asthma was well controlled using this type of drug before pregnancy.

Intranasal corticosteroids are recommended for the treatment of allergic rhinitis, given the limited systemic effect. The current nonsedating antihistamines of choice are loratadine and cetirizine.

Patients at risk for fatal asthma are those with a large bronchodilator response, overreliance on short-acting bronchodilators, marked circadian variation in lung function, history of hospitalization or intubation, and frequent systemic steroid use. There are specific considerations in pregnant patients who require airway intubation, based on pregnancy physiology.

Pregnant patients have a low functional residual capacity and oxygen reserve, a more profound response to sedatives, airway edema, and larger airways. Intubation failure is much higher in pregnant women, so intubation should be performed by the most experienced professional available.

Breast-feeding should be encouraged in all patients with asthma, as there is some evidence that it decreases atopy in offspring. Data are conflicting regarding the development of asthma in offspring.

● DIABETES (CHAPTERS 236 AND 237)

Diabetes affects 1.85 million women of reproductive age, and it is estimated that preconception management could reduce the risk for 113,000 births per year. All women of reproductive age with diabetes should be counseled about the relationship between glucose control and congenital anomalies. Hyperglycemia is a teratogen, and the incidence of congenital anomalies is directly related to the hemoglobin A_{1C} level at conception (Fig. 247-3). The anomaly rate was as high as 11% in women without preconception care, including cardiac anomalies, neural tube defects, and sacral agenesis. The single most important contribution an internist can make to the prevention of congenital anomalies is to address pregnancy risk with all women of childbearing age with diabetes. The responsibility to normalize hemoglobin A_{1C} before conception falls to the medical care provider; once pregnancy is diagnosed and the patient is seen by her obstetrician, the teratogenic effects of glucose have already occurred.

DEFINITION

Gestational diabetes mellitus (GDM) is defined as glucose intolerance that first occurs or is first identified during pregnancy. Either type 1 or type 2 diabetes in a pregnant patient is referred to as preexisting or pregestational diabetes.

EPIDEMIOLOGY

The frequency of GDM is rising in the United States; it now occurs in 4 to 14% of all pregnancies, depending on patient characteristics. The epidemic of type 2 diabetes has resulted in a higher prevalence at a younger age; in the United States, there has been a 70% increase in the prevalence of diabetes in the 30- to 39-year-old age group, versus 33% overall. The proportion of women with type 2 versus type 1 pregestational diabetes has also increased, from 26% in 1980 to 65% in 2000, and it is still increasing. The perinatal morbidity and mortality associated with type 2 diabetes is at least as great as that associated with type 1 during pregnancy.

PATHOBIOLOGY

Type 1 diabetes is caused by autoimmune destruction of pancreatic beta cells, resulting in an absolute insulin deficiency. Ninety percent of cases are diagnosed before age 25 years and are often associated with other autoimmune illnesses or a family history of autoimmune illness, including thyroid disorders, Addison's disease, and celiac disease. Type 2 diabetes is part of the metabolic syndrome, which includes insulin resistance, hyperinsulinemia, dyslipidemia, abdominal obesity, and hypertension with premature atherosclerosis and likely has a genetic component. GDM may also be a manifestation of the metabolic syndrome, unmasked by the insulin-resistant state of pregnancy. Patients with GDM have a 50% chance of developing type 2 diabetes in the ensuing 5 to 10 years and a long-term risk of approximately 70%.

Pregnancy is a state of accelerated starvation and marked insulin resistance. Lower fasting glucose levels are seen early in the first trimester, and nocturnal hypoglycemia is common. There is blunted hypoglycemic awareness owing to decreased epinephrine and norepinephrine release, with falls in blood sugar and increased ketogenesis, resulting in an increased risk for diabetic ketoacidosis. Insulin requirements may decrease 20% in weeks 7 to 12 but then gradually rise later in gestation, such that insulin doses need to be increased by 16 weeks' gestation. Marked insulin resistance is related to the presence of elevated levels of cortisol, prolactin, human placental lactogen, and human placental growth hormone. Insulin sensitivity is decreased by about 50% in the third trimester, resulting in increased serum insulin and postprandial glucose levels, explaining the timing of the onset of GDM.

DIAGNOSIS

The diagnosis of pregestational diabetes is based on the finding of a fasting blood sugar level greater than 125 mg/dL or a 2-hour or random blood sugar level 200 mg/dL or greater. The American Diabetes Association recently added a hemoglobin A_{1C} level of 6.5% or greater as an acceptable alternative diagnostic criterion. GDM is based on the results of a blood sugar screen after a 50-g glucose challenge test ($\geq$140 mg/dL), followed by a 3-hour confirmatory 100-g oral glucose tolerance test. Positive results are any two of the following: fasting, 95 or greater, 1 hour, 180; 2 hours, 155; and 3 hours, 140 mg/dL. It may be difficult to distinguish between GDM and type 2 diabetes that was not diagnosed before pregnancy. Elevated fasting glucose levels before 24 weeks' gestation and elevated hemoglobin A_{1C} are both suggestive of type 2 diabetes. Any diabetes diagnosed during pregnancy is referred to as GDM; if it persists post partum, it is reclassified as type 2.

TREATMENT ⟨Rx⟩

Dietary recommendations are for 30 kcal/kg, with 40 to 50% carbohydrates, divided into three meals and three snacks. Aerobic exercise may decrease insulin resistance and reduce maternal glucose levels and may be an effective adjunct to diet in patients with GDM. Adjustment of medications should include the discontinuation of ACE inhibitors, ARBs, and statins and the institution of folate and prenatal vitamins. An assessment of baseline disease status in all patients with diabetes should include hemoglobin A_{1C}, ophthalmologic examination, electrocardiogram, assessment of urine protein excretion, serum creatinine, and thyroid-stimulating hormone. Baseline preeclampsia laboratory studies are also recommended.

The fetal assessment plan includes ultrasound to confirm dates and viability; this is done by the patient's obstetric care provider. There will also be a quad screen, looking for serum markers that suggest neural tube defects or Down syndrome, a level 2 ultrasound to assess for congenital anomalies, and a fetal echocardiogram.

Control of Blood Glucose

The goal of treatment for pregestational diabetes is the best hemoglobin A_{1C} level possible, without excessive hypoglycemia.**5** This is achieved by frequent insulin adjustments and self-monitoring of blood glucose at least four times a day. The specific goals for both GDM and pregestational diabetes are fasting glucose of 65 to 95 mg/dL, 1-hour postprandial glucose less than 140, and 2-hour less than 120. This is best achieved by multiple doses of insulin, including basal, intermediate, or long-acting insulin, with prandial bolus rapid-acting insulin to cover the anticipated carbohydrate load. This regimen requires self-monitoring of blood glucose six or seven times a day, so it may be difficult to comply with. Further, the risk of serious hypoglycemia may limit these glycemic targets, particularly in women with type 1 diabetes. Extreme vigilance is required to avoid serious hypoglycemia, particularly in weeks 7 to 12, when insulin requirements are the lowest during pregnancy. In patients with decreased glycemic awareness, the risk of nighttime hypoglycemia is significant, and patients' partners should be counseled about this risk.

Insulin analogues are being used with increasing frequency. Of the rapid-acting analogues, there are data that lispro does not cross the placenta; there are no data yet on aspart. Although long-acting glargine is being used in pregnancy, its placental transfer is unknown, and there are theoretical concerns about its binding to the insulin-like growth factor receptor and its mitogenic potential.

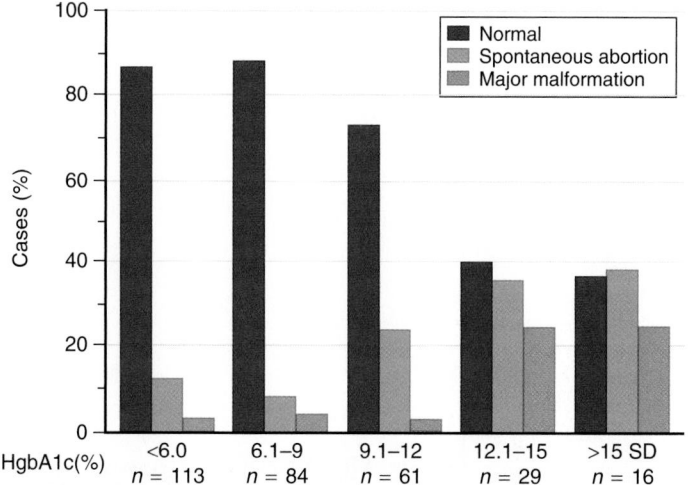

FIGURE 247-3. Relationship of hemoglobin A_{1c} (HgbA$_{1c}$), congenital anomalies, and spontaneous abortion.

Of the oral agents for which there are data, glyburide is safe and efficacious in women with GDM. A recent trial comparing it with metformin concluded that the failure rate was twice as high in the metformin group.[6] Oral agents are less useful with significant insulin resistance and type 2 diabetes, so insulin continues to be the "gold standard" in this group. Metformin does not appear to increase the risk of congenital anomalies or spontaneous abortion, but it does cross the placenta. It is important to recognize that women with polycystic ovary syndrome treated with metformin may regain their fertility and should be advised to use contraception. Recent trials support the safety of metformin in the second and third trimesters. In the United States, metformin is not yet recommended for the treatment of type 2 diabetes in pregnancy or for GDM. There are inadequate pregnancy data for the meglitinides and glitazones.

Maternal and Fetal Monitoring

During pregnancy, increased vigilance and continual assessment for the development of complications, including hypertension, preeclampsia, worsening nephropathy, and retinopathy, are required. The incidence of retinopathy in pregnant women with type 1 and type 2 diabetes is 34 to 50% and 3 to 5%, respectively. Nephropathy is found in 4% of diabetic pregnancies and is associated with increased maternal and perinatal morbidity. Most studies agree that pregnancy may accelerate the progression of nephropathy, but the reversibility of this complication is unclear. Most studies show a worsening of retinopathy in pregnant patients similar to that occurring over the same period in nonpregnant patients. The level of severity of retinopathy before pregnancy is most predictive of worsening during pregnancy, and treatment is recommended before conception.

Labor and Delivery

During labor and delivery, tight glucose control is necessary to avoid neonatal hypoglycemia due to hyperinsulinemia at birth. The goal is to maintain serum glucose levels of 72 to 144 mg/dL. The use of an insulin drip with dextrose infusion in active labor is recommended. Immediately after delivery, insulin requirements decrease to prepregnancy levels. Insulin needs should be one half to two thirds prepregnancy requirements, with a further decreased need found in breast-feeding patients.

Postpartum Considerations

Fifteen percent to 25% of type 1 diabetics develop postpartum thyroiditis, so all patients require postpartum measurements of thyroid-stimulating hormone and follow-up for 6 months. Other postpartum recommendations are to restart ACE inhibitors and to monitor closely for infection. It is important to discuss diabetes prevention in the offspring and to address contraception. It is most important to recommend an effective contraceptive method that is acceptable to the patient. Oral estrogens can increase triglycerides, and both oral and injectable progesterone-only contraceptives may increase insulin resistance. Low-dose combined oral contraceptives and the progesterone-releasing intrauterine device appear to have little effect on glucose.

Insulin is acceptable in breast-feeding women, and limited data suggest that glyburide and metformin are safe as well. One small study found that glyburide is not excreted in breast milk and that metformin is excreted in a small amount that is probably not clinically significant.

PROGNOSIS AND COMPLICATIONS

The maternal complications of diabetes may be impacted by pregnancy and may affect the course of the pregnancy. Patients with nephropathy experience an increase in proteinuria and a risk for progression of renal disease, especially if the serum creatinine is greater than 1.4 mg/dL. There is an increased risk for hypertension, which is seen in 30% during the first trimester and 75% of patients by the third trimester. Autonomic neuropathy may worsen, as manifested by increasing gastroparesis, orthostatic hypotension, and decreased hypoglycemic awareness. Patients with long-standing diabetes may need to be evaluated for ischemic heart disease, which may impair the heart's ability to meet the cardiovascular demands of pregnancy. Pregnant patients are also at risk for hyperlipidemia and for preeclampsia. Diabetes increases the risk for operative delivery and for infections, the most common of which are wound, urinary tract, and respiratory.

Diabetic ketoacidosis may be precipitated by steroid use for fetal lung maturity, hyperemesis, infection, and noncompliance with insulin regimens. Acidosis may occur more quickly and at lower glucose levels in pregnant than in nonpregnant patients. There is a very high fetal mortality associated with diabetic ketoacidosis (9 to 10%), and patients should be monitored in an intensive care setting.

Fetal and Neonatal Effects (Fig. 247-4)

There is an increased risk of spontaneous abortion, fetal loss, congenital anomalies, preeclampsia, and preterm delivery in patients with diabetes. Poor glycemic control during pregnancy, especially in type 2 diabetes and GDM, is also associated with macrosomia (baby weighing >4000 g) and fetal intraventricular septal hypertrophy. Poor control is also associated with the effects of maternal vascular and renal disease and ketoacidosis, which include fetal loss, preeclampsia, and low birthweight.

Neonatal complications include respiratory distress syndrome, hypoglycemia, hypocalcemia, cardiac hypertrophy, hyperbilirubinemia, and polycythemia. The risk of hypoglycemia may be ameliorated by careful control of maternal glucose during labor and delivery. Normalization of maternal glucose prevents hyperinsulinemia in the fetus and mitigates the risk of neonatal hypoglycemia.

Maternal Effects

GDM is a marker for type 2 diabetes: 50% of patients will develop type 2 diabetes within 7 to 10 years, and overall, 70% will develop the disease. Patients who have had GDM need directed testing at their 6-week postpartum visit, annual screening, and recommendations for lifestyle modification and cardiovascular risk reduction. Offspring of patients with GDM and type 2 diabetes are at increased risk for obesity and glucose intolerance.

FIGURE 247-4. Fetal, neonatal, and childhood effects of exposure to hyperglycemia. CNS = central nervous system; RDS = respiratory distress syndrome.

SUMMARY

Women of childbearing age with chronic medical conditions benefit greatly from preconception counseling and interventions that address control of their disease and safety of their medications. Pregnant patients with acute or chronic medical illnesses require a multidisciplinary team that understands the maternal and fetal risks related to both the underlying illness and untreated disease. Pregnancy is a window of opportunity to address maternal health, and the maternal response to pregnancy may be predictive of future risk. The 6-week postpartum visit, rather than being the end of pregnancy care, should represent the beginning of a woman's long-term health care.

Grade A

1. Koopmans CM, Bijlenga D, Groen H, et al. Induction of labour versus expectant monitoring for gestational hypertension or mild pre-eclampsia after 36 weeks' gestation (HYPITAT): a multicentre, open-label randomised controlled trial. *Lancet*. 2009;374:979-988.
2. Belfort MA, Anthony J, Saade GR, et al. A comparison of magnesium sulfate and nimodipine for the prevention of eclampsia. *N Engl J Med*. 2003;348:304-341.
3. Roberts JM, Myatt L, Spong CY, et al. Vitamins C and E to prevent complications of pregnancy-associated hypertension. *N Engl J Med*. 2010;362:1282-1291.
4. Duley L, Henderson-Smart DJ, Knight M, et al. Meta-analysis for ASA for prevention of preeclampsia. Antiplatelet agents for preventing pre-eclampsia and its complications. *Cochrane Database Syst. Rev.* 2004;1:CD004659.
5. Landon MB, Spong CY, Thom E, et al. A multicenter, randomized trial of treatment for mild gestational diabetes. *N Engl J Med*. 2009;361:1339-1348.
6. Moore LE, Clokey D, Rappaport VJ, et al. Metformin compared with glyburide in gestational diabetes: a randomized controlled trial. *Obstet Gynecol*. 2010;115:55-59.

SUGGESTED READINGS

Berg CJ, MacKay A, Cheng Q, et al. Overview of maternal morbidity during hospitalization for labor and delivery in the United States: 1993-1997 and 2001-2005. *Obstet Gynecol*. 2009;113:5. *Review of U.S. data confirming that there has been an increase in the rate of pregnancies complicated by medical conditions.*

Bourjeily G, Paidas M, Khalil H, et al. Pulmonary embolism in pregnancy. *Lancet*. 2010;375:500-512. *Well-referenced, comprehensive review of available data on the diagnosis of pulmonary embolism in pregnancy.*

Joshi D, James A, Quaglia A, et al. Liver disease in pregnancy. *Lancet*. 2010;375:594-605. *Review.*

Landon MB, Mele L, Spong CY, et al. The relationship between maternal glycemia and perinatal outcome. *Obstet Gynecol*. 2011;117:218-224. *A monotonic relationship exists between increasing maternal glycemia and perinatal morbidity.*

Mathiesen ER, Ringholm L, Damm P. Therapeutic management of type 1 diabetes before and during pregnancy. *Expert Opin Pharmacother*. 2011;12:779-786. *Review emphasizing tight glycemic control with rapid-acting insulin analogues to reduce the risk of hypoglycemia.*

Murphy VE, Gibson PG. Asthma in pregnancy. *Clin Chest Med*. 2011;32:93-110. *Review of management.*

Niebyl JR. Clinical practice: nausea and vomiting in pregnancy. *N Engl J Med*. 2010;363:1544-1550. *Clinical review.*

Smith G, Walker M, Liu A, et al. A history of preeclampsia identifies women who have underlying cardiovascular risk factors. *Am J Obstet Gynecol*. 2009;200:58.e1-58.e8. *Women with preeclampsia have a 2- to 3-fold higher cardiovascular risk at 1 year postpartum.*

Steegers EA, von Dadelszen P, Duvekot JJ, et al. Pre-eclampsia. *Lancet*. 2010;376:631-644. *Comprehensive review.*

TERIS. http://depts.washington.edu/terisweb/teris. *Online subscription and diskette containing more than 1000 agents and including Shepard's Catalogue of Teratogenic Agents. Summary of all human and animal data on individual medications by an expert panel.*

248

MENOPAUSE

DEBORAH GRADY AND ELIZABETH BARRETT-CONNOR

DEFINITION

All healthy women transition from a reproductive or premenopausal period marked by regular ovulation and cyclic menstrual bleeding to a postmenopausal period marked by infertility and amenorrhea (Fig. 248-1). The onset of the menopausal transition is generally marked by subtle changes in the length of the menstrual cycle and in the duration or amount of menstrual flow. As the menopausal transition progresses, menstrual cycles are missed until complete amenorrhea occurs, but the pattern of missed cycles is not predictable. Amenorrhea for a few months is not a good indicator of menopause because one half to three fourths of middle-aged women who are amenorrheic for 6 months resume cycles. Thus, menopause is typically defined retrospectively after 12 months of amenorrhea.

EPIDEMIOLOGY

The menopausal transition usually begins in the middle to late 40s and lasts approximately 4 years, with menopause occurring at a median age of 51 years and ranging in age from approximately 45 to 57 years. Age at menopause has not changed significantly over the past century. However, a century ago, most women in the United States did not live beyond menopause. A gradual increase in life expectancy to the low 80s now means that the average woman is postmenopausal for more than one third of her life. Age at menopause does not vary significantly by race or ethnicity, but on average, cigarette smokers experience menopause approximately 2 years earlier than nonsmokers.

BIOLOGY

During the early menopausal transition, estrogen levels are generally normal (50 to 200 pg/mL, depending on the stage of the menstrual cycle) or even slightly elevated, whereas the levels of follicle-stimulating hormone (FSH) and luteinizing hormone (LH) begin to increase (see Fig. 248-1). As the menopause transition progresses, estrogen levels fall markedly, and FSH continues to increase. After menopause, women do not ovulate, and their ovaries do not produce estradiol or progesterone. However, a small amount of estrogen may be produced by metabolism of adrenal steroids to estradiol in peripheral fat tissue. In the early postmenopausal period, mean estradiol levels average approximately 40 pg/mL, and they fall to less than 15 pg/mL in the late postmenopausal period. Depending on the measurement method, approximately 15 to 30% of older postmenopausal women have unmeasurable estradiol levels. Testosterone levels after menopause are similar to premenopausal levels.

It is not clear what causes menopause, but two leading theories have been proposed. Age-related depletion of ovarian follicles may lead to decreased production of estrogen and inhibin and may thus cause altered hypothalamic-pituitary feedback that results in menopause. Alternatively, age-related changes in hypothalamic production of gonadotropin-releasing hormone and subsequent effects on FSH and LH may be responsible for the increased rate of loss of ovarian follicles, declining ovarian function, and menopause.

MENOPAUSAL SYMPTOMS

Menopause is a very positive occurrence in the life of many women. It marks the end of cyclic bleeding and the need for birth control. It occurs at an age when children generally have become independent adults, thereby reducing family and child care responsibilities. Conversely, menopause is a notable sign of aging in a culture that values youth. In addition, it often occurs with other stresses, such as caring for elderly or ill parents. Women in the menopausal transition commonly report a wide variety of symptoms, including hot flushes, night sweats, vaginal dryness, trouble sleeping, sexual dysfunction, depression, anxiety, labile mood, memory loss, fatigue, headache, joint pains, weight gain, and urinary incontinence.

Only vasomotor symptoms, vaginal dryness, and sleep disturbance are consistently associated with the menopausal transition. Other reported symptoms may result from aging or stress associated with menopause. Some symptoms, such as depression, anxiety, memory loss, and fatigue, may be the consequence of frequent hot flushes or poor sleep.

Vasomotor Symptoms

DEFINITION

Vasomotor symptoms include hot flushes, chills, and sweats. A *hot flush* is a sudden feeling of warmth, generally most intense over the face, neck, and chest. The duration is variable, but it averages approximately 4 minutes. It is often accompanied by sweating that can be profuse and followed by a chill.

EPIDEMIOLOGY

The prevalence of hot flushes is maximal in the late menopausal transition, occurring in approximately 50% of women (Fig. 248-2). However, prevalence varies markedly, depending on the definition of flushing (any flushing, daily flushing, troublesome flushing) and the population studied. Lower

Final menstrual period

	Reproductive			Menopause Transition		Postmenopause	
Reproductive stage	Early	Peak	Late	Early	Late	Early	Late
				Perimenopause			
Menstrual cycle	Variable or regular	Regular		Cycle length variable, 1 or 2 missed cycles per year	3 or more missed cycles	None	
Age (duration)	Puberty to mid-40s			Mid-40s to mid-50s (4 yr)		Mean of 51 years to death	
Steroid hormones	Estradiol 50 to 200 pg/mL			Same or slightly higher		40 pg/mL	0-15 pg/mL
	Testosterone 400 pg/mL			Same		same	same
Pituitary hormones	FSH 10 mIU/mL day 2-4			Same or higher		>100 mIU/mL	
	LH 10 mIU/mL day 2-4			Same or higher		>100 mIU/mL	

FIGURE 248-1. Stages of the menopause transition. FSH = follicle-stimulating hormone; LH = luteinizing hormone.

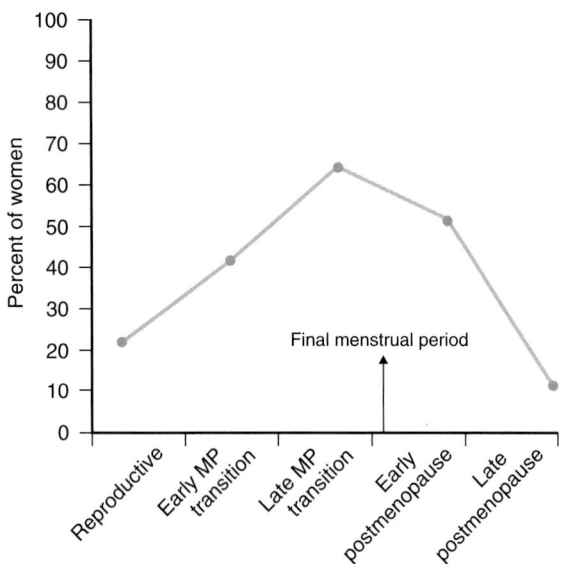

FIGURE 248-2. Prevalence of hot flushes during the menopause (MP) transition.

prevalence is reported among women in China, Japan, and other Asian countries. The reason for this variation is not clear, but investigators have suggested that it may result from differences in biology, cultural influences on experiencing or reporting flushes, or diet and lifestyle. In the United States, flushes are more common in African American and Latina women and less common in Chinese and Japanese women compared with white women. Approximately 15% of women with menopausal symptoms consult a physician.

Cigarette smoking increases the likelihood of flushing, but other potential risk factors, including surgical menopause, physical activity, body mass index, alcohol consumption, and socioeconomic status, have been inconsistently associated with hot flushes. Currently, there is no way to predict whether an individual woman will suffer from hot flushes.

NATURAL HISTORY

In most women, hot flushes are transient. Approximately 50% of women report resolution of symptoms within a few years, and symptoms resolve in about 90% within 8 years. However, some women continue to have frequent and severe flushes many years after menopause. Approximately 10% of women in their middle to late 60s report significant flushing. It is not clear why flushes persist for many years in some women and resolve in others.

PATHOBIOLOGY

In humans, body temperature is regulated by inducing vasodilation and sweating to release heat and vasoconstriction and shivering to conserve heat. Thermoregulation is complex and depends on central stimuli from the anterior hypothalamus and local changes in cutaneous vasoconstriction or dilation (Chapters 230 and 427). A hot flush is very similar to a heat dissipation response because both result in vasodilation, sweating, and reduction in core body temperature. The core body temperature at which postmenopausal women with hot flushes vasodilate and sweat is lower than in premenopausal women or in postmenopausal women without hot flushes. Variability in core body temperature does not appear to be greater in postmenopausal women with hot flushes than in premenopausal women or in postmenopausal women without hot flushes, but normal small fluctuations in core body temperature may exceed the lowered threshold for vasodilation and result in hot flushes.

The cause of altered thermoregulation in postmenopausal women with hot flushes is not clear. One theory suggests that changes in estrogen levels associated with menopause alter central nervous system adrenergic neurotransmission. This theory is supported by studies showing that metabolites of norepinephrine increase during spontaneous and experimentally induced hot flushes, and that systemic administration of yohimbine, an α_2-adrenergic antagonist that increases norepinephrine release, provokes hot flushes, whereas administration of clonidine, an α_2-adrenergic agonist that decreases norepinephrine release, reduces the frequency of hot flushes. Alternatively, some evidence indicates that declining estrogen levels during the menopause transition result in changes in serotonergic neurotransmission that could cause hot flushes. Lower estrogen levels are associated with lower levels of serotonin (5-hydroxytryptamine) in blood, resulting in increased sensitivity of 5-hydroxytryptamine-2A receptors in the hypothalamus. Stimulation of these receptors can alter the thermoregulatory set point in animals. Mild stressors, such as heat or anxiety, cause a brief release of 5-hydroxytryptamine that may stimulate central 5-hydroxytryptamine-2A receptors, lower the thermoregulatory set point, and cause flushing. This hypothesis is supported by the finding that drugs that increase central serotonin levels may be effective in the treatment of hot flushes.

Estrogen treatment effectively relieves hot flushes, but the exact role of estrogen in flushing is not clear. Fluctuations in estrogen levels in an individual woman do not correlate with the onset of flushes. Prepubertal girls with very low levels of endogenous estrogen, premenopausal women with marked fluctuations in estrogen during the menstrual cycle, and most postmenopausal women with low, constant levels of estradiol do not experience flushing. However, women with gonadal dysgenesis (Chapter 241) who are treated with estrogen for several months experience flushing when treatment is discontinued. Thus, withdrawal of estrogen, rather than the absolute estrogen level, appears to play a key role in the etiology of hot flushes.

In addition to changes in estradiol, menopause is associated with multiple other hormonal changes. In the Study of Women's Health Across the Nation (SWAN), a large cohort study in the United States, lower estradiol was

TABLE 248-1 DIFFERENTIAL DIAGNOSIS OF HOT FLUSHES

Alcohol consumption
Carcinoid syndrome
Dumping syndrome
Hyperthyroidism
Narcotic withdrawal
Pheochromocytoma
Medications
    Aromatase inhibitors
    Gonadotropin-releasing hormone agonists or antagonists
    Nicotinic acid
    Nitrates
    Selective estrogen receptor modulators (tamoxifen and raloxifene)

associated with flushing in middle-aged women in univariate models. However, higher FSH was the only measure independently associated with flushing after adjustment for other hormone levels. Hot flushes correlate with pulsatile increases in LH, but suppression of LH with gonadotropin-releasing hormone agonists does not eliminate flushing. Androgens may also play a role because men who are treated with androgen deprivation therapy for prostate cancer frequently report severe flushing.

DIAGNOSIS

Vasomotor symptoms are classic manifestations of the menopause transition, and the diagnosis is generally obvious from a woman's age and description of the symptoms. No abnormal physical findings are associated with hot flushes. Estradiol, FSH, and LH levels may be in the normal premenopausal range during the menopausal transition (see Fig. 248-1). A woman in her middle 40s to middle 50s who complains of classic hot flushes does not require any specific physical or laboratory evaluation unless there is good reason to suspect another cause of flushing (Table 248-1). However, an FSH determination may be helpful in assessing the risk for pregnancy. A woman in her middle 40s to middle 50s with an FSH level obtained on the third day after menses that is higher than 20 IU/L is not at risk of becoming pregnant.

TREATMENT   Rx

Because self-reported frequency and severity of hot flushes improve markedly with placebo, conclusive evidence of efficacy of treatments requires randomized, blinded trials. Clinical trials of treatments for hot flushes have typically been small and of short duration, limiting information about potential adverse effects.

General Measures
Behavioral and Alternative Therapies

Many women have mild flushes and obtain adequate relief with simple measures such as lowering ambient temperature and wearing lighter clothing. Moderate exercise does not improve flushing.

There is no convincing evidence that acupuncture, Chinese herbs, dong quai, evening primrose oil, ginseng, kava, or red clover extract improve hot flushes.[1][2] Evidence regarding black cohosh is mixed but primarily negative.[1][2] Multiple trials have been performed using different phytoestrogen preparations. Although some of these studies have reported benefit, the weight of evidence, especially from good-quality trials with blinded comparisons, suggests little benefit.[1-3] One trial of vitamin E supplementation found an improvement in flushes, but the decrease was only one hot flush per day. Many women prefer alternative medications because they believe that these treatments are harmless, but phytoestrogens and, possibly, black cohosh bind estrogen receptors and theoretically could cause adverse outcomes similar to those observed with estrogen. No studies of these preparations have been of adequate size or duration to document safety.

Medical Therapy
Estrogens

Multiple randomized trials have demonstrated that estrogen markedly improves the frequency and severity of hot flushes.[4] All types, preparations, and routes of administration of estrogen are effective. Estrogen reduces the frequency of hot flushes 60 to 95%, depending on the dose. Higher doses of estrogen may control symptoms more rapidly, but they are also associated with a higher rate of side effects, including uterine bleeding, breast tenderness, and headache.

At similar biologically active doses, oral and transdermal estrogens are approximately equally effective for treatment of vasomotor symptoms. Oral estrogens undergo "first-pass" metabolism in the liver that results in changes in hepatic proteins and enzymes. Hepatic effects are responsible for the beneficial effects of estrogen on lipoproteins (reduced low-density lipoprotein cholesterol and increased high-density lipoprotein cholesterol) but also for potentially adverse effects such as increases in clotting factors. The transdermal route may be safer because it minimizes these changes.

Many estrogen preparations are approved for treatment of vasomotor symptoms (Table 248-2). To individualize treatment, physicians should become familiar with several of these preparations.

Treatment with estrogen alone increases the risk for uterine hyperplasia and cancer. The risk for endometrial abnormalities appears not to be increased with the use of vaginal estrogens that deliver low systemic doses, especially if they are used only a few times per week, as is generally recommended (Table 248-3).

Adding a progestin to the estrogen regimen prevents the increased risk for uterine cancer. For this reason, a woman with a uterus who takes estrogen should also be given a progestin. There is no reason to add progestins to the hormone regimen in women who have had a hysterectomy. Several progestins are approved by the U.S. Food and Drug Administration (FDA) for this purpose and are available either to add to estrogen or in preparations combined with estrogen (see Table 248-2). Two general approaches are used to prescribing progestins to protect the endometrium. Sequential therapy (estrogen given daily with a progestin added on the last 10 to 14 days of a 28-day cycle) results in endometrial shedding and cyclic bleeding resembling a menstrual period in approximately 80% of women. Alternatively, the progestin can be added to the estrogen every day. This continuous regimen results in endometrial atrophy and unpredictable uterine spotting or bleeding that can be difficult for the woman to anticipate and manage. Bleeding occurs in approximately 80% of women in the first 6 months of continuous treatment. Amenorrhea becomes more common with prolonged use, but some women continue to bleed or spot for many years.

The most commonly used progestins in sequential regimens in women using standard doses of estrogens (0.625 mg oral conjugated estrogens, 1 mg oral estradiol, or 0.05 mg transdermal estradiol) are medroxyprogesterone acetate, 5 mg, and micronized progesterone, 200 mg, for 10 to 14 days per month. Continuous regimens generally include half these progestin doses given daily. In some situations, it may be slightly less costly to prescribe estrogen and progestins separately, but the convenience of taking a single pill and the assurance that the estrogen is adequately opposed by progestin make combination preparations preferred.

The use of "bioidentical hormones" is based on the concept that estrogens (estradiol, estrone, and estriol) and progestins (progesterone) made from plant products are identical to women's endogenous hormones and more natural, safe, and effective than FDA-approved hormone preparations. Bioidentical hormone therapy often uses doses and combinations of steroid hormones guided by patient symptoms or hormone levels, and prescriptions are generally filled by Internet-based compounding pharmacies. There is little scientific rationale for the mixtures and ratios of hormones employed, and there are no adequate clinical trial data to support the safety or efficacy of these regimens, some of which include very large doses of estradiol. Bioidentical hormones are not approved by the FDA for treatment of menopausal symptoms.

Side Effects and Risks of Postmenopausal Hormone Therapy

Estrogen is generally well tolerated, but it may cause headache (especially in women with a history of migraine) and breast tenderness. Added progestins tend to make these side effects more severe and also cause uterine bleeding.

The effects of hormone therapy on disease outcomes have been evaluated among postmenopausal women in the Women's Health Initiative (WHI) randomized trials[5-8] (Table 248-4). Both estrogen and estrogen in combination with progestin reduced the risk for hip fracture by 35 to 40%. Neither estrogen alone nor estrogen with a progestin reduced the risk for coronary events, and both increased the risk for stroke by approximately 40%.

Compared with estrogen alone, added progestin appears to increase the risk for coronary events, pulmonary embolism, breast cancer, and dementia (see Table 248-4). This finding suggests that adding a progestin should be avoided, but treatment with unopposed estrogen in women with a uterus markedly increases the risk for uterine hyperplasia and cancer as well as the rate of gynecologic procedures and hysterectomy.

The excess risk of any one of the adverse events listed in Table 248-4 in the WHI trials was about 2 per 1000 women treated for 1 year with estrogen in combination with progestin (4.3 per 1000 per year in women older than 65 years if dementia is included), and 0.6 strokes per 1000 women treated with unopposed estrogen. These risks are relatively small, but they cumulate such that treatment for 5 years is associated with an excess risk of one event per 100 women treated with estrogen in combination with progestin and three strokes per 1000 women treated with unopposed estrogen. Based on the findings of the WHI trials and the availability of other effective and safe drugs for prevention of osteoporotic fractures, postmenopausal hormone therapy currently has no role for prevention of disease. Some investigators have proposed that estrogen treatment, if started very soon after menopause, would reduce risk for coronary disease events. However, careful subgroup analyses of data from the WHI randomized trials do not support this hypothesis.[9]

The mean age of the women included in the WHI trials was 63 years, whereas the average age of women treated for menopausal vasomotor symptoms is approximately a decade younger. Because the risk for most diseases approximately doubles with each decade of age, the absolute risk for the outcomes listed in Table 248-4 is less for younger than for older women, and the absolute risk increase is proportionately smaller. However, hormone therapy is relatively contraindicated in women with a history of stroke, breast cancer, or venous thromboembolic events and should be avoided in women at high risk for these conditions.

Stopping Hormone Therapy

Given the possible adverse effects of hormone therapy, current guidelines recommend that women use the lowest effective dose for the shortest time necessary. Vasomotor symptoms improve or resolve spontaneously within a few years of onset in most women, a finding suggesting that most women should be able to discontinue hormone therapy within a few years of starting. Women using hormone therapy for treatment of symptoms should stop every 6 to 12 months to determine whether symptoms have improved to the point that treatment is no longer needed. A small percentage of women are unable to stop hormone therapy because vasomotor symptoms persist.

Women experiencing intolerable symptoms after stopping hormone treatment can be told to resume therapy and either to begin a slow taper or to wait 6 months before trying again to stop. Tapering can be accomplished by decreasing the dose of hormone therapy, but it may be easier to decrease slowly the number of days per week that hormone therapy is used. The *dose taper* involves progressively reducing the dose of hormone therapy, for example by reducing the dose of conjugated estrogens from 0.625 mg/day to 0.45 to 0.3 mg/day and then discontinuing therapy. If changing to a lower dose is associated with symptoms, the next reduction in dose should not occur until symptoms improve and are easily tolerable, which may require 3 to 6 months in some women. The *day taper* involves decreasing the number of days per week of hormone therapy use and effectively decreasing the weekly dose. For example, therapy with the same dose may be continued, but only Monday through Friday. If this reduced weekly dose is tolerated, therapy may be discontinued on Thursday, and so on. As with the dose taper, if symptoms develop, the weekly dose should be maintained until symptoms improve. Both these approaches to tapering can require many months or even years until therapy is discontinued. The day taper has the advantages of allowing smaller reductions in weekly dose, ensuring that the estrogen dose is appropriately opposed by a progestin in women using continuous therapy and does not require multiple new prescriptions for different doses of hormone therapy. For women who cannot tolerate even a slow taper, the value of symptom relief likely outweighs the risks of hormone therapy.

Other Prescription Drugs

A drug that appears to be as effective as estrogens for treatment of hot flushes is tibolone, a steroid hormone that is not marketed in the United States but is widely available elsewhere (Table 248-5). Tibolone preserves bone density, reduces the risks for fracture and breast cancer, but increases risk for uterine cancer and stroke. [10] The progestins megestrol and medroxyprogesterone acetate are effective for the treatment of hot flushes, but they have frequent side effects, and progestin use was associated with increased risk for adverse effects in the WHI trials. Several selective serotonin and serotonin-norepinephrine reuptake inhibitors and gabapentin have been studied. [11] Paroxetine and gabapentin appear to have modest efficacy in relieving hot flushes (see Table 248-5). Recently, the selective serotonin reuptake inhibitor escitalopram (10 to 20 mg per day) was shown to reduce the number and intensity of menopausal hot flashes. [12] However, clinical trials have not been adequately large or prolonged to detect uncommon adverse effects.

Summary of Approach to Treatment of Vasomotor Symptoms

Women with mild vasomotor symptoms may find adequate relief by wearing layered clothing and keeping the home and bedroom cool. Women with moderate symptoms may choose a low dose of estrogen or a nonestrogen therapy. Paroxetine is modestly effective and probably has the best side-effect profile of the nonhormonal drugs. For women with severe symptoms, hormone therapy is the most effective treatment.

Vaginal Dryness

EPIDEMIOLOGY

The prevalence of vaginal dryness, discomfort, itching, and dyspareunia increases as women transition through the menopause. Up to 30% of perimenopausal and early postmenopausal women and a higher proportion of older menopausal women express these complaints. Urologic symptoms, including urgency, frequency, dysuria, and incontinence, are not clearly correlated with the menopause transition.

TABLE 248-2 ESTROGEN AND PROGESTIN PREPARATIONS FOR TREATMENT OF MENOPAUSAL VASOMOTOR SYMPTOMS

HORMONES	GENERIC NAME	BRAND NAME	DOSE (mg/day)
ESTROGENS*			
Oral	Conjugated estrogens	Premarin	0.3, 0.45, **0.625**, 0.9, 1.25
	17β-Estradiol	Estrace/generics	0.5, **1.0**, 2.0
Transdermal	17β-Estradiol	Alora patch[†]	0.025, **0.05**, 0.075, 0.1
		Climara patch[‡]	0.025, 0.0375, **0.05**, 0.075, 0.1
		Menostar patch[‡]	0.014
		Evamist spray	1.53/spray
		Elestrin gel	0.025/pump
Vaginal	Estradiol acetate	Femring vaginal ring[§]	**0.05**, 0.1
PROGESTINS			
Oral	Medroxyprogesterone acetate	Provera/generics	2.5, 5.0, 10.0
	Micronized progesterone	Prometrium	100, 200 (in peanut oil)
Vaginal	Progesterone	Prochieve 4%	45 every other day
COMBINATION PREPARATIONS			
Oral sequential[ǁ]	Conjugated estrogens and medroxyprogesterone acetate	Premphase	0.625 + 5.0
Oral continuous[¶]	Conjugated estrogens and medroxyprogesterone acetate	Prempro	0.625 + 5.0; 0.45 + 2.5 or 1.5; 0.3 + 1.5
	17β-Estradiol and norethindrone acetate	Activella	1.0 + 0.5
Transdermal continuous[¶]	17β-Estradiol and levonorgestrel	Climara Pro[‡]	0.045 + 0.015
	17β-Estradiol and norethindrone acetate	CombiPatch[†]	0.05 + 0.14 or 0.25

*Approximately equivalent doses of estrogens are shown in **bold**.
[†]Patch applied twice per week.
[‡]Patch applied once per week.
[§]Vaginal ring inserted every 90 days; note that Femring, as opposed to the vaginal preparations listed in Table 248-3, delivers systemic levels of estrogen and should be opposed by a progestin in women with a uterus.
[ǁ]Each pill contains estrogen days 1 to 14 and estrogen with progestin days 15 to 28.
[¶]Each pill or patch contains estrogen and progestin.

TABLE 248-3 ESTROGEN VAGINAL PREPARATIONS FOR TREATMENT OF VAGINAL DRYNESS*

PREPARATION	GENERIC NAME	BRAND NAME	DOSE
Vaginal cream	Conjugated estrogens	Premarin	0.625 mg/2 g cream: 2 g/day for 2 wk, then 1-2 g 2 to 3 times/wk
	17β-Estradiol	Estrace	0.1 mg/2 g cream: 2 g/day for 2 wk, then 1-2 g 2 to 3 times/wk
Vaginal tablet	Estradiol hemihydrate	Vagifem	0.025 mg tablet: 1 tablet/day for 2 wk, then 1 tablet twice/wk
Vaginal ring	17β-Estradiol	Estring[†]	0.0075 mg/day

*Most oral, transdermal, and vaginal products listed in Table 248-2 for treatment of vasomotor symptoms are also approved for treatment of vaginal dryness.
[†]Vaginal ring is inserted every 90 days.

TABLE 248-4 RESULTS OF THE WOMEN'S HEALTH INITIATIVE RANDOMIZED TRIALS OF THE EFFECTS OF POSTMENOPAUSAL HORMONE THERAPY ON DISEASE OUTCOMES

| | Relative Risk and 95% Confidence Interval | |
OUTCOMES	ESTROGEN AND PROGESTIN*[5,6]	ESTROGEN†[7,8]
Coronary heart disease events	1.29 (1.02-1.63)	0.91 (0.75-1.12)
Stroke	1.41 (1.07-1.85)	1.39 (1.10-1.77)
Pulmonary embolism	2.13 (1.39-3.25)	1.34 (0.87-2.06)
Breast cancer	1.26 (1.00-1.59)	0.77 (0.59-1.01)
Colon cancer	0.63 (0.43-0.92)	1.08 (0.75-1.55)
Hip fracture	0.66 (0.45-0.98)	0.61 (0.41-0.91)
Dementia	2.05 (1.21-3.48)	1.49 (0.83-2.66)
Death	0.98 (0.82-1.18)	1.04 (0.88-1.22)

*Results of the Women's Health Initiative estrogen plus progestin randomized trial: 16,608 postmenopausal women without hysterectomy randomized to 0.625 mg conjugated estrogen plus 2.5 mg medroxyprogesterone acetate per day or identical placebo and followed for 5.2 years.
†Results of the Women's Health Initiative estrogen-only randomized trial: 10,739 postmenopausal women with hysterectomy randomized to 0.625 mg conjugated estrogen per day or identical placebo and followed for 6.8 years.

PATHOBIOLOGY

Vaginal symptoms generally correlate with findings (often called vaginal atrophy) including pallor, dryness, friability, and decreased rugosity of the vaginal mucosa. Vaginal fluid in premenopausal women is acidic, ranging from a pH of approximately 4.5 to 5.5 with mild alkalinization to approximately 6.0 before ovulation. Acidity is produced by proton excretion from the vaginal epithelial cells and by metabolism of glycogen stored in vaginal epithelial cells by *Lactobacillus* species, the normal vaginal flora. The acid environment of the vagina inhibits growth of *Escherichia coli* and other enteric gram-negative bacteria that are a potential cause of urinary tract infections. Vaginal pH can easily be measured from lateral vaginal wall fluid.

In postmenopausal women, vaginal pH is generally neutral, and the predominant flora are often *E. coli* and other gram-negative bacteria. This appears to occur because estrogen deficiency associated with menopause causes vaginal epithelial cell dysfunction, including decreased storage of glycogen, less ability to acidify the vaginal fluid, and lowered production of vaginal lubrication. Vaginal epithelial cells, which are primarily superficial and intermediate cells in premenopausal women, shift to predominately immature parabasal cells in postmenopausal women. Treatment with estrogen improves

TABLE 248-5 EVIDENCE FROM RANDOMIZED, CONTROLLED CLINICAL TRIALS OF THE EFFICACY OF NONESTROGEN DRUGS FOR TREATMENT OF MENOPAUSAL HOT FLUSHES

TREATMENT	EVIDENCE OF BENEFIT	COMMENTS	REFERENCES	SIDE EFFECTS*
ANTIDEPRESSANTS				
Citalopram	No	No benefit of 30 mg citalopram compared with placebo	Suvanto-Luukkonen E, Koivunen R, Sundstrom H, et al. *Menopause.* 2005;12:18-26.	Selective serotonin reuptake inhibitors citalopram, escitalopram, fluoxetine, paroxetine, and sertraline: nausea, vomiting, diarrhea, insomnia or somnolence, anxiety, decreased libido, dry mouth, worsening depression, mania, suicidality, serotonin syndrome, withdrawal syndrome, and possible decreased tamoxifen effectiveness.
Escitalopram	Yes	Among generally healthy women, frequency of hot flushes reduced 47% with escitalopram 10 to 20 mg/day compared with 33% with placebo.	Freeman EW, Guthrie KA, Caan B, et al. *JAMA.* 2011;305:267-274.	
Fluoxetine	Mixed	Among breast cancer survivors, frequency of hot flushes reduced 50% with fluoxetine 20 mg/day compared to 36% with placebo. No benefit among women with breast cancer treated with 30 mg fluoxetine compared with placebo	Loprinzi CL, Sloan JA, Perez EA, et al. *J Clin Oncol.* 2002:20:1578-1583. Suvanto-Luukkonen E, Koivunen R, Sundstrom H, et al. *Menopause.* 2005;12:18-26.	
Paroxetine	Yes	Among generally healthy women, frequency of hot flushes reduced 62% with 12.5 mg and 65% with 25 mg paroxetine CR compared with 38% in placebo. In a crossover trial in which 81% of participants had a history of breast cancer, paroxetine 10 mg reduced hot flush frequency by 41% compared with 14% with placebo, and paroxetine 20 mg reduced hot flush frequency by 52% compared with 27% placebo.	Steans V, Beebe KL, Lyengar M, et al. *JAMA.* 2003;289:2827-2834. Stearns V, Slack R, Greep N, et al. *J Clin Oncol.* 2005;23:6919-6930.	
Sertraline	No	Among women with a history of breast cancer, no benefit of treatment with 50 mg of sertraline compared with placebo. Among generally healthy women, no benefit of 100 mg of sertraline compared with placebo.	Kimmick GG, Lovato J, McQuellon R, et al. *Breast J.* 2006;12:114-122. Grady D, Cohen B, Tice J, et al. *Obstet Gynecol.* 2007;109:823-830.	
Venlafaxine	Mixed	Among breast cancer survivors, frequency of hot flushes reduced 61% with 75 or 150 mg venlafaxine compared with 27% placebo. Among women without breast cancer, no effect on frequency of flushes with 75 mg venlafaxine, but women treated with venlafaxine were more likely to report that flushes improved compared with placebo.	Loprinzi CL, Kugler JW, Sloan JA, et al. *Lancet.* 2003:356:2059-2063. Evans ML, Pritts E, Vittinghoff E, et al. *Obstet Gynecol.* 2005;105:161-166.	In addition to the side effects noted above, the selective serotonin-norepinephrine reuptake inhibitors venlafaxine and desvenlafaxine can also cause hypertension.

TABLE 248-5 EVIDENCE FROM RANDOMIZED, CONTROLLED CLINICAL TRIALS OF THE EFFICACY OF NONESTROGEN DRUGS FOR TREATMENT OF MENOPAUSAL HOT FLUSHES—cont'd

TREATMENT	EVIDENCE OF BENEFIT	COMMENTS	REFERENCES	SIDE EFFECTS*
Desvenlafaxine	Yes	Frequency of hot flushes reduced by 60% with 100 mg per day and 66% with 150 mg per day compared with 47% in placebo.	Archer DF, Seidman L, Constatine GD, et al. *Am J Obstet Gynecol.* 2009;200:238.	
ANTIHYPERTENSIVES				
Clonidine	Mixed	Small trials suggest little or no benefit.	Nelson HD, Haney E, Humphrey L, et al. AHRQ Publication No. 05-E016-2. Rockville, MD: Agency for Healthcare Research and Quality; 2005. Goldberg RM, Loprinzi CL, O'Fallon JR, et al. *J Clin Oncol.* 1994;12:155-158. Pandya KJ, Raubertas RF, Flynn PJ, et al. *Ann Intern Med.* 2000;132:78-93.	α-Adrenergic antagonists clonidine and methyldopa: dry mouth, drowsiness, dizziness, hypotension, rebound hypertension
Methyldopa	No		Nelson HD, Haney E, Humphrey L, et al. AHRQ Publication No. 05-E016-2. Rockville, MD: Agency for Healthcare Research and Quality; 2005.	
HORMONES				
Medroxyprogesterone acetate	Yes	Frequency of hot flushes was reduced 74% with 20 mg medroxyprogesterone acetate compared with 26% with placebo.	Schiff I, Tulchinsky D, Cramer D, et al. *JAMA.* 1980;244:1443-1445.	Progestins medroxyprogesterone and megestrol: nausea, vomiting, constipation, somnolence, depression, breast tenderness, uterine bleeding; possible increased risk for venous thromboembolism, cardiovascular events, and breast cancer
Megestrol	Yes	Among breast cancer survivors, frequency of hot flushes reduced 74% with 20 mg megestrol twice a day compared with 27% with placebo	Loprinzi CL, Michalak JC, Quella SK, et al. *N Engl J Med.* 1994;331:347-352.	
Tibolone†	Yes	Several trials reported improved hot flushes compared with placebo and efficacy equivalent to standard doses of estrogens with 1.25-5.0 mg tibolone	Modelska K, Cummings S. *J Clin Endocrinol Metab.* 2002;87:16-23. Nelson HD, Haney E, Humphrey L, et al. AHRQ Publication No. 05-E016-2. Rockville, MD: Agency for Healthcare Research and Quality; 2005.	Steroid hormone: headache, weight gain, uterine bleeding; effects on venous thromboembolism, cardiovascular disease, and breast and uterine cancer
OTHER DRUGS				
Gabapentin	Yes	Among healthy women, frequency of hot flushes was reduced 45% with gabapentin 300 mg three times/day compared with 29% with placebo. Frequency of hot flushes was reduced 31% more than placebo among breast cancer survivors	Guttuso TJ, Kurlan R, McDermott MP, et al. *Obstet Gynecol.* 2003;101:337-345. Pandya JK, Morrow GR, Rosco JA, et al. *Lancet.* 2005;366:818-824.	Nausea, vomiting, somnolence, dizziness, rash, ataxia, fatigue, leukopenia

*Side effects were reported in clinical trials of the therapy or from Epocrates RX drug reference (available at *http://www.epocrates.com*).
†This drug had not been approved by the U.S. Food and Drug Administration at the time of publication.

or relieves vaginal dryness, lowers vaginal pH, and increases the proportion of superficial cells in the vaginal epithelium.

DIAGNOSIS

Diagnosis is primarily based on typical complaints of vaginal dryness, discomfort, itching, or dyspareunia in women undergoing the menopause transition or older postmenopausal women. Pelvic examination should exclude other causes of discomfort, including infections, lesions, and trauma. Physical findings of vaginal dryness, pallor, friability, and vaginal pH greater than 5.5 support the diagnosis. Cytologic examination of the proportion of superficial, intermediate, and parabasal cells from a scraping of the lateral vaginal wall (vaginal maturation index) showing primarily parabasal cells also supports the diagnosis. In clinical practice, measurement of pH and vaginal maturation index are not necessary to make the diagnosis.

TREATMENT Rx

Many women with vaginal symptoms obtain adequate relief with use of over-the-counter vaginal moisturizers, such as Replens. Estrogen therapy is highly effective. Topical therapy is efficacious and is preferred because it generally results in smaller increases in systemic estrogen levels than oral or transdermal therapy.[13] Estrogen vaginal creams, tablets, and rings approved for treatment of vaginal dryness are listed in Table 248-3.

Most clinicians do not add a progestin to protect the uterus in women treated with vaginal estrogen, but evidence to support the uterine safety of vaginal estrogen is limited to short-term studies. Low-dose, intermittent treatment (e.g., 1 to 2 g conjugated estrogen cream or 0.025 mg estradiol tablet twice a week) results in very small increases in systemic estrogen levels that appear not to cause endometrial stimulation. However, full-dose daily treatment has been shown to increase estradiol levels to 50 pg/mL or higher in approximately half of treated women and has been associated with uterine bleeding and hyperplasia.

Sleep Disturbance

The prevalence of self-reported sleep disturbance increases from about 40% of premenopausal women to approximately 60% of postmenopausal women. Sleep disturbances, including trouble falling asleep and early awakening, are reported by menopausal women, but awakening during the night appears to be most bothersome.

The etiology of sleep disturbance associated with menopause is unclear. Postmenopausal women with hot flushes are more likely to report sleep disturbance than are those without flushes, and women commonly report that they are awakened by hot flushes. However, studies using polysomnography find that nocturnal hot flushes do not consistently occur at the same time as sleep disturbance. Thus, disturbed sleep appears to be part of a menopausal syndrome, but it may not be caused by flushing.

Menopause-related sleep disturbance can be treated using standard approaches to sleep hygiene and prescription medications. Both oral and transdermal estrogen preparations improve sleep in perimenopausal and postmenopausal women with hot flushes.

1. Nelson HD, Haney E, Humphrey L, et al. *Management of Menopause-Related Symptoms.* AHRQ Publication No. 05-E016-2. Rockville, MD: Agency for Healthcare Research and Quality; 2005.
2. Kronenberg F, Fugh-Berman A. Complementary and alternative medicine for menopausal symptoms: a review of randomized, controlled trials. *Ann Intern Med.* 2002;137:805-813.
3. Krebs EE, Ensrud KE, MacDonald R, et al. Phytoestrogens for treatment of menopausal symptoms: a systematic review. *Obstet Gynecol.* 2004;104:824-836.
4. MacLennan A, Lester S, Moore V. Oral estrogen replacement therapy versus placebo for hot flushes: a systematic review. *Climacteric.* 2001;4:58-74.
5. Rossouw JE, Anderson GL, Prentice RL, et al. Risks and benefits of estrogen plus progestin in healthy postmenopausal women: principal results from the Women's Health Initiative randomized controlled trial. *JAMA.* 2002;288:321-333.
6. Shumaker SA, Legault C, Thal L, et al. Estrogen plus progestin and the incidence of dementia and mild cognitive impairment in postmenopausal women: the Women's Health Initiative Memory Study. A randomized controlled trial. *JAMA.* 2003;289:2651-2662.
7. Shumaker SA, Legault C, Kuller L, et al. Conjugated equine estrogens and incidence of probable dementia and mild cognitive impairment in postmenopausal women. *JAMA.* 2004;291:2947-2958.
8. Women's Health Initiative Steering Committee. Effects of conjugated equine estrogen in postmenopausal women with hysterectomy: the Women's Health Initiative Randomized Controlled Trial. *JAMA.* 2004;291:1701-1712.
9. Prentice RL, Manson JE, Langer RD, et al. Benefits and risks of postmenopausal hormone therapy when it is initiated soon after menopause. *Am J Epidemiol.* 2009;170:12-23.
10. Cummings SR, Ettinger B, Delmas PD, et al. The effects of tibolone in older postmenopausal women. *N Engl J Med.* 2008;359:697-708.
11. Nelson HD, Vesco KK, Haney E, et al. Nonhormonal therapies for menopausal hot flashes: systematic review and meta-analysis. *JAMA.* 2006;295:2057-2071.
12. Freeman EW, Guthrie KA, Caan B, et al. Efficacy of escitalopram for hot flashes in healthy menopausal women: a randomized controlled trial. *JAMA.* 2011;305:267-274.
13. Suckling J, Lethaby A, Kennedy R. Local oestrogen for vaginal atrophy in postmenopausal women. *Cochrane Database Syst Rev.* 2006;4:CD001500.

SUGGESTED READINGS

Chlebowski RT, Anderson GL, Gass M, et al. Estrogen plus progestin and breast cancer incidence and mortality in postmenopausal women. *JAMA.* 2010;304:1684-1692. *Estrogen plus progestin is associated with greater breast cancer incidence, and the cancers are more commonly node positive.*

Mac Bride MB, Rhodes DJ, Shuster LT. Vulvovaginal atrophy. *Mayo Clin Proc.* 2010;85:87-94. *Approach to diagnosis and treatment, including the controversies surrounding local estrogen treatment.*

Pollycove R, Naftolin F, Simin JA. The evolutionary origin and significance of menopause. *Menopause.* 2011;18:336-342. *Review emphasizing opportunities for disease prevention and morbidity reduction in postmenopausal women.*

Santen RJ, Allred DC, Ardoin SP, et al. Postmenopausal hormone therapy: an Endocrine Society scientific statement. *J Clin Endocrinol Metab.* 2010;95:s1-s66. *Consensus guidelines based on randomized trials.*

Taylor HS, Manson JE. Update in hormone therapy use in menopause. *J Endcrinol Metab.* 2011;96:255-264. *Review of adverse effects of estrogen and the potential for possible hormone therapies with more favorable benefit-to-risk ratios.*

249

INTIMATE PARTNER VIOLENCE

GENE FEDER AND HARRIET MACMILLAN

DEFINITION

Intimate partner violence (IPV) is defined as any behavior within an intimate relationship or ex-relationship that causes physical, psychological, or sexual harm. This includes physical aggression, such as hitting, kicking, and beating; psychological violence, such as intimidation, constant humiliation; various controlling behaviors, such as isolation from family and friends, monitoring movements, financial control, and restricting access to services; and sexual violence, including forced intercourse and other sexual coercion. Lifetime prevalence of isolated violent acts within relationships is comparable for men and women, but repeated coercive, sexual, or severe physical violence is perpetrated largely against women by men. Although IPV also occurs in same-sex relationships, research evidence on the health consequences of IPV and the care of survivors is largely confined to women in heterosexual relationships.

Historically, there has been the stereotype of a male batterer as one who uses severe, repeated, and unilateral violence against a nonviolent female victim. It is now recognized that *bilateral violence* is a common form of IPV, even though the overwhelming burden of morbidity and mortality related to IPV is experienced by women. Bilateral violence, sometimes referred to as *common couple violence*, is considered less severe that the pattern of abuse known as *battering* or *intimate terrorism*—a severe and escalating form of IPV characterized by threats, terrorization, multiple forms of abuse, and controlling behavior on the part of the abuser. Current research suggests that women rarely subject men to battering.

IPV is a risk factor for a wide range of medical and psychiatric conditions and therefore can be understood as an epidemiologic exposure. Yet violence perpetrated by an intimate partner or ex-partner is essentially a violation of human rights and a preventable psychosocial issue that needs to be addressed through social and educational policies.

EPIDEMIOLOGY

The prevalence of IPV against women varies internationally but is universally high, comparable to chronic conditions like diabetes and asthma. The most robust comparative study (24,097 women from 15 sites in 10 countries), conducted by the World Health Organization (WHO) found a lifetime prevalence of physical or sexual violence, or both, ranging from 15 to 71%. Prevalence of physical or sexual violence during the past year ranged from 15 to 54%. In all sites but one, women were more at risk for violence from a partner or ex-partner than from violence by other people.

A Canadian survey highlights a comparable prevalence of physical violence against men by their female partners (6% 5-year prevalence), which is replicated in most community surveys, but with substantially less serious violence (beaten, choked, or threatened with or had a weapon used against them), sexual violence, or fear of their partner.

Causation

Several theories about the causes of IPV have been proposed over the years. Social learning theory suggests that IPV is a learned behavior. The fact that male perpetrators and female victims are more likely to report histories of exposure to violence in childhood supports this theory. However, most individuals exposed to violence in childhood do not go on to commit violence as adults, and not all abusers have violent upbringings. Furthermore, the link between poor parenting generally, including neglect, and subsequent IPV in adulthood suggests that the effect is not simply one of modeling abusive behavior. Exposure to rejecting or neglectful parenting is associated with adverse effects on intrapersonal (e.g., poor self-worth) and interpersonal development, which are associated with IPV.

A feminist perspective views IPV against women as a form of social control that results from society's patriarchal structure leading to inequality in power relationships between men and women. Lending support to this perspective is the finding that IPV appears to be less common in more democratic and less economically polarized societies. Although IPV occurs more often in contexts in which there is support for male authority in the family and women have less access to economic security, it is not clear why some individuals are more likely to be violent under such conditions than others.

With regard to psychological theory, there are conflicting views about the association between IPV and psychopathology. Some researchers argue that abusive males have deficits in one or more coping mechanisms, anger control, and communication skills, whereas others suggest that IPV results from dysfunctional interactional patterns between partners. Because types of IPV are not the same for all couples, there are likely multiple causes for its occurrence. Most of the research has focused on factors associated with increased risk of men abusing women (Table 249-1); however, whether these factors are "causal" is unknown.

TABLE 249-1   FACTORS ASSOCIATED WITH A MAN'S RISK FOR ABUSING HIS PARTNER

INDIVIDUAL	RELATIONSHIP	COMMUNITY	SOCIETAL
Young age	Poor family	Weak community	Traditional
Heavy drinking	functioning	sanctions	gender norms
Depression	Marital instability	against intimate	Social norms
Personality disorders	Marital conflict	partner violence	supportive of
Low academic	Male dominance	Poverty	violence
achievement	Economic stress	Economic	
Low income		inequality	
Exposure to violence		Low social capital	
in childhood			

Adapted from WHO. *World Report on Violence and Health.* Geneva: WHO; 2002.

CLINICAL MANIFESTATIONS

The information in this section pertains to female patients because most of the research examining clinical manifestations associated with IPV exposure has focused on women. However, recent studies of male victims suggest that they also experience increased risk for poor health as well as chronic physical and emotional health problems and injuries.

Patients seldom present with a chief complaint of IPV. Injuries are the most obvious manifestation; a clinician should have increased suspicion for IPV if there are multiple injuries, the presenting history of injuries is not consistent with the physical examination, and there is a delay in seeking medical care for injuries. Patients exposed to physical violence may present with injuries that vary from minor abrasions to life-threatening trauma. Although there can be overlap between injuries resulting from IPV and injuries from other causes, the former typically involve trauma to the head, face, and neck, whereas the latter are more typically injuries of the extremities. Multiple facial injuries are suggestive of IPV rather than from other causes, and those that are more specific for IPV include zygomatic complex fractures, orbital blow-out fractures, and perforated tympanic membrane. Although facial injuries are the most common injuries associated with IPV, they have low specificity. Musculoskeletal injuries are considered the second most common type of injuries, including sprains, fractures, and dislocations. Blunt-force trauma to the forearms should raise suspicion of IPV because these can occur when trying to block being struck.

Victims of IPV often experience multiple mechanisms of injury; being struck by a hand is the most common, followed by use of a household object. Injuries from weapons such as knives and guns are far less common (<1%) but are associated with higher risk for mortality. Strangulation also occurs frequently, but less is known about the types of clinical manifestations that result from this form of IPV. Other injuries that raise suspicion of IPV include fractures of the spine or trunk, bites, hair pulling, and open wounds. Those exposed to sexual abuse may show signs of trauma to the genital area, but sexual assault is associated with signs of injury in less than one third of cases.

Most victims of IPV presenting to health care settings do not have signs of obvious trauma, but rather a constellation of overlapping physical and mental health problems. A patient presenting with vague signs and symptoms or chronic somatic complaints, including pain, suggests the possibility of IPV. Other behaviors that suggest IPV include delay in seeking medical care or multiple cancellations of medical appointments.

There are no systematic reviews of studies on the overall physical health consequences of IPV, but a recent overview of studies reported increased rates of chronic physical conditions, particularly gynecologic, gastrointestinal, and nervous system disorders, as well as increased cardiovascular risk, although most of the studies were small and poorly adjusted for other risk factors. The overview also found that women with a history of abuse, particularly physical and sexual violence, were more likely to experience chronic pain and nonspecific symptoms, although an association between abuse and number of physical symptoms is also found in women who experience emotional abuse without any physical abuse. The WHO study reported significant associations between women's lifetime experiences of partner violence and self-reported poor health and specific health problems in the previous 4 weeks, such as difficulty walking, difficulty with daily activities, pain, memory loss, dizziness, and vaginal discharge. Other physical conditions that should raise suspicion of IPV include chronic gynecologic or gastrointestinal symptoms, such as irritable bowel syndrome or chronic pelvic pain. It should not be assumed, however, that there is a specific association between functional disorders such as irritable bowel syndrome or fibromyalgia over and above

the greater reporting of physical syndromes in general. IPV exposure is associated with an increased risk for sexually transmitted infections, including human papillomavirus.

Exposure to any type of IPV can be associated with a wide range of emotional and behavioral symptoms; depression and post-traumatic stress disorder (PTSD) are the two most commonly associated emotional conditions, but other anxiety disorders and substance abuse are also associated with IPV exposure. In the WHO study, women who reported IPV at least once in their life reported three to four times more emotional distress, suicidal thoughts, and suicide attempts than nonabused women. There is strong evidence of increased risk for depression, anxiety, substance abuse, and PTSD, with longitudinal studies reporting increased morbidity following violence. The cross-sectional design of most studies examining associated impairment precludes conclusions about the causal role of IPV in these conditions, but the few published longitudinal studies show the onset or worsening of depression, PTSD, and substance abuse *after* exposure to IPV.

Pregnant women deserve special mention because IPV can threaten the health of both mother and fetus. Injury patterns during pregnancy are more likely to be central, including blunt trauma to the head, torso, abdomen, breasts, and genitalia. Abuse directed to the abdomen may lead to poor pregnancy outcomes and perinatal death. Although the evidence regarding a direct association between IPV in pregnancy and low birthweight has been conflicting, the increased risk for preterm birth as well as other factors such as psychosocial stress may play a role in adverse outcomes for infants, but more investigation is required.

Although beyond the scope of this chapter, there is increasing recognition that children's exposure to IPV shows a significant association with children's internalizing and externalizing problems, including trauma symptoms, developmental delay, educational problems, and long-term mental health conditions.

Identification

Screening for IPV can be performed by interview or with computer assistance,[1] but there is insufficient evidence for a policy of universal IPV screening of women presenting to health care settings. For example, a multisite randomized trial that evaluated the effectiveness of screening and communication of a positive result to clinicians in health care settings compared with no screening concluded that the benefits were too small to justify screening.[2] However, it is important to be alert to the signs and symptoms associated with IPV, including those associated with the broad range of physical and mental health conditions referred to previously. Risk indicators that point to a higher likelihood of IPV include symptoms of depression, somatization and PTSD in the female patient, and a history of alcohol or drug abuse and unemployment in the male partner (or ex-partner). It is important when asking about exposure to IPV, to do so privately, with no one else present, including a child (beyond infancy) or partner; if the inquiry or response is overheard, it could put the patient at risk for further IPV. A recent meta-analysis of qualitative studies of women's expectations and experiences reported that when the topic of IPV is raised, patients want questioning that is nonjudgmental, compassionate, and caring. Women want to be asked about IPV with confidentiality assured, but do not want to be pressured to disclose. In some jurisdictions, however, disclosure of IPV when a patient has children in the home can lead to mandatory reporting to child protection services. It is important that patients be advised about the limits of confidentiality before being asked about IPV exposure.

Possible questions to ask if IPV is suspected include the following: (1) Sometimes partner or ex-partners use physical force. Has this ever happened to you? (2) Have you felt humiliated or emotionally harmed by your partner or ex-partner? (3) Are you now or have you ever been afraid of your partner or ex-partner? (4) Have you ever been physically threatened or hurt by your partner or ex-partner? (5) Have you been forced to have any kind of sexual activity by your partner or ex-partner? (6) Has your partner or ex-partner ever tried to control your behavior; for example, control where you go or whom you see?

The initial clinical response when IPV is identified should include validation of the experience (e.g., everyone deserves to feel safe at home); affirmation that violence is unacceptable; and expression of support. The clinician needs to acknowledge the complexity of IPV and respect the patient's individual concerns and decisions. The assessment should include an evaluation of safety; the patient should be asked if it is safe for her (or him or any children) to return home. The following are examples of safety considerations: (1) Has the frequency or severity of the violence increased? (2) Is the partner or ex-partner obsessed with the patient? (3) How safe does she (he) feel? (4) Does the partner or ex-partner have a weapon or access to one? (5) Has she (he) been threatened with a weapon? Although a general discussion of gun violence is beyond the scope of this section, having firearms in the home is associated with an increased risk for homicide associated with IPV. Another predictor of domestic homicide is threats of deadly violence.

TREATMENT · Rx

The initial response of clinicians to the disclosure of IPV by female patients, whether the disclosure is spontaneous or the result of clinical inquiry, routine inquiry, or screening, is crucial in gaining trust and is the basis of further management. IPV is a highly stigmatized condition, akin to sexually transmitted infection or substance abuse, with the added dimension of risk for further harm from breach of confidentiality. A meta-analysis of 25 qualitative studies of women's expectations and experiences (847 informants) reported consistent messages about how clinicians can respond appropriately to disclosure. *Before disclosure or questioning*, they should understand the problem, including knowing about the available community services and appropriate referral systems; ensure that the clinical environment is supportive, welcoming, and nonthreatening; place brochures and posters in the clinical setting; try to ensure continuity of care; assure abused women about matters of privacy, safety, and confidentiality; be alert to the signs of abuse and raise the matter when indicated; use verbal and nonverbal communication skills to develop trust; and be compassionate, supportive, and respectful toward abused women. *When the topic of IPV is raised*, they should be nonjudgmental, compassionate, and caring when questioning about abuse; be confident and comfortable asking about domestic violence; not pressure women to disclose abuse because simply raising the topic may be helpful to women; ask about abuse over the course of several interviews because a woman may disclose abuse at a later date; ensure that the environment is private and confidential; and provide time. *Immediate response to disclosure* should be nonjudgmental, with compassion, support, belief of experiences; acknowledge the complexity of the problem and respect the woman's unique concerns and decisions; put the needs identified by the woman first and help to ensure that social and psychological needs are met; take time to listen, provide information, and offer referrals to specialist help; validate her experiences, challenge assumptions, and provide encouragement; and respond to any concerns about safety. *Response in later interactions* should be patient and supportive, allowing her to progress at her own therapeutic pace; understand the chronicity of the problem and provide follow-up and continued support; respect the woman's wishes and not pressure her into making any decisions; be nonjudgmental if a woman does not follow up with referrals immediately; give abused women an opportunity to disclose abuse at a later date.

Beyond their initial response and managing the medical sequelae of abuse, most generalists have neither the expertise nor the capacity to meet the specific needs of women experiencing IPV, which include legal, financial, housing, and safety needs. A key step, particularly in the context of current or recent violence, is an offer of referral to some sort of specialist support. Two main types of services have been evaluated: advocacy programs and psychological interventions (individual or group based). Generally, advocates engage with individual clients who are being abused, aiming to empower them and linking them to community services. Core activities of advocacy include provision of legal, housing, and financial advice, facilitating access to and use of community resources, such as refuges (shelters, safe houses), emergency housing, and provision of safety planning advice. Advocates can also provide ongoing support and informal counseling. A Cochrane review of 10 randomized controlled trials (1527 participants) of domestic violence advocacy concluded that there was equivocal evidence that advocacy for women recruited in domestic violence shelters (refuges) had a beneficial effect on their physical and psychosocial well-being and were unable to draw any conclusions for women receiving advocacy in or referred from health care settings.**3** A broader systematic review that included all controlled studies of domestic violence advocacy concluded that most showed a reduction in abuse, increased social support, and improved quality of life as well as increased use of safety behaviors and accessing of community resources. Only two of the studies had participants referred from health care settings. Clinicians should be able to refer patients to specialist IPV advocacy and are more likely to ask about abuse if they have the support of these services. If such services are not immediately available, shelters and refuges often provide these kinds of services for women both in residences and on an outreach basis.

A systematic review of controlled studies of psychological interventions for survivors of IPV identified 17 studies, 7 of individual and 10 of group interventions. There was a wide range of individual psychological interventions that demonstrated improvements in psychological outcomes, including depression, PTSD, and self-esteem. Two well-executed trials**4,5** of individual cognitive therapy–based interventions for women with PTSD who were no longer experiencing violence provided reasonable evidence for this intervention, but this cannot be extrapolated to women still in an abusive relationship. All the studies of group psychological interventions showed improvement in one or more psychological or mental health outcomes, but with the exception of one study, they were poorly executed. Consequently, the effectiveness of this type of intervention remains uncertain, particularly for women who are still experiencing IPV.

Although the assessment and treatment of the abuser should be carried out by mental health professionals with expertise in this area, it can be helpful for general clinicians to have some awareness of the effects of treatment. The evidence for batterer treatment is mixed, with the better-designed studies generally indicating little or no benefit**6** or potential harm (i.e., increased recidivism). The evidence for couple therapy is mixed, with trial-level evidence indicating no benefit in a military sample. Most authors caution that these couple therapy programs are not safe for many abused women, particularly those experiencing "intimate terrorism." Furthermore, when abusers are enrolled in treatment programs, it is important that women are provided with concurrent advocacy and support. There is some evidence to suggest that permanent, but not temporary, civil protection orders may be effective in reducing future violence.

PREVENTION

From a public health perspective, primary prevention of IPV is desirable, although most of the available research focuses on the health care response to the survivors of IPV, both while a woman is still exposed to abuse (secondary prevention) and when she is experiencing the long-term health problems associated with IPV (tertiary prevention).

Efforts aimed at primary prevention of IPV through educational programs have focused on changes in attitude and knowledge rather than actual reduction in IPV. In one study of adolescent dating violence, considered a precursor to IPV in adulthood, an interactive curriculum for grade 9 students that included information about dating violence and healthy relationships was associated with a statistically significant reduction in self-reported physical dating violence, but the differences were small (9.8% in control versus 7.4% in experimental group).**7**

There is no clinical trial evidence for the effectiveness of interventions provided in general medical settings with the aim of secondary prevention. However, an advocacy and empowerment program in antenatal clinics reduced psychological and minor physical violence,**8** and a program for pregnant African American women based on individual counseling sessions reduced violence and improved pregnancy outcomes.**9** Outside of health care settings, intensive advocacy (12 hours or more duration) may reduce physical abuse among women leaving shelters or refuges after 12 to 24 months of follow-up, but not for shorter or longer follow-up.**10**

PROGNOSIS

The prognosis of IPV with and without intervention is uncertain. Trials of interventions have small samples and short follow-up, and most have substantial attrition of participants. As far as the "natural history" of the condition is concerned, cohort studies are rare, and cross-sectional studies are potentially misleading. In a 3-year follow-up of participants who received an advocacy intervention after leaving a shelter, 36% had been assaulted by their original partner or a new partner in the 6 months before the interview. The difference in re-victimization at 2 years between intervention and control arms did not persist, but there was still a significant difference in quality of life and social support among women receiving advocacy. In a U.S. cohort study, 44% of participants were still being abused after 3½ years.

1. Ahmad F, Hogg-Johnson S, Stewart DE, et al. Computer-assisted screening for intimate partner violence and control: a randomized trial. *Ann Intern Med.* 2009;151:93-102.
2. MacMillan HL, Wathen CN, Jamieson E, et al. Screening for intimate partner violence in health care settings: a randomized trial. *JAMA.* 2009;302:493-501.
3. Ramsay J, Carter Y, Davidson L, et al. Advocacy interventions to reduce or eliminate violence and promote the physical and psychosocial well-being of women who experience intimate partner abuse. *Cochrane Database Syst Rev.* 2009;3:CD005043.
4. Kubany ES, Hill EE, Owens JA. Cognitive trauma therapy for battered women with PTSD: preliminary findings. *J Trauma Stress.* 2003;16:81-91.
5. Kubany ES, Hill EE, Owens JA, et al. Cognitive trauma therapy for battered women with PTSD (CTT-BW). *J Consult Clin Psychol.* 2004;72:3-18.
6. Babcock JC, Green CE, Robie C. Does batterers' treatment work? A meta-analytic review of domestic violence treatment. *Clin Psychol Rev.* 2004;23:1023-1053.
7. Wolfe DA, Crooks C, Jaffe P, et al. A school-based program to prevent adolescent dating violence: a cluster randomized trial. *Arch Pediatr Adolesc Med.* 2009;163:692-699.
8. Tiwari A, Leung WC, Leung TW, et al. A randomised controlled trial of empowerment training for Chinese abused pregnant women in Hong Kong. *Br J Obstet Gynaecol.* 2005;112:1249-1256.
9. Kiely M, El-Mohandes AA, El-Khorazaty MN, et al. An integrated intervention to reduce intimate partner violence in pregnancy: a randomized controlled trial. *Obstet Gynecol.* 2010;115:(2 pt 1)273-283.

10. Bybee D, Sullivan CM. Predicting re-victimization of battered women 3 years after exiting a shelter program. *Am J Community Psychol.* 2005;36:85-96.

SUGGESTED READINGS

Bhandari M, Sprague S, Dosanjh S, et al. The prevalence of intimate partner violence across orthopaedic fracture clinics in Ontario. *J Bone Joint Surg Am.* 2011;93:132-141. *The overall prevalence of intimate partner violence in the past year was 32%, including 3% whose fracture was directly related to physical abuse.*

Feder G, Ramsay J, Dunne D, et al. How far does screening women for domestic (partner) violence in different health-care settings meet criteria for a screening programme? Systematic reviews of nine UK National Screening Committee criteria. *Health Technol Assess.* 2009;13:iii-iv, xi-xiii, 1-113, 137-347. *Review.*

Hewitt LN, Bhavsar P, Phelan HA. The secrets women keep: intimate partner violence screening in the female trauma patient. *J Trauma.* 2011;70:320-323. *About 11% of female trauma patients report IPV.*

Roberts AL, McLaughlin KA, Conron KJ, et al. Adulthood stressors, history of childhood adversity, and risk of perpetration of intimate partner violence. *Am J Prev Med.* 2011;40:128-138. *Individuals with recent stressors and histories of childhood adversity are at particularly higher risk.*

Vives-Cases C, Ruiz-Cantero MT, Escribà-Agüir V, et al. The effect of intimate partner violence and other forms of violence against women on health. *J Public Health (Oxf).* 2011;33:15-21. *Victims of abuse had higher rates of neck and back pain, mental health problems, and coronary disease.*

Wu V, Huff H, Bhandari M. Pattern of physical injury associated with intimate partner violence in women presenting to the emergency department: a systematic review and meta-analysis. *Trauma Violence Abuse.* 2010;11:71-82. *Unwitnessed head, neck, and facial injuries suggest IPV, whereas extremity injuries are less likely to be the consequence of IPV.*

XX

DISEASES OF BONE AND MINERAL METABOLISM

MINERAL AND BONE HOMEOSTASIS

MURRAY J. FAVUS

HOMEOSTATIC SYSTEMS FOR CALCIUM, MAGNESIUM, AND PHOSPHATE

Metabolic bone diseases and mineral disorders may arise from excesses or deficiencies of the calciotropic hormones, vitamin D and its metabolites, and parathyroid hormone (PTH), or of the steroid or peptide hormones that have direct actions on bone (estrogens, androgens, glucocorticoids, thyroid hormone, insulin-like growth factor-I [IGF-I]), and excessive or deficient intake of the key minerals that form the bone mineral phase (calcium, magnesium, and phosphorus). Genetic or acquired defects in osteoblast or osteoclast function, bone matrix synthesis, mineralization, bone turnover, or repair may also cause metabolic bone diseases. Maintenance of Ca, Mg, and P (biologic forms of P are mostly in the form of inorganic phosphate, and P is expressed as PO_4) homeostasis is achieved through a coordinated trafficking of the ions across intestine and kidney to ensure delivery of sufficient amounts to support mineralization of the bone matrix. Disorders that impair intestine, kidney, parathyroid, or bone may disturb homeostasis and may cause bone loss and fractures. Measurements of blood levels of PTH, the vitamin D metabolites 25-hydroxyvitamin D [25(OH)-D], and 1,25-dihydroxyvitamin D_3 [$1,25(OH)_2D_3$], other key steroid and peptide hormones, biomarkers of bone turnover, and the blood and urine levels of Ca, Mg, and PO_4 are critical for accurate diagnosis. Mineral levels in blood and urine permit inferences about mineral balance, intestinal absorption, renal handling, and bone mineralization and resorption. This chapter reviews the homeostatic systems for Ca, Mg, and PO_4. Bone cellular functions and turnover and matrix composition are discussed in Chapter 251. Details of parathyroid gland function and regulation of PTH secretion are discussed in Chapter 253.

Total Body Divalent Elements

Calcium

In a healthy 70-kg man, the total body Ca content is 25 mmol (mg/40 = mmol), of which 99% exists in the mineral phase of bone as the hydroxyapatite [$Ca_{10}(PO_4)_6(OH)_2$] crystal. The molar ratio of Ca to P in $Ca_{10}(PO_4)_6(OH)_2$ is approximately 2:1, so as bone is resorbed, Ca and P ions are released into the extracellular fluid (ECF) at a ratio of 2:1. The serum total Ca concentration is 10^{-3} mol/L. Ca is present in the freely ionized state (48%) or protein bound (46%) largely to albumin. Clinical laboratories measure total serum Ca. The blood ionized Ca fraction is the most informative measurement because the ionized Ca fraction is readily exchangeable with pools of Ca in bone, blood, and intracellular sites. Errors in drawing and processing blood samples may compromise the accuracy of ionized Ca; therefore, automated measurements of total Ca are more reliable if the albumin level is not reduced and blood pH is normal.

Magnesium

The average adult body contains 1.0 mol of Mg, of which 54% is located within the skeleton and 45% is intracellular in soft tissues. Mg is not consistently incorporated into the $Ca_{10}(PO_4)_6(OH)_2$ crystal structure of bone. Mg is the most abundant intracellular divalent cation (cytosolic concentration 5×10^{-4} M). Blood ionic Mg is the fraction that most closely correlates with Mg-dependent biologic actions. Serum total and ionic Mg levels are not accurate estimates of Mg concentrations in the intracellular, soft tissue, or total body spaces.

Phosphate

P exists in tissues and blood primarily as PO_4. In bone, PO_4 is a major constituent of the $Ca_{10}(PO_4)_6(OH)_2$ crystal structure and accounts for 85% of total body PO_4. The soft tissue contains 15% of total body PO_4. Serum PO_4 levels fluctuate depending on age, sex, dietary intake, and growth rate. Serum levels of PTH, $1,25(OH)_2D_3$, growth hormone, IGF-I, and phosphotonins, which include fibroblast growth factor-23 (FGF-23), control serum PO_4 levels primarily by regulating the efficiency of renal proximal tubule

reabsorption of filtered PO_4, $1,25(OH)_2D_3$ increases serum PO_4 through stimulation of intestinal PO_4 absorption, and PTH and $1,25(OH)_2D_3$ release bone PO_4 through stimulation of bone resorption.

Normal serum PO_4 contributes to the maintenance of the Ca × PO_4 ion product, which, through physicochemical forces, drives bone mineralization. Low serum PO_4 lowers the Ca × PO_4 ion product and may thus impair mineralization. A high serum and ECF Ca × PO_4 product may result in extraskeletal soft tissue calcification.

Maintenance of Blood Levels

Calcium

Ca homeostasis has two goals: (1) sufficient delivery of Ca to support skeletal mineralization; and (2) maintenance of blood ionized Ca (Ca^{2+}) within a narrow normal range. A decline in blood Ca^{2+} is defended against by the actions of PTH (Chapter 253). $1,25(OH)_2D_3$ increases serum PO_4 levels by stimulating both intestinal PO_4 absorption and bone resorption with mineral dissolution that releases bone Ca and PO_4. A large PO_4 load could increase blood PO_4 and lower Ca^{2+}, but PTH decreases renal proximal tubule PO_4 reabsorption and dissipates the PO_4 load by increased urinary excretion.

Magnesium

Mg blood levels are influenced by the influx and efflux of Mg across intestine, bone, and kidney with the major influence being the regulation of renal proximal tubular Mg reabsorption. Like Ca^{2+}, Mg may downregulate PTH secretion but is less potent than Ca^{2+}. Serum Mg levels are regulated by renal proximal tubular reabsorption.

Phosphate

Serum PO_4 levels decline rapidly during periods of low dietary PO_4 intake, but proximal tubular reabsorption becomes more efficient and thereby lowers urine PO_4 losses to 1 to 2% of the filtered load within 2 to 4 days of ingesting a diet low in PO_4.

Mineral Intake and Intestinal Absorption

Calcium

Dietary Ca is incompletely absorbed with an efficiency of absorption between 25 and 60%. The range reflects the influence of age, habitual Ca intake, skeletal requirements, vitamin D status, the state of the homeostatic system, and the bioavailability of Ca contained in foods. Fractional Ca absorption is positively correlated with circulating $1,25(OH)_2D_3$ levels. Conditions of increased Ca requirements, such as during growth, pregnancy, and lactation, or when dietary Ca intake is low, stimulate its intestinal adaptive increase though increased renal $1,25(OH)_2D_3$ production. The intestinal adaptation is lost with aging, and the practice of increasing dietary Ca or using Ca supplements in postmenopausal women and in older men is an attempt to compensate for this age-related decline. Negative Ca balance (urine Ca + fecal Ca > net intestinal Ca absorption) occurs as Ca net absorption falls to less than 5.0 mmol/day. Fecal Ca is the sum of unabsorbed dietary Ca, Ca in secreted pancreatic and biliary juices, and mucosal secretions. Fecal Ca losses are between 2.5 and 5.0 mmol/day and are not regulated by Ca^{2+}, PTH, or $1,25(OH)_2D_3$.

Sites and Mechanisms of Absorption

The large surface areas of duodenum and jejunum are responsible for 90% of Ca absorbed. The physiologic adaptation to low Ca intake increases fractional Ca absorption from 25 to 45% to 55 to 70%. The increases are largely in the duodenum and ileum.

There are two absorptive mechanisms: (1) cell-mediated, active transport that dominates absorption at low luminal Ca concentrations; and (2) a passive, diffusional absorption driven by transepithelial electrochemical gradients that dominates at normal and high luminal Ca concentrations (>1.0 mmol/L) when serum $1,25(OH)_2D_3$ levels are low. Intestinal epithelial transcellular Ca transport is stimulated by high ambient $1,25(OH)_2D_3$ levels and by upregulation of the vitamin D receptor, which in turn mediates expression of vitamin D–dependent genes encoded for proteins that are required for Ca active transport (e.g., the brush border Ca transport protein TRPV6). Once within the cell, Ca is bound to the high-affinity Ca-binding protein, calbindin.

Phosphate

PO_4 absorption increases linearly with dietary PO_4 intake. At normal to high intake, absorption occurs by passive diffusion and is driven by the luminal

PO$_4$ concentration. During low PO$_4$ intake, PO$_4$ absorption largely occurs through an active, cell-mediated transport process that is stimulated by 1,25(OH)$_2$D$_3$. During adequate intake (25 to 60 mmol/day), PO$_4$ absorption is highly efficient, with 60 to 80% of dietary PO$_4$ absorbed. Transcellular PO$_4$ transport begins with influx across the brush border by overcoming the electrochemical gradients through either an energy-dependent transport process or a secondary active transport process coupled to the influx of a cation such as Na. 1,25(OH)$_2$D$_3$ stimulates net PO$_4$ absorption by increasing saturable brush border PO$_4$ uptake. The saturable active transport mechanism is present primarily in the proximal duodenum and jejunum.

Magnesium

Mg is abundant in highly cellular foods. During usual Mg intake of 7 to 30 mmol (mg/24 = mmol)/day, fractional Mg absorption averages 35 to 40%, and net intestinal Mg absorption increases in direct relation to dietary Mg. 1,25(OH)$_2$D$_3$ does not stimulate Mg absorption, and serum 1,25(OH)$_2$D$_3$ and net Mg absorption do not co-vary. Dietary PO$_4$ and other dietary anionic constituents may form nonabsorbable complexes with luminal Mg and reduce Mg absorption.

Renal Handling and Urinary Excretion

The fine tuning adjustments of Ca, Mg, and PO$_4$ balances occur at the level of the kidney, where filtered loads and tubular reabsorptions are highly regulated under changing body mineral requirements and wide variations in intakes and net absorptions.

Calcium

Approximately 98% of Ca in the glomerular ultrafiltrate undergoes tubular reabsorption that permits precise regulation of serum Ca^{2+}. Ultrafilterable Ca contains serum complexed and ionized Ca fractions and undergoes complete filtration when Ca concentration is 1.5 mmol/L. The amount of Ca filtered each day, more than 270 mmol, is far in excess of the Ca content contained in the ECF and exceeds net intestinal Ca absorption. Therefore, 98% of the filtered Ca must be reabsorbed to maintain neutral Ca balance. Seventy percent of filtered Ca is reabsorbed in the proximal tubule. Another 20% is reabsorbed in the thick ascending limb of the loop of Henle (TALH). The collecting duct is the final site of Ca reabsorption (5%). The urine contains only 2% of the filtered Ca load.

Volume expansion increases and volume contraction decreases urine Ca and Na excretion, respectively. Hypercalcemia decreases glomerular filtration rate (GFR) and proximal tubule, TALH, and distal convoluted tubule Ca reabsorption, resulting in a greater urinary excretion of Ca than Na. In the TALH, Ca sensing receptor (CaR) activation by hypercalcemia decreases Ca reabsorption; Ca may also alter paracellin-1-regulated Ca and Mg permeability with decreased reabsorption of both ions. PTH is also the principal regulator of Ca reabsorption by reducing GFR and stimulating tubule reabsorption. Acute and chronic metabolic acidosis increases and alkalosis decreases urine Ca excretion.

Thiazide diuretics (hydrochlorothiazide, chlorthalidone), indapamide, and amiloride increase urine Na excretion and decrease urine Ca through an increase in distal tubule Ca reabsorption. Loop diuretics increase urine Ca and Na excretion by inhibiting the Na-K-2Cl transporter in the TALH. Hypercalciuria continues as long as urinary Na losses are replaced.

Magnesium

Urine Mg averages 24 mmol/day, indicating that approximately 95% of Mg filtered in the glomerulus is reabsorbed. The proximal tubule reabsorbs only 15% of the Mg ultrafiltrate. Seventy percent of Mg is reabsorbed in the cortical TALH, and 10% of filtered Mg is reabsorbed in the distal convoluted tubule. High serum Mg may decrease Mg reabsorption.

Urine Mg reabsorption is highly regulated by ECF volume expansion and high serum Mg, which increase urine Mg excretion. Hypomagnesemia increases TALH Mg reabsorption. Hypercalcemia decreases Mg reabsorption in the proximal tubule and TALH. Loop diuretics markedly increase urine Mg excretion.

Phosphate

Ultrafilterable PO$_4$ represents 85% of total serum PO$_4$, and 12.5% of the filtrate appears in the final urine. Eighty-five percent of PO$_4$ reabsorption occurs in the proximal tubule through an Na-PO$_4$ cotransporter, which reabsorbs PO$_4$ against the brush border electrochemical PO$_4$ gradients. Three genes encode for related Na gradient-dependent PO$_4$ transporters

(Npt1-Npt3), with the apical brush border membrane Npt2 accounting for 85% of proximal tubule PO$_4$ reabsorption. The *Npt2* gene is regulated by FGF-23.

Mineral Balance and Adaptation to Changing Requirements

Mineral balance (retention or loss) is maintained by the calciotropic hormones PTH and 1,25(OH)$_2$D$_3$. Insufficient dietary mineral supply stimulates an adaptation of the homeostatic systems through hormonal changes to maintain external balance (balance = net absorption − [fecal excretion + urine excretion]). Mineral balance becomes positive (intake and retention exceed urinary and intestinal losses) during rapid skeletal growth in childhood and adolescence and during pregnancy and lactation. Negative balance (gastrointestinal or urinary losses, or both, exceed intake and retention) may occur during high rates of bone remodeling, as seen during estrogen deficiency, aging, and accompanying diseases such as hyperthyroidism and primary hyperparathyroidism. PTH and 1,25(OH) increase intestinal Ca and PO$_4$ absorption and regulate renal tubule Ca, PO$_4$, and Mg reabsorption. The Ca homeostatic system maintains blood ionized Ca within the normal range despite wide variations in dietary Ca intake and changing rates of bone mineralization.

SUGGESTED READINGS

Confavreux CB. Bone: from a reservoir of minerals to a regulator of energy metabolism. *Kidney Int.* 2011;121:S14-S19. *Review of how energy metabolism affects osteoblasts through the central control of bone mass involving leptin, serotoninergic neurons, the hypothalamus, and the sympathetic nervous system.*

Ferron M, Wei J, Yoshizawa T, et al. Insulin signaling in osteoblasts integrates bone remodeling and energy metabolism. *Cell.* 2010;142:296-308. *Insulin signals in osteoblasts activate a hormone, osteocalcin, that promotes glucose metabolism.*

Karsenty G, Oury F. The central regulation of bone mass, the first link between bone remodeling and energy metabolism. *J Clin Endocrinol Metab.* 2010;95:4795-4801. *Review of recent findings on the link of bone metabolism with energy metabolism.*

O'Toole JF. Disorders of calcium metabolism. *Nephron Physiol.* 2011;118:22-27. *Review of the molecules that regulate calcium homeostasis via the intestine, kidney, and bone.*

251

OSTEOPOROSIS

CLIFFORD ROSEN

DEFINITION

Osteoporosis is a disorder characterized by enhanced skeletal fragility as a result of reduced bone quantity and quality. The clinical symptoms of this disease may include back pain, height loss, and a history of fractures. Bone mineral density (BMD), which can be determined by several techniques, is often markedly reduced in osteoporotic patients with fractures. The World Health Organization (WHO) defines osteoporosis as a condition in which a BMD is less than −2.5 standard deviations (SD) below peak bone mass (i.e., a T-score measured as the units of SD below the normative mean of a 35-year-old woman). However, several large observational studies have shown that osteoporotic fractures can occur across a wide spectrum of BMDs. These events are likely related to altered bone quality, as a result of microarchitectural changes in the trabecular and cortical skeleton. Qualitative determinants of osteoporotic fractures include trabecular perforations, microcracks, mineralization defects, changes in bone size, and rapid bone turnover (Fig. 251-1). Unfortunately, most of these qualitative changes in the skeleton cannot be captured by clinical measurements, even though they strongly influence overall fracture risk. Recently, introduction of extreme high-resolution computed tomography (CT) and more refined quantitative CT measurements have allowed investigators to measure trabecular size, number, and shape accurately, although to date fracture prediction is not markedly enhanced with these new tools. Hence, although low BMD defines osteoporosis, this diagnosis should not be excluded in susceptible individuals, particularly those with a history of a low-impact fracture. Finally, although the WHO defined *osteopenia* as a condition with a T-score between −1.0 and −2.5, and therefore places a given individual at a greater risk for fracture, the clinical significance of this term remains nebulous. Introduction of the FRAX

FIGURE 251-1. Microcomputed tomography images of trabecular bone from the vertebrae of an osteoporotic individual (*left*) and a healthy age-matched normal woman (*right*).

TABLE 251-1	FACTORS THAT MAY AFFECT PEAK BONE MASS

Gender
Race
Genetic factors
Gonadal steroids
Growth hormone
Timing of puberty
Calcium intake
Exercise

Internet tool, which weighs clinical risk factors with BMD of the hip, may provide greater insight into the long-term fracture risk in individuals with low bone mass. In sum, low BMD is a strong risk factor for subsequent fractures, but there is no threshold BMD above or below which fractures occur. Other risk factors, such as a previous fracture history, age greater than 65 years, a strong family history, and recent significant weight loss must be considered.

EPIDEMIOLOGY

By the age of 50 years, the lifetime risk of developing a fracture resulting from osteoporosis in a white woman is nearly 40%, similar to that for coronary heart disease; in men, the corresponding figure is 13%. In the United States, approximately 350,000 hip fractures, close to 1 million vertebral fractures, and 200,000 wrist fractures occur every year. In addition, other fragility-related fractures, particularly those of the pelvis and humerus, are significant causes of morbidity in elderly persons. The incidence of osteoporotic fractures increases markedly with age. In women, this increase is seen after the age of 45 years and is mainly the result of forearm fractures. After the age of 65 years, the incidence of hip fractures rises exponentially. In men, the incidence of fragility-related fractures increases after the age of 75 years, and in both sexes the hip is the most common fracture site after the age of 85 years. The incidence of vertebral fractures in both men and women is less well documented because many such patients are asymptomatic. Clinical vertebral fractures increase dramatically with age in men, whereas a more linear age-related increase is noted in women. This age-related increase in fracture prevalence is independent of the change in BMD and almost certainly relates to qualitative changes in trabecular and cortical bone. Hence, age alone is an independent risk factor for fracture.

Marked geographic variations in the incidence of osteoporotic fractures are reported. This characteristic may partly be explained by racial differences in skeletal size; osteoporosis is most common in Asian and white populations and is less frequent in African and American blacks. In many parts of the world, evidence indicates that osteoporotic fractures have increased considerably, even allowing for aging of the population. However, a recent report in Canadian individuals demonstrated that in the past 10 years, there has been a decline in hip fractures. Notwithstanding, greater life expectancy alone is expected to increase the number of hip fractures over the next 50 years.

Ethnic and gender differences play a major role in the epidemiology of fractures. Men have higher bone density than women, and African Americans have significantly greater BMD during their adult life than whites, both in the cortical and trabecular compartments. These differences are related in part to the effects of body composition, including muscle strength, body fat distribution, and bone size. Hence, significantly fewer fractures occur in African Americans than in Asians or whites, particularly whites of European descent. However, the role of fat mass relative to BMD has recently undergone reexamination. Clearly, low body mass index (<20) is associated with low BMD and a greater risk for fracture. This in part is due to lower peripheral conversion of testosterone to estrogen and less insulation during impact. On the other hand, the relationship of bone mass to increased fat mass (BMI > 30) is less clear-cut. Increased subcutaneous fat positively affects cortical bone area, but several recent reports suggest that visceral fat may have a negative impact on bone mass and may be associated with a higher fracture risk.

Although often considered protective, it is now established that obesity does not prevent fractures and in some circumstances may increase risk.

BIOLOGY
Bone Remodeling

Even though trauma is the principal cause of fracture, factors that alter the quality or quantity of bone predispose an individual to osteoporotic fractures. Thus, an understanding of bone remodeling is essential for determining how bone mass can be altered by heritable and environmental influences. Briefly, skeletal remodeling preserves serum calcium and bone strength in adults through *remodeling* or *basic multicellular units*. Bone remodeling begins with bone dissolution or resorption and ends with new bone formation, leaving no net change in bone mass. In adulthood, each remodeling unit is balanced—resorption equals formation—and lasts between 90 and 130 days. Remodeling preserves bone mass, ensures a ready source of calcium for bodily function, and maintains bone strength through changes in architecture. However, remodeling units can become imbalanced, and over several cycles, this scenario can result in significant bone loss. These imbalances are a result of greater bone resorption relative to bone formation and can be traced to changes in systemic hormones, environmental factors, and mechanical loading.

Peak Bone Mass

Acquisition of peak bone mass occurs between 12 and 15 years of age but is highly dependent on gender (i.e., girls reach peak earlier than boys) and type of bone (i.e., trabecular versus cortical). During this time, there is a rapid increase in bone mass as a result of growth and modeling of the skeleton, which favors formation over resorption. Pubertal surges of gonadal steroids and growth hormone are critical to propel this increase in bone mass with adolescence. Longitudinal studies suggest that several factors regulate peak bone density, including dietary intake of specific nutrients, physical activity, and most importantly, genetic determinants (Table 251-1). The latter view was established in several ways in both humans and animal models. Daughters of mothers with severe osteoporosis have low BMD. Monozygotic twins have much greater concordance in bone mass than dizygotic pairs, and inbred strains of mice differ significantly in peak BMD. However, despite intense efforts over the past decade to identify the heritable determinants of bone mass, minimal progress has been made. Polymorphic differences in the most promising candidate genes, including the vitamin D and estrogen receptors, insulin-like growth factor-I (IGF-I), parathyroid hormone (PTH), collagen A1a, Lrp5, and others are associated with bone mass. But these genetic determinants individually contribute only 1 to 3% to the variance in BMD. It is likely, although not yet proved, that nucleotide polymorphisms in multiple genes contribute more to bone mass than changes in single genes.

Bone Formation

Investigators have uncovered two new pathways in the osteoblast that are genetically regulated and affect the rate of bone formation: (1) the Wnt/Lrp5/β-catenin signaling system, and (2) the lipoxygenase pathways. In the former, activating mutations of the low-density lipoprotein receptor–related protein 5 (LRP5) leads to high bone mass, whereas inactivating mutations lead to the osteoporosis pseudoganglioma syndrome, a condition related to low bone mass in children. The canonical LRP5 signaling pathway is stimulated by Wnt ligands and leads directly to greater osteoblast proliferation and differentiation. In the latter system, two critical enzymes determine when and how stromal cells enter into either the fat or bone lineage: *12,15-lipoxygenase* (*12 LO* or *Alox 12,15*) produces prostaglandins and other endogenous ligands that bind to the nuclear receptor peroxisome proliferator activator receptor-γ (PPARG) and stimulate adipocyte differentiation; *5'LO*, or *Alox 5*, generates leukotrienes that can also activate PPARG through generation of prostaglandin J2. Polymorphisms in these two genes in mice and humans have been associated with differences in peak bone mass. Twin studies have shown that the genetic regulation of peak bone mass can be modified by both hormonal and environmental factors. In particular, adequate and timely secretion of sex steroids, balanced nutrient intake, and physical activity can optimize peak BMD even in people with a genetic predisposition to low bone mass. It is likely that disturbances in peak bone acquisition contribute to osteoporosis later in life. For example, men with constitutionally delayed puberty have lower BMD in their 30s and 40s than do men who went through puberty at the appropriate age. Women with anorexia nervosa during their teen years have significantly lower BMD at the time of menopause than do healthy adolescents who do not develop amenorrhea. Women with delayed menarche also have lower BMD in adulthood than do women with a normal timing of menses onset. One area of controversy relates to whether childhood fractures are a sign of subsequent osteoporosis. At least two studies have shown that adolescent radial fractures are associated with lower area bone density and reduced cortical bone size compared with findings in children who do not have fractures. These determinants could predispose children to fractures with relatively low impact and may provide some indication of future risk, although more studies are needed. Interestingly, obesity in children is a risk factor for future radial fractures.

PATHOBIOLOGY

Adult BMD is determined both by the acquisition of peak bone mass during adolescence and by the degree of subsequent bone loss over a lifetime (Fig. 251-2). These two processes are regulated at the level of the bone remodeling unit, which is composed of bone-forming osteoblasts, bone-resorbing osteoclasts, and deeply imbedded cortical osteocytes capable of sensing gravitational forces. The remodeling sequence is tightly orchestrated at several levels by the interaction of genetic, environmental, and hormonal factors (Chapter 250). Even small changes in bone formation or bone resorption can result in bone loss or impairment in the capacity to acquire peak bone mass during adolescence. Although an osteoporotic fracture inevitably occurs as a result of trauma—major or minor—to a bone with reduced bone quantity or quality, a strong inverse relationship exists between BMD and fractures. Hence, changes in remodeling that lead to lower bone mass are major factors in determining the overall risk for osteoporosis.

Bone loss occurs when the bone remodeling unit is uncoupled such that bone resorption exceeds formation. The timing of bone loss is a critical determinant of future fracture risk. For example, rapid bone loss in elderly persons is rarely recouped and leaves these individuals at very high risk for fracture independent of BMD. Conversely, accelerated bone turnover over a short period (such as that related to transient glucocorticoid excess in childhood or adolescence) may be reversible. Once the inciting event (i.e., pituitary tumor) has been removed or the treatments have stopped, fracture risk returns to baseline, and BMD can be restored. However, bone loss can also be incessant, particularly in postmenopausal women, in whom estrogen

deprivation results in markedly increased osteoclastic activity and high-turnover remodeling. Although the basic multicellular unit is tightly coupled, rapid bone resorption over a prolonged period results in an imbalance because formation cannot be maintained at the same accelerated rate as resorption. During the first few years of menopause (and possibly during the latter phases of premenopause), as estrogen levels decline, trabecular bone loss occurs first. This is followed by cortical thinning. Both conditions are a result of a mismatch between resorption and formation. Surprisingly, during adult bone loss, periosteal expansion occurs in an attempt to preserve bone strength.

In menopause, bone loss averages about 1% per year, but in a few women, loss of spine BMD can be as great as 5% per year. At present, it is impossible to identify those women prospectively. Moreover, premature menopause, chemotherapeutically induced ovarian dysfunction, and amenorrhea related to heavy exercise result in even higher rates of bone resorption that cannot be matched by any increase in bone formation. However, tremendous heterogeneity exists in the response to estrogen deprivation among postmenopausal women. A few women during their first few years of menopause may lose bone at a rate of 2 to 4% per year. Even among "fast losers," this decline slows over time. Estrogen replacement prevents postmenopausal bone loss even among fast losers, although the popularity of this type of prevention has waned in the years following publication of the Women's Health Initiative (WHI).

Bone Loss in Elderly Persons

Later in life, particularly in the eighth and ninth decades, bone loss can accelerate dramatically. Several potential mechanisms are responsible for this change. First and foremost, elderly individuals generally have reduced vitamin D and calcium intake, as well as less sun exposure. This, combined with a reduced capacity to generate pre-vitamin D in the skin, results in secondary hyperparathyroidism and enhanced bone resorption. Remarkably, more than 50% of women who are older than 70 years and who live in northern latitudes have insufficient or deficient levels of vitamin D (i.e., serum 25-hydroxyvitamin D < 20 ng/mL). Other factors also play a role in the accelerated bone turnover of senescence. Increasing levels of homocysteine may enhance bone resorption or may alter the nature of reactive oxygen species within the skeletal milieu. Inflammatory cytokines such as interleukin-6 (IL-6) and tumor necrosis factor (TNF) also increase with age and can stimulate bone turnover.

The uncoupling of the bone remodeling unit in an older person may be associated with a defect in bone formation because both osteoblast number and function decline with age. These changes may be related to low levels of circulating or skeletal IGF-I or to other trophic factors that either enhance osteoblast survival or stimulate stromal cell recruitment. Alterations in lineage allocation among stromal cells can lead to increased marrow adipogenesis at the expense of osteoblast differentiation. The process of fatty infiltration of the bone marrow, particularly in the vertebrae of older individuals, is due in part to an age-related increase in activation of PPARG, a nuclear receptor and transcription factor essential for adipocyte differentiation. Drugs may also enhance PPARG activation, and these include the thiazolidinediones (e.g., rosiglitazone and pioglitazone) and glucocorticoids. Interestingly, PPARG activation may also stimulate new osteoclast development resulting in a marked uncoupling between resorption and formation. Thus, as a result of impaired osteoblast function, the remodeling deficit becomes more pronounced, particularly in the setting of greater bone resorption. Irrespective of the cause of bone loss with aging, estrogen and other antiresorptive therapies are effective in inhibiting bone resorption and in resetting the bone remodeling units, so the two processes are now coupled.

Classification of Osteoporosis

Earlier work proposed two types of osteoporosis, based on age of onset: type I, or postmenopausal, osteoporosis, caused by estrogen deprivation around the time of menopause; and type II osteoporosis, related to high turnover from calcium and vitamin D insufficiency. However, it is clear that this type of classification is outdated and has little clinical purpose. Many younger postmenopausal women can have vitamin D deficiency, and elderly individuals may suffer just as much from bone loss as a result of progressive estrogen insufficiency as younger women. Similarly, even though wrist fractures are more common, as are vertebral fractures, in younger, healthy postmenopausal women, these fractures are very characteristic of any type of osteoporosis, and they represent skeletal failure related to impaired bone quantity or quality, or both, irrespective of age.

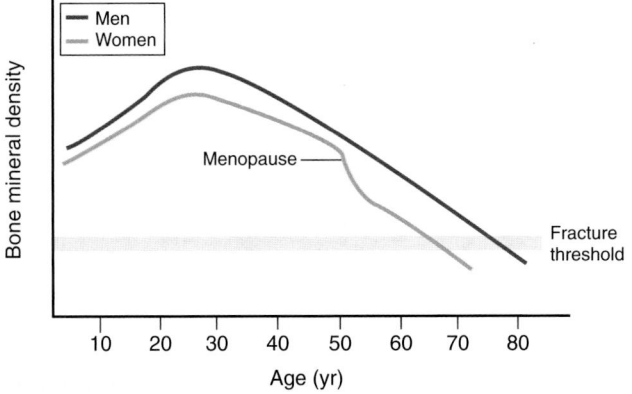

FIGURE 251-2. Cortical bone mineral density versus age in men and women. Women have lower peak cortical bone density than men and experience a period of rapid bone loss at menopause, thus reaching the fracture threshold (the level of bone density at which the risk of developing osteoporotic fractures begins to increase) earlier than men.

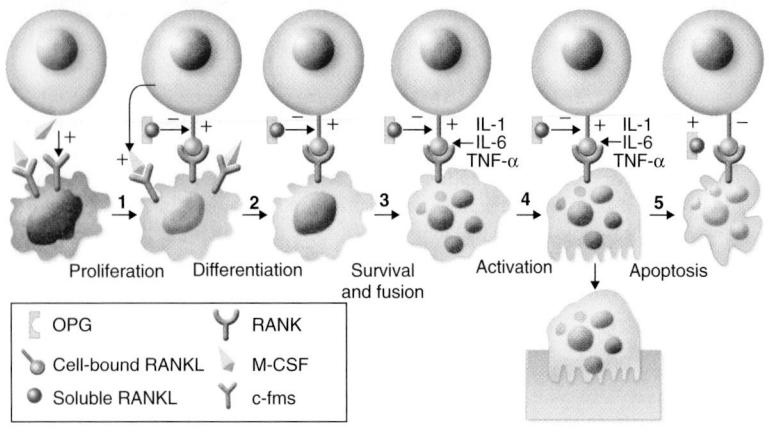

FIGURE 251-3. Regulation of osteoclast development by receptor activator of nuclear factor-κB ligand (RANKL), receptor activator of nuclear factor-κB (RANK), and osteoprotegerin (OPG). c-fms = receptor for M-CSF; IL = interleukin; M-CSF = macrophage colony-stimulating factor; TNF-α = tumor necrosis factor-α. (From Hofbaurer LC, Heufelder AE. The role of receptor activator of nuclear factor-κ ligand and osteoprotegerin in the pathogenesis and treatment of metabolic bone diseases. *J Clin Endocrinol Metab.* 2000;85:2355-2363.)

Molecular and Cellular Mechanisms of Normal Remodeling

To understand the pathophysiologic mechanisms of bone loss more fully, it is necessary to define the key molecular and cellular events that occur during normal adult remodeling. Mesenchymal stromal cells (MSCs), or osteoblast precursor cells, undergo a series of differentiation stages that culminate in a mature osteoblast capable of laying down matrix and secreting growth factors. These cells, as noted previously, are multipotent, and under the influence of various factors, they may become adipocytes, muscle cells, chondrocytes, or osteoblasts. The ultimate fate of the stromal cells is a critical determinant of normal remodeling. During MSC differentiation, stromal cells release a series of cytokines that target osteoclast progenitors, resulting in the differentiation of multinucleated cells from the macrophage lineage. Once these cells become osteoclasts, they have the capacity to cause bone resorption by secreting hydrogen ions and enzymes that dissolve the bone matrix. Within the matrix are several key trophic factors, activated by bone dissolution; as these enter the skeletal milieu, cells of the osteoblast lineage are pushed into differentiation. In this manner, bone resorption is coupled to bone formation.

Several cytokines, including IL-1, IL-6, TNF, receptor activator of nuclear factor-κB ligand (RANKL), and osteoprotegerin (OPG), a soluble decoy receptor for RANKL, are secreted by preosteoblasts during their differentiation. RANKL is expressed on the surface of the osteoblast precursors, and its receptor RANK is the receptor for RANKL on the surface of the osteoclast, a convenient match that actually permits cell-cell interaction (Fig. 251-3). Binding of RANKL to RANK in the presence of permissive levels of another cytokine, macrophage colony-stimulating factor, stimulates the differentiation of osteoclasts into mature bone resorbing cells. In contrast, OPG, a circulating protein also produced by stromal cells, can bind to RANKL and can prevent its occupation of RANK, thereby reducing osteoclastogenesis.

PATHOGENESIS

Cellular and Molecular Mechanisms of Bone Loss

Osteoporosis results from an imbalance in bone remodeling. Changes in bone turnover can be due to a number of factors that target both osteoblasts and osteoclasts and result in greater resorption than formation. For example, declining estrogen levels during menopause or after oophorectomy result in an upregulation of all the stromal cytokines, particularly RANKL. Conversely, OPG secretion is suppressed. This scenario results in greater osteoclastogenesis and accelerated bone resorption. Because bone formation is coupled to resorption, the entire remodeling unit is activated. Bone resorption is a rapid process, taking about 2 weeks for the osteoclasts to attach and resorb matrix. Formation is much more deliberate, meaning that with the release of soluble cytokines, an imbalance in remodeling immediately occurs, and this favors bone resorption. Eventually, this imbalance leads to increased breakdown of collagen and matrix and an inability to match this loss with increased formation. Estrogen administration can prevent bone loss by enhancing OPG production as well as by suppressing RANKL expression. Other systemic and local factors can cause imbalanced remodeling. High levels of PTH for long periods can stimulate RANKL expression and cause bone loss. Glucocorticoid excess from exogenous steroids or Cushing's disease also stimulates RANKL production, but in addition shifts stromal cell differentiation away from the osteoblast lineage and toward adipogenesis.

Immobilization suppresses bone formation and enhances bone resorption. Aging in general leads to a reduction in several osteoblastic trophic factors such as IGF-I, as well as increased PPARG activation, and these changes can impair the rate of new bone formation.

Secondary Causes of Bone Loss in the Adult

Although most cases of osteoporosis can be labeled idiopathic and result from the cellular and molecular processes that are related to estrogen deprivation and aging, it is important to exclude secondary causes, primarily because these disorders are sometimes reversible with resolution of the underlying disease (Table 251-2). Hypogonadism of any cause, in either men or women, is probably the most frequent secondary cause of osteoporosis, particularly in younger patients. Anorexia nervosa, hypothalamic amenorrhea, hyperprolactinemia, and exercise-induced amenorrhea lead to early and rapid bone loss that can result in subsequent osteoporotic fractures if these conditions are sustained over a prolonged period. In male patients, primary or secondary hypogonadism results in low peak bone mass and can cause significant bone loss during middle life. Hormonal disorders that interfere with the normal hypothalamic gonadal axis, such as hypercortisolemia, also lead to reduced bone mass. Glucocorticoid excess dampens gonadotropin-releasing hormone signaling, thereby lowering estrogen or androgen levels and enhancing bone resorption; these changes are accompanied by alterations in osteoblast recruitment and function, increased marrow adiposity, reduced IGF-I signaling, and impaired calcium absorption. As the remodeling unit is uncoupled, bone loss occurs rapidly, and fractures are a frequent component of this syndrome. Other endocrine disorders are associated with low bone mass or high bone turnover (see Table 251-2). These include severe hyperthyroidism, primary hyperparathyroidism, and growth hormone deficiency. In primary hyperparathyroidism, bone loss is principally confined to cortical bone sites and is reversible with surgical removal of the tumor.

Other systemic diseases can cause osteoporosis (see Table 251-2). Patients with hepatobiliary disorders often have osteoporosis or osteomalacia, or both, resulting from impaired absorption of vitamin D and secondary hyperparathyroidism. Gluten enteropathy is one of the most common heritable diseases, and patients frequently present in adult life with low bone mass (Chapter 252). These patients often have low 25-hydroxyvitamin D levels and markedly increased PTH concentrations with modest elevations in total alkaline phosphatase. The definitive diagnosis is made by small bowel biopsy, and tissue transglutaminase levels can be very helpful when screening individuals with low bone mass. Patients with systemic disorders such as lupus erythematosus (Chapter 274), scleroderma (Chapter 275), rheumatoid arthritis (Chapter 272), and mixed connective tissue disease may also present with low bone mass independent of whether they have been treated with glucocorticoids. This form of secondary osteoporosis most likely results from a combination of immobility, malabsorption, and the release of inflammatory cytokines both locally and systemically as well as the use of other medications that may be detrimental to the skeleton, such as heparin, ethanol, cyclosporine, tacrolimus, and anticonvulsant agents. Chronic alcohol ingestion (Chapter 32) may be particularly detrimental to the skeleton because it can suppress osteoblast function, increase stromal cell differentiation into adipocytes, and enhance bone resorption. Many patients who suffer from chronic alcoholism are hypogonadal (either primary or secondary) and frequently have low vitamin D levels. Male patients with hypercalciuria or

TABLE 251-2 SECONDARY CAUSES OF OSTEOPOROSIS

ENDOCRINE DISEASES

Female hypogonadism
    Hyperprolactinemia
    Hypothalamic amenorrhea
    Anorexia nervosa
    Premature and primary ovarian failure
Male hypogonadism
    Primary gonadal failure (e.g., Klinefelter's syndrome)
    Secondary gonadal failure (e.g., idiopathic hypogonadotropic hypogonadism)
    Delayed puberty
Hyperthyroidism
Hyperparathyroidism
Hypercortisolism
Growth hormone deficiency
Vitamin D deficiency
Idiopathic hypercalciuria
Diabetes mellitus

GASTROINTESTINAL DISEASES

Subtotal gastrectomy
Malabsorption syndromes
Chronic obstructive jaundice
Primary biliary cirrhosis and other cirrhoses
Alactasia

BONE MARROW DISORDERS

Multiple myeloma
Lymphoma
Leukemia
Hemolytic anemias
Systemic mastocytosis
Disseminated carcinoma

CONNECTIVE TISSUE DISEASES

Osteogenesis imperfecta
Ehlers-Danlos syndrome
Marfan syndrome
Homocystinuria

DRUGS

Alcohol
Heparin
Glucocorticoids
Thyroxine
Anticonvulsants
Gonadotropin-releasing hormone agonists
Cyclosporine
Tacrolimus
Chemotherapy
Selective serotonin reuptake inhibitors (?)
Thiazolidinediones
Proton pump inhibitors

MISCELLANEOUS CAUSES

Immobilization
Rheumatoid arthritis
Renal tubular acidosis

kidney stones are also at risk for low bone mass and osteoporotic fractures. The pathogenesis of this relationship is not entirely clear, but secondary hyperparathyroidism in patients with hypercalciuria leads to enhanced bone resorption and gradual bone loss. Finally, drug-induced bone loss is a major cause of secondary osteoporosis. Besides glucocorticoids, chronic heparin therapy, some anticonvulsants, the thiazolidinediones, and some second-generation antipsychotics can cause osteoporosis. Recently, use of second-generation selective serotonin reuptake inhibitors (SSRIs) and proton pump inhibitors has been linked to both bone loss and osteoporotic fractures in older women and men. If confirmed in prospective trials, these agents may become the most common cause of secondary osteoporosis.

Malignancy

Metastatic neoplasms to the skeleton can sometimes manifest as an osteoporotic fracture or as a lytic lesion of uncertain significance. Usually, these lesions are atypical in location (e.g., midshaft of long bones, or pelvis), and the underlying disease frequently is obvious. Less commonly confused with osteoporosis are osteoblastic lesions of vertebrae or long bones. However, primary hematopoietic and lymphoproliferative disorders are often insidious and can be associated with low bone mass and fractures. Multiple myeloma (Chapter 193) is the most common hematologic malignancy related to osteoporosis because patients with this disease often have diffuse osteopenia, occasionally with classic osteoporotic fractures of the spine or long bones. Unlike other metastatic processes to bone, multiple myeloma is associated with very high rates of bone resorption but no change or suppression in bone formation. This situation can lead to rapid bone loss. Plasma cells release cytokines, particularly TNF-α, IL-1, and IL-6, that stimulate osteoclastogenesis. Simultaneously, these cells produce Dickopf I and III, soluble factors that block the Wnt/LRP5/β-catenin canonical network. Hence patients have dramatic uncoupling of bone remodeling, rapid bone loss, and fractures. Debate is ongoing about the relationship of osteoporosis to monoclonal gammopathies of uncertain significance (MGUS), although osteopenia is often reported in these patients. Other secondary causes of osteoporosis are noted in Table 251-2.

CLINICAL MANIFESTATIONS

Although osteoporosis is often considered a silent disease, its presentation has changed dramatically in the past two decades. Previously, fractures of the vertebrae, with or without height loss, were the most frequent presenting complaints. Until recently, hip fractures in elderly patients, which can be a late manifestation of osteoporosis, were frequently considered traumatic but not metabolic. Similarly, wrist fractures in early postmenopausal women are a sentinel indication of underlying osteoporosis. They were treated in the past by orthopedic surgeons without regard for any underlying skeletal pathologic processes. However, these patterns began to change in the early 21st century, particularly with the availability of dual-energy x-ray absorptiometry (DXA), the method of choice for measuring BMD. Now, the most frequent presenting complaint to a provider regarding osteoporosis is a low BMD measurement, done either routinely or for screening purposes. Because bone mass is only one of several risk factors for osteoporosis, other clinical manifestations of this disease must be considered. Loss of more than 2 inches in height is a reasonable surrogate of previous vertebral fractures. A clinical history of wrist or ankle fractures is another indication of underlying osteoporosis and may be the first manifestation of the disease in younger postmenopausal women. Compression fracture of the spine with minimal stress is another presenting complaint of osteoporosis. Such fractures cause significant midlumbar and lower thoracic back pain that may radiate to the flanks or anteriorly. Sharp, knifelike back pain after an acute injury is disabling, frequently requires narcotics, and often subsides over a period of weeks to months unless a new fracture intervenes. Patients have an approximately 20% likelihood of a new vertebral fracture in the first year after a spinal fracture. In addition, some patients have chronic back pain as a result of one or more vertebral fractures. Low bone mass in and of itself does not result in back pain, and other diagnoses should be considered in that situation. Cervical lordosis and dorsal kyphosis are the classic manifestations of "dowager's hump" but are less frequently seen in young women. Hip fractures resulting in femoral neck, trochanteric, or cervical injuries generally occur following a fall. The direction and height of the fall are critical elements in determining the type of hip fracture, the ensuing surgery, and disability. Hip fractures can be extremely catabolic, both because of the trauma and because of the resultant major surgery. These factors, combined with underlying illnesses, enhance the mortality of hip fractures in older individuals to approximately 20% in the first year alone.

Osteoporosis can also be diagnosed by a radiologist or a primary care provider from plain radiographs, as shown in Figure 251-4. Most often, patients have an obvious loss of bone mass, resulting in the radiographic term *osteopenia*, although at that stage BMD by DXA is usually well below −2.5 SD. Radiographs of the spine can demonstrate kyphosis, osteopenia, and compression fractures in the thoracic or lumbar vertebrae. For the upper lumbar or lower thoracic areas that are the most vulnerable to injury, compression fractures can frequently be visualized. Collapse of either the anterior or posterior elements is often visible on lateral radiographs of the spine; anterior wedging or the so-called codfish deformity results from weakening of the subchondral plates and expansion of the intervertebral discs (see Fig. 251-4). CT scanning of the spine for other reasons will sometimes be able to detect fractures and can be used clinically to measure density. Magnetic resonance imaging (MRI) is now more frequently used as a diagnostic tool; it may demonstrate a compression fracture with or without marrow edema resulting in a bright signal on T1-weighted images. Technetium-99m bone scans are

FIGURE 251-4. Radiograph showing radiolucency, compression fractures, and kyphosis in the spine of a patient with osteoporosis.

very sensitive to fracture and can be used to detect stress fractures in the pelvis, femur, or tibia. However, because of its high sensitivity, this test is not a useful tool for diagnosis of osteoporosis. In fact, it is rare for the bone scan to be the initial clue to osteoporosis, and in the setting of a positive bone scan, alternative diagnoses, including malignant disease, should be considered.

DIAGNOSIS

A recent fragility-related fracture of the spine, hip, wrist, ankle, shoulder, or other appendicular sites in postmenopausal women or men should lead to a diagnosis of osteoporosis. However, secondary causes of this condition (as discussed earlier and listed in Table 251-2) should be excluded before therapy is initiated. Similarly, because the WHO has established that a BMD at any site lower than −2.5 SD from the young normal value meets the definition of osteoporosis, a diagnosis can be made from a densitometry report or measurement. However, this finding must be interpreted in relation to the patient's age, ethnicity, fracture history, family background, previous medications, timing of menopause, and other concomitant disorders. Based on the WHO criteria, most providers make the diagnosis of osteoporosis by measuring bone density with or without biochemical markers of bone turnover. Recently the introduction of the FRAX Internet tool by WHO has made long-term fracture risk prediction an important and easy tool for the patient and the provider.

Bone Densitometry

Several techniques are available for measuring areal BMD (i.e., two-dimensional measurements expressed as g/cm^2) in the axial and appendicular skeleton. Multiple prospective studies have convincingly shown that a low BMD at virtually any site (i.e., hip, spine, radius, total body, calcaneus) predicts subsequent osteoporotic fractures whether these are in the same area or elsewhere. In general, regardless of the technology, for every 1 SD below a young (i.e., 35-year-old) normal value (i.e., T-score), the risk for future osteoporotic fractures increases by nearly 50%. However, site-specific measurements, for example, spine BMD, usually predict spine fractures better than a hip BMD. Because of the inverse relationship between fracture risk and BMD, a very strong rationale exists for measuring bone mass at least once during the lifetime of every postmenopausal woman.

Dual-Energy X-Ray Absorptiometry Measurements of Bone Mineral Density

Techniques for measuring bone mass include the following: DXA of the spine, hip, radius, or total body; CT of the spine; ultrasound scanning of the calcaneus or wrist; finger DXA; and peripheral quantitative CT of the wrist or tibia. Other experimental techniques that are being tested for evaluating trabecular bone and bone quality include MRI of the calcaneus and radius, virtual MRI using computerized reconstructions of trabecular bone, and

"extreme CT" with high-resolution imaging of the radius. The most popular, least expensive, and most precise tool is DXA. Results from DXA measurements are traditionally expressed as either the T-score or the Z-score. The T-score is the number of SDs below or above which the patient's BMD differs from peak bone density of an individual of the same gender and ethnicity. The Z-score is the number of SDs by which the patient's bone density differs from that of an individual matched for age, gender, and ethnicity. Not surprisingly, there can be disparity in absolute BMD by skeletal site within the same individual. This disparity can be attributed to the relative proportion of trabecular and cortical bone at a particular site. For example, the vertebra is 85% trabecular bone, whereas the femoral shaft or neck is principally cortical bone. Several studies have shown that nearly one in three subjects has disparate hip and spine T-scores. This finding can be attributed to the differences in skeletal composition; in other words, cortical or outer shell bone is thicker and remodels less frequently, whereas trabecular bone, which is the inner spongiform bone bathed by marrow elements, is metabolically very active. DXA integrates both skeletal compartments as an areal measurement. However, because skeletal sites often differ in composition and function, this disparity is frequently noted. Furthermore, age-related changes in the two skeletal compartments differ, and their genetic determinants may be completely distinct. In general, it is recommended that the lowest BMD measurement at any site be used for fracture risk assessment.

The two most common skeletal sites recommended for measuring BMD by DXA are spine and hip. For the spine, both anteroposterior and lateral spine DXAs can be obtained, although most providers use the anteroposterior spine, which is both a sensitive indicator of early bone loss and a precise measure. However, anteroposterior spine DXA can often show high bone mass resulting from increases in degenerative arthritis, disc collapse, vertebral fracture, or calcification of the aorta. Hence, in patients who are more than 65 years old, femoral neck and total hip BMD measurements are preferable. Both have good precision, are accurate, and are not complicated by those processes. Either site has strong predictive value for subsequent fractures.

Other Tools for Measuring Bone Mass

Other means of measuring BMD are available, and each provides T-score equivalents, although these cannot easily be translated across technologies. Quantitative CT scanning of the vertebrae provides a true volumetric measure of bone mass (mg/cm^3), can detect early bone loss, is accurate, and is available at many centers. However, its reproducibility is not as good as that of DXA, and T-scores can be quite disparate from DXA measurements. Moreover, significantly greater radiation exposure occurs with CT than DXA, and CT requires more time. Ultrasound scanning of peripheral sites has the advantages of portability and ease of operation, and the technique enables the clinician to predict fractures; however, the parameters used to measure sound transmission do not change much with age, or with treatment, thereby making this tool difficult to use for follow-up examination. Peripheral quantitative CT is expensive but accurate; it has greater radiation exposure but provides information about both cortical and trabecular elements. Fewer data on fracture risk are available with this technique, which is primarily a research tool.

In summary, DXA provides the most accurate and precise tool to assess fracture risk. The DXA measurement, combined with age, history of previous fracture, and family history, gives the clinician the most accurate assessment of osteoporotic risk. For follow-up, BMD measurements by DXA are preferable to other technologies because of the low precision error and greater reproducibility.

Risk Assessment Using FRAX

Since the introduction of widespread bone density measurements, it has become clear that BMD alone is not sufficient to define overall fracture risk and that consideration of clinical risk factors is essential. Often this is done at the point-of-care using age (>65 years), previous fracture, and family history. However, this combination does provide an estimate of 10-year risk, which clinicians often use to assess other diseases such as myocardial infarction. Hence, the WHO in collaboration with international osteoporosis foundations developed a virtual tool, FRAX, that can be used alongside the patient to determine his or her 10-year fracture risk. On any computer, BMD by DXA of the hip is entered into a box along with age, height, gender, country, and responses to queries about family history, use of glucocorticoids or alcohol, previous fracture, and weight loss. A 10-year fracture risk in percent is then calculated for a major osteoporotic fracture (i.e., spine, hip, wrist, and humerus) as well as hip fracture alone. Current guidance suggests that high-risk individuals are those with a 10-year risk of more than 3% for hip fracture and 20% for major osteoporotic fracture.

The FRAX tool has been widely praised, and its use has increased significantly since its introduction in 2007. Its strengths lie in the point-of-care nature of performing risk assessment, the country-specific assessment (e.g., United States vs. England vs. France), the recent revisions that incorporate new data sets providing more up-to-date fracture incidences for the United States, and ease of use. Concerns persist about several limitations, including that only hip BMD can be entered for fracture risk; FRAX should not be used in patients already receiving treatment; and in some populations, risk is overestimated, particularly in the younger postmenopausal female. Notwithstanding, fracture risk evaluation provides a reliable estimate for both the patient and provider and is preferred over a single BMD measurement to establish risk.

Biomarkers: Biochemical Markers of Bone Turnover

Newer methods of measuring bone breakdown and synthesis products have been developed since the mid-1980s. Previously, urinary calcium and hydroxyproline were the two urinary markers used to assess bone resorption; both were nonspecific, and their precision was poor. Subsequently, serum and urine biochemical markers have been perfected and tested in large clinical trials and are now available for clinical use. Markers of bone resorption mediated by osteoclasts include urinary pyridinoline and deoxypyridinoline as well as urine cross-links of the C- and N-terminal peptides of type I collagen. The latter can be measured either in urine or in serum. Markers of osteoblast-mediated bone formation include bone-specific alkaline phosphatase, osteocalcin, type I procollagen amino-terminal propeptide, and type I procollagen carboxy-terminal propeptide. Increases in markers of formation or resorption, or both, imply accelerated remodeling. For example, immediately after estrogen production ceases, markers of bone formation and bone resorption increase significantly. Similarly, later in life, and during states of secondary hyperparathyroidism, these markers can be extremely elevated. In addition, antiresorptive drugs such as estrogen or the bisphosphonates significantly lower urinary and circulating concentrations of these markers. Both longitudinal and cross-sectional studies have demonstrated that high turnover markers predict fracture in elderly women. These markers are independent of BMD and imply that accelerated bone turnover itself is a risk for fracture. Such indices of bone turnover provide a current estimate of the state of the skeleton, whereas bone density measurements are stoichiometric and reflect all the events leading up to the measurement.

In addition its potential for defining risk for fracture, several groups have shown that suppression in turnover markers with bisphosphonates or estrogens can predict fracture risk reduction in older postmenopausal women. Notwithstanding, the use of markers in clinical practice has been disappointing for several reasons. First, the variability in individual measurements, particularly for urine studies, is quite high. Therefore, even a single measurement has significant measurement error; follow-up to assess change from baseline is often even more confusing because of the variability issue. Second, most women have turnover marker values within the normal range, making interpretation difficult. Third, the number of older women with high bone turnover has probably been overestimated, particularly in the early postmenopausal period. These issues have limited enthusiasm for a single blood or urine test to help determine risk and assist in management once therapy has commenced. Occasionally, these tests can be helpful: in the young woman who undergoes premature menopause resulting from chemotherapy, for example, knowledge not just of the BMD but also of the rate of bone turnover could help in managing her condition with either aggressive antiresorptive therapy or a more measured approach using calcium and vitamin D. It is not recommended that these markers be used routinely to assess compliance with antiresorptive therapies.

Diagnostic Evaluation

The diagnosis of osteoporosis is usually made by bone mass measurements and a history of previous osteoporotic fractures. Secondary causes of osteoporosis must be excluded, and follow-up is required to ensure that the disease is not rapidly progressive. Routine profiles for renal and thyroid function are indicated. A serum 25-hydroxyvitamin D measurement in an older individual, particularly in northern latitudes, is recommended because deficiencies can be corrected with vitamin D supplementation. At present, DXA, combined with fracture risk assessment such as performed in the FRAX model, represents the best tool for assessing overall fracture risk and determining the course of therapy. Biochemical markers may be helpful in some cases.

TREATMENT   Rx

Treatment Plan

A comprehensive management plan for osteoporosis includes diagnosing those at highest risk, excluding secondary causes of low BMD, and selecting appropriate treatment. Decision making should also take into account several caveats. First, osteoporosis therapy can reduce fracture risk by as much as 50%, but some women will continue to have fractures despite treatment. Identifying those women at greatest risk for progressive disease is mandatory. Second, lifestyle and pharmacologic interventions are lifetime commitments such that cost, compliance, and safety must be factored into therapeutic decisions. Studies suggest that even with weekly or monthly bisphosphonate therapy, more than 40% of individuals treated will not continue therapy beyond 1 year. Third, it is not uncommon for women with T-scores higher than −2.5 to have fractures. In fact, in the National Osteoporosis Risk Assessment cohort of more than 140,000 postmenopausal women in the United States, almost one third of the women who had fractures also had BMD scores in the "osteopenic" range. Thus, treatment decisions should not be based solely on BMD.

Therapy for postmenopausal osteoporosis is framed in terms of *primary prevention* when it is prescribed for those at risk who do not have low bone mass (T-score < −2.5) or fractures or in terms of *treatment* for those with established disease, including previous osteoporotic fractures or markedly reduced BMD, or both. Thus, selection of an appropriate treatment regimen depends on whether the therapy is designed principally to prevent bone loss or to reduce the likelihood of a new spine or nonvertebral fracture in high-risk individuals.

General Measures

Diet

Calcium

Calcium supplementation should be an adjunct to drug treatments for women with established osteoporosis and must be part of any prevention strategy to ameliorate bone loss independent of other treatment choices. Increased calcium intake reduces the secondary hyperparathyroidism often seen with advancing age and can enhance mineralization of newly formed bone. Evidence that calcium and vitamin D together or individually reduce fracture risk in the osteoporotic individual remains somewhat controversial. However, a recent meta-analysis of calcium and vitamin D intervention trials demonstrated a consistent albeit small increase in BMD and a reduction in nonvertebral fractures when at least 1200 mg of calcium is combined with more than 400 units of vitamin D. Calcium supplementation alone has not been shown to reduce the incidence of nonvertebral fractures in high-risk women. A very large calcium intervention trial from WHI did not demonstrate hip fracture reduction with 1000 mg of daily calcium supplements and 400 IU of vitamin D for all postmenopausal women. However, for those older than 60 years, the risk reduction was statistically significant.[1] Interestingly, calcium supplementation in this cohort was associated with a 17% greater risk for kidney stones. This may have been due to the finding that baseline calcium intake in these women averaged 1100 mg per day. New Institute of Medicine (IOM) guidelines recommend 1200 mg per day of calcium in women over age 70 and 800 IU of vitamin D per day in that same age group. Certainly, with intakes greater than 2000 mg per day, the risk for nephrocalcinosis increases.

Vitamin D

Vitamin D is essential for skeletal maintenance and for enhancement of calcium absorption. Insufficiency of this vitamin is a growing problem; as many as two thirds of all patients who have hip fractures are classified as vitamin D deficient (Chapter 252). However, the results from randomized trials are conflicted. Elderly people in chronic care living situations are particularly vulnerable to vitamin D deficiency and may benefit from supplementation. One large randomized placebo-controlled trial (RPCT) demonstrated a 33% reduction in hip fractures for nursing home residents who received calcium and vitamin D compared with those receiving placebo.[2] In another trial, high-dose intermittent vitamin D reduced nonvertebral fractures by nearly one third among ambulatory elderly persons.[3] In older New England men and women, the combination of calcium citrate and 700 IU of vitamin D was shown to lessen by one third the risk for nonvertebral fractures.[4] However, in a large population-based study with calcium and vitamin D, supplementation had no effect on nonvertebral fractures,[5] although compliance and assessment of vitamin D levels were not sufficiently well documented to exclude an effect. Several recent meta-analyses suggest that 800 IU per day of vitamin D is needed to have fracture efficacy. Besides the potentially positive effects of vitamin D supplementation on the skeleton, particularly in older women, vitamin D may also enhance muscle strength and has been shown to reduce the risk for falling. Therefore, for most individuals with osteoporosis, 800 IU/day of vitamin D is sufficient to maintain adequate levels of 25-hydroxyvitamin D. However, in those patients with low bone mass and insufficient or deficient 25-hydroxyvitamin D levels (i.e., <20 ng/mL), administration of 50,000 IU of ergocalciferol (vitamin D₂) or cholecalciferol (vitamin D₃) given once weekly is a safe and effective way to restore vitamin D levels to the normal range. Upper limits of vitamin D supplementation are currently being reviewed to determine whether there is toxicity at higher doses.

Vitamin D analogues have been used in the treatment of osteoporosis since the early 1980s. However, this remains a controversial area. High doses of 1,25-dihydroxyvitamin D increase bone mass, but many patients develop hypercalciuria or hypercalcemia, or both. At doses of 0.5 µg/day, calcitriol reduced the rate of both vertebral and nonvertebral fractures, and it increased bone density in a very small trial. Other studies have found little benefit with a narrow therapeutic window, particularly in relation to renal function and hypercalcemia. Currently, vitamin D analogues are not recommended for the routine treatment of osteoporosis. A subset of patients with renal insufficiency (chronic kidney disease > 3) and high PTH levels may benefit from supplementation with calcitriol.

Physical Activity

Bedrest or immobility, particularly in elderly persons, can result in rapid bone loss. Moreover, the number of falls increases with age, and the number of falls that result in fractures also rises. A meta-analysis by the Cochrane Review Group demonstrated that muscle strengthening, balance retraining, home hazard assessment, withdrawal of psychotropic medications, and use of a multidisciplinary risk factor assessment program are beneficial in protecting against falls. An additional approach is to reduce loads applied to the hip during a fall by padding. Hip protectors have been shown to reduce the risk for hip fractures in at least one population, although compliance is generally poor. A more recent study failed to demonstrate the efficacy of these devices in older women in an assisted living facility. Regular physical activity, including aerobic, weight-bearing, and resistance exercises, is effective in increasing spine BMD and in strengthening muscle mass in postmenopausal women, but no large-scale studies have established whether these interventions reduce fracture risk.

Lifestyle

Other interventions, including smoking cessation and reduction of alcohol intake, should be considered within the framework of an individual's preventive health strategy. However, studies to date have been inconclusive in respect to understanding how changes in these lifestyles affect overall fracture risk.

Medical Therapy

Abundant evidence indicates that an aggressive intervention program can be successful in reducing fracture risk and in improving quality of life among postmenopausal women with preexisting osteoporosis. Several pharmacologic options are available, and these can be classified by their mechanism of action. The two major classes of osteoporosis drugs are (1) *antiresorptives* (i.e., agents that block bone resorption by inhibiting osteoclasts), and (2) *anabolics* (i.e., drugs that stimulate bone formation by primarily acting on osteoblasts).

Antiresorptive Agents

Antiresorptives inhibit bone resorption by suppressing osteoclast activity. Slowing the remodeling cycle allows bone formation to catch up to resorption, thereby enhancing matrix mineralization and stabilizing trabecular microarchitecture. The antiresorptives increase BMD and reduce fracture risk, but their efficacy varies.

Estrogen

Estrogen replacement therapy was long considered the cornerstone of therapy for postmenopausal women with osteoporosis. It works by slowing bone resorption through inhibition of cytokine signaling including RANKL from the osteoblast to the osteoclast, thereby increasing BMD. Estrogen replacement inhibits both cortical and trabecular bone loss, and BMD generally increases by 3 to 5% after 3 years.[6] There does not appear to be an additive effect from progesterone on bone mass in women also receiving estrogen. Conversely, progesterone is a necessary part of hormone replacement therapy in women with a uterus because it prevents the development of endometrial hyperplasia and carcinoma. In the WHI, estrogen and progesterone lowered hip fracture risk by one third.[7] Low-dose conjugated estrogens (0.3 or 0.45 mg/day) and ultralow-dose estradiol increase BMD and have been approved for the prevention of bone loss, but antifracture efficacy for these preparations has not been established. Discontinuation of estrogen results in measurable bone loss (3 to 5% in the first year), although whether that translates into a greater fracture risk is not clear.

Significant concern has been expressed about the nonskeletal risks associated with long-term estrogen and estrogen in combination with progesterone (Chapter 248). Particularly troublesome is the increased risk for breast cancer with the long-term use of estrogen and progesterone. In the WHI, there was a 26% increase in risk for invasive breast cancer over a 5.2-year period of follow-up.[7] Hence, estrogen replacement is contraindicated in any woman with a history of breast cancer; yearly mammograms are indicated in all women receiving hormone replacement therapy. Previous case-control and retrospective studies suggested that estrogen could reduce the risk for coronary artery disease; however, in the WHI, the risk for myocardial infarction or death from coronary artery disease was 29% higher in women receiving combination therapy.[7] Thromboembolic disease is also increased more than three-fold by hormone replacement therapy.[7] Hence, the use of estrogen or estrogen in combination with progestins for the prevention or treatment of osteoporosis has fallen dramatically. Moreover, the availability of newer and effective antiresorptive drugs for the treatment of osteoporosis has lessened enthusiasm for primary hormonal therapy in osteoporotic women.

Selective Estrogen Receptor Modulators

Selective estrogen receptor modulators such as tamoxifen and raloxifene also inhibit bone resorption by blocking cytokine release from the osteoblast. Both have been shown to reduce bone loss in postmenopausal women with breast cancer, but only raloxifene is approved by the U.S. Food and Drug Administration (FDA) for the prevention and treatment of osteoporosis.

Both these agents block the actions of estrogen on the breast but act like an estrogen agonist in bone; tamoxifen, but not raloxifene, has estrogen agonistic properties on the uterus and is associated with a greater risk for endometrial carcinoma with long-term use. Both agents have been associated with a reduction in new cases of breast cancer when they are administered as prophylaxis for high-risk patients.[8] Low-density lipoprotein cholesterol levels are also reduced in patients receiving these selective estrogen receptor modulators. Raloxifene increases spine BMD slightly (as does tamoxifen) and lowers the risk for vertebral fracture by 40%, although it has no effect on nonvertebral fracture risk.[9] Hot flashes, leg cramps, and a greater risk for deep venous thrombosis can occur with raloxifene therapy. The recommended dose of raloxifene is 60 mg once daily.

Tissue selectivity with these selective estrogen receptor modulators and others being investigated is a subject of great scientific interest. Raloxifene and estrogen both bind to the same region of the estrogen receptor, but they induce different conformational changes in that receptor. Coactivating and co-repressing proteins are recruited to the receptor-ligand complex, and it is thought that these transcription factors ultimately determine the activity of the nuclear complex. Because recruitment also depends on location, it is highly likely that significant tissue selectivity exists for these partners. Newer agents have been designed to facilitate particular complexes and rearrangements within the nucleus; these are being studied at both the preclinical and the clinical levels.

Bisphosphonates

The bisphosphonates are the most widely prescribed antiresorptives and are often considered first-line therapy for the treatment of severe postmenopausal osteoporosis. These drugs are carbon-substituted analogues of pyrophosphate that bind tightly to hydroxyapatite crystals. It is thought these agents directly suppress resorption by inhibiting osteoclast attachment and enhancing programmed cell death. The first-generation bisphosphonates include etidronate and clodronate. Neither is approved for the treatment of osteoporosis, although etidronate is widely used "off label" and in Europe. The dose of etidronate is 400 mg/day for 2 weeks every 3 months. The drug has few gastrointestinal side effects, and vertebral fracture risk reduction is significant with this agent. Alendronate and risedronate, two second-generation nitrogen-containing bisphosphonates, are effective in suppressing bone resorption and increasing BMD. In postmenopausal women with established osteoporosis, alendronate and risedronate reduced vertebral, hip, and nonvertebral fractures by nearly 50%, particularly during the first year of treatment.[10,11] Like other antiresorptive drugs, increases in BMD with alendronate or risedronate account for a small fraction of their antifracture efficacy. Hence, follow-up DXA measurements may significantly underestimate fracture risk reduction. Recent clinical trials have shown that these drugs can be safely administered for at least 7 years without adversely affecting bone strength. Moreover, discontinuation of alendronate after 5 years results in minimal bone loss over the ensuing 5 years. Both drugs have excellent safety profiles, although erosive esophagitis is a serious complication of all nitrogen-containing bisphosphonates. Once-weekly administration of alendronate has been shown to reduce the prevalence of drug-induced esophagitis, and currently both bisphosphonates are marketed as once-weekly treatments. Recently, the FDA approved the use of once-monthly risedronate (150 mg) for the treatment of osteoporosis.

Two new bisphosphonates have been approved by the U.S. FDA and have reached the market in the past 5 years: ibandronate and zoledronate. Ibandronate is given in a single monthly dose of 150 mg or intravenously (3 mg) every 3 months. It suppresses bone resorption and reduces the rate of spine fractures, but its efficacy in nonspine fractures is somewhat less than that of alendronate or residronate.[12,13] Compliance with the once-monthly regimen is higher than the weekly dosing, although long-term data are not encouraging. Zoledronate is also approved for the prevention and treatment of osteoporosis.[14] It is administered as a single intravenous infusion over 15 minutes (5 mg) once yearly. Large randomized controlled trials have unequivocally established its antifracture efficacy for hip, spine, and other nonspine fractures. Recently, the FDA approved the use of zoledronate for prevention of osteoporosis by administration of the drug once every 2 years. Both newer bisphosphonates can cause first-dose side effects, including joint pain, stiffness, and low-grade fevers. These do not persist with recurrent administration. However, the FDA has cautioned that zoledronic acid should be administered over 1 hour rather than 15 minutes to lessen any risk, albeit small, of renal damage.

Intravenous zoledronic acid is also approved for the treatment of hypercalcemia of malignancy (Chapter 186) and multiple myeloma, and as palliative therapy for metastatic disease.

Other bisphosphonates are available for off-label use or are being studied for the treatment of osteoporosis. Intravenous pamidronate has been available since the mid-1990s for the treatment of Paget's disease (Chapter 255) and malignant hypercalcemia (Chapter 186). It is currently also used to treat osteoporotic women who cannot tolerate oral bisphosphonates, although it has not been formally approved by the FDA for this indication, and its antifracture efficacy has not been established. The dose ranges from 30 to 90 mg given every 3 to 9 months. Acute and delayed-type hypersensitivity reactions can occur with this drug, and its use is contraindicated in patients who are vitamin D deficient because it can precipitously drop serum calcium.

In regard to the bisphosphonates, two rare side effects have been reported. Osteonecrosis of the jaw is a devastating condition associated with mandibular destruction following dental intervention (Chapter 256). It has been seen in patients taking bisphosphonates, particularly those receiving intravenous therapy who also have associated conditions such as multiple myeloma or metastatic breast cancer. Its true prevalence is unknown but is likely about 1 in 250,000 cases, and it is rare in women and men treated for osteoporosis who are otherwise healthy. Nevertheless, caution must be exercised in recommending dental surgery to patients taking a bisphosphonate. Subtrochanteric fracture is the other condition that may be associated with long-term bisphosphonate use. These midshaft fractures usually occur in middle-aged women taking an oral bisphosphonate for several years, frequently accompanied by treatment with glucocorticoids or use of an additional antiresorptive agent. The patient typically complains of leg pain before the fracture, and cortical thickening is noted in the subtrochanteric region on radiograph before the fracture. The true prevalence of this is unknown, but it is likely extremely uncommon, and the etiology is thought to be related to oversuppression of bone turnover. Treatment does not differ from any surgical management, although discontinuation of the bisphosphonate is recommended.

Calcitonin

Calcitonin is a 32–amino acid peptide normally produced by the thyroid C cells. Osteoclasts have calcitonin receptors, and calcitonin can rapidly inhibit bone resorption. Salmon calcitonin is more potent than human and is the preferred treatment choice. Nasal and subcutaneous calcitonin are both approved for the treatment of postmenopausal osteoporosis. However, the evidence favoring a strong effect from this hormone on either bone loss or fracture efficacy is lacking. In an RPCT of women with postmenopausal osteoporosis, 200 IU/day of nasal calcitonin reduced vertebral fracture incidence by one third.[15] However, methodologic flaws in that trial have limited enthusiasm for this agent as a primary treatment for osteoporosis. In at least one placebo-controlled study, nasal calcitonin reduced the pain associated with new spine fractures. The recommended dose of nasal calcitonin is 200 IU/day, and that of subcutaneous calcitonin is 100 IU/day. Side effects are uncommon with intranasal calcitonin and include nasal stuffiness and flushing. With subcutaneous administration, nausea is not infrequent.

Strontium Ranelate

Strontium ranelate is orally administered and stimulates calcium uptake in bone while it inhibits bone resorption. It is thought to have some anabolic activity, although the precise mechanism of action in the skeleton, where it is incorporated, is not known. In an RPCT of postmenopausal women with established disease, daily strontium reduced the risk for vertebral fractures by 40%.[16] However, a statistically significant effect on nonvertebral fractures was limited to a small subset of women in a post hoc analysis. This drug is approved by European regulatory agencies but not by the FDA.

Anabolic Agents

A new class of antiosteoporosis drugs was introduced in 2002. These are the so-called anabolics, agents that stimulate bone formation more than bone resorption. As such, these agents enhance bone remodeling and contrast sharply with the antiresorptives, which slow bone turnover. PTH_{1-34} (teriparatide) was the first of this class of drugs to be approved by the FDA.

The prototypical anabolic drug was sodium fluoride, which saw widespread use in the 1970s and 1980s because of its ability to stimulate new bone formation. However, an RPCT in 1990 established that although there were dramatic increases in BMD, nonvertebral fracture risk actually increased. Unlike sodium fluoride, synthetic PTH (PTH_{1-34}) was approved by the FDA for the treatment of postmenopausal osteoporosis because it not only increases bone mass but also reduces fractures. In the largest RPCT using teriparatide in postmenopausal women with severe osteoporosis, 20 μg/day of PTH, administered subcutaneously, reduced spinal and nonvertebral fractures by more than 50% while it substantially increased (i.e., 8% per year) lumbar BMD.[17] Similar findings were noted in men with osteoporosis who were treated for 11 months. Unfortunately, the PTH trial in postmenopausal women was stopped after 20 months because of concerns related to the development of osteosarcoma in rats treated with high doses of PTH_{1-34}. However, retrospective studies have found no association between osteosarcoma and primary or secondary hyperparathyroidism, and only two cases of osteosarcoma in PTH-treated patients

have been reported. More recently, recombinant human PTH (PTH_{1-84}) has shown similar benefits.[18] Currently, it is recommended that PTH therapy should be limited to those individuals with moderate to severe osteoporosis, and then taken only for 2 years.

Despite the appeal of using an anabolic with an antiresorptive, no evidence indicates that combinations of classes of drugs are additive or synergistic. Unlike the bisphosphonates, discontinuation of PTH can result in bone loss of 3 to 4% in the first year after PTH cessation. This post-treatment effect is prevented by adding an antiresorptive drug after PTH is stopped. In general, PTH is well tolerated, although nausea, flushing, hypotension, and mild but asymptomatic hypercalcemia (i.e., serum calcium < 11.0 mg/dL) can occur. Cost and compliance have been major limiting factors.

Vertebroplasty/Kyphoplasty

Vertebroplasty (percutaneous injection of cement into a collapsed vertebra to stabilize it) and kyphoplasty (use of a balloon to inflate the vertebral body prior to injection of the cement, in an attempt to restore the height and angle of the vertebral body) are widely used to treat the pain of vertebral compression fracture. Despite promising results for pain relief compared with standard care, benefits have not been seen when compared with a sham procedure.[19]

GLUCOCORTICOID-INDUCED OSTEOPOROSIS

The most common secondary cause of osteoporosis is glucocorticoid induced. This is often a result of pharmacologic doses of steroids used to treat inflammatory or autoimmune disorders. Generally, it is considered that glucocorticoids (Chapter 34) have a dose-dependent effect on the skeleton, such that longer duration and higher doses of steroids are most likely to cause bone loss and fractures. However, there clearly are subsets of individuals who are more or less sensitive to the skeletal effects of high doses of glucocorticoids. As a general clinical rule, those individuals with a cushingoid appearance and fat redistribution almost always have low bone mass or fractures, or both.

The effects of glucocorticoids on the skeleton are multifaceted and are particularly devastating because these agents cause uncoupling in the remodeling unit. Besides the indirect suppressive effects of glucocorticoids on the hypothalamic-gonadal axis, and inhibition of calcium absorption in the gut, high doses of steroids can stimulate osteoclastogenesis, increase RANKL production, and decrease OPG. This situation results in higher rates of bone resorption. Additionally, glucocorticoids also have a strong negative effect on bone formation by suppressing expression of IGF-I in bone cells and by shifting marrow stromal cells into the fat lineage and away from the osteoblast differentiation pathway. It is presumed that just as fat redistribution syndrome in the supraclavicular and mediastinal area is a clinical hallmark of Cushing's syndrome, enhanced adiposity in the bone marrow is a characteristic feature, almost certainly as a function of increased stromal cell differentiation into adipocytes. Bone strength is markedly compromised by the uncoupling in remodeling, and bone loss can be rapid over a short time period, particularly with high doses of glucocorticoids. Although there is no true dose-dependent effect on bone resorption, it is thought that prednisone doses as low as 5 mg/day may increase fracture risk. Indeed, in this syndrome, baseline BMD is not predictive of fractures and can often be normal even in the presence of ongoing resorption and recurrent fractures. Trabecular bone suffers the most in this syndrome, and spine DXA is the most sensitive indicator of bone loss. Markers of bone turnover are not helpful in the management of these patients.

Therapy for steroid-induced bone loss centers on treating the underlying disease or reducing the dose of glucocorticoids to the lowest possible regimen, or both. Barring that, several interventions have been shown to retard bone loss and prevent fractures. Adequate calcium and vitamin D intake is critical for every patient receiving glucocorticoids. However, these measures alone are not sufficient. Three bisphosphonates have been shown to have efficacy in glucocorticoid-induced osteoporosis—etidronate, alendronate,[20] and risedronate—and they are now considered the standard of care for this disease. These drugs are administered either weekly or cyclically to prevent bone loss and to reduce the risk for fractures. Some anecdotal data support the use of gonadal steroids in this condition, but clearly the bisphosphonates are superior. In a randomized trial, synthetic PTH (teriparatide, 20 mg daily subcutaneously for 18 months) significantly increased hip and spine bone mass density and reduced new vertebral fractures (from 7.2 to 3.4%), but not other fractures, compared with alendronate.[21] More studies are needed to establish its long-term efficacy in this disease, particularly because secondary hyperparathyroidism is a frequent accompaniment of steroid-induced osteoporosis.

FUTURE DIRECTIONS

Denosumab, a synthetic RANKL antibody that works like OPG, prevents bone loss in women with severe disease and, in large randomized placebo-controlled trials, reduced hip, spine, and nonspine fractures when administered as a single subcutaneous injection (60 mg) once every 6 months. This drug is not associated with osteonecrosis of the jaw, but lower extremity cellulitis occurs three times more often with this therapy than with placebo. Currently, denosumab is not approved by the FDA. PTH-related protein (PTHrp), a peptide that is structurally similar to PTH, binds to the same receptor, is responsible for some cases of hypercalcemia of malignancy, and has significant anabolic properties when administered intermittently. It is not approved yet by the FDA for the treatment of osteoporosis.

OSTEOPOROSIS IN MEN

EPIDEMIOLOGY

Osteoporosis in men is now more frequently recognized. This may stem from greater awareness in respect to the clinical presentation, the role of bone density screening, and a better understanding of the pathogenesis of osteoporosis, particularly in older men. Thirty percent of all hip and vertebral fractures occur in men, and one in six men in later life will suffer a hip fracture.

CLINICAL MANIFESTATIONS

The clinical presentation is often different from that in women, especially in relation to the time to diagnosis after symptoms begin. Back pain with vertebral compression is the most common presenting complaint. Bone density measurements are less frequently obtained in men, but they are performed after symptoms occur, a far different situation than in postmenopausal women.

PATHOPHYSIOLOGY

Secondary causes of osteoporosis dominate this disease in men. Hypogonadism and hypercortisolemia are the major etiologic factors in male osteoporosis and must be considered regardless of the phenotypic presentation. However, certain other conditions, including gluten enteropathy, gastric resection or bypass, and ethanol abuse, are more common in men than women with osteoporosis. Hypercalciuria (with or without kidney stones) that is associated with secondary hyperparathyroidism occurs in men and is a frequent cause of low bone mass in young men. In contrast, anorexia in male patients is extremely rare, and the athlete's triad so characteristic of women runners (i.e., exercise, hypogonadism, and low bone mass) is infrequent, although not unheard of, in men.

Lack of androgens results in a skeletal deficit. Peak bone mass is clearly reduced in androgen-insufficient young male patients whether the condition results from idiopathic hypogonadotropic hypogonadism, Klinefelter's syndrome, or constitutional delayed puberty. The use of long-acting gonadotropin-releasing hormone analogues that block androgen production and are administered in the treatment of prostate cancer is also associated with significant bone loss and fractures in later life. Men with primary gonadal failure, hemochromatosis, hyperprolactinemic hypogonadism, and other disorders of the hypothalamus or pituitary often have very low bone mass. Androgens act by directly stimulating bone formation because osteoblasts have androgen receptors. However, testosterone probably also blocks bone resorption and can dampen the release of TNF, IL-6, and IL-1. Not surprisingly, estrogen also plays an important role in the male skeleton. Inhibition of aromatization of testosterone (i.e., aromatase P-450) to estrogen, whether caused by a genetic mutation or drugs, leads to significant bone loss. Investigators have also shown that men with low estradiol levels are at greater risk for osteoporosis. Thus, it appears that both estrogen and androgen are necessary for the development and maintenance of the male skeleton.

TREATMENT   Rx

Therapies for osteoporosis in male patients center on identifying any underlying cause and then treating with drugs that are also used in women. Hypogonadism can be effectively treated with androgen replacement, although caution must be used in elderly men because of the risk for prostate cancer. Hypercalciuria can be diminished by use of hydrochlorothiazide, which may

also enhance bone density in men. Alendronate has been shown to prevent bone loss and to reduce fractures in men with idiopathic osteoporosis or osteoporosis resulting from androgen deficiency states.[22] PTH_{1-34} has also been approved for the treatment of male osteoporosis because it too can enhance bone density and prevent fractures. In a large randomized trial of men with limited prostate cancer taking gonadotropin-releasing agonists, denosumab reduced fractures and prevented bone loss. This agent, if approved by the FDA, may be the most appropriate therapy for a growing cohort of men receiving aggressive anticancer therapy. Selective androgen receptor modulators are under development and may offer a new approach to male osteoporosis.

Grade **A**

1. Jackson RD, LaCroix AZ, Gass M, et al. Calcium plus vitamin D supplementation and the risk of fractures. *N Engl J Med.* 2006;354:669-683.
2. Chapuy MC, Arlot ME, Duboeuf F, et al. Vitamin D3 and calcium to prevent hip fractures in the elderly woman. *N Engl J Med.* 1992;327:1637-1642.
3. Trivedi DP, Doll R, Khaw KT. Effect of four monthly oral vitamin D3 (cholecalciferol) supplementation on fractures and mortality in men and women living in the community: randomised double blind controlled trial. *BMJ.* 2003;326:469.
4. Dawson-Hughes B, Harris SS, Krall EA, et al. Effect of calcium and vitamin D supplementation on bone density in men and women 65 years of age or older. *N Engl J Med.* 1997;337:670-676.
5. Grant AM, Avenell A, Campbell MK, et al, for the RECORD Trial Group. Oral vitamin D3 and calcium for secondary prevention of low-trauma fractures in elderly people (Randomised Evaluation of Calcium Or vitamin D, RECORD): a randomised placebo-controlled trial. *Lancet.* 2005;365:1621-1628.
6. Writing Group for the PEPI. Effects of hormone therapy on bone mineral density: results from the Postmenopausal Estrogen/Progestin Interventions (PEPI) trial. *JAMA.* 1996;276:1389-1396.
7. Rossouw JE, Anderson GL, Prentice RL, et al. Risks and benefits of estrogen plus progestin in healthy postmenopausal women: principal results from the Women's Health Initiative randomized controlled trial. *JAMA.* 2002;288:321-333.
8. Cummings S, Eckert S, Krueger K, et al. The effect of raloxifene on risk of breast cancer in postmenopausal women: results from the MORE randomized trial. *JAMA.* 1999;281:2189-2197.
9. Ettinger B, Black D, Mitlak B, et al. Reduction of vertebral fracture risk in postmenopausal women with osteoporosis treated with raloxifene. *JAMA.* 1999;282:637-645.
10. McClung MR, Geusens P, Miller PD, et al. Effect of risedronate on the risk of hip fracture in elderly women: Hip Intervention Program Study Group. *N Engl J Med.* 2001;344:333-340.
11. Black D, Cummings S, Karpf D, et al. Randomised trial of effect of alendronate on risk of fracture in women with existing vertebral fractures: Fracture Intervention Trial Research Group. *Lancet.* 1996;348:1535-1541.
12. Chesnut IC, Skag A, Christiansen C, et al. Effects of oral ibandronate administered daily or intermittently on fracture risk in postmenopausal osteoporosis. *J Bone Miner Res.* 2004;19:1241-1249.
13. Felsenberg D, Miller P, Armbrecht G, et al. Oral ibandronate significantly reduces the risk of vertebral fractures of greater severity after 1, 2, and 3 years in postmenopausal women with osteoporosis. *Bone.* 2005;37:651-654.
14. Eastell R, Black DM, Boonen S, et al, for the HORIZON Pivotal Fracture Trial. Effect of once-yearly zoledronic acid five milligrams on fracture risk and change in femoral neck bone mineral density. *J Clin Endocrinol Metab.* 2009;94:3215-3225.
15. Chesnut CH 3rd, Silverman S, Andriano K, et al. A randomized trial of nasal spray salmon calcitonin in postmenopausal women with established osteoporosis: the prevent recurrence of osteoporotic fractures study. PROOF Study Group. *Am J Med.* 2000;109:267-276.
16. Meunier PJ, Roux C, Seeman E, et al. The effects of strontium ranelate on the risk of vertebral fracture in women with postmenopausal osteoporosis. *N Engl J Med.* 2004;350:459-468.
17. Neer RM, Arnaud CD, Zanchetta JR, et al. Effect of parathyroid hormone (1-34) on fractures and bone mineral density in postmenopausal women with osteoporosis. *N Engl J Med.* 2001; 344:1434-1441.
18. Greenspan SL, Bone HG, Ettinger MP, et al. Effect of recombinant human parathyroid hormone (1-84) on vertebral fracture and bone mineral density in postmenopausal women with osteoporosis: a randomized trial. *Ann Intern Med.* 2007;146:326-339.
19. Kallmes DF, Comstock BA, Heagerty PJ, et al. A randomized trial of vertebroplasty for osteoporotic spinal fractures. *N Engl J Med.* 2009;361:569-579.
20. de Nijs RNJ, Jacobs JWG, Lems WF, et al. Alendronate or alfacalcidol in glucocorticoid-induced osteoporosis. *N Engl J Med.* 2006;355:675-684.
21. Saag KG, Shane E, Boonen S, et al. Teriparatide or alendronate in glucocorticoid-induced osteoporosis. *N Engl J Med.* 2007;357:2028-2039.
22. Orwoll ES, Ettinger M, Weiss S, et al. Alendronate for the treatment of osteoporosis in men. *N Engl J Med.* 2000;343:604-610.

SUGGESTED READINGS

Cummings SR, Ensrud K, Delmas PD, et al. Lasofoxifene in postmenopausal women with osteoporosis. *N Engl J Med.* 2010;362:686-696. *In a randomized trial of postmenopausal women with osteoporosis, lasofoxifene (0.5 mg per day) decreased the risk of fractures, breast cancer, strokes, and coronary heart disease but increased the risk of venous thromboembolic events.*

Donaldson MG, Cawthon PM, Lui LY, et al. Estimates of the proportion of older white men who would be recommended for the pharmacologic treatment by the new U.S. National Osteoporosis Foundation guidelines. *J Bone Miner Res.* 2010;25:1506-1511. *Estimates that about 35% of U.S. white men aged 65 years and older and 50% of those aged 75 years and older would be recommended for drug treatment.*

Favus MJ. Bisphosphonates for osteoporosis. *N Engl J Med.* 2010;363:2027-2035. *Review.*

Grossman JM, Gordon R, Ranganath VK, et al. American College of Rheumatology 2010 recommendations for the prevention and treatment of glucocorticoid-induced osteoporosis. *Arthritis Care Res (Hoboken).* 2010;62:1515-1526. *Consensus guidelines.*

Papaioannou A, Morin S, Cheung AM, et al. 2010 clinical practice guidelines for the diagnosis and management of osteoporosis in Canada: summary. *CMAJ.* 2010;182:1864-1873. *Consensus guidelines.*

Rachner TD, Khosla S, Hofbauer LC. Osteoporosis: now and the future. *Lancet.* 2011;377:1276-1287. *Review.*

Sanders KM, Stuart AL, Williamson EJ, et al. Annual high-dose oral vitamin D and falls and fractures in older women: a randomized controlled trial. *JAMA.* 2010;303:1815-1822. *In a randomized controlled trial, high-dose vitamin D surprisingly increased the risk of falls and fractures.*

U.S. Preventive Services Task Force. Screening for osteoporosis: U.S. Preventive Services Task Force recommendation statement. *Ann Intern Med.* 2011;154:356-364. *Clinical guidelines recommend screening in women but not clearly in men.*

Watts NB, Bilezikian JP, Camacho PM, et al. American Association of Clinical Endocrinologists Medical Guidelines for Clinical Practice for the diagnosis and treatment of postmenopausal osteoporosis. *Endocr Pract.* 2010;16:1-37. *Consensus guidelines.*

252

OSTEOMALACIA AND RICKETS

ROBERT S. WEINSTEIN

DEFINITION

Rickets refers to impaired mineralization of the cartilaginous growth plate and abnormal endochondral bone formation and therefore cannot occur in adults after epiphyseal closure. *Osteomalacia,* literally meaning softening of bone, refers to defective or delayed mineralization of the organic matrix of bone, or osteoid, at the interface between calcified bone and osteoid, and may occur at any age. Both rickets and osteomalacia may be present in a growing child, but defective mineralization can cause only osteomalacia in adults; therefore, this chapter focuses on osteomalacia. Despite advances in our understanding of vitamin D metabolism and the increased sensitivity of measurements of serum 25-hydroxyvitamin D, osteomalacia remains a common but frequently overlooked disorder in the Western world. Optimal therapy requires precise identification of the etiology of the abnormal mineralization, which may present a problem because there are numerous causes (Table 252-1). However, once a correct diagnosis is made, therapy is usually gratifying and often spectacular. Early recognition of osteomalacia depends on familiarity with the typical clinical manifestations and settings. It is helpful to appreciate that the bone disease almost always manifests in the same manner regardless of the cause of the osteomalacia.

EPIDEMIOLOGY

About 20% of North American women receiving treatment for osteoporosis have 25-hydroxyvitamin D levels below 20 ng/mL (adequate values are greater than 30 ng/mL), and 8% have levels below 15 ng/mL, indicating that at the least, impaired bone mineralization could be a confounding factor in their osteoporosis treatment and, at worst, osteomalacia is the correct diagnosis (a defect in mineralization) rather than osteoporosis (a reduced amount of normally mineralized bone). Vitamin D deficiency is more common in elderly people, especially in nonaffluent elderly people during the winter and at higher latitudes. Vitamin D deficiency is also commonly found in medical inpatients and in postmenopausal women with acute hip fracture.

The prevalence of osteomalacia due to vitamin D deficiency varies with the referral source. The disorder is far more frequent when patients are referred from geriatricians, gastroenterologists (osteomalacia may be found in up to 30% of patients with gastric surgery or bypass for obesity), nursing homes, or orthopedists concerned about symmetrical or nonhealing fractures. The most common hypophosphatemic osteomalacia is the inherited disease X-linked hypophosphatemia, but affected adults infrequently present to internists and then only when troubled by severe bone pain or nonunion of fractures.

PATHOBIOLOGY

A review of normal bone remodeling and the mineralization of osteoid (bone matrix) serves as a background to understanding the abnormal mineralization characteristic of osteomalacia. Bone remodeling or turnover is carried

TABLE 252-1	CAUSES OF OSTEOMALACIA
VITAMIN D DEFICIENCY	
Dietary deprivation and lack of sunlight exposure	
VITAMIN D MALABSORPTION	
Postgastrectomy	
Gastric bypass for obesity	
Gluten enteropathy	
Small bowel disease or resection	
Pancreatic insufficiency	
Cholestyramine therapy for cholestatic liver disease	
Laxative abuse	
IMPAIRED 1-HYDROXYLATION OF 25-HYDROXYVITAMIN D	
Vitamin D–dependent rickets type I	
X-linked hypophosphatemia	
Oncogenic osteomalacia	
IMPAIRED TARGET-ORGAN RESPONSE TO 1,25-DIHYDROXYVITAMIN D	
Vitamin D–dependent rickets type II	
HYPOPHOSPHATEMIA	
X-linked hypophosphatemia	
Sporadic hypophosphatemia	
Oncogenic osteomalacia	
Antacid-induced osteomalacia	
Chronic metabolic acidosis	
Paraproteinemia	
Saccharated ferric oxide	
Tenofovir	
Cadmium	
INHIBITORS OF MINERALIZATION	
Etidronate	
Fluoride	
Aluminum	
Iron	
MISCELLANEOUS	
Hypophosphatasia	
Axial osteomalacia	
Fibrogenesis imperfecta ossium	

out by teams of juxtaposed osteoclasts and osteoblasts, comprising temporary anatomic structures known as basic multicellular units (BMUs). In cortical bone, the BMUs drill tunnels or "cutting cones" through the compact tissue; while in spongy, cancellous bone, they gouge across the trabecular surface, forming serpiginous trenches. Bone turnover begins by conversion of a quiescent skeletal surface to a remodeling site, a process referred to as activation. Activation involves proliferation of new blood vessels needed to bring recruited osteoclast progenitors to the remodeling site and retraction of the flat, pavement-like bone-lining cells that cover the quiescent surfaces to expose the mineralized bone surface. The recruited cells become multinucleated osteoclasts, which attach to the newly exposed bone surface with a ring of contractile proteins sealing off a subosteoclastic resorption compartment. Lysosomal enzymes, hydrogen ions, and collagenase are secreted through the microvilli of the ruffled underside border of the osteoclasts, and these chemicals excavate a resorption cavity. The osteoclasts remove both the bone mineral and matrix. It is a misunderstanding to attribute to these cells or to metabolic acidosis the ability to remove only the mineral leaving behind demineralized osteoid. Demineralized bone in vivo is a misnomer. Demineralized or decalcified bone only occurs when bones are placed in acid (1 N HCl) or chelating solutions (ethylenediaminetetraacetate, or EDTA). Osteoclasts are motile cells, capable of resorbing more than just the cavity within which they are identified. After an osteoclast digs a cavity, it may detach from bone and move on to a new resorption site or die by apoptosis and be quickly removed by phagocytes. When the osteoclasts have moved on, osteoblasts assemble to reconstitute the previously resorbed cavity with new bone. In any established BMU, both events are happening at the same time; bone formation begins to occur while bone resorption advances.

Between the end of bone resorption and the beginning of bone formation is the reversal phase, when mononuclear phagocytes smooth out the jagged erosion bays. During this phase, the old bone is coated by a thin layer of cement substance, a collagen- and mineral-poor matrix rich in glycosaminoglycans, glycoproteins, and acid phosphatase, to which the new osteoblasts attach. In adults, new osteoblasts assemble only at sites where osteoclasts have recently been eroding bone, a phenomenon referred to as coupling. The arrival of the osteoblasts in the right place at the right time and in sufficient numbers to reconstitute the cavity is referred to as remodeling balance and is likely due to proportional production of osteoblasts and osteoclasts in the bone marrow, release of osteoblast recruiting substances from the resorbed bone, and chemotaxis by the cement substances. As osteoblasts complete their bone matrix synthesis and move away from the cement line, they gradually flatten. Some osteoblasts become bone-lining cells, and some become osteocytes, but as many as 65% of the osteoblasts that originally assembled at the remodeling site die by apoptosis. It is the balance between cell proliferation and apoptosis that determines the amount of work performed by these cells.

Normally, up to 70% of the mineralization of the osteoid deposited by the osteoblasts starts within 4 to 12 days and proceeds at about 1 μm per day; but in osteomalacia, mineral deposition in the osteoid slows or stops completely, while the osteoblasts continue to make osteoid, which then accumulates in excessive amounts. Therefore, normal osteoid width is about 4 to 12 μm, but in osteomalacia, the osteoid width may become dramatically augmented. Depending on the extent of the delay in mineralization, overt osteomalacia may take many years to develop. In normal subjects, further mineralization proceeds slowly over months to years and at the cost of displacement of the water in the hydroxyapatite crystals resulting in increased brittleness and the eventual need for another round of remodeling. Even though a million BMUs are undergoing remodeling every day, bone mass in a healthy adult is preserved, owing to a remarkably tight balance between the amount of bone resorbed and formed during each cycle of remodeling. By this means, the adult skeleton is almost completely regenerated every 10 years.

Mineralization requires the availability of sufficient calcium and phosphorus at the remodeling site, the presence of a normal bone collagen matrix, the absence of inhibitors of mineralization, and an adequate amount of skeletal alkaline phosphatase activity. Defects in these requirements are the cause of most forms of osteomalacia. Deficiency of vitamin D per se has traditionally been incriminated as the cause of the osteomalacia, but today, considerable evidence indicates that the abnormal mineralization associated with vitamin D deficiency depends more on the deficiency of calcium and phosphorus than from the absence of a direct effect of vitamin D on bone cells. The primary function of vitamin D is to provide adequate levels of calcium and phosphorus by increasing their intestinal absorption. Chronic metabolic acidosis has also been identified as a cause of osteomalacia, but evidence suggests that the bone disease associated with chronic metabolic acidosis is primarily due to the associated hypophosphatemia.

CLINICAL MANIFESTATIONS

The clinical presentation of osteomalacia depends on three overlapping manifestations. Those due to the underlying disorder such as gastrointestinal disease or surgery (especially troublesome are gastric resection, stapling, or bypass for obesity and intestinal malabsorption); those due to hypocalcemia or hypophosphatemia; and those directly due to the bone disease. The most common symptoms and signs are bone pain, muscle weakness, and bone tenderness. The bone pain is usually nonspecific and poorly localized. Because of the paucity of findings, the pains are often attributed to rheumatism or neurosis. They may be worse at night and after sudden movements such as turning in bed or the change from sitting to standing. Most often, the pain is in the lower back, pelvis, and legs and is worse on weight bearing, resulting in a characteristic flat-footed, springless, waddling gait made worse by proximal muscle weakness. The gait has been referred to as "mother penguin's walk." Patients may complain that they can only climb stairs by pulling themselves up with the hand rail or rise from sitting in a chair or on the toilet by using their hands to push off. The decrease in strength is usually far greater than the degree of muscle wasting. Fasciculations are absent, and both reflexes and sensation remain normal. The bulbar, facial, and ocular muscles are always spared. However, muscle weakness is conspicuously absent when the osteomalacia is due to X-linked hypophosphatemia. Often, bone tenderness can be elicited by rib cage compression or pressing on the tibiae, wrists, pubic rami, or iliac crests. Hypocalcemia is usually mild to moderate but, rarely, can be severe enough to present with paresthesias, muscle cramps, a positive Chvostek's sign, or seizures. If the osteomalacia is mistaken for osteoporosis and treatment is started with a bisphosphonate, the patient may experience new-onset paresthesias, muscle cramps, and palpitations. This not uncommon scenario occurs because the antiresorptive treatment interferes

with the compensatory secondary hyperparathyroidism and aggravates the hypocalcemia.

DIAGNOSIS

Biochemical changes depend on the stage of the disease and its etiology. In vitamin D deficiency, hypophosphatemia precedes and is more severe than the hypocalcemia because of the secondary hyperparathyroidism (Chapter 253) that almost invariably accompanies the disorder by the time that osteomalacia has occurred. In malabsorption, hypomagnesemia may contribute to the hypocalcemia, and hypoalbuminemia may lead to a spurious diagnosis of hypocalcemia. Increased serum alkaline phosphatase activity is classically associated with osteomalacia due to vitamin D deficiency but is not an early or reliable clue because some patients may have normal or borderline levels. The serum 25-hydroxyvitamin D levels are often less than 10 to 15 ng/mL. In contrast, serum 1,25-dihydroxyvitamin D levels are usually elevated owing to the concomitant hyperparathyroidism and do not contribute to the diagnosis of osteomalacia except in the rare abnormalities of vitamin D resistance (when 1,25-dihydroxyvitamin D levels may be extraordinarily high) or when 1-hydroxylation is defective (and 1,25-dihydroxyvitamin D levels are low). Quite a different pattern occurs with the inherited disease hypophosphatasia: serum 25-hydroxyvitamin D and calcium are normal, phosphorus is high normal or elevated, and alkaline phosphatase activity is below the normal range. Radiographic findings may be absent with early osteomalacia, and only blurred margins of the cancellous bone with thin cortices may be noted. The presence of bilateral, thin (2 to 3 mm), radiolucent bands known as pseudofractures (Fig. 252-1) found perpendicular to the periosteal surface in ribs, pubic and ischial rami, the neck of the femur, metatarsals, and below the glenoid fossa on the outer border of the scapulae are generally considered to be pathognomonic of osteomalacia, but this classic radiographic sign is infrequent today. Rarely, it may be seen in disorders lacking excessive osteoid. These pseudofractures (sometimes called Looser's zones or Milkman's fractures) show increased uptake on bone scans (Fig. 252-2) and may lead to an inappropriate search for a primary malignancy. Bone mineral density T-scores are often −3 or −4, with the radial diaphyseal density lower than that of the lumbar spine or total proximal femur.

Although characteristic clinical, radiographic, and biochemical findings may suggest osteomalacia, the absence of these findings cannot exclude the diagnosis. Quantitative histologic examination of undecalcified bone is, therefore, required to establish the unequivocal presence of osteomalacia (Fig. 252-3). Rigorous kinetic criteria for the histologic recognition of osteomalacia are necessary to preserve the traditional clinical, biochemical, and therapeutic connotations of the term. Therefore, a review of the quantitative bone histologic findings or histomorphometry in osteomalacia is useful. The histomorphometric diagnosis of osteomalacia requires the simultaneous presence of three findings: excessive osteoid (osteoid area greater than 10%;

FIGURE 252-1. Radiographic evidence of a pseudofracture of the femoral neck is suspicious for osteomalacia (*arrow*).

FIGURE 252-2. In osteomalacia, focal increased uptake of radionuclide on a bone scan may erroneously suggest metastatic disease (*arrows*).

FIGURE 252-3. An undecalcified bone biopsy specimen shows the characteristic abundant osteoid and flattened osteoblasts (*arrows*) of osteomalacia. (Normally, mineralized bone appears gray and osteoid is black.)

normal is less than 4%), augmentation of the osteoid width (more than 15 μm; normal is 4 to 12 μm), and prolongation of the mineralization lag time (greater than 100 days; normal is 9 to 20 days), as determined by the osteoid width divided by the distance between and linear extent of double tetracycline labels observed in the bone after the patient receives two time-spaced courses of oral tetracycline. Tetracycline is deposited early in the course of hydroxyapatite crystal formation and generates bright stripes at the interface of mineralized bone and osteoid when viewed with fluorescent microscopy. If the two time-spaced courses of tetracycline (1 g/day for 3 days) are separated by a 14-day interval, the rate of mineralization (μm/day) can be calculated by measuring the average distance between the double labels divided by the number of days between the two courses. When the double labels are numerous and widely spaced, mineralization is intact, and excess osteoid must be due to increased bone turnover. A paucity of tetracycline labels that are narrowly spaced indicates that if excessive osteoid is present, it must be due to the delayed or ceased mineralization of osteomalacia.

Therefore, it follows that excessive osteoid can occur from two distinct mechanisms. Osteomalacia is the consequence of defective mineralization while osteoid production continues. However, osteoid will also accumulate with accelerated bone formation if the rate of osteoid deposition exceeds the rate of mineralization as occurs in states of increased bone turnover, such as hyperparathyroidism (Chapter 253), Paget's disease, or thyrotoxicosis. Although osteoblasts in osteomalacia are usually sparse and flattened, whereas they are numerous, plump, and cuboidal with high bone turnover, these two groups of disorders can be reliably distinguished only with the use of tetracycline markers. The treatment of increased bone turnover and

of defective mineralization is completely different and that is why the three histomorphometric criteria are necessary. Additionally, evaluation of each of the criteria in isolation has limitations. Regarding the first requirement, a small increase in the osteoid area relative to the total bone area may occur in osteoporosis with a decrease in the amount of mineralized bone. In the second requirement, wide osteoid seams may be seen in some specimens obtained from patients with severe secondary hyperparathyroidism, such as those on maintenance hemodialysis therapy. In the third requirement, reduced mineral appositional rate and increased mineralization lag time are nonspecific indices of impaired matrix synthesis by osteoblasts, as is often found in patients with involutional osteoporosis. Only when all three requirements are fulfilled is the diagnosis of osteomalacia irrefutable.

Several presumed causes of osteomalacia (anticonvulsant drugs, metabolic acidosis without hypophosphatemia, pseudohypoparathyroidism, and chronic renal failure) have not fulfilled all of these requirements and primarily represent secondary hyperparathyroidism. Patients with the nephrotic syndrome lose albumin and vitamin D metabolites in the urine, but evidence indicates that serum ionized calcium and parathyroid hormone levels are normal and that metabolic bone disease in adults with the nephrotic syndrome is absent. Muscle weakness and bone pain are significantly more common in patients in whom the rigorous histologic diagnosis of osteomalacia has been proved. However, bone biopsy is not always necessary to be reasonably certain of the diagnosis. When biopsy is necessary, the local pathologist must be familiar with the processing of undecalcified bone specimens and plastic embedding; otherwise, the best solution is to refer the patient to a bone histomorphometry center for biopsy. This ensures satisfactory communication among the clinician, operator, and pathologist and is the best insurance against the incomplete, broken, fragmented, or accidentally decalcified bone specimens. Such referral may be indispensable in the evaluation of a patient with unusually painful disease or progressive loss of bone mineral density, particularly when the results of the physical examination, radiographs, and biochemical findings are ambiguous. Biopsy may also be indicated in patients with unexplained chronic hypophosphatemia.

The best approach is to avoid overlooking the diagnosis of osteomalacia by maintaining a high degree of suspicion in the typical clinical settings. This is especially important because osteomalacia can usually be successfully treated. An investigation for osteomalacia is indicated in elderly patients with bone pain and muscle weakness, in patients with gastric surgery and low bone mineral density or bone pain, and in patients with persistent hypophosphatemia. Unexplained elevations of the serum alkaline phosphatase activity are usually due to drugs (e.g., anticonvulsants, anabolic steroids, phenothiazines, or antibiotics) or Paget's disease of bone (Chapter 255) but rarely may be the only biochemical clue to osteomalacia in a patient with variable skeletal discomfort. Bilateral or slowly healing fractures also warrant an investigation for osteomalacia.

TREATMENT   Rx

Understanding the treatment of osteomalacia is facilitated by dividing the disease into four subgroups. The first subgroup is osteomalacia due to disorders of vitamin D absorption or metabolism; the second is osteomalacia due to chronic hypophosphatemia. Most patients with osteomalacia will be in these first two subgroups. The third subgroup includes osteomalacia caused by inhibitors of mineralization such as etidronate (the first oral bisphosphonate, now rarely used in North America); high doses of fluoride; and accumulation of a skeletal burden of aluminum from water used for dialysis or as a contaminant in solutions used for parenteral nutrition (now rarely seen), iron overload as in thalassemia, and cadmium or tenfovir, which induce the proximal tubular lesion of Fanconi's syndrome and cause osteomalacia due to the resultant hypophosphatemia. The fourth subgroup includes miscellaneous causes of osteomalacia that lack specific therapy but are fortunately quite rare. This last subgroup includes the variable forms of the heritable disorder hypophosphatasia, caused by a deficiency of the tissue-nonspecific (liver, bone, kidney) isoenzyme of alkaline phosphatase; axial osteomalacia, a sporadic osteosclerotic disorder primarily affecting middle-aged men and presenting with mild to moderate pain in the spine and pelvis (but without fractures), apparently from the production of an abnormal and poorly mineralized bone matrix by osteoblasts; and fibrogenesis imperfecta ossium, another sporadic disorder presenting with intractable bone pain and fractures mainly in middle-aged men and woman, apparently also due to production of an abnormal bone matrix by osteoblasts. In axial osteomalacia and fibrogenesis imperfecta ossium, serum calcium, phosphorus, and vitamin D levels are normal, but serum alkaline phosphatase activity may be increased. General measures for this last subgroup include routine nutritional advice and avoidance of further bone loss due to postmenopausal or involutional osteoporosis. High-dose vitamin D therapy in these disorders has caused nephrocalcinosis, nephrolithiasis, and renal insufficiency and must be avoided.

Osteomalacia Due to Vitamin D Disorders

Iron deficiency anemia, hypocalcemia, weight loss, glossitis or rash, and bone discomfort in a patient with low bone mineral density point to celiac disease (Chapter 142), even without gastrointestinal symptoms. These signs suggest the need to test for antiendomysial immunoglobulin A antibodies. Cholestyramine therapy for cholestatic liver disease may increase malabsorption of vitamin D by binding bile salts. Laxative abuse may cause osteomalacia and severe resistance to vitamin D supplementation, including treatment with calcitriol. Advice on nutrition and sun exposure, discontinuation of offending drugs, adherence to a gluten-free diet, and pancreatic enzyme replacement may cure the mineralization defect in mild cases without the need for additional treatment.

Patients with severe disease usually require vitamin D and calcium supplementation. Replacement doses depend on the serum 25-hydroxyvitamin D level, as shown in Table 252-2. Because pharmacologic doses of any vitamin D preparation carry the risk for vitamin D intoxication, increases in the dose must be made carefully. The interval between increments in dosage should be at least the time required to reach maximal effects plus about 50%. However, experience with the doses given in Table 252-2 indicates that serum 25-hydroxyvitamin D levels rarely reach 80 to 100 ng/mL. Vitamin D intoxication is unlikely even with of levels of 100 to 110 ng/mL. The goal is to raise the serum 25-hydoxyvitamin D level well above 30 ng/mL and restore the elevated parathyroid hormone concentration to normal without hypercalcemia or hypercalciuria. Urinary calcium excretion should be monitored when treatment has normalized the serum calcium level. The urinary calcium-to-creatinine ratio (mg/mg) should be kept below 0.22. Approximately 1 to 1.5 g per day of oral elemental calcium is a reasonable initial dose. Frequent small doses (three times a day) are more effective and tolerable than fewer larger ones, and the absorbability of calcium supplements is enhanced with meals. Most patients do well with the calcium preparations used for osteoporosis, such as calcium carbonate (40% calcium as in Os-Cal or the equivalent) or calcium citrate (21% calcium as in Caltrate or the equivalent). Some patients who cannot tolerate calcium carbonate or citrate experience fewer adverse gastrointestinal symptoms with the use of the chocolate- or coffee-flavored formulations known as Viactiv (500 mg calcium per tablet). The vitamin D content of these calcium supplements is trivial in the treatment of osteomalacia.

In patients with malabsorption, vitamin D requirements may increase during periods of increased diarrhea, and calcitriol may be easier for these patients to absorb. Its rapid onset of action and disappearance after cessation add to the safety of treatment, albeit at far greater cost. Calcium, phosphorus, potassium, magnesium, multivitamins, and gonadal steroids may also be beneficial in patients with malabsorption. Some patients do not tolerate any form of oral vitamin D, and the parenteral ergocalciferol preparations in North America are ineffective. These patients can be improved, although not restored to normal, by the use of weekly tanning bed treatments to areas of their bodies not normally exposed to the sun, with an attempt to minimize solar-induced skin cancer. Calcitriol is the drug of choice in patients with the autosomal recessive disease vitamin D–dependent rickets type I, in which the 1α-hydroxylase enzyme necessary to convert 25-hydroxyvitamin D to 1,25-dihydroxyvitamin D is deficient. In vitamin D–dependent rickets type II, another rare autosomal recessive disease presenting with alopecia, diminished target sensitivity to 1,25-dihydroxyvitamin D may require extraordinarily high doses of calcitriol. If oral treatment fails, nocturnal infusions of calcium and phosphorus have been successful, providing additional evidence that the osteomalacia is due to inadequate calcium and phosphorus rather than from the defect in vitamin D metabolism.

An increase in the serum alkaline phosphatase activity (the healing "flare") and a small increase in the serum and urine calcium levels are the earliest signs of effective treatment. Thereafter, the serum alkaline phosphatase activity level falls progressively as healing occurs. At the start of therapy, serum calcium levels should be measured at weekly intervals. If hypoalbuminemia is present, serum ionized calcium determinations are more useful. When therapy appears stabilized, biweekly or monthly intervals are usually sufficient for the first 3 or 4 months, but even with long-term therapy, measurements should be at least three times a year. In some patients with severe osteomalacia, bone pain and paresthesias may increase and the serum calcium levels decrease during the first few weeks of therapy. This is due to the increased skeletal avidity for mineral during healing and indicates the need for additional calcium supplementation.

Osteomalacia Due to Hypophosphatemia

Therapy of chronic hypophosphatemia is aimed at maintaining normal concentrations of serum phosphorus without inducing secondary hyperparathyroidism or nephrocalcinosis. This considerably difficult task requires divided doses of phosphorus supplements (1 to 3 g/day) and calcitriol (1 to 4 μg/day) to increase the absorption of phosphorus and calcium to prevent the increase in parathyroid hormone. If phosphorus-induced secondary

hyperparathyroidism develops, the phosphorus supplements are rapidly excreted, and therapy not only is futile but also causes the additional bone disease of hyperparathyroidism (Chapter 253). Baseline and yearly renal ultrasound examinations are necessary to recognize early nephrocalcinosis or nephrolithiasis.

A rare form of acquired hypophosphatemic osteomalacia is called oncogenic osteomalacia. This disorder is associated with a variety of small, hard to find mesenchymal tumors that secrete phosphaturic proteins. Fibroblast growth factor 23 (FGF23) is the most frequently documented protein, but others are also incriminated. The muscle pain, weakness, fractures, and osteomalacia characteristic of this syndrome are due to hypophosphatemia made worse by inappropriately low levels of 1,25-dihydroxyvitamin D. Oncogenic osteomalacia is also treated with phosphorus supplementation and calcitriol until the offending tumor can be located and resected. Surgical correction of deformities should be postponed until medical management achieves persistently normal levels of calcium, phosphorus, and alkaline phosphatase activity. An exception to this rule is an acute fracture of the femoral neck. Prompt surgical repair may be essential to avoid osteonecrosis. In addition to the X-linked form of hypophosphatemia, adult hypophosphatemia may also occur sporadically, but a search for an offending mesenchymal tumor is still indicated. Antacid-induced hypophosphatemia due to the ingestion of large quantities of phosphate-binding antacids has become rare with the increased availability of proton pump inhibitors but still occurs occasionally.

PREVENTION

Advice about vitamin D supplementation should help to prevent osteomalacia caused by vitamin D deficiency, but this has proved to be difficult because routine supplements may be inadequate and compliance with nutritional supplements is poor. The optimal vitamin D supplementation dosage is not clear, but most bone and mineral problems are avoided by 50,000 units of ergocalciferol given once monthly. Notable exceptions occur in patients with celiac disease, gastric surgery, or bypass for obesity, who often require much larger amounts (see Table 252-2). In patients with osteomalacia due to hypophosphatemia, the need for phosphorus supplementation may be lifelong (Table 252-3). Exceptions occur in oncogenic osteomalacia when surgical removal of the tumor is accomplished.

TABLE 252-2 VITAMIN D PREPARATIONS FOR TREATMENT OF OSTEOMALACIA

	VITAMIN D₂ (ERGOCALCIFEROL)	CALCITRIOL [1,25(OH)₂D₃]
Trade name (generic name)	Drisdol (ergocalciferol)*	Rocaltrol (calcitriol)
Dosage form	Caps: 50,000 U = 1.25 mg	Caps: 0.25 and 0.50 μg
Dosage:		0.50-2.0 μg/day
If 25(OH)D = 20 to 30 ng/mL	50,000 once a week × 10 weeks† and once a month thereafter	
If 25(OH)D = 10 to 20 ng/mL	50,000 twice a week × 10 weeks† and twice a month thereafter	
If 25(OH)D = less than 10 ng/mL	50,000 three times a week × 10 weeks† and three times a month thereafter	
Dosage in resistant cases	Up to 50,000 units per day	5-20 μg/day
Time to reach maximal effects	4-10 weeks	3-7 days
Persistence of effects after cessation	6-30 weeks	3-7 days
Cost	$150/100 capsules of 50,000 units	$130/100 capsules of 0.25 μg $150/100 capsules of 0.5 μg

*The soft, gel capsule formulations are best because the hard, coated tablet preparations are unreliable.
†If not >30 ng/mL after 10 weeks, exclude malabsorption, gluten enteropathy, and noncompliance. Weekly tanning bed treatments may be used if oral vitamin therapy fails, or a switch to the more costly calcitriol may be necessary.
25(OH)D = 25-hydroxyvitamin D.

TABLE 252-3 PHOSPHATE PREPARATIONS FOR TREATMENT OF OSTEOMALACIA

PREPARATION	SODIUM CONTENT (mEq)	POTASSIUM CONTENT (mEq)	AMOUNT THAT CONTAINS 1 GRAM OF ELEMENTAL PHOSPHORUS
Neutra-Phos	28.5	28.5	4 unit dose caps*
Neutra-Phos-K	—	57.0	4 unit dose caps*
K-Phos Neutral	50.4	4.6	4 tabs
K-Phos Original	—	33.0	9 tabs

*Each unit dose cap is reconstituted with 75 mL of water, fruit juice, or cola. The unit dose cap contains the powder concentrate and is not to be swallowed undiluted.

PROGNOSIS

The response to appropriate treatment in most forms of osteomalacia is usually excellent. Improvements in bone pain and muscle weakness usually occur within 2 or 3 months and healing of skeletal lesions within 6 to 18 months. Depending on the quantity of excess osteoid, repeat bone mineral density determinations may show as much as 20% gains at the lumbar spine and total proximal femur. However, bone density at the radial diaphysis may not improve owing to the irreversible loss of cortical bone resulting from prolonged secondary hyperparathyroidism. Furthermore, if decreased bone volume is present in addition to excess osteoid, skeletal recovery may be incomplete, and the risk for fractures remains increased.

SUGGESTED READINGS

Bhan A, Rao AD, Rao DS. Osteomalacia as a result of vitamin D deficiency. *Endocrinol Metab Clin North Am.* 2010;39:321-331. *Review noting increase in nutritional causes and need for aggressive vitamin D repletion.*

Binkley N, Ramamurthy R, Krueger D. Low vitamin D status: definition, prevalence, consequences, and correction. *Endocrinol Metab Clin North Am.* 2010;39:287-301. *Review.*

Farrow EG, White KE. Tumor-induced osteomalacia. *Expert Rev Endocrinol Metab.* 2009;4:435-442. *Emphasizes the role of renal phosphate wasting, typlically owing to phosphatonins produced by mesenchymal tumors.*

Gifre L, Peris P, Monegal A, et al. Osteomalacia revisited: a report on 28 cases. *Clin Rheumatol.* 2011;30:639-645. *Of 28 patients, 13 had vitamin D deficiency and 15 had hypophosphatemia; the main symptom was polyarthralgias (89%), and 75% of patients had fractures.*

Quarles LD. Endocrine functions of bone in mineral metabolism regulation. *J Clin Invest.* 2008;118:3820-3828. *A review of new signaling pathways for phosphate excretion and vitamin D metabolism.*

Rosen CJ. Clinical practice: vitamin D insufficiency. *N Engl J Med.* 2011;364:248-254. *Practical review.*

Russell LA. Osteoporosis and osteomalacia. *Rheum Dis Clin North Am.* 2010;36:665-680. *Comprehensive review.*

253

THE PARATHYROID GLANDS, HYPERCALCEMIA, AND HYPOCALCEMIA

JOHN J. WYSOLMERSKI AND KARL L. INSOGNA

CALCIUM AND CALCIUM METABOLISM

Calcium serves two principal physiologic functions. First, insoluble calcium salts (primarily hydroxyapatite) provide the structural characteristics that allow bones to protect internal organs, to bear weight, and to function as the levers on which muscles act during locomotion. Second, soluble calcium ions in the extracellular fluid (ECF) and cytosol are critical for myriad biochemical reactions, signaling cascades, and electrical systems that are necessary for life. An adult human contains about 1000 g of calcium, the majority of which (≈99%) is found in bone. Approximately 1% of total body calcium is contained within the ECF and soft tissues. Therefore, the skeleton is called on as a source of calcium when the ECF concentration falls, and it acts as a storehouse for excess calcium. Of the total circulating calcium, the ionized fraction

is 50%; the remainder is bound to serum proteins, primarily albumin, and, to a lesser extent, is complexed with anions such as citrate or sulfate. Only the ionized fraction is physiologically important, and this component is regulated on a minute-to-minute basis. Although it is possible to measure ionized calcium, the specimen must usually be obtained anaerobically and analyzed promptly. Therefore, total serum calcium is often used as an indirect assessment of the ionized calcium fraction.

A complicated homeostatic system involving multiple organs and several hormones regulates both the calcium concentration of the ECF and the calcium content of the skeleton. The organs involved in the regulation of calcium metabolism are the parathyroid glands, kidneys, skeleton, and gut. The hormones include parathyroid hormone (PTH), vitamin D, and PTH-related protein (PTHrP). Abnormalities in these organs, the hormones, or their receptors can cause disturbances in calcium metabolism and lead to hypercalcemia or hypocalcemia. In this chapter, we review calcium homeostasis in humans and then discuss the most common causes of hypercalcemia and hypocalcemia.

Calcium Homeostasis

Parathyroid Glands and Parathyroid Hormone

The four parathyroid glands are located in the neck. The pair of glands located at the upper poles of the thyroid is derived from the fourth branchial pouch, whereas those located at the lower poles migrate downward from the third branchial pouch, along with the thymus gland. Extra parathyroids or parathyroid glands in aberrant locations are not uncommon, especially along the path of embryologic migration.

The parathyroid glands make PTH, an 84–amino acid protein. PTH is synthesized initially as a single-chain, pre-proparathyroid peptide. The 25-residue presequence is cleaved twice to generate the mature, 84–amino acid, full-length protein (PTH 1–84). Full-length PTH is the biologically active form of the hormone. It has a very short half-life (minutes) in the circulation and is degraded by the liver and kidney. This degradative process releases carboxy-terminal (C-terminal) fragments of PTH into the circulation. In addition, in response to hypercalcemia, proteases found within parathyroid secretory granules digest the amino-terminal portion of PTH, and these inactive C-terminal fragments are secreted. Therefore, the concentration of circulating inactive C-terminal species is a product of both parathyroid cell secretion and peripheral metabolism of full-length PTH. These fragments accumulate in the circulation in renal failure.

PTH secretion is regulated by the extracellular ionized calcium concentration. A steep inverse sigmoidal relationship exists between PTH secretion and calcium concentration, which can be defined by four parameters (Fig. 253-1). The steep part of this curve encompasses the physiologic range for extracellular calcium, over which small changes in the concentration of ionized calcium elicit large changes in the rate of PTH secretion.

For parathyroid cells to regulate PTH secretion, they must sense changes in extracellular calcium concentration. This is accomplished through a G protein–coupled receptor (GPCR) known as the *calcium-sensing receptor* (CaR). Calcium binding to the CaR activates downstream signaling pathways (primarily the induction of phospholipases and intracellular calcium transients). This process, in turn, suppresses PTH secretion. If calcium levels are persistently elevated, activation of this receptor also reduces PTH messenger RNA levels and inhibits parathyroid cell proliferation. In addition to parathyroid cells, the CaR is prominently expressed in the kidney, where it regulates calcium handling by the renal tubules. Hypercalcemia activates the CaR, suppressing renal calcium reabsorption. In this way, hypercalcemia directly promotes the excretion of calcium in the urine, and hypocalcemia directly enhances its reabsorption.

The actions of PTH are mediated by the type 1 PTH/PTHrP receptor (PTH1R). The calcium-regulating effects of the receptor appear to be primarily the result of activation of adenylyl cyclase. During usual conditions, this receptor is activated equally well by the amino-terminal portions of PTH and PTHrP (see later). The PTH1R is most abundant in bone and kidney, where it mediates the systemic functions of PTH. However, PTH1R is also expressed in many other cells in the body, where it serves as a PTHrP receptor. In this capacity, PTH1R has important functions during bone and mammary development and mediates many of PTHrP's effects on cellular proliferation, apoptosis, and differentiation (see later).

PTH exerts direct effects on kidney and bone cells and indirect effects on enterocytes. The integrated action of PTH on these organs results in an increase of ionized calcium. In the kidney, PTH has three principal effects.

FIGURE 253-1. Regulation of parathyroid hormone (PTH) secretion in response to changes in extracellular calcium. **A,** PTH secretion by dispersed normal human parathyroid cells in culture in response to varying concentrations of extracellular calcium. **B,** The four-parameter model describing the inverse sigmoidal relationship between extracellular calcium and PTH secretion. Parameter 1 is the maximal secretory rate, parameter 2 is the slope of the curve at the midpoint, parameter 3 is the set point, and parameter 4 is the minimum secretory rate. (From Brenner BM, Stein H. Divalent ion homeostasis. *Contemp Issues Nephrol.* 1997;2:479-499.)

First, it acts on proximal tubular cells to inhibit the reabsorption of phosphate. Phosphate transport depends on the actions of sodium-phosphate cotransporters 2a and 2c (NPT2a, NPT2c), which are located in the luminal membranes of proximal tubular cells. PTH acts to inhibit phosphate reabsorption by causing NPT2a and NPT2c to be removed from the luminal membrane and degraded. Second, PTH stimulates the activity of renal 1α-hydroxylase in proximal tubular cells. This leads to the formation of biologically active 1,25(OH)$_2$ vitamin D from its circulating precursor 25(OH) vitamin D. PTH also inhibits 24-hydroxylase, thus preventing the formation of the inactive metabolite 24,25(OH)$_2$ vitamin D. Both these actions increase the circulating concentrations of 1,25(OH)$_2$ vitamin D, an increase that stimulates intestinal calcium absorption. Finally, PTH acts to increase the reabsorption of calcium by the kidney. The majority of calcium is reclaimed from the glomerular filtrate in the proximal tubule through a PTH-independent paracellular process linked to the reabsorption of sodium. PTH helps promote some calcium reabsorption in the cortical thick ascending loop of Henle by increasing the net positive charge on the luminal side of the tubule, which enhances paracellular calcium and magnesium reabsorption. The distal tubule is the primary target of PTH's actions to promote calcium transport. In these cells, PTH leads to the insertion of calcium channels into the apical membrane of the cell and stimulates the activity of basolateral sodium-calcium exchangers. The net result is to stimulate directional, transcellular calcium transport from the tubule lumen, across the cell, and into the ECF.

In the skeleton, PTH activates bone turnover and liberates stored calcium. The immediate action of PTH is to stimulate the transport of calcium across bone lining cells from an easily mobilized pool of calcium at the surface of bone. A more delayed action of PTH is to increase the number and activity of bone-forming osteoblasts and bone-resorbing osteoclasts. PTH acts directly on cells within the osteoblast lineage. Overall, in vivo, PTH increases the size of the osteoblast precursor pool and increases the bone-forming activity of mature osteoblasts. PTH acts indirectly on osteoclasts. The hormone stimulates osteoblasts to release cytokines, such as colony-stimulating factor 1 and receptor activator of nuclear factor-κB (NF-κB) ligand (RANKL), which stimulate the formation of new osteoclasts and activate mature osteoclasts. PTH also inhibits osteoblast production of osteoprotegerin, a soluble decoy receptor for RANKL that inhibits osteoclast development. Through mechanisms that are still not entirely understood, persistent elevations of PTH increase osteoclast activity more than osteoblast activity, whereas intermittent elevations in PTH do the opposite, stimulating osteoblasts more than osteoclasts. As a result, continuous exposure to PTH causes net bone resorption, and intermittent exposure to PTH causes net bone formation.

Vitamin D

In response to ultraviolet light, keratinocytes in the epidermis convert 7-dehydrocholesterol, the immediate precursor of cholesterol, into vitamin D$_3$. Cutaneous production of vitamin D$_3$ is affected by a variety of factors such as latitude, season, use of sunscreen, concentration of melanin, and type of clothing, all of which vary the amount of ultraviolet light that penetrates the skin. Aging also reduces the ability of the skin to synthesize vitamin D. Most foods contain little vitamin D, although some is found in oily fish and in fish liver oils. In the United States, vitamin D is also found in fortified foods, including certain cereals, milk, and bread. Given these restrictions on its production and availability, vitamin D deficiency is very common in the winter months in elderly populations living at higher latitudes.

Vitamin D$_3$ produced in the skin is biologically inert and must be hydroxylated in two successive steps to become active. The first hydroxylation is performed in the liver by vitamin D 25-hydroxylase and generates 25-hydroxyvitamin D$_3$. This has little biologic activity, but it is metabolized by cells in the proximal renal tubule to form the active hormone 1,25(OH)$_2$ vitamin D$_3$. The 25(OH)D-1α-hydroxylase (1α-hydroxylase) enzyme catalyzes this final hydroxylation step. PTH stimulates the activity of renal 1α-hydroxylase. This enzyme is also stimulated by phosphate and is inhibited by hypercalcemia. Although renal conversion of 25(OH)D to 1,25(OH)$_2$ vitamin D is the reaction most relevant to calcium homeostasis, it is worth noting that this reaction occurs in other tissues and cells in the body, such as macrophages, where 1,25(OH)$_2$ vitamin D may serve different roles.

Vitamin D is a steroid hormone that interacts with specific nuclear receptors to regulate gene expression. The vitamin D receptor is a member of the steroid hormone receptor family of ligand-binding transcription factors. It heterodimerizes with the retinoic acid X receptor, and, in the presence of 1,25(OH)$_2$ vitamin D, the vitamin D receptor–retinoic acid X receptor complex binds to specific DNA recognition sequences within target genes. The main function of 1,25(OH)$_2$ vitamin D is to support the circulating calcium concentration through two actions. The first is to stimulate calcium absorption from the gut lumen by enterocytes. The active vitamin D metabolite stimulates the expression of calcium channels within intestinal cells that allow calcium to enter the apical surface of the cell. It also enhances the production of proteins that shuttle calcium through the cytoplasm and stimulates the activity of calcium pumps that extrude calcium across the basolateral membrane of the cells. These functions enhance the transcellular transport of calcium across enterocytes. Vitamin D also enhances paracellular calcium absorption by the gut. In addition to calcium, vitamin D stimulates the absorption of phosphorus from the diet. The second important action of 1,25(OH)$_2$ vitamin D in calcium homeostasis is to increase bone resorption by stimulating osteoblastic production of RANKL. This latter effect is clinically important only when production of 1,25(OH)$_2$ vitamin D is elevated to pathologic levels.

Parathyroid Hormone–Related Protein

PTHrP was discovered in the course of studies exploring the pathogenesis of humoral hypercalcemia of malignancy (see later). In humans, the gene is located on chromosome 12. The PTH and PTHrP genes share structural features that suggest they arose from a common ancestor. In particular, of the first 13 amino-terminal amino acids in each protein, 8 are identical; after this, the sequences of the two proteins diverge. The amino-terminal homology allows both PTH and PTHrP to bind to PTH1R with equal affinity and to activate the same signaling pathways. PTH is made only in the parathyroid glands, is secreted into the systemic circulation, and activates PTH1R in bone and kidney to regulate calcium metabolism. In contrast, PTHrP is made in a variety of cell types, is secreted locally, and acts in a paracrine or autocrine fashion to activate PTH1R on neighboring cells. Important sites of action include developing cartilage, bone, breast tissue, and various types of smooth muscle. During lactation, PTHrP is secreted by the breast into the circulation and acts like PTH to regulate systemic calcium metabolism.

Integrated Regulation of Calcium Metabolism

Hormones and organ systems coordinate to regulate the ECF ionized calcium concentration such that it is maintained within a very narrow physiologic range. As illustrated in Figure 253-2, if the calcium level falls below the physiologic range, PTH is rapidly secreted from the parathyroid glands and activates the release of calcium and phosphate from the skeleton. In the kidney, PTH increases the reabsorption of calcium from the urine while simultaneously inhibiting phosphate reabsorption to dispose of the phosphate released from the skeleton. This process prevents serum phosphate from rising, an action that would otherwise inhibit a rise in serum calcium by inducing the precipitation of calcium phosphate salts in soft tissues. In addition, alterations in CaR signaling within the kidney activate calcium reabsorption independent of changes in PTH. Combined, these actions return the calcium concentration back toward normal, thus inhibiting further PTH release. When hypocalcemia persists, PTH also stimulates the renal production of 1,25(OH)$_2$ vitamin D, which increases intestinal calcium absorption. In the presence of hypercalcemia, PTH secretion is suppressed, and the various organs alter their calcium handling in an opposite fashion so circulating calcium levels fall. Data in animals suggest that CaR-mediated calcium

excretion by renal tubules may be a particularly important defense against hypercalcemia.

HYPERCALCEMIA

PATHOBIOLOGY

The long list of potential causes of hypercalcemia is provided in Table 253-1. However, most cases of hypercalcemia (>90%) are caused by either primary hyperparathyroidism or malignancy-associated hypercalcemia (MAHC). These two diseases, along with a few others, are discussed in detail. Several of the less common causes of hypercalcemia are worth noting briefly. First, abnormalities in serum proteins and severe thrombocytosis (platelet count >700,000) can cause pseudohypercalcemia, defined as elevations in total calcium without elevations in ionized calcium. Several endocrine disorders, including thyrotoxicosis, pheochromocytoma, adrenal insufficiency, and islet cell tumors of the pancreas, can manifest with mild to moderate hypercalcemia. An increasingly common cause of hypercalcemia is the milk-alkali syndrome. Patients with this disorder present with a triad of hypercalcemia, systemic alkalosis, and renal insufficiency associated with the ingestion of large amounts of calcium and absorbable alkali. The disorder was originally described in the 1930s as a complication of the treatment of peptic ulcer disease, but in its modern form, it is associated with the ingestion of calcium carbonate for the treatment or prevention of osteoporosis. In some patients, this syndrome can be precipitated by the daily intake of as little as 2 g of calcium. Immobilization uncouples bone turnover by inhibiting bone formation. Thus, in patients with elevated rates of bone resorption, immobilization can worsen or precipitate hypercalcemia. Patients at greatest risk include adolescents with physiologic elevations in bone turnover and patients with preexisting Paget's disease (Chapter 255) or subtle primary

FIGURE 253-2. Homeostatic response to a fall in serum calcium (Ca^{2+}). Pi = inorganic phosphate; PTH = parathyroid hormone.

TABLE 253-1 CAUSES OF HYPERCALCEMIA IN ADULTS

HYPERPARATHYROIDISM
Adenoma
Hyperplasia
Carcinoma
Familial hypocalciuric hypercalcemia
Tertiary hyperparathyroidism of renal failure

MALIGNANCY-ASSOCIATED HYPERCALCEMIA
Humoral hypercalcemia of malignancy
Local osteolytic hypercalcemia

GRANULOMATOUS DISORDERS
Tuberculosis
Leprosy
Cryptococcosis
Histoplasmosis
Cytomegalovirus infection
Sarcoidosis
Wegener's granulomatosis

ENDOCRINE DISORDERS
Hyperthyroidism
Adrenal insufficiency
Pheochromocytoma
Vasoactive intestinal polypeptide tumor (VIPoma)

MEDICATIONS
Vitamin D preparations
Thiazides
Lithium
Aminophylline
Vitamin A
Tamoxifen
Total parenteral nutrition

MISCELLANEOUS CAUSES
Milk-alkali syndrome
Immobilization
Aluminum toxicity
Acute renal failure
Rhabdomyolysis (recovery phase)
Systemic lupus erythematosus
Breast hyperplasia

hyperparathyroidism. Finally, several medications other than calcium carbonate can cause hypercalcemia. The most commonly implicated drugs include thiazide diuretics, lithium carbonate, and vitamin D preparations. Several well-documented episodes of vitamin D intoxication have been caused by errors in the fortification of dairy products or the preparation of dietary supplements.

CLINICAL MANIFESTATIONS

Patients with mild hypercalcemia (<1 mg/dL above normal) are usually asymptomatic unless they have concomitant cerebral dysfunction. The likelihood of developing symptoms from hypercalcemia is related to both the degree of elevation in serum calcium and the rapidity with which the calcium level rises. When present, symptoms are caused by dehydration secondary to urinary losses of calcium, water, and other electrolytes and to an increase in membrane potential caused by the elevation in ECF ionized calcium concentration. Dehydration develops because an increase in the filtered load of calcium leads to variable degrees of hypercalciuria. Loss of calcium in the urine obligates the loss of anions and water. In addition, hypercalcemia causes nephrogenic diabetes insipidus because stimulation of the CaR in the collecting ducts of the kidney interferes with the trafficking of aquaporin water channels in response to vasopressin. Consequently, patients with hypercalcemia frequently report symptoms of polyuria and polydipsia. If significant dehydration ensues, hypercalcemia can worsen quickly because any impairment of glomerular filtration reduces the ability of the kidneys to excrete excess calcium. Patients with moderate to severe hypercalcemia often complain of nausea and vomiting, symptoms likely related to dehydration as well as to the effects of hypercalcemia on central nervous system function. Because hypercalcemia tends to hyperpolarize membranes, a range of neurologic and neuromuscular signs and symptoms can occur. Patients with mild hypercalcemia often complain of fatigue, depressed affect, and asthenia. With further increases in serum calcium, these complaints progress to impaired concentration and memory, difficulty with cognitive function, stupor, and coma. Muscle weakness can be seen, which occasionally progresses to flaccid paralysis if hypercalcemia becomes severe. Gastrointestinal motility is impaired; this commonly results in constipation and likely contributes to nausea and

vomiting. Occasionally, pancreatitis can be the cause of abdominal pain in patients with hypercalcemia. Finally, cardiovascular function can be impaired, as manifested by bradycardia and sensitivity to the effects of digitalis. Electrocardiographic changes include shortening of the QT interval, varying degrees of atrioventricular block, and bradyarrhythmias and tachyarrhythmias.

DIAGNOSIS

As noted previously, most patients with hypercalcemia have either hyperparathyroidism or MAHC (Fig. 253-3). If the patient has hyperproteinemia or hypoproteinemia, or if the platelet count is markedly elevated, hypercalcemia should be confirmed by measuring the serum ionized calcium concentration. Otherwise, the first test should be a serum intact PTH level. Elevated PTH in the presence of hypercalcemia establishes the diagnosis of hyperparathyroidism. If PTH levels are suppressed and the patient has a known malignant disease, the diagnosis of MAHC is entertained. If the patient has a suppressed PTH level in the absence of a known malignant disease, the serum PTHrP level should be measured, and a careful screen for occult malignant disease should be performed. If the PTHrP level is normal in this setting, a careful history of prescription and over-the-counter medications should be taken, and laboratory tests to investigate other causes of hypercalcemia should be performed.

Primary Hyperparathyroidism

DEFINITION

Primary hyperparathyroidism is a disorder of calcium metabolism caused by the overproduction of PTH by the parathyroid glands. It is therefore characterized by simultaneous elevations in both circulating PTH and calcium levels.

EPIDEMIOLOGY

Historically, hyperparathyroidism was thought to be a rare disorder associated with severe complications. However, with the introduction of routine serum calcium measurements in the 1970s, it was recognized that many

FIGURE 253-3. Algorithmic approach to the diagnosis of hypercalcemia. PTH = parathyroid hormone; PTHrP = PTH-related protein; vit = vitamin.

patients had milder forms of the disease. The incidence of hyperparathyroidism is currently estimated to be between 1 in 500 and 1 in 1000 persons. After age 50 years, women are more frequently affected than men; the female-to-male ratio in that age group is 3:1. Although hyperparathyroidism can manifest at any age, it is more common in older individuals, and the peak incidence is in the sixth decade. Typically, hyperparathyroidism occurs sporadically, but in a few patients it is part of a familial syndrome. Apart from these genetic disorders, the only other known risk factor is exposure to external neck irradiation during childhood.

PATHOBIOLOGY

In 80 to 85% of cases, hyperparathyroidism is caused by a solitary adenoma arising in one of the four parathyroid glands. These adenomas are benign, clonal neoplasms of parathyroid chief cells that tend to remain remarkably stable in size once they become clinically apparent. Although the molecular origins of parathyroid adenomas are only partly understood, these tumors presumably arise from somatic mutations in a single cell. Approximately 20 to 40% of adenomas have been reported to overexpress cyclin D1, a cell-cycle regulatory protein that can act as a dominant oncogene. An additional 25 to 30% of sporadic adenomas reportedly have somatic mutations in the multiple endocrine neoplasia 1 (MEN1; menin) tumor suppressor gene on chromosome 11 (Chapter 239). Approximately 15% of patients with hyperparathyroidism have diffuse enlargement of all four parathyroid glands caused by chief cell hyperplasia. The most common cause of four-gland hyperplasia is long-standing renal failure, which leads to chronic hypocalcemia, hyperphosphatemia, and low serum $1,25(OH)_2$ vitamin D levels, all of which stimulate parathyroid cell growth. This hyperplasia can eventually lead to hypercalcemia, so-called tertiary hyperparathyroidism. Most cases of inherited parathyroid hyperplasia result from one of the two MEN syndromes (Chapter 239). Hyperparathyroidism is a prominent feature of the MEN 1 syndrome (Chapter 239), which is caused by mutations in the menin gene, a tumor suppressor. In contrast, hyperparathyroidism associated with the MEN 2 syndrome (Chapters 239 and 254) is usually mild and occurs in fewer affected individuals. MEN 2 is caused by mutations in the ret proto-oncogene. Both syndromes have an autosomal dominant mode of inheritance. Hyperplasia in these syndromes can be asynchronous, with unequal enlargement of the individual glands over time, giving the misimpression of single-gland disease. Approximately 0.5% of all patients with hyperparathyroidism have parathyroid carcinoma. Typically, these patients have severe hypercalcemia and hyperparathyroidism that recurs following initial therapy. It can be very difficult to distinguish a parathyroid carcinoma from an adenoma by pathologic evaluation alone, but local tissue invasion, local lymph node involvement, and the presence of mitotic figures are clues to the diagnosis. Parathyroid carcinoma occurs with increased frequency in a rare genetic syndrome known as hyperparathyroid jaw-tumor syndrome, which is characterized by primary hyperparathyroidism in association with mesenchymal tumors of the mandible. This syndrome is caused by mutations in the gene encoding the tumor suppressor parafibromin; mutations in this gene may also cause a significant proportion of sporadic cases of parathyroid carcinoma.

CLINICAL MANIFESTATIONS

The presentation of hyperparathyroidism includes the characteristic symptoms of hypercalcemia combined with the variable occurrence of skeletal and renal complications. Hypercalcemia is caused by the chronic overproduction of PTH by the abnormal parathyroid cells. An important component of this abnormal secretion is a shift of the set point and slope of the calcium-PTH response curve; that is, adenoma cells become less sensitive to calcium's ability to suppress PTH production. Parathyroid adenomas still respond to calcium, but only at higher ambient levels of the ion, resulting in the establishment of a new equilibrium at abnormally high levels of calcium and PTH.

The most common complication of hyperparathyroidism besides hypercalcemia is nephrolithiasis. Approximately 20% of patients present with kidney stones. Nephrocalcinosis, which is the diffuse deposition of calcium phosphate complexes in the renal parenchyma, is seen less commonly. The most common stone type is calcium oxalate. However, stones of mixed chemical composition (calcium oxalate and calcium phosphate) are often observed. The risk factors for stone disease in patients with hyperparathyroidism are hypercalciuria (calcium excretion >4 mg/kg lean body weight over 24 hours) and a tendency to waste bicarbonate, which leads to a relatively alkaline urine. Precipitation of calcium phosphate is favored in an alkaline urine. Whether mild hyperparathyroidism directly impairs renal function is unclear. In the

majority of patients with this disease followed conservatively, renal function remains stable.

The classic skeletal presentation of hyperparathyroidism is osteitis fibrosa cystica, which is defined as the combination of subperiosteal bone resorption, especially in the distal phalanges and skull; bone cysts; brown tumors of the long bones; osteoporosis; and fractures. This form of bone disease is now uncommon, occurring in less than 5% of patients. However, more than 50% of otherwise asymptomatic patients with hyperparathyroidism eventually develop progressive bone loss and are at risk for osteoporosis. Thus, bone mineral density should be measured in all patients with hyperparathyroidism. Cortical bone is more sensitive to the effects of hyperparathyroidism, so bone mineral density in the distal forearm and hip is typically more severely affected than is bone mineral density in the spine.

Patients with severe hyperparathyroidism can develop muscle weakness and myopathy. Patients with mild disease often complain of weakness, fatigue, listlessness, and trouble concentrating. However, the specificity and origin of these symptoms are debated. Occasionally, patients with hyperparathyroidism develop acute or subacute monarticular inflammatory arthritis resulting from calcium pyrophosphate dihydrate crystal arthropathy. Finally, some reports suggest that patients with hyperparathyroidism have excess body fat, are insulin resistant, and suffer from an increased incidence of cardiovascular events. Serum levels of the inflammatory cytokine interleukin-6 (IL-6), which has been linked to insulin resistance and adverse cardiac outcomes, are elevated in patients with hyperparathyroidism. Thus, it is possible that IL-6 provides a pathogenic link between hyperparathyroidism and these complications.

DIAGNOSIS

The diagnosis of hyperparathyroidism is made by documenting simultaneous elevations in the circulating levels of calcium and PTH in a patient with normal renal function. If abnormalities of serum proteins are noted, it may be necessary to measure ionized calcium to be certain that hypercalcemia is present. Again, C-terminal fragments of PTH are excreted by the kidney and may accumulate in renal failure. Historically, this was a problem in assays that used antisera directed at the mid-region or C-terminal portions of PTH and therefore gave falsely elevated results in patients with renal insufficiency. Newer, "biointact" PTH assays avoid this problem and should be used to measure PTH in any patient with abnormal renal function. Patients with hyperparathyroidism also may have slightly low or low-normal serum phosphorus concentrations and mild hyperchloremic metabolic acidosis. Alkaline phosphatase levels may be elevated in patients with overt bone disease.

Once a diagnosis of hyperparathyroidism is made, patients should be screened for end-organ complications. Renal ultrasonography or spiral computed tomography (CT) scans can be used to determine whether the patient has kidney stones. Bone mineral density should be measured to detect skeletal disease, preferably using dual-energy x-ray absorptiometry, at the spine, hip, and wrist. A 24-hour urine collection should be performed to determine whether hypercalciuria is present. Hyperparathyroid myopathy can be diagnosed by electromyography.

TREATMENT   Rx

Surgery is the only curative treatment for hyperparathyroidism. Traditionally, this involved bilateral neck exploration, during which the surgeon identified all four parathyroid glands before resecting the abnormal gland. However, minimally invasive parathyroidectomy has been supplanting traditional neck exploration in referral centers. This requires preoperative localization of the offending adenoma. Technetium-99m-sestamibi scans, ultrasonography, four-dimensional CT scans, and magnetic resonance imaging can all be used as preoperative localization studies; we prefer the first two. If parathyroid hyperplasia is suspected, a minimally invasive approach is not appropriate because the surgeon must remove either three and a half parathyroid glands or all four glands, with autotransplantation of some parathyroid tissue to the forearm. Complications of parathyroid surgery include damage to the recurrent laryngeal nerve and permanent hypoparathyroidism. Activity of the unaffected parathyroid glands is suppressed by the hypercalcemia associated with hyperparathyroidism, and the remaining glands take several days to recover normal secretory activity after removal of an adenoma. This can result in postoperative hypocalcemia in the first 24 to 48 hours. If significant bone disease is present, the influx of calcium into the skeleton as it heals following parathyroid adenomectomy can lengthen the duration and increase the severity of hypocalcemia. This phenomenon is known as the hungry bones syndrome. Operative and postoperative complications are much less frequent when parathyroidectomy is performed by an experienced surgeon. Therefore, patients should be referred to centers that perform this operation frequently.

Many patients with mild hyperparathyroidism are asymptomatic and have no evidence of end-organ damage. In addition, many patients with mild forms of the disease do not develop more severe disease over time. Therefore, not all patients necessarily benefit from surgery. However, concern lingers over the possibility of excess vascular disease in these patients, as well as the subtle neurocognitive effects ascribed to hyperparathyroidism in some studies. In addition, the most recent studies found that up to 59% of initially asymptomatic patients developed a greater than 10% decline in bone mineral density at one or more sites over a 15-year period of observation. Given the ongoing uncertainty about this topic, a group of international experts met for the third time in 2008 to review and update guidelines for parathyroidectomy first formulated by a National Institutes of Health consensus conference in 1990. Table 253-2 lists the criteria for surgery in otherwise asymptomatic patients, and Table 253-3 provides the guidelines for managing nonsurgical patients as suggested by the 2008 international workshop. These guidelines are not rigid, and each patient must be approached with his or her unique circumstances in mind. Studies have demonstrated that most patients who do not meet the criteria for surgery remain stable from the standpoint of biochemical parameters, although many patients develop progressive cortical bone loss after 10 to 15 years of follow-up. Up to 37% of asymptomatic patients eventually develop signs of progressive disease. Therefore, patients who do not undergo surgical treatment should have annual measurements of serum calcium and serum creatinine and bone density measurements every year or every other year. If patients demonstrate worsening of hypercalcemia, deterioration of renal function, or progressive bone loss, they should be referred for surgery.

Medical management of hypercalcemia is discussed further in the Treatment section for Hypercalcemia of Malignancy. Several adjunct medical therapies exist for patients who meet the criteria for surgery but either decline parathyroidectomy or are poor operative candidates. Maintenance of hydration and physical activity are important in all patients. Bisphosphonates and estrogen replacement therapy have been shown to prevent and even reverse, to a limited extent, low bone mass in patients with hyperparathyroidism. Finally, cinacalcet can lower serum calcium levels in patients with primary hyperparathyroidism. This drug is an allosteric activator of CaR and directly inhibits PTH release by parathyroid adenomas. Cinacalcet showed good efficacy in controlling serum calcium in a 1-year randomized clinical trial in patients with this disease. Normalization of serum calcium continued for up to 5 years of therapy in an open-label extension of this trial.[1] However, cinacalcet does not normalize PTH levels or prevent bone loss, so its role in the long-term management of primary hyperparathyroidism remains uncertain.

Hypercalcemia of Malignancy

DEFINITION

The most common cause of elevated calcium levels in hospitalized patients is MAHC. MAHC has two pathophysiologic subgroups: humoral hypercalcemia of malignancy (HHM), which is caused by tumor cell secretion of a bone-resorbing factor (usually PTHrP) into the systemic circulation; and local osteolytic hypercalcemia (LOH), which is caused by localized bone resorption surrounding tumor cells within the skeleton. HHM is also discussed in Chapter 186.

TABLE 253-2	GUIDELINES FOR PARATHYROID SURGERY IN ASYMPTOMATIC PRIMARY HYPERPARATHYROIDISM: THIRD INTERNATIONAL WORKSHOP, 2008

Serum calcium >1.0 mg/dL above upper limit of normal
Reduction of creatinine clearance to <60 mL/min
Bone mineral density T-score <−2.5 at any site and/or previous fragility fracture
Age <50 yr

TABLE 253-3	GUIDELINES FOR MONITORING PATIENTS WITH ASYMPTOMATIC HYPERPARATHYROIDISM NOT MEETING CRITERIA FOR SURGERY: THIRD INTERNATIONAL WORKSHOP, 2008

Measurement of serum calcium annually
Measurement of serum creatinine annually
Measurement of bone density at spine, hip, and forearm every 1-2 yr

EPIDEMIOLOGY

Hypercalcemia, a frequent complication of cancer, occurs in up to 20 to 30% of patients during the course of their malignant disease. MAHC is usually a manifestation of advanced disease, and investigators have estimated that patients with MAHC have a 50% 30-day mortality. HHM is classically associated with squamous cell tumors of the lung, head and neck, esophagus, and cervix; urothelial malignant diseases (both renal cell and transitional cell); and breast cancers. However, almost every tumor type has been reported to secrete PTHrP and to cause HHM. LOH is most frequently diagnosed in patients with multiple myeloma or breast cancer.

PATHOBIOLOGY

The principal cause of hypercalcemia in MAHC is increased bone resorption. In HHM, patients have a generalized increase in osteoclast number and activity, whereas in LOH, osteoclast number and activity are increased only in the vicinity of skeletal metastases. In both instances, hypercalcemia develops when the efflux of calcium from the skeleton exceeds the kidneys' ability to excrete the excess calcium that enters the ECF. Patients with MAHC often suffer from nausea and anorexia and have hypercalcemia-induced polyuria. Therefore, dehydration is an important component of the presentation of all patients with MAHC.

In most cases, HHM is caused by the secretion of PTHrP into the systemic circulation by tumor cells. As noted earlier, PTH and PTHrP bind and activate PTH1R with equal affinity. Thus, when PTHrP gains access to the systemic circulation, it activates the PTH1R in the bone and stimulates bone resorption throughout the skeleton, as occurs in hyperparathyroidism. However, in contradistinction to patients with hyperparathyroidism, patients with HHM have suppressed bone formation. Because no compensatory increase in bone formation occurs, patients with HHM tend to be more severely hypercalcemic than are patients with hyperparathyroidism. Another important biochemical difference between these two diseases is that in HHM, $1,25(OH)_2$ vitamin D levels are either low-normal or low, so intestinal calcium absorption is not increased. Therefore, bone is the main and often the sole source of the excess calcium in this disease.

In LOH, tumor cells within the skeleton secrete various cytokines into the local microenvironment, which recruit new osteoclasts into the area surrounding the tumor cells. This process leads to osteolysis, which releases growth factors from the bone matrix that stimulate the growth of the adjacent tumor cells. This pernicious positive feedback loop sustains the pathologic bone resorption, leads to expansion of the bone metastasis, and can ultimately result in local pain and pathologic fracture. Once the size and number of metastases reach a point at which the amount of calcium released from the skeleton exceeds the kidneys' ability to excrete it, systemic hypercalcemia ensues. Much research has been directed at elucidating the nature of the osteoclast-activating factors secreted by bone metastases. In the case of multiple myeloma, several cytokines, including MIP-1α, transforming growth factor-α, IL-1, IL-3, IL-6, and CD47, have been implicated. More recent work has suggested that myeloma cells also secrete Dickkopf 1 (DKK-1), an inhibitor of the Wnt signaling pathway that suppresses osteoblast activity and bone formation. In the case of breast cancer, local production of PTHrP, IL-8, and IL-11 may be important in mediating osteolysis.

DIAGNOSIS

Patients with HHM typically present with moderate to severe elevations in serum calcium levels, low to low-normal levels of serum phosphorus, low levels of $1,25(OH)_2$ vitamin D, suppressed levels of PTH, and elevated circulating levels of PTHrP. These patients, by definition, have no (or only a few) skeletal metastases. In contrast, patients with LOH have many skeletal metastases. They have moderate to severe hypercalcemia, but they do not have elevations in PTHrP; they also have normal serum phosphorus concentrations. Because MAHC is a late manifestation of malignant disease, the offending tumor is usually clinically obvious, and detailed laboratory investigations are not needed. However, because hyperparathyroidism is common in the general population, it should be ruled out by measuring PTH levels in all hypercalcemic patients, even those with cancer. In patients with suspected HHM, documentation of elevated PTHrP levels confirms the diagnosis. This approach is not needed in all cases, but it can be helpful in patients with unusual tumor types and for the rare occurrence of HHM in association with benign tumors.

TREATMENT

Rehydration is the first step in the acute treatment of MAHC. This often requires the infusion of isotonic saline at rates of 200 to 300 mL/hour, and it should be accompanied by close monitoring of electrolytes and cardiovascular status. Once volume depletion is corrected, treatment with loop diuretics can be initiated to induce natriuresis, which increases renal calcium excretion. Rehydration and forced saline diuresis can result in a lowering of the serum calcium on the order of 1 to 1.5 mg/dL. The only cure for MAHC is successful treatment of the underlying malignant disease; hypercalcemia resolves with successful surgery or chemotherapy. If the tumor cannot be successfully treated, pharmacologic therapy can be used to lower calcium levels transiently. Because the principal cause of MAHC is increased bone resorption, antiresorptive drugs have the greatest efficacy in this condition. Calcitonin is the most rapidly acting antiresorptive agent. It can be given in doses of 4 to 8 IU/kg subcutaneously or intramuscularly every 6 to 12 hours. This treatment can lower serum calcium levels by 1 to 2 mg/dL within several hours, but tachyphylaxis to calcitonin occurs within 24 to 48 hours. Bisphosphonates are now the standard treatment for MAHC. Pamidronate was once the most commonly used medication for this purpose. The intravenous infusion of 60 or 90 mg pamidronate begins to lower serum calcium after 24 to 72 hours, and nadir calcium levels are reached within 5 to 6 days. Up to 70% of patients experience a normalization of calcium levels that can last up to 18 days. More recently, zoledronate has become the treatment of choice. Intravenous infusions of 4 to 8 mg zoledronate result in the normalization of calcium within 3 to 5 days in approximately 90% of patients, with a duration of response up to 32 days. In a head-to-head trial, zoledronate resulted in more rapid and more durable remission of hypercalcemia in patients with MAHC than did pamidronate. The use of a humanized, neutralizing monoclonal antibody to RANKL (denosumab) for the treatment of MAHC is currently under investigation. Dialysis against a calcium-free bath can be useful in patients with MAHC and renal failure or in patients who cannot tolerate bisphosphonates.

TABLE 253-4 CAUSES OF HYPOCALCEMIA

HYPOCALCEMIA RESULTING FROM REDUCED OR ABSENT PTH SECRETION

Surgical damage or destruction of parathyroid glands
Infiltrative diseases and deposition of heavy metals
High-dose radiation
Failure of organogenesis: DiGeorge sequence
Idiopathic hypoparathyroidism
Molecular abnormalities in PTH gene (loss-of-function mutations)
Molecular abnormalities in calcium-sensing receptor gene (gain-of-function mutations)
Autoimmune polyglandular syndrome type 1
Functional defects in PTH secretion

HYPOCALCEMIA RESULTING FROM RESISTANCE TO THE ACTIONS OF PTH

Pseudohypoparathyroidism
Hypomagnesemia

HYPOCALCEMIA IN THE SETTING OF NORMAL OR INCREASED SERUM PTH LEVELS AND NORMAL PTH RECEPTOR FUNCTION

Hypocalcemia induced by hyperphosphatemia
Nutritional vitamin D deficiency
Vitamin D malabsorption
Loss-of-function mutations in 1α-hydroxylase enzyme
Hereditary resistance to 1,25(OH)$_2$ vitamin D
Hypocalcemia resulting from accelerated skeletal mineralization (hungry bones syndrome)
Medical illness (sepsis)
Medications

PTH = parathyroid hormone.

● HYPOCALCEMIA

DEFINITION

Hypocalcemia is defined as an abnormally low serum concentration of ionized calcium.

PATHOBIOLOGY

Hypocalcemia can be caused by abnormalities of PTH availability, result from PTH resistance due to PTH receptor or postreceptor defects, or occur in the setting of normal or increased PTH activity and normal PTH receptor function. A full listing of the causes of hypocalcemia is given in Table 253-4. Selected disorders are discussed in the following subsections.

Hypocalcemia Resulting from Abnormalities of Parathyroid Hormone Availability

Various congenital or acquired disorders can lead to developmental failure of the parathyroid glands, failure of functional hormone production, or destruction of the glands. These disorders all manifest as hypocalcemia, usually with attendant hyperphosphatemia and undetectable or inappropriately low levels of circulating PTH.

Destruction of the Parathyroid Glands

Surgical destruction of the parathyroid glands is the most common cause of hypoparathyroidism. Given the close anatomic relationship of the parathyroid glands with the thyroid, complete or near-complete extirpation of the thyroid gland (Chapter 233) for the management of either Graves' disease or thyroid cancer can be complicated by the destruction or vascular compromise of parathyroid tissue and varying degrees of hypoparathyroidism. Aggressive surgical treatment of head and neck cancer can also cause parathyroid damage. Permanent destruction of the parathyroid glands should be a rare complication of neck surgery; for experienced surgeons, it occurs with a frequency of less than 10%. More common is transient parathyroid dysfunction—so-called stunned parathyroids—which can cause a decline in total serum calcium of 1 mg/dL in the first 24 to 48 hours postoperatively. The presumed cause is temporary vascular compromise or mechanical damage to the glands.

Infiltrative diseases, granulomatous diseases, metastases to the parathyroids, and deposition of heavy metals are all uncommon but recognized causes of parathyroid destruction and hypoparathyroidism. Although the

parathyroid glands are quite resistant to radiation, hypoparathyroidism following radioactive iodine treatment for hyperthyroidism has been described.

Hypomagnesemia

Magnesium is an important cofactor for PTH secretion; it is apparently required for the release of stored hormone from secretory granules. In severe cases of hypomagnesemia (i.e., serum levels <1 mg/dL), suppressed parathyroid secretion can occur. This is most often seen in chronic gastrointestinal disease; in nutritional deficiency, especially alcoholism; or with cis-platinum therapy. Resistance to the actions of PTH at the level of bone and kidney may also contribute to the hypocalcemia seen with magnesium deficiency. Replenishment of magnesium stores promptly restores parathyroid function to normal.

Idiopathic Hypoparathyroidism

Isolated failure of parathyroid gland development is a rare genetic cause of hypoparathyroidism. Molecular abnormalities in PTH biosynthesis can cause genetic absence of the hormone in the presence of apparently normal parathyroid glands. In addition, activating mutations in the CaR can lead to inappropriate suppression of PTH secretion, a condition referred to as autosomal dominant familial hypocalcemia. In affected individuals, the mutant receptor constitutively signals and leads to the continuous suppression of PTH secretion, despite hypocalcemia.

Autoimmune Polyglandular Syndrome Type 1

This autoimmune disorder is characterized by the early development of hypoparathyroidism in association with Addison's disease and mucocutaneous candidiasis. Most affected individuals manifest hypocalcemia by age 10 years. In addition to Addison's disease, one third of these patients develop other endocrine disorders such as diabetes mellitus, pernicious anemia, or premature ovarian failure. This disorder is now known to be caused by mutations in the gene encoding an autoimmune regulatory protein (AIRE).

Autoimmune Hypoparathyroidism Caused by Antibodies to the Calcium-Sensing Receptor

Following cloning of the CaR, a few cases have been reported in which the presence of antibodies to the CaR appeared to cause hypoparathyroidism. In this situation, the antibody is thought to directly activate the CaR, thereby suppressing parathyroid secretion. These cases are rare. Although antibodies to the CaR have also been reported with variable and usually low frequency in autoimmune polyglandular syndrome type 1, it remains unclear what role, if any, these antibodies play in the pathogenesis of the hypoparathyroidism seen in that disorder.

Hypocalcemia Resulting from Resistance to the Actions of Parathyroid Hormone

Pseudohypoparathyroidism

Peripheral tissue resistance to PTH was classically termed *pseudohypoparathyroidism* (PHP). The characteristic biochemical manifestations of PHP are hypocalcemia and hyperphosphatemia, just as in parathyroprivic hypoparathyroidism; however, circulating levels of PTH are elevated, rather than low or undetectable. The renal tubule is the primary site of PTH resistance, although variable degrees of skeletal resistance have also been reported. When the skeleton retains sensitivity to PTH, lesions characteristic of hyperparathyroidism, including osteitis fibrosa cystica, can develop. PTH stimulates renal cyclic adenosine monophosphate (cAMP) production, and levels of cAMP increase in the urine following administration of the hormone. A direct correlation has been demonstrated between the degree of PTH resistance (as assessed by the magnitude of the change in cAMP excretion or renal phosphate threshold) and the ambient circulating PTH level.

The renal cAMP response is the basis of a diagnostic test that allows the partial classification of this heterogeneous group of disorders. Individuals with PHP who demonstrate a blunted urinary cAMP response have type I PHP. Those who generate a normal cAMP response have type II PHP.

PHP type I has been further characterized as types Ia, Ib, and Ic. Type Ia describes those individuals with the Albright's hereditary osteodystrophy phenotype, defined by short stature and large frame, broad facies, and shortened fourth metacarpals (Fig. 253-4). Soft tissue calcifications and multiple endocrine abnormalities are often present. These individuals frequently have

a mutation in the α-subunit of the stimulatory guanine nucleotide binding regulatory protein G_s. This regulatory protein couples membrane receptors to adenylate cyclase, thereby regulating receptor-dependent cAMP production. The presence of G_s in various cell types accounts for the generalized hormone resistance that may occur. Affected patients often have elevated thyrotropin levels with a compensated euthyroid state. Variable degrees of gonadotropin, antidiuretic hormone, adrenocorticotropic hormone, and glucagon resistance have been described. Patients with type Ib PHP have only PTH resistance, without the Albright's hereditary osteodystrophy phenotype. It has been suggested that this phenotype may result from abnormalities in the tissue-specific imprinting of the G_s α gene, such that $G_{s\alpha}$ function is specifically lost in the kidney but retained in other tissues. Patients without a mutation in $G_{s\alpha}$ but with associated hormonal abnormalities and/or Albright's hereditary osteodystrophy have been classified as having type Ic PHP. The catalytic subunit of adenylate cyclase is a possible site for the defect in this latter condition.

Type II PHP appears to result from a variety of defects distal to cAMP generation in the intracellular PTH signaling cascade. No distinct phenotype exists, although various autoimmune findings have been described in some patients. Other investigators have suggested that a circulating PTH inhibitor may play a role in the pathogenesis of PHP, indicating that this inhibitor may be generated by parathyroid tissue itself. Resistance to PTH has also been described in hypomagnesemia, as noted earlier.

Hypocalcemia in the Setting of Normal or Increased Parathyroid Hormone Activity and Normal Receptor Function

Despite normal PTH function and downstream signaling from its receptor, hypocalcemia can still result from disturbances in skeletal homeostasis, vitamin D metabolism, and a variety of medical illnesses.

FIGURE 253-4. Patients with Albright's hereditary osteodystrophy. **A,** Note the short stature and round facies in this patient. **B,** Hands of the patient shown in **A.** Note that the third and fourth fingers are shorter than the second. This is because of short metacarpals. **C,** Hand radiograph of another patient; note the short fourth and fifth metacarpals *(arrows).* (**A** and **B,** From Albright F, Burnett CH, Smith PH, Parson W. Pseudoparathyroidism—an example of Seabright-Bantam syndrome. *Endocrinology.* 1942;30:922; **C,** From Kolb FO, Steinbach HL. Pseudohypoparathyroidism with secondary hyperparathyroidism and osteitis fibrosa. *J Clin Endocrinol Metab.* 1962;22:59-70.)

Hypoproteinemia

The most common cause of a low serum calcium level in hospitalized patients is a reduction in the concentration of serum proteins (particularly albumin). In these patients, the ionized calcium is unaffected, and signs and symptoms of hypocalcemia are absent. Low serum albumin concentrations are often seen in patients with nephrotic syndrome, chronic illness, malnutrition, cirrhosis, and volume overexpansion. One commonly cited rule of thumb for correcting the effects of decreased serum albumin on total serum calcium concentration is to add 0.8 mg/dL to the total serum calcium for every 1 g/dL decline in serum albumin to less than 4 g/dL. However, this estimate is somewhat inaccurate, and it is preferable to determine the ionized calcium concentration directly in this setting.

Vitamin D Deficiency

Vitamin D synthesis in the skin requires adequate exposure to ultraviolet light. Thus, vitamin D deficiency is less common where sunlight exposure is abundant. In extremes of latitude (e.g., northern climates in North America) and where industrial pollution can interfere with the transmission of ultraviolet light, normal vitamin D status depends on adequate dietary intake. Supplementation of milk products with vitamin D has reduced the incidence of vitamin D deficiency in North America. Elderly persons in particular are at risk for this complication because of their general nutritional compromise and limited sunlight exposure.

Overt hypocalcemia is seen only in severe vitamin D deficiency. PTH levels are high in this setting. Serum levels of alkaline phosphatase (of bone origin) can be elevated as a result of associated osteomalacia, which is manifested by painful pseudofractures, particularly in weight-bearing long bones. The best way to assess vitamin D status is to measure circulating levels of 25(OH) vitamin D. Levels of this metabolite are low in vitamin D deficiency. Levels lower than 20 ng/mL indicate frank vitamin D deficiency; levels below 30 ng/mL are considered insufficient. However, hypocalcemia is usually not seen until serum levels are very low, often less than 10 ng/mL. Circulating 1,25(OH)$_2$ vitamin D levels may be low, normal, or elevated in the setting of vitamin D deficiency. This finding may appear paradoxical, but 1,25(OH)$_2$ vitamin D circulates in 1000-fold lower concentrations than 25(OH) vitamin D.

Because vitamin D is a fat-soluble vitamin, generalized fat malabsorption can also lead to vitamin D deficiency. Gastrointestinal diseases such as Crohn's disease, celiac sprue, and pancreatic insufficiency can be accompanied by hypocalcemia resulting from vitamin D malabsorption. Interruption of the enterohepatic circulation of both 25(OH) vitamin D and 1,25(OH)$_2$ vitamin D may lower body vitamin D stores in these diseases. Mild hypocalcemia and secondary hyperparathyroidism are also seen in cholestatic liver diseases such as primary biliary cirrhosis. Circulating levels of 25(OH) vitamin D are reduced in this setting because of impaired hydroxylation of vitamin D in the liver and intestinal malabsorption of vitamin D.

Hyperphosphatemia

Oral or parenteral phosphate can induce a decline in serum calcium concentrations, and hyperphosphatemia can lead to frank hypocalcemia. Clinical settings in which this can occur include excessive enteral or parenteral phosphate administration, the tumor lysis syndrome, and rhabdomyolysis-induced acute renal failure. Hypocalcemia induced by either oral or parenteral phosphate administration is often associated with soft tissue calcifications. Such ectopic calcification has been observed during the treatment of hypophosphatemia resulting from either diabetic ketoacidosis or acute alcoholism. Adults receiving phosphate-containing enemas may also become hypocalcemic. Under most circumstances, with the discontinuation of exogenous phosphate intake, the serum calcium level promptly returns to normal. Hypocalcemia in the setting of massive tumor lysis results from the release of intracellular phosphate as a consequence of chemotherapy-induced cell death, usually during the treatment of rapidly proliferating neoplasms. The hypocalcemia may continue beyond the period of hyperphosphatemia and appears to be aggravated by suppressed 1,25(OH)$_2$ vitamin D levels. Rhabdomyolysis-induced acute renal failure occurs with trauma and drug or alcohol abuse. Marked hypocalcemia can occur in the early oliguric phase, and moderate to severe hypercalcemia is noted in the subsequent polyuric phase. The appearance of hypercalcemia and high serum 1,25(OH)$_2$ vitamin D levels during the diuretic phase may result from the rapid development of secondary hyperparathyroidism during the initial hypocalcemic period.

Pancreatitis

Hypocalcemia and tetany were first reported in patients with pancreatitis (Chapter 146) in the early 1940s. Pancreatic lipase released from the damaged gland is believed to liberate free fatty acids that chelate calcium, thereby removing it from the ECF. Hypomagnesemia resulting from poor oral intake, alcohol use, or vomiting may contribute to the hypocalcemia. Hypocalcemia in the setting of pancreatitis often suggests a poor clinical course. Treatment consists of parenteral calcium and magnesium when indicated.

Chronic Kidney Disease

Progressive renal disease (Chapter 132) is associated with a decline in serum calcium resulting from several factors. Important among these are a rise in serum phosphate as the kidneys' ability to clear absorbed phosphate declines, and a fall in serum levels of 1,25(OH)$_2$ vitamin D because of both diminishing renal production of this metabolite and a rise in circulating levels of fibroblast growth factor 23, which directly suppresses 1α-hydroxylase activity. Hypocalcemia leads to chronic parathyroid stimulation, which can lead to severe secondary and even tertiary hyperparathyroidism. Early intervention with phosphate binders and calcitriol or calcitriol analogues is now the standard of care for patients with significantly impaired renal function. The challenges of managing hypocalcemia in a patient treated with dialysis are beyond the scope of this chapter (Chapter 133).

Sepsis

Up to 20% of septic patients (Chapter 108) have reductions in ionized serum calcium. Hypocalcemia is associated with a worse prognosis. This phenomenon is most often reported with gram-negative sepsis, but it has occurred in toxic shock syndrome caused by staphylococcal infection. The pathophysiology of hypocalcemia in this setting is unknown.

CLINICAL MANIFESTATIONS

Manifestations of hypocalcemia are related primarily to increased neuromuscular irritability. Tetany is the classic sign of hypocalcemia, but it is not always present. Paresthesias are more common and often occur around the mouth or in the fingertips. They may progress to overt muscle spasm in the face and extremities, the latter typified by carpopedal spasm. The term *latent tetany* refers to signs elicited by provocative stimuli such as ischemia or percussion. A positive Trousseau's test is the induction of carpal spasm within 3 minutes of inflating a sphygmomanometer above systolic blood pressure. A positive Chvostek's sign is percussion of the facial nerve to induce involuntary contraction of the facial muscles, including the corner of the mouth, nose, and eye. Neither the degree of hypocalcemia nor the rapidity with which it develops necessarily correlates with clinical manifestations, although the frequency of overt signs increases when serum calcium falls to less than 7.5 mg/dL.

Patients with hypomagnesemia or hyperkalemia may present with similar findings, which can be exacerbated by hypocalcemia. In contrast, hypermagnesemia or hypokalemia can mask symptoms in a hypocalcemic individual. Abnormalities of cardiac repolarization are seen in hypocalcemic individuals, reflected by a prolonged QT interval on the electrocardiogram.

Basal ganglia calcifications are typical findings in long-standing hypoparathyroidism. Osteopetrosis and dental abnormalities have also been reported in chronic untreated hypoparathyroidism. Dry skin, coarse hair, and a form of psoriasis that responds to correction of hypocalcemia have all been described in this clinical setting.

DIAGNOSIS

The initial step in evaluating hypocalcemia is to confirm that the ionized calcium level is low (Fig. 253-5). If the serum albumin concentration is within the normal range, total serum calcium can be considered an accurate reflection of the ionized fraction. Otherwise, ionized serum calcium must be measured. Once it has been established that the patient is hypocalcemic, a serum PTH level should be measured. A low or undetectable PTH level in the presence of hypocalcemia confirms the diagnosis of hypoparathyroidism. The diagnostic focus in this setting is on destructive, infiltrative, and autoimmune diseases of the parathyroid glands, as well as genetic disorders leading to the absence of the parathyroid glands or (as in the case of activating mutations of the CaR) their functional absence. If the serum PTH level is elevated, the differential diagnosis should focus on factors inducing resistance to the actions of PTH. The presence of hyperphosphatemia suggests concomitant renal failure or excessive ingestion or administration of phosphate salts. A low serum phosphorus level in the setting of hypocalcemia and an elevated PTH

FIGURE 253-5. Algorithmic approach to the diagnosis of hypocalcemia. PTH = parathyroid hormone; vit = vitamin.

suggests the possibility of vitamin D deficiency, and a serum 25(OH) vitamin D level should be checked early in the evaluation. The presence of vitamin D deficiency indicates nutritional deficiency or intestinal malabsorption. The diagnosis of hypomagnesemia should be excluded. In the absence of any of these accompanying changes, phenotypic abnormalities such as those seen in Albright's hereditary osteodystrophy should be sought because PHP is a likely diagnostic possibility.

TREATMENT   Rx

Acute Management

Hypocalcemia-induced seizures, laryngospasm, and tetany are examples of clinical settings in which the immediate correction of hypocalcemia is required. In these emergencies, 10 to 20 mL of 10% calcium gluconate should be infused over a 10- to 15-minute period. This treatment can be followed, if necessary, by an infusion of calcium. For this purpose, 10 ampules of calcium gluconate can be diluted in 1 L of 5% dextrose, and, beginning at a rate of 50 mL/hour, the infusion rate can be titrated to maintain the serum calcium in the low-normal range.

In patients with hypomagnesemia, magnesium therapy may be required to restore PTH secretion and peripheral activity. Before the administration of magnesium salts, adequate renal function and urinary output should be ensured. In the acute setting, elemental magnesium can be infused slowly, with up to 2.4 mg/kg body weight given over a 20-minute period (to a maximum of 180 mg). The length of parenteral therapy must be individualized, and maintenance with oral magnesium salts should be implemented when ongoing hypomagnesemia is anticipated.

The administration of intravenous calcium or magnesium should be carefully monitored. The patient's cardiac status should be followed and the infusions stopped if electrocardiographic changes occur. Deep tendon reflexes can be used to monitor for magnesium toxicity, and therapy should be halted if reflexes diminish. Intravenous calcium gluconate is a useful antidote for magnesium intoxication and should be available at the bedside.

Long-Term Treatment

Many of the causes of hypocalcemia discussed earlier are corrected by treating the underlying disorder (e.g., vitamin D deficiency, tumor lysis syndrome). However, some patients require maintenance therapy for hypocalcemia, including those with hypoparathyroidism, PHP, and vitamin D–resistant states.

Hypoparathyroidism, whether primary or secondary to trauma or surgery, is the most frequently encountered condition that requires long-term therapy to support circulating calcium concentrations. In these individuals, the goal is to maintain serum calcium in the low-normal range (8.5 to 9.2 mg/dL). This approach reduces the likelihood of symptoms such as circumoral tingling, signs such as carpopedal spasm, and long-term complications such as cataracts. Increasing the serum calcium level to the middle to high-normal range can result in significant hypercalciuria, nephrocalcinosis, and nephrolithiasis.

There is no single best way to achieve target calcium levels, although the combination of a vitamin D metabolite and calcium supplements is generally preferred. Many different preparations of both are available. Because of the prolonged toxicity that occurs with excessive ingestion of either ergocalciferol or 25(OH) vitamin D, the use of rapid-acting preparations of vitamin D is generally preferred for the treatment of hypoparathyroidism. Calcitriol [1,25(OH)$_2$D$_3$] and dihydrotachysterol are two preparations suited to this purpose. Both are fully active in vivo. In general, it is best to establish a stable dose for one of these agents and refine the serum calcium level by adjusting the intake of supplemental calcium, rather than by making repeated changes in vitamin D metabolite therapy. Calcitriol can be used in most patients. The dose of calcitriol can range from as little as 0.25 up to 2.0 µg/day. The biologic half-life of the drug is 12 to 14 hours. When hypercalcemia develops during therapy with calcitriol, it usually resolves within 3 to 4 days after discontinuing the drug, although it can persist for more than 1 week. In addition to a high-calcium diet, calcium supplements are important for the treatment of hypoparathyroidism, and doses of 1000 to 2000 mg/day may be necessary. Calcium preparations including the carbonate, citrate, lactate, gluconate, and glucobionate salts are suitable for this purpose. In some patients with hypoparathyroidism, a thiazide diuretic may be useful in augmenting serum calcium levels and reducing the hypercalciuria that can occur with the institution of treatment. Long-term treatment of hypoparathyroidism with synthetic human PTH is not yet practical, although therapy for up to 3 years was well tolerated in a clinical trial. Various stresses such as trauma, infection, and pregnancy can increase the therapeutic requirements of patients with chronic hypocalcemia, and the clinician should be alert to this possibility.

1. Peacock M, Bolognese MA, Borofsky M, et al. Cinacalcet treatment of primary hyperparathyroidism: biochemical and bone densitometric outcomes in a five-year study. *J Clin Endocrinol Metab.* 2009;94:4860-4867.

SUGGESTED READINGS

Augustine MM, Bravo PE, Zeiger MA. Treatment of primary hyperparathyroidism. *Endocr Pract.* 2011;17:75-82. *Review including imaging for preoperative localization and the use of minimally invasive and endoscopic-, video-, and robot-assisted parathyroidectomy.*

Bilezikian JP, Khan AA, Potts JT Jr. Guidelines for the management of asymptomatic primary hyperparathyroidism; summary statement from the third international workshop. *J Clin Endocrinol Metab.* 2009;94:335-339. *Summary of the latest expert recommendations for the management of hyperparathyroidism.*

Felger EA, Kandil E. Primary hyperparathyroidism. *Otolaryngol Clin North Am.* 2010;43:417-432. *Review emphasizing the role of surgery, including preoperative localization and intraoperative parathyroid hormone measurement.*

Sankaran S, Gamble G, Bolland M, et al. Skeletal effects of interventions in mild primary hyperparathyroidism: a meta-analysis. *J Clin Endocrinol Metab.* 2010;95:1653-1662. *Surgical and antiresorptive treatments increase bone mineral density in mild primary hyperparathyroidism to a similar degree.*

Sharretts JM, Kebebew E, Simonds WF. Parathyroid cancer. *Semin Oncol.* 2010;37:580-590. *This uncommon malignancy is a rare and serious cause of primary hyperparathyroidism.*

254

MEDULLARY THYROID CARCINOMA AND CALCITONIN

SAMUEL A. WELLS JR.

MEDULLARY THYROID CARCINOMA

DEFINITION

Medullary thyroid carcinoma (MTC) is a relatively uncommon form of thyroid cancer that occurs either sporadically or as part of multiple endocrine neoplasia (MEN) type 2.

EPIDEMIOLOGY

MTC accounts for 5 to 10% of thyroid cancers, and there are 1500 to 3000 new cases in the United States each year. In 25% of cases, MTC occurs as a uniform component of MEN 2 or related syndromes: MEN 2A, (80%), MEN 2B (5%), and familial MTC (15%) (Table 254-1). The incidence of the hereditary forms of MTC is 1 in 30,000 persons.

PATHOBIOLOGY

MTC originates from the neural crest–derived C cells, which localize within the upper poles of the thyroid lobes during embryogenesis as the lateral thyroid complex closes. Even though MTC occurs within the thyroid parenchyma, it is actually a neuroendocrine tumor, as it does not arise from the thyroid follicular cells. Sporadic MTC occurs as a solitary tumor, whereas in the hereditary forms of MTC, the tumor involves both thyroid lobes and is multifocal. In patients with hereditary MTC, the first manifestation of this

TABLE 254-1	MULTIPLE ENDOCRINE NEOPLASIA (MEN) TYPE 2 AND RELATED SYNDROMES
MEN 2A	
Medullary thyroid carcinoma (≈100%)	
Pheochromocytoma (50%)	
Hyperparathyroidism (20–30%)	
VARIANTS OF MEN 2A	
MEN 2A with cutaneous lichen amyloidosis	
MEN 2A with Hirschsprung's disease	
FAMILIAL MEDULLARY THYROID CARCINOMA	
MEN 2B	
Medullary thyroid carcinoma (≈100%)	
Pheochromocytoma (50%)	
Mucosal neuroma, ganglioneuromatosis, marfanoid habitus, colonic abnormalities, characteristic phenotype (100%)	

C-cell disorder is C-cell hyperplasia, which progresses over time to microinvasive MTC and then invasive MTC.

The C cells have diverse biosynthetic activity and secrete calcitonin, carcinoembryonic antigen (CEA), chromogranin-A, histaminase, somatostatin, gastrin-releasing peptide, and adrenocorticotropin. Of these markers, calcitonin and CEA are the most useful clinically, and both are excellent serum markers for MTC. The hormone calcitonin was once thought to be important in calcium homeostasis; however, its physiologic importance has recently been called into question. Histologically, the MTC cells are spindle shaped, and special staining demonstrates calcitonin and CEA. With age, the central portion of the tumor calcifies, which can be seen on radiographic imaging studies.

Dominant-negative, activating, germline, missense, and point mutations in the *RET* proto-oncogene are present in virtually all cases of hereditary MTC. Somatic *RET* mutations are demonstrated in at least half of sporadic MTCs. *RET* is located in the pericentromeric region of chromosome 10q11.2 and spans 21 exons, including more than 60 kb of genomic DNA. *RET* is highly conserved, and homologues have been found in lower vertebrates and the fruit fly. *RET* plays a central role in various intracellular signaling cascades that regulate cellular differentiation, proliferation, migration, and survival. The RET protein is expressed in developing neuroendocrine cells (including thyroid C cells; adrenal medullary cells; parathyroid cells; neural cells, including parasympathetic and sympathetic ganglion cells; and cells of the testis and urogenital tract).

MEN 2A, MEN 2B, and familial MTC (FMTC) are inherited as autosomal dominant traits with near-complete penetrance and, in the case of MEN 2A and MEN 2B, variable expressivity. Approximately 75 *RET* mutations have been reported in association with MEN 2A, MEN 2B, and FMTC, and 95% of families with one of the forms of hereditary MTC have demonstrated *RET* mutations. The mutations for MEN 2A are located mostly in the extracellular, cysteine-rich region of exon 10 (including codons 609, 611, 618, and 620) and exon 11 (including codons 630 and 634). Approximately 85% of the mutations associated with MEN 2A involve *RET* codon 634, approximately half of which are *C634R RET* mutations. The mutations characteristic of FMTC also occur in exons 10 and 11; however, noncysteine point mutations have also been found in exon 8 (codons 532 and 533), exon 13 (codons 768, 790, and 791), exon 14 (codons 804 and 844), exon 15 (codon 891), and exon 16 (codon 912).

Unlike the mechanism in MEN 2A and FMTC, MEN 2B mutations occur in the kinase domain and cause constitutive RET activation in a monomeric form of RET, thereby altering substrate specificity, presumably due to a conformational change in the binding pocket of the kinase. Approximately 95% of mutations causing MEN 2B are in codon 918 (exon 16), and 5% are located in codon 883 (exon 15).

It is estimated that the disease arises de novo in 50% of patients with MEN 2B and in 10% of patients with MEN 2A and FMTC. In all founder cases studied thus far, the de novo mutation arose from the paternal allele.

CLINICAL MANIFESTATIONS

The peak incidence of sporadic MTC is in the fifth decade of life, and most patients present with a solitary thyroid nodule and lymph node metastases, although the latter may not be evident on physical examination. Clinically, the tumors are more aggressive than papillary thyroid carcinoma and follicular thyroid carcinoma, and overall, the 10-year survival rate is 75%.

MTC occurs in virtually all patients with MEN 2A, MEN 2B, and FMTC and is the most common cause of death in affected patients. Approximately 50% of patients with MEN 2A and MEN 2B develop pheochromocytomas (Chapters 235 and 239). An undiagnosed pheochromocytoma, which makes itself known during induction of anesthesia for thyroidectomy or childbirth, can be catastrophic and often lethal. Thus, pheochromocytoma must be excluded in all patients with a confirmed or presumptive diagnosis of hereditary MTC (Chapter 235).

Parathyroid hyperplasia occurs in 30% of patients with MEN 2A and usually involves all four glands. The disease is frequently asymptomatic, with the only abnormality being an elevated serum calcium concentration.

There is a strong relationship between genotype and phenotype in patients with MEN 2A. For example, pheochromocytomas are most common in patients with mutations in exon 11 (particularly codon 634). Also, the presence of hyperparathyroidism is associated with codon 634 mutations, especially the C634R mutation. The clinical aggressiveness of MTC (age of onset, tumor size, frequency of regional and distant metastases) is related to the form of hereditary MTC. For example, MTC associated with MEN 2B is much more aggressive than that occurring with MEN 2A or FMTC. The primary basis for the difference is that MEN 2B mutations are associated with greater basal kinase activity and thus are more highly activating compared with mutations occurring in MEN 2A and FMTC.

Patients with MEN 2A may also develop one of two associated disorders: cutaneous lichen amyloidosis or Hirschsprung's disease. Cutaneous lichen amyloidosis occurs in about 25% of patients with MEN 2A and involves the interscapular region of the back, corresponding to dermatomes T2 through T6. Pruritus, the dominant symptom, leads to repetitive scratching and secondary skin changes characterized by the deposition of amyloid. The lesion may be evident in infancy, thus serving as a precursor marker of MEN 2A. Cutaneous lichen amyloidosis is associated with a RET codon 634 mutation.

Hirschsprung's disease, manifested by the absence of intrinsic ganglion cells in the distal gastrointestinal tract, has been reported in 30 or more families with MEN 2A or FMTC and is associated with mutations in exon 10 of RET involving codons 609 (15%), 611 (4%), 618 (30 to 35%), and 620 (50%). In functional studies, the cell surface expression of RET with these codon mutations is lower than that found with codon 634 mutation, suggesting a novel mechanism whereby the mutations have a dual effect: causing the transformation of C cells, leading to MTC, and interfering with transportation of the protein to the plasma membrane, resulting in the absence of ganglion cells and the development of Hirschsprung's disease.

Patients with MEN 2B develop mucosal neuromas, ganglioneuromatosis throughout the aerodigestive tract, hypotonia, and medullated corneal nerves. They also develop colonic dysfunction manifested by abdominal pain and occasionally intestinal obstruction requiring surgery. Patients have a characteristic physical appearance, which may not be evident very early in life. The failure to diagnose MEN 2B at a young age can be catastrophic because MTC develops early; it is often evident soon after birth, and regional or distant metastases occur soon thereafter.

Patients with FMTC develop only MTC, which, relative to the tumors in patients with MEN 2A and MEN 2B, is slow growing. There has been some question whether FMTC is a distinct disease entity or a form of MEN 2A.

DIAGNOSIS

Once it was discovered that C cells secrete calcitonin, the measurement of serum levels of this hormone, either in the basal state or following the intravenous administration of the secretagogues calcium or pentagastrin, became the primary method of establishing the diagnosis of a C-cell disorder. With the discovery that MEN 2A, MEN 2B, and FMTC are caused by mutations in the RET proto-oncogene, direct DNA analysis to detect a mutated RET allele replaced serum calcitonin measurement as the method of choice for identifying affected family members. At present, the measurement of serum calcitonin is used to evaluate disease progression, either after thyroidectomy for MTC or during the course of medical treatment for advanced disease. In European countries it is common practice to measure basal serum calcitonin in patients with nodular thyroid disease; this technique has proved more effective than fine-needle aspiration cytology in detecting patients with MTC.

The Gene Tests directory currently lists 38 laboratories that perform DNA analysis for RET in MEN 2A, MEN 2B, FMTC, and sporadic MTC (http://www.genetests.org). Almost all the laboratories use direct sequence analysis to evaluate mutations in exons 10, 11, 13, 14, 15, and 16, and some laboratories include exon 8. If no mutations are found in these exons, the entire coding region of RET can be sequenced. RET mutations in exons 10 or 11 are identified in more than 95% of families demonstrating a germline transmission of MEN 2A or FMTC.

Approximately 7% of patients with presumed sporadic MTC actually have MEN 2A or FMTC; therefore, it is important to perform direct DNA analysis on all patients with "sporadic" disease. The diagnosis of hereditary MTC widens the disease spectrum to be considered by the responsible physician, and it also creates the obligation to screen family members, some of whom will have early-stage MTC.

TREATMENT   Rx

The primary treatment for patients with MTC is total thyroidectomy and resection of lymph nodes in the central compartment of the neck, an area bounded by the hyoid bone superiorly, the thoracic inlet inferiorly, and the carotid sheaths laterally (levels I through VI). Total thyroidectomy is indicated because the incidence of intrathyroid lymphatic spread is 10 to 20%, and even though the disease appears to be sporadic, the patient's hereditary status is usually unknown at the time of thyroidectomy. If lymph nodes are palpable in the ipsilateral or contralateral neck or are evident on preoperative ultrasound examination, the respective lymph node compartments (levels II through V) are cleared. During the procedure, great care must be taken to preserve the parathyroid glands, the recurrent laryngeal nerve, and the external branch of the superior laryngeal nerve.

The preoperative serum levels of calcitonin and CEA are important predictors of nodal metastases. Half of patients with serum calcitonin levels greater than 3000 pg/mL and 30% of patients with CEA levels greater than 10 ng/nL have lymph node metastases. Spread to regional nodes is associated with treatment failure, indicated by normalization of the serum calcitonin in only 10% of patients with node-positive disease, compared with 60% of patients with node-negative disease. Even though surgical resection seldom cures patients with regional lymph node metastases, many have a good prognosis, with 5- and 10-year survival rates of 80 and 70%, respectively.

Repeat neck operation following initial thyroidectomy is indicated in patients with serious complications from recurrent tumor compressing or invading vital structures, such as the spinal cord, airway, or esophagus. Relief often follows tumor excision or debulking. Also, patients who have intractable diarrhea due to markedly elevated tumor hormone secretions, presumably calcitonin, may obtain symptom relief by tumor ablation. Rarely, patients with MTC develop Cushing's syndrome due to the inappropriate secretion of adrenocorticotropin or corticotropin-releasing hormone. Such patients usually have advanced disease, and bilateral adrenalectomy may be required if steroidogenesis inhibitors are ineffective. This is a poor prognostic sign and is associated with an average survival of 2 years.

Patients who develop persistent or recurrent MTC following thyroidectomy, as indicated by elevated serum levels of calcitonin or CEA, are also candidates for reoperation; however, the benefit of such surgical procedures is open to question, with a lack of long-term data on quality of life and survival.

The treatment of pheochromocytoma is adrenalectomy, as described in Chapter 235. Hyperparathyroidism is managed by either three-and-a-half-gland parathyroidectomy or total parathyroidectomy and heterotopic autotransplantation.

For patients with locally advanced or metastatic MTC, single-agent or combined chemotherapeutic regimens have been minimally effective, and chemotherapy does not play a major role in those with advanced disease. Similarly, external beam radiotherapy has little effect on primary tumors or soft tissue metastases and is indicated only for the treatment of central nervous system or bone metastases.

With the demonstration that the tyrosine kinase inhibitor imatinib induced remissions in patients with chronic myelogenous leukemia and gastrointestinal stromal tumors, there was hope that similar small-molecule therapeutics would be developed for patients with MTC. The tyrosine kinase inhibitor vandetanib inhibits vascular endothelial growth factor signaling, angiogenesis, tumor growth, KDR tyrosine kinase activity, and oncogenic RET kinases. A phase II clinical trial of vandetanib in locally advanced or metastatic hereditary MTC resulted in partial remissions in 20% of patients and a disease control rate of 80%. Similar results have been observed with other tyrosine kinase inhibitors. Thus, there is hope that effective systemic therapies will be available for patients with advanced disease and perhaps for patients with minimal disease after primary thyroidectomy for MTC.

PREVENTION

There are several hereditary cancer syndromes for which the causative abnormality has been identified. In many of these syndromes, removal of the organ at risk for malignancy is considered a preventive strategy. Patients with MEN 2A, MEN 2B, and FMTC are ideal candidates for prophylactic thyroidectomy because the genetic mode of inheritance is characterized by near-complete penetrance, and direct DNA analysis identifies carriers of a mutated RET allele who are destined to develop MTC. Furthermore, the thyroid is easily removed, with minimal morbidity and virtually no mortality; there is a suitable replacement for the organ's function; and there is a reliable serologic test to determine whether the patient has been rendered disease free.

Apparently normal, young members of kindreds with hereditary MTC who are found to have a mutated *RET* allele on genetic screening have the greatest likelihood of being cured by prophylactic thyroidectomy. Surgeons in several countries have reported success with this operative procedure, and the question is no longer should it be done but at what age.

The Consensus Committee of the 7th International Workshop on MEN, the EUROMEN group, and the International Guideline Committee of the American Thyroid Association have all proposed guidelines for the timing of prophylactic thyroidectomy in patients with MEN 2A, MEN 2B, and FMTC. The recommendations of the three groups are similar, in that children with MEN 2B (or with mutations in codons 918 or 882) should have thyroidectomy at the time of diagnosis, even during the first months of life. Children with mutations in codons 611, 618, 620, or 634 should have the thyroid removed at or before 5 years of age. In children with mutations in other *RET* codons, the recommended timing of thyroidectomy is less clear but is generally between 5 and 10 years of age. Some clinicians use basal or stimulated calcitonin levels to determine the timing of thyroidectomy.

PROGNOSIS

A poor prognosis is associated with the following findings: a large primary tumor, metastases to regional lymph nodes, markedly elevated serum levels of calcitonin and CEA preoperatively, extrathyroidal invasion of the trachea or soft tissues intraoperatively, elevated and increasing serum levels of calcitonin and CEA postoperatively, and radiographic evidence of distant metastases. Generally, MTC is more aggressive in patients with sporadic disease than in those with hereditary disease. Also, patients with MEN 2B and patients with MEN 2A who have *RET* mutations in codon 634 have a poorer prognosis than those with *RET* mutations in other codons. Patients apparently cured by thyroidectomy are followed at 6-month intervals by the measurement of serum levels of calcitonin. The doubling time of serum calcitonin is very useful in predicting the course of the disease; calcitonin doubling times less than 6 months (vs. those >24 months) are associated with a poor prognosis.

SUGGESTED READINGS

Ahmed SR, Ball DW. Incidentally discovered medullary thyroid cancer: diagnostic strategies and treatment. *J Clin Endocrinol Metab.* 2011;96:1237-1245. *Patients with persistently elevated serum calcitonin levels, positive RET test, or nodal disease are good candidates for thyroidectomy, whereas patients with undetectable calcitonin, negative RET testing, and no sonographic abnormalities often may be watched conservatively.*

Kloos RT, Eng C, Evans DB, et al. Medullary thyroid cancer: management guidelines of the American Thyroid Association. *Thyroid.* 2009;19:565-612. *Recommendations for managing patients with MEN 2 and related syndromes.*

Romei C, Cosci B, Renzini G, et al. RET genetic screening of sporadic medullary thyroid cancer (MTC) allows the preclinical diagnosis of unsuspected gene carriers and the identification of a relevant percentage of hidden familial MTC (FMTC). *Clin Endocrinol (Oxf).* 2011;74:241-247. *RET genetic screening in apparently sporadic cases is a major tool for the preclinical diagnosis and early treatment of unsuspected affected family members.*

255

PAGET'S DISEASE OF BONE

G. DAVID ROODMAN

DEFINITION

Paget's disease is a focal disorder of the skeleton that is the second most common bone disease, exceeded only by osteoporosis. It affects approximately 1 to 2% of adults older than 55 years in the United States and up to 4 to 6% of adults 55 years old or older in certain areas of the United Kingdom. Paget's disease is the most exaggerated form of bone remodeling, involving increases in all phases of the bone remodeling process. The initial phase is characterized by markedly increased bone resorption, followed by exuberant new bone formation. The new bone is abnormal and woven, with disorganized collagen. This increased bone formation results in bone enlargement and deformity because of the poor quality of the bone.

EPIDEMIOLOGY AND ETIOLOGY

The cause of Paget's disease is unknown. However, a genetic predisposition has been clearly established. Approximately 40% of patients with Paget's disease have an affected first-degree relative, and many families with vertical transmission of Paget's disease and an autosomal dominant pattern of inheritance have been described. At least six genetic loci have been linked to Paget's disease, and mutations in the sequestosome-1 gene (*SQSTM1*), also known as p62, are the most frequent. *SQSTM1* mutations have been detected in 30% of patients with familial Paget's disease and in 10% of patients with sporadic Paget's disease. Although the penetrance for Paget's disease is high, it can vary in families with a genetic predisposition. Elderly patients with *SQSTM1* mutations may have no evidence of Paget's disease, even though they are homozygous for the mutation.

The primary cellular abnormality in Paget's disease resides in the osteoclast. These cells contain nuclear inclusions that resemble paramyxoviral nucleocapsids. Both measles virus and respiratory syncytial virus nucleocapsid proteins and transcripts have been detected in osteoclasts from patients with Paget's disease, but some studies have not detected paramyxoviral transcripts or proteins in pagetic osteoclasts. Furthermore, a cause-and-effect relationship between Paget's disease and paramyxovirus infection has not been definitively established. Nevertheless, in vitro studies in which normal osteoclast precursors were transfected with measles virus transcripts or infected with measles virus have demonstrated that osteoclast precursors containing the measles virus nucleocapsid gene can form pagetic-like osteoclasts. Furthermore, transgenic mice in which expression of the measles virus nucleocapsid gene was targeted to cells of the osteoclast lineage developed bone lesions and osteoclasts characteristic of Paget's disease.

Although Paget's disease is the second most common bone disease, its prevalence varies among different populations. In the United Kingdom, for instance, Paget's disease affects up to 6% of the population older than 55 years. Further, the frequency of symptomatic Paget's disease increases with age. Paget's disease occurs with similar prevalence in western Europe and in the white populations of New Zealand and Australia. However, Paget's disease is extremely rare in Scandinavia and the Far East, and it does not affect indigenous populations in either Australia or New Zealand. The prevalence of Paget's disease appears to have decreased since the early 1980s. Its prevalence has reportedly decreased from approximately 8 to 4% in England and from 5 to 3% in New Zealand. In addition, the severity of Paget's disease in these populations has decreased. The basis for these changes is unknown.

PATHOBIOLOGY

Bone remodeling is increased 5- to 10-fold in patients with Paget's disease. Paget's disease is highly localized, with focal areas of involvement. In pagetic lesions, osteoclast numbers are increased, and the osteoclasts are hyper-multinucleated, with up to 100 nuclei per cell. In contrast, normal osteoclasts contain 3 to 20 nuclei per cell. The bone resorbing capacity of pagetic osteoclasts on a per nucleus basis is decreased compared with normal osteoclasts. However, because of the large numbers of osteoclasts in the pagetic lesion, overall bone resorption is markedly increased (Fig. 255-1). The increased bone resorption phase is followed by new bone formation. As the disease progresses, bone formation begins to predominate, and the bones become enlarged (Fig. 255-2). Large numbers of osteoblasts are often found near areas of resorbed bone, and they may even be prominent in a lesion that appears to be purely osteolytic by roentgenogram. The osteoblasts contain abundant rough endoplasmic reticulum, mitochondria, and a well-developed Golgi zone. These features of heightened cellular activity are consistent with the increased bone formation in active lesions. In addition to the increased numbers of osteoclasts and osteoblasts, the marrow in pagetic lesions is often grossly abnormal. The normal hematopoietic elements are usually absent and are replaced by mononuclear cells of indeterminate origin, intermixed with highly vascular connective tissue. The bone matrix structure in Paget's disease is extremely abnormal and arises as a consequence of disordered bone resorption and formation. The matrix consists of a "mosaic" of irregularly shaped pieces of lamellar bone with an erratic pattern of cement lines. The matrix is interspersed with numerous foci of woven bone, which, in adults, is ordinarily associated with fracture healing. After a long time, the lesions become sclerotic. This rapid and abnormal deposition of bone results in the characteristic irregular cement lines that give rise to the mosaic appearance on radiographs and in tissue sections. Marrow vascularity is markedly increased in pagetic

FIGURE 255-1. Sequential radiographs of the distal end of the femur at the dates shown. **A,** Distinction between pagetic and normal bone *(arrows)*, the osteolytic front, and expansion of bone diameter at the affected site. **B,** Treatment with a bisphosphonate induced filling in of the resorption front. **C,** Relapse after treatment was associated with a new area of osteolysis *(thick arrow)* and progression of the resorption front. (From Kanis JA. *Pathophysiology and Treatment of Paget's Disease of Bone*, 2nd ed. London: Martin Dunitz; 1998.)

FIGURE 255-2. Advanced involvement of the skull with Paget's disease. Note the marked thickening of the entire vault, areas of osteolysis, and patchy new bone formation, resulting in a "cotton-wool" appearance.

lesions, such that involved bones often feel warm to the touch. Electron microscopy studies of pagetic osteoclasts show nuclear inclusions that resemble paramyxovirus nucleocapsids. However, these nuclear inclusions are not unique to Paget's disease and have been reported in rare cases of osteopetrosis and other bone diseases, such as giant cell tumors of bone.

CLINICAL MANIFESTATIONS

Most patients with Paget's disease are elderly, and the age at diagnosis is usually older than 50 years. Paget's disease affects both men and women, with a slight male predominance. Although Paget's disease is often asymptomatic, 10 to 30% of patients experience pain, skeletal deformity, neurologic symptoms, pathologic fractures, or deafness. Patients may have only one affected bone or pagetic lesions in multiple bones. Patients with familial Paget's disease tend to have more bones affected and more deformity than those with sporadic Paget's disease. Paget's disease remains highly localized, and patients rarely develop new lesions in previously unaffected bones after diagnosis. Table 255-1 lists the common clinical features and complications of Paget's disease.

DIAGNOSIS

The biochemical findings in Paget's disease reflect the cellular events occurring throughout the skeleton of affected patients. Measurement of collagen cross-link degradation products in urine provides a specific measure of skeletal matrix degradation. Urinary *N*-telopeptide, pyridinoline, and deoxypyridinoline have all been used as measures of skeletal matrix resorption.

TABLE 255-1 CLINICAL FEATURES AND COMPLICATIONS OF PAGET'S DISEASE

COMMON

Pagetic or articular bone pain
Fracture of long bones and vertebral bodies
Neurologic deafness
Deformity and enlargement of bones

UNCOMMON

Spinal neurologic syndromes
Hypercalciuria of immobilization or fracture
Vascular bleeding from bone during surgery
Extraskeletal (aortic) calcification
Osteosarcoma and other bone tumors

RARE

Cardiovascular disease
Cranial nerve lesions (except VIII)
Brain stem and cerebellar lesions
Hypercalcemia of immobilization
Extramedullary hematopoiesis
Epidural hematoma

SIGNIFICANCE UNCERTAIN

Gout
Pseudogout
Angioid streaks
Hyperparathyroidism
Urolithiasis

Serum tartrate-sensitive acid phosphatase, released by osteoclasts, is another index of bone resorption in Paget's disease.

Osteoblast activity can be assessed by measuring total serum alkaline phosphatase activity, serum bone-specific alkaline phosphatase concentration, serum osteocalcin concentration, and serum type 1 carboxy-terminal procollagen peptide concentration. The most useful are total serum alkaline phosphatase and bone-specific alkaline phosphatase determinations. Total serum alkaline phosphatase measurements are routinely used to monitor disease activity in the clinic.

TREATMENT   Rx

Medical Therapy

Symptomatic patients with Paget's disease require treatment. No data support the treatment of asymptomatic patients, except in the presence of rapidly advancing osteolytic lesions in weight-bearing long bones, in which case the risk of pathologic fractures is increased. Because the osteoclast is the primary cell involved in Paget's disease, medical treatment that inhibits osteoclast activity—in particular, the use of bisphosphonates, calcitonin, and mitomycin—has been successful. Salmon calcitonin by injection, which has been used since the early 1980s, is an effective treatment for Paget's disease, suppressing the biochemical parameters of the disease by 50%. Bisphosphonates can inhibit osteoclast formation, but they predominantly induce osteoclast apoptosis; they are the most frequently used treatment for Paget's disease. Bisphosphonates, which contain nitrogen, are pyrophosphate derivatives with a high affinity for bone. They are incorporated into sites of bone resorption, released during the resorption process, and taken up by osteoclasts. This process results in the death of osteoclasts. Osteoclasts were recently reported to be angiogenic, and bisphosphonates affect angiogenesis as well as cytokine production by osteoclasts. Because biochemical markers strongly correlate with disease activity, following serum alkaline phosphatase levels is a simple method for monitoring the activity of Paget's disease. Some treatments may result in a high degree of normalization of both skeletal abnormalities and bone scan findings in these patients. With the availability of more potent bisphosphonates, the prognosis has greatly improved (Table 255-2). A single intravenous dose of 5 mg of zoledronic acid can provide a 96% response rate for the next 6 months and is more effective than 2 months of oral risedronate.[1]

Patients treated with bisphosphonates can usually attain remission. Symptomatic bisphosphonate treatment for pagetic bone pain unresponsive to analgesics or anti-inflammatory drugs is as good as repeat courses of bisphosphonates, irrespective of symptoms, in reducing and maintaining normal alkaline.[2] However, after variable periods of time, patients suffer relapse and require further treatment. Bisphosphonates by themselves have not been shown to "cure" Paget's disease. However, treatment with zoledronate can result in very long remissions.

TABLE 255-2	BISPHOSPHONATES USED IN THE TREATMENT OF PAGET'S DISEASE		
AGENT	**ROUTE**	**DOSE (mg/day)**	**DURATION OF EFFECT**
Alendronate	Oral	40	6 mo
Clodronate*	Oral	1600	3-6 mo
	Intravenous	300	5 days
Etidronate	Oral	400	6 mo
Pamidronate	Intravenous	30-60†	3 days
Risedronate	Oral	30	2 mo
Tiludronate	Oral	400	3 mo
Zoledronate	Intravenous	5 mg as a single injection	>2 yr

*Has not been approved by the Food and Drug Administration at the time of publication.
†Lower dose has been approved; higher dose is used by investigators.

Surgical Therapy

Surgery is used to treat fractures, correct the deformity of bowed bones, and treat bone disease in the hip. In addition, surgical treatment may relieve the neurologic complications of the overgrowth of pagetic bone, with resultant nerve root compression. Before elective surgery, patients with Paget's disease are usually treated with bisphosphonates to decrease the vascularity and activity of the bone and to prevent increased bleeding.

PROGNOSIS

Pagetic bone pain responds to medical treatment. Much of the bone pain associated with the disease results from arthritis or joint pain arising from the bone deformity, rather than pain from the pagetic bone per se. Unless treated, pagetic lesions continue to increase in size, but patients rarely if ever develop new lesions in previously unaffected bones. In patients for whom analgesic or other specific treatments are unsuccessful, joint replacement can be performed. The most dreaded complication in Paget's disease is the development of osteosarcoma in the pagetic lesion. Although it is an extremely rare complication, affecting less than 1% of patients, Paget's disease is the most common cause of osteosarcoma in adults. Once patients develop osteosarcoma, their prognosis is extremely poor, and the outcome is usually fatal. Active treatment of Paget's disease decreases the biochemical abnormalities, with near normalization of alkaline phosphatase activity, and improves the neurologic syndromes associated with this disease.

1. Reid IR, Miller P, Lyles K, et al. Comparison of a single infusion of zoledronic acid with risedronate for Paget's disease. N Engl J Med. 2005;353:898-908.
2. Langston AL, Campbell MK, Fraser WD, et al. Randomized trial of intensive bisphosphonate treatment versus symptomatic management in Paget's disease of bone. J Bone Miner Res. 2010;25:20-31.

SUGGESTED READINGS

Goode A, Layfield R. Recent advances in understanding the molecular basis of Paget disease of bone. J Clin Pathol. 2010;63:199-203. *Review emphasizing the newly defined functions of the p62 protein. SQSTM1 gene mutations on this protein may affect the development of the pagetic phenotype.*
Seton M, Moses AM, Bode RK, et al. Paget's disease of bone: the skeletal distribution, complications and quality of life as perceived by patients. Bone. 2011;48:281-285. *Patients report substantially lower levels of physical health, and there is a reasonable correlation of complications with radiographic abnormalities, except for headache or hearing loss.*

256

OSTEONECROSIS, OSTEOSCLEROSIS/HYPEROSTOSIS, AND OTHER DISORDERS OF BONE

MICHAEL P. WHYTE

OSTEONECROSIS

DEFINITION

Osteonecrosis (aseptic, avascular, or ischemic necrosis of bone) refers to skeletal infarction. Bone infarcts may be asymptomatic, cause self-limited discomfort, or engender painful collapse of subarticular bone that leads to joint destruction.

PATHOBIOLOGY AND PATHOGENESIS

Many conditions are associated with osteonecrosis (Table 256-1). In adults, the most common causes are ethanol abuse and long-term glucocorticoid therapy, both of which have dose-dependent effects.

Skeletal infarction may result from blood vessel destruction (e.g., joint dislocation, fracture), obstruction (e.g., thromboemboli, sickle cell disease, fat emboli, caisson disease), or, hypothetically, compression from local expansion of fatty tissue (e.g., ethanol abuse, glucocorticoid treatment, diabetes mellitus). However, symptoms may not occur unless, weeks later, resorption of dead bone during skeletal repair leads to pathologic fracture. Certain skeletal sites (often subarticular) are predisposed to osteonecrosis, but the sites differ for traumatic and nontraumatic processes and for children and adults. *Osteochondrosis* refers to necrosis of ossification centers; more than 50 eponymic types have been recorded. The susceptibility of children to osteochondrosis and its pathogenesis are poorly understood. At all ages, however, the femoral head is especially prone to infarction. Nontraumatic osteonecrosis commonly affects the femoral condyles, distal end of the tibia, humeral head, and talus.

CLINICAL MANIFESTATIONS

Pain occurs acutely on skeletal collapse. Chronic arthralgia results from desquamated necrotic tissue and articular destruction. Although the pathogenesis is uncertain, intravenous administration of amino-bisphosphonates, especially to patients with malignancy, has been associated with osteonecrosis of the jaw (Fig. 256-1).

TABLE 256-1	CAUSES OF ISCHEMIC NECROSIS OF CARTILAGE AND BONE

Endocrine/metabolic
    Ethanol abuse
    Glucocorticoid therapy
    Cushing's disease
    Diabetes mellitus
    Hyperuricemia
    Osteomalacia
    Hyperlipidemia
    Bisphosphonate therapy (osteonecrosis of the jaw)
Storage diseases (e.g., Gaucher's disease)
Hemoglobinopathies (e.g., sickle cell disease)
Trauma (e.g., dislocation, fracture)
Human immunodeficiency virus (HIV) infection
Dysbaric conditions (e.g., caisson disease)
Collagen vascular disorders
Irradiation
Pancreatitis
Organ transplantation
Hemodialysis
Burns
Intravascular coagulation
Idiopathic, familial
Pregnancy

FIGURE 256-1. Exposed dead bone characterizes osteonecrosis of the jaw.

DIAGNOSIS

Magnetic resonance imaging (MRI) that demonstrates bone marrow edema is especially sensitive for detecting early osteonecrosis. Bone scintigraphy discloses skeletal reconstitution with or without fracture. Relatively late in the pathologic process, radiographs first show patchy areas of osteopenia and osteosclerosis that reflect skeletal repair. A linear subchondral radiolucency (crescent sign) indicates bony collapse.

TREATMENT   Rx

Non–weight bearing is advisable for the affected limb. Decompression by trephine insertion is used at some sites. Arthrotomy to remove debris, transpositional osteotomy, arthroplasty, or joint replacement may be necessary.

● OSTEOSCLEROSIS/HYPEROSTOSIS

Many conditions are associated with radiographic evidence of increased bone density. Skeletal dysplasias, metabolic disturbances, and various other disorders can cause generalized or focal increases in bone mass (Table 256-2). Aberrations in skeletal growth, modeling (shaping), and/or remodeling (turnover) may be at fault. *Osteosclerosis* refers to thickening of trabecular (spongy, cancellous) bone. *Hyperostosis* describes widening of cortical (compact) bone. Increases in trabecular bone, cortical bone, or both may augment skeletal density.

Osteosclerosis

Neoplastic, hematologic, and metabolic disorders may preferentially cause sclerosis in trabecular bone because it houses marrow and remodels more rapidly than cortical bone.

FIBROGENESIS IMPERFECTA OSSIUM

DEFINITION

This rare, sporadic condition features generalized osteopenia, but coarsening of the remaining trabeculae places it among disorders of increased bone mass.

PATHOBIOLOGY

The cause is unknown. Subperiosteal bone formation and collagen synthesis in nonosseous tissues seem to be normal.

CLINICAL MANIFESTATIONS

Typically, intractable skeletal pain begins gradually during middle age or later and then rapidly increases, with a debilitating course and eventual immobility. Spontaneous fractures are a prominent complication. Physical examination reveals marked bone tenderness.

TABLE 256-2 DISORDERS THAT CAUSE DENSE BONES

DYSPLASIAS

Central osteosclerosis with ectodermal dysplasia
Craniodiaphyseal dysplasia
Craniometaphyseal dysplasia
Dysosteosclerosis
Endosteal hyperostosis
   Van Buchem's disease
   Sclerosteosis
   Worth type (LRP5 activation)
Frontometaphyseal dysplasia
Infantile cortical hyperostosis (Caffey's disease)
Juvenile Paget's disease
Lenz-Majewski syndrome
Melorheostosis
Metaphyseal dysplasia (Pyle's disease)
Mixed sclerosing bone dystrophy
Oculodento-osseous dysplasia
Osteodysplasia of Melnick and Needles
Osteopathia striata
Osteopetrosis (several types)
Osteopoikilosis
Progressive diaphyseal dysplasia (Engelmann's disease)
Pyknodysostosis

METABOLIC CONDITIONS

Carbonic anhydrase II deficiency
Fluorosis
Heavy metal poisoning
Hepatitis C–associated osteosclerosis
Hyperparathyroidism, hypoparathyroidism, pseudohypoparathyroidism
Hypervitaminosis A, D
Hypophosphatemic rickets or osteomalacia
Milk-alkali syndrome
Renal osteodystrophy

OTHER DISORDERS

Axial osteomalacia
Fibrogenesis imperfecta ossium
High bone mass (with or without torus palatinus): LRP5 activation
Ionizing radiation
Lymphoma
Mastocytosis
Multiple myeloma
Myelofibrosis
Osteomyelitis
Osteonecrosis
Paget's bone disease
Sarcoidosis
Skeletal metastases
Tuberous sclerosis

From Whyte MP. Skeletal disorders characterized by osteosclerosis or hyperostosis. In: Avioli LV, Krane SM, eds. *Metabolic Bone Disease*, 3rd ed. San Diego: Academic Press; 1998.

DIAGNOSIS

On radiography, only the skull is spared. Initially, osteopenia and a slightly abnormal appearance of trabecular bone are noted. Subsequently, the changes suggest osteomalacia. Corticomedullary junctions become indistinct as compact bone is replaced by an abnormal cancellous pattern. Generalized osteopenia causes the remaining spongy bone to appear coarse and dense, in a fishnet pattern of mixed lytic and sclerotic areas. Alkaline phosphatase activity in serum is increased.

The skeletal lesion is a localized form of osteomalacia that varies considerably in severity from area to area.

Hyperostosis
PROGRESSIVE DIAPHYSEAL DYSPLASIA (CAMURATI-ENGELMANN DISEASE)
PATHOBIOLOGY

Progressive diaphyseal dysplasia (Camurati-Engelmann disease) affects all races and is inherited as an autosomal dominant trait with variable penetrance. New bone formation gradually envelops both the periosteal and endosteal surfaces of long bone diaphyses. In patients with severe disease, osteosclerosis also occurs in the axial skeleton.

Mutations alter the gene that encodes transforming growth factor-β1. Osteoblast differentiation may be deranged.

CLINICAL MANIFESTATIONS

During childhood, limping or a broad-based, waddling gait is noted. Muscular dystrophy can be diagnosed erroneously. Severely affected individuals may have a characteristic body habitus featuring an enlarged head with a prominent forehead, proptosis, and thin limbs with little subcutaneous fat or muscle mass and tender, thickened bones. Cranial nerve palsies and raised intracranial pressure can occur. Some patients have hepatosplenomegaly and Raynaud's phenomenon. Symptoms may remit after puberty.

DIAGNOSIS

Irregular hyperostosis of the diaphyses of the major long bones slowly develops as a result of periosteal and endosteal new bone formation. The femur and tibia are most commonly affected. Metaphyses may be involved. The age of onset, rate of progression, and severity are variable. Clinical, radiographic, and bone scan findings are generally concordant. Serum alkaline phosphatase activity, urinary hydroxyproline levels, and erythrocyte sedimentation rate may be elevated. Histopathologic study reveals newly formed woven bone that matures and becomes incorporated into cortical bone. Electron microscopy of muscle may show myopathic changes and vascular abnormalities.

TREATMENT

Glucocorticoid therapy (typically a low dose of prednisone on alternate days) can relieve bone pain and may normalize skeletal histology. Bisphosphonates are sometimes useful.

ENDOSTEAL HYPEROSTOSIS

PATHOBIOLOGY

Sclerosteosis and van Buchem's disease, autosomal recessive disorders, are the principal types of endosteal hyperostosis. Sclerosteosis and van Buchem's disease both map to chromosome 17q12-q21. Sclerosteosis is caused by deactivating mutations in a gene called *SOST*. Van Buchem's disease involves a downstream deletion. Enhanced osteoblast activity with failure of osteoclasts to compensate for the increased bone formation seems to explain the skeletal changes.

CLINICAL MANIFESTATIONS

Sclerosteosis (cortical hyperostosis with syndactyly) occurs primarily in patients of Dutch ancestry. The gender distribution appears to be equal. Patients are tall and heavy beginning in childhood; have a prominent, square mandible; and are deaf and experience facial nerve palsy from cranial nerve entrapment. Raised intracranial pressure and headache may reflect a small cranial cavity that can shorten life expectancy. Van Buchem's disease causes progressive asymmetrical enlargement of the jaw during puberty. Patients may be symptom free, or, beginning as early as infancy, they may have recurrent facial nerve palsy, deafness, and optic atrophy from the narrowing of cranial foramina. Long bones may hurt with applied pressure but are not fragile.

DIAGNOSIS

In sclerosteosis, the skeleton is radiographically normal in early childhood except for syndactyly, which is common and most often involves the index and third fingers. Progressive bony thickening widens the skull and causes prognathism. Long bones have thickened cortices. The pelvis, vertebral pedicles, ribs, and tubular bones may become dense. Computed tomography has shown fusion of ossicles and narrowing of the internal auditory canals and cochlear aqueducts. Endosteal thickening homogeneously widens diaphyseal cortices and narrows medullary canals. Osteosclerosis involves the skull base, facial bones, vertebrae, pelvis, and ribs. Serum alkaline phosphatase activity can be increased from enhanced skeletal formation.

TREATMENT

Surgical decompression of narrowed foramina may alleviate cranial nerve palsies.

PACHYDERMOPERIOSTOSIS

PATHOBIOLOGY

Pachydermoperiostosis (hypertrophic osteoarthropathy, primary or idiopathic) is an autosomal dominant disorder that features clubbing of the digits, hyperhidrosis with thickening of the skin (especially of the face), and periosteal new bone formation, most prominently in the distal ends of the limbs. Autosomal recessive inheritance also seems to occur. Not all patients manifest all three principal features. A loss-of-function mutation is found in the gene that encodes 15-hydroxyprostaglandin dehydrogenase.

CLINICAL MANIFESTATIONS

Men seem to be more severely affected than women, and blacks more commonly than whites. Symptoms typically begin during adolescence, intensify during the next decade, but then become quiescent. Arthralgia and fatigue are common. Stiffness and limited mobility occur in both the appendicular and the axial skeleton. Clubbing, with slowly progressive enlargement of the hands and feet, results in a pawlike appearance. Cutaneous changes include thickening, furrowing, pitting, and oiliness, especially of the scalp and face.

DIAGNOSIS

Periostitis thickens the distal portions of the tibia, fibula, radius, and ulna. Clubbing is obvious, and acro-osteolysis can occur. Periosteal proliferation is exuberant, with an irregular texture, and it often involves the epiphyses, whereas secondary hypertrophic osteoarthropathy (pulmonary or otherwise) typically causes a smooth and undulating periosteal reaction. Ankylosis of the joints, especially in the hands and feet, may trouble older patients. Bone scanning reveals symmetrical, diffuse, regular uptake along the cortical margins of long bones, especially in the legs—the "double-stripe" sign.

TREATMENT

Patients with painful synovial effusions may respond to nonsteroidal anti-inflammatory drugs. Contractures or neurovascular compression by osteosclerotic lesions may require surgical intervention.

● OSTEOSCLEROSIS WITH HYPEROSTOSIS
Osteopetrosis
DEFINITION

Osteopetrosis (marble bone disease) is a group of rare disorders characterized by an increase in bone mass due to dysfunction in or lack of osteoclasts. There are two major clinical forms: the autosomal recessive or "malignant" type, which results in death during early childhood if untreated; and the autosomal dominant or "benign" type, which causes fewer problems. Other autosomal recessive types feature intermediate severity, neuronal storage disease, stillbirth, or renal tubular acidosis with cerebral calcification secondary to carbonic anhydrase II isoenzyme deficiency. Bisphosphonate-induced osteopetrosis has been reported.

PATHOGENESIS

The defective gene causing autosomal dominant osteopetrosis encodes a chloride channel important for osteoclast activity. Abnormalities in this gene or one that encodes a subunit of a vacuolar proton pump can also result in malignant disease. Carbonic anhydrase II deficiency is caused by deactivating mutations in the gene that encodes this isoenzyme. Rare autosomal recessive cases involve loss-of-function mutations within the genes that encode either receptor activator of nuclear factor kappa-B (RANK) or its ligand (RANKL).

Histopathologic studies show that all true forms of osteopetrosis feature profound deficiency of osteoclast action. Primary spongiosa (calcified cartilage deposited during endochondral bone formation) persists away from growth plates and constitutes the pathognomonic finding. Defective endosteal bone resorption impairs the formation of marrow space. Quiescent skeletal remodeling leads to bone fragility from the diminished interconnection of osteons and the delayed conversion of immature (woven) bone to mature (compact) bone. Neuronal storage disease (ceroid-lipofuscin) could reflect a lysosomal defect. Deficient superoxide production (necessary for bone resorption) may also be a pathogenetic factor.

FIGURE 256-2. Osteopetrosis. Anteroposterior radiograph of the distal end of the femur shows a widened metadiaphyseal region, with characteristic alternating dense and lucent bands. (From Whyte MP, Murphy WA. Osteopetrosis and other sclerosing bone disorders. In: Avioli LV, Krane SM, eds. *Metabolic Bone Disease*, 2nd ed. Philadelphia: WB Saunders; 1990.)

CLINICAL MANIFESTATIONS

Malignant osteopetrosis can manifest during infancy as nasal "stuffiness" from underdeveloped mastoid and paranasal sinuses. Small cranial foramina may cause optic, oculomotor, or facial nerve palsy. Failure to thrive, delayed dentition, and fractures are common. Hypersplenism and recurrent infection, bruising, and bleeding reflect myelophthisis. Short stature, large head, frontal bossing, nystagmus, hepatosplenomegaly, and genu valgum are characteristic physical features. Untreated children usually die during the first decade of life of hemorrhage, pneumonia, severe anemia, or sepsis. Benign osteopetrosis occasionally causes fracture, facial palsy, deafness, mandibular osteomyelitis, bone marrow failure, impaired vision, psychomotor delay, carpal tunnel syndrome, or osteoarthritis. Carbonic anhydrase II deficiency can result in failure to thrive, fracture, developmental delay, mental subnormality, and short stature. Cerebral calcification develops during childhood, but defective skeletal modeling and osteosclerosis may correct spontaneously. Both proximal and distal renal tubular acidosis have been described.

DIAGNOSIS

A generalized increase in bone density is the radiographic hallmark. In severe disease, modeling defects in long bones produce an "Erlenmeyer flask" deformity (Fig. 256-2). Alternating dense and lucent bands commonly occur in the metaphyses and pelvis. The cranium is usually thickened and dense, especially at the base, and the paranasal and mastoid sinuses are underpneumatized. Vertebrae may show, on a lateral view, a "bone-in-bone" (endobone) configuration or end plate sclerosis causing a "rugger jersey" appearance. Skeletal scintigraphy can disclose fractures and osteomyelitis. MRI helps monitor the response to bone marrow transplantation.

Serum levels of acid phosphatase and creatine kinase (brain isoenzyme) are often increased. In malignant osteopetrosis, hypocalcemia with secondary hyperparathyroidism and elevated serum concentrations of calcitriol can accompany radiographic changes that resemble rickets. In benign osteopetrosis, biochemical indices of mineral homeostasis are typically unremarkable, although serum parathyroid hormone levels may be elevated.

TREATMENT   Rx

Because the origin, pathogenesis, and prognosis of the osteopetroses differ, correct classification is crucial. It may be necessary to evaluate disease progression and to study the family. For the malignant form, human leukocyte antigen (HLA)–identical bone marrow transplantation to supply functional osteoclasts has remarkably benefited some children. Calcium-deficient diets have been tried, but their use may be limited by hypocalcemia and rickets. Massive oral doses of calcitriol (1,25-dihydroxyvitamin D_3), together with dietary calcium restriction (to prevent hypercalciuria and hypercalcemia) or human interferon-γ, which enhances superoxide production, have successfully stimulated osteoclast activity. Prednisone alone or with a low-calcium, high-phosphate diet

may also be effective. Glucocorticoid therapy stabilizes pancytopenia and hepatosplenomegaly. Hyperbaric oxygenation helps in the treatment of osteomyelitis. Surgical decompression of optic and facial nerves can be beneficial. Mutation analysis is recommended for nearly all patients.

Pyknodysostosis

EPIDEMIOLOGY

Pyknodysostosis is believed to have affected French impressionist painter Henri de Toulouse-Lautrec (1864–1901). Most descriptions have come from Europe and the United States, but the disorder seems to be especially common in Japan.

PATHOBIOLOGY

This autosomal recessive condition is caused by defects in *CTSK*, the gene that encodes cathepsin K. Diminished rates of collagen degradation and skeletal turnover are reported. In chondrocytes and osteoblasts, abnormal inclusions have been described.

CLINICAL MANIFESTATIONS

Characteristic features seen during infancy or early childhood are disproportionate short stature, relatively large cranium, fronto-occipital prominence, proptosis, bluish sclerae, beaked and pointed nose, small facies and chin, obtuse mandibular angle, high-arched palate, and dental malocclusion with retention of primary teeth. Cranial sutures remain open. Fingers are short and clubbed from acro-osteolysis or aplasia of the terminal phalanges, and the hands are small and square. Repeated fractures cause knock-knee deformity. Mental retardation is noted in approximately 10% of patients. Adult height ranges from 4 feet 3 inches to 4 feet 11 inches. Life expectancy can be shortened by recurrent respiratory infections and right-sided heart failure from chronic upper airway obstruction secondary to micrognathia.

DIAGNOSIS

Osteosclerosis is uniform, first becoming apparent in childhood and increasing with age. Skeletal modeling defects do not occur, although long bones appear to have thick cortices because of narrow medullary canals. Clavicles are gracile and hypoplastic at their lateral segments. The calvaria and base of the skull are sclerotic, orbital ridges are dense, and wormian bones are present.

TREATMENT

No effective medical therapy has been documented. Fractures of the long bones usually mend satisfactorily. Internal fixation of long bones is formidable because of their hardness. Tooth extraction is difficult. Osteomyelitis of the mandible may require antibiotic, surgical, and/or hyperbaric therapy.

Hepatitis C–Associated Osteosclerosis

Rarely, achy and tender limbs develop in individuals who are infected with hepatitis C virus. Radiographic studies reveal a marked generalized increase in bone mass from osteosclerosis and hyperostosis. Disturbances in the insulin-like growth factor system may explain the enhanced bone formation. Calcitonin or bisphosphonate therapy has benefited some patients.

● FOCAL OSTEOSCLEROSIS/HYPEROSTOSIS
Osteopoikilosis

Osteopoikilosis ("spotted bones") is a radiologic curiosity inherited as a highly penetrant autosomal dominant trait resulting from a deactivating mutation of the *LEMD3* gene. The bony lesions are asymptomatic. However, incorrect diagnosis may lead to confusion with serious conditions, including metastatic disease. Some patients have connective tissue nevi called *dermatofibrosis lenticularis disseminata* (or Buschke-Ollendorff syndrome). Radiologically, numerous small, round or oval foci of bony sclerosis appear in cancellous bone in the tarsal, carpal, pelvic, and metaepiphyseal regions of tubular bones.

Osteopathia Striata

This autosomal dominant curiosity features linear striations in the metaphyseal regions of long bones and in the ilium. Clinically important syndromes include osteopathia striata with cranial sclerosis or with focal dermal hypoplasia (Goltz's syndrome). Goltz's syndrome is an X-linked dominant disorder featuring widespread linear areas of dermal hypoplasia and various bony defects in the limbs of female patients due to mutation in the *PORCN* gene.

Melorheostosis

DEFINITION

Melorheostosis causes bony changes likened to wax that has dripped down a candle. No mendelian basis for this disorder has been established. The anatomic distribution suggests a segmentary embryogenic defect.

CLINICAL MANIFESTATIONS

Usually, monomelic involvement is noted; bilateral disease is generally asymmetrical. Cutaneous changes over affected bones are common (e.g., linear scleroderma-like areas and hypertrichosis). Soft tissue abnormalities often appear before the hyperostosis. Symptoms typically begin during childhood, with pain and stiffness as the major complaints. Joints may become contracted and deformed. Leg length inequality results from soft tissue contractures and premature fusion of epiphyses. Skeletal changes seem to progress most rapidly throughout childhood. During adult life, melorheostosis may or may not gradually spread, but pain is especially common.

DIAGNOSIS

As seen radiographically, irregular, very dense, eccentric periosteal and endosteal hyperostosis affects a single bone or several adjacent bones. The lower limbs are most commonly involved. Endosteal thickening predominates during infancy and childhood, and periosteal new bone formation is prominent during adulthood. Ectopic bone formation may occur, particularly near joints.

TREATMENT · Rx

Surgical correction of contractures is difficult. Recurrent deformity is common.

Mixed Sclerosing Bone Dystrophy

This typically sporadic disorder features combinations of osteopoikilosis, osteopathia striata, melorheostosis, cranial sclerosis, and other skeletal defects in one individual. Problems are associated with the individual patterns of osteosclerosis or hyperostosis, such as nerve palsy with cranial sclerosis and bone pain with melorheostosis.

● OTHER DISORDERS OF BONE
Fibrous Dysplasia

This sporadic developmental disorder features an expansile fibrous lesion within bone. Polyostotic disease (with multiple bone lesions) is typically seen before age 10 years; monostotic disease (with solitary bone lesions) begins in adolescence or early adulthood. *McCune-Albright syndrome* refers to a condition characterized by polyostotic fibrous dysplasia, cafe au lait spots (Fig. 256-3), and endocrine hyperfunction.

PATHOBIOLOGY

Postzygotic mosaicism for an activating mutation in the gene that encodes the α subunit of the receptor subunit/adenylate cyclase–coupling G protein, *GNAS*, causes fibrous dysplasia and McCune-Albright syndrome. Imperfect bone forms because mesenchymal cells do not fully differentiate to osteoblasts.

CLINICAL MANIFESTATIONS

Monostotic fibrous dysplasia is more common than polyostotic disease. The skull and long bones are affected most often. The skeletal lesions can deform bones, cause fractures, and occasionally entrap nerves. Sarcomatous degeneration is rare (<1%), but it typically occurs within the facial bones or femur and is more frequent with polyostotic disease. Pregnancy may reactivate previously quiescent lesions. McCune-Albright syndrome usually causes pseudo–precocious puberty in girls. Less commonly, one sees pseudo–precocious puberty in boys or thyrotoxicosis, Cushing's disease, acromegaly,

FIGURE 256-3. McCune-Albright syndrome. Typical rough-border ("coast of Maine"), pigmented cafe au lait spots. (From Whyte MP. Metabolic and dysplastic disorders. In: Coe FL, Favus MJ, eds. *Disorders of Bone and Mineral Metabolism*. New York: Raven Press; 1992.)

FIGURE 256-4. Fibrous dysplasia. A characteristic expansile lesion with a ground-glass appearance has caused thinning of the cortex in the mid-diaphysis of the fibula. (From Whyte MP. Fibrous dysplasia. In: Favus MJ, ed. *Primer on the Metabolic Bone Diseases and Disorders of Mineral Metabolism*, 3rd ed. Philadelphia: Lippincott-Raven; 1996.)

hyperprolactinemia, or hyperparathyroidism. In some patients, acquired renal phosphate wasting causes hypophosphatemic rickets or osteomalacia.

DIAGNOSIS

As seen radiographically, lesions are found in either the metaphysis or diaphysis of long bones. They are typically well defined, with thin cortices, and have a ground-glass appearance (Fig. 256-4). Occasionally, the defects are lobulated, with trabeculated areas of radiolucency.

TREATMENT · Rx

In patients with mild disease, bone lesions may not expand. In severe cases, individual defects can progress, and new ones may appear. Spontaneous healing does not occur, but pathologic fractures generally mend well. Stress fractures, however, can be difficult to detect and treat. When the skull is involved, nerve compression may require surgical intervention. In McCune-Albright syndrome, pharmacologic control of pseudo–precocious puberty can be beneficial in girls. Intravenous infusions of the bisphosphonate pamidronate can help some patients.

Hereditary Multiple Exostoses

This relatively common, highly penetrant autosomal dominant disorder features irregular bony excrescences that protrude from expanded metaphyses. Osteocartilaginous exostoses arise from growth plates and increase in size until linear growth ceases. Lesions may or may not become detached from the parent bone. Their structure is relatively unremarkable, with an outer cortex and an inner spongiosa. Disability results primarily from limb length discrepancies when linear bone growth suffers at the expense of transverse expansion. Compression of nerves, the spinal cord, or the vascular system occurs occasionally. Sarcomatous degeneration (0.5 to 2% of patients) should be suspected when an exostosis enlarges rapidly, especially in an adult.

Enchondromatosis (Dyschondroplasia, Ollier's Disease)

This sporadic disorder features cartilaginous masses within the trabecular bone that arise from growth plates. The condition begins in childhood with localized swelling and interferes with linear bone growth. At puberty, expansion of cartilage masses ceases, and these masses can be replaced by mature bone. Enchondromas appear radiographically as lucent defects in flat bones or in metaphyses of tubular bones, often with central calcific stippling. When enchondromatosis occurs with multiple hemangiomas (Maffucci's syndrome), the enchondromas or hemangiomas undergo malignant transformation in 15% of cases.

Achondroplasia

Chondrodystrophies are disorders of cartilage growth that result in disproportionate short stature. Achondroplasia is the most common. A defect occurs in the gene that encodes fibroblast growth factor receptor type 3; 80% of cases are the result of new autosomal dominant mutations, which increase in frequency with increasing paternal age. Short tubular bones form because of abnormal endochondral ossification in the limbs. In the chondrocranium, membranous ossification is undisturbed; hence the skull vault is normal. However, the cranial base and foramen magnum are small. Lumbar lordosis is greatly exaggerated, and the spinal canal narrows from the upper to lower segments of the vertebral column. This disturbance is revealed radiographically by a decreasing interpediculate distance. The head is large, with frontal bossing and midface hypoplasia. The trunk length is relatively normal, but the limbs show rhizomelic shortening, and the hands have a trident configuration. The long bones appear massive owing to their disproportionately normal width. Growth plates are not grossly disorganized, and chondrocytes appear normal. Complications can include hydrocephalus or compression of the brain stem, spinal cord, or nerve roots. Minimal impingement by a disc or osteophyte on the small spinal canal can cause neurologic disturbances. Despite these problems, achondroplasia is compatible with good health and a normal lifespan.

SUGGESTED READINGS

de Vernejoul MC, Kornak U. Heritable sclerosing bone disorders: presentation and new molecular mechanisms. *Ann N Y Acad Sci.* 2010;1192:269-277. *Review including osteopetrosis, osteosclerosis, osteopoikilosis, and the rare autosomal recessive and dominant sclerosing disorders.*

Fukushima W, Fujioka M, Kubo T, et al. Nationwide epidemiologic survey of idiopathic osteonecrosis of the femoral head. *Clin Orthop Relat Res.* 2010;468:2715-2724. *The peak age is in the 40s, with systemic corticosteroids (50%), habitual alcohol use (30%), and systemic lupus erythematosus (30%) as the most common associated factors.*

Hoff AO, Toth B, Hu M, et al. Epidemiology and risk factors for osteonecrosis of the jaw in cancer patients. *Ann N Y Acad Sci.* 2011;1218:47-54. *The frequency ranges from 0.6 to 6.2% in breast cancer and from 1.7 to 15% in multiple myeloma, but it is also reported in prostate cancer and benign bone disease, especially in relation to dental extractions.*

Ruggiero SL. Bisphosphonate-related osteonecrosis of the jaw: an overview. *Ann N Y Acad Sci.* 2011;1218:38-46. *Review including stage-specific management strategies and guidelines.*

Scaramuzzo L, Messuti L, Mancione PF, et al. Clinical and histological modifications in osteopetrotic bone: a review. *J Biol Regul Homeost Agents.* 2009;23:59-63. *Review of the cause, pathogenesis, and mechanisms of abnormal bone remodeling in osteopetrosis, one cause of diffuse osteosclerosis and bone fragility.*

XXI

DISEASES OF ALLERGY AND CLINICAL IMMUNOLOGY

257

APPROACH TO THE PATIENT WITH ALLERGIC OR IMMUNOLOGIC DISEASE

STEPHEN I. WASSERMAN

Allergic diseases and disorders of the immune system affect multiple organ systems and may arise in a variety of manners. The reader is directed to Section VII for a detailed discussion of the immune system and specific autoimmune and acquired immune disorders. This chapter addresses allergic disorders, the most common manifestation of immune system dysfunction, and primary immune deficiencies, which are uncommon manifestations of immune dysfunction. For clarity, these two issues are treated separately.

ALLERGIC DISEASE

DEFINITION

Allergic disorders are common, and their prevalence is increasing, particularly in urbanized, Western societies. It is said that allergic diseases are the most common disorders seen by primary care physicians. Moreover, even in nonallergic patients, consideration of allergy frequently enters the differential diagnosis of a problem under consideration. Therefore, an appreciation of how to approach the diagnosis and treatment of allergic patients is of major importance to the practice of internal medicine. Allergic disorders are those caused by the interaction of a sensitized host (one who has made immunoglobulin E [IgE] antibody recognizing a specific antigen) with a specific allergen. Not all patients possessing specific IgE antibody react adversely on interaction with the allergen, and such individuals are termed *sensitized* but not *allergic*. The primary allergic conditions are seasonal allergic rhinoconjunctivitis (hay fever), perennial allergic rhinitis or sinusitis, asthma, anaphylaxis (especially secondary to foods, medications, and hymenopteran stings), urticaria or angioedema, atopic dermatitis (eczema), and food allergy.

EPIDEMIOLOGY

It is currently estimated that more than 50% of the population is atopic (i.e., able to mount an IgE immune response and to exhibit an immediate positive prick-puncture hypersensitivity response to common aeroallergens). Clinically, 10 to 20% of the general population will develop allergic rhinoconjunctivitis, 5 to 7% will have active asthma, and 20% will experience urticaria at some time.

The increase in allergic diseases noted in the past 2 decades is thought to result from better hygienic conditions, decreases in infant and childhood infections, and an increasingly sedentary and indoor lifestyle. These changes appear to be associated with a less effective activation of the innate immune system, thereby altering the protective maturation of the acquired immune system. The immune bias in utero and in infancy is toward a type 2 helper T-lymphocyte (T_H2)–directed immune response, which is the immune pathway required for the expression of allergic disease. Ineffective generation of regulatory T lymphocytes underlies the genesis and persistence of allergy. It is therefore postulated that without sufficient early childhood infection to induce a switch to an effective and protective T_H1 immune response, allergic disease is more likely to emerge during childhood. Substantial epidemiologic evidence has been gathered to support this concept, now termed the *hygiene hypothesis*. Thus, allergy is more prevalent in individuals of higher socioeconomic status, among those living in urban areas, in less polluted communities (e.g., western Germany), in first-born children compared with later siblings, in multiply immunized individuals, and in those free of mycobacterial disease. Conversely, children living on farms, in rural communities, and in more highly polluted areas (e.g., eastern Germany), as well as children with mycobacterial infection and those who have experienced multiple early childhood infections, are less likely to develop allergic disorders. A concentration-effect relationship appears to exist between exposure to endotoxin (as a marker for hygiene) and the incidence of allergic sensitization. Low and very high levels of exposure to endotoxin are associated with abnormal immune maturation and allergic expression, whereas moderate levels of exposure predispose to a nonallergic phenotype.

PATHOBIOLOGY

The persistence or aberrant activation of T_H2 lymphocytes leads to the generation of cytokines (e.g., interleukins-4, -5, -13), which stimulate B-lymphocyte synthesis of IgE antibody and the production of eosinophilic polymorphonuclear leukocytes. The expression of allergic disorders results from the interaction of a specific allergen with allergen-reactive IgE bound to high-affinity receptors on mast cells and basophils. This interaction leads to activation of these target cells and to their release of preformed, granule-associated mediators (exemplified by histamine); the synthesis of lipid mediators from membrane lipids (sulfidopeptide leukotrienes); and the transcription and secretion of cytokines, including tumor necrosis factor-α and interleukins-4, -5, and -13. These mediators directly induce smooth muscle contraction, vascular dilation, and endothelial leakage; they also cause vascular adhesion molecule expression, and they attract and activate inflammatory leukocytes, particularly CD4$^+$ T lymphocytes, basophils, and eosinophils. These and other IgE-dependent mediators are thought to be responsible for stimulating smooth muscle proliferation and tissue remodeling.

DIAGNOSIS

Allergy is a systemic immune disorder, so its expression can be multifocal. It is essential to remember this fact when examining a patient with suspected allergic problems because a focus on only the major presenting symptom may be insufficient to identify all the pertinent medical issues in a given patient.

History

Allergic disease has a high degree of heritability, with a great degree of concordance in identical twins. The risk of expressing allergic disease is highest if both parents are atopic. The inheritance of specific manifestations of allergy and of the specific allergen to which a patient is sensitized is less simple. Quite often, the diagnosis of allergic disorders is straightforward and can be made by asking about the nature of the patient's complaints, when and where reactions occur, and what exposures the patient believes are relevant to symptom induction or exacerbation (Table 257-1).

Seasonal and Perennial Rhinitis

Patients with seasonal and perennial rhinitis (Chapter 259) commonly present with complaints of itchy nose and palate; sneezing; watery rhinorrhea; itching, watery, and burning eyes; and nasal obstruction, which, when severe, may cause anosmia. In the evaluation of possible causes of seasonal rhinoconjunctivitis or sinusitis, the time of the year when symptoms occur is pertinent. Symptoms may be associated with the pollination of trees (early spring), grasses (late spring and summer), or weeds (fall). In some patients with perennial symptoms, the multiple overlapping pollen seasons are responsible for their symptoms. Indoor exposures at home, school, work, or

TABLE 257-1 SYMPTOMS, SIGNS, AND TREATMENT OF ALLERGIC DISEASE

SYMPTOMS AND SIGNS	APPROACH TO TREATMENT
SYMPTOMS	
Cutaneous: itch, rash	H_1-antihistamine
Ocular: gritty sensation, itch	Topical H_1-antihistamine or mast cell stabilizing agent
Upper respiratory: palatal pruritus, clear rhinorrhea, sneeze, nasal obstruction	Topical corticosteroid, oral H_1-antihistamine, leukotriene receptor antagonist, topical nasal H_1-antihistamine
Lower respiratory: wheeze, cough, dyspnea	β_2-agonist, inhaled corticosteroid, inhaled β_2-agonist, leukotriene receptor antagonist, oral methylxanthine, parenteral corticosteroid, parenteral anti-IgE
Gastrointestinal: nausea, vomiting, cramping pain	Epinephrine (if caused by anaphylaxis), oral corticosteroid, oral cromolyn
SIGNS	
Cutaneous: flushing, urticaria, angioedema, eczema	
Ocular: conjunctival erythema, chemosis	
Upper respiratory: pallor, edema, clear rhinorrhea, polyps	
Lower respiratory: wheeze	

recreational sites to furred animals, dust mites or insects, and mold should be addressed in the search for additional causes of perennial symptoms. Mold and mites are to be expected in humid environments, and mites are nearly ubiquitous in bedding and in homes with pets, carpeting, and overstuffed furnishings. Additional occupational or recreational exposures may be pertinent in selected situations (e.g., bakers, health care workers, food handlers, horse fanciers, laboratory animal handlers) in which specific inciting allergens may be identified. Because many patients with rhinitis have concomitant asthma, it is important to obtain information about the presence of this disease in patients with rhinitis.

Asthma

Patients with asthma (Chapter 87) may present with cough or wheeze with dyspnea, which is reversible spontaneously or with treatment. In addition to the association with rhinitis, the influence of exercise, exposure to tobacco smoke, effect of respiratory infection (particularly viral), occupational exposures (e.g., ≤30% of atopic animal handlers develop asthma), and medication use (e.g., β-adrenergic blocking drugs) are pertinent. Because most patients with asthma have concurrent rhinitis, it is essential that the physician evaluate this issue in all asthmatic patients. Wheezing may accompany other disorders, including pulmonary edema in congestive heart failure.

Urticaria and Angioedema

Patients with urticaria (Chapter 260) describe pruritic, erythematous cutaneous lesions with regular or irregular borders occurring anywhere on the body; they may vary in size from small (1×1 mm) to extremely large. Skin lesions are often preceded by intense intertriginous pruritus. Individual urticarial lesions generally persist for a few hours and rarely last for more than 24 hours. However, many disorders can cause a sensation of itching; skin and systemic diseases associated with pruritus are listed in Table 443-1 in Chapter 443. Angioedema (Chapter 260) is most frequently appreciated in the face, hands, and other soft tissues and is generally accompanied by symptoms of stretching, tingling, and tightness of the skin rather than pruritus. Lesions, especially in the face, typically last 24 to 36 hours. Although most cases of urticaria or angioedema are not IgE mediated, it is important to identify foods and medications used by patients with acute urticaria or angioedema, particularly those substances ingested within 2 to 4 hours of the development of lesions, and to inquire about insect stings. Chronic urticaria is less often IgE mediated; questions about medications, especially nonsteroidal anti-inflammatory drugs, recent infection (especially with Epstein-Barr virus), and the presence of autoantibodies to the IgE receptor must be addressed. Approximately one half to two thirds of patients with such autoantibodies also have antibodies to thyroid antigens. In angioedema, the use of angiotensin-converting enzyme inhibitors must be sought. Atopic dermatitis is another allergic cutaneous disorder in which patients complain of intense pruritus, especially in flexural surfaces. In adults, foods (IgE mediated) and cutaneous infection with *Staphylococcus aureus* (superantigen mediated) are the most commonly identified precipitating events for atopic dermatitis.

Anaphylaxis

Anaphylaxis (Chapter 261) is the most important allergic emergency and is potentially fatal. It is an acute allergic response associated with cutaneous (urticaria, angioedema, flushing), respiratory (laryngeal edema, asthma), cardiovascular (arrhythmia, hypotension, extravascular fluid loss), gastrointestinal (nausea, vomiting, abdominal pain, diarrhea), and nonspecific symptoms (metallic taste, sense of impending doom) that may occur singly or together. Historical information of note includes all medications, foods, and other encounters occurring within 2 hours of the reaction. Epidemiologic data suggest that foods (especially peanuts, tree nuts, shellfish, milk, and eggs), hymenoptera stings, and medications (antibiotics, muscle relaxants, radiocontrast media) are the most frequently identified causes of this important problem.

Food Allergy

Patients presenting with food allergy often complain of oral pruritus and nausea, vomiting, diarrhea, and abdominal pain. Eczema, urticaria, and anaphylaxis, as noted previously, may also be consequences of food allergy. In general, allergic symptoms consequent to foods occur within minutes to 2 hours of ingestion of the causative food; delayed symptoms are unlikely to be mediated by an IgE-allergen interaction. Other symptoms attributable to foods are less easily explained by allergic mechanisms and are termed *food intolerance*.

Physical Examination

The physical examination of a patient with suspected allergic disease should emphasize the organ systems pertinent to the patient's complaints. The skin should be examined for the presence of urticarial or angioedematous lesions and for signs of atopic dermatitis, including flexural papules, excoriations, and lichenification. Keratosis pilaris, particularly on the outer aspect of the upper arm, commonly accompanies atopic dermatitis. Urticaria typically consists of small, pink, irregular lesions that blanch on pressure and then clear, leaving normal skin. In a patient with urticaria, a simple test for dermatographism should be undertaken. Angioedematous lesions are larger, more diffuse, and pale, and they are found most often on the face and in acral areas.

The eyes, ears, nose, and throat should be examined in all patients suspected of having allergic disease, particularly those whose symptoms suggest seasonal or perennial allergic rhinoconjunctivitis-sinusitis or asthma. In allergic disease, the conjunctivae are often injected and may be edematous. "Cobblestoning" of the epithelium may be present. The periorbital tissues may be swollen and darkened. Examination of the nares may show pale and edematous nasal mucous membranes and swollen turbinates, and polyps may be seen. Secretions, generally clear, may be seen in the nasal passages or in the posterior pharynx. Such secretions generally contain copious numbers of eosinophils (see later), and their absence is a point against an allergic cause. Fever and discolored secretions, particularly those that are thick and yellow or green, in the presence of neutrophilic polymorphonuclear leukocytes suggest infection. Percussion over the maxillary or frontal sinuses may elicit tenderness in acute sinusitis, and in this case, transillumination of the sinus (albeit a test of low sensitivity) may be impaired. In chronic sinusitis, the physical examination may be unrevealing. In acute otitis media, patients may have erythema and bulging or perforation of the tympanic membrane, with fluid in the canal; in chronic cases the drum may be scarred and retracted. Alteration in airborne conduction may be noted as well.

Patients with acute asthma may display tachypnea and auditory wheezes, and they may be unable to speak in full sentences because of shortness of breath. Use of accessory muscles of respiration and evidence of cyanosis should be sought. Examination of the chest includes inspection for evidence of chronic hyperinflation and auscultation for wheezing (which, if unilateral, may suggest a foreign body or tumor). In mild asthma, the examination may be normal, or the only physical finding may be wheezing on forced expiration and a slight prolongation of the expiratory phase.

Patients experiencing acute anaphylaxis usually demonstrate flushing, and concomitant urticaria and angioedema are often present. Assessment of vital signs may disclose hypotension and tachycardia. In some situations, hoarseness or stridor related to laryngeal edema or wheezing secondary to asthma can be identified. Hyperactive bowel sounds may be noted. Progressive hypoxia and cyanosis may ensue. In severe anaphylaxis, cardiovascular collapse secondary to hypoxia and hypotension may result in death.

Laboratory Evaluation

In the evaluation of patients with allergic disorders, the laboratory may be of assistance in both the identification and the quantification of specific organ dysfunction, as well as in the assessment of the presence and specificity of IgE antibody.

Assessment of Total and Allergen-Specific Immunoglobulin E

Essentially all (>95%) IgE antibody is bound to specific high-affinity receptors on tissue mast cells and circulating peripheral blood basophils. The small amount of free serum IgE antibody circulates in nanogram quantities and can be identified only with techniques of sufficient sensitivity. A large proportion of IgE in a given individual may be directed toward a single antigen, so total IgE levels may be normal in the presence of allergic disease. Therefore, the measurement of total serum IgE is rarely of help in making a diagnosis. In a few situations, such as adult atopic dermatitis or allergic bronchopulmonary aspergillosis, measurement of total serum IgE levels may provide insight into disease severity or risk of disease exacerbation.

Of more importance is the identification of allergen-specific IgE in a patient with suspected allergic disease (Table 257-2). Such specific IgE may be identified in vitro or in vivo. A search for allergen-specific IgE is particularly useful in the evaluation of patients with suspected allergic rhinitis, asthma, eczema, food reactions, and anaphylaxis. In vitro assessment is similar to the quantification of total IgE, except the initial capture reagent bound to a solid phase is a specific pollen, mold, insect, venom, food, or other allergen. Development of the assay is identical to that used to quantify total

TABLE 257-2   ADVANTAGES AND DISADVANTAGES OF DIFFERENT ALLERGY TESTING METHODS

METHOD	PATIENT SELECTION	CLINICAL ADVANTAGES	CLINICAL DISADVANTAGES
Skin testing	Clinical indication suggesting allergic disease	Rapid (15-30 min) turnaround Sensitive and specific; prick-puncture for aeroallergens, prick-puncture followed by intradermal testing for drugs, sera, and venoms	Patient must not be taking H$_1$-antihistamine agents for 5-7 days Not interpretable in the presence of dermatographism Requires sufficient normal skin to enable testing
In vitro testing	Clinical indication suggesting allergic disease	Antihistamine therapy not contraindicated Dermatographism not a problem Sensitive and specific; equal to prick-puncture skin testing	Requires blood drawn Slow turnaround (7-14 days)

IgE, and results are generally reported in a semiquantitative manner. The magnitude of the reaction is weakly correlated with the degree of sensitization and expression of allergy, although for certain foods, more precise correlative data exist on the risk of allergy and the amount of allergen-specific IgE detected. To assess allergen-specific IgE in vivo, a minute quantity of the allergen in question is introduced into the skin by a prick-puncture technique, and the cutaneous response is assessed 15 to 30 minutes thereafter. A positive response is one in which a wheal and flare at least 2 mm larger than those caused by a saline control occur at the injection site. In vivo tests are rapid and inexpensive; their use requires the absence of dermatographism, that patients not be taking antihistamine medications, and that patients exhibit a positive response to a control using histamine. In some situations (e.g., penicillin allergy or hymenopteran sting), a more diluted allergen is injected intradermally, and wheal and flare responses are assessed similarly. The presence of allergen-specific IgE antibody and a clear temporal correlation between exposure to allergen and genesis of symptoms are required to conclude that a patient is allergic to a specific allergen. In the absence of symptoms, a patient with allergen-specific IgE is termed *sensitized* but not allergic.

Specific in vivo challenge tests can also be used to identify allergen responsiveness. Such tests in the presence of specific IgE antibody may be useful in research settings, or they may be used clinically to clarify the exact relationship between exposure and symptoms. Such tests can be dangerous, however, because they introduce the allergen to which the patient is presumed allergic. In the case of food allergy, such challenges are best done in a double-blind and placebo-controlled manner; they may be useful to distinguish allergy from sensitization or to eliminate a suspect food from consideration. However, food challenge tests are unnecessary in the case of anaphylaxis and a positive test for IgE antibody to the putative allergen. Because many patients falsely believe that foods are responsible for their symptoms, such double-blind challenges may be useful in directing patients' concerns to more productive areas. Inhalation tests employing specific allergens or chemicals have been helpful in elucidating some cases of occupational allergy or asthma.

Other Laboratory Aids in Allergic Disease
In a patient with acute asthma, chest radiographs generally demonstrate hyperinflation. In some instances, evidence of bronchiectasis may be present, a finding that raises the specter of allergic bronchopulmonary aspergillosis. The presence of a tumor or radiopaque foreign body may be noted on a chest radiograph and should be sought in a patient with unilateral localized wheezing. In the examination of a patient with asthma, assessment of both airflow and volumes can provide a clear picture of the severity of asthma and its response to treatment. Flow-volume loops can also identify the presence of vocal cord dysfunction. When patients with airway obstruction are evaluated, their response to an inhaled β$_2$-adrenergic agonist medication can be helpful in elucidating the reversible nature of their disorder. Essentially all asthmatic patients exhibiting bronchoconstriction display a bronchodilatory response to the inhalation of such agents. In suspected cases of asthma in which pulmonary function is normal, a histamine or methacholine challenge can be performed. These agents take advantage of the nonspecific bronchial hyperresponsiveness that is characteristic of patients with asthma. Failure to develop bronchoconstriction on inhalation of either of these agents strongly argues against the diagnosis of asthma.

Other laboratory tools may be of clinical benefit in the identification and classification of allergic disorders. Audiometry may clarify the degree of hearing loss caused by otitis media in a patient with allergic rhinitis. When sinusitis is suspected, computed tomography of the sinuses provides the most complete image and has the highest degree of sensitivity for the identification

of mucosal thickening, opacification of air spaces, and presence of polyps and bone erosions. Computed tomography is particularly useful in the examination of the ethmoid and sphenoid sinuses, which are often affected in chronic allergic disease and are difficult to assess on physical examination or with plain radiographs.

The quantification of blood, sputum, nasal mucus, or tissue eosinophilia and the response to corticosteroid therapy are useful correlates in the identification and management of allergic disease. The quantification of tryptase, a mast cell–specific protease with a serum half-life of 2 hours, can assist in the diagnosis of anaphylaxis if performed on serum or plasma obtained within hours of a systemic response with associated hypotension.

IMMUNOLOGIC DISEASE

EPIDEMIOLOGY

Diseases related to disordered immune function (immunodeficiency) are far less common than allergic disorders. The most frequent is IgA deficiency, which occurs in approximately 1 in 1000 individuals and is often asymptomatic. Next most frequent are disorders of B and T lymphocytes, such as common variable hypogammaglobulinemia, and other disorders, including DiGeorge syndrome and severe combined immunodeficiency (Chapter 258). Much less common are defects in neutrophil function or complement.

DIAGNOSIS

The clinical expression of immunodeficiency disorders is primarily infection, related to impaired host defense. Thus, the diagnosis of suspected immunodeficiency involves the evaluation of recurrent, persistent, severe, and otherwise unexplained infections. Many, but not all, immune disorders arise in early childhood, and with improved management, many patients presenting in childhood live into adulthood. It is important for the general internist and internal medicine subspecialist to be cognizant of the presentation of these disorders.

History
The most important historical information includes the following: age at onset of the problem in question; family history of frequent infection or death at an early age from infection; number, site, and type of infections; and presence of other physical abnormalities (Table 257-3). The earlier the onset of infections, the more severe the immune defect is likely to be. T-lymphocytic defects, with or without B-cell deficiencies, usually arise in the first 3 to 5 months of life, whereas B-cell function is supported by maternal antibody until after 6 months of age. Many of the immune disorders are X-linked, and a careful family history is critical in such situations. Infection-related death of a patient's male sibling or the patient's mother should lead to the search for such an X-linked disorder.

In a patient with a T-cell disorder, viral, fungal, mycobacterial, and other opportunistic infections (*Pneumocystis jirovecii, Toxoplasma gondii*) are most commonly noted, and live virus vaccination may be associated with disseminated and progressive viral disease. Persistent thrush, diarrhea, malabsorption, and failure to thrive occurring in early childhood may suggest the presence of T-cell abnormalities.

In B-cell or antibody deficiency, pyogenic bacterial infections predominate, particularly infections involving encapsulated microorganisms. Usually such infections affect the upper and lower respiratory tract and the skin and are severe and persistent. Infections with unusual organisms, with unexpected complications, or involving multiple sites (lung, sinus, joint, bone, or

TABLE 257-3 KEY POINTS REGARDING IMMUNOLOGIC DISORDERS

ANTIBODY DEFICIENCY DISORDERS

Onset after 6 mo of age
Recurrent respiratory infection
Infection with bacteria, especially encapsulated organisms
Absence of isohemagglutinins
Evaluation of B-cell function, not numbers

CELLULAR IMMUNE DEFECTS

Onset before 6 mo of age
Recurrent viral, fungal, or parasitic (opportunistic) infection
Defective delayed hypersensitivity skin responses
Malabsorption or diarrhea

COMPLEMENT DEFICIENCIES

Recurrent bacterial infection
Recurrent neisserial infection (deficiency of late components)
Associated rheumatic disorder (especially systemic lupus erythematosus)

FACTORS SUGGESTING NEUTROPHIL DYSFUNCTION

Late separation of umbilical cord
Persistent neutrophilic leukocytosis
Recurrent or persistent gingivitis or periodontitis
Recurrent bacterial infection with granuloma formation

meninges, with abscess formation or sepsis) should raise the index of suspicion. In adults, the most common disorder in this class is termed *common variable immunodeficiency.*

As in any patient with infection, information should be sought about exposure to ill individuals or to irritants such as tobacco smoke, the hygiene of the environment to which the patient has been exposed, and the presence of an anatomic abnormality or allergy that could predispose to infection.

Physical Examination

Physical examination beyond that necessary to assess the extent and severity of a particular infection should focus on immune organs. Assessment of tonsillar tissue and determination of the presence and size of lymph nodes, spleen, and liver are important. Patients with common variable immunodeficiency often present with hepatosplenomegaly and lymph node hyperplasia, whereas in X-linked hypogammaglobulinemia, lymph tissue is absent. Telangiectasia (ataxia-telangiectasia), cardiac defects (DiGeorge syndrome), chronic eczema (Wiskott-Aldrich syndrome), and chronic periodontitis (neutrophil defects) all suggest immunodeficiency syndromes.

Laboratory Evaluation

The proper use of the laboratory is essential to elucidate a suspected immunodeficiency disorder. Screening tests appropriate to the generalist's initial approach include complete blood count, total neutrophil and lymphocyte enumeration, quantitative immunoglobulin levels, and assessment of isohemagglutinins (especially when common variable immunodeficiency is suspected). In some situations, quantification of IgG subclasses may be warranted to identify a specific subclass deficiency. When considering T-lymphocyte defects, it is important to enumerate total T cells and specific T-cell subsets. Delayed hypersensitivity skin testing to recall antigens is also helpful in assessing cellular immunity. When neutrophil defects are suspected, a nitroblue tetrazolium test or measurement of phagocytic potency can be performed. Complement defects are best addressed by obtaining a CH_{50} level. CH_{50} is the amount of patient serum required to cause lysis of 50% of test erythrocytes. It is compared with the amount of pooled normal serum required to cause the same degree of lysis. Tests for specific individual components of complement, or of complement regulatory proteins, can also be obtained under special circumstances.

Additional tests of antibody production in response to defined stimuli, including vaccinations, may be helpful when selective antibody deficiency is suspected or when borderline immunoglobulin levels are encountered in the presence of frequent infection. In some situations, assessment of T-cell proliferation to mitogens or antigen may be of benefit. Further testing might include the assessment of natural killer–cell function and the production of cytokines by activated lymphocytes. In general, such additional laboratory

tests should be performed in consultation with an expert in immune disorders.

SUGGESTED READINGS

Alqudah M, Graham SM, Ballas ZK. High prevalence of humoral immunodeficiency patients with refractory chronic rhinosinusitis. *Am J Rhinol Allergy.* 2010;24:409-412. *Among patients with three episodes in one year, nearly 25% had low levels of one or more immunoglobulins, and one of 67 patients was diagnosed with common variable immunodeficiency.*

Boyce JA, Assa'ad A, Burks AW, et al. Guidelines for the diagnosis and management of food allergy in the United States: summary and the NIAID-sponsored expert panel report. *Nutr Res.* 2011;31:61-75. *Consensus guidelines.*

Nelson KS, Lewis DB. Adult-onset presentations of genetic immunodeficiencies: genes can throw slow curves. *Curr Opin Infect Dis.* 2010;23:359-364. *Review including adult-onset X-linked agammaglobulinemia and other conditions that usually present in childhood but can present in adults.*

Samson M, Audia S, Lakomy D, et al. Diagnostic strategy for patients with hypogammaglobulinemia in rheumatology. *Joint Bone Spine.* 2011;78:241-245. *Drugs, the nephritic syndrome, and protein-losing enteropathy are leading causes, but common variable immunodeficiency is the most usual primary immunodeficiency.*

Sastre J. Molecular diagnosis in allergy. *Clin Exp Allergy.* 2010;40:1442-1460. *New approaches to diagnosis.*

258

PRIMARY IMMUNODEFICIENCY DISEASES

MARK BALLOW

DEFINITION

Although immunodeficiency diseases are relatively uncommon, more than 165 primary immunodeficiency diseases have been described. Immunodeficiencies are generally divided into several categories: B-cell or antibody immunodeficiencies (55% of all immune deficiencies), T-cell or cellular immunodeficiencies (20%), immunodeficiencies associated with the phagocytic system (20%), immune defects of the innate immune system, and immune abnormalities associated with the complement system (5%). Although many primary immunodeficiencies are first noticed in infants and young children, the most frequent B-cell (humoral) immunodeficiencies become evident later in life, especially in young adults; the characteristic presentations of these diseases should be recognized by the physician so diagnosis and treatment can be initiated. The purpose of this chapter is not to present an encyclopedic list of all the known immunodeficiencies but to identify the most common presenting clinical characteristics, define the initial laboratory evaluation, and briefly discuss the approach to treatment.

PATHOBIOLOGY

Genetics

Many of these disorders are caused by mutations of genes required for the development of T cells or B cells or genes needed for the development of precursor cell lineages that differentiate into various types of immune cells. Other genetic abnormalities are widely expressed in many tissues, resulting in complex multisystem disorders along with the immunodeficiency. Some gene mutations that occur in the same immunologic pathway (e.g., cytokine receptor and signaling pathway) result in similar clinical phenotypes and laboratory findings. Conversely, depending on the nature and location of the mutation, defects in other genes may result in immune defects associated with compound heterozygous mutations with complex variable (hypomorphic) clinical phenotypes.

CLINICAL MANIFESTATIONS

This chapter presents the important details of the history and physical examination and the common clinical signs when evaluating a patient with recurrent infections. The association of particular sites of infection and specific pathogens with certain immunodeficiencies is also helpful in directing the physician toward a differential diagnosis and the appropriate screening laboratory tests.

Clues from the Infecting Pathogen and the Organ System Involved

The organ systems affected by infection and the identity of the isolated pathogens provide clues to the nature of the possible defect. A patient presenting with lymphadenitis or recurrent abscesses caused by low-virulence gram-negative organisms such as *Escherichia coli, Serratia,* or *Klebsiella* may have an abnormality in phagocyte function (Chapter 172). Infections with unusual pathogens such as *Staphylococcus epidermidis* or *Pseudomonas* species, especially *Burkholderia cepacia,* also suggest a phagocytic disorder. Another characteristic presentation of patients with a phagocyte defect is a history of recurrent skin infections with catalase-positive *Staphylococcus aureus,* a finding underscoring the importance of effective phagocytosis and intracellular superoxide-mediated killing in controlling these infections. A history of delayed separation of the umbilical cord exceeding 6 to 8 weeks or poor wound healing suggests the diagnosis of a leukocyte adhesion defect. Suppurative adenitis is common in patients with chronic granulomatous disease, and it can be an important clue in the diagnosis when gram-negative bacteria are recovered from the tissues. Gingivostomatitis and dental erosions are characteristic of patients with a phagocytic cell defect such as leukocyte adhesion deficiency (Chapter 172). Recurrent oral ulcers are characteristic of patients with cyclic neutropenia (Chapter 170). Defects in the late complement components C5 through C9 (Chapter 49) are associated with infections caused by *Neisseria* species, such as meningitis caused by *Neisseria meningitidis* or septic arthritis caused by *Neisseria gonorrhoeae.* Patients with C3 deficiency can present with overwhelming septicemia, especially with gram-negative organisms; this finding is consistent with the important role of complement, particularly C3b, in opsonization and the facilitation of phagocytosis.

B-cell abnormalities most commonly lead to recurrent sinopulmonary infections that are frequently caused by encapsulated bacteria such as *Streptococcus pneumoniae* or *Haemophilus influenzae.* Examination of the pharynx and nasal cavities for signs of sinusitis, including posterior pharyngeal cobblestoning, postnasal drainage, or purulent nasal discharge, is important. Tympanic membranes can appear scarred and disfigured as a result of recurrent or chronic infection of the middle ear. Rales on auscultation of the chest may suggest bronchiectasis as a complication of recurrent lung infections. Digital clubbing points to significant lung disease. A characteristic feature of patients with X-linked agammaglobulinemia (XLA) is an unusual susceptibility to a viral meningoencephalitis caused by enteroviruses (e.g., coxsackievirus, echovirus). Chronic gastrointestinal symptoms caused by *Giardia lamblia* are likely related to impaired mucosal immunity and lack of secretory immunoglobulin (Ig) A. Small bowel bacterial overgrowth and infections with *Yersinia* and *Campylobacter* can lead to chronic gastrointestinal symptoms; diarrhea and occasionally malabsorption may be presenting symptoms in patients with common variable immunodeficiency (CVID).

T cells are essential not only in controlling viral, fungal, mycobacterial, and protozoal infections but also in providing crucial signals to help B cells produce immunoglobulins. Extensive mucous membrane candidiasis suggests a T-cell defect. Patients with cellular immune defects often present with opportunistic infections such as *Mycobacterium avium-intracellulare* and *Pneumocystis jirovecii.*

Lymphatic System in Patients with Immunodeficiency

Assessing the lymphatic system for hepatosplenomegaly and for the presence or absence of lymphoid tissue is an important aspect of the physical examination in a patient suspected of immunodeficiency (Chapter 171). Patients with severe combined immunodeficiency disease (SCID) or infantile XLA do not have palpable lymphoid tissue or visible tonsils. However, the presence of lymphoid tissue can be misleading: adult patients with CVID or IgA deficiency may actually have enlarged lymphoid tissue and even hepatosplenomegaly. This occurs because the reticuloendothelial system undergoes hyperplasia in the absence of opsonic antibody.

Immunodeficiency and Autoimmunity

Deficiencies of the early complement components, such as C4 and C2, often present in adults as an associated autoimmune disease that manifests first with arthritis, frequently in conjunction with dermal vasculitis. A lupus-like rash with negative or low-titer antinuclear antibodies may occur in deficiencies of the early components of the classical complement pathway. Patients with some primary immunodeficiencies present with features of autoimmunity involving hematopoietic or other organ systems. For example, the diagnosis of CVID can be preceded by autoimmune hemolytic anemia (Chapter 163).

Immunodeficiency and Gastrointestinal Disease

Many patients with primary immunodeficiency disease have symptoms and clinical findings referable to the gastrointestinal tract. In a survey of 248 patients with CVID, 21% had significant gastrointestinal disease. Liver disease occurred in an additional 12%. Bacterial overgrowth of the small bowel, including infections with *Yersinia* and *Campylobacter,* parasitic infestations with such organisms as *G. lamblia,* and chronic viral enteritis caused by enteroviruses and cytomegalovirus are relatively common in patients with B- or T-cell immune defects. The incidence of lactose intolerance is high in patients with immunodeficiency. Similarly, patients with IgA deficiency often present with gastrointestinal manifestations.

Immunodeficiency and Family History

A detailed family history in patients with suspected immunodeficiency can add valuable information. Numerous immunodeficiencies are X-linked; therefore, a family history of maternal male relatives with unusually frequent infections or who died in early infancy should suggest the possibility of an X-linked form of immunodeficiency. The mother in these cases would be expected to be a carrier, although the rate of new mutations for X-linked disorders is significant; therefore, a negative family history may not exclude this inheritance pattern. CVID and IgA deficiency are familial disorders and often occur in a setting of other family members with autoimmune disorders.

● DEFECTS IN THE INNATE IMMUNE SYSTEM: COMPLEMENT AND PHAGOCYTE DEFICIENCIES
Deficiencies of Complement Proteins

DEFINITION

The complement (C) system is important in host defense and is composed of a complex system of plasma proteins and cell surface receptors (Chapter 49). Important functions of the complement system include opsonization to enhance phagocytosis, clearance of immune complexes, induction of the humoral immune response, and clearance of apoptotic cells.

EPIDEMIOLOGY

Approximately 5% of patients with primary immunodeficiency diseases have complement deficiencies. Although rare, C2 deficiency is the most common of the early complement component diseases; it occurs in 1 in 10,000 whites. C6 deficiency is the most common of the late complement component disorders. The frequency of complement deficiency in sporadic cases of systemic meningococcal infection has been estimated at 15%. In patients with recurrent meningococcal disease, the prevalence is as high as 40%.

CLINICAL MANIFESTATIONS

These disorders are usually inherited as autosomal codominant traits: the parents of the patient have half-normal levels of the involved complement component, and the patient has a complete absence of the component in question. The complement deficiencies can be broadly divided into those of the early classical complement pathway (C1, C2, and C4), the components of the alternative complement pathway (factors B, D, and P), the mannose-binding proteins and their associated proteases (MASP-1 and MASP-2), and the late complement components (C5, C6, C7, C8, and C9). Persons deficient in C3 share characteristics of both early and late complement component deficiencies. Patients lacking one of the early complement components frequently present as adults with a rheumatologic disease. These patients may exhibit the typical features of systemic lupus erythematosus, except they often are seronegative; that is, anti-DNA antibodies are absent, and antinuclear antibodies are present in only low titers. Individuals with C2 deficiency may have either systemic lupus erythematosus or discoid lupus. Other rheumatologic disorders associated with early complement component deficiencies include dermatomyositis, scleroderma, vasculitis, and membranoproliferative glomerulonephritis. Homozygous deficiency of factor H, a complement regulatory protein, may manifest as hemolytic-uremic syndrome (Chapter 175). Likewise, deficiencies of the late complement components are occasionally associated with vasculitis or other lupus-like illnesses. Less frequently, patients with late component deficiencies develop Raynaud's syndrome, scleroderma, or dermatomyositis.

Patients with deficiencies in the late complement components usually present with recurrent, invasive meningococcal or gonococcal infections caused by *Neisseria* species, such as meningococcal meningitis, gonococcal arthritis, or gonococcal septicemia. However, patients with deficiencies of early or alternative pathway complement components, such as properdin deficiency, may also present with recurrent or invasive neisserial infections.

DIAGNOSIS

Individuals with recurrent blood-borne infection with encapsulated bacteria (e.g., *S. pneumoniae*, *H. influenzae*, invasive meningococcal or gonococcal disease) or immune complex disease should be screened for complement deficiency by determining the total hemolytic complement activity (CH_{50}) in the serum, a test of classical pathway activity. The CH_{50} should be undetectable. If the CH_{50} is normal, alternative pathway function should be tested with the AH_{50}. Hemolytic activity is very sensitive to heat degradation, so blood samples must be handled appropriately, and the serum should be separated and frozen at $-70°$ C as soon as possible. Abnormalities in CH_{50} or AH_{50} may be followed by a determination of specific component concentrations in serum.

TREATMENT Rx

Patients with late complement defects should be immunized with the conjugate meningococcal vaccine. There is controversy over the use of prophylactic antibiotics because this could lead to the emergence of resistant strains of *Neisseria*.

Phagocytic Cell and Other Innate Immune Defects

Patients with defects in phagocyte function (Chapter 172) experience repeated infections where the body surface interfaces with the environment. Because of defective phagocyte function, the manifestations of infection may be blunted; erythema, swelling, and pus formation may be limited or absent. Phagocyte defects frequently manifest as infections caused by bacteria of relatively low virulence, such as *S. aureus*; fungi; and gram-negative enteric bacteria, including *Klebsiella*, *E. coli*, *B. cepacia*, and *Serratia* species. These infections often fail to respond optimally to the usual courses of antimicrobial agents. Many patients also have a history of poor wound healing, reflecting the critical role of phagocytes in tissue repair. The clinical features of phagocytic cell defects are shown in Table 258-1.

Normal function of the phagocyte compartment requires adequate numbers of neutrophils and monocytes, as well as the full performance of a number of closely integrated functions that result in the effective killing of a pathogen by the leukocyte. Defects in neutrophil number (severe congenital neutropenia, cyclic neutropenia, Kostmann's syndrome, Shwachman-Diamond syndrome; Chapter 170), adherence, deformability, locomotion, chemotaxis, recognition of foreign particles, phagocytosis, oxidative respiratory metabolism, and intracellular microbial killing (Chapter 172) have all been reported. Data from the history and physical examination can help the clinician focus on which phagocyte function is most likely defective.

A critical aspect of host defense is the accumulation of neutrophils at the site of infection. Absence of pus at the site of infection, for example, suggests that the patient has a decreased number of granulocytes or that these cells have an impaired ability to concentrate at the site of bacterial invasion, that is, defective chemotaxis or adhesion. Conversely, a history of persistent

abscesses with exudates suggests that the phagocytes can migrate to the appropriate site but are defective in intracellular bacterial killing. A history of recurrent gingivitis, skin infections with furunculosis, abscesses of the viscera or perirectal tissues, and lymphadenitis should prompt an evaluation of the phagocyte host immune defenses.

INTERFERON-γ/INTERLEUKIN-12 PATHWAY DEFICIENCIES

These patients have increased susceptibility to infections with nontuberculous mycobacteria, *Salmonella*, and certain viruses, as well as disseminated infection following bacille Calmette-Guérin vaccination. Several genetic defects of the monocyte-macrophage-T_H1 T-cell pathway have been identified. Patients with complete interferon-γ receptor defects have severe impairment in interferon-γ signaling and fail to form tuberculoid granulomas. Patients with a partial defect have a better prognosis. Other patients with a similar clinical phenotype have an interleukin (IL)-12p40 deficiency or a mutation in the IL-12 receptor.

There is significant redundancy in the innate immune system, such that mutations in genes that are important in host defense, such as the defects in the interferon/IL-12 pathway, lead to an increased susceptibility to a variety of pathogens. In contrast, mutations in UNC-93B and TLR3 lead to a pathogen-specific predisposition to herpes simplex viral encephalitis. Undoubtedly there will be more discoveries of primary immune deficiencies associated with gene mutations that lead to specific single-pathogen–associated diseases.

DEFICIENCIES OF T-CELL IMMUNITY

DEFINITION

Profound defects in T-lymphocyte function, or defects arresting the development of T cells early in ontogeny, not only affect cell-mediated immunity but also impair the development of B-lymphocyte function (humoral immunity) owing to the absence of T-cell help and T-cell–derived cytokines. The clinical syndromes resulting from these more profound immune defects are referred to as SCID. Recurrent infections with organisms of relatively low virulence in an immunologically normal host (i.e., opportunistic infections) occur. Patients with T-cell immunodeficiency may develop infection with *Candida albicans* involving the mucous membranes and skin, but this infection is not invasive. Other fungal infections, severe viral diseases, and infection with opportunistic pathogens such as *P. jirovecii* or *M. avium-intracellulare* should prompt an evaluation for disorders in T-cell function. Graft-versus-host disease can be a significant problem in patients with severe T-cell immunodeficiency, either after the transfusion of lymphocyte-containing blood products or as a result of intrapartum or prenatal maternal-fetal transfusion. The clinical characteristics of patients with T-cell deficiency are shown in Table 258-2.

DIAGNOSIS

Patients are evaluated for T-cell deficiency by enumerating peripheral blood T-cell subsets and natural killer (NK) cells by flow cytometry; in addition, lymphocyte proliferative responses to mitogens and specific antigens can be assessed in vitro. Delayed hypersensitivity skin testing can be an initial screening test for T-cell immunity, using the intracutaneous injection of 0.1 mL of recall antigens (i.e., *Candida*) at 1:100 dilution weight/volume, tetanus toxoid at 1:100 dilution weight/volume, or *Trichophyton* at 1:30 dilution. Negative results are seen in patients with impaired T-cell responses, but they can also occur because of the lack of prior antigen exposure. Severe illness or the use of immunosuppressive drugs or systemic corticosteroids can also diminish delayed hypersensitivity responses (anergy).

TABLE 258-1	CLINICAL CHARACTERISTICS OF DISEASES OF PHAGOCYTIC CELL DYSFUNCTION

Can range from mild skin infections to severe systemic infections
  Skin infections, furunculosis, visceral or perirectal abscess with granuloma formation, lymphadenitis, gingivitis
  Poor wound healing, lack of pus
Mainly susceptible to low-grade virulent bacterial infections
  Staphylococcus species
  Gram-negative organisms

TABLE 258-2	CLINICAL CHARACTERISTICS OF T-CELL DEFICIENCIES

Onset of symptoms often in early infancy (4-5 mo)
Recurrent infections with fungi (*Candida*), viruses, and mycobacterial pathogens
Infections with opportunistic organisms: *Pneumocystis jirovecii*
Failure to thrive, often fatal in childhood
Fatal infections from live virus vaccines or bacille Calmette-Guérin vaccination
Graft-versus-host disease from transfusion of blood products containing viable T lymphocytes

● B-CELL IMMUNODEFICIENCIES

Unlike patients with SCID, who first manifest symptoms at 4 to 5 months of age, patients with severe B-cell deficiencies usually do not have problems with infections until 7 to 9 months of age. The onset of infection is later in this group of patients because they are protected initially by maternal antibodies that pass through the placenta during the third trimester of pregnancy. Patients with B-cell immunodeficiencies usually develop infections with encapsulated bacterial organisms such as pneumococci and *H. influenzae*. The types of infection, as discussed previously, include otitis media, meningitis, septicemia, sinusitis, pneumonia, abscess, and osteomyelitis. Occasionally, these patients have problems with fungal or viral pathogens. Male patients with infantile XLA are unusually susceptible to enteroviruses and may develop chronic enteroviral encephalomyelitis. Generally, one does not see severe growth failure in patients with B-cell deficiency, as occurs in T-cell–deficient patients. Patients with antibody deficiency can survive into adulthood and can lead normal lives with the use of replacement intravenous immunoglobulin (IVIG) therapy.

Patients with severe B-cell deficiency, such as infantile XLA, typically have a paucity of lymphoid tissue (tonsils, adenoids, and peripheral lymph nodes). In contrast, patients with CVID often have lymphoid hypertrophy or hepatosplenomegaly. The incidence of allergy and autoimmune disease is increased, particularly in patients with IgA deficiency and CVID. The clinical characteristics of patients with B-cell deficiency are shown in Table 258-3.

X-Linked Agammaglobulinemia

DEFINITION

XLA is an X-linked recessive B-cell immunodeficiency with agammaglobulinemia and absent circulating B cells.

EPIDEMIOLOGY

Worldwide, the incidence appears to be approximately 1 in 100,000 to 200,000, or 5 to 10 cases per 1 million population.

PATHOBIOLOGY

The gene responsible for XLA is located on the X chromosome, and it encodes for a cytoplasmic tyrosine kinase (i.e., Bruton's tyrosine kinase [Btk]), which is expressed mainly in lymphocytes of the B-cell lineage. Btk

TABLE 258-3 CLINICAL CHARACTERISTICS OF B-CELL DEFICIENCIES

Recurrent infections with encapsulated organisms
Sinopulmonary infections, otitis media, meningitis, sepsis, abscess, osteomyelitis, cellulitis
No problems with fungal or viral infections (except enteroviral infection in XLA)
Lymphoid tissues: absent in patients with XLA, hypertrophied in those with CVID
Increased incidence of atopy and autoimmune disease
Granulomatous lung disease in CVID
Gastrointestinal disease
   Celiac disease
   Lactose intolerance
   Bacterial overgrowth of small bowel
   Nodular lymphoid hyperplasia in CVID
Higher incidence of malignancy in CVID

CVID = common variable immunodeficiency; XLA = X-linked agammaglobulinemia.

is critical in B-lymphocyte signal transduction pathways and B-cell differentiation. Numerous mutations of the *BTK* gene have been described in patients with XLA, most involving the kinase domain. Mutations in the *BTK* gene lead to a block in B-cell maturation from pro-B cells to pre-B cells.

Some patients with *BTK* mutations do not present until later in life. This variation may reflect different types of *BTK* mutations. In fact, the block in B-cell differentiation may be "leaky," leading to a low level of immunoglobulin synthesis. A study of one family with XLA showed marked phenotypic variation among the male members who had the same gene mutation; serum immunoglobulin levels were also variable. Investigators have estimated that approximately 10% of adult patients with a diagnosis of CVID may be misdiagnosed and may actually have XLA with deficient Btk.

CLINICAL MANIFESTATIONS

Infections in patients with XLA occur predominantly in the sinopulmonary tract (60% of patients) and include otitis media, chronic sinusitis, and pneumonia. Other types of infections include pyoderma (25%), chronic conjunctivitis (8%), gastroenteritis (35%), arthritis (20%), meningitis or encephalitis (16%), and, less commonly, osteomyelitis (3%) and septicemia (10%). The most common pathogens are *H. influenzae* and *S. pneumoniae*. Patients who are untreated experience repeated pulmonary tract infections, leading eventually to bronchiectasis (Chapter 90). Infections may also occur with *G. lamblia*. Because cellular immunity is intact, most viral infections, fungal infections, and tuberculosis do not present a problem in patients with XLA. Exceptions to this include viral hepatitis, disseminated polio, and chronic enteroviral encephalitis.

Physical findings are related to repeated bacterial infections of susceptible target organs, such as the middle ear, sinuses, and lungs. Patients have a paucity of lymphoid tissues (e.g., adenoids, lymph nodes, spleen), unlike patients with CVID, who often have lymphoid hyperplasia. Unusual complications of XLA include a dermatomyositis-like syndrome and enteroviral meningoencephalitis.

Arthritis occurs in less than half the patients with XLA. In some patients, joint inflammation results from infection with enteroviruses or *Ureaplasma urealyticum.* Joint symptoms usually improve or resolve with IVIG therapy. Patients with XLA are highly susceptible to poliovirus infection; vaccine-associated poliomyelitis has been reported in XLA.

Unlike patients with CVID, autoimmune disorders are not a frequent problem in patients with XLA. Although a predisposition to various cancers is common with many types of immunodeficiencies, it is unclear whether patients with XLA have the same predisposition. The primary immunodeficiency registry reported that only 4.2% of registry patients with malignancies had XLA; lymphoreticular and gastrointestinal malignant diseases were more common.

Patients with XLA have a total absence or marked deficiency of serum immunoglobulins, and they fail to make antibodies to even potent protein antigens. Circulating B cells or surface membrane immunoglobulin-positive lymphocytes are extremely low (≤2%) or absent. T lymphocytes and other lymphoid subpopulations and delayed skin reactivity to recall antigens are normal. The response of peripheral blood lymphocytes to mitogens and allogeneic cells is normal. Lymphoid tissues show an absence of plasma cells, lymphoid follicles, and germinal centers.

DIAGNOSIS

Serum immunoglobulin levels should be quantified; as noted, patients with XLA usually have a profound hypogammaglobulinemia or agammaglobulinemia and fail to make antibodies even to potent protein antigens. Flow cytometry for B-cell numbers shows absent or very low numbers of CD19⁺ B cells (e.g., <2%). Molecular analysis for *BTK* gene mutations can be very helpful in diagnostic evaluations. T-cell number and function are normal.

Immunodeficiency with Hyper–Immunoglobulin M (Immunoglobulin Class Switch Defects)

DEFINITION

Immunodeficiency with hyper-IgM is characterized by severe recurrent bacterial infections and decreased serum levels of IgG, IgA, and IgE but normal or elevated levels of IgM. The X-linked form of this syndrome (type 1) is most common, but a similar phenotype with an autosomal recessive inheritance occurs in female patients (type 3).

PATHOBIOLOGY

Immunodeficiency with hyper-IgM is primarily a disorder of B-cell isotype switching. Mutations in the CD40 ligand (CD40L or CD154) on T cells are responsible for the X-linked form of hyper-IgM (type 1), whereas mutations in the CD40 ligand receptor (e.g., CD40) on B cells are responsible for hyper-IgM type 3.

CLINICAL MANIFESTATIONS

Recurrent bacterial infections of the sinopulmonary tract usually begin in the first or second year of life. Stomatitis and mouth ulcers may occur in association with the neutropenia. *P. jirovecii* has been reported in patients with X-linked hyper-IgM. Other opportunistic pathogens include cytomegalovirus, *Cryptococcus,* and mycobacteria. Patients are susceptible to opportunistic organisms and have a high incidence of autoimmune diseases such as thrombocytopenia, hemolytic anemia, neutropenia, nephritis, and arthritis. Diarrhea is a frequent finding, occurring in more than 50% of patients, often as a result of cryptosporidiosis. Hepatitis B and hepatitis C viral infections produce chronic hepatitis in these patients. Unlike patients with XLA, these patients have marked hypertrophy of the lymphoid tissues, including the tonsils, lymph nodes, and spleen. However, the lymph nodes are poorly organized, with an absence of germinal centers. Proliferation of IgM-producing plasma cells, with extensive invasion of the gastrointestinal tract and liver, may occur by the second decade of life. Patients also have an increased risk of malignant diseases, especially lymphomas. An increased incidence of liver and biliary tumors is a unique feature of X-linked hyper-IgM.

DIAGNOSIS

Serum levels of IgM are often markedly increased and may exceed 1000 mg/dL; however, early in life the serum level of IgM may be normal. Patients can produce IgM antibody, but the secondary IgG response is usually markedly diminished or absent. Surface immunoglobulin–positive lymphocytes in the peripheral blood are primarily positive for IgM; IgA- and IgG-bearing lymphocytes are decreased or absent. T-lymphocyte numbers and mitogen responses are normal. Patients with X-linked hyper-IgM type 1 lack CD40L on activated T cells as a result of mutations in the gene for CD40L. Patients with hyper-IgM type 3 lack the receptor for CD40 ligand (CD40) on B cells and antigen-presenting cells.

TREATMENT   Rx

Supportive care, prophylactic antibiotics for *P. jirovecii*, and recognition and treatment of other opportunistic infections are important. Parenteral nutrition may be necessary for patients with severe gastrointestinal disturbances. Treatment consists of IVIG replacement therapy. The commonly associated autoimmune neutropenia responds well to treatment with IVIG and granulocyte colony-stimulating factor. Bone marrow transplantation has been used to treat patients with this disease.

OTHER FORMS OF HYPER–IMMUNOGLOBULIN M PHENOTYPES

Other patients with a hyper-IgM phenotype have been described with normal CD40L and CD40 expression; these patients may possess mutations in the activation-induced cytidine deaminase (type 2) gene (*AICDA*) or the uracil DNA glycosylase (type 5) gene (*UNG*). These patients differ from those with the X-linked form by exhibiting marked lymph node hyperplasia, enlarged germinal centers with highly proliferating B cells, and the absence of T-cell defects or opportunistic infections.

Another rare form of X-linked hyper-IgM syndrome (sometimes called NEMO syndrome) is associated with ectodermal dysplasia characterized by the absence or hypoplasia of hair, teeth, and sweat glands and by the presence of immunodeficiency. These patients exhibit increased susceptibility to bacterial infections, including atypical mycobacteria, encapsulated bacteria, and herpes viral infections. Most patients have low serum levels of IgG, variable levels of IgM and IgA, and poor antibody production; NK cell function is also defective. This disorder is related to mutations in the gene that encodes the nuclear factor-κB (NF-κB) essential modulator (NEMO or IKKγ), which is required for activation of the transcription factor NF-κB. Treatment consists of IVIG and mycobacterial prophylaxis.

DISEASES OF IMMUNE DYSREGULATION AND IMMUNODEFICIENCY

DEFINITION

The majority of autoimmune diseases have a complex, multifactorial, polygenic cause in which environmental triggers play an important role in their pathogenesis. A separate group of immune disorders affects patients with monogenic defects that impact processes of immune tolerance. These immune deficiencies include autoimmune polyendocrinopathy with candidiasis and ectodermal dystrophy (APECED); immunodysregulation with polyendocrinopathy, enteropathy, and X-linked inheritance syndrome (IPEX); and autoimmune lymphoproliferative syndrome (ALPS).

PATHOBIOLOGY

APECED is an autosomal recessive disorder with a higher frequency in individuals of Finnish, Sardinian, and Iranian Jewish origin. This disorder is caused by mutations in the gene encoding the autoimmune regulator protein (AIRE), a transcription factor that is important in controlling the ectopic expression of self-antigens in the thymus. Mutations in the *AIRE* gene lead to a breakdown in central tolerance and the development of multiorgan autoimmune diseases. IPEX is an X-linked disorder that involves mutations in the *FOXP3* gene, which is important in peripheral tolerance and the function of T-regulatory cells. ALPS is a disorder of programmed cell death, with several different gene mutations leading to defective Fas-mediated lymphocyte apoptosis (Table 258-4).

CLINICAL MANIFESTATIONS

Chronic mucocutaneous candidiasis, hypoparathyroidism, and adrenocortical failure are the classic triad of findings in APECED, with only two of the three required to make the diagnosis. Associated autoimmune disorders include insulin-dependent diabetes mellitus, thyroiditis, premature ovarian failure, hepatitis, and hypergonadotropic hypogonadism. IPEX patients typically present during the first few months of life, most commonly with diabetes mellitus, intractable diarrhea, and failure to thrive. Eczema, hemolytic anemia, thyroiditis, and serious infections are also classic features of the syndrome. Patients with ALPS may present with splenomegaly and lymphadenopathy (Chapter 171), as well as with various autoimmune manifestations, including hemolytic anemia, thrombocytopenia, and neutropenia.

DIAGNOSIS

There are no specific diagnostic tests for APECED; if the disease is suspected based on the clinical presentation, establishing the diagnosis depends on sequencing the *AIRE* gene. For IPEX, evaluating T cells for *FOXP3* expression is helpful. In ALPS, flow cytometry for the presence of double-negative T cells (CD4 and CD8 negative), along with the clinical presentation, is useful to screen for the disorder.

TABLE 258-4	**IMMUNE DISORDERS WITH ABNORMALITIES IN IMMUNE REGULATION**

Autoimmune polyendocrinopathy, candidiasis, ectodermal dystrophy (APECED): mutations in autoimmune regulator gene (*AIRE*)

Immune dysregulation, polyendocrinopathy, enteropathy, X-linked disorder (IPEX): mutations in *FOXP3* gene

Autoimmune lymphoproliferative syndrome (ALPS)
   ALPS type Ia: mutations in Fas (*TNFRSF6*)
   ALPS type Im: somatic mutation in the gene encoding Fas
   ALPS type Ib: mutations in Fas ligand (*TNGSF6*)
   ALPS type II: mutation in caspase 10 (*CASP10*)
   ALPS type III: unknown mutation
   ALPS type IV: mutation in *NRAS*

TREATMENT   Rx

Therapy for APECED is directed at the autoimmune processes and the candidiasis. In IPEX, immunosuppression with calcineurin inhibitors is the most frequent approach. Bone marrow transplantation early in the disease can arrest the progression of diabetes. In ALPS, thrombocytopenia secondary to hypersplenism may respond to splenectomy, although the autoimmune cytopenias may require immunosuppressive therapy. Pneumococcal infections are frequent, and prophylactic antibiotics may be helpful. The increased risk of lymphoma in ALPS patients and family members requires careful vigilance.

COMMON VARIABLE IMMUNODEFICIENCY

DEFINITION

CVID comprises a heterogeneous group of disorders involving both B-cell and T-cell immune dysfunction in which the predominant manifestation is hypogammaglobulinemia. CVID is characterized by recurrent bacterial infections, decreased serum immunoglobulin levels (at least two immunoglobulin isotypes more than 2 standard deviations lower than normal for age), and abnormal specific antibody responses. These patients may present in early childhood, during adolescence, or as young adults. In most patients, the onset of symptoms occurs in the second or third decade of life. In a large study, the average age at onset of symptoms was 25 years, and the average age at diagnosis was 28 years.

EPIDEMIOLOGY

The estimated incidence of CVID ranges from 1 in 10,000 to 1 in 50,000. These figures may underestimate the true numbers of CVID patients because of the late onset of symptoms and underdiagnosis of this immunodeficiency disorder.

PATHOBIOLOGY

The number of immune deviations described in patients with CVID underscores the heterogeneous nature of the immune defects in this syndrome. A homozygous deletion in the gene encoding ICOS, a T-cell costimulatory molecule of the CD28 family that enhances the activation of T cells and is important in T-cell–B-cell interactions, was found in two German families of CVID patients. The clinical phenotype of ICOS deficiency is similar to that of other patients with CVID. Other genetic mutations associated with CVID include the CD19 receptor TACI (*TNFRSF13B*, a receptor for the B-cell growth factor cytokines BAFF and APRIL), the BAFF receptor (*TNFRSF13C*), and *MSH5*.

Family members of patients with CVID exhibit an unusually high incidence of IgA deficiency, autoimmune diseases, autoantibodies, and malignant disease. An inheritance pattern of autosomal dominance with variable penetrance has been suggested.

CLINICAL MANIFESTATIONS

The most frequent presenting infections in adults with CVID involve the respiratory tract, including recurrent otitis media, chronic sinusitis, and recurrent pneumonia, often resulting in bronchiectasis. The bacterial pathogens are similar to those described in XLA. The gastrointestinal tract is affected in approximately half the patients with CVID; patients often present with malabsorption or chronic diarrhea. These symptoms can be related to numerous underlying abnormalities, including lactose intolerance, protein-losing enteropathy, superimposed infection of the small bowel with bacteria such as *Campylobacter* or *Yersinia* or the parasite *G. lamblia*, or infection of the large bowel with normal flora (small bowel bacterial overgrowth syndrome). Atrophic gastritis with achlorhydria may lead to pernicious anemia.

Approximately 5 to 10% of patients with CVID present with noncaseating granulomatous lesions that infiltrate the liver, lymph nodes, skin, and, more commonly, lung. These lesions are often confused with sarcoidosis (Chapter 95). Chronic gastrointestinal disease is often associated with nodular lymphoid hyperplasia, characterized by hypertrophy of the Peyer's patches in the small bowel and diffuse lymphoid infiltration. Hypertrophy of other lymphoid tissues, including the peripheral lymph nodes, the spleen, and occasionally the liver, is also seen. Rarely, hepatosplenomegaly may be severe enough to result in secondary neutropenia or thrombocytopenia. The pathogenesis of this process is not known but may be related to increased production of tumor necrosis factor-α. Patients with granulomatous-lymphocytic interstitial lung disease have a worse prognosis, often developing a restrictive pulmonary pattern with a low-normal diffusing lung capacity for carbon monoxide and diminished T-cell function. High-resolution computed tomography of the chest is helpful in identifying these patients, who require higher replacement doses of IVIG and sometimes treatment with corticosteroids.

Autoimmune disorders occur frequently in CVID (20 to 25% of patients), including rheumatic diseases, hematologic disorders, neurologic diseases, chronic active hepatitis, and endocrinopathies. The incidence of malignant disease is increased (11 to 13%) in patients with CVID during the fifth and sixth decades of life. Most of these malignant diseases involve the gastrointestinal tract and the lymphoid tissues (e.g., non-Hodgkin's lymphoma).

DIAGNOSIS

The serum immunoglobulin levels are markedly diminished in patients with CVID; however, a large variability is seen in the degree of hypogammaglobulinemia. Specific antibodies are usually lacking, and isohemagglutinin titers are generally diminished. The proportions of circulating B cells in the peripheral blood are usually normal, but a subset of patients may lack circulating B lymphocytes. T-cell function can be quite variable, being normal in half of patients. The other half of patients with CVID may exhibit depressed T-cell function, with absent delayed hypersensitivity skin reactivity to recall antigens, low numbers of circulating peripheral blood CD4$^+$ T cells, often a decrease in the CD4/CD8 ratio, and depressed in vitro responses to mitogens and specific antigens. Other recent laboratory findings associated with CVID include the lack of isotype-switched memory B cells (e.g., CD27$^+$, IgM$^-$, IgD$^-$ B cells).

TREATMENT   Rx

Patients with CVID are treated with doses of IVIG ranging from 400 to 600 mg/kg every 4 weeks. Generally, this regimen should achieve a trough serum IgG level higher than 500 mg/dL. Patients who continue to experience recurrent infections or who develop bronchiectasis should be treated with higher doses of IVIG to achieve higher trough levels (e.g., >750 mg/dL).

PROGNOSIS

The prognosis is generally good for patients with CVID whose illness is diagnosed early and who undergo replacement IVIG therapy. The reported mortality rate over a 25-year period was 24%, mostly because of lymphoma (18%) and chronic pulmonary disease (11%). The mean age at the time of death was 45.5 years in women and 40 years in men. The patients who died were more likely to have lower levels of IgG at the time of diagnosis and poorer T-cell proliferative responses to phytohemagglutinin. Twenty-year survival after the diagnosis of CVID was 64% for men and 67% for women, compared with 92 to 94% for the general population. With early diagnosis and replacement IVIG therapy, survival is much improved.

Immunodeficiency with Thymoma

Immunodeficiency with thymoma (Good's syndrome) is a disorder of adults. It typically presents between the ages of 40 and 70 years with recurrent sinopulmonary infections. Affected individuals have adult-onset hypogammaglobulinemia, which may affect all major immunoglobulin isotypes. During the initial investigation of hypogammaglobulinemia, a thymoma (Chapter 99) may be detected as a mediastinal mass on the chest radiograph. Occasionally, the thymoma predates the hypogammaglobulinemia. Thymic tumors are predominantly of the spindle cell type and are usually benign. The clinical symptoms are similar to those found in patients with CVID. In contrast to CVID, however, frequently associated disorders include aregenerative (pure red cell) anemia, agranulocytosis, and myasthenia gravis. These conditions may improve after thymectomy, but the immunodeficiency may persist; CD4$^+$ T-cell lymphopenia and a decreased CD4$^+$/CD8$^+$ ratio are commonly seen. Infections associated with T-cell abnormalities can be seen in these patients, including mucocutaneous candidiasis, cytomegalovirus infection, herpes zoster, and *P. jirovecii* pneumonia.

IMMUNOGLOBULIN A DEFICIENCY

DEFINITION

IgA deficiency is defined as a serum IgA concentration lower than 7 mg/dL, with normal serum levels of IgM and IgG. It is one of the most common

B-cell immunodeficiencies, with an approximate incidence of 1 in 400 to 2000 individuals in the general population.

PATHOBIOLOGY

The genetic defect responsible for IgA deficiency is not known. IgA deficiency shares with CVID the inheritance of a restricted major histocompatibility complex extended haplotype. Although the pathogenesis of IgA deficiency is still unknown, it may share a common origin with CVID because these two disorders have many immune aspects in common. In fact, some patients with IgA deficiency have mutations in *TACI*, similar to the defects described in patients with CVID. IgA deficiency may occur in association with the administration of drugs such as phenytoin, sulfasalazine, hydroxychloroquine, and D-penicillamine. IgA deficiency has also been described in association with partial deletion of the long arm of chromosome 18 (18q syndrome) or with a ring chromosome 18.

CLINICAL MANIFESTATIONS

Many individuals with selective IgA deficiency do not have symptoms. The variability in clinical expression may be related to two factors. First, the IgA-deficient patients who are relatively asymptomatic appear to have a compensatory increase in secretory monomeric IgM in their saliva, upper respiratory tract secretions, and gastrointestinal fluids. Second, the association of IgG2/IgG4 or IgG4 subclass deficiencies with IgA deficiency may predispose IgA-deficient patients to more severe and recurrent sinopulmonary infections.

Symptoms of IgA deficiency include sinopulmonary infections and involvement of the gastrointestinal tract with giardiasis, nodular lymphoid hyperplasia, ulcerative colitis, Crohn's disease, or a sprue-like disease. An increased frequency of autoimmune disorders has also been associated with IgA deficiency, including arthritis, a lupus-like illness, endocrinopathies, chronic active hepatitis, and hematologic disorders. IgA-deficient patients are at risk for the development of anti-IgA antibodies on receipt of blood products. Caution must be exercised in the administration of IVIG for the treatment of IgG subclass deficiency in IgA-deficient patients because most of these preparations contain small amounts of IgA. However, this risk does not appear to be significant in patients with partial IgA deficiency.

DIAGNOSIS

Despite very low serum levels of IgA, the peripheral blood B cells of IgA-deficient patients coexpress IgA, IgM, and IgD, an immature phenotype. However, the lymphoid tissues are deficient in IgA-producing plasma cells. Studies of T-cell function have been normal in most patients with selective IgA deficiency.

TREATMENT   Rx

No specific treatment for IgA deficiency exists. Prophylactic antibiotics may be helpful in patients with recurrent sinopulmonary tract infections. Patients with chronic lung disease should receive conventional therapy to prevent the development of bronchiectasis (Chapter 90). IVIG is not indicated in patients with isolated IgA deficiency. Other supportive treatments are aimed at associated diseases. Patients should be transfused only with washed red cells to avoid sensitization to the IgA in blood products.

PROGNOSIS

The prognosis is good in most cases. Respiratory infections and autoimmune disease are more common in IgA-deficient patients. A few patients with IgA deficiency presenting in childhood may recover spontaneously; other patients may develop CVID.

IMMUNOGLOBULIN G SUBCLASS DEFICIENCIES AND SELECTIVE ANTIBODY DEFICIENCY

DEFINITION

Considerable controversy exists over the biologic significance of IgG subclasses and the clinical significance of an isolated IgG subclass level outside of the normal range. Because healthy individuals without recurrent infections may have abnormally low serum IgG subclass concentrations, immunologists

have questioned whether IgG subclass deficiency represents a true immunodeficiency disease. Deficiency in an IgG subclass is defined as a serum IgG subclass concentration more than 2 standard deviations lower than the normal mean for age. The age at which each of the IgG subclasses reaches adult levels varies. In adults, IgG3 deficiencies are most common, whereas in children, IgG2 deficiencies are most prevalent. IgG subclass deficiency may be seen in conjunction with other primary immunodeficiency disorders such as ataxia-telangiectasia and IgA deficiency. IgG subclass deficiency occurs in approximately 18% of IgA-deficient patients. An IgG subclass deficiency may occur as an isolated immune defect, or two or more IgG subclass deficiencies may coexist (e.g., IgG2 and IgG4 deficiency).

Patients with *selective antibody deficiency* exhibit low responses to immunization with polysaccharides such as *H. influenzae* type b (Hib) capsular antigen or to the pneumococcal polysaccharide antigens, but they have normal serum immunoglobulin isotypes and IgG subclass concentrations. However, these patients respond normally to immunization with Hib-conjugate vaccine, in that the antibody response to the vaccine falls principally within the IgG1 subclass instead of the IgG2 subclass.

CLINICAL MANIFESTATIONS

The most frequent clinical problems associated with IgG subclass deficiency and selective antibody deficiency are recurrent infections of the upper and lower respiratory tracts. Pathogens are generally limited to encapsulated bacteria and respiratory viruses. Because IgG2 is important in the response to polysaccharide antigens, patients with IgG2 deficiency may have increased infections with *H. influenzae* or *S. pneumoniae*. Patients may be unable to produce specific antibodies after immunization with purified polysaccharide antigens (e.g., Pneumovax). Some patients with IgG2 subclass deficiency may be asymptomatic. In part, this may result from a shifting of the antibody response to another IgG subclass or immunoglobulin isotype to compensate for the IgG2 deficiency. IgG3 deficiency, more common in adults, has been associated with recurrent upper and lower respiratory tract infections and may occur in combination with IgG1 deficiency. Several studies have suggested that IgG3 is especially important in the primary response to viral respiratory agents. IgG3 is also the predominant antibody response in *Moraxella catarrhalis,* an organism frequently isolated from patients with chronic sinusitis. IgG4 deficiency occurs in the general population at a rate of approximately 10 to 15%. The clinical significance of IgG4 deficiency is not known.

DIAGNOSIS

Serum immunoglobulin concentrations should be measured by quantitative techniques (nephelometry). Levels in children must be compared with laboratory normals for age. Immunoelectrophoresis is semiquantitative and should not be used to evaluate patients with suspected antibody deficiency. Immunoelectrophoresis should be used only to examine serum for paraproteins such as those found in Waldenström's macroglobulinemia or multiple myeloma. IgG subclass quantification may be helpful, although controversy exists over the utility of these measurements. A careful history and physical examination, and the measurement of functional or specific antibodies, are important in determining the clinical relevance of an IgG subclass deficiency.

Patients may have normal levels of total serum immunoglobulins and normal IgG subclasses yet may fail to make specific antibodies to bacterial or common viral pathogens. Therefore, the assessment of specific antibody formation following vaccine administration is an important part of the laboratory evaluation in patients with suspected B-cell deficiency. Usually, specific antibody titers are obtained at baseline and at 4 weeks after immunization to assess the specific antibody response. Isohemagglutinins are naturally occurring IgM antibodies to the ABO blood group substances. Responses to protein antigens generally fall in the IgG1 subclass, whereas the immune response to the polysaccharide antigens resides in the IgG2 subclass. The antibody responses to conjugate vaccines for Hib and pneumococcal polysaccharides occur primarily in the IgG1 rather than IgG2 subclass. Therefore, these conjugate vaccines may not be helpful in the functional evaluation of an IgG2 subclass deficiency or a selective polysaccharide antibody deficiency. Because recurrent upper respiratory tract infections are common in these patients, one can test the serum for the presence of antibodies to common respiratory agents such as influenza A and B, mycoplasma, respiratory syncytial virus, adenovirus, and the parainfluenza viruses.

TREATMENT   Rx

Replacement IVIG should be considered *only* if patients demonstrate poor antibody responses to vaccine immunization such as Pneumovax. Often, prophylactic antibiotics are useful in this group of patients, at least during the winter months.

SUGGESTED READINGS

CEREDIH: The French PID study group. The French national registry of primary immunodeficiency diseases. *Clin Immunol.* 2010;135:264-272. *The prevalence is 4.4 cases per 100,000 inhabitants, with B-cell immunodeficiencies accounting for 43% of cases.*

Fried AJ, Bonilla FA. Pathogenesis, diagnosis and management of primary antibody deficiencies and infections. *Clin Microbiol Rev.* 2009;22:396-414. *Review emphasizing predisposition to sinopulmonary infections.*

Kobrynski LJ. Primary immunodeficiencies presenting in adolescence. *Adolesc Med.* 2009;20:121-148. *Review.*

Lucas M, Lee M, Lortan J, et al. Infection outcomes in patients with common variable immunodeficiency disorders: relationship to immunoglobulin therapy over 22 years. *J Allergy Clin Immunol.* 2010;125: 1354-1360. *Case series showing trough IgG levels needed to avoid serious clinical manifestations.*

Netea MG, van der Meer JW. Immunodeficiency and genetic defects of pattern-recognition receptors. *N Engl J Med.* 2011;364:50-70. *Gene mutations associated with deficiencies in the innate immune system.*

Notarangelo LD. Primary immunodeficiencies. *J Allergy Clin Immunol.* 2010;125:S182-S194. *Review of diagnosis and treatment.*

Shapiro RS. Malignancies in the setting of primary immunodeficiency; implications for hematologists/oncologists. *Am J Hematol.* 2011;86:48-55. *Since patients with primary imunodeficiency disorders are living longer as a result of advances in recognition and treatment, cancer vigilance is important.*

259

ALLERGIC RHINITIS AND SINUSITIS

LARRY BORISH

DEFINITION

Allergic rhinitis (AR) refers to the nasal and ocular symptoms that occur as a result of an inflammatory hypersensitivity reaction to aeroallergens deposited on the nasal mucosa and conjunctiva.

EPIDEMIOLOGY

AR, the most common chronic disease in the United States, affects between 10 and 30% of adults and up to 40% of children. Each year, nearly 80 million people in the United States experience 7 or more days of nasal or ocular symptoms as a result of AR. Although it is not a severe disorder, the socio-economic costs of AR are substantial. AR is one of the chief reasons for visiting a primary care physician; it adversely affects work productivity and school performance, and it limits socialization. The impact of AR also reflects its association with a variety of comorbid conditions, including asthma (Chapter 87), acute and chronic sinusitis, nasal polyposis, secretory otitis media, and sleep disorders. Adequately addressing AR requires a thorough understanding of its pathophysiology, its relation to these comorbid conditions, and the effects of various therapeutic options on AR and its associated comorbidities.

PATHOBIOLOGY
Airborne Allergens

Allergic respiratory diseases result from a hypersensitivity immune reaction to airborne allergens. These include the pollens and molds that are responsible for seasonal AR (SAR) and the indoor allergens, such as dust mites and animal proteins, that are responsible for perennial AR (PAR) (Table 259-1).

In any area, the specific pollens that are likely to cause symptoms can be predicted from the number of days a pollen is airborne in large numbers. All these pollens use a windborne mechanism to achieve fertilization. Insect-borne pollens, specifically those produced by flowers, are not significantly airborne and therefore are not inhaled in sufficient concentrations to generate immune responses. In the United States, grass pollens (May to June) and ragweed (mid-August to October) are the most important causes of SAR. Tree pollens vary locally but typically start in late February and continue

TABLE 259-1	ALLERGENS CAUSING ALLERGIC RHINITIS
COMMON NAME	**SEASON**
SEASONAL ALLERGENS	
Trees	
Birch	March–May
Cottonwood	April–May
Elm	February–May
Cedar	March–May
Oak	May–June
Maple	March–May
Grasses	
Kentucky blue	Mid-May–June
Timothy	Mid-May–June
Orchard	Mid-May–June
Sweet vernal	Mid-May–June
Fescue	Mid-May–June
Bermuda	Mid-May–June
Weeds	
Ragweed	August–September
Kochia	July–September
Russian thistle	July–September
Sage	July–September
Marsh elder	July–September
English plantain	July–September
Outdoor Molds	
Alternaria	Spring–fall
Cladosporium	Spring–fall
PERENNIAL ALLERGENS	
Household Allergens	
Cockroaches (German and American)	
Dust mites: *Dermatophagoides farinae, D. pteronyssinus, Blomia tropicalis*	
Other insects (spiders, ladybugs)	
Animals	
Cats	
Dogs	
Other pets (guinea pigs, ferrets, hamsters, horses)	
Rodents	
? Chicken feathers	
Indoor Molds	
Aspergillus	
Cladosporium	
Penicillium	

through April. The major trees implicated in allergy include birch in the North, oak in the mid-Atlantic region, live oak in the South, and mountain cedar in the Southwest. In addition to pollens, outdoor molds, particularly *Alternaria* and *Cladosporium,* can produce symptoms. These molds have variable seasons, depending on the weather; high levels of airborne fungi may be common at any time between March and October. In recent years, climate change has influenced both the length and the region of pollen seasons.

PAR may occur year-round, but the term is applied to any rhinitis that does not have a clearly defined seasonal association. The most common causes include (1) indoor fungi, which are related to periods of high indoor humidity; (2) animal danders, particularly cats, but rodents (mice, rats, guinea pigs, ferrets, hamsters), rabbits, dogs, and birds may also be significant; (3) dust mites of the genus *Dermatophagoides,* which grow in bedding and pillows and are semiseasonal, with maximal levels from August to December; and (4) other insects (the best studied is the cockroach, but gypsy moths, crickets, ladybugs, spiders, and beetles may be locally important). Dust mites and cats produce the most important indoor allergens. Dust mites grow well only with a relative humidity higher than 50%. Dust mite allergy is probably relevant in all areas with more than 6 humid months in the year.

Immunoglobulin E, Mast Cell, and Basophil Activation

The traditional view is that AR is caused by the triggering of mast cell degranulation resulting from the cross-linking of surface-bound immunoglobulin

(Ig) E molecules by the aeroallergen. As with all antibody-mediated immune responses, the initial exposure to the antigen results in B-lymphocyte secretion of low-affinity IgM antibodies. Subsequent exposure to the allergen in genetically predisposed subjects leads to a secondary immune response characterized by the isotype switch to IgE. The resulting release of IgE antibodies into the circulation does not cause allergic symptoms; only after these IgE antibodies bind to their high-affinity receptors on basophils and mast cells do symptoms develop with subsequent allergen exposure. It takes the cross-linking of approximately 300 IgE receptors and cells to stimulate degranulation; therefore, it often requires several allergy seasons before sufficient numbers of allergen-specific IgE molecules are present on the mast cell surface to drive degranulation. This means that the development of symptomatic AR is a protracted process, generally requiring at least three or four exposures. As a result, SAR is generally not observed in children until they are approximately 4 years of age. Similarly, in adults, symptomatic responses to local allergens may not develop until approximately 4 years after moving to a region. PAR, however, can develop much faster.

Within minutes of allergen exposure, IgE-sensitized mast cells degranulate and release preformed and newly synthesized mediators, including histamine, proteases (tryptase and chymase), cysteinyl leukotrienes, prostaglandins, and cytokines. Some of these mediators produce the characteristic early-phase symptoms of AR—namely, sneezing, pruritus, rhinorrhea, and, to some extent, congestion. Other mediators stimulate infiltration of the nasal mucosa with inflammatory cells, including basophils, eosinophils, neutrophils, additional mast cells, and mononuclear cells. This infiltration of inflammatory cells and their subsequent release of a secondary wave of mediators sustain the inflammatory reaction and produce the late-phase response of AR. This slowly developing inflammatory response is characterized primarily by nasal congestion. The inflammation that develops over the course of an allergy season is associated with an approximately 10-fold increase in the number of mast cells present in nasal epithelial and submucosal tissue. This reflects the migration of preexisting mast cells into the epithelium and the differentiation and influx of newly synthesized mast cells under the influence of cytokine growth factors. During the course of chronic allergen stimulation, these mast cells also display increased *priming*, which reflects increases in the number of IgE receptors and surface-bound IgE, as well as enhancement of signal transduction pathways. As a result, as the allergen season progresses, less and less allergen is required to trigger mast cell degranulation.

Antigen-Presenting Cell and Helper T-Lymphocyte Activation

In addition to their interaction with mast cells, allergens behave like any other foreign antigen and are processed and presented by antigen-presenting cells to helper T (T_H) lymphocytes. Activation of these antigen-presenting cells, including mononuclear phagocytic cells, B lymphocytes, and especially dendritic cells, is an important source of cytokines, especially those associated with innate immunity such as interleukin (IL)-1, IL-6, and tumor necrosis factor-α (TNF-α). With the development of allergic inflammation, there is an increased presence of B cells expressing allergen-specific surface immunoglobulin and dendritic cells expressing surface-bound IgE. These antibodies can function as receptors that "capture" allergen and increase these cells' effectiveness in antigen processing. The newly activated T lymphocytes tend to resemble T_H2 cells, characterized by the production of IL-4, IL-5, IL-9, IL-13, and granulocyte-macrophage colony-stimulating factor (GM-CSF). These cytokines are also major components of the inflammatory response in AR and contribute to the increased production, recruitment, and activation of eosinophils, mast cells, and basophils. A milieu rich in IL-4 and IL-13 drives the IgE isotype switch and contributes to the further production of allergen-specific IgE.

As a result of these inflammatory processes, over the course of allergen exposure, rhinitis evolves and becomes more dependent on mediators associated with the infiltration of eosinophils, basophils, neutrophils, mononuclear cells, and T_H lymphocytes, as well as the increasingly primed mast cells. The symptoms of acute rhinitis, such as sneezing, itching, and rhinorrhea, largely reflect vasoactive mediator release, especially histamine. As SAR or PAR persists, however, these infiltrating cells continue to produce cytokines and other inflammatory mediators, leading to the mucous hypersecretion, tissue edema, goblet cell hyperplasia, and tissue damage that become the primary sources of allergy patients' symptoms. Because the role of histamine diminishes as AR progresses (discussed later), antihistamines become less effective.

Eosinophils represent an important component of the inflammation that develops in AR. Eosinophils release a wide variety of pro-inflammatory mediators, including cysteinyl leukotrienes (leukotrienes C4, D4, and E4), eosinophil cationic protein, eosinophil peroxidase, major basic protein, IL-3, IL-5, GM-CSF, and platelet-activating factor. Eosinophil-derived mediators are major components of the chronic allergic response and produce many of the symptoms of AR, especially nasal congestion. The natural history of AR is for symptoms to worsen inexorably over several weeks in the presence of ongoing allergen exposure. Symptoms often do not peak until well after the peak in pollen counts, and then they persist after pollen counts have declined. These observations reflect the time frame of the onset of nasal inflammation and tissue damage. The influx of eosinophils into the nasal mucosa correlates with the development and progression of symptoms. In summary, the natural history of AR represents an evolution from an acute, primarily mast cell–mediated process that is responsive to antihistamines to a chronic inflammatory process that is primarily eosinophil mediated and is much less responsive to antihistamines.

CLINICAL MANIFESTATIONS

The diagnosis of AR is based on a history of sneezing, which is often paroxysmal; rhinorrhea with clear, watery secretions; nasal congestion; and itching in the nares and palate. These symptoms are generally associated with allergic conjunctivitis manifested by ocular itching, lacrimation, and conjunctival injection. Severe conjunctivitis is less common in PAR than in SAR. The best explanation for this difference is that pollen grains affect the eyes when they are blown into them. Indoor allergens are less likely to be blown into the eyes because the air is relatively still. Indoor aeroallergens are drawn into the nose by breathing.

What is less well appreciated is that AR is a systemic disease associated with circulating activated T lymphocytes and mononuclear phagocytic cells. The activation of these cells is demonstrated by their production of cytokines associated with innate immunity, such as IL-1, TNF-α, and IL-6. These cytokines are responsible for the lethargy, fatigue, arthralgias, myalgias, and cognitive impairment that frequently accompany AR. These systemic symptoms, which are often the chief complaints of allergy sufferers, contribute to a diminished quality of life and are often severe enough to make normal activities difficult, including work or school. Although fever is not a feature of AR, it is intriguing that the lay terminology for this condition is *hay fever*, a designation reflecting the pronounced flu-like nature of this disease.

DIAGNOSIS

AR is primarily a clinical diagnosis based on symptoms and exposure history. It is a complex genetic disorder, and affected patients generally give a positive family history. Vasoactive mediators induce glandular secretions and vascular leakage, along with engorgement of capacitance nasal venous sinusoids. Physical examination therefore reveals the nasal mucosa to be cyanotic and swollen, with clear secretions. Nasal smears (Hansel stains) of nasal secretions are seldom required, but when performed, they typically reveal eosinophils.

The diagnosis of AR is confirmed by the demonstration of specific IgE antibodies reactive to the relevant allergen through either positive allergy skin tests or IgE immunoassays. Identification of the specific triggering allergen is essential for the institution of appropriate environmental controls. Prick skin testing is safe, specific, and rapid, and it is the diagnostic test of choice for identifying relevant allergens. A positive intradermal test in the presence of a negative prick skin test is often a false-positive result. Intradermal testing is therefore rarely indicated and is associated with potentially life-threatening systemic reactions. If prick skin testing is not available or if the test cannot be performed (e.g., in patients with eczema or dermatographism or in those using antihistamines or antipsychotic agents), IgE immunoassays are an appropriate alternative. As with prick skin tests, positive IgE immunoassays correlate with symptoms caused by natural exposure, establish the diagnosis of AR, and can form the basis for environmental therapy; these assays should therefore be used extensively by primary care physicians who manage patients with AR. However, a negative IgE immunoassay with a strong clinical suspicion suggests the need for referral.

Differential Diagnosis

Other causes of rhinitis are shown in Table 259-2, and the approach to patients with sneezing and rhinorrhea is illustrated in Figure 259-1.

Viral rhinitis may be difficult to distinguish from SAR. Viral rhinitis is not associated with the release of mast cell mediators. The main mediators present in nasal secretions from patients with the common cold are kinins; histamine, leukotrienes, and prostaglandins are less prevalent. The presence of these different mediators is in keeping with the observation that pruritus, paroxysmal sneezing, and clear secretions help distinguish SAR from viral rhinitis, along with the distinct recurrent, seasonal nature of SAR. Viral rhinitis produces thicker, purulent secretions, with neutrophils present on the nasal smear. Conjunctival symptoms are less pronounced, and on physical examination, the nasal mucosa is erythematous and swollen.

Hormonal influences that may produce chronic nasal congestion and rhinorrhea include hypothyroidism, birth control pill use, pregnancy, and menopause. Abuse of topical nasal decongestants (e.g., oxymetazoline), with chronic reflex vasodilation, has historically been the most common cause of rhinitis medicamentosa; however, cocaine abuse is another frequent cause of this condition. Chronic unilateral nasal blockage suggests an anatomic defect, typically a deviated or fractured septum, but such blockage can also result from polyps, tumors, and foreign bodies. This history necessitates computed tomography (CT) of the nose and sinuses and rhinoscopy. Nasal septum deviation hardly ever causes bilateral nasal congestion, and surgical therapy has little role in the treatment of rhinitis that is producing symptomatic congestion.

An abnormal neurogenic response to irritants (e.g., cold air, pollutants, cigarette smoke, strong odors, alcohol, foods) is the predominant feature of vasomotor rhinitis. This disorder is characterized by nasal autonomic nerve dysfunction. Patients with vasomotor rhinitis typically have chronic nasal congestion and posterior pharyngeal drainage, but they lack the paroxysmal sneezing, rhinorrhea, pruritus, conjunctivitis, and systemic complaints typical of patients with AR. In addition, eosinophils are absent in nasal mucus. Topical antihistamines (nasal azelastine, olopatadine) are often effective in vasomotor rhinitis. Patients with this condition also respond to therapy with topical corticosteroids or atropine (nasal ipratropium).

TABLE 259-2 DIFFERENTIAL DIAGNOSIS OF RHINITIS

ALLERGIC
Seasonal allergic rhinitis (SAR)
Perennial allergic rhinitis (PAR)

INFLAMMATORY
Infectious rhinitis (viral)
Nonallergic rhinitis with eosinophilia syndrome (NARES)
Chronic sinusitis with or without nasal polyposis

HORMONAL
Pregnancy, oral contraceptives, perimenopause
Hypothyroidism
Hyperthyroidism

RHINITIS MEDICAMENTOSA
Topical decongestants
Antihypertensives
Antidepressants
Cocaine

VASOMOTOR
Irritant induced (pollution, cigarette smoke)
Cold air induced
Gustatory (food induced)

ANATOMIC
Nasal septal deviation
Tumor, neoplasm
Foreign body
Cerebrospinal fluid leak
Atrophic (post-surgical or trauma)

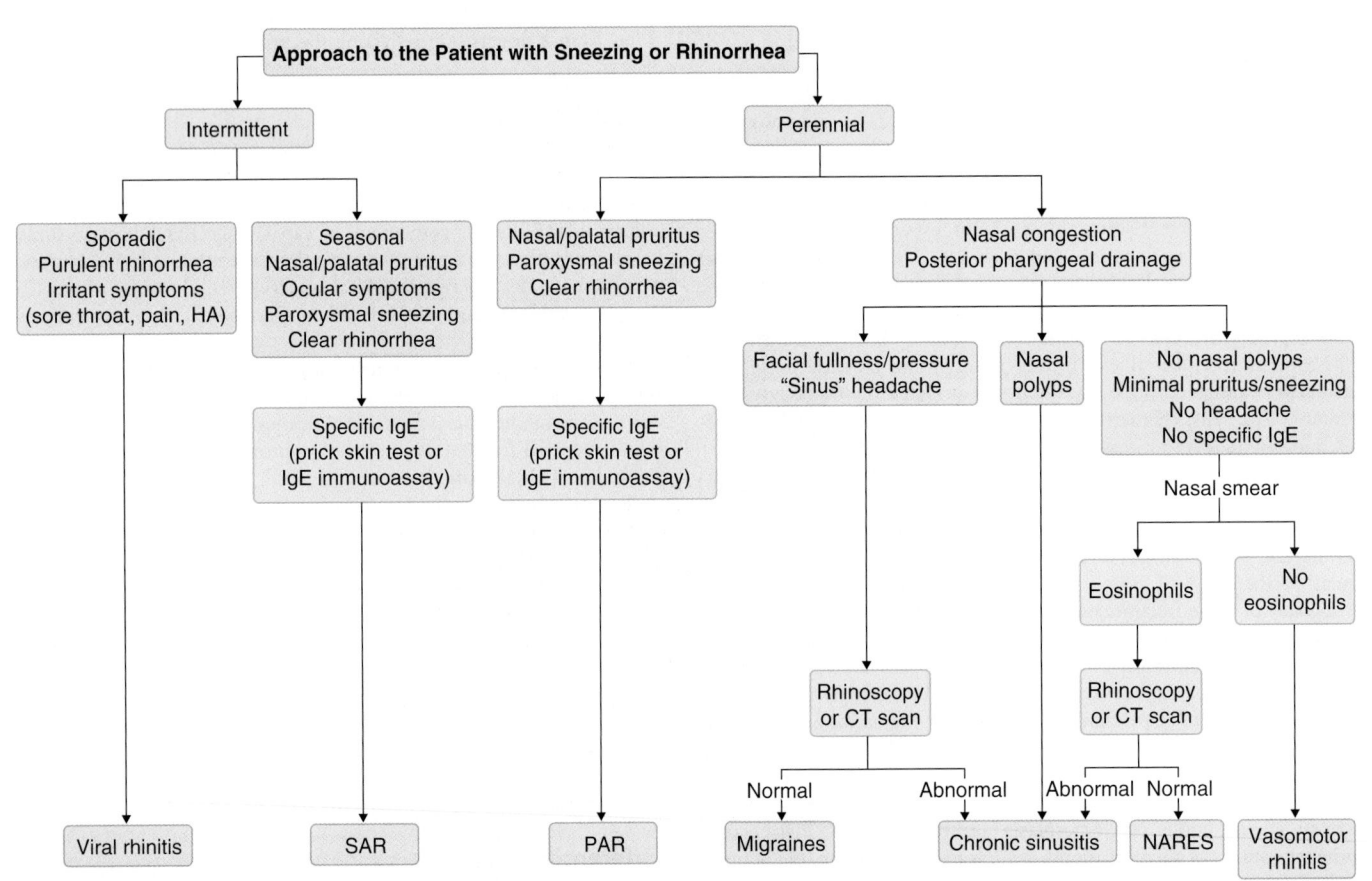

FIGURE 259-1. Approach to the patient with rhinitis symptoms. CT = computed tomography; HA = headache; IgE = immunoglobulin E; NARES = nonallergic rhinitis with eosinophilia syndrome; PAR = perennial allergic rhinitis; SAR = seasonal allergic rhinitis.

Chronic sinusitis with or without nasal polyposis can produce a spectrum of symptoms, including rhinorrhea, mucopurulent posterior pharyngeal drainage, and nasal congestion, that can be mistaken for PAR. However, chronic sinusitis, particularly when it is eosinophilic (discussed later), is often asymptomatic, and a reduced or absent sense of smell may be the only complaint. In contrast to acute sinusitis, headaches are an unusual manifestation of either perennial rhinitis (allergic or nonallergic) or chronic sinusitis, and virtually all patients who complain of "sinus headaches" suffer from atypical migraines or other headache syndromes. Atypical migraines routinely produce headaches that occur in a bilateral distribution involving the maxillary or ophthalmic branches of the trigeminal nerve; this distribution, especially when combined with vasomotor symptoms such as nasal congestion, rhinorrhea, and conjunctival injection, often leads to their misdiagnosis as chronic sinusitis or rhinitis. Because of this overlap in symptoms among chronic sinusitis, perennial rhinitis, and atypical migraines, objective evaluation with either CT or rhinoscopy is usually required to establish the diagnosis of chronic sinusitis.

Atrophic rhinitis is characterized by atrophy of the nasal epithelium and is associated with complaints of nasal congestion and a perceived bad odor. It is observed in elderly patients, but the most common cause is devascularization secondary to nasal surgery or trauma.

Finally, a nonallergic nasal disease characterized by prominent eosinophilic inflammation has been described and termed *non-AR with eosinophilia syndrome* (NARES). On further analysis, many of these patients prove to have chronic sinusitis and nasal polyps. Patients with NARES present with symptoms similar to those of vasomotor rhinitis. NARES is diagnosed by performing a nasal smear (Hansel stain) for eosinophils; however, a CT scan or rhinoscopy is required to rule out chronic sinusitis or nasal polyposis because these conditions may be minimally symptomatic. In contrast to vasomotor rhinitis, NARES is more responsive to intranasal cromolyn and intranasal corticosteroids.

SYSTEMIC MANIFESTATIONS

Allergic inflammation associated with AR can lead to obstruction of the sinus ostia and is an important cause of acute (bacterial) sinusitis. More important is the association between AR and chronic sinusitis. Chronic sinusitis represents many disease processes, including those caused by chronic bacterial infections, cystic fibrosis, immotile cilia syndrome, immune deficiencies, nonspecific inflammation (Fig. 259-2A), hypersensitivity to colonized fungi (allergic fungal sinusitis), aspirin-exacerbated respiratory disease (Samter's triad), and a disorder termed *chronic hyperplastic eosinophilic sinusitis* (CHES) (Table 259-3). In the absence of immunodeficiency or cystic fibrosis, infection is a very unusual cause of chronic sinusitis. Approximately half of all patients with chronic sinusitis have CHES, and this discussion focuses on the underlying allergic mechanisms.

CHES, which generally occurs in association with nasal polyposis, is an inflammatory disorder characterized by the accumulation of eosinophils, fibroblasts, goblet cells, and T_H2-like lymphocytes. The prominent accumulation of eosinophils, however, is the diagnostic feature of this condition (Fig. 259-2B). The inflamed tissue expresses cytokines responsible for eosinophil hematopoiesis (IL-5), survival (IL-3, IL-5, and GM-CSF), recruitment (CCL11 [eotaxin]), and activation (CCL11, CCL5 [RANTES], IL-3, IL-4, IL-5, GM-CSF, and TNF-α). Sensitivity to allergens increases the risk of developing CHES, and more than 50% of individuals with AR have abnormal sinus radiographs. Allergens are unable to gain access to the sinus cavities in healthy subjects (they are not inhaled into the sinuses with breathing, and diffusion is not efficient), and they are even less likely to do so in the presence of occlusion of the sinus openings, which is characteristic of sinusitis. Nevertheless, nasal allergen challenges in sensitive individuals produce radiographic changes and eosinophilic infiltration within the sinuses, and worsening of CHES can be demonstrated during seasonal exacerbations of AR.

The link between AR and sinusitis is thought to involve a systemic inflammatory process (Fig. 259-3). AR is not just a localized inflammatory disorder of the nasal mucosa; it is associated with systemic inflammation. Consequently, it is often seen with other inflammatory conditions such as asthma (Chapter 87), secretory otitis media, and CHES. For example, in patients with SAR who also have asthma, nasal allergen provocation, performed so that the allergen does not gain access to the lungs, leads to increased adhesion molecule expression, eosinophil infiltration, and bronchial hyperreactivity. As illustrated in Figure 259-3, in sensitized subjects, allergen exposure activates immune cells, including T_H lymphocytes, dendritic cells, mononuclear

A

B

FIGURE 259-2. Immunohistochemical analysis of nasal polyp biopsies. **A,** Chronic inflammatory sinusitis displays prominent glandular hypertrophy, collagen bundles, and scattered mononuclear infiltrates. **B,** Chronic hyperplastic eosinophilic sinusitis demonstrates edematous tissue, basement membrane thickening, and prominent eosinophilia (original magnification × 200). (From Payne S, Early SB, Huyett P, et al. Histology and cytochemical profile of nasal polyposis: evidence for distinct eosinophilic and non-eosinophilic diseases distinguished by edema, collagen content, and growth factor expression. In press.)

cells, mast cells, and others, both within the nares and in nasal-associated lymphatic tissues. These cells also include locally produced eosinophil precursors. Some of these T_H cells migrate to the bone marrow, where they stimulate the marrow to produce inflammatory cells, including basophils, eosinophils, and mast cell precursors. Thus, allergen challenges increase the bone marrow concentrations of both cytokines and eosinophil and basophil progenitor cells. Ultimately, these newly generated inflammatory cells enter the circulatory system and are selectively recruited to the sinuses in CHES (and to the lungs in asthma). This selective recruitment of inflammatory cells into the sinuses occurs only in individuals with preexisting CHES in whom specific adhesion molecules, such as vascular cell adhesion molecule-1

TABLE 259-3 HETEROGENEITY OF CHRONIC SINUSITIS

PHENOTYPE	CHARACTERISTIC
Infectious	Very unusual as a cause of chronic sinusitis Occurs in association with cystic fibrosis, immune deficiency
Inflammatory	Reflects remodeling secondary to frequent, recurrent acute sinusitis Develops secondary to anatomic obstruction of the sinus ostia; often responds to surgical correction Pathology demonstrates dense collagen fibrils and glandular hypertrophy and a chronic mononuclear infiltrate, with or without neutrophils Bacterial biofilms contribute to presence and severity Often associated with nasal polyps
Hyperplastic eosinophilic	Prominent eosinophilic infiltrate with systemic eosinophilia Pathology demonstrates edema, sub-basement thickening Frequent association with allergies and asthma Usually associated with nasal polyps
Allergic fungal	Often unilateral; presents as expansive infiltrate on CT scan Associated with elevated total IgE and specific IgE to colonizing fungi
Aspirin-exacerbated respiratory disease (Samter's triad)	Intense eosinophilic infiltrate Usually associated with nasal polyps and asthma Exacerbations of upper and lower respiratory disease (asthma) after ingestion of aspirin and nonselective COX1 inhibitors

COX1 = cyclooxygenase 1; CT = computed tomography; IgE = immunoglobulin E.

(VCAM-1), and chemoattractants, such as CCL11 (eotaxin), are already present. Persons without CHES do not have these addressins in their sinuses and thus do not have the machinery in place to recruit inflammatory cells in response to AR. This model explains the absence of CHES in approximately half of AR sufferers, but it does not explain the event that initiates CHES. Similar systemic mechanisms could produce an interaction between AR and secretory otitis media or asthma. It is not known whether treating AR can lessen the severity of CHES, but the observation that nasal-directed therapies can attenuate bronchial inflammation and symptoms of asthma suggests that such a linkage is plausible.

PREVENTION

Avoidance and Environmental Control

When feasible, avoidance or elimination of the source of the allergen is the treatment of choice for patients with AR. Avoidance studies in AR are limited, and the amount of allergen reduction needed to alleviate symptoms is unknown. Avoidance studies in asthma (Chapter 87) provide compelling evidence of a beneficial effect on bronchial hyperreactivity, symptom severity, and need for β-agonist rescue therapy.

Dust mite avoidance involves four principles: (1) remove reservoirs for mite growth (i.e., use allergen-impermeable mattress and pillow covers and remove fitted carpets), (2) keep the relative humidity lower than 50%, (3) wash bedding in hot water (130° F) to kill mites, and (4) wear a simple mask when dust is being disturbed. Many of the measures suggested for mites are also helpful for fungi, especially dehumidification. Windows, shower curtains, and indoor plants are important sites for fungal growth and can be treated with mild fungicides (dilute household bleach).

In some houses, and particularly urban apartment blocks, large numbers of cockroaches are present, and IgE sensitivity is common. Although it may be difficult to kill cockroaches in an apartment, it is usually possible to keep a house clear of cockroaches by using chemical sprays and traps. Care must be taken when using chemical sprays because they be an irritant to asthmatic patients.

Air-conditioning with closed windows is useful for reducing seasonal allergens, and the dehumidification provided by air-conditioning also mitigates the mite and indoor mold load.

Pets, especially cats, are the most preventable source of allergic diseases. Animal dander accumulates in houses over a prolonged period and takes many months to eliminate after the pet is removed. Although it is difficult to persuade patients to get rid of their animals, it may be possible to move the pet outside into the garage or to restrict the pet's access to certain parts of the house. Dogs kept outside and allowed into the house only occasionally do not appear to be an important cause of symptoms. Cat allergy is a much more serious problem because a single cat can deposit a huge concentration of allergen. Cat owners, in turn, deposit sufficient concentrations of allergen in classrooms and work environments to induce symptoms in their allergic colleagues. The dominant rodent allergen is a urinary protein, and rodents, like cats, can deposit large quantities of allergen in a house.

EVIDENCE-BASED TREATMENTS   Rx

Although avoidance interventions can reduce allergen levels, they often fail to produce clinically significant improvement.[1][2] As a result, pharmacotherapy is frequently required.

Antihistamines

Antihistamines are the oldest drugs used to treat AR and are considered first-line therapy. Antihistamines compete with histamine for the H_1-receptor sites that contribute to sneezing, itching, rhinorrhea, and conjunctivitis. Oral antihistamines ameliorate these symptoms of AR but generally do not improve nasal congestion. They also inhibit mast cell activation as manifested by diminished histamine, cysteinyl leukotrienes, and mast cell tryptase secretion. First-generation antihistamines cross the blood-brain barrier and have significant sedative and anticholinergic effects. In addition to causing sleepiness, they interfere with school, work, driving, or use of machinery. Whereas only 10 to 15% of treated patients complain of sedation, virtually all subjects demonstrate decreased motor skills, diminished driving ability, and reduced cognition when they are given first-generation antihistamines (e.g., chlorpheniramine, diphenhydramine, clemastine). Therefore, use of these drugs is no longer recommended. Second-generation antihistamines have a longer duration of action, do not cross the blood-brain barrier, and are nonsedating. These agents include fexofenadine, descarboxyloratadine, and loratadine. Although less sedating than their parent compound hydroxyzine, cetirizine and levo–cetirizine may occasionally produce sedation. The intranasal antihistamines azelastine and olopatadine do not have a significantly more rapid onset of action than currently available oral antihistamines, but they do have decongestant efficacy and are useful in nonallergic forms of rhinitis. No studies have convincingly demonstrated the superiority of one oral antihistamine over another.

As discussed earlier, the role of histamine diminishes over the course of an allergy season or with PAR, making antihistamines less effective. Antihistamines are quite effective for acute allergic reactions that are mediated prominently by mast cell–derived histamine; as such, they are most beneficial in patients with intermittent allergen exposures, such as occasional outdoor exposure during pollen season. In patients with continuous allergen exposures, however, such as PAR caused by indoor allergens or after several days of continuous exposure to seasonal allergens, these drugs often prove to be little better than placebo.[3][4]

Decongestants

Decongestants such as pseudoephedrine treat nasal stuffiness but are mild stimulants. These drugs are usually used in combination with antihistamines to control the full spectrum of AR symptoms. Antihistamines and decongestants alone generally do not provide satisfactory relief in patients with moderate to severe AR.

Leukotriene Modifiers

Leukotriene modifiers (zileuton, zafirlukast, montelukast) have confirmed efficacy in AR comparable to that of antihistamines.[3][4] This efficacy reflects the presence and importance of these pro-inflammatory vasoactive mediators in AR. Zafirlukast significantly reduces sneezing, rhinorrhea, and—in contrast to antihistamines—nasal congestion in patients with SAR. Similarly, montelukast significantly improves nasal and ocular symptoms as well as quality of life in patients with SAR and PAR.[3] No studies have been performed to determine whether, in contrast to antihistamines, leukotriene modifiers have additive effects when combined with intranasal corticosteroids in patients with refractory AR.

Nasal Cromolyn

Nasal cromolyn stabilizes mast cells and mediates additional anti-inflammatory activities toward macrophages and T lymphocytes. Although not as effective as intranasal corticosteroids, cromolyn provides relief in patients with mild to moderate symptoms,[4] and it may be effective in combination with corticosteroids in the treatment of refractory symptoms. The

FIGURE 259-3. In sensitized subjects, allergen exposure activates immune cells, including helper T (Th) lymphocytes, dendritic cells, mononuclear phagocytic cells, mast cells, and others, both within the nares and in nasal-associated lymphatic tissues. These cells may also include locally produced CD34⁺ interleukin-5 receptor-positive (IL-5R⁺) eosinophil/basophil (Eo/B) progenitors. These newly activated Th lymphocytes have the phenotype of Th2-like cells, characterized by their production of IL-3, IL-4, IL-5, IL-9, IL-13, CCL11 (eotaxin), and granulocyte-monocyte colony-stimulating factor (GM-CSF). Some of these T_H cells migrate to the bone marrow, where they stimulate the marrow to produce inflammatory cells, including basophils, mast cells, and—most important—eosinophils. Ultimately, these newly generated inflammatory cells enter the circulatory system and are selectively recruited back to the nose as well as to the sinuses (and lungs), thus exacerbating inflammation. This selective recruitment of inflammatory cells into the sinuses and lungs occurs only in individuals with preexisting chronic hyperplastic eosinophilic sinusitis and asthma in whom specific adhesion molecules, such as vascular cell adhesion molecule-1 (VCAM-1), and chemoattractants, such as CCL11, already exist. VLA-4 = α4B1 integrin; very late antigen-4. (From Borish L. Allergic rhinitis: systemic inflammation and implications for management. *J Allergy Clin Immunol.* 2003;112:1021-1032.)

value of cromolyn is mitigated by the need for frequent doses (four times/day), a lack of efficacy in approximately 30 to 40% of recipients, and the superior efficacy of intranasal corticosteroids in controlled studies. Cromolyn (one to two sprays in each nostril every 3 to 4 hours) may be especially useful preventatively (e.g., immediately before cat exposure or before the start of the allergen season). Unlike antihistamines, cromolyn controls nasal congestion. Ocular cromolyn has been especially useful in the treatment of allergic conjunctivitis. No significant side effects are associated with its use.

Intranasal Corticosteroids

Intranasal corticosteroids (fluticasone [Flonase, Veramyst], triamcinolone [Nasacort], flunisolide [Nasarel], budesonide [Rhinocort], mometasone [Nasonex], and ciclesonide [Omnaris]) are the most effective AR treatments and are considered the treatments of choice for patients with moderate to severe SAR or PAR.[4,5] Comparative studies of antihistamines and intranasal corticosteroids consistently favor the corticosteroids and show insignificant additive effects when antihistamines are combined with optimal topical corticosteroids.[4,6] In well-performed placebo-controlled studies, intranasal corticosteroids provided a 50 to 90% reduction in symptoms (compared with 20 to 30% for antihistamines). In contrast to antihistamines, topical corticosteroids reduce nasal congestion in addition to relieving itching, rhinorrhea, sneezing, and allergic conjunctivitis. Few studies have directly addressed the influence of corticosteroids on the systemic effects of AR—including missed work and school, poor productivity, reduced cognition, and fatigue—which are often the dominant complaints of patients with AR; however, intranasal corticosteroids significantly improve quality of life, reflecting relief from these complaints. Corticosteroid therapy must be given for up to 1 week before it is fully effective, so ideally, it should be started before exposure or the start of the allergy season. However, intranasal corticosteroids produce some clinical improvement in less than 24 hours and possibly as quickly as 6 to 8 hours. Although efficacy is greatest with continuous administration, as-needed intranasal corticosteroids have proved efficacious.

Topical corticosteroid therapy does not inhibit IgE synthesis or mast cell degranulation, traditionally considered the two determinants for the development of AR. However, corticosteroids do inhibit T-lymphocyte proliferation, chemokine and cytokine production, recruitment of eosinophils and basophils, mucous secretion, vascular permeability, and mast cell proliferation. Intranasal corticosteroid use is therefore associated with diminished nasal eosinophilia, mast cell numbers, and cytokine expression. The efficacy of intranasal corticosteroids emphasizes the importance of these nonhistamine mechanisms to the pathophysiology of AR.

Several intranasal corticosteroid preparations are currently available and differ according to dose, approval age, and propellant (Table 259-4). No studies have demonstrated superior efficacy for any of the nasal corticosteroid preparations. Clinical experience with asthma (Chapter 87) suggests that patients refractory to one intranasal corticosteroid may be switched to a higher-potency corticosteroid; however, the best evidence is that all these agents are comparably valuable when patients are willing to comply with their use. Choices should be based primarily on patient preference.

There is no convincing evidence of clinically significant systemic absorption or the production of systemic side effects from intranasal corticosteroids. Given these drugs' hydrophobicity, local metabolism, and lack of absorption from lung tissue, systemic absorption from the nasal passages is unlikely. Intranasal corticosteroids, even at greater than recommended doses, do not significantly suppress serum or urinary cortisol levels or adrenocorticotropic hormone stimulation tests. Studies have reported a small but statistically significant effect on short-term growth velocity in children with PAR but no impact on ultimate adult height. Nasal corticosteroids cause minimal topical side effects, including local irritation, dryness, and epistaxis. Adverse side effects may differ based on the drug's formulation; aqueous formulations usually produce fewer adverse reactions than aerosols. Nasal biopsy studies do not demonstrate nasal atrophy. Nasal perforation has been reported, but primarily in the setting of underlying devascularization (previous trauma, surgery, or cocaine abuse).

TABLE 259-4 INTRANASAL CORTICOSTEROIDS*

GENERIC NAME	DOSE (PER ACTUATION)	MINIMUM APPROVED AGE	USUAL DOSING
Flunisolide	25 μg	6 yr	Twice daily
Triamcinolone	55 μg	6 yr	Once daily
Budesonide	32 μg	6 yr	Twice daily
Fluticasone	50 μg	4 yr	Once daily
Mometasone	50 μg	12 yr	Once daily
Ciclesonide	50 μg	6 yr	Once daily

*Intranasal corticosteroids are generally administered at 2 sprays per nostril.

Immunotherapy

The clinical efficacy of immunotherapy for AR caused by grass, ragweed, many other pollens, cat and dog dander, and dust mites has been categorically established in innumerable well-designed, controlled studies. Immunotherapy decreases the severity of AR, reduces the need for pharmacotherapy, and significantly improves quality of life. In patients with severe AR and conjunctivitis poorly controlled by antihistamines and intranasal corticosteroids, immunotherapy can reduce allergen sensitivity by more than 10-fold, as well as significantly decreasing total symptoms and reducing total antiallergic drug usage.[7][8] The efficacy of immunotherapy has also been convincingly established in allergen-exacerbated (extrinsic) asthma (Chapter 87), with studies showing decreased symptoms and less need for β-agonist rescue therapy. Efficacy depends on delivery of the correct antigen, regular injections for 3 to 5 years, and administration of an adequate dose of the allergen (10 to 15 μg), a dose significantly higher than those used historically.

Immunotherapy is indicated primarily in patients with refractory rhinitis or in those experiencing unacceptable side effects from standard medications. Because intranasal corticosteroids are not universally effective and do not provide complete relief in all patients, consideration of immunotherapy is necessary. In addition, despite the excellent safety profile of intranasal corticosteroids, many patients are reluctant to use them. Patients should normally go through at least one full pollen season before considering immunotherapy. Immunotherapy is the only treatment that produces long-term immune modulation. Both avoidance and pharmacotherapy are effective only if they are sustained. The effects of immunotherapy, in contrast, persist for many years after a 3- to 5-year course of treatment has been discontinued, and they could be lifelong.[9] A 5-year course of immunotherapy also has cost advantages over lifelong pharmacotherapy. Many patients are attracted to immunotherapy by this potential for long-term immune modulation, remission of symptoms, and ability to discontinue daily pharmacotherapy.

Immunotherapy is associated with a small risk of fatal anaphylaxis (about 3 fatalities/year in the United States, out of 2 million people receiving this form of treatment). Because of this risk, immunotherapy must be administered only in a facility where resuscitation equipment and trained personnel are available. Asthmatic patients are uniquely at risk for fatal anaphylaxis, so immunotherapy should be recommended with caution in these patients.

Summary

Many patients have multiple antigen sensitivities, and specific immunotherapy at effective doses may not be practical. Furthermore, immunotherapy has poor efficacy for many antigens, such as molds. These issues have led to a search for new immune-based therapies capable of attenuating allergic inflammation. Many experimental approaches being developed for asthma, including various anticytokine therapies, may have efficacy for AR.

In general, however, currently available therapies provide adequate relief for virtually all AR sufferers. The persistence of nasal symptoms in the face of adequate AR-directed pharmacotherapies should suggest the diagnosis of an alternative form of rhinitis (see Fig. 259-1) or the presence of sinusitis or atypical migraines. Given the high frequency of AR in the population (and the even higher prevalence of allergic sensitization), treatment becomes particularly challenging when a patient presents with nonallergic nasal symptoms and either concomitant AR or evidence of allergic sensitization (IgE) in the absence of AR.

Grade **A**

1. Woodcock A, Forster L, Matthews E, et al. Control of exposure to mite allergen and allergen-impermeable bed covers for adults with asthma. *N Engl J Med.* 2003;349:225-236.
2. Terreehorst I, Hak E, Oosting AJ, et al. Evaluation of impermeable covers for bedding in patients with allergic rhinitis. *N Engl J Med.* 2003;349:237-246.
3. Meltzer EO, Malmstrom K, Lu S, et al. Concomitant montelukast and loratadine as treatment for seasonal allergic rhinitis: a randomized, placebo-controlled clinical trial. *J Allergy Clin Immunol.* 2000;105:917-922.
4. Wallace DV, Dykewicz MS, Bernstein DI, et al. The diagnosis and management of rhinitis: An updated practice parameter. *J Allergy Clin Immunol.* 2008;122:S1-S84.
5. Vaidyanathan S, Barnes M, Williamson P, et al. Treatment of chronic rhinosinusitis with nasal polyposis with oral steroids followed by topical steroids: a randomized trial. *Ann Intern Med.* 2011;154:293-302.
6. Weiner JM, Abramson MJ, Puy RM. Intranasal corticosteroids versus oral H₁ receptor antagonists in allergic rhinitis: systematic review of randomized controlled trials. *BMJ.* 1998;317:1624-1629.
7. Nanda A, O'Connor M, Anand M, et al. Dose dependence and time course of the immunologic response to administration of standardized cat allergen extract. *J Allergy Clin Immunol.* 2004; 114:1339-1344.
8. Cox L, Li JT, Nelson H, et al. Allergen immunotherapy: A practice parameter second update. *J Allergy Clin Immunol.* 2007;120:S25-S85.
9. Durham SR, Walker SM, Varga EM, et al. Long-term clinical efficacy of grass-pollen immunotherapy. *N Engl J Med.* 1999;341:468-475.

SUGGESTED READING

Brozek JL, Bousquet J, Baena-Cagnani CE, et al. Allergic rhinitis and its impact on asthma (ARIA) guidelines: 2010 revision. *J Allergy Clin Immunol.* 2010;126:466-476. *Focused update on the prevention of allergic diseases and the use of oral and topical medications.*

URTICARIA AND ANGIOEDEMA

STEPHEN C. DRESKIN

● URTICARIA

Urticaria (hives) consists of pruritic, edematous, erythematous, blanching papules that are round or oval in shape; have pale, raised centers (wheals); are several millimeters to a few centimeters in size; and are transient, lasting minutes to days (Fig. 260-1). Angioedema appears as a brawny, nonpitting edema, typically without well-defined margins and without erythema. Angioedema can be accompanied by a sense of burning, pressure, or aching but not pruritus; it is distinguished from other edematous states by its frequent involvement of the lips, tongue, eyelids, hands, feet, or genitalia and its rare occurrence in dependent areas of the body. Episodes (daily or almost daily symptoms) of recurrent hives and/or angioedema over a period of less than 6 weeks are considered acute, and those lasting longer are said to be chronic. Patients typically present with urticaria alone or urticaria with angioedema. Rarely, patients present with angioedema alone. The terms *urticaria* and *urticaria/angioedema* are used interchangeably here to refer to illnesses characterized by urticaria and/or angioedema in which mast cells are activated.

EPIDEMIOLOGY

Urticaria/angioedema occurs in 15 to 25% of individuals at some time during their lives and can affect both genders and all races. Acute urticaria is more common in young adults and children. Chronic urticaria is more common in adults, affecting women (75% of cases) more often than men.

PATHOBIOLOGY

Mast cells, the primary effector cells in urticaria/angioedema, are found in high numbers throughout the body, particularly within the subcutaneous tissue. After activation of mast cells there is a rapid (<10 minutes) release of histamine, leukotriene C₄ (LTC₄), and prostaglandin D₂ (PGD₂), leading to vasodilation, subcutaneous and intradermal leakage of plasma from postcapillary venules, and pruritus. In addition, there is the delayed (4 to 8 hours) production and secretion of inflammatory cytokines such as tumor necrosis factor-α (TNF-α), interleukin (IL)-4, and IL-5, leading to an inflammatory infiltrate and perpetuation of longer-lived lesions. Angioedema is formed by a similar extravasation of fluid, not superficially in the skin but in deeper dermal and subdermal sites.

Lesions of acute urticaria typically show subcutaneous edema with widened dermal papillae, swollen collagen fibers, and rare inflammatory cells. Most episodes of acute urticaria/angioedema are caused by immediate hypersensitivity reactions to drugs or foods or result from inflammatory

FIGURE 260-1. Extensive urticaria. Many presentations are more subtle. (From Roitt I, Brostoff J, Male D, eds. *Immunology*, 6th ed. London: Mosby; 2001: figure 21-2.)

processes initiated by viral illnesses. The most common drugs that cause acute urticaria/angioedema are penicillins, sulfonamides, muscle relaxants, diuretics, and nonsteroidal anti-inflammatory drugs (NSAIDs), although any drug acting as a hapten can generate an allergic response. The predominant allergenic foods are milk, eggs, and peanuts for children and peanuts, tree nuts, fish, and shellfish for adults, although sensitization can occur to many other foods as well. These allergens cross-link immunoglobulin (Ig) E bound to the high-affinity receptor for IgE (FcεRI), leading to activation of mast cells. Some drugs (e.g., opioids, vancomycin, NSAIDs) and radiocontrast dye can activate mast cells by an IgE-independent (pseudoallergic) mechanism. Ingestion of fish contaminated with bacteria that produce histamine leads to hives as part of a toxic reaction to the histamine (scombroid food poisoning).

Lesions of chronic urticaria are characterized by similar edematous findings, with the addition of a dense perivascular inflammatory infiltrate consisting of CD4⁻ and CD8⁺ T lymphocytes, eosinophils, basophils, and neutrophils. A minority of patients exhibit urticarial vasculitis, with lesions characterized by vascular destruction with leukocytoclasis.

The largest subgroup of chronic urticaria/angioedema is idiopathic urticaria, accounting for approximately 80% of cases. These patients have symptoms in the absence of a specific physical trigger, allergen exposure, or coexistent disease. Half the patients with idiopathic urticaria have evidence of autoimmunity based on the presence of IgG antibodies that can cross-link FcεRI and/or antithyroid antibodies. Some experts consider these patients to have a separate entity called *autoimmune urticaria,* whereas others consider these patients to have idiopathic urticaria with evidence of autoimmunity.

Physical stimuli activate mast cells by unknown mechanisms and account for about 20% of cases of chronic urticaria. The most common of the physical urticarias is dermographism (also called dermatographism), in which wheals can be "written on the skin" by simple stroking or scratching. Cholinergic urticaria is often included as a physical urticaria, although the trigger leading to mast cell activation is related to cholinergic stimuli occurring after exposure to heat or after exercise. Other physical stimuli can cause urticaria, including cold, solar radiation, pressure, vibration, and water. Cold-induced urticaria is rarely caused by cryoglobulins.

In approximately 5% of patients with chronic urticaria/angioedema, symptoms appear to be caused by ingestants (e.g., foods, medications, dietary supplements), contactants (e.g., soaps, detergents, cosmetics, hair or nail products, latex), concomitant infections, hormonal changes, or systemic illnesses. A food must be consumed regularly to cause chronic urticaria. Wheat is occasionally found to be a trigger. Multicellular parasites (e.g., those causing strongyloidiasis or filariasis) elicit strong IgE responses and are important causes of chronic urticaria in endemic areas. Rare patients report that their urticaria occurs only during menses or is worsened by menses. Some of these patients have immediate hypersensitivity to progesterone (positive skin tests), and others may be reacting to NSAIDs taken for uterine cramping. Chronic urticaria/angioedema can be associated with flares of rheumatic conditions, other autoimmune conditions (including Hashimoto's thyroiditis), or neoplastic conditions. Occult neoplasia is exceedingly unlikely to be the cause of chronic urticaria.

CLINICAL MANIFESTATIONS

Patients often report that the first sensation of urticaria is poorly localized pruritus that quickly develops into the typical lesions of urticaria. The intensity of the pruritus varies from a minor inconvenience to an unbearable sensation that can lead to self-inflicted abrasion of the skin. Groups of hives often appear together over a short period, and episodes of hives can come in waves starting several times a day. Patients with cholinergic urticaria usually have a distinctive clinical presentation of diffuse urticarial lesions measuring a few millimeters in diameter on exertion sufficient to cause sweating. The pruritus is particularly intense, and all the symptoms are generally limited to the skin. A self-rated quality-of-life survey of patients with chronic urticaria revealed dramatic impairment in terms of loss of sleep, fatigue, and emotional discomfort. Angioedema can originate near a wheal or independently in other parts of the body. Symptoms vary from minor discomfort to an intense sense of pressure and may lead to other symptoms, such as severe shortness of breath if there is compromise of the airway.

DIAGNOSIS

The first episode of acute urticaria/angioedema may occur in the absence of an identifiable stimulus. If hives occur 5 to 30 minutes after ingestion of a drug or a food, the patient often can identify the association. If a physician is consulted, the best approach is to take a careful history, with attention to ingestants and intercurrent illnesses. Unnecessary drugs and food supplements should be discontinued, and any recently added medication should be changed to a structurally different agent. Most often no causative agent is identified, and the hives are treated symptomatically (see the later discussion) for days or weeks before they resolve spontaneously.

Differential Diagnosis

The differential diagnosis of chronic urticaria/angioedema includes the subgroups of urticaria discussed earlier: idiopathic, autoimmune, physical, ingestant-mediated, and associated with a variety of systemic illnesses. Other conditions that can be confused with chronic urticaria/angioedema include diffuse pruritus complicated by dermographism, flushing disorders, urticarial vasculitis, urticaria pigmentosa, systemic mastocytosis, exercise-induced anaphylaxis, exercise-induced food-associated anaphylaxis, idiopathic anaphylaxis, hereditary angioedema, acquired angioedema, and angioedema associated with angiotensin-converting enzyme (ACE) inhibitors (Table 260-1).

Approximately 95% of patients with urticaria/angioedema are not reacting to an ingestant and do not have another illness that is causing their hives. However, it is sometimes difficult for patients (and some physicians) to accept this fact, prompting an extensive, invasive, expensive, and unnecessary investigation. The best "test" to identify patients with a specific underlying cause (i.e., physical trigger, autoimmune condition, allergen, or systemic disease) is a careful and detailed history and physical examination by a specialist knowledgeable in urticarial disease.

A good place to begin is by excluding possible physical triggers. Specific tests are available to establish the diagnosis of most physical urticarias, including scratching the skin and exposing the skin to heat, ice, vibration, pressure, ultraviolet radiation, or water. Acquired cold urticaria must be distinguished from the familial cold autoinflammatory syndrome, which is characterized by a cold-induced papular rash (not urticaria) and is now classified in the family of hereditary periodic fever syndromes. Solar urticaria must be distinguished from other types of light sensitivity, including metabolic abnormalities (e.g., erythrogenic porphyria) and photosensitivity due to drugs.

Even though foods and drugs are infrequent causes of chronic urticaria, many patients focus on ingestants and are not satisfied until these causes are ruled out. As in the evaluation of acute urticaria, the patient must discontinue all food supplements and medications that are not absolutely necessary and, if possible, change essential medications to structurally unrelated compounds. The patient then keeps a food diary to identify suspect foods that

TABLE 260-1 CLASSIFICATION OF URTICARIA AND ANGIOEDEMA

I. Acute urticaria/angioedema
  A. Hypersensitivity reactions
    1. Drug allergy
    2. Food allergy
    3. Insect allergy
  B. Idiopathic
  C. Pseudoallergic reactions
    1. Drugs
    2. Radiocontrast dye
  D. Toxic reactions
  E. Immune complex
    1. Serum sickness
    2. Transfusion related
    3. Postviral
II. Chronic urticaria/angioedema
  A. Idiopathic
    1. Autoantibody associated
      a. Anti-IgE receptor (FcεRI)
      b. Anti-IgE
      c. Antithyroid
      d. Other
    2. Not associated with autoantibodies
  B. Physical
    1. Dermographism
    2. Cholinergic
    3. Delayed pressure
    4. Solar
    5. Cold
    6. Vibratory
    7. Aquagenic
  C. Immune complex
    1. Urticarial vasculitis
    2. Collagen vascular disease associated
III. Urticaria pigmentosa and systemic mastocytosis
IV. Complement-related and kinin-mediated angioedema
  A. Hereditary angioedema
  B. Acquired angioedema
  C. Angiotensin-converting enzyme inhibitor–induced angioedema
  D. Renin inhibitor–induced angioedema
V. Urticaria pigmentosa and systemic mastocytosis

can be eliminated. Some allergists use skin tests with foods to identify "suspects." For highly motivated patients, 2 weeks of a severely restricted diet, often based on lamb and rice, is recommended. Antihistamines and other medications used to control the urticaria must be discontinued. If the urticaria resolves, it is critical to reintroduce foods in a controlled fashion to identify the specific food causing the urticaria and to reinstate a healthy diet.

Chronic infections, including sinus infection, dental abscess, *Helicobacter pylori* gastric infection, cholecystitis, onychomycosis, and tinea pedis, have been associated with urticaria. Case reports indicate the resolution of urticaria after treatment of these infections, although rigorous proof of an association is lacking. The natural history of chronic urticaria probably accounts for coincidental spontaneous improvement after treatment of these conditions, at least in some cases.

Laboratory evaluation in a patient with typical urticaria should always include a complete blood count with differential, basic metabolic panel, liver enzymes, and urinalysis. Specialists are not in full agreement regarding the necessity of additional laboratory testing. Levels of thyroid-stimulating hormone and antithyroid antibodies may be measured in otherwise euthyroid-appearing patients to screen for occult hypothyroidism and for antithyroid autoantibodies. Skin tests for immediate hypersensitivity to foods may be ordered for patients with a suggestive history. Some specialists order no screening tests at all. As in vitro tests for anti-FcεRI autoantibodies become more widely available, it is likely that many specialists will perform this test. A positive test for anti-FcεRI autoantibodies is useful, because this reassures the patient that the urticaria is being driven by an internal process and is not caused by an ingestant or occult illness. Also, this finding helps direct the physician toward immunomodulatory therapies. Other tests should be ordered only as a result of positive findings in the history and physical examination.

Although not routinely indicated in every case of chronic urticaria, a skin biopsy can provide useful information. The most common indication for this procedure is to rule out urticarial vasculitis when the hives are more painful than pruritic, last longer than 24 hours, or leave discolored skin. The presence of vascular destruction, fibrinoid necrosis, and immune complex deposition on microscopic examination (including immunofluorescence) should lead to a consideration of the specific causes of urticarial vasculitis (e.g., systemic lupus erythematosus) and the rapid initiation of more aggressive treatment.

Primary mast cell disorders rarely manifest as chronic urticaria (Chapter 263). Systemic mastocytosis is a very rare condition resulting in increased numbers of atypical mast cells in the bone marrow, skin, and other organs. Levels of tryptase (an enzyme specific for mast cells) are usually elevated in the serum. This condition is frequently accompanied by episodic flushing, urticaria pigmentosa, prominent gastrointestinal symptoms, neuropsychiatric symptoms, and/or recurrent anaphylaxis. Urticaria pigmentosa is characterized by distinctive pigmented cutaneous lesions containing nests of mast cells and is not easily confused with urticaria/angioedema.

Hereditary angioedema, acquired angioedema, and angioedema associated with ACE inhibitors are discussed later in this chapter. Briefly, these syndromes are characterized by episodic swelling without urticaria and are best identified by a careful history, physical examination, and focused laboratory evaluation.

TREATMENT   Rx

Acute urticaria is usually self-limited and responds well to histamine 1 (H_1)-type antihistamines. Antihistamines work better if they are taken prophylactically rather than after histamine has been released and is bound to the receptor. Patients often self-medicate with or are prescribed diphenhydramine (25 to 50 mg every 6 hours) and hydroxyzine (25 to 50 mg every 6 hours), but they may experience significant sedation. Second-generation antihistamines such as cetirizine (10 mg nightly at bedtime), fexofenadine (180 mg/day), and loratadine (10 mg/day) are much better tolerated and can be effective, although doses two to three times the standard doses are sometimes necessary. Occasionally, a brief course of corticosteroids is warranted to control severe symptoms. Epinephrine (0.3 mL of 1 : 1000 intramuscularly) quickly (but transiently) reverses the signs and symptoms of urticaria and angioedema. Patients who have experienced potentially life-threatening angioedema or anaphylaxis should have ready access to epinephrine and be knowledgeable about its indications, administration, and brief duration of action. β-Blockers not only can aggravate urticaria but also can interfere with the action of epinephrine. NSAIDs and codeine can lead to IgE-independent mast cell activation. These medications should be discontinued if it is clinically safe to do so.

H_1 antihistamines are the cornerstone of therapy for chronic urticaria/angioedema but are frequently inadequate to control symptoms. Certain H_1 antihistamines have been proposed as "preferred" for particular subtypes of chronic urticaria, such as hydroxyzine (25 to 50 mg three to four times daily) for cholinergic urticaria or cyproheptadine (2 to 4 mg every 6 hours) for cold-induced urticaria. Some have advocated using multiple H_1 antihistamines, changing or "rotating" agents, or using them in dosages well above those approved by U.S. Food and Drug Administration (FDA) labeling procedures.

Approximately 15% of histamine receptors in the skin are of the H_2 subtype; therefore, the addition of an H_2 antihistamine, such as ranitidine (150 mg twice daily) or famotidine (20 mg twice daily), is a logical adjunct to H_1 antihistamine therapy, providing additional clinical benefit. The tricyclic antidepressant doxepin (10 to 100 mg nightly at bedtime) has highly potent H_1 and H_2 antihistamine activity, with an H_1-receptor affinity almost 800 times that of diphenhydramine and an H_2-receptor affinity 6 times that of cimetidine, but its use can be limited by significant sedation.

Symptoms often persist despite the use of maximal or supramaximal doses of antihistamines. This is not surprising, considering the number of vasoactive and pruritogenic mediators released by mast cells, of which histamine is only one. Antileukotriene medications, such as montelukast (10 mg/day) or zafirlukast (20 mg twice daily) can be added to antihistamines, with some success. Especially severe symptoms may require systemic corticosteroids (prednisone 10 to 60 mg/day) to achieve symptomatic control, but concerns about side effects limit their usefulness.

Refractory symptoms have been treated with a wide variety of other medications. Some of these medications (adrenergic agents, calcium-channel blockers) are thought to decrease the ability of mast cells to release mediators. Others drugs are anti-inflammatory (hydroxychloroquine, sulfasalazine, dapsone, colchicine), immunomodulatory (cyclosporine, tacrolimus, mycophenolate), or antimetabolic (azathioprine, cyclophosphamide, methotrexate). Other treatments of refractory autoimmune chronic urticaria include intravenous immunoglobulin, plasmapheresis, and omalizumab (anti-IgE).

Evidence-Based Treatments

Multiple randomized, placebo-controlled studies of chronic urticaria/angioedema have shown the efficacy of both sedating and nonsedating antihistamines. If sedating antihistamines must be used, doxepin is more effective than diphenhydramine, but it must be titrated carefully to avoid significant sedation. Prednisone is generally accepted as a mainstay of therapy in difficult cases but has not been formally studied. Cyclosporine (4 mg/kg/day) was shown to be effective in a randomized, placebo-controlled, parallel study of 30 patients with autoimmune urticaria.[1] LTC$_4$ receptor antagonists (montelukast, zafirlukast) do not provide any incremental benefit when added to an antihistamine. Although well described in case studies and used by experts, sulfasalazine, hydroxychloroquine, dapsone, colchicine, methotrexate, azathioprine, intravenous gamma globulin, and omalizumab have not been formally studied.

PREVENTION

It is essential to encourage patients with chronic urticaria to accept the chronicity of their illness and to focus on achieving reasonable symptomatic control with effective treatments that cause the fewest side effects. Many patients with physical urticaria can learn to avoid or minimize triggers. The few patients whose chronic urticaria is a feature of systemic illness may find relief if the underlying condition is appropriately treated. An excellent example is that chronic urticaria in patients with clinically apparent thyroid disease often resolves once the thyroid disease is treated. For many patients, other factors that exacerbate their specific symptoms can be identified, including stress or anxiety, hormonal fluctuations, aspirin and other NSAIDs, and agents that cause cutaneous vasodilation (e.g., alcohol, hot baths or showers, exercise, heated waterbeds). Psychosocial stress is a commonly reported trigger of worsening symptoms. A plausible biochemical mechanism may include increased release of cutaneous neuropeptides known to lower the threshold for mast cell degranulation.

PROGNOSIS

The prognosis for most patients with chronic urticaria/angioedema is excellent. Spontaneous resolution occurs within 12 months in 50% of patients and within 5 years in an additional 20%. However, 10 to 20% of patients, particularly those with physical or autoimmune urticaria, continue to have symptoms for as long as 20 years. Patients who had one episode of chronic urticaria that lasted for months or years and then resolved may experience one or more similar recurrences later in life.

FUTURE DIRECTIONS

The current trend in the treatment of urticaria/angioedema is to use multiple antihistamines and other agents that block the actions of the mediators produced by mast cells. In the near future, it is likely that patients will be treated earlier with anti-inflammatory and immunomodulatory drugs. Some agents under development for asthma and rhinitis may be useful for the treatment of urticaria/angioedema, including 5-lipoxygenase inhibitors, PGD receptor antagonists, and more potent nonsedating antihistamines. Agents that decrease the sensitivity of mast cells to degranulation, such as phosphodiesterase 4 inhibitors and syk kinase inhibitors, may also find a role in the treatment of this condition. In spite of the fact that chronic urticaria/angioedema is not thought to be an IgE-mediated disease, omalizumab, a humanized antibody to IgE, appears to have therapeutic activity. This may be due to unexpected effects of IgE on mast cell activation. This finding could have a significant impact on future therapies.

● HEREDITARY ANGIOEDEMA AND RELATED DISEASES

DEFINITION

Hereditary angioedema (HAE) and related illnesses are characterized by recurrent attacks of angioedema mediated by vasoactive peptides such as bradykinin.

EPIDEMIOLOGY

HAE affects approximately 1 in 50,000 people. It is an autosomal dominant disease and therefore affects 50% of offspring of both genders. Frequently, a history of several generations with this disease is obtained, but new mutations do occur, and a negative family history is not uncommon. Acquired angioedema (AAE) is rarer, affecting older persons who often have paraproteinemia or malignancies such as lymphoma. Angioedema associated with ACE inhibitors occurs in 0.1 to 0.2% of treated patients.

PATHOBIOLOGY

HAE and AAE are caused by either low levels or abnormal function of a regulatory protein in the plasma, C1 inhibitor (C1 INH deficiency), which exerts control of the complement, fibrinolytic, and kinin-generating pathways. Because there is one normal gene, levels of C1 INH are detectable but are not sufficient to control the generation of kinins. The C1 esterase enzyme, when activated, cleaves two complement products, C4 and C2; without proper inhibition, this leads to low levels of circulating C4 and C2. C1 INH is also a critical modulator of the bradykinin pathway, and decreased C1 INH function leads to increased levels of bradykinin. Increased generation of bradykinin, not mediators from mast cells or activation of complement, leads to capillary leakage and angioedema.

In HAE type I (85% of patients), the abnormal gene does not produce C1 INH. In HAE type II (15%), an antigenically detectable C1 INH protein is produced, but it is not functional. In HAE type III (very rare), C1 INH is present and functional, but there is a yet-to-be-defined abnormality in the generation of vasoactive compounds. In AAE, unknown factors activate C1 and deplete the C1 INH activity in plasma, or there is an autoantibody to C1 INH that interferes with its function. ACE inhibitor–associated angioedema is due to unintended inhibition of the enzyme that inactivates bradykinin; the complement pathway is unaffected.

CLINICAL MANIFESTATIONS

Children with HAE can have attacks shortly after birth, but these tend to be mild. For most patients, the severity of the attacks worsens at puberty, with episodes of swelling that can affect any external body surface, including the genitalia. Mucosal surfaces are also affected, and patients can have life-threatening swelling of the uvula and posterior pharynx, leading to asphyxiation. Swelling of the submucosa of the gastrointestinal tract can cause symptoms of an "acute abdomen," leading to unnecessary exploratory laparotomy. About half of patients report that trauma, particularly trauma associated with local pressure, precipitates an attack, and about half note an increased frequency of attacks during times of emotional stress. Attacks in patients with AAE are clinically similar to those in patients with HAE. In patients taking ACE inhibitors, angioedema may manifests as severe swelling or simply as a chronic cough beginning days to months after ACE inhibitor therapy is initiated.

DIAGNOSIS

The best tests to support the diagnosis of HAE or AAE are measurements of C1 INH levels, C1 INH function, and C4 levels, particularly during an attack. The distinguishing features of AAE are onset later in life and the presence of a malignancy or paraproteinemia. However, in addition to having low levels of C2 and C4, patients with AAE can have profound depressions in the level of C1, a protein that is commonly normal in HAE. Patients with ACE inhibitor–associated angioedema can present within hours after initiation of therapy or after many months. The angioedema seen in urticaria/angioedema is distinctive, in that it is usually associated with urticaria and is pruritic, responding to antihistamines, steroids, and epinephrine.

TREATMENT Rx

Acute Attacks of HAE

C1 INH concentrate (20 units/kg intravenously) is the treatment of choice for acute attacks.[2] Another new agent, ecallantide, an inhibitor of the bradykinin B$_2$ receptor, is also approved for treatment of acute attacks (30 mg SC).[3] If C1 INH concentrate or ecallantide is not available, treatment of angioedema of the airway should include racemic epinephrine (1:1000) delivered in the airway by nebulization and by intramuscular injections (0.2 to 0.3 mL of 1:1000 at intervals of 20 to 30 minutes). The addition of antihistamine for sedation may be helpful. Treating physicians must be prepared to perform nasotracheal intubation, preferably in the operating room under conditions in which tracheostomy can be performed if needed. Acute attacks can be terminated by administering 2 units of fresh-frozen plasma (FFP) to supply the missing C1 INH, but in rare instances, patients may become more edematous, presumably reflecting the increased availability of substrates for the generation of kinins. Therefore, although FFP can be useful for treating non–life-threatening acute attacks, it is not recommended for life-threatening laryngeal edema. At this time, C1 INH concentrate and ecallantide are the recommended treatments for acute abdominal or facial attacks.

Long-Term Treatment of HAE

Attenuated androgens, such as danazol (100 to 200 mg up to twice daily), increase the production of C1 INH and lead to a marked amelioration of symptoms in patients with HAE. Masculinizing side effects are usually mild but can be problematic. C1 INH concentrate (1000 units IV every 3 to 4 days) is approved for long-term treatment but is very expensive.

Prophylaxis

Patients should be treated prophylactically before dental work or other procedures that involve trauma to tissue. Those treated with attenuated androgens, antifibrinolytic agents, FFP (2 units intravenously), or C1 INH concentrate (500 units subcutaneously) have fewer attacks.

Acquired Angioedema

Treatment of AAE is similar to that for HAE, but definitive treatment requires amelioration of the underlying disease. Treatment of angioedema associated with the use of an ACE inhibitor includes antihistamines, epinephrine, or both, as appropriate, and discontinuation of the ACE inhibitor. The direct renin inhibitor aliskiren is also associated with a significant risk of angioedema. Rare patients develop angioedema when taking angiotension receptor blockers. An approach to the evaluation and treatment of patients with urticaria and angioedema is summarized in Figure 260-2.

Evidence-Based Treatments

Current therapy for HAE in the United States is directed toward prophylactic treatment, including attenuated androgens, antifibrinolytics, and FFP. C1 INH concentrate and danazol were shown in a double-blind, placebo-controlled trial to significantly reduce the number of acute attacks; they are also used for prophylaxis. In a study of 193 episodes of laryngeal edema treated with C1 INH concentrate, 192 responded within 60 minutes, and the remaining 1 case responded at 4 hours.

FIGURE 260-2. Evaluation and treatment of urticaria/angioedema. Treatment of urticaria with or without angioedema (AE) is similar. Treatment of AE without urticaria depends on the cause. If the AE is caused by an angiotensin-converting enzyme (ACE) inhibitor, discontinuation of the medication is required. Treatment of AE caused by a deficiency or dysfunction of C1 inhibitor (C1 INH) is discussed in the text. Idiopathic AE often responds to treatments described for urticaria/angioedema. CBC = complete blood count; ESR = erythrocyte sedimentation rate; FcεRI = high-affinity receptor for IgE; H & P = history and physical examination; H_1 = histamine 1; H_2 = histamine 2; IgE = immunoglobulin E; IgG = immunoglobulin G; TSH = thyroid-stimulating hormone; UA = urinalysis; UTI = urinary tract infection.

PROGNOSIS

The long-term outlook for patients with HAE is largely dependent on the phenotype of the illness (frequency of laryngeal attacks), the patient's access to C1 INH concentrate, and how well the patient tolerates attenuated androgens. For most patients, life expectancy should be normal. AAE usually resolves with treatment of the underlying condition, but the ultimate prognosis depends on the nature of that illness. Angioedema associated with the use of an ACE inhibitor resolves after the medication is removed.

FUTURE DIRECTIONS

For the treatment of HAE and related disorders, there is a strong effort to have C1 INH concentrate approved for use in the United States. New therapies are also being developed, including kallikrein inhibitors, bradykinin receptor antagonists, and recombinant C1 INH.

Grade Ⓐ

1. Grattan CE, O'Donnell BF, Francis DM, et al. Randomized double-blind study of cyclosporin in chronic "idiopathic" urticaria. *Br J Dermatol.* 2000;143:365-372.
2. Zuraw BL, Busse PJ, White M, et al. Nanofiltered C1 inhibitor concentrate for treatment of hereditary angioedema. *N Engl J Med.* 2010;363:513-522.
3. Cicardi M, Levy RJ, McNeil DL, et al. Ecallantide for the treatment of acute attacks of hereditary angioedema. *N Engl J Med.* 2010;363:523-531.

SUGGESTED READINGS

Morgan M, Khan D. Therapeutic alternatives for chronic urticaria: an evidence-based review, part 1. *Ann Allergy Asthma Immunol.* 2008;100:403-412. *Contains references to many earlier double-blind, placebo-controlled studies of antihistamines as treatment for urticaria.*

Morgan M, Khan D. Therapeutic alternatives for chronic urticaria: an evidence-based review, part 2. *Ann Allergy Asthma Immunol.* 2008;100:517-526. *Contains references to immunomodulatory treatments for urticaria.*

Riedl MA. Update on the acute treatment of hereditary angioedema. *Allergy Asthma Proc.* 2011;32:11-16. *Review of the newly approved acute treatments and others currently being evaluated.*

Tai S, Mascaro M, Goldstein NA. Angioedema: a review of 367 episodes presenting to three tertiary care hospitals. *Ann Otol Rhinol Laryngol.* 2010;119:836-841. *The mean age was 52 years, and about 50% of patients were taking an ACE inhibitor or angiotensin receptor blocker.*

261

SYSTEMIC ANAPHYLAXIS, FOOD ALLERGY, AND INSECT STING ALLERGY

LAWRENCE B. SCHWARTZ

DEFINITION

Systemic anaphylaxis, a form of immediate hypersensitivity, arises when mast cells and possibly basophils are provoked to secrete mediators with potent vasoactive and smooth muscle contractile activities that evoke a systemic response. Although mast cells in any organ system may be involved, depending on the distribution of the instigating stimulus, the principal targets are the cardiovascular, cutaneous, respiratory, and gastrointestinal systems, sites where mast cells are most abundant. Systemic anaphylaxis can occur when these cells are activated by an allergen that binds immunoglobulin (Ig) E, resulting in classic immediate hypersensitivity, or when they are activated by alternative pathways.

EPIDEMIOLOGY

Assessments of the annual incidence of systemic anaphylaxis and the prevalence of those at risk for it are compromised by imprecise diagnostic measures. Data analyzed retrospectively in Rochester, Minnesota, indicate that the incidence of systemic anaphylaxis has increased from about 48 per 100,000 person years in 1990 to about 60 in 2000. In the United States, approximately 1500 to 2000 deaths occur each year from systemic anaphylaxis. Nonfatal cases are much more common, estimated to occur at an incidence of between 10 and 100 cases per 100,000 person years. Further analyses suggest that between 3 million and 43 million people (1 to 15% of the U.S. population) may be at risk for such reactions. Drug reactions

(Chapter 262) account for many of these cases. β-Lactam antibiotics and radiocontrast media provoke most such events, but the list of offending agents is lengthy and ever-increasing. During general anesthesia, systemic anaphylactic reactions occur with a frequency of about 1 in 3500, and muscle relaxants, latex, and induction drugs are the three classes of agents most commonly implicated.

Anaphylaxis to foods and insect stings each account for about 100 deaths per year. Most fatal anaphylactic reactions to injected venom proteins begin within 30 minutes after the sting. Most fatal food and insect sting reactions and many drug reactions are preceded by an immediate mild hypersensitivity reaction to the same allergen. Recognition that these earlier events are important risk factors for future fatal anaphylaxis should lead to the implementation of an action plan to prevent and deal with such reactions.

Food allergy is found in about 6% of children younger than 3 years and in half that percentage of adults; these individuals are at risk for food-induced anaphylaxis. Most children lose their allergic sensitivities to cow's milk, egg, wheat, or soy by 5 years of age, whereas sensitivities to peanuts, tree nuts, or seafood are typically long-lasting. About 20% of children lose peanut sensitivity by school age, but a small portion of them regain peanut sensitivity later in life, particularly if they continued to avoid this food.

Latex provokes anaphylaxis in a small but significant group of individuals, particularly patients who have undergone multiple surgical procedures early in life, such as those with spina bifida or congenital urinary tract disorders, and those with frequent exposure later in life, such as medical personnel. Estimates of the prevalence of latex hypersensitivity range from 1 to 6% in the general population and about 10% among regularly exposed health care workers. Over a 5-year period, the Food and Drug Administration (FDA) collected approximately 1100 reports of latex-induced anaphylaxis, including 15 deaths. The elimination of powder latex gloves and the use of nonlatex gloves have diminished the prevalence of this problem. Contact hypersensitivity is diagnosed by patch testing, and immediate hypersensitivity is diagnosed by latex-specific IgE tests performed in vitro. Latex allergen skin test reagents have not yet received FDA approval.

PATHOBIOLOGY

Etiology

The mediators produced by activated mast cells and basophils initiate many of the signs and symptoms of anaphylaxis. These cells constitutively express the high-affinity receptor for IgE, FcεRI, on their cell surfaces. Consequently, these cells are always armed by the antigen-specific IgE being produced by sensitive individuals and respond to antigens that aggregate IgE-FcεRI complexes on their cell surfaces. Therapeutic interventions aim to prevent the activation of these cells and to block the production or actions of their mediators. Cells other than mast cells and basophils also undoubtedly participate in systemic anaphylaxis, particularly those expressing FcεRI. Eosinophils, monocytes, antigen-presenting cells, and epithelial cells may be induced to express this receptor and thereby affect the intensity, duration, or character of anaphylactic reactions.

Most IgE-dependent mast cell activation events occur at local sites and result in local disease. For example, allergic conjunctivitis, allergic rhinitis, or allergic asthma typically occurs when allergen lands on the corresponding mucosal surface of a sensitive individual and diffuses into the tissue where mast cells reside. Systemic anaphylaxis presumably requires the allergen (or nonallergen agonist) to be distributed systemically to activate mast cells at remote sites. This is most likely to occur when allergen is administered parenterally; it is less likely after oral ingestion, inhalation, or cutaneous or ocular topical contact. Activation of mast cells in perivascular locations should have the greatest effect on systemic vascular responses. Although mediators released at one tissue site could, in theory, spill into the circulation and affect remote sites, most vasoactive mediators are rapidly metabolized. Accordingly, intravenous penicillin is more likely than oral penicillin to elicit a severe anaphylactic reaction. However, the precise distribution of mast cells activated during anaphylactic reactions is undetermined.

Allergens

The most common allergens causing systemic anaphylactic reactions include drugs, insect venoms, foods, radiocontrast media, allergen immunotherapy injections, and latex (Table 261-1). Most allergens are typically proteins or glycoproteins that serve as complete antigens, capable of eliciting immediate hypersensitivity reactions in a sensitized subject without further processing. The protease activity of some allergens may facilitate their penetration at

TABLE 261-1 CAUSES OF SYSTEMIC ANAPHYLAXIS	
IgE-MEDIATED (ANAPHYLAXIS)	**NON-IgE-MEDIATED (ANAPHYLACTOID)**
Insect stings	Aspirin
Foods	Radiocontrast media
Drugs	Exercise
Latex	Narcotics/vancomycin
Allergen extracts	Autoimmune
	Idiopathic

mucosal sites. Others have lipid binding domains that may increase their antigenic potency. Anaphylactic reactions to a humanized monoclonal antibody, cetuximab, have occurred owing to IgE recognizing a nonhuman carbohydrate moiety made by the animal cells expressing the antibody. In contrast to complete antigens, most drugs act as haptens. They become covalently linked to self-proteins in the circulation, in tissues, or on cells, emerging as multivalent allergens. Multivalency is important for immediate hypersensitivity because the cross-linking of at least two IgE molecules on the surface of cells aggregates FcεRI molecules, which then transmit an activating signal into the cell. Monovalent antigens fail to elicit mediator release because they bind IgE molecules without cross-linking them.

An allergen exposure must lead to sensitization before an immediate hypersensitivity reaction can occur. This process, which takes 1 to 2 weeks, involves antigen processing by antigen-presenting cells, which then present peptide antigens to T_H2 cells (helper T lymphocytes), which in turn select, nurture, and instruct allergen-specific B cells to switch from the production of IgM or IgG to IgE. This involves the production of interleukin (IL)-4 or IL-13 by T_H2 cells and the binding of T_H2 CD40 ligand to B-cell CD40. Consequently, anaphylaxis does not occur on first exposure to an allergen (sensitization phase) but may occur after subsequent exposures.

Most cases of food-induced anaphylaxis in children occur in response to eggs, peanuts, cow's milk, wheat, or soy, whereas peanuts, tree nuts, and seafood account for most reactions in adults. Reactions to seeds such as sesame seem to be growing in importance, and a variety of different foods have proved to be important allergens in specific individuals. Some individuals have the oral allergy syndrome, in which allergic reactions result from food contact but rarely progress to systemic reactions. Many of these reactions are associated with cross-reactivities between food and pollen allergens, such as melon with ragweed pollen and peach or apple with birch pollen. Also, the food epitopes associated with this syndrome are typically conformational (rather than linear) and are therefore more easily destroyed by heating (cooking) and by protease degradation and acid denaturation in the stomach and intestines.

Food allergy–associated, exercise-dependent anaphylaxis occurs when a sensitive subject exercises within several hours after eating a food to which he or she is sensitive, but not when the food is eaten without exercise. Shrimp and wheat are most commonly implicated. Exercise appears to increase intestinal permeability to food antigens, which then enter the systemic circulation. Aspirin and nonsteroidal anti-inflammatory drugs (NSAIDs) can act similarly to exercise. Avoiding the implicated food for at least 4 to 6 hours before exercising is recommended.

The Hymenoptera families primarily responsible for anaphylactic reactions are the Apidae (honeybees and bumblebees), Vespidae (hornets, yellow jackets, and paper wasps), and Formicidae (fire ants). Major allergens of honeybees include phospholipase A_2 (Api m 1), hyaluronidase (Api m 2), and melitin (Api m 4). Bumblebee venom proteins exhibit immunologic cross-reactivity with those of the honeybee, even though melitin is lacking. Vespid venoms cross-react among themselves and include a protein called antigen 5, phospholipase, and hyaluronidase; the latter allergen cross-reacts with bee hyaluronidase. Fire ant venom toxicity is caused principally by various alkaloids, which are not allergenic. Immediate hypersensitivity reactions to fire ant venom target a phospholipase that cross-reacts with the comparable vespid enzyme and various other proteins that are unique antigens. Allergens in fire ant venom cross-react with those in scorpion venom. A person may exhibit an anaphylactic reaction on first exposure to an insect's sting if he or she was previously sensitized to cross-reactive venom from a different insect. In contrast to stinging insects, allergens from biting insects of the Diptera order (mosquitoes, gnats, midges, true flies) are salivary in origin and do not cross-react with Hymenoptera venom allergens.

Anaphylaxis to these salivary proteins appears to be uncommon, but precise epidemiologic data are problematic because people are often unaware of mosquito bites, and high-quality commercial diagnostic reagents are not yet available.

Latex allergens are derived from the rubber tree *Hevea brasiliensis*. Irritant dermatitis is the most frequent contact reaction and does not involve acquired immunity. Contact hypersensitivity, which results from cell-mediated immunity to haptenic chemicals added to latex during processing, produces a poison ivy–like local reaction that may appear the day after a sensitive subject is exposed. In contrast, immediate hypersensitivity occurs when IgE is made against proteins naturally found in this plant-derived product. Cutaneous (elastic materials), mucosal or intravascular (catheters), oral (balloon), and inhaled (powdered latex gloves) routes of exposure have been well documented and generally elicit signs and symptoms within minutes of exposure. IgE-mediated cross-reactivities between latex proteins and allergens in certain fresh foods such as banana, chestnut, avocado, kiwi, peach, bell pepper, and tomato have been reported and may necessitate avoidance of these foods.

Non-IgE-Dependent Agonists

Most non-IgE-dependent foreign agents do not require antigen processing and can elicit a mast cell activation response on first exposure. These include radiocontrast dyes, narcotics such as codeine and morphine, and vancomycin (see Table 261-1). The dose and rate of administration and individual variations in sensitivity determine severity. For radiocontrast dyes, media of low ionic strength are less likely than those of high ionic strength to elicit a systemic reaction. Vancomycin produces a mast cell activation event known as "red man syndrome," typically involving urticaria without cardiovascular compromise; this can usually be avoided by reducing the rate of administration of the antibiotic.

Endogenous mast cell activators include neuropeptides such as substance P, neurokinin A, calcitonin gene-related peptide, and the complement anaphylatoxins C3a and C5a. Whether mast cell activation of sufficient magnitude to cause systemic anaphylaxis can result from endogenous secretion or generation of these peptides by themselves is unproved.

Aspirin hypersensitivity typically manifests as either a respiratory or a cardiovascular reaction, although overlap is sometimes observed. Respiratory reactions include bronchospasm, nasal congestion, and rhinorrhea and may extend beyond the respiratory tract to include abdominal cramping, watery diarrhea, and urticaria. Cardiovascular reactions that are clinically identical to allergen-induced systemic anaphylaxis and shock can also occur. In most cases, such reactions appear to be pharmacologically (not IgE) mediated, and in sensitive subjects they can occur in response to any of the cyclooxygenase 1 (COX1) inhibitors (Chapter 36). Although COX inhibitors may shunt arachidonic acid metabolism to the lipoxygenase pathway, a mechanism to explain mast cell activation has not yet emerged. COX2-selective inhibitors appear to be relatively safe in aspirin-intolerant asthmatics, but they may still cause cardiovascular reactions in those who present with this manifestation. Less commonly, sensitivity occurs to only one of the drugs in this class and is caused by IgE against an associated unique chemical moiety on that particular drug.

Physical stimuli may precipitate systemic anaphylaxis in certain individuals. Episodes can occur in response to exercise, heat, solar radiation, vibration, pressure, or cold. Exercise-dependent anaphylaxis is sometimes associated with the ingestion of any food, regardless of whether sensitivity to the food can be documented; it occurs within several hours of ingestion and may be avoided by delaying exercise until several hours after eating.

Autoimmunity and Activating Kit Mutations

Some patients experience spontaneous bouts of anaphylaxis without an obvious stimulus. Those with systemic mastocytosis are particularly prone to systemic anaphylaxis, perhaps because they have too many mast cells and because those mast cells harbor an activating mutation of Kit tyrosine kinase that primes their activation status. A related disorder, mast cell activation syndrome, occurs in patients with clonal mast cell disease, reflected by these same Kit mutations, who have recurrent bouts of anaphylaxis but do not meet the diagnostic criteria for systemic mastocytosis.

Some cases of chronic urticaria are known to be associated with IgG and IgM antibodies against FcεRI or IgE. In such cases, complement activation leading to the generation of complement anaphylatoxins at the surface of mast cells has been postulated to synergize with FcεRI-mediated activation. These reactions may occur preferentially in the skin because the anaphylatoxin receptors are expressed on the type of mast cell predominant in the skin but not on the type predominant in the lung. An analogous, albeit speculative, autoimmune process might activate mast cells localized in blood vessel walls, resulting in anaphylaxis.

Autoimmune progesterone-mediated anaphylaxis, which tends to occur just before menses, is uncommon but well documented and may respond to oral conjugated estrogens.

Pathophysiology

Mast cells participate in both acquired and innate forms of immunity. They develop in peripheral tissues from bone marrow progenitors (Chapter 159), primarily under the influence of stem cell factor, the ligand for the tyrosine kinase receptor called Kit. Armed with allergen-specific IgE, mast cells are activated by multivalent allergens that cross-link IgE and aggregate FcεRI molecules on the cell surface. This may be important in the defense against certain parasites that elicit a strong IgE response. Experiments performed in rodents suggest that mast cells can also be directly activated by certain bacterial products, leading to the secretion of mediators that recruit neutrophils. This innate immune response may restrain bacterial dissemination until a more potent acquired immune response develops. Activation of mast cells by endogenous peptides such as substance P or calcitonin gene-related peptide may influence basic biologic processes such as wound healing and angiogenesis. Whether human mast cells have a critical, nonredundant role in these biologic and immunologic processes remains controversial. However, their central role in immediate hypersensitivity is clear.

Mediators released by mast cells include preformed mediators stored in secretory granules, newly generated products of arachidonic acid, and an array of cytokines and chemokines. Histamine, formed from histidine by histidine decarboxylase, is the sole biogenic amine stored in all granules of human mast cells and basophils. Histamine released by mast cells or basophils diffuses freely and interacts with H_1, H_2, H_3, and H_4 receptors. H_1 receptors are found on endothelial cells, smooth muscle cells, and sensory nerves; when stimulated, they lead to bronchial and gastrointestinal smooth muscle contraction, vascular smooth muscle relaxation, increased permeability of postcapillary venules, coronary artery vasoconstriction, and pruritus—signs and symptoms often associated with systemic anaphylaxis. In the central nervous system (CNS), blockade of H_1 receptors appears to cause drowsiness. H_2 receptors reside on gastric parietal cells and at lower levels on inflammatory cells, bronchial epithelium, and endothelium and in the CNS. An H_2-receptor-mediated increase in acid production in the stomach, albeit transient, may occur during systemic anaphylaxis, but it is more likely to become clinically significant if histamine levels are chronically elevated, as observed in patients with systemic mastocytosis. H_3 receptors are found primarily on cells in the CNS. H_4 receptors are found on hematopoietic cells such as mast cells, basophils, eosinophils, and lymphocytes and may modulate certain aspects of inflammation, such as eosinophil recruitment, as well as pruritus. Histamine, after its secretion from mast cells and basophils, is rapidly metabolized to inactive methyl histamine and indole acetic acid.

Prostaglandin D_2 (PGD_2) is the principal COX-catalyzed product of arachidonic acid secreted by activated mast cells, but it is not made by basophils. It binds to the G protein–coupled receptors CRTH2 and DP. Both COX1 and COX2 are involved in PGD_2 production by mast cells. Consequently, a bipotent COX inhibitor might be better than a selective one at blocking PGD_2-mediated responses during anaphylaxis, which may include hypotension, bronchospasm, and inhibition of platelet aggregation.

Leukotriene (LT) C_4 is released by both mast cells and basophils after its formation from arachidonic acid and glutathione; its formation is sequentially catalyzed first by 5-lipoxygenase and 5-lipoxygenase-activating protein and then by LTC synthase. Conversion to LTD_4 and LTE_4, which are also bioactive, occurs in the extracellular space. These sulfidopeptide leukotrienes bind to the G protein–coupled receptors cysteinyl leukotriene 1 ($CysLT_1$), on bronchial smooth muscle, epithelial and endothelial cells, and leukocytes, and $CysLT_2$, on vascular smooth muscle, endothelial and epithelial cells, leukocytes, and heart muscle. Sulfidopeptide leukotrienes cause bronchoconstriction, mucus secretion, eosinophil recruitment, vasopermeability, diminished cardiac contractility, vasoconstriction of coronary and peripheral arteries, and vasodilation of venules. Antagonists of $CysLT_1$ (montelukast, zafirlukast) but not of $CysLT_2$, as well as a 5-lipoxygenase inhibitor (zileuton), are currently available for patients.

Platelet-activating factor (PAF) is generated from 2-lyso-glycero-3-phosphorylcholine when an acetyl group is placed on the sn-2 carbon of glycerol by acetyltransferase. PAF activates platelets, but it is also a potent vasoactive mediator that enhances vasodilation and vasopermeability and a smooth muscle constrictor that is capable of inducing bronchospasm. PAF is generated by both mast cells and basophils, as well as by other cell types. Elevated levels of PAF and low levels of circulating PAF acetylhydrolase, which converts PAF back to inactive lyso-PAF by removing the sn-2 acetyl moiety, have been associated with more severe food-induced systemic anaphylaxis.

Sphingosine-1-phosphate (S1P) is generated from sphingosine by sphingosine kinase in activated mast cells as well as in other cell types, and it may affect the vascular response during systemic anaphylaxis.

Mast cells are also the sole or principal source of heparin proteoglycan and certain proteases. All express β-tryptase, and a subset also expresses chymase, mast cell carboxypeptidase, and cathepsin G (like neutrophils and monocytes). Mast cells that express only tryptase are called MC_T cells; those that also express the other proteases are called MC_{TC} cells. Mature tryptase is stored in the secretory granules of all mast cells and is released during the degranulation of activated cells; levels in serum serve as a clinical marker of mast cell activation. In contrast, precursor forms of tryptase (protryptase) are spontaneously secreted by mast cells at rest; levels in serum serve as a clinical marker of the total body burden of mast cells and of anaphylactic risk in allergen-sensitized subjects. MC_{TC} cells express CD88 and therefore are activated by C5a generated during complement activation. Basophils are relatively deficient in these proteases, but they also express CD88.

Cytokines (tumor necrosis factor-α [TNF-α]; IL-4, -5, -6, -8, -13, and -16; granulocyte-macrophage colony-stimulating factor [GM-CSF]; basic fibroblast growth factor [bFGF]; vascular endothelial growth factor [VEGF]) and chemokines (IL-8, monocyte chemotactic protein-1, monocyte inflammatory protein-1α) represent another dimension of the mediators released by mast cells and basophils. Although these mediators are not selectively produced by mast cells and basophils, their vasoactive and inflammatory potential can affect the severity and duration of anaphylaxis. As selective antagonists of the relevant cytokines and chemokines become available and are tested for therapeutic benefits, the roles of these mediators in the pathogenesis of anaphylaxis will be better understood.

DIAGNOSIS

Systemic anaphylaxis can be diagnosed clinically by consensus criteria outlined in Figure 261-1. The acute onset of cutaneous signs of immediate hypersensitivity, along with either hypotension or respiratory compromise in the apparent absence of allergen exposure; the rapid onset of hypersensitivity signs involving at least two organs from among the cutaneous, gastrointestinal, respiratory, and cardiovascular systems after exposure to a likely allergen; or the rapid onset of hypotension after exposure to a known allergen can be used to diagnose systemic anaphylaxis. This can sometimes be precisely confirmed in the laboratory by demonstrating antigen-specific IgE (sensitization) and an acute serum level of total (mature plus pro-) tryptase (mast cell activation) that is greater than a baseline level obtained at least 24 hours after all signs and symptoms have resolved. Skin testing or in vitro measurements of antigen-specific IgE should be delayed for at least 2 weeks after the precipitating event to prevent false-negative results. Insect venom allergies have also been assessed by experimental sting challenges, but these are not recommended for routine evaluation. For food allergies, larger wheal-and-flare responses to prick skin tests and higher IgE titers to specific allergens are associated with more severe reactions. Oral food challenges are performed under certain circumstances, taking care to minimize the risk of systemic anaphylaxis. These food-allergic reactions involve IgE sensitization and IgE-dependent mechanisms and should be distinguished from a variety of other types of adverse food reactions, including lactose intolerance due to a deficiency in lactase, food-induced enterocolitis in infants (in reaction to cow's milk, soy, or grains), and celiac disease associated with the ingestion of gluten in wheat and other grains.

An increased level of total tryptase in serum, which peaks 15 to 60 minutes after the onset of anaphylaxis and then declines, with a half-life of about 2 hours (normal levels being undetectable), indicates that mast cell activation has occurred. The magnitude of mast cell activation is a primary determinant of clinical severity. Although an increased serum total tryptase level during putative systemic anaphylaxis may be useful for distinguishing anaphylaxis from other conditions in the differential diagnosis, elevations do not occur in some cases of anaphylaxis, particularly after food ingestion. This observation raises questions of whether there are anaphylactic pathways that bypass mast cells, perhaps involving basophil activation. Plasma histamine, because it is rapidly metabolized, is not as practical as serum or plasma mature tryptase for detecting anaphylaxis. Urinary histamine or methylhistamine levels

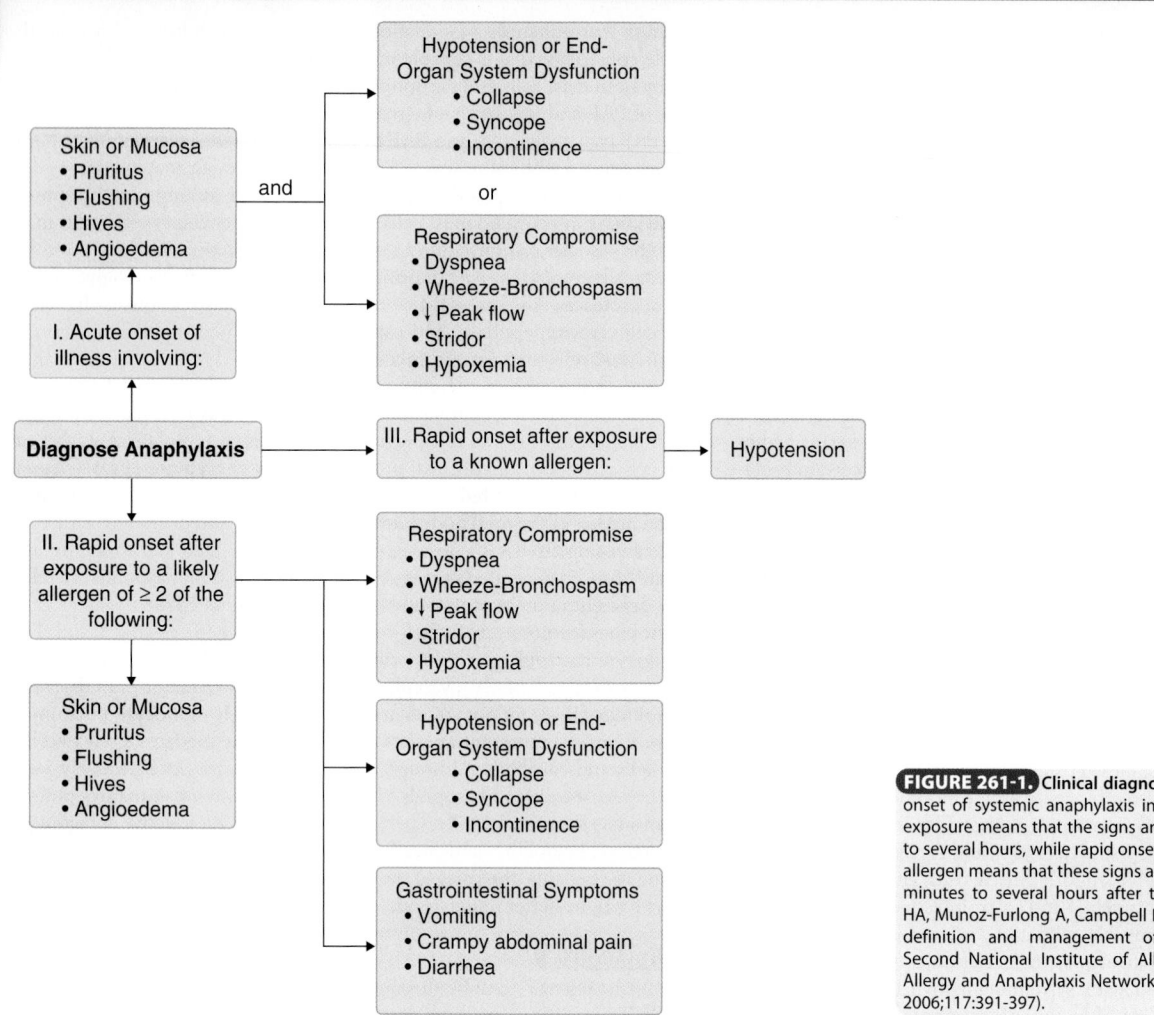

FIGURE 261-1. Clinical diagnosis of systemic anaphylaxis. Acute onset of systemic anaphylaxis in the apparent absence of allergen exposure means that the signs and symptoms develop over minutes to several hours, while rapid onset after exposure to a likely or known allergen means that these signs and symptoms begin to occur within minutes to several hours after that exposure. (Based on Sampson HA, Munoz-Furlong A, Campbell RL, et al. Second symposium on the definition and management of anaphylaxis: summary report—Second National Institute of Allergy and Infectious Disease/Food Allergy and Anaphylaxis Network symposium. *J Allergy Clin Immunol.* 2006;117:391-397).

also may reflect overall levels of released histamine, but they are affected by ingested histamine-containing foods, histamine-producing mucosal bacteria, and variability in histamine metabolism. PGD$_2$ is also rapidly metabolized and is made by several cell types, including mast cells, and urinary metabolites of this mediator are elevated during anaphylaxis.

Elevated baseline levels of serum total tryptase also appear to be a risk factor for increasing severity of insect venom–mediated systemic anaphylaxis. Future studies will determine whether baseline serum tryptase levels should guide therapy for venom-sensitive subjects as well as for those with other allergic sensitivities. Other risk factors for severe systemic anaphylaxis include a prior allergic event to that allergen and high blood pressure, particularly if the latter is being treated with nonspecific β-blockers or angiotensin-converting enzyme (ACE) inhibitors.

Low serum levels of PAF acetylhydrolase, which metabolizes PAF, and of ACE, which metabolizes bradykinin, have been associated with more severe food-induced systemic anaphylaxis. Whether slow metabolism of PAF and bradykinin might allow these mediators to play a role in such reactions, and whether mediator-specific therapies would be clinically useful in such reactions, remains to be determined.

Differential Diagnosis

Anaphylaxis should be distinguished from a variety of disorders with overlapping presentations. Vasovagal syncope (Chapter 62) causes diaphoresis, nausea, hypotension, and bradycardia, but without urticaria. Flushing disorders may be benign and unrelated to anaphylaxis, or they could be a manifestation of pathologic conditions such as the carcinoid syndrome (Chapter 240), which is typically not associated with urticaria and profound hypotension, or pheochromocytoma (Chapter 235), which causes episodic hypertension. Precise detection of these latter conditions involves the determination of serum levels of serotonin and urinary levels of 5-hydroxyindole acetic acid, catecholamines, and vanillylmandelic acid. Panic attacks and vocal cord dysfunction can be a challenge to distinguish from anaphylaxis, especially by

history alone, but they must be considered. Acute attacks of hereditary and acquired angioedema caused by C1 esterase inhibitor deficiency (Chapter 260) are not associated with pruritic urticaria and persist longer than anaphylaxis. Shock due to complement activation by contaminated hemodialysis tubing or to activation of the contact system by an oversulfated chondroitin sulfate contaminant in heparin preparations, presumably leading to the production of bradykinin, has occurred without involving mast cell activation. Scombroidosis occurs 5 to 90 minutes after the ingestion of histamine in poorly stored fish and manifests with flushing, palpitations, headache, and gastrointestinal symptoms. The condition lasts several hours, with both duration and severity dependent on the amount of histamine ingested; it usually responds to H$_1$-receptor and H$_2$-receptor antihistamines but occasionally requires epinephrine and intravenous fluids. Acute serum sickness, various cell activation syndromes, endotoxin-mediated septic shock, and superantigen-mediated toxic shock syndromes manifest with fever, which is not characteristic of anaphylaxis by itself. Also, hypoglycemia, seizure, and primary pulmonary or cardiac events should be considered.

The systemic capillary leak syndrome is a rare condition that may present with shock and mimic anaphylaxis or sepsis (Chapter 108). Patients may report preceding fatigue, weakness, and myalgias before presenting with shock and massive edema, accompanied by hemoconcentration and hypoalbuminemia owing to reversible plasma extravasation. About 80% of patients have an underlying monoclonal gammopathy of undetermined significance (Chapter 193), but the role of paraproteins in precipitating the syndrome is unknown. The syndrome is distinguished from anaphylaxis by the presence of hypoalbuminemia and the absence of allergic signs or symptoms; it is distinguished from hereditary angioedema by the presence of severe hypotension. The syndrome typically responds to intravenous vasopressors and fluid replacement, but unlike anaphylaxis, it may be resistant to even high doses of vasopressors. When the syndrome resolves, usually rapidly, the re-entry of plasma into the systemic circulation can cause pulmonary edema. Other acute complications include compartment syndromes, acute tubular necrosis, rhabdomyolysis, and venous and arterial thrombosis. Most patients survive the acute attack, but recurrences are common and can be prevented or reduced by the administration of terbutaline (20 to 25 mg/day in divided doses, as tolerated) and theophylline (400 to 1600 mg/day to achieve a peak serum concentration between 55.5 and 111 µmol/L).

In some cases, systemic anaphylaxis occurs together with another disorder. For example, severe hypotension or its treatment with epinephrine may precipitate an acute myocardial infarction.

Systemic mastocytosis is an important condition to consider in the setting of anaphylaxis. In adults, a somatic activating mutation in the gene for Kit in mast cell progenitors results in mast cell hyperreactivity and an excessive body burden of mast cells. The disease may regress spontaneously in children, but regression is uncommon in adults. Patients with an elevated baseline level of tryptase, one of the diagnostic criteria for systemic mastocytosis, are at increased risk for anaphylaxis, and anaphylaxis may be a presenting manifestation of an underlying clonal mast cell disorder such as the mast cell activation syndrome or systemic mastocytosis. For example, anaphylaxis in response to an insect sting, particularly in the absence of venom-specific IgE (due to direct mast cell agonists), should raise the possibility of such disorders. Diagnostic criteria for systemic mastocytosis and the mast cell activation syndrome are discussed in detail in Chapter 263.

FIGURE 261-2. Acute treatment of systemic anaphylaxis. H1R = histamine-1 receptor; H2R = histamine-2 receptor.

TREATMENT Rx

Fatal outcomes in anaphylaxis are principally the result of either airway constriction or hypotension. Accordingly, the acute treatment of systemic anaphylaxis requires that airway patency, blood pressure, and cardiac status be addressed (Fig. 261-2). Intubation, tracheostomy, volume expanders, and vasopressors may be needed. Patients exhibiting any signs or symptoms of hypotension should immediately assume the Trendelenburg position, which may prevent progression to anaphylactic shock or what has been called in postmortem examinations the "empty ventricle syndrome," because almost all hypotensive anaphylactic deaths are preceded by syncope occurring in a sitting or upright posture. Epinephrine injected intramuscularly into the thigh (0.2 to 0.5 mg for adults and 0.01 mg/kg [up to 0.3 mg] for children, repeated every 5 to 30 minutes, as indicated) is the most critical drug to administer; the earlier during the course of an anaphylactic event it is administered, the better. Alternatively, intravenous administration of a solution of epinephrine (1 mg/100 mL solution starting at 30 to 100 mL/hour and titrated to the lowest effective rate of infusion) can be considered. Epinephrine relaxes bronchial smooth muscle and improves vasomotor tone and vasopermeability, thereby counteracting bronchospasm, hypotension, and tissue edema. However, the benefits of epinephrine need to be weighed against its disadvantages in elderly subjects and in those with cerebrovascular or coronary artery disease, hypertension, diabetes, hyperthyroidism, cardiomyopathy, or narrow-angle glaucoma, in whom adverse events such as myocardial infarction, stroke, or pulmonary edema can be precipitated. Also, patients taking a β-blocker may be resistant to epinephrine; in such cases, glucagon (1 mg IV, or 1 to 5 mg/hour IV) or vasopressin (5 to 40 IU IV) may be used. Oxygen should be administered by nasal cannula. Inhaled bronchodilators can relieve bronchospasm. Parenteral administration of H₁-receptor (diphenhydramine 1 to 2 mg/kg, up to 50 mg) and H₂-receptor (ranitidine 300 mg IV over 5 minutes) antihistamines may prevent the progression of some signs and symptoms, particularly urticaria and pruritus, but it is not likely to reverse hypotension or tissue edema. Prednisone (40 mg PO) or Solu-Medrol (40 mg IV) may reduce the risk of a protracted reaction or the late phase of biphasic anaphylaxis, but it is unlikely to be of benefit acutely.

PREVENTION

Patients who have experienced an anaphylactic reaction are at greatest risk for another episode. Such individuals should wear a Medic-Alert bracelet and be instructed in the use of epinephrine (e.g., EpiPen), which they should carry. Avoidance of nonspecific β-blockers and ACE inhibitors is recommended because either may worsen the severity of an anaphylactic episode, and β-blockers clearly interfere with β-agonist treatment. In subjects with recurrent anaphylaxis, prophylactic use of H₁- and H₂-receptor antihistamines is beneficial. A leukotriene antagonist and COX inhibitor would theoretically provide additional benefit, but this has not been well studied. Finally, cyclosporine (3 to 5 mg/kg/day) might be considered in difficult cases of recurrent anaphylaxis because of its ability to inhibit mast cell activation in vitro and in vivo in chronic urticaria. Glucocorticosteroids do not inhibit mast cell activation in vitro or immediate skin test responses to allergens

in vivo, but they may be beneficial in selected patients with recurrent anaphylaxis.

Specific anaphylactic syndromes have unique considerations. Anti-IgE therapy in peanut-allergic subjects can increase the threshold of sensitivity from the equivalent of half a peanut to almost nine peanuts. Insect venom sensitivity can be selectively treated by venom immunotherapy, which dramatically decreases the risk of anaphylaxis in response to future stings. Reactions to radiocontrast media can be prevented or attenuated by prior administration of prednisone and H₁- and H₂-receptor antihistamines. Patients who are hypersensitive to penicillin should avoid β-lactam antibiotics in general but can be desensitized if an antibiotic in this class is critically needed (e.g., penicillin for neurosyphilis). However, desensitization is temporary; once the drug has cleared, sensitivity is likely to return. Progesterone-induced anaphylaxis may respond to the luteinizing hormone–releasing hormone analogue leuprolide acetate (Lupron), oophorectomy, or conjugated estrogens. Patients with systemic mastocytosis, in addition to instituting prophylactic pharmacologic measures, should avoid using direct mast cell agonists such as codeine, morphine, and vancomycin. Aspirin-intolerant subjects can be desensitized, but they must continue to ingest a daily dose of aspirin to maintain their desensitization status. Food- and latex-sensitive subjects must practice avoidance of the provocative agent, although preliminary data on anti-IgE neutralization therapy and oral immunotherapy indicate that these measures might provide some protection against small inadvertent food allergen exposures. Future research should yield therapies that produce more effective and long-lasting clinical tolerance.

FUTURE DIRECTIONS

Ongoing research will provide more precise diagnostic tools for delineating different pathways of anaphylaxis, indicating which cell types and biochemical pathways are involved, and thereby dictating appropriate treatments. Predictors for anaphylactic risk will be better understood. Consequently, interventions that reduce anaphylactic risk (including better desensitization regimens) and that more effectively reverse the signs and symptoms of this potentially fatal disorder will be developed.

SUGGESTED READINGS

Bonadonna P, Perbellini O, Passalacqua G, et al. Clonal mast cell disorders in patients with systemic reactions to Hymenoptera stings and increased serum tryptase levels. *J Allergy Clin Immunol.* 2009;123:680-686. *Most patients who experience a systemic allergic reaction to an insect sting and also have a baseline serum tryptase level of at least 11.5 ng/mL have an underlying clonal mast cell disorder.*

Boyce JA, Assa'ad A, Burks AW, et al. Guidelines for the diagnosis and management of food allergy in the United States: summary of the NIAID-sponsored expert panel report. *Nutr Res.* 2011;31:61-75. *Consensus guidelines.*

Druey KM, Greipp PR. Narrative review: the systemic capillary leak syndrome. *Ann Intern Med.* 2010;153:90-98. *Review of the fewer than 150 reported cases of this syndrome.*

Lieberman P, Nicklas RA, Oppenheimer A, et al. The diagnosis and management of anaphylaxis practice parameter: 2010 update. *J Allergy Clin Immunol.* 2010;126:477-480. *Consensus guidelines.*

Pansare M, Kamat D. Peanut allergy. *Curr Opin Pediatr.* 2010;22:642-646. *Clinical review.*

Robson-Ansley P, Toit GD. Pathophysiology, diagnosis and management of exercise-induced anaphylaxis. *Curr Opin Allergy Clin Immunol.* 2010;10:312-317. *Review.*

Wang J, Sampson HA. Food allergy. *J Clin Invest.* 2011;121:827-835. *Review.*

Waserman S, Chad Z, Francoeur MJ, et al. Management of anaphylaxis in primary care: Canadian expert consensus recommendations. *Allergy.* 2010;65:1082-1092. *Consensus guidelines.*

262

DRUG ALLERGY

LESLIE C. GRAMMER

DEFINITION

Adverse drug reactions (ADRs) are recognized as an important public health problem, in that they may be life-threatening. An ADR is defined by the World Health Organization (WHO) as an unintended, noxious response to a drug that occurs at a dose usually prescribed for human patients. The classic pharmacologic definition of ADRs by Rawlins and Thompson separates these into two major types: type A reactions, which are predictable and dose dependent, and type B reactions, which are unpredictable and not dose dependent. Type B reactions account for 10 to 25% of all ADRs and include drug allergy. The WHO Nomenclature Review Committee defines *drug allergy* as a hypersensitivity reaction for which a definite immunologic mechanism, either a B-cell– (antibody) or a T-cell–mediated process, is documented. Most published epidemiologic studies refer to ADRs in general and not to drug allergy specifically because the demonstration of drug-specific B-cell– or T-cell–mediated mechanisms is often quite difficult, and the immunologic culprit may be a drug metabolite.

EPIDEMIOLOGY

Drug allergy is responsible for significant mortality, morbidity, and socioeconomic costs that are probably underestimated. Current data must be evaluated carefully, because they involve different populations, different definitions of ADRs and drug allergy, and different methodologies, especially in terms of data analysis. The Boston Collaborative Drug Surveillance Program collected information on all ADRs in 4031 hospitalized patients during a period of 6 months. An incidence of 6.1% was reported, of which 42% were severe; 1% of the severe reactions resulted in the patient's death. Using an automatic detection system in a Salt Lake City hospital, Claussen and coinvestigators identified 731 ADRs among 36,653 hospitalized patients. Of note, only 12.3% of these were reported by physicians in the hospital. In a meta-analysis of 33 U.S. prospective studies from 1966 to 1996, Lazarou reported that 15% of hospitalized patients experienced ADRs and that the frequency of drug-related hospital admissions varied from 3 to 6%. Most other subsequent studies reported similar data. Epidemiologic information on drug allergy in nonhospitalized people and in the general population is even more limited and is confined mainly to studies of antibiotics.

Risk Factors

Some risk factors have been identified for the development of drug allergy. Certain drugs more commonly cause adverse reactions, and some drugs lead to more severe reactions (Table 262-1). The dosage and route of administration of a drug can also be risk factors; intermittent, repeated administrations of a drug can be more sensitizing than uninterrupted therapy. Drug allergy is more common in women, the elderly, and patients with AIDS. Some ethnic groups appear to be more prone to certain ADRs. White Americans are at a higher risk for hypersensitivity reactions to abacavir than other ethnic groups. In a study of drug allergy caused by angiotensin-converting enzyme (ACE) inhibitors, the vulnerable population was African American.

TABLE 262-1	DRUGS FREQUENTLY IMPLICATED IN ALLERGIC DRUG REACTIONS
Allopurinol	
Amiodarone	
Anesthetic agents (muscle relaxants, thiopental)	
Antiarrhythmic drugs (procainamide, quinidine)	
Antibiotics (β-lactams, sulfas, nitrofurans)	
Anticonvulsants (hydantoin, phenobarbital, carbamazepine)	
Antihypertensive agents (angiotensin-converting enzyme inhibitors)	
Antipsychotic tranquilizers	
Antisera (antitoxins, monoclonal antibodies)	
Antituberculous drugs (isoniazid, rifampicin)	
Aspirin and nonsteroidal anti-inflammatory drugs	
Chemotherapy agents (cisplatin, doxorubicin, taxanes)	
Enzymes (L-asparaginase, streptokinase, chymopapain)	
Heavy metals (gold salts)	
Monoclonal antibodies (anti–tumor necrosis factor, anti-CD20, epidermal growth factor receptor inhibitors)	
Radiocontrast media	
Recombinant proteins (insulin, other hormones)	
Vaccines (egg-based, gelatin)	

In the United States, approximately 10% of individuals who seek health care have a history of penicillin allergy. However, if tested with an appropriate panel of skin tests, less than 10% of those individuals would be deemed to have a penicillin allergy. Individuals with a positive history and negative skin tests tolerate penicillin-type antibiotics at the same rate as the general population with a negative history; in addition, there is a very low rate of resensitization.

PATHOBIOLOGY

Hypersensitivity reactions to drugs can be classified according to the type of immunologic reaction. An immunologic response to any antigen may be diverse, and the resulting reaction complex: drugs are no exception. Drugs that are more frequent perpetrators of significant allergy are listed in Table 262-1.

Most pharmacologic agents are simple structures with molecular weights of less than 1000 D. Alone, they are unable to induce hypersensitivity-type immunologic responses. However, most of these agents have the ability to covalently bind to proteins and form hapten-carrier complexes, with the low-molecular-weight agent acting as the hapten and the protein being the carrier. Hapten-carrier complexes can induce immunologic responses, with most responses being directed at the hapten.

A well-known example of such an agent is penicillin. Benzylpenicillin has a molecular weight of approximately 300 D and is metabolized into a penicilloyl hapten moiety. The penicilloyl moiety, which constitutes about 95% of all penicillin metabolites, is referred to as the major determinant because it is the major metabolite in terms of quantity. It has been conjugated to poly-D-lysine to form penicilloyl-polylysine, which is now commercially available as Pre-Pen (Alk-Abello, Round Rock, TX) for skin testing. The other 5% of penicillin metabolites are referred to as the minor determinants. Although they are minor in quantity, these determinants actually cause most of the immediate-type anaphylactic reactions, whereas the major determinant is associated with later and less severe reactions. Minor determinant reagents have never been commercially available in the United States. Penicillin skin testing is not widely used by U.S. physicians; annually, only 40,000 doses of the major determinant are sold. The potential market for a complete set of penicillin skin test reagents is estimated to be approximately 30 million tests in the United States alone.

In contrast to simple low-molecular-weight drugs, therapeutic agents that are proteins with molecular weights exceeding 5000 D can be recognized by the human immune system and can result in sensitization and hypersensitivity reactions on subsequent exposure. Because these proteins are complete antigens, they can be used as skin testing reagents or as antigens or allergens in in vitro assays. Included among therapeutic protein reagents that reportedly cause hypersensitivity are antithymocyte globulin (rabbit or equine), chymopapain, streptokinase, latex, and vaccines such as tetanus toxoid, influenza, yellow fever, pertussis, rubella, and MMR (measles, mumps, rubella). Unexpectedly, a variety of human recombinant proteins, including insulin and fully humanized monoclonal antibodies, can cause hypersensitivity reactions. In addition to hypersensitivity reactions, biologics such as monoclonal antibodies can cause other immunologic reactions (Chapter 35). One such reaction is the cytokine release syndrome, in which high cytokine levels result in systemic symptoms, including fever, arthralgia, and capillary leak; interleukin-2 is the original biologic agent in which this was described. Immune imbalance is another immunologic reaction, exemplified by anti–tumor necrosis factor therapy that results in immune dysregulation consisting of increased susceptibility to infection or autoimmunity.

CLINICAL MANIFESTATIONS

The clinical manifestations of drug allergy often include a dermatologic component (Chapter 448). It is estimated that 80 to 90% of drug allergies result in one of the following cutaneous manifestations: exanthematous or morbilliform eruption; urticaria, angioedema, or both; contact dermatitis; fixed drug eruption; erythema multiforme–like eruption; or photosensitivity. There are, however, organ-specific drug hypersensitivity reactions that do not include cutaneous manifestations (Table 262-2).

DIAGNOSIS

The diagnosis of drug allergy may be quite simple if a patient has recently started therapy with a single agent known to cause hypersensitivity, such as a β-lactam antibiotic. In contrast, in a hospitalized patient in whom multiple drugs have been started and stopped, identifying the offending drug may be difficult, requiring a complete and exhaustive history along with a physical examination. It also requires compatible clinical manifestations and temporal relationships. In vitro tests are rarely useful clinically. In vivo testing, such as cutaneous tests and provocative test dosing, may be indicated in some situations.

TABLE 262-2 ORGAN-SPECIFIC REACTIONS AND IMPLICATED DRUGS

REACTION	IMPLICATED DRUG
PULMONARY MANIFESTATIONS	
Pulmonary infiltrates with eosinophilia	Nitrofurantoin
Pneumonitis and fibrosis	Bleomycin, amiodarone
Noncardiogenic pulmonary edema	Hydrochlorothiazide, cocaine, heroin, methadone
AUTOIMMUNE MANIFESTATIONS	
Drug-induced lupus	Hydralazine, procainamide
DRUG-INDUCED IMMUNE CYTOPENIAS	
Thrombocytopenia	Quinidine, gold salts, sulfonamides, heparin
Hemolytic anemia	Penicillin, methyldopa
Agranulocytosis	Sulfonamides, propylthiouracil, quinidine, procainamide, phenytoin
HEPATIC MANIFESTATIONS	Aminosalicylic acid, dapsone
Cholestasis	Phenothiazines, erythromycin
Hepatocellular damage	Halothane, isoniazid, phenytoin
Mixed pattern	Phenytoin, sulfonamides
RENAL MANIFESTATIONS	
Nephrotic syndrome	Gold salts, captopril, NSAIDs, penicillamine
Acute interstitial nephritis	β-Lactam antibiotics, NSAIDs, sulfonamides
LYMPHOID SYSTEM MANIFESTATIONS	
Pseudolymphoma	Phenytoin
Infectious mononucleosis–like syndrome	Aminosalicylic acid, dapsone
CARDIAC MANIFESTATIONS	Sulfonamides, β-lactam antibiotics
NEUROLOGIC MANIFESTATIONS	
Peripheral neuritis	Colchicine, nitrofurantoin, sulfonamides

NSAIDs = nonsteroidal anti-inflammatory drugs.

Differential Diagnosis

To distinguish drug allergy from other ADRs, several criteria are helpful. Allergic reactions occur in a tiny fraction of individuals who receive the drug, and they cannot be predicted. The observed clinical effects do not resemble known pharmacologic actions of the drug. In the absence of prior exposure to the drug, allergic or hypersensitivity symptoms rarely appear before 1 week of continuous therapy. In general, drugs used with no reactions for several months or longer are rarely responsible.

Drug allergy often resembles other allergic or hypersensitivity reactions, such as anaphylaxis, urticaria, and serum sickness–like illness. Although most drug reactions include cutaneous manifestations, some involve only other organ systems—for example, pulmonary infiltrates with eosinophilia, hepatitis, and acute interstitial nephritis. A list of drugs that cause organ-specific reactions is provided in Table 262-2. Drug-specific antibodies or T-cell receptors or T lymphocytes have been identified that react with the suspected drugs or relevant drug metabolites. As with ADRs in general, the reaction often subsides after the drug is discontinued. However, a hypersensitivity reaction may persist because of the formation of drug metabolites, which act as haptens and bind to carrier proteins such as human serum albumin.

TREATMENT   Rx

Evidence-Based Treatments

There is a paucity of evidence-based information regarding drug allergy. One study, evaluating the evidence related to premedication before the administration of antivenom snakebite toxins, concluded that routine prophylactic adrenaline for polyvalent antivenom, known to have high adverse event rates, seems sensible, based on one clinical trial.[1] Antihistamines have no obvious benefit in preventing acute reactions from antivenoms. A second study, evaluating treatment for toxic epidermal necrolysis, concluded that there are no randomized controlled trials of the most commonly used therapies (i.e., systemic steroids, cyclosporin A, intravenous immunoglobulins).

There are published clinical guidelines for the management of infusion-related hypersensitivity reactions caused by the administration of chemotherapeutic or biologic therapy. These guidelines were developed as part of a performance improvement initiative and resulted in a standardized approach to the management and reporting of ADRs.

PREVENTION

Although the outcome of allergic drug reactions is generally favorable, prevention is the obvious goal. The physician should prescribe medications only if they are clinically appropriate and, if possible, should avoid drugs that are known to produce significant hypersensitivity reactions (see Table 262-1). Before starting a medication, the patient should be asked about prior ADRs to the medication or to other pharmacologically related medications. If appropriate, oral administration is probably preferable to parenteral administration; anaphylaxis is less likely, as is sensitization. Protocols for skin testing to foreign antisera and for management of medication hypersensitivity reactions (e.g., premedication, test dosing, desensitization) are available in Suggested Readings. Therapeutic guidelines regarding treatment of the most important and common allergic drug reactions are also reviewed in those references. A general algorithm is provided in Figure 262-1.

The risk of an anaphylactic reaction to a drug such as penicillin is a function of the history of onset, severity, and proximity (Table 262-3). If an individual experienced an immediate-type reaction that was rapid in onset, involved life-threatening symptoms or signs, and occurred relatively recently, that individual is at high risk for a severe anaphylactic reaction on subsequent exposure.

Even with a negative Pre-Pen skin test, a patient could have reactivity against minor determinants;, therefore, the approach to a patient who needs a β-lactam antibiotic depends on the risk as listed in Table 262-3. Risks and benefits should be thoroughly discussed and documented. In a high-risk individual, cautious test dosing can be performed. If a reaction occurs, desensitization can be considered if the clinical risks and benefits so warrant. In the case of HIV/AIDS patients with a previous history of mild hypersensitivity to cotrimoxazole, evidence-based rechallenge protocols are available.[2]

PROGNOSIS

Most drug allergies involve cutaneous eruptions that are self-limited and resolve shortly after the offending agent has been discontinued. However,

FIGURE 262-1. Guidelines for the treatment of patients with a history of drug allergy. In patients with a suspected or known drug allergy, the first choice is to use an appropriate non–cross-reacting drug. If such a drug is not available, or if the patient does not respond to it, further evaluation is based on the availability of a reliable immunologic test to detect drug hypersensitivity.

TABLE 262-3	RISK OF ANAPHYLACTIC REACTION TO PENICILLIN OR OTHER PHARMACOTHERAPEUTIC AGENT	
FACTOR	LOW RISK	HIGH RISK
Onset of previous reaction	>24 hr	<30 min
Signs and symptoms of previous reaction	Morbilliform eruption Urticaria alone	Life-threatening symptoms: hypotension, upper airway angioedema, bronchospasm
Time elapsed since previous reaction	>20 yr	<1 yr

severe, life-threatening reactions occur in approximately 1 in every 1000 hospitalized patients. In 1998, the death rate for hospitalized Medicare patients was 20% higher in those who experienced an ADR. The proportion of ADRs that were allergic reactions was not determined in this study, but it can be estimated at about one fourth. The incidence of adverse cutaneous reactions to drugs is higher in women than in men. There is also an increased incidence of ADRs in the elderly.

One of the most severe reactions associated with drug allergy is anaphylactic shock. It is usually immunoglobulin E (IgE) mediated, but it may occur with non-IgE-mediated reactions to drugs such as nonsteroidal anti-inflammatory drugs or radiocontrast media. It is estimated that approximately 1500 people die annually in the United States owing to anaphylaxis from medications. In the United Kingdom, drugs are the leading cause of anaphylactic fatalities (88 of 202 fatalities in 2001).

Anaphylaxis is not the major cause of mortality due to allergic drug reactions, however. Erythema multiforme major, also known as Stevens-Johnson syndrome, has a mortality rate of about 5%, and toxic epidermal necrolysis has a mortality rate of about 30%, mostly due to sepsis. The estimated incidence of Stevens-Johnson syndrome or toxic epidermal necrolysis is approximately five cases per million.

Pharmacogenomics will be an important method of identifying those individuals at risk for a significant allergic reaction to a given drug. Human leukocyte antigen (HLA) genotyping can reportedly identify individuals who are at increased risk for drug hypersensitivity. For example, individuals with HLA-B*5701 are at greater risk for a drug hypersensitivity reaction to abacavir, an HIV transcriptase inhibitor. Severe cutaneous adverse reactions to allopurinol are highly associated with the genetic marker HLA-B*5801. In patients of Asian ancestry, HLA-B*1508 is highly associated with development of Stevens-Johnson syndrome if carbamazepine is prescribed. Why this genetic variant is not a risk factor in patients of African or European ancestry is unclear. Other avenues by which susceptible individuals may be identified include polymorphisms in genes for immune recognition molecules, drug-metabolizing enzymes, and macromolecular adduct repair systems.

1. Nuchpraryoon I, Garner P. Interventions for preventing reactions to snake antivenom. *Cochrane Database Syst Rev.* 2000;2:CD002153.
2. Lin D, Li WK, Rieder MJ. Cotrimoxazole for prophylaxis or treatment of opportunistic infections of HIV/AIDS in patients with previous history of hypersensitivity to cotrimoxazole. *Cochrane Database Syst Rev.* 2007;2:CD005646.

SUGGESTED READINGS

Classen DC, Jaser L, Budnitz DS. Adverse drug events among hospitalized Medicare patients: epidemiology and national estimates from a new approach to surveillance. *Jt Comm J Qual Patient Saf.* 2010;36:12-21. *Documents the persistently high rate in U.S. hospitals.*
Fox S, Park MA. Penicillin skin testing in the evaluation and management of penicillin allergy. *Ann Allergy Asthma Immunol.* 2011;106:1-7. *Skin testing is safe, and a negative test predicts a 97-99% probability of being able to use penicillin safely.*
Gangemi S, Guameri C, Romeo P, et al. Safety and reliability of the drug tolerance test: our experience in 739 patients. *Pharmacology.* 2011;87:90-95. *Drug tolerance tests are generally safe and predictive, but physicians often do not trust their results.*
Reisfeld S, Goldberg A, Confino-Cohen R. Management of patients with known drug hypersensitivity in an emergency department in Israel. *Int Arch Allergy Immunol.* 2011;155:361-366. *About 10% of patient-reported hypersensitivities were overlooked, especially those related to NSAIDs.*
Um SJ, Lee SK, Kim YH, et al. Clinical features of drug-induced hypersensitivity syndrome in 38 patients. *J Investig Allergol Clin Immunol.* 2010;20:556-562. *The most common causative drugs were anticonvulsants (47%), antibiotics (18%), and NSAID (13%).*
Walsh SA, Creamer D. Drug reaction with eosinophilia and systemic symptoms (DRESS): a clinical update and review of current thinking. *Clin Exp Dermatol.* 2011;36:6-11. *Review of the severe medication-induced adverse reaction.*

263

MASTOCYTOSIS

CEM AKIN

DEFINITION

Mastocytosis is a heterogeneous group of disorders characterized by pathologic accumulation of mast cells in tissues such as skin and bone marrow. According to the classification of the World Health Organization (WHO), based on clinical presentation and pathologic findings, there are seven distinct categories of mastocytosis (Table 263-1). The term *cutaneous mastocytosis* describes skin disease alone without any evidence of internal organ involvement, whereas the term *systemic mastocytosis* describes the disorder when it involves internal organs (most commonly the bone marrow) with or without skin disease.

EPIDEMIOLOGY

Mastocytosis can be diagnosed at any age. Pediatric-onset and adult-onset forms are distinguished based on the age of the patient at initial diagnosis. These forms display differences in their clinical course, molecular pathology, and prognosis. The most common clinical scenario leading to diagnosis in the pediatric population is a child presenting with skin lesions of cutaneous mastocytosis within the first year of life. Patients with a later onset of skin lesions are more likely to have systemic mastocytosis, as are most patients with adult-onset mastocytosis. The disease has been diagnosed in all ethnic populations. Pediatric-onset mastocytosis appears to be diagnosed more

TABLE 263-1	WORLD HEALTH ORGANIZATION CLASSIFICATION OF MASTOCYTOSIS

Cutaneous mastocytosis
Indolent systemic mastocytosis
Systemic mastocytosis with associated clonal hematologic non–mast cell lineage disease
Aggressive systemic mastocytosis
Mast cell leukemia
Mast cell sarcoma
Extracutaneous mastocytoma

From Horny HP, Metcalfe DD, Bennett JM, et al. Mastocytosis. In: Swerdlow SH, Campo E, Harris NL, et al, eds. *WHO Classification of Tumours of Haematopoietic and Lymphoid Tissues.* Lyon, France: IARC Press; 2008:54-63.

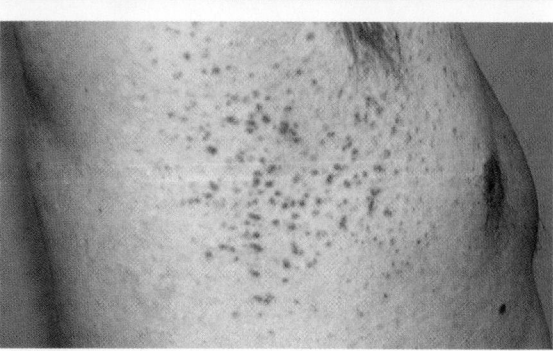

FIGURE 263-1. Urticaria pigmentosa.

commonly in males (approximately 60%). Estimates of the prevalence of patients with cutaneous mastocytosis range from 1 in 500 to 1 in 8000 patients presenting in dermatology clinics. The prevalence of systemic mastocytosis is more difficult to estimate because the diagnosis requires biopsy of an involved tissue and a high degree of clinical suspicion. Systemic mastocytosis is likely to be underdiagnosed, considering the fact that there are neither physical examination findings nor routine hematologic or chemistry laboratory abnormalities specifically associated with the disease. Consequently, it is not unusual to encounter several years' delay after the onset of symptoms in many patients before a diagnosis of mastocytosis is reached. The disease is sporadic, although rare cases of familial occurrence have been described.

PATHOBIOLOGY

Pathogenesis

The pathogenesis of mastocytosis involves the accumulation of mast cells in tissues, with mediators released by activated mast cells. The primary reason for the increased mast cell numbers in tissues appears to be defective apoptosis rather than uncontrolled proliferation. It is unusual to see increased mitotic activity in biopsy specimens from patients with mastocytosis, and, in most patients, the disease follows an indolent course. Tissue microenvironment and altered chemotaxis may also contribute to the final level of tissue mast cell burden.

Genetics

Mast cells are derived from hematopoietic progenitors. Systemic mastocytosis is associated with somatic gain-of-function point mutations in the *KIT* (formerly *c-kit*) gene of the mast cell progenitor, leading to a clonal neoplastic expansion of mast cells. *KIT* encodes a transmembrane receptor (Kit), whose intracellular portion functions as a tyrosine kinase enzyme. The extracellular portion of Kit binds the cytokine stem cell factor (SCF or Kit ligand). The interaction between SCF and Kit provides the single most important growth and differentiation stimulus for mast cells from their progenitors. Under physiologic conditions, homodimeric SCF binds and cross-links two Kit receptor molecules, which leads to autophosphorylation of the tyrosine amino acids of the intracellular portion of the Kit molecule. Phosphorylated tyrosine residues in turn act as docking sites for downstream adaptor and signal transduction molecules that regulate the differentiation, proliferation, chemotaxis, and functional activation of mast cells.

Most of the mutations reported in systemic mastocytosis involve codon 816 in *KIT,* resulting in the replacement of an aspartic acid by a valine residue (D816V) in the Kit protein. D816 is a critical residue involved in the kinase activity of Kit. Substitution of the wild-type aspartic acid residue in this location by another amino acid results in constitutive activation and autophosphorylation of the receptor molecule without the need for cross-linking by its ligand, SCF. The D816V mutation has been shown in lesional mast cells from the skin and bone marrow tissue of patients with mastocytosis, as well as from other hematopoietic lineages in patients with extensive disease. This aspect of the pathobiology of systemic mastocytosis is similar to the multilineage involvement observed in myeloproliferative disorders (Chapter 169). The sensitivity of detecting the mutation is much higher when a lesional tissue such as bone marrow or skin is analyzed compared with peripheral blood. Other pathogenetic factors, some yet to be determined, appear to be responsible for the final disease phenotype because the presence of the D816V *KIT* mutation alone does not explain the remarkable heterogeneity in the clinical presentation and prognosis of the disease.

Symptomatology

The symptomatology of mastocytosis is primarily manifested by the release of mast cell mediators and rarely by a destructive infiltration of mast cells into tissues. Mast cell activation results in the release of various preformed mediators stored in mast cell granules, de novo synthesis of sulfidopeptide leukotrienes such as LTC_4 and prostaglandins (mostly PGD_2) from membrane lipids, and cytokine synthesis. Preformed mediators stored in mast cell granules include histamine; proteases such as tryptase, chymase, and carboxypeptidase A; and proteoglycans such as heparin and chondroitin sulfate. Vasoactive mediators such as histamine, LTC_4, and PGD_2 at local or distant tissues cause vasodilation, which may lead to flushing, tachycardia, hypotension, presyncope, and syncope. Histamine also causes pruritus and stimulates gastric acid hypersecretion from parietal cells. Mast cells are rich sources of cytokines. Elevated serum levels of tumor necrosis factor-α (TNF-α) and interleukin-6 (IL-6) have been found in patients with mastocytosis and may contribute to the pathophysiology of fatigue and accelerated osteoporosis observed in some patients. Rare aggressive categories of mastocytosis may be associated with an extensive destructive infiltration of mast cells into tissues such as the gastrointestinal tract, which may result in malabsorption, and the liver, which may cause portal fibrosis with associated portal hypertension.

Mast cell activation and mediator release may occur after triggers such as temperature changes (e.g., hot showers); exercise; ingestion of alcohol or spicy foods; emotional stress; insect stings; exposure to certain drugs such as opioid analgesics, nonsteroidal anti-inflammatory drugs (NSAIDs), or muscle relaxants; and sometimes spontaneously without an obvious trigger. The prevalence of atopic disease in patients with mastocytosis is similar to that in the general population, and the serum immunoglobulin E (IgE) level is often found to be low. However, patients with anaphylactic sensitivity to hymenoptera venoms appear to have a disproportionately high incidence of mastocytosis.

Clinical Manifestations

Mastocytosis is a disease with protean clinical manifestations. Although in some patients the only complaint is the cosmetic appearance of urticaria pigmentosa lesions, others suffer from frequent episodes of vascular instability or have life-threatening hematologic disease. In general, patients with mastocytosis belong to one of two broad categories, according to the site of tissue involvement: those with cutaneous disease alone, or those with systemic disease with or without skin involvement. Cutaneous mastocytosis (i.e., disease limited to the skin in the absence of internal organ involvement) is commonly diagnosed in children within the first year of life, whereas systemic mastocytosis is mostly diagnosed in adults by a bone marrow biopsy and aspirate.

Cutaneous Manifestations

Skin lesions of urticaria pigmentosa are the most common presentation of cutaneous mastocytosis (Fig. 263-1). They are also present in 50 to 90% of patients with systemic mastocytosis, depending on the disease category. Remarkably different in appearance from urticaria or hives, lesions of urticaria pigmentosa are fixed, tan- to salmon-colored, maculopapular lesions varying in size from a few millimeters to a few centimeters. They are most prominently observed on the trunk and extremities and tend to spare the face and the sun-exposed areas of the skin, although facial involvement may be seen in children. Blistering of the lesions may occur in children in the first 3 years of life. The lesions are generally not pruritic at rest but may urticate after exposure to a number of triggers (see Pathobiology). Many patients note that the skin lesions become more prominent after exposure to heat or after physical irritation such as rubbing. The lesions may be found concentrated in skin areas that are prone to irritation, such as the axillae and groin.

Uncommon presentations of cutaneous mastocytosis include mastocytomas, diffuse cutaneous mastocytosis, and telangiectasia macularis eruptiva perstans (TMEP). Mastocytomas are benign and generally solitary mast cell tumors, although they have been known to precede urticaria pigmentosa lesions in some cases. They occur almost exclusively in children, and physical irritation of the lesion may result in generalized flushing and other symptoms of mast cell mediator release. Diffuse cutaneous mastocytosis (DCM) is another form of skin involvement seen exclusively in children. It is characterized by diffuse thickening of the skin and appendages with a peau d'orange appearance without individual urticaria pigmentosa lesions. TMEP is a rare form of cutaneous mastocytosis characterized by the presence of diffuse telangiectatic macules. Because TMEP lesions are generally seen in the presence of urticaria pigmentosa, there is debate about whether TMEP represents a distinct form of cutaneous mastocytosis.

Patients with cutaneous mastocytosis may manifest systemic symptoms such as abdominal pain, diarrhea, and flushing.

Systemic Manifestations

Symptoms caused by mast cell degranulation may be experienced as brief, recurrent, and self-limited episodes with multiorgan manifestations or as chronic complaints over a prolonged time course. A typical mast cell degranulation episode may variably involve flushing, conjunctival hyperemia, nausea, vomiting, abdominal cramping, diarrhea, tachycardia, and lightheadedness. Hypotension may develop, and the episode may progress to full loss of consciousness in some patients. Therefore, mastocytosis should be ruled out in all patients with recurrent anaphylaxis before a diagnosis of idiopathic anaphylaxis can be made. Tryptase, a protease stored in mast cell granules, may be elevated above the patient's baseline level in the serum or plasma if measured within 3 hours after the onset of the episode in patients with suspected mast cell degranulation or anaphylaxis, regardless of the cause. Angioedema, hives, and wheezing are uncommon in mastocytosis, in contrast to idiopathic anaphylaxis. Flushing usually involves the face and upper chest area. A consistent trigger can be identified in only a small number of patients (see Pathobiology). The episodes usually last 30 minutes to a few hours. Hypotensive episodes can be life-threatening, particularly in the presence of comorbidities such as cardiac or pulmonary disease.

Gastrointestinal Symptoms

Gastrointestinal symptoms are observed in more than 50% of patients with mastocytosis. Epigastric pain, lower abdominal cramping, nausea, vomiting, or diarrhea can occur episodically in the context of an acute mast cell degranulation episode or on a chronic basis. Gastric acid hypersecretion induced by mast cell–derived histamine may lead to esophagitis, gastritis, and peptic ulcer disease, although measurements of basal acid output have shown great variability in different studies, ranging from hypersecretion in the range of Zollinger-Ellison syndrome to achlorhydria. Mucosal edema, thickened gastric or duodenal mucosal folds, or nodular lesions may be observed in radiographic or endoscopic evaluations. Diarrhea alternating with constipation may be seen. Severe persistent diarrhea may be complicated by clinically significant malabsorption in patients with aggressive systemic mastocytosis. Hematochezia, hematemesis, and melena are uncommon symptoms and should prompt endoscopic evaluation to rule out coexisting pathology. Mast cells are constituents of the normal lamina propria in gastrointestinal mucosa, and their numbers may be increased in inflammatory states affecting the gastrointestinal tract. However, quantitation of mast cell numbers in gastrointestinal biopsy specimens is generally not helpful, and diagnosis of mast cell disease by a gastrointestinal biopsy, solely based on increased mast cell numbers without evidence for other WHO criteria, should be avoided. Mild to moderate hepatomegaly with or without abnormalities in serum transaminases may be observed, although portal hypertension and ascites are rare and indicate the presence of advanced categories of mastocytosis. Jaundice and findings on cholangiography resembling those of primary sclerosing cholangitis have been reported in some patients.

Musculoskeletal Symptoms

Musculoskeletal pain is common in patients with mastocytosis and is mostly caused by soft tissue pain resembling fibromyalgia. Accelerated osteoporosis may be seen in a subgroup of patients, particularly those with other risk factors, such as postmenopausal women, and those receiving glucocorticoid therapy. Pathologic compression fractures may be the initial finding in some patients. A bone densitometry measurement should be recommended as part of the standard evaluation of women with mastocytosis and of any patient with a history of pathologic fractures. Radiographic abnormalities have been reported in up to 75% of patients with mastocytosis. In addition to generalized osteoporosis, bone surveys may show a mixture of sclerotic or lytic lesions, and skeletal scintigraphy may reveal focal or diffuse radiotracer uptake.

Hematologic Manifestations

Peripheral blood abnormalities have been noted in up to 50% of patients with systemic mastocytosis. Mild normochromic normocytic anemia is the most common abnormality, followed by thrombocytopenia, eosinophilia, monocytosis, and leukopenia. Eosinophilia in mastocytosis rarely causes organ damage, as is observed in chronic eosinophilic leukemia or idiopathic hypereosinophilic syndrome (Chapter 173). It is important to differentiate a primary eosinophilic disorder from mastocytosis with eosinophilia. Some cases of chronic eosinophilic leukemia are associated with the *FIP1L1-PDGFRA* fusion gene and respond to the drug imatinib, whereas systemic mastocytosis is associated with codon 816 point mutations of the *KIT* gene, which confers resistance to this drug.

Approximately 20% of patients with systemic mastocytosis have been reported to display evidence of another clonal non–mast cell hematologic disease. Non–mast cell clonal hematologic neoplasms associated with mastocytosis are commonly myeloid in nature (myeloproliferative disorders, myelodysplastic syndromes, or myeloid leukemias) but may also involve lymphoproliferative disorders such as lymphomas, myelomas, and lymphocytic leukemias.

DIAGNOSIS

The diagnosis and classification of mastocytosis is carried out according to the guidelines published by the WHO. A suggested algorithm for the diagnosis of mastocytosis is shown in Figure 263-2.

Cutaneous Mastocytosis

Diagnosis of cutaneous mastocytosis is made by observing the typical hyperpigmented maculopapular lesions of urticaria pigmentosa and is confirmed by skin biopsy, which shows infiltration of mast cells in the upper dermis, particularly in perivascular locations. It should be noted that mild increases in mast cell numbers can be observed in inflammatory and neoplastic skin diseases, and establishing a diagnosis of cutaneous mastocytosis by a blind skin biopsy or biopsy of a lesion that does not have the typical appearance of urticaria pigmentosa should be avoided. A localized wheal-and-flare reaction limited to the lesional skin within a few minutes after rubbing or scratching the skin is known as Darier's sign. Diagnosis of urticaria pigmentosa in adults should always prompt investigation of possible systemic mastocytosis.

Systemic Mastocytosis
Biopsy

A bone marrow biopsy and aspiration is the recommended diagnostic procedure to evaluate the presence of WHO diagnostic criteria for systemic disease (discussed later). This procedure is recommended for all patients with adult-onset urticaria pigmentosa, patients with recurrent symptoms suggestive of mast cell degranulation (such as flushing and hypotension accompanied by abdominal complaints), patients with unexplained osteoporosis, and patients with suspected hematologic disease (see Clinical Manifestations). Children with an onset of lesions within the first year of life usually do not require a bone marrow biopsy unless they have an abnormal complete blood count, lymphadenopathy, hepatomegaly, or splenomegaly. Children with late-onset skin lesions and those who experience persistence of urticaria pigmentosa into adulthood should be considered for diagnostic evaluation for systemic disease.

World Health Organization Diagnostic Criteria

WHO guidelines for diagnosis of systemic mastocytosis consist of one major and four minor criteria (Table 263-2). Presence of the major criterion with at least one minor criterion, or demonstration of three minor criteria in the

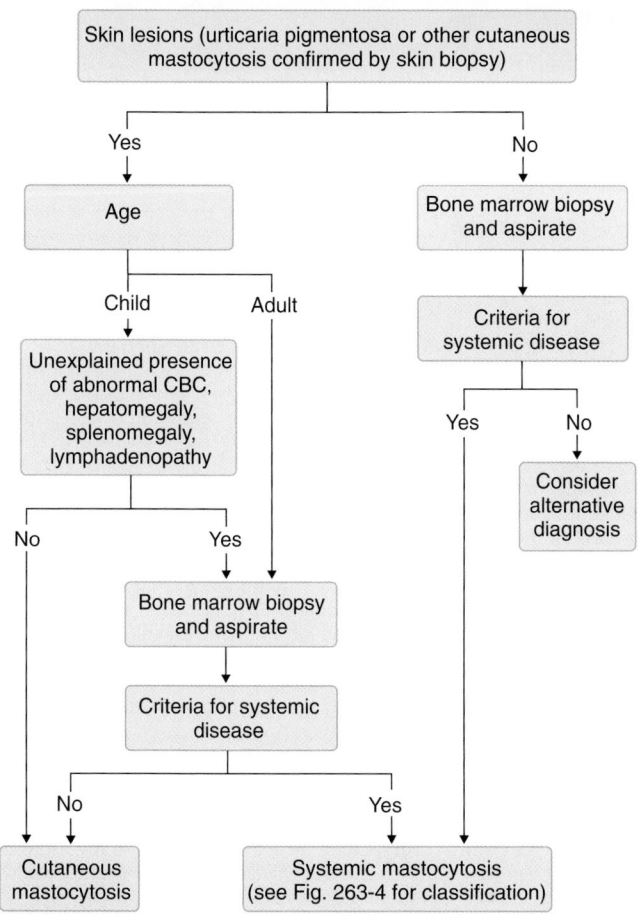

FIGURE 263-2. Suggested diagnostic algorithm for mastocytosis. CBC = complete blood count.

FIGURE 263-3. Diagnostic findings in the bone marrow biopsy and aspirate. **A,** Characteristic mast cell aggregates on tryptase staining (major criterion) in biopsy section *(arrow)*. **B,** Mast cells with atypical spindle shapes in aspirate smear *(arrow)*.

TABLE 263-2	WORLD HEALTH ORGANIZATION DIAGNOSTIC CRITERIA FOR SYSTEMIC MASTOCYTOSIS

MAJOR

Multifocal, dense infiltrates of mast cells consisting of 15 or more mast cells in aggregates detected in sections of bone marrow and/or other extracutaneous organs, confirmed by tryptase immunohistochemistry or other special stains

MINOR

More than 25% of mast cells in biopsy sections or bone marrow aspirate smears showing spindle shape or atypical morphology
Detection of a *KIT* codon 816 point mutation in bone marrow, blood, or other extracutaneous organs
Expression of CD2 and/or CD25 by mast cells in bone marrow, blood, or extracutaneous organs
Persistent elevation of serum total tryptase >20 ng/mL*

*Criterion not valid if there is an associated clonal myeloid disorder.
From Horny HP, Metcalfe DD, Bennett JM, et al. Mastocytosis. In: Swerdlow SH, Campo E, Harris NL, et al, eds. *WHO Classification of Tumours of Haematopoietic and Lymphoid Tissues.* Lyon, France: IARC Press; 2008:54-63.

absence of the major criterion, is needed to establish a diagnosis of systemic mastocytosis and distinguish it from reactive mast cell hyperplasia. The major diagnostic criterion is the presence of multifocal, dense aggregates of 15 or more mast cells in bone marrow or other extracutaneous tissue biopsy sections (Fig. 263-3A). Such clusters are frequently observed around blood vessels and next to bone trabeculae in bone marrow biopsies. Immunohistochemical staining for tryptase is the recommended method for visualization of mast cells. Routine hematoxylin and eosin or metachromatic stains such as toluidine blue are not sufficiently sensitive to demonstrate subtle mast cell infiltrates or abnormal morphologic features of mast cells within the infiltrates in decalcified bone marrow biopsy sections.

Mast cell morphology in bone marrow provides important clues to the diagnosis of systemic mastocytosis. Bone marrow mast cells in systemic mastocytosis often display atypical morphology, such as an elongated (spindle) shape, hypogranularity, and an eccentric or lobulated nucleus (see Fig. 263-3B). These atypical mast cells are usually observed in close association with bone marrow spicules in the aspirate smear. Mast cells in mast cell leukemia (MCL) may be very sparsely granulated.

Flow cytometric analysis of the mast cells in a bone marrow aspirate, when performed appropriately, is a very sensitive diagnostic aid. The mean percentage of mast cells in a healthy bone marrow aspirate is approximately 0.02%, and it does not exceed 1% in most patients with mastocytosis. Therefore, to visualize the mast cell population correctly, the total cell numbers analyzed by flow cytometry should be significantly higher than those in other, more routine evaluations (e.g., leukemia phenotyping). The characteristic flow cytometric finding of systemic mastocytosis is the aberrant expression of CD25 and/or CD2 on CD117+ mast cells. Serum tryptase level may be elevated in patients with mastocytosis. Currently available commercial tryptase immunoassays measure levels of total tryptase, the sum of mature tryptase and tryptase precursors. Mature tryptase enzyme is a serine protease stored in mast cell granules and is transiently elevated in serum or plasma after mast cell degranulation episodes such as anaphylaxis. In contrast, tryptase precursor proenzymes (α and β protryptases) are constitutively secreted outside the cell, and their serum levels at baseline correlate with mast cell burden. The median serum tryptase level in a healthy population is approximately 5 ng/mL. A serum tryptase level higher than 20 ng/mL raises suspicion for systemic mastocytosis in the appropriate clinical setting. It should be noted that a normal tryptase level does not rule out a diagnosis of mastocytosis and that increased tryptase levels can be seen in other conditions, such as myelodysplastic syndromes, acute myeloid leukemias, chronic eosinophilic leukemia, and chronic renal insufficiency. Metabolites of histamine, such as *N*-methylhistamine, are found to be elevated in a 24-hour urine specimen but are neither more sensitive nor more specific than the baseline serum tryptase measurement in mastocytosis.

Demonstration of a codon 816 *KIT* mutation (D816V) may be necessary to fulfill the diagnostic criteria in patients lacking the major criterion (see Pathobiology). Examination of lesional tissues such as skin and bone marrow affords the highest sensitivity. Codon 816 *KIT* mutations have been detected in a variety of other neoplastic diseases, such as core binding factor acute myeloid leukemias, sinonasal lymphomas, and seminomas, in addition to mastocytosis.

World Health Organization Disease Categories

Each patient diagnosed with mastocytosis should be assigned a category of disease according to the WHO classification (see Table 263-1). *Cutaneous mastocytosis* in the absence of bone marrow and internal organ involvement is the most common category in patients with pediatric-onset disease.

Systemic mastocytosis is divided into the categories of indolent systemic mastocytosis, systemic mastocytosis with associated clonal hematologic non–mast cell lineage disease (SM-AHNMD*)*, aggressive systemic mastocytosis, and MCL. An algorithm for classification of systemic mastocytosis is presented in Figure 263-4. *Indolent systemic mastocytosis* is the most common category in adults. Patients in this category usually do not have a decreased life expectancy owing to the mast cell disease, although they experience symptoms related to release of mast cell mediators. Indolent systemic mastocytosis follows a persistent course, and progression to a more advanced category is unusual. *SM-AHNMD* is the second most common category in adults, and a non–mast cell hematologic disease is usually diagnosed at the time that the diagnosis of mastocytosis is made. Therefore, bone marrow biopsy and aspirate specimens should be carefully evaluated for the presence of other hematologic disease in every patient with newly diagnosed systemic mastocytosis. *Aggressive systemic mastocytosis* is a rare category characterized by the presence of organ dysfunction resulting from destructive mast cell infiltration. Aggressive systemic mastocytosis may involve the hematopoietic, gastrointestinal, and skeletal systems in the form of cytopenias, hypersplenism, malabsorption with weight loss, hepatomegaly with portal hypertension and ascites, and large osteolytic lesions with pathologic fractures. MCL is characterized by 10% or more mast cells in the peripheral circulation or 20% or more mast cells in bone marrow aspirate smears, or both. To diagnose MCL, the mast cell percentage in bone marrow aspirate smears should be assessed in an area of the slide that is sufficiently distant from the spicules. *Mast cell sarcoma* and *extracutaneous mastocytoma* are rare diagnoses characterized by malignant and benign solid mast cell collections, respectively.

Recent studies identified a subset of patients with recurrent idiopathic or hymenoptera venom-induced anaphylaxis who had evidence of clonal mast cells carrying the D816V *KIT* mutation or aberrantly expressing surface CD25, without fully meeting the WHO diagnostic criteria and without displaying urticaria pigmentosa skin lesions. Such patients are provisionally referred to as having a "monoclonal mast cell activation syndrome."

FIGURE 263-4. An algorithm for classification of systemic mastocytosis. ASM = aggressive systemic mastocytosis; ISM = indolent systemic mastocytosis; MDS = myelodysplastic syndromes; MPD = myeloproliferative disorders; SM-AHNMD = systemic mastocytosis with associated clonal hematologic non–mast cell lineage disease.

TREATMENT

The major goal of treatment for all categories of mastocytosis is symptom control. A reduction in mast cell numbers is considered only in disease categories with a poor prognosis (i.e., SM-AHNMD, aggressive systemic mastocytosis, MCL, and mast cell sarcoma). Current treatment modalities have not been shown to change the natural course of the disease.

Medical Therapy

Patients with cutaneous and indolent systemic mastocytosis are treated symptomatically. Pruritus in mastocytosis usually responds to scheduled doses of histamine-1 antihistamines such as fexofenadine or cetirizine, or both. Sedating antihistamines such as hydroxyzine or diphenhydramine may be used before bedtime. Photochemotherapy (oral psoralen plus ultraviolet A) or phototherapy may be helpful in patients with refractory pruritus; it results in symptomatic improvement and temporary fading of the pigmented skin lesions in up to 50% of patients. The side effects of phototherapy, including increased risk of skin cancer, should be taken into account when this treatment is considered.

Histamine-2 antihistamines such as ranitidine or famotidine are usually prescribed as a first-line treatment for patients with gastrointestinal complaints such as heartburn, nausea, and abdominal pain. Proton pump inhibitors may be added in patients whose abdominal symptoms are refractory to histamine-2 antihistamines. Oral cromolyn sodium (adult dose, 200 mg four times daily) has been effective in reducing abdominal pain, diarrhea, nausea, vomiting, and pruritus in various studies, although the beneficial effects are variable among patients. Finally, low to moderate doses of systemic glucocorticoids can be beneficial in unusual cases of aggressive mastocytosis presenting with recalcitrant diarrhea associated with malabsorption or hepatomegaly with ascites.

Cysteinyl leukotrienes, such as LTC$_4$, that are produced after mast cell activation are thought to contribute to symptoms in mastocytosis. Therefore, drugs targeting the synthesis or receptor binding of leukotrienes are usually added to the treatment regimens of patients who derive suboptimal relief of itching and abdominal pain from histamine receptor–blocking therapy. However, there have been no controlled studies evaluating the clinical efficacy of this class of drugs in patients with mastocytosis.

Self-administered epinephrine should be considered for all patients even if they do not have any history of hypotensive or anaphylactic episodes resulting in presyncope or syncope from acute mast cell degranulation. These episodes should be treated like systemic anaphylaxis (Chapter 261).

Cytoreductive therapy, considered in aggressive disease variants associated with poor prognosis, has yielded disappointing results thus far. Approaches to cytoreductive treatment of mastocytosis have included interferon-α2b (IFN-α2b) and the nucleoside analogue 2-chlorodeoxyadenosine (2-CDA). IFN-α2b (0.5 to 5 million units, three to five times per week), alone or with prednisone, has been reported to improve partially clinical and laboratory abnormalities in approximately 50% of patients with aggressive systemic mastocytosis, patients with osteoporosis and pathologic fractures, and patients with recalcitrant recurrent anaphylaxis, although complete histopathologic and molecular remissions appear to be rare. IFN-α is difficult to tolerate because of its many side effects, including flu-like symptoms, bone pain, and depression. A regimen of 2-CDA (0.10 to 0.17 mg/kg/day for 5 days, repeated at intervals of 4 to 8 weeks) has been reported to result in partial and transient responses in patients with advanced categories of disease in case reports and small series. MCL usually is treated with polychemotherapy as acute myeloid leukemia (Chapter 189), although a successful treatment regimen has not yet been identified.

Imatinib, a tyrosine kinase inhibitor with activity against wild-type *KIT*, *PDGFR*, and *abl*, has been effective in a small number of patients without D816V *KIT* mutation or with the *FIP1L1-PDGFRA* fusion gene, who present with chronic eosinophilic leukemia (Chapter 173) with a modest increase in bone marrow mast cells. However, most patients with mastocytosis have the D816V *KIT* mutation, which confers resistance to imatinib, and therefore are not appropriate candidates for this therapy.

Ancillary and Other Therapies

Avoidance of the triggers of mast cell degranulation is an important adjunct to the pharmacologic treatment of symptoms. These show remarkable individual variation among patients (see Pathobiology), and the individual medical history can be helpful in identifying such triggers. General anesthesia and surgery impose an additional risk to patients with mastocytosis because several agents that are used perioperatively, such as muscle relaxants, opioid analgesics, and NSAIDs, can induce acute mast cell degranulation. Prior surgical and anesthesia records should be obtained if available, and an appropriate strategy for the anesthetic management of the patient should be determined, with close communication involving the patient, anesthesiologist, surgeon, and an allergist.

Non–mast cell clonal hematologic disorders associated with mastocytosis should be treated according to the standard-of-care guidelines for that disorder, regardless of the presence of mastocytosis. Bone marrow transplantation

(Chapter 181) has yielded generally disappointing results for the treatment of mast cell disease, although occasional cases resulting in complete remission have been reported.

PROGNOSIS

The prognosis for mastocytosis varies by the category of disease. At least 50% of patients with pediatric-onset cutaneous mastocytosis have complete resolution of the disease by adolescence, and the rest of those patients experience improvement or fading of the skin lesions. Indolent systemic mastocytosis is a persistent disease but has a good prognosis without a decrease in life expectancy, and progression to a more aggressive disease category is rare. Factors associated with poorer prognosis have been reported as the absence of urticaria pigmentosa, older age at onset of symptoms, elevated serum lactate dehydrogenase or alkaline phosphatase, thrombocytopenia, anemia, peripheral blood smear abnormalities, and detectability of the D816V *KIT* mutation in peripheral blood. The prognosis for SM-AHNMD is determined by the prognosis for the associated hematologic disorder. Aggressive systemic mastocytosis and MCL have poor prognoses, with median survival times of less than 3 years and less than 1 year, respectively.

SUGGESTED READINGS

Akin C. Anaphylaxis and mast cell disease. What is the risk? *Curr Allergy Asthma Rep.* 2010;10:34-38. *Discussion of increased risk of anaphylaxis, especially venom-induced and idiopathic, associated with mastocytosis.*

Bodemer C, Hermine O, Palmérini F, et al. Pediatric mastocytosis is a clonal disease associated with D816V and other activating c-KIT mutations. *J Invest Dermatol.* 2010;130:804-815. *Pediatric mastocytosis is a clonal disease even though it can spontaneously regress.*

Escribano L, Alvarez-Twose I, Sánchez-Muñoz L, et al. Prognosis in adult indolent systemic mastocytosis: a long-term study of the Spanish Network on Mastocytosis in a series of 145 patients. *J Allergy Clin Immunol.* 2009;124:514-521. *Generally low disease progression rate and majority with normal life expectancy with this disease; laboratory markers that predict transformation into more aggressive form.*

Pardanani A, Tefferi A. Systemic mastocytosis in adults: a review on prognosis and treatment based on 342 Mayo Clinic patients and current literature. *Curr Opin Hematol.* 2010;17:125-132. *Comprehensive review emphasizing that patients with indolent disease have a normal life expectancy.*

Valent P, Sperr WR, Akin C. How I treat patients with advanced systemic mastocystosis. *Blood.* 2010;116:5812-5817. *Review emphasizing interferon-alpha and 2-chlorodeoxyadenosine.*

XXII

RHEUMATIC DISEASES

264

APPROACH TO THE PATIENT WITH RHEUMATIC DISEASE

WILLIAM P. AREND AND GEORGE V. LAWRY

Diseases of the musculoskeletal system are common and may be both disabling and costly. This chapter provides an approach to the evaluation of patients with rheumatic diseases by outlining the components necessary for identifying the patient's problems, formulating a diagnosis, and initiating treatment.

Musculoskeletal disorders may manifest as acute, subacute, or chronic problems. Pain and interference with daily activities are what bring the patient to a physician and determine the impact of the condition. A general medical approach to the patient with rheumatic complaints is paramount, with particular reliance on an accurate history and a thoughtful physical examination. Usually, only limited additional testing is required to diagnose most musculoskeletal disorders, but in some instances, assessment with a number of laboratory analyses, imaging studies, and other disciplines may be necessary.

PATHOBIOLOGY

Categories of Musculoskeletal Diseases

Musculoskeletal diseases can be practically classified into nine categories, defined by the predominantly affected tissues (Table 264-1). At each point in the evaluation (history, physical examination, and laboratory testing), it is important to consider what tissues are involved. Recognition of the pattern of predominant tissue involvement can direct attention toward the disease primarily associated with that tissue. Before consideration of clinical approaches to the evaluation of patients with musculoskeletal problems, it is useful to first review the anatomy and pathophysiology of the affected structures.

Anatomy

The structures that may be involved in musculoskeletal diseases are shown in Figure 264-1A. Foremost is the joint cavity. The lining membrane, known as the *synovium*, consists of a thin layer of macrophages (type A cells) and fibroblasts (type B cells) with a sublining of rich, vascular, loose connective tissue. Hyaline cartilage overlies the bony end plates and provides a cushion to joint motion. The cartilage has high water content and obtains its nutrition solely from the synovial fluid, which is derived from the synovium primarily as an ultrafiltrate of plasma. The synovium also secretes specialized molecules into the synovial fluid, such as hyaluronic acid. An intact bony end plate is required to support the cartilage. The joint capsule and ligaments provide further support and blend with the periosteum. Periarticular anatomy is equally important and includes the tendons, bursae, and muscles associated with each joint.

Pathophysiology

The etiology of musculoskeletal problems is usually inflammatory, metabolic, degenerative, tumor, or some combination thereof. The disorders associated with musculoskeletal tissues are summarized in Table 264-1 and Figure 264-1B. Periarticular inflammation may involve tendons or bursae, and these structures are common causes of pain and stiffness, often misinterpreted as arising from the joint itself. The noninflammatory, degenerative disease osteoarthritis (OA) begins in the cartilage and leads to cartilage loss, subchondral new bone formation, and marginal bony overgrowth. Cartilage loss may also occur secondarily to synovial inflammation or trauma. Synovial inflammatory disorders, such as rheumatoid arthritis (RA), begin in the synovium and secondarily damage the cartilage, joint capsule, and bone. Crystal deposition disorders, such as gout or pseudogout, may also cause articular inflammation. Inflammation at entheses (enthesopathy), the insertion sites of tendons or ligaments on bone, is characteristic of the spondyloarthropathies, such as ankylosing spondylitis. Infections primarily involve the joint cavity (septic arthritis) or bone (osteomyelitis). Osteonecrosis of bone may be associated with secondary cartilage damage after collapse of the bony end plate. Inflammatory diseases of the muscle usually manifest with painless proximal weakness. Lastly, the common clinical problem of fibromyalgia is characterized by soft tissue and joint pain with local tenderness in specific points but without objective evidence of inflammation or swelling.

DIAGNOSIS

History

Demography

An appreciation of the age, gender, and personal history of the patient is helpful, including marital status, occupation, and psychosocial factors.

Age

The age of the patient is the first step in considering a differential diagnosis. For example, arthritis is a major manifestation of hemophilia with onset during childhood. The term *juvenile idiopathic arthritis* refers to three different forms of arthritis with onset before the age of 16 years. In young adults, inflammatory and septic arthritic conditions may be seen, but OA is exceptional. The onset of RA is often in the middle years, whereas elderly people are more prone to OA. Arthritis in elderly people is often assumed to be degenerative, when in fact the patient may have an inflammatory process such as polymyalgia rheumatica, RA, or systemic lupus erythematosus (SLE) (Chapter 274).

Gender

RA and other autoimmune diseases are more common in women, whereas ankylosing spondylitis and the other spondyloarthropathies (Chapter 273) associated with the human leukocyte antigen HLA-B27 are more common in men. Gouty arthritis is more common in men and rarely attacks women before menopause.

Occupation and Recreation

Occupation and recreational activities are also important because of associated physical and psychological stresses. The clinician should inquire about the patient's job to determine how demanding it is. Occupational factors such as repetitive joint trauma may contribute to the development of OA in susceptible individuals. Musculoskeletal symptoms may also be associated with jogging or with trauma from sports activities.

Family History

It is important to obtain a complete family history because autoimmune diseases, spondyloarthropathies, and gout occur with an increased incidence in families.

Onset and Evolution of Symptoms

Knowledge of the pattern of onset, location, and evolution of musculoskeletal symptoms is essential for accurate diagnosis. The development of symptoms over hours to days is characteristic of *acute arthritis* and usually represents an inflammatory or traumatic process. The persistence of symptoms for more than 6 weeks is considered *chronic arthritis*, whereas an intermediate duration of days to weeks is referred to as *subacute arthritis*. Musculoskeletal pain can be further characterized using the mnemonic "OPQRST" where O = onset, P = precipitating (and ameliorating) factors, Q = quality, R = radiation, S = severity, and T = timing. The most common symptom of musculoskeletal disease is pain; a diagnostic approach to the evaluation of patients presenting with musculoskeletal pain is presented in Figure 264-2.

Pattern of Joint Involvement

The distribution of joint involvement is one of the most essential aspects of diagnosis of musculoskeletal diseases. Monoarthritis describes symptoms in a single joint; oligoarthritis (or pauciarthritis), symptoms in two to four joints; and polyarthritis, involvement of five or more joints. Arthritis in an extremity is called *peripheral joint disease*, whereas spinal involvement is termed *axial disease*. It is important to elicit a history of symmetrical versus asymmetrical peripheral joint disease. The predominant involvement of the small joints of the hands and feet or of large joints such as the shoulder, hip, and knee also has diagnostic importance.

A critical feature in clinical diagnosis is the distinction between arthralgia (subjective joint pain) and arthritis (objective joint swelling, deformity, or impaired function). Objective findings on physical examination must be found for a diagnosis of arthritis to be made.

TABLE 264-1 CLASSIFICATION OF MUSCULOSKELETAL DISEASES

CATEGORY	PROTOTYPES	USEFUL TESTS	TREATMENTS
Local and regional conditions	Tendonitis or bursitis	Aspirate bursa if infection is suspected	Local injections
Cartilage degeneration	Osteoarthritis	Radiographs of affected area	NSAIDs, analgesics, and physical therapy
Inflammatory synovitis	Rheumatoid arthritis Autoimmune diseases	Rheumatoid factor, ESR Antinuclear antibody test	DMARDs and biologic agents Prednisone and immunosuppressive drugs
Crystal-induced synovitis	Gout CPPD (pseudogout)	Joint fluid crystal examination Radiographic chondrocalcinosis	NSAIDs NSAIDs
Enthesopathy	Ankylosing spondylitis and biologic agents	Sacroiliac radiographs	NSAIDs, MTX, and spondyloarthropathies
Joint space disease	Septic arthritis	Joint fluid culture	Antibiotics
Osteoarticular disease	Osteonecrosis	Radiographs, magnetic resonance imaging	Core decompression or prosthetic joint replacement
Inflammatory myopathy	Polymyositis Dermatomyositis Inclusion body myositis	Muscle enzymes, electromyography, muscle biopsy	Corticosteroids and immunosuppressive drugs
General conditions	Polymyalgia rheumatica Fibromyalgia	Elevated ESR Normal ESR	Corticosteroids Aerobic exercise, stretches, and sleep medications

Biologic agents = anti-tumor necrosis factor (anti-TNF) drugs and others; CPPD = calcium pyrophosphate dehydrate disease; DMARDs = disease-modifying antirheumatic drugs; ESR = erythrocyte sedimentation rate; MTX = methotrexate; NSAIDs = nonsteroidal anti-inflammatory drugs.

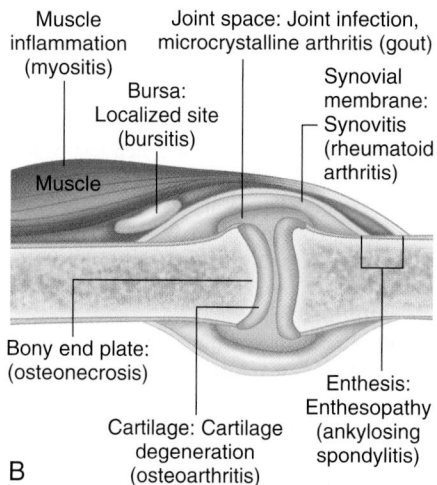

FIGURE 264-1. Structures involved in musculoskeletal diseases. **A,** Anatomic structures of the musculoskeletal system. **B,** Location of rheumatic disease processes.

Inflammatory versus Noninflammatory Conditions

An important initial step in the evaluation of musculoskeletal symptoms is the differentiation of inflammatory versus noninflammatory disease. A history of warmth and erythema over a joint suggests inflammatory disease. Morning stiffness lasting longer than 60 minutes, a "gel" phenomenon (stiffness after rest that is more than transient), and improvement in pain and stiffness with activity all suggest the presence of inflammatory disease. In contrast, minimal morning stiffness and worsening pain with activity suggest noninflammatory joint disease.

Extra-articular and Systemic Features

A careful history may reveal important systemic and extra-articular manifestations, including fever, fatigue, weakness, dry eyes, ocular inflammation, pulmonary symptoms, or Raynaud's phenomenon (Chapter 80). The finding of musculoskeletal complaints in the setting of systemic symptoms and multiorgan involvement strongly suggests the possibility of a diffuse autoimmune disease such as SLE.

Functional Disability Indices

A number of self-report questionnaires such as the Stanford Health Assessment Questionnaire, Functional Disability Index, and Arthritis Impact Measurement Scales, or modifications of these, have been developed for ongoing evaluation of patients with arthritis. These instruments document patient-reported functional status with results comparable to those of traditional physician-reported measures of joint disease activity, such as tender joint count, or to a radiographic joint erosion score and erythrocyte sedimentation rate.

Physical Examination
Essential Concepts

The physical examination includes a record of the patient's gait and posture as well as examination of the spine and skeletal muscles. The joints shown in Figure 264-3 should be examined systematically, region by region, with a side-to-side comparison to determine whether any are inflamed or damaged. The pattern of joint involvement, whether symmetrical, axial, or peripheral, should be recorded using the diagram. The abnormalities detected in each joint should be recorded as deformity, tenderness, erythema, swelling, and altered range of motion (ROM) to allow comparison between the same or different examiners over time.

Examination Components

There are four essential steps in musculoskeletal physical examination.

Inspection

Inspect for asymmetry, deformity, erythema, and swelling.

Palpation

Palpate for tenderness, warmth, synovial thickening and effusion, bony hypertrophy, and crepitus.

Range of Motion

Take the joint through passive or active ROM (or a combination of both).

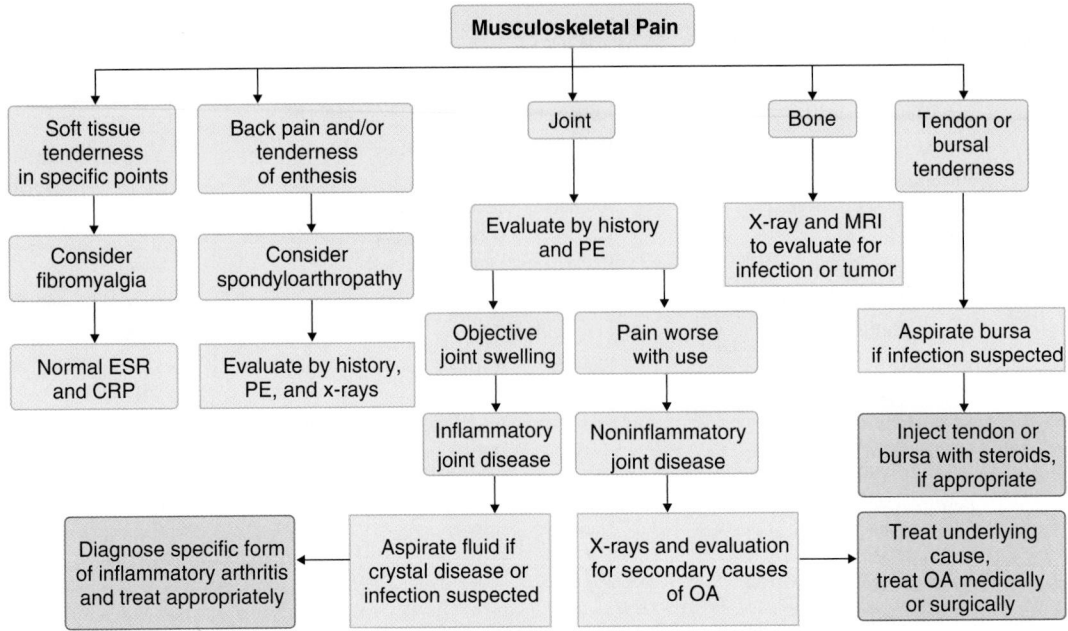

FIGURE 264-2. Diagnostic approach to musculoskeletal pain. CRP = C-reactive protein; ESR = erythrocyte sedimentation rate; MRI = magnetic resonance imaging; OA = osteoarthritis; PE = physical examination.

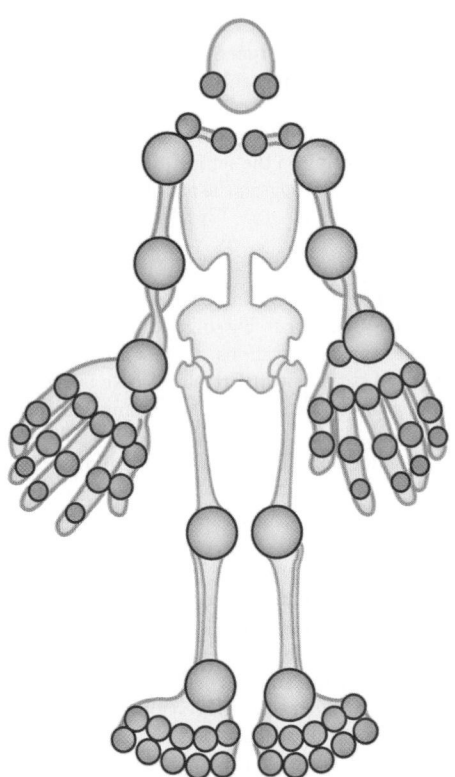

FIGURE 264-3. A pictorial method for recording joint disease activity or destruction. The sketch can be used on a printed form or rubber stamp to chart which joints are active or deformed at the time of each assessment. (Courtesy of Dr. Hugh A. Smythe, Toronto.)

Special Testing

Perform an assessment of supporting structures (such as ligaments and tendons) or for conditions particular to a single region (such as Tinel's sign at the wrist for detection of carpal tunnel syndrome; Chapter 428).

Objective Joint Findings

A careful examination is critical in distinguishing articular from periarticular conditions.

Joint tenderness alone is insufficient for diagnosis and must be correlated with the finding of an objective, visible, or palpable abnormality for a diagnosis of arthritis to be made. Joint redness (erythema) depends on the acuteness and severity of the underlying inflammation, and its presence may suggest the possibility of infection or crystalline arthritis. Joint warmth also depends on the acuteness of the underlying inflammation. Joint swelling is a definitive sign of arthritis and may be caused by either a joint effusion (excess synovial fluid) or an inflamed and swollen synovial membrane (synovitis). Bony hypertrophy around a joint (osteophytic swelling) is characteristic of osteoarthritis. *Crepitus* refers to a continuous grating sensation that is felt by the examiner's hand during joint motion. Fine or velvety crepitus may denote chronic proliferative synovitis, whereas coarse crepitus may indicate either roughening of the cartilage surface or complete loss of hyaline cartilage. Joint damage and deformity are usually signs of prior arthritis or injury (ligamentous laxity, joint subluxation, tendon rupture, or contracture).

Range of Motion

Both active and passive ROM are important in assessing joint function. Active ROM is patient-initiated movement of the joint; it tests integrated function and requires intact innervation and muscle and tendon function, as well as joint mobility. Passive ROM is examiner-initiated movement of a joint; it tests only joint mobility. The combined use of passive and active ROM minimizes the need for patient instruction and maximizes the speed and efficiency of the examination. Whenever joint motion is anticipated to be painful, it is best first to observe active ROM, to appreciate the degree of pain and dysfunction, before gently attempting passive ROM.

Extra-articular Findings

Because many rheumatic diseases are multisystem disorders, physical examination may document the presence of important extra-articular features. In RA, for example, these include subcutaneous nodules, digital vasculitis, and other systemic features as described in Chapter 272.

Classification

Clinical evaluation enables the establishment of which anatomic structures are inflamed, which are damaged, and how function is impaired. Seven types of rheumatic involvement can be identified as a framework for various diagnostic possibilities or hypotheses to be considered (see Fig. 264-1B). The nine categories presented in the following paragraphs are listed in Table 264-1 along with typical diseases, examples of useful diagnostic tests, and treatments. Table 264-1 and the descriptions in this section provide the basis for more detailed information contained in the following chapters.

Local and Regional Conditions

Nonarticular disorders such as tendonitis, bursitis, and neck and low-back strains are very common regional problems. They usually respond to analgesics or nonsteroidal anti-inflammatory drugs, physical therapy, protective splints, or injection of corticosteroids.

Cartilage Degeneration

OA is defined as loss of articular cartilage with a bony response leading to the formation of osteophytes. Primary OA is thought to be caused by biochemical abnormalities in the cartilage that predispose to microfissures in the surface with subsequent degeneration of the cartilage. Secondary OA may develop as a consequence of inflammatory conditions such as RA, ankylosing spondylitis, septic arthritis, and calcium pyrophosphate deposition disease (CPPD). Previous trauma and joint hypermobility are other mechanical factors that may predispose to OA.

Inflammatory Synovitis

Inflammation of the synovial membrane lining of the joint is typical of inflammatory polyarthritides such as RA and other autoimmune diseases. Synovial inflammation is the dominant clinical feature of RA and may lead to irreversible joint damage. Synovial inflammation may also be present in conditions such as SLE, but the presence of multiorgan involvement should lead to the clinical suspicion of a systemic autoimmune disease.

Crystal-Induced Synovitis

Crystals of monosodium urate (gout), calcium pyrophosphate (pseudogout), or hydroxyapatite are capable of inducing an acute inflammatory reaction in both synovial fluid and synovium. Acute crystalline arthritis usually affects only one or at most a few joints at a time. Joint aspiration and synovial fluid analysis for crystals using polarized light microscopy establish the diagnosis. CPPD is often associated with the radiologic appearance of chondrocalcinosis of hyaline cartilage.

Enthesopathy

The enthesis is the anatomic transition zone where tendons, ligaments, and joint capsules attach to bone. Inflammation in this region is the hallmark of the family of spondyloarthropathies (Chapter 273), of which ankylosing spondylitis is the prototype. Other members of this group include reactive arthritis associated with enteric or urethral infection, the arthropathy associated with inflammatory bowel disease, and psoriatic arthritis. In ankylosing spondylitis, the sacroiliac joints and apophyseal joints of the spine show characteristic inflammation with a tendency to bony ankylosis (axial predominance), whereas in psoriatic arthritis, there is frequently enthesitis with an oligopolyarthritis (peripheral predominance).

Joint Space Disease

Septic arthritis (Chapter 280) may develop from hematogenous spread of microorganisms into the joint space, through local extension from adjacent soft tissues or by joint penetration. Joint infections are usually associated with intense pain even at rest, and the diagnosis is confirmed by joint aspiration with Gram stain and culture of the synovial fluid. A joint prosthesis increases susceptibility to infection in that joint. Blood in the joint space, known as *hemarthrosis,* may result from microfractures, coagulopathy, or tumor.

Osteoarticular Disease

Osteopenia/osteoporosis may complicate many rheumatic conditions and are dealt with in Chapter 251. Osteonecrosis (Chapter 256), which results from collapse of the bony end plate due to vascular insufficiency, causes secondary crushing and fragmentation of the overlying articular cartilage. Osteonecrosis may be idiopathic or associated with systemic conditions such as sickle cell disease or ethanol abuse; it may also occur after treatment with high-dose corticosteroids. Inflammation of the periosteum, known as *periostitis,* may be associated with hypertrophic pulmonary osteoarthropathy and clubbing (Chapter 283). This syndrome may be a clue to underlying lung cancer.

Inflammatory Myopathy

Inflammation and (usually painless) weakness of the proximal skeletal muscles are characteristic of inflammatory myopathies (Chapter 277): polymyositis, dermatomyositis, and inclusion body myositis. Elevated creatine kinase levels, electromyographic abnormalities, and characteristic histologic abnormalities on muscle biopsy are present in inflammatory myopathies.

General Conditions

These nonarticular or extra-articular disorders are not usually associated with arthritis. This group includes polymyalgia rheumatica, complex regional pain syndrome/reflex sympathetic dystrophy, and fibromyalgia. Polymyalgia rheumatica usually affects whites older than 50 years of age and causes proximal muscle pain in the neck, shoulders, and hips, with significant morning stiffness and a high erythrocyte sedimentation rate. It is sometimes associated with giant cell (temporal) arteritis (Chapter 279). Fibromyalgia usually manifests in individuals younger than 50 years; is associated with widespread arthralgia and myalgia (deceptively inflammatory sounding), morning stiffness, significant fatigue, and nonrestorative sleep. It is accompanied by the presence of tender points in characteristic locations, as described in Chapter 282.

TREATMENT

Effective treatment must be based on accurate diagnosis (see Table 264-1).

If a formal diagnosis is not apparent, generation of a prioritized problem list can be very helpful in suggesting a differential diagnosis and creating an initial management strategy. The acuteness and severity of presentation dictate whether immediate intervention is required or further observation is more appropriate. For example, an acute monarthritis (possible septic or crystalline arthritis) requires immediate attention, whereas a widespread smoldering polyarthritis may not. However, a patient with polyarthritis who is systemically ill requires prompt investigation to exclude a diffuse autoimmune disease, underlying infection, or hidden malignancy.

Arthrocentesis is helpful diagnostically, and aspiration of synovial fluid is also helpful therapeutically in relieving symptoms and permitting injection of corticosteroids when appropriate. *Photographs showing important landmarks for needle aspiration and injection of common joints are present in the online version of this text.*

Regardless of the diagnosis, educating the patient and family is crucial to successful management of any chronic musculoskeletal problem. Informed patients are more likely to comply with treatment and develop more realistic expectations of outcome. The goal of management for patients with musculoskeletal diseases is to control pain, prevent joint destruction, and maintain independence. For this reason, treatment should be individualized and based on early, accurate identification of symptoms and signs, a firm diagnosis, prompt administration of appropriate therapy, and vigilant monitoring of response.

SUGGESTED READINGS

Candelas G, Abasolo L, Leon L, et al. Diagnostic concordance between primary care physicians and rheumatologists in patients with work disability related to musculoskeletal disorders. *Rheumatol Int.* 2011. [Epub ahead of print.] *Agreement was modest—highest for tendinitis and lowest for peripheral osteoarthritis.*

Machado P, Castrejon I, Katchamart W, et al. Multinational evidence-based recommendations on how to investigate and follow up undifferentiated peripheral inflammatory arthritis: integrating systematic literature research and expert opinion of a broad international panel of rheumatologists in the 3E Initiative. *Ann Rheum Dis.* 2011;70:15-24. *Consensus recommendations for evaluation.*

Raza SH, Pattanaik D, Egerman RS. Painful, swollen hands in a young woman. *Obstet Gynecol.* 2010;116:983-988. *Case-based differentiated diagnosis.*

265

LABORATORY TESTING IN THE RHEUMATIC DISEASES

DAVID S. PISETSKY

The rheumatic diseases are a heterogeneous group of conditions that result from diverse pathophysiologic mechanisms and involve the musculoskeletal system as well as other organs. These conditions range from mild, diffuse joint and muscle pain to severe life-threatening kidney failure and stroke. Although the rheumatic diseases have many origins, immune disturbances resulting in local and systemic inflammation are frequently the underlying cause. The approach to diagnosis therefore entails specific laboratory tests to assess functional disturbances of individual organs and their relationship to inflammation and autoimmunity.

Laboratory testing in patients with rheumatic disease has two main purposes. The first is diagnostic, and the second is prognostic. Some tests are useful in both contexts, but others have different performance characteristics related to their specificity and pattern of expression during disease. Prognostic tests provide critical information to help distinguish activity that is reversible from damage that is fixed and irreversible. In general, the assessment of damage relies on specific tests of end-organ function or structure rather than process markers. Distinguishing activity from damage is important in patient management, especially with respect to the use of therapies associated with toxicity.

MARKERS OF INFLAMMATION

For many patients, the initial goal of evaluation is to determine the presence of inflammation. Inflammation is the body's response to injury and is characterized by a cascade of cellular and molecular events that arise irrespective of stimulus or locale (Chapter 47). The immediate response to inflammatory stimuli is termed the *acute phase response* and includes a set of proteins produced primarily in the liver in response to cytokines such as interleukin-6 (IL-6), tumor necrosis factor-α (TNF-α), and IL-1. These cytokines are produced by macrophages and dendritic cells after stimulation of pattern recognition receptors (PRRs) that include both toll-like receptors (TLRs) and other non-TLR sensing systems that trigger a system called the *inflammasome*; PRRs recognize intracellular as well as extracellular bacterial and viral products as well as large and small (e.g., uric acid crystals) molecules released from damaged cells. The result is stimulation of innate immunity (Chapters 44 and 47). Many proteins in the acute phase response show dramatic increases in serum levels, although some show a reduction. Because the levels of these proteins can increase hundreds to thousands of times in magnitude, they provide a sensitive and powerful set of markers for inflammation, whether induced by infection, trauma, or autoimmunity.

Of the proteins stimulated during the acute phase response, C-reactive protein (CRP) has received the most attention as a marker of inflammation in both rheumatic and nonrheumatic disease. CRP is a member of the pentraxin family; although its function is not fully known, its ability to bind to phosphocholine suggests a scavenger function to eliminate bacterial products or damaged cells and to attenuate the consequences of infection or tissue injury. Other molecules, such as serum amyloid protein (SAP), fibrinogen, and complement, also show marked elevations in levels during the acute phase response, signifying a broad-based effort at host defense.

The CRP level provides a very useful measure of inflammation and can convey information for categorization of a clinical process (e.g., inflammatory versus noninflammatory arthritis) as well as assessment of disease activity or prognosis (e.g., activity of rheumatoid arthritis [RA] or likelihood of joint erosion). The advantage of measuring CRP in the blood, rather than cytokines, is that the protein levels are much higher. Furthermore, CRP levels remain elevated for a longer period (days) than cytokines; the latter may appear only transiently in the blood and thereby evade detection.

Another simple laboratory test reflecting the acute phase response is the erythrocyte sedimentation rate (ESR). In this test, commonly called the *sed rate*, anticoagulated blood is drawn into a long, thin tube and allowed to settle under the influence of gravity for 1 hour. The distance the blood falls depends on a number of factors, including the concentration of serum proteins such as immunoglobulins and fibrinogen, an acute phase reactant. The sedimentation rate is nonspecific with respect to disease association and also depends on age and gender. The upper limits of normal vary between women and men.

Other simple laboratory tests point to an acute phase response. For example, patients with inflammation frequently exhibit a leukocytosis or thrombocytosis, most likely reflecting the action of cytokines and other mediators, including glucocorticoids, during this process. With chronic inflammation, anemia of chronic disease can also occur, with the hematocrit, in conjunction with the white blood cell and platelet counts, pointing to the presence of an inflammatory process. In systemic lupus erythematosus (SLE), lymphopenia, thrombocytopenia, and low CRP values often characterize active disease, with the discordance between laboratory and clinical findings a clue to diagnosis.

LABORATORY EVALUATION OF MUSCULOSKELETAL DISEASE

The most common presentation of musculoskeletal disease is pain in and around the joints in association with functional impairment. Collectively, diseases causing joint symptoms are called arthritis, implying inflammation. The extent of inflammation in these diseases varies markedly, however, with some forms such as osteoarthritis (Chapter 270) showing scant evidence of inflammation either locally or systemically.

Arthritis results from many different diseases and occurs in various patterns defined by the number and size of joints affected, symmetry, and involvement of the axial as well as peripheral joints. For each pattern (e.g., chronic polyarthritis), a key issue in diagnosis concerns its place in the spectrum of inflammatory versus noninflammatory arthritis. Furthermore, although many diseases can cause arthritis, their prevalence varies enormously, with osteoarthritis or degenerative joint disease being the most common form of noninflammatory arthritis and RA the most common form of inflammatory arthritis.

The differential diagnosis of arthritis is based on a comprehensive history and physical examination to assess symptoms suggesting inflammation (e.g., morning stiffness and fatigue), the presence of synovitis, and results of laboratory tests indicative of inflammation. Of these tests, the ESR and CRP are nonspecific indicators of inflammation. Two autoantibody tests, rheumatoid factor (RF) and antibodies to citrullinated proteins, provide more specific diagnostic information. Given the demographics of inflammatory arthritis, testing for antinuclear antibodies is often part of this evaluation as well.

Rheumatoid Factor

RF comprises a family of specificities that bind to the immunoglobulin G (IgG) molecule. These RFs target primarily the constant region or Fc portion of IgG, reacting with antigenic determinants that are most likely conformational in origin. IgM RFs are the most abundant of these antibodies and have been easiest to measure, using agglutination assays with red blood cells or latex beads coated with IgG. More recently, enzyme-linked immunosorbent assay (ELISA) and nephelometry have been used to detect RFs.

RFs occur in approximately 80% of patients with RA (Chapter 272) and represent one criterion for the classification or diagnosis of this disease. Furthermore, high levels of RFs are often associated with a worse prognosis, the occurrence of joint erosion as measured by radiographs, and deformity. Despite these associations, RFs occur in the sera of patients with a wide range of autoimmune and inflammatory diseases as well as in normal individuals, especially with age (Table 265-1). The frequent occurrence of RFs may reflect their etiology and role in innate immune responses to promote the binding of IgG to antigen by Fc cross-linking. Although RFs may occur in many

TABLE 265-1 RHEUMATIC DISEASES AND NONRHEUMATIC CONDITIONS ASSOCIATED WITH A POSITIVE RHEUMATOID FACTOR

DISEASES	FREQUENCY
Rheumatoid arthritis	50-90%
Systemic lupus erythematosus	15-35%
Sjögren's syndrome	75-95%
Systemic sclerosis	20-30%
Polymyositis/dermatomyositis	5-10%
Cryoglobulinemia	40-100%
Mixed connective tissue disease	50-60%
Aging (>70 yr)	10-25%
Infection	
Bacterial endocarditis	25-50%
Liver disease	15-40%
Tuberculosis	8%
Syphilis	Up to 13%
Parasitic diseases	20-90%
Leprosy	5-58%
Viral infection	15-65%
Pulmonary disease	
Sarcoidosis	3-33%
Interstitial pulmonary fibrosis	10-50%
Silicosis	30-50%
Asbestosis	30%
Miscellaneous diseases	
Primary biliary cirrhosis	45-70%
Malignancy	5-25%

Modified from Shmerling RH, Delbanco TL. The rheumatoid factor: an analysis of clinical utility. *Am J Med.* 1991;91:530.

settings other than RA, depending on the pretest probability, the test nevertheless remains useful in the evaluation of patients with inflammatory arthritis.

Antibodies to Citrullinated Proteins

Antibodies to citrullinated proteins are other autoantibody specificities important in the diagnosis of RA (Chapter 272). Citrulline is a posttranslational modification of the amino acid arginine that results from deimidation. This chemical reaction is catalyzed by the enzyme peptidylarginine deiminase (PAD) and may occur in the setting of inflammation; the function of this modification is unknown. Citrullination can affect many different proteins, creating antigenic sites on proteins that include keratin, fibrinogen, and filaggrin. This antibody system can be detected by Western blotting, ELISA, or cellular immunofluorescence.

Although antibodies are directed to citrullinated residues on intact proteins, they can be conveniently measured using synthetic peptides containing citrulline. Among these synthetic antigens, a citrulline-containing protein with a cyclic structure provides sensitive and specific assays in an ELISA format. Antibodies directed to this type of antigen are known as anti-CCP (cyclic citrullinated peptide) and can be formally distinguished from antibodies to the citrullinated proteins themselves (ACPA, or anti–citrullinated protein antibodies). The term *anti-CCP* is commonly used for these specificities, although it is not formally synonymous with ACPA.

Anti-CCP antibodies are highly associated with RA. They occur in 60 to 70% of patients with RA and uncommonly in those with other forms of inflammatory arthritis, making their presence important in diagnosis. Significantly, anti-CCP antibodies can occur before the onset of other signs and symptoms of RA, suggesting utility for screening of at-risk patients. Because anti-CCP antibodies are more specific markers than RFs, their presence in patients with early inflammatory arthritis may indicate the diagnosis of RA and allow more prompt initiation of therapy.

Joint Fluid Analysis

Analysis of joint fluid can provide decisive data in the evaluation of arthritis and, in some instances, a definitive diagnosis. This analysis is essential in the setting of acute monoarthritis to investigate the possibility of infection; for chronic forms of arthritis, joint fluid should be analyzed if there is uncertainty about the diagnosis and involvement of one joint out of proportion to others. Joint aspiration is a sterile procedure performed with a local anesthetic. Although fluid can be analyzed by tests to assess viscosity and mucin content, the cell count, examination of crystals, and stains and cultures to evaluate infection are the most informative.

On the basis of cell counts, joint fluids can be categorized into four main types: noninflammatory, inflammatory, septic, and hemorrhagic. A noninflammatory fluid has fewer than 2000 cells/mm³ with mononuclear cell predominance. An inflammatory fluid has more than 2000 cells/mm³, with 50,000 cells/mm³ frequently used as the upper limit for this type of fluid. In an inflammatory fluid, polymorphonuclear cells predominate. A septic fluid is an inflammatory fluid in which culture or staining for microorganisms demonstrates infection. Suspicion of infection is especially high for fluids with cell counts greater than 50,000/mm³. However, crystal-induced arthritis can produce cell counts of this magnitude, and an infected fluid can have counts below this level. Hemorrhagic fluids have red cell predominance that can approximate that of blood.

In the setting of an acute monoarthritis, crystal-induced disease is much more common than infection, with the presence of crystals demonstrated by polarization microscopy. With this technique, monosodium urate crystals in gout appear needle-shaped and are negatively birefringent. In contrast, calcium pyrophosphate dihydrate crystals in pseudogout are rhomboidal in shape and are weakly positively birefringent. Infection can coexist with crystal-induced disease, necessitating microbiologic evaluation even when crystals are found. Hemorrhagic fluids can also result from infection, although their presence suggests malignancy or trauma. Figure 265-1 provides an algorithm for the analysis of joint fluid.

Depending on the clinical findings and the results of initial laboratory testing, other studies may be performed to investigate less common diagnostic possibilities such as metabolic disease or malignancy. The laboratory evaluation of inflammatory arthritis may also include serologic tests for infections such as Lyme disease, human immunodeficiency virus (HIV) infection, or hepatitis.

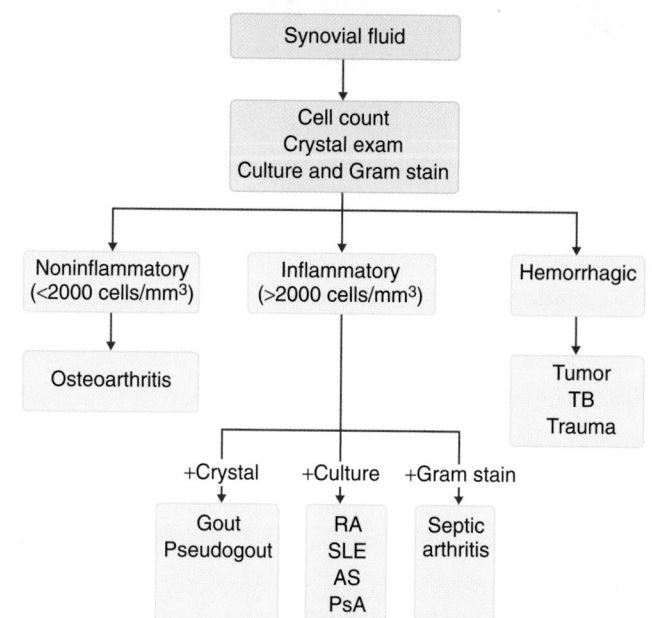

FIGURE 265-1. **Algorithm for analysis of joint fluid.** Examples of inflammatory arthritis are indicated, although many conditions can produce these findings. AS = ankylosing spondylitis; PsA = psoriatic arthritis; RA = rheumatoid arthritis; SLE = systemic lupus erythematosus; TB = tuberculosis.

⬤ LABORATORY EVALUATION OF SYSTEMIC INFLAMMATORY DISEASE

Among rheumatic diseases, some are characterized by severe systemic inflammation that can cause organ-threatening and life-threatening manifestations. These diseases can have arthritis as a component and presenting complaint, although the prominence of extra-articular manifestations, especially as they develop over time and involve organs such as the kidney, points to their systemic nature. These diseases can be categorized on the basis of clinical, serologic, and pathologic findings, with the presence of vasculitis, irrespective of blood vessel size, providing a unifying feature in disease classification.

The terms *connective tissue disease* (CTD) and *collagen vascular disease* are both used to denote a group of diseases that includes RA, SLE, Sjögren's syndrome, polymyositis, dermatomyositis, and progressive systemic sclerosis. Diseases in this group can share common or overlapping clinical features, especially early in their course, when their presentations may be similar. In this stage of disease, the condition may be called *undifferentiated CTD*, with serologic markers sometimes predictive of the eventual diagnosis.

Antinuclear Antibodies

The expression of antibodies to components of the cell nucleus (antinuclear antibodies, or ANAs) is characteristic of CTD and is essentially invariable in patients with SLE (Chapter 274). These antibodies target a host of nuclear macromolecules, including DNA, RNA, and proteins as well as complexes of proteins with nucleic acid. These antigens are ubiquitously expressed in cells and subserve critical processes related to chromosomal structure, cell division, transcription, and translation. The basis for the antigenicity of these molecules is unknown, although DNA and RNA both have intrinsic immunologic activities and can stimulate cytokine production through action on both TLR and non-TLR PRRs, especially when in the form of immune complexes. ANAs are commonly measured by immunofluorescence (IF) assays in which sera are incubated with tissue culture cells (e.g., Hep2 cells) fixed to a glass slide. Antibody binding is revealed by fluorescence microscopy after incubation of the slide with a fluoresceinated anti-immunoglobulin reagent. Results are reported in terms of the pattern of fluorescence as well as the end-point titer of sera at which fluorescence can be observed. The patterns of binding differ depending on the location of the particular macromolecular target, although a few patterns predominate. These patterns include homogeneous, rim, nucleolar, and speckled; in addition, ANA tests can detect antibodies to cytoplasmic antigens. Despite some disease associations, these patterns do not have diagnostic significance. Table 265-2 presents a list of major ANAs with their pattern and disease associations.

A major limitation in the assays of ANA concerns the frequency of positive reactivity in the sera of otherwise normal individuals who lack evidence of a

TABLE 265-2 SELECTED ANTINUCLEAR ANTIBODIES AND RHEUMATIC DISEASES

DISEASE PATTERN	ANTIBODY	ANTIGEN	ASSOCIATION
Homogeneous	Antihistone	Histones H1, H2A, H2B, H3, H4	Drug-induced lupus (>95%)
Rim	Anti-double-stranded DNA	Double-stranded DNA snRNP proteins	SLE (50%)
Speckled	Anti-Sm	snRNP proteins	SLE (30%)
	Anti-U1-RNP	U1 snRNP proteins	SLE (30%); MCTD (>95%)
	Anti-Ro (SS-A)	Two proteins complexed to small RNAs Y1-Y5	SLE (30%); Sjögren's syndrome (70-80%)
	Anti-La (SS-B)	Single protein plus RNA polymerase III transcript	SLE (15%); Sjögren's syndrome (50-70%)
	Anti-Ku	DNA binding protein	SLE (10%)
	Anti-SCL-70	DNA topoisomerase I	PSS (40-70%); CREST (10-20%)
Nucleolar	Anti-PM-Scl	Nucleolar protein complex	PSS (3%); PM (8%)
	Anti-Mi-2	Nuclear protein complex	DM (15-20%)
	Anti-RNA polymerase	Subunits of RNA polymerase I	PSS (4%)
Dividing cell	Anticentromere	Centromere/kinetochore protein	CREST (80%); PSS (30%)
	Antiproliferating cell nuclear antigen	Auxiliary protein of DNA polymerase δ	SLE (3%)
Cytoplasmic	Anti-Jo-1	Histidyl tRNA synthetase	ILD in PM/DM (18-25%)
	Anti-PL-7	Threonyl tRNA synthetase	PM/DM (3%)
	Anti-PL-12	Alanyl tRNA synthetase	PM (4%)
	Anti-SRP	Signal recognition particle	SLE (10%)
	Anti-ribosomal P	Large ribosomal subunit	PM/DM (3%)

CREST = calcinosis, Raynaud's phenomenon, esophageal dysmotility, sclerodactyly, and telangiectasia; DM = dermatomyositis; ILD = interstitial lung disease; MCTD = mixed connective tissue disease; PM = polymyositis; PSS = progressive systemic sclerosis (diffuse scleroderma); SLE = systemic lupus erythematosus; snRNP = small nuclear ribonucleoprotein; tRNA = transfer RNA.

CTD. The sera of as many as 5% of normal individuals express reactivity in the IF ANA test. The basis of this reactivity is not well understood, although it may reflect a predisposition to autoimmunity that is manifest in ANA production in the absence of other immunopathologic disturbances for the complete development of a CTD. Because ANA testing is often performed to evaluate nonspecific complaints such as arthralgias, fatigue, and fever, a positive test must be interpreted with caution and not used as proof of a CTD in the absence of correlative clinical or laboratory findings.

Because of detailed biochemical studies, the molecular identity of many ANAs is now known, allowing for the development of specific immuno-chemical assays using technologies that can eliminate the need for visual inspection of a slide stained for fluorescence. These tests (e.g., ELISA) can be performed individually, although multiplex assays provide simultaneous assessment of multiple specificities. With multiplex assays, the equivalent of an ANA test can be generated by measuring antibodies to a select set of more commonly targeted autoantigens, with positive binding to any one antigen considered indicative of a positive value for an ANA. Because sera of patients with SLE and other systemic inflammatory diseases contain numerous ANAs, focus on a limited set of specificities may fail to detect many positive sera. In addition, because immunochemical assays may detect low levels of antibody binding, the significance of this reactivity is not certain. Thus, although multiplex assays are operationally easier than conventional ANA testing by immunofluorescent staining, in clinical situations, the IF assay remains an important laboratory test for patient evaluation.

Among many ANA specificities now identified, only a few are performed routinely because of their value for diagnosis and prognosis. For several CTDs, diagnosis can be readily determined from clinical findings or other laboratory tests. In these instances, the ANA determination provides confirmatory information as well as clues to the occurrence of certain clinical manifestations.

Antibodies to DNA

Antibodies to DNA (anti-DNA) are serologic markers of SLE and represent a criterion in the classification of patients with this disease (Chapter 274). These antibodies bind sites on both single-stranded (ss) and double-stranded (ds) DNA, although anti-dsDNA antibodies are more specific for SLE and therefore routinely measured. Although these antibodies can bind free DNA, DNA in the cell occurs in association with histones to form a structure called the *nucleosome*, with DNA wrapped around a histone core. Anti-DNA may therefore be considered a subset of antibodies to nucleosomes, with nucleo-somes probably serving as the driving antigen for this response.

In clinical practice, the measurement of anti-DNA antibodies is an important element in the evaluation of patients with a broad array of clinical complaints, given the heterogeneity and multisystemic nature of SLE. Anti-DNA determinations, in addition to their value in diagnosis, also convey prognostic information and serve as an index of disease activity. The association with disease activity appears strongest with glomerulonephritis, most likely because of the role of DNA–anti-DNA immune complexes in immunopathogenesis. The association of anti-DNA antibodies with other disease manifestations is less certain, limiting the use of this marker as a measure of overall disease activity.

Several immunochemical approaches can be used to detect anti-DNA antibodies, although solid-phase ELISA assays are convenient and sensitive and eliminate the need for radioactivity. The assays vary in regard to the spectrum of anti-DNA antibodies detected, and results between assays may not correlate. Nevertheless, for each assay, the dynamic range for testing is large. With treatment and disease quiescence, anti-DNA antibodies may essentially disappear; with flare, levels may increase dramatically. This property distinguishes anti-DNA antibodies from other ANAs in SLE, levels of which tend to be more consistent over time.

As is the case for other ANAs, the appearance of anti-DNA antibodies in the serum may precede other manifestations of SLE, suggesting vigilance if these antibodies are present in patients who have symptoms that suggest a CTD but lack other evidence to establish a firm diagnosis.

Other Antinuclear Antibodies

Anti-Sm and anti-RNP antibodies are related specificities that commonly occur together in the sera of patients with SLE, a phenomenon called *linkage*. These antibodies bind proteins on subcellular particles called *snRNPs* (small nuclear ribonucleoproteins) that are composed of a set of proteins and uridine-rich RNAs. Anti-Sm and anti-RNP antibodies differ in protein specificity and in the ability to cause immunoprecipitation of the bound RNA molecules. Anti-Sm antibodies occur only in patients with SLE and represent a serologic marker in disease classification. In contrast, anti-RNP antibodies can appear in the sera of patients with other clinical presentations and, in the absence of anti-Sm, may characterize patients with overlapping CTD features, so-called mixed CTD. In SLE, the frequencies of anti-Sm and anti-RNP antibodies vary among racial and ethnic groups, although a clear association with particular clinical manifestations has not been established.

Anti-Ro and anti-La antibodies (or anti-SS-A and anti-SS-B), another set of linked ANAs, are directed to protein-RNA complexes that are involved in cellular metabolism of RNA. These antibodies are expressed more widely in patients with CTD and appear in the sera of patients with SLE, RA, and

Sjögren's syndrome, among others. Assessment of these antibodies is important because of their association with the neonatal lupus syndrome, which results from the transplacental passage of antibodies and causes congenital heart block as well as rash in the neonate.

Although ANAs are directed to ubiquitous antigens, they nevertheless are expressed in disease-specific patterns and may show association with particular organ-specific manifestations. These associations include anti–ribosomal P antibodies with central nervous systemic involvement in SLE, antibodies to DNA topoisomerase 1 (anti-SCL-70) with progressive systemic sclerosis (diffuse scleroderma), antibodies to centromeres with CREST syndrome (calcinosis, Raynaud's phenomenon, esophageal dysmotility, sclerodactyly, and telangiectasia), and antibodies to histidyl transfer RNA synthetase (anti-Jo-1) with interstitial lung disease in scleroderma (Chapter 275).

In addition to their association with specific disease manifestations, antibodies to both DNA- and RNA-binding proteins such as Sm and RNP may contribute to overall immune dysregulation in patients with autoimmune disease because of their formation of immune complexes containing DNA or RNA. These complexes can stimulate the production of type 1 interferon by triggering both TLR and non-TLR nucleic acid sensors as well as other cellular receptors (e.g., Fc receptors). Because immunoassays of interferon with patient sera are limited, the presence of interferon is observed more clearly in the pattern of gene expression known as the interferon signature in peripheral blood cells. Because antibodies to RNA-binding proteins in particular may promote this pattern, the serologic assay of these ANAs may allow assessment of the likelihood of both nonspecific and specific immunologic disturbances.

Antibodies to Phospholipids

Originally defined by their effects on in vitro clotting tests, antibodies to phospholipids (APLs) are associated with in vivo thrombosis and have been termed *lupus anticoagulants* (LACs). Patients with these antibodies display a clinical condition, termed the *antiphospholipid antibody syndrome*, which is characterized by arterial or venous thrombosis, thrombocytopenia, and first-trimester spontaneous abortions (Chapter 179). This syndrome may occur by itself or in the context of SLE, where it may contribute to the acceleration of atherosclerosis, premature stroke, and myocardial infarction. The laboratory evaluation of this condition involves specific assays of antibodies to phospholipids and related proteins as well as functional assays of clotting. Because expression of these antibodies may vary over time, testing must be performed on more than one occasion at least 6 weeks apart. Furthermore, the results of immunochemical and functional assays may not be congruent, because it is likely related to the heterogeneity of antibodies.

The serology of APLs is complicated because it is related to their antigenic targets as well as heterogeneity. Of phospholipids, cardiolipin is a common antigen for these assessments. Although they are designated as antibodies to cardiolipin or phospholipids, these antibodies may be actually directed to the protein β_2-glycoprotein 1; in the format of an ELISA, this protein may bind to phospholipids to create antigenic sites. ELISA determinations of anticardiolipin (aCL) antibodies can provide quantitative assessment of different isotypes (IgG, IgM, and IgA), although the association with thrombosis appears strongest with IgG antibodies. Importantly, patients with the clinical syndrome may lack antibodies to phospholipids when measured in these assays.

Functional assays for LACs involve tests directed at inhibition of in vitro clotting (e.g., activated partial thromboplastin time, dilute Russell's viper venom time), recognizing the discordance between in vivo thrombosis and in vitro anticoagulation. Functional assays to detect lupus anticoagulants involve a mixing step in which patient plasma is mixed with normal plasma to determine the presence of an inhibitor (i.e., an antibody) as opposed to a deficiency state. The mechanism by which antibodies to phospholipids and related proteins may cause thrombosis in vivo is unknown, although these antibodies may interact with the surface of cells (e.g., endothelium) to promote a prothrombotic state.

Complement

Assessment of the complement system provides valuable information on the presence of activity of diseases in which immune complex deposition may promote inflammation and tissue injury (Chapter 49). This system involves a large number of proteins that function in enzyme cascades to generate degradation products that amplify immunologic reactions and promote the destruction or removal of foreign organisms as well as damaged cells. In the setting of SLE and in certain forms of vasculitis and glomerulonephritis, immune complexes activate complement to promote local inflammation.

This activation can be measured in terms of the total complement level in the blood by functional assays of hemolytic activity; by measurement of individual complement components such as C3 and C4, whose levels are reduced by cleavage during activation; by measurement of split products of cleaved complement components; and by measurement of complement fragments bound to red blood cells during complement activation. Proteins of the complement system are acute phase reactants and can increase with inflammation, including active disease. Correspondingly, low levels may reflect inherited complement deficiency rather than consumption; genetic deficiency of C1q, for example, is highly associated with SLE.

Antineutrophil Cytoplasmic Antibodies

Antineutrophil cytoplasmic antibodies (ANCAs) are autoantibodies that react to determinants in the neutrophil and occur prominently in patients with certain forms of necrotizing vasculitis or rapidly progressive glomerulonephritis. Two main forms of ANCA have been distinguished on the basis of the target antigens and pattern of immunofluorescence staining of fixed neutrophils: PR3-ANCA (C-ANCA), which reacts with proteinase-3 (PR3), and MPO-ANCA (P-ANCA), which reacts with myeloperoxidase (MPO). By immunofluorescence, PR3-ANCA shows staining in the cytoplasm; staining by MPO-ANCA localizes in the perinuclear area. ANCAs to other proteins have also been identified, but these may also occur in conditions other than vasculitis.

In the evaluation of severe, multisystem inflammatory disease, ANCA testing is necessary to distinguish possible etiologies. PR3-ANCA occurs commonly in patients with Wegener's granulomatosis, whereas MPO-ANCA marks the course of vasculitis caused by microscopic polyangiitis, polyarteritis nodosa, and Churg-Strauss disease, among others (Chapter 278). In patients with ANCA-associated glomerulonephritis, the kidney lacks evidence of immune deposits, as indicated by the lack of staining for immunoglobulins or complement. Kidney disease of this kind is termed *pauci-immune glomerulonephritis*. Although ANCA testing is useful in initial diagnosis, its role for assessing disease activity is less certain. Occasionally, in patients who are desperately ill and cannot tolerate a lung or kidney biopsy, the presence of an ANCA can be used as preliminary evidence for diagnosis to allow the initiation of immunosuppressive therapy.

Cryoglobulins

Cryoglobulins are serum immunoglobulins that precipitate in the cold and promote the pathogenesis of systemic inflammatory disease through tissue deposition. The presence of a cryoglobulin is detected by allowing blood, collected warm, to remain cool at 2° to 4° C for 1 or more days. After centrifugation, the amount of cryoprecipitate is measured and expressed as a cryocrit. Subsequent analysis of the cryoprecipitate by immunochemical assays allows determination of its components. Cryoglobulins can be classified into three main types on the basis of their composition: (1) single, or type I; (2) mixed, type II; and (3) mixed, type III. A type I cryoglobulin consists of only a monoclonal immunoglobulin that precipitates in the cold. A mixed-type cryoglobulin contains RFs bound to polyclonal IgG to form an immune complex. In type II cryoglobulins, the IgM RF is monoclonal, and in type III, the IgM RF is polyclonal.

Type I cryoglobulins occur in patients with lymphoproliferative disorders such as Waldenström's macroglobulinemia, multiple myeloma, or chronic lymphocytic lymphoma (Chapters 190 and 193). In contrast, patients with mixed cryoglobulins can present with a wide range of signs and symptoms resulting from vasculitis. These manifestations include purpura (a sign of leukocytoclastic vasculitis), weakness, arthritis, and neuropathy; they represent a syndrome known as *essential mixed cryoglobulinemia*. Most patients with this condition have infection with hepatitis C virus, with viral components present in the complexes. These patients have serologic evidence of this infection as well as manifestations attributable to the underlying liver disease. As in the case of other CTDs and systemic inflammatory diseases, the evaluation of patients with essential mixed cryoglobulinemia demands attention to the entire patient and the impact of disease on multiple organs.

SUGGESTED READINGS

Eriksson C, Kokkonen H, Johansson M, et al. Autoantibodies predate the onset of systematic lupus erythematosus in northern Sweden. *Arthritis Res Ther.* 2011;13:R30. *Autoantibodies against nuclear antigens were detected several years before the onset of symptoms and diagnosis.*

Giannakopoulos B, Passam F, Ioannou Y, et al. How we diagnose the antiphospholipid syndrome. *Blood.* 2009;113:985-994. *As described in this review, the diagnosis of antiphospholipid antibody syndromes is* complicated and involves a variety of serologic and functional assays whose results have to be interpreted in the context of the clinical situation.

Janssens HJ, Fransen J, va de Lisdonk EH, et al. A diagnostic rule for acute gouty arthritis in primary care without joint fluid analysis. *Arch Intern Med.* 2010;170:1120-1126. *Key predictive factors are male sex, a previous patient-reported arthritis attack, onset within 1 day, joint redness, first metatarsophalangeal joint involvement, and serum uric acid level exceeding 5.88 mg/dL.*

Meroni PL, Schur PH. ANA screening: an old test with new recommendations. *Ann Rheum Dis.* 2010;69:1420-1422. *Review.*

Pascual E, Sivera F, Andrés M. Synovial fluid analysis for crystals. *Curr Opin Rheumatol.* 2011;23:161-169. *How to identity crystals.*

Van der Linden MPM, van der Woude D, Ioan-Facsinay A, et al. Value of anti-modified citrullinated vimentin and third-generation anti-cyclic citrullinated peptide compared with second-generation anti-cyclic citrullinated peptide and rheumatoid factor in predicting disease outcome in undifferentiated arthritis and rheumatoid arthritis. *Arthritis Rheum.* 2009;60:2232-2241. *Antibodies to citrullinated proteins (ACPA) have emerged as important markers for rheumatoid arthritis and its distinction from other forms of inflammatory arthritis.*

266

IMAGING STUDIES IN THE RHEUMATIC DISEASES

LYNNE S. STEINBACH

FIGURE 266-1. Rheumatoid arthritis is demonstrated on a posteroanterior radiograph of a hand. Findings include joint space narrowing at the radiocarpal and metacarpophalangeal joints, with subluxation of the metacarpophalangeal joints and interphalangeal joint of the thumb as well as erosions of the metacarpal heads and proximal interphalangeal joints.

Imaging of the rheumatic diseases is essential to diagnosis and assessment of progression of arthropathy. The mainstay for imaging has always been the radiograph. This continues to be the case because radiographs provide a relatively low-cost baseline evaluation of the bones, joints, and soft tissues. Frequently, the information provided is adequate for diagnosis and treatment. Other imaging modalities, such as magnetic resonance imaging (MRI), computed tomography (CT), ultrasound, and bone scintigraphy, can aid in characterization and follow-up of rheumatic disease. This chapter discusses the various imaging options for evaluation of rheumatic disease, providing the reader with their capabilities and appropriate use.

RADIOGRAPHY

The radiographic image represents a map of radiation attenuation through different tissues along the course of the x-ray beam. A white structure such as bone attenuates more radiation than a darker structure such as cartilage, muscle, or joint effusion. An analogue detector with a film cassette has been used to image the body for more than a century.

Digital radiography is being used increasingly for imaging. It employs a photostimulated phosphor imaging plate and an image reader-writer that processes the latent image information. When the plate absorbs x-rays, the energy is converted to light energy by fluorescence, with the intensity of light being proportional to the energy absorbed by the phosphor. The stimulated light is used to create a digital image. This type of image is then transferred to x-ray film or to a picture-archiving system (PACS) that is used for viewing by the clinician. Digital images have advantages over conventional radiography in that they can be manipulated by the technologist or by the clinician at the PACS station for contrast and brightness as well as window width and level. Magnification and quantification are also possible. The images can be easily stored and retrieved from a server.

The radiograph is the initial imaging technique used for evaluation of arthritis. Radiographs are affordable and available, and they render high spatial resolution images of the joint. Frequently, a radiograph is all that is needed to assess joint damage. Radiographs demonstrate joint changes with high resolution down to approximately 0.05 mm in size. No other imaging study is able to accomplish this degree of spatial resolution. The radiograph can provide detailed evaluation of osseous cortex. Features such as joint space narrowing, erosion, subluxation, calcification, new bone formation, subchondral cyst formation, subchondral sclerosis, and soft tissue swelling all can be evaluated on radiographs (Fig. 266-1).

Radiographs should be obtained with at least two views of the involved bone at 90-degree angles to each other in order to detect and characterize abnormalities such as erosion, effusion, soft tissue swelling, subluxation, dislocation, and fracture. Standard views usually comprise frontal and lateral views, but occasionally, oblique and special views are needed, particularly in assessing the elbow, wrist, fingers, ankle, foot, toes, pelvis, and sacroiliac joints. Weight-bearing views of joints may be of value for assessing joint space narrowing. This is particularly true in the knee. Although there is no universal consensus on routine views for the different joints, recommended screening views are listed in Table 266-1.

Because they have poor contrast resolution, radiographs do not reveal all aspects of arthropathy. Unlike MRI, radiography lacks the ability to show early cartilage loss and erosion, especially in the larger joints. Soft tissue pathology and muscle abnormalities cannot be assessed on radiographs as they can with MRI. Radiographs are also not as sensitive for evaluating activity of the disease. Other imaging techniques that will be discussed later in the chapter have these advantages and are considered complementary to radiographs in the assessment of joint and soft tissue disease.

Fluoroscopy, which employs x-ray in real time, is a quick and precise method for needle placement during aspirations and injections, particularly for joints that are deep or complex and difficult to enter with the blind technique, such as the hip, shoulder, and sacroiliac joints. It can also be used to evaluate joint motion and stress. Videotaping of joint motion is useful for recording the kinematics of the joint. Because of the high dose of radiation, one must keep fluoroscopic time to a minimum. CT and ultrasound are other imaging methods that are helpful for joint aspiration and injection and are discussed subsequently in this chapter.

MAGNETIC RESONANCE IMAGING

The demands of imaging are increased in this age of therapeutic approaches designed to halt the progression of arthritis. During the past two decades, MRI has become the imaging modality of choice for evaluation of joint soft tissue, marrow structures, and muscle pathology. This is because MRI has high contrast resolution that enables the differentiation of various soft tissues from each other. Abnormal joint structures usually display different signal intensities than their normal counterparts. Morphologic changes resulting from destruction of tissue by joint and muscle inflammation are also identified.

MRI applies a strong magnetic field with radiofrequency pulses that pass through the different body tissues to produce varying signal intensities. Each soft tissue structure contains unique properties that provide a characteristic signal intensity based on the proton density, T1 relaxation time, and spin density of the tissue. Various pulse sequences can be used to evaluate the joint.

Multiple factors can influence spatial resolution and thus the quality of the MRI. These include field strength and coil selection. Most imaging is done

TABLE 266-1	ROUTINE RADIOGRAPHIC SCREENING VIEWS OF THE SKELETON
UPPER EXTREMITY	
Fingers	PA, lateral (separate fingers)
Hand	PA, oblique, lateral
Wrist	PA, lateral (both with neutral positioning); "ball catcher" oblique useful for inflammatory arthritis
Forearm	AP, lateral
Elbow	AP (supinated), lateral (90-degree flexed), obliques as needed
Humerus	AP, lateral
Glenohumeral joint	AP internal and external rotation (axillary, Grashey, or transthoracic view)
Acromioclavicular joint	AP, 15-degree cephalad AP (bilateral weight-holding if dislocation)
Sternum	AP, oblique AP (also Hobbs view or lordotic view)
LOWER EXTREMITY	
Hip	AP internal rotation, frog-leg lateral (or cross-table)
Femur	AP, lateral
Knee, arthritis	PA flexed and AP weight-bearing views, lateral
Knee, patellofemoral joint	Merchant view (45-degree flexion)
Tibia/fibula	AP, lateral
Ankle	AP, lateral, mortise
Foot	AP, lateral, medial oblique (simulated weight-bearing lateral for foot alignment abnormality)
Subtalar joint	Lateral, Harris-Beath view
Calcaneus	Lateral, AP craniocaudal angulated view
Toes	AP, lateral, AP oblique
AXIAL SKELETON	
Cervical spine	AP, lateral, open mouth (odontoid), swimmer's view for lower C spine, obliques or pillar views for facet joints
Thoracic spine	AP, lateral, swimmer's view for upper T spine
Lumbar spine	AP, lateral; obliques for pars interarticularis, flexion-extension laterals for subluxation
Sacrum	30-degree cephalad angulated AP, lateral
Coccyx	10-degree caudal angulated AP, lateral
Sacroiliac joints	30-degree cephalad angulated AP
Pelvis	AP, Judet views and/or inlet-outlet views for pelvic ring fractures

Modified from Lee JHE. Imaging modalities. In: Johnson T, Steinbach L, eds. *Essentials of Musculoskeletal Imaging*. Rosemont, IL: American Academy of Orthopaedic Surgeons; 2004:6.

on high-field superconducting magnets. Permanent or resistive magnets are also in use at lower field strengths. Field strength is measured in Tesla (T). In general, the higher the field strength, the better the signal from the tissue and the shorter the imaging time.

There are five types of magnets used for clinical imaging of joints: (1) ultra-high-field (3.0 T); high-field (1.0-2.0 T); midfield (0.3-1.0 T); low-field (< 0.1 to 0.2 T); and ultra-low-field (<0.1 T). Most clinical MRI scanners operate between 0.3 and 3 T. Open MRI scanners are less confining for claustrophobic patients but are not usually available at the high-field range above 1.0 T that provides increased resolution. Ultra-high-field 3 T scanners offer the highest spatial resolution and are being increasingly used for imaging small joints and cartilage.

Coils are also important for proper joint imaging in MRI. These are electrical devices that can generate or detect a magnetic field. They are placed over the body region of interest, keeping the field of view as low as possible, and improve spatial resolution. Many types of coils are available for different joint sizes and configurations, including shoulder, extremity, wrist, and flex coils. Phased array coils use several coils in one component, allowing for a larger field of view. These are often used in spine imaging.

The widely used contrast for MRI studies is a neutral, hydrophilic salt of the gadolinium chelate, gadolinium diethylenetriamine-penta-acetic acid (Gd-DTPA). Gadolinium can be injected intravenously or directly into the joint. Intravenous injection (indirect magnetic resonance arthrography) carries the contrast in the vascular system to areas of hyperemia and inflammation. It is recommended for assessment of synovial activity in inflammatory joint diseases. Gadolinium is taken up in inflamed synovium and is able to demonstrate thickened pannus. The slope of the time-signal intensity curve is useful for showing inflammatory activity, and gadolinium is commonly employed in research and clinical trials.

Patients with renal disease who receive intravenous injection of gadolinium can develop nephrogenic systemic fibrosis (NSF). When the kidney cannot sufficiently clear out the gadolinium, it produces fibrosis of many tissues, including the skin, muscle, heart, nerves, and pleura. To date, NSF has been seen only in patients who have been given intravenous gadolinium with acute or chronic renal insufficiency and a glomerular filtration rate (GFR) of less than 30 mL/minute/1.73 m^2, with acute renal insufficiency of any severity due to the hepatorenal syndrome, or in the perioperative liver transplantation period. The changes in the skin with NSF are usually bilateral and symmetrical, primarily involving the extremities and the trunk. These changes can mimic systemic sclerosis but, unlike that disease, the face is usually spared. If renal function improves, the skin lesions may stabilize or get better, although in some patients, the process progresses, affecting mobility and causing severe pain.

Injection of dilute gadolinium into the joint (direct magnetic resonance arthrography) is helpful for outlining structures to determine whether there is morphologic damage. This technique is particularly effective for visualization of small structures such as the labrum of the hip or shoulder if there is no joint effusion. It is also helpful for demonstrating breakdown of soft tissue structures that normally prevent communication between joint compartments such as the rotator cuff, triangular fibrocartilage of the wrist, and ligaments in the various joints.

With special regard to rheumatic disease, MRI demonstrates joint effusion, intra-articular masses, synovitis, damage to hyaline and fibrocartilage, tendons, ligaments, bone, muscle, and surrounding soft tissue (Fig. 266-2). MRI is sensitive for marrow abnormalities such as reactive edema and erosion from arthritis, although it can be nonspecific. Infectious processes can have a similar appearance. Hemosiderin demonstrates a low signal intensity on MRI, which allows for characterization of joint diseases such as pigmented villonodular synovitis and hemophilic arthritis. MRI is useful for early detection of osteonecrosis, particularly when radiographs are normal. It is also used to evaluate the spine for disc disease, nerve root compression, and inflammatory changes.

Disadvantages of MRI include the fact that it is more costly than CT and other imaging modalities and can be claustrophobic. Calcification is not easily identified by MRI, and radiographs and CT are often complementary in this regard. MRI is contraindicated in patients who have certain devices implanted into their tissues. These include cochlear implants, some heart valves, cardiac pacemakers, and spinal implants. Metal implants, such as joint prostheses and spinal hardware, do not represent contraindications for MRI. Although metallic devices can cause some distortion of the image, newer materials such as cobalt-chrome cause less artifact. Various imaging parameters can also be adjusted to improve the visibility of tissues surrounding metallic devices, allowing for diagnostic interpretation.

⬤ ULTRASOUND

Ultrasound pulses sound waves through tissues to obtain an image that can localize and characterize pathology. Through the years, resolution has increased markedly. Portable scanners are also being used, especially by nonradiologists. They are adequate for injections and detection of fluid collections and tenosynovitis, but do not provide the detailed anatomy of their high-end counterparts.

Ultrasound provides a less expensive, noninvasive method to visualize joint structures such as tendons, ligaments, and fibrocartilage as well as muscles and soft tissue masses without ionizing radiation. Areas of pain and swelling can be scanned in real time with the opposite side for comparison. Fluid within tendon sheaths can be easily assessed. Fluid, blood, pus, and mucin in ganglia, cysts, bursae (e.g., a popliteal [Baker's] cyst [Chapter 271]), hematomas, seromas, and abscesses can be differentiated from solid masses based on echogenicity (Fig. 266-3). Areas around metallic hardware or other implants are easily assessed for such masses without the artifact that might limit MRI or CT evaluation.

Hypervascularity is a component of inflammatory joint disease. Angiofibroblastic response in tendons can be assessed by Doppler imaging, a

FIGURE 266-2. Sausage digit in psoriatic arthritis demonstrated on radiographs, scintigraphy, and magnetic resonance imaging. **A,** Anteroposterior radiograph of the forefoot demonstrates soft tissue swelling of the second toe without obvious bone involvement *(arrow).* **B,** There is increased tracer uptake of technetium-99m methylene diphosphonate *(arrow)* in the entire second toe from the metacarpophalangeal joint to the distal phalanx on the bone scan, suggesting osteitis and soft tissue inflammation. **C,** A coronal fat-suppressed T1-weighted magnetic resonance image of the second toe obtained after intravenous gadolinium administration reveals high signal intensity uptake *(arrow)* in the bone and surrounding soft tissues consistent with osteitis and soft tissue inflammation.

sonographic method that assesses vascular flow. This information can be used for diagnosis and assessment of therapeutic response as well as to identify locations for anesthetic or steroid injections.

Ultrasound can demonstrate dynamic properties of tendons and other structures. The real-time capability allows for identification of subluxation and impingement, pinpointing causes of pain with certain movements. Ultrasound is a quick and inexpensive method to perform accurate aspirations and injections of joints and soft tissue structures such as tendon sheaths and bursae. Areas of hydroxyapatite crystal deposition disease can be aspirated and injected.

Ultrasound is an operator-dependent technique with a steep learning curve. It can be time-consuming for the person scanning the patient. Some important joint structures are in sonographically inaccessible areas, such as those obscured by bone. This would include portions of the menisci and the cruciate ligaments of the knee, labra of the hip and shoulder, and some hyaline cartilage that are well seen with MRI.

COMPUTED TOMOGRAPHY

CT employs an x-ray source with multiple detectors housed in a circular gantry that rotates 360 degrees around the patient lying on a table surrounded by the gantry. The computer processes the data that are displayed tomographically in multiple planes with thin slices. There is also a capability to render a three-dimensional reconstruction of the body part. Newer CT scanners have increased numbers of detectors and are able to image more quickly and with thinner slices. They employ spiral or helical scanning through continuous rotation of the x-ray source and the detectors while the patient moves on the table through the gantry.

CT is useful for evaluating vertebral alignment and fractures as well as abnormalities of the flat bones and pelvis. Complex fractures are best evaluated with CT. Joints that are difficult to assess on radiographs, including the sacroiliac, temporomandibular, wrist, and sternoclavicular joints, are well seen with CT. However, internal derangement of these joints is better appreciated on MRI, which has superior soft tissue contrast.

There are many different iodinated contrast agents that can be injected intravenously to enhance the CT study. The contrast has higher attenuation and spreads hematogenously to areas of increased vascularity and inflammation. MRI with gadolinium is the preferred method for demonstrating pannus and joint inflammation and for characterizing a soft tissue mass. CT with contrast can be used to determine whether the mass is cystic or solid in patients in whom MRI is contraindicated (e.g., those with claustrophobia, aneurysm clips, or cardiac pacemakers). Ultrasound can also be used for this purpose. Fluid collections, such as abscesses, seromas, bursae, and ganglia, are identified on all three imaging modalities.

CT arthrography may also be performed. This is useful when MRI is contraindicated. Intra-articular injection of iodinated contrast or room air, or both, coats the joint structures and can be useful to see small and large cartilage defects, fibrocartilage, tendon and ligament tears, and ossified and cartilaginous bodies.

The radiation dose from CT is high, especially when using the newer scanners. Repeated imaging with CT or requesting a CT in children or pregnant women must be carefully considered as far as risk versus benefit. Algorithms to reduce tissue dose are used for children and other vulnerable patients. These images are lower resolution but usually provide adequate information for diagnosis.

ARTHROGRAPHY

Arthrography involves placement of a needle intra-articularly with aspiration of joint fluid and injection of a contrast agent to enhance imaging. It is often performed to exclude an infection in patients with hip pain or in patients with total joint prostheses. It is also occasionally used to determine whether there is a full-thickness tear of the rotator cuff, triangular fibrocartilage and ligaments of the wrist, or collateral ligaments of the elbow and ankle. However,

FIGURE 266-3. Knee ganglion demonstrated on magnetic resonance imaging and ultrasound. **A,** A fat-suppressed T2-weighted axial magnetic resonance image of the knee demonstrates a high signal intensity mass in the posterior aspect of the knee. Without intravenous gadolinium to show enhancement pattern, it is difficult to determine whether this is cystic or solid. **B,** An ultrasound demonstrates that this mass is hypoechoic—a finding consistent with a ganglion. This hypoechogenic appearance is also seen with bursae, such as a popliteal cyst, but a popliteal cyst lies between the gastrocnemius and semimembranosus tendons, unlike this ganglion.

MRI has replaced conventional arthrography for these indications in most centers.

Arthrography can be combined with MRI or CT to evaluate more precisely the internal structures through joint distention and contrast coating of structures along the articular surface, including the labrum, ligaments, and capsule. This is discussed in the sections of those imaging modalities.

● SCINTIGRAPHY

Scintigraphy employs detectors in the form of a gamma camera that can identify the decay of radioactive isotopes that have been injected intravenously. Bone scintigraphy is used to identify sites of activity in the rheumatic diseases. The bone scan employs technetium-99m methylene diphosphate as the radioactive tracer. The isotope goes to areas of high bone turnover and vascular flow as well as areas of calcium or bone deposition. Three-phase bone scans are obtained at different intervals following injection. Images are obtained at three time points: the early vascular phase, the intermediate blood pool phase, and the late phase. Each phase allows for further characterization of the disease process. Abnormal tracer uptake is seen in areas of inflammation, infection, neoplasm, osteonecrosis, and fracture (see Fig.

266-2). The scan is most useful to identify the location of lesions within the skeleton but is nonspecific. Further imaging of the abnormal areas is often necessary to characterize the pathology.

SUGGESTED READINGS

Douis H, Gillett M, James SL. Imaging in the diagnosis, prognostication, and management of lower limb muscle injury. *Semin Musculoskelet Radiol.* 2011;15:27-41. *Review of biomechanical and imaging features of common acute muscle injuries.*

Douis H, James SL, Davies AM. Musculoskeletal imaging: current and future trends. *Eur Radiol.* 2011;21:478-484. *Review.*

French SD, Green S, Buchbinder R, et al. Interventions for improving the appropriate use of imaging in people with musculoskeletal conditions. *Cochrane Database Syst Rev.* 2010;1:CD006094. *Most interventions improved the use of radiographic procedures.*

Hayashi D, Guermazi A, Crema MD, et al. Imaging in osteoarthritis: what have we learned and where are we going? *Minerva Med.* 2011;102:15-32. *Review focusing on conventional radiography and MRI but also including ultrasound, scintigraphy, and computed tomography.*

Jain M, Samuels J. Musculoskeletal ultrasound in the diagnosis of rheumatic disease. *Bull NYU Hosp Jt Dis.* 2010;68:183-190. *Overview of this increasingly useful procedure.*

Turecki MB, Taljanovic MS, Stubbs AY, et al. Imaging of musculoskeletal soft tissue infections. *Skeletal Radiol.* 2010;39:957-971. *Review including septic bursitis, tenosynovitis, fasciitis, and abscesses.*

267

CONNECTIVE TISSUE STRUCTURE AND FUNCTION

RICHARD F. LOESER

Connective tissue provides the architectural framework of the musculoskeletal system and serves as a reservoir for the storage of growth factors, cytokines, and undifferentiated mesenchymal precursor cells that regulate repair and remodeling in response to injury and disease. Articular joints are formed by several common types of connective tissue, including muscle, bone, tendon, ligament, cartilage, meniscus, and synovium, which function as a unit during joint movement. These tissues demonstrate distinct characteristics when imaged by magnetic resonance because of their unique cellular and matrix composition (Fig. 267-1). In this type of image, tissues with greater water content, such as adipose tissue and cartilage, appear lighter than very dense tissues, such as the subchondral bone, which appear dark.

Despite their diversity, connective tissues have in common cells, usually of mesodermal origin, that have an abundant extracellular matrix. The cells within a particular type of connective tissue control the composition of the extracellular matrix, which, in turn, determines the physical properties of the tissue. The many types of connective tissue cells range from fibroblasts, which are present in the connective tissue found in skin, synovium, tendons,

FIGURE 267-1. Magnetic resonance image of a knee joint demonstrating the diversity of connective tissue structures. The image was obtained with a 1.5-Tesla magnet using a fast spin-echo T2-weighted imaging protocol. Tissues with a higher water content, such as adipose and articular cartilage, appear lighter, as does the synovial fluid. The subchondral bone is dark because of a high mineral and low water content and can be seen just below the very thin layer of articular cartilage. (Courtesy of Dr. Carol Muehleman, Rush Medical College, Chicago.)

TABLE 267-1 DIVERSITY OF CONNECTIVE TISSUE–CONTAINING STRUCTURES

STRUCTURE	FUNCTION	CELLS	KEY MATRIX COMPONENTS
Adipose tissue	Energy storage, organ protection	Adipocytes, fibroblasts	Fine reticular fibers
Basement membrane	Support and filtration barrier	Epithelial and endothelial cells	Type IV collagen, laminin
Bone	Skeletal support, blood cell production, mineral storage	Osteoblasts, osteoclasts, osteocytes	Type I collagen, osteocalcin, bone sialoprotein, hydroxyapatite
Cartilage	Allows joint motion, transmits loads	Chondrocytes	Type II collagen, aggrecan
Dermis	Support and resiliency	Fibroblasts	Type I collagen, elastin
Ligament	Connects bone to bone	Fibroblasts	Type I collagen, small proteoglycans
Tendon	Connects muscle to bone	Fibroblasts	Type I collagen, small proteoglycans
Stroma	Support of organs	Fibroblasts, organ-specific cells	Type I, VI collagen, fibronectin
Synovium	Joint lining, produces synovial fluid	Fibroblasts, macrophages	Type I, III collagen
Vessel wall	Structural support of blood vessels	Vascular smooth muscle cells	Type III collagen, elastin

ligaments, and fascia, to more specialized cells such as chondrocytes and osteoblasts, which are found in cartilage and bone, respectively (Table 267-1). Basement membranes are a more special form of connective tissue produced by epithelial and endothelial cells, rather than by mesenchymal cells. The connective tissue matrix consists of an intricate mixture of proteins and other macromolecules, which are responsible for the unique function of each particular type of connective tissue. Connective tissues that must withstand high tensile loads, such as tendons, have a high content of collagen fibers, whereas tissues that must resist compression, such as cartilage, have a high content of proteoglycans.

Because of the wide distribution of connective tissues within the human body, diseases that affect connective tissue cells or extracellular matrix proteins often have systemic effects. These connective tissue disorders can be divided into three general types: those that arise from a mutation within a gene encoding a connective tissue protein (e.g., Marfan syndrome); those that are the result of an inflammatory, sometimes autoimmune, process centered in connective tissues (e.g., rheumatoid arthritis); and those that are the result of a degenerative type of process often associated with aging (e.g., osteoarthritis). A basic understanding of the composition of the various connective tissues and of the way in which this composition relates to structure and function is important for understanding the clinical presentation, as well as management, of the spectrum of musculoskeletal and connective tissue disorders.

CONNECTIVE TISSUE PROTEINS AND MACROMOLECULES

Connective tissues are composed of various types of collagens, proteoglycans, elastins, and matrix glycoproteins. Collagen is the most abundant protein in the body; it accounts for about 25 to 30% of the total protein mass. Collagens are triple-helical proteins formed when three polypeptide chains, called α *chains*, wind around each other to form a collagen molecule. More than 30 collagen genes code for the collagen α chains, which combine to form more than 20 different collagen types. The types of collagen can be grouped by structure and function and include fibrillar collagens (collagen types I, II, III, V, and XI), fibril-associated collagens (types IX, XII, XIV), basement membrane collagen (type IV), and network-forming collagens (types VI, VIII, and X). Others include anchoring fibrils (VII) and multiplexin collagens (types XV and XVIII). Tissues such as bone, tendon, and cartilage, which must withstand high biomechanical loads, are packed with large amounts of long fibrillar collagens, primarily type I collagen in bone and tendons and type II collagen in cartilage. The loose connective tissues, such as basement membranes and organ stroma, experience much less mechanical force but require a matrix that allows more rapid diffusion of molecules and so contain a higher content of aggregating or anchoring types of collagen and less fibrillar collagen. Recent work correlating mutations in particular collagen genes with disease phenotypes in humans and studies of phenotype after gene disruption in transgenic mice have added to our knowledge of collagen function. Some examples include "brittle-bone disease" or osteogenesis imperfecta resulting from type I collagen mutations, severe premature osteoarthritis from type II collagen mutations, and fragile blood vessel and visceral walls in Ehlers-Danlos syndrome type IV from mutations in type III collagen. Excess collagen production can also disrupt tissue function, usually by causing tissue fibrosis, as seen in scleroderma. Finally, fragile connective tissues can result from inadequate collagen production and cross-linking, as occurs in scurvy from vitamin C deficiency. Vitamin C (ascorbic acid) serves as a cofactor for the hydroxylation reaction necessary to modify specific prolyl and lysyl residues in procollagen, and a deficiency in ascorbic acid reduces collagen secretion, stability, and cross-linking.

Proteoglycans consist of a protein core to which short oligosaccharides and longer chains of glycosaminoglycans are covalently attached. The composition and length of the glycosaminoglycan chains, as well as the sequence and length of the protein core, determine the size and function of each specific proteoglycan type. Chondroitin sulfate, keratan sulfate, heparan sulfate, and dermatan sulfate are four different forms of glycosaminoglycans that consist of repeating disaccharide units. The sulfates present on the glycosaminoglycans create a highly negatively charged environment that is hydrophilic. Aggrecan is an example of a very large (>200,000 kD) proteoglycan found in cartilage that contains a protein core of more than 2000 amino acids to which are attached approximately 100 long chondroitin sulfate chains, approximately 30 shorter keratan sulfate chains, and approximately 50 short oligosaccharides. The structure of aggrecan is responsible for the high water content in cartilage, which makes up 75 to 80% of the tissue. Decorin, biglycan, fibromodulin, asporin, and lumican are examples of small proteoglycans that have much shorter protein cores (30 to 60 kD) and fewer glycosaminoglycan side chains, and they contain leucine-rich repeats. These small proteoglycans form β-sheets and interact with collagen to regulate the formation of collagen fibrils and help to stabilize the collagen network. In addition to binding water and interacting with collagens, proteoglycans bind cationic proteins, which in some cases include growth factors, resulting in a mechanism by which tissues can store growth factors in the matrix. Recent studies have shown that polymorphisms in asporin that increase its binding of transforming growth factor-β can contribute to the development of osteoarthritis.

In addition to collagens and proteoglycans, other important groups of matrix proteins include the noncollagenous fibrillar proteins and glycoproteins. Fibrillar proteins include elastin and microfibrils, such as fibrillin. Elastic fibers must withstand repeated stretching and deformation and must be capable of returning to a relaxed state. Tropoelastin is the precursor to elastin and is synthesized by several cell types, including vascular smooth muscle cells and dermal fibroblasts, where it contributes to the elasticity of the blood vessel wall and skin, respectively. Fibrillin is found in several elastic tissues and is particularly abundant in the aorta, the suspensory ligament of the lens, and the periosteum. Fibrillin was a little-known protein until investigators discovered that fibrillin mutations are the cause of most cases of Marfan syndrome. Glycoproteins include fibronectin, vitronectin, osteopontin, laminin, and thrombospondin. Fibronectin is found in most connective tissues throughout the body. Laminin is particularly prominent in basement membranes, and osteopontin is found in greater amounts in cartilage and bone. All these proteins bind to cells through specific cell surface receptors to promote attachment of cells to the matrix. The proteins also interact with other matrix proteins, such as collagen and proteoglycans, to integrate the cells further with the extracellular matrix. Through the interactions with cell receptors and other matrix proteins, the noncollagenous glycoproteins function in regulating tissue morphogenesis as well as in tissue repair and remodeling. They also appear to play a role in other diverse processes, including tumor growth and metastasis.

Extracellular Matrix Protein Receptors

Connective tissue cells use specific receptors to bind to extracellular matrix (ECM) proteins, and these cell-matrix interactions are an important mechanism for the regulation of connective tissue growth and remodeling. The major types of ECM receptors include integrins, CD44, discoidin domain receptors (DDRs), and proteoglycan family receptors such as the syndecans. CD44 is expressed by several different connective tissue cell types as well as by nonconnective tissue cells such as lymphocytes. On connective tissue cells, CD44 is the principal receptor for hyaluronan. CD44 binding of hyaluronan is particularly important in forming a gel-like pericellular coat found around certain connective tissue cells such as chondrocytes. DDR1 and DDR2 are receptor tyrosine kinases found on epithelial and mesenchymal cells. DDR1 can bind types I through VI and type VIII collagen, whereas DDR2 is activated only by fibrillar collagens. Syndecans contain a transmembrane protein core to which heparan sulfate proteoglycans are attached to the extracellular domain. The proteoglycans bind growth factors such as fibroblast growth factor. Syndecans also appear to interact with integrins and may modulate integrin function.

The integrins represent the largest family of cell surface matrix receptors and have been found to be the primary receptors for many matrix proteins, including collagens, fibronectin, laminin, vitronectin, osteopontin, and thrombospondin. The specificity of ECM protein binding is determined by specific integrin α- and β-subunits. Each connective tissue cell expresses a combination of integrins that is regulated, at least in part, by the mix of proteins present in the ECM. Binding of ECM proteins to integrins activates signal transduction pathways that regulate cell responses to the matrix, including changes in gene expression. Research in bone has found that the αvβ3 integrin present on osteoclasts plays an important role in the ability of these cells to resorb bone. For this reason, chemical inhibitors of αvβ3 are being developed for the treatment of osteoporosis.

⬤ SPECIALIZED CONNECTIVE TISSUE STRUCTURES

Articular Cartilage, Tendons, and Ligaments

Normal pain-free joint movement is dependent on the function of articular cartilage, tendons, and ligaments. Articular cartilage, present on bones at the ends of diarthrodial joints (see Fig. 267-1), is a form of hyaline cartilage that is responsible for the normal smooth gliding motion of the joints. The surface of cartilage has an extremely low coefficient of friction (less than that of ice on ice), owing to a protein called *lubricin* (also known as *superficial zone protein* or PRG4), produced by chondrocytes and synovial cells. The articular cartilage matrix contains large amounts of type II collagen, which is responsible for the tensile strength of the tissue, and aggrecan, which provides the cartilage with resiliency. In the superficial region of cartilage, the collagen fibers are arranged parallel to the surface of the tissue to withstand the shear forces occurring at the joint surface during movement, whereas in the deep zone of cartilage, collagen fibrils are oriented perpendicular to the surface in order to withstand compressive forces better. Degradation and loss of articular cartilage in people with arthritis severely impairs joint function and causes pain. However, because articular cartilage lacks nerve innervations, pain in arthritis occurs from damage or inflammation in other joint tissues, such as bone, synovium, and the joint capsule.

Tendons connect muscle to bone, and ligaments connect bone to bone. Both are composed of connective tissue that must withstand the high tensile loads occurring during movement. Tendons transmit the force from muscle contraction to bone, and the result is movement. Ligaments serve to stabilize joints, thereby allowing for a certain degree and direction of movement but resisting excessive displacement between bones. Tendon and ligament fibroblasts are responsible for synthesis and maintenance of the matrix. Tendons and ligaments contain a very high content of type I collagen, which is found in long and densely packed parallel fibers. The noncollagenous proteins include proteoglycans such as decorin and biglycan; these are much smaller than the aggrecan found in cartilage, a feature giving them a comparatively reduced water content.

Synovium

The synovium lines diarthrodial joints and is composed of loose connective tissue. In most places within normal joints, the surface area of synovium is only a few cell layers thick. Unlike cartilage, synovium contains blood vessels, lymphatics, and nerves. It is the major source of nutrients for the cartilage and produces many of the major constituents found in the synovial fluid,

including hyaluronic acid. The two types of cells in the synovial matrix are fibroblasts (sometimes called *type B synovial cells*) and macrophages (type A cells). The synovial fibroblasts are responsible for matrix protein production. The macrophages are responsible for removing cell debris and any microorganisms that could gain entrance. The synovium is a major site of inflammation in arthritic diseases, where it becomes thickened by proliferation of resident cells and by an influx of inflammatory cells from the circulation. In inflammatory arthritis, activated synovial fibroblasts produce enzymes, including the matrix metalloproteinases (MMPs), which degrade joint structures, whereas inflammatory cells produce cytokines, such as tumor necrosis factor-α and interleukin-1 among others, which stimulate MMP production and drive the inflammatory process.

Intervertebral Discs

The intervertebral discs, which assist in movement and provide flexibility to the spine, have distinct regions consisting of the inner nucleus pulposus and an outer fibrotic rim, the annulus, along with an intermediate area between the two. Blood vessels are present in the outer region of the annulus but not in the nucleus pulposus, which must obtain its nutrients by diffusion. The annulus contains denser connective tissue to provide structural support, whereas the nucleus pulposus has a higher water content and is more gel-like. Discs contain both types I and II collagen along with proteoglycans, including aggrecan, found predominantly in the nucleus pulposus. The cells in this region more closely resemble chondrocytes, whereas those in the outer fibrotic regions are more similar to fibroblasts. By adulthood, very few cells are present in the nucleus pulposus. This scarcity, along with the changes associated with aging discussed in the next section, make discs very susceptible to degeneration, with an inability to repair damaged matrix.

⬤ CONNECTIVE TISSUE DEGRADATION

Connective tissues need to repair and remodel in response to injury, growth, and changes in the biomechanical demands at specific tissue sites. Repair and remodeling of connective tissues require that components of the tissue be removed by matrix-degrading enzymes and replaced with new components. When the balance of degradation and synthesis is disrupted, connective tissue destruction occurs, such as in osteoarthritis and rheumatoid arthritis. The largest family of matrix-degrading enzymes, the MMP family, consists of enzymes that share functional domains, require zinc for activity, and are active at neutral pH. The MMPs either are released into the extracellular matrix or, in some cases, such as the membrane-type MMPs, are directly anchored to the cell where they serve to activate other MMPs, and sometimes growth factors at the cell surface. MMP-1, MMP-8, and MMP-13 are collagenases, which are the primary enzymes capable of degrading native collagen, whereas MMP-2 and MMP-9 are gelatinases, which degrade denatured collagen. MMP-3, MMP-10, and MMP-11 are stromelysins responsible for degrading noncollagen proteins such as proteoglycans and fibronectin, whereas MMP-12 functions as an elastase. More recently discovered members of the MMP family include the ADAMs (a *d*isintegrin *a*nd a *m*etalloproteinase) and the ADAMTSs (a *d*isintegrin *a*nd a *m*etalloproteinase with a *t*hrombospondin motif). Enzymes of the ADAMS family are localized to the cell surface, at least in part through the disintegrin domain. ADAM-17 is also known as TACE (tumor necrosis factor-α–converting enzyme) because of its ability to cleave tumor necrosis factor-α to an active form. Finally, the ADAMTSs use the thrombospondin motif to interact with proteoglycans, which can serve as substrates for these enzymes. ADAMTS-4 and ADAMTS-5 are aggrecanases that have been shown to cleave the large proteoglycan aggrecan. Studies have suggested that ADAMTS-5 may play an important role in matrix degradation in osteoarthritis.

Other matrix-degrading enzymes are the serine proteases, which include plasmin and elastase, the aspartic proteases, which include pepsin and cathepsin D, and the cysteine proteases, including papain and cathepsins B, C, K, L, and S. Plasmin, the cleavage product of plasminogen, can cleave MMP propeptides and can result in MMP activation. Elastase, often a product of neutrophils, can degrade elastin and some fibrillar collagens. Cathepsin K has been recognized as a key mediator of bone resorption, where it functions to cleave collagen under the acidic conditions found at the osteoclast ruffled border. As with the MMPs, production and secretion of these proteases are controlled by signals from growth factors, cytokines, and matrix components. Thus, an intricate balance within connective tissues controls the integrity of the tissue and the response to injury. This balance is disturbed in disease states that result in connective tissue destruction.

Visit expertconsult.com for e-expanded chapter

SUGGESTED READINGS

Agarwal SK, Wu M, Livingston CK, et al. Toll-like receptor 3 upregulation by type I interferon in healthy and scleroderma dermal fibroblasts. *Arthritis Res Ther.* 2011;13:R3. *Type I interferons increase the inflammatory potential of dermal fibroblasts through the upregulation of TLR3.*

Anderson MB, Pingel J, Kjaer M, et al. Interleukin-6: a growth factor stimulating collagen synthesis in human tendon. *J Appl Physiol.* 2011. [Epub ahead of print.] *Local concentration of IL-6 in peritendinous tissue is a growth factor of the connective tissue in healthy human tendons.*

Legate KR, Wickstrom SA, Fassler R. Genetic and cell biological analysis of integrin outside-in signaling. *Genes Dev.* 2009;23:397-418. *Review of the integrin family of matrix receptors including how integrins regulate cell signaling.*

Orgel JP, San Antonio JD, Antipova O. Molecular and structural mapping of collagen fibril interactions. *Connect Tissue Res.* 2011;52:2-17. *Review of collagen's molecular packing, fibrillar structure, domain organization, and extracellular matrix.*

Shoulders MD, Raines RT. Collagen structure and stability. *Annu Rev Biochem.* 2009;78:929-958. *Extensive review of collagen structure and function and how mutations in collagen genes can lead to disease.*

Symoens S, Renard M, Bonod-Bidaud C, et al. Identification of binding partners interacting with the α1-N-propeptide of type V collagen. *Biochem J.* 2010;433:371-381. *Describes how these interactions are involved in extracellular matrix homeostasis.*

268

INHERITED DISEASES OF CONNECTIVE TISSUE

REED E. PYERITZ

MUCOPOLYSACCHARIDOSES

DEFINITION

Proteoglycans are ubiquitous components of the extracellular matrix (ECM) and the surfaces of cells, and they are among the largest and most complex of human molecules. Proteoglycans consist of a protein core to which are covalently bound glycosaminoglycans (GAGs; formerly called *mucopolysaccharides*) of several types: dermatan sulfate, heparan sulfate, keratan sulfate, and chondroitin sulfate. These four polymeric molecules are cleaved from their protein core in lysosomes; then they, plus hyaluronan (a GAG lacking a protein core), are catabolized further in lysosomes in a stepwise fashion by more than a dozen enzymes. Genetic defects in any one of these enzymes lead to the accumulation of GAG metabolites in lysosomes, with profound disruption of cellular physiology. The phenotypes resulting from deficiencies of these catabolic enzymes are termed *mucopolysaccharidoses* (MPSs) and are classified into seven types (Table 268-1). Several additional storage disorders, termed *mucolipidoses* (MLs), are caused by a genetic defect in post-translational modification of lysosomal enzymes and share features with the MPS.

EPIDEMIOLOGY

All MPS disorders are rare, each with an incidence of 1 or fewer cases per 100,000 births, and are without ethnic predilection.

PATHOBIOLOGY

With the exception of MPS II (Hunter's syndrome), which is X-linked, each of these disorders is autosomal recessive. All MPSs are caused by deficiency of a single lysosomal enzyme responsible for a specific step in GAG metabolism. Catabolism of GAG proceeds normally until the step requiring the defective enzyme, when further normal metabolism halts. Although a minor degree of nonspecific breakdown occurs, resulting in urinary excretion of cleaved GAG that can be useful diagnostically, the accumulation of GAG within lysosomes of cells of mesenchymal origin, endothelium, and, in most cases, neurons causes widespread, progressive cellular dysfunction and clinical effects. Lysosomal enzymes are targeted to lysosomes by post-translational addition of mannose 6-phosphate. Deficiency of the phosphotransferase that catalyzes the first step in this reaction results in an inability to catabolize any GAG molecules. The catabolic enzymes, which normally would be transported into lysosomes, instead are secreted from the cell and are found in unusually high concentrations in plasma, providing one diagnostic test for ML.

TABLE 268-1   MUCOPOLYSACCHARIDOSES AND MUCOLIPIDOSES

TYPE	EPONYM OR COMMON NAME	CLINICAL FEATURES	INHERITANCE	OMIM*	ENZYMATIC DEFECT
MPS IH	Hurler's syndrome	DM and short stature; MR; corneal clouding; HS; heart disease; death in childhood	AR	252800	α-L-iduronidase
MPS IS	Scheie's syndrome	Coarse facies; stiff joints; corneal clouding; aortic valve disease; normal intelligence and lifespan	AR	252800	α-L-iduronidase
MPS II	Hunter's syndrome	Severe form: coarse facies, DM, and short stature; HS; MR; no corneal clouding; death by late adolescence Mild form: coarse facies, short stature; normal intelligence; survival to adulthood	XL	309900	Iduronate sulfatase
MPS IIIA	Sanfilippo's A	Severe MR and hyperactivity; mild somatic changes	AR	252900	Heparan N-sulfatase
MPS IIIB	Sanfilippo's B	Same as MPS IIIA	AR	252920	α-N-acetylglucosaminidase
MPS IIIC	Sanfilippo's C	Same as MPS IIIA	AR	252930	Acetyl-coenzyme A: α-glucosaminide acetyltransferase
MPS IIID	Sanfilippo's D	Same as MPS IIIA	AR	252940	N-acetylglucosamine 6-sulfatase
MPS IVA	Morquio's A	Short stature and distinct skeletal dysplasia with odontoid hypoplasia and myelopathy; corneal clouding; normal intelligence; valvular heart disease	AR	253000	Galactose 6-sulfatase
MPS IVB	Morquio's B	Same as MPS IVA	AR	253010	β-Galactosidase
MPS VI	Maroteaux-Lamy	DM and short stature; corneal clouding; normal intelligence; aortic stenosis; leukocyte inclusions; hydrocephalus in severe form	AR	253200	N-acetylgalactosamine 4-sulfatase
MPS VII	Sly's syndrome	DM; HS; widely variable, including MR	AR	253220	β-Glucuronidase
MPS IX	—	Short stature; periarticular soft tissue masses	AR	601492	Hyaluronidase
ML II	I-cell disease	Similar to but more severe than MPS IH but with cellular inclusions; no mucopolysacchariduria	AR	252500	UDP-N-acetylglucosamine: lysosomal enzyme N-acetylglucosaminyl-1-phosphotransferase
ML III	Pseudo-Hurler polydystrophy	Short stature and mild DM; stiff joints, arthropathy, coarse facies; variable but mild MR; survival to adulthood	AR	252500	Same as ML II

*Entries in Online Mendelian Inheritance in Man, OMIM. Bethesda, MD, National Center for Biotechnology Information, National Library of Medicine. http://www.ncbi.nlm.nih.gov/omim. Accessed Sept. 11, 2009.

AR = autosomal recessive; DM = dysostosis multiplex; HS = hepatosplenomegaly; MR = mental retardation; XL = X-linked.

Pathology

All pathologic manifestations of MPS and ML disorders worsen with age, and some are present from early developmental stages. Gross anatomic hallmarks are hepatosplenomegaly, marked skeletal alterations (termed *dysostosis multiplex*) that result in short stature and thoracic cage deformity, thickening and narrowing of airways and arteries, and coarsening of facial features. Although mental retardation is a prominent feature of some of these conditions, the brain may show only ventriculomegaly secondary to communicating hydrocephalus. On microscopy, mesenchymal cells show a cytoplasm full of apparently empty vacuoles; these are lysosomes from which GAG has been removed by fixation. Cells cultured from patients show greatly enlarged lysosomes filled with granular material. In the severe form of ML, dense inclusions are present, which gave rise to the common name, *I-cell disease*.

CLINICAL MANIFESTATIONS

Each of the disorders in Table 268-1 shows a wide spectrum of clinical severity. This wide spectrum has led to a classification that gives the impression of separate disorders within some of the MPS and ML types, but these represent the apparent ends of the continuum. Some of the disorders result in death by adolescence (Hurler's syndrome, severe Hunter's syndrome, ML II), whereas others are commonly compatible with survival to adulthood. The latter group of disorders is emphasized here.

The milder end of the MPS I spectrum, Scheie's syndrome, may not be diagnosed until adulthood; patients present with stiffened joints, corneal clouding and glaucoma, carpal tunnel syndrome, and aortic valvular disease. Stature and intelligence are not affected. The main health risks are valvular involvement, thickening of meninges that can produce a myelopathy, and thickening of the upper airways that can produce obstructive symptoms and sleep apnea.

The milder form of MPS II, Hunter's syndrome, is distinctive because it is X-linked (affecting males almost exclusively), and the cornea shows little overt clouding. Cervical myelopathy, obstructive airway disease, and cor pulmonale are important concerns. A combined conductive-neurosensory hearing loss is common.

Neither MPS IV (Morquio's syndrome) nor MPS VI (Maroteaux-Lamy syndrome) affects intelligence. Both syndromes often are associated with severe skeletal changes, which are distinct radiographically but produce similar problems of kyphoscoliosis, pectus carinatum, restrictive lung disease, severe short stature, and joint degeneration. Cervical myelopathy resulting from a thickened dura is common to both disorders and is accentuated by odontoid hypoplasia in MPS IV. Thickening of the aortic and mitral valves may produce severe dysfunction necessitating their replacement. General anesthesia is especially hazardous because of the narrow upper and middle airways and cervical instability.

Patients with ML III (pseudo-Hurler's polydystrophy) resemble patients with MPS VI but often have mild-to-moderate mental retardation. Aortic regurgitation is common.

DIAGNOSIS

Differential Diagnosis

Diagnosis of these conditions is difficult in the young child, before most of the clinical features have progressed, but should be considered in any person with hepatosplenomegaly and coarsening of the facial features. Evaluation requires a pedigree analysis, skeletal radiographic survey, echocardiogram, and analysis of the urine for excretion of GAGs. Often the specific MPS is evident from radiographs, the presence or absence of corneal clouding, and the pattern of mucopolysacchariduria. Enzymatic analysis of leukocytes confirms the diagnosis. Patients with MLs do not show mucopolysacchariduria but have marked elevation of all the GAG catabolic lysosomal enzymes in plasma.

TREATMENT ℞

Ventriculoperitoneal shunting is necessary if intracranial pressure is elevated. Close attention to hearing and visual problems is essential throughout life. Many adults with MPS or ML require surgery for carpal tunnel syndrome. Cardiovascular surgery for valvular or coronary disease may be necessary. All use of anesthesia is high risk because of the narrow airways and, in the case of MPS IV, atlantoaxial instability. For patients who remain ambulatory, selective joint replacement can be beneficial. Because of the morbidity associated with thoracic cage deformity, consideration should be given to stabilizing the spinal deformity before it becomes severe.

Replacement of the deficient enzyme by intravenous infusion is being studied for most of the MPS disorders. Laronidase (Aldurazyme) has been approved in the United States for treatment of MPS I. An infusion every 2 weeks for 1 year in adolescent and adult patients resulted in substantial reduction in hepatosplenomegaly and modest improvement in pulmonary function, sleep apnea, and joint mobility. Whether early institution of therapy in young children modulates mental retardation in the Hurler's variant of MPS I is uncertain. Galsulfase (Naglazyme) has been approved for the treatment of MPS VI, in which somatic rather than neurologic problems predominate. Bone marrow transplantation has been attempted in many of the MPS disorders, with mixed success. The earlier transplantation occurs, the better the outcome in terms of somatic problems, but prevention of mental retardation has not occurred.

⬤ MARFAN SYNDROME

DEFINITION

Marfan syndrome is an autosomal dominant, pleiotropic disorder caused by defects in the principal component of the extracellular microfibril, the large glycoprotein fibrillin-1. The disease manifests in multiple systems, especially the eye, skeleton, heart, aorta, lung, and integument. Notable features include dislocation of the ocular lens, tall stature with particularly long limbs and digits, deformity of the thoracic cage from pectus carinatum or excavatum with abnormal curvature of the spine, mitral and tricuspid valve prolapse, dilation of the sinuses of Valsalva and predisposition to aortic dissection, spontaneous pneumothorax, abnormal skin stretch marks, hernias, and dural ectasia. If untreated, patients often die before 30 or 40 years of age from aortic dissection or congestive heart failure.

EPIDEMIOLOGY

Marfan syndrome is a common mendelian disorder, with an estimated incidence of about 1 per 5000 births. Marfan syndrome is found throughout the world, without ethnic or geographic predilection.

PATHOBIOLOGY

Pathogenesis

Mutations in *FBN1*, which maps to human chromosome 15q21.1 and encodes fibrillin-1, cause Marfan syndrome and related connective tissue disorders. More than 800 distinct mutations have been found, and few occur in more than one family. Patients are heterozygous for mutations in *FBN1*, leading to autosomal dominant inheritance. Extracellular microfibrils are polymers of many fibrillin-1 molecules and are ubiquitous in the ECM of most tissues. Latent transforming growth factor-β (TGF-β) binding protein, which keeps the cytokine inactive, bears striking homology to regions of fibrillin. Abnormalities of either the quality or the quantity of microfibrils disrupt normal signaling by TGF-β, especially during embryonic development and postnatal growth. Studies in mice engineered to harbor human mutations in *FBN1* showed that excessive TGF-β signaling causes abnormal lung septation (the precursor to pneumothorax), mitral valve prolapse, muscular hypoplasia, and aortic dilation. This fundamental shift in understanding of the pathogenesis of Marfan syndrome has suggested novel therapies, such as with small molecules that affect the activity of TGF-β.

The features of Marfan syndrome are highly variable, even among relatives who share the same mutation in *FBN1*. This variability persists after accounting for the effects of age. Men tend to be affected more severely, for unclear reasons.

Pathology

The features of Marfan syndrome are age dependent. Some severely affected infants have flagrant features and often die of mitral regurgitation and heart failure despite aggressive management. At the other end of the clinical spectrum, Marfan syndrome merges with several related disorders, and patients may not come to medical attention, let alone receive a definitive diagnosis, until adulthood.

None of the gross or microscopic pathologic changes is specific for Marfan syndrome. The medial degeneration of the aortic wall, characterized by disarray and fragmentation of the elastic fibers and increased proteoglycan (often inappropriately termed *cystic medial necrosis*) also can be seen in other disorders and in older people with hypertension. Aortic dissection (Chapter 78) usually begins just superior to the aortic valve (type A) and often progresses to the bifurcation. Death usually results from retrograde dissection and hemopericardium. About 10% of dissections begin in the descending thoracic aorta (type B).

CLINICAL MANIFESTATIONS

The lens tends to be displaced superiorly, and usually the zonules remain intact. The retina is at increased risk for detachment, especially in patients who are highly myopic. Tubular bones overgrow, accounting for the disproportionate tall stature (dolichostenomelia), long digits (arachnodactyly), and sternal deformity. Ligaments may be lax, causing scoliosis and joint hypermobility. Alternatively, congenital contractures are common, especially of the elbows and digits. The palate typically is highly arched, and the dentition can be crowded and maloccluded. Mitral valve prolapse occurs in about 80% of cases, and the valve leaflets become progressively thickened (myxomatous on histopathology) (Chapter 75). The mitral annulus may dilate and calcify. Aortic root dilation begins in the sinuses of Valsalva and progresses with age, albeit at highly variable rates (Chapter 78). Most males with Marfan syndrome have an aortic root dimension above the upper limit of normal for their body surface area by adolescence. Some females show a slower progression and may have a root diameter near the upper limit of normal well into adulthood. The dilation usually does not involve the distal ascending aorta. Spontaneous pneumothorax, resulting from rupture of apical blebs, occurs in about 5% of patients. Stretch marks (striae atrophicae) occur over areas of flexural stress, such as the shoulders, breasts, and lower back. The neural canal in the lumbosacral region is enlarged in most people with Marfan syndrome; this may be visible on plain radiographs, especially if the neuroforamina are widened. Computed tomography or magnetic resonance imaging is diagnostic and should be used in patients with back pain and radicular symptoms. Large anterior meningoceles in the pelvis are a severe manifestation of dural ectasia. Simple cysts in the liver and kidneys are common, increase with age, and seldom cause clinical problems.

DIAGNOSIS

Differential Diagnosis

The conditions that overlap clinically and genetically with Marfan syndrome include familial aortic aneurysm, familial ectopia lentis, MASS phenotype (which includes many families with mitral valve prolapse syndrome), and Loeys-Dietz syndrome. Most of these conditions are diagnosed clinically, so differentiating among them is arbitrary. A careful family history is essential to this process. Molecular genetic testing has a limited role. However, if the mutation in *FBN1* is known in a family, analysis of DNA can be used effectively for presymptomatic or prenatal diagnosis. Loeys-Dietz syndrome, which is associated with generalized arterial tortuosity and susceptibility to dissection, is caused by mutation in either of two receptors for TGF-β, *TGFBR1* and *TGFBR2*, and molecular analysis is clinically available.

A question of Marfan syndrome arises most commonly in the tall, lanky adolescent who has several minor skeletal features, nearsightedness, and athletic desires. A detailed ophthalmologic examination with full pupillary dilation and a transthoracic echocardiogram are essential components in the evaluation. If these tests are negative and no one in the family has a history of Marfan syndrome or aortic dissection, the patient probably can be reassured.

TREATMENT   Rx

Life expectancy in Marfan syndrome has improved markedly, to the point that many patients can expect survival to advanced years. All patients should be seen at least annually by a physician who manages the overall care. Most patients require annual ophthalmologic and cardiologic consultation and orthopedic consultation as required by specific problems. A number of studies, but only one randomized clinical trial, support the prophylactic use of β-adrenergic blockade from an early age to slow the rate of aortic root dilation and protect against aortic dissection.▪ Prophylactic surgical repair of the aortic root has had the greatest beneficial impact. The composite graft, involving a prosthetic valve in a Dacron tube and implantation of the coronary ostia into the graft, was the first approach to produce markedly improved survival in these patients. More recently, replacement of the aneurysm and preservation of the native aortic valve have shown promise and should be considered first. For the adult, aortic root surgery should be recommended when the maximal aortic diameter reaches 50 mm, and a strong family history of aortic dissection should prompt earlier repair.

● EHLERS-DANLOS SYNDROMES

DEFINITION

The Ehlers-Danlos syndromes (EDSs) are clinically variable and genetically heterogeneous. Diagnoses still are based largely on the bedside examination. The unifying themes among these disorders are fragility of tissues, joint hypermobility, and skin hyperextensibility.

EPIDEMIOLOGY

No accurate data exist, but an incidence of about 1 in 5000 births is a reasonable estimate of how many individuals qualify for one of the EDS diagnoses. Each type represents something of a clinical spectrum, with the mild end merging with what might be considered normal variation. Just as the diagnostic criteria are arbitrary, so would be any determination of prevalence based on phenotypic criteria. The extent to which normal variation in joint hypermobility, skin elasticity, and tissue fragility represents genetic variation at loci that encode collagen or other ECM genes requires considerable research.

PATHOBIOLOGY

Pathogenesis

Defects in collagen and other proteins in the ECM of various tissues underlie all forms of EDS that have been elucidated so far. The specific mutations occur in a variety of genes, with the effect of altering the structure, synthesis, post-translational modifications, or stability of the collagens involved. The known molecular defects are listed in Table 268-2.

Pathology

Few findings in the routine pathologic evaluation distinguish among the various types of EDS or even distinguish individual types from normal. Thickness of the dermis is decreased in some forms, especially the vascular type, and the walls of arteries are reduced in thickness in this type. By electron microscopy, the classic, hypermobile, and kyphoscoliotic types have abnormal collagen fibers, especially when viewed in cross section (variable and often increased fiber diameter with an irregular outline). In the vascular type, some patients have dilated endoplasmic reticulum consistent with aberrant secretion of type III collagen molecules.

CLINICAL MANIFESTATIONS

The major and minor features of each EDS are detailed in Table 268-2. Infants with classic EDS often are born prematurely by 4 to 8 weeks because of rupture of fetal membranes. Diagnosis of the vascular and kyphoscoliotic types is important because of their cardiovascular features. The vascular type, previously termed *EDS IV*, is characterized by a troublesome tendency toward spontaneous rupture of large arteries and hollow organs, especially the colon and uterus. Because these events carry considerable morbidity, life expectancy is reduced, on average, by more than half. During pregnancy, women with this form of EDS are especially vulnerable to rupture of major arteries and the uterus. In the kyphoscoliotic type, aortic root dilation and aortic regurgitation can develop. Patients with most forms of EDS are prone to develop mitral valve prolapse, and progression to mitral regurgitation (Chapter 75) occurs more often than in the common form of mitral valve prolapse.

DIAGNOSIS

Differential Diagnosis

By careful adherence to the clinical features shown in Table 268-2 and judicious use of laboratory tests, the various defined types of EDS can be differentiated. Many specific non-EDS syndromes need to be excluded. The kyphoscoliotic type of EDS in infants shares some features with severe Marfan syndrome. Patients with Larsen's syndrome may resemble patients with the arthrochalasis type of EDS. The skin redundancy and loss of elasticity of the dermatosparaxis type of EDS are reminiscent of autosomal dominant cutis laxa, which is not associated with easy bruising or tissue fragility.

The most difficult decision is whether any diagnosis of EDS is warranted. Patients who have only joint hypermobility without skin changes should not be labeled with EDS; a diagnosis of familial joint hypermobility might be more appropriate. Familial joint instability involves a predisposition to dislocations of major joints that is rare in most types of EDS except for arthrochalasis.

TABLE 268-2 EHLERS-DANLOS SYNDROMES

TYPE	FORMER NAME	CLINICAL FEATURES*	INHERITANCE	OMIM†	MOLECULAR DEFECT
Classic	EDS I and II	Joint hypermobility; skin hyperextensibility; atrophic scars; smooth, velvety skin; subcutaneous spheroids	AD	130000 130010	Structure of type V collagen due to mutations in COL5A1, COL5A2
Hypermobility	EDS III	Joint hypermobility; some skin hyperextensibility, with or without smooth, velvety texture	AD AR	130020 225320	? Tenascin-X (TNX)
Vascular	EDS IV	Thin skin; easy bruising; pinched nose; acrogeria; rupture of large-caliber and medium-caliber arteries, uterus, and large bowel	AD	130050 (225350) (225360)	Deficient type III collagen (COL3A1)
Kyphoscoliotic	EDS VI	Joint hypermobility; congenital, progressive scoliosis; scleral fragility with globe rupture; tissue fragility, aortic dilation, MVP	AR	225400	Deficiency of lysyl hydroxylase
Arthrochalasis	EDS VII A and B	Joint hypermobility, severe, with subluxations, congenital hip dislocation; skin hyperextensibility; tissue fragility	AD	130060	No cleavage of amino terminus of type I procollagen due to mutations in COL1A1 or COL1A2
Dermatosparaxis	EDS VII C	Severe skin fragility; decreased skin elasticity, easy bruising; hernias; premature rupture of fetal membranes	AR	225410	No cleavage of amino terminus of type I procollagen due to deficiency of peptidase
Unclassified types	EDS V	Classic features	XL	305200	?
	EDS VIII	Classic features and periodontal disease	AD	130080	?
	EDS X	Mild classic features, MVP	?	225310	?
	EDS XI	Joint instability	AD	147900	?
	EDS IX	Classic features; occipital horns	XL	309400	Allelic to Menkes' syndrome
	EDS, progeroid form	Classic features and premature aging	AR	130700	Deficiency of galactosyltransferase I

*Listed in order of diagnostic importance.

†Entries in Online Mendelian Inheritance in Man, OMIM. Bethesda, MD, National Center for Biotechnology Information, National Library of Medicine. http://www.ncbi.nlm.nih.gov/omim. Accessed Sept. 11, 2009.

AD = autosomal dominant; AR = autosomal recessive; EDS = Ehlers-Danlos syndrome; MVP = mitral valve prolapse; XL = X-linked.

TREATMENT Rx

Management of most skin and joint problems should be conservative and preventive. Sutures need to be placed with careful attention to approximating the margins and avoiding tension; removable sutures should be left in place for twice the usual time. Most instances of joint hypermobility and pain in EDS do not require surgical treatment. Benefit often is derived from physical therapy designed to strengthen the muscles that provide support for the loose ligaments. All patients should receive genetic counseling about the mode of inheritance and their risk of having children affected with EDS. The possibility of prenatal diagnosis exists for all of the EDS types with defined molecular or biochemical defects.

The vascular type of EDS requires particular surgical care; the ruptured arteries are difficult to repair because of the pronounced vascular fragility. Rupture of the bowel is a surgical emergency. Because the risk for uterine and vascular rupture is especially high during pregnancy in women with the vascular form, affected women should be advised that there is a substantial risk for death related to pregnancy and delivery. Patients should be advised to avoid contact sports and to treat blood pressure elevations aggressively. Arteriography and arterial lines should be avoided if possible. Biochemical and genetic screening holds the potential for reassuring relatives at risk that they do not have a defect in type III collagen.

The kyphoscoliotic type of EDS may improve with large doses of vitamin C (1 to 4 g/day) because ascorbate is a cofactor for the enzyme that is deficient. Celiprolol, a cardioselective β1-blocker with β2 agonist vasodilatory properties (titrated up by 100 mg every 6 months up to a maximum of 400 mg twice daily), reduced cardiovascular events by 64% in patients with EDS.[2] No other metabolic or genetic therapy is effective in other forms of EDS.

⬤ OSTEOGENESIS IMPERFECTA SYNDROMES

DEFINITION

The heterogeneous group of disorders called *osteogenesis imperfecta* (OI) includes, at one end of the severity spectrum, a type that is lethal prenatally or in the neonatal period and, at the other, such mild features that distinguishing affected individuals from the general population is difficult. The unifying feature is hereditary osteopenia (insufficient bone), with primary defects in the protein matrix in bone and other tissues. The clinical syndromes all involve osteoporosis with liability to fracture (Chapter 251).

EPIDEMIOLOGY

No careful epidemiologic study has been performed, and the milder forms of type I OI merge with the phenotypes of familial osteoporosis, fracture susceptibility, and joint hypermobility found in the general population. A crude estimate of the overall prevalence of OI is 1 to 2 per 20,000 births. The neonatal lethal form (type II), which is almost always caused by a new mutation in a parental gamete, has an incidence of about 1 in 50,000 births.

PATHOBIOLOGY

Pathogenesis

Most patients in whom mutations have been found usually have defects in the two genes that encode the procollagen chains of type I collagen, *COL1A1* and *COL1A2*. Type I collagen is composed of two α1(I) and one α2(I) procollagen chains; the mature fiber requires considerable post-translational modification, which occurs appropriately only if the three procollagen chains have intertwined to form a triple helix that is perfect and completed at the right speed. A mutation that affects formation of the triple helix, such as substitution of one of the mandatory glycine residues that occurs at every third position, also has adverse effects on the modifications that render the molecule capable of forming effective mature fibers. As a result, a single nucleotide change resulting in a missense mutation can have profound effects on the ECM and produce a severe condition. Alternatively, and at first glance paradoxically, a mutation that eliminates an entire allele, or at least production of any product capable of intertwining with normal procollagen chains, has a much milder effect on the ECM and on the severity of OI. Examples of the most common classes of mutations are shown in Table 268-3. Hundreds of mutations have been described. Patients with mutations in *COL1A1* or *COL1A2* are heterozygous, and thus the most common forms of OI are inherited as autosomal dominant traits. Several autosomal recessive forms of OI occur because of mutations in genes that encode enzymes that process type I collagen into mature fibrils.

Pathology

Other than the gross pathology associated with the clinical manifestations, the most characteristic pathology is a primary reduction in bone matrix with secondary undermineralization.

CLINICAL MANIFESTATIONS

The major phenotypic features of OI are shown in Table 268-3. Among the most common forms, the most severe type is type II, followed in decreasing order by types III, IV, and I. In type II, infants either are stillborn or die soon after birth of pulmonary failure secondary to the small thorax, which usually is compromised further by myriad rib fractures. A few infants have survived for at least a few years but require enormous attention to their medical needs.

Type III OI may be confused with type II at birth, but survival alone helps make the distinction. Bony deformity is pronounced and not necessarily due

TABLE 268-3   OSTEOGENESIS IMPERFECTA

TYPE	CLINICAL FEATURES	INHERITANCE	OMIM*	BASIC DEFECTS
I	Fractures variable in number; little deformity; stature normal or nearly so; blue sclerae; hearing loss common but not always present; DI uncommon	AD	166200	Typically, one nonfunctional *COL1A1* allele
II	Lethal in utero or shortly after birth; many fractures at birth typically involving ribs (may appear "beaded") and other long bones; little calvaria; pulmonary hypertension	AD	166210	*COL1A1* or *COL1A2*: substitution of glycyl residues; occasionally deletions of a portion of the triple-helical domain
		AR	259400	Deletion in *COL1A2* plus a nonfunctional allele
III	Fractures common, but long bones progressively deform starting in utero; stature markedly reduced; sclerae often blue but become lighter with age; DI and hearing loss common	AD	259420	One single–amino acid substitution
		AR (rare)	259440	Two mutations in *COL1A1* and/or *COL1A2* (rarely)
IV	Fractures common; stature usually reduced; bone deformity common but rarely severe; scleral hue normal to grayish; hearing loss variable; DI common	AD	166220	Point mutations in *COL1A1* or *COL1A2*
			166240	Exon skipping mutations in *COL1A2*
V	Similar to type IV without DI or blue sclerae; fractures develop hyperplastic callus; calcification of the interosseous membrane between the radius and ulna	AD	610967	?
VI	Similar to type IV without DI, blue sclerae or wormian bones; excess osteoid present in bone	?	610968	?
VII	Similar to types II or III with fractures at birth, blue sclerae, no DI; presence of rhizomelic limb shortening and coax vara	AR	610682	Mutations in *CRTAP*
VIII	Similar to types II or III with fractures at birth	AR	610915	Mutations in *LEPRE1*
IX	Similar to types II or III with fractures at birth	AR	259440	Mutations in *PPIB*

*Entries in Online Mendelian Inheritance in Man, OMIM. Bethesda, MD, National Center for Biotechnology Information, National Library of Medicine. http://www.ncbi.nlm.nih.gov/omim/. Accessed June 11, 2009.

AD = autosomal dominant; AR = autosomal recessive; DI = dentinogenesis imperfecta.

to fractures. Mobility is impaired, and most patients require a wheelchair at an early age. Stature may be severely compromised. Because of progressive vertebral column deformity and rib fractures, restrictive lung disease is a common problem as patients age; many die of pulmonary complications. Basilar impression causing compression of the brain stem and the craniocervical junction can produce central sleep apnea, headache, and upper motor neuron signs.

Patients with type IV OI generally have reduced stature, some bony deformity, and abnormal teeth that are opalescent and wear easily (dentinogenesis imperfecta). As in type I OI, the tendency to fracture is highest in childhood and lessens with adolescence. A distinguishing characteristic of type IV OI is a normal scleral hue.

Type I OI is probably the most common form and is associated with a bluish or blue-gray scleral hue. People with type I OI who also have dentinogenesis imperfecta tend to have more severe skeletal problems. The risk of fracture diminishes during adulthood but reemerges as a major concern for women after menopause. Hearing impairment in all forms of OI is common and age related, being rare before adolescence. The deficits are of either a mixed or a predominantly conductive form.

The recessive forms of OI (types VI to IX) range in severity from type IV to type II and may have distinctive radiologic or histopathologic findings.

DIAGNOSIS

Differential Diagnosis

The range of diagnostic possibilities in a person with multiple fractures largely depends on age. In infancy, the genetic conditions hypophosphatasia, severe osteochondrodysplasias (e.g., achondrogenesis and forms of spondyloepiphyseal dysplasia), and Menkes' syndrome need to be excluded when a diagnosis of type II or type III OI is considered. The radiographic features eventually become entirely diagnostic, but often the neonatologist has to arrive at a definitive answer in short order. Analysis of serum alkaline phosphatase and copper can be helpful. In childhood, the most common situation leading to consideration of a mild form of OI is child abuse. In this situation, the pattern of fracture is usually distinct, and bone mineralization should be normal if the child is the object of nonaccidental or repeated accidental trauma. Abnormal scleral hue, dentinogenesis imperfecta, and wormian bones (microfractures along the cranial sutures) all support the diagnosis of OI. The legal and child-protective systems often request exclusion of OI by analysis of collagen production from cultured skin fibroblasts.

In older children, the disorder idiopathic juvenile osteoporosis should be considered in any patient seen initially with repeated fractures. Occasionally, studies of skin fibroblasts are needed to document whether a defect in type I collagen (which would be characteristic of OI) is present. Many

osteochondrodysplasias are associated with short stature, skeletal deformity, and a tendency to fracture. Pyknodysostosis and osteopetrosis are associated with sclerotic bones rather than osteoporotic ones. In adulthood, early-onset osteoporosis may be confused with OI (Chapter 251). Mutations in type I collagen also cause familial osteoporosis, and the skeletal phenotypes merge; patients with true OI may have scleral, hearing, or dental abnormalities and a positive family history.

Analysis of the specific enzymes defective in the recessive forms of OI is useful for establishing the diagnosis and enabling reproductive counseling and prenatal diagnosis if desired.

TREATMENT

Management of the skeletal complications largely depends on orthopedic, physical, and occupational therapy approaches. Although no medical treatment has yet been demonstrated to improve the quality of the bone, studies of mesenchymal stem cell transplantation and bisphosphonates are underway. The latter treatment clearly can increase bone mineral density. The long-term goals are for the patient to maintain function and independence as an individual. These goals can be advanced in some patients by judicious use of intramedullary rods in the long bones of the legs; if mobility and especially ambulation can be maintained, the demineralization associated with inactivity can be avoided.

Unaffected parents of a child with OI and all affected individuals should have genetic counseling. For the parents of a child with type II OI, the possibility of germinal mosaicism (which has been well documented in this condition) should not be overlooked. If one parent has a "new" mutation in one of the type I procollagen genes and multiple gonadal cells carry this mutation, the risk for recurrence in future children is not negligible. If the mutation in the affected child can be defined, the risk for recurrence can be quantified (through molecular analysis of sperm) if the mutation arose in the father.

PSEUDOXANTHOMA ELASTICUM

DEFINITION

Pseudoxanthoma elasticum (PXE) is a heritable disorder of connective tissue with pleiotropic manifestations wherever elastic fibers are found but primarily in the skin, eye, and vasculature. Life expectancy is reduced, on average, because of a predisposition to myocardial infarction and gastrointestinal hemorrhage.

EPIDEMIOLOGY

The exact frequency of PXE is unknown, but it is probably underdiagnosed. Rough approximations suggest a prevalence of 1 in 25,000 to 100,000 births.

Males and females are equally affected, although women are more likely to seek medical attention out of concern for the skin changes.

PATHOBIOLOGY

Pathogenesis

In most families, PXE occurs as an autosomal recessive trait, which means, given relatively small sibships, that many patients will have no affected relatives. Apparent autosomal dominant inheritance may reflect expression in occasional heterozygotes. The gene for PXE maps to human chromosome 16 and encodes one of the adenosine triphosphate–binding cassette transporters (*ABCC6*). Because of the prominent histopathologic feature of calcification of elastic tissue, this gene may be important in calcium homeostasis. It is unclear, however, whether calcification is a primary or a secondary phenomenon in PXE.

Pathology

The hallmark of PXE, and an important diagnostic clue, is the histopathologic finding of hyperproliferated elastic fibers in the mid-dermis; these fibers become fragmented, clumped, and calcified. An arteriolar sclerosis develops in the media of muscular arteries and arterioles; the lumen may become progressively and concentrically narrowed. Alternatively, microaneurysms can form. Thickening of the endocardium, especially the atrial endocardium, develops in some patients. In the eye, Bruch's membrane becomes calcified and fragmented.

CLINICAL MANIFESTATIONS

Because of the pleiotropic nature of PXE, the diagnosis initially may be suspected by any of a variety of clinicians, especially dermatologists, ophthalmologists, cardiologists, and gastroenterologists. The condition gains its name from the dermatologic feature of yellowish papules that appear at areas of flexural stress, especially the neck, groin, and popliteal and cubital fossae; in periumbilical regions; and on the buccal mucosa. The appearance of affected skin has been likened to that of a "plucked chicken." Over time, affected areas coalesce and become thickened.

Changes in the eye begin as a generalized, subtle, mottled pattern in the retina (peau d'orange) and progress to the characteristic angioid streaks. The latter changes are not specific for PXE and can be seen in diabetes mellitus, sickle cell disease, and a variety of other conditions. Streaks represent breaks in Bruch's membrane, an elastic lamina that lies between the retinal vasculature and the choroid. Spontaneous hemorrhages, especially those involving the macula, lead to progressive visual loss.

Involvement of arteries of various calibers produces problems because of occlusion and hemorrhage. The lifetime risk of serious gastrointestinal hemorrhage from any site, but especially the stomach, is about 10%. Hypertension is relatively common, in part because of involvement of the renal vasculature. Progressive occlusion of peripheral arteries leads to absence of pulses; acral ischemia is rare because of the development of collaterals. The risk for stroke, myocardial infarction, abdominal angina, and intermittent claudication is increased independent of other risk factors.

DIAGNOSIS

Differential Diagnosis

An acquired form of PXE has been reported and is also of unclear etiology. This form is difficult to differentiate from a sporadic case in a family due to heterozygosity in the parents, but it tends to affect only the skin. As suggested by the name, the cutaneous features of PXE need to be differentiated from those of true xanthoma, which results from a disorder of lipid metabolism (Chapter 213). The dermatologic manifestations need to be differentiated from those of Miescher's elastoma, elastic tissue nevi (Buschke-Ollendorff syndrome), and solar elastosis.

TREATMENT Rx

No cure for or means of preventing PXE is known. In many instances, careful attention to the ocular features by a retinal specialist experienced in PXE can delay but not prevent loss of vision. The risk of gastrointestinal hemorrhage suggests that patients should avoid gastric irritants such as aspirin, nonsteroidal anti-inflammatory drugs, and excessive alcohol. Stool should be checked regularly for occult blood, and angiography may be necessary to detect the source of bleeding. All standard risk factors for atherosclerosis should be managed aggressively. Complaints of chest pain should prompt a rigorous investigation for coronary artery disease. Angioplasty has not been reported to be effective, and the coronary lesions tend to be diffuse. Coronary artery bypass graft surgery has been performed, but long-term results have not been reported. It may be theoretically advantageous to use vein grafts rather than the internal mammary artery for bypass. The excessive wrinkling and pseudoxanthoma in exposed areas can be ameliorated by plastic surgery.

FUTURE DIRECTIONS

Each of these disorders poses special considerations in clinical diagnosis, utility of molecular testing, genetic counseling, and management. For the storage disorders, the clinical utility of enzyme replacement therapy is actively being pursued by several pharmaceutical companies. For several of the other conditions, somatic stem cell therapy offers some promise but is years away from routine clinical use. In Marfan syndrome, clinical trials of drugs that modulate activity of TGF-β are under way. Considerable progress will be made over the next few years in delineating the milder ranges of the phenotypes in Marfan syndrome, OI, and EDS. Molecular testing will have an increasing role in specific circumstances, especially as the costs of screening large genes for mutations decreases. Additionally, close medical management for individuals detected as being at heightened risk for cardiovascular, skeletal, and ocular complications will remain a mainstay.

1. Shores J, Berger KR, Murphy EA, et al. Chronic β-adrenergic blockade protects the aorta in the Marfan syndrome: a prospective, randomized trial of propranolol. *N Engl J Med.* 1994;330: 1335-1341.
2. Ong KT, Perdu J, De Backer J, et al. Effect of celiprolol on prevention of cardiovascular events in vascular Ehlers-Danlos syndrome: a prospective randomised, open, blinded-endpoints trial. *Lancet.* 2010;376:1476-1484.

SUGGESTED READINGS

Benedetto U, Melina G, Takkenberg JJ, et al. Surgical management of aortic root disease in Marfan syndrome: a systematic review and meta-analysis. *Heart.* 2011;97:955-958. *Review of surgical options.*
Brooke BS, Arnaoutakis G, McDonnell NB, et al. Contemporary management of vascular complications associated with Ehlers-Danlos syndrome. *J Vasc Surg.* 2010;51:131-138. *Review of vascular procedures, which were almost always done electively.*
Cañadas V, Vilacosta I, Bruna I, et al. Marfan syndrome. Part 1: pathophysiology and diagnosis. *Nat Rev Cardiol.* 2010;7:256-265. *Review including the role of genetic testing.*
Finger RP, Charbel IP, Ladewig MS, et al. Pseudoxanthoma elasticum: genetics, clinical manifestations and therapeutic approaches. *Surv Ophthalmol.* 2009;54:272-285. *The exact pathogenesis remains unclear, but therapies directed at the retina can retain vision.*
Keane MG, Pyeritz RE. Medical management of Marfan syndrome. *Circulation.* 2008;117:2802-2813. *A review of nonsurgical approaches to therapy.*

269

THE SYSTEMIC AUTOINFLAMMATORY DISEASES

DANIEL L. KASTNER

DEFINITION

The systemic autoinflammatory diseases (Table 269-1) are a group of illnesses characterized by seemingly unprovoked inflammation, without evidence of high-titer autoantibodies or antigen-specific T cells, thus distinguishing them from the more classic autoimmune diseases. The first conditions recognized as autoinflammatory were the hereditary recurrent fevers, a group of mendelian disorders characterized by episodic or fluctuating degrees of fever and localized inflammation. The scope of autoinflammatory disease has been broadened to include other heritable illnesses, including disorders in which purulent or granulomatous inflammation predominates, as well as inherited disorders of the complement system (Chapter 49). In addition, in numerous autoinflammatory conditions, some of which present in childhood and others that occur later in life, there is a complex interaction

TABLE 269-1 THE SYSTEMIC AUTOINFLAMMATORY DISEASES: A PARTIAL LISTING

INHERITED AUTOINFLAMMATORY DISEASES	INHERITANCE/ETIOLOGY	GENES OR RISK FACTORS	OMIM*
HEREDITARY RECURRENT FEVER SYNDROMES			
Familial Mediterranean fever (FMF)	Autosomal recessive	*MEFV*†	249100
Tumor necrosis factor receptor–associated periodic syndrome (TRAPS)	Autosomal dominant	*TNFRSF1A*†	142680
Hyperimmunoglobulinemia D with periodic fever syndrome (HIDS)	Autosomal recessive	*MVK*†	260920
Familial cold autoinflammatory syndrome (FCAS)	Autosomal dominant	*NLRP3* (formerly *CIAS1*)†	120100
Muckle-Wells syndrome (MWS)	Autosomal dominant	*NLRP3* (formerly *CIAS1*)†	191900
Neonatal-onset multisystem inflammatory disease (NOMID)/chronic infantile neurologic cutaneous and articular (CINCA) syndrome	Sporadic, autosomal dominant	*NLRP3* (formerly *CIAS1*)†	607115
GRANULOMATOUS DISORDERS			
Granulomatous inflammatory arthritis, dermatitis, and uveitis (Blau's syndrome)	Autosomal dominant	*NOD2/CARD15*†	186580
Early-onset sarcoidosis	Sporadic, autosomal dominant	*NOD2/CARD15*†	609464
Crohn's disease	Complex inheritance	*NOD2/CARD15*†	266600
PYOGENIC DISORDERS			
Syndrome of pyogenic arthritis with pyoderma gangrenosum and acne (PAPA)	Autosomal dominant	*PSTPIP1*†	604416
AUTOINFLAMMATORY DISORDERS OF SKIN AND BONE			
Deficiency of IL-1 receptor antagonist (DIRA)	Autosomal recessive	*IL1RN*	612852
Chronic recurrent multifocal osteomyelitis (CRMO)	Sporadic, autosomal recessive	*LPIN2*†, when associated with congenital dyserythropoietic anemia (Majeed's syndrome)	259680
Synovitis acne pustulosis hyperostosis osteitis syndrome (SAPHO)	Idiopathic	—	—
COMPLEMENT DISORDERS			
Hereditary angioedema	Autosomal dominant	*C1NH*	106100
Hemolytic-uremic syndrome	Autosomal dominant, sporadic	HF1 (complement factor H)	235400
Age-related macular degeneration	Complex inheritance	HF1 (complement factor H)	603075
OTHER AUTOINFLAMMATORY SYNDROMES			
Syndrome of periodic fever with aphthous stomatitis, pharyngitis, and cervical adenopathy (PFAPA)	Idiopathic	—	—
Systemic-onset juvenile idiopathic arthritis (SOJIA)	Complex inheritance	IL-6, *MIF* polymorphisms	604302
Adult-onset Still's disease	Idiopathic	—	—
Schnitzler's syndrome	Idiopathic	—	—
Behçet's disease	Complex inheritance	HLA-B51, polymorphisms in *IL10, IL23R*	109650
Crystalline arthropathies	Complex inheritance	*SLC2A9/GLUT9, ABCG2*	—

*Online Mendelian Inheritance in Man, an online catalog of genetic disorders, available at http://www.ncbi.nlm.nih.gov/entrez/query.fcgi?db=OMIM.
†An updated listing of disease-associated mutations is available online at http://fmf.igh.cnrs.fr/infevers.

of genetic susceptibilities and environmental factors. These illnesses include systemic-onset juvenile idiopathic arthritis (Still's disease), Behçet's disease, and even the crystalline arthritides. Recent advances in the genetics and pathophysiology of the inherited autoinflammatory diseases suggest that these conditions are inborn errors of innate immunity, the phylogenetically more primitive part of the immune system that uses germline membrane and intracellular receptors expressed in granulocytes and macrophages to mount the body's first line of defense against pathogens (Chapters 44 and 47).

● HEREDITARY RECURRENT FEVER SYNDROMES
Familial Mediterranean Fever

DEFINITION

Familial Mediterranean fever (FMF) is a recessively inherited illness that typically manifests with 12- to 72-hour episodes of fever and localized serosal, synovial, or cutaneous inflammation. Between attacks, patients usually feel completely well, although biochemical evidence of inflammation may remain, and some patients eventually develop systemic amyloidosis. Before the identification of the causative gene, FMF was defined purely clinically; clinical features remain an important part of the diagnosis, because some patients with typical disease have only one, or sometimes no, demonstrable mutation in *MEFV*, the only known causative gene.

EPIDEMIOLOGY

FMF is most common in individuals of Jewish, Arab, Armenian, Turkish, and Italian ancestry. The frequency of asymptomatic carriers of a single *MEFV* mutation in these populations is as high as 1 in 5, a finding that suggests a selective advantage for heterozygotes. With genetic testing, FMF is now frequently recognized in both Ashkenazi (eastern European) and non-Ashkenazi Jewish populations, as well as in Mediterranean populations previously thought not to be at risk. Mutation-positive individuals with typical symptoms have been documented worldwide. FMF usually manifests in childhood, sometimes even in infancy, although approximately 10% of patients experience their first attack as adults; infrequently, FMF first occurs in persons older than 40 years.

PATHOBIOLOGY

MEFV, the gene for FMF, was identified by positional cloning in 1997, and it encodes a 781–amino acid protein denoted pyrin (or marenostrin) that is expressed in granulocytes, monocytes, and dendritic cells, as well as in peritoneal, synovial, and dermal fibroblasts. The N-terminal 92 amino acids of pyrin are the prototype for a motif, the PYRIN domain, that is involved in protein-protein interactions; this domain defines a family of more than 20 human proteins, including pyrin itself, involved in the regulation of cytokine production (particularly the interleukin-1 [IL-1] family), nuclear factor kappa B (NF-κB) activation, and apoptosis. More than 50 FMF-associated mutations in pyrin have been identified, many of which reside in the C-terminal domain encoded by exon 10 of *MEFV.*

CLINICAL MANIFESTATIONS

Episodes of FMF are more properly termed recurrent than periodic, and some patients associate attacks with psychological stress or physical exertion. Women of childbearing age sometimes experience their attacks with menses, with remissions during pregnancy. Some patients are unaware of fever during the attacks, but it is almost always observed when sought.

Serosal involvement in FMF is usually peritoneal or pleural. Abdominal attacks are the most frequent, and they may vary from mild discomfort to frank peritonitis, with board-like rigidity, direct and rebound tenderness, and air-fluid levels on upright films of the abdomen. Regardless of the severity of the abdominal attack, constipation is much more common than diarrhea. When a laparotomy or laparoscopy is performed during an attack, a small amount of sterile exudate rich in polymorphonuclear leukocytes is found. Except for serosal inflammation, the appendix is normal. Repeated abdominal attacks may cause peritoneal adhesions, but ascites is rare. Pleurisy, usually unilateral, may accompany abdominal pain, or it may occur independently. Physical findings, if present, may include diminished breath sounds and a friction rub, whereas radiographs may show a small effusion or atelectasis. With multiple attacks, pleural thickening may develop. Symptomatic nonuremic pericardial involvement in FMF has been reported but is unusual.

In adults, the arthritis of FMF typically manifests as monoarticular involvement of the knee, hip, or ankle, and attacks of arthritis may persist for up to 1 week at a time. In children, oligoarticular or polyarticular joint involvement may occur. Large joint effusions are sometimes present, and the synovial fluid may have as many as 100,000 leukocytes/mm^3. In approximately 5% of patients who are not treated with prophylactic colchicine, chronic arthritis (usually of the hip or knee) may develop, often necessitating joint replacement surgery. Regardless of colchicine treatment or a particular human leukocyte antigen (HLA-B27) status, some patients with FMF develop sacroiliitis. Arthralgia without frank arthritis is common in FMF.

Cutaneous manifestations of FMF tend to be less common than serosal or synovial involvement. The characteristic skin lesion of FMF is erysipeloid erythema, a painful, demarcated erythematous area most often seen on the lower leg, ankle, or dorsum of the foot. This rash may occur independently, or it may accompany an episode of arthritis. Histologically, one sees a mixed perivascular cellular infiltrate. Other acute manifestations of FMF include unilateral scrotal inflammation (the tunica vaginalis is an embryologic remnant of the peritoneal membrane) and myalgia, either with fever or, especially in children, without fever and induced by vigorous exercise. Various forms of vasculitis have also been associated with FMF; Henoch-Schönlein purpura may occur in children with FMF; less frequently, polyarteritis nodosum is seen.

COMPLICATIONS

Before the widespread use of colchicine prophylaxis, systemic AA amyloidosis (Chapter 194) was a frequent complication of FMF, caused by the ectopic deposition of a misfolded fragment of serum amyloid A (SAA), an acute phase reactant, in the gastrointestinal tract, kidneys, spleen, lung, testes, and adrenals. Malabsorption and nephrotic proteinuria leading to renal failure are the most common manifestations of AA amyloidosis. Cardiomyopathy is less common, and neuropathy and arthropathy are rare. Several risk factors for amyloidosis development in FMF have been identified, including late diagnosis of FMF, colchicine noncompliance, male gender, and specific genotypes of the *MEFV* and *SAA* genes. Amyloidosis in FMF is less common in the United States than in the Middle East. Abdominal fat aspirates are much less sensitive than rectal or renal biopsy in detecting the amyloidosis of FMF. The latter procedure may be preferred, because of the increasing recognition of nonamyloid glomerular disease in FMF. With early diagnosis, aggressive suppression of the acute phase response with colchicine or adjunctive agents may lead to improvement, but for patients with renal failure, early renal transplantation is preferred.

DIAGNOSIS

Based on a simple recessive model of inheritance, two mutations in *MEFV,* in *trans,* should be identified to establish the genetic diagnosis of FMF. Nevertheless, the interpretation of genetic testing is complicated by complex alleles consisting of various combinations of mutations in *cis,* as well as by the

observations that as many as one third of patients with clinically typical FMF have only one demonstrable mutation in *MEFV,* and a few patients with typical disease have no identifiable *MEFV* mutations. These latter two findings suggest that, under some circumstances, one *MEFV* mutation may be sufficient for symptoms or that additional genes for FMF exist.

For these reasons, clinical data remain an essential part of the diagnosis of FMF, and genetic testing plays an adjunctive role in settings where clinical experience is limited. Clinical criteria emphasize attack duration (12 to 72 hours); recurrence of symptoms (three or more episodes); documented fever (rectal temperature >38° C); painful manifestations in the abdomen, chest, joints, or skin; and the absence of other causative factors. The differential diagnosis includes the other hereditary recurrent fever syndromes (Table 269-2), as well as other conditions specific to the clinical setting. For patients with recurrent abdominal pain, considerations include gynecologic disorders, porphyria (Chapter 217; which can be distinguished by hypertension during attacks, dominant inheritance, and urine porphyrins), and hereditary angioedema (Chapter 260; which usually does not cause fever). The syndrome of periodic fever with aphthous stomatitis, pharyngitis, and cervical adenopathy is probably the most common cause of unexplained recurrent fever in children and is also included in the differential diagnosis. In patients presenting primarily with recurrent monoarthritis, joint aspiration for cultures and crystals may aid in excluding bacterial and crystalline arthritis, respectively.

Still's disease in children (systemic-onset juvenile idiopathic arthritis) and adults (adult-onset Still's disease) is also considered in the differential diagnosis. Adult-onset Still's disease (see Table 269-1) is an uncommon autoinflammatory condition of unknown cause that is not considered to be hereditary. It is characterized by spiking fever, an evanescent salmon-pink maculopapular rash, arthritis, and neutrophilic leukocytosis. It can be clinically distinguished from FMF by the pattern of fever (intermittent quotidian in Still's disease vs. discrete episodes in FMF), the pattern of arthritis (chronic polyarthritis vs. intermittent monoarthritis), the characteristic skin involvement (evanescent rash vs. erysipeloid erythema), and the presence of lymphadenopathy (more common in Still's disease).

TREATMENT   **Rx**

The mainstay of therapy for FMF is daily oral colchicine, which can prevent both acute attacks of FMF and the development of systemic amyloidosis. Colchicine probably works by several mechanisms, including its effects on inhibiting leukocyte adhesion and modulating cytokine production. In adults, the therapeutic dose is 1.2 to 1.8 mg/day, and nearly 90% of patients note significant improvement at this dose. The major side effects are gastrointestinal, and they can usually be minimized by gradually increasing the dosage and avoiding milk products in patients who develop lactose intolerance. Most experts continue to prescribe colchicine to patients during pregnancy, with the recommendation that amniocentesis be performed to exclude trisomy 21, for which there may be a slightly increased risk. Use of colchicine in lactating women is considered safe. Intravenous colchicine should be used with extreme caution, if at all, in FMF, because fatal toxicity has been reported in patients already receiving oral colchicine who are given the drug intravenously. IL-1 inhibitors are investigational in patients who are poorly responsive to colchicine or who cannot tolerate therapeutic doses.

Tumor Necrosis Factor Receptor–Associated Periodic Syndrome

DEFINITION

Worldwide, the tumor necrosis factor (TNF) receptor–associated periodic syndrome (TRAPS) is the second most frequently diagnosed hereditary recurrent fever syndrome, behind FMF. TRAPS is defined by recurrent episodes of fever and localized inflammation, in many ways resembling FMF, but differing in key details (noted later) and caused by mutations in the 55-kD receptor for TNF (TNFRSF1A, TNFR1, p55, CD120a). Whereas a positive genetic test is not necessary to diagnose FMF, the diagnosis of TRAPS requires the identification of a TNF receptor mutation. One of the first well-characterized families with what was later defined as TRAPS was of Irish ancestry, and the condition was termed *familial Hibernian fever* to emphasize the ethnic background and clinical differences from FMF. However, with the discovery of TNF receptor mutations in families of other ancestries, the ethnically neutral TRAPS nomenclature was proposed.

TABLE 269-2 CLINICAL FEATURES OF THE HEREDITARY RECURRENT FEVER SYNDROMES

CLINICAL FEATURE	FMF	TRAPS	HIDS	FCAS	MWS	NOMID/CINCA
Typical ethnicity	Arab, Armenian, Italian, Jewish, Turkish	Any ethnicity	Dutch, other North European	European	European	Any
Attack duration	12-72 hr	Days to weeks	3-7 days	12-24 hr	1-2 days	Continuous, with flares
Abdominal attacks	Sterile peritonitis, constipation more often than diarrhea	Severe pain, vomiting, peritonitis	Sterile peritonitis, diarrhea, rarely constipation	Nausea	Abdominal pain	Not common
Pleural attacks	Common	Common	Rare	Not seen	Rare	Rare
Joint/bone involvement	Monoarthritis, rarely protracted arthritis in knee or hip	Arthritis in large joints, arthralgia	Arthralgia, symmetrical polyarthritis	Polyarthralgia	Polyarthralgia, oligoarthritis, clubbing	Epiphyseal overgrowth, contractures, intermittent or chronic arthritis, clubbing
Skin rash	Erysipeloid erythema on lower leg, ankle, foot	Migratory rash, underlying myalgia	Diffuse maculopapular rash, urticaria	Cold-induced urticaria-like rash	Urticaria-like rash	Urticaria-like rash
Lymphatic involvement	Splenomegaly, occasional lymphadenopathy	Splenomegaly, occasional lymphadenopathy	Cervical adenopathy in children	Not seen	Rare	Hepatosplenomegaly, adenopathy
Neurologic involvement	Aseptic meningitis?	Controversial	Headache	Headache	Sensorineural deafness	Sensorineural deafness, chronic aseptic meningitis, mental retardation, headache
Ophthalmologic involvement	Rare	Conjunctivitis, periorbital edema, rarely uveitis	Uncommon	Conjunctivitis	Conjunctivitis, episcleritis	Uveitis, conjunctivitis, progressive vision loss
Vasculitis	Henoch-Schönlein purpura (HSP), polyarteritis nodosa	HSP, lymphocytic vasculitis	Cutaneous vasculitis common, rarely HSP	Not seen	Not seen	Occasional
Systemic amyloidosis	Risk depends on *MEFV* and *SAA* genotypes; more common in Middle East	Occurs in ~10%; risk increased with cysteine mutations	Rare	Rare	Occurs in ~25%	May develop in some, usually in adulthood

FCAS = familial cold autoinflammatory syndrome; FMF = familial Mediterranean fever; HIDS = hyperimmunoglobulinemia D with periodic fever syndrome; MWS = Muckle-Wells syndrome; NOMID/CINCA = neonatal-onset multisystem inflammatory disease/chronic infantile neurologic cutaneous and articular syndrome; TRAPS = tumor necrosis factor receptor–associated periodic syndrome.

PATHOBIOLOGY

The p55 TNF receptor is composed of four cysteine-rich extracellular domains, a transmembrane region, and an intracellular death domain. To date, all of the more than 60 mutations described are in the extracellular domains, and approximately half are missense substitutions of cysteine residues that abolish highly conserved disulfide bonds. The initial description of TRAPS documented a defect in activation-induced ectodomain cleavage of the p55 receptor in patients with the C52F *TNFRSF1A* mutation, possibly leading to a defect in homeostasis by impaired downregulation of membrane receptors and diminished shedding of potentially antagonistic soluble receptor molecules. More recent studies indicate a more complex pathogenetic picture, because not all mutant receptors exhibit this shedding defect. Additional mechanisms by which p55 mutations may lead to autoinflammation include impaired leukocyte apoptosis and impaired intracellular receptor trafficking, with possible constitutive activation of mitogen-activated protein (MAP) kinases by intracellular aggregates of mutant receptors.

DIAGNOSIS

Although genetic testing is necessary for the diagnosis of TRAPS, certain clinical clues can help distinguish TRAPS from FMF. These include ethnicity (FMF is seen predominantly in Mediterranean and Middle Eastern populations, whereas TRAPS has a more widespread distribution), mode of inheritance (autosomal recessive in FMF, dominant in TRAPS), and duration of attacks, which tends to be longer in TRAPS and sometimes approaches continuous symptoms. The rash of FMF is typically erysipeloid erythema on the lower extremity, whereas patients with TRAPS often have a distinctive erythematous rash, often with underlying myalgia, which may migrate on the trunk or centrifugally on the extremities. Ocular involvement, with periorbital edema, conjunctivitis, and occasionally even uveitis, is observed in TRAPS but not in FMF. Finally, whereas colchicine is much more effective than corticosteroids in FMF, the opposite is true in TRAPS. Nevertheless, aside from the difference in duration and susceptibility to pharmacologic intervention, the abdominal, pleural, synovial, and even scrotal manifestations of the two diseases are rather similar. The usual age of onset for TRAPS is also in childhood, and systemic AA amyloidosis is seen in about 10% of untreated patients with TRAPS. As in FMF, life expectancy in TRAPS is normal in patients whose disease is not complicated by amyloidosis.

As noted earlier, the diagnosis of TRAPS is established by the identification of *TNFRSF1A* mutations in the appropriate clinical setting. One variant, the substitution of glutamine for arginine at residue 92 (R92Q), is present in more than 1% of whites and may be associated with a broader spectrum of symptoms than is typically seen in TRAPS, including early inflammatory arthritis or, in some cases, no symptoms at all. The substitution of lysine for proline at residue 46 (P46L) is common among African American patients with TRAPS and is associated with a receptor shedding defect, but it is also seen among healthy African American controls. These findings establish a "gray zone" for the diagnosis of TRAPS and emphasize the potential role of polymorphisms in the recurrent fever genes in other more common phenotypes.

TREATMENT   Rx

The treatment of TRAPS depends on the frequency and severity of attacks. Patients with relatively infrequent, mild episodes may respond to nonsteroidal anti-inflammatory drugs. Patients with more severe attacks that occur infrequently may be treated with corticosteroids, although increasing doses may be required as the episodes become more frequent, and toxicities may become limiting. For patients with severe attacks occurring once a month or more frequently, treatment with etanercept, the soluble p75 TNF receptor:Fc fusion protein, may be warranted. More recently, some patients with TRAPS who did not respond to TNF inhibition did respond to anakinra, the IL-1 receptor antagonist.

Hyperimmunoglobulinemia D with Periodic Fever Syndrome

DEFINITION AND EPIDEMIOLOGY

Hyperimmunoglobulinemia D with periodic fever syndrome (HIDS) was first described in 1984 as an FMF-like illness seen in six patients of Dutch ancestry. Besides the difference in ethnicity, a key distinction was the observation of extremely high levels of immunoglobulin D (IgD) in the serum of the Dutch patients, thus prompting the HIDS nomenclature. HIDS is now recognized in a broader ethnic distribution, although northern Europeans still predominate. Overall, HIDS is still quite rare.

PATHOBIOLOGY

Family studies documented autosomal recessive inheritance. In 1999, patients with HIDS were found to have mutations in *MVK*, which encodes the mevalonate kinase enzyme involved in the biosynthesis of cholesterol and nonsterol isoprenes. Enzyme activity in patients is markedly reduced, but not absent.

The elevated IgD levels seen in HIDS appear to be an epiphenomenon. They do not correlate with disease severity either among patients or in a given patient over time, although IgD may contribute to the release of proinflammatory cytokines in vitro. Moreover, modest elevations of IgD are seen in several inflammatory conditions, including chronic infections, and can be observed in other hereditary recurrent fever syndromes. Up to 20% of patients (particularly young children) with typical recurrent fevers and *MVK* mutations have normal serum IgD levels. Current data suggest that isoprenoid deficiency may play a more important pathogenic role in the pathophysiology of HIDS. In vitro studies suggest that isoprenoid deficiency may lead to excessive IL-1β production, and increased body temperature can further decrease mevalonate kinase enzymatic activity, thereby creating a vicious circle in which infection or immunization can precipitate HIDS attacks.

CLINICAL MANIFESTATIONS

One of the well-recognized clinical characteristics of HIDS is the provocation of attacks by immunizations. Other distinguishing clinical features include a very early age of onset (average age, 6 months), a duration of attacks intermediate between FMF and TRAPS (3 to 7 days), prominent cervical lymphadenopathy during attacks, polyarticular joint involvement, a diffuse maculopapular rash, the predominance of diarrhea over constipation with abdominal attacks, and the infrequency of pleuritic attacks or systemic amyloidosis.

DIAGNOSIS

Based on our current understanding of the genetics and pathophysiology of HIDS, the diagnosis can be established in a patient with recurrent episodes of fever and typical associated findings by documenting either two mutations in *MVK* or elevated levels of mevalonic acid, the substrate for mevalonate kinase, in the urine during attacks. Approximately 10% of patients with otherwise typical disease have only a single identifiable *MVK* mutation. The significance of elevated IgD without genetic or biochemical findings remains unknown.

TREATMENT AND PROGNOSIS **Rx**

Nonsteroidal anti-inflammatory drugs or corticosteroids are sometimes useful in the treatment of the arthritic manifestations of HIDS. Colchicine is generally not effective. Numerous agents are investigational in HIDS, including the statins, TNF inhibitors, and IL-1 receptor antagonists. Patients with HIDS have a normal lifespan, and attacks may become somewhat less frequent in adulthood.

Cryopyrin-Associated Periodic Syndromes: The Cryopyrinopathies

Three rare, recurrent febrile disorders usually beginning early in life have been associated with mutations in *NLRP3* (formerly *CIAS1*), the gene encoding a protein variously named cryopyrin, NLRP3, NALP3, PYPAF1, or CATERPILLER 1.1. The least severe clinical phenotype is familial cold autoinflammatory syndrome (FCAS; formerly called familial cold urticaria), which is dominantly inherited and is notable for day-long attacks of chills, fever, headache, diffuse urticarial skin rash, arthralgia, and conjunctivitis, precipitated by generalized cold exposure. Amyloidosis is rare in FCAS. Of intermediate severity is Muckle-Wells syndrome (MWS), also dominantly inherited, in which 1- to 2-day episodes of chills, fever, urticarial rash, limb pain, and arthritis occur independently of cold exposure. Sensorineural hearing loss is common in MWS, and systemic amyloidosis may also occur. The most severe *NLRP3*-associated phenotype is neonatal-onset multisystem inflammatory disease (NOMID), known in Europe as chronic infantile neurologic cutaneous and articular (CINCA) syndrome. It is usually sporadic owing to the reduced reproductive fitness of most affected individuals. Fever and constitutional symptoms occur almost daily, often from birth, with generalized urticarial skin rash, a peculiar arthropathy characterized by epiphyseal overgrowth of the long bones, and central nervous system involvement that includes chronic aseptic meningitis, uveitis, and cochlear inflammation, which may lead to mental retardation, blindness, and deafness. In all three cryopyrinopathies, the rash is not true urticaria because there is a neutrophilic rather than a mast cell infiltrate, and serum histamine levels are normal.

The protein mutated in all three disorders is a critical component of a newly recognized macromolecular complex termed the *inflammasome*, which serves as an intracellular scaffold for the processing of IL-1β from its 31-kD precursor form to the biologically active 17-kD form. Cryopyrin is so named because it has an amino-terminal PYRIN domain; thus it bears a structural and functional relationship to the protein mutated in FMF. Disease-associated cryopyrin mutations are thought to decrease the threshold for inflammasome activation, thereby increasing IL-1β production. In vitro studies also suggest a role for cryopyrin/NALP3 in NF-κB activation and apoptosis.

Because there are patients with FCAS, MWS, and NOMID/CINCA without demonstrable *NLRP3* mutations, these diagnoses remain clinical, although genetic testing serves as a valuable adjunct and has greatly increased the recognition of all three conditions. In addition, overlap syndromes that are intermediate between FCAS and MWS and between MWS and NOMID/CINCA have been reported.

Data indicate that IL-1 blockade with anakinra, the IL-1 receptor antagonist, appears to be effective in controlling fever and acute phase reactants in all three cryopyrinopathies. Moreover, in a large series completed at the National Institutes of Health, anakinra markedly decreased central nervous system inflammation in NOMID/CINCA. Recent studies have also documented the efficacy of two other IL-1 inhibitors, rilonacept and canakinumab, in FCAS and MWS. Such data suggest that the major biologic effect of cryopyrin in humans is mediated through IL-1β rather than by other distinct inflammatory pathways.

OTHER INHERITED SYSTEMIC AUTOINFLAMMATORY DISEASES

Deficiency of Interleukin-1 Receptor Antagonist

Deficiency of the IL-1 receptor antagonist (DIRA) is a newly described clinical entity characterized by the neonatal onset of a pustular skin rash, multifocal osteomyelitis, periostitis, and, rarely, vasculitis. Fever is not a prominent finding, although acute phase reactants are markedly elevated. DIRA is caused by recessively inherited loss-of-function mutations in *IL1RN*, which encodes the IL-1 receptor antagonist (IL-1Ra). Patients usually present within the first 2 weeks of life with skin lesions ranging from discrete crops of pustules to generalized severe pustulosis or ichthyosiform lesions. Histologic examination demonstrates extensive neutrophilic infiltrates in the dermis and epidermis. Typical radiographic findings include multifocal osteolytic lesions, periosteal elevation of the long bones, heterotopic ossification of the proximal femurs, and widening of the anterior rib ends. Bone biopsies demonstrate sterile purulent osteomyelitis, fibrosis, and sclerosis. To date, four different *IL1RN* mutations have been identified, three of which are truncating point mutations that drastically reduce IL-1Ra messenger RNA and protein levels. The fourth is a 175-kilobase genomic deletion in chromosome 2q that subsumes *IL1RN* and five other genes in the IL-1 family. In DIRA, the lack of IL-1Ra leads to unopposed IL-1β and IL-1α signaling, whereas in the cryopyrinopathies, *NLRP3* mutations lead to inflammasome activation and increased IL-1β production. DIRA patients respond dramatically to anakinra, the recombinant form of the protein they lack.

Syndrome of Pyogenic Arthritis with Pyoderma Gangrenosum and Acne

The syndrome of pyogenic arthritis with pyoderma gangrenosum and acne (PAPA) is a rare, dominantly inherited autoinflammatory disease characterized by intermittent episodes of sterile pyogenic arthritis, pyoderma gangrenosum, and severe cystic acne. It is caused by mutations in proline-serine-threonine phosphatase–interacting protein 1 (PSTPIP1), also known as CD2BP1. PSTPIP1 is a cytoskeletal protein that interacts with certain other proteins involved in the immune response, including CD2; the

Wiskott-Aldrich syndrome protein (WASP); a phosphatase denoted PTP-PEST; and pyrin, the FMF protein. PAPA mutations abrogate the binding of PSTPIP1 to PTP-PEST, leading to hyperphosphorylation of PSTPIP1 and increased binding to pyrin. Both in patients and in cell lines, this finding is associated with markedly increased IL-1β production. Early in life, PAPA tends to present with monoarticular or pauciarticular pyogenic arthritis, sometimes induced by trauma. In the absence of treatment, arthritis may progress to severe joint damage and ankylosis. As patients reach puberty, skin manifestations begin to predominate, including disfiguring cystic acne. Pathergy may also develop, and extensive pyoderma gangrenosum may require opiates for pain control. The diagnosis of PAPA syndrome is made by documenting *PSTPIP1* mutations in the appropriate clinical setting. High doses of corticosteroids have been used in PAPA, with varying success, and patients with arthritis sometimes require aspiration, intra-articular corticosteroids, or open drainage. Newer investigational approaches for PAPA syndrome focus on the use of targeted cytokine inhibitors. Anecdotal evidence supports the use of anakinra for the arthritis and infliximab for the pyoderma gangrenosum of PAPA.

Granulomatous Inflammatory Arthritis, Dermatitis, and Uveitis (Blau's Syndrome)

Blau's syndrome is a rare, dominantly inherited illness characterized by the following features: early-onset granulomatous synovitis often complicated by cyst formation and camptodactyly (flexion contractures of the fingers and toes); granulomatous anterior and posterior uveitis, sometimes causing retinal detachment, glaucoma, cataracts, and blindness; and an intermittent papular rash with noncaseating granulomas. Lung or other visceral involvement is generally not present. However, visceral involvement of the liver and spleen is observed in early-onset sarcoidosis (Chapter 95), which is phenotypically quite similar to Blau's syndrome. Both Blau's syndrome and some cases of early-onset sarcoidosis are caused by mutations in *NOD2/CARD15*. Distinct variants of *NOD2/CARD15* have been associated with susceptibility to Crohn's disease, which manifests as granulomatous inflammation of the gastrointestinal tract (Chapter 143). The protein encoded by this gene is thought to be an intracellular sensor of bacterial products. Crohn's disease–associated mutations in the ligand-binding, leucine-rich repeat region of the protein may require bacterial contact in the gastrointestinal tract to cause inflammation, whereas Blau's syndrome mutations in the nucleotide binding domain may lead to constitutive extraintestinal inflammation. Topical and systemic corticosteroids are currently the mainstay of treatment of Blau's syndrome.

SUGGESTED READINGS

Henderson C, Goldbach-Mansky R. Monogenic autoinflammatory diseases: new insights into clinical aspects and pathogenesis. *Curr Opin Rheumatol.* 2010;22:567-578. *Comprehensive review.*

Jacobs Z, Ciaccio CE. Periodic fever syndromes. *Curr Allergy Asthma Rep.* 2010;10:393-404. *Consensus review.*

Shohat M, Halpern GJ. Familial Mediterranean fever—a review. *Genet Med.* 2011. [Epub ahead of print.] *Review of types 1 and 2, including recommendations of lifelong treatment with colchicines for homozygotes and compound heterozygotes.*

Wurster VM, Carlucci JG, Edwards KM. Periodic fever syndromes. *Pediatr Ann.* 2011;40:48-54. *Review.*

270

OSTEOARTHRITIS

NANCY E. LANE AND THOMAS J. SCHNITZER

DEFINITION

Osteoarthritis (OA) is a disorder of diarthrodial joints that is characterized clinically by pain and functional limitations, radiographically by osteophytes and joint space narrowing, and histopathologically by alterations in cartilage and subchondral bone integrity. OA is the most common of all joint diseases, and its importance derives from its economic impact, in terms of both productivity (single greatest cause of days lost from work) and cost of treatment (chronic use of analgesics and anti-inflammatory drugs). Although the etiology of OA is still not clearly understood, it has been shown to be a family of disorders with cartilage as a target organ in which biomechanical factors play a central role and risk factors such as age, weight, and occupation are also of major importance. Because there is currently no treatment to prevent or ameliorate the basic disease process, medical treatment is aimed primarily at relieving pain and improving joint function, with orthopedic intervention largely reserved for those situations that cannot be controlled with more conservative therapy.

EPIDEMIOLOGY

OA is by far the most common joint disorder, one of the most common chronic diseases in elderly people, and a leading cause of disability. Because OA can be defined both radiographically and clinically, with little correlation between the two, the prevalence of this condition has been variously estimated in epidemiologic studies. Using radiographic criteria, the prevalence of the joint findings of OA steadily increases, from less than 2% in women younger than 45 years of age, to 30% in those aged 45 to 64 years, and to 68% in those older than 65 years of age. Prevalence in men is slightly higher in the younger age groups (<45 years of age), whereas women are affected more commonly at ages older than 55 years, except for disease of the hip.

The pattern of joint involvement in OA is strikingly affected by age, gender, previous joint injury, and occupational history. Before age 55 years, there is little difference in joint pattern between men and women. In older men, hip OA is more common, whereas older women tend to have more involvement of the proximal interphalangeal (PIP) joints and the base of the thumb (first carpometacarpal [CMC] joint). Joints subjected to repeated trauma or overuse demonstrate a higher prevalence of OA. Cotton and mill workers have increased OA of the hand and involved fingers; miners and warehouse workers who bend, squat, and lift heavy loads frequently demonstrate increased knee and spine involvement; and pneumatic drill workers experience increased elbow and wrist disease.

Racial and genetic factors are also important in OA prevalence and pattern. Chinese, Jamaican blacks, South African blacks, and Asian Indians have a lower incidence of OA of the hip than whites, whereas Japanese have an increased incidence, apparently related to the more frequent occurrence of congenital hip dysplasia. Black women have a higher prevalence of knee OA than white women but a lower prevalence of involvement of the distal interphalangeal (DIP) joints of the hand (Heberden's nodes). Involvement of the DIP joints of the hands is particularly common in women and is often found to have a familial pattern of inheritance; female relatives of a proband have similar joint findings with a two- to five-fold increased prevalence.

Large cohort studies of subjects with radiographic evidence of OA report a significant genetic contribution to the disorder. A heritable component of OA is reported from family and twin studies to be between 60 and 65%, and the genetic predisposition appears to differ by OA site. Single nucleotide polymorphisms in genes that code for structural proteins in the extracellular matrix (e.g., collagen type II), hormones and growth factors that influence cartilage and bone metabolism (vitamin D receptor, estrogen receptor a, insulin-like growth factor-1, and frizzled-related protein), and cell signaling proteins involved with joint development increase the risk of OA in weight-bearing joints.

Modifiable risk factors for OA have also been identified in recent studies. Increased weight is the most significant independent predictor of both incidence and progression of OA in weight-bearing joints, and weight reduction has been shown to reduce the development and progression of knee OA. Certain types of high-impact repetitive activities are associated with an increased risk for development of OA in the stressed joint (see earlier discussion), whereas other activities are not. In particular, there appears to be an increased risk of hip and knee OA in elite, highly competitive runners, but no increased prevalence in participants in low-impact activities such as marathon running. However, this difference may be the result of a self-selection process in which those individuals who experience knee pain are unable to continue the activity. Smoking and osteoporosis have both been shown to be negatively associated with OA, but the explanations for these associations are unknown.

PATHOBIOLOGY
Pathology

The hallmarks of OA on gross or arthroscopic examination are focal ulcerated areas of cartilage exposing underlying eburnated (ivory-appearing) bone that occur at the load-bearing areas of the joint surface, as well as juxta-articular osteophytes that grow at the joint margins. These states represent the end stage of the continuum of OA as a pathologic process. At its earliest stage, it manifests as softening of the cartilage surface, progressing to fibrillation of the surface layers, loss of cartilage thickness, development of clefts into the depth of cartilage, and eventual loss of cartilage integrity with release of shards of cartilage. Bone participates in this process as well, with reactive changes (bony subchondral sclerosis) underlying the areas of cartilage loss, development of subchondral bone cysts that may communicate with the joint space and expand into geodes, and marginal osteophytes (new cartilage and bone growth) at non–weight-bearing areas. Magnetic resonance imaging (MRI) has identified additional alterations in bone associated with OA progression accompanied by pain.

The earliest histologic changes in OA reveal loss of extracellular cartilage matrix, loss of chondrocytes in the surface layers of articular cartilage, and reactive changes in the deeper chondrocytes manifested by cellular division and "cloning" in an apparent attempt at repair. Later, there is progressive loss of chondrocytes at all levels, with marked thinning of the cartilage matrix and, in some instances, development of fibrocartilage in place of lost hyaline articular cartilage. The surrounding synovium is largely unaffected, although in later disease, cartilage fragments may incite focal inflammatory lesions without the progressive and destructive pannus seen in typical inflammatory arthropathies.

Pathogenesis

Articular cartilage serves two major functions: (1) to permit nearly frictionless joint motion; and (2) to act as a "shock absorber" and transmit loads across joint surfaces to the surrounding tissues. The requisite properties of elasticity and high tensile strength are imparted by proteoglycans and collagen of the extracellular matrix, which comprise more than 90% of the cartilage macromolecules. The proteoglycan elements of the matrix are actively metabolized and turned over, with a half-life of weeks. The highly negatively charged sulfated glycosaminoglycan components of the proteoglycans impart the elastic properties to cartilage. The collagen component of cartilage matrix is characterized by a unique structure (type II collagen) that provides the tensile strength and tightly constrains the proteoglycan molecules in a three-dimensional framework. The collagen fibers are covalently linked by other matrix molecules, which are believed to provide the "glue" to hold the matrix intact. Collagen itself is metabolized very slowly (half-life of many years) in the normal state.

In OA, there is an initial phase in which chondrocyte metabolic activity is upregulated (enhanced proteoglycan synthesis), followed by eventual chondrocyte loss (apoptosis). The reason for failure of repair is unclear but may relate to the inability to re-form, once it is disrupted, the three-dimensional architecture of cartilage in mature individuals.

Degradation of collagen and proteoglycans in OA is carried out by proteolytic enzymes (matrix metalloproteinases [MMPs]) that are synthesized by and released from the chondrocytes themselves. A number of cytokines and other mediators of inflammation, including interleukin-1β (IL-1β), tumor necrosis factor-α (TNF-α), IL-6, IL-8, nitric oxide (NO), and prostaglandins, can be produced by the chondrocyte and act within the cartilage to promote a catabolic state by activating MMPs. The subsequent activation of these potent enzymes overwhelms the natural matrix defenses and ultimately results in collagen breakdown and proteoglycan cleavage. Fragments from these molecules are then released into the synovial fluid and enter the circulation, where they provide "markers" of degradation and can be used as a means to detect and measure disease activity.

The factors responsible for activating chondrocytes to release MMPs are currently being elucidated. However, those conditions that cause alteration in biomechanical loading of cartilage are known to lead to OA: joint injury; abnormal joint loading due to neuropathic changes (Charcot's joint); ligamentous damage (anterior cruciate ligament [ACL]) or meniscus injuries; altered joint surface congruity, as in dysplasias or malalignment or joint laxity; and muscle atrophy in elderly people. A number of metabolic conditions are known to predispose to the early onset of OA, including ochronosis with the deposition of homogentisic acid (Chapter 212) and hemochromatosis with the deposition of iron (Chapter 219). Gene defects affecting matrix structures might be expected to lead to OA, but thus far genetic factors have been shown to play a role only in the development of dysplasias with secondary OA. The pathogenetic mechanisms and feedback loops associated with structural damage to the cartilage structure and associated alteration in chondrocyte function are demonstrated in Figure 270-1.

FIGURE 270-1. Summary of the pathophysiology of osteoarthritis with emphases on structural damage to the cartilage and alteration in chondrocyte function. MMP = metalloproteinase.

CLINICAL MANIFESTATIONS

The initial stages of the OA disease process are clinically silent, which explains the high prevalence of radiographic and pathologic signs of OA in clinically asymptomatic patients. Even in later stages of OA, there is a poor correlation between clinical symptoms and alterations in cartilage and bone integrity, defined arthroscopically or by indirect imaging techniques (radiography, MRI). The factors or events that make the OA disease process clinically apparent are unknown but are likely to be heterogeneous in nature and invoke changes within the synovium, bone, and surrounding supporting structures (muscle, ligaments) that produce pain. Pain does not derive from cartilage, a tissue without any innervation.

Pain is the predominant symptom that prompts the diagnosis of OA; often only one joint is involved initially, with others becoming painful subsequently. The pain of OA is most often described as a deep ache, accompanied frequently by joint stiffness after periods of inactivity (on arising in the morning or after sitting). Pain is aggravated by use of the involved joints, may radiate, and may be referred to surrounding structures. In the early stages of the disease, pain is commonly relieved by rest. With more severe disease, pain may be persistent, interfering with normal function and preventing sleep, even with medical management. Even in severe disease, however, systemic manifestations such as fever, weight loss, anemia, and elevated erythrocyte sedimentation rate (ESR) are not present.

The joints most commonly involved in OA are the metatarsophalangeal (MTP) joint of the great toe (hallux valgus or "bunion"); the PIP and DIP joints of the fingers, the CMC joint of the thumb, hips, knees, and the lumbar and cervical spine (Fig. 270-2). Other joints, even major weight-bearing joints such as the ankle, are typically spared unless involved in secondary forms of OA (Table 270-1). On physical examination, the joints may demonstrate tenderness, crepitus, and a limited range of motion. Joint swelling may be caused by an accompanying synovial effusion or by bony enlargement and the presence of osteophytes. Joint instability is seen only in severe disease or after internal derangement of the knee with disruption of one or more of the major supporting structures (e.g., ACL, medial collateral ligament). Patients with far-advanced disease exhibit gross deformity with subluxation of the involved joints. Although OA is thought to be a uniformly progressive disease that invariably leads to joint replacement, this is not the case. The disease appears to stabilize in many patients, with no worsening of signs or symptoms, and there may be actual improvement in some patients.

Specific Joint Involvement
Hand

Firm, slowly progressive bony enlargements of the DIP joints are called *Heberden's nodes* and represent marginal osteophytic spurs (Fig. 270-3). Occasionally, the onset of symptoms in the hand is acute, with sudden

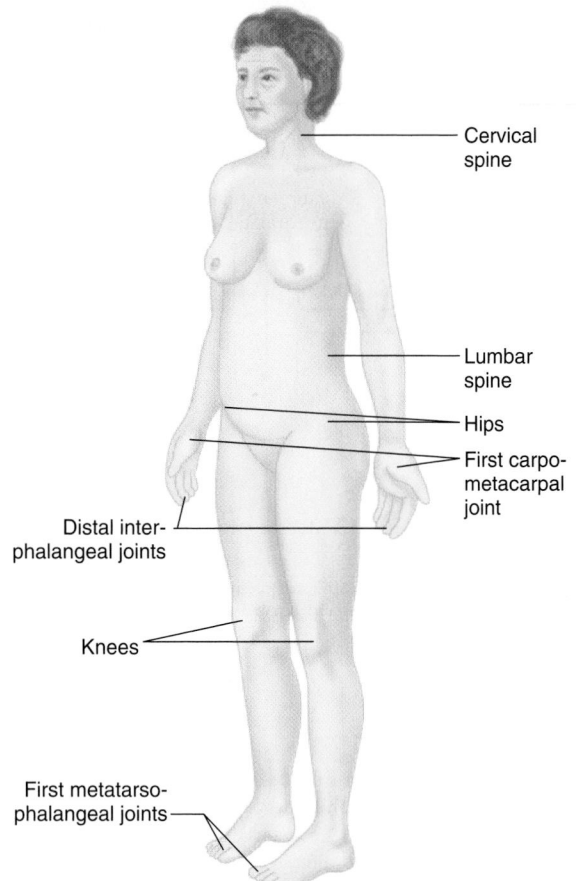

Cervical spine

Lumbar spine

Hips

First carpo-metacarpal joint

Distal inter-phalangeal joints

Knees

First metatarso-phalangeal joints

FIGURE 270-2. Joints commonly affected by osteoarthritis.

TABLE 270-1	**ETIOLOGIC CLASSIFICATION OF OSTEOARTHRITIS**

IDIOPATHIC (PRIMARY)

Localized
  Hands: Heberden's nodes, erosive interphalangeal arthropathy
  Feet: hallux valgus, hammer toes; talonavicular
  Knees: medial, lateral, patellofemoral compartments
  Hips: sites of cartilage loss—eccentric (superior), concentric (axial, medial), diffuse, and femoral osteophytes
  Spine: zygapophyseal joints, intervertebral discs (spondylosis); ligaments (e.g., disseminated idiopathic skeletal hyperostosis) with osteophytes as most common radiographic findings
  Other single sites: shoulder, temporomandibular joints, carpometacarpal joints
Generalized—includes three or more areas listed above
Mineral deposition diseases
  Calcium pyrophosphate deposition disease
  Hydroxyapatite arthropathy
Destructive disease (e.g., Milwaukee shoulder)

SECONDARY

Post-traumatic
Congenital or developmental
  Legg-Calvé-Perthes hip dislocation
  Epiphyseal dysplasias
  Articular cartilage disorders associated with a gene deficiency (e.g., association with type II procollagen gene mutation)
Disturbed local tissue structure by primary disease (e.g., ischemic necrosis, tophaceous gout, hyperparathyroid cysts, Paget's disease, rheumatoid arthritis, osteopetrosis, osteochondritis)
Miscellaneous additional diseases
  Endocrine: diabetes mellitus, acromegaly, hypothyroidism
  Metabolic: hemochromatosis, ochronosis, Gaucher's disease
  Neuropathic arthropathies
  Miscellaneous: frostbite, Kashin-Beck disease, caisson disease
  Mechanical: obesity, unequal lower extremity length; valgus/varus deformities, ligamentous laxity (including associations with type I procollagen gene mutations of Ehlers-Danlos syndrome)

Compiled in part by Osteoarthritis Diagnostic Criteria Committee, American Rheumatism Association, 1983.

FIGURE 270-3. **Typical hand deformities in osteoarthritis.** Heberden's nodes are seen on the distal interphalangeal joints, and Bouchard's nodes are at the proximal interphalangeal joints. (From Forbes CD, Jackson WF. *Color Atlas and Text of Clinical Medicine*, 3rd ed. London: Mosby; 2003).

redness and tenderness in the involved joint. These changes can lead to deformity, with lateral and flexor deviation at these joints. A related disorder, erosive OA, is associated with repetitive episodes of acute symptoms and is differentiated by the additional finding of erosive changes on radiographs of the involved joints and a tendency to bony ankylosis. A genetic basis for Heberden's nodes appears to exist, the condition demonstrating a distinct female-dominant familial tendency (women are affected 10 times more commonly than men).

Changes similar to those in the DIP joints occur in the PIP joints and are termed *Bouchard's nodes* (see Fig. 270-3). The only other hand joint to be commonly involved is the CMC joint of the thumb. Patients often complain of pain on use of the thumb, as in wringing out clothes (washerwoman's hands) or grasping objects such as screwdrivers and doorknobs. The condition leads to a squared appearance of the base of the hand.

Knee

Idiopathic knee OA is a leading cause of painful ambulation and is more common in women than in men. The medial compartment of the femorotibial joint space is most commonly affected, resulting in varus deformity (bow legs). Lateral compartment disease may lead to valgus deformity (knock-knee). Patellofemoral disease is also common and may represent a substantial portion of knee pathology in patients presenting with knee pain. It is important to exclude other causes of knee pain, such as internal derangements of the knee (e.g., meniscal tears, ligament tears) that may lead to secondary knee OA; soft tissue sprains; bursal inflammation; and Baker's cysts (which may coexist with knee OA). In young women, the possibility of chondromalacia patellae should always be considered. Its cause is not known; it is almost always self-limited and is not thought to lead to OA. In idiopathic knee OA, physical examination of the involved joint often elicits crepitation of the tibiofemoral joint, pain, and decreased range of motion. Effusions are not infrequently present but are often small and may be difficult to appreciate.

Hip

Although congenital (Legg-Calvé-Perthes disease) and developmental (slipped femoral capital epiphysis) abnormalities have long been implicated in secondary hip OA, most cases of primary hip OA are now believed to be the consequence of mild dysplasia of the femoral head or acetabulum resulting in incongruity of the articulating surfaces. With use of the joint, there is progressive cartilage degeneration and secondary bony productive changes typical of OA. Pain is usually referred to the groin, with anterior thigh and knee symptoms occasionally predominant. Many patients presenting with pain in their "hip" may have referred pain from degenerative disc disease or OA of the lumbar spine. The earliest physical finding in hip OA is loss of internal rotation; with progressive disease, range of motion is limited further in all directions, the affected leg shortens, and significant functional limitation occurs, often necessitating surgery.

Foot

The first MTP joint is the primary foot joint involved in OA, with associated bony swelling and deformity (bunion). Significantly more common in women than men, these changes have been attributed to abnormal stresses imposed on the joint by footwear. In extreme cases, the joint space may be destroyed, leading to a condition known as *hallux rigidus*, which may interfere with normal ambulation and necessitate surgical correction.

Spine

Technically, OA of the spine relates strictly to changes in synovium-lined joints (apophyseal and uncovertebral joints) that can lead to localized pain as well as irritation of adjacent nerve roots with referred pain in the form of radiculopathy. Nerve root compression resulting from apophyseal joint subluxation, prolapse of an intervertebral disc, or osteophytic spurring may occur, and the patient may present with muscle weakness, hyporeflexia, and paresthesia or hypesthesia. In the cervical region, spinal involvement can lead to cord impingement with long tract signs, or it may affect the vertebral artery, producing insufficiency of the posterior circulation with associated symptoms (Chapter 414). OA of the spine should be differentiated from diffuse skeletal hyperostosis, in which there is marked calcification of the paraspinous ligaments and sparing of the arthrodial spinal joints.

Primary Generalized Osteoarthritis

The pattern of involvement of three or more joints or joint groups with OA has been given the name *primary generalized osteoarthritis*; it is seen most commonly in older women. Typically, the DIP and PIP joints of the hand, the knees, and the spine are involved. Whether this represents a distinct subset of OA is not known but has been suggested.

DIAGNOSIS

Laboratory Findings

OA involves a pathologic process that appears largely limited to the joint and associated tissues, with no evidence of systemic involvement. Typically, the ESR is normal, and there is no elevation of acute phase reactants. The hemoglobin and leukocyte counts remain within normal limits. The synovial fluid itself demonstrates no evidence of an inflammatory reaction, with few leukocytes (typically fewer than $2000/mm^3$) and good viscosity. Occasionally, fragments of cartilage and crystals of calcium hydroxyapatite or calcium pyrophosphate dihydrate are seen in the synovial fluid. Rheumatoid factor is absent in most patients with OA, but a significant number of older individuals exhibit low-titer elevations that are not diagnostic of rheumatoid arthritis but are a common accompaniment of aging.

Cartilage matrix components unique to the joints have been identified, and sensitive assays have been developed to detect these "biomarkers" in synovial fluid, serum, and urine. Further clinical correlations need to be performed to determine the relationship of these biomarkers to the disease process, activity, and state, and their possible use for earlier diagnosis and management of OA.

Radiology Findings

Pathognomonic findings of OA on plain radiography include the presence of osteophytes at the margins of involved joints, associated joint space narrowing representing areas of cartilage thinning or loss, and evidence of bony reaction marked by subchondral sclerosis and bone cysts in more progressive disease. Some patients may lack one or more of these findings.

Radiography has been shown to be insensitive to the pathologic processes occurring in the cartilage. Many patients exhibit normal radiographs with destructive cartilage changes documented by arthroscopy. However, performing a weight-bearing knee radiograph with the knee flexed to 20 degrees allows a more reliable assessment of joint space narrowing, and repeat radiographs in this view can be used to assess changes in joint space narrowing over time.

Imaging

Other techniques have been developed with greater potential sensitivity to detect cartilage and bone changes. In particular, MRI has the advantage of demonstrating cartilage as a positive image and has been used widely to document major cartilage injuries such as meniscal tears and to provide a quantitative estimate of cartilage volume. MRI has identified distinctive changes in bone, often adjacent to cartilage lesions, which are associated with pain, altered mechanical loading, and enhanced disease progression. Further refinement of this technology will be important in the future for assessing disease progression and the efficacy of therapeutic interventions.

Other technologies being developed to evaluate the OA joint include scintigraphy and ultrasonography.

TREATMENT   Rx

People with OA seek pain relief and improved physical function. Because at this time there is no known therapy in humans that affects the basic disease process (i.e., to inhibit cartilage degradation or enhance synthesis), medical therapy has focused on providing symptomatic relief. Largely because of ease of administration and acceptance by patients, an unwarranted reliance has been placed on pharmacologic intervention, particularly nonsteroidal anti-inflammatory drugs (NSAIDs), as initial therapy, at the expense of physical measures that have less morbidity and may provide longer-term benefit. The American College of Rheumatology and the American Academy of Orthopedic Surgeons have formulated evidence-based guidelines for progressive, stepwise treatment of patients with knee and hip OA that incorporate this approach.

Physical Measures

Although often overlooked, physical therapy and exercise programs provide important benefit and should be prescribed as baseline therapy for all patients with OA. Muscle atrophy commonly accompanies OA. Because muscles serve to reduce load on cartilage, maintaining muscle function is crucial for cartilage integrity and pain reduction. Both muscle strength and range of motion can be improved with appropriate physical therapy. Isometric exercises are preferred to isotonic ones because they place less stress on the involved joint.

Heat and cold are both used, with varying effectiveness, to provide symptomatic relief to patients with OA and as an important adjunct to physical therapy regimens. Transcutaneous nerve stimulation, particularly to relieve back pain, and acupuncture are effective in some patients and sometimes may provide an alternative to pharmacologic intervention.

Periods of rest throughout the day may be an important adjunct in the routine of patients with OA. Reduction in joint loading, either by rest or by appropriate use of a cane, often permits increased periods of activity with reduced pain. Use of cushioned shoes (commercial running or walking shoes) also may ameliorate lower extremity joint symptoms. Back pain may be reduced by muscle-strengthening exercises and by a well-fitted brace. However, the fitted brace should be used only intermittently to prevent abdominal and paraspinal muscle atrophy.

Medical Therapy

Symptomatic relief of joint pain in patients with OA may be achieved with simple analgesic agents such as acetaminophen (Table 270-2). Particularly in elderly patients with decreased renal reserve and an increased incidence of upper gastrointestinal bleeding, acetaminophen and other simple analgesics should be the drugs of initial choice. If inflammation is present (erosive OA) or symptoms are not well controlled with simple analgesics, NSAIDs are generally more effective. **1**

A second class of NSAIDs, the cyclooxygenase-2 (COX2) inhibitors, inhibit inflammatory-mediated production of prostaglandins (COX2 mediated) but permit constitutive prostaglandin production (COX1 mediated) (Chapter 36). Although they produce less gastrointestinal toxicity than traditional nonselective NSAIDs, they have been associated with an increase in cardiovascular risk, a property that may be shared with nonselective NSAIDs as well. **2** Therefore, only one selective COX2 inhibitor, celecoxib, is currently marketed in the United States. COX2 inhibitors may be preferred to nonselective NSAIDs, particularly in patients at high risk for gastrointestinal side effects, but each patient should be carefully informed of the cardiovascular risks associated with this class of medications.

Oral glucosamine and chondroitin are referred to as *nutriceuticals*; their use has been shown in some randomized clinical trials to reduce pain in subjects with knee OA but more recent, larger trials have been negative. **3 4** The time to onset of pain relief and the magnitude of this response have not been well characterized. Studies are still underway to determine whether these nutriceuticals alter the structural deterioration of the knee joint in OA.

Controlled studies of intra-articular steroid injections have demonstrated safety and benefit when injections were given every 3 months for up to 2 years at both the knee and the hip. **5** Intra-articular injections of steroids should not be repeated more than three or four times per year in any given joint because of the possibility of potentiating cartilage breakdown. Systemic use of steroids has no place in the treatment of OA. Intra-articular hyaluronate can improve joint symptoms and appears to be effective in subgroups of subjects with knee OA. Topical treatment with capsaicin, a substance P inhibitor, has been shown to relieve localized pain in some patients with OA. The development of compounds that can stimulate cartilage synthesis or prevent degradation is actively being pursued as disease modifying agents, whereas a number of novel agents are currently in development for the treatment of pain from OA, including inhibitors of nerve growth factors.

Surgical Therapy

Joint replacement surgery has been the most important advance in the treatment of OA in the past half-century (Chapter 285). Patients for whom optimal medical management has failed, who continue to have pain that interferes with sleep or activity or have significant limitations of joint function,

TABLE 270-2 RECOMMENDATIONS FOR PHARMACOLOGIC MANAGEMENT OF OSTEOARTHRITIS OF THE HIP AND KNEE*

ORAL

Acetaminophen
Nonselective NSAID plus misoprostol or a proton pump inhibitor[†]
COX2-selective inhibitor
Nonacetylated salicylate
Other pure analgesics
Glucosamine and/or chondroitin sulfate
Tramadol
Opioids

INTRA-ARTICULAR

Glucocorticoids
Hyaluronan

TOPICAL

Capsaicin
Methylsalicylate

*The choice of pharmacologic therapy should be individualized for each patient.
[†]Misoprostol and proton pump inhibitors may be used in patients who are at increased risk for upper gastrointestinal adverse events.
COX2 = cyclooxygenase-2; NSAID = nonsteroidal anti-inflammatory drug.
From the American College of Rheumatology Subcommittee on Osteoarthritis Guidelines. *Arthritis Rheum.* 2003;43:1905-1915.

---

are candidates for an operation. Those individuals with altered limb alignment and early OA of a hip or knee may benefit from osteotomy. Most patients have more advanced disease and require total joint replacement. Ideal candidates for total joint arthroplasty exhibit well-maintained muscle strength and should be older than 60 years of age. Younger patients are discouraged from undergoing joint replacement because of the small but real incidence of long-term failure of joint implants, mainly due to loosening. Revision arthroplasty is possible but has a higher failure rate and can be avoided by delaying the initial arthroplasty as long as possible and putting less load on the replaced joint.

Arthroscopic surgery is useful for removing loose bodies and repairing intrinsic defects of the knee, and in shoulder (rotator cuff) and ankle disease. In patients with knee OA without such findings, arthroscopy has not been shown to provide superior outcomes compared with medical management.[6] Total shoulder arthroplasty appears to be preferred over alternative techniques in terms of shoulder function.[7] Abrasion arthroplasty (chondroplasty) has been widely used in patients with knee OA, but no data exist to demonstrate its efficacy, and it cannot be recommended currently.

FUTURE DIRECTIONS

Novel agents to treat the pain of OA are actively being evaluated, including those acting at the level of the peripheral nervous system, such as inhibitors of nerve growth factor, and a number of centrally acting drugs thought to act at a supraspinal level to alter pain pathways and pain perception, such as serotonin and noradrenaline reuptake inhibitors. Potential disease-modifying agents under investigation include systemic agents inhibiting cartilage degradation (calcitonin, vitamin D, inhibitors of MMPs, inducible nitric oxide synthases, cathepsin K, IL-1β, and TNF-α), local intra-articular anticatabolic agents (lubricin, tissue inhibitor of metalloproteinase-3 inhibitors of IL-1β, TNF-α, and MMP-13), and potential anabolic agents administered through intra-articular injections (fibroblast growth factor-18, osteogenic protein-1, and mesenchymal stem cells). In addition, current research involves biosynthetic cartilage replacement and improved materials for total joint replacement. Therefore, the future holds promise not only to slow the joint degeneration in OA but possibly also to reverse it.

1. Towheed TE, Maxwell L, Judd MG, et al. Acetaminophen for osteoarthritis. *Cochrane Database Syst Rev.* 2006;1:CD004257
2. Kearney PM, Baigent C, Godwin J, et al. Do selective cyclo-oxygenase-2 inhibitors and traditional non-steroidal anti-inflammatory drugs increase the risk of atherothrombosis? Meta-analysis of randomised trials. *BMJ.* 2006;332:1302-1308.
3. Rozendaal RM, Koes BW, van Osch GJ, et al. Effect of glucosamine sulfate on hip osteoarthritis: a randomized trial. *Ann Intern Med.* 2008;148:268-277.
4. Clegg DO, Reda DJ, Harris CL, et al. Glucosamine, chondroitin sulfate, and the two in combination for painful knee osteoarthritis. *N Engl J Med.* 2006;354:795-808.
5. Raynauld JP, Buckland-Wright C, Ward R, et al. Safety and efficacy of long-term intraarticular steroid injections in osteoarthritis of the knee: a randomized, double-blind, placebo-controlled trial. *Arthritis Rheum.* 2003;48:370-377.
6. Kirkley A, Birmingham TB, Litchfield RB, et al. A randomized trial of arthroscopic surgery for osteoarthritis of the knee. *N Engl J Med.* 2008;359:1097-1107.
7. Singh JA, Sperling J, Buchbinder R, et al. Surgery for shoulder osteoarthritis. *Cochrane Database Syst Rev.* 2010;10:CD008089.

SUGGESTED READINGS

Lane NE, Schnitzer TJ, Birbara CA, et al. Tanezumab for the treatment of pain from osteoarthritis of the knee. *N Engl J Med.* 2010;363:1521-1531. *Treatment with tanezumab (humanized monoclonal antibody that binds and inhibits nerve growth factor at 10,250 μg/kg on days 1 and 56) was associated with a reduction in joint pain and improvement in function in patients with moderate-to-severe osteoarthritis of the knee.*
Rannou F, Poiraudeau S. Non-pharmacological approaches for the treatment of osteoarthritis. *Best Pract Res Clin Rheumatol.* 2010;24:93-106. *Evidence-based approach to nonpharmacologic treatments available for knee, hip, and hand OA.*
Reeves ND, Bowling FL; Medscape. Conservative biomechanical strategies for knee osteoarthritis. *Nat Rev Rheumatol.* 2011;7:113-122. *Review of nonoperative interventions including changes in gait, valgus knee braces, and muscle strengthening.*
Richmond J, Hunter D, Irrgang J, et al. American Academy of Orthopaedic Surgeons clinical practice guideline on the treatment of osteoarthritis (OA) of the knee. *J Bone Joint Surg Am.* 2010;92:990-993. *Consensus guidelines.*
Zhang W, Nuki G, Moskowitz RW, et al. OARSI recommendations for the management of hip and knee osteoarthritis: part III: changes in evidence following systematic cumulative update of research published through January 2009. *Osteoarthritis Cartilage.* 2010;18:476-499. *Review.*

271

BURSITIS, TENDINITIS, AND OTHER PERIARTICULAR DISORDERS AND SPORTS MEDICINE

JOSEPH J. BIUNDO

DEFINITION

An entire array of painful and sometimes disabling musculoskeletal syndromes exist that are not articular in origin but arise from tendons and bursae. These conditions are referred to by various names, in addition to *tendinitis* and *bursitis*, including the terms *nonarticular rheumatism, soft tissue diseases, regional rheumatic pain syndromes, overuse syndromes,* and *repetitive use syndromes* (Tables 271-1 and 271-2). These entities are often ignored, misdiagnosed as arthritis, or attributed to the aging process; awareness of the existence of these conditions and knowledge of basic musculoskeletal anatomy (Figs. 271-1 and 271-2) are the fundamental requirements for diagnosis. This knowledge is coupled with brief but specific physical diagnosis techniques. The accurate diagnosis and successful treatment of these conditions is gratifying to the clinician because many people can be relieved of their chronic painful syndromes.

Various terms regarding tendon injuries are used and may be confusing. The main term used is *tendinitis. Tendinosis* has been proposed as the correct terminology because there are degenerative changes in the tendon but very few inflammatory cells. In addition, fatty mucoid degeneration and hyaline features occur in these tendon syndromes. These tendon conditions are described by some as a *tendinopathy* because use of this term avoids the need

TABLE 271-1 MUSCULOSKELETAL CONDITIONS BY ETIOLOGY

TENDINITIS	TENDON RUPTURE	BURSITIS
Rotator cuff	Rotator cuff	Subacromial
Bicipital	Bicipital	Olecranon
Volar flexor	Quadriceps	Trochanteric
de Quervain's	Patellar	Ischial
Patellar	Posterior tibialis	Iliopsoas
Posterior tibialis	Achilles	Pes anserine
Achilles		Prepatellar
Epicondylitis		Retrocalcaneal

to decide whether or not inflammation is a factor. Also, tendons may *rupture* or *tear,* partially or completely. The term *tendon insufficiency* is used when the tendon is stretched or is partially or even completely torn. The terms *tenosynovitis* and *peritendinitis* refer to an inflammatory response of the tenosynovium or peritendon, respectively.

Tendon syndromes are basically "overuse" injuries. Tendinitis may occur when the tendon repeatedly bears more load than it can withstand. This may result from excessively high loads across normal tendons or from normal loads across degenerated tendons. In addition to load and repetitiveness, tendon changes resulting from immobility and from aging may play a role, as may the use of certain medications such as floxins and corticosteroids.

Bursae are closed sacs that are lined by a synovial membrane and serve as a cushion. They are located between tendon and bone, tendon and tendon, or bone and skin and allow smooth gliding between these structures. A bursa, which normally has a small amount of bursal fluid, can become inflamed from trauma or overuse, or become infected, producing a bursitis. When this occurs, some swelling and pain of the bursa may be present.

EPIDEMIOLOGY

The incidence of the nonarticular syndromes of bursitis and tendinitis is high. They are more common than both rheumatoid arthritis (RA) and systemic lupus erythematosus (SLE). For example, the incidence of shoulder pain, largely due to rotator cuff tendinitis and rotator cuff tear, was about 20% in a population older than 70 years of age.

DIAGNOSIS

A precise history is needed to identify the conditions present, and more than one syndrome can occur concomitantly. A working knowledge of regional anatomy and an approach that uses a regional differential diagnosis will help in obtaining a specific diagnosis. A complete neuromusculoskeletal examination should be performed, emphasizing careful palpation, passive range of motion (ROM), and active ROM alone or sometimes with resistance. Systemic and infectious causes must be considered. Diagnostic ultrasonography and magnetic resonance imaging (MRI) are sometimes useful in confirming a diagnosis.

TABLE 271-2	TENDINITIS AND BURSITIS CONDITIONS BY REGION

SHOULDER

Rotator cuff tendinitis
Rotator cuff tear
Bicipital tendinitis
Subacromial bursitis
Adhesive capsulitis

ELBOW

Olecranon bursitis
Medial epicondylitis
Lateral epicondylitis

WRIST AND HAND

de Quervain's tenosynovitis
Volar flexor tenosynovitis
Ganglion

HIP

Trochanteric bursitis
Iliopsoas bursitis
Ischial bursitis
Coccydynia

KNEE

Prepatellar bursitis
Pes anserine bursitis
Popliteal cyst (Baker's cyst)
Patellar tendinitis
Patellar/quadriceps tendon tear

ANKLE AND FOOT

Achilles tendinitis
Achilles tendon tear
Posterior tibial tendinitis
Posterior tibial tendon tear
Retrocalcaneal bursitis
Plantar fasciitis

TREATMENT Rx

Treatment of tendinitis and bursitis includes use of nonsteroidal anti-inflammatory drugs (NSAIDs), relative rest of the injured site, stretching and strengthening exercises, friction massage, use of modalities (heat, ice, and ultrasound), splinting, corticosteroid injections, and surgery. A comprehensive management of these regional syndromes should be undertaken, rather than relying on oral medications alone. The causative aspects should be evaluated, and activity modification should be advised as needed. The goals of therapeutic exercise are to increase flexibility by stretching, increase muscle strength by resistive exercises, and improve muscle endurance by some repetitive regimen. Caution should be exerted in performing corticosteroid injections; the injections should not be placed into the tendon proper, but rather into the peritendinous sheath. The injection should be placed beneath the subcutaneous tissue, to avoid skin and subcutaneous fat atrophy, and injections should not be given too frequently, to avoid the possibility of weakening and rupture of the tendon. The accuracy of injections may be improved with concomitant use of diagnostic ultrasonography to assist with determining the correct needle site. Also, fluoroscopically guided injections can be used to increase accuracy.

● SPORTS MEDICINE INJURIES

An overlap exists between commonly occurring conditions of tendinitis and bursitis and those attributed to sports injuries (Table 271-3). For example, lateral epicondylitis, frequently referred to as *tennis elbow,* occurs more commonly secondary to non–sports-related causes. In contradistinction, iliotibial band syndrome is usually related to sports. Other entities that occur more often in relation to sports include ligamentous knee injuries, patellar

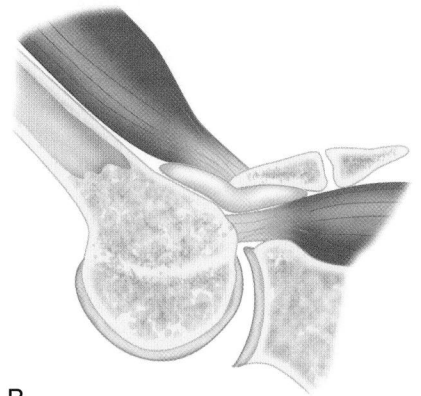

FIGURE 271-1. Relationship of subacromial bursa (shown in *blue*) to supraspinatus muscle and acromion process. **A,** In the position of adduction of the humerus. To show this bursa more clearly, the synovial membrane of the glenohumeral joint is not shown in blue. **B,** In the position of abduction of the humerus, the acromion impinges on the subacromial bursa and the insertion of the supraspinatus tendon. (From Polley HF, Hunder GG, eds. *Rheumatologic Interviewing and Physical Examination of the Joints,* 2nd ed. Philadelphia: WB Saunders; 1978:65.)

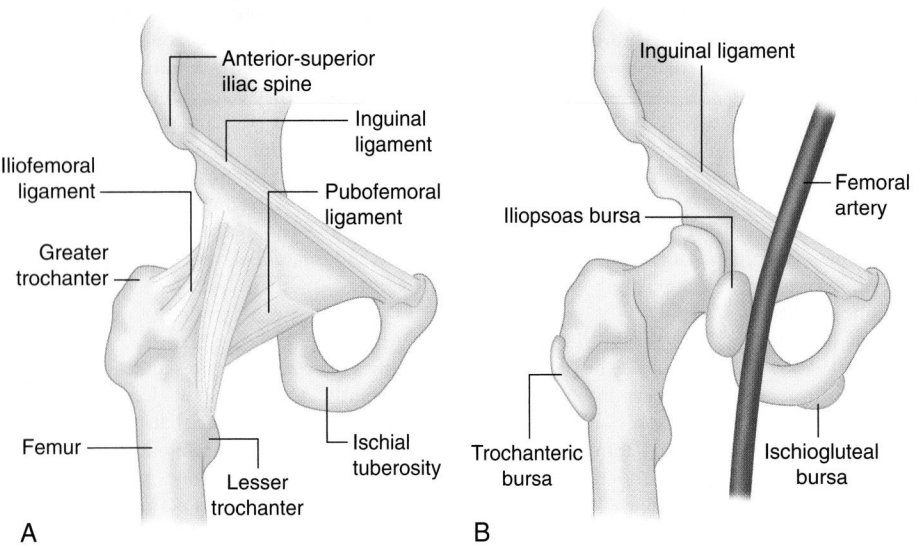

FIGURE 271-2. Musculoskeletal anatomy of the hip. **A,** Anterior aspect of the hip joint and bony structures. **B,** Relationship of the distended iliopsoas, trochanteric, and ischiogluteal bursae (shown in *blue*) to the hip joint and adjacent structures. (From Polley HF, Hunder GG, eds. *Rheumatologic Interviewing and Physical Examination of the Joints,* 2nd ed. Philadelphia: WB Saunders; 1978:183.)

TABLE 271-3	ADDITIONAL CONDITIONS THAT ARE SPORTS RELATED

SHOULDER

Acromioclavicular separation
Glenoid labial tear (SLAP lesion)
Glenohumeral instability with dislocation

ELBOW

Triceps tendinopathy
Little League elbow (apophysitis)
Distal biceps tendinitis

WRIST AND HAND

Gamekeeper's thumb (skier's thumb)
Mallet finger (baseball finger)
Extensor carpi ulnaris tendinitis
Rupture of flexor digitorum profundus tendon
Injury to triangular fibrocartilage

HIP

Adductor strain (groin pull)
Hip pointer
Hamstring strain

KNEE

Anterior cruciate tear
Posterior cruciate tear
Medial collateral ligament tear/strain
Lateral collateral ligament tear/strain
Popliteal tendinitis
Medial and lateral meniscal tears
Patellar tendinitis
Iliotibial band syndrome

ANKLE AND FOOT

Ankle sprain
Turf toe
Stress fracture

FIGURE 271-3. The impingement sign is elicited by forced forward elevation of the arm. Pain results as the greater tuberosity impinges on the acromion. The examiner's hand prevents scapular rotation. This maneuver may be positive in other periarticular disorders. (From Neer CS II. Impingement lesions. *Clin Orthop.* 1983;173:70-77.)

tendinitis, ankle sprains, turf toe, and acromioclavicular separations. It is important in both categories to know the anatomy and biomechanics of the condition, so as to better diagnose and treat the problem. Sports-related injuries are helped with the classic RICE treatment, consisting of *rest, ice, compression,* and *elevation.* Often, anti-inflammatory and analgesic drugs are used. However, there is less use of corticosteroid injections in athletic injuries than in routine cases of tendinitis and bursitis.

DISORDERS OF THE SHOULDER REGION

Shoulder pain is one of the most common musculoskeletal complaints in people older than 40 years of age. In younger people, athletic injuries are a frequent source of such pain.

Rotator cuff tendinitis, or impingement syndrome, is the most common cause of shoulder pain. Tendinitis (and not bursitis) is the primary cause of pain, but secondary involvement of the subacromial bursa occurs in some cases. The condition may be acute or chronic and may or may not be associated with calcific deposits within the tendon. The key finding is pain in the rotator cuff on active abduction, especially between 60 and 120 degrees, and sometimes when lowering the arm. In more severe cases, pain may begin on initial abduction and continue throughout the ROM. Typically, chronic rotator cuff tendinitis manifests as an ache in the shoulder, usually over the lateral deltoid, and occurs with various movements, especially abduction and internal rotation. Other symptoms include difficulty in dressing oneself and night pain due to difficulty in positioning the shoulders. The physical findings include pain and loss of active abduction and internal rotation, less pain on passive motion, tenderness of the area of supraspinatus insertion, and a positive impingement sign (Fig. 271-3, Neer's sign), which is pain occurring in forced flexion. The causes of rotator cuff tendinitis are multifactorial, but relative overuse, especially from overhead activity causing impingement of the rotator cuff, is commonly implicated. Treatment consists of rest and modalities such as hot packs, ultrasound, or cold applications, with specific ROM exercises as soon as tolerated. NSAIDs are often beneficial, but the most frequent treatment is injection of a depot corticosteroid into the subacromial bursa, the floor of which is contiguous with the rotator cuff. Disodium EDTA administered by phonophoresis and mesotherapy to patients with calcific tendinitis of the shoulder has been found to be effective in pain reduction, improvement in shoulder function, and disappearance of calcifications.∎

In a rotator cuff tear, an acute tear after trauma is usually easily recognized. The trauma may be superimposed on an already degenerative and possibly even partially torn cuff. In cases of trauma resulting in a ruptured cuff, fracture of the humeral head and dislocation of the joint should also be considered. However, most patients with a tear recall no trauma. In these cases, degeneration of the rotator cuff occurs gradually, resulting ultimately in a complete tear. Rotator cuff tears are classified as small (≤1 cm), medium (1 to 3 cm), large (3 to 5 cm), or massive (>5 cm). Shoulder pain, weakness on abduction, and loss of motion occur in varying degrees, ranging from severe pain and mild weakness to no pain and marked weakness. A positive drop-arm sign with inability to maintain actively 90 degrees of passive shoulder abduction may be present in patients with large or massive tears. Small complete tears and incomplete tears of the rotator cuff are treated conservatively with rest, physical therapy, and NSAIDs. Although its role has not yet been established by careful studies, a subacromial injection of a corticosteroid may relieve pain. Surgical repair is indicated in younger patients.

Bicipital tendinitis is manifested by pain, most often in the anterior region of the shoulder and occasionally more diffusely. The pain may be acute but is usually chronic and is related to impingement of the biceps tendon by the acromion. Tenosynovitis of the long head of the biceps is present, and the tendon may be frayed and fibrotic. Palpation over the bicipital groove reveals localized tenderness. The patient's response should be compared with the response to palpation of the opposite side (i.e., tendon with normal tenderness). Pain may be reproduced over the bicipital tendon in some cases by supination of the forearm against resistance (Yergason's sign), shoulder flexion against resistance (Speed's test), or extension of the shoulder. Treatment of bicipital tendinitis consists of rest, hot packs, ultrasound, and, as pain subsides, passive and then active ROM exercises. NSAIDs may be helpful, and occasionally a small amount of corticosteroid carefully injected into the tendon sheath may be of benefit. Rupture of the biceps tendon can occur at the superior edge of the bicipital groove, producing a characteristic bulbous enlargement of the lateral half of the muscle belly.

Adhesive capsulitis (frozen shoulder) is associated with generalized pain and tenderness and severe loss of active and passive motion in all planes. It is rare before 40 years of age but may occur secondary to any type of shoulder problem. However, not every stiff and painful shoulder is necessarily adhesive capsulitis. Inflammatory arthritis and diabetes can cause adhesive capsulitis. Additional factors such as immobility, low pain threshold, depression, and neglect or improper initial treatment also favor the development of a frozen shoulder. Many cases, however, are idiopathic. The joint capsule adheres to the anatomic neck, and the axillary fold binds to itself, causing restricted motion. The capsule becomes thickened and contracted. Arthrography can help confirm this diagnosis by showing a decrease in volume of the shoulder joint capsule. Oral steroids improve pain and range of motion in the short term, but a frozen shoulder is probably best treated with a comprehensive program involving NSAIDs and corticosteroid injections into the glenohumeral joint and the subacromial bursa. Physical therapy consists of ice packs, ultrasound, transcutaneous electrical nerve stimulation, and gentle ROM exercises, beginning with pendulum exercises and wall climbing with the fingers and progressing to active ROM and strengthening exercises.

DISORDERS OF THE ELBOW REGION

Olecranon bursitis occurs frequently and involves the subcutaneous olecranon bursa, either secondary to trauma or as an idiopathic condition. The bursa is characteristically swollen and tender on pressure, but pain may be minimal and usually no motion is lost. Aspiration may yield clear or blood-tinged fluid with a low viscosity, or grossly hemorrhagic fluid. Inflammatory olecranon bursitis may be caused by gout, RA, or calcium pyrophosphate deposition disease, and infection can also cause a bursitis. Aspiration alone and protection from trauma are usually sufficient to resolve the condition. A small dose of corticosteroid may be injected into the bursa. With septic olecranon bursitis, localized erythema is the major clue. Heat, pain, and a positive culture are also frequently present.

Lateral epicondylitis, or tennis elbow, is a common condition in those who overuse their arms. Localized tenderness directly over or slightly anterior to the lateral epicondyle is the hallmark of this disorder. Pain may occur during handshakes, while lifting a briefcase, or with other similar activities. Probably fewer than 10% of patients actually acquire lateral epicondylitis through playing tennis. Job and recreational activities, including gardening and athletics, are the usual causes. Pathologically, the condition consists of degeneration of the common extensor tendon, particularly of the extensor carpi radialis brevis tendon. Treatment is aimed at altering activities and preventing overuse of the forearm musculature. Ice packs, heat, and NSAIDs are of some benefit. A forearm brace can also be used. A local corticosteroid injection with a 25-gauge needle over the lateral epicondyle often produces satisfactory initial relief. Isometric strengthening is important as the initial part of a rehabilitation program.

Medial epicondylitis, or golfer's elbow, which mainly involves the flexor carpi radialis, is less common and less disabling than lateral epicondylitis. Local pain and tenderness over the medial epicondyle are present, and resistance to wrist flexion exacerbates the pain.

DISORDERS OF THE WRIST AND HAND

A ganglion is a cystic swelling that arises from a joint or tendon sheath and occurs most commonly over the dorsum of the wrist. It is synovial lined and contains thick, jelly-like fluid. Ganglia apparently develop secondary to trauma or prolonged wrist extension. Usually, the only symptom is swelling, but occasionally a large ganglion produces discomfort on wrist extension.

De Quervain's tenosynovitis may result from repetitive activity that involves pinching with the thumb while moving the wrist. The symptoms are pain, tenderness, and occasionally swelling over the radial styloid. Pathologic findings include inflammation and narrowing of the tendon sheath around the abductor pollicis longus and extensor pollicis brevis. A positive Finkelstein test result is usually seen: pain increases when the thumb is folded across the palm and the fingers are flexed over the thumb as the examiner passively deviates the wrist toward the ulnar side. However, this test may also be positive in patients with osteoarthritis (OA) of the first carpometacarpal (CMC) joint and must be differentiated from this common condition. Treatment involves splinting, local corticosteroid injection (Fig. 271-4), and NSAIDs as indicated. Rarely, surgical removal of the inflamed tenosynovium is needed.

Volar flexor tenosynovitis consists of inflammation of the tendon sheaths of the flexor digitorum superficialis and flexor digitorum profundus tendons in the palm. It is extremely common but often unrecognized. Pain in the palm is felt on finger flexion, but in some cases the pain radiates to the proximal interphalangeal (PIP) and metacarpophalangeal (MCP) joints on the dorsal side, misleading the examiner. The diagnosis is made by palpation and identification of localized tenderness and swelling of the volar tendon sheaths. The middle and index fingers are most commonly involved, but the ring and little fingers can also be affected. Often a nodule composed of fibrous tissue can be palpated in the palm just proximal to the MCP joint on the volar side. The nodule interferes with the normal tendon gliding and can cause a triggering or locking, which may be intermittent and may produce an uncomfortable sensation. Similar involvement can occur at the flexor tendon of the thumb. The most common cause is overuse trauma of the hands from gripping with increased pull on the flexor tendons. It may be part of inflammatory conditions, such as RA, psoriatic arthritis, or apatite crystal deposition disease. It is seen frequently in conjunction with OA of the hands. Injection of a long-acting steroid into the tendon sheath usually relieves the problem, although surgery on the tendon sheath may be needed in unremitting cases.

Gamekeeper's thumb (skier's thumb) is caused by trauma to the thumb resulting in instability of the first MCP joint. This instability is due to laxity or rupture of the ulnar collateral ligament. It is treated by immobilization, but surgical repair may be necessary.

Avulsion of flexor digitorum profundus (jersey finger) may result from trauma, usually in football, when a player grabs onto a jersey. The distal phalanx, usually the fourth, is hyperextended while the digitorum profundus

FIGURE 271-4. Injection of de Quervain's tenosynovitis.

is contracting maximally. The avulsion of the tendon results in an inability to flex the distal phalanx of that digit. Surgery is required to correct the problem.

DISORDERS OF THE HIP REGION

Although trochanteric bursitis is common, it frequently goes undiagnosed. It occurs predominantly in middle-aged to elderly people, and somewhat more often in women than in men. The main symptom is aching over the trochanteric area and lateral thigh. Walking, various movements, and lying on the involved hip may intensify the pain. Onset may be acute, but more often it is gradual, with symptoms lasting for months. In chronic cases, the patient may fail to locate or describe the pain adequately, or the physician may fail to note the symptoms or interpret them correctly. Occasionally, the pain has a pseudoradiculopathic quality, radiating down the lateral aspect of the thigh. In a few cases, the pain is so severe that the patient cannot walk and complains of diffuse pain of the entire thigh. The best way to diagnose trochanteric bursitis is to palpate over the trochanteric area and elicit point tenderness. In addition to specific pain on deep pressure over the trochanter, other tender points may be noted throughout the lateral aspect of the thigh muscle. Pain may be worse with external rotation and abduction against resistance. Although bursitis is usually described as the principal problem, the condition may actually arise at the insertions of the gluteus maximus and gluteus medius tendons. Local trauma and degeneration play a role in the pathogenesis. Conditions that may contribute to trochanteric bursitis, apparently by adding stress to the area, include OA of the lumbar spine or of the hip, leg-length discrepancy, and scoliosis. Treatment consists of local injection of depot corticosteroid using a 22-gauge, 3.5-inch needle to ensure that the bursal area is reached (Fig. 271-5). NSAIDs, weight loss, and strengthening and stretching of the gluteus medius muscle and iliotibial band help in management.

Coccydynia is manifested by pain in the coccyx area when pressure is applied to the area. This most notably occurs on sitting. The patient squirms from buttock to buttock to relieve the pressure and consequent pain, and often chooses to sit on a cushion. The symptoms may be chronic and severe. The condition may relate to a fall on the coccyx, dropping to a hard chair when sitting, or some related trauma to the coccyx. However, at times no obvious cause can be detected. Women are much more frequently affected, perhaps because the lordosis that often occurs in women exposes the coccyx to more trauma. The diagnosis is confirmed by finding localized tenderness over the coccyx on palpation. A plain x-ray can be obtained to exclude a fracture or dislocation of the coccyx. Treatment with a local injection of 1 mL of a long-acting corticosteroid and 2 mL of a 2% lidocaine solution is usually very effective. The exact nature of the pathology of coccydynia has not been studied, but it is presumed to be a bone bruise.

In iliopsoas bursitis, groin and anterior thigh pain are present and worsen on passive hip hyperextension and sometimes on flexion, especially with resistance. Tenderness is palpable over an involved bursa. The patient may hold the hip in flexion and external rotation to eliminate pain and may limp to prevent hyperextension of the hip. The iliopsoas bursa lies behind the iliopsoas muscle, anterior to the hip joint and lateral to the femoral vessels. It communicates with the hip in 15% of cases. The diagnosis is more apparent if a cystic mass is seen (about 30% of the cases); however, other causes of cystic swelling in the femoral area must first be excluded. A bursal mass can

FIGURE 271-5. Injection of trochanteric bursitis.

cause femoral venous obstruction or femoral nerve compression. As with most cases of bursitis, acute or recurrent trauma and inflammatory conditions such as RA may lead to iliopsoas bursitis (also called *iliopectineal bursitis*). The diagnosis is confirmed by plain x-ray with injection of a contrast medium into the bursa, or by computed tomography or MRI. Iliopsoas bursitis usually responds to conservative treatment including corticosteroid injections. With recurrent involvement, excision of the bursa may be necessary.

Ischial or ischiogluteal bursitis is caused by trauma or by prolonged sitting on hard surfaces, as evidenced by the name *weaver's bottom*. Pain is often exquisite when sitting or lying down. Because the ischiogluteal bursa is located superficial to the ischial tuberosity and separates the gluteus maximus from the tuberosity, the pain may radiate down the back of the thigh. Point tenderness over the ischial tuberosity is present. Use of cushions and local injection of a corticosteroid are helpful.

DISORDERS OF THE KNEE REGION

Anserine bursitis is seen predominantly in overweight, middle-aged to elderly women with large legs and OA of the knees. The symptoms are pain and tenderness over the medial aspect of the knee about 2 inches below the joint margin with the pain worsened by climbing stairs. The pes anserinus (Latin for "goose foot") is composed of the conjoined tendons of the sartorius, gracilis, and semitendinosus muscles. The bursa extends between the tendons and the tibial collateral ligament. The diagnosis is made by eliciting exquisite tenderness over the bursa. Anserine bursitis is often overlooked because it frequently occurs concomitantly with OA of the knee, which, when present, is the assumed cause of pain; however, in some cases of dual involvement, anserine bursitis is the principal source of pain. The treatment is rest, stretching of the adductor and quadriceps muscles, and a corticosteroid injection into the bursa.

Prepatellar bursitis is manifested as a swelling superficial to the kneecap and results from trauma such as frequent kneeling, leading to the name *housemaid's knee*. The prepatellar bursa lies anterior to the lower half of the patella and the upper half of the patellar ligament. The pain is generally slight unless pressure is applied directly over the bursa. The infrapatellar bursa, which lies between the patellar ligament and the tibia, is also subject to trauma and swelling. Chronic prepatellar bursitis can be treated by protecting the knee from the irritating trauma.

Patellar tendinitis (jumper's knee) is seen predominantly in athletes engaging in activities such as repetitive running, jumping, or kicking. Pain and tenderness are present over the patellar tendon.

Iliotibial band syndrome is manifested by lateral knee pain caused by friction between the iliotibial band and the lateral femoral condyle. It is an overuse injury and is seen in runners, cyclists, and other athletes performing repetitive knee flexion activities.

Popliteal cysts, also known as Baker's cysts, are not uncommon, and the clinician should be well aware of the possibility of their dissection or rupture. A cystic swelling behind the knee with mild or no discomfort can be the only initial finding. With further distention of the cyst, however, a greater awareness and discomfort are experienced, particularly on full flexion or extension. The cyst is best seen when the patient is standing and examined from behind. Any knee disease having a synovial effusion can develop into a popliteal cyst. Popliteal cysts are most common secondary to RA, OA, or internal derangements of the knee. There are a few reported cases secondary to gout and Reiter's syndrome. A syndrome of pseudothrombophlebitis may occur as a result of cyst dissection into the calf or actual rupture of the cyst. Findings include diffuse swelling of the calf, pain, and sometimes erythema and edema of the ankle. An ultrasound or arthrogram of the knee confirms both the cyst and the possible dissection or rupture. A cyst related to an inflammatory arthritis is treated by injection of a depot corticosteroid into the knee joint, and possibly into the cyst itself, which usually resolves the problem. If the cyst results from OA or an internal derangement of the knee, surgical repair of the underlying joint lesion is usually necessary to prevent a recurrence of the cyst.

In the knee area, tendon ruptures may occur, and quadriceps tendon rupture is involved about 50% of the time; otherwise, patellar tendon rupture occurs. Quadriceps tendon rupture is generally caused by sudden violent contractions of the quadriceps muscle when the knee is flexed. A hemarthrosis of the knee joint may follow. Patients with chronic renal failure, RA, hyperparathyroidism, or gout, and patients with SLE taking steroids have been reported to have spontaneous ruptures of the quadriceps tendon. The patient experiences a sudden sharp pain and cannot extend the leg.

Radiographic studies may show a high-riding patella. The tendon is usually found to be degenerated, and surgical repair is often indicated. Rupture of the patellar tendon has been associated with a specific episode of trauma, repetitive trauma from sporting activities, and systemic diseases.

● DISORDERS OF THE ANKLE AND FOOT REGION

Achilles tendinitis usually results from trauma, athletic overactivity, or improperly fitting shoes with a stiff heel counter, but it can also be caused by inflammatory conditions such as ankylosing spondylitis, Reiter's syndrome, gout, RA, and calcium pyrophosphate dihydrate crystal deposition disease. Pain, swelling, and tenderness occur over the Achilles tendon at its attachment and in the area proximal to the attachment. Crepitus on motion and pain on dorsiflexion may be present. Management includes NSAIDs, rest, shoe corrections, heel lift, gentle stretching, and sometimes a splint with slight plantar flexion. Local injection of platelet-rich plasma (PRP) has become an increasingly used treatment for releasing growth factors into degenerative tendons; however, a randomized controlled trial for treatment of chronic Achilles tendinopathy was found to be ineffective in improving pain and activity.**3** The Achilles tendon is vulnerable to rupture when involved with tendinitis, and treatment with a corticosteroid injection could increase this possibility.

Achilles tendon rupture is well known and occurs with a sudden onset of pain during forced dorsiflexion. An audible snap may be heard, followed by difficulty in walking and standing on toes. Swelling and edema over the area usually develop. Diagnosis can be made with the Thompson test, in which the patient kneels on a chair with the feet extending over the edge and the examiner squeezes the calf and pushes toward the knee. Normally this produces plantar flexion, but in a ruptured tendon, no plantar flexion occurs. Achilles tendon rupture usually occurs during athletic events or with trauma from jumps or falls. The tendon is more prone to tear in people with preexisting Achilles tendon disease and in those taking corticosteroids. Orthopedic consultation should be obtained, and immobilization or surgery may be selected, depending on the situation.

For acute, severe ankle sprain, a below-knee cast or Aircast produces a faster recovery than a tubular compression bandage, but there is no difference in outcomes at 9 months.**4**

Plantar fasciitis, which is seen primarily in persons between 40 and 60 years of age, is characterized by pain in the plantar area of the heel. The onset may be gradual, or it may occur with trauma or overuse from some activity, such as athletics, prolonged walking, using improper shoes, or striking the heel with some force. Plantar fasciitis may be idiopathic; it also is likely to be present in younger patients with spondyloarthritis (Chapter 273). The pain characteristically occurs in the morning on arising and is most severe for the first few steps. After an initial improvement, the pain may worsen later in the day, especially after prolonged standing or walking. The pain is burning, aching, and occasionally lancinating. Palpation typically reveals tenderness anteromedially on the medial calcaneal tubercle at the origin of the plantar fascia. Treatment includes relative rest with a reduction in stressful activities, NSAIDs, use of heel pad or heel cup orthosis, arch support, and stretching of the heel cord and plantar fascia. A local corticosteroid injection, using a 25-gauge needle, is often of help.

In posterior tibial tendinitis, pain and tenderness occur just posterior to the medial malleolus; it can be caused by trauma, excessive pronation, RA, or spondyloarthropathy. Extension and flexion may be normal, but pain is present on resisted inversion or passive eversion. The discomfort is usually worse after athletic activity, and swelling and localized tenderness may be present. Treatment usually includes rest, NSAIDs, and possibly a local injection of corticosteroid. Immobilization with a splint is sometimes needed.

Posterior tibialis tendon rupture, which is not commonly recognized, is a cause of progressive flat foot. It can result from trauma, chronic tendon degeneration, or RA. An insidious onset of pain and tenderness may be noted along the course of the tendon just distal to the medial malleolus, along with swelling medial to the hind foot. The unilateral deformity of hind foot valgus and forefoot abduction is an important finding. The forefoot abduction can best be seen from behind; more toes are seen from this position than would be seen normally. The result of the single heel rise test is positive when the patient is unable to rise onto the ball of the affected foot while the contralateral foot is off the floor. Treatment usually includes rest, NSAIDs, and possibly a local injection of corticosteroid. Immobilization with a splint is sometimes needed.

Manifestations of retrocalcaneal bursitis include pain at the back of the heel, tenderness of the area anterior to the Achilles tendon, and pain on dorsiflexion. Local swelling is present, with bulging on the medial and lateral aspects of the tendon. Retrocalcaneal bursitis, also called sub-Achilles bursitis, may coexist with Achilles tendinitis, and distinguishing the two is sometimes difficult. This condition may be secondary to RA, spondylitis, a reactive arthritis, gout, or trauma.

Turf toe is an injury of the big toe originally described during play on artificial turf. It results from hyperextension of the first metatarsophalangeal (MTP) joint when a fixed, dorsiflexed foot is forced into the ground. The plantar capsular ligament may be sprained or torn.

Stress fracture is also known as march fracture or fatigue fracture because it was associated with spontaneous fracture after long marches in army recruits. Pain, swelling, tenderness, and occasionally erythema develop over the metatarsal area, usually without any clear history of trauma. On questioning, however, the episode of spontaneous pain related to onset of the fracture can be identified in some cases. The neck of the second metatarsal bone is most frequently involved, but the third metatarsal is also a site of fracture. Aside from prolonged marching, other athletic events with overactivity, including jogging, are common causes. Stress fractures may be seen in patients with RA and in elderly people. The difficulty in diagnosing stress fractures is that the initial radiographs usually show no abnormalities or, at most, only a faint fracture line. A repeat radiograph several weeks later shows healing with callus formation. Bone scans aid the early diagnosis of stress fractures by showing an increase in uptake over the fracture site. Usually these fractures heal spontaneously, and rest and strapping of the foot are helpful. Occasionally, a cast is needed.

1. Cacchio A, De Blasis E, Desiati P, et al. Effectiveness of treatment of calcific tendinitis of the shoulder by disodium EDTA. *Arthritis Rheum.* 2009;61:84-91.
2. Buchbinder R, Green S, Youd JM, et al. Oral steroids for adhesive capsulitis. *Cochrane Database Syst Rev.* 2006;4:CD006189.
3. de Vos RJ, Weir A, van Schie HT, et al. Platelet-rich plasma injection for chronic Achilles tendinopathy: a randomized controlled trial. *JAMA.* 2010;303:144-149.
4. Lamb SE, Marsh JL, Hutton JL, et al. Mechanical supports for acute, severe ankle sprain: a pragmatic multicentre, randomised controlled trial. *Lancet.* 2009;373:575-581.

SUGGESTED READINGS

Coombes BK, Bisset L, Vicenzino B. Efficacy and safety of corticosteroid injections and other injections for management of tendinopathy: a systematic review of randomised controlled trials. *Lancet.* 2010;376:1751-1767. *For management of tendinopathy, corticosteroid infections reduce short-term but not long-term pain, and platelet-rich plasma is no better than placebo.*

Frick MA, Murthy NS. Imaging of the elbow: muscle and tendon injuries. *Semin Musculoskelet Radiol.* 2010;14:430-437. *Review.*

House J, Mooradian A. Evaluation and management of shoulder pain in primary care clinics. *South Med J.* 2010;103:1129-1135. *Review including supraspinatus tendinitis, subdeltoid bursitis, frozen shoulder, biceps tendinitis, and acromioclavicular joint arthritis.*

Maffulli N, Longo UG, Loppini M, et al. Current treatment options for tendinopathy. *Expert Opin Pharmacother.* 2010;11:2177-2186. *Review.*

272

RHEUMATOID ARTHRITIS

JAMES R. O'DELL

DEFINITION

Rheumatoid arthritis (RA) is a chronic systemic inflammatory disease of unknown etiology that primarily targets synovial tissues. It is relatively common, with a prevalence of slightly less than 1% in adults all over the world. RA shortens survival and significantly affects quality of life in most patients. Essentially all patients exhibit some systemic features such as fatigue, low-grade fevers, anemia, and elevations of acute phase reactants (erythrocyte sedimentation rate [ESR] or C-reactive protein [CRP]). The primary target of RA is the synovium, and this is responsible for most of the protean clinical features. Synovial tissues proliferate in an uncontrolled fashion, resulting in excess fluid production, destruction of cartilage, erosion of marginal bone, and stretching and damage of the tendons and ligaments.

In the past decade, the landscape of treatment of RA has changed dramatically. Current therapies result in substantial clinical benefit for most patients, particularly with early diagnosis, and 50% of patients can achieve remissions with treatment with an appropriate disease-modifying antirheumatic drug (DMARD).

EPIDEMIOLOGY

RA is present all over the world, with a remarkably consistent prevalence of 0.5 to 1% of adults, and with some differences in certain population groups. For reasons that are still unclear, the prevalence in women is two or three times greater than that in men. RA can occur at any age, but onset before the age of 45 years in men is uncommon. The relatively few well-done inception cohorts that are available suggest that the yearly incidence of RA is approximately 40 per 100,000 for women, and about half that for men. These figures vary significantly based on the age of the cohort. The best available data suggest that the incidence of RA in women increases with age until approximately 50 years of age and then reaches a plateau. The incidence rate is much lower in young men, approximately one third that in women, but increases steadily with age and approaches that of women older than 65 years. Because the incidence of RA increases or is stable with age and RA is a lifelong disease, the prevalence of RA increases with each decade. Recent data suggest that the incidence of RA, particularly rheumatoid factor (RF)-negative RA, may be decreasing. The reasons for this are unclear, but, if elucidated, they could provide valuable insights into the etiology and pathogenesis of RA and might allow the implementation of strategies to prevent clinical disease.

RA has a significant genetic component; therefore, it is not surprising that RA is reportedly very unusual in certain populations and more common in others. Most notably, cohorts have been described in rural Nigeria in which no individuals are affected with RA; in contrast, a prevalence of RA of 5% has been found in some studies of Chippewa, Yakima, and Inuit Native American tribes.

PATHOBIOLOGY

Genetics

Genetics plays a significant role in determining both the risk of developing RA and the severity of the disease. Twin studies reveal a concordance rate for RA that averages 15% for monozygotic twins and approximately 5% for dizygotic twins. These data in monozygotic twins simultaneously reveal both the significance of genetic factors and the fact that they are clearly not the only important factor, or else the concordance rate would approach unity.

It has now been clearly shown that RA is a multigene disease with important contributions from both human leukocyte antigen (HLA) and non-HLA genes. The association of certain HLA alleles, specifically HLA-DR4, with an increased risk of developing RA and of having more severe disease has long been recognized. This association is explained by a particular amino acid sequence in the third hypervariable region on the DRβ1 chain. HLA-DR molecules are present on the surface of antigen-presenting cells and allow T cells to recognize antigen in the context of DR. Hypervariable regions on the DR molecule are particularly important for antigen recognition. Table 272-1

details the amino acid sequence of several DRβ1 chains that are associated with RA and some that are not. The amino acid sequence associated with RA has been called the *shared epitope* or the *at-risk allele*. It has been shown by a number of investigators that patients with the shared epitope have more severe RA and more extra-articular manifestations than those who are negative for the shared epitope. Furthermore, individuals with two copies of the shared epitope, particularly those with HLA-DR4, have a further increased risk for the development of severe RA. This association with a particular antigen recognition site may ultimately aid understanding of the antigen or antigens that are important for triggering RA. Recently, proteins in which arginine has been converted to citrulline were shown to be bound with greater avidity by the shared epitope. The importance of certain DRβ1 alleles in RA supports the concept that T cells are integrally involved in the pathogenesis.

Population-based studies have suggested that only about one third of the genetic risk for RA is explained by genes located in the HLA region. A functional polymorphism for the gene that encodes intracellular protein tyrosine phosphatase nonreceptor 22 (*PTPN22*) has been reproducibly associated with RA and with a number of other autoimmune diseases, including type 1 diabetes, systemic lupus erythematosus, Graves' disease, and Hashimoto's thyroiditis. Recent genome-wide association studies (GWAS) have identified at least 20 other candidate genes that are associated with RA, including polymorphisms for signal transducer and activator of transcription (STAT4), tumor necrosis factor receptor–associated factor 1 (TRAF-1), and CD40.

The shared epitope is present in approximately 25 to 35% of the white population, but the chance of developing RA among individuals who carry this allele is only about 1 in 25. Therefore, despite identifying the most important genetic risk factor for RA, this test has little or no clinical utility. In addition to genetics, a number of other factors have been associated with the incidence, and in some cases the severity, of RA, including estrogen use (protective), smoking, and silica exposure.

ETIOLOGY

Clearly, other factors, in addition to genetics, are active in precipitating or triggering RA. RA appears to require the complex interaction of genetic and environmental factors with the immune system, and ultimately in the synovial tissues throughout the body (Fig. 272-1). Serum collected before the development of clinical RA show that immunologic changes predate clinical manifestations by years. Autoantibodies, particularly anti–citrullinated peptide antigen (ACPA) antibodies and RF, are present in the sera of many individuals 5 to 10 years before the clinical onset of disease. By following cohorts of people at high risk for RA, investigators are learning much about these early immunologic changes and ultimately about the triggers for the disease.

The use of oral contraceptives has been associated with a decrease in the incidence of RA; because the effect appears to be strongest for oral contraceptives that have high estrogen content, it is postulated that estrogen is

---

TABLE 272-1 HUMAN LEUKOCYTE ANTIGEN ASSOCIATIONS WITH RHEUMATOID ARTHRITIS

HLA Types (Alleles) and Methods of Detection			Third Hypervariable Region Amino Acid Sequences					MOST COMMON ETHNIC GROUPS
ALLOANTISERA (DR)	MLC (Dw)	DNA (DRβ1)	70	71	72	73	74	
ASSOCIATED WITH RA								
DR4	Dw4	*0401	Q	K	R	A	A	Whites (Western Europe)
DR4	Dw14	*0404		R				Whites (Western Europe)
DR4	Dw15	*0405		R				Japanese, Chinese
DR1	Dw1	*0101		R				Asian Indians, Israelis
DR6 (14)	Dw16	*1402		R				Yakima Native Americans
DR10	—	*1001	R	R				Spanish, Greeks, Israelis
NOT ASSOCIATED WITH RA								
DR4	Dw10	*0402	D	E				Whites (Eastern Europe)
DR4	Dw13	*0403		R			E	Polynesians
DR2	Dw2	*1501	D	A				Whites
DR3	Dw3	*0301				G	R	Whites

A = alanine; D = aspartic acid; E = glutamic acid; HLA = human leukocyte antigen; K = lysine; MLC = mixed leukocyte cultures; Q = glutamine; R = arginine; · = the same amino acid in that position as for DRB1*0401.

responsible for this protective effect. Studies that have tried to address the question of postmenopausal estrogen use and its effect on RA have yielded conflicting results.

Smoking has long been associated with a significant increase in the risk of developing RA but recently it has been shown that this is true only for ACPA-positive patients and is not associated with ACPA-negative disease. Furthermore, smoking appears to be a risk factor for RA only in those patients who are shared-epitope positive. Smoking has also been associated with poor responses to treatment. Purported triggers in addition to smoking have included bacteria (*Mycobacteria, Streptococcus, Mycoplasma, Escherichia coli, Helicobacter pylori*), viruses (rubella, Epstein-Barr virus, parvovirus), superantigens, and other undefined factors.

PATHOGENESIS

The pathogenesis of RA is complex, and there are almost certainly multiple triggering mechanisms including but not limited to smoking, infection, molecular mimicry, immune complexes, altered T-cell repertoire, and T-cell reactivity. Furthermore, it is likely that the triggers may be different based on the genetic background. As mentioned previously, smoking is a well-known trigger for some individuals but appears to be a risk factor only in those patients who possess the shared epitope.

Rheumatic fever, reactive arthritis (formerly known as *Reiter's syndrome*), and, more recently, Lyme arthritis are examples of arthritic syndromes for which infectious triggers have clearly been demonstrated, but these triggering agents are often difficult or impossible to isolate at the time when the arthritic syndromes occur. Many other examples exist in animal models of arthritis,

FIGURE 272-1. Initiation of rheumatoid arthritis (RA). HLA = human leukocyte antigen.

including syndromes induced by mycobacteria and streptococci. Reactive arthritis has clearly been shown to occur when any one of a myriad of different but specific infectious triggers is presented to a specific location in the body (the gastrointestinal or genitourinary tract) of individuals with a certain genetic background, in most cases HLA-B27. Additionally, in this syndrome, the age and gender of the individual and hence the maturity of the immune system may be critical in the development of clinical disease, which occurs primarily between the ages of 15 and 40 years in males. Once unraveled, the pathophysiology of RA is likely to be similarly complex.

Despite the absence of clear evidence linking any infectious agent to RA, it is widely believed that ultimately an important triggering role will be elucidated for infectious or other environmental agents. Once triggers for RA are identified, strategies for prevention can be addressed, but this information may not help individuals with established disease. Possibly infections involving the innate immune system are causative in an early subclinical phase of the rheumatoid disease process, with the agents being absent once clinical disease develops.

The relative roles of the cellular versus the humoral immune system in the initiation and perpetuation of RA are much debated; both appear to be important. Most likely, the mechanisms of initiation of the disease process are different from those that perpetuate the chronic disease. T cells, particularly of the activated T_H1 and T_H17 types, appear to predominate in synovial tissues. These T cells, presumably activated by some as yet unknown antigen presented by macrophages, B cells, or synoviocytes in the context of HLA-DR, secrete cytokines that drive further synovial proliferation. It is believed by many that, although RA may initially be triggered by exogenous antigens, the process, once initiated, may be perpetuated by autoantigens. Macrophage-derived cytokines, particularly interleukin-1 (IL-1) and tumor necrosis factor-α (TNF-α), play central roles in this ongoing inflammatory process. As definitive proof, biologic products directed against these cytokines have shown significant efficacy in the treatment of RA.

The humoral immune system also plays a role. RF has long been a serologic marker of RA and is well known to correlate with more severe disease, including erosions of bone, and with the presence of extra-articular features. The reason that RF is produced in excess and the exact role that it plays remains elusive. RF production may increase complement activation and result in the release of lysosomal enzymes, kinins, and oxygen free radicals. ACPA antibodies exhibit a high specificity (95 to 99%) for RA, although their sensitivity for RA with currently available assays is only about 70%. Even though both RF and ACPA antibodies also correlate with more aggressive erosive disease, this link is strongest for ACPA antibodies.

PATHOLOGY

The synovial tissues are the primary target of the autoimmune inflammatory process that is RA; the reason for this remains elusive. Once RA is initiated, the synovial tissues throughout the body become the site of a complex interaction of T cells, B cells, macrophages, and synovial cells (Fig. 272-2). The resultant proliferation of the synovial tissues (synovitis) causes the production of excessive amounts of synovial fluid and the infiltration of pannus into adjacent bone and cartilage. Synovitis results in the destruction of cartilage

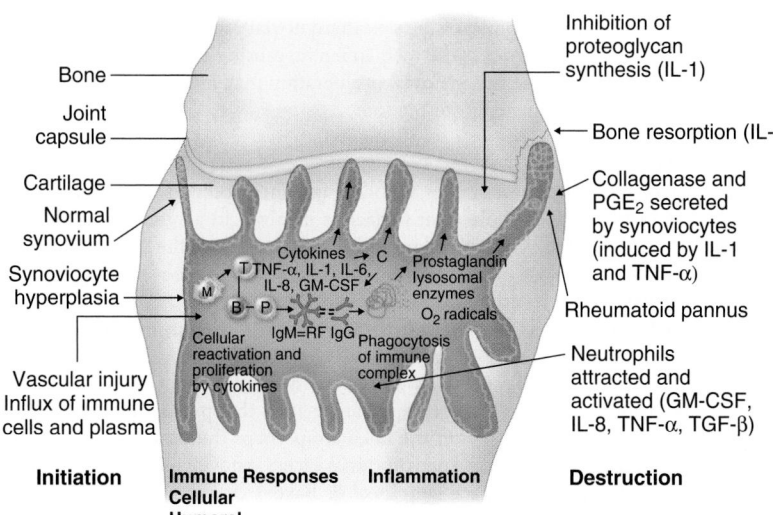

FIGURE 272-2. Events involved in the pathogenesis of rheumatoid synovitis (progressing from left to right). B = B lymphocyte; C = complement; GM-CSF = granulocyte-macrophage colony-stimulating factor; IgG, IgM = immunoglobulin G, M; IL = interleukin; M = macrophage; P = plasma cell; PGE₂ = prostaglandin E₂; RF = rheumatoid factor; T = T lymphocyte; TGF-β = transforming growth factor-β; TNF-α = tumor necrosis factor-α.

FIGURE 272-3. Severe advanced rheumatoid arthritis of the hands. There is massive tendon swelling over the dorsal surface of both wrists, severe muscle wasting, ulnar deviation of the metacarpophalangeal joints, and swan-neck deformity of the fingers. (From Forbes CD, Jackson WF. *Color Atlas and Text of Clinical Medicine*, 3rd ed. London: Mosby; 2003.)

FIGURE 272-4. Distribution of involved joints in the two most common forms of arthritis: rheumatoid arthritis and osteoarthritis. *Shaded circles* are shown over the involved joint areas.

and marginal bone and in the stretching or rupture of the joint capsule as well as tendons and ligaments. In patients, these effects are manifested by the deformities (Fig. 272-3 and E-Fig. 272-1) and disabilities that make up the clinical picture of RA.

CLINICAL MANIFESTATIONS
Articular Manifestations

RA can affect any of the synovial (diarthrodial) joints (Fig. 272-4). Most commonly, the disease starts in the metacarpophalangeal (MCP), proximal interphalangeal (PIP), and metatarsophalangeal (MTP) joints, followed by the wrists, knees, elbows, ankles, hips, and shoulders, in roughly that order. Early treatment helps limit the number of joints involved. Less commonly, and usually later, RA may involve the temporomandibular, cricoarytenoid, and sternoclavicular joints. RA may involve the upper part of the cervical spine, particularly the C1-C2 articulation, but, unlike the spondyloarthropathies, it does not involve the rest of the spine. However, RA patients are at an increased risk for osteoporosis, and this risk should be considered and dealt with early.

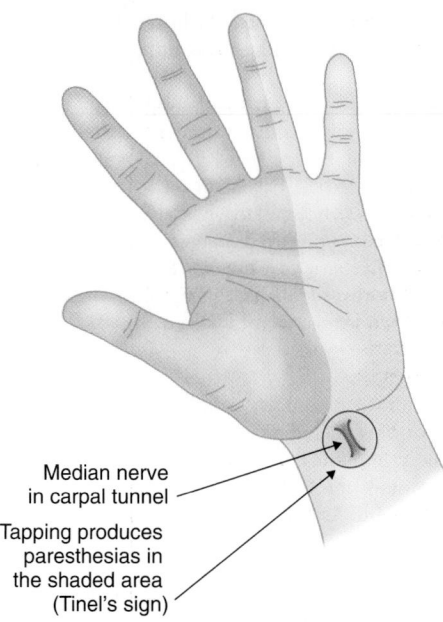

FIGURE 272-5. Carpal tunnel syndrome. Distribution of pain and/or paresthesias (*shaded area*) when the median nerve is compressed by swelling in the wrist (carpal tunnel).

Hands

The hands are a major site of involvement, and a significant portion of the disability that RA causes is because of damage and dysfunction of the hands. Typical early disease starts with swelling of the PIPs and MCPs. The distal interphalangeal (DIP) joints are rarely involved; significant involvement of the DIP joints should suggest the possibility of a different diagnosis (i.e., osteoarthritis or psoriatic arthritis). Figure 272-3 illustrates the classic ulnar deviation of the MCP joints and swan-neck deformities (hyperextension of the PIP joints) that are commonly seen in late, more established disease. Boutonniere (or buttonhole) deformities also occur as a result of hyperflexion of the PIP joints. If the clinical disease remains active, hand function deteriorates. Sudden loss of function of individual fingers may occur as a result of tendon rupture, which requires the expertise of a carefully selected hand surgeon to repair.

Feet

Feet, particularly the MTP joints, are involved early in most patients with RA. Radiographic erosions occur at least as early in the feet as in the hands. Subluxation of the toes is common and leads to the dual problem of breakdown of the skin and ulcers on the top of the toes. Painful ambulation may also develop owing to loss of the cushioning pads that usually protect the heads of the MTP joints.

Wrists

The wrist joints are involved in most patients with RA; radial deviation is the rule, and patients with severe involvement may progress to volar subluxation. Even early in the course of the disease, synovial proliferation in and around the wrists may compress the median nerve, causing carpal tunnel syndrome (Fig. 272-5). Later, this synovial proliferation may invade tendons and lead to rupture of some extensor tendons.

Large Joints

Involvement of knees, ankles, elbows, hips, and shoulders is common. Characteristically, the whole joint surface is involved in a symmetrical fashion. Therefore, RA is symmetrical not only from one side of the body to the other but also within the individual joint. In the case of the knee (Fig. 272-6A), the medial and lateral compartments are both severely narrowed in RA; in contrast, in patients with osteoarthritis (see Fig. 272-6B), only one compartment of the knee may be involved.

Synovial cysts may occur around any of the joints (large or small), and they occasionally manifest as soft, fluctuant masses that present diagnostic challenges. Synovial cysts from the knee are perhaps the best examples of this phenomenon. When the knee produces excess synovial fluid, it may accumulate in the popliteal space (popliteal or Baker's cyst) (E-Fig. 272-2). These cysts can cause problems by pressing on the popliteal nerve, artery, or veins.

A   B

FIGURE 272-6. Radiographs of the knees in the two most common forms of arthritis: rheumatoid arthritis and osteoarthritis. **A,** Severe involvement in rheumatoid arthritis, with almost complete symmetrical loss of joint space in both the medial and the lateral compartment, but with little subchondral sclerosis or osteophyte formation. **B,** Typical osteoarthritis, with severe, near-total loss of joint space of one compartment and a normal or actually increased joint space of the other compartment. Note also the significant subchondral sclerosis in the involved area, typical of osteoarthritis.

FIGURE 272-7. Rheumatoid nodules. Large rheumatoid nodules are seen in a classic location along the extensor surface of the forearm and in the olecranon bursa.

FIGURE 272-8. Rheumatoid nodulosis. In this patient, multiple rheumatoid nodules are present over joints. In some cases, nodules may dominate the clinical picture. Rarely, this may be seen as a side effect of methotrexate therapy.

Baker's cysts may dissect into the tissues of the calf (usually posteriorly), or they may rupture into the upper calf. Dissection may produce only minor symptoms, such as a feeling of fullness; rupture of the cyst with extravasation of the inflammatory content produces significant pain and swelling and may be confused with thrombophlebitis, the so-called pseudothrombophlebitis syndrome. Ultrasonography of the popliteal fossa and calf is useful to establish the correct diagnosis and to rule out thrombophlebitis, which may be precipitated by popliteal cysts. Treatment of popliteal (Baker's) cysts should be directed at interrupting the inflammatory process through an intra-articular injection of corticosteroid into the knee.

Neck

Although most of the axial skeleton is spared in RA, the cervical spine is commonly involved, particularly the C1-C2 articulation. Bony erosions and ligament damage can occur in this area and may lead to subluxation (see E-Fig. 272-1). Most often, subluxation at C1-C2 is minor and without accompanying symptoms; patients and caregivers need only be cautious and avoid forcing the neck into positions of flexion. Occasionally, subluxation at C1-C2 is severe and leads to compromise of the cervical cord with symptoms and in some cases death.

Other Joints

Wherever synovial tissue exists, RA can cause problems. The temporomandibular, cricoarytenoid, and sternoclavicular joints are examples of other joints that may be involved in RA. The cricoarytenoid joint is responsible for abduction and adduction of the vocal cords. Involvement of this joint may lead to a feeling of fullness in the throat, to hoarseness, and, rarely, when the cords are essentially fused in a closed position, to a syndrome of acute respiratory distress with or without stridor. In this latter situation, emergent tracheotomy may be life-saving.

Extra-articular Manifestations

Systemic features of RA such as fatigue, weight loss, and low-grade fevers occur frequently. As with all the other extra-articular features, they are more common in those patients who possess RF or ACPA antibodies, or both (Table 272-2).

Skin

Subcutaneous nodules are seen in approximately one fourth of patients with RA, almost exclusively in those who are RF positive. Patients with nodules who are RF negative should be carefully scrutinized for a different diagnosis, such as chronic tophaceous gout. Nodules may occur almost anywhere (e.g., lungs, heart, eye), but most commonly they occur subcutaneously on

TABLE 272-2	EXTRA-ARTICULAR MANIFESTATIONS OF RHEUMATOID ARTHRITIS
Skin	Nodules, fragility, vasculitis, pyoderma gangrenosum
Heart	Pericarditis, premature atherosclerosis, vasculitis, valve disease, and valve ring nodules
Lung	Pleural effusions, interstitial lung disease, bronchiolitis obliterans, rheumatoid nodules, vasculitis
Eye	Keratoconjunctivitis sicca, episcleritis, scleritis, scleromalacia perforans, peripheral ulcerative keratopathy
Neurologic	Entrapment neuropathy, cervical myelopathy, mononeuritis multiplex (vasculitis), peripheral neuropathy
Hematopoietic	Anemia, thrombocytosis, lymphadenopathy, Felty's syndrome
Kidney	Amyloidosis, vasculitis
Bone	Osteopenia

extensor surfaces (particularly the forearms) (Fig. 272-7), over joints, or over pressure points. Rheumatoid nodules are firm on examination, usually are not tender, have a characteristic histologic picture, and are thought to be initiated by small vessel vasculitis. A syndrome of increased nodulosis, despite good control of the joint disease, has been described with methotrexate therapy (Fig. 272-8).

Small vessel vasculitis, manifested as digital infarcts or leukocytoclastic vasculitis, may occur in RA (Fig. 272-9) and should prompt more aggressive

FIGURE 272-9. Small vessel vasculitis. A and B, Rheumatoid vasculitis with small brown infarcts of palms and fingers in chronic rheumatoid arthritis. (Courtesy of Dr. Martin Lidsky, Houston, TX.)

DMARD treatment. A vasculitis of small and medium arteries that is indistinguishable from polyarteritis nodosa also can be seen with RA and requires aggressive systemic therapy. Finally, pyoderma gangrenosum occurs with increased frequency in association with RA.

Cardiac Involvement

Cardiac involvement directly related to RA is uncommon; however, patients with RA have a significantly increased morbidity and mortality from coronary artery disease. The reasons are not clear, but chronic inflammation may be the major cause. Some of the medications used to treat RA and a sedentary lifestyle may be additional risk factors for the development of coronary artery disease. Pericardial effusions are common in RA (50% by echocardiography) but usually are asymptomatic. Rarely, long-standing pericardial disease may result in a fibrinous pericarditis, and patients may present clinically with constrictive pericarditis (Chapter 77). Uncommonly, rheumatoid nodules occur in the conduction system and cause heart block.

Pulmonary Manifestations

Pulmonary manifestations of RA include pleural effusions, rheumatoid nodules, and parenchymal lung disease (Chapters 84 and 92). Pleural effusions occur more commonly in men and are usually small and asymptomatic. Of interest, pleural fluid in RA is characterized by low levels of glucose and low pH and, therefore, may at times be confused with empyema. Rheumatoid nodules may occur in the lung, especially in men (Fig. 272-10); these are usually solid but may calcify, cavitate, or become infected. Rarely, pulmonary nodules rupture and produce a pneumothorax. If RA patients are exposed to coal dust, diffuse nodular densities may occur (Caplan's syndrome). Differentiating rheumatoid nodules from lung cancer can be problematic, particularly if the lesion is solitary. Therefore, the presence of pulmonary nodules in a patient with RA should precipitate an aggressive diagnostic evaluation.

Diffuse interstitial fibrosis occurs in RA and may progress to a honeycomb appearance on radiography with increasing dyspnea. Rarely, bronchiolitis obliterans can be seen with or without organizing pneumonia. Bronchiolitis obliterans carries a poor prognosis and may occur more often in association with D-penicillamine or gold therapy.

Ophthalmologic Manifestations

The most common manifestation of RA in the eye is keratoconjunctivitis sicca (dry eyes) from secondary Sjögren's syndrome. Patients may have associated xerostomia (dry mouth), parotid gland swelling, or, occasionally, lymphadenopathy. Scleritis can also occur and may be painful, with progression to thinning of the sclera (with deep pigment showing through on physical examination). Scleritis may progress to perforation of the orbit (scleromalacia perforans). Rarely, tendonitis of the superior oblique muscles can result in double vision (Brown's syndrome).

Neurologic Manifestations

Peripheral nerve entrapment syndromes, including carpal tunnel syndrome (median nerve at the wrist), and tarsal tunnel syndrome (anterior tibial nerve at the ankle), are common in RA. Vasculitis can lead to mononeuritis multiplex and a host of additional neurologic problems. Subluxations at C1-C2 may produce myelopathy (see E-Fig. 272-1). Rheumatoid nodules in the central nervous system have been described but are rare and usually asymptomatic.

Felty's Syndrome

Felty's syndrome is the triad of RA, splenomegaly, and neutropenia. This complication is seen in patients with severe, RF-positive disease and may be

FIGURE 272-10. Rheumatoid nodules in the lung. Chest radiograph demonstrates discrete rheumatoid nodules in both right and left lower lobes. (Courtesy of Dr. Martin Lidsky, Houston, TX.)

accompanied by hepatomegaly, thrombocytopenia, lymphadenopathy, and fevers. Most patients with Felty's syndrome do not require special therapy; instead, treatment should be directed toward their severe RA. If severe neutropenia (Chapter 170) exists (<500 cells/μL) and is accompanied by recurrent bacterial infections or chronic, nonhealing leg ulcers, splenectomy may be indicated.

Some patients with RA, who were previously thought to have Felty's syndrome, have peripheral white blood cell counts dominated by large granular lymphocytes with almost complete absence of neutrophils. This condition is known as the *large granular lymphocyte syndrome* and is thought to be a variant of T-cell leukemia. In the setting of RA, this syndrome has a good prognosis, with the neutropenia often responding dramatically to methotrexate therapy.

Clinical Course

Although the presentation is variable, most patients with RA have an insidious onset of pain, stiffness, or swelling, or a combination of these, in multiple joints over the course of weeks to months. Systemic features such as fatigue, low-grade fevers, and weight loss may accompany the joint manifestations of RA. Less commonly, the onset can be fulminant, occurring almost overnight, or patients may exhibit persistent monoarthritis or oligoarthritis for prolonged periods before manifesting the more typical pattern of joint involvement. Rarely, some patients, particularly men, develop extra-articular features of RA before the joint problems appear.

The distribution of involved joints is a critical clue to the underlying diagnosis. The joints that are involved in patients with RA at presentation are also variable; typically, the symptoms start in the small joints of the hands (PIP and MCP joints) and in the toes (MTP joints). Importantly, RA usually spares the DIP joints and the small joints of the toes (see Fig. 272-4). Later, RA moves, or some would say "metastasizes," to larger joints: wrists, knees, elbows, ankles, hips, and shoulders (roughly in that order). Although the patient's history of joint symptoms (arthralgia) is important, the diagnosis of RA requires the presence of inflammation (swelling, warmth, or both) on examination of the joints.

Morning stiffness is a hallmark of inflammatory arthritis and is a prominent feature of RA. Patients with RA are characteristically at their worst in the morning or after prolonged periods of rest (called *gel phenomenon*). This stiffness in and around joints often lasts for hours, and quantifying it is one way to measure improvement. Stiffness is relieved by warmth and activity, and reducing or eliminating joint stiffness is a clear goal of therapy.

DIAGNOSIS

All current treatment paradigms for RA stress the early and aggressive use of DMARDs. Therefore, the importance of accurate early diagnosis of RA cannot be overemphasized. However, there is no one single finding on physical examination or laboratory testing that is pathognomonic of RA. Instead, the diagnosis of RA requires a collection of historical and physical features as well as an alert and informed clinician.

TABLE 272-3 CLASSIFICATION CRITERIA FOR RHEUMATOID ARTHRITIS*

Morning stiffness (≥1 hr)
Swelling (soft tissue) of three or more joints
Swelling (soft tissue) of hand joints (PIP, MCP, or wrist)
Symmetrical swelling (soft tissue)
Subcutaneous nodules
Serum rheumatoid factor
Erosions and/or periarticular osteopenia in hand or wrist joints seen on radiograph

*Criteria 1 through 4 must have been continuously present for 6 wk or longer, and criteria 2 through 5 must be observed by a physician. A classification of rheumatoid arthritis requires that four of the seven criteria be fulfilled.
MCP = metacarpophalangeal; PIP = proximal interphalangeal.

Classification

Table 272-3 lists the current classification criteria for RA; although they are not designed specifically for the purpose of diagnosis, these criteria are widely used as a diagnostic aid. The first five criteria are all clinical; in other words, they are established by physical examination or by talking with the patient. Only the last two criteria require laboratory tests or radiographs. The first four criteria must be present for at least 6 weeks before a diagnosis of RA can be made. This caveat is necessary because a host of conditions, including many virus-related syndromes, can cause self-limited polyarthritis syndromes that look identical to RA, including at times the presence of RF. Such conditions usually last only 2 to 3 weeks. Therefore, inflammatory arthritis that is present for at least 6 weeks should not be considered a postviral condition, except for parvovirus arthritis, and the diagnosis of RA should be strongly considered, with the early initiation of appropriate treatment. The goal for most RA patients should be to establish a diagnosis and to start DMARD therapy within 3 months of disease onset. The presence of ACPA antibodies, even in the first few weeks of disease, is strongly suggestive of ongoing aggressive RA. New classification criteria for RA have been developed and, once validated, may prove more useful in diagnosis.

Laboratory Findings

Historically, the most characteristic laboratory abnormality in RA is the presence of RF, which is found in approximately 80% of patients. RF was first described in the 1930s and is an antibody that recognizes the Fc portion of immunoglobulin G as its antigen. The presence of RF is strongly associated with more severe articular disease as well as with essentially all the extra-articular features previously discussed. Importantly, RF is seen in association with many diseases other than RA, particularly in disease processes that provide chronic stimulation of the immune system (Table 272-4). ACPA antibodies, found in approximately 70% of patients with RA, have a high specificity (93 to 98%), are often present before clinical disease is diagnosed, and are associated with aggressive erosive disease. RA is associated with many other autoantibodies, including antinuclear antibodies (~30%) and antineutrophil cytoplasmic antibodies, particularly of the perinuclear type (~30%).

Most patients with RA have an anemia of chronic disease. The degree of anemia is proportional to the activity of the disease, and therapy that controls the disease will normalize the hemoglobin levels. Other causes of anemia should also be considered in RA, particularly iron deficiency anemia from gastrointestinal blood loss. Thrombocytosis is common, with platelet counts returning to normal as the inflammation is controlled. Acute phase reactants and ESR and CRP levels also parallel the activity of the disease, and their persistent elevation portends a poor prognosis in terms of both joint destruction and mortality. White blood cell counts may be elevated, normal, or, in the case of Felty's syndrome, profoundly depressed. Eosinophilia is present in some patients with RA.

Synovial fluid in RA is characterized by white blood cell counts in the range of 5000 to 100,000/mm³, with approximately two thirds of the cells being polymorphonuclear leukocytes. There are no synovial fluid findings that are pathognomonic of RA.

Differential Diagnosis

The accurate diagnosis of RA early in its course, although challenging, is critical if patients are to benefit maximally from therapeutic intervention. Once disease has been present and active for years and the characteristic deformities and radiographic changes have occurred, the diagnosis is all too obvious.

TABLE 272-4 DIFFERENTIAL DIAGNOSIS OF RHEUMATOID ARTHRITIS

DISORDER	SUBCUTANEOUS NODULES	RHEUMATOID FACTOR
Viral arthritis (hepatitis B and C, parvovirus, rubella, others)	−	±
Bacterial endocarditis	±	+
Rheumatic fever	+	−
Sarcoidosis	+	+
Reactive arthritis	−	−
Psoriatic arthritis	−	−
Systemic lupus erythematosus	±	+
Primary Sjögren's syndrome	−	+
Chronic tophus gout	+	−
Calcium pyrophosphate disease	−	−
Polymyalgia rheumatica	−	−
Osteoarthritis (erosive)	−	−

− = Not present; + = frequently present; ± = occasionally present.

Unfortunately, once RA has progressed to that point, many of the deformities no longer are amenable to medical therapy.

Many diseases can mimic RA (see Table 272-4). Early in the course of disease, self-limited viral syndromes need to be considered, especially hepatitis B and C, parvovirus, rubella (infection or vaccination), and Epstein-Barr virus. At any time, systemic lupus erythematosus, psoriatic arthritis, and reactive arthritis may present diagnostic challenges. In the case of these three mimics, a targeted history and examination to elucidate their associated clinical features, such as rashes, oral ulcers, nail changes, dactylitis, urethritis, and renal, pulmonary, gastrointestinal, or ophthalmologic problems, is critical. Especially in elderly patients with fulminant-onset RA, remitting RF-negative symmetrical synovitis with pitting edema (the so-called RS3PE syndrome) and paraneoplastic syndromes should be considered. Chronic tophaceous gout may also mimic severe nodular RA. Hypothyroidism not only causes many rheumatic manifestations but also occurs commonly in conjunction with RA and, therefore, should be kept in mind.

TREATMENT   Rx

General Measures

RA is a lifelong disease process that has no known cure; the diagnosis is made based on clinical criteria, and many different options exist for treatment. All these factors magnify the importance of the patient-physician relationship and place a premium on the art rather than the science of medicine. Optimal care for patients with RA requires effective ongoing interactions between primary care physicians and rheumatologists, and, in some cases, physical therapists, occupational therapists, and orthopedic surgeons. Because of the serious nature of the disease, the rapid introduction of new treatments, and the need for expertise in monitoring these therapies, all patients with RA should be evaluated early by a rheumatologist and followed closely.

The goal of therapy is disease remission (Table 272-5). When RA is treated early, remission is possible in 40 to 50% of patients. However, remissions require the ongoing use of DMARDs and, even then, are not always durable. Essentially all RA patients should be treated with DMARDs. Some combination of nonsteroidal anti-inflammatory drugs (NSAIDs), steroids, and DMARDs is necessary in most patients. In many, or perhaps most, patients with RA, combinations of different DMARDs (conventional and biologic) are necessary for optimal control. Therapy should be escalated rapidly to ensure maximal suppression of disease while minimizing toxicity and expense. Patients with RA should be educated about their disease and its treatment. In most cases, patients should have an opportunity to spend time with physical therapists and occupational therapists to learn about range-of-motion exercises, joint protection, and assistive devices.

Medical Therapy

In the treatment of RA, three types of medical therapies are used: NSAIDs, glucocorticoids, and DMARDs (both conventional and biologic). Initial therapy should include at least one DMARD, whereas combinations of the three types of medications is the rule.

Nonsteroidal Anti-inflammatory Drugs

NSAIDs are important for the symptomatic relief they provide to RA patients; however, they play only a minor role in altering the underlying disease process (Chapter 36). Therefore, NSAIDs should rarely, if ever, be used to treat RA without the concomitant use of DMARDs. Many clinicians waste valuable time switching from one NSAID to another before starting DMARD therapy.

Much has been written about the gastrointestinal toxicity of NSAIDs, and these concerns are particularly relevant to RA patients who often have significant risk factors, including age and concomitant steroid use. Therefore, cyclooxygenase-2 (COX2)–selective agents have been a popular choice for patients with RA. The recent evidence linking these agents to increased cardiovascular toxicity has been particularly troubling for patients with RA, who are already at high risk for myocardial infarction. Therefore, if COX2-selective agents are used, they should be kept at a low dose. Consideration should be given to low-dose aspirin prophylaxis in RA, but this may increase the gastrointestinal toxicity of NSAIDs. The use of concomitant misoprostol or proton pump inhibitors should be considered in all patients with RA who are taking NSAIDs. Additionally, the potential for NSAIDs to decrease renal blood flow and to increase blood pressure should be kept in mind.

Glucocorticoids

Glucocorticoids have had a significant role in the treatment of RA for more than half a century (Chapter 34). Indeed, RA was chosen as the first disease to be treated with this new therapy, partly because it was thought that RA was a disease of glucocorticoid deficiency (an issue that remains unresolved). As was the case with the first patient treated in 1948, glucocorticoids are dramatically and rapidly effective in patients with RA. Not only are glucocorticoids useful for symptomatic improvement, but they also significantly decrease the radiographic progression of RA. However, the toxicities of long-term therapy are extensive and potentially devastating. Therefore, the optimal use of these drugs requires an understanding of several principles (Table 272-6).

Glucocorticoids remain among the most potent anti-inflammatory treatments available; for this reason, and because of their rapid onset of action, they are ideally suited to help control the inflammation in RA while the much slower-acting DMARDs are starting to work. Prednisone, the most commonly used glucocorticoid, should rarely be used in doses higher than 10 mg/day to treat the stiffness and articular manifestations of RA. This dose should be slowly tapered to the lowest effective dose, and the concomitant DMARD therapy should be adjusted to make this possible. Glucocorticoids should rarely, if ever, be used to treat RA without concomitant DMARD therapy. The paradigm is to shut off inflammation rapidly with glucocorticoids and then to taper them as the DMARD is taking effect ("bridge therapy"). In all patients receiving glucocorticoids, strong measure should be taken to prevent osteoporosis. Bisphosphonates have been shown to be particularly effective in this regard. Higher doses of glucocorticoids may be necessary to treat extra-articular manifestations, especially vasculitis and scleritis.

Disease-Modifying Antirheumatic Drugs

DMARDs are a group of medications that have the ability to inhibit greatly the disease process in the synovium and to modify or change the disabling potential of RA. In most cases, these drugs have the ability to halt or slow the radiographic progression of RA.

Conventional DMARDs

Included in this group of medications are methotrexate, sulfasalazine (Azulfidine), gold, antimalarials (Plaquenil and others), leflunomide (Arava), azathioprine (Imuran), and minocycline. It is critically important that clinicians and patients understand that conventional DMARDs take 2 to 6 months to exert their maximal effect, and all require some monitoring (Table 272-7). Therefore, other measures, such as glucocorticoid therapy, may be needed to control the disease while these medications are starting to work.

All these DMARDs have been shown to be effective in treating both early and more advanced RA that remains active. Until additional research elucidates factors that allow selection of the best initial therapy for each patient, the choice will depend on patient and physician concerns about toxicity and monitoring issues, as well as the activity of disease and presence of comorbid conditions. The critical factor is not which DMARD to start first but rather getting the DMARD therapy started early in the disease process.

Methotrexate

Methotrexate is the preferred DMARD of most rheumatologists, in part because patients have a more durable response, and because, with correct monitoring, serious toxicities are rare. Methotrexate is dramatically effective in slowing radiographic progression and is usually given orally in doses ranging from 5 to 25 mg/week as a single dose. This once-a-week administration is worthy of emphasis; prior experience with daily therapy in psoriasis has demonstrated the importance of allowing the liver time to recover between doses. Oral absorption of methotrexate is variable; subcutaneous injections of methotrexate may be effective if oral treatment is not. Side effects of methotrexate include oral ulcers, nausea, hepatotoxicity, bone marrow suppression, and pneumonitis. With the exception of pneumonitis, these toxicities respond to dose adjustments. Monitoring of blood counts and liver blood tests (albumin and aspartate aminotransaminase [SGOT] or alanine aminotransferase [SGPT]) should be done every 4 to 8 weeks initially and, when stable, every 3 months thereafter, with adjustments in the dose of methotrexate as needed. Renal function is critical for clearance of methotrexate; previously stable patients may experience severe toxicities when renal function deteriorates. Pneumonitis, although rare, is less predictable and can be fatal, particularly if the methotrexate is not stopped or is restarted. Folic acid, 1 to 4 mg/day, can significantly decrease most methotrexate toxicities without apparent loss of efficacy. If methotrexate alone does not sufficiently control disease, it is combined with other DMARDs. Methotrexate in combination with virtually any of the other DMARDs (conventional or biologic) has been shown to be more effective than either drug alone. [2]

Leflunomide

Leflunomide, a pyrimidine antagonist, has a very long half-life and is most commonly started at 10 to 20 mg/day orally. Diarrhea is the most common toxicity and responds to dose reduction, and doses of leflunomide of 10 to 20 mg three to five times per week are frequently used. Also, because of the long half-life and teratogenic potential of leflunomide, women wishing to become pregnant who have previously received leflunomide, even if therapy was stopped years ago, should have blood levels drawn. If toxicity occurs or if pregnancy is being considered, leflunomide can be rapidly eliminated from the body by treatment with cholestyramine. Laboratory monitoring for hematologic and hepatic toxicity should be done during treatment with leflunomide, as recommended for methotrexate.

Antimalarial Drugs

The antimalarial drugs hydroxychloroquine (Plaquenil) and chloroquine are frequently used for the treatment of RA. They have the least toxicity of any of the DMARDs and do not require monitoring of blood tests. Yearly monitoring by an ophthalmologist is recommended to detect any signs of retinal toxicity (rare). Hydroxychloroquine is the most commonly used preparation and is given orally at 200 to 400 mg/day. These drugs are frequently used in combination with other DMARDs, particularly methotrexate.[2] Hydroxychloroquine has recently been shown to decrease the incidence of diabetes in patients with RA.

Sulfasalazine

Sulfasalazine is an effective treatment when given in doses of 1 to 3 g/day. Monitoring of blood counts, particularly white blood cell counts, in the first 6 months is recommended. Sulfasalazine and hydroxychloroquine are often combined with methotrexate,; this is referred to as triple therapy.

Minocycline

Minocycline, 100 mg twice daily, has been shown to be an effective treatment for RA, particularly when used in early, RF-positive disease. Chronic therapy (>2 years) with minocycline may lead to cutaneous hyperpigmentation. Minocycline has been associated with drug-induced lupus.

Gold

Gold, the oldest DMARD, when given intramuscularly remains an extremely effective therapy for a small percentage of patients. It is less commonly used because of its slow onset of action, need for intramuscular administration, frequent monitoring required (complete blood count and urinalysis), and frequent toxicities. Toxicities include skin rashes, bone marrow suppression, and proteinuria.

Biologic DMARDs

Recent research has continued to elucidate the central role that cytokines, most notably TNF-α and IL-1, play in the pathophysiology of RA (Chapter 35). This has led directly to the development and clinical use of biologic agents directed against TNF-α1 (etanercept[3] [Enbrel], infliximab[4] [Remicade], adalimumab[5] [Humira], golimumab [Simponi], and certolizumab [Cimzia]) and IL-1 (anakinra [Kineret]). Three new monoclonals have been approved for RA: an anti-CD20, rituximab (Rituxan); a T-cell agent, abatacept (Orencia); and an anti–IL-6 receptor antibody, tocilizumab (Actemra).[6-8] All RA patients receiving biologic therapies should be monitored by a rheumatologist, and their physicians should be aware of the risk for infections that are often atypical. Essentially all the biologicals, when combined with methotrexate, have been shown to decrease disease activity and slow radiographic progression in RA patients with active disease despite methotrexate. Currently, biologic agents should not be used in combination with each other because all studies to date have shown a significant increase in infections. See Chapter 35 for further details on the use of biologic agents in the treatment of RA.

Treatment of Underlying Conditions

Optimal care of patients with RA requires recognition of the associated comorbid conditions, including an increased risk of cardiovascular death, osteoporosis, infections (especially pneumonia), and certain cancers.

Cardiovascular Disease

Increasingly, cardiovascular disease is being recognized as the cause of much of the excess mortality in RA. A number of factors contribute to this mortality, including sedentary lifestyle, glucocorticoid therapy, and treatments that increase homocysteine levels, such as methotrexate and sulfasalazine. However, recently a strong association between chronic inflammation and cardiovascular disease was identified, and it is likely that this may be the most significant factor. Therapies that control RA earlier and better can be expected to decrease cardiovascular morbidity and mortality. Clinicians should consider RA a risk factor for cardiovascular disease and should aggressively address other cardiovascular risk factors (Chapter 51) in their rheumatoid patients.

Other Associated Diseases

Osteoporosis is common in patients with RA, and early treatment results in long-term dividends. Patients with RA are at an increased risk for infections, and some forms of treatment further increase this risk. Patients should be cautioned to seek medical attention early for even minor symptoms suggestive of infection, especially if receiving anti-TNF therapy. All patients with RA should receive a pneumococcal vaccine at appropriate intervals and yearly influenza vaccinations. Finally, patients with RA have an increased risk of lymphoma. Occasionally, B-cell lymphomas are associated with immunosuppression and regress after immunosuppression is discontinued. RA patients have significantly decreased risk (odds ratio, 0.2) of developing colon cancer. This is thought to be secondary to chronic inhibition of COX by NSAIDs.

PROGNOSIS

Until recently, RA was thought to be a relatively benign disease. It is now clear that, once established, RA is a lifelong progressive disease that produces significant morbidity in most patients and premature mortality in many. Long-term studies have found that 50% of patients with RA have had to stop working after 10 years (approximately 10 times the average rate). Patients who are RF or ACPA positive and those who are positive for the shared epitope have a worse prognosis, with more erosions and more extra-articular disease (see Table 272-2). Once deformities are found on examination or erosions on radiography, the damage is largely irreversible. It has been clearly shown that erosions occur in most patients in the first 1 to 2 years and that the rate of radiographic damage can be affected by early therapy. Therefore, early DMARD therapy is critical. Although limited long-term data are available, the current information strongly suggests that patients have the opportunity to benefit greatly if the newer principles of therapy are practiced.

FUTURE DIRECTIONS

Significant advances in the effective treatment of RA have come from an understanding of the cytokine imbalance that accompanies this disease. Much research is focused on the further development of biologic products to modulate this balance. Biologic therapies that modulate B-cell and T-cell function have been shown to be effective in the treatment of RA. There remains a critical need for a cytokine thermostat that would allow titration of the desired cytokine balance to control disease without altering critical immune functions.

Even with existing therapies, there are many different effective options for patients with RA. The challenge for the clinician is to pick the right option for each patient. Few data are currently available to aid in this choice, and the establishment of parameters, genetic or otherwise, that would allow selection of the best initial option for each patient would be a major breakthrough. Finally, elucidation of the trigger or triggers for RA may allow the development of strategies to prevent the onset of clinical disease.

1. Goekoop-Ruiterman YP, de Vries-Bouwstra JK, Allaart CF, et al. Comparison of treatment strategies in early rheumatoid arthritis: a randomized trial. *Ann Intern Med.* 2007;146:406-415.
2. O'Dell JR, Haire CE, Erickson N, et al. Treatment of rheumatoid arthritis with methotrexate alone, sulfasalazine and hydroxychloroquine, or a combination of all three medications. *N Engl J Med.* 1996;334:1287-1291.
3. Bathon JM, Martin RW, Fleischmann RM, et al. A comparison of etanercept and methotrexate in patients with early rheumatoid arthritis. *N Engl J Med.* 2000;343:1586-1593.
4. Lipsky PE, Van der Heijde D, St. Clair EW, et al. Infliximab and methotrexate in the treatment of rheumatoid arthritis. *N Engl J Med.* 2000;243:1594-1602.
5. Weinblatt ME, Keystone EC, Furst DE, et al. Adalimumab, a fully human anti-tumor necrosis factor alpha monoclonal antibody, for the treatment of rheumatoid arthritis in patients taking concomitant methotrexate: the ARMADA trial. *Arthritis Rheum.* 2003;38:35-45.
6. Lee YH, Bae SC, Song GG. The efficacy and safety of rituximab for the treatment of active rheumatoid arthritis: a systematic review and meta-analysis of randomized controlled trials. *Rheumatol Int.* 2011. [Epub ahead of print.]
7. Genovese MC, Becker JC, Schiff M, et al. Abatacept for rheumatoid arthritis refractory to tumor necrosis factor inhibition. *N Engl J Med.* 2005;353:1114-1123.
8. Genovese MC, McKay JD, Nasonov EL, et al. Interleukin-6 receptor inhibition with tocilizumab reduces disease activity in rheumatoid arthritis with inadequate response to disease-modifying antirheumatic drugs: the tocilizumab in combination with traditional disease-modifying antirheumatic drug therapy study. *Arthritis Rheum.* 2008;58:2968-2980.

SUGGESTED READINGS

McInnes IB, O'Dell JR. State-of-the-art: rheumatoid arthritis. *Ann Rheum Dis.* 2010;69:1898-1906. *Review of pathophysiology and treatment.*

Scott DL, Wolf F, Huizinga TW. Rheumatoid arthritis. *Lancet.* 2010;376:1094-1108. *Comprehensive review.*

Singh JA, Wells GA, Christensen R, et al. Adverse effects of biologics: a network meta-analysis and Cochrane overview. *Cochrane Database Syst Rev.* 2011;2:CD008794. *Biologics are associated with significantly higher rates of adverse events and TB reactivation.*

Whiting PF, Smidt N, Sterne JA, et al. Systematic review: accuracy of anti-citrullinated peptide antibodies for diagnosing rheumatoid arthritis. *Ann Intern Med.* 2010;152:456-464, W155-66. *Anti-citrullinated peptide antibodies are useful for the early diagnosis of rheumatoid arthritis.*

273

THE SPONDYLOARTHROPATHIES

ROBERT D. INMAN

COMMON FEATURES OF THE SPONDYLOARTHROPATHIES

DEFINITION

The spondyloarthropathies (SpAs) encompass a group of clinical syndromes that are linked in terms of disease manifestations and genetic susceptibility. The clinical subsets most commonly recognized are ankylosing spondylitis (AS), reactive arthritis (ReA), psoriatic arthritis (PsA), and enteropathic arthritis (EA) (Fig. 273-1). In addition, a sizable number of patients do not fit into one of these distinct diagnostic categories but share some of the common clinical features described in this chapter. This syndrome is termed *undifferentiated spondyloarthropathy* (USpA); it may evolve over time into a classic pattern such as AS, or it may retain an undifferentiated pattern in long-term follow-up studies.

PATHOBIOLOGY

Family studies involving multiple individuals with SpA have emphasized some of the common features among the four distinct subsets. The impression from such studies is that there is a shared common path of immunogenetic susceptibility, with further genetic and environmental influences that lead to characteristic clinical subsets. Thus, EA may occur in one such family, but in another family the disease may be PsA. In this sense, the SpAs seem to "breed true." It should be recognized, however, that some distinct clinical features can be very similar in their manifestations (e.g., guttate psoriasis and keratoderma blennorrhagicum), making simple discrimination difficult.

CLINICAL MANIFESTATIONS

There are several common features in the family of SpAs that serve to both link them with and distinguish them from the other major contributor to chronic polyarthritis—rheumatoid arthritis (RA) (Chapter 272). The SpAs have a strong predilection for the spine, in particular the sacroiliac joints. There is a shared tendency for new bone formation at sites of chronic inflammation, with joint ankylosis as a consequence. When peripheral arthritis occurs, it is commonly in the lower extremity and asymmetrical. There is a predilection for sites of tendon insertion into bone (entheses), so enthesitis is one of the most specific clinical manifestations of the SpAs. Theories

postulating the basis for this target organ involvement have invoked biomechanical factors, innervation, local vascularity, and bone marrow–derived inflammatory mediators, but the precise mechanism remains incompletely defined. Whatever the reason, inflammation in the enthesis and contiguous subchondral bone is a characteristic feature of this form of arthritis, and the appearance of this inflammation on magnetic resonance imaging (MRI) is distinct enough to lead some investigators to use MRI for diagnostic purposes.

A predilection for ocular inflammation, particularly acute anterior uveitis, is a common feature of all SpA subsets. Indeed, some investigators consider anterior uveitis to be a feature of SpA in its own right because it may occur in the same susceptible population of patients even in the absence of joint involvement, and it may have a unique genetic predisposition. Finally, all SpA subsets have an association with the class I human leukocyte antigen (HLA) allele B27, with the strength of the association varying somewhat among them.

DIAGNOSIS

Increasingly, diagnostic criteria (Table 273-1) are emphasizing the common clinical features—namely, inflammatory spinal pain or asymmetrical lower extremity synovitis. Several distinct features differentiate the SpAs from RA, the other main contributor to the differential diagnosis of chronic polyarthritis (Table 273-2). These features include sex predilection, HLA association, pattern of joint involvement, and presence of rheumatoid factor, which becomes the serologic distinction between seropositive disease (RA) and seronegative disease (SpAs).

At the level of joint histopathology, sites of chronic inflammation in RA are associated with erosions, but in the SpAs such sites are associated with new bone formation. This distinction suggests a fundamental difference in the cytokine profile in the microenvironment of the joint, but this issue has not been resolved, and the mediators of neo-ossification await identification. Dysregulation of the wnt/β-catenin pathway may play a key role in the ankylosing process. Synovial histopathology in SpA is characterized by abundant neutrophils, macrophages, and hypervascularity, whereas in RA the prominent features are lymphoid aggregates, dendritic cells, lining cell hyperplasia, and citrullinated proteins. These differences suggest that SpA reflects a fundamental alteration in innate immunity, whereas RA reflects dysregulation of adaptive immunity.

TREATMENT

General Measures

The SpAs necessitate a global approach to management in which education of patients is the cornerstone. Because the typical onset is during young adulthood, with a male preponderance, these patients may experience significant frustration or depression if their acute arthritis evolves into a chronic disease that significantly impairs their functional capabilities and quality of life. A clinician managing patients with SpA should be aware that these psychosocial aspects are an important part of the burden of illness. Similarly, there may be important implications for the workplace, particularly if a job demands significant bending or twisting. It is important to include the mechanical demands of the workplace in the global assessment of patients with SpAs.

Exercise is an important part of the treatment plan for patients with AS. Generally, high-impact sports should be avoided, whereas swimming is an

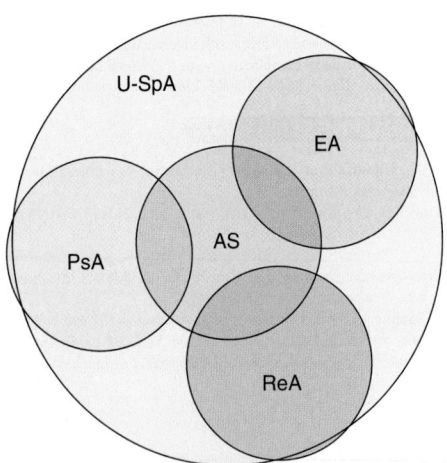

FIGURE 273-1. Schematic relationships among the different spondyloarthropathy (SpA) subsets. Ankylosing spondylitis (AS), considered the classic SpA, encompasses the essential features of this family of diseases. AS may overlap with psoriatic arthritis (PsA), enteropathic arthritis (EA), or reactive arthritis (ReA). Many patients have clinical features of SpA that do not meet the diagnostic criteria for any of the four defined subsets. Such cases are termed *undifferentiated SpA* (U-SpA).

TABLE 273-1	EUROPEAN SPONDYLOARTHROPATHY STUDY GROUP CRITERIA FOR SPONDYLOARTHROPATHY

Inflammatory spinal pain
OR
Synovitis (asymmetrical or predominantly in the lower limb)
PLUS
Any one of the following:
  Positive family history
  Psoriasis
  Inflammatory bowel disease
  Urethritis, cervicitis, or acute diarrhea within 1 mo before arthritis
  Alternating buttock pain
  Enthesopathy
  Sacroiliitis

TABLE 273-2 COMPARISON OF RHEUMATOID ARTHRITIS AND THE SPONDYLOARTHROPATHIES

FEATURE	RHEUMATOID ARTHRITIS	ANKYLOSING SPONDYLITIS	ENTEROPATHIC ARTHRITIS	PSORIATIC ARTHRITIS	REACTIVE ARTHRITIS
Male-female ratio	1 : 3	3 : 1	1 : 1	1 : 1	10 : 1
HLA association	DR4	B27	B27 (axial)	B27 (axial)	B27
Joint pattern	Symmetrical, peripheral	Axial	Axial and peripheral	Axial and asymmetrical peripheral	Axial and asymmetrical peripheral
Sacroiliac	0	Symmetrical	Symmetrical	Asymmetrical	Asymmetrical
Syndesmophyte	0	Smooth, marginal	Smooth, marginal	Coarse, nonmarginal	Coarse, nonmarginal
Eye	Scleritis	Iritis	+/−	0	Iritis and conjunctivitis
Skin	Vasculitis	0	0	Psoriasis	Keratoderma
Rheumatoid factor	>80%	0	0	0	0

HLA = human leukocyte antigen.

ideal exercise. Stretching to maintain mobility and maintenance of posture should be emphasized, and an experienced physiotherapist can greatly assist in instructing patients in daily exercises. Long car trips and air travel should include periodic stretching. Sleep position should emphasize a straight back position rather than one curled on the side. Deep breathing exercises and avoidance of cigarettes should be stressed.

One key area of concern for patients is prognosis, because the SpAs, particularly ReA, often occur in young, active individuals for whom athletic activity is a priority. There is general recognition that ReA has a greater propensity for chronicity than was previously appreciated, and this should temper an overly optimistic projection of the disease's natural history. At the 5-year follow-up of a cohort of patients with *Salmonella*-induced ReA, two thirds continued to have subjective complaints, and one third demonstrated objective changes in their joints. The variability in prognosis for the large group of patients falling into the USpA group is perplexing. At present, there is a lack of reliable predictors of progression in patients with this heterogeneous cluster of articular and extra-articular features.

Medical Therapy
Nonsteroidal Anti-inflammatory Drugs

In general, joint inflammation in the SpAs improves significantly after the introduction of nonsteroidal anti-inflammatory drugs (NSAIDs). Indomethacin and diclofenac (up to 200 mg/day in divided doses) or naproxen (up to 1000 mg/day in divided doses) are generally well tolerated in this population. These agents have to be used with caution in EA because of concern about exacerbating the underlying inflammatory bowel disease. In the case of AS, the goal with anti-inflammatory treatment is to achieve sufficient relief of pain and stiffness to allow an active, sustained program of exercise and physical activity that maintains posture and improves quality of life. Whether NSAIDs have disease-modifying capability has not been definitively resolved.

Corticosteroids

The response to the intra-articular injection of steroids in the peripheral joints of patients with SpA is often neither as dramatic nor as sustained as in those with RA. Corticosteroid injection into the sacroiliac joints is usually performed under imaging guidance (fluoroscopy or computed tomography [CT]). One study found that such injections resulted in a good response in 79% of patients and that the improvement could persist for many months. Systemic corticosteroids (either orally or via an intravenous bolus protocol) have been used for severe symptomatic flares, but controlled trials to validate their effectiveness are lacking. The goal should be prompt tapering of the dose when symptomatic control is achieved. The recognition that osteoporosis (Chapter 251) is a significant problem in AS provides further impetus to use corticosteroids sparingly. Topical steroids are usually effective for the treatment of the mucous membrane and skin manifestations of ReA. For uveitis, topical corticosteroid eye drops are an integral component of management, and treatment should be monitored jointly with an ophthalmologist.

Sulfasalazine

Randomized, placebo-controlled trials have provided some support for the use of sulfasalazine (SSZ), particularly in PsA. Three 36-week, randomized, double-blind multicenter studies of patients with AS, PsA, and ReA, respectively, were undertaken to compare SSZ (2 g/day) with placebo in each case. The different response rates in the placebo arms of these trials highlight the variability in the clinical course of the SpAs. An analysis of these studies stratified the patients into those having axial disease and those having peripheral disease. In patients with only axial disease, response criteria were met equally in the SSZ group and the placebo group. In patients with peripheral arthritis, responses were seen in 59% of the SSZ group and 43% of the placebo group (*P* < .0005).[1] These findings are useful in guiding the selection of patients for SSZ treatment.

Methotrexate

Concurrent with the widespread use of methotrexate (MTX) in patients with RA, there has been increasing use of MTX in patients with SpA. Generally, responses have been good, particularly for peripheral joint disease, but few controlled trials have been conducted to substantiate these clinical impressions. There is no evidence that MTX changes the course of axial diseases in AS. Experience with long-term MTX therapy in 38 patients with PsA has been reported, and despite an improvement in joint count, there was no evidence of a slowing of radiographic progression. Long-term follow-up may be required to resolve whether MTX has a joint-sparing effect in PsA.

Other Disease-Modifying Agents

There have been several therapeutic approaches to the control of PsA, including chloroquine, intramuscular gold, and cyclosporine, all of which show some clinical efficacy; however, long-term studies are needed to evaluate these drugs more comprehensively. The response of SpA patients to SSZ may be attributable to the antibiotic moiety of this compound (sulfapyridine) or to the anti-inflammatory moiety (5-aminosalicylic acid). An open study of intravenous pamidronate for refractory AS showed significant improvement in disease activity scores, but the current impression is that this agent is less effective than the anti–tumor necrosis factor agents (see later).

Antibiotic Therapy

The current concept of the pathogenesis of ReA postulates that a bacterial infection, usually gastrointestinal (GI) or genitourinary (GU), is the triggering event in an immunogenetically susceptible host. For the other SpAs, there is less compelling evidence that infection plays a causal role. It is sound clinical practice to treat any culture-proven chlamydial urethritis in conjunction with treatment of the sexual partner. For this indication, a single 1-g dose of azithromycin is as effective as doxycycline 100 mg twice a day for 7 days. The role of antibiotics in the management of SpA has been controversial. An earlier retrospective review concluded that 37% of episodes of urethritis not treated with anti-*Chlamydia* agents were associated with subsequent ReA, whereas only 10% of such episodes progressed to ReA when treated with tetracycline. In a 3-month, double-blind, placebo-controlled study of chronic ReA, lymecycline significantly decreased the duration of illness in patients with *Chlamydia*-induced ReA but not in patients with ReA triggered by enteric pathogens. Two controlled trials demonstrated no significant difference between ciprofloxacin and placebo in ReA and undifferentiated oligoarthritis. Ciprofloxacin was not effective in *Yersinia*- or *Salmonella*-induced ReA, but there was a trend toward a response in *Chlamydia*-induced ReA. A study examining azithromycin in the treatment of SpA found no convincing evidence of disease-modifying potential.[2] A recent report compared rifampin/azithromycin, rifampin/doxycycline, and placebo for chronic *Chlamydia*-induced ReA and observed that tender and swollen joint counts responded more significantly to the combination antibiotics than to placebo.[3] The precise role of antibiotic agents in this clinical situation has not yet been finalized.

Anti–Tumor Necrosis Factor Therapy

The role of immunomodulatory cytokines in the pathogenesis of SpA has been controversial. Some studies have implicated a genetic polymorphism associated with the relative impairment of tumor necrosis factor-α (TNF-α) production as an AS susceptibility marker, but not all studies have supported this notion. Biologic agents, such as monoclonal antibodies to TNF-α (infliximab, adalimumab, golimumab) or the soluble TNF receptor (etanercept), have been used in the treatment of SpA. So far, these four anti-TNF agents have been comparably effective in trials of AS and PsA[4-7] and appear to be better than antibiotics.[8] These studies generally reported a prompt response in clinical outcome measures and in laboratory indicators of inflammation, and MRI evaluations have shown improvement in local inflammation in the sacroiliac joints and spine. The anti-TNF treatments have been well tolerated, with no significant incidence of serious adverse events, but patients appear to relapse when treatment is discontinued. Experience with longer-term treatment with anti-TNF agents (>2 years) has been encouraging with regard to the persistence of the therapeutic effect and the infrequency of late adverse events. These biologic agents have been shown to retard radiographic progression in PsA, but whether anti-TNF treatments can alter the progressive ankylosis of AS over the long term awaits further study. The objective improvements seen on MRI provide hope that these agents may alter the long-term outcomes of AS structurally as well as functionally.

GENETIC SUSCEPTIBILITY

DEFINITION

The major histocompatibility complex (MHC), on the short arm of chromosome 6 in humans, is one of the most polymorphic regions of the human genome (Chapter 45). This is particularly so for the B locus, which constitutes part of the class I MHC genes in this complex. More than 200 different alleles have been detected at this locus, of which B27 is just one. As with all HLA alleles, there is codominant expression of B locus genes, such that most individuals who are B27 positive are heterozygous for the B locus. There appears to be little clinical or prognostic significance associated with the less common homozygous B27 state. The conventional role of class I HLAs is to present a processed peptide to the T-cell receptor of a specific CD8$^+$ cytotoxic T cell, thereby initiating an immune response against the pathogen from which that peptide was derived by intracellular proteolysis and processing. This function gives the HLAs a critical role in host defense against pathogens, and the heterogeneity of cellular immune responses is alleged to be an advantage for a species (such as humans) with an extensive polymorphism region of the genome. This idea has led to the concept that infectious diseases have driven allelic polymorphisms in the MHC. Such a hypothesis postulates a selective advantage in the extensive peptide-binding capabilities conferred by different alleles of the B locus, but there may also be disadvantages.

Recent genome-wide association studies in AS have identified additional genetic markers of susceptibility for AS. Polymorphisms in the *IL-23R* gene are associated with AS, and these particular variants are the same as those seen in inflammatory bowel disease and psoriasis. Thus the clinical convergence of these different diseases, well known to clinicians, now appears to have a common genetic element. Polymorphisms in the endoplasmic reticulum aminopeptidase (ERAP) gene constitute the strongest genetic risk factor for AS after HLA-B27. ERAP plays a key role in trimming peptides in the endoplasmic reticulum before loading these peptide complexes onto a nascent class I MHC molecule. This finding continues to attribute a central role to MHC class I peptide presentation in the pathogenesis of AS.

EPIDEMIOLOGY

It is clear that HLA is strongly associated with the SpAs, yet the prevalence of HLA-B27 varies widely in different racial and ethnic clusters around the world. It is virtually absent in aboriginal populations in Australia, occurs in 1% of the population in Japan, in 7% in northern European countries, and in 50% in some of the native tribes in western Canada. The environmental-genetic interaction that may account for the expansion or restriction of this gene in human populations is unknown, but some evidence indicates that B27 may confer a more effective host response to some viruses. This variability has a practical impact for the clinician. Because the relative risk conferred by a gene reflects the prevalence of the gene in affected individuals versus its prevalence in the normal population, the relative risk for SpAs is higher in a population in which the gene is uncommon (e.g., Japan) than in a population in which B27 is more common (e.g., Scandinavia). In the North American white population, the prevalence of the gene is approximately 7%. Thus, there is a 7% "false-positive" rate if one is attempting to use the gene as a diagnostic marker to decipher the cause of chronic back pain in an unselected population of patients. In contrast, 90% of patients with AS are B27 positive, so there is a 10% "false-negative" rate when using the test diagnostically. The key factor is pretest probability. In a patient with chronic back pain that is clearly inflammatory in character, the addition of B27 positivity combines to strengthen the likelihood of AS accounting for the back problem. The presence of distinctive extra-articular features (e.g., uveitis) further increases this likelihood.

It is believed that the prevalence of AS in various parts of the world closely parallels the prevalence of B27 in that population, and in general, this pattern is valid. What introduces complexity into this concept is the recognition that there are more than 30 subtypes of B27. HLA-B2705 is regarded as the primordial subtype, with variability developing over time on the basis of alterations in genomic DNA. Some subtypes, notably B2706 and B2709, do not seem to confer increased susceptibility to the development of AS. This observation has led to a search for "arthritogenic peptides" that are presented by the disease-associated subtypes such as B2705 and B2704 but not by the non-disease-associated subtypes. To date, no simple peptide-susceptibility relationship has been demonstrated, but this is an important clue to the pathogenic role of B27, and studies are ongoing to explore this relationship.

Other steps have also been taken to define the mechanism whereby B27 confers disease susceptibility in addition to that of uniquely presenting an arthritogenic peptide to T cells. According to the theory of molecular mimicry, an autoimmune response can ensue after an infection if the immune response against the pathogen cross-reacts with host antigens. There is a degree of sequence homology between B27 and several candidate gram-negative enteric bacteria, and there is evidence for cross-reacting monoclonal antibodies, but the significance of such homology for disease pathogenesis remains unresolved. It has also been argued that B27 is distinctive in its propensity to misfold in the endoplasmic reticulum, which may induce a pro-inflammatory cascade called the *unfolded protein response*. Furthermore, B27 may have a distinct tendency to form heavy chain homodimers at the cell surface, and the possible consequences of this change for the immune response are under investigation. There has also been investigation into the alteration of primary host-pathogen interactions, such as modulation of pathogen invasion, intracellular replication, and clearance. However, no definitive allele-specific relationships have been demonstrated in these studies.

In B27 transgenic rats, the spontaneous development of pathology strikingly similar to human SpAs has supported the notion that B27 itself is the critical genetic factor in disease pathogenesis. These animals demonstrate pathology similar to that of Crohn's disease in the GI tract, spondylitis, peripheral arthritis, uveitis, and psoriasiform skin and nail changes. Of interest, if such animals are raised in a germ-free environment, there is a marked reduction in joint and gut disease, implying a dynamic interrelationship between microbial triggers and background host genes that seems to recapitulate the situation seen clinically.

Genome-wide screening studies of multiplex families with SpAs, particularly AS, are ongoing in several countries to identify other genes involved in the predisposition to these diseases. The strongest association of SpA to date remains with the HLA complex, so at least in familial AS, B27 may to a certain extent be necessary (but not sufficient) to confer disease susceptibility. MRI studies in asymptomatic B27-positive individuals indicate that there is a much higher prevalence of sacroiliitis than previously recognized, and studies are continuing to define that prevalence and indeed the prevalence of SpAs in the general population. Some investigators have concluded that SpAs are as common as RA.

CLINICAL SUBSETS OF THE SPONDYLOARTHROPATHIES
Ankylosing Spondylitis

EPIDEMIOLOGY

AS is the most common inflammatory disorder of the axial skeleton. The following is a useful rule of thumb: AS occurs in 0.2% of the general population, in 2% of the B27-positive population, and in 20% of B27-positive individuals with an affected family member. There is a male preponderance in the disease, with the male-to-female ratio ranging from 2.5 : 1 to 5 : 1; however, recent epidemiologic studies have found less female involvement than these estimates indicate. The basis for the gender bias has not been resolved. It is held, however, that AS is underrecognized in women, perhaps because of milder axial disease and a more delayed disease onset, but alternative diagnoses of pelvic and low back pain in women may hinder clinician awareness of the disease in female patients.

CLINICAL MANIFESTATIONS

AS typically begins in young adulthood, but symptoms may arise in adolescence or earlier. Up to 15% of children with juvenile chronic polyarthritis are classified as having juvenile AS. Such children may have a pauciarticular pattern, with a predilection for the tarsal joints and frequently minimal axial complaints. During the adolescent years there is an increasing prevalence of radiographic sacroiliitis, with a significant proportion of patients manifesting this feature by the end of the teenage years. At the other end of the age spectrum, a small number of patients with late-onset AS may have sacroiliitis and oligoarthritis. The axial involvement and asymmetrical lower extremity

TABLE 273-3	MODIFIED NEW YORK CRITERIA FOR ANKYLOSING SPONDYLITIS (1984)

CLINICAL CRITERIA

Low back pain and stiffness for >3 mo that improve with exercise but are not relieved by rest
Limitation of motion of the lumbar spine in both sagittal and frontal planes
Limitation of chest expansion

RADIOLOGIC CRITERIA

Sacroiliitis: grade ≥2 bilateral *or* grade 3 or 4 unilateral

GRADING

Definite AS if the radiologic criterion is associated with at least one clinical variable
Probable AS if:
    The three clinical criteria are present
    The radiologic criterion is present without the clinical criteria

AS = ankylosing spondylitis.

FIGURE 273-2. Bilaterally symmetrical sacroiliitis in ankylosing spondylitis.

involvement may serve to differentiate such patients from those with late-onset RA, although there may be overlapping clinical features. Recent studies indicate that the rate of radiographic progression may be less in juvenile-onset AS than in adult-onset AS.

The classic manifestation of AS is the onset of low back pain that persists for more than 3 months, is accompanied by early-morning stiffness, and is typically improved by exercise (Table 273-3). An extensive discussion of the differential diagnosis of low back pain is presented in Chapter 407. Some investigators would include a response to NSAID therapy as an additional feature differentiating AS from mechanical low back pain. Back pain that awakens the patient from sleep is often a clue to inflammatory back pain that may have been misdiagnosed as the pain of degenerative disc disease, the latter being a much more common cause of low back pain in the population at large. The pain typically occurs in the region of the sacroiliac joints, with or without slight radiation to the buttock area. Mid-thoracic pain and cervical pain, particularly at night, are less common but strongly suggest inflammatory back pain when they occur. Fatigue is also a suggestive symptom and is often highlighted by the typical young male patient, who sets a high functional norm in terms of sports and recreation. If the inflammation is inadequately controlled, there is increasing stiffness, which may persist most of the day, as well as progressive loss of mobility and flexibility.

Peripheral oligoarthritis is seen in up to 30% of patients with AS. Typically, it is an asymmetrical oligoarthritis with a predilection for the lower extremities. It is important to ask about concurrent or previous tendinitis (e.g., Achilles tendinitis) or heel pain (e.g., plantar fasciitis) because either may reflect an enthesitis that is part of the clinical picture. Involvement of the hip can occur at any point in the course of AS and can follow a course to joint destruction. A hip flexion contracture on this basis may contribute to increasing stoop on standing and walking, which may otherwise be attributed to spinal involvement in the disease.

Extra-articular features primarily involve the eye. Ocular involvement may occur in up to 40% of AS patients, most typically acute anterior uveitis (iritis). The uveitis often manifests as a slight impairment in visual acuity, with accompanying photophobia and eye pain. Typically, it is unilateral and recurrent. Inflammatory bowel disease and psoriasis occur in approximately 10% of AS cohorts. Less common manifestations include aortic insufficiency, cardiac conduction defects, and pulmonary fibrosis.

DIAGNOSIS

Physical Examination
Physical examination of the spine characteristically indicates restricted movement, which in the early stages may reflect paraspinal muscle spasm in part; late in the course it reflects ankylosis of the zygapophyseal joints and syndesmophyte bridging of the vertebral bodies. Forward flexion is restricted and can be monitored by measuring the finger to floor distance on bending forward. Schober's test is used to measure mobility in the lower part of the back: with the patient standing upright, a 10-cm span is marked from the fifth lumbar vertebra upward. On maximal forward flexion, the distance between the marks is remeasured. With normal spinal mobility, the flexed distance should register as 15 cm, or an increment of 5 cm. Thoracic involvement is measured in chest expansion, with the chest circumference at maximal

inspiration being more than 5 cm greater than the circumference at maximal expiration. Changes in cervical mobility can be measured as the occiput to wall distance, with the patient's heels against the wall as the patient attempts to touch the back of the head to the wall. Restricted spinal mobility early in the course of the disease may best be detected by lateral spinal flexion, measured as the difference in the finger to floor distance when standing erect compared with maximal bending to the side. Inflammation in the sacroiliac joint may be reflected by joint line tenderness to direct pressure or by the fabere or Gaenslen maneuver. In the former, the patient lies supine while the examiner flexes and externally rotates the hip. In the latter, the examiner extends the hip by letting the leg dangle off the side of the examining table. In both cases, stress is placed on the sacroiliac joint and may reproduce the back pain if it derives from this site.

Laboratory Findings
Laboratory tests in the evaluation of inflammatory back pain are relatively nonspecific. The erythrocyte sedimentation rate and C-reactive protein are typically elevated, but normal levels do not exclude inflammatory back pain, and the degree of elevation is typically less than would be seen in acute RA. Anemia of chronic disease may be observed if the condition is long-standing. Serum immunoglobulin A levels may be elevated, but autoantibodies are notable for their absence. HLA-B27 is rarely the definitive factor for diagnosis, and the false-positive and false-negative rates have already been discussed; however, in the setting of characteristic back symptoms, the test has reasonably high sensitivity and specificity.

Imaging
Radiographic assessment is important for confirmation of disease, but early in the course there may be no radiographic changes in the sacroiliac joints. If the clinician has a high index of suspicion in such cases, MRI may improve the sensitivity of the plain radiograph because inflammatory changes on MRI predate radiographic changes. When ordering x-rays, specific views of the sacroiliac joints should be requested because the obliquity of the joint renders it difficult to assess on a routine anteroposterior pelvic radiograph. The classic findings are bilateral changes in the sacroiliac joints (Fig. 273-2). Abnormalities include erosions in the joint line, pseudowidening, subchondral sclerosis, and, finally, ankylosis, reflecting complete bony replacement of the sacroiliac joints.

Radiographs of the spine may reveal squaring of the vertebral bodies (loss of the normal anterior concavity of the lumbar vertebra) and "shiny corners" (subchondral sclerosis at the upper edge of the vertebral body), both of which are manifestations of enthesitis. Syndesmophytes, which represent marginal bridging of the vertebrae (Figs. 273-3 and 273-4), eventually develop and make the diagnosis clear. Because ankylosis of the apophyseal joints may occur without syndesmophyte formation, it is important to assess the posterior joints on the lateral lumbosacral spine views, as well as the anterior margin of the vertebrae. Eventually, the changes may result in a "bamboo spine," so called because the bridging syndesmophytes can mimic the appearance of bamboo. It is now appreciated that osteoporosis (Chapter 251) is a significant feature of AS, probably reflecting both the local chronic

FIGURE 273-3. *Left,* Lumbar spondylitis in ankylosing spondylitis with symmetrical, marginal bridging syndesmophytes and calcification of the spinal ligament. *Right,* The bulky, nonmarginal, asymmetrical syndesmophytes of reactive arthritis with lumbar spondylitis.

FIGURE 273-4. A 34-year-old man who has had ankylosing spondylitis for 9 years and neck pain. Radiographs demonstrate narrowing of the C2-C3 apophyseal joints posteriorly and anterior bridging marginal syndesmophytes extending from C2 to C5.

inflammation and the abnormal biomechanical loading of the vertebrae as the disease progresses.

Differential Diagnosis

The differential diagnosis of AS includes the other SpAs; osteitis condensans ilii; diffuse idiopathic skeletal hyperostosis; the syndrome of synovitis, acne, pustulosis, hyperostosis, and osteomyelitis (SAPHO); and some induced hyperostotic states (vitamin A intoxication, fluorosis). New bone formation occurs in degenerative disc disease, but the bulky, horizontal appearance of osteophytes is easily distinguished from that of syndesmophytes, and narrowing of the disc space is not a feature of AS. Osteoarthritis of the sacroiliac joint has recently been recognized as having a higher prevalence than previously appreciated.

The clinical course and severity of AS are highly variable. Inflammatory back pain and stiffness dominate the picture in the early stages, whereas chronic pain and deformity may develop over time. In both early and late phases of the disease there may be a significant impact on work disability and

quality of life. In only a minority of patients does the full-blown picture of a bamboo spine eventually develop, but there are few variables that can reliably aid in prognosticating the course. At present, the strongest predictor of new syndesmophyte formation is the presence of syndesmophytes at baseline. In AS patients in whom new, refractory spinal pain develops, an intervertebral fracture should be considered, which can occur after only minimal trauma.

Additional late complications may include cauda equina syndrome, osteoporotic compression fractures, spondylodiscitis, and restrictive lung disease.

Reactive Arthritis

DEFINITION

ReA is an aseptic arthritis that occurs subsequent to an extra-articular infection, most typically of the GI or GU tract. In the former, the key pathogens are *Salmonella typhimurium, Yersinia enterocolitica, Shigella flexneri,* and *Campylobacter jejuni.* In the latter, *Chlamydia trachomatis* is the most common offender.

EPIDEMIOLOGY

The true incidence and prevalence of ReA are not well defined. In epidemics involving *Salmonella* (Chapter 316) or *Yersinia* (Chapter 320), it is estimated that ReA develops in 2 to 7% of infected individuals but in as many as 20% of B27-positive infected individuals. In such epidemic studies, B27 confers risk not only for the onset of arthritis but also for axial involvement and chronicity. Genetic variants in Toll-like receptor 2 (TLR-2) are associated with acute ReA, thus implicating host innate immunity as central in ReA. The variability in the rate of ReA is determined by the heterogeneity of the cohorts reported, which introduces confounding variables of different genetic backgrounds in the population and different species of pathogens. Even in the setting of an epidemic point source outbreak, the inoculum varies widely among the exposed individuals, and the genetic makeup of the population at risk (e.g., the prevalence of B27) may differ greatly among different studies. Case ascertainment and relative risk are even more difficult to determine for post-*Chlamydia* ReA. Young adults in the United States have a high prevalence of asymptomatic *Chlamydia* carriage in the GU tract, and establishing a causal link between *Chlamydia* and synovitis can be difficult. Nevertheless, it is with *Chlamydia* that ReA has been most intensively studied.

PATHOBIOLOGY

Although immunofluorescence studies have identified bacterial antigens in the joints of patients with ReA after both GI and GU infections, it is primarily in post-*Chlamydia* ReA that results of polymerase chain reaction studies on synovial tissues have most consistently been positive, suggesting that viable *Chlamydia* may persist in the joints of such patients, albeit in a metabolically altered state.

Typically, the onset of arthritis occurs 1 to 3 weeks after the GI or GU infection, but the temporal details are often difficult to define precisely.

Although the definition of aseptic arthritis after an extra-articular infection may include a broader range of pathogens (e.g., *Chlamydia pneumoniae*), sites of infection (e.g., streptococcal pharyngitis), and types of infections (e.g., *Giardia* infections of the GI tract), these clinical scenarios have not generally been included in the category of ReA. They lack the other associated clinical features of the SpA group of diseases, and they lack an association with B27.

DIAGNOSIS

The pattern of joint involvement in ReA is one of asymmetrical oligoarthritis with a predilection for the lower extremity, a pattern shared by most SpA syndromes. Enthesitis may present as Achilles tendinitis or plantar fasciitis. Dactylitis, appearing as a sausage digit, may also be seen. Dactylitis is the net result of inflammatory changes affecting the joint capsule, entheses, periarticular structures, and periosteal bone. Sacroiliitis may be seen in the acute phase, but radiographic changes are seen largely in patients with a more chronic course.

When ReA is accompanied by certain extra-articular features such as urethritis, conjunctivitis, or mucocutaneous lesions, the term *Reiter's syndrome* has been applied historically, but it is no longer in common use. The urethritis may manifest as dysuria or discharge and the rash as circinate balanitis, which appears as vesicles or shallow ulcerations on the glans penis. Painless lingual or oral ulcerations may also be seen. The fact that the cervicitis may be less symptomatic could partially account for the underdiagnosis in women. The classic skin manifestation of ReA is keratoderma blennorrhagicum, a painless papulosquamous eruption on the palms or soles (Fig. 273-5). Occasionally, nail dystrophy with pitting and onycholysis or subungual keratosis can be seen. The conjunctivitis can be bilateral and painful; in contrast, the acute anterior uveitis that can also be seen in this setting tends to be less painful and unilateral.

Radiographic changes of ReA can be seen in the involved peripheral joints, with early findings consisting of soft tissue swelling and juxta-articular osteopenia. Areas of periostitis and new bone formation may develop in peripheral joints. When changes in the sacroiliac joints are seen, they are typically asymmetrical (Fig. 273-6), in contrast to the symmetrical pattern seen in AS. In the chronic phase, syndesmophytes may develop, but they are described as bulky, nonmarginal, often asymmetrical formations that differ from the classic syndesmophytes of AS. The frequency with which ReA evolves into bona fide AS has not been determined definitively.

Differential Diagnosis

The most important differential diagnosis for such reactive arthropathies is septic arthritis. Both *Yersinia* and *Salmonella* can induce septic arthritis, so an appropriate culture of synovial fluid should precede the diagnosis of ReA whenever possible. The course of ReA is variable, and few prognostic markers are available for the clinician to predict the course in an individual case. The majority of patients have an initial episode lasting 2 to 3 months, but synovitis may persist for a year or longer. In one 5-year follow-up of a point source cohort of post-*Salmonella* ReA, 20% of patients had ongoing inflammatory joint disease, and some degree of functional disability was observed in 30% of patients 5 years after the onset of disease.

FIGURE 273-5. Keratoderma blennorrhagicum of the feet in reactive arthritis.

FIGURE 273-6. Bilaterally asymmetrical sacroiliitis in reactive arthritis. Erosions, pseudowidening, and ileal sclerosis are present.

REACTIVE ARTHRITIS AND HUMAN IMMUNODEFICIENCY VIRUS

An aggressive form of SpA may be seen in patients who are concomitantly infected with human immunodeficiency virus (HIV). There is no increased frequency of ReA in patients with HIV, but HIV may alter the course of these arthropathies, with a tendency for a more aggressive and more refractory joint disease. Aggressive skin and joint disease may be seen in patients in whom PsA develops in the setting of HIV infection. Most North American patients with the HIV-ReA constellation are B27 positive, but studies of comparable patients in Africa have found a sizable B27-negative component in such patients. The arthritis in these patients falls into two clinical patterns: (1) an additive, asymmetrical polyarthritis or (2) an intermittent oligoarthritis that most commonly affects the lower extremities. Enthesitis, fasciitis, conjunctivitis, and urethritis can all be seen in such patients. Sacroiliitis can occur, although extensive spinal syndesmophyte formation is not common.

Psoriatic Arthritis

EPIDEMIOLOGY

PsA develops in 5 to 7% of patients with psoriasis. Although most cases arise in patients with established cutaneous disease, some patients (particularly children) have arthritis that antedates the appearance of the skin lesions. Although the extent of psoriatic skin disease correlates poorly with the development of arthritis, the risk for PsA increases with a family history of SpA. The age at onset can range from 30 to 55 years, with an equal predilection for PsA in women and men. Psoriatic spondylitis has a slight male preponderance.

PATHOBIOLOGY

The genetic associations with PsA are complex. Psoriasis itself is associated with several HLA loci; some B alleles have been reported, but the dominant element is HLA-Cw6. HLA-B39 and HLA-B27 have been associated with sacroiliitis and axial involvement. No etiologic agent has been proved in PsA, although some investigators have proposed that the disease process represents ReA in response to cutaneous bacteria. The histopathology of the synovitis of PsA is comparable to that of the other SpAs, with the absence of the local production of immunoglobulin and rheumatoid factor differentiating this disease from RA. There is the potential for aggressive osteolysis, fibrous ankylosis, and heterotopic new bone formation to occur in PsA. As mentioned earlier, the coexistence of HIV and PsA seems to set the stage for an aggressive course of joint destruction in some patients.

DIAGNOSIS

PsA has a variable manifestation and disease course, but several clinical patterns have been identified in prospectively monitored cohorts of patients. The clinical subsets are not mutually exclusive, nor are they static over time. The most common form, which affects 30 to 50% of patients, is an asymmetrical oligoarthritis that may involve both large and small joints. Dactylitis, arising as sausage digits, can be seen in fingers and toes and actually represents an enthesitis. In the second subset there is selective targeting of the distal interphalangeal joints, seen in 10 to 15% of patients. These changes are strongly associated with nail dystrophy, of which the features are onycholysis, subungual keratosis, pitting, and oil drop–like staining (Fig. 273-7). The third

FIGURE 273-7. Nail pitting in psoriasis. The pits are more discrete and regular compared with pits affecting the nail plate in dermatitis.

subset (15 to 30% of patients) has a symmetrical polyarthritis that mimics RA in many ways, except for the absence of rheumatoid nodules and rheumatoid factor. The fourth clinical variant is psoriatic spondylitis, which occurs in 20% of patients; 50% of such patients are B27 positive. Finally, arthritis mutilans (5% of patients) is a destructive, erosive arthritis that affects large and small joints and can be associated with marked deformities and significant disability.

Radiographic changes in PsA involve soft tissue swelling (particularly in the case of dactylitis), erosions, and periostitis. Axial involvement may lead to the appearance of asymmetrical sacroiliitis with syndesmophytes that are bulky, asymmetrical, and nonmarginal. The classic "pencil-in-cup" deformity may be seen in patients with distal interphalangeal joint disease or arthritis mutilans. Acro-osteolysis is noted in a minority of patients and reflects an aggressive erosive process.

Differential Diagnosis

The diagnosis of PsA depends on finding the typical skin or nail changes in association with one of the articular variants described previously. The differential diagnosis for the skin lesions can include seborrheic dermatitis, dyshidrotic eczema, fungal infection, keratoderma blennorrhagicum, and palmoplantar pustulosis.

TREATMENT   Rx

Patients typically receive aggressive treatment for psoriasis (Chapter 446). The advent of biologic agents has had a major impact on the treatment of PsA. The anti-TNF agents have been studied most extensively, indicating the efficacy of infliximab, etanercept, adalimumab, and golimumab. In a study of patients with PsA, ustekinumab, a monoclonal antibody against interleukin-12/23, was well tolerated, reduced the extent and severity of psoriasis, and was safe.[9]

Enteropathic Arthritis

DEFINITION

EA refers to the arthritis associated with Crohn's disease (CD) or ulcerative colitis (UC) (Chapter 143; Table 273-4).

PATHOBIOLOGY

All extraenteric manifestations, including arthritis, occur more commonly in CD than in UC. Peripheral arthritis occurs in 10 to 20% of CD patients and in 2 to 7% of UC patients. This pattern of arthritis occurs more commonly in patients with other extraenteric features (e.g., erythema nodosum, iritis). It is typically an inflammatory, nonerosive polyarthritis, predominantly of large joints. In general, the clinical activity of the peripheral arthritis parallels the activity of the gut inflammation, and measures that control the GI disease usually control the joint disease as well. The peripheral arthritis of EA is not associated with B27. As mentioned earlier, both inflammatory bowel disease and AS share genetic susceptibility associated with genetic variants of *IL23-R*.

In contrast, the sacroiliitis or spondylitis of EA follows a pattern in which the joint inflammation waxes and wanes independently of the bowel inflammation. Axial disease occurs in 2 to 7% of both CD and UC patients. HLA-B27 is found in 50% of patients with axial arthritis. The course tends to be chronic, as opposed to the transient course of peripheral arthritis.

The association of bowel inflammation and arthritis is supported by ileocolonoscopic studies in which subclinical inflammation of the bowel has been demonstrated in diseases covering the entire spectrum of SpAs. Histologic evaluation demonstrates that changes of acute ileitis are seen in postdysenteric ReA, whereas chronic inflammatory changes are more likely to be seen in patients with AS. As mentioned earlier, the abnormalities in the bowel of B27 transgenic rats have strong similarity to the lesions of CD, and a germ-free environment minimizes inflammatory changes in both the gut and the joints. This finding argues that altered bowel permeability, with enhanced bacteremia or antigenemia, may provide the link in both cases.

DIAGNOSIS

It is important to recognize that the musculoskeletal features of EA may precede any GI symptoms or signs. Conversely, the diarrhea preceding the onset of peripheral or axial arthritis in a young patient could just as likely represent a food-borne pathogen (e.g., *Salmonella*, *Yersinia*), with secondary ReA as inflammatory bowel disease and accompanying EA. In the initial assessment of such a patient, it is important to carry out careful and complete stool cultures. If the GI symptoms persist, diagnostic colonoscopy is often required to resolve the issue.

Undifferentiated Spondyloarthropathy

Despite careful clinical and radiographic assessment, there are still a substantial number of patients who do not fall into one of the classic diagnostic subsets of SpA outlined previously. These patients are often defined as having USpA with peripheral enthesitis, asymmetrical arthritis or sacroiliitis, or iritis in the absence of identifiable antecedent infection or concurrent inflammatory bowel disease or psoriasis. The natural history of USpA has not been well defined, and case heterogeneity and diagnostic dilemmas plague a systematic or multicenter approach to the problem. When the clinical course is examined, a number of patients may finally meet the diagnostic criteria for AS, but many retain a distinct USpA pattern for prolonged periods.

1. Clegg DO, Reda DJ, Abdellatif M. Comparison of sulfasalazine and placebo for the treatment of axial and peripheral articular manifestations of the seronegative spondylarthropathies: a Department of Veterans Affairs cooperative study. *Arthritis Rheum.* 1999;42:2325-2329.
2. Kvien TK, Gaston JS, Bardin T, et al. Three month treatment of reactive arthritis with azithromycin: a EULAR double blind, placebo controlled study. *Ann Rheum Dis.* 2004;63:1113-1119.
3. Carter JD, Espinoza LR, Inman RD, et al. Combination antibiotics as a treatment for chronic Chlamydia-induced reactive arthritis. *Arthritis Rheum.* 2009;60:S430.
4. Braun J, Brandt J, Listing J, et al. Treatment of active ankylosing spondylitis with infliximab: a randomised controlled multicentre trial. *Lancet.* 2002;359:1187-1193.
5. Braun J, Davis J, Dougados M, et al: First update of the International ASAS Consensus Statement for the use of anti-TNF agents in patients with ankylosing spondylitis. *Ann Rheum Dis.* 2006;65: 316-320.
6. van der Heijde D, Kivitz A, Schiff MH, et al. ATLAS Study Group. Efficacy and safety of adalimumab in patients with ankylosing spondylitis: results of a multicenter, randomized, double-blind, placebo-controlled trial. *Arthritis Rheum.* 2006;54:2136-2146.
7. Inman RD, Davis JC, van der Heijde D, et al. Efficacy and safety of golimumab in patients with ankylosing spondylitis: results of the randomized, double-blind, placebo-controlled GO-RAISE trial. *Arthritis Rheum.* 2008;58: 3402-3412.
8. Braun J, van der Horst-Bruinsma F, Huang F, et al. Clinical efficacy and safety of etanercept versus sulfasalazine in ankylosing spondylitis patients: a randomized, double-blind study (ASCEND Trial). *Arthritis Rheum.* 2011. [Epub ahead of print.]
9. Gottlieb A, Menter A, Mendelsohn A, et al. Ustekinumab, a human interleukin 12/23 monoclonal antibody, for psoriatic arthritis: randomised, double-blind, placebo-controlled, crossover trial. *Lancet.* 2009;373:633-640.

SUGGESTED READINGS

Cantini F, Niccoli L, Nannini C, et al. Psoriatic arthritis: a systematic review. *Int J Rheum Dis.* 2010;13:300-317. *Review of clinical characteristics and treatment, emphasizing that sulphasalazine and methotrexate are effective in peripheral psoriatic arthritis.*

Heldmann F, Dybowski F, Saracbasi-Zender E, et al. Update on biologic therapy in the management of axial spondyloarthritis. *Curr Rheumatol Rep.* 2010;12:325-331. *TNF antagonists are effective therapies but do not substantially inhibit radiographic progression.*

TABLE 273-4	ENTEROPATHIC ARTHRITIS	
FEATURE	**PERIPHERAL ARTHRITIS**	**SACROILIITIS, SPONDYLITIS**
CROHN'S DISEASE (CD)		
Frequency in CD	10–20%	2–7%
HLA-B27 associated	No	Yes
Pattern	Transient, symmetrical	Chronic
Course	Related to activity of CD	Unrelated to activity of CD
Effect of surgery	Remission of arthritis uncommon	No effect
Effect of anti-TNF therapy	Effective	Effective
ULCERATIVE COLITIS (UC)		
Frequency in UC	5–10%	2–7%
HLA-B27 associated	No	Yes
Pattern	Transient	Chronic
Course	More common in pancolitis than proctitis; related to activity of UC	Unrelated
Effect of surgery	Remission of arthritis	No effect

HLA = human leukocyte antigen; TNF = tumor necrosis factor.

Jang JH, Ward MM, Rucker AN, et al. Ankylosing spondylitis: patterns of radiographic involvement—a re-examination of accepted principles in a cohort of 769 patients. *Radiology.* 2011;258:192-198. *Symmetrical sacroiliitis was seen in 86% of patients with lumbar predominance during the first 20 years, after which the cervical lumbar spine was equally involved.*

Passalent LA. Physiotherapy for ankylosing spondylitis: evidence and application. *Curr Opin Rheumatol.* 2011;23:142-147. *Physiotherapy is an effective intervention.*

274

SYSTEMIC LUPUS ERYTHEMATOSUS

MARY K. CROW

DEFINITION

Systemic lupus erythematosus (SLE) is a multisystemic autoimmune disease that results from immune system–mediated tissue damage. Manifestations of SLE can involve the skin, joints, kidney, central nervous system (CNS), cardiovascular system, serosal membranes, and the hematologic and immune systems. The disease is highly heterogeneous, with individual patients manifesting variable combinations of clinical features. In most patients with SLE, the disease is characterized by a waxing and waning clinical course, although some demonstrate a pattern of chronic activity. The molecular triggers of the disease are not known, but the pathogenesis is understood to involve the production of autoantibodies exhibiting multiple specificities, with reactivity with nucleic acid–binding proteins being a common feature. Immune complexes, along with immune system cells and soluble mediators, generate inflammation and tissue damage. Therapeutic approaches generally involve immunosuppression.

EPIDEMIOLOGY

A notable feature of SLE is that it occurs much more frequently in females than in males. Like Hashimoto's thyroiditis and Sjögren's syndrome, the female-to-male ratio is approximately 8 : 1 to 9 : 1 in adults, and most cases are diagnosed between the ages of 15 and 44 years. In children and women older than 55, the ratio is closer to 2 : 1. The prevalence of SLE is estimated to be approximately 124 per 100,000 in the United States, and the incidence of new cases is 1.8 to 7.6 per 100,000 per year. The prevalence, severity, and characteristics of disease differ in different ethnic groups, with SLE being three to four times more frequent in African Americans than in the white population. The severity of disease is also greater in Hispanics than in whites, although data for Hispanic populations are less abundant. Asians may also have a higher prevalence of disease than whites. Recent studies of lupus in minority populations indicate that socioeconomic factors are major contributors to the increased prevalence and severity of disease in African Americans and Hispanic Americans.

PATHOBIOLOGY

Current understanding of lupus pathogenesis incorporates roles for genetic susceptibility based on a threshold model involving multiple genes; environmental triggers, including microbial infection, sunlight, and certain drugs; and altered immune system function. Recent advances in immunology have focused attention on the mechanisms that account for innate immune system activation. At least some of the genetic and environmental contributions to lupus are likely to promote innate immune system activation and subsequent autoimmunity. Others may contribute to inflammation and tissue damage.

Murine models have proved useful in identifying genes that could contribute to lupus susceptibility or define patterns of disease. Production of autoantibodies characteristic of SLE and development of nephritis and accelerated death have been demonstrated in numerous murine strains in which immune system genes have been modified. In most cases, no alterations have been noted in the homologous human genes. The ease of induction of lupus-like disease in murine models suggests that there are numerous possible pathogenic paths that might lead to the clinical manifestations of lupus. It is not known which of these molecular pathways is responsible for human SLE.

Genetics

An important role for a genetic contribution to lupus susceptibility is suggested by the high concordance of disease in monozygotic twins (14 to 57%).

TABLE 274-1 GENES ASSOCIATED WITH SYSTEMIC LUPUS ERYTHEMATOSUS

GENE*	PROTEIN
BANK1	B-cell scaffold protein with ankyrin repeats 1
BLK	B-lymphocyte–specific tyrosine kinase
C1QA, B, and C	Complement component C1q
C2	Complement component 2
C4A and C4B	Complement component C4
CRP	C-reactive protein
DRB11501	MHC class II (DR2)
DRB10301	MHC class II (DR3)
FCGR2A	Activating FcγRIIA
FCGR3A	Activating FcγRIIIA
IRF5	Interferon regulatory factor 5
ITGAM	Mac1/complement receptor 3
IRAK1	Interleukin-1 receptor–associated kinase 1
LYN	Lyn tyrosine kinase
PTPN22	Protein tyrosine phosphatase nonreceptor type 22
STAT4	Signal transducer and activator of transcription 4
TNFAIP3	A20
TNFSF4	Ox40 ligand
TREX1	DNase III

*Genes listed have an odds ratio of ≥1.3.
MHC = major histocompatibility complex.

Genes that might account for increased lupus susceptibility or severity include those encoding components of the complement pathway, including C1q, C2, and C4A (Table 274-1). Impaired production of these early complement components may decrease the clearance of apoptotic cells, thereby augmenting the pool of available autoantigens, or decrease the solubility of immune complexes. Polymorphic variants in components of the toll-like receptor (TLR) pathways that regulate type I interferon production, including interferon regulatory factor 5 (*IRF5*), have been associated with a diagnosis of SLE and increased plasma interferon activity in some populations. Association of SLE with the major histocompatibility complex (MHC) class II alleles human leukocyte antigen (HLA)-DR2 and HLA-DR3 has been documented in many studies and is most striking in patients expressing particular autoantibody specificities. Polymorphisms in the Fc receptor genes *FCGR2A* and *FCGR3A* have been associated with SLE nephritis, possibly based on altered clearance of immune complexes. Variants of the *PTPN22* gene, which encodes a phosphatase that regulates T-cell activation, are also associated with SLE. Genome-wide association studies have expanded the list of lupus-associated gene variants to include regulators of innate immune system activation (*TNFAIP3, ITGAM, IRAK1*) and signaling molecules important in lymphocyte activation (*STAT4, BANK1, BLK,* and *LYN*). Rare mutations in the *TREX1* gene, encoding a DNase, have been documented in some patients with lupus-like disease and high levels of interferon. The available data suggest a common theme: the genes that have been associated with lupus confer either increased activation or impaired regulation of the innate or adaptive immune responses, with increased type I interferon often observed in association with the risk genotype.

Environmental Triggers

Several classes of potential environmental triggers for lupus have been studied. Although the female preponderance of SLE implies a role for hormonal factors in the disease, recent concepts describe a possible contribution of epigenetic modification or dosage effects of the X chromosome as accounting for at least some of the sex skewing. A role for microbial triggers, particularly virus infection, has been postulated consistent with the constitutional symptoms that often characterize the earliest stage of the disease. Epstein-Barr virus has garnered particular interest among investigators because the frequency of previous infection in SLE patients is significantly higher than in the general population (99 vs. 94%). Evidence of exposure to other viruses, including cytomegalovirus, is equivalent between SLE patients and healthy control subjects. Ultraviolet light exposure is a well-described trigger of lupus flares. Possible mechanisms include DNA damage and induction of apoptosis of skin cells, which result in concentration of nucleic acids and associated proteins in cell membrane blebs and increased processing by antigen-presenting cells. Data also support an association between current tobacco use and anti-double-stranded DNA antibodies and lupus disease activity. Certain drugs, including procainamide and hydralazine, can induce a lupus-like syndrome, but the symptoms usually abate after discontinuing use of the drug. These agents may promote demethylation of DNA, thereby increasing the availability of immunostimulatory DNA. Sulfa antibiotics have been reported to induce lupus flare in some patients. Administration of recombinant interferon-α to patients with hematologic malignancies or hepatitis C infection has been associated with induction of a lupus-like syndrome. In addition, anti–tumor necrosis factor agents have induced lupus autoantibodies and occasionally clinical lupus in patients with rheumatoid arthritis.

Immunologic Triggers

Genetic and environmental factors that increase the probability of development of SLE are likely to act on the immune system to induce autoimmunity and consequent tissue inflammation and damage. In addition to mechanisms that increase the availability of self-antigens, such as ultraviolet light, altered expression of gene products that mediate or regulate apoptosis, or impaired clearance of apoptotic debris, results in generalized activation of the immune system and contributes to autoimmunity in lupus. In parallel with the events that account for effective immune responses directed at exogenous microbes, the autoimmunity that occurs in SLE patients is likely to require activation of both innate and adaptive immune responses. The innate immune response is first activated by common molecular patterns expressed on the microbe and results in augmented antigen-presenting cell capacity and successful generation of an antigen-specific adaptive immune response. The characterization of the TLR family of pattern recognition receptors has provided new understanding of the mechanisms through which the innate immune system is activated by exogenous and endogenous stimuli, including nucleic acid–containing immune complexes, and promotes induction of a self-directed adaptive immune response.

Type I Interferon

Recent studies of gene expression in peripheral blood mononuclear cells of SLE patients using microarray technology have demonstrated that activation of genes regulated by type I interferon is a common feature in patients with active disease and may represent innate immune system activation. Interferon-α is gaining attention as a soluble mediator that may be responsible for many of the immunologic alterations that have been observed in SLE and is identified as a potential therapeutic target. Immune complexes containing DNA or RNA are postulated to contribute to the production of type I interferon in SLE. Demethylated CpG-rich DNA or RNA associated with nucleic acid–binding proteins can activate plasmacytoid dendritic cells and other immune system cells through TLRs and thereby result in the production of type I interferon (interferon-α or -β) and other proinflammatory cytokines (E-Fig. 274-1). Diverse effects of type I interferon on immune system function are consistent with the altered immune responses observed in SLE patients, including maturation of dendritic cells, increased immunoglobulin (Ig) class switching to mature immunoglobulin isotypes (IgG and IgA), and induction of soluble mediators that increase B-cell differentiation and inflammatory responses, such as B-lymphocyte stimulator (BLyS) and interferon-γ. Induction of an immunostimulatory microenvironment by interferon-α may support the development of a humoral immune response directed at self-antigens, particularly intracellular particles that contain nucleic acids and nucleic acid–binding proteins. It is not known why some individuals initiate immune system activation directed at self-antigens and others do not.

Autoantibodies

The most characteristic lupus autoantibodies target intracellular particles containing both nucleic acid and nucleic acid–binding proteins. Understanding the significance of induction of these particular autoantibody specificities may provide clues to the etiology of SLE. A recent analysis of the spectrum of autoantibodies present in the sera of individuals in whom SLE is later diagnosed has suggested that autoantibodies reactive with certain RNA-binding proteins, including the Ro protein, occur early in the preclinical stage of the disease, along with a positive antinuclear antibody (ANA) test. These are often followed by anti-DNA antibodies and, finally, by the development

FIGURE 274-1. Proportion of patients with positive antibody tests relative to the time of diagnosis or appearance of the first clinical manifestation of systemic lupus erythematosus (SLE). For each autoantibody, the proportion of patients testing positive relative to the time of diagnosis or to the time of appearance of the first clinical criterion was assessed. In analyses of the time from antibody development to the diagnosis of SLE, antinuclear antibodies (ANAs) appeared significantly earlier than anti-Sm antibodies ($Z = 3.22$, $P < .001$) and antinuclear ribonucleoprotein (anti-nRNP) antibodies ($Z = 4.18$, $P < .001$), but not significantly earlier than anti-Ro, anti-La, antiphospholipid (APL), or anti-double-stranded DNA antibodies (anti-dsDNA). (From Arbuckle MR, McClain MT, Rubertone MV, et al. Development of autoantibodies before the clinical onset of systemic lupus erythematosus. N Engl J Med. 2003;349:16.)

of antibodies specific for the spliceosomal proteins Smith (Sm) and ribonucleoprotein (RNP) at approximately the time of diagnosis (Fig. 274-1). These observations suggest that individuals who demonstrate progression from a narrow focus of humoral immunity to proteins associated with RNA to antibodies that bind DNA and other specificities are those in whom sufficient autoimmunity develops to manifest clinical symptoms. Approximately one third of SLE patients have autoantibodies reactive with phospholipids or the proteins associated with them, particularly β₂-glycoprotein I (β₂GPI). These autoantibody specificities can also be present independently of SLE in primary antiphospholipid antibody syndrome (Chapter 177).

Immune Complexes and Complement

Tissue and organ damage in SLE is mediated by the deposition or in situ formation of immune complexes and subsequent complement activation and inflammation. The complement system (Chapter 49), composed of more than 30 proteins that act in concert to protect the host against invading organisms, initiates inflammation and tissue injury. Complement activation promotes chemotaxis of inflammatory cells and generates proteolytic fragments that enhance phagocytosis by neutrophils and monocytes. The classic pathway is activated when antibodies bind to antigen and generate potent effectors. Alternative pathway activation mechanisms differ in that they are initiated by the binding of spontaneously activated complement components to the surfaces of pathogens or self-tissues. C3a, an anaphylatoxin that binds to receptors on leukocytes and other cells, causes activation and release of inflammatory mediators. C5a is a potent soluble inflammatory, anaphylatoxic, and chemotactic molecule that promotes recruitment and activation of neutrophils and monocytes and mediates endothelial cell activation through its receptor. The release of reactive oxygen and nitrogen intermediates is an additional mechanism that contributes to tissue damage.

Tissues targeted by immune system activity in lupus include the skin, where immune complexes and complement are deposited in a linear pattern (as demonstrated in the lupus band test, in which deposited antibodies are identified by a fluorescent tag), the glomeruli, and heart valves. Recent data also suggest that antibodies reactive with hippocampal neurons in the brain can mediate excitotoxic death. Immune and inflammatory mechanisms responsible for the vasculopathy of lupus are multifactorial and not clearly defined. Microvascular damage is observed in splenic arteries and is characterized by the typical onion-skin pattern of concentric connective tissue deposition. In addition to vascular damage mediated by inflammation, thrombosis, including microthrombi, contributes to ischemia and cell necrosis in the brain and other organs.

CLINICAL MANIFESTATIONS

Symptoms and Signs

Constitutional Symptoms

SLE is a disease that involves virtually all components of the immune system and can be accompanied by constitutional symptoms similar to those seen in the setting of microbial infection. Fatigue, headaches, weight loss, and fevers are common, along with generalized arthralgias, myalgias, and lymphadenopathy. The level of activity of lupus typically follows a pattern of flares and remissions, although some patients sustain active disease for prolonged periods. Careful monitoring for the development of major organ system disease is important to ensure timely adjustments in medical therapy.

Cutaneous and Mucous Membranes

The skin and mucous membranes are affected in most lupus patients (Table 274-2). The erythematous facial rash with a butterfly distribution across the malar and nasal prominences and sparing of the nasolabial folds is the classic rash of SLE and is seen in 30 to 60% of patients (Fig. 274-2). The butterfly rash is often triggered by sun exposure, but photosensitivity can also be demonstrated diffusely in other areas of the body.

TABLE 274-2	CLINICAL MANIFESTATIONS OF SYSTEMIC LUPUS ERYTHEMATOSUS	
MANIFESTATION	**APPROXIMATE FREQUENCY (%)**
Cutaneous	88
Arthritis/arthralgias	76
Neuropsychiatric	66
Pleurisy/pericarditis	63
Anemia	57
Raynaud's phenomenon	44
Vasculitis	43
Atherosclerosis	37
Nephritis	31
Thrombocytopenia	30
Sensorimotor neuropathy	28
Cardiac valvar disease	18
Pulmonary alveolar hemorrhage	12
Pancreatitis	10
Myositis	5
Myocarditis	5

FIGURE 274-2. Malar rash in a patient with systemic lupus erythematosus. Note that the rash does not cross the nasolabial fold. (From Gladman DD, Urowitz MB. Systemic lupus erythematosus: clinical features. In: Klippel JH, Dieppe PA, eds. *Rheumatology*, 2nd ed. London: Mosby; 1998.)

The discoid skin lesions are erythematous plaques with central scarring and may be covered with scale. These lesions are seen in about 25% of patients, involve the scalp or the face and ears, and may be associated with alopecia. Discoid lesions can be present in the absence of systemic manifestations of SLE (*discoid lupus*). In addition to the scarring alopecia of discoid lupus, more transient alopecia may be a clinical sign of increased disease activity and is associated with apoptosis of cells in the hair follicle.

Inflammation of the deep dermis and subcutaneous fat can result in lupus panniculitis, with firm painful nodules that sometimes adhere to the epidermis causing irregularities in the superficial skin. Subacute cutaneous lupus erythematosus is seen in sun-exposed areas and can involve erythematous plaques or psoriasiform lesions. It is associated with autoantibodies to the Ro (SSA) RNA-binding protein. Mucosal ulcerations, especially of the buccal mucosa and upper palate, result from mucositis and are typical of SLE. Manifestations of vasculopathy are also common in SLE, including arteriolar spasm or infarcts in the nail folds, a diffuse lacey pattern over the skin described as livedo reticularis, and petechial-purpuric or urticarial lesions on the extremities. Vasculopathy in SLE is often associated with the presence of antiphospholipid antibodies.

Musculoskeletal System

Arthralgias and nonerosive arthritis are among the most common clinical features of SLE and are experienced by more than 85% of patients. The proximal interphalangeal and metacarpophalangeal joints of the hand are most commonly symptomatic, along with the knees and wrists. In some patients (about 10%), deformities resulting from damage to periarticular tissue can occur, a condition termed *Jaccoud's arthropathy*. The heavy use of corticosteroids in many lupus patients can be accompanied by the development of osteoporosis, including osteoporotic fractures, or osteonecrosis, most commonly of the hips, although the underlying vasculopathy can also contribute to joint damage.

Inflammation of the muscles with elevated creatine phosphokinase can occur rarely in SLE, and myopathy may be observed as a consequence of corticosteroid therapy. Fibromyalgia, characterized by painful trigger points at characteristic locations, commonly accompanies SLE and can contribute to fatigue and depression.

Renal System

Kidney involvement in SLE is common, with 74% of patients being affected at some time in the course of disease, and is a poor prognostic indicator. Renal pathology is generally attributed to the deposition of circulating immune complexes or in situ formation of these complexes in glomeruli and results in the activation of complement and subsequent recruitment of inflammatory cells. In addition to glomerular inflammation, necrosis, and scarring, renal pathology is characterized by vascular lesions, including thrombotic microangiopathy and extraglomerular vasculitis, and tubulointerstitial disease, including tubular atrophy and interstitial fibrosis. Hypertension may be a consequence of significant renal involvement.

Most cases of lupus nephritis present a complex immunopathologic picture, but, in general, the pattern of renal disease reflects the site of deposition of immunoglobulins and the quality of the effector mechanisms they induce. Mesangial deposition of immunoglobulin induces mesangial cell proliferation and is associated with microscopic hematuria and mild proteinuria (Fig. 274-3). Subendothelial deposition of immune complexes results in proliferative and exudative inflammation, together with hematuria, mild to moderate proteinuria, and reduced glomerular filtration rate. Subepithelial deposition of immune complexes adjacent to podocytes and along the glomerular basement membrane can result in membranous nephritis with nephrotic-range proteinuria. In addition, antiphospholipid antibodies may support the development of thrombotic or inflammatory vascular lesions within or external to glomeruli.

A World Health Organization classification of lupus nephritis lesions was first published in 1975 with subsequent revisions. These classifications were reviewed and rigorously reexamined in the revised International Society of Nephrology and Renal Pathology Society classification criteria for lupus glomerulonephritis (GN) (Table 274-3). Class I and II GN involves mesangial deposition of immune complexes (class I without and class II with mesangial hypercellularity), class III describes focal GN involving less than 50% of total glomeruli, class IV includes diffuse GN involving 50% or more of glomeruli, class V designates membranous lupus nephritis, and class VI is characterized by advanced sclerotic lesions. Classes III and IV have subdivisions for active and sclerotic lesions, and class IV also has subdivisions for segmental and

FIGURE 274-3. Histopathology of lupus nephritis. **A,** Lupus nephritis class II. A light micrograph of a glomerulus shows mild mesangial hypercellularity (periodic acid–Schiff). **B,** Lupus nephritis class III (A). Light micrograph showing a glomerulus with segmental endocapillary hypercellularity, mesangial hypercellularity, capillary wall thickening, and early segmental capillary necrosis (methenamine silver). **C,** Lupus nephritis class IV-G (A/C). A glomerulus manifests global endocapillary proliferation, leukocyte influx and apoptotic bodies, double contours, crescent formation with tubular transformation, early sclerosis, and disruption of Bowman's capsule (periodic acid–Schiff). **D,** Thrombotic microangiopathy in a patient with systemic lupus erythematosus and circulating anticoagulant. A glomerulus shows severe capillary and arteriolar thrombosis, endothelial cell swelling and necrosis, neutrophil influx, and stasis of erythrocytes. No signs of immune deposits were found (methenamine silver). (From Wenning JJ, D'Agati VD, Schwartz MM, et al. The classification of glomerulonephritis in systemic lupus erythematosus revisited. *J Am Soc Nephrol.* 2004;15:241.)

TABLE 274-3	INTERNATIONAL SOCIETY OF NEPHROLOGY/RENAL PATHOLOGY SOCIETY 2003 CLASSIFICATION OF LUPUS NEPHRITIS
Class I	**Minimal mesangial lupus nephritis** Normal glomeruli by light microscopy, but mesangial immune deposits by immunofluorescence
Class II	**Mesangial proliferative lupus nephritis** Purely mesangial hypercellularity of any degree or mesangial matrix expansion by light microscopy, with mesangial immune deposits. May be a few isolated subepithelial or subendothelial deposits visible by immunofluorescence or electron microscopy, but not by light microscopy
Class III	**Focal lupus nephritis*** Active or inactive focal, segmental, or global endocapillary or extracapillary glomerulonephritis involving <50% of all glomeruli, typically with focal subendothelial immune deposits, with or without mesangial alterations
Class III (A)	Active lesions: focal proliferative lupus nephritis
Class III (A/C)	Active and chronic lesions: focal proliferative and sclerosing lupus nephritis
Class III (C)	Chronic inactive lesions with glomerular scars: focal sclerosing lupus nephritis
Class IV	**Diffuse lupus nephritis†** Active or inactive diffuse, segmental or global endocapillary or extracapillary glomerulonephritis Involving ≥50% of all glomeruli, typically with diffuse subendothelial immune deposits, with or without mesangial alterations. This class is divided into diffuse segmental (IV-S) lupus nephritis when ≥50% of the involved glomeruli have segmental lesions and into diffuse global (IV-G) lupus nephritis when ≥50% of the involved glomeruli have global lesions. Segmental is defined as a glomerular lesion that involves less than half of the glomerular tuft. This class includes cases with diffuse wire loop deposits but with little or no glomerular proliferation.
Class IV-S (A)	Active lesions: diffuse segmental proliferative lupus nephritis
Class IV-G (A)	Active lesions: diffuse global proliferative lupus nephritis
Class IV-S (A/C)	Active and chronic lesions: diffuse segmental proliferative and sclerosing lupus nephritis Active and chronic lesions: diffuse global proliferative and sclerosing lupus nephritis
Class IV-S (C)	Chronic inactive lesions with scars: diffuse segmental sclerosing lupus nephritis
Class IV-G (C)	Chronic inactive lesions with scars: diffuse global sclerosing lupus nephritis
Class V	**Membranous lupus nephritis** Global or segmental subepithelial immune deposits or their morphologic sequelae by light microscopy and by immunofluorescence or electron microscopy, with or without mesangial alterations Class V lupus nephritis may occur in combination with class III or IV, in which case both will be diagnosed Class V lupus nephritis shows advanced sclerosis
Class VI	**Advanced sclerosis lupus nephritis** ≥90% of glomeruli globally sclerosed without residual activity

*Indicate the proportion of glomeruli with active and with sclerotic lesions.
†Indicate the proportion of glomeruli with fibrinoid necrosis and/or cellular crescents.
From Weening JJ, D'Agati VD, Schwartz MM, et al. The classification of glomerulonephritis in systemic lupus erythematosus revisited. *J Am Soc Nephrol.* 2004;15:241.

global involvement. Pathologic diagnosis should include descriptions of tubulointerstitial and vascular disease as well as glomerular involvement.

The prognosis of class I and class II disease is usually good, whereas class IV, the most common form of lupus nephritis, has the worst prognosis, particularly when the serum creatinine level is elevated at the time of diagnosis.

Class V nephritis occurs in 10 to 20% of patients, and the implication for long-term outcome depends on the degree of proteinuria, with mild proteinuria having a good prognosis and nephrotic syndrome with chronic edema having a more negative prognosis. It should be noted that renal veins can occasionally become involved with thrombosis, which then contributes to nephrotic syndrome. This complication can be evaluated by renal ultrasound.

Cardiovascular System

Pericarditis and valve nodules were among the first clinical manifestations described in SLE. It is only recently that the extent of premature atherosclerotic disease has been well documented. Pericarditis (Chapter 77) is the most common cardiac manifestation, but it is sometimes recognized only on imaging studies or at autopsy. It is a component of the generalized serositis that is often a feature of SLE and is associated with local autoantibodies and immune complexes. Pericarditis is usually manifested as substernal chest pain that is improved by bending forward and can be exacerbated by inspiration or coughing. The symptoms and effusions associated with pericarditis are quite responsive to moderate-dose (20 to 30 mg/day of prednisone) corticosteroid treatment.

Structural valve abnormalities in SLE range from sterile nodules originally described by Libman and Sacks to nonspecific valve thickening. The nodules are immobile and usually located on the atrial side of the mitral valve and sometimes on the arterial side of the aortic valve. Right-sided lesions are rare. These structural changes may in some cases result in valvular regurgitation. Although valve nodules are detected in most patients with SLE at autopsy, clinically significant valvular heart disease is much less common (1 to 18%). The verrucous valvular lesions of Libman and Sacks are most likely inflammatory in nature and may be associated with the presence of antiphospholipid antibodies.

Premature and accelerated atherosclerosis is increasingly recognized as being prevalent in lupus patients, and preclinical atherosclerotic carotid plaque has been documented in 37% of SLE patients as opposed to 15% of age- and sex-matched controls. Traditional cardiovascular risk factors apply, but the diagnosis of SLE is itself a significant risk factor for premature atherosclerosis. Although the lupus-specific mechanisms that confer additional risk for atherosclerosis have not been defined, it is likely that chronic inflammation associated with immune system activation contributes to the accumulation of vascular damage. Mortality from atherosclerosis may be up to 10 times greater in patients with SLE than in age- and sex-matched controls.

Although not specific to SLE, Raynaud's phenomenon (Chapter 80), characterized by episodic vasospasm and occlusion of the digital arteries in response to cold and emotional stress, is a feature in up to 60% of SLE patients and contributes to pain and sometimes necrosis of the distal ends of extremities. The character of the digits classically changes from pallor to cyanosis and then to rubor as vascular perfusion becomes impaired. In addition, small arteries, arterioles, and capillaries can be affected by vasculitis and fibrinoid necrosis with clinical manifestations that include periungual telangiectases, abdominal pain, and neuropsychiatric symptoms.

Pulmonary System

Pleuritis is the most frequent manifestation of pulmonary involvement in SLE and occurs in about 30% of patients at some point in their disease course. Pleuritis is characterized by pain on respiration and exudative effusions. Parenchymal disease is less common but may be based on several distinct mechanisms, including pneumonitis in the absence of documented infection and sometimes involving alveolar hemorrhage (in up to 12% of patients), pulmonary embolism secondary to peripheral thrombosis, or pulmonary hypertension with increased pulmonary resistance and impaired diffusing capacity.

Neuropsychiatric Involvement

Clinical features of SLE that involve the nervous system include both neurologic and psychiatric manifestations. The central and peripheral nervous systems can be affected by the disease. The American College of Rheumatology has identified 19 neuropsychiatric syndromes that can be associated with SLE, and validation of these neuropsychiatric findings has been substantiated in several independent studies (Table 274-4). The most common manifestations that are probably attributable to SLE cerebritis include cognitive dysfunction, present in 17 to 66% of SLE patients; psychosis or mood disorder, the former reported in up to 8% of patients; cerebrovascular disease in 5 to 18% of patients; and seizures, present in 6 to 51% of patients. Headaches are also common. Because none of these CNS manifestations are found exclusively in SLE, it can be difficult to be certain that a neuropsychiatric complaint or symptom can be attributed to SLE.

Evaluation of neuropsychiatric lupus depends on a careful clinical history and physical and laboratory examinations and, in some cases, imaging studies

TABLE 274-4	NEUROPSYCHIATRIC SYNDROMES OBSERVED IN SYSTEMIC LUPUS ERYTHEMATOSUS

CENTRAL NERVOUS SYSTEM

Aseptic meningitis
Cerebrovascular disease
Demyelinating syndrome
Headache (including migraine and benign intracranial hypertension)
Movement disorder (chorea)
Myelopathy
Seizure disorders
Acute confusional state
Anxiety disorder
Cognitive dysfunction
Mood disorder
Psychosis

PERIPHERAL NERVOUS SYSTEM

Acute inflammatory demyelinating polyradiculoneuropathy (Guillain-Barré syndrome)
Autonomic disorder
Mononeuropathy, single/multiplex
Myasthenia gravis
Neuropathy, cranial
Plexopathy
Polyneuropathy

From The American College of Rheumatology nomenclature and case definitions for neuropsychiatric lupus syndromes. *Arthritis Rheum.* 1999;42:599-608.

and analysis of cerebrospinal fluid to rule out infection. Magnetic resonance imaging is useful for detecting intracranial abnormalities, which are seen in 19 to 70% of patients and include white matter lesions, cerebral infarction, venous sinus thrombosis, and sometimes atrophy. More sophisticated imaging techniques such as magnetic resonance angiography and magnetic resonance spectroscopy can be used to assess cerebral blood flow or neuronal metabolism.

Cranial nerve and ocular involvement, most likely based on vasculopathy and focal ischemia, can sometimes affect vision. Ocular examination of the retina can reveal cotton-wool spots as a result of retinal ischemia or necrosis. Although rare, transverse myelopathy, frequently associated with antiphospholipid antibodies, can have devastating consequences, including paraplegia. Sensorimotor neuropathies, often asymmetrical, are more common (up to 28%) and are based on damage to small nerve fibers with vasculopathy in the small arteries that supply the nerve fibers.

As is the case with lupus nephritis, the pathophysiologic mechanisms that account for the neuropsychiatric manifestations of SLE are diverse and complex. Recent data suggest that autoantibodies cross-reactive with neuronal cell surface glutamate receptors and DNA may mediate excitotoxic death of neurons and are proposed to contribute to cognitive dysfunction. Antibodies directed against ribosomal P protein have also been associated with neuropsychiatric lupus, and antiphospholipid antibodies can contribute to a procoagulant state, vascular thrombosis, and cerebral ischemia. Cerebral vasculopathy has been clearly demonstrated by angiographic and pathologic studies. Noninflammatory small vessel vasculopathy is the most common lesion and can be associated with microinfarcts. Inflammatory mediators, including the cytokines interleukin-6 and interferon-α, and matrix metalloproteinases may also contribute to the neuropsychiatric manifestations of SLE.

Gastrointestinal System

Although uncommon, vasculitis of the gastrointestinal tract or mesentery can result in pain and bowel necrosis. Less common than pleuritis and pericarditis, peritonitis can manifest as peritoneal effusion and abdominal pain. Pancreatitis occurs in less than 10% of patients but may also be due to vascular pathology. Lupoid hepatitis, a syndrome that was named for the presence of positive ANAs in patients with chronic active hepatitis, is a misnomer because elevated transaminases are only rarely seen in lupus patients.

Lymphadenopathy

About one third of SLE patients demonstrate diffuse lymphadenopathy at some time during the course of their disease. The nodes are often nontender, and lymphoma is sometimes considered in the differential diagnosis. Biopsy usually reveals follicular hyperplasia, although some histopathologic findings appear similar to the histiocytic necrotizing lymphadenitis that is a feature of Kikuchi's disease, a self-limited syndrome characterized by fever and lymphadenopathy. Recent multicenter studies have determined the frequency of malignancies in patients with SLE and have found a significant increase in hematologic malignancies, particularly non-Hodgkin's lymphoma. Splenomegaly is sometimes seen in SLE, and spleen pathology is characterized by a classic onion-skin histology that appears as concentric circles of collagen matrix surrounding splenic arteries and arterioles.

Hematologic System

In addition to autoantibody specificities that are fairly specific for SLE (anti-DNA, anti-Sm), antibodies that target each of the cellular blood elements are also common. Anemia is present in about 50% of patients and is multifactorial. It can be associated with a positive Coombs' test or microangiopathic hemolysis (Chapter 163) or reflect chronic disease (normochromic, normocytic) (Chapter 161). Leukopenia, particularly lymphopenia, is observed, with the lymphocyte count decreasing in the setting of increased disease activity. Antibodies that bind to lymphocytes and neutrophils have been described, and an increased tendency for lymphocytes to undergo spontaneous apoptosis may contribute to lymphopenia. Idiopathic thrombocytopenic purpura (Chapter 175) can be an early manifestation of SLE, and thrombocytopenia, induced by antiplatelet antibodies, can sometimes lead to a life-threatening risk for hemorrhage. Antibodies to clotting factors can also occur and contribute to impaired clot formation and hemorrhage.

Lupus Pregnancy and Neonatal Lupus

Whether pregnancy increases the likelihood of lupus exacerbation has been debated, with differences on this point presented by different investigators. However, abundant data indicate that patients with SLE have worse fetal outcomes than healthy individuals. Gestational hypertension, fetal growth restriction, and fetal distress are increased in patients with SLE and may lead to fetal loss or premature delivery. Preeclampsia can contribute to a poor outcome in both the mother and fetus and can be difficult to distinguish from a lupus flare associated with lupus nephritis.

Neonatal lupus is a distinct entity that can occur in infants of mothers with or without a diagnosis of SLE. The syndrome is characterized by cutaneous lesions and congenital heart block in the infant and the presence of antibodies to the Ro (SSA) or La (SSB) RNA-binding proteins (or both) in the mother. Mortality in babies with a congenital heart block is 15 to 31%. Deposition of anti-Ro IgG in the fetal heart, indicative of transplacental transfer of maternal autoantibody, and dense connective tissue encompassing the conduction system have been demonstrated in autopsy specimens. Prenatal testing of lupus mothers for the presence of anti-Ro and anti-La antibodies is appropriate, and careful monitoring with fetal echocardiography starting at week 16 of pregnancy can detect conduction defects. Fluorinated corticosteroids such as dexamethasone have been effective in reversing heart block in some cases.

Antiphospholipid Antibody Syndrome

Antiphospholipid antibodies represent a distinct class of autoantibodies that are seen in about one third of SLE patients but can also be present in individuals who do not carry a diagnosis of SLE (Chapter 174). Although these antibodies were initially thought to be specific for phospholipids exposed in cell membranes, particularly after "flipping" of the membranes of apoptotic cells, extensive data support their primary reactivity with phospholipid-binding proteins, particularly β_2GPI. Whether in primary antiphospholipid syndrome or in SLE, antiphospholipid antibodies have been associated with venous and arterial thromboses. In addition to vascular thromboses, clinical manifestations of antiphospholipid syndrome include thrombotic microangiopathic glomerular disease, cardiac valve lesions, livedo reticularis, thrombocytopenia, hemolytic anemia, and CNS disease. Recent data indicate that these autoantibodies can contribute to fetal loss and growth restriction by binding to the placenta, activating the complement system, and inducing inflammation. Catastrophic antiphospholipid syndrome, triggered by the acute onset of multisystemic (three or more organs) thrombosis, is resistant to anticoagulation treatment and is fatal in approximately 50% of cases.

DIAGNOSIS

Classification

Criteria for the classification of patients with SLE for the purpose of clinical studies were developed by the American College of Rheumatology, with the most recent full revision published in 1982 and an update published in 1997 (Table 274-5). The criteria include 11 features that encompass manifestations of skin and mucosal involvement, arthritis, serositis, renal disorder, neurologic disorder, hematologic disorder, immunologic disorder, and an abnormal titer in the ANA test, with at least four criteria required for classification as SLE. ANA has low specificity but strengthens the sensitivity of the

---

TABLE 274-5   UPDATE OF THE 1982 REVISED CRITERIA FOR CLASSIFICATION OF SYSTEMIC LUPUS ERYTHEMATOSUS

CRITERION*	DEFINITION
1. Malar rash	Fixed erythema, flat or raised, over the malar eminences that tends to spare the nasolabial folds
2. Discoid rash	Erythematous raised patches with adherent keratotic scaling and follicular plugging; atrophic scarring may occur in older lesions
3. Photosensitivity	Rash as a result of unusual reaction to sunlight, by history or physician observation
4. Oral ulcers	Oral or nasopharyngeal ulceration, usually painless, observed by a physician
5. Arthritis	Nonerosive arthritis involving 2 or more peripheral joints and characterized by tenderness, swelling, or effusion
6. Serositis	A. Pleuritis—convincing history of pleuritic pain or rubbing heard by a physician or evidence of pleural effusion *or* B. Pericarditis—documented by electrocardiography, a rub, or evidence of pericardial effusion
7. Renal disorder	A. Persistent proteinuria greater than 0.5 g/day or greater than 3+ if quantitation is not performed *or* B. Cellular casts—may be red cell, hemoglobin, granular, tubular, or mixed
8. Neurologic disorder	A. Seizures—in the absence of offending drugs or known metabolic derangements; e.g., uremia, ketoacidosis, or electrolyte imbalance *or* B. Psychosis—in the absence of offending drugs or known metabolic derangements; e.g., uremia, ketoacidosis, or electrolyte imbalance
9. Hematologic disorder	A. Hemolytic anemia—with reticulocytosis *or* B. Leukopenia—less than 4000/mm³ total on 2 or more occasions *or* C. Lymphopenia—less than 1500/mm³ on 2 or more occasions *or* D. Thrombocytopenia—less than 100,000/mm³ in the absence of offending drugs
10. Immunologic disorder	A. Deleted in 1997 update B. Anti-DNA: antibody to native DNA in abnormal titer *or* C. Anti-Sm: presence of antibody to Sm nuclear antigen *or* D. Positive finding of antiphospholipid antibodies based on (1) an abnormal serum level of IgG or IgM anticardiolipin antibodies, (2) a positive test for lupus anticoagulant using a standard method, or (3) a false-positive serologic test for syphilis known to be positive for at least 6 months and confirmed by *Treponema pallidum* immobilization or the fluorescent treponemal antibody absorption test (modified in the 1997 update)
11. Antinuclear antibody	An abnormal titer of antinuclear antibody by immunofluorescence or an equivalent assay at any point in time and in the absence of drugs known to be associated with "drug-induced lupus" syndrome

*The proposed classification is based on 11 criteria. For the purpose of identifying patients in clinical studies, a person shall be said to have systemic lupus erythematosus if any 4 or more of the 11 criteria are present, serially or simultaneously, during any interval of observation.

From Tan EM, Cohen AS, Fries JF, et al. The 1982 revised criteria for the classification of systemic lupus erythematosus. *Arthritis Rheum.* 1982;25:1271.

criteria because it is positive in virtually all lupus patients. These criteria are not intended for use as diagnostic criteria because more than 50% of patients with SLE do not meet four criteria at any point in time, although all do meet these criteria at some point during the course of the disease. The criteria are useful in reminding the clinician of the most characteristic features of SLE, but a careful history with detailed review of systems and triggering factors, as well as a family history, is essential in raising suspicion for a diagnosis of SLE. Because drugs can trigger a lupus-like syndrome, a careful drug history should be taken. Procainamide and hydralazine present the greatest risk for development of lupus, with quinidine, isoniazid, minocycline, and recombinant interferon-α presenting a lower risk. At the onset of clinical symptoms, the diagnosis of SLE can be uncertain because many of the systemic manifestations of lupus can mimic other conditions, particularly viral infections or malignancy, and only some of the typical clinical symptoms may be expressed at any one point in time. Important features of SLE are its multisystemic nature and characteristic serology. The differential diagnosis of SLE includes other rheumatic disorders, such as rheumatoid arthritis and vasculitis; infections, including gonococcal arthritis, parvovirus B19, and mononucleosis; inflammatory bowel disease; thrombotic thrombocytopenic purpura; drug reactions; and malignancies, particularly lymphoma.

Laboratory Findings

Laboratory tests can be very helpful in supporting the diagnosis of SLE. All cellular elements of blood can be affected in lupus, so the complete blood count is an essential test that aids in diagnosis and management. A prolonged activated partial thromboplastin time (aPTT) can indicate the presence of pathogenic antiphospholipid antibodies (Chapter 174). These antibodies are also associated with a false-positive result in the serologic test for syphilis, an observation that is mainly of historical interest.

Evaluation of renal disease in SLE includes urinalysis with microscopic analysis of urine sediment, serum blood urea nitrogen and creatinine, and 24-hour urine collection for protein and creatinine clearance. Low serum albumin would be consistent with persistent proteinuria and membranous GN, whereas red and white blood cell casts in the urinary sediment suggest proliferative GN. Although a renal biopsy is usually performed only when the result may influence therapeutic decisions, pathologic classification of the features of renal disease can provide prognostic information.

The erythrocyte sedimentation rate (ESR), although a very nonspecific indicator of systemic inflammation, is often monitored and in many patients can provide an indication of disease activity. Interestingly, C-reactive protein, an acute phase reactant, is relatively uninformative in SLE because it is often low in comparison to an ESR performed on the same occasion.

Assaying and monitoring characteristic lupus serologic tests can strongly support the diagnosis of SLE and, in some cases, can assist in the assessment of disease activity. The ANA test is positive in virtually all patients and does not need to be repeated once it has been documented to be positive (Table 274-6). Anti-double-stranded DNA antibodies are common in SLE, and some studies have found that monitoring their titer can be useful in assessing the activity of lupus nephritis. Autoantibodies specific for proteins that associate with nucleic acids in intracellular particles are present in many patients and can provide support for a diagnosis of SLE. Anti-Sm antibodies are highly specific for SLE and, along with anti-RNP antibodies, react with the spliceosome particle. Anti-Ro (SSA) and anti-La (SSB) antibodies are specific for proteins in an RNA-containing particle and are common in patients with Sjögren's syndrome and in mothers of babies with neonatal lupus, as well

as being a feature of SLE. It is useful to document the presence of anti-Sm, anti-RNP, anti-Ro, and anti-La antibodies when the diagnosis of SLE is being made, but the titers of these autoantibodies are not helpful in monitoring disease activity.

Proteins of the complement system are activated by immune complexes, such as those that form in patients with SLE. The activation products that result from enzymatic cleavage of the complement components promote inflammation directly, by binding to cell surface receptors on mononuclear phagocytes, and indirectly, by acting as chemotactic agents to recruit inflammatory cells. Decreased levels of two of the more stable complement components, C3 and C4, are typically measured in serum, and decreased C3 and C4 levels are often indicators of enhanced consumption and increased disease activity. Some laboratories also use a functional measure of total hemolytic complement activity (CH_{50}).

It is the global picture provided by a careful history, physical examination, and blood, urine, and serologic data that supports a diagnosis of SLE. It should be recognized that there is considerable heterogeneity among patients and that different combinations of clinical features will characterize any one individual. As is the case with many systemic diseases, infection and some malignancies may have a similar picture and should be included in the differential until the diagnosis of SLE is secure.

TREATMENT Rx

Although current knowledge of genetic risk factors for SLE is not sufficient to predict those in whom the disease will develop, once the diagnosis has been made, regular counseling and education are fundamental to the treatment of SLE patients. Patients should be advised to avoid known triggers of disease exacerbation, such as ultraviolet light, and should be instructed regarding the need for adequate rest. Pregnancy should be undertaken with caution and with careful monitoring. Lupus patients can be informed that data indicate that oral contraceptive agents[1] and estrogen replacement therapy[2] do not contribute to disease exacerbations.

Conventional Medical Therapy

Clinical manifestations of lupus that do not involve major organ systems can often be managed with nonsteroidal anti-inflammatory drugs, low-dose corticosteroids, and antimalarials. Corticosteroids are immunosuppressive agents that modulate many functions of lymphocytes and monocytes, including the production of proinflammatory cytokines. Oral prednisone in doses ranging from 5 to 30 mg daily is effective in treating constitutional symptoms, arthralgias, pericarditis and pleuritis, and skin disease. Topical corticosteroids are sometimes applied to cutaneous lesions. For more serious disease, particularly active nephritis, CNS disease, or systemic vasculitis, prednisone at 60 mg daily or 1 g of intravenous methylprednisolone administered daily for 3 days can often gain control of disease activity. Although effective, corticosteroids also have toxicities that add to the morbidity associated with lupus. The broad immunosuppression mediated by these drugs contributes to the susceptibility to infection that is an inherent feature of SLE. Osteonecrosis, osteoporotic fractures, posterior subcapsular cataracts, diabetes, myopathy, hypertension, hypoadrenalism, and emotional disturbance are additional deleterious effects of corticosteroids.

Antimalarial agents, most commonly hydroxychloroquine administered at 200 to 400 mg/day, have long been used to control skin involvement and arthralgias and are now routinely used in most lupus patients. An important Canadian study demonstrating an increased frequency of disease flare in patients who discontinued hydroxychloroquine contributed to its recent use in lupus for a broader range of clinical manifestations. Hydroxychloroquine has been associated with a decreased incidence of thrombosis, a mechanism that could affect vasculopathy and end-organ damage. An additional potential mechanism of action implicates the TLR pathway, which is responsible for activation of the innate immune response. The effects of antimalarial agents on acidification of the intracellular vesicles where TLRs associate with their ligands may inhibit immune cell activation mediated by stimulatory nucleic acids. Antimalarials are well tolerated. Because they can rarely cause eye toxicity, ophthalmologic examinations should precede initiation of therapy and take place every 6 to 12 months.

In addition to controlling autoimmunity and inflammation in SLE, it is essential to control hypertension adequately when it occurs. In patients with a history of thrombosis, who will usually have antiphospholipid antibodies, warfarin is recommended.

Immunosuppressive Agents
Alkylating Agents

Approximately 33% of lupus patients receive cytotoxic therapy during the course of their disease. Cyclophosphamide is a cytotoxic agent that has been one of the more reliable and studied treatments for severe organ system manifestations of lupus, particularly lupus nephritis and CNS involvement.

TABLE 274-6	AUTOANTIBODIES ASSOCIATED WITH SYSTEMIC LUPUS ERYTHEMATOSUS
TARGET ANTIGEN	**APPROXIMATE FREQUENCY**
Nuclear antigens	99
dsDNA	70
Sm	38
RNP (U1-RNP)	33
Ro (SSA)	49
La (SSB)	35
Phospholipids	21
Ribosomal P	10

Studies performed at the National Institutes of Health in the 1980s led to recommendations of a standard regimen of cyclophosphamide, 0.5 to 1.0 g/m² body surface area administered intravenously monthly for 6 months, followed by quarterly doses through 2 years. Cyclophosphamide is usually given with oral prednisone in tapering doses or sometimes with pulse methylprednisolone. Although this regimen is often effective in controlling GN, overall patient survival has not been demonstrated to be increased, and cyclophosphamide is associated with significant toxicity, including cytopenia, infection, gonadal failure, and malignancy. Recent clinical studies have included modified immunosuppressive regimens, such as a 6-month induction followed by maintenance with less toxic immunosuppressive agents, including azathioprine❸ or mycophenolate mofetil (MMF). Cyclophosphamide is relatively contraindicated in pregnant women.

Purine Synthesis Inhibitors

Azathioprine has been used for the treatment of lupus nephritis and as a steroid-sparing agent in SLE for many years. Azathioprine inhibits DNA synthesis and inhibits key signaling pathways in T lymphocytes. Azathioprine is commonly dosed at 2 to 3 mg/kg/day administered as a tablet. Toxicities of azathioprine target the bone marrow and result in cytopenias, as well as the liver, occasionally resulting in transaminitis. Its use is rarely associated with non-Hodgkin's lymphoma (Chapter 191). It has been used safely in pregnant women.

MMF is an inhibitor that binds to the isoform of inosine monophosphate dehydrogenase that mediates purine synthesis in activated lymphocytes. It has a good track record of utility in inhibiting allograft rejection. Recent clinical trials have compared MMF with intravenous cyclophosphamide for induction therapy in lupus nephritis; the results demonstrated equivalence of MMF and cyclophosphamide in patients with lupus nephritis.❹ As noted, MMF may also be useful for maintenance treatment of lupus nephritis after induction with cyclophosphamide.

Methotrexate

Methotrexate is a folate antagonist that is commonly used in rheumatoid arthritis. A double-blind, randomized, placebo-controlled trial of oral methotrexate (15 to 25 mg/week for 6 months) in SLE controlled disease and allowed tapering of prednisone. The most responsive clinical manifestations were cutaneous and articular.

Ancillary and Other Therapies

Intravenous Gamma Globulin

Although positive data from controlled trials of intravenous gamma globulin are not available, case reports and clinical experience indicate that administration of pooled IgG fractions can sometimes be efficacious in gaining control of lupus disease activity that is refractory to other therapies. A common regimen is 2 g/kg in divided doses over a 3- to 5-day period. Several mechanisms have been proposed for this therapy, including blockade of Fc receptors, modulation of lymphocyte function through Fc receptors, increased catabolism of pathogenic immunoglobulin, and actions of the anti-idiotype antibody that is a component of the administered IgG.

Plasmapheresis

Removal of pathogenic antibodies and immune complexes is the goal of plasmapheresis, but there are scant data supporting the utility of this therapy. Nonetheless, plasmapheresis has been occasionally useful in lupus patients with life-threatening complications in which the clinical manifestations can be clearly attributed to pathogenic autoantibodies. In particular, plasmapheresis has been effective in cases of thrombotic thrombocytopenic purpura associated with SLE (Chapter 175).

Biologic Therapies

Biologic therapies (Chapter 35) are being actively investigated in clinical trials, but only one agent has been successful as yet in phase III studies. Belimumab, a monoclonal antibody, blocks a B-cell survival and differentiation signal. At a dose of 1 to 10 mg intravenously on days 1 and 28 and then every 28 days for 48 weeks, belimumab reduces disease activity by both validated measures and physician global assessment, and decreases autoantibody levels.❺ The clinical settings that are most appropriate for the use of belimumab, which was recently approved by the U.S. Food and Drug Administration, will be determined by future clinical trials and clinical experience. Additional agents under investigation target B cells, T-cell activation, and cytokines. Rituximab, a monoclonal antibody specific for the cell surface B-cell molecule CD20, is approved for use in B-cell lymphomas and has been used in some patients with SLE who are poorly responsive to other therapies. Rituximab depletes B cells, often for many months, and may limit T-cell activation by eliminating activated B cells that can serve as antigen-presenting cells. However, controlled clinical trials of rituximab in lupus have not shown efficacy. Other agents that block B-cell survival and differentiation factors or target B-cell surface molecules are under study. T-cell targets include CD28 and inducible costimulator (ICOS), a T-cell surface molecule in the same molecular family as CD28 and CTLA4. Blockade of T-cell activation by CTLA4-Ig, a soluble inhibitor of CD28 ligation, or inhibition of ICOS-ICOS ligand interaction might inhibit B-cell differentiation in the germinal center. Monoclonal antibodies specific for most

isoforms of interferon-α are under study and represent a rational approach in view of the increased interferon in many SLE patients. IL-6 and interferon-γ represent additional cytokine targets under study.

Future Directions

Recent advances in basic immunology, together with detailed molecular and clinical characterization of cohorts of SLE patients, have directed attention to the role that adjuvant-like factors play in activating the innate immune response through TLRs. The primary triggers of that response are not known, but abundant data support production of type I interferon as an important consequence of immune activation that has an impact on many aspects of lymphocyte function, probably including induction of self-antigen-specific immune responses. In addition to the biologic therapies currently under study that target T and B lymphocytes, future therapies may be designed that can inhibit TLR activation, signaling components downstream from TLRs, or type I interferon itself. Recognition that the complement system is an essential contributor to inflammation triggered by antiphospholipid antibodies, as well as by immune complexes, provides additional targets that might be inhibited therapeutically and limit tissue damage. Continued investigation of the genetic and environmental factors that contribute to disease susceptibility may permit identification of individuals at risk for the development of SLE and may elucidate the primary stimuli that lead to autoimmunity. Identification of informative biomarkers that reflect or even predict disease flares would improve medical management of lupus patients.

PROGNOSIS

Although survival of patients with a diagnosis of SLE is good, lupus remains a disease that is potentially fatal. SLE demonstrates a bimodal pattern of death, with deaths within the first year attributable to active lupus and infection and late deaths attributable to atherosclerotic cardiovascular disease. Recent cohort studies have estimated 5-year survival rates greater than 90%, with improvement in medical management probably contributing to improved outcomes as opposed to earlier studies, and 85% survival rates at 10 years. However, once a diagnosis of SLE has been made, prolonged remission is rare. Of 702 patients registered in a lupus clinic in Canada, 6.5% achieved complete remission (score of 0 on the SLE Disease Activity Index), and only 1.7% maintained remission for at least 5 years with no treatment. The presence of any permanent organ damage within the first year after a diagnosis of SLE is associated with poorer survival at 10 years (a 75 vs. 95% rate in those without permanent organ damage). Regarding renal outcome, an elevated level of serum creatinine at the time of diagnosis has been correlated with an adverse outcome.

Recent studies of minority populations in the United States have indicated that predictors of high lupus disease activity include Hispanic Texan and African American ethnicities, lack of health insurance, and poor social support. African admixture and anti-double-stranded DNA antibodies also predicted high levels of disease activity, as did previous disease activity.

Data from a multicenter study of nearly 10,000 patients has supported an increased risk for hematologic malignancies in SLE patients, particularly non-Hodgkin's lymphoma. Prognostic factors for an adverse fetal outcome in pregnant lupus mothers are maternal renal disease and hypertension.

1. Petri M, Kim MY, Kalunian KC, et al. Combined oral contraceptives in women with systemic lupus erythematosus. N Engl J Med. 2005;353:2550-2558.
2. Sanchez-Guerrero J, Gonzalez-Perez M, Durand-Carbajal M, et al. Menopause hormonal therapy in women with systemic lupus erythematosus. Arthritis Rheum. 2007;56:3070-3079.
3. Houssiau FA, Vasconcelos C, D'Crus D, et al. The 10-year follow-up data of the Euro-Lupus Nephritis Trial comparing low-dose and high-dose intravenous cyclophosphamide. Ann Rheum Dis. 2010;69:61-64.
4. Appel GB, Contreras G, Dooley MA, et al, for the Aspreva Lupus Management Study Group. Mycophenolate mofetil versus cyclophosphamide for induction treatment of lupus nephritis. J Am Soc Nephrol. 2009;20:1103-1112.
5. Navarra SV, Guzmán RM, Gallacher AE, et al. Efficacy and safety of belimumab in patients with active systemic lupus erythematosus: a randomised, placebo-controlled, phase 3 trial. Lancet. 2011;377:721-731.

SUGGESTED READINGS

Bomback AS, Appel GB. Updates on the treatment of lupus nephritis. J Am Soc Nephrol. 2010;21:2028-2035. Review emphasizing cyclophosphamide, mycophenolate mofetil, and azathioprine.

Chang C, Gershwin ME. Drugs and autoimmunity: a contemporary review and mechanistic approach. J Autoimmunity. 2010;34:j266-j275. A comprehensive review of the drugs associated with induction of lupus, including consideration of potential pathogenic mechanisms.

Crispin JC, Liossis SN, Kis-Toth K, et al. Pathogenesis of systemic lupus erythematosus: recent advances. Trends Mol Med. 2010;16:47-57. Recent understanding of genetic, immunologic, and environmental contributions to SLE pathogenesis and their potential as biomarkers and therapeutic targets.

Elbirt D, Sthoeger D, Asher I, et al. The management of systemic lupus erythematosus: facts and controversies. *Clin Dermatol.* 2010;28:330-336. *Review of anti-inflammatory, antimalarial, and immunosuppressive agents, as well as new biologic agents.*

Kozora E, Filley CM. Cognitive dysfunction and white matter abnormalities in systemic lupus erythematosus. *J Int Neuropsychol Soc.* 2011;17:385-392. *Clinico-pathologic correlation in SLE neuropsychiatric disease.*

Ronnblom L, Elkon KB. Cytokines as therapeutic targets in SLE. *Nat Rev Rheumatol.* 2010;6:338-347. *Review of promising candidate therapeutic targets, with a focus on B-cell activating factor, interferon-alpha and tumor necrosis factor.*

Skamra C, Ramsey-Goldman R. Management of cardiovascular complications in systemic lupus erythematosus. *Int J Clin Rheumatol.* 2010;5:75-100. *Review of the link between SLE and atherosclerotic cardiovascular disease and SLE-specific variables that contribute to cardiovascular risk.*

275

SYSTEMIC SCLEROSIS (SCLERODERMA)

JOHN VARGA

DEFINITION

Systemic sclerosis (SSc) is an acquired rheumatic disease of unknown cause. It most commonly affects middle-aged women and is associated with considerable morbidity and mortality. Systemic sclerosis has protean clinical manifestations and follows a chronic and often progressive course. The hallmark of SSc is thickening and hardening of the skin (scleroderma), but most patients also manifest characteristic abnormalities in the lungs, gastrointestinal tract, kidneys, and heart. In its earliest stages, SSc is associated with prominent autoimmune and inflammatory features and altered vascular function. Over time, structural alterations in small blood vessels and progressive fibrosis in multiple organs ensue and cause organ failure. Although there is no cure for SSc, current treatment strategies can effectively control symptoms, slow disease progression, and improve quality of life. The presence of scleroderma (hard skin) distinguishes SSc from other autoimmune and rheumatic diseases, but skin induration is also a prominent feature of localized forms of scleroderma and multiple unrelated conditions (Table 275-1).

Classification

Systemic Sclerosis

Systemic sclerosis is commonly classified into two principal subsets: diffuse cutaneous SSc (dcSSc) and limited cutaneous SSc (lcSSc). These disease subsets are defined by the pattern of skin involvement and are associated with distinct clinical and laboratory manifestations (Table 275-2). In lcSSc, skin involvement is restricted to the fingers, toes, distal extremities, and face, and the trunk is spared. Diffuse cutaneous SSc is characterized by involvement of the skin proximal to the elbows and knees, including the trunk, as well as distal extremities. Diffuse cutaneous SSc is generally rapidly progressive with early pulmonary fibrosis and acute renal failure. In contrast, patients with lcSSc develop Raynaud's phenomenon long before other manifestations appear. A subset of patients with lcSSc have a constellation of calcinosis cutis, Raynaud's phenomenon, esophageal dysmotility, sclerodactyly (scleroderma of the fingers), and telangiectasia, which is termed *CREST syndrome*. Patients with the CREST syndrome generally have an indolent course and a good prognosis. In some patients, Raynaud's phenomenon and other characteristic clinical and laboratory findings of SSc occur in the absence of obvious skin thickening. This entity is designated *SSc sine scleroderma*.

Mixed Connective Tissue Disorder

Mixed connective tissue disorder (MCTD) is an overlap syndrome first described in 1971 that is characterized by features of systemic lupus erythematosus (SLE), SSc, and myositis, all occurring in the same patient. In the early phase, most patients have Raynaud's phenomenon in association with edema of the hands and evidence of inflammatory muscle disease. Over time, these patients sequentially manifest other features of connective tissue diseases, including pericarditis, esophageal dysmotility, sclerodactyly, neuropathy, and pulmonary arterial hypertension. Erosive arthritis does not occur. On the other hand, some patients develop acute renal involvement similar to scleroderma renal crisis. In the early stage of this disorder, it is often difficult to predict whether the patient will progress to develop a distinct connective tissue disease such as SSc or SLE, or will be ultimately diagnosed with MCTD. A diagnostic hallmark of MCTD is the presence in the serum of a highly characteristic autoantibody specificity against U1-ribonuclear protein (U1-RNP). Most MCTD patients have a very high titer (often greater than 1 : 1,000) of anti-U1-RNP autoantibody. Some of the features of MCTD might respond to corticosteroid therapy. Overall, patients with MCTD generally have a better prognosis than those with SSc.

Localized Scleroderma

Localized scleroderma refers to a family of generally benign skin conditions primarily affecting children. These conditions are characterized by discreet areas of skin induration in the absence of Raynaud's phenomenon or systemic involvement. Lesional skin is discolored and indurated and histologically may be indistinguishable from SSc. Localized scleroderma may occur as single or multiple solitary patches of induration (morphea) or as a coalescence of multiple patches (generalized morphea). The lesions are generally asymmetrical in distribution and spare the digits. Some individuals have extensive and disabling induration (pansclerotic morphea). Induration of the skin may follow in a linear distribution, most commonly on the lower extremities (linear scleroderma). In children, linear scleroderma can be complicated by growth retardation and joint contractures.

EPIDEMIOLOGY

SSc occurs as a sporadic disease with a worldwide distribution and affects all races. The incidence is 9 to 19 cases per million per year, with an estimated 100,000 cases in the United States. Studies from several countries suggest that the incidence of SSc is increasing, particularly among women. Like other connective tissue diseases, SSc shows a marked female predominance in the childbearing years and declines after menopause. The most common age of

TABLE 275-1 CONDITIONS WITH SCLERODERMA-LIKE SKIN INDURATION

Systemic sclerosis (SSc)
    Limited cutaneous SSc
    Diffuse cutaneous SSc
Localized scleroderma
    Morphea (plaque, guttate, generalized)
    Pansclerotic morphea
    Linear scleroderma, "coup de sabre"
Scleredema and diabetic scleredema
Scleromyxedema (papular mucinosis)
Nephrogenic fibrosing syndrome (nephrogenic fibrosing dermopathy, nephrogenic systemic fibrosis)
Chronic graft-versus-host disease
Diffuse fasciitis with eosinophilia (Shulman's disease, eosinophilic fasciitis)
Eosinophilia-myalgia syndrome
Chemically induced scleroderma-like conditions
    Vinyl chloride–induced disease, other solvents
    Pentazocine-induced skin fibrosis
    Other drug associations
Paraneoplastic syndrome

TABLE 275-2 CLASSIFICATION OF SYSTEMIC SCLEROSIS

FEATURES	LIMITED CUTANEOUS SYSTEMIC SCLEROSIS	DIFFUSE CUTANEOUS SYSTEMIC SCLEROSIS
Skin induration	Limited to fingers, distal to elbows, face; slow progression	Diffuse: fingers, extremities, face, trunk; rapid progression; tendon rubs
Raynaud's phenomenon	Precedes skin involvement; associated with critical ischemia	Onset may be coincident with or subsequent to skin changes
Pulmonary fibrosis	Occasional, moderate	Frequent, early and severe
Pulmonary arterial hypertension	Frequent, late, may be isolated	May occur, often in association with pulmonary fibrosis
Scleroderma renal crisis	Very rare	Occurs in 15%; early
Calcinosis cutis	Frequent, prominent	Infrequent
Characteristic autoantibodies	Anticentromere	Antitopoisomerase I (Scl-70), anti-RNA polymerase III

onset is 30 to 50 years for both the limited and diffuse cutaneous forms. African Americans have a higher incidence than whites and an earlier age of onset, and are more likely to exhibit the diffuse cutaneous form of SSc associated with interstitial lung involvement and a worse prognosis.

Etiology and Environmental and Occupational Exposures

Although the cause of SSc is unknown, the onset is commonly ascribed to an interplay between environmental factors and genetic susceptibility. Suspected environmental triggers include infectious agents and occupational, dietary, medical, and lifestyle exposures. Patients with SSc possess elevated serum levels of antibodies to cytomegalovirus and parvovirus B19. Because some SSc autoantibodies cross-react with certain virus-associated epitopes, molecular mimicry has been considered a possible pathogenetic link between viral infection and SSc.

Epidemic outbreaks of SSc-like syndromes have been linked with specific toxic exposures. An outbreak of toxic oil syndrome in the 1980s affected more than 20,000 individuals in Spain. The syndrome was characterized by chronic skin induration and neuropathy, and the outbreak was linked to ingestion of contaminated rapeseed oils used for cooking. An outbreak of eosinophilia-myalgia syndrome (EMS) a decade later was linked to ingestion of over-the-counter L-tryptophan dietary supplements used for insomnia, weight loss, and other indications. The syndrome was characterized by peripheral blood eosinophilia and severe myalgia in the acute stage, followed by intractable scleroderma-like diffuse skin induration. Neither toxic oil syndrome nor EMS was associated with Raynaud's phenomenon or SSc-specific autoantibodies.

Occupational exposures tentatively linked with SSc include silica (in miners), polyvinyl chloride, epoxy resins, and aromatic hydrocarbons including toluene and trichloroethylene. Certain drugs, including bleomycin, pentazocine, hormone replacement therapy, cocaine, and appetite suppressants, have been linked with SSc or pulmonary arterial hypertension. Although earlier studies implied a possible association of SSc with silicone breast implants, large-scale epidemiologic investigations failed to establish an increased risk.

Genetic Factors

A genetic contribution to SSc susceptibility is indicated by the fact that 1.6% of patients have a first-degree relative with SSc, a prevalence rate substantially higher than in the general population (0.026). Indeed, a family history is the strongest identified risk factor for SSc. The risk for other autoimmune diseases is also increased among relatives of SSc patients. Genetic investigations in SSc to date have used the candidate gene approach. Case-control studies of genes for autoimmune susceptibility have indicated an association of SSc with *STAT4, IRF4, PTPN22,* and *BANK1,* and with the genes from human leukocyte antigen (HLA) class II, angiotensin-converting enzyme (ACE), endothelin-1, growth factors and their receptors, and extracellular matrix proteins. These findings suggest that SSc is a complex polygenic disease in which multiple genetic loci exert minor individual effects on disease susceptibility. A recent genomewide association study (GWAS) in a population of European ancestry identified multiple susceptibility loci associated with SSc. One of these is CD247, a component of the T-cell receptor-CD3 complex that has previously been associated with susceptibility to SLE. Additional SSc susceptibility loci confirmed in this GWAS included *MHC, IRF5,* and *STAT4,* each of which is involved in immune regulation, highlighting the role of autoimmunity in the pathogenesis of SSc.

PATHOBIOLOGY

The protean clinical and pathologic manifestations of SSc reflect a highly complex pathobiology encompassing three cardinal processes: autoimmunity and inflammation, vascular injury and obliteration, and fibrosis and matrix deposition in multiple organs (Fig. 275-1). This triad of distinct yet

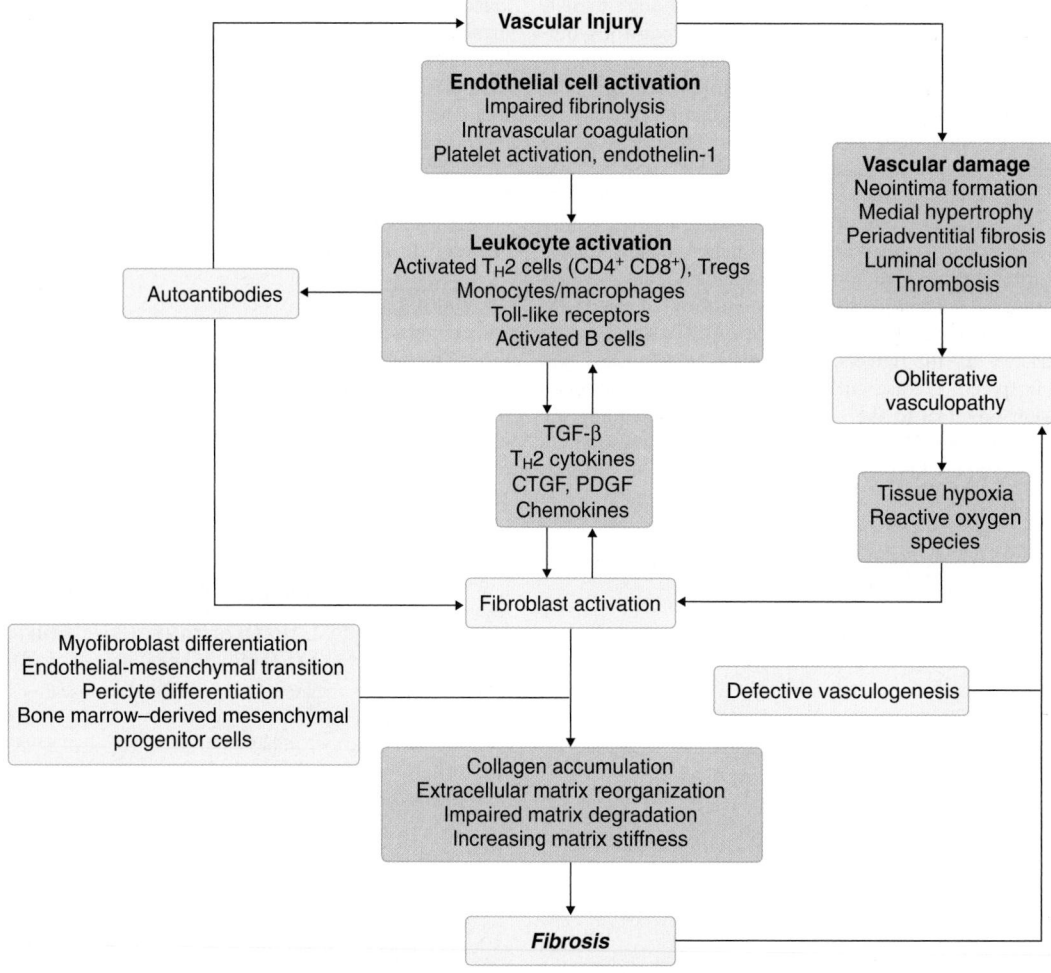

FIGURE 275-1. The pathogenetic triad of systemic sclerosis: vasculopathy, autoimmunity, fibrosis. Initial endothelial injury in a genetically susceptible individual leads to vascular damage, inflammation, and autoimmunity. The inflammatory and immune responses initiate fibroblast activation, resulting in intractable fibrosis. Vasculopathy, loss of microvasculature and reduced blood flow result in ischemia and generation of reactive oxygen species that contribute to, and further aggravate, tissue fibrosis and atrophy. CTGF = connective tissue growth factor; PDGF = platelet-derived growth factor; TGF-β = transforming growth factor-β.

interrelated processes is operative to a greater or lesser extent in every patient, and their variable relative contributions to the individual clinical phenotype account for the observed disease heterogeneity.

PATHOLOGY

The distinguishing pathologic hallmark of SSc is the constellation of capillary loss and obliterative vasculopathy coexisting with acellular fibrosis in the skin and internal organs. In early disease, perivascular inflammation can be detected in multiple organs before the appearance of fibrosis. The vascular lesion is characterized by intimal proliferation in the small and medium-sized arteries, resulting in luminal narrowing and obliteration. In later-stage SSc, fibrosis is prominent in the skin, lungs, gastrointestinal tract, heart, tendon sheath, perifascicular tissue surrounding skeletal muscle, and some endocrine organs. Accumulation of connective tissue rich in collagens, fibronectin, cartilage oligomeric matrix protein, and proteoglycans disrupts normal architecture, resulting in functional impairment of affected organs.

In the dermis, collagen deposition causes obliteration of the hair follicles, sweat glands, and other appendages as well as invasion of the subjacent adipose layer with entrapment of fat cells. The epidermis is atrophic, and the rete pegs are effaced. In late-stage disease, there is a paucity of vascular and lymphatic endothelium, and there is capillary rarefaction in the skin. In the lungs, the interstitium and alveolar spaces are infiltrated with inflammatory cells in early disease. With progression, interstitial fibrosis and vascular damage, often coexisting within the same lesions, dominate the pathologic picture. The most common histologic pattern in SSc lung is nonspecific interstitial pneumonitis. Progressive thickening of the alveolar septae results in obliteration of the air spaces, honeycombing, and loss of pulmonary blood vessels. Intimal thickening of the pulmonary arteries, best seen with elastin stain, underlies pulmonary hypertension. The lesions resemble those of, but are distinct from, idiopathic pulmonary arterial hypertension, with frequent vascular fibrosis but an absence of plexiform lesions. Pathologic changes in the gastrointestinal tract can be found at any level from the mouth to the rectum. Fibrosis of the lamina propria and submucosa with atrophy of the muscular layers are prominent changes in the lower esophagus, whereas striated muscle in the upper third of the esophagus is generally spared. Replacement of the normal intestinal tract architecture leads to disordered peristaltic activity with gastroesophageal reflux and dysmotility, gastroparesis, and small bowel obstruction. Chronic reflux is associated with esophageal inflammation, ulcerations, stricture formation, and Barrett's metaplasia.

Pathologic changes are common in the heart in SSc, with involvement of the myocardium and pericardium. Characteristic microvascular lesions are seen with concentric intimal hypertrophy and luminal narrowing, but not affecting epicardial coronary arteries. Contraction band necrosis reflecting ischemia-reperfusion injury in the myocardium is prominent and may be accompanied by patchy myocardial fibrosis. In the kidneys, noninflammatory lesions occur in the interlobular arteries. Scleroderma renal crisis is associated with striking changes in small renal arteries with reduplication of elastic lamina, marked intimal proliferation, and concentric narrowing of the lumen (onion-skin appearance), frequently accompanied by thrombosis and microangiopathic hemolysis (Fig. 275-2).

FIGURE 275-2. Pulmonary arterial obliterative vasculopathy. Striking intimal hyperplasia and narrowing of the lumen of a small pulmonary artery, coexisting with interstitial pulmonary fibrosis, in a patient with diffuse cutaneous systemic sclerosis.

Animal Models of Disease

Although no single animal model fully recapitulates the tripartite pathobiology of SSc, certain models exhibit particular disease features and are useful in investigating pathogenesis and therapy. The tight-skin mouse (Tsk1) spontaneously develops diffuse skin thickening and fibrosis. This phenotype is due to a duplication mutation in the gene for fibrillin-1, a component of extracellular microfibrils that provides a scaffold for elastin fibers but is also involved in the storage and regulation of transforming growth factor-β (TGF-β) and other growth factors. Different mutations in the fibrillin-1 gene cause Marfan syndrome, but such mutations have not been described in SSc. Scleroderma-like skin changes and fibrosis of the lungs and kidneys can be induced in mice by subcutaneous injection of bleomycin, or by transplantation of HLA-mismatched bone marrow or spleen cells. Increasingly, targeted genetic modifications such as deletion or transgenesis are used to create novel animal models for dissecting the interaction of molecules and pathways in fibrosis and for preclinical evaluation of novel therapies. For instance, mice transgenic for transcription factors Egr-1 and Fra-2, or for certain growth factors (TGF-β, connective tissue growth factor [CTGF], platelet-derived growth factor [PDGF], or Wnt10), spontaneously develop scleroderma-like features, whereas genetic targeting of Smad3 yields mice that are resistant to bleomycin-induced scleroderma.

Pathophysiologic Triad: Vasculopathy, Autoimmunity, and Fibrosis

Vasculopathy

Vasculopathy occurs early in SSc, involves multiple vascular beds, and accounts for major clinical complications. The process affects primarily the small and medium-sized arteries and arterioles and over time causes their obliteration. Factors thought to be responsible for triggering the initial vascular injury include viruses, oxygen radicals, circulating cytotoxic factors, complement activation, and autoantibodies. Endothelial cell injury and activation result in altered production of endothelium-derived vasodilatory (nitric oxide and prostacyclin) and vasoconstricting (endothelin-1) substances. Dysfunctional endothelium causes enhanced vascular permeability, upregulation of adhesion molecules with transendothelial leukocyte diapedesis, platelet aggregation, activation of intravascular coagulation, and defective fibrinolysis. Small blood vessels show intimal hyperplasia with thickening and reduplication of the basement membrane. In the vascular media, myointimal cells proliferate, whereas fibrosis develops in the adventitial layers; the net result is progressive narrowing and obliteration of capillaries, arterioles, and even large vessels. Impaired blood flow results in widespread tissue ischemia. Recurrent ischemia-reperfusion is associated with the generation of reactive oxygen species that further damage the endothelium. Paradoxically, despite the presence of tissue hypoxia and sometimes dramatically elevated levels of angiogenic factors, compensatory vasculogenesis is impaired. The combination of widespread capillary loss, obliterative vasculopathy of small and medium-sized arteries, and failure to regenerate damaged vessels are hallmarks of SSc.

Raynaud's Phenomenon

The earliest vascular complication of SSc, Raynaud's phenomenon, can precede other disease manifestations by years. Raynaud's phenomenon in SSc is characterized by an initially reversible altered blood flow response to cold challenge and is associated with autonomic and peripheral nervous system changes leading to impaired production of calcitonin gene–related peptide from sensory afferent nerves and heightened sensitivity of α_2-adrenergic receptors on vascular smooth muscle cells. In contrast to primary Raynaud's phenomenon, a common and relatively benign condition, Raynaud's phenomenon in SSc is generally progressive and complicated by irreversible structural changes in the blood vessels with tissue damage due to recurrent ischemia-reperfusion.

Inflammation and Autoimmunity

Cellular Immunity

Evidence of inflammation and autoimmunity is an invariable feature that SSc shares with other rheumatic diseases such as systemic lupus erythematosus and rheumatoid arthritis. The association of SSc with autoimmunity genes such as *IRF5* and *STAT4* provides strong support for the autoimmune basis of the disease. In early SSc, activated T cells and monocyte-macrophages accumulate in the skin, lungs, and other affected organs. Infiltrating T cells display restricted receptor signatures indicative of oligoclonal expansion in

TABLE 275-3 CHARACTERISTIC AUTOANTIBODIES IN SYSTEMIC SCLEROSIS

AUTOANTIBODY	SYSTEMIC SCLEROSIS SUBSET	CLINICAL ASSOCIATION
Topoisomerase-I	Diffuse cutaneous	Tendon friction rubs, ILD, cardiac involvement, scleroderma renal crisis
Centromere	Limited cutaneous	Digital ischemia, calcinosis, isolated PAH; scleroderma renal crisis rare
RNA polymerase III	Diffuse cutaneous	Extensive skin involvement; tendon friction rubs, scleroderma renal crisis
U3-RNP0	Diffuse cutaneous	PAH, ILD, scleroderma renal crisis, myositis
Th/T0	Limited cutaneous	ILD, PAH
PM/Scl	Limited cutaneous	Calcinosis, myositis
U1-RNP	MCTD	PAH

ILD = interstitial lung disease; MCTD = mixed connective tissue disease; PAH = pulmonary arterial hypertension.

response to unknown antigens and show T_H2 polarization with secretion of interleukin-4 (IL-4) and IL-13. T_H2 cytokines induce TGF-β and promote the synthesis of collagen and other extracellular matrix molecules. The frequency of circulating regulatory T cells is elevated, but their immunosuppressive function is defective. Macrophages show evidence of alternative activation associated with pathologic fibrogenesis. A role is emerging for innate immunity through toll-like receptors, which could provide a link of environmental triggers to the disease.

Humoral Autoimmunity and B Lymphocytes
Although autoantibodies have well-established clinical utility as diagnostic and prognostic markers in SSc, their role in pathogenesis and tissue damage remains speculative. In addition to antinuclear antibodies (ANAs), a number of highly disease-specific and mutually exclusive autoantibodies occur (Table 275-3). Some autoantibodies are directed against intracellular proteins (topoisomerase-I, centromere, and the RNA polymerases I and III), whereas others are directed against cell surface antigens (platelet-derived growth factor receptor) or secreted proteins (fibrillin-1 and matrix metalloproteases) and may directly contribute to vascular injury or fibrosis. B cells are implicated in both the autoimmune and fibrotic responses in SSc. In addition to their role in antibody production, B cells also present antigen, produce profibrotic cytokines such as IL-6 and TGF-β, and modulate the function of T cells and dendritic cells. In SSc, B cells show elevated CD19 expression, and the numbers of memory B cells and early plasma cells are reduced. Gene expression profiling has identified messenger RNA expression signatures characteristic of B-cell activation in the lesional skin.

Fibrosis
Fibrosis of the skin and multiple internal organs is the distinguishing feature of SSc. It characteristically follows, and is thought to be a consequence of, inflammation and vascular injury. Fibrosis is characterized by progressive replacement of normal tissue architecture with an acellular collagen-rich extracellular matrix secreted and remodeled by resident fibroblasts. Under physiologic conditions, fibroblasts that are activated by TGF-β and related factors can proliferate, migrate, elaborate collagens and extracellular matrix, and transdifferentiate into contractile myofibroblasts, enabling them to execute prompt repair of damaged tissue. When this highly regulated and self-limited physiologic repair program becomes sustained and amplified, excessive intractable scar tissue formation ensues.

Effector Cells in Fibrosis
Myofibroblasts are contractile connective tissue cells that display smooth muscle cell–like features and contribute to scar formation through production of collagen and TGF-β and contraction of the surrounding extracellular matrix. In SSc, activated myofibroblasts appear in tissue due to in situ activation of quiescent resident fibroblasts, through transdifferentiation from damaged epithelial cells, endothelial cells, or pericytes, or by migration and terminal differentiation of bone marrow-derived mesenchymal progenitor cells. Fibroblasts explanted from patients with SSc display cell-intrinsic

abnormalities that persist during in vitro passage. For instance, cultured SSc fibroblasts exhibit increased rates of collagen gene transcription, secretion of cytokines and growth factors, expression of cell surface adhesion molecules, and evidence of constitutive autocrine TGF-β signaling.

CLINICAL MANIFESTATIONS

Overview
Multiple organs are affected in SSc, but the frequency, tempo, and severity of their involvement show substantial patient-to-patient variability. Patients with dcSSc characteristically develop extensive skin induration and early progressive internal organ involvement. Patients with lcSSc commonly present with long-standing Raynaud's phenomenon, modest skin changes, and indolent internal organ disease. However, many patients with SSc defy easy subclassification, and others show an overlap of typical SSc features coexisting with clinical and laboratory evidence of another autoimmune disease such as polymyositis, Sjögren's syndrome, polyarthritis, or systemic lupus erythematosus.

Initial Clinical Presentation
Diffuse Cutaneous Systemic Sclerosis
Patients with dcSSc typically present with soft tissue swelling, erythema, and pruritus, often accompanied by fatigue, stiffness, and malaise. Although arthralgia, muscle weakness, and carpal tunnel syndrome are common, Raynaud's phenomenon may not be present until later in the disease. In the ensuing weeks to months, the inflammatory edematous phase evolves into a chronic "fibrotic" phase with skin induration accompanied by hyperpigmentation, loss of body hair, and impaired sweating. The wrists, elbows, shoulders, knees, and ankles become stiff owing to fibrosis of the joint structures. Advancing skin changes are commonly accompanied by onset of internal organ involvement that is most rapidly progressive during the initial 4 years from disease onset. The risk for new organ involvement declines thereafter.

Limited Cutaneous Systemic Sclerosis
In lcSSc, the diagnosis is generally made at a more advanced stage of the disease. These patients give a history of long-standing Raynaud's phenomenon, sometimes complicated by ischemic ulcerations. The course of disease is indolent, with delayed onset and slow progression of gastroesophageal reflux, telangiectasia, or cutaneous calcinosis. Vascular manifestations tend to be more pronounced compared with dcSSc, and digital ischemia, cutaneous telangiectasia, and progressive pulmonary artery hypertension (PAH) are frequent late manifestations. In contrast, scleroderma renal crisis is uncommon in lcSSc.

Organ Involvement
Skin
Skin thickening, the distinguishing hallmark of SSc, is symmetrical and bilateral. It typically starts in the fingers and advances from distal to proximal extremities. The skin generally becomes hyperpigmented, but dark-skinned individuals may develop vitiligo-like hypopigmentation or "salt-and-pepper" changes most prominently on the upper back and chest. Obliteration of sweat glands and sebaceous glands results in decreased sweating and dry skin. The face gradually assumes a characteristic appearance with a beaklike nose, thinning and retraction of the lips, fine wrinkles (radial furrowing) around the mouth, and occasionally a masklike facies due to reduced mobility of the eyelids, cheeks, and mouth (Fig. 275-3). Decreased oral aperture (microstomia) interferes with eating and oral hygiene.

In patients with established SSc, the skin is atrophic and tethered to the subcutaneous tissue. Telangiectasia, similar to the skin lesions of hereditary hemorrhagic telangiectasia, is prominent on the face, hands, lips, and oral mucosa. Breakdown of atrophic skin leads to painful ulcerations at the extensor surfaces of the interphalangeal joints, fingertips, and bony prominences such as the elbows and malleoli. Ulcers may become secondarily infected, resulting in osteomyelitis. Ischemic fingertip ulcerations show slow healing that results in characteristic digital "pits." Ischemic loss of soft tissue at the fingertips is associated with resorption of the terminal phalanges (acroosteolysis) (Fig. 275-4).

Calcium deposits varying in size from tiny punctate lesions to large conglomerate masses develop in the skin and soft tissues. They are composed of calcium hydroxyapatite crystals and can be readily visualized on plain radiographs. Frequent locations include the finger pads, extensor surfaces of the forearms, and olecranon and prepatellar bursae. Calcific deposits can ulcerate

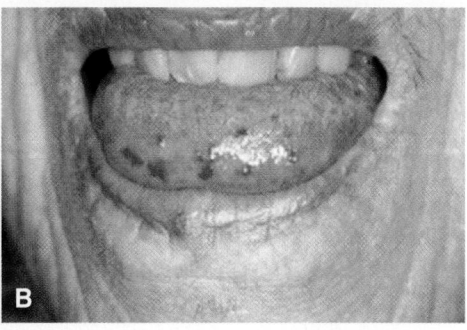

FIGURE 275-3. Facial features in systemic sclerosis. **A,** Perioral furrowing. Note vertical lines of furrowing around the mouth in a patient with diffuse cutaneous systemic sclerosis. **B,** Telangiectasia on the lips and tongue in a patient with long-standing limited cutaneous systemic sclerosis.

FIGURE 275-4. Vascular complications of systemic sclerosis in the fingers. **A,** Nail fold microvascular changes. **B,** Digital infarction. Sharply demarcated necrosis of the fingertip in a patient with limited cutaneous systemic sclerosis associated with severe Raynaud's phenomenon. **C,** Digital tip ulceration and pitting.

through the overlying skin, producing drainage of chalky white material, pain, and local inflammation.

Raynaud's Phenomenon

Raynaud's phenomenon (Chapter 80) is an episodic vasoconstriction in the digits that occurs in virtually all patients with SSc. Typical attacks start with pallor (vasoconstriction), followed by cyanosis (ischemia) and erythema (reperfusion). Attacks are commonly triggered by exposure to cold or emotional stress. Primary Raynaud's phenomenon, a benign condition representing an exaggerated physiologic response to cold, occurs in 3 to 5% of the population and is more frequent in women. Secondary Raynaud's phenomenon occurs not only in SSc but also in other connective tissue diseases, hematologic and endocrine conditions, and occupational disorders, and with the use of β-blockers and anticancer drugs such as cisplatin and bleomycin.

Distinguishing primary from secondary Raynaud's phenomenon can present a challenge. Secondary Raynaud's phenomenon typically develops at an older age (>30 years), tends to be more severe, and is frequently complicated by critical ischemia. Nailfold capillaroscopy allows cutaneous capillaries to be viewed under a drop of immersion oil using an ophthalmoscope. Patients with primary Raynaud's phenomenon have normal nailfold capillaries that appear as regularly spaced parallel vascular loops, whereas in SSc, capillaries are distorted with widened and irregular loops, dilated lumen, and areas of vascular "dropout."

Gastrointestinal Involvement

The gastrointestinal tract is commonly affected in both limited and diffuse cutaneous forms of SSc. A pathologic picture of smooth muscle atrophy and fibrosis and obliterative small vessel vasculopathy is seen throughout the length of the gastrointestinal tract.

Upper Gastrointestinal Tract

Oropharyngeal manifestations of SSc include xerostomia, reduced oral aperture, periodontal disease, and resorption of the mandibular condyles. The frenulum of the tongue may be shortened. Gastroesophageal reflux disease (GERD) with heartburn, regurgitation, and dysphagia is very common (Chapter 140). Reduced lower esophageal sphincter pressure resulting in gastroesophageal reflux frequently coexists with impaired esophageal clearance of refluxed gastric contents due to diminished motility in the distal two thirds of the esophagus. Delayed gastric emptying further aggravates the problem. On chest computed tomography scans, the esophagus is dilated with intraluminal air. Severe erosive esophagitis may be found on endoscopy

in patients with minimal GERD symptoms. Esophageal strictures and Barrett's esophagus (Chapter 140) complicate chronic GERD. Because Barrett's esophagus is associated with an increased risk for adenocarcinoma, SSc patients require periodic endoscopy with mucosal biopsy. Hoarseness and chronic cough may be extraesophageal manifestations of GERD. Aspiration pneumonitis may aggravate underlying interstitial lung disease.

Stomach

Gastroparesis contributes to delayed gastric emptying with early satiety, abdominal distention, and aggravated reflux symptoms. Gastric vascular ectasia (GAVE) develops in 5% of patients, and is equally prevalent in limited and diffuse cutaneous disease. On endoscopy, parallel longitudinal mucosal folds resembling the stripes of a watermelon are seen in the antrum. The histologic features of dilated mucosal capillaries and fibromuscular dysplasia of the lamina propria reflect the diffuse small vessel vasculopathy of SSc. Patients with GAVE may develop recurrent gastrointestinal bleeding and typically present with unexplained anemia.

Lower Gastrointestinal Tract

Impaired small bowel motility in SSc can cause chronic diarrhea due to bacterial overgrowth. Fat and protein malabsorption, vitamin B$_{12}$ and D deficiency, and occasionally severe malnutrition may ensue. Disturbed intestinal motor function can also cause recurrent episodes of intestinal pseudo-obstruction with acute abdominal pain, nausea, and vomiting. Differentiating pseudo-obstruction, which responds to supportive care and intravenous nutritional supplementation, from mechanical bowel obstruction, is a diagnostic challenge. Colonic involvement can cause constipation, rectal prolapse, and fecal incontinence. In late-stage SSc, wide-mouth colonic sacculations can occur and cause perforation and bleeding. An occasional radiologic finding is pneumatosis cystoides intestinalis due to air trapping in the bowel wall. These lesions can rupture and cause pneumoperitoneum. The liver is rarely affected in SSc. However, primary biliary cirrhosis associated with antimitochondrial antibodies may occur.

Lung Involvement

The two principal types of pulmonary diseases are interstitial lung disease and PAH. Many patients develop some degree of both complications. Less frequent pulmonary manifestations include aspiration pneumonitis complicating gastroesophageal reflux, pulmonary hemorrhage, obliterative bronchiolitis, pleural reactions, restrictive ventilatory disease due to chest wall fibrosis, spontaneous pneumothorax, and drug-induced lung toxicity. The incidence of lung cancer, particularly bronchoalveolar carcinoma (Chapter 197), is increased.

Interstitial Lung Disease and Pulmonary Fibrosis

Interstitial lung disease (Chapter 92) in SSc can remain asymptomatic until quite advanced. The most frequent presenting symptoms are exertional dyspnea, fatigue, and reduced exercise tolerance. A chronic dry cough may be present. Physical examination may reveal "Velcro" crackles at the lung bases. Pulmonary function testing (Chapter 85) is a sensitive method for detecting early interstitial lung disease. The most common abnormalities are reductions in forced vital capacity (FVC) or single breath diffusing capacity (DLCO). However, a reduction in DLCO that is significantly out of proportion to the reduction in FVC (FVC/DLCO ratio >1.6) suggests pulmonary vascular disease.

Evidence of interstitial lung disease can be found in almost all patients and is clinically significant in up to 50%. Risk factors for interstitial lung disease include male gender, African American race, diffuse skin involvement, severe gastroesophageal reflux, and the presence of topoisomerase-I autoantibodies. The most rapid progression in interstitial lung disease occurs within the first 3 years of the disease.

Chest radiography is useful for ruling out infection and other causes of pulmonary involvement but is relatively insensitive for detection of early interstitial lung disease. In contrast, high-resolution computed tomography (HRCT) is highly sensitive (Chapter 84). Prominent HRCT features include reticular linear interstitial opacities, predominantly in the lower lobes. These may occur in isolation or in combination with ground-glass opacification. Additional findings include mediastinal lymphadenopathy and, rarely, honeycombing. The extent of lung disease on HRCT at initial evaluation correlates with progression and prognosis. Bronchoalveolar lavage (Chapter 85) can be useful for ruling out occult infection. Lung biopsy is only rarely indicated.

Pulmonary Arterial Hypertension

PAH is defined as a mean pulmonary arterial pressure of more than 25 mm Hg with a pulmonary capillary wedge pressure of less than 15 mm Hg (Chapter 68). Approximately 15% of SSc patients develop PAH, which can occur as an isolated abnormality or coexist with interstitial lung disease. The natural history of SSc-associated PAH is variable. However, many patients follow a downhill course with development of right heart failure and increased mortality. Risk factors for PAH in SSc include limited cutaneous disease, late age of disease onset, large number of cutaneous telangiectasias, and the presence of anticentromere autoantibodies, or antibodies to U1-RNP, U3-RNP (fibrillarin), B23, and β_2-glycoprotein I.

Early PAH is often clinically silent. The initial symptoms are exertional dyspnea and reduced exercise capacity. With progression, angina, syncope, and symptoms and signs of right-sided heart failure may appear. Physical examination shows tachypnea, a prominent pulmonic S_2 heart sound, palpable right ventricular heave, elevated jugular venous pressure, and dependent edema. Pulmonary arterial systolic pressures exceeding 40 mm Hg determined by Doppler echocardiography suggest the presence of PAH, as does an FVC/DLCO ratio of more than 1.6 on pulmonary function testing. Right heart catheterization is typically required for confirming the diagnosis of PAH, assessing its severity, and evaluating ventricular function. The serum levels of N-terminal brain natriuretic peptide (pro-BNP) are elevated and correlate with the severity of PAH and with survival.

Kidney Involvement

The kidneys are frequently involved in SSc. Scleroderma renal crisis is an uncommon but life-threatening acute complication, but chronic and indolent kidney disease also occurs.

Scleroderma Renal Crisis

Scleroderma renal crisis, the most dreaded complication of SSc, develops in 10 to 15% of patients, and almost always occurs within 4 years of the onset of SSc. Before the advent of ACE inhibiting drugs in the 1980s, scleroderma renal crisis was invariably fatal, with most patients dying within weeks. The pathogenesis involves obliterative vasculopathy and luminal narrowing of the renal arcuate arteries. Progressive reduction in renal blood flow, aggravated by vasospasm, leads to juxtaglomerular hyperplasia and increased renin secretion, with further renal vasoconstriction resulting in a vicious cycle that culminates in malignant hypertension (Chapters 67 and 127).

Scleroderma renal crisis is a medical emergency. Although most patients present with abrupt onset of hypertension and progressive renal insufficiency,

in some, the blood pressure remains normal or only modestly elevated. Normotensive renal crisis is associated with a poor outcome. Hypertensive encephalopathy and retinopathy, pericarditis, and arrhythmias may occur. Urinalysis shows mild proteinuria, granular casts, and microscopic hematuria. When thrombocytopenia and microangiopathic hemolysis with fragmented red blood cells is detected, the diagnosis of thrombotic thrombocytopenic purpura (Chapter 175) is sometimes entertained. In many patients, oliguric renal failure develops over a period of weeks. Kidney biopsy can be useful for diagnosis and prognosis, but the characteristic lesions of intimal and medial proliferation and luminal narrowing are indistinguishable from the changes of accelerated hypertension.

Risk factors for scleroderma renal crisis include rapidly progressive skin involvement and the presence of tendon rubs, African American race, male gender, and autoantibodies to RNA polymerases I and III. In contrast, the presence of anticentromere antibodies is associated with a low risk for scleroderma renal crisis. Pericardial effusion, new-onset anemia, and thrombocytopenia may be harbingers of impending scleroderma renal crisis, and a history of recent corticosteroid use is associated with a more than ten-fold increased risk. Accordingly, SSc patients with early and progressive cutaneous disease should be counseled to determine their blood pressure daily. In these patients, corticosteroids should be used only when absolutely required, and at low doses.

Once scleroderma renal crisis occurs, prompt hospitalization and treatment with short-acting ACE inhibitors is essential. The goal is adequate blood pressure control before the onset of renal failure. Despite appropriate timely intervention, more than half of patients with scleroderma renal crisis require hemodialysis, although many recover sufficient renal function to discontinue hemodialysis. Oliguria or a serum creatinine level higher than 3 mg/dL at presentation predict poor outcome. The "prophylactic" use of ACE inhibitors to prevent scleroderma renal crisis is associated with a worse outcome and is not recommended.

Chronic Kidney Disease

Kidney biopsy specimens from SSc patients who have not developed scleroderma renal crisis commonly show chronic lesions such as reduplication of elastic fibers, sclerosed glomeruli, tubular atrophy, and interstitial fibrosis. In one study, evidence of abnormal renal function or proteinuria was found in more than one third of patients, but none progressed to end-stage renal disease. Patients with SSc may rarely develop glomerulonephritis associated with lupus serologies or antineutrophil cytoplasmic antibody–positive renal vasculitis.

Cardiac Involvement

Primary cardiac involvement is frequently detected using sensitive diagnostic tools but can be clinically silent. Cardiac involvement occurs more frequently in dcSSc and generally develops early in the disease. Clinically evident cardiac involvement is a poor prognostic factor. The endocardium, myocardium, and pericardium may be affected separately or together. Clinical manifestations include tachycardias, conduction abnormalities, valvular regurgitation, diastolic heart failure, and pericardial effusion. Systemic and pulmonary arterial hypertension and lung and renal involvement also affect the heart. Conventional echocardiography has a low sensitivity for detecting SSc heart involvement. Newer modalities such as tissue Doppler echocardiography, single-photon emission computed tomography, and especially cardiac magnetic resonance imaging (MRI) reveal a high prevalence of myocardial abnormalities such as abnormal ventricular relaxation and reversible perfusion defects (Chapter 56). Elevated serum level of NT-pro-BNP is a sensitive marker for increased pulmonary artery pressure but may also indicate primary cardiac involvement. Myocarditis can develop in association with muscle inflammation. Pericardial effusion occurs in more than 15% of SSc patients but is rarely significant.

Musculoskeletal Complications

Carpal tunnel syndrome (Chapter 428) occurs frequently and may be a presenting manifestation of SSc. Joint mobility is progressively impaired, especially in the hands. Large joint contractures can be accompanied by tendon friction rubs that can be heard or palpated on passive movement. Tendon rubs are due to extensive fibrosis and adhesion of the tendon sheaths and fascial planes at the affected joint. Joint inflammation is uncommon in SSc; however, erosive polyarthritis in the hands can occur. Muscle weakness may be a sign of deconditioning, disuse atrophy, and malnutrition. Less commonly, inflammatory myositis indistinguishable from idiopathic polymyositis (Chapter 277) occurs in early disease. A noninflammatory myopathy characterized by atrophy and fibrosis in the absence of elevated muscle enzyme levels may occur in late disease. Bone resorption can affect the distal tufts of terminal phalanges (acro-osteolysis), mandibular condyles, ribs, and distal clavicles.

Other Manifestations of Systemic Sclerosis

Many SSc patients develop dry eyes and dry mouth, but in contrast to Sjögren's syndrome (Chapter 276), salivary gland biopsy shows fibrosis rather than focal lymphocytic infiltration. Hypothyroidism due to thyroid fibrosis is common and may be associated with antithyroid autoantibodies. The central nervous system is generally spared in SSc. However, a primarily sensory neuropathy of the trigeminal nerve due to fibrosis or vasculopathy can occur. Pregnancy in SSc is associated with an increased rate of adverse fetal outcomes. Furthermore, cardiopulmonary involvement may worsen, and scleroderma renal crisis can occur with pregnancy. Inability to attain or maintain penile erection is due to vascular insufficiency and fibrosis is frequent and may be the presenting disease manifestation. Cancer of the lung, tongue, and breast occur more frequently in patients with SSc. Barrett's esophagus is associated with increased risk for adenocarcinoma.

Laboratory Features

Anemia is common in SSc and may reflect chronic inflammation, gastrointestinal bleeding caused by GAVE or chronic esophagitis, or a maturation disorder caused by folate and vitamin B_{12} deficiency due to small bowel bacterial overgrowth and malabsorption. Microangiopathic hemolytic anemia (Chapter 163) caused by mechanical trauma and red blood cell fragmentation is a hallmark of scleroderma renal crisis. In contrast to other connective tissue diseases, the erythrocyte sedimentation rate and C-reactive protein are generally not elevated.

Antinuclear autoantibodies (ANAs) are present in virtually all patients with SSc at disease onset. Characteristic autoantibodies in SSc are described in Table 275-3. Autoantibodies against topoisomerase-I (Scl-70) are detected in 31% of patients with dcSSc but in only 13% of patients with lcSSc; conversely, anticentromere antibodies are detected in 38% of patients with lcSSc but in less than 2% of patients with dcSSc. Anticentromere antibodies are associated with PAH but are rarely seen with cardiac involvement, significant pulmonary fibrosis, or scleroderma renal crisis. Topoisomerase-I antibody–positive patients have reduced survival compared with those without this antibody, whereas anticentromere antibody–positive patients have improved survival compared with those without this antibody. Antibodies to RNA polymerase III (often recognized based on a speckled pattern of immunofluorescence) are associated with increased risk for scleroderma renal crisis. Antibodies to β_2-glycoprotein I are not specific but in SSc identify increased risk for critical ischemia.

DIAGNOSIS

Skin induration and Raynaud's phenomenon associated with typical visceral organ manifestations are sufficient to establish the diagnosis of SSc. Occasionally, full-thickness skin biopsy may be required for diagnosing scleroderma mimics such as scleredema, scleromyxedema, or nephrogenic systemic fibrosis (see Table 275-1). Primary Raynaud's phenomenon is differentiated from SSc by nailfold capillaroscopy and by testing for autoantibodies. Making the diagnosis of SSc can be difficult in early disease because initial symptoms are often nonspecific and can be mistaken for rheumatoid arthritis, systemic lupus erythematosus, myositis, or undifferentiated connective tissue disease. Rarely, SSc may present with accelerated hypertension or gastrointestinal bleeding caused by watermelon stomach as the initial manifestation. Laboratory features, including autoantibodies, are discussed in the previous section.

TREATMENT AND PREVENTION   Rx

With the exception of ACE inhibitors for scleroderma renal crisis, no therapy has been shown to alter significantly the natural history of SSc. In contrast, effective treatments are available for alleviating symptoms of SSc and for slowing the progression of the cumulative organ damage. A significant reduction in disease-related mortality has occurred during the past 25 years. Because of the marked heterogeneity in clinical presentation, a thorough and individualized evaluation at baseline is indicated. Treatment must be tailored to each patient's unique needs. Optimal management incorporates prompt diagnosis, accurate classification and risk stratification, early recognition of organ-based complications, and regular monitoring for assessing progression,

disease activity, and response to therapy. Management of complications should be proactive, with regular screening and initiation of appropriate intervention at the earliest possible opportunity. Given the multisystemic nature of SSc, an integrated team-based management approach is optimal. The team should incorporate appropriate medical specialists. Patients are empowered by learning about potential complications, therapeutic options, and natural history of their disease.

Disease-Modifying Therapy
Immunosuppressive Agents

Immunosuppressive agents effective in the treatment of other connective tissue diseases have generally shown modest or no benefit in SSc. Corticosteroids may alleviate stiffness and aching in early-stage dcSSc but do not slow the progression of skin or internal organ involvement and are associated with an increased risk for scleroderma renal crisis. Therefore, corticosteroids should be avoided if possible; when absolutely necessary, they should be given at the lowest dose possible and for brief periods only.

The use of cyclophosphamide in SSc has been evaluated in retrospective and controlled clinical trials.**[1][2]** Cyclophosphamide was shown to reduce the progression of symptomatic interstitial lung disease in early SSc. Compared with placebo, patients treated with cyclophosphamide showed stabilization and, rarely, modest improvement in respiratory symptoms, pulmonary function, and abnormalities on chest HRCT after 1 year of treatment.**[1]** The beneficial effect of oral cyclophosphamide on lung function was short-lived. Its use in SSc needs to be balanced against its potential for side effects, including bone marrow suppression, opportunistic infections, hemorrhagic cystitis, bladder cancer, and premature ovarian failure.

In small clinical trials, methotrexate and mycophenolate mofetil treatment were associated with a modest improvement in skin involvement. These drugs are generally well tolerated in SSc. There is some support in the literature for the use of immunomodulatory agents and interventions such as cyclosporine, azathioprine, intravenous immunoglobulin, and extracorporeal photophoresis for the treatment of SSc. Recent reports suggest that rituximab might be effective in ameliorating skin and lung involvement. Immune ablation using high-dose chemotherapy, with or without irradiation, followed by autologous stem cell reconstitution, has been reported to induce dramatic and durable remission in some patients with SSc and is currently being evaluated in randomized clinical trials. In light of its potential morbidity and mortality and its substantial cost, autologous stem cell transplantation is presently considered an experimental therapy in SSc.

Antifibrotic Therapy

Because tissue fibrosis causes progressive organ damage and contributes to the mortality of SSc, drugs that block the fibrotic process represent a rational approach to therapy. D-Penicillamine has been extensively used as an antifibrotic agent. In retrospective studies, D-penicillamine stabilized and improved skin induration, prevented new internal organ involvement, and improved survival of SSc. However, in a randomized controlled clinical trial of early active SSc, there was no difference in the extent of skin involvement between patients treated with standard-dose (750 mg/day) or very low-dose (125 mg every other day) D-penicillamine. Minocycline, bosentan, recombinant relaxin, interferon-γ, and inhibitors of tumor necrosis factor are putative antifibrotic agents that have failed to show meaningful benefit in SSc clinical trials. Small-molecule inhibitors of protein tyrosine kinases used successfully for the treatment of malignancies, such as imatinib, nilotinib, and dasatinib, block signaling by TGF-β and PDGF and thereby prevent fibrotic responses in vitro and in vivo. These agents are currently in clinical trials for the treatment of SSc.

Treatment of Organ-Specific Complications
Gastrointestinal Complications

Because significant gastroesophageal reflux may occur in the absence of symptoms, all patients with SSc should be treated for this complication. Proton pump inhibitors may need to be given in relatively high doses, and patients should be instructed to elevate the head of the bed and eat frequent small meals. Recurrent gastrointestinal bleeding from GAVE can be successfully treated with laser photocoagulation. Bacterial overgrowth due to small bowel hypomotility causes bloating and diarrhea and may lead to malabsorption, weight loss, and malnutrition. Treatment with short courses of rotating broad-spectrum antibiotics such as metronidazole, erythromycin, and tetracycline can eradicate bacterial overgrowth. Parenteral hyperalimentation may be indicated. Chronic hypomotility of the small bowel may respond to octreotide injections.

Vascular Therapy and the Treatment of Raynaud's Phenomenon

The goal of therapy is to reduce the frequency and duration of vasospastic episodes, prevent ischemic complications and enhance their healing, and slow the progression of obliterative vasculopathy. Patients should dress warmly, minimize cold exposure, and avoid drugs that could precipitate or exacerbate vasospastic episodes. The calcium-channel blockers nifedipine and diltiazem are commonly used but show only moderate benefit, and their use is often limited by side effects (palpitations, dependent edema, light-headedness). ACE inhibitors do not reduce the frequency or severity of episodes, but angiotensin II receptor blockers such as losartan are effective and generally well tolerated. Some patients with Raynaud's phenomenon might require α1-adrenergic receptor blockers (e.g., prazosin), 5-phosphodiesterase inhibitors (e.g., sildenafil), topical nitroglycerine, or intravenous prostaglandins. Low-dose aspirin and dipyridamole prevent platelet aggregation and may have a role as adjunctive agents. The endothelin-1 receptor antagonist bosentan reduces development of new ischemic ulcers. Intravenous prostacyclin infusion and digital sympathectomy are options for some patients with severe Raynaud's phenomenon associated with digital ischemia. Empirical long-term therapy with statins and antioxidants may delay the progression of vascular damage.

Pulmonary Arterial Hypertension

Patients with SSc should be screened for PAH at initial evaluation and, for high-risk patients, on a yearly basis. When symptomatic PAH is detected, treatment should be started with an endothelin-1 receptor antagonist or a 5-phosphodiesterase inhibitor. Diuretics, oral anticoagulation, and digoxin may be used when appropriate. If hypoxemia is documented, supplemental oxygen should be given. If clinical response is inadequate, 5-phosphodiesterase inhibitors may be used in combination with endothelin-1 receptor antagonists. Prostacyclin analogues can be administered intravenously, by continuous subcutaneous infusion, or by frequent inhalations. Lung transplantation remains an option for selected SSc patients with PAH who fail medical therapy.

Treatment and Prevention of Scleroderma Renal Crisis

Prompt recognition of impending or early scleroderma renal crisis is essential. Because patients with early-stage SSc and progressive skin involvement are at highest risk, they should monitor their blood pressure daily and report significant alterations immediately. Corticosteroids should be used at the lowest possible doses and only when absolutely necessary. When scleroderma renal crisis occurs, patients should be hospitalized and treatment with short-acting ACE inhibitors started immediately to achieve prompt blood pressure normalization. There is no evidence that "prophylactic" use of ACE inhibitors can prevent the development of scleroderma renal crisis or ameliorate its severity. Although up to two thirds of patients who develop renal crisis require dialysis, delayed recovery of renal function can occur. Kidney transplantation is appropriate for patients unable to discontinue dialysis after 2 years. Survival with renal transplantation in SSc is comparable to that in other connective tissue diseases, and recurrence of scleroderma renal crisis is rare.

Skin Care

Skin involvement in early SSc is inflammatory and can be controlled with systemic antihistamines or short-term low-dose corticosteroids. Because of the increased risk for scleroderma renal crisis, blood pressure should be carefully monitored. Cyclophosphamide, methotrexate, D-penicillamine, and mycophenolate have been associated with modest improvement in skin induration in early-stage SSc. Skin dryness can be managed with the use of hydrophilic ointments and emollient bath oils. Fingertip ulcerations should be protected by occlusive dressing to promote healing and prevent infection. Infected skin ulcers are treated with topical or oral antibiotics and may necessitate surgical débridement. No medical therapy has been shown to be effective in preventing soft tissue calcification or in promoting its dissolution, and surgical therapy is only occasionally effective.

PROGNOSIS AND NATURAL HISTORY

Compared with patients with lcSSc, patients with dcSSc have a more rapidly progressive disease, greater internal organ involvement, and worse prognosis. However, the course of the disease is difficult to predict in early stages when the specific SSc subset—diffuse or limited cutaneous—is not clear.

Early inflammatory symptoms of dcSSc such as fatigue, edema, arthralgia, and pruritus subside after 2 to 4 years, and skin thickening reaches a plateau. Subsequently, the skin changes generally show slow regression, which characteristically occurs in an order that is the reverse of initial involvement, with softening on the trunk followed by proximal and finally the distal extremities. Sclerodactyly and finger contractures generally persist. Relapse or recurrence of skin thickening is rare. Visceral organ involvement develops and shows most rapid progression during the initial 2 to 4 years of the disease, and new organ involvement is rare after the skin involvement has reached a plateau. Scleroderma renal crisis almost invariably occurs within the first 4 years of disease. In patients with lcSSc, Raynaud's phenomenon typically precedes other manifestations by years or even decades, whereas visceral organ involvement such as PAH and GERD generally occurs late in the course of the disease.

Age- and gender-adjusted mortality rates in patients with SSc are more than five-fold higher than in the general population. The ten-year survival rate of patients with dcSSc is 55%, and 75% with lcSSc. Survival correlates with the extent of skin involvement, which represents a surrogate for visceral organ involvement. The leading causes of death are pulmonary fibrosis, PAH, gastrointestinal involvement, and cardiac disease. Markers of poor prognosis include male gender, African American race, older age of disease onset, a low body mass index, extensive skin thickening with truncal involvement, evidence of significant or progressive visceral organ involvement, the presence of antibodies to topoisomerase-I or RNA polymerase III, or the absence of anticentromere antibodies. In one study, SSc patients who had extensive skin involvement, vital capacity less than 55% of predicted, significant gastrointestinal involvement, and clinically evident cardiac involvement or scleroderma renal crisis had a less than 40% 10-year survival rate. The severity of PAH is correlated with mortality, and SSc patients who demonstrated a mean pulmonary arterial pressure of 45 mm Hg or greater had a 33% 3-year survival rate. Therapy with ACE inhibitors has had a dramatic affect on survival in scleroderma renal crisis, increasing from less than 10% at 1 year in the pre-ACE inhibitor era to a more than 70% 3-year survival rate at the present time.

● NEPHROGENIC SYSTEMIC FIBROSIS

Nephrogenic systemic fibrosis (NSF) is a novel complication of renal insufficiency with certain clinical features resembling systemic sclerosis. The condition was initially described in 2000 and is now recognized as an emerging problem in patients with chronic renal failure. It is estimated that 2% of patients on long-term hemodialysis might develop NSF. Originally considered a purely dermatologic scleromyxedema-like condition and termed *nephrogenic fibrosing dermatopathy*, NSF is now recognized to be associated with visceral organ involvement and is therefore more accurately termed *nephrogenic systemic fibrosis*. The cutaneous manifestations of NSF share histopathologic and clinical features with other scleroderma-spectrum disorders, notably fasciitis and scleromyxedema. In most patients with NSF, the condition develops while undergoing long-term dialysis. However, no association with a particular route or type of renal replacement therapy has been demonstrated. Furthermore, NSF has also been described in patients who have never received dialysis. Histologic hallmarks include cutaneous fibrosis with mucin deposition and accumulation of spindle-shaped cells, including numerous CD34-positive cells, in the lesional skin.

The clinical hallmark of NSF is thickening and "woody" tightness of skin over the lower and, less commonly, upper extremities and contractures at large joints. Raynaud's phenomenon and hallmark SSc autoantibodies do not occur. A link between NFS and exposure to gadolinium-containing MRI contrast agents was suggested in 2006, leading to a warning by the U.S. Food and Drug Administration regarding the use of these agents in patients with renal insufficiency. This was followed by a substantial decline in the incidence of NSF. The pathogenesis of the syndrome remains unknown, but several studies described the detection of gadolinium in tissues from patients with NFS. Other studies report increased expression of fibrogenic cytokines, including TGF-β and CTGF, and evidence of activated TGF-β signaling in lesional NFS tissues. Of note, it has been observed that hemodialysis patients without NFS also had elevated levels of these cytokines in the skin. The course of NFS is generally progressive, and the prognosis is poor. Some patients show improvement with adjustment to renal replacement therapy, and others respond to renal transplantation. Anecdotal reports describe treatment with phototherapy, imatinib mesylate, and immunosuppressive agents. However, in most patients with NSF, the induration is resistant to therapy and leads to progressive induration, joint contractures, and reduced mobility. Many patients become wheelchair dependent.

1. Tashkin DP, Celli B, Senn S, et al. Cyclophosphamide versus placebo in scleroderma lung disease. *N Engl J Med.* 2006;354:2655-2666.
2. Hoyles RK, Ellis RW, Wellsbury J, et al. A multicenter, prospective, randomized, double-blind, placebo-controlled trial of corticosteroids and intravenous cyclophosphamide followed by oral azathioprine for the treatment of pulmonary fibrosis in scleroderma. *Arthritis Rheum.* 2006;54:3962-3970.

SUGGESTED READINGS

Bussone G, Bérezné A, Pestre V, et al. The scleroderma kidney: progress is risk factors, therapy, and prevention. *Curr Rheumatol Rep.* 2011;13:37-43. *Review emphasizing use of ACE inhibitors and avoidance of corticosteroids.*

Chen AY, Zirwas MJ, Heffernan MP. Nephrogenic systemic fibrosis: a review. *J Drugs Dermatol.* 2010;9:829-834. *Review of epidemiology, pathogenesis, clinical manifestation, diagnosis, histolopathology, differential diagnosis, and treatment.*

Gabrielli A, Avvedimento EV, Krieg T. Scleroderma. *N Engl J Med.* 2009;360:1989-2003. *A comprehensive up-to-date review of SSc.*

Rosenbloom J, Castro SV, Jimenez SA. Narrative review. Fibrotic diseases: cellular and molecular mechanisms and novel therapies. *Ann Intern Med.* 2010;152:159-166. *Recent knowledge about the pathogenesis of the fibrotic process providing opportunities for novel therapeutic agents capable of modifying the deleterious effects of fibrotic diseases, including SSc and pulmonary, liver, and kidney fibrosis.*

276

SJÖGREN'S SYNDROME

STANLEY NAGUWA AND M. ERIC GERSHWIN

DEFINITION

Sjögren's syndrome (SS) is an autoimmune disease characterized by the immune-mediated destruction of exocrine glands, particularly salivary and lacrimal glands, with secondary development of keratoconjunctivitis and xerostomia. Primary and secondary forms of SS have been defined. Primary SS occurs in the absence of a connective tissue disease; secondary SS occurs most commonly in association with a systemic connective tissue disorder, particularly rheumatoid arthritis but also systemic sclerosis, systemic lupus erythematosus, and polymyositis.

EPIDEMIOLOGY

SS was first described in detail in 1933, but there was in fact an earlier description in 1892, where the disease was termed *Mikulicz's syndrome*. For more than 3 decades after the 1933 description, SS was considered a relatively uncommon diagnosis of older women. However, more recent data, obtained by the use of standardized criteria, suggest that SS may affect 0.5 to 2% of women. The incidence of SS increases with age, and SS is virtually absent in children. Nearly 2% of women older than 60 years have features of primary SS, particularly dry eyes and dry mouth. Other exocrine glands can also be affected, with subsequent development of pancreatic dysfunction, vaginal dryness, and dry cough. SS occurs in 10 to 25% of patients with systemic lupus erythematosus (Chapter 274) and in 30 to 50% of patients with rheumatoid arthritis (Chapter 272).

PATHOBIOLOGY

Multiple viral agents have been incriminated as etiologic factors for either the development or the modulation of SS; these include Epstein-Barr virus, retroviruses, and coxsackieviruses, but in all cases, the data remain controversial. SS does have a strong immunogenetic basis, however, and it was one of the first autoimmune diseases associated with specific major histocompatibility complex genes. Several genetic alleles have been found to occur more commonly in patients with SS, particularly human leukocyte antigen (HLA) class II antigens. As with other autoimmune diseases, the specific HLA gene association varies according to the ethnic background of the individual. The responsible mechanisms are unknown, and more extensive studies are required to map class II genes precisely, particularly in the DQB1 first hypervariable region. The following sequence of events has been proposed and is summarized in E-Figure 276-1: (1) viral stimulation of Toll-like receptors (TLRs); (2) stimulation of interferon-α (IFN-α)–associated genes, with modification by interferon regulatory factor 5 (*IRF5*) gene polymorphisms; (3) stimulation of the B-cell activation factor (BAFF); and (4) production of autoantibodies, including anti-M3 muscarinic receptor (M3R) antibodies; leading to (5) glandular dysfunction.

The significance of anti-Ro and anti-La antibodies in SS is speculative. These antibodies are found deposited in the salivary glands of affected patients. The Ro proteins colocalize to the blebs of apoptotic cells and may become an immune target or function as a primary immunogen. Nonetheless, serum levels of antibodies to Ro and La do not correlate with disease activity. A pathologic role of anti-Ro antibodies has been described because their passive transfer in pregnancy leads to neonatal congenital heart block. In fetuses of mothers with anti-Ro antibodies and heart block, therapy with dexamethasone, which readily passes across the placenta, is preferred to prednisone.

CLINICAL MANIFESTATIONS

The differential diagnosis of xerophthalmia (dry eyes) and xerostomia (dry mouth) is noted in Table 276-1; presentation is most common in women in their 30s to 50s. Dry mouth leads to difficulty swallowing, recurrent and unique dental infections, pain on eating salty or spicy foods, and difficulty talking. In many patients, impairment of fluid secretion within the nasal and throat passages predisposes to oral erythematous thrush. Dry eyes result in complaints of ocular itching, a sense of grittiness, eyelid symptoms, and an exaggerated sensitivity to ocular insults such as smoke. Other upper and lower respiratory symptoms are secondary to dryness and include a nonproductive cough and occasionally tracheobronchitis.

Classically, SS manifests with painless enlargement of the salivary glands, generally beginning unilaterally. This enlargement may be dramatic and cyclic in nature and is generally absent in patients with coincidental rheumatoid arthritis. The symptoms of SS develop insidiously, and often the diagnosis is not considered for several years because the complaints of sicca are attributed to medications (e.g., antihistamines, antidepressants), a dry

TABLE 276-1	DIFFERENTIAL DIAGNOSIS OF DRY EYES AND MOUTH

Aging
Diabetes mellitus
Hepatitis C
Acquired immunodeficiency syndrome (AIDS)
Parkinson's disease
Head and neck radiation therapy
Sarcoidosis
Graft-versus-host disease
Medications
    Antidepressants
    Antihistamines
    Antipsychotics
    Incontinence medications
    Isotretinoin
    Diuretics

TABLE 276-2	SYMPTOMS OF SJÖGREN'S SYNDROME SECONDARY TO EXOCRINE GLAND DYSFUNCTION

EYE (XEROPHTHALMIA)

Burning
Blurring
Foreign body sensation
Photosensitivity
Blepharitis

ORAL (XEROSTOMIA)

Burning (especially with atypical thrush)
Difficulty chewing
Dysphonia
Inability to "spit"
Increased dental caries
Nocturnal awakening to drink water
Pain with "spicy" and salty food (e.g., mustard)
Sialadenitis

NOSE, THROAT

Difficulty swallowing (especially dry foods)
Epistaxis, dry nares
Hoarseness

CARDIOPULMONARY

Tracheobronchitis, including a dry cough

GENITOURINARY

Dyspareunia
Dysuria
Vaginal dryness

SKIN

Xerosis

environment, or aging. The neurologic components of SS include peripheral and cranial neuropathies and a multiple sclerosis "look-alike" central nervous system disease. Skin manifestations include palpable or nonpalpable purpura, papules, urticarial lesions, and annular lesions. Xerosis is frequently found on examination. A nonerosive arthritis, polyarthralgia, and Raynaud's phenomenon are typically seen in SS. In addition to tracheobronchitis, lung involvement in SS may include bronchiectasis, interstitial pneumonitis, and fibrosis. Smoking is an additional major risk factor for pulmonary disease in patients with SS. Renal involvement may include interstitial nephritis, renal tubular acidosis, and hyposthenuria with glomerulonephritis, a more recently recognized problem. Autoimmune liver disease and pancreatitis are seen occasionally.

The classic exocrine symptoms of SS are listed in Table 276-2, but theoretically, SS can affect all major organ systems (Table 276-3). Patients may initially present with only extraglandular symptoms, especially a nonerosive rheumatoid factor–positive arthritis. In addition, as a component of the inflammatory process and pro-inflammatory cytokine release, patients may manifest chronic fatigue and low-grade fevers. Finally, mucosa-associated lymphoid tissue (MALT) and B-cell lymphomas (Chapter 191) have been described as secondary events in SS. The incidence of lymphoma in SS varies among studies and may depend on local referral patterns (selection bias); lymphoma develops in approximately 5% of patients.

Laboratory Findings

The most commonly used test for the diagnosis of SS is the Schirmer test, performed without anesthetic eye drops. This involves measuring the wetting of standardized tear test strips applied between the eyeball and the lateral inferior lid. Tear osmolarity may be a better test for SS. Salivary flow and labial salivary biopsy are also commonly used for diagnosis. Patients with SS have antinuclear antibodies of either homogeneous or speckled patterns (80 to 90% frequency), antibodies to Ro (SSA; 60 to 75% frequency) and La (SSB; 40% frequency), presence of rheumatoid factor (70 to 90% frequency), mixed cryoglobulin with rheumatoid factor activity (type II; <5%), and antibodies to centromere (<5%). The presence of mixed cryoglobulinemia suggests hepatitis C infection; these complexes contain rheumatoid factor, hepatitis C antigen, and complement. Antibodies to mitochondria have likewise been described in SS, but they are found reliably only in patients with coexistent primary biliary cirrhosis. It has been reported that patients with SS develop antibodies to three new autoantigens called IFI16, KLHL12, and KLHL7. These autoantigens represent a family of transcription regulators; KLHL12 and KLHL7 are kelch-like proteins of unknown physiologic function. Although diagnostic tests for these autoantigens are not widely available, we believe they will become important biomarkers for the clinical diagnosis of SS.

TABLE 276-3 EXTRAGLANDULAR MANIFESTATIONS OF PRIMARY SJÖGREN'S SYNDROME

CONSTITUTIONAL SYMPTOMS

Fatigue
Low-grade fever

SKIN AND VASCULAR

Small vessel vasculitis
Raynaud's phenomenon
Photosensitivity reactions similar to subacute cutaneous systemic lupus erythematosus
Xerosis

UPPER AND LOWER AIRWAYS

Pyogenic sialadenitis or parotitis
Interstitial pneumonitis or fibrosis
Chronic bronchitis
Bronchiectasis
Bronchiolitis obliterans with organizing pneumonia
Pseudolymphoma with intrapulmonary nodules
Chronic obstructive pulmonary disease

MUSCULOSKELETAL

Polyarthralgia, polyarthritis
Myopathy, polymyositis

RENAL

Type I renal tubular acidosis
Tubular interstitial nephritis
Hyposthenuria
Glomerulonephritis

NEUROLOGIC

Peripheral motor sensory neuropathy
Multiple sclerosis–like focal lesions
Transient ischemic attacks, including cerebrovascular accident
Cognitive dysfunction
Spinal cord dysfunction, including transverse myelitis

GASTROINTESTINAL

Hepatomegaly
Primary biliary cirrhosis

ENDOCRINE

Hashimoto's thyroiditis with possible hypothyroidism
Other endocrine dysfunctions secondary to autoimmune endocrinopathy

NEOPLASIA

Lymphadenopathy, pseudolymphoma, MALT lymphoma

MALT = mucosa-associated lymphoid tissue.

TABLE 276-4 CLASSIFICATION CRITERIA FOR SJÖGREN'S SYNDROME

I. OCULAR SYMPTOMS

A positive response to at least one of these three questions:
1. Have you had daily, persistent, troublesome dry eyes for more than 3 months?
2. Do you have a recurrent sensation of sand or gravel in the eyes?
3. Do you use tear substitutes more than three times a day?

II. ORAL SYMPTOMS

A positive response to at least one of these three questions:
1. Have you had a daily feeling of dry mouth for more than 3 months?
2. Have you had recurrent or persistently swollen salivary glands as an adult?
3. Do you frequently drink liquids to aid in swallowing dry food?

III. OCULAR SIGNS

Objective evidence of ocular involvement, defined as a positive result in at least one of the following two tests:
1. Schirmer test (≤5 mm in 5 min)*
2. Rose bengal score (≥4 according to van Bijsterveld scoring system)

IV. HISTOPATHOLOGY

A focus score ≥1 in a minor salivary gland biopsy specimen (a focus is defined as an agglomerate of at least 50 mononuclear cells; the focus score is defined by the number of foci in 4 mm² of glandular tissue)

V. SALIVARY GLAND INVOLVEMENT

Objective evidence of salivary gland involvement, defined by a positive result in at least one of the following three diagnostic tests:
1. Salivary scintigraphy
2. Parotid sialography
3. Unstimulated salivary flow (≤1.5 mL in 15 min)*

VI. AUTOANTIBODIES

Presence in the serum of the following autoantibodies: antibodies to Ro (SSA) or La (SSB) antigens, or both

RULES FOR CLASSIFICATION

In patients without any potentially associated disease, primary Sjögren's syndrome is diagnosed if: four of six criteria are met, including IV or VI; or three of four criteria from III, IV, V, and VI are met
For secondary Sjögren's syndrome, criteria I or II plus any two from criteria III, IV, and V should be met

EXCLUSION CRITERIA

Preexisting lymphoma, AIDS, sarcoidosis, graft-versus-host disease, past head and neck radiation treatment, use of anticholinergic drugs, and hepatitis C

*Because it has been shown that this test may be reduced in normal subjects older than 60 years, it should be excluded from the criteria or not considered indicative for a diagnosis of Sjögren's syndrome in elderly subjects.
From Vitali C, Bombardieri S, Jonsson R, et al. Classification criteria for Sjögren's syndrome: a revised version of the European criteria proposed by the American-European Consensus Group. *Ann Rheum Dis.* 2002;61:554-558.

Dry eyes for >3 mo, recurrent sensation of sand or gravel in the eyes, or use of tear substitutes >3× per day

—or—

Daily feeling of dry mouth for >3 mo, recurrent or persistent swollen salivary glands, or use of liquids to aid in swallowing dry food

Negative → No SS

Positive → Positive Shirmer's test (≤ 5 mm in 5 min), or a Rose Bengal score of ≥ 4 according to von Bijsterveld scoring system

Negative → Focus score ≥ 1 in a minor salivary gland biopsy

Negative → No SS

Positive → Positive result in one of the following tests: salivary scintigraphy, parotid sialography, or unstimulated salivary flow (≤ 5 mL in 15 min)

Negative → No SS

Positive → SS

Positive → Focus score ≥ 1 in a minor salivary gland biopsy

Negative → Antibodies to Ro(SS-A) or La(SS-B), antinuclear antibodies, or rheumatoid factors

Positive → SS

Negative → Positive result in one of the following tests: salivary scintigraphy, parotid sialography, or unstimulated salivary flow (≤ 5 mL in 15 min)

Positive → SS

Negative → No SS

Positive → SS

FIGURE 276-1. Algorithm for the diagnosis of Sjögren's syndrome (SS). (From Tzioufas AG, Moutsopoulos HM. Sjögren's syndromes. In: Klippel JH, Dieppe PA, eds, *Rheumatology*, 2nd ed. London: Mosby; 1998.)

Patients with SS exhibit a dramatic polyclonal B-cell activation. Several other autoantibodies have been described with variable frequencies, including antibodies to carbonic anhydrase, α-fodrin, proteosomal subunits, and the muscarinic M3 receptor (M3R); the last-mentioned protein is found on salivary glands and may explain glandular dysfunction in SS. There is also evidence for altered B-cell differentiation. An SS-like disorder develops in mice transgenic for BAFF (a member of the tumor necrosis factor-α [TNF-α] superfamily that regulates B-cell proliferation). Anemia (including autoimmune hemolytic anemia), leukopenia, and thrombocytopenia occur in SS and are most commonly found in patients with chronic disease.

The serious immune system abnormalities in SS include lymphadenopathy, pseudolymphoma, and lymphoma. The transition from a rheumatoid factor–positive MALT polyclonal gammopathy to a rheumatoid factor–negative oligoclonal or monoclonal gammopathy augurs a change from a benign to a malignant process. This process can be enhanced if the V_K3b-related and the G6 (V_H1-related) idiotypes are present. On histologic examination, the intense lymphoid infiltration includes germinal centers in the exocrine glands; the intense lymphocytic infiltrate is predominantly CD4+ T-cell TCRαβ CD45RO cells. Finally, the degree of inflammation seems to be associated with a T_H1 response, with striking production of IFN-γ, interleukin-2, and interleukin-10. The development of severe histologic changes may be a prodrome of lymphoma. The migration of mononuclear cells to exocrine glands is mediated by chemokines and their cognate receptors, particularly macrophage inflammatory protein-1 (MIP-1) and RANTES.

DIAGNOSIS

Diagnostic Criteria

The diagnostic criteria of SS continue to evolve, but revised American-European classification criteria are currently employed (Table 276-4 and Fig. 276-1). These criteria cannot be used if the patient has compounding medical problems, including preexisting lymphoma, acquired immunodeficiency syndrome, sarcoidosis, graft-versus-host disease, past head and neck irradiation, use of anticholinergic drugs, and hepatitis C—diseases commonly included in the differential diagnosis. A Sjögren's-like disorder is associated with graft-versus-host disease. Diffuse infiltrative lymphocytosis syndrome (DILS) is a Sjögren's-like syndrome occurring in HIV-positive patients, characterized by salivary gland enlargement, peripheral CD8+ lymphocytosis, and the presence of sicca and extraglandular features. The diagnosis of graft-versus-host disease is clinically obvious on the basis of the history. DILS occurs more commonly in males in the absence of the unique autoantibody profile of SS. The classification criteria are helpful in distinguishing between SS and sicca syndrome secondary to medications. An abnormal finding on lip biopsy and the presence of autoantibodies suggest a systemic autoimmune disease. SS is more commonly associated with several other autoimmune diseases, including Hashimoto's thyroiditis, primary biliary cirrhosis, chronic active hepatitis, celiac sprue, myasthenia gravis, and pernicious anemia. The development of universally accepted classification criteria has been hampered by small sample sizes; a National Institutes of Health–funded Sjögren's International Collaborative Clinical Alliance has begun an International Sjögren's Syndrome Registry to acquire a sufficiently large database to develop such classification criteria.

TREATMENT Rx

The primary treatment of SS is to minimize discomfort by the use of substitutes for the dysfunctional exocrine secretions (e.g., artificial tears, artificial saliva, increased oral fluids, ocular lubricants, vaginal lubricants). Ocular steroids are not recommended because they predispose to serious secondary infections. Goggles and punctal occlusion are also used to slow the loss of tears. Topical cyclosporine is a recently added treatment, although there is a concern about herpesvirus infections. Oral pilocarpine and cevimeline may stimulate functional exocrine glands and improve symptoms, but the response varies greatly among patients. The appearance of thrush warrants prompt treatment because it severely aggravates oral symptoms; nystatin is generally effective for this complication. Finally, regular dental examinations and oral hygiene are crucial for reducing subsequent oral health issues (i.e., caries and periodontal disease associated with xerostomia). TNF-α inhibitors have proved largely disappointing, likely due to increases of IFN-α and BAFF. Rituximab is reportedly beneficial in SS-associated lymphoma (Chapter 191) and for sicca symptoms in early disease. Multiple other biologic agents are under development, including belimumab and bortezomub.

Extraglandular manifestations of SS are also managed in a symptomatic fashion. Treatment of arthritis includes nonsteroidal anti-inflammatory drugs, prednisone, hydroxychloroquine, methotrexate, and TNF-α inhibitors. Constitutional symptoms are treated with hydroxychloroquine or prednisone. Inflammatory organ system disease (involving the lung, liver, neurologic system, hematologic system, and kidney) is treated individually with prednisone, methotrexate, azathioprine, or TNF-α inhibitors. Careful surveillance for infectious complications and neoplasia is crucial because the risk of both is increased in SS. Intravenous immunoglobulin has been suggested as a treatment of SS, but there is no evidence to support its use. The mortality of patients with SS has been estimated to be 2.7-fold greater than that of a control population.

TABLE 277-1 CRITERIA FOR THE DIAGNOSIS OF POLYMYOSITIS AND DERMATOMYOSITIS AFTER EXCLUSION OF ALL OTHER FORMS OF MYOPATHY*

1. Symmetrical, often progressive, proximal muscle weakness
2. Characteristic electromyographic triad:
   Short-duration, small, low-amplitude polyphasic potentials
   Fibrillation potentials, seen even at rest
   Bizarre high-frequency repetitive discharges
3. Elevations of serum activities of myositis-associated enzymes:
   Creatine kinase
   Aldolase
   Lactate dehydrogenase
   Transaminases—aspartate transaminase and alanine transaminase
4. Evidence of chronic inflammation in muscle biopsy specimen:
   Necrosis of type I and type II muscle fibers
   Degeneration and regeneration of myofibers, with variation in myofiber size
   Focal collections of interstitial or perivascular mononuclear cells
5. Characteristic rashes of dermatomyositis:
   Scaly, erythematous, palpable eruptions over the metacarpophalangeal or interphalangeal joints, knees, elbows, or medial malleoli (Gottron's papules)
   Scaly, erythematous macules over the metacarpophalangeal or interphalangeal joints, knees, elbows, or medial malleoli (Gottron's sign)
   Periorbital purplish discoloration (heliotrope rash)

*Criteria originally proposed by Bohan and Peter in 1975:
Definite disease: for polymyositis, all of the first four criteria; for dermatomyositis, any three of the first four criteria plus the rash.
Probable disease: for polymyositis, any three of the first four criteria; for dermatomyositis, any two of the first four criteria plus the rash.
Possible disease: for polymyositis, any two of the first four criteria; for dermatomyositis, any one of the first four criteria plus the rash.

FUTURE DIRECTIONS

It is ironic that although much has been learned about the effector mechanisms of SS, little is known about the inductive mechanisms. It is likely that future therapy will focus on interrupting the inflammatory pathways, even without understanding how the disease begins. If the latency time for the development of an autoimmune disease is measured in years, it will be extremely difficult to identify the etiologic agents involved. Future work will focus on specific cytokines, chemokines, and their cognate receptor interactions in efforts to block the exocrine gland destruction. Topical glandular secretagogue use (e.g., diquafosol) is under development. It is also likely that more specific therapy for the anti-Ro-mediated complete heart block of newborns will be developed, again focusing on the abrogation of effector inflammatory pathways. Finally, it is anticipated that newer biologic agents will directly influence effector mechanisms, but they will probably be effective only if they are given to patients early in the disease course.

Grade A

1. Ramos-Casals M, Tzioufas AG, Stone JH, et al. Treatment of primary Sjögren syndrome: a systematic review. *JAMA*. 2010;304:452-460.

SUGGESTED READINGS

Kittridge A, Routhouska SB, Korman NJ. Dermatologic manifestations of Sjögren syndrome. *J Cutan Med Surg*. 2011;15:8-14. *About 50% of patients develop skin symptoms, including xeroderma, purpura, and urticaria.*

Sene D, Jallouli M, Lefaucheur JP, et al. Peripheral neuropathies associated with primary Sjögren syndrome: immunologic profiles of nonataxic sensory neuropathy and sensorimotor neuropathy. *Medicine (Baltimore)*. 2011;90:133-138. *About 25% of patients present with peripheral neuropathy, predominantly sensory.*

277

POLYMYOSITIS AND DERMATOMYOSITIS

FREDERICK W. MILLER

DEFINITION

Polymyositis and dermatomyositis are the most common forms of a family of acquired, systemic, connective tissue diseases known as the *idiopathic inflammatory myopathies*. These disorders are characterized by the clinical and pathologic effects of chronic muscle inflammation of unknown cause. Other forms of idiopathic inflammatory myopathy include inclusion body myositis and myositis seen in association with cancer or with other connective tissue diseases (e.g., scleroderma, systemic lupus erythematosus, rheumatoid arthritis) as a myositis overlap syndrome. The idiopathic inflammatory myopathies, also known as the *myositis syndromes*, are diagnosed on the basis of a combination of clinical, laboratory, and pathologic findings (Table 277-1).

EPIDEMIOLOGY

Polymyositis and dermatomyositis are rare disorders that were first described more than a century ago in Europe; they are now known to be worldwide in distribution and are likely to be increasing in frequency. The estimated annual incidence ranges from 5 to 10 per million, and the estimated prevalence is 50 to 110 per million. Polymyositis and dermatomyositis peak in prevalence in childhood (7 to 15 years) and in midlife (30 to 50 years), whereas the malignancy-associated forms and inclusion body myositis are more common after 50 years of age. Current studies suggest, however, that the prevalence, frequency of clinical forms, and risk factors for development of the idiopathic inflammatory myopathies are likely to differ in different parts of the world. There is an approximately 3 : 1 female predominance in all forms except for inclusion body myositis, in which the female-to-male ratio is inverted (approximately 1 : 3). Certain ethnic groups, including persons of African or Latino descent, may be at increased risk for idiopathic inflammatory myopathies and have poorer outcomes compared with those of European ancestry. Anecdotal clusterings in time and space suggest strong environmental influences on polymyositis and dermatomyositis, but the specific agents involved remain elusive.

PATHOBIOLOGY

An immune-mediated component to the myositis syndromes is suggested by (1) the inflammatory process, (2) the frequent finding of autoantibodies and other immune abnormalities, (3) the overlap with autoimmune diseases such as systemic lupus erythematosus in some patients, (4) the immunogenetic risk factors, and (5) the clinical response to anti-inflammatory agents. Nonetheless, by definition, the pathogenesis remains unknown. Many lines of evidence suggest that chronic immune activation in genetically susceptible individuals, after exposure to environmental triggers, plays a pivotal role in the development of idiopathic inflammatory myopathies.

The pathologic change in the muscle, skin, and other affected tissues is characterized by focal collections of mononuclear cells. Lymphocytes are the most common cells in the infiltrates, but macrophages, plasma cells,

TABLE 277-2 CLASSIFICATIONS OF THE IDIOPATHIC INFLAMMATORY MYOPATHIES

CLASSIFICATION GROUP	ASSOCIATED CLINICAL FEATURES	SEVERITY OF MYOSITIS	RESPONSE OF MYOSITIS TO THERAPY	PROGNOSIS (5-YR SURVIVAL)
CLINICAL GROUPS				
Polymyositis	None of the features below	Variable	Variable	Moderate (~80%)
Dermatomyositis	Gottron's papules or heliotrope rash	Mild to moderate	Good	Moderate (~85%)
Connective tissue myositis	Overlap with other connective tissue diseases	Mild	Excellent	Good (~90%)
Cancer-associated myositis	Cancer diagnosed within 2 yr of idiopathic inflammatory myopathy	Variable	Moderate to poor	Poor, secondary to cancer (~60%)
Juvenile myositis	Diagnosis before age 18 yr
Dermatomyositis » polymyositis
Subcutaneous calcifications
Gastrointestinal vasculitis	Variable	Moderate to good	Good (>95%)
Inclusion body myositis	Insidious onset in older white men
Distal involvement, atrophy, and asymmetrical weakness
Poor response to therapy	Mild but progressive	Poor	Few deaths, but significant morbidity (>85%)
SEROLOGIC GROUPS				
Antisynthetases	Acute onset in polymyositis or dermatomyositis
Interstitial lung disease, fever, dyspnea on exertion, arthritis, mechanic's hands, Raynaud's phenomenon	Moderate to severe	Moderate, but flares with taper	Poor (~75%)
Anti–signal recognition particle	Acute onset in black female
Palpitations, cardiac disease, severe weakness
No rash (clinically polymyositis)	Severe	Poor	Very poor (~30%)
Anti-Mi-2	Classic dermatomyositis "V" and "shawl" rashes, cuticular changes	Mild	Good	Good (>95%)

basophils, and neutrophils are sometimes present. In certain variants, eosinophils (eosinophilic myositis) or granulomas (granulomatous myositis) predominate. The muscle cells (myocytes) show evidence of necrosis, with degeneration and regeneration (E-Fig. 277-1), and there is often increased connective tissue or fibrosis in the interstitial areas around the myocytes.

Immunohistochemical and other studies implicate different mechanisms of pathogenesis in the various forms of myositis. In polymyositis and inclusion body myositis, the pathologic change suggests a cytotoxic T lymphocyte-mediated process with CD8$^+$ T cells surrounding and invading otherwise normal-appearing myocytes in endomysial areas. In dermatomyositis, however, the infiltrate is composed predominantly of B lymphocytes, dendritic cells, and CD4$^+$ helper T cells in perimysial areas around the fascicles and small blood vessels. Blood vessel pathology, with endothelial cell damage from complement deposition, and atrophy of the myofibers at the periphery of the fascicle (called *perifascicular atrophy*) are also characteristic findings in dermatomyositis. A type I interferon signature is present in the blood cells and in muscle and skin biopsies from a majority of dermatomyositis patients and in some polymyositis patients, although its role in pathogenesis remains to be elucidated. Inclusion body myositis differs from polymyositis and dermatomyositis by the presence of characteristic reddish inclusions and vacuoles, rimmed by purple granules, inside the myocytes, as demonstrated in trichrome-stained frozen muscle sections. Additional features of inclusion body myositis include frequent endomysial fibrosis, amyloid deposition, marked variation in myofiber diameter, and characteristic intranuclear and intracytoplasmic filamentous tubules seen on electron microscopy.

Autoantibodies are found in more than 90% of patients with polymyositis and dermatomyositis, although it remains unclear what role, if any, they play in pathogenesis. The most frequent of these are antinuclear antibodies, but many others are commonly seen, including rheumatoid factor, anti-U1RNP, anti-La, anti-Ro, anti-PM/Scl, and anti-Ku autoantibodies. None of these is diagnostic for polymyositis or dermatomyositis, but if present, they do assist in distinguishing the idiopathic inflammatory myopathies from other forms of myopathy. More than one third of patients with idiopathic inflammatory myopathy have autoantibodies that are diagnostic, known as myositis-specific autoantibodies. The most common of these are antisynthetase autoantibodies (and the most common antisynthetases are anti-Jo-1 autoantibodies), anti–signal recognition particle autoantibodies, and anti-Mi-2 autoantibodies that are directed against a nuclear helicase. Each of these autoantibodies is strongly associated with a distinct clinical presentation, response to therapy,

and prognosis, suggesting that each autoantibody may be representative of a truly different myositis syndrome (Table 277-2). The myositis-specific autoantibodies are available commercially, but they need not be obtained in all patients. They may be particularly useful in the diagnosis of perplexing cases or in predicting prognosis. Several other autoantibodies, called *anti-p155* and *anti-MJ autoantibodies*, have recently been identified in association with dermatomyositis and appear to be common in children with the disease.

As is the case for other autoimmune conditions, polymyositis and dermatomyositis are complex disorders that are likely caused by the interaction of multiple genetic and environmental risk factors. The strongest genetic risk factors identified to date are the polymorphic human leukocyte antigen (HLA) genes that regulate the immune responses in the major histocompatibility complex (Chapter 45). In patients of European descent, the ancestral HLA haplotype containing A1, B8, DRB1*0301, and DQA1*0501 alleles is most strongly associated with all forms of myositis. The major clinical and autoantibody groups, however, each have additional HLA risk and protective alleles. In other ethnic groups, such as Koreans and Mesoamericans, HLA genes are not risk factors. In these ethnic groups, alleles of the genes encoding immunoglobulin proteins, which regulate levels of antibody responses to infectious agents and are known as *GM and KM loci*, are the major genetic risk factors for polymyositis and dermatomyositis. Alleles of other polymorphic genes, including those that regulate cytokine responses to environmental exposures, such as alleles of tumor necrosis factor-α and interleukin-1 receptor antagonist genes, have recently been associated with the childhood myositis syndromes. The environmental triggers for polymyositis and dermatomyositis are not known, but selected viral and bacterial infections, as well as certain drugs, cytokines, dietary supplements, vaccines, medical implants, and occupational exposures, have been implicated in case reports and in some epidemiologic studies. In the first worldwide study of myositis, global surface ultraviolet light intensity was found to correlate with the proportion of dermatomyositis compared with polymyositis cases and with the proportion of patients with anti-Mi-2 autoantibodies at the referral centers in the study. In a U.S. study, similar associations were seen only in women, suggesting that men and women may have inherently different responses to ultraviolet radiation.

CLINICAL MANIFESTATIONS

Myositis may present acutely, subacutely, or insidiously, and patients can exhibit single or multiple episodic attacks or persistent disease activity. The idiopathic inflammatory myopathies can be divided into groups on the basis of clinical-pathologic or serologic features, and each of these groups has characteristic clinical and prognostic associations (see Table 277-2). Therefore, the manner in which the disease presents can suggest the form of idiopathic inflammatory myopathy present. For example, an acute, severe onset of polymyositis with pulmonary fibrosis may herald a difficult course with persistent disease, as is often seen in patients with anti-Jo-1 and other antisynthetase autoantibodies. In contrast, a slowly progressive onset associated with proximal and distal weakness and thigh muscle atrophy in an older man suggests inclusion body myositis.

Symmetrical, proximal muscle weakness is present in most cases and results in difficulty arising from chairs, getting out of cars, reaching overhead, or combing hair. Many patients also report generalized fatigue or muscle pain. Patients with dermatomyositis may present with a variety of photosensitive rashes over the face, chest, and hands. Gottron's papules are raised, often scaly, palpable lesions overlying an erythematous base on extensor surfaces such as the metacarpophalangeal and proximal interphalangeal joints, elbows, and knees; these are virtually pathognomonic for dermatomyositis (Fig. 277-1). Other characteristic rashes of dermatomyositis are Gottron's sign (macules in a distribution similar to Gottron's papules) and a characteristic purplish rash over and sometimes surrounding the upper eyelids known as the *heliotrope rash*. Patients may also develop a rash in the V of the neck (V sign) or in the distribution of a shawl (shawl sign). Other findings in dermatomyositis include cuticular overgrowth, periungual capillary changes, and dilated capillaries in the gingiva, the latter of which are especially common in juvenile dermatomyositis (see Fig. 277-1). A roughening, scaling, and erythematous fissuring of the palmar and lateral aspects of the fingers, known as *mechanic's hands*, may be seen in patients with either polymyositis or dermatomyositis and is common in those with antisynthetase autoantibodies. On occasion, patients may develop classic dermatomyositis rashes without apparent muscle weakness or elevated muscle enzymes in a syndrome called *dermatomyositis sine myositis*. Some of these individuals, however, have subclinical myositis, as demonstrated by magnetic resonance imaging studies of muscle or muscle biopsy; in others, clinical myositis develops over time. Children with dermatomyositis are particularly at risk for the development of subcutaneous calcifications and occasionally present with life-threatening intestinal vasculitis.

Although the patient and physician often focus on skeletal muscle involvement, the idiopathic inflammatory myopathies are systemic diseases with frequent extramuscular manifestations that can become the most troubling aspects of the disease (Table 277-3). Patients may suffer from arthralgias and arthritis, a variety of skin disorders, and general symptoms such as fatigue, weight loss, Raynaud's phenomenon, or fever. The gastrointestinal, pulmonary, and cardiac systems may be involved, which can both complicate therapy and adversely affect prognosis. These extramuscular manifestations may precede or follow the development of myositis, and their severity may be independent of the degree of myositis.

DIAGNOSIS

Muscle pain and weakness are frequent complaints that can arise from many causes, including intrinsic muscle diseases (myopathies), disorders of the nerves innervating the muscle (neuropathies), or the effects of drugs, toxins, or infectious agents. All these entities must be carefully considered and excluded to allow the diagnosis of polymyositis or dermatomyositis (Table 277-4). A careful medical and family history, exposure history, complete physical examination, and directed laboratory testing with electromyography and muscle biopsy should reveal the cause of muscle weakness in most cases. Given that the pathologic changes of muscle in idiopathic inflammatory myopathy are often focal and not evenly distributed, magnetic resonance imaging of the muscle can be useful to identify where inflammation is present and to increase the yield of muscle biopsy.

Population-based studies have confirmed a two- to three-fold increased relative risk of a variety of cancers within 2 years of the development of dermatomyositis and, to a lesser extent, polymyositis and inclusion body myositis. Patients with myositis at disease onset should therefore be carefully assessed for malignant neoplasms, especially cancers for which they have other risk factors. The cancer work-up should be directed and should include a thorough history for any changes in habits that might suggest a neoplasm, careful physical examination and screening rectal examination, fecal occult blood test, urinalysis, blood chemistry studies, chest radiograph, and prostate-specific antigen testing in men. Women should undergo serial breast and gynecologic examinations with Papanicolaou's stain. Physicians should have a low threshold for performing pelvic ultrasonography or computed tomography to exclude ovarian cancer, given its frequency in women with dermatomyositis. Any abnormalities in these initial studies should be followed by appropriate investigations to conclusively exclude malignant disease.

FIGURE 277-1. Clinical findings in dermatomyositis. **A,** Erythematous to violaceous raised papules overlying the metacarpal and interphalangeal joints, known as *Gottron's papules*. These are considered the hallmark finding in dermatomyositis. **B,** Cuticular overgrowth and periungual capillary changes, which include dilated and tortuous blood vessels with areas of atrophy, telangiectasia, vessel dropout, and bushy loop formation along the fingernail bed. **C,** Erythema and minimal edema involving the upper eyelids, with occasional telangiectasia, known as the heliotrope rash. **D,** Dilated capillaries and bushy loop formations are sometimes seen in the gingiva, especially in juvenile dermatomyositis.

TABLE 277-3 EXTRAMUSCULAR MANIFESTATIONS OF POLYMYOSITIS AND DERMATOMYOSITIS

GENERAL

Fatigue
Malaise
Weight loss
Raynaud's syndrome

MUSCULOSKELETAL

Arthralgias, usually symmetrical and involving the hand joints
Nonerosive polyarthritis, usually symmetrical and involving the hand joints
Deforming arthropathy of hand joints
Joint contractures
Carpal tunnel syndrome
Osteopenia and osteoporosis

CUTANEOUS

Characteristic dermatomyositis rashes: Gottron's papules, Gottron's sign, heliotrope rash
Other rashes: V sign and shawl sign rashes; linear extensor erythema; roughening, scaling, and erythematous fissuring of the palmar and lateral aspects of the fingers (mechanic's hands)
Photosensitivity
Periungual abnormalities, including telangiectasias and cuticular overgrowth
Bleeding gums from dilated capillaries in the gingiva
Irregular indurated plaques over the fingers, with mucin accumulation in the dermis
Subcutaneous and intradermal calcification, which may ulcerate with secondary infection
Vasculitis with infarcts and digital ulcers
Subcutaneous inflammation (panniculitis)
Alopecia

GASTROINTESTINAL

Abnormal pharyngeal and cricopharyngeal function, often leading to dysphonia
Esophageal dysphagia with occasional nasal regurgitation or aspiration
Delayed gastric emptying and reflux
Dysmotility of the small and large intestines, sometimes leading to chronic abdominal pain
Malabsorption
Vasculitis with infarcts and necrosis of the bowel

PULMONARY

Ventilatory insufficiency due to respiratory muscle weakness
Atelectasis
Aspiration pneumonia
Interstitial lung disease (pulmonary fibrosis)
Pulmonary hypertension
Drug-related pneumonitis
Opportunistic infections in immunocompromised patients

CARDIAC

Myocarditis with arrhythmias and congestive failure
Cardiomyopathy
Cor pulmonale
Rare pericarditis and pericardial effusions

TABLE 277-4 DIFFERENTIAL DIAGNOSIS OF MUSCLE WEAKNESS

DRUG- AND TOXIN-INDUCED MYOPATHIES

Corticosteroids
Ethanol
Lipid-lowering agents (HMG-CoA reductase inhibitors and fibrates)
D-Penicillamine
Colchicine
Cocaine
Cyclosporine
Ipecac
Chloroquine, hydroxychloroquine
Zidovudine (AZT)
L-Tryptophan (eosinophilia-myalgia syndrome)

ENDOCRINE DISEASES

Hypothyroidism
Hyperthyroidism
Acromegaly
Diabetes mellitus

NEUROLOGIC DISORDERS

Amyotrophic lateral sclerosis
Myasthenia gravis
Eaton-Lambert syndrome
Multiple sclerosis
Guillain-Barré syndrome
Motor neuron disease

OTHER IMMUNOLOGIC OR CONNECTIVE TISSUE DISEASES

Hypereosinophilic syndrome
Polyarteritis nodosa and other forms of vasculitis
Polymyalgia rheumatica
Still's disease
Rheumatoid arthritis
Systemic lupus erythematosus
Systemic sclerosis
Tendinitis and overuse syndromes

ACQUIRED METABOLIC ABNORMALITIES

Hypokalemia
Hypercalcemia
Hypocalcemia

INHERITED METABOLIC MYOPATHIES

Acid maltase deficiency
Phosphorylase deficiency (McArdle's disease)
Lipid metabolic defects (primary and secondary carnitine deficiency)
Palmityltransferase deficiency
Phosphofructokinase deficiency

MITOCHONDRIAL MYOPATHIES

Mitochondrial encephalomyopathy, lactic acidosis, stroke (MELAS)
Neuropathy ataxia, retinitis pigmentosa (NARP)
Myoclonic epilepsy, ragged red fibers (MERRFs)
Kearns-Sayre syndrome

INHERITED MUSCLE STRUCTURAL PROTEIN DEFECTS (MUSCULAR DYSTROPHIES)

Duchenne's and Becker's dystrophies
Facioscapulohumeral dystrophy
Dysferlinopathies and other limb-girdle dystrophies
Myotonic dystrophy
Emery-Dreifuss dystrophies
Other dystrophies

INFECTIOUS MYOPATHIES

Bacterial (pyomyositis, gangrene, Lyme disease)
Parasitic (trichinosis, toxoplasmosis, sarcosporidiosis, trypanosomiasis)
Fungal (candidiasis, cryptococcosis, sporotrichosis, actinomycosis, histoplasmosis)
Viral (influenza; adenovirus; coxsackievirus; echovirus; Epstein-Barr virus; retroviruses, including human immunodeficiency virus and human T-lymphotropic viruses 1 and 2; hepatitis B and C viruses)

TREATMENT ℞

Therapy for polymyositis and dermatomyositis is directed at decreasing inflammation in target tissues, relieving symptoms, and rebuilding endurance and muscle strength. It is important to distinguish the level of disease activity (reversible active inflammation in tissues) from the amount of disease damage (irreversible scarring or fibrotic changes that result from prior inflammation) present in all affected organ systems because the therapeutic approaches are very different. For active inflammation, corticosteroids are the initial and primary therapy for these diseases (Chapter 34). Several factors are important in determining corticosteroid responses. In addition to the patient's clinical and serologic groups, these factors include an adequate initial dose (at least 1 mg/kg/day of prednisone or equivalent), the continuation of prednisone until after the serum creatine kinase activity normalizes, and a slow rate of prednisone tapering (approximately 10 mg/month, or about 15% of the existing dose per month). High-dose intravenous corticosteroids (1 g/day for 3 days) and additional immunosuppressive therapy are probably useful as initial treatments in severe cases or for those in poor prognostic groups.

There is no consensus on the best treatment of corticosteroid-resistant patients. Intravenous immunoglobulin was successful in one short-term study,[1] but it is expensive and neither proven nor practical for long-term use. Oral methotrexate (7.5 to 25 mg/week, depending on disease severity and body

weight) and azathioprine (50 to 200 mg/day, depending on disease severity and body weight) are the major therapeutic options used in practice, but cyclosporin A, tacrolimus, mycophenolate mofetil, cyclophosphamide, anti–tumor necrosis factor agents, anti-B-cell agents such as rituximab, or combinations of these may also be beneficial in difficult cases (Chapters 34 and 35). With the exception of the use of topical corticosteroids, hydroxychloroquine, and sunscreens to treat the dermatomyositis rash, no specific treatment other than that for the underlying myositis improves the systemic manifestations of the idiopathic inflammatory myopathies. Rehabilitation and physical therapy are important in maintaining range of motion and preventing contractures during active disease and are the primary treatment approaches for patients with only disease damage. Exercise probably improves strength and endurance when it is initiated in a graded way during periods of disease control.

The treatment of inclusion body myositis is controversial. Retrospective reviews of corticosteroid and cytotoxic therapy, as well as several prospective trials, suggest that the rate of deterioration may be decreased or stabilized and strength improved by treating patients with evidence of active myositis. Physical therapy, however, plays the most important role in the long-term care of those with inclusion body myositis.

PROGNOSIS

The prognosis of polymyositis and dermatomyositis has been poorly studied, but current information suggests that each clinical and serologic group may differ in response to therapy and outcome (see Table 277-2). Patients with myositis who also have another connective tissue disease (the overlap group) tend to have the mildest myositis, the best clinical responses, and the fewest exacerbations of myositis over time. Patients with dermatomyositis have more severe disease, followed by patients with polymyositis. Patients with inclusion body myositis do not respond to therapy as well as patients in the other clinical groups do. The serologic groups are also different in terms of disease courses and prognosis. Patients with anti-Mi-2 autoantibodies tend to have mild myositis with good responses to therapy and few disease exacerbations with tapering of therapy. Patients with antisynthetase autoantibodies have more severe disease with moderate therapeutic responses, and they exhibit frequent exacerbations with tapering of therapy. As a group, patients with anti–signal recognition particle autoantibodies have the most acute onset, the most severe myositis, the least response to therapy, and the most persistent disease. Other clinical features associated with a poor prognosis include delay from disease onset to therapy; pulmonary, cardiac, or gastrointestinal involvement; and poor responses to immunosuppressive therapy. Any patient with an unexpectedly unresponsive or perplexing clinical course should be reevaluated for possible misdiagnosis or the development of another cause of muscle weakness.

FUTURE DIRECTIONS

Given the incurable nature of the myositis syndromes and the poor outcomes in many patients, future directions are likely to focus on improved classification criteria to separate the idiopathic inflammatory myopathies from dystrophies and metabolic myopathies through the use of genetic, pathologic, and immunologic information. A more complete understanding of the molecular pathogenesis of these disorders may result in more focused therapies. A clearer understanding of which groups of patients have poor prognoses or respond to specific agents differently would also allow more effective treatments. Because these complex diseases probably arise from the interactions of genetic and environmental risk factors, defining these elements may provide insight into the mechanisms leading to the development of myositis. This knowledge might allow the future prevention of some myositis cases by the avoidance of certain environmental exposures in genetically susceptible individuals or by gene therapy.

1. Choy EH, Hoogendijk JE, Lecky B, et al. Immunosuppressant and immunomodulatory treatment for dermatomyositis and polymyositis. *Cochrane Database Syst Rev.* 2005;3:CD003643.

SUGGESTED READINGS

Aggarwal R, Oddis CV. Therapeutic approaches in myositis. *Curr Rheumatol Rep.* 2011;13:182-191. *Steroids are generally first-line therapy despite the absence of randomized trials; intravenous immunoglobulin is effective in the short term, but its long-term benefit is unknown.*

Distad BJ, Amato AA, Weiss MD. Inflammatory myopathies. *Curr Treat Options Neurol.* 2011;13:119-130. *Review.*

Dugan EM, Huber AM, Miller FW, et al. International Myositis Assessment and Clinical Studies Group. Photoessay of the cutaneous manifestations of the idiopathic inflammatory myopathies. *Dermatol Online J.* 2009;15:1. *Comprehensive review of skin manifestations of myositis.*

Gunawardena H, Betteridge ZE, McHugh NJ. Myositis-specific autoantibodies: their clinical and pathogenic significance in disease expression. *Rheumatology (Oxford).* 2009;48:607-612. *Enumeration of autoantibodies in myositis and their clinical usefulness.*

Hengstman GJ, van den Hoogen FH, van Engelen BG. Treatment of the inflammatory myopathies: update and practical recommendations. *Expert Opin Pharmacother.* 2009;10:1183-1190. *Useful review of therapeutic approaches in polymyositis and dermatomyositis.*

Mammen AL. Dermatomyositis and polymyositis: clinical presentation, autoantibodies, and pathogenesis. *Ann N Y Acad Sci.* 2010;1184:134-153. *Comprehensive review.*

Zahr ZA, Baer AN. Malignancy in myositis. *Curr Rheumatol Rep.* 2011;13:208-215. *Dermatomyositis is associated with an underlying malignancy in about 25% of cases.*

278

THE SYSTEMIC VASCULITIDES

JOHN H. STONE

DEFINITION

The vasculitides are a heterogeneous group of disorders linked by the common finding of destructive inflammation within blood vessel walls. On the basis of current classification schemes, approximately 20 different forms of primary vasculitis are recognized (Table 278-1).

CLASSIFICATION

Classification by Vessel Size

The cause of most forms of vasculitis remains unknown, and major gaps exist in our understanding of the pathophysiologic processes. The most valid basis for classifying the vasculitides is the size of the predominant blood vessels involved: large, medium, or small (see Table 278-1). Within individual cases, however, there is frequently overlap in the size of the blood vessels affected.

Additional Considerations in Classification

Several considerations other than blood vessel size are relevant to the classification of vasculitis (E-Table 278-1): (1) age, gender, and ethnic background of the patient; (2) tropism for particular organs; (3) presence or absence of granulomatous inflammation; (4) participation of immune complexes in the pathophysiologic process; and (5) detection of characteristic autoantibodies in the patients' serum, such as antineutrophil cytoplasmic antibodies (ANCAs).

Age, gender differences, and ethnic variation are discussed later in the section on epidemiology. The organ tropisms of these disorders are illustrated by the following examples. Henoch-Schönlein purpura typically affects the skin, joints, kidneys, and gastrointestinal tract, whereas Wegener's granulomatosis classically involves the upper airways, lungs, and kidneys. In contrast, Cogan's syndrome involves the eyes, the audiovestibular apparatus of the inner ear, and the large arteries (in 10 to 15% of cases). The granulomatous features of some forms of vasculitis resemble fungal and mycobacterial infections or the inflammation induced by the presence of a foreign body, suggesting a role for chronic antigenic stimulation.

Immune complexes are essential to the pathophysiologic mechanism of some forms of small- and medium-vessel vasculitis. Complexes of immunoglobulin (Ig) A1 are found in Henoch-Schönlein purpura. Immune complexes consisting of IgG, IgM, complement components, and the hepatitis C virion characterize most cases of mixed cryoglobulinemia. In contrast, "pauci-immune" types of small- and medium-vessel vasculitis, such as Wegener's granulomatosis and microscopic polyangiitis, have little immunoglobulin or complement deposition within diseased tissues. Many but not all patients with pauci-immune forms of vasculitis are ANCA positive.

EPIDEMIOLOGY

The epidemiologic features of individual forms of systemic vasculitis vary tremendously by geography (Table 278-2). This may reflect genetic influences, variation in environmental exposures, and other unknown disease risk factors. For example, Behçet's syndrome is rare in North Americans, affecting only 1 in approximately 300,000 persons; this condition is several hundred times more common among inhabitants of countries bordering the ancient Silk Route. Similarly, although Takayasu's arteritis is rare in the United States—on the order of 3 new cases per million people per year—this disease is reportedly the most common cause of renal artery stenosis in India, where the incidence may be as high as 200 to 300 per million per year.

Age is an important consideration in the epidemiology of vasculitis. Eighty percent of patients with Kawasaki disease are younger than 5 years. In contrast, giant cell arteritis virtually never occurs in patients younger than 50 years, and the mean age of patients with this disease is 72 years. Age may also have an impact on disease severity and outcome. In the overwhelming majority of children with Henoch-Schönlein purpura (who represent 90% of all cases), the disease is self-limited, resolving within several weeks. In adults, however, Henoch-Schönlein purpura has a higher likelihood of chronicity and a poor renal outcome.

The gender distribution varies across many forms of vasculitis. Buerger's disease is the only form of vasculitis with a striking male predominance. The greater prevalence of smoking among males in most societies probably explains this predilection. In contrast, Takayasu's arteritis has an overwhelming tendency to occur in females (a 9:1 female-to-male ratio). The pauci-immune forms of vasculitis, such as Wegener's granulomatosis, microscopic polyangiitis, and Churg-Strauss syndrome, occur in males and females with approximately equal frequencies, but the phenotypic expression of these conditions may be affected by both age and gender.

The strongest link between any single gene and vasculitis is the association of HLA-B51 with Behçet's syndrome. Eighty percent of Asian patients with Behçet's syndrome have the HLA-B51 gene. The prevalence of HLA-B51 is significantly higher among patients with Behçet's syndrome in Japan than among control subjects without the disease (55% vs. <15%). Among the sporadic cases of Behçet's syndrome involving whites in the United States, however, HLA-B51 occurs in less than 15% of cases.

With the exception of Buerger's disease and smoking, no definitive associations have been confirmed between disease development and environmental or occupational exposures. Associations between exposure to silica and some types of pauci-immune vasculitis have been reported but not confirmed. Studies of potential associations between any type of exposure and vasculitis are complicated by the difficulty of obtaining reliable measurements of the levels of exposure, the likelihood of recall bias among patients who are diagnosed with vasculitis, and the choice of appropriate control groups.

PATHOBIOLOGY

Table 278-3 illustrates the pathologic characteristics of selected forms of vasculitis. Specific pathologic features are discussed in the subsections on each disease. The type of inflammatory cell infiltrate in vasculitis is independent of the size of blood vessels involved. Mixed cell infiltrates in vasculitis are the rule rather than the exception, and histopathologic patterns of vasculitis may include leukocytoclasis (degranulation and destruction of neutrophils within blood vessel walls), granulomatous findings (with or without giant cells), lymphoplasmacytic infiltrates, varying degrees of eosinophilic infiltration, necrosis, and combinations of all these findings.

PATHOPHYSIOLOGY

Regardless of the size of the predominant blood vessels involved, some pathophysiologic mechanisms are common to many different forms of vasculitis. Immune complex deposition, for example, is present in several types of vasculitis that involve both medium-sized and small blood vessels. In this section, the general concepts related to the pathogenesis of large-vessel vasculitides are discussed separately from those of medium- and small-vessel vasculitides.

Large-Vessel Vasculitides

The pathologic process in large-vessel vasculitis appears to begin in the adventitia. In both Takayasu's arteritis and giant cell arteritis, abundant numbers of activated T lymphocytes are found within inflamed arterial walls, centering on the adventitia. In Takayasu's arteritis, most of these T cells appear to be of the CD8$^+$ subtype. Current evidence suggests that the cytotoxic functions of these cells, mediated by perforin and granzyme B, contribute to smooth muscle cell damage in this disease. CD4$^+$ T-cell responses in Takayasu's arteritis have not been well defined.

In giant cell arteritis, much evidence now suggests an antigen-driven disease, with the site of immunologic recognition events being the adventitia. CD4$^+$ T cells that secrete interferon-γ appear to be recruited to the adventitia by a specific antigen, the identity of which remains unknown. Both the T cells that orchestrate the transmural inflammation and the inciting antigens are theorized to reach the adventitia through the vasa vasorum. Subsequently, T-cell signals from the adventitia stimulate macrophages and multinucleated giant cells to elaborate an array of downstream mediators, such as metalloproteinases and platelet-derived growth factor. The results of this inflammatory cascade are granulomatous inflammation, destruction of the internal elastic lamina, arterial wall hyperplasia, smooth muscle cell proliferation, intimal thickening, vascular occlusion, and, in some cases, weakening of the vessel wall, leading to dilation and aneurysm formation.

TABLE 278-1	CLASSIFICATION SCHEME OF VASCULITIDES ACCORDING TO SIZE OF PREDOMINANT BLOOD VESSELS INVOLVED

PREDOMINANTLY LARGE-VESSEL VASCULITIDES

Takayasu's arteritis
Giant cell arteritis
Cogan's syndrome
Behçet's syndrome*

PREDOMINANTLY MEDIUM-VESSEL VASCULITIDES

Classic polyarteritis nodosa
Cutaneous polyarteritis nodosa
Rheumatoid vasculitis†
Buerger's disease
Kawasaki disease
Primary angiitis of the central nervous system

PREDOMINANTLY SMALL-VESSEL VASCULITIDES

Immune complex mediated
  Cutaneous leukocytoclastic angiitis ("hypersensitivity" vasculitis)
  Henoch-Schönlein purpura
  Urticarial vasculitis
  Cryoglobulinemia†
"ANCA-associated" disorders
  Wegener's granulomatosis†
  Microscopic polyangiitis†
  Churg-Strauss syndrome†
Miscellaneous small-vessel vasculitides
  Connective tissue disorders†
  Paraneoplastic diseases
  Infection
  Inflammatory bowel disease

*May involve small, medium, and large blood vessels.
†Frequent overlap of involvement of small and medium-sized blood vessels.
ANCA = antineutrophil cytoplasmic antibody.

TABLE 278-2	EPIDEMIOLOGY OF SELECTED VASCULITIDES		
DISEASE	**UNITED STATES**	**ELSEWHERE**	**AGE, GENDER, AND ETHNIC PREDISPOSITIONS**
Giant cell arteritis	Incidence: 240/million (Olmsted County, MN)	220-270/million (Scandinavian countries)	Age >50 yr, mean age 72 yr; females 3:1; northern European ancestry
Takayasu's arteritis	Incidence: 3/million	200-300/million (India)	Age <40 yr; females 9:1; Asian
Behçet's syndrome	Prevalence: 3/million	3000/million (Turkey)	Silk Route countries
Polyarteritis nodosa	Incidence: 7/million	7/million (Spain)	Slight male predominance
Kawasaki disease	Incidence: 100/million*	900/million (Japan)	Children of Asian ancestry
Wegener's granulomatosis	Incidence: 4/million	8.5/million (United Kingdom)	Whites ≫ blacks

*Among children younger than 5 years.
From Gonzalez-Gay MA, Garica-Porrua C. Epidemiology of the vasculitides. *Rheum Clin North Am.* 2001;27:729-749.

TABLE 278-3 PATHOLOGIC CHARACTERISTICS OF SELECTED FORMS OF VASCULITIS

	TAKAYASU'S ARTERITIS	POLYARTERITIS NODOSA	WEGENER'S GRANULOMATOSIS	CHURG-STRAUSS SYNDROME	HENOCH-SCHÖNLEIN PURPURA	CUTANEOUS LEUKOCYTOCLASTIC ANGIITIS
Vessels involved	Elastic (large) or muscle (medium-sized) arteries	Medium-sized and small muscle arteries	Small arteries and veins; sometimes medium-sized vessels	Small arteries and veins; sometimes medium-sized vessels	Capillaries, venules, arterioles	Capillaries, venules, arterioles
Organ involvement	Aorta, aortic arch and major branches, pulmonary arteries	Skin, peripheral nerve, gastrointestinal tract, other viscera	Upper respiratory tract, lungs, kidneys, skin, eyes	Upper respiratory tract, lungs, heart, peripheral nerves	Skin, joints, gastrointestinal tract, kidneys	Skin, joints
Type of vasculitis and inflammatory cells	Granulomatous with some giant cells; fibrosis in chronic stages	Necrotizing, with mixed cellular infiltrate	Necrotizing or granulomatous (or both); mixed cellular infiltrate plus occasional eosinophils	Necrotizing or granulomatous (or both); prominent eosinophils and other mixed infiltrate	Leukocytoclastic, with some lymphocytes and variable eosinophils; IgA deposits in affected tissues	Leukocytoclastic, with occasional eosinophils

Medium- and Small-Vessel Vasculitides

Several different pathophysiologic mechanisms are operative among the medium- and small-vessel vasculitides. In many cases, the mechanisms outlined in the following sections overlap.

Immune Complex–Mediated Vascular Injury

Immune complex–mediated tissue injury does not produce a single clinical syndrome; rather, it applies to many forms of vasculitis and overlaps with injuries caused by other immune mechanisms. Numerous variables influence immune complex–mediated injury, including the physical properties of the immune complexes (e.g., their size), the ability of the immune complexes to activate complement, the antigen-to-antibody ratio, and the hemodynamic features of specific vascular beds. Immune complexes participate in the pathophysiologic process of some forms of both medium- and small-vessel vasculitis, including polyarteritis nodosa, cryoglobulinemia, Henoch-Schönlein purpura, cutaneous leukocytoclastic angiitis, and rheumatoid vasculitis.

Role of ANCAs

ANCAs are directed against antigens that reside within the primary granules of neutrophils and monocytes. Two types of ANCAs are relevant to vasculitis: (1) those directed against proteinase 3 (PR3), known as *PR3-ANCAs*; and (2) those directed against myeloperoxidase (MPO), termed *MPO-ANCAs*. ANCAs interact with cytokines, neutrophils, monocytes, and other elements of the immune system to amplify ongoing inflammation in certain forms of vasculitis. A striking and still unexplained feature of ANCA-associated vasculitis is that patients virtually never have antibodies to both PR3 and MPO. Despite the specificity of these antibodies, however, evidence of ANCA's primary role in causing human disease is still absent.

In Wegener's granulomatosis, abnormal cytokine regulation interacts with the production of ANCA to fuel the inflammatory response. T_H1 cytokines such as interferon-γ, interleukin-12, and tumor necrosis factor (TNF) appear to play important roles. Under the direction of interleukin-12, CD4$^+$ T cells from patients with Wegener's granulomatosis produce elevated levels of TNF, and peripheral blood mononuclear cells secrete increased amounts of interferon-γ. Serum levels of soluble receptors for TNF are elevated in patients with active Wegener's granulomatosis and normalize with the induction of remission. In vitro priming of activated neutrophils with TNF markedly enhances the ability of ANCA to stimulate neutrophil degranulation. Despite the strong rationale for anti-TNF strategies in Wegener's granulomatosis, however, a randomized trial of etanercept showed no efficacy in the maintenance of disease remission.

B-cell depletion was recently shown to be a more effective approach than intravenous cyclophosphamide to treat Wegener's granulomatosis and microscopic polyangiitis, particularly in relapsing disease,[1] although another study did not demonstrate the superiority of a rituximab-based regimen.[2] The efficacy of this treatment strategy probably relates to the removal of several B-cell functions beyond their evolution into plasma cells and the production of ANCA. These other B-cell functions include cytokine production, antigen presentation, and B cell–T cell crosstalk.

Superantigen Model

The degree of immune activation in Kawasaki disease and the acute but generally self-limited nature of this illness imply a potential role for superantigens. Superantigens are proteins produced by microbial pathogens (e.g., *Staphylococcus aureus* or *Streptococcus* species) that are capable of stimulating large populations of T cells in a manner unrestricted by the class II major histocompatibility complex (MHC). Superantigens bind directly to conserved amino acid residues outside the antigen-binding groove on class II MHC molecules, thereby selectively stimulating T cells that express particular β-chain variable gene segments. Through the binding of this MHC-superantigen complex to its cognate T-cell receptors, as many as 20% of circulating lymphocytes may become activated, leading to a potentially enormous outpouring of cytokines. With regard to the etiology of Kawasaki disease, substantial attention has focused on toxic shock syndrome toxin 1, an exotoxin produced by *S. aureus*. Superantigens have also been postulated to play roles in the susceptibility to disease flares in Wegener's granulomatosis. Nasal carriage of *S. aureus* and superantigens associated with these organisms has been linked to a greater likelihood of disease flares in some studies.

Antiendothelial Cell Antibodies

Antiendothelial cell antibodies can induce endothelial cell injury and lysis through either complement-mediated cytotoxicity or antibody-dependent cellular cytotoxicity. Both these mechanisms have been demonstrated to cause endothelial injury in in vitro assays employing sera from patients with systemic vasculitis. The ability of these antibodies to damage endothelial cells is an appealing argument for their potential role in forms of vasculitis in which the endothelium is the focus of inflammation (as opposed to the more external vessel wall layers). However, the true relevance of antiendothelial cell antibodies to human disease and their importance within the larger context of other disease mechanisms remain unclear.

CLINICAL MANIFESTATIONS

Large-Vessel Vasculitides

Takayasu's Arteritis

Takayasu's arteritis affects the aorta and its major branches. In contrast to atherosclerosis, which is characterized by focal, irregular lesions, the lesions of Takayasu's arteritis are long, smooth, tapered stenoses (E-Fig. 278-1A). The most commonly involved arteries are the subclavian and innominate arteries. Takayasu's arteritis has been termed *pulseless disease* because of its ability to obliterate peripheral pulses (particularly in the upper extremities). Exuberant collateral circulation develops over time in response to the gradual narrowing of major arteries, making the loss of digits or limbs from ischemia extremely rare. The pulmonary circulation is involved in approximately 50% of cases of Takayasu's arteritis.

Patients with severe narrowing of the aortic arch vessels supplying the head may develop Takayasu's retinopathy, a hypotension retinopathy leading to neovascularization. In contrast, patients with prolonged hypertension associated with renal artery stenosis demonstrate the classic ocular features of hypertension: copper wiring and multiple retinal infarctions. This complication is particularly difficult to diagnose, and it is dangerous because vascular narrowings of large arteries to the arms and legs can cause underestimation of the true central aortic pressure. When Takayasu's arteritis involves the ascending aorta, it may lead to aortic dilation, aortic regurgitation, aneurysm formation, and aortic rupture (E-Fig. 278-1B).

The cornerstone of treatment of Takayasu's arteritis is glucocorticoids. For patients with marked symptoms and signs of an inflammatory phase, prednisone (1 mg/kg/day) is usually effective in controlling the disease. This dose should be tapered within 8 to 12 weeks to less than 20 mg/day and ultimately to less than 10 mg/day as a maintenance dose. Methotrexate (up to 25 mg/week), mycophenolate mofetil (1500 mg twice daily), and infliximab (3 to 5 mg/kg every 6 weeks) have been employed as steroid-sparing agents. Tocilizumab, an inhibitor of the interleukin-6 receptor, also shows significant potential as a treatment modality.

Cogan's Syndrome

The combination of inflammatory eye disease and vestibuloauditory dysfunction is the sine qua non of Cogan's syndrome. In addition to inflammatory disease of the eyes and ears, up to 15% of patients with Cogan's syndrome have vasculitis involving medium-sized to large blood vessels. Although the ocular manifestations vary, the classic presentation is the combination of interstitial keratitis and sensorineural hearing loss. Cogan's syndrome may first appear in either the eyes or the ears. Although intervals as long as 1 to 2 years have been described between the onset of disease in one organ and the appearance of disease in the other, it is usually only a matter of months. Patients usually present with photophobia and blurry vision, sometimes accompanied simultaneously by auditory or vestibular dysfunction. The vascular disease in Cogan's syndrome resembles Takayasu's arteritis.

Rapidly progressive sensorineural hearing loss requires early, aggressive therapy with high doses of systemic glucocorticoids. Cytotoxic agents can be considered for patients with suboptimal responses to glucocorticoids who still have salvageable hearing. Many Cogan's syndrome patients become candidates for cochlear implants.

Behçet's Syndrome

Behçet's syndrome may affect small, medium, and large vessels in either the venous or the arterial circulation. The most typical lesions in Behçet's syndrome are mucocutaneous, reflecting the involvement of small blood vessels. The triad of recurrent mouth ulcers, genital ulcers, and eye inflammation is the classic presentation. The diagnostic criteria of the International Study Group for Behçet's Syndrome consist of one required manifestation—recurrent oral ulceration—plus at least two of the following: recurrent genital ulceration, characteristic eye or skin lesions, or a pathergy reaction (see later). However, the spectrum of Behçet's syndrome encompasses many manifestations not included in these criteria.

Large-vessel complications of Behçet's syndrome may include aneurysms in the pulmonary and systemic arterial systems. Venous complications include thromboses of the deep venous system, vena cava, portohepatic vein, and cerebral sinus. Pathergy—the development of pustules at the sites of sterile needle pricks—is a distinctive feature in many patients with Behçet's syndrome, particularly those of Turkish origin. The arthritis of Behçet's syndrome is a nondeforming, oligoarticular, asymmetrical arthritis of large joints. Gastrointestinal lesions in Behçet's syndrome typically consist of ulcerations of the distal ileum or cecum. Crohn's disease, which can cause genital ulcers as well as gastrointestinal tract disease, may be particularly difficult to distinguish from Behçet's syndrome.

Colchicine (up to 1.5 to 2 mg/day) is sometimes effective for the treatment of mild oral and genital ulcers in Behçet's syndrome. Thalidomide (100 mg/day) is also useful for mucocutaneous disease manifestations. Low-dose glucocorticoids are also effective for intransigent mucocutaneous disease and may have a better side effect profile than thalidomide. Intermittent courses of glucocorticoids during periods of particular mucocutaneous disease activity are also effective.

Severe disease in any organ system almost always requires high doses of prednisone (e.g., 1 mg/kg/day). TNF inhibition with infliximab or adalimumab has largely replaced cyclophosphamide or chlorambucil as the treatment of choice for patients with the most severe forms of uveitis or meningoencephalitis. Azathioprine (2 mg/kg/day), cyclosporine (3 to 5 mg/kg/day in two divided doses), methotrexate (up to 25 mg/week), and interferon-α (3 million to 5 million units three times a week) are also appropriate therapies for many complications of Behçet's syndrome.

Medium-Vessel Vasculitides
Polyarteritis Nodosa

Polyarteritis nodosa has a striking predilection for certain organs, particularly the skin, peripheral nerves, gastrointestinal tract, and kidneys. This disease usually begins with nonspecific symptoms that may include malaise, fatigue, fever, myalgias, and arthralgias. Overt signs of vasculitis may not occur until weeks or months after the onset of the first symptoms. Skin lesions of polyarteritis nodosa include livedo reticularis, subcutaneous nodules, ulcers, and digital gangrene. A majority of patients with polyarteritis nodosa (>80% in some series) have vasculitic neuropathy, typically in the pattern of a mononeuritis multiplex (Chapter 428).

The classic gastrointestinal manifestation of polyarteritis nodosa is "intestinal angina," the occurrence of postprandial abdominal pain. Polyarteritis nodosa can also affect individual gastrointestinal tract organs such as the gallbladder or appendix, presenting as cholecystitis or appendicitis. The typical renal manifestation of polyarteritis nodosa is vasculitic involvement of the medium-sized intrarenal arteries, leading to renin-mediated hypertension and renal infarctions. Cardiac lesions, which usually remain subclinical, may lead to myocardial infarction or congestive heart failure. Polyarteritis nodosa usually spares the lungs.

The diagnosis of polyarteritis nodosa requires either a tissue biopsy or an angiogram that demonstrates microaneurysms (Fig. 278-1). Simultaneous nerve and muscle biopsies (e.g., sural nerve and gastrocnemius muscle) have a high yield if there is clinical suspicion of vasculitic neuropathy. Symptoms suggestive of a neuropathy can be confirmed by electrodiagnostic studies that demonstrate a sensorimotor axonal neuropathy, often in a mononeuritis multiplex pattern. The pathologic changes in polyarteritis nodosa are limited to the arterial circulation; the lesions are segmental and favor the branch points of arteries. In gross pathologic specimens, aneurysmal bulges of the arterial wall may be visible. Histologic sections reveal infiltration and destruction of the blood vessel wall by inflammatory cells, accompanied by fibrinoid necrosis. Granulomatous inflammation is absent.

Approximately half of patients with polyarteritis nodosa achieve remissions or cures with high doses of glucocorticoids alone. Cyclophosphamide (2 mg/kg/day, adjusted for renal dysfunction) is indicated for patients whose disease is refractory to glucocorticoids or who have serious involvement of

FIGURE 278-1. Vasculitis of medium-sized arteries in polyarteritis nodosa. **A,** Mesenteric angiogram showing numerous aneurysms in medium-sized arteries. **B,** Fibrinoid necrosis in a jejunal artery from a patient who required surgical resection of necrotic bowel.

major organs. In recent years, therapeutic regimens involving lamivudine or entecavir and plasma exchange have substantially improved the treatment of hepatitis B virus (HBV)–associated polyarteritis nodosa. Because of increasing use of the HBV vaccine, less than 10% of polyarteritis nodosa cases are now associated with HBV infections.

Buerger's Disease

Buerger's disease, also known as *thromboangiitis obliterans*, has a remarkably strong yet poorly understood association with cigarette smoking. Buerger's disease does not occur in the absence of exposure to tobacco. The vessels affected by Buerger's disease are the distal medium-sized arteries and veins, particularly vessels at the levels of the ankles and wrists. The disease is characterized by thrombotic obliterations that begin distally and proceed proximally. Buerger's disease tends to be segmental in nature, involving 5- to 10-cm lengths of blood vessels. Arterial obliteration leads to the development of collateral vessels with a "corkscrew" appearance on angiography. Vascular occlusion in Buerger's disease often leads to the loss of digits and, if smoking persists, to the loss of greater amounts of tissue (e.g., hands or feet). Despite the intense involvement of the extremities in Buerger's disease, internal organ disease almost never occurs.

Complete abstinence from tobacco is essential to the treatment of Buerger's disease. Failure to stop smoking is associated with a dramatic increase in the risk of limb loss by amputation. No other therapeutic interventions, including glucocorticoids and anticoagulation, have dramatic effects on Buerger's disease.

Kawasaki Disease

Kawasaki disease occurs exclusively in young children. Because of its striking mucocutaneous findings and lymphadenopathy, Kawasaki disease is also known as *mucocutaneous lymph node syndrome*. Features of Kawasaki disease include high fevers, cervical adenopathy, conjunctival congestion, buccal erythema, prominence of the tongue papillae ("strawberry tongue"), polymorphous truncal rash, erythema of the palms and soles, and desquamation of skin from the fingertips occurring days to weeks into the illness. In its acuity and severity, Kawasaki disease resembles toxic shock syndrome and scarlet fever, both of which are mediated by superantigens (see Pathophysiology).

In a small number of patients with Kawasaki disease, panvasculitis in the coronary vessels leads to acute cardiac complications. Coronary arteritis leads to narrowing of the vessel lumen by the migration of myointimal cells from the media through the fragmented internal elastic lamina. Direct complications include aneurysmal dilation and thrombosis of the coronary arteries, leading to myocardial infarction and possibly death (in 1 to 2% of patients with Kawasaki disease during the acute illness). Late mortality from myocardial infarction may occur from the thrombosis of coronary artery aneurysms formed during the initial inflammatory stage. Such myocardial infarctions have been reported in middle-aged individuals who had febrile illnesses consistent with Kawasaki disease in childhood.

The recommended therapeutic regimen in Kawasaki disease is the combination of intravenous immune globulin (IVIG; 400 mg/kg/day on 4 consecutive days) and acetylsalicylic acid (100 mg/kg/day, lowered to 3 to 5 mg/kg/day after resolution of the fever). IVIG prevents the formation of coronary aneurysms in most cases. Glucocorticoids are reserved for salvage therapy in patients in whom treatment with IVIG and acetylsalicylic acid has failed. **3**

Vasculitis of the Central Nervous System

Central nervous system (CNS) vasculitis includes two major categories of disease, one of which is not a true vasculitis: primary angiitis of the CNS (PACNS) and reversible cerebral vasoconstriction syndrome (RCVS). The diagnosis and management of these two conditions differ dramatically. The clinical, radiologic, and pathologic characteristics of PACNS and RCVS are shown in Table 278-4.

PRIMARY ANGIITIS OF THE CENTRAL NERVOUS SYSTEM. PACNS typically develops in a subacute fashion, with the evolution of multifocal strokes, encephalopathy, headache, and other clinical features over months. Headache is often the first symptom. As the condition progresses, most patients develop lethargy, confusion, and memory loss. Some patients develop multifocal strokes, seizures, evidence of increased intracranial pressure, or myelopathy. The results of routine laboratory tests (e.g., erythrocyte sedimentation rate) are often normal in PACNS. Lumbar puncture demonstrates abnormalities of the cerebrospinal fluid in approximately 80% of cases, usually

TABLE 278-4	PRIMARY ANGIITIS OF THE CENTRAL NERVOUS SYSTEM (PACNS) VERSUS REVERSIBLE CEREBRAL VASOCONSTRICTION SYNDROME (RCVS)	
	PACNS	**RCVS**
Gender ratio (female to male)	1:1	2–3:1
Onset	Subacute (weeks to months)	Sudden (seconds to minutes)
Headache	Insidious, dull	Thunderclap
Typical lumbar puncture findings	Abnormal in 50-80%: lymphocytic pleocytosis, elevated protein	Normal
Typical MRI findings	Multifocal subacute infarctions	Normal; watershed infarcts in minority
Typical angiogram findings	Normal in up to 40% of cases; abnormal angiographic features, when present, cannot be distinguished from RCVS	Multifocal stenoses/dilations
Utility of brain biopsy	Reasonable sensitivity in appropriately selected patients; important for excluding disease mimickers	Little to no role; helpful if confusing clinical situation confounds differentiation from PACNS or PACNS mimickers

MRI = magnetic resonance imaging.

a modest monocytosis and elevated protein. Lumbar punctures should be performed in all patients in whom the diagnosis of PACNS is being seriously considered. Although the findings in PACNS patients are nonspecific, a normal lumbar puncture argues against PACNS, and the procedure frequently identifies important PACNS mimickers such as infection or malignancy.

Magnetic resonance imaging (MRI) is the critical imaging modality in PACNS. Because of the subacute nature of the disorder, MRI studies reveal multifocal CNS infarctions in most cases. Strokes, hemorrhagic lesions, and mass lesions typically occur in more than one vascular territory. A normal brain MRI argues strongly against the diagnosis of PACNS. Angiography is less helpful in the evaluation of patients with PACNS, for two main reasons. First, the blood vessels involved in PACNS are often too small to be visualized adequately, even by conventional angiography. The false-negative rate of angiography in PACNS is on the order of 35%. Second, the classic "string of beads" abnormality on angiography, produced by segmental arterial narrowing alternating with dilations, is entirely nonspecific and is mimicked perfectly by a host of nonvasculitic conditions (the most common of which is RCVS). No angiographic pattern is pathognomonic for PACNS, and there is a significant tendency to overdiagnose "vasculitis" on angiographic grounds alone. A normal brain MRI in the setting of an abnormal angiogram should make one think first of RCVS, not PACNS.

When employed in appropriately selected patients whose history and radiologic studies suggest PACNS, brain biopsy is associated with reasonable positive and negative predictive values and frequently identifies important PACNS mimickers. Prednisone and cyclophosphamide are appropriate treatments for patients with abnormal findings on brain biopsy. Treatment courses of 6 to 12 months are recommended.

REVERSIBLE CEREBRAL VASOCONSTRICTION SYNDROME. Eighty percent of patients with RCVS are women. RCVS is probably far more common than PACNS. Overtreatment of patients with RCVS who are misdiagnosed as having PACNS leads to substantial morbidity.

A careful history is the most important part of the evaluation. In contrast to the subacute course that typifies PACNS, RCVS usually begins in a more dramatic fashion with a thunderclap headache. Compared with PACNS, the neurologic signs are less severe (encephalopathy is less common). RCVS frequently occurs in the setting of precipitants associated with vasospasm, such as the postpartum setting or the use of vasoactive agents such as nasal decongestants and recreational drugs.

The lumbar puncture is usually normal in RCVS, and brain MRI usually does not show multifocal CNS infarctions, with the exception of watershed infarctions. The typical angiographic findings in RCVS—vascular narrowing and beading—are generally indistinguishable from those of PACNS and conditions that mimic PACNS. Multifocal vascular narrowing is particularly characteristic of RCVS. The most distinctive angiographic feature of RCVS is that the abnormalities are completely reversible, usually within 4 to 8 weeks. These abnormalities in RCVS are caused by vasospasm rather than true vasculitis. In the evaluation of patients with potential RCVS, a diagnostic strategy that can clinch the diagnosis is a follow-up angiogram 4 to 8 weeks after the first. Angiographic abnormalities due to RCVS resolve during this interval.

Several approaches to the treatment of RCVS are reasonable. First, one may opt for watchful waiting. It is not clear that immunosuppression is either necessary or helpful. Moreover, attempts to treat vasospasm with calcium-channel blockers may lead to vascular steal phenomena, potentially causing more harm than good. However, because it is frequently difficult to do nothing for a patient with possibly serious CNS disease, calcium-channel blockers (e.g., nifedipine 30 mg three times daily) may be tried. Finally, because of the frequent diagnostic uncertainty at the time of presentation, some clinicians opt to treat empirically with glucocorticoids (prednisone 1 mg/kg/day) for 1 month, followed by a taper over several weeks. Cytotoxic therapy is not indicated in RCVS.

Small-Vessel Vasculitides

Wegener's Granulomatosis

Classic Wegener's granulomatosis involves the upper respiratory tract, the lungs, and the kidneys. Distinctive features may also occur in the eyes, ears, and other organs. The three pathologic hallmarks of Wegener's granulomatosis are (1) granulomatous inflammation in the upper or lower respiratory tract, (2) necrotizing vasculitis affecting arteries or veins, and (3) segmental glomerulonephritis associated with necrosis and thrombosis of capillary loops, with or without granulomatous lesions.

Approximately 90% of patients with Wegener's granulomatosis have nasal involvement, including crusting, bleeding, and obstruction. Cartilaginous inflammation may lead to nasal septal perforation and collapse of the nasal bridge ("saddle nose" deformity). Erosive sinus disease and subglottic stenosis (narrowing of the trachea just below the vocal cords) are highly characteristic of Wegener's granulomatosis.

Both conductive and sensorineural hearing loss can occur in Wegener's granulomatosis, although conductive lesions caused by middle ear disease are more common. Orbital masses ("pseudotumors" that develop behind the eye), scleritis, and peripheral ulcerative keratitis are the most dangerous ocular lesions. Episcleritis and conjunctivitis also occur. Anterior uveitis is rare. The clinical manifestations of Wegener's granulomatosis in the lung range from asymptomatic nodules to fulminant alveolar hemorrhage. The most common radiographic findings are pulmonary infiltrates, nodules, and cavitary lesions. Disease of the large airways leading to bronchial narrowing is a challenging diagnosis to make because patients present with few symptoms until advanced disease is present.

The clinical presentation of renal disease in Wegener's granulomatosis is usually rapidly progressive glomerulonephritis: hematuria, red blood cell casts, and proteinuria (usually non-nephrotic). Without appropriate therapy, end-stage renal disease may ensue within weeks.

Sixty percent of patients with Wegener's granulomatosis have musculoskeletal symptoms during the disease course. The presenting complaint is frequently arthralgias or an oligoarthritis that is migratory in nature. Skin lesions in Wegener's granulomatosis include the full panoply of lesions associated with cutaneous vasculitis, including purpura (Fig. 278-2). Cutaneous nodules over the extensor surfaces of joints, particularly the elbow, may mimic rheumatoid nodules. These lesions are known as *cutaneous extravascular necrotizing granulomas* or *Churg-Strauss lesions*. Meningeal inflammation, presenting with headaches, cranial neuropathies, and a clinical picture compatible with chronic meningitis, is perhaps the most common CNS manifestation of Wegener's granulomatosis. Mononeuritis multiplex may affect the peripheral nervous system.

Wegener's granulomatosis is the prototype of the conditions associated with ANCA. Positive results of immunofluorescence tests for ANCA in either the cytoplasmic (C-ANCA) or perinuclear (P-ANCA) pattern should be confirmed by enzyme immunoassays for antibodies to either PR3 or MPO. An ANCA-negative assay sample does not exclude Wegener's granulomatosis because a substantial minority of patients (between 15 and 40% overall) lack these antibodies. Furthermore, ANCA titers do not correlate reliably with disease activity.

FIGURE 278-2. Cutaneous small-vessel vasculitis showing palpable purpuric lesions with necrosis and crusting.

Manifestations of Wegener's granulomatosis that constitute immediate threats to either the function of a vital organ or the patient's life require urgent treatment. From the late 1960s until 2010, the combination of cyclophosphamide (2 mg/kg/day orally) and high doses of glucocorticoids (prednisone 1 mg/kg/day orally, tapered over 6 to 12 months) was the standard of care for Wegener's granulomatosis.[4] Intermittent administration of cyclophosphamide by intravenous infusion is also effective in remission induction.[5] However, based on the results of a multicenter clinical trial that compared rituximab with cyclophosphamide in patients with ANCA-associated vasculitis (either Wegener's granulomatosis or microscopic polyangiitis), rituximab (375 mg/m^2/week for 4 weeks) appears to be at least as effective for most patients with severe ANCA-associated vasculitis.[1] In addition, rituximab seems to be more effective for patients who present with disease flares. An alternative dosing regimen, rituximab 1 g times two separated by 2 weeks, may also be effective. Limited forms of Wegener's granulomatosis may respond to the combination of methotrexate (up to 25 mg/week) and glucocorticoids. The role of rituximab in the treatment of limited Wegener's granulomatosis is not yet clear. Azathioprine and methotrexate both appear to be effective remission agents for maintenance therapy,[6] and azathioprine is better than mycophenolate mofetil in this situation.[7]

Microscopic Polyangiitis

Microscopic polyangiitis is characterized by (1) nongranulomatous, necrotizing vasculitis, with few or no immune deposits; (2) involvement of small (and possibly medium-sized) blood vessels in the arterial or venous circulation; and (3) tropism for the kidneys and lungs. Many cases of small-vessel vasculitis once regarded as polyarteritis nodosa are now more properly classified as microscopic polyangiitis. In contrast to polyarteritis nodosa, an ANCA-negative disorder, 70% of microscopic polyangiitis patients are ANCA positive. Thus, microscopic polyangiitis is often considered to fall within the spectrum of ANCA-associated vasculitis. The ANCAs in microscopic polyangiitis are usually directed against MPO, leading to a perinuclear pattern of staining on immunofluorescence testing (P-ANCA). Upper respiratory tract symptoms in microscopic polyangiitis, if present at all, are much milder than those associated with Wegener's granulomatosis.

The approach to the treatment of microscopic polyangiitis is similar to that of Wegener's granulomatosis. The combination of rituximab and glucocorticoids is the treatment regimen of choice for most patients with microscopic polyangiitis.[1]

Churg-Strauss Syndrome

Churg-Strauss syndrome is an eosinophil-rich form of granulomatous inflammation that involves the respiratory tract and other organs. The disease is associated with necrotizing vasculitis of small to medium-sized vessels. Two hallmarks of Churg-Strauss syndrome are asthma and eosinophilia. Several phases of Churg-Strauss syndrome are described, as follows:

- A prodromal phase, characterized by the presence of allergic disease (typically asthma or allergic rhinitis), which may last months to many years;
- An eosinophilia–tissue infiltration phase, in which remarkably high peripheral eosinophilia may occur and tissue infiltration by eosinophils is observed in the lung, gastrointestinal tract, and other tissues; and
- A vasculitic phase, in which systemic necrotizing vasculitis afflicts a wide range of organs, ranging from the heart and lungs to peripheral nerves and skin.

Patients with mild disease may be treated with prednisone. Those with evidence of neurologic, cardiac, renal, or gastrointestinal involvement should be treated with cyclophosphamide in addition to glucocorticoids. Although clinical remissions are obtained in more than 90% of patients with Churg-Strauss syndrome, disease recurrence is seen in 25%. In most cases, relapses are heralded by the return of eosinophilia. Approximately 50% of cases of Churg-Strauss syndrome are associated with ANCA, usually directed against MPO, but the percentage may be higher among untreated patients.

Henoch-Schönlein Purpura

Henoch-Schönlein purpura (HSP) is characterized by nonthrombocytopenic purpura, arthritis, abdominal pain, and glomerulonephritis. The histopathologic findings are those of a leukocytoclastic vasculitis with IgA deposition. HSP can develop at any age, but 80 to 90% of cases occur in children. Although the cause is unknown, the disease's seasonal variation and the fact that two thirds of patients with HSP experience antecedent acute upper respiratory illnesses suggest an infectious trigger. Medications (e.g., antibiotics) can trigger HSP, and other environmental triggers are also likely. The diagnosis of HSP can be confirmed only by demonstration of IgA deposition within and around blood vessel walls.

The classic HSP patient presents with the acute onset of fever, palpable purpura on the lower extremities and buttocks, abdominal pain, arthritis, and hematuria. The clinician must be alert to the possibility of HSP even when only parts of the syndrome are present. Most patients with HSP, especially children, have a self-limited disease that lasts an average of 4 weeks. Glucocorticoids ameliorate the joint and gastrointestinal symptoms in most cases and improve the cutaneous manifestations in some. The efficacy of glucocorticoids in the glomerulonephritis of HSP is controversial. Uncontrolled studies suggest that methylprednisolone pulses (1 g/day for three doses), followed by oral prednisone combined with azathioprine or cyclophosphamide, may be useful in severe glomerulonephritis associated with HSP.

Cutaneous Leukocytoclastic Angiitis

Also termed *hypersensitivity vasculitis*, *cutaneous leukocytoclastic angiitis* is the preferred name because no hypersensitivity or allergy is evident in many cases. Histories of exposure to new medications or infections may be elicited, however, and immune complex deposition is central to the pathophysiologic process. Although it is occasionally associated with synovitis, other signs of systemic involvement are absent.

The skin lesions in cutaneous leukocytoclastic angiitis occur in "crops" following exposure to the inciting antigen. The usual interval between the exposure and the onset of clinically evident vasculitis is 10 to 14 days. The lesions typically occur first in dependent regions, such as on the lower extremities or buttocks. The rash may be asymptomatic but is usually accompanied by burning or tingling sensations.

Keys to the management of cutaneous leukocytoclastic angiitis include the exclusion of any underlying form of vasculitis that may cause subclinical involvement of other organs and removal of any agent (e.g., medication) that may have triggered the vasculitis. For patients in whom a precipitant can be identified, removal of the offending agent usually leads to resolution of the vasculitis within days to weeks. The type, intensity, and duration of therapy for cutaneous leukocytoclastic angiitis are based on the disease severity. Mild cases may be treated simply with leg elevation and the administration of nonsteroidal anti-inflammatory agents or H₁ antihistamines. For persistent disease not associated with cutaneous gangrene, colchicine, hydroxychloroquine, or dapsone may be tried. For severe cases, immunosuppressive agents may be indicated, generally beginning with glucocorticoids. Azathioprine is commonly used as a steroid-sparing agent.

Urticarial Vasculitis

At least three subtypes of urticarial vasculitis are known: (1) normocomplementemic, a form that is generally idiopathic and benign (and may be viewed as a manifestation of cutaneous leukocytoclastic angiitis); (2) hypocomplementemic, a form that is often associated with a systemic inflammatory disease; and (3) hypocomplementemic urticarial vasculitis syndrome (HUVS), a potentially severe condition usually associated with autoantibodies to the collagen-like region of C1q. Most patients with the hypocomplementemic subtype have an underlying systemic disorder, such as systemic lupus erythematosus (Chapter 274) or Sjögren's syndrome (Chapter 276). Many HUVS patients have C1q "precipitins," that is, IgG autoantibodies to the collagen-like region of C1q that trigger the classical pathway of complement activation. The role of anti-C1q antibodies in disease pathogenesis remains unclear.

The lesions of urticarial vasculitis must be distinguished from the far more common chronic idiopathic urticaria (Chapters 260 and 448). Unlike idiopathic urticaria, the lesions of urticarial vasculitis last more than 48 hours, often have a purpuric component (i.e., they do not blanch), and resolve with postinflammatory hyperpigmentation. In urticarial vasculitis, lesions associated with vasculitis are often accompanied by stinging or burning. Urticarial vasculitis affects the capillaries and postcapillary venules, showing leukocytoclastic vasculitis on light microscopy. Direct immunofluorescence studies reveal both immunoglobulin and complement deposition in or around blood vessels of the upper dermis or the dermoepidermal junction.

Patients with urticarial vasculitis whose serum complement levels remain normal during attacks often have self-limited disease and require little therapy. Other cases, especially HUVS, may cause life-threatening involvement of the lungs or other organs and require periods of intensive immunosuppression. Treatment decisions in HUVS must be individualized according to the patient's clinical status.

Cryoglobulinemia

Cryoglobulins are antibodies that precipitate from serum under conditions of cold and resolubilize on rewarming. Cryoglobulins are classified into types I, II, and III on the basis of whether monoclonality and rheumatoid factor activity (the ability to bind to the Fc portion of IgG) are present. Type I cryoglobulins, which are monoclonal but lack rheumatoid factor activity, are associated with certain hematopoietic malignant neoplasms (e.g., multiple myeloma) and often lead to hyperviscosity rather than to vasculitis (Chapter 193). In contrast, type II and type III cryoglobulins may be associated with systemic vasculitis involving small (and often medium-sized) blood vessels. Vasculitis results from the deposition of cryoglobulin-containing immune complexes within blood vessel walls and the activation of complement.

Cryoglobulin types II and III are termed mixed cryoglobulins because they consist of both IgG and IgM antibodies. The IgM components in both type II and type III cryoglobulinemia possess rheumatoid factor activity (i.e., assays for rheumatoid factor are positive, indicating binding of the IgM antibody to the Fc portion of IgG). Whereas the IgM component in type II cryoglobulin is monoclonal, the IgM in type III cryoglobulin is polyclonal. Ninety percent of patients with vasculitis secondary to mixed cryoglobulins are hypocomplementemic, with C4 levels characteristically more depressed than C3 levels. Infection with hepatitis C virus (HCV) accounts for at least 80% of the vasculitis cases associated with mixed cryoglobulins.

The optimal therapy for most cases of cryoglobulinemic vasculitis is successful treatment of the underlying HCV infection. For cryoglobulinemic patients with relatively mild disease (e.g., frequent purpuric lesions, shallow cutaneous ulcers), pegylated interferon-α2b (1 μg/kg/week) combined with ribavirin (1000 to 1200 mg/day) may be effective. For patients with mononeuritis multiplex or other manifestations of severe disease, glucocorticoids and possibly cyclophosphamide are required. Plasmapheresis may be a useful adjunctive therapy. Small case series also suggest that rituximab is an effective intervention.

▶ DIAGNOSIS

Differential Diagnosis

The major categories of diseases that can mimic vasculitis are listed in Table 278-5. Certain features of a patient's case should raise the diagnostic suspicion for vasculitis. First, most cases of vasculitis do not begin suddenly; rather, they unfold subacutely during weeks or months. Second, pain is usually a prominent feature of vasculitis, resulting from arthritis or arthralgias, myalgias, headaches, neuropathy, testicular infarction, digital ischemia, sinusitis, otalgia, back pain (caused by aortic inflammation), postprandial abdominal pain (caused by mesenteric vasculitis), or other disease manifestations. Third, signs of inflammation, such as fever, rash, weight loss, and elevated acute phase reactants, are highly characteristic. Finally, multiorgan system involvement is the rule in vasculitis.

TABLE 278-5	MAJOR DISEASE CATEGORIES IN THE DIFFERENTIAL DIAGNOSIS OF VASCULITIDES

Other forms of vasculitis
Simultaneous occurrence of common medical problems in the same patient
Infections
    Bacterial, viral, mycobacterial, fungal
Occlusive processes
    Hypercoagulable states
    Livedoid vasculopathy (atrophie blanche)
    Atheroembolic disease
Malignant neoplasms
    Lymphoma (including lymphomatoid granulomatosis)
    Castleman's disease
    Amyloidosis
    Paraproteinemias
Connective tissue disorders
    Systemic lupus erythematosus, mixed connective tissue disease
    Systemic sclerosis
    Rheumatoid arthritis
Miscellaneous
    Atrial myxoma
    Calciphylaxis
    Fibromuscular dysplasia
    Neutrophilic dermatoses
    Pyoderma gangrenosum
    Sarcoidosis
    Reversible cerebral vasoconstriction syndrome

Ideally, the diagnosis of vasculitis is established through biopsy of an involved organ. Diagnoses based on angiography alone have many potential pitfalls, as discussed in the sections on PACNS and RCVS. Angiographic findings that are "consistent with vasculitis" must be interpreted in the proper context. A diverse array of other diseases, ranging from atherosclerosis to vasospasm to pheochromocytoma, may mimic the angiographic appearance of vasculitis. Systemic vasculitis is frequently mimicked by two or more common medical problems or treatment complications occurring simultaneously in the same patient. Finally, prominent in the differential diagnosis of any individual form of vasculitis are other forms of vasculitis. For example, digital ischemia and splinter hemorrhages may be secondary to idiopathic polyarteritis nodosa. They may also be caused by polyarteritis nodosa associated with HBV infection, Wegener's granulomatosis, cryoglobulinemia, microscopic polyangiitis, Churg-Strauss syndrome, Buerger's disease, or some other form of vasculitis. Because the appropriate interventions for these conditions vary widely, careful distinction among these potential causes is essential.

TREATMENT   Rx

The intensity of treatment in patients with vasculitis must be guided by the degree of disease activity. Specifically, the treatment of vasculitis should be predicated not only on abnormal laboratory test results but also on clear evidence of active disease. In addition, the intensity of treatment must be adapted to the type of vasculitis. For example, giant cell arteritis responds to high doses of glucocorticoids in essentially all cases, but Wegener's granulomatosis nearly always requires an additional agent (rituximab, cyclophosphamide, or methotrexate) for disease control. In contrast, despite the dramatic fashion in which they sometimes present, most cases of HSP and cutaneous leukocytoclastic angiitis require no immunosuppressive treatment at all. In a randomized trial of patients with ANCA-associated vasculitis, azathioprine (2 mg/kg/day) and methotrexate (0.3 mg/kg/week, progressively increased to 25 mg/week) were equally effective for the maintenance of disease remission.

Conventional therapies such as glucocorticoids, immunomodulating agents, and cytotoxic drugs induce remissions and control vasculitis in most cases. Moreover, in some cases—a variable percentage, depending on the type of vasculitis—the disease is curable. Unfortunately, the treatments of vasculitis have enormous potential for toxicity. Regular monitoring of patients' bone marrow, renal, and hepatic function is essential to avoid treatment-induced toxicity. Prophylaxis against opportunistic infections, particularly *Pneumocystis* pneumonia (Chapter 349), is an important part of many vasculitis treatment regimens. During the tapering of immunosuppressive medications, disease flares are common in many forms of vasculitis.

A common error is treating patients with high doses of immunosuppressive agents for too long. The most appropriate use of medications such as cyclophosphamide and glucocorticoids is to induce remission as quickly as possible with early, aggressive treatment regimens and then convert patients to safer treatments for the maintenance of remission. Rituximab is replacing cyclophosphamide as the drug of choice for some forms of vasculitis, particularly severe ANCA-associated vasculitides. In such patients, the appropriate timing of re-treatment is not clear. Current treatment approaches to the specific vasculitides are described under Clinical Manifestations.

PROGNOSIS

Assuming that the diagnosis is made before the patient has become catastrophically ill, the prognosis in systemic vasculitis is determined largely by the answers to four questions:

1. Was the diagnosis established before the occurrence of major, irreversible organ damage?
2. Was aggressive (but appropriately dosed) treatment begun in a timely fashion?
3. Was there careful monitoring during treatment, and were specific steps taken to avoid drug-induced toxicity (e.g., opportunistic infection)?
4. Were the potentially toxic medications that induced remission stopped at an appropriate juncture and replaced with less dangerous medications (or was treatment stopped altogether)?

For most forms of vasculitis, the factors that determine long-term, drug-free remissions remain poorly understood. The likelihood of achieving sustained remission after the discontinuation of all medications (or cures) varies according to the specific type of vasculitis.

FUTURE DIRECTIONS

Compelling laboratory and spontaneously occurring animal models of disease, combined with the known associations among HBV, HCV, and vasculitis in humans, suggest that additional links between infection and systemic vasculitis may be established in the future. Important strides have been made in the description of cytokine and chemokine pathways that are operative in vascular inflammation, but relevant anticytokine interventions remain to be defined for clinical therapies. B-cell depletion is rapidly emerging as the treatment of choice for some forms of severe vasculitis. Additional studies are required to define the full spectrum of the clinical utility of B-cell depletion strategies for remission induction, as well as to understand the appropriate timing of re-treatment.

Grade **A**

1. Stone JH, Merkel PA, Spiera R, et al. Rituximab versus cyclophosphamide for remission induction in ANCA-associated vasculitis. *N Engl J Med.* 2010;363:221-232.
2. Jones RB, Tervaert JWC, Hauser T, et al. Rituximab versus cyclophosphamide in ANCA-associated renal vasculitis. *N Engl J Med.* 2010;363:211-220.
3. Newburger JW, Sleeper LA, McCrindle BW, et al. Randomized trial of pulsed corticosteroid therapy for primary treatment of Kawasaki disease. *N Engl J Med.* 2007;356:663-675.
4. Jayne D, Rasmussen N, Andrassy K, et al. A randomized trial of maintenance therapy for vasculitis associated with antineutrophil cytoplasmic autoantibodies. *N Engl J Med.* 2003;349:36-44.
5. De Groot K, Harper L, Jayne DR, et al. Pulse versus daily oral cyclophosphamide for induction of remission in antineutrophil cytoplasmic antibody-associated vasculitis: a randomized trial. *Ann Intern Med.* 2009;150:670-680.
6. Pagnoux C, Mahr A, Hamidou MA, et al. Azathioprine or methotrexate maintenance for ANCA-associated vasculitis. *N Engl J Med.* 2008;359:2790-2803.
7. Hiemstra TF, Walsh M, Mahr A, et al. Mycophenolate mofetil vs azathioprine for remission maintenance in antineutrophil cytoplasmic antibody–associated vasculitis: a randomized controlled trial. *JAMA.* 2010;304:2381-2388.

SUGGESTED READINGS

Chen M, Kallenberg CG. ANCA-associated vasculitides—advances in pathogenesis and treatment. *Nat Rev Rheumatol.* 2010;6:653-664. *Review of Wegener's granulomatosis, microscopic polyangiitis, Churg-Strauss syndrome, and renal-limited vasculitis.*

Holle JU, Gross WL, Latza U, et al. Improved outcome in 445 patients with Wegener's granulomatosis in a German vasculitis center over four decades. *Arthritis Rheum.* 2011;63:257-266. *Mortality has declined from a two-fold increase in mortality to a mortality close to the average population, probably due to more rapid diagnosis and better treatment.*

Ideguchi H, Suda A, Takeno M, et al. Behçet disease: evolution of clinical manifestations. *Medicine (Baltimore).* 2011;90:125-132. *In a case series of 412 patients, oral ulcer, the most common initial manifestation, preceded the diagnosis by an average of 7-8 years.*

279

POLYMYALGIA RHEUMATICA AND TEMPORAL ARTERITIS

ROBERT F. SPIERA AND STEPHEN A. PAGET

DEFINITION

Polymyalgia rheumatica (PMR) and temporal arteritis, also called *giant cell arteritis* (GCA), are systemic inflammatory disorders of unknown cause that represent a spectrum from severe proximal aches and pains and constitutional symptoms to an occlusive granulomatous vasculitis of medium and large vessels that can lead to permanent blindness or other organ and tissue damage. These disorders occur primarily in patients older than 50 years, in women more than in men; they are propagated by antigen-driven, cell-mediated (T_H1) immune mechanisms that may be associated with specific genetic markers, and they are highly responsive to corticosteroids.

EPIDEMIOLOGY

In the United States, the average annual incidence of PMR is 52.5 per 100,000 patients aged 50 years and older, and it increases with age. The prevalence is about 0.5 to 0.7%. Internationally, the frequency varies according to country, with the highest rates occurring in the Scandinavian countries. The incidence and prevalence of GCA are approximately one third those of PMR.

PATHOBIOLOGY

The cause of PMR and GCA is unknown, but both demonstrate familial aggregation, have a genetic association with human leukocyte antigen (HLA)-DR4, and are associated with a sequence polymorphism encoded within the hypervariable region of the HLA-DRβ1*04 gene. In genetically predisposed patients, disease may be triggered by environmental factors such as viruses or by internal antigens such as elastin. The inflammatory manifestations are directed by specific patterns of cell-mediated, T_H1-associated cytokines. Cytokine production by the mononuclear cells in the involved tissues appears to influence the clinical phenotype. Cytokine profiles characterized in temporal artery biopsy specimens obtained from patients with PMR and GCA differ. GCA tissue contains the T-lymphocyte products interferon (IFN)-γ and interleukin (IL)-2 and the macrophage products IL-1β, IL-6, and transforming growth factor-β. In PMR vascular tissue, transcripts are found for transforming growth factor-β, IL-1, and IL-2 but not for IFN-γ. Patients with GCA who present with fever of unknown origin and who do *not* have ischemic symptoms, such as visual loss, exhibit low IFN-γ levels in the arteries. Arteries that express high IFN-γ levels typically have multinucleated giant cells present; these cells remove debris and secrete cytokines that stimulate intimal hyperplasia and lead to angiogenesis.

The adventitia is considered the immunologic center in the pathogenesis of GCA. Macrophages and T lymphocytes enter the vessel wall through the vasa vasorum with the aid of adhesion molecules and come into contact with an inciting antigen. Here, it is likely that clonal proliferation of CD4$^+$ T cells is triggered by the presentation of unknown antigens by antigen-presenting cells. The activated CD4 cells produce IFN-γ, which attracts macrophages to the arterial wall. Some of these macrophages fuse at the intima-media junction to form multinucleated giant cells. These cells produce vascular endothelial growth factor, which triggers neovascularization both in the intima-media junction and at the level of the vasa vasorum, sprouting from the adventitia to the media. The subsequent immunologic events lead to a characteristic topography of mononuclear cells throughout the vessel wall. Products of giant cells and macrophages at the intima-media junction include collagenase and nitric oxide, both of which probably contribute to tissue damage. The pathologic impact of cytokines leads not only to the characteristic medial damage but also to the significant intimal hyperplasia that, if not treated, may eventually cause luminal narrowing and tissue ischemia.

In GCA, a transmural (involving all layers of the vessel) inflammatory infiltrate comprising predominantly mononuclear cells, and commonly with giant cells, is found in the superficial temporal arteries as well as in other large and medium-sized arteries. In elderly patients, fragmentation of the internal elastica is characteristic and helps differentiate this vascular lesion from that

of atherosclerosis. Often, macrophages containing fragments of elastic tissue are found at the intima-media junction, the histologic center of the inflammatory process. As mentioned earlier, immunochemical techniques demonstrate differing patterns of cells and their pro-inflammatory and pro-fibrotic products in the adventitia, media, and intima. Intimal proliferation may be prominent and lead to luminal narrowing. Fibrinoid necrosis, a common histologic feature in polyarteritis nodosa, is not seen in GCA.

In PMR, mononuclear cell inflammation can be found not only in the proximal joints, such as the shoulders, but also in the surrounding tendons, bursae, and soft tissues, consistent with enthesitis. Although muscle pain may be present, no muscle inflammation is found.

CLINICAL MANIFESTATIONS

PMR and GCA are systemic inflammatory disorders that occur primarily in patients older than 50 years, in women more than in men (2 : 1), and in whites. PMR and GCA are particularly uncommon in African Americans.

Shared characteristics of the two disorders include significant cytokine-driven constitutional symptoms such as fever, fatigue, and weight loss, as well as a markedly elevated erythrocyte sedimentation rate (ESR), anemia, and thrombocytosis. The musculoskeletal hallmark of PMR is proximal, severe, and symmetrical morning or even day-long stiffness, soreness, and pain in the shoulder, neck, and pelvic girdles. Fifty percent of patients with GCA share this characteristic proximal pain syndrome. Carpal tunnel syndrome and hand and knee synovitis may be seen in patients with PMR, but the overall presentation remains predominantly proximal, as opposed to the presentation of rheumatoid arthritis, in which distal synovitis dominates. Although patients with PMR may appear to have proximal muscle weakness, this is invariably due to pain and not muscle inflammation. Magnetic resonance imaging and ultrasound studies in patients with PMR have confirmed the presence of inflammation of extra-articular synovial structures, in particular, subacromial and subdeltoid bursae in the shoulders.

Specific signs and symptoms of GCA are best appreciated in their anatomic and physiologic contexts. GCA preferentially affects certain blood vessels, including the branches of the external carotid artery; the ophthalmic artery and, in particular, its posterior ciliary branches; and the large arteries that arise from the aortic arch and abdominal aorta. Headache and scalp pain are probably the most frequent symptoms, occurring in 50 to 75% of patients. Headache is often the first manifestation of GCA and is described as boring, severe, and constant; unresponsive to simple pain medications; and persisting through the night. Classically, patients complain of persistent and prominent temporal headaches, but occipital pain can also occur. Ear, pinna, or parotid gland pain may occur secondary to involvement of the posterior auricular artery. Jaw claudication and pain due to masseter muscle ischemia on chewing occur in 50% of patients. Lingual and maxillary artery involvement can lead to jaw or tongue pain on chewing or talking. The superficial temporal artery may become tortuous, prominent, nodular, or tender, but these findings are not invariable, and an abnormal temporal artery may be found on biopsy in vessels that appear to be normal on examination.

Fixed or intermittent symptoms related to vasculitic involvement of the ophthalmic arteries and its branches are the most dreaded manifestation of this illness and demand immediate therapeutic intervention. These symptoms are related to vascular narrowing due to both active inflammation and endothelial injury–derived vasospasm. Decreased vision secondary to arteritis is the most common serious consequence of GCA, occurring in 20 to 50% of patients who present to ophthalmologists. It is the presenting symptom in 60% of patients with GCA who develop visual loss. A careful history obtained from patients who present with "sudden" visual loss reveals that headache, constitutional symptoms, and PMR preceded the visual loss in approximately 40% of patients. Even the evolution of the visual loss is often staggered, with amaurosis fugax in 10% and a partial field defect progressing to complete blindness over days. If GCA remains untreated, the second eye may become involved within 1 to 2 weeks. The posterior ciliary arteries are the most frequently involved; thus, anterior ischemic optic neuropathy is the most common lesion, which can be easily defined by an ophthalmologist. Occlusion of the central retinal artery and its branches is uncommon; thus, exudates, hemorrhages, and frank vasculitis are infrequent. Five percent of patients with GCA may present with diplopia or ptosis, which may precede visual loss. The final visual abnormality can be a composite of many ischemic events occurring together in the optic nerve, the extraocular muscles, the chiasm, and the brain itself. Because GCA primarily involves arteries that contain elastica, and the elastic lamina is lost as vessels pierce the dura, intracerebral lesions such as strokes are uncommon but may occur.

Large artery involvement most commonly presents as arm or leg claudication; rarer manifestations are stroke, subclavian steal syndrome, intestinal infarction, and symptomatic aortic aneurysm. Thus, a subclinical arteritis can exist and demands long-term monitoring.

Steroid-treated PMR and GCA are self-limited illnesses lasting 1 to 2 years in most patients. However, a subgroup of patients with both disorders can have active inflammatory disease, as manifested by persistent symptoms and blood test signs of active inflammation, for 7 to 10 years. Of note is the fact that thoracic aneurysms with giant cells in the tissue can develop as long as 15 years after the diagnosis, successful treatment, and discontinuation of steroids. Indeed, the incidence of thoracic and aortic aneurysms is markedly higher in patients with prior history of presumably successfully treated GCA than in age-matched control subjects. Conversely, in studies of repaired aortic aneurysms, pathologic findings consistent with GCA have been found in approximately 2% of specimens from individuals without previously recognized or suspected arteritis. In most studies, survival in those with PMR and GCA is similar to that of unaffected persons of the same age. However, one study showed that survival was decreased in a group of patients with GCA who had permanent visual loss and required more than 10 mg/day of prednisone at 6 months. This probably supports the observation that morbidity and mortality are caused by steroid-related treatment complications in this high-risk, elderly group of patients possessing many comorbid conditions.

DIAGNOSIS

The diagnoses of PMR and GCA are based on clinical facts, with support from laboratory tests and temporal artery biopsy (Fig. 279-1). No physician should await an abnormal finding on temporal artery biopsy or demand the presence of an elevated ESR before making the definitive diagnosis of GCA in the setting of a characteristic clinical picture. That said, the laboratory hallmark of PMR and GCA is an elevation in IL-6-stimulated acute phase reactants such as the ESR and C-reactive protein. The ESR is usually in excess of 50 mm/hour and may exceed 100 mm/hour. An ESR in the low 20s or 30s, however, does not exclude a diagnosis of PMR or GCA if other characteristic clinical features are present, and especially if the patient is already taking steroids.

Normocytic, normochromic anemia and thrombocytosis occur in approximately 50% of patients with both disorders and are excellent guides to the state of inflammation. In both PMR and GCA, the frequency of rheumatoid factor, antinuclear antibody, complement levels, monoclonal proteins, and cryoglobulins is no higher than in age-matched control subjects. Alkaline phosphatase activity may be elevated in one third of patients, primarily those with GCA. Although these tests are not indicated in PMR and GCA, muscle enzymes and electromyography are normal, and muscle biopsy shows type II fiber atrophy but no inflammation.

Superficial Temporal Artery Assessment

Temporal artery tenderness, nodularity, and diminished pulsation are typical findings on physical examination in a patient with GCA. Color duplex ultrasonography has been used as an adjunctive noninvasive diagnostic tool in GCA. A hypoechoic halo around the superficial temporal artery has been reported in 73% of patients with biopsy-proven GCA. The halo, representing edema in the arterial wall, was observed bilaterally in a significant subset of patients and disappeared at a mean of 16 days after the initiation of steroids. The presence of the halo had a sensitivity of 73% and was 100% specific for GCA in one study. Other groups have been unable to replicate this experience, however, and have found Doppler ultrasonography to be no more sensitive or specific than physical examination in patients thought to have the disease. Findings of stenosis or occlusion of temporal arteries by Doppler ultrasound have also been recognized as modestly sensitive and specific for the diagnosis of GCA in some studies. Operator dependency remains a challenge to the more widespread use of this modality diagnostically. [^{18}F]Fluorodeoxyglucose positron emission tomography may be helpful in identifying large-vessel inflammation suggestive of GCA, but it is not helpful in assessing the temporal arteries themselves, given their relatively small size and high background uptake in that area. Recent studies have suggested that magnetic resonance imaging or magnetic resonance angiography may be a helpful noninvasive diagnostic modality. Superficial cranial arteries can be visualized, and mural inflammatory changes and luminal narrowing can be identified. Large-vessel involvement can also be assessed. Studies have suggested that the sensitivities and specificities of magnetic resonance imaging and angiography are similar to those of biopsy in the diagnosis of GCA. Nevertheless, temporal artery biopsy remains the diagnostic "gold standard" in GCA, and given the relatively easy accessibility of the artery and potentially significant morbidity of therapy in GCA, histologic confirmation is favored in most cases.

Although temporal artery biopsy continues to be an important diagnostic test for the presence of GCA, a few caveats must be stated. First, in a patient

FIGURE 279-1. Diagnostic algorithm for polymyalgia rheumatica (PMR). GCA = giant cell arteritis.

in whom the clinical diagnosis is likely, treatment with steroids should be instituted immediately, without waiting for the biopsy results. Second, because of the skipped nature of the pathologic inflammatory lesions in the vessel wall, as many as 20 to 30% of biopsy specimens may be normal despite an overwhelming diagnostic likelihood of GCA. However, because the biopsy is helpful in confirming the diagnosis of GCA, in which high doses of steroids are used, the following guidelines are given: Patients with pure PMR and no GCA signs or symptoms do not need a biopsy. However, because 10% of these patients may develop clinical manifestations of GCA within the next year, they should be told to report such symptoms immediately. When GCA is likely, an outpatient biopsy should be performed on the symptomatic side of the head, preferably including inflamed areas with tenderness or nodularity and incorporating 2 to 3 cm of vessel. Multiple sections should be requested because of the segmental nature of the disease process. Some rheumatologists routinely perform bilateral biopsies, which may increase the likelihood of obtaining an abnormal finding by up to 5%, whereas others perform a contralateral biopsy if the first specimen is normal. Diagnostic biopsy findings continue to be present for as long as 2 to 4 weeks after the clinical diagnosis is made and steroid treatment is instituted.

Differential Diagnosis

The systemic nature of these disorders and the fact that they occur in the elderly demand careful diagnostic scrutiny to avoid missing a malignant neoplasm or major infection and possibly treating patients inappropriately with high-dose steroids. This is true in PMR because there is no diagnostic test, and it is true in GCA because the biopsy findings may be normal in the face of active, vision-threatening vasculitis. Infections that must be considered and ruled out if clinically appropriate include tuberculosis, endocarditis, and hepatitis B and C. Malignant neoplasms such as lymphoma and multiple myeloma may mimic PMR, and an age-appropriate cancer evaluation is always indicated in this age group. Autoimmune disorders such as elderly-onset rheumatoid arthritis and systemic lupus erythematosus, as well as dermatomyositis and other types of vasculitis, must be considered in the differential diagnosis and evaluated by clinical information and serologic testing. There is support for the concept that elderly-onset rheumatoid arthritis is the same disorder as PMR with a negative rheumatoid factor, a more proximal focus of joint inflammation, and a good response to low-dose prednisone. The distinction may be semantic, because neither disorder tends to evolve into an erosive arthritis. A more protracted clinical course, however, is often seen in patients in whom distal synovitis is a prominent feature, and these patients are classified as having elderly-onset rheumatoid arthritis. PMR and GCA should always be considered in the setting of a fever of unknown origin, because symptoms and signs may be occult or the history may be incomplete.

TREATMENT   Rx

Both PMR and GCA are highly responsive to corticosteroids, which are the preferred treatment choice. This response is so characteristic that an immediate and dramatic improvement in PMR and GCA symptoms within 1 to 3 days after steroid institution supports the diagnosis. Conversely, the lack of a rapid and significant improvement in signs, symptoms, and function within 5 to 7 days should be considered a major point against the diagnosis. The physician should then consider an alternative diagnosis (e.g., tumor, infection) or the presence of GCA in PMR patients, which might demand a higher steroid dose. Because the inflammatory set point of the two disorders is different, different doses of steroids are used at the onset of treatment. Whereas PMR usually responds to 15 mg/day of prednisone, GCA usually requires 60 to 80 mg/day of prednisone in divided doses or higher doses if organ or tissue damage is present or threatened. In GCA, if visual symptoms such as a fixed loss or amaurosis fugax are present, the patient should be treated with high-dose intravenous methylprednisolone at doses ranging from 40 mg every 8 hours to 1 g/day for 3 days, followed by high-dose oral steroids in divided doses.

Within 2 to 3 days after the institution of steroids, most symptoms of PMR or GCA clear rapidly, and patients describe a miraculous improvement. The steroid dose is then maintained for 2 to 3 weeks, during which time the ESR, C-reactive protein, hemoglobin, and platelet counts normalize. Steroid taper is then instituted and is guided by the clinical response. In PMR, the dose is commonly tapered by 1 mg every 7 to 10 days; in GCA, it is tapered by 5 to 10 mg every 7 to 10 days. In GCA, the use of alternate-day corticosteroid regimens to minimize steroid side effects is generally not recommended because randomized controlled trials have demonstrated higher rates of treatment failure with alternate-day dosing schedules. It is important that the taper be guided primarily by clinical findings (e.g., PMR stiffness, headache, fatigue) and that the level of ESR elevation be considered within that clinical context. One

should never "chase the ESR," because this would inappropriately subject an elderly patient to a dangerously high cumulative dose of steroids, with the attendant side effects. An increased dose of prednisone should be based on a change in symptoms, not solely on an increase in the ESR. One possible exception is a patient with a history of GCA and prior abrupt vision loss in one eye, in whom any further compromise of vision would be catastrophic. The effective dose demanded for a flare is often as low as 5 to 10 mg of prednisone; uncommonly, up to 60 mg/day may be needed to control symptoms (e.g., visual abnormalities). A persistently elevated ESR (>50 mm/hour) without PMR or GCA symptoms should alert the physician to look for alternative causes, such as infection. Treatment is a careful balancing act between disease control and avoidance of steroid-related toxicity. The overall goal is to attain the best disease control with the lowest dose of steroids. In most patients, prednisone can be tapered safely in 1 to 2 years. However, some patients may need to take low doses of steroids for 2 years or more. Appropriate immunizations, osteoporosis regimens (calcium, vitamin D, and bisphosphonates), and metabolic monitoring are mandatory in all patients prescribed chronic steroid therapy.

The major feared outcome in GCA is ischemic complications of the disease, most often vision loss or, less frequently, cerebrovascular accidents. Vision loss is usually irreversible, and although it is uncommon once the diagnosis is suspected and glucocorticoid therapy is instituted, it can occur early in the course of treatment. Aspirin is known to be protective against ischemic events in patients with atherosclerosis and has anti-inflammatory effects in inflamed blood vessels, including inhibition of IFN-γ. Two retrospective studies have suggested that low-dose aspirin may be protective against cranial ischemic complications in GCA. Adjunctive therapy with low-dose aspirin should be considered unless there is a strong contraindication to its use.

Alternative immunosuppressive agents have been tested in both PMR and GCA patients in an attempt to "spare steroids" and control the inflammatory state. Studies examining the efficacy of methotrexate in GCA have yielded mixed results, with the largest, most recent study showing no incremental benefit from combined therapy.[1] One meta-analysis of three randomized placebo-controlled trials suggested a modest benefit to the use of methotrexate in GCA in terms of its steroid-sparing benefit and a reduced likelihood of flares.[2] Given the modest nature of the benefit demonstrated, the methodologic issues with such a meta-analysis, and the potential toxicities of methotrexate in this elderly population, methotrexate is not routinely incorporated as first-line therapy in GCA. In PMR, one study found that methotrexate provided a steroid-sparing benefit and possibly reduced the number of flares.[3] The magnitude of the benefit appears to be modest, however, and no reduction in corticosteroid-related side effects was demonstrated. At present, methotrexate is not standard in the management of either disease, but in individual patients with refractory disease or excessive corticosteroid morbidities, rheumatoid arthritis–type doses of methotrexate (7.5 to 20 mg/week) or azathioprine (2 mg/kg/day) are added in some instances.

Tumor necrosis factor inhibition has been of interest as a potential therapeutic strategy in GCA and PMR. Tumor necrosis factor has been demonstrated in the inflamed arteries of patients with GCA, and inhibition of this cytokine has a known clinical benefit in other inflammatory granulomatous disorders, such as Crohn's disease. Randomized controlled trials of infliximab in GCA[4] and PMR,[5] however, failed to demonstrate a benefit in terms of preventing relapses or offering a steroid-sparing effect.

FUTURE DIRECTIONS

Better understanding of the disease-causing roles of immunologically active cells and their cytokine products, along with genetics and correlations with clinical subsets, will lead to more focused treatment modalities and the avoidance of long-term treatment with steroids.

1. Hoffman GS, Cid MC, Hellmann DB, et al. A multicenter, randomized, double-blind, placebo-controlled trial of adjuvant methotrexate treatment for giant cell arteritis. *Arthritis Rheum.* 2002;46:1309-1318.
2. Mahr AD, Jover JA, Spiera RF, et al. Adjunctive methotrexate for treatment of giant cell arteritis: an individual patient data meta-analysis. *Arthritis Rheum.* 2007;56:2789-2797.
3. Caporali R, Cimmino MA, Ferraccioli G, et al. Prednisone plus methotrexate for polymyalgia rheumatica: a randomized, double-blind, placebo-controlled trial. *Ann Intern Med.* 2004;141:493-500.
4. Hoffman GS, Cid MC, Rendt-Zagar KE, et al. Infliximab for maintenance of glucocorticosteroid-induced remission of giant cell arteritis: a randomized trial. *Ann Intern Med.* 2007;146:621-630.
5. Salvarani C, Macchioni P, Manzini C, et al. Infliximab plus prednisone or placebo plus prednisone for the initial treatment of polymyalgia rheumatica: a randomized trial. *Ann Intern Med.* 2007; 146:631-639.

SUGGESTED READINGS

Assie C, Janvresse A, Pilssonnier D, et al. Long-term follow-up of upper and lower extremity vasculitis related to giant cell arteritis: a series of 36 patients. *Medicine (Baltimore).* 2011;90:40-51. *Review of manifestations noting that the median chronic prednisone dose was 6 mg, and prednisone could be discontinued in only one third of patients.*

Gonzalez-Gay MA, Martinez-Dubois C, Agudo M, et al. Giant cell arteritis: epidemiology, diagnosis, and management. *Curr Rheumatol Rep.* 2010;12:436-442. *Review.*

Marie I, Proux A, Duhaut P, et al. Long-term follow-up of aortic involvement in giant cell arteritis: a series of 48 patients. *Medicine (Baltimore).* 2009;88:182-192. *Review showing that 65% of patients required chronic low-dose prednisone.*

Meisner RJ, Labropoulos N, Gasparis AP, et al. How to diagnose giant cell arteritis. *Int Angiol.* 2011;30:58-63. *Ultrasound and MRI may be alternatives to biopsy.*

Walvick MD, Walvick MP. Giant cell arteritis: laboratory predictors of a positive temporal artery biopsy. *Ophthalmology.* 2011. [Epub ahead of print.] *Predictors included ESR >45 mm/hr, CRP >2.45 mg/dL, and platelets >400,000/μL.*

Waqar S, Salman R, Sleep T. Ophthalmic manifestations of giant cell arteritis. *Br J Hosp Med (Lond).* 2011;72:26-30. *Review.*

280

INFECTIONS OF BURSAE, JOINTS, AND BONES

ERIC L. MATTESON AND DOUGLAS R. OSMON

INFECTION OF BURSAE
Septic Bursitis

DEFINITION

Bursae are the satellite structures that form to protect tissues from bony prominences. The superficial bursae, including the olecranon, prepatella, infrapatella, and bursae over the first metatarsophalangeal bunions, are more likely to become infected than are the deep bursae, such as the subacromial, trochanteric, and iliopsoas bursae.

EPIDEMIOLOGY

Olecranon bursitis may occur in as many as 10 in 100,000 persons. The majority of cases occur in men, and antecedent trauma to the skin is frequent.

PATHOBIOLOGY

Septic bursitis of superficial bursae is most commonly due to direct inoculation through the overlying skin; less commonly, it is secondary to overlying cellulitis. Most cases of deep septic bursitis are due to contiguous spread from adjacent infected joints or hematogenous seeding.

Predisposing risk factors for septic bursitis include trauma to the skin, as may occur in plumbers, athletes, and patients with chronic obstructive pulmonary disease (COPD) who frequently lean on the elbows; pre- or infrapatellar septic bursitis occurs in housecleaners, gardeners, and carpet layers. At least one third of patients with septic bursitis have an underlying comorbid illness such as diabetes mellitus, rheumatoid arthritis, gout, COPD, or alcoholism.

CLINICAL MANIFESTATIONS

In immune-competent patients, septic bursitis often but not always presents with fever and erythema and warmth of the overlying skin; there may be swelling of the bursae. In contrast to those with septic arthritis, patients with septic bursitis of superficial bursae have intact range of motion of the joints, which may be limited only at the extremes of flexion. Pain on motion of the joint and restriction of joint range of motion are highly suggestive of septic arthritis. Acute phase reactants such as C-reactive protein, the sedimentation rate, and the white blood cell count (WBC) may be elevated.

DIAGNOSIS

Radiography should be performed to look for a foreign body and to evaluate the surrounding bones. Aspiration of bursal fluid is helpful in the diagnosis of patients who have pain, erythema, and/or swelling of an affected area. However, given the risk of contaminating the bursa if the aspiration occurs through cellulitic skin, many clinicians choose to aspirate a bursa only if empirical antimicrobial therapy has failed. Ultrasound or computed tomography (CT) guidance greatly enhances the successful aspiration of superficial bursae. Care must be taken not to violate the joint space when aspirating a bursa to avoid inoculating the joint space.

The leukocyte count of the bursal fluid is generally lower than that seen in septic arthritis, with a mean of 13,500 cells/mm^3. Even in immune-competent hosts, cell counts can range from less than 1500 to greater than 100,000/mm^3. A leukocyte count greater than 2000/mm^3 has a sensitivity of 94% and a specificity of 79% for superficial (olecranon or prepatellar) bursitis. Bacterial culture and in vitro susceptibilities must be obtained; if additional fluid is available, a Gram stain may be obtained, although its sensitivity may be as low as 15%. The presence of crystals does not exclude the possibility of septic bursitis.

Staphylococcus aureus (Chapter 296) is the most common cause of septic bursitis, present in more than 80% of culture-proved cases, followed by β-hemolytic streptococci. Aerobic gram-negative bacilli, including *Escherichia coli, Campylobacter jejuni,* and *Pseudomonas* species, are rare causes of septic bursitis. Chronic bursitis may be associated with systemic infections due to *Brucella abortus,* atypical mycobacteria, or *Mycobacterium tuberculosis,* as well as fungi; the presence of these infections should raise the possibility of systemic infection.

Differential Diagnosis

In the immune-competent host, nonseptic bursitis (Chapter 271) may have a somewhat more indolent presentation than septic bursitis. The differential diagnosis includes gout, pseudogout, arthritis, and trauma with hemobursa. An overlying cellulitis may be confused with bursitis. Fever is usually not present in nonseptic bursitis due to mechanical or friction trauma.

TREATMENT Rx

Treatment of septic bursitis is guided by knowledge of the putative underlying organisms, in most cases, *S. aureus*. Because the Gram stain is positive in less than two thirds of patients and cultures may be delayed, empirical therapy is guided by the clinical presentation. Most patients can be treated as outpatients, but those who are immunocompromised may require hospitalization for intravenous antibiotic therapy. Initial ambulatory treatment in patients without comorbidities may consist of an oral antistaphylococcal penicillin or first-generation cephalosporin. If community-acquired methicillin-resistant *S. aureus* (MRSA) is suspected, co-trimoxazole or minocycline may be added to one of these agents. In patients who are allergic to penicillin, oral clindamycin or linezolid may be used. Patients who have severe inflammation, are septic, or are immunocompromised may require hospitalization for initiation of treatment with intravenous nafcillin, oxacillin, or cefazolin; if MRSA is suspected, intravenous vancomycin, daptomycin, or linezolid should be used. Vancomycin can also be used in patients who are allergic to penicillin.

The duration of antimicrobial therapy is guided by the clinical response and comorbid states. It should be continued until there is no longer bursal inflammation. This may require several weeks of intravenous or oral therapy and multiple aspirations. Failure of the septic bursitis to respond to initial antibiotic therapy mandates a second course of therapy; recurrence thereafter or inability to adequately drain the bursa with needle aspiration is an indication for surgical intervention.

PREVENTION

Because superficial septic bursitis is often associated with occasional or avocational activities involving kneeling or resting on the elbows, using protective padding may be helpful.

PROGNOSIS

The optimal duration of therapy is unknown, but prognosis of superficial bursitis is generally excellent. The presence of comorbid conditions, especially those associated with deep bursal infections, including septic arthritis, bacteremia, and osteomyelitis, is associated with more intractable and difficult disease.

INFECTION OF JOINTS
Septic Arthritis

DEFINITION

Septic arthritis refers to infection of a joint by a microorganism. It is associated with increased morbidity and mortality, as well as loss of articular integrity and function. Septic arthritis is usually caused by a bacterial infection. Other microorganisms can cause infections with clinical characteristics that differ from those of bacterial infections; these are reviewed separately.

NONGONOCOCCAL SEPTIC ARTHRITIS

EPIDEMIOLOGY

The incidence of septic arthritis affecting native joints is about 5 to 8 in 100,000 patient years. Among patients presenting with an acutely swollen and painful joint, the prevalence of bacterial arthritis ranges widely, from less than 10 to as high as 27%, depending on the source population. Nongonococcal septic arthritis is the most common form of septic arthritis and is somewhat more common in men than in women.

PATHOBIOLOGY

More than 90% of cases of septic arthritis are due to staphylococci or streptococci (Table 280-1). Septic arthritis can result from direct inoculation (e.g., accidents, bites, surgery) or by extension from infected bone into an adjacent joint space. Approximately 75% of cases are due to hematogenous spread, particularly in patients with indwelling catheters and immunocompromised patients. Septic arthritis due to needle arthrocentesis (<1 in 10,000 procedures) or arthroscopy (4 cases per 1000 to 10,000 procedures) is very rare.

Bacteria causing septic arthritis produce an acute inflammatory reaction in the synovial membrane. Synovial hyperplasia and inflammatory cell immigration with the release of pro-inflammatory and cartilage-destroying cytokines and proteases result in damage to cartilage and bone. Bacterial toxins and DNA and superantigens, such as those seen in staphylococcal toxic shock syndrome, also contribute to cartilage and bone damage.

Risk factors for the development of septic arthritis include diabetes, alcoholism, cutaneous ulcers, intravenous drug use, prosthetic joints, rheumatoid arthritis, osteoarthritis, and low socioeconomic status, as well as advanced age, skin infection, indwelling intravenous catheters, cancer, and immunosuppressive therapies, including biologic response modifiers used in the management of autoimmune diseases such as rheumatoid arthritis and inflammatory bowel disease.

CLINICAL MANIFESTATIONS

Most patients with bacterial arthritis feel ill and have fever. Immunocompromised and elderly patients may not have a marked febrile response. Most cases (>80%) of septic arthritis are monoarticular; the knee is involved in more than 50% of cases. Polyarticular joint sepsis may be seen in immunocompromised patients and those with rheumatoid arthritis or systemic lupus erythematosus. Such patients frequently lack typical signs and symptoms of infection and may not appear to be particularly ill at presentation, but they may have rapid cardiovascular decompensation. This is particularly true for patients who are taking glucocorticosteroids, other immunosuppressive agents, and biologic response modifiers, including tumor necrosis factor-α (TNF-α) inhibitors.

Patients with septic arthritis affecting nondiarthrodial joints, such as the acromioclavicular or sacroiliac joints, may have a history of intravenous drug use or may have intravenous catheters in place to treat other medical conditions. Infection of the symphysis pubis is associated with previous urinary tract surgery, pelvic malignancy, intravenous drug use, or vigorous weight-bearing physical activity, such as long-distance running, in female athletes.

A finding of microorganisms in the joint should lead to an appropriate history and physical examination to identify a source of hematogenous infection, such as cellulitis, pneumonia, or urinary tract infection. Staphylococci and β-hemolytic streptococci may enter directly through open wounds, whereas gram-negative infection may be associated with bowel or bladder disease.

DIAGNOSIS

Plain radiography should be performed to evaluate the surrounding bones and joint space and to provide a baseline for comparison after therapy is completed. Imaging modalities such as magnetic resonance imaging (MRI), CT, and plain radiography are useful to determine whether there is associated osteomyelitis and in cases of diagnostic uncertainty. Blood cultures are positive in up to 50% of patients with bacterial septic arthritis and should be obtained in all patients in whom this diagnosis is suspected. If septic arthritis is suspected, synovial fluid arthrocentesis is indicated, and the fluid should be examined for bacterial culture and Gram stain; the latter is positive in only about 50% of patients. The choice of culture method is not critical, whether blood culture or conventional agar plate. Specific cultures and stains for fungal and mycobacterial organisms should be done if there is a history of exposure or if antibacterial therapy has failed. Polymerase chain reaction

| TABLE 280-1 | MICROORGANISMS RESPONSIBLE FOR ACUTE SEPTIC ARTHRITIS AND ACUTE AND CHRONIC OSTEOMYELITIS |

Septic Arthritis		Osteomyelitis: Acute and Chronic	
MICROORGANISM	**FREQUENCY (%)**	**MICROORGANISM**	**FREQUENCY (%)**
GRAM-POSITIVE	**60-90**	**GRAM-POSITIVE**	**80-90**
Staphylococcus aureus	50-70	*Staphylococcus aureus*	60-80
Group A, B, C streptococci	15-30	Group A, B, C streptococci	10-20
Coagulase-negative staphylococci	6-20	*Staphylococcus epidermidis*	10-15
Streptococcus pneumoniae	1-3	*Streptococcus pneumoniae*	<1
Enterococcus sp	<1	*Enterococcus* sp	1-2
Corynebacterium sp	<1	*Corynebacterium* sp	1-2
GRAM-NEGATIVE	**5-25**	**GRAM-NEGATIVE**	**5-20**
Salmonella sp		*Salmonella* sp	
Pseudomonas aeruginosa		*Enterobacter* sp	
Escherichia coli		*Pseudomonas aeruginosa*	
Klebsiella pneumoniae		*Brucella* sp	
Enterobacter sp		*Pasteurella multocida*	
Kingella kingae		*Bartonella henselae*	
Haemophilus influenzae	<1-3*	*Propionibacterium* sp	
ANAEROBES	**1-2**	**ANAEROBES**	
Fusobacterium sp		*Bacteroides* sp	
Bacteroides fragilis			
MISCELLANEOUS	**<5**	**MISCELLANEOUS**	**5-7**
Mycoplasma		*Mycobacterium* sp	
Mycobacterium sp		Fungi (candidiasis, coccidioidomycosis, blastomycosis, histoplasmosis)	
Fungi			
Viruses			
Algae			

*Children.

(PCR) assays may be helpful for diagnosing less common joint infections such as *Borrelia,* but the value of PCR over standard culture for the diagnosis of staphylococcal or streptococcal joint infection has not been demonstrated. Other helpful examinations include leukocyte count and differential, as well as evaluation of the synovial fluid for the presence of crystals. The presence of gout or pseudogout crystals does not exclude the possibility of septic arthritis, particularly in patients whose WBC is above 50,000/mm³.

A frequent clinical scenario is the patient who is anticoagulated. Because of the rapidly destructive nature of septic arthritis and the often profound systemic consequences, anticoagulation is not a contraindication to arthrocentesis. The procedure may be assisted by ultrasound guidance, especially when only small amounts of joint fluid are present or when the joint is difficult to aspirate. CT-guided arthrocentesis is particularly useful for aspiration of deep joints such as the hips and nondiarthrodial joints.

The total WBC and differential in synovial fluid is helpful in distinguishing infected from noninfected joints in immunocompetent patients. A diagnosis of septic arthritis is present in 47% of patients with a synovial WBC greater than 50,000/mm³ and in 77% of patients with a WBC greater than 100,000/mm³. It is important to realize that a WBC less than 50,000/mm³, especially in immunocompromised patients, can be associated with septic arthritis, so the absolute WBC in synovial fluid is not, by itself, a reliable way to confirm or exclude a diagnosis of septic arthritis.

Differential Diagnosis

Symptoms of septic arthritis, such as acute joint pain, swelling, and even fever, with an increase in acute phase reactants, can be caused by crystalline arthritis (Chapter 281), especially pseudogout and gout, as well as psoriatic arthritis and reactive arthritis (Chapter 273). In patients who have preexisting inflammatory joint disease, such as rheumatoid arthritis, septic arthritis may be suspected if there is a sudden onset of acute or subacute monoarticular or pauciarticular joint swelling when the disease is otherwise well controlled. The presence or absence of fever is not a reliable indicator of an infected joint (Fig. 280-1).

TREATMENT **Rx**

As soon as the joint has been aspirated and, ideally, after blood cultures have been obtained, prompt treatment with antibiotics must be instituted. Removal of purulent material and, where appropriate, débridement are essential. The choice of empirical antimicrobial therapy is based on which organisms are the likely cause of the septic arthritis and on the results of Gram stain and culture. No advantage of one antibiotic regimen over another has been demonstrated. If the initial Gram stain of the synovial fluid reveals gram-positive cocci, vancomycin is recommended, given the increasing frequency of infection due to MRSA and the need to initiate effective antimicrobial therapy as soon as possible. Daptomycin and linezolid are alternative agents. If the initial

---

Clinical Evaluation of Infections of Soft Tissues, Joints, and Bone

FIGURE 280-1. Clinical evaluation of infections of soft tissues, joints, and bone. CBC = complete blood count; CT = computed tomography; ESR = erythrocyte sedimentation rate; GA = gonococcal arthritis; HIV = human immunodeficiency virus; IV = intravenous; MRI = magnetic resonance imaging; NGSA = nongonococcal septic arthritis; OA = osteoarthritis; PCR = polymerase chain reaction; PET = positron emission tomography; PMN = polymorphonuclear leukocyte; RA = rheumatoid arthritis.

Gram stain reveals gram-negative bacilli, an agent with broad coverage, including activity against *Pseudomonas aeruginosa*, is recommended. Such agents include ceftazidime, cefepime, imipenem, meropenem, piperacillin-tazobactam, and intravenous ciprofloxacin. If the Gram stain is negative, vancomycin alone in immunocompetent patients or in those unlikely to have gram-negative infection based on history and examination, or vancomycin plus one of the gram-negative antibacterials listed, is reasonable. Once culture and in vitro susceptibility results are available, therapy can be modified. The duration of antibacterial therapy usually ranges from 2 to 6 weeks, with data suggesting that one aspiration and 2 weeks of therapy are usually adequate, at least in children.[1]

The role of arthroscopic versus needle versus open drainage of the joint is unsettled. Surgical management is appropriate for septic arthritis of the hip, for patients who fail to respond to serial needle aspiration and antibiotic therapy, and for patients who appear to be developing life-threatening complications such as necrotizing fasciitis. No studies have demonstrated the utility of lavage with or without synovectomy by arthroscopy versus arthrotomy or débridement. Patients should be mobilized as rapidly as possible to prevent joint contractures. In children, concomitant oral dexamethasone for 4 days can lead to more rapid symptomatic improvements.[2]

PREVENTION

In patients requiring immunosuppression or glucocorticosteroid therapy to manage their underlying diseases, every effort should be made to use the lowest possible dose of these medications.

PROGNOSIS

Up to one third of patients with septic arthritis have a poor functional outcome, particularly older patients, patients with preexisting diseases of the joints such as osteoarthritis or rheumatoid arthritis, and patients with prosthetic joints. Poor joint outcome is associated with *S. aureus* infection in more than 50% of patients; mortality may be as high as 10 to 15%, particularly in patients who are immunocompromised or have polyarticular sepsis.

GONOCOCCAL SEPTIC ARTHRITIS

EPIDEMIOLOGY

Neisseria gonorrhoeae (Chapter 307) is a common cause of polyarthralgias and arthritis as well as oligoarticular arthritis and tenosynovitis in young, healthy patients. Disseminated gonococcal infection occurs in 0.5 to 3% of patients with gonorrhea (Chapter 307). Many of of these patients have arthritis. Disseminated gonococcal infection and septic arthritis due to *N. gonorrhoeae* occur two to three times more often in women than in men. Most patients do not have a recent history of a symptomatic genital infection. The incidence of gonococcal arthritis is 133 cases per 100,000 population per year. Predisposing factors for disseminated gonococcal infection with arthritis include pregnancy, recent menstruation, complement deficiencies (C5, C6, C7, or C8), and systemic lupus erythematosus.

CLINICAL MANIFESTATIONS

Patients with gonococcal arthritis usually present with one of two clinical syndromes. The first is a purulent arthritis without skin lesions; the second is the triad of tenosynovitis, dermatitis, and polyarthralgias without purulent arthritis. The latter patients may have bacteremia and fever as well as maculopapular, vesicular, necrotic, pustular skin lesions anywhere on the integument. The arthritis is usually asymmetrical and may involve large or small joints, typically the elbows and knees or joints distal to these.

DIAGNOSIS

A high degree of clinical suspicion is required for diagnosis because many patients are asymptomatic for the primary infection. A thorough joint evaluation is important, as is an evaluation of soft tissues, particularly for tenosynovitis affecting the hands and feet. Cultures of blood, endocervix, and urethra are essential; cultures of the pharynx and rectum may be very helpful. *N. gonorrhoeae* is isolated in less than 30% of patients with the tenosynovitis-dermatitis syndrome and in about 50% of those with monoarthritis. PCR may be used to detect the gonococcal DNA in synovial fluid, skin lesions, urine, and throat samples, which are culture negative. Cultures should be submitted on Thayer-Martin media. Patients with suspected gonococcal arthritis should be screened for other coexisting sexually transmitted diseases (Chapter 293) such as syphilis, HIV, and chlamydia, as well as hepatitis B and C.

Viral Arthritis

Patients with viral syndromes may have polyarthralgias or inflammatory polyarthritis, which can mimic rheumatoid arthritis (Chapter 272). The most common viral infections associated with arthritis include hepatitis A, B, and C; cytomegalovirus; parvovirus B19; rubella; measles; and HIV. Other forms of viral arthritis are caused by adenovirus, echovirus, Epstein-Barr virus, and herpes zoster in North America and Europe; chikungunya and o'nyong-nyong viruses, especially in Africa; and Ross River virus in Australia. Arthritis related to viral infections is likely principally reactive in nature, rather than being caused by direct synovial infection.

Other Forms of Infectious Arthritis

FUNGAL ARTHRITIS

Fungal arthritis is unusual and most commonly occurs in immunocompromised patients. Treatment with high doses of immunosuppressants, anti-TNF agents, and possibly other biologic response modifiers used in the treatment of rheumatoid arthritis and other autoimmune diseases may increase the risk for fungal infections. The infections are often systemic and may be indolent. An understanding of the epidemiology of the organisms as well as the patient's risk factors, including occupational and avocational risk factors, is essential to the diagnosis. The most common fungi in the United States include *Blastomyces dermatitidis*, *Coccidioides immitis*, and *Histoplasma capsulatum*. *Sporothrix schenckii* fungal infections may be seen, especially in gardeners. More unusual infections occur in immunocompromised patients, including *Aspergillus*, *Candida*, *Cryptococcus*, and *Nocardia*.

LYME ARTHRITIS

Lyme disease (Chapter 329) usually causes oligoarticular arthritis, most commonly affecting the knee. Antibiotic treatment, initially with a second-generation cephalosporin, is effective. Polyarticular disease affecting the small joints has been associated with HLA-DR4, which is found in greater frequency in patients with rheumatoid arthritis.

MYCOPLASMA ARTHRITIS

Mycoplasma hominis (Chapter 325) causes an oligo- or monoarticular arthritis. Risk factors include an immunocompromised state and hypogammaglobulinemia. The treatment of choice is tetracyclines, usually doxycycline; alternatively, clindamycin or fluoroquinolones can be used.

TUBERCULOUS ARTHRITIS

Most cases of tuberculosis (TB; Chapter 332) in Canada, the United States, western Europe, Australia, and New Zealand occur in immigrants. The arthritis is usually monoarticular or oligoarticular, affecting larger joints, and TB should be suspected in patients who have refractory mono- or pauciarticular arthritis thought to be secondary to another bacterial infection or to a systemic inflammatory disease such as rheumatoid arthritis. TB screening is mandatory for all patients before beginning treatment with immunosuppressive drugs or biologic response modifiers.

The diagnosis of TB may be delayed because of a lack of suspicion because patients may not have pulmonary disease. Atypical mycobacterial infection may occur in fishermen and immunocompromised patients. Appropriate treatment for septic arthritis due to TB is based on guidelines and in vitro susceptibility testing, but it often includes isoniazid, ethambutol, or rifampin and pyrazinamide as empirical therapy (Chapter 332). Atypical mycobacteria are often not susceptible to traditional antituberculous agents, and infectious disease consultation is recommended. Patients with a history of TB in whom anti-TNF therapies are being considered should be appropriately treated for TB before these drugs are started. Patients with a positive purified protein derivative (PPD) test or QuantIFERON assay for TB without a history of diagnosed tuberculosis should be treated prophylactically for several months before starting anti-TNF therapy. Clinical suspicion and culture of synovial fluid or synovial membrane obtained at biopsy are essential to the diagnosis.

SYPHILIS

Musculoskeletal involvement by syphilis infections (Chapter 327) is manifold and includes mono- or oligoarticular arthritis, polyarthralgias, tenosynovitis, sacroiliitis, spondylitis, chondritis, osteitis, and periostitis. Charcot's joints, osteitis, and chronic arthritis are typical of tertiary syphilis. Most patients with syphilis-related arthritis can be treated successfully. Arthritis may complicate congenital, secondary, and tertiary syphilis.

PROSTHETIC JOINT INFECTION

More than 1 million joint replacements (Chapter 285) are done each year in the United States, and this number continues to increase. Infection occurs in 0.3 to 1.7% of hip arthroplasties and 0.8 to 1.9% of knee arthroplasties, and the infection risk is two- to three-fold higher in patients with rheumatoid arthritis. Prosthetic joint infections are classified as (1) early infections, occurring within 3 months of joint replacement; (2) delayed infections, occurring 3 months to about 1 year after joint replacement; and (3) late infections, occurring more than 1 to 2 years after joint replacement. Infections occurring within the first year are usually related to the implantation surgery itself, and late infections are usually due to hematogenous spread.

The development of a bacterial biofilm on the prosthetic joint is characteristic of prosthetic joint infection, increasing the susceptibility to infection in experimental animal models with as few as 100 colony-forming units. These biofilms are formed by bacterial glycocalyx, which increases the organisms' resistance to antimicrobial agents and likely accounts for the difficulty in obtaining viable organisms from the infected joint. More than half of all prosthetic joint infections of hips and knees are caused by staphylococci. Other organisms, including gram-negative bacilli, anaerobes, and *Candida* species, may also cause infection. In particular, *Propionibacterium* species are associated with infected shoulder arthroplasties. About 20% of cases are polymicrobial, and in 7%, cultures are negative.

Risk factors associated with the development of prosthetic joint infection include wound healing complications, prior superficial surgical site infection, prior infection of the joint, previous surgery on the joint, rheumatoid arthritis, advanced age, obesity, smoking, cancer, and diabetes mellitus. Other risk factors include simultaneous bilateral arthroplasty, prolonged operative time, requirement for blood transfusion, and infection occurring elsewhere in the body that can hematogenously seed the prosthesis.

Patients with early-onset infection may have classic symptoms and signs of septic arthritis, including joint pain, effusion, erythema, and fever. Patients with delayed infection may have only joint pain, with or without implant loosening, requiring a high degree of suspicion for the presence of infection.

The definitive diagnosis of prosthetic joint infection is based on the recovery of organisms from multiple specimens of synovial fluid and periprosthetic tissue, sonication of the prosthesis itself, acute inflammation suggestive of infection on pathologic examination of periprosthetic tissue obtained at surgery, or the presence of a sinus track communicating with the prosthesis, even in the absence of microorganisms.

An elevated sedimentation rate or C-reactive protein without another obvious cause, such as inflammatory arthritis or recent surgery, is very suggestive of infection in a patient with a painful, loose prosthesis. Plain radiographs may show loosening, new bone formation, and lucencies along the implant margin but are often nonspecific. Technetium-based scintigraphy combined with indium-labeled white blood cell scanning is suggestive of established infection but is often not performed owing to the expense. MRI and CT have low utility in diagnosing prosthetic joint infection.

Surgical treatment of prosthetic joint infection typically consists of débridement with retention of the prosthesis for acute infection, resection arthroplasty with or without staged reimplantation for chronic infection, or amputation in a few limited instances. Systemic antibiotic therapy in a patient with a prosthetic joint infection is pathogen directed and driven by the surgical therapy used to manage the infection. Following an attempt at salvage of the prosthesis with 2 to 6 weeks of effective intravenous antibiotic therapy, chronic suppressive therapy with oral antimicrobial agents is often used. In rifampin-susceptible staphylococcal infections, its addition to a companion intravenous or oral antimicrobial is recommended to avoid the emergence of resistance, to treat biofilm organisms, and to improve the chance of salvaging the prosthesis. Following resection arthroplasty, 4 to 6 weeks of pathogen-directed intravenous therapy is typical before an attempt at reimplantation several weeks later. The use of depot local antimicrobial therapy with antibiotic-impregnated polymethylmethacrylate spacers following resection arthroplasty is also very common.

PREVENTION

In addition to optimizing comorbidities such as diabetes mellitus and discontinuing tobacco use preoperatively, careful screening for infection, including asymptomatic urinary tract infection, is prudent when considering joint surgery. Perioperative antibiotic treatment with cephalosporin in patients undergoing prosthetic joint replacement reduces the risk of infection by approximately three-fold. **3** Antimicrobial therapy should be given within 60 minutes of the initial incision, ideally before tourniquet application. Cefazolin or cefuroxime can be given to patients with normal renal function, and vancomycin can be used in patients who are allergic to penicillin.

Whether an antirheumatic agent should be stopped before joint replacement surgery is unclear. The usual practice is to hold drugs such as methotrexate and anti-TNF agents for one to four half-lives before and after surgery. The impact of this strategy on reducing prosthetic joint infections is unknown.

● OSTEOMYELITIS

DEFINITION

Osteomyelitis is a bacterial infection of bone that causes destruction and can occur through a variety of mechanisms.

EPIDEMIOLOGY

Osteomyelitis of the bones of the foot in adult patients with diabetes, neuropathy, and arterial insufficiency is very common. Hematogenous seeding of the spine also occurs, but less frequently. The incidence of osteomyelitis due to trauma and surgery is increasing.

PATHOBIOLOGY

Osteomyelitis can develop from (1) hematogenous seeding from a distant infection, (2) contiguous spread from nearby skin and joints, and (3) penetration of microorganisms into bone at the time of trauma or surgery. Unless there is trauma or the presence of a foreign body, bone is typically very resistant to infection. Organisms such as *S. aureus* cause disease more frequently because they colonize the skin in up to 30 to 40% of individuals, frequently cause cellulitis and bacteremia, and have the ability to bind to bone through the expression of receptors for fibronectin and collagen.

Hematogenous causes of osteomyelitis typically present in the elderly; it usually involves two or more vertebrae and their intervening disc spaces. Bacteria gain access to these structures through the arterial and venous systems (Batson's venous plexus). Bacteremia from any source can cause osteomyelitis of the spine, but cellulitis, urinary tract infection, and pneumonia are the most common sources.

Contiguous focus osteomyelitis is common in adults, typically occurring in the elderly. It results from the spread of infection from nearby skin, often in the feet of patients with diabetes, neuropathy, or vascular insufficiency, or in pelvic bones in patients with decubitus due to impaired sensation from spinal cord injury or disease. Alternatively, it can occur at the time of orthopedic surgery, from contamination at the time of an open fracture, or from a human or animal bite.

Acute osteomyelitis has a duration of less than 10 days, whereas chronic infection has a duration of more than 10 days. *S. aureus* is the most common cause of hematogenous and contiguous osteomyelitis in adults. Osteomyelitis due to β-hemolytic streptococci and aerobic gram-negative bacilli is much less common, but it can occur if infections due to these organisms result in hematogenous seeding, if nosocomial contiguous osteomyelitis occurs due to surgical site infection, or if contamination occurs at the time of traumatic open fracture. Polymicrobial infection, including infection due to anaerobes, is very common in osteomyelitis of the bones of the feet associated with diabetes and vascular insufficiency. Coagulase-negative staphylococci can be pathogenic in patients with orthopedic implants.

CLINICAL MANIFESTATIONS

Localized pain over the affected bones is a hallmark of osteomyelitis. A sinus tract or swelling and erythema due to concomitant soft tissue infection or abscess may be present in osteomyelitis due to contiguous infection. Constitutional symptoms, including fever, are present in the minority of cases and more often in hematogenous osteomyelitis. If neurologic structures are involved, neurologic signs and symptoms may be present. Signs and symptoms due to a coexisting infection that has caused hematogenous osteomyelitis may be present as well. The differential diagnosis of osteomyelitis includes diseases that can cause acute and chronic bone pain in adults, including osteoarthritis, metastatic malignancy, fractures, and SAPHO (synovitis, acne, pustulosis, hyperostosis, and osteitis) syndrome, as well as postoperative pain and soft tissue infection without concomitant osteomyelitis.

DIAGNOSIS

The WBC is often elevated in hematogenous and acute osteomyelitis. Serum inflammatory markers such as the sedimentation rate and C-reactive protein are often abnormal, particularly in cases of hematogenous infection, but may be normal in chronic contiguous osteomyelitis. Blood cultures are positive in 25 to 50% of cases of hematogenous infection but are almost always negative in chronic osteomyelitis unless concomitant soft tissue infection is present. In the setting of chronic contiguous osteomyelitis, plain radiographs often show specific abnormalities; in vertebral osteomyelitis, they are often not helpful in confirming the diagnosis of infection.

The ability to percutaneously probe or palpate bone with a probe is a simple, effective diagnostic test in patients with diabetes mellitus and possible contiguous osteomyelitis of the feet. In one prospective study, the ability to palpate bone through a contiguous ulcer had a sensitivity of 66% and a specificity of 85% for osteomyelitis.

MRI is the most sensitive and diagnostic imaging technique to identify osteomyelitis, except when orthopedic implants are present. Gallium scans are more sensitive and specific than three-phase technetium (^{99m}Tc) bone scans or indium-labeled leukocyte scans for the diagnosis of vertebral osteomyelitis. Gallium scans are used when spinal hardware is present that degrades the magnetic resonance images and in cases of skull bone osteomyelitis due to malignant external otitis.

Multiple specimens of involved bone, contiguous soft tissue, and purulence should be sent for Gram stain, aerobic and anaerobic culture, and pathologic examination at the time of bone biopsy or surgical débridement. If the history, examination, or imaging is suggestive of atypical infection, culture for fungi and mycobacteria or other unusual organisms should be performed.

TREATMENT   Rx

There are no large randomized studies comparing antimicrobial therapy for osteomyelitis.[4] Antimicrobials for specific pathogens based on in vitro susceptibility testing are recommended, and examples of antimicrobials used to treat common pathogens causing osteomyelitis and septic arthritis are shown in Table 280-2.

The duration of antimicrobial therapy is almost always dictated by surgical therapy in chronic osteomyelitis. For example, if an amputation is performed, a short course of antimicrobial therapy may be required, whereas if an extensive débridement of chronic osteomyelitis is performed, prolonged intravenous antimicrobial therapy for 4 to 6 weeks is typically recommended. If the surgical therapy could lead to a worse outcome than no surgery, chronic oral antimicrobial suppression may be recommended. Acute hematogenous vertebral osteomyelitis in adults is typically treated with 6 weeks of intravenous antimicrobial therapy, without surgical intervention, after identification of the pathogen through percutaneous or open biopsy. Hyperbaric oxygen therapy for chronic osteomyelitis is controversial.

PREVENTION

Improving the control of diabetes and decreasing the incidence of peripheral vascular disease will reduce the incidence of diabetic foot bone infection. Optimal strategies to prevent surgical site infection after orthopedic procedures will prevent orthopedic implant infection after surgery and open fractures.

PROGNOSIS

The success of osteomyelitis management depends on the medical and surgical therapy employed and the ability to improve comorbidities such as arterial insufficiency. The ability of orthopedic surgeons to perform more

TABLE 280-2 ANTIMICROBIAL THERAPY FOR SELECTED MICROORGANISMS IN OSTEOMYELITIS OR SEPTIC ARTHRITIS IN ADULTS

MICROORGANISM	FIRST CHOICE*	ALTERNATIVE CHOICE
Methicillin/oxacillin/nafcillin–sensitive staphylococci	Nafcillin sodium or oxacillin sodium 1.5–2 g IV q4–6h for 4–6 wk or cefazolin 1–2 g IV q8h	Vancomycin 15 mg/kg IV q12h for 4–6 wk
Methicillin/oxacillin/nafcillin–resistant staphylococci (MRSA)	Vancomycin[†] 15 mg/kg IV q12h or daptomycin 6 mg/kg IV q24h	Linezolid 600 mg PO/IV q12h or levofloxacin[†] 500–750 mg PO/IV daily
Penicillin-sensitive streptococci	Aqueous penicillin G 20 × 10⁶ U/24 hr IV either continuously or in 6 equally divided daily doses or ceftriaxone 1–2 g IV q24h or cefazolin 1–2 g IV q8h	Vancomycin 15 mg/kg IV q12h
Enterococci	Aqueous crystalline penicillin G 20 × 10⁶ U/24 hr IV either continuously or in 6 equally divided daily doses or ampicillin sodium 12 g/24 hr IV either continuously or in 6 equally divided daily doses; the addition of gentamicin sulfate 1 mg/kg IV or IM q8h for 1–2 wk is optional	Vancomycin[†] 15 mg/kg IV q12h; the addition of gentamicin sulfate 1 mg/kg IV or IM q8h for 1–2 wk is optional
Enterobacteriaceae	Ceftriaxone 1–2 g IV q24h	Ciprofloxacin[†] 500–750 mg PO q12h
Pseudomonas aeruginosa	Cefepime 2 g IV q12h	Ciprofloxacin[†] 750 mg PO q12h or ceftazidime 2 g IV q8h

*Antimicrobial selection should be based on in vitro sensitivity data, as well as allergies, intolerances, and drug interactions in individual patients.
†Doses shown are based on normal renal and hepatic function and may need to be adjusted or serum levels monitored (vancomycin).
MRSA = methicillin-resistant *Staphylococcus aureus*.
Adapted from Berbari EF, Steckelberg JM, Osmon DR. Osteomyelitis. In: Mandell GL, Bennett JE, Dolin R, eds. *Mandell, Douglas, and Bennett's Principles and Practice of Infectious Diseases*, 7th ed. Philadelphia: Churchill Livingstone/Elsevier; 2010:1457-1467.

extensive reconstructive surgery has allowed more extensive débridement and higher success rates, as well as restoration of function. Treatment failure can lead to relapse of infection or progression of infection to involve more of the affected bone. Long-standing osteomyelitis can be complicated by amyloidosis, squamous cell carcinoma of the skin in a chronic sinus tract, or primary bone malignancy.

1. Peltola H, Pääkkönen M, Kallio P, et al. Prospective, randomized trial of 10 days versus 30 days of antimicrobial treatment, including a short-term course of parenteral therapy, for childhood septic arthritis. *Clin Infect Dis.* 2009;48:1201-1210.
2. Harel L, Prais D, Bar-On E, et al. Dexamethasone therapy for septic arthritis in children: results of a randomized double-blind placebo-controlled study. *J Pediatr Orthop.* 2011;31:211-215.
3. American Academy of Orthopedic Surgeons (AAOS). Advisory Statement. Recommendations for the Intravenous Antibiotic Prophylaxis in Primary Total Joint Arthroplasty, 2004. http://www.aaos.org/about\papers\advistmt\1027.asp.
4. Conterno LO, da Silva Filho CR. Antibiotics for treating chronic osteomyelitis in adults. *Cochrane Database Syst Rev.* 2009;3:CD004439.

SUGGESTED READINGS

Del Pozo JL, Patel R. Infection associated with prosthetic joints. *N Engl J Med.* 2009;361:787-794. *Review of diagnostic approach to and management of prosthetic joint infections.*
Johannsson B, Taylor J, Clark CR, et al. Treatment approaches to prosthetic joint infections: results of an Emerging Infections Network survey. *Diagn Microbiol Infect Dis.* 2010;66:16-23. *Recent Infectious Diseases Society of America survey.*
Matthews CJ, Weston VC, Jones A, et al. Bacterial septic arthritis in adults. *Lancet.* 2010;375:846-855. *Review of the changing epidemiology of septic arthritis of native joints and its evolving antibiotic resistance.*
Torralba KD, Quismorio FP Jr. Soft tissue infections. *Rheum Dis Clin North Am.* 2009;35:46-62. *Review of potentially serious soft tissue infections in patients with rheumatic disease, including septic bursitis and tenosynovitis.*
Zimmerli W. Vertebral osteomyelitis. *N Engl J Med.* 2010;362:1022-1029. *Strategies for evaluation and treatment.*

281

CRYSTAL DEPOSITION DISEASES

N. LAWRENCE EDWARDS

The pro-inflammatory and destructive characteristics of intrasynovial crystals have been recognized for over a century. The mechanisms of crystal-induced inflammation and joint destruction have become much better clarified over the past several decades. The three most common crystal-induced arthropathies are caused by precipitation of monosodium urate monohydrate (MSU), calcium pyrophosphate dihydrate (CPPD), and basic calcium phosphate (BCP) and are termed *gout, pseudogout,* and *hydroxyapatite arthropathy,* respectively.

GOUT AND HYPERURICEMIA

DEFINITION

Gout is an inflammatory arthritis of metabolic origin that is caused by crystallization of MSU within joints. It is the most common inflammatory joint disease in men and older women. Its incidence and prevalence are increasing markedly worldwide. The metabolic derangement responsible for gout is the supersaturation of blood and body fluids with the urate ion to the point that crystal formation is possible. At physiologic pH and at normal body temperature, urate is considered to be supersaturated at concentrations of 6.8 mg/dL or greater. Therefore, from a biologic perspective, hyperuricemia is defined as any serum urate level greater than 6.8 mg/dL in both men and women. Although hyperuricemia is a prerequisite for developing gout, only a small percentage (15 to 25%) of all hyperuricemic subjects ultimately develop gout.

Gout is a progressive arthritis that begins as an intermittent mono- or oligoarthritis in the lower extremities and can progress over years to decades into a chronic, destructive, and debilitating polyarthritis involving almost any peripheral joint in the body. Also considered within the definition of gout is the spectrum of clinical conditions resulting from the deposition of MSU crystals in the subcutaneous tissues and kidney manifesting as tophaceous deposits, inflammatory cellulitis, urate nephropathy, and kidney stones.

EPIDEMIOLOGY

An elevation of serum urate that is sustained over a prolonged period is the primary risk factor for the development of gout. Hyperuricemia is very common in Western culture, with a prevalence as high as 15 to 20% reported in some recent population-based studies. This rate of hyperuricemia is more than twice that observed just 3 decades ago. A number of factors have been proposed to explain this dramatic rise, including the overall increase in longevity; the greater prevalence of hypertension, metabolic syndrome, and obesity; the ubiquitous use of thiazide diuretics and low-dose aspirin; changes in dietary trends, including the greater use of high-fructose corn syrup as a sweetener; and the increased survival of patients with end-stage renal disease and recipients of organ transplants.

There is a direct correlation between the degree of serum urate elevation and the likelihood of developing gout. The reported annual incidence of gout in subjects with baseline serum urate levels of 9 mg/dL or greater is 4.9%, compared with only 0.5% for those with serum urate levels of 7.0 to 8.9 mg/dL.

Multiple studies have reported that men are three to six times more likely to develop gout than women, and age has a decided impact on the prevalence of gout (Fig. 281-1). Overall, the prevalence of gout in the United States has been estimated at 13.6 per 1000 adult men and 6.4 per 1000 adult women. This prevalence varies from country to country; there is also marked variation within countries, depending on sociodemographic factors other than gender and age. In New Zealand, for example, the prevalence of gout among Maori men is 2.4 times higher than in men of European ancestry.

PATHOBIOLOGY

Uric acid is the end product of purine metabolism in humans. In most mammals, purine catabolism is taken one step further via the enzyme uric acid oxidase or uricase, with the purine end product in these species being the very soluble allantoin. Humans and most other hominoids lost the ability

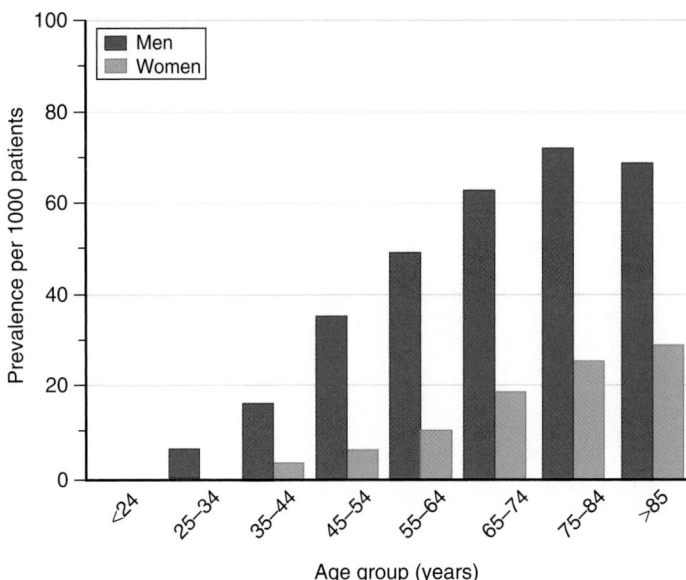

FIGURE 281-1. Prevalence of gout in men and women of different age groups. The overall prevalence in this 1999 study from the United Kingdom was 1.4%, and the male-female ratio was 3.6:1. The prevalence in women continues to rise with age, whereas the prevalence in men appears to peak in the 75 to 84 age group.

to produce the enzyme uricase nearly 18 million years ago. As a result, uric acid accumulation is possible. Whether caused by overproduction of uric acid or underexcretion by the kidneys (Table 281-1), this accumulation leads to the supersaturation of urate ion in blood and the precipitation of MSU crystals in synovial fluid, soft tissues, and organs. Urate is produced by the conversion of a very soluble molecule, hypoxanthine, to the less soluble xanthine, which in turn is converted to the very insoluble uric acid by progressive purine ring oxidations catalyzed by the enzyme xanthine oxidase. Xanthine oxidase is present in several organs, but most activity occurs in the liver and intestines. Because of its potential for causing disease, urate elimination is very important. The total daily accumulation of uric acid from de novo synthesis, nucleotide degradation, and dietary consumption is between 800 and 1200 mg/day and is balanced by the renal excretion of approximately two thirds of the total amount and intestinal elimination of the remaining one third.

Simply put, hyperuricemia occurs when urate production is not balanced by renal excretion. In 90% of all gout patients, the cause of this imbalance is renal underexcretion. The remaining 10% of gout cases are caused by purine overproduction or a combination of overproduction and underexcretion.

Renal Urate Underexcretion

The underexcretion of urate by the kidney may be caused by genetic factors (primary hyperuricemia), by clinical renal disorders (renal insufficiency or diminished glomerular filtration), by endogenous organic acid accumulation (lactate, β-hydroxybutyrate, acetoacetate), or by exogenous substances (low-dose aspirin, thiazides, β-blockers, cyclosporine, tacrolimus).

Because uric acid is small and not protein bound, it is completely filtered by the glomerulus. In normal persons, approximately 8 to 10% of the filtered load is ultimately cleared in the urine. The various renal tubular transporters responsible for determining how much of the filtered uric acid is actually excreted are located in the proximal convoluted tubules (Fig. 281-2). Both reabsorption and secretion occur in this segment through the actions of several organic acid transporters (OATs), with the net effect being the reabsorption of nearly 90% of the uric acid filtered at the glomerulus. These OATs are also responsible for eliminating organic acids other than uric acid, as well as many commonly used medications. The most important tubular transporter for handling uric acid is urate transporter 1 (URAT1). This transporter swaps urate ions for other monocarboxylate organic ions in both directions across the luminal membrane of proximal tubular cells. This system can be driven to reabsorb more uric acid from the tubular lumen by raising the tubular intracellular concentration of lactate, pyruvate, or the ketoacids acetoacetate and β-hydroxybutyrate. Certain drugs, when present in the tubular lumen, can displace uric acid from the transporter, causing more uric acid to be lost in the urine. These compounds, which include probenecid, losartan, and high-dose aspirin, are considered uricosuric.

TABLE 281-1   CLASSIFICATION OF HYPERURICEMIA AND GOUT

IMPAIRED URIC ACID EXCRETION

Primary gout with decreased uric acid clearance
Secondary gout
    Clinical conditions
        Reduced GFR
        Hypertension
        Obesity
        Systemic acidosis
        Familial juvenile hyperuricemic nephropathy
        Medullary cystic kidney disease
        Lead nephropathy
    Drugs
        Diuretics
        Ethanol
        Low-dose salicylates (0.3-3.0 g/day)
        Cyclosporine
        Tacrolimus
        Levodopa

EXCESSIVE URATE PRODUCTION

Primary metabolic disorders
    HPRT deficiency
    PRPP synthetase overactivity
    Glucose-6-phosphatase deficiency
    Fructose-1-phosphate aldolase deficiency
Secondary causes
    Clinical conditions
        Myelo- and lymphoproliferative disorders
        Obesity
        Psoriasis
        Glycogenoses III, V, VII
    Drugs and dietary components
        Nicotinic acid
        Pancreatic extract
        Cytotoxic drugs
        Red meat, organ meat, shellfish
        Alcoholic beverages (especially beer)
        Fructose

GFR = glomerular filtration rate; HPRT = hypoxanthine-guanine phosphoribosyltransferase; PRPP = phosphoribosylpyrophosphate.

When the renal clearance of uric acid by normal adult men and gouty men is compared, the gouty subjects excrete only 70% as much uric acid as normal individuals at any given serum urate concentration. In general, gouty subjects require a serum urate concentration 1.7 mg/dL higher to obtain the same level of excretion seen in normals. This is apparently not related to a difference in the transport kinetics of the URAT1 protein in gouty subjects versus normal individuals but rather to the relative abundance of these transporters in the proximal convoluted tubule.

Hyperuricemia is also associated with type 2 diabetes mellitus (Chapter 237) in the fully expanded metabolic syndrome. Elevated insulin levels, like those seen in insulin-resistant states, stimulate the sodium-hydrogen exchanger, ultimately leading to increased reabsorption of sodium in certain organic acids, including uric acid.

Urate Overproduction

In approximately 10% of gouty subjects, hyperuricemia is caused by uric acid overproduction rather than reduced renal excretion. In most of these people, the hyperuricemia reflects accelerated cell turnover (e.g., lymphoproliferative and myeloproliferative diseases, psoriasis, chronic hemolytic states, and certain muscle glycogenoses) or other causes of enhanced purine nucleotide breakdown, such as that seen with alcohol abuse or fructose ingestion. In addition to these secondary causes of urate overproduction, some primary disease processes are responsible for urate overproduction. These are inborn errors of metabolism that result in increased de novo purine synthesis, as seen in phosphoribosylpyrophosphate synthetase overactivity, or decreased purine salvage, as seen in hypoxanthine-guanine phosphoribosyltransferase deficiency (Lesch-Nyhan syndrome). Regardless of the cause, urate overproduction is determined by a 24-hour urine collection showing greater than 1000 mg of uric acid while eating a standard Western diet.

Pathogenesis of MSU Crystals and Inflammation

MSU crystals in joints, soft tissues, and organs are the cause of pain and destruction in gout. Urate crystals form only when physiologic conditions permit. In plasma, urate becomes insoluble at concentrations of 6.8 mg/dL (408 µmol/L), with a pH of 7.40 and normal body temperature. A reduction in pH or temperature lowers the solubility threshold further. Not all people who are hyperuricemic form crystals. There appears to be an additional requirement of a "nucleation factor" that is still poorly defined for gout, along with other local factors that either promote or inhibit crystal growth.

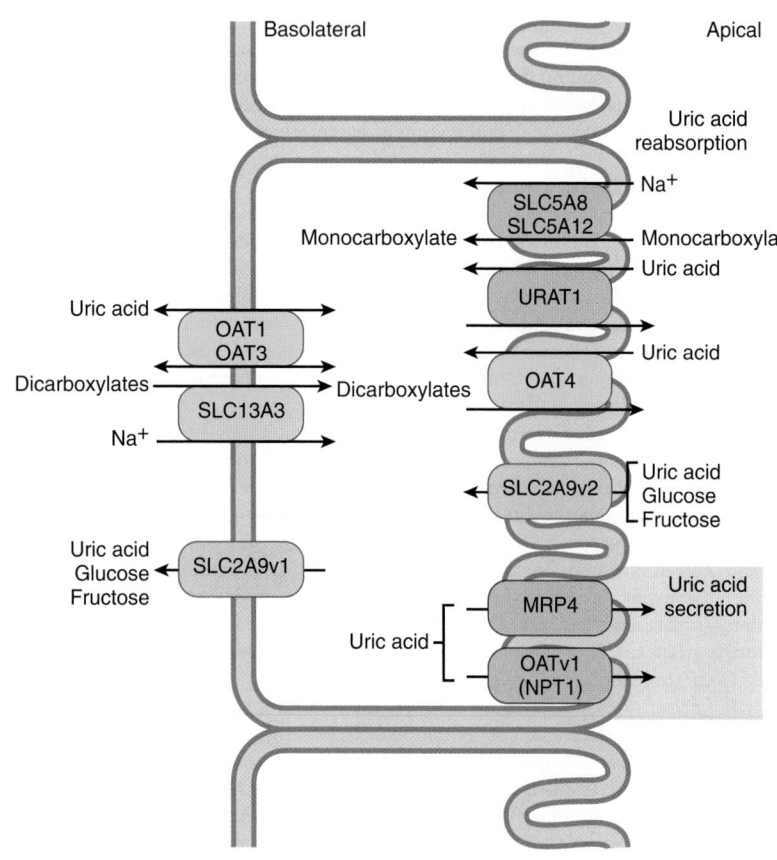

FIGURE 281-2. Urate transport in the proximal convoluted tubule. The proximal convoluted tubule is the major site of urate handling in the kidney. Urate reabsorption and secretion occur through the actions of a series of organic acid transporters (OATs; gene family *SLC22A*) that are linked directly to organic acid movement and indirectly to sodium reabsorption. The OATs are critical in the renal excretion of drugs and their metabolites. The predominant urate reuptake transporter in this system is URAT1 *(SLC22A-12)*, which is located on the luminal (apical) side of the tubular epithelium. Polymorphisms in this gene can lead to urate retention and have been reported in German families. A URAT1 mutation in a Japanese cohort appears to increase uric acid excretion by the kidney. The *SLC2A9* glucose-fructose transporter (GLUT-9) is also a urate transporter, and polymorphisms in this gene are associated with gout.

MSU crystals form in joints and soft tissues of individuals long before they have any symptoms of gout. They deposit in small lattice structures called *microtophi* on the surface of cartilage and in the synovial lining. These microtophi grow slowly but are generally stable as long as the surrounding environment does not change drastically with regard to pH, urate concentration, or temperature. At the time of the first and subsequent clinical flares, something changes in the joint environment to cause these crystal lattice structures to break apart and shed a massive number of crystals into the joint space. These newly released and nonopsonized crystals activate receptors on synovial macrophages; they are then phagocytized by monocytes and macrophages, leading to interaction with the NALP3 inflammasome. This results in the rapid production of interleukin-1 (IL-1), which is responsible for all the cardinal features of severe inflammation associated with acute gout. The gout flare is self-limited, probably caused by a physical change in the MSU crystals after they have been repeatedly phagocytized and partially digested. A maturation of the resident monocytes in the inflamed joint also appears to help terminate the gouty flare. Even after the acute attack subsides, low-grade inflammation persists in the asymptomatic joint. It is this persistent, ongoing inflammatory process that eventually leads to bony erosion, cartilage destruction, and synovial hypertrophy if the hyperuricemia is not treated and the MSU crystals dissolved.

CLINICAL MANIFESTATIONS

Classic Gout

The natural course of classic gout passes through three stages: asymptomatic hyperuricemia, acute intermittent gout, and chronic advanced gout. The rate of progression from asymptomatic hyperuricemia to chronic advanced gout varies considerably from one person to another and is dependent on numerous factors, the most important being the degree of increase in serum urate levels.

Asymptomatic hyperuricemia refers to a state in which serum urate exceeds the level of solubility (6.8 mg/dL) but symptoms of crystalline deposition have not occurred. Only 15 to 20% of all hyperuricemic people are prone to develop MSU crystals, and for this group, the period of asymptomatic hyperuricemia begins a stage of subclinical structural changes. In men, asymptomatic hyperuricemia frequently begins at puberty, whereas in women, it is usually delayed until menopause.

The initial episode of acute gout usually follows decades of asymptomatic hyperuricemia. In men, the first attack usually occurs between the fourth and sixth decades of life. In women, the age of onset is older and varies with several factors, the most important being the age at menopause. The classic acute gout attack is characterized by the rapid development of warmth, swelling, erythema, and exquisite pain in one or occasionally two joints. The characteristically severe pain evolves from its faintest twinge to its most intense level over an 8- to 12-hour period. Initial attacks are usually monoarticular and involve lower extremity joints. The most common joint involved is the first metatarsophalangeal joint (termed *podagra*), followed by the ankle, midfoot, and knee (Fig. 281-3). After years of acute intermittent attacks, upper extremity joints, including the wrists, elbows, and small joints of the hands, can also become involved. Systemic symptoms of fever, chills, and malaise may accompany acute attacks, along with an intense erythema extending beyond the area of the involved joint. This may lead to confusion with a septic process.

Factors capable of provoking episodes of acute gout are those that cause fluctuations in serum urate levels, including trauma, surgery, starvation, overindulgence in certain high-purine foods, and the ingestion of any medication that raises or lowers serum urate.

The other characteristic of classic gout flares is the self-remitting nature. For the first several acute flares, the duration of the attack is 5 to 8 days. The resolution of symptoms is gradual but complete, even if no anti-inflammatory therapy is administered. The periods between acute attacks are devoid of articular pain, although synovial fluid aspirates during this stage continue to show low-grade inflammation and the presence of MSU crystals.

Eventually the untreated patient progresses to chronic polyarticular gout, also referred to as *advanced gout*. This stage usually develops after 10 or more years of acute intermittent gout and is evident when the pain-free intercritical periods have disappeared. Gouty flares can continue to occur against this constantly painful background. The intensity of the chronic pain is not nearly as severe as that experienced with acute flares.

The subcutaneous tophus is the most characteristic lesion of advanced gout. The development of tophaceous deposits of MSU is a function of the duration and severity of hyperuricemia. Subcutaneous tophi can occur anywhere in the body but are most common in the fingers, wrists, ears, knees, and olecranon bursa and at pressure points under the ulnar aspect of the forearm and at the Achilles tendon (Fig. 281-4). Gout at this stage can be confused with rheumatoid arthritis, especially if tophi are confused with rheumatoid nodules.

Atypical Gout Presentations

Approximately 5% of patients with gout experience the onset of symptoms before age 25. These individuals with early-onset gout represent a special subset that generally has a genetic component (see Table 281-1). They have a more accelerated clinical course and require more aggressive antihyperuricemic therapy.

Gout develops in approximately 15% of heart transplant patients taking cyclosporine to prevent allograft rejection. A slightly lower frequency of gout is seen in kidney and liver transplant recipients. Cyclosporine-induced gout has a marked shortening of the asymptomatic and acute intermittent stages, with a rapid appearance of tophi in 1 to 4 years.

In most large reviews, women account for no more than 5% of all gout subjects. This demographic is changing as gout is becoming more common in older women. Most women with gout are postmenopausal. Women with premenopausal gout usually have renal insufficiency, are taking thiazide diuretics for hypertension, or have a strong genetic predilection. Gout in older women may differ from classic gout in its propensity to occur in joints previously damaged by osteoarthritis (Chapter 270), such as the knees or the distal interphalangeal joints with Heberden's nodes.

Saturnine gout is the term used to describe gout caused by chronic lead exposure (Chapter 21). In the middle of the 20th century, this was most commonly observed in consumers of "moonshine" whiskey. Occupational exposure in plumbers and environmental exposure from lead-based paints are other potential causes of this unusual form of gout.

DIAGNOSIS

Hyperuricemia is a critical risk factor for developing gout, but it is not a reliable diagnostic test because many people with elevated serum urate levels never develop gout. Serum urate levels during an acute flare of gout are also

FIGURE 281-3. The intense inflammation of acute gouty arthritis. **A,** Marked swelling of the first metatarsophalangeal joint (podagra) is demonstrated. A dusky blue hue over an intense erythema is characteristic. **B,** Ankle swelling with erythema extending beyond the area of the tibiotalar joint.

FIGURE 281-4. Characteristic locations of gouty tophi. **A,** At the elbow, tophi present as hard nodules along the ulnar ridge or as multiple nodules within the olecranon bursa. **B,** Ear tophi are uncommon but may be an easy source of crystal confirmation when present. **C,** Small subcutaneous tophi can occur along the ventral creases of fingers. **D,** Tophi over the proximal interphalangeal or distal interphalangeal joints may be confused with Bouchard's or Heberden's nodes, respectively.

unreliable because they may be suppressed by as much as 1.5 to 2.0 mg/dL from baseline values. The definitive diagnosis of gout is made by polarized compensated microscopy of a synovial fluid aspirate from the affected joint. The presence of intracellular needle-shaped crystals with strong negative birefringence is the diagnostic "gold standard" (Fig. 281-5). Similar microscopic results from a tophus aspirate or spontaneously draining fluid also confirm the diagnosis of gout.

Synovial fluid confirmation is obtained in as few as 10% of patients with gout. The presumptive diagnosis of gout is based on a pattern of acute joint symptoms coupled with the patient's own medical history or a family history. The patient's medical history may reveal comorbidities frequently associated with gout or the use of medications associated with urate retention.

The characteristic clinical presentation is the rapid onset (over 8 to 12 hours) of severe pain in one or several lower extremity joints (especially the great toe, midfoot, or ankle). The presumptive diagnosis has much greater credence if there have been similar previous attacks that spontaneously resolved to a symptom-free state.

Radiographic evaluation is not helpful in early attacks of gout, except to rule out fracture. In advanced gout, affected joints may show punched out periarticular erosions with classic overhanging edges. Ultrasonography can detect MSU crystals layered over articular cartilage in early disease and may be diagnostic. Magnetic resonance imaging is not part of the standard evaluation, but it can reveal soft tissue and intra-articular tophi long before they become clinically evident.

The differential diagnosis of acute gout includes bacterial infection, trauma, sarcoidosis, and CPPD arthropathy (pseudogout). Diseases occasionally confused with advanced gout include rheumatoid arthritis, reactive arthritis, and CPPD arthropathy.

FIGURE 281-5. Comparison of calcium pyrophosphate dihydrate (CPPD) crystals (A) and monosodium urate crystals (B) by means of compensated polarized light microscopy of synovial fluid. Both crystal types are found within leukocytes, and both can be extracellular, as shown here for CPPD crystals. CPPD crystals are weakly birefringent and are more variable in shape, with rhomboid, square, or rod-like structures that can resemble urate crystals. Urate crystals are uniformly needle shaped and more brightly birefringent than are CPPD crystals. The arrows indicate the axis of slow rotation of light of the first-order red plate compensator used in compensated polarized light microscopy. Urate crystals are negatively birefringent (i.e., yellow when the long axis of the crystal is parallel to the red plate compensator axis, and blue when the long axis of the crystal is perpendicular to the compensator axis). CPPD crystals are positively birefringent (i.e., blue when the long axis of the crystal is parallel to the axis of slow rotation of the red plate compensator, and yellow when the long axis of the crystal is perpendicular to the axis of the compensator), as seen for the two CPPD crystals in **A**. These findings indicate the need to use compensated polarized light microscopy to both identify urate and CPPD crystals and to accurately distinguish between these crystal types. (**A,** Available at http://www.emedicine.com/med/topic1938.htm; **B,** ACR Clinical Slide Collection on the Rheumatic Diseases, American College of Rheumatology, 1998.)

TREATMENT AND PREVENTION Rx

Weight loss, dietary modification to reduce animal-derived purine intake, reduction in alcohol intake, and regular exercise should be encouraged in all patients with gout. Soft drinks sweetened with fructose can increase serum urate levels and should also be restricted. Increased consumption of low-fat dairy products may be recommended for their urate-lowering impact. Such modifications may lower urate levels and help many comorbid conditions associated with gout, but they are rarely sufficient to obviate the need for pharmacologic intervention in acute and chronic gout.**1**

Acute Gout

The treatment goal for acute gout is to relieve pain and terminate the attack as quickly as possible. Resting the painful joint and applying topical ice are generally helpful, but pharmacologic intervention is usually necessary. The therapeutic options include nonsteroidal anti-inflammatory drugs (NSAIDs), oral colchicine, and corticosteroids. NSAIDs are the most widely used approach, but they may be inappropriate in subjects with renal insufficiency or peptic ulcer disease. Oral colchicine 1.8 mg/24 hours in divided doses for the first several days may also be effective. A recent randomized, double-blind, placebo-controlled study showed that self-administered low-dose colchicine (1.8 mg total over 1 hour) was comparable in efficacy to high-dose colchicine (4.8 mg total over 6 hours) for acute gout flare, and the safety profile of low-dose colchicine was indistinguishable from that of placebo.**2** Corticosteroids administered orally, intramuscularly, or intra-articularly are a valuable option in patients with poor renal function or intolerance to colchicine. Issues critical to treatment success are rapid initiation, adequate dosing, and continuation of therapy until the flare has resolved. Anti–IL-1 therapies may also be beneficial in treating acute gout symptoms. During the acute gout flare, subjects already taking urate-lowering therapy should continue the drug; those not receiving this therapy should not be started on it.

Recurrent and Advanced Gout

The goal of therapy in subjects with multiple recurrent gout flares or advanced gout is to prevent disease progression. This is done by lowering serum urate levels to less than 6.0 mg/dL, resulting in the mobilization and depletion of MSU crystals so that recurrent flares are prevented and joint destruction is halted. Urate-lowering therapy is recommended for patients with two or more attacks of gout per year, tophi or urate kidney stones, joint damage, polyarticular attacks, or persistent synovitis. Urate-lowering therapy falls into three categories—uricostatic, uricosuric, and uricolytic agents. Allopurinol and febuxostat are uricostatic drugs, the most widely used approach. Both drugs work by inhibiting the enzyme xanthine oxidase to prevent urate formation. This class of drugs is effective in both overproducers and underexcreters of uric acid. Probenecid is a uricosuric agent that works by increasing the renal excretion of uric acid. This drug is not appropriate for subjects who are urate overproducers because of the risk of nephrolithiasis. Renal function is an issue with allopurinol and probenecid; dose adjustment is recommended if allopurinol is used in patients with chronic kidney disease, and probenecid is generally ineffective in anyone with a creatinine clearance less than 50 mL/minute. Allopurinol causes a rash in about 2% of patients, and allopurinol and febuxostat cause hepatic transaminase elevations in 5%. Allopurinol can also cause a rare (2 to 3 per 1000) but potentially fatal hypersensitivity syndrome that manifests with fever, severe exfoliative rash, eosinophilia, and hepatic and renal failure. All patients taking allopurinol should be cautioned to discontinue this drug at the first sign of rash. Pegloticase is a pegylated recombinant mammalian urate oxidase currently being studied in patients for whom conventional therapy with allopurinol, febuxostat, or probenecid is either ineffective or inadequate. This form of therapy is termed *uricolytic* because it degrades uric acid into a very soluble end product, allantoin. This is an intravenous therapy requiring infusions every 2 weeks.

CPPD DEPOSITION DISEASE

DEFINITION

The heterogeneous group of clinical conditions associated with CPPD crystals is collectively called *CPPD deposition disease*. Within this spectrum is the common radiographic finding of chondrocalcinosis, which is frequently asymptomatic. The acute synovitis associated with intra-articular CPPD crystals can closely mimic the findings of gout and is thus referred to as *pseudogout*. The more chronic changes associated with CPPD-induced bone and cartilage destruction is referred to as *pyrophosphate arthropathy*. These conditions are further classified as familial (genetic), metabolic, and sporadic.

EPIDEMIOLOGY

The true prevalence of CPPD deposition disease is unknown, but it is generally thought to be underdiagnosed because of its confusion with other forms of arthritis. The prevalence of radiographic chondrocalcinosis has been studied extensively and is clearly an age-related phenomenon (Fig. 281-6). Chondrocalcinosis of the meniscal and articular cartilage of the knee is seen in 4% of people between the ages of 55 and 59, in 18% of those aged 80 to 84 years, and in approximately 27% of those older than 85.

PATHOBIOLOGY

Clinical CPPD deposition disease is divided into three categories, based on the cause of the altered inorganic pyrophosphate (PPi) metabolism: hereditary (familial), sporadic (idiopathic), and metabolic. All three types are associated with extracellular PPi accumulation around chondrocytes, and extracellular PPi is necessary for the formation of CPPD crystals. Intracellular PPi is a common byproduct of many synthetic reactions, and if it is allowed to accumulate intracellularly, it impedes the further synthesis of proteins, nucleotides, and lipids. Therefore, there are multiple mechanisms for removing PPi from the cellular cytoplasm, including specific and nonspecific membrane transporters in both intracellular and extracellular (ecto-) pyrophosphate hydrolysis.

Hereditary forms of CPPD deposition disease may be caused by increased transmembrane transport of chondrocyte intracellular PPi to its extracellular matrix owing to diminished activity of the protective pyrophosphate hydrolases, or because of altered influences of factors that lead to increased extracellular PPi, including transforming growth factor-β, bone morphogenetic proteins 2 and 4, ascorbic acid, and osteopontin. The best characterized of the hereditary causes is a gain-of-function mutation of the *ANK* anion transporter gene on the chondrocyte plasma membrane. These types of mutations are rarely observed in the sporadic form of CPPD disease. Aging chondrocytes in culture produce considerably more PPi than do younger chondrocytes, although the exact mechanism for this is unclear.

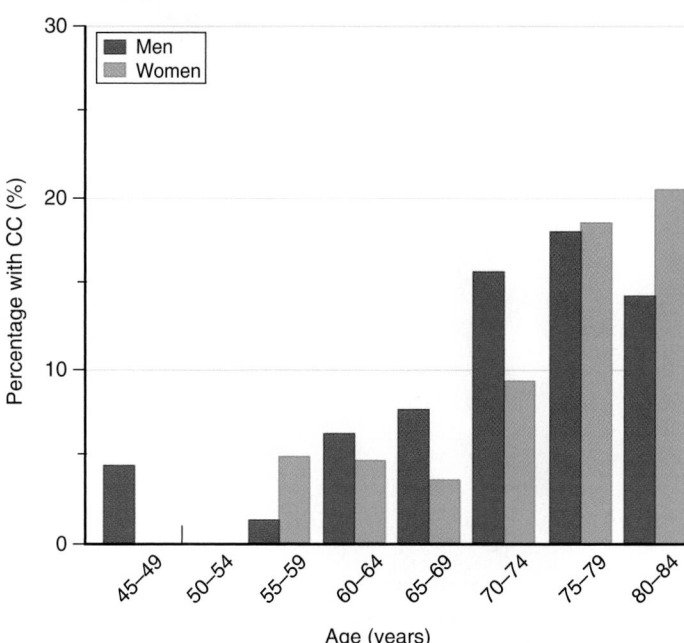

FIGURE 281-6. Prevalence of chondrocalcinosis (CC) in men and women of different age groups. The overall prevalence of chondrocalcinosis in this study from the United Kingdom was 7%. The strong association of age and gender with chondrocalcinosis of the knee is demonstrated. Fibrocartilage (meniscal) was affected in 95% of cases, and hyaline (articular) cartilage in 45%. Chondrocalcinosis was observed bilaterally in the knees in 72% of cases and in both medial and lateral knee compartments in 38%.

The metabolic diseases that predispose to CPPD deposition disease include hemochromatosis (Chapter 219), hyperparathyroidism (Chapter 253), hypomagnesemia (as in Gitelman's syndrome; Chapter 130), and hypophosphatasia (Chapter 121). All these metabolic conditions result in increased concentrations of extracellular PPi or in other alterations in the cartilage matrix that permit CCPD crystal formation.

CLINICAL MANIFESTATIONS

CPPD deposition disease can present in a variety of ways. It is frequently asymptomatic (lanthanic) and is recognized only by the appearance of chondrocalcinosis on radiographs. The most common clinical manifestation, accounting for approximately 60% of cases of CPPD disease, is a polyarticular, noninflammatory arthritis affecting joints not typically involved in primary osteoarthritis, including the wrists, shoulders, and metacarpophalangeal joints (particularly the second and third). This form of CPPD disease is called *pseudo-osteoarthritis,* and it may lead to occasional inflammatory attacks. The acute monoarticular presentation is known as *pseudogout*. The pain and swelling of pseudogout can be similar to that seen in gout; however, the onset is usually not as abrupt as in gout, and the attacks tend to last longer—frequently months. Pseudogout occurs more often in the large joints than in small joints. CPPD deposition disease occasionally presents as a chronic polyarticular inflammatory disease that may mimic rheumatoid arthritis or polymyalgia rheumatica.

DIAGNOSIS

CPPD disease is diagnosed by identifying chondrocalcinosis by radiography in a patient with a clinical history suggestive of the disease (Fig. 281-7). The diagnosis should be confirmed by aspiration of synovial fluid and examination for CPPD crystals by compensated polarized light microscopy (see Fig. 281-5).

TREATMENT AND PREVENTION   Rx

There are no specific therapies for CPPD deposition disease. In patients with CPPD disease associated with a metabolic disease, treatment and control of the metabolic disease can afford some improvement in the arthritis. For both acute and chronic forms of CPPD deposition disease, therapy is directed at symptoms. NSAIDs are the mainstay of treatment. Low-dose oral colchicine can be used in both acute and chronic settings. Intra-articular steroids have also proved to be beneficial for symptomatic CPPD deposition disease. However, intra-articular viscosupplementation (hyaluronic acid) may exacerbate joint symptoms.

FIGURE 281-7. CPPD arthropathy of the hand. Chondrocalcinosis of the triangular fibrocartilage of the wrist is demonstrated by the *large arrow*. Joint space narrowing, sub-chondral cysts, and large palmar (parrot-beak) osteophytes of the second and third meta-carpophalangeal joints *(arrowheads)* are also characteristic of CPPD hand involvement. (From Jacobson JA, Girish G, Jiang Y, Sabb BJ. Radiographic evaluation of arthritis: degenerative joint disease and variations. *Radiology.* 2008;248:737-747.)

FIGURE 281-8. Diffuse idiopathic skeletal hyperostosis (DISH) in the lumbar spine. Thick, flowing anterior osteophytes at multiple levels in the thoracic and lumbar spine are characteristic of DISH. (From Nakhoda K. eMedicine Radiology. Medscape. Updated Aug. 17, 2009.)

APATITE-ASSOCIATED (BASIC CALCIUM PHOSPHATE) ARTHROPATHY

BCP crystals include several different crystal species. The most common of these is hydroxyapatite. The BCP crystals are unlike MSU or CPPD crystals, in that they are not identifiable by polarized microscopy. These very tiny crystals are responsible for several important clinical conditions. Although BCP crystals are found in 50% of osteoarthritic synovial fluids, the incidence and prevalence of the individual apatite-associated clinical manifestations have not been established. This is especially true of the most severe and destructive apatite syndromes, such as Milwaukee shoulder and tumoral calcinosis. The prevalence of the most common apatite-associated condition, calcific periarthritis of the shoulder, was 3% in a large North American study.

PATHOBIOLOGY

Like MSU and CPPD crystals, BCP crystals exert their pro-inflammatory effects by being phagocytized by resident synoviocytes and influxing leukocytes. Unlike MSU and CPPD crystals, apatite crystals apparently do not act through the NALP3 inflammasome. Rather, BCP crystals are dissolved in the acidic phagosome, raise intracellular calcium levels, and then activate the calcium-dependent signaling pathways. The synoviocytes are stimulated by these pathways to increase the production of tumor necrosis factor-α and IL-6, and influxing neutrophils are stimulated to increase pro-inflammatory oxygen radicals. The fibroblasts in the joint lining and surrounding soft tissues are stimulated to increase the production of many of the matrix metalloproteinases, such as collagenase 1, collagenase 3, and stromolysin 1.

CLINICAL MANIFESTATIONS

The clinical manifestations of BCP deposition can be acute or chronic, idiopathic, hereditary, or secondary to other diseases that cause hypercalcemia (Table 281-2). BCP crystals can be found in 50% of synovial fluids from osteoarthritic knees. The presence of BCP crystals correlates with more severe radiographic changes secondary to more rapid deterioration in these osteoarthritic knees. Acute inflammatory arthritis associated with BCP deposition is similar in many ways to that of gout and pseudogout and has been referred to as *pseudo-pseudogout*. The patients tend to be younger and usually have evidence of soft tissue BCP deposition elsewhere in the body. Periarticular calcifications are often asymptomatic. However, BCP deposition can cause an acute and severe inflammation of the ligaments, tendons, and bursae surrounding a joint, termed *acute calcific periarthritis*. This frequently occurs

TABLE 281-2	CLINICAL MANIFESTATIONS OF BCP DEPOSITION DISEASE
Osteoarthritis and BCP deposition	
Acute inflammatory arthritis	
Acute calcific periarthritis	
Chronic noninflammatory arthropathy	
Diffuse idiopathic skeletal hyperostosis (DISH)	
Tumoral calcinosis	
Calcifications associated with hypercalcemic states	
Hyperparathyroidism	
Hypervitaminosis D	
Sarcoidosis	
Metastatic cancer	
Myeloma	
Leukemia	

BCP = basic calcium phosphate.

around the shoulders and hips but can also occur in fingers, toes, wrists, and ankles.

The most destructive BCP-associated arthropathy is Milwaukee shoulder, which is characterized by large noninflammatory effusions containing BCP crystals with or without CPPD crystals. The process results in destruction of the rotator cuff, leading to marked instability and glenohumeral cartilage dissolution. This process can also affect the knees. Like acute calcific periarthritis, Milwaukee shoulder is observed four times more frequently in women than in men.

Diffuse idiopathic skeletal hyperostosis (DISH) predominates in men and the elderly. The radiographic appearance of this condition is flowing ossifications along the anterolateral aspect of spinal vertebrae, especially in the thoracic spine (Fig. 281-8). DISH is usually asymptomatic, but very large bridging osteophytes can cause pain and, in the cervical spine, can even result in dysphagia.

Idiopathic tumoral calcinosis is a rare disease most prevalent in young people of African descent. These patients have large, irregular calcifying masses in the soft tissues surrounding the shoulders, hips, and elbows. Some cases exhibit a familial occurrence and medical conditions associated with hyperphosphatemia.

Finally, metastatic calcifications can arise in any medical condition associated with hypercalcemia (Chapter 253), including hyperparathyroidism, hypervitaminosis D, sarcoidosis, metastatic cancer, myeloma, and leukemia.

TREATMENT AND PREVENTION **Rx**

The treatment of most BCP-associated syndromes is conservative. For acute inflammatory arthritis and periarthritis, low-dose oral colchicine and NSAIDs are the mainstays of symptomatic therapy. The persistent large effusion seen in Milwaukee shoulder should be serially aspirated to decrease intracapsular pressure. The added effectiveness of corticosteroid injections in this setting is unproved. The calcinosis associated with abnormal calcium and phosphate metabolism is best managed by treating the underlying metabolic process.

Grade Ⓐ

1. Zhang W, Doherty M, Bardin T, et al. EULAR evidence based recommendations for gout. Part II: management. Report of a task force of the EULAR Standing Committee for International Clinical Studies Including Therapeutics (ESCISIT). *Ann Rheum Dis.* 2006;65:1312-1324.
2. Terkeltaub RA, Furst DE, Bennett K, et al. High versus low dosing of oral colchicine for acute gout flare. *Arthritis Rheum.* 2010;62:1060-1068.

SUGGESTED READINGS

Burns CM, Wortmann RL. Gout therapeutics: new drugs for an old disease. *Lancet.* 2011;377: 165-177. *Review of current options.*
Busso N, So A. Mechanisms of inflammation in gout. *Arthritis Res Ther.* 2010;12:206-213. *Review of the basic mechanisms of an acute attack of gout as a paradigm of acute sterile (as opposed to pyogenic) inflammation.*
Neogi T. Gout. *N Engl J Med.* 2011;364:443-452. *Case-based review.*
Sundy JS. Progress in the pharmacotherapy of gout. *Curr Opin Rheumatol.* 2010;22:188-193. *Summary of new knowledge about approved and emerging drugs.*

282

FIBROMYALGIA AND CHRONIC FATIGUE SYNDROME

ROBERT M. BENNETT

Fibromyalgia (FM) and chronic fatigue syndrome (CFS) are multisymptomatic syndromes defined by the core features of chronic widespread pain and chronic unexplained fatigue, respectively. The 1990 American College of Rheumatology (ACR) classification criteria are universally used to diagnose FM (Table 282-1). The 1994 Centers for Disease Control and Prevention (CDC) criteria are widely used to diagnose CFS (see Table 282-1). According to these definitions, FM and CFS are separate entities, but in practice, there is great overlap, with many patients being given both labels. Myofascial pain is a universal experience that is usually self-limited; when it becomes persistent, it may accentuate and perpetuate the experience of chronic fatigue and FM.

● FIBROMYALGIA

EPIDEMIOLOGY

Chronic musculoskeletal pain is commonly encountered in the general population with an estimated prevalence of about 35%. It is subdivided into chronic regional pain, with a prevalence of about 25%, and chronic widespread pain, with a prevalence of about 10%.

FM is considered to be a subset of chronic widespread pain and has a prevalence of about 2% in women and 0.5% in men. There is a steady increase in FM with age, with about 12% of women in their 60s being affected. Chronic musculoskeletal pain is associated with a reduction in overall health status, and FM patients have more impairment than do patients with chronic widespread pain or chronic regional pain. The prevalence of FM in the medical setting is much greater, with about 20 to 30% of rheumatology visits in the United States being made for FM.

PATHOBIOLOGY

There is persuasive evidence that FM pain results from abnormal sensory processing within the central nervous system. This is commonly referred to as *central sensitization* and results from an amplification of peripheral sensory stimuli and a deficit of descending inhibitory control from the midbrain. The magnification of peripheral sensory input is readily visualized as increased activity in somatosensory areas of the brain on magnetic resonance imaging in FM subjects versus healthy controls. Central sensitization is the result of a persistent neuronal hyperexcitability that continues long after the original sensitizing input has waned. The pathophysiology of this phenomenon is based, in part, on temporal summation of neural impulses. This occurs when pain fibers (unmyelinated C) are repetitively stimulated at a rate greater than one impulse every 3 seconds. At a biochemical level, such stimulation results in depolarization of N-methyl-D-aspartate (NMDA) receptors, which causes transcriptional changes that affect pain processing. Experimentally, this has been demonstrated in FM patients after repetitive thermal stimulation of the skin and after intramuscular electrical stimulation. Thus, persistent pain input may eventually give rise to central sensitization in some individuals, probably based, in part, on a genetic predisposition.

The frequent development of FM from focal pain states, such as in rheumatoid arthritis, post-traumatic injuries, and endometriosis, is thought to be a result of chronic nociceptive input stimulating central neuroplastic changes. However, the occurrence of FM in relation to persistent psychological stressors and infections cannot be so readily explained by temporal summation. FM developing in these settings is now thought to involve the activation of glial cells by cytokines, chemokines, and other neuronal activators. Several studies have reported elevated blood levels of interleukin-8 and a two- to three-fold increase in cerebrospinal fluid levels of substance P, glutamate, and nerve growth factor in patients with FM.

The descending pain system, originating in the periaqueductal gray nucleus of the midbrain and terminating in the dorsal horn, is important in modulating the transmission of nerve impulses to the brain. Activation of the nuclei in the midbrain involved in this system occurs in response to opioids, endorphins, emotions, and the placebo response. This modulation may upregulate or downregulate sensory processing, and in part, it underlies the influence of the psyche on the pain experience.

Understanding the biologic basis for central sensitization has provided an explanation for the common association of FM with other conditions such as irritable bowel syndrome, overactive bladder, multiple chemical hypersensitivity, and chronic daily headaches. Other common symptoms in FM, such as fatigue and cognitive dysfunction, cannot currently be explained by central sensitization. These symptoms are also common features of CFS, and their pathobiologic basis remains ill defined.

CLINICAL MANIFESTATIONS

Signs and Symptoms

Pain

The core symptom of FM is chronic widespread pain and stiffness. Characteristically, the pain is described as a constant dull ache that is worsened by muscle overactivity. FM-related pain is usually perceived as arising from muscle; however, many patients also report joint pain but have no objective evidence of arthritis.

Fatigue

Easy fatigability from physical exertion, mental exertion, and psychological stressors is typical of FM. Patients with CFS and FM share many similarities; about 75% of patients meeting the diagnostic criteria for CFS also meet the criteria for FM.

Disordered Sleep

FM patients have nonrestorative sleep. Even if they sleep continuously for 8 to 10 hours, they awake feeling tired. Many exhibit an alpha-delta electroencephalographic pattern that explains their failure to achieve restorative stages 3 and 4 of non–rapid eye movement sleep. A poor night's sleep is often followed by a worsening of FM symptoms the next day. Restless leg syndrome and the associated periodic limb movement disorder occur in up to 60% of FM patients.

Cognitive Dysfunction

Cognitive dysfunction is a prominent complaint of many FM patients. They commonly describe difficulties with working memory, semantic memory, concentration, logical analysis, and motivation. It has been estimated that the working memory deficit in FM is comparable to 20 years of aging. Recent studies have documented that these neurocognitive deficits correlate

TABLE 282-1 COMPARISON OF CLASSIFICATION CRITERIA FOR FIBROMYALGIA AND CHRONIC FATIGUE SYNDROME

	FIBROMYALGIA	CHRONIC FATIGUE SYNDROME
Primary symptom	Persistent, unexplained, widespread pain of ≥3 mo duration (*Widespread* is defined as pain in ≥3 quadrants of the body plus pain in an axial distribution, such as the neck, front of the chest, thoracic spine, or low back.)	Unexplained persistent or relapsing chronic fatigue of new or definite onset (not lifelong) that is not the result of ongoing exertion; is not substantially alleviated by rest; and results in a substantial reduction in previous levels of occupational, educational, social, or personal activities
Secondary features	None	Concurrent occurrence of 4 or more of the following symptoms, all of which must have persisted or recurred during 6 or more consecutive months of illness and must not have predated the fatigue: Sore throat; Tender cervical or axillary lymph nodes; Muscle pain; Multijoint pain without swelling or redness; Headaches of a new type, pattern, or severity; Nonrefreshing sleep; Postexertional malaise lasting >24 hr
Physical examination	The finding of ≥11 of 18 designated tender points examined at a palpation pressure of 4 kg	None
Exclusionary diagnoses	None	Any active medical condition that might explain the presence of chronic fatigue. Any previous condition that might explain fatigue and is still ongoing. Any past or current diagnosis of a major depressive disorder with psychotic or melancholic features, bipolar affective disorders, schizophrenia disorders, delusional disorders, dementias, anorexia nervosa, bulimia, or substance abuse within 2 yr before onset, or morbid obesity

with local brain morphology in the frontal lobe and anterior cingulate gyrus.

Psychological Distress

Having a chronic, painful disorder for which there is no generally accepted cure often produces an existential crisis. Approximately 30% of FM patients have significant depression at any given time, and about 60% have a lifetime prevalence of depressive illness. Although psychiatric disorders are common in FM patients, they do not seem to be intrinsically related to the pathophysiology of FM; effective treatment of depression with a selective serotonin re-uptake inhibitor (SSRI) does not eliminate FM pain. However, FM and depression show familial clustering, suggesting an underlying genetic susceptibility.

Associated Problems

FM patients often have a spectrum of other pain disorders that share similar features, such as not having a well-defined cause, being associated with mood disorders, and having no definitive cure. These accompanying disorders are often referred to as *central sensitivity syndromes* and include irritable bowel syndrome, painful bladder syndrome, temporomandibular pain disorder, chronic pelvic pain, chronic daily headaches, and chemical hypersensitivity syndrome.

History

Initiation and Maintenance of Fibromyalgia

FM seldom emerges "out of the blue." Many patients report an acute injury, repetitive workload, persistent stress, infections, and toxins related to the onset of FM. It is not uncommon for a regional pain state to evolve into FM. FM is commonly found as an accompaniment of other painful disorders, such as rheumatoid arthritis, low back pain, systemic lupus erythematosus, Sjögren's syndrome, inflammatory bowel disease, endometriosis, and osteoarthritis. There is increasing evidence that FM is a common occurrence in victims of post-traumatic stress disorder; for instance, both FM and CFS were common diagnoses after Operation Desert Storm in 1991.

DIAGNOSIS

The diagnosis of FM is usually based on the 1990 classification criteria recommended by the ACR (see Table 282-1). Following are the locations of the nine paired tender points:

- Occiput: bilateral, at the suboccipital muscle insertions
- Low cervical: bilateral, at the anterior aspects of the intertransverse spaces at C5-C7
- Trapezius: bilateral, at the midpoint of the upper border

TABLE 282-2 MAJOR ISSUES IN THE MANAGEMENT OF PATIENTS WITH FIBROMYALGIA

Education
Pain
Fatigue
Sleep
Mood disorders
Deconditioning
Associated "central sensitization" disorders

- Supraspinatus: bilateral, at the origins, above the scapular spine near the medial border
- Second rib: bilateral, at the second costochondral junctions just lateral to the junctions on the upper surfaces
- Lateral epicondyle: bilateral, 2 cm distal to the epicondyles
- Gluteal: bilateral, in the upper outer quadrants of the buttocks in the anterior fold of muscle
- Greater trochanter: bilateral, posterior to the trochanteric prominence
- Knee: bilateral, at the medial fat pad proximal to the joint line

There is some recent evidence that the FM tender points are in fact typical myofascial trigger points, thus providing an important link to a peripheral source of pain input to the central nervous system. FM is not a diagnosis of exclusion; thus, laboratory tests and imaging studies play no role in establishing the diagnosis according to the 1990 ACR criteria, although they are often indicated in the evaluation of accompanying peripheral pain generators.

TREATMENT

Successful management of FM requires a thorough analysis in terms of the biopsychosocial model of disease. The major management issues that require attention are listed in Table 282-2.

Education

There is evidence that higher educational attainment is associated with a better prognosis in many chronic disorders such as FM. Education has a positive effect through cognitive behavioral strategies, such as goal setting and reassessment of priorities. Educated patients are more likely to take an active role in self-management.

Pain

In considering the management of pain in FM, it is logical to focus on the major sites of pain processing, namely, peripheral pain generation and central pain pathways. There is no specific tissue pathology, at least in peripheral tissues, that is characteristic of FM. However, once the central nervous system is sensitized, not only are peripheral pain generators perceived as being more painful, but they also prolong and amplify the central neuroplastic changes. Thus, a critical first component of treating FM pain is to identify and effectively treat all peripheral pain generators, which commonly include peripheral arthritis, axial arthritis, spinal stenosis, myofascial trigger points, neuropathic pain, vascular headaches, visceral pain (e.g., irritable bowel syndrome, overactive bladder), postsurgical pain, and pelvic pain syndromes (e.g., endometriosis).

Management of central sensitization is typically initiated with heterocyclic antidepressant (HCA) medications such as amitriptyline, trazodone, cyclobenzaprine, or nortriptyline. There is good evidence that antidepressant medications with both re-uptake inhibition of serotonin and norepinephrine (e.g., venlafaxine, duloxetine, milnacipran) are more effective in treating FM pain. Both duloxetine and milnacipran have been approved by the Food and Drug Administration (FDA) for use in FM.[1,2] Importantly, the mechanism of action of these drugs is independent of any antidepressant effect and results from upregulation of the descending pain system that originates in the brain stem and uses serotonin and norepinephrine as neurotransmitters at dorsal horn synapses. Anticonvulsant medications such as gabapentin, pregabalin, and topiramate are increasingly being used in FM and other chronic pain states; they inhibit the presynaptic release of glutamate and thus modulate the activation of NMDA receptors.[3] Pregabalin has FDA approval for use in FM. Sedative-hypnotics such as zolpidem and zopiclone often help with nonrestorative sleep but not with pain. Sodium oxybate, an FDA-approved drug for narcolepsy, has been shown to improve not only sleep but also pain, stiffness, and fatigue in FM patients.[4]

Opioids are often used in the treatment of FM, but long-term trials are lacking. Although they should not be the first choice of analgesia, they should not be withheld if less powerful analgesics have failed. Tramadol (both Ultram and Ultracet) proved useful in reducing FM pain in two controlled trials.[5] Tramadol is a weak opioid agonist that also inhibits the re-uptake of serotonin and norepinephrine at the level of the dorsal horn. It is metabolized by CYP2D6, as are many antidepressant medications. FM patients who are taking tramadol or any of several antidepressants that are eliminated by CYP2D6 are at risk for developing a serotonin syndrome. Thus, careful review of concomitant medications is an important prerequisite before prescribing new medications, especially in difficult-to-treat patients who are often taking multiple medications.

Fatigue

A search for a treatable cause of fatigue is always indicated (Table 282-3). Common treatable causes of chronic fatigue in FM patients are inappropriate dosing of medications, depression, aerobic deconditioning, a primary sleep disorder (e.g., sleep apnea), nonrestorative sleep, a coexisting inflammatory disorder, and neurally mediated hypotension. As in CFS, the underlying cause of *primary* fatigue in FM is not known. Sodium oxybate, methylphenidate, and modafinil have improved fatigue in some FM patients.

Sleep

Low-dose HCAs are the mainstay of sleep pharmacotherapy in FM patients. Some patients cannot tolerate HCAs because of unacceptable levels of daytime drowsiness or weight gain. In these patients, short-acting benzodiazepine-like medications such as zolpidem, zapelon, and eszopiclone may be beneficial. Sodium oxybate is proving to be a useful medication in improving the nonrestorative sleep of FM. About 25% of male and 15% of female FM patients have sleep apnea, which usually requires treatment with continuous positive airway pressure or surgery. By far the most common sleep disorder in FM patients is restless leg syndrome or periodic limb movement disorder. Treatment is with dopamine agonists such as L-dopa/carbidopa (Sinemet), pramipexole (Mirapex), or ropinirole (Requip).[6]

Psychological Distress

Stressors related to psychosocial, economic, and health issues often develop in FM patients. Psychological intervention in terms of improving the internal locus of control and more effective problem solving is important in such patients. Cognitive-behavioral therapy is particularly well suited to effect these changes.[7] Although antidepressant medications are commonly used in the treatment of pain and disordered sleep in FM patients, the doses are often suboptimal for treating depressive illness.

Deconditioning

A carefully graded program of aerobic conditioning and stretching is a critical component of an effective FM treatment program.[8] The benefits of exercise are based on good scientific evidence, but overzealous exercise usually aggravates pain. Tai chi also may be an effective treatment for fibromyalgia.[9] In general, exercise needs to be added incrementally to the program *after* some control of pain, sleep, and depression has been achieved.

Endocrine Dysfunction

There is no good evidence that FM is primarily due to an endocrine disorder. However, common problems such as hypothyroidism and menopausal symptoms often aggravate pain and fatigue, and appropriate replacement therapy is often worth a trial.

TABLE 282-3 DIFFERENTIAL DIAGNOSIS OF CHRONIC FATIGUE

CHRONIC INFECTIONS	CHRONIC INFLAMMATION
Hepatitis C	Rheumatoid arthritis
Lyme disease	Systemic lupus erythematosus
Parasitic and fungal infections	Sjögren's syndrome
Tuberculosis	Polymyositis/dermatomyositis
Human immunodeficiency virus	Vasculitis
Xenotropic murine leukemia retrovirus	Sarcoidosis
SLEEP DISORDERS	**CARDIOPULMONARY**
Obstructive sleep apnea	Congestive heart failure
Restless leg syndrome	Neurally mediated hypotension
Circadian rhythm disorder	Postural orthostatic tachycardia syndrome
Upper airway resistance syndrome	Pulmonary hypertension
Narcolepsy/parasomnias	Chronic obstructive pulmonary disease
Alpha-delta sleep disorder	Mitral valve prolapse
ENDOCRINE/METABOLIC DISORDERS	**GASTROINTESTINAL**
Addison's disease	Celiac disease
Cushing's syndrome	Inflammatory bowel disease
Poorly controlled diabetes	Autoimmune hepatitis
Thyroid disorders	Hepatic cirrhosis
Hemochromatosis	**MALIGNANCY**
Hypopituitarism	Lymphoma and occult malignancies
Diabetes insipidus	Postchemotherapy syndrome
GENERAL MEDICAL DISORDERS	**NEUROLOGIC DISORDERS**
Anemia (any cause)	Multiple sclerosis
Chronic renal/hepatic failure	Myasthenia gravis
Malnutrition	Muscular dystrophies
Medication side effects	Parkinson's disease
Chronic pain disorders	Early dementia
PSYCHOLOGICAL	**LIFESTYLE FACTORS**
Mood disorders (depression, anxiety, bipolar)	Chronic overwork
Schizophrenia	Persistent unresolved stress
Post-traumatic stress disorder	Inadequate exercise
Anorexia nervosa/bulimia	Morbid obesity (body mass index >40)
Childhood abuse and/or neglect	Alcoholism/drug abuse

PROGNOSIS

FM symptoms usually persist for many years. However, patients seen in the community rather than at tertiary care centers reportedly have a 24% remission rate after 2 years. The consequences of pain, fatigue, and cognitive dysfunction negatively influence the sustained performance of physical and mental tasks. Everyday activities take longer for FM patients, who need more time to get started in the morning and often require extra rest periods during the day. A survey of FM patients seen at academic centers reported that 70% perceived themselves as being disabled, and 16% were receiving Social Security benefits.

CHRONIC FATIGUE SYNDROME

EPIDEMIOLOGY

Fatigue is a common symptom; indeed, some 50% of individuals report "feeling fatigued" in population surveys. Fatigue is one of the most common problems reported to primary care doctors. In a series of 1000 consecutive patients seen in primary care settings, 8.5% reported debilitating fatigue lasting 6 months or longer without apparent cause; only 15% satisfied the clinical definition for CFS shown in Table 282-1. In many cases, fatigue is self-limited or the causes are self-evident (e.g., insufficient rest, a medical illness, depression, insomnia). The prevalence of CFS has ranged from 0.006 to 3.0% in various population surveys. CFS is diagnosed predominantly in women aged 30 to 45 years. They are typically highly functional before the onset of the illness.

PATHOBIOLOGY

The cause of CFS remains poorly defined. There are many reports linking CFS with chronic infections; most have not stood up to careful scrutiny. The latest such study reported that 67% of patients with CFS versus 3.7% of healthy controls were infected with a retrovirus—the xenotropic murine leukemia virus (XMRV); two other studies failed to find an association with XMRV infection. Although many CFS patients complain of nonrestorative sleep, polysomnographic studies have been inconclusive. The similarity between CFS and early Addison's disease has prompted numerous neuroendocrine studies, which have failed to show a clinically treatable endocrine deficiency; however, subtle changes in the hypothalamic-pituitary-adrenal response to acute stressors is found in about 30% of patients. A similar proportion of CFS patients have abnormal results on tilt-table testing, with evidence of autonomic dysfunction in terms of neurally mediated hypotension or postural orthostatic tachycardia syndrome. This may be relevant in a subpopulation of patients, but treatment with fludrocortisone had no overall benefit in one large placebo-controlled study. Many studies have suggested a low level of immune stimulation in CFS, the most common abnormalities being reduced natural killer cell function and increased numbers of cytotoxic T cells. However, these findings are not diagnostically useful, and clinical improvement has not been associated with any significant change in immune markers. Extensive psychological testing in CFS patients has failed to reveal a common psychiatric denominator. Nevertheless, it is generally accepted, as in FM and other chronic illnesses, that psychosocial distress and maladaptive coping strategies play a role in symptom attribution and perpetuation.

CLINICAL MANIFESTATIONS

The chief complaint of patients in whom CFS is diagnosed is an abrupt onset of debilitating fatigue that causes significant impairment in daily activities, work ability, and social relationships. Typically, these patients report an excellent health status just before the onset of fatigue, which is often preceded by a flu-like prodrome. Symptoms suggestive of an infectious etiology include low-grade fever, night sweats, tender cervical lymph nodes, sore throat, myalgias, and headaches. As in FM, many CFS patients complain of generalized musculoskeletal pain, cognitive dysfunction, irritable bowel syndrome, temporomandibular pain disorders, nonrestorative sleep, and multiple chemical sensitivities.

DIAGNOSIS

The current diagnosis of CFS is based on the recommendations of the 1994 international CFS study group (see Table 282-1). This revision added the minor criteria of postexercise fatigue and cognitive dysfunction to the CDC's original 1988 working case definition. Unlike the criteria for FM, there are no physical findings in the CFS criteria. Furthermore, whereas the definition of FM contains no exclusionary criteria, the definition of CFS excludes patients with fatiguing medical disorders, melancholic depression, psychotic disorders, substance abuse, and severe obesity (body mass index >40). Because CFS is not a diagnosis of exclusion, it is important to systematically evaluate the patient for treatable causes of fatigue (see Table 282-3).

TABLE 282-4	DIAGNOSTIC FEATURES OF A MYOFASCIAL TRIGGER POINT

Focal point of tenderness on palpation of involved muscle
Reproduction of pain complaint by trigger point palpation (≈3 kg pressure)
Palpation reveals induration of adjacent muscle ("taut band")
Often pseudoweakness of muscle involved (no atrophy)
Often referred pain on continued pressure (≈5-sec duration) over trigger point

● MYOFASCIAL PAIN

Pain arising from muscle is a universal human experience. In most instances, it is due to muscle *macrotrauma* (i.e., muscle tear or sprain) or muscle *microtrauma* (i.e., injury at the sarcomere level resulting from repetitive muscle use or overexertion). After appropriate rest, the pain usually dissipates over a period of a few days to weeks. In some cases, a persistent pain focus develops that has the characteristics of a myofascial trigger point. This diagnosis should be considered if the patient complains of focal pain that is aggravated by muscle use or psychological stressors that cause increased muscle tension. Myofascial trigger points often play a role in poorly characterized focal pain syndromes such as low back pain, jaw pain, pelvic pain, and headache.

A myofascial trigger point is a well-defined point of focal tenderness within a muscle. Palpation usually reveals a rope-like induration referred to as a *taut band*. In many instances, firm palpation of this area causes pain in a referred distribution that reproduces the patient's symptoms. Importantly, referred pain from a trigger point does not follow a nerve root distribution (i.e., it is not dermatomal). Trigger points frequently cause dysfunction in terms of restricted range of movement and weakness; the involved muscle or muscles often demonstrate easy fatigability (Table 282-4).

Electromyographic recordings from trigger points show spontaneous low-voltage activity resembling end plate spike potentials. In normal muscle, depolarization of the motor end plate initiates the release of calcium ions from the sarcoplasmic reticulum, which in turn results in activation of the myosin-actin contractile elements ("contraction coupling"). It is thought that the areas of electrical hyperexcitability in trigger points result from a nonphysiologic focal contraction caused by an influx of calcium ions into the damaged sarcomeres. If this process is not "switched off," excessive utilization of adenosine triphosphate may result in a focal energy crisis in the injured muscle, thus perpetuating the problem. Functional magnetic resonance imaging studies have confirmed the hyperalgesic features of myofascial trigger points in terms of increased activity of brain regions involved in processing stimulus intensity and negative affect. Microdialysis of trigger point foci have shown a more acidic pH and an increase of inflammatory cytokines, bradykinin, substance P, and calcitonin gene–related peptide compared with adjacent muscle.

Factors commonly cited as predisposing to trigger point formation include deconditioning, poor posture, repetitive mechanical stress, mechanical imbalance (e.g., leg length inequality), joint disorders, and nonrestorative sleep. The muscle pain experienced by FM patients is often the result of pain originating from myofascial trigger points and amplified by central sensitization. Interestingly, FM tender points were recently reported to have the clinical and electromyographic features typical of myofascial trigger points. It is hypothesized that myofascial pain is an important peripheral pain generator that may, in some FM patients, perpetuate and accentuate the process of central sensitization.

TREATMENT   Rx

Management of CFS follows the general management guidelines for FM. Patients with presumed CFS should have a general medical work-up to exclude treatable causes of fatigue (e.g., hypothyroidism, anemia), and consideration should be given to more specialized studies such as polysomnography and tilt-table testing in selected cases. Currently, there is no generally accepted pharmacologic intervention for patients with CFS. Antidepressants (HCAs and SSRIs) are of minimal benefit, although two studies reported a modest benefit with the use of monoamine oxidase inhibitors in patients with significant vegetative symptoms. Inconsistent benefits have been described with fludrocortisone and low-dose corticosteroids. The mainstay of treating CFS is to engage the patient in a gently graded program of aerobic exercise.■10■ Cognitive-behavioral therapy may correct dysfunctional thought patterns but seldom improves fatigue. Management of pain and psychological distress in CFS is the same as for FM.

TREATMENT   Rx

Management of myofascial trigger points is based on the following principles.

Posture and Ergonomics

An important issue in the effective management of myofascial pain syndromes is correction of predisposing factors (see earlier). These factors interfere with the muscle's ability to fully recover and are the most common reason for treatment failure.

Stretching

Restoration of a muscle to its full stretch length breaks the link between the energy crisis and the contraction of injured sarcomeres (see earlier). Commonly used stretching techniques include spray and stretch with ethyl chloride, acupressure, post-isometric relaxation, and deep stroking massage.

Strengthening

Muscles harboring trigger points usually become weak because of the inhibitory effects of pain. A program of slowly progressive strengthening is essential to restore full function and minimize the risk of recurrence and perpetuation of satellite trigger points.

Trigger Point Injections

Needling the myofascial trigger point with a "peppering technique" often provides a worthwhile and long-lasting benefit. Although dry needling is effective, the use of a local anesthetic (1% lidocaine or 1% procaine) helps confirm the accuracy of the injection and provides immediate relief. Validation of the accuracy of the injection is suggested by the patient's report that the pain is reproduced on entry of the needle into the trigger point; in superficial muscles, a local twitch response may be observed, providing further evidence of an accurate injection. Both injections and lidocaine patches have shown effectiveness in controlled trials. **11**

Medications

Treatment of myofascial trigger points is mainly nonpharmacologic. Nonsteroidal anti-inflammatory drugs and other analgesics often provide moderate symptomatic relief. As in FM, drugs that modulate pain at the central level are a useful adjunct in difficult-to-treat patients, especially if central sensitization is suspected.

FUTURE DIRECTIONS

Both FM and CFS represent a major challenge to modern medicine in terms of understanding a constellation of common, often disabling symptoms that originate in the central nervous system but cannot be explained by a classic psychological disorder. The central sensitization demonstrated in FM patients has provided important insight into the physiologic basis for the complaint of widespread pain, but no such breakthrough has occurred in the comprehensive understanding of fatigue in either FM or CFS. Current research suggests that both these conditions have a genetic predisposition that interacts with environmental insults such as infections, trauma, myofascial foci, and psychological stressors. One common denominator being actively explored in both conditions is the activation of glial cells within the central nervous system by cytokines and chemokines. Both these disorders are prime examples of the need to integrate the classic biomedical model of disease with psychosocial influences (i.e., the biopsychosocial model of disease). The challenge that faces investigators in the 21st century is to discern whether mental processes can influence and interact with environmental stressors and focal pain generators to change the epigenetic expression of genes involved in pain processing and fatigue.

1. Arnold LM. Duloxetine and other antidepressants in the treatment of patients with fibromyalgia. *Pain Med.* 2007;8(Suppl 2):S63-S74.
2. Mease PJ, Clauw DJ, Gendreau RM, et al. The efficacy and safety of milnacipran for treatment of fibromyalgia. A randomized, double-blind, placebo-controlled trial. *J Rheumatol.* 2009;36:398-409.
3. Crofford LJ, Rowbotham MC, Mease PJ, et al. Pregabalin for the treatment of fibromyalgia syndrome: results of a randomized, double-blind, placebo-controlled trial. *Arthritis Rheum.* 2005;52:1264-1273.
4. Russell IJ, Perkins AT, Michalek JE. Sodium oxybate relieves pain and improves function in fibromyalgia syndrome: a randomized, double-blind, placebo-controlled, multicenter clinical trial. *Arthritis Rheum.* 2009;60:299-309.
5. Bennett RM, Kamin M, Karim R, et al. Tramadol and acetaminophen combination tablets in the treatment of fibromyalgia pain: a double-blind, randomized, placebo-controlled study. *Am J Med.* 2003;114:537-545.
6. Ferini-Strambi L. Treatment options for restless legs syndrome. *Expert Opin Pharmacother.* 2009;10:545-554.
7. Vazquez-Rivera S, Gonzalez-Blanch C, Rodriguez-Moya L, et al. Brief cognitive-behavioral therapy with fibromyalgia patients in routine care. *Compr Psychiatry.* 2009;50:517-525.
8. Brosseau L, Wells GA, Tugwell P, et al. Ottawa Panel evidence-based clinical practice guidelines for strengthening exercises in the management of fibromyalgia. *Phys Ther.* 2008;88:873-886.
9. Wang C, Schmid CH, Rones R, et al. A randomized trial of tai chi for fibromyalgia. *N Engl J Med.* 2010;236:743-754.
10. White PD, Goldsmith KA, Johnson AL, et al. Comparison of adaptive pacing therapy, cognitive behaviour therapy, graded exercise therapy, and specialist medical care for chronic fatigue syndrome (PACE): a randomised trial. *Lancet.* 2011;377:823-836.
11. Affaitati G, Fabrizio A, Savini A, et al. A randomized, controlled study comparing a lidocaine patch, a placebo patch, and anesthetic injection for treatment of trigger points in patients with myofascial pain syndrome: evaluation of pain and somatic pain thresholds. *Clin Ther.* 2009;31:705-720.

SUGGESTED READINGS

Avellaneda Fernández A, Pérez-Martín A, Izquierdo Martínez M, et al. Chronic fatigue syndrome: aetiology, diagnosis and treatment. *BMC Psychiatry.* 2009;9(Suppl 1):S1-11. *Comprehensive description of the clinical, diagnostic, investigational, and psychosocial features of CFS.*
Bennett RM. Clinical manifestations and diagnosis of fibromyalgia. *Rheum Dis Clin North Am.* 2009;35:215-232. *Up-to-date review of the clinical spectrum of fibromyalgia and diagnostic considerations.*
Menéndez-Arias L. Evidence and controversies on the role of XMRV in prostate cancer and chronic fatigue syndrome. *Rev Med Virol.* 2011;21:3-17. *Review of the current controversy on a possible link to a retrovirus.*
Yunus MB. Central sensitivity syndromes: a new paradigm and group nosology for fibromyalgia and overlapping conditions, and the related issue of disease versus illness. *Semin Arthritis Rheum.* 2008;37:339-352. *Well-referenced article on the common clinical and physiologic aspects of syndromes that overlap with FM.*

283

SYSTEMIC DISEASES IN WHICH ARTHRITIS IS A FEATURE

STERLING G. WEST

Arthritis, arthralgias, and myalgias can be significant features of several systemic diseases and may be the presenting symptoms for some of these disorders (Table 283-1). Appropriate evaluation of these musculoskeletal symptoms, including selected laboratory tests and radiographs, can provide clues to the early diagnosis of these diseases. Synovial biopsies are rarely necessary but can be diagnostic. Brief descriptions of the arthritic manifestations of some of these systemic disorders follow; a more detailed discussion of each entity is found in the chapters devoted to these diseases. Because of the rarity of many of these diseases, evidence-based treatments with Food and Drug Administration–approved medications are lacking.

AUTOIMMUNE HEPATITIS

Patients with type I autoimmune hepatitis (Chapter 151) may present with a syndrome resembling systemic lupus erythematosus (SLE; Chapter 274). Patients with the early-onset subset are frequently young and female, with complaints of polyarthralgia and occasionally fever. Laboratory examination may show leukopenia, a positive antinuclear antibody (70 to 90%), elevated erythrocyte sedimentation rate, polyclonal gammopathy, and elevated liver-associated enzymes. Antibodies against double-stranded DNA are usually not seen, whereas antibodies against the smooth muscle antigen (F1 actin) support the diagnosis. Joint radiographs show soft tissue swelling without erosions or deformity. Joint pain resolves with corticosteroid therapy for the liver disease.

PRIMARY BILIARY CIRRHOSIS

Up to 50% of patients with primary biliary cirrhosis (Chapter 158) have other autoimmune disorders, including rheumatoid arthritis (RA), Sjögren's syndrome, limited scleroderma, and autoimmune thyroiditis. In addition to antimitochondrial antibodies, rheumatoid factor, antinuclear antibodies, and anticentromere antibodies are often present. More than 10% of patients with primary biliary cirrhosis have a symmetrical or asymmetrical small joint inflammatory arthritis. Unlike RA, it can involve distal interphalangeal joints and is rarely erosive or deforming. Other musculoskeletal manifestations include osteomalacia related to vitamin D deficiency, osteoporosis related to renal tubular acidosis, and hypertrophic osteoarthropathy associated with liver disease.

WHIPPLE'S DISEASE

An inflammatory arthritis occurs in 60 to 90% of patients with Whipple's disease (Chapter 142) and may precede other clinical manifestations by

TABLE 283-1 SYSTEMIC DISEASES ASSOCIATED WITH ARTHRITIS

DISEASE	TEST*
GASTROINTESTINAL DISEASES	
Autoimmune hepatitis	Liver-associated enzymes, *ASMA*
Primary biliary cirrhosis	Alkaline phosphatase, *antimitochondrial Ab*
Pancreatitis-arthritis syndrome	Lipase, amylase, *abdominal CT scan*
Whipple's disease	*Tissue biopsy, PCR for Tropheryma whippelii DNA*
Gluten-sensitive enteropathy	*Antitransglutaminase antibody, small bowel biopsy*
Inflammatory bowel disease	Stool guaiac, *colonoscopy*
Hepatitis B/hepatitis C	Liver-associated enzymes, *hepatitis serology, cryoglobulins*
Intestinal bypass arthritis	*Cryoglobulins*
HEMATOLOGIC DISORDERS	
Hemophilia	PTT, *factor VIII and IX levels*
Hemoglobinopathies	CBC, *hemoglobin electrophoresis*
Hypogammaglobulinemia	Low total protein, *SPEP, immunoglobulins*
Plasma cell dyscrasias	High total protein, *SPEP, UPEP, IEF*
ENDOCRINE DISORDERS	
Diabetes mellitus	Glucose, *hemoglobin A$_{1c}$*
Thyroid disorders	TSH, *thyroxine*
Parathyroid disorders	Calcium, phosphorus, *PTH*
Acromegaly	Radiographs, *growth hormone*
Hyperlipoproteinemia	Lipid panel
Paget's disease	Alkaline phosphatase, radiographs, *bone scan*
MALIGNANT DISORDERS	
Hypertrophic osteoarthropathy	Radiographs (hands, wrists, chest)
Leukemia and lymphoma	CBC, LDH, *bone marrow/tissue biopsy*
Carcinomatous polyarthritis	*Cancer screen*
Palmar fasciitis and arthritis	*CA-125, pelvic CT scan*
OTHER DISEASES	
Hemochromatosis	Iron studies, radiographs, *HFE gene*
Multicentric reticulohistiocytosis	Radiographs, *skin/synovial biopsy*
Sarcoidosis	Chest radiograph, *ACE level, tissue biopsy*
Alkaptonuria	Radiographs, *homogentisic acid level*
Fabry's disease	Angiokeratomas, *α-galactosidase A level or gene mutation*
Relapsing polychondritis	*Cartilage biopsy*
Cystic fibrosis	Chest radiograph, *sweat chloride*
Pigmented villonodular synovitis	Synovial fluid analysis, *MRI, synovial biopsy*
Systemic infections	Cultures, serologies (RPR, HIV, parvovirus)

*Tests listed are common laboratory tests and radiographs that are frequently ordered; this information should provide a clue that a systemic disease is a possible cause of the patient's musculoskeletal symptoms. These tests, coupled with the history and physical examination, should be followed by more specific serologies and biopsies (listed in italics) to confirm the diagnosis.

Ab = antibody; ACE = angiotensin-converting enzyme; ASMA = anti–smooth muscle antibody; CBC = complete blood cell count; CT = computed tomography; HIV = human immunodeficiency virus; IEF = immunoelectrophoresis; LDH = lactate dehydrogenase; MRI = magnetic resonance imaging; PCR = polymerase chain reaction; PTH = parathyroid hormone; PTT = partial thromboplastin time; RPR = rapid plasmin reagin; SPEP = serum protein electrophoresis; TSH = thyroid-stimulating hormone; UPEP = urine protein electrophoresis.

years. The joint involvement is typically an intermittent, migratory oligoarthritis affecting large joints more than small joints or the spine, lasting from several hours to days. The synovial fluid is inflammatory, with a predominance of mononuclear cells. Subcutaneous nodules are occasionally seen, contributing to an erroneous diagnosis of rheumatic fever or RA. However, patients consistently test negative for rheumatoid factor and antinuclear antibodies. Synovial biopsies show rod-shaped bacilli on electron microscopy, which have been identified as *Tropheryma whippelii*. Diagnosis is typically made by duodenal, synovial, or lymph node biopsy showing periodic acid–Schiff–positive macrophages. Polymerase chain reaction to detect DNA of the organism in peripheral blood, cerebrospinal fluid, synovial fluid, or tissue biopsy specimens is under investigation and is not universally available. Typically, the arthritis does not cause radiographic changes or deformities. Prolonged antibiotic therapy results in resolution of musculoskeletal as well as other symptoms of this disease.

GLUTEN-SENSITIVE ENTEROPATHY (CELIAC DISEASE)

An asymmetrical oligoarthritis or symmetrical polyarthritis occurs in up to 25% of adults with celiac disease (Chapter 142). It may precede the enteropathic symptoms by months to years. Large joints such as knees and ankles, more than hips and shoulders, are most commonly involved. Axial involvement is reported. The arthritis does not cause deformities or radiographic changes and resolves with a gluten-free diet in 40 to 50% of cases. Another musculoskeletal manifestation is osteomalacia related to vitamin D malabsorption, which may mimic diffuse fibromyalgia.

PANCREATIC-ARTHRITIS SYNDROME

Pancreatic panniculitis is a systemic syndrome occurring in some patients with pancreatic acinar cell carcinoma and less commonly in patients with pancreatitis or hematologic malignancies. This syndrome is characterized by tender red nodules, usually on the extremities; these are frequently misdiagnosed as erythema nodosum, but biopsy shows areas of lobular panniculitis with fat necrosis. Arthritis occurs in 60% of patients and usually involves the ankles and knees. Synovial fluid is typically noninflammatory and creamy in color. It contains multiple lipid droplets because of necrosis of fat in the synovial membrane. Other manifestations include osteolytic lesions (10%) from bone marrow fat necrosis, pleuropericarditis, fever, and eosinophilia. The prominent fat necrosis is due to the release of lipase, amylase, and trypsin from the diseased pancreas. Another musculoskeletal manifestation resulting from pancreatic disease is osteomalacia from vitamin D deficiency related to malabsorption.

HEMOPHILIA

Hemophilia A (factor VIII deficiency) and hemophilia B (factor IX deficiency) (Chapter 177) are associated with hemarthrosis. Almost all patients with factor levels less than 1% of normal experience recurrent hemarthroses spontaneously or after minor trauma. Large joints (knees, elbows, ankles) are most commonly involved. Intramuscular hemorrhage can also occur. Recurrent hemarthrosis can lead to proliferative synovitis and cartilage degradation, resulting in both erosive and degenerative changes on radiographs. Physical examination shows bone enlargement, crepitus, atrophic muscles, and joint contractures. Treatment of acute monoarthritis consists of factor replacement to achieve a level of 30% or greater, given at the first sign of joint swelling. Patients with fever (temperature >38° C) or who fail to respond to factor replacement need joint aspiration to rule out septic arthritis, which occurs with an increased incidence in hemophilia. Chronic arthritis is treated with nonsteroidal anti-inflammatory drugs (NSAIDs), which do not inhibit platelet function; arthroscopic or radiation synovectomy for chronic synovitis; and total joint arthroplasty for end-stage joint disease. The regular prophylactic administration of factor replacement has reduced the risk of developing chronic arthropathy. Acute and chronic arthritis is less frequent and less severe in patients with hemophilia B compared with hemophilia A.

HEMOGLOBINOPATHIES

Patients with sickle cell anemia (Chapter 166) or the heterozygous state of sickle β-thalassemia, sickle-C disease, and sickle-D disease frequently experience polyarthralgia. Local sickling of cells leads to obstruction of the microcirculation and to bone infarctions. Patients most commonly experience painful crises causing chest, back, and joint pain. A painful large joint arthritis (usually in the knees), often with noninflammatory synovial effusions, lasting days to 2 to 3 weeks can also occur. Infarcts in the metaphyses of bones are commonly found on joint radiographs. Vertebral bodies have a characteristic "Lincoln log" appearance or a central cup-like indentation ("codfish vertebrae"). Femoral and humeral head osteonecrosis can occur in up to 33% of sickle cell anemia and sickle-C disease cases. Because of splenic dysfunction, septic arthritis and osteomyelitis (50% caused by *Salmonella*) have been associated with sickle cell disease. In adults, gout has been reported, whereas in children younger than 2 years, an acute, painful, nonpitting swelling of the hands and feet (hand-foot syndrome) associated with fever and leukocytosis may be the first manifestation of sickle cell anemia. Treatment includes intravenous hydration, oxygen, and analgesics. Hydroxyurea can reduce the frequency of painful crises. In patients with β-thalassemia major (Cooley's anemia; Chapter 165), significant expansion of bone marrow develops as a result of increased erythroid precursors, leading to osteoporosis and microfractures that affect primarily the lower extremities.

HYPOGAMMAGLOBULINEMIA

Patients with congenital X-linked hypogammaglobulinemia (Bruton's disease) or acquired common variable immunodeficiency (CVID; Chapter 258) can develop a nonerosive, noninfectious large joint oligoarthritis that responds to intravenous gamma globulin therapy. However, septic arthritis caused by common pathogens or *Mycoplasma* can also occur and must be rigorously excluded. In adults with acquired CVID, autoimmune conditions are common (22%), including autoimmune cytopenias, RA, and pernicious anemia. Selective immunoglobulin A (IgA) deficiency (Chapter 258) is associated with various rheumatic manifestations, including positive autoantibodies, in the absence of clinical disease. Systemic autoimmune disorders, including SLE, juvenile RA, and others, as well as organ-specific autoimmune disorders such as type 1 diabetes mellitus and myasthenia gravis, also occur in IgA-deficient individuals.

DIABETES MELLITUS

Diabetic stiff hand syndrome of limited joint mobility (diabetic cheiroarthropathy) occurs in more than 30% of patients with long-standing, poorly controlled type 1 or type 2 diabetes mellitus (Chapters 236 and 237). Patients present with the insidious development of flexion contractures and thickened skin of the fingers, which may be confused with scleroderma. These changes may be due to excess glycosylation of tendinous structures and accumulation of sugar alcohols, producing excess water content in the tissues and leading to increased stiffness. As a result of the inability to extend the fingers fully, the "prayer sign" is observed on physical examination. Unlike diabetic stiff hand syndrome, Dupuytren's contractures are due to a chronic thickening of the palmar aponeurosis, causing flexion deformities of the third and fourth digits. It is a frequent musculoskeletal complication, occurring in more than 20% of type 2 diabetics. A less common manifestation is Charcot's, or neuropathic, joints, occurring in less than 1% of all patients with long-standing diabetes. All patients have a diabetic peripheral neuropathy and typically present with painless swelling of the feet caused, most commonly, by destruction of the tarsometatarsal joints. Deformities can occur with midtarsal collapse ("rocker bottom" feet), predisposing to ulceration and infection of the skin over desensate bony prominences. Radiographs are diagnostic, and treatment should include supportive footwear and protected weight bearing.

Unlike Charcot's joint, diabetic osteolysis and diabetic amyotrophy are unique to diabetes. The osteolysis is characterized by resorption of the distal metatarsal bone and proximal phalanges of the feet, giving radiographs a characteristic "licked candy" appearance. Pain is variable, and treatment is conservative because the process may terminate on its own. Diabetic amyotrophy is a lumbar polyradiculopathy (L2-L4) that arises with severe pain, dysesthesias, and rapid atrophy of the proximal muscles of one or both thighs. Carpal tunnel syndrome (25%), adhesive capsulitis of the shoulder (frozen shoulder), flexor tenosynovitis (trigger finger) of the hands, diffuse idiopathic skeletal hyperostosis (type 2 diabetes), osteopenia (type 1 diabetes), diabetic muscle infarction (usually of the thigh), osteomyelitis of the foot, and septic joints are all musculoskeletal conditions that occur with increased frequency in diabetic patients. Aggressive control of blood glucose helps prevent some of these musculoskeletal complications.

THYROID DISORDERS

Musculoskeletal symptoms occur in 33% of patients with clinical hypothyroidism (thyroid-stimulating hormone levels >20 µU/mL) (Chapter 233). Patients can present with carpal tunnel syndrome, Raynaud's phenomenon, or muscle aching and stiffness similar to fibromyalgia and polymyalgia rheumatica. Patients with severe hypothyroidism can experience a noninflammatory myopathy with proximal muscle weakness and elevated creatine kinase, which may be confused clinically with polymyositis. Similarly, myxedematous patients can develop a symmetrical arthropathy of the large joints, especially the knees, associated with noninflammatory synovial fluid with increased viscosity. The association of hypothyroidism with chondrocalcinosis is controversial, but clearly patients beginning thyroid replacement therapy can experience an acute attack of pseudogout. Patients with hyperthyroidism can develop proximal myopathy (70%), adhesive capsulitis of the shoulder (10%), osteoporosis, or thyroid acropachy. Thyroid acropachy occurs in less than 1% of patients with Graves' disease and consists of soft

tissue swelling of the hands, digital clubbing, and periostitis, particularly involving the metacarpal and phalangeal bone shafts. Pain is usually mild, radiographs are characteristic, and there is no effective therapy. Patients with autoimmune thyroid disease have an increased prevalence of positive antinuclear antibodies and an increased association with systemic connective tissue diseases such as Sjögren's syndrome.

PARATHYROID DISORDERS

Primary hyperparathyroidism (Chapter 253) can arise with osteoporosis and fractures or with chondrocalcinosis and episodes of acute pseudogout. In severe hyperparathyroidism, which is rare, vague myalgias and arthralgias resembling fibromyalgia; a reversible, painless, proximal myopathy with normal creatine kinase; and osteitis fibrosa cystica with bone pain can be seen. Osteitis fibrosa cystica occurs primarily in patients with secondary hyperparathyroidism associated with renal failure and has a characteristic radiographic appearance, with subperiosteal resorption on the radial side of the phalanges, small erosions in the hands and distal clavicles, and discrete lytic bone lesions (brown tumors). Ectopic calcifications, joint laxity, and tendon ruptures have been reported in patients with severe hyperparathyroidism. Hypoparathyroidism has also been associated with myopathy and ectopic calcifications. Patients with type Ia pseudohypoparathyroidism and pseudo-pseudohypoparathyroidism have a shortened fourth metacarpal bone bilaterally.

ACROMEGALY

Up to 75% of patients with acromegaly (Chapter 231) develop an atypical form of osteoarthritis. The knees, shoulders, hips, and lumbosacral and cervical spine are the most frequently symptomatic areas, although the hands reveal the most characteristic radiographic changes, with widened joint spaces due to cartilage hypertrophy. Carpal tunnel syndrome (50%), Raynaud's phenomenon (33%), and proximal muscle weakness with normal creatine kinase can also occur.

HYPERLIPOPROTEINEMIA

Type IIa familial hyperlipidemia (Chapter 213) is associated with tendinous and tuberous-osseous xanthomas as well as episodic Achilles tendinitis. An acute migratory, inflammatory arthritis persisting up to a month and resembling rheumatic fever occurs in up to 50% of patients. Predominantly large joints are affected. In addition, a self-limited, acute monoarticular or oligoarticular arthritis involving the knee or ankle can occur. Patients with type III familial hyperlipoproteinemia can develop tendon and bone xanthomas. Patients with human immunodeficiency virus (HIV) infection taking protease inhibitor drugs can develop dyslipidemia leading to tendon xanthomas. In all hyperlipidemias, gout must be excluded before ascribing the symptoms to hyperlipoproteinemia. Therapy with NSAIDs and treatment of the underlying lipid disorder should be pursued. Notably, some of the therapies used to treat hyperlipidemia can cause musculoskeletal symptoms, including hyperuricemia and gout from nicotinic acid and myalgias (with or without elevated creatine kinase) from statin therapy.

PAGET'S DISEASE

Paget's disease (Chapter 255) can cause bone pain and deformity. An elevated bone-specific alkaline phosphatase and characteristic radiographic changes can help make the diagnosis. Joint pain caused by secondary osteoarthritis in areas of bone involvement by Paget's disease most commonly occurs in the hips, knees, or vertebrae. Spinal stenosis from Paget's disease of the spine has been reported. Bisphosphonate therapy is highly effective.

HYPERTROPHIC OSTEOARTHROPATHY

Hypertrophic osteoarthropathy is a syndrome that includes clubbing of the fingers and toes, periostitis of long bones (distal tibia, femur, radius), and arthritis (Fig. 283-1). Hypertrophic osteoarthropathy is classified into primary (hereditary) and secondary forms. Between 80 and 90% of secondary hypertrophic osteoarthropathy is associated with non–small cell lung cancer. Other causes include other neoplasms (mesothelioma), chronic pulmonary infections, congenital heart disease, cirrhosis, HIV infection, and inflammatory bowel disease. Patients with secondary hypertrophic osteoarthropathy can present with acute, severe, burning bone pain and a noninflammatory arthritis caused by periarticular periostitis. Pain is accentuated by dependency of the limbs. Pitting edema, warmth, and tenderness of the legs and forearms can be seen. Radiographs show diagnostic changes of periosteal elevation, new bone formation, or both along the distal ends of long bones.

A   B

FIGURE 283-1. Hypertrophic osteoarthropathy. **A,** Severe clubbing of the nails. **B,** Radiograph demonstrating periosteal elevation of the distal radius and ulna.

Therapy is symptomatic, and hypertrophic osteoarthropathy improves with successful treatment of the underlying primary disease. In resistant cases, treatment with intravenous bisphosphonate has been effective in modulating symptoms.

LEUKEMIA AND LYMPHOMA

Leukemia can arise as an asymmetrical or migratory polyarthritis, monoarthritis (rare), back pain (10%), or nocturnal bone pain. Articular manifestations occur in 14 to 50% of children and 4 to 16% of adults with acute leukemia and can precede the diagnosis by months. Joint pain is attributed to leukemic synovial infiltration and usually involves the ankle or knee, but it can be polyarticular, resembling juvenile or adult RA. The joint pain is disproportionately more severe than the clinical findings. Synovial effusions are uncommon, and evidence of leukemic cells in the synovial fluid is rare. Bone pain occurs in up to 50% of patients with leukemia and is more common in the lower extremities. The peripheral white blood cell count may be normal initially, but serum lactate dehydrogenase is always elevated, frequently to very high levels. Radiographs are normal in 50% of cases. The musculoskeletal symptoms are poorly responsive to NSAIDs but can resolve with successful therapy of the leukemia. Musculoskeletal symptoms occur in 25% of patients with non-Hodgkin's lymphoma. Nocturnal bone pain is the most common presenting musculoskeletal complaint. A seronegative monoarthritis or polyarthritis can occur and should be suspected in patients with severe constitutional symptoms or lymphadenopathy out of proportion to the degree of arthritis. Patients with angioimmunoblastic T-cell lymphoma (Chapter 191) may occasionally develop a chronic, nonerosive polyarthritis with erythroderma.

CARCINOMATOUS POLYARTHRITIS

Polyarthritis can rarely be the presenting manifestation of an occult malignancy; it may precede the discovery of the malignancy by several months. Breast, colon, lung, ovarian, and lymphoproliferative malignancies are the most commonly associated cancers. Clinical features suggesting carcinomatous polyarthritis include the explosive onset of a rheumatoid factor–negative, asymmetrical polyarthritis involving predominantly the lower extremities and sparing the hands and wrists in a patient older than 60 years. Polymyalgia rheumatica and RA must be excluded. Treatment of the underlying malignancy results in improvement of the arthritis.

PALMAR FASCIITIS AND ARTHRITIS SYNDROME

Ovarian carcinoma (Chapter 205) is the most common malignancy found in patients with palmar fasciitis and arthritis. Patients present with a severe, painful, symmetrical inflammatory polyarthritis and fasciitis causing contractures primarily of the hands and, less commonly, the feet. Patients may have vasomotor instability, causing diagnostic confusion with reflex sympathetic dystrophy syndrome or RA. This syndrome portends a poor prognosis because it typically manifests after tumor metastasis. Response to treatment is poor, although clinical improvement can occur with successful eradication of the underlying tumor.

FIGURE 283-2. Hemochromatotic arthropathy. Radiograph demonstrating degenerative changes, with hook-like osteophytes of the second and third metacarpophalangeal joints bilaterally.

HEMOCHROMATOSIS

Joint involvement occurs in 40 to 75% of patients with hereditary hemochromatosis (Chapter 219) and may be the presenting symptom (Fig. 283-2). The metacarpophalangeal (MCP) joints (especially the second and third MCP joints), wrists, knees, hips, shoulders, and ankles are most often involved in a symmetrical pattern. The arthropathy resembles osteoarthritis, with joint swelling resulting from bone enlargement, but it is distinguished clinically by the involvement of atypical joints, such as MCP joints, wrists, and ankles. Radiographs show joint space narrowing, subchondral cysts, sclerosis, and osteophytes that are hook-like at the MCP joints. Chondrocalcinosis is present in up to 50% of patients. It is typically asymptomatic, but in some patients it leads to attacks of acute inflammatory synovitis (pseudogout), which may result in the misdiagnosis of RA. The prevalence of overt arthritis increases with age, and it may be only minimally symptomatic when the disease arises in other organs. However, it is not uncommon for articular pain to be the initial presenting complaint. Consequently, all patients (especially male) presenting with premature osteoarthritis occurring in atypical joints, especially MCP joints and wrists, should be screened for hereditary hemochromatosis with iron studies. The mechanism whereby iron causes arthritis is unclear, but it may be related to hemosiderin deposits in the synovial membrane and chondrocytes activating degradative enzymes. Treatment is symptomatic with NSAIDs and, when severe, total joint arthroplasties. Phlebotomy for iron removal does not alter the course of the arthritis. Additional rheumatic manifestations in patients with hemochromatosis include osteoporosis related to hypogonadotropic hypogonadism, osteomalacia related to vitamin D deficiency when liver disease is severe, and an increased susceptibility to *Yersinia* septic arthritis.

MULTICENTRIC RETICULOHISTIOCYTOSIS

Multicentric reticulohistiocytosis (MRH) is a chronic, symmetrical, inflammatory polyarthritis most commonly affecting the hands and cervical spine. It may resemble RA but can be differentiated by its prominent distal interphalangeal joint synovitis. Joint involvement remits and relapses initially, but in 50% of cases it worsens into a severely deforming arthritis mutilans. Firm, nonpruritic, reddish brown or yellow papulonodular lesions ("coral beads") that wax and wane occur around the nail beds and on the face, hands, ears, and other areas predominantly above the waist. The skin lesions have a diagnostic histology. However, in 50 to 66% of patients, these diagnostic nodules follow the onset of arthritis by months to years. Additional associations include xanthelasma (33%) and malignancies of various types (25%), which may precede or follow the onset of MRH. MRH usually remits spontaneously in 8 to 10 years but often leaves permanent cutaneous and joint damage. Treatment may include cytotoxic therapy if the arthritis is aggressive. Anti–tumor necrosis factor-α (TNF-α) therapy is reportedly beneficial in resistant cases.

SARCOIDOSIS

Joint manifestations including arthritis, periarthritis, and arthralgias occur in 4 to 38% of patients with sarcoidosis (Chapter 95). Rheumatic involvement is divided into acute and chronic types. The first consists of the triad of arthritis, erythema nodosum, and hilar adenopathy on chest radiographs (Löfgren's syndrome), which may be accompanied by fever. Arthritis arises most often in the knees and ankles, and periarticular pain can be severe. Treatment is with NSAIDs, colchicine, or both, and symptoms usually remit spontaneously over several weeks. The less common type of joint involvement in sarcoidosis consists of synovitis that accompanies the slower-onset, more chronic, systemic form of sarcoidosis. Polyarthritis, oligoarthritis, or monoarthritis can affect the small or large joints; it is typically nondestructive but in some cases can be aggressive. Dactylitis resulting from sarcoid bone and soft tissue involvement can occur (Fig. 283-3). In contrast to the acute type, chronic sarcoid arthropathy is characterized by inflammatory synovial fluid and histologic granulomas on synovial biopsy. Treatment consists of NSAIDs, low-dose corticosteroids, hydroxychloroquine, and methotrexate or azathioprine. In refractory cases, anti–TNF-α therapy has been successful. Other musculoskeletal manifestations of sarcoidosis include lytic or sclerotic bone lesions (3 to 13%) and symptomatic acute or chronic myopathy (3%).

ALKAPTONURIA (OCHRONOSIS)

Although an inherited disorder, alkaptonuria is usually not diagnosed until the patient presents with progressive premature osteoarthritis as a young

FIGURE 283-3. Sarcoid bone involvement. Punched-out lytic lesions of the middle phalanx, with soft tissue swelling.

adult (before age 30 to 35 years) (Chapter 212). The spine is initially involved, followed by the knees, shoulders, and hips. Small peripheral joints are spared. Radiographs show multiple vacuum discs, disc space ossification, and osteoarthritic changes in the spine. Nonarticular features include bluish brown discoloration of ear pinna, sclera, and nasal cartilage. Deposition of ochronotic pigment onto collagen fibers causes the articular cartilage to become brittle and fragmented. The noninflammatory synovial fluid may show tiny shards of pigmented cartilage ("ground pepper"). The diagnosis of alkaptonuria is suspected when a patient gives a history of passing dark urine or when fresh urine turns dark brown or black on standing. The diagnosis is confirmed by quantitative measurement of increased homogentisic acid in urine or blood. There is no effective therapy for alkaptonuria. The arthritis is treated symptomatically with analgesics.

FABRY'S DISEASE

Most patients with hereditary lysosomal storage diseases present and are diagnosed during childhood (Chapter 215). However, female heterozygotes and atypical variants of Fabry's disease may have a milder and later-onset phenotype. Fabry's disease is an X-linked lipid storage disease caused by a deficiency of lysosomal α-galactosidase A. Males with classic Fabry's disease usually develop neuromuscular symptoms in childhood, including painful crises with burning paresthesias of the distal extremities, often accompanied by fever. However, in female heterozygotes and males with low residual α-galactosidase A levels, disease manifestations may occur for the first time in adulthood. Neuromuscular manifestations can range from painful acroparesthesias to fibromyalgia. Progressive or isolated cardiac, cerebrovascular, and renal disease can develop later. Fabry's disease should be suspected in any patient with a paternal family history of early-onset renal failure. Patients should be examined for characteristic ocular stigmata (cornea verticillata) and dermal signs (angiokeratomas). The diagnosis is confirmed in males by determining α-galactosidase A activity in plasma or peripheral leukocytes. In contrast, female carriers must be tested for one of the specific gene mutations. Early diagnosis is important because enzyme replacement therapy can prevent irreversible organ damage.

RELAPSING POLYCHONDRITIS

Relapsing polychondritis is an uncommon multisystem disorder characterized by recurrent episodes of inflammation of cartilaginous tissues. Patients with relapsing polychondritis typically present with the sudden onset of pain and erythema involving the cartilage of the external ear, larynx, trachea, or nose. A nonerosive, seronegative polyarthritis or oligoarthritis affecting small, large, or parasternal joints (23 to 47%); ocular inflammation, including episcleritis or scleritis; and audiovestibular disturbances may also be presenting symptoms. The arthritis is typically acute, migratory, and episodic and resolves spontaneously over days to weeks. Rarely, it can become chronic. Tenosynovitis is also common. Relapsing polychondritis is presumably due to a cell-mediated immune response against cartilage components; biopsies showing acute and chronic inflammation destroying cartilage support the diagnosis. Late sequelae of relapsing polychondritis include deformity of the pinnae or nose, reduced vision or hearing, tracheal narrowing or collapse, and aortic insufficiency resulting from aortic ring dilation as well as other cardiovascular abnormalities. Patients with relapsing polychondritis frequently have associated coexisting diseases, such as systemic vasculitis, various connective tissue diseases (e.g., RA), myelodysplastic syndromes and other cancers, and thyroid disease. Treatment depends on the severity of the presentation and whether major organs are involved. Mild episodes of inflammation are treated with NSAIDs, colchicine, dapsone, and low-dose corticosteroids. Life-threatening or organ-threatening complications are treated with high-dose corticosteroids and immunosuppressive agents such as methotrexate or cyclophosphamide. Infliximab has been anecdotally effective in treatment-resistant cases.

CYSTIC FIBROSIS

In up to 10% of patients with cystic fibrosis (Chapter 89), an episodic, nondestructive, inflammatory oligoarthritis develops, most commonly involving the fingers and lower extremity joints. This arthritis is thought to be due to immune complex deposition caused by chronic lung infections. Attacks last for a few days and may be associated with fever and painful nodular skin lesions and purpura. Other musculoskeletal manifestations include osteoporosis and osteomalacia related to malabsorption and, more rarely, hypertrophic osteoarthropathy (5%) and a small-vessel vasculitis.

PIGMENTED VILLONODULAR SYNOVITIS

Pigmented villonodular synovitis occurs most commonly in the third and fourth decades of life. It is characterized by the onset of unilateral pain and swelling of a joint, typically the knee (80%). Unusually, a tendon, bursa, or another joint can be involved. The synovial fluid is characteristically brown or hemorrhagic, and radiographs may show soft tissue swelling, osteolysis, subchondral cysts, and bone erosions. Pigmented villonodular synovitis is a nonmalignant condition that is best diagnosed by synovial biopsy. Microscopic examination reveals a characteristic histology, including marked synovial cell hyperplasia and subsynovial invasion by masses of polygonal cells, multinucleated giant cells, and lipid-filled macrophages. Hemosiderin deposits are between and within cells and have a characteristic appearance on magnetic resonance imaging scans, with nodular foci of decreased signal on both T1- and T2- weighted images. The treatment for pigmented villonodular synovitis is synovectomy.

FUTURE DIRECTIONS

With the advances being made in immunology and genetics, there will be an increased understanding of the pathogenesis of many of these diseases. Treatments such as immunomodulating biologic agents or cartilage-preserving therapy with metalloproteinase inhibitors will be developed on the basis of new discoveries elucidating the etiology of these unusual disorders.

SUGGESTED READINGS

Carroll GJ, Breidahl WH, Bulsara MK, et al. Hereditary hemochromatosis is characterized by a clinically definable arthropathy that correlates with iron load. *Arthritis Rheum.* 2011;63:286-294. *An arthropathy is present in about 25% of patients.*

Dunn AL. Pathophysiology, diagnosis and prevention of arthropathy in patients with haemophilia. *Haemophilia.* 2011. [Epub ahead of print.] *Review including the benefits of prophylactic factor infusion regimens.*

Izumi M, Takayama K, Yabuuchi H, et al. Incidence of hypertrophic pulmonary osteoarthropathy associated with primary lung cancer. *Respirology.* 2010;15:809-812. *About 4.5% of patients had evidence by bone scintigraphy, but only 1% had clubbing and pain.*

Lagier JC, Lepidi H, Raoult D, et al. Systemic *Tropheryma whipplei*: clinical presentation of 142 patients with infections diagnosed or confirmed in a reference center. *Medicine (Baltimore).* 2010;89:337-345. *The main presenting symptom was arthralgia in 78% of patients.*

Nguyen S, Hojjati M. Review of current therapies for secondary hypertrophic pulmonary osteoarthropathy. *Clin Rheumatol.* 2011;30:7-13. *Other than treatment of the tumor or infection, no therapy is proven to be beneficial.*

Sweiss NJ, Patterson K, Sawaqed R, et al. Rheumatologic manifestations of sarcoidosis. *Semin Respir Crit Care Med.* 2010;31:463-473. *Overview of etiology and treatment.*

Vereckei E, Mester A, Hodinka L, et al. Back pain and sacroiliitis in long-standing adult celiac disease: a cross-sectional and follow-up study. *Rheumatol Int.* 2010;30:455-460. *Sacroiliac joint involvement was confirmed in 70% of patients.*

Vergani D, Longhi MS, Bogdanos DP, et al. Autoimmune hepatitis. *Semin Immunopathol.* 2009;31:421-435. *Comprehensive review of the spectrum of autoimmunity and pathology in autoimmune hepatitis.*

284

IDIOPATHIC MULTIFOCAL FIBROSCLEROSIS

WILMER L. SIBBITT JR.

DEFINITION

Idiopathic multifocal fibrosclerosis (IMF) is an inflammatory disease characterized by the development of inflammatory pseudotumors, resulting in some combination of retroperitoneal fibrosis, mediastinal fibrosis, orbital pseudotumor, Dupuytren's contracture, lymphoid hyperplasia, Peyronie's disease, vasculitis, thyroiditis, primary biliary cirrhosis, testicular fibrosis, and pachymeningitis. Retroperitoneal fibrosis (Ormond's disease) is a subset of IMF and is characterized by fibrosis of the retroperitoneum that entraps and distorts retroperitoneal structures, including the great vessels, ureters, nerves, kidneys, and biliary tree.

EPIDEMIOLOGY

IMF is a rare condition with a prevalence estimated at less than 20 in 100,000 and an annual incidence of 1.3 to 3 per 100,000. However, in relevant populations with predisposing conditions, the incidence is higher. IMF is epidemiologically associated with cigarette smoking, asbestos exposure, aortic atherosclerosis, aortic aneurysm, systemic inflammation, drugs (Table

TABLE 284-1 DRUGS ASSOCIATED WITH IDIOPATHIC MULTIFOCAL FIBROSCLEROSIS

HIGH-RISK DRUGS

Ergot-derived dopaminergic agonists (pergolide, pramipexole, lisuride, bromocriptine, cabergoline)
Other ergot-derived alkaloids (methysergide, ergotamine, lysergic acid diethylamide [LSD])
Adrenergic agents (amphetamines, cocaine, ephedrine)
Strychnine
Chemotherapeutic agents (carboplatin, mitoxantrone, 5-fluorouracil, cisplatin, floxuridine)

LOW-RISK DRUGS

Non-ergot dopaminergic agents and agonists (levodopa, carbidopa)
β-Adrenergic blockers (atenolol, metoprolol, timolol, sotalol, propranolol, oxprenolol, labetalol)
Diuretics (furosemide, hydrochlorothiazide, chlorthalidone)
Other antihypertensive drugs (methyldopa, hydralazine, prazosin, clonidine)
Acetaminophen

284-1) and toxins, elevated immunoglobulin (Ig) G4, malignant tumors (metastatic carcinoma, carcinoid, lymphoma), retroperitoneal injury (hemorrhage, infection, radiation, surgery, stenting, angioplasty), autoimmune disease, Erdheim-Chester disease, tuberculosis, sarcoidosis, biliary tract disease, gonorrhea, and ascending lymphangitis. T-cell receptor gene rearrangements have been reported, as well as a 40% association with HLA-B27; however, these associations have not been proved. Mean age at presentation is 56 to 64 years, and the male-female ratio is 3:1.

PATHOBIOLOGY

The histopathology of IMF is characterized by multifocal fibrosis, granulation tissue, B cells, T helper cells, large numbers of spindle-shaped cells expressing macrophage markers, and activated fibroblasts. Degenerative and inflammatory diseases of the aorta (atherosclerosis, aortitis, inherited diseases of collagen, trauma, infection, aortic aneurysm) cause the shedding of inflammatory lipids and oxidized lipoproteins through the aortic adventitia into the retroperitoneum, resulting in an intense inflammatory and fibrotic process. Thus, the presence of IMF should trigger an evaluation for aortic disease. Recently, elevated levels of IgG4 have been reported in IMF, suggesting a direct immune causation. Confounding syndromes, including lymphoma, crystal-storing histiocytosis, immunocytoma, neuroblastoma, diffuse retroperitoneal carcinoma (pancreatic, scirrhous gastric, prostate, ovarian, renal, uterine cervix, carcinoid), Wegener's granulomatosis, xanthogranulomatous pyelonephritis, chronic pyelonephritis, tuberculosis, guinea worm infestation, sarcoidosis, and aortic graft infection, should be excluded by appropriate imaging, biopsy, aspiration, and/or serologies.

CLINICAL MANIFESTATIONS

IMF commonly presents as (1) isolated retroperitoneal fibrosis; (2) retroperitoneal, mesenteric, pulmonary, and periarticular fibrosis accompanied by subcutaneous panniculitis; (3) a triad of sclerosing cholangitis, retroperitoneal fibrosis, and Riedel's thyroiditis (Chapter 233); or (4) other less common combinations. The retroperitoneal form of IMF typical presents as (1) ill-defined pain in the lower abdomen, lumbosacral region, or flank; (2) visceral obstruction resulting in vomiting, diarrhea, or dehydration; (3) hydronephrosis or renal insufficiency; (4) severe peripheral edema and venous varicosities; or (5) claudication, pain, dysesthesias, weakness, or spasticity secondary to nerve entrapment and epidural cord compression. Pulmonary emboli, deep vein thrombosis, and obstruction of the bowel, bladder, or bronchi can occur. Mediastinal fibrosis may result in a lymphoma-like mass and superior vena cava syndrome, with edema and venous dilation of the arms, neck, and head. Extrahepatic portal vein obstruction, portal hypertension, esophageal varices, and uveitis may occur. A definitive diagnosis should be made rapidly, and therapy should be seriously considered.

DIAGNOSIS

Computed tomography (CT), magnetic resonance imaging (MRI), and urography with appropriate contrast demonstrate a retroperitoneal inflammatory reaction; obstruction of the ureters, great vessels, biliary tree, or pancreatic ducts; or the presence of diffuse or discrete unifocal or multifocal retroperitoneal masses. Fibrosis may extend into the root of the mesentery, the bladder, and peribronchial areas, resulting in traction, distortion, and obstruction of the gut, urethra, and bronchi. Indium-111–labeled leukocyte, gallium, and technetium-99m methylene diphosphonate radionuclide scans, and F-18 fluorodeoxyglucose positron emission tomography (PET), are useful to exclude abscess and tumor, demonstrate inflammatory processes, and follow disease activity. Appropriate questioning and testing should exclude autoimmune diseases, drug use, and toxin exposure. After suspicious masses are identified, a biopsy is usually essential to confirm the diagnosis and exclude confounding conditions, especially neoplasia and infection. Biopsy may be guided by CT, MRI, ultrasound, fluoroscopy, mediastinoscopy, laparoscopy, or retroperitoneal exploration, and it can often be accomplished by percutaneous needle biopsy.

PREVENTION AND TREATMENT — Rx

Surgical interventions are often necessary to preserve organ function. These include surgical lysis of fibrotic masses and stenting or catheter drainage of ureteral, biliary, venous, and arterial obstructions to preserve organ function. Surgical repair or stenting of an abdominal aortic aneurysm may be either an exacerbating or an ameliorating factor for IMF; thus, therapy for an aneurysm must be individualized. The most important treatment for IMF is removal of the cause, most commonly an offending drug. Otherwise, treatment for IMF is largely empirical, but it may be necessary because the disease can be progressive and fatal. There are no controlled trials; however, first-line therapy consists of pulse methylprednisolone initially, followed by high-dose oral corticosteroids for 6 months. Long-term maintenance is necessary with azathioprine, cyclophosphamide, colchicine, cyclosporine, tamoxifen, or mycophenolate, with the latter two drugs used most commonly. Statin drugs may also be of benefit. Lifelong anticoagulation is required for those patients with large vein involvement and associated deep vein thrombosis.

PROGNOSIS

The cumulative actuarial survival rate is 86% at 1 year and 78% at 2 years, suggesting that therapy is often indicated.

FUTURE DIRECTIONS

It is anticipated that further research in fibrosing diseases, including the role of inflammation, vascular injury, cholesterol pathways, chronic periaortitis, IgG4-secreting plasma cells, collagen-producing spindle-shaped macrophages, transforming growth factor-β, connective tissue growth factor, bone morphogenetic protein 7, the interleukins, and viral infections, will provide new avenues for the prevention and therapy of IMF.

SUGGESTED READINGS

Li KP, Zhu J, Zhang JL, et al. Idiopathic retroperitoneal fibrosis (RPF): clinical features of 61 cases and literature review. *Clin Rheumatol.* 2011;30:601-605. *Mean age was 56 years, with 3% requiring dialysis.*

Scheel PJ Jr, Feeley N. Retroperitoneal fibrosis: the clinical, laboratory, and radiographic presentation. *Medicine (Baltimore).* 2009;88:202-207. *New cohort study with a logical classification scheme.*

Scheel PJ Jr, Feeley N, Sozio SM. Combined prednisone and mycophenolate mofetil treatment for retroperitoneal fibrosis: a case series. *Ann Intern Med.* 2011;154:31-36. *Prednisone (40 mg per day tapered over 6 months) with mycophenolate mofetil (1000 mg daily for about 2 years) was effective for 28 consecutive patients with retroperitoneal fibrosis, although two subsequently relapsed.*

Swartz RD. Idiopathic retroperitoneal fibrosis: a review of the pathogenesis and approaches to treatment. *Am J Kidney Dis.* 2009;54:546-553. *Excellent review of the therapy of IMF.*

van Bommel EF, Jansen I, Hendriksz TR, et al. Idiopathic retroperitoneal fibrosis: prospective evaluation of incidence and clinicoradiologic presentation. *Medicine (Baltimore).* 2009;88:193-201. *Excellent epidemiologic study of IMF.*

285

SURGICAL TREATMENT OF JOINT DISEASE

C. RONALD MACKENZIE AND EDWIN P. SU

Estimates of the prevalence of arthritis and other rheumatic diseases demonstrate the enormous impact these conditions have on the U.S. populace and the health care system in general. More than 21% of U.S. adults (46 million people) currently report physician-diagnosed arthritis. Although the majority of this health burden arises as a consequence of osteoarthritis, the full span of rheumatic diseases contributes to the impact. Arthritis is already the leading cause of disability in the nation, and the number of adults with arthritis and arthritis-attributable limitations in activity is anticipated to approach 67 million by the year 2030. Ultimately, surgical intervention is required in many of these individuals. Factors such as increased patient awareness of the benefits of surgery, the desire for higher activity levels, and improvements in surgical techniques have, in concert with the increasing prevalence of chronic arthritis, fueled the growth in orthopedic surgery performed for the treatment of arthritis. In 2007 it was estimated that 270,000 primary total hip replacements and 507,000 primary total knee replacements were performed in the United States. It is predicted that by 2030, more than 500,000 hip replacements and 3 million knee replacements will be performed each year.

PATHOBIOLOGY

The pathobiology of joint arthritis leading to surgical intervention is essentially that of articular cartilage damage resulting in the loss of mechanical properties, accompanied by inflammation of the joint lining. With continued cartilage deterioration, stiffness and pain ensue. Without the protective layer of articular cartilage, the nociceptive and proprioceptive receptors in the periosteum are activated, leading to unremitting pain (Chapter 29).

Osteoarthritis is the most common cause of end-stage arthritis (Chapter 270). Osteoarthritis may be primary, due to biochemical changes in the cartilage, or it may be secondary to systemic disease affecting the cartilage, joint damage from preexisting inflammatory joint disease, or trauma. Mechanical overload and imbalances lead to further cartilage degradation. Important adaptive processes such as subchondral sclerosis and osteophyte formation occur in response to joint overload; if these become chronic, cyst formation in the subarticular bone may also result. Over time, the osteophytes or bone spurs lead to restricted range of motion (Fig. 285-1).

Inflammatory arthritis, by contrast, is a constellation of diseases involving the synovium. Included in this class of disorders are such important conditions as rheumatoid arthritis (Chapter 272), psoriatic arthritis, and the seronegative spondyloarthropathies (Chapter 273). On a pathologic level, all involve the release of inflammatory mediators in the adjacent synovium, leading secondarily to cartilage destruction. In contrast to osteoarthritis, there is no mechanical overload as a primary mechanism, and no bone sclerosis or osteophyte formation is seen. Rather, the inflammatory synovitis leads to characteristic loss of cartilage matrix, marginal bony erosions, destruction of the joint capsule, and osteopenia (Fig. 285-2).

Trauma is another important cause of joint destruction. Post-traumatic arthritis is initiated by cartilage damage at the time of injury or by secondary mechanical imbalances that result from fractures of juxta-articular bone. Abnormal loading conditions subsequently lead to a wear-and-tear form of cartilage damage.

FIGURE 285-1. Radiograph of an osteoarthritic left hip. Note the asymmetrical joint space narrowing and subchondral sclerosis, which are characteristic of a wear-and-tear pattern of joint deterioration.

FIGURE 285-2. Radiograph of a left hip with end-stage inflammatory arthritis. Note the symmetrical pattern of cartilage loss and the presence of osteopenia.

Osteonecrosis (Chapter 256) is another entity that may lead to joint arthritis. In this process, the blood supply to the bone is compromised, leading to necrosis of the bone supporting the articular surface. The most commonly affected joints are the hip, shoulder, and knee. As the disease progresses, the necrotic bone may collapse, resulting in the loss of articular integrity and progressive cartilage deterioration.

Other causes of arthritis that may lead to joint damage include metabolic disorders (chondrocalcinosis, gout), tumor (synovial chondromatosis), infections (post-septic), and bleeding disorders (hemophilia; Chapter 177).

PREOPERATIVE CONSIDERATIONS

The indications for orthopedic surgery are refractory joint pain and disability. Ultimately, the patient and his or her physicians need to agree that the possible benefits of surgery outweigh the risks. The decision to proceed with surgery therefore reflects a consensus among the patient, the orthopedic surgeon, and the patient's primary physician or rheumatologist. Achieving the necessary decision-making balance may be complicated, especially given the increasing burden of comorbidity in aging patients.

In the elective setting, joint replacement and spine surgery are the most common procedures under consideration. With the former, severe pain and functional limitation unrelieved by conservative treatment are the most common indications for surgical intervention. In the case of spine surgery, severe radiculopathy, nerve dysfunction (e.g., acute footdrop), or myelopathy are additional considerations. In contrast to elective surgery, there are circumstances when a deliberative approach is not possible owing to the development of more urgent, occasionally life-threatening clinical problems. Examples include hip fracture, acute myelopathy, or an infected native or prosthetic joint. In these settings, the patient's general health is at risk, so the medical-surgical team must stabilize the patient as quickly as possible to optimize the outcome. Owing to the coupling of medical advances with increasing financial and resource constraints, a trend to perform surgery in the ambulatory setting has emerged. Indeed, the percentage of all surgical procedures performed on an outpatient basis in the United States rose from 20% in 1982 to 60% in 1995, a phenomenon particularly relevant to the arthroscopic techniques of orthopedic surgery. Among the benefits of these developments has been the opportunity to move the preoperative medical evaluation to the outpatient arena. This change in practice allows time for discourse with the other physicians involved in the patient's care, for supplementary consultation and investigation, and, when necessary, for the institution of therapy directed at optimizing the patient's medical status before the contemplated surgery. Approached in this manner, the preoperative evaluation becomes a focal point of communication among all members of the medical team, enhancing the collaborative nature of the consultative process and, ultimately, the patient's care.

Although the efficacy of preoperative assessment has not been definitively established, the aging and increasing complexity of modern-day surgical patients justifies this clinical practice. Although no consensus exists regarding what constitutes the optimal preoperative medical evaluation, a growing literature pertaining to perioperative medicine supports various core principles that underlie effective medical consultation in this clinical setting.

ANESTHESIA IN THE ORTHOPEDIC PATIENT

Given the protean clinical features that accompany chronic arthritis and the connective tissue diseases, a variety of issues, including airway considerations, the surgical site (joint region), the anticipated duration of surgery, and comorbidities, are important determinants of the type of anesthesia to be used, whether invasive monitoring will be necessary, and the length of time the patient will require intensive monitoring after surgery.

General and regional anesthesia are commonly used in the orthopedic patient. General anesthesia with endotracheal intubation may present a particular danger in patients with rheumatoid arthritis or ankylosing spondylitis. Patients with cervical spine instability or a rigid airway may require fiberoptic intubation. Regional anesthesia may involve local anesthesia or peripheral nerve block for minor procedures or epidural/spinal anesthesia for total joint arthroplasty.

Although the debate concerning the relative merits of regional versus general anesthesia remains unresolved, many procedures, particularly orthopedic surgery, are well suited for regional anesthetic techniques. Advantages of regional anesthesia include a reduction in blood loss, deep vein thrombosis, pulmonary embolism, adverse postoperative respiratory events, and death. Further, postoperative pain, a significant problem for patients with a painful rheumatic disease, may be best managed with regional anesthetic approaches. For example, peripheral nerve blocks using longer-acting anesthetics and infusion methodologies are often employed because they provide excellent intraoperative anesthesia and postoperative pain relief.

A number of options exist for the control of postoperative pain (Chapter 29), including the traditional intravenous or intramuscular routes (systemic) versus the administration of epidural analgesia. Patient-controlled analgesia (PCA) via an epidural route of administration is an effective method of pain control after surgery. Further, PCA facilitates postoperative physical therapy, which is important for the restoration of range of motion in patients undergoing orthopedic procedures. PCA also reduces the systemic absorption of analgesics, thereby minimizing the problem of narcotic-induced respiratory depression. Parenterally administered nonsteroidal anti-inflammatory drugs (NSAIDs) are also useful and can reduce narcotic requirements after major surgery. However, the common contraindications to NSAID therapy, such as peptic ulcer, renal disease, and ischemic heart disease, should be observed in the postoperative setting.

SURGICAL MANAGEMENT

Surgical treatment of joint disease is focused primarily on the relief of pain; secondary objectives are improvement in joint motion and swelling, return to function, and prevention of continued cartilage destruction. Realizing that surgical treatment has limitations and complications, the decision to move forward must be individualized for each patient. Factors such as disease severity, the patient's desired activity level, and the anticipated longevity of the patient are all relevant to decision making. Typically, patients who are candidates for the surgical treatment of joint diseases have failed conservative measures (NSAIDs, physical therapy, intra-articular injections) and have daily pain that affects their quality of life.

ORTHOPEDIC PROCEDURES

Osteotomy

When a structural abnormality around a joint has led to mechanical overload, an osteotomy may be an option to correct alignment problems. The most common sites for osteotomy are the hip, to treat acetabular dysplasia, and the tibia, to realign the knee. In acetabular dysplasia, the hip socket is excessively shallow, leading to abnormal stresses on the articular cartilage and premature osteoarthritis. An acetabular osteotomy can be performed in patients in whom cartilage still remains. By rotating the pelvic bones, a deeper socket can be formed, reducing stresses on the cartilage and thereby slowing the arthritic process. With tibial osteotomy, the knee joint can be realigned to direct forces away from the region of cartilage damage. Usually, a varus (bowlegged) deformity indicates that the medial compartment of the knee is excessively worn, so a tibial osteotomy realigns the joint to direct forces to the uninvolved lateral compartment. Typically, osteotomy is considered an option for patients younger than 40 years; beyond this age, the extent of cartilage loss generally means that total joint arthroplasty would achieve more beneficial results.

Arthroscopy

Arthroscopic surgery is performed by inserting a camera and specialized instruments into a joint via small, puncture-type incisions. Arthroscopic surgery is effective in the treatment of intra-articular pathology such as meniscal tears of the knee, labral tears of the hip, cartilage flaps, small chondral defects, and loose bodies. However, once the articular cartilage is significantly damaged, arthroscopic débridement is usually ineffective in the absence of mechanical symptoms such as locking and clicking. In some instances, underlying joint arthritis may lead to tears in the meniscus or labrum; if such a tear results in new mechanical symptoms, arthroscopic surgery may be helpful in selected cases. For osteoarthritis, arthroscopic knee surgery is no better than medical therapies.[1]

In the assessment of the hip, there has been an increased focus on the femoral head and neck architecture as a cause of osteoarthritis. In certain patients, the anatomy of the femoral head and neck may lead to impingement of the femoral neck on the acetabular rim, typically in flexion and internal rotation. This condition, known as *femoroacetabular impingement*, results in repetitive contact between the femoral neck and acetabular rim and is believed to cause labral tears, cartilage damage, and eventual arthritis. Thus, there is currently great interest in reshaping the bones of the femur and acetabulum by so-called osteochondroplasty. This technique is being performed as an open procedure or arthroscopically and provides good symptomatic relief in the short term. The long-term effects and the influence of the procedure on the development of arthritis have yet to be demonstrated.

Synovectomy

Synovectomy refers to removal of the synovial lining of the joint, via either an open or an arthroscopic approach. In conditions such as rheumatoid arthritis, where the disease process involves an actively inflamed synovium, debulking the pathologic tissue may reduce symptoms and slow the destruction of cartilage. In practice, synovectomy can be effective for relieving pain, as long as there is remaining cartilage. However, the procedure has not been predictable in terms of regaining joint motion. Further, once the cartilage is completely worn through, the joint deterioration is too advanced for synovectomy to be helpful. Therefore, synovectomy is generally performed in patients with rheumatoid arthritis (or other forms of inflammatory arthritis) who have active synovitis in the presence of relatively preserved articular cartilage. The most common joints that benefit from synovectomy are the knee and elbow. However, synovectomy should be considered a procedure that merely "buys time," because the synovium will reappear.

Arthrodesis

Arthrodesis, or fusion of a joint, achieves the goal of pain relief by creating a nonmobile joint. Rather than have the arthritic joint surfaces elicit pain with movement, a surgical fusion (arthrodesis) of the articulating bones creates a construct that can bear weight and is stable. This is achieved by removing the articular surfaces from the joint and immobilizing the bones such that they heal in a solid union. This procedure was formerly the treatment of choice for hip and knee arthritis in young, active laborers because of its durability and the avoidance of implants, with their propensity to wear. However, creating stiffness at one joint increases stresses on the joints above and below the fused joint.

Hip fusion may be performed in young patients to treat the sequelae of slipped capital femoral epiphysis, Legg-Calvé-Perthes disease, post-septic arthritis, or osteonecrosis of the femoral head. Fusion surgery can achieve a painless, supportive joint that is capable of bearing heavy loads while avoiding artificial implants. However, the gait mechanics after fusion are altered, requiring more energy for ambulation. Further, the lack of motion at the hip increases stresses on the joints above and below it. Thus, the natural history of a hip fusion is the development of ipsilateral knee arthritis and low back pain after 20 to 25 years, necessitating conversion of the fused hip to a hip replacement (fusion takedown). Although hip arthrodesis is still a viable option in young arthritic patients, the desire to maintain hip mobility in order to sit and drive has made this largely a treatment of the past.

Fusion of the knee joint is performed less commonly than hip fusion. In addition to the lack of motion, which may make it difficult to sit or climb stairs, knee fusion cannot be successfully converted to total knee replacement. Thus, knee fusion is generally considered a salvage procedure, employed mainly when replacement is not possible (e.g., lack of muscle function or persistent infection).

Ankle fusion is still commonly performed as the treatment of choice for tibiotalar arthritis. Historically, the results of ankle replacement have not been durable; therefore, fusing the ankle is the best method of creating a pain-free joint. Further, the ability of the knee and the subtalar joints to compensate for a stiff ankle has made this procedure more tolerable.

Total Joint Arthroplasty

Joint arthroplasty refers to the re-creation of congruent joint surfaces, typically with artificial parts. In certain patients and in non-load-bearing joints such as the elbow, interpositional arthroplasty can be performed by placing a tissue graft between the arthritic surfaces. In the case of weight-bearing joints such as the hip and knee, however, metal and plastic materials produce the most durable results. In such circumstances, the articular surfaces are replaced by shaped materials designed to re-create the joint kinematics; thus, the procedures are commonly called *total hip, knee, and shoulder replacements*.

In general, once the articular cartilage is completely worn or destroyed on both sides of the joint, arthroplasty is the most predictable way to relieve pain. After total joint arthroplasty, it is advisable to reduce stresses on the joint to promote implant longevity. This includes weight loss and avoidance of impact activities; walking, cycling, and gliding-type activities are permitted, but in general, running and jumping should be avoided. Because a total joint arthroplasty involves artificial, moving components, the replaced joints are subject to the same wear and tear as native joints. Thus, they have a finite lifespan that is dependent on the patient's weight and activity level and the implant materials. Subsequent revisions of joint replacements can be difficult and less durable; thus, it is wise to defer joint arthroplasty until there are no other options.

Total hip replacement (THR) was first developed in the 1950s in the United Kingdom using metal and plastic components attached to the bone with cement. The early results were so beneficial and reproducible that the technique rapidly spread worldwide. The National Institutes of Health published a consensus statement in 1994, noting that THR "is one of the most successful surgical procedures and provides immediate and substantial improvement in a patient's pain, mobility, and quality of life. Compared to treatments for other chronic debilitating diseases, THR is highly cost effective."

THR is the treatment of choice for end-stage arthritis caused by any of the aforementioned pathobiologic processes. It involves exposure of the joint, removal of the arthritic femoral head at the level of the femoral neck, and removal of enough acetabular bone to place a prosthetic socket. The femoral implant is inserted into the intramedullary canal and anchored with bone-ingrowth techniques or bone cement. The choice of bearing material (metal, plastic, ceramic) is based on the patient's age and activity level and the surgeon's preference (Fig. 285-3).

FIGURE 285-3. Radiograph of a total hip replacement consisting of uncemented acetabular and femoral components. The articulating materials are a metal ball and a polyethylene liner.

FIGURE 285-4. Radiograph of a total knee replacement. The components are metal, with a polyethylene insert between the tibial and femoral components.

Using modern implant materials and surgical techniques, the implant survival rates are 90 to 95% at 15 years; however, longevity varies, depending on patient factors such as weight and activity. There have been cases in which THR implants lasted more than 30 years.

A major cause of failure of THR is wearing of the implant materials, coupled with the body's reaction to the particulate debris shed into the joint space over time. In the process of immunologic uptake of the debris, inflammatory cytokines are released, causing osteoclasts to resorb periprosthetic bone. The end result of this osteolytic process is that the implant attachments to bone may be compromised, causing loosening of the prosthesis and pain. The hope is that the current generation of implant materials will reduce the amount of particulate wear debris, extending longevity further.

Total knee replacement (TKR) was developed in the United States shortly after THR. The surgery involves removal of the arthritic surfaces of the tibia and femur, followed by their replacement with a metal femoral implant and a metal and/or polyethylene tibial component (Fig. 285-4). It is termed *total* knee replacement to distinguish it from a unicompartmental or *partial* knee replacement.

The recovery from TKR is more difficult than that from THR because of greater postoperative pain and the emphasis on regaining motion. Nonetheless, pain relief and function are usually excellent once recovery is complete. Current studies demonstrate modern implant survival to be 90 to 95% at 15 years, again depending on patient factors.

Although less commonly performed than hip and knee replacement, total shoulder replacement (TSR) is an excellent pain-relieving procedure for glenohumeral arthritis and is preferred over hemiarthroplasty.[2] Developed from experience gained with THR and TKR, TSR uses a stemmed humeral implant with a metal ball and a metal and/or polyethylene glenoid socket. TSR requires an extensive rehabilitation protocol to regain range of motion and strength; however, at 1 year after surgery, 95% of patients have pain-free use of the shoulder.

In general, smaller joints such as the wrist and ankle are better treated with arthrodesis, because the implants necessary for arthroplasty in these joints have limited bone surfaces on which to attach the prosthesis. Additionally, the location of these joints allows the adjacent joints to compensate more effectively.

Surgical Innovations in Joint Arthroplasty
Minimally Invasive Surgery
As in all surgical subspecialties, there has been a movement toward "minimally invasive surgery." This may be a misnomer, because the actual work done inside the joint has not changed. Some surgeons have suggested that the terminology be changed to "smaller incision surgery" or "less invasive surgery." In any case, the idea is to use the smallest incision possible to perform the operation, resulting in less tissue trauma. The interest in this type of surgery has resulted in improvements in instrument design and surgical training. Typically, a hip replacement, until recently performed via a 10-inch incision, can now be done through a 4- to 5-inch incision. Similarly, knee replacement incisions are about half their former length. Despite these surgical advances, even larger benefits have resulted from the increased attention to various nonsurgical modalities directed at more rapid recovery. Examples include the increased use of peripheral nerve blocks and preemptive analgesia and a more expeditious approach to rehabilitation. Such approaches have reduced the average hospital stay to 2 to 3 days after THR and 3 to 4 days after TKR.

Improvements in Implant Technology
As the average age of patients undergoing hip and knee replacement decreases and their activity level increases, the number of revision surgeries is projected to grow. Therefore, much research is being performed to improve the longevity of implant materials. The "gold standard" of arthroplasty is to use a cobalt-chome (metal) implant against a polyethylene (plastic) surface. Unfortunately, the harder metal surface eventually wears away the softer plastic surface. Therefore, biomechanical engineers have developed a more resistant, highly cross-linked polyethylene that demonstrates greater wear resistance in laboratory simulators. Such highly cross-linked polyethylene has been in clinical use for about 7 years, and the early experience suggests significantly less wear compared with standard polyethylene. Other materials such as ceramics and metals are also being used in an attempt to improve longevity. Nonetheless, to date, there is no consensus concerning the optimal weight-bearing surfaces.

Bone-preserving implants have also been developed to provide more options when revision surgery becomes a necessity. Such procedures may require removal of the implant and placement of a new prosthetic device; thus, with more bone available, surgical options are enhanced. One such bone-preserving implant is the hip resurfacing device introduced in the United States in 2006 (discussed more fully later).

Unicompartmental knee replacement is a bone-preserving implant for the knee. As suggested by its name, it involves replacing only one of the three knee compartments with a prosthetic device (Fig. 285-5). Therefore, candidates for unicompartmental knee replacement must have arthritis limited to a single compartment. Because the surgical trauma and dissection are significantly reduced compared with TKR, the patient's recovery tends to be less painful and quicker. However, there is a higher failure rate for unicompartmental knee replacement than for TKR because of the possibility of developing arthritic changes elsewhere in the joint.

Resurfacing Arthroplasty
Hip resurfacing is quickly becoming an alternative treatment to THR in younger, more active patients. In countries where the procedure has been established for a decade or longer, it represents approximately 8% of all primary total hip arthroplasties. The main benefit is preservation of proximal femoral bone in the event that future (revision) surgery is necessary. Rather than removing the femoral head and a portion of the femoral neck, as in THR, the bone is sculpted to accept a metal resurfacing cap (like a tooth), preserving an additional 4 to 5 cm of bone (Fig. 285-6). Preservation of the proximal femoral bone raises an additional risk of failure (i.e., femoral neck fracture below the resurfacing implant), which is estimated to occur in 1% of cases. Although there are no defined age limits for hip resurfacing, the best candidates have been men younger than 55 years, probably because the bone quality in this group is the strongest and most robust. In this age group, the 7-year results of hip resurfacing in Australia have demonstrated a greater than 97% rate of implant survival (free of revision), which is comparable to THR. However, concerns regarding longevity, a greater short-term failure rate than THR, poorer results in women, and metal ion release have led to questions concerning the superiority of this procedure.

Computer Navigation
An orthopedic surgeon relies on visualization, instrument jigs, and experience to re-create the proper joint mechanics. Although the surgeon may know exactly how the artificial components are to be placed, it may be difficult to achieve perfect alignment in every operation. Computer navigation is a tool that can aid in the reproducible positioning of implants. Although some errors are inherent in the precision of computer navigation, such techniques have reliably diminished outlier results. It has yet to be determined whether the longevity of hip and knee replacements inserted with the aid of computer navigation differs from the longevity of those inserted by conventional approaches. For this reason, as well as the expense and time associated with its use, computer navigation is not universally practiced.

FIGURE 285-5. **A,** Radiograph of a knee with arthritis limited to the medial compartment. **B,** A medial unicompartmental knee replacement.

FIGURE 285-6. **Radiograph of a patient with a right total hip replacement and a left hip resurfacing.** The total hip replacement consists of a longer stem placed in the medullary canal of the femur. The hip resurfacing implant preserves the proximal femoral bone.

ORTHOPEDIC PROCEDURES ON OTHER JOINTS

Elbow, Ankle, Wrist, and Hand

The elbow, ankle, and wrist are less frequently replaced than the hip, knee, and shoulder. With the exception of the rheumatoid wrist, these joints are less commonly afflicted by chronic arthritis. Further, the smaller bones making up these joints translates to a diminished surface area for implant fixation, thus lowering the durability of surgical procedures. Although total joint arthroplasty can be successful at relieving pain in the short term, 10-year results do not approach those of THR or TKR. Synovectomy remains an effective surgical option in selected patients with inflammatory arthritis of the elbow, ankle, or wrist. Patients who develop dysfunctional hand deformities from rheumatoid arthritis may benefit from replacement of the metacarpophalangeal joints with Silastic prostheses and realignment of the small joints of the thumb and fingers with arthrodeses.

Spine

The spine consists of multiple levels of articulating bones, discs, and facets. Although not a "joint" in the typical sense of the word, various spinal segments may be differentially involved in chronic arthritis. Generally, the lumbar spine is most affected, although a similar process can occur in the cervical spine; more than 95% of patients older than 50 years exhibit degenerative changes in the lumbar spine. With aging, the nucleus pulposus of the intervertebral disc loses water content and elasticity, resulting in disc space collapse and increased forces across the vertebral facets. As a consequence

of the increased pressure, bone spurs develop, leading to stenosis (narrowing) of the neural foramen. As a result of the degenerative process, or *spondylosis*, patients may experience mechanical back pain with bending, extending, and twisting. Pain, numbness, or weakness radiating down the extremities in a radicular distribution can result from the neural foraminal stenosis.

Mechanical back pain is the most common affliction of the spine. Unfortunately, this constellation of back symptoms is not reliably relieved by surgical intervention. Physical therapy and use of proper back mechanics are the mainstay of treating mechanical back pain.

The advanced sequelae of spinal arthritis is spinal stenosis, which can result in lower extremity pain and weakness. This disorder can reliably benefit from decompressive surgery with or without instrumented fusion. The spinal unit must be evaluated for stability to determine whether spinal fusion is necessary.

Newer surgical treatments, such as lumbar disc replacement, may be used in certain cases to treat spinal disorders. Whereas the "gold standard," vertebral fusion, eliminates painful motion at degenerative disc levels, disc replacement attempts to preserve motion of the spinal unit. As in hip and knee arthrodesis, fusion of the spinal unit increases forces at the levels above and below the fused segment, and further degeneration often occurs. Disc replacement surgery aims to eliminate the progression of arthritis at adjacent levels by retaining motion. Long-term studies comparing disc replacement and spinal fusion are not yet available.

MANAGEMENT ISSUES IN PATIENTS WITH ARTHRITIS UNDERGOING SURGERY

Prevention of Postoperative Infection

Efforts to prevent and detect any infectious processes pre- and postoperatively are of utmost importance. The skin and urinary tract are sites of specific concern, and infection can be ruled out by a careful physical examination and routine preoperative urine culture. In addition, dental consultation may be appropriate in patients with poor oral hygiene and dentition.

Prophylactic antibiotic therapy for total joint arthroplasty patients should begin less than 2 hours before surgery and continue for 24 hours. A common protocol involves cefazolin (Ancef) 1 g every 8 hours (total of three doses) or, in penicillin-allergic patients, vancomycin 1 g every 12 hours (total of two doses).

Peripheral Nerve Injuries

Peripheral nerve injuries arise more often after upper and lower extremity surgery because they generally result from excessive traction on the nerve or, alternatively, nerve compression resulting from prolonged positioning of the extremity during surgery or while in a cast. Early detection and intervention are critical. Patients with chronic neurologic conditions, such as neuropathies in the setting of diabetes or spinal stenosis, are at increased risk of nerve injury from surgery.

Venous Thromboembolism

Venous thromboembolic phenomena after orthopedic surgery are the most thoroughly studied postoperative complications, and pulmonary embolism remains an important cause of mortality (Chapter 98). The orthopedic literature has concentrated on lower extremity arthroplasty, although a recent study suggests that similar approaches should also be considered after total shoulder arthroplasty, where the risk of thromboembolism may be higher than generally appreciated.

After orthopedic surgery, a complicated balance exists between preventing a possibly life-threatening pulmonary embolus and reducing the potential for postoperative bleeding. Numerous protocols have documented the effectiveness of prophylaxis, which should begin at the time of the procedure. Short intraoperative time reduces the risk of deep vein thrombosis, as does the type of anesthesia. Epidural anesthesia reduces the risk of proximal deep vein thrombosis following THR by two- to three-fold and also reduces the overall risk of deep vein thrombosis by at least 20%. Other intraoperative interventions, such as hypotensive anesthesia and intraoperative heparin administration, further reduce thrombogenesis. Mechanical methods can also reduce the risk of thromboembolism. These include compression methodologies such as stockings and various pneumatic devices, foot flexion-extension exercises, and early ambulation. These are safe, effective approaches that do not increase the risk of bleeding.

The mainstay of prevention is prophylactic anticoagulation, which should begin immediately following surgery. Regimens include aspirin, warfarin, and low-molecular-weight heparin, often used in combination with various mechanical compression devices.

Fat Embolism Syndrome

Fat embolization, a well-described complication of skeletal trauma, can also occur after procedures involving instrumentation of the femoral medullary canal. Although the embolization of fat is believed to occur in almost all patients who sustain hip or femoral fractures, 1 to 3% of patients undergoing joint replacement surgery (particularly simultaneous bilateral procedures) develop fat embolism syndrome (FES).

The signs and symptoms of FES involve the respiratory, neurologic, and hematologic systems, as well as the skin. The time of onset is variable, with hemodynamic instability developing almost immediately in some patients or insidiously over the first 2 to 3 postoperative days in others. The latter patients gradually become hypoxemic, may be hypotensive, and are often confused. Transient thrombocytopenia is common. Respiratory signs are the most common manifestation. The majority of patients develop mild to moderate hypoxemia or radiographic changes (mainly bilateral alveolar infiltrates), but only a minority develop life-threatening adult respiratory distress syndrome. Neurologic manifestations range from mild drowsiness to acute confusional states to severe obtundation and coma, all consequences of the hypoxemia and the direct effect of fat embolization on the brain. The skin eruption, which is rare in total joint arthroplasty patients, takes the form of a petechial rash involving the conjunctiva and oral mucosa and may be distributed over the folds of the neck and axilla. Retinal edema and hemorrhage are also common.

Although patients suspected of having FES need to be closely monitored, in most cases, FES that develops after total joint arthroplasty is relatively benign. Treatment is supportive and includes the administration of oxygen and the prevention of pulmonary hypertension (by fluid restriction and the use of diuretics and venodilators). Corticosteroids are not effective. In the majority of patients, the condition resolves within 3 to 7 days, although in severe cases, the mortality rate is 5 to 15%, even with modern aggressive therapy.

Cervical Spine Involvement

In rheumatoid patients who exhibit advanced destructive disease, the presence of cervical spine instability should be ruled out before surgery with flexion-extension films. Patients with neck instability from rheumatoid arthritis may or may not exhibit symptoms such as neck pain, neck crepitus on range of motion testing, radicular symptoms, arm and/or leg weakness, or bladder and bowel dysfunction. Affected patients should wear a soft cervical collar to the operating room. When possible, epidural or spinal anesthesia should be used.

Conversely, in patients with ankylosing spondylitis, the rigid cervical spine may present technical challenges for the anesthesiologist during intubation. Fiberoptic methods are often employed in this clinical setting.

Immunosuppressive and Anti-inflammatory Therapy

The potential contributions of corticosteroids, disease-modifying antirheumatic drugs (DMARDs), and newer biological agents (Chapters 34 and 35) to the genesis of postoperative infection and wound dehiscence are well recognized by clinicians, although the debate concerning how to manage these medications in the perioperative setting is not settled. The primary challenge in this context is to achieve an optimal balance between maintaining control of the underlying disease and minimizing the risk of postoperative wound infection and/or wound breakdown.

Methotrexate is the most commonly used DMARD for the treatment of rheumatoid and other forms of inflammatory arthritis, so it is frequently seen in the perioperative setting. Given its importance in disease control, coupled with low rates of postoperative wound infection and dehiscence associated with its use, it appears to be safe—indeed, desirable—to continue methotrexate throughout the perioperative period.

With respect to the biological (anti–tumor necrosis factor) agents (etanercept, infliximab, adalimumab), recommendations formulated by international groups suggest that such agents be discontinued for short periods before surgery, generally 2 to 4 weeks. Some favor the longer 4-week interval for infliximab and adalimumab owing to the longer half-life of these agents. There is virtually no information concerning postoperative infection and wound healing with the newer agents such as anakinra, rituximab, and abatacept. Recommendations similar to those for the other biological agents must suffice until more data can be gathered.

The other important drugs commonly encountered in the perioperative setting are corticosteroids. In addition to problems related to the wound, there is concern about postoperative adrenal insufficiency. Traditionally, steroids have been shown to increase the rate of wound infection and dehiscence in surgical patients, although data derived from the orthopedic setting remain scant. Similarly, the published experience concerning postoperative adrenal insufficiency is scant. In contrast to methotrexate and the biological therapies, however, the question is not whether to stop corticosteroids before surgery, because this is generally not feasible. Rather, management considerations pertain to how much steroid augmentation (stress dosing) will be required, and for how long. In this regard, a nuanced approach, premised on patient-specific considerations, is required. For the patient managed with low doses of corticosteroid (≤7.5 mg/day) or on any dosage for less than 3 weeks, stress-dose steroid therapy is unnecessary, and maintenance of the patient's usual daily dosage should be sufficient. In contrast, for patients taking larger doses (≥20 mg/day) for longer periods (>3 weeks), it is prudent to assume that secondary adrenal suppression exists, justifying the use of stress-dose steroid therapy. For those taking intermediate doses (7.5 to 20 mg/day), decision making must be individualized. In addition to the dosage and duration of steroid therapy, other considerations include the presence of diabetes, the use of other immunosuppressive therapy, the presence of hypoalbuminemia, the patient's nutritional status, and the magnitude of the surgical procedure.

1. Kirkley A, Birmingham TB, Litchfield RB, et al. A randomized trial of arthroscopic surgery for osteoarthritis of the knee. *N Engl J Med.* 2008;359:1097-1107.
2. Singh JA, Sperling J, Buchbinder R, et al. Surgery for shoulder osteoarthritis. *Cochrane Database Syst Rev.* 2010;10:CD008089.

SUGGESTED READINGS

Del Pozo JL, Patel R. Clinical practice: infection associated with prosthetic joints. *N Engl J Med.* 2009;361:787-794. *Case-based review.*

Labek G, Thaler M, Janda W, et al. Revision rates after total joint replacement: cumulative results from worldwide joint register datasets. *J Bone Joint Surg Br.* 2011;93:293-297. *Rates of revision are about 6% after 5 years and 12% after 10 years.*

Seida JC, LeBlanc C, Schouten JR, et al. Nonoperative and operative treatments for rotator cuff tears. *Ann Intern Med.* 2010;153:246-255. *Review indicating that there is not definitive evidence on the superiority of any specific therapy or procedure.*

XXIII

§ INFECTIOUS DISEASES

286

INTRODUCTION TO MICROBIAL DISEASE: HOST-PATHOGEN INTERACTIONS

W. MICHAEL SCHELD

Infectious diseases have profoundly influenced the course of human history. The "black death" (caused by *Yersinia pestis*) changed the social structure of medieval Europe, in the process eliminating approximately a third of the population. The outcomes of military campaigns have been altered by outbreaks of diseases such as dysentery and typhus. Examples include Napoleon's retreat from Russia, after typhus did more damage to his army than the opposition forces did; the decision by the French to sell the Louisiana Territory after French soldiers died from yellow fever in Cuba and the Gulf Coast; and the introduction of smallpox to the nonimmune population of the New World by Europeans, thus facilitating the "conquest" and the dawn of the colonial age. Malaria influenced the geographic and racial pattern and distribution of hemoglobins and erythrocyte antigens in Africa. The development of *Plasmodium falciparum* is inhibited by the presence of hemoglobin S, and Duffy blood group–negative erythrocytes are resistant to infection with *Plasmodium vivax*. Thus, populations with these erythrocyte factors are found in areas where malaria is common.

Infections are a major cause of morbidity and mortality in the world. Of the approximately 53 million deaths worldwide in 2009, at least a third were due to infectious diseases. In the United States, pneumonia is the fifth leading cause of death overall and the most common cause of death related to infection. In addition, invasive disease caused by *Streptococcus pneumoniae* and community-acquired pneumonia overall have increased in incidence over the past decade. Acquired immunodeficiency syndrome (AIDS) threatens to disrupt the social fabric in many countries of Africa and is severely distressing the health care system in the United States and other parts of the world. The year 2006 marked the 25th "anniversary" of the AIDS epidemic. Approximately 33 million people worldwide are currently infected with human immunodeficiency virus (HIV), and since 1981, approximately 25 million have died ($\approx$ 600,000 in the United States alone). AIDS is now the leading cause of death in sub-Saharan Africa.

Infection can be defined as the multiplication of microbes (from viruses to multicellular parasites) in the tissues of the host. The host may or may not be symptomatic. For example, HIV infection may cause no overt signs or symptoms of illness for years. The definition of infection should also include the multiplication of microbes on the surface or in the lumen of the host that causes signs and symptoms of illness or disease. For example, toxin-producing strains of *Escherichia coli* may multiply in the gut and cause a diarrheal illness without invading tissues. Microbes can cause diseases without actually coming in contact with the host by virtue of toxin production. *Clostridium botulinum* may grow in certain improperly processed foods and produce a toxin that can be lethal on ingestion. A relatively trivial infection such as that caused by *Clostridium tetani* in a small puncture wound can cause devastating illness because of a toxin released from the organism growing in tissues. It has now become apparent that multiple virulence factors of microorganisms can be carried in tandem on so-called pathogenicity islands of the genome (the "virulome").

We live in a virtual sea of microorganisms, and all our body surfaces have indigenous bacterial flora. This normal flora actually protects us from infection. Reduction of gut colonization increases susceptibility to infection by pathogens such as *Salmonella enteritidis* serovar *typhimurium*. Bacteria that constitute the normal flora are thought to exert their protective effect by several mechanisms: (1) utilizing nutrients and occupying an ecologic niche, thus competing with pathogens; (2) producing antibacterial substances that inhibit the growth of pathogens; and (3) inducing host immunity that is cross-reactive and effective against pathogens. These conclusions appear to be oversimplistic, however. For example, colonization of the gastrointestinal tract with *Bacteroides fragilis* expressing an immunodominant bacterial polysaccharide, through dendritic cell activation and induction of a T_H1-mediated response, leads to a splenic response characterized by normal numbers of $CD4^+$ T cells, lymphoid architecture, and systemic lymphocytic

expansion. Thus, a single bacterial molecule in our gut is necessary to make us "immunologically fit." In addition to the normal flora, transient colonization may be seen with known or potential pathogens. This may be a special problem in hospitalized patients because it can lead to nosocomial infection (Chapter 290).

Only a small proportion of microbial species can be considered primary or professional pathogens, and even among these species, a relatively small number of clones have been shown to cause disease. For example, epidemic meningococcal meningitis and meningococcemia are due to a small number of clones of *Neisseria meningitidis*, and the worldwide explosion of penicillin-resistant *S. pneumoniae* can be traced to a few clones originating in South Africa and Spain. This observation supports the concept that pathogenic organisms are highly adapted to the pathogenic state and have developed characteristics that enable them to be transmitted, attach to surfaces, invade tissue, avoid host defenses, and thus cause disease. In contrast, opportunistic pathogens cause disease principally in impaired hosts, and these organisms, which may be harmless members of normal flora in healthy persons, can act as virulent invaders in patients with severe defects in host defense mechanisms. Although opportunistic infection has traditionally been viewed as the exploitation of a weakened host through physiologic stress or immunocompromise (or both) by relatively "avirulent" pathogens, this is an oversimplification. For example, *Pseudomonas aeruginosa* recognizes host immune activation, specifically by binding interferon-γ to a cell surface protein OprF, which in turn, through a quorum-sensing signaling system, leads to the overexpression of virulence determinants such as PA-I (lecA) and pyocyanin. Thus, bacteria have developed a "contingency system" that recognizes immunologic perturbations in the host and counters this response by the expression of virulence factors.

Pathogenic organisms may be acquired by several routes. Direct contact has been implicated in the acquisition of staphylococcal disease. Airborne spread, usually by droplet nuclei, occurs in respiratory diseases such as influenza and in severe acute respiratory syndrome (SARS). Contaminated water is the usual vehicle in *Giardia* infection and typhoid fever. Food-borne toxic illnesses may be caused by extracellular toxins produced by *Clostridium perfringens* and *Staphylococcus aureus*. Blood and blood products may be vectors for transmitting hepatitis B and C viruses, as well as HIV. Sexual transmission is also important for these agents and for a variety of other pathogens, including *Treponema pallidum* (syphilis), *Neisseria gonorrhoeae* (gonorrhea), and *Chlamydia trachomatis* (nonspecific urethritis). The fetus may be infected in utero, and the infection may be devastating if the agent is rubella virus or cytomegalovirus. Arthropod vectors may be important, as illustrated by mosquitoes for malaria and dengue, ticks for Lyme disease and ehrlichiosis, and lice for typhus.

Pathogens are able to cause disease because of a finely tuned array of adaptations, including the ability to attach to appropriate cells, often mediated by specialized structures such as the pili on Gram-negative rods. Microbes such as *Shigella* species have the ability to invade cells and cause damage. Toxins may act at a distance or may intoxicate only infected cells. Pathogens have the ability to thwart host defenses by a variety of ingenious maneuvers. The antiphagocytic coat of the pneumococcus is an example. Organisms may change their surface antigen display at an astonishingly rapid rate to outmaneuver the host immune system. Examples include influenza virus and trypanosomes. Certain pathogens have the ability to inhibit the respiratory burst of phagocytes (*Toxoplasma gondii*), and others can destroy phagocytic cells that have engulfed them (e.g., *Streptococcus pyogenes*). The environment plays an important role in infection, both in transmission and in the host's ability to combat the invader. The humidity and temperature of air may affect the infectivity of airborne pathogens. The sanitary state of food and water, woefully lacking in many areas of the developing world, is an important factor in the acquisition of enteric pathogens, one of the major causes of mortality and morbidity, such as physical and mental developmental delay leading to poor performance in school and other consequences. The malaria associated with the "bad air" of swamps is, in fact, due to the mosquitoes there, but the environmental association was appropriate. The nutritional status of the host is clearly a significant factor in certain infectious diseases. It is likely that micronutrient deficiency contributes to the invasion and multiplication of certain pathogens. A new concept is the possibility that infectious diseases cause malnutrition through a vicious circle of diarrhea leading to dehydration and poor oral intake, resulting in secondary diarrhea with a propensity for "stunting" and delaying intellectual development. Establishment of infection is a complicated interplay of factors involving the microbe, the host, and the environment.

Host reaction to infection may result in illness. For example, previous infection with *Campylobacter jejuni* is responsible for about 40% of cases of Guillain-Barré syndrome. The mechanism is thought to be the production of antibodies against *C. jejuni* lipopolysaccharides that cross-react with gangliosides in peripheral nerves. Similarly, much of the damage resulting from meningitis is due to the host's response to invading bacterial pathogens.

With some exceptions, infectious diseases are often treatable and curable. Thus, it is important to make an accurate etiologic diagnosis and institute appropriate therapy promptly. In acute infections such as pneumonia, meningitis, or sepsis, rapid institution of therapy may be life-saving; thus, a presumptive etiologic diagnosis should be established before a definitive diagnosis. This presumptive diagnosis is based on the history, physical examination, epidemiology of illness in the community, and rapid techniques such as microscopic examination of appropriate Gram-stained specimens. Antimicrobial therapy can then be instituted for the presumptive etiologic agents, but it must be reevaluated as more definitive diagnostic information becomes available.

The study as well as the understanding of infectious diseases is a dynamic process. A number of factors or themes of current interest contribute to this conclusion, including the following:

EMERGING INFECTIONS. The most obvious is AIDS, but recent examples with a major impact on the public health in the United States include community-associated methicillin-resistant *S. aureus*, a hypervirulent strain of *Clostridium difficile*, and the 2009 H1N1 influenza. More than 300 new, emerging infectious diseases have been described in the last 70 years; approximately 60% are zoonoses associated with geographic "hotspots." Their emergence is driven largely by ecologic, socioeconomic, and environmental factors.

GENOMICS AND OTHER "OMICS." The exact sequence of the genome of more than 2000 microbes relevant to humans has been determined. This new information, in concert with genomic information from multicellular organisms such as the *Anopheles* mosquito, offers significant promise for the development of new therapies and vaccines. Careful analysis of the genomes of pathogens will continue to yield important information about the pathogenesis of infection. For example, genome sequencing of group A streptococci, collected over time with relevant robust clinical information, has detected the acquisition of new determinants (often by prophage) responsible for increased virulence and resulting in toxic shock syndrome, necrotizing fasciitis, or both. Proteomics, transcriptomics, metabolomics, and virulomics have transformed research on infectious diseases and promise significant improvements in diagnostics and therapeutics in the future.

GENETIC FACTORS ALTERING SUSCEPTIBILITY TO INFECTION AND THE RESPONSE TO INFECTIOUS DISEASES. This field promises new and significant information relevant to the wide variety of responses to infectious diseases in humans. For example, an overvigorous response, with generation of tumor necrosis factor-α, may accentuate the development of cerebral complications in falciparum malaria. Analysis of single-nucleotide polymorphisms of the human genome will lead to an enhanced understanding of two fundamental issues in infectious diseases: why invasive, overt disease develops in only a small fraction of individuals colonized with a given microbe, and why infections are more severe in some people than in others. Variants in genes that encode molecules that mediate attachment, pathogen recognition, inflammatory cytokine response, and innate and adaptive immunity are being identified at an astonishing rate.

INNATE IMMUNITY. This is the most active field in immunology. The identification of pattern recognition receptors (e.g., Toll-like receptors [TLRs] and nucleotide oligomerization domain [NOD]-like receptors) that recognize pathogen-associated molecular patterns, as well as endogenous substances reflecting tissue injury (e.g., alarmins), has revolutionized our understanding of the early host response to infection. Agonists or antagonists of TLRs have already entered clinical trials as adjuvant therapies (e.g., editoran for sepsis) or to improve the immunogenicity of vaccines. The other area that has exploded recently is the study of antimicrobial peptides (e.g., defensins, cathecidins, histatins, galectins) and their role in the early response to infectious disorders.

ANTIMICROBIAL RESISTANCE. The development of new antimicrobial agents has slowed despite the burgeoning problem of antimicrobial resistance. This disconnect has been the focus of meetings among the pharmaceutical industry, the Infectious Diseases Society of America, the Food and Drug Administration, and others. Multiresistant pneumococci, vancomycin resistance in *S. aureus,* vancomycin-resistant enterococci, and, perhaps most important, multidrug-resistant gram-negative bacilli (MDR-GNB) are

just a few examples. Some MDR-GNB are susceptible to only a few agents of "last resort," such as colistin or tigecycline; others are truly untreatable (Chapter 313). Unfortunately, new agents active against these strains are years, if not decades, away from introduction.

THE ROLE OF INFECTIOUS AGENTS IN CHRONIC DISEASES. Many so-called idiopathic diseases may in fact have an infectious basis. Conditions for which there is some evidence (but not conclusive proof) of an infectious basis include diabetes, atherosclerosis, acute leukemia, collagen vascular diseases, and inflammatory bowel disease. Detection of "uncultivatable" microorganisms by newer techniques, such as 16S RNA analysis, may uncover agents responsible for "noninfectious" diseases or suggest a role in conditions that are considered infectious but in which the pathogen or pathogens are controversial (e.g., bacterial vaginosis). In addition, we know that hepatitis C virus, human papillomavirus, and *Helicobacter pylori* cause human cancers. Furthermore, changes in our own microbiome may lead to disease. Alterations in the gut microbiome are associated with obesity. Another recent example comes from experiments with mice lacking TLR5. These mice develop hyperphagia and hallmark features of the metabolic syndrome, including hyperlipidemia, hypertension, insulin resistance, and increased adiposity, associated with an altered gut microbiome. Further, transfer of this changed microbiota into germ-free wild-type mice induces most features of the metabolic syndrome in the recipients.

SUGGESTED READINGS

Gibson DG, Glass JI, Lartigue C, et al. Creation of a bacterial cell controlled by a chemically synthesized genome. *Science.* 2010;329:52-56. *Report of the design, synthesis, assembly, and transfer of a 1.08–megabase pair* Mycoplasma *genome, with retention of donor characteristics by the recipient.*

Monsalvo AC, Batelle JP, Lopez MF, et al. Severe pandemic 2009 H1N1 influenza disease due to pathogenic immune complexes. *Nat Med.* 2011;17:195-199. *Suggests a previously unknown biologic mechanism for the unusual age distribution of severe cases during influenza pandemics.*

Sogaard OS, Lohse N, Harboe ZB, et al. Improving the immunogenicity of pneumococcal conjugate vaccine in HIV-infected adults with a Toll-like receptor 9 agonist adjuvant: a randomized controlled trial. *Clin Infect Dis.* 2010;51:42-50. *Example of the use of Toll-like receptor agonists as adjuvants to enhance vaccine immunogenicity.*

Turvey SE, Broide DH. Innate immunity. *J Allergy Clin Immunol.* 2010;125:S24-S32. *Excellent review of recent advances, and how innate immunity interacts with adaptive immunity.*

Vijay-Kumar M, Aitken JD, Carvalho FA, et al. Metabolic syndrome and altered gut microbiota in mice lacking Toll-like receptor 5. *Science.* 2010;328:228-231. *The salient findings of these experiments are discussed in the text.*

287

PRINCIPLES OF ANTI-INFECTIVE THERAPY

GEORGE M. ELIOPOULOS

Among the pharmaceutical agents used in the treatment of human disease, antimicrobial agents are distinctive because they target invading microorganisms rather than abnormal human cellular functions. As a result, to select an appropriate antimicrobial regimen, it is necessary to consider both the activity of the agent against the known or suspected pathogen and the effects that agent might have on the individual under treatment. Although the term *anti-infective agent* can be used more broadly to include substances that ameliorate infection by altering the virulence of the pathogen or modulating the host's response to infection, for purposes of this chapter, *anti-infective agent* and *antimicrobial agent* are used interchangeably to refer to drugs that inhibit the growth of microbial pathogens. This chapter focuses primarily on agents directed against bacterial pathogens, although many parallels can be drawn to the use of antimicrobial agents for the treatment of fungal, viral, or parasitic infections.

On the time scale of human history, the modern antibiotic era is short. Since the introduction of penicillin for general clinical use in the mid-1940s, the numerous antimicrobial agents developed for human use have saved countless lives and have led to amazing advances in cancer chemotherapy, organ transplantation, and implant surgery that have improved and extended the lives of many others. Unfortunately, over time, resistance to available antibiotics has become widespread among many common bacterial pathogens, making the selection of appropriate antimicrobial regimens ever more challenging and threatening to thrust an unfortunate few into a situation resembling the pre-antibiotic era.

SELECTING ANTIMICROBIAL THERAPY TARGETING THE PATHOGEN

Empirical Antimicrobial Therapy

In most instances, selection of the initial antimicrobial therapy proceeds empirically, before a causative organism is identified or tested for susceptibility to antimicrobial agents. The clinician's first decision is whether a patient's symptoms are likely to represent infection. Fever may result from neoplastic, rheumatologic, or other noninfectious processes and does not necessarily imply the presence of infection. Noninfectious causes of fever, such as deep vein thrombophlebitis, drug reaction, or vasculitis, may pose just as great a risk to the patient as infection and must not be overlooked.

Additional symptoms, signs, and laboratory or radiographic data usually help define whether infection is likely and, if so, localize the organ systems involved. This information allows an initial prediction about the organisms likely to be involved. For example, if the initial data cause one to suspect a diagnosis of community-acquired pneumonia in a previously healthy person who does not have any unusual exposures, *Streptococcus pneumoniae* and atypical bacteria such as *Mycoplasma pneumoniae* or *Chlamydophila pneumoniae* would be prominent on the list of potential pathogens to be targeted when selecting antimicrobial therapy. Examination of a Gram-stained slide of expectorated sputum may provide valuable information. The prominent appearance of gram-positive cocci in clusters, for example, would alert the clinician to the possible presence of *Staphylococcus aureus,* many isolates of which are now methicillin resistant.

Guidance regarding the probable pathogens for site-specific infections and the susceptibility of these organisms to antimicrobial agents is available from a number of sources. In some cases, the susceptibility of suspected pathogens can be predicted with a high degree of certainty. For example, *Streptococcus pyogenes* remains uniformly susceptible to penicillin G. In other instances, resistance has emerged to antimicrobials previously considered to be highly active against a species. Resistance rates for a given organism may vary widely by region, by health care institution, or even by patient care area within a hospital. For this reason, access to periodically updated, cumulative antibiotic susceptibility profile data specific to an institution can be very important. Typically presented in tabular form, these "antibiograms" show the percentage of recently isolated bacterial pathogens that proved "susceptible" to the antibiotics tested and can help guide the selection of appropriate empirical regimens at that practice site.

There is mounting evidence that selection of an appropriate regimen (i.e., one that contains an antimicrobial that can be expected to inhibit the causative pathogen at the site of infection) and the prompt initiation of that empirical treatment result in improved clinical outcomes in those with serious infections. Published guidelines for the treatment of community-acquired pneumonia advise administration of the first dose of appropriate antimicrobial therapy while the patient is still in the emergency room.

Whenever possible, samples of purulent exudates, blood, or other body fluids suspected to be infected should be obtained for culture before starting antimicrobial therapy. Identification and susceptibility testing of the microorganisms detected can be used to direct subsequent definitive treatment. At times, however, this principle must be overridden. For example, when bacterial meningitis is suspected, antibiotic therapy (often with adjunctive corticosteroids) must not be delayed when a lumbar puncture cannot be performed promptly to obtain material for culture. In such instances, blood samples taken for culture before the administration of antibiotics often reveal the causative organism, or the pathogen may grow from spinal fluid even if lumbar puncture is delayed.

Definitive Antimicrobial Therapy

Identification of the causative microorganism and determination of its susceptibility to available drugs are the basis for optimizing definitive antimicrobial regimens. Often, the antibiotics used for empirical therapy are appropriate for definitive therapy and can be continued. At other times, the results allow one to switch to a narrower spectrum, better tolerated, or less expensive antimicrobial. In some instances, test results indicate the need to broaden the spectrum of an anti-infective regimen by adding or substituting agents active against pathogens inadequately targeted by the initial empirical regimen.

In almost all cases, it is desirable to test an infecting organism's susceptibility to antimicrobials that may be useful. To extend the example cited earlier,

although it is not necessary to test the susceptibility of *S. pyogenes* to penicillin G, some isolates are resistant to macrolide antibiotics (e.g., erythromycin, azithromycin) and other drugs, so the testing of alternative agents might be useful for patients who are intolerant of β-lactam antibiotics. Even when the activity of certain antimicrobials can be predicted with great confidence, susceptibility testing is still useful. For example, surveillance studies examining hundreds of isolates have predicted that vancomycin or linezolid would inhibit virtually all *S. aureus* strains recovered from initial clinical specimens. Therefore, on statistical grounds, testing these agents would not seem warranted; however, rare isolates resistant to these agents have now been encountered, and it is advantageous to detect such isolates for both therapeutic and epidemiologic purposes. For most bacterial pathogens, resistance to commonly used agents is sufficiently frequent that testing of antimicrobials being considered for definitive therapy is essential. Organisms of the family Enterobacteriaceae that are resistant to multiple antibiotics are isolated often enough, even among outpatients, that susceptibility to agents previously considered broadly active, including third-generation cephalosporins, fluoroquinolones, and aminoglycosides, is no longer assured. Even more challenging problems of drug resistance are encountered among isolates of species such as *Pseudomonas aeruginosa, Acinetobacter baumannii,* and *Stenotrophomonas maltophilia.*

Susceptibility Testing

Several methods are available for determining the susceptibility of a bacterial isolate to antimicrobial agents being considered for therapy. Tests used in clinical microbiology laboratories today are variations of three methods: serial dilution, disc diffusion, and gradient diffusion. The minimal inhibitory concentration (MIC) represents the lowest concentration of an antimicrobial tested that inhibits growth of the microorganism in test media.

In the dilution method, the antimicrobial is diluted in broth or agar to span a range of (usually) two-fold decreasing concentrations, and the medium is then inoculated with a standardized number of organisms. After incubation for a specified period (usually 16 to 24 hours) at 35 to 37° C, the series of dilution tubes or microtiter wells (for broth dilution) or agar plates (for agar dilution) is examined for growth. The MIC is determined by direct inspection as the lowest concentration that prevents turbidity of the broth or colony formation on agar. Modifications of this method allow the automation of many steps in the process, permitting more efficient test performance in clinical laboratories.

In the disc diffusion method, paper discs impregnated with a standardized amount of the antimicrobial are placed on an agar plate, the surface of which has been seeded with the bacterium to be tested. During incubation, the antimicrobial diffuses from the disc into the surrounding agar and inhibits growth of the seeded organism. After a specified period of incubation, the zone of growth inhibition around the disc is measured. By this method, the MIC is not determined directly. Instead, relying on accumulated data correlating inhibition zones with MICs, the measured zone is used to predict the susceptibility of the organism to the drug tested.

The gradient diffusion method is similar to the disc diffusion method, except that instead of using a round paper disc impregnated with a single concentration of the antimicrobial, this test uses a strip impregnated with the antimicrobial applied in a concentration gradient along its length. The strip is laid on the surface of an agar plate that has been inoculated with a suspension of the organism to be tested, and the plate is then incubated. By visually inspecting where the zone of growth inhibition on the agar surface intersects the strip (which is marked at intervals corresponding to MIC equivalents), it is possible to determine the MIC value directly.

To perform and interpret the results of susceptibility studies, it is necessary to identify the organism to be tested. This knowledge allows the selection of appropriate interpretive criteria to determine whether an organism is "susceptible," "intermediate," or "resistant" to an antimicrobial based on measurement of the MIC or the inhibition zone diameter. To illustrate this point, consider that an enterococcus is determined to be susceptible to penicillin if the MIC is less than or equal to 8 μg/mL, whereas for viridans streptococci, the corresponding breakpoint for susceptibility to penicillin is a MIC of 0.12 μg/mL. Thus, knowledge that the MIC of a gram-positive coccus growing in short chains is 2 μg/mL does not allow the determination of whether it is susceptible to penicillin unless the organism has been identified.

Additional tests are sometimes required to fully assess susceptibility to an antimicrobial. For oxacillin-susceptible *S. aureus,* a test for penicillinase production is performed to assess susceptibility to penicillin G. For erythromycin-resistant, clindamycin-susceptible *S. aureus,* the laboratory may perform a supplementary D-zone test before reporting the clindamycin result. A positive D-zone test (i.e., blunting of the inhibition zone around a clindamycin disc in proximity to an erythromycin disc) predicts the presence of *erm* genes. Their product, a ribosomal methylase, can confer resistance to clindamycin if expressed; however, clindamycin is a poor inducer of this resistance trait (in contrast to erythromycin, which is a good inducer). Mutants with constitutive production of methylase can be selected during treatment, resulting in the emergence of clindamycin resistance and an increased risk of clinical failure when this drug is used to treat serious staphylococcal infections caused by strains with the *erm* gene.

In principle, tests for the presence of resistance genes, their products, or both can be used in place of phenotypic resistance testing. Such methods have the potential to provide answers more rapidly than can be obtained with the usual susceptibility tests of growth inhibition, which generally require several hours of incubation. However, at present, these tests have not been widely adopted, with the exception of testing for methicillin resistance by detection of the *mecA* gene or its product, penicillin-binding protein 2a.

Bactericidal Activity

In some circumstances, an antimicrobial regimen that kills pathogenic microorganisms would be preferable to an alternative regimen that only inhibits growth of the pathogen. Bactericidal activity is desirable in the treatment of endocarditis or meningitis; in these infections, bacteriostatic agents have generally performed poorly, possibly because of inadequate host responses to infection at these sites. Tests to measure the bactericidal activity of an antibiotic in vitro have been developed. Bactericidal activity is usually defined as a 99.9% reduction in the number of viable colony-forming units relative to the inoculum density at a specified incubation time, which is usually 20 to 24 hours.

Despite the theoretical benefit of determining the bactericidal activity of an antibiotic or drug regimen, these tests are rarely used clinically because of several factors, including (1) the labor-intensive nature of the tests, (2) the potential for discordant results owing to the various methods and criteria for determining bactericidal activity, and (3) imperfect correlation between bactericidal activity measured in vitro and clinical outcomes observed.

● SELECTING ANTIMICROBIAL THERAPY APPROPRIATE TO THE INFECTION AND PATIENT

Nature of the Infection

Determination that a pathogenic microorganism is susceptible to an antibiotic in vitro does not ensure that treatment with that drug will result in a successful clinical outcome. The antimicrobial must reach the site of infection in adequate concentration, which is generally assumed to be some multiple of the MIC, and it must demonstrate activity in the infection milieu. For some infections and antimicrobials, these requirements cannot easily be met.

A number of antimicrobials fail to penetrate into cerebrospinal fluid sufficiently well to permit their use for the treatment of bacterial meningitis in adults. First-generation cephalosporins or aminoglycosides given intravenously do not enter the subarachnoid space well enough to allow their use as primary agents for treatment of this disease. Aminoglycosides have been administered by intrathecal or intraventricular instillation when needed for the treatment of gram-negative meningitis, but the availability of newer β-lactams with broad activity, high potency, and reasonable penetration represents a major advance.

In other situations, antimicrobials may penetrate to the site of infection, only to be inactivated by local factors. For example, daptomycin is inactivated by interaction with pulmonary surfactant, so this antibiotic is not indicated for the treatment of bronchopneumonia, even though it is highly active against *S. pneumoniae* isolates in vitro. Antibiotics can also be inactivated by cellular debris or macromolecules present within abscesses, and some exhibit reduced potency at the low pH and reduced oxygen tensions prevailing at these sites. Finally, high densities of microorganisms within abscesses may elaborate sufficiently high concentrations of β-lactamases to inactivate some relatively labile β-lactam antibiotics. All these factors provide a rationale for the drainage of large abscesses as an adjunct to antimicrobial therapy.

Bacterial infections associated with foreign bodies such as artificial joints, cardiac pacemakers, or prosthetic heart valves can be particularly difficult to eradicate without removing the foreign material. The reasons are not completely understood, but they relate, at least in part, to the presence of biofilm,

which is composed of bacteria embedded within extracellular material that is adherent to the foreign body. Bacteria recovered from biofilms are metabolically different from and less susceptible to antimicrobial agents than planktonic cells (i.e., those freely suspended in liquid medium) of the same organism. Rifampin is often added to antimicrobial regimens for the treatment of infections involving prosthetic material. This inhibitor of RNA polymerase rapidly penetrates into biofilms and demonstrates relatively similar activity against both biofilm-associated and planktonic cells of a susceptible organism. However, because resistance to rifampin emerges rapidly, it is not used as a single agent in these circumstances; rifampin must be combined with a second active drug to minimize the risk that resistance will emerge. Despite such approaches, many infections involving implanted devices prove refractory to antimicrobial therapy alone and require removal of the foreign material for eradication.

Host Factors

After considering the nature of the infection and the antimicrobials determined in vitro to be active against a bacterial isolate (or likely to be active against probable pathogens when an isolate is not yet available), the ultimate choice of an antimicrobial regimen must take into account a number of additional patient-specific factors, some examples of which are examined in the following paragraphs.

Allergies

It is imperative to obtain a history of previous allergic reactions to antimicrobial agents. Some reactions are by nature so severe and potentially life-threatening that one must avoid using the same agent or drugs within the same class for which cross-reactivity is likely to occur. Examples of such reactions include an immediate hypersensitivity reaction to penicillin (e.g., hives, lip swelling, laryngeal edema, circulatory collapse) or a mucocutaneous bullous eruption from a sulfonamide (e.g., Stevens-Johnson syndrome).

In cases in which the allergic reaction was mild, such as a faint, self-limited rash in a patient receiving penicillin, the clinician may elect to use a related antimicrobial, such as a cephalosporin, when the probability of cross-sensitivity and the risk for a severe adverse outcome if a reaction were to occur are both assessed to be low. In these instances, careful monitoring of the patient for adverse reactions is essential. Rarely, for patients with significant allergies to potentially life-saving antimicrobial agents for which no alternative exists, desensitization of the patient to the antimicrobial is attempted so that the agent can be used. For example, desensitization protocols are available for penicillin and for trimethoprim-sulfamethoxazole. Because of the risks involved, these procedures may need to be performed in intensive care unit settings.

Pregnancy

A number of antimicrobial agents have the potential to cause fetal harm if administered to a pregnant woman. For example, tetracyclines can cause tooth discoloration and hypoplasia of dental enamel and are thus avoided in pregnant women and young children. Streptomycin given during pregnancy can cross the placenta, and evidence of eighth nerve toxicity has been reported. A few other antimicrobials are labeled by the Food and Drug Administration (FDA) as pregnancy category D (evidence of human risk) or are contraindicated because of fetal harm (category X). Many more antimicrobials, however, are assigned to category C; for these drugs, the potential risk to the fetus is based on animal studies. When designing antimicrobial regimens, the possibility of pregnancy should be considered in any woman of childbearing age so that the risks of candidate agents can be individually reviewed and the safest possible therapy selected.

It should also be noted that many antibiotics used to treat lactating women can be found in breast milk. Thus, it may be necessary to suspend breast-feeding during treatment if exposure of the infant to the drug must be avoided.

Pregnant women may be particularly susceptible to certain antimicrobial-associated toxicities. Death resulting from hepatic failure has been described in pregnant women receiving large doses of tetracycline. Potentially life-threatening hepatic steatosis has been observed in patients treated with a combination of the antiretroviral agents didanosine plus stavudine; pregnant women may be especially vulnerable to this toxic effect.

Age

For reasons discussed earlier, tetracycline antibiotics are avoided in children during tooth development to prevent discoloration and enamel hypoplasia of the permanent teeth. Because fluoroquinolone antimicrobials produce erosion of cartilage and arthropathy in juvenile animals, they are avoided in children when alternative agents are available. Recently, limited pediatric indications were added for ciprofloxacin (for complicated urinary tract infection and pyelonephritis and, along with levofloxacin, for treatment after inhalational exposure to anthrax). Musculoskeletal complaints appear to be more frequent in children treated with ciprofloxacin than with nonfluoroquinolone antimicrobials.

Pediatric dosing regimens differ from those appropriate for adults. Some agents, such as linezolid, are eliminated much more rapidly in young children (excluding preterm neonates) than in older children and adults, so higher doses are required. In premature infants and neonates, renal function has not yet reached full capacity, and drug elimination may be delayed. Similarly, hepatic clearance activity is not fully developed in the very young, which has led to cardiovascular collapse and fatalities from chloramphenicol treatment. Absorption of oral antimicrobials may also differ with age if their absorption is dependent on gastric pH. The gastric pH of young children is higher than that of adults, and achlorhydria resulting in higher gastric pH is more common in adults older than 60 years than in younger adults. Thus, in young children and older adults, the absorption of oral drugs that are unstable in acid, such as penicillin G, may be higher than that in younger adults. In contrast, antimicrobials such as ketoconazole require gastric acid for absorption and may be less bioavailable in persons with reduced gastric acid production.

A curious association between the appearance of a rash and the patient's age and sex was noted during development of the fluoroquinolone antimicrobial gemifloxacin. In clinical studies, rash was more common in young women than in men and older women, suggesting there may be hormonal influences on the risk of developing a rash.

Renal and Hepatic Function

Renal excretion and hepatobiliary excretion are the major routes of elimination for antimicrobial agents. Relatively few antibacterial agents can be administered without dosage adjustments in patients with renal dysfunction. Included among these drugs are nafcillin, ceftriaxone, doxycycline, azithromycin, and linezolid. Although linezolid exposure is not significantly altered, microbiologically inactive metabolites of the compound do accumulate in end-stage renal disease; what, if any, effect this has is unknown.

A number of antimicrobial agents require major dosage adjustments in the presence of renal dysfunction. The dosing interval for ceftazidime, usually administered every 8 hours in patients with normal renal function, is extended to once every 48 hours in persons with creatinine clearance below 10 mL/minute. Vancomycin is also administered at substantially increased dosing intervals or at smaller doses as renal function declines. Because of the increased efficiency of newer hemodialysis membranes in removing vancomycin, dosages are usually based on measured serum drug concentrations, and dosing may be required after each dialysis session.

In some instances, clearance of the antimicrobial agent is not affected by renal dysfunction, but excipients may accumulate, with the potential for toxic effects. For example, clearance of the antifungal agent voriconazole is not dependent on renal function. However, its intravenous preparation contains the solubilizing agent sulfobutyl ether β-cyclodextrin, which does accumulate in the presence of renal insufficiency. The intravenous preparation should not be used in those with renal dysfunction, but the oral formulation, which does not contain β-cyclodextrin, can be administered. A number of other antimicrobials may accumulate in the presence of severe liver disease, with the possibility of an increased risk for adverse events. Antimicrobials requiring dose adjustments for various levels of hepatic insufficiency include metronidazole, chloramphenicol, tigecycline, caspofungin, and voriconazole. For ceftriaxone, dosage adjustments or careful monitoring may be required in patients with both hepatic and renal dysfunction. Several of the newer antimicrobials, such as daptomycin, linezolid, and micafungin, have not been studied sufficiently to determine whether dosing modifications are required in patients with severe liver disease.

Drug-Drug Interactions

One of the most important considerations in the selection of an appropriate antimicrobial regimen is to determine whether the drug or drugs will interact with other medications the patient is taking. Some drug-drug interactions can have severe or even fatal consequences. There are too many potential interactions to list comprehensively, but some examples are provided in this section. Fortunately, resources are now available that allow the clinician to check for potential drug-drug interactions when an antimicrobial agent is ordered.

A large number of antimicrobials are eliminated via cytochrome P-450 pathways. As a result, they may interfere with the elimination of other drugs cleared by these pathways, leading to their accumulation to potentially dangerous levels. Several macrolide antibacterials, some fluoroquinolones, and human immunodeficiency virus (HIV) protease inhibitors are among the most likely antimicrobials to inhibit the clearance of other drugs. For example, use of the protease inhibitor nelfinavir is contraindicated with several drugs, including the antiarrhythmics amiodarone and quinidine, ergot derivatives, the neuroleptic drug pimozide, and certain sedative-hypnotic agents. Macrolides may result in increased levels of 3-hydroxy-3-methylglutaryl coenzyme A (HMG-CoA) reductase inhibitors, which can lead to rhabdomyolysis. Although quinupristin-dalfopristin is not eliminated by the cytochrome P-450 system, this drug inhibits the elimination of various agents cleared by this pathway, including cyclosporine, midazolam, nifedipine, and others.

In contrast, administration of rifampin induces the cytochrome P-450 system and may enhance the clearance of other drugs, some of which have narrow therapeutic windows. This may result in a number of important effects, including reduced effectiveness of oral contraceptives and increased warfarin requirements to maintain desired levels of anticoagulation. It is very important to consider these potential interactions not only when starting rifampin therapy but also when *stopping* treatment. When rifampin is stopped, unless the previously increased dose of warfarin is adjusted downward accordingly, excessive anticoagulation and possibly serious bleeding can occur.

A number of other drug interactions have been described. Linezolid has weak monoamine oxidase inhibitor activity. As such, it has the potential to enhance the hypertensive effect of adrenergic agonists and has been associated with the development of serotonin syndrome in patients taking selective serotonin re-uptake inhibitors (SSRIs). Patients with this syndrome can exhibit a number of signs and symptoms, including fever, tachycardia, tremulousness, agitation, confusion, and clonus, occasionally with fatal results. Serotonin syndrome (Chapter 442) has been described in patients taking linezolid together with drugs other than SSRIs; in principle, it could occur when linezolid is combined with any of a large number of agents that increase serotonin concentrations in the central nervous system.

Other Host Factors

Several additional host factors may influence the choice of a suitable antimicrobial regimen. Some antimicrobials have the potential to induce hemolysis in persons with glucose-6-phosphate dehydrogenase deficiency (Chapter 164). Among the drugs that should be avoided in these individuals are primaquine, nitrofurantoin, and various sulfonamides.

Coexisting diseases should also be taken into account. Use of fluoroquinolones has been associated with abnormalities in glucose homeostasis. Hyperkalemia has been observed in patients with renal insufficiency during treatment with trimethoprim-sulfamethoxazole because trimethoprim blocks the renal excretion of potassium in the distal tubule.

In some cases, the patient's occupation might play a role in the selection of a treatment regimen. Antibiotics that can cause transient (minocycline) or permanent (streptomycin) dizziness or unsteadiness may create hazardous situations in those whose occupations require excellent balance. Antimicrobial agents with the potential to cause photosensitivity, such as tetracyclines, fluoroquinolones, trimethoprim, and sulfonamides, may be problematic in persons with significant sun exposure during outdoor employment or other activities.

● ANTIMICROBIAL COMBINATIONS

It is very common for hospitalized patients to receive more than one antimicrobial agent simultaneously. The rationale for using antimicrobials in combination is not always clearly defined, and there are a number of potential disadvantages to combination therapy. The basis for using combination therapy is considered in this section.

Reasons to Use Combination Antimicrobial Therapy

The clinical indications for using combination antimicrobial therapy can be divided into five categories. Two of these categories (empirical therapy and polymicrobial infections) relate to maximizing the likelihood that at least one agent in the combination will be active against known or suspected pathogens. The other three reasons (minimizing toxicity, preventing the emergence of resistance, and obtaining synergistic inhibition or killing) attempt to exploit the unique advantages of combinations versus any component drug alone.

Provide Broad Coverage during Empirical Therapy

A common reason for using more than one antimicrobial in hospitalized patients is to provide broad coverage against potential pathogens and to maximize the likelihood of delivering an active antimicrobial agent as quickly as possible to seriously ill patients. When the pathogen is unknown, the antimicrobial regimen often includes an agent broadly active against gram-positive bacteria, including methicillin-resistant *S. aureus* (MRSA), such as vancomycin, as well as an agent active against aerobic or facultative gram-negative bacteria. Selection of the latter is strongly influenced by local patterns of antimicrobial resistance specific to the institution and might include an extended-spectrum cephalosporin, an aminoglycoside, a fluoroquinolone, a β-lactam–β-lactamase inhibitor drug, or a carbapenem. The latter two choices also provide activity against gram-negative anaerobes. Alternatively, one could add an agent such as metronidazole to provide anaerobic activity. Because of the high frequency of antibiotic resistance in *Pseudomonas aeruginosa* isolates, in settings in which that pathogen is encountered frequently, empirical use of two agents with antipseudomonal activity may be justified to maximize the likelihood that at least one of the agents will inhibit the organism.

Combination therapy is widely used in the initial treatment of hospitalized patients with community-acquired pneumonia. Commonly used regimens include a third-generation cephalosporin such as ceftriaxone with a macrolide or fluoroquinolone. The cephalosporin provides antimicrobial activity against *S. pneumoniae, Haemophilus influenzae, Moraxella catarrhalis,* and several other "typical" bacterial pathogens associated with community-acquired pneumonia, with the notable exception of MRSA. The macrolide azithromycin is commonly used, or a fluoroquinolone that inhibits "atypical" bacteria that cause pneumonia, including *M. pneumoniae, C. pneumoniae,* and *Legionella* species. Although fluoroquinolones approved for respiratory tract infections are likely to cover most or all of the organisms targeted by the cephalosporin, isolates of *S. pneumoniae* resistant to fluoroquinolones do exist, so guidelines recommend combination therapy in patients with severe pneumonia requiring hospitalization.

Treat Documented Polymicrobial Infections

For many infections from which two or more pathogens are recovered, it is possible to provide adequate coverage with a single, broadly active antimicrobial agent. Switching to a single agent reduces the patient's exposure to potential antibiotic toxicities, is usually more convenient for nursing staff, and may be less expensive. For some patients, susceptibility profiles or allergies to broad-spectrum agents justify the use of antibiotic combinations for the treatment of polymicrobial infections.

Attempt to Reduce Toxicity

It is theoretically possible to use two or more drugs of different classes with additive antimicrobial activities and independent toxicities, each at relatively low doses, to achieve sufficient potency while avoiding toxicity. However, there are no situations in which the approach of using submaximal doses of multiple agents is predictably effective in accomplishing this goal. This does not exclude the possibility that, in isolated instances, a successful response might be attained when drugs with marginal activities are combined.

Prevent the Emergence of Drug Resistance

The treatment of tuberculosis provides the paradigm for using combinations of drugs in an attempt to prevent the emergence of resistance to any one agent. The basis for this approach is that if resistance to two different agents occurs by independent mechanisms, the probability of resistance developing to both drugs is the product of the probability of resistance developing to each drug, which is likely to be very low, so resistance should not emerge. Similar reasoning has justified the use of combination regimens when rifampin is required for the treatment of nonmycobacterial infections. Rifampin is not used alone (with rare exceptions, such as brief courses for the eradication of meningococcal carriage) because resistance to this agent emerges quickly. As mentioned earlier, rifampin is particularly useful in the treatment of infections related to foreign devices because of its activity against biofilm-associated bacteria. In such cases, it is combined with another active antimicrobial, such as vancomycin for coagulase-negative staphylococcal prosthetic valve endocarditis (usually with a brief course of gentamicin as well to reduce the bacterial inoculum further at the beginning of therapy) or a fluoroquinolone for orthopedic device–related infections.

It has been difficult to show unequivocally that combination therapy protects against the emergence of resistance to antimicrobial drugs in other situations, including infections caused by *P. aeruginosa* or *Enterobacter* species. There are two plausible explanations of why combinations do not prevent resistance predictably. First, there may be differential penetration of the two antimicrobials at an infected site or differences in activity at the site of infection. Thus, a more readily penetrating agent may be left relatively unprotected in a privileged site of infection. Second, for many commonly encountered bacteria, resistance mechanisms against unrelated antimicrobial classes may not be truly independent. Some bacterial efflux pumps recognize chemically unrelated substrates, so upregulation of pump activity may confer resistance to several classes of antimicrobials. In other instances, there may be coordinated upregulation of efflux mechanisms and downregulation of outer membrane protein channels (porins), again potentially conferring resistance simultaneously to two or more antimicrobial classes.

Attain Synergism

Decades ago, the surprising benefits of using penicillin and streptomycin together for the treatment of enterococcal endocarditis were discovered empirically. Penicillin alone usually inhibits but does not kill enterococci, and failure rates were high when penicillin G was used alone to treat enterococcal endocarditis. Streptomycin has no significant activity against enterococci at clinically relevant concentrations. However, the combination results in bactericidal synergism in vitro and high cure rates in patients with enterococcal endocarditis. Detailed studies of this phenomenon demonstrated that in the presence of a cell wall–active antibiotic, uptake of the aminoglycoside into the bacterial cell increases substantially. Unfortunately, increasing rates of high-level resistance to streptomycin (MIC > 2000 μg/mL), gentamicin (MIC > 500 μg/mL), or both have nullified the benefit of such combinations against a substantial number of enterococcal isolates today. An example of bactericidal synergism between vancomycin and gentamicin against an *Enterococcus* isolate is illustrated in Figure 287-1A.

Combinations of cell wall–active agents plus aminoglycosides have been shown to achieve synergistic killing against a broad range of gram-positive and gram-negative bacteria when tested in vitro. Modest clinical benefits were shown when short courses of gentamicin were added to nafcillin for the

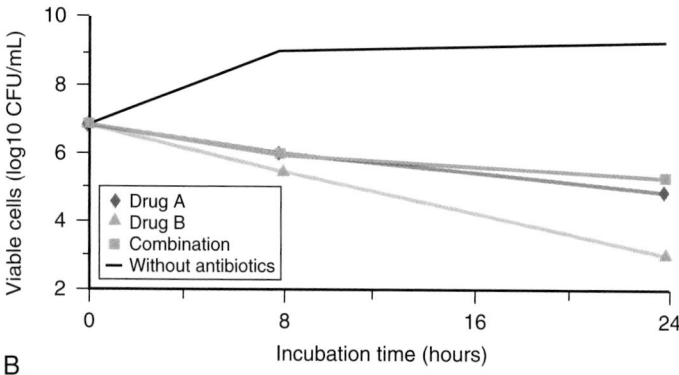

FIGURE 287-1. Bactericidal synergism and antagonism. **A,** Bactericidal synergism between vancomycin and gentamicin against an isolate of *Enterococcus* species. Killing by the combination of drugs is substantially greater than that by each agent alone. **B,** Antagonism of the bactericidal activity of drug B by the more slowly bactericidal drug A. Killing by the combination of drugs is less than that by drug B alone. Growth in the absence of antibiotics is also shown. CFU = colony-forming unit.

treatment of *S. aureus* endocarditis, but at the cost of added nephrotoxicity. Against strains of viridans streptococci that are relatively insensitive to penicillin, the addition of an aminoglycoside for the first 2 weeks of a 4-week course of penicillin G is believed to result in a higher likelihood of cure.

Although it was once considered important in the treatment of gram-negative bacterial infections, especially in immunocompromised (e.g., neutropenic) patients, the clinical value of a synergistic combination of a cell wall–active agent and an aminoglycoside has been difficult to prove in recent experience. To a large extent, the introduction of agents with very potent activity against gram-negative bacteria has diminished the perceived value of synergistic combinations. Nevertheless, there is some evidence that administering two or more active drugs for empirical therapy may achieve a better outcome than is possible with a single active agent for *P. aeruginosa* infections, especially in neutropenic patients. The major value of combination therapy in this setting is to ensure that at least one active agent is administered promptly (Chapter 289). The combination of sulfamethoxazole and trimethoprim, agents that block sequential steps in folic acid synthesis, can also achieve bactericidal (or bacteriostatic) synergism against a number of important gram-positive and gram-negative pathogens. Quinupristin and dalfopristin are streptogramin antibiotics that display inhibitory activity against gram-positive organisms. Combining these two agents, as is done in the commercial formulation, results in bactericidal synergism against organisms susceptible to both.

β-Lactam–β-lactamase inhibitor antimicrobials represent another example of synergistic combinations. Four drugs in this category are currently marketed in the United States: amoxicillin-clavulanate, ampicillin-sulbactam, ticarcillin-clavulanate, and piperacillin-tazobactam. The β-lactamase inhibitors themselves, clavulanic acid, sulbactam, and tazobactam, are devoid of significant antimicrobial activity, with rare exceptions. However, by inhibiting common β-lactamases that are sensitive to these agents, the inhibitors restore the activity of the hydrolyzable companion penicillins against many target pathogens elaborating these enzymes.

Antagonism

Antibiotic combinations can sometimes result in microbiologic antagonism, such that the combination may have *reduced* activity when compared with the most active single agent of the treatment regimen. Time-kill curves illustrating in vitro antagonism are shown in Figure 287-1B. In this example, the more slowly bactericidal drug A antagonizes the killing effect of the intrinsically more bactericidal drug B. Antagonistic interactions against *S. aureus* between less bactericidal (linezolid) and more bactericidal (vancomycin) antimicrobials have also been demonstrated in vivo in experimental endocarditis. In vitro antagonism can be demonstrated when certain β-lactams are tested in combination against gram-negative bacteria with inducible β-lactamases. Here, exposure to one β-lactam can de-repress the synthesis of inducible β-lactamases, which then degrade the second antibiotic.

It is uncommon to encounter clinically apparent antagonism between antibiotics in the patient care setting, in part because offending combinations are not likely to be used in routine clinical care today. However, if unusual antimicrobial combinations are used, in desperation, against isolates exhibiting multiple drug resistance, it is possible that clinically relevant antagonism will be encountered more often in the future. Antagonism of bactericidal activities may also be difficult to detect in clinical practice because most common infections (with the exception of endocarditis and meningitis) do not unequivocally benefit from bactericidal therapy. As long as one agent maintains inhibitory activity, it is unlikely that failure resulting from antagonism will be observed.

⬤ CONSIDERATIONS IN ANTIMICROBIAL ADMINISTRATION

Route of Administration

In almost all instances, antimicrobial therapy for infections of mild to moderate severity that are treated in the outpatient setting can be undertaken with oral agents. There are notable exceptions, such as the use of intramuscular injections of benzathine penicillin for the treatment of syphilis or ceftriaxone for the treatment of otitis media or gonorrhea caused by strains resistant to oral agents.

Drugs such as levofloxacin and linezolid demonstrate virtually complete bioavailability when administered by the oral route in persons with normally functioning gastrointestinal tracts, and they can be used as an alternative to intravenous therapy in many patients with more serious infections. Even for these well-absorbed antimicrobials, however, treatment of seriously ill patients in the hospital is often initiated with intravenous formulations because of the uncertainty of gastrointestinal tract function under conditions of hemodynamic instability.

Antimicrobial therapy can be administered by other routes, including topical administration for the treatment of infected skin lesions (e.g., mupirocin ointment) and intravaginal administration for candidiasis (e.g., azole creams) or for bacterial vaginosis (e.g., metronidazole gel). Topical administration *onto* the eye is used to treat conjunctivitis or as adjunctive therapy for deeper infections; administration *into* the globe itself is a component of regimens for the treatment of endophthalmitis. Infections associated with peritoneal dialysis are frequently treated by intraperitoneal instillation of antimicrobials admixed with the dialysis solution. Rarely, direct administration into the thecal space or into the cerebral ventricles is necessary for the treatment of meningitis when the required antimicrobials do not achieve adequate concentrations in cerebrospinal fluid after systemic administration. Vancomycin is almost always given orally, but it is occasionally administered directly into the intestine for the intraluminal treatment of *Clostridium difficile*–associated diarrhea.

The availability of protocols for the outpatient use of long venous catheters, whether inserted centrally or peripherally, has made it possible to administer antimicrobial agents that are not well absorbed orally. Thus, many patients who require long-term antibiotic treatment for infections such as endocarditis, osteomyelitis, neuroborreliosis, and other conditions can be treated as outpatients after an initial period of hospitalization for a full assessment of the infection, initiation of therapy, and stabilization of the medical condition. In addition to monitoring for adverse effects from the antibiotic itself, patients treated via indwelling intravenous devices require close observation for complications related to the catheter, such as thrombophlebitis, entry site infections, or line-related blood stream infections.

Pharmacodynamic Considerations

In recent years, the scientific basis for selecting a dosing regimen has extended well beyond empirical dosing strategies based primarily on the pharmacokinetic characteristics of antimicrobial agents. Pharmacodynamics relate the time course of antibiotic concentrations after dosing, the observed antimicrobial effects against likely pathogens, and the potential adverse effects of the agent.

Studies of the pharmacokinetic and pharmacodynamic properties of antimicrobial agents allow the prediction of their activities with various dosing regimens. For β-lactam antibiotics, the time during which the concentration of free drug (i.e., the non-protein-bound fraction) exceeds the MIC of the pathogen best relates to antimicrobial effectiveness in animal models. This provides the rationale for the frequent dosing schedules of β-lactams with short half-lives, such as penicillin G and the antistaphylococcal penicillins.

In contrast, the aminoglycosides and fluoroquinolones demonstrate concentration-dependent killing of bacteria. For these drugs, animal models show that the ratio of either peak concentration to MIC or the area under the 24-hour drug concentration curve to MIC better predicts effectiveness. With these agents, less frequent, higher dosing would be optimal. For the aminoglycosides, less frequent dosing may also allow more time for washout of the drug from the kidney, thus potentially minimizing the risk for nephrotoxicity; however, the advantages of this approach are not striking.

For daptomycin, the adoption of once-daily dosing largely mitigated the muscle toxicity that had been seen with more frequent dosing and allowed the use of this agent for serious gram-positive infections.

⬤ MONITORING ANTIMICROBIAL CONCENTRATIONS

From a practical point of view, there are few situations in which assays to determine concentrations of antimicrobials in blood or body fluids are readily available. Commercial assays for the measurement of serum aminoglycoside concentrations are available and, because of these agents' great potential for toxicity, are used frequently. Commercial assays to measure vancomycin concentrations are also widely available. It may be prudent to monitor serum concentrations of vancomycin in patients with unstable renal function, those undergoing hemodialysis, patients at the extremes of body composition, or those with particularly serious infections in which high concentrations may be desirable. In some young adults, clearance of vancomycin may be so great that unexpectedly low concentrations result with the usual dosing regimens.

ADMINISTRATIVE ASPECTS OF ANTIMICROBIAL THERAPY

Formularies

In most practice settings today, the choice of antimicrobials is constrained in some way. For example, in hospitals and other facilities, institutional formularies may limit the choice of antimicrobial agents available, require special approval for the use of selected agents, or both. Such policies can, in principle, enhance efficiency by avoiding the need to stock and dispense multiple agents with very similar antimicrobial activities, minimize costs by allowing purchase of the most cost-effective alternatives, and potentially increase patient safety by encouraging clinical personnel to become familiar with a manageable number of agents. In the outpatient setting, it is common practice for health insurers to assign oral drugs to various tiers of coverage and copayment; as a result, there may be dramatic financial benefits or disincentives for the patient to receive specific agents. In both health care settings, the practitioner must be familiar with the options available to patients under these constraints.

Interchangeability

It is important to remember that although two drugs may have antimicrobial spectra that are so similar that only one need be included on a formulary, it is not always safe to assume that the activity of either agent can be predicted perfectly by susceptibility to the other. For example, for most bacterial species, the percentage of isolates susceptible to meropenem and imipenem will be roughly comparable. However, there are differences in mechanisms of resistance to these two carbapenems, so it is possible that a specific strain will be susceptible to one but resistant to the other. For serious infections, even when two drugs are considered interchangeable, one should determine susceptibility to the specific antimicrobial used.

Impact on the Institutional Environment

In contrast to other medications, which almost always affect only the patient receiving them, antimicrobial use can have a significant impact on the institutional environment as well. As a result, it is sometimes necessary or desirable to manage the use of antimicrobial agents on an administrative level to avoid selective pressure leading to the spread of antibiotic resistance. Within institutions, antimicrobial-resistant organisms not only threaten the patient treated with the antimicrobial but can also be transmitted to other vulnerable persons, including those who have not been exposed to the drug.

SUGGESTED READINGS

Costelloe C, Metcalfe C, Lovering A, et al. Effect of antibiotic prescribing in primary care on antimicrobial resistance in individual patients: systematic review and meta-analysis. *BMJ.* 2010;340:c2096. *Individuals who are prescribed an antibiotic develop resistance that may persist for up to 1 year.*

Gilbert DN, Moellering RC Jr, Eliopoulos GM, et al, eds. *The Sanford Guide to Antimicrobial Therapy.* 40th ed. Sperryville, VA: Antimicrobial Therapy; 2010. *General information for selecting and properly using antimicrobials in clinical care.*

Kopterides P, Siempos II, Tsangaris I, et al. Procalcitonin-guided algorithms of antibiotic therapy in the intensive care unit: a systematic review and meta-analysis of randomized controlled trials. *Crit Care Med.* 2010;38:2229-2241. *Implementation of a procalcitonin-based algorithm may reduce antibiotic exposure in critically ill patients without compromising outcome.*

Rybak MJ, Lomaestro BM, Rotschafer JC, et al. Therapeutic monitoring of vancomycin in adults: summary of consensus recommendations from the American Society of Health-System Pharmacists, the Infectious Diseases Society of America, and the Society of Infectious Diseases Pharmacists. *Pharmacotherapy.* 2009;29:1275-1279. *Recommendations for monitoring serum concentrations during vancomycin therapy.*

288

APPROACH TO FEVER OR SUSPECTED INFECTION IN THE NORMAL HOST

JAMES LEGGETT

We are constantly exposed to microorganisms via our skin or mucous membranes. Most microorganisms are adapted to niches in the environment that make them avirulent to humans. Pathogens in a normal host are relatively few, and most of the time, exposure results in only transient or stable colonization. Infection can be defined as invasion of a pathogen that triggers an immune response, whether the infection is asymptomatic or symptomatic. Manifestations of infection are protean and are due as much to our immune response as to the attributes of the particular pathogen.

The inflammatory response that accompanies infection is usually marked by fever. Fever is a tightly controlled elevation in body temperature above the normal range in response to a central nervous system change in the set point. Defining normal body temperature is somewhat problematic because it is dependent on both physiology and the method of measurement. Normal oral temperature in 99% of the population ranges from 36.0 to 37.7° C, with a circadian variation of 1° C or more between the morning nadir and the evening peak. Mean oral temperature in healthy adults is 36.8 ± 0.4° C, with women exhibiting slightly higher values than men (36.9 vs. 36.7° C). In menstruating women, the morning temperature may rise by 0.6° C with ovulation and remain higher until menses occur. Measured rectal temperatures are 0.4° C higher than oral and 0.8° C higher than aural (tympanic membrane) temperatures. However, considerable individual variability exists. Clinicians generally define significant fever as a temperature higher than 38.3° C (101.0° F). Despite historical claims, fever patterns are not especially helpful in establishing a specific diagnosis.

The vast majority of acute febrile illnesses lasting less than 2 weeks have an infectious cause. These infections occur predominantly where body surfaces interact with the environment, such as the upper and lower respiratory tracts, gastrointestinal and genitourinary systems, and skin. The majority of acute respiratory and gastrointestinal infections are viral in nature. As the duration of the febrile illness lengthens beyond 3 weeks, other inflammatory illnesses become more prominent in the differential diagnosis. Most chronic febrile illnesses are not caused by infection.

PATHOBIOLOGY OF INFECTION AND FEVER

Infection ensues only when a pathogen overcomes both nonspecific innate and specific adaptive humoral and cellular immune responses. The normal indigenous microflora, host physical barriers (e.g., skin, mucous membranes, cilia), and soluble factors (e.g., cytokines, complement) provide important barricades to pathogen invasion. Disruption of these barriers, which provide a first line of defense, permits the invasion of pathogens. The acute phase response triggered by such disruption provides direct antimicrobial activity and prompts the development of adaptive immunity mediated by lymphocytes and macrophages. This inflammatory response plays an important role in containing infection. Unfortunately, an exaggerated response may worsen the clinical condition. It is the neutrophil response that causes the damage seen in septic arthritis, and it is the unchecked immune response that precipitates the systemic inflammatory response syndrome.

Body temperature is regulated both physiologically and behaviorally. Basal metabolic processes, governed especially by thyroid hormones but also by catecholamines and growth hormone, are responsible for the normal resting body temperature. Thermogenesis may be increased up to 80% by hyperthyroidism and decreased as much as 50% by hypothyroidism. Moderate activity increases thermogenesis and results in a transiently increased temperature until heat-dissipating processes are engaged. Each 1° F increase in temperature results in a 7% increase in the basal metabolic rate. Vaporization from the lungs and skin accounts for a third of basal body heat loss and for as much as all heat loss at ambient dry temperatures above 36° C. The elderly have a decrease in basal metabolism, as well as blunted responses to thermogenetic stimuli, but they have the same average core temperature as young people.

The hypothalamus contains temperature-sensitive neurons that have receptors for pro-inflammatory and anti-inflammatory cytokines, which are continuously balanced to maintain a homeothermic set point. When body temperature becomes elevated, cutaneous vasodilation and sweating occur, and people may reduce activity and seek a cooler environment. In contrast, low body temperature is increased by shivering, piloerection, cutaneous vasoconstriction, adding clothes, and seeking a warmer environment. In a febrile illness, symptoms may be due to the underlying disease or to the fever itself. Malaise is the rule, and many febrile patients experience myalgia secondary to the muscle contractions used to generate temperature elevation. Although it was once thought that the back and thigh pain related to rigors suggests bacteremia, any febrile stimulus can produce such symptoms. The chill associated with rigors may be related to the surface vasoconstriction that accompanies the increase in core temperature.

Fever is a complex physiologic process involving metabolic and immunologic responses (Fig. 288-1). Exogenous pyrogens cause fever largely mediated by endogenous pro-inflammatory pyrogenic cytokines produced by

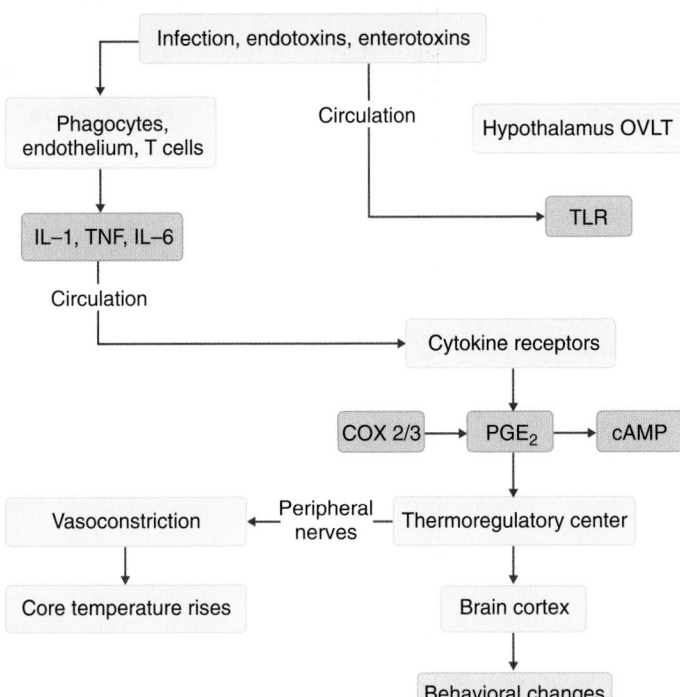

FIGURE 288-1. Pathways leading to the production of fever in bacterial infection, whether local or systemic. Bacteria release cell wall products such as peptidoglycans and endotoxin, as well as enterotoxins, which bind to Toll-like receptors (TLRs) on phagocytes (neutrophils, macrophages) and endothelial cells. As a result, pyrogenic cytokines such as interleukin (IL)-1 and IL-6 or tumor necrosis factor (TNF)-α are released into the circulation and bind to cytokine receptors in the hypothalamic organum vasculosum of lamina terminalis (OVLT). Bacterial products may also directly bind to TLRs on the OVLT. Activation of TLRs and cytokine receptors induces cyclooxygenase 2 (COX2), which leads to the production of prostaglandin E_2 (PGE$_2$) and elevates cyclic adenosine monophosphate (cAMP) in the brain. This, in turn, triggers neurons in the thermoregulatory center to raise the hypothalamic thermostatic set point. In addition, neuronal signals to the cortex prompt behavioral changes to conserve heat (e.g., posturing, adding clothing). The hypothalamus also triggers sympathetic peripheral efferent nerves that constrict peripheral blood vessels and conserve central heat until hypothalamic PGE$_2$ levels fall.

TABLE 288-1 SELECTED EXAMPLES OF FEVER ASSOCIATED WITH RECENT TRAVEL

	Incubation Period	
DISEASE	**<2-3 wk**	**>3-4 wk**
COMMON		
Dengue	+	
Dysentery	+	
Entamebic liver abscess		+
Enteric fever	+	
Malaria	+	+
Pulmonary tuberculosis		+
Viral hepatitis		+
LESS COMMON		
Ehrlichiosis	+	
Leptospirosis	+	
Schistosomiasis		+
Viral (hemorrhagic, encephalitic)	+	
Visceral leishmaniasis		+

phagocytic leukocytes, including interleukin (IL)-1, IL-2, IL-6, tumor necrosis factor-α, and interferon-γ. These cytokines stimulate the immune responses of T and B cells, macrophages, and polymorphonuclear leukocytes. They appear to act via a common mechanism involving the induction of prostaglandin synthesis. Feedback inhibitory responses are mediated by adrenocorticotropic hormone, arginine vasopressin, serotonin, dopamine, and other homeostatic mechanisms, thus emphasizing the orchestrated nature of fever production and response to infection. These thermoregulatory mechanisms rarely allow fevers to exceed 41° C (106° F). Temperatures exceeding 41° C are often due to a drug-induced imbalance in these mechanisms and may cause direct cellular damage.

Failure of fever to develop during severe bacterial infection has, in some studies, been associated with higher morbidity and mortality. Whether this is due to the absence of fever per se or to associated conditions such as chronic renal failure or corticosteroid use has not been determined. Favorable effects of fever on host-microbe interactions are suggested by inhibited multiplication of some pathogens such as *Streptococcus pneumoniae* and *Treponema pallidum,* reduced proliferation of pathogens in the presence of hypoferremia, augmented complement-mediated lysis, and increased neutrophil entry into inflammatory sites. Temperature-pulse dissociation, in which there is relative bradycardia compared with the usual increase of about 10 beats/minute/1° F, has been described in typhoid fever, leptospirosis, rickettsiosis, dengue, legionellosis, and babesiosis, for unclear reasons.

No laboratory abnormalities accompany typical benign acute viral infections. Leukocytosis (Chapter 170) of various lineages is usually seen in other infections in immunocompetent adults. Neutrophilia is the norm in most acute infections, whatever the cause. The elderly, though not mounting a neutrophilic response, generally display bandemia during an acute bacterial infection. Neutropenia (Chapter 170) may be seen in rickettsial, severe viral, and overwhelming bacterial infections. Eosinophilia (Chapter 173) is typical

of invasive helminthic and some protozoal infections. Lymphocytosis may accompany many viral and rickettsial infections and is common during convalescence from acute bacterial infection. Monocytosis may be seen in tuberculosis. Virtually all infections have an impact on the erythroid system, but given the long half-life of erythrocytes, usually only chronic infections or other inflammatory diseases result in anemia (Chapter 161). Few acute infections rapidly produce anemia. For instance, *Helicobacter pylori* may induce a bleeding ulcer, *Plasmodium falciparum* may directly lyse erythrocytes, overwhelming clostridial and other bacterial infections associated with disseminated intravascular coagulopathy may cause hemolytic anemia, and *Mycoplasma pneumoniae* may induce immunologically mediated hemolysis.

APPROACH TO FEBRILE ILLNESS IN OUTPATIENTS AND INPATIENTS

Infectious disease epidemiology depends on the interaction among pathogens, susceptible hosts, and environmental conditions allowing exposure. Most infections are transmitted horizontally between people via contact (e.g., hands, fomites), a common vehicle (e.g., food, water), air (e.g., tuberculosis), or vectors (e.g., mosquitoes). Evaluation of a patient with a known or possible infection should determine whether the condition might be due to a transmissible agent and its source; whether the patient has done any recent traveling; whether there are secondary causes; and what measures need to be taken to contact health department officials and prevent additional infections.

The age of a patient influences which illnesses should be considered. Natural exposure or immunization generally limits certain illnesses, such as rubeola, rubella, or varicella. Waning of immunity may likewise lead to pertussis in young adults or reactivation of tuberculosis in the elderly. Other physiologic effects of aging, such as impaired bladder emptying, lead to increased rates of urinary tract infection in the elderly.

A patient's occupation and travel history should be noted. An abattoir worker is more likely to have been exposed to *Brucella* (Chapter 318) than someone with another occupation. Indiana residents are more likely be infected with histoplasmosis (Chapter 340), whereas those from the Southwest desert may have coccidioidomycosis (Chapter 341), despite having a similar febrile illness. Many other illnesses are likewise directly related to specific geographic exposure, with varying incubation times before their onset (Chapter 294). Typhoid fever should manifest within a few weeks, whereas amebic liver abscess might not cause symptoms until months after a traveler's return from an endemic area (Table 288-1). The Centers for Disease Control and Prevention website and many others provide more specific information about prevalent infections in all parts of the world (see *http://www.cdc.gov*).

Many travelers return home with fever after a variable incubation time, generally with other symptoms and signs as well. The first consideration in evaluating such a patient is that an infection unrelated to travel is more likely to be the cause of the illness. Once such routine infections have been ruled out, the differential diagnosis should include infections related to travel, whether within a region of the United States (e.g., ehrlichiosis, Colorado tick fever, hantavirus) or abroad (e.g., visceral leishmaniasis, tick-borne encephalitis in Europe) (Chapter 294). For example, prompt evaluation of a patient who has traveled to a malaria-endemic area should be undertaken and blood tests performed to determine the presence of parasites.

The setting in which a febrile illness occurs influences both the diagnostic approach and the differential diagnosis. In the ambulatory arena, with a generally healthy febrile patient, the clinician should not necessarily pursue a diagnosis as aggressively as with a hospitalized or chronically ill patient. Empirical treatment of a presumed urinary tract infection is warranted for an outpatient, where the cost of a culture is often more than that of the antibiotic. However, the cost of a urine culture in a hospital setting is minimal in comparison to the daily cost of care, and accurately identifying the pathogen may speed hospital discharge. Likewise, the pathogens commonly causing febrile illness in health care facilities, including nursing homes, may differ from those seen in ambulatory settings. Most patients in the ambulatory setting have noncritical, self-limited infections.

Higher temperatures are usually due to invasive visceral disease such as community-acquired pneumonia or pyelonephritis. Common viral respiratory infections and gastroenteritis, as well as some cases of subacute bacterial endocarditis, are accompanied by fevers below 102° F. Moreover, many infections may not be associated with fever, such as Lyme disease, osteomyelitis, and most sexually transmitted diseases. The clinician must always keep in mind that certain infections, such as sexually transmitted diseases (Chapter 293) or herpes zoster, occur normally in immunocompetent hosts and may signal a higher risk for infection with human immunodeficiency virus (HIV) or an already established immunodeficiency.

FEVER IN OUTPATIENTS. In the ambulatory setting, an acutely febrile patient represents a common problem and only infrequently presents an enigmatic diagnostic challenge. In most instances, a febrile illness is accompanied by localizing symptoms and signs suggesting a specific diagnosis. For instance, leg erythema, pain, and fever in a patient with tinea pedis or a saphenous vein graft incision immediately suggests streptococcal cellulitis. If the patient has had a gradual onset and does not appear toxic, only clinical observation and follow-up are required. If the patient appears toxic, with tachypnea and apprehension or confusion accompanying localized findings, clinically focused diagnostic studies should be performed immediately, and hospitalization should be considered. When a patient has fever and only nonspecific constitutional symptoms, it may be more difficult to address the problem in a single ambulatory clinic visit, requiring a balance between observation and investigation.

FEVER IN INPATIENTS. Fever and leukocytosis are probably the main clinical parameters for evaluating potential infections in hospitalized patients. However, about 10% of nosocomial bacteremias occur without fever, and health care–associated infections occur without fever in a substantial proportion of patients who are elderly or have significant comorbid conditions. Most cases of hospital-associated fever represent nosocomial infection, which typically involves the lower respiratory tract, urinary tract, or surgical wounds (Table 288-2). Some important causes of nosocomial fever may not exhibit easily discernible localizing symptoms or signs. Antibiotic-induced colitis secondary to *Clostridium difficile* (Chapter 304) is increasing in prevalence and may be characterized by little or no diarrhea. It is probably the most common cause of a leukemoid reaction in hospitalized patients. Other intra-abdominal processes involving the hepatobiliary system, bowel infarction, viscus perforation, or abscesses may have little in the way of localizing symptoms or signs.

Given the greater severity of illness and comorbid conditions in intensive care unit (ICU) patients, it is logical that fever and infection are more frequent in the ICU than elsewhere. Infection was recently found to be present in more than 80% of febrile ICU patients, although both infectious and noninfectious causes of fever may coexist. Indeed, ischemia or devitalization of tissue provokes an inflammatory response similar to that prompted by infection. About half of patients with acute myocardial infarction have a temperature between 38.0 and 38.5° C within 2 to 3 days of their infarction. Similarly, about half of patients with deep vein thrombosis and pulmonary embolism have a temperature in the same range, most commonly in the first 3 days after diagnosis. A third or more of patients with stroke demonstrate fever, which is also a common consequence of subarachnoid hemorrhage and subdural hematoma, especially within 72 hours of onset. The fever in such cases may result from damage to the hypothalamus or pulmonary aspiration secondary

TABLE 288-2	SELECTED CAUSES OF HOSPITAL-ASSOCIATED FEVER	
COMMON	**LESS COMMON**
Infectious	**Infectious**
Clostridium difficile enterocolitis	Biliary tract disease
Pneumonia	Endometritis
Surgical wound	Intra-abdominal abscess
Urinary tract	Mediastinitis
Vascular catheter	Sinusitis
Noninfectious	**Noninfectious**
Drug-induced fever	Adrenal insufficiency
Hematoma	Gout
Immediate postoperative state	Myocardial infarction
Transfusion reaction	Organ infarction
Venous thromboembolism	Pancreatitis

to obtundation. Iatrogenic causes of fever should be considered. Fever and chills may be seen in up to a quarter of patients receiving platelet transfusions, although the frequency is much less with other blood products.

SYNDROMIC APPROACH: FEVER AND RASH

A syndromic approach is valuable to narrow the many possible causes of a suspected infection. Two approaches must be juxtaposed in this evaluation, and both are key in recognizing patterns. The clinician must be aware of (1) the differential diagnosis of the particular type of lesion observed and (2) the constellation of findings produced by individual pathogens. Because of the variety of possible manifestations and the often overlapping symptoms and signs, both elements are key in arriving at a probable diagnosis. Moreover, fever and associated findings such as exanthem, lymphadenopathy, or jaundice may be due to noninfectious systemic diseases as well as infectious ones. For instance, leukocytoclastic vasculitis and fever may be found in meningococcemia, Rocky Mountain spotted fever, and hepatitis C, but they are also seen in noninfectious inflammatory diseases. Likewise, fever and adenopathy may be due to lymphoma or to cat-scratch disease.

A recognizable exanthem may lead to the immediate recognition of a particular pathogen (Chapter 449), but often a larger differential diagnosis must be entertained. The clinician must recognize the type or types of skin lesions present, the distribution of the exanthem, and the chronologic progression with respect to the onset of fever and other symptoms (Table 288-3). Morphologic variations in skin lesions help in the differential diagnosis. Maculopapular exanthems are frequently seen in viral illness, hypersensitivity drug reactions, and immune complex–mediated diseases. Some of the most common viral causes include the many enteroviruses, but similar lesions may also be seen with hepatitis B and West Nile viruses. Erythema multiforme, a subset of maculopapular exanthem, can result from various viral infections or drug eruptions (Chapter 448). It may have a spectrum of disease that ranges from benign to the life-threatening Stevens-Johnson syndrome/toxic epidermal necrolysis complex. Herpes simplex virus is perhaps the most common cause of erythema multiforme. Although drugs, especially antibiotics, are the major precipitating factor in the Stevens-Johnson syndrome/toxic epidermal necrolysis complex, *M. pneumoniae* has been associated with it as well. Evolution of the cutaneous findings over time may give clues to the cause; for example, the initial blanching, erythematous, maculopapular lesions may later evolve into petechiae, as seen in meningococcemia, Rocky Mountain spotted fever, and dengue. Secondary syphilis may manifest with a multitude of morphologic skin lesions. Sometimes, many different manifestations occur simultaneously in the same patient. Most vesiculobullous skin exanthems are immunologically mediated. The few infections associated with these eruptions include herpes simplex and varicella-zoster viruses and enteroviruses such as echovirus and coxsackievirus. The poxviruses, which can also cause such exanthems, are much rarer or are associated with bioterrorism. Pustules, or vesicles containing leukocytes, are usually associated with psoriasis or infections with *Pseudomonas, Staphylococcus,* or *Neisseria.* Bullous exanthems in the presence of sepsis suggest severe streptococcal cellulitis or necrotizing fasciitis, staphylococcal impetigo, or *Vibrio* infections.

TABLE 288-3 SELECTED INFECTIONS WITH FEVER AND RASH

ETIOLOGY	MACULES, PAPULES	VESICLES, BULLAE	PETECHIAE, PURPURA
BACTERIA			
Borrelia burgdorferi	+ (annular)		
Neisseria meningitidis			+
Rickettsia rickettsii	+		+
Treponema pallidum	+ (secondary)		
Vibrio vulnificus		+	
FUNGI AND MYCOBACTERIA			
Disseminated disease	+ (nodular)		
PROTOZOA			
Plasmodium falciparum			+
VIRUSES			
Enteroviruses	+	+	+
Epstein-Barr	+		+
Hemorrhagic fever			+
Herpes		+	
HIV	+		

TABLE 288-4 FEVER AND RASH INVOLVING THE PALMS AND SOLES

Erythema multiforme
Hand-foot-and-mouth disease
Neisseria infection
Rocky Mountain spotted fever
Streptobacillus moniliformis infection
Subacute bacterial endocarditis
Syphilis (secondary)
Toxic shock syndrome
Varicella-zoster infection

TABLE 288-5 COMMON CAUSES OF FEVER AND LYMPHADENOPATHY

REGIONAL	GENERALIZED
Cervical	Cytomegalovirus
Streptococci	Epstein-Barr virus
Tuberculosis	HIV
Viral upper respiratory tract infection	Lymphoma
	Sarcoidosis
Peripheral	Syphilis (secondary)
Bartonella henselae	Toxoplasmosis
Herpesviruses	Viral hepatitis
Lymphoma	
Metastatic cancer	
Sporotrichosis	
Streptococci	
Inguinal	
Chancroid	
Herpes	
Lymphogranuloma venereum	
Syphilis (primary)	

Petechial and purpuric eruptions are due to the extravasation of red blood cells and should always lead to consideration of a potentially serious illness. Pathogens creating such lesions most commonly include *Neisseria meningitidis*, *Rickettsia*, and *Capnocytophaga canimorsus*, but these eruptions may be seen with a variety of other pathogens, including *Staphylococcus aureus*, group B streptococci, and other gram-negative bacilli. A petechial exanthem may also be seen with enteroviruses and viral hemorrhagic fevers. The most common causes of petechiae not attributable to infections include thrombocytopenia and vasculitis.

The presence of fever and rash involving the palms and soles allows considerable narrowing of the differential diagnosis (Table 288-4). In addition to the diffuse erythema associated with toxic shock syndrome, illnesses such as Rocky Mountain spotted fever, secondary syphilis, hand-foot-and-mouth disease, *Neisseria* infections, and rat-bite fever should be considered in patients with maculopapular exanthems involving these areas.

Nodular skin lesions may be either noninfectious, as seen in malignancy or with certain drugs (e.g., sulfonamides), or infectious, as seen in a variety of inflammatory diseases. Atypical mycobacteria and disseminated fungi often produce skin nodules. The tender nodules of erythema nodosum usually occur in crops located pretibially, but they may be solitary or occur on other parts of the body. They do not typically suppurate, and they heal without scarring. Infectious agents are the most likely cause of erythema nodosum. Diffuse erythema may be seen with scarlet fever, toxic shock syndrome, Kawasaki disease, Stevens-Johnson syndrome, and toxic epidermal necrolysis, with desquamation occurring late in all these syndromes. Sweet's syndrome, a febrile neutrophilic dermatosis, represents a hypersensitivity reaction often preceded by an upper respiratory tract infection.

⬤ SYNDROMIC APPROACH: FEVER AND MUSCULOSKELETAL COMPLAINTS

Fever and localized tenderness, swelling, or erythema generally accompany septic arthritis and often accompany osteomyelitis (Chapter 280). Septic bacterial arthritis in adults usually manifests acutely and involves a single large joint such as the knee, hip, or shoulder, unless the infection is directly inoculated by trauma or surgery. Septic oligoarthritis may be seen with endocarditis and rat-bite fever. Disseminated gonococcal disease is the usual cause of arthritis involving small joints of the wrist, ankle, and digits, often with tenosynovitis. Acute or subacute polyarthritis may be seen in several viral diseases, including parvovirus B19 and hepatitis B, and in Lyme disease, but it is more typical of immunologic disorders. Rheumatologic diseases generally have more subacute manifestations, with more symmetrical polyarthritis. Hematogenous osteomyelitis in adults frequently involves the vertebrae and

is almost always initiated by discitis with symmetrical involvement of adjacent vertebrae (as opposed to malignant metastasis, which is asymmetrical and does not involve the disc).

Myositis secondary to clostridia, streptococci, *Aeromonas*, or mixed aerobic-anaerobic infections usually causes an acutely septic picture with painful, edematous involvement of the limb or torso. Pyomyositis frequently involves deep muscles such as the psoas or gluteus and is usually due to *S. aureus*. Diffuse myositis may be seen with leptospirosis or toxoplasmosis, and rhabdomyolysis occurs with a variety of viral infections and legionellosis.

⬤ SYNDROMIC APPROACH: FEVER AND LYMPHADENOPATHY OR HEPATOSPLENOMEGALY

Fever and lymphadenopathy may suggest a variety of illnesses, both infectious and noninfectious (Table 288-5). Lymphadenopathy (Chapter 171) may be regional or generalized. Local enlargement can occur with either a local infection or some systemic illnesses (e.g., posterior cervical lymphadenopathy with Epstein-Barr virus and other viral illnesses). Generalized lymphadenopathy usually suggests a systemic disorder, which may itself be either infectious or noninfectious. Although the combination of fever and lymphadenopathy secondary to infection is especially common during childhood, it is also frequently seen in adults. As in other syndromes, acute versus chronic adenopathy tilts the diagnosis toward different broad categories of illness. In the latter, histopathologic evaluation of enlarged lymph nodes may point to a particular diagnosis. For instance, toxoplasmosis or cat-scratch disease can be easily differentiated from mycobacterial disease or sarcoidosis.

Fever and hepatosplenomegaly (Chapter 171) may provide an important clue to the cause of a febrile illness, which is typically either an infection or a malignancy arising from bone marrow or the reticuloendothelial system. Jaundice may also limit the differential diagnosis (Table 288-6). Aside from the viral hepatitides and other diseases affecting primarily the liver, many pathogens producing sepsis can cause hyperbilirubinemia.

APPROACH TO FEVER OF UNKNOWN ORIGIN

The majority of febrile illnesses are short-lived, but fever may be prolonged for weeks or months as part of an infectious disease, inflammatory disorder, or occult neoplasm. When fever is caused by infection, the site is an area not easily controlled by host defenses, leading to the continued release of inflammatory cytokines. Likewise, macrophage and lymphocyte involvement in inflammatory disorders causes persistent cytokine production, as do certain neoplasms. Given this final common pathway, it is easy to understand why the majority of cases of classic fever of unknown origin (FUO), loosely defined as lasting longer than 3 weeks despite routine investigation, are found in these three broad categories. Two other categories round out the bulk of FUO cases: miscellaneous illnesses and cases in which the fever remains undiagnosed (Table 288-7). The proportion of patients in each category varies by geographic locale, age, duration of fever, and immune status. As more effective methods of diagnosing viral and bacterial infections have become available, and with improved serologic studies to detect connective tissue disorders and better imaging techniques to detect occult malignancies, the proportion of patients with FUO in the miscellaneous and undiagnosed categories has increased to about a third of the total in developed countries. The longer a febrile illness persists without a diagnosis or appropriate therapy, the less likely it is to be due to an infection. In one study, only 6% of patients who had persistent FUO beyond 6 months were found to have infection. Most such cases resolve spontaneously, with a mortality rate of less than 3% at 5 years.

Bacterial species, particularly *Mycobacterium tuberculosis*, make up the largest category of infections that cause prolonged FUO. *M. tuberculosis* and other bacterial pathogens causing FUO have adapted to survive intracellularly or frequently change their surface antigens so that they are not readily eradicated by host defenses. Other infections causing FUO are localized in cryptic abscesses, especially intra-abdominally, or reside on heart valves, where the inflammatory response is blunted. Persistent viral infections constitute a small and shrinking subset of patients with FUO because modern techniques can more readily detect infection with Epstein-Barr virus, cytomegalovirus, and others. Among the pathogens likely to be characterized initially by fever alone, cytomegalovirus is the most common cause of mononucleosis in adults, and malaria is a common cause of fever in returning travelers. Malignancy may result in persistent fever owing to the production of inflammatory cytokines, necrosis, or the presence of a complicating infection. The most common malignancies manifesting as FUO are lymphomas, leukemias, and solid tumors with metastases to the liver. Connective tissue disorders may lead to tissue inflammation, which produces fever as a prominent feature of the illness. In a recent series, adult Still's disease (Chapter 269) was the leading rheumatologic disorder manifesting as FUO. Temporal arteritis and polymyalgia rheumatica (Chapter 279) are seen almost exclusively in patients older than 50 years. Systemic lupus erythematosus (Chapter 274) is an occasional cause of FUO, especially if it manifests in an atypical fashion.

The miscellaneous category of FUO includes several disparate groups of diseases. Granulomatous diseases such as granulomatous hepatitis, Crohn's disease, or sarcoidosis may incite cellular immune responses that result in fever. Granulomatous hepatitis was present in up to 6% of National Institutes of Health cases with fever lasting longer than 6 months. Chronic pancreatitis may occasionally cause FUO, as may recurrent pulmonary embolism.

Drug-induced fever (Table 288-8) may be the only manifestation of an adverse drug event in up to 5% of cases of drug hypersensitivity. Recognizing drug-induced fever is important to avoid extra tests, additional therapy, and prolonged hospitalization. The mechanisms by which drugs incite fever are not well understood in many cases. These events may result from hypersensitivity reactions, altered thermoregulatory homeostasis directly related to either drug administration or the drug's pharmacologic action, or idiosyncratic reactions. Hypersensitivity reactions are usually accompanied by an exanthem or enanthem and hepatic, renal, or pulmonary dysfunction, in addition to fever. Antimicrobial agents appear to be the most common cause of drug-induced fever and are responsible for approximately a third of episodes in some studies. β-Lactams and sulfonamides account for most cases because they are among the most frequently administered antimicrobials. Anticonvulsants are also common causes of drug-induced fever secondary to hypersensitivity reactions. Altered thermoregulation is possible with a variety of drugs, including those with anticholinergic activity such as phenothiazines and tricyclic antidepressants. Sympathomimetic agents such as amphetamines and cocaine may also cause fever. Drug administration itself may cause fever if the vehicle of the drug is contaminated with exogenous pyrogens or chemical phlebitis occurs. Some drugs appear to have intrinsic pyrogenic properties, such as amphotericin B and bleomycin. Others cause fever as a result of their pharmacologic activity, such as interferon-α or IL-2. With antibiotics, drug-induced fever occurs with the rapid lysis of spirochetes or other bacteria, known as the Jarisch-Herxheimer reaction. Idiosyncratic drug-induced febrile reactions include malignant hyperthermia, neuroleptic malignant syndrome, and serotonin syndrome. Drugs implicated in these reactions are inhaled anesthetic agents, central nervous system dopamine-depleting agents, and serotonin re-uptake inhibitors, among others. Drug-induced fever is usually a diagnosis of exclusion. The duration of drug exposure before the onset of fever, the clinical appearance of the patient, and the pattern of the fever are not particularly useful. Elimination of a single drug at a time, beginning with the one most likely to be implicated, is the usual means of identifying the causative agent. The fever abates once the drug has been eliminated from the body, usually within 3 to 4 days of discontinuing use of the drug.

Laboratory evaluation and diagnostic imaging studies should be chosen according to information derived from a detailed history and physical examination. These may initially include a complete blood count and blood chemistry determinations, erythrocyte sedimentation rate, blood cultures, and antibody tests (antinuclear antibody, cytomegalovirus, Epstein-Barr virus, HIV), as well as a chest radiograph and computed tomography of the abdomen. Despite the recent focus on "emerging" infectious diseases, the cause of FUO is still more likely to be a common pathogen presenting atypically.

INITIAL MANAGEMENT OF SUSPECTED INFECTION IN THE AMBULATORY SETTING

An acutely febrile patient in the ambulatory setting presents a common but often demanding diagnostic problem. In most cases, the history and physical

---

TABLE 288-6	COMMON INFECTIOUS CAUSES OF FEVER AND JAUNDICE

Bacterial sepsis
Cholangitis
Hepatic abscess
Leptospirosis
Malaria
Viral hepatitis
Yellow fever

TABLE 288-7   FREQUENCY OF SELECTED CHRONIC FEBRILE ILLNESSES

INFECTION, 25-50%	MALIGNANCY, 20-30%	CONNECTIVE TISSUE DISEASE, 15-30%	MISCELLANEOUS, 10-20%	UNDIAGNOSED, 10-30%
Cytomegalovirus	Carcinomatosis	Polyarteritis nodosa	Drug-induced fever	
Endocarditis	Leukemia	Rheumatoid arthritis	Granulomatous hepatitis	
Intra-abdominal	Local tumor	Still's disease	Inflammatory bowel disease	
Mycoses	Lymphoma	Systemic lupus erythematosus	Pancreatitis	
Occult abscess		Temporal arteritis	Pulmonary embolism	
Tuberculosis				

TABLE 288-8 SELECTED AGENTS ASSOCIATED WITH DRUG-INDUCED FEVER

COMMON	LESS COMMON
Antimicrobial	
Amphotericin B	Clindamycin
β-Lactams	Fluoroquinolones
Sulfonamides	Rifampin
Cardiovascular	
Procainamide	Diltiazem
Quinidine	Hydralazine
Central Nervous System	
Carbamazepine	Haloperidol
Phenytoin	Serotonin re-uptake inhibitors
Miscellaneous	
Bleomycin	Allopurinol
Interferon-α	Cimetidine
Interleukin-2	Tacrolimus

examination reveal diagnostic clues and may guide decisions about additional studies or therapy. More difficult to diagnose is a fever that occurs without localizing symptoms or is accompanied only by nonspecific symptoms such as malaise or anorexia. Fortunately, most such acute, undifferentiated febrile illnesses are benign and resolve spontaneously within 1 or 2 weeks without a specific diagnosis being made. In such cases, no further evaluation beyond the initial visit is warranted. If symptoms persist, the history and physical examination should be repeated, looking for previously unsought clues and new physical findings. Laboratory studies might be required.

In patients with a cough illness of less than 3 weeks' duration, the evaluation should focus on ruling out serious illness. Normal vital signs and a normal chest examination effectively rule out most cases of pneumonia. Such cough illnesses are caused by viral pathogens in more than 90% of cases. Antibiotics are ineffective in such patients, and antimicrobial therapy does not prevent bacterial complications such as pneumonia. The presence of sputum and its characteristics are not helpful in distinguishing bacterial from viral infections. Adults with prolonged coughing lasting longer than 3 weeks or with recurrent episodes should be evaluated for reactive airway disease, gastroesophageal reflux, and other illnesses. Infections rarely causing prolonged cough include *Bordetella pertussis, M. pneumoniae,* and *Chlamydia pneumoniae.* Clinicians in this case should obtain a chest radiograph; treat for exacerbation of chronic obstructive pulmonary disease (fever, leukocytosis, purulent sputum), if present; treat a confirmed bacterial infection; and direct therapy to a specific underlying cause or other causes.

Symptoms and signs of pharyngitis include fever, tonsillar exudates, tender anterior cervical lymph nodes, and absence of cough. If fewer than two of these criteria are present, the patient should be managed as though viral pharyngitis were the cause. With two or more of these criteria, one should consider obtaining a rapid streptococcal antigen test. Because of the low incidence of streptococcal infection and acute rheumatic fever in adults, a negative rapid test alone is sufficient to rule out infection with *Streptococcus pyogenes.* If the antigen test is positive, the patient can be managed with a β-lactam antibiotic if not allergic. Ninety percent of cases of pharyngitis in adults are viral in origin. In a patient with symptoms of upper respiratory tract infection and a mucopurulent nasal discharge of less than 10 days' duration, it is important to remember that purulent nasal secretions do not predict bacterial infection. Most cases of acute rhinosinusitis seen in the outpatient setting are caused by uncomplicated upper respiratory viral infection. If symptoms have been present for more than 10 days without improvement, or if there are specific symptoms of sinusitis of any duration (purulent nasal discharge lasting 3 to 4 days, unilateral facial pain and pressure, maxillary toothache, or worsening of symptoms after initial improvement), amoxicillin or another β-lactam should be considered, with other antimicrobial classes used in penicillin-allergic patients.

Community-acquired pneumonia (Chapter 97) should be suspected in a patient with cough, sputum production, or dyspnea, especially if accompanied by fever and altered breath sounds. A chest radiograph should be performed to confirm the diagnosis. Determining where to care for the patient is the most important immediate decision. Outpatient care generally suffices for patients younger than 50 years with no cardiopulmonary disease, no comorbid conditions (including malignancy, heart failure, diabetes, hospitalization within the last year), and no physical examination findings such as altered mental status, pulse of 125 beats/minute or greater, or respiratory rate of 30/minute or greater. Recent guidelines developed by the American Thoracic Society and the Infectious Diseases Society of America suggest a β-lactam, macrolide, or doxycycline. Fluoroquinolones should be used for outpatients only when the patient has failed first-line therapy, has a significant comorbidity, or has a known allergy to a first-line agent.

Skin and soft tissue infections are caused, for the most part, by streptococci; a minority are due to *S. aureus* and, rarely, other bacteria whose presence may be suggested by epidemiologic considerations (e.g., swimming in fresh water, where *Aeromonas* may be the pathogen). Pain may be present for 12 hours or more before skin discoloration is noted. A furuncle or abscess formation should prompt consideration of *S. aureus* and, rarely, *Streptococcus milleri.* Incision and drainage may be sufficient for a skin abscess, although the rapidly expanding, virulent, community-acquired methicillin-resistant *S. aureus* phenotype may require antimicrobial therapy. Septic bursitis is nearly always due to *S. aureus,* and the infected bursa should be aspirated and drained, in addition to using antibiotics.

Gastrointestinal infections may be due to ingested toxins, viruses, or, less commonly, bacteria, with or without associated toxin production. The appropriate approach depends on the epidemiologic setting, such as improper food storage, travel abroad, or contact with another ill person. Symptoms of cystitis in a young, sexually active woman can be treated with empirical antibiotics, but when fever and flank pain are present and the patient is nauseated, consideration of a brief hospital admission or an initial intravenous dose of antibiotics may be necessary. The possibility of pelvic inflammatory disease should also be entertained.

In the initial evaluation of a patient with a more chronic, persistent fever, a careful history and physical examination provide important diagnostic clues, directing further investigation. The initial goal is to characterize the illness accurately, in addition to eliciting important host and epidemiologic factors. A careful review of systems is necessary to understand the extent of involvement of various organ systems, as well as to note previous medical conditions. The examination should be broader than for an acute febrile illness with localizing symptoms and signs. Laboratory tests may also play a more important role in guiding further investigation. Repeat evaluations are the norm rather than the exception in these cases. Blindly initiating empirical therapy in febrile patients with no imminent risk of serious clinical harm or death should be discouraged because it may impede a timely diagnosis affording definitive care.

INITIAL MANAGEMENT OF SUSPECTED NOSOCOMIAL INFECTION

Determination of the nature of a febrile illness in a hospitalized patient must take into account the host, the setting, and the timing of recent trauma or type and duration of surgery, in addition to the general approach taken for ambulatory patients. A classic mnemonic—the six Ws—may help guide the evaluation: wind, water, wound, walk, wonder drug, and what we did. "Wind" refers to fever within the first 24 hours of surgery, when it is unusual to have an infection. A fever at this time is often thought to be related to the anesthetic agent or to surgical trauma. The only bacteria believed to cause significant infections within 24 hours of surgery are *S. pyogenes* and *Clostridium* species, both of which are unusual in the typical hospital patient. "Water" refers to a urinary tract infection occurring after the third day of urinary tract catheterization. Because nearly all nosocomial urinary tract infections occur in patients with indwelling urinary catheters or in those who have undergone urologic instrumentation, urinalysis or culture (or both) should be performed routinely only in febrile patients with such risk factors. There is a high prevalence of bacteriuria in patients who have been catheterized for 3 days or longer, and there is a relatively low incidence of true infection attributable to bacteriuria. "Wound" infections commonly occur about 5 to 7 days postoperatively, whether they are surface wounds or complications of dehiscence of gastrointestinal anastomoses. Some of the highest rates of skin and soft tissue infections in the National Nosocomial Infection Surveillance database are seen with gastrointestinal procedures. Toxin-producing *C. difficile* is the only significant nosocomial gastrointestinal infection seen in hospitalized patients, so a routine bacterial culture is not necessary. "Walk" refers to possible deep vein thrombosis or pulmonary embolism in someone who has not received appropriate prophylaxis or who is otherwise at risk for thrombosis.

Fever induced by a "wonder drug" is typically seen after approximately 7 to 10 days of use if the patient does not already have an allergy to that medication, in which case it recurs immediately. An exception to this rule is sulfamethoxazole, in which approximately half of hypersensitivity reactions occur within 3 days of initiation. Finally, "what we did" alerts the clinician to the possibility of an iatrogenic infection, such as intravenous catheter–related bacteremia.

CONCLUSION

The initial management of patients with febrile illnesses requires three major considerations. First, is the illness more likely to be infectious or more likely to be related to some other process? Excessive antibiotic use when not warranted, such as for viral infections or collagen vascular disease, may cause an adverse reaction, in addition to contributing to the worldwide increase in antimicrobial resistance. However, an empirical antibiotic is appropriate in many cases of fever and localizing signs of bacterial infection. Second, the clinician must rapidly assess the severity of the illness and determine whether it is likely to cause significant organ damage or even death. In a febrile patient with signs of sepsis, the clinician must quickly decide which specific therapy is indicated, because a delay in initiating antimicrobial therapy is correlated with increased morbidity and mortality. Finally, the clinician needs to determine whether supportive care alone, including antipyretic therapy, is warranted.

The nearly universal prevalence of febrile adaptive responses to microbial challenge suggests that fever has a net benefit to the host. In addition to clinical studies correlating elevated core temperature and improved prognosis during infection, investigations of principal endogenous mediators have provided evidence of a protective effect of pyrogenic cytokines. Although the use of antipyretic medications is a long-established and widespread practice, the actual benefit of temperature reduction in febrile patients is uncertain. Antipyretic therapy does not protect against the recurrence of childhood febrile seizures, nor has its risk-benefit ratio been determined in patients with cardiopulmonary and other underlying disorders. In summary, fever is usually not harmful, and antipyretics may confuse the clinical picture by dampening it, although their anti-inflammatory effects are often beneficial.

SUGGESTED READINGS

Affronti M, Mansueto P, Soresi M, et al. Low-grade fever: how to distinguish organic from nonorganic forms. *Int J Clin Pract.* 2010;64:316-321. *Low-grade fever (37.5° to 38.3° C) has the same differential diagnosis as higher fever of unknown origin.*

Balink H, Collins J, Bruyn GA, et al. F-18 FDG PET/CT in the diagnosis of fever of unknown origin. *Clin Nucl Med.* 2009;34:862-868. *F-18 FDG PET/CT identified the source in about 55% of patients.*

Chandra A, Nicks B, Maniago E, et al. A multicenter analysis of the ED diagnosis of pneumonia. *Am J Emerg Med.* 2010;28:862-865. *Among patients admitted with an initial diagnosis of community-acquired pneumonia, 27% ultimately had other diagnoses established.*

Lampland KB. Fever in the critically ill medical patient. *Crit Care Med.* 2009;37:S273-S278. *Review of determinants and management of fever in the ICU.*

O'Grady NP, Barie PS, Bartlett JG, et al. Guidelines for evaluation of new fever in critically ill adult patients: 2008 update from the American College of Critical Care Medicine and the Infectious Diseases Society of America. *Crit Care Med.* 2008;36:1330-1349. *Practice parameters to determine whether an infection is present.*

289

APPROACH TO FEVER AND SUSPECTED INFECTION IN THE COMPROMISED HOST

KIEREN A. MARR

DEFINITION

This chapter focuses on the approach to suspected infection and fever in compromised hosts. There are multiple states (e.g., burns, intensive care unit hospitalization) that can fulfill the general definition of *compromised*, specifically with consideration of heightened risks for infection, but focus here will be placed on the immunocompromised host who has acquired defects in immune function, secondary to medical therapies. Examples include

treatment of conditions such as neoplastic diseases (particularly hematologic disorders such as leukemia and lymphoma), organ transplantation, and treatment of collagen vascular or autoimmune diseases. Management of people with the acquired immunodeficiency syndrome (AIDS) is discussed in Chapters 392 through 402.

APPROACH TO THE PATIENT

The approach to the immunosuppressed patient requires detailed knowledge of the type of immune defect and related risks. Table 289-1 is an attempt to outline general defects in host responses with the types of agents or conditions that characterize the three general groups of "medically immunosuppressed" patients discussed in the context of this chapter (treatment of neoplastic diseases, transplantation, and treatment of autoimmune and collagen vascular diseases).

Patients with Malignancy

In patients with neoplastic diseases, particularly hematologic malignancies, the underlying condition plays a role in dictating infectious risks. For instance, the absolute number of phagocytic cells belonging to the polymorphonuclear leukocyte series may be reduced or the function of those cells impaired in the setting of specific malignancies (e.g., acute or chronic leukemias). In conditions such as acute leukemia, in which the cells are abnormal in morphology and function, and only a small proportion of normally functioning cells circulate, risks for bacterial infections are enhanced, even in the absence of administered cytotoxic therapies. In certain conditions, such as in the setting of chronic lymphocytic leukemia, there may be quantitative defects in humoral factors that are critical in host defense, such as circulating immunoglobulin G (IgG) and IgM antibodies, secretory IgA antibodies, and components of the complement cascade that can directly lyse some bacteria and viruses. Another component of the population of phagocytic cells includes circulating monocytes and tissue macrophages and the fixed mononuclear cells of the reticuloendothelial system. These cells collaborate with helper T cells in defense against pathogens that can survive intracellularly, such as mycobacteria, fungi, and some viruses and parasites. The spectrum of infectious risks is further enhanced and prolonged after treatment with cytotoxic drugs (Chapter 182). These therapies affect other organ functions that are critical to defense, especially the integrity of the gastrointestinal tract mucosal barrier and airway innate clearance mechanisms, posing additional innate susceptibilities to bacterial and fungal pathogens. In this manner, the neoplastic disorder itself, as well as the specific therapies used to treat it, combine to define both acute and chronic risks for infection.

Transplant Recipients

Hematopoietic stem cell transplantation (HSCT) (Chapter 181) posits additional risks to the patient as a result of the agents used for conditioning therapy in preparation for the stem cell transplantation, variable rate and magnitude of cellular engraftment, and, in recipients of allogeneic HSCT, administration of additional agents to modulate risks for and treatment of graft-versus-host disease (GVHD). Thus, risks for specific infections can be roughly divided on a time scale relative to engraftment. Organ dysfunction, loss of natural barriers (skin and gut), and neutropenia dictate enhanced early risks for bacteria and fungi that inhabit the gastrointestinal tract; impaired humoral and secondary immunity enhance late risks for infections caused by viruses, fungi, and encapsulated bacteria, especially in people treated aggressively for GVHD.

Immunodeficiency in solid organ transplant recipients (Chapter 48) is largely related to the acute initiation and chronic maintenance requirements of therapies to suppress T- and B-cell function in order to minimize impact of allosensitization and decrease risks for early and late graft rejection. Therapies have evolved over time, with increased use of targeted biologic therapies, but in general, risks are largely related to those associated with acute and chronic cellular and humoral dysfunction. Type and amount of therapy differ according to immunologic risk of recipients. Additional variables modulating overall risks for infection include the altered anatomy, surgical intervention, and potential of infection transmitted from the graft itself (i.e., donor derived).

Transplant recipients have increased risks both for acute infection and for reactivation of latent infections after initiation of immunosuppression. Hence, pretransplantation evaluation should be focused on detection of latent herpes viruses (e.g., cytomegalovirus [CMV]) and other pathogens (e.g., *Mycobacterium tuberculosis*) that can be transferred or reactivated with transplantation and immunosuppression.

Two important concepts regarding immunosuppression that have emerged from the field of transplantation include observations of the

TABLE 289-1 CONDITIONS, INTERVENTIONS, AND IMMUNE DEFECTS TYPICALLY ENCOUNTERED IN THREE GROUPS OF COMPROMISED HOSTS

UNDERLYING CONDITION	INTERVENTION	TYPE OF DEFECT
Treatment of neoplastic diseases (particularly hematologic malignancies)	Cytotoxic chemotherapies	Bone marrow suppression. Defects in primary and secondary humoral and cellular immunity. Breach in mucosal barriers (skin, gut). Impairment in mucociliary clearance. Defects in other organ function (e.g., kidney, liver)
Transplantation: hematopoietic stem cell transplantation (HSCT)	Underlying disease (e.g., hematologic malignancies)	Defects in primary and secondary humoral and cellular immunity. Defects in phagocytic cell quantity and function
	Cytotoxic conditioning therapy (± total body irradiation)	Bone marrow suppression. Defects in primary and secondary humoral and cellular immunity. Breach in mucosal barriers. Defects in organ function
	Stem cell manipulation (e.g., T-cell depletion)	Delay in cellular engraftment
	Prophylaxis and treatment of graft-versus-host disease (e.g., corticosteroids, calcineurin inhibitors, antimetabolites, TNF-α antagonists)	Defective function in phagocytic cells and dysfunction of primary and secondary humoral and cellular immunity
Solid organ transplantation (SOT)	Underlying disease (e.g., diabetes, end-stage liver disease)	Organ dysfunction and miscellaneous immune dysfunction
	Induction therapies (e.g., corticosteroids, antilymphocyte globulin, splenectomy, anti-IL-2 Ab, anti-CD52 Ab, calcineurin inhibitors	Depletion and impairment in primary and secondary cellular and humoral immunity
	Surgical intervention and altered anatomy	Breach in mucosal barriers. Defects in organ function.
	Acute and chronic rejection prophylaxis and treatment (e.g., corticosteroids, calcineurin inhibitors, antimetabolites and alkylating agents, plasmapheresis, antithymocyte globulin, monoclonal antibodies to B and T cells, anticytokine therapies, T-cell costimulation blockers)	Defective function in phagocytic cells, primary and secondary humoral and cellular immunity
Treatment of collagen vascular and autoimmune diseases	Anti-inflammatory and immunosuppressive agents (corticosteroids, nonsteroidal anti-inflammatory drugs, calcineurin inhibitors, sirolimus, mycophenolate mofetil)	Defective function in phagocytic cells, primary and secondary humoral and cellular immunity
	Antimetabolite and alkylating agents	Bone marrow suppression, defects in primary and secondary humoral and cellular immunity
	Biologic immune response modifiers (e.g., antithymocyte globulin, monoclonal antibodies to B and T cells, anticytokine therapies, T-cell costimulation blockers)	Defective function in primary and secondary humoral and cellular immunity

Ab = antibody; TNF = tumor necrosis factor.

immunomodulatory effects of viral reactivation and infection, and the "net state of immunosuppression." It was long ago noted that viral infections (both reactivation and disease) and, in many models, seropositivity alone enhance risks for other infections. This has been particularly well documented for CMV (Chapter 384), which is recognized as a risk for other infections in both recipients of hematopoietic stem cell and solid organ transplant grafts. Overall risks for infection are largely related to epidemiologic exposures and the net state of immunosuppression, dictated by multiple host, donor, and medical variables. This net state is variable both in quantity and changes in character over time, largely influenced by therapies to prevent rejection or GVHD, and other complications, such as viral reactivation. This concept, which originated toward an understanding of solid organ transplantation, can perhaps be applied to the care of all immunosuppressed patients in general.

Patients Treated for Autoimmune Disease

Table 289-1 also outlines the types of immunosuppressive therapies frequently administered to patients for the control of connective tissue diseases and autoimmune conditions. This is detailed here in order to emphasize that this group of patients is growing in importance in both hospitalized and outpatient populations, with increased use of biologic immune response modifiers (Chapters 34 and 35) enhancing risks for both reactivation of latent infection (e.g., *M. tuberculosis*) and severe manifestations of acute infection.￭ Infectious risks should be considered when balancing need for these therapies, designing preventative regimens, and creating differential diagnoses of suspected infection.

● **FEVER DURING NEUTROPENIA: CONSIDERATIONS AND DIAGNOSTIC EVALUATION**

The onset of fever in a compromised patient can be an ominous development, and depending on the nature and magnitude of the impaired host defenses,

a febrile response can herald the onset of a life-threatening systemic infection. If fever occurs in the setting of chemotherapy-induced neutropenia, the risk for bacterial infection increases proportionally with the decline in neutrophil count, especially with prolonged durations of significant neutropenia. Early pivotal studies documented that infection rates increase with neutrophil levels lower than 1000 cells/mm^3, progressively increasing as counts decline to less than 100 cells/mm^3. The duration of significant neutropenia is also an important determinant of the type of infection most likely to occur, with the risk for bacterial and fungal infections increasing with each successive week in which leukocyte counts are less than 500 cells/mm^3. In these studies, neutropenia and lymphopenia played significant roles in influencing infection rates in the setting of acute leukemia; however, neutropenia alone was more important than lymphopenia alone. This study marked some of the earliest efforts that laid the foundation for our current approach to treatment of fever during neutropenia.

Historically, the most common causes of fever during neutropenia were gram-negative bacteria arising from the gastrointestinal tract. These observations drove establishment of empirical and prophylactic antibiotic practices designed to prevent primary development and to treat unrecognized infection caused by the most common predicted pathogens. In the 1990s, concurrent with increased use of prophylactic and empirical antibiotics, especially quinolones and extended spectrum β-lactams, reported rates of gram-negative bacteremias declined, with proportional increases in the numbers of bacteremias caused by gram-positive organisms. The precise reason, such a change in epidemiology occurred, is a matter of debate and likely multifactorial; in addition to increased use of effective preventive antibacterials, there has likely been a role played by increased use of indwelling intravascular devices. It has also been recognized that fever that persists despite administration of broad-spectrum antibacterial therapy may herald the onset or presence of undiagnosed invasive fungal infections.

The importance of mucositis in influencing both the occurrence of primary inflammation and the development of bacterial or fungal infection through mucosal barrier injury cannot be overemphasized in patients administered

TABLE 289-2	APPROACH TO FEVER DURING CHEMOTHERAPY-INDUCED NEUTROPENIA

PAST AND CURRENT CLINICAL CONSIDERATIONS

What is the type and duration of immunologic deficiency?

Does the patient have any organ dysfunction that would predispose to particular infection?

Does the patient have any unique environmental or epidemiologic exposures?

What are the patient's prior infections and colonizing organisms?

What are the current and recently administered antimicrobial agents?

Are there any specific presenting signs or symptoms that suggest a particular type of infection or syndrome?

TABLE 289-3	MULTINATIONAL ASSOCIATION OF SUPPORTIVE CARE IN CANCER (MASCC) RISK SCORING INDEX FOR IDENTIFICATION OF LOW-RISK PATIENTS WITH FEBRILE NEUTROPENIA

CHARACTERISTIC	SCORE
Extent of illness	
No symptoms	5
Mild symptoms	5
Moderate symptoms	3
No hypotension	5
No chronic obstructive lung disease	4
Solid tumor or no fungal infection	4
No dehydration	3
Outpatient at onset of fever	3
Age < 60 yr*	2

*Does not apply to age < 16 yr.

cytotoxic therapy for treatment of malignancies or HSCT. Studies have shown that mucositis can produce inflammation adequate to drive development of fever. It is also likely that a reasonable percentage of patients develop fever due to transient seeding of the blood stream with colonizing bacterial or fungal pathogens. Some of these infections may be caused by organisms that are less well adapted toward growth using standard microbiologic methods. These concepts support liberal use of empirical antimicrobials in the febrile neutropenic setting, with the focus on administering a compound that is active against the most likely pathogens, considering the patients' epidemiologic exposures and colonizing organisms and the hospital environment.

Table 289-2 lists multiple questions and considerations that the clinician should entertain when approaching fever in the neutropenic patient. The differential diagnosis of fever in the setting of chemotherapy-induced neutropenia is influenced by local and hospital exposure and the type of preventive antibiotics administered to the patient, which serve to alter microbial epidemiology within the gastrointestinal tract (see Table 289-2). Importantly, the type and the duration of immunodeficiency can alter overall risks, with "latent" infections presenting at development of first fever. Specific organ dysfunction, such as underlying pulmonary disease or renal impairment, can predispose to unique infectious syndromes (see later). Epidemiologic exposures should be thoroughly solicited; for instance, diagnostic evaluation should consider whether the patient previously or currently resides in areas endemic for *M. tuberculosis* or other infections that become latent (e.g., histoplasmosis). Current and previously administered antimicrobial drugs both affect risks for specific infections and can alter host microbial epidemiology. With this in mind, it is useful to have some information on colonizing organisms that may display complex resistance profiles, such as vancomycin-resistant enterococci and bacteria that express extended spectrum β-lactamases. Knowledge of recent colonization with these organisms should tailor initial antibiotic management, especially in patients who present severely ill.

One early consideration in treatment of fever during neutropenia is whether the patient requires hospitalization for therapy. Risk assessment is an integral part of early evaluation to determine whether outpatient therapy is feasible. Two risk-assessment systems have been developed, with the Multinational Association of Supportive Care in Cancer (MASCC) score validated to serve as a useful predictor of outcome, potentially assisting in identifying patients who can be treated with oral antibiotics and close monitoring rather than inpatient therapy (Table 289-3). In this model, a calculated index of more than 21 identifies low-risk patients who have a less than 5% risk for complications. Although the score is useful as a general guide to risk stratification, other variables that are important to consider when making risk assessment are underlying disease (e.g., lymphoma vs. leukemia), past and anticipated duration of neutropenia, symptoms and signs of infection foci, other comorbidities, and perhaps most importantly, whether the patient has access to immediate and reliable medical attention if discharged from the medical facility.

The onset of fever should trigger a prompt and thorough bedside evaluation of the patient. Beginning with examination of the head and neck, there should be a specific examination for evidence of central nervous system (CNS) infection as well as a general evaluation of mental status. The oropharynx must be examined for evidence of pharyngitis and focal tenderness. Sinus membranes should be evaluated for the presence of erythema or necrosis. Complete examination of the heart, lung fields, and abdomen is critical, with attention to the potential presence of new murmurs, pneumonia, and intra-abdominal tenderness. The perirectal area and the entire integument should be examined. Intravenous catheter exit sites and tunnels should be carefully examined, and blood should be drawn through all catheter channels for culture. Because catheter exit sites and tunnels can be infected in neutropenic patients without showing early signs of inflammation and erythema and with classic signs of infection presenting only after return of neutrophils, examination should be performed daily and with close scrutiny for evolving localized infection that may necessitate catheter removal.

Laboratory studies should be undertaken, with emphasis placed on procedures that can yield prompt results, such as Gram stain of body fluids, exudates, or aspirates. Routine blood work should include a complete blood count with differential, serum creatinine, and screening liver function studies. A chest radiograph should be part of the initial evaluation, as should routine urinalysis. Because routine radiographs are insensitive for detection of small nodular lesions, especially those caused by filamentous fungi, computed tomography (CT) should be performed when evaluating persistent fever, especially in the presence of airway symptoms.

Although fever is the hallmark of infection, it is not specific for the presence of an infectious process. The development of fever may be a result of multiple causes, including medications, reaction to blood components, and GVHD. The fundamental principle is that infection should be suspected as the most likely cause of fever in a compromised host, and therapy should be applied empirically, even as diagnostic tests are being performed. Multiple episodes of fever during prolonged hospitalization and neutropenia are not uncommon; each episode requires comprehensive assessment. After a documented infection, it should not be assumed that a subsequent episode of fever is caused by the same recrudescent pathogen; the law of diagnostic parsimony tends to be less reliable in immunosuppressed patients.

FEVER DURING NEUTROPENIA: MANAGEMENT

Progression of infection can occur rapidly in neutropenic hosts. Observation of very high mortality rates associated with bacteremia, especially those caused by gram-negative bacteria, triggered the introduction of routine empirical therapies (i.e., treatment of fever before diagnosis of infection). There are now many options for initial antibiotic therapy; choice should be tailored according to patient and institutional variables, as outlined in Table 289-1 and Figure 289-1. The first therapeutic distinction is whether a patient is at high risk, warranting inpatient management and intravenous antibiotic therapy, or low risk, potentially treated with oral regimens as an outpatient. In low-risk patients, the combination of a fluoroquinolone such as ciprofloxacin with amoxicillin-clavulanate, or levofloxacin alone, has been shown to be effective. In high-risk patients, admission for treatment and prompt administration of a broad-spectrum antibiotic regimen is necessary. Early studies demonstrated that the combination of an antipseudomonal β-lactam and an aminoglycoside is effective. Extended-spectrum agents, such as third- and fourth-generation cephalosporins and carbapenems, were then shown to be effective options administered as monotherapy. Meta-analyses have now shown that the routine use of an aminoglycoside in combination may result in more toxicities and no better outcomes.

One major choice in early therapy involves the decision to use vancomycin initially in high-risk patients. Advocates point to the risk for gram-positive infections that may carry a higher morbidity in neutropenic patients, including those caused by *Staphylococcus aureus* and viridans streptococci. However,

FIGURE 289-1. Algorithm for the initial management of febrile neutropenic patients. Risk assessment discussed in text and summarized in Table 289-3. "Vancomycin needed" is also discussed in text. (Modified from Hughes WT, Armstrong D, Bodey GP, et al. 2002 Guidelines for the use of antimicrobial agents in neutropenic patients with cancer. *Clin Infect Dis.* 2002;34: 730-751.)

because initiation of vancomycin with fever does not affect outcomes except in the case of treating breakthrough viridans streptococcal infection, general guidelines for initiation of vancomycin include documented or suspected catheter-related infection, colonization with penicillin and cephalosporin-resistant pneumococci or methicillin-resistant *S. aureus*, positive blood cultures for gram-positive bacteria, and hemodynamic instability. A meta-analysis of randomized controlled trials showed that addition of a glycopeptide to an initial empirical regimen did not result in improved treatment success, and adverse effects, including nephrotoxicity, were more common.[2] These observations, combined with increased use of broad-spectrum empirical agents, support a strategy of applying glycopeptides with persistent fever or in select situations of high risk for gram-positive infections, as described previously.

The median time to defervescence is shorter (2 days) in low-risk patients and longer (5 to 7 days) in high-risk patients. Clinical response to the first few days of therapy is a critical determinant of the course of extended antimicrobial therapy. Therapy should be tailored to the diagnostic findings. If patients are stable yet still febrile during a period of prolonged and severe neutropenia, clinical judgment must be used in deciding whether to maintain the initial regimen or switch to an alternative regimen. If patients become afebrile after 3 to 5 days of antibacterial treatment but cultures are negative, some authorities recommend continuing the broad-spectrum intravenous coverage until recovery of the neutrophil count. This, however, may not be practical for patients with leukemia in blast crisis or refractory aplastic anemia, in whom periods of aplasia lasting weeks or more are common. Others believe that a switch to oral treatment is justifiable (e.g., a fluoroquinolone possibly paired with a ß-lactam) if the patient becomes afebrile and appears to be clinically stable. If the patient remains afebrile, there is rapid improvement in the underlying condition, such as with recovery of the circulating neutrophil count to higher than 500 cells/mm³, and no focus of infection is identified, discontinuation of treatment is an option. If the neutrophil count recovers to above 500 cells/mm³ and fever persists, clinical judgment must be used to define needs for antimicrobial therapy while a search for the cause of the fever is continued. If the patient was initially treated with vancomycin and no confirmatory cultures supporting continued vancomycin use are obtained after 3 days (e.g., no coagulase-negative staphylococci from blood or methicillin-resistant *S. aureus*), intravenous vancomycin therapy should be discontinued.

Clinical deterioration should trigger consideration of infections resistant to the empirical regimen. Classic examples include breakthrough streptococcal bacteremia in patients not receiving vancomycin, breakthrough extended-spectrum β-lactamase–producing gram-negative bacteria in patients taking single-agent β-lactams, *Stenotrophomonas* species infections occurring in the setting of carbapenem monotherapy, and, especially more recently, infections with multidrug-resistant pathogens, such as *Acinetobacter* species and organisms that produce carbapenemases.

There are many causes of persistent fever, both noninfectious and infectious. Noninfectious causes include hematomas, drug reactions, transfusion reactions, pulmonary emboli, splenic infarcts, and the underlying malignancy. The possibility of infection caused by nonbacterial pathogens, such as fungi (especially *Candida* and *Aspergillus* species) prompted evaluation and widespread adoption of routine antifungal empirical therapies in the setting of fever that persists more than 4 to 7 days. Many drugs have been evaluated and shown to be effective in this setting, including azole drugs, echinocandins, and polyenes.[3,4] Choice should be tailored to current antifungal prophylaxis, diagnostic findings, suspicion of *Candida* versus *Aspergillus* infection, and organ function.

There are no hard and fast rules for duration of therapies; the simplest recommendation is to treat documented pathogens until the signs and symptoms of infection subside. On the other hand, persistently compromised hosts may remain febrile for weeks without identification of the cause. For a patient with persistent fever in whom no pathogen is identified, the duration of therapy must be based on integration of clinical data and the best estimate of the direction of the host's status. As mentioned previously, therapy can be discontinued in stable, afebrile patients, assuming that the absolute neutrophil count exceeds 500 cells/mm³. Clearly, if broad-spectrum antibacterial therapy is to be discontinued, the patient must be monitored carefully thereafter. For patients whose neutrophil counts remain at levels less than 500 cells/mm³, particularly the subset with severe profound neutropenia of less than 100 cells/mm³, it is prudent to continue empirical antibacterial and antifungal therapy, with reappraisal of all diagnostic measures. The decision to stop therapy at whatever arbitrary interval may be justified if the patient's condition is stable.

The use of granulocyte colony-stimulating factors (G-CSFs) for the prevention of febrile neutropenia is discussed in Chapter 170. For the management of established fever in neutropenic patients, evidence-based guidelines have been published by the American Society of Clinical Oncology[5] and by the Infectious Disease Society of America. The guidelines generally agree, and they support the use of CSFs in similar circumstances that indicate high risk for infection-associated complications and poor clinical outcomes, such as in patients with anticipated long and profound durations of neutropenia,

TABLE 289-4   INFECTIOUS AND NONINFECTIOUS SYNDROMES IN IMMUNOCOMPROMISED HOSTS

PRIMARY ORGAN SYSTEM	BACTERIA	FUNGI	VIRUSES	NONINFECTIOUS
Cutaneous	Disseminated gram-positive and gram-negative bacteria, e.g., *Staphylococcus aureus* *Pseudomonas aeruginosa* *Mycobacterium* spp. *Nocardia* spp.	*Candida* spp. Filamentous fungi, e.g., *Aspergillus* species Zygomycetes *Fusarium* spp. *Scedosporium* spp. *Cryptococcus* spp.	Herpes simplex Varicella-zoster CMV HHV-6 Adenovirus Parvovirus B19	Drug eruptions GVHD Sweet's syndrome
Sinopulmonary	Gram-positive and gram-negative causes of sinusitis and pneumonia *S. aureus* *Streptococcus pneumoniae* *P. aeruginosa* *Haemophilus influenzae* Anaerobes Legionella *Nocardia* spp. *Mycobacterium* spp.	Filamentous fungi, e.g., *Aspergillus* spp. Zygomycetes *Fusarium* spp. *Scedosporium* spp. *Cryptococcus* spp. Endemic fungi, e.g., *H. capsulatum* *C. immitis* *B. dermatitidis* *P. jirovecii*	Respiratory viruses, e.g., RSV Parainfluenza Influenza Adenovirus Reactivation herpes viruses, e.g., VZV	Drug-related pulmonary toxicities Pneumonitis (sirolimus) Diffuse alveolar damage Bronchiolitis obliterans syndromes
Gastrointestinal	Bacterial enterocolitis ("typhlitis") Mixed gram-positive, gram-negative *Clostridium difficile* colitis Enteric diarrheal pathogens *Salmonella* spp. *Shigella* spp. *Escherichia coli* *Campylobacter* spp.	*Candida* spp.	CMV EBV-PTLD Adenovirus Coxsackievirus Rotavirus Norovirus	Drug-related toxicities, e.g., MMF
Neurologic	Gram-positive and gram-negative bacteria *Listeria* spp. *Pneumococcus* spp. *Meningococcus* spp. *Mycobacterium tuberculosis*	Filamentous fungi *Cryptococcus* spp.	Herpes viruses HSV HHV-6 VZV JC virus West Nile virus Misc. viral encephalitides	Drug-related toxicities, e.g., carbapenem-related seizures PRES

EBV-PTLD = Epstein-Barr virus–post-transplantation lymphoproliferative disorder; GVHD = graft-versus-host disease; HHV-6 = human herpes virus-6; HSV = herpes simplex virus; MMF = mycophenolate mofetil; PRES = posterior reversible encephalopathy; RSV = respiratory syncytial virus; VZV = varicella-zoster virus.

age greater than 65 years, uncontrolled primary disease, pneumonia, hemodynamic compromise, and invasive fungal infections.

The remainder of this chapter discusses diagnosis and evaluation of specific syndromes that are common in neutropenic hosts and individuals who are immunocompromised because of other therapies, including transplantation. Table 289-4 summarizes some of the most common infectious and noninfectious syndromes that involve the skin, lungs, gastrointestinal tract, and nervous system, as discussed later.

CUTANEOUS SYNDROMES

Cutaneous abnormalities can provide a clue to bacteremia, and aspiration and culture of suspicious lesions can be as valuable as a blood culture. Ascending streptococcal or staphylococcal cellulitis can occur in both immunocompromised and normal patients. Metastatic abscesses are a well-recognized part of the *S. aureus* bacteremia syndrome. Necrotizing vasculitis is classically associated with *Pseudomonas aeruginosa* infections (the cutaneous lesion of ecthyma gangrenosum is an erythematous, indurated target or "bull's eye" lesion with an area of central necrosis that can appear in crops) (Fig. 289-2). However, other gram-negative endotoxin-producing bacteria have been associated with similar cutaneous lesions.

In the neutropenic host, disseminated fungal infections may be initially recognized by characteristic cutaneous lesions. Disseminated candidiasis in neutropenic patients can present with diffuse maculopapular, erythematous, and sometimes tender lesions. Disseminated infections caused by filamentous organisms such as *Aspergillus* species cause similar lesions, but usually fewer in number and more often with some component of central necrosis. Other filamentous fungi, namely those with which infection is characterized by a high fungal burden, such as *Fusarium* species, typically cause more skin lesions in multiple stages of evolution, ranging from papules to larger erythematous lesions with central necrosis. Multiple filamentous fungi such as *Aspergillus* species and Zygomycetes can also cause primary cutaneous lesions, especially with a breech in skin integrity, associated with catheter sites, trauma, and surgery. Infection with *Cryptococcus neoformans*

can be accompanied with cutaneous involvement, with manifestations ranging from molluscum-like lesions to primary cutaneous cellulitis, which may be especially common in solid organ transplant recipients. Cutaneous lesions are an opportunity to establish diagnosis through aspiration, biopsy, and culture.

Morbilliform eruptions or maculopapular exanthems are frequent in neutropenic patients and transplant recipients, and they can be caused by drug reactions, GVHD, and numerous viral infections. Primary infection and reactivation with herpes viruses such as CMV and Epstein-Barr virus (EBV) can be accompanied by rashes, and diagnostics should be considered in the appropriate context. Human herpesvirus-6 (HHV-6), the primary cause of roseola infantum in childhood, leads to latency and can cause disease in immunocompromised hosts both by reactivation and primary infection. Disease can be accompanied by fever, rash, myelosuppression, and involve other organ systems (e.g., CNS). In immunocompromised patients, adenovirus can be both primarily acquired, usually through the respiratory tract, and reactivated, and it causes fever, rash, and potentially disease involving multiple organ systems (lungs, gastrointestinal tract, kidneys, liver, CNS). In HSCT recipients, the constellation of fever, rash, diarrhea, and hepatitis may be confused for severe GVHD. Parvovirus B19 infection can be severe in immunocompromised hosts and associated with fever, rash, and manifestations of hemophagocytosis, although there are other infectious causes of hemophagocytic syndromes as well. The characteristic vesicular rashes of varicella reactivation are frequent in stem cell and solid organ transplant recipients with chronic T-cell deficiencies, especially in the absence of antiviral prophylaxis; an important therapeutic consideration is to recognize and aggressively treat disease that involves viscera because disseminated disease is associated with high mortality rates. Antivirals administered as prophylaxis in high-risk HSCT and solid organ transplant recipients can decrease both early morbidity and late mortality associated with herpes simplex virus (HSV), varicella-zoster virus (VZV), and CMV disease, although drug-related toxicities need to be measured in risk-benefit calculations.[6,7]

FIGURE 289-2. Ecthyma gangrenosum. A 28-year-old woman with fever and neutropenia while on chemotherapy for acute leukemia developed several tender edematous papules on her thighs. **A,** Central crust and surrounding erythema are shown. **B,** The papula becomes necrotic over 1 to 2 days, with the formation of black, well-demarcated eschar. Cultures from blood and the necrotic eschar grew *Pseudomonas aeruginosa*. (© DermAtlas; http://www.DermAtlas.org.)

There are numerous noninfectious causes of skin rashes and lesions that are common in immunocompromised individuals. Drug-induced hypersensitivity syndromes can be both mild and severe, potentially associated with life-threatening toxic epidermal necrolysis. As in other populations, antimicrobial agents are frequently implicated as causative agents. GVHD, especially during the acute phase, frequently presents as suspected infection, with fever, nonspecific skin rashes, and frequently, disease involving the gastrointestinal tract (diarrhea, hepatitis).

Sweet's syndrome, or acute febrile neutrophilic dermatosis, is characterized by skin lesions with neutrophilic infiltration in the dermis (see Fig. 448-22 in Chapter 448). This presents a diagnostic dilemma in neutropenic patients and has been described in the setting of impending neutrophil recovery or treatment with G-CSF. It is also associated with numerous drugs and can appear as a paraneoplastic phenomenon. Biopsy with appropriate microbial stains and culture is essential to distinguish these lesions from infectious causes of ecthyma gangrenosum and other disseminated infections such as those caused by fungi.

RESPIRATORY SYNDROMES

The lungs are a challenging site in evaluating fever in a compromised patient because detection of abnormalities is easy but obtaining lung secretions or infected tissues can be difficult. Pneumonia should be suspected in a patient who has respiratory symptoms as manifested by cough, shortness of breath, chest pain, and hypoxia. In the early stages of pneumonitis, routine chest radiographs may be negative, whereas more expensive imaging procedures such as computed axial tomography can reveal pulmonary infiltrates or abscesses. Both community-acquired pathogens such as pneumococci and *Haemophilus influenzae* can cause lobar or diffuse pneumonia. Gram-negative bacilli can cause pneumonia of a necrotizing type in severely neutropenic patients. All patients who are receiving ventilator support are at risk for secondary gram-negative bacillary pneumonia or staphylococcal pneumonia. Clusters of outbreaks of *Legionella pneumophila* infection have occurred in immunocompromised patients maintained in dialysis, transplant, or intensive care units; these outbreaks reflect institutional environmental contamination. Pulmonary involvement is primary with tuberculosis but may be secondary with nontuberculous mycobacteria such as *Mycobacterium avium*, which usually originates from the gastrointestinal tract.

Opportunistic fungi have been increasingly recognized as causes of lung infection in compromised neutropenic patients and transplant recipients. A travel history is essential in a compromised patient who has evidence of lung disease; epidemic mycoses such as blastomycosis, coccidioidomycosis, and histoplasmosis may present as acute pneumonia after recent exposure (although more typically, initial exposure in a normal host leads to containment in an initial focus of fungal lung disease). After immune suppression, the primary focus can be the source of reactivated disease. *Candida* species, in contrast, are uncommon primary lung pathogens. Although *Candida* species commonly colonize indwelling vascular and urinary catheters, candidal pneumonia is unusual in the absence of systemic candidiasis. Systemic candidiasis usually originates from the gastrointestinal or genitourinary tract if not secondary to vascular catheter dissemination. Although traditionally

associated with an "interstitial pattern" of lung infiltration, *Pneumocystis* species pneumonia can be manifested as local consolidation or pulmonary nodules, frequently exhibiting granulomatous inflammation on pathology. Filamentous fungi, which include *Aspergillus*, Zygomycetes, and less frequently diagnosed *Fusarium* species and *Scedosporium* species, are difficult to treat. These infections may be accompanied by chest pain and occasionally hemoptysis. From an initial focus, *Aspergillus* infection can spread through the pulmonary vasculature, which sets the stage for localized hemorrhage, creating a halo sign on CT scan, and infarction and necrosis, which can progress to cavitary lesions. Non-neutropenic hosts frequently also develop less specific radiographic findings, such as bronchopneumonia. These organisms can also cause primary airway disease, presenting with features typical of tracheobronchitis, with or without findings apparent on CT scan. This infection is particularly well described in lung transplant recipients, who may also have involvement of the bronchial anastomosis.

Recently, attention has been drawn to the high risks for severe pulmonary infection caused by reactivation *M. tuberculosis* in people who are treated with biologic immune response modifiers (Chapter 35) in the setting of autoimmune or other inflammatory diseases, such as with rheumatoid arthritis, psoriasis, and inflammatory bowel diseases. High risks are particularly well described in the setting of treatment with tumor necrosis factor antagonists, justifying enhanced vigilance, including routine screening for prior infection, and consideration of preventive chemotherapy. These patients are also at increased risk for invasive fungal infections, including reactivation of endemic infections such as histoplasmosis, warranting enhanced screening and high suspicion for disease.

Viral infections that involve the lung are difficult to diagnose in immunocompromised patients. Particularly common concerns are reactivation pneumonitis caused by members of the herpesvirus family, especially CMV, which occur most frequently in the setting of chronic T-cell depression associated with transplantation. Respiratory viruses, which infect immunocompromised hosts with the same frequency as in the general population, cause lower tract disease and pneumonitis more frequently in hosts with suppressed cellular immunity. Essentially any respiratory virus can cause upper and lower tract disease, depending on geographic and seasonal epidemiology; most frequently recognized are respiratory syncytial virus, parainfluenza viruses, influenza viruses, and adenoviruses. Patients who have defects in cellular immunity typically exhibit higher viral loads and prolonged shedding, presenting considerations with regard to enhanced therapy, emergence of antiviral resistance, and infection control. The transplant population has served as a sentinel population in recognizing multiple emerging viral pathogens, including human metapneumovirus, bocavirus, and the KI and WU polyomaviruses.

There are numerous recognized noninfectious causes of pulmonary infiltrates in immunosuppressed hosts. These include early complications of chemotherapy administration, such as diffuse alveolar damage and hemorrhage, as well as late complications of GVHD and organ rejection (e.g., bronchiolitis obliterans syndromes). Certain drugs that are frequently administered in these patient populations can cause direct lung toxicity; classic examples include the proliferation signal inhibitor sirolimus.

GASTROINTESTINAL SYNDROMES

There are multiple causes of diarrhea in a compromised host, including conventional enteric pathogens such as *Salmonella* (Chapter 316), *Shigella* (Chapter 317), and *Campylobacter* (Chapter 311). In patients who have been in the hospital and have been receiving multiple courses of antibiotic treatment, *C. difficile* (Chapter 304) is a common occurrence, and colitis can be both severe and persistent in immunosuppressed hosts. Two acid-fast staining parasites are *Isospora belli* and *Cryptosporidium* species, and they are associated with predisposing impairments in cell-mediated immunity. More recently recognized are the microsporidians. *Giardia lamblia* is classically associated with hypogammaglobulinemia. Individuals who have received long courses of chemotherapy, radiation, and antibiotics commonly experience *Candida* mucosal overgrowth in the mouth and esophagus. HSV and CMV can cause symptoms identical to those of *Candida* esophagitis. In severely neutropenic patients, anaerobic streptococci and gram-negative pathogens such as *P. aeruginosa* can cause severe mucositis and pharyngitis. In cancer patients, these organisms take advantage of the cytotoxic effects of chemotherapy, which promotes sloughing of mucosal surfaces and subsequently predisposes to infection.

Neutropenic patients may develop enterocolitis that can be of mixed anaerobic and aerobic bacterial origin. Neutropenic enterocolitis, also known as typhlitis or ileocecal syndrome, results from chemotherapeutic damage to the intestinal mucosa in the setting of neutropenia. Presentation usually includes fever, abdominal pain, nausea, vomiting, and diarrhea. Because neutropenic enterocolitis can rapidly progress to intestinal perforation, sepsis, and multisystem organ failure, prompt diagnosis and aggressive medical or surgical intervention are required.

CMV colitis can be focal or diffuse; in some solid organ transplant recipients, disease can be present without demonstration of a positive blood polymerase chain reaction for CMV, so endoscopy is required for diagnosis. Norovirus gastroenteritis can be severe and protracted and is frequently misdiagnosed as gastrointestinal GVHD in allogeneic HSCT recipients. Because the differential diagnosis of colitis and diarrhea is broad and includes multiple infections, focal EBV-associated post-transplantation lymphoproliferative disorder, GVHD, and drug-induced toxicities such as that caused by mycophenolate mofetil, these patients should be evaluated with endoscopy to reach definitive diagnosis.

NEUROLOGIC SYNDROMES

Both gram-positive and gram-negative bacteria (including anaerobes) can cause brain abscess or meningitis. *Listeria monocytogenes* is a common cause of meningitis in a compromised host. This pathogen is a gram-positive pleomorphic bacillus that may be difficult to identify on routine Gram stain of cerebrospinal fluid. Encapsulated bacteria such as pneumococci and staphylococci can cause metastatic CNS disease and meningitis. In patients with impaired cell-mediated immunity, *C. neoformans* is also a leading cause of CNS infection. Other fungal pathogens such as *Aspergillus* and other molds can invade the CNS, both by direct sinus invasion and by hematogenous spread. Focal brain lesions and meningoencephalitis in individuals who have chronic deficiency in cellular immunity can be caused by reactivation or acute severe infection by typically latent organisms such as *Toxoplasma gondii, M. tuberculosis,* and *Histoplasma capsulatum*. Reactivated or quiescent CNS syphilis should also be considered in patients with severe immunologic impairment.

There are numerous viral causes of meningoencephalitis; similar to other populations, one needs to consider enteroviruses, measles, and, neurotropic herpesviruses (HSV-1, CMV, VZV). HHV-6 is a common cause of encephalitis and post-transplantation acute limbic encephalitis in transplant recipients, characterized by seizures, anterograde amnesia, and neuroimaging abnormalities involving the temporal lobes. Progressive multifocal leukoencephalopathy caused by JC polyomavirus occurs in patients with chronic CD4 deficiency, such as with human immunodeficiency virus type 1 (HIV-1) infection. Recent studies have emphasized that solid organ transplant recipients are at increased risk for meningoencephalitis caused by West Nile virus compared with the general population. Anyone presenting early after transplantation should be considered at risk for potentially severe infections acquired from the donor; West Nile virus, rabies, HIV, HSV, and multiple other viruses have been documented to be transmitted through organ donation.

There are multiple noninfectious causes of neurological symptoms, which include drug toxicities and immunologic disorders, such as paraneoplastic syndromes and Guillain-Barré syndrome. Particularly relevant in the transplant recipient, patients with autoimmune diseases, and recipients of high-doses of cancer chemotherapy is the posterior reversible encephalopathy syndrome (PRES). The classic presentation of PRES encompasses a sudden onset of severe "thunderclap" headache, seizures, confusion, and visual disturbance, accompanied by a CT or magnetic resonance imaging pattern of predominantly posterior cerebral edema and angiographic evidence of reversible vasoconstriction. It may be caused by endothelial injury, vasospasm, or edema associated with drugs such as calcineurin inhibitors (cyclosporine, tacrolimus).

CONCLUSION

Infections are a major cause of mortality in immunocompromised hosts. The approach to fever and suspected infection requires knowledge of specific risks inherent to the type and duration of immunodeficiency, diagnostic diligence, and tailored therapeutics designed to avoid rapid progression and poor outcomes.

1. Leombruno JP, Einarson TR, Keystone EC. The safety of anti-tumour necrosis factor treatments in rheumatoid arthritis: meta and exposure-adjusted pooled analysis of serious adverse events. *Ann Rheum Dis.* 2009;68:1136-1145.
2. Vardakas KZ, Samonis G, Chrysanthopoulou SA, et al. Role of glycopeptides as part of initial empirical treatment of febrile neutropenic patients: a meta-analysis of randomised controlled trials. *Lancet Infect Dis.* 2005;5:431-439.
3. Walsh TJ, Teppler H, Donowitz GR, et al. Caspofungin versus liposomal amphotericin B for empirical antifungal therapy in patients with persistent fever and neutropenia. *N Engl J Med.* 2004;351:1391-1402.
4. Freifeld AG, Bow EJ, Sepkowitz KA, et al. Clinical practice guideline for the use of antimicrobial agents in neutropenic patients with cancer: 2010 update by the Infectious Diseases Society of America. *Clin Infect Dis.* 2011;52:427-431.
5. Smith TJ, Khatcheressian J, Lyman GH, et al. 2006 Update of recommendations for the use of white blood cell growth factors: an evidence-based clinical practice guideline. *J Clin Oncol.* 2006;24:3187-3205.
6. Yahav D, Gafter-Gvili A, Muchtar E, et al. Antiviral prophylaxis in haematological patients: systematic review and meta-analysis. *Eur J Cancer.* 2009;45:3131-3148.
7. Kalil AC, Freifeld AG, Lyden ER, et al. Valganciclovir for cytomegalovirus prevention in solid organ transplant patients: an evidence-based reassessment of safety and efficacy. *PLoS One.* 2009;4:e5512.

SUGGESTED READING

Bow EJ. Neutropenic fever syndromes in patients undergoing cytotoxic therapy for acute leukemia and myelodysplastic syndromes. *Semin Hematol.* 2009;46:259-268. *Review of discrete neutropenic fever syndromes to help the clinician make better clinical judgments and management plans.*

Kumar D. Emerging viruses in transplantation. *Curr Opin Infect Dis.* 2010;23:374-378. *Review of the emergence of "new" viruses and manifestations in the solid organ transplant population.*

Mebis J, Goossens H, Berneman ZN. Antibiotic management of febrile neutropenia: current developments and future directions. *J Chemother.* 2010;22:5-12. *Review of changing microbial epidemiology in the heterogeneous population of patients with febrile neutropenia.*

Wallis RS. Infectious complications of tumor necrosis factor blockade. *Curr Opin Infect Dis.* 2009;22:403-409. *Review of the biology of TNF-α blockade and resultant infectious risks, with a focus on tuberculosis.*

PREVENTION AND CONTROL OF HEALTH CARE–ASSOCIATED INFECTIONS

NEIL FISHMAN AND DAVID P. CALFEE

Health care–associated infections, often referred to as *nosocomial* (from the Greek word *nosocomium*, meaning hospital), have been traditionally defined as infections that occur after hospital admission and that were neither present nor incubating at the time of admission. Because the site of health care delivery and management has increasingly shifted to the ambulatory setting, the relevance of traditional "hospital-associated" infections has diminished. An increasing number of patients are intermittently exposed to the health care environment and may become colonized or infected with health care–associated pathogens without ever being admitted to the hospital and thus may acquire health care–associated infections before admission. For example, patients may receive ablative chemotherapy for a stem cell transplantation and then be seen only as outpatients until substantial medical problems occur, including infections. Similarly, an increasing number of patients who have malignancies are being treated in "day hospital" settings and may never get admitted unless problems occur with respect to their care, including health care–associated infections.

Additionally, some health care–associated infections become manifested after hospital discharge. Delayed manifestations of these infections usually occur within days of discharge but may occasionally not become clinically apparent for months or even years. Development of these infections is dependent on the incubation period of the particular pathogen, the individual immunologic response to the infection, and the various specific risk factors for the infection. For example, operative insertion of prosthetic devices (such as joints) can impair the immune response to infection and allow an insidious infection to continue developing and finally be manifested months after insertion of the device. Similarly, hepatitis B or C infection acquired during surgery often does not become evident for weeks to months after discharge. Health care–related infections are associated with increased patient morbidity and mortality, substantial inconvenience for the patient and institution, and striking increases in the cost of care that are primarily absorbed by the institution in which they occur.

IMPORTANCE OF HEALTH CARE–ASSOCIATED INFECTIONS

The literature from the 1970s suggests that six to eight health care–associated infections occurred for every 100 patients admitted to the hospital. During the 1990s, the total number of health care–associated infections remained essentially unchanged, but because there was a decrease in hospital admissions, the rate of health care–associated infections actually increased. The number and rates of these infections increased in great measure because the most severely ill patients continued to be admitted. Because of both their underlying disease states and the aggressive and invasive therapies used to manage their illnesses, seriously ill patients often have the highest risks for health care–associated infections. For a variety of reasons, discussed in more detail later, the numbers and types of antimicrobial-resistant organisms continued to increase, and these antibiotic-resistant infections have spread with facility throughout health care institutions. During the 1990s, the Centers for Disease Control and Prevention (CDC) estimated that the number of deaths directly or indirectly related to health care–associated infections increased from 80,000 to 88,000 annually.

Health care–associated infections are important because they cause additional inconvenience, suffering, and mortality for patients. Furthermore, these infections prolong hospitalization and significantly increase the cost of care, thus having a significant adverse effect on the health care system. The CDC has estimated the annual cost of health care–associated infections to be 28.4 to 45 billion dollars. Both the mildest (e.g., urinary tract infections) and the most severe (e.g., septic shock) infections are associated with unnecessary increases in cost and inconvenience for patients. Moreover, in the era of prospective payment plans, third-party payers will not reimburse for approximately 95% of the cost of nosocomial infections. For a variety of reasons, then, health care institutions must focus on prevention of these infections not only to increase patient survival and satisfaction but also to save money.

The attributable cost of nosocomial infections relates in part to prolonged duration of intensive care unit (ICU) or total hospital stays and in part to costs associated with the management of specific infections (e.g., additional diagnostic tests, antimicrobial therapy, personal protective equipment for isolation, and sometimes surgery). Studies have demonstrated that nosocomial blood stream infections result on the average in a 7-day prolongation of hospitalization associated with $40,890 in additional cost for surviving ICU patients and an attributable mortality rate as high as 30%. Generally, surgical site infections result in prolongation of hospitalization for an additional week. Health care–associated pneumonia usually occurs in patients who have been receiving mechanical ventilation and often results in 7 or more excess days in the hospital, frequently in the ICU. These patients often require ventilator support and expensive antimicrobial agents. Cases of health care–associated pneumonia result in increases in cost similar to those incurred by blood stream and surgical site infections (Table 290-1).

Urinary tract infection, the most frequent and least severe health care–related infection, has been associated with a 3-day increase in length of stay in two large case-control studies from different countries. A recent economic analysis estimated the cost per catheter-associated urinary tract infection to be $749 to $1007 (in 2007 U.S. dollars). Although urinary tract infections

SITE	NO. OF INFECTIONS PER 100 ADMISSIONS	% OF ALL NI	DIRECT COD	EXTRA DAYS	% OF NI EXTRA DAYS
Urinary tract	2.5	30	<1%	1-3	15
Surgical site	1.4	15	1-2%	7	23
Lung	1.4	15	5-10%	7	23
Blood stream					
Primary	1.4	15	3%	7	23
Secondary	0.3	3	25%	10	5
Others	2.2	24	<1%	2	11

TABLE 290-1 RATE AND IMPACT OF NOSOCOMIAL INFECTIONS IN ACUTE CARE HOSPITALS

COD = cause of death; NI = nosocomial infection.

are generally milder infections, they can cause more severe illness when infection ascends to the kidney or when secondary blood stream infection occurs. Blood stream infection secondary to urinary tract infection is associated with a crude case-fatality rate of 13 to 30%.

RESERVOIRS AND TRANSMISSION OF HEALTH CARE–ASSOCIATED INFECTIONS

Health care–associated infections occur for a wide variety of reasons and are caused by a broad spectrum of pathogens. In some cases (particularly in instances in which patients are severely immunocompromised by disease or treatment), a microbe that would rarely produce an infection may colonize and ultimately infect a hospitalized patient. Hospitalization and the diagnostic and therapeutic interventions associated with hospitalization may provide access to some normally protected parts of the body (e.g., insertion of a percutaneous catheter through the skin provides a portal of entry into the blood stream). Other pathogens that cause these infections are not present in or on the host at the time of hospital admission but colonize the host after admission (frequently after spending just 24 hours in the hospital). After variable periods of colonization, these health care–associated pathogens may produce active infections. Because many patients become colonized or infected with health care–associated pathogens, spread from one patient to another in a health care institution may occur by direct contact between patients, by contact with contaminated environmental surfaces, and perhaps most commonly by the contaminated hands, clothing, or equipment of health care providers. Health care workers move from patient to patient and, in the absence of appropriate hand hygiene, may easily transmit hospital pathogens. Studies have found that health care workers, on average, follow hand hygiene recommendations after only 40% of patient contacts that should prompt the use of hand hygiene. Nurses and allied health professionals comply more often than physicians, but no category of health care provider achieves rates of compliance greater than 70%. Poorest compliance has been observed in areas at highest risk for transmission, such as the ICU, where the number, types, and immediacy of invasive interventions are the highest and where, unfortunately, patients at the highest risk for adverse outcomes of these infections are often housed. Nevertheless, in recent years, substantial efforts have been made in many health care facilities to improve adherence to hand hygiene recommendations among health care personnel.

ANTIBIOTIC-RESISTANT INFECTIONS

Resistant microorganisms became a significant problem in health care institutions within only a few years after the introduction of antibiotics for clinical therapy. Infections caused by antibiotic-resistant organisms are important because they are generally associated with prolonged illnesses, longer hospital stays, increased risk for death, and greater cost to the health care system than infections caused by antibiotic-susceptible strains of the same species. Antimicrobial resistance to new agents occurs rapidly and is often identified within months of the introduction of a new antimicrobial agent into the pharmacologic armamentarium (Table 290-2). Resistance is often first identified in hospitals and later in the general community. PRSA emerged in just this fashion at the time of discovery of penicillin, even before its widespread clinical use. For some antibiotics (e.g., vancomycin), resistance did not appear until three decades after its introduction. VRE first appeared in the

TABLE 290-2 ANTIBIOTIC DISCOVERY AND DEVELOPMENT OF RESISTANCE

ANTIBIOTIC	DISCOVERY	CLINICAL USE	RESISTANCE IDENTIFIED
Penicillin	1940	1943	1940
Streptomycin	1944	1947	1947
Tetracycline	1948	1952	1956
Erythromycin	1952	1955	1956
Vancomycin	1956	1972	1987
Gentamicin	1963	1967	1970

TABLE 290-3 ANTIMICROBIAL RESISTANCE AMONG PATHOGENS CAUSING HEALTH CARE–ASSOCIATED INFECTIONS IN U.S. HOSPITALS, 2006-2007

ORGANISM	ANTIMICROBIAL AGENT	Percentage of Isolates Resistant to Antimicrobial			
		CLABSI	CAUTI	VAP	SSI
Staphylococcus aureus	Oxacillin	56.8	65.2	54.4	49.2
Enterococcus faecium	Vancomycin	78.9	81.0	NR	56.5
Escherichia coli	Ceftriaxone or ceftazidime	8.1	5.5	11.0	5.3
	Fluoroquinolones	30.8	24.8	22.7	22.7
Klebsiella pneumoniae	Ceftriaxone or ceftazidime	27.1	21.2	23.7	14.8
	Carbapenems	10.8	10.1	3.6	5.2
Pseudomonas aeruginosa	Fluoroquinolones	30.5	33.8	27.8	15.9
	Piperacillin or piperacillin-tazobactam	20.2	17.1	17.0	7.9
	Cefepime	12.6	10.8	11.1	5.7
	Carbapenems	23	25.1	26.4	11.8
Acinetobacter baumannii	Carbapenems	29.2	25.6	36.8	30.6

CLABSI = central line–associated blood stream infection; CAUTI = catheter-associated urinary tract infection; SSI = surgical site infection; VAP = ventilator-associated pneumonia.
From Hidron AI, Edwards JR, Patel J, et al. Antimicrobial-resistant pathogens associated with healthcare-associated infections: annual summary of data reported to the National Healthcare Safety Network at the Centers for Disease Control and Prevention, 2006-2007. *Infect Control Hosp Epidemiol.* 2008;29:996-1011.

mid-1980s. The organism appears to have different origins in the United States and Europe. In the United States, emergence of resistance is thought to be due to clinical overuse of vancomycin, but in Europe, it is attributed to the use of a related compound (avoparcin) as a nutritional supplement and growth enhancer in farm animals.

Two predominant risk factors have been identified for infection with antibiotic-resistant pathogens in hospitals: the volume of antimicrobial agents (especially broad-spectrum agents) used in the institution and spread from patient to patient in an institution (frequently by health care personnel). The reason that the prevalence of antibiotic-resistant pathogens has grown so rapidly in hospitals was perhaps most clearly explained by Charles Darwin, who noted that nature selects the strain or species most suited to survive within each environment. Because up to half of all patients in U.S. hospitals and almost all patients in ICUs receive antibiotics, a microbe that is resistant to currently administered antimicrobials has a selective advantage to survive, proliferate, and spread. For some combinations of microbe and antibiotic, the probability of a spontaneous mutation to resistance to that particular drug is so high that giving that drug alone for infections caused by that microbe invariably results in antimicrobial resistance. Two prime examples of the risk for development of resistance when using a single agent are tuberculosis and human immunodeficiency virus (HIV) infection.

For example, the risk for mutation to isoniazid resistance among *Mycobacterium tuberculosis* isolates is so high that monotherapy for active tuberculosis with isoniazid results in the development of resistance in 70% of patients. For other combinations of microbes and antibiotics, however, the probability of a spontaneous mutation to resistance is much lower, and administration of that drug alone does not result in an increased risk for resistance of that microbe to that drug. The latter pattern is true for combinations such as enterococci and vancomycin or *S. aureus* and methicillin, which correspond to two of the most frequent antibiotic-resistant infections in U.S. hospitals. In these two examples, antimicrobial resistance is due to acquisition of a genetic resistance determinant (e.g., the *vanA* and *mecA* genes, respectively) rather than spontaneous mutation within the organisms' genome. The pattern mentioned earlier (i.e., that large proportions of hospital patients are taking antibiotics and that microbes are routinely transported from patient to patient) has resulted in a steadily growing prevalence of antibiotic-resistant pathogens such as methicillin-resistant *S. aureus* (MRSA), VRE, and multidrug-resistant gram-negative bacilli inside U.S. hospitals (Table 290-3).

Widespread and sometimes injudicious use of antibiotics along with the ready transmission of bacteria between patients in the hospital has resulted in an alarming trend in the emergence of antimicrobial-resistant organisms. Table 290-3 illustrates the most recent data reported by the CDC's National Healthcare Safety Network (NHSN), formerly known as the National Nosocomial Infection Surveillance (NNIS) system. Not only are both gram-positive and gram-negative organisms becoming increasingly resistant to available agents, but many bacteria are also acquiring multiple genes that render them resistant to multiple antibiotics (i.e., multidrug-resistant organisms).

GENERAL STRATEGIES EFFECTIVE IN PREVENTING SPREAD OF RESISTANCE IN HOSPITALS

Antibiotic Stewardship

Many experts believe that improving or shortening the duration of antibiotic use (or both) may be among the most cost-effective means of controlling antibiotic-resistant infections. Bacteria naturally acquire chromosomal mutations or, in other instances, acquire genetic material from other bacteria that

confer resistance to antibacterial drugs. Subsequent survival of the resistant organisms depends on a number of factors. Extensive use of antimicrobial agents can promote selective pressure for the survival of resistant pathogens. The risk for emergence of antimicrobial resistance increases markedly after the administration of antibiotics for just 7 days. Thus, inappropriate or unnecessarily prolonged use of antimicrobial agents can select for antimicrobial-resistant isolates. Such strains can colonize and cause infection and can be transmitted between patients.

Several prospective studies have documented a clear association between the use of antimicrobial agents and colonization or infection with resistant organisms in health care institutions, including an association with the use of broad-spectrum agents. In many studies, other interventions were implemented at the same time as restriction of antibiotic use, thus making interpretation of the relative importance of antibiotic restriction problematic. Antibiotic stewardship may be a more effective means of preventing the emergence of resistance in certain organisms (such as gram-negative bacteria), whereas prevention of transmission may be the more important intervention for others (such as MRSA).

Hand Hygiene

Proper use of hand hygiene clearly reduces nosocomial transmission of resistant organisms. Adherence to hand hygiene recommendations is associated with a reduced risk for health care cross-contamination, and failure to perform appropriate hand hygiene is generally considered to be the leading cause of patient-to-staff-to-patient transmission of health care–associated infections. Hands that are visibly dirty or contaminated should be washed with soap and water, and hands that are not visibly soiled should be decontaminated with an alcohol-based hand rub before contacting patients or engaging in clinical procedures. Similarly, health care workers should use an alcohol-based rub after contacting patients' intact or nonintact skin, mucous membranes, or body fluids. Finally, hand hygiene should be used after removing gloves and after any contact with inanimate objects or medical equipment in the vicinity of patients. Alcohol-based hand hygiene products have been demonstrated to be superior to soap and water for general hand hygiene. These products are rapidly bactericidal, are easier to use, do not require a sink, save time, and are less irritating to the skin than handwashing with soap and water. However, soap and water appears to be the preferable mode of hand hygiene when providing care for patients with *Clostridium difficile* infection because *C. difficile* spores are not reliably killed by alcohol.

FIGURE 290-1. Percentage of *Staphylococcus aureus* bacteremias caused by strains resistant to antimicrobials in Danish hospitals from 1960 to 1995. (From Bager F, ed. *DANMAP 98—Consumption of Antimicrobial Agents and Occurrence of Antimicrobial Resistance in Bacteria from Food Animals, Food, and Humans in Denmark.* Copenhagen: Danish Zoonosis Centre; 1999.)

Staffing Strategies

Cohorting care means having staff dedicated solely to providing care for patients known to be infected or colonized with resistant pathogens. When cohorting, staff do not cross-cover both infected or colonized and noncolonized patients. In an outbreak setting, keeping infected and colonized patients separate from uninfected and uncolonized patients, as well as managing them with separate staff, provides a powerful mechanism to prevent transmission. Understaffing clearly contributes to the spread of resistant organisms, particularly in epidemic settings. An association among understaffing, patient overcrowding, and the spread of infectious diseases has been established in several studies.

Decreasing Hospital and Intensive Care Unit Stay

Decreasing the length or the frequency of hospital stay, or both, as well as the length and frequency of stay in critical care units, has been suggested to be an effective mechanism to decrease the risk for spread of resistant organisms, and the results from a number of clinical studies provide support for this concept. Several studies conducted over the past 10 years provide evidence that shortening the hospital or ICU stay decreases rates of infection with resistant organisms.

Microbiologic Surveillance

Although interventions aimed at controlling institutional use of antimicrobials have been associated with modest control of resistance, their success has been far from uniform. Some experts argue for aggressively identifying colonized patients (i.e., an important reservoir for institutional spread) by performing prospective surveillance cultures and then implementing contact isolation precautions to limit opportunity for transmission. This latter strategy has been shown to decrease the spread of resistant pathogens, in some instances even in the absence of antibiotic control measures. The relative efficacy of these interventions—antimicrobial stewardship versus aggressive identification and isolation—probably varies from organism to organism, if not from institution to institution.

A controversial issue in the health care epidemiology community is whether to use aggressive microbiologic surveillance (called active surveillance) as an intervention in an attempt to minimize transmission of resistant microorganisms. By microbiologically screening all patients admitted to a health care setting, one can prospectively identify those who are colonized or infected with these organisms. Such patients can then be managed aggressively with isolation precautions, cohorting, or even attempts at decolonization. Active surveillance is labor-intensive and costly, and from a practical standpoint only specific organisms can be targeted. Conversely, active surveillance is likely to identify problematic pathogens sooner and thus enable measures to be taken to prevent their spread within the health care environment. Many experts believe that tight control is reasonably important to prevent cross-contamination with multiply resistant organisms. To date, no studies have definitively demonstrated the efficacy of this strategy as an independent intervention. Similar to the investigations of antimicrobial stewardship interventions, although many studies have demonstrated a benefit of prospective surveillance cultures, most of them introduced several infection control interventions simultaneously. Because of the simultaneous use of several strategies, one cannot determine the individual contribution of any single intervention. Some European and Scandinavian countries have implemented policies of restrictive antibiotic use and aggressive surveillance. The Netherlands uses an aggressive surveillance approach for the prevention of MRSA transmission as well as a policy of restrictive antibiotic use. In the Netherlands, prospective surveillance cultures of all admissions are performed, strict barrier precautions are required for patients who carry the identified resistant organisms, temporary furloughs are provided for colonized health care workers, and hospital wards—and sometimes even entire institutions—are closed when the prevalence starts to rise. As an example of the efficacy of this approach, the prevalence of staphylococcal isolates resistant to methicillin and causing infection in the Netherlands is currently less than 2%. Similar approaches have been used in Denmark (Fig. 290-1) and other Scandinavian countries. Many U.S. hospitals have not implemented the aggressive surveillance approach because of the cost of both the microbiologic procedures and the requisite isolation gear.

Contact Isolation

Most major infection control guidelines for multiply resistant organisms recommend some kind of isolation for patients who harbor these organisms; the category of isolation most frequently used is contact isolation. In studies in which contact isolation has been used as part of a program designed to limit the spread of resistant pathogens, the overall approach has been reasonably effective. One report described a 16-fold reduction in MRSA transmission associated with the use of contact precautions. However, as previously discussed, contact isolation has typically been implemented concurrently with other (usually several) infection control measures. Therefore, determining the benefits of any single intervention is often not possible. Using contact isolation as an infection control strategy does have the potential for unintended, adverse consequences. Some recent studies have found that isolated patients were more likely to experience adverse events during their hospitalizations and were less likely to have narrative notes from physicians or nurses in their charts. Additionally, isolated patients in this study were substantially more likely than controls to experience failure of supportive care, including falls, pressure ulcers, and fluid and electrolyte imbalances. Because these adverse outcomes appear to be due to changes in health care worker activities and behavior, health care personnel must make a conscious effort to ensure that their patients in isolation receive the same level of care as those who are not in isolation. Similarly, the potential benefits associated with the use of isolation in an attempt to limit spread of resistant pathogens must be evaluated in the context of the potential adverse impact on patient care.

Antibiotic Cycling

Antibiotic cycling—that is, rotating or cycling the use of different antimicrobials or antimicrobial combinations over time—has been advocated as a possible approach to limiting resistance in health care institutions. To date, the data are quite limited and somewhat contradictory about this approach. Furthermore, this approach has been studied only in the ICU setting and may not be generalizable throughout the health care institution. In short, the verdict is not yet in concerning the relative efficacy of this approach.

Combinations of Strategies

Based on mathematical modeling, strategies that might be expected to be effective in preventing or reducing the prevalence of resistant bacteria in hospitals include reducing antibiotic use, decreasing the length of hospital stays (i.e., increasing patient turnover), and instituting infection control measures to disrupt the spread of bacteria. These infection control measures include restriction of contact between patients and health care workers carrying resistant bacteria, improved hand hygiene, and the use of personal protective equipment (e.g., gloves, masks, protective eyewear or face shields, and gowns). These models also suggest that an important byproduct of these interventions is that interdictions that reduce transmission of all bacteria within a hospital will disproportionately reduce the prevalence of colonization with resistant bacteria. These interventional strategies based on mathematical models need to be subjected to empirical testing to confirm their veracity and utility in clinical settings.

At a more pragmatic level, educating the staff about the epidemiology, pathogenesis, and general routes of transmission of resistant bacteria within the hospital environment, as well as the role that antibiotic use plays in the emergence and spread of bacterial resistance, is of paramount importance. Staff knowledge is required both to understand the rationale for interventions and to encourage compliance with infection control measures.

● CATEGORIES OF HEALTH CARE–ASSOCIATED INFECTIONS

Urinary Tract Infections

Nosocomial urinary tract infection usually follows instrumentation of the urinary tract, most often with a catheter. Infection occurs in about 1% of individuals who undergo a single in-and-out catheterization. For patients who have an indwelling urinary catheter, the risk for infection remains relatively constant at about 3 to 6% per catheter day (higher for female than for male patients and increased by manipulation of the catheter). After 10 to 14 days, about half of catheterized patients have bacteriuria. Thus, infection develops at some point in virtually all patients who have long-dwelling urinary catheters. Because enteric flora are the usual cause of urinary tract infection and because diarrhea predisposes to contamination of the catheter-urethra interface, diarrhea is an independent risk factor for catheter-associated urinary tract infection. Urinary tract infections (Chapter 292) account for between 30 and 40% of all health care–associated infections.

According to data from the CDC's NHSN, the pathogens most frequently responsible for health care–associated, catheter-associated urinary tract infections are (in order of decreasing relative frequency) *Escherichia coli*, *Candida* species, *Enterococcus* species, *Pseudomonas aeruginosa*, *Klebsiella pneumoniae*, *Enterobacter* species, coagulase-negative staphylococci, *S. aureus*, *Acinetobacter baumannii*, and *Klebsiella oxytoca*. Recommended measures for the prevention of catheter-associated urinary tract infections include the use of indwelling urinary catheters only for appropriate indications and durations, aseptic insertion and maintenance techniques, securing the catheter, and keeping the collection system below the level of the bladder. Device technology that has been associated with preventing catheter-associated urinary tract infections includes closed drainage systems and antiseptic-impregnated (e.g., silver alloy) urinary catheters.

Pneumonia

Infection of the pulmonary parenchyma can occur after the aspiration of either microbe-laden secretions from the upper respiratory tract or regurgitated gastric contents. Infection at a distant site in the body, such as *S. aureus* infection of a central venous catheter or an arteriovenous fistula used for hemodialysis, can sometimes result in hematogenously spread septic pulmonary emboli, which in turn can produce infection in the pulmonary parenchyma (often with a radiographically distinct pattern of multiple diffuse expanding pneumatoceles throughout the lungs). Another rare source of health care–associated pneumonia is direct inhalation of a microbe from the air. Examples of microbes that usually cause pneumonia by inhalation include *M. tuberculosis* (Chapter 332) and *Aspergillus fumigatus* (Chapter 347). Infection with the former occurs by contagion through small-particle droplet nuclei from a coughing patient. These droplet nuclei float in the air for hours and may infect patients several rooms away, although those closer to the coughing patient are at greater risk. Infection with *A. fumigatus* occurs by inhalation of its spores, which may be liberated from the surface of almost any organic material on which it can grow (e.g., an orange). These spores are virtually ubiquitous and may be present in both outdoor and indoor air.

Because of the increase in airborne fungal spores that can occur in association with construction and demolition activities, implementation of effective dust control measures when such projects are performed in health care facilities is needed to minimize the risk for nosocomial transmission of these pathogens. *Legionella* infection (Chapter 322) was originally thought to result from inhalation, but it may occur more frequently after the aspiration of *Legionella*-contaminated potable water. Viruses such as respiratory syncytial virus, parainfluenza virus, and adenovirus have also been described as causes of health care–associated pneumonia, particularly in severely immunocompromised patients.

Most patients who acquire nosocomial pneumonia have been maintained on mechanical ventilators in an ICU. The most frequent microbial agents causing ventilator-associated pneumonia, according to NHSN data, are *S. aureus*, *P. aeruginosa*, *Enterobacter* species, *Acinetobacter baumannii*, *K. pneumoniae*, and *E. coli* (in decreasing order of relative frequency). Rates of pneumonia in mechanically ventilated patients range from 6 to 30%, with a risk of 1 to 3% per day of intubation and mechanical ventilation. A number of factors influence the risk for nosocomial pneumonia in these patients. In a critically ill, supine, ventilated patient, oropharyngeal secretions pool in the oropharynx and subglottic space above the tracheal tube cuff and form a reservoir of contaminated secretions. These secretions often get aspirated into the pulmonary parenchyma along the endotracheal tube. Using a device that provides continual subglottic suction to prevent pooling of these secretions has been associated with lower rates of clinical aspiration and early ventilator-associated pneumonia (defined as pneumonia occurring within 3 to 5 days of intubation).

The inner lumen of an endotracheal tube rapidly becomes covered with a biofilm containing high concentrations of microorganisms. Pieces of this biofilm (carrying large numbers of bacteria) can be inoculated directly into the lower respiratory tract, either by ventilatory flow or by inserting devices through the tube (such as might occur during suctioning or therapeutic bronchoscopy). These pieces of biofilm can seed the pulmonary parenchyma with microorganisms and serve as a nidus for ongoing infection.

The use of either continuous or intermittent enteral feeding also increases gastric pH and, at least in some studies, has been associated with an 80% risk for gram-negative colonization of the stomach. Conversely, maintenance of adequate nutritional status is clearly associated with a reduced risk for ventilator-associated pneumonia, and enteral nutrition is clearly the route of choice for supplementing the nutritional status of these patients.

Abnormal elevation of gastric pH related to the patient's underlying disease or to the use of histamine-2 (H_2)-blockers, proton pump inhibitors, or antacid therapy is associated with an increased risk for infection because of the resulting microbial overgrowth in stomach fluids. When these fluids are regurgitated and aspirated, they may rapidly produce pneumonia because of the large bacterial inocula involved. Use of sucralfate, which does not affect gastric pH as substantially as H_2-blockers or proton pump inhibitors, to prevent stress ulceration during mechanical ventilation has been associated with lower rates of nosocomial pneumonia in some studies; however, other studies have suggested that this agent may not be as effective in preventing gastrointestinal bleeding as H_2-blockers.

Aspiration of gastric contents occurs four times more frequently when the patient is in the supine position than when the head of the patient's bed is elevated at a 45-degree angle. Studies have demonstrated that isolation of the same organisms from the stomach, pharynx, and endobronchial samples occurs extremely uncommonly in semirecumbent patients compared with patients placed in the supine position. Nonetheless, gastric reflux occurs frequently, irrespective of body position, in mechanically ventilated patients who have nasogastric tubes. Current recommendations for the prevention of ventilator-associated pneumonia include elevating the head of the bed 30 to 45 degrees unless medically contraindicated.

Selective digestive tract decontamination with antibiotics (e.g., swabbed onto the teeth as a paste or squirted into the stomach through a nasogastric tube, or both) has also been shown to result in significantly lower health care–associated pneumonia rates and mortality,[2] but this approach has not generally been used in the United States because of potential for the rapid development of antimicrobial resistance among the gut flora in these patients. However, good oral hygiene does help prevent health care–associated pneumonia without introducing the risk for antimicrobial resistance.

Surgical Site Infections

Historically, surgical site infection was almost inevitable because of the inhospitable environment in early hospitals. Today, the reverse is true for "clean," elective procedures (e.g., coronary bypass graft or total hip replacement). Most of these operations are not complicated by infection because of the use of strict aseptic technique (i.e., antiseptic preparation of the surgeon's hands and the patient's skin),**3** the use of sterile barriers (e.g., surgical gown and gloves), timely administration of prophylactic antibiotics before (and when appropriate, additional doses during) the procedure, and sterilization of surgical instruments used for the procedure. Despite these major improvements, infections still do occur. In the 21st century, the occurrence of these infections is most highly dependent on the technical skills of the surgeon and the presence of comorbid conditions in the patient who is undergoing the procedure.

The most frequent microbial pathogens causing surgical site infections (according to NHSN data) are, in decreasing order of relative frequency, *S. aureus*; coagulase-negative staphylococci; enterococci; gram-negative bacilli such as *E. coli*, *P. aeruginosa*, *Enterobacter* species, *Klebsiella* species, and *A. baumannii*; and *Candida* species.

Both surgery-related and patient-related factors contribute to the risk for surgical site infections. Despite equivalent provision of care and preventive measures, differences in postoperative infection rates can still occur for a variety of reasons. A higher prevalence of comorbid conditions in patients being referred for care (i.e., obesity, diabetes mellitus, severe peripheral vascular disease) inevitably results in higher surgical site infection rates. A variety of factors related to the technical aspects of surgery also influence the risk for infection. For example, the presence of dead space and the presence of dead tissue in the wound (e.g., as might occur through the excessive use of electrocautery) are both associated with an increased risk for infection. Other technical factors also influence this risk; for example, shaving to remove hair the day before the operation is associated with higher infection risk than is using clippers to remove hair within the hour before the operation.

The timing of antimicrobial prophylaxis is an important variable for surgical site infections. Making certain that agents with the appropriate antimicrobial spectrum are administered in time to ensure adequate blood levels of the drug or drugs at the time of scalpel entry into the skin and that adequate levels are maintained throughout the procedures is key to the success of perioperative prophylaxis. Antibiotics should be administered within 1 hour before incision to guarantee adequate serum levels. Recent studies suggest that, within this 1-hour period, administering antibiotics 30 to 60 minutes before the surgical incision may be associated with the lowest risk for surgical site infection. Antibiotics should be redosed if the procedure lasts longer than 4 hours. Finally, antibiotics administered for prophylaxis should not be continued for longer than 24 hours after the procedure and frequently are not required at all postoperatively.

Patients who have intrinsically contaminated wounds (e.g., a ruptured appendix) have a much higher risk for intra-abdominal infection, despite modern preventive measures, primarily because high-inoculum microbial exposure occurs and infection may already be established before surgery begins. Gut decontamination before surgery remains an important, effective option to reduce the risk for postoperative infection in some settings. For example, elective colon surgery after appropriate antimicrobial prophylaxis and mechanical cleansing is associated with much lower infection rates.

Serum glucose control has also been shown to decrease the risk for surgical site infections. Other strategies for the prevention of surgical site infections for which some evidence exists include maintenance of normothermia during surgery, screening for *S. aureus* colonization before surgery with decolonization therapy provided to identified carriers,**4** and preoperative bathing or showering with an antiseptic soap (e.g., chlorhexidine). Most of these approaches, however, have not yet been included in published guidelines or have been recommended for use only in certain procedures owing to the absence of definitive evidence of their effectiveness. Finally, surgical infection rates can also be reduced by providing information about postoperative infectious complications to the surgeons.

Blood Stream Infections

Blood stream infections may result from primary infection within the cardiovascular system (e.g., from an infected vascular catheter) or may be secondary to a local infection in another organ (e.g., *E. coli* infection of the urinary tract). Approximately 80% of health care–associated blood stream infections are primary, and the overwhelming preponderance of them are due to vascular catheter infections. Approximately 20% are secondary to infections in other organs. According to NHSN data, the most frequent microbial causes of primary blood stream infection in hospitalized patients with central venous catheters are (in decreasing order of frequency) coagulase-negative staphylococci, enterococci, *Candida* species, *S. aureus*, and gram-negative bacilli such as *K. pneumoniae* and *Enterobacter* species. Although coagulase-negative staphylococci definitely do cause such infections, a large proportion of blood cultures growing this organism actually represent contamination and not true infection. By contrast, *S. aureus* and *Candida* species are more virulent and associated with a much higher probability of true blood stream infection.

Microorganisms can reach the circulation through three separate pathways associated with the use of intravascular catheters. They can colonize the catheter insertion site and subsequently move along the catheter through the tissues; they can colonize hubs, junctions, and other connectors and gain access to the system when these sites are manipulated and through intrinsic or extrinsic contamination of the infusion fluid.

Catheter-related blood stream infection most frequently begins with colonization of the catheter. Because vascular catheters are usually placed through the patient's skin, most such colonizing microbes come from the patient's resident skin flora. Studies using electron microscopy have shown that microbial contamination of catheters is virtually universal from the first day after insertion. Organisms migrate from skin along the insertion tract by capillary action. Colonization often occurs at time of insertion but may also take place days afterward. Initially, organisms colonize along the external surface of the catheter. By contrast, after 10 days of placement, ultrastructural studies demonstrate an increasing relative frequency of intraluminal contamination, and most long-term catheters appear to become colonized and produce blood stream infection by the intraluminal route. Colonization is facilitated by the formation of a fibrin sheath around the catheter as a result of platelet deposition and is also facilitated by organism-produced biofilm.

The reason that all vascular catheters do not uniformly result in clinical infection relates to the body's innate immune response and its ability to kill microbial invaders and limit their growth and spread. Because most colonizing and infecting flora come from the patient's skin, use of antiseptics to prepare the site before catheter insertion and every few days thereafter to decrease the microbial burden has been a successful strategy for decreasing the risk for infection. In several clinical trials, chlorhexidine gluconate skin preparation has been shown to reduce the risk for catheter colonization significantly when compared with alcohol or povidone-iodine preparation of the skin. Although most such trials were designed to have statistical power only to be able to detect a reduction in catheter colonization, two of the studies demonstrated significant reductions in catheter-related blood stream infections as well. The use of maximal barriers to create a large sterile field during catheter insertion has also been shown to decrease the risk for infection.

A number of other factors, such as the type of dressing, the composition of the catheter, the number of lumens, and the type of intravenous administration system used, all influence the risk for catheter-associated primary blood stream infection. Either cotton gauze dressings covered by tape or semipermeable transparent membrane dressings can be used to protect the insertion site; however, the cutaneous microbial burden increases substantially underneath the semipermeable dressing. Conversely, the semipermeable dressing requires less frequent changes and manipulations and anchors the device in place more securely than gauze and tape dressing. These two types of dressings have been shown to be equivalent with respect to infection rate and local complications. Again, preparation of the site with chlorhexidine gluconate during dressing changes also decreases the infection rate. However, gauze dressings may be preferable if the insertion site is oozing. Use of chlorhexidine-impregnated dressings at the catheter-insertion site has been associated with reduced catheter-associated infection rates.**5** Several catheter characteristics or properties have been suggested to be associated with an increased risk for catheter-associated infection. For example, catheters made of stiff materials traumatize the vascular endothelium and move around in the insertion site—both facilitating colonization. Larger-bore catheters are also probably associated with increased risk for colonization and infection. Finally, the manner in which catheters are used may influence the risk for infection. In critically ill patients, for example, pulmonary artery catheters are frequently repositioned to obtain accurate readings (increasing local endothelial trauma, as well as the likelihood for catheter colonization).

Health care–related factors also contribute to the risk for catheter-associated primary blood stream infection. For example, antimicrobial therapy may alter the patient's skin flora, thereby facilitating colonization with an aggressive pathogen. Furthermore, health care workers who do not practice appropriate hand hygiene may inadvertently colonize a patient's catheter insertion site with health care–associated pathogens (e.g., MRSA). Manipulating the intravascular delivery system (e.g., to reposition the catheter, obtain a blood sample, administer medications) also increases the likelihood of catheter colonization. Techniques used for insertion and maintenance of catheters likewise influence the risk for infection. Inserting central venous catheters with less than maximal sterile barriers increases the risk for infection. The site chosen for insertion of a central venous catheter also influences the risk; insertion into the femoral vein is associated with a greater risk for colonization and infection than is insertion into either the subclavian or internal jugular vein. Although guidelines from the Healthcare Infection Control Practices Advisory Committee have recently recommended the subclavian route of insertion over the internal jugular approach, the data that support this recommendation are quite limited, and the risk for mechanical complications associated with insertion at each of these two sites must be considered for each patient.

One approach to attempt to reduce the risk for catheter-associated infections has been to bond antimicrobial substances (antiseptics or antibiotic agents) to the catheter. A catheter impregnated with antiseptic (chlorhexidine-silver sulfadiazine) reduced both colonization and blood stream infection by nearly 50%. Antibiotic-coated catheters (e.g., minocycline-rifampin-coated catheters) may be associated with even greater risk reduction. Minocycline-rifampin catheters are coated on both the internal and external surfaces of the catheters, whereas first-generation chlorhexidine–silver sulfadiazine catheters were coated only on their external surfaces. Compared with first-generation chlorhexidine–silver sulfadiazine, antibiotic-impregnated central venous catheters substantially reduced catheter-related blood stream infections in head-to-head comparisons. Second-generation chlorhexidine–silver sulfadiazine catheters are coated on both the internal and external surfaces but have not yet been compared with minocycline-rifampin catheters. Antimicrobial agent–coated catheters are associated with at least a theoretical risk for the development of antimicrobial resistance to the agents coating the catheters, although such resistance has not yet been documented in studies including hundreds of patients.

Recently, studies have demonstrated that the use of needleless administration systems also contributes to the risk for intravascular device–associated infections. When these devices were initially marketed, they had two primary goals—health care worker safety and device patency. They were not intended to reduce infection rates. Unfortunately, some recent studies suggest that these devices actually increase the risk for infection. The care and use practices of staff who are unfamiliar with these systems often do not follow the manufacturer's recommendations. Staff may not disinfect the device properly, or the device may be intrinsically difficult to disinfect. Nonetheless, several studies have documented increased risk for health care–related primary blood stream infections associated with the use of these devices.

Prevention of primary blood stream infections should be an important focus for all health care institutions. The Institute for Healthcare Improvement (IHI) has advocated bundling five infection prevention strategies—each of which is known to be independently effective—to prevent primary blood stream infections. The five techniques are effective hand hygiene; maximal barrier precautions at insertion; cutaneous antisepsis with chlorhexidine; optimal insertion site selection; and daily review of the necessity for maintaining the catheter, with prompt removal when it is no longer needed. Recently, the Joint Commission, formerly known as the Joint Commission on Accreditation of Healthcare Organizations (JCAHO), has adopted the IHI recommendation and requires implementation of these five strategies as a standard for continued accreditation.

Other Nosocomial Infections

During a national study of nosocomial infections conducted by the CDC in the 1970s, only about 6% of recognized infections did not involve the four main body sites listed earlier (see Table 290-1); currently, about 25% of all infections acquired in hospitals conducting hospital-wide surveillance are of this miscellaneous type. This category includes gastrointestinal infections caused by organisms such as C. difficile, rotavirus, and Salmonella species; viral infections caused by varicella, influenza, and respiratory syncytial virus; and candidal infections of the mouth, esophagus, and vagina. C. difficile–associated diarrhea and enterocolitis are of particular concern because of the emergence of a new, highly virulent strain associated with epidemic spread in the United States. This strain, which was previously quite uncommon, has variations in its toxin genes and is distinguishable, at least in part, by its increased resistance to fluoroquinolones. The highly virulent strain has emerged as an increasingly common cause of health care–associated epidemics.

INFECTION CONTROL PROGRAMS

Formal infection control programs did not exist in most hospitals until the 1970s. These programs were introduced into U.S. hospitals at that time, based on recommendations from the CDC, the American Hospital Association (AHA), and JCAHO. The primary rationale for the creation of these programs was to attempt to control antibiotic-resistant infections, which had soared out of control in most hospitals during the 1950s and 1960s.

As hospitals began to implement such programs, the CDC conducted a national study of the effectiveness of these efforts, titled the Study of the Efficacy of Nosocomial Infection Control (SENIC). The largest study of infection control ever conducted, SENIC used a probability sample of general hospitals nationwide, determined nosocomial infection rates, and assessed predictors in multivariate analysis. The size and intensity of work by the infection control program were found to predict infection rates. The most important predictors of success in decreasing health care–associated infection rates were (in decreasing order of importance) the intensity of surveillance, the intensity of control measures, the ratio of infection control practitioners to number of patient beds, the presence of a trained hospital epidemiologist on staff, and provision of surgical site infection rates to surgeons. The most effective programs (i.e., those with all these predictors) experienced a 32% relative reduction in the nosocomial infection rate compared with hospitals that did not have infection control programs.

Although programs vary from institution to institution, depending on the needs and resources available, most programs share certain essential functions, among which are surveillance for health care–associated infections; investigation of outbreaks, problematic trends, or distinctive or unusual infections; and education of staff about the epidemiology, pathogenesis, and prevention of health care–associated infections. In addition, hospital epidemiology programs work closely with other professionals in the health care setting who share similar interests. Specifically, infection control programs routinely form working partnerships with the clinical medical and nursing staffs, the infectious diseases service, the occupational medicine service, clinical microbiology, and the hospital safety program. The work of each of these services is complementary to the hospital epidemiology program. Communication among these groups is essential for success of the program.

The most likely reason that surveillance for nosocomial infections was important in SENIC is straightforward. By understanding what is happening microbiologically in an institution, specific control measures can be fashioned to intervene and thereby limit outbreaks and reduce high endemic rates of infection.

Initially, many hospitals implemented continual hospital-wide surveillance. Because some infections appeared to be more important than others in analyses from the SENIC database in terms of prolongation of stay and extra cost, and because interhospital comparison of crude hospital rates was thought to be difficult given the differences in severity of underlying illness in patients admitted to hospitals of different types in different regions, some authorities advocated targeted surveillance programs with a focus on the most significant problems for each hospital. Even though such a strategy does allow an institution to focus its efforts on its most pressing problem, the strategy may also cause institutions to overlook significant problems. For instance, outbreaks in ICUs may be missed for months in hospitals targeting only surgical site infections.

Infection control programs in U.S. hospitals today are often underfunded and understaffed. A consensus report from the CDC, Joint Commission, AHA, and a variety of other agencies and national societies concluded that infection control is more difficult in the hospital now than it was during the 1970s and 1980s when SENIC was conducted. That consensus report also concluded that more than one infection control practitioner per every 250 hospital beds (the ratio found to be essential by SENIC) is needed to do an effective job of controlling infections. This report has had limited impact, however, because many hospitals continue to reduce support for infection control activities, and others are now requiring infection control personnel to work on other adverse effects associated with health care, thus again increasing the infection control program workload without increasing program resources.

OCCUPATIONAL AND NOSOCOMIAL INFECTIONS IN HEALTH CARE WORKERS

Nosocomial infection can affect health care workers as well as patients. Health care workers in facilities that pay limited attention to the rising prevalence of colonization of patients with antibiotic-resistant pathogens are more likely to become colonized at a higher rate than the general population. Casually contagious viral infections such as influenza, varicella, rubella, and measles occur more frequently in health care workers because they are exposed to sick people in the community as well as to patients who are not always recognized and placed on appropriate isolation precautions. Several infectious diseases are worthy of more detailed consideration with respect to occupational exposure and infection, among which are hepatitis B, hepatitis C, HIV, and tuberculosis.

Occupational Risk for Human Immunodeficiency Virus Infection

The risk for acquiring HIV infection from a patient in the health care setting is small (Chapter 395). Fewer than 75 documented occupational infections with HIV have occurred in more than 5 million health care workers in the United States during the nearly three decades since acquired immunodeficiency syndrome (AIDS) and HIV entered the health care workplace. The routine use of universal or standard infection control precautions, development and implementation of safer devices and other engineered controls, and education and training of staff have all contributed to additional risk reduction.

A multinational case-control study conducted by the CDC and collaborators showed that deep percutaneous injuries, visibly bloody sharp instruments, devices that had been used in blood vessels, and exposure to source patients who had end-stage HIV disease (i.e., who died within 2 months after exposure—presumably a surrogate marker for high viral burden) were independent predictors of HIV transmission. In this study, administration of postexposure antiretroviral chemoprophylaxis with zidovudine was associated with an almost 80% relative reduction in the risk for infection in multivariate analysis. This finding led to a U.S. Public Health Service recommendation for the routine administration of postexposure chemoprophylaxis after occupational exposure to HIV. The CDC updates its recommended guidelines for the use of postexposure antiretroviral prophylaxis periodically.

Because the long-term consequences of taking antiretroviral agents for a month are unknown, and because significant adverse effects such as nausea, vomiting, and diarrhea develop in more than 70% of health care workers who take these agents for postexposure prophylaxis, they should not be administered casually or unnecessarily. Institutions should have defined protocols for determining whether an exposure has occurred, for encouraging reporting of exposures, and for facilitating access to antiretroviral agents when they are needed.

Occupational Risk for Hepatitis

Before development of the hepatitis B vaccine, hepatitis B (Chapter 150) represented the largest occupational risk to health care providers who were exposed to blood in the health care workplace. Standard precautions and OSHA requirements to offer free hepatitis B vaccine to health care workers have resulted in a dramatic decrease in hepatitis B infection in health care workers. However, approximately 10% of those vaccinated do not respond to vaccine, and some workers decline to be vaccinated because of concerns about side effects. Studies have shown the vaccine to be safe, and compliance has probably increased with dissemination of this information.

No vaccine is available as yet for hepatitis C (Chapter 150), the most common blood-borne viral infection and the most frequent indication for severe chronic liver disease requiring liver transplantation in the United States. An open trial of early interferon therapy for acute hepatitis C virus infection, as well as a National Institutes of Health consensus conference, documented higher cure rates for patients treated for acute hepatitis C than had been demonstrated for the treatment of established chronic infection. Although no formal recommendations have been issued for the management of health care workers who sustain occupational exposure to hepatitis C, one approach is to monitor the health care worker by polymerase chain reaction for hepatitis C virus RNA. Those who become PCR positive are then monitored for a brief period to make certain that the PCR findings are reproducible and to see whether individuals can clear their infections immunologically (which is thought to occur in as many as 50% of cases). Those who do not clear their infections spontaneously can be treated for acute hepatitis infection as described earlier.

Occupational Risk for Tuberculosis

Rates of tuberculosis (Chapter 332) in the United States declined for more than a century, and this decline was accelerated in the 1950s in association with the discovery and clinical use of effective antituberculous therapy. In 1985, tuberculosis rates once again began to increase and continued to do so until 1992. Epidemiologic analysis of the increase suggested that increased immigration of persons with tuberculosis and the expanding pool of immunocompromised patients produced by the HIV epidemic were the two predominant factors influencing this increase. The increase in case rates was compounded by a simultaneous, marked increase in resistance to antituberculous agents among isolates during this period.

Both these factors contributed substantially to health care–associated tuberculosis outbreaks in New York, New Jersey, and Florida. Major factors contributing to these outbreaks included (1) inadequate administrative controls (e.g., index of suspicion for the diagnosis, policies for placing patients in appropriate isolation, policies requiring that isolation patients remain in isolation), (2) inadequate engineering controls (i.e., lack of appropriate negative-pressure ventilation rooms for the isolation of patients with possible or known tuberculosis), and (3) inadequate use of personal protective equipment (e.g., respirators). These outbreaks resulted in the development of new CDC recommendations and OSHA requirements mandating administrative and engineering controls, as well as a program of respirator fit testing, annual or semiannual purified protein derivative testing, and regular retraining regarding tuberculosis. Tuberculosis case rates and health care–associated spread of tuberculosis were controlled before these guidelines were issued, thus leaving the question of the relative importance of respirators and respirator fit testing to the overall tuberculosis control effort in health care institutions unanswered. Since 1992, the rate of tuberculosis has steadily decreased in the United States, and nosocomial outbreaks have been reported much less frequently.

 Visit expertconsult.com for e-expanded chapter

Grade A

1. Meddings J, Rogers MA, Macy M, et al. Systematic review and meta-analysis: reminder systems to reduce catheter-associated urinary tract infections and urinary catheter use in hospitalized patients. *Clin Infect Dis.* 2010;51:550.
2. de Smet AM, Kluytmans JA, Cooper BS, et al. Decontamination of the digestive tract and oropharynx in ICU patients. *N Engl J Med.* 2009;360:20-31.
3. Darouiche RO, Wall MJ Jr, Itani KM, et al. Chlorhexidine-alcohol versus povidone-iodine for surgical-site antisepsis. *N Engl J Med.* 2010;362:18-26.
4. Bode LG, Kluytmans JA, Wertheim HF, et al. Preventing surgical-site infections in nasal carriers of *Staphylococcus aureus*. *N Engl J Med.* 2010;362:9-17.
5. Timsit JF, Schwebel C, Bouadma L, et al. Chlorhexidine-impregnated sponges and less frequent dressing changes for prevention of catheter-related infections in critically ill adults: a randomized controlled trial. *JAMA.* 2009;301:1231-1241.

SUGGESTED READINGS

Alangaden GJ. Nosocomial fungal infections: epidemiology, infection control, and prevention. *Infect Dis Clin North Am.* 2011;25:201-225. *Comprehensive review.*

Edwards JR, Peterson KD, Banerjee S, et al. National Healthcare Safety Network (NHSN) report: data summary for 2006 through 2008, issued December 2009. *Am J Infect Control.* 2009;37:783-805. *A summary of health care–associated infection data reported by hospitals in the United States.*

Goff DA. Antimicrobial stewardship: bridging the gap between quality care and cost. *Curr Opin Infect Dis.* 2011 Feb;24(Suppl 1):S11-S20. *Emphasizes what works and what may not work.*

Huskins WC, Huckabee CM, O'Grady NP, et al. Intervention to reduce transmission of resistant bacteria in intensive care. *N Engl J Med.* 2011;364:1407-1418. *In a cluster-randomized study, surveillance and barrier precautions did not reduce MRSA infections.*

Jain R, Kralovic SM, Evans ME, et al. Veterans Affairs initiative to prevent methicillin-resistant *Staphylococcus aureus* infections. *N Engl J Med.* 2011;364:1419-1430. *Strict surveillance and precautionary protocols can reduce MRSA infections.*

Peleg AY, Hooper DC. Hospital-acquired infections due to gram-negative bacteria. *N Engl J Med.* 2010;362:1804-1813. *Review.*

Rebmann T, Greene LR. Preventing catheter-associated urinary tract infections: an executive summary of the Association for Professionals in Infection Control and Epidemiology, Inc, Elimination Guide. *Am J Infect Control.* 2010;38:644-664. *Executive summary of consensus guidelines.*

Toth NR, Chambers RM, Davis SL. Implementation of a care bundle for antimicrobial stewardship. *Am J Health Syst Pharm.* 2010;67:746-749. *An antimicrobial stewardship program was associated with an increased rate of appropriate de-escalation of empirical antimicrobial therapy and improved compliance with quality indicators.*

291

APPROACH TO THE PATIENT WITH SUSPECTED ENTERIC INFECTION

HERBERT L. DUPONT

EPIDEMIOLOGY

Enteric infections are second only to respiratory tract infections as common medical problems. In certain populations, enteric infections are hyperendemic: poorly nourished infants living in developing tropical countries showing excessive rates of mortality; infants in certain daycare centers; unhygienic residents of custodial institutions for the mentally retarded; immunosuppressed persons; and visitors from industrialized areas to developing regions with traveler's diarrhea.

ETIOLOGY

In approaching a patient with an enteric infection, epidemiologic (Table 291-1) and clinical features (Table 291-2) are used to identify the type of etiologic agent responsible for illness and to develop a plan for evaluation (Table 291-3) and management (Table 291-4).

Recent travel (Chapter 294) to mountainous regions or recreational lakes of North America should raise the suspicion of infection caused by *Giardia* species. Travel to Russia, particularly St. Petersburg, is associated with an increased risk for infection by *Cryptosporidium* and *Giardia* species because there the protozoa can be found in drinking water. When diarrhea occurs during or after travel to a developing tropical region, a bacterial enteropathogen should be suspected. The leading causes of traveler's diarrhea worldwide are the diarrheogenic *Escherichia coli*: enterotoxigenic *E. coli* (ETEC) and enteroaggregative *E. coli* (EAEC). The invasive bacteria (*Shigella*, *Salmonella*, and *Campylobacter* species) cause diarrhea among travelers to all regions but are more common in Asia. Infection with *Cyclospora* species should be suspected when persistent or recurrent diarrhea follows travel to Nepal, Haiti, or Peru (travel-related infections are discussed in detail in Chapter 294).

A specific food or water vehicle cannot be suspected unless multiple cases of illness with a common exposure occur. All too frequently, persons assume the last food consumed before an illness onset is responsible for the symptoms. The highly variable incubation period for diarrheal disease, which may be as short as 2 hours after eating a food, for preformed toxins, to a week or even longer for microbial enteropathogens, makes the determination of a specific food or beverage in a single case of illness impossible. When an outbreak of diarrhea results in multiple cases, a category of etiology often can be determined by calculating the incubation period after looking at timing of the common exposure. Short incubation periods are associated with food poisoning associated with enterotoxins (2 to 7 hours for cases caused by *Staphylococcus aureus*, 2 to 4 hours for *Bacillus cereus* enterotoxin food poisoning). Longer incubation periods (usually 12 to 48 hours) are associated with most cases of intestinal infection.

The clinical expression of diarrheal illness will give clues to the etiologic agent (see Table 291-2). In the patient with diarrhea who is receiving or

TABLE 291-1 EPIDEMIOLOGIC FEATURES IMPORTANT IN DETERMINING POTENTIAL CAUSE OF ENTERIC INFECTION IN A PERSON OR PERSONS WITH DIARRHEA

EPIDEMIOLOGIC FEATURE	ETIOLOGIC AGENT TO SUSPECT
Travel to mountainous areas of North America	*Giardia* spp
Travel to Russia (especially St. Petersburg)	*Cryptosporidium, Giardia* spp
Travel to Nepal	*Cyclospora* spp
Travel to the developing tropical/semitropical world from an industrialized region	Enterotoxigenic *Escherichia coli*, enteroaggregative *E. coli*; *Shigella, Campylobacter, Salmonella* spp.; other bacterial causes; *Giardia, Cyclospora, Cryptosporidium* spp and noroviruses
Presence of associated cases (an outbreak)	Use incubation period and clinical features to determine probable cause
Antibiotic, chemotherapy, or proton pump inhibitor use in the past 2 months, particularly with a history of recent or current hospitalization	*Clostridium difficile*
Contact with day care centers	Any enteropathogen, often the low-dose organisms: *Giardia, Cryptosporidium, Shigella* spp or viral pathogens
Homosexual person practicing unprotected sex	Any organism spread by fecal-oral route; in those with proctitis, suspect *Neisseria gonorrhoeae, Chlamydia trachomatis,* herpes simplex, or *Treponema palladium*
Immunosuppressed person	Any agent, especially *Cryptosporidium, Cyclospora, Isospora, Shigella,* and *Salmonella* spp, *C. jejuni, C. difficile, Mycobacterium avium-intracellulare,* microsporidia, herpes simplex virus, and cytomegalovirus
Recent or current cruise ship travel	Norovirus

TABLE 291-2 CLINICAL FEATURES OF ENTERIC INFECTION

CLINICAL SYNDROME	ETIOLOGIC AGENTS SUSPECTED	SPECIAL CONSIDERATIONS
Sustained fever, often with systemic toxicity (enteric or typhoid fever)	*Salmonella typhi,* nontyphoid *Salmonella* spp, *Campylobacter* spp, *Shigella* spp, *Yersinia enterocolitica*	Stool and blood cultures; empirical antibiotics generally indicated
Acute watery (secretory) diarrhea	Any agent. Consider *Vibrio cholerae* (if water losses are major), enterotoxigenic or enteroaggregative *Escherichia coli, Shigella* spp, *Salmonella* spp, *Campylobacter jejuni,* viral or parasitic protozoal pathogen	Fluid and electrolyte therapy crucial for recovery in dehydration
Recurrent vomiting (gastroenteritis)	Viral agents (rotavirus or noroviruses) or preformed toxin (*Staphylococcus aureus* or *Bacillus cereus*)	In case of an outbreak, incubation period suggests the etiology
Bloody diarrhea (dysentery)	*Shigella* spp, *C. jejuni, Salmonella* spp, Shiga toxin–producing *E. coli* (e.g., O157:H7 or other serotype) or invasive *E. coli, Aeromonas hydrophilia,* noncholera *Vibrio* spp, *Yersinia enterocolitica, Entamoeba histolytica,* or inflammatory bowel disease	Stool culture and occasionally parasite examination important to determining cause; hemolytic-uremic syndrome may complicate diarrheal disease caused by Shiga toxin–producing *E. coli* or rarely *Shigella dysenteriae*
Diarrhea lasting ≥2 wk (persistent diarrhea)	*Giardia* spp and other protozoal parasites, bacterial overgrowth, bacterial diarrhea, lactase deficiency, Brainerd diarrhea, postinfectious irritable bowel syndrome (PI-IBS), unmasked inflammatory bowel disease (IBD), or celiac sprue	Stool culture and parasite exam indicated; empirical anti-*Giardia* therapy may be useful; remove milk from diet; raw milk or untreated (well or surface) water consumption or international travel may predispose to Brainerd diarrhea; illness not responding to antimicrobial therapy suggests the possibility of Brainerd diarrhea, PI-IBS, or IBD

recently has completed a course of an antimicrobial drug, a proton pump inhibitor, or an anticancer drug, particularly with recent or current hospitalization, *Clostridium difficile* (Chapter 304) should be suspected. An increasing number of cases of *C. difficile* diarrhea are occurring in the community. When a person has close contact with an infant or infants attending a daycare center, a number of low-dose pathogens found in this setting (e.g., *Giardia, Cryptosporidium,* or *Shigella* species or viral pathogens) should be suspected. Some homosexuals may show high rates of enteric infection acquired through fecal-oral contamination, often associated with infection by multiple pathogens or through the practice of unprotected receptive anal intercourse leading to proctitis due to sexually transmitted organisms. When persons experience advanced acquired immunodeficiency syndrome (AIDS) or other forms of severe immunodeficiency associated with metastatic malignancy or chronic use of immunosuppressive drugs, depressed intestinal immunity may lead to enteric infection with a variety of parasitic, bacterial, or viral pathogens (see Table 291-1) (Chapter 397).

Enteric infection syndromes may be divided into at least five groups based on the clinical presentation: (1) febrile systemic disease (enteric fever); (2) acute watery diarrhea (secretory diarrhea); (3) recurrent vomiting as the primary manifestation of enteric disease (gastroenteritis); (4) passage of many small-volume stools containing blood and mucus (dysentery); and (5) diarrhea lasting 2 weeks or longer (persistent diarrhea). Table 291-2 lists the major syndromes along with the expected cause.

Noroviruses (Chapter 388) have become the major cause of foodborne gastroenteritis and the most commonly identified cause of waterborne enteric disease in the United States. *Campylobacter* species (Chapter 311) is the most common reportable bacterial enteropathogen in industrialized countries and is the most important definable cause of Guillain-Barré syndrome (Chapter 428), often resulting in severe disease requiring assisted ventilation, intensive care unit confinement, and permanent neurologic sequelae. *E. coli* O157:H7 and other Shiga toxin–producing *E. coli* (Chapter 312) are important causes of food-borne and waterborne colitis complicated

TABLE 291-3   LABORATORY TESTS AND PROCEDURES USEFUL IN THE DIAGNOSIS OF INFECTIOUS DIARRHEA

SPECIFIC TEST OR PROCEDURE	WHEN INDICATED	CLINICAL SIGNIFICANCE
Fecal leukocyte test	For moderate to severe cases	When present, indicates diffuse colonic inflammation, often due to *Shigella, Salmonella, Campylobacter* spp, Shiga toxin–producing *Escherichia coli*, or *Clostridium difficile*
Fecal lactoferrin	For moderate to severe cases to help identify inflammatory forms of enteric infection, to use in health care–associated diarrhea to help determine whether *C. difficile* toxin test should be performed	More sensitive test than fecal leukocytes and will pick up less striking degrees of inflammation seen in enteroaggregative *E. coli* (EAEC) and *C. difficile* diarrhea
C. difficile toxins A and B	Diarrhea associated with use of antibiotics, chemotherapy, or proton pump inhibitors, especially associated with current or recent hospitalization	Most sensitive tests are culture, tissue culture assay, and polymerase chain reaction; most specific tests are enzyme immunoassay for toxins A and B; a two-step procedure can be used: sensitive but nonspecific *C. difficile* glutamate dehydrogenase antigen test followed by toxin assay
Stool culture for *Shigella, Salmonella,* and *Campylobacter* spp	Moderate to severe diarrhea and when stools are positive for inflammatory markers or contain gross blood and mucus (dysentery)	The three principal invasive bacteria are the only ones routinely sought by most laboratories.
Specialized stool culture for *Vibrios* spp and *E. coli* O157:H7 and other Shiga toxin–producing *E. coli*	For cases of profuse watery diarrhea in cholera-endemic areas or in outbreaks of diarrhea especially associated with dysenteric illness	Cholera cases may need aggressive fluid therapy. Outbreaks of dysenteric diarrhea should be evaluated for Shiga toxin–producing *E. coli.*
Parasite examination: (1) trichome stain; (2) acid-fast stain for *Cyclospora* or *Cryptosporidium* spp; or (3) enzyme immunoassay (EIA) for *Giardia* spp, *Cryptosporidium* spp, and/or *Entamoeba histolytica*	In any patient with persistent diarrhea and when diarrhea follows visits to mountainous or recreational lakes in North America, Nepal, Haiti, Peru, or Russia (particularly St. Petersburg)	If microscopic evaluation is performed, experience of the laboratory personnel is important. The commercially available EIA tests are sensitive.
Esophagogastroduodenoscopy and flexible sigmoidoscopy	Persistent diarrhea in patients without evidence of cause of illness	Identified cause of diarrhea is treated; without diagnosis, subjects may be treated symptomatically.

TABLE 291-4   THERAPY AND PREVENTION OF INFECTIOUS DIARRHEA

THERAPEUTIC OPTION	INDICATION	PHARMACOLOGIC AGENT
Oral fluid and electrolyte therapy	For infants, elderly patients, and anyone with profuse watery diarrhea	Soups, soft drinks, and saltine crackers are sufficient; formal oral replacement therapy may be needed with dehydrating forms of diarrhea
Diet	In all forms of diarrhea to facilitate enterocyte renewal and recovery	Soups and broth, saltine crackers, steamed vegetables, baked or broiled meats
Nonspecific therapy	For temporary (≤48 hr) control of diarrhea in older children and adults without evidence of severe diarrhea caused by an invasive or inflammatory bacterial or parasitic pathogen	Loperamide is the most effective symptomatic treatment and will decrease number of stools passed by 60%; bismuth subsalicylate is much less effective and will reduce number of stools by 40%; new antisecretory agents are being developed
Empirical antibacterial drugs	Enteric fever with toxicity Febrile dysenteric diarrhea Traveler's diarrhea	Fluoroquinolones for 7-10 days Azithromycin for 3 days Rifaximin for 3 days, fluoroquinolone or azithromycin for 1-3 days
Specific antibacterial therapy	Shigellosis, campylobacteriosis, cholera	See Chapters 310, 311, and 317
Antiparasitic drugs	Giardiasis, amebiasis, cryptosporidiosis, cyclosporiasis,	See Chapters 358, 359, and 361
Prophylaxis in traveler's diarrhea	Persons traveling to developing areas on tight schedules, those with history of prior traveler's diarrhea, persons with unstable underlying medical disorders, and those interested in prophylaxis	Rifaximin, 200 mg twice daily with meals, while in a high-risk region

by hemolytic-uremic syndrome in children and occasionally in elderly people.

DIAGNOSIS
Laboratory Findings

Laboratory tests (Fig. 291-1; see Table 291-3) can be useful and are of particular value in the more severely ill patients when subjects are forced by their illness to alter activities or are totally disabled and confined to bed, or when many patients are afflicted during an outbreak. In each of these situations, the laboratory may help establish cause and allow development of a proper plan of treatment (see Table 291-3). Useful laboratory tests include procedures looking for fecal inflammatory markers such as microscopic detection of fecal leukocytes or the more sensitive, commercially available test, fecal lactoferrin. These tests are particularly helpful to suggest the presence of the invasive bacterial pathogens, *Shigella*, *Salmonella*, and *Campylobacter* species or the noninvasive but inflammatory *C. difficile*. Stool culture is performed in more severe cases of sporadic diarrhea and in disease outbreaks and is carried out with blood culture in a patient with fever and systemic toxicity. Other indications for stool culture are presence of dysentery (passage of grossly bloody stools) and when fecal inflammatory markers are found. In dysenteric diarrhea, particularly in the presence of an outbreak, the laboratory should also be instructed to look for *E. coli* O157:H7 and other Shiga toxin–producing *E. coli*. Parasite examination is indicated by diarrhea and persistent ($\geq$14 days) illness; a recent trip to Nepal, Haiti, Peru, or Russia; evidence the subject practices oral-anal sex or unprotected receptive anal intercourse; or associated immunosuppression. Other tests are indicated in special situations, including stool culture for *Vibrio cholerae* in a patient with severe watery diarrhea with excessive fluid losses in a cholera-endemic area and culture for *Mycobacterium avium-intracellulare*, herpes simplex virus, and cytomegalovirus in those with immunosuppression. For patients with persistent diarrhea without etiologic diagnosis when routine tests are employed, endoscopy (esophagogastroduodenoscopy and flexible sigmoidoscopy, or colonoscopy) may be indicated in attempting to determine the nature and cause of illness.

TABLE 291-5   NONINFECTIOUS CAUSES OF DIARRHEA

Running	Small bowel bacterial overgrowth
Fecal impaction	Systemic mastocytosis and eosinophilic
Drugs and laxatives	gastroenteritis
Enteral feeding	Tropical sprue
Irradiation	Celiac sprue
Pancreatic insufficiency	Dermatitis herpetiformis
Intestinal lymphangiectasia	Whipple's disease
Foods (especially dietetic)	Thyrotoxicosis
Cirrhosis and biliary obstruction	Adrenal insufficiency
Diabetic diarrhea	Factitious
Alcoholism	Inflammatory bowel disease
Collagenous colitis	Food allergy
VIPoma	Carcinoid
Ischemic bowel disease	Villous adenoma
Irritable bowel syndrome	Stress with autonomic stimulation

TREATMENT   Rx

Treatment of diarrhea should be tailored to the clinical syndrome. Oral rehydration with fluids and electrolytes is used to treat acute watery diarrhea and gastroenteritis and all forms of enteric infection complicated with any degree of dehydration. ORT is particularly important in infants; it can be life-saving in developing countries for infants with severe diarrhea. Patients with diarrhea should be fed easily digestible foods to facilitate enterocyte renewal and to speed up disease recovery. In afebrile, nondysenteric diarrhea, symptomatic drugs may allow older children and adults with illness to return earlier to school or work. Loperamide is the most active drug for improvement of

FIGURE 291-1. Laboratory tests to diagnose cause of diarrhea. **A,** Dysenteric stool. **B,** Stool culture and biochemical tests confirm *Salmonella.* **C,** *Giardia* trophozoites. **D,** Many leukocytes in diffuse colonic inflammation.

FIGURE 291-1, cont'd. **E,** *Entamoeba histolytica* trophozoite with ingested red blood cells. **F,** Oocysts of *Cryptosporidium* (*left*) and *Cyclospora* (*right*). (From the CDC Public Health Information Library. http://phil.cdc.gov/phil/home.asp: images 7829 and 7827.)

symptoms. Bismuth subsalicylate can reduce diarrhea and is mildly effective in reducing nausea and vomiting associated with viral gastroenteritis.

For enteric fever, febrile dysenteric disease, and moderate to severe cases of traveler's diarrhea, empirical antimicrobial therapy is indicated (see Table 291-4). For outbreaks of dysenteric diarrhea, particularly in children in whom fever is not significant, antibacterial and antimotility drugs should be initially withheld while the etiology of the outbreak is being established in order to prevent patients infected by Shiga toxin–producing *E. coli* from being predisposed to hemolytic-uremic syndrome. For bacterial and parasitic pathogen-specific diarrhea, antimicrobial therapy is often advised (see other chapters in the text for specific treatments). Because of the importance of diarrhea when persons travel from industrialized regions to developing countries, prophylaxis with the orally administered, poorly absorbed rifaximin can be employed for some groups (see Table 291-4), with expected protection rates exceeding 70%.

In sporadic cases of acute or persistent diarrhea, infectious agents are not always responsible. Table 291-5 offers a partial list of the noninfectious causes of diarrhea that should be considered.

SUGGESTED READINGS

DuPont HL. Clinical practice: bacterial diarrhea. *N Engl J Med.* 2009;361:1560-1569. *The article is a recent clinical review of the causes and recommended therapy of pathogen-specific acute diarrhea and provides estimates for the number of cases of each seen in the United States on an annual basis.*

Eckardt AJ, Baumgart DC. Viral gastroenteritis in adults. *Recent Pat Antiinfect Drug Discov.* 2011;6:54-63. *Review emphasizing noroviruses, astroviruses, and rotaviruses.*

Sherman PM, Ossa JC, Wine E. Bacterial infections: new and emerging enteric pathogens. *Curr Opin Gastroenterol.* 2010;26:1-4. *Concise review focusing on enterohemorrhagic* Escherichia coli *O157:H7 and* Campylobacter jejuni *infections.*

292

APPROACH TO THE PATIENT WITH URINARY TRACT INFECTION

S. RAGNAR NORRBY

DEFINITION

This chapter addresses bacterial and fungal infections of the normally sterile urine, including asymptomatic bacteriuria, cystitis, pyelonephritis, and urosepsis (dissemination of microorganisms from the urine to blood). Urethritis caused by *Chlamydia trachomatis, Ureaplasma urealyticum* (Chapter 293), or *Neisseria gonorrhoeae* (Chapter 307); prostatitis (Chapter 131); and renal tuberculosis (Chapter 332) are addressed elsewhere in this text.

In the 1950s, Kass studied patients with or without bacterial colonization of the bladder urine. He defined *significant bacteriuria* as 10^5 or more colony-forming units (CFUs; where 1 CFU is one or more bacterial cells forming a colony when growing on an agar plate) per milliliter in two consecutive samples of midstream urine (i.e., urine obtained during voiding, discarding the first and last urine portions). Since then, *significant bacteriuria* has been redefined to optimize the sensitivity and specificity of diagnostic tests. In women with symptoms of uncomplicated cystitis, significant bacteriuria is now defined as 10^2 or more CFU/mL midstream urine plus pyuria (≥ 5

leukocytes/mm^3 of urine). In women with uncomplicated pyelonephritis and men with urinary tract infections (UTIs), significant bacteriuria is defined as 10^4 CFU/mL plus pyuria. In patients with complicated UTIs, the definition is 10^5 or more CFU/mL with or without pyuria.

CLASSIFICATION

It is clinically important to classify UTIs by type of infection, presence or absence of symptoms, tendency to recur, and presence or absence of complicating factors (Table 292-1). Recurrent infections can be subdivided into reinfections caused by new bacterial strains and relapses caused by the same strains that caused preceding infections. Complicating factors are host factors facilitating the establishment and maintenance of bacteriuria or worsening the prognosis of UTIs engaging the kidneys. The most common ones are listed in Table 292-2.

EPIDEMIOLOGY

Worldwide, at least 150 million cases of symptomatic UTIs occur each year. Because many UTI patients have recurrent infections, the number of individuals who have UTIs each year is lower than the number of cases.

In general, 90% of patients have cystitis and 10% have pyelonephritis. The infections are sporadic in about 75% of patients and recurrent in 25%. About 2% have complicated infections related to factors that increase the risk of the establishment and maintenance of bacteriuria. These patients typically have frequently recurring UTIs. If factors that can increase the severity of a renal infection are included, the frequency of complicated infections is about 8%.

UTIs are somewhat more common in very young boys than in very young girls because of the higher frequency of urethral malformations in boys. Later in childhood, symptomatic UTIs are more common in girls, who are also more likely to have asymptomatic bacteriuria. In most cases, this is due to the short urethra, but it may also be the result of sexual abuse. Symptomatic UTIs are most common in sexually active women. In young men, bacterial UTIs are rare and are often the result of underlying infections of the prostate. In elderly people, both symptomatic UTIs and asymptomatic bacteriuria are common. In women, this is often the result of an atrophic vaginal mucosa, whereas in men, it is often a consequence of prostate hyperplasia or prostate cancer.

UTI is also the most common type of hospital-acquired infection because of the frequent use of bladder catheters.

PATHOBIOLOGY

In a majority of patients, UTIs are the result of colonization of the urine with fecal bacteria, which grow aerobically. Growth of anaerobic bacteria, such as *Bacteroides fragilis*, in the urine indicates a communication between the intestines and the urinary tract. This is seen in rare cases of fistulas between the intestines and the renal tract and following reconstructive surgery in the urinary tract, which involves the intestines. Growth of fungi in the urine may be seen in patients with bladder catheters and in immunocompromised patients with hematologic dissemination of *Candida* species from infections at other sites.

In women, bacteria colonize the periurethral area; from there, they reach the distal part of the urethra. Atrophic vaginal mucosa with altered vaginal flora after menopause and the use of diaphragms and spermicides in sexually active women are factors that increase the risk of colonization with large numbers of uropathogenic bacteria. Sexual intercourse results in increased numbers of bacteria in the periurethral area of the vagina and the distal part of the urethra, increasing the risk of bacteriuria.

In the normal male urethra, the distance between the end of the urethra and the bladder is too long to allow ascending transport of bacteria to the bladder. Therefore, bacteriuria in men should always be considered an abnormal finding, and men cannot have uncomplicated infections. However, transport of bacteria to the bladder urine through the male urethra is possible when there is turbulent urine flow, such as with a stricture or obstruction of the urethra, as a result of prostatic hyperplasia, and when the patient has a bladder catheter.

The female urethra is short and allows transport of bacteria to the bladder in healthy individuals. With many uropathogens, such transport is facilitated by adherence of the bacteria to urethral epithelial cells. Bacterial cells, such as *Escherichia coli* strains causing uncomplicated pyelonephritis, have fimbriae that adhere to α-D-Gal-4-β-D-Gal receptors (the P blood group) on the mucosal cells in the urethra and the ureters, thus facilitating the establishment of bacteriuria and further transport to the kidneys. Such adhesion

TABLE 292-1	CLASSIFICATION OF URINARY TRACT INFECTIONS
Type of UTI	Cystitis
	Pyelonephritis
	Asymptomatic bacteriuria
Symptoms	Symptomatic
	Asymptomatic
Recurrences	Sporadic (≤1 UTI/6 mo and ≤2 UTIs/yr)
	Recurrent (≥2 UTIs/6 mo or ≥3 UTIs/yr)
	Relapse
	Reinfection
Complicating factors	Uncomplicated
	Complicated (see text)

UTI = urinary tract infection.

TABLE 292-2	HOST FACTORS COMPLICATING BACTERIURIA
OUTCOME	**FACTORS**
Facilitated establishment and maintenance of bacteriuria	Residual bladder urine after voiding
	Physiologic
	Neurogenic bladder
	Prostate hyperplasia/tumor
	Turbulent urethral urine flow
	Strictures
	Foreign bodies
	Catheters
	Calculi
	Tumors
	Atrophic vaginal mucosa after menopause
	Vesicoureteral reflux
	Anatomic defects
	Pregnancy
Worse prognosis of urinary tract infections involving the kidneys	Childhood pyelonephritis
	Diabetic nephropathy
	Malignant hypertension
	Chronic pyelonephritis

stimulates mucosal cells to release cytokines such as interleukin-6, which causes fever and increases C-reactive protein, and interleukin-8, which mobilizes leukocytes. Individuals who lack the receptors for bacterial adhesion (those who do not have the P blood group) are less likely to have acute pyelonephritis. In patients with complicated UTIs, bacterial adhesion seems to be of less importance. The role of other bacterial virulence factors, such as the O and K antigens of *E. coli*, in the pathogenesis of UTIs is less well known.

When bacteria have reached the bladder, the establishment of bacteriuria is facilitated by incomplete bladder emptying. Even with residual urine volumes as low as 10 mL, which are not uncommon in healthy individuals, bacterial growth in the urine may be established. Pyelonephritis results from ascending bacteriuria from the bladder through the ureter to the renal pelvis and the renal parenchyma. This transport may be facilitated by host factors such as anatomic defects of the ureters or the kidneys, vesicoureteral reflux, or, in patients without anatomic defects, adhesion to the ureter mucosa. About one third of patients with pyelonephritis are also bacteremic.

In rare cases, bacteriuria and funguria may result from the hematogenous dissemination of bacteria to the kidneys, causing a renal abscess. The primary focus of the infection is usually an infection at a site outside the renal tract, such as endocarditis.

Patients with asymptomatic bacteriuria frequently harbor organisms that are less virulent than those causing symptomatic infections. Such organisms are often killed by normal human plasma or serum ("serum bactericidal effect"). Patients with persistent asymptomatic bacteriuria may be protected from symptomatic UTIs by large numbers (≥10^6 CFU/mL) of less virulent bacteria in the urine. However, in pregnant women and in patients with type

2 diabetes, asymptomatic bacteriuria is a strong predictor of subsequent symptomatic infection. Pyelonephritis is common during pregnancy because vesicoureteral reflux often occurs during the second and third trimesters. In children and adults, asymptomatic bacteriuria may be a sign of underlying urinary tract malformations.

Bladder catheterization leads to bacteriuria or funguria in all patients who have had their catheters for more than 1 week. Formation of a biofilm on the catheter surfaces facilitates the growth of microorganisms. Urosepsis, resulting from dissemination of bacteria from the urine to the blood in a patient with bacteriuria, is often the consequence of removing or changing a bladder catheter during the preceding 24 to 48 hours. This risk is further increased if the catheter has been in place for more than 1 week and the softener in the plastic material of the catheter is eluted, rendering the catheter stiff. The urethral mucosa may also be damaged by crystals that form on the catheter surface.

ETIOLOGY

The microbiologic etiology of a UTI depends on several factors. Table 292-3 summarizes the most common findings. In all types of UTI, *E. coli* is the dominating bacterial species, causing up to 85% of all symptomatic UTIs in women with community-acquired, sporadic, uncomplicated infections. In most countries, the second most common species causing such infections is *Staphylococcus saprophyticus,* which, at least in northern Europe, has a pronounced seasonal pattern, accounting for up to 40% of all uncomplicated cases of cystitis and pyelonephritis in July and August and virtually no infections in January and February. In patients with recurrent infections, species such as *Enterococcus faecalis, Enterococcus faecium, Klebsiella* species, *Proteus* species, *Providencia stuartii,* and *Morganella morganii* become more common. In patients with very frequent recurrences or with bladder catheters, especially in hospital and nursing home settings, where antimicrobials are frequently used, *Pseudomonas aeruginosa, Acinetobacter baumannii, Serratia marcescens,* and *Stenotrophomonas maltophilia* are important organisms. In such patients, *E. coli* accounts for less than 50% of infections. Findings of *Proteus mirabilis* or other *Proteus* species may indicate that the patient has renal calculi or a tumor because these organisms grow in an alkaline environment. Calculi in the renal pelvis, ureter, or bladder may also form as a result of the growth of ammonia-producing organisms such as *Proteus* species. Because *Proteus* species are common in the male preputial flora, the finding of such organisms in a voided urine sample from uncircumcised men or young boys could represent contamination and not bacteriuria.

CLINICAL MANIFESTATIONS

Typical symptoms of cystitis, pyelonephritis, and urosepsis are listed in Table 292-4. The onset of cystitis is rapid, and symptoms develop over less than 24 hours. Clinically, it is often impossible to differentiate between cystitis and urethritis caused by chlamydia, ureaplasma, or gonococci, especially when there is no urethral discharge. Fever is unusual among patients with cystitis. In sexually active women, cystitis commonly occurs 24 to 48 hours after intercourse, especially if the practice of postcoital bladder emptying has not been followed. Cystitis patients normally have symptoms for 3 to 5 days. Antimicrobial therapy does not markedly reduce the duration.

Pyelonephritis also has a rapid onset, with or without preceding cystitis symptoms. About one third of patients develop bacteremia. The typical flank pain, resulting from inflammation and edema of the renal parenchyma, may be masked by the intake of analgesic drugs such as acetaminophen, which may also reduce the fever. An important differential diagnosis is renal calculi, which may result in a similar location of the pain but characteristically do not cause fever. Also, patients with appendicitis and cholecystitis can present with flank pain similar to that in a patient with right-sided pyelonephritis.

Urosepsis is a life-threatening condition caused by dissemination of bacteria from the urine in a patient with bacteriuria. The most common reason for urosepsis is withdrawal (and sometimes insertion) of a bladder catheter. Thus, uroseptic patients do not always have a renal infection.

DIAGNOSIS

Laboratory Findings

The hallmark of the types of UTIs dealt with here is demonstration of bacteriuria in a urine sample that has been incubated in the bladder for at least 2 hours to allow the growth of bacteria. The most reliable result is obtained if the sample is taken by suprapubic aspiration, a technique frequently used in infants but rarely in older children and adults. It is superior to sampling by bladder catheterization, which carries about a 2% risk of introducing bacteria into the bladder and subsequently causing bacteriuria. The normal procedure for quantitative cultures is to collect a midstream urine sample. This requires the patient to be well informed about the sampling procedure. Men should withdraw the foreskin, and women should keep the labia apart. Washing of the genital tract before sampling is not recommended. During voiding, the first and last parts of the urine should not be sampled. After sampling, the urine should be chilled (but not frozen) to prevent growth during transportation to the laboratory. At the laboratory, the sample is streaked onto agar plates using a loop, which delivers a known amount of urine. The result is obtained after incubation overnight, providing a determination of the bacterial species present in the sample and the number of organisms per milliliter of urine. The presence of more than one species in a sample usually indicates defective sampling procedures and contamination.

A simplified quantitative urine culture can be obtained outside the microbiologic laboratory by using a dip slide. With that technique, a plastic slide

TABLE 292-3	MICROBIAL ETIOLOGY OF URINARY TRACT INFECTIONS
ORGANISMS	**CLINICAL CHARACTERISTICS**
GRAM-NEGATIVE BACTERIA	
Escherichia coli	Typical
Klebsiella pneumoniae	Often reinfection
Enterobacter spp	Often reinfection and/or health care–associated infection*
Proteus spp	May indicate tumor or calculi
Providencia stuartii	Often reinfection and/or health care–associated infection*
Morganella morganii	Often reinfection and/or health care–associated infection*
Serratia marcescens	Often health care–associated infection*
Acinetobacter baumannii	Often health care–associated infection*
Burkholderia spp	Often health care–associated infection*
Pseudomonas aeruginosa	Often health care–associated infection*
Stenotrophomonas maltophilia	Often health care–associated infection*
GRAM-POSITIVE BACTERIA	
Staphylococcus saprophyticus	Most common during summer
Staphylococcus aureus	May indicate focus outside the genitourinary tract
Enterococcus spp	Often reinfection
Other gram-positive bacteria	In most cases contaminants
FUNGI	
Candida spp	May indicate focus outside the genitourinary tract

*Includes hospital and nursing home care.

TABLE 292-4	CLINICAL SYMPTOMS OF URINARY TRACT INFECTIONS
TYPE OF URINARY TRACT INFECTION	**TYPICAL SYMPTOMS**
Cystitis	Frequent voiding Burning during and after voiding Suprapubic pain Hematuria and/or cloudy urine
Pyelonephritis	Fever Chills Flank pains Cystitis symptoms (may be absent)
Urosepsis	Fever Chills Septic shock

with agar media on both surfaces is dipped in the urine sample, or the urine sample is poured over the slide's surfaces. After overnight incubation at room temperature or in a simple incubator, the culture allows highly reliable quantification of bacteriuria. Because gram-negative, but not gram-positive, bacteria grow on both sides of the slide, the method also allows quick classification. However, if a determination of the species or the antimicrobial sensitivity pattern is required, the dip slide must be transported to a regular laboratory. The dip slide is most suitable for use in outpatient settings, especially when laboratories are unavailable locally.

All culture techniques require overnight incubation. For screening of bacteriuria, a nitrite test can be used. It is a stick test that demonstrates the presence of nitrite in the urine. Gram-negative bacteria, with the exception of *P. aeruginosa*, metabolize nitrate to nitrite, which can be demonstrated by a color reaction on a paper stick. Gram-positive bacteria and fungi do not metabolize nitrate. The technique is rapid (<1 minute) and inexpensive. It has a high degree of specificity but is rather insensitive because it does not detect infections caused by gram-positive organisms. Thus, it is not suitable for use in patients with recurrent infections (in whom an enterococcal cause is common) or when the frequency of *S. saprophyticus* infection is high.

Pyuria should be demonstrated in patients with UTIs. This is best done by staining uncentrifuged urine and counting leukocytes in a Bürker chamber. The second best technique is to use a leukocyte esterase stick test, which is highly sensitive and allows a crude quantification of pyuria. The technique of counting leukocytes in the sediment obtained after centrifugation of a urine sample was once used routinely, but it is imprecise and is not recommended. Persistent pyuria with negative routine bacteriologic cultures should lead to the suspicion of renal tuberculosis, and a sample should be obtained for direct microscopy and culture for *Mycobacterium tuberculosis* (Chapter 332).

Blood cultures should be obtained in all patients with suspected pyelonephritis or urosepsis. It is recommended that at least two cultures be obtained.

Imaging

Radiography and ultrasound examination are normally not helpful in the acute phase of suspected pyelonephritis unless there is suspicion of a blockage of the urine flow, which may indicate formation of a renal abscess. When the patient has recovered, such investigations are recommended in those with recurrent infections to exclude complicating factors. Normally, a simple pyelography or ultrasound examination is performed. For the diagnosis of vesicoureteral reflux, special radiographic techniques are used.

Differential Diagnosis

Although clinical manifestations should lead to a relatively clear differentiation of acute cystitis and acute pyelonephritis, it is often difficult to diagnose the latter. Laboratory tests may offer some help and should be used. Patients with acute pyelonephritis, but not those with acute cystitis, have increased levels of C-reactive protein in blood. That acute phase parameter increases rapidly in patients with acute pyelonephritis. It is also a useful test for determining response to therapy and diagnosing recurrences. The erythrocyte sedimentation rate is a less useful test because it takes several days to increase in a patient with acute pyelonephritis. In patients with acute pyelonephritis, leukocyte casts can often be demonstrated in urine sediment. When a patient has become afebrile, the diagnosis of acute pyelonephritis can be supported by testing urine osmolality, which is markedly reduced for at least 1 month after the onset of symptoms. Although not routinely indicated, the osmolality of urine is checked in a sample obtained after 12 hours of fasting and no fluid intake or 1 to 8 hours after intramuscular or subcutaneous injection of a small dose of desmopressin, a vasopressin analogue. Urine osmolality in individuals with normal renal concentrating ability is 850 to 1000 mOsm/L and varies with age. Demonstration of antibody-coated bacteria in the urine is neither sensitive nor specific for diagnosing pyelonephritis and is no longer recommended.

TREATMENT   Rx

All symptomatic UTIs should be treated. The purpose of early treatment of cystitis is to reduce the risk of progression to pyelonephritis. Treatment does not affect the duration of symptoms, which is 3 to 4 days. In patients with pyelonephritis, early treatment is important to reduce the duration of symptoms, eliminate microorganisms from the renal parenchyma, and reduce the risk of dissemination to the blood.

Because verifying the microbial etiology and determining the susceptibility to antimicrobial drugs take at least 1 day and often more than 2 days, initial treatment is empirical. The best guide is the antimicrobial susceptibility pattern of organisms obtained from comparable patients. For example, if the patient is a woman with sporadic, uncomplicated cystitis or pyelonephritis, antimicrobial susceptibility patterns generated from outpatients with sporadic UTIs are the appropriate reference. If the patient is hospitalized and has hospital-associated pyelonephritis, susceptibility patterns generated from samples collected in the hospital, preferably in the department or ward where the patient acquired the infection, are the appropriate reference. Large national or international surveillance studies have limited value when choosing antimicrobial treatments for individual patients. Susceptibility patterns developed from large reference laboratories may overestimate antimicrobial resistance because patients with uncomplicated infections are less likely to have cultures. However, there has recently been a marked increase of multidrug-resistant bacteria causing UTIs. Examples of such organisms are *E. coli* and *Klebsiella* species producing extended-spectrum β-lactamases and vancomycin-resistant enterococci. Due to this trend, the use of urine cultures and antibiotic resistance tests in patients with UTIs is recommended. Should multidrug resistance be demonstrated, the choice of antibiotics depends on resistance patterns.

Cystitis

Table 292-5 lists possible choices for the antimicrobial treatment of cystitis. Ideally, the antimicrobial should be excreted renally to achieve high concentrations in the renal parenchyma and in the urine. The safety profile is also important because cystitis is common and is associated with low mortality. The treatment time varies with the type of antimicrobial. Trimethoprim, trimethoprim-sulfamethoxazole, and fluoroquinolones are effective treatments,[1] even in pregnant women,[2] because they reduce uropathogenic bacteria in the periurethral flora and the fecal flora; a 3-day course is recommended. β-Lactam antimicrobials and nitrofurantoin generally have shorter elimination times and do not affect the periurethral and fecal flora; treatment for 5 to 7 days is required to eliminate bacteriuria in most patients. Single-dose treatment is recommended only for a high dose of trimethoprim-sulfamethoxazole and for fosfomycin (which is licensed only for single-dose treatment). Although these single-dose regimens may seem preferable to treatment for several days, 3-day regimens seem to have the best acceptance among patients. When patients have recurrent or complicated cystitis, the treatment duration should be at least 7 days.

Fluoroquinolones are not recommended for routine use in sporadic cystitis, although many of them have well-documented efficacy when used at relatively low doses for 3 days or even as a high single dose. The reason is that widespread use in cystitis patients is likely to lead to overuse and the emergence of resistance.

Patients with frequently recurring cystitis can benefit from early self-treatment if they are well informed and compliant. If treatment is started very shortly after the onset of symptoms, a 3-day course or even a single dose of antimicrobial provides rapid relief of symptoms.

Pyelonephritis

For antimicrobial treatment of pyelonephritis, the primary decision is whether the patient needs initial treatment with a parenteral antimicrobial or whether oral treatment alone will suffice. Table 292-6 lists antimicrobials suitable for the treatment of pyelonephritis. Oral formulations of penicillins or cephalosporins should be used only after initial parenteral therapy. After initial treatment with a parenteral drug, a transition to oral treatment is normally possible after 24 to 48 hours unless the patient does not improve. The recommended treatment time is still 14 days, although recent information indicates that in patients with uncomplicated pyelonephritis, treatment for 7 days may suffice.

Only fluoroquinolones and trimethoprim-sulfamethoxazole can be used for initial oral treatment of pyelonephritis, if the patient's general condition allows it. Because both these alternatives are unsuitable for use in pregnant women, pyelonephritis during pregnancy should be treated with a parenteral antimicrobial, preferably a cephalosporin, followed by oral step-down therapy.

Bacteriuria

Bacteriuria in patients with catheters should not be treated unless the patient is febrile or has other evidence of systemic infection. Administration of antimicrobials to catheterized patients with asymptomatic bacteriuria inevitably results in multiresistant and difficult-to-treat organisms.

Urosepsis

In patients with suspected urosepsis, antimicrobial treatment must start as early as possible. Antimicrobials should be given intravenously, and those recommended for injectable treatment of pyelonephritis should be used. Previous antimicrobial treatment should always be ascertained in patients with urosepsis because such treatment may have resulted in resistant organisms. A relatively new cause of urosepsis is vancomycin-resistant enterococci (*E. faecium* or *E. faecalis*), which usually occurs in immunocompromised patients.

TABLE 292-5 ANTIMICROBIALS USED TO TREAT CYSTITIS

ANTIMICROBIAL	DOSE* AND DURATION
Trimethoprim	100-150 mg q12h for 3 days
Trimethoprim/sulfamethoxazole	80/400 mg q12h for 3 days or 320/1600 mg single dose
Nitrofurantoin	50 mg q8h for 5-7 days
Amoxicillin/clavulanic acid	250 mg (amoxicillin dose) q8h for 5-7 days
Cefuroxime axetil	250 mg q8h for 5-7 days
Cefpodoxime proxetil	200 mg q8h for 5-7 days
Cefixime	400 mg/day for 5-7 days
Ceftibuten	400 mg/day for 5-7 days
Cefprozil	250 mg/day for 5-7 days
Norfloxacin[†]	200 mg q12h for 7 days
Ciprofloxacin[†]	100 mg q12h for 7 days
Levofloxacin[†]	250 mg/day for 7 days
Fosfomycin	400 mg single dose

*Doses given are for adults with normal renal function. The need to reduce dosages because of renal impairment related to infection in the kidneys, other renal diseases, or advanced age should always be considered.
[†]Should be reserved for recurrent and/or complicated cystitis.

TABLE 292-6 ANTIMICROBIALS USED TO TREAT PYELONEPHRITIS

ROUTE OF ADMINISTRATION AND ANTIMICROBIAL	DOSE*	COMMENTS
INJECTABLE		
Cefepime	2 g q12h	Health care–associated infections[†]
Cefotaxime	1 g q12h	Community-acquired infections
Ceftazidime	1 g q12h	Health care–associated infections[†]
Ceftriaxone	2 g/day	Community-acquired infections
Cefuroxime	750 mg q8h	Community-acquired infections
Amikacin	15 mg/kg/day	Monitor renal function
Gentamicin	4.5 mg/kg/day	Monitor renal function
Netilmicin	4.5 mg/kg/day	Monitor renal function
Tobramycin	4.5 mg/kg/day	Monitor renal function
Ciprofloxacin	200 mg q12h	
Levofloxacin	250 mg/day	
Trimethoprim/ sulfamethoxazole	160/800 mg q12h	Community-acquired infections
ORAL		
Amoxicillin/clavulanic acid	500 mg (amoxicillin dose) q8h	Only step-down therapy
Cefuroxime axetil	250 mg q12h	Only step-down therapy
Cefpodoxime proxetil	200 mg q8h	Only step-down therapy
Cefixime	400 mg/day	Only step-down therapy
Ceftibuten	400 mg/day	Only step-down therapy
Cefprozil	250 mg/day	Only step-down therapy
Norfloxacin	400 mg q12h	
Ciprofloxacin	100 mg q12h	
Levofloxacin	250 mg/day	

*Doses given are for adults with normal renal function. The need to reduce dosages because of renal impairment related to infection in the kidneys, other renal diseases, or advanced age should always be considered.
[†]Includes hospital and nursing home care.

Funguria

Funguria can be treated with fluconazole 400 mg once daily for 1 day, followed by 200 mg once daily for 7 to 14 days. Funguria in catheterized patients should be treated only when there is a symptomatic UTI.

Follow-up

Patients with sporadic, uncomplicated cystitis do not require follow-up. Patients with symptomatic recurrences, pyelonephritis, or complicated UTI should be observed. Table 292-7 lists some examinations that may be considered. Follow-up cultures are important because bacteriuria may persist and cause renal damage in afebrile pyelonephritis patients. The decision process for upper (pyelonephritis) and lower (cystitis) UTIs appears in Table 292-8.

PREVENTION

There are well-known measures that markedly reduce the risk of UTI recurrence. The most important is for sexually active women to urinate shortly after sexual intercourse. In doing so, they wash out the increased number of bacteria in the distal urethra. Another useful suggestion is for patients with recurrent UTIs to practice double or triple voiding. This means that the patient should make an extra effort to empty the bladder at each urination, thus decreasing the volume of residual urine. Increased fluid intake was

TABLE 292-7 FOLLOW-UP PROCEDURES IN PATIENTS WITH URINARY TRACT INFECTIONS OTHER THAN SPORADIC CYSTITIS

PROCEDURE	RECOMMENDATION
Urine culture	All patients with pyelonephritis, complicated infections, or frequent recurrences; 4-5 days and 3-4 wk after treatment
Pyuria test	Always perform together with urine culture
C-reactive protein	4-5 days and 3-4 wk after treatment of pyelonephritis
Radiography or ultrasonography	After pyelonephritis to exclude scars from childhood infections in patients with recurrent infections and to exclude complications
Serum creatinine	Before treatment in elderly; 3-4 wk after treatment in patients with pyelonephritis
Urine osmolality	Verification of suspected pyelonephritis

TABLE 292-8 DECISION PROCESS FOR UPPER (PYELONEPHRITIS) AND LOWER (CYSTITIS) URINARY TRACT INFECTIONS

	CYSTITIS	PYELONEPHRITIS
SIGNS AND SYMPTOMS		
Fever	No	Yes
Dysuria	Yes	May be present
Frequency	Yes	May be present
Flank pain	No	Yes
DIAGNOSIS		
Pyuria	Yes	Yes
Nitrite test	Normally positive	Normally positive
Bacteriuria	Yes	Yes
C-reactive protein	Normal	Increased
Blood cultures	Negative	Positive in ≈30%
TREATMENT		
First line	Trimethoprim or trimethoprim-sulfamethoxazole for 3 days	Fluoroquinolone or trimethoprim-sulfamethoxazole for 2 wk orally
Second line	Fluoroquinolone for 3 days or cephalosporin for 5-7 days	Injectable cephalosporin until afebrile, followed by oral step-down for total of 2 wk
Pregnant women	Nitrofurantoin or cephalosporin for 5-7 days	Injectable cephalosporin until afebrile, followed by oral cephalosporin for 2 wk

previously advocated, probably because of the risk of crystalluria with older sulfonamides; however, there are no obvious benefits of excessive diuresis.

Today, antimicrobial prophylaxis of UTIs is restricted to just a few groups of patients. One group in which it is still recommended is pregnant women with asymptomatic bacteriuria. Thus, screening for bacteriuria at regular intervals during pregnancy is recommended. Another group in which screening of bacteriuria and prophylaxis have been proposed is patients with diabetes mellitus, especially those with type 2.

Cranberry products have been proposed for the prevention of recurrent UTIs. Analyses of studies suggest that these products might have a low preventive effect in young and middle-aged women, but the use of cranberries as prophylaxis of UTI is not recommended.

Prophylaxis is sometimes used in patients with frequently recurring UTIs, especially when there are no defined, treatable complications. In such patients, one daily dose of nitrofurantoin 50 to 100 mg or trimethoprim 150 to 200 mg, taken at bedtime, is recommended.

Antimicrobial prophylaxis should not be used in catheterized patients because it results in the selection of microbes resistant to the antimicrobial used.

In postmenopausal women with atrophic vaginal mucosa and recurrent symptomatic UTIs, replacement therapy with oral or vaginal estriol should be considered. Such treatment restores the normal premenopausal vaginal and periurethral microbial flora and reduces the incidence of symptomatic UTIs.

PROGNOSIS

The prognosis of uncomplicated cystitis and pyelonephritis is generally good unless urosepsis occurs. Secondary morbidity is rare.

In patients with complications such as renal scars from childhood pyelonephritis, chronic pyelonephritis or glomerulonephritis, or other chronic renal diseases, acute pyelonephritis may lead to a further reduction of renal function. As mentioned earlier, infections with *Proteus* species or other ammonia-producing organisms may lead to the formation of calculi or the worsening of existing ones.

Patients with urosepsis have a poor prognosis, with fatality rates of about 30% or higher. Factors increasing the risk of death are advanced age and underlying diseases, as well as inadequate antimicrobial treatment. It has been demonstrated that in patients with sepsis caused by gram-negative bacteria, the death rate increases drastically if the organisms are resistant to the empirical treatment given.

1. Zalmanovici Trestioreanu A, Green H, Paul M, et al. Antimicrobial agents for treating uncomplicated urinary tract infection in women. *Cochrane Database Syst Rev.* 2010;10:CD007182.
2. Vazquez JC, Abalos E. Treatments for symptomatic urinary tract infections during pregnancy. *Cochrane Database Syst Rev.* 2011;1:CD002256.

SUGGESTED READINGS

Barbosa-Cesnik C, Brown MB, Buxton M, et al. Cranberry juice fails to prevent recurrent urinary tract infection: results from a randomized placebo-controlled trial. *Clin Infect Dic.* 2011;52:23-30. *Cranberry juice twice daily did not decrease the incidence of a second UTI.*

Brown PD. Management of urinary tract infections associated with nephrolithiasis. *Curr Infect Dis Rep.* 2010;12:450-454. *Review with an emphasis on the high risk of infection with an antimicrobial-resistant pathogen.*

Chenoweth CE, Saint S. Urinary tract infections. *Infect Dis Clin North Am.* 2011;25:103-115. *Review with an emphasis on catheter-associated urinary tract infections.*

Gupta K, Hooton TM, Naber KG, et al. Executive summary: international clinical practice guidelines for the treatment of acute uncomplicated cystitis and pyelonephritis in women: a 2010 update by the Infectious Diseases Society of America and the European Society for Microbiology and Infectious Diseases. *Clin Infect Dis.* 2011;52:561-564. *Consensus guidelines.*

Swaminathan S, Alangaden GJ. Treatment of resistant enterococcal urinary tract infections. *Curr Infect Dis Rep.* 2010;12:455-464. *Potential parenteral agents include daptomycin, linezolid, and quinipristin-dalfopristin.*

293

APPROACH TO THE PATIENT WITH A SEXUALLY TRANSMITTED DISEASE

MYRON S. COHEN

SEXUALLY TRANSMITTED DISEASES

DEFINITION

Sexually transmitted diseases (STDs) include a wide variety of organisms that are transmitted through intimate contact involving skin and/or mucosal surfaces of the oropharynx, vagina, penis, and rectum. STDs can generally be divided into five broad categories (Table 293-1).

ETIOLOGY

The interaction between the host and the STD pathogen plays a critical role, and characteristic tissue changes offer exceptionally strong clues about etiology. Several STD pathogens cause local inflammation only (*Neisseria gonorrhoeae, Chlamydia trachomatis, Trichomonas vaginalis*), with the potential for local tissue invasion (*N. gonorrhoeae, C. trachomatis*) or systemic dissemination (*N. gonorrhoeae*). Some STD pathogens cause tissue ulceration (*Treponema pallidum, Haemophilus ducreyi*, herpes simplex viruses 1 and 2). Human papillomaviruses (HPVs) cause epithelial cell changes and predispose to neoplasm. And several STDs (human immunodeficiency virus [HIV], hepatitis B and C, cytomegalovirus) routinely use the genital tract for access without causing any local changes.

EPIDEMIOLOGY

STDs are among the most common infections worldwide, and most are never reported. Each year there are more than 9 million new STD infections among persons aged 15 to 24 years in the United States, and many infections are asymptomatic during the time they are transmissible. The incidence of syphilis declined in the 1990s, but since 2000, rates have been increasing among women (from 0.8 cases per 100,000 in 2004 to 1.5 cases per 100,000 in 2008) and men who have sex with men (from 3.0 cases per 100,000 in 2001 to 7.6 cases per 100,000 in 2008). Following years of decline, gonorrhea rates have been stable over the past 12 years (111.6 cases per 100,000 in 2008). Approximately 20% of the U.S. population is already infected with herpes simplex virus type 2 (HSV-2), and many newly acquired genital ulcers are now due to HSV-1. It is estimated that 26.8% of U.S. women aged 14 to 59 have had HPV infection (including high- and low-risk serotypes), and 5.6% of sexually active 14- to 59-year-old women have reported genital warts.

The spread of STDs depends on the organism and the host, the length of time an infected person remains contagious, and the number of people exposed. These parameters have been reduced to the following formula:

$$R_o = B \times D \times C$$

where R_o is the basic reproductive rate of an infection, or the mean number of secondary cases a typical single infected person will cause in a population; B is the efficiency of transmission; D is the duration of infectiousness; and C is the number of sexual partners.

PATHOGENESIS

The STD pathogens depend entirely on human-human transmission, although *T. vaginalis* may have some inanimate sources. The efficiency of transmission reflects the infectiousness of the host (which depends on the concentration and phenotype of the organism in the genital tract) and the susceptibility of the sexual partner (which reflects the resistance of the host and can be hereditary, acquired, or innate). Because immunity to STDs is rare, reinfections are common, and vaccine development has been difficult; the only STD vaccines available target hepatitis B and HPV.

STDs produce syndromes precisely because each pathogen has a proclivity for one or more tissues and (when symptomatic) can evoke a predictable inflammatory response. For example, gonococci that infect the male urethra generally produce an intense neutrophil response that leads to a purulent discharge and pain with urination, whereas *C. trachomatis* is less likely to

TABLE 293-1 SYNDROMES OF SEXUALLY TRANSMITTED DISEASES

SYNDROME	ORGANISM
Urethritis	
Gonococcal	*Neisseria gonorrhoeae*
Nongonococcal	*Chlamydia trachomatis*
	Trichomonas vaginalis
	Mycoplasma genitalium
	Ureaplasma urealyticum
	Herpes simplex (primary infection)
Genital Ulcers	
Syphilis	*Treponema pallidum*
Genital herpes	Herpes simplex
Chancroid	*Haemophilus ducreyi*
Epithelial Cell Infections	
Genital warts	Human papillomavirus
Molluscum	*Molluscum contagiosum*
Cervical neoplasia	Human papillomavirus types 16, 18
Female Genital Discharge	
Cervicitis	*Neisseria gonorrhoeae*
	Chlamydia trachomatis
	Trichomonas vaginalis
	Herpes simplex
Pelvic inflammatory disease	*Neisseria gonorrhoeae*
	Chlamydia trachomatis
Vaginitis	*Trichomonas vaginalis*
	Candida albicans
Bacterial vaginosis	*Gardnerella vaginalis*, anaerobes
Ectoparasites	
Pubic lice	*Phthirus pubis*
Scabies	*Sarcoptes scabiei*

TABLE 293-2 SYNDROMIC TREATMENT OF URETHRITIS

GONOCOCCAL*

Recommended

Ceftriaxone 250 mg injected intramuscularly once, or
Cefixime 400 mg orally (single dose)

NONGONOCOCCAL

Recommended

Azithromycin 1 g orally (single dose), or
Doxycycline 100 mg orally twice daily for 7 days

Alternative

Erythromycin base 500 mg orally four times daily for 7 days, or
Erythromycin ethylsuccinate 800 mg orally four times daily for 7 days, or
Ofloxacin 300 mg orally twice daily for 7 days, or
Levofloxacin 500 mg orally once a day for 7 days

*Uncomplicated anorectal and genital disease.

produce such a response in the same tissue and is more likely to produce a mild, watery discharge or no symptoms at all.

STDs serve as markers for sexual risk-taking behavior, and coinfections are common. The detection of an STD should lead to a variety of other (seemingly unrelated) tests. STD pathogens move together: gonorrhea and chlamydia cause urethritis; genital ulcers greatly increase the probability of HIV acquisition.

DIAGNOSIS AND TREATMENT

Syndromic Strategies

For a variety of common STD syndromes, treatment of the index case based on signs and symptoms is empirical, as is treatment of sexual partners. This approach reflects the facts that the diagnostic accuracy of some tests is imperfect, coinfection demands concomitant therapy that overrides the search for individual pathogens, and patients who are not treated immediately may not return for therapy. Empirical therapy is so successful that follow-up care ("proof of cure") is usually unnecessary.

The syndromic approach is particularly critical in resource-constrained countries or in areas of the United States where laboratory tests are not available or their cost is prohibitive. In the United States, concomitant microbiologic diagnosis is preferred because it (1) confirms the choice of empirical therapy or redirects subsequent care; (2) permits the detection and monitoring of resistance to treatment; and (3) enables specific diagnoses to be reported to public health authorities, which is required by state law for many STDs. However, even when laboratory tests are ordered, the most appropriate agents should be provided empirically at the point of care to resolve infection and to reduce the spread of STDs.

Relationship of STDs to HIV

Diagnosis of an STD demonstrates increased sexual risk-taking behavior and inconsistent condom use and serves as a marker for potential HIV infection.

Genital ulcers disrupt the epithelium and allow the entry of HIV, and inflammation recruits macrophages and lymphocytes, increasing the number of targets for HIV. Any patient undergoing evaluation or treatment for an STD should be tested for HIV. Early diagnosis of HIV has very great personal and public health benefits.

● SYNDROMES
Urethritis

Urethritis is characterized by some combination of urethral discharge and dysuria, but prostatitis can cause similar complaints. Urethritis is caused by a limited group of pathogens (see Table 293-1) that may be difficult to visualize microscopically or grow in culture. Accordingly, empirical therapy is provided to treat a spectrum of potentially causative organisms.

Urethritis is diagnosed when one or more of the following are demonstrated: (1) mucopurulent or purulent urethral discharge, (2) Gram stain of urethral secretions demonstrating 5 or more leukocytes per oil immersion microscopic field, (3) positive leukocyte esterase test on first-void urine, or (4) microscopic examination of first-void urine demonstrating 10 or more leukocytes per high-power field. If no discharge can be expressed from the urethral meatus, a calcium alginate swab can be inserted 5 mm into the urethra; the material collected is transferred to a slide by rolling the swab along the glass.

A Gram stain of urethral discharge is a simple and rapid diagnostic test to document both urethritis and gonococcal infection (Chapter 307), characterized by the detection of leukocytes containing intracellular gram-negative diplococci. Confirmation of gonococcal urethritis does not rule out concomitant infection with *Chlamydia* or *Mycoplasma*. As culture and Gram stain have become less popular or less available, nucleic acid amplification tests (NAATs) that are highly sensitive and specific for the detection of organisms have been used routinely. NAATs for gonorrhea, *Chlamydia*, and *Trichomonas* can be applied to first-voided urine samples (the meatus is intentionally not cleaned so that the urine is contaminated with these organisms) and/or urethral swab material. Specific diagnosis may enhance the management of sexual partners, and the results from such tests should be reported to the health department. However, in practice, patients and (in most cases) sexual partners must be treated before the results of these tests are available.

Treatment for urethritis should be initiated as soon as possible after the clinical diagnosis and should be directly observed if feasible (Table 293-2). *N. gonorrhoeae* (Chapter 307) has become resistant to many antimicrobials, including quinolones, so the choice of optimal therapies is limited.🔳 Dual therapy with azithromycin and ceftriaxone increases the cure rate of uncomplicated urogenital, anorectal, and pharyngeal gonorrhea. Azithromycin can also be expected to cure most causes of nongonococcal urethritis (NGU), including those caused by *Mycoplasma genitalium*, an increasingly recognized cause of NGU.🔳 *T. vaginalis*, which is susceptible to metronidazole or tinidazole, also causes urethritis and should be considered in the face of NGU treatment failure.

Women with urethritis present with some combination of dysuria and pyuria, which must be differentiated from bacterial cystitis. Because treatment for urinary tract pathogens may also resolve urethritis, the clinician treating a presumed bladder infection should consider an STD as well.

Genital Ulcers

In the United States, HSV-1 and HSV-2 (Chapter 382) and *T. pallidum* are responsible for virtually all the ulcers encountered, and HSV-1 and -2 are by far the most common cause.

GENITAL HERPES

Genital herpes usually develops after an incubation period of less than 21 days and arises as clustered vesicles on an erythematous base. The vesicles become pustular and then rupture to form shallow, painful ulcers, which may coalesce. The ulcers heal by crusting over, and the process is usually completed 2 to 3 weeks after the initial lesions. Recurrences proceed through the same stages but generally last only about 5 to 7 days. The first (incident) episode of HSV-2 may be accompanied by systemic signs and symptoms including fever and headache, the latter reflecting the spread of HSV to the central nervous system. About 20% of infected individuals manifest the classic presentation, 60% have mild and atypical signs and symptoms, and at least 20% are completely asymptomatic. Individuals who have acquired HSV-2 shed the virus approximately 3 to 4% of the time (even while asymptomatic), posing an ongoing risk to sexual partners.

SYPHILIS

The ulcerative lesion of syphilis (Chapter 327)—the chancre—is indurated and painless, and in many cases it escapes detection. Secondary syphilis results when the spirochetes spread systemically, leading to a characteristic rash, alopecia, oral mucous patches, or condyloma latum. These skin manifestations should prompt testing for syphilis. The serologic screening test of choice for syphilis is based on the formation of antibodies to cardiolipin, a constituent of the spirochetal cell wall (e.g., rapid plasma regain [RPR], Venereal Disease Research Laboratory [VDRL], TRUST tests). Confirmatory testing requires the search for an antitreponemal antibody (e.g., microhemagglutination assay–*T. pallidum* [MHA-TP], FTA-Ab). The anticardiolipin test provides a titer that must be used to monitor the response to treatment. Some larger commercial laboratories have reversed the order of testing, using an antitreponemal test followed by an anticardiolipin test, which allows automation and may be cost-effective in areas of low endemicity. Dark-field microscopy of ulcer scrapings suspended in normal saline or touch preparations of moist lesions reveals motile spirochetes. A patient who had a negative syphilis test in the past year and now has a positive test is said to have early latent syphilis. This patient may not recall any of the signs or symptoms of primary or secondary syphilis.

Later stages of syphilis may be identified only serologically or on pathologic specimens. Late latent syphilis and syphilis of unknown duration are managed similarly. Neurosyphilis can occur at any stage of infection and should be suspected in any patient with a positive serologic test who also has findings suggestive of nervous system involvement, including ocular and vestibular symptoms.

Worldwide, syphilis infection has been detected in a substantial number of people with recognized or unrecognized HIV infection, especially men who have sex with men. Accordingly, the diagnosis of syphilis requires HIV testing.

CHANCROID

Chancroid (Chapter 309), infection with *H. ducreyi*, produces ragged, dirty ulcers and tender inguinal lymphadenopathy, which may be fluctuant. Unlike the lesions of HSV, these genital ulcers are likely to vary in size.

Epithelial Cell Infections
HUMAN PAPILLOMAVIRUS

HPV infection (Chapter 381) is generally transient and asymptomatic, but some patients develop visible genital warts. These warts are painless, soft, moist, pink, or flesh-colored swellings that vary in shape and can be raised or flat, single or multiple, small or large, and sometimes cauliflower shaped. Warts occur in the vulva, vagina, and anus; on the cervix; and on the penis, scrotum, groin, or thigh. Genital warts are diagnosed by visual inspection. Treatment is primarily with topical agents but is generally not curative.

Two oncogenic HPV genotypes (16 and 18) are responsible for at least 85% of all cervical neoplasia, and HPV types 6 and 11 are responsible for most cases of genital warts. HPV vaccines are available that target these genotypes. Pap smears are recommended for sexually active women beginning at age 21 or 3 years after they become sexually active; the frequency of rescreening is influenced by normal examinations and risk factors.

Female Genital Discharge

Infections of the female genitourinary tract produce several syndromes with overlapping symptoms (dysuria, vaginal discharge, vulvar irritation), the cause of which can usually be established with a careful history, examination, and laboratory tests. The initial approach depends on the primary anatomic site of infection—urinary tract, endocervix, or vagina. The columnar epithelium of the endocervix is susceptible to infection with *N. gonorrhoeae*, *C. trachomatis*, and *T. vaginalis*, and the vagina is susceptible to infection with *Candida albicans*, *T. vaginalis*, and the syndrome of bacterial vaginosis. The cervix may appear completely normal in women with cervical infection, whereas mucopurulence at the cervical os or mucosal friability suggests infection. Vaginitis is associated with a visible discharge, and the characteristics of the vaginal fluid offer diagnostic clues.

Female genital discharge is a condition in which syndromic management strategies often lack sensitivity and specificity. In women with vaginal discharge, microscopic examination of a wet mount preparation substantially enhances the effectiveness of syndromic treatment.

BACTERIAL VAGINOSIS

Bacterial vaginosis (BV) is the most common cause of vaginal discharge in the United States. Affected women are often minimally symptomatic but may note mild vaginal discharge and vaginal odor (which is often increased after coitus). The normal vaginal flora contains hydrogen peroxide–producing lactobacilli such as *Lactobacillus crispatus* and *Lactobacillus jensenii*, which probably help "defend" the vagina against a number of pathogens (an example of innate immunity). *Lactobacillus acidophilus* is rarely found in the normal vagina, which explains the failure of yogurt to serve as a remedy or a preventive. BV begins with the unexplained disappearance of the normal vaginal flora and its replacement with *Gardnerella vaginalis* and many species of anaerobic bacteria. The precise mechanism causing this shift in vaginal flora is poorly understood. Most recently, previously unrecognized anaerobic bacterial species (BV-associated bacteria) have been described as causative and potentially transmissible. The discharge of BV is homogeneous and may contain bubbles. Vaginal pH is elevated above the normal 4.0 to 4.5. Adding 10% potassium hydroxide to the vaginal discharge on the microscope slide or to the discharge present in the extracted speculum elicits an amine-like, fishy odor, yielding a positive "whiff" test because of the elaboration of amines from the anaerobic flora. Examination of vaginal material as a wet mount reveals the absence of bacilli and their replacement with clumps of coccobacilli. Some vaginal epithelial cells are coated with coccobacilli, which may obscure their edges (clue cells) or the normally clear appearance of the cytoplasm. Relatively few polymorphonuclear leukocytes are observed; large numbers of leukocytes in the wet mount of a woman with BV suggest a coincident infection, possibly trichomoniasis or bacterial cervicitis.

BV is not necessarily a benign change in flora. It is associated with an increased rate of upper tract infection (endometritis, salpingitis) and, on occasion, with complications of pregnancy, including premature rupture of the membranes and preterm delivery. However, treating asymptomatic women with BV who are not at high risk for preterm delivery appears to confer no benefit. Women with BV appear to have increased risk for the acquisition of HIV. Treatment is generally directed against the anaerobic flora and consists of metronidazole or clindamycin for 7 days. A single oral dose of metronidazole is not recommended for BV because of the high failure rate. The BV relapse rate is about 30%, and treating male sexual partners offers no benefit.

CANDIDIASIS

Vulvovaginal candidiasis (Chapter 346) is common and is seen most frequently in women taking antibiotics or using oral contraceptives when endogenous *Candida* species outgrow normal bacterial flora. Women usually complain of vulvar itching and discomfort and may or may not notice an accompanying discharge. The vagina generally maintains normal numbers of lactobacilli, so the vaginal pH is usually normal; this is very helpful in discriminating between candidiasis and other vaginal infections. The labia and vaginal walls may be erythematous. Although classically described as "curdy," the discharge of candidiasis is frequently loose and is difficult to distinguish from other discharges. Vaginal material may be treated with 10% potassium hydroxide to destroy other cellular elements and make the fungi easier to observe. Wet mount, however, has a sensitivity of only about 50%, and a woman with a classic presentation should be treated even if fungal elements are not observed.

A wide range of topical antifungal medications are available (many without a prescription), and all these drugs are approximately equally effective, although the cure rate with some single-dose therapies appears to be lower than that with longer regimens. Fluconazole administered as a single oral dose of 150 mg is highly effective. Infection with yeasts other than *C. albicans* may require longer therapy. Recurrent vulvovaginal candidiasis is a problem for many women, and optimal management has not been defined. Recurrent infection should lead the clinician to consider underlying diabetes mellitus or HIV. Treatment of sexual partners of women with candidiasis confers no benefit.

Women with *T. vaginalis* infection complain of a purulent discharge and vulvar irritation. The vaginal walls are red, and the vagina may contain excessive yellow or green discharge displaying large bubbles. The ectocervix may also be inflamed or have punctate microhemorrhages, causing the pathognomonic "strawberry cervix" (colpitis macularis). Vaginal pH is elevated, but the whiff test is generally negative. Wet mount reveals large numbers of polymorphonuclear leukocytes as well as motile protozoa about the same size as the leukocytes, with visible flagellae; motile organisms may be recognized in about two thirds of cases. Therapy for trichomoniasis requires metronidazole or tinidazole, but resistant organisms are encountered with increasing frequency.

CERVICITIS

The diagnosis of cervicitis is suggested by tenderness on bimanual examination, visible inspection revealing inflammation, and/or discharge. The specific diagnosis can be made only by detecting microorganisms from the cervix. *N. gonorrhoeae* and *C. trachomatis* have tropism for cervical tissue, whereas other pathogens (including HIV) can apparently infect the vaginal tissues as well.

PELVIC INFLAMMATORY DISEASE

Each year, 250,000 to 500,000 women develop salpingitis in the United States. *N. gonorrhoeae, C. trachomatis,* and *Mycoplasma* species ascend from the cervix into the uterine cavity, producing endometritis, and then extend to the fallopian tubes, causing salpingitis. The STD pathogens cause inflammatory changes that allow the tissues to become coinfected with bowel and vaginal anaerobic bacteria. Chlamydial salpingitis may be mild, and patients may not seek medical attention. Some intrauterine devices have been associated with an increased risk of salpingitis, and some data suggest that vaginal douching is a predisposing factor.

Adnexal tenderness on bimanual examination leads to the clinical diagnosis of salpingitis. Cervical tenderness, fever, leukocytosis, and an elevated sedimentation rate are sometimes observed. The clinical diagnosis is confirmed laparoscopically in only about 70% of cases. Vaginal ultrasonography or computed tomography is often helpful in defining the cause of pelvic pain syndromes. Pregnant women with evidence of salpingitis should be hospitalized. Infertility complicates approximately 15% of initial attacks of salpingitis and affects about 75% of women who suffer three or more attacks. Ectopic pregnancy and tubo-ovarian abscess are long-term complications of salpingitis.

▌PREVENTION▐

STDs are preventable.**2** The Centers for Disease Control and Prevention recommends five strategies as the foundation for an effective prevention program: (1) education and counseling of persons at risk to motivate the adoption of safer sexual behavior; (2) identification of asymptomatic infected persons and symptomatic persons unlikely to seek diagnostic and treatment services; (3) rapid and effective diagnosis and treatment of infected persons; (4) evaluation, treatment, and counseling of exposed sexual partners; and (5) pre-exposure vaccination of persons at risk for vaccine-preventable STDs.

Abstinence or Monogamy

Abstaining from sexual intercourse or being in a long-term, mutually monogamous relationship with an uninfected partner is the most reliable way to prevent STDs. Abstinence should be recommended during treatment for an STD and for anyone who wants to avoid STDs and unintended pregnancy. Both partners should be tested for STDs, including HIV, before initiating sexual intercourse.

Barrier Methods

When used consistently and correctly, male latex condoms are effective in preventing the sexual transmission of HIV infection and can reduce the risk of other STDs (gonorrhea, chlamydia, trichomoniasis). However, because condoms do not cover all exposed areas, they are likely to be more effective in preventing infections transmitted by fluids from mucosal surfaces (e.g., gonorrhea, chlamydia, trichomoniasis, HIV) than in preventing those transmitted by skin-to-skin contact (e.g., HSV, HPV, syphilis, chancroid). Male condom failure usually results from inconsistent or incorrect use rather than condom breakage. Non-latex condoms (those made of polyurethane or other synthetic material) can be used by persons with latex allergy. There is less information available on the effect of female condoms on the incidence of STDs. Although cervical caps and diaphragms cover the cervix, there is little evidence that they can prevent STDs or HIV.

Male Circumcision

Male circumcision reduces mucosal tissue susceptible to HIV and STD pathogens. Circumcision reduces the acquisition of HIV by more than 50% and appears to reduce the acquisition of viral STDs, including HSV-2 and HPV.**3**

Counseling

Counseling is essential for people with STDs. Interactive counseling, video presentations, peer groups, and other formats that emphasize correct condom use have reduced the incidence of subsequent infections among STD clinic patients and adolescents. Randomized controlled trials demonstrate that structured risk-reduction counseling can reduce the incidence of infections by 25 to 40% among some STD clinic populations. HIV testing is preceded by a counseling session, but there is little evidence of a preventive benefit from this communication.

Partner Services

The detection of an STD demands consideration of the infected person's sexual partners, who may have undetected and serious disease. In addition, in the absence of partner treatment, reinfection of the index case can be expected.**4** The probability that a sexual partner is also infected reflects the efficiency of transmission of the STD pathogen, as described earlier. For example, most men with gonococcal urethritis infect their partners, whereas only about half of patients with HIV infection have infected their partners at the time of outreach; partners who differ in terms of STD or HIV infection status are referred to as "discordant."

Sexual partners can be notified directly by the infected person or by health care workers, sometimes through proactive contact tracing. In general, dependence on the infected person is a less reliable way to get partners treated. However, in many states it is legal to pursue expedited care by providing the infected patient with the appropriate treatment for his or her partners. Expedited partner care appears to work well for the treatment of gonorrhea and chlamydia infections.

Pre-exposure Interventions

Pre-exposure vaccination is the most effective method for preventing the transmission of certain STDs. For example, because hepatitis B virus is frequently transmitted sexually, hepatitis B vaccination is recommended for all unvaccinated persons being evaluated for an STD. In addition, hepatitis A vaccine is recommended for men who have sex with men and for drug users (both injection and noninjection). Vaccines for HPV are now available for both females and males.**5**

Antiretroviral agents are in development to prevent HIV acquisition. Topical antivirals are considered "microbicides" and can be used in gel form or as slow-release cervical rings. Oral antiretroviral agents are considered pre-exposure prophylaxis. Clinical trials to evaluate the antiretroviral agent tenofovir or tenofovir plus emtricitabine are in progress.

Post-Exposure Prophylaxis

After consensual or nonconsensual sexual exposure, a variety of STDs can be prevented with empirical antibiotics. Prevention of HIV appears to require several antiretroviral agents that must be used in combination for 28 days.

Contraception

All methods of birth control can influence the acquisition and outcome of an STD. In addition, pregnancy itself (in the absence of effective birth control) affects STD acquisition and the health of the pregnancy and the neonate. Accordingly, STD management demands consideration of the reproductive health of both partners, as well as family planning issues.

● TOWARD A COMPREHENSIVE MANAGEMENT STRATEGY

Although most STDs are self-limited and readily treated, the comprehensive and proper management of the patient with an STD requires considerable skill. First, the correct syndrome must be recognized, and a decision about specific diagnostic tests must be made. Second, empirical therapy must be provided and must be sufficiently broad to promise cure or reduced duration of illness. Third, the clinician is obligated to search for other STDs of public health or personal significance. Fourth, the clinician must deal with the patient's sexual partners, through either referral or expedited partner therapy. Fifth, the patient needs counseling and adjunctive preventive measures, where appropriate. Such measures might include vaccination for hepatitis B or HPV or antibiotics to prevent another STD such as incubating syphilis or HIV.

1. Workowski KA, Berman S; Centers for Disease Control and Prevention (CDC). Sexually transmitted diseases treatment guidelines, 2010. *MMWR Recomm Rep.* 2010;59:1-110.
2. Mena LA, Mroczkowski TF, Nsuami M, et al. A randomized comparison of azithromycin and doxycycline for the treatment of *Mycoplasma genitalium* positive urethritis in men. *Clin Infect Dis.* 2009;48:1649-1654.
3. Tobian AA, Serwadda D, Quinn TC, et al. Male circumcision for the prevention of HSV-2 and HPV infections and syphilis. *N Engl J Med.* 2009;360:1298-1309.
4. Centers for Disease Control and Prevention. Recommendations for Partner Services Programs for HIV Infection, Syphilis, Gonorrhea, and Chlamydial Infection. *MMWR.* 2008;57(RR09):1-63.
5. Koutsky LA, Ault KA, Wheeler CM, et al. A controlled trial of a human papillomavirus type 16 vaccine. *N Engl J Med.* 2002;347:1645-1651.

SUGGESTED READINGS

Jaiyeoba O, Lazenby G, Soper DE. Recommendations and rationale for the treatment of pelvic inflammatory disease. *Expert Rev Anti Infect Ther.* 2011;9:61-70. *Review of outpatient treatment for appropriate patients and inpatient treatment for severe cases, which must be evaluated for possible tubo-ovarian abscess.*

Wetmore CM, Manhart LE, Wasserheit JN. Randomized controlled trials of interventions to prevent sexually transmitted infections: learning from the past to plan for the future. *Epidemiol Rev.* 2010;32:121-136. *Comprehensive overview including behavioral interventions, vaginal microbicides, vaccines, partner services, physical barriers, and male circumcision.*

294

APPROACH TO THE PATIENT BEFORE AND AFTER TRAVEL

PAUL ARGUIN

According to the World Tourism Organization, approximately 700 million international trips are taken each year. This estimate includes travel to and from developed and developing countries and exotic vacation destinations as well as travel for business, government, or humanitarian activities in remote areas of the world. International travelers encompass a wide variety of unique subsets, including children, the elderly, the immunocompromised, missionaries, military personnel, immigrants, and refugees. Some of these subsets of travelers may be particularly vulnerable to certain problems while traveling and may require more specialized counseling. In fact, first- and second-generation immigrants to developed countries who return to their countries of origin to visit friends and relatives have some of the highest risk for acquiring infectious diseases during travel.

● PRETRAVEL HEALTH CARE AND RISK ASSESSMENT

Destination country–based recommendations are not applicable to everyone. To determine the best health advice for prospective travelers, the approach should be tailored both to the individual and to the itinerary. Thus, the practice of travel medicine has become a new specialty; its practitioners include primarily physicians in internal medicine, primary care, family medicine, pediatrics, emergency medicine, and occupational health, as well as nurses, physicians' assistants, and pharmacists. These health care providers review the entire itinerary with the traveler to characterize potential risks and exposures along the route. These risks are dependent on the destination city, the style of travel, specific activities, the length of stay, the altitude of the destination, and the season of travel. The underlying health of the traveler is also important. Previous and current medical problems must be considered, as must potential immunodeficiency, current prescription and over-the-counter medications, previous vaccinations, and pregnancy. It is essential to determine whether the traveler has medical conditions that would affect the ability to complete the planned itinerary or would alter any prophylactic measures.

● PREVENTION AND RISK REDUCTION

Based on assessment of the risk, travelers should be advised about and provided with appropriate vaccinations, medications for prevention or self-treatment of certain diseases such as malaria and traveler's diarrhea, and prevention counseling about behavioral modifications that can help reduce the risk for injuries, infections, and other adverse health events. Specific advice should include information on hand washing. Hand washing is one of the most important practices in preventing illness from infections at home and while traveling. Travelers should wash their hands often with soap and water or use an alcohol-based hand rub to remove potentially infectious material from the skin and help prevent transmission of diseases. Finally, all travelers should be given some guidance about common over-the-counter items (in addition to their prescription medications) that they should remember to carry with them in their travel health kit: pain relievers and antipyretics, cold and motion sickness medicines, antacids, laxatives, sunscreen, and insect repellent. Unless security regulations demand it, travelers should be told to keep these kits with them at all times and not to place them in checked baggage.

Some primary care providers are comfortable in giving some pretravel health advice and are encouraged to learn the basics. However, patients who have more complicated travel itineraries or multiple medical problems should be referred to a travel health specialist. International travelers should contact health care providers who provide pretravel health advice at least 4 to 6 weeks before departure to obtain vaccinations and prophylactic medications. Travel to developed countries (e.g., United States, Canada, Australia, New Zealand, Japan, and Western Europe) involves lower risk than travel to developing countries. Travelers visiting urban tourist areas and staying in first-class accommodations may also have a lower risk for exposure to infectious diseases. Thus, additional vaccines and protective measures may be recommended for the more adventuresome travelers.

After their pretravel visit but before departure, travelers should continue to assess both their health status and the conditions at their destination. It is advisable for persons to postpone travel if they are not feeling well, particularly if they have febrile illnesses. By delaying travel, persons who are ill avoid potential emergencies and are courteous toward other travelers who may not wish to be exposed to someone with a transmissible illness. Travelers should be aware of the occurrence of any disease outbreaks, natural disasters, political unrest, or other major events at their international destinations. Current travel notices on diseases of international concern are posted on the Travelers' Health home page on the Centers for Disease Control and Prevention (CDC) website at *www.cdc.gov/travel*.

Injury Prevention

Most international travel health guidelines concentrate on the prevention of exotic infectious diseases. However, injuries, especially those caused by motor vehicle crashes, are the leading cause of preventable mortality among travelers. Trauma from motor vehicle crashes accounts for 21 to 26% of travel-associated deaths. Accidents tend to occur more frequently at dusk, in poor weather conditions, at crossroads, while speeding, while passing other drivers, and when the participants are impaired by alcohol consumption. Other factors such as failure to use safety measures, including seat belts and helmets, contribute not only to increased accidents but also to increased injuries. Travelers should always try to choose safe vehicles equipped with seat belts and use them. If their vehicle has only two wheels, they should always wear a helmet.

Protection against Mosquitoes and Other Arthropods

In addition to being nuisances, the bites of mosquitoes and other arthropods such as ticks can transmit a variety of infectious diseases, many of which are associated with specific travel itineraries (e.g., malaria, dengue fever, Japanese encephalitis, and African tick bite fever). Thus, no matter where they travel, patients should be counseled on avoidance of arthropod bites. Health care providers should remind travelers of some commonsense prevention tips, such as wearing long sleeves and pants, sleeping under an insecticide-treated mosquito net if not in air-conditioned quarters, and using appropriate insect repellents.

For the prevention of malaria, the CDC recommends the use of one of the four insect repellents approved by the U.S. Environmental Protection Agency; these are DEET (*N,N*-diethyl-*m*-toluamide), picaridin, oil of lemon eucalyptus, and IR3535. The efficacy and duration of protection are affected by factors such as temperature, perspiration, exposure to water, and abrasive removal. In general, higher concentrations of the active ingredients in these repellents provide longer duration of protection. Products with 10% or less of the active ingredient may offer only limited protection, often from 1 to 2 hours. However, products that offer sustained release or controlled release (i.e., microencapsulated) formulations may provide longer protection times. Note that DEET efficacy tends to plateau at about 50%, so higher concentrations are not recommended. Regardless of what product is used, if travelers start to get mosquito bites, they should reapply the repellent according to the label instructions or leave the area with biting insects if possible.

To avoid overexposure to the repellents, these products should be applied only to exposed skin, not under the clothing. They should not be applied to mucous membranes or sprayed in enclosed spaces. Parents should also apply the repellent to young children rather than allowing them to do it themselves. In addition, certain insect repellents, such as those containing permethrin, are recommended for use on clothing, shoes, bed nets, and camping gear. Permethrin-treated clothing repels and kills ticks, mosquitoes, and other arthropods and retains this effect after repeated laundering, but it should be reapplied after every five washings.

Immunizations

Immunizations for international travel can be categorized as routine, recommended, and required (Table 294-1). Routine vaccinations are childhood and adult vaccinations recommended for all persons regardless of travel. Recommended vaccinations are those that are prescribed according to the traveler's risk for infection. Required vaccinations are those needed to cross international borders, as required by international health regulations or specific countries. The specifics of vaccine administration are provided in package inserts and should be consulted before giving any vaccine. It is the responsibility of the health care provider to ensure that travelers are not allergic to any of the vaccine components. Multiple vaccines may be given at the same time at different sites, depending on patient tolerance. Live-virus vaccines should be administered simultaneously or at a 4-week interval to avoid immune interference.

Routine Immunizations

A consultation before travel is an excellent opportunity to update routine immunizations, especially because adults are often not up to date on these. The CDC recommends that most adults have a tetanus and diphtheria toxoid (Td) booster vaccine every 10 years; have two recorded doses of measles, mumps, and rubella (MMR) vaccine (if born after 1956); and have evidence of previous varicella infection or vaccination. Finally, the pretravel visit is also a great opportunity to provide additional routine vaccines such as pertussis (Tdap), human papillomavirus (HPV), varicella-zoster virus, and pneumococcal vaccines to patients for whom these vaccines would be recommended but have not yet received them from their primary care providers.

Recommended Immunizations
Hepatitis A

Hepatitis A (Chapter 150), transmitted through contaminated food or water or intimate contact with another infected person, is one of the most

TABLE 294-1	VACCINATIONS THAT MAY BE INDICATED FOR TRAVELERS*
ROUTINE VACCINES: RECOMMENDED REGARDLESS OF TRAVEL	
Tetanus, diphtheria, and pertussis (Td or Tdap)	Every 10 years; substituting a tetanus and diphtheria toxoid and acellular pertussis (Tdap) booster once for the next Td booster is now recommended as well
Measles, mumps, and rubella (MMR)	Persons without two documented doses if born after 1956
Varicella	Persons without evidence of previous infection or vaccination
Human papillomavirus	Females between the ages of 11 and 26 years
Pneumococcal	Older and chronically ill persons if not already appropriately vaccinated
Varicella-zoster virus	Persons 60 years of age and older
RECOMMENDED VACCINES: PRESCRIBED IF TRAVEL POSES AN EXPOSURE RISK	
Hepatitis A	First dose before travel to developing countries; second dose 6 to 12 months later
Hepatitis B	Three dose series for those with indications or at risk for exposure
Influenza	Travel at any time during the year, especially to tropical latitudes
Japanese encephalitis	Travel to rural southern and eastern Asia with extensive outdoor exposure
Meningococcal disease	Travel to the sub-Saharan meningitis belt during the dry season or to areas experiencing outbreaks
Poliomyelitis	Single adult booster for travel to countries where disease is present or where outbreaks have recently occurred
Rabies	Travel to countries where rabies is common and exposure to animals is anticipated
Typhoid fever	Travel to developing countries
Yellow fever	Travel to yellow fever–endemic zones in sub-Saharan Africa and South America, unless contraindicated (older age, thymus disease)
REQUIRED VACCINES: REQUIRED BY INTERNATIONAL HEALTH REGULATIONS OR SPECIFIC COUNTRIES TO CROSS INTERNATIONAL BORDERS	
Meningococcal vaccine	Travel to Saudi Arabia during Hajj and Umrah pilgrimages
Yellow fever	Travel to countries where vaccination is required by international health regulations unless waived for medical contraindications by an official vaccine provider; primary dose at least 10 days before departure, administered by a World Health Organization Yellow Fever Vaccinating Center and documented on the international certificate of vaccination to be carried by the traveler

*Vaccine recommendations continue to evolve, so always check http://wwwnc.cdc.gov/travel for the most current advice for travelers and other information about indications, contraindications, dosing, and side effects.

frequently reported vaccine-preventable, travel-related illnesses. In 2006 in the United States, among cases for which information regarding exposures during the incubation period was collected, the most frequently identified risk factor for hepatitis A was international travel (reported by 15% of case-patients overall). Although not usually fatal, acute hepatitis A infection can result in weeks of lost work time and early repatriation of travelers. The hepatitis A vaccine is indicated for most travelers to the developing world unless they are known to be immune. One dose should be administered before travel; a second dose 6 to 12 months later increases protection to long term. Before the introduction of hepatitis A vaccine, immune globulin injections were used to provide short-term protection against hepatitis A. They are still recommended for children younger than 1 year.

Hepatitis B

Hepatitis B (Chapter 150) is transmitted through infected blood and body fluids, has a case-fatality rate of 1%, and can result in chronic infection in up to 5% of adults. Almost one fourth of international travelers have pretravel indications for hepatitis B vaccine, including occupational risk for exposure to blood and body fluids or a history of a recent sexually transmitted disease, and 10% of travelers experience exposures that would be categorized as high risk for hepatitis B infection during travel. However, less than one third of persons who should be immunized against hepatitis B receive the full three-dose series before travel. Travelers should be advised to avoid behavior that is high risk for the acquisition of hepatitis B, although it is clear that it is difficult to identify travelers at risk during the pretravel encounter. Travelers going to areas with intermediate to high levels of endemic hepatitis B transmission should receive the three-dose series. The usual schedule for this vaccine is a dose at 0, 1, and 6 months, which is often difficult to complete for last-minute travelers. There are also accelerated schedules with doses at 0, 7, and 14 days; however, these have not been approved by the U.S. Food and Drug Administration. The CDC recommends that persons who receive vaccinations on an accelerated schedule also receive a booster dose 6 months after the start of the series to promote long-term immunity. A combination vaccine that provides protection against hepatitis A and B infections is also available.

Influenza

Recently, the influenza situation has become more complicated. It is no longer appropriate to consider this a single entity with a single set of prevention recommendations for travelers. Consideration should be given to the prevention of seasonal influenza, the long-standing clusters of H5N1 avian influenza, and pandemic influenza such as the H1N1 novel influenza A that emerged in 2009. Seasonal influenza tends to circulate predominantly in the respective winter months in the Northern and Southern hemispheres and year round in the tropical latitudes. Thus, all travelers, especially those at high risk for complications, should be considered candidates for seasonal influenza vaccination. Travelers visiting areas with active outbreaks of H5N1 avian influenza are advised to avoid direct contact with live birds, particularly in venues such as farms or live bird markets. In the event of a circulating pandemic influenza virus, specific and rapidly evolving guidance on appropriate prevention measures will be promulgated by national and international health authorities, including recommendations on vaccination.

Japanese Encephalitis

Japanese encephalitis (Chapter 391) is transmitted by infected mosquitoes in rural parts of southern and eastern Asia. Travelers to endemic areas who will have extensive rural outdoor exposure, such as campers and hikers, should consider receiving this vaccination series and be very vigilant in their mosquito avoidance measures. For persons 18 years and older, a new two-dose cell culture–derived vaccine has become the standard. For persons younger than 18 years, the three-dose inactivated mouse brain–derived vaccine is still available.

Meningococcal Disease

The sub-Saharan African "meningitis belt," which extends from Mali to Ethiopia, experiences increased rates of transmission of *Neisseria meningitidis* (Chapter 306) regularly during the dry season, which is usually December through June. Travelers to an area where there is an ongoing outbreak of meningococcal disease and those traveling to the meningitis belt of sub-Saharan Africa during the dry season should receive one of the two quadrivalent (A, C, Y, and W-135) meningococcal vaccines that are currently available: the polysaccharide and the conjugate vaccine.

Poliomyelitis

The global polio eradication effort has reduced the number of countries with ongoing transmission to just a few, specifically, Afghanistan, Pakistan, India, and Nigeria. However, occasional outbreaks of polio (Chapter 423) still occur in countries that had previously eradicated it. A single adult booster for polio is recommended for travel to all of these countries.

Rabies

Rabies is a fatal disease transmitted by the bite of infected mammals; however, effective prevention strategies are available. The three-dose preexposure vaccination series is indicated for persons with a higher likelihood of encountering animals such as stray dogs in countries where both rabies transmission is known to occur and access to antirabies biologics, including human rabies immune globulin and cell culture–produced vaccines, may not be available. Travelers who will be spending extended periods outdoors, such as hikers, spelunkers, and small children, are examples of persons who may be at higher risk for rabies. Health care providers should counsel travelers on appropriate behavior around stray, wild, or domesticated animals not known to be vaccinated against rabies to try to prevent rabies exposure. Travelers should always avoid contact with these animals and not feed or pet them. In the event of an animal bite, all travelers should be instructed to seek appropriate rabies postexposure prophylaxis. Previously unimmunized persons will need to receive the full postexposure regimen, including vaccine and rabies immune globulin. It is important to realize that persons who received the preexposure series still need two booster doses of rabies vaccine if they are bitten by a rabid animal. Health care providers should be strongly discouraged from deviating from these established preexposure and postexposure regimens in an attempt to reduce costs or for the convenience of the traveling patient.

Since 2007, the United States has been experiencing a limitation in the supply of rabies vaccines. To ensure sufficient availability of vaccine for postexposure use, preexposure vaccine has not been available to international travelers. Thus, there should be increased emphasis on educating travelers on the importance of animal bite avoidance and the correct steps to take if they are exposed to rabies while traveling.

Typhoid Fever

Annually in the world, 22 million cases of typhoid fever result in 200,000 deaths (Chapter 316). In the United States, approximately 400 travel-associated cases are reported each year, mostly among travelers visiting friends and relatives and returning from their home countries. Although typhoid fever is a treatable bacterial infection, prevention is preferable because of increasing rates of antibiotic resistance. Travelers to certain developing countries should be vaccinated against typhoid fever with either of the two types of typhoid vaccine: the live oral vaccine (Ty21a) or the inactivated injectable vaccine (Vi capsular polysaccharide).

Yellow Fever

Yellow fever (Chapter 389) is transmitted by the bite of infected mosquitoes in sub-Saharan Africa and tropical South America, where it is endemic and intermittently epidemic. All persons traveling to the yellow fever–endemic zones without contraindications should be vaccinated with the live viral vaccine. In rare but severe instances, yellow fever–like syndromes develop from the attenuated live vaccine virus; these adverse events are characterized as either viscerotropic disease or neurotropic disease. Being older than 60 years and having a history of thymus disease have been identified as independent risk factors for development of one of these severe but rare adverse events. Persons with contraindications should reconsider their travel itinerary. If they choose to travel to yellow fever–endemic areas despite contraindications, they should be very vigilant in their mosquito avoidance measures.

Required Immunizations
Meningococcal Meningitis

Vaccination against meningococcal disease is not a requirement for entry into any country except Saudi Arabia for travelers to Mecca during the annual Hajj and Umrah pilgrimage.

Yellow Fever

In addition to vaccination for protection of the traveler, yellow fever vaccine may be required by some countries as a condition of entry, as outlined in the International Health Regulations. Vaccination becomes valid for the purpose of entry 10 days after primary inoculation, and it must be administered at an approved World Health Organization Yellow Fever Vaccinating Center. Receipt of the vaccine must be documented on an international certificate of vaccination that should be carried with the passport. A national registry of such providers in the United States is available on the CDC website at *wwwnc.cdc.gov/travel/yellow-fever-vaccination-clinics-search.aspx*. Persons for whom the vaccine is contraindicated should be issued a vaccination waiver letter bearing the official yellow fever vaccine provider stamp.

Malaria Protection

As many as 30,000 travelers from industrialized countries acquire malaria annually (Chapter 353). On average, 1400 cases of malaria (including about four fatalities) are diagnosed in the United States and reported to the CDC each year. The CDC also maintains a country-by-country listing, often with regional- or subcountry-level recommendations for malaria prevention. All travelers to malaria-endemic countries should be counseled to avoid mosquito bites by the appropriate use of repellents and insecticide-treated mosquito nets. An individual risk assessment should be conducted for every traveler, taking into account not only the destination country but also the detailed itinerary, including specific cities, types of accommodation, season, and style of travel. In addition, conditions such as pregnancy or the presence of antimalarial drug resistance at the destination may modify the risk assessment. Depending on level of risk, it may be appropriate to recommend mosquito avoidance measures only, or mosquito avoidance measures plus chemoprophylaxis. Depending on the destination, there are usually several medication options so that travelers who may not have tolerated one type of medication in the past because of unpleasant side effects can still be prescribed one of the others. For travel to areas with predominantly *Plasmodium vivax*, primaquine can be used for primary prophylaxis (provided that the person does not have glucose-6-phoshate dehydrogenase deficiency). For travel to areas of risk where chloroquine-resistant malaria has *not* been reported, chloroquine can still be used. For areas with chloroquine resistance, the CDC currently recommends mefloquine, doxycycline, or the combination of atovaquone and proguanil as equal alternatives. The choice of one or the other is usually based on the side effects, cost, and duration of the trip.

Travelers should also be warned about trying to acquire malaria medications while overseas, either for reasons of cost or for convenience. Medicines with similar-sounding names, such as Malarone, Malasone, or Maloprim, do not contain the same active ingredients. In addition, counterfeit medicines that contain either smaller amounts or none of the active ingredient stated on the box are increasingly prevalent in many developing countries. Travelers should also be counseled to be alert for symptoms consistent with malaria after returning and to seek prompt evaluation and treatment if indicated.

Traveler's Diarrhea

A diarrheal illness develops in about 50% of travelers to developing countries, with an average duration, if untreated, of approximately 4 days. All travelers should be instructed on ways to avoid illnesses transmitted through food and water. Although diarrheal illness is sometimes very difficult to avoid, travelers should be taught when possible to make safer choices to reduce the chance of acquiring a food-borne or waterborne illness. They should avoid tap water or ice made with tap water in favor of beverages that have been boiled or placed in sealed containers, such as bottled water or carbonated items. Selecting foods freshly prepared rather than eating from communal vessels or buffets is also a safer choice.

Frequently, despite the best efforts, diarrhea occurs, and travelers should be taught how manage the situation by drinking abundant fluids to avoid dehydration and by trying to manage symptoms with over-the-counter medications such as bismuth subsalicylate or loperamide. The current standard of care also includes prescribing an antibiotic for the traveler to carry—not to take to prevent diarrhea, but rather to have readily available for use when needed to treat a moderate to severe case of diarrhea acquired while traveling. Fluoroquinolone antibiotics are generally used for self-treatment of diarrhea, although azithromycin is now also being used for travel to areas with high rates of antibiotic resistance (e.g., parts of Southeast Asia) and for treatment of children and pregnant women.

POST-TRAVEL CARE

Travelers may be exposed to a variety of pathogens and risks, both exotic and mundane. Approximately half of all travelers will experience some health problems while traveling. Overall, during international travel, 5 to 8% of travelers seek medical attention, some requiring emergency medical evacuation. Health care providers who see returned travelers should be aware that most ailments diagnosed during the post-travel period are not necessarily travel related. However, providers should also be able to recognize important syndromes in returned travelers that may be travel related and require prompt treatment or referral for definitive management. A thorough history, including a review of the travel itinerary and specific exposures (e.g., insect bites, unprotected sexual contact, and consumption of untreated water), is an essential first step. The most frequent health problems in ill returned travelers are chronic diarrhea, rashes, and respiratory infections. Although gastrointestinal ailments are the most frequent problem, fever is the most serious. Fever in a traveler who has recently returned from a malaria-endemic region should be immediately evaluated so that antimalarial treatment can be initiated rapidly if indicated. Finally, certain long-term travelers should be evaluated by a travel or tropical medicine specialist when they return to screen for conditions that may be asymptomatic, such as schistosomiasis or strongyloidiasis.

SUGGESTED READINGS

Ansart S, Perez L, Thellier M, et al. Predictive factors of imported malaria in 272 febrile returning travelers seen as outpatients. *J Travel Med.* 2010;17:124-129. *In France, malaria accounted for 56% of cases, with other leading causes being bacterial enteritis, bacterial pneumonia, infectious cellulitis, pyelonephritis, prostatitis, dengue fever, primary viral infection, and tuberculosis.*

Centers for Disease Control and Prevention. Health Information for International Travel, 2010. Atlanta: U.S. Department of Health and Human Services, Public Health Service; 2010. *Also known as "the Yellow Book," this text is updated and published every 2 years and is considered the "gold standard" source of prevention guidelines for international travelers' health.*

Centers for Disease Control and Prevention. Travelers' health website. http://wwwnc.cdc.gov/travel. Accessed March 3, 2011. *An up-to-date source of travel health information searchable by disease and geographic region, as well as timely travel-related notices such as information on disease outbreaks or vaccine shortages.*

Mirzaian E, Durham MJ, Hess K, et al. Mosquito-borne illnesses in travelers: a review of risk and prevention. *Pharmacotherapy.* 2010;30:1031-1043. *Overview.*

Ravel A, Nesbitt A, Marshall B, et al. Description and burden of travel-related cases caused by enteropathogens reported in a Canadian community. *J Travel Med.* 2011;18:8-19. *The main causes were campylobacter, salmonella, and giardia, with about 40% if cases becoming symptomatic before return.*

295

ANTIBACTERIAL CHEMOTHERAPY

GEORGE L. DRUSANO AND WILLIAM A. CRAIG

Antibiotics have been classified as "miracle drugs" since their introduction and have transformed our expectations regarding the outcome of infection. More recently, they have been the backbone of modern interventional medicine. Barriers not meant to be breached have been. Catheters have been inserted into veins and arteries, the bladder, and the tracheal tree. These interventions support the seriously ill patient, but they also give bacteria access to normally sterile areas. Therapies for cancer and immune-mediated disease often leave patients severely immunosuppressed. Bacterial infections in such patients are serious and, when untreated or treated late, frequently result in death. Antibacterial agents allow critical life-saving support for such patients.

What is clear is that the overuse and poor use of antibiotics have allowed many pathogens to develop resistance to drugs. Multiresistant *Staphylococcus aureus* has become a plague both in the hospital and, of late, in the community. Extended-spectrum β-lactamases and *Klebsiella pneumoniae* carbapenemase enzymes have mediated resistance to many of our most potent and broad-spectrum β-lactam agents, including the carbapenems. Consequently, it is important to understand the principles of antibacterial chemotherapy to obtain the best clinical outcomes for our patients but also, in a broader sense, to lower the probability of the emergence of resistance and maintain the potency of the drugs we currently have in our therapeutic armamentarium.

CHOICE OF ANTIBIOTIC, ANTIBIOTIC DOSE, AND SCHEDULE TO OPTIMIZE CLINICAL OUTCOME

As in all of clinical medicine, a well-done history and physical examination are central to proper decision making and to the achievement of optimal therapeutic outcomes in patients with infections. Key to choosing the correct drug, dose, and schedule is recognition that an infection exists. The next step is to document where the infection exists, and then to identify the dominant organisms present at each site of infection. The next step is to determine whether there are any risk factors that might predict the presence of drug-resistant pathogens.

As an example, we know that community-acquired pneumonia is caused by certain traditional pathogens. *Streptococcus pneumoniae, Haemophilus influenza*, and perhaps *Moraxella catarrhalis* are the "classic" bacterial pathogens associated with this entity. "Atypical" pathogens such as *Legionella* species, *Mycoplasma pneumoniae*, and *Chlamydophila pneumoniae* may also be seen. In contrast, intra-abdominal infections are dominated by *Escherichia coli* and other Enterobacteriaceae and anaerobic organisms such as *Bacteroides* species. Consequently, it is important to understand the dominant pathogens present at different infection sites so that the best drug or combination of drugs can be chosen to treat the infection.

Knowing the source of infection is also critical because drugs penetrate differently into different spaces. Classically, penetration is poorer into spaces

TABLE 295-1	PRIMARY INFECTION SITES AND THE DOMINANT BACTERIAL SPECIES PRESENT
SITE	**BACTERIA**
Complicated skin/skin structure infection	*Staphylococcus aureus* and *Streptococcus* spp
Diabetic foot ulcer	Organisms above plus Enterobacteriaceae
Intra-abdominal infections	*Escherichia coli* and other Enterobacteriaceae plus anaerobes
Community-acquired bacterial pneumonia	*Streptococcus pneumoniae, Haemophilus influenzae, Moraxella catarrhalis,* "atypical" pathogens
Hospital-acquired pneumonia	*S. aureus, Klebsiella pneumoniae, Enterobacter* spp, *Pseudomonas aeruginosa, Acinetobacter* spp
Meningitis	*S. pneumoniae, H. influenzae* (nontypable), meningococci; in hospital settings, *S. aureus* and gram-negatives may be seen
Urinary tract infections	Enterobacteriaceae, particularly in sexually active women; multiresistant gram-negatives in patients with complicated urinary tract infections or those instrumented; enterococci, particularly in elderly men
Prostatitis	Enterobacteriaceae, enterococci, atypical pathogens

where there are tight junctions, such as the central nervous system, the eye, and the prostate. Generally, the penetration of many classes of antibacterial agents is quite good into complicated skin and skin structure infection sites. What is often not appreciated is the divergent penetrations of different agents and even agents within the same class into the lung to treat bacterial pneumonia. For instance, the penetration by macrolide antibiotics into skin infection sites is modest, but their penetration into the lung is quite good, with penetration ratios (area under the concentration-time curve [AUC] in epithelial lining fluid/AUC in plasma) ranging from 4 to 20. The penetration of β-lactam drugs can range from 15 to 100%, but there is no set of variables (at least to date) that explains such a range of penetrations. Table 295-1 presents a partial list of infection sites and their dominant pathogens. The point is not to have an encyclopedic knowledge of infection sites or of pathogens but to appreciate that different infection sites require different drugs to provide adequate coverage for the most likely pathogens present.

It is also important to understand other factors that increase the probability that a resistant organism is present at the primary infection site. An example is a patient who has recently taken antibiotics before acquiring the present infection. Other examples are the acquisition of an infection in the hospital or in an extended care facility or in a patient who is immunosuppressed. In such patients, the choice of antimicrobial agents must be carefully considered to cover more resistant pathogens.

CULTURE AND GRAM STAIN

Once the site of infection has been definitively identified or the most likely source of infection has been determined, it is critical to obtain cultures from that site as well as to obtain blood cultures. Coordination with the microbiology laboratory is key to make sure that culture specimens are handled appropriately. Also of great importance is the performance and interpretation of a Gram stain on the specimen. This can be straightforward if the specimen is from a normally sterile space, or it may require considerable skill in interpretation if the specimen is from an area where mixed flora is normally present, such as sputum.

Although it is not possible to make a definitive diagnosis based on the cellular morphology of the organism, it is quite possible to combine information on the morphology, the organism's gram positivity or negativity, the infection site, and the most likely pathogens to make an initial antimicrobial choice with the highest probability of producing effective chemotherapy. It should be noted that the initial antibiotic chosen to cover organisms present at the primary infection site has a significant influence on the outcome of therapy. Initial choices should err on the side of caution. When definitive cultures are available, the chemotherapy can be "streamlined" to provide the most effective and least toxic antimicrobial for the patient. As the seriousness of the infection increases, providing the correct initial coverage becomes more important with regard to the ultimate outcome.

SUSCEPTIBILITY

Because infections occur at a specific place, it is important to have an understanding of the antimicrobial susceptibility patterns in one's particular hospital. Most frequently, the microbiology susceptibility patterns are different in the cultures taken from patients on the general wards as opposed to those in intensive care units (ICUs), because the former are generally (but not always) infected with pathogens derived from the community setting. In severely infected patients, particularly those whose infections were acquired in the ICU, it is critical to know the susceptibility patterns for these pathogens, which are likely to be multiply resistant to different classes of agents.

After the definitive culture, the identified pathogen must be examined in an antimicrobial susceptibility test. This can be automated, in which case the information returned is the minimal inhibitory concentration (MIC), or it can be reported from a disc diffusion test, where the results are typically reported as "S" (susceptible), "I" (intermediate), or "R" (resistant). The MIC is often misunderstood as the concentration of drug that prevents the pathogen from growing, but it is actually the concentration of drug that allows a tube (or well) containing the pathogen to remain clear by visual examination after 18 to 24 hours. If one starts with an organism concentration of 1 to 5×10^5 colony-forming units (CFUs)/mL, this criterion can actually allow almost a $1 \log_{10}$ (CFU/mL) increase in bacterial count over this time frame and still be read as the MIC. With all its limitations, the MIC provides critical information regarding drug choice. For several infections, such as meningitis, endocarditis, and perhaps bacteremia, knowing the minimal bactericidal concentration (defined as the concentration required to kill 99.9% of organisms over 18 to 24 hours) is valuable. In these cases, it is important to obtain multilog killing of the organism to ensure a high probability of a good clinical outcome. For meningitis and endocarditis, there is also the confounding problem of penetration of the drug to the primary infection site. In other circumstances (e.g., ventilator-associated pneumonia) in which bacterial burdens are very high, optimizing the probability of cure requires highly bactericidal therapy.

DETERMINING THE "CORRECT" DRUG DOSE

The correct drug dose is the one that produces a high likelihood of achieving a good clinical response with a low probability of causing a concentration-driven adverse event. Another consideration is that the optimal dose should have a high probability of suppressing the emergence of resistant mutants. To be confident that a drug dose has a high likelihood of producing a good clinical outcome requires an understanding of the relationship between the measure of drug exposure and infection outcome—that is, pharmacodynamics (Chapter 28).

When we administer a drug either intravenously or orally, the drug concentration starts low, increases to a maximal value, then declines over time until another dose of the drug is given (in a multidose regimen). This drug concentration–time profile should be seen relative to a measure of drug potency against the pathogen in question: the MIC (or minimal bactericidal concentration). It is also critical to note that protein binding is important because in almost all cases, it is the free or non-protein-bound drug that kills the causative pathogen. So understanding the pharmacodynamics of a drug or class of agents first requires knowledge of the concentration-time profile, protein binding, and MIC (Fig. 295-1). For drugs that kill organisms much faster as their concentrations rise (e.g., fluoroquinolones, aminoglycosides), the free drug AUC/MIC ratio is most closely linked to drug effect. For other drugs (e.g., penicillins, carbapenems, cephalosporins, monobactams), the rate of organism kill rises slowly with concentration and plateaus quickly, in which case the free drug time greater than MIC is most closely linked to drug effect. Occasionally, the free drug peak concentration/MIC ratio is linked to drug effect. This is seen when there is a rapid and frequent emergence of resistance and the peak concentration helps suppress the amplification of resistant mutant subpopulations.

These measures of drug exposure need to be linked to drug effect. There are a number of ways to do this, but two are most common. In the first and most valuable way, patients are studied during the course of a clinical trial. Multiple plasma samples are taken for documentation of the drug's pharmacokinetics and corrected for protein binding. The MIC of the infecting pathogen is determined for the drug being administered, and the three measures of drug exposure cited earlier are calculated. The outcome of the patient is then determined (usually success or failure, but in some instances, time to success or failure serves as the outcome measure). If the outcome is success or failure, the appropriate measure of drug exposure is linked to the outcome

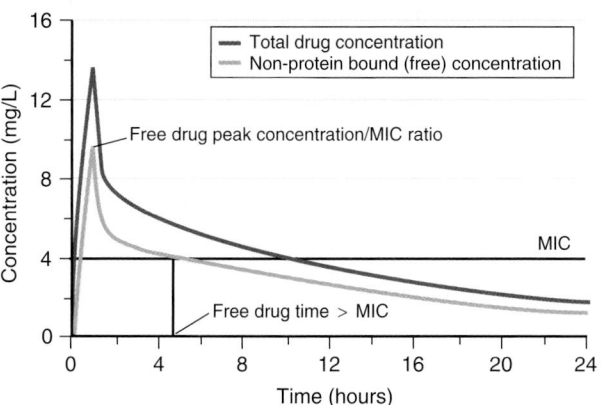

FIGURE 295-1. Three measures of drug exposure are important to the measure of potency, or the minimal inhibitory concentration (MIC). Free drug peak concentration/ MIC ratio, free drug time greater than MIC, and free drug area under the curve (AUC)/ MIC ratio.

through logistic regression analysis. By creating such a relationship, we can directly estimate the probability of a patient having a successful outcome if a certain measure of drug exposure is achieved. For example, if a patient receiving a drug that is a concentration-dependent killing agent achieves a free drug AUC/MIC ratio of 88, the logistic regression relationship allows the calculation that the probability of a good outcome is a specific number (perhaps 91%). Over the past 10 years, we have been able to generate such relationships for a great number of drugs and across drug classes. The most common relationships are for the fluoroquinolone antimicrobials, but examples can be found for the aminoglycosides, oxazolidinones, β-lactams, and glycylcyclines, among others.

The second way to link exposure to antibacterial effect is through preclinical animal models of infection. Here, the end point is microbiologic. We observe the drug concentration–time profile in the animals and at the end of the experiment determine the number of organisms left after therapy at the infection site (the baseline number of organisms having been previously determined). We can then link the measure of drug exposure (as earlier) to the number of bacterial cells killed by a specific regimen. In this way, we can determine whether free drug peak concentration/MIC ratio, free drug AUC/MIC ratio, or free drug time greater than MIC is the best measure of drug exposure for the class of drug being studied.

How does knowing the relationship between drug exposure and microbiologic effect in an animal infection model help in treating patients? Based on experience with different drugs and drug classes, it has become possible to link a drug's microbiologic effect in an animal model to clinical outcome. For instance, in the therapy of complicated skin and skin structure infections, a drug exposure in the animal model that stops organisms from growing for 24 hours or reduces their number by approximately 1 $\log_{10}$ (CFU/g) is adequate to generate a high probability of a good clinical outcome. This has been documented for oxazolidinones and glycylcyclines. For severe community-acquired pneumonia or for hospital-acquired pneumonia, a greater cell kill—generally 2 $\log_{10}$ (CFU/g)—is required for a high likelihood of a good clinical outcome.

Thus, when we have clinical data with a logistic regression function, it is possible to identify an exposure target that is associated with a specific probability of a good outcome (e.g., a free drug AUC/MIC ratio of 88 generates a 91% probability of a good outcome). In the case of the animal model, it is possible to identify a target drug exposure that will achieve a certain microbiologic effect associated with a good clinical outcome (the logic is one step removed). In both cases, we have a target drug exposure, and this is used to identify the "correct" dose.

It is important to remember that when the same dose of a drug is administered to a number of patients, no two concentration-time curves will be identical. Indeed, it is not unusual to have a 10-fold range in measures of drug exposure (e.g., peak concentration, trough concentration, AUC). When these are transformed by incorporating MIC values, ranges of 100- to 1000-fold are commonly encountered. As part of the drug development process, the pharmacokinetics of new agents are now identified in a large number of patients with the infection of interest. As part of this process, the interpatient variability in important pharmacokinetic parameters (e.g., drug clearance = $10 \pm$

4 L/hour) is determined. This information is then used with a tool called the Monte Carlo simulation to ask and answer a key question: If I give this specific drug dose to a large number of patients and I recognize that the MIC values I am likely to encounter will range (for example) between 0.06 and 8 mg/L, how many patients will achieve the desired measure of drug exposure to give them a high likelihood of a good clinical outcome? This can be calculated directly from the data indicated earlier plus the MIC distribution for the drug and the type of infection one wishes to treat. Indeed, many of the dosage recommendations for new drugs are calculated in this manner and validated in large phase III clinical trials. It provides the clinician with a degree of confidence that the recommended doses are likely to work if the infecting pathogen is still susceptible to the drug.

● EMERGENCE OF RESISTANCE

If the drug is properly chosen, the organism should have a high probability of being susceptible to it. However, during the course of therapy, the organism has many mechanisms available to make it less susceptible (the MIC increases) to the drug being used. This leads to less effect than was originally envisioned, which results in a lower probability of cure.

When are organisms likely to become resistant? There are many determinants, but five factors account for the majority of cases of resistance emerging during therapy. The first is the mutational frequency of the organism being treated. Because mistakes are made by the organism during replication, mutations occur in the genome at a specific rate, which is organism dependent. For antibiotic resistance, the mutational frequency rate is generally around $1/10^8$ to $1/10^6$. There are organisms, however—referred to as hypermutators—that have mutations in other places in the genome (often mutS) that alter their DNA replication error-checking mechanisms. These organisms' mutational frequencies are generally 10- to 100-fold higher than those of organisms without these other mutations.

The second factor is related to the bacterial burden. The higher the bacterial burden, the more likely it is that a preexistent mutant is already extant in the bacterial population. Antibiotic pressure then provides this mutant with a selective advantage, and it amplifies in the population while its more susceptible cousins are killed by the antibiotic. As the bacterial burden increases and ultimately surpasses the inverse of the mutational frequency to resistance, it becomes more and more likely that a resistant mutant exists in the population. For instance, if the mutational frequency to resistance is $1/10^7$ (1 resistant organism per a population of 10^7), and the patient has a bacterial infection in which the total bacterial burden is 10^9 organisms, it is highly likely that a resistant organism is present in the population a priori. A calculation of the actual probability can be performed using a Poisson distribution, the bacterial burden, and the mutational frequency to resistance. Consequently, infections in which the bacterial burden is high are more likely to generate resistance during therapy. For example, in clinical trials of ventilator-associated pneumonia, single-agent β-lactam drugs or fluoroquinolones allowed the emergence of resistance during therapy 33 to 50% of the time.

The third issue is drug penetration. There are circumstances (e.g., empyema) in which the bacterial burden is high but the drug's penetration to the infection site is reduced. In this case, the emergence of resistance is more likely. In contrast, poor penetration with relatively low bacterial burdens (e.g., meningitis) generally does not result in a high probability of the emergence of resistance.

The fourth issue has to do with error-prone replication in bacterial pathogens. When resistance occurs relatively late in therapy and the bacterial burden is modest, error-prone replication is often to blame. Antibiotics differ greatly with respect to their ability to induce the bacterial isolate to perform error-prone replication. Perhaps the best example is the fluoroquinolone antimicrobials, because these drugs strike at the heart of DNA replication. The organism senses the attack of the antibiotic, and a whole cascade of events takes place, the most important of which is the induction of error-prone polymerases (e.g., pol V). These polymerases markedly increase the error rate in DNA replication. Most of these errors are lethal to the organism and therefore unhelpful to it. But because this is a totally random process, by chance, a mutation can occur in a spot that provides protection from the onslaught of the antibiotic (e.g., a mutation in the DNA gyrase when the patient is receiving a fluoroquinolone). We perceive this as the organism having a selective replication advantage (emergence of resistance), and we see an increase in the MIC of the mutant organism relative to the baseline organism.

The fifth factor has to do with mechanisms other than antibacterial target site mutations that allow the organisms to survive in the face of appropriate antibiotic chemotherapy. One extremely common mechanism seen in the vast majority of both gram-positive and gram-negative organisms is the upregulation of efflux pumps. These pumps are quite indiscriminate in their ability to pump molecules; they can eject multiple classes of antibacterials from the organism, as well as natural substances that can harm it. These pumps keep drug concentrations at their target sites much lower than they would be in the absence of the pumps. The pumps can be induced and then downregulated once the threat has passed, or occasionally, the organism can pick up a mutation in the part of the genome where the pump is expressed, so the pump is always expressed (constitutive expression).

A similar process is seen with the production of β-lactamases. Often, these enzymes are situated on plasmids and are produced all the time. Sometimes, as with the efflux pumps, they sense the attack by the β-lactam, and their production is markedly increased (the phenomenon of induction, seen with ampC-type enzymes, which reside on the chromosome). Sometimes, also like the pumps, the organisms pick up a mutation in the part of the genome that regulates production of the β-lactamase. This is referred to as stable de-repression, and the enzyme is made all the time. The enzyme hydrolyzes its substrate (the β-lactam drug), thus preventing its binding to the target sites, the β-lactam binding proteins.

Finally, in gram-negative organisms, the drug must cross the diffusional barrier of the outer membrane before binding to β-lactam binding proteins (if the drug is a β-lactam) in the periplasm of the organism, or it must cross the inner membrane if its target site is actually inside the organism. For many agents, particularly those that are water soluble, a large percentage of their influx is due to passage through porin proteins. These proteins are water-filled channels that pass through the entirety of the outer membrane of gram-negative bacteria. Part of their function is to provide access to nutrients for the organism and allow the easy diffusion of waste products. These channels are also used to obtain passage by water-soluble antibacterial agents. The organism has the ability to downregulate these channels, either temporarily or permanently (by mutation). An example is *Pseudomonas aeruginosa*, in which downregulation of the porin channel oprD markedly diminishes the penetration of carbapenem antibiotics (β-lactam agents), with a resultant two- to eight-fold rise in MIC. With all these mechanisms that can be brought to bear, it is no surprise that poor dosing and prolonged courses of therapy often lead to the emergence of resistance.

These mechanisms also interact. In the case of fluoroquinolone antimicrobials, where error-prone replication almost always occurs under pressure, the upregulation of efflux pumps relieves some of the antibiotic pressure, allowing the organisms to undergo more rounds of replication per unit of time, giving the error-prone replication mechanism more time to find a mutation that is not lethal and provides protection against the drug at the primary target site.

SUPPRESSING THE EMERGENCE OF RESISTANCE

Suppressing the emergence of resistance is an end point that is different from achieving a good clinical or microbiologic outcome. It should be recognized that the antimicrobial exposure (free drug peak concentration/MIC ratio, free drug AUC/MIC ratio, or free drug time greater than MIC) necessary to suppress resistance is always at least as high as that required to attain maximal killing of bacterial cells, and in the vast majority of instances, it is substantially higher.

Recently, it has been shown experimentally that it is possible to identify doses and schedules of drugs that suppress the emergence of resistance as well as provide optimal killing of bacterial cells. Unfortunately, many of the exposures necessary to achieve such an outcome are high enough to result in increased drug toxicity. Nevertheless, as new agents are developed, it will become important to identify resistance-suppressive exposures and ascertain whether they are too toxic to be used clinically, as a way of retaining the potency of the antibacterial therapeutic armamentarium.

The other way to help suppress the emergence of resistance is to employ combination chemotherapy. Combination therapy has major advantages, but there are significant disadvantages as well. Among the advantages are that combination therapy can improve the spectrum of coverage in the setting of empirical treatment, as well as help suppress the emergence of resistance. This is best seen in the treatment of *Mycobacterium tuberculosis*, although there is growing evidence that this may also be true for difficult-to-treat pathogens such as *P. aeruginosa* and *Acinetobacter* species. Combination therapy can be effective against some pathogens in serious infections for which a single agent would not be adequate. Enterococcal endocarditis is the classic example: Ampicillin or vancomycin is generally static and not up to the task of curing this disease, and the second agent (an aminoglycoside, streptomycin, or gentamicin) is somewhat resistant when used alone (MIC values <500 mg/L). Yet the combination produces excellent bacterial kill in the endocarditic vegetation, with a high probability of cure if the patient can tolerate the combination for the requisite period of time. Some authors have discussed reducing drug doses in combination as a way of ameliorating toxicity, but this theoretical advantage is difficult to demonstrate convincingly in the clinical setting.

The disadvantages of combination therapy are also well known. At full doses of each, there may be added toxicity, and there are certainly greater costs associated with combinations. Finally, combinations of agents may interact antagonistically instead of either additively or synergistically. For example, the combination of tetracycline and penicillin is somewhat antagonistic and caused a number of failures in the treatment of pneumococcal meningitis in the 1950s. However, there are circumstances in which weak antagonism is tolerable. It has been shown that isoniazid plus rifampin, part of the standard therapy for *M. tuberculosis*, is somewhat antagonistic with respect to cell killing, but the combination provides superb protection against the emergence of resistance. Consequently, when discussing drug interactions (synergy, additivity, antagonism), it is important to be specific about the end point to which one is referring.

MECHANISM OF ACTION

The search for new antimicrobials begins with the principle that the target that affects pathogens must not be in the human genome or must be sufficiently different that the agent in question does not cause appreciable human toxicity. β-lactam antibiotics are a good example: the inhibition of peptidoglycan synthesis has no effect on humans, because this target is simply not present. An example of differing susceptibility to inhibition because of poor sequence homology between bacteria and humans can be seen in the inhibitors of the bacterial ribosome. The bacterial ribosome is much smaller than that in humans and has differing affinities for such drugs as aminoglycosides, tetracyclines, macrolides, and clindamycin. Consequently, such agents are an important part of the therapeutic armamentarium and cause only minor adverse effects related to their primary mode of action. It should be recognized that in some cases so-called off-target toxicity may take place. Again, an example is the β-lactams: a major toxicity is accelerated allergic reaction, even though the target for the agents is not present in humans. Table 295-2 lists the sites of action and the effects of many antimicrobial agents.

Often, antimicrobials are thought of as either *bacteriostatic* or *bactericidal*, for which there are standard definitions. An agent that causes a 1000-fold decline (3 $\log_{10}$ [CFU/mL] decrease) in an in vitro test system over 18 to 24 hours is defined as being bactericidal. Any agent that causes a smaller decline is defined as bacteriostatic. It is clear that these definitions are arbitrary; however, there is a clinical connection. In some circumstances, such as meningitis and endocarditis, it is critical to kill every last organism with the combination of drugs employed and the immune system. Obviously, the more organisms the antimicrobial kills, the easier this is to accomplish. In other circumstances, such as multilobar pneumonia, it is critical to kill as many of the organisms as possible so as not to overwhelm the body's immunologic defenses. For these reasons, clinicians generally prefer bactericidal to bacteriostatic agents.

MECHANISMS OF RESISTANCE

Earlier, we examined how to suppress the emergence of resistance. Here we examine the mechanisms by which organisms can become less susceptible to antimicrobial agents. As stated earlier, in the vast majority of cases, resistance is caused by an alteration in the target site; by an enzyme that alters the drug, resulting in a lack of activity; by the drug's being pumped out of the organism; or, in the case of gram-negative pathogens, by the loss or downregulation of a transmembrane porin protein. These mechanisms, along with error-prone replication, can interact to cause large increases in the MIC. For example, a gram-negative pathogen that acquired a mutation in its gyrase enzyme would generally have only a 4-fold increase in its MIC value for a fluoroquinolone antimicrobial; however, if this isolate also had an efflux pump upregulated, the MIC could change 8- to 16-fold. Table 295-3 shows the mechanisms of resistance for multiple drug classes, as well as the most common organisms in which these mechanisms are seen.

EFFECTS OF PHARMACOKINETIC CHANGES

Whereas antimicrobial pharmacodynamics is the study of the effect of a drug on an infecting organism, pharmacokinetics is the study of the effect of the

TABLE 295-2 MECHANISMS OF ACTION OF ANTIMICROBIAL AGENTS

AGENT	SITE OF ACTION	EFFECT	BACTERICIDAL	BACTERIOSTATIC
β-Lactams (penicillins, cephalosporins, carbapenems, aztreonam)	Cell wall: penicillin binding proteins	Inhibit cross-linking of peptidoglycan (transpeptidation), impair cell wall synthesis	+	Occasionally (enterococci)
Vancomycin, teicoplanin, dalbavancin, telavancin	Cell wall: terminal D-alanyl-D-alanine of pentapeptide peptidoglycan precursor	Inhibit polymerization of disaccharide precursors to peptidoglycan (transglycosylation), impair cell wall synthesis	+	Occasionally (enterococci)
Daptomycin	Cell membrane	Rapid depolarization of membrane potential	+	Occasionally (enterococci)
Aminoglycosides	Protein synthesis: 30S ribosome subunit	Inhibit peptide elongation, cause misreading of genetic code, inhibit protein synthesis	+	
Tetracyclines, glycylcyclines	Protein synthesis: 30S ribosome subunit	Inhibit binding of transfer RNA, inhibit protein synthesis	Occasionally	+
Chloramphenicol	Protein synthesis: 30S ribosome subunit	Block attachment of aminoacyl transfer RNA, inhibit protein synthesis	Occasionally	+
Macrolides, azalides, ketolides	Protein synthesis: 50S ribosome subunit	Block transfer of amino acids to peptide chain, inhibit protein synthesis	Occasionally	+
Clindamycin	Protein synthesis: 50S ribosome subunit	Block transfer of amino acids to peptide chain, inhibit protein synthesis	Occasionally	+
Quinupristin/dalfopristin	Protein synthesis: 50S ribosome subunit	Block extrusion of peptide chains, inhibit protein synthesis	+	+ (with quinupristin resistance)
Linezolid	Protein synthesis: 50S ribosome subunit	Block formation of 70S initiation complex, inhibit protein synthesis	Occasionally	+
Rifampin	Nucleic acid synthesis: β-subunit of DNA-dependent RNA polymerase	Inhibit RNA synthesis	+	
Metronidazole	Nucleic acid synthesis	Damage nucleic acids, inhibit DNA synthesis	+	
Quinolones	Nucleic acid synthesis: DNA gyrase, topoisomerase IV	Impair supercoiling of DNA, prevent decatenation of DNA molecules after replication, inhibit DNA synthesis	+	
Sulfonamides	Folic acid synthesis: dihydropteroate synthetase	Competitive inhibition of synthesis of dihydrofolate from p-aminobenzoic acid, pteroate, and glutamic acid	Occasionally (when used with trimethoprim)	+
Trimethoprim	Folic acid synthesis: dihydrofolate reductase	Inhibit reduction of dihydrofolate to tetrahydrofolic acid	Occasionally (when used with sulfonamide)	+

body's processes on the drug concentration–time profile and the drug's ability to penetrate to the infection site (or the toxicity site). As such, it is a prime determinant of whether a drug will be able to kill or inhibit the offending pathogen and, because many toxicities are concentration related, whether a serious drug-related toxicity will occur.

Earlier, the algorithm for identifying appropriate drug doses and schedules was outlined. Table 295-4 shows recommended doses and schedules of important antimicrobial agents, as well as their protein binding ability and whether alterations in renal or hepatic function generate major changes in the concentration-time profile. As in all chemotherapy, the aim is to generate a concentration-time profile in the plasma to generate a concentration-time profile at the infection site that allows the drug to inhibit or kill the pathogen without causing toxicity.

Although there is almost always a guide to the concentration-time profile that results in an appropriate antimicrobial effect, it is more difficult to identify a linkage between drug exposure and the occurrence of toxicity. Data in this regard are available for the aminoglycosides, including a considerable amount of information on the association between drug concentrations and the likelihood of nephrotoxicity, and for daptomycin, for which a link between exposure and the likelihood of creatine phosphokinase (CPK) elevation has been elucidated.

For aminoglycosides, the relationships between drug exposure and the likelihood of a good clinical outcome and between drug exposure and the likelihood of nephrotoxicity have been determined. These are in the form of logistic regression functions, so the actual probability of both outcomes can be calculated. The one difference is that for the relationship with good outcome, the MIC value is part of the evaluation, whereas it does not figure in the toxicity relationship. Nevertheless, it is possible to derive appropriate

information by making the outcome relationship MIC specific. Figure 295-2 illustrates the effect and toxicity relationships for aminoglycosides at three different MIC values. As shown, it is relatively easy to achieve a high probability of good clinical outcomes with aminoglycosides when the MIC is 0.25 mg/L, but it is virtually impossible to do so when the MIC rises to a value of 1.0 mg/L. The evaluation in the figure is based on twice daily dosing; daily aminoglycoside dosing markedly improves this circumstance. Also, it should be noted that these relationships permit one to calculate the probabilities of effect and toxicity when, for example, aminoglycoside AUC is increased owing to renal dysfunction, because these agents are largely eliminated renally.

When no toxicity relationship is available, there is still a target for good clinical effect. Achievement of this target should be paramount, and alterations for renal or hepatic impairment should strive to maintain the high likelihood of effect seen in patients with a relatively normal clearance function. One can change the dose or schedule of a drug to decrease its accumulation in the presence of renal or hepatic impairment (depending on the drug) and then recalculate the impact on the likelihood of attaining a good clinical outcome. One can also calculate the amount of accumulation with the proposed dose reduction or extension of the dosing interval. For the increase in exposure (relative to that in normally clearing patients), there is no clear guidance, but one can accept a certain maximal amount of accumulation as long as the proposed dose adjustment maintains a high likelihood of a good outcome. The acceptability of the increased drug exposure after dosage adjustment is usually based on a combination of preclinical toxicology and the largest exposures seen in phase I and phase II clinical trials. However, the overarching issue is that the proposed dose or schedule alteration maintains a high probability of a good clinical outcome.

TABLE 295-3 MECHANISMS OF ANTIMICROBIAL RESISTANCE

ANTIBACTERIAL AGENT	MECHANISM	REPRESENTATIVE ORGANISM
β-Lactams (penicillins, cephalosporins, carbapenems, aztreonam)	Altered target (penicillin binding proteins)	Methicillin-resistant *Staphylococcus aureus* (MRSA), penicillin-resistant *Streptococcus pneumoniae*, *Enterococcus faecium*
	Reduced permeability	*Enterobacter* spp, *Pseudomonas aeruginosa*
	Enhanced efflux	*P. aeruginosa*
	β-Lactamases	*S. aureus*, Enterobacteriaceae (includes ESBLs), *Haemophilus influenzae*, *Moraxella catarrhalis*, *Neisseria gonorrhoeae*, *Enterococcus faecalis*
Aminoglycosides	Inactivating enzymes (acetylation, adenylation, phosphorylation)	*S. aureus*, enterococci, *P. aeruginosa*, Enterobacteriaceae
	Reduced permeability	Enterobacteriaceae, *P. aeruginosa*, enterococci
	Enhanced efflux	*P. aeruginosae*
	Decreased ribosomal binding	*S. aureus*, *E. faecalis*, mycobacteria (streptomycin)
Chloramphenicol	Enhanced efflux	*H. influenzae*
	Reduced permeability	Enterobacteriaceae
	Inactivating enzyme (acetylation)	*S. aureus*, *S. pneumoniae*, enterococci
Daptomycin	Altered target	*S. aureus*
Glycylcyclines	Enhanced efflux	Enterobacteriaceae, especially *Proteus*
Macrolides, clindamycin, ketolide, quinupristin	Altered target (methylation of ribosomal RNA)	*S. aureus*, *S. pneumoniae* (not ketolide), streptococci, *Bacteroides fragilis*
	Enhanced efflux (not clindamycin or ketolide)	*S. pneumoniae*, streptococci
	Reduced permeability	Enterobacteriaceae
	Inactivating enzymes	*Escherichia coli*, *Klebsiella pneumoniae*, *S. aureus*
Linezolid	Altered target	Enterococci, *S. aureus*
Quinolones	Altered target (DNA gyrase, topoisomerase IV)	Enterobacteriaceae, *P. aeruginosa*
	Reduced permeability	Enterobacteriaceae, *P. aeruginosa*
	Enhanced efflux	*E. coli*, *P. aeruginosa*
Tetracyclines	Altered target (ribosome)	*N. gonorrhoeae*, streptococci
	Enhanced efflux	*E. coli*, *S. pneumoniae*
	Reduced permeability	Enterobacteriaceae
	Drug inactivation	*B. fragilis*
Rifampin	Altered target (β-subunit of polymerase)	*E. coli*, *S. aureus*
Sulfonamides, trimethoprim	Altered target (dihydropteroate synthetase or dihydrofolate reductase)	Enterobacteriaceae, *M. catarrhalis*
	Enhanced *p*-aminobenzoic acid production	*S. aureus*, *N. gonorrhoeae*
	Reduced permeability	*P. aeruginosa*, Enterobacteriaceae
Vancomycin	Altered target (peptidoglycan precursor binding site)	*E. faecium*, *E. faecalis*, *S. aureus*

ESBL = extended-spectrum β-lactamases.

DRUG CLASSES AND THEIR PROPERTIES

Over the past 70 years, a large number of different classes of antimicrobial agents have been developed. These classes differ in their mechanisms of action, mechanisms of emergence of resistance, and whether they kill substantial numbers of organisms or only shut off bacterial growth. The following sections examine some of the properties of the major classes of antimicrobial agents in use today.

β-Lactam Agents

This class of drugs is arguably the most important group of antimicrobials. With chemical modification, they have an exceptionally broad spectrum of activity and, in general, an excellent safety profile. The major toxicity is related to allergic reactions to a degradation product of the drug. There are a number of different types of β-lactams, including the penicillins, the cephalosporins, the monobactams, and the carbapenems.

These agents bind to their target, the β-lactam binding proteins (sometimes referred to as penicillin binding proteins). These binding proteins have an active site serine, and the drug forms a covalent bond with this site through the carbonyl of the β-lactam ring. Sometimes, the binding has direct effects on the organism's shape. For example, in gram-negative organisms, binding to penicillin binding protein (PBP)-2 causes the organism to assume a spherical shape, whereas binding to PBP-3 causes the formation of long chains of organisms. Generally, high-affinity binding to PBP-1 leads to the rapid death of the organism, sometimes accompanied by lysis. The classic response of *S. pneumoniae* to penicillin G is rapid lysis of the organism. Binding to PBP-1

(1a or 1b) leads to activation of N-acetylmuramic acid amidase, which destroys the bacterial cell wall, resulting in lysis.

The most common way for pathogens to protect themselves from β-lactams is by elaborating β-lactamases. The genes for these enzymes may be on plasmids or other bits of transmissible DNA, or they may reside on the bacterial chromosome. Some drugs, such as the carbapenems, are resistant to hydrolysis by many enzymes (but certainly not all of them—especially the metallo-β-lactamases and *K. pneumoniae* carbapenemase–type β-lactamases). One of the ways developed to protect these drugs is to add a second agent, the β-lactamase inhibitor. Examples include K-clavulanate, sulbactam, tazobactam, and, most recently, NXL-104 (an experimental drug). These agents inhibit different types of β-lactamases, with NXL-104 being the only one able to inhibit the ampC-type enzymes carried by *P. aeruginosa*, *Enterobacter* species, *Citrobacter* species, *Serratia marcescens*, and indole-positive *Protea* (SPICE organisms).

All β-lactams are relatively non–concentration dependent in their kill rate, and free drug time greater than MIC is the important factor for increased organism killing. The classes differ somewhat, with carbapenems requiring approximately 40% free drug time greater than MIC for near-maximal cell killing. For penicillins, this percentage is approximately 50%, and for cephalosporins and monobactams, it is 60 to 70%.

Aminoglycosides

These important agents were discovered in the late 1940s for the treatment of *M. tuberculosis* (streptomycin). Screening of natural products identified a

TABLE 295-4 DOSAGE REGIMENS OF ANTIBACTERIALS, PHARMACOKINETICS, AND DOSE ADJUSTMENT IN PATIENTS WITH RENAL OR HEPATIC FAILURE

CLASS/AGENT	DOSE* FOR SYSTEMIC INFECTION	ORAL FORMULATION	PEAK SERUM CONCENTRATION (MG/ML)	PROTEIN BINDING (%)	NORMAL SERUM HALF-LIFE (HR)	HEPATIC FAILURE	RENAL FAILURE	SERUM LEVELS AFFECTED BY DIALYSIS
AMINOGLYCOSIDES								
Amikacin	5 mg/kg q8h or 15 mg/kg q24h	—	35	0	2-3	No	Major	Yes (H, P)
Gentamicin	1.7 mg/kg q8h or 5 mg/kg q24h	—	7	0	2-3	No	Major	Yes (H, P)
Netilmicin	1.7 mg/kg q8h or 5 mg/kg q24h	—	7	0	2-3	No	Major	Yes (H, P)
Tobramycin	1.7 mg/kg q8h or 5 mg/kg q24h	—	7	0	2-3	No	Major	Yes (H, P)
ANTITUBERCULOUS AGENTS								
Ethambutol	15 mg/kg q24h (PO)	Yes	2	10	3.3	No	Major	Yes (H, P)
Isoniazid	5 mg/kg q24h or 300 mg q24h (PO)	Yes	4.5	10	3	Yes	Major	Yes (H, P)
Pyrazinamide	10 mg/kg q8h (PO)	Yes	12	10	10	Yes	Yes	Yes (H)
Rifampin	10 mg/kg or 600 mg q24h (PO)	Yes	7	81-89	3	Yes	Minor	No (H)
CARBAPENEMS								
Doripenem	0.5-1.0 g q8h	—	23	<10	1	No	Yes	Yes (H)
Ertapenem	1 g q24h	—	155	95	4-5	Unknown	Yes	Yes (H)
Imipenem	0.5-1 g q6-8h	—	40	15	1	No	Avoid in severe renal dysfunction	Yes (H)
Meropenem	0.5-2 g q8h	—	50	<10	1	No	Yes	Yes (H)
FIRST-GENERATION CEPHALOSPORINS								
Cefadroxil	1000 mg q12h (PO)	Yes	16	20	1.5	No	Yes	Yes (H)
Cefazolin	0.5-2 g q8h	—	180	80	2	No	Major	Yes (H) No (P)
Cephalexin	250-500 mg q6h (PO)	Yes	18	15	1	No	Yes	Yes (H, P)
Cephradine	500-1000 mg q6-12h	Yes+	140	10	103	No	Yes	Yes (H, P)
SECOND-GENERATION CEPHALOSPORINS								
Cefaclor	250-500 mg q8h (PO)	Yes+	10	25	0.8	No	Yes	Yes (H)
Cefoxitin	1-2 g q6-8h	—	220	70	0.8	No	Yes	Yes (H) No (P)
Cefprozil	250-500 mg q12h (PO)	Yes	10	35	1.4	No	Yes	Yes (H)
Cefuroxime	750-1500 mg q8h	—	100	50	1.5	No	Yes	Yes (H, P)
Cefuroxime axetil	250-500 mg q12h (PO)	Yes	9	50	1.5	No	Yes	Yes (H, P)
THIRD-GENERATION CEPHALOSPORINS								
Cefdinir	300 mg q12h (PO)	Yes	2	65	1.7	Unknown	Minor	Yes (H)
Cefditoren pivoxil	400 mg q12h (PO)	Yes	4	88	1.6	No	Yes	Yes (H)

TABLE 295-4 DOSAGE REGIMENS OF ANTIBACTERIALS, PHARMACOKINETICS, AND DOSE ADJUSTMENT IN PATIENTS WITH RENAL OR HEPATIC FAILURE—cont'd

CLASS/AGENT	DOSE* FOR SYSTEMIC INFECTION	ORAL FORMULATION	PEAK SERUM CONCENTRATION (MG/ML)	PROTEIN BINDING (%)	NORMAL SERUM HALF-LIFE (HR)	HEPATIC FAILURE	RENAL FAILURE	SERUM LEVELS AFFECTED BY DIALYSIS
THIRD-GENERATION CEPHALOSPORINS—cont'd								
Cefixime	400 mg q24h (PO)	Yes	3-5	67	3	No	Yes	No (H, P)
Cefotaxime	1-2 g q6-8h	—	200	50	1.5	Minor	Minor	Yes (H) No (P)
Cefpodoxime proxetil	200-400 mg q12h (PO)	Yes	3	25	2.5	No	Yes	Yes (H)
Ceftazidime	1-2 g q8h	—	160	60	2	No	Major	Yes (H, P)
Ceftibuten	400 mg q24h (PO)	Yes	15	65	2.5	Unknown	Yes	Yes (H)
Ceftizoxime	1-2 g q6-8h	—	130	30	1.3	No	Major	Yes (H) No (P)
Ceftriaxone	1-2 g q12-24h	—	250	90-95	8	No	No	No (H)
FOURTH-GENERATION CEPHALOSPORINS								
Cefepime	1-2 g q8h	—	193	20	2	No	Major	Yes (H, P)
PENICILLINS								
Amoxicillin	500 mg q8h (PO)	Yes	10	20	1	No	Yes	Yes (H) No (P)
Amoxicillin-clavulanic acid‡	875/125 mg q8-12h	Yes	2.7	25	1.3	Unknown	Moderate	Yes (H, P)
Ampicillin	1 g q6h	Yes†	200	20	1	No	Yes	Yes (H) No (P)
Aztreonam	1-2 g q8h	—	250	60	2	No	Major	Yes (H, P)
Cloxacillin	500 mg q6h (PO)	Yes†	9	95	0.5	No	No	No (H, P)
Dicloxacillin	500 mg q6h (PO)	Yes†	18	97	0.5	No	No	No (H, P)
Nafcillin	1-2 g q4-6h	—	160	90	0.5	Yes	No	No (H, P)
Oxacillin	1-2 g q4-6h	—	200	90	0.5	Yes	No	No (H, P)
Penicillin G	3-4 million units q4-6h	Yes†	60	60	0.5	No	Yes	Yes (H) No (P)
Penicillin V	500 mg q6h (PO)	Yes	5	80	1	No	No	Yes (H) No (P)
Piperacillin/tazobactam	3.375-4.5 g q6-8h	—	240	50	1	Minor	Minor	Yes (H)
Ticarcillin/clavulanate	3.1 g q4-8h	—	220	50	1	Minor	Major	Yes (H, P)
QUINOLONES								
Ciprofloxacin	400 mg q8-q12h 500-750 mg q12h (PO)	Yes†	2-3	30	4	No	Minor	No (H, P)
Gemifloxacin	320 mg q24h (PO)	Yes	1.6	60-70	7	No	Minor	No (H, P)
Levofloxacin	250-750 mg q24h (IV or PO)	Yes	6-9	30	7	No	Yes	No (H, P)
Moxifloxacin	400 mg q24h (IV or PO)	Yes	4-5	50	10	No–minor	No	No (H, P)

TETRACYCLINES, GLYCYLCYCLINES

Drug	Dose							
Doxycycline	100 mg q12-24h (PO) after 200-mg loading dose	Yes	1.5-2.1	93	15-20	Avoid	No	No (H, P)
Minocycline	100 mg q12-24h (PO) after 200-mg loading dose	Yes	2.2	75	15	No	Avoid	No (H, P)
Tetracycline	500 mg q6h (PO)	Yes[†]	4	50	7	Avoid	Avoid	No (H, P)
Tigecycline	100 mg, then 50 mg q12h	—	0.6-0.9	70	37-38	Minor	No	No (H, P)
SULFONAMIDES								
Sulfadiazine	15 mg/kg q6h	Yes	30	50	3	Avoid	Avoid	Unknown
Sulfamethoxazole	0.5-1 g q6-8h (PO)	Yes	100	50	9	Avoid	Major	Yes (H) No (P)
Trimethoprim (with sulfamethoxazole)	3-5 mg/kg q6-8h (based on trimethoprim component)	Yes	3-9	60	10	No	Avoid	Yes (H) No (P)
MACROLIDES, LINCOSAMIDES, KETOLIDES								
Azithromycin	500 mg first dose, followed by 250 mg q24h or 500 mg ×3 days (PO) Single-dose therapy of 1-2 g for STDs	Yes[†]	0.4	25	12-50	Unknown	No	No (H, P)
Clarithromycin	500 mg q12h (PO)	Yes	2-3	70	7	No	Minor	Yes (H) No (P)
Clindamycin	0.3-0.9 g q8h	Yes	15	90	2.5	Minor	No	No (H, P)
Erythromycin	500 mg q6h (PO)	Yes[†]	1.8	70	2	Minor	No	No (H, P)
Telithromycin	800 mg q24h (PO)	Yes	2	65	10	No	No	No (H)
OTHER AGENTS								
Chloramphenicol	0.25-1 g q6h	Yes	8-14	60	1.5	Minor	No	Yes (H) No (P)
Daptomycin	4-6 mg/kg q24h	—	58-100	90	8-9	No	Minor	No (P) Minor (H)
Linezolid	600 mg q12h	Yes	18	30	5	No–minor	No	Yes (H)
Metronidazole	500 mg q6h (anaerobes) 250 mg q8h (trichomoniasis) 750 mg q8h (amebiasis) (IV or PO)	Yes	25	20	8	Yes	No	Yes (H) No (P)
Nitrofurantoin	100 mg q6h (PO)	Yes	Nil	60	0.3	No	Avoid	Yes (H)
Quinupristin/dalfopristin (30:70)	7.5 mg/kg q8-12h	—	3.2/8§	90/30	3/1§	Minor	No	No (P)
Spectinomycin	2 g/24hr	—	100	0	2	No	Avoid	Unknown
Vancomycin	15 mg/kg q12h	Yes§	35	50	6	No	Major	No (H, P)

*Dose in milligrams per kilogram body weight at hour intervals and/or oral dose in milligrams in patients with normal renal function; all doses are parenteral unless specified PO.
†Significant decrease or delay in absorption when administered with food.
‡Refers to information for clavulanic acid.
§Includes parent compound and active metabolites.
¶Oral vancomycin is not absorbed; it is used for intraluminal therapy only.
H = hemodialysis; P = peritoneal dialysis; STD = sexually transmitted disease.

FIGURE 295-2. Probability of clinical effect versus nephrotoxicity as a function of aminoglycoside area under the curve (AUC). **A,** Minimal inhibitory concentration (MIC) = 0.25 mg/L. **B,** MIC = 0.5 mg/L. **C,** MIC = 1.0 mg/L.

bacterial cell killing. Therefore, large doses administered daily to patients with normal renal function would be expected to optimize bacterial cell killing while minimizing the probability of inducing an aminoglycoside-related toxic event.

The older aminoglycosides (streptomycin and gentamicin) have the best profile for synergizing with drugs active against gram-positive streptococci (particularly enterococci). Tobramycin generally has the most potent activity against *P. aeruginosa* (depending on the aminoglycoside-modifying enzymes present in a specific locale), and less resistance is generally seen with amikacin (again, depending on the locale). Streptomycin and amikacin, because of the number of amino groups carried, are usually about four-fold less potent than gentamicin or tobramycin. Consequently, their dosages are approximately three- to four-fold higher.

These agents should be thought of as components of combination regimens for seriously ill patients, particularly those thought to be infected by gram-negative organisms, in the empirical therapy setting.

Quinolones

These agents are completely synthetic and do not exist in nature. They are inhibitors (depending on the drug and the organism) of topoisomerases II and IV. This means that they strike at the heart of DNA replication, making them rapidly bactericidal. The use of fluorination markedly enhanced the microbiologic activity of these drugs, so they became useful for both community-acquired infections (especially urinary tract infections and pneumonia) and hospital-acquired gram-negative infections.

These drugs penetrate well into most spaces, with substantial concentrations inside cells. This makes them active against obligate intracellular pathogens such as *Chlamydophila*, *Legionella*, and *Mycoplasma*. They also penetrate well into spaces with tight junctions (prostate, eye, central nervous system) and into epithelial lining fluid.

Typically, the toxicities associated with these drugs are "off target." A number of these drugs were either withdrawn from the marketplace or given black box warnings by health authorities because of the infrequent occurrence of torsades de pointes (Chapter 65) or other serious and life-threatening toxicities, such as eosinophilic hepatitis.

These agents are concentration-dependent bacterial killers, indicating that the free drug AUC/MIC ratio is best associated with a regimen's ability to kill bacterial cells. Of interest, particularly for a drug that is completely synthetic, there are a number of resistance mechanisms that allow bacterial escape from drug pressure. The combination of efflux pump overexpression and error-prone replication, resulting in target site mutants as well as serious underdosing for some of the earlier drugs in the class, has resulted in the emergence of considerable resistance, particularly among gram-negative isolates and in the ICU setting.

Macrolides, Tetracyclines, Ketolides, Clindamycin, and Linezolid

These agents all bind to different places in the bacterial ribosome, making them inhibitors of protein synthesis and, for the most part, drugs with limited bactericidal activity. An exception may be their activity against *S. pneumoniae*.

Macrolides (particularly clarithromycin and azithromycin) are most useful for community-acquired respiratory tract infections, for two reasons. First, their spectrum is well suited to the classic and atypical pathogens encountered in these patients. Second, they concentrate quite well in the epithelial lining fluid, with accumulations that range from 6-fold to almost 20-fold that in plasma. This accumulation also partially explains why these agents have fared much better in the respiratory tract setting than in the skin and skin structure setting. Telithromycin, a ketolide, retains activity against many (but not all) macrolide-resistant isolates.

The macrolides and telithromycin are free drug AUC/MIC ratio–driven drugs with respect to bacterial activity, but for different reasons. Telithromycin is somewhat concentration dependent with regard to its microbiologic activity, whereas classic macrolides are not. Telithromycin is more like aminoglycosides or quinolones in terms of the association between exposure indices and bacterial effect. Classic macrolides, especially azithromycin, induce a long persistent or post-antibiotic effect and are *not* concentration dependent in their bacterial effect. This post-antibiotic effect suppresses bacterial regrowth after the drug concentration declines below the MIC until the next dose of drug is administered. In this way, we perceive the linkage to be driven by the free drug AUC/MIC ratio, but with a different mechanism from agents whose bacterial kill rate is concentration dependent.

number of different aminoglycosides such as kanamycin, neomycin, gentamicin (actually a combination of three congeners), and tobramycin. Other semisynthetic agents such as amikacin, netilmicin, and arbekacin (among others) have been discovered and used for therapy in the United States and elsewhere.

Nephrotoxicity and middle ear toxicity (hearing loss or loss of balance) are these drugs' defining dose-limiting toxicities and resulted in aminoglycosides going out of favor in the 1990s and early in the first decade of the 21st century. It has now been recognized that most (but not all) of the nephrotoxic potential can be ameliorated by intermittent dosing of these drugs (usually once daily). Even with daily therapy, however, prolonged use can still result in nephro- or ototoxicity.

The recent rise in resistance, particularly among gram-negative isolates, and new resistance mechanisms, such as the advent of *K. pneumoniae* carbapenemase enzymes mediating resistance to even our best β-lactam agents, has resulted in renewed interest in existing aminoglycosides and a search for new ones that are more resistant to inactivation by the aminoglycoside-modifying enzymes.

These drugs are concentration dependent in terms of their kill rate and are quite rapid killers. Hence, the AUC/MIC ratio (or, as sometimes reported, peak concentration/MIC ratio) is the factor most closely associated with

Most of the toxicities seen here are off target and gastrointestinal. However, there is also some elongation of the QT interval (Chapter 54).

Tetracyclines have an exceptionally broad spectrum of activity, including both gram-positive and gram-negative pathogens, and are quite active against atypical pathogens. The latest incarnation of a tetracycline-type agent (tigecycline, a glycylcycline) has good activity against methicillin-resistant *S. aureus* (MRSA) as well. Tigecycline differs from previous tetracyclines (e.g., doxycycline, minocycline) in that its structure prevents many efflux pumps from removing the drug from the bacteria and also provides a degree of ribosomal protection.

The lincosamide antibiotic clindamycin has a spectrum that covers most clinically significant anaerobes, including many in the *Bacteroides* group (although some resistance is being seen). It is thus a useful agent for infections in which anaerobes play a prominent role, such as lung abscesses and intra-abdominal infections. In many areas of the country, it retains activity against MRSA, but this should be verified with a D-test (inducible macrolide-lincosamide-streptogramin resistance) in the microbiology laboratory. It also has good activity against many streptococci. Because it is a protein synthesis inhibitor, it may provide improved results when the staphylococcal or streptococcal isolate elaborates a great deal of toxin.

Again, most toxicity is off target, with gastrointestinal symptoms being most frequent. Antibiotic-associated diarrhea and the more serious *Clostridium difficile* colitis can occur.

Linezolid is a member of the oxazolidinone class of antibiotics and is a protein synthesis inhibitor. It is distinguished by having excellent gram-positive activity and robust activity against MRSA. It has been used in skin and skin structure infections and is being evaluated in MRSA nosocomial pneumonia. Linezolid penetrates well into skin as well as the epithelial lining fluid, which is the reason for its evaluation in hospital-acquired MRSA against vancomycin. It is also distinguished by having an oral formulation that is highly bioavailable.

The free drug AUC/MIC ratio is the pharmacodynamic index most associated with cell killing for linezolid. Its toxicity is reflected by dropping counts of bone marrow–derived cells, particularly platelets, seen most frequently with prolonged use. Resistance occurs rarely and is seen with enterococci more frequently than with *S. aureus*. There are five or six gene copies of the target site. As more and more copies become mutated, the MIC increases almost linearly. Because these mutated targets have some biofitness cost, there is a slow reversion to wild-type targets when therapy is discontinued. If all copies become mutated, however, they cannot revert to wild type. The early detection of MIC changes should lead to the consideration of changing or stopping therapy.

Vancomycin, Quinupristin/Dalfopristin, and Daptomycin

Though structured differently, these agents (along with linezolid) are distinguished by having reliable activity against MRSA.

Vancomycin acts at the cell wall and is bactericidal. The free drug AUC/MIC ratio is the driver of antimicrobial effect. Vancomycin has activity against many gram-positive pathogens and has lately become distinguished for its activity against *C. difficile* when administered orally. As with most drugs, wide use has caused the emergence of vancomycin resistance in both enterococci and *S. aureus* (although the latter is rare).

Although vancomycin has a reputation for being a somewhat slow killer, no new agent has significantly outperformed it, at least in trials of skin and skin structure infections. MIC creep has been documented. Although many *S. aureus* isolates were once susceptible with MIC values of 0.25 and 0.5 mg/L, these are now in the distinct minority; 1.0 mg/L represents the modal value, with a few isolates having values of 2.0 mg/L. The higher MICs make these isolates more difficult to treat reliably with standard dosing (1 g IV every 12 hours). Also, it has recently become clear that higher vancomycin doses are associated with a significantly higher risk of nephrotoxicity, even when the agent is administered alone. In addition to nephrotoxicity, vancomycin causes histamine release ("red man syndrome") when administered too quickly intravenously. Infusion times of approximately 1 hour are recommended for standard doses.

Quinupristin/dalfopristin is a combination of streptogramin A and streptogramin B antibiotics. Although each is bacteriostatic, the combination can produce some cell killing because the two drugs are synergistic. The synergy is lost, however, with the emergence of resistance to either drug. Further, the amount of bacterial cell killing is modest because of the drugs' rapid half-lives and the imposition of a 12-hour dosing interval. This combination product has activity against resistant enterococci as well as MRSA. Its toxicity includes

relatively severe muscle pain in some patients. It is also quite phlebitogenic and has to be administered with a central venous catheter, limiting its utility.

Daptomycin is a lipopeptide antibiotic discovered in the 1980s and resurrected in the 1990s with a greater understanding of the relationship between exposure and effect versus exposure and toxicity. It was discovered that the antibacterial effect against MRSA was driven by the free drug AUC/MIC ratio. Muscle effects were seen early in its development that limited therapy. Trough concentrations of daptomycin drive this toxicity and can be ameliorated by once-daily dosing (thus minimizing trough concentrations).

This agent has been licensed for skin and skin structure infections and, of note, for complicated *S. aureus* bacteremia and right-sided endocarditis. It also has activity against enterococci. The drug is bound up in epithelial lining fluid by surfactant, excluding its use in the therapy of pneumonia.

Daptomycin may cause muscle toxicity, which is quite rare, but this may be preceded by the harbinger of an elevated CPK level. The muscle damage is driven by daptomycin trough concentrations, generally above a concentration of about 25 mg/L. Monitoring of CPK is useful in the management of patients on daptomycin therapy.

TOXICITIES

All antimicrobials have toxicities. The most common observed toxicities for many antimicrobial agents are presented in Table 295-5.

DURATION OF THERAPY

Relatively little is known about the optimal duration of therapy. Some work has been done to define certain circumstances in which short courses of chemotherapy are effective. For instance, gonorrhea is highly likely to be cured by a single dose of drug (ceftriaxone, cefixime, fluoroquinolones), as long as the organism is susceptible to the drug given.

For trimethoprim-sulfamethoxazole and fluoroquinolones, controlled trials have shown that 3 days of therapy is adequate for uncomplicated urinary tract infections. For β-lactam antimicrobials, a somewhat longer duration is required.

In community-acquired pneumonia, controlled trials with fluoroquinolones have demonstrated optimal results with 5 days of therapy, most likely because of concentration-dependent killing. For bacterial sinusitis, direct sampling from the infected sinus has demonstrated that bacterial pathogens were eradicated by day 3 of therapy or earlier, particularly for *S. pneumoniae* infections.

In ventilator-associated pneumonia, a double-blind comparison of 8 versus 15 days of therapy demonstrated that, with a single exception, clinical outcomes were just as good, there was less emergence of resistance, fewer antibiotics were administered, and there was less toxicity in the group receiving 8 days of therapy. The single exception was when a nonfermenting gram-negative rod was recovered (*P. aeruginosa* or *Acinetobacter* species). In this circumstance, there were significantly more relapses with 8-day versus 15-day treatment, but clinical outcomes were no different.

In some infections, the organisms are slow growing and require more time for control. Both endocarditis and osteomyelitis are examples. Therapy durations of 4 to 6 weeks and occasionally longer may be required for cure in this circumstance.

Finally, one of the longest durations of therapy is seen in the treatment of tuberculosis. In this case, some organisms are in the "non-replicative persister" (NRP) state, indicating that they are not growing or metabolically active. When recovered, they are still fully susceptible to the antimicrobials being used, but while in the NRP state, they cannot be readily killed with current chemotherapy (phenotypic, not genotypic resistance). Therapy durations of 6 months for wild-type organisms and 18 to 24 months for multidrug-resistant tuberculosis are required because of the need to use suboptimal regimens. Indeed, it is a major research goal to find drugs that will readily kill organisms in the NRP state and thus substantially shorten the therapeutic course for *M. tuberculosis*.

FAILURE OF ANTIMICROBIAL THERAPY

Occasionally, antimicrobial therapy fails, with failure defined as the persistence of signs and symptoms of infection or the persistence of fever. When one is confronted with failure after what was thought to be adequate antimicrobial therapy, it should set off a sequence of investigations: (1) Did resistance emerge, or did superinfection occur? (2) Is there an obstructed hollow viscus (e.g., urinary or gastrointestinal tract)? (3) Is there an undrained abscess or infected collection (e.g., empyema)? (4) Is there an infected foreign body (e.g., intravenous catheter or prosthesis), or is there devitalized

TABLE 295-5   ADVERSE EFFECTS OF ANTIMICROBIAL AGENTS

AGENT	GENERAL	SKIN	GI TRACT	BLOOD CELLS	KIDNEY	NERVOUS SYSTEM	OTHER
Penicillins	Hypersensitivity, anaphylaxis, serum sickness	Rash, urticaria, erythema multiforme	Diarrhea (ampicillin, amoxicillin-clavulanate), hepatitis (oxacillin)	Coombs-positive hemolytic anemia, impaired platelet function (ticarcillin), leukopenia, thrombocytopenia	Nephritis (methicillin), hypokalemia (carboxy- and ureido-penicillins)	Seizures, twitching (high doses, renal failure)	Inactivates aminoglycosides when admixed; possible with concurrent therapy in renal failure
Cephalosporins	Serum sickness (cefaclor), hypersensitivity, anaphylaxis (rare)	Rash, urticaria	Diarrhea, hepatic dysfunction, precipitates in bile (ceftriaxone), mild increase in LFTs	Neutropenia, increased prothrombin time, bleeding (due to MTT side chain), positive Coombs test	Enhances aminoglycoside toxicity, acute renal failure (rare), interstitial nephritis		Disulfiram-like reaction with alcohol use (MTT side chain)
Carbapenems	Hypersensitivity	Rash, urticaria, erythema multiforme	Vomiting with rapid infusion (imipenem), abnormal LFTs	Bone marrow suppression, positive Coombs test	Renal dysfunction	Seizures, myoclonus	
Aminoglycosides	Fever	Rash			Reversible renal failure	Irreversible vestibular toxicity and/or auditory damage, muscular blockade (with anesthetics and myasthenia gravis)	Histamine release with flushing and hypotension (infusion <1 hr, antihistamines can prevent)
Vancomycin	Allergy, fever	Rash		Leukopenia, thrombocytopenia	Nephrotoxic with aminoglycoside	Decreased hearing, neuropathy	
Quinolones	Headache, allergy, anaphylaxis (rare)	Rash (gemifloxacin), urticaria, photosensitivity (lomefloxacin)	GI distress, abnormal LFTs			Dizziness, insomnia, nervousness, tremors, visual changes, seizures	Tendon rupture arthropathy in young animals
Sulfonamides	Hypersensitivity, anaphylaxis, serum sickness, fever	Rash, Stevens-Johnson syndrome, photosensitivity	Hepatitis	Hemolysis (G6PD deficiency), agranulocytosis, marrow suppression	Crystalluria	Neuropathy	Vasculitis
Trimethoprim ± sulfamethoxazole	Fever	Rash, erythema multiforme, Stevens-Johnson syndrome, TEN	Hepatitis, pancreatitis	Marrow suppression	Hyperkalemia, acute renal failure		
Chloramphenicol	Fever			Marrow suppression (dose related), aplastic anemia		Optic neuritis, neuropathy	Circulatory collapse (gray baby syndrome in neonates)
Tetracyclines	Hypersensitivity	Photosensitization (doxycycline)	GI discomfort, hepatotoxicity in azotemia or pregnancy		Antianabolic aggravation of azotemia (except doxycycline)	Vertigo (minocycline)	Deposition in bone (dysplasia) and teeth (staining)
Macrolides	Fever	Rash	GI discomfort			Reversible decreased hearing	Phlebitis (IV erythromycin), metallic taste (clarithromycin)
Clindamycin	Fever	Rash	Diarrhea, pseudomembranous colitis				
Metronidazole	Headache, hypersensitivity	Rash	Nausea, metallic taste, pancreatitis	Leukopenia		Peripheral neuropathy, ataxia	Mutagenic, carcinogenic in rodents, disulfiram-like reaction with alcohol

GI = gastrointestinal; G6PD = glucose-6-phosphate dehydrogenase; LFT = liver function test; MTT = methylthiotetrazole; TEN = toxic epidermal necrolysis.

tissue (e.g., sequestrum in osteomyelitis)? (5) Is the fever (if present) attributable to a drug being administered? Thoughtful re-examination should sort out the cause in many instances.

SUGGESTED READINGS

Grayson ML, Crowe SM, McCarthy JS, et al, eds. The Use of Antibiotics: A Clinical Review of Antibacterial, Antifungal and Antiviral Drugs, 6th ed. London: Hodder Arnold; 2010. *The latest edition of an extensively referenced textbook on antimicrobial agents.*

Tamma PD, Cosgrove SE. Antimicrobial stewardship. *Infect Dis Clin North Am.* 2011;25:245-260. *Review of the ways in which such programs can reduce the overuse and misuse of antimicrobial agents, as well as how to establish them.*

296

STAPHYLOCOCCAL INFECTIONS

HENRY CHAMBERS

TABLE 296-1 COMPARISON OF COMMUNITY AND HOSPITAL CLONES OF METHICILLIN-RESISTANT *STAPHYLOCOCCUS AUREUS* (MRSA)

PROPERTY	COMMUNITY MRSA	HOSPITAL MRSA
Methicillin-resistance gene cassette	*SCCmecIV**	*SCCmecI, II, III*
Common genotypes[†]	USA300 (ST8) USA400 (ST1)	USA100 (ST5) USA500 (ST8) USA800 (ST5)
Panton-Valentine leukocidin	Present in ≈95%	Present in <5%
Antimicrobial resistances	β-Lactams, macrolides, fluoroquinolones	β-Lactams, macrolides, clindamycin, tetracycline, fluoroquinolones, aminoglycosides
Doubling time[‡]	30 min	45-60 min
agr Mutants	Uncommon	Common

*Staphylococcal chromosomal cassette type; this element contains the methicillin resistance gene *mecA*.
[†]Pulsed field gel electrophoresis type with the sequence type (ST) in parentheses.
[‡]Time for the number of cells to double in broth culture.

Staphylococci are well adapted as both commensals and pathogens. Coagulase-negative species constitute a significant proportion of the normal human cutaneous microbiome. *Staphylococcus aureus*, a coagulase-positive species, is present in nasopharyngeal flora in a third of individuals, most of whom will not become infected. As a pathogen, *S. aureus* is one of the most common causes of bacterial infections, which range in severity from relatively trivial skin infections to lethal invasive disease. Coagulase-negative species are intrinsically less virulent and less invasive than *S. aureus* but are responsible for one in four health care–associated infections, almost always involving an indwelling medical device. Antibiotic-resistant strains of staphylococci are quite prevalent, which has a profound impact on therapy.

THE PATHOGEN

The genus *Staphylococcus* consists of more than 30 distinct species. These organisms have co-evolved as normal flora of mammals and birds. They are gram-positive spherical cells (i.e., cocci) 0.5 to 1.5 μm in diameter that divide in multiple planes to form clusters resembling grapes (*staphylo* is derived from the Greek word for "bunch of grapes") when viewed under the microscope. Staphylococci are nonmotile, nonsporulating, hardy organisms that are resistant to desiccation, extremes of pH, and high salt concentrations and are capable of growth under aerobic or anaerobic conditions. Staphylococci produce catalase, an enzyme that degrades hydrogen peroxide into water and oxygen, which definitively distinguishes them biochemically from streptococci and enterococci. The coagulase test is the basis for differentiating *S. aureus* from the numerous other nonpathogenic, coagulase-negative species. Coagulase is a secreted cell surface protein that, in the presence of a prothrombin-like plasma protein, converts fibrinogen to fibrin, forming a clot. *S. aureus* produces a variety of other species-specific surface proteins that differentiate it from other species.

The staphylococcal chromosome is circular; approximately 75% of the genes constitute a core genome common to all staphylococcal species. The remaining 25% contains species-defining elements and mobile genetic elements acquired by horizontal gene transfer. The *S. aureus* genome is abundant in genes encoding toxins, superantigens, and adhesins, whereas coagulase-negative species contain few adhesin and no toxin or superantigen genes. Genetically, *S. aureus* is sufficiently uniform to classify it as a single species; greater diversity among coagulase-negative species merits their classification as distinct species.

STAPHYLOCOCCUS AUREUS

EPIDEMIOLOGY

S. aureus is maintained in the human population primarily through asymptomatic colonization of the anterior nares, mucous membranes, and other moist areas of the body, as well as the groin, perineum, and perianal area in healthy children and adults. Infants become colonized by strains from their mothers within weeks of birth. Carriage rates are higher in children than in adults. Higher-than-average *S. aureus* carriage rates are associated with atopic dermatitis, eczema, chronic skin ulcers, and other acute and chronic skin conditions; insulin-dependent diabetes; dialysis; human immunodeficiency virus (HIV) infection; and recreational injection drug use. Carriers have a several-fold higher risk of developing a subsequent *S. aureus* infection compared with noncarriers. The principal mode of transmission of *S. aureus* is direct contact with an infected individual or an asymptomatic carrier, probably via transient hand carriage. *S. aureus* may also contaminate environmental surfaces, where it can persist for days. The role of environmental contamination in transmission is not well defined, but it may be important if heavily contaminated surfaces or materials are contacted. Droplet and aerosol transmission of *S. aureus* plays little if any role.

S. aureus is responsible for millions of infections in the United States each year, most of which are community-acquired skin infections. Approximately 5 to 10% of *S. aureus* infections are invasive and are often associated with bacteremia. *S. aureus* also causes hundreds of thousands of health care–associated infections each year, 50 to 60% of which are caused by methicillin-resistant *S. aureus* (MRSA). Prior to the mid-1990s, MRSA strains were almost exclusively hospital or health care associated, but they have now become prevalent in the community. Community-associated MRSA strains are distinct from classic health care–associated MRSA strains in several ways (Table 296-1).

PATHOBIOLOGY

Virulence Factors

S. aureus is highly adapted to humans through millions of years of co-evolution with hominids. Well over 50 virulence factors, including adhesins, toxins, enzymes, surface-bound proteins, and capsule polysaccharides, may be produced (E-Table 296-1). Genes encoding these factors may be located on the chromosome either as part of the core genome or within mobile genetic elements (or their remnants), including bacteriophages, pathogenicity islands, and cassettes, or on plasmids. Biofilm formation occurs in the presence of foreign material such as vascular catheters or implanted devices. Biofilm is a complex network of extracellular polysaccharides, DNA, and protein in which bacterial cells become embedded, rendering them inaccessible to clearance by host defense mechanisms. Organisms within biofilms tend to be metabolically inactive and tolerant to killing by antimicrobial agents.

Virulence factors serve to promote binding to host tissues; to evade, circumvent, or disrupt host immune responses; and to facilitate cell injury and tissue invasion. Variability in both the presence of virulence determinants and their expression among strains allows extreme diversity among clinical isolates and the remarkable adaptability of *S. aureus* as a pathogen. An extensive network of two component response systems, DNA binding proteins and regulatory RNAs, controls the expression of virulence (and other) factors in response to environmental conditions. Principal among these is the accessory gene regulator *agr*, a two-component quorum sensing and global gene regulator that controls the expression of numerous surface and secreted proteins. Mutations in *agr* are associated with reduced susceptibility to vancomycin and with loss of virulence.

Mechanisms of Disease

Pathogenesis of *S. aureus* disease occurs by two mechanisms: tissue invasion, which may be local or systemic; and toxin mediated. The characteristic lesion of tissue invasion is the abscess, a focal collection of pus (liquefied and necrotic host tissue, blood, inflammatory cells, DNA, and cellular debris) and bacterial cells surrounded by an ill-defined, surrounding layer of edematous and inflamed tissue infiltrated by acute and chronic inflammatory cells.

Host defenses against *S. aureus* infection consist of an intact, normal skin barrier and the innate immune system. Conditions in which these defenses are impaired are associated with increased risk of *S. aureus* infection. Among these conditions are injection drug use, presence of vascular access devices, burns, chronic skin diseases, use of systemic steroids, traumatic wounds, minor skin abrasions or trauma, surgical procedures, insulin-dependent and non-insulin-dependent diabetes, peritoneal dialysis, hemodialysis, subcutaneous and intramuscular injections, acupuncture, prosthetic implants, and congenital or acquired neutrophil disorders (e.g., chronic granulomatous disease, Job's syndrome). Once the cutaneous barrier has been breached, the next line of defense is the innate immune system. Neutrophils recruited to the site of infection ingest and kill staphylococci. Staphylococci elaborate numerous virulence factors specifically designed to thwart each step of the host response. If large numbers of organisms are present, the host response is overwhelmed, infection is not contained, and dissemination occurs. Endothelial cell injury and invasion can also occur. Intracellular organisms within phagocytes and endothelial cells may play a role in relapse and persistent bacteremia. High tissue burdens of organisms and bacteremia are usually, but not always, accompanied by fever, tachycardia, and other signs of the systemic inflammatory response syndrome, including frank septic shock.

Three toxin-mediated syndromes, which can occur in the absence of invasive disease, are staphylococcal food poisoning, staphylococcal toxic shock syndrome, and staphylococcal scalded skin syndrome. Staphylococcal food poisoning is caused by the ingestion of a preformed heat-stable enterotoxin. The emetic activity of enterotoxin is mediated by the intestinal release of 5-hydroxytryptamine and the stimulation of receptors present on afferent vagal neurons. Toxic shock syndrome is caused by a specific toxin, TSST-1, or other staphylococcal enterotoxins, acting as superantigens, promiscuously binding to major histocompatibility complex (MHC) class II molecules of antigen-presenting cells and T-cell receptors, stimulating the massive release of cytokines from T cells and resulting in septic shock and death. Staphylococcal scalded skin syndrome and bullous impetigo are caused by either of two exfoliative toxins, A or B. These toxins are serine proteases that specifically cleave desmoglein 1, a desmosomal protein that anchors the overlying superficial epidermis to the stratum granulosum.

CLINICAL MANIFESTATIONS

Skin and Soft Tissue Infections

Skin and soft tissue infections are by far the most common infections caused by *S. aureus*; millions of cases occur annually in the United States. Community MRSA strains have been associated with a 50% increase in the rates of skin and soft tissue infections in the United States. This heterogeneous group of skin diseases includes impetigo, folliculitis, furuncle, abscess, erysipelas and cellulitis, mastitis (cellulitis of the breast), necrotizing fasciitis, and wound infections.

Impetigo, folliculitis, and furuncle are superficial infections; fever and other systemic signs of infection are not present. Impetigo is a focal infection of the epidermis that occurs most commonly in children. The typical lesion, which may be multiple or in clusters, is about 1 cm in diameter, with erythema surrounding a bulla or bullae (caused by the production of exfoliative toxin) containing cloudy fluid or with a crusty or scabbed-over appearance. Gram stain of the fluid or drainage from the lesion shows the organism. Folliculitis is a superficial infection with tender, erythematous, maculopapular or pustular lesions centered around hair follicles. Both impetigo and folliculitis readily respond to local measures such as application of soap and water, topical antibiotics, or antiseptics; systemic antimicrobial therapy may be indicated for extensive or refractory infections.

A furuncle is simply a boil—an erythematous, suppurative infection measuring 1 to 2 cm that extends through the dermis into the subcutaneous tissue. It may drain spontaneously; if not, hot compresses can be applied to encourage drainage, or the furuncle can be incised and drained. Antimicrobial therapy is not needed. The distinction between a furuncle and an abscess is somewhat arbitrary; abscesses tend to be larger and deeper and may be associated with systemic signs of infection and bacteremia. Furuncles may

extend to fascia or deeper tissues and coalesce into carbuncles, a more severe form of infection that may be accompanied by bacteremia. Large abscesses and carbuncles, particularly in the presence of fever and the systemic inflammatory response syndrome, require surgical drainage and systemic antimicrobial therapy.

Erysipelas and cellulitis, which are similar in appearance, are painful, warm, indurated, erythematous, nonlocalized infections that may be accompanied by lymphangitis. Cellulitis extends into the dermis and subcutaneous fat; erysipelas is more superficial. Surrounding cellulitis is often associated with an obvious cutaneous abscess, but it may also overlie a deeper abscess; the primary therapy is surgical drainage. Cellulitis without an associated abscess should be treated with systemic antimicrobial therapy. Cellulitis due to streptococci (Chapter 298) cannot reliably be distinguished from that caused by *S. aureus*, owing to their similar appearance; the presence of an associated purulent lesion suggests staphylococcal infection, and culture should be performed to make a microbiologic diagnosis.

Necrotizing fasciitis is an infection of the deep layers of skin and subcutaneous tissues, extending to muscle and along fascial planes. It is associated with systemic toxicity, leukocytosis, and severe pain, often out of proportion to the physical findings. The overlying skin may appear to be uninvolved, belying the serious nature of this infection, which requires immediate surgical intervention for débridement of involved tissue. Necrotizing fasciitis, which is more typically caused by group A streptococci (Chapter 298) or occurs as a mixed infection, has been associated with community MRSA infection.

Pyomyositis (also termed *tropical myositis*) is an infection of the skeletal muscle; *S. aureus* is the most common cause. The patient presents with fever, pain, and swelling and induration that can be felt on deep palpation; the overlying skin and soft tissue may appear normal. There is often a history of trauma to the infected area. Although it can occur in otherwise normal children and adults, acquired immunodeficiency syndrome (AIDS) and other immunocompromising conditions are predisposing factors. This infection is thought to occur as a consequence of metastatic seeding from a subclinical bacteremia; blood cultures may not be positive at the time of diagnosis. The diagnosis is established by culture of pus collected by needle aspirate. Surgical or percutaneous drainage should be performed, and systemic antimicrobial therapy is indicated.

S. aureus causes 30% of surgical site infections overall in the United States, and approximately 50% of those follow neurosurgical or orthopedic procedures. These infections occur at the site of incision, typically after the second or third postoperative day. Signs and symptoms are fever accompanied by erythema, edema, induration, drainage, pain, and tenderness at the surgical site. Superficial infections respond to removal of stitches, débridement of devitalized tissue, opening of the wound to allow drainage, and a short course of antimicrobial therapy. Deeper infections may require more extensive débridement and longer courses of therapy (4 to 6 weeks), particularly if bone or a prosthetic device is involved. Removal of infected prosthetic material or a foreign body greatly increases the chance of cure.

Bacteremia

Bacteremia, the presence of bacteria in the blood stream, exemplifies the pathogenicity of *S. aureus*. It is virtually synonymous with invasive disease, present in approximately 75% of cases. The most common sources of bacteremia are skin and soft tissue infections, central venous catheters and other intravascular devices, bone and joint infections, pneumonia, and endocarditis. Bacteremia can emanate from any source, which may not be obvious in 25% of cases. Invasion of the blood stream allows the organism to disseminate widely throughout the body, establishing multiple metastatic sites of infection and thereby perpetuating bacteremia. Fever is usually, but not always, present. Sepsis syndrome and septic shock are common, and death occurs in 10 to 20% of cases.

The presence of bacteremia dictates the approach to the diagnosis, management, and therapy of *S. aureus* infection. When blood cultures are positive, even if the primary source is known, there is always the possibility of endocarditis or other secondary foci of infection. Echocardiography is recommended to look for evidence of endocarditis. Source control is the cornerstone of management and therapy; both primary and secondary foci of infection should be identified and removed whenever possible, because these may lead to treatment failure or relapse once therapy is discontinued. Computed tomography (CT) or magnetic resonance imaging (MRI) should be considered if signs and symptoms point to deep tissue abscesses or osteomyelitis. Follow-up blood cultures should be obtained to document clearance. Persistent bacteremia is suggestive of endovascular infection, and failure to clear

TABLE 296-2	CRITERIA FOR DIAGNOSIS OF UNCOMPLICATED *STAPHYLOCOCCUS AUREUS* BACTEREMIA*

Resolution of fever and systemic signs of infection by day 3 of therapy
Sterile blood cultures within 2–3 days of initiation of antimicrobial therapy
Presence of an identifiable and easily removable focus of infection
Prompt removal of the primary focus of infection
No echocardiographic or clinical signs of endocarditis
No osteomyelitis
No hematogenous secondary foci of infection
No preexisting valve abnormalities predisposing to endocarditis (e.g., prosthetic
   valve, rheumatic heart disease, bicuspid aortic valve)
No implanted prosthetic device (e.g., prosthetic hip)

*Uncomplicated *S. aureus* bacteremia can be treated with a shorter course of antibiotics (see text).

FIGURE 296-1. Chest radiograph shows multiple nodular pulmonary lesions, suggestive of septic embolization, in a patient with tricuspid valve *S. aureus* endocarditis. The red circle shows a lesion with signs of cavitation.

blood cultures after 3 to 4 days of appropriate therapy is a strong predictor of complicated bacteremia, necessitating a longer course of therapy. Antimicrobial therapy should always be administered. A shorter duration of therapy (i.e., 14 days) is appropriate for uncomplicated bacteremia (Table 296-2). Longer courses of 4 to 6 weeks are recommended for the treatment of endocarditis or bacteremia complicated by slow resolution or the presence of metastatic infection.

Endocarditis

S. aureus is the leading cause of endocarditis (Chapter 76), accounting for approximately 30% of all cases. Most are community-acquired infections, often occurring as a complication of injection drug use. The number of health care–associated infections has been increasing in recent years; risk factors are diabetes mellitus, hemodialysis, and presence of a prosthetic valve. The presentation is that of an acute febrile illness, with high fever developing over a few days. The patient may appear toxic and septic. A source of infection may not be evident at first; a minority of patients have an associated infection of bone, joint, or skin and soft tissue. The aortic and mitral valves are most commonly involved, except in injection drug users (discussed later); however, a pathologic murmur may not be evident when the patient first presents. Systemic embolization to the brain, kidneys, spleen, gut, or other large vessels is clinically evident in about one third of cases. Peripheral manifestations, including Roth's spots, Osler's nodes, Janeway's lesions, and petechiae, occur with a similar frequency. Morbidity and mortality are high, in part due to the occurrence of this infection in older patients, many of whom have medical comorbidities. Strokes occur in approximately 20% of patients, and congestive heart failure occurs in 40 to 50%; 25 to 30% do not survive the initial hospitalization.

Endocarditis in injection drug users involves the tricuspid valve in approximately three quarters of cases. Patients typically have fever, cough, hemoptysis, and pleuritic chest pain as a consequence of hematogenous seeding of the lung and septic emboli from the valve. The chest radiograph may show pulmonary infiltrates; signs of consolidation or pleural effusion; or multiple, often peripheral nodular pulmonary infiltrates with cavitation, hallmark features of septic embolization (Fig. 296-1). Patients tend to be young and otherwise healthy, so mortality is relatively low—5% or less. Injection drug users can also have aortic valve or mitral valve endocarditis, in which case the presentation is similar to that described earlier. Conversely, patients who are not injection drug users may have tricuspid valve endocarditis with pulmonary findings.

Pericarditis

S. aureus is the most common cause of purulent pericarditis in children and following cardiac surgery in adults. It may occur by contamination at the time of surgery; bacteremic seeding from another site of infection; as a complication of endocarditis, paravalvular abscess, or myocardial abscess; or by direct extension of infection from pneumonia, lung abscess, or empyema. The presentation is that of acute pericarditis (Chapter 77), with fever and severe chest pain, tachycardia, and hemodynamic instability. The clinical course may be extremely rapid, terminating in septic shock or cardiac tamponade. Immediate drainage of the infected pericardial space and administration of systemic antimicrobial therapy are indicated. Needle pericardiocentesis is useful for confirming the diagnosis and providing temporary decompression of the pericardial space, but definitive therapy requires surgical or continuous tube drainage.

FIGURE 296-2. Noncontrast, non–fat-saturated, T1-weighted, sagittal sequence shows discitis, osteomyelitis, prevertebral and epidural abscess, and cord compression in a patient with *S. aureus* infection of the cervical spine.

Osteomyelitis

S. aureus is the most common cause of osteomyelitis, both acute and chronic (Chapter 280). The primary mode of infection is hematogenous seeding. Up to a quarter of cases of bacteremia are complicated by osteomyelitis, and bacteremia is present in 50 to 75% of osteomyelitis cases. Acute osteomyelitis—defined as an initial episode with a clinical course of days to weeks, but not months—presents with fever and pain at the site of infection. Long bones are more commonly infected in children, whereas vertebrae are more commonly infected in adults. Adults can also have long bone osteomyelitis, however, usually from a contiguous focus of infection or at a site of fracture or prior trauma. Vertebral osteomyelitis is frequently accompanied by paravertebral or epidural abscess (Fig. 296-2). Back pain accompanied by signs of cord compression, such as radicular pain, sensory loss, lower extremity weakness, urinary retention, and bowel or bladder incontinence, is an emergency. MRI should be performed as soon as possible to define the location and extent of infection, and neurosurgical consultation should be obtained in anticipation of surgical decompression and drainage.

Septic Arthritis

S. aureus is the most common cause of septic arthritis (Chapter 280), usually as a consequence of bacteremic seeding, trauma, or a surgical procedure. Risk factors include diabetes, recent joint surgery or joint prosthesis (Chapter

285), and rheumatoid arthritis (Chapter 272). Cardinal features are joint pain, history of joint swelling, and fever. The diagnosis is established by analysis of synovial fluid. The white blood cell count exceeds 25,000/mm³, with 90% neutrophils. Organisms are usually present on Gram stain, and the culture is virtually always positive. Hip, knee, ankle, and wrist are most commonly affected. *S. aureus* also has a predilection for infecting the sternoclavicular, sacroiliac, and symphysis pubis joints. Multiple joints are involved in 5% of cases. Both antimicrobial therapy and drainage of the infected joint (by repeated needle aspiration, arthrotomy, or arthroscopically) are required to prevent destructive arthritis.

Central Nervous System Infections

S. aureus is an uncommon cause of community-acquired central nervous system infections such as bacterial meningitis, primary brain abscess, or subdural empyema. These infections are often associated with endocarditis or a contiguous focus of infection, such as cavernous sinus thrombosis. Mortality of these infections is as high as 30 to 50%. *S. aureus* is an important cause of nosocomial meningitis following head trauma, craniotomy, or implantation of intraventricular or extraventricular catheters.

Pulmonary Infections

S. aureus is an uncommon cause of community-acquired pneumonia (Chapter 97). It is typically a severe, often fatal, fulminant necrotizing pneumonia accompanied by evidence of cavitation on chest radiographs. Production of Panton-Valentine leukocidin has been associated with severe pneumonia. Community-acquired staphylococcal pneumonia should be considered, and coverage for MRSA strains should be included in the empirical regimen, in two clinical settings: severe pneumonia requiring admission to an intensive care unit, and pneumonia in a patient with influenza.

The most common hospital-acquired and ventilator-associated pneumonias are caused by *S. aureus,* and MRSA in particular. Mortality is in the range of 40 to 50%, reflecting the virulence of the organism and the comorbid conditions that contribute to poor outcomes. The diagnosis is readily established by examination of a Gram stain of sputum, tracheal aspirate, or lavage (obtained to avoid oropharyngeal contamination), which typically shows organisms and numerous neutrophils. The culture is less specific than the Gram stain because it is positive in colonized patients, but it is highly sensitive. Coverage for MRSA can be discontinued if the organism is not isolated in culture or not seen on Gram stain.

Lung abscess and pleural empyema, infections most commonly caused by oral anaerobic bacteria, are occasionally caused by *S. aureus.* The clinical course may be subacute or even indolent. Empyema occurs as a complication of prior chest tube placement, surgery, trauma, staphylococcal pneumonia, or tricuspid valve endocarditis. These infections are treated with drainage and antimicrobial therapy.

Prosthetic Device Infections

Prosthetic device– and implant-associated infections occurring within the first 12 weeks of surgery are most commonly caused by *S. aureus. S. aureus* is second only to coagulase-negative staphylococci as a cause of later infections. The presentation may be acute, with joint pain, evidence of arthritis, fever, and systemic signs of infection; alternatively, the infection may run a more chronic course, with pain and loosening of the prosthesis but little or no fever. Formation of biofilm makes treating these infections a challenge. In most cases, the infection is incurable if the infected hardware is not removed. Débridement and removal of the prosthesis or implant in conjunction with antimicrobial therapy offer the best chance of cure. This can be accomplished either as a one-stage procedure, in which the infected prosthesis or implant is removed and immediately replaced, or as a two-stage procedure, in which the device is removed and replaced after completion of a 4- to 6-week course of antimicrobial therapy.

Genitourinary Infections

Genitourinary infections arise by hematogenous dissemination or as an ascending infection, usually as a result of instrumentation, urinary catheterization, or surgery. These infections include cystitis, pyelonephritis, microabscess, perinephric abscess, prostatitis, and prostatic abscess. *S. aureus* can also be a contaminant introduced during the collection of urine from a patient with asymptomatic vaginal or perineal colonization. Contamination should be suspected if the urine colony counts are low, repeat urine cultures are negative, pyuria is absent, and there are no signs or symptoms of urinary tract infection. If contamination seems unlikely and there is no well-documented

history of an event that could lead to ascending infection, hematogenous dissemination has to be assumed. Blood cultures should be obtained to determine whether there is ongoing bacteremia, and appropriate imaging studies should be performed to identify a deep focus of infection and the presence of renal and perinephric abscesses.

Toxin-Mediated Diseases

These diseases are caused by the ingestion of preformed toxin or the elaboration of toxin by *S. aureus* from a site of colonization or infection. Staphylococcal food poisoning is a gastroenteritis caused by the ingestion of a preformed enterotoxin produced in food contaminated by *S. aureus* from an infected or colonized food handler. When contaminated food is kept at room temperature for several hours, organisms replicate and produce a heat-stable toxin that is not inactivated by cooking or digestive enzymes. Nausea, vomiting, abdominal pain, and diarrhea occur within 2 to 6 hours of eating the contaminated food. There is no fever, and the illness is self-limited, generally lasting about a day. Antibiotics have no role in therapy, which consists of fluid replacement to prevent dehydration. Infants, small children, and the elderly are more severely affected and may require intravenous fluids.

Toxic shock syndrome is caused by colonization or infection with a strain that elaborates a specific toxin, TSST-1, or certain staphylococcal enterotoxins. TSST-1 is responsible for 100% of menstrual cases due to its ability to cross the vaginal mucosa and achieve systemic concentrations. TSST-1 and the staphylococcal enterotoxins SEA, SEB, and SEC are responsible for nonmenstrual toxic shock syndrome, which is characteristically associated with an identifiable focus of infection, usually of the skin. The diagnosis is clinical, defined by fever, erythroderma, hypotension, involvement of three of more organ systems (renal, hematologic, hepatic, pulmonary, gastrointestinal, muscle, central nervous system, mucous membranes), and desquamation, especially of the palms and soles, 1 to 2 weeks after the onset of illness. Bacteremia is rare, present in only 5% of cases. The case fatality rate is about 5%. Treatment consists of systemic antimicrobial therapy, removal of the source of toxin production, and treatment of septic shock (streptococcal toxic shock syndrome is discussed in Chapter 298).

Colonization or infection with an *S. aureus* strain that produces exfoliative toxin A or B may cause staphylococcal scalded skin syndrome, a disease primarily of infants but occasionally seen in adults (Fig. 296-3), and bullous impetigo, a pustular skin lesion. The appearance is that of a scald, burn, or blister. The differential diagnosis of staphylococcal scalded skin syndrome includes drug reaction (Chapter 448), toxic epidermal necrolysis (Chapter 447), Kawasaki disease (Chapter 447), and pemphigus foliaceus (Chapter 443).

DIAGNOSIS

S. aureus infection is diagnosed by isolating the organism in cultures of blood, tissue, or pus. Non–culture-based methods such as nucleic acid amplification tests are becoming available, but their utility is still being defined; culture remains the "gold standard." Gram stain is very useful for making a presumptive diagnosis of staphylococcal infection and should be performed whenever possible to look for gram-positive cocci in tetrads or clusters in pus, bone or tissue samples, respiratory secretions, or body fluids such as cerebrospinal

FIGURE 296-3. Scalded skin–type lesions with multiple ruptured bullae and desquamation in a patient with aortic valve endocarditis caused by an exfoliative toxin–producing strain of *S. aureus.*

fluid, pleural or pericardial fluid, synovial fluid, or urine. Failure to isolate the organism in culture is strong evidence against *S. aureus* infection unless a patient is being actively treated with an antibiotic; even then, several days of therapy would be needed to render an infected site culture negative. The specificity of isolating *S. aureus* from blood or other sterile body sites is essentially 100%. Because of nasopharyngeal colonization in some uninfected individuals, isolation of *S. aureus* from culture of a respiratory specimen lacks specificity; however, if Gram stain also shows gram-positive cocci in tetrads and clusters and many neutrophils, this is very suggestive of *S. aureus* pneumonia.

Susceptibility Testing

Susceptibility testing should be performed for clinically significant isolates to guide antimicrobial therapy. The critical determination is whether the isolate is methicillin resistant (i.e., resistant to β-lactam antibiotics). Resistance to macrolides and fluoroquinolones is common, and these drugs should not be used to treat suspected staphylococcal infection without confirmation of in vitro susceptibility. Clindamycin is usually active, although macrolide-resistant strains that produce a ribosomal methylase, inducibly or constitutively, are cross-resistant. Tetracyclines and trimethoprim-sulfamethoxazole are active against 80 to 90% of strains. Resistance to vancomycin, daptomycin, telavancin, or linezolid, though rare, may occur, particularly when there has been prior exposure to the drug, making susceptibility testing important for these antibiotics.

TREATMENT Rx

The two principles of therapy for *S. aureus* infections are (1) elimination of focal infection and infected foreign material whenever feasible, and (2) administration of systemic antimicrobial therapy. For boils and cutaneous abscesses, incision and drainage may be all that is required. Antimicrobial therapy is indicated if the infection is not amenable to removal (e.g., cellulitis, pneumonia), drainage is impossible or inadequate, systemic signs and symptoms of infection are present, or there is invasive disease (i.e., secondary sites of infection; involvement of deep tissues, vital organs, sterile sites) and in all cases of bacteremia. An undrained focus of infection or retention of an infected foreign body is the most common reason for unsatisfactory clinical response, treatment failure, or relapse.

The most important consideration when selecting an antibiotic is susceptibility of the *S. aureus* isolate to β-lactams. A penicillinase-resistant penicillin, such as nafcillin (1 to 2 g every 4 to 6 hours IV, depending on the severity of the infection), oxacillin, or flucloxacillin, or a cephalosporin (e.g., cefazolin 1 to 2 g every 8 hours IV) is the agent of choice for the treatment of methicillin-susceptible (MSSA) infections; no other antibiotic is as safe or as effective as a β-lactam. An orally administered β-lactam (e.g., dicloxacillin 500 mg four times daily or cephalexin 500 mg four times daily) is appropriate for most cutaneous infections; a parenteral agent is recommended, at least initially, for invasive infections. Only if the patient is allergic or has a serious reaction is an agent other than a β-lactam preferred for the treatment of infection caused by an MSSA strain.

Methicillin-resistant strains are cross-resistant to all currently available β-lactams, except for ceftaroline, recently FDA approved at a dose of 600 mg intravenously every 12 hours for treatment of skin and skin structure infections caused by methicillin-resistant strains. Otherwise, a β-lactam should not be used to treat infection caused by a methicillin-resistant strain or as empirical therapy when the prevalence of methicillin-resistant strains is high. The prevalence of methicillin resistance in *S. aureus* isolates from hospital-acquired and health care–associated infections in most hospitals in the United States and in many European countries is 25 to 50% or higher. MRSA also causes a substantial proportion of community-onset infections in individuals lacking other risk factors, especially in the United States. Trimethoprim-sulfamethoxazole (one or two 80/160-mg tablets twice a day), clindamycin (300 mg three times a day), and doxycycline or minocycline (100 mg twice a day) are active in vitro against most community-acquired MSSA and MRSA strains and are effective when administered orally for the treatment of skin and soft tissue infections in outpatients. Fluoroquinolones should not be used because most methicillin-resistant strains are also fluoroquinolone resistant. For invasive infections, vancomycin is still the drug of choice. It must be administered intravenously; doses of 30 to 60 mg/kg/day, adjusted based on creatinine clearance, are recommended to achieve trough serum concentrations of 15 to 20 µg/mL for patients with bacteremia, endocarditis, or other serious infections. Treatment failures are not uncommon; approximately a quarter of patients with bacteremia or endocarditis remain persistently bacteremic (≥7 days) or relapse, even when the strain is susceptible (minimal inhibitory concentration [MIC] ≤2 µg/mL) in vitro. Other than the presence of an undrained focus of infection, the reasons for this are unclear. Possible explanations include vancomycin's slowly bactericidal activity; tolerance, in which the isolate is inhibited at low concentrations but not killed; or so-called heteroresistance, in which a small fraction of the population of organisms has a higher MIC. Treatment failures have also been associated with isolates having MICs of 2 µg/mL. Isolates with intermediate susceptibility to vancomycin (MICs of 4 or 8 µg/mL) in vitro are in fact "nonsusceptible" and should be considered resistant because this is highly predictive of treatment failure. Approximately 1 to 3% of clinical isolates have intermediate susceptibility to vancomycin. Vancomycin-resistant strains (MIC >8 µg/mL) are rare. Alternatives to vancomycin include quinupristin-dalfopristin (7.5 mg/kg every 8-12 hours), linezolid (600 mg every 12 hours), daptomycin (4 mg/kg once daily for complicated skin and soft tissue infections; 6 mg/kg once daily for bacteremia,■ although some authorities recommended higher doses of 10 mg/kg), and telavancin (10 mg/kg once daily for complicated skin and soft tissue infection).■

The role of combination therapy is ill defined. Aminoglycoside combination regimens have not been shown to improve outcomes, but there are good data demonstrating increased toxicity and adverse events with aminoglycoside combinations. Aminoglycoside combinations should not be used routinely; if used at all, they should be reserved for patients who have failed first-line therapy. Rifampin combination therapy may have a role in the treatment of osteomyelitis, particularly that caused by methicillin-resistant strains. Rifampin (300 to 450 mg twice daily) must always be administered in combination with a second active agent because resistance emerges rapidly during therapy.

COAGULASE-NEGATIVE STAPHYLOCOCCI

More than 30 different species of coagulase-negative staphylococci have been identified, and about half of these colonize humans. *Staphylococcus epidermidis* is the species that most commonly causes infection. Coagulase-negative staphylococci rarely cause infection unless there is a foreign body in place, and although bacteremia occurs, metastatic seeding of secondary sites of infection is distinctly uncommon. Coagulase-negative staphylococci are typically resistant to methicillin and multiple other antibiotics, and they are an important reservoir of drug-resistance elements that are horizontally transferrable to *S. aureus*. They are the most common cause of health care–associated infections overall in the United States (Chapter 290); they account for one third of central line–associated blood stream infections; and they are the second most common cause of surgical site infections, particularly when a prosthetic device or other foreign material has been implanted. Infections are often indolent, causing little in the way of fever or systemic signs of infection, but they may also be acute and life-threatening, as in the case of prosthetic valve endocarditis. Coagulase-negative staphylococci are proficient biofilm producers; consequently, débridement and removal of the infected prosthetic device or foreign body are paramount. Antimicrobial therapy of these infections is similar to that for *S. aureus*, except that hematogenous seeding rarely occurs, so attention is focused primarily on source control.

Coagulase-negative staphylococci, because they are normal skin flora, are the most common blood culture contaminant. In approximately 75% of cases, when the blood culture is positive for coagulase-negative staphylococci, this reflects contamination rather than infection. Sorting out whether a positive culture represents contamination or true infection can be a challenge. A single positive blood culture or blood cultures in which more than one strain is present are likely to be due to contamination. Time to blood culture positivity, quantitative blood cultures, and the presence of multiple positive cultures can be useful in determining whether a positive blood culture represents true infection. Isolation of coagulase-negative staphylococci from the blood of a patient with a prosthetic valve, intravenous pacemaker, or vascular graft can be especially problematic because these patients are at high risk for true infection. Unless the patient is hemodynamically unstable or otherwise seriously ill, it is advisable to withhold antibiotics until additional cultures are obtained to document the presence of true bacteremia. Isolation of coagulase-negative staphylococci from cultures of deep tissue, bone, prosthetic devices, or other normally sterile sites, especially if multiple cultures are positive, strongly suggests true infection.

PREVENTION

The emergence of community MRSA and the large burden of hospital-acquired and health care–associated staphylococcal infections have stimulated renewed interest in prevention strategies. The organisms that cause these infections are usually resident flora (either *S. aureus* or coagulase-negative staphylococci), or they are acquired by direct contact with a contaminated source, such as a wound or dressing, the skin or hands of an asymptomatically colonized individual, or a contaminated health care provider. The most effective strategy is adherence to principles of basic infection control, the key component of which is hand hygiene, whether it be handwashing or use of an alcohol-based hand rub. This disrupts transmission of organisms via the hands of care providers, a well-documented source of bacterial contamination. Barrier precautions (gloves and gowns) are important for minimizing contact with infected wounds, contaminated secretions, and dressings. Isolation precautions and screening for asymptomatic carriage are more controversial and less well documented in terms of their efficacy. For patients undergoing surgical procedures, surgical hand and surgical site antisepsis, aseptic surgical technique, and antimicrobial prophylaxis are important preventive measures.

Screening and decolonization of *S. aureus* carriers is another potentially effective means of preventing infection. Studies to determine whether decolonization actually prevents infection, however, have had mixed results. Nevertheless, decolonization may be considered in two settings: prevention of recurrent infection in individuals who have had several prior episodes, and prevention of surgical site infections. The best-studied regimens are topically applied mupirocin nasal ointment (0.5 g twice daily in each nostril for 5 days), with or without bathing with chlorhexidine soap, and orally administered rifampin (600 mg in one or two divided doses) in combination with another active agent (e.g., a fluoroquinolone if the isolate is susceptible, trimethoprim-sulfamethoxazole, doxycycline). In a recent randomized, double-blind, placebo-controlled, multicenter trial, the number of surgical site *S. aureus* infections acquired in the hospital was reduced by the rapid screening of nasal carriers using a real-time polymerase chain reaction assay and the decolonization of carriers with mupirocin nasal ointment and chlorhexidine soap.**3** Several antistaphylococcal vaccine candidates are currently in phase I and phase II clinical trials; the availability of an effective vaccine would be an important tool in preventing staphylococcal infections.

1. Fowler VG Jr, Boucher HW, Corey GR, et al. Daptomycin versus standard therapy for bacteremia and endocarditis caused by *Staphylococcus aureus*. *N Engl J Med.* 2006;355:653-665.
2. Stryjewski ME, Graham DR, Wilson SE, et al. Telavancin versus vancomycin for the treatment of complicated skin and skin-structure infections caused by gram-positive organisms. *Clin Infect Dis.* 2008;46:1683-1693.
3. Bode LG, Kluytmans JA, Wertheim HF, et al. Preventing surgical-site infections in nasal carriers of *Staphylococcus aureus*. *N Engl J Med.* 2010;362:9-17.

SUGGESTED READINGS

Corey GR. *Staphylococcus aureus* bloodstream infections: definitions and treatment. *Clin Infect Dis.* 2009;48(suppl 4):S254-S259. *Excellent guide to the principles of therapy for patients with S. aureus bacteremia.*
Deleo FR, Otto M, Kreiswirth BN, et al. Community-associated methicillin-resistant *Staphylococcus aureus.* Lancet. 2010;375:1557-1568. *Review of the epidemiology of community MRSA, its pathogenesis, and options for antimicrobial therapy.*
Liu C, Bayer A, Cosgrove SE, et al. Clinical practice guidelines by the Infectious Diseases Society of American for the treatment of methicillin-resistant *Staphylococcus aureus* infections in adults and children: executive summary. *Clin Infect Dis.* 2011;52:285-292. *Consensus guidelines.*
Otto M. *Staphylococcus epidermidis*—the "accidental" pathogen. *Nat Rev Microbiol.* 2009;7:555-567. *Authoritative review of the biology of S. epidermidis and diseases caused by it.*

297

STREPTOCOCCUS PNEUMONIAE INFECTIONS

LIONEL A. MANDELL

DEFINITION

The term *pneumococcal pneumonia* refers to infection of the pulmonary parenchyma and its associated structures by *Streptococcus pneumoniae*. The estimated 500,000 cases that occur annually in the United States result in approximately 50,000 deaths.

The Pathogen

S. pneumoniae is a gram-positive coccus that typically grows in pairs or short chains. Careful examination of the diplococcal form reveals slightly tapered ends that give rise to its lancet-shaped appearance. It is a facultative anaerobe

that grows best on blood agar plates in a 5% carbon dioxide ambient environment. The colonies are typically surrounded by a greenish zone of hemolysis resulting from degradation of hemoglobin by a pneumococcal toxin. The organism can be distinguished from other streptococci by its susceptibility to ethyl hydrocuprein (optochin) and bile solubility.

The surface of the pneumococcus consists of a capsule and a cell wall. The capsule, which helps prevent phagocytosis, is composed of polysaccharides that define the 90 pneumococcal serotypes. The cell wall is a dynamic structure composed of more than a dozen distinct glycopeptides.

EPIDEMIOLOGY

The pneumococcus causes about two thirds of cases of community-acquired pneumonia (CAP) and is responsible for a corresponding percentage of deaths; it can cause hospital-acquired and health care–associated pneumonia as well. The false impression that *S. pneumoniae* is uncommon has arisen because at least one third of patients with CAP are unable to produce sputum and, even if they do, often provide an inadequate sample. Moreover, if the patient has recently taken just one dose of a drug to which the pneumococcus is susceptible, it may not be possible to isolate the organism.

The ecologic niche of the pneumococcus is the nasopharynx, and up to 80% of infants and 20% of healthy adults may be colonized. Simultaneous colonization with more than one capsular type has been reported. Asymptomatic colonization is an immunizing experience because homologous anticapsular antibodies may be demonstrated in individuals after colonization with a specific serotype.

A particular serotype may colonize the nasopharynx for varying periods, but the average duration in infants is 7 weeks. Carriage rates are highest during the late fall, winter, and early spring. Although each of the 90 serotypes is potentially pathogenic, the most frequently encountered are types 3, 4, 6, 7, 9, 12, 14, 18, 19, and 23.

Person-to-person transmission results from close interpersonal contact. Although pneumococcal pneumonia is typically a sporadic illness, epidemics can occur in crowded settings such as daycare centers, barracks, nursing homes, or prisons.

The incidence of pneumococcal pneumonia is about 18 per 100,000 people per year. For persons 5 years or younger and 75 years or older, rates are about 23 and 35.8 per 100,000 people, respectively. For pneumococcal bacteremia, the incidence is about 7.5 per 100,000 people per year and increases with age; the case-fatality rate is 21%.

Risk factors for pneumococcal pneumonia include dementia, seizure disorders, heart failure, cerebrovascular disease, chronic obstructive pulmonary disease, human immunodeficiency virus (HIV) infection, previous viral respiratory illness, alcoholism, malnutrition, diabetes, cirrhosis, and renal insufficiency.

Certain ethnic groups such as Native Americans, particularly Alaskan natives, and Australian Aboriginals appear to be particularly susceptible to invasive pneumococcal infection. Any individual who has a defect in immunoglobulin G (IgG) synthesis (Chapter 258) or phagocyte function (Chapter 172) or who has undergone splenectomy is also at increased risk for invasive pneumococcal infection.

PATHOBIOLOGY

Pneumonia is the result of a breakdown in the interplay between colonizer and host. In pneumococcal pneumonia, the microorganism first colonizes the nasopharynx. Aspiration of small amounts of oropharyngeal contents occurs in deep sleep, even in normal individuals, but if the oropharyngeal material includes pneumococcal serotypes associated with invasive infection and if normal clearance mechanisms fail, the colonizers may become pathogens. The risk for infection is increased by any process or condition that exposes the host to the pathogen, that allows oropharyngeal secretions to bypass upper airway defenses, or that interferes with the host's ability to ingest and kill the pneumococci (Table 297-1).

It appears that aspirated pneumococci adhere to type II cells in the alveolus if they are not cleared by normal defense mechanisms. Attachment to resting cells is mediated by two classes of glycoconjugates, but local inflammatory mediators upregulate host cell receptors, such as those for platelet-activating factor (PAF), and provide a site of attachment for the bacteria. This interaction between PAF receptor and pathogen appears to be an important step in internalization of the bacteria by means of an endocytic vacuole and may promote invasion.

Once in the lung, the pneumococci are able to activate complement and stimulate the cytokine response. Initially, the alveoli fill with fluid exudate

TABLE 297-1	PREDISPOSING FACTORS FOR PNEUMOCOCCAL PNEUMONIA

INCREASED EXPOSURE TO *STREPTOCOCCUS PNEUMONIAE*

Prisons
Military barracks
Daycare centers
Shelters for the homeless

DECREASED HOST DEFENSES

Complement deficiency
Antibody deficiency
Functional or anatomic asplenia
Decreased numbers or function of phagocytes

SPECIFIC DISEASE ENTITIES

Multiple myeloma
Lymphoma
Chronic lymphocytic leukemia
Human immunodeficiency virus infection

RESPIRATORY AND PULMONARY PROBLEMS

Chronic obstructive pulmonary disease
Smoker
Allergies
Previous viral infection

FIGURE 297-1. **Pneumonia. A,** Low-power magnification (× 100) of hematoxylin and eosin (H&E) stain of tissue section from left lower lobe of lung. Note intact alveolar walls and alveoli filled with edema and thick cellular exudates. **B,** Higher magnification (× 500) H&E stain of same section shown in **A.** Note heavy infiltrate of polymorphonuclear cells and intact alveolar walls.

(Fig. 297-1), which allows the infection to spread to adjacent uninfected alveoli. In healthy lungs, polymorphonuclear leukocytes (PMNs) constitute less than 1 to 2% of alveolar cells and normally reside in the interstitial areas of the lung and in adjacent capillaries. Recruitment of PMNs into alveoli depends on the generation of chemoattractants necessary for the directed migration of neutrophils.

The pneumococcal polysaccharides of the bacterial capsule help the organism resist phagocytosis, and absence of anticapsular antibody limits the ability to opsonize and ingest pathogens. Ultimately, the signs and symptoms of disease are due both to the pathogens themselves and to the body's response to them. The bacterial cytotoxin pneumolysin and pneumococcal cell wall components, such as teichoic acid and peptidoglycan, are able to induce a variety of effects that initiate and then enhance the inflammatory response, thereby resulting in the various signs and symptoms of pneumonia.

The effects of pneumococcal infection are ultimately manifested as changes in lung mechanics secondary to reductions in lung volumes and lung compliance, as well as gas exchange problems resulting from intrapulmonary shunting and subsequent arterial hypoxemia. If severe enough, death may ensue.

Antibiotic Resistance

The phenotypic expression of antibiotic resistance corresponds to genetic alterations resulting from horizontal acquisition of foreign genetic information or from mutations in the microbial genome. With *S. pneumoniae*, resistance may be acquired by direct DNA incorporation and remodeling from closely related oral commensal bacteria by the process of natural transformation. Pneumococcal resistance to β-lactams such as penicillin is due solely to the presence of low-affinity penicillin-binding proteins (PBPs). The PBPs themselves are *trans* and carboxypeptidase enzymes that are involved in bacterial cell wall synthesis and represent the primary sites of action for β-lactam drugs.

Resistance to macrolides, in contrast, can occur through multiple mechanisms, including target site modification or an efflux pump. Target site modification is caused by a ribosomal methylase encoded by the *ermB* gene. A change in 23S recombinant RNA mediated by this gene can result in resistance to macrolides, lincosamides, and streptogramin B–type antibiotics (MLS$_B$ phenotype). The efflux mechanism is encoded by the *mefA* gene, which results in an M phenotype. The former is typically associated with high-level resistance with minimal inhibitory concentrations (MICs) of 64 μg/mL or higher, whereas the latter is usually associated with low-level resistance with MICs of 1 to 32 μg/mL. These two mechanisms account for approximately 45 and 55%, respectively, of resistant isolates. Some pneumococcal isolates have been found with both the *erm* and *mef* gene, but the significance of such a finding is unknown.

Resistance to fluoroquinolones may be mediated by changes in one or both target sites (topoisomerase II and IV), which usually result from mutations in the *gyrA* and *parC* genes, respectively. An efflux pump may have a role as well. Of concern is the fact that the incidence of multidrug-resistant isolates is increasing.

CLINICAL MANIFESTATIONS

The clinical features of pneumococcal pneumonia depend on factors such as whether the patient is immunocompetent or immunosuppressed, the severity of illness, and whether the patient has taken antibiotics. Temperatures can vary from 101° F to higher than 103° F (38 to 39.5°C), can be accompanied by chills and rigors, and are usually associated with a tachycardic response. A cough, typically productive of purulent and occasionally blood-tinged sputum, is often present, and as many as 46% of patients report chest pain. About 20% have gastrointestinal symptoms such as nausea, vomiting, or diarrhea. In elderly people, symptoms and signs may be more subtle; for example, older patients may have predominantly confusion.

On examination, the patient is often listless and may be cyanotic. The respiratory rate is increased; if pleuritic pain is marked, the patient may be splinting the affected side. Dullness to percussion over a lung segment suggests consolidation, whereas a flat percussion note is typically associated with a pleural effusion. Breath sounds may be "distant" if there is an overlying effusion, but they are bronchial in nature if the underlying lung is consolidated. Rales may be noted. If the patient has pleurisy without much pleural fluid, a friction rub may be heard.

No radiographic appearance is characteristic of pneumococcal pneumonia (Chapter 97). Typically, however, involvement is limited to one or more segments within a single lobe. Involvement is unilateral approximately 80% of the time, and the presence of cavitation or lung abscess is uncommon. Forty-five percent of patients have an associated pleural effusion, but only 15% have an effusion of sufficient size to warrant drainage (>10 mm on lateral decubitus views).

Patients with lobar consolidation are more likely to be bacteremic, but there are no consistently significant differences in the radiologic manifestations of bacteremic and nonbacteremic pneumococcal pneumonia. Bacteremic pneumococcal pneumonia may seed distant sites and cause meningitis (Chapter 420), endocarditis (Chapter 76), or septic arthritis (Chapter 280).

With sepsis, sepsis syndrome, or septic shock (Chapter 108), the patient may be hypotensive, and the findings of organ failure vary depending on the target organ involved. For example, oliguria, anuria, and acidosis suggest renal failure; myocardial impairment suggests heart failure; and jaundice is consistent with hepatic failure. Systemic activation of coagulation together with consumption of clotting proteins can result in simultaneous clotting and bleeding (Chapter 178). In some cases, peripheral gangrene and purpura fulminans may be seen.

DIAGNOSIS

Despite extensive testing, a specific etiologic agent is not found in half or more of patients with CAP. The history, physical examination, chest radiograph, sputum Gram stain, and blood and sputum cultures are insensitive and lack specificity, whereas more invasive methods (e.g., endotracheal

TABLE 297-2	INDICATIONS FOR MORE EXTENSIVE DIAGNOSTIC TESTING

Intensive care unit admission for community-acquired pneumonia
Failure of outpatient treatment
Radiographic appearance of cavities on initial evaluation
Infection resulting in neutropenia
Alcohol abuse
Chronic severe liver disease
Severe chronic obstructive lung disease
Asplenia (anatomic or functional)
Recent travel (within 2 weeks)
Positive rapid *Legionella* species or pneumococcal urinary antigen test
Pleural effusion

aspirate, bronchoscopy techniques, pleural fluid aspiration, and lung biopsy) require special expertise and are infrequently indicated. As a general rule, routine diagnostic tests to identify a pathogen are optional for outpatients with CAP, but more extensive testing is recommended for hospitalized patients (Table 297-2).

Ultimately, the diagnosis should be based on suggestive clinical features plus a chest radiograph with or without corroborating microbiologic data. Because *S. pneumoniae* is the most common etiologic agent of CAP, virtually any recommended treatment regimen must provide adequate coverage for it, so documentation of its presence has little or no effect on ultimate clinical outcomes. From the point of view of epidemiology and antimicrobial susceptibility, however, documentation of a pathogen is desirable.

The sputum Gram stain is a relatively simple and inexpensive procedure to document the presence of certain pathogens. The adequacy of the specimen is based on the relative number of PMNs and squamous epithelial cells (SECs). There should be at least 25 PMNs and less than 10 SECs per low-power field ($\times$ 100 magnification). The sensitivity of sputum Gram stain for *S. pneumoniae* is 55%, whereas the specificity is higher than 80%. Unfortunately, approximately 30% of patients overall are unable to produce an appropriate sputum sample. In elderly patients, this figure reaches almost 70%. Overall, only 28% at best of sputum samples are of good quality. Sputum cultures are neither sensitive nor specific, particularly when dealing with relatively fastidious pathogens such as *S. pneumoniae*.

Blood cultures are positive in only 5 to 14% of patients with CAP. If patients have taken a previous dose of antibiotic, culture results are even less useful. As a result, sputum Gram stain, sputum culture, and blood cultures are generally recommended only in patients with selected clinical indications (see Table 297-2). In patients with severe CAP, an expectorated sputum sample should be replaced by an endotracheal aspirate sample if the patient is intubated.

Pneumococcus can also be detected by polymerase chain reaction (PCR), but this is not done routinely. An increased pneumococcal bacterial load demonstrated by real-time PCR is associated with an increased risk for septic shock, need for mechanical ventilation, and death, suggesting that such a test may be of help in identifying patients suitable for care in the intensive care unit. Pneumococcal capsular polysaccharide can be detected in urine, and this may occasionally be helpful for diagnosis after antibiotic therapy has been started. The overall sensitivity of the pneumococcal urinary antigen test is less than 80% but can reach 90% or higher in patients with pneumococcal bacteremia and those with high-risk pneumonia. The specificity in adult patients with CAP can exceed 95%. Detection of antibody to pneumococcal polysaccharide is not useful.

PREVENTION
Polysaccharide Vaccine

A polysaccharide vaccine contains 25 μg of each of the 23 capsular polysaccharides that account for 90% of invasive infections (Chapter 17). Polysaccharide vaccines stimulate B-cell responses, thereby resulting in type-specific antibody production that enhances ingestion and killing of the pathogens by phagocytes. The antigens, however, are T-cell independent and therefore do not result in long-lasting immunity. Two types of polysaccharide vaccine have been available—Pneumovax (Merck) and Pnu-Imune (Lederle).

The effectiveness of the pneumococcal polysaccharide vaccine ranges from 56 to 81%. It is not effective in immunocompromised patients, such as those with sickle cell disease, chronic renal failure, immunoglobulin deficiency, Hodgkin's disease, non-Hodgkin's lymphoma, leukemia, and multiple

myeloma. It is also not effective in preventing nonbacteremic pneumonia. The vaccine is recommended for (1) persons 65 years or older; (2) persons 2 to 64 years old with chronic illnesses such as cardiovascular disease, chronic pulmonary disease (not asthma), diabetes mellitus, alcoholism, chronic liver disease, or cerebrospinal fluid leaks; (3) persons 2 to 64 years old with functional or anatomic asplenia; and (4) persons 2 to 64 years old living in special environments or social settings (Alaskan natives, certain Native American populations, residents of long-term care facilities).

Although the effectiveness of the vaccine is less in these subgroups, the following immunocompromised patients 2 years or older should also be immunized: (1) persons with HIV infection, leukemia, lymphoma, or Hodgkin's disease; and (2) those with multiple myeloma, generalized malignancy, chronic renal failure, nephrotic syndrome, or organ or bone marrow transplants and individuals being treated with immunosuppressive chemotherapy, including steroids.

The lack of an anamnestic response with polysaccharide vaccines means that antibody levels decrease over time and revaccination is required. Although the exact timing is unclear, most experts suggest revaccination at 5 years. For immunocompetent persons 65 years or older, a second dose is suggested if the patient was given the first vaccine 5 years earlier at an age younger than 65 years. For persons 2 to 64 years of age with asplenia, a single revaccination is suggested 5 years after the initial dose if the patient is older than 10 years. However, if the patient is younger than 10 years, revaccination should be given 3 years after the first dose. For immunocompromised patients, revaccination should be given 5 years after the first dose if the patient is older than 10 years and 3 years after the first dose if the patient is younger than 10 years.

Conjugated Vaccine

A seven-valent pneumococcal conjugate vaccine (Prevenar, Wyeth-Lederle) has also been approved for use. The basis of this newer vaccine is that pneumococcal polysaccharide is conjugated to a carrier protein, thereby producing T-cell-dependent antigens, which results in long-term immunologic memory. In this case, the carrier protein is CRM 197, which is similar to diphtheria toxoid. The seven serotypes (4, 6B, 9V, 14, 18C, 19F, 23F) are found most commonly in children and account for approximately 80% of invasive infections in children younger than 6 years. Use of this vaccine has resulted in an overall decrease in the prevalence of antimicrobial resistant pneumococci and in the incidence of invasive pneumococcal disease in both children and adults. Vaccine use can result in replacement with nonvaccine serotypes such as 19A and 35B. As a result, in 2010 the U.S. Food and Drug Administration licensed a new 13-valent pneumococcal conjugate vaccine to replace the 7-valent vaccine. For recommendations in children, see the policy statement of the American Academy of Pediatrics in Suggested Readings.

TREATMENT

Empirical therapy is usually used for CAP.[1] If pneumococcal infection can be documented, however, antibiotic therapy can be targeted against this specific pathogen.

Treatment Regimens
Directed Therapy against Known *S. pneumoniae*

S. pneumoniae can be treated with a number of antimicrobials, including various β-lactams, macrolides, and selected fluoroquinolones (Table 297-3). Resistance has been described for virtually all these agents. For nonmeningeal infections such as pneumonia, susceptibility is now defined by a penicillin MIC of 2 μg/mL or less, intermediate as an MIC of 4 μg/mL, and resistant as an MIC of more than 8 μg/mL. Multidrug-resistant pathogens, which are resistant to three or more antimicrobial agents with different mechanisms of action, have been seen in a number of countries. Risk factors for drug-resistant pneumococcal infection include recent antimicrobial therapy, age younger than 2 years or older than 65 years, attendance at a daycare center, recent hospitalization, and HIV infection.

If a good-quality Gram stain of sputum reveals sheets of PMNs with lancet-shaped gram-positive diplococci as the only organism, if the patient has no risk factors for infection with resistant *S. pneumoniae*, and if the patient is not living in an area endemic for penicillin-resistant *S. pneumoniae*, it is reasonable to initiate parenteral treatment with penicillin G, 2.4 million U/day. For outpatients, oral therapy is usually given in the form of amoxicillin, 500 mg three times daily. For infection with *S. pneumoniae* with penicillin MICs of up to 1 μg/mL, penicillin is still an appropriate agent. For strains with penicillin MICs of 2 to 4 μg/mL, data regarding efficacy are conflicting, and higher doses may be

TABLE 297-3 ANTIMICROBIAL DOSES AND FREQUENCY OF ADMINISTRATION

ANTIMICROBIAL	DOSE AND ROUTE	FREQUENCY
MACROLIDE		
Azithromycin	500 mg × 1 then 250 mg PO	q24h
Clarithromycin	500 mg PO	q12h
Erythromycin	500 mg PO	q6h
TETRACYCLINE		
Doxycycline	100 mg PO	q12h
FLUOROQUINOLONE		
Moxifloxacin	400 mg PO or IV	q24h
Gemifloxacin	320 mg PO	q24h
Levofloxacin	750 mg PO or IV	q24h
Ciprofloxacin	400 mg IV	q12h
β-LACTAMS		
Amoxicillin	1 g PO	q8h
Amoxicillin-clavulanate	2 g PO	q12h
Ampicillin-sulbactam	2 g IV	q6h
Aztreonam	2 g IV	q8-12h
Cefepime	1-2 g	q12h
Cefixime	400 mg PO	q12h
Cefotaxime	1-2 g IV	q8h
Ceftriaxone	1-2 g IV	q24h
Cefpodoxime	100-200 mg	q12h
Cefuroxime	500 mg PO	q12h
Ertapenem	1 g IV	q24h
Imipenem	500 mg IV	q6h
Meropenem	1 g IV	q8h
Piperacillin-tazobactam	3.375 g IV	q6h
AMINOGLYCOSIDE		
Amikacin	15 mg/kg	q24h
Gentamicin	1.7 mg/kg	q24h
Tobramycin	1.7 mg/kg	q24h
MISCELLANEOUS		
Linezolid	600 mg PO or IV	q12h
Vancomycin	0.75-1 g IV	q12h

that even in patients younger than 50 years, only 60% of cases will have resolved radiologically by 1 month. In patients older than 50 years or those with more severe infection or chronic obstructive pulmonary disease, only 25% may clear radiographically by 1 month.

A patient who fails to respond or deteriorates after initial treatment must be carefully reassessed with a detailed review of the history and treatment course, plus appropriate radiographic studies and cultures. If the diagnosis is incorrect, other infectious causes of pneumonia, such as *Haemophilus influenzae* (Chapter 308) or the atypical agents (Chapter 97), must be considered. Noninfectious illnesses must also be considered: heart failure (Chapter 58), pulmonary embolism (Chapter 98), neoplasm (Chapter 197), radiation injury (Chapter 19), drug reaction (Chapter 262), and inflammatory lung disease, to name a few. If the original diagnosis was correct, metastatic infection, lung abscess (Chapter 90) or empyema, and unsuspected drug resistance must be considered. Drug factors such as errors in selection, dose, or route of administration are possible explanations, especially in patients who receive oral medication.

1. Levy ML, Le Jeune I, Woodhead MA, et al. Primary care summary of the British Thoracic Society Guidelines for the management of community acquired pneumonia in adults: 2009 update. Endorsed by the Royal College of General Practitioners and the Primary Care Respiratory Society UK. *Prim Care Respir J.* 2010;10:21-27.

SUGGESTED READINGS

Committee on Infectious Diseases. Policy statement. Recommendations for the prevention of *Streptococcus pneumoniae* infections in infants and children: use of 13-valent pneumococcal polysaccharide vaccine (PPSV23). *Pediatrics.* 2010;126:186-190. *Consensus guidelines.*

Dagan R. Impact of pneumococcal conjugate vaccine on infections caused by antibiotic-resistant *Streptococcus pneumoniae. Clin Microbiol Infect.* 2009;15:16-20. *A review of the effect of pneumococcal conjugate vaccine on pneumococcal resistance.*

Feldman C, Anderson R. Bacteraemic pneumococcal pneumonia: current therapeutic options. *Drugs.* 2011;71:131-153. *Review emphasizing the use of either a β-lactam/macrolide combination or fluoroquinolone monotherapy.*

Lynch JP III, Zhanel GG. *Streptococcus pneumoniae*: epidemiology and risk factors, evolution of antimicrobial resistance, and impact of vaccines. *Curr Opin Pulm Med.* 2010;16:217-252. *Review.*

Musher DM, Sampath R, Rodriguez-Barradas MC. The potential role for protein-conjugate pneumococcal vaccine in adults: what is the supporting evidence? *Clin Infect Dis.* 2011;52:633-640. *Though very effective in children, this new vaccine may not be cost-effective in adults.*

Van der Poll S, Opal SM. Pathogenesis, treatment and prevention of pneumococcal pneumonia. *Lancet.* 2009;374:1543-1556. *Comprehensive review.*

better. If the patient is allergic to penicillin, a macrolide such as azithromycin (500 mg on day 1, then 250 mg/day) or clarithromycin (500 mg twice daily) may be used. Five days is the minimal recommended duration of treatment of CAP that is not complicated, severe, or associated with bacteremia.

For patients who are hospitalized because of CAP, higher doses of parenteral antibiotics are generally used: penicillin in the range of 12 million U (2 to 3 million every 4 hours) or ampicillin, 4 g/day (1 g every 6 hours). Third-generation cephalosporins such as ceftriaxone (1 to 2 g every 24 hours) and cefotaxime (1 to 2 g every 8 hours) are other alternatives.

The patient can be switched to an oral regimen when cough and shortness of breath are improving, the white blood cell count is normalizing, and oral intake and gastrointestinal tract absorption are adequate. Febrile patients are frequently treated outside the hospital, so absence of a fever is not a prerequisite for switching to an oral regimen.

Some studies have suggested that initial combination antimicrobial treatment of bacteremic pneumococcal pneumonia that includes a macrolide is associated with lower mortality rates possibly because of an immunomodulatory effect of the macrolides.

Drotrecogin alfa activated (Chapters 108 and 178) used as adjunctive immunomodulatory therapy in selected cases of CAP provides a survival advantage in those with severe sepsis due to pneumococcal infection.

Empirical Treatment

This is discussed in the chapter dealing with CAP (Chapter 97).

PROGNOSIS

In an otherwise well, relatively young patient with no comorbid conditions and with mild to moderate infection, the elevated temperature and white blood cell count usually resolve by days 2 to 4 and 4, respectively. The patient looks and feels better within a few days, but it is important to keep in mind

298

NONPNEUMOCOCCAL STREPTOCOCCAL INFECTIONS, RHEUMATIC FEVER

DONALD E. LOW

THE PATHOGENS

The *Streptococcus* genus contains a number of species that inhabit a broad range of hosts, including humans and domesticated animals, where they often colonize as part of the normal flora and cause infection. They are gram-positive cocci that grow in chains. The two most useful methods of classifying streptococci are by the type of hemolytic reaction displayed on blood agar on which they are grown and the serologic reactivity of the cell wall polysaccharide antigens as originally described by Rebecca Lancefield (Table 298-1). On blood agar plates, streptococci may cause complete (β), incomplete (α), or no (γ) hemolysis. Hemolytic streptococci from humans can be classified into Lancefield groups A, B, C, F, G, and L on the basis of carbohydrate antigens of the cell wall and can be subdivided into large-colony and small-colony (<0.5 mm in diameter) formers. The β-hemolytic group A and group B streptococci are considered the major pathogenic β-hemolytic

TABLE 298-1 IDENTIFICATION OF THE β-HEMOLYTIC STREPTOCOCCI

SPECIES	LANCEFIELD GROUP	COLONY SIZE	ORIGIN
S. pyogenes	A	Large	Human
S. agalactiae	B	Large	Human, bovine
S. dysgalactiae subsp. equisimilis	A, C, G, L	Large	Human, animals
S. equi subsp. zooepidemicus	C	Large	Animals, human
S. canis	G	Large	Dog, human
S. anginosus (group)*	A, C, G, F, none	Small	Human

*Group carbohydrate antigen.

FIGURE 298-1. Acute streptococcal pharyngitis. Pus is present in the tonsillar crypts, and some palatal petechiae are seen. (From Forbes CD, Jackson WF. Color Atlas and Text of Clinical Medicine. 3rd ed. London: Mosby; 2003.)

streptococci. The β-hemolytic large-colony-forming species, *Streptococcus dysgalactiae* subspecies *equisimilis,* may possess Lancefield group A, C, G, or L antigens. The small-colony-forming β-hemolytic strains with Lancefield group A, C, F, or G or no group antigens belong to the anginosus (or previously termed *Streptococcus milleri*) group. Members of the anginosus group (*Streptococcus anginosus, Streptococcus constellatus,* and *Streptococcus intermedius*) are considered part of the viridans group streptococci, most of which display α-hemolytic or nonhemolytic reactions.

STREPTOCOCCUS PYOGENES (GROUP A STREPTOCOCCUS)

The most clinically significant of the streptococcal human pathogens are *Streptococcus pyogenes* (also referred to as group A streptococci), which contain the Lancefield group A antigen on their cell surface. Group A streptococcus (GAS) causes primarily infections of the upper respiratory tract and the skin. It is also responsible for a toxic shock–like syndrome, necrotizing fasciitis, and delayed nonsuppurative sequelae including acute rheumatic fever and poststreptococcal glomerulonephritis. The major virulence factor of the organism is the M protein. This protein, a stable dimer, is anchored to the cell membrane and traverses and penetrates the cell wall. The proximal portion of the molecule is highly conserved among GAS, whereas the distal portions contain type-specific epitopes localized on the tips that protrude from the cell surface. This variation in the distal region of the M proteins provides the basis of widely used epidemiologic typing schemes that employ serologic methods (M type) or nucleotide sequence analysis of the M protein gene (*emm* type). There are more than 150 distinct *emm* and *emm*-like genes recognized. Epidemiologic studies have revealed that certain disease manifestations are commonly associated with particular M types, such as M1 and M3 types, which are associated with the most severe invasive manifestations such as toxic shock syndrome and necrotizing fasciitis. Humans are the natural host, and there is no animal or environmental reservoir. The throat and skin of the human host are the principal reservoirs for GAS. GAS is transmitted primarily person to person by either contact or droplet transmission.

EPIDEMIOLOGY

All GAS infections have the highest incidence in children younger than 10 years. The asymptomatic prevalence is also higher (15 to 20%) in children than in adults. Age is not the only factor; crowded conditions in temperate climates during the winter months are also associated with epidemics of pharyngitis in school children as well as in military recruits. The peak incidence for streptococcal pharyngitis and impetigo varies with season and locale. In many temperate regions of the world, the incidence of pharyngitis peaks in winter, whereas impetigo, although less common, peaks during the summer months. In contrast, for many tropical host populations, impetigo is hyperendemic year round, whereas throat infection, whether pharyngitis or asymptomatic carriage, ranges from very low to moderate levels.

CLINICAL MANIFESTATIONS
Respiratory Tract Infections
Pharyngitis
GAS is a major cause of pharyngitis and remains the only agent of this syndrome requiring etiologic diagnosis and treatment. The burden and

TABLE 298-2 SCORE FOR USE IN BOTH CHILDREN AND ADULTS WITH SORE THROAT TO ESTIMATE PROBABILITY OF POSITIVE CULTURE AND GUIDE MANAGEMENT APPROACH

Diagnostic Criteria		Management		
FINDINGS	POINTS	SCORE	RISK FOR STREPTOCOCCAL INFECTION	RECOMMENDATION
Temperature >38° C	+1	≤0	1 to 2.5%	No culture or antibiotics
Absence of cough	+1	1	5 to 10%	
Swollen, tender anterior cervical nodes	+1	2	11 to 17%	Culture: antibiotics only if culture positive
Tonsillar swelling or exudate	+1	3	18 to 35%	
Age		≥4		Antibiotics
3 to 14 yr	+1			
>44 yr	−1			

Adapted from McIsaac WJ, Kellner JD, Aufricht P, et al. Empirical validation of guidelines for the management of pharyngitis in children and adults. *JAMA.* 2004;291:1587-1595.

economic costs of GAS pharyngitis are great. It has been estimated that in the United States alone more than 7 million cases of acute pharyngitis are diagnosed by pediatricians annually. *S. pyogenes* is the cause in only 15% to 30% of them, but antibiotics are prescribed in 55% to 75% of the cases. Although a major consequence of GAS pharyngitis, acute rheumatic fever (see later), is much less common now than in the past, it is still a considerable problem in the developing world. The World Health Organization (WHO) estimates that there are about half a million cases of acute rheumatic fever worldwide annually. On clinical grounds, streptococcal pharyngitis (Fig. 298-1) is strongly suggested by the presence of fever, tonsillar exudate, tender enlarged anterior cervical lymph nodes, and absence of cough.

Because these findings are nonspecific and commonly found in cases of viral origin, however, even experienced physicians may accurately diagnose streptococcal pharyngitis based on the clinical findings alone in no more than 75% of the cases. Treatment of suspected GAS pharyngitis at the time of initial clinical evaluation has only a modest effect on relieving acute symptoms and perhaps on preventing suppurative complications. However, antibacterial treatment may be delayed for several days and still achieve the goal of preventing rheumatic fever and spread of disease. Prospective studies to compare the impact of various pharyngitis management strategies on clinically relevant outcomes have been recommended. A particular focus of recent guidelines has been to reduce overall use of antibiotics for treatment of pharyngitis in both children and adults in order to limit antibiotic resistance (Table 298-2).

Throat culture is the conventional method for establishing the diagnosis of GAS pharyngitis. In an untreated patient with GAS pharyngitis, a properly obtained throat culture (by vigorous swabbing of both tonsils and posterior pharynx) is almost always positive; however, a positive throat culture may reflect chronic colonization by GAS, and the acute illness may be caused by another agent. Quantitation of GAS from the throat swab culture cannot be used to differentiate carriage from infection because sparse growth may be associated with true infection. A negative throat culture permits the physician to withhold antibiotic therapy from most patients with sore throats.

Many GAS antigen detection tests are available commercially. These tests vary in method. Most of these tests have a high degree of specificity, but their sensitivity in clinical practice can be unacceptably low. Therefore, treatment is indicated for the patient with acute pharyngitis who has a positive rapid antigen detection test.

Otitis Media and Rhinosinusitis

During the past several decades, a number of studies have reported isolation of GAS from 2 to 5% of cultures of middle ear fluid specimens obtained from children with acute otitis media (AOM). Thus, in contrast to the very striking role of GAS as the major bacterial agent of acute pharyngitis, GAS has been fairly consistently the fourth most predominant pathogen causing pediatric AOM, after *Streptococcus pneumoniae, Haemophilus influenzae,* and *Moraxella catarrhalis.* GAS AOM is associated with increased risk for development of mastoiditis. Although the risk is small (<1%), it is much greater than with AOM due to *S. pneumoniae, H. influenzae,* or *M. catarrhalis.* GAS is the etiologic agent of acute bacterial rhinosinusitis in 2 to 7% of cases.

Pneumonia

The occurrence of pneumonia has increased with the resurgence of invasive GAS disease during the past several decades, with 10% of patients with invasive GAS disease presenting with pneumonia. Small outbreaks of GAS pneumonia have been described in chronic care facilities and within families, as well as sporadic cases occurring in the community. GAS pneumonia now occurs with a frequency similar to that of other well-recognized causes, such as *Staphylococcus aureus* or *Klebsiella pneumoniae.* A Canadian population-based surveillance program of invasive GAS disease confirmed that GAS pneumonia is a severe illness of sudden onset frequently associated with local and systemic complications, particularly empyema (19%), toxic shock (32%), and death (38%).

Skin and Soft Tissue Infections

Scarlet Fever

Scarlet fever is a diffuse erythematous eruption that generally occurs in association with pharyngitis, most commonly in children 5 to 15 years of age. Development of the scarlet fever rash requires prior exposure to *S. pyogenes* and occurs as a result of delayed-type skin reactivity to pyrogenic exotoxin (erythrogenic toxin, usually types A, B, or C) produced by the organism. The rash of scarlet fever is a diffuse erythema that blanches with pressure, with numerous small (1 to 2 mm) papular elevations, giving a sandpaper quality to the skin. It usually starts on the head and neck and is accompanied by circumoral pallor and a strawberry tongue. Subsequently, the rash expands rapidly to cover the trunk, followed by the extremities, and then ultimately desquamates; the palms and soles are usually spared. The rash is most marked in the skinfolds of the inguinal, axillary, antecubital, and abdominal areas and about pressure points. It often exhibits a linear petechial character in the antecubital fossae and axillary folds, known as Pastia's lines.

Erysipelas

Erysipelas is an acute, superficial, non-necrotizing dermal or hypodermal infection that is mainly caused by streptococci. The definitive diagnosis is based on clinical findings that usually include a sharply demarcated shiny erythematosus plaque associated with pain, swelling, and fever. Erysipelas affects predominantly adult patients in the sixth or seventh decade and is located on the lower limb in more than 80% of cases. A female predominance exists, except in young patients. Risk factors include disruption of the cutaneous barrier (leg ulcer, wound, fissured toe-web intertrigo, and pressure ulcer), lymphedema, chronic edema, or local surgical operations (lymph node dissection, saphenectomy). Toe-web intertrigo appears to be a major portal of entry whether or not due to dermatophytes. Erysipelas is less commonly caused by group B, C, or G streptococci and rarely by staphylococci. Bulla formation is considered as a relatively severe but frequent local complication of the disease. Although most cases of erysipelas are caused by β-hemolytic streptococci, many other bacteria can produce non-necrotizing cellulitis, which can often occur in particular circumstances, such as *Pasteurella multocida* following cat or dog bites, *Aeromonas hydrophila*

following immersion in fresh water, *Vibrio* species after saltwater exposure, or *H. influenzae* in periorbital cellulitis in children. Recurrence is the main complication of erysipelas; it occurs in about 20% of cases. Measures to reduce recurrences of erysipelas include treatment of any predisposing factor, such as toe-web intertrigo or wound, and reducing any underlying edema. If frequent infections occur despite such measures, prophylactic antibiotics may be warranted.

Impetigo

Impetigo is a highly contagious infection of the superficial epidermis that most often affects children 2 to 5 years of age, although it can occur in any age group. Impetigo is classified as bullous or nonbullous impetigo; the latter is the most common form. Bullous impetigo simply means that the skin eruption is characterized by bullae (blisters). The infection usually heals without scarring, even without treatment. *S. aureus* is the most important causative organism, especially in bullous impetigo. GAS causes fewer cases, either alone or in combination with *S. aureus,* and is more often found in nonbullous impetigo. The diagnosis usually is made clinically and can be confirmed by Gram stain and culture, although this is not usually necessary. Culture may be useful to identify patients with nephritogenic strains of GAS during outbreaks of poststreptococcal glomerulonephritis. Impetigo usually is transmitted through direct contact. Patients can further spread the infection to themselves or others after excoriating an infected area. Infections often spread rapidly through schools and daycare centers.

The Cochrane Collaboration reviewed interventions for impetigo. There was little evidence found for the use of disinfecting measures, such as chlorhexidine. There was good evidence that topical mupirocin and topical fusidic acid are equally or more effective than oral antibiotics for people with limited disease. Fusidic acid and mupirocin were of similar efficacy. It was found to be unclear whether oral antibiotics are superior to topical antibiotics for people with extensive impetigo.

Cellulitis

Bacterial cellulitis refers to a diffuse, spreading skin infection. Associated regional lymphadenopathy and lymphatic streaking are variable, and local complications (abscesses, necrosis) are more frequent than in erysipelas. Petechiae and ecchymoses with frequent bullae may develop in inflamed skin resulting in hemorrhagic cellulitis. Cellulitis usually refers to a more deeply situated skin infection than erysipelas. However, the distinction between these entities is not clear-cut, and the two conditions share the typical clinical features, including sudden onset, usually with a high fever, and the tendency to recur. GAS has been considered the main causative agent of cellulitis, although groups B, C, and G streptococcus and *S. aureus* can also be a cause.

The predominant infection site for cellulitis is on the lower extremities. Lymphedema and disruption of the cutaneous barrier, which serves as a site of entry for the pathogens, are risk factors for infections. Twenty to 30% of patients have a recurrence during a 3-year follow-up period. Blood cultures are positive for β-hemolytic streptococci in less than 5% of cases.

Invasive Group A Streptococcus Disease

Invasive disease is defined as the isolation of GAS from an otherwise sterile site. Since the late 1980s, a resurgence of severe invasive infections due to GAS, including streptococcal toxic shock syndrome and necrotizing fasciitis, has been reported worldwide. Both manifestations are associated with high morbidity and mortality. The clinical spectrum of disease may vary from mild to severe, resulting in streptococcal toxic shock or necrotizing fasciitis, or both.

Toxic Shock Syndrome

Streptococcal *toxic shock syndrome* is defined as hypotension accompanied by multiple organ failure, indicated by two of the following signs: renal impairment, coagulopathy, liver involvement, adult respiratory distress syndrome, a generalized rash, and soft tissue necrosis. In contrast to the other major form of toxic shock syndrome that is caused by toxin-producing *S. aureus* (Chapter 296), in which blood cultures are positive in less than 5% of cases, most (60%) patients with streptococcal toxic shock syndrome have positive blood cultures. A focus of infection in staphylococcal toxic shock syndrome, if present at all, tends to be superficial, a complication of surgical wounds or burns or a foreign body (e.g., tampons). Streptococcal toxic shock syndrome can originate from an unknown focus or from a deep-seated soft tissue infection (e.g., necrotizing fasciitis, myositis, cellulitis). Mortality rates are much higher with streptococcal than staphylococcal toxic shock, reported at up to 80% when associated with myositis.

Necrotizing Fasciitis

Necrotizing fasciitis is defined by infection of the subcutaneous tissue and fascia that often results in necrosis with relative sparing of the underlying muscle. Histopathology demonstrates both necrosis of superficial fascia and polymorphonuclear infiltrates as well as edema of the reticular dermis, subcutaneous fat, and superficial fascia. GAS organisms in this disorder secrete proteases that disrupt host tissue and exotoxins that can cause local tissue injury or systemic manifestations as the result of an excessive and inappropriate inflammatory response leading to a life-threatening infection.

In the early stages of necrotizing fasciitis due to GAS, the clinical findings can be nondescript, with as many as one third of patients initially being given a diagnosis other than necrotizing fasciitis. The only feature that might alert the clinician is a complaint of pain out of proportion to that expected on examination, even for those patients who report previous trauma to the area. Necrotizing fasciitis has been found to occur more frequently during the winter months and in older men. More then half of patients give a history of an antecedent skin lesion or injury at the site of infection. In adults, most cases occur in persons with at least one chronic underlying illness, and in children, the most frequent underlying illness is an infection due to varicella-zoster virus (Chapter 383). The most common primary site of infection is the lower extremity, followed by the upper extremity, trunk, and groin or perineum.

Streptococcal exotoxins, which are superantigens, have been recognized as central mediators of the systemic effects associated with severe GAS infections. As superantigens, they have the ability to stimulate a large proportion of the T-cell population and yield an intense, uncontrolled immune response with excessive amounts of cytokines, leading to hyperinflammation, tissue destruction, and shock syndrome. Twelve distinct superantigens produced by GAS have been identified, and many GAS strains harbor genes encoding four to six different superantigens. The magnitude of the inflammatory response is determined by the patient's human leukocyte antigen (HLA) class II type. Another important risk factor for invasive GAS infections is lack of opsonic anti-M1 protein and neutralizing antisuperantigen antibodies.

Treatment of either streptococcal toxic shock or necrotizing fasciitis has not been critically studied because of the low incidence of disease and difficulty in patient recruitment for clinical trials. The importance of aggressive surgical treatment with adequate débridement or amputation has been based on observational studies of patients with necrotizing fasciitis due to a number of different etiologies and underlying diseases. The finding that lack of protective antibodies against streptococcal M protein and superantigens correlates with risk for developing invasive streptococcal diseases, highlights the importance of antibodies in protection against these infections, and suggests that intravenous immune globulin might be a potential adjunctive therapy. Intravenous immune globulin exhibits high polyspecificity generated by antibodies pooled from several thousands of donors and has been shown to contain broad-spectrum antibodies against streptococcal superantigens and M proteins. In addition, intravenous immune globulin has a general anti-inflammatory effect due in large part to Fc receptor–mediated mechanisms. The documentation of clinical efficacy of intravenous immune globulin includes several case reports and two observational cohort studies, one case-control study, and one multicenter placebo-controlled trial.

Nonsuppurative Sequelae of Streptococcal Infections

Acute Rheumatic Fever

Acute rheumatic fever is a delayed, nonsuppurative sequela of a pharyngeal infection with the GAS. Following the initial pharyngitis, a latent period of 2 to 3 weeks occurs before the first signs or symptoms of acute rheumatic fever appear. The disease presents with various manifestations that may include arthritis, carditis, chorea, subcutaneous nodules, and erythema marginatum. In developing areas of the world, acute rheumatic fever and rheumatic heart disease are estimated to affect nearly 20 million people and are the leading causes of cardiovascular death during the first five decades of life. Worldwide, there are 470,000 new cases of rheumatic fever and 233,000 deaths attributable to rheumatic fever or rheumatic heart disease each year; most occur in developing countries and among indigenous groups. The observation in some studies that only a few M serotypes (types 3, 5, 6, 14, 18, 19, 24, and 29) were implicated in outbreaks of rheumatic fever suggested

a particular "rheumatogenic" potential of certain strains of GAS. The decrease in the incidence of acute rheumatic fever in developed countries with the replacement of rheumatogenic types by nonrheumatogenic types is not solely responsible for the decrease in acute rheumatic fever, and the issue of potential rheumatogenic strains remains unresolved. A streptococcal strain capable of causing a well-documented pharyngitis almost always is potentially capable of causing rheumatic fever. The lack of specific rheumatogenic strains also can explain the relatively high risk for recurrent disease with new streptococcal infections, in contrast to poststreptococcal glomerulonephritis, in which only a few "nephritogenic" strains appear to be capable of inducing the disease (e.g., type 12 with pharyngitis and type 49 with impetigo), and recurrent disease is uncommon.

Modified Jones criteria were first published in 1944 to be able to define persons with acute rheumatic fever. They have been periodically revised by the American Heart Association in collaboration with other groups. According to revised Jones criteria, the diagnosis of rheumatic fever can be made when two of the major criteria, or one major criterion plus two minor criteria, are present along with evidence of streptococcal infection. Exceptions are chorea and indolent carditis, each of which by itself can indicate rheumatic fever. Major criteria include the following:

1. Migratory polyarthritis: a temporary migrating inflammation of the large joints, usually starting in the legs and migrating upward
2. Carditis: inflammation of the heart muscle, which can manifest as congestive heart failure, pericarditis with a rub, or a new heart murmur
3. Subcutaneous nodules: painless, firm collections of collagen fibers over bones or tendons, commonly appearing on the back of the wrist, the outside elbow, and the front of the knees
4. Erythema marginatum: a long-lasting rash that begins on the trunk or arms as macules and spreads outward to form a snakelike ring while clearing in the middle. This rash never starts on the face, and it is made worse with heat.
5. Sydenham's chorea (St. Vitus's dance): a characteristic series of rapid movements of the face and arms without purpose, generally occurring late in the disease

Minor criteria include the following:

1. Fever
2. Arthralgia: joint pain without swelling
3. Raised erythrocyte sedimentation rate or C-reactive protein
4. Leukocytosis
5. Electrocardiogram showing features of heart block, such as a prolonged PR interval
6. Supporting evidence of streptococcal infection: elevated or rising anti-streptolysin O titer or anti-DNAse B
7. Previous episode of rheumatic fever or inactive heart disease

The pathogenic mechanisms that lead to the development of acute rheumatic fever remain incompletely understood. Clearly, streptococcal pharyngeal infection is required, and genetic susceptibility may be present. On the other hand, evidence is sparse that toxins produced by the streptococcus are important. Molecular mimicry is thought to play an important role in the initiation of the tissue injury. As a result of molecular mimicry, antibodies directed against GAS antigens cross-react with host antigens. In addition to the role of antibody, observations suggest a role for cellular immunity in molecular mimicry.

Primary prevention of acute rheumatic fever is accomplished by proper identification and adequate antibiotic treatment of GAS tonsillopharyngitis. Diagnosis of GAS pharyngitis is best accomplished by combining clinical judgment with diagnostic test results, the criterion standard of which is the throat culture. Penicillin (either oral penicillin V or injectable benzathine penicillin) is the treatment of choice because it is cost-effective, has a narrow spectrum of activity, and has long-standing proven efficacy. In addition, GAS resistant to penicillin has not been documented. For penicillin-allergic individuals, acceptable alternatives include a narrow-spectrum oral cephalosporin, oral clindamycin, or various oral macrolides. The individual who has had an attack of rheumatic fever is at very high risk of developing recurrences after subsequent GAS pharyngitis and needs continuous antimicrobial prophylaxis to prevent such recurrences (secondary prevention). The recommended duration of prophylaxis depends on the number of previous attacks, the time elapsed since the last attack, the risk for exposure to GAS infections, the age of the patient, and the presence or absence of cardiac involvement. Penicillin is again the agent of choice for secondary prophylaxis, but sulfadiazine or a macrolide is an acceptable alternative in penicillin-allergic individuals.∎

Post-streptococcal Reactive Arthritis

The term *poststreptococcal reactive arthritis* was first used to describe patients with arthritis after documented GAS infection but who failed to meet the Jones criteria for the diagnosis of acute rheumatic fever. Since then, the differentiation of post-streptococcal reactive arthritis from acute rheumatic fever has remained unsettled. Compared with acute rheumatic fever, the arthritis of post-streptococcal reactive arthritis is more likely to occur within 10 days after infection, be symmetrical and nonmigratory, last longer than 3 weeks, and be poorly responsive to aspirin or other nonsteroidal anti-inflammatory drugs (NSAIDs). Periarticular findings, such as tenosynovitis, have not been considered to be part of the clinical spectrum of acute rheumatic fever but have been described with poststreptococcal reactive arthritis. However, some studies have reported that an additive and prolonged pattern of arthritis, as well as aspirin unresponsivity, may be seen in 19 to 36% of patients with acute rheumatic fever. Some have suggested that patients with higher erythrocyte sedimentation rate, C-reactive protein, and shorter duration of joint symptoms after NSAID therapy, and without relapse when NSAIDs were stopped, were diagnosed as having acute rheumatic fever rather than post-streptococcal reactive arthritis. Although all patients with post-streptococcal reactive arthritis have serologic evidence of a recent GAS infection, no more than half of these patients who have a throat culture performed have GAS isolated. Because a small proportion of patients with poststreptococcal reactive arthritis have been reported to develop subsequent valvular heart disease, these patients should be observed carefully for several months for clinical evidence of carditis. If valvular disease is detected, the patient should be classified as having had acute rheumatic fever and should continue to receive secondary prophylaxis.

Post-streptococcal Glomerulonephritis

Acute post-streptococcal glomerulonephritis (PSGN) is a disease characterized by the sudden appearance of edema, hematuria, proteinuria, and hypertension (Chapter 123). It is now known to follow infection by nephrogenic strains of GAS; M types 1, 2, 4, 12, 18, 25, 49, 55, 57, and 60. These may cause skin or throat infections, but specific M types, such as 49, 55, 57, and 60, are most commonly associated with skin infections. In addition, nontypeable GAS is frequently isolated from the skin or throat of patients with glomerulonephritis, representing presumably unclassified nephritogenic strains. The overall risk of developing acute PSGN after infection by these nephritogenic strains is about 15%. The risk for nephritis may also be related to the M type and the site of infection. The risk of developing nephritis infection by M type 49 is 5% if it is present in the throat. This risk increases to 25% if infection by the same organism is present in the skin. The time lapse between infection and onset of PSGN symptoms is typically 1 to 3 weeks following a throat infection and 3 to 6 weeks after a skin infection.

The pathogenic mechanism of PSGN remains largely unknown (Chapter 123). Diffuse glomerular hypercellularity, C3 and immunoglobulin G (IgG) deposition, as well as proteinuria and hematuria are cardinal features. However, it can occur without all these signs present concurrently. For a reliable diagnosis of PSGN, clear evidence that a streptococcal infection preceded the glomerulonephritis is required. However, streptococcal infection has often cleared by the time the patient appears in the clinic because the symptoms generally arise 1 to 3 weeks after the patient was infected. Acute PSGN most often follows upper respiratory tract GAS infections in colder climates and skin infections in warmer climates. Occasionally, it may also be seen following group C or G streptococcal infections. A high incidence of PSGN is noted in other parts of the world, especially in areas with tropical climates where skin infections are common. Epidemic episodes tend to occur in highly populated areas where poor hygiene, malnutrition, anemia, and parasites are common, and episodes are separated by periods of 5 to 7 years in certain communities. Epidemics occur also in the Western world, especially in closed communities. Acute PSGN affects all age groups but most commonly children and young adults. Males are affected more often than females, often in the ratio of 2 : 1. Acute PSGN rarely strikes the same individual twice. Thus, it appears likely that protective immunity is acquired as a result of an infection with a nephritogenic strain.

Although penicillin treatment of the antecedent streptococcal infections is highly efficacious in preventing acute rheumatic fever, it does not appear to be the case in PSGN. Studies carried out during epidemics of nephritis found that prior antibiotics had little, if any, effect in preventing PSGN. Penicillin is, nevertheless, effective in epidemiologic attempts to eradicate nephritogenic strains by treatment of acute glomerulonephritis patients and their colonized family contacts. Because recurrent episodes of acute glomerulonephritis are so rare, continuous antibiotic prophylaxis, such as is used in the secondary prevention of rheumatic fever, is unnecessary.

The ultimate prognosis in persons with acute glomerulonephritis depends largely on the severity of the initial insult. In an extremely small proportion of patients, the initial injury is so severe that either persistent renal failure or progression to renal failure occurs. However, in most patients, histologic regression of the disease is the rule, and the ultimate prognosis is good.

DIAGNOSIS

Streptococcal Antibody Tests

Antistreptococcal antibody titers reflect past and not present immunologic events and therefore cannot be used to determine whether an individual with pharyngitis and GAS in the pharynx is truly infected or merely a streptococcal carrier. When present, elevated or rising antistreptococcal antibody titers provide reliable confirmation of a recent GAS infection and are of value in identifying a preceding GAS infection in a patient suspected of having rheumatic fever. The most commonly used and commercially available antibody assays are antistreptolysin O and anti-DNAse B. These tests are valuable in patients who have possible nonsuppurative complications of GAS infections (acute rheumatic fever or acute glomerulonephritis). The antistreptolysin O test is usually obtained first, and if it is not elevated, an anti-DNAse B test may be performed. Antistreptolysin O titers begin to rise approximately 1 week and peak 3 to 6 weeks after the infection. Anti-DNAse B titers begin to rise 1 to 2 weeks and peak 6 to 8 weeks after the infection. Elevated titers for both tests may persist for several months after even uncomplicated GAS infections.

It is not uncommon for laboratory personnel and physicians to misinterpret streptococcal antibody titers because of a failure to appreciate that the normal levels of these antibodies are higher among school-aged children than among adults. Single antibody titers are often misleading. Sequential samples more accurately define infection, allowing correlation of titer increases with temporal confirmation of GAS acquisition.

TREATMENT ℞

Antimicrobial Susceptibility

Penicillin and the cephalosporins continue to be the drugs of first choice for the treatment of most GAS infections.■ The continued susceptibility of *S. pyogenes* to β-lactams is remarkable, especially when compared with the emergence of resistance to β-lactams among pneumococci and viridans group streptococci over the past decade. A limited ability to acquire foreign DNA and a physiologic fitness cost associated with β-lactam resistance are possible explanations for this organism's continued susceptibility to penicillin. The macrolides are the second-line drug of choice and are used in penicillin-hypersensitive patients. Clindamycin is also the drug of choice for chronic, recurrent pharyngitis. However, resistance has emerged in this organism. Elevated rates of macrolide resistance (>25%) among GAS reported in Korea, Taiwan, Spain, and Italy are causes of concern. Limited surveillance data suggest that the overall rate of macrolide-resistant GAS in North America is 3 to 9%. There are two primary mechanisms of macrolide resistance in GAS: efflux (encoded by *mefA*) and target modification due to ribosomal methylation (encoded by *ermB* or *ermA*). Isolates with the *mefA* gene have a pattern of resistance known as the M phenotype: they are macrolide resistant but clindamycin susceptible. GAS isolates with the *ermB* gene are usually resistant to macrolides and clindamycin. Isolates with the *ermA* gene typically have an inducible phenotype that requires exposure to a macrolide inducer before clindamycin resistance becomes evident. There are rare reports of L4 ribosomal protein and 23S recombinant RNA mutations in macrolide-resistant GAS isolates.

Fluoroquinolones are a useful therapeutic alternative for the treatment of skin and soft tissue infections in adults. Although strains of GAS nonsusceptible to the fluoroquinolones have been reported, they are rare. The mechanisms of decreased susceptibility to the fluoroquinolones among *Streptococcus* species are mainly mediated by point mutations in the quinolone resistance–determining region of the bacterial topoisomerase II enzymes, namely, DNA gyrase and topoisomerase IV. DNA gyrase and topoisomerase IV enzymes are homologues, with each enzyme consisting of a tetramer with two subunits (two *gyrA* and two *gyrB* molecules in DNA gyrase, two *parC* and two *parE* molecules in topoisomerase IV). In the last few years, *S. pyogenes* isolates that are resistant or have reduced susceptibility to fluoroquinolones have been reported by several authors, but isolates with a high level of resistance have been detected very infrequently.

PREVENTION

Tetracycline resistance in GAS is quite common. In gram-positive organisms, resistance to tetracycline is typically conferred by ribosome protection genes, such as *tet*(M) and *tet*(O). Tetracycline resistance is usually acquired by GAS through horizontal gene transfer. A global sample of GAS revealed 80 or more separate acquisitions of tetracycline resistance. Of 244 clones, 38 and 25% displayed resistance to tetracycline and erythromycin, respectively; a relatively high proportion (15%) were resistant to both classes of drugs. *tet*(M) displayed a highly significant association with *erm*(B). Trimethoprim-sulfamethoxazole is not active against GAS and therefore should not be used as monotherapy for infections potentially caused by GAS.

STREPTOCOCCUS AGALACTIAE (GROUP B STREPTOCOCCUS)

EPIDEMIOLOGY

Group B streptococcus (GBS), also known as *Streptococcus agalactiae*, was once considered a pathogen of only domestic animals, causing mastitis in cows. Although asymptomatic vaginal carriage of GBS was described in 1935, the first report of GBS sepsis in a neonate was not reported until 1964. Since the 1970s, GBS is recognized as one of the most common causes of neonatal infectious morbidity and mortality in developed countries. GBS causes significant maternal and perinatal morbidity, asymptomatic bacteriuria in pregnancy, and urinary tract and other infections in the adult nonpregnant population. The virulence of *S. agalactiae* is related to the polysaccharide toxin it produces. Immunity is mediated by antibodies to the capsular polysaccharide and is serotype specific. Several serotypes are known, including Ia, Ib, Ic, II, III, IV, V, VI, VII, and VIII.

CLINICAL MANIFESTATIONS

Neonatal Group B Streptococcus Disease

GBS colonizes the vaginal and gastrointestinal tracts in healthy women, with carriage rates ranging from 15 to 45%. Neonates can acquire the organism vertically in utero or during delivery from the maternal genital tract. Although the transmission rate from mothers colonized with *S. agalactiae* to neonates delivered vaginally is approximately 50%, only 1 to 2% of colonized neonates go on to develop invasive GBS disease. Neonatal GBS disease is divided into early and late disease. Early GBS neonatal sepsis often presents within 24 hours of delivery but can become apparent up to 7 days postpartum. Pneumonia with bacteremia is common, whereas meningitis is less likely. Late GBS neonatal sepsis is defined as infection that presents between 1 week postpartum and age 3 months. Late disease commonly involves GBS serotype III, typically characterized by bacteremia and meningitis.

PREVENTION

The current approach to the prevention of early-onset GBS infection in pregnancy requires intrapartum antimicrobial prophylaxis in term women with culture evidence of recent vaginal or rectal GBS infection.⬛ Women without a known GBS status delivering before 37 weeks' gestation with premature rupture of the membranes or intrapartum fever are also candidates for intrapartum antimicrobial prophylaxis. Penicillin or ampicillin is the initial approach. Clindamycin and macrolides are standard in individuals with penicillin allergy, but GBS infections are no longer always sensitive to these two drugs. Despite these recommendations, there is lack of evidence from well-designed and well-conducted trials to recommend intrapartum antibiotic prophylaxis to reduce neonatal early-onset GBS disease.

Invasive Group B Streptococcus Disease

S. agalactiae infection is extremely rare in healthy adults and is almost always associated with underlying abnormalities. Bacteremia with an unknown source accounts for approximately 25% of all cases of invasive GBS disease. Diabetes mellitus and malignancy are the most common underlying diseases associated with infection. Urinary tract infections are a common manifestation of GBS disease and are observed in both pregnant and nonpregnant adults. Other presentations of GBS infection include pneumonia, skin and soft tissue infections, septic arthritis, osteomyelitis, meningitis, peritonitis, and endo-ophthalmitis.

Invasive GBS disease is a major cause of illness and death in older adults and is even more frequent among long-term care facility residents, possibly because of concurrent conditions such as advanced age, diabetes, cirrhosis, and stroke, which are known risk factors for GBS infection. Case-fatality rates are about 13% for persons 65 years and older. An increased prevalence of serogroup V has been reported in adult populations. Serotype V has been associated with higher rates of antimicrobial drug resistance.

TREATMENT   Rx

Although β-lactams remain the preferred therapy for GBS infections, strains with elevated penicillin minimal inhibitory concentrations have been reported but are rare.

STREPTOCOCCUS DYSGALACTIAE SUBSPECIES EQUISIMILIS (HUMAN GROUP C AND G STREPTOCOCCI)

EPIDEMIOLOGY

Non–group A or B β-hemolytic streptococci that are frequently normal inhabitants of the oropharynx, skin, and gastrointestinal and genitourinary tracts are also capable of causing significant disease. These include groups C, G, F, and L, of which the most common are groups G and C (see Table 298-1). According to recent taxonomic studies, large-colony-forming human groups C and G streptococci are currently classified as *Streptococcus dysgalactiae* subspecies *equisimilis* (SDSE). Few laboratories identify groups C and G streptococci to the species level; therefore, exact numbers of human SDSE infections are not available. Infections due to SDSE are transmitted person to person; an animal reservoir for these strains has not been reported. Zoonotic group C or G streptococcal infections are comparatively rare and are mostly caused by other streptococcal species after animal contact or are associated with the consumption of unpasteurized dairy food products. Non-human large-colony-forming β-hemolytic group G streptococci usually belong to *Streptococcus canis*, an animal pathogen that has been found only rarely in humans.

CLINICAL MANIFESTATIONS

A population-based study carried out in North America demonstrated a substantial morbidity and mortality associated with infections due to SDSE, comparable to that caused by invasive GAS infection during the same study period. Both SDSE and GAS affected similar adult populations, tended to be community acquired, and affected primarily persons with underlying medical conditions. The mortality rate was similar to that (8 to 21%) reported in other studies. SDSE primarily presented as skin and soft tissue infection in older patients, whereas individuals with invasive *S. anginosus* group infections were more likely to be younger patients with intra-abdominal infections; these were typically polymicrobial and represented sequelae of perforated appendicitis and associated peritonitis. This finding is supported by the fact that *S. anginosus* group isolates have been recovered from 20 to 40% of healthy appendices.

Pharyngitis is a classic presentation in adult patients, and SDSE has clearly been responsible for epidemic outbreaks of pharyngitis in children. The etiologic role of SDSE in pharyngitis is supported by reports on acute poststreptococcal glomerulonephritis and, more recently, on acute rheumatic fever after SDSE isolation from the upper respiratory tract.

In a 1-year study of 90 patients presenting with 98 disease episodes of acute bacterial cellulitis in Finland, SDSE instead of GAS was strikingly the most common finding. Some patients and household members also carried SDSE in the pharynx, whereas it was not detected in the control subjects. SDSE was isolated either from skin lesion or blood from 22% of patients, whereas GAS was isolated from 7% of patients.

TREATMENT

The non–group A or B β-hemolytic streptococci are typically susceptible to penicillins and cephalosporins, although α-hemolytic viridans group streptococci have shown increasing resistance to penicillin and other β-lactams. In contrast, the resistance to erythromycin and tetracycline among SDSE is similar to rates found in GAS.

VIRIDANS GROUP STREPTOCOCCI

There are more than 20 streptococcal species that have the phenotypic characteristics of typical viridans streptococci and are divided into the mutants group, salivarius group, anginosus group, sanguineous group, and mitis group. Although often found as commensals whose pathogenic abilities appear to be much more subtle than those of the pyogenic streptococci, they may also participate in various infections such as subacute bacterial endocarditis, catheter-related and neutropenia-related blood stream infections, and purulent abdominal, hepatobiliary, brain, and dental infections. Antimicrobial resistance is substantial in the viridans streptococci as a group. Penicillin resistance is from 30 to 50% in strains isolated from patients in North America. *S. mitis* and *S. oralis* are the most common strains found in blood cultures of cancer patients and are commonly resistant to β-lactam antimicrobials. *S. sanguinis*, *S. oralis*, and *S. gordonii*, in descending order, are the most common strains isolated from cultures of blood of endocarditis patients. In the *S. anginosus* group, resistance to ß-lactam antimicrobial is only at the intermediate level, but resistance to macrolides has been found in 17% of the strains. In addition, *S. anginosus* plays a significant role as a reservoir of antimicrobial resistance genes, transferring different resistance traits to more pathogenic organisms such as *Streptococcus pneumoniae* and *S. pyogenes*.

ZOONOTIC STREPTROCOCCI

Streptococcus suis

S. suis is a pathogen in pigs that can cause severe infection in humans. *S. suis* was first reported by veterinarians in 1954, after outbreaks of meningitis, septicemia, and purulent arthritis occurred among piglets. Fourteen years later, the first human *S. suis* cases were diagnosed in Denmark, and subsequently, other cases were reported in more than 30 countries, including Canada, the United States, Japan, Vietnam, and Thailand. It can be clinically manifested with meningitis, arthritis, and septicemia. *S. suis* is the name assigned to streptococci that were formally called Lancefield groups R, S, and T. Of the 35 known serotypes, the most frequent serotype identified from humans has been serotype 2 (group R). Human *S. suis* infections are most often reported from countries where pig rearing is common. The relatively high mean patient age (47 to 55 years) and almost complete absence of children in case series, as well as the high male-to-female patient ratio (3.5 : 1 to 6.5 : 1), support the notion that infection with *S. suis* is generally an occupational disease. The annual risk of developing *S. suis* meningitis among abattoir workers and pig breeders has been estimated to be 3 cases per 100,000 population; the risk is lower for butchers, at 1.2 cases per 100,000 population in developed countries. The incubation period of *S. suis* is from hours to 14 days (median, 2.2 days). A very short incubation time is consistent with direct entry of *S. suis* into the blood through skin wounds. Patients have generally been healthy before infection with *S. suis*, although predisposing factors, such as splenectomy, diabetes mellitus, alcoholism, malignancy, and structural heart diseases have been reported. An outbreak in China was associated with an overall case-fatality rate of 18%, but this reached 63% among patients with septicemia and septic shock.

Data from Vietnam show that *S. suis* is susceptible to penicillin, ceftriaxone, and vancomycin. Resistance was seen to tetracycline (83%), erythromycin (20%), and chloramphenicol (3%). In a European study, 384 *S. suis* strains from diseased pigs were susceptible to penicillin, but resistance was detected to gentamicin (1.0%), trimethoprim-sulfamethoxazole, (6.0%), and tetracycline (75%). There may be a role for the use of dexamethasone as an adjunctive treatment to reduce mortality and improve the outcome of bacterial meningitis due to *S. suis*. In a randomized, double-blind, placebo-controlled clinical trial in Vietnam, dexamethasone (0.4 mg/kg twice daily for 4 days) resulted in a significant reduction in the risk for death at 1 month and in the risk for death and disability at 6 months in patients with confirmed bacterial meningitis: *S. suis* accounted for 25% of pathogens.[4]

Currently, a human vaccine is not available, but simple preventive measures, such as wearing gloves during processing pig meat or slaughtering, hand washing after handling raw pork meat, and thorough cooking of pork, should prevent most cases. Travelers should be aware that dietary habits in some countries may pose a risk for infectious diseases, including *S. suis* infection.

Streptococcus canis

S. canis is an organism that was described in 1986 as having the Lancefield group G antigen and was isolated from animals, most frequently dogs. Extensive phenotypic testing of isolates from dogs was described in 1994, and the isolation of *S. canis* from a human with sepsis was reported in 1997. Despite its name, *S. canis* has been isolated from animals other than dogs, including

cats, harbor porpoises, cows, mice, rats, and rabbits. In healthy dogs, *S. canis* is found as commensal flora of the skin, oropharynx, genital urinary tract, and anus. Rare cases of *S. canis* infection in humans have been reported in the literature. Resistance to erythromycin and tetracycline is common. In the clinical laboratory, group G streptococci are not usually identified to the species level. In addition, laboratory tests have only recently been able to identify *S. canis* accurately. Thus, the true incidence of *S. canis* infection is unknown.

Streptococcus bovis Group

Members of the *Streptococcus bovis* group have long been regarded as opportunistic pathogens in humans causing up to 11 to 14% of all endocarditis cases and 24% of streptococcal endocarditis. *S. bovis* group isolates from human infections are divided into three biotypes, designated biotype I, biotype II/1, and biotype II/2. Most *S. bovis* group endocarditis isolates belong to biotype I, for which a reclassification as *Streptococcus gallolyticus* subspecies *gallolyticus* was recently proposed. The human intestinal tract is a major natural reservoir of *S. bovis* group strains with a reported carriage rate of about 10%. There is a strong association between the presence of malignant or premalignant lesions in the gastrointestinal tracts of patients and isolation of *S. bovis* as a causative agent of bacteremia or endocarditis.

Streptococcus iniae

S. iniae is a β-hemolytic streptococcus without a group antigen. It is a major fish pathogen in many regions of the world. These bacteria are also zoonotic, with infections in humans associated with the handling and preparation of infected fish. The first human infections were reported in 1996. Most cases of human *S. iniae* infections have been in persons of Asian descent, who are elderly and commonly have underlying conditions such as diabetes mellitus, chronic rheumatic heart disease, cirrhosis, or other conditions.

Carrier fish have been implicated in fish-to-fish transmission of *S. iniae*, and these carriers may be responsible for human infection because fish with overt signs of disease are unmarketable. Soft tissue injuries that occur during the preparation of fresh fish from wet markets usually result in bacteremic cellulitis of the hand, followed by one or more of the following conditions: endocarditis, meningitis, arthritis, sepsis, pneumonia, osteomyelitis, and toxic shock. *S. iniae* is susceptible to penicillin and other antimicrobials. The expression of a suite of virulence factors, many of them similar to those found in GAS, is responsible for successful entry, propagation, and evasion of immune defenses of the host by this bacterium. Underreporting of human cases is likely because identification of *S. iniae* is based on biochemical testing of isolates with commercial kits; the use of kits is associated with problems because *S. iniae* is not listed in commercial or clinical databases, and many atypical strains are assigned low matches.

1. Gerber MA, Baltimore RS, Eaton CB, et al. Prevention of rheumatic fever and diagnosis and treatment of acute streptococcal pharyngitis: a scientific statement from the American Heart Association Rheumatic Fever, Endocarditis, and Kawasaki Disease Committee of the Council on Cardiovascular Disease in the Young, the Interdisciplinary Council on Functional Genomics and Translational Biology, and the Interdisciplinary Council on Quality of Care and Outcomes Research: endorsed by the American Academy of Pediatrics. *Circulation*. 2009;119:1541-1551.
2. van Driel ML, De Sutter AI, Keber N, et al. Different antibiotic treatments for group A streptococcal pharyngitis. *Cochrane Database Syst Rev*. 2010;10:CD004406.
3. Ohlsson A, Shah VS. Intrapartum antibiotics for known maternal group B streptococcal colonization. *Cochrane Database Syst Rev*. 2009;3:CD007467.
4. Nguyen TH, Tran TH, Thwaites G, et al. Dexamethasone in Vietnamese adolescents with bacterial meningitis. *N Engl J Med*. 2007;357:2431-2440.

SUGGESTED READINGS

Johansson L, Thulin P, Low DE, et al. Getting under the skin: the immunopathogenesis of *Streptococcus pyogenes* deep tissue infection. *Clin Infect Dis*. 2010;51:58-65. *Review including streptococcal toxic shock syndrome and necrotizing fasciitis.*

Kothari NJ, Morin CA, Glennen A, et al. Invasive group B streptococcal disease in the elderly, Minnesota, USA, 2003-2007. *Emerg Infect Dis*. 2009;15:1279-1281. *Defines an important cause of infection in elderly patients.*

Lappin E, Ferguson AJ. Gram-positive toxic shock syndromes. *Lancet Infect Dis*. 2009;9:281-290. *Clinical review of this multisystem, toxin-mediated disease that often results in multiorgan failure.*

van der Helm-van Mil AH. Acute rheumatic fever and poststreptococcal reactive arthritis reconsidered. *Curr Opin Rheumatol*. 2010;22:437-442. *Differentiates the two separate disease entities.*

Wessels MR. Clinical practice: streptococcal pharyngitis. *N Engl J Med*. 2011;364:648-655. *Review.*

299

ENTEROCOCCAL INFECTIONS

ELI N. PERENCEVICH AND TRISH M. PERL

DEFINITION

Enterococci, formerly called group D streptococci, are endogenous human flora that had been considered pathogens with low virulence. However, more recently they have emerged as increasingly important health care–associated (nosocomial) pathogens. This emergence is primarily due to their inherent resistance to commonly used antimicrobials, acquisition of high-level resistance to vancomycin, persistence in the environment, and transmission from patient to patient by way of the contaminated hands of health care workers. The emergence of vancomycin-resistant enterococci (VRE) has limited therapeutic options in confirmed enterococcal infections and in empirical therapy for infections in severely ill hospitalized patients. One third of enterococcal isolates from hospitalized patients are now reported to be highly resistant to vancomycin. Additionally, there have been several reported cases of vancomycin-resistant *Staphylococcus aureus* (VRSA). In each case, the staphylococcus acquired a vancomycin resistance gene (*VanA*) from a VRE isolate that colonized the same VRSA-infected patient. This highlights that resistance in one species can affect the evolution of resistance in another pathogenic species and that failure to control one species can negatively affect patient outcomes in those infected with another bacteria.

Enterococci are common residents of the human gastrointestinal tract and the female genitourinary tract and act as opportunistic pathogens in severely ill patients. They are known to cause urinary tract infections, intra-abdominal abscesses, bacteremia, including catheter-associated blood stream infections, and endocarditis; less commonly, they cause osteoarticular infections and meningitis.

The Pathogen

Members of the genus *Enterococcus* were long classified within group D of the genus *Streptococcus*. However, in the past 25 years, they have been reclassified based on new molecular and genetic analyses. Enterococci are catalase-negative gram-positive cocci that can appear singly or in pairs or short chains. They are facultative anaerobes that grow optimally at 35° C in broth containing 6.5% NaCl and hydrolyze esculin in the presence of 40% bile salts (bile-esculin medium). Demonstration of the group D antigen may assist the identification of enterococci; however, it is not a particularly sensitive test because it is present in about 80% of enterococcal strains. *Enterococcus faecalis,* the most common cause of enterococcal infections in humans, is the causative agent for 80 to 90% of the enterococcal infections, followed by *Enterococcus faecium,* which is found in 5 to 10% of the infections. *Enterococcus casseliflavus* and *Enterococcus raffinosus* have been reported in clusters of infections. Other species reported to cause infections in humans include *Enterococcus avium, Enterococcus cecorum, Enterococcus dispar, Enterococcus durans, Enterococcus gallinarum, Enterococcus glivus, Enterococcus hirae, Enterococcus mundtii,* and *Enterococcus pallens.*

EPIDEMIOLOGY

The proportion of infections caused by enterococci in hospitalized patients has been increasing over the past several decades. Overall, urinary tract infections (UTIs) are the most common clinical condition caused by enterococci. *Enterococcus* species are now the third most common isolate from UTIs in hospitalized patients, causing 14 to 16% of these infections in North America and can be involved in both complicated and uncomplicated UTIs. Enterococci are the second most common cause of central line–associated blood stream infections and are involved in approximately 5 to 15% of all cases of infective endocarditis. They are also the third most frequent pathogen recovered in surgical site infections. Overall, they are the third most common pathogen in the United States, causing 12% of all health care–associated infections.

Enterococci are part of the normal human gut flora, and infections in both hospitalized and nonhospitalized patients can arise from an endogenous source. However, most infections are health care associated and appear to result from an exogenous source, meaning that transmission from the environment, another patient, or on the hands of a health care worker has

occurred before infection. Nearly all infections are preceded by some period of colonization, and although most colonized patients do not develop infections, they are still able to shed and transmit bacteria to other hospitalized patients. The organism, including VRE, contaminates the hospital environment and equipment and has been associated with outbreaks. Increasingly, hospitalized patients, if they are colonized or infected with an *Enterococcus* species, tend to have a strain resistant to vancomycin (i.e., VRE).

VRE was first reported in Europe in 1986. Since the mid-1990s, the proportion of enterococcal strains resistant to vancomycin has risen steadily. According to the Centers for Disease Control and Prevention (CDC) National Healthcare Safety Network (NHSN), 80% of *E. faecium* isolates and 7% of *E. faecalis* isolates were resistant to vancomycin in 2006 to 2007. There are two major phenotypes for acquired vancomycin resistance, VanA and VanB. The genes encoding the VanA phenotype result in high-level resistance to vancomycin and teicoplanin and are carried on a transposon usually found on a plasmid that is transferable to other gram-positive cocci, including *Staphylococcus aureus.* VanB is associated with variable resistance to vancomycin, but isolates are usually susceptible to teicoplanin. Linezolid resistance is increasingly reported even in patients without previous exposure to the antibiotic. Daptomycin resistance is also reported in both *E. faecalis* and *E. faecium* after prolonged courses of therapy. *E. faecalis* is intrinsically resistant to the streptogramin combination quinupristin-dalfopristin, and resistance exists in *E. faecium* or can develop during therapy.

The epidemiology of VRE differs between Europe and North America. In Europe, VRE is often detected in farm animals, likely due to the use of the antibiotic avoparcin in animal feeds until it was banned in 1997. The proportion of VRE among enterococcal clinical isolates in hospitalized Europeans has been historically lower than in the United States; however, these rates are increasing. In the United States, avoparcin was never used in animal feeds, and therefore VRE is not usually found in farm animals or healthy humans. In contrast, the proportion of enterococcal isolates resistant to vancomycin is higher in U.S. hospitals than European hospitals.

The most common mode of nosocomial transmission of VRE is patient-to-patient cross-transmission by the hands of health care workers who become transiently colonized with the organism. Enterococci with genetic relatedness by pulse-field gel electrophoresis (PFGE) have been cultured on the hands of health care workers caring for infected patients. A study in a U.S. hospital's medical intensive care unit (ICU) found that the number of patients already colonized with VRE in a defined geographic area ("colonization pressure") was the most significant variable in predicting new acquisition of VRE. This finding was significant in that it highlights the important role that patient-to-patient transmission has had in the emergence of VRE. Similarly, a study on hemodialysis patients found the only significant predictor of VRE colonization was hospitalization in the prior year, suggesting the importance of nosocomial transmission in VRE acquisition. A study of hospitalized patients recently admitted to non-ICU wards found that the most sensitive factor for predicting VRE colonization on surveillance culture was previous admission to an acute care hospital in the past year. Importantly, once colonized with VRE, patients may harbor the strain in their gastrointestinal tract for years.

Apart from preexisting gastrointestinal colonization, risk factors for enterococcal infections, particularly VRE infections, include severe underlying conditions such as renal failure, previous solid organ or bone marrow transplantation, solid and hematologic malignancy, diabetes mellitus, and neutropenia. Other factors associated with infection include prior surgical or gastrointestinal procedures, presence of a vascular or urinary indwelling catheter, hospital factors such as location in the ICU or oncology ward, proximity to colonized patients, prolonged length of hospitalization, and recent antimicrobial exposure.

Numerous epidemiologic investigations have revealed that most classes of antimicrobials have been associated with VRE infections. In particular, vancomycin, cephalosporins, and drugs with anaerobic organism coverage use have been linked to VRE acquisition. However, measuring the attributable impact of a particular antibiotic on VRE acquisition is difficult. Increasingly, an association between VRE colonization and *Clostridium difficile* infection is reported in high-risk patients such as those with hematologic malignancies.

PATHOBIOLOGY

Enterococci are commensal organisms that colonize the human gastrointestinal tract and female genital tract. Although they are not as intrinsically virulent as other gram-positive pathogens, under certain conditions, the commensal relationship is disrupted, and serious infections occur. Several adhesion factors have been identified, including aggregation substance, which allow binding to epithelial surfaces and enhance the ability for colonization. The ability to adhere to heart valves and urinary tract epithelium enables the enterococcus to cause endocarditis and UTIs. Enterococci are also known to secrete potential virulence factors. These include cytolysin/hemolysin, which is a bacterial toxin that is produced in a higher proportion of infecting strains compared with stool-colonizing strains. Infecting strains also possess the ability of intestinal translocation, although the exact mechanisms of this process have yet to be determined. To this point, little is known about the host defense mechanisms in enterococcal infections. In addition, the exact role of capsular polysaccharides in colonization or infection is unknown. Strains have been shown to survive within phagocytic cells, yet it is unclear whether this represents successful host defense or evasion by the enterococci. The intrinsic resistance to multiple antimicrobials that enterococci possess, along with their ability to acquire new resistance mechanisms through mutation or acquisition of new genes, enhances their ability to survive and multiply in the many hospitalized patients treated with broad-spectrum antimicrobials.

CLINICAL MANIFESTATIONS

There are no specific clinical manifestations to help distinguish enterococcal infections from infections caused by other bacteria. Enterococci are not thought to cause lower respiratory tract infections or ventilator-associated pneumonia and, if found in these settings, likely represent colonization and not infection.

Urinary Tract Infections

UTIs are the most frequent type of infection caused by enterococci. Most infections are nosocomial in origin and include uncomplicated cystitis, pyelonephritis, prostatitis, and perinephric abscess. These infections are typically secondary to urinary catheterization or instrumentation. In contrast to nosocomial UTI, enterococci cause less than 5% of uncomplicated cystitis or pyelonephritis cases in otherwise healthy nonhospitalized women. Patients with diabetes mellitus appear to be at increased risk for enterococcal UTI. Bacteremia is only infrequently associated with enterococcal UTI.

Bacteremia

The incidence of bacteremia caused by enterococci continues to increase. Specific risk factors include prolonged hospitalization, preexisting urethral catheters or intravascular lines, recent surgery, malignancy, neutropenia, and biliary pathology. Secondary bacteremia without endocarditis usually arises from the urinary tract, hepatobiliary tract, or soft tissue infection. Bacteremia secondary to an intra-abdominal source carries a high mortality rate. Risk factors for VRE bacteremia parallel those mentioned previously but additionally include severe preexisting comorbid conditions, including hematologic malignancy, human immunodeficiency virus (HIV) infection, chronic renal insufficiency, and liver transplantation. Prior exposure to broad-spectrum antimicrobials, including those with antianaerobic activity such as clindamycin or metronidazole and exposure to multiple and prolonged antimicrobial therapy are consistent risk factors. Enterococcal bacteremia is frequently polymicrobial, and the clinical picture is often influenced by whether it is isolated alone or with other bacteria. When enterococci are isolated alone, the course is typically indolent, and frequently fever is the only sign. In contrast, polymicrobial bacteremia is more severe, often presenting with shock or disseminated intravascular coagulation. VRE bacteremia is associated with higher mortality rates than bacteremia due to vancomycin-susceptible strains, and early treatment with an appropriate antibiotic within the first 48 hours of presentation has been associated with improved outcomes.

Endocarditis

Enterococci, particularly *E. faecalis*, are an increasingly frequent cause of endocarditis even though most enterococcal bacteremias are not complicated by endocarditis. The disease occurs most frequently in older patients, with a male predominance. Most cases appear to arise in the community. Patients with preexisting valvular heart disease, including prosthetic valves, are at highest risk, yet many patients lack underlying heart disease. Enterococci more commonly cause left-sided endocarditis primarily affecting the mitral valve. Clinically, these patients present with symptoms that closely resemble a subacute bacterial endocarditis caused by viridans streptococci. Many patients have symptoms for weeks or months before seeking medical care.

Intra-abdominal Infections

In intra-abdominal infections, enterococci are often detected as part of a polymicrobial process. These infections typically arise from a hepatobiliary source, including postoperative infection in liver transplantation, and are complicated by secondary bacteremia.

Skin and Soft Tissue Infections

Enterococci rarely cause cellulitis or other soft tissue infections alone but are often isolated in mixed surgical site infections, diabetic foot infections, and decubitus ulcers along with other gram-negative bacilli, gram-positive cocci, and anaerobic bacteria. Their clinical significance in these situations has not been adequately determined. Enterococci are not thought to be primary pathogens in chronic osteomyelitis. When they are identified, it is thought they may solely represent superinfection, and thus adequate therapy may not require antibiotics directed at enterococcal eradication.

DIAGNOSIS

The diagnosis of an *Enterococcus* infection is made by isolating the organism through culture of a sterile site, such as blood culture or urine culture. The diagnosis and differential diagnosis of specific conditions are the same as discussed for UTIs (Chapter 292) and endocarditis (Chapter 76).

TREATMENT   Rx

Therapy for enterococcal infections is complicated by the fact that strains exhibit inherent resistance to many commonly used antibiotics, including cephalosporins. In addition, enterococci have acquired resistance to a wide-range of antibiotic classes, including aminoglycosides, β-lactams, fluoroquinolones, lincosamides, macrolides, oxazolidinones (linezolid), quinupristin/dalfopristin, rifampin, tetracyclines, and vancomycin. Thus, effective directed therapy for any severe enterococcal infection requires susceptibility testing by experienced microbiology laboratories, with therapy adjusted based on the results. However, even when enterococcus appears susceptible to trimethoprim-sulfamethoxazole in vitro, it should not be used in therapy because clinical failures have been reported secondary to the ability of enterococci to utilize exogenous folate. Recently, there has been increasing isolation of *E. faecium* strains with intrinsic resistance to penicillins. Importantly, *E. faecalis* is intrinsically resistant to quinupristin/dalfopristin, which therefore should not be used in therapy for infections caused by this species. However, most *E. faecalis* strains remain susceptible to ampicillin and the related piperacillin, in contrast to most *E. faecium* strains, which are resistant to ampicillin. Optimal therapy for most infections includes intravenous ampicillin, penicillin, or vancomycin. Given the resistance or tolerance to cell wall–targeting antibiotics, including penicillins and vancomycin, standard therapy with these antibiotics, except in UTIs, should include the addition of a synergistic aminoglycoside (i.e., streptomycin or gentamicin), as long as high-level resistance is not detected. This strategy of two-drug therapy has been associated with improved outcomes. If the VRE strains are known to be susceptible, potential therapy in these infections includes linezolid, quinupristin/dalfopristin, and daptomycin. Although daptomycin is not approved by the U.S. Food and Drug Administration (FDA) to treat VRE, it has been used to treat skin and soft tissue infections and bacteremia. Newly licensed tigecycline is FDA approved to treat complicated skin and soft tissue infections and complicated intra-abdominal infections caused by vancomycin-susceptible isolates of *E. faecalis*. Quinupristin/dalfopristin use is associated with myalgias and arthralgias, and linezolid use is associated with bone marrow suppression including thrombocytopenia; both have only bacteriostatic activity against the enterococci. Linezolid, when used in combination with selective serotonin reuptake inhibitors, can be associated with serotonin syndrome (Chapter 442). Given the complexity of enterococcal infections, an infectious disease consult should be considered for therapeutic guidance.

Urinary Tract Infections

A single agent can usually be used to treat enterococcal UTIs, including ampicillin, amoxicillin, penicillin, or vancomycin. Vancomycin is typically reserved for penicillin-allergic patients or if the strain has high-level penicillin resistance. β-Lactam/β-lactamase inhibitor combinations are usually reserved for polymicrobial infections. Nitrofurantoin is also occasionally used because most strains remain susceptible.

Bacteremia without Endocarditis

Many cases of enterococcal bacteremia are transient or self-limited, yet antibiotic therapy with penicillin or ampicillin has been shown to improve outcomes. Unlike in endocarditis therapy, it is not known whether patients benefit from combination therapy (penicillin or ampicillin or vancomycin plus an aminoglycoside), except perhaps when an indwelling intravascular catheter is present. In the setting of an indwelling intravascular catheter, especially for VRE, removal of the catheter is recommended.

Endocarditis

Combination therapy (intravenous penicillin, ampicillin, or vancomycin plus an aminoglycoside) is the standard therapy for enterococcal endocarditis. Doses and durations are found in Chapter 76. Importantly, the aminoglycoside is used to provide synergistic killing of the organism. Duration of therapy is typically 4 weeks, with 6-week duration given to patients who had prolonged symptoms before seeking therapy, prosthetic valve infection, or relapsed after initial treatment. If the causative enterococcal strain is highly resistant to both gentamicin and streptomycin, then alternative agents and durations must be explored, and surgery to excise infected valves should be considered. Optimal therapy of VRE strains that are resistant to ampicillin is not known but includes combination therapy under the guidance of an infectious disease consultant. Several newly approved agents, including quinupristin/dalfopristin, linezolid, and daptomycin, could be considered if the strain is found to be susceptible. VRE endocarditis may require early surgery because outcomes with antibiotic therapy can be poor. Careful microbiologic and clinical assessment of all patients with enterococcal endocarditis and VRE in particular is helpful in deciding when surgery is necessary. If repeated blood cultures grow for more than 7 days after the initiation of medical therapy or other signs of uncontrolled infection (persistent fever or leukocytosis) are present, surgical repair of the valve or valve replacement should be considered early in the treatment course if there are no absolute contraindications for surgery.

Optimal infection prevention for VRE, like many multidrug-resistant bacteria, includes proper use and compliance with hand hygiene, proper management and timely removal of urinary and vascular catheters, reduction of antibiotic selective pressure through antimicrobial stewardship, use of Contact Precautions, and environmental cleaning of equipment and patient rooms. The latter is particularly important for VRE. Decontamination of patients' skin, called source control, may broadly control transmission of resistant pathogens and reduce device-related infections such as central venous catheter–associated blood stream infections. Source control using daily bathing of patients with chlorhexidine gluconate (CHG)-saturated cloths has been associated with reduced VRE contamination of patients' skin and health care workers' hands. A multicenter quasi-experimental study in six ICUs found daily bathing with CHG solution reduced VRE acquisition by 50% and decreased the risk for VRE bacteremia in known VRE-colonized patients by one third.

The methods for VRE-specific prevention are directed at preventing incident colonization in high-risk hospitalized patients. Nearly all enterococcal infections, including VRE infections, are preceded by gastrointestinal colonization, and although most colonized patients do not develop infections, they are still able to shed and transmit bacteria to other hospitalized patients. At least with VRE, a colonization-to-infection ratio of 10:1 has been reported, suggesting for every 1 clinical infection in an ICU, there may be 10 colonized patients lurking undetected in the unit. Thus, the unrecognized colonized patients represent the target population for infection prevention and control efforts such as active surveillance. Active surveillance programs use rectal or perirectal surveillance swabs to detect previously unrecognized, colonized patients and isolate them to prevent further transmission. Currently, surveillance cultures are recommended at the time of hospital admission for patients at high risk for carriage of VRE, and colonized patients or infected patients should be placed in isolation using Contact Precautions. Contact Precautions typically entail private rooms, dedicated equipment such as stethoscopes, and gloves and gowns for all patient contact. Implicit in this is the continued use of standard precautions that requires cleaning and disinfection of equipment that is used in patient rooms. Many hospitals do use active surveillance in the ICU and other wards with a high prevalence of VRE, although the overall adoption of this strategy has been hindered by the perceived high costs of surveillance programs and lack of available randomized control trial data.

Enterococcal bacteremia is associated with prolonged hospitalization and added costs compared with similar patients without enterococcal bacteremia. Still, apart from enterococcal endocarditis, the attributable mortality of enterococcal infections is difficult to quantify owing to its predilection to infect patients with preexisting comorbid conditions and high levels of illness severity. In certain patient populations, including those with liver and bone marrow transplants, studies have suggested increased morbidity, length of stay, and mortality associated with vancomycin resistance. Furthermore, a

recent meta-analysis reported that the odds of dying from a vancomycin-resistant enterococcal blood stream infection were 2.5 times higher than dying from an infection caused by a susceptible enterococcus. The unadjusted mortality in susceptible enterococcal bacteremia was 20%. It is unclear why resistance is associated with higher mortality, although it is thought that delayed adequate empirical therapy may play a role. These studies should be interpreted cautiously because the clinical impact of resistance in enterococci was assessed before the availability of newer antimicrobials with activity against VRE.

SUGGESTED READINGS

Climo MW, Sepkowitz KA, Zuccotti G, et al. The effect of daily bathing with chlorhexidine on the acquisition of methicillin-resistant *Staphylococcus aureus*, vancomycin-resistant *Enterococcus*, and healthcare-associated bloodstream infections: results of a quasi-experimental multicenter trial. *Crit Care Med.* 2009;37:1858-1865. *An important study demonstrating both reduced VRE transmission and infection in intensive care unit patients.*

Heintz BH, Halilovic J, Christensen CL. Vancomycin-resistant enterococcal urinary tract infections. *Pharmacotherapy.* 2010;30:1136-1149. *Ampicillin, nitrofurantoin, fosfomycin, and doxycycline are options for UTI, with linezolid and daptomycin reserved for confirmed or suspected pyelonephritis or bacteremia.*

Kinney KK. Treatment of infections caused by antimicrobial-resistant gram-positive bacteria. *Am J Med Sci.* 2010;340:209-217. *Review including linezolid, daptomycin, tigecycline, and telavancin.*

Lin MY, Hayden MK. Methicillin-resistant *Staphylococcus aureus* and vancomycin-resistant enterococcus: recognition and prevention in intensive care units. *Crit Care Med.* 2010;38:S335-S344. *Review evidence for ICU interventions.*

Solomkin JS, Mazuski JE, Bradley JS, et al. Diagnosis and management of complicated intra-abdominal infection in adults and children: guidelines by the Surgical Infection Society and the Infectious Disease Society of America. *Clin Infect Dis.* 2010;50:133-164. *Includes recommendations for covering for potential enterococcal infection.*

300

DIPHTHERIA AND OTHER CORYNEBACTERIA INFECTIONS

ROLAND W. SUTTER

DIPHTHERIA

Diphtheria is an acute infectious disease caused by *Corynebacterium diphtheriae*, a gram-positive bacillus. The organism infects primarily the respiratory tract, where it causes tonsillopharyngitis, laryngitis, or both (typically with a pseudomembrane), as well as the skin, where it is responsible for a variety of indolent lesions. If the infecting strain produces exotoxin, myocarditis and neuritis may ensue.

The Pathogen

C. diphtheriae is a member of a group of aerobic, nonmotile, unencapsulated, nonsporulating, pleomorphic gram-positive bacilli. Its name comes from the Greek *korynee* (meaning "club"), which describes the shape of the organism on stained smears—with one end usually being wider—and *diphtheria* (meaning "leather hide"), for the characteristic adherent membrane. The genus *Corynebacterium* is characterized by bacilli that line up in parallel groups and bend when dividing to create "Chinese character" arrangements. Both nontoxigenic and toxigenic *C. diphtheriae* strains exist. Toxigenicity is conferred when a nontoxigenic organism is infected with a beta-phage carrying the gene for the toxin (*tox*). *C. diphtheriae* has three biotypes—*gravis, mitis,* and *intermedius*—that are distinguished by colonial morphology and varying biochemical and hemolytic reactions. Strains can be distinguished for epidemiologic purposes by molecular techniques. Diphtheria toxin–producing strains of *Corynebacterium ulcerans* can produce classic diphtheria, including local respiratory tract and distal toxic complications.

Humans are the only natural reservoir of *C. diphtheriae*, although the organism has occasionally been isolated from a variety of domestic and other animals. Spread occurs in close-contact settings through respiratory droplets or by direct contact with respiratory secretions or skin lesions. The organism survives for weeks and possibly months on environmental surfaces and in dust, and fomite transmission may occur. The majority of nasopharyngeal *C. diphtheriae* infections result in asymptomatic carriage, with clinical disease developing in only about one in seven individuals. However, asymptomatic carriers are important in maintaining transmission.

Diphtheria immunization protects against disease but does not prevent carriage. In the prevaccine era, respiratory disease dominated in temperate climates, with a fall/winter peak in incidence. Most individuals acquired natural immunity by the midteen years. Cutaneous disease was the predominant form of the disease in tropical countries, but the current contribution of cutaneous diphtheria in inducing or maintaining diphtheria immunity in tropical countries is not known. Over the past 3 decades, outbreaks of this form of diphtheria have occurred in the United States and Europe, typically in homeless and alcoholic inner-city adults.

Vaccination with diphtheria toxoid (formalin-treated toxin) was introduced in the 1920s. Immunization of children in an era when the majority of older individuals had natural immunity resulted in a dramatic drop in the incidence of diphtheria and an even more rapid decline in the proportion of toxigenic strains isolated, presumably because the selective advantage of the *tox* gene—promotion of greater replication and spread of the organism—is lost in an immune host. In most Western countries, toxigenic *C. diphtheriae* has been virtually eliminated. In the United States, reported cases fell from 147,991 in 1920 to 15,536 in 1940 to a total of 40 cases from 1980 to 1993. The absence of reported diphtheria cases in the United States in recent years, however, does not indicate that circulation of toxigenic *C. diphtheriae* has ceased. Investigations in a Northern Plains Indian community in North Dakota and First Nations communities in Ontario, Canada, suggest that *C. diphtheriae* strains might have circulated independently for more than 2 decades in these communities, despite the absence of reported respiratory diphtheria cases.

Vaccine-induced immunity to diphtheria wanes with time, and there is a growing cohort of individuals with no natural diphtheria immunity. Serosurveys indicate that 20 to 60% of adults in industrialized countries have diphtheria antitoxin levels below minimal protective levels. A level of 0.01 IU/mL from an in vitro neutralization assay, the "gold standard" test, is considered the lower limit of protection. Long-term protection against diphtheria requires a level of greater than 0.1 IU/mL. As long as a high proportion of the population remains susceptible, the danger of reintroduction or reemergence of toxigenic strains exists.

Large outbreaks of diphtheria have occurred in the vaccine era. In the 1990s there was a major resurgence of diphtheria in several countries of the former Soviet Union. In Russia, the number of reported cases rose from 593 in 1989 to 39,582 in 1994, with more than two thirds of cases occurring in adults. Large-scale campaigns to administer diphtheria toxoid to virtually the entire population in the affected states of the former Soviet Union led to significant decreases in the incidence of diphtheria, from a peak of 50,449 cases in 1995 to 7197 cases in 1997 to pre-resurgence levels by the later 1990s (Fig. 300-1). In general, outbreaks of diphtheria may occur in susceptible populations due to clonal spread of the organism or transfer of the bacteriophage to nontoxigenic strains of *C. diphtheriae*.

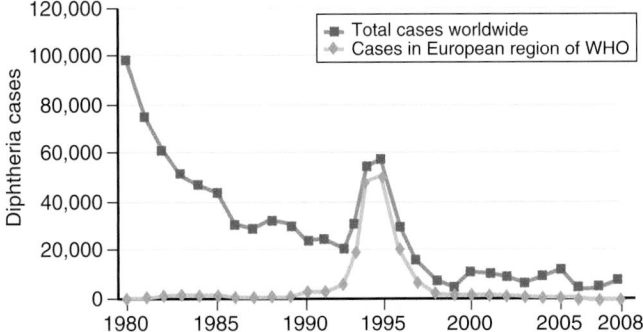

FIGURE 300-1. Reported diphtheria cases worldwide and by European region of the World Health Organization (WHO), 1980 to 2008. (Data from the World Health Organization.)

PATHOBIOLOGY

In classic respiratory diphtheria, *C. diphtheriae* colonizes the mucosal surface of the nasopharynx and multiplies locally without blood stream invasion. Released toxin causes local tissue necrosis, with the formation of a tough, adherent pseudomembrane composed of a mixture of fibrin, dead cells, and bacteria. The membrane usually begins on the tonsils or posterior to the pharynx. In more severe cases, it spreads by progressively extending over the pharyngeal wall, fauces, and soft palate into the larynx, which may result in respiratory obstruction. Toxin entering the blood stream causes tissue damage at distant sites, particularly the heart (myocarditis), nerves (demyelination), and kidney (tubular necrosis). Nontoxigenic strains may cause mild local respiratory disease, sometimes including a membrane.

Diphtheria toxin is an extremely potent inhibitor of protein synthesis, and the estimated human lethal dose is 0.1 mg/kg. The extent of toxin absorption varies with the site of infection, being much less from the skin or nose than from the pharynx.

CLINICAL MANIFESTATIONS

Respiratory Diphtheria

Infection limited to the anterior nares manifests as a chronic serosanguineous or seropurulent discharge without fever or significant toxicity. A whitish membrane may be observed on the septum. The faucial (pharyngeal) form is most common. After an incubation period of 1 to 7 days, the illness begins with a sore throat, malaise, and mild to moderate fever. Initially there is mild pharyngeal erythema, usually followed by progressive formation of a whitish tonsillar exudate; over 24 to 48 hours, this exudate changes into a grayish membrane that is tightly adherent and bleeds on attempted removal. In more severe cases, the patient appears toxic, and the membrane is more extensive. Cervical adenopathy and soft tissue edema may occur and result in the typical "bull neck" appearance and stridor. Laryngeal involvement, which may develop on its own or as a result of membrane extension from the nasopharynx, manifests as hoarseness, stridor, and dyspnea. The following clinical classification has been proposed by the World Health Organization: (1) catarrhal form (erythema of pharynx, no membrane); (2) follicular form (patches of exudate, no pharyngeal or tonsillar involvement); (3) spreading form (membranes covering the tonsils and the posterior pharynx); and (4) combined form (more than one anatomic site involved, such as the throat and skin). The more severe clinical manifestations are associated with increasing toxin absorption levels.

The likelihood of toxic complications depends primarily on the interval between disease onset and administration of antitoxin. The severity of disease at the initial evaluation closely predicts the likelihood of a severe clinical course, complications, and death. Myocarditis typically occurs in the first or second week after the onset of respiratory symptoms and develops either suddenly or insidiously with signs of low cardiac output and congestive failure. Conduction disturbances, which may occur without other signs of myocarditis, include ST-T wave abnormalities, arrhythmias, and heart block. Neurologic impairment manifests as cranial nerve palsies and peripheral neuritis. Palatal or pharyngeal paralysis (or both) occurs during the acute phase; peripheral neuritis, which is symmetrical and predominantly motor, occurs 2 to 12 weeks after the onset of the disease. Motor deficits may range from minor proximal weakness to complete paralysis. Complete recovery is the rule. In fulminant, sometimes called "hypertoxic," diphtheria, toxic circulatory collapse with hemorrhagic features occurs.

Cutaneous Diphtheria

Cutaneous diphtheria lesions are classically indolent, deep, punched-out ulcers that may have a grayish white membrane. However, the lesions may be indistinguishable from impetigo, or *C. diphtheriae* may infect chronic dermatoses such as stasis dermatitis. Coinfection with *Streptococcus pyogenes, Staphylococcus aureus,* or both occurs frequently. Toxic complications of only cutaneous diphtheria are rare.

DIAGNOSIS

The decision to initiate therapy should be based on clinical grounds because delayed treatment, especially delay in the administration of antitoxin, is associated with worse outcomes. A high index of suspicion is required. Specimens for culture should be taken from beneath the membrane, from the nasopharynx, and from any suspicious skin lesions. Because special media are required, the laboratory should be alerted to the possibility of diphtheria. *C. diphtheriae* is best isolated on selective media that inhibit the growth of other nasopharyngeal organisms; one containing potassium tellurite is generally used. Based on colonial morphology and Gram stain appearance, a presumptive diagnosis may be possible within 18 to 24 hours. Cultures may be negative if the patient previously received antibiotics. Toxigenicity testing should be performed on all *C. diphtheriae* isolates. Because both nontoxigenic and toxigenic strains may be isolated from the same patient, more than one colony should be tested. Traditional methods include guinea pig inoculation and the Elek test, in which the isolate and appropriate controls are streaked on a culture plate in which a filter strip soaked with antitoxin has been embedded; toxin production is confirmed by an immunoprecipitation line in the agar. Identification of the diphtheria *tox* gene has allowed the development of rapid and accurate polymerase chain reaction–based methods for identifying toxigenic strains.

Differential Diagnosis

The differential diagnosis includes streptococcal and viral tonsillopharyngitis, infectious mononucleosis, Vincent's angina, candidiasis, and acute epiglottitis. A history of travel to a region with endemic diphtheria or a history of contact with a recent immigrant from such an area increases the possibility of diphtheria, as does a serum antitoxin level of less than 0.01 IU/mL before antitoxin treatment.

TREATMENT   Rx

The goals of treatment are to neutralize the toxin rapidly, eliminate the infecting organism, provide supportive care, and prevent further transmission (Table 300-1). The mainstay of therapy is equine diphtheria antitoxin. Because only unbound toxin can be neutralized, treatment should commence as soon as the diagnosis is suspected because each day of delay in administration increases the likelihood of a fatal outcome. A single dose is given, ranging from 20,000 units for localized tonsillar diphtheria to 100,000 units for extensive disease with severe toxicity. Antitoxin can be administered intramuscularly or intravenously; particularly for more severe cases, the intravenous route is preferred. Tests for sensitivity to antitoxin should be performed according to package insert instructions before administering it, and desensitization should be carried out if necessary. Antibiotic therapy, by eliminating the organism, halts toxin production, limits local infection, and prevents transmission. Parenteral penicillin (4 to 6 million U/day) and erythromycin (40 mg/kg/day in four divided doses to a maximum of 2 g/day, usually orally if the patient can swallow) are the drugs of choice. General supportive care includes ensuring a secure airway (with tracheotomy, if necessary), monitoring the electrocardiogram for evidence of myocarditis, treating heart failure and arrhythmias, and preventing secondary complications of neurologic impairment such as aspiration pneumonia. The patient should be in strict isolation until follow-up cultures are negative. Convalescing patients should receive diphtheria toxoid.

The local health department must be notified. Close contacts should have cultures performed and should be given prophylactic antibiotics. A positive culture in a contact may confirm the diagnosis if the patient is culture negative. All contacts without full primary immunization and a booster within the preceding 5 years should receive diphtheria toxoid. Because U.S. manufacturers discontinued diphtheria antitoxin production, no licensed product is available. However, diphtheria antitoxin for therapeutic purposes can be obtained from the Centers for Disease Control and Prevention (CDC; call the National Immunization Program at 1-404-639-8257 during working hours and 1-770-488-7100 at other times), which distributes a Brazilian-produced antitoxin (Instituto Butantan, Sao Paulo, Brazil) under an investigational new drug protocol.

TABLE 300-1	GOALS AND PROPOSED INTERVENTIONS FOR THE MANAGEMENT OF SUSPECTED DIPHTHERIA CASES	
GOALS	**PROPOSED INTERVENTIONS**
Neutralize toxin as soon as possible to reduce severe complications, including death	After a presumptive diagnosis of diphtheria, immediately obtain and administer antitoxin, initiate antimicrobial treatment, and arrange for appropriate supportive care
Prevent further spread of *C. diphtheriae* to close contacts, including hospital staff	Isolate the patient; strictly observe respiratory barrier procedures Notify the health department Review the vaccination status of the family and other close contacts, and initiate postexposure prophylaxis
Confirm the diagnosis	Collect appropriate specimens for culture (alert the laboratory to ensure that it can prepare specific culture media)
Induce long-term protection against *C. diphtheriae* in case and close contacts	Complete the primary series with diphtheria toxoid as needed

PREVENTION

Immunization with diphtheria toxoid is the only effective means of primary prevention. The primary series is four doses of diphtheria toxoid (given with tetanus toxoid and pertussis vaccine) at 2, 4, 6, and 15 to 18 months of age; a preschool booster dose is given at 4 to 6 years of age. Thereafter, a booster should be given as part of the adolescent immunization schedule (i.e., between 11 and 13 years of age), followed by doses administered every 10 years. Since 2005, the CDC recommends the routine use of tetanus toxoid, reduced diphtheria toxoid, and acellular pertussis vaccine, adsorbed (Tdap), in adolescents aged 11 to 18 years in place of tetanus and diphtheria toxoid (Td) vaccines. In addition, the CDC recommends the routine use of a single

TABLE 300-2	CORYNEBACTERIA AND RELATED ORGANISMS ASSOCIATED WITH HUMAN DISEASE		
SITE OF INFECTION	**PATHOGEN**	**CLINICAL SYNDROME**	**COMMENT**
Respiratory tract	*C. diphtheriae*	Classic diphtheria	
	C. ulcerans	Diphtheria	Zoonotic infection; may produce diphtheria toxin
	C. pseudodiphtheriticum	Pharyngitis Rarely, pneumonia in patients with advanced AIDS	
	Arcanobacterium haemolyticum	Pharyngitis, tonsillar abscess, rash	Clinically indistinguishable from streptococcal pharyngitis
Skin and soft tissue	*C. pseudotuberculosis*	Granulomatous lymphadenitis	Zoonotic infection, especially in sheep; occupational risk for veterinarians and butchers
	C. minutissimum	Erythrasma	
	C. kroppenstedtii	Granulomatous breast abscess	
Genitourinary tract	*C. glucuronolyticum*	Urinary tract infection in men; chronic prostatitis	
	C. urealyticum	Chronic and recurrent urinary tract infection	More common in the elderly, chronically ill, immunosuppressed patients and those with indwelling catheters
	C. riegelli	Encrusted cystitis	
Health care–associated infections	*C. jeikeium* and, less commonly, many others, including *C. amycolatum*, *C. striatum*, and *C. urealyticum*	Catheter- and device-associated infection Postprocedure wound and soft tissue infection Prosthetic valve, joint infection Nosocomial pneumonia Cerebrospinal fluid shunt infection	*C. jeikeium* is the most common corynebacterial pathogen in hospitals and causes severe infections in immunosuppressed patients and those with indwelling devices

dose of Tdap for adults 19 to 64 years of age to replace the next booster dose of Td.

Genetically altered, fully immunogenic mutants of diphtheria toxin have been created (e.g., CRM197) and could be used as potentially less reactogenic alternatives to immunization with the toxoid. CRM197 is used as a protein carrier in several polysaccharide-protein conjugate vaccines.

PROGNOSIS

In the 21st century, diphtheria remains a serious disease associated with a high case-fatality rate. In the United States, the diphtheria case-fatality rate has remained virtually unchanged (between 5 and 10%) over recent decades.

OTHER *CORYNEBACTERIUM* SPECIES

Corynebacteria other than *C. diphtheriae* are ubiquitous in the environment and are among the normal flora colonizing humans and animals. The pathogenic potential of many of these organisms was not appreciated in the past, but many are now known to be associated with specific and often serious infectious diseases, especially in immunosuppressed, chronically ill, and hospitalized patients (Table 300-2). In general, these organisms remain susceptible to vancomycin, but resistance to other classes of antimicrobials is not uncommon and varies among species.

SUGGESTED READINGS

Gautret P, Wilder-Smith A. Vaccination against tetanus, diphtheria, pertussis and poliomyelitis in adult travelers. *Travel Med Infect Dis.* 2010;8:155-160. *Review emphasizing that diphtheria has been reported in travelers without adequate protection.*

Mokrousov I. *Corynebacterium diphtheriae*: genome diversity, population structure and genotyping perspectives. *Infect Genet Evol.* 2009;9:1-15. *With the epidemic reemergence of diphtheria in the former Soviet Union in the 1990s and the reemergence of new toxigenic variants, more high-resolution typing schemes and databasing are needed.*

Wagner KS, Stickings P, White JM, et al. A review of the international issues surrounding the availability and demand for diphtheria antitoxin for therapeutic use. *Vaccine.* 2009;28:14-20. *Review of its role in treatment.*

Wagner KS, White JM, Crowcroft NS, et al. Diphtheria in the United Kingdom, 1986-2008: the increasing role of *Corynebacterium ulcerans. Epidemiol Infect.* 2010;138:1519-1530. *An average of four cases of toxigenic corynebacteria infection per year, with a 5% fatality rate.*

Wagner KS, White JM, Neal S, et al. Screening for *Corynebacterium diphtheriae* and *Corynebacterium ulcerans* in patients with upper respiratory tract infections 2007-2008: a multicentre European study. *Clin Microbiol Infect.* 2011;17:519-525. *Six toxigenic and 28 non-toxigenic strains were identified.*

Wei SC, Tatti K, Cushing K, et al. Effectiveness of adolescent and adult tetanus, reduced-dose diphtheria, and acellular pertussis vaccine against pertussis. *Clin Infect Dis.* 2010;51:315-321. *Review.*

301

LISTERIOSIS

BENNETT LORBER

DEFINITION

Listeriosis is a food-borne infection caused by the gram-positive rod *Listeria monocytogenes*. Most patients have impaired cell-mediated immunity and are seen with life-threatening bacteremia or meningitis, although a self-limited, febrile gastroenteritis in healthy persons also occurs.

The Pathogen

Widely distributed in nature, *L. monocytogenes* may be found in soil, on vegetation, and in the stool of healthy mammals, including humans. It causes disease in animals, especially herd animals, and in humans. The organism has been isolated from many foods, including raw vegetables, raw milk, fish, poultry, and meat.

EPIDEMIOLOGY

Ingestion of contaminated foods appears to be the source of most human infection. Outbreaks have been documented in association with coleslaw, milk, soft cheese, pâté, ready-to-eat pork products, deli counter meats, smoked fish, and butter. Sporadic cases have been traced to contaminated cheese, milk, deli counter meats, turkey frankfurters, and alfalfa tablets. Molecular epidemiologic tools such as pulsed-field gel electrophoresis are important resources when tracking outbreaks.

Information on annual incidence comes from active surveillance studies performed by the Centers for Disease Control and Prevention. The annual incidence of listeriosis in the United States decreased by 44% between 1989 and 1993, possibly related to more stringent regulations in the food-processing industry. Presently, the annual incidence of listeriosis is 3 cases per million population, and it accounts for 1800 cases per year and about 400 deaths. Neonates and adults older than 60 years have the highest infection rates. Pregnant women represent 30% of all affected individuals; other adults at increased risk for invasive listeriosis (bacteremia, meningitis) include those with hematologic malignancy, advanced acquired immunodeficiency syndrome (AIDS), a solid organ transplant, or iron overload and anyone treated with corticosteroids or an anti–tumor necrosis factor (TNF) agent. However, as many as a fourth of all cases of invasive listeriosis occur in apparently healthy persons, particularly those older than 60 years.

PATHOBIOLOGY

L. monocytogenes enters the human body through the intestine, most often after the ingestion of contaminated food. The bacterium induces its own uptake by gastrointestinal cells and macrophages. Mother-to-child transmission occurs transplacentally or through an infected birth canal. Within the host cell the bacterium is enclosed in a phagolysosome, but through the production of an exotoxin called listeriolysin O, it destroys the phagolysosome membrane and gains access to the cytoplasm. All pathogenic strains of *L. monocytogenes* produce listeriolysin O, the major virulence factor. Listeriae actively divide in the cytoplasm, migrate to the periphery of the cell by polymerization of host cell actin, and then push out the cell membrane to form pseudopods, which are taken up by adjacent host cells. The bacteria move from cell to cell in this fashion and repeat their life cycle.

After invasion through the gastrointestinal tract, listeriae may disseminate hematogenously to any body site but show a particular tropism for the central nervous system (CNS). Less commonly, listeriae may spread intra-axonally through cranial nerves to reach the CNS.

Immunity to listerial infection is handled through the cell-mediated arm of the immune system; persons with abnormalities solely of humoral immunity or leukocytes are not at increased risk for infection.

CLINICAL MANIFESTATIONS

The incubation period for invasive listeriosis (time from ingestion of contaminated food to illness) averages about 30 days. Invasive listeriosis in an immunocompromised adult is most often manifested as bacteremia without an obvious focus. In such cases, patients have nonspecific complaints such as fever, malaise, myalgia, and back pain. Bacteremia is the form of invasive listeriosis that complicates pregnancy; CNS infection is extremely rare in the absence of other risk factors. Listeriosis during pregnancy may lead to spontaneous abortion or neonatal sepsis, but early antimicrobial therapy may result in the birth of a healthy child. Endocarditis with *L. monocytogenes* can occur on both native and prosthetic valves and carries a high rate of septic complications. Endocarditis, but not bacteremia per se, may be a clue to underlying colon cancer; colonoscopy should be considered in all cases of listerial endocarditis.

Persons in whom *L. monocytogenes* bacteremia develops may progress to CNS infection, most commonly manifested as meningitis. *Listeria* has a predilection for infecting brain tissue, as well as the meninges, and unlike other common bacterial causes of meningitis, it not infrequently causes encephalitis or brain abscess. Brain abscess as a result of infection by *L. monocytogenes* exhibits unusual features when compared with other bacteria: listerial brain abscess coexists with bacteremia in nearly all cases and with meningitis in a fourth; in addition, abscesses are often subcortical.

L. monocytogenes is the most common cause of bacterial meningitis in patients with lymphomas, organ transplant recipients, and patients treated with corticosteroids for any reason. Affected persons usually have the classic acute symptoms of meningitis but may also have a subacute disease course more characteristic of tuberculous meningitis. Most have a stiff neck, but 25% may not. Focal neurologic findings, including ataxia, tremors, myoclonus, and seizures, may be seen consistent with the tropism of *Listeria* for brain parenchyma. The glucose content in cerebrospinal fluid (CSF) is normal in more than 60% of cases. Gram stain of CSF reveals *L. monocytogenes* in only about 40% of cases, and even when seen, the organisms may be mistaken for pneumococci.

Listerial rhombencephalitis is an unusual form of listerial encephalitis that involves the brain stem. Unlike other listerial CNS infections, rhombencephalitis usually occurs in healthy adults. The typical clinical picture is one of a biphasic illness with a prodrome of fever, headache, nausea, and vomiting lasting about 4 days, followed by the abrupt onset of asymmetrical cranial nerve deficits, cerebellar signs, and hemiparesis or hemisensory deficits, or both. Respiratory failure develops in about 40% of patients. Nuchal rigidity is present in about half, and CSF findings are only mildly abnormal, with a positive CSF culture in about 40%. Almost two thirds of patients are bacteremic. Magnetic resonance imaging is superior to computed tomography for demonstrating rhombencephalitis. Mortality is high, and serious sequelae are common in survivors.

Localized infection may occur after hematogenous seeding (e.g., liver abscess, septic arthritis) or, rarely, after direct inoculation (e.g., conjunctivitis, cellulitis).

Well-documented reports of food-borne outbreaks have demonstrated that ingestion of *L. monocytogenes* in a sufficiently large inoculum can result in a self-limited illness consisting of fever, chills, diarrhea, abdominal cramps, and sometimes nausea and vomiting. Symptoms follow exposure by 1 to 2 days and last for about 2 days.

DIAGNOSIS

Differential Diagnosis

Clinical situations in which a diagnosis of listeriosis should be considered include (1) neonatal sepsis or meningitis; (2) meningitis or parenchymal brain infection in the following: patients with hematologic malignancies, AIDS, organ transplantation, corticosteroid immunosuppression, treatment with anti-TNF agents, and age older than 50 years; (3) simultaneous infection of the meninges and brain parenchyma; (4) subcortical brain abscess; (5) fever during pregnancy, particularly in the third trimester; (6) blood, CSF, or other normally sterile specimen reported to have "diphtheroids" on Gram stain or culture; and (7) food-borne outbreak of febrile gastroenteritis when routine cultures fail to identify a pathogen. The differential diagnosis of listerial CNS infection includes the more common causes of bacterial meningitis and brain abscess; indolent listerial meningitis or rhombencephalitis may mimic CNS tuberculosis.

Laboratory Findings

The diagnosis of listeriosis is best made by routine bacterial culture of specimens from usually sterile sites such as blood or CSF. The laboratory must exercise caution because *L. monocytogenes* may be mistaken for diphtheroids, streptococci, enterococci, or *Haemophilus influenzae*. Specific stool culture is recommended only when routine stool cultures are negative in the setting of an outbreak of gastroenteritis; many people have enteric colonization with *L. monocytogenes* without invasive disease. The laboratory must be advised that listerial infection is suspected because the organism is unlikely to be identified with routine stool culture media.

Serologic testing (antibody to listeriolysin O) is not useful for invasive disease but may be helpful in the retrospective identification of food-borne outbreaks of febrile gastroenteritis when routine cultures are negative.

PREVENTION

Guidelines for preventing listeriosis are similar to those for preventing other food-borne illnesses. In general, one should thoroughly cook raw food from animal sources, wash raw vegetables thoroughly before eating, keep uncooked meats separate from vegetables and from cooked and ready-to-eat foods, avoid raw (unpasteurized) milk or foods made from raw milk, and wash hands, knives, and cutting boards after each handling of uncooked foods.

People at high risk for listeriosis (those immunocompromised by illness or medications, pregnant women, and the elderly) may choose to avoid soft cheeses such as feta, Brie, Camembert, blue-veined, and Mexican-style cheese such as queso fresco. Hard cheeses, processed cheeses, cream cheese, cottage cheese, and yogurt are safe. Leftover foods or ready-to-eat foods such as hot dogs should be cooked until steaming hot. It is best to avoid foods from delicatessen counters, such as prepared salads, meats, and cheeses, or at least to reheat cold cuts thoroughly until they are steaming hot before eating.

Listeriosis is effectively prevented by trimethoprim-sulfamethoxazole given as *Pneumocystis* prophylaxis to organ transplant recipients or to

individuals infected with human immunodeficiency virus. In areas with a high prevalence of AIDS, the widespread use of trimethoprim-sulfamethoxazole for *Pneumocystis* prophylaxis appears to have resulted in a marked decline in nonperinatal listeriosis.

Second episodes of neonatal listerial infection are virtually unheard of, and intrapartum antibiotics are not recommended for women with a history of perinatal listeriosis.

Except from infected mother to fetus, human-to-human transmission of listeriosis does not occur; patients do not need to be isolated.

TREATMENT   Rx

Recommendations for the treatment of infection with *L. monocytogenes* derive from in vitro data, animal models, and clinical experience with small numbers of patients; no controlled trials have been performed to prove the efficacy of one drug over another. Many antimicrobials show in vitro activity against *L. monocytogenes*. Clinical utility is more relevant than in vitro susceptibility test results because cephalosporins and other drugs to which the bacterium appears to be susceptible are inadequate to treat infection.

Twenty percent of cases of bacterial meningitis in those older than 50 years are due to *L. monocytogenes*. Therefore, empirical therapy for bacterial meningitis in all adults older than 50 years should include either ampicillin or trimethoprim-sulfamethoxazole, especially in the absence of associated pneumonia, otitis, sinusitis, or endocarditis, which would suggest a cause other than *L. monocytogenes*. Cephalosporins, commonly used for the treatment of bacterial meningitis, should not be used alone when *Listeria* is a diagnostic consideration.

Ampicillin is generally considered the drug of choice for treating confirmed cases of listeriosis. In cases of meningitis and endocarditis and in patients with severely impaired T-cell function, many authorities recommend the addition of gentamicin to ampicillin for synergy based on in vitro testing and animal models. For meningitis, therapy should be continued for at least 3 weeks; bacteremic patients without CNS involvement may be treated for 2 weeks. Endocarditis and brain abscess should be treated for at least 6 weeks. Meningitis doses should be used to treat all cases of invasive listeriosis, even in the absence of CNS or CSF abnormalities.

In patients with penicillin hypersensitivity, trimethoprim-sulfamethoxazole is the preferred agent. It is bactericidal and appears to be as effective as the combination of ampicillin and gentamicin. Drugs that should be avoided because of treatment failure and relapse include cephalosporins, chloramphenicol, tetracycline, and erythromycin.

Corticosteroids appear to be important adjunctive agents in treating the most common forms of bacterial meningitis. Their role in the treatment of listerial CNS infection is unknown.

Iron is a virulence factor for *L. monocytogenes,* and clinically, iron overload states are risk factors for listerial infection. Therefore, in patients with listeriosis and iron deficiency, it may be prudent to withhold iron replacement until antimicrobial therapy is complete.

PROGNOSIS

Listeria meningitis carries a mortality of about 25%, and mortality is higher in those with underlying malignancy. Mortality from brain abscess and endocarditis is about 50%; survivors of brain abscess commonly have significant neurologic residua.

SUGGESTED READINGS

Allerberger F, Wagner M. Listeriosis: a resurgent foodborne infection. *Clin Microbiol Infect*. 2010;16:16-23. *Review of sources of infection and clinical manifestations, including febrile gastroenteritis, sepsis, and meningitis.*

Bortolussi R. Listeriosis: a primer. *CMAJ*. 2008;179:795-797. *Review of clinical features, diagnosis, and management.*

Guevara RE, Mascola L, Sorvillo F. Risk factors for mortality among patients with nonperinatal listeriosis in Los Angeles County, 1992-2004. *Clin Infect Dis*. 2009;48:1507-1515. *The case fatality rate of 20% was associated with nonhematologic malignancy, alcoholism, and steroid medication and was higher with sepsis than with isolated meningitis.*

Martins IS, Faria FC, Miguel MA, et al. A cluster of *Listeria monocytogenes* infections in hospitalized adults. *Am J Infect Control*. 2010;38:e31-e36. *An outbreak from the hospital kitchen.*

Morvan A, Moubareck C, Leclercq A, et al. Antimicrobial resistance of *Listeria monocytogenes* strains isolated from humans in France. *Antimicrob Agents Chemother*. 2010;54:2728-2731. *Resistance to tetracyclines and fluoroquinolones was common, whereas resistance to trimethoprim and higher dose penicillin was rare.*

Schuppler M, Loessner MJ. The opportunistic pathogen *Listeria monocytogenes*: pathogenicity and interaction with the mucosal immune system. *Int J Inflam*. 2010;2010:704321. *Review.*

ANTHRAX

DANIEL R. LUCEY

DEFINITION

Anthrax is caused by *Bacillus anthracis*, a spore-forming, gram-positive rod that is aerobic or facultatively anaerobic. The name comes from the Greek word for "coal," a reference to the black eschar that eventually forms in the cutaneous form of anthrax. Anthrax is primarily a disease of animals, but it has also been developed in past decades by some nations as a biowarfare weapon and was used by one or more persons as a bioterrorist weapon in 2001 in the United States.

The Pathogen

The bacterium is a large (1 to 1.5 by 3 to 5 μm), gram-positive rod. It has a "ground-glass appearance" of growth on sheep blood agar, with 2- to 5-mm, nonhemolytic, tenacious ("beaten egg white") colonies after 15 to 24 hours of culture; oval, central to subterminal spores; and a capsule that can be visualized by India ink staining and that may also be seen in smears of blood or cerebrospinal fluid.

EPIDEMIOLOGY

Human infection with *B. anthracis* is usually linked to a zoonotic source such as goats, sheep, cattle, antelope, kudu, pigs, horses, zebu, and other animals. Animal-related products that can transmit the infection include meat, wool, hides, bones, and hair. Soil contaminated with spores, which can persist for many years, is also a source of infection. The spores can infect humans or animals, after which they germinate into the vegetative form of the bacterium and then cause clinical disease.

The World Health Organization makes available online an extensive global epidemiology database for anthrax and offers guidelines on epidemiologic and ecologic control issues in both humans and animals. From 1900 to 2005, at least 82 patients with inhalational anthrax were reported in detail in the worldwide medical literature, including 18 from the United States with naturally acquired disease diagnosed before 1977. Many of these 18 patients had environmental exposure to spores, such as in goat hair–processing plants in New England. In 2006, the first patient with naturally acquired inhalational anthrax in the United States in 30 years was hospitalized in Pennsylvania; the source was dried African animal hides used in making drums. Of note, this patient was the first to have a component of anthrax toxin, specifically "lethal factor," assayed for and found in high concentration in pleural fluid. In 2009 the first case of naturally acquired, culture-confirmed, gastrointestinal anthrax in the United States was diagnosed in a patient in New Hampshire. Again, the source of the infection was linked to drums.

Between December 2009 and June 2010, anthrax, mainly severe soft tissue infection, was diagnosed in at least 48 patients in the United Kingdom, primarily Scotland. Approximately 30% (15/48) of infections were fatal, including some patients with central nervous system (CNS) hemorrhage. The source was linked to the injection of heroin contaminated by *Bacillus anthracis*.

Clinical experience with inhalational anthrax in the United States is primarily related to events in 2001, when 11 persons were infected after spores were sent in letters that arrived in several locations, including Florida, New York, New Jersey, Washington, DC, and Virginia (Chapter 20). A previous attempt to use anthrax as a bioterrorist weapon, by releasing it from a Tokyo rooftop in 1993, failed to cause any human illness.

In 1979, accidental release of anthrax from a military facility in Sverdlovsk (now Yekaterinburg), Russia, resulted in the deaths of many dozens of humans and animals. Eventually, epidemiologic and clinical data revealed that the deaths followed the probable airborne path ("plume") of the anthrax spores downwind from the military facility. At autopsy, 50% of 42 patients who died had anthrax meningitis in addition to inhalational anthrax.

Some of the largest outbreaks of anthrax in humans have involved the cutaneous form. For example, an estimated 10,000 human infections with cutaneous anthrax occurred in Zimbabwe from 1979 to 1985, primarily attributed to human exposure to an outbreak in cattle that had not been

vaccinated against anthrax. In the United States, bioterrorism via anthrax in mailed letters caused 11 cases of cutaneous anthrax in addition to the 11 inhalational cases.

Notably, *B. anthracis* is not transmitted from person to person through the air. There is, however, evidence of spores being able to re-aerosolize under some experimental indoor and outdoor conditions.

PATHOBIOLOGY

The major virulence factors of *B. anthracis* include its two binary toxins, "edema factor" (EF) and "lethal factor" (LF), and its antiphagocytic poly-D-glutamic acid capsule. Both EF and LF must first bind a third anthrax toxin component, "protective antigen" (PA), following binding of PA to a cellular "anthrax toxin receptor" (ATR). For example, edema toxin consists of EF bound to PA (EF-PA binary toxin), and lethal toxin consists of LF bound to PA (LF-PA binary toxin). EF, LF, and PA are all encoded on one plasmid ("pX-01"), and the immune system–evading, antiphagocytic capsule is encoded on a second plasmid ("pX-02").

The pathogenesis of anthrax is linked to its two binary toxins. Two cellular receptors serve as the ATR: tumor endothelial marker 8 (TEM-8) and capillary morphogenesis protein 2 (CMG-2). Once the PA component of edema toxin and lethal toxin binds to a cellular receptor, the toxin complex can enter the target cell, first going into the acidic endosome and then the cytosol.

EF is a calmodulin-dependent, adenylate cyclase enzyme that catalyzes excessive production of cyclic adenosine monophosphate from adenosine triphosphate and results in water and calcium dysregulation, which is manifested as the characteristic edema of anthrax (sometimes described as "gelatinous"). Edema toxin is also reported to impair the function of polymorphonuclear leukocytes.

LF is a zinc-dependent metalloproteinase that impairs the immune system by interfering with the function of macrophages and other antigen-presenting cells, such as dendritic cells, that are essential for normal T-cell function. Dendritic cell function is inhibited by blockade of costimulatory molecules that are required for the presentation of antigen to T cells, such as CD40, CD80, and CD86, and by blockade of the activation of cytokines that help prime naïve T cells, such as interleukin-12.

The primary mechanism of action of lethal toxin is to inhibit the mitogen-activated protein kinase (MAP kinase) intracellular signal transduction pathway. Lethal toxin is linked to excessive production of inflammatory cytokines and dysregulation of the cytokine network, possibly leading to a "cytokine storm" that contributes to rapid multiorgan clinical failure, shock, and death. Lethal toxin is also reported to impair platelets, again by inhibiting MAP kinase pathways, such as p38 MAP kinase. In addition, lethal toxin can impair human whole blood clotting in vitro. Thus, lethal toxin may contribute in several ways to the striking bleeding diathesis, including bleeding into lymph nodes, the pleural space, the meninges, the intestines, and ascitic fluid.

CLINICAL MANIFESTATIONS

Four major clinical manifestations of anthrax infection—inhalational, cutaneous, gastrointestinal, and meningeal—are related to the three routes by which *B. anthracis* can enter the body: inhalation, ingestion, or via the skin. An apparent fifth major clinical manifestation, "injection anthrax," which causes "serious soft tissue infection," has been described in 2010 in heroin-injecting drug users in the United Kingdom.

Inhalational anthrax typically causes mediastinal adenopathy that results in mediastinal widening (Fig. 302-1), as well as pleural effusions that are often bloody, can expand rapidly, recur if drained by thoracentesis rather than by chest tube, and can be rapidly fatal if not treated with multiple antibiotics and pleural drainage. In 2005, a new clinical staging system for inhalational anthrax (Table 302-1) added an "intermediate progressive stage" based on clinical, microbiologic, and radiologic information acquired from the 11 patients in 2001. Radiography demonstrated either pulmonary infiltrates or consolidation in 8 of the 11 patients. The incubation period of inhalational anthrax is generally 3 to 14 days, with a range of 2 to 43 days in humans. In all six of the patients who survived the anthrax attacks in 2001, anthrax was diagnosed during the "intermediate progressive stage," and prompt therapy prevented progression of disease beyond this stage.

Cutaneous anthrax is the most common form of the disease (95%). The incubation period is usually 1 to 12 days. Cutaneous anthrax typically progresses from a papule that is pruritic, to a central vesicular or bullous lesion with surrounding nonpitting edema, and finally to a necrotic and hemorrhagic central lesion that evolves into the classic painless black eschar with surrounding edema (Fig. 302-2). This sequence of progressive cutaneous

FIGURE 302-1. Clinical features of anthrax. **A**, A portable chest radiograph in a 56-year-old man with inhalational anthrax depicts a widened mediastinum *(arrowheads)*, bilateral hilar fullness, right pleural effusion, and bilateral perihilar air space disease. **B**, A non–contrast-enhanced spiral computed tomography scan depicts an enlarged and hyperdense right hilar lymph node *(white arrowhead)*, bilateral pleural effusions *(black arrowheads)*, and edema of mediastinal fat. (From Mayer TA, Bersoff-Matcha S, Murphy C, et al. Clinical presentation of inhalational anthrax following bioterrorism exposure. *JAMA.* 2001;286: 2549-2543.)

TABLE 302-1 CLINICAL STAGING SYSTEM FOR INHALATIONAL ANTHRAX

I. EARLY PRODROMAL STAGE

Nonspecific illness sometimes described as "flulike" and including any of the following: fever, cough, headache, chills, nausea, chest pain, or abdominal pain. Laboratory tests and radiographs are nondiagnostic. The prognosis for cure is good with appropriate therapy, but the diagnosis is difficult to confirm acutely in this stage.

II. INTERMEDIATE PROGRESSIVE STAGE

Any of the following findings are defining inclusion criteria for this stage:
1. Positive blood cultures (typically positive in <24 hours)
2. Mediastinal adenopathy
3. Pleural effusions: bloody, often large, require drainage, and may recur

Findings in this stage may include high fever, dyspnea, confusion or syncope, or increasing nausea and vomiting. Exclusion criteria for this stage include the following:
1. Meningitis
2. Respiratory failure requiring intubation and mechanical ventilation or
3. Shock

Importantly, patients in the "intermediate-progressive" stage can still be cured with appropriate antibiotics *and* drainage of pleural effusions by thoracentesis and/or chest tube to reduce the adverse mechanical effect on respiration by large-volume effusions and to remove potentially toxin-producing *Bacillus anthracis* from the pleural space.

III. LATE FULMINANT STAGE

Inclusion criteria include any one of the following findings:
1. Meningitis
2. Respiratory failure requiring intubation and mechanical ventilation
3. Shock: end-organ hypoperfusion

Findings in this stage may also include any of those from previous stages, so there are no exclusion criteria. The probability of survival is lowest in this stage. Novel therapeutics that safely and effectively neutralize anthrax toxin may be needed to increase survival.

FIGURE 302-2. The lesion of cutaneous anthrax. (From Freedman A, Freedman A, Afonja O, et al. Cutaneous anthrax associated with micro-angiopathic hemolytic anemia and coagulopathy in a 7-month-old infant. *JAMA.* 2002;287:869-874.)

lesions can still occur even if appropriate antibiotics are given, and total resolution can take up to 2 months. The differential diagnosis includes brown recluse spider bites (which typically cause a painful lesion, unlike the painless anthrax lesion; Chapter 367), cutaneous leishmaniasis (Chapter 356), plague (Chapter 320), tularemia (Chapter 319), typhus (Chapter 335), and warfarin (Coumadin) or heparin necrosis (Chapter 37), among others.

Gastrointestinal anthrax can be divided into an oropharyngeal form and an intestinal form. Extremely rare in the United States, gastrointestinal anthrax in other nations is often linked to consumption of the meat of infected animals, thereby suggesting that the vegetative form of the bacteria can cause gastrointestinal disease in humans. The oropharyngeal form is accompanied by painful cervical adenopathy and fever. The incubation period ranges from 2 to 144 hours. Oral lesions can ulcerate and progress to cause a white pseudomembrane, hoarseness, and dysphagia. Three phases of intestinal disease have been noted: an initial prodromal phase with fever, malaise, and syncope; a second progressive phase with abdominal pain, nausea, vomiting,

abdominal distention, ascites, and severe weakness; and a fulminant third phase with suddenly increasing abdominal girth and expanding ascites, paroxysmal abdominal pain, and shock.

Anthrax meningoencephalitis can occur in association with inhalational, cutaneous, or gastrointestinal anthrax, and in rare cases it occurs without a known portal of entry. Anthrax meningitis is nearly always fatal. Cerebral edema, parenchymal brain hemorrhages, vasculitis, and subarachnoid hemorrhages can be seen.

DIAGNOSIS

Most importantly, if anthrax is suspected, blood should be obtained immediately for culture before any antibiotics are started; blood from patients with inhalation anthrax will grow the typical large, gram-positive rods in less than 24 hours. Surprisingly, even one dose of an effective antibiotic can sterilize the blood cultures. Nasal cultures should not be performed as a clinical diagnostic test for individual patients but might be useful as part of an epidemiologic investigation. If the initial culture is suggestive, three additional tests that should be performed in a biosafety cabinet are motility (nonmotile), catalase (positive), and hemolysis (negative). If these characteristics are found, *B. anthracis* is suspected but not proved until a sample is sent to a reference laboratory where polymerase chain reaction can identify *B. anthracis* and gamma-phage lysis of the encapsulated bacteria can provide confirmation. In addition, the Anthrax Quick ELISA (enzyme-linked immunosorbent assay) test can detect the eventual presence of antibodies to anthrax in blood.

A non–contrast-enhanced computed tomography scan can be a valuable adjunctive diagnostic tool for inhalational anthrax and is better than chest radiography for demonstrating the characteristic hyperattenuating mediastinal adenopathy and pleural effusions seen with inhalational anthrax. The hyperattenuation is consistent with bleeding into lymph nodes and thus is helpful in distinguishing anthrax from tularemia (Chapter 319), histoplasmosis (Chapter 340), tuberculosis (Chapter 332), sarcoidosis (Chapter 95), and most other causes of hilar or mediastinal adenopathy.

Anthrax meningitis is typically bloody and neutrophilic. Large gram-positive rods distinguish it from other causes of gram-positive rod meningitis, such as the smaller *Listeria monocytogenes* (Chapter 301).

TREATMENT   Rx

Treatment of clinical anthrax includes antibiotics and, in the case of inhalational anthrax, pleural fluid drainage. The Centers for Disease Control and Prevention (CDC) recommendations for treatment include a multidrug regimen with either ciprofloxacin (400 mg intravenously every 12 hours) or doxycycline (100 mg intravenously every 12 hours) plus one or more additional antimicrobials for inhalational or gastrointestinal anthrax: rifampicin, vancomycin, penicillin, ampicillin, chloramphenicol, imipenem, clindamycin, or clarithromycin. Penicillin (or ampicillin) should not be used as a single agent in the initial therapy for inhalational anthrax because of the risk that resistance will develop. A detailed algorithm for the management of cutaneous anthrax is posted on the website of the American Academy of Dermatology (available at www.aad.org/professionals/educationcme/bioterrorism/CutaneousAnthrax. htm). Initial treatment of suspected anthrax meningitis should be combination therapy with a fluoroquinolone given intravenously and one or two other antibiotics that penetrate well into the CNS and are active against *B. anthracis*, such as penicillin, ampicillin, meropenem, vancomycin, or rifampicin.

If persons are potentially exposed to aerosolized anthrax spores, they should also receive three doses of anthrax vaccine at 0, 2, and 4 weeks under a Food and Drug Administration (FDA) Investigational New Drug (IND) or Emergency Use Authorization (EUA) protocol, according to CDC recommendations.

A 60-day course of antibiotic therapy is recommended for inhalational anthrax because of concern that residual spores may germinate into vegetative bacteria if antibiotic therapy is stopped sooner. When clinically appropriate, intravenous therapy can be changed to oral therapy, and multiple antibiotics might be reduced to only ciprofloxacin or doxycycline. Cutaneous anthrax is usually treated for 7 to 10 days rather than 60 days if inhaled spores are not an issue.

Adjunctive corticosteroids have been used historically for anthrax meningitis and for severe airway compromise caused by cutaneous anthrax of the neck. However, steroids have not been shown in a randomized clinical trial to be beneficial in any clinical forms of anthrax.

Another critical treatment modality for inhalational anthrax is pleural drainage via chest tube or by thoracentesis initially performed when the patient is still in the intermediate progressive stage, if possible. Thoracentesis may need to be repeated if the typically bloody fluid reaccumulates.

As of 2009, there are two types of anthrax toxin antibodies in the Strategic National Stockpile (SNS). One is polyclonal, called Anthrax Immune Globulin (AIG), and is derived from the plasma of persons who have received the anthrax vaccine. The other is a humanized monoclonal antibody called raxibacumab. Neither is licensed by the FDA as of June 2010. AIG has been given as adjunctive therapy to several patients, including two in the United States in 2006 and 2009 and several in the U.K. heroin-contaminated outbreak in 2009-2010.

PREVENTION

Clinical anthrax can be prevented by pre-exposure vaccination or by postexposure antibiotic prophylaxis. The current FDA-licensed anthrax vaccine contains PA as the vaccine antigen and alum as an adjuvant. It requires five shots over an 18-month period when given before exposure. In contrast, postexposure prophylaxis, which is an off-label use of this same vaccine and thus needs an IND or EUA protocol, requires only three shots given over a 1-month period. This vaccine is in limited supply and is dedicated primarily to use by the military, so it is not available for routine use by civilian populations.

Antibiotics that are approved by the FDA for postexposure prophylaxis include ciprofloxacin, doxycycline, and procaine penicillin G, as well as levofloxacin. In addition, in certain situations (children, pregnant women, and breast-feeding mothers), the CDC has advised that amoxicillin is another option for postexposure prophylaxis. Either doxycycline or ciprofloxacin is recommended by the CDC for initial prophylaxis when the antibiotic susceptibility of an anthrax strain is unknown. The CDC website on anthrax (available at http://www.bt.cdc.gov/agent/anthrax) is the best source for detailed recommendations regarding the choice of antibiotics, doses, and durations for both prevention and treatment of anthrax. Recommendations currently include either ciprofloxacin, 500 mg orally every 12 hours, or doxycycline, 100 mg orally every 12 hours, for a total of 60 days. Levofloxacin has the potential for once-daily 500-mg dosing, but safety data beyond 28 consecutive days in adults are very limited. The 2001 recommendations from the CDC on antibiotic use for prevention and treatment have not yet been officially updated as of May 2010. The CDC did, however, convene a multidisciplinary conference to address updating the clinical guidelines in March 2006 and published the conference report in April 2008 in their journal *Emerging Infectious Diseases*.

Prevention of anthrax secondary to bioterrorism remains a priority. Evolving approaches for detecting and responding to any future bioterrorism attacks with anthrax include the BioWatch antiterrorist system and the Autonomous Detection System. The "Cities Readiness Initiative" was initially described on the CDC website in June 2004 as a program for multiple U.S. cities and metropolitan areas to help prepare them for large-scale public health emergencies, including bioterrorism attacks (e.g., with aerosolized anthrax or another organism). Large volumes of medical supplies, including but not limited to antibiotics, could be delivered rapidly from the SNS to one or multiple locations across the nation, followed by local and regional distribution.

PROGNOSIS

The inhalational anthrax of all six patients who survived the attacks of 2001 was diagnosed during the "intermediate progressive stage," and prompt therapy prevented progression beyond this stage. The 45% case-fatality rate in 2001 was much improved over the 88% rate seen in the United States from 1900 to 1976. Survival is more likely in patients who undergo pleural drainage, receive multidrug antibiotic regimens, do not require intubation or tracheotomy, and do not progress to anthrax meningoencephalitis. The mortality from cutaneous anthrax is approximately 20% if untreated, including patients in whom upper airway compression develops from a lesion on the neck or in whom secondary bacteremic anthrax meningitis develops. In 2009-2010, an approximate 30% mortality (15/48 cases) in U.K. heroin-injecting drug users with serious soft tissue infections occurred despite surgical débridement, multiple antibiotics, and in some cases antitoxin (AIG). Anthrax meningitis remains fatal in more than 95% of victims, and thus better, more rapid therapies are needed.

FUTURE DIRECTIONS

Research is ongoing in an attempt to develop a commercially available, clinically validated, rapid test for the diagnosis of infection with *B. anthracis*, either before symptoms start, in the early prodromal stage of the illness, or in later clinical stages if the patient may have received antibiotics before blood or cerebrospinal fluid was obtained for culture. Anthrax toxin inhibitors, in conjunction with antibiotics, could be particularly useful in treating patients who have progressed into the systemic stages of anthrax as a result of inhalational, gastrointestinal, or injection anthrax causing serious soft tissue infection; however, whether antitoxins cross the blood-brain barrier and can treat human neurologic anthrax remains to be determined.

In addition, antitoxin could be useful in the setting of infection with an engineered form of multidrug-resistant (MDR) or extremely drug-resistant (XDR) anthrax. Currently, however, the best hope for the treatment of MDR/XDR anthrax is to find licensed or investigational antibiotics (or both) to which such an organism is susceptible. New anthrax vaccines are also still being tested.

SUGGESTED READINGS

Centers for Disease Control and Prevention. Conference Report on Public Health and Clinical Guidelines for Anthrax. www.cdc.gov/eid 2008 (April) vol. 14. No 4. *Multidisciplinary recommendations, including pleural fluid drainage and optimizing CNS antibiotic coverage, for updating the 2001 CDC guidelines.*

Chitlaru T, Altboum Z, Reuveny S, et al. Progress and novel strategies in vaccine development and treatment of anthrax. *Immunol Rev.* 2011;239:221-236. *Review including post-exposure anti-toxemic and anti-bacteremic treatment.*

Health Protection Scotland. Anthrax Outbreak Information. www.hps.scot.nhs.uk/anthrax. *Best source for detailed data and new guidelines for the ongoing 2010 anthrax outbreak in U.K. injection drug users.*

Infectious Diseases Society of America (IDSA). Anthrax: current, comprehensive information on pathogenesis, microbiology, epidemiology, diagnosis, treatment, and prophylaxis. Infectious Disease Society of America (IDSA) website: www.cidrap.umn.edu/idsa/bt/anthrax/biofacts/anthraxfactsheet.html. *Detailed and updated online source.*

303

ERYSIPELOTHRIX INFECTIONS

ANNETTE C. REBOLI

FIGURE 303-1. Erysipeloid with its characteristic purple, nonpurulent swelling of the finger. Also known as whale finger or pork finger, this form of cellulitis caused by *Erysipelothrix rhusiopathiae* should not be confused with streptococcal or staphylococcal erysipelas (see Fig. 449-4 in Chapter 449). (From Farrar WE, Wood MJ, Innes JUA, Tubbs H. *Infectious Diseases: Text and Color Atlas,* 2nd ed. New York: Gower Medical Publishing, 1992.)

DEFINITION

Erysipelothrix rhusiopathiae causes three well-defined patterns of human infection: (1) erysipeloid, a cellulitis of the fingers and hands (also known as whale finger or pork finger), which is the most common manifestation of infection with *E. rhusiopathiae;* (2) a diffuse cutaneous form; and (3) a bacteremic form, with or without cutaneous involvement, usually complicated by endocarditis.

The Pathogen

E. rhusiopathiae is a thin, pleomorphic, nonsporulating, microaerophilic gram-positive rod. It may be confused with other gram-positive bacillary organisms, particularly *Listeria monocytogenes* and *Corynebacterium* species. It can be differentiated from *L. monocytogenes* by its lack of motility, lack of catalase and coagulase production, and resistance to neomycin. Most strains of *E. rhusiopathiae* produce hydrogen sulfide on triple sugar iron agar slants, a feature that distinguishes *E. rhusiopathiae* from *L. monocytogenes* and from corynebacteria. Because α-hemolysis may be seen after 48 hours of incubation of *E. rhusiopathiae*, confusion with streptococci may also occur. The term *erysipeloid* refers to cutaneous infection by *E. rhusiopathiae* and should not be confused with erysipelas, which is a superficial cellulitis caused by streptococci or staphylococci.

EPIDEMIOLOGY

E. rhusiopathiae is found worldwide as a commensal or as a pathogen in a variety of wild and domestic animals, including swine, sheep, cattle, horses, dogs, rodents, chickens, ducks, turkeys, penguins, and parrots, as well as in flies, ticks, mites, and lice. The greatest commercial impact of *E. rhusiopathiae* infection is due to disease in swine, but infection of sheep and poultry is also important economically. Environmental surfaces in contact with infected animals or their products are potential sources of *E. rhusiopathiae*. It can persist for prolonged periods in contaminated soil. *E. rhusiopathiae* is killed within 15 minutes by heating to 55° C and by several commercially available home disinfectants.

The incidence of cutaneous infection in humans seems to be decreasing because of technologic advances in animal industries. It is usually the result of contact with infected animals or their products. Persons at greatest risk for infection include fishers, fishmongers, farmers, butchers, slaughterhouse workers, and veterinarians. The organism gains entry through cuts and abrasions on the skin. The seasonal incidence of erysipeloid parallels that of swine erysipeloid and is highest in the summer and early fall. The rare instances of systemic infection that do not have an occupational link tend to occur in immunocompromised hosts, suggesting that oropharyngeal or gastrointestinal colonization with the organism may occur. Chronic alcoholism has been acknowledged as a common underlying condition. Erysipeloid and erysipeloid with bacteremia have been reported rarely after cat and dog bites, suggesting that *E. rhusiopathiae* may be part of the oral flora of these animals.

PATHOBIOLOGY

The virulence of *E. rhusiopathiae* is associated, at least in part, with resistance to phagocytosis by polymorphonuclear leukocytes. This antiphagocytic ability results from the organism's possession of a capsule. In the absence of specific antibodies, *E. rhusiopathiae* evades phagocytosis, but even if phagocytized, it is able to replicate intracellularly in these cells. Other virulence factors include enzymes (neuraminidase and hyaluronidase) and surface proteins.

CLINICAL MANIFESTATIONS

Because of the mode of acquisition (contact with infected animals or their products, with organisms inoculating abrasions on the skin), lesions are usually confined to the fingers and hands (Fig. 303-1). A well-defined, slightly elevated, violaceous lesion accompanied by a very painful, throbbing, burning, or itching sensation develops within 2 to 7 days of traumatic dermal inoculation. The infected area is swollen. Vesicles may be present, but suppuration is absent. The lesion spreads slowly to other fingers but rarely involves the fingertips or the skin above the wrist. As the lesion spreads peripherally, the central area clears. Systemic signs and symptoms are rare. There may be sterile arthritis of an adjacent joint. Regional lymphadenopathy or lymphadenitis occurs in about 20% of cases, and low-grade fever develops in approximately 10%. Lesions usually resolve within 3 weeks without treatment. Relapse occurs in 1% of cases.

The diffuse cutaneous form is rare. The cutaneous lesion progresses proximally from the site of inoculation or appears at remote areas. Patients often have fever and arthralgias, but blood cultures are generally negative.

Systemic infection with *Erysipelothrix* is uncommon. Approximately 90 cases of bacteremia have been reported; most of the patients had endocarditis. Although cases of prosthetic valve endocarditis have been reported, most cases have involved native valves. In 60% of cases, infection developed on apparently normal heart valves. One third of patients had an antecedent or concurrent skin lesion of erysipeloid. The clinical manifestations of endocarditis secondary to *E. rhusiopathiae* and other microorganisms are similar. *E. rhusiopathiae* endocarditis correlates highly with occupation, exhibits a tropism for the aortic valve, affects more males than females, and is associated with high mortality. The latter may reflect a delay in appropriate therapy because of the empirical use of vancomycin, which is not an effective treatment of *E. rhusiopathiae*. Cases of *E. rhusiopathiae* endocarditis have been complicated by paravalvular and myocardial abscess formation, cerebral emboli, congestive heart failure, valve perforation, and acute renal failure. *E. rhusiopathiae* bacteremia without endocarditis occurs more frequently than was previously believed. Bacteremia is occurring with increased frequency in immunocompromised patients, whereas endocarditis usually occurs in immunocompetent patients. Focal infections, including brain abscess, meningitis, endophthalmitis, osteomyelitis, septic arthritis, liver abscess, necrotizing fasciitis, intra-abdominal abscess, and peritonitis, have been reported. Some of these infections were complications of bacteremia. Septic arthritis has occurred in native joints, in prosthetic joints, and after arthroscopic surgery. Peritonitis has complicated peritoneal dialysis.

DIAGNOSIS

E. rhusiopathiae grows on routine laboratory media. Because *E. rhusiopathiae* is located only in deeper parts of the skin in cases of erysipeloid, biopsy of the entire thickness of the dermis from the edge of the lesion yields maximal recovery of the organism. Routine blood culture techniques are adequate for growth and isolation of the organism in suspected cases of bacteremia or endocarditis. Various selective media have been used to improve the isolation of *E. rhusiopathiae* from contaminated specimens. Molecular techniques such as polymerase chain reaction with primers specific for *E. rhusiopathiae* have been developed and improve the efficiency of detection and identification.

Most isolates of *E. rhusiopathiae* are susceptible to penicillin, cephalosporins, imipenem, clindamycin, ciprofloxacin, ofloxacin, and daptomycin. Some resistance has been observed with erythromycin, tetracycline, and chloramphenicol. *E. rhusiopathiae* is resistant to vancomycin, aminoglycosides, trimethoprim-sulfamethoxazole, and sulfonamides. Penicillin G is the treatment of choice. Uncomplicated cutaneous lesions generally respond well to a 5- to 7-day course of oral penicillin. Treatment hastens healing, although relapse may still occur. Bacteremia should be treated with intravenous penicillin; cases of endocarditis should be treated with 12 million to 20 million units of penicillin G daily or ceftriaxone 1 g daily for 4 to 6 weeks. Two weeks of intravenous therapy followed by 2 weeks of oral therapy has been successful. The use of quinolones or daptomycin may be considered for *Erysipelothrix* infections when the patient is allergic to β-lactams. Oral linezolid was used to complete therapy in a case of bacteremia complicated by endophthalmitis. Valve replacement may be necessary in patients with endocarditis.

PREVENTION

Proper cleaning and disinfection of work surfaces and attention to hygienic work practices, including the use of gloves and hand hygiene, reduce the risk for infection. Vaccines are available for commercial use in animals only.

SUGGESTED READINGS

Nassar IM, de la Llana R, Garrido P, et al. Mitral-aortic infective endocarditis produced by *Erysipelothrix rhusiopathiae*: case report and review of the literature. *J Heart Valve Dis.* 2005;14:320-324. *Review of clinical features of endocarditis.*

Pal N, Bender JS, Opriessnig T. Rapid detection and differentiation of *Erysipelothrix* spp. by a novel multiplex real-time PCR assay. *J Appl Microbiol.* 2010;108:1083-1093. *The assay is simple, rapid, reliable, specific, and highly sensitive.*

Shimoji Y. Pathogenicity of *Erysipelothrix rhusiopathiae*: virulence factors and protective immunity. *Microbes Infect.* 2000;2:965-972. *Recent advances in our understanding of pathogenicity and protective immunity are discussed.*

Veraldi S, Girgenti V, Dassoni F, et al. Erysipeloid: a review. *Clin Exp Dermatol.* 2009;34:859-862. *Review of clinical manifestations, with an emphasis on skin lesions.*

Wang Q, Chang BJ, Riley TV. *Erysipelothrix rhusiopathiae.* *Vet Microbiol.* 2010;140:405-417. *Comprehensive review, including nomenclature, epidemiology, clinical manifestations in animals and humans, diagnosis, and treatment.*

304

CLOSTRIDIAL INFECTIONS

DALE N. GERDING AND STUART JOHNSON

Clostridial infections are characterized by disease produced by toxins. They include tetanus and botulism, both caused by neurotoxins, and clostridial myonecrosis or gas gangrene, caused by the toxins of *Clostridium perfringens* as well as those of other clostridial species. Although these clostridial infections remain important clinically, their frequency has declined markedly with the advent of vaccines and better public health measures. Several previously little known species of clostridia that produce very large clostridial cytotoxins (LCCs) that vary in size from 250 to 308 kD have become increasingly prominent. They include, in particular, *Clostridium difficile,* which is responsible for one of the most common health care–associated infections and for increasing mortality among elderly patients. Another LCC-producing organism, *Clostridium sordellii,* has caused devastating infections in young women in association with pregnancy and medical abortion, in injection drug users, and in patients with traumatic wounds. *Clostridium novyi* type A is a third LCC organism that has also caused severe infections in injection drug users.

⬤ *CLOSTRIDIUM DIFFICILE* INFECTION

DEFINITION AND PATHOGEN

C. difficile infection (CDI) is a gastrointestinal infection characterized by diarrhea (three or more loose or unformed stools in ≤24 hours) and a positive test for *C. difficile* toxin A or toxin B in stool, evidence of a toxin-producing strain of *C. difficile* in stool, or evidence of pseudomembranous colitis on direct visualization of the colon. *C. difficile* is a spore-forming, anaerobic, gram-positive organism that survives well in water, soil, and animals and has a worldwide distribution.

EPIDEMIOLOGY

CDI occurs most frequently in health care settings, particularly in long-term care facilities and acute care hospitals, and is most frequent and lethal among the elderly, especially those older than 75 years. Rates in U.S. hospitals have nearly tripled in the decade since 2000, and it is now estimated that there are 500,000 to 750,000 CDIs each year. A specific strain of *C. difficile*—identified as the restriction endonuclease group BI, pulse field gel type NAP1, PCR ribotype 027 (BI/NAP1/027) strain—is thought to be responsible for much of the epidemic that has extended to Canada and Europe. Rates of CDI in the community have also increased somewhat during the past decade, in association with the rising rates in hospitals and nursing homes. However, it is unlikely that community cases account for more than 15 to 20% of all CDIs. Risk factors for CDI include antimicrobial use, advanced age, and stay in an acute or chronic care facility. Hospitals are considered a particularly high-risk environment because patients are elderly, antimicrobial use is frequent, the environment is contaminated with *C. difficile* spores (which are difficult to eradicate), asymptomatic patients carry *C. difficile* in their stools, and health care workers carry *C. difficile* on their hands if they do not practice good hand hygiene. In about 2 to 3% of healthy adults, *C. difficile* can be cultured from their stools, but the frequency in asymptomatic hospitalized patients increases with the duration of hospitalization and may reach 20% or more. Exposure to nearly all antimicrobials has been associated with subsequent CDI, but those with the highest risk are clindamycin, the cephalosporins, and the fluoroquinolones. CDI is rare in children and young adults, despite their frequent exposure to antimicrobials. However, children younger than 1 year are commonly colonized with *C. difficile* but remain asymptomatic, an observation that remains largely unexplained.

PATHOBIOLOGY

CDI risk appears to be minimal in the absence of antimicrobial therapy. When antimicrobials are administered, they have the unintended consequence of disrupting the normal protective bowel flora, which may persist for days to weeks after the antimicrobial is stopped. If *C. difficile* is ingested during this time, the spores germinate in the gut, and the vegetative form of the organism multiplies and begins to make toxins. At this point, whether the patient will develop diarrhea is dictated by the status of his or her immunity to the toxins, which is best correlated with serum immunoglobulin G (IgG) antibodies directed at toxin A and toxin B of *C. difficile.* Those with good antibody responses will be asymptomatic but will remain colonized with *C. difficile,* whereas those with little or no antibody response will develop diarrhea and CDI. Toxin A is primarily an enterotoxin, and toxin B is a cytotoxin. Both act by glucosylation that disrupts the cell cytoskeleton, resulting in colonic epithelial cell rounding, fluid leakage, and cell death. In the presence of pseudomembranous colitis, the colon appears to be covered in yellow to white pseudomembranes that vary in size from punctate to completely confluent and covering the entire colon in advanced cases. Histologically, the colon demonstrates a marked neutrophil infiltration throughout the colon wall, with mucosal necrosis and volcano-like lesions from which the pseudomembrane is seen to "erupt." The pseudomembrane is composed of proteinaceous material and cellular debris.

CLINICAL MANIFESTATIONS

Clinical symptoms of CDI range from asymptomatic carriage to severe and sometimes life-threatening pseudomembranous colitis complicated by major fluid losses and systemic complications. With mild CDI, patients may simply have "nuisance diarrhea" that resolves when the implicated drug is discontinued. Others with more severe CDI have substantial fluid and protein losses combined with fever, cramps, hypoalbuminemia, leukocytosis, and hypotension. Leukocytosis is common (occurring in up to 50% of patients) and is a marker of severe CDI when it exceeds 15,000/mm³. Extremely high levels greater than 50,000/mm³ are an indication of fulminant and potentially fatal illness. Other factors that may be indicative of severe or late-stage disease include toxic megacolon, high fever, renal failure, hypotension, and a lactic acidosis greater than 5.0 mmol/L.

DIAGNOSIS

The diagnosis should be suspected in any patient who has otherwise unexplained diarrhea (three or more loose or unformed stools in ≤24 hours) in association with recent or concurrent antibiotic use. Only about 10 to 20% of patients in this category actually have CDI, but this is the patient group that should be tested. The standard test to establish the diagnosis is to detect toxins A and B in stool or to detect a toxin-producing strain of *C. difficile* in stool. Tests that detect only toxin A are not acceptable because about 1 to 3% of strains that cause CDI produce toxin B but not toxin A. The most common laboratory method is an enzyme immunoassay (EIA), but its sensitivity is only 50 to 80%. Repeat testing does not improve the diagnostic accuracy because EIAs also have specificity deficiencies that increase the rate of false-positive test results with repeated testing. A number of polymerase chain reaction (PCR) tests for *C. difficile* are available commercially and markedly improve test sensitivity to 90 to 95% (compared with the "gold standard" of culture for a toxigenic strain). The PCR tests are more expensive, but when they become more widely used, they should increase the sensitivity and specificity of diagnosis and eliminate the common practice of ordering *C. difficile* tests "times 3," which has no justification. When a negative test result does not confirm the diagnosis in a patient whose clinical symptoms are highly suggestive of CDI, empirical treatment for CDI should be given rather than repeating the test. The standard cell cytotoxin assay is more sensitive than EIA but has the disadvantages of a 24- to 48-hour turnaround and the requirement for tissue culture facilities, which may not be available in clinical laboratories. Stool culture for *C. difficile*, which is the most sensitive test available, is likewise slow and requires confirmation of toxin production by the organism before reporting. Testing stools for glutamate dehydrogenase, or "common antigen," can be used as a screening test, but it is only about 50% specific and requires confirmation with a toxin test, which increases the turnaround time for reporting positive results. CDI can also be diagnosed by observing pseudomembranous colitis directly via sigmoidoscopy or colonoscopy or at surgery. The cause of diarrhea in an adult patient with an onset longer than 48 hours after hospital admission is almost always CDI because other infectious enteric pathogens are extremely rare in the hospital setting. Also common in the differential diagnosis are noninfectious causes of diarrhea, such as antibiotic or other drug-associated diarrhea, ischemic colitis, and idiopathic inflammatory bowel disease. For patients with antibiotic-associated diarrhea and no evidence of colitis, the cause of diarrhea with a negative *C. difficile* toxin assay is usually not defined.

PREVENTION

Two major prevention strategies are employed. The first is traditional infection control in which barriers to transmission (gowns, gloves, isolation, hand hygiene, environmental cleaning) are used to prevent the spores of *C. difficile* from reaching the patient. The second strategy is to reduce the likelihood of infection if the patient does encounter *C. difficile* while in the hospital. The most efficacious strategy, also known as antimicrobial stewardship, is to avoid or minimize exposure to antimicrobials, especially those with a high CDI risk such as clindamycin, cephalosporins, and fluoroquinolones. Interventions to restrict exposure to clindamycin and to cephalosporins have been highly effective in interrupting outbreaks of CDI in hospitals.

TREATMENT   Rx

Treatment of CDI begins with discontinuation of the implicated antibiotic, supportive care, and avoidance of antiperistaltic agents. Mildly ill patients may recover with these simple conservative measures, but most require specific treatment. Continuation of the offending antibiotics while treating CDI with vancomycin and other agents results in lower cure rates and higher CDI recurrence rates in patients. Metronidazole, at a dose of 500 mg orally three times a day for 10 to 14 days, is the recommended treatment for patients with mild CDI. It provides response rates comparable to those for vancomycin, is much less expensive, and avoids some of the concern about vancomycin-resistant enterococcus colonization.**[1,2]** Patients with severe CDI (variously defined as a white blood cell count >15,000 or a creatinine increase to >1.5-fold over baseline) should be treated with vancomycin 125 mg orally four times a day for 10 days.**[1,2]** Vancomycin can be substituted for metronidazole if there is a delayed response in patients with mild illness. A newer option is fidaxomicin (200 mg orally twice daily), which is as efficacious as vancomycin.**[3]** The anticipated response to these drugs is rapid defervescence, with gradual normalization of bowel habits. Mean time to resolution of diarrhea is about 3 days; if symptoms have not resolved by day 5 or 6 of treatment, a change in therapy should be considered. However, there are no data to support the use of more than one drug at a time to treat CDI. Failure to respond often means that either the disease has progressed too far or another condition is causing the symptoms. For patients with severe complicated or fulminant CDI, medical management includes vancomycin at a higher dose (500 mg four times a day) orally or by nasogastric tube; if ileus is present, metronidazole (500 mg IV every 8 hours) is added, with vancomycin administered by enema. If symptoms progress with this therapy, colectomy may be life-saving and should be performed before the white blood cell count reaches 50,000/mm³ or lactate reaches 5.0 mmol/L.

Other antibiotic options include oral fusidic acid, teicoplanin, nitazoxanide, rifaximin, and bacitracin, but most of these drugs have been evaluated in only a small number of patients, and none (like metronidazole) has Food and Drug Administration approval for the treatment of CDI. There is no convincing evidence that toxin-binding agents such as cholestyramine or probiotics such as lactobacillus are useful in preventing or treating CDI. About 20% of patients treated with either vancomycin or metronidazole have a recurrence of symptoms when treatment is stopped because of the persistence of *C. difficile* spores or acquisition of a new strain. Treatment is readministration of either vancomycin or metronidazole, depending on the severity of the recurrence. Patients with multiple recurrences of CDI are extremely difficult to treat and may benefit from consultation with an infectious disease specialist or gastroenterologist.

PROGNOSIS

The majority ($\approx$70%) of patients respond to simple withdrawal of the implicated antibiotic combined with a single course of metronidazole or vancomycin. Some patients with fulminant disease eventually require colectomy. The attributable mortality rate is as high as 7% in large series, and the majority of lethal cases occur in patients older than 65 years. Patients with multiple recurrences require repeated courses of antibiotics, usually vancomycin with tapering and pulse-dose regimens that may need to be continued for weeks to months.

NECROTIZING CLOSTRIDIAL TISSUE INFECTION
Clostridium sordellii

DEFINITION AND PATHOGEN

C. sordellii is another clostridial species that produces LCCs, and it has become more common as a cause of septic shock and necrotizing fasciitis in association with trauma, childbirth, medical abortion, and injection drug use. *C. sordellii* antitoxin cross-neutralizes the cytotoxic effect of *C. difficile* toxins, indicating the similarity of these LCCs.

EPIDEMIOLOGY

The organism is commonly found in soil and in the intestines of animals and occasionally humans worldwide. Soil contamination of wounds is the usual suspected route of infection. Infections have been described following traumatic wounds, childbirth, medical abortion, and intramuscular or subcutaneous injection drug use.

PATHOBIOLOGY

C. sordellii produces up to seven identified toxins; of these, lethal toxin and hemorrhagic toxin, which are both LCCs, are considered major virulence factors. The toxins produce local necrosis, progressive edema, and shock that results in high mortality. The toxins are glycosyltransferases that glycosylate the Rho, Rac, or Ras proteins, causing impaired cytoskeletal organization and massive capillary leakage, leading to the progressive edematous state.

CLINICAL MANIFESTATIONS

Initial symptoms are nonspecific and include nausea, lethargy, dizziness, and tenderness at the infection site. Tachycardia and hypotension follow within hours. Laboratory tests show a marked leukocytosis or leukemoid reaction. Hypotension and tachycardia are refractory to treatment. Edema secondary to capillary leakage is prominent, resulting in hemoconcentration but little or no fever. Peritoneal and pleural effusions are common. White blood cell elevations greater than 75,000/mm³ are associated with a fatal outcome.

INFECTION ASSOCIATED WITH CHILDBIRTH AND MEDICAL ABORTION. This is a rare infection in which patients present 4 to 7 days following the administration of oral mifepristone and vaginal misoprostol for medical abortion with nausea, vomiting, weakness, abdominal pain, hypotension, and tachycardia but little or no fever and, often remarkably, a lack of findings on pelvic examination. The presentation is similar to toxic shock syndrome. There is rapid progression to vascular collapse and cardiac arrest. Leukocytosis is dramatic, with white blood cell counts near 100,000/mm³ in most patients. Following delivery, the presentation is similar, but localized swelling and discoloration of the labia and perineum may be evident if the episiotomy site is infected. All patients to date have died.

INFECTION ASSOCIATED WITH INJECTION DRUG USE. Black tar heroin (a dark, gummy, less refined and cheaper form of heroin) has been associated with necrotizing fasciitis at the subcutaneous or intramuscular injection site, presumably a result of the contaminants mixed with the heroin. Patients present with 2 to 7 days of symptoms of necrotizing fasciitis of the upper or lower extremity where they injected heroin, in some cases accompanied by hypotension. Aggressive surgical débridement is required at the infection site, together with fluids and pressors. Cultures of débrided tissue reveal multiple organisms in addition to *C. sordellii*. Mortality in these patients is 50%.

DIAGNOSIS

Diagnosis is difficult due to the lack of specific symptoms, but it is usually made by identifying the likely source of infection and isolating *C. sordellii* from the infection site or blood cultures. PCR for *C. sordellii* in infected tissues may be required to make the diagnosis when cultures are negative. Other bacteria are also commonly found at the infection site. Computed tomography or magnetic resonance imaging may be helpful in identifying localized infections, which can then be excised or drained surgically, providing material for microbiologic diagnosis.

PREVENTION

C. sordellii infections are very rare, and the exact mechanism of infection, especially following medical abortion, is not known. However, careful attention to wound cleansing, avoidance of injecting drugs into skin or muscle, and good hygiene during childbirth are likely to help prevent *C. sordellii* infection.

TREATMENT Rx

Definitive treatment information is lacking. The infection progresses so rapidly that therapeutic interventions are rarely successful. Surgery to remove necrotic sites of infection and administration of intravenous fluids and pressors to treat hypotension and tachycardia are supportive. Antibiotic susceptibility suggests that β-lactams, clindamycin, tetracyclines, and chloramphenicol are active, but no clinical treatment efficacy data are available. Theoretically, use of an antibiotic such as clindamycin to suppress toxin synthesis could be a useful adjunct to treatment. At present, there is no antitoxin available.

PROGNOSIS

Infections following childbirth or medical abortion have been uniformly fatal. Mortality in injection drug users or patients following trauma or surgery is about 50%.

Clostridium novyi Infection in Injecting Drug Users

C. novyi α-toxin causes an LCC-producing disease in humans. *C. novyi* has long been recognized as a cause of fatal toxemia in animals with contaminated wounds. An extended outbreak of human infections occurred in Scotland, Ireland, and elsewhere in the United Kingdom in 2000 among persons injecting heroin extravascularly (skin or muscle popping). A localized necrotizing infection with sepsis and significant mortality was recognized. The findings include soft tissue inflammation, edema and necrosis at the injection sites, circulatory collapse, leukocytosis, and pleural effusions. Treatment usually involves débridement and antibiotic administration (gentamicin, flucloxacillin, penicillin, metronidazole, and clindamycin were used during this outbreak).

Clostridial Myonecrosis

DEFINITION

Clostridial myonecrosis, or gas gangrene, can be caused by several *Clostridium* species, most commonly *C. perfringens* following trauma or tissue injury and *Clostridium septicum* following dissemination from a colonic source.

EPIDEMIOLOGY

Gas gangrene has historically been a complication of battlefield injuries and of trauma in noncombat settings. The estimated number of cases in the United States is about 1000 per year. Traumatic injuries account for about 50% of cases, with vehicular accidents accounting for the majority; the remaining cases develop in patients after crush injuries, industrial accidents, gunshot wounds, and burns. Minor injuries such as puncture wounds, intramuscular injections, simple lacerations, and subcutaneous injections with epinephrine may occasionally precipitate clostridial myonecrosis. Postoperative complications account for about 30% of cases and are most frequently associated with surgery on the appendix, biliary tract, or intestine. Approximately 20% are "spontaneous" or nontraumatic and are invariably associated with an occult colonic malignancy.

PATHOBIOLOGY

Clostridia are widely distributed in nature and can be cultured from nearly all soil samples, from environmental sites in the hospital, and from the human intestine. A critical factor is a physiologic state of the wound with conditions that support germination and toxin production by toxigenic clostridia. Particularly critical are a low oxidation-reduction potential, hypoxia, appropriate substrates, and calcium ions. The probability of infection is substantially increased by devitalized muscle and the presence of foreign material such as dirt. *C. perfringens* elaborates at least 12 recognized toxins, most importantly α-toxin and θ-toxin of *C. perfringens* type A. Although the interaction is complex, good evidence supports a central role for α-toxin, a phospholipase C, and θ-toxin or perfringolysin O, a cholesterol-dependent cytolysin, in the extensive cell death and disruption of microvascular perfusion that are characteristic of clostridial myonecrosis. The vascular perfusion changes are likely mediated by toxin-induced platelet aggregation and leukocyte margination. The α-toxin of *C. septicum*, a spore-forming cytolysin unrelated to α-toxin of *C. perfringens*, also causes cell death and microvascular perfusion changes.

CLINICAL MANIFESTATIONS

Initial symptoms of traumatic myonecrosis usually occur 1 to 4 days after the precipitating event, although the range is 8 hours to 3 weeks. The initial symptom is pain that is often sudden and severe at the site of surgery or trauma. The involved skin has intense edema and is initially pale before progressing to a bronze or magenta color, followed by the formation of bullae. The bullae contain fluid that may be clear or hemorrhagic. The discharge has an odor that is described as "foul-sweet."

Circulatory collapse and hypotension unresponsive to fluid challenge are common and may reflect the effect of α-toxin, which suppresses cardiac contractility. About 15% of patients have bacteremia that is usually complicated by rapid hemolysis with a dramatic drop in the hematocrit, which may even decrease to 0%. Common complications include jaundice, hypotension, hepatic failure, and renal failure. The renal failure is often due to hemoglobulinuria and myoglobulinuria, but it may also be due to acute tubular necrosis from hypotension. Despite the severity of the illness, the patient's mental status is usually remarkably good until very late in the disease. Surgical intervention shows necrotic muscle that does not contract with stimulation. Deeper dissection reveals beefy red necrotic muscle that becomes black and extremely friable in the late stages.

Uterine gas gangrene, which was once common after septic abortions, is now rare but may complicate normal delivery, amniocentesis, cesarean section, or abortion. The onset is usually sudden, with fever, tachycardia, hypotension, renal failure, and jaundice. Radiography may show gas in the uterine wall. The urine is often "port wine" in color as a result of hemoglobulinuria, and there is often jaundice because of massive intravascular hemolysis. The usual causes are *C. perfringens* and *C. sordellii*.

Spontaneous myonecrosis occurs in the absence of trauma and is usually caused by *C. septicum*. One distinctive association is colon cancer or neutropenic enterocolitis, which represent portals of entry for hematogenous seeding of *C. septicum*. This infection is also seen with acute leukemia and is most common with chemotherapy for solid tumors and after stem cell transplantation. The usual portals of entry are the terminal ileum, cecum, and ascending colon, hence the term *typhlitis*. The usual manifestation is a necrotizing infection in an extremity or in the abdominal wall, accompanied by hypotension and renal failure. Examination shows spreading crepitations with rapid clinical deterioration over a period of hours, and imaging reveals gas.

DIAGNOSIS

The diagnosis of gas gangrene is usually based on a constellation of characteristic clinical features, including myonecrosis, shock, and renal failure. The patient typically complains of very severe pain. Early recognition is important, because early institution of treatment may strongly influence the prognosis. The diagnosis is established by examination of the muscle, which shows putrid discharge, characteristic bullae, and crepitations. Gram stain demonstrates abundant gram-positive bacilli and no inflammatory cells. Histopathologic examination of the lesion shows myonecrosis without polymorphonuclear leukocytes, a finding that is remarkably different from most soft tissue infections, which do not feature necrosis and have abundant inflammatory cells. Gas is present in the tissue and may be detected by physical examination, radiography, or other imaging methods.

PREVENTION

The basic principle of prevention is adequate management of traumatic wounds—establishing adequate drainage, removing foreign bodies, draining hematomas, and ensuring good hemostasis.

TREATMENT — Rx

The most important facet of treatment is prompt surgical débridement. Many cases require extensive, often mutilating surgery. Penicillin and clindamycin are recommended but are rarely adequate without radical surgery, except in patients with neutropenic enterocolitis, who can often be managed with antibiotics. The rationale for penicillin combined with clindamycin is that some strains of clostridia are resistant to clindamycin, but clindamycin is probably the superior drug for reducing toxin formation. Other antibiotics that are generally effective include metronidazole and chloramphenicol. The use of hyperbaric oxygen is controversial, in part because the therapeutic trials have been either of poor quality or not convincing.

PROGNOSIS

Factors associated with a poor prognosis include elderly age, location on the trunk, association with severe underlying disease, leukopenia, renal failure, hemolysis, and shock. The best results are seen in young patients with involvement of a single extremity. Management plays an important role, particularly the use of early and aggressive surgery, as well as antibiotics. The overall mortality rate of patients with traumatic gas gangrene in tertiary centers is about 25%.

NEUROTOXIC CLOSTRIDIAL INFECTIONS
Botulism
DEFINITION

Botulism is a severe neuroparalytic disease characterized by a descending flaccid motor neuron paralysis. It is caused by botulinum toxin produced by *Clostridium botulinum.*

The Pathogen

C. botulinum is a gram-positive, spore-forming obligate anaerobe that is widely distributed in nature and is frequently found in soil, marine environments, and agricultural products. Each strain produces one of seven toxins designated by the letters A to G. Botulinum toxin may also be produced by related clostridial species, *Clostridium baratii* and *Clostridium butyricum.* All these neurotoxins produce the same syndrome, and the causes of disease in humans are types A, B, and E, with rare cases caused by type F.

EPIDEMIOLOGY

Botulism in humans is generally one of three types: food-borne botulism, infant botulism, or wound botulism. Rarely, botulism may be acquired as a result of iatrogenic misadventures with botulinum toxin, which is a potential bioterrorism agent if inhaled or ingested.

Food-borne botulism is the most common form of botulism in the world, but it is a distant second to infant botulism in the United States, with only 19 food-borne cases occurring in the United States in 2006. Foods most frequently implicated are home canned vegetables or fermented foods, and most cases are sporadic single cases occasionally involving two or three people. Commercially preserved and restaurant-prepared foods are also rare causes of food-borne botulism. Type A toxin is predominant in the United States. Alaska has the highest rate of any state, with approximately 35% of all cases; 80 to 90% of events and cases in Alaska are caused by type E and are most often associated with fermentation methods used to prepare fish and marine mammals by native Alaskans. Meat and meat products are frequently implicated in Europe, where the predominant toxin is type B. In China, the most frequent vehicle is a vegetable product, and type A predominates.

Infant botulism is the most frequently recognized form in the United States and is the most recently discovered type of botulism, first described in 1976. It is caused by production of botulinum toxin in the intestine after presumed spore ingestion and colonization in 2- to 36-week-old infants. Honey has been identified as the source of *C. botulinum* spores, but in most cases the source is never identified. Nearly all cases are caused by type A or B toxin. The symptoms usually begin with constipation followed by poor feeding, weak cry, lethargy, and generalized weakness characterized as the "floppy baby syndrome" due to loss of head control. This form of botulism is rare in adults, occurring most often in patients with anatomic or functional abnormalities of the intestines.

Wound botulism, first described in 1943, is the least frequent form of the disease and is usually caused by either type A or B toxin. Sporadic cases in traumatic wounds contaminated by soil are rarely reported. Outbreaks have been described in black tar heroin users in the western United States, particularly if they inject the drug intramuscularly or subcutaneously (skin popping). These drug users also develop other clostridial infections, including necrotizing fasciitis caused by *C. sordellii* and *C. novyi,* and tetanus caused by *Clostridium tetani.*

Inhalation or ingestion of botulinum toxin is considered one of the top six bioweapon agents in terms of probability of use. The presumed method would be contamination of the food supply, water supply, or commercial beverages or aerosolization in a highly populated area to cause inhalational botulism. It is estimated that a point-source aerosol release of the toxin could incapacitate or kill 10% of people within a 0.5-km radius.

Iatrogenic botulism results from the misuse of botulinum toxin for cosmetic or therapeutic purposes. Cosmetic treatment doses are far too low to cause systemic disease, but the use of unlicensed products with high concentrations of botulinum toxin can cause systemic symptoms. Higher doses used for the management of muscle movement disorders have caused occasional cases with systemic botulism-like symptoms.

PATHOBIOLOGY

Pathologic findings are due to absorption of toxins from the intestine (ingested preformed toxin in foods or in situ production in the intestine in infants), inhalation (aerosol from bioterrorism), absorption from cutaneous infection sources (wounds), or iatrogenic injection. The toxin is disseminated by the systemic circulation and causes flaccid paralysis by binding presynaptic motor neuron terminals and blocking acetylcholine transmission across the neuromuscular junction. The estimated lethal doses of purified botulinum toxin A for a 70-kg human are 0.09 to 0.15 μg when given intravenously, 0.8 to 0.9 μg when inhaled, and 70 μg when given orally.

CLINICAL MANIFESTATIONS

In contrast to Guillain-Barré syndrome (Chapter 428), which is an ascending paralysis, botulism is characterized by generalized weakness and a descending paralysis. Symptoms are due to absorption of botulinum toxin from the gut, lung, or a wound. Clinical symptoms consist of highly distinctive and usually symmetrical cranial nerve palsies, followed by a symmetrical descending flaccid paralysis. Prominently involved cranial nerves III, IV, and VI cause blurred vision and diplopia; involvement of cranial nerve VII causes the characteristic expressionless facies and dysphagia; and involvement of cranial nerve IX causes dysarthria. Thus, the initial symptoms include the "four Ds"—diplopia, dysarthria, dysphagia, and dysphonia—although the last is rarely reported, and blurred vision is reported more commonly than diplopia. These findings are followed by a descending upper extremity paralysis and respiratory paralysis. Neurologic examination shows bilateral cranial nerve VI paresis, ptosis, dilated pupils with a sluggish reaction, and diminished gag reflex, followed by descending involvement of motor neurons. Deep tendon reflexes are diminished or absent. Mentation remains clear, vital signs are normal, and the neurologic findings are symmetrical. The most common cause of death is respiratory failure. The tempo of the disease and the extent of paralysis in the absence of treatment are highly variable. The symptoms may be restricted to a few cranial nerves, or there may be complete paralysis of all voluntary muscles. Progression may occur over a period of hours or days. The timing and extent of neurologic deficits depend on the size of the botulinum toxin inoculum.

DIAGNOSIS

Botulism should be suspected in patients with an acute flaccid paralysis involving the cranial nerves, particularly in the presence of bilateral cranial nerve VI dysfunction, associated neurologic findings, and a 10-hour to 5-day history of consuming suspect food, such as preserved or home-canned foods. Nausea, vomiting, abdominal pain, and diarrhea are common early in the illness, with constipation present when paralysis develops. The finding of two or more cases that are epidemiologically linked is virtually diagnostic of food-borne botulism because other causes of paralysis are rare and sporadic. In the absence of a history of suspect food ingestion, potentially infected wounds should be sought, including injection sites in users of black tar heroin. With bioterrorism, the epidemiology may reflect a common source exposure, such as a local water supply or an aerosolized toxin, but it could also be widely distributed with a contaminated food source, such as the milk supply.

Laboratory tests for suspected food-borne botulism include analysis of serum, stool, gastric contents, or food for botulinum toxin and culture of stool and suspect food or wounds for *C. botulinum*. Toxin assay specimens should be collected before treatment with antitoxin. With wound botulism, recovery of *C. botulinum* from wound cultures or detection of toxin in serum is diagnostic. The toxin assays are generally available only at public health laboratories. The standard is a mouse bioassay for detection and quantifica-tion of toxin. Toxin type is determined by type-specific antibody neutraliza-tion. In general, adult patients with clinical evidence of botulism have detectable toxin in sera in a third of cases and detectable toxin in stool in a third of cases, but the organism is recovered from stool in about 60%.

The differential diagnosis includes myasthenia gravis, Guillain-Barré syn-drome, tick paralysis, cerebrovascular accident, trichinosis, Eaton-Lambert syndrome, hypocalcemia, hypermagnesemia, organophosphate poisoning, atropine poisoning, and paralytic poisoning by shellfish or puffer fish. Elec-tromyography using repetitive stimulation at 2 to 50/second may be helpful in distinguishing causes of flaccid paralysis. Electromyography patterns with slow and rapid supramaximal stimulation show similar responses in botulism and Eaton-Lambert syndrome. Cerebrospinal fluid analysis and cranial imaging are normal in botulism.

PREVENTION

The disease can be prevented by destroying spores in the original food source, inhibiting germination, or destroying preformed toxin, as detailed in the online version of this chapter.

TREATMENT   Rx

Clinicians who suspect botulism should immediately seek clinical consulta-tion, notify public health authorities, and administer antitoxin. The agency to contact in the United States is the state health department or the Centers for Disease Control and Prevention (24-hour emergency service at 404-329-2888); similar public health agencies should be contacted in other coun-tries. Treatment consists of supportive care and passive neutralization with equine botulinum antitoxin.

The standard treatment of adults is trivalent antitoxin if the toxin type is not known or type-specific antitoxin for types A, B, or E; the standard dose is one vial (5500 to 8500 IU) diluted 1:10 in saline and delivered by slow intravenous infusion. An experimental heptavalent vaccine (A to G) from the U.S. Army may be available for unusual types associated with bioterrorism. The antitoxin should be given as early as possible and should not be delayed while awaiting microbiologic results. This treatment does not reverse paralysis or neutralize toxin already bound to nerve endings, but it does neutralize unbound toxin in the circulation to prevent progression. The antitoxin is horse serum, which is associated with anaphylaxis in 2% and other hypersensitivity reactions in 9% of patients when larger doses are used; patients should be given small doses to screen for reaction before receiving the full dose.

Respiratory failure is a major risk, and patients must be monitored carefully with liberal criteria for ventilatory support. The requirement for mechanical ventilation varies from about 20% in adults with food-borne disease to 60% in patients with infant botulism. Other forms of supportive care include enteral or parenteral feeding and positioning in the reverse Trendelenburg position.

Toxin can be removed from the gastrointestinal tract by gastric lavage, cathartics, and enemas early in the course. Antibiotic treatment is unnecessary, except for wound botulism.

PROGNOSIS

The case-fatality rate for untreated food-borne botulism was once 60 to 70% but is currently 3 to 5% with treatment. Infant botulism in the United States now has a mortality rate of less than 1%; the use of human antitoxin has reduced the median duration of hospitalization from 6 to 3 weeks. Patients who survive any form of botulism generally have a complete recovery.

Tetanus

DEFINITION

Tetanus is a neurologic syndrome characterized by generalized rigidity and convulsive spasm of skeletal muscles caused by a neurotoxin elaborated at the site of injury by *C. tetani*.

The Pathogen

C. tetani is an anaerobic, gram-positive, slender, motile bacillus. When it sporulates, the terminal spore gives the organism a characteristic "drumstick" or "tennis racket" shape. The vegetative form produces tetanospasmin, a protein neurotoxin with a molecular weight of approximately 151 kD, includ-ing a heavy chain (100 kD) that binds neuronal cells and a light chain that blocks the release of neurotransmitters.

EPIDEMIOLOGY

C. tetani can be found in 2 to 23% of soil samples, with the highest yield in manure-treated soil. The organism can also be found in stool from a variety of domestic and farm animals and poultry. Tetanus is most common in warm climates and in highly cultivated rural areas. The greatest problem occurs in resource-limited countries because of high numbers of unimmunized mothers and unhygienic practices. The estimated annual toll from neonatal tetanus in developing countries is greater than 257,000, mostly secondary to inadequate passive immunity caused by absence of immunity in the mother. In the United States, an average of 31 cases of tetanus are reported annually, and almost all occur in unimmunized or inadequately immunized persons. The age of these patients is near 60 years in 58% and younger than 20 years in 6%; this age distribution reflects the impact of waning immunity with aging.

PATHOBIOLOGY

Tetanospasmin ranks with botulinum toxin as one of the most potent known microbial toxins; 2.5 ng/kg is a lethal human dose. Clinical tetanus usually results from entry of the organism into a wound and low oxygen conditions that allow spore germination and survival of the vegetative organism to produce toxin. Entry is usually through a traumatic or surgical wound, injec-tion site, burn, skin ulcer, or infected umbilical cord. Tetanospasmin binds the peripheral nerve terminals and is then carried intra-axonally within mem-brane-bound vesicles to spinal neurons at a transport rate of approximately 75 to 250 mm/day. The light chain passes to the presynaptic terminals, where it blocks the release of neurotransmitters in inhibitory afferent motor neurons. Loss of the inhibitory influence results in sustained muscular contraction. Binding of the toxin is irreversible, so recovery requires the generation of new axon terminals.

CLINICAL MANIFESTATIONS

Forms of tetanus include generalized, local, cephalic, and neonatal. General-ized tetanus, which is the most common form, accounts for 80 to 90% of reported cases in the United States. The usual incubation period is 3 to 21 days (mean, 8 days), depending largely on the distance between the site of injury and the central nervous system. A short incubation period is associated with more severe symptoms. Generalized tetanus is characterized by a per-sistent tonic spasm with brief exacerbations. The neck and jaw are almost always involved. Trismus is the initial complaint in 75% of cases, so the patient is often initially seen by a dentist or oral surgeon. Other early features include irritability, restlessness, diaphoresis, and dysphagia with hydrophobia and drooling. Persistent spasm of the back musculature may cause opisthoto-nos. These early manifestations reflect involvement of the paraspinous muscles. With progression, all muscles contract, with stronger muscles over-taking weaker muscles. Noise or tactile stimuli may precipitate spasms and generalized convulsions. Involvement of the autonomic nervous system may result in severe arrhythmias, blood pressure oscillation, profound diaphore-sis, hyperthermia, rhabdomyolysis, laryngeal spasm, and urinary retention. In most cases, the patient remains lucid and afebrile. The condition may continue for 3 to 4 weeks, despite antitoxin therapy, because of the time required for intra-axonal toxin transport. Complications include fractures from sustained contractions, pulmonary emboli, bacterial infections, and dehydration.

Local tetanus, in which the patient has persistent muscle contractions in the extremity involving a contaminated wound, is rare and shows consider-able variation in severity. In mild cases, a patient may simply have spasms of the involved extremity; in more severe cases, local painful spasms progress to generalized tetanus. This relatively unusual form of tetanus has an excellent prognosis, with only about 1% mortality.

Cephalic tetanus is also rare and generally follows a head injury or occurs with *C. tetani* infection of the middle ear. Clinical symptoms consist of isolated or combined dysfunction of the cranial motor nerves, most frequently cranial nerve VII. This dysfunction may remain localized or progress to generalized tetanus. The incubation period is only 1 or 2 days, and the prognosis for survival is usually poor.

Neonatal tetanus is generalized tetanus resulting from *C. tetani* infection in neonates and occurs primarily in underdeveloped countries, where it accounts for up to half of all neonatal deaths.

DIAGNOSIS

The diagnosis of tetanus is usually based on clinical observations. The putative agent, *C. tetani*, is recovered from wound culture only about 30% of the time. Results of cerebrospinal fluid analysis are entirely normal. Diagnostic testing is usually not necessary except in cases lacking an identified portal of entry. The differential diagnosis depends on the dominant clinical features and includes dystonic reactions as a result of neuroleptic toxicity, seizure disorders, hypocalcemic or alkalotic tetany, alcohol withdrawal, and strychnine poisoning. Strychnine also antagonizes glycine, and strychnine poisoning is the only condition that truly mimics tetanus. Strychnine levels in blood and urine establish the diagnosis. Dystonic reactions may resemble tetanus and are distinguished by rapid response to anticholinergic agents.

PREVENTION

Immunization with tetanus toxoid is virtually 100% effective, so nearly all cases of tetanus occur in unimmunized or inadequately immunized individuals. The Immunization Practices Advisory Committee recommends active immunization of infants and children with DPT (diphtheria, tetanus toxoids, and pertussis adsorbed) at 2 months, 4 months, 6 months, 15 to 18 months, and 4 to 6 years of age. Protective levels of serum antitoxin in persons who complete the primary series persist for at least 10 years. Td (tetanus and diphtheria toxoids adsorbed for adult use) is recommended every 10 years, but this recommendation is commonly neglected, as demonstrated by serosurveys showing that 40% of persons older than 60 years in the United States lack protective levels of tetanus antitoxin. The recommended primary immunization series for unimmunized persons older than 7 years is Td at time 0, 4 to 8 weeks, and 6 to 12 months after the second dose, and then every 10 years. Nearly all states now require DPT immunization for school enrollment. Immunization of childbearing women confers protection to their infants through transplacental maternal antibody.

Prevention of tetanus after injury (Table 304-1) requires appropriate wound management, assurance of adequate immunity, and consideration of antibiotic prophylaxis. The aim of surgery is to eliminate necrotic tissue, purulent collections, and foreign bodies that promote the environmental conditions necessary for spore germination. Passive immunization with tetanus immune globulin (TIG) is recommended only for "tetanus-prone" wounds in patients with an inadequate or unknown primary immunization status. The determination of whether a wound is tetanus prone depends on the interval between injury and treatment, the degree of contamination, the extent of devitalized tissue or foreign bodies at the site of injury, and the depth of injury. Antimicrobial agents such as penicillin or metronidazole may be given to inhibit replication of the vegetative forms of *C. tetani*, but immunization and wound cleansing are considered more important.

TREATMENT

Patients with tetanus require intensive care, with particular attention to respiratory support; treatment with benzodiazepines; autonomic nervous system support; passive and active immunization; surgical débridement; and antibiotics directed against *C. tetani*. There may be clinical progression for 2 to 4 weeks, despite antitoxin treatment, because of the time required to complete the transport of toxin. The severity of disease may be reduced by partial immunity, so some patients have mild disease with minimal mortality, whereas others have mortality rates as high as 60% despite expert care.

Supportive Care

It is most important to assess airway function. Many patients require endotracheal intubation with benzodiazepine sedation and neuromuscular blockade; a tracheostomy should be placed if the endotracheal tube causes spasms. A feeding tube is usually required for nutritional support.

Control of Muscle Spasms

Benzodiazepines have become the mainstay of therapy to control spasms and provide sedation. The most extensively studied is diazepam given in 5-mg increments; lorazepam and midazolam are equally effective. Patients with tetanus may have high tolerance for the sedative effects of these drugs and may require exceptionally high doses. When tetanus symptoms resolve, the drugs must be tapered over at least 2 weeks to prevent withdrawal reactions. If control of spasms cannot be achieved by benzodiazepines, long-term neuromuscular blockade is performed with vecuronium (6 to 8 mg/hour).

Passive Immunization

Human TIG should be given as soon as possible to neutralize toxin that has not entered neurons. The usual dose is 500 IU intramuscularly. Higher doses or intrathecal administration does not appear to be more effective. An alternative to TIG is pooled intravenous immunoglobulin. Equine TIG is equally effective, but the rate of allergic reactions is high because of the equine source; this preparation should not be used if human TIG is available.

Active Immunization

The standard three-dose schedule of immunization with tetanus toxoid should be given at an injection site separate from that used for immunoglobulin.

Antibiotic Therapy

C. tetani is susceptible in vitro to penicillins, cephalosporins, imipenem, macrolides, metronidazole, and tetracyclines. Clinical studies favor the use of metronidazole, which should be given in an intravenous dose of 2 g/day for 7 to 10 days.

Autonomic Nervous System Dysfunction

This complication generally reflects excessive catecholamine release and is usually treated with labetalol (0.25 to 1.0 mg/minute) for blood pressure control. Hypotension may require norepinephrine infusion. Bradycardia may require a pacemaker.

Surgery

Any wounds should be appropriately débrided.

PROGNOSIS

The overall mortality rate for generalized tetanus is 20 to 25%, even in modern medical facilities with extensive resources. Patients with moderate or severe generalized tetanus generally require treatment for 3 to 6 weeks. The highest mortality rates are at the extremes of age. The most frequent cause of death is pneumonia, but many patients have no obvious findings at autopsy, suggesting that death was directly due to the neurotoxin. Patients who recover usually recover completely.

● OTHER CLOSTRIDIAL INFECTIONS
Clostridium perfringens Type C Enteritis

C. perfringens type C enteritis, also called enteritis necroticans, is a necrotizing disease involving the proximal small intestine caused by β-toxin–producing strains of *C. perfringens*. Enteritis necroticans occurs as

TABLE 304-1	GUIDE TO TETANUS PROPHYLAXIS IN ROUTINE WOUND MANAGEMENT			
HISTORY OF ADSORBED TETANUS TOXOID (NO. OF DOSES)	**Clean Minor Wounds**		**All Other Wounds***	
	TDAP OR TD†	**TIG‡**	**TDAP OR TD†**	**TIG‡**
<3 or unknown	Yes	No	Yes	Yes
≥3	No§	No	No¶	No

*Such as (but not limited to) wounds contaminated with dirt, feces, soil, and saliva; puncture wounds; avulsions; and wounds resulting from missiles, crushing, burns, and frostbite.
†For children younger than 7 years, DTaP (pediatric diphtheria–tetanus toxoid plus acellular pertussis vaccine) is recommended; if pertussis vaccine is contraindicated, DT (pediatric diphtheria–tetanus toxoid) is given. For persons aged 7 to 9 years or 65 years or older, Td (adult tetanus–diphtheria toxoid) is recommended. For persons 10 to 64 years, Tdap (adult tetanus–diphtheria toxoid plus acellular pertussis vaccine) is preferred to Td if the patient has never received Tdap and has no contraindication to pertussis vaccine. For persons 7 years and older, if Tdap is not available or not indicated because of age, Td is preferred to TT (tetanus toxoid alone). Note that pediatric formulations (DT and DTaP) contain a similar amount of tetanus toxoid as adult Td, but they contain three to four times as much diphtheria toxoid. DTaP and Tdap vaccines do not contain thimerosal as a preservative.
‡TIG is human tetanus immune globulin. Equine tetanus antitoxin should be used when TIG is not available.
§Yes, if more than 10 years since the last dose.
¶Yes, if more than 5 years since the last dose.

sporadic cases or in outbreaks, most often in underdeveloped countries. There were outbreaks among Khmer refugees in Thailand in the 1980s and in Sri Lanka in 2007. Enteritis necroticans also occurs rarely in isolated cases in the developed world, particularly among patients with diabetes mellitus.

PATHOBIOLOGY

Experimental and clinical evidence supports infection with *C. perfringens* type C and β-toxin as the causative agent of and key virulence factor in enteritis necroticans. The organism has been identified at the site of necrotic lesions, the disease can be reproduced in guinea pigs, isogenic β-toxin gene null mutants are avirulent, and vaccination with a toxoid preparation of β-toxin is protective. Intestinal helminthic coinfection is common in patients at risk for enteritis necroticans, and the proximal small intestine is the preferential site of infection with helminths such as *Strongyloides* (Chapter 365). This has led to a hypothesis of subclinical helminthic infestation facilitating local clostridial infection or intoxication with β-toxin following the ingestion of a contaminated meal.

CLINICAL MANIFESTATIONS

In Papua New Guinea, affected patients usually develop severe abdominal pain 12 hours to several days after a ritual pork feast (or, presumably, other infected food). Vomiting and bloody diarrhea are frequently associated findings. The abdomen becomes distended, and thickened bowel loops are sometimes appreciated on palpation. Disease severity and whether the patient experiences spontaneous recovery or bowel perforation and death depend on the extent of intestinal involvement.

DIAGNOSIS

Recognition of the clinical syndrome is critical to making the diagnosis. Culture to identify specific β-toxin–producing strains of *C. perfingens* remains a research tool and is not helpful in the management of patients. Plain radiographs of the abdomen may show dilated small bowel loops and ileus.

PREVENTION

An effective toxoid vaccine is available and has been used in Papua New Guinea (where the disease is endemic) as well as in the Khmer refugee camp outbreak in 1986.

TREATMENT Rx

Treatment is primarily supportive, including nasogastric suction and intravenous hydration. Surgical resection of the infected bowel is often required for those who do not initially respond to supportive measures. Antibiotics (penicillin, chloramphenicol, metronidazole) are almost always given empirically, but their role has not been defined. Prognosis depends on the extent of disease and the availability of surgery for those with more extensive intestinal involvement.

Clostridium perfringens **Type A Diarrhea**

C. perfringens type A is a well-recognized cause of food poisoning due to the ingestion of food, usually meat, heavily contaminated with enterotoxin-producing *C. perfringens*. The incubation period is 7 to 15 hours following ingestion, and the most prominent symptoms are diarrhea and abdominal pain. The syndrome is usually mild and self-limited.

In contrast to food poisoning due to *C. perfringens* type A, a more severe and protracted infectious diarrhea syndrome due to this organism has been recognized among hospitalized or institutionalized patients. These patients often have a history of prior or concomitant antibiotic use, and an EIA for *C. perfringens* enterotoxin is commercially available for investigative use. Metronidazole treatment is recommended for those with protracted diarrhea. As with CDI, diarrhea may recur following successful treatment.

 Visit expertconsult.com for e-expanded chapter

Grade **A**

1. Cohen SH, Gerding DN, Johnson S, et al. Clinical practice guidelines for *Clostridium difficile* infection in adults: 2010 update by the Society for Healthcare Epidemiology of America (SHEA) and the Infectious Diseases Society of America (IDSA). *Infect Control Hosp Epidemiol.* 2010;31:431-455.
2. Zar FA, Bakkanagari SR, Moorthi KM, et al. A comparison of vancomycin and metronidazole for the treatment of *Clostridium difficile*-associated diarrhea, stratified by disease severity. *Clin Infect Dis.* 2007;45:302-307.
3. Louie TJ, Miller MA, Mullane KM, et al. Fidaxomicin versus vancomycin for *Clostridium difficile* infection. *N Engl J Med.* 2011;364:422-431.

SUGGESTED READINGS

Bauer MP, Notermans DW, van Benthem BH, et al. *Clostridium difficile* infection in Europe: a hospital-based survey. *Lancet.* 2011;377:63-73. *C. difficile was frequently found in European hospitals.*
Peterson LR, Robicsek A. Does my patient have *Clostridium difficile* infection? *Ann Intern Med.* 2009;151:176-179. *Clinical review.*

305

DISEASES CAUSED BY NON–SPORE-FORMING ANAEROBIC BACTERIA

ITZHAK BROOK AND ELLIE J GOLDSTEIN

DEFINITION

Anaerobic bacteria are the main members of the indigenous, normal human flora, including the skin and the oral, gastrointestinal, and vaginal mucosa (Fig. 305-1; Table 305-1). However, the types of predominant anaerobes are different at each site.

The Pathogens

Recent advances in taxonomics have led to reclassification of many anaerobic species (E-Table 305-1). The genus *Bacteroides* is used only for species of the *Bacteroides fragilis* group. The "oral" *Bacteroides* and "pigmented" *Bacteroides* species have been reclassified as *Prevotella* (saccharolytic, pigmented species), *Porphyromonas* (asaccharolytic species), and other genera. Capnophilic organisms (which require an elevated concentration of carbon dioxide for growth), sometimes referred to as microaerophiles, are not true anaerobes and are often more related to *Campylobacter*, *Capnocytophaga*, and other genera. In addition, many new genera and several new species have been created to accommodate pathogens such as *Bilophila wadsworthia*, *Sutterella wadsworthensis*, *Centipeda periodontii*, and *Anaerobiospirillum thomasii*. *Fusobacterium nucleatum* is the predominant *Fusobacterium* species from clinical specimens.

TABLE 305-1 LOCATION OF VARIOUS GROUPS OF ANAEROBES AS NORMAL MICROFLORA IN HUMANS

LOCATION	No. of Organisms Per Gram		PREDOMINANT ANAEROBIC BACTERIA
	AEROBES	ANAEROBES	
Skin	—	—	*Propionibacterium acnes* *Peptostreptococcus* spp
Mouth/upper respiratory tract (in saliva)	10^8-10^9	10^9-10^{11}	Pigmented *Prevotella* and *Porphyromonas* spp *Fusobacterium* spp *Peptostreptococcus* spp *Actinomyces* spp
Gastrointestinal tract (in fecal material)			
Upper	10^2-10^5	10^3-10^7	*Bacteroides fragilis* group *Clostridium* spp
Lower	10^5-10^9	10^{10}-10^{12}	*Peptostreptococcus* spp *Bifidobacterium* spp *Eubacterium* spp
Female genital tract (in vaginal secretions)	10^8	10^9	*Peptostreptococcus* spp *Prevotella bivia* *Prevotella disiens*

Skin
  Propionibacterium acnes
  Gram-positive cocci

Oral cavity and upper respiratory passages
  Prevotella melaninogenica
  Prevotella oralis
  Other *Prevotella* sp
  Porphyromonas sp
  Fusobacterium nucleatum
  Anaerobic cocci—peptostreptococci, *Veillonella*, microaerophilic streptococci
  Actinomyces

Female genital tract
  Prevotella melaninogenica
  Other *Prevotella*
  Other *Bacteroides*
  Peptostreptococcus
  Clostridium
  Porphyromonas

Colon
  Bacteroides fragilis group
  Anaerobic cocci—peptostreptococci, *Veillonella*
  Clostridium
  Eubacterium
  Bifidobacterium

FIGURE 305-1. Anaerobes as the predominant normal microflora of the human body by general anatomic location. (Adapted from Finegold SM, Sutter VL. *Diagnosis and Management of Anaerobic Infections.* Kalamazoo, MI: Upjohn; 1976. Copyright by Dr. Finegold.)

EPIDEMIOLOGY

Although these organisms perform beneficial functions as part of the gastrointestinal flora, they are also consummate opportunistic pathogens that can cause serious infections, typically in synergistic infections in combination with aerobic bacteria. Because the microbiology of these infections is often complex and culture results may be delayed, knowledge of the normal flora at the location of infection is an indispensable guide for selecting and instituting empirical antimicrobial therapy.

PATHOBIOLOGY

Anaerobic bacteria range from those that die with very brief exposure to oxygen to those that can survive even in the presence of atmospheric oxygen (e.g., *B. fragilis*). Most anaerobes require an environment with a low oxidation-reduction potential (E_h gradient), which can be achieved in association with low pH, tissue destruction, byproducts from aerobic bacterial metabolism, or low oxygen content. Though not true anaerobes, some organisms such as microaerophilic streptococci and other capnophilic or hard-to-grow organisms are sometimes lumped together with anaerobes because of their fastidious nature. Some genera such as *Lactobacillus* and *Actinomyces* contain both aerobic and anaerobic species.

Anaerobic bacteria possess a variety of virulence factors that differ among species (Table 305-2).

CLINICAL MANIFESTATIONS

Bacteremia

Transient anaerobic bacteremia occurs in approximately 85% of patients immediately after dental cleaning or manipulation. More than 200 cases of endocarditis from anaerobes are reported annually in the United States, usually in association with anatomic abnormalities or damaged cardiac valves (Chapter 76). The majority of anaerobic bacteremias are intermittent and associated with serious intra-abdominal or female genital tract, skin, and soft tissue infections, often near the fecal stream. Which organisms are involved depends on their portal of entry and the underlying disease. The common isolates are the *B. fragilis* group (60 to 75% of isolates). Overall, about 5 to 15% of bacteremias are due to anaerobes, and they are the sole isolates in two thirds of such infections. *B. fragilis* group bacteremia is associated with a 15 to 30% mortality rate. Bacteremia with the *B. fragilis* group is mostly associated with a gastrointestinal source; bacteremia with pigmented *Prevotella, Porphyromonas,* and *Fusobacterium* spp, with oropharyngeal and pulmonary sources; *Fusobacterium* spp with the female genital tract; and *Propionibacterium acnes* with foreign bodies. Bacteremia with peptostreptococci is associated with all sources, but especially with the oropharyngeal, pulmonary, and female genital tracts.

TABLE 305-2   POTENTIAL VIRULENCE FACTORS IN VARIOUS ANAEROBES

FACTOR	SPECIES
ADHESION	
Capsule	*Bacteroides fragilis* group, *Prevotella melaninogenica*
Pili/fimbriae	*B. fragilis* group
	Porphyromonas gingivalis
Hemagglutinin	*P. gingivalis*
Lectin	*Fusobacterium nucleatum*
INVASION/TISSUE DAMAGE	
Proteases	*Fusobacterium necrophorum*
	Bacteroides spp
	Porphyromonas spp
Hemolysins	Many species
Endotoxin	*B. fragilis*
Fibrinolysin	*B. fragilis* group
	Porphyromonas spp
Heparinase	*B. fragilis* group
	Porphyromonas spp
Neuraminidase	*B. fragilis* group
	Porphyromonas spp
ANTIPHAGOCYTIC	
Capsule	*B. fragilis* group
	P. gingivalis
Lipopolysaccharide	*B. fragilis* group
	F. necrophorum, P. gingivalis
Metabolic products	Most anaerobes
TOXINS	
Endotoxin	*B. fragilis*
	F. necrophorum
Enterotoxin	*B. fragilis*

Adapted from Duerden BI. Virulence factors in anaerobes. *Clin Infect Dis.* 1994;18(Suppl. 4):253.

Central Nervous System Infections

Anaerobes can cause brain abscess, subdural empyema, epidural abscess, and meningitis. The main source of brain abscess is an adjacent, generally chronic infection in the ears, mastoids, sinuses, oropharynx, teeth, or lungs. Rarely, bacteremia of another origin or endocarditis can lead to such infection.

Meningitis caused by anaerobes is rare and can follow respiratory infection or develop as a complication of a cerebrospinal fluid shunt. The isolates generally recovered from brain abscesses that complicate respiratory and dental infections include *Prevotella, Porphyromonas, Bacteroides, Fusobacterium,* and *Peptostreptococcus* spp. Microaerophilic and other streptococci are also often isolated. *P. acnes* is common in shunt infections.

Head and Neck

Dental infections (Chapter 433) associated with a variety of oral anaerobic bacteria include periodontal disease, gingivitis, pulpitis, acute necrotizing ulcerative gingivitis, localized juvenile periodontitis, adult periodontitis, pericoronitis, endodontitis, periapical and dental abscesses, and postextraction infection. Peritonsillar, retropharyngeal, and parapharyngeal abscesses (Chapter 437) are deep-seated, potentially life-threatening infections that may extend into the various potential spaces of the neck or mediastinum and cause jugular vein thrombosis. Oral anaerobes may be isolated in more than 50% of such cases, usually in mixed culture with aerobes. Other regional infections include cervicofacial actinomycosis (Chapter 337), Ludwig's angina, *Fusobacterium necrophorum* sepsis with metastatic infection (Lemierre's syndrome), suppurative sialoadenitis (including parotitis), neck space infections, thyroiditis and chronic sinusitis (Chapter 434), otitis media (Chapter 434), and mastoiditis. Management involves surgical drainage and appropriate antimicrobial therapy.

Pleuropulmonary

Anaerobes are the predominant "normal flora" of the oral cavity and upper respiratory tract, and most pneumonias are due to aspiration of this flora (Chapter 97). Aspiration may be a result of altered consciousness, dysphagia, or mechanical devices such as intubation equipment. Poor oral hygiene is associated with an increased anaerobic bacterial burden, and the presence of aerobes or necrotic tissue lowers the pH, which in turn facilitates the growth of anaerobes. Anaerobes are involved in 90% of patients with community-acquired aspiration pneumonia and in about a third of patients with nosocomial aspiration pneumonia, empyema, lung abscess, and pneumonia associated with tracheostomy. If the anaerobic component of aspiration pneumonia is not treated, the anaerobes can cause a lung abscess. Management requires good pulmonary toilet and antimicrobial therapy.

Intra-abdominal

Anaerobes outnumber aerobes by 1000 : 1 in the large intestine, so it is not surprising that they play an important role in almost all intra-abdominal infections. Most visceral abscesses (e.g., hepatic; Chapter 154), chronic cholecystitis (Chapter 158), perforated and gangrenous appendicitis (Chapter 144), postoperative wound infections and abscesses, diverticulitis (Chapter 144), and any infection associated with fecal contamination of the abdominal cavity involve both aerobes and anaerobes. *B. fragilis* group members are especially important pathogens because they are encapsulated and resist phagocytosis, are often resistant to many commonly used antibiotics, and promote abscess formation. They may also be associated with concomitant bacteremia and sepsis.

Obstetric-Gynecologic

A variety of obstetric-gynecologic diseases involve anaerobes (Table 305-3). These infections are polymicrobial and include the following: bacterial vaginosis; soft tissue perineal, vulvar, and Bartholin gland abscesses; endometritis; pyometra; salpingitis; tubo-ovarian abscesses; adnexal abscess; pelvic inflammatory disease, which may include pelvic cellulitis and abscess; chorioamnionitis; vaginal cuff cellulitis; septic pelvic thrombophlebitis; intrauterine contraceptive device–associated infection; septic abortion; and postsurgical obstetric and gynecologic infections. Bacterial vaginosis has been associated with preterm labor or delivery, chorioamnionitis, low birthweight, postpartum endometritis, and postabortal pelvic inflammatory disease. Bacterial vaginosis can increase the risk for infection with human immunodeficiency virus (HIV) type 1 and the development of other sexually transmitted diseases (Chapter 293).

Skin and Soft Tissue

Cutaneous infections include infected ulcers, cellulitis (including synergistic necrotizing cellulitis), pyoderma, paronychia, hidradenitis suppurativa, and a variety of secondarily infected sites. Such sites include secondarily infected gastrostomy or tracheostomy site wounds, subcutaneous sebaceous or inclusion cysts, eczema, psoriasis, poison ivy, atopic dermatitis, eczema herpeticum, scabies or kerion, and postsurgical wounds.

Subcutaneous infections include abscesses, decubitus ulcers, infected diabetic (vascular or trophic) ulcers, human and animal bite wounds, anaerobic cellulitis and gas gangrene, bacterial synergistic gangrene, Fournier's gangrene, infected pilonidal cyst or sinus, and burn wounds. Anaerobic soft tissue infections that occur deeper are necrotizing fasciitis, necrotizing

TABLE 305-3	CLINICAL INDICATORS OF ANAEROBIC INFECTION

Infection adjacent to a mucosal surface
Foul-smelling discharge
Necrotic gangrenous tissue and abscess formation
Free gas or crepitus in tissue
Bacteremia or endocarditis with no growth on aerobic blood cultures
Infection related to the use of antibiotics effective against aerobes only (e.g., trimethoprim-sulfamethoxazole, aminoglycosides, older quinolones)
Infection related to tumors or other destructive processes
Infected thrombophlebitis
Infection after bites
Black discoloration of exudates containing *Prevotella melaninogenica*, which may fluoresce under ultraviolet light
"Sulfur granules" in discharges caused by actinomycosis
Clinical finding of gas gangrene or necrotizing fasciitis
Clinical condition predisposing to anaerobic infection (e.g., after maternal amnionitis, fistulous tracts, bites, dental infection, bowel perforation)

synergistic cellulitis, and gas gangrene. These infections can involve the fascia and can induce myositis and myonecrosis.

Cultures frequently yield isolates that are members of the "normal flora" of the region of the infection. In addition to oral and skin flora, human bite infections often contain *Eikenella* species and animal bites harbor *Pasteurella multocida*.

The infections are generally polymicrobial, and some (e.g., decubitus ulcers, diabetic foot ulcers) are often complicated by osteomyelitis or bacteremia. Deep tissue infections such as necrotizing cellulitis, fasciitis, and myositis often involve *Clostridium* species, *Streptococcus pyogenes*, or a polymicrobic aerobic and anaerobic flora. They are often associated with gas in the tissues and putrid-like pus with a gray thin quality and have a high rate of bacteremia and mortality. Management of deep-seated soft tissue infection includes surgical débridement, drainage, and vigorous surgical management.

Osteomyelitis and Septic Arthritis

Anaerobes are notable in osteomyelitis of the long bones after trauma and fracture, osteomyelitis related to peripheral vascular disease, decubitus ulcers, and osteomyelitis of the cranial and facial bones. Most of these infections are polymicrobial.

Cranial and facial bone osteomyelitis is generally caused by spread from a contiguous soft tissue source or from sinus, ear, or dental infection. Intestinal anaerobes originating from decubitus ulcers are involved in pelvic osteomyelitis. Osteomyelitis of long bones and septic arthritis are generally caused by hematogenous spread, trauma, or the presence of a prosthetic device.

The predominant isolated anaerobes are peptostreptococci and *P. acnes* (often in prosthetic joint infection), *B. fragilis* group and fusobacteria (often of hematogenous origin), and clostridia (associated with trauma).

DIAGNOSIS

Anaerobic infections should be suspected in a number of specific clinical scenarios (Table 305-3). An appropriately collected microbiologic specimen (Table 305-4) is critical for accurate diagnosis.

TREATMENT

General principles of treatment (Table 305-5) include appropriate antimicrobial therapy coupled with prompt drainage, decompression of closed-space infections, relief of obstructions, and surgical débridement. The various clinically important anaerobes can be characterized by reasonably predictable susceptibility patterns to antimicrobial agents (Table 305-6), but culture and sensitivity results should ultimately guide therapy. The efficacy of hyperbaric oxygen is unproved, but its use in conjunction with other therapeutic measures is not contraindicated.

When choosing antimicrobials for the treatment of mixed infections, their aerobic and anaerobic antibacterial spectra and their availability in oral or parenteral form should be considered. Some antimicrobials have a limited range of activity. For example, metronidazole is active only against anaerobes and therefore cannot be administered as a single agent for the treatment of mixed infections. Others (i.e., carbapenems, tigecycline) have wide spectra of activity against aerobes and anaerobes.

Aside from susceptibility patterns, other factors influencing the choice of antimicrobial therapy include the pharmacologic characteristics of the various drugs, their toxicity, their effect on normal flora, and their bactericidal activity. Although identification of the infecting organisms and their antimicrobial susceptibility may be needed for selection of optimal therapy, the clinical setting and Gram stain preparation of the specimen may indicate the types of anaerobes present in the infection and the nature of the infectious process.

Even though the duration of therapy for anaerobic infections is generally longer than that for aerobic and facultative infections, the length of treatment must be individualized, depending on the response. In some cases, treatment may require 6 to 8 weeks, but therapy may be shortened with proper surgical drainage. An anti–gram-negative enteric agent is generally added to treat Enterobacteriaceae when managing intra-abdominal infections.

The available parenteral antimicrobials for most infections are clindamycin, metronidazole, chloramphenicol, cefoxitin, a penicillin (i.e., ticarcillin, ampicillin, piperacillin) and a β-lactamase inhibitor (i.e., clavulanic acid, sulbactam, tazobactam), a carbapenem (i.e., imipenem, meropenem, doripenem, ertapenem), or tigecycline.[1-4]

An agent effective against gram-negative enteric bacilli (e.g., an aminoglycoside, fluoroquinolone) or an antipseudomonal cephalosporin (e.g., cefepime) is generally added to metronidazole and, occasionally, cefoxitin when treating intra-abdominal infections. Penicillin can be added to metronidazole for the treatment of intracranial, pulmonary, or dental infections to cover microaerophilic streptococci and *Actinomyces* species. Penicillin is added to clindamycin to supplement its coverage against *Peptostreptococcus* species and other gram-positive anaerobic organisms. For *Chlamydia* and *Mycoplasma* species, doxycycline is added to most regimens when treating pelvic infections. Oral therapy is often substituted for parenteral therapy. The agents available for oral therapy are clindamycin, amoxicillin and clavulanate, and metronidazole.

TABLE 305-4　SPECIMEN ACCEPTABILITY FOR ANAEROBIC CULTURE

SPECIMENS THAT SHOULD NOT BE CULTURED FOR ANAEROBES

Feces or rectal swabs
Throat or nasopharyngeal swabs
Sputum or bronchoscopic specimens
Routine or catheterized urine
Vaginal or cervical swabs
Material from superficial wounds or abscesses not collected properly to exclude surface contamination
Material from abdominal wounds obviously contaminated with feces, such as an open fistula

SPECIMENS APPROPRIATE FOR ANAEROBIC CULTURE

All normally sterile body fluids other than urine, such as blood, pleural, and joint fluids
Urine obtained by suprapubic bladder aspiration
Percutaneous transtracheal aspiration, direct lung puncture, or double-lumen catheter bronchial brushing and bronchoalveolar lavage (both cultured quantitatively)
Culdocentesis fluid obtained after decontamination of the vagina
Material obtained from closed abscesses
Material obtained from sinus tracts or draining wounds

TABLE 305-5　GENERAL PRINCIPLES OF THERAPY FOR ANAEROBIC INFECTIONS

Decompression of closed spaces
Débridement
Drainage
Relief of obstructions
Irrigation
Provision of adequate circulation when possible
Removal of foreign bodies
Antimicrobials
　Activity against most likely pathogen or pathogens: location dependent, minimal effect on normal flora
　Absorption, appropriate route of administration (intravenous, oral)
　Penetration into site of infection
　Dosage appropriate for local tissue levels, body mass of patient, renal and liver function
　Duration appropriate for condition
　Susceptibility testing of isolate to guide specific therapy

TABLE 305-6　ANTIMICROBIAL SUSCEPTIBILITY PATTERNS FOR ANAEROBIC BACTERIA*

BACTERIA	PENICILLIN	β-LACTAMASE†	CEFOXITIN	CEFOTETAN	CARBAPENEMS, TIGECYCLINE	MOXIFLOXACIN	CLINDAMYCIN	METRONIDAZOLE
Bacteroides fragilis	−	+	+	+	+	+	V	+
Bacteroides thetaiotaomicron	−	+	V	V	+	V	V	+
B. fragilis group, other	−	+	V	V	+	+	V	+
Prevotella spp	V	+	+	+	+	+	+	+
Fusobacterium nucleatum	V	+	+	+	+	V	+	+
Fusobacterium necrophorum	+	+	+	+	+	V	+	+
Porphyromonas spp	+	+	+	+	+	+	+	+
Peptostreptococcus	+	+	+	+	+	+	+	V
Propionibacterium acnes	+	+	+	+	+	+	+	−
Veillonella	+	+	+	+	+	+	+	+
Actinomyces	+	+	+	+	+	+	+	−

*Based on a variety of in vitro susceptibility studies from different laboratories and using different techniques.
†β-Lactamase inhibitor–β-lactam combination (e.g., ticarcillin-clavulanate, ampicillin-sulbactam, piperacillin-tazobactam).
+ = Susceptible; − = resistant; V = variable.

1. Ott SR, Allewelt M, Lorenz J, et al. Moxifloxacin vs ampicillin/sulbactam in aspiration pneumonia and primary lung abscess. *Infection*. 2008;36:23-30.
2. Goldstein EJ, Citron DM, Merriam CV, et al. Infection after elective colorectal surgery: bacteriological analysis of failures in a randomized trial of cefotetan vs. ertapenem prophylaxis. *Surg Infect (Larchmt)*. 2009;10:111-118.
3. Malangoni MA, Song J, Herrington J, et al. Randomized controlled trial of moxifloxacin compared with piperacillin-tazobactam and amoxicillin-clavulanate for the treatment of complicated intra-abdominal infections. *Ann Surg*. 2006;244:204-211.
4. Lucasti C, Jasovich A, Umeh O, et al. Efficacy and tolerability of IV doripenem versus meropenem in adults with complicated intra-abdominal infection: a phase III, prospective, multicenter, randomized, double-blind, noninferiority study. *Clin Ther*. 2008;30:868-883.

SUGGESTED READINGS

Dahlén G, Ebenfelt A. Necrobacillosis in humans. *Expert Rev Anti Infect Ther*. 2011;9:227-236. *Review of a rare infectious disease that responds to metronidazole in combination with penicillin or amoxicillin.*

Lee CS, Lee J. Evaluation of new gyrB-based real-time PCR system for the detection of B. fragilis as an indicator of human-specific fecal contamination. *J Microbiol Methods*. 2010;82:311-318. *A new method for rapid detection.*

Mazuski JE, Solomkin JS. Intra-abdominal infections. *Surg Clin North Am*. 2009;89:421-437. *Review of the diagnosis and treatment of intra-abdominal polymicrobial infections.*

Sullivan DC, Chapman SW. Bacteria that masquerade as fungi: actinomycosis/nocardia. *Proc Am Thorac Soc*. 2010;7:216-221. *Review emphasizing chronic progression, abscess formation with fistulous tracks, and draining sinuses.*

Takayanagi N, Kagiyama N, Ishiguro T, et al. Etiology and outcome of community-acquired lung abscess. *Respiration*. 2010;80:98-105. *Emphasizes importance of anaerobic species, which are the most common cause of community-acquired lung abscess in the West.*

Wick EC, Sears CL. Bacteroides spp. and diarrhea. *Curr Opin Infect Dis*. 2010;23:470-474. *The leading anaerobe in human disease is emerging as an important cause of diarrhea.*

306

NEISSERIA MENINGITIDIS INFECTIONS

DAVID S. STEPHENS

DEFINITION

Neisseria meningitidis (the meningococcus) is the cause of epidemic meningitis, a fulminant sepsis (meningococcemia), milder bacteremia, and, less commonly, other focal infections.

The Pathogen

N. meningitidis is an aerobic, gram-negative β-proteobacterium and a member of the family Neisseriaceae, which also includes *Neisseria gonorrhoeae* (Chapter 307), another important human pathogen. The meningococcus is a common commensal of the human upper respiratory tract, but it can also cause local and devastating invasive human disease. Human mucosal surfaces, most commonly the nasopharynx, are the only known reservoir. There are 13 known serogroups of *N. meningitidis*, based on different capsular polysaccharide structures, but only 6 serogroups (A, B, C, W-135, X, and Y) cause the majority of invasive meningococcal disease (Fig. 306-1). Highly pathogenic meningococci are also distinguished by genetically defined clonal complexes that can emerge and spread worldwide. Dissecting the basis of meningococcal disease has provided important scientific lessons for bacterial emergence and pathogenesis, antibiotic resistance mechanisms, innate and adaptive human immune responses, and vaccine strategies.

EPIDEMIOLOGY

For at least 200 years, *N. meningitidis* has inflicted rapid death, disability, and fear on disparate human populations. Beginning with the initial descriptions of outbreaks in Geneva in 1805 and New Bedford, Massachusetts, in 1806, the meningococcus has caused endemic cases, case clusters, epidemics, and pandemics of meningitis and septicemia. An estimated 500,000 cases occur worldwide each year. The greatest burden of disease occurs in Africa and in parts of Asia, where endemic rates of disease are 5 to 10 per 100,000 population. Especially in sub-Saharan Africa, seasonal epidemics occur yearly, and cyclic pandemics have occurred every 8 to 10 years since 1905. During the

epidemics and cyclic pandemics, the incidence can climb to 1 per 1000 population for weeks before the frequency of disease declines in the immediate outbreak area. For example, despite partially effective vaccines, the dry seasons in Burkina Faso, located in the sub-Saharan meningitis belt, can be accompanied by more than 5000 cases of meningitis per week (>680/100,000 population), an almost yearly occurrence in the country. Meningococcal epidemics in developing countries cause catastrophic expense, which contributes to the cycle of poverty and hence the disorganization of social structures.

The disease remains endemic, with focal outbreaks, in the United States, Canada, Europe, Japan, Australia, and other industrialized countries, with a lower overall incidence of 0.3 to 2 per 100,000 population. The introduction and widespread use of new meningococcal conjugate vaccines in North America, Australia, and Europe have lowered the incidence. Endemic disease and outbreaks continue to occur in China, eastern Europe, Russia, South America, India, and Southeast Asia. Before and during World War II, large epidemic outbreaks (mainly due to serogroup A) affected the United States, Europe, Japan, and Australia; after the war these outbreaks disappeared, for reasons that are not clear. Meningococcal disease has the highest incidence in children younger than 4 years and in adolescents, but in endemic settings, half of all cases occur in adults.

PATHOBIOLOGY

N. meningitidis is transmitted among humans through close contact via large respiratory droplets. Colonization of the upper respiratory mucosal surfaces (e.g., nasopharynx) by *N. meningitidis* is the first step in establishment of a human carrier state and invasive meningococcal disease. Acquisition of meningococci through contact with respiratory secretions or saliva can be transient, lead to colonization (carriage), or result in invasive disease. The inoculum size needed for transmission is unknown. Meningococcal disease usually occurs within 1 to 14 days of acquisition. Rarely, meningococci are transmitted sexually.

Initial contact of meningococci with mucosal epithelial cells is mediated by type IV pili. These structures provide mobility to penetrate mucus and are the initial adhesins for epithelial cells; the receptor for pili may be the I-domain of integrin α chains or possibly CD46. Meningococci proceed to proliferate on the surface of human nonciliated epithelial cells, forming small microcolonies at the site of attachment; they can disseminate from colonies by post-translational modification of pili and migrate to adjacent cells via pili-mediated "twitching" motility. Meningococci can also spread from the nasopharynx to adjacent epithelial surfaces and can infrequently cause local infections, including pneumonia, sinusitis, or otitis media. Close adherence of meningococci to the host epithelial cells results in the formation of epithelial cell cortical plaques and leads to the recruitment of factors ultimately responsible for the formation and extension of pseudopodia that can surround the meningococcus. Intimate meningococcal association with the epithelial cell is mediated by the bacterial opacity proteins Opa and Opc with CD66/carcinoembryonic antigen–related cell adhesion molecules (CEACAMs) and integrins, respectively, on the surface of the cell. However, other meningococcal epithelial cell mediators include the meningococcal adhesin NadA and meningococcal lipo-oligosaccharide. The formation of epithelial cell membrane protrusions and pseudopodia stems from the organization of specific molecular complexes involving the linkers ezrin and moesin, along with the clustering of several membrane-integral proteins, including CD44, intracellular adhesion molecule 1, and cortical actin polymerization. These events can lead to internalization of *N. meningitidis* in epithelial cells (Fig. 306-2). Intracellular meningococci reside within a membranous vacuole and are capable of translocating through the epithelial layers within 18 to 40 hours. Meningococci are capable of intracellular replication, due in part to the protective capsule and the organism's capacity to acquire iron through specialized transport systems.

Meningococci cross mucosal surfaces, enter the blood stream, and, in some individuals, produce systemic infection. Damage to the mucosal surface by coinfection, drying (e.g., very low humidity), or smoke exposure may increase this risk of invasion. The molecular interactions noted for epithelial cells also occur with endothelial cells, and meningococci can translocate across the blood-meninges barrier, possibly at the choroid plexus or by opening of intercellular junctions, and proliferate in the subarachnoid space, resulting in meningitis. In vasculature and cerebrospinal fluid (CSF), high levels of multiplying bacteria lead to an intense inflammatory response, with pronounced increases in concentrations of tumor necrosis factor-α (TNF-α), interleukins (IL-1β, IL-6, IL-8, and IL-10), different chemokines, and other inflammatory mediators.

Resistance to complement-mediated lysis and phagocytosis is due to the expression of the capsule and lipo-oligosaccharide. Meningococcal endotoxin released in blebs plays a major role in the inflammatory events of meningococcemia and meningococcal meningitis. Meningococcal lipid A is responsible for much of the biologic activity and toxicity of meningococcal endotoxin. The Toll-like receptor 4 (TLR4) is critical to the innate immune response to bacterial endotoxins, and meningococcal endotoxin is no exception. Activation of TLR4 by endotoxin requires association with the accessory protein MD-2, an *N*-glycosylated 19- to 27-kD protein expressed in both a soluble and a membrane-bound form. Binding of endotoxin to MD-2 in association with TLR4 leads to dimerization or oligomerization of two or more TLR4s, subsequent cellular activation, and cytokine and chemokine release.

In contrast, an asymptomatic *N. meningitidis* carrier state is found in 8 to 25% of healthy individuals. Meningococcal carriage is affected by age, intimate personal contact, crowding (e.g., bars, dormitories), and vaccination or chemoprophylaxis interventions in the community. Variable carriage rates have been reported, even during epidemics. Meningococcal carriage is a dynamic process, is less common in young children than in adults (<3%; *N. lactamica* predominates), is highest in adolescents (7 to 37%), and increases in closed populations (e.g., military recruits, hajj pilgrims). Rates as high as 36 to 71% have been reported in military recruits. Damage to the

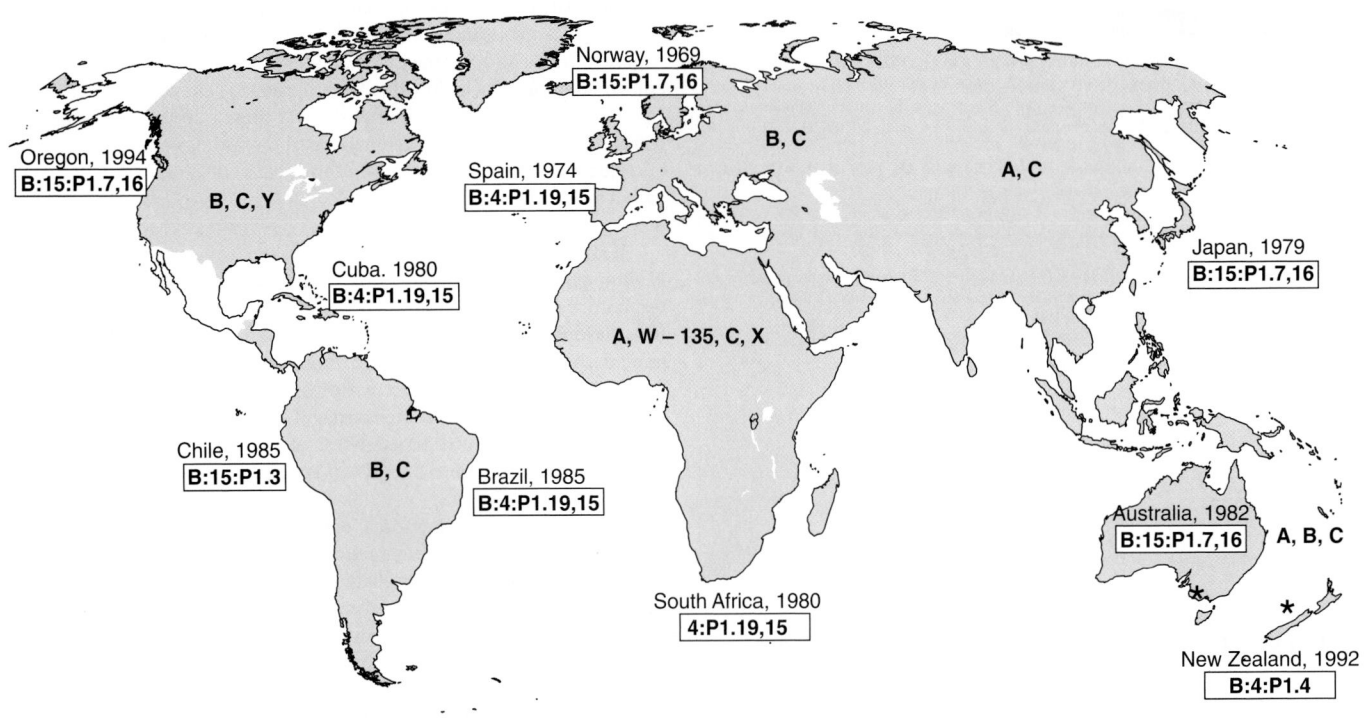

*Group B by serotype, modified from Caugant, APMIS 1998; 106:505-525

FIGURE 306-1. **Epidemiology of meningococcal disease** (major serogroups causing disease and serogroup B epidemics). (Modified from Stephens DS, Greenwood B, Brandtzaeg P. Epidemic meningitis, meningococcemia and *Neisseria meningitidis*. Lancet. 2007;369:2196-2210.)

Invasion and dispersion

Microcolony formation

FIGURE 306-2. **Steps in initiating meningococcal colonization and invasion at the human nasopharynx. A,** Adhesion and introduction of cell microvilli. **B,** Microcolony formation. **C,** Cortical plaque formation and close adherence. **D,** Human epithelial cell invasion. (Modified from Stephens DS. Biology and pathogenesis of the evolutionarily successful, obligate human bacterium *Neisseria meningitidis*. Vaccine. 2009;27S:B71-B77.)

upper respiratory tract by coinfections (e.g., mycoplasma, influenza, other respiratory viral infections), smoking, very low humidity, drying of mucosal surfaces, and trauma induced by dust predisposes to both carriage and meningococcal disease. Carriage has been linked to status as a secretor of glycoprotein ABO blood group antigens, which are water soluble, and to ethnic background. In a large U.K. study, social behavior (e.g., attendance at pubs or clubs, intimate kissing, cigarette smoking or exposure to passive smoke) was highly associated with the risk of meningococcal carriage. Carriage can last for days, weeks, or months and is an immunizing event leading to protective immunity against the organism.

The absence of protective bactericidal antibodies is the most important predisposing factor for systemic meningococcal disease, but genetic polymorphisms and other host cofactors can contribute to disease and disease severity. Disappearance of protective maternal antibodies increases the risk in older infants and young children. Congenital and acquired antibody deficiencies also increase risk. Opsonization and phagocytic function are important host defense mechanisms, as shown by disease reduction after polysaccharide vaccination in individuals with complement deficiencies. Rapidly progressive, fatal meningococcemia can arise in patients without properdin, and there is an increased risk of recurrent meningococcal infections in those with defects in the terminal complement pathway (C5–C9).

Polymorphisms in genes coding for the Fcγ-receptor II (CD32), Fcγ-receptor III (CD16), mannose-binding lectin, and TLR4 have been associated with increased risk. Mannose-binding lectin is a plasma opsonin that initiates complement activation; specific polymorphisms in the gene are identified more frequently in children with meningococcal disease than in controls. Plasminogen activator inhibitor-1 concentrations appear to affect the severity and mortality of meningococcal sepsis, suggesting that impaired fibrinolysis is an important factor in its pathophysiology. Meningococcal disease is occasionally linked to immunosuppressive disorders such as nephrotic syndrome, congenital or acquired hypogammaglobulinemia, splenectomy, and HIV/AIDS (about a 10-fold increased risk for sporadic disease). However, there has been no documented increase in epidemic outbreaks of meningococcal disease in countries with very high rates of HIV infection.

Meningococci can multiply rapidly in the vascular compartment, with an estimated doubling time of 30 to 45 minutes in some patients, or in the CSF. The release of high levels of inflammatory mediators such as endotoxin in the circulation or the CSF triggers an exaggerated release of chemokines, cytokines, bradykinin, and nitric oxide. Vascular dilation, hypovolemia, capillary leak, and a pronounced reduction in myocardial function are the result. At a later stage, substantial complement activation contributes to the altered endothelial barrier function and relaxation of the smooth muscles in the vessel wall through the generation of high levels of anaphylatoxins (C3a and C5a). The capillary leak syndrome results in an increased flux of albumin and water across the altered capillary wall to the extravascular space. A patient with fulminant meningococcemia accumulates a large amount of fluid in the extravascular tissue. Circulatory collapse and multiorgan dysfunction are the primary causes of death due to meningococcemia. In meningitis, morbidity and death are due predominantly to cerebral edema.

Unraveling the pathogenic mechanisms of this devastating, evolutionarily successful obligate human pathogen has significance for other new vaccines directed at mucosal pathogens and vaccine adjuvants, as well as for the understanding of human sepsis and the design of sepsis antagonists.

CLINICAL MANIFESTATIONS

The meningococcus causes meningitis (~50% of cases); septicemia (meningococcemia) or, less commonly, a mild bacteremia pneumonia; and much less commonly (<5% of cases), septic arthritis, pericarditis, chronic bacteremia, or conjunctivitis. Very rarely, meningococci can cause urethritis. In endemic and epidemic disease outbreaks, hemorrhagic skin lesions (petechiae, purpura; Fig. 306-3) are present in 28 to 77% of patients with invasive meningococcal disease on admission; these lesions can be difficult to see in patients with dark skin. Hemorrhagic lesions sometimes occur on mucous membranes and sclera, but they are especially prevalent on the limbs. Petechiae of meningococcemia are usually larger and bluer than the pinpoint petechiae caused by thrombocytopenia, leukocytoclastic vasculitis induced by other infections or drugs, or vomiting or coughing. A nonblanching macular rash can also be a manifestation of meningococcal bacteremia. Evolving ecchymoses or purpura (diameter >10 mm) are noted mainly in patients with meningococcemia and disseminated intravascular coagulation (Chapter 178), but they may not appear until 12 hours into the illness. In addition to vasculitis, other conditions in the differential diagnosis of meningococcemia include Rocky Mountain spotted fever and enteroviral infections.

Meningitis is the most common clinical presentation of invasive meningococcal disease. Headache, fever, and rash with meningismus and altered mental status are the characteristic features; however, the rash may be absent, and the presentation can resemble pneumococcal or bacterial meningitis of other causes, viral meningitis, or early-stage encephalitis. Bacteremic meningococcal pneumonia has been linked most often to serogroup Y and is more common in adolescents, adults, and especially older adults (approximately one third of cases occur in those older than 65 years). Isolated septic pericarditis or septic arthritis can also be a presentation, and an autoimmune- or antibody-mediated polyarthritis can be seen in the recovery phase following invasive meningococcal disease. Chronic meningococcemia can present with low-grade fever and a polyarticular arthritis that can be confused with rheumatoid arthritis.

DIAGNOSIS

The clinical diagnosis of meningococcal meningitis relies on the recognition of fever, rash, meningeal signs, and altered mental status and is confirmed by CSF pleocytosis; Gram stain and/or polymerase chain reaction (PCR) of CSF, with or without growth in culture; or culture of blood or skin lesions.

FIGURE 306-3. Clinical manifestations of meningococcal disease. **A** and **B,** Macular and petechial rashes of meningococcal bacteremia. **C,** Fulminant meningococcal sepsis with ecchymoses. **D,** Digital necrosis of meningococcemia sepsis. **E,** Hemorrhagic adrenals in fulminant meningococcal sepsis. (Modified from Stephens DS, Greenwood B, Brandtzaeg P. Epidemic meningitis, meningococcemia and *Neisseria meningitidis. Lancet.* 2007; 369:2196-2210.)

The early clinical diagnosis of meningococcemia is a challenge because a rash, meningeal signs, and high fever may not be present. Blood cultures are diagnostic, but the course can be quite fulminant (<24 hours), and the early stages of disease can mimic viral infections such as influenza. Thus, it can be difficult to identify and treat the disease quickly. General symptoms of sepsis (nausea and vomiting, drowsiness, irritability, leg pains, cold hands and feet, abnormal skin color) are present. However, these symptoms (in contrast to fever and rash) are not likely to be specific markers. Parents and relatives should be instructed to undress and inspect a febrile child, adolescent, or young adult for a rash, and physicians and other health care providers should be alert to the concerns of parents or relatives about the abrupt or rapid deterioration of a patient.

PCR is increasingly used for the diagnosis of meningococcal meningitis, including serogrouping and genomic typing. Improved antigen and nucleic acid detection systems are leading to better meningococcal disease surveillance and molecular epidemiology. Biopsy samples from dermis show that meningococci are present in and around the microvascular endothelial cells. Meningococci in these lesions can be cultured up to 12 hours after effective antibiotic treatment is started. In two studies, the sensitivity of culture and Gram stain of the aspiration and biopsy samples of skin lesions was 62 and 56%, respectively.

TREATMENT   Rx

Early antibiotic administration is most important because effective antibiotics immediately stop the growth of *N. meningitidis*. Ceftriaxone, cefotaxime, and penicillin are all effective antibiotics, as are meropenem and chloramphenicol. Fluoroquinolones have excellent in vitro activity, but clinical experience is limited, and meningococcal resistance is now emerging to quinolones. Meningococci in CSF are killed within 3 to 4 hours after intravenous treatment with an adequate dose of a third-generation cephalosporin or penicillin, and concentrations of endotoxin in plasma fall by 50% within 2 hours. The concentrations of key cytokines and chemokines fall in parallel. Antibiotic treatment does not induce a large release of meningococcal endotoxin or lead to an increased inflammatory response.

Prehospital antibiotic treatment is advocated if the disease is suspected. One goal is to reduce the case-fatality rate for patients with fulminant meningococcal sepsis or meningitis with rapidly increasing concentrations of meningococci and inflammatory mediators in the circulation or CSF. If antibiotic treatment is initiated before admission, ceftriaxone or another effective antibiotic should be injected intravenously or intramuscularly. During epidemics in developing countries, a single injection of ceftriaxone or long-acting chloramphenicol may be sufficient for patients with meningitis,[1] and this simple treatment has saved many thousands of lives. Although the sensitivity of meningococci to penicillin is decreasing worldwide because of a reduced affinity for penicillin–binding protein 2, high-level penicillin resistance remains rare. Ceftriaxone and cefotaxime can achieve CSF concentrations 45- to 8750-fold higher than the minimal inhibitory concentrations for meningococci.

Patients with suspected bacterial meningitis of unknown cause are often given ceftriaxone or cefotaxime, often combined with vancomycin, until the causative agent has been identified. When *N. meningitidis* is identified, antibiotic treatment can be continued with a third-generation cephalosporin or penicillin alone. Traditionally, patients were treated for 7 days, but 3 or 4 days of intravenous treatment can provide a cure without relapses.

Recognition of the different pathophysiologic processes associated with meningococcal meningitis (which causes death and morbidity predominantly by cerebral edema) and meningococcal septic shock (which causes death and morbidity predominantly through hypovolemia, capillary leak, myocardial dysfunction, and multiorgan failure) has led to improved management strategies for these two different forms of disease. Early and aggressive management of shock through the use of volume expansion, intensive care monitoring, and inotropic support can reduce fatality rates of meningococcal sepsis from higher than 30% to 5 to 10%. In meningococcemia with hypotension, the primary goal is to increase the circulating blood volume by aggressive fluid treatment. Both colloids and crystalloids (saline 0.9%) can be used. Adults are given saline starting with 1 L infused intravenously over 15 to 20 minutes, followed by several liters at a reduced rate. Some patients require two to three times their own blood volume during the first 24 hours. The total fluid volume needed per 24 hours is determined by response to treatment—tissue perfusion, blood pressure, urine output, and evidence of intravascular volume overload. The volume treatment may be combined with a vasopressor such as dopamine, norepinephrine, epinephrine, or dobutamine. Fluid treatment may be complicated in patients with reduced renal function. They may need dialysis or hemofiltration to compensate for renal failure and to reduce the substantial edema that accumulates.

Patients with meningitis or mild meningococcemia should be given the normal daily fluid requirement, supplemented with the volume lost before admission. Excessive volume treatment in patients with meningitis can induce fatal brain edema and herniation. Management of raised intracranial pressure (hyperosmolar solutions, diuretics, mechanical ventilation), seizures, and hyponatremia is indicated.

Anticoagulant treatment of patients with meningococcemia and disseminated intravascular coagulation has not been documented to improve outcome. A phase III study of recombinant activated protein C in children with sepsis of all causes, including meningococcemia, was stopped because no benefit was noted.[2] Administration of activated protein C is associated with an increased risk of cerebral hemorrhage. The use of recombinant human tissue plasminogen activator does not appear to be beneficial. Randomized controlled clinical trials using hyperimmune serum, antibodies, or recombinant bactericidal or permeability-increasing protein designed to inactivate *N. meningitidis* endotoxin have not demonstrated a beneficial effect on survival. Blockade of other specific inflammatory mediators has not been adequately tested in meningococcal septic shock.

Patients with fulminant meningococcal septicemia can develop adrenal hemorrhage (Waterhouse-Friderichsen syndrome). The corticotropin concentration is higher, the cortisol concentration is lower, and the corticotropin to cortisol ratio is higher in patients with fatal meningococcal shock than in survivors. Adults with septic shock and indications of inadequate adrenal function are given low doses of steroids.[3] Although the benefit has not been documented in children, many intensive care specialists use stress replacement doses of hydrocortisone in children with shock caused by *N. meningitidis*.

Plasmapheresis, blood exchange, and extracorporeal membrane oxygenation have been used in patients with meningococcemia; however, no controlled trial to assess the results has been done. Plasmapheresis and blood exchange appear to have little additive effect on the endogenous clearance of endotoxin and cytokines from the circulation. Extracorporeal membrane oxygenation has been used in several centers, with better results in children with acute pulmonary failure than in those with refractory septic shock. The use of insulin to control mild hyperglycemia in critically ill adults has not shown benefits (Chapter 108).

Pharmacologic doses of dexamethasone have been shown to reduce morbidity in pneumococcal and *Haemophilus influenzae b* meningitis.[4] The use of dexamethasone to reduce death caused by brain edema or to prevent sequelae such as deafness in patients with meningococcal meningitis remains unproved based on randomized controlled trials, but large studies have not been performed, and its early use in suspected bacterial meningitis is a consideration.

PREVENTION

Chemoprophylaxis to eliminate meningococcal carriage is recommended for close contacts of patients to prevent further transmission and disease (Table 306-1). The occurrence of meningococcal disease in household contacts is approximately 100-fold higher than in the general population.

TABLE 306-1 **CHEMOPROPHYLAXIS AGAINST MENINGOCOCCAL DISEASE***

DRUG	AGE GROUP	DOSAGE	DURATION AND ROUTE OF ADMINISTRATION
Rifampin[†]	Children <1 mo	5 mg/kg body weight q12h	2 days, oral
	Children ≥1 mo	10 mg/kg body weight q12h	2 days, oral
	Adults	600 mg q12h	2 days, oral
Azithromycin	<15 yr	10 mg/kg body weight	Single oral dose
	>15 yr	500 mg	Single oral dose
Ceftriaxone	<15 yr	125 mg	Single IM dose
	>15 yr	250 mg	Single IM dose
Ciprofloxacin[‡]	Adults	500 mg	Single oral dose

*Modified from guidelines issued by the Centers for Disease Control and Prevention.
†Not recommended for pregnant women; teratogenic in laboratory animals. Because the reliability of oral contraceptives might be affected by rifampin therapy, consider alternative contraceptive measures while rifampin is being administered. Secretions (e.g., tears) may be stained red.
‡Not usually recommended for persons younger than 18 years or for pregnant or lactating women because it causes cartilage damage in immature laboratory animals; however, it may be considered for chemoprophylaxis in children when no acceptable alternative is available. Note that meningococcal resistance to quinolones has been reported in the United States, India, and other locations.
IM = intramuscular.

Chemoprophylaxis can be helpful to control localized outbreaks in residential schools and barracks, but it is generally not recommended for the control of large epidemics (see the discussion of vaccines, later). Rifampin, ceftriaxone, azithromycin, and quinolones (but not penicillin) all have the ability to eradicate meningococci in the nasopharynx. Most meningococci are now resistant to sulfonamides; resistance to rifampin can develop rapidly, and quinolone resistance in meningococci is occurring.

Prevention through vaccination is the best option for the long-term control of meningococcal disease. Capsular polysaccharide vaccines to decrease serogroup A, C, Y, and W-135 meningococcal disease were introduced in the 1970s and 1980s. These vaccines are safe, with mild local adverse events; they are effective (>85%) in children older than 2 years and adults but are less immunogenic in younger children. Immunity to the polysaccharide vaccines is limited to 3 to 5 years of protection, and immunologic hyporesponsiveness is induced by repeated doses of the polysaccharide. Meningococcal polysaccharide vaccines do not induce immunologic memory and have little or no effect on nasopharyngeal carriage. Although these vaccines have been used extensively to control epidemics in the African meningitis belt, they are usually deployed too late in the course of an outbreak to achieve maximal effect. There is no evidence that widespread use of polysaccharide vaccines has reduced the frequency of epidemics in Africa.

A major advance in the past decade has been the development of meningococcal polysaccharide-protein conjugate vaccines and their introduction into the United Kingdom, other parts of Europe, Canada, Australia, and the United States.**5** These vaccines are safe and immunogenic in young children, induce immunologic memory, and can decrease nasopharyngeal carriage of meningococci. In the United Kingdom, introduction of the C conjugate meningococcal vaccine in 2000 to all children and young adults greatly reduced the rate of serogroup C disease (90% vaccine effectiveness at 3 years for patients aged 11 to 18 years). A major protective effect of the C conjugate vaccine is mediated through herd immunity. Rates of serogroup C carriage and disease in nonvaccinated individuals were reduced by more than 50%. Serogroup A, C, Y, and W-135 polysaccharide-protein conjugate meningococcal vaccines were introduced for adolescents in the United States in 2005 and extended to children aged 2 to 10 years at increased risk for meningococcal disease. In addition to children and adolescents, populations that should benefit from the new conjugate vaccines are military recruits, patients with immunoglobulin or complement deficiencies (inherited or chronic deficiencies such as C3, properdin, factor D, or late complement components), anatomic or functional asplenia, microbiologists who are routinely exposed to isolates of *N. meningitidis*, and people who travel to or reside in countries where *N. meningitidis* is epidemic. The development of additional meningococcal conjugate vaccines holds great promise for controlling meningococcal disease in highly endemic and epidemic areas (e.g., sub-Saharan Africa), where serogroup A, C, and W-135 epidemics continue to occur. Further, serogroup X outbreaks have recently appeared in Africa.

The development of vaccines for serogroup B *N. meningitidis* remains a challenge. Serogroup B has caused prolonged outbreaks, such as those seen over the past 2 decades in the Pacific Northwest (Oregon, parts of Washington), Brazil, Norway, and New Zealand. The serogroup B capsule has an identical structure to polysialic structures expressed in fetal neural tissue and does not induce a protective bactericidal immunoglobulin G response. Thus, strategies are focused on noncapsular antigens, such as outer membrane proteins and vesicles and lipo-oligosaccharides. The diversity of major outer membrane structures in meningococci has limited these approaches, but success in controlling serogroup B epidemics that are strain specific (e.g., in New Zealand), the identification of conserved novel surface proteins for use in combination vaccines, and the discovery of novel group B capsule-specific epitopes are paths for new vaccines to prevent serogroup B meningococcal disease.

PROGNOSIS

Historically, the mortality of untreated systemic meningococcal disease was 70 to 90%. Despite highly effective antibiotics and aggressive supportive care, the mortality of invasive meningococcal disease remains at about 10%. The failure to recognize disease early and the very rapid development of disease, especially meningococcemia, remain the most significant challenges. The chance of surviving shock is directly correlated to plasma concentrations of endotoxin, and half the nonsurviving patients with shock die within the first 12 hours of hospital admission.

Morbidity includes limb loss (single amputation, 2%; multiple amputations, 1%), hearing loss (≈9%), and significant long-term neurologic disability (>2%), including cognitive dysfunction, visual impairment, educational difficulties, developmental delays, motor nerve deficits, seizure disorders, and behavioral problems. If parents and health care professionals recognize the importance of fever and headache with a nonblanching rash and seek treatment early, morbidity and mortality can be reduced with prehospital antibiotic treatment, rapid transportation to medical facilities, and stabilization in an intensive care unit. Prevention of meningococcal disease with new vaccines and vaccine strategies remains the major worldwide goal.

1. Nathan N, Borel T, Djibo A, et al. Ceftriaxone as effective as long-acting chloramphenicol in short-course treatment of meningococcal meningitis during epidemics: a randomised non-inferiority study. *Lancet.* 2005;366:308-313.
2. Nadel S, Goldstein B, Williams MD, et al. Drotrecogin alfa (activated) in children with severe sepsis: a multicentre phase III randomised controlled trial. *Lancet.* 2007;369:836-843.
3. Annane D, Sébille V, Charpentier C, et al. Effect of treatment with low doses of hydrocortisone and fluorocortisone on mortality in patients with septic shock. *JAMA.* 2002;288:862-871.
4. de Gans J, van de Beek D, European Dexamethasone in Adulthood Bacterial Meningitis Study Investigators. Dexamethasone in adults with bacterial meningitis. *N Engl J Med.* 2002;347:1549-1556.
5. Centers for Disease Control and Prevention (CDC). Updated recommendations for use of meningococcal conjugate vaccines—Advisory Committee on Immunization Practices (ACIP), 2010. *MMWR Morb Mortal Wkly Rep.* 2011;60:72-76.

SUGGESTED READINGS

Brouwer MC, Read RC, van de Beek D. Host genetics and outcome in meningococcal disease: a systematic review and meta-analysis. *Lancet Infect Dis.* 2010;10:262-274. *A clear association exists.*
Bryant CE, Spring DR, Gangloff M, et al. The molecular basis of the host response to lipopolysaccharide. *Nat Rev Microbiol.* 2010;8:9. *Review of endotoxin and host interactions.*
CDC. Emergence of fluoroquinolone-resistant *Neisseria meningitidis*—Minnesota and North Dakota, 2007-2008. *MMWR.* 2008;57:173-175. *Emergence of quinolone resistance in meningococci.*
Chamot-Rooke J, Mikaty G, Malosse C, et al. Posttranslational modification of pili upon cell contact triggers *N. meningitidis* dissemination. *Science.* 2011;331:778-782. *Molecular mechanisms of colonization and dissemination.*
Harrison LH. Epidemiological profile of meningococcal disease in the United States. *Clin Infect Dis.* 2010;50:S37-S44. *Review of epidemiology and how vaccines are changing it.*
Tan LK, Carlone GM, Borrow R. Advances in the development of vaccines against *Neisseria meningitidis. N Engl J Med.* 2010;362:1511-1520. *Review.*
Virji M. Pathogenic neisseriae: surface modulation, pathogenesis and infection control. *Nat Rev Microbiol.* 2009;7:274-286. *Cell surface modulation and niche establishment as challenges to Neisseria vaccine development.*

307

NEISSERIA GONORRHOEAE INFECTIONS

MATTHEW R. GOLDEN AND H. HUNTER HANDSFIELD

DEFINITION

Neisseria gonorrhoeae is a sexually transmitted organism that infects primarily the columnar epithelia of mucosal surfaces and causes urethritis in men and endocervicitis and urethritis in women. Other sites of primary infection include the rectum, pharynx, and conjunctiva, and vulvovaginitis can occur in prepubertal girls. The most common complication of gonococcal infection is pelvic inflammatory disease (PID), which can lead to infertility, ectopic pregnancy, and chronic pelvic pain. Other much less common complications include epididymitis, posterior urethritis, urethral stricture, Bartholin's gland abscess, and perihepatitis. Bacteremia may occur, with the production of characteristic cutaneous lesions, arthritis, and, rarely, endocarditis or meningitis. Neonatal conjunctivitis (ophthalmia neonatorum) was formerly a common cause of blindness. Gonococcal infections are also thought to increase the risk of human immunodeficiency virus (HIV) transmission from persons dually infected with HIV and *N. gonorrhoeae* and to increase the risk of HIV acquisition among persons with gonorrhea who are exposed to HIV.

The Pathogen

The gonococcal envelope is similar in its basic structure to that of other gram-negative bacteria and is composed of an inner cytoplasmic membrane, a middle peptidoglycan cell wall, and an outer membrane. The outer membrane contains several surface components that play a central role in the organism's interaction with the host and its pathogenicity. Pili, hair-like projections also referred to as fimbriae, are composed of several different protein subunits and, along with other outer membrane adhesins (i.e., opacity-related proteins), facilitate attachment and invasion of host cells. Gonococci vary the composition of these proteins and surface lipo-oligosaccharides over time, allowing the organism to elude host defenses. This phase variation has also been a barrier to successful vaccine development.

EPIDEMIOLOGY

Gonorrhea is the second most commonly reported infectious disease in the United States, with 336,742 cases reported to the Centers for Disease Control and Prevention (CDC) in 2008. The incidence of gonorrhea in the United States in 2008 was 111.6 per 100,000 population, although this number, which is based on cases reported to U.S. health departments, is certainly an underestimate. The overall incidence of gonorrhea in the United States has been relatively stable for more than a decade, and current rates are more than 70% lower than the incidence observed in the mid-1970s. The prevalence of gonorrhea varies widely, depending on the population tested. The Ad Health study tested a representative sample of U.S. 18- to 26-year-olds in 2001 and 2002 and found that 0.43% were infected, with wide variations geographically and among population groups. Among women aged 15 to 24 tested for gonorrhea in family planning clinics in 43 U.S. states and territories in 2008, the overall prevalence of gonorrhea was 0.9%, but it varied from 0 to 3.8%. By comparison, the prevalence of chlamydial infection in the Ad Health study was 4.19%, and among 15- to 24-year-old females tested in U.S. family planning clinics in 2008, it was 7.4% (range, 3.1 to 15%).

Like virtually all other sexually transmitted infections (STIs; Chapter 293), gonorrhea rates vary widely with age, geographic location, sexual orientation, and race or ethnicity. In the United States, the rate of reported infection is highest among 15- to 24-year-olds, and rates in the South are more than twice those observed in the West and Northeast. However, the most glaring disparities are observed when comparing rates of infection among different racial and ethnic groups and when comparing heterosexuals to men who have sex with men (MSM).

Rates of reported gonorrhea among U.S. African Americans are more than 20 times higher than those among non-Hispanic whites, and rates among American Indians/Alaska Natives and Hispanics are 3.6 and 2.2 higher, respectively, than those among non-Hispanic whites. Variations in reporting probably account for some of these observed differences, because low socioeconomic status is associated with receiving care in public health clinics and other venues where there is more complete reporting than in the private health care sector. However, the marked disparity in reported rates is also apparent in population-based studies, clearly establishing that the different rates of infection in different racial and ethnic groups are not simply a result of reporting bias. The reasons for this profound disparity are certainly multifactorial and are not entirely clear. Different racial groups in the United States vary little in terms of their number of sex partners, so this cannot explain the different rates of STIs. Although inadequate access to medical care likely plays a role in the racial disparities in STI rates, profound racial and ethnic disparities are also observed in the United Kingdom and the Netherlands, nations with nationalized health care systems in which access to care should be more uniform than it is in the United States. Recent research has highlighted the importance of concurrency (i.e., partnerships that overlap in time) and patterns of sexual mixing based on age, race, and level of sexual activity as critical determinants of a population's risk of STI. These factors are thought to be shaped by social factors (e.g., poverty, incarceration, joblessness, racism) that play a central role in defining the epidemiology of all STIs worldwide.

Gonorrhea also disproportionately affects gay and bisexual men and other MSM. Numerous cities in the United States, western Europe, and Australia have reported increases in the rate and number of gonorrhea cases among MSM since the mid-1990s.

Gonorrhea is highly transmissible. Though not precisely defined, the risk of transmission from a man to a woman during a single episode of unprotected vaginal intercourse is thought to be 50 to 70%, and the risk of transmission from a woman to a man is 20%. The transmission risks associated with anal sex, fellatio, or cunnilingus are not well defined, but anal intercourse is likely a relatively efficient mode of transmission. Gonococci die rapidly on drying, and with the exception of occasional acquisition by laboratory personnel working with the organism, nonsexual transmission does not occur in adults. Perinatal transmission causing neonatal ophthalmitis or pharyngeal infection is now rare.

PATHOBIOLOGY

Following attachment to host epithelial cells, gonococci are endocytosed into the cell in a process thought to be facilitated by Por (or protein 1). Gonococci then replicate within the host cell and are released into the subepithelial space.

Typical urethral infections result in prominent inflammation, probably as a result of the release of toxic lipo-oligosaccharide and peptidoglycan fragments, as well as the release of chemotactic factors that attract neutrophilic leukocytes. The reasons why some gonococcal strains selectively cause asymptomatic genital infection are poorly understood, but this propensity may be related to differences in the organism's ability to bind complement-regulatory proteins that downregulate the production of chemotactic peptides. In particular, gonococcal strains that express PorB1A appear to bind factor H and complement-binding protein and have an increased propensity for causing disseminated gonococcal infections.

Although the gonococcus is not highly mutable, many gonococci possess conjugative plasmids and are consequently able to efficiently transfer other, nontransferable plasmids, such as those conferring resistance to penicillin and tetracycline. Gonococci are also capable of efficiently transferring naked DNA (transformation). These characteristics are important in the organism's ability to develop resistance to antimicrobials.

CLINICAL MANIFESTATIONS

Gonococcal infections can result in a number of specific clinical syndromes, each of which has its own manifestations, differential diagnosis, and recommended evaluation. The major clinical manifestations of gonococcal infection are discussed separately later. Gonococcal ophthalmia, which occasionally results from autoinoculation in individuals with anogenital gonorrhea, presents as an acute, purulent conjunctivitis that can result in corneal ulceration if not treated promptly. This syndrome is now rare and is not discussed further.

DIAGNOSIS

Microscopy

Microscopy of a Gram-stained smear is positive when polymorphonuclear neutrophils are observed to contain intracellular gram-negative diplococci of typical morphology (Fig. 307-1). Gram-stained urethral smears are 90 to 98% sensitive in the diagnosis of symptomatic gonococcal urethritis in men and have a specificity greater than 95%. However, Gram stain is only approximately 50% sensitive for cervical or rectal infection and for asymptomatic urethral gonorrhea. Although Gram stain is often considered highly specific for such infections, the actual performance varies with the skill and experience of the examiner, and rectal and cervical smears are

FIGURE 307-1. Histopathology in an acute case of gonococcal urethritis with Gram stain technique. This slide is used to demonstrate the nonrandom distribution of gonococci among polymorphonuclear neutrophils. Note that there are both intracellular and extracellular bacteria in the field of view.

unreliable in many clinical settings. Smears are both insensitive and nonspecific for pharyngeal gonococcal infection and are not recommended.

Culture

Isolation of *N. gonorrhoeae* by culture, generally using antibiotic-containing selective media, is the historic mainstay of the diagnosis of gonorrhea. Ideally, growth media should be inoculated directly and placed promptly into a humid atmosphere with increased carbon dioxide, such as a candle extinction jar. However, standard transport systems (e.g., Culturette) are acceptable if specimens are kept moist, are not refrigerated, and are processed within 6 hours. When testing specimens not likely to be colonized by competing flora (e.g., synovial fluid), nonselective chocolate agar should be used.

Nucleic Acid Amplification Tests

In most settings in the United States, nucleic acid amplification tests (NAATs) have now supplanted culture as the dominant laboratory test used to diagnose gonorrhea. NAATs approved by the Food and Drug Administration (FDA) include polymerase chain reaction (PCR), transcription-mediated amplification (TMA), and DNA strand displacement (SDA). The advantages of NAATs include a slight increase in sensitivity over culture, the ability to test urine specimens and self-obtained vaginal swabs, and the fact that most NAATs are now marketed as combination assays that allow simultaneous testing for *N. gonorrhoeae* and *Chlamydia trachomatis*. The disadvantages of NAATs include the inability to perform antimicrobial susceptibility testing and the poor or inadequately defined positive predictive value of some NAATs when used to test low-prevalence populations. Because the prevalence of *N. gonorrhoeae* in family planning clinics in many parts of the United States and other nations is now well below 1%, the risk of false-positive screening results may be high, and reliable results depend on the use of assays with exquisite specificity. Existing evidence suggests that TMA has a high positive predictive value even in very low-prevalence settings, and the Roche PCR has a low positive predictive value when used as a screening test in low-prevalence populations; the positive predictive value of SDA is not well defined.

Although NAATs have been approved by the FDA only for the testing of genital tract and urine specimens, increasing evidence suggests that at least some NAATs (e.g., TMA, SDA) are substantially more sensitive than culture in detecting *N. gonorrhoeae* in pharyngeal and rectal specimens and that these NAATs are sufficiently specific to screen high-risk populations for rectal and pharyngeal gonorrhea (owing to low specificity, the Roche PCR should not be used to test rectal or pharyngeal specimens). Given the decreasing availability of gonococcal culture, the poor sensitivity of culture on non–genital tract specimens, and the high prevalence of asymptomatic rectal and pharyngeal infections in some populations (particularly MSM), clinicians caring for patients at high risk for nongenital gonococcal infections should be able to use NAATs. Recent studies suggest that self-obtained rectal and pharyngeal specimens yield accurate results and are acceptable to MSM.

● CLINICAL SYNDROMES
Urogenital Gonorrhea in Males

CLINICAL MANIFESTATIONS AND DIAGNOSIS

Gonococcal urethritis in men is typically characterized by a purulent urethral discharge and dysuria. The usual incubation period is 2 to 6 days. A small minority of men who acquire urethral infection—generally estimated at 1 to 10%, and varying with the auxotype or serotype of the infecting strain—remain asymptomatic.

Physical examination typically reveals a purulent urethral exudate (Fig. 307-2); this is usually readily apparent, but sometimes compression of the urethra is required to express the exudate. Erythema of the meatus is sometimes present. Nongonococcal urethritis (Chapter 293) is typically characterized by less copious and less purulent discharge.

The diagnosis of gonococcal urethritis is usually suspected clinically, confirmed preliminarily by a Gram-stained smear showing leukocytes with intracellular gram-negative diplococci (see Fig. 307-1), and made definitively when *N. gonorrhoeae* is identified by culture or NAAT.

PROGNOSIS

With prompt treatment, urethral gonorrhea seldom results in significant long-term morbidity. Acute epididymitis complicates gonococcal urethritis

FIGURE 307-2. Male with a purulent penile discharge from gonorrhea and an overlying penile pyodermal lesion. Pyoderma involves the formation of a purulent skin lesion, which in this case is located on the glans penis.

in less than 1% of cases. Patients with epididymitis usually present with unilateral testicular pain and swelling, often with fever. Posterior urethritis or prostatitis, typically manifesting as pelvic or perineal pain and urinary retention, was once fairly common but is now rare. Urethral stricture, another formerly common complication, is now very rare. Although it is not a direct effect of gonorrhea, having gonorrhea is associated with an elevated risk of future HIV acquisition among MSM, so the diagnosis of gonorrhea should alert clinicians to counsel such patients about their sexual risk and to encourage them to seek frequent HIV testing.

Lower Genital Tract Gonorrhea in Females

CLINICAL MANIFESTATIONS, DIAGNOSIS, AND PROGNOSIS

The primary site of infection in women is the endocervical canal. The proportion of infected women who develop symptoms is not precisely known, although one study of 19 recently infected women found that 50% had symptoms. More certain, however, is that most prevalent infections among women are asymptomatic. Although gonorrhea is sometimes associated with an abnormal vaginal discharge, bacterial vaginosis, trichomonas vaginitis, and candidal vaginitis are much more common causes of this symptom, and gonorrhea does not cause vaginitis in sexually mature women. Lower genital tract gonorrhea in women can be associated with abnormal vaginal bleeding, which typically manifests as metrorrhagia, scant intermenstrual bleeding, or postcoital spotting. *N. gonorrhoeae* sometimes causes dysuria and can be isolated from the urethra in up to 80% of women with gonorrhea; however, the urethra is rarely the only infected site, except in women who have had hysterectomies. In a minority of women, physical examination is notable for a purulent or mucopurulent cervical discharge, cervical edema, or easily induced cervical bleeding, signs of mucopurulent cervicitis. In uncomplicated infections, purulent exudate can sometimes be expressed from a Bartholin's gland duct, near the vaginal introitus laterally, or from Skene's glands, adjacent to the urethral meatus.

Microbiologic diagnosis usually rests on identifying *N. gonorrhoeae* in cervical secretions by culture or NAAT. Gram-stained smears are insensitive and are seldom used.

The most important common complication of lower genital tract gonorrhea in women is PID (see later). Much rarer complications include Bartholin's gland abscess, which manifests as a tender introital mass and may involve superinfection with facultative and anaerobic bacteria.

Pelvic Inflammatory Disease

CLINICAL MANIFESTATIONS

PID refers to an infection of the lower female genital tract and can involve the uterus (endometritis), fallopian tubes (salpingitis), and ovaries (oophoritis), as well as neighboring pelvic structures. An estimated 10 to 40% of women with endocervical gonococcal infections develop PID, and gonorrhea is thought to be the cause of approximately 10 to 30% of all diagnosed cases of PID in the United States, although this percentage varies with overall rates of gonorrhea and other (e.g., chlamydial) infections in the population.

Low abdominal pain is the dominant symptom of PID. Pain is variable in intensity and is often mild; it is usually bilateral, typically present for days to weeks before clinical presentation, and can be exacerbated by coitus. Symptoms often coincide with the onset or cessation of menses. Approximately one third of women have abnormal vaginal bleeding. Fever, chills, anorexia, vaginal discharge, urethritis, and proctitis occur, but they are neither sensitive nor specific in identifying women with PID.

The physical examination is typically notable for diffuse abdominal tenderness that is greatest in the lower quadrants and for tenderness of the pelvic organs on bimanual examination, with or without manipulation of the cervix. Most women have signs of cervicitis or bacterial vaginosis. Fever is present in a minority of cases. Abdominal or adnexal signs are occasionally unilateral, and this finding can cause confusion with appendicitis (Chapter 144), ectopic pregnancy, and other conditions. Right upper quadrant abdominal tenderness is sometimes present due to Fitz-Hugh-Curtis syndrome, in which intra-abdominal extension of infection results in perihepatitis, which can mimic acute cholecystitis or viral hepatitis. Sometimes perihepatitis occurs in the absence of other abdominal or pelvic findings typical of PID, especially when caused by *C. trachomatis*. Severe PID may be accompanied by signs of generalized peritonitis.

DIAGNOSIS

The clinical diagnosis of PID is imprecise. Published studies, which have used somewhat variable criteria in populations with different prevalences of the syndrome, have reported positive predictive values of 65 to 95% compared with the "gold standard" of laparoscopically defined PID. Although nonspecific, the presence of neutrophils on a saline wet mount of vaginal secretions was 91% sensitive for endometritis in one study. The absence of white blood cells on a wet mount, particularly if mucopurulent cervicitis is also absent, should prompt the consideration of alternative diagnoses. The differential diagnosis of PID includes ectopic pregnancy; appendicitis; rupture, bleeding, or torsion of an ovarian cyst; endometriosis; urinary tract infection or pyelonephritis; renal or ureteral stones; inflammatory bowel disease; and, rarely, viral hepatitis or cholecystitis.

Because of the potential seriousness of the infection and the relative simplicity, low cost, and low toxicity of treatment, clinical diagnostic criteria emphasize sensitivity at the cost of specificity. The CDC recommends that all sexually active women with pelvic or lower abdominal pain and uterine, adnexal, or cervical motion tenderness be treated for possible PID if no other cause for their symptoms and signs is readily apparent. Factors such as fever, an elevated erythrocyte sedimentation rate or C-reactive protein, and concurrent bacterial vaginosis or mucopurulent cervicitis further support the clinical diagnosis, but these are frequently absent. Definitive diagnosis requires histologic evidence of endometritis on endometrial biopsy, transvaginal ultrasound or other diagnostic imaging showing thickened or fluid-filled fallopian tubes or tubo-ovarian abscess, or laparoscopic findings of a purulent tubal exudate, erythema, or edema.

PROGNOSIS

Fallopian tube scarring secondary to PID often results in tubal factor infertility (TFI), ectopic pregnancy, and chronic pelvic pain. Previous gonococcal and chlamydial infections are among the most common antecedents of these complications. Each episode of PID, whether due to *N. gonorrhoeae*, *C. trachomatis*, or neither of these organisms, significantly increases the risk for recurrent salpingitis.

The natural history of clinically apparent PID is well defined. In what is probably the best single study on the subject, TFI occurred in 8% of women following a single episode of laparoscopically proved PID, in 20% after two such episodes, and in 40% after three or more episodes. The first pregnancy after an episode of PID was ectopic in almost 8% of women, and like TFI, the risk of ectopic pregnancy increased with each successive episode of the syndrome. Chronic pelvic pain, sometimes disabling in its severity, occurs in almost 20% of women after one or more episodes of PID. Importantly, these outcomes were best studied in women with clinically apparent PID, and the pertinent studies were undertaken at a time when clinical recognition and treatment were likely delayed. Many women suffer clinically mild or silent PID. The risk of sequelae associated with silent PID is not well defined, but more clinically severe PID is associated with a higher risk of sequelae. Most women with TFI deny a history of PID, and it seems likely that silent PID, particularly silent PID associated with *C. trachomatis*, is responsible for most cases of severe STI-related reproductive tract sequelae. For example, *C. trachomatis* seropositivity is strongly associated with TFI, independent of clinical or historical evidence of PID.

Rectal Infection

CLINICAL MANIFESTATIONS

Gonococcal infection of the rectum is common in women and in MSM. In women, infection is acquired either through perineal contamination with cervicovaginal secretions or by anal intercourse; the latter is the exclusive route of infection in MSM. In women with cervical gonorrhea and in MSM with gonorrhea at any anatomic site, about 40% have rectal infection. More than 80% of infections are subclinical, but symptomatic proctitis sometimes manifests as varying combinations of anal pruritus, mucopurulent discharge (often characterized by the patient as mucus-coated feces), pain, tenesmus, and bleeding. Symptomatic proctitis seems to be more common in MSM than in women with rectal gonorrhea, which suggests that the size of the infecting inoculum or the trauma of anal intercourse may influence the clinical manifestations. Among MSM, rectal gonorrhea, particularly recurrent episodes, is a potent risk factor for the acquisition of HIV.

DIAGNOSIS

Diagnosis of rectal gonorrhea depends on the identification of *N. gonorrhoeae* by culture or, increasingly, by NAAT. The Gram-stained smear is insensitive and nonspecific. The differential diagnosis of symptomatic proctitis includes other traditional STIs, (herpes, syphilis, and chlamydial infection, including lymphogranuloma venereum; Chapter 326), as well as ulcerative colitis, Crohn's colitis, anal fissure, rectal lacerations, and proctocolitis caused by *Shigella, Campylobacter, Yersinia enterocolitica*, and other enteric pathogens. Recent studies using NAAT among STI clinic patients suggest that approximately 5% of tested MSM and 1% of tested women have rectal infections without concurrent genital tract infections, findings that support the routine screening of MSM, but not women, for rectal gonorrhea.

Pharyngeal Infection

CLINICAL MANIFESTATIONS

Pharyngeal gonococcal infection results from orogenital exposure. It is more efficiently acquired by fellatio than by cunnilingus and is typically found in 3 to 7% of heterosexual men, 10 to 30% of women, and 10 to 30% of MSM with genital tract gonorrhea. Asymptomatic infection is the rule, although rare cases may exhibit exudative pharyngitis and cervical lymphadenopathy. Isolated pharyngeal infection is common is MSM and may also be common in at least some populations of heterosexuals. Complications are infrequent, and most cases resolve spontaneously or in response to therapy for genital or rectal infection. Although the modest morbidity associated with pharyngeal infections probably does not justify extensive screening efforts, the oropharynx may be an important reservoir for infection in some populations, particularly MSM. Current guidelines suggest that MSM at risk for STIs be tested periodically for pharyngeal gonorrhea.

Gonorrhea in Children

Gonococcal conjunctivitis may develop in infants born to mothers with gonorrhea, a condition termed *ophthalmia neonatorum*. Formerly a common cause of blindness, gonococcal ophthalmia is now rare in industrialized countries because of both improved control of gonorrhea and routine use of neonatal ocular prophylaxis with topical antibiotics or 1% silver nitrate. Neonates may also acquire pharyngeal or rectal infection and, rarely, gonococcal pneumonia or sepsis. Beyond the neonatal period, purulent vaginitis is the most common manifestation of gonorrhea or chlamydial infection in girls, and rectal or pharyngeal infection is the most common manifestation in prepubertal boys. Most cases are acquired through sexual abuse, but occasional cases in young children may be acquired from fomites or by nonsexual personal exposure in crowded conditions, especially in tropical climates.

Disseminated Gonococcal Infection

CLINICAL MANIFESTATIONS

Disseminated gonococcal infection (DGI) usually manifests with various combinations of polyarticular tenosynovitis, dermatitis secondary to focal septic embolization, and septic arthritis. Studies undertaken in the 1960s and

1970s estimated that DGI occurred in 1 to 3% of adults with gonorrhea, but the risk depends on characteristics of the particular strains of *N. gonorrhoeae* circulating in the population. Today, DGI probably occurs in well under 1% of gonococcal infections in most geographic areas. Women may be somewhat more susceptible to DGI than men, and the onset often coincides with menstruation. Severity varies from a mild illness with slight joint discomfort, a few skin lesions, and little or no fever to a fulminant illness with overt polyarthritis, innumerable skin lesions, high fever, and prostration. Most persons with DGI have no symptoms of genital gonorrhea, probably because the strains of *N. gonorrhoeae* that are prone to disseminate are also associated with subclinical mucosal infections. The absence of clinical symptoms and signs of mucosal infection in these strains is probably due to their ability to bind complement downregulatory molecules, thereby diminishing the local inflammatory response.

The presentation of DGI can be divided into the clinical syndromes of tenosynovitis-dermatitis or mono- or oligoarticular arthritis, although these presentations sometimes overlap. Tenosynovitis-dermatitis is thought to predominate early in the course of dissemination, and approximately 70% of DGI cases in published series present with this syndrome. These patients usually suffer migratory polyarthralgias without purulent arthritis. There is often tendon inflammation affecting the wrists, fingers, ankles, or toes. Skin lesions are typically painless, are few in number (5 to 30), affect predominantly the extremities, and are pustular or vesiculopustular (Fig. 307-3), although petechiae, hemorrhagic macules, papules, bullae, and nodules rarely occur (see Fig. 449-5 in Chapter 449). Axial skeletal involvement is uncommon, a feature that can help differentiate DGI from reactive arthritis (Chapter 273). The tenosynovitis-dermatitis syndrome often subsides spontaneously, or it may evolve over a period of several days into an overt septic arthritis with purulent synovial fluid, usually involving only one or two joints. Approximately 30 to 40% of persons with DGI present initially with purulent oligoarthritis. A sequential evolution from arthritis-dermatitis syndrome is often not observed, so some patients present initially with septic arthritis. This form of DGI typically affects the knee, ankle, elbow, or wrist, but any joint may be involved.

FIGURE 307-3. Cutaneous gonococcal lesion secondary to disseminated *Neisseria gonorrhoeae* infection. Although gonorrhea is a sexually transmitted disease, if it remains untreated, the *N. gonorrhoeae* bacteria responsible for the infection can disseminate throughout the body and form lesions in extragenital locations (also see Fig. 449-5 in Chapter 449).

DIAGNOSIS

Sexually active young persons with arthritis, tenosynovitis, or papulopustular skin lesions should be tested for *N. gonorrhoeae* at all potentially exposed anatomic sites. The diagnosis of DGI is secure when gonococci are identified by culture or NAAT in the blood, a skin lesion, or synovial fluid, but it is often made presumptively when genital, rectal, or pharyngeal gonorrhea is present in a patient with a compatible clinical syndrome that responds promptly to antibiotics.

Blood, synovial fluid, and mucosal tract cultures are positive in approximately 4 to 35%, 10 to 34%, and 80% of patients, respectively. However, the yield from culture varies with the clinical presentation. The performance of NAAT versus culture has not been studied in patients with DGI. Patients with tenosynovitis-dermatitis more frequently have bacteremia, whereas patients with septic gonococcal arthritis are seldom bacteremic, and close to 50% have positive synovial fluid cultures; it is reasonable to suspect that the yield might be higher with NAAT. Because bacteremia is intermittent, clinicians should obtain more than one set of blood cultures to maximize the likelihood of isolating the organism. Similarly, culture or NAAT should be obtained from all potentially exposed anatomic sites (genital tract, pharynx, rectum). Cultures of skin lesions are generally negative despite demonstrable gonococci by fluorescent antibody, but NAATs may be positive in persons with negative blood and mucosal site cultures. The peripheral blood leukocyte count is generally elevated but may be normal. The synovial fluid leukocyte count is usually 20,000 to 60,000/mm^3, with higher numbers of white cells seen in persons with clinically apparent arthritis than in those with tenosynovitis-dermatitis. Liver function tests often show elevations in aminotransferase levels, suggestive of mild hepatitis.

The differential diagnosis of DGI includes reactive arthritis (Chapter 273), meningococcemia (Chapter 306), other kinds of septic arthritis (Chapter 280), rheumatoid arthritis (Chapter 272), systemic lupus erythematosus (Chapter 274), acute HIV (Chapter 393), syphilis (Chapter 327), and other rheumatologic conditions and infectious diseases. Reactive arthritis, often triggered by sexually acquired chlamydial infection, is the principal consideration in young adults. The skin lesions of the two conditions, when present, are generally distinct and often pathognomonic for one syndrome or the other. In addition, conjunctivitis and involvement of the axial skeleton (e.g., sacroiliitis) are common in Reiter's syndrome and infrequent in DGI.

PROGNOSIS

Endocarditis, meningitis, and myocarditis have been reported in 0 to 10% of DGI case series. Gonococcal endocarditis usually involves the aortic valve and often progresses rapidly, leading to valve destruction and heart failure. Many cases of arthritis-dermatitis syndrome resolve spontaneously, but untreated septic arthritis can lead to contiguous osteomyelitis or joint destruction.

PREVENTION

Control of gonorrhea depends on prompt diagnosis and effective treatment of infected persons, screening of sexually active women and MSM in settings where gonorrhea is prevalent, treatment of patients' partners, rescreening of persons with a recent history of gonorrhea, and efforts to promote safer sexual behaviors (e.g., condom use, abstinence, fewer partners). Sexually active MSM outside of mutually monogamous relationships, including HIV-infected men, are at high risk for gonorrhea and should be tested at least annually for rectal and pharyngeal gonococcal infection and for other STIs. The value of screening asymptomatic males for urethral infection (by NAAT of urine) is uncertain; the yield is low in most settings. Gonococcal screening criteria for woman are not well defined. However, because virtually all current NAATs for *C. trachomatis* also test for gonorrhea, most young women tested for STIs are tested for gonorrhea.

Public education and personal counseling of persons with gonorrhea or at risk of contracting it should emphasize the effectiveness of mutual monogamy and condoms. Every patient with gonorrhea should be counseled about the risks for HIV infection and should be tested for HIV, *C. trachomatis,* and syphilis. Because accurate epidemiologic data are essential to generate and maintain resources for the prevention and control of STIs, all cases of gonorrhea, chlamydial infection, syphilis, and HIV infection should be promptly reported to the health department in accordance with local laws. Ultimate control of gonorrhea may require immunization, but no effective vaccine is on the horizon, despite intensive research for more than 4 decades.

TREATMENT

Antimicrobial Susceptibility

Gonococci with chromosomal or plasmid-borne mutations that confer relative or absolute resistance to the penicillins, tetracyclines, and sulfonamides are prevalent worldwide, and none of these drugs is acceptable as empirical therapy anywhere in the world. The prevalence of β-lactamase (penicillinase) plasmids, which confer absolute resistance to penicillin, ampicillin, and amoxicillin, varies from about 10% of gonococci in the United States and western Europe to almost 50% in some developing countries. Strains with relative resistance to some but not all cephalosporins are common in parts of Japan, and ongoing surveillance for cephalosporin resistance remains a high priority in all areas. All gonococci were highly susceptible to the fluoroquinolones when these drugs were introduced 3 decades ago, but resistant strains are now widespread. These agents were in common use in the United States until 2007, by which time 7% of gonococcal isolates obtained from heterosexual men and 36% of isolates from MSM in the CDC's Gonococcal Isolate Surveillance Project were resistant to ciprofloxacin. Approximately 5% of gonococcal isolates in the United Kingdom are azithromycin resistant, and azithromycin-resistant *N. gonorrhoeae* has recently been identified in the western United States, although such strains were rare as recently as 2008. Clinicians who treat patients for gonorrhea and other STIs should keep abreast of regional trends in resistance and be alert to modified therapeutic recommendations.

Principles of Treatment

Gonorrhea almost always responds to single-dose treatment with an appropriate antibiotic. Because of the need to curtail transmission, therapy is usually based on clinical or epidemiologic suspicion before the diagnosis is confirmed microbiologically. Even when *N. gonorrhoeae* is isolated by culture, antimicrobial susceptibility testing is generally not performed. Accordingly, routine treatment is dictated by local or regional patterns of antimicrobial susceptibility, without knowledge of susceptibility in individual patients. However, susceptibility testing should be used to guide the treatment of gonococcal septic arthritis, endocarditis, or other serious complications.

In North America, 5 to 10% of MSM, 15 to 25% of heterosexual men, and 35 to 50% of women with gonorrhea are also infected with *C. trachomatis,* so routine treatment of chlamydial infection is advised in addition to specific therapy for gonorrhea.

Treatment Regimens

Ceftriaxone, 250 mg intramuscularly, or cefixime, 400 mg orally, should be given as a single dose for uncomplicated gonorrhea (Table 307-1).**1** Cefpodoxime, 400 mg orally, and cefuroxime, 1 g orally, are also options, but they may be less effective than other regimens, particularly in the treatment of pharyngeal gonococcal infection. Because of the high prevalence of concurrent pharyngeal infection in women and in MSM, and because of concerns related to the possible increased number of *N. gonorrhoeae* isolates with decreased susceptibility to cephalosporins, ceftriaxone is the drug of choice for the routine treatment of gonorrhea. All persons with gonorrhea should routinely be treated with an oral regimen active against *C. trachomatis,* usually azithromycin in a single oral dose of 1 g or doxycycline 100 mg twice daily for 7 days. Such treatment is warranted even in persons who test negative for *C. trachomatis* because observational data suggest that dual therapy may enhance the efficacy of treatment for pharyngeal gonorrhea, and using more than one drug may retard the selection of antimicrobial resistance in *N. gonorrhoeae*. Azithromycin 2 g should be used in persons with β-lactam allergies.

Women with acute PID should be treated with antibiotics active against *N. gonorrhoeae, C. trachomatis,* and a broad range of facultative and anaerobic pathogens, regardless of whether gonococcal or chlamydial infection is documented. Suggested outpatient regimens include an intramuscular dose of a cephalosporin (ceftriaxone 250 mg or cefoxitin 1 g) and doxycycline 100 mg twice daily, with or without metronidazole (500 mg twice daily) for 14 days.**2** Although oral regimens containing levofloxacin (500 mg once daily) or ofloxacin (400 mg twice daily) plus metronidazole (500 mg twice daily) for 14 days were recommended in the past, the CDC no longer recommends these regimens because of quinolone-resistant *N. gonorrhoeae*. For hospitalized patients or others who require parenteral therapy, the CDC recommends intravenous cefotetan or cefoxitin plus oral doxycycline, or parenteral therapy with clindamycin plus gentamicin. Parenteral therapy is continued until improvement is observed, after which oral therapy is prescribed to complete 14 days' total treatment.

Most persons with DGI should be hospitalized and treated with a parenteral third-generation cephalosporin such as ceftriaxone, cefotaxime, or ceftizoxime, or with ciprofloxacin, ofloxacin, or levofloxacin if the infecting strain is known to be sensitive. Joint irrigation or drainage appears to be unnecessary for septic arthritis, although repeated aspiration of synovial fluid may speed clinical improvement. Oral treatment (e.g., cefixime, cefpodoxime, or a fluoroquinolone) can usually be substituted after improvement begins and then continued to complete 7 days' therapy. More prolonged parenteral treatment and higher doses are indicated for the treatment of gonococcal meningitis or

TABLE 307-1 ANTIBIOTIC REGIMENS FOR THE TREATMENT OF GONORRHEA IN THE UNITED STATES*

PREFERRED	ALTERNATIVE
UNCOMPLICATED GONORRHEA OF THE URETHRA, CERVIX, OR RECTUM	
Ceftriaxone 250 mg IM single dose	Cefpodoxime 400 mg PO single dose
Cefixime 400 mg PO single dose	Cefuroxime 1 g PO single dose
	Azithromycin 2 g PO single dose
	Ceftizoxime 500 mg IM single dose
	Cefotaxime 500 mg IM single dose
	Cefoxitin 2 g IM with probenecid 1 g PO
INFECTION OF THE PHARYNX	
Ceftriaxone 250 mg IM single dose	
CONJUNCTIVITIS (NOT OPHTHALMIA NEONATORUM)	
Ceftriaxone 1 g IM single dose	
DISSEMINATED GONOCOCCAL INFECTION	
Ceftriaxone 1 g IM or IV q24h[†]	Cefotaxime 1 g IV q8h
	Ceftizoxime 1 g IV q8h

*Treatment of gonorrhea in adults should always include treatment for chlamydial infection, treatment of sex partners, and advice to abstain from sex for 7 days.
[†]Treat with intravenous therapy until the patient has been clinically improved for 24 to 48 hours. Then switch to cefixime 400 mg orally twice a day to complete a 7-day course.

endocarditis, although modern data are lacking. Gonococcal epididymitis, bartholinitis, and other localized complications should generally be treated for 7 to 14 days with drugs active against both *N. gonorrhoeae* and *C. trachomatis*. Gonococcal conjunctivitis in adults can be managed with a single dose of ceftriaxone, 1 g intramuscularly, with optional saline lavage.

Management of Sex Partners

Failure to ensure treatment of patients' sex partners contributes to the continued transmission of gonorrhea and often results in reinfection of the index case. For gonorrhea and chlamydia, all partners in the preceding 2 months should be treated (if the patient has not had sex in the preceding 2 months, the most recent partner should be treated). Because very few U.S. health departments routinely make an effort to ensure that sex partners receive treatment, the responsibility lies jointly with the patient and the diagnosing clinician. Optimally, the partners of persons with gonorrhea should undergo diagnostic testing for gonorrhea, chlamydial infection, syphilis, and HIV infection. However, clinicians should not wait to obtain the results of diagnostic testing before treating a potentially exposed sex partner; all partners of infected persons should be treated when they initially present for evaluation.

In most settings, approximately 50% of potentially exposed sex partners are not treated. In an effort to address this problem, the CDC and several state health departments recommend that clinicians offer heterosexual patients with gonorrhea or chlamydial infection medication to give to their sex partners. This practice, termed patient-delivered partner therapy (PDPT), is supported by three randomized controlled trials showing that treating sex partners without requiring their examination can decrease the risk of reinfection and increase the proportion of partners treated.**3-5** As of 2010, PDPT was legal in most of the United States, and clinicians should offer most heterosexual patients PDPT. The CDC website maintains up-to-date information on the legality of PDPT in U.S. states and territories (*http://www.cdc.gov/std/ept/legal/default.htm*). Clinicians who give patients medication for their sex partners should also provide written information about the medication and STI prevention, as well as advice to seek clinical care in addition to taking the medication provided. Examples of forms that can be dispensed with PDPT can be found at the following websites: *http://www.doh.wa.gov/cfh/std/ept.htm, http://www.cdph.ca.gov/HealthInfo/discond/Pages/SexuallyTransmittedDiseases.aspx.*

Follow-up

The recommended regimens cure 96 to 100% of uncomplicated cases of genital or rectal gonorrhea caused by susceptible strains. Retesting of infected patients to ensure resolution ("test of cure") is not recommended except in pregnant women, when adherence with therapy is in doubt, or when atypical treatment regimens are employed. When test of cure is indicated, culture can be performed a week after treatment is completed, but retesting by NAAT should be delayed at least 3 weeks after treatment to reduce the possibility of detecting persistent gonococcal DNA despite the eradication of viable organisms.

Although test of cure per se is generally not advised, all persons diagnosed with gonorrhea should be rescreened 3 to 4 months after treatment. In prospective studies, 10 to 20% of both men and women with gonorrhea or chlamydial infection are infected when retested in the 3 to 4 months following therapy; however, in one trial, PDPT decreased that risk by 70% in persons with gonorrhea. in Rescreening can be done using urine or self-obtained vaginal swab testing by NAAT and does not require a second visit with a clinician.

 Visit expertconsult.com for e-expanded chapter

1. Uemo M, Shipitsyna E, Domeika M; Eastern European Sexual and Reproductive Health (EE SRH) Network Antimicrobial Resistance Group. Recommended antimicrobial treatment of uncomplicated gonorrhoea in 2009 in 11 East European countries: implementation of *Neisseria gonorrhoeae* antimicrobial susceptibility programme in this region is crucial. *Sex Transm Infect.* 2010;86:442-444.
2. Ness RB, Soper DE, Holley RL, et al. Effectiveness of inpatient and outpatient treatment strategies for women with pelvic inflammatory disease: results from the Pelvic Inflammatory Disease Evaluation and Clinical Health (PEACH) randomized trial. *Am J Obstet Gynecol.* 2002;186:929-937.
3. Golden MR, Whittington WL, Handsfield HH, et al. Effect of expedited treatment of sex partners on recurrent or persistent gonorrhea or chlamydial infection. *N Engl J Med.* 2005;352:676-685.
4. Schillinger JA, Kissinger P, Calvet H, et al. Patient-delivered partner treatment with azithromycin to prevent repeated *Chlamydia trachomatis* infection among women: a randomized, controlled trial. *Sex Transm Dis.* 2003;30:49-56.
5. Kissinger P, Mohammed H, Richardson-Alston G, et al. Patient-delivered partner treatment for male urethritis: a randomized, controlled trial. *Clin Infect Dis.* 2005;41:623.

SUGGESTED READINGS

Gorgos L, Newman L, Satterwhite C, et al. Gonorrhoea positivity among women aged 15-24 years in the USA, 2005-2007. *Sex Transm Infect.* 2011;87:202-204. *The prevalence is about 1.3%.*
Judlin P. Current concepts in managing pelvic inflammatory disease. *Curr Opin Infect Dis.* 2010;23:83-87. *Reviews changes in the management of PID.*
Stupiansky NW, Van Der Pol B, Williams JA, et al. The natural history of incident gonococcal infection in adolescent women. *Sex Transm Dis.* 2011. [Epub ahead of print.] *Bacterial load does not decline for at least several weeks.*
Workowski KA, Berman S; Centers for Disease Control and Prevention (CDC). Sexually transmitted diseases treatment guidelines, 2010. *MMWR Recomm Rep.* 2010;59:1-110. *National recommendations.*

308

HAEMOPHILUS AND *MORAXELLA* INFECTIONS

MICHAEL S. SIMBERKOFF

HAEMOPHILUS INFECTIONS

DEFINITION

The name *Haemophilus* is derived from the Greek nouns *haima*, meaning "blood," and *philos*, meaning "lover." *Haemophilus* species colonize the respiratory tract, cause infections of the respiratory tract, skin, or mucous membranes of humans, and from these sites can invade and cause bacteremia, meningitis, epiglottitis, endocarditis, septic arthritis, or cellulitis.

The Pathogen

Haemophilus species are small, nonmotile, aerobic or facultative anaerobic, pleomorphic, gram-negative bacilli. The prototype of this genus, *Haemophilus influenzae*, was originally recovered from patients with influenza by Pfeiffer in 1893, and it was considered the cause of that disease for many years. Primary isolation of *Haemophilus* species is best accomplished on chocolate agar medium in a CO_2-enriched atmosphere.

EPIDEMIOLOGY

The precise prevalence and incidence of *H. influenzae* infections are unknown. This organism can be detected in the nasopharynx of both children and adults. Before the introduction of an effective vaccine, between 3 and 5% of infants harbored *H. influenzae* type b in their nasopharynx. Children who have been immunized against *H. influenzae* type b are far less likely to be colonized and infected with this organism. However, the risk for infection in

nonimmune household contacts of a patient with invasive *H. influenzae* disease is approximately 600-fold greater than the risk in the age-adjusted general population. Nontypeable *H. influenzae* can be detected in the nasopharyngeal cultures of more than 70% of young children, but infection occurs in only a small proportion of colonized individuals.

H. influenzae type b was the most common cause of meningitis in young children before effective vaccines were introduced in the 1980s. Vaccination has had a dramatic impact on the incidence of infection in this group. In a population-based study in Atlanta over a 1-year period, invasive *H. influenzae* disease occurred in only 5.6 per 100,000 children and 1.7 per 100,000 adults. Forty of the 47 strains associated with invasive disease from adult patients in this study were serotyped. Twenty of these isolates (50%) were *H. influenzae* type b, 19 (47.5%) were nontypeable, and 1 (2.5%) was type f. Other studies have shown that the proportion of invasive infections caused by other encapsulated *H. influenzae* serotypes (particularly a and f) and by nontypeable (unencapsulated) *H. influenzae* strains has increased and now exceeds those caused by *H. influenzae* serotype b.

Patients with human immunodeficiency virus (HIV) infection are at increased risk for *H. influenzae* infection. Rates of invasive *H. influenzae* infection in men aged 20 to 49 with HIV infection and acquired immunodeficiency syndrome (AIDS) were 14.6 and 79.2 per 100,000, respectively. The majority of these infections were caused by nontypeable *H. influenzae* strains, although in a second study, 10 of 15 bacteremic *H. influenzae* type b infections observed in adults occurred in patients at risk for HIV infection, and AIDS was documented in 7 of these patients.

Other factors also increase the risk for *H. influenzae* infection, including globulin deficiencies, sickle cell disease, splenectomy, malignancy, pregnancy, cerebrospinal fluid (CSF) leaks, head trauma, alcoholism, chronic obstructive pulmonary disease (COPD), and race. Eskimo, Navajo, and Apache children have *H. influenzae* type b infection rates that are significantly greater than those in comparable non-native populations. In addition, daycare attendance, crowding, the presence of siblings, prior hospitalizations, and previous otitis media have been shown to increase the risk for *H. influenzae* type b disease in young children, whereas breast-feeding decreases this risk.

PATHOBIOLOGY

H. influenzae consists of encapsulated (typable) and nonencapsulated (nontypeable) forms. The former are responsible for most of the invasive infections in children and acute epiglottitis in both children and adults, whereas the latter cause respiratory mucosal infections, conjunctivitis, female genital tract infections, and invasive disease in adults. The capsules of *H. influenzae* consist of polysaccharide antigens. Six capsular serotypes (a through f) exist and are important virulence factors that inhibit opsonization, clearance, and intracellular killing of the organisms. *H. influenzae* type b, formerly the most common cause of meningitis in infancy and childhood worldwide, contains a pentose capsular polysaccharide consisting of polyribosyl ribitol phosphate (PRP). Other serotypes contain hexose polysaccharides. *H. influenzae* type b is more virulent than the other serotypes, probably because it is highly resistant to clearance once bacteremia has been initiated.

Fimbriae are important virulence factors that enhance the adherence of *H. influenzae* to mucosal surfaces. Both typable and nontypeable *H. influenzae* isolates contain fimbriae. The lipo-oligosaccharides (LOSs) of *H. influenzae* also contribute to their virulence. LOSs appear to play a crucial role in facilitating the survival of *H. influenzae* on mucosal surfaces within the nasopharynx and in initiating invasive disease (blood stream invasion) from these sites.

Outer membrane proteins (OMPs) also serve as virulence factors in *H. influenzae* disease. At least 15 different *H. influenzae* OMPs have been identified. One of these (P2, 39 to 40 kD) functions as a porin, and others are associated with iron binding. Successful scavenging of iron within the human host is crucial for multiplication of *H. influenzae*.

Antibodies have been recognized for decades as an important part of host defenses against *H. influenzae* diseases. The classic studies of Fothergill and Wright in 1933 demonstrated that most cases of *H. influenzae* meningitis occur in young children after they lose passively acquired maternal antibodies and before active humoral immunity to the organism develops. These protective antibodies function primarily to opsonize and facilitate clearance of *H. influenzae* rather than to kill virulent organisms directly.

Complement is also an essential component of host defenses against some *H. influenzae* diseases. Children with congenital deficiencies of C2, C3, and factor I have an increased incidence of *H. influenzae* infections. Patients who lack a functional spleen or who have undergone splenectomy also are at risk for the development of overwhelming infection with *H. influenzae* type b.

CLINICAL MANIFESTATIONS

Meningitis

H. influenzae meningitis commonly occurs in children younger than 5 years and in adults with a history of skull trauma or CSF leaks. *H. influenzae* type b strains cause the overwhelming majority of these cases. A review of 493 episodes of acute bacterial meningitis in adults over a 27-year period showed that 19 cases (4%) were due to *H. influenzae*.

H. influenzae meningitis is clinically indistinguishable from other forms of acute bacterial meningitis. Most patients with *H. influenzae* meningitis have CSF white blood cell counts greater than 1000/mm^3 and hypoglycorrhachia. CSF Gram stain shows pleomorphic gram-negative bacilli in 60 to 70% of untreated cases. In some patients, however, the bipolar staining may result in a mistaken diagnosis of pneumococcal meningitis. Thus, Gram stain is neither sensitive nor specific for diagnosing *H. influenzae* meningitis.

A diagnosis of *H. influenzae* type b meningitis can be rapidly and reliably established by detecting PRP capsular antigens in CSF. The diagnosis can be established in most cases even when antibiotics have been given before CSF is obtained. Other serotypes (most commonly type f) can also cause meningitis in adults. Therefore, serologic tests for type b antigen in CSF cannot be relied on to rule out *H. influenzae* meningitis in all cases.

Epiglottitis

H. influenzae type b is the most common cause of acute epiglottitis in both children and adults. Epiglottitis is a life-threatening infection in children that usually occurs in those younger than 5 years. The symptoms are fever, drooling, dysphagia, and respiratory distress or stridor, which appear over the course of hours. In adults, fever, sore throat, dysphagia, and odynophagia occur. Cervical tenderness and lymphadenopathy can be found at all ages. Laryngoscopy demonstrates a swollen, cherry-red epiglottis. However, this procedure should be avoided or undertaken only by experts because it may precipitate acute airway obstruction and thus make emergency tracheotomy necessary. A lateral radiograph of the neck more safely confirms the diagnosis of acute epiglottitis. The patient must be maintained in an upright position during this procedure, however, to avoid additional compromise of the airway. The cause is usually established by blood culture. Cultures of the pharynx and other mucosal surfaces are less useful because *H. influenzae* may be part of the normal flora. One review suggests that although vaccination has effectively reduced the incidence of this disease in children, it may be increasing in adults.

Pneumonia

H. influenzae is a common cause of pneumonia in both children and adults. These organisms can also cause nosocomial infections, including ventilator-associated pneumonia. The clinical features of *H. influenzae* pneumonia include fever, cough, and signs and radiographic findings of lobar consolidation. Parapneumonic effusions or empyema occur commonly in patients with *H. influenzae* pneumonia. Gram-negative bacilli in sputum suggest the diagnosis, but isolation of *H. influenzae* from sputum culture alone is inadequate to prove a cause because of the high frequency with which this organism colonizes the respiratory tract. A diagnosis can be established by isolating *H. influenzae* from either blood or pleural fluid. Most isolates are nontypeable.

Tracheobronchitis

Tracheobronchitis is a condition characterized by fever, cough, and purulent sputum that occurs in the absence of radiographic infiltrates suggestive of pneumonia. It frequently develops in patients with known chronic lung disease. Blood cultures are rarely positive. A combination of pleomorphic gram-negative bacilli predominating in purulent sputum, antibody titers to *H. influenzae* that rise after infection, and a response, at least transiently, to treatment of *H. influenzae* infection strongly suggests this diagnosis.

Sinusitis

H. influenzae and *Streptococcus pneumoniae* are the most frequent bacterial isolates from antral punctures or surgical specimens of patients with acute purulent sinusitis. Most *H. influenzae* isolates are nontypeable. Although patients may respond initially to treatment directed against *H. influenzae*, the response is transient if the sinus obstruction is not relieved. *H. influenzae* is not an important pathogen in patients with chronic sinusitis.

Otitis Media

H. influenzae is the most frequent cause of otitis media in young children. Approximately 90% of the *H. influenzae* isolates obtained by tympanocentesis are nontypeable; *H. influenzae* type b causes most of the remaining 10% of infections. Patients with otitis media may have ear pain or exhibit irritability. Drainage can be present. An inflamed, opaque, bulging, or perforated tympanic membrane is usually demonstrated. The cause can be proved by Gram stain and culture of purulent fluid obtained by tympanocentesis. Otitis caused by *H. influenzae* type b may occur in association with bacteremia and meningitis.

Cellulitis

H. influenzae type b is the cause of 5 to 15% of cases of cellulitis in young children. Most of the infections occur on the face or neck. *H. influenzae* cellulitis is often described as causing a distinctive blue or violaceous discoloration of the skin. However, the fever, erythema, and tenderness observed may not be distinguishable from those attributable to other causes. The diagnosis is established by culture of blood or tissue aspirates from the involved area, or both.

Bacteremia without a Primary Focus of Infection

H. influenzae causes primary bacteremia in both children and adults. In infants or children, occult meningitis or epiglottitis can be present. Rigorous clinical and laboratory evaluation is essential to avoid missing a diagnosis of life-threatening focal infection in these patients. In adults, primary *H. influenzae* type b bacteremia often occurs in those with underlying diseases such as lymphoma, leukemia, or alcoholism.

Obstetric and Gynecologic Infection

Pregnancy is associated with a significant risk for *H. influenzae* infection. In the Atlanta study, 7 of 47 adult *H. influenzae* invasive infections occurred in pregnant women. Nontypeable *H. influenzae* is also an important cause of tubo-ovarian abscess and salpingitis in women.

Pericarditis

H. influenzae type b is an important cause of primary bacterial pericarditis in children. It rarely causes this infection in adults; however, pericarditis can occur in association with pneumonia, probably as a result of contiguous spread of the infection.

Endocarditis

H. influenzae is a very unusual cause of endocarditis in view of the frequency with which invasive disease occurs. Most infections occur in patients with preexisting valvular heart disease. Because of its slow initial growth in blood culture media, diagnosis of this infection may be delayed or missed. Patients with *H. influenzae* endocarditis are at high risk for arterial embolic phenomena.

Septic Arthritis

H. influenzae type b is a common cause of septic arthritis in young children; it is rare in adults. *H. influenzae* type b arthritis is clinically indistinguishable from other causes of pyogenic arthritis.

Purulent Conjunctivitis and Brazilian Purpuric Fever

H. influenzae, biogroup *aegyptius* (Koch-Weeks bacillus), causes epidemic purulent conjunctivitis in children. This disease commonly occurs in hot climates or in the summer season.

The infection is characterized by conjunctival erythema, edema, mucopurulent exudate, and varying discomfort in the eyes. An unusually virulent clone of *H. influenzae*, biogroup *aegyptius*, causes an invasive infection called Brazilian purpuric fever, which is characterized by petechial or purpuric skin lesions and vascular collapse; it occurs days to weeks after an initial episode of conjunctivitis in infants and children younger than 10 years.

TREATMENT

Third-generation cephalosporins are considered the treatment of choice for serious *H. influenzae* infections, such as meningitis or epiglottitis. Treatment with ceftriaxone (adult dose, 1 to 2 g intravenously every 12 hours) or cefotaxime (adult dose, 2 g intravenously every 6 hours) should be started in patients with proven or suspected *H. influenzae* infection, and it should be continued at least until full susceptibility data are available.

Ampicillin was effective treatment of all *H. influenzae* infections until the mid-1970s. Since the first reports of ampicillin-resistant *H. influenzae* isolates in 1972, however, the prevalence of resistance has increased dramatically. Most resistance is due to a plasmid-mediated, R-factor enzyme (tumor endothelial marker 1 [TEM-1]), β-lactamase, which can be detected rapidly in the laboratory. A small number of isolates, however, have altered penicillin-binding proteins that have decreased binding affinity to penicillin and other β-lactam antibiotics. As a consequence, the isolates may be resistant to some cephalosporins, such as cefaclor, cefamandole, and cefuroxime, in addition to ampicillin. Therefore, patients with proven or suspected *H. influenzae* infections should not be treated with ampicillin or second-generation cephalosporins until susceptibility to these antibiotics has been proved. Chloramphenicol resistance also occurs in *H. influenzae*; an inactivating enzyme, chloramphenicol acetyltransferase, causes resistance. A small number of *H. influenzae* isolates are resistant to both ampicillin and chloramphenicol.

Oral antibiotics are commonly used to treat tracheobronchitis in patients with COPD and otitis media in children, in whom *H. influenzae* isolates are common. Because of resistance, ampicillin and amoxicillin cannot be recommended for the more serious of these infections unless the susceptibility of isolates is known. Most *H. influenzae* isolates are susceptible to amoxicillin-clavulanate. They are also susceptible to azithromycin and clarithromycin, the newer macrolide antibiotics. Fluoroquinolones, such as ciprofloxacin, ofloxacin, levofloxacin, and gatifloxacin, are active against these organisms. Trimethoprim-sulfamethoxazole is also effective for most isolates.

PREVENTION

The first *H. influenzae* type b vaccines were licensed for use in the United States in 1985. They contained purified PRP antigens. However, postlicensing studies of PRP vaccines in the United States showed variable efficacy. The PRP vaccines elicit a type 2, thymus-independent B-cell response, generate few (if any) memory B cells, and fail to stimulate a response in neonates and infants.

Protein-conjugated PRP vaccines were developed to overcome the problem of lack of immune response in the most susceptible infants and some young children. Several are now licensed for use in infants. At present, protein-conjugated PRP vaccines are recommended for use in all infants older than 2 months but not earlier than 6 weeks of age. Recent studies have shown that protein-conjugated vaccines are effective in diverse populations, including adults with COPD.

Antibiotic prophylaxis should be used for the nonimmunized household or daycare contacts of patients with invasive *H. influenzae* type b disease. Rifampin is the treatment of choice. It should be given in a dosage of 10 mg/kg once daily for 4 days to neonates younger than 1 month, 20 mg/kg (up to a maximum of 600 mg) once daily for 4 days to older children, and 600 mg/day for 4 days to adults.

Other *Haemophilus* Species

Haemophilus parainfluenzae can be found as part of the normal flora of the mouth and pharynx (Table 308-1). It is a rare cause of meningitis in children and an even rarer cause of meningitis in adults. It may cause dental infections or dental abscesses. Cases of brain abscess, epidural abscess, liver abscess, osteomyelitis, pneumonia, empyema, epiglottitis, peritonitis, septic arthritis,

and bacteremia have been reported to be caused by this organism. *H. parainfluenzae* also causes subacute endocarditis, often in young adults. *Haemophilus* species are responsible for approximately 1% of cases of infective endocarditis in non–drug-abusing patients. *H. parainfluenzae*, *Haemophilus aphrophilus*, and *Haemophilus paraphrophilus* are the species most frequently recovered from these patients. *H. parainfluenzae* forms bulky vegetations on heart valves. Arterial embolization is common in patients with *H. parainfluenzae* endocarditis. Most isolates are sensitive to ampicillin, but some produce β-lactamases.

MORAXELLA INFECTIONS

DEFINITION

Moraxella species are associated with a variety of infections, the most common of which is exacerbation of chronic bronchitis by *Moraxella catarrhalis*.

The Pathogen

Moraxella organisms are small, gram-negative bacteria that grow well on blood or chocolate agar. They are catalase and oxidase positive. These small diplococci are morphologically difficult to distinguish from *Neisseria*. Some *Moraxella* species are gram-negative bacilli. *M. catarrhalis* is the most important pathogen of this genus (Table 308-2).

PATHOBIOLOGY

The organism is isolated exclusively from humans and is found predominantly in the respiratory tract. *M. catarrhalis* adheres to mucosal cells with the aid of pili. Infection is believed to result from contiguous spread of the organism from sites of colonization, possibly as a result of the introduction of new, more virulent strains to which the host lacks immunity.

M. catarrhalis can often be found in respiratory secretions together with *H. influenzae*. Although the mechanism for coexistence of these pathogens is not known, recent evidence suggests that the outer membrane vesicles of *M. catarrhalis* inactivate complement, thus enhancing survival of the latter.

CLINICAL MANIFESTATIONS

M. catarrhalis is associated with exacerbations of chronic bronchitis. Studies indicate that this organism can be isolated from 0.2 to 8.1% of the sputum aspirates of patients with this disease. It is the third most common pathogen isolated from these patients behind *S. pneumoniae* and *H. influenzae*.

M. catarrhalis can cause pneumonia, particularly in elderly patients with COPD and other underlying conditions such as diabetes mellitus. Sir William Osler is believed to have died as a result of *M. catarrhalis* pneumonia. Cases of bacteremic pneumonia have been reported. In addition, *M. catarrhalis* can cause nosocomial pneumonia with evidence of patient-to-patient spread of the organism.

M. catarrhalis is a common cause of otitis media in young children. Microbiologic studies indicate that this organism is present in approximately 15% of the aspirates from such patients. The organism also causes sinusitis and is a rare cause of bacteremia in children and adults.

Serious infections with other *Moraxella* species are uncommon. However, these organisms are associated with chronic conjunctivitis. Furthermore, case

TABLE 308-1   SITES OF COLONIZATION AND INFECTIONS BY *HAEMOPHILUS INFLUENZAE*

SPECIES	NORMAL FLORA	ASSOCIATED DISEASES
H. influenzae	Nasopharynx Upper respiratory tract	Meningitis Epiglottitis Sinusitis Otitis Pneumonia Cellulitis Arthritis Osteomyelitis Obstetric infections Endocarditis
H. influenzae type b, *aegyptius*	No	Purulent conjunctivitis Brazilian purpuric fever

TABLE 308-2   SITES OF COLONIZATION AND INFECTION BY *MORAXELLA* SPECIES

SPECIES	NORMAL FLORA	ASSOCIATED DISEASES
M. catarrhalis	Oral cavity and upper respiratory tract	Chronic bronchitis exacerbation Otitis media Pneumonia Sinusitis Bacteremia, endocarditis Arthritis, osteomyelitis, epiglottitis (all extremely rare)
M. lacunata	Upper respiratory tract	Chronic conjunctivitis
Other *Moraxella*	Upper respiratory tract	Rare cases of bacteremia, endocarditis, arthritis, meningitis

reports have documented the rare occurrence of invasive infections, including bacteremia, endocarditis, arthritis, pericarditis, and meningitis. The latter may occur in patients with complement deficiency.

TREATMENT

Oral antibiotics are sufficient for the treatment of most *M. catarrhalis* infections. Inducible β-lactamases are present in many isolates. Therefore, treatment with a β-lactamase–stable antibiotic such as amoxicillin-clavulanate (usual adult dose, 500 mg every 12 hours), a cephalosporin (e.g., cefaclor, usual adult dose, 500 mg every 8 hours), or a non–β-lactam antibiotic such as trimethoprim-sulfamethoxazole (usual adult dose, 1 double-strength tablet every 12 hours) should be initiated pending susceptibility test results.

SUGGESTED READINGS

Bender JM, Cox CM, Mottice S, et al. Invasive *Haemophilus influenzae* disease in Utah children: an 11-year population-based study in the era of conjugate vaccine. *Clin Infect Dis.* 2010;50:e41-e46. *This article details the continued problem of invasive* H. influenzae *disease in children and the emergence of type a as the predominant serotype.*

Laupland KB, Schønheyder HC, Ostergaard C, et al. Epidemiology of *Haemophilus influenzae* bacteremia: a multi-national population-based assessment. *J Infect.* 2011;62:142-148. *The annual incidence was 1.31 per 100,000 population, mostly in the very young and very old, with a 30-day case-fatality rate of 18%.*

Murphy TF, Parameswaran GI. *Moraxella catarrhalis,* a human respiratory tract pathogen. *Clin Infect Dis.* 2009;49:124-131. *M. catarrhalis causes otitis media in young children and exacerbations of respiratory tract infection in adults with chronic obstructive pulmonary disease.*

Okada F, Ando Y, Nakayama T, et al. Pulmonary thin-section CT findings in acute *Moraxella catarrhalis* pulmonary infection. *Br J Radiol.* 2011. [Epub ahead of print.] *Major findings were ground-glass opacity, bronchial wall thickening, and centrilobular nodules in the peripheral parenchyma of elderly patients with preexisting emphysema.*

Okada F, Ando Y, Tanoue S, et al. Radiological findings in acute *Haemophilus influenzae* pulmonary infection. *Br J Radiol.* 2011. [Epub ahead of print.] *Findings were mainly ground-glass opacity, bronchial wall thickening, centrilobular nodules, and consolidation, usually in the peripheral lung parenchyma, and only 5% of patients had pleural effusions.*

Prymula R, Kriz P, Kaliskova E, et al. Effect of vaccination with pneumococcal capsular polysaccharides conjugated to *Haemophilus influenzae*–derived protein D on nasopharyngeal carriage of *Streptococcus pneumoniae* and *H. influenzae* in children under 2 years of age. *Vaccine.* 2010;28:71-78. *A pneumococcal–*H. influenza *protein D (PD) conjugate vaccine in children younger than 2 years reduced the nasopharyngeal carriage rates of vaccine-type pneumococcal and* H. influenzae *strains, as well as the risk for acute otitis media caused by these organisms.*

309

CHANCROID

STANLEY M. SPINOLA

DEFINITION

Chancroid is a sexually transmitted disease characterized by painful genital ulcers and inguinal lymphadenitis. Chancroid is caused by *Haemophilus ducreyi,* a gram-negative coccobacillus that is not a true *Haemophilus* species. *H. ducreyi, Mannheimia haemolytica,* and *Actinobacillus pleuropneumoniae* form a distinct lineage within the Pasteurellaceae. *H. ducreyi* likely diverged from these animal respiratory pathogens to occupy its niche in the human genital epithelium.

EPIDEMIOLOGY

Chancroid is endemic in resource-poor regions of Africa and Asia and plays a major role in facilitating the transmission of human immunodeficiency virus (HIV-1). In the 1990s the World Health Organization estimated the annual global prevalence of chancroid to be 4 million to 6 million cases. The prevalence of chancroid is now unknown owing to an emphasis on the syndromic management of genital ulcers, which consists of treatment for syphilis and chancroid without diagnostic testing. Chancroid can be maintained only in networks with high sex partner change rates, and female sex workers play an important role in its epidemiology. Where clinical services have been provided to sex workers, chancroid prevalence has declined. However, reports of chancroid persist from several regions. Urban outbreaks of chancroid associated with sex work occurred in the United States in the 1980s and

1990s. Owing to contact tracing and treatment efforts, the number of domestic cases of chancroid has decreased steadily, with a 60-year low of 17 cases in 2005 and 25 cases in 2008.

The male to female ratio of chancroid is 3 : 1. The excess number of male cases is usually attributed to the infection of multiple partners by sex workers. However, human inoculation experiments indicate that men are twice as susceptible to disease progression compared with women.

PATHOBIOLOGY

Much of what is known about the pathogenesis of *H. ducreyi* is derived from experiments in which bacteria are inoculated into the skin of the upper arm of human volunteers. Puncture wounds are required to initiate infection, and the estimated infectious dose is as low as one bacterium. Papules develop within 24 hours and either spontaneously resolve or evolve into pustules in 2 to 5 days. Neutrophils and macrophages surround the organism and form an abscess that erodes the epidermis. Below the abscess, there is a dermal infiltrate of macrophages, CD4 and CD8 T cells, natural killer (NK) cells, Langerhans cells, and myeloid dendritic cells. This histopathology is identical to that of natural ulcers. In both experimental and natural infection, *H. ducreyi* associates with neutrophils and macrophages, which fail to ingest the organism. In addition to revealing the bacterial components required for infection, the human model has shown that different hosts are differentially susceptible to disease progression versus resolution. Differential host susceptibility is associated with distinct dendritic cell responses to the organism, which may shape T-cell and NK-cell responses that influence the ability of phagocytes to ingest the organism.

CLINICAL MANIFESTATIONS

H. ducreyi enters the skin through breaks in the epithelium that occur during intercourse. Papules form within hours to days and evolve into pustules in 2 to 3 days. After a few days to 2 weeks, the pustules ulcerate. Patients typically develop one to four painful ulcers (Fig. 309-1) and do not seek treatment until they have had ulcerative symptoms for 1 to 3 weeks. By this time, 10 to 40% have suppurative inguinal lymphadenopathy or buboes (see Fig. 309-1).

Natural ulcers are classically very painful and nonindurated, with ragged edges. The ulcer may be covered by a yellow or gray necrotic exudate and bleeds when scraped. However, this presentation occurs in a minority of patients, and chancroid is frequently indistinguishable from syphilis and genital herpes. Lesions in men are usually on the foreskin, coronal sulcus, or penile shaft. Lesions in women are usually on the labia, but women may have

FIGURE 309-1. Typical chancroidal ulcer and lymphadenitis in a male. (From Herpes-Coldsores.com. http://www.herpes-coldsores.com/std/chancroid_pictures.htm.)

internal vaginal and cervical ulcers that are painless. Lesions also occur on the thighs and buttocks or at distant sites; extragenital lesions are thought to be due to autoinoculation. Untreated, chancroid persists for months and causes giant ulcers, erosion of the infected area, or fibrosis, leading to phimosis in men.

H. ducreyi also causes chronic limb ulcers in the western Pacific. Close contact with family members with leg ulcers is implicated in these cases. The epidemiology of this syndrome has yet to be defined.

DIAGNOSIS

Diagnosis requires either a positive culture or a polymerase chain reaction (PCR) test. In research settings, PCR has a resolved sensitivity of 95 to 98% and a specificity of 99% for *H. ducreyi*. In comparison, the sensitivity for culture is approximately 75%, but clinical diagnosis is neither sensitive (range, 50 to 75%) nor specific (range, 50 to 75%). Unfortunately, PCR-based tests are not commercially available. Most sexually transmitted disease clinics do not routinely test patients for chancroid, and the diagnosis is typically made by the exclusion of genital herpes and syphilis. If patients with genital ulcers and lymphadenitis or treatment failure for primary syphilis appear in a community, public health authorities should be notified so that specific diagnostic testing can be initiated.

The differential diagnosis includes syphilis, genital herpes, lymphogranuloma venereum, and granuloma inguinale. Mixed infections with herpes simplex virus and/or syphilis are common, occurring in approximately 17% of chancroid cases diagnosed by PCR. Patients with suspected chancroid should be tested for genital herpes and have serologic tests for syphilis and HIV-1 and a dark-field examination.

TREATMENT   Rx

Little is known about the prevalence of antibiotic resistance in *H. ducreyi*. Most strains have acquired plasmid-mediated resistance to ampicillin, tetracyclines, and sulfonamides. The only reliable treatment regimens are macrolides, quinolones, or third-generation cephalosporins. The fact that some Enterobacteriaceae harbor plasmids that encode extended-spectrum ß-lactamases and quinolone resistance is a concern. Current treatment recommendations include single-dose azithromycin 1 g orally or ceftriaxone 250 mg intramuscularly, ciprofloxacin 500 mg orally twice a day for 3 days, or erythromycin base 500 mg orally three times a day for 7 days. Thiamphenicol, which is not available in the United States, is effective as a single 2.5-g dose.

Repeated aspiration of buboes may be required to effect a cure. In a randomized study comparing repeated aspiration versus incision and drainage, the latter was considered preferable. However, incision and drainage may cause excessive scarring, especially in persons of African descent, and should be avoided according to some experts.

Initial reports on coinfection with HIV and chancroid indicated that such individuals have a greater number of ulcers that do not heal as readily after antibiotic treatment compared with patients infected with *H. ducreyi* alone. Antibiotic treatment failures were reported in HIV-seropositive patients given single-dose regimens. Subsequent studies failed to show that HIV status had any influence on the efficacy of single-dose antibiotic regimens.

PROGNOSIS

Clinical cure correlates with a reduction in pain and purulence and re-epithelialization of the ulcer within 7 days. Patients who do not show improvement within 7 days should be regarded as treatment failures and given an alternative agent. Even if *H. ducreyi* is eradicated, ulcers may persist if genital herpes or syphilis is present and not treated. Most ulcers heal in 2 weeks; large ulcers may take 4 weeks to heal.

PREVENTION

Circumcision protects against chancroid in men. Condoms are likely protective. There is no vaccine, although several antigens that may afford protection have been identified. Contacts of patients with chancroid should be treated with an approved regimen.

SUGGESTED READINGS

Belda W Jr, Di Chiacchio NG, Di Chiaccio N, et al. A comparative study of single-dose treatment of chancroid using thiamphenicol versus azithromycin. *Braz J Infect Dis.* 2009;13:218-220. *Not available in the United States, thiamphenicol 2.5 g orally (89% cure rate) was better than azithromycin (73% cure rate), especially among HIV-positive patients.*

Centers for Disease Control and Prevention. Sexually transmitted diseases treatment guidelines, 2010. *MMWR.* 2010;59(RR 12):1-116. *Current treatment and management recommendations for chancroid.*

Janowicz DM, Li W, Bauer ME. Host-pathogen interplay of *Haemophilus ducreyi*. *Curr Opin Infect Dis.* 2010;23:64-69. *Study of regulatory genes that may coordinate virulence.*

Janowicz DM, Ofner S, Katz BP, et al. Experimental infection of human volunteers with *Haemophilus ducreyi*: fifteen years of clinical data and experience. *J Infect Dis.* 2009;199:1671-1679. *Comprehensive review of human inoculation experiments and the role of bacterial virulence determinants in human disease.*

Peel TN, Bhatti D, De Boer JC, et al. Chronic cutaneous ulcers secondary to *Haemophilus ducreyi* infection. *Med J Aust.* 2010;192:348-350. *Two unusual cases of non–sexually transmitted infection, spread from Papua New Guinea and Samoa, that led to chronic lower limb ulcers.*

Yeung A, Cameron DW, Desjardins M, et al. Use of signature-tagged mutagenesis to identify virulence determinants in *Haemophilus ducreyi* responsible for ulcer formation. *J Microbiol Methods.* 2011;84:290-298. *Genome screening found two virulence determinants, hgbA and IspA1.*

310

CHOLERA AND OTHER *VIBRIO* INFECTIONS

EDUARDO GOTUZZO AND CARLOS SEAS

CHOLERA

DEFINITION

Cholera is a feared epidemic diarrheal disease caused by *Vibrio cholerae* serogroup O1 and, since 1992, by the new serogroup O139. The disease is characterized by acute watery diarrhea. In its more severe form, a person may be severely dehydrated and in hypovolemic shock; the patient may die in a matter of a few hours after contracting the infection if treatment is not provided. Cholera is endemic today in Africa and Asia, and cases are also reported from Latin America, North America, and Europe. Seven pandemics have been registered in history since 1816; the most recent has lasted more than 4 decades since its recognition in Indonesia in 1961.

The Pathogen

V. cholerae is a curved gram-negative bacillus that belongs to the family Vibrionaceae and shares common characteristics with the family Enterobacteriaceae. *V. cholerae* O1 can be classified into three serotypes according to the presence of somatic antigens and into two biotypes, classic and El Tor, according to specific phenotypic characteristics. There is no evidence of different clinical spectra among the three serotypes of *V. cholerae*. The classic biotype, responsible for the first six pandemics of cholera, causes an approximately equal number of symptomatic and asymptomatic cases, whereas the El Tor biotype causes more asymptomatic infections. The classic biotype is confined to the south of Bangladesh, and the El Tor biotype is responsible for the current pandemic. The O139 serogroup is composed of a variety of genetically diverse strains, both toxigenic and nontoxigenic; it is genetically closer to El Tor *V. cholerae*.

EPIDEMIOLOGY

Cholera has both a predisposition to cause epidemics with pandemic potential and an ability to remain endemic in all affected areas. People of all ages are at risk to contract the infection in epidemic settings, whereas children older than 2 years are mainly affected in endemic areas. *V. cholerae* lives in riverine, brackish, and estuarine ecosystems, where both O1 and non-O1 strains coexist, with non-O1 and nontoxigenic O1 strains predominating over toxigenic O1 strains. In its natural environment, *V. cholerae* lives attached to algae or to crustacean shells and copepods, with which it coexists in a symbiotic manner. Several conditions, such as temperature, salinity, and availability of nutrients, determine the survival of *V. cholerae*; when these conditions are adverse, vibrios survive in a viable, but non-culturable state. More recent data suggest that cholera phages modulate the abundance of *V. cholerae* in the environment and determine the beginning and end of epidemics. Phages may also play a role in the emergence of new *V. cholerae* serogroups by transferring genetic material to non-toxigenic strains.

From its aquatic environment, *V. cholerae* is introduced to humans through contamination of water sources and food. Once humans are infected, very high attack rates may take place, particularly in previously naïve populations. Acquisition of the disease by drinking contaminated water from rivers, ponds, lakes, and even tube well sources has been documented. Drinking unboiled water, introducing hands into containers used to store drinking water, drinking beverages from street vendors, drinking beverages to which contaminated ice has been added, and drinking water outside the home are risk factors; these factors contributed to the acquisition of cholera during the large Peruvian epidemic of 1991. Drinking boiled water, acidic beverages, and carbonated water and using narrow-necked vessels for storing water are protective measures. Epidemics of cholera associated with the ingestion of leftover rice, raw fish, cooked crabs, seafood, raw oysters, and fresh vegetables and fruits have been documented. Person-to-person transmission is less likely to occur because a large inoculum is necessary to transmit disease. High transmission rates (approximately 50%) are reported among household contacts of patients with cholera in endemic areas.

Epidemics of cholera tend to occur during the hot season. Factors affecting climate change and climate variability have an impact on the incidence of cholera. The El Niño-southern oscillation (ENSO), a periodic phenomenon representative of global climate variability, affects the transmission of cholera and vector-borne diseases. ENSO causes the warming of normally cool waters in the Pacific coastline of Peru, thereby promoting phytoplankton bloom, zooplankton bloom, and *V. cholerae* proliferation.

Some host factors are important in the transmission of cholera. The chronic gastritis associated with *Helicobacter pylori* predisposes to cholera by inducing hypochlorhydria, which reduces the ability of the stomach to contain the infection. An unexplained predisposition to severe disease in persons with the O blood group has been observed in Asia and more recently in Latin America. Thus, complex associations among climatic, seasonal, bacterial, and human factors affect cholera transmission. Although for the most part developing countries are affected by cholera, several developed countries

such as the United States, Canada, and Australia have reported indigenous and imported cases. Figure 310-1 shows the distribution of cholera in the world from 1990 to 2008.

PATHOBIOLOGY

V. cholerae O1 and O139 cause clinical disease by secreting an enterotoxin that promotes the secretion of fluids and electrolytes by the small intestine. The infectious dose of bacteria varies with the vehicle. When water is the vehicle, more bacteria are needed to cause disease (10^3 to 10^6), but when the vehicle is food, lower amounts are needed (10^2 to 10^4). The incubation period varies from 12 to 72 hours. Cholera toxin (CTX) has two subunits, a pentamer B subunit and a monomer A subunit. The B subunit allows binding of the toxin to a specific receptor, a ganglioside (GM_1) located on the surface of cells lining the mucosa along the intestine of humans and certain suckling mammals. The active, or A, subunit has two components, A1 and A2, linked by a disulfide bond. Activation of adenylate cyclase by the A1 component results in an increase in cyclic adenosine monophosphate in intestinal epithelial cells, which blocks the absorption of sodium and chloride by microvilli and promotes the secretion of chloride and water by crypt cells. These events lead to the production of watery diarrhea with electrolyte concentrations similar to those of plasma, as shown in Table 310-1. A few other toxins have been isolated from pathogenic *V. cholerae*, but their roles in genesis of the disease are less clear.

The genetic material of El Tor *V. cholerae* O1 is included in two circular chromosomes, the larger containing 3 megabases and the smaller containing 1.07 megabases. The main virulence genes are *ctx*A and *ctx*B, which encode for CTX subunits A and B, respectively, and *tcp*A, which codes for toxin coregulated pilus. Regulation of expression of these genes is complex. Recent data suggest that vibrios are able to upregulate the expression of CTX in response to intestinal fluid components, as well as in the presence of certain

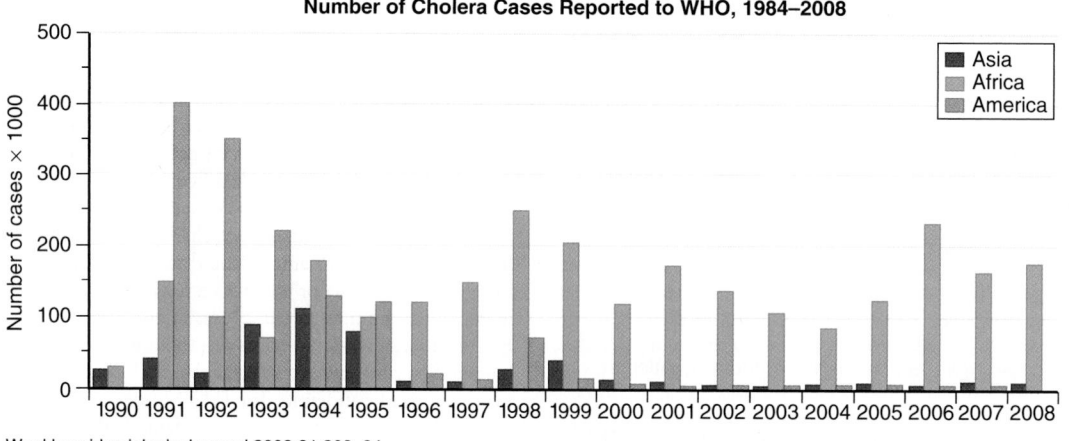

Number of Cholera Cases Reported to WHO, 1984–2008

Weekly epidemiological record 2009;31:309–24.

FIGURE 310-1. World distribution of cholera in 2008 based on reports to the World Health Organization (WHO). (Reprinted with permission from the World Health Organization: Cholera, 2008. *Wkly Epidemiol Rec.* 2009;31:309-324.)

TABLE 310-1 ELECTROLYTE COMPOSITION OF CHOLERA STOOLS AND SOLUTIONS RECOMMENDED FOR TREATMENT

	Na$^+$	Cl$^-$	K$^+$	HCO$_3^-$	GLUCOSE	OSMOLARITY
Stools of adults with severe cholera	130	100	20	44		
Intravenous lactated Ringer's solution	130	109	4	28*	0	271
Intravenous normal saline	154	154	0	0	0	308
Standard oral rehydration solution promoted by the WHO	90	80	20	10†	111	311
Reduced-osmolarity oral rehydration solution promoted by the WHO	75	65	20	10†	75	245
Rice-based oral rehydration solution	90	80	20	10†		270

Glucose concentration is in mg/dL, electrolyte concentrations are in mEq/L, and osmolarity is in mOsm/L.
*Lactated Ringer's solution contains citrate instead of bicarbonate.
†Bicarbonate is replaced by trisodium citrate.
WHO = Word Health Organization.
Modified with permission from Seas C, DuPont HL, Valdez LM, et al. Practical guidelines for the treatment of cholera. *Drugs.* 1996;51:966-973.

environmental factors. Genes unique to El Tor *V. cholerae* may encode for specific features that allow this biotype to better survive in the environment, as well as to be more infectious to humans.

CLINICAL MANIFESTATIONS

Cholera is characterized by watery diarrhea and dehydration, which ranges from mild to severe and life-threatening. Patients with mild dehydration cannot be differentiated from those infected by other enteric pathogens causing watery diarrhea. In contrast, patients with severe dehydration secondary to cholera are easy to identify in that their stools have the appearance of rice water and no other clinical illness produces such severe dehydration as quickly (in a matter of a few hours) as cholera. Onset of the disease is abrupt and characterized by watery diarrhea, vomiting, generalized cramps, and oliguria. Physical examination shows a feeble pulse, fever is rarely present, patients look anxious and restless, the eyes are very sunken, mucous membranes are dry, the skin has lost its elasticity and when pinched retracts very slowly, the voice is almost nonaudible, and intestinal sounds are prominent. Although watery diarrhea is the hallmark of cholera, some patients do not have diarrhea but instead have abdominal distention and ileus, a relatively rare type of cholera called cholera "sicca."

Laboratory findings in patients with severe dehydration consist of an increase in hematocrit, urine specific gravity, and total serum protein; azotemia; metabolic acidosis with a high anion gap; normal or low serum potassium levels; and normal or slightly low sodium and chloride levels. The calcium and magnesium content in plasma is high as a result of hemoconcentration. Leukocytosis is observed in patients with severe cholera. Hyperglycemia, caused by high concentrations of epinephrine, glucagon, and cortisol stimulated by hypovolemia, is more commonly seen than hypoglycemia. Acute renal failure is the most severe complication of cholera. Incidence rates of 10.6 cases per 1000 were reported in Peru during the first months of the 1991 epidemic. Patients with acute renal failure almost always have a history of improper rehydration. Cholera in pregnant women carries a bad prognosis. Pregnant women have more severe clinical illness, especially when the disease is acquired at the end of the pregnancy. Fetal loss occurs in as many as 50% of these pregnancies. Cholera in the elderly also carries a bad prognosis because of an increase in complications, particularly acute renal failure, severe metabolic acidosis, and pulmonary edema.

DIAGNOSIS

Chaotic movement under darkfield microscopy and a high number of bacteria in a stool sample from patients with diarrhea are characteristic of *V. cholerae* infection. Specific antisera against the serotype block the movement of vibrios and allow confirmation of the diagnosis. Under epidemic conditions, observing bacteria with a darting movement in a stool sample from a suspected patient under darkfield microscopy is adequate to make the diagnosis. Definitive confirmation requires isolation of the bacterium in culture. Specific medium is needed to isolate *V. cholerae* from stool. Higher sensitivity and specificity have been reported with DNA amplification by polymerase chain reaction for detection of vibrios in stool and environmental samples.

TREATMENT   (Rx)

The objectives of therapy are to restore the fluid losses caused by diarrhea and vomiting, correct the metabolic acidosis, restore potassium deficits, and replace continuous fluid losses. Treatment of patients with milder forms of dehydration is easy, but treatment of patients with severe dehydration requires experience and proper training. The intravenous route should be restricted to patients with some dehydration who do not tolerate the oral route, those who purge more than 10 to 20 mL/kg/hr, and all patients with severe dehydration. Rehydration should be accomplished in two phases: the rehydration phase and the maintenance phase. The purpose of the rehydration phase is to restore normal intravascular volume, and it should last no longer than 4 hours. Intravenous fluids should be infused at a rate of 50 to 100 mL/kg/hr in severely dehydrated patients. Lactated Ringer's solution is preferred, but other solutions may be used as well (see Table 310-1). All signs of dehydration should have disappeared and the patient should pass urine at a rate of 0.5 mL/kg/hr or greater after finishing the rehydration phase. The maintenance phase follows immediately. During this phase the objective is to maintain normal hydration status by replacing ongoing losses. The oral route is preferred during this phase, and the use of oral rehydration solutions is highly recommended. Oral rehydration therapy uses the principle of common transportation of solutes, electrolytes, and water by the intestine not affected by cholera toxin. People with diarrhea can undergo successful rehydration with simple solutions containing glucose and electrolytes. The World Health Organization recommends an oral rehydration solution with reduced osmolarity (245 mOsm/L) to treat all diarrheal diseases. This solution contains lower sodium than the standard oral rehydration solution promoted since 1975 (75 vs. 90 mEq/L). No more symptomatic hyponatremia is observed with the reduced-osmolarity than with the standard solution. The addition of L-histidine to rice-based oral rehydration solutions has recently been shown to reduce the volume and duration of diarrhea and the unscheduled use of intravenous therapy in adult cholera patients.[1] Patients without severe dehydration who tolerate the oral route can be rehydrated with oral rehydration solutions exclusively and discharged promptly from the health center. Recommendations for treating cholera patients are shown in Table 310-2. Treatment of cholera caused by *V. cholerae* O139 is the same as described earlier.

Antimicrobial agents are not life-saving and always need to be accompanied by fluid therapy. Effective antibiotics in patients with severe dehydration decrease the duration of diarrhea and the volume of stool by nearly half. Oral tetracycline and doxycycline are the agents of choice in areas of the globe where sensitive strains predominate A single dose of doxycycline (300 mg) is the preferred regimen. Pregnant women can be treated with erythromycin or furazolidone. Because of the emergence of resistance to tetracyclines and other antimicrobials in many endemic areas, the quinolones and, more recently, azithromycin have been tested in clinical trials. A single-dose regimen of azithromycin (20 mg/kg) showed clinical and bacteriologic results that in children were comparable to a 3-day regimen with erythromycin and, in adults, comparable to a single-dose regimen of ciprofloxacin (1 g).[2,3] The addition of oral zinc (30 mg/day) to an erythromycin regimen in children reduced the duration of diarrhea in 12%, with an additional 11% reduction in the volume of diarrhea in comparison to placebo.[4] Antimotility agents such as loperamide or diphenoxylate, adsorbents, analgesics, and antiemetics are not recommended. Antisecretory drugs, including racecadotril, an encephalinase inhibitor, are not useful in patients with severe cholera. Chemoprophylaxis of household contacts of cholera cases is not routinely recommended.

PREVENTION

Access to potable water and ensuring proper management of excreta to avoid contamination of other water sources are important measures to reduce transmission of cholera. Alternative ways to prevent cholera transmission are necessary in developing countries. Water can be made safer to drink by boiling, adding chlorine, or filtering it with cloth made of cotton. An inability to implement these measures to curtail cholera transmission has prompted a search for vaccines. An ideal vaccine against cholera should elicit a fast and long-lasting immune response with minimal side effects. Parenteral vaccines are no longer recommended. Two oral vaccines, the two-dose regimen of the inactivated vaccine WC-BS (whole cell plus B subunit) and a single dose of the live attenuated CVD 103-HgR vaccine, have been tested extensively in epidemic settings and in field trials in endemic areas. Although the WC-BS vaccine showed good short-term protective efficacy (85% at 6 months), the results at 3 and 5 years were less impressive (60%), particularly in children. A large effectiveness study in Mozambique confirmed the high short-term

TABLE 310-2   RECOMMENDATIONS FOR TREATING CHOLERA PATIENTS

1. Determine the degree of dehydration on arrival.
2. Rehydrate the patient in two phases:
   Rehydration phase—lasts 2 to 4 hours
   Maintenance phase—lasts until the end of the diarrheal episode
3. Register and periodically review input and output in predesigned charts.
4. Use the intravenous route in the following situations:
   In all severely dehydrated patients, in whom the speed of infusion varies from 50 to 100 mL/kg/hr
   Patients with some dehydration who are unable to tolerate the oral route
   Patients with high stool output (>10 mL/kg/hr) during the maintenance phase
5. Use oral rehydration solutions, glucose or rice based, during the maintenance phase to match ongoing losses. Volumes of 800 to 1000 mL/hr are usually required. Low-osmolarity solutions are not recommended.
6. Start an oral antimicrobial agent in patients with severe cholera when full rehydration has been achieved and oral tolerance is confirmed. Single-dose doxycycline, 300 mg, is the preferred regimen. Erythromycin or a quinolone is a suitable alternative.
7. Discharge patients only if oral tolerance is adequate (≥1000 mL/hr), urine output is satisfactory (≥40 mL/hr), and stool volume is low (≤400 mL/hr).

Modified with permission from Seas C, DuPont HL, Valdez LM, et al. Practical guidelines for the treatment of cholera. *Drugs.* 1996;51:966-973.

protection against cholera (80%) by this vaccine, especially against severe dehydration (90%). Additionally, reanalysis of data on this vaccine in field trials has shown that it may also confer herd protection in the unvaccinated population. A large field trial of the live attenuated vaccine showed no protective efficacy. Indications for use of the currently available cholera vaccines include travel to endemic areas and situations in which high attack rates of cholera are expected, such as after environmental disasters, in refugee camps, and in urban slums in highly endemic areas. New oral vaccines including both killed and live *Vibrio* are being evaluated in endemic areas, with promising preliminary reports.

PROGNOSIS

Patients with severe cholera left untreated or improperly treated carry a poor prognosis, with mortality rates higher than 50%. However, case-fatality rates during epidemics may be reduced to values below 1% even in disaster situations, provided that adequate access to health care centers and proper management of patients can be ensured. In contrast, figures higher than 10% have been reported in epidemic settings when patients had no access to health care or received improper treatment.

OTHER *VIBRIO* INFECTIONS

Noncholera vibrios have worldwide distribution and coexist in environments in which *V. cholerae* lives. They cause a spectrum of clinical syndromes, including acute diarrhea, soft tissue infections, and sepsis, especially in immunocompromised hosts. In the United States, 549 patients with disease attributable to non-*cholerae Vibrio* were reported in 2007 to the Cholera and Other Vibrio Illness Surveillance System. Complete information was available for 199 patients; 39% were hospitalized and 7% died. The most frequently reported species were *Vibrio parahaemolyticus*, *Vibrio vulnificus*, and nontoxigenic *Vibrio cholerae*. *Vibrio* illnesses in the United States are seasonal and peak during the summer (Fig. 310-2). The incubation period for noncholeragenic *Vibrio* infection is usually 12 to 72 hours but can be as long as 1 week.

Nontoxigenic *V. cholerae* causes gastroenteritis, but unlike toxigenic *V. cholerae* O1 or O139, nontoxigenic *V. cholerae* does not cause epidemics. Illness ranges in severity from mild diarrhea to severe watery diarrhea. Fever and bloody diarrhea are unusual, but immunocompromised persons and those with liver disease can experience more severe illness, including fever, chills, and septic shock.

V. parahaemolyticus lives in marine environments and is a source of intestinal illness associated with the ingestion of contaminated shellfish. Certain serovars have shown pandemic spread (O3:K6 and O4:K68). It is not well known how this *Vibrio* causes infection in humans, but the clinical illness may mimic cholera, although the vast majority of cases are milder and self-limited forms of acute watery diarrhea. Acute dysentery is reported rarely.

In the United States, *V. parahaemolyticus* and *V. vulnificus*, as well as other noncholeragenic vibrios, caused skin and soft tissue infections in victims and responders affected by the Gulf Coast hurricane disasters in fall 2005. *V. parahaemolyticus* wound infections are generally less severe than those caused by *V. vulnificus*. However, in persons with liver disease or those who are immunocompromised, fatal infections can occur.

V. vulnificus is associated with wound infections in persons in contact with contaminated water, as well as with primary sepsis in immunocompromised hosts. Wound infections follow trauma and are characterized by rapid

progression of skin and soft tissue involvement, with necrosis and bulla formation occurring in more severe cases. Fever, chills, and sepsis syndrome may ensue rapidly. Primary sepsis with bacteremia and metastatic lesions on the skin, characterized by disseminated erythematous lesions that may evolve to necrotic lesions, is a distinctive clinical manifestation in patients with chronic liver illnesses, alcoholics, and patients with blood disorders such as thalassemia. A history of seafood ingestion, usually oysters, is typical. Patients are acutely ill with high fever and need to be managed aggressively with fluid resuscitation, surgical débridement, general supportive care, and antibiotic coverage. An intravenous combination of cefotaxime, 2 g four times a day, plus doxycycline, 100 mg two times a day, is recommended. This combination is synergistic in vitro. Alternative antimicrobials are ceftazidime and ciprofloxacin.

1. Sur D, Lopez AL, Kanungo S, et al. Efficacy and safety of a modified killed-whole-cell oral cholera vaccine in India: an interim analysis of a cluster-randomised, double-blind, placebo-controlled trial. *Lancet.* 2009;374:1694-1702.
2. Saha D, Karim MM, Khan WA, et al. Single-dose azithromycin for the treatment of cholera in adults. *N Engl J Med.* 2006;354:2452-2462.
3. Roy SK, Hossain MJ, Khatun W, et al. Zinc supplementation in children with cholera in Bangladesh: randomised controlled trial. *BMJ.* 2008;336:266-268.
4. Jeuland M, Whittington D. Cost-benefit comparisons of investments in improved water supply and cholera vaccination programs. *Vaccine.* 2009;27:3109-3120.

SUGGESTED READINGS

Centers for Disease Control and Prevention (CDC). Update on cholera—Haiti, Dominican Republic, and Florida, 2010. *MMWR Morb Mortal Wkly Rep.* 2010;59:1637-1641. *Review of over 120,000 cases.*
Reyburn R, Deen JL, Grais RF, et al. The case for reactive mass oral cholera vaccinations. *PLoS Negl Trop Dis.* 2011;5:e952. *The reactive vaccination approach can prevent cholera cases in outbreak settings.*
Tena D, Arias M, Alvarez BT, et al. Fulminant necrotizing fasciitis due to *Vibrio parahaemolyticus*. *J Med Microbiol.* 2010;59:235-238. *Systematic review of sepsis caused by* V. parahaemolyticus.
Weil AA, Khan AI, Chowdhury F, et al. Clinical outcomes in household contacts with cholera in Bangladesh. *Clin Infect Dis.* 2009;49:1473-1479. *About 50% of contacts developed diarrhea.*

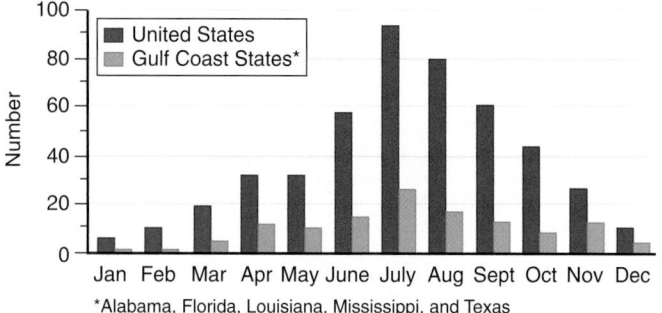

100
80
Number
60
40
20
0
Jan Feb Mar Apr May June July Aug Sept Oct Nov Dec

■ United States
▨ Gulf Coast States*

*Alabama, Florida, Louisiana, Mississippi, and Texas

FIGURE 310-2. Cases of noncholeragenic *Vibrio* infection, 2000 to 2004, United States. (From Centers for Disease Control and Prevention [CDC]. Vibrio illnesses after Hurricane Katrina—multiple states, August-September 2005. *MMWR Morb Mortal Wkly Rep.* 2005;54(37):928-931.)

311

CAMPYLOBACTER INFECTIONS

BAN MISHU ALLOS

DEFINITION

Campylobacter jejuni is one of the most commonly recognized bacterial causes of diarrhea in developed nations. More than 95% of the campylobacters isolated in developed countries are *C. jejuni* or *Campylobacter coli*. However, other *Campylobacter* species are also associated with human disease.

The Pathogen

Campylobacters are motile, curved, gram-negative rods that are found in domestic and wild animals—especially poultry—all over the world. *C. jejuni* is microaerophilic, requires 3 to 15% oxygen for growth, and is oxidase and catalase positive. It grows best at 42° C; however, other *Campylobacter* species that may also be pathogenic grow best at 37° C. Currently, the entire genome sequences for eight *Campylobacter* species have been determined.

EPIDEMIOLOGY

C. jejuni infections are endemic in young children in developing nations, where they may be isolated in up to 20% of children younger than 5 years with diarrhea. In developed nations, *Campylobacter* infections are among the most common bacterial causes of diarrhea in children and adults, but the incidence of *C. jejuni* infection in the United States fell by more than 40% from 21.7 per 100,000 population in 1998 to 12.7 in 2008. The actual burden of disease caused by *Campylobacter* is probably much higher because even active surveillance systems substantially underreport the true incidence of infection. Epidemiologic studies have estimated that more than 2 million people in the United States are infected with *C. jejuni* each year. For reasons that are not clear, the incidence is highest in western states such as California and Hawaii. Similarly high rates of infection are observed in Europe. In the United States, Europe, and Australia, *C. jejuni* infections show a substantial peak in warmer months. Such seasonality is not observed in tropical developing countries, perhaps because of the absence of extreme temperature variations.

The incidence of *Campylobacter* infections is highest in early childhood—an epidemiologic feature common to many food-borne bacterial pathogens. However, in the United States and other industrialized countries, the incidence of *Campylobacter* infections peaks again in early adulthood. The incidence of infection is also higher in men, a gender difference most pronounced in young adults.

Most human *C. jejuni* infections occur sporadically, with only a tiny fraction occurring as part of outbreaks. The dominant source of sporadic infections in both developed and developing countries is consumption or handling of poultry. Other sources of transmission in developed nations include foreign travel, contact with pets and other animals, contaminated drinking water, and consumption of unpasteurized milk. Cross-contamination within a kitchen (e.g., use of the same utensils or cutting boards to prepare uncooked chicken and to chop fruit) has led to a variety of foods being implicated as sources of human *C. jejuni* infection. In contrast to sporadic infections, the most common source of *C. jejuni* outbreaks is unpasteurized milk; occasionally, large waterborne outbreaks occur. Transmission of *C. jejuni* infection from ill food handlers is uncommon. Even in households in which an individual has culture-proven *C. jejuni* gastroenteritis, secondary transmission to other family members is unusual.

PATHOBIOLOGY

Persons become infected with *C. jejuni* as a result of orally ingesting the organism, usually in food or water. Factors that affect whether *Campylobacter* infection leads to illness include the dose of bacteria ingested, the virulence of the organism, and the specific immunity of the host to the ingested organism. The minimum number of bacteria needed to cause illness varies between people, but it may be quite low, especially in water; because *C. jejuni* is susceptible to gastric acidity, ingestion of very few organisms may cause illness if gastric pH is elevated as a result of illness or medication. The median incubation period is 2 to 4 days, although it may range from 1 to 7 days.

In early infection, *C. jejuni* multiplies in the bile-rich upper intestines; subsequently, tissue injury is seen in the jejunum, ileum, and colon. Gross inspection of the bowel shows a diffuse, bloody, edematous enteritis. Microscopic examination reveals an inflammatory infiltrate consisting of neutrophils, mononuclear cells, and eosinophils in the lamina propria. The mucosal epithelium is ulcerated, and crypt abscesses may be seen. The pathologic appearance is nonspecific and may mimic ulcerative colitis or Crohn's disease.

Invasion of the epithelium by *C. jejuni* appears to be central to its pathogenesis, and many factors influence how *C. jejuni* adheres to and invades intestinal tissues. A superficial conserved antigen, PEB1, appears to be a major adhesin and is a target of the immune response to *C. jejuni* infection. Other factors that contribute to *C. jejuni*'s invasiveness and pathogenicity, which may be encoded by a virulence plasmid, include type IV secretion systems and mechanisms that disrupt microtubules in host cells. The presence of the plasmid pVir in clinical isolates is significantly associated with bloody stools. Glycolipids and glycoproteins on the surface of *C. jejuni* are important for the organism's survival in the intestinal lumen and in pathogenesis because they have an impact on cell-to-cell interactions, as well as the host's immune response to infection. The bacterium's flagella facilitate its ability to colonize the gastrointestinal tract by promoting motility and chemotaxis of the organism. *C. jejuni* may produce extracellular toxins, but their role in pathogenesis has not been confirmed, with the possible exception of the cytoskeletal distending toxin (cdt), which may facilitate intracellular activities that lead to apoptosis.

Regardless of the organism's virulence, host factors are pivotal in affecting the clinical outcome of infection. In healthy volunteers fed a fixed dose of a single *C. jejuni* strain, a spectrum of illnesses develops. Patients infected with *C. jejuni* excrete the organism in feces for 2 to 3 weeks. In developing nations, where the level of immunity to *C. jejuni* is higher because of recurrent exposure, the period of convalescent excretion of *C. jejuni* is shorter.

After recovery from *Campylobacter* infection, at least short-term immunity develops. The decreasing illness-to-infection ratio with age seen in

developing nations also suggests that individuals are acquiring immunity. Specific IgA, IgG, and IgM antibodies in serum and IgA antibodies in intestinal secretions develop in patients infected with *C. jejuni*. Patients with congenital or acquired hypogammaglobulinemia are at risk for severe or recurrent *C. jejuni* infections. Because the incidence of *C. jejuni* infection is markedly higher in persons infected with human immunodeficiency virus (HIV), cell-mediated immunity might also play a role in preventing and terminating infection.

CLINICAL MANIFESTATIONS

The clinical consequences of *Campylobacter* infection range from complete absence of symptoms to fulminant sepsis and death. In most cases, however, illnesses are brief and do not require hospitalization. In developed nations, detection of *C. jejuni* in the stool of asymptomatic persons is rare. However, in developing nations, where infections are endemic and recurrent infections occur frequently, asymptomatic infections are more common. In both developing and developed nations, persons infected with *C. jejuni* typically contract a diarrheal illness that resolves within a week. The case-fatality rate associated with this infection is low, about 0.05 deaths per 1000 infections, and not surprisingly is highest in the elderly and persons with comorbid conditions.

The gastroenteritis that is caused by infection with *C. jejuni* is clinically indistinguishable from that caused by other enteric bacterial pathogens, such as *Salmonella* (Chapter 316), *Shigella* (Chapter 317), and *Escherichia coli* O157:H7 (Chapter 312). The most common symptoms are diarrhea, malaise, fever, and abdominal pain (Table 311-1). Most patients with *C. jejuni* gastroenteritis experience at least 1 day with 10 or more stools; the diarrhea may be loose, watery, or bloody. Nausea is reported by some patients, but vomiting is less common. More than half the patients describe subjective fever. The abdominal cramping may be severe and is sometimes the predominant symptom. Although in most patients the symptoms resolve within 7 days, symptoms may persist in 10 to 20% of patients, and another 5 to 10% may experience a relapse.

Almost regardless of the nature of the symptoms, fecal leukocytes are found in 75% of infected patients; gross or occult blood is seen in 50%. Peripheral white blood cell counts may be elevated, but liver function test results, the hematocrit, and serum electrolytes are usually normal. Sigmoidoscopic examination reveals diffuse colonic inflammation, which is nonspecific.

Local complications of *C. jejuni* gastroenteritis are rare. In its most severe form, infection may lead to massive gastrointestinal hemorrhage or toxic megacolon. Infection of the biliary tract may result in obstructive hepatitis, cholecystitis (Chapter 158), or pancreatitis (Chapter 146). Other reported local complications include peritonitis (Chapter 144), splenic rupture, and exacerbations of inflammatory colitis. Bacteremia is detected in 1.5 per 1000 intestinal infections, with higher rates in persons who are immunocompromised or elderly, but transient bacteremia may be more common because blood cultures are infrequently obtained in patients with diarrhea and the bacteria are killed rapidly by normal human serum. Other extraintestinal complications such as meningitis, endocarditis, osteomyelitis, and purulent arthritis are rare.

TABLE 311-1	CLINICAL FEATURES OF *CAMPYLOBACTER* ENTERITIS DERIVED FROM OUTBREAKS IN WHICH MORE THAN 50 PATIENTS WERE INFECTED	
SYMPTOM	**MEDIAN FREQUENCY (%)**	**RANGE (%)**
Fever	50	6-75
Diarrhea	84	52-100
Headache	41	6-69
Abdominal pain	79	56-99
Myalgia	42	28-59
Vomiting	15	1-42
Blood in feces	15	0.5-32

Modified from Blaser MJ, Engberg J. Clinical aspects of *Campylobacter jejuni* and *Campylobacter coli* infections. In: Nachamkin I, Szymanski CM, Blaser MJ, eds. *Campylobacter*, 3rd ed. Washington, DC: ASM Press; 2008:99-121.

Guillain-Barré syndrome (Chapter 428), which is a postinfectious complication of *C. jejuni* infection, occurs about once in every 2000 infections; between 30 and 50% of all cases may be triggered by a preceding *C. jejuni* infection. Because the onset of neurologic symptoms occurs about 1 to 3 weeks after the onset of gastrointestinal symptoms, cross-reactivity between antibodies formed against the lipopolysaccharide and capsule of *C. jejuni* and proteins in peripheral nerve myelin or other glycolipids in peripheral nerves is probably the cause. Certain *C. jejuni* serotypes (O type 19, O type 41) are overrepresented in patients in whom Guillain-Barré syndrome develops after culture-documented *C. jejuni* infection. Other postinfectious complications of *C. jejuni* infection include reactive arthritis (seen mostly in persons with HLA-B27 histocompatibility antigens), uveitis, hemolytic-uremic syndrome, erythema nodosum, encephalitis, carditis, and hemolytic anemia.

DIAGNOSIS

The diagnosis of *C. jejuni* infection should be considered in any patient with an acute febrile diarrheal illness. The diagnosis is established by culturing the organism from stool or tissue. Primary isolation of *Campylobacter* species from blood may take up to 14 days.

The presence of curved gram-negative rods on a Gram stain of stool is specific but only 50 to 75% sensitive for detecting *C. jejuni*. Examination of fecal specimens by darkfield microscopy is useful if done within 2 hours of passage; the characteristic darting motility of *Campylobacter* provides a presumptive diagnosis. Serum serologic studies and polymerase chain reaction of stool are currently available only as research tools.

Differential Diagnosis

In patients with acute colitis and bloody diarrhea, especially those whose symptoms last longer than 1 week, *Campylobacter* enteritis may be mistaken for ulcerative colitis or Crohn's disease (Chapter 143). In such cases, it is critical to exclude infectious colitis before starting immunosuppressive therapy. In patients with severe abdominal pain, appendicitis may be suspected and unnecessary appendectomy may result (Chapter 144).

PREVENTION

Because the most common source of transmission of *C. jejuni* infection to humans in developed countries is through the consumption and handling of poultry, interrupting this route of infection will probably have the greatest effect on reducing the burden of disease caused by *Campylobacter*. The nearly universal colonization of poultry flocks with *C. jejuni* makes eradication of the organism in chickens unlikely, but improvements in slaughtering plants appear to be reducing the level of contamination of products reaching humans. For the consumer, careful food preparation methods are critical; chicken must be cooked thoroughly. To avoid cross-contamination in the kitchen, cutting boards, knives, and other utensils used to prepare raw chicken should be washed with hot soapy water before being used to prepare foods eaten uncooked such as fruits or vegetables. Person-to-person transmission of *Campylobacter* is not common; nevertheless, all persons with diarrhea, especially those who handle food, should wash their hands after using the bathroom. Travelers and campers should be cautioned against drinking untreated water. Many outbreaks of *C. jejuni* infection might also be avoided if persons abstain from drinking unpasteurized milk. Antibiotic prophylaxis for travelers is not advised. An effective anti-*Campylobacter* vaccine has not yet been developed.

TREATMENT   Rx

As is true of most patients with infectious or noninfectious diarrhea, the most important principle of treatment of *Campylobacter* gastroenteritis is restoration of proper hydration and electrolyte balance, typically with oral fluids. Occasionally, intravenous fluids are needed, especially in elderly patients or young children. Most *C. jejuni* infections are self-limited and resolve without specific antibiotic treatment. Furthermore, treatment with antibiotics shortens the duration of illness by less than 48 hours.■ Prompt antimicrobial therapy is indicated for patients with high fever (>38.5°C), prolonged illness (>1 week), bloody stools, or worsening symptoms or for those who have relapsed. Antimicrobial treatment is also warranted in the elderly, infants, pregnant women, and persons who are immunocompromised, including those infected with HIV.

The antibiotic of choice for the treatment of *C. jejuni* gastroenteritis is erythromycin (500 mg twice daily for 5 days); azithromycin and clarithromycin are equally effective but considerably more expensive. One concern with erythromycin, which is primarily metabolized by CYP3A4, is the risk for sudden cardiac

death. The risk is increased five-fold when erythromycin is given with medications that inhibit CYP3A4. In patients taking one or more of these medications, azithromycin may be substituted for erythromycin.

Fluoroquinolones, carbapenems, aminoglycosides, and clindamycin may also be effective, but resistance to quinolones is now common in many parts of the world. In general, rates of resistance to ampicillin, amoxicillin, and cephalosporins are too high for them to be useful in the treatment of *C. jejuni* infections.

Critically ill or septic persons with *Campylobacter* infection may benefit from imipenem or aminoglycosides, agents to which campylobacters are exquisitely susceptible, with resistance rates consistently less than 1%. In contrast, persons with persistent or relapsing infection, especially those who are immunocompromised, may require prolonged use (sometimes months) of antibiotics. In the absence of continuing sepsis, oral agents may be used.

OTHER *CAMPYLOBACTER* SPECIES

Campylobacter fetus may cause systemic and diarrheal illnesses in compromised hosts and diarrheal illnesses in normal hosts. Most *C. fetus* strains, unlike *C. jejuni*, are not susceptible to the lethal effect of normal human serum because they possess a protein capsule (S layer). In immunocompromised persons, *C. fetus* can cause extraintestinal illnesses such as bacteremia, vascular infections, and meningitis. *C. fetus* infection may also cause perinatal infection and fetal loss. Prolonged treatment with erythromycin plus either imipenem, meropenem, an aminoglycoside, or a third-generation cephalosporin is indicated for serious *C. fetus* infections.

Campylobacter upsaliensis may cause acute or chronic diarrhea in healthy or immunocompromised persons. The organism is frequently isolated from dogs with diarrhea, which could be a source of transmission to humans. Some *C. upsaliensis* strains are resistant to erythromycin, but most are susceptible to fluoroquinolones, doxycycline, third-generation cephalosporins, and amoxicillin-clavulanate.

Campylobacter hyointestinalis was first recognized as a cause of proliferative enteritis in swine; *Campylobacter lari* is most often cultured from gulls and other birds. Both organisms have now been identified as rare causes of watery diarrhea and abdominal cramping in immunocompetent children and adults. Most infected patients do not require antimicrobial therapy; all isolates studied in vitro have been susceptible to erythromycin.

Helicobacter cinaedi and *Helicobacter fennelliae*, once called "*Campylobacter*-like organisms," are causes of proctocolitis or enterocolitis and have also been reported to cause bacteremia in immunocompromised patients. The organisms are frequently resistant to erythromycin; fluoroquinolones are considered the treatment of choice in patients who require antimicrobial therapy. The organisms are also susceptible to third-generation cephalosporins, aminoglycosides, and carbapenems.

Other *Campylobacter* or related species that have been associated with human illness include *Campylobacter mucosalis*, *Campylobacter doylei*, *Campylobacter curvus*, *Campylobacter concisus*, *Campylobacter insulaenigrae*, *Campylobacter rectus*, *Campylobacter helveticus*, *Arcobacter butzleri*, and *Arcobacter cryaerophila*. Illnesses include diarrhea and localized infections, presumably as a result of transient bacteremia from intestinal sources. New pathogenic species of *Campylobacter* are being identified with some regularity.

PROGNOSIS

Even in critically ill patients, 1 week of therapy is generally sufficient to eradicate infection.

Campylobacter infections in HIV-positive patients may be more severe, persist, recur, and be resistant to antibiotics. More severe and extraintestinal illness is also more likely to occur in patients with acquired or congenital hypogammaglobulinemia. Most *C. jejuni* gastrointestinal infections in pregnant women are mild and self-limited, with no severe consequences for the mother or baby. However, if bacteremia develops in the mother, placental infection and fetal death may ensue. Infection during the third trimester can also cause neonatal sepsis and death if the woman is excreting *Campylobacter* in her stool at the time of delivery.

1. Ternhag A, Asikainen T, Giesecke J, et al. A meta-analysis on the effects of antibiotic treatment on duration of symptoms caused by infection with *Campylobacter* species. *Clin Infect Dis.* 2007; 44:696-700.

SUGGESTED READINGS

Bessède E, Delcamp A, Sifré E, et al. New methods for detection of campylobacters in stool samples in comparison to culture. *J Clin Microbiol*. 2011;49:941-944. *Culture had only a 60% sensitivity compared with immunoenzymatic and molecular tests.*

Drenthen J, Yuki N, Meulstee J, et al. Guillain-Barré syndrome subtypes related to *Campylobacter* infection. *J Neurol Neurosurg Psychiatry* 2011;82:300-305. *C jejuni explained 14% of Guillain-Barré syndrome.*

Poly F, Guerry P. Pathogenesis of *Campylobacter*. *Curr Opin Gastroenterol*. 2008;24:27-31. *Summarizes the pathogenic mechanisms of Campylobacter infections.*

312

ESCHERICHIA COLI ENTERIC INFECTIONS

THEODORE S. STEINER AND RICHARD L. GUERRANT

DEFINITION

Escherichia coli, which is the predominant aerobic coliform species in the normal colon, can be an enteric pathogen and cause intestinal disease, usually diarrhea. The diarrhea associated with *E. coli* may be watery, inflammatory, or bloody, depending on the organism's genetic codes for virulence traits. These virulence traits and the clinical syndromes that they cause form the basis for six major categories of *E. coli*: enterotoxigenic (ETEC), enteroinvasive (EIEC), enterohemorrhagic (EHEC), enteropathogenic (EPEC), enteroaggregative (EAEC), and diffusely adherent (DAEC). Each of these categories can be further defined by the type of enterotoxin (e.g., the cholera-like heat-labile toxin [LT] or the heat-stable toxin [ST]) or adherence (e.g., localized and effacing, aggregative, or diffuse) that it produces. Taken

together, the various types of diarrheagenic *E. coli* not only constitute the major category of bacterial enteric pathogens but also illustrate the many ways in which enteric pathogens can cause disease.

The Pathogen

E. coli is a small catalase-positive, oxidase-negative, gram-negative bacillus in the family Enterobacteriaceae. It characteristically reduces nitrates, ferments glucose and usually lactose, and is either motile (with peritrichate flagella) or nonmotile. It exhibits a positive methyl red reaction and negative reactions with Voges-Proskauer, urease, phenylalanine deaminase, and citrate agents. *E. coli* is the predominant facultative gram-negative bacillus in the intestinal tract of humans and other mammals. As with other gram-negative organisms, the lipopolysaccharide cell wall contains lipid A and 2-keto-3-deoxyoctanate, a core glycolipid that has been used to develop vaccines that provide cross-protection against systemic infections with other gram-negative organisms. Smooth (S) forms of *E. coli* have O-specific carbohydrate chains attached to this core glycolipid to produce 173 O serogroups, as well as at least 56 heat-labile protein flagellar (H) antigens, by which strains are currently serotyped. Historically, some 80 variably heat-labile capsular (K) antigens have also been described (L, B, and A), not including the numerous adherence, entero-toxic, cytotoxic, and invasiveness factors that may be gained or lost by a particular serotype because they are characteristically encoded on transmis-sible genetic elements such as plasmids or bacteriophages. Consequently, this common inhabitant of the normal human intestinal tract becomes a pathogen when it houses one or more specific traits contributing to its colonization and virulence in the intestinal tract. Other traits such as the O and H serogroups may also be important for certain enteropathogenic and enteroinvasive organisms. For reasons that remain obscure, only a few O serogroups tend to predominate in the normal human colon (O groups 1, 2, 4, 6, 7, 8, 18, 25, 45, 75, and 81), whereas others (Table 312-1) tend to be associated with specific virulence traits and thus different types of pathogenesis in the intestine.

Well-established mechanisms of *E. coli* pathogenesis include cholera-like intestinal fluid secretion because of at least three different types of enterotox-ins (ETEC), *Shigella*-like tissue invasion (EIEC), and epithelial necrosis as a

TABLE 312-1 DIFFERENT TYPES OF ENTERIC *ESCHERICHIA COLI* INFECTIONS

TYPE	MECHANISM	PREDOMINANT O SEROGROUPS	GENETIC CODE	DETECTION	CLINICAL SYNDROMES
ENTEROTOXIGENIC *E. COLI* (ETEC)					
1. Heat-labile toxin (LT)	Activates intestinal adenylate cyclase	6, 8, 11, 15, 20, 25, 27, 63, 80, 85, 139	Plasmid	Gene probe, PCR	Watery diarrhea, traveler's diarrhea
2. Heat-stable toxin (STa: STh or STp)	Activates intestinal guanylate cyclase	12, 78, 115, 148, 149, 153, 155, 166, 167	Plasmid (transposon)	ELISA, suckling mice, 6-hr ileal loop assay, gene probes, PCR	Watery diarrhea, traveler's diarrhea
3. Heat-stable toxin (STb)	Calcium-dependent HCO$_3^-$ secretion and cytotoxicity		Plasmid	Piglet loops, gene probe	Colibacillosis (diarrhea) in piglets, ?human infections
ENTEROINVASIVE *E. COLI*					
4. Enteroinvasive (EIEC)	Cell invasion and spread	11, 28ac, 29, 124, 136, 144, 147, 152, 164, 167	Plasmid (140 Md, pWR110)	Sereny test, gene probe, (lys⁻, NM, often lactose⁻)	Inflammatory dysentery
ENTEROHEMORRHAGIC *E. COLI*					
5. Enterohemorrhagic (EHEC)	Shiga-like toxin(s) (SLT) and attaching/effacing ability	26, 39, 113, 121, 128, 139, 145, 157, occ 55, 111	Phage(s) and adhesin plasmid(s); type III secretion system	ELISA for SLT, serotype, HeLa, Vero cells, cytotoxicity, sorbitol agar, SLT or *eae* gene probes	Afebrile, bloody diarrhea, hemolytic-uremic syndrome
ENTEROPATHOGENIC *E. COLI*					
6. Focal attaching and effacing (EPEC)	Attach, then efface the mucosa	55, 111, 119, 125, 126, 127, 128, 142, 158	Plasmid (60 Md, pMAR2) + chromosomal type III secretion system and effectors	Serotype, focal HEp2 adhesion, gene probes for *EAF* or *eae*	Infantile diarrhea
ENTEROADHERENT *E. COLI*					
7. Enteroaggregative (EAEC)	Colonize; toxins (EAST, Pet), biofilm formation	3, 15, 44, 51, 77, 78, 91	Plasmid (AA) chromosome (Pic/ShET)	HEp2 cell adherence; AA probe; PCR for *aggR* or other virulence genes; biofilm formation	Endemic persistent diarrhea, acute traveler's diarrhea, sporadic acute diarrhea
8. Diffusely adherent (DAEC)	Colonize (F 1845 afimbriate adhesin)	75 (F 1845), 15 (57-1), ?(189)	Chromosomal/ plasmid	HEp2 cell adherence; DA gene probe/PCR	Persistent diarrhea in children >18 mo old

AA = aggregative adherence; DA = diffuse adherence; ELISA = enzyme-linked immunosorbent assay; NM = nonmotile; PCR = polymerase chain reaction.

result of *Shiga*-like toxins (SLTs) causing food-borne hemorrhagic colitis (EHEC) (see Table 312-1). By comparison, the classically recognized EPEC serotypes are neither enterotoxigenic nor invasive but rather attach and efface the epithelium. Still other types of enteroadherent *E. coli* exhibit aggregating (EAEC) or diffuse adherence (DAEC) traits, and the former in particular is associated with prolonged diarrhea in children in tropical developing areas, in patients infected with human immunodeficiency virus (HIV), and in acute diarrhea in outbreak settings and travelers from developed areas.

EPIDEMIOLOGY

Enteric *E. coli* infections are acquired by the fecal-oral route, although the fecal sources differ among the pathotypes. It is believed that a human reservoir is required for most recognized types of EPEC and ETEC. ETEC is also an important veterinary pathogen, especially in calves and piglets. However, the attachment traits of animal strains are different from those of strains that infect humans. EHEC colonizes commercial livestock but does not infect them; human cases can originate from food or water contaminated by manure or through person-to-person spread in secondary cases. The natural reservoir of EAEC is not known, but outbreaks have been traced to contaminated food, and live organisms can be found in drinking water, table salsa, and other consumable items.

The infectious doses of ETEC, EIEC, and EAEC have been determined in volunteers to be 10^6 to 10^{10}, numbers that usually require multiplication in contaminated food or water vehicles for their transmission. Heavy contamination with ETEC has been documented in foods prepared in homes and restaurants and by street vendors, as well as in drinking water in many tropical areas, and contaminated water and food probably represent the major sources of their acquisition, primarily in warm or wet seasons. In the United States, a large waterborne outbreak of diarrhea at a popular national park was caused by ETEC, and a widespread outbreak of EIEC enteritis was traced to the consumption of French Camembert cheese. Many EHEC (O157:H7 and others) infections have been attributed to eating undercooked hamburgers, and large outbreaks have been associated with contamination of unpasteurized apple juice, spinach, or seed sprouts. Approximately 600 people were infected in a large outbreak caused by contamination of the domestic water supply in Walkerton, Ontario, in 2000. EHEC infections are especially alarming because they are increasing in frequency and may cause hemolytic-uremic syndrome (HUS) (Chapter 175). HUS can be fatal despite antimicrobial therapy, which in some instances may actually induce phage and toxin production. Patients (generally children) who recover from HUS may also suffer chronic kidney injury as a result. Occasional nosocomial outbreaks of EAEC, ETEC, and EPEC serotypes have also occurred in hospitalized infants in the United States and other industrialized countries.

As with most diarrheal illnesses, the highest age-specific attack rates of ETEC are found in young children, especially at the time of weaning, when ETEC accounts for 15 to 50% of illnesses. Like immunologically inexperienced young children, a traveler visiting tropical areas has a 30 to 50% chance of acquiring traveler's diarrhea (Chapters 142 and 291) over a 2- to 3-week stay unless untreated water or ice and uncooked foods such as salads are strictly avoided. The most commonly recognized pathogen associated with traveler's diarrhea in most tropical areas of the world is ETEC that produces either the heat-stable toxin STa, the heat-labile toxin LT, or both. A close second to ETEC as a cause of traveler's diarrhea is EAEC, now reported in 19 to 33% of affected travelers to India or Mexico.

Of potential immunologic significance is the continued occurrence of symptomatic infections with *E. coli* that produce the less immunogenic STa in adult residents of tropical or other areas endemic for ETEC infection. In contrast, adult residents in endemic areas often carry LT-producing *E. coli* asymptomatically, thus suggesting that they may be protected from symptoms, if not from colonization.

Limited data on invasive *E. coli* suggest that infectious doses are relatively high. As with ETEC infections, such large numbers have readily been spread in food with high attack rates. EPEC has been recognized primarily in urban areas, especially among hospitalized infants in their first year of life, with apparent cross-infection in hospital nurseries. Although sporadic cases still occur, nosocomial outbreaks of EPEC diarrhea during the summer appear to have become less common and less severe in industrialized countries in the past few decades. EAEC increasingly appears to be an important cause of persistent diarrhea and malnutrition, especially in children in tropical areas and in patients with HIV infection. It was also recently shown in several studies to be a major cause of sporadic diarrhea in the United States and the United Kingdom.

PATHOBIOLOGY

The pathogenesis of enteric *E. coli* infection begins with ingestion of the organism in contaminated food or water, which then faces the normal gastric acid barrier. Both ETEC and EIEC appear to be sensitive to gastric acid; neutralization of gastric acid reduces the infectious dose by 100- to 1000-fold. Ingestion is followed by an incubation period of 2 to 7 days, during which colonization of the involved part of the intestinal tract, toxin production, and invasion or other disruption of cell function take place. For example, colonization by ETEC in the upper portion of the small bowel involves one of at least five major colonization factor antigen groups (which are fimbriate or fibrillar protein structures on the surface of the organism). The colonization fimbriae bind the organism to cell surface receptors in the upper part of the small bowel, where the enterotoxin is delivered to reduce normal absorption and cause net electrolyte and water secretion. LT, with a molecular weight of about 86,000, has a binding and active subunit and, like cholera toxin, binds to a monosialoganglioside (GM_1) receptor. Also like cholera toxin, the active subunit adenosine diphosphate ribosylates the regulatory subunit of adenylate cyclase to activate adenylate cyclase. The consequently increased chloride secretion and reduced sodium absorption combine to cause net isotonic electrolyte loss that must be replaced to prevent severe dehydration, hypotension, and their potential consequences. Other strains produce the heat-stable toxin (STa), which is a much smaller molecule than LT (18 to 19 amino acids) and activates intestinal particulate guanylate cyclase. Like cyclic adenosine monophosphate, the cyclic guanosine monophosphate thus formed also causes net secretion. The roles of other enterotoxins such as LTII, EAST, EIET, and others seen in ETEC, EAEC, and EIEC, respectively, are unclear at present. Both the colonization traits and production of enterotoxin are encoded on transmissible plasmids. Besides the complications of dehydration, the only significant pathologic change with ETEC is depletion of mucus from intestinal goblet cells.

EIEC, often of certain serogroups (see Table 312-1), has the capacity, analogous to *Shigella*, to invade and multiply in epithelial cells, cause conjunctivitis in guinea pigs (Sereny test), and produce inflammatory colitis and dysenteric or bloody diarrhea. As seen with shigellosis, a striking inflammatory response occurs, with numerous polymorphonuclear leukocytes in stool. The colon shows patchy, acute inflammation in the mucosa and submucosa with focal denuding of the surface epithelium, usually without deeper invasion or systemic spread. Although epithelial cell invasiveness in both EIEC and *Shigella* appears to be encoded on a large 120- to 140-Md plasmid, several chromosomal determinants, including the O antigen, are crucial for full invasive virulence.

The classically recognized EPEC serotypes often fail to produce known enterotoxins or to be invasive. Nevertheless, they are well-established causes of infantile diarrhea and exhibit a remarkable array of chromosome- and plasmid-encoded traits that orchestrate their initial attachment and subsequent effacement of the brush border epithelium. The majority of classically recognized EPEC serotypes, such as O55 and O111, exhibit both plasmid-encoded localized adherence to epithelial cells (via specialized bundle-forming pili) and chromosomally mediated attachment and effacement of microvilli. The latter is characterized by the formation of pedestals that hold the bacteria intimately to the cell surface and is mediated via effectors secreted directly into host cells by a specialized type III secretion system. There is also villous atrophy, mucosal thinning, inflammation in the lamina propria, and variable crypt cell hyperplasia. These morphologic changes are associated with a reduction in mucosal brush border enzymes and may contribute to the impaired absorptive function and diarrhea.

EHEC, most notably serotype O157:H7 but also serogroups O26, O39, and others, cause type III secretion–dependent intimate adherence and microvillous effacement like EPEC, but they also produce SLTs that are responsible for the characteristic colonic mucosal disruption and hemorrhage, as well as the complication of HUS. Organisms that produce SLTs without intimate adherence and pedestal formation are known as STEC or VTEC (Shiga-toxigenic or verotoxigenic *E. coli*), and their clinical importance remains uncertain. However, the terms EHEC, STEC, and VTEC were often used interchangeably in the older literature.

EAEC is defined by a characteristic aggregative adherence pattern to cells and the substrata associated with biofilm formation. This adherence requires a large plasmid known as the AA plasmid, which encodes specialized aggregative adherence fimbriae and other virulence genes, including a serine protease autotransporter toxin known as Pet and an antiaggregative protein called dispersin. Chromosomal virulence traits include a mucinase, Pic, and a second enterotoxin, ShET. Limited studies on human infections with EAEC suggest that the organisms do not intimately adhere or invade but reside within a biofilm and that secreted factors contribute to a damaging host inflammatory response.

The fundamental pathogenesis of DAEC is still an area of active investigation but appears to depend on direct interactions between specialized adhesins (Afa/Dr) with host CD55 (decal accelerating factor).

Host risk factors for diarrheagenic *E. coli* infection differ among the various bacterial pathotypes but in general include age, recent antibiotic use, and loss of gastric acid. Recent studies suggest that specific single nucleotide polymorphisms in the lactoferrin, osteoprotegerin, and interleukin-8 genes are associated with traveler's diarrhea caused by ETEC, EAEC, or both.

CLINICAL MANIFESTATIONS

The clinical manifestation of enteric *E. coli* infections vary among the pathotypes. ETEC infections generally produce watery diarrhea, particularly in young children and travelers to tropical or developing areas. Diarrhea may range from mild to severe and cholera-like; it may be life-threatening, especially in small children and elderly patients, who are particularly prone to dehydration, undernutrition, and electrolyte imbalance (especially hypokalemia and acidosis). Other characteristic symptoms include malaise, abdominal cramping, anorexia, and occasionally nausea, vomiting, or low-grade fever. The illness is generally self-limited to 1 to 5 days and rarely extends beyond 10 days or 2 weeks. Infections with *E. coli* that produce both ST and LT or ST alone may be more severe than those caused by *E. coli* strains that produce only LT. The persistence of impaired mucosal absorptive capacity for 1 to 3 weeks may further compound the cycle of malnutrition that complicates diarrheal illnesses in children in developing, tropical areas.

Infection with EIEC is characterized by inflammatory colitis, often with abdominal pain, high fever, tenesmus, and bloody or dysenteric diarrhea, essentially like that seen with *Shigella*, to which this organism is closely related. The incubation period is usually 1 to 3 days, with the duration generally self-limited to 7 to 10 days.

Outbreaks of EPEC infection in newborn nurseries have ranged from mild transient diarrhea to severe and rapidly fatal diarrheal illnesses, especially in premature or otherwise compromised infants. The more severe illnesses appear to have been more common in industrialized countries before 1950. However, more recent outbreaks and sporadic cases are well documented.

Hemorrhagic colitis associated with EHEC is characterized by grossly bloody diarrhea, often with remarkably little fever or inflammatory exudate in stool but with significant abdominal pain. Although this diarrheal illness is self-limited, potentially fatal HUS or thrombotic thrombocytopenic purpura subsequently develops in a significant number of children and older adults (Chapter 175). Outbreaks of hemorrhagic colitis secondary to EHEC in nursing homes or other institutions may be common and quite severe. The incubation period in two outbreaks has been 3 to 4 days (range, 1 to 7 days), and the illness is characteristically self-limited to 5 to 12 days (mean, 7.8 days).

EAEC has been associated with persistent diarrhea and malnutrition in children in developing areas, in HIV-positive patients, and in travelers who experience diarrhea (especially those genetically predisposed to greater inflammatory responses). Elevated inflammatory markers in stool are fairly common. DAEC has also been associated with diarrhea with no particular identifying features in children older than 18 months.

DIAGNOSIS

With the exception of EHEC (which should be sought by enzyme-linked immunosorbent assay or other testing for SLT and growth of sorbitol-negative EHEC O157:H7 in all patients with bloody diarrhea), definitive etiologic diagnosis of *E. coli* diarrhea requires documentation of a specific virulence trait—such as enterotoxin, invasiveness, enteroadherence—or serotype, which requires specialized immunologic tests, tissue culture, animal bioassay, or gene probes that are usually available only in research and reference laboratories. Other than for EHEC, such tests are rarely cost-effective or clinically indicated, except in outbreak or research situations. Fortunately, a probable diagnosis can often be suspected by the clinical and epidemiologic setting.

In the case of EHEC, sigmoidoscopy, which is rarely indicated, generally reveals only moderately hyperemic mucosa, and barium enema may show a thumbprint pattern of submucosal edema in the ascending and transverse colon. Some patients have superficial ulceration with mild neutrophil infiltration in the edematous submucosa. These changes are not pathognomonic.

Differential Diagnosis

Numerous other causes of diarrhea must be considered, depending on the clinical circumstances (Chapters 142 and 291). For example, self-limited, noninflammatory diarrhea in tropical, developing areas is most likely due to ETEC, rotaviruses (young children), or noroviruses (older children and adults) (Chapter 388). Noninflammatory diarrhea in older children or younger adults in the winter months in temperate areas is more likely to be due to noroviruses. *Vibrio* infections (Chapter 310) are common in areas endemic for cholera or in any coastal area where inadequately cooked seafood may be eaten. If noninflammatory diarrhea persists, especially with weight loss, other possibilities include *Giardia lamblia* (Chapter 359), *Cryptosporidium* (Chapter 358), *Cyclospora* (Chapter 361), and microsporidial infection (Chapter 361). In outbreaks of food poisoning, *Staphylococcus aureus* (Chapter 296), *Clostridium perfringens* (Chapter 304), and *Bacillus cereus* should be considered.

Inflammatory colitis with high fever and tenesmus, as well as leukocytes, mucus, and blood in the stool, may well be due to EIEC but should prompt a stool culture for more common invasive pathogens such as *Campylobacter jejuni* (Chapter 311), *Shigella* (Chapter 317), *Salmonella* (Chapter 316), *Yersinia enterocolitica* (Chapter 320), or noncholera *Vibrio* (Chapter 310). Any patient with a history of recent antibiotic use, gastrointestinal surgery, or parturition should be screened for toxigenic *Clostridium difficile* (Chapter 304). EHEC should be strongly considered in any case of bloody diarrhea, particularly in the absence of fever; many laboratories now routinely screen for this pathogen in all stool cultures, and most will screen any grossly bloody samples.

TREATMENT   Rx

As with all diarrheal illnesses, the primary treatment is replacement and maintenance of water and electrolytes, usually with a simple oral rehydration solution that uses the intact, sodium-coupled glucose or amino acid absorption (or both) to replace the fluid losses. Oral rehydration solution should be given ad libitum with free water, and in breast-fed infants, continued breast-feeding and early refeeding can compensate for the nutritional losses. Zinc supplementation is also recommended for diarrhea in infants in developing areas.

Because most *E. coli* diarrhea is self-limited, the role of antimicrobial agents is debated and remains of secondary importance to rehydration. In areas where ETEC remains sensitive, early initiation of sulfamethoxazole-trimethoprim, tetracycline, azithromycin, rifaximin, or a quinolone antibiotic may reduce a 3- to 5-day illness to a 1- to 2-day illness if the agent is started with the first loose stool in travelers to endemic, tropical areas. The use of antimotility agents should be tempered by the potential added risk of worsening or prolonging inflammatory diarrheas and increasing the risk for HUS (Chapter 175) with EHEC infections and their lack of effectiveness in reducing fluid loss, even though abdominal cramping and overt diarrhea may be temporarily reduced. Bismuth subsalicylate may reduce symptoms in traveler's diarrhea but should be used with caution to avoid toxic doses of salicylate.

PREVENTION

Prevention of many *E. coli* enteric infections is ultimately related to basic economic development, adequate sanitary facilities, and sufficient availability of safe water. In the interim, especially in areas where adequate water supplies and sanitary facilities are not available, measures such as breast-feeding for at least 6 to 12 months and handwashing reduce the likelihood of acquiring *E. coli* enteric infections. Travelers to developing or tropical areas should avoid drinking untreated or unboiled water or ice and eating uncooked fruits or vegetables that may have been "freshened" with highly contaminated water. Although a number of antimicrobial agents are effective over short periods when taken prophylactically, their effectiveness is sharply limited by rapidly emerging resistance to antimicrobial drugs, as well as by the potential side effects of their indiscriminate, widespread use. For example, tetracycline resistance among ETEC is common, and resistance to trimethoprim-sulfamethoxazole and even some quinolones is rapidly emerging around the world. More useful is the inactivated *Vibrio* cholera toxin B subunit vaccine (Dukoral), which provides transient protection against ETEC in travelers. EHEC infections can be reduced by adequately cooking beef, especially hamburger, and by careful handwashing and other hygienic measures in daycare centers and nursing homes.

PROGNOSIS

The overall prognosis of the various types of *E. coli* diarrhea is generally excellent if they are treated adequately. However, the impact of *E. coli* and other common diarrheas on mortality and morbidity (particularly with repeated infections compounding malnutrition in young children) remains one of the major health problems on a global scale. The one exception is EHEC-associated HUS, which causes significant morbidity and even mortality.

SUGGESTED READINGS

Du Pont HL. Bacterial diarrhea. *N Engl J Med.* 2009;361:1560-1569. *Case-based review, with good discussion of enterotoxigenic, enteropathogenic, enteroinvasive, Shiga toxin–producing, enteroaggregative, and diffusely adherent E. coli strains that cause diarrhea.*

Mercado EH, Ochoa TJ, Ecker L, et al. Fecal leukocytes in children infected with diarrheagenic *E. coli*. *J Clin Microbiol.* 2011;49:1376-1381. *Fecal leukocytes were present in 8% of cases.*

Pennington H. *Escherichia coli* O157. *Lancet.* 2010;376:1428-1435. *Review, including the link to the hemolytic-uremic syndrome.*

TABLE 313-1 MEDICALLY IMPORTANT MEMBERS OF THE ENTEROBACTERIACEAE FAMILY

GENUS	IMPORTANT SPECIES
Enterobacter	*E. cloacae*
Escherichia	*E. coli*
Klebsiella	*K. pneumoniae, K. oxytoca*
Morganella	*M. morganii*
Plesiomonas	*P. shigelloides*
Proteus	*P. mirabilis, P. vulgaris*
Providencia	*P. stuartii*
Salmonella	*S. enterica*
Serratia	*S. marcescens*
Shigella	*S. sonnei*
Yersinia	*Y. pestis, Y. enterocolitica*

313

INFECTIONS DUE TO OTHER MEMBERS OF THE ENTEROBACTERIACEAE, INCLUDING MANAGEMENT OF MULTIDRUG-RESISTANT STRAINS

DAVID L. PATERSON

DEFINITION

The Pathogens

The Enterobacteriaceae is a family of gram-negative bacilli that are responsible for a broad range of infections in humans and animals. They may be motile or nonmotile, depending on the species. They are aerobic or facultatively anaerobic in growth and have a predilection for inhabiting the gastrointestinal tract. Only extra-gastrointestinal manifestations of disease are discussed in this chapter. Enteric infections caused by *Escherichia coli* are discussed in Chapter 312.

From a microbiologic perspective, members of the Enterobacteriaceae ferment sugars. They grow on a variety of solid media and are usually readily identified by clinical microbiology laboratories. A number of subtleties can arise in the detection of antibiotic resistance mechanisms, however, sometimes affecting the reporting of antibiotic susceptibilities. There is a worldwide trend toward the development of multidrug resistance in all gram-negative bacilli, including the Enterobacteriaceae. This chapter emphasizes the treatment and prevention of these multidrug-resistant strains.

Medically important members of the Enterobacteriaceae are listed in Table 313-1. Infections due to *Salmonella*, *Shigella*, and *Yersinia* are discussed in Chapters 316, 317, and 320, respectively.

EPIDEMIOLOGY

Members of the Enterobacteriaceae are among the most common pathogens that infect humans worldwide. They are responsible for community-acquired, hospital-acquired, and health care–associated infections. Examples of the last category include infections acquired in nursing homes and those associated with outpatient management of cancers or hematologic malignancies. It is also important to note that, as resident components of the gastrointestinal tract flora, isolates of Enterobacteriaceae may represent colonization rather than true infection. This applies to isolates from rectal swabs, urine, or respiratory secretions. Although most infections due to the Enterobacteriaceae arise sporadically, outbreaks of infection may occur. This is most common in hospitals or nursing homes with *Klebsiella* species. Less commonly, outbreaks may be due to *E. coli*, *Enterobacter* species, or *Serratia marcescens*. Typically, outbreaks are due to multiply resistant strains, compounding the difficulties of infection control.

E. coli is the most common cause of urinary tract infection (UTI), accounting for more than 80% of isolates from urine in most clinical situations. Any of the remaining members of the Enterobacteriaceae can cause this infection, with *Klebsiella* species and *Proteus mirabilis* being other common causes of UTI. *Providencia stuartii* is a notable cause of UTI among chronically catheterized patients. The Enterobacteriaceae can cause uncomplicated UTI in healthy women, acute pyelonephritis, and UTI complicating renal tract abnormalities or catheterization. As previously mentioned, the Enterobacteriaceae may colonize the urine or be found in contaminated, improperly collected samples.

Antibiotic-resistant, uropathogenic *E. coli* may spread clonally. In other words, *E. coli* isolates from multiple people with UTIs may be identical or closely related at a genetic level. Trimethoprim/sulfamethoxazole–resistant *E. coli* is notable for its spread in a clonal fashion in the United States (e.g., "clonal group A" and *E. coli* O15:K52:H1). A widely spread *E. coli* clone, defined serologically as O25:H4 and by multilocus sequence typing as sequence type (ST) 131, is associated with the production of extended-spectrum β-lactamases (ESBLs). This clone is typically associated with community-acquired UTI. It has been detected in every inhabited continent and is particularly prominent in the United Kingdom, Canada, and India. In evaluations from New Zealand and Canada, the isolation of ESBL-producing ST131 *E. coli* has been associated with travel to India, Bangladesh, or Pakistan. The presence of ST131 *E. coli* has been confirmed in the United States.

Given the niche of most Enterobacteriaceae in the gastrointestinal tract, it is not surprising that these bacteria are prominent as causes of peritonitis. *E. coli* is the most common cause of both spontaneous bacterial peritonitis (occurring in cirrhotic patients) and bacterial peritonitis arising from visceral perforation. Pyogenic liver abscess and intra-abdominal abscess may be due to *E. coli* as well. Other members of the Enterobacteriaceae may also cause these intra-abdominal infections, especially in patients with "tertiary" peritonitis occurring after prior surgery for intra-abdominal pathology.

Enterobacteriaceae members may also be the causative pathogens of pneumonia. They are more frequently the cause of hospital-acquired and health care–associated pneumonia than community-acquired pneumonia. *Klebsiella pneumoniae* was once a renowned cause of community-acquired pneumonia in alcoholics, but it has declined in significance over the past few decades. One exception is the finding of pneumonia, liver abscess, or meningitis in Asia due to highly mucoid strains of *K. pneumoniae*. Hospital-acquired pneumonia due to the Enterobacteriaceae may be ventilator associated. Enterobacteriaceae members rank as some of the most common causes of ventilator-associated pneumonia, after *Staphylococcus aureus*, *Pseudomonas aeruginosa*, and *Acinetobacter baumannii*. The Enterobacteriaceae may also cause hospital-acquired pneumonia in non–mechanically ventilated patients, such as those with neurologic impairment from head injury or cerebrovascular accident.

Outbreaks of antibiotic-resistant *K. pneumoniae* infection in hospitals have been prominent for more than 3 decades. In the hospital setting, *K. pneumoniae* is usually the cause of peritonitis, pneumonia, or complicated UTI. Blood stream infection arising from these sites of infection, from vascular catheters, or associated with neutropenia may also occur. In the 1970s, outbreaks occurred due to gentamicin-resistant strains. In the 1980s and 1990s, hospital outbreaks of ESBL-producing *K. pneumoniae* became commonplace. Finally, in the past decade, *K. pneumoniae* carbapenemase (KPC)–producing *K. pneumoniae* became a substantial infection control issue. The KPC-producing organisms are discussed in detail later in this chapter.

PATHOBIOLOGY

The virulence factors associated with *E. coli* causing enteric infections are discussed in detail in Chapter 312. At least 40 different virulence genes have been described in *E. coli* causing extraintestinal infections. Among the virulence properties of these strains is the renowned ability of *E. coli* to adhere to uroepithelial cells. It is noteworthy that the ST131 *E. coli* clone is typically highly virulent. It belongs to phylogenetic group B2, which is known for extraintestinal pathogenic infections. In an evaluation of the ST131 clone, 46 extraintestinal virulence genes were assessed, and 35% of these genes were found in at least one isolate. Five virulence genes were uniformly present in ST131 *E. coli*. A recently published clinical case documented the occurrence of severe recurrent pyelonephritis with multiple renal abscesses in a man whose daughter was infected with the same ST131-positive *E. coli* strain. The daughter developed emphysematous pyelonephritis with bacteremia and septic shock. Enterobacteriaceae other than *E. coli* also possess a number of virulence mechanisms.

As previously noted, many members of Enterobacteriaceae are now multidrug resistant. Their resistance to aminoglycosides is usually mediated by the production of aminoglycoside-modifying enzymes. However, 16S ribosomal RNA methylation is a more recently described mechanism that results in resistance to gentamicin, tobramycin, and amikacin. Resistance of the Enterobacteriaceae to fluoroquinolones is a growing problem. In most areas, more than 20% of *E. coli* strains are resistant to fluoroquinolones. Resistance is usually mediated by mutation at target sites. However, other mechanisms, such as efflux pump overexpression or expression of the plasmid-mediated *qnr* genes, may play a role. The mechanisms of resistance of the Enterobacteriaceae to β-lactam antibiotics are worthy of detailed description (Table 313-2).

Narrow-Spectrum β-Lactamases

Ampicillin was introduced into clinical practice in the early 1960s. Enterobacteriaceae, with genes encoding β-lactamases inherent to their chromosome, were found to be intrinsically resistant to this antibiotic. Examples include the production of the SHV-1 β-lactamase by *K. pneumoniae* or the AmpC β-lactamase by *Enterobacter cloacae*. Other Enterobacteriaceae (e.g., *E. coli, P. mirabilis, Salmonella*) did not produce substantial amounts of chromosomally encoded β-lactamase. However, within months of the release of ampicillin, a plasmid-mediated β-lactamase, leading to *E. coli's* resistance to the antibiotic, was discovered. This β-lactamase was called the *TEM β-lactamase*, in honor of the patient (Temoneira) from whom it was first isolated. Plasmids encoding resistance to ampicillin have now become widespread, with at least 40% of *E. coli* in most parts of the world being TEM β-lactamase producers.

Extended-Spectrum β-Lactamases

Third-generation cephalosporins (e.g., ceftriaxone) were active against Enterobacteriaceae producing narrow-spectrum β-lactamases. However, mutant genes encoding β-lactamases capable of inactivating third-generation cephalosporins were discovered in the 1980s. The genes encoding these β-lactamases were identical to TEM or SHV, except for point mutations that led to an altered amino acid sequence. The subsequent structural change led to an ability to hydrolyze and thus inactivate third-generation cephalosporins. In view of the extended antibiotic-hydrolyzing abilities compared with the parent TEM and SHV enzymes, these β-lactamases were called *extended-spectrum β-lactamases*. In addition to the TEM- and SHV-type ESBLs, many new ones have now been described, most notably the CTX-M–type ESBL.

Typically, the ST131 *E. coli* clone mentioned earlier produces a CTX-M–type ESBL (especially CTX-M-15). Although ESBLs are typically susceptible to β-lactamase inhibitors (e.g., clavulanic acid), many ST131 *E. coli* isolates produce an additional β-lactamase (OXA-1) that confers resistance to β-lactamase inhibitors. The antibiotic resistance phenotype of the ST131-positive *E. coli* means that the organisms are typically resistant to ceftriaxone, cefotaxime, fluoroquinolones, trimethoprim, trimethoprim/sulfamethoxazole, penicillin/β-lactamase inhibitor combinations, and tetracyclines. Resistance to aminoglycosides is variable. The clone confers multidrug resistance by the presence of multiple antibiotic resistance genes. These are usually encoded on plasmids.

AmpC β-Lactamases

A number of genera within the Enterobacteriaceae have a chromosomally encoded β-lactamase capable of producing resistance to all penicillins and all cephalosporins except cefepime. Additionally, these β-lactamases are not affected by β-lactamase inhibitors such as clavulanic acid or tazobactam. These β-lactamases are known as *AmpC β-lactamases*. They are not derived from narrower spectrum parent β-lactamases, so it is not correct to call them ESBLs. These AmpC β-lactamases may be overproduced in the presence of certain antibiotics (i.e., the genes encoding the AmpC β-lactamases are "inducible"). *Enterobacter* species, *Citrobacter freundii, S. marcescens,* and *Morganella morganii* have inducible, chromosomally encoded AmpC β-lactamases. The genes encoding these β-lactamases have now been found on plasmids in *E. coli, Salmonella,* and other gram-negative bacteria.

Klebsiella pneumoniae Carbapenemase and Other Carbapenemases

In 2001, a novel carbapenem-hydrolyzing β-lactamase from a carbapenem-resistant strain of *K. pneumoniae* was first described: KPC. KPC-producing organisms are typically resistant to penicillins, cephalosporins, and carbapenems and are not inhibited by clavulanic acid or other commonly used β-lactamase inhibitors such as sulbactam and tazobactam. KPC production has been documented in *E. coli* and in many genera of the Enterobacteriaceae, such as *Enterobacter, Citrobacter, Proteus,* and *Salmonella.*

The epicenter of KPC-producing *K. pneumoniae* has been New York City. By 2004, approximately one quarter of *K. pneumoniae* isolates in a surveillance study in Brooklyn, New York, were KPC producing. The Centers for Disease Control and Prevention has reported KPC-producing organisms in numerous cities across the United States. International spread of KPC-producing organisms has been well described, with outbreaks in Israel and Greece being particularly problematic. Individual patients with KPC-producing organisms in France and the United Kingdom had traveled in the United States, Israel, or Greece. Investigators in China and South America have also reported KPC-producing organisms.

Other β-lactamase types have been linked to resistance of the Enterobacteriaceae to carbapenems. The most significant have been metallo-β-lactamases. These also result in resistance to penicillins and cephalosporins. A new metallo-β-lactamase (termed the *New Delhi metallo-β-lactamase,* or NDM) in *K. pneumoniae* from India, with subsequent spread to the United Kingdom, Sweden, and Australia, is particularly concerning.

CLINICAL MANIFESTATIONS

The clinical manifestations of UTI, peritonitis, pneumonia, and blood stream infection due to the Enterobacteriaceae are described in other chapters devoted to specific microbial pathogens.

TABLE 313-2	ANTIBIOTIC RESISTANCE ISSUES IN ENTEROBACTERIACEAE	
ORGANISM	**β-LACTAMASE**	**COMMENTS**
NARROW-SPECTRUM β-LACTAMASES		
Escherichia coli	TEM-1	Present in at least 40% of strains globally
Klebsiella pneumoniae	SHV-1	Found universally
EXTENDED-SPECTRUM β-LACTAMASES		
E. coli	CTX-M-15	International clone causing community-acquired urinary tract infection
K. pneumoniae	SHV, TEM, CTX-M	Hospital outbreaks
AmpC β-LACTAMASES		
Enterobacter cloacae	AmpC	Found universally
E. coli	AmpC	Occasional plasmid-mediated strains
CARBAPENEMASES		
K. pneumoniae	KPC	Hospital outbreaks in the United States
K. pneumoniae	NDM	Hospital outbreaks in India

DIAGNOSIS

Infection with Enterobacteriaceae is readily diagnosed in clinical microbiology laboratories after the collection of appropriate specimens. Examination of the Gram stain enables the rapid differentiation of gram-negative bacilli from other pathogens. However, it is frequently difficult to differentiate infection with the Enterobacteriaceae from infection with other gram-negative bacilli, such as *P. aeruginosa,* based on clinical findings and Gram stain results.

Once a member of the Enterobacteriaceae has been identified, it is important to perform appropriate antibiotic susceptibility testing. In some instances, specialized tests need to be performed by the clinical microbiology laboratory to detect ESBL or KPC production. Molecular epidemiologic assessment may be required to determine whether an isolate belongs to an outbreak strain.

TREATMENT   Rx

Treatment depends on the site of infection and the extent of antibiotic resistance. Empirical antibiotic choices for orally administered therapy for UTI due to *E. coli* and the other Enterobacteriaceae may include fluoroquinolones, trimethoprim/sulfamethoxazole, amoxicillin/clavulanate, or nitrofurantoin. It is noteworthy that *P. mirabilis* is resistant to nitrofurantoin. Empirical parenteral choices may include third-generation cephalosporins, penicillin/β-lactamase inhibitor combinations, aminoglycosides, fluoroquinolones, or carbapenems.

The advent of antibiotic resistance in the Enterobacteriaceae may have a huge impact on the treatment of common infections. UTI is a pertinent example. Orally administered drugs such as fluoroquinolones, trimethoprim/sulfamethoxazole, and amoxicillin/clavulanate are typically inactive against the ST131 *E. coli* strain. Because of this resistance, some patients may need to be admitted for parenteral antibiotics. Worse still, some patients with hospital-acquired infections may need "last-line" antibiotics such as colistin or polymyxin B. Specific treatment choices for antibiotic-resistant Enterobacteriaceae are given in the following paragraphs and in Table 313-3.

Treatment of ESBL-Producing Organisms

In vitro, the carbapenems (including imipenem, meropenem, doripenem, and ertapenem) have the most potent activity against ESBL-producing organisms. This is not surprising, given that these antibiotics are not inactivated by ESBLs. Carbapenems should be regarded as the drugs of choice for serious infections with ESBL-producing organisms, based on extensive positive clinical experience. No randomized trials have been performed comparing carbapenems with other antibiotic classes against ESBL producers. Prospective, observational studies have shown a significantly lower mortality from carbapenem-treated blood stream infections due to ESBL-producing *K. pneumoniae* compared with other antibiotic classes. Although synergy has occasionally been exhibited between carbapenems and other antibiotic classes, there is no evidence that combination therapy is superior to the use of a carbapenem alone.

The choice among the different carbapenems for serious infections with ESBL producers is difficult. In general, minimal inhibitory concentrations (MICs) are slightly lower for meropenem and doripenem than for imipenem and ertapenem, although the clinical significance of this in vitro difference is not clear. The ability to administer ertapenem once daily makes it potentially useful for serious infections due to ESBL producers in nursing home residents or patients continuing parenteral therapy outside the hospital. However, some ESBL-producing strains are resistant to ertapenem.

The advent of KPC, NDM, and other carbapenemases threatens the future utility of the carbapenems. Tigecycline and colistin are active against most ESBL-producing strains and, as non-β-lactams, are not inactivated by β-lactamases. Clinical experience with tigecycline or colistin to treat ESBL producers is sparse. Fluoroquinolones and aminoglycosides are obviously not affected by β-lactamases either, but the coexistence of resistance mechanisms affecting these antibiotics and ESBLs is frequent. Three observational clinical studies have assessed the relative merits of quinolones and carbapenems for serious infections due to ESBL-producing organisms. Two of these studies found that carbapenems were superior to quinolones, and one study found that they were equally effective. It is possible that suboptimal dosing of quinolones in the presence of strains with elevated quinolone MICs (yet remaining in the "susceptible" range) accounts for these differences.

Nitrofurantoin is an option for the oral treatment of cystitis due to ESBL-producing *E. coli* or *Klebsiella* species. It is important to note that nitrofurantoin is not useful in patients with upper tract infections or with moderate to severe renal impairment. Oral pivmecillinam and fosfomycin are available in some countries for the treatment of cystitis due to ESBL producers.

Treatment of KPC Producers

Treatment of KPC-producing organisms is difficult because they may lack susceptibility to all β-lactam antibiotics, fluoroquinolones, and aminoglycosides. KPC-producing organisms sometimes appear to be susceptible to carbapenems such as meropenem and imipenem (although they are always recognized as resistant to ertapenem), but these antibiotics should not be used against KPC producers.

Susceptibility to polymyxins (colistin, polymyxin B) and tigecycline is typically present. However, neither of these drug classes is a perfect solution. The pharmacokinetics of the polymyxins is not well understood, especially in critically ill or renally impaired patients. Nephrotoxicity and neurotoxicity are potential adverse effects of the polymyxins, although they are less common than when 30 to 50 years ago, when the polymyxins first came into widespread use. Of concern is that increased polymyxin MICs have been observed during the treatment of KPC producers. Tigecycline attains low serum, urine, and cerebrospinal fluid concentrations relative to MICs of the drug with KPC producers. For this reason, tigecycline should be used with great caution in blood stream infection, UTI, and meningitis.

Antibiotics that may not be widely available, such as fosfomycin and temocillin, may have activity against KPC producers. Clinical experience with these antibiotics against KPC-producing organisms is limited. Combination therapy (e.g., colistin plus a carbapenem or rifampin) is an option, but it has not been evaluated in randomized controlled trials. Novel inhibitors of KPC may hold some promise, but their clinical availability is years away.

PREVENTION

Prevention of hospital-acquired outbreaks caused by ESBL or KPC producers rests on a number of basic infection control principles (Chapter 290). First, if a focus of infection exists in the hospital environment, it should be removed. Examples include contamination of ultrasonography coupling gel or bronchoscopes. Outbreaks have been dramatically curtailed when these sources of contamination have been properly cleaned or removed.

Evidence suggests that transient carriage on the hands of health care workers is the most important means of transferring ESBL- or KPC-producing Enterobacteriaceae from patient to patient. The hands of health care workers are presumably colonized by contact with the colonized skin of patients or by contact with a contaminated environment around the patient. It is important to recognize that many patients may have asymptomatic colonization with ESBL- or KPC-producing organisms and thus exhibit no signs of overt infection. These patients represent an important reservoir of organisms. In some hospital wards with ongoing issues related to ESBL or KPC producers, more than 30% of patients have gastrointestinal tract colonization with these organisms at any given time. These patients should be subject to contact precautions. Hand carriage by health care workers is usually eliminated by hand hygiene with alcohol-based agents. Compliance with contact isolation precautions and hand hygiene must be high to maximize the effectiveness of these interventions.

Changes in antibiotic policy may play a role in controlling outbreaks attributed to ESBL and KPC producers, but this concept remains controversial. In one reported outbreak of ESBL producers, no effort was made to change infection control procedures. Instead, ceftazidime use decreased, and piperacillin-tazobactam was introduced to the hospital's formulary. This coincided with curtailment of the outbreak. In another institution, the entire class of cephalosporins was removed to gain control over endemic ESBL producers. The difficulty with this approach is that the replacement of one antibiotic class with another may result in the replacement of one antibiotic resistance issue with another. No study has demonstrated that removing carbapenems from a hospital formulary leads to the elimination of KPC producers. This is not surprising, because no study has shown an independent association between prior carbapenem use and the isolation of KPC producers. These

TABLE 313-3   TREATMENT OPTIONS FOR MULTIPLY RESISTANT ENTEROBACTERIACEAE

ESBL PRODUCERS

Carbapenems (first choice, serious infections)
Piperacillin/tazobactam, cefepime (second choice, serious infections)
Nitrofurantoin, fosfomycin (first choice, UTI)
Ciprofloxacin, amoxicillin/clavulanate (second choice, UTI)

KPC PRODUCERS

Colistin, polymyxin B, tigecycline

ESBL = extended-spectrum β-lactamase; KPC = *Klebsiella pneumoniae* carbapenemase; UTI = urinary tract infection.

organisms are resistant to multiple antibiotic classes, and it is more common for patients to receive β-lactam/β-lactamase inhibitor combinations and fluoroquinolones than carbapenems prior to colonization or infection with KPC producers. Prudent use of all antibiotic classes, with an emphasis on reducing the duration of antibiotic use, may be more useful than the restriction of individual antibiotic classes.

PROGNOSIS

The prognosis of infection with the Enterobacteriaceae depends on multiple factors, including site of infection, presence of underlying diseases, and adequacy of empirical antibiotic therapy. At one extreme, inadequate orally administered antibiotic therapy for uncomplicated UTI due to an ESBL producer may have no impact on mortality, although it may have an impact on the duration of symptoms and the need for parenteral therapy due to treatment failure. At the other extreme, patients in the intensive care unit with serious infections due to KPC producers may have an in-hospital mortality rate exceeding 70%. In contrast, comparable patients without infection due to a KPC producer have in-hospital mortality rates of 20 to 30%.

SUGGESTED READINGS

Boucher HW, Talbot GH, Bradley JS, et al. Bad bugs, no drugs: no ESKAPE! An update from the Infectious Diseases Society of America. *Clin Infect Dis.* 2009;48:1-12. *Underscores the relative importance of antibiotic resistance issues among the Enterobacteriaceae and the paucity of new agents being developed to meet this threat.*

Kanj SS, Kanafani ZA. Current concepts in antimicrobial therapy against resistant gram-negative organisms: extended-spectrum β-lactamase-producing Enterobacteriaceae, carbapenem-resistant Enterobacteriaceae, and multidrug-resistant *Pseudomonas aeruginosa. Mayo Clin Proc.* 2011;86:250-259. *Review of the current approach to infections with resistant organisms.*

Peleg AY, Hooper DC. Hospital-acquired infections due to gram-negative bacteria. *N Engl J Med.* 2010;362:1804-1813. *Comprehensive review of resistance mechanisms, clinical manifestations, and limited management options.*

Yong D, Toleman MA, Giske CG, et al. Characterization of a new metallo-beta-lactamase gene, bla(NDM-1), and a novel erythromycin esterase gene carried on a unique genetic structure in *Klebsiella pneumoniae* sequence type 14 from India. *Antimicrob Agents Chemother.* 2009;53:5046-5054. *First report of the NDM β-lactamase, which threatens patients in India and poses a major antibiotic resistance issue.*

314

PSEUDOMONAS AND RELATED GRAM-NEGATIVE BACILLARY INFECTIONS

GERALD B. PIER

DEFINITION

The *Pseudomonas*-related group of organisms comprises a set of gram-negative rods, including *Pseudomonas aeruginosa*, the most commonly encountered human pathogen in the family Pseudomonadaceae. Also included in this group are relatively low-virulence, uncommon pathogens such as members of the genera *Burkholderia* and *Stenotrophomonas* and two highly pathogenic species, *Burkholderia mallei* and *Burkholderia pseudomallei*, which can cause serious infections in the limited parts of the world where they occur naturally. On occasion, some non–*P. aeruginosa* organisms in the genus *Pseudomonas* or the related genus *Ralstonia* cause human infection, although such infection is almost always due to improper decontamination of a medication or device used to treat humans.

The Pathogen

P. aeruginosa is readily identified as a gram-negative, straight or slightly curved rod with a length ranging from 1 to 3 μm and a width of 0.5 to 1.0 μm. Major morphologic characteristics on laboratory media include the production of pigments, notably a soluble blue phenazine pigment called *pyocyanin*. Some strains produce red or black colonies because of synthesis of the pigments pyorubin and pyomelanin, respectively. Another diffusible yellow-green to yellow-brown pigment produced by *P. aeruginosa* is called *pyoverdin*, which when produced along with pyocyanin gives rise to a typical green to green-blue colony on solid media. The name *aeruginosa* stems from the green-blue hue seen within colonies of many clinical isolates.

EPIDEMIOLOGY

In adult clinical medicine, *P. aeruginosa* is primarily encountered as a nosocomial pathogen. However, as patients with cystic fibrosis (CF) survive longer and their medical care as adults is increasingly shifted away from pediatric providers, treatment of chronic *P. aeruginosa* CF lung disease by adult practitioners has become common (Chapter 89). This organism is able to survive in environments that have only minimal nutritional components. Within the hospital, *P. aeruginosa* can colonize moist surfaces of the axilla, ear, and perineum. It is also isolated from other moist, inanimate environments, including water in sinks and drains, toilets, and showers, with the source being *P. aeruginosa*–containing biofilms formed in plumbing fixtures. Pathogenic strains have likewise been isolated from the water used for flowers in patients' rooms. Hospital equipment that comes in contact with water, such as mops, respiratory ventilators, cleaning solutions, and food and food-processing machines, can be sources of *P. aeruginosa*.

Infections with *P. aeruginosa* have remained relatively constant in terms of incidence and tissue sites of occurrence over the past 30 to 40 years, and relative frequencies of hospital-acquired pneumonia and ventilator-associated pneumonia (VAP) can vary significantly among health care settings in different countries. In intensive care units in the United States in 2003, *P. aeruginosa* accounted for 18.1% of hospital-acquired pneumonias and a significant percentage of urinary tract infections (16.3%), surgical site infections (9.5%), and blood stream infections (3.4%). With increasing problems because of infections with strains of *P. aeruginosa* resistant to multiple antibiotics, it can be anticipated that therapeutic difficulties with this organism will remain a major cause of morbidity and mortality for some time to come.

Though much less of a problem than nosocomial infection, community-acquired *P. aeruginosa* infection does occur in certain settings, and such infection is often associated with exposure to moist environments. *P. aeruginosa* infections in the community are related to the use of hot tubs, whirlpools, swimming pools, and other types of baths, as well as the use of contact lenses, particularly the extended-wear variety. It is also a cause of otitis externa. Puncture wounds through tennis shoes can give rise to serious *P. aeruginosa* infection. *P. aeruginosa* endophthalmitis after surgery or eye trauma can result in serious visual compromise, and *P. aeruginosa* endocarditis is frequently found in injection drug users, a problem that often recurs within individual communities as a result of sharing of contaminated needles and drugs.

PATHOBIOLOGY

Host Factors in Pathogenesis

Although many factors contribute to host susceptibility to *P. aeruginosa* infection, one overarching factor for community-acquired and nosocomial *P. aeruginosa* infection appears to be neutropenia. Even in settings in which polymorphonuclear neutrophil (PMN) numbers are normal but their recruitment and activation in responses to infection are impaired, such as those associated with the constitutive inflammation in the lung of patients with CF, *P. aeruginosa* infections readily develop. Other host factors known to be associated with increased susceptibility to infection include dead or poorly perfused tissue in burns and wounds, loss of mucosal barrier function, such as occurs in the tracheobronchial tree of mechanically ventilated patients, and disruption of the normal bacterial flora in the gastrointestinal tract and oropharynx. The panoply of cytokines and chemokines that humans can produce in response to infection, with their additive, synergistic and complementary, or antagonistic effects, makes it difficult to ascribe a role in resistance to *P. aeruginosa* infection to a single cytokine. In transgenic mice, some cytokines and chemokines serve as key elements in both resistance and enhancement of pathology related to *P. aeruginosa* infection.

Although all known monocytic, granulocytic, and lymphocytic cell types have shown some effect in having an impact on *P. aeruginosa* infection in both human and experimental animal infections, it is clear that the major cellular mediators of resistance to *P. aeruginosa* infection are PMNs. Even though the incidence of serious *P. aeruginosa* infection in neutropenic hosts seems to have declined in the past 10 to 15 years when compared with the incidence in the 1970s, neutropenia in humans is still a major risk factor for *P. aeruginosa* infection. Signaling via the MyD88 adaptor protein used by such cytokine receptors as those for interleukin-1 and tumor necrosis factor-α to induce translocation of nuclear factor κB is essential for PMN recruitment to the lung. In the absence of MyD88, lethal pneumonia and sepsis can be induced by fewer than 60 bacterial cells applied to the noses of mice. Thus, MyD88-mediated cellular responses provide essentially all of the resistance to *P. aeruginosa* lung infection.

Epithelial cells, particularly in the lung, are among the first cell types to encounter *P. aeruginosa* after exposure. Principally through studies directed at elucidating why CF patients are so commonly infected with *P. aeruginosa* (>80% of patients are infected by 15 to 20 years of age), much has been learned about the role of epithelial cells in orchestrating innate immunity to *P. aeruginosa* infection (Chapter 89). The major challenge has been to correlate the genetic defect leading to the synthesis of either no cystic fibrosis transmembrane conductance regulator (CFTR) protein or dysfunctional CFTR to the pathogenesis of *P. aeruginosa* infection. Lack of functional CFTR compromises the host's ability to respond rapidly to *P. aeruginosa* with a protective inflammatory response involving such diverse factors as epithelial uptake of bacteria via binding to CFTR, which in turn leads to rapid cytokine responses and PMN infiltration to protect against further bacterial spread within the bronchial mucosa. Delays in these responses, particularly the rapid recruitment of PMNs to the site of infection, could underlie the ability of *P. aeruginosa* to survive in the lung of CF patients and ultimately lead to destructive inflammation.

Bacterial Factors in Pathogenesis

P. aeruginosa is a formidable pathogen in humans because of the multitude, diversity, and complexity of its virulence factors. Virtually all major classes of bacterial virulence systems are found in this organism (Table 314-1), including exotoxins, endotoxins, type III secreted toxins, pili, flagella, proteases, phospholipases, iron-binding proteins, exopolysaccharides, the ability to form biofilms, and elaboration of toxic small molecules such as pyocyanins. The potential of *P. aeruginosa* to cause infection in virtually any body site is probably due to the array of factors that it can call on from its large genome to establish itself at a specific site and use a wide variety of nutrients for growth, along with the ability to produce a panoply of factors to counteract host defenses.

Bacterial factors produced to counter host defenses include the expression of long O side chains on bacterial lipopolysaccharide to prevent lysis by complement and production of a variety of proteases that can inactivate host immune effectors and kill immune effector cells, as well as degrade tissue components, thereby allowing the organism to advance the infectious process. *P. aeruginosa* uses typical siderophore systems to acquire iron, specifically involving factors referred to as *pyoverdin* and *pyochelin*.

A major cellular toxin is exotoxin A, an adenosine diphosphate–ribosylating toxin with activity very similar to that of diphtheria toxin. Purified exotoxin A is lethal to experimental animals in small doses, and its production is affected by iron levels. *P. aeruginosa* can induce hemolysis of red blood cells as a result of the production of PlcHR, a hemolytic phospholipase C. A second, nonhemolytic phospholipase C, PlcN, is also made by *P. aeruginosa* strains. Type III secretion systems are highly conserved features of bacterial pathogens, including *P. aeruginosa*. This system allows direct injection of bacterial toxins into eukaryotic cells, which disrupts cellular trafficking by inhibiting the actin cytoskeleton and also by affecting protein synthesis. For *P. aeruginosa*, clinical isolates expressing type III toxins are isolated significantly more frequently from patients who have poor clinical outcomes. Four major effector proteins are known: ExoS, ExoT, ExoU, and ExoY.

As bacterial counts increase in a tissue, the organisms reach a critical mass that is thought to allow them to effectively communicate with each other through the system of quorum sensing (QS). For *P. aeruginosa*, three major, interrelated QS systems are known to date, designated the las, rhl, and *Pseudomonas* quinolone system (PQS). The molecular mediators of the QS system are known as autoinducers because of their self-regulatory effects on bacterial responses to the environment. These three systems, along with some other regulatory factors, have a complex interaction in the context of regulation of gene transcription and production of virulence factors.

Another major bacterial phenotype regulated by the QS system is the formation of *P. aeruginosa* biofilms, a well-studied area but with some important limitations in terms of applicability to clinical infection and disease. Although biofilms are thought to play a role in chronic infections such as osteomyelitis or CF lung infection, the structured communities typical of biofilms are not really observed in infected tissues, notably the CF lung. Rather, microcolonies or aggregates of bacteria are present, and these microcolonies contain not only bacterial factors but also host factors, including host DNA, mucus, actin, and probably other products from dead and dying bacterial and host cells. How these in vivo microcolonies are actually related to the QS-controlled biofilms studied in vitro on abiotic surfaces is still unclear.

CLINICAL MANIFESTATIONS

Bacteremia

The clinical manifestations of *P. aeruginosa* blood stream infection are rarely different from those of bacteremia in general. Patients are usually febrile, but more severely ill patients in shock may be hypothermic. The only point differentiating this entity from other causes of gram-negative sepsis may be the occurrence of distinctive skin lesions known as *ecthyma gangrenosum* (Chapter 449), which occur almost exclusively in markedly neutropenic

TABLE 314-1 VIRULENCE FACTORS FOR *PSEUDOMONAS AERUGINOSA*

LOCATION OR CLASS	EXAMPLES	ACTIVITY/EFFECTS ON HOST
Cell surface	Alginate	Antiphagocytic, resists opsonic killing
	LPS	Endotoxic, antiphagocytic, evades preformed antibody to previously encountered O antigens
	Pili (produced by type IV secretion)	Twitching motility, biofilm formation, adherence to host tissues
	Flagella	Motility, biofilm formation, adherence to host tissues and mucin components
	Injection of type III secretion factors	PcrG, PcrV, PcrH, PopB, and PopD proteins form injection bridge for type III effectors
Outer membrane	Siderophore receptors	Provide iron for microbial growth and survival
	Efflux pumps	Remove antibiotics
Secretion systems		
Type II	Elastase, lipase, phospholipases, chitin-binding protein, exotoxin A, and others	Variety of proteolytic, lipolytic, and toxic factors. Degrade host immune effectors
Type III	ExoS, ExoT, ExoU, ExoY	Intoxicate cells (ExoS/ExoT); cytotoxic (ExoU), disrupt actin cytoskeleton
Type VI	Cytoplasmic and membrane-associated proteins, ATPases, lipoproteins, Hcp1 protein	Poorly characterized but found in animal studies to be needed for optimal virulence, particularly in chronic infection
Iron acquisition	Pyoverdin, pyochelin	Scavenge iron from the host for bacterial use
Secreted toxins	Exotoxin A, leukocidin, phospholipases, hemolysins, rhamnolipid phospholipases	Kill leukocytes, hemolysis of red cells, degrade host cell surface glycolipids
Secreted oxidative factors	Pyocyanin, ferripyochelin	Produce reactive oxygen species: H_2O_2, O_2^- Inflammatory, disrupts epithelial cell function
Quorum sensing	LasR/LasI, RhlR/RhlI, PQS	Biofilm formation, regulation of virulence factor secretion

ATPases = adenosine triphosphatases; LPS = lipopolysaccharide; PQS = *Pseudomonas* quinolone signal.

patients. These small, painful, reddish, maculopapular, well-circumscribed lesions have a geographic margin and begin pink, darken to purple, and finally become black and necrotic. Histopathology indicates that the lesions are caused by vascular invasion after bacteremia and are teeming with bacteria.

Acute Pneumonia

The respiratory tract remains the most frequent site of infection by *P. aeruginosa*. This organism ranks either first or second in most lists as the causative pathogen in VAP. However, much debate centers on the actual role of the organism in VAP because the conclusion that *P. aeruginosa* plays a major role in VAP is based on results of cultures of sputum or endotracheal tube aspirates. Frequently, these culture results represent only nonpathogenic colonization of the tracheobronchial tree, formation of an innocuous biofilm on the endotracheal tube, or simple tracheobronchitis. In the absence of radiologic evidence of pneumonia, the question remains whether *P. aeruginosa* is the cause of anything more than purulence in tracheobronchial secretions (i.e., tracheobronchitis). At the current time there is an emerging consensus that an invasive procedure such as bronchoalveolar lavage or protected brush sampling of the distal airways should be used to perform quantitative culture of the lung to substantiate the occurrence of *P. aeruginosa* pneumonia in a ventilated patient. However, the results of treatment when endotracheal aspirates are used as the diagnostic procedure appear to be just as good as those when bronchoalveolar lavage is used.

Chronic Respiratory Tract Infections

P. aeruginosa is responsible for chronic infections of the airways associated with a number of underlying or predisposing conditions, the most prevalent being CF. A description and management of *P. aeruginosa* infection in patients with CF can be found in Chapter 89. A somewhat similar state of chronic colonization is seen in some Asian populations in a disease of unknown cause called *chronic* or *diffuse panbronchiolitis*. The disease is most often described in Japan but is not restricted to that country. However, not unlike CF, there is a chronic relapsing infection by *P. aeruginosa* that is characterized by increased sputum production, fever, and focal lung infiltrates. Strains of *P. aeruginosa* isolated from these patients also undergo the same type of mucoid conversion as do strains from patients with CF, which reflects overproduction of an exopolysaccharide called *alginate,* a clear pathogenic factor in chronic CF lung disease.

Bone and Joint Infections

P. aeruginosa is not a frequent cause of bone or joint infections. Such infections result from at least three different mechanisms: bacteremia, direct inoculation into bone, or spread from contiguous infection. Bacteremia secondary to either injection of contaminated illicit drugs or infective endocarditis in the addict population has been well documented to cause vertebral osteomyelitis and septic arthritis of then sternoclavicular joint. The clinical manifestation of vertebral *P. aeruginosa* osteomyelitis is more indolent than that of staphylococcal osteomyelitis. The duration of symptoms in the addict population with vertebral osteomyelitis is from weeks to months. Fever is not uniformly present but, when present, tends to be low grade. Sternoclavicular septic arthritis from *P. aeruginosa* is seen almost exclusively in intravenous drug addicts. It may occur with or without endocarditis, but a primary site of infection is often not found.

Pseudomonas osteomyelitis of the foot most frequently follows puncture wounds through sneakers. The organism has been found between the rubber sole layers of sneakers in many cases. Most of these cases are reported in children, but it is also seen in adults. The main manifestation is pain in the foot, and there may be superficial cellulitis around the puncture wound and tenderness on deep palpation of the wound.

Central Nervous System Infections

Primary central nervous system (CNS) infections by *P. aeruginosa* are a relative rarity. Involvement is almost always secondary to a surgical procedure or head trauma and is occasionally noted following bacteremia. The entities seen most often are postoperative or post-traumatic meningitis and occasionally subdural or epidural infections resulting from initial contamination of access areas. Brain abscess secondary to embolic disease from endocarditis has also been described in intravenous drug addicts. The cerebrospinal fluid (CSF) profile of *P. aeruginosa* meningitis is no different from that of pyogenic meningitis. Other forms of *P. aeruginosa* CNS infection, such as brain abscess and epidural and subdural empyema, generally require surgical drainage in addition to antibiotics.

Eye Infections

Eye infections by *P. aeruginosa* occur from direct inoculation into tissue as a result of trauma or surface injury caused by contact lenses. Keratitis is the most frequent type of disease seen, and its association with contact lens wear, especially extended-wear lenses, is well established. However, any form of trauma may predispose to this type of infection, including surgery and burns. Keratitis can be slowly or rapidly progressive, but the classic description is that of disease progressing over a 48-hour period and leading to involvement of the entire cornea with opacification and sometimes perforation. *P. aeruginosa* keratitis should be considered a medical emergency because of the rapidity with which it can progress and lead to loss of sight. Prevention of contact lens–associated infections by proper use of daily-wear disposable lenses would probably drastically reduce the incidence of keratitis in lens users.

P. aeruginosa endophthalmitis is one of the most feared of *P. aeruginosa* infections. Loss of sight or very much reduced visual acuity is the most common outcome of these infections. This entity may result from penetrating injuries, surgery, perforation of a corneal ulcer, or seeding from bacteremia. The disease is fulminant, with severe pain, chemosis, decreased visual acuity, anterior uveitis, vitreous involvement, and panophthalmitis. *P. aeruginosa* also causes a number of uncommon eye infections, including orbital cellulitis in neutropenic patients and gangrene necrosis of the eyelids, both of which result from bacteremia.

Ear Infections

P. aeruginosa ear infections vary from the mild swimmer's ear, to chronic persistent draining ears, to serious life-threatening infections that lead to neurologic sequelae or even death. Swimmer's ear is commonly seen in children and results from infection of moist, macerated skin of the external ear canal. The source of the organism is likely to be hot tubs or swimming pools, particularly if not sufficiently chlorinated. The natural history of most of these cases is resolution without sequelae, but chronic drainage occurs in some patients. Systemic symptoms such as fever develop in a small minority of patients. The diagnosis is made easily as long as there is a high index of suspicion, which should be the case in diabetics and patients with acquired immunodeficiency syndrome.

Another poorly understood form of *P. aeruginosa* ear infection is a chronic middle ear drainage called *chronic suppurative otitis media*. *P. aeruginosa* is isolated from a large percentage of these draining middle ears. Frequently, it is found in mixed culture, but in about 30% of cases it is the sole organism isolated from aerobic cultures. The pathogenesis of this condition is unclear. It is possible that it begins with external otitis similar to swimmer's ear, with subsequent middle ear involvement followed by chronic mastoiditis.

Urinary Tract Infections

P. aeruginosa urinary tract infections generally occur as a complication of the presence of a foreign body such as a stone, stent, or catheter in the urinary tract or an obstruction within the genitourinary system or after instrumentation or surgery on the urinary tract. Paraplegic patients are at high risk for *P. aeruginosa* urinary tract infections, and frequent use of antibiotics in this setting may select for *P. aeruginosa*. Notwithstanding the relationship between obstructive lesions and *P. aeruginosa* urinary tract infections, there have been descriptions of *P. aeruginosa* urinary tract infections in outpatient children without stones or evident obstruction. *P. aeruginosa* urinary tract infection frequently serves as the nidus for *P. aeruginosa* bacteremia by ascending infection.

Skin and Soft Tissue Infections, Including Burns

P. aeruginosa causes ecthyma gangrenosum in neutropenic patients, an entity described earlier in this chapter. Secondary infection of chronic skin ulcers or burns (see later) can also occur. Maceration of normal skin, such as from soaking in a hot tub, can lead to superficial infection. Folliculitis and other papular or vesicular lesions attributed to *P. aeruginosa*, collectively called *dermatitis*, have now been described extensively. Multiple outbreaks have been linked to whirlpools, spas, and swimming pools. Thus, control of growth of this organism in the home or recreational environment by proper antibacterial treatment of water is essential, comparable to the control commonly practiced in hospitals.

Burn wound infections by *P. aeruginosa* constituted one of the most significant problems caused by this organism during the 1960s and 1970s in countries with advanced medical care. A specific clinical picture of sepsis, with high colony counts of *P. aeruginosa* exceeding 10^5 organisms per gram of tissue, was the defining feature. Patients generally exhibited progressive formation of a black necrotic eschar and sepsis, with or without bacteremia. The occurrence of *P. aeruginosa* burn wound sepsis does not appear to be as frequent as reported in the past in countries with advanced medical care, when as many as 10% of burn patients had *P. aeruginosa* sepsis. However, *P. aeruginosa* remains a major pathogen in settings where burn patients have high rates of infection. The diagnosis may be made by culture of blood or by the pathognomonic clinical picture of an expanding burn lesion caused by infection with *P. aeruginosa*. Clinicians usually rely on isolation of *P. aeruginosa* from wounds or blood along with the finding of sepsis in diagnosing burn wound sepsis secondary to *P. aeruginosa*.

Endovascular Infections

P. aeruginosa may cause endovascular infections, including infective endocarditis. In intravenous drug addicts, the source is generally contaminated paraphernalia or illicit drugs. This organism has also been reported to cause prosthetic heart valve endocarditis. Outbreaks of *P. aeruginosa* endocarditis on native heart valves have been described in drug addicts residing in particular cities, probably resulting from local contamination of illicit drugs. The manifestations of *P. aeruginosa* endocarditis resemble those of other forms of acute endocarditis in addicts except that it appears to be more indolent than *Staphylococcus aureus* endocarditis.

Febrile Neutropenia

P. aeruginosa infections during febrile neutropenia occupy a historical place as the organism against which empirical coverage must always be included. Currently, the organism does not appear to be as common in neutropenic patients as it once was. However, the importance of *P. aeruginosa* infection in neutropenic patients has not diminished simply because when it does cause pneumonia or bacteremia, mortality is likely to be high if not appropriately treated by empirical therapy. Additionally, in some parts of the world, *P. aeruginosa* continues to be responsible for the largest proportion of infections caused by a single organism in neutropenic patients. The classic clinical syndromes in febrile neutropenic patients were bacteremia, pneumonia, and soft tissue infection, mainly manifested as ecthyma gangrenosum.

Uncommon *P. aeruginosa* Infections

In addition to the entities just described, *P. aeruginosa* can cause a number of infrequently seen syndromes, including noma neonatorum, a necrotizing mucosal and perianal infection of newborns, toe web infections (especially in the tropics), and the "green nail syndrome" caused by *P. aeruginosa* paronychia as a result of frequent submersion of the hands in water. In the last entity, the green discoloration results from diffusion of pyocyanin into the nail bed.

TREATMENT   Rx

Treatment of Bacteremia

Removal of an infected vascular catheter may be needed to control device-related bacteremia. The standard of care for *P. aeruginosa* bacteremia is usually an effective β-lactam antibiotic combined with an aminoglycoside. Monotherapy with an aminoglycoside has generally resulted in very poor outcomes. There have been at least four studies, none of which have been prospective, double-blinded studies, indicating that *P. aeruginosa* bacteremia has the same outcome when treated with a single antipseudomonal β-lactam or such an agent combined with an aminoglycoside.

Depending on the antibiotic susceptibility of *P. aeruginosa* isolates routinely found in a specific setting, one of the following regimens would be appropriate for *P. aeruginosa* bacteremia, pending return of susceptibility testing results. Adult, nonazotemic patients may be given ceftazidime, 2 g intravenously every 8 hours, cefepime, 2 g intravenously every 12 hours, meropenem, 1 g every 8 hours, or imipenem, 0.5 g every 6 hours. Aztreonam, 1.5 to 2.0 g every 6 to 8 hours, has been used for patients with serious β-lactam allergy. If piperacillin-tazobactam is used empirically, it should be given at a dose of 3.375 g every 4 hours, or if administration of a second drug is indicated, amikacin, 15 mg/kg every 24 hours, may be added to the piperacillin-tazobactam therapy. The addition of an aminoglycoside to the other regimens is perhaps less critical and probably depends on the level of resistance to β-lactam antibiotics seen in any given institution. At the current time, the highest levels of susceptibility are to amikacin in most regions of the world.

Treatment of Pneumonia

Optimal therapy for *P. aeruginosa* pneumonia has not been determined by rigorous studies.**1** As with bacteremia, high failure rates were seen when aminoglycosides were used as single agents. The drugs of choice for *P. aeruginosa* pneumonia would appear to be similar to those just mentioned for bacteremia. A strong case cannot be made for inclusion of the aminoglycoside component for the treatment of fully susceptible organisms, given the evidence that aminoglycosides are not optimally active in the lungs at concentrations normally used for intravenous administration. Aerosolized aminoglycoside might provide adequate drug levels in the tracheobronchial tree, but there is no reason to believe that the drug would penetrate into the consolidated lung. The usually recommended drug is tobramycin, 300 mg inhaled daily. Inhaled aztreonam lysine (75 mg three times daily for 28 days) has shown safety and efficacy for CF patients with moderate to severe lung disease.**2** Patients with nosocomial pneumonia may have *P. aeruginosa* isolates resistant to many of the usual drugs, a problem that appears to be becoming progressively worse. Doripenem is a new carbapenem reportedly with a lower rate of seizures and with activity against a small percentage of meropenem- or imipenem-resistant *P. aeruginosa* isolates. Doripenem has been shown to have activity for treating lower respiratory tract infections if given as a 500-mg dose every 8 hours via a 1-hour infusion, with adjustments in dose needed in patients with impaired renal clearance. A longer infusion time (up to 4 hours) shows somewhat improved pharmacodynamic profiles.

Patients with diffuse panbronchiolitis respond clinically to antipseudomonal therapy, but the organism is not eradicated. Significant advances have, however, been made in its management with the long-term use of macrolides, a class of drugs that have no antibacterial activity against *P. aeruginosa* but are thought to suppress the inflammatory response and perhaps suppress production of *P. aeruginosa* virulence factors. The most commonly used agents have been clarithromycin and azithromycin. Recent clinical studies in *P. aeruginosa*–infected patients with CF have demonstrated benefits in clinical status from the use of macrolides, with a single weekly dose based on weight showing efficacy over a placebo-treated group.**3**

Treatment of Other Infections

With the exception of osteomyelitis after puncture wounds, which occurs mainly in children, antibiotic therapy for other *P. aeruginosa* infections is difficult. The choices are single-drug therapy with an antipseudomonal β-lactam antibiotic or ciprofloxacin. However, resistance of *P. aeruginosa* to ciprofloxacin has increased dramatically worldwide and may preclude its use in many cases.

For the treatment of meningitis, the general principles involved in the treatment of this infection apply, that is, the need for high doses of bactericidal agents to attain high levels within CSF. The agent with which there is some published experience for *P. aeruginosa* meningitis is ceftazidime, but other antipseudomonal β-lactam agents that achieve high CSF concentrations, such as cefepime and meropenem, have also been used successfully.

The usual therapy for keratitis is topical antibiotics. Fortified aminoglycoside preparations or fluoroquinolones are recommended. In cases in which involvement is extensive, ceftazidime or gentamicin may be given by subconjunctival injection.

Therapy for endophthalmitis includes both systemic antibiotics at high doses to achieve better concentrations in the eye and intravitreal antibiotics. Ceftazidime has been the most frequently used antibiotic for this entity, but little is written about outcomes. Its penetration into the vitreous is excellent. Aminoglycosides are also injected subconjunctivally and by intraocular routes and sometimes given intravenously. Adjunctive surgery is generally performed to remove infected vitreous.

Management of otitis externa involves the use of topical antibiotic agents (otic solutions). Aminoglycoside-containing solutions are the most frequently used. Recurrences are frequent and can lead to chronically draining ears that may require more intensive topical therapy.

Treatment of malignant external otitis has undergone significant changes since it was first described in 1960. At the current time, the approach appears to be débridement of the ear canal, including any necrotic tissue cartilage and adjacent bone, rather than extensive bone débridement or facial nerve decompression. Treatment with a single agent, usually ceftazidime or ciprofloxacin, has been successful.

Most *P. aeruginosa* urinary tract infections fit into the category of complicated urinary tract infections, with therapy being more prolonged than the usual course recommended for cystitis. There are no real comparative data on proper therapies. Foley catheters, stents, or stones should be removed if possible to prevent relapse. Generally, 7 to 10 days of antibiotic treatment will suffice, with up to 2 weeks for pyelonephritis. Antipseudomonal β-lactams, ciprofloxacin, levofloxacin, gatifloxacin, and aminoglycosides given once daily are all equally acceptable, given their normally high levels of urinary excretion. Alternative antibiotics that may be used for the oral treatment of *P. aeruginosa* urinary tract infections include doxycycline, to which many strains are sensitive; in cases of multiple antibiotic resistance or in patients with very low urinary output, bladder irrigation with 0.25% acetic acid may be useful. Relapse is common, and it may not be due to antibiotic resistance but to host factors.

Management of *P. aeruginosa*–infected burn wounds is both surgical and medical. Extensive débridement of colonized eschar or necrotic tissue is required. The general principle is to reduce the organism count, which would probably diminish the sepsis response, but importantly, it would reduce the risk of resistance developing during therapy given the extremely high microbial burden of such wounds. At the current time, true burn wound sepsis secondary to *P. aeruginosa* is probably best managed with a combination of antibiotics.

For treatment of *P. aeruginosa* infections in febrile, neutropenic patients, antipseudomonal β-lactams such as cefepime, ceftazidime, or a carbapenem can be used either alone or in combination with an aminoglycoside. Alternatively, an antipseudomonal penicillin such as piperacillin can be used in combination with an aminoglycoside if so preferred.

Antibiotic Resistance and Antibiotic Therapy for Multiresistant *Pseudomonas* Infections

P. aeruginosa strains that occur worldwide and carry multiple resistance determinants that mediate β-lactam multiresistance, along with fluoroquinolone and aminoglycoside resistance, have emerged as significant causes of infection. The medical community is now turning to drugs such as colistin and polymyxin, which were discarded decades ago but are now being considered as antimicrobials for the "21st century." Alternative approaches to the management of multiresistant *P. aeruginosa* began some time ago because of the complexity of management of such organisms in patients with CF. Colistin (polymyxin E) is used intravenously, not withstanding its toxicity. Use of this agent—or the related peptide antibiotic polymyxin B—is now rapidly becoming the therapy of choice of last resort in non-CF patients infected with multiresistant *P. aeruginosa*. The dose of either agent needs to be adjusted for renal insufficiency. One recommended schedule for colistin is as follows: for patients with creatinine clearance greater than 20 mL/min, 75 to 100% of the daily dose given in two divided doses; for creatinine clearance of 5 to 20 mL/min, 50% of the daily dose given in two divided doses; and for creatinine clearance less than 5 mL/min, 30% of the daily dose given in two divided doses every 12 to 18 hours. Addition of rifampicin to colistin has been suggested to have a synergistic effect.

Infections Caused by Organisms at One Time Classified As Pseudomonads

Most of these infections are due to members of the genus *Burkholderia*, including *Burkholderia cenocepacia*, a complex of about 10 related species previously referred to as *genomovars* that are phenotypically similar but distinguished primarily by nucleic acid sequences, as well as *B. mallei* and *B. pseudomallei*, causes of glanders and melioidosis, respectively. Infections caused by members of the genus *Ralstonia* and non–*P. aeruginosa* pseudomonads such as *Pseudomonas fluorescens* are generally rare and often iatrogenically induced by accidental contamination of solutions or medications delivered to patients. *Stenotrophomonas maltophilia* is an uncommon cause of a variety of diseases and often occurs as part of a polymicrobial infection; it can be involved in pneumonia, endocarditis, bacteremia, and urinary tract infections. This organism is generally resistant to many types of common antibiotics used for *P. aeruginosa* but is frequently sensitive to trimethoprim-sulfamethoxazole, ticarcillin-clavulanate, many fluoroquinolones, and rifampin.

Organisms in the *B. cenocepacia* complex are usually pathogenic for immunocompromised hosts and individuals with long-standing underlying serious disease. It infects the lungs of about 4% of CF patients, most commonly after many years of tissue destruction from chronic *P. aeruginosa* infection. Some strains of *B. cenocepacia* and *Burkholderia dolosa* are known to cause precipitous deterioration in the clinical condition of CF patients who acquire these hypervirulent strains and, though relatively rare, can still cause focal outbreaks in CF centers. Outside of CF, *B. cenocepacia* infection can either be acquired from hospital surfaces or be brought in from outside the hospital because of its ubiquity in the environment. As with *P. aeruginosa*, *B. cenocepacia* is found in moist or water-based environments. Pseudobacteremia caused by contamination of blood culture bottles has to be suspected when *B. cenocepacia* organisms are reported. Treatment of *B. cenocepacia* infections can be highly problematic because the organisms are at times naturally resistant to almost all commonly used antibiotics. Nonetheless, combinations of meropenem with ciprofloxacin and tobramycin appear to be successful, and in CF patients with β-lactam hypersensitivity, meropenem monotherapy has been effective. In vitro susceptibility profiles can be used to guide initial therapy.

Melioidosis from *B. pseudomallei* can occur in humans and animals and is endemic in parts of Southeast Asia and northern Australia. Findings range from asymptomatic infection to localized skin infections, chronic lung infection, and even fulminant septicemia with multiple organ failure. *B. pseudomallei* infections can occur in individuals who have recently traveled to endemic areas and is also a category B bioterrorism agent. Infection with *B. pseudomallei* can remain latent for long periods and then become reactivated, so lack of recent exposure or travel to an infected area may be insufficient to exclude a diagnosis of melioidosis. Underlying conditions such as diabetes, excessive alcohol consumption, and renal disease are found in more than half of such patients. Initial intensive therapy for 10 to 14 days can include ceftazidime, meropenem, or imipenem, to which trimethoprim-sulfamethoxazole can be added. For eradication therapy, 3 months or more of trimethoprim-sulfamethoxazole with or without doxycycline is used.

Glanders, caused by *B. mallei*, is primarily a disease of horses and is thus an occupational risk for those who come in contact with these animals. Glanders has been eliminated from enzootic foci in most countries, but some pockets remain in South America, Asia, Africa, and the Middle East. A history of contact with horses or similar species such as donkeys in one of these areas is consistent with a diagnosis of glanders. Incubation periods can be short (1 to 2 days after inhalation) or up to a few months, and as with *B. pseudomallei*, latent foci can be reactivated years after primary exposure. Clinical manifestations include an acute febrile illness and necrosis in the tracheobronchial tree accompanied by mucopurulent discharge from the eyes, nose, or lips. Systemic infections along with lymphadenopathy, respiratory tract involvement, and skin lesions are also manifestations of this disease. Untreated, the infection is lethal within 10 to 14 days. Antibiotic susceptibility and treatment are similar to that for *B. pseudomallei*, although newer macrolides appear to be effective against glanders, but they are not effective against melioidosis, as is gentamicin. *B. mallei* is also a category B bioterrorism agent and was used during World War I by German agents to infect and incapacitate horses in the United States, Europe, and Argentina.

Grade A

1. Langton Hewer SC, Smyth AR. Antibiotic strategies for eradicating *Pseudomonas aeruginosa* in people with cystic fibrosis. *Cochrane Database Syst Rev.* 2009;4:CD004197.
2. Retsch-Bogart GZ, Quittner AL, Gibson RL, et al. Efficacy and safety of inhaled aztreonam lysine for airway *Pseudomonas* in cystic fibrosis. *Chest.* 2009;135:1223-1232.
3. Steinkamp G, Schmitt-Grohe S, Döring S, et al. Once-weekly azithromycin in cystic fibrosis with chronic *Pseudomonas aeruginosa* infection. *Respir Med.* 2008;102:1643-1653.

SUGGESTED READINGS

Berra L, Sampson J, Wiener-Kronish J. *Pseudomonas aeruginosa*: acute lung injury or ventilator-assisted pneumonia? *Minerva Anestesiol.* 2010;76:824-832. *An important compendium of information about the epidemiologic, pathogenic, and clinical outcomes associated with* Pseudomonas aeruginosa *ventilator-associated pneumonia.*

Miliani K, L'hériteau F, Lacavé L, et al. Imipenem and ciprofloxacin consumption as factors associated with high incidence rates of resistant *Pseudomonas aeruginosa* in hospitals in northern France. *J Hosp Infect.* 2011;77:343-347. *Imipenem and ciprofloxacin use play a major role in driving* P. aeruginosa *resistance.*

Paul M, Yahav D, Bivas A, et al. Anti-pseudomonal beta-lactams for the initial, empirical, treatment of febrile neutropenia: comparison of beta-lactams. *Cochrane Database Syst Rev.* 2010;11:CD005197. *Evidence-based recommendations.*

Rybtke MT, Jensen PØ, Høiby N, et al. The implication of *Pseudomonas aeruginosa* biofilms in infections. *Inflamm Allergy Drug Targets.* 2011;10:141-157. *The extracellular matrix encasing the biofilm-associated bacteria is a major contributor to antibiotic resistance.*

Silby MW, Winstanley C, Godfrey SA, et al. *Pseudomonas* genomes: diverse and adaptable. *FEMS Microbiol Rev.* 2011. [Epub ahead of print.] *The versatile metabolic capacity explains adaptation to fluctuating environmental conditions.*

Williams BJ, Dehnbostel J, Blackwell TS. *Pseudomonas aeruginosa*: host defence in lung diseases. *Respirology.* 2010;15:1037-1056. P. aeruginosa *rarely infects healthy human lungs, thereby suggesting the importance of the mechanical barriers, including mucus clearance, innate immunity, and neutrophilic response.*

315

DISEASES CAUSED BY *ACINETOBACTER* AND *STENOTROPHOMONAS* SPECIES

ROBERT BONOMO

ACINETOBACTER SPECIES

DEFINITION

The Pathogen

Acinetobacter species are gram-negative aerobic bacteria that are coccobacillary in shape and are generally described as aerobic, non–lactose fermenting, nonfastidious, nonmotile, catalase positive, and oxidase negative. Unique among microbial pathogens, the appearance of *Acinetobacter* species is highly dependent on the life cycle. In the early growth phases, *Acinetobacter* species appear rod shaped. In the stationary phase, they acquire a coccobacillary morphology.

There are now more than 30 different species in the genus *Acinetobacter*, and their classification and identification remain problematic for clinicians. Automated and biochemical systems are sometimes inaccurate for the identification of *Acinetobacter* species. In the context of this chapter, the term *Acinetobacter* species refers specifically to *Acinetobacter baumannii* and *Acinetobacter baumannii-calcoaceticus* complex. A full list of *Acinetobacter* species is provided in E-Table 315-1. Molecular methods used to identify and classify *Acinetobacter* are listed in E-Table 315-2.

An increasing number of strains of *Acinetobacter* species are resistant to all antibiotics, and these strains are often responsible for outbreaks in large hospitals. These multidrug-resistant (MDR) strains are often resistant to three or more classes of antibiotics. Among the resistance genes found in *Acinetobacter* species are a large collection of genes for β-lactamase, aminoglycoside-modifying enzymes, and many efflux pumps. Unfortunately, resistance to "last-line" agents, such as the cationic antimicrobial peptides colistin (polymyxin E) and its close relative polymyxin B, also occurs.

CLINICAL MANIFESTATIONS

Acinetobacter species can colonize all body surfaces and cause infection in almost any organ system. Consequently, there are a number of common clinical syndromes associated with infection by *Acinetobacter*. The most common infections are respiratory (pneumonia), blood stream (bacteremia), urinary tract, wound, skin and soft tissue, and burn infections; osteomyelitis secondary to trauma; and meningitis. In general, infection is observed only in immunocompromised or injured hosts. Overall, there are few distinguishing features of *Acinetobacter* infection except for skin manifestations.

Pneumonia

Because of colonization of the oropharynx and tracheostomy tubes in patients on ventilators, the upper respiratory tract is the most common site for infection by *Acinetobacter* species. The distinct syndromes associated with respiratory tract infection due to *Acinetobacter* are community-acquired pneumonia (CAP) and hospital-acquired pneumonia (HAP). In tropical regions of China, Asia, Australia, and the South Pacific, CAP due to *Acinetobacter* species is increasingly recognized. In some locations the incidence can be as high as 10%. The common comorbid conditions seen in CAP due to *Acinetobacter* species are mainly chronic obstructive pulmonary disease (emphysema), renal disease, diabetes mellitus, and alcoholism. CAP due to *Acinetobacter* species appears to be associated with a high incidence of bacteremia, acute respiratory distress syndrome, sepsis, and death (mortality rates ≥50%). The reasons for these fulminant presentations are still unknown. Rarely, CAP due to *Acinetobacter* species can present with consolidation and multiple lung abscesses.

More frequently, *Acinetobacter* species are a cause of HAP. In the United States, *Acinetobacter* species are the third leading cause of nosocomial pneumonia. This disease largely resembles the clinical spectrum of gram-negative pneumonias (bilateral infiltrates, pleural effusion, cavitations, hypoxemia, and bacteremia). Most cases are described in patients on ventilators. The main factors associated with HAP due to *Acinetobacter* species are intubation, previous antibiotic use, intensive care unit stay, surgery, and underlying pulmonary disease. Moreover, *Acinetobacter* species can be acquired occupationally. The major challenge complicating nosocomial pneumonia due to *Acinetobacter* species is the frequent recovery of MDR strains. When isolates are MDR, the options for treatment are limited, and complications quickly arise. *Acinetobacter* HAP is associated with excess length of stay and excess mortality.

Bacteremia

Blood stream infection due to *Acinetobacter* species is often a consequence of infection or colonization of intravenous catheters or of HAP. Less commonly, wound infections cause bacteremia. In most series, mortality associated with blood stream infection ranges from 17 to 46%.

Urinary Tract Infection

Commonly, urinary tract infections are caused by enteric gram-negative bacilli; only rarely are these infections caused by *Acinetobacter* species. The indwelling bladder catheter has been implicated as the major risk factor for urinary tract infection (cystitis and pyelonephritis) due to *Acinetobacter* species.

Wound, Burn, and Skin and Soft Tissue Infections

In most clinical series to date, traumatic or postoperative wounds, burns, and skin and soft tissue infections (SSTIs) are the most common causes of *Acinetobacter* infections. Most likely, the combination of antibiotic use, colonization, and compromised or devitalized tissues is responsible. The spectrum of infection can extend from cellulitis to necrotizing fasciitis.

As a result of the outbreak of *A. baumannii* among military personnel in Iraq and Afghanistan, reports of severe wound infections and SSTIs caused by this pathogen are increasing in frequency. Necrotizing SSTI associated with *A. baumannii* occurs in hosts with underlying comorbidities (e.g., trauma, cirrhosis) and is often accompanied by bacteremia. Multiple drug resistance and the presence of co-pathogens frequently complicate treatment. Most cases require surgical débridement and lead to substantial mortality (≈30%). In addition, the use of central venous catheters and total parenteral nutrition is more common among patients with SSTIs. *Acinetobacter* species–associated SSTIs can present with a peau d'orange appearance, with overlying tiny vesicles (Fig. 315-1) and, when untreated, progress to necrotizing infection with bullae (hemorrhagic and nonhemorrhagic).

Osteomyelitis

The conflicts in Iraq and Afghanistan highlighted the first cases of osteomyelitis due to *Acinetobacter* species. Before this time, rare cases of osteomyelitis occurring in soldiers were reported during the Korean and Vietnam wars. Most of the initial reports from the Middle East described "contiguous focus" osteomyelitis. These patients had open fractures or exposed bone, with gross findings of infection: purulence, necrotic tissue, or environmental contamination with exposed bone; temperature higher than 38° C; leukocyte count greater than 12,000/µL; and *Acinetobacter* species identified from culture of deep wound tissue obtained intraoperatively. Antibiotic treatment of these infections also requires multiple surgical débridements of necrotic bone.

Meningitis

Acinetobacter meningitis is usually found in the post-neurosurgical setting, with mortality exceeding 15%. Although an uncommon cause of meningitis from the community, the frequency is almost 4% in cases of hospital-acquired meningitis. Treatment is problematic because cephalosporins do not achieve high enough levels in cerebrospinal fluid to be effective (see later).

FIGURE 315-1. Cellulitis caused by *Acinetobacter baumannii*. There is characteristic edematous peau d'orange erythema, with associated vesicles that may coalesce to form nonhemorrhagic bullae. (From Guerrero DM, Perez F, Conger NG, et al. *Acinetobacter baumannii*–associated skin and soft tissue infections: recognizing a broadening spectrum of disease. *Surg Infect [Larchmt].* 2010;11:49-57.)

TREATMENT Rx

Increasing resistance to a variety of antimicrobial agents complicates the treatment of *Acinetobacter* species infections. Evidence is emerging that mortality in patients with *Acinetobacter* blood stream infection is significantly greater than that due to other gram-negative pathogens, *Pseudomonas*, *Staphylococcus aureus*, and *Candida* species. In addition, infection with MDR *Acinetobacter* species is associated with increased mortality and length of hospitalization.

Infection with MDR *Acinetobacter* species is often treated, largely empirically, with colistin (2.5 to 5 mg/kg/day IV, which is equivalent to 6 to 12 mg/kg/day colistimethate sodium), sulbactam (ampicillin/sulbactam 3 g IV every 6 hours), imipenem (500 to 1000 mg IV every 6 hours), or tigecycline (100 mg loading dose, then 50 mg every 12 hours). The duration of treatment is generally similar to that for infections caused by other gram-negative pathogens and is dependent on the site of infection. Often clinicians add rifampin (10 mg/kg/day, not to exceed 600 mg) to either colistin or sulbactam. Unfortunately, too few patients have been studied properly, and animal models may have significant limitations in helping to determine the best form of therapy. In cases of meningitis due to *Acinetobacter* species, treatment should be intravenous meropenem (2000 mg every 8 hours) plus the intraventricular administration of an aminoglycoside (gentamicin, depending on susceptibilities, or amikacin). Intraventricular gentamicin is administered at a dose of 4 mg once daily every 1 to 3 days until clinical and microbiologic improvement occurs. Amikacin can be used in place of gentamicin at the dose of 30 mg once a day, if required. For cases of meningitis due to carbapenem-resistant *Acinetobacter*, intravenous colistin supplemented with intraventricular or intrathecal administration of 5 to 10 mg in 1 to 2 mL sterile normal saline, after the removal of a greater or equal volume of cerebrospinal fluid, plus removal of infected neurosurgical material, appears to be the therapeutic strategy most likely to succeed.

STENOTROPHOMONAS MALTOPHILIA

DEFINITION

S. maltophilia has attracted significant attention because it is often MDR owing to intrinsic and acquired factors, and it contributes significantly to morbidity, but usually not mortality, in immunocompromised patients. The role of *S. maltophilia* in infections in patients with cystic fibrosis (Chapter 89) increases with age and appears to be linked to antibiotic exposure history.

The Pathogen

S. maltophilia are gram-negative bacteria that need methionine for growth and, like *Pseudomonas aeruginosa* and *Acinetobacter* species, are non–lactose fermentors. *S. maltophilia* possess flagellae that are multitrichous (more than one flagellum arising from the pole) and are distinguished from *P. aeruginosa* as oxidase negative. Colonies of *S. maltophilia* may appear pale yellow or lavender-green on blood agar plates. The organism emits a mild ammonia-like odor that is used for preliminary identification.

CLINICAL MANIFESTATIONS

Despite harboring many resistance genes, little is known about the virulence of *S. maltophilia*. Nevertheless, a number of risk factors are associated with infection by *S. maltophilia* (Table 315-1). Although *S. maltophilia* is regarded as primarily a nosocomial pathogen, community-acquired infection can occur.

Respiratory Tract

The respiratory tract is the most common site of isolation of *S. maltophilia* in hospitalized patients, accounting for the origin of 70% of isolates. Nosocomial pneumonia due to *S. maltophilia* is often associated with significant pulmonary disease such as emphysema, bronchiectasis, lung transplantation, or endobronchial obstruction. In addition, many of these patients are on mechanical ventilators, have tracheostomy tubes in place, or are receiving broad-spectrum antibiotics. Respiratory tract involvement with *S. maltophilia* is associated with significantly increased mortality; late-onset ventilator-associated pneumonia due to *S. maltophilia* has a mortality rate of 65%. In patients with neutropenia, mortality is as high as 40%; however, CAP due to *S. maltophilia* is very rare.

The incidence of respiratory tract infection due to *S. maltophilia* in patients with cystic fibrosis (Chapter 89) is increasingly being reported. There may

TABLE 315-1 RISK FACTORS FOR INFECTION BY *STENOTROPHOMONAS MALTOPHILIA*

Central venous catheters
Prolonged hospitalization or intensive care unit stay
Neutropenia or cytotoxic chemotherapy
Mechanical ventilation
Malignancy
Corticosteroids
Antibiotic exposure
Exposure to other patients with *S. maltophilia*

be clear links with antipseudomonal antibiotics (tobramycin, imipenem, ceftazidime) used to treat these patients and the duration of hospitalization. The prognostic significance of *S. maltophilia* in the respiratory tract of patients with cystic fibrosis is unclear. Although some studies have shown progressive deterioration in pulmonary function, particularly in patients who are chronically colonized, recent data show that patients who acquire *S. maltophilia* have more advanced disease than those who do not. Moreover, detection of this species in sputum culture does not independently affect the rate of deterioration or survival.

Blood Stream Infection and Endocarditis

Bacteremia may be secondary to a respiratory, urinary, or gastrointestinal source or to an indwelling intravascular device. In many cases, except for those involving intravenous catheters, the portal of entry is not apparent. Despite the inability to demonstrate virulence, attributable mortality in blood stream infection is between 40 and 60%. On occasion, an environmental reservoir or contaminated vascular access device is linked to the presence of bacteremia. Intravenous drug users are at especially high risk for contaminating prosthetic valves with *S. maltophilia*. In the case of endocarditis, favorable outcomes are reported with antimicrobial therapy, but surgery may also be required.

Urinary Tract Infection

Although *S. maltophilia* is frequently recovered from urine specimens in patients with urinary catheters, the role of this organism is unclear.

Meningitis

Rarely, cases of central nervous system infection are reported due to *S. maltophilia*. Often these are associated with central nervous system devices or antecedent neurosurgery.

Skin and Soft Tissue Infection

S. maltophilia can be isolated form postoperative wounds, but its role in this setting is unclear. In contrast, *S. maltophilia* can cause burn wound sepsis, presenting as a syndrome very similar to ecthyma gangrenosum (Chapter 449) in immunocompromised oncology patients.

TREATMENT Rx

As a pathogen that is an increasingly important cause of nosocomial infections, *S. maltophilia* exhibits intrinsic resistance to many antibiotics. The complexity of resistance genes and mechanisms is summarized in Table 315-2. Resistance to imipenem, piperacillin/tazobactam, ceftazidime, and aminoglycosides is very common. Despite significant resistance to many agents, trimethoprim-sulfamethoxazole remains the drug of choice (one DS tablet orally twice a day, or 12 to 15 mg/kg/day IV, based on the trimethoprim dose). Treatment duration is uncertain, but it is usually 14 days or longer. In addition, in vitro studies indicate that ticarcillin–clavulanic acid (3.1 g every 6 hours), minocycline (200 mg followed by 100 mg every 12 hours, not to exceed 400 mg in 24 hours), some of the new fluoroquinolones (ciprofloxacin 400 mg IV every 8 hours), and tigecycline may be useful agents. Colistin and rifampin (see earlier) may serve as alternatives in the face of resistance to trimethoprim-sulfamethoxazole. Aztreonam is effective against strains exhibiting resistance to β-lactams by metallo-β-lactamases.

TABLE 315-2 MECHANISMS OF RESISTANCE IN *STENOTROPHOMONAS MALTOPHILIA*

DRUG	MECHANISM OF RESISTANCE
β-lactams, including imipenem	L1 and L2 β-lactamases Outer membrane permeability/efflux
Aminoglycosides	Aminoglycoside-modifying enzymes, transport

SUGGESTED READINGS

Garnacho-Montero J, Amaya-Villar R. Multiresistant *Acinetobacter baumannii* infections: epidemiology and management. *Curr Opin Infect Dis.* 2010;23:332-339. *Colistin and tigecycline are newer options.*

Michalopoulos A, Falagas ME. Treatment of *Acinetobacter* infections. *Expert Opin Pharmacother.* 2010;11:779-788. *Comprehensive review of all antimicrobial agents available for the treatment for these commonly multidrug-resistant infections.*

Munoz-Price LS, Weinstein RA. *Acinetobacter* infection. *N Engl J Med.* 2008;358:1271-1281. *Review of the emergence of nosocomial* Acinetobacter *infections, including in-depth discussion of multidrug resistance and specific treatment regimens.*

Neonakis IK, Spandidos DA, Petinaki E. Confronting multidrug-resistant *Acinetobacter baumannii*: a review. *Int J Antimicrob Agents.* 2011;37:102-109. *Review of treatment options.*

316

SALMONELLA INFECTIONS (INCLUDING TYPHOID FEVER)

JOHN A. CRUMP

DEFINITION

A member of the family Enterobacteriaceae, *Salmonella enterica* subspecies *enterica* includes more than 2400 serotypes found in humans and other warm-blooded animals. These serotypes may be associated with human asymptomatic intestinal carriage, intestinal infection, and invasive disease with extraintestinal infection. Each serotype designation follows the species name (e.g., *Salmonella enterica* subspecies *enterica* serotype Typhmurium) and is frequently abbreviated as simply *Salmonella* followed by the serotype name (e.g., *Salmonella* Typhimurium).

The Pathogen

Salmonellae are gram-negative, non–spore-forming bacilli. They are differentiated from other Enterobacteriaceae by biochemical tests. They ferment glucose, maltose, and mannitol but typically not lactose or sucrose. They reduce nitrates and do not produce cytochrome oxidase. Almost all salmonellae produce acid and gas with fermentation. Most *Salmonella* serotypes cannot be distinguished by biochemical reactions. However, *S.* Typhi may be preliminarily identified by its production of only trace amounts of hydrogen sulfide and diminished biochemical activity compared with other serotypes.

Salmonellae can be differentiated into more than 2400 serotypes (also called *serovars*) by their somatic (O) antigens, which are composed of lipopolysaccharides and are part of the cell wall, and by their flagellar (H) and capsular (Vi) antigens. *Salmonella* serogroups were traditionally designated by letters based on O antigens (e.g., A, B, C1, C2). More recently, the growing number of serogroups has made it necessary to move to a numeric designation. During the transition, the traditional letter-based serogroup may be retained in brackets after the numeric designation (e.g., O:2 [A], O:4 [B], O:6,7 [C1], O:8 [C2]). Some of the important serotypes and their serogroups are Typhi (group O:9 [D1]), Choleraesuis (group O:7 [C1]), Typhimurium (group O:4 [B]), and Enteritidis (group O:9 [D1]). *Salmonella* Enteritidis and Typhimurium are the most common nontyphoidal serotypes causing human disease.

EPIDEMIOLOGY

S. Typhi, *S.* Paratyphi *A, S.* Paratyphi *B, S.* Paratyphi *C*, and *S.* Sendai are either solely or almost exclusively pathogens of humans; they cause primarily enteric fever rather than diarrhea, and human-to-human transmission is important. As a result of modern sewage and water treatment facilities and improved food safety practices, typhoid fever and paratyphoid fever have become rare in developed countries but remain a problem in countries that lack adequate sanitation and a safe water supply. There are usually fewer than 500 cases of typhoid fever each year in the United States, mainly acquired abroad; in contrast, an estimated 21 million cases occur elsewhere in the world.

Other serotypes of *Salmonella* (described here as nontyphoidal *Salmonella*) have reservoirs in warm-blooded animals and cause human food-borne illness following the consumption of contaminated meat or animal products, contamination of produce or water by animal feces or animal products, or contact with animals and their environments. Some nontyphoidal *Salmonella* serotypes appear frequently in particular animal species, and human illness is often associated with exposure to these animals and their products. For example, *S.* Enteritidis has a reservoir in chickens, and infection is often linked to the consumption of undercooked eggs, poultry products, or exposure to live chicks. Such a relationship is less clear for some other nontyphoidal serotypes (e.g., *Salmonella* Typhimurium). The annual incidence of nontyphoidal *Salmonella* infections in the United States is estimated at 16.2 per 100,000 persons, and most infections are sporadic (i.e., not linked to outbreaks). A disproportionate number of infections occur in July through October, probably related to warm weather. *Salmonella* infections are most common in infants and children younger than 5 years.

Antimicrobial Resistance

Salmonellae have become increasingly resistant to antimicrobial agents, usually by acquiring resistance transfer factors (e.g., plasmid mediated). It is thought that antimicrobial resistance in the human-restricted salmonellae (e.g., *S.* Typhi) is driven primarily by antimicrobial use in humans, whereas antimicrobial resistance among the nontyphoidal salmonellae (e.g., *S.* Typhimurium) is associated with the widespread use of antimicrobial agents in farm animals. A multidrug-resistant strain of *S.* Typhimurium (definitive phage type 104 [DT 104]) has emerged as an important cause of infection in the world. These salmonellae are resistant to ampicillin, chloramphenicol, streptomycin, sulfonamides, and tetracycline. In addition, decreased susceptibility and, more recently, resistance to fluoroquinolones has been increasing worldwide, particularly in Asia.

Etiology

Salmonellae are transmitted by the ingestion of fecally contaminated food or water; contact with animals, their environments, and other fomites; and, rarely, close contact with infected persons (e.g., oral-anal intercourse). The ultimate sources of contamination are humans or animals that are acutely ill or are asymptomatic carriers.

Contaminated Animal Products

Nontyphoidal *Salmonella* are widely spread in the animal kingdom. *Salmonella* infection in humans usually occurs from ingesting contaminated animal food products, most often eggs, poultry, and meat. *S.* Choleraesuis is associated with pig products, *S.* Dublin with cattle and unpasteurized milk from cattle, and *S.* Enteritidis is associated with poultry and poultry products, including eggs. Eggs may become contaminated from feces on the surface of the eggshell that enter through small cracks; by infection of the ovary, resulting in primary incorporation of salmonellae into the egg; or by penetration of the intact shell. Fecal material on poultry and other animal carcasses can spread at slaughterhouses, such as when many poultry carcasses are placed in the same hot water tank to remove feathers. *Salmonella* contaminating carcasses can multiply to high levels if meat or other animal products are not refrigerated. Human illness may result if such animal products are inadequately cooked or if utensils or other uncooked foods are cross-contaminated during preparation. A wide range of foods can be contaminated with animal or human feces, from production on the farm through consumption in the home. Reports of produce-associated *Salmonella* outbreaks, due to contamination by animal or human feces during production, are increasing. *Salmonella* outbreaks have occurred from contaminated cheese, ice cream, vegetables, fruit, juice, and alfalfa sprouts.

Contaminated Food and Water

CONTAMINATION BY PETS. *Salmonella* infections may be acquired after contamination of food or water with the feces of pet turtles, chicks, ducks, birds, dogs, cats, and many other species.

CONTAMINATION BY HUMANS. *Salmonella* infection can also be acquired by eating food or by drinking water contaminated by human carriers who have not adequately washed their hands. Infection has been spread by the fecal-oral route among children, by contaminated enema and fiberoptic instruments, by diagnostic and therapeutic preparations made from animal or insect products (e.g., pancreatic extract, carmine dye), and from intentional or unintentional contamination of restaurant salad bars. Outbreaks of salmonellosis may occur in institutionalized patients, who are probably more prone to the development of *Salmonella* infections for three reasons. First, within institutionalized populations there is an increased prevalence of underlying diseases that decrease host defense mechanisms against salmonellae, such as disorders of gastric acidity and intestinal motility; second, the use of antimicrobial agents modifies the normal, protective intestinal flora; and third, institutional food prepared in bulk is more likely to be contaminated than are individually prepared meals. Outbreaks in nurseries and among the elderly in nursing homes are associated with the highest mortality rates (>5%).

Contact with Animals and Their Environments

Both healthy and sick animals may harbor and shed *Salmonella*. Transmission of *Salmonella* from animals and their environment to humans occurs primarily by the fecal-oral route. Animal fur, hair, skin, and saliva often harbor fecal organisms, and transmission can occur when persons pet, touch, feed, or are licked by animals. Transmission has also been associated with contaminated animal bedding, flooring, barriers, other environmental surfaces, and clothing and shoes. Contact with calves, turtles and other reptiles, rodents, and young poultry and their environments have all been associated with *Salmonella* outbreaks. Humans may also become infected when animals come into contact with their food or water. Both animals and humans can acquire nontyphoidal *Salmonella* from pet food or animal feed. Infections can be prevented by education, supervision of animal contact, provision and promotion of handwashing facilities, and separation of food handling and consumption from animal areas.

Contact with Infected Persons

Close contact with persons shedding *Salmonella* is an occasional source of infection. Transmission has been documented among persons handling feces (e.g., parents changing the diapers of an infected infant) and is associated with certain sexual practices (e.g., oral-anal intercourse).

PATHOBIOLOGY

After the ingestion of organisms, the likelihood of infection developing, as well as the severity of infection, is related to the dose, the virulence of the *Salmonella* strain, and the status of host defense mechanisms. Usually at least 10^2 to 10^3 bacteria are required to produce clinical infection in a normal host. Higher inocula are associated with increased disease severity, whereas smaller inocula are more likely to result in transient intestinal carriage. Gastric acid serves as a host defense mechanism by killing many of the ingested organisms, and intestinal motility is probably another host defense mechanism. In the absence of or a decrease in gastric acidity (e.g., in infants and the elderly; following gastrectomy, vagotomy, or gastroenterostomy; or with the use of drugs that reduce gastric acidity) and with decreased intestinal motility (e.g., the use of antimotility drugs), much smaller inocula can produce infection, and the infection tends to be more severe.

Administration of antimicrobial agents before the ingestion of salmonellae can markedly reduce the size of the inoculum needed to produce infection, presumably by reducing the concentration of protective bowel flora.

Although any *Salmonella* serotype can produce any of the *Salmonella* syndromes (transient asymptomatic carrier state, enterocolitis, enteric fever, bacteremia, and chronic carrier state), each serotype tends to be associated with certain syndromes much more frequently than others. For example, S. Anatum usually causes asymptomatic intestinal infection, whereas S. Typhimurium generally causes enterocolitis. S. Choleraesuis is more likely to produce bacteremia (often with metastatic infection) than asymptomatic infection or enterocolitis, and some serotypes such as S. Typhi and S. Paratyphi are most likely to cause enteric fever as well as the chronic carrier state. Fortunately, most *Salmonella* serotypes are of relatively low pathogenicity for

humans. Therefore, although food products are commonly contaminated, large outbreaks tend to involve the more virulent serotypes.

To produce infection, invasion must occur across the mucosa of the intestine. When the organisms reach the lamina propria, an influx of polymorphonuclear leukocytes serves as a host defense mechanism to prevent invasion of the lymphatics. Certain serotypes seem to have a greater ability than others to invade the lymphatics and subsequently produce bacteremia (e.g., S. Choleraesuis and S. Dublin, which commonly produce bacteremia after intestinal infection). Both the small intestine and the colon are involved in the inflammatory process.

In the case of S. Typhi and other causes of enteric fever, salmonellae invade the mononuclear phagocytes in Peyer's patches in the ileum and mesenteric lymph nodes, multiply intracellularly, and are carried through the lymphatic system and blood stream to the liver, spleen, bone marrow, and other parts of the reticuloendothelial system. Once in the reticuloendothelial system, they multiply intracellularly in mononuclear phagocytes and produce the systemic manifestations of enteric fever. The onset of fever is associated with bacteremia and the release of cytokines (e.g., tumor necrosis factor and interleukins) from mononuclear phagocytes. Ulcerations over Peyer's patches are responsible for the intestinal manifestations of enteric fever such as pain, perforation, and bleeding.

In *Salmonella* enterocolitis, the organisms remain localized in the intestinal mucosa, and diarrhea results from the inflammation produced by polymorphonuclear leukocytes. In addition, watery diarrhea may occur, apparently the result of the secretion of water and electrolytes by small intestinal epithelial cells in response to an enterotoxin secreted by some of the *Salmonella* strains, or in response to tissue mediators of inflammation.

Patients with diseases that impair host defense mechanisms seem to have an increased frequency of severe *Salmonella* infection. For many years, a striking association has been recognized between diseases producing hemolysis and *Salmonella* bacteremia. Specifically, *Salmonella* bacteremia is common in patients with sickle cell disorders, malaria, and bartonellosis. In fact, because of the frequency of *Salmonella* bacteremia in sickle cell diseases and the underlying bone disease in these patients to which salmonellae localize, these organisms are the most common cause of osteomyelitis in patients with sickle cell disorders (Chapter 166). Prolonged *Salmonella* bacteremia may occur in patients with hepatosplenic schistosomiasis, possibly related to localization on and in the intravascular schistosomes. Patients with lymphoma and leukemia are also more prone to the development of *Salmonella* bacteremia. A markedly increased frequency and severity of *Salmonella* infections in general have been observed in patients with human immunodeficiency virus (HIV) infection, particularly those with CD4+ T-lymphocyte counts less than 200 cells/mm^3. Prolonged and recurrent, refractory *Salmonella* bacteremia is common among these patients. Other risk factors that increase the frequency and severity of *Salmonella* infection are extremes of age, immunocompromised states (e.g., from immunosuppressive agents), malnutrition, and probably diabetes. Nontyphoidal *Salmonella* species are a leading cause of community-acquired blood stream infection in sub-Saharan Africa, where children younger than 3 years and HIV-infected adults carry most of the burden of invasive disease.

CLINICAL MANIFESTATIONS

Asymptomatic Intestinal Carrier State

The asymptomatic intestinal carrier state may result from inapparent infection (which is the most common form of *Salmonella* infection), or it may follow clinical disease (in which case the patient becomes a convalescent carrier). The carrier state is usually self-limited to several weeks to months, with the incidence of positive stool cultures rapidly decreasing over time. By 1 year, far less than 1% of carriers still have positive stools. The main exception is S. Typhi; about 3% of those infected excrete the organism for life. Women and older men are most likely to become chronic carriers of S. Typhi, related to the presence of biliary tract disease, especially calculi. A patient who has had salmonellae in stool for 1 year (chronic carrier) is likely to become a lifelong carrier; the reservoir is in the biliary tree, usually in calculi in the gallbladder. Patients with *Schistosoma haematobium* infection are predisposed to become chronic urinary carriers of salmonellae.

Enterocolitis

After an incubation period of usually 12 to 48 hours, the illness starts suddenly with crampy abdominal pain and diarrhea. Nausea and vomiting may occur but are usually not prominent or persistent. The diarrhea may be watery and of large or small volume. Stools may contain mucus and are occasionally bloody. Polymorphonuclear leukocytes are present in the stool. Diarrhea may be mild or severe, with up to 20 to 30 stools a day. Fever is present in most patients, and the temperature may reach 40° C (104° F) or higher. The abdomen is tender to palpation. Transient bacteremia may occur and is most commonly seen in infants, the elderly, and patients with impaired host defense mechanisms.

Symptoms generally improve over a period of days, with fever lasting no more than 2 to 3 days and diarrhea lasting no more than 5 to 7 days. However, these symptoms occasionally persist for up to 14 days. More severe disease is seen with malnutrition, inflammatory bowel disease, and HIV infection. Reactive arthritis may follow enterocolitis in up to 7% of cases, especially among those with the HLA-B27 phenotype.

Enteric Fever

Enteric fever is produced by *S.* Typhi (typhoid fever), *S.* Paratyphi *A, B,* and *C* (paratyphoid fever), and occasionally other serotypes. Sometimes it immediately follows classic enterocolitis caused by the same organism. The syndrome is characterized by prolonged, sustained fever and may be associated with relative bradycardia, splenomegaly, rose spots, and leukopenia.

Therapy aborts the course of the disease. The following is a description of untreated illness. After an incubation period of 5 to 21 days (generally 7 to 14 days), fever and malaise develop, often associated with cough. A small proportion of patients may have diarrhea during the incubation period. The fever tends to rise in a stepwise fashion over the first few days to a week and then becomes sustained, usually at 39.4 to 40° C (103 to 104° F) or higher. Relative bradycardia is seen in up to half of patients. Apathy, confusion, delirium, and even psychosis may occur. Abdominal distention, pain, and tenderness may occur in the first week and may be associated with diarrhea or constipation; these symptoms are generally more pronounced during the second week of fever. Most patients have abdominal tenderness during the course of the illness.

In about 30% of patients, rose spots develop on the abdomen or chest (or both) toward the end of the first week or during the second week of fever. These faint, salmon-colored maculopapular lesions are subtle and may be difficult to see, particularly in dark-skinned patients. Salmonellae can be cultured from punch biopsies of these lesions. Hepatosplenomegaly occurs in about half of patients. Leukopenia and neutropenia are seen in about 20%. Abnormal liver function test results are common.

After 2 weeks of illness, the severe complications of intestinal hemorrhage or perforation related to necrosis of Peyer's patches may be observed in about 5% of patients. These perforations may require surgical as well as medical therapy and can occur even in a patient treated with antimicrobials. Intestinal perforation is the leading cause of death from enteric fever.

The illness usually resolves by the end of the fourth week in an untreated patient. Relapse may occur in untreated as well as treated patients, but the illness is milder than the original episode.

Rarely, some of the following complications may occur: pancreatitis, cholecystitis, infective endocarditis, meningitis, pneumonia, hepatic or splenic abscess, orchitis, or focal infection at virtually any site.

Bacteremia

Patients with the syndrome of *Salmonella* bacteremia usually complain of fever and chills lasting days to weeks. Gastrointestinal symptoms are unusual, but in some patients the syndrome of *Salmonella* bacteremia follows classic enterocolitis. Other symptoms are nonspecific, such as malaise, anorexia, and weight loss. Metastatic infection of bones, joints, aneurysms (particularly of the abdominal aorta), meninges (mainly in infants), pericardium, pleural space, lungs, heart valves, cysts, uterine myomas, malignancies, and other sites is common, and symptoms may be related to the site of metastatic infection. Stool cultures are often negative for salmonellae, but blood cultures are positive.

Although any *Salmonella* serotype can produce bacteremia, *S.* Dublin, *S.* Choleraesuis, *S.* Heidelberg, *S.* Oranienburg, *S.* Panama, and *S.* Sandiego are associated with increased likelihood of bacteremia.

Salmonella bacteremia occurs with increased frequency in infants, the elderly, and patients with diseases associated with hemolysis (e.g., sickle cell diseases, malaria, bartonellosis), HIV, lymphoma, leukemia, disseminated histoplasmosis, and perhaps systemic lupus erythematosus. Localization to bone is common in patients with sickle cell diseases (Chapter 166).

Prolonged *Salmonella* bacteremia lasting for months may occur in patients with hepatosplenic schistosomiasis. In patients with HIV infection,

recurrent, relapsing *Salmonella* bacteremia may develop, which may be difficult to cure with antimicrobial agents.

DIAGNOSIS

Although *Salmonella* enterocolitis is an invasive disease, the differential diagnosis includes all causes of acute diarrhea, including invasive bacteria such as *Campylobacter jejuni, Shigella* species, invasive *Escherichia coli, Yersinia enterocolitica,* and *Vibrio parahaemolyticus;* toxigenic bacteria such as *Vibrio cholerae,* enterotoxigenic *E. coli,* enterohemorrhagic *E. coli* (e.g., *E. coli* O157:H7), *Staphylococcus aureus, Bacillus cereus, Clostridium perfringens,* and *Clostridium difficile;* viruses; and protozoa such as *Entamoeba histolytica, Giardia intestinalis,* and *Cryptosporidium* species. Invasive bacterial causes of diarrhea, enterohemorrhagic *E. coli,* and *C. difficile* infection are also associated with polymorphonuclear leukocytes in stool, whereas bacterial toxigenic causes (other than *C. difficile* and enterohemorrhagic *E. coli*), viruses, and protozoa generally are not. The bacterial toxigenic causes of diarrhea other than *C. difficile* and enterohemorrhagic *E. coli* do not produce fever.

Stool culture is definitive for the diagnosis of *Salmonella* enterocolitis, but by the time the results of stool culture are available, most patients are recovering. A stained smear of the stool usually demonstrates polymorphonuclear leukocytes. Serologic studies are of little clinical value in *Salmonella* enterocolitis, but they may be of use in epidemiologic studies.

The differential diagnosis of *Salmonella* bacteremia includes all acute infectious and noninfectious causes of fever, including bacteremia caused by other organisms. The diagnosis is proved by isolation of the microorganism from blood or from another normally sterile site.

The differential diagnosis of enteric fever is very broad and depends in part on the area of the world where the infection was acquired. All causes of sustained fever are in the differential diagnosis, including infective endocarditis, disseminated tuberculosis, brucellosis, tularemia, *Mycoplasma pneumoniae* infection, rickettsial infections, Q fever, and viral infections such as infectious mononucleosis. Depending on the site of acquisition, diseases such as malaria, amebic abscesses of the liver, and visceral leishmaniasis enter into the differential diagnosis.

The diagnosis of enteric fever is best proved by isolation of the microorganism from blood, stool, or bone marrow. During the first week of illness, blood cultures are positive in about 90% of patients, but culture positivity decreases over the next 2 weeks to less than 50% during the third week of illness. Stool cultures are usually negative during the first week but are generally positive by the third week. Bone marrow cultures give the highest yield, with up to 95% being positive; they should be considered in suspected cases with negative blood cultures. Bone marrow cultures may be positive even after several days of antimicrobial treatment, when blood cultures have become negative. Urine cultures and cultures of punch biopsies of rose spots may also be positive. The string test to obtain samples of bile from the duodenum has also yielded positive cultures.

The peripheral leukocyte count is usually normal, but leukopenia, which occurs in about 20% of cases, may be suggestive of enteric fever. Fecal leukocytes are generally present.

The Widal and other serologic tests that detect serum antibodies against *S.* Typhi are limited by shortcomings of both sensitivity and specificity and rarely provide useful information to guide patient management. Polymerase chain reaction and other molecular techniques have not proved useful for diagnosis from blood and other specimens, but they have been used to determine the *Salmonella* serotype of bacterial isolates.

TREATMENT

Enterocolitis

The primary approach to the treatment of *Salmonella* enterocolitis is fluid and electrolyte replacement. Drugs with antiperistaltic effects such as loperamide or diphenoxylate with atropine can relieve cramps, but they should be used sparingly because they can prolong the diarrhea.

Salmonella enterocolitis is self-limited, and antimicrobial therapy is usually not indicated, except perhaps in patient groups at high risk for invasive disease. Antimicrobial therapy reportedly has little effect on the clinical course, and in some studies, it has prolonged the duration of salmonellae excretion in stool. In addition, most patients are improving by the time salmonellae or other bacterial pathogens are isolated from stool.

The fluoroquinolones are active against virtually all bacterial pathogens that cause diarrhea (including salmonellae), except for *C. difficile* and many *Campylobacter* organisms. Thus, it is reasonable to use fluoroquinolones for patients with suspected or known *Salmonella* enterocolitis who are severely ill and suspected of being bacteremic. The threshold for antimicrobial treatment is also decreased in those at increased risk for severe illness (e.g., infants, the elderly, patients with sickle cell disease, immunosuppressed individuals). As an example, in adults, ciprofloxacin, 500 mg every 12 hours orally or 400 mg every 12 hours intravenously for 3 to 5 days, or until defervescence, has been widely used. An extended-spectrum cephalosporin such as ceftriaxone is an alternative. In the presence of gross bloody diarrhea, antimicrobial therapy should be withheld until the possibility of *E. coli* O157:H7 infection has been eliminated because antimicrobial therapy may increase the frequency of hemolytic-uremic syndrome.

Other agents, such as amoxicillin and trimethoprim-sulfamethoxazole, have also been widely used in severely ill adults. However, many strains of *Salmonella* are now resistant to these agents.

Enteric Fever

Resistance to the traditional first-line antimicrobial agents (ampicillin, chloramphenicol, trimethoprim-sulfamethoxazole) has emerged worldwide among the salmonellae causing enteric fever. Consequently, alternative antimicrobial agents are now preferred.

The fluoroquinolones have become the agents of choice for the treatment of enteric fever, for several reasons.[1] They can be administered orally and have high bioavailability, they concentrate in bile and the bowel, and they often retain activity against multidrug-resistant strains of *S.* Typhi and other causes of enteric fever. Most important, the fluoroquinolones have proved to be effective in the treatment of enteric fever, even with short courses (e.g., 3 to 7 days). Cure rates exceed 95%, and relapse and chronic fecal carriage after therapy are uncommon. Ciprofloxacin (500 mg orally twice a day) for 7 to 14 days has been the fluoroquinolone of choice for enteric fever. If a patient cannot tolerate oral therapy, the fluoroquinolones can be administered intravenously. Reduced susceptibility to fluoroquinolones, often associated with nalidixic acid resistance, is increasingly reported in *S.* Typhi strains both in the United States and elsewhere and is associated with treatment failure. Consequently, it is recommended that all isolates be tested in vitro against nalidixic acid; ideally, the minimal inhibitory concentration of the fluoroquinolone to be used should also be determined. If decreased fluoroquinolone susceptibility is suspected or demonstrated, an extended-spectrum cephalosporin (e.g., intravenous ceftriaxone) or azithromycin is indicated.

Extended-spectrum cephalosporins such as ceftriaxone are reliable agents for the treatment of enteric fever. Ceftriaxone dosed at 1 to 2 g every 12 to 24 hours for adults and 75 mg/kg/day for children, given intravenously or intramuscularly for 10 to 14 days, results in cure rates of 95%. Resistance to ceftriaxone has been described in clinical strains of *S.* Typhi, but this occurs rarely.

If the *Salmonella* isolate is shown to be susceptible by antimicrobial susceptibility testing, ampicillin, chloramphenicol, or trimethoprim-sulfamethoxazole may be considered. The ampicillin dose is 25 mg/kg intravenously every 6 hours. The use of chloramphenicol should be weighed against the risk of bone marrow toxicity. The chloramphenicol dose is 50 mg/kg/day orally, divided into four doses. Chloramphenicol can be given intravenously at the same dose if oral therapy is not possible. Trimethoprim-sulfamethoxazole (4/20 mg/kg intravenously or orally every 12 hours) is given for 10 to 14 days.

Azithromycin (10 mg/kg/day orally for 7 days) is effective in the treatment of patients with uncomplicated typhoid fever caused by multidrug-resistant strains.[2] The oral route of administration makes it a particularly attractive choice in settings where multidrug resistance is common and intravenous extended-spectrum cephalosporins are impractical, unavailable, or too expensive.

Patients often require supportive care with intravenous saline, correction of electrolyte and acid-base disturbances, and, in the setting of intestinal bleeding, blood transfusion. If perforation is suspected, abdominal imaging should be performed to evaluate for free air. If perforation seems likely, laparotomy should be performed as soon as possible to repair the perforation. In the setting of perforation, antimicrobial therapy should be broadened to cover bowel flora.

Steroid therapy is beneficial in some patients with severe enteric fever and coma, delirium, or shock. Dexamethasone is administered at doses of 3 mg/kg initially, followed by 1 mg/kg every 6 hours for 48 hours. Steroids can mask the signs and symptoms of abdominal perforation and should not be continued for more than 48 hours. Salicylates should be avoided.

Relapses of typhoid fever may be treated with the same antimicrobial regimen as the initial attack.

Bacteremia

The agents of choice to treat *Salmonella* bacteremia are the fluoroquinolones, such as ciprofloxacin, and the extended-spectrum cephalosporins, such as ceftriaxone. Typical doses are ciprofloxacin 400 mg every 12 hours intravenously and ceftriaxone 1 to 2 g every 12 to 24 hours intravenously. When the salmonellae are known to be susceptible, ampicillin 1 to 2 g intravenously every 4 to 6 hours or trimethoprim-sulfamethoxazole 8 mg/kg/day (of the trimethoprim component) intravenously can be used. Chloramphenicol is another option. Antimicrobial susceptibility testing is necessary because of

the emergence of infections resistant to the fluoroquinolones or extended-spectrum cephalosporins.

In cases of sustained bacteremia, the possibility of endovascular infection should be investigated. For transient bacteremia or bacteremia without localization, therapy is continued for 7 to 14 days. With localization to bone, aneurysms, heart valves, and various other sites, antimicrobial therapy should be given for much longer periods (e.g., 6 weeks). Surgical drainage, removal of foreign bodies, or resection of an aneurysm is often necessary to cure localized infection. The possibility of schistosomiasis should be considered and treated, when present, in patients with sustained *Salmonella* bacteremia. Patients with HIV infection tend to experience repeated relapses after treatment courses for *Salmonella* bacteremia. In this group, initial treatment with ciprofloxacin for 2 weeks or longer is recommended. Long-term suppressive therapy has been suggested for those experiencing frequent relapses.

Carriers

Chronic carriers (i.e., >1 year) of salmonellae other than *S.* Typhi are rare. Stools of convalescent carriers spontaneously become negative over a period of weeks to months, and no therapy should be given. The rare chronic carrier of nontyphoidal serotypes (usually infected with *S.* Paratyphi *A*, *B*, or *C*) may be treated with a fluoroquinolone, amoxicillin, or trimethoprim-sulfamethoxazole in the doses listed later for 4 to 6 weeks. Patients who experience relapse usually have gallbladder disease (most often calculi) and will not be cured with antimicrobial therapy alone. Cholecystectomy plus antimicrobial therapy may cure these patients, but it is doubtful that the carrier state per se is a sufficient indication for cholecystectomy.

Chronic fecal carriers of *S.* Typhi can be treated with ciprofloxacin (500 to 750 mg twice daily) for 6 weeks or with amoxicillin at doses of 6 g/day in three to four divided doses plus probenecid 2 g/day in divided doses for 6 weeks. Trimethoprim-sulfamethoxazole (160/800 mg twice daily) plus rifampicin (300 mg twice daily) for 6 weeks may be considered as an alternative regimen. Patients with persistent urinary carriage and *S. haematobium* infection should be treated with praziquantel before eradication of *S.* Typhi is attempted. For patients with persistent carriage and anatomic abnormalities (e.g., gallstones), cholecystectomy combined with antimicrobial therapy is often necessary. For patients with persistent carriage despite adequate antimicrobial therapy and without an identifiable anatomic abnormality, chronic suppressive therapy may be considered. It should be noted that chronic carriers who do not prepare food and who practice adequate personal hygiene usually do not constitute a public health hazard. Therefore, after the institution of appropriate personal hygienic precautions, and in the absence of evidence of a chronic carrier infecting others, cholecystectomy is probably not indicated to eradicate the carrier state.

PREVENTION

Salmonella infection is best prevented by protecting the water supply, preventing fecal contamination during food production, cooking and refrigerating foods, pasteurizing milk and milk products, and handwashing before preparing foods. Travelers should judiciously avoid consuming untreated water, including ice, raw vegetables, and fruits. Food should be cooked or peeled, and drinks should be boiled, carbonated, or commercially bottled. The widespread presence of salmonellae in the animal kingdom means that reducing the risk for *Salmonella* infections requires a multifaceted approach.

There is no vaccine for *Salmonella* infection other than that for *S.* Typhi. Travelers should be vaccinated before going to areas that are endemic for typhoid fever. Two vaccines are available in the United States. One is the typhoid Vi capsular polysaccharide vaccine, which is administered as a single intramuscular injection, with booster doses given every 2 years if needed. This vaccine provides a degree of herd protection against typhoid fever when used at the population level. The other licensed typhoid fever vaccine is the oral live attenuated Ty21a vaccine. Revaccination is necessary every 5 years, if indicated. Ty21a vaccine should not be used in immunocompromised persons or those receiving antimicrobials. Both these vaccines confer greater than 75% protective efficacy. Efforts are under way to develop oral typhoid vaccines that are effective in young children.

Vaccines afford only partial immunity to typhoid fever. Persons who have been vaccinated should still restrict their diets to avoid potentially contaminated food and fluids. When cases of imported typhoid are identified in the United States, the local health department should be informed and will monitor stool cultures. Typhoid fever acquired in the United States is typically investigated by the public health department to identify potential sources and chronic carriers.

PROGNOSIS

Mortality in patients with *Salmonella* enterocolitis is rare; infants and the elderly are at greatest risk, with death occurring as a result of dehydration and electrolyte imbalance. Mortality from *Salmonella* bacteremia is not uncommon and is most likely to occur in the very young, the very old, the malnourished, and the immunocompromised. *S.* Choleraesuis bacteremia has a very high case-fatality rate (20 to 30% if untreated) compared with other *Salmonella* serotypes.

Before the advent of antimicrobial therapy, typhoid fever had a case-fatality rate of 15 to 20%. This rate has been reduced to less than 1% in industrialized countries. However, the case-fatality rate remains high in some developing countries. In treated patients, the temperature usually returns to normal after 3 to 5 days of therapy, but this may take longer in patients treated with extended-spectrum cephalosporins than in those treated with fluoroquinolones and in those infected with isolates with decreased fluoroquinolone susceptibility who are treated with ciprofloxacin.

In the era before antimicrobial therapy, 5 to 10% of patients who recovered from typhoid fever had relapses. Relapses continued to occur in 10 to 15% of patients treated with chloramphenicol, ampicillin, and trimethoprim-sulfamethoxazole, but this seemed to be much less frequent (<5%) in those treated with ceftriaxone and fluoroquinolones. Intestinal bleeding or perforation occurs in about 5% of patients. With perforation, mortality rates of 10 to 30% have been reported. Up to 3% of patients recovering from *S.* Typhi infection become chronic fecal carriers.

1. Thaver D, Zaidi AK, Critchley JA, et al. Fluoroquinolones for treating typhoid and paratyphoid fever (enteric fever). *Cochrane Database Syst Rev.* 2008;4:CD004530.
2. Effa EE, Bukirwa H. Azithromycin for treating uncomplicated typhoid and paratyphoid fever (enteric fever). *Cochrane Database Syst Rev.* 2008;4:CD006083.

SUGGESTED READINGS

Barton Behravesh C, Mody RK, Jungk J, et al. 2008 Outbreak of *Salmonella* Saintpaul infections associated with raw produce. *N Engl J Med.* 2011;364:918-927. *An outbreak associated with raw tomatoes, jalapeños, and Serrano peppers.*

Centers for Disease Control and Prevention. Preliminary FoodNet Data on the Incidence of Infection with Pathogens Transmitted Commonly through Food—10 States, 2008. *MMWR Morb Mortal Wkly Rep.* 2009;58:333-337. *U.S. population-based surveillance of* Salmonella *and other pathogens commonly transmitted by food.*

Crump JA, Medalla FM, Joyce KW, et al. Antimicrobial resistance among invasive nontyphoidal *Salmonella enterica* isolates in the United States, National Antimicrobial Resistance Monitoring System, 1996-2007. *Antimicrob Agents Chemother.* 2011;55:1148-1154. *Patterns of antimicrobial resistance to be anticipated in invasive nontyphoidal* Salmonella *in the United States.*

Lynch MF, Blanton EM, Bulens S, et al. Typhoid fever in the United States, 1999-2006. *JAMA.* 2009;302:859-865. *Review of sources and patterns of antimicrobial resistance seen in contemporary U.S.* Salmonella typhi *strains.*

317

SHIGELLOSIS

GERALD T. KEUSCH

DEFINITION

Shigellosis is an acute infection of the large bowel characterized by mucosal inflammation and fever. Clinical disease ranges from watery diarrhea to bloody diarrhea or dysentery and a triad of signs and symptoms: multiple small-volume bloody stools per day, abdominal cramping, and tenesmus, a painful straining with the urge to defecate.

The Pathogen

The etiologic agents of shigellosis are gram-negative bacilli of the family Enterobacteriaceae, tribe Escherichieae, and genus *Shigella*. The organism is so closely related to *Escherichia coli* (Chapter 312) that if it were discovered today, *Shigella* would be classified as distinct serotypes of *E. coli*.

EPIDEMIOLOGY

In the United States, approximately 10,000 to 15,000 confirmed cases of shigellosis are reported to the Centers for Disease Control and Prevention (CDC) each year. The incidence has been slowly diminishing for the past 3 decades, from 6.4 per 100,000 per year between 1968 and 1988 to 5.6 per 100,000 per year between 1989 and 2002; an all-time low of 3.5 per 100,000 was reported in 2006 (the most recent year for which statistics are available). About one third of cases occur in infants and children younger than 5 years, commonly associated with daycare centers, where hygiene is difficult to maintain. The majority of infections are due to *Shigella sonnei*, which is true in other developed countries but not in most developing countries. Because most cases are not diagnosed microbiologically, most infections go unreported. The CDC estimates that 450,000 cases of *Shigella* infection occur each year in the United States, primarily in the form of self-limited watery diarrhea. The small inoculum required to cause infection and disease, from 10 to 10,000 organisms, has been demonstrated in experimental human infections. This is why shigellosis is most often transmitted from person to person via organisms from stool carried on the hands and transmitted to another person or an object subsequently handled by a susceptible individual. It also explains why one case in a family is associated with transmission to 20 to 40% of household members, with children more likely to develop clinical illness than adults as a result of their more limited prior experience with the organism. Fecal contamination of food or water can also be involved, and in settings where there is open defecation and no sanitary disposal of feces, flies can transmit the organism to food or water, resulting in larger outbreaks. In the United States, food-borne shigellosis appears to be increasing in frequency, generally related to an infected food handler. Several recent multicountry outbreaks of *S. sonnei* due to contaminated fresh foods shipped from Africa or Southeast Asia demonstrate how globalization of the food supply can readily globalize infection with particular strains of *Shigella*. This has important implications for the importation of antibiotic-resistant strains from areas of the world where the prevalence is particularly high. In the United States, contamination of swimming pools or bathing areas, usually by young children harboring the organism who defecate in the water, can result in common source outbreaks. All these routes are involved in complex humanitarian emergencies such as floods, landslides, earthquakes, or the gathering of refugees of conflict into crowded camps with limited sanitary facilities.

Shigella dysenteriae and *Shigella flexneri* often cause more severe illness, resulting in bloody diarrhea or dysentery. The majority of shigellosis cases in developing countries are due to *S. flexneri* strains, with an important component due to *S. dysenteriae* type 1. *Shigella boydii* is found primarily in the Indian subcontinent and resembles *S. sonnei* more than *S. dysenteriae* type 1 or *S. flexneri* in terms of virulence. These four species cause disease of different severity, with *S. dysenteriae* type 1 being most severe, *S. flexneri* next, *S. boydii* distinctly less so, and *S. sonnei* the least severe, presenting primarily as watery diarrhea. Whenever there is severe underlying childhood malnutrition, however, even *S. sonnei* can cause lethal illness.

In the United States, the incidence peaks in summer and fall. There is no gender difference except among young adults, where females are infected more often, presumably because of closer contact with sick children. In young adults, shigellosis is also transmitted through anal-oral sex practices, most often among men who have sex with men, and it is more commonly due to *S. flexneri* than *S. sonnei*, the reverse ratio observed in the general population. In developing countries, seasonal peaks occur in the rainy season, when organisms from open defecation can be washed into the water used for drinking, or in the dry season, when water for personal hygiene is scarce. Asymptomatic carriage of organisms is limited to a few weeks. However, because an etiologic diagnosis of *S. sonnei* is rarely made, except in common source outbreaks investigated by local, state, or federal public health officials, convalescent carriers often return to their normal activities while still able to transmit infection. This may account for the predilection for outbreaks to occur in daycare centers.

PATHOBIOLOGY

When *Shigella* exit an infected host in feces, they are resistant to acid pH. This facilitates their ability to survive gastric acid and accounts in large part for the small inoculum required. Once past the stomach, the organisms turn off the genes governing acid resistance and turn on the genes that allow them to invade the host's colon. *Shigella* appear to first gain entry into M cells overlying the lymphoid Peyer's patches; they are then transcytosed to the lamina propria, where they are ingested by macrophages and induce inflammatory cytokines, leading to the migration of polymorphonuclear leukocytes, which force open the tight junctions between epithelial cells. This allows many more organisms to gain access to the basolateral membrane of the colonic epithelial cells, where they induce the host cells to ingest them by a mechanism resembling phagocytosis. *Shigella* then lyse the phagocytic vesicle to enter the cytoplasm and multiply; although they are nonmotile, they use their capacity to cross-link actin to propel themselves to the host cell surface. There, by the induced phagocytosis-like mechanism, they pass laterally from one epithelial cell to another. The inflammation and death of contiguously invaded host epithelial cells lead to mucosal ulcerations and further exudation of blood and leukocytes into the colonic lumen. Mucosal inflammation and ulceration are the characteristic pathology caused by *Shigella*. The difference between infection by one species versus another is the severity of the process, which is proportional to the severity of the illness they cause.

The attributes of virulence are present in a large virulence plasmid present in all *Shigella* and in enteroinvasive *E. coli* serotypes capable of causing a similar clinical illness. The virulence plasmid encodes the proteins for a type 3 secretion system that is capable of transferring microbial effector proteins into the host cell; these proteins regulate the cytoskeleton of the host cell to ingest the organism. Once inside the epithelial cell, shigellae are sequestered from host immune responses. *S. dysenteriae* type 1 also produces a chromosomally encoded toxin, Shiga toxin, which inhibits protein synthesis and directly causes cell death. It is one important reason why infection due to this species is so severe. Structurally and antigenically similar toxins are produced by certain *E. coli*, notably serotype O157:H7, responsible for cases of hemorrhagic colitis (Chapter 312). All Shiga toxin–producing organisms are known causes of hemolytic-uremic syndrome (HUS; Chapter 175), a potentially lethal complication of infection due to the toxin's effects on vascular endothelium within the kidneys.

CLINICAL MANIFESTATIONS

Infections due to *S. sonnei* or *S. boydii* typically present after an incubation period of 1 to 3 days with fever and mild to moderate watery diarrhea (Table 317-1). They do not cause serious dehydration and resolve without treatment in 3 to 5 days. However, if the stool is examined under the microscope, many white and red blood cells are visible, indicative of the underlying inflammation of the mucosa. When the inflammation is more severe, as with *S. flexneri*, the watery diarrhea turns bloody and may progress to dysentery, with its characteristic small-volume bloody, mucoid stool passed many (10 to >40) times per day, abdominal cramps, and tenesmus. The most severe infections due to *S. dysenteriae* type 1 progress rapidly from watery to bloody diarrhea and frequently to frank dysentery. Bacteremia with the infecting strain or other enteric flora occurs in up to 10% of cases of severe dysentery due to *S. dysenteriae* type 1 and in some patients with *S. flexneri* infection. Intense mucosal inflammation can result in toxic megacolon, associated in many patients with leukemoid reactions and HUS. Colonic perforation and pancolitis are rare complications and may require surgical intervention. In resource-limited settings, where post-colectomy management may be difficult to ensure, conservative management with fluids and antibiotics or limited surgery to oversew a perforation is the prudent choice; however, mortality may still be as high as 50%. In young children, rectal prolapse may occur due to the intense proctitis, straining to pass stool, and less well developed mesenteric support for the rectosigmoid colon. A rapid rise in temperature can lead to a seizure, distinguished from typical febrile seizures by the older age of the child and the fact that more than one seizure is very uncommon. Patients may become obtunded or comatose, usually with *S. dysenteriae* type

1 or *S. flexneri* infections. This is often associated with hypoglycemia, due to poor food intake and inadequate gluconeogenesis, or hyponatremia, due to inappropriate secretion of antidiuretic hormone. Anorexia may be intense and prolonged. Combined with ongoing catabolism of host muscle protein associated with excessive pro-inflammatory cytokine production and protein-losing enteropathy due to colitis, this always results in some degree of protein-energy malnutrition (Chapter 222). Even with adequate protein-containing and energy-dense diets post infection, replacement of nutrient stores may take as long as four times the duration of the clinical illness. This is more problematic in developing countries where the diet is poor. Hence, full nutritional recovery may not occur before the next infection develops, causing further nutritional deterioration. Because of its prolonged metabolic effects, shigellosis is often the precipitating cause of severe protein-energy malnutrition or kwashiorkor. *Shigella* infection is also associated with reactive arthritis and other autoimmune inflammatory manifestations such as tendinitis, conjunctivitis, uveitis, urethritis, or erythema nodosum, a constellation of findings previously termed *Reiter's syndrome* (Chapter 273). This is most common in individuals positive for HLA-B27 antigen and may be a consequence of molecular mimicry. Routine laboratory studies document leukocytosis with many immature "band" forms, especially in patients with bloody diarrhea or dysentery, and this may progress to a leukemoid reaction with thrombocytopenia and microangiopathic hemolytic anemia. With the development of HUS (Chapter 175), the biochemical manifestations of renal failure are present.

DIAGNOSIS

Shigellosis presenting with fever and watery diarrhea is clinically indistinguishable from the many other causes of watery diarrhea unless the stool is examined microscopically to demonstrate the presence of red and white blood cells or *Shigella* infection is confirmed microbiologically. Bloody diarrhea or dysentery in patients in the developed world is most commonly due to *S. flexneri* or a Shiga toxin–producing *E. coli*, such as serotype O157:H7, and less commonly due to *Campylobacter jejuni*, nontyphoid *Salmonella* species, or, rarely, *Yersinia enterocolitica* or *Entamoeba histolytica*. In patients who have recently received antibiotics, bloody diarrhea is often the consequence of *Clostridium difficile* (Chapter 304). In developing countries, *S. flexneri* and *S. dysenteriae* type 1 are the most common causes of bloody diarrhea or frank dysentery. Although more sophisticated methods of diagnosis are available, including polymerase chain reaction or enzyme-linked immunoassay (ELISA) or other rapid immunoassays, the standard method remains microbiologic culture. For a genus capable of causing such severe illness, *Shigella* species are remarkably fragile outside the intestine. Culture is most often positive when stool is processed rapidly; this is best done at the bedside, and stool samples are better than rectal swabs. Using more than one selective culture medium (e.g., MacConkey and xylose-lysine-deoxycholate or *Salmonella-Shigella* agar) and obtaining multiple cultures can increase the yield. Initially, laboratory screening is based on the failure of *Shigella* species to ferment lactose. Subculture to differential media such as triple sugar iron confirms lactose negativity and the ability to ferment glucose anaerobically, while the lack of motility or production of H_2S distinguishes the putative isolate from *Salmonella* species. Specific diagnosis can then be made using standard serologic methods for *Shigella* O antigens. In the case of mild watery

TABLE 317-1	CLINICAL SYNDROMES AND COMPLICATIONS IN SHIGELLOSIS		
STAGE	**TIME OF APPEARANCE AFTER ONSET OF ILLNESS**	**SYMPTOMS AND SIGNS**	**PATHOLOGY AND PATHOGENESIS**
Prodrome	Earliest findings	Fever, chills, myalgias, anorexia	None or early colitis
Watery diarrhea	0-3 days	Fever, abdominal cramps, loose stools	Colitis with fecal leukocytes and erythrocytes
Bloody diarrhea	1-3 days	Frequent stools containing blood and mucus, abdominal cramps and tenderness, fever, anorexia	Colitis with fecal leukocytes and erythrocytes
Dysentery	1-5 days	Frequent small-volume stools consisting of blood, mucus, and pus; severe abdominal cramps; tenesmus	More extensive colitis with crypt abscesses and mucosal ulcerations
Acute complications	3-7 days	Seizures, obtundation, bacteremia, colonic obstruction, mucosal perforation, peritonitis	Severe colitis, terminal ileitis
Additional acute complications due to infection with *Shigella dysenteriae* type 1	3-7 days	Toxic megacolon, leukemoid reaction, hemolytic-uremic syndrome	Severe colitis, expression of Stx toxin
Postinfectious syndromes	1-3 wk	Reactive arthritis, with or without urethritis and conjunctivitis	Autoimmune inflammatory response, most common in individuals expressing HLA-B27 antigen

diarrhea due to *S. sonnei*, the patient is often recovered by the time the laboratory results are available, so they are of little use in guiding treatment. Yields are maximized when patients with bloody diarrhea or dysentery are studied. These results are valuable for the patient, to select empirical treatment, and for epidemiologic purposes when antibiotic sensitivity is also determined, to track the emergence of antibiotic resistance.

TREATMENT   Rx

Because of the mild nature of *S. sonnei* infection in well-nourished children, cultures are not obtained, the specific diagnosis is typically unknown, and no treatment is required. Although it might be sensible from a public health perspective to eliminate convalescent carriers with antibiotic treatment to prevent subsequent transmission, such as in the setting of daycare centers, it cannot be justified because of *Shigella*'s predilection to acquire antibiotic resistance, resulting in the loss of valuable therapeutics to treat more severe illness. The CDC notes that because of the emergence of drug resistance, antibiotics should be reserved for more severe cases, even in outbreak settings. Some authorities have suggested that culture-positive patients—particularly food handlers, caretakers in daycare or clinical care settings, teachers or other school employees, and the immunocompromised—should be kept at home until three consecutive stool cultures are negative; however, this recommendation is unlikely to be followed in the vast majority of instances.

In the case of bloody diarrhea or dysentery, antibiotics are the mainstay of treatment. This is particularly problematic in developing countries, where many of the inexpensive, safe, and useful oral drugs, such as ampicillin and trimethoprim-sulfamethoxazole, have become ineffective because of drug resistance. Presently, a fluoroquinolone such as ciprofloxacin or azithromycin is reliable in most settings, but these drugs are expensive (particularly azithromycin). Parenteral ceftriaxone is very useful in severe illness. However, intravenous treatment requires hospitalization and monitoring and seriously increases the cost of treatment in both developed and developing countries.

In severe shigellosis, the prompt initiation of effective antibiotic treatment shortens the duration of illness and achieves a more rapid improvement in symptoms such as fever, cramps, and tenesmus. Evidence from Bangladesh in patients with *S. dysenteriae* type 1 infection also demonstrates that prompt treatment reduces the complication of HUS and presumably other complications due to colonic inflammation, such as megacolon, perforation, and rectal prolapse. In the United States and other developed countries, HUS is virtually exclusively associated with Shiga toxin–producing *E. coli*. The toxin genes in these *E. coli* are present on plasmids, in contrast to the chromosomal location of the *stx* gene in *S. dysenteriae* type 1, and are upregulated by commonly used antibiotics. Hence, most experts recommend withholding antibiotic treatment in patients with these *E. coli* infections.

Given the known epidemiology of antibiotic resistance among *Shigella* species, empirical therapy of adults with bloody diarrhea or dysentery can be initiated with ciprofloxacin 500 mg orally twice daily for 3 to 5 days. There is increasing evidence that shorter courses are sufficient, except perhaps for known or suspected *S. dysenteriae* type 1 infections, which should be treated with a full 5-day course. A reliable oral alternative is azithromycin, with an initial dose of 500 mg followed by 250 mg/day for 4 additional days. Depending on the epidemiology of resistance in specific geographic areas, ampicillin (500 mg orally four times daily for 3 days) or trimethoprim-sulfamethoxazole (160/800 mg combination twice daily for 3 days) may still be effective. Doses for young children are ciprofloxacin 10 mg/kg twice daily for 3 days; azithromycin 10 mg/kg on day 1, followed by 5 mg/kg for 4 more days; ampicillin 25 mg/kg four times daily for 5 days; and a pediatric syrup of trimethoprim-sulfamethoxazole containing 4/20 mg, respectively, twice daily for 5 days. Newer β-lactam antibiotics, such as amoxicillin or oral cephalosporins, are not recommended because initial studies have shown that they are less effective in vivo than predicted by in vitro drug sensitivity studies. This may be due to absorption and insufficient amounts in the intestinal lumen. Pivamdinocillin (mecillinam; marketed as Coactin) is effective but is not marketed in the United States. Nonabsorbable antimicrobial agents are contraindicated because effective treatment requires therapeutic levels of the drugs in both the lumen and the mucosal compartments.

In more severe infections, complications such as hypoglycemia or hyponatremia can be managed with appropriate glucose or saline given intravenously, but patients must be monitored by trained clinical staff. Colitis with toxic megacolon and intestinal perforation represent difficult problems, especially in the resource-poor settings where these complications are most likely to occur. Conservative medical or surgical management is best, even if not optimal. Renal failure due to HUS can generally be managed conservatively or with peritoneal dialysis, if available. Seizures are usually self-limited, and other neurologic complications respond to fluid and electrolyte management and correction of hypoglycemia and hyponatremia. Reactive arthritis is a greater problem, as it is an autoimmune response that occurs primarily in genetically susceptible individuals positive for HLA-B27 antigen. In addition to effective antibiotic treatment to eliminate the causative organism, chronic arthritis may require nonsteroidal anti-inflammatory agents, steroids, or inflammatory

cytokine inhibitors. In the susceptible host, infection-induced reactive arthritis can result in troublesome destructive joint disease and requires ongoing medical management. Some evidence suggests that antimotility agents are contraindicated in shigellosis, particularly in cases of bloody diarrhea or dysentery in young children; these drugs may prolong contact between the organisms and the mucosa, thereby increasing microbial invasion and pathology, including toxic megacolon.

Because of the prolonged anorexia and catabolic responses in shigellosis, attention to nutrition is an important component of treatment.

PREVENTION

Personal hygiene, in particular handwashing after handling the diapers of infected children and before food preparation, the sanitary disposal of feces, and protection of food and water sources, is essential to limit the spread of shigellosis. Preventing fecal contamination of hands in daycare settings is particularly problematic because it is so difficult to stop young children from constantly exploring their world by bringing their fingers and potentially contaminated fomites to their mouths. In such settings, it is particularly important for the adult caretakers to observe good personal hygiene. Soap and water are sufficient for handwashing, but hand sanitizers work and may be more convenient. In places where soap is unavailable, even the use of water with sand or ash for scrubbing is useful. When the cause of an outbreak is known, keeping children away from daycare until their stool is negative, or separating infected children from the susceptible, is recommended but is not easy to ensure. Hygiene in the household of an index case, including handwashing and caution in the handling of soiled garments, caring for children with diarrhea, and food preparation, is essential to limit intrahousehold spread.

Vaccines, particularly for the more virulent species, would be useful. However, despite much effort, a safe and effective vaccine has not been developed or approved for general use. It is doubtful whether a vaccine for *S. sonnei* infection would be recommended for children in a developed country such as the United States, even if safe and effective, because the illness is so mild and self-limited and because other vaccines are more important to administer in the context of an increasingly antivaccine public. Such a vaccine might, however, be useful for travelers or those in the military who are deployed overseas. In contrast, effective and safe vaccines for *S. flexneri* or *S. dysenteriae* type 1 would be extremely useful in developing countries, where shigellosis accounts for a significant portion of the 1.5 million to 2.5 million deaths each year due to enteric infections. Our current understanding of immunity in shigellosis indicates that serotype-specific immunity is most important; however, whether this is best conveyed by antibody, whether immunoglobulin G or A, or by cell-mediated mechanisms remains uncertain. This has limited vaccine development efforts, which have focused on attenuated live oral vaccines; unfortunately, the vaccines most effective in inducing immunity have also been the most reactogenic, causing fever and often diarrhea in recipients. Current efforts are also directed toward killed whole cells, O antigen–protein conjugates, and subunit vaccines. Unless common protective antigens are identified, the most likely vaccine strategy will be based on a combination of serotype-specific antigens from the most common *S. flexneri* strains and *S. dysenterieae* type 1. We are a long way from having an approved vaccine for shigellosis.

PROGNOSIS

S. sonnei infection and most cases of *S. boydii* infection are mild and self limited, with no sequelae. Infection with *S. flexneri* or *S. dysenteriae* responds to proper treatment with antibiotics. When treatment is not effective, either a drug-resistant strain or another etiologic agent should be suspected. In some instances, severe shigellosis with pancolitis has been misdiagnosed as inflammatory bowel disease. This can be a disaster if the patient is treated with steroids. Early and effective treatment reduces the risk of complications such as HUS and probably megacolon and bowel perforation. Because of the autoimmune nature of reactive arthritis, early treatment might not prevent its occurrence but could mitigate its severity. Infection with one serotype of *Shigella* generally provides durable immunity to reinfection with the same strain, but it leaves the individual susceptible to other antigenically distinct strains and serotypes.

SUGGESTED READINGS

Arvelo W, Hinkle CJ, Nguyen TA, et al. Transmission risk factors and treatment of pediatric shigellosis during a large daycare center-associated outbreak of multidrug resistant *Shigella sonnei*: implications for the management of shigellosis outbreaks among children. *Pediatr Infect Dis J.* 2009;28:976-980. *Characteristics of daycare-associated shigellosis in the United States, and its management.*

Bardhan P, Faruque AS, Naheed A, et al. Decrease in shigellosis-related deaths without *Shigella* spp-specific interventions, Asia. *Emerg Infect Dis.* 2010;16:1718-1723. *Nonspecific interventions (measles vaccination, vitamin A supplementation, and improved nutrition) may explain the reduction in shigellosis-related deaths.*

Prince Christopher R H, David KV, John SM, et al. Antibiotic therapy for *Shigella* dysentery. *Cochrane Database Syst Rev.* 2010;1:CD006784. *Antibiotics reduce the duration of* Shigella *dysentery by 70 to 80%.*

Rahman KM, Arifeen SE, Zaman K, et al. Safety, dose, immunogenicity, and transmissibility of an oral live attenuated *Shigella flexneri* 2a vaccine candidate (SC602) among healthy adults and school children in Matlab, Bangladesh. *Vaccine.* 2011;29:1347-1354. *Early testing of an oral vaccine.*

Soofi SB, Habib MA, von Seidlein L, et al. A comparison of disease caused by *Shigella* and *Campylobacter* species: 24 months community based surveillance in 4 slums of Karachi Pakistan. *J Infect Public Health.* 2011;4:12-21. *Shigellosis is a more severe illness than* Campylobacter *infection, with 31% of patients presenting with dysentery.*

318

BRUCELLOSIS

ROBERT A. SALATA

DEFINITION

Bacteria of the genus *Brucella* cause disease with protean manifestations. Infection is transmitted to humans from animals as a consequence of occupational exposure or ingestion of contaminated milk products. Despite the attempt to institute effective control measures, brucellosis remains a significant health and economic burden in many countries.

The Pathogen

Brucellae are slow-growing, small, aerobic, nonmotile, nonencapsulated, non-spore-forming, gram-negative coccobacilli. *Brucella abortus, Brucella suis, Brucella melitensis,* and *Brucella canis* are best known to infect humans and are typed on the basis of biochemical, metabolic, and immunologic criteria. DNA hybridization analysis shows a high degree of homology among strains.

EPIDEMIOLOGY

Etiology

There are differences in virulence among the four major species. *B. abortus,* with a reservoir in cattle, is usually associated with mild to moderate sporadic disease; suppurative or disabling complications are rare. *B. suis* infection, resulting from swine contact, is often associated with destructive, suppurative lesions and may have a prolonged course. *B. melitensis,* with a reservoir in sheep, goats, and camels, may cause severe, acute disease and disabling complications. *B. canis,* spread to humans from infected dogs, causes disease with an insidious onset, frequent relapse, and a chronic course that is indistinguishable from that of infection related to *B. abortus.* Studies indicate that there are two new species, *Brucella pinnipediae* and *Brucella cetaceae,* related to seals and cetaceans, respectively. Two human cases of marine-associated *Brucella* infection have been reported. *Brucella microti,* with high pathogenicity, was recently isolated from the common vole, red fox, and soil. No instances of human infection have been reported. Brucellae are also potential agents for bioterrorism.

Incidence and Prevalence

More than 500,000 cases of brucellosis are reported yearly to the World Health Organization from 100 countries. *B. melitensis* infection accounts for the majority of cases, distributed primarily in the Mediterranean region (particularly Spain and Greece), Latin America, the Arabian Gulf, and the Indian subcontinent. *B. abortus* infection occurs worldwide but has been effectively eradicated in several European countries, Japan, and Israel. *B. suis* occurs mainly in the Midwestern United States, South America, and Southeast Asia, whereas *B. canis* infection is most common in North America, South America,

Japan, and central Europe. Identification of the *Brucella* species recovered in humans can provide clues to the likely source of infection.

In animals, brucellosis is a chronic infection that persists for life. In association with effective control programs in animals, human brucellosis has decreased dramatically in the United States, from more than 6000 cases in 1947 to fewer than 200 cases each year since 1980. States reporting the greatest number of cases include Texas, California, Virginia, and Florida. In North America, brucellosis occurs mainly in the spring and summer and is more common in men, usually related to occupational exposure.

Brucella infection in the United States occurs mostly through direct contact with animals or their secretions in high-risk groups, including slaughterhouse workers, farmers and dairy workers, veterinarians, travelers to endemic areas, and laboratory workers handling the organisms. More than half the reported cases are associated with the meat-processing industry, particularly the kill areas, where infection is spread through abraded or lacerated skin; the conjunctiva, possibly by aerosolization; and, rarely, by ingestion of infected tissue. Many cases of *B. abortus* infection in veterinarians have resulted accidentally through exposure to the strain 19 vaccine used to immunize cattle. In the southern United States, 20% of feral swine are positive for *B. suis,* and human infections in hunters have been reported. *B. melitensis* infection, transmitted through the ingestion of goat's milk cheese, has been seen in U.S. travelers to and immigrants from Mexico. Brucellosis contracted abroad may not become symptomatic until the patient returns to the United States. Although persons with human immunodeficiency virus (HIV) infection are at risk for intracellular pathogens, the clinical manifestations of brucellosis in HIV-infected and noninfected individuals are similar in the few cases reported. There are increased reports of sexually transmitted brucellosis.

Brucellosis in pregnancy has been associated with spontaneous abortions, possible congenital abnormalities, and neonatal infections. Brucellosis in children accounts for only 3 to 10% of all reported cases worldwide; it is common in endemic areas (where it may account for 20 to 25% of cases) and is often a mild, self-limited process. Infection occurs most frequently in school-aged children and in familial outbreaks.

PATHOBIOLOGY

Pathogenesis

After penetrating the epithelial cells of human skin, conjunctiva, pharynx, or lung, *Brucella* organisms initially induce an exuberant polymorphonuclear neutrophil response in the submucosa. After ingestion of organisms by neutrophils and tissue macrophages, spread to regional lymph nodes occurs. If host defenses within the lymph nodes are overwhelmed, bacteremia follows. The usual incubation period between infection and bacteremia is 1.5 to 3 weeks. Bacteremia is accompanied by phagocytosis of free *Brucella* organisms by neutrophils and localization of bacteria primarily to the spleen, liver, and bone marrow, with the formation of granulomas.

If the inoculum is large and the patient receives no treatment, large granulomas may form, suppurate, and serve as a source of persistent bacteremia, with the potential for multiorgan spread. The primary virulence factor of *Brucella* appears to be cell wall lipopolysaccharide.

Both virulent and attenuated strains of *Brucella* are readily phagocytized by neutrophils after opsonization with normal human serum. Whole bacteria and extracts of *Brucella* species may inhibit neutrophil oxidative burst activity and degranulation. Intracellular killing of ingested bacteria has been demonstrated with *B. abortus* but not *B. melitensis;* this may explain differences in pathogenicity between these species. The major cell wall antigen and virulence factor of *Brucella* is the smooth lipopolysaccharide containing A and M antigens, which also dominates antibody production.

Immunity

Humoral factors may be important in the host defense against *Brucella.* Even in the absence of specific agglutinating antibody, normal human serum is bactericidal for *Brucella* organisms; *B. abortus* is more susceptible to serum lysis than is *B. melitensis.* The intracellular location within macrophages of the organism may provide a means for the bacteria to escape the lethal effects of serum. Specific serum agglutinating antibody has opsonic activity but does not correlate with the development of protective immunity.

A role for mononuclear phagocytes and cell-mediated immunity in brucellosis has been demonstrated. Protection against *Brucella* infection in animals is associated with preceding infection with *Listeria monocytogenes* or *Mycobacterium tuberculosis,* both of which stimulate cell-mediated immune mechanisms. Skin testing with *Brucella* proteins elicits a typical delayed hypersensitivity response in infected individuals. Macrophages, activated

TABLE 318-1   CLINICAL CLASSIFICATION OF HUMAN BRUCELLOSIS

CLASSIFICATION	DURATION OF SYMPTOMS BEFORE DIAGNOSIS	MAJOR SYMPTOMS AND SIGNS	DIAGNOSIS	COMMENTS
Subclinical	—	Asymptomatic	Positive (low titer) serology, negative cultures	Occurs in abattoir workers, farmers, and veterinarians
Acute and subacute	Up to 2-3 mo and 3 mo–1 yr	Malaise, chills, sweats, fatigue, headache, anorexia, arthralgias, fever, splenomegaly, lymphadenopathy, hepatomegaly	Positive serology, positive blood or bone marrow cultures	Presentation can be mild, self-limited (*B. abortus*) or fulminant with severe complications (*B. melitensis*)
Localized	Occurs with acute or chronic untreated disease	Related to involved organs	Positive serology, positive cultures in specific tissues	Bone or joint, genitourinary, hepatosplenic involvement most common
Relapsing	2-3 mo after initial episode	Same as acute illness but may have higher fever and more fatigue, weakness, chills, and sweats	Positive serology, positive cultures	May be extremely difficult to distinguish relapse from reinfection
Chronic	>1 yr	Nonspecific presentation but neuropsychiatric symptoms and low-grade fever most common	Low titer or negative serology, negative cultures	Most controversial classification; localized disease may be associated

with T helper 1 (T_H1)–type cytokines (e.g., interferon-γ, tumor necrosis factor-α, interleukin-1, interleukin-12), kill *Brucella*. Recent studies have shown that, despite high levels of T_H1 cytokine production, including interferon-γ, deficient effector phagocytic activity persists.

CLINICAL MANIFESTATIONS

Clinically, human brucellosis can be conveniently but arbitrarily divided into subclinical illness, acute or subacute disease, localized disease and complications, relapsing infection, and chronic disease (Table 318-1).

Subclinical Illness

Detected only by serologic testing, asymptomatic or clinically unrecognized human brucellosis often occurs in high-risk groups, including slaughterhouse workers, farmers, and veterinarians. More than 50% of abattoir workers and up to 33% of veterinarians have high anti-*Brucella* antibody titers but no history of recognized clinical infection. Children in endemic areas frequently have subclinical illness.

Acute and Subacute Disease

After an incubation period of several weeks or months, acute brucellosis may occur as a mild, transient illness (*B. abortus* or *B. canis*) or as an explosive, toxic illness with the potential for multiple complications (*B. melitensis*). Approximately 50% of patients have an abrupt onset over days, whereas the remainder have an insidious onset over weeks. Symptoms in brucellosis are protean and nonspecific. More than 90% of patients experience malaise, chills, sweats, fatigue, and weakness. More than 50% of patients have myalgias, anorexia, and weight loss. Fewer patients complain of arthralgias, cough, testicular pain, dysuria, ocular pain, or visual blurring. Likewise, few localizing physical signs are apparent. Fever, with temperatures often greater than 39.4° C (103° F), occurs in 95% of patients. An undulating or intermittent fever pattern is unusual. A pulse-temperature deficit (i.e., relative bradycardia) may occur. Splenomegaly is present in 10 to 15% of cases, and lymphadenopathy occurs in up to 14% (axillary, cervical, and supraclavicular locations are most frequent, related to hand wound or oropharyngeal routes of infection); hepatomegaly is less frequent. Other laboratory findings in acute or subacute disease may include mild anemia, lymphopenia or neutropenia (especially with bacteremia), lymphocytosis, thrombocytopenia, or (rarely) pancytopenia. The majority of infected individuals recover completely without sequelae if the appropriate diagnosis is made and prompt therapy is initiated.

Localized Disease and Complications

Brucella organisms can localize in almost any organ, but they most commonly localize in bone, joint, central nervous system, heart, lung, spleen, testis, liver, gallbladder, kidney, prostate, pancreas, and skin. Localized disease may occur simultaneously at multiple sites. Localized complications most often appear in association with a more chronic course of illness, although complications may occur with acute disease caused by *B. melitensis* or *B. suis*. In the United States, localized disease is most frequently related to *B. suis*. Osteoarticular complications are most frequent and are reported in 10 to 80% of series. The most common site is sacroiliitis in younger persons and spondylitis in older

persons. Vertebral osteomyelitis (most often in the lumbar area) is also well recognized and can be associated with paravertebral, epidural, and psoas abscesses.

Relapsing Infection

Up to 10% of patients with brucellosis experience relapses after antimicrobial therapy. Relapses usually occur 3 to 6 months after completion of therapy but may be seen up to 2 years after treatment. Relapses are often associated with antimicrobial resistance and the intracellular location of organisms, which protects the bacteria from certain antibiotics and host defense mechanisms. Relapsing infection is difficult to distinguish from reinfection in high-risk groups with continued exposure. Studies have shown that relapses are associated with inappropriate or insufficient antimicrobial therapy, positive blood cultures on initial presentation, and an acute onset of disease.

Chronic Disease

Disease with a duration of more than 1 year has been called *chronic brucellosis*. A majority of patients classified as having chronic brucellosis really have persistent disease caused by inadequate treatment of the initial episode, or they have focal disease in bone, liver, or spleen. About 20% of patients diagnosed with chronic brucellosis complain of persistent fatigue, malaise, and depression; in many respects, this condition resembles chronic fatigue syndrome. These symptoms are frequently not associated with clinical, microbiologic, or serologic evidence of active infection and may represent a preexisting psychoneurosis.

DIAGNOSIS

Culture

Many more common illnesses mimic the clinical presentation of brucellosis, and a thorough history is needed, including occupation, travel to endemic areas, avocations, and ingestion of at-risk food and beverages. The most conclusive means of establishing the diagnosis of brucellosis is positive culture from normally sterile body fluid or tissue. Rates of positive cultures have ranged from 15 to 90%, depending on the methods employed and the specimen type. The culture of *Brucella* organisms is potentially hazardous to laboratory personnel.

In acute brucellosis, positive blood cultures are obtained in 10 to 30% of cases (as high as 85% with *B. melitensis*). Blood culture positivity decreases with increasing duration of illness. With *B. melitensis* infection, bone marrow cultures are of higher yield than blood cultures. Blood processed in radiometric detection or isolator systems may yield positive cultures in less than 10 days. With localized brucellosis (e.g., lymph nodes, spleen, liver, skeletal system), cultures of purulent material or tissues usually yield *Brucella* organisms. Culture of cerebrospinal fluid is positive in 45% of patients with meningitis. Antibody against *Brucella* may be demonstrated in cerebrospinal fluid by enzyme-linked immunosorbent assay (ELISA).

Standard Tube Agglutination

In the absence of microbiologic confirmation, a presumptive diagnosis can be made by history and serology. The most frequently used test is the standard tube agglutination (STA) test, measuring antibody to *B. abortus* antigen.

TABLE 318-2 TREATMENT FOR BRUCELLOSIS

	TREATMENT	COMMENTS
Acute, with no endocarditis or central nervous system involvement	Doxycycline (200 mg/day) plus rifampin (600-900 mg/day) for 6 wk	Treatment of choice by World Health Organization; widely used; low rate of relapse; intramuscular administration of streptomycin may be difficult
	or	
	Tetracycline (2 g/day) for 6 wk plus streptomycin (1 g/day) or gentamicin for 1 wk	Combination therapy still preferred; fluoroquinolones plus rifampin is an alternative
	Alternative agents: chloramphenicol, fluoroquinolones, trimethoprim-sulfamethoxazole, imipenem	
In children	Trimethoprim-sulfamethoxazole plus rifampin	
Central nervous system	Doxycycline plus rifampin and trimethoprim-sulfamethoxazole	Third-generation cephalosporin can be substituted if susceptible in vitro
Localized	Surgically drain abscesses plus antimicrobial therapy for ≥6 wk	
Brucella endocarditis	Bactericidal drugs; early valve replacement may be necessary	Possible aortic valve destruction and/or major arterial emboli

A four-fold or greater rise in titer to 1 : 160 or higher is considered significant. A presumptive case is one in which the agglutination titer is positive (1 : 160) in single or serial specimens, with symptoms consistent with brucellosis. By 3 weeks of illness, more than 97% of patients demonstrate serologic evidence of infection. This test detects antibodies to *B. abortus*, *B. suis*, and *B. melitensis* but not to *B. canis*. Serologic confirmation of *B. canis* infection requires *B. canis* or *Brucella ovis* antigen. Despite adequate antibiotic treatment, significant STA titers can persist for up to 2 years in 5 to 7% of cases. Because the STA titer may remain elevated, it is not useful in differentiating relapsing infection from other febrile illnesses in patients with past *Brucella* infections. Individuals with subclinical infection may demonstrate significant STA titers. In chronic localized brucellosis, STA titers may appear absent or low owing to a prozone phenomenon. This prozone effect appears to be related to the presence of immunoglobulin G or immunoglobulin A blocking antibodies; it can be eliminated if dilutions are carried out to at least 1 : 1280. False-positive STA titers related to immunologic cross-reactivity have been associated with *Brucella* skin testing, cholera vaccination, or infection with *Vibrio cholerae*, *Francisella tularensis*, or *Yersinia enterocolitica*.

Other Tests

Certain newer antibody tests, including ELISA, are more sensitive and specific than STA and are being used more widely. Preliminary studies of the diagnosis of brucellosis using polymerase chain reaction with random or selected primers of blood and other fluids or tissues have been promising, but additional evaluation is necessary, and access to this diagnostic technology is still limited.

TREATMENT **Rx**

Effective treatment of *Brucella* infection requires antibiotics that can penetrate intracellularly, are available for prolonged therapy to prevent relapse, and are bactericidal in order to treat central nervous system infection and endocarditis. There is still considerable debate over which antibiotic regimen is superior, but the combination of oral doxycycline for 45 days or 8 weeks plus intramuscular gentamicin for 5 to 7 days is equally effective as traditional therapy using doxycycline for 45 days plus streptomycin for 14 days.[1] The World Health Organization recommends doxycycline plus rifampin orally for 6 weeks. This regimen is less effective for cases of spondylitis. Monotherapy with fluoroquinolones has been disappointing, and if these agents are used, they should always be combined with another active agent. Recent in vitro studies have demonstrated significant activity and synergy of tigecycline with gentamicin and rifampin; these observations must be supported in clinical trials. Recommendations are given in Table 318-2.

PREVENTION

The control of human brucellosis is directly related to prevention programs in domestic animals and the avoidance of unpasteurized milk and milk products. In slaughterhouses, important means of prevention include careful wound dressing, the wearing of protective glasses and clothing, the prohibition of raw meat ingestion, and the use of previously infected (immune) individuals in high-risk areas. Work is ongoing to find an effective vaccine for

humans. There is controversy about the effectiveness of postexposure antimicrobial prophylaxis.

PROGNOSIS

Brucellosis that is treated appropriately within the first month of symptom onset is curable. Acute brucellosis often produces severe weakness and fatigue, and patients are frequently unable to work for up to 2 months. Immunity to reinfection follows initial *Brucella* infection in the majority of individuals. With early antimicrobial therapy, cases of chronic brucellosis or localized disease and complications are rare. Of the patients who die of brucellosis, 84% have endocarditis involving a previously abnormal aortic valve, often associated with severe congestive heart failure.

Grade **A** ————————————————O

1. Roushan MR, Amiri MJ, Janmohammadi N, et al. Comparison of the efficacy of gentamicin for 5 days plus doxycycline for 8 weeks versus streptomycin for 2 weeks plus doxycycline for 45 days in the treatment of human brucellosis: a randomized clinical trial. *J Antimicrob Chemother.* 2010;65: 1028-1035.

SUGGESTED READINGS

Buzgan T, Karahocagil MK, Irmak H, et al. Clinical manifestations and complications in 1028 cases of brucellosis: a retrospective evaluation and review of the literature. *Int J Infect Dis.* 2010;14:e469-e478. *About 50% of patients were engaged in raising livestock, and the main risk factor in others was consumption of raw milk and dairy products; the STA was positive in 99% of cases.*

Eales KM, Norton RE, Ketheesan N. Brucellosis in northern Australia. *Am J Trop Med Hyg.* 2010;83:876-887. *Fever (94%), fatigue (78%), and arthralgia (78%) were the main features, with a median 2-week diagnostic delay.*

Seleem MN, Boyle SM, Sriranganathan N. Brucellosis: a re-emerging zoonosis. *Vet Microbiol.* 2010;140:392-398. *Review of the epidemiology of the more than 500,000 human cases reported annually.*

319

TULAREMIA AND OTHER *FRANCISELLA* INFECTIONS

WILLIAM SCHAFFNER

DEFINITION

Tularemia is an infectious zoonosis caused by *Francisella tularensis*, a small aerobic, pleomorphic, gram-negative bacillus. Many animal species harbor the organism, most prominently rabbits, squirrels, and muskrats. Humans acquire the infection through various means: direct contact with infected animal tissues, ingestion of contaminated water or meat, the bite of an infected tick or deer fly, or breathing an aerosol of bacteria. Although *F. tularensis* is highly infectious and is a well-recognized risk to laboratory personnel manipulating culture plates of the organism, it is a paradox that the illness is not communicable from person to person. Edward Francis established that deer flies can transmit the infection from animals to humans and provided detailed descriptions of its clinical manifestations. Colloquially, the disease is often referred to as *rabbit fever* or *deer fly fever.*

The Pathogen

The organism occurs in two major subspecies (biovars). *F. tularensis* biovar *tularensis* (type A) is more virulent in animals and humans, has distinctive biochemical reactions (it produces acid from glycerol and has citrulline ureidase activity), and is the common North American biovar. In contrast, *F. tularensis* biovar *holarctica* (type B) is less virulent and occurs commonly in Europe and Asia. Type B is most frequently isolated from rodent species, including muskrats *(Ondatra zibethicus)*, mice *(Mus musculus)*, beavers *(Castor canadensis)*, voles *(Microtus* species*)*, and water voles *(Arvicola terrestris)*, and has been associated with an outbreak of infection in wild-caught prairie dogs. Specific virulence factors for *F. tularensis* have not been identified.

EPIDEMIOLOGY

Tularemia has been reported in the United States, Canada, Mexico, Japan, and Europe, particularly Scandinavia. It has not been reported in the United Kingdom or the Southern Hemisphere. In the United States, reported cases diminished during the second half of the 20th century from a high of 2291 cases in 1939 to the approximately 125 cases reported annually at present. Tularemia has occurred in all the continental states, but four states account for 56% of reported cases: Arkansas, Missouri, Oklahoma, and South Dakota. The island of Martha's Vineyard off the coast of Massachusetts is also a focus of tularemia.

In the United States, tularemia is usually acquired from tick bites or from contact with infected animals, especially rabbits. Tick-associated cases now constitute the majority and occur during the summer. The most common vectors in the United States are the wood tick *(Dermacentor andersoni)*, the dog tick *(Dermacentor variabilis)*, and the Lone Star tick *(Amblyomma americanum)*. A smaller peak of autumn-winter cases is a consequence of rabbit hunters skinning and eviscerating their game. Public health education materials aimed at decreasing the hazards of handling wild animals have contributed to the reduction of tularemia in hunters. Mosquitoes are the common vectors in northern Europe. Occasional individuals acquire infection from the bite of an infected animal or, more likely, from the bite of an animal whose mouth was contaminated from recently eating a diseased animal. The latter probably explains most instances of cat-bite tularemia.

Males experience a higher incidence of disease than females in all age groups, probably as a consequence of their greater exposure to the outdoors and animal-related activities and less use of protective measures against tick bites. Persons in all age groups are affected, with children 5 to 14 years of age and older adults most prominently represented. In the United States, American Indians/Alaska natives experience the highest annual incidence (0.5 per 100,000); whites have a lower risk (0.04 per 100,000), and African Americans and Asians/Pacific Islanders have the lowest occurrence of tularemia (≤0.01 per 100,000).

Although tularemia is usually a sporadic infection, outbreaks of disease have been traced to laboratory exposure, contaminated groundwater, muskrat handling, lawn mowing, and brush cutting. In the latter two cases, primary pneumonic tularemia apparently occurred when the affected individuals created an environmental aerosol by mowing grass and cutting brush that had been contaminated with *F. tularensis* excreted in the urine and feces of infected rodents. The organism can survive in water, mud, and straw for weeks to months.

Recently, interest in tularemia has been enhanced because of its potential use as a bioterrorism agent. Its high infectivity (as few as 10 organisms have induced pneumonic disease), its ease of dissemination, and the difficulty of rapidly diagnosing acute illness are characteristics that merit its inclusion among threat agents. Thus, tularemia must be reported immediately to local public health authorities. Unusual patterns of disease will be investigated for both conventional and bioterrorist sources.

PATHOBIOLOGY

F. tularensis can infect humans through several portals of entry, including the skin, mucous membranes, and gastrointestinal and respiratory tracts. It

requires intracellular residence and can multiply within macrophages and other cells. After inoculation into the skin and subcutaneous tissue, local bacterial multiplication occurs and evokes a suppurative necrotic reaction characterized by an initial polymorphonuclear response, followed by an influx of macrophages and lymphocytes. These suppurative lesions evolve into granulomas. Bacteremia can occur both early and late during this process. The infection can disseminate to the lymph nodes, liver, spleen, lungs, and pleura. Viable *F. tularensis* can persist in tissues for long periods, contributing to the tendency to relapse after treatment.

CLINICAL MANIFESTATIONS

Classically, the clinical manifestations of tularemia have been separated into six categories: ulceroglandular, glandular, oculoglandular, typhoidal, oropharyngeal, and pneumonic. Although this classification has historic roots, it should not be used rigidly because many patients have features of several types. The course of illness is determined by the portal of entry, the degree of systemic involvement, and the dose and virulence of the infecting strain of *F. tularensis.*

The general features of tularemia are similar, regardless of the portal of entry. After exposure, the usual incubation period is 3 to 5 days (range, 1 to 21 days). The disease begins abruptly with the onset of fever (≥101° F), chills, malaise, and headache. Myalgia, vomiting, sore throat, and abdominal pain can also occur. Almost half the patients have a pulse rate that is substantially slower than would be anticipated based on the degree of fever (pulse-temperature dissociation). The fever may abate somewhat after 1 to 3 days, only to recur and continue along with other symptoms for 2 to 3 weeks. Untreated, weight loss, easy fatigue, and lymphadenopathy may persist for weeks longer.

Ulceroglandular Disease

Ulceroglandular disease is the form of infection most readily recognized by physicians. Along with fever and other constitutional symptoms, the patient calls attention to tender, swollen lymph nodes that drain an inoculation site. The nodes are usually axillary or inguinal, and a local lesion appears concurrently or 1 or 2 days before or after the lymphadenopathy. The lesions at the site of inoculation begin as small, red, tender, or painful papules that progress to pustules and then undergo necrosis to produce an ulcer with sharp, somewhat elevated edges and a flat base that becomes black. Untreated, the ulcers heal over a period of weeks and leave scars. Tick-induced infections produce lesions on the trunk, about the waist, and in the perineum, along with the expected local adenopathy. Children typically have occipital and cervical adenopathy from tick bites on the neck and in the hair. Animal exposure often produces lesions on the hands and forearms. Lesions may be multiple. Because the organisms evoke a localized granulomatous response, frank lymphangitis does not occur in uncomplicated tularemia, but an occasional patient manifests a chain of nodules in "sporotrichoid" fashion along the lymphatic drainage.

Patients with such apparently "localized" disease often have symptoms and findings indicating a more widespread infection. Sore throat with or without an erythematous pharynx occurs, as well as chest radiographic findings of patchy infiltrates in the lower lobes, pleural effusions, and hilar adenopathy.

Glandular and Typhoidal Disease

Glandular disease is essentially the same clinical syndrome as ulceroglandular disease, but without the local lesion. Thus, the patient has fever, constitutional symptoms, and lymphadenopathy. The local lesion may have been on a part of the body where it was not seen, or it may have been small and already healed by the time the patient sought medical care. Glandular disease accounts for only 3 to 20% of cases. Typhoidal disease does not show evidence of lymphadenopathy and is essentially characterized by fever of unknown cause. These illnesses evade diagnosis unless the physician specifically considers the possibility of tularemia and inquires about tick or animal exposure. Occasionally, the diagnosis is made fortuitously when a positive blood culture is reported.

Oculoglandular Disease

Oculoglandular disease is rare (<5% of cases) and occurs when the conjunctival sac is the portal of entry via an aerosol, splash, or contaminated fingers. It is almost always unilateral and can have a dramatic manifestation with inflamed, swollen eyelids, chemosis, and painful conjunctivitis. The palpebral conjunctiva often shows small yellow nodules and ulcers, counterparts to the skin lesions of ulceroglandular disease. The affected regional lymph nodes are those of the head and neck.

Oropharyngeal Disease

Oropharyngeal disease is also uncommon in the United States and occurs when the mucous membranes of the mouth and pharynx are the portal of entry. Contaminated water or food (inadequately cooked game meat) is the source. Painful exudative pharyngitis and tonsillitis, pharyngeal ulcers, and swollen retropharyngeal and cervical lymph nodes are seen.

Pneumonic Disease

Although pneumonia may be one aspect of the other tularemic syndromes, *pneumonic tularemia* refers to an illness that manifests as a distinctive pneumonia. It accounts for about 10% of reported cases and occurs from inhalational exposure. This is the form of the disease that would result from bioterrorism. In addition to fever and malaise, patients may have a dry cough, substernal discomfort, pleural pain, dyspnea, and sore throat. These pulmonary symptoms may not be very prominent in the context of the systemic illness. Hemoptysis is unlikely. The results of physical examination reflect the extent and distribution of the pneumonic process, which may range from barely evident to frank consolidation with pleural effusion. Radiographic findings range from modest peribronchial infiltrates early in the illness to distinctive bronchopneumonia with effusion. Hilar adenopathy is present in more than a third of cases. Sputum examination is not helpful. Pleural effusions generally contain more than 1000 lymphocytes/mm^3. Gram stains are negative, and pleural biopsies occasionally contain granuloma, thus inviting confusion with tuberculosis. Without a suggestive history of tick or animal exposure, patients with tularemic pneumonia may be thought to have poorly responding community-acquired pneumonia. Fluoroquinolone antibiotics are commonly used as empirical therapy in this circumstance to treat some patients with undiagnosed tularemia pneumonia.

DIAGNOSIS

The diagnosis of tularemia usually involves serologic testing with tube agglutination or microagglutination techniques. Antibody concentrations do not reach diagnostic levels until after the 11th day of illness. A single acute titer of 1:160 is considered presumptive; a confirmed diagnosis requires a fourfold rise in titer between acute and convalescent specimens. Titers of both immunoglobulin M and immunoglobulin G antibodies may remain elevated for many years after the illness.

Differential Diagnosis

The differential diagnosis of patients with tularemia is substantial. The local lesions can be confused with cat-scratch disease, brown recluse spider bites, *Mycobacterium marinum* infection, herpes simplex infection (Chapter 382), and even syphilis (Chapter 327) and chancroid (Chapter 309) when the lesions are in the perineum or on the penis. Pneumonic tularemia resembles common community-acquired pneumonia (Chapter 97), as well as less common infections such as psittacosis, legionellosis, and Q fever. The glandular and typhoidal forms can resemble typhoid fever (Chapter 316), brucellosis (Chapter 318), ehrlichiosis, and other illnesses accompanied by nonspecific fevers.

Routine laboratory studies do not provide specific results. Leukocyte counts may be within normal limits or elevated; thrombocytopenia, elevated liver enzymes, and sterile pyuria occur with some frequency. *F. tularensis* may be isolated from blood cultures and tissue specimens when media containing cysteine are used. Laboratory personnel should be notified when tularemia is suspected so that appropriate media can be used and to ensure that safeguards are in place to protect against the production of hazardous aerosols.

TREATMENT   Rx

Because tularemia is a relatively uncommon disease, therapeutic recommendations are based on a combination of in vitro studies and accumulated clinical experience. The preferred antimicrobials are streptomycin and gentamicin; either one is given for 10 days. Streptomycin is given at a dose of 1 g intramuscularly twice daily. Gentamicin may be more readily available and is administered at a dose of 5 mg/kg intramuscularly or intravenously once daily. Both chloramphenicol and the tetracyclines have been used in the past to treat tularemia; however, use of both these bacteriostatic agents has resulted in higher rates of relapse than treatment with streptomycin or gentamicin. Because chloramphenicol may produce bone marrow toxicity, it is rarely used today. Doxycycline is administered at a dose of 100 mg intravenously twice daily for 14 days. In recent years, ciprofloxacin has been used successfully in a growing number of patients; the dosage is 400 mg intravenously twice daily for 10 days. Both these drugs can be switched to oral administration of the same doses as soon as tolerated by the patient.

PREVENTION

Prevention of tularemia entails minimizing exposure to ticks and avoiding direct exposure to wild animals. Tick protection includes clothing that extends to the wrists and ankles, regular inspection for attached ticks, and the use of insect repellents containing diethyltoluamide (DEET). Gloves should be worn when skinning and dressing game animals, especially rabbits, and all wild rabbit and other game meats should be cooked thoroughly.

A live, attenuated vaccine has been used in the past to provide some protection to researchers working with *F. tularensis*. The vaccine is not available commercially.

PROGNOSIS

Before treatment became available, acute tularemia often lasted as long as a month, followed by several months of debility. Mortality approached 10%. When appropriately diagnosed and treated, the mortality from tularemia is now 1% or less.

SUGGESTED READINGS

Foley JE, Nieto NC. Tularemia. *Vet Microbiol.* 2010;140:332-338. *Review of epidemiology, including the rabbit as a vector.*

Hofinger DM, Cardona L, Mertz GJ, et al. Tularemic meningitis in the United States. *Arch Neurol.* 2009;66:523-527. *Case report and literature review.*

Snowden J, Stovall S. Tularemia: retrospective review of 10 years' experience in Arkansas. *Clin Pediatr (Phila).* 2011;50:64-68. *Seventeen patients presented with ulceroglandular tularemia and 13 with glandular disease, usually with a 10- to 14-day delay in diagnosis.*

Thomas LD, Schaffner W. Tularemia pneumonia. *Infect Dis Clin North Am.* 2010;24:43-55. *Pneumonia can occur either from direct inhalation or as a secondary manifestation of ulceroglandular disease.*

320

PLAGUE AND OTHER *YERSINIA* INFECTIONS

KENNETH L. GAGE

The genus *Yersinia* currently contains more than 15 species, only 3 of which are known to be significant human pathogens (*Yersinia pestis, Yersinia enterocolitica,* and *Yersinia pseudotuberculosis*). The remaining species are normally considered nonpathogenic and are most frequently isolated from environmental specimens, including fish, water, and fecal samples. Although these minor yersiniae have been identified primarily from environmental samples, they are occasionally recovered from patient samples, suggesting a possible role as human pathogens.

YERSINIA PESTIS

DEFINITION

Plague is a highly fatal flea-borne disease that is best known as the cause of the Black Death of the Middle Ages. Its etiologic agent, *Y. pestis,* is a gram-negative coccobacillus belonging to the family Enterobacteriaceae.

The Pathogen

Y. pestis is microaerophilic, nonmotile, and nonsporulating; it can exist as a facultative intracellular pathogen and exhibits bipolar staining with Wayson, Giemsa, and Wright stains (Fig. 320-1). It is fragile outside its hosts or vectors but can be grown within 24 to 48 hours on a variety of bacteriologic media at temperatures ranging from 4 to 40° C. *Y. pestis* lacks a true capsule but has a carbohydrate-protein envelope referred to as the *capsular* or *fraction 1 antigen.* Production of this antigen occurs only at temperatures above 33° C. Wild-type strains typically bear three plasmids with sizes of approximately 100 to 110 kilobases (kb), 70 to 75 kb, and 9.5 kb (19 kb if present as a

FIGURE 320-1. Wayson-stained blood smear from a fatal case of human septicemic plague. (Courtesy Centers for Disease Control and Prevention archives.)

Plague cases in the Western U.S., 1970–2006

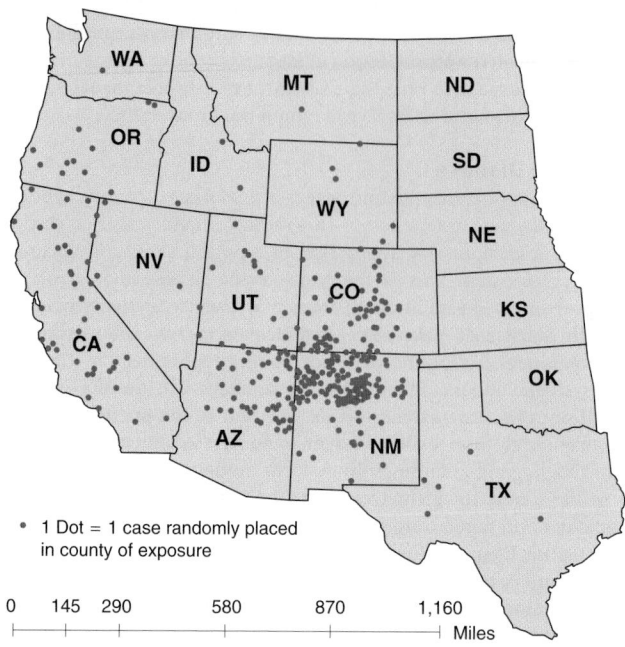

* 1 Dot = 1 case randomly placed in county of exposure

| 0 | 145 | 290 | 580 | 870 | 1,160 |

Miles

FIGURE 320-2. Distribution of human plague cases in the United States. Case points were randomly placed within counties where exposures occurred to indicate the general distribution and clustering of cases by region. (Courtesy John Montenieri, Centers for Disease Control and Prevention.)

dimer). Although only one serotype is thought to exist, strains can be classified into biotypes. The three classic biotypes (antiqua, mediaevalis, and orientalis) differ in their ability to ferment glycerol and reduce nitrates. All three biotypes occur in Asia, which is generally accepted as the site where plague originated. Two biotypes exist in Africa (antiqua and orientalis), but only the orientalis biotype occurs in the Americas. Although these three biotypes have historical and biogeographic significance, all are highly virulent and appear to cause virtually identical signs and symptoms in humans. Recently, a fourth biotype (microtus), which is purportedly nonpathogenic for humans, was reported from east-central Asia. More modern typing methods, including ribotyping, multiple-locus variable-number tandem repeat assays, and single-nucleotide polymorphism analysis, are useful for molecular epidemiology studies, identification of probable environmental sources of human infection, and phylogenetic analysis.

EPIDEMIOLOGY

Y. pestis is maintained in nature through transmission cycles involving certain rodent species and their fleas, which act as vectors. Although other mammals often become infected with *Y. pestis* and occasionally succumb to plague, the only non-rodent species thought to be important hosts for infecting vector fleas are some species of rabbits and hares, the steppe pika of central Asia, and the house shrew of southeastern Asia and Madagascar. Rodent-consuming carnivores and raptors might play indirect roles in spreading plague by transporting infected rodent fleas from one area to another.

Foci of *Y. pestis* infection occur in rodent populations in many regions of Africa, Asia, and the Americas, although only about 2000 to 5000 human cases were reported each year to the World Health Organization (WHO) in the period 1987 to 2009. In the 1960s and 1970s, the majority of human cases occurred in Southeast Asia, which was the site of civil wars and political unrest. However, beginning in the 1980s, this situation began to change, and most cases now occur in Africa and nearby Madagascar. According to the most recently released WHO statistics for 2004 to 2009, 96.6% of the world's cases occurred in the Democratic Republic of Congo, Madagascar, Uganda, and other countries in Africa. Asian countries reported only 1.6% of the total cases, and another 1.8% were reported from countries in the Americas, including the United States. Since 1970, evidence of *Y. pestis* infection has been identified in animals or their fleas in 17 western states, and human cases have been identified in 13 of these states (Fig. 320-2).

Humans most frequently acquire plague as a result of being bitten by infectious fleas. On a worldwide basis, the risk of flea bite exposure is highest in poverty-stricken areas that are situated near natural plague foci and have large infestations of commensal rats (*Rattus* sp) heavily infested with fleas, particularly the oriental rat flea (*Xenopsylla cheopis*). *X. cheopis* readily feeds on humans and is an efficient vector of *Y. pestis* to people as well as to rats. Persons are most likely to be bitten by infectious *X. cheopis* when plague epizootics cause massive mortality among susceptible rats, forcing these fleas to seek new hosts. Currently, certain regions of central and southern Africa (including Madagascar), southeastern Asia and India, and a few areas in South America remain at high risk for rat-associated plague outbreaks. The spread of rat-associated plague from one region to another, perhaps by

the natural movement of rats or their transport along with trade goods, poses a threat of major epidemics in large rat-infested cities. The appearance of bubonic cases acquired via flea bite in large cities also greatly increases the possibility that pneumonic plague will develop in untreated bubonic cases and that the infection will spread to others through coughing and the expulsion of infectious respiratory droplets (primary pneumonic plague). Though rare in the United States, primary pneumonic plague still poses a threat in developing countries, with outbreaks occurring in the past 20 years in India, Ecuador, Madagascar, the Democratic Republic of Congo, and Uganda.

At present, rat-associated plague poses little risk to persons in the United States, with the last cases being reported in 1925. Since that time, most cases have occurred as a result of being bitten by infectious wild rodent fleas (79% in one case series), although a significant number (19%) were exposed while handling *Y. pestis*–infected animals, including rabbits, domestic cats, wild rodents, and wild carnivores. These direct-contact exposures occurred primarily in persons who had been bitten or scratched by infected cats or had skinned infectious rabbits or rodents for meat or certain wild carnivores for their fur. The risk of exposure to infectious wild rodent fleas or animals is typically greatest when epizootics cause high mortality in certain rodent species in the western United States, particularly ground squirrels, prairie dogs, wood rats, and chipmunks. Epizootics appear to progress most rapidly during late spring to early fall, when human cases also peak, probably because this is the period of greatest flea vector activity. The few human cases reported during the winter months are typically acquired through direct contact with infected animals, and affected individuals have a history of hunting or trapping wild animals or handling domestic cats. The exposure sites for most U.S. cases are peridomestic environments, with smaller numbers of exposures occurring during recreational activities such as hunting or camping. Occupational exposure has also rarely occurred among veterinary staff, biologists, and trappers. Rarely, primary pneumonic plague has been acquired in the United States through the inhalation of infectious materials (2% of cases) by means of close face-to-face contact with *Y. pestis*–infected cats that had oral lesions or signs of plague pneumonia, including cough.

Recently, concern has been raised that plague could be used as an agent of bioterrorism (Chapter 20). In most projected scenarios, bioterrorists would spread plague in an aerosol form, potentially resulting in numerous primary pneumonic cases, high mortality, and widespread panic, especially if the *Y. pestis* strains released had been engineered to be resistant to antimicrobial agents commonly used to treat plague.

PATHOBIOLOGY

Few bacteria rival the pathogenicity of *Y. pestis* for humans. *Y. pestis* usually enters the body at the site of a flea bite or perhaps as a result of contact between abraded or cut skin and blood or other body fluids from a *Y. pestis*–infected animal. On entering the body, plague bacteria come under attack by host phagocytes and other host defenses. The ability to escape from these defenses and disseminate to regional lymph nodes depends in part on a protease (Pla) that helps degrade fibrin clots and promote the production of excess plasmin, which can affect inflammatory exudates, break down extracellular proteins and basement membranes, and reduce levels of chemoattractants, possibly because of the inhibition of interleukin-8 production at the site of initial infection. Another virulence factor, YopM, is one of many *Yersinia* outer proteins (Yops), encoded by genes on the mid-sized (70 to 75 kb) plasmid of *Y. pestis*. Although most other Yops are degraded by the Pla protease, YopM is resistant to its activity and probably aids in the dissemination of *Y. pestis* by competing with platelets for thrombin, a factor that not only reduces clotting but also inhibits the activation of platelets, thereby lowering local inflammatory responses and promoting the dissemination of *Y. pestis* to regional lymph nodes. Initial invasion and dispersal to regional lymph nodes also depend on the ability of *Y. pestis* to survive for at least brief periods in host phagocytes. Survival in such environments is promoted by other Yops that work in concert with a type III secretory apparatus to deliver into host phagocytes those Yops that act as intracellular effectors. These effector Yops disturb the cytoskeletal dynamics of phagocytic cells and block their production of pro-inflammatory cytokines. Affected phagocytes are rendered incapable of killing the invading *Y. pestis,* thereby allowing this bacterium to survive extracellularly in lymphoid tissues. Survival of *Y. pestis* in mammalian hosts also depends on its ability to acquire sufficient quantities of iron for growth. The most important means of iron uptake in *Y. pestis* is a siderophore (yersiniabactin) system that can effectively compete with host iron-binding molecules for this essential nutrient. Although the ability of *Y. pestis* to resist host phagocytic killing and survive intracellularly in phagocytes is thought to be particularly important during the early stages of infection, plague bacteria also express a glycoprotein capsular antigen (caf1 or fraction 1 antigen) that confers resistance to phagocytosis. Expression of caf1 is temperature dependent, being repressed at the cooler temperatures found in the flea vector and upregulated at mammalian host body temperatures.

Infected lymph nodes, termed *buboes,* can appear edematous and congested early in the course of illness but exhibit little evidence of inflammatory infiltrates or vascular injury. These buboes represent the most obvious manifestation of the lymphatic system's efforts to arrest the spread of *Y. pestis,* and within a few days after infection, they contain massive numbers of *Y. pestis* and heavy neutrophil infiltrates, which causes them to swell to the size of a hen's egg and become surrounded by serous fluid. As the illness progresses, hemorrhagic necrosis and vascular damage in the node become apparent; some nodes spontaneously rupture, and abscesses appear. Although *Y. pestis* can be present in small quantities in blood samples taken relatively early in the course of infection, large quantities of plague bacteria usually appear in the blood of patients with bubonic plague only after the lymph node defenses are overwhelmed.

As the bacteria escape from the node and proliferate in blood, patients with bubonic plague begin to exhibit evidence of plague septicemia (secondary septicemic plague). Patients with inadequately treated septicemic plague can experience widespread and overwhelming destruction of tissues as *Y. pestis* spreads to various organs, eventually resulting in their failure. Patients who die of plague often experience diffuse interstitial myocarditis, cardiac dilation, diffuse hemorrhagic splenic necrosis, renal glomeruli containing fibrin thrombi, and multifocal necrosis in the liver. Disseminated intravascular coagulation can lead to thrombosis within capillaries, vascular necrosis, ecchymoses, acral gangrene, and cutaneous, mucosal, and serosal petechiae. In a small proportion of cases, septicemia occurs in the absence of buboes or other signs of localized infection, a condition referred to as *primary septicemic plague.* Septicemic plague can also occur secondary to primary pneumonic plague.

Rarely, plague can be acquired through the inhalation of infectious respiratory droplets or other materials. Patients with primary pneumonic plague typically experience a rapidly progressing lung infection that is initially lobular, then lobar, and finally multilobar, with large numbers of *Y. pestis* being present in the alveoli and pulmonary secretions of affected sites. Pneumonic plague can also occur secondary to bubonic or primary septicemic plague. In these instances, *Y. pestis* invades the lungs in a diffuse manner, with

FIGURE 320-3. Young Malagasy boy with a bubo. (Courtesy Brook Yockey, Centers for Disease Control and Prevention.)

most bacilli appearing in interstitial spaces. The most common pathologic findings are edema, diffuse pulmonary congestion, limited neutrophilic infiltration, and hemorrhagic necrosis. Cavitation and liquefaction necrosis can also occur and result in scarring of the lungs, particularly at sites of consolidation.

CLINICAL MANIFESTATIONS

The three most commonly observed forms of plague (in order of decreasing occurrence) are bubonic, septicemic, and pneumonic. Unusual manifestations of plague include meningitis and pharyngitis. In rare instances, *Y. pestis* has been inoculated through the conjunctiva, resulting in oculoglandular plague. The incubation period is 2 to 6 days for bubonic plague and 1 to 3 days for primary pneumonic plague.

The characteristic swollen and tender lymph nodes (buboes) of bubonic plague usually appear in the node or nodes located closest to the site of initial infection (Fig. 320-3). Most cases of bubonic plague in the United States are thought to be acquired from flea bites on the legs, as indicated by the appearance of inguinal or femoral lymph node involvement on the side where the flea bite occurred. Axillary buboes are also common, often indicating the handling of an infected animal or other flea-infested object. Cervical buboes are much less common in the United States than in many developing countries, perhaps because persons in the latter are more likely to sleep on dirt floors in flea-infested huts, thus increasing their chances of being bitten about the head and neck by infectious fleas. Rarely, a skin lesion appears at the site of an infectious flea bite or other source of inoculation.

Symptoms of bubonic plague include fever, chills, myalgia, arthralgia, headache, malaise, and prostration. Untreated patients with bubonic plague become increasingly toxic, remain febrile, and experience tachycardia, agitation, confusion, delirium, and convulsions.

Septicemic plague manifests as a rapidly progressive, overwhelming endotoxemia. Patients often complain of gastrointestinal symptoms, including nausea, vomiting, diarrhea, and abdominal plain. Disseminated intravascular coagulation can also occur with the appearance of petechiae, ecchymoses, bleeding, and ischemia in the tips of the extremities. Later-stage septicemic patients are likely to experience refractory hypotension, renal shutdown, obtundation, and other signs of shock. Patients with late-stage septicemic plague can also exhibit acute respiratory distress syndrome (Chapter 104), which has occasionally been confused with hantaviral pulmonary syndrome (Chapter 389) in the American Southwest. Because septicemic plague is likely to be fulminant and fatal, favorable outcomes depend on rapid diagnosis and prompt treatment with appropriate antimicrobials.

Pneumonic plague can be accompanied by fever, cough, chest discomfort that becomes increasingly painful, tachycardia, dyspnea, bacteria-laden sputum, chills, headache, achiness, weakness, and dizziness. As the illness progresses, patients may experience increasing respiratory distress, hemoptysis, cardiopulmonary insufficiency, and circulatory collapse. In the early stages of illness, patients with primary pneumonic plague may have signs of localized pulmonary involvement, beginning in a single lung and rapidly progressing to segmental consolidation and later bronchopneumonia, with death ensuing within 24 hours of the onset of symptoms. Localized infection is unlikely to be observed in the lungs of patients with secondary pneumonic plague because the lung tissues are infected initially through circulatory spread, which results in a diffuse interstitial pneumonitis. The appearance of sputum also differs in primary versus secondary pneumonic plague, being watery or mucoid, frothy, and perhaps tinged with blood in primary pneumonic cases but scanter, thicker, and more tenacious in secondary pneumonic cases.

DIAGNOSIS

Plague fatalities are typically related to delay in seeking treatment or misdiagnosis. The differential diagnosis of plague in its various clinical forms includes staphylococcal (Chapter 296) or streptococcal adenitis (Chapter 298) or pneumonia (Chapter 97); cat-scratch disease (Chapter 323); tularemia (Chapter 319); chancroid (Chapter 309); acute filarial lymphadenitis (Chapter 366); mycobacterial infection (Chapter 333); septicemia caused by other bacteria; meningococcemia; bacterial endocarditis; mycoplasmal pneumonia and other community-acquired pneumonias; legionnaires' disease (Chapter 322); Q fever; influenza pneumonitis (Chapter 372); hantaviral pulmonary syndrome (Chapter 389); viral pneumonia caused by respiratory syncytial virus (Chapter 370), cytomegalovirus (Chapter 384), or other viruses; and strangulated inguinal hernia.

Laboratory confirmation relies on bacterial culture accompanied by specific bacteriophage lysis tests or detection of a four-fold rise in antibody titer to the *Y. pestis* F1 capsular antigen over a period of 2 to 4 weeks. Although the procedures for confirming the laboratory diagnosis of *Y. pestis* infection are relatively simple, delays can occur because the relevant expertise and reagents are often limited to a few public health or reference laboratories. Because cases of plague can rapidly progress to a life-threatening illness, and because culture of *Y. pestis* on bacteriologic media may require 48 hours or longer before colonies become visible, it is essential that patients suspected of having plague receive appropriate antimicrobial therapy immediately after samples have been taken. Direct fluorescent antibody assays can be used to identify *Y. pestis* bacteria in bubo aspirates, sputum samples, and tracheal washes; this procedure requires about 1 hour and provides strong presumptive evidence of infection. A presumptive diagnosis can also be obtained rapidly by detecting *Y. pestis* DNA in polymerase chain reaction (PCR) assays or *Y. pestis*–specific antigens in immunologic assays, but these tests are not widely available. Recently, rapid immunochromatographic tests have been developed that can detect plague antigen or antibodies. The potential advantages of these tests are that they require few laboratory resources, can be done in field settings, and yield results in less than an hour. One such test designed to detect *Y. pestis* antigens in patient samples has been used in some developing countries to diagnose plague, but these assays are still being evaluated and are not widely available. Preferred laboratory samples include blood, serum, bubo aspirates, tracheal washes, and swabs of skin lesions or pharyngeal mucosa. Cerebrospinal fluid can also be collected from patients in whom plague meningitis is suspected.

PREVENTION

No commercially available plague vaccine exists in the United States. Newer recombinant vaccines designed to stimulate immune responses to the F1 and V antigens of *Y. pestis* are undergoing clinical trials and have yielded promising results, but they are unlikely to be available in the near future.

Human plague risk can be reduced through the implementation of effective surveillance programs to rapidly identify human cases and threatening epizootics. When appropriate, affected areas can be treated with insecticides to reduce the risk for flea bite exposure. Appropriate steps should be taken to reduce the amount of food and shelter available to rodents. In rare instances, rodenticides can be used to reduce host numbers, but their use is not recommended before the implementation of effective flea control measures. Persons living in or visiting areas endemic for plague should avoid sick or dead animals and use insect repellents to reduce the risk for infectious flea bites. Dogs and cats should be prevented from roaming freely in rodent-infested areas, and these animals should be treated with flea control agents that safely and effectively kill fleas. Although most dogs appear to be somewhat resistant to plague, cats are highly susceptible, often experience severe illness, and can serve as sources of infection for their owners or veterinary staff. Cats that roam outside in endemic areas and suddenly become seriously ill should be taken to a veterinarian for evaluation.

Persons with pneumonic plague should be held in respiratory isolation for at least 48 hours after the initiation of appropriate antimicrobial therapy, and persons caring for such patients should follow respiratory droplet precautions (mask, gloves, gown, eye protection). Although human-to-human transmission has not been reported in the United States for many decades, rare cases of primary pneumonic plague have occurred after face-to-face contact with infected cats that had oral lesions or symptoms of pneumonic plague. Veterinary staff from plague-enzootic areas should take appropriate precautions (mask, gloves, gown, eye protection) when handling sick cats with illnesses suggestive of plague.

Prophylactic antimicrobial therapy is generally recommended for persons with possible plague exposure only in relatively high-risk situations, such as after close contact with pneumonic plague patients, handling of *Y. pestis*–infected animals, or being bitten by rodent fleas in an area with a recent history of epizootic activity. The most recently recommended prophylactic antimicrobials are doxycycline and ciprofloxacin (Table 320-1).

TREATMENT   Rx

The most commonly recommended agent for treating plague is streptomycin (see Table 320-1), but a randomized trial in Tanzania concluded that gentamicin and doxycycline are effective for treating plague in adults and children and cause few adverse responses.■ A review of human cases treated in New Mexico also strongly suggests that gentamicin is effective and can be substituted for streptomycin. Tetracyclines are effective for treating uncomplicated cases of bubonic plague, and chloramphenicol is believed to be effective, particularly for plague meningitis. Although antimicrobial resistance is not believed to be a problem in the United States, strains resistant to tetracyclines and other agents have been described occasionally, and resistance to streptomycin and chloramphenicol may also occur. The occasional persistence of *Y. pestis* in necrotic or partially necrotic tissues emphasizes the importance of adequately excising these tissues.

PROGNOSIS

Patients with uncomplicated bubonic plague respond quickly to appropriate antimicrobial therapy and typically defervesce, with relief from most other systemic manifestations within 2 to 5 days. Large buboes can remain swollen, however, for more than a week after the *Y. pestis* infection has been eliminated, and some patients require many weeks of convalescence before feeling fully recovered. In rare instances, ischemic necrosis in septicemic cases has resulted in the amputation of digits.

● ENTEROPATHOGENIC YERSINIAE

DEFINITION

Y. enterocolitica and *Y. pseudotuberculosis* differ significantly from *Y. pestis*, in that they are enteropathogenic, rarely cause death, and are spread via the fecal-oral route. Like *Y. pestis*, both of these bacteria are gram-negative members of the family Enterobacteriaceae.

The Pathogens

Y. enterocolitica is genetically quite distinct from *Y. pseudotuberculosis* and *Y. pestis*; the plague bacterium is thought to have arisen as a recent clone of *Y. pseudotuberculosis*, and the chromosomal DNA of these two species is extremely similar. All three species share an approximately 70-kb plasmid that encodes for various proteins (Yops) that are key virulence factors. Unlike *Y. pestis*, the enteropathogenic yersiniae are urease positive and motile at temperatures lower than 30° C. *Y. pseudotuberculosis* is rhamnose positive, thereby distinguishing it from the closely related *Y. pestis* and the more distantly related *Y. enterocolitica*. The enteropathogenic yersiniae are genetically more diverse than the more recently evolved plague bacterium. *Y. enterocolitica* contains 6 biogroups and more than 50 serogroups, whereas *Y. pseudotuberculosis* has been classified into 6 distinct serogroups (O groups 1 to 6).

EPIDEMIOLOGY

Enteropathogenic yersiniae are transmitted via the fecal-oral route, and successful infection of the host requires large doses of bacteria (median infective dose of 10^8 to 10^9 bacteria). Typical sources of infection include the consumption of contaminated foods such as dairy products, inadequately cooked meat, and certain vegetables. Both *Y. enterocolitica* and *Y. pseudotuberculosis*

TABLE 320-1 RECOMMENDATIONS FOR THE TREATMENT OF PATIENTS WITH PNEUMONIC PLAGUE IN CONTAINED AND MASS CASUALTY SETTINGS AND FOR POSTEXPOSURE PROPHYLAXIS*

PATIENT CATEGORY	RECOMMENDED THERAPY
CONTAINED CASUALTY SETTING	

Adults	Preferred choices:
	  Streptomycin 1 g IM twice daily
	  Gentamicin 5 mg/kg IM or IV once daily or 2 mg/kg loading dose followed by 1.7 mg/kg IM or IV 3 times daily
	Alternative choices:
	  Doxycycline 100 mg IV twice daily or 200 mg IV once daily
	  Ciprofloxacin 400 mg IV twice daily†
	  Chloramphenicol 25 mg/kg IV 4 times daily‡

Children§	Preferred choices:
	  Streptomycin 15 mg/kg IM twice daily (maximum daily dose, 2 g)
	  Gentamicin 2.5 mg/kg IM or IV 3 times daily¶
	Alternative choices:
	  Doxycycline: if ≥45 kg, give adult dosage; if <45 kg, give 2.2 mg/kg IV twice daily (maximum, 200 mg/day)
	  Ciprofloxacin 15 mg/kg IV twice daily†
	  Chloramphenicol 25 mg/kg IV 4 times daily‡

Pregnant women¶	Preferred choice:
	  Gentamicin 5 mg/kg IM or IV once daily or 2 mg/kg loading dose followed by 1.7 mg/kg IM or IV 3 times daily¶
	Alternative choices:
	  Doxycycline 100 mg IV twice daily or 200 mg IV once daily
	  Ciprofloxacin 400 mg IV twice daily†

MASS CASUALTY SETTING AND POSTEXPOSURE PROPHYLAXIS**	

Adults	Preferred choices:
	  Doxycycline 100 mg PO twice daily††
	  Ciprofloxacin 500 mg PO twice daily†
	Alternative choices:
	  Chloramphenicol 25 mg/kg PO 4 times daily‡‡

Children§	Preferred choices:
	  Doxycycline††: if ≥45 kg, give adult dosage; if <45 kg, give 2.2 mg/kg PO twice daily
	  Ciprofloxacin 20 mg/kg PO twice daily
	Alternative choice:
	  Chloramphenicol 25 mg/kg PO 4 times daily‡‡

Pregnant women¶	Preferred choices:
	  Doxycycline 100 mg PO twice daily††
	  Ciprofloxacin 500 mg PO twice daily
	Alternative choice:
	  Chloramphenicol 25 mg/kg PO 4 times daily‡‡

*These are consensus recommendations of the Working Group on Civilian Biodefense and are not necessarily approved by the Food and Drug Administration. One antimicrobial agent should be selected, and therapy should be continued for 10 days. Oral therapy should be substituted when the patient's condition improves.
†Other fluoroquinolones can be substituted at doses appropriate for age. The ciprofloxacin dosage should not exceed 1 g/day in children.
‡The concentration should be maintained between 5 and 20 μg/mL. Concentrations >25 μg/mL can cause reversible bone marrow suppression.
§In children, the ciprofloxacin dose should not exceed 1 g/day, and the chloramphenicol dose should not exceed 4 g/day. Children younger than 2 years should not receive chloramphenicol.
¶Aminoglycoside dosages must be adjusted based on renal function. Evidence suggests that gentamicin 5 mg/kg IM or IV once daily would be efficacious in children, although this is not yet widely accepted in clinical practice. Neonates up to 1 week of age and premature infants should receive gentamicin 2.5 mg/kg IV twice daily.
¶In neonates, a gentamicin loading dose of 4 mg/kg should be given initially.
**The duration of treatment of plague in a mass casualty setting is 10 days. The duration of postexposure prophylaxis to prevent plague infection is 7 days.
††Tetracycline can be substituted for doxycycline.
‡‡Children younger than 2 years should not receive chloramphenicol. An oral formulation is available only outside the United States.
Adapted from Inglesby TV, Dennis DT, Henderson DA, et al. Plague as a biological weapon: medical and public health management. Working Group on Civilian Biodefense. *JAMA.* 2000; 283:2281-2290.

can survive and proliferate slowly at refrigerator temperatures. Though far less common, person-to-person transmission has been reported, as has transmission via blood transfusion. Pigs, rodents, rabbits, sheep, goats, cattle, horses, dogs, cats, and sometimes birds serve as reservoirs for these yersiniae. Most hosts act as asymptomatic carriers, but a few human cases have been associated with handling sick animals. Symptomatic patients shed large amounts of yersiniae for as long as 2 to 3 weeks. Untreated, infected persons can become carriers and shed for 2 to 3 months.

Yersiniosis is a reportable disease in many countries. Most cases result from *Y. enterocolitica* infection, and this agent reportedly accounts for 1 to 3% of all cases of acute enteritis in some areas. The overall annual incidence is about 0.9 cases per 100,000 persons in the United States, but the incidence rates vary among ethnic groups, being highest in African Americans (3.2 cases per 100,000) and lower in Asian Americans (1.5 cases per 100,000), Hispanics (0.6 cases per 100,000), and whites (0.4 cases per 100,000). The highest incidence occurs in African American infants (141.9 cases per 100,000). Regardless of ethnicity, the incidence decreases with age. High rates among African American populations have been associated with the home preparation of chitterlings made from contaminated pork intestines.

Y. enterocolitica serotypes O:3, O:8, O:9, and O:5,27 have been associated with human disease. Serotype O:3 predominates in most countries and is found most commonly in swine. Serotype O:9 has been isolated from sheep, cows, and goats. Although serotype O:8 infections appear to be decreasing in incidence in the United States, they are becoming increasingly important in Japan, Italy, and France. In Europe, most cases involve serotype O:3 infections, although a few are associated with serotypes O:9 and O:5,27. Biotype 1A appears to be nonpathogenic, and biotype 5 has been isolated only from hares. Strains pathogenic in humans are esculin, salicin, and pyrazinamidase negative.

Y. pseudotuberculosis has been isolated from rodents, cattle, sheep, cats, dogs, and birds. It occurs worldwide but is most common in northern Europe and in Asia, including Japan. O group 1, 2, and 3 strains are associated with human disease, with most cases being attributed to O:1 or O:2 strains. Infected animals serve as chronic carriers and sources for the infection of water and foods such as meat, dairy products, and stored vegetables. Some cases have been associated with the handling of kittens and puppies. Recent outbreaks of *Y. pseudotuberculosis* in Finland were traced to eating iceberg lettuce and carrots (serotypes O:3 and O:1, respectively). A large Canadian outbreak was associated with milk that had been pasteurized but nevertheless became contaminated. Outbreaks in the former Soviet Union have been associated with the consumption of root vegetables that were stored underground for winter consumption and presumably became contaminated with rodent excreta containing *Y. pseudotuberculosis*.

PATHOBIOLOGY

On reaching the ileum, *Y. enterocolitica* adheres to the mucosa, where intracellular infections in Peyer's patches, mucosal cells, and macrophages can occur. Invasion of the ileal mucosa is favored by the presence of invasin, an outer membrane protein, and a 17-kD surface factor (Ail). An inflammatory response causes abdominal pain and diarrhea, as well as ulcerative ileitis, mesenteric adenitis, and necrosis within Peyer's patches. If the regional defenses are breached, the bacteria can disseminate and cause sepsis and hepatic and splenic abscesses. Polyarthritis can also occur later in the course of illness, particularly in human leukocyte antigen (HLA)-B27–positive individuals.

Like *Y. pestis*, the enteropathogenic yersiniae attack host lymphoid tissues. Invasion of these tissues and resistance against host defenses depend on the possession of an approximately 70-kb plasmid that bears genes encoding for various Yops and the so-called V antigen. The products of this plasmid work in concert to inhibit phagocytosis and reduce inflammation, thereby suppressing the host immune response and favoring persistence of these microbes.

Once *Y. enterocolitica* and *Y. pseudotuberculosis* become established in the lymph nodes, they can resist phagocytosis, which allows them to replicate extracellularly and form aggregates in the nodes. The ability to acquire host iron can be a significant factor contributing to the virulence of *Y. enterocolitica* strains. O:8 serotypes, which are virulent for mice, have the *irp2* (iron repressible 2) gene that encodes for a pair of high-molecular-weight outer membrane proteins, whereas the mouse avirulent O:3 and O:9 serotypes lack *irp2*. O:3 and O:9 serotypes typically remain confined to the guts of their hosts, except when iron overload is present or patients are being treated with an iron chelator.

Patients with reactive arthritis (Chapter 273) are more likely to have fewer gastrointestinal symptoms, lower T-cell proliferative responses to *Yersinia* antigens, lower initial immunoglobulin (Ig) M responses, higher and more persistent IgG and IgA responses, and increased levels of IgA with a secretory component. *Yersinia*-specific antibody responses are also more likely to persist in patients with reactive arthritis than in those with uncomplicated gastrointestinal disease. *Yersinia* antigens thought to contribute to reactive arthritis include Yops and released proteins, which stimulate host CD4 cells, and heat shock protein 60, which has been hypothesized to work in conjunction with other antigens to modulate the host immune response. Evidence exists that hosts can maintain chronic *Y. enterocolitica* infections for years after the initial infection, a factor that may induce the inflammation associated with reactive arthritis (Chapter 273).

CLINICAL MANIFESTATIONS

After an incubation period of about 3 to 7 days, a gastroenteritis typically develops that can be difficult to distinguish from *Salmonella* (Chapter 316) or *Campylobacter* (Chapter 311) gastroenteritis. The most common clinical syndromes associated with *Y. enterocolitica* infection are acute enteritis with fever, diarrhea, vomiting, right lower quadrant pain suggestive of appendicitis (Chapter 144), erythema nodosum, and reactive arthritis. Other common symptoms include associated pharyngitis, rash, joint pain, and headache. Stool examination reveals leukocytes or erythrocytes, and one fourth of patients experience bloody diarrhea.

Y. pseudotuberculosis infections most commonly manifest as acute mesenteric adenitis with diarrhea, fever, vomiting, and bloody stools.

Enterocolitis is most likely to occur in young children, whereas older children more frequently experience acute terminal ileitis, mesenteric adenitis, and systemic disease. Pseudoappendicitis has been reported in patients with mesenteric lymphadenitis. Sepsis is uncommon and is most likely to occur in persons with underlying conditions such as diabetes mellitus, cirrhosis, immunosuppression, older age, and hemochromatosis. Splenic abscesses, meningitis, or endocarditis can develop in septic patients, and mortality can approach 50%. Erythema nodosum is identified in about a third of all patients and in 10% of adults.

DIAGNOSIS

Yersiniosis should be suspected in patients with abdominal pain and fever, especially if they live in endemic areas. Diagnosis is best accomplished by isolation of the bacterium from stool, blood, or other appropriate samples. Recovery of *Y. enterocolitica* and *Y. pseudotuberculosis* from clinical and environmental samples can be greatly complicated by the presence of other bacteria that are likely to predominate. The preferred selective agar for isolation from stool specimens is CIN (cefsulodin-irgasan-novobiocin) agar prepared with relatively low cefsulodin concentrations. Isolation of yersiniae is also helped by culture at 25 to 30°C, which results in better growth than when cultures are kept at 35°C and favors growth of the more cold-tolerant yersiniae over other bacteria that require higher temperatures. Once obtained, isolates can be confirmed as enteropathogenic *Yersinia* by biochemical tests. Biotyping and serotyping, which are often available only in research or reference laboratories, can provide useful epidemiologic information. Isolation difficulties and the reported low sensitivity (about 10^3 to 10^6 colony-forming units per gram of sample) of current isolation techniques have led some to suggest that PCR or other DNA-based methods are likely to result in the more rapid and sensitive detection of these bacteria.

Tube or microagglutination tests can identify antibodies to the pathogenic *Y. enterocolitica* serogroups O:3, O:9, O:5,27, and O:8, but cross-reactivity can be a problem, particularly between *Y. enterocolitica* O:9 and *Brucella* species. PCR for O genotyping of *Y. pseudotuberculosis* could eventually replace traditional serotyping methods. Immunologically mediated *Yersinia* illnesses, including reactive arthritis, are associated with the production of IgA antibodies that can be detected by enzyme-linked immunosorbent assay (ELISA) or immunoblotting. IgG antibodies can persist for many years, but persistence of IgA antibodies for more than a few months could indicate a chronic *Yersinia* infection.

PREVENTION

Prevention depends on measures intended to protect persons from contact with contaminated environments, foods, and wastes. These include using proper sewage disposal methods, protecting water supplies from contamination with human or animal wastes, following appropriate procedures for animal husbandry and slaughtering, thoroughly cooking meats (especially pork), avoiding long-term storage of meats at temperatures higher than 39° F, and consuming only pasteurized milk. Individuals should thoroughly wash their hands after handling potentially contaminated pork or other foods. Diarrheic persons should not work in food-handling areas, care for young children, or work with patients, and hospital staff should follow enteric precautions. Vaccines are not available.

TREATMENT

Antibiotics do not improve the course of uncomplicated enterocolitis or mesenteric adenitis, and the use of antimicrobial therapy is not recommended for intestinal forms of the disease. Such therapy is, however, recommended for immunocompromised patients, patients with septicemia, and those with systemic disease or extraintestinal foci of infection. It should be noted that in vitro susceptibility does not necessarily indicate efficacy in vivo.

Broad-spectrum cephalosporins, sometimes accompanied by aminoglycosides, have resulted in successful outcomes in patients with extraintestinal forms of yersiniosis, including septicemia. Ciprofloxacin, cefotaxime, and ceftriaxone are considered the most effective agents for treating *Y. enterocolitica* serogroup O:3 infection. In addition, *Y. enterocolitica* serogroup O:3 and O:9 isolates possess chromosomally determined β-lactamases that can confer resistance to ampicillin, carbenicillin, and cephalothin. Although serogroup O:8 strains, which produce type A β-lactamase, show resistance to the latter two agents, they are susceptible to ampicillin. It has yet to be determined whether antimicrobial therapy is useful for treating immunologically mediated forms of yersinial illness, including reactive arthritis.

PROGNOSIS

Cases of *Y. enterocolitica* enteritis are generally mild and self-limited after a 2- to 3-week course of illness. Sequelae most commonly include reactive arthritis and erythema nodosum. Glomerulonephritis and myocarditis have also been reported, particularly with serogroup O:3, biotype 4, phage type 8 infections. Other sequelae can include endocarditis, pericarditis, and osteitis. *Y. enterocolitica*–induced reactive arthritis, which can appear 1 to 3 weeks after infection, is oligoarticular, asymmetrical, and peripheral; it occurs most frequently in the lower limbs and eventually resolves over a period of a few weeks to months. HLA-B27–positive patients are more likely to experience severe and prolonged arthritis.

Y. pseudotuberculosis infections are also generally mild and self-limited. Reported complications include erythema nodosum, iritis, reactive arthritis, and nephritis.

1. Mwengee W, Butler T, Mgema S, et al. Treatment of plague with gentamicin or doxycycline in a randomized trial in Tanzania. *Clin Infect Dis.* 2006;42:614-621.

SUGGESTED READINGS

Bertherat E, Thullier P, Shako JC, et al. Lessons learned about pneumonic plague diagnosis from 2 outbreaks, Democratic Republic of the Congo. *Emerg Infect Dis.* 2011;17:778-784. *Review emphasizing the utility of rapid diagnostic testing.*

Butler T. Plague into the 21st century. *Clin Infect Dis.* 2009;49:736-742. *Update focusing on epidemiologic trends, bacterial virulence, diagnosis, and treatment of plague.*

Zheng H, Sun Y, Lin S, et al. *Yersinia enterocolitica* infection in diarrheal patients. *Eur J Clin Microbiol Infect Dis.* 2008;27:741-752. *Review of 118 cases.*

321

WHOOPING COUGH AND OTHER *BORDETELLA* INFECTIONS

ERIK L. HEWLETT

DEFINITION

Pertussis (whooping cough), an acute respiratory illness with a potentially protracted clinical course, is caused by infection with *Bordetella pertussis* or related members of the genus, especially *Bordetella parapertussis*. The infection is highly contagious and can have both endemic and epidemic features in a population, but there are no chronic carriers of the organism. Pertussis is not solely a pediatric illness, and the greatest increases in incidence in recent years have been in adolescents and adults. Although death is rare except in infants, in whom mortality approaches 1% in the United States, almost 300,000 people are believed to die of pertussis worldwide each year.

The Pathogen

There are now eight species in the genus *Bordetella*, but *B. pertussis, B. parapertussis,* and *B. bronchiseptica* (primarily a veterinary pathogen) are most likely to cause respiratory infections in humans. Recently identified species such as *B. holmesii* and *B. trematum* have been associated with bacteremia and wound infections. The organisms are fastidious, gram-negative, coccobacillary in shape, and particularly small relative to other gram-negative organisms. *B. pertussis* was first isolated by Bordet and Gengou in 1906, and the medium used for culture (Bordet-Gengou agar) still bears their names.

EPIDEMIOLOGY

In the pre-vaccine era (before the mid-1950s), pertussis was primarily a childhood illness; as a result, the disease has received little attention in adult medicine. The extensive use of pertussis vaccines in the United States and other parts of the world resulted in a marked reduction of pertussis in the population and a change in the age-specific incidence of disease, with the majority of cases now occurring in infants too young to be vaccinated and in adolescents and adults who become susceptible because of waning immunity after childhood vaccination. In recent years, this shift has been particularly notable, with 25,827 cases of pertussis reported in the United States in 2004, the highest number since 1959. Approximately 60% of those cases occurred in adolescents and adults. The annual incidence of reported cases in the United States has remained above 10,000 since that time. In fact, seroepidemiologic data suggest that 25% of adolescents and adults with a cough lasting more than 1 week have pertussis. The disease is endemic in the United States, but epidemics occur every 3 to 4 years.

B. pertussis is highly contagious and is believed to be spread primarily by large droplets. Although there is no classic "carrier" state such as that recognized for many other infectious organisms, the organism can be cultured for a brief time from exposed individuals who remain asymptomatic. Although these subjects could, in theory, spread the organism, they are unlikely to do so because they are not coughing. Dissemination in a community is often due to symptomatic adolescents, who spread the organism during school attendance and social events. Health care personnel are also important sources of transmission, and health care–associated outbreaks can affect both vulnerable patients and their care providers.

PATHOBIOLOGY

Although *B. pertussis* and related organisms produce a number of interesting toxins, and pertussis has been described as a "toxin-mediated" disease, there is no clear pathophysiologic link between the known virulence factors and clinical manifestations of disease. The infection is localized to the respiratory tract, where organisms adhere to the ciliated surface of epithelial cells, many of which are damaged and lost from the mucosa. Mucous secretion is prominent, especially during later stages of the illness. Intracellular *B. pertussis* organisms have been demonstrated both in vitro and in samples collected from patients, but this is not an obligate intracellular organism, and the significance of these observations remains unknown.

The toxins and adhesins are important both for their potential role in the pathogenesis of disease and for their use as antigens in acellular pertussis vaccines. Filamentous hemagglutinin (FHA), pertactin, and fimbriae are adhesins that are components of some acellular vaccines, and all currently available vaccines include pertussis toxin (PT). In addition to being an adhesin, FHA has been shown to modulate the functions of cells in the host immune system. PT is a member of the family of adenosine diphosphate–ribosylating toxins that includes cholera toxin and diphtheria toxin, and its intracellular target consists of several guanosine triphosphate–binding proteins such as $G_{i\alpha}$. Although PT causes lymphocytosis and enhances insulin secretion, its target cell or cells and its contribution to the clinical manifestations of pertussis are still a mystery. Bordetellae also possess an adenylate cyclase (AC) toxin, which is a bacterial AC that enters host cells to produce supraphysiologic levels of cyclic adenosine monophosphate (cAMP). AC toxin acts against phagocytic cells, such as polymorphonuclear leukocytes and alveolar macrophages, whose antibacterial functions are inhibited by the

increased cAMP. Additional "toxins," including the tracheal cytotoxin BrkA, tracheal colonization factor, and heat-labile or dermonecrotic toxin, have been identified by virtue of their activities in vitro or in animals. The relationship of these toxins to disease also remains ill defined.

CLINICAL MANIFESTATIONS

Although the classic paroxysmal cough of pertussis is striking and unforgettable, not all patients experience the typical cough. Infants may have apnea as an early manifestation, and only sometimes does the characteristic cough develop subsequently.

Incubation Period

After exposure to a patient with active pertussis (typically by way of aerosol from an infected patient who is coughing), an infected individual does not experience the onset of symptoms until 1 to almost 3 weeks later. This relatively long incubation period makes it difficult to track transmission and increases the time necessary for intervention and the institution of control measures.

Catarrhal Phase

Importantly, the symptoms that initiate the catarrhal phase (rhinorrhea, increased lacrimation, conjunctival injection, and sometimes low-grade fever) are nonspecific and do not suggest pertussis, except in the setting of an ongoing hospital or community outbreak. This phase, which can last from a few days to as long as a week, is often associated with the onset of nonproductive cough.

Paroxysmal Phase

A patient's transition to the paroxysmal phase and initiation of the typical cough can suggest the diagnosis of pertussis. This striking cough consists of a series of uncontrollable expirations, followed by gasping inhalation, which, depending on the airway anatomy, can be responsible for the "whooping" sound. Whoop is more frequent in children than in adults. It is not uncommon for each episode of coughing to be associated with cyanosis and end with gagging and vomiting, which in an infant can result in dehydration and malnutrition. The paroxysmal stage can last up to 4 weeks, and the development of fever or worsening pulmonary function during this time should suggest the possibility of secondary pneumonia. Eighty percent or more of adolescents and adults with pertussis have paroxysmal cough, but the frequency of whoop and post-tussive vomiting in this population is quite variable. In addition, during the paroxysmal stage, adults experience symptoms not described in children, such as a scratchy throat, other pharyngeal symptoms, and episodes of sweating.

Convalescent Phase

A reduction in the frequency and severity of coughing attacks marks the transition to the convalescent phase, which can last weeks to months. It is often during this time that adults present to the health care system with "chronic cough" and may be evaluated for conditions such as asthma, tuberculosis, other chronic lung diseases, malignancies, and gastroesophageal reflux. After the coughing spells have ended, patients may experience a return of the paroxysmal cough in conjunction with an unrelated upper respiratory illness; this is often incorrectly interpreted as a recurrence of pertussis. Eighty percent of adults with pertussis have an illness of at least 3 weeks' duration, and 27% are still coughing after 90 days.

Complications

In infants and children younger than 5 years, hospitalization is common; 5 to 10% have pneumonia, nearly 1% of infants experience seizures, and encephalopathy is seen in 0.1%. Pertussis pneumonia in infants and small children can be complicated by pulmonary hypertension. Adolescents and adults have these same complications with a lower frequency, but adults can experience other problems associated with underlying medical conditions. For example, there are anecdotal reports of cough syncope, herniated intervertebral disc, sudden-onset hearing loss, angina episodes, and carotid artery dissection.

DIAGNOSIS

Several methods can be used to detect *B. pertussis,* its products, and the host response to them, but each has its limitations. Culture of a nasopharyngeal swab or aspirate (Fig. 321-1) is the "gold standard" (specificity approaching 100% in symptomatic patients), but even with the use of specialized transport

Posterior nasopharynx

FIGURE 321-1. Technique for obtaining a nasopharyngeal specimen for the isolation of *Bordetella pertussis*. Dacron or calcium alginate swabs are recommended to obtain culture specimens. Dacron swabs are appropriate if polymerase chain reaction testing will be performed. (Redrawn from Cornia PB, Lipsky BA, Saint S, Gonzales R. Clinical problem solving: nothing to cough at. *N Engl J Med.* 2007;357:1432-1437.)

medium and processing in a careful, interested laboratory, recovery rates are often less than 50% and are completely dependent on the duration of illness and whether antimicrobial treatment was initiated before specimen collection. Polymerase chain reaction (PCR)–based diagnostic tests of nasopharyngeal swabs or aspirates are much more sensitive than culture and can remain positive for several days after the initiation of antimicrobial treatment. In addition, appropriately designed PCR assays can identify and distinguish among *B. pertussis, B. parapertussis,* and *B. bronchiseptica.* However, several apparent "outbreaks" of pertussis were later found to represent false-positive PCR results. Detection of serum antibodies to products of *B. pertussis* can be used to identify patients during infection, but care must be taken to distinguish an acute response from residual antibodies from prior immunization.

In view of the limited resources and equipment available for the diagnosis of pertussis, the World Health Organization has established a clinical case definition: 21 or more days of paroxysmal coughing with laboratory confirmation or epidemiologic linkage. Although this definition is often used for clinical trials, it is now clear that its application can result in cases of lesser severity or shorter duration being missed.

TREATMENT   Rx

Supportive Therapy
Because infants and young children have the highest risk for complications and death, supportive therapy is often the most important component of their medical care. Close observation (preferably in the hospital) is essential to ensure adequate feeding, oxygenation, and hydration to minimize complications in this age group. None of the pharmacologic interventions tested for the amelioration of cough and other symptoms is effective in pertussis.[1]

Antimicrobial Agents
There are two reasons to use antimicrobials in a patient with pertussis: first, to eliminate the causative organism and reduce transmission, and second, to limit the course of illness in the treated patient by eliminating the infection. Because individuals can remain culture positive and can potentially transmit *B. pertussis* for several weeks after the onset of symptoms, it is appropriate to treat patients who are seen within that time frame. Whether antimicrobials provide symptomatic relief is controversial, but they can do so only when treatment is started within the first week of symptoms.

The recommendation of the Centers for Disease Control and Prevention for the treatment of pertussis in adults is azithromycin (500 mg on day 1, followed by 250 mg/day on days 2 to 5), clarithromycin (1 g/day in two divided doses for 7 days), erythromycin (2 g/day in four divided doses for 14 days), or trimethoprim-sulfamethoxazole (trimethoprim 320 mg/day, sulfamethoxazole 1600 mg/day, in two divided doses for 14 days). It has now been shown that treatment with erythromycin for 7 days is as effective as treatment for 14 days. The newer macrolides (azithromycin and clarithromycin) are better tolerated but more expensive.[2]

PREVENTION
Chemoprophylaxis
Chemoprophylaxis with the aforementioned antimicrobial agents is an important mechanism for controlling outbreaks in hospitals or in the community.[3] This approach is effective when initiated before the onset of symptoms and is recommended for individuals exposed within the preceding 3 weeks; high-risk persons with underlying health problems, particularly infants; or those who might have occupational or other contact with susceptible hosts.

Immunization
A killed, whole cell vaccine was introduced in the late 1940s. Use of that product had a dramatic effect on the incidence of pertussis, with the number of reported cases in the United States falling from more than 200,000 annually to less than 2000 in 1980. In the 1970s and 1980s, recognition of the adverse events associated with the whole cell product and public concern led to the development of the purified acellular pertussis vaccines that are in use today.

Current acellular pertussis vaccines, which contain one or more purified protein antigens (all contain PT and other combinations of FHA, pertactin, and fimbriae types 2 and 3), are administered to infants and children up to the age of 6 years. They are safe and efficacious and cause significantly fewer adverse reactions compared with the whole cell vaccines. In recognition of the significant incidence of pertussis in adolescents and adults and their role in transmitting the disease to infants and small children, several vaccines are now licensed for administration to these age groups. Use of these vaccines is now routinely recommended to boost immunity in adolescents 11 to 18 years old who completed the recommended childhood vaccination series. An important group for whom adult booster immunization is not yet available is pregnant women, who can acquire *B. pertussis* and transmit it to their neonates.

Future work will be directed at improving and standardizing diagnostic methods and increasing vaccine coverage to include pregnant women and other adults.

PROGNOSIS
Most patients will eventually clear *B. pertussis,* even without antimicrobial treatment, but in most cases the illness lasts weeks to months. Antimicrobials are of limited effectiveness in altering the course of the illness unless they are started before the paroxysmal phase. The introduction of booster doses of vaccines for adolescents and adults has the potential to control pertussis in well-immunized populations.

Grade A

1. Bettiol S, Thompson MJ, Roberts NW. Symptomatic treatment of the cough in whooping cough. *Cochrane Database Syst Rev.* 2010;1:CD003257.

2. Centers for Disease Control and Prevention. Recommended antimicrobial agents for the treatment and post-exposure prophylaxis of pertussis: 2005 CDC guidelines. *MMWR Recomm Rep.* 2005;54(RR-14):1-16.
3. Langley JM, Halperin SA, Boucher FD, et al. Azithromycin is as effective and better tolerated than erythromycin estolate for treatment of pertussis. *Pediatrics.* 2004;111:e96-e101.

SUGGESTED READINGS

Centers for Disease Control and Prevention. Health Topic: Pertussis. http://www.cdc.gov/ncidod/dbmd/diseaseinfo/pertussis_t.htm. *Extensive compilation of recommendations on all aspects of pertussis from both the National Immunization Program and the National Center for Infectious Diseases.*

Cornia PB, Hersh AL, Lipsky BA, et al. Does this coughing adolescent or adult patient have pertussis? *JAMA.* 2010;304:890-896. *Post-tussive emesis and an inspiratory whoop modestly increase the likelihood of pertussis but are not conclusive to exclude or establish the diagnosis.*

Crespo I, Cardeñosa N, Godoy P, et al. Epidemiology of pertussis in a country with high vaccination coverage. *Vaccine.* 2011. [Epub ahead of print.] *Review of over 500 cases, including in persons over age 35 years.*

Hong JY. Update on pertussis and pertussis immunization. *Korean J Pediatr.* 2010;53:629-633. *Review emphasizing continued cases despite a 94% vaccination rate.*

Vincent M, Rodeghiero C, Eylenbosch R, et al. Pertussis serodiagnosis in Belgium in the period 1990-2009. *Clin Vaccine Immunol.* 2011;18:588-594. *Between 50 and 150 cases were diagnosed annually, with a peak at the ages of 10 to 20 yr and at the ages of 35 to 50 yr.*

322

LEGIONELLA INFECTIONS

THOMAS J. MARRIE

FIGURE 322-1. **A,** Direct fluorescent antibody stain of *Legionella pneumophila.* **B,** Colonies of *L. pneumophila* growing on a BCYE plate. **C,** Thin section of replicative form of *L. pneumophila.* **D,** Freeze-fracture replica of the mature infectious form obtained after growth in ameba. The latter shows prominent cytoplasmic inclusions (I) and a polar distribution of membrane proteins (*arrow*). **E,** Electron micrograph of *L. pneumophila* growing within *Acanthamoeba castellani.* (**A,** Courtesy Dr. Paul Hoffman, University of Virginia; **B,** Courtesy Dr. Sharon Berk, Tennessee Technical University; **C** to **E,** Courtesy Drs. Rafel Garduno and Gary Faulkner, Dalhousie University.)

DEFINITION

Legionellosis is the term for infection due to bacteria in the *Legionella* genus, of which there are two main manifestations—pneumonia (legionnaires' disease) and Pontiac fever (named after Pontiac, Michigan, where it was first recognized). The latter is usually a mild febrile illness presumed to be a reaction to lipopolysaccharide of *Legionella* species.

The 58th annual convention of the American Legion was held at a hotel in Philadelphia from July 21 to 24, 1976. Subsequently, 182 of the delegates became ill (hence the name legionnaires' disease), and 146 were hospitalized at 87 institutions across the United States. Most had radiographic evidence of pneumonia, and 29 (16%) died. Within about 6 months of the outbreak, a new microorganism, *Legionella pneumophila,* was isolated from the pulmonary tissue of some of those who had died in the Philadelphia outbreak. In retrospect, the organism had first been isolated in 1943.

The Pathogen

Legionellae are small, gram-negative, aerobic, non-spore-forming bacilli that measure 0.3 to 0.9 μm wide by 2 to 20 μm long (Fig. 322-1A to D). These organisms require special media for growth, and many laboratories are unable to isolate legionellae; thus, when laboratory expertise is uncertain, a negative culture is meaningless. They usually do not stain with Gram stain, and in tissue specimens, Dieterle or Warthin-Starry stain is used to visualize these organisms. *Legionella micdadei* retains the modified acid-fast stain and can appear as acid-fast bacilli in clinical specimens. Legionellae are aquatic organisms that thrive in both natural and man-made waterways and distribution systems, especially hot water pipes, water heaters (electrical more so than gas heaters), cooling towers, and water fountains. In these systems, they are found in biofilms that help confer resistance to biocides and chlorine. They are also found in moist soil and mud. They can survive in these environments for long periods and can tolerate temperatures of 0 to 68° C and a pH range of 5 to 8.5. In their natural environments, they are intracellular parasites of protozoa such as the freshwater ameba *Acanthamoeba* and *Hartmanella* species (Fig. 322-1E). Humans are accidental hosts who become infected by inhaling *Legionella* bacteria or ameba laden with these bacteria. Genomes of four different strains of *L. pneumophila* have been sequenced, and they range in size from 3.3 to 3.5 Mb. Legionellae have many eukaryotic-like proteins, which may help the intracellular growth of these organisms in human macrophages by mimicking host proteins. *Legionella* species have type I, II, IV, and V secretion systems, which allow the efficient and rapid delivery of molecules into the phagocytic host cell.

The number of new *Legionella* species continues to grow; there are now at least 56 *Legionella* species and 73 or more serogroups, including 15 serogroups of *L. pneumophila.* A variety of typing systems can be used to further refine the isolates so that individual strains can be identified, a factor that is important for determining the source of an outbreak or understanding the difference between environmental and clinical isolates. It is noteworthy that *L. pneumophila* and all its serotypes cause disease in humans, whereas only about 50% of the remaining species of *Legionella* cause such disease.

EPIDEMIOLOGY

The incubation period for Legionnaires' disease (LD) is most commonly cited as 2 to 10 days, with extremes of 1 to 28 days. Person-to-person transmission does not occur. Legionellosis is found worldwide, predominantly in developed countries owing to the frequent use of cooling towers and complex plumbing systems. Underdiagnosis may be a feature in developing countries owing to the laboratory facilities required. From 1990 to 2005, 23,076 cases of LD were reported in the United States. Only 1.7% of these cases occurred in children, whereas 63% occurred in those aged 45 to 64 years. The number of cases has increased over time. Males account for 61% of cases, and rates are highest in the eastern United States, where most cases occur in the summer or fall. There is an association between increased rainfall and cases of LD. The connection may be aerosolization of *Legionella* from rain puddles on roads. Eastern Canada also has higher rates of LD than the rest of that country. In a U.S. study, 20 to 25% of cases were travel related, whereas in Europe, 390 of 656 (59%) outbreaks reported from 1995 to 2005 were travel related. Travel to Italy, France, Spain, and Turkey accounted for more than 50% of the cases.

The most common risk factors for the acquisition of LD are listed in Table 322-1. *Legionella* species account for 1 to 5% of community-acquired pneumonia requiring admission to a hospital. In some areas, *Legionella* accounts for about the same percentage of pneumonia treated on an ambulatory basis. Nosocomial LD is usually due to contamination of the hospital's water supply. Colonization of 30% or more of the distal water outlets by *Legionella* is almost always associated with cases of LD. Most patients who are infected with non-*pneumophila Legionella* infections are immunocompromised. Nosocomial legionellosis has occurred with *L. pneumophila, L. micdadei, L. bozemanii, L. dumoffi,* and *L. sainthelensis.*

Legionella infections can be sporadic or occur in outbreaks. Outbreaks have been associated with exposure to a variety of aerosol-producing devices, including showers, a grocery store mist machine, cooling towers, whirlpool spas, decorative fountains, and evaporative condensers. LD can be acquired

TABLE 322-1　RISK FACTORS FOR LEGIONNAIRES' DISEASE

RISK FACTOR	APPROXIMATE INCREASED RISK (-FOLD) OVER PERSONS WITHOUT THIS RISK FACTOR
HOST FACTORS	
Renal failure requiring dialysis	20
Corticosteroid therapy	5-10
Hairy cell leukemia	20
Lung or hematologic cancer	7-20
Cytotoxic chemotherapy	5
>3 Alcoholic drinks/day	3-4
Cigarette smoking	2-10
Male gender	—
Age older than 50 yr	2
Diabetes mellitus	2
Solid organ transplantation (immunosuppression)	2
Anti–tumor necrosis factor treatment	16-21
Chronic heart or lung disease	>1
Splenectomy (non-*pneumophila* strains only)	—
ENVIRONMENTAL FACTORS	
Travel	2
Recent plumbing work in home or at work	2
Hospitalization	—
Exposure to contaminated water sources—cooling towers, hot tubs, decorative fountains	—
Exposure to potting soil (Australia)—*Legionella longbeachae*	—

up to 10 km away from contaminated cooling towers. Aspiration of contaminated potable water by immunosuppressed patients is another mechanism by which *Legionella* is acquired.

Pontiac fever occurs predominantly in outbreaks with very high attack rates. *L. pneumophila, L. micdadei,* and *L. anisa* have been implicated in outbreaks of Pontiac fever. Among residents of nursing homes, Pontiac fever has been associated with *L. pneumophila* concentrations greater than 10^4 colony-forming units/L in shower water. Those receiving corticosteroid therapy have a six-fold higher risk of developing Pontiac fever.

PATHOBIOLOGY

After being inhaled, legionellae are phagocytized in the lungs by alveolar macrophages. Legionellae abrogate phagosome-lysosome fusion and replicate in an endosome surrounded by the endoplasmic reticulum. Once it is intracellular, the bacteria-laden endosome recruits small vesicles, mitochondria, and ribosomes, and within 4 to 6 hours it becomes enveloped by the endoplasmic reticulum, thereby establishing the replicative endosome. Bacterial growth then begins and continues in the macrophages for approximately 24 hours, at which time the macrophage disintegrates by apoptosis and the bacteria are released. The released bacteria are often phagocytized by other macrophages, dendritic cells, and epithelial cells, perpetuating the infection. Cell-mediated immunity is necessary for recovery from *Legionella* infection. Production of type 1 interferons has a protective effect by promoting the activation of macrophages. Activated macrophages limit the intracellular replication of legionellae by decreasing the expression of transferrin receptors and limiting the availability of iron to the bacteria. Toll-like receptor (TLR) 2, TLR4, TLR5, and TLR9 are activated during infection with *L. pneumophila*. Interleukin (IL)-1α, IL-1β, IL-4, IL-6, IL-12, and IL-18 are detected during *Legionella* infection. Vaccination of guinea pigs with the purified major outer membrane protein OmpS protects against an LD100 lethal challenge, whereas immunization with purified Hsp60 provides little protection. Polymorphonuclear leukocytes are present in abundance in the infected lung, but their role in clearing the infection is unclear. Bacteria can spread beyond the lung and cause metastatic infection. However, many extrapulmonary effects of LD, such as cerebellar ataxia and confusion, are not due to metastatic infection; they are presumably due to as yet unidentified toxins. The infected lung is consolidated, and there is usually no parenchymal damage once recovery occurs. Abscess formation and bronchiolitis obliterans or fibrosing alveolitis are occasionally seen.

The pathogenesis of Pontiac fever is unclear. The onset of illness occurs within 12 to 36 hours after the inhalation of, presumably, endotoxin. This period is too short for bacterial multiplication to cause the symptoms.

CLINICAL MANIFESTATIONS

Most of our knowledge of the clinical features of LD comes from studying patients who have been hospitalized with this illness—that is, those with the most severe manifestations. Fever (often quite high), malaise, and cough are present in most patients. Chills occur in about 75%, and dyspnea in just over half the patients. Other features include myalgias, headache, chest pain, and diarrhea. The cough is nonproductive in 50% of patients; others have scant sputum production that is usually mucoid, rarely purulent, and very rarely bloody. There are no clinical features that distinguish individual patients with LD from those with pneumonia caused by other pathogens. However, when patients with LD are compared with those with community-acquired pneumonia due to other agents, the patients with LD are more likely to have myalgias, headache, diarrhea, and a higher mean oral temperature at the time of presentation. They also present to the hospital sooner after the onset of symptoms—4.7 days versus 7.7 days. When patients with LD were compared with patients with bacteremic pneumococcal pneumonia, the following features were associated with *Legionella* pneumonia: male sex (odds ratio [OR] 4.6), heavy drinking (OR 4.8), previous β-lactam therapy (OR 19.9), axillary temperature greater than 39° C (OR 10.3), myalgias (OR 8.5), and gastrointestinal symptoms (OR 3.5). Pleuritic chest pain and purulent sputum were less likely to be present. In a young, otherwise healthy person with rapidly progressive pneumonia (especially if the progression occurs in the setting of β-lactam therapy), LD should be strongly suspected. Mental confusion is common, and on occasion, the presentation is dominated by extrapulmonary manifestations such as cerebellar ataxia, seizures, or encephalitis. Rarely, extrapulmonary infection such as prosthetic valve endocarditis, sinusitis, dialysis shunt infection, or abscess formation occurs.

Physical findings include fever, tachypnea, relative bradycardia, and initially only a few crackles on chest examination. Later the findings of pulmonary consolidation are not uncommon. Abdominal examination is usually unremarkable. Rash as a manifestation of LD is very rare. Progression of the illness is not uncommon, even following the institution of antibiotic therapy. This is more likely in immunocompromised patients, who may require up to a week to respond to therapy. About half the patients with LD who require hospitalization have a complicated course.

Pontiac fever has an incubation period of about 36 hours. Fever, severe myalgia, headache, and extreme fatigue are the dominant manifestations. The illness is of short duration, lasting, on average, 3 days.

DIAGNOSIS

It is most important to have a high index of clinical suspicion that a patient might have LD. Routine laboratory tests are nonspecifically abnormal. Leukocytosis is common; leukopenia, thrombocytopenia, and disseminated intravascular coagulation also occur. Other laboratory abnormalities can include hyponatremia (in about half the patients, sometimes severe), hypophosphatemia (also common, occurring early and resolving within a few days of the initiation of treatment), mild liver function test abnormalities (except for alkaline phosphatase, which is occasionally very elevated), elevated creatine kinase (occasionally with rhabdomyolysis), microscopic hematuria, and mild proteinuria. High procalcitonin levels exceeding 1.5 are associated with a higher rate of admission to intensive care units and death.

There are a number of specific tests for the diagnosis of LD. Tests to detect *L. pneumophila* SG 1 antigen in urine are available commercially. These are easy to use, but there is a false-negative rate of up to 26%.■ LD is now usually diagnosed with a urinary antigen test, and it is often diagnosed earlier in the course of the illness than previously. This may be a factor in the lower mortality rates from LD compared with historic rates. Sputum culture has a low sensitivity but is 100% specific. It should be performed on all patients suspected of having LD. Serologic tests are not clinically useful because of the long time (6 to 12 weeks) required to seroconvert; however, they do have a role in the work-up of outbreaks of LD. Polymerase chain reaction (PCR) can be used to amplify *Legionella* DNA in sputum, bronchoalveolar lavage fluid, pleural fluid, pulmonary tissue, or serum. However, PCR tests are not sufficiently developed to be used in most diagnostic laboratories.

FIGURE 322-2. Posteroanterior chest radiograph of a patient with community-acquired pneumonia due to *Legionella pneumophila.* Note the dense consolidation of the right upper lobe, with bulging of the fissure. Such dense consolidation is a common radiographic appearance of legionnaires' disease.

FIGURE 322-3. Posteroanterior chest radiograph of a patient with community-acquired legionnaires' disease (*L. pneumophila*) manifesting as a right lower lobe nodular opacity.

FIGURE 322-4. Posteroanterior chest radiograph of a patient with community-acquired *Legionella feeleii* pneumonia. There is patchy consolidation of the right upper lobe.

FIGURE 322-5. Posteroanterior chest radiograph of a patient with community-acquired pneumonia due to *Legionella pneumophila*. There is patchy consolidation at the right base, with subsegmental atelectasis and elevation of the right hemidiaphragm.

A chest radiograph is necessary to establish a diagnosis of pneumonia. About half the patients with LD have unilateral pulmonary involvement. The lower lobes are involved most commonly. About one third of patients have a pleural effusion. Dense opacification is common, but interstitial and nodular opacities also occur. Cavitation is uncommon. Figures 322-2 through 322-5 illustrate some of the radiographic findings in LD.

The diagnosis of Pontiac fever is based on demonstration of *Legionella* in water to which the patient was exposed, seroconversion to *Legionella*, and a compatible clinical course.

Differential Diagnosis

LD should be considered in any patient with pneumonia who is admitted to the hospital, especially those who require treatment in an intensive care unit. If *Legionella* is present in a hospital's water supply, LD should be considered in all patients with nosocomial pneumonia.

TREATMENT   **Rx**

If the diagnosis of LD is known, levofloxacin and moxifloxacin are first-choice agents (Table 322-2). Unfortunately, no randomized controlled trials have studied the therapy of LD. Data from a prospective, nonrandomized study indicate that levofloxacin is superior to macrolides for the treatment of

severe LD. In this study carried out in Murcia, Spain, 3.4% of the patients receiving levofloxacin had complications, compared with 27.2% of those receiving macrolides; the levofloxacin patients had a shorter length of stay—5.5 versus 11.3 days. The addition of rifampin to levofloxacin produced no additional benefit. In one clinical trial, 20 of 21 patients with LD were cured when treated with azithromycin. In another study, the authors selected 139 cases of *L. pneumophila* pneumonia in a prospective series of 1934 consecutive cases of community-acquired pneumonia. The overall mortality rate was 5%. Eighty patients received initial therapy with a macrolide, and 40 received levofloxacin. Those who received levofloxacin had a faster time to defervescence (2 vs. 4.5 days) and to clinical stability (3 vs. 5 days) and a shorter median length of stay (8 vs. 10 days); there were no significant differences in complications or mortality. In a review of data from six clinical trials, 75 patients with *Legionella* infection were treated with levofloxacin, and 90% of these infections had resolved clinically at the post-therapy visit 2 to 14 days after the termination of treatment. The authors concluded that treatment with levofloxacin 500 mg/

TABLE 322-2 TREATMENT FOR LEGIONNAIRES' DISEASE

SEVERITY OF LEGIONELLA PNEUMONIA	DRUG	DOSAGE
Mild pneumonia in a non-immunocompromised person treated at home	Azithromycin	500 mg once daily for 5 days
	Clarithromycin	500 mg bid for 10 days
	Doxycycline	200 mg loading dose, then 100 mg bid for 10 days
	Levofloxacin	500 mg once daily for 10 days
	Moxifloxacin	400 mg once daily PO for 10 days
Pneumonia requiring hospitalization and/or pneumonia in an immunocompromised person	Levofloxacin	750 mg once daily (IV initially) for 10-14 days*
	Azithromycin	500 mg once daily for 10 days*
	Moxifloxacin	400 mg once daily for 10 days*
	Ciprofloxacin	400 mg q8h IV for 14 days*
	Erythromycin	1000 mg IV qid for 3 days; then 500 mg qid for a total of 21 days
	plus	
	Rifampin	600 mg PO bid for 5 days

*Increase duration of treatment to 21 days for immunocompromised persons.

day for 7 to 14 days or 750 mg/day for 5 days was effective. In a study of 33 patients admitted to an intensive care unit with LD, fluoroquinolone administration within 8 hours of arrival was associated with decreased mortality. There are no good data on the duration of treatment of LD. The consensus is that 7 to 10 days of treatment with azithromycin or a quinolone is sufficient. However, longer treatment is required if there is lung abscess, empyema, or endocarditis. In immunosuppressed patients, therapy should last for 21 days.

A meta-analysis of 24 trials involving 5015 patients with pneumonia showed that for patients with LD, there was a significant benefit when empirical therapy for pneumonia included agents active against *Legionella*.[3] All patients who are severely ill with pneumonia should receive empirical therapy that treats *Legionella* as well as other pathogens. This is in line with the pneumonia guidelines issued by the American Thoracic Society and the Infectious Diseases Society of America.

PROGNOSIS

The case-fatality rate from LD has been decreasing. In one study from Spain, the case-fatality rate fell from 35% in 1993 to 5.6% in 2004. In general, the fatality rate is higher in sporadic cases than in outbreak cases, and it is higher in nosocomial cases compared with community-acquired cases. The highest fatality rate is seen in nosocomial LD, where it is still about 30%. Earlier diagnosis using the urinary antigen test and more effective antibiotic therapy account for much of the reduction in mortality. Factors associated with mortality are older age, immunosuppression, and severity of pneumonia.

Cases of LD should be reported to local health officials. An investigation is often required to determine the source of the *Legionella*.

1. Shimada G, Noguchi Y, Jackson JL, et al. Systematic review and meta-analysis: urinary antigen tests for Legionellosis. *Chest.* 2009;136:1576-1585.
2. Blázquez Garrido RM, Espinosa Parra FJ, Alemany Francés L, et al. Antimicrobial chemotherapy for Legionnaires' disease: levofloxacin versus macrolides. *Clin Infect Dis.* 2005;40:800-806.
3. Shefet D, Robenshtock E, Paul M, et al. Empiric antibiotic coverage of atypical pathogens for community-acquired pneumonia in hospitalized adults. *Cochrane Database Syst Rev.* 2005;2: CD004418.

SUGGESTED READINGS

Carratalà J, Garcia-Vidal C. An update on *Legionella*. *Curr Opin Infect Dis.* 2010;23:152-157. *Review emphasizing the key role of diagnostic laboratory tests, including the urinary antigen.*
Cunha BA. Legionnaires disease: clinical differentiation from typical and other atypical pneumonias. *Infect Dis Clin North Am.* 2010;24:73-105. *Good review of the more uncommon manifestations of Legionnaires' disease. The differential diagnosis of signs such as relative bradycardia and many of the laboratory findings, such as hypophosphatemia and lymphopenia, will be of use to the reader.*

Hilbi H, Jarraud S, Hartland E, et al. Update on Legionnaires' disease: pathogenesis, epidemiology, detection and control. *Mol Microbiol.* 2010;76:1-11. *Summarizes key information presented at the seventh international* Legionella *conference held in Paris in October 2009.*
Joseph CA, Ricketts KD, European Working Group for *Legionella* Infections. Legionnaires' disease in Europe 2007-2008. *Euro Surveill.* 2010;15:19683. *Up-to-date account of the epidemiology of legionellosis in Europe.*
Sakamoto R, Ohno A, Nakahara T, et al. Legionella pneumophila in rain water on roads. *Emerg Infect Dis.* 2009;15:1295-1297. Legionella *was isolated from rain puddles on roads in Japan. Because aerosolization occurs when cars and trucks pass through puddles, this represents a potential source of transmission.*

323

BARTONELLA INFECTIONS

JEAN-MARC ROLAIN AND DIDIER RAOULT

DEFINITION

Bartonella species belong to the alpha 2 subgroup of *Proteobacteria* and are closely related to the genera *Brucella*, *Agrobacterium*, and *Rhizobium*. Since 1993 the genus *Bartonella* has been reorganized by adding the genera *Rochalimaea* and *Grahamella* to the family Bartonellaceae. More than 30 known *Bartonella* species and 3 subspecies have been isolated from both animals and humans. These bacteria are considered emerging pathogens that are associated with zoonosis and/or human infections. Among them, 13 validated species have been implicated in human diseases: *B. henselae*, *B. quintana*, *B. bacilliformis*, *B. elizabethae*, *B. clarridgeiae*, *B. vinsonii* subsp. *arupensis*, *B. vinsonii* subsp. *berkhoffii*, *B. alsatica*, *B. tamiae*, *B. grahamii*, *B. washoensis*, *B. rochalimae*, and *B. koehlerae* (Table 323-1). The other *Bartonella* species have been isolated only from the blood of animals, including rodents, felids, canids, dolphins, and ruminants. The route of transmission of *Bartonella* species in mammals and humans is via fleas, ticks, mites, and lice (see Table 323-1).

Bartonella infections are emerging infectious diseases that lead to a wide spectrum of either acute or chronic diseases. The status of the host immune response plays an important role in the development of the different manifestations. Four different clinical syndromes may occur with *Bartonella* infections: infection of red blood cells and erythrophagocytosis, granulomatous disease controlled by the immune response, blood culture–negative endocarditis and bacteremia, and vasculoproliferative diseases. A single *Bartonella* species can cause either acute or chronic infections and either vasculoproliferative or suppurative manifestations, but with different pathogenetic mechanisms that mainly depend on the patient's immune status. For example, *B. quintana* is responsible for trench fever as well as endocarditis, bacteremia in the homeless population, and vasculoproliferative diseases, whereas *B. bacilliformis* is the agent of Carrion's disease, which corresponds to either an acute intra-erythrocytic bacteremic disease (Oroya fever) or a chronic vasculoproliferative disease (verruga peruana). Infection of red blood cells has been well established for *B. bacilliformis* (Oroya fever) and *B. quintana* (trench fever and bacteremia in the homeless), whereas *B. henselae* and *B. koehlerae* have been seen in erythrocytes of infected cats. *B. henselae* can cause granulomatous disease—that is, cat-scratch disease (CSD)—which affects lymph nodes but can also be responsible for other clinical manifestations and/or complications such as endocarditis. Vasculoproliferative diseases include bacillary angiomatosis caused by *B. henselae* and *B. quintana*, peliosis hepatis caused by *B. henselae*, and verruga peruana caused by *B. bacilliformis*. The immune status of the host plays a critical role in the development of these different forms of the disease. *B. henselae* usually causes CSD (a self-limited disease) in immunocompetent hosts, whereas it is responsible for bacillary angiomatosis in immunocompromised patients. In patients with a previous valvulopathy, any *Bartonella* infection may lead to endocarditis.

The Pathogen

Bartonella species are small, gram-negative, fastidious, pleomorphic coccobacilli or slightly curved rods (0.5 by 1 to 2 µm). Because of the slow growth of these bacteria and the lack of reproducible biochemical methods for their

TABLE 323-1 *BARTONELLA* SPECIES CAUSING HUMAN DISEASE

BARTONELLA SPECIES	First Cultivation		YEAR OF DESCRIPTION	RESERVOIR HOST/VECTOR	HUMAN DISEASE
	MAMMAL	**COUNTRY**			
B. alsatica	Wild rabbit (*Oryctolagus cuniculus*)	France	1999	Rabbit	Endocarditis, lymphadenopathy
B. bacilliformis	Human		1909	Human/sandfly	Carrion's disease, Oroya fever, verruga peruana
B. clarridgeiae	Cat		1996	Cat/cat flea	Cat-scratch disease
B. elizabethae	Endocarditis patient	United States	1993	Rat	Endocarditis, neuroretinitis
B. grahamii	Woodland mammal (*Clethrionomys glareolus*)	United Kingdom	1995	Rat, insectivore	Neuroretinitis
B. henselae	Cat		1990	Cat/cat flea	Cat-scratch disease, endocarditis, bacillary angiomatosis, bacillary peliosis, Parinaud's oculoglandular syndrome, neuroretinitis, osteomyelitis, arthropathy, bacteremia with fever
B. koehlerae	Domestic cat	United States	1999	Cat	Endocarditis
B. mayotimonensis	Endocarditis patient	United States	2009	Unknown	Endocarditis
B. quintana	Human		1920	Human/body louse	Trench fever, endocarditis, bacillary angiomatosis
B. rochalimae	Human	United States	2007		Bacteremia, fever, splenomegaly
B. tamiae	Human	Thailand	2008		Febrile illness
B. vinsonii arupensis	Cattle rancher	United States	1999	Dog, rodent/ticks	Bacteremia with fever
B. washoensis			2000	Ground squirrel	Myocarditis

identification, they are usually identified using molecular methods. Recently, matrix-assisted laser desorption/ionization time-of-flight mass spectrometry has emerged as a new technique for species identification and is an accurate and reproducible method for the rapid and inexpensive identification of *Bartonella* species. The bacteria can grow on enriched blood-containing media with a 5% carbon dioxide atmosphere after 5 to 15 days to up to 45 days on primary culture. The optimal growth temperature ranges from 28° C for *B. bacilliformis* to 35 to 37° C for the other species. *Bartonella* species can also be cocultured with endothelial cells. *Bartonella* species are either flagellated or nonflagellated cells. *B. bacilliformis* uses flagella for binding and deforming into the surface of erythrocytes. Bacteria can either persist in the blood stream of the host as intra-erythrocytic parasites or colonize human endothelial cells.

EPIDEMIOLOGY

Almost all *Bartonella* species are vector-borne bacteria (see Table 323-1). Some are limited geographically, such as *B. bacilliformis*, which is only found in the Andes Mountains in South America at high altitudes, where its principal vector *Lutzomia verrucarum* is distributed; others have a worldwide distribution, such as *B. henselae* and *B. quintana*. Each *Bartonella* species is highly adapted to its mammalian reservoir, in which bacteria usually cause a long-lasting intra-erythrocytic bacteremia that may be asymptomatic. Humans are the hosts and reservoirs for *B. bacilliformis* and *B. quintana*. *B. quintana* is transmitted via the human body louse by inoculation of arthropod feces through broken skin (Chapter 367). Cats represent the main reservoir hosts for *B. henselae* infection; this pathogen is the agent of CSD in humans, caused by cat bites or scratches. *B. henselae* infection is transmitted from cat to cat by the cat flea. Cat fleas may also be infected by *B. quintana*. The role of dogs as reservoir hosts has been documented for several species, including *B. vinsonii* subsp. *arupensis*, *B. vinsonii* subsp. *berkhoffii*, and *B. henselae*. Wild rabbits are the reservoir hosts for *B. alsatica*, which was recently reported to be an agent of endocarditis and lymphadenopathy in humans in close contact with rabbits. For other *Bartonella* species known to cause diseases in humans (see Table 323-1), their pathogenic role and mode of transmission are not fully understood.

● INFECTION OF RED BLOOD CELLS: OROYA FEVER AND TRENCH FEVER

PATHOBIOLOGY

In Oroya fever, *B. bacilliformis* invades up to 80% of erythrocytes and produces their massive lysis, which results in severe hemolytic anemia, the major symptom of the disease. Similarly, trench fever is characterized by an

FIGURE 323-1. Section of human red blood cell infected with *Bartonella quintana* as viewed by confocal microscopy.

intracellular erythrocyte parasitism by *B. quintana*, with the percentage of infected red blood cells ranging from 0.001 to 0.005% (Fig. 323-1). Bacteria can also be seen extracellularly and in erythroblasts. This intracellular erythrocyte parasitism can presumably preserve the pathogens for efficient transmission by body lice, protect *B. quintana* from the host immune response, and contribute to decreased antimicrobial efficacy. During bacteremia in the homeless, *B. quintana* can also be seen in red blood cells.

CLINICAL MANIFESTATIONS

The main clinical manifestations of infection by *Bartonella* species are summarized in Table 323-2.

Oroya fever is the acute or hemolytic phase of Carrion's disease, caused by *B. bacilliformis*; it usually develops 3 to 12 weeks after inoculation. Oroya fever results from the massive invasion of erythrocytes by *B. bacilliformis*, and without antibiotic treatment, it causes death in up to 85% of infected humans by hemolysis or when complicated by opportunistic infections such as salmonellosis. The onset is usually abrupt, with high fever, chills, headache, and anorexia. Patients have intense myalgias and arthralgias, abdominal pain, and jaundice. Complications are frequent, including meningoencephalitis, dyspnea, delirium, and superinfection leading to death. Asymptomatic persistent bacteremia may serve as the reservoir of the organism.

Trench fever is transmitted by lice (Chapter 367) and is the clinical manifestation of *B. quintana*. Trench fever affected more than 1 million people

TABLE 323-2 CLINICAL MANIFESTATIONS ASSOCIATED WITH *BARTONELLA* SPECIES

CLINICAL MANIFESTATION	*B. BACILLIFORMIS*	*B. QUINTANA*	*B. HENSELAE*	*B. ALSATICA*	OTHERS
Intra-erythrocytic bacteremia	+	+			
Chronic bacteremia	+	+	+		+
Infective endocarditis		+	+	+	+
Verruga peruana	+				
Bacillary angiomatosis		+	+		
Peliosis hepatis			+		
Lymphadenopathy		+	+ (CSD)	+	+
SENLAT with skin lesion			+		
Meningoencephalitis			+		
Uveitis-retinitis		+	+		+

CSD = cat-scratch disease; SENLAT = scalp eschar and neck lymphadenopathy.

during World War I; more recently, *B. quintana* has been recognized in immunocompromised hosts, homeless people, and chronic alcoholics. Clinical manifestations of trench fever may range from asymptomatic infection to severe, life-threatening illness. After an incubation period of 2 to 3 weeks, there is a sudden onset of fever that lasts 1 to 3 days associated with headache, shin pain, and dizziness. Although fatal cases have not been reported, the disease may persist for 4 to 6 weeks and result in prolonged disability. Relapses may occur years later, and in some cases there may be bacteremia with no clinical signs.

CAT-SCRATCH DISEASE

PATHOBIOLOGY

Little is known about the pathogenesis of the long-lasting lymphadenopathy in CSD. Immunopathogenesis is assumed to play an important role in CSD because bacteria have only rarely been isolated from affected lymph nodes. Thus, the disease is usually controlled by the host immune response, and there are few or no viable bacteria when lymph node biopsy specimens are analyzed; they are necrotic by pathology.

CLINICAL MANIFESTATIONS

Typical CSD is the most common manifestation of infection with *B. henselae* and usually presents as a self-limited regional lymphadenitis. Transmission from cat to human occurs directly by a cat scratch or cat bite or possibly by a cat flea or tick bite. A typical papule or pustule may be seen 3 to 10 days after the scratch or bite at the site of inoculation and may last for 1 to 3 weeks. The subsequent lymphadenopathy is localized mainly to the axillary, cervical, or submaxillary nodes that drain the area where the cat scratch occurred. The enlarged lymph node is often painful and tender. Lymphadenopathy sometimes lasts for months, and in a few cases it can persist for as long as 1 to 2 years. In some cases the lymph node may suppurate if it is not drained. Most patients are not febrile during the course of typical CSD. Systemic or severe disease may occur in about 5 to 14% of patients, with most of them suffering severe systemic symptoms due to disseminated infection. *B. alsatica* was recently reported as a cause of lymphadenitis in a woman scratched on the finger while butchering a wild rabbit. Interestingly, it has recently been demonstrated that following exposure to *B. henselae*, patients may develop bacteremia with or without clinical signs of typical CSD, and in patients with valvular lesions, this may result in infective endocarditis. Thus, CSD represents the primary infection of *B. henselae*, and endocarditis may follow in patients with heart valve lesions.

Approximately 10% of patients with CSD have atypical clinical manifestations, including prolonged fever (>2 weeks), malaise, neuroretinitis, encephalitis, erythema nodosum, hepatitis, fatigue, weight loss, and splenomegaly. A recent clinical study showed that musculoskeletal manifestations (myalgia, arthritis, arthralgia, tendinitis, osteomyelitis, neuralgia) were present in more than 10% of patients with CSD, demonstrating that these clinical manifestations are not as rare as might be expected from the cases reported in the past. In this series of 913 patients, myalgia and arthropathy were the most common manifestations, with an incidence of 5.8% and 5.5%, respectively. Moreover, these occurred primarily in adults whose ages ranged from 20 to 59 years. Myalgia had a mean duration of 4 weeks and was often severe. Arthropathy had a mean duration of 5.5 weeks, was more common in female patients older than 20 years, affected large and medium joints (half of those involved being weight-bearing joints), and was associated with symmetrical erythema nodosum early in the course of CSD. These musculoskeletal manifestations are often severe and may evolve into chronic forms that persist for more than a year. Tendinitis, neuralgia, and osteomyelitis are less common, with incidences lower than 1%.

Ocular and Neurologic Manifestations

Parinaud's oculoglandular syndrome is a self-limited conjunctivitis associated with preauricular lymphadenopathy. Other atypical manifestations include neurologic syndromes (meningoencephalitis, meningitis, neuroretinitis). Encephalopathy may occur in 2 to 4% of CSD patients, mainly adolescents and adults. Patients usually have persistent headaches with or without fever and may develop seizures. Acute neurologic disorders range from self-limited nuchal rigidity to pupillary dilatation or aphasia and hemiplegia; they may last for several weeks to months. Neuroretinitis has been associated with CSD in patients experiencing a sudden unilateral loss of visual acuity. The most common picture remains papilledema associated with macular exudates causing stellar retinitis. A few reports have now established that *B. henselae* can be responsible for uveitis, along with *B. grahamii* and *B. quintana*. Patients present with either nongranulomatous or granulomatous uveitis.

Finally, tick-borne *B. henselae* infection has been described, including scalp eschar and neck lymphadenopathy after tick bites in three patients during the colder months in France. *B. henselae* was detected using molecular tools both in skin biopsy (cervical and occipital) and in a *Dermacentor marginatus* tick removed from the scalp of one patient. All three patients had asthenia, but none had alopecia.

ENDOCARDITIS

PATHOBIOLOGY

B. quintana, *B. henselae*, *B. alsatica*, *B. vinsonii* subsp. *berkhoffii*, *B. elizabethae*, and "*Candidatus Bartonella mayotimonensis*" have been associated with blood culture–negative endocarditis, whereas *B. vinsonii* subsp. *arupensis* has been detected in a patient with fever and bacteremia; *B. washoensis* has been identified in one patient with myocarditis; *B. rochalimae* was recently reported in a patient with fever, bacteremia, and splenomegaly; and *B. tamiae* has been isolated in a patient with a febrile illness. Patients with endocarditis usually have preexisting heart valve disease that promotes the development of infective endocarditis and, in some cases, a definite risk factor for infection specifically with *Bartonella*. Endocarditis caused by *Bartonella* species exhibits slight inflammation, with a few inflammatory mononuclear cells and small vegetations; the bacteria are seen extracellularly in dense immunopositive clusters that are mainly included in vegetations and in neutrophil and macrophage cytoplasm.

CLINICAL MANIFESTATIONS

The most commonly identified agents of *Bartonella* endocarditis are *B. quintana*, followed by *B. henselae* and other *Bartonella* species. Patients appear to have chronic, blood culture–negative endocarditis, usually with fever (90%). Echocardiography reveals vegetations (in 90%) that should be removed by surgery in the majority of patients. Infections with *B. henselae* are epidemiologically linked to close contact with cats or cat fleas and previous valvular heart disease, whereas *B. quintana* endocarditis is frequently described in homeless and alcoholic patients with body lice infection and can be observed in patients without previous valve lesions. The onset is usually subacute, with some patients being afebrile at the time of admission. About half the patients have embolic phenomena. Interestingly, there is a north (Europe) to south (North Africa) gradient for the proportion of *Bartonella* endocarditis in humans; thus *Bartonella* is apparently a very common cause of endocarditis in North Africa. Sporadic cases of endocarditis have been also associated with *B. koehlerae*, *B. vinsonii* subsp. *berkhoffii*, *B. vinsonii* subsp. *arupensis*, *B. elizabethae*, *B. alsatica*, and "*Candidatus Bartonella mayotimonensis.*"

VASCULOPROLIFERATIVE DISEASE: VERRUGA PERUANA, BACILLARY ANGIOMATOSIS, AND PELIOSIS HEPATIS

PATHOBIOLOGY

Bartonella species have the ability to cause vasculoproliferative lesions through a process of pathologic angiogenesis resulting in the formation of new capillaries from preexisting ones. These typical vasoproliferations can be expressed as skin lesions called bacillary angiomatosis, which are caused by *B. quintana* and *B. henselae*; there is also a cystic form in the liver and spleen called peliosis hepatis, which is caused only by *B. henselae*. Skin lesions are very similar to those reported for verruga peruana, the chronic form of Carrion's disease. Bacillary angiomatosis is a neovascular proliferation that has been reported most commonly in AIDS patients and involves the skin (Fig. 323-2) and lymph nodes; it occurs less frequently in patients with other causes of immunosuppression and exceptionally in immunocompetent patients. In bacillary angiomatosis, lesions comprise proliferating endothelial cells, bacteria, and mixed infiltrates of macrophages/monocytes and polymorphonuclear neutrophils, leading to chronic inflammation. Bacteria are clustered as aggregates both surrounding and within endothelial cells, indicating that the vascular endothelium represents a target tissue for intra- and extracellular colonization in vivo. Histologically, bacillary angiomatosis is a lobular proliferation of small blood vessels containing endothelial cells and bacteria, usually seen in clusters when stained with Warthin-Starry. As in bacillary angiomatosis, lesions of verruga peruana are characterized by lobular proliferations and atypical endothelial cells forming both relatively solid sheets and small, well-formed vessels with patent lumens. Lesions are typically infiltrated, indicating a chronic inflammatory process.

CLINICAL MANIFESTATIONS

As already noted, bacillary angiomatosis is seen most often in AIDS patients. Cutaneous lesions often arise in crops and can be subcutaneous or dermal nodules with red or purple papules millimeters to centimeters in diameter. When cutaneous lesions are absent, the diagnosis is often difficult and delayed because signs of visceral involvement are usually nonspecific. The potentially systemic nature of bacillary angiomatosis is reflected by the involvement of brain, bone, lymph node, bone marrow, skeletal muscle, conjunctiva, and mucosal surfaces of the gastrointestinal and respiratory tracts. Peliosis hepatis affects solid internal organs, primarily the liver, with reticuloendothelial elements; in the liver it is defined as a vascular proliferation of sinusoidal hepatic capillaries resulting in blood-filled spaces. The spleen, abdominal lymph nodes, and bone marrow may also be involved.

Following acute Oroya fever, patients usually develop angioproliferative cutaneous tumors called verruga peruana after a latent period ranging from weeks to months. The infection is characterized by benign cutaneous vascular lesions that typically consist of round papules that are frequently pruritic and bleeding. The infection is accompanied by malaise and arthralgias. Skin lesions may change over time from miliary to nodular subcutaneous lesions to large mulaire lesions. These large lesions are often engorged with blood and prone to ulceration and bleeding. This eruptive phase clinically resembles Kaposi's sarcoma or bacillary angiomatosis. However, it has a low morbidity, and there are no reports of mortality.

DIAGNOSIS OF *BARTONELLA* INFECTION

Methods used for the diagnosis of *Bartonella* infection include serology, microscopy, culture, molecular amplification of *Bartonella* species genes, direct immunofluorescence, and immunohistochemistry. The usefulness of these techniques may vary according to the disease involved (Table 323-3).

Serologic Tests

Serology remains the most widely used method for the diagnosis of CSD and *Bartonella* endocarditis because culture and isolation are difficult and time-consuming, and molecular methods are not available in all laboratories. There are currently two classic serologic methods for the diagnosis of *Bartonella* infections: enzyme-linked immunosorbent assay (ELISA) and immunofluorescence assay (IFA). By IFA, an immunoglobulin G titer of 1:64 or greater should be considered positive for CSD, whereas patients with endocarditis

FIGURE 323-2. Skin lesion of bacillary angiomatosis.

TABLE 323-3 LABORATORY METHODS FOR THE DIAGNOSIS OF *BARTONELLA* INFECTIONS

CLINICAL MANIFESTATION	SEROLOGY	CULTURE	MOLECULAR METHODS	IMMUNOHISTOCHEMISTRY (WARTHIN-STARRY STAIN)	MICROSCOPY FOR INTRA-ERYTHROCYTIC ORGANISM (GIEMSA OR IF)
Oroya fever	–	+	+	–	+++
Verruga peruana	–	–	+	+	–
Trench fever	+/–	+	+	–	+
Chronic bacteremia	+/–	+++	+	–	–
Infective endocarditis	+++	+++	+++	+++	–
Bacillary angiomatosis	+/–	++	+++	+++	–
Peliosis hepatis	+/–	++	+++	+++	–
Cat-scratch disease	+	–	+++	+/–	+/–
SENLAT with skin lesion	+	+	+++	+	–
Meningoencephalitis	++	–	++	–	–
Uveitis-retinitis	++	–	++	+	–

IF = immunofluorescence; SENLAT = scalp eschar and neck lymphadenopathy.

usually have higher antibody titers (≥1:800). In homeless patients, bacteremia has been associated with serologic tests that were positive for *B. quintana*. However, reported sensitivities of IFA vary considerably, from nearly 100% to less than 30%, depending on the nature of the antigens used and the selected patients. Moreover, owing to cross-reactive antibodies between *Bartonella* species, the diagnosis of *Bartonella* infection at the species level is usually not possible. More sophisticated methods should be used, especially Western blot with cross-adsorption analysis. Western blot is also useful for the differential diagnosis of endocarditis because the profile obtained for endocarditis is specific compared with that for CSD or chronic bacteremia.

Microscopy, Immunofluorescence, and Immunohistochemistry

The diagnosis of Oroya fever is based on examination of a peripheral blood smear stained by Giemsa; the percentage of infected red blood cells is sufficiently high so that bacteria are visible. Similarly, *B. quintana* can be seen within red blood cells using specific monoclonal antibody by immunofluorescence and confocal microscopy (see Fig. 323-1). Microscopic examination after Warthin-Starry silver staining or immunohistochemistry of cardiac valve or skin biopsy is also useful for the detection of *Bartonella* organisms in patients with endocarditis and bacillary angiomatosis.

Culture

Bartonella species can be recovered from the blood of bacteremic patients as well as from cardiac valves, skin and liver biopsies, and, rarely, lymph nodes. Bacteria can be isolated directly from these specimens after plating onto blood agar solid media, blood culture in broth, and cocultivation in endothelial cells. Cultures are usually positive after 2 weeks of incubation, but up to 45 days may be necessary for primary isolation.

Molecular Detection Methods

Direct detection and final identification of *Bartonella* species from blood and tissue specimens, including lymph node, cardiac valve, skin, and liver, can be achieved using polymerase chain reaction (PCR) amplification and sequencing of various housekeeping genes. Real-time PCR with Taqman probes has been added to the panel of molecular techniques for the specific detection of *Bartonella* at the species level from lymph nodes in CSD, directly from cardiac valves in patients with endocarditis, and in patients with bacillary angiomatosis or peliosis hepatis.

Differential Diagnosis

The differential diagnosis of bacillary angiomatosis is Kaposi's sarcoma, but visualization of bacteria in the tissue specimen can help distinguish between these two entities. Trench fever may be confused mainly with typhus group rickettsiosis, relapsing fever, and malaria. CSD may be confused with tularaemia, pyogenic lymphadenitis, mycobacterial infection, and neoplasia.

TREATMENT   **Rx**

Trench Fever

Before the advent of antibiotics, acetylsalicylic acid was the most effective drug for the pain caused by trench fever. However, a randomized clinical trial in homeless persons with episodes of bacteremia demonstrated that the combination of gentamicin and doxycycline is more effective in stopping bacteremia compared with no treatment or the use of β-lactams or doxycycline alone.**1** Because the intra-erythrocytic presence of *B. quintana* decreases antimicrobial efficacy, the duration of treatment is critical in trench fever. Patients with *B. quintana* bacteremia should be treated with gentamicin (3 mg/kg body weight/day IV for 14 days), in combination with doxycycline (200 mg/day PO) for 28 days.

Oroya Fever and Verruga Peruana

In Oroya fever, treatment with penicillin, streptomycin, fluoroquinolones, tetracycline, or erythromycin produces rapid defervescence and disappearance of the organisms from the blood, usually within 24 hours. As an alternative treatment, chloramphenicol can be used alone or in combination with a β-lactam. Treatment with chloramphenicol may also have the advantage of covering commonly associated *Salmonella* species. Patients with Oroya fever should be treated with chloramphenicol (500 mg PO four times a day) for 14 days in combination with another antibiotic (especially a β-lactam compound). Streptomycin (15 to 20 mg/kg/day for 10 days) was the traditional treatment for verruga peruana. However, its use is problematic, especially in children, and rifampin has become the drug of choice for the treatment of eruptive-phase bartonellosis. Failures of rifampin treatment have been reported in verruga

peruana. Finally, ciprofloxacin (500 mg PO twice daily for 7 to 10 days) has been used successfully for the treatment of multiple eruptive-phase lesions in adults and has been proposed as an appropriate alternative. Doxycycline in association with gentamicin may be used to treat the eruptive phase of Carrion's disease.

Cat-Scratch Disease

Typical CSD is a self-limited illness that resolves within 2 to 6 months and usually does not respond to therapy because the bacteria within necrotic lymph nodes are not alive. In cases of long-lasting lymphadenopathy, patients should be reassured that it is benign and will probably subside spontaneously within 2 to 4 months. Management consists of analgesics for pain and prudent follow-up. However, azithromycin (500 mg PO on day 1 and 250 mg PO on days 2 to 5 as single daily doses) is an alternative for patients with large, bulky lymphadenopathy. If lymphadenopathy does not resolve, lymph nodes can surgically be removed. For atypical presentations of CSD, there are no data regarding the benefit of specific antimicrobial therapy for immunocompetent patients. For neuroretinitis, the combination of doxycycline (100 mg PO or IV twice daily) with rifampin (300 mg PO twice daily) seems to promote disease resolution, improve visual acuity, reduce optic disc edema, and decrease disease duration.

Endocarditis

Patients with *Bartonella* endocarditis have a higher death rate and undergo valvular surgery more frequently than patients with endocarditis caused by other pathogens. Patients with suspected (but culture-negative) *Bartonella* endocarditis or proved *B. quintana* endocarditis should be treated with oral doxycycline 100 mg twice a day for 6 weeks in combination with gentamicin 3 mg/kg/day in one intravenous daily dose for 14 days. The American Heart Association consensus on treating infective endocarditis is ceftriaxone plus gentamicin, with or without doxycycline, when *Bartonella* is suspected, and doxycycline plus gentamicin when *Bartonella* endocarditis is confirmed. However, there is direct evidence that patients receiving an aminoglycoside are more likely to fully recover, and those treated with aminoglycosides for at least 14 days are more likely to survive than those receiving a shorter duration of therapy. In the absence of any prospective study for the treatment of *Bartonella* endocarditis, the same regimen as in *B. henselae* and *B. quintana* should be used for endocarditis when another *Bartonella* species has been identified as the causative agent.

Bacillary Angiomatosis and Peliosis Hepatis

Without appropriate therapy, infection spreads systemically and can involve virtually any organ, and the outcome is sometimes fatal. Thus, antibiotic treatment is warranted in all cases of *Bartonella*-associated vasculoproliferative disease. Based on empirical clinical reports, erythromycin remains the treatment of choice and has been used successfully to treat many patients with bacillary angiomatosis. The response to treatment in bacillary angiomatosis can be dramatic in immunocompromised patients, with resolution of palpable subcutaneous lesions within hours. Erythromycin also has an antiangiogenic effect on microvascular endothelial cells that could explain this quick disappearance of lesions. Erythromycin (500 mg four times daily) for 3 months is first-line therapy. Doxycycline (100 mg PO or IV twice daily) is currently proposed as an appropriate alternative. In patients with serious infections, erythromycin or doxycycline can be used in combination with rifampin (300 mg PO twice daily). The duration of therapy is critical. We recommend that treatment be given for at least 3 months for bacillary angiomatosis and 4 months for peliosis hepatis. Peliosis hepatis responds slowly, and hepatic lesions continue to improve after several months of treatment, whereas cutaneous bacillary angiomatosis demonstrates improvement after 4 to 7 days of treatment and resolves after about 1 month of treatment. Relapses of peliosis hepatis and bacillary angiomatosis lesions after antibiotic treatment have been reported frequently, especially in immunocompromised patients with a shorter duration of therapy. Patients who relapse after the recommended treatment should probably be retreated for 4 to 6 months with erythromycin (500 mg PO four times daily) or doxycycline (100 mg PO twice daily), and those with repeated relapses should receive antibiotic therapy as long as they are immunocompromised.

PREVENTION

Because arthropods play an important role in the transmission of feline *Bartonella* species to humans, rigorous arthropod control (Chapter 367) should be recommended by health care workers, particularly when advising immunocompromised individuals on the risks related to pet ownership. Cat fleas live on both cats and dogs and are best controlled by fumigating areas where these animals live.

PROGNOSIS

Mortality in those with Oroya fever was as high as 50% before the antibiotic era but is now limited by the use of antibiotics. Trench fever should be treated with antibiotics to avoid more severe disease, especially in patients with valvulopathy who are at risk of developing endocarditis. CSD usually resolves spontaneously without any treatment in immunocompetent patients. In the case of complications or in immunocompromised patients, antibiotic therapy should be given, and patients usually respond well to treatment. Finally, for vasculoproliferative diseases, antibiotics are usually effective if given for a long time, but cutaneous lesions in verruga peruana may benefit from surgery.

1. Foucault C, Raoult D, Brouqui P. Randomized open trial of gentamicin and doxycycline for eradication of *Bartonella quintana* from blood in patients with chronic bacteremia. *Antimicrob Agents Chemother.* 2003;47:2204-2207.

SUGGESTED READINGS

Gan JJ, Mandell AM, Otis JA, et al. Suspecting optic neuritis, diagnosing *Bartonella* cat scratch disease. *Arch Neurol.* 2011;68:122-126. *Cat-scratch disease should be in the differential diagnosis for patients with blurred vision and headache, even in the absence of fever and lymphadenopathy.*

Guptill L. Bartonellosis. *Vet Microbiol.* 2010;140:347-359. *Public health implications of animal bartonellosis.*

Kaiser PO, Riess T, O'Rourke F, et al. *Bartonella* spp: throwing light on uncommon human infections. *Int J Med Microbiol.* 2011;301:7-15. *Review of infections from asymptomatic to Oroya fever.*

Maguina C, Guerra H, Ventosilla P. Bartonellosis. *Clin Dermatol.* 2009;27:271-280. *Reviews the distinct clinical syndromes of Carrion's disease, trench fever, cat-scratch disease, bacillary angiomatosis, and peliosis hepatis.*

Piérard-Franchimont C, Quatresooz P, Piérard GE. Skin diseases associated with *Bartonella* infection: facts and controversies. *Clin Dermatol.* 2010;28:483-488. *Review.*

FIGURE 324-1. Typical primary lesion of granuloma inguinale. (Reproduced with permission from Herpes-Coldsores.com. http://www.herpes-coldsores.com/std/lymphogranuloma_pictures.htm.)

324

GRANULOMA INGUINALE (DONOVANOSIS)

EDWARD W. HOOK III

DEFINITION

Granuloma inguinale, also known as donovanosis, is a slowly progressive ulcerative disease that involves principally the skin and subcutaneous tissues of the genital, inguinal, and anal regions.

The Pathogen

The causative organism is *Klebsiella granulomatis* (formerly *Calymmatobacterium granulomatis*), a facultative intracellular parasite. The organism is challenging to cultivate but can be grown in yolk sacs, and successful cell culture has been reported from South Africa and Australia. Successful culture, in turn, has permitted the development of polymerase chain reaction (PCR) assays for research purposes.

EPIDEMIOLOGY

The organism is primarily transmitted sexually, but it can probably be transmitted by nonsexual contact as well. Transmission efficiency is relatively low, and multiple sexual contacts with an infected partner seem to be necessary for the transmission of infection. The disease is uncommon in the United States, with fewer than 50 recorded cases annually. Historically, however, it is more common in other areas of the world, including India, Papua New Guinea, southern Africa, and parts of Australia. Even in these endemic areas, the limited data available suggest that the disease may be becoming less common.

CLINICAL MANIFESTATIONS

The initial lesion usually appears as a subcutaneous nodule that erodes through the surface and develops into a beefy, elevated granulomatous lesion (Fig. 324-1). The lesion is painless and unassociated with systemic symptoms. Lesion exudate is often described as foul smelling. Secondary bacterial infection may cause a necrotic, painful, ulcerative lesion that may be rapidly

destructive. A cicatricial form may also occur, with a depigmented elevated area of keloid-like scar containing scattered islands of granulomatous tissue. Genital lesions are commonly associated with pseudobuboes in the inguinal region; these swellings are usually not due to involvement of the inguinal lymph nodes but rather to granulomatous involvement of subcutaneous tissue. Metastatic infection of bones or viscera is occasionally seen. Clinical experience suggests that secondary carcinomas may be a rare complication of granuloma inguinale.

DIAGNOSIS

The diagnosis is made by demonstrating intracellular Donovan's bodies in histiocytes or other mononuclear cells from lesion scrapings or biopsy samples. Wright stain and Giemsa stain of fresh impression smears or unfixed biopsy specimens usually demonstrate the bacilli relatively easily, although multiple biopsies may be necessary in chronic cases. Histologic examination of biopsy specimens shows mononuclear cells with some infiltration by polymorphonuclear leukocytes but no giant cells. In infected lesions, *K. granulomatis* is found primarily in histiocytes or other mononuclear cells. Cell culture and PCR methods are primarily research tools. No serologic test is clinically available.

Differential Diagnosis

The differential diagnosis includes squamous cell carcinoma, chancroid (Chapter 309), lymphogranuloma venereum (Chapter 326), syphilis (Chapter 327), and other ulcerative granulomatous diseases. In the absence of therapy, patients may not present until lesions have been present for months, long after the lesions of syphilis and other ulcerative sexually transmitted diseases have resolved. Chancroid is usually differentiated by its irregular undermined borders, which are not seen in typical cases of granuloma inguinale. Dark-field examination and serologic tests should help distinguish syphilis. Biopsy of lesions may be necessary to distinguish granuloma inguinale from certain tumors.

TREATMENT

There are no recent clinical trials of therapy for granuloma inguinale. Recommended treatment consists of doxycycline 100 mg twice daily. Azithromycin 1.0 g weekly, ciprofloxacin 750 mg twice daily, or erythromycin base 500 mg four times daily, and one double-strength trimethoprim-sulfamethoxazole tablet twice daily, are all recommended as alternative therapies. An aminoglycoside (e.g., gentamicin 1 mg/kg intravenously every 8 hours) may be added if these regimens do not result in clinical improvement within a few days. Treatment should be administered for at least 3 weeks and until lesions are completely healed. Patients should be monitored for at least several weeks after treatment is discontinued because of the possibility of relapse. Although the risk of communicability appears to be low, sexual contacts should also be examined; at present, treatment of contacts is not indicated in the absence of clinically evident disease.

SUGGESTED READINGS

Belda W Jr, Velho PE, Arnone M, et al. Donovanosis treated with thiamphenicol. *Braz J Infect Dis.* 2007:11:388-389. *A commonly successful treatment in Brazil.*

O'Farrell N, Moi H; IUSTI/WHO European STD guidelines Editorial Board. European guideline for the management of donovanosis. 2010. *Int J STD AIDS.* 2010;21:609-610. *Consensus guidelines including diagnosis by stained tissue smears or PCR and treatment with azithromycin (1 g weekly) until complete healing is achieved.*

Velho PE, de Souza EM, Belda W Jr. Donovanosis. *Braz J Infect Dis.* 2008;12:521-525. *Comprehensive review of the microbiology, epidemiology, clinical manifestations, and management of granuloma inguinale.*

325

MYCOPLASMA INFECTIONS

STEPHEN G. BAUM

DEFINITION

Mycoplasma organisms of the class Mollicutes are ubiquitous as pathogens and colonizing agents in the plant, animal, and insect kingdoms. They represent the smallest known free-living forms, but because they have fastidious growth requirements, they are difficult to culture. However, the presence of several species of *Mycoplasma* as commensals in animals and on human oral and genital mucosa frequently resulted in contamination of cell cultures. Such contamination led to the false implication of mycoplasmas as causative agents in many human diseases, both trivial and life-threatening. Of the human diseases proved to be due to mycoplasmas, pneumonia caused by *Mycoplasma pneumoniae* is by far the most clinically important. This infection constitutes a significant proportion of cases previously classified as "atypical pneumonia," a nonspecific term for patchy pneumonias that generally do not respond to β-lactam antibiotics and have etiologic agents that are not easily cultured or visible on Gram stain. The term *atypical pneumonia* persists despite our increasing ability to identify specific etiologic agents such as viruses, *Legionella*, and *Chlamydophila*. Other proven *Mycoplasma* infections include those in the urogenital tract caused by *Ureaplasma* species, *Mycoplasma hominis*, and *Mycoplasma genitalium*; wound infections caused by *M. hominis*; and overwhelming systemic infection in immunocompromised patients caused by *Mycoplasma fermentans* (*incognitus* strain).

The Pathogen

Mycoplasmas are short rods (10 × 200 nm) that have no cell wall and are bounded by a sterol-containing membrane; thus, they are unaffected by cell wall–inhibiting antimicrobials such as β-lactams. In tissue culture, mycoplasmas are intracellular, but in vivo, infection is primarily extracellular and affects epithelial cells and their organelles, such as cilia. Attachment to respiratory epithelium is by way of terminal adhesin proteins. Mycoplasmas are active in stimulating several components of the immune system. They can act as polyclonal T-cell and B-cell activators and can cause capping of lymphocytes.

EPIDEMIOLOGY

M. pneumoniae infection is spread person to person by respiratory droplets produced by coughing. Relatively close association with the index case appears to be required. The disease is usually introduced into families by a young child; in some studies, most of the infected adults were the parents of young children. As opposed to most viral respiratory infections, which manifest 1 to 3 days after infection, *Mycoplasma* has an incubation period of 2 to 3 weeks. Therefore, a careful history showing several weeks between cases within a family may be an important clue to the mycoplasmal etiology. Organisms can be cultured from the sputum of infected individuals for weeks to months after clinically efficacious treatment, and it is unclear how the treatment of an index case affects subsequent transmission to family members.

Most cases of *Mycoplasma* respiratory infection occur singly or as family outbreaks. However, in closed populations, such as military recruit camps and boarding schools, *Mycoplasma* can cause mini-epidemics and may be responsible for 25 to 75% of cases of pneumonia in such settings. Serologically based epidemiologic studies have documented the high incidence of *Mycoplasma* respiratory infection throughout the world. In the United States, it is estimated that each year at least one case of *Mycoplasma* pneumonia occurs for every 1000 persons, or more than 2 million cases annually. The incidence of *Mycoplasma* nonpneumonic respiratory infection may be 10 to 20 times greater. The highest attack rates are in individuals 5 to 20 years old, but *M. pneumoniae* infection can occur at any age and may cause particularly severe disease in neonates.

As opposed to viral respiratory infections that peak in winter in temperate climates, a few studies have reported a peak incidence of *M. pneumoniae* outbreaks in the fall. Most surveys, however, show little or no seasonal predominance in sporadic cases. There is an age-related relationship of upper versus lower respiratory tract infection caused by *M. pneumoniae*. In children younger than 3 years, primarily upper respiratory tract infection develops, whereas in those 5 to 20 years old, bronchitis and pneumonia tend to occur. In older adults, pneumonia predominates.

The prevalence and incidence of clinical urogenital disease caused by *Ureaplasma urealyticum*, *Ureaplasma parvum*, *M. hominis*, and *M. genitalium* are much less well documented (Table 325-1). These organisms are rarely cultured outside the realm of clinical studies, and they exist as clinically inapparent commensals of the genitourinary tract. Diseases attributed to *Ureaplasma* species include urinary tract infection with and without calculus formation. The organism has been implicated as a cause of low birthweight in neonates. *M. hominis* is a common genitourinary and oral commensal as well and has been documented as a cause of endometritis and postpartum fever.

M. hominis has also caused sternal wound infection after cardiothoracic surgery and has been implicated in arthritis in immunocompromised patients. *Mycoplasma salivarium* may be involved in periodontal disease, and *M. genitalium* is implicated in some cases of nongonococcal urethritis and vaginitis. *M. fermentans*, *incognitus* strain, was identified about 3 decades ago as an infectious agent in immunocompromised patients, in whom it causes overwhelming multisystem involvement.

PATHOBIOLOGY

Because of the low fatality of most *Mycoplasma* infections, there is little human pathologic material. Inoculation onto animal tracheal organ cultures is followed by ciliary damage and desquamation of surface epithelium. This latter effect is probably responsible for the hacking cough in *Mycoplasma* respiratory infection.

Several characteristics of *M. pneumoniae* probably play a direct role in the respiratory pathogenicity of this organism. The first is the affinity of *M. pneumoniae* for respiratory epithelial cells. Attachment appears to be between a terminal organelle at one end of the filamentous organism and a sialated glycoprotein (I-FI) on the surface of both respiratory epithelium and erythrocytes that acts as a receptor. The mycoplasmal terminal adhesin

TABLE 325-1   SITES AND INFECTIONS RELATED TO HUMAN MYCOPLASMAS

SUBGROUP	SITES OF ISOLATION	DISEASES	OCCURRENCE
M. hominis	GU tract (F > M)	Cervicitis, vaginitis, ?prostatitis	Common
	Conjunctivae (neonate)	Conjunctivitis	
	Blood (peripartum)	Peripartum sepsis	
	Surgical wounds, joints	Sternotomy infection, arthritis	
M. orale	Oropharynx	?	Common
M. pneumoniae	Respiratory tract	URI, pneumonia	Common
M. salivarium	Oropharynx, gingiva	?Periodontal disease	Common
M. fermentans	GU tract, blood, tissues	Multisystem disease in AIDS	Uncommon
M. genitalium	GU tract	Urethritis, cervicitis, PID	Uncommon
Ureaplasma spp	GU tract	Urethritis, upper GU infection	Common

AIDS = acquired immunodeficiency syndrome; F = female; GU = genitourinary; M = male; PID=pelvic inflammatory disease; URI = upper respiratory tract infection.

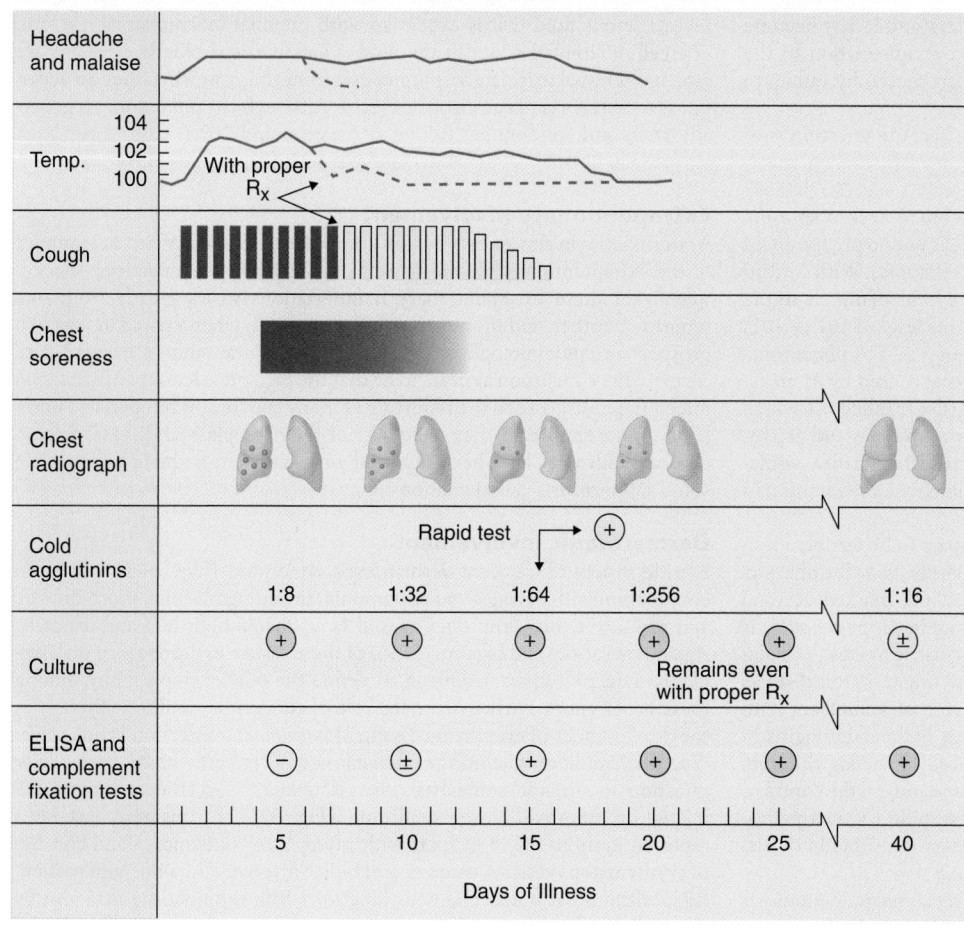

FIGURE 325-1. Major clinical and laboratory manifestations of mycoplasmal pneumonia. ELISA = enzyme-linked immunosorbent assay. (Adapted from Baum SG. Mycoplasmal infections. In: Wyngaarden JB, Smith LH Jr, eds. *Cecil Textbook of Medicine,* 17th ed. Philadelphia: Saunders; 1985:1506.)

proteins (P1, P30, P116, and HMW1-3) have been purified, and adherence-deficient mutants are avirulent. *M. pneumoniae* attaches to ciliated epithelial cells at the base of cilia and appears to produce most of its physiologic and cytolytic changes while remaining extracellular. Hydrogen peroxide produced by *M. pneumoniae* (the only human mycoplasma to do so) may be responsible for some in vivo cell damage, as it is for the hemolysis seen when the organisms are grown on blood agar plates. *Mycoplasma* infection activates T and B cells and induces many pro-inflammatory and anti-inflammatory cytokines and chemokines that may play a role in inflammation-related cell destruction.

In the course of *M. pneumoniae* infection, some patients produce cold agglutinins. These oligoclonal M-type immunoglobulins (IgM) cross-react with I antigens, one of the blood group antigens common to almost all mature human erythrocytes, and high titers may cause hemolysis (presumably as a result of complement-activated, Coombs-positive erythrocyte destruction) and lead to some of the complications described in the Clinical Manifestations section. Like other IgM antibodies, the *Mycoplasma*-induced cold agglutinins (Chapter 163) develop early in the disease (7 to 10 days) and are often present by the time the patient seeks medical attention. The titer of these agglutinins peaks at 2 to 3 weeks, and they persist for 2 to 3 months (Fig. 325-1).

Several theories about the factors triggering the formation of cold agglutinins in *Mycoplasma* pneumonia have been proposed. One is that the organism alters the I antigen such that it becomes antigenic to the patient. The hydrogen peroxide elaborated by *M. pneumoniae* could be responsible for this alteration. One study indicated that the I antigen in a sialated state may serve as a receptor for *M. pneumoniae* and that the cold agglutinins are directed at the modified receptor. Other studies indicate that the cold agglutinins are directed at mycoplasmal substructures themselves and merely cross-react with the I antigen (altered or native) on red cells. Given their apparent target, these antibodies could either contribute to cytolysis and exacerbate infection or interfere with cell-to-cell spread by blocking or disrupting the cell receptor for the mycoplasma. High titers of cold agglutinins have also been associated with hemolysis, presumably as a result of the activation of complement-mediated erythrocyte destruction (Chapter 163). Although clinically significant

hemolysis is uncommon, subclinical levels of red cell destruction are common.

Sickle cell disease, sickle-related hemoglobinopathies, and hypogammaglobulinemia predispose to increased severity and mortality. Therefore, some of the available pathologic data may be influenced by the pathophysiology of these underlying conditions. Deaths have occurred in patients with diffuse pneumonia, acute respiratory distress syndrome, thromboembolism, and disseminated intravascular coagulation.

In nonfatal cases in which lung biopsy was performed, the inflammatory process involved primarily the trachea, bronchioles, and peribronchial tissue. The lumen of the respiratory tree was filled with a purulent exudate rich in polymorphonuclear leukocytes. The lining of the bronchial and bronchiolar walls showed metaplastic cells, and the walls themselves were infiltrated with monocytic elements, especially plasma cells. There was widening of the peribronchial septa and hyperplasia of type II pneumocytes.

CLINICAL MANIFESTATIONS

In view of the very high incidence of *Mycoplasma* respiratory infection when studied epidemiologically in large populations, versus the rarity of individual sporadic diagnoses, it appears that a specific, confirmed diagnosis of this entity is seldom accomplished in routine clinical practice. There are probably four reasons for this. The first is that *Mycoplasma* pneumonia is usually self-limited and rarely fatal. This fact dampens the zeal to establish the cause of infection. Second, mycoplasmas are relatively fastidious and slow growing; therefore, culture results, if obtained at all, often return after the patient is well. Third, *M. pneumoniae* responds to the empirical antimicrobial therapy suggested for community-acquired pneumonia. Finally, knowledge of the epidemiology and clinical manifestations of infection is deficient, so the diagnosis is often not considered outside the classic age group.

Respiratory Infection

The majority of *M. pneumoniae* infections involve only the upper respiratory tract. After a 2- to 3-week incubation period, the disease has an insidious onset consisting of fever, malaise, headache, and cough (see Fig. 325-1). Cough is the clinical hallmark of *M. pneumoniae* infection. The frequency and severity of the cough increase over the next 1 to 2 days, and it may become debilitating. The gradual onset of symptoms is in contradistinction to the often fulminant manifestation of respiratory infection caused by influenza virus or adenovirus.

In 5 to 10% of patients, depending somewhat on age, the infection progresses to tracheobronchitis or pneumonia. In these cases, the original manifestations persist, and the cough becomes more severe. It is usually relatively nonproductive but may yield white or occasionally blood-flecked sputum. Gram staining of this sputum reveals inflammatory cells but no predominant bacterial species (part of the definition of atypical pneumonia). With continued cough, parasternal chest soreness may develop as a result of muscle strain, but true pleuritic pain is unusual. Fever is usually at the level of 101 to 102° F and may be associated with chilly sensations. As opposed to pneumonia caused by *Streptococcus pneumoniae* (Chapter 297), that caused by *M. pneumoniae* rarely produces true shaking chills. In comparison to influenza, which can also manifest as an atypical pneumonia syndrome, myalgias and gastrointestinal complaints of nausea and vomiting are unusual. Diarrhea, sometimes a concomitant of adenoviral or *Legionella* pneumonia, is uncommon in *Mycoplasma* infection.

On physical examination, the patient does not appear to be terribly ill. In fact, this disease is the paradigm of the term *walking pneumonia*. The pharynx may be injected and erythematous, usually without the marked cervical adenopathy seen with group A streptococcal pharyngitis. *M. pneumoniae* is not a common cause of isolated pharyngitis in the pediatric or adult population. Much has been made of the finding of bullous myringitis in this disease. Although this abnormality was present in about 20% of volunteers with experimentally induced *M. pneumoniae* infection, true bullous myringitis in naturally occurring *Mycoplasma* disease is rare. In a study involving children, otitis was rarely associated with isolation of *Mycoplasma* and, on the contrary, was often associated with bacterial and viral upper respiratory tract pathogens. Thus, the absence of myringitis, bullous or otherwise, should not dissuade one from a diagnosis of *Mycoplasma* pneumonia.

Examination of the chest in patients with *Mycoplasma* pneumonia is often unrevealing, even in those with severe, productive cough. There may be no auscultative or percussive findings, or only minimal rales may be present. The disparity between physical findings and radiographic evidence of pneumonia in this condition may be the greatest of any of the atypical pneumonia syndromes (Fig. 325-2). Although wheezing can occur in this disease, in one study of asthmatic patients, the presence of wheezing had a negative correlation with isolation of *M. pneumoniae* compared with isolation of viral respiratory pathogens such as respiratory syncytial virus (Chapter 370). *M. pneumoniae* does not seem to be a common pathogen in patients with preexisting chronic obstructive lung disease, either. Bacterial superinfection after *M. pneumoniae* respiratory infection is rare. The radiographic finding of interstitial or patchy alveolar pneumonia does not allow differentiation from any of the other causes of the atypical pneumonia syndrome.

Pleural effusion (usually small) occurs in 5 to 20% of patients with *M. pneumoniae* infection. This low incidence of pleural inflammation is consistent with the rarity of pleuritic pain. If effusion is present, thoracentesis reveals serous fluid that is exudative, with minimal inflammatory reaction. The cell differential count in the fluid is variable, and bloody effusions are rare. It is unusual to isolate *M. pneumoniae* from effusions when they do occur, but several reports of such isolation exist. Although the pneumonia is generally mild and self-limited, fulminant, severe, and lethal cases have been reported in normal young adults and may be underdiagnosed.

Extrapulmonary Involvement

Abnormalities in almost every organ system have been described as examples of the extrapulmonary manifestations of *M. pneumoniae* infection. The frequency of these extrapulmonary manifestations varies greatly from one report to another, and they are much less common when viewed as part of a prospective epidemiologic study rather than as the sum of isolated case reports. The conclusion appears to be that the high prevalence of *Mycoplasma* infection predisposes to the reporting of many concurrent but perhaps unrelated events as though they were part of the mycoplasmal disease. Several clinical syndromes have been reported with sufficient frequency to provide some support for a causal relationship.

Dermatologic Involvement

A wide variety of transient dermatologic conditions have been reported in conjunction with *Mycoplasma* pneumonia, including macular, morbilliform, and papulovesicular eruptions, as well as erythema nodosum and urticaria. Again, the variety and high incidence of these rashes in the absence of *Mycoplasma* infection make it difficult to define the relationships, if any, among these occurrences. Furthermore, the role of concurrent antibiotic therapy in the development of exanthems during *M. pneumoniae* infection is unknown. One skin condition that occurs often enough in concert with *M. pneumoniae* infection to provide some basis for relatedness is erythema multiforme majus, or Stevens-Johnson syndrome (Fig. 325-3). This rash has been reported in up to 7% of patients with *Mycoplasma* pneumonia and consists of erythematous vesicles, plaques, and bullae involving the skin, with particular localization at mucocutaneous junctions. The conjunctivae may also be involved, as well as organs of the gastrointestinal and genitourinary tracts and the joints. Stevens-Johnson syndrome has been associated with isolated cases of many other infections, including some that can manifest as atypical pneumonia syndrome, such as legionnaires' pneumonia, adenovirus respiratory-conjunctivitis syndrome, and influenza B infection. However, the association with *M. pneumoniae* infection is by far the most common. Stevens-Johnson syndrome tends to occur in younger patients with *Mycoplasma* pneumonia and has a definite male preponderance (2:1 to 4:1).

The pathogenesis of Stevens-Johnson syndrome is unclear. It has long been supposed that immunity plays a major role, but several reports have noted the culture of *M. pneumoniae* from the lesions. The relationship to the level of cold agglutinins in this disease is variable. It has been suggested that the development of Stevens-Johnson syndrome may be the result of augmented sensitivity to antibiotics in the presence of *M. pneumoniae* infection, but erythema multiforme majus develops in some patients in the absence of previous or concurrent antibiotic therapy. Most patients clear the lesions in 1 to 2 weeks without scarring unless impetiginization supervenes.

FIGURE 325-2. Chest radiograph showing moderate interstitial pneumonia due to *Mycoplasma pneumoniae* infection in a patient with a paucity of findings on chest auscultation.

FIGURE 325-3. Stevens-Johnson syndrome in a child with *Mycoplasma* pneumonia. (From Baum SG. *Mycoplasma pneumoniae* and atypical pneumonia. In: Mandell GL, Bennett JE, Dolin R, eds. *Mandell, Douglas, and Bennett's Principles and Practice of Infectious Diseases*, 6th ed. Philadelphia: Churchill Livingstone; 2005:2274.)

Raynaud's syndrome (Chapter 80), a transient, reversible vasospasm of the digits that develops on exposure to cold, is not technically a dermatologic syndrome; however, it manifests in the skin. This phenomenon occurs in many people, usually women, without any association with infection. It has been reported in patients with acute *Mycoplasma* pneumonia, regardless of whether they exhibited the syndrome before infection. Although the pathophysiology of this condition in *M. pneumoniae* infection is unclear, it may be related to the in vivo action of cold agglutinins (see Diagnosis, later). Other vascular complications reported in *M. pneumoniae* infection include internal carotid artery occlusion and cerebral infarction.

Cardiac Complications

Cardiac abnormalities are among the most commonly reported extrapulmonary manifestations of *M. pneumoniae* infection. Signs and symptoms suggesting involvement of the heart are arrhythmia, congestive failure, chest pain, and electrocardiographic abnormalities, particularly conduction defects. Although cardiac abnormalities have been reported in as many as 10% of cases of *M. pneumoniae* infection, other reports indicate a much lower prevalence. Cardiac complications are more common with increasing age. They prolong the illness but rarely lead to death. The mechanism of heart damage is unknown, but *M. pneumoniae* has been isolated from the pericardial fluid of at least one patient.

Neurologic Complications

There are increasing reports of neurologic complications of *Mycoplasma* infection, but proof of the cause of central nervous system involvement is somewhat tenuous. Aseptic meningitis and meningoencephalitis, transverse myelitis, brain stem dysfunction, Guillain-Barré syndrome, and peripheral neuropathy have all been reported. In the aggregate, these central nervous system manifestations occur in no more than 1 per 1000 patients. Cerebrospinal fluid findings in these cases are variable, but the cellular response is usually minimal, with slightly elevated protein and normal to slightly depressed glucose. Most often, the diagnosis of *Mycoplasma*-related central nervous system involvement is based on the exclusion of other causes, the presence of an antecedent or intercurrent respiratory illness, and a rise in antibody titer to *M. pneumoniae* in serum. Occasionally, *Mycoplasma*-specific antibodies have been demonstrated in cerebrospinal fluid, but these titers have paralleled serum antibody titers. Neurologic complications are usually reversible; however, mortality in patients with central nervous system involvement is higher than in those without such involvement. Although *M. pneumoniae* has been isolated from a few of these patients, polymerase chain reaction (PCR) failed to detect *M. pneumoniae* DNA in the cerebrospinal fluid of 11 patients deemed to have *M. pneumoniae*–related central nervous system disease on serologic grounds. Therefore, immune mechanisms of neural damage have been suggested. Some mycoplasmas elaborate a neurotoxin, but this has not been described for *M. pneumoniae*.

Musculoskeletal, Renal, and Hematopoietic Complications

Polyarthralgias are common in *Mycoplasma* pneumonia, but monoarticular or migratory arthritis is rare. Immune mechanisms have been postulated, but there have been a few reports of the isolation of *M. pneumoniae* from joint fluid. Several of the cases of frank arthritis were reported in patients with hypogammaglobulinemia. Nonhuman mycoplasmas probably cause arthropathy in several animal species, and *M. hominis* has been associated with human arthritis. Rhabdomyolysis has also been reported.

Renal complications associated with immune complex deposition and high-titer cold agglutinins have been reported. There are several case reports of *M. pneumoniae*–associated aplastic anemia.

Conditions Leading to Increased Susceptibility

Several reports have emphasized the unusual severity of *M. pneumoniae* infection in patients with sickle cell disease or sickle-related hemoglobinopathies (Chapter 166). Large pleural effusions and marked respiratory distress may develop in these patients. Functional asplenia and its attendant opsonization deficiencies may contribute to overwhelming infection with *M. pneumoniae*, as they do with *S. pneumoniae* infection. Some patients with sickle cell disease and *M. pneumoniae* infection in whom extremely high cold agglutinin titers develop may experience digital necrosis, as they do with *S. pneumoniae*. A hypothesis about the pathogenesis is provided in the discussion on cold agglutinins in the Diagnosis section. Children with immunodeficiency syndromes have been the subjects of case reports of *M. pneumoniae* infection. Because *Mycoplasma* infections are so common in normal children, the

contribution of immunodeficiency is unclear. *M. pneumoniae* is not a very common opportunistic agent in patients with acquired immunodeficiency syndrome (AIDS), but *M. fermentans* (*incognitus* strain) has been identified in these patients. Unusually severe but nonlethal *M. pneumoniae* infection has also been reported in children with Down syndrome.

DIAGNOSIS

The diagnosis of *Mycoplasma* pneumonia is made primarily on clinical grounds. The organism can be grown in cell-free media, but most hospital diagnostic laboratories are not prepared to culture mycoplasmas. Because of this, there is considerable interest in developing rapid diagnostic tests with high sensitivity and specificity. These assays fall into three categories: detection of *M. pneumoniae*–specific immunoglobulins in serum, and detection of *M. pneumoniae*–specific antigens or nucleotide sequences directly in clinical specimens. Diagnostically, the most useful *M. pneumoniae*–specific immunoglobulin to detect is IgM because it is most likely to indicate recent infection. Enzyme-linked immunoassays have been developed to detect IgM and IgG directed against *M. pneumoniae*. When used in patients with positive assays for complement-fixing antibodies, the enzyme immunoassay had a specificity of more than 99% and a sensitivity of 98%. Specificity was retained, but sensitivity dropped to only 46% when IgG alone was the target. Variations on this theme detect IgM antibodies directed at specific *M. pneumoniae* antigens. The tests are simple to perform and have high sensitivity and specificity, but because all these tests are designed to detect IgM antibody, they may be negative early in the course of infection (<7 to 10 days). Therefore, they do not provide the desired confirmation early enough to guide initial therapy.

Detection of *M. pneumoniae* antigens directly in sputum specimens has been accomplished with the use of an antigen-capture, indirect enzyme immunoassay. The specificity of the assay was high, the reagents reacting only with *M. pneumoniae* and *M. genitalium*. Sensitivity was also relatively high (91%) when the assay was used on sputum and nasopharyngeal aspirates from patients who were shown by culture or serologically to have *M. pneumoniae* infection.

The high sensitivity and specificity of real-time PCR performed on sputum, nasopharyngeal aspirate, or throat swab material suggest that this test could serve as a specific and rapid diagnostic method. Detection of *M. pneumoniae*–specific nucleotide sequences directly in clinical material has been accomplished with the use of tests developed locally or by large reference laboratories. These tests, which can be completed in a few hours, detect either *M. pneumoniae* DNA (PCR) or ribosomal RNA (reverse transcriptase nucleic acid amplification). When compared with PCR as the "gold standard" of proven infection, very few of the available antibody assays have acceptable sensitivity and specificity. Although the nucleic acid probe assays show excellent specificity, they fail to detect infection in some antibody-positive patients, and their sensitivity varies considerably, depending on the source of the specimen tested: highest for sputum, but lower for nasopharyngeal aspirate or throat swab material. This latter point is very important when evaluating comparative studies, many of which use different specimen sources for their assays.

In the course of *M. pneumoniae* infection, several classes of antibody are produced. Some of these fulfill the desired role of antibody production—neutralization of the agent—and others appear to be autoantibodies. The latter include agglutinins to lung, brain, cardiolipins, and smooth muscle. The best studied of these autoagglutinins are the cold isohemagglutinins. These agglutinins were found to be capable of clumping erythrocytes at 4° C. Agglutination was reversible by warming the serum-erythrocyte mixture to 37° C and, unlike hemagglutination by myxoviruses and paramyxoviruses, was repeatable with the same sample, indicating that receptor-destroying enzyme (neuraminidase) plays no role in the dissociation at 37° C.

The cold agglutinin phenomenon, when positive, occurs early, but it is neither very sensitive nor specific. Other diseases that can give rise to cold agglutinins are mononucleosis caused by Epstein-Barr virus (anti-i), cytomegalovirus (anti-I), some other viral diseases, and lymphoma. A titer of 1:32 or greater is highly suggestive of infection with *M. pneumoniae*.

When performed in a laboratory, the results of this test will not be available for at least a day and in some cases a week, but a rapid version can be done at the bedside. In this test, 1 mL of the patient's blood is drawn into a tube containing anticoagulant. The type of tube used to collect specimens for prothrombin determination is preferred. Before cooling, examination shows a smooth coating of the tube by red cells. The blood is cooled to 4° C by placing it on liquid ice or in a standard refrigerator. After several minutes, the tube is examined for the presence of macroscopic erythrocyte agglutination.

The tube is then rewarmed to 37° C in an incubator or by exposure to body heat and reexamined. The agglutination should dissociate at 37° C, and the appearance should be as it was before cooling. This temperature-associated agglutination and dissociation can be repeated many times on the same sample. A positive result in the bedside test correlates with a laboratory titer of 1:64 or greater and is therefore less sensitive than the laboratory test. It can be accomplished in minutes, however, and if positive, it is highly suggestive of *Mycoplasma*-related cold agglutination. The presence of cold agglutinins can also artifactually give rise to macrocytic indices secondary to in vitro clumping of erythrocytes, as measured by the Coulter counter method. In this case, the red cell distribution width would be high, indicative of heterogeneity in measured red cell size.

Finally, although PCR should become the gold standard for diagnosis because of its high sensitivity and specificity and the rapidity with which results can be obtained, the test is not available or is rarely ordered, even in microbiology laboratories serving major children's hospitals. There is no commercially available kit for this test, and specimens are generally sent out to large diagnostic laboratories. Even when a home-grown test is available on-site, the low frequency of requests forces only periodic testing of bundled specimens. Both these situations undermine the inherent timeliness of PCR diagnostic results.

TREATMENT

Despite the number and variety of tests for the rapid diagnosis of *M. pneumoniae* infection, most cases are encountered in the ambulatory setting, and the institution of antimicrobial therapy is empirical and based on clinical recognition of the syndrome.

Antimicrobial therapy is not necessary for mycoplasmal upper respiratory tract infection, and the mycoplasmal cause of this syndrome most often goes undiagnosed. The pneumonia caused by *Mycoplasma* is self-limited and not life-threatening in most cases. However, treatment with effective antimicrobials can shorten the duration of illness and, by reducing cough and the number of organisms per unit volume of sputum, may reduce the spread of infection to contacts.

As would be predicted by the lack of a cell wall, all mycoplasmas, including *M. pneumoniae,* are unaffected by β-lactam antibiotics such as the penicillins and cephalosporins. Aminoglycosides are effective in vitro but have not been evaluated for efficacy in vivo. The mainstays of treatment of *M. pneumoniae* respiratory tract infection are macrolides and tetracyclines. Use of either drug class significantly shortens the duration of illness. The radiographic findings may take a week or longer to resolve, even with appropriate therapy (see Fig. 325-1), and organisms may continue to be cultured from sputum for several weeks after a complete course of clinically effective treatment. This may be a result of the fact that although *M. pneumoniae* causes respiratory disease as an extracellular parasite, it has the capacity to reside intracellularly as well, thus making it difficult to eradicate the organism in vivo as opposed to cell cultures. The effect of therapy on extrapulmonary manifestations is unknown. *M. hominis* is not sensitive to erythromycin.

Although the tetracyclines are very active against *M. pneumoniae,* their use is precluded in young children because of adverse effects on developing teeth and bones. Erythromycin is poorly tolerated by many people because of its gastrointestinal side effects, including nausea, vomiting, abdominal pain, and diarrhea. Erythromycin also raises theophylline levels, a consideration in the few asthmatic patients who may still be taking this drug.

Because of the adverse effects of erythromycin and tetracycline, there is considerable interest in the antimycoplasmal efficacy of other agents. Doxycycline is somewhat better tolerated than tetracycline and can be administered in two daily doses rather than three. In vitro, doxycycline is as effective as tetracycline against *M. pneumoniae,* but it is contraindicated in young children.

Several other classes of antimicrobials have significant in vitro and in vivo activity against *M. pneumoniae* and other *Mycoplasma* species, including the fluoroquinolones, broad-spectrum macrolides (azithromycin, clarithromycin), and members of the macrolide-lincomycin-streptogramin-ketolide (MLSK) class of antimicrobials. There are no good data on the optimal duration of therapy needed to minimize carriage and relapse with these agents.

The macrolides are more active in vitro than the tetracyclines are. Fluoroquinolones have adequate activity for the treatment of these infections. They are more active than the tetracyclines but are at least 100 times less active than the macrolides. The streptogramins are also less active than the macrolides but more active than the tetracyclines. There is a significant cost differential in the use of these drugs. The newer macrolides and quinolones are 50 to 60 times more expensive than the tetracyclines and 6 to 10 times more costly than erythromycin.

Taking all this into account, recommended therapy includes doxycycline 100 mg every 12 hours in older children and adults, or azithromycin 500 mg on day 1 and then 250 mg every 24 hours. Young children should be given erythromycin (10 mg/kg every 6 hours) or an extended-spectrum macrolide (10 to 12 mg/kg on day 1, followed by 5 mg/kg/day). The usual duration of therapy is 14 days; shorter courses may lead to relapse. *M. hominis* is not sensitive to macrolides, but it is sensitive to the other antimicrobials recommended for *M. pneumoniae* infection. Azithromycin (1 g single dose) achieves a significantly higher cure rate for *Mycoplasma genitalium*–associated urethritis than does multi-dose doxycycline.

PREVENTION

Outbreaks of *M. pneumoniae* respiratory infection among military recruits led to great interest in producing a vaccine to protect against this organism. The resulting vaccines induced specific antibody responses, but protection was limited to no more than 50% of vaccine recipients. Live vaccines using attenuated wild-type and temperature-sensitive mutant mycoplasmas have proved no more effective. In one study, volunteers who received vaccine but did not mount an antibody response had more severe disease when rechallenged with wild-type *Mycoplasma* than did nonvaccinated personnel.

Although *M. pneumoniae* is perhaps the leading cause of atypical pneumonia syndrome in closed populations, the enthusiasm for developing a vaccine for this disease has waned. New technology involving DNA expression library immunization has proved successful in animal studies with nonhuman mycoplasmas, and these methods may breathe new life into *M. pneumoniae* vaccine development.

Secondary Prevention

Prophylactic antibiotic use in family members exposed to *Mycoplasma* decreases clinical disease in these patients, but seroconversion is not prevented. One study showed that azithromycin prophylaxis, given as a 500-mg loading dose and 250 mg/day on days 2 through 5, significantly reduced the secondary attack rate of *M. pneumoniae* infection in a long-term care facility.

Grade Ⓐ ─────────────────────────────────○

1. Mena LA, Mroczkowski TF, Nsuami M, et al. A randomized comparison of azithromycin and doxycycline for the treatment of *Mycoplasma genitalium*–positive urethritis in men. *Clin Infect Dis.* 2009;48:1649-1654.

SUGGESTED READINGS

Goto H. Multicenter surveillance of adult atypical pneumonia in Japan: its clinical features, and efficacy and safety of clarithromycin. *J Infect Chemother.* 2011;17:97-104. Mycoplasma *was a common cause of relatively mild infections in young adults.*

Patel MA, Nyirjesy P. Role of *Mycoplasma* and ureaplasma species in female lower genital tract infections. *Curr Infect Dis Rep.* 2010;12:417-422. *No convincing evidence that they cause disease or should be treated.*

Smith LG. *Mycoplasma* pneumonia and its complications. *Infect Dis Clin North Am.* 2010;24:57-60. *Brief review.*

326

DISEASES CAUSED BY CHLAMYDIAE

WILLIAM M. GEISLER

DEFINITION

Chlamydiae are obligate intracellular bacteria that cause a variety of human and animal diseases and much morbidity. Chlamydiae were originally classified taxonomically into one genus, *Chlamydia*. However, revision of the chlamydial taxonomy based on sequence analysis of 16S rRNA genes has led to the proposal of two genera: *Chlamydia* and *Chlamydophila*. Within the family are four species: *Chlamydia trachomatis, Chlamydophila pneumoniae, Chlamydophila psittaci,* and *Chlamydophila pecorum*. *C. trachomatis* is classified into three biovars: the trachoma biovar, the lymphogranuloma venereum (LGV) biovar, and the mouse pneumonitis biovar. This chapter is limited to human diseases caused by chlamydiae.

The Pathogen

Chlamydiae have a gram-negative cell wall structure consisting of an outer membrane that contains lipopolysaccharide and an inner cytoplasmic membrane. The outer membrane contains a single 40-kD major outer membrane protein, OmpA (also known as MOMP), and two cysteine-rich minor outer membrane-associated proteins (OmcA and OmcB); through intermolecular and intramolecular disulfide bonding, these proteins form a complex that provides structural rigidity.

Chlamydiae grow only within intracellular membrane-bound vacuoles, termed inclusions, that seclude the organism from extracellular and cytoplasmic environments. They share a distinct biphasic developmental cycle (Fig. 326-1) that includes an extracellular, metabolically inactive, infectious form (an elementary body) and an intracellular replicative form (a reticulate body). In vitro studies have shown that chlamydiae may enter a persistent state under certain conditions (penicillin treatment, challenge with certain cytokines, restriction of select nutrients) in which they have reduced metabolic activity and may be more refractory to antibiotic treatment; whether this occurs in vivo is unclear. Knowledge of chlamydial cell biology has emerged with the sequencing of several chlamydial genomes.

PATHOBIOLOGY

Macrophages are the principal host cells for *C. psittaci* and *C. trachomatis* LGV biovar, whereas the principal host cells for *C. trachomatis* trachoma biovar and *C. pneumoniae* strains are columnar epithelial cells at mucosal sites.

Host cell tropism correlates with the type of inflammation elicited by chlamydiae. The LGV biovar and *C. psittaci* produce granulomatous inflammation, characteristic of delayed hypersensitivity reactions. The trachoma biovar produces neutrophilic exudate during acute infection and submucosal mononuclear infiltration with lymphoid follicle formation during later stages of infection.

Chlamydiae elicit both humoral and cellular immune responses. Infection persists or recurs even after an adaptive immune response develops, suggesting that the organism has evolved strategies for immune evasion. Persistent or recurrent infections elicit inflammatory cellular immune responses that cause tissue injury.

● CHLAMYDIAL DISEASES

Table 326-1 summarizes the diseases caused by chlamydiae in humans and the associated clinical and laboratory characteristics.

Chlamydia trachomatis

C. trachomatis infection is a common bacterial infection in humans and accounts for significant morbidity worldwide. *C. trachomatis* isolates have been differentiated into 18 major serovars (i.e., OmpA types) based on variations in OmpA that are identified on antigen cross-reactivity in the microimmunofluorescence test. The major diseases caused by *C. trachomatis* are (1) trachoma, caused by serovars A, B, Ba, and C; (2) sexually and perinatally transmitted diseases, caused by serovars D through K (and, rarely, serovars B and Ba); and (3) sexually transmitted LGV, caused by serovars L_1, L_2, L_{2a}, and

8 hrs			40-60 hrs		
Attachment	Endocytosis	Differentiation EB → RB	Binary fission	Differentiation RB → EB	Release

FIGURE 326-1. Developmental cycle of chlamydiae. The *top panel* shows the developmental cycle common to all chlamydiae. The *red circles* represent elementary bodies (EBs), and the *blue circles* represent reticulate bodies (RBs). Chlamydiae infect eukaryotic cells through multiple attachment mechanisms. After attachment, EBs enter the cell within a membrane-bound vacuole that remains unfused with lysosomes. EBs reorganize into RBs and asynchronously replicate 8 to 12 times, with a doubling time of 2 to 3 hours. At the conclusion of the growth cycle, RBs differentiate back to EBs, and each inclusion yields 100 to 1000 new infectious EBs. The *bottom left panel*, a transmission electron micrograph taken 40 hours after infection, shows the large RBs and the smaller EBs, which have a condensed nucleoid structure within their cytoplasm. The *bottom right panel*, a scanning electron micrograph taken 60 hours after infection, shows a membrane-bound vacuole containing many EBs exiting from an infected HeLa cell.

TABLE 326-1 MAJOR DISEASES CAUSED BY CHLAMYDIAE IN HUMANS AND ASSOCIATED CLINICAL AND LABORATORY FEATURES

SPECIES	SEROVAR	DISEASE	TRANSMISSION ROUTE	DIAGNOSIS	PREVENTION
C. trachomatis	A–C	Trachoma	Fomites, eye-seeking flies	Clinical criteria or culture/NAAT	SAFE strategy
	D–K	Urethritis, cervicitis, proctitis, epididymitis, PID	Sexual contact	NAAT	Abstinence/monogamy, education, condoms, partner treatment
	D–K	Inclusion conjunctivitis, infant pneumonia	Perinatal contact	Culture/DFA/NAAT or serology (for pneumonia)	Prenatal chlamydia screening: treat infected mothers
	L1–L3	Lymphogranuloma venereum	Sexual contact	Serology or culture/NAAT + OmpA typing	Abstinence/monogamy, education, condoms, partner treatment
C. pneumoniae	One	Upper respiratory infections, atypical pneumonia, asthma exacerbations	Respiratory droplet	Serology or culture/PCR	None
C. psittaci	Multiple	Psittacosis, atypical pneumonia, febrile illness	Aerosolized bird secretions, dust	Serology	Quarantine and chlortetracycline for imported birds, avoidance or precautions for at-risk subjects

DFA = direct fluorescent antibody test; NAAT = nucleic acid amplification test; PCR = polymerase chain reaction; PID = pelvic inflammatory disease; SAFE = World Health Organization's recommended strategy: acronym for *surgery (for trichiasis), antimicrobials (periodic community-wide treatment), facial cleanliness, and environmental improvement.*

L_3. Sequencing of the *ompA* gene has led to the recognition of more OmpA variants. Trachoma and LGV are endemic in developing areas of the world (although LGV outbreaks have also occurred in populations of men who have sex with men in developed countries), whereas sexually and perinatally transmitted chlamydial infections occur worldwide.

TRACHOMA

EPIDEMIOLOGY

Trachoma is a chronic follicular conjunctivitis. The overall incidence is unknown, but is has been estimated to occur in more than 100 million people worldwide, most of whom are young children. Trachoma is endemic in more than 50 countries and is especially common in poor areas of sub-Saharan Africa, where the disease prevalence in children may exceed 40%. It is a major public health problem because scarring from trachoma causes blindness in an estimated 6 million people, and trachoma is the most common preventable cause of blindness worldwide. Active trachoma often occurs in the first few years of life. The inflammation from recurrent and/or persistent trachoma can lead to conjunctival scarring, which can ultimately cause corneal damage and blindness later in life. The *C. trachomatis* serovars that produce trachoma are spread by direct contact with fingers or fomites (e.g., washcloths, handkerchiefs) contaminated with eye discharge from an infected person or by eye-seeking flies. Because of this mode of transmission, trachoma often clusters in households. Risk factors for trachoma include poor facial hygiene, limited access to water, poor sanitation, and close proximity to other infected persons or to a heavy density of eye-seeking flies.

CLINICAL MANIFESTATIONS

There are two stages of trachoma disease, and they can overlap. Initially, trachoma begins as an inflammatory follicular conjunctivitis (i.e., active trachoma). Upon everting the upper eyelid, white to pale yellow lymphoid follicles can be visualized on the superior tarsal conjunctival surface, and papillae may be noted between follicles. Minimal watery or mucoid ocular discharge may also be seen. In more severe active trachoma, the conjunctiva can be thickened and edematous. Subsequently, conjunctival inflammation can progress to cause scarring of the upper tarsal conjunctiva (the cicatricial stage of disease). Scarring deforms the eyelid and can lead to an inward turning of the eyelashes, which can result in corneal abrasion (trichiasis). Over time, trichiasis causes corneal edema, ulceration, vascularization (pannus), scarring, and opacification. The corneal damage leads to decreased vision or blindness, occurring mostly in young adults and middle-aged persons. Viral conjunctivitis (e.g., adenovirus) presents in a similar clinical fashion as active trachoma, but it is self-limited and usually resolves within a week. Trachoma can be complicated by superinfection with other bacterial pathogens (e.g., *Haemophilus influenzae*), which should be considered when purulent ocular discharge or significant inflammation of the bulbar conjunctiva is present.

DIAGNOSIS

Because the majority of trachoma cases occur in developing countries without access to laboratory testing or the necessary resources, trachoma is often diagnosed clinically based on findings of active trachoma (follicles on the upper tarsal conjunctiva or pronounced inflammatory thickening of the tarsal conjunctiva) or cicatricial disease. When laboratories are available, detection of *C. trachomatis* provides definitive evidence of active trachoma and may identify infection in subjects with minimal clinical evidence of active trachoma. Isolation of the organism in cell culture is one means to detect *C. trachomatis*, but the test's sensitivity is less than 50% and the methods are labor intensive. Nonculture tests have higher sensitivities in active trachoma. For instance, nucleic acid amplification tests (NAATs) are the most sensitive diagnostic tests, but they are not widely available in many trachoma-endemic areas. It is uncommon for adults with late scarring to have *C. trachomatis* detected by any of these assays.

TREATMENT   Rx

Active trachoma can be treated with a tetracycline eye ointment twice daily for 6 weeks or oral macrolide therapy. The latter is preferred in part because extraocular sites such as the nasopharynx may be infected in young children. Single-dose oral azithromycin (20 mg/kg; maximum of 1 g) is as effective as tetracycline ointment and is more advantageous in terms of compliance and side effect profile; tetracycline application can irritate the ocular surface.

Surgical intervention is the only effective management for trichiasis. Eyelid rotation surgery prevents the eyelashes from abrading the cornea, preventing blindness and other nonvisual symptoms. Trichiasis recurrence following surgery is a major concern, and recurrence rates are highly variable across studies. Other concerns include accessibility to surgery and patient acceptance.

PREVENTION

The World Health Organization is committed to eliminating blinding trachoma by 2020 and recommends that all countries with endemic trachoma adopt the SAFE strategy: surgery (for trichiasis), antimicrobials (periodic community-wide treatment), facial cleanliness, and environmental improvement. Mass treatment of a community with single-dose oral azithromycin is safe and has dramatically reduced the prevalence of infection for up to 1 year after treatment, without an increase in antimicrobial resistance; it has also been shown to reduce mortality in children.[1] Annual azithromycin treatment is recommended for trachoma-endemic areas. Reintroduction of trachoma following mass treatment has been demonstrated, which may be due in part to decreased herd immunity. Repeated mass treatment (every few months) provides herd protection to the entire community.[2]

Mass antibiotic treatment as the sole intervention for eliminating trachoma is unlikely to be successful if other factors that facilitate transmission are not addressed. Face washing and good hygiene help reduce the risk of transmission through contact with fingers and flies. Although the promotion of facial cleanliness through educational campaigns may be one of the most important interventions, sustaining such behavioral changes can be challenging. Achieving better environmental conditions through measures that reduce household and community fly density and improve waste management and access to clean water can also limit transmission. Improvement in socioeconomic conditions in a community correlates with a decline in trachoma prevalence.

SEXUALLY AND PERINATALLY TRANSMITTED CHLAMYDIAL INFECTIONS

EPIDEMIOLOGY

Chlamydia is the most prevalent bacterial sexually transmitted infection in the United States. Currently, more than 1.2 million infections are reported to the Centers for Disease Control and Prevention (CDC) annually. The number of reported cases is increasing each year; this may reflect increased chlamydia screening efforts rather than a true increase in infection burden, but this remains unclear. Taking into account underreporting and underscreening, it is estimated that more than 3 million new chlamydial infections occur annually in the United States. Higher chlamydia prevalence rates have been associated with younger age (sexually active adolescents and young adults), select minority ethnic groups (especially African Americans), and new or multiple sexual partners. Chlamydia prevalence is higher in women than in men; it is unclear whether this is due to higher screening rates in women or whether women may be more susceptible to infection acquisition or persistence. Chlamydia prevalence is highest in the southeastern United States. The estimated total cost attributable to chlamydial disease in the United States exceeds $2.4 billion annually. From a global perspective, there are an estimated 90 million new chlamydial infections annually. In addition to the adverse effects on the reproductive health of women, chlamydia has a substantial impact on perinatal outcomes and facilitates the transmission of human immunodeficiency virus (HIV).

CLINICAL MANIFESTATIONS
Urethritis

C. trachomatis is the most common cause of nongonococcal urethritis in men, being responsible for 20 to 55% of cases. Although the majority of men with chlamydial urethritis are asymptomatic, studies in high-prevalence venues (e.g., sexually transmitted disease clinics) have reported that 40 to 60% of men with chlamydial urethritis are symptomatic. The most frequent symptoms are urethral discomfort (itching or pain) with urination and urethral discharge. On examination, a mild to moderate amount of clear or cloudy/mucoid (rarely purulent) urethral discharge may be visualized (Fig. 326-2A). Urethral discharge sometimes becomes apparent only after stripping the urethra from the base of the penis to the glans; this should be considered in men reporting urethral symptoms but without urethral discharge on initial inspection. Gram stain from a urethral swab specimen demonstrates five or more polymorphonuclear leukocytes (PMNs) per oil

FIGURE 326-2. Clinical manifestations of genital *Chlamydia trachomatis* infection. **A,** Cloudy urethral discharge of urethritis. **B,** Urethral specimen Gram stain revealing nongonococcal urethritis findings: five or more polymorphonuclear cells per oil field (1000×) and the absence of intracellular gram-negative diplococci. **C,** Purulent endocervical discharge of mucopurulent cervicitis. (**A,** Courtesy James Sizemore, MD; **B** and **C,** From *Practitioner's Handbook for the Management of Sexually Transmitted Disease*. http://depts.washington.edu/nnptc/online_training/std_handbook. Accessed May 12, 2011.)

field (1000×) in the majority of chlamydial infections (Fig. 326-2B). Chlamydial organisms cannot be visualized on Gram stain. Up to 20% of men with chlamydial urethritis have fewer than five PMNs per oil field on urethral Gram stain, reflecting the fact that minimal inflammation may be elicited in some cases of chlamydial urethritis. Urethral inflammation can also be detected by a positive urinary leukocyte esterase test on unspun first-void urine.

C. trachomatis urethritis also occurs in women, who may be asymptomatic or present with an acute urethral syndrome characterized by dysuria, urinary frequency, and pyuria. This acute urethral syndrome mimics a urinary tract infection, and chlamydia should be suspected in women with pyuria but negative urine nitrite or negative urine culture, especially in sexually active adolescents and young adults. Mild urethral discharge may be seen. Pelvic examination should be performed in women with suspected chlamydia urethritis to search for other clinical findings of chlamydia (e.g., cervicitis).

Epididymitis

Chlamydia can spread from the urethra to the epididymis, causing epididymitis in up to 1 to 3% of infected men. Symptoms include testicular pain and scrotal erythema and swelling that are typically unilateral. On examination, there is palpable swelling and tenderness of the epididymis; accompanying findings may include testicular tenderness, scrotal erythema and swelling, urethral discharge, or hydrocele. In men younger than 35 years, *C. trachomatis* is the principal cause of epididymitis, whereas in men older than 35 years, complicated urinary tract infection with uropathogens is a more common cause, especially in those with prostate disorders. Up to 15% of epididymitis cases are complicated by chronic pain that is usually idiopathic and often unresponsive to antibiotics. Other complications include decreased fertility and, rarely, testicular abscess.

Cervicitis

C. trachomatis is the most common cause of cervicitis, being responsible for up to 50% of cases. The majority of women with endocervical chlamydial infection are asymptomatic. Symptoms, when present, are often mild and nonspecific for chlamydia and include the following: vaginal discharge, intermenstrual vaginal bleeding, dysuria, and pain during intercourse (dyspareunia). Approximately 10% of women with asymptomatic cervical chlamydial infection have mucopurulent cervicitis detected on pelvic examination (Fig. 326-2C); this is characterized by a purulent or cloudy endocervical discharge visible in the endocervical canal or on the tip of an endocervical swab. A similar proportion may have endocervical bleeding that is easily induced with passage of a swab through the cervical os. Nonspecific findings may include vaginal discharge and edematous ectopy (a darker red area of columnar epithelium visible on the face of the cervix). Gram stain of an endocervical sample usually shows more than 10 PMNs per oil field. A vaginal wet mount often shows more than 5 to 10 PMNs per 400× field.

Pelvic Inflammatory Disease

Chlamydia can spread from the cervix to the endometrium (causing endometritis), fallopian tubes (causing salpingitis), and peritoneum (causing peritonitis or perihepatitis). These upper genital tract infections are collectively referred to as pelvic inflammatory disease (PID). Estimates of the proportion of cervical chlamydial infections that progress to PID vary greatly but are most commonly around 10 to 20%. The majority of PID cases are subclinical or silent. PID symptoms include pelvic or lower abdominal pain (especially during menses or the first 2 weeks of the menstrual cycle) and nausea. Fever is less common. Examination findings include cervical motion tenderness or tenderness of the uterus or adnexa. Although most cases of chlamydial PID are due to the natural progression of infection, they may also occur post partum or following pregnancy termination. The long-term consequences of PID include infertility, ectopic pregnancy, and chronic pelvic pain.

Complications during Pregnancy

There is conflicting evidence on whether genital chlamydial infection during pregnancy leads to adverse outcomes. Reported adverse outcomes include preterm labor, low birthweight, miscarriage, and stillbirth.

Reactive Arthritis

Reactive arthritis, characterized by the classic triad of trigger infection (e.g., chlamydia), conjunctivitis, and arthritis, can complicate chlamydial infection (Chapter 273). There is a male predominance in reactive arthritis cases triggered by chlamydia, and it has been estimated that reactive arthritis occurs in about 1% of men presenting with chlamydial urethritis.

Proctitis

Proctitis caused by non-LGV *C. trachomatis* OmpA types is usually asymptomatic. Subjects with acute symptomatic proctitis may report rectal pain and/or bleeding, tenesmus, pruritus, rectal discharge, or diarrhea. Anoscopy or sigmoidoscopy may reveal friable mucosa and a mucoid or mucopurulent discharge. A rectal swab Gram stain often reveals many PMNs per oil field.

Conjunctivitis

An acute follicular conjunctivitis may rarely occur in adolescents or adults with genital chlamydial infection. The presumed mode of acquisition is auto-inoculation with infected genital secretions. The typical clinical presentation is subacute or chronic infection characterized by unilateral conjunctival redness, mucoid or mucopurulent ocular discharge, a foreign body sensation, and preauricular adenopathy.

Oropharyngeal Infection

C. trachomatis has been detected in the oropharynx of sexually active subjects, but the clinical significance and transmissibility of *C. trachomatis* detected at this site are unclear.

Infant Inclusion Conjunctivitis and Pneumonia

Because the prevalence of chlamydia in pregnant adolescents and young adults in the United States can be high (>5%), the morbidity associated with perinatally transmitted chlamydia is considerable. Neonates exposed to *C. trachomatis* during passage through the birth canal may develop inclusion conjunctivitis (≈20 to 40%) or pneumonia (≈10 to 20%). The conjunctivitis—termed *inclusion conjunctivitis* because the cytoplasmic chlamydia inclusion bodies demonstrated in neonatal conjunctival scrapings are the same as those seen in genital scrapings from adults with genital chlamydia—usually develops 5 to 12 days after birth but may occur as long as 4 to 6 weeks after birth. Clinical manifestations include conjunctival injection and thickening, a clear or mucopurulent ocular discharge, and eyelid swelling. Chlamydia pneumonia in infants usually occurs subacutely between 1 and 3 months of age. Characteristic clinical features include a repetitive staccato cough and absence of fever. Other clinical findings may include tachypnea, crackles on auscultation of the lungs, nasal discharge, and eosinophilia. Chest radiographs may reveal bilateral diffuse infiltrates.

Lymphogranuloma Venereum

LGV is a sexually transmitted infection caused by *C. trachomatis* LGV OmpA types. In contrast to infection with non-LGV strains, LGV is a more invasive systemic infection that involves lymphoid tissue (causing lymphadenitis) and can be ulcerative. LGV is endemic in Africa, India, Southeast Asia, South America, and the Caribbean. LGV is uncommon in the United States, with fewer than 100 cases reported annually. Since 2003, LGV outbreaks have occurred in Europe and Canada, primarily involving HIV-positive men who have sex with men who also had proctitis and were infected with LGV OmpA variant L2b.

The clinical manifestations of LGV differ in early versus later stages of infection. In the early stage (3 to 30 days after acquisition) of genital LGV, a primary skin lesion or lesions may develop on the genital mucosa or adjacent skin in the form of a papule, ulcer, or herpetiform lesion. The lesion is usually asymptomatic and goes unnoticed, but it may be erosive; it heals quickly without scarring. Early genital LGV may also present as a nonspecific inflammatory syndrome (e.g., urethritis and cervicitis), similar to infection with non-LGV strains. Genital LGV can progress to an inguinal syndrome 2 to 4 weeks later, characterized by painful, erythematous inguinal

lymphadenopathy (buboes; see Fig. 320-3 in Chapter 320) and systemic manifestations including fever, headache, arthralgias, myalgias, and leukocytosis. The buboes are commonly unilateral, and about one third spontaneously rupture and drain pus, which can be complicated by fistulas or sinus tracts; unruptured buboes usually heal. In later stages, genital tract fibrosis can lead to complications such as infertility, elephantiasis, strictures, fistulas, and subcutaneous sclerosis.

LGV may also present as an anogenital syndrome with invasive proctitis. Symptoms include fever, tenesmus, anal pruritus, and a rectal discharge that may be mucoid or, less commonly, mucopurulent or bloody. The rectal mucosa is friable, with multiple superficial ulcerations, and biopsy may reveal submucosal granulomas and crypt abscesses; these clinical and histopathologic findings resemble Crohn's disease (Chapter 143). Late complications include rectal strictures, anal fistulas, and lymphorrhoids (perianal growths of lymphatic tissue).

Natural History

The natural history of untreated genital *C. trachomatis* infection has not been fully elucidated, in part because ethical considerations limit such research. Outcomes of untreated genital chlamydia include spontaneous resolution (i.e., immune-mediated clearance) and persisting infection; the latter may be subclinical or progress to clinical manifestations (e.g., urethritis cervicitis), which can remain uncomplicated or progress to a complication (e.g., PID). Based on limited evidence in subjects with chlamydia detected initially by a screening test who returned within weeks to months for treatment and were retested, anywhere from 10 to 40% of infections resolve spontaneously before treatment. Some patients with persisting infection develop clinical manifestations before returning for treatment, including a small proportion of females (up to 4%) who develop symptomatic PID. Other sparse data in females suggest that up to 50% of genital chlamydial infections resolve after a year, but a small percentage (<10%) could persist for several years. An improved understanding of the natural history of chlamydia could impact screening and treatment recommendations.

DIAGNOSIS

C. trachomatis infections are difficult to diagnose clinically because the majority are asymptomatic, and even when symptoms or signs are present, they are nonspecific. Therefore, a definitive diagnosis relies on detecting the organism. Laboratory diagnosis confirms the clinical diagnosis in those with clinical manifestations and detects infection in asymptomatic individuals (i.e., screening). The CDC recommends annual chlamydia screening for sexually active women aged 25 years and younger, as well as for older women with risk factors (e.g., new or multiple sexual partners). Select studies have demonstrated that chlamydia screening reduces the prevalence of chlamydia in women and the rate of PID. Universal chlamydia screening in men is not recommended; selective screening is appropriate in venues with high prevalences (e.g., sexually transmitted disease clinics, correctional facilities), for high-risk men, or for symptomatic men.

The reference standard for the detection of *C. trachomatis* has been isolation of the organism in cell culture. Development of nonculture tests was important because culture is technically demanding, expensive, and not widely available. Earlier nonculture tests included enzyme immunoassay, direct fluorescent antibody, and nucleic acid hybridization. These tests were less expensive and less technically demanding than culture but had lower sensitivities (lower limit of detection ≥10^3 elementary bodies) and therefore detected fewer infections. These earlier tests have been replaced in most laboratories by nucleic acid amplification tests (NAATs), which are now the recommended diagnostic tests for chlamydia. NAATs have the highest sensitivity (detecting a small number of elementary bodies) and can be performed on genital swabs and on noninvasively collected specimens (first-void urine or self-collected vaginal swabs) with similar accuracy. The CDC's recommended specimens for NAATs are first-void urine in males and vaginal swabs in females. NAATs have not been cleared by the Food and Drug Administration for use with rectal, oropharyngeal, or conjunctival swab specimens; however, some laboratories have validated the assays to meet Clinical Laboratory Improvement Amendments (CLIA) requirements.

The role of serology in diagnosing *C. trachomatis* infection is limited primarily to two indications: (1) infant pneumonia syndrome, the diagnosis of which is suggested by a *C. trachomatis* immunoglobulin M antibody titer of 1:32 or greater using the microimmunofluorescence (MIF) assay, and (2) LGV, the diagnosis of which is suggested by a complement fixation (CF) antibody titer greater than 1:64 or MIF antibody titer greater than 1:256 in the appropriate clinical context; MIF has a higher specificity than CF. LGV can also be diagnosed by demonstrating an LGV OmpA type on *C. trachomatis* DNA from infected material.

TREATMENT Rx

C. trachomatis is susceptible to tetracyclines, macrolides, and select quinolones (ofloxacin and levofloxacin, but not ciprofloxacin). The CDC's recommended treatment for uncomplicated genital chlamydia is either doxycycline 100 mg orally twice daily for 7 days or azithromycin 1 g orally in a single dose. A meta-analysis of clinical trials that used primarily chlamydia culture revealed that these regimens are equally efficacious, with cure rates around 97 to 98%.[3] Recent studies in women using the more sensitive NAATs suggest that the cure rate may be a slightly lower (≈92%). Azithromycin is a little more expensive than doxycycline, but treatment compliance is higher. Alternative treatment regimens include erythromycin base 500 mg orally four times a day for 7 days, ofloxacin 300 mg orally twice daily for 7 days, or levofloxacin 500 mg orally once a day for 7 days. Azithromycin is the recommended treatment for chlamydia-infected pregnant women. *C. trachomatis* epididymitis and PID should be treated with doxycycline for 10 and 14 days, respectively. Treatment of these syndromes is usually empirical before test results are available; therefore, ceftriaxone 250 mg intramuscularly in a single dose is added to doxycycline to cover gonorrhea. LGV should be treated with doxycycline for 3 weeks; some experts recommend azithromycin 1 g orally weekly for 3 weeks as an alternative. Infant chlamydial infections are treated with erythromycin base 50 mg/kg/day divided into four daily doses for 14 days; data on other macrolides are limited.

A test of cure (approximately 3 weeks after completion of chlamydia treatment) is recommended only for pregnant women. Sexual partners (including current partners and those with contact in the preceding 60 days) and parents of chlamydia-infected infants should be evaluated and treated empirically. Expedited partner therapy, whereby chlamydia-infected patients are offered medication or a prescription to give to their sexual partners, or clinicians provide medication to contacts without an examination, may reduce the risk for recurrent chlamydia. Patients and their partners should remain abstinent until treatment is completed.

PREVENTION

Education and the provision of condoms are preventive measures that should accompany chlamydia treatment. Recurrent chlamydia occurs in approximately 10 to 20% of chlamydia-infected subjects within a few months of treatment, so repeat chlamydia testing is recommended approximately 3 months after treatment.

Chlamydophila pneumoniae

In 1986 a new chlamydial pathogen that caused acute respiratory tract infections was identified and designated *Chlamydia* strain TWAR. It was initially thought to be a novel *C. psittaci* strain but was later recognized as the species *C. pneumoniae* in 1989. Pneumonia and upper respiratory tract infections (bronchitis, pharyngitis, and sinusitis) are the most frequently identified diseases caused by *C. pneumoniae*. However, *C. pneumoniae* may also contribute to exacerbations of chronic bronchitis and asthma. Recent evidence suggests that *C. pneumoniae* may contribute to atherosclerosis and possibly to select central nervous system disorders.

EPIDEMIOLOGY

The majority of adults in the United States and other developed countries are seropositive for *C. pneumoniae*, exceeding 80% in some populations. Seroconversion often occurs during childhood or adolescence and may be subclinical. Studies incorporating culture or polymerase chain reaction (PCR) suggest that infection is not uncommon in children younger than 5 years. *C. pneumoniae* causes an atypical pneumonia syndrome, with an estimated annual incidence of 1 case per 1000 population; epidemiologic studies suggest a 4-year cycle of increased pneumonia incidence. Approximately 10% of community-acquired pneumonias are attributed to *C. pneumoniae*, and coinfection with other respiratory pathogens such as *Streptococcus pneumoniae* and *Mycoplasma pneumoniae* is not uncommon. The organism is believed to be acquired through the inhalation of infected respiratory droplets from persons with disease and possibly asymptomatic carriers. This mode of transmission can facilitate the spread of infection among household members and can cause epidemics in enclosed populations, such as persons in military barracks, nursing homes, and schools.

CLINICAL MANIFESTATIONS

Most *C. pneumoniae* infections occur in children, who often have mild clinical manifestations or are asymptomatic. Clinical manifestations are more evident in adults, especially the elderly, who have the highest incidence of *C. pneumoniae* pneumonia. *C. pneumoniae* causes an atypical pneumonia that is usually of mild to moderate severity. The incubation period may be several weeks, and the disease onset is gradual. A nonproductive cough is usually present and is often preceded or accompanied by nasal congestion, sore throat, and hoarseness. Headache may occur in up to half of patients. Fever and dyspnea occur less commonly. On examination, localized pulmonary crackles or rhonchi are often heard. Chest radiography shows pneumonitis, most often evident as a single subsegmental lower lobe infiltrate. The leukocyte count is usually normal. *C. pneumoniae* may also present as isolated bronchitis, sinusitis, laryngitis, or nonexudative pharyngitis. The clinical course of these upper respiratory tract infections may be protracted over several weeks.

DIAGNOSIS

C. pneumoniae infection is usually diagnosed by serology or direct detection of the organism in respiratory specimens using cell culture or other nonculture methods. Serology is the test used in most clinical settings, with the MIF assay considered the reference standard for serodiagnosis. However, serology is limited by its specificity, reproducibility, and clinical correlation. *C. pneumoniae* can be isolated in cell culture, but culture is technically challenging and time-consuming. Antigen detection using fluorescent monoclonal antibodies has a lower sensitivity than culture and is also technically challenging. *C. pneumoniae* PCR is more sensitive than culture, and real-time PCR appears to have advantages over conventional PCR. Although there are still issues involving the standardization of PCR methods for *C. pneumoniae* detection, PCR is promising and will likely become the test of choice.

TREATMENT Rx

C. pneumoniae is susceptible to tetracyclines, macrolides, and fluoroquinolones. Treatment trials using culture have demonstrated that select macrolide and fluoroquinolone regimens eradicate *C. pneumoniae* in approximately 70 to 85% of subjects with pneumonia. The clinical response to treatment may be slow, and some patients may need re-treatment. The suggested treatment duration for most regimens is typically 10 to 14 days, except that shorter courses may be effective for azithromycin (10 mg/kg on day 1, followed by 5 mg/kg over the next 4 days; up to 1.5 g orally over 5 days). Chronic *C. pneumoniae* infections may require even longer courses of treatment (e.g., 6 weeks), and macrolides are suggested in this setting.

Chlamydophila psittaci

EPIDEMIOLOGY

C. psittaci naturally infects a variety of mammals and birds. *C. psittaci* strains appear to be host specific, and most human infections are linked to contact with an infected bird. *C. psittaci* infection in humans is termed *psittacosis*, in part because exposure to psittacine birds (parrots, parakeets, and budgerigars) is commonly implicated in infections. However, because human cases have been linked to exposure to finches, pigeons, pheasants, ducks, turkeys, chickens, seagulls, and other birds, *ornithosis* may be a more appropriate term. Psittacosis disease in birds ranges from an asymptomatic carriage state to a mild symptomatic illness manifested by ruffled feathers, anorexia, shivering, dyspnea, diarrhea, and/or depression. Infected birds shed *C. psittaci* in urine, feces, or secretions from their beaks or eyes. Their feathers and surrounding environment become contaminated. Transmission to humans is primarily by inhalation of aerosolized bird secretions or dust. Infected birds may shed the organism for months. Person-to-person transmission rarely occurs.

Human psittacosis is a rare infection, due in part to antibiotic-laced bird feed and a mandated quarantine for imported birds. The number of cases of psittacosis in the United States has been stable for the past 10 years, with fewer than 50 confirmed cases reported annually; a larger number of cases are reported but not confirmed.

CLINICAL MANIFESTATIONS

Psittacosis initially involves the lungs and then spreads to the reticuloendothelial system. The clinical spectrum of infection ranges from asymptomatic to fulminant, and clinical manifestations may resemble Q fever, typhoid fever, or legionnaires' disease. After an incubation period of 5 to 14 days, some patients may present with a nonspecific virus-like illness or a mononucleosis-like syndrome. The presentation most suggestive of psittacosis is an acute febrile atypical pneumonia. Patients initially have an abrupt onset of shaking chills and a fever as high as 40.5° C. Temperature-pulse dissociation (i.e., elevated temperature with a normal pulse) may occur. Constitutional symptoms, including headache, myalgias, and arthralgias, are prominent. A cough, usually nonproductive, appears early in the illness and may accompany chest pain, which is usually nonpleuritic. Auscultation may be normal or reveal bilateral crackles. Chest radiograph findings are usually more dramatic than lung examination findings; the most common finding is single lower lobe consolidation, but multiple localized bronchopneumonic patches, diffuse ground-glass changes, or a miliary pattern have been described. Small pleural effusions may be seen. In contrast to *C. pneumoniae* pneumonia, psittacosis is more severe, with high fever and absent or minimal upper respiratory complaints.

Extrapulmonary findings frequently occur in psittacosis. Splenomegaly is common. A faint erythematous, blanching, maculopapular rash (Horder's spots), resembling the rose spots of typhoid fever, can occur, as can erythema nodosum. Signs of hepatitis, endocarditis (culture negative), pericarditis, myocarditis, meningoencephalitis, hemolytic anemia, or disseminated intravascular coagulation may be noted.

DIAGNOSIS

Psittacosis should be suspected in patients with a febrile illness (especially atypical pneumonia) who report exposure to sick or imported birds or who have regular exposure to birds, including bird owners, pet shop workers, veterinarians, zookeepers, and poultry processing plant workers. The diagnosis can be made with serology or by isolating the organism in cell culture. *C. psittaci* is a biocontainment level 3 agent owing to its stability in the environment and aerosol transmission. Because laboratory-acquired *C. psittaci* infections are well documented, culture is discouraged and serology is preferred. If culture is attempted, laboratory staff should be notified in advance so that appropriate precautions can be taken. A serologic diagnosis of psittacosis is made by demonstrating (1) a four-fold or greater rise in CF or MIF antibody against *C. psittaci* to a titer of at least 1:32 from acute to convalescent sera collected at least 2 weeks apart (3 to 6 weeks is recommended), or (2) an immunoglobulin M titer of 1:16 or greater against *C. psittaci* by MIF.

TREATMENT Rx

Untreated psittacosis can be fatal, but mortality is rare with prompt antimicrobial treatment. Because of the delay in laboratory diagnosis of psittacosis, empirical therapy should be provided based on clinical suspicion. *C. psittaci* susceptibility has been demonstrated to tetracyclines, macrolides, and some of the newer fluoroquinolones. The recommended treatment regimen, based on clinical experience, is either tetracycline 500 mg four times a day or doxycycline 100 mg twice a day for 10 to 21 days. Further studies on the clinical efficacy of azithromycin and newer fluoroquinolones are needed. The initial treatment response can be dramatic, with defervescence and marked clinical improvement within 24 to 48 hours. Full recovery may take several weeks, and relapse or reinfection can occur. Endocarditis treatment includes prolonged antibiotic treatment and consideration of valve replacement.

PREVENTION

Epidemic psittacosis is preventable by a 30-day period of quarantine for all imported psittacine birds and their treatment with feed containing chlortetracycline. The U.S. Department of Agriculture recommends extending treatment for an additional 15 days after quarantine. Prevention of epidemic and endemic psittacosis also relies on avoidance of or protection from exposure to dust or body secretions from birds or their living areas, as well as avoiding the handling of sick birds. Environmental sanitation is another important preventive measure, considering the organism's resistance to drying.

Visit expertconsult.com for e-expanded chapter

Grade **A**

1. Porco TC, Gebre T, Ayele B, et al. Effect of mass distribution of azithromycin for trachoma control an overall mortality in Ethiopian children: a randomized trial. *JAMA.* 2009;302:962-968.
2. House JI, Ayele B, Porco TC, et al. Assessment of herd protection against trachoma due to repeated mass antibiotic distributions: a cluster-randomised trial. *Lancet.* 2009;373:1111-1118.
3. Lau CY, Qureshi AK. Azithromycin versus doxycycline for genital chlamydial infections: a meta-analysis of randomized clinical trials. *Sex Transm Dis.* 2002;29:497-502.

SUGGESTED READINGS

Batteiger BE, Tu W, Ofner S, et al. Repeated *Chlamydia trachomatis* genital infections in adolescent women. *J Infect Dis.* 2010;201:42-51. *Novel longitudinal study in adolescent women that used clinical, laboratory, and behavioral data to evaluate the rate of repeat versus persistent genital chlamydial infections.*
Geisler WM. Duration of untreated, uncomplicated *Chlamydia trachomatis* genital infection and factors associated with chlamydia resolution: a review of human studies. *J Infect Dis.* 2010;201(Suppl 2):S104-S113. *Recent review of studies on the natural history of untreated genital chlamydial infections and discussion of study limitations and future directions.*
Hu VH, Harding-Esch EM, Burton MJ, et al. Epidemiology and control of trachoma: systematic review. *Trop Med Int Health.* 2010;15:673-691. *Currently, 40 million people are thought to have active disease and 8.2 million to have trichiasis.*
Land JA, Van Bergen JE, Morre SA, et al. Epidemiology of *Chlamydia trachomatis* infection in women and the cost-effectiveness of screening. *Hum Reprod Update.* 2010;16:189-204. *Overview of the epidemiology of chlamydia infection and the risk estimates of its late complications, including pelvic inflammatory disease and infertility.*
Paavonen J. *Chlamydia trachomatis* infections of the female genital tract: state of the art. *Ann Med.* 2011. [Epub ahead of print.] *Review emphasizing that single-dose azithromycin remains effective.*
Stewardson AJ, Grayson ML. Psittacosis. *Infect Dis Clin North Am.* 2010;24:7-25. *Review of the clinical manifestations, diagnosis, and treatment of this systemic zoonotic infection with protean clinical features.*

327

SYPHILIS

EDWARD W. HOOK III

DEFINITION

Syphilis, which is a chronic infectious disease caused by the bacterium *Treponema pallidum,* is usually acquired by sexual contact with another infected individual. Syphilis is remarkable among infectious diseases for its large variety of clinical manifestations. It progresses, if untreated, through primary, secondary, and tertiary stages. The early stages (i.e., primary and secondary) are infectious. Spontaneous healing of early lesions occurs, followed by a long latent period. In about 30% of untreated patients, late disease of the heart, central nervous system (CNS), or other organs may develop years after the initial infection. Although the disease is less common now than previously, it remains a challenge to clinicians because of its protean manifestations, and it is of interest to biologists because of the prolonged, tenuous balance between the host and the invading spirochete.

The Pathogen

The causative agent of syphilis, *T. pallidum,* is closely related to other pathogenic spirochetes (Chapter 328), including those causing yaws (*T. pallidum* subspecies *pertenue*) and pinta (*Treponema carateum*). *T. pallidum* is a thin, helical bacterium approximately 0.15 μm wide and 6 to 15 μm long. The organism has 6 to 14 spirals and is tapered on either end. It is too thin to be seen by ordinary Gram stain microscopy but can be visualized in wet mounts by dark-field microscopy or in fixed specimens by silver stain or fluorescent antibody methods.

Unlike most bacteria, which have protein-rich outer membranes, the *T. pallidum* outer membrane appears to be composed of predominantly phospholipids, with few surface-exposed proteins. It has been hypothesized that because of this structure, syphilis can progress despite the brisk antibody response to non–surface-exposed internal antigens, which is the basis for serologic tests for the diagnosis and management of syphilis. Between the outer membrane and the peptidoglycan cell wall are six axial fibrils; three are attached at each end, and they overlap in the center of the organism. They are structurally and biochemically similar to flagella and are in part responsible for the organism's motility.

It is possible to culture *T. pallidum,* but sustained in vitro cultivation is not yet possible, and yields are very low. Culture is of limited use in research and of no use in clinical practice. All isolates studied have been susceptible to penicillin and are antigenically similar. The only known natural hosts for *T. pallidum* are humans and certain monkeys and higher apes.

EPIDEMIOLOGY

With the exception of congenital syphilis, syphilis is acquired almost exclusively by intimate contact with the infectious lesions of primary or secondary syphilis (e.g., chancres, mucous patches, condylomata lata). Disease is usually acquired through sexual intercourse, including anogenital and orogenital intercourse. Health care workers are sometimes infected during the unsuspecting examination of patients with infectious lesions. Infection by contact with fomites is extremely uncommon. Before the advent of modern blood banking techniques, syphilis was occasionally transmitted through the transfusion of blood from persons with *T. pallidum* bacteremia, and occasional parenteral transmission still occurs as a result of the sharing of contaminated needles.

Syphilis is most common in large cities and in young, sexually active individuals. The highest rate is found in men between the age of 20 and 29 years. In 2008, 69% of the 3141 U.S. counties reported no cases of primary or secondary syphilis, and just 26 locales accounted for about 50% of all reported infections. The disease is most prevalent in the Southeast.

Syphilis spares no class, race, or group but is more prevalent among persons living on the margins of society. U.S. syphilis rates are about eightfold greater in African Americans than in non-Hispanic whites (17.3 vs. 2.2 cases per 100,000 people). Increased numbers of different sexual partners and perhaps the indiscriminate choice of partners increase the risk of acquiring sexually transmitted disease (Chapter 293). Patients with primary and secondary syphilis name, on average, nearly three different sexual contacts within the previous 90 days. A traditional cornerstone of syphilis control has been the epidemiologic investigation and treatment of sexual contacts of patients with primary or secondary lesions and patients with early latent disease. As syphilis has become associated with drug use and anonymous sex, epidemiologic investigations have become less efficacious.

The incidence of syphilis has generally declined worldwide for more than 100 years, with the exception of periods of war or social upheaval. With the introduction of penicillin, there was a rapid decline in primary and secondary syphilis, to approximately 4 cases per 100,000 people in 1957. This decline was followed by reductions in federal expenditures for syphilis control, which resulted in a resurgence of infectious primary and secondary syphilis in the United States; peaks of more than 12 cases per 100,000 people were attained several times from 1965 through the mid-1990s. Because many cases of syphilis are not reported, the true incidence is much higher.

Over the past 40 years, syphilis epidemics have occurred serially in at least three U.S. population subgroups. In the 1970s and 1980s, men who had sex with other men accounted for a disproportionate number of the total cases of infectious syphilis. Similar trends occurred in other countries. Then, after a period of decline, U.S. syphilis rates nearly doubled from 1986 to 1990, with 50,578 cases reported in 1990 in an epidemic disproportionately affecting multiracial heterosexual men and women and occurring contemporaneously with an epidemic of crack cocaine use. After 1990, syphilis rates again declined; in 2001, there were 6103 cases of primary and secondary syphilis reported, one of the lowest numbers since 1959. The epidemic of the late 1980s probably contributed to the spread of human immunodeficiency virus (HIV) infection (see Syphilis-HIV Interactions) and to dramatic increases in the rate of congenital syphilis. Since 2000, syphilis rates have begun to increase in men, especially men infected with HIV, and they have been increasing since 2005 in women.

Patients with clinically evident late syphilis, particularly those with cardiovascular or gummatous syphilis, are becoming less common, perhaps as a result of the effectiveness of penicillin therapy for early syphilis. However, surveys indicate that there are still significant numbers of patients with untreated neurologic syphilis, especially in older age groups.

Natural Course of Untreated Syphilis

The incubation period from the time of exposure to development of the primary lesion averages approximately 21 days (range, 10 to 90 days). Initially, a painless papule develops at the site of inoculation and soon breaks down to form a clean-based ulcer—the chancre—with raised, indurated margins (Fig. 327-1A). The chancre persists for 2 to 6 weeks and then heals spontaneously. Several weeks later, a secondary stage characterized by low-grade fever, headache, malaise, generalized lymphadenopathy, and a mucocutaneous rash typically develops. There may be involvement of visceral organs. The secondary eruption may occur while the primary chancre is still healing

FIGURE 327-1. Syphilis lesions. **A,** Chancre in primary syphilis. **B,** Palmar lesions of a coppery color in secondary syphilis. **C,** Mucous patch in secondary syphilis. **D,** Condylomata lata in secondary syphilis (**A, C,** and **D,** From Forbes CD, Jackson WF. *Color Atlas and Text of Clinical Medicine,* 3rd ed. London: Mosby; 2003; **B,** From Habif TP, Cambell JI, Quitadamo MJ, et al. *Skin Disease: Diagnosis and Treatment.* St. Louis: Mosby; 2001.)

or up to several months after disappearance of the chancre. Secondary lesions also heal spontaneously within 2 to 6 weeks, and the infection then becomes latent. In more than 20% of patients with untreated latent syphilis, relapsing lesions later develop, similar to those of the secondary stage; rarely, the relapse takes the form of recurrence of the primary chancre. In the era before antibiotics, late, destructive tertiary lesions involving the eyes, the CNS, the heart, and other organs, including the skin, eventually developed in about a third of untreated patients. These lesions may occur a few years to as long as 25 years after infection.

The incidence of late complications of untreated syphilis is currently unknown, but it seems to be less than that seen previously. Cases of gumma are now so rare as to be reportable.

PATHOBIOLOGY

T. pallidum may penetrate through normal mucosal membranes and minor abrasions on epithelial surfaces. The first lesions appear at the site of primary inoculation. The minimal number of treponemes needed to establish infection is not known but may be as low as one. Multiplication of organisms is slow, with a division time in rabbits of approximately 33 hours. The slow growth of treponemes in humans probably accounts in part for the protracted nature of the illness and for the relatively long incubation period.

Syphilis is a systemic disease from the onset. Treponemes are capable of specific attachment to host cells, but it is not known whether attachment results in damage to the host cells. Most treponemes are found in the intercellular spaces, but they are occasionally seen within phagocytic cells. However, there is no evidence of prolonged intracellular survival of treponemes. *T. pallidum* is not known to produce toxins.

The primary pathologic lesion of syphilis is a focal endarteritis with an increase in adventitial cells, endothelial proliferation, and the presence of an inflammatory cuff around affected vessels. Lymphocytes, plasma cells, and monocytes predominate in the inflammatory lesion, and polymorphonuclear cells are seen in some cases. The vessel lumen is frequently obliterated. With healing, there is considerable fibrosis. Treponemes may be seen in most early lesions of syphilis and in some of the late lesions, such as the meningoencephalitis of general paresis.

Granulomatous reaction is common in secondary and late syphilis. The granulomas are histologically nonspecific, and cases of syphilis have been incorrectly diagnosed as sarcoidosis or other granulomatous diseases. Human inoculation studies suggest that the pathogenesis of the gumma, which is a granulomatous lesion, involves hypersensitivity to small numbers of virulent treponemes introduced into a previously sensitized host.

Intracutaneous inoculation of partially purified antigens of *T. pallidum* into patients with syphilis in various stages has shown that delayed cellular hypersensitivity develops only late in secondary syphilis but is uniformly present in latent syphilis. There may be temporary hyporesponsiveness of lymphocytes to treponemal antigens in patients with primary and secondary syphilis. It is possible that the waxing and waning of lesions in early syphilis depend on the balance between the development of effective cellular immunity and the suppression of thymus-derived lymphocyte function.

The host also responds to infection by producing numerous antibodies; in some instances, circulating immune complexes may be formed as well. For example, nephrotic syndrome has occasionally been recognized in secondary syphilis, and renal biopsy specimens from such patients have shown membranous glomerulonephritis characterized by focal subepithelial basement membrane deposits containing immunoglobulin G (IgG), C3, and treponemal antibody.

CLINICAL MANIFESTATIONS

Primary Syphilis

The typical lesion of primary syphilis, the chancre, is a painless, clean-based, indurated ulcer (see Fig. 327-1A). The chancre starts as a papule, but then superficial erosion results in ulceration. The borders of the ulcer are raised, firm, and indurated. Occasionally, secondary infections change the appearance and cause a painful lesion. Most chancres are single, but multiple ulcers are sometimes seen, particularly when skin folds are apposed (i.e., kissing chancres). An untreated chancre heals in several weeks and leaves a faint scar. The chancre is usually associated with regional adenopathy, which may be unilateral or bilateral. The regional nodes are movable, discrete, and rubbery. If the chancre occurs in the cervix or the rectum, the affected regional iliac nodes are not palpable.

Chancres can occur at any site of potential inoculation by direct contact, with most occurring in anogenital locations. Chancres may also be seen in the pharynx, on the tongue, around the lips, on the fingers, on the nipples, and in other diverse areas. The morphology depends in part on the area of the body where they occur and on the host's immune response. Chancres in previously infected individuals may be small and remain papular. Chancres of the finger may appear more erosive and can be quite painful. Chancres of the anal canal may be missed in men who have sex with men unless a careful examination is undertaken.

Secondary Syphilis

Between 4 and 8 weeks after the appearance of the primary chancre, signs and symptoms of secondary syphilis typically develop. Symptoms may include malaise, fever, headache, sore throat, and other systemic complaints. Most patients have generalized lymphadenopathy, including involvement of the epitrochlear nodes. Approximately 30% of patients have evidence of a healing chancre, although many patients (including a disproportionate number of women and of men who have sex with men) give no history of a primary lesion.

At least 80% of patients with secondary syphilis have cutaneous or mucocutaneous lesions at some point in their illness. The diagnosis is generally first suspected on the basis of the cutaneous eruption. The rash is often minimally symptomatic, and many patients with late syphilis do not recall primary or secondary lesions. The rashes are quite varied in appearance but have certain characteristic features. The lesions are usually widespread, are symmetrical in distribution, and are frequently pink, coppery, or dusky red (particularly the earliest macular lesions). They are generally nonpruritic, although occasional exceptions have been reported, and they are rarely vesicular or bullous in adults. They are indurated, except for the very earliest macular lesions, and frequently have a superficial scale (i.e., papulosquamous lesions). The lesions tend to be polymorphic and rounded, and on healing, they may leave residual pigmentation or depigmentation. They may be quite faint and difficult to visualize, particularly on dark-skinned individuals.

The earliest pink macular lesions are typically seen on the trunk, with later spread to the rest of the body. The face is often spared, except around the mouth. Subsequently, a papular rash appears that is usually generalized but is quite marked on the palms and soles (Fig. 327-1B). These rashes are often associated with a superficial scale and may be hyperpigmented. When the rash occurs on the face, it may be pustular and resemble acne vulgaris. Occasionally, the scale may be so great that it resembles psoriasis. Ulceration may occur and produce lesions resembling ecthyma. In malnourished or debilitated patients, extensive and destructive ulcerative lesions with a heaped-up crust may occur, the so-called rupial lesions. Lesions around the hair follicles may result in patchy alopecia of the beard or scalp.

Ringed or annular lesions may occur, especially around the face, and particularly on dark-skinned individuals. A lesion at the angle of the mouth or the corner of the nose may have a central linear erosion, the so-called split papule.

The palate and pharynx may be inflamed. In approximately 30% of secondary syphilis patients, so-called mucous patches (Fig. 327-1C) develop; these slightly raised, oval areas are covered by a grayish white membrane that, when raised, reveals a pink base that does not bleed. These lesions may be seen on the genitalia, in the mouth, or on the tongue; like condylomata lata, they are highly infectious.

In warm, moist areas such as the perineum, large, pale, flat-topped papules may coalesce to form condylomata lata (Fig. 327-1D). Papules may also be seen in the axilla and rarely occur in a generalized form. They are extremely infectious. These papules are not to be confused with the common venereal warts (i.e., condylomata acuminata), which are small, often multiple, and more sharply raised than condylomata lata.

Other manifestations of secondary syphilis include hepatitis, which has been reported in up to 10% of patients in some series. Jaundice is rare, but an elevated alkaline phosphatase level is common. Liver biopsy reveals small areas of focal necrosis and mononuclear infiltrate or periportal vasculitis. Spirochetes can often be visualized with silver stains. Periostitis with widespread lytic lesions of bone has been reported occasionally; bone scanning appears to be a sensitive test for early syphilitic osteitis. An immune complex type of nephropathy with transient nephrotic syndrome has been documented rarely. There may be iritis or an anterior uveitis. Between 10 and 30% of patients have pleocytosis in cerebrospinal fluid (CSF), but symptomatic meningitis is seen in less than 1% of patients. Symptomatic gastritis may occur.

Relapsing Syphilis

After resolution of the primary or secondary skin lesions, 20 to 30% of patients experience cutaneous recurrences. Recurrent lesions may be fewer or more firmly indurated than the initial lesions. Like the typical lesions of primary or secondary syphilis, they are infectious for exposed sexual partners.

Latent Syphilis

By definition, latent syphilis is the stage at which there are no clinical signs of syphilis and the CSF is normal. Latency, which begins when the first attack of secondary syphilis has passed and may last for a lifetime, is usually detected by reactive serologic tests for syphilis (see Diagnosis). Congenital syphilis must also be excluded before the diagnosis of latent syphilis can be made. Patients may or may not have a clinical history of earlier primary or secondary syphilis.

Latency has been divided into two stages: early and late. Most infectious relapses occur in the first year, and epidemiologic evidence shows that the most infectious period is during the first year of infection. Early latency is therefore defined as the first year after resolution of the primary or secondary lesions, or as a newly reactive serologic test for syphilis in an otherwise asymptomatic individual who has had a negative serologic test within the preceding year. Late latent syphilis is ordinarily not infectious, except for pregnant women, who can transmit infection to the fetus after many years. Most cases of latent syphilis are most accurately called latent syphilis of unknown duration and should be treated in the same manner as late latent syphilis (see later).

Late Syphilis

Late syphilis (Table 327-1) is usually slowly progressive, although certain neurologic syndromes may have a sudden onset because of endarteritis and CNS thrombosis. Late syphilis is not infectious through sexual contact. Any organ of the body may be involved, but three main types of disease can be distinguished: late benign (gummatous), cardiovascular, and neurosyphilis.

TABLE 327-1	NEWLY DIAGNOSED TERTIARY SYPHILIS IN 105 PATIENTS IN DENMARK, 1961-1970
TYPE OF TERTIARY SYPHILIS	**NO. OBSERVED***
Neurosyphilis	72
Asymptomatic	45
Tabes dorsalis	11
General paresis	13
Meningovascular	1
Optic atrophy	2
Cardiovascular syphilis	44
Aortic insufficiency	16
Aortic aneurysm	13
Uncomplicated aortitis[†]	15
Late benign syphilis (gumma)	4

*Some patients had more than one form of late syphilis.
[†]Autopsy diagnoses only.

Late Benign Syphilis

In the penicillin era, gummas are rare. They typically develop 1 to 10 years after initial infection and may involve any part of the body. Although gummas may be destructive, they respond rapidly to treatment and are therefore relatively benign. Histologically, the gumma is a granuloma.

Gummas may be solitary or multiple and most often come to medical attention as space-occupying lesions. They are usually asymmetrical and are often grouped. Gummas may start as a superficial nodule or as a deeper lesion that breaks down to form punched-out ulcers. They are ordinarily indolent, slowly progressive, and indurated on palpation. There is often central healing, with an atrophic scar surrounded by hyperpigmented borders. Cutaneous gummas may resemble other chronic granulomatous ulcerative lesions caused by tuberculosis, sarcoidosis, leprosy, and other deep fungal infections. Precise histologic diagnosis may not be possible. However, syphilitic gummas are the only such lesions to heal dramatically with penicillin therapy.

Gummas may also involve deep visceral organs, particularly the respiratory tract, gastrointestinal tract, and bones. In addition, they may involve the larynx or the pulmonary parenchyma. Gummas of the stomach may masquerade as carcinoma of the stomach or lymphoma. Gummas of the liver were once the most common form of visceral syphilis and often manifested as hepatosplenomegaly and anemia and occasionally as fever and jaundice. Skeletal gummas typically produce lesions in the long bones, skull, and clavicle; a characteristic symptom is nocturnal pain. Radiologic abnormalities, when present, include periostitis and lytic or sclerotic, destructive osteitis.

Cardiovascular Syphilis

The primary cardiovascular complications of syphilis are aortic insufficiency (Chapter 75) and aortic aneurysm (Chapter 78), usually of the ascending aorta. Less commonly, other large arteries may be affected, and involvement of the coronary ostia rarely results in coronary insufficiency. All these complications are caused by obliterative endarteritis of the vasa vasorum, with resultant damage to the intima and media of the great vessels. This damage results in dilation of the ascending aorta, but the valve cusps remain normal. An aneurysm occasionally manifests as a pulsating mass bulging through the anterior chest wall. Syphilitic aortitis may also involve the descending aorta proximal to the renal arteries.

Cardiovascular syphilis usually begins within 5 to 10 years of the initial infection but may not manifest clinically until 20 to 30 years later. Cardiovascular syphilis does not occur after congenital infection—a phenomenon that remains unexplained.

Asymptomatic aortitis is best diagnosed by visualizing linear calcifications in the wall of the ascending aorta by radiography. The signs of syphilitic aortic insufficiency are the same as for aortic insufficiency of other causes. In aortic insufficiency resulting from dilation of the aortic ring, the decrescendo murmur is often loudest along the right sternal margin. Syphilitic aneurysms may be fusiform but are more typically saccular and do not lead to aortic dissection. Between 10 and 20% of patients with cardiovascular syphilis have coexistent neurosyphilis.

Neurosyphilis

CNS involvement occurs throughout the natural history of syphilis. Neurosyphilis can be divided into five groups: asymptomatic, syphilitic meningitis, meningovascular syphilis, tabes dorsalis, and general paresis. Asymptomatic neurosyphilis can occur at any time, whereas syphilitic meningitis is most common during the secondary stage of infection. Meningovascular syphilis, tabes dorsalis, and general paresis are typically manifestations of late syphilis. The divisions are not absolute, and overlap between syndromes is typical. Current cases of neurosyphilis are likely to be variants of the classic syndromes, possibly as a result of the use of antimicrobial agents for other diseases.

Syphilitic Meningitis

Acute to subacute aseptic meningitis can occur at any time after the primary stage, but it usually occurs within the first year of infection. It frequently involves the base of the brain and may result in unilateral or bilateral cranial nerve palsies. Mild aseptic meningitis may be relatively common in patients with early syphilis, but severe disease occurs in only about 1.5% of untreated patients. Syphilitic meningitis typically resolves without treatment.

Meningovascular Syphilis

Some patients have sufficient endarteritis and perivascular inflammation to result in cerebrovascular thrombosis and infarction, generally 5 to 10 years after the initial infection. Patients frequently have associated aseptic meningitis. Most cerebrovascular accidents are not caused by syphilitic arteritis, even in patients with a reactive serologic test result for syphilis. However, syphilis should be considered a potential cause in relatively young patients with a history of syphilis and without other risk factors for cerebrovascular accidents.

Tabes Dorsalis

Tabes dorsalis, which appears to be far less common than in the pre-penicillin era, is a slowly progressive, degenerative disease that involves the posterior columns and posterior roots of the spinal cord and results in progressive loss of peripheral reflexes, impairment of vibration and position sense, and progressive ataxia. There may be chronic destructive changes in the large joints of the affected limbs in far-advanced cases (i.e., Charcot's joints). Incontinence of the bladder and impotence are common. Sudden and severely painful crises of uncertain origin are a characteristic part of the syndrome. These features typically involve the lower extremities but can occur at any site. Severe, sharp abdominal pain may lead to exploratory surgery. These attacks may be triggered by exposure to cold or other stresses or may arise with no obvious precipitating cause.

Optic atrophy is seen in 20% of cases. In 90% of patients, the pupils are bilaterally small and fail to constrict further in response to light, but they do respond normally to accommodation (i.e., Argyll Robertson pupils).

The onset of tabes dorsalis is usually first noticed 20 to 30 years after the initial infection. Its cause is unclear, and spirochetes cannot be demonstrated in the posterior column or dorsal root.

General Paresis

This form of neurosyphilis is a chronic meningoencephalitis resulting in the gradual and progressive loss of cortical function. It typically occurs 10 to 20 years after the initial infection. Pathologically, there is a perivascular and meningeal chronic inflammatory reaction, with thickening of the meninges, granular ependymitis, degeneration of the cortical parenchyma, and abundant spirochetes in tissues. In the United States, first admissions to mental hospitals because of syphilitic psychosis declined from 7694 in 1940 to 154 in 1968, the last year for which definite figures are available.

In its early stages, general paresis results in nonspecific symptoms of early dementia, such as irritability, fatigability, headaches, forgetfulness, and personality changes. Later, there is impaired memory, defective judgment, lack of insight, confusion, and often depression or marked elation. Patients may be delusional, and seizures sometimes occur. There may also be loss of other cortical functions, including paralysis or aphasia.

Physical signs are primarily those of the altered mental status. Cranial nerve palsies are uncommon, and optic atrophy is rare. The complete Argyll Robertson pupil is also uncommon, but irregular or otherwise abnormal pupils are not infrequent. Peripheral reflexes are often somewhat increased.

Syphilis-HIV Interactions

Syphilis, like other genital ulcer diseases, is associated with a three- to five-fold increased risk for acquisition of HIV infection. Presumably, genital ulcers act as portals of entry through which HIV may more readily infect exposed individuals. As a result, HIV serologic testing 3 months after a diagnosis of syphilis is recommended for all patients. Conversely, in individuals with HIV infection who acquire syphilis, the natural history of the infection may be modified. HIV-infected syphilis patients are somewhat more likely than non-HIV-infected patients to present initially with secondary syphilis. HIV-infected secondary syphilis patients are also more likely than HIV-negative secondary syphilis patients to have coexistent chancres, suggesting that the healing of chancres is delayed or the appearance of secondary manifestations is accelerated in the presence of HIV coinfection.

Congenital Syphilis

Congenital syphilis results from the transplacental, hematogenous spread of syphilis from the mother to the fetus. The incidence of congenital syphilis diagnoses in the United States fell below 1000 per year for the first time in 1975, and fewer than 500 cases occurred each year until 1988, when the epidemic of syphilis in adults led to parallel increases in congenital infections. From 1990 through 1993, more than 3000 new cases of congenital syphilis were reported each year. A Venereal Disease Research Laboratory (VDRL) test should be performed in all expectant mothers at the beginning of pregnancy and should be repeated near the end of pregnancy in women living in areas where syphilis is relatively common.

The risk for fetal infection is greatest in the early stages of untreated maternal syphilis and declines slowly thereafter, but the mother can infect her fetus during at least the first 5 years of her infection. Adequate treatment of the mother before the 16th week of pregnancy usually prevents clinical illness in the neonate. Later treatment may not prevent late sequelae of the disease in the child. Untreated maternal infection may result in stillbirth, neonatal death, prematurity, or syndromes of early or late congenital syphilis in surviving infants.

Manifestations of early congenital syphilis are often seen in the perinatal period but may not develop until the infant has been discharged from the hospital. The disease resembles secondary syphilis in adults, except that the rash may be vesicular or bullous. The child often has rhinitis, hepatosplenomegaly, hemolytic anemia, jaundice, and pseudoparalysis (i.e., immobility of one or more extremities) as a result of painful osteochondritis. There may be thrombocytopenia and leukocytosis. The early stages of congenital syphilis must be differentiated from congenital rubella, cytomegalovirus infection, toxoplasmosis, bacterial sepsis, and other diseases.

Late congenital syphilis is defined as congenital syphilis diagnosed more than 2 years after birth. The disease may remain latent, with no manifestations of late damage. Cardiovascular alterations have not been observed in patients with congenital syphilis. Neurologic manifestations are common and may include eighth cranial nerve deafness and interstitial keratitis. Periostitis may result in prominent frontal bones of the skull, depression of the bridge of the nose (saddle nose), poor development of the maxilla, and anterior bowing of the tibias (saber shins). There may be late-onset arthritis of the knees (Clutton's joints). The permanent dentition may show characteristic abnormalities known as Hutchinson's teeth; the upper central incisors are widely spaced, centrally notched, and tapered in the manner of a screwdriver. The molars may show multiple poorly developed cusps (mulberry molars).

DIAGNOSIS

Dark-Field Examination

The most definitive means of syphilis diagnosis is finding spirochetes of typical morphology and motility in lesions of early acquired or congenital syphilis. Dark-field examination is often positive in cases of primary syphilis and in patients with the moist mucosal lesions of secondary and congenital syphilis. The result may occasionally be positive for aspirates of lymph nodes in secondary syphilis. False-negative results may occur in primary syphilis because of the application of soaps, antiseptics, or other compounds toxic to *T. pallidum* to the lesions. A single negative result is therefore insufficient to exclude syphilis. For high-risk individuals (e.g., drug users, homosexually active men), it is appropriate to treat presumptively based on suspicious lesions after performing serologic tests. Confusion may also arise because of the presence of spirochetes that are morphologically indistinguishable from *T. pallidum* organisms in the mouth, particularly around the gingival margins. Living *T. pallidum* organisms demonstrate gradual motion to and fro, rotational movement around the long axis, and rather sudden 90-degree flexing near the center of the organism. Because most physicians do not have the proper equipment and are not familiar with dark-field microscopy techniques, public health authorities can be called for assistance. *T. pallidum* may also be demonstrated in biopsy or pathologic specimens by fluorescent antibody stains or by silver stains.

TABLE 327-2	SEROLOGIC TESTS FOR SYPHILIS
TYPE	**USE**
NONTREPONEMAL (ANTICARDIOLIPIN) ANTIBODIES	
VDRL (slide flocculation)	Screening, quantitation of response to treatment
RPR (circle card) (agglutination)	Screening, quantitation of response to treatment
SPECIFIC TREPONEMAL ANTIBODIES	
FTA-ABS (immunofluorescence with absorbed serum)	Confirmatory, diagnostic; not for routine screening
TP-PA (microhemagglutination)	Similar to FTA-ABS but can be quantified and automated
EIA	Confirmatory and increasingly used for screening; automated

EIA = enzyme immunoassay; FTA-ABS = fluorescent treponemal antibody absorption test; RPR = rapid plasma regain test; TP-PA = *Treponema pallidum*—particle agglutination; VDRL = Venereal Disease Research Laboratory.

TABLE 327-3	FREQUENCY OF POSITIVE SEROLOGIC TESTS IN UNTREATED SYPHILIS		
STAGE	**VDRL (%)**	**FTA-ABS (%)**	**TP-PA (%)**
Primary	70	85	50-60
Secondary	99	100	100
Latent or late	70	98	98

FTA-ABS = fluorescent treponemal antibody absorption test; TP-PA = *Treponema pallidum*–particle agglutination; VDRL = Venereal Disease Research Laboratory.

Serologic Tests

Two basic types of serologic tests (Table 327-2) are widely used to diagnose infection with *T. pallidum*: (1) nontreponemal tests that detect antibodies reactive with diphosphatidylglycerol (cardiolipin), which is a normal component of many tissues, and (2) tests that detect antibodies to specific treponemal antigens.

Nontreponemal Tests

The standard tests to detect anticardiolipin antibody are the VDRL and rapid plasma reagin (RPR) tests, which are slide flocculation tests. The VDRL and RPR are readily quantified, so they are the tests of choice for monitoring patients' responses to treatment. The relative proportion of patients with a false-positive VDRL result depends on the prevalence of syphilis in the community; the lower the prevalence of syphilis, the higher the proportion of reactive VDRL test results from nonsyphilitic causes.

The VDRL test begins to turn positive less than 1 week after onset of the chancre; thus, a nonreactive VDRL test does not exclude primary syphilis, particularly if the lesion is less than 1 week old. The VDRL test result is positive in 99% of patients with secondary syphilis (Table 327-3). Patients with advanced HIV infection may have negative test results, and some patients have such high titers of antibody that they are in antibody excess; dilution of their serum paradoxically results in conversion of a negative test result to a positive one, the so-called prozone reaction. VDRL reactivity tends to diminish in later stages of syphilis, and only about 70% of patients with cardiovascular or neurosyphilis have positive VDRL test results.

The *quantitative titer* of the VDRL or RPR test is somewhat useful in diagnosis and is quite useful for monitoring the therapeutic response. The titer is reported as the highest dilution that gives a positive response. Most patients with secondary syphilis have titers of at least 1:16. Most patients with false-positive VDRL test results have titers of less than 1:8. No single titer is diagnostic by itself. Significant rises (four-fold or greater) in paired sera, however, strongly indicate acute syphilis.

Treponemal Tests

Several types of treponemal tests are widely used. Agglutination of particles to which *T. pallidum* antigens have been fixed is the basis of the *T. pallidum* particle agglutination (TP-PA) test. More recently, treponemal enzyme immunoassays (EIAs) have become available from several manufacturers and have gained favor because of their low cost and ease of use.

The treponemal tests are best used to confirm that persons with reactive nontreponemal tests have antibodies to *T. pallidum*. Results of treponemal tests are not reliably quantified. They are sensitive and have a high degree of specificity, in that only approximately 1% of normal individuals have reactive treponemal tests. They are reactive in 85% of patients with primary syphilis, 99% with secondary syphilis, and at least 95% with late syphilis. They may therefore be the only test with a positive result in patients with cardiovascular or neurologic syphilis. For patients with late syphilis, treponemal tests often remain reactive for life, despite adequate therapy. The fluorescent treponemal antibody absorption (FTA-ABS) test is reported in terms of relative brilliance of fluorescence, from borderline to 4 plus, and most laboratories report only tests with 2 plus or greater reactivity as positive. For patients lacking historical or clinical evidence of syphilis but with a reactive FTA-ABS test result, the test should be repeated. Use of another treponemal test, such as the TP-PA test, may be helpful in problem cases. The TP-PA test is slightly less sensitive than the VDRL or FTA-ABS test in primary syphilis. Its sensitivity and specificity are otherwise nearly identical to those of the FTA-ABS test.

EIAs for the detection of antitreponemal antibodies use cloned *T. pallidum* antigens generated from bacterial expression systems. EIA serologic tests permit the screening of large numbers of sera and have performance characteristics (sensitivity, specificity, predictive values) similar to those of other treponemal tests. Persons with syphilis diagnosed by treponemal antigen EIAs should be tested with quantitative nontreponemal tests such as the VDRL or RPR for confirmation and to permit the use of these tests to evaluate the subsequent response to therapy.

Differential Diagnosis

The differential diagnosis of a genital ulcer (Chapter 293) includes genital herpes (Chapter 382), chancroid (Chapter 309), lymphogranuloma venereum (Chapter 326), and a number of other ulcerative processes. Classically, herpetic ulcers are multiple, painful, superficial, and, if seen early, vesicular. However, atypical manifestations may be indistinguishable from a syphilitic chancre. Genital herpes is much more common than syphilis and is now the most common cause of a "typical chancre" in North America. Syphilitic chancres may also be coinfected with herpes simplex virus in about 15% of cases. The ulcers of chancroid are usually painful, often multiple, and frequently exudative and nonindurated. Lymphogranuloma venereum may produce a small, papular lesion associated with regional adenopathy. Other conditions that must be distinguished include granuloma inguinale (Chapter 324), drug eruptions, carcinoma, superficial fungal infections (Chapter 446), traumatic lesions, and lichen planus (Chapter 446). In most cases, the final distinction is based on dark-field examination, which is positive only in syphilis, and on serologic test results.

The differential diagnosis of the skin lesions of secondary syphilis includes pityriasis rosea (Chapter 446), which can be differentiated by the occurrence of lesions along lines of skin cleavage and frequently by the presence of a herald patch. Drug eruptions, acute febrile exanthems, psoriasis, lichen planus, scabies, and other diseases must also be considered in some cases. A mucous patch may superficially resemble oral candidiasis (i.e., thrush). Infectious mononucleosis (Chapter 385) may appear very similar to secondary syphilis, with sore throat, generalized adenopathy, hepatitis, and a generalized rash. Hepatitis (Chapter 150) may also cause confusion.

False-Positive Serologic Test Results for Syphilis

The VDRL or RPR test is reactive in patients with other treponemal diseases such as pinta, yaws, and endemic syphilis (Chapter 328). These tests may also be falsely reactive in persons who do not have treponemal infections based on a negative clinical history or negative results of serum treponemal tests.

Acute (<6 months) false-positive VDRL test results occur with low frequency in patients with atypical pneumonia, malaria, and other bacterial or viral infections, and they may occur after smallpox or other vaccinations as well. Chronic false-positive VDRL test results (persisting >6 months) are relatively common in patients with autoimmune disorders such as systemic lupus erythematosus (SLE; Chapter 274), parenteral drug users, HIV-infected patients, patients with leprosy, and the aged. Between 8 and 20% of patients with SLE have false-positive VDRL test results. Chronic false-positive VDRL test results in female patients 20 years or younger indicate a significant risk for the future development of SLE, thyroiditis, or other autoimmune disorders. As many as a third of parenteral drug users have

false-positive VDRL test results. More than 1% of persons 70 years old and 10% of those older than 80 also have low-titer, false-positive VDRL test results. In most cases of false-positive VDRL tests, the titer is less than 1:8, although a few patients with lymphoma and other diseases have very high-titer, false-positive results.

There is also an increased incidence of false-positive treponemal test results in other chronic inflammatory diseases associated with hyperglobulinemia, including rheumatoid arthritis and biliary cirrhosis. Occasionally, reproducible positive FTA-ABS results are obtained in patients with no clinical or historical evidence of syphilis and no evidence of diseases typically associated with false-positive FTA-ABS results. If the diagnosis is in doubt and if the patient is not allergic to penicillin, it is often prudent to treat for possible syphilis.

Neurosyphilis

Asymptomatic neurosyphilis is diagnosed when there are CSF abnormalities, such as lymphocytic pleocytosis, protein elevation, or a reactive VDRL test result, in a syphilis patient in the absence of signs and symptoms of neurologic disease. Although numerous other processes can cause CSF pleocytosis or protein elevations, false-positive CSF VDRL test results are rare in the absence of a traumatic tap. If the CSF is normal 2 years or longer after the initial infection, a positive CSF finding is not likely to develop later. Routine lumbar punctures to examine CSF are not indicated in early syphilis unless the patient is known to have HIV infection. Lumbar puncture in HIV-infected persons with early syphilis is the subject of controversy. Although a nonreactive CSF FTA-ABS result may be useful to rule out the diagnosis, no diagnosis of neurosyphilis should be based solely on the CSF FTA-ABS test.

In syphilitic meningitis, the CSF shows a lymphocytic pleocytosis, with increased protein and usually normal glucose concentrations. The CSF VDRL test is nearly always reactive. Rarely, the CSF glucose concentration is decreased. Without treatment, syphilitic meningitis generally resolves, similar to the course of other manifestations of early syphilis. This syndrome can mimic tuberculous or fungal meningitis or nonpurulent meningitis of various causes.

In tabes dorsalis, the VDRL test for serum is nonreactive in as many as 30 to 40% of patients, and 10 to 20% of patients (even before the advent of penicillin) have normal CSF VDRL results. The FTA-ABS test for serum is nearly always reactive.

In general paresis, the CSF is nearly always abnormal, with lymphocytic pleocytosis and an increased total protein concentration. The VDRL test is usually reactive for CSF and serum.

Congenital Syphilis

Because many infants with congenital syphilis may be clinically normal at birth but develop serious, symptomatic disease some weeks later, it is important to determine whether a newborn with a reactive VDRL or FTA-ABS test result has passively transferred maternal antibody or is actively infected. If the mother has been adequately treated for syphilis during pregnancy and the infant is clinically normal at birth, one option is to monitor the infant carefully by serial examinations and VDRL titers. If the reactive VDRL result for the infant is caused by passively transferred maternal antibody, the titer will fall markedly in the first 2 months of life; a rising titer indicates active disease and the need for treatment. However, the risk of improper follow-up of VDRL-positive but clinically normal neonates makes the immediate empirical administration of effective therapy an attractive alternative.

TREATMENT

T. pallidum is inhibited by less than 0.01 µg/mL of penicillin G. Because treponemes divide slowly and penicillin acts only on dividing cells, it is necessary to maintain serum levels of penicillin for many days (Table 327-4).

Early Infectious Syphilis

Early syphilis (<1 year) can be treated with a single injection of 2.4 million U of benzathine penicillin G, which provides low but effective serum levels for more than 2 weeks and cures approximately 95% of patients. It is not necessary to examine CSF at this stage because penicillin prevents the later development of neurosyphilis.

Individuals with other sexually transmitted diseases may have been exposed to syphilis at the time they became infected. Treatment with a single dose of β-lactam antibiotics (penicillins, cephalosporins), which provide relatively high

TABLE 327-4 PENICILLIN TREATMENT FOR SYPHILIS AS RECOMMENDED BY THE U.S. PUBLIC HEALTH SERVICE

INDICATIONS FOR SYPHILIS THERAPY*	Dosage and Administration†	
	BENZATHINE PENICILLIN G	AQUEOUS BENZYLPENICILLIN G OR PROCAINE PENICILLIN G
Primary, secondary, and early latent syphilis (<1 yr); epidemiologic treatment	Total of 2.4 million U; single IM dose of two injections of 1.2 million U in one session	Total of 4.8 million U IM in doses of 600,000 U/day for 8 consecutive days
Late latent (>1 yr) or when CSF was not examined in "latency"; cardiovascular syphilis, late benign (cutaneous, osseous, visceral gumma)	Total of 7.2 million U IM in doses of 2.4 million U at 7-day intervals over a 21-day period	Total of 9 million U IM in doses of 600,000 U/day over a 15-day period
Symptomatic or asymptomatic neurosyphilis	2-4 million U aqueous (crystalline) penicillin G IV q4h for at least 10 days	2-4 million U procaine penicillin IM daily and probenecid 500 mg orally four times daily, for 10-14 days
Congenital		
Infants	CSF normal: Total of 50,000 U/kg IM in a single or divided dose at one session	CSF abnormal: Total of 50,000 U/kg/day IM for 10 consecutive days‡
Older children	CSF normal: Same as for early congenital syphilis, up to 2.4 million U	CSF abnormal: 200,000-300,000 U/kg/day aqueous crystalline penicillin IV for 10-14 days

*In *pregnancy,* treatment depends on the stage of syphilis.
†Individual doses can be divided for injection in each buttock to minimize discomfort.
‡For aqueous penicillin, give in two divided intravenous doses per day; for procaine penicillin, give as one daily dose intramuscularly.
CSF = cerebrospinal fluid.

serum levels for a brief period, is ineffective in established early syphilis but is curative if the disease is still in the incubating stage. The ceftriaxone regimen used for gonorrhea (Chapter 307) is probably curative for incubating syphilis, but careful follow-up is indicated if there is reason to suspect exposure to syphilis in a patient treated for gonorrhea with ceftriaxone. Single-dose therapy with 2.0 g of azithromycin administered orally was as effective as benzathine penicillin therapy in several studies of early syphilis, but treatment failures have been reported in persons with coexistent HIV infection.■ Currently, azithromycin should not be used for the treatment of early syphilis unless close follow-up can be ensured.

For patients allergic to penicillin, 100 mg of doxycycline orally twice daily for 14 days is recommended. Particularly careful follow-up is necessary for patients treated with drugs other than penicillin because they may not be fully compliant with these prolonged courses of oral therapy and these regimens have been less fully evaluated clinically. Ceftriaxone, given in doses of 500 mg to 1.0 g intramuscularly daily for 10 days, may be effective but has been studied only in small numbers of patients with syphilis. Quinolone antibiotics have essentially no effect on syphilis.

Syphilis of More than 1 Year's Duration

Prolonged therapy with intramuscular injections of 2.4 million U of benzathine penicillin G weekly for 3 weeks is recommended for the treatment of late latent syphilis and latent syphilis of unknown duration. Limited evidence suggests that treating latent syphilis with a total dose of 7.2 million U of benzathine penicillin over a 3-week period is curative, even if the patient has asymptomatic neurosyphilis. However, because of the possible lack of efficacy of benzathine penicillin G in some patients with CNS syphilis, CSF examination should be considered in those with latent syphilis to exclude asymptomatic neurosyphilis, particularly HIV-positive patients, in whom the prevalence of asymptomatic neurosyphilis is higher. Alternatively, a lumbar puncture can be performed at the conclusion of the follow-up period (2 years); if the CSF is normal, the patient can be reassured that neurosyphilis will not develop.

Larger doses of penicillin are recommended for persons with proven neurosyphilis (see Table 327-4). General paresis responds well to penicillin therapy if administered early, although progressive neurologic decline may develop later in as many as a third of treated patients. Carbamazepine in doses of 400 to 800 mg/day reportedly treats the lightning pains of tabes dorsalis effectively. Published studies show that a total of 6.0 to 9.0 million U of penicillin G results in a satisfactory clinical response in approximately 90% of patients with neurosyphilis who do not have HIV infection. There are anecdotal reports of increased treatment failures in patients with concomitant HIV infection, and there is considerable rationale to treat these patients with intravenous penicillin G (20 million U/day for at least 10 days). Therapy for neurosyphilis can result in increased CSF pleocytosis for 7 to 10 days after starting treatment and may transiently convert a normal CSF to abnormal.

Although there is no evidence that therapy with antimicrobial drugs is clinically beneficial in patients with cardiovascular syphilis, treatment is recommended to prevent further progression of disease and because approximately 15% of patients with cardiovascular syphilis have associated neurosyphilis. If patients are allergic to penicillin, it is mandatory that the CSF be examined before therapy is undertaken; if the CSF is abnormal, desensitization to penicillin is generally recommended. With a normal CSF, tetracycline (500 mg orally four times a day) or doxycycline (100 mg orally two times a day) taken for 4 weeks is probably effective.

Syphilis in Pregnancy

Because of the risk to the fetus, evaluation and treatment of a pregnant VDRL-positive patient must be rapid, particularly those first seen in the later stages of pregnancy. If a confirmatory FTA-ABS test is positive and the patient has not been treated, penicillin should be administered in doses appropriate for early or late syphilis, as outlined earlier. For penicillin-allergic patients, penicillin desensitization is preferred; patients should not be treated with tetracycline or erythromycin because of toxicity (tetracycline) or lack of efficacy (erythromycin). For patients who are VDRL positive but FTA-ABS negative and have no clinical signs of syphilis, treatment may be withheld; a quantitative VDRL test and another FTA-ABS test should be repeated in 4 weeks. If the VDRL titer has risen four-fold or more, or if clinical signs of syphilis have developed, the patient should be treated. If, after repeat examination, the diagnosis remains equivocal, the patient should be treated to prevent possible disease in the neonate. After treatment, a quantitative VDRL titer should be monitored monthly; if it rises four-fold, the patient should be treated a second time.

Congenital Syphilis

Proper treatment of the mother usually prevents active congenital syphilis in the neonate. However, infected infants may be clinically normal at birth, and the infant may be seronegative if the mother's infection was acquired late in pregnancy. The infant should be treated at birth if the mother has received no treatment or inadequate treatment or has been treated with drugs other than penicillin, if the mother has not yet responded to possibly effective therapy, or if the infant cannot be carefully monitored for several months after birth. The infant's CSF should be examined before treatment. If the CSF is normal, the child can be treated with a single intramuscular injection of 50,000 U/kg (up to 2.4 million U) of benzathine penicillin G. If the CSF is abnormal, the infant should be treated with 50,000 U/kg of aqueous penicillin G given intramuscularly or intravenously twice daily for a minimum of 10 days. Alternatively, a single daily intramuscular injection of 50,000 U/kg of procaine penicillin may be given for 10 days. Antimicrobial agents other than penicillin are not recommended for treating congenital syphilis.

Jarisch-Herxheimer Reactions

Up to 60% of patients with early syphilis and a significant proportion of patients with later stages of syphilis experience a transient febrile reaction after therapy for syphilis. The pathogenesis is unclear, but it may be caused by the liberation of antigens from spirochetes.

This reaction usually occurs in the first few hours after therapy, peaks at 6 to 8 hours, and disappears within 12 to 24 hours of therapy. Occasionally, Jarisch-Herxheimer reactions are mistaken for allergic reactions to syphilis therapy. Temperature elevation is usually low grade, and there is often associated myalgia, headache, and malaise. The skin lesions of secondary syphilis are frequently exacerbated during the Jarisch-Herxheimer reaction, and cutaneous lesions that were not visible may become visible. The reaction is generally of no clinical significance and in most cases can be treated with salicylates. Corticosteroids have been used to prevent adverse effects of the Jarisch-Herxheimer reaction, but there is no evidence that they are clinically beneficial (other than reducing fever) or necessary. Institution of treatment with small doses of penicillin does not prevent the reaction.

PREVENTION

All patients with syphilis should be reported to public health authorities. In the absence of an effective vaccine, control of syphilis depends on finding and treating persons with infectious lesions of primary and secondary syphilis before they can transmit the disease, as well as finding and treating individuals with incubating syphilis before infectious lesions develop. All patients with early syphilis (primary, secondary, or early latent) should be carefully interviewed by qualified persons to determine the nature of their recent sexual contacts. Approximately 16% of the named recent contacts of patients with early syphilis are found to have active, untreated syphilis on examination, and a similar proportion of individuals named as suspects or associates also have active syphilis.

Treatment of the sexual contacts of patients with early syphilis with 2.4 million U of benzathine penicillin G intramuscularly is recommended even if the contacts are clinically and serologically normal on examination. This is because syphilis eventually develops in 30% of clinically normal contacts who are untreated. In general, preventive treatment is given to all sexual contacts in the past 90 days, although nearly all cases of syphilis in contacts develop within 60 days of exposure.

PROGNOSIS

Follow-up Examinations

All HIV-seronegative patients with early or congenital syphilis should return for quantitative VDRL titers and clinical examination 6 and 12 months after treatment. For HIV-positive patients, serologic tests should be repeated at 1, 2, 3, 6, 9, and 12 months. Patients with late latent syphilis should also be examined 24 months after therapy.

In about 85% of patients with early (i.e., primary, secondary, or early latent) syphilis, quantitative VDRL titers decline two or more dilutions (four-fold) by 6 and 12 months after therapy. Prolonged reactive VDRL test results are associated with higher initial VDRL titers, prolonged infection, more advanced stage (primary < secondary < early latent), or repeated infection. Chronic, low-titer VDRL reactivity after therapy is much more common in cases of late syphilis and should not be viewed with alarm. Treponemal tests may remain positive for years despite adequate therapy. A four-fold or greater rise in VDRL titer after therapy is sufficient evidence for repeat treatment. Patients with treated early syphilis are susceptible to reinfection, and many clinical and serologic relapses after therapy are probably reinfections. As such, they represent failures of proper epidemiologic case finding and preventive therapy for the patient's sexual contacts.

Patients with neurosyphilis should be monitored with serologic tests for at least 3 years and with repeat CSF examinations at 6-month intervals. CSF pleocytosis is the first abnormality to disappear, but cell counts may not be normal for 1 to 2 years. Elevated CSF protein levels fall even more slowly, followed by a change in the positive CSF VDRL test, which may take years to become negative. It is not known whether high-dose intravenous penicillin therapy accelerates the return of CSF to normal. Rising CSF cell counts, protein, and VDRL titer obtained at follow-up are an indication for repeat treatment.

Antibiotic therapy should ultimately cure essentially all patients with early or secondary syphilis, although treatment failures may occur in patients with concomitant HIV infection. In tabes dorsalis, penicillin usually arrests progression but does not reverse the symptoms. Meningovascular syphilis generally responds well, except for residual damage resulting from ischemic infarcts.

Visit expertconsult.com for e-expanded chapter

1. Hook EW, Behets F, Van Damme K, et al. A phase III equivalence trial of azithromycin versus benzathine penicillin G for treatment of early syphilis. *J Infect Dis.* 2010;201:1729-1735.

SUGGESTED READINGS

French P, Gomberg M, Janier M, et al. IUSTI: 2008 European guidelines on the management of syphilis. *Int J STD AIDS.* 2009;20:300-309. *Consensus guidelines.*

Tucker JD, Bu J, Brown LB, et al. Accelerating worldwide syphilis screening through rapid testing: a systematic review. *Lancet Infect Dis.* 2010;10:381-386. *Review of several available rapid tests, with a focus on the best evaluated immunochromatographic strip test to detect* Treponema *antibody.*

Wolff T, Shelton E, Sessions C, et al. Screening for syphilis infection in pregnant women: evidence for the U.S. Preventive Services Task Force reaffirmation recommendation statement. *Ann Intern Med.* 2009; 150:710-716. *New evidence to support universal screening of pregnant women for syphilis.*

Workowski KA, Berman S; Centers for Disease Control and Prevention (CDC). Sexually transmitted diseases treatment guidelines, 2010. *MMWR Recomm Rep.* 2010;59:1-110. *National recommendations.*

328

NONSYPHILITIC TREPONEMATOSES

EDWARD W. HOOK III

DEFINITION

The nonsyphilitic treponematoses—yaws, endemic syphilis (previously known as bejel), and pinta—are the spirochetal diseases caused by *Treponema pallidum* subspecies (yaws and endemic syphilis) or by the closely related organism *Treponema carateum* (pinta). Like syphilis, the nonsyphilitic treponematoses are usually transmitted through direct contact with an infectious cutaneous or mucosal lesion. The natural history of the nonsyphilitic treponematoses also has a number of similarities to that of syphilis (Chapter 327).

The Pathogen

Yaws is caused by *T. pallidum* subspecies *pertenue,* pinta is caused by *T. carateum,* and endemic syphilis is caused by *T. pallidum* subspecies *endemicum.* The *T. pallidum* subspecies causing nonsyphilitic treponematoses are closely related to *T. pallidum* subspecies *pallidum,* which causes venereal syphilis; there is a high degree of DNA homology, and they share unique pathogen-restricted antigens. Analyses of recently described genetic sequence variations among *T. pallidum* subspecies promise the eventual clarification of pathophysiologic differences among the subspecies, as well as answers to the age-old question of the origins of syphilis. Like *T. pallidum,* these treponemes are spirochetal bacteria with helical structures and measure about 0.2 µm in diameter and 10 µm in length. They are visible by dark-field microscopy but cannot be cultivated for prolonged periods in vitro.

EPIDEMIOLOGY

Worldwide, the nonsyphilitic treponematoses are rare. However, rates appear to be increasing (particularly for yaws) in some regions where previous World Health Organization (WHO)–coordinated control programs had dramatically reduced disease prevalence. Yaws is prevalent in moist, humid regions, including rural areas of tropical Africa, the Americas, Southeast Asia, and Oceania. The highest incidence occurs in children between 2 and 5 years of age. Endemic syphilis occurs in more arid climates, including Africa, eastern Mediterranean countries, the Arabian peninsula, central Asia, and Australia. Pinta occurs in rural areas of tropical Central and South America and affects mostly older children and adolescents. Humans are the only known carriers of the nonsyphilitic treponematoses. The spirochete enters the skin only after it is broken, such as by a scratch or an insect bite. Transmission is believed to occur by contacting the skin directly or by indirect contamination through hands or fomites; it is facilitated by conditions of poor personal hygiene and crowding.

PATHOBIOLOGY

Primary nodular or ulcerative lesions typically develop at sites of inoculation after an incubation period of several weeks. Untreated primary lesions serve as a source for local spread through scratching or for hematogenous dissemination, which gives rise to a secondary stage of infection characterized by the development of widespread manifestations involving the skin, lymph nodes, and bone or cartilage. Without therapy, the primary and secondary manifestations of infection resolve, and the infection becomes latent; however, periodic recurrent secondary manifestations may occur for several years. A proportion of persons with long-standing untreated infection are at risk for late sequelae, which may include bony deformity, destruction of nasal cartilage, or chronic skin changes. Unlike syphilis, the nonsyphilitic treponematoses are primarily diseases of children, are not transmitted across the placenta, and do not invade the central nervous system.

CLINICAL MANIFESTATIONS

Yaws, the most common nonsyphilitic treponematosis, produces a skin papule at the inoculation site after an incubation period of 3 to 4 weeks. The most common sites are the legs and buttocks. The papule enlarges, ulcerates, and forms a serous crust from which treponemes can be recovered. Regional lymphadenitis may accompany the papule, which heals spontaneously within

6 months. A generalized secondary rash occurs before or after the initial lesion heals; this rash is also papular and is often covered with brown crusts. Relapsing crops of lesions can occur. Papillomas may result, and the plantar surfaces of the feet are involved with hyperkeratotic lesions. Periostitis of the long bones leads to tenderness, and fever may be present. Relapsing lesions of early yaws may occur over a period of several years and result in chronic ulcerations and destructive gummatous lesions affecting the skin and bones.

Endemic syphilis produces patches on the mucous membranes of the oral cavity and pharynx and can cause split papules at the mucocutaneous junction of the oral angles. Anal, genital, and other intertriginous skin areas can be affected by lesions that resemble secondary syphilis. Regional lymphadenitis is common, and generalized rashes are rare. Healing of these early lesions is followed by latency, manifested as seropositivity, or by late lesions that resemble gummatous tertiary syphilis. Lesions include nodular skin ulcers, bone deformities, and ulcerative lesions that can perforate the palate.

Pinta starts similarly as a cutaneous papule with regional lymphadenitis, followed by a generalized maculopapular eruption. One to 3 years after healing of the initial lesion, large hyperpigmented brown or blue macules develop; they subsequently lose their pigment and become white. The time required for lesions to pass through these stages varies, so the same patient may have coexisting areas of increased pigment and loss of pigment.

DIAGNOSIS

The clinical differentiation of the nonsyphilitic treponematoses from one another and from syphilis may be challenging, requiring the integration of epidemiologic features, clinical findings, and supportive but not diagnostic laboratory test results. The skin lesions of the endemic treponematoses may resemble other cutaneous processes, including impetigo (Chapter 447), cutaneous fungal infections (Chapter 446), and other diseases. By dark-field microscopy, the causative spirochetes from early skin lesions can be observed directly. There is no specific test for any of the nonsyphilitic treponematoses, but serologic tests for syphilis detect cross-reacting antibodies in these diseases. The rapid plasma reagin (RPR) test, the Venereal Disease Research Laboratory (VDRL) test, and the fluorescent treponemal antibody absorption (FTA-ABS) test, as well as other specific treponemal tests, give positive results if serum is obtained at least 2 weeks after the lesions initially appear.

PREVENTION

The prevalence of these diseases was reduced in the 1950s by mass penicillin treatment campaigns in areas where they were prevalent. The WHO treated about 53 million cases of yaws and 350,000 cases of pinta in the 1950s, with good results. These campaigns, however, were not adequate to eradicate the disease, and in recent years, the prevalence of yaws has increased, with foci of infection now reported in sub-Saharan Africa; several Pacific islands, including Indonesia; and the Amazon region of South America. Current estimates are that as many as 2.5 million persons are infected worldwide, 75% of whom are younger than 15 years. Although penicillin is effective for the prevention of infection in exposed persons, it has been suggested that reduction in transmission requires improvements in sanitation and in the economic standards of people living in endemic areas.

TREATMENT AND PROGNOSIS   Rx

Single-dose, long-acting benzathine penicillin G, 1.2 million U intramuscularly, is the preferred treatment in patients with early lesions. For patients with late manifestations, this therapy should be repeated twice at approximately 7-day intervals. The early lesions heal rapidly, and most seropositive cases convert to seronegative status. Late destructive lesions take longer to show improvement.

SUGGESTED READINGS

Fegan D, Glennon MJ, Thami Y, et al. Resurgence of yaws in Tanna, Vanuatu: time for a new approach? *Trop Doct.* 2010;40:68-69. *The disease has a prevalence of almost 30% but remains sensitive to intramuscular benzathine penicillin or oral azithromycin.*

Mitjà O, Hays R, Ipai AS, et al. Osteoperiostitis in early yaws: case series and literature review. *Clin Infect Dis.* 2011;52:771-774. *A complication occurring weeks after the primary infection but responding to benzyl-penicillin therapy.*

Satter EK, Tokarz VA. Secondary yaws: an endemic treponemal infection. *Pediatr Dermatol.* 2010;27:364-367. *This endemic condition in some locales may be brought to the U.S. by travelers.*

329

LYME DISEASE

GARY P. WORMSER

DEFINITION

Lyme disease (also known as Lyme borreliosis) is a zoonotic infection transmitted by certain *Ixodes* tick species and caused by a group of related spirochetes referred to formally as *Borrelia burgdorferi* sensu lato or, more simply, as Lyme borrelia. Lyme disease was first described in 1977 following the investigation of a cluster of cases of arthritis among children living in the area of Lyme, Connecticut. With more than 25,000 cases reported annually, it is the most common vector-borne infection in the United States; Lyme disease is also an infection of public health importance in both Europe and Asia. The most common clinical manifestation is a characteristic skin lesion called erythema migrans. This lesion is a result of inflammation associated with the centrifugal spread of the spirochete within the skin from the site where the tick deposited the microorganism. The spirochete may also spread hematogenously to other skin locations, resulting in secondary erythema migrans skin lesions, or to nonskin sites such as the joints, nervous system, or heart, leading to a variety of extracutaneous clinical manifestations.

The Pathogen

In the United States, the only species of Lyme borrelia known to cause human infection is *B. burgdorferi* (also referred to as *B. burgdorferi* sensu stricto). Although *B. burgdorferi* also causes Lyme disease in Europe, collectively, other species of Lyme borrelia that can be distinguished genotypically account for the majority of infections there, especially *Borrelia afzelii* and *Borrelia garinii*. The fact that at least six species of Lyme borrelia cause infection in Europe has created serodiagnostic challenges and accounts for a wider variety of clinical manifestations there than occur in the United States (see later). *B. garinii* appears to be the most neurotropic and *B. burgdorferi* the most arthritogenic among the species of Lyme borrelia.

Lyme borrelia are motile, microaerophilic, spirochetal bacteria with 3 to 10 loose coils arranged in a helical shape. The cells are 10 to 30 μm long and 0.2 to 0.5 μm wide and contain at least seven periplasmic flagella that are responsible for the organism's motility. Borrelia are too thin to be seen by Gram stain, but live organisms can be visualized by dark-field or phase-contrast microscopy. In tissues they can be recognized by light microscopy after application of silver stains or by fluorescent microscopic methods. *B. burgdorferi* was the first spirochete for which the complete genome was sequenced. Genetic studies suggest the nearly complete absence of biosynthetic pathways, making the microorganism dependent on its environment for nutritional requirements. Lyme borrelia can be grown in vitro in a highly enriched culture medium.

EPIDEMIOLOGY

In the United States, more than 90% of human cases are concentrated in just 10 middle Atlantic, northeastern, and north-central states. New York and the nearby states of Connecticut, Pennsylvania, and New Jersey have the largest number of cases. *Ixodes scapularis* (also known as the deer tick or black-legged tick) is the tick vector in these 10 states. *Ixodes pacificus* is the vector for the cases that occur in the northwestern United States. Lyme disease also occurs in limited areas of Canada. Cases of Lyme disease occur throughout the temperate regions of Europe and are especially common in Scandinavia and the countries of central Europe such as Slovenia, Austria, and Germany. *Ixodes ricinus* transmits the infection in Europe, and *Ixodes persulcatus* is the vector in Asian Russia, China, and Japan.

The principal reservoirs for Lyme borrelia (i.e., the source of infection for ticks) in the United States and Eurasia are small mammals such as mice and certain species of birds. Deer play an essential role in the life cycle of the *I. scapularis* tick, but they are not a competent reservoir for *B. burgdorferi*.

Although Lyme borrelia exist in enzootic cycles in the southern United States, cases of Lyme disease arising indigenously have not been well documented in states south of Virginia. A skin lesion that resembles erythema migrans does occur in the southern United States, but it is associated with the bite of the *Amblyomma americanum* tick, a species that is not a competent

FIGURE 329-1. From left to right is an unfed nymphal stage *Ixodes scapularis* tick, a nymphal stage *I. scapularis* tick after about 48 hours of feeding, a nymphal stage *I. scapularis* tick after about 126 hours of feeding, and a sesame seed. The distance between the ruler marks is 1 mm. (Courtesy Kam Truhn, Fordham University.)

vector for *B. burgdorferi*. This condition, whose cause is unknown, is referred to as southern tick-associated rash illness (STARI).

The likelihood of acquiring Lyme disease is directly related to exposure to environments where infected ticks are present. Of the three feeding stages in the life cycle of *I. scapularis*, the second, or nymphal, stage is most important epidemiologically for the transmission of infection to humans. Ticks in the first, or larval, stage are uninfected and cannot transmit the infection because transovarian transmission of this spirochete does not occur. Although ticks in the third, or adult, stage are more likely to be infected with *B. burgdorferi* than those in the nymphal stage, they are less important in terms of transmission to humans because they are present in smaller numbers in the environment and there is less human activity outdoors during the periods in the spring and fall when the ticks are seeking blood meals. In addition, adult ticks are larger, and their bites cause more skin irritation than the bites of nymphal ticks, thereby increasing the likelihood that they will be noticed and detached by a person who has been bitten. If not removed, *Ixodes* ticks usually feed for at least 3 days (Fig. 329-1). Transmission of *B. burgdorferi* by *I. scapularis* or *I. pacificus* ticks is typically delayed for more than 36 hours from the start of the blood meal, providing the opportunity to prevent infection simply by finding and removing the tick. Transmission of *B. afzelii* by the European tick *I. ricinus* is considerably faster, often occurring within the first 24 hours of feeding.

Most cases of erythema migrans in the United States occur from June through August, coinciding with exposure to the nymphal stage of the tick. Like most tick-borne infections, there is a slight male predominance. There is a bimodal age distribution, with the highest incidences in children aged 5 to 9 years and in adults aged 55 to 59 years, but individuals of all ages are at risk. The reported incidence of Lyme disease in the United States is rising, partially as a result of an expansion of the deer population and the spread of infected *I. scapularis* ticks to new geographic areas.

Extracutaneous manifestations are somewhat less likely than erythema migrans to occur in June through August because the interval between infection and the onset of these manifestations is longer. Because adult *I. scapularis* ticks may become active on warm days during the winter, cases of erythema migrans occasionally occur in the colder months.

PATHOBIOLOGY

B. burgdorferi resides in the midgut of the *Ixodes* tick through attachment of its outer surface protein A (OspA) to the cells lining this site. With the onset of the blood meal, changes in pH, temperature, and probably other factors induce the spirochete to increase in number and undergo a sequence of phenotypic changes, including downregulation of OspA expression and upregulation of another outer surface protein, OspC. This series of events releases the spirochete from the midgut and permits its migration to the salivary gland. At that site, OspC binds Salp 15, a salivary protein induced during the blood meal in borrelia-infected ticks; this protects the spirochete from antibody-mediated killing and aids in transmission to a vertebrate host. *Ixodes* tick saliva also contains other components with anti-inflammatory and immunomodulatory effects that serve to promote infection with Lyme

borrelia and other tick-transmitted pathogens. Expression of OspC by the spirochete in the mammalian host is essential for infection to be established; in some manner, this protein protects the microorganism from immediate elimination by the innate immune system.

The spirochete is deposited by the tick into the skin rather than directly into the blood stream. Hematogenous dissemination seems to be responsible for spread of the spirochete to other sites, but much remains to be learned about the precise properties of the microorganism-host interaction that enable this event to take place. One important factor is the strain of Lyme borrelia causing the infection. Unlike patients who are bacteremic with more conventional pathogens, patients with spirochetemia rarely appear septic. In one study, only 5% of 93 spirochetemic patients were febrile when the blood culture was obtained, and almost no one was found to have leukocytosis. The lack of fever and other clinical signs of sepsis may be due to the absence of lipopolysaccharide within the borrelial cell wall.

Infection of humans or animals elicits innate and adaptive immune responses resulting in both macrophage- and antibody-mediated killing of the spirochete. The inflammatory response in tissue typically shows an infiltration of lymphocytes, macrophages, and plasma cells, although granulocytes predominate in synovial fluid samples of Lyme arthritis patients. The potential for persistence of infection despite a robust humoral and cellular immunologic response is typical of infection with Lyme borrelia, as it is with *Treponema pallidum* infection. The virulence factors responsible for the persistence of infection include the spirochete's ability to downregulate the expression of certain immunogenic surface-exposed proteins, including OspC, and to rapidly and continually alter by recombination the antigenic properties of a surface lipoprotein known as variable major protein-like sequence expressed (VlsE). In addition, the ability of the spirochete to bind avidly to various components of the extracellular matrix may contribute to persistence.

All the objective clinical manifestations of Lyme disease are thought to be due to an inflammatory response to live spirochetes or to their undegraded antigens. Obliterative endarteritis has been seen histologically in synovial tissue, but its importance in pathogenesis is unclear. Lyme borrelia are not known to produce toxins. So far, the only role established for host genetic factors in humans is in the development of antibiotic-refractory Lyme arthritis, which is seen most often in patients with certain human leukocyte antigen (HLA) DR alleles, some of which coincide with those associated with rheumatoid arthritis.

CLINICAL MANIFESTATIONS

The clinical manifestations are often categorized as follows:

- Early localized infection, typically manifested by a single erythema migrans skin lesion, with or without viral infection–like symptoms, but without objective extracutaneous manifestations.
- Early disseminated infection, usually manifested by multiple erythema migrans skin lesions or by an objective manifestation of early neurologic Lyme disease or Lyme carditis.
- Late disease, usually manifested by arthritis but possibly including certain rare neurologic manifestations or the skin condition known as acrodermatitis chronica atrophicans.

Children and adults have similar clinical manifestations. The expected frequency of the various clinical presentations is well illustrated by a study of 313 cases of Lyme disease diagnosed in Wurzburg, Germany, over a 12-month period. In this series, erythema migrans by itself was seen in 89% of cases, early neurologic manifestations in 3%, cardiac manifestations in less than 1%, borrelial lymphocytoma in 2%, arthritis in 5%, and acrodermatitis chronica atrophicans in 1%. None of the patients had late neurologic Lyme disease. A similar distribution has been seen in recent case series in the United States, except for the absence of borrelial lymphocytoma and acrodermatitis chronica atrophicans. In earlier U.S. studies from the 1980s, a much higher proportion of patients had neurologic, cardiac, or joint manifestations. This may have been due to a bias of ascertainment in the older studies or to improved recognition and treatment of patients with erythema migrans more recently, thereby preventing the development of the extracutaneous complications that occur later.

Early Localized Infection
Single Erythema Migrans Skin Lesion
As indicated earlier, erythema migrans is by far the most common clinical manifestation of Lyme disease. Although the appearance of the skin lesion is often rather distinctive (Fig. 329-2), it is not pathognomonic for Lyme

FIGURE 329-2. Erythema migrans skin lesion on the posterior aspect of the right thigh.

TABLE 329-1 CLINICAL SYMPTOMS AND SIGNS PRESENT IN AT LEAST 20% OF PATIENTS WITH ERYTHEMA MIGRANS

CHARACTERISTIC	Percentage Exhibiting the Characteristic (95% CI)	
	UNITED STATES	**EUROPE**
Viral infection–like symptoms	65 (52-76)	37 (27-49)
Fatigue	47 (37-58)	—
Headache	36 (27-46)	20 (14-29)
Myalgias	35 (26-45)	—
Arthralgias	35 (25-46)	—
Fever	33 (23-43)	—
Stiff neck	31 (21-43)	—
Lymphadenopathy	22 (13-33)	—
Dysesthesia	20 (12-32)	35 (25-47)

CI = confidence interval.
Modified from Tibbles CD, Edlow JA. Does this patient have erythema migrans? *JAMA.* 2007;297:2617-2627.

disease. Erythema migrans appears 7 to 14 days (range, 3 to 30 days) after tick detachment and is characterized by an expanding, flat to slightly raised, erythematous skin lesion (usually ≥5 cm in diameter) that is round or oval in shape. The mark from the preceding tick bite can sometimes be identified at or near the center of the lesion and is called a punctum. Approximately 80% of patients in the United States with erythema migrans have a single skin lesion. Nonspecific viral infection–like symptoms or signs such as malaise, neck pain, headache, fatigue, migratory arthralgias, or chills and fever may be present (Table 329-1) but are more common in patients infected with *B. burgdorferi* or *B. garinii* than with *B. afzelii.* Prominent respiratory or gastrointestinal symptoms are highly atypical for Lyme disease. An acute febrile illness in the absence of a skin lesion or other objective clinical manifestation has been attributed to early Lyme disease, but the possibility of misdiagnosis is greater in this situation owing to the potential for false-positive serologic testing.

Erythema migrans skin lesions can vary in appearance. Some lesions (especially those of short duration) are nearly uniform in color, whereas others may show central clearing or have a target-like appearance. About 5% have a vesicular-pustular center. Erythema migrans on the lower extremities is sometimes purpuric. Erythema migrans lesions may be scaly when they are long-standing and fading or if topical corticosteroid creams have been applied. The most common locations include the thigh, back, shoulder, and calf. Lesions are often asymptomatic but can be mildly painful or pruritic, and tender regional lymphadenopathy may be present. The majority of U.S. patients with erythema migrans do not recall a preceding tick bite.

Certain signs and symptoms described in small numbers of patients with erythema migrans in early case series, such as hepatomegaly, splenomegaly, sore throat, conjunctivitis, or testicular swelling, may have been coincidental findings. There has been no microbiologic confirmation of borrelia infection at these sites.

Borrelial Lymphocytoma

Borrelial lymphocytoma is a rare cutaneous manifestation of Lyme disease that almost never occurs in the United States. It often presents at or near a preceding tick bite as a solitary bluish red swelling up to a few centimeters in diameter. The most common locations are the earlobe in children and the breast in adults. Histologic examination shows a dense polyclonal infiltration of the cutis and subcutis by predominantly B lymphocytes, frequently with germinal center formation. Histologic evaluation may be necessary to exclude malignancy for patients with suspected borrelial lymphocytoma at a location other than the earlobe.

Early Disseminated Infection
Multiple Erythema Migrans Skin Lesions

In the United States, approximately 20% of patients with erythema migrans have multiple skin lesions at the time of presentation. Secondary erythema migrans skin lesions can be smaller than 5 cm, do not have a punctum, and are usually not tender or pruritic. They arise from hematogenous dissemination to the skin rather than from additional tick bites.

Early Neurologic Lyme Disease

Within weeks to several months after infection, patients may develop neurologic manifestations, the most common of which are cranial neuropathy, particularly peripheral seventh nerve palsy, which may be bilateral; lymphocytic meningitis; and sensory (often painful) radiculopathy. Less common manifestations include mononeuritis multiplex (multifocal involvement of anatomically unrelated nerves) and brachial or lumbosacral plexopathies. A pseudotumor cerebri–like picture has occasionally been reported in children. The presence of a concomitant erythema migrans lesion or the patient's recollection of a recent lesion consistent with erythema migrans may be helpful diagnostically. Studies suggest that approximately 90% of children with Lyme meningitis in the United States have at least one of the following three findings: concomitant erythema migrans, cranial nerve palsy, or papilledema.

Cardiac Lyme Disease

Weeks to months after infection, patients may develop cardiac manifestations of Lyme disease, most often fluctuating degrees of atrioventricular heart block or other manifestations of a myopericarditis, which may cause complaints of lightheadedness, palpitations, dyspnea, chest pain, or syncope. Heart block is typically at or above the atrioventricular node. Erythema migrans is often but not invariably present concurrently. Valvular dysfunction is not known to occur, and chronic cardiomyopathy has only rarely been reported in Europe.

Late Lyme Disease
Lyme Arthritis

If patients with erythema migrans are not treated with antibiotics, approximately 60% will develop a mono- or oligoarticular arthritis at a mean time of 6 months after disease onset (range, 4 days to 2 years). In untreated patients, Lyme arthritis is characterized by intermittent attacks of synovitis that last for a few weeks to several months. One or two joints are involved at a time. Primarily large joints are affected, but there may be involvement of the temporomandibular joint, small joints, and periarticular sites. The most commonly involved joint is the knee. Baker's cysts may form and rupture. Joint swelling is often pronounced, but pain is usually relatively modest. Particularly in children there may be concomitant fever, but adults are often minimally symptomatic aside from the arthritis.

In about 10% of adult patients with Lyme arthritis in the United States, involvement of a large joint (almost always the knee) may persist despite appropriate antibiotic treatment. Erosion of cartilage or bone may develop in such cases.

Late Neurologic Lyme Disease

After months to years of infection, late neurologic manifestations may develop. These include encephalomyelitis, peripheral neuropathy, or encephalopathy. Because most patients with Lyme disease are now diagnosed and treated early in the course of infection, these more indolent forms of neurologic Lyme disease are quite rare.

In untreated patients, encephalomyelitis is monophasic and slowly progressive, mainly involving white matter. It is the most severe neurologic manifestation and is more common (though still infrequent) in Europe (where it most often affects the spinal cord) than in the United States. Cerebrospinal fluid (CSF) examination typically shows a lymphocytic pleocytosis, a moderately elevated protein level, and a normal glucose level, with evidence of intrathecal production of antibody to borrelia. Magnetic resonance imaging of the affected part of the brain or spinal cord can demonstrate areas of inflammation, typically with increased signal on T2 and FLAIR imaging and enhancement following contrast administration.

In the United States, peripheral neuropathy typically presents as a mild, diffuse "stocking-glove" process. Patients typically complain of intermittent limb paresthesias and sometimes radicular pain. The most common abnormality on neurologic examination is reduced vibratory sensation of the distal lower extremities. Electrophysiologic studies show a patchy axonal neuropathy. Nerve biopsy shows axonal loss and small perivascular collections of lymphocytes without spirochetes. CSF findings are often normal, without evidence of intrathecal antibody production.

Encephalopathy is an imprecisely defined clinical entity characterized by mild abnormalities of memory and/or other cognitive functions that are demonstrable on either a careful mental status examination or formal neuropsychological testing. CSF examination may be completely normal or may show intrathecal antibody production, mild protein elevation, or a mild pleocytosis. Cranial imaging studies occasionally demonstrate focal areas of presumed parenchymal inflammation, but findings are usually normal.

Acrodermatitis Chronica Atrophicans

Acrodermatitis chronica atrophicans is a late skin manifestation of Lyme disease that is most commonly seen in women older than 40 years. This skin lesion develops insidiously several years after the initial infection, usually on the extensor surfaces of the hands and feet. Early lesions are characterized by a slight bluish red discoloration and doughy swelling. Histologic examination shows lymphocytes and plasma cells in the skin and sometimes in the subcutis, with or without atrophy. Initially unilateral, the lesion may later become bilateral. Over time, the edema resolves, and the skin atrophies. Nodules may develop over bony prominences. About two thirds of patients have an associated peripheral neuropathy of the affected extremity, manifesting primarily as local sensory loss.

Although presumably any species of Lyme borrelia can cause acrodermatitis chronica atrophicans, by far the most common etiologic agent is *B. afzelii*. Therefore, this manifestation is rarely seen in the United States.

DIAGNOSIS

General Laboratory Testing

White blood cell count, hemoglobin and hematocrit levels, and platelet count are usually normal in Lyme disease, unless coinfection with *Anaplasma phagocytophilum*, *Babesia microti*, or a tick-borne encephalitis virus is present (see later). Lymphopenia may be found in the absence of a recognized coinfection. In approximately 35% of patients with erythema migrans, abnormal liver function tests (particularly mild elevations of aspartate and alanine aminotransferase levels) are seen. The erythrocyte sedimentation rate may be modestly elevated in all stages of Lyme disease, but values greater than 80 mm/hour are distinctly uncommon.

CSF examination in Lyme meningitis typically shows a pleocytosis with greater than 90% lymphocytes, a modestly elevated protein level, and a normal glucose level. Synovial fluid examination in Lyme arthritis typically shows approximately 25,000 white cells/mm^3 (range, 500 to 110,000/mm^3), with a polymorphonuclear predominance.

Skin Examination

Erythema migrans skin lesions may go unnoticed owing to the absence of prominent local symptoms and their occurrence on parts of the body that are difficult for the patient to visualize. Therefore, a complete skin examination should be performed in any patient suspected of having early localized or disseminated Lyme disease. Erythema migrans is the only clinical manifestation sufficiently distinctive to allow a clinical diagnosis in the absence of a supporting laboratory test. Erythema migrans is diagnosed based on the characteristic appearance of the skin lesion in a person who lives in or recently traveled to a Lyme disease–endemic area. Owing to the short duration of infection at this stage, serologic assays for antibodies to Lyme borrelia are seldom positive and should be obtained only in atypical cases, followed by convalescent-phase serologic testing 2 to 4 weeks after obtaining the acute sample (Table 329-2).

TABLE 329-2	DIAGNOSIS OF LYME DISEASE	
DIAGNOSTIC MODALITY	**APPLICATION**	**COMMENT**
Visual inspection	Erythema migrans	Usually seronegative at time of presentation
Two-tier serology with a positive IgM and/or IgG immunoblot	Lyme carditis	Look for concomitant erythema migrans
	Early neurologic Lyme disease	Intrathecal antibody may be detectable before serum antibody in Europe; PCR sometimes positive on CSF
	Borrelial lymphocytoma	Biopsy may be needed to exclude malignancy
Two-tier serology with a positive IgG immunoblot	Lyme arthritis	PCR often positive on synovial fluid
	Late neurologic Lyme disease	Intrathecal antibody positivity expected in Lyme encephalomyelitis
	Acrodermatitis chronica atrophicans	

CSF = cerebrospinal fluid; Ig = immunoglobulin; PCR = polymerase chain reaction.

Serologic Testing

For non–erythema migrans presentations of Lyme disease, the mainstay of laboratory diagnosis is two-tier serologic testing in which the first-tier test is usually a sensitive enzyme immunosorbent assay (EIA). If the EIA is positive or equivocal, separate immunoglobulin (Ig) M and IgG immunoblots are performed on the original serum sample. If symptoms have persisted for at least 4 weeks, the IgG immunoblot should be positive for the results to be interpreted as evidence of seropositivity. Untreated patients who remain seronegative for 6 to 8 weeks are unlikely to have Lyme disease, and other diagnoses should be pursued.

Omitting the first-tier EIA or interpreting the immunoblot using alternative criteria that are not evidence based can decrease the specificity of testing and is not recommended. False-positive results on the IgM immunoblot may be due to cross-reactive antibodies that arise from polyclonal B-cell stimulation. Probably the most common cause of false-positive results, however, is the overreading of nonspecific weak bands. Background rates of seropositivity, which may exceed 4% in highly endemic areas of the United States and may be even higher in Europe, can also confound the interpretation of seroreactivity. Therefore, a positive serologic test does not necessarily mean that the patient has active Lyme disease. The positive predictive value is most informative when the pretest probability based on clinical features is at least 20%. Serologic testing is not indicated in the routine follow-up of patients after treatment because either IgM or IgG borrelial antibodies can persist for many years in successfully treated patients.

Testing for borrelial antibody produced locally in the central nervous system (i.e., intrathecal antibody) may be helpful in the diagnosis of neurologic Lyme disease and has been reported to precede the detection of serum antibody in a minority of European patients. Positive tests for intrathecal antibody may persist, however, for long periods after successful antibiotic treatment.

Other Diagnostic Modalities

Culture for Lyme borrelia is not routinely performed or available to diagnose Lyme disease. It is unnecessary for patients with erythema migrans and too insensitive for patients with extracutaneous manifestations of Lyme disease. In contrast, polymerase chain reaction (PCR) for the detection of borrelial DNA is positive on synovial fluid specimens in up to 80% of untreated patients with Lyme arthritis, and a positive result supports this diagnosis in a patient who is IgG seropositive. The sensitivity of PCR in CSF tends to be much lower, however, and was only about 5% in a recent study of children from the United States with early neurologic Lyme disease. A negative PCR result on either type of fluid does not exclude Lyme disease.

Differential Diagnosis
Erythema Migrans

Tick-bite hypersensitivity reactions can be mistaken for erythema migrans, but these reactions occur within 48 hours of a tick bite, are usually pruritic, and tend to wane within a few days. In contrast, erythema migrans skin lesions in untreated patients last for a median of approximately 4 weeks in the United States and even longer in Europe. Bacterial cellulitis rarely occurs at the most common sites of erythema migrans and does not demonstrate central clearing or a target-like appearance. Erythema migrans, unlike erythema multiforme, does not involve the mucous membranes, palms, or soles. STARI is the most likely diagnosis in patients with erythema migrans–like skin lesions who were bitten by an *A. americanum* tick or developed this lesion in the southern United States. Other conditions that can usually be readily distinguished include tinea (often pruritic, with a thin, raised, scaly border), nummular eczema (symmetrical pruritic lesions with a tendency to scale and crust), granuloma annulare (acral location, especially on the dorsum of hands and feet; relatively fixed in size and <5 cm in diameter), contact dermatitis (pruritic, with streaking along the area of contact and a vesicular component), urticaria (raised, pruritic, and usually <5 cm in diameter), fixed drug eruption (usually on the genitalia, hands, feet, or face and fixed in size), pityriasis rosea (multiple, moderately pruritic lesions with peripheral scale and relatively fixed in size), and spider bite (often very painful and necrotic with a central eschar).

Extracutaneous Lyme Disease

Included in the differential diagnosis of early neurologic Lyme disease is Bell's palsy. Even in highly endemic areas of the United States, other causes of seventh nerve palsy outnumber Lyme disease by a margin of three to one. Viral meningitis and mechanical radiculopathy may be confused with manifestations of early neurologic Lyme disease. Viral or other causes of myopericarditis may resemble cardiac Lyme disease. Many causes of synovitis might be considered in the differential diagnosis of Lyme arthritis, but the pattern of joint involvement, such as symmetrical small joint involvement in rheumatoid arthritis, is often distinctly different from that found in Lyme arthritis. Lyme encephalomyelitis may occasionally be confused with a first episode of relapsing-remitting multiple sclerosis or primary progressive multiple sclerosis. Testing for borrelial antibody in serum (and in CSF, for the last condition) usually suffices to differentiate these conditions from Lyme disease.

TREATMENT (Rx)

In vitro studies have shown that Lyme borrelia are highly susceptible to tetracyclines, most penicillins, and many second- and third-generation cephalosporins. *B. burgdorferi* is resistant to certain fluoroquinolones, rifampin, and first-generation cephalosporins. Whether macrolides are active in vitro depends on the borrelial strain tested and the assay technique used. Although most manifestations of Lyme disease resolve spontaneously without treatment, antibiotic therapy may hasten resolution and prevent progression.

Oral antibiotic therapy is used to treat patients with erythema migrans (Table 329-3). Doxycycline, amoxicillin, and cefuroxime axetil are each highly effective and are the preferred agents for this indication. Macrolides such as azithromycin are somewhat less effective than other oral antibiotics and are not recommended as first-line therapy.

Among the first-line agents, only doxycycline is effective against *A. phagocytophilum* coinfection, and it is the only agent for which a prospective clinical trial demonstrated that just 10 days of treatment is effective.[1] Doxycycline may cause photosensitivity, however, which is a concern because early Lyme disease occurs most commonly during the summer months; in addition, this drug is relatively contraindicated in children younger than 8 years and in women who are pregnant or breast-feeding. When erythema migrans cannot be reliably distinguished from community-acquired bacterial cellulitis, either cefuroxime axetil or amoxicillin/clavulanate potassium (Augmentin) is preferred because these antimicrobials are generally effective against both infections.

Within 24 hours of the initiation of antimicrobial therapy, up to 15% of patients treated for erythema migrans experience a Jarisch-Herxheimer–like reaction characterized by an increase in the size or intensity of erythema in the skin lesion and more intense viral infection–like systemic symptoms. Fever, if present, should resolve within 48 hours, and the skin lesion should resolve within 7 to 14 days. Other symptoms, such as fatigue or arthralgia, tend to improve but do not invariably resolve within this time frame, lasting for more than 3 months in one quarter of patients. Extending the initial course of treatment does not result in the faster relief of symptoms. Oral antibiotic therapy is also used as first-line treatment for the other cutaneous manifestations of Lyme disease and as the initial treatment for patients with Lyme arthritis.

The preferred parenteral agent for Lyme disease is ceftriaxone because it is highly active against Lyme borrelia in vitro, crosses the blood-brain barrier well, and has a long serum half-life, allowing the convenience of once daily administration. Alternative parenterally administered antibiotics are cefotaxime and penicillin. Parenteral antibiotic therapy is recommended for patients with late neurologic Lyme disease and those with cardiac Lyme disease who are admitted to the hospital for monitoring (see Table 329-3). Parenteral antibiotics are often given to patients with Lyme arthritis who have failed to respond to one or more courses of oral antibiotic treatment.

In the United States, parenteral therapy has been preferred for early neurologic Lyme disease, especially for meningitis and radiculitis, with oral therapy reserved for patients with uncomplicated seventh nerve palsy. Studies conducted in Europe, however, have provided convincing evidence that oral doxycycline is just as effective as ceftriaxone for any of the primary manifestations of early neurologic Lyme disease.[2] Although the same may be true in the United States, studies are lacking. Other oral antibiotics such as amoxicillin have been used successfully to treat patients with uncomplicated seventh nerve palsy, but published data on efficacy are much more limited for these agents. Because seventh nerve palsy resolves with or without antibiotic treatment at identical rates, the primary reason to treat such patients is to prevent the subsequent development of complications, particularly Lyme arthritis.

The presence of either papilledema or sixth cranial nerve palsy may indicate the presence of increased intracranial pressure in patients with neurologic Lyme disease. The elevated pressure typically falls in response to antibiotic therapy, but other measures conventionally used to lower pressure may need to be considered in individual cases.

Symptomatic patients with cardiac Lyme disease and those with high-grade first-degree atrioventricular heart block (PR interval ≥300 msec) or second- or third-degree block should be hospitalized and closely monitored. Temporary cardiac pacing may be required. In treated patients, complete heart block generally resolves within 1 week, and lesser conduction disturbances resolve within 6 weeks.

Lyme arthritis typically responds to antibiotic treatment. Patients whose arthritis is improved but not resolved after an initial course of oral therapy can be re-treated with a second course of oral antibiotics, reserving parenteral antibiotic therapy for those without any significant clinical response. Approximately 10% of adult patients in the United States do not respond clinically to antibiotic therapy and are said to have antibiotic-refractory Lyme arthritis; this condition has been defined as persistent synovitis for at least 2 months after completion of a course of intravenous ceftriaxone (or 1 month after completion of two 4-week courses of an oral antibiotic), in conjunction with negative PCR testing on synovial fluid and synovial tissue, if available. Because these patients are no longer believed to be actively infected, they are customarily treated with nonsteroidal anti-inflammatory drugs, intra-articular injections of corticosteroids, or disease-modifying antirheumatic drugs. Arthroscopic synovectomy has also been used successfully in patients with this condition.

Pregnant patients with Lyme disease are generally treated similarly to nonpregnant patients, except that doxycycline should be avoided because of the potential adverse effects on both the fetus and the mother. No published data convincingly support a congenital Lyme disease syndrome.

Post–Lyme Disease Symptoms and Syndrome

The outcome of treatment in the vast majority of patients with erythema migrans is excellent. Studies show, however, that when questioned 6 months or longer after treatment of erythema migrans, approximately 5 to 15% of patients report purely subjective symptoms such as fatigue or musculoskeletal pain. These subjective symptoms are typically mild and may wax and wane in intensity. Patients with these complaints are said to have post–Lyme disease symptoms or syndrome, depending on the symptom duration and severity. The cause of these symptoms is currently unknown. Careful microbiologic evaluations have failed to find evidence of either persistent *B. burgdorferi* infection or coinfection with a second *Ixodes*-transmitted pathogen. Furthermore, re-treatment provides no measurable benefit or a benefit so modest or ambiguous that it is outweighed by the risks associated with antibiotic therapy. Therefore, symptomatic treatment is recommended for such patients. Two prospective studies conducted in Europe that incorporated healthy control groups have challenged the notion that such a syndrome even exists. In each of these studies, the frequency of unexplained subjective symptoms in the Lyme disease group was no higher than that in the control group at 6 months into follow-up.

Chronic Lyme Disease

The term *chronic Lyme disease* is poorly defined but widely used. In Europe, it has been used to refer to the objective manifestations that most authorities prefer to call late Lyme disease. Others have used the term to refer to patients with post–Lyme disease subjective complaints. Most often, the term *chronic Lyme disease* is used as a diagnosis for patients with persistent pain, neurocognitive complaints, and/or fatigue, without objective clinical or serologic

THERAPY	MANIFESTATION	DURATION (DAYS)
Doxycycline 100 mg PO bid *or*	Erythema migrans	14
	Borrelial lymphocytoma	14
Amoxicillin 500 mg PO tid *or*	Acrodermatitis chronica atrophicans	21
Cefuroxime axetil 500 mg PO bid	Lyme arthritis	28
	Lyme carditis—mild	14
	Cranial neuropathy[†]	14
Doxycycline 100 mg PO bid	Lyme meningitis or radiculopathy in Europe and possibly in U.S.	14
Ceftriaxone 2 g IV daily	Lyme arthritis that failed oral therapy	14-28
	Late neurologic Lyme disease	14-28
	Lyme carditis requiring hospitalization	14
	Lyme meningitis or radiculopathy in U.S.	14
Azithromycin 500 mg PO daily	Erythema migrans in a patient intolerant of doxycycline and β-lactam antibiotics	6-10

TABLE 329-3 RECOMMENDED THERAPY FOR ADULT PATIENTS WITH LYME DISEASE*

*Regardless of the clinical manifestations of Lyme disease, complete response to treatment may be delayed beyond the treatment duration. Relapse may occur with any of these regimens; patients with objective signs of relapse may need another course of treatment.

[†]Although any one of the first-line oral antibiotics appears to be effective in patients with cranial neuropathy, there is only limited experience in patients with a cranial neuropathy other than seventh nerve palsy or with agents other than doxycycline.

Modified from Wormser GP, Dattwyler RJ, Shapiro ED, et al. The clinical assessment, treatment, and prevention of Lyme disease, human granulocytic anaplasmosis, and babesiosis: clinical practice guidelines by the Infectious Diseases Society of America. *Clin Infect Dis.* 2006;43:1089-1134.

evidence of past or present *B. burgdorferi* infection. In this usage, the term is a misnomer and has become the latest in a series of postulated syndromes that attempt to attribute medically unexplained symptoms to particular infections.

Coinfections

Ixodes ticks may be coinfected with and transmit Lyme borrelia along with other pathogens such as *A. phagocytophilum; B. microti,* the primary cause of babesiosis; or a tick-borne encephalitis virus. The likelihood of coinfection is dependent on the particular species of *Ixodes* tick and on the geographic area. Thus, bites from *I. scapularis* ticks in certain areas may lead to the development of Lyme disease, human granulocytic anaplasmosis, or babesiosis as a single infection or, less frequently, as a coinfection. In addition, this tick species can very rarely transmit a Powassan-like encephalitis virus. In Europe, the most common coinfection is Lyme disease with tick-borne encephalitis virus infection.

Coinfection should be considered in patients from geographic areas endemic for these pathogens who present with more severe initial symptoms than are commonly observed with Lyme disease alone. This is especially true for those who have high-grade fever for more than 48 hours despite antibiotic therapy appropriate for Lyme disease, those who develop recurrent fever, and those who have unexplained leukopenia, thrombocytopenia, or anemia. Coinfection might also be considered when the erythema migrans skin lesion has resolved but there has been either no improvement or worsening of the viral infection–like symptoms.

Reinfection

Patients treated for early Lyme disease do not appear to develop an immunologic response that is adequate to protect against reinfection. Therefore, patients with erythema migrans may become reinfected at a different skin site if they are bitten by another infected tick. Reinfection has been well documented only in patients who were treated for early infection (nearly always erythema migrans), but not after late manifestations of Lyme disease such as Lyme arthritis. Clinical manifestations of reinfection appear to be similar to those of the primary infection.

PREVENTION

Lyme disease can be prevented by avoiding tick-infested environments and by covering bare skin and using tick repellents on skin and clothing when in

such environments. The tick density around individual residences can be reduced by removing leaf litter, placing wood chips where lawns abut forests, applying acaricides to property, and constructing fences to keep out deer. Bathing within 2 hours of tick exposure has been shown to decrease the risk of Lyme disease. Daily inspections of the entire skin surface (including scalp) to remove attached ticks is recommended because of the grace period between tick attachment and transmission of *B. burgdorferi*. Removal is accomplished by grasping the tick as close to its mouth parts as possible with a forceps (or tweezers) and gently pulling it out. Clinical studies have demonstrated that without any other intervention, more than 96% of individuals who find and remove an attached *I. scapularis* tick do not develop Lyme disease, even in highly endemic geographic regions. If the tick is not found or removed, the probability of infection approaches the infection rate in the regional tick population (typically, >20% of nymphal stage *I. scapularis* ticks are infected in highly endemic areas of the northeastern and Midwestern United States).

Evidence shows that doxycycline chemoprophylaxis can further reduce the chance of developing Lyme disease after removing an *I. scapularis* tick. A single 200-mg dose of doxycycline was found to be 87% effective in preventing erythema migrans at the tick bite site.[3] A single dose of doxycycline within 72 hours of tick removal should be considered for persons in highly endemic areas who are known to have been bitten by a nymphal or adult *I. scapularis* tick estimated to have been attached for at least 36 hours. Given the uncertain efficacy of a short course of amoxicillin in this situation, observation rather than chemoprophylaxis has been recommended for individuals in whom doxycycline is contraindicated. No vaccine is currently available to prevent Lyme disease in humans.

1. Wormser GP, Ramanathan R, Nowakowski J, et al. Duration of antibiotic therapy for early Lyme disease. A randomized, double-blind, placebo-controlled trial. *Ann Intern Med.* 2003;138: 697-704.
2. Ljostad U, Skogvoll E, Eikeland R, et al. Oral doxycycline versus intravenous ceftriaxone for European Lyme neuroborreliosis: a multicentre, non-inferiority, double-blind, randomised trial. *Lancet Neurol.* 2008;7:690-695.
3. Nadelman RB, Nowakowski J, Fish D, et al. Prophylaxis with single-dose doxycycline for the prevention of Lyme disease after an *Ixodes scapularis* tick bite. *N Engl J Med.* 2001;345:79-84.

SUGGESTED READINGS

Cerar D, Cerar T, Ruzic-Sabjlic E, et al. Subjective symptoms after treatment of early Lyme disease. *Am J Med.* 2010;123:79-86. *The frequency of subjective complaints 6 months after treatment of erythema migrans did not exceed that in a healthy control group.*

Mygland A, Ljostad U, Fingerle V, et al. EFNS guidelines on the diagnosis and management of European Lyme neuroborreliosis. *Eur J Neurol.* 2010;17:8-16. *Treatment guidelines for neurologic Lyme disease in Europe.*

Poland GA. Vaccines against Lyme disease: what happened and what lessons can we learn? *Clin Infect Dis.* 2011;3:s253-s258. *Review of the licensing and withdrawal of the vaccine to prevent Lyme disease.*

Smith BG, Cruz AI Jr, Milewski MD, et al. Lyme disease and the orthopaedic implications of Lyme arthritis. *J Am Acad Orthop Surg.* 2011;19:91-100. *Practical review.*

330

RELAPSING FEVER AND OTHER *BORRELIA* INFECTIONS

WILLIAM A. PETRI, JR.

DEFINITION

Relapsing fever is a spirochetal infection with bacteria of the genus *Borrelia*. There are two modes of transmission: epidemic louse-borne and endemic tick-borne relapsing fever. Disease is characterized by recurrent bouts of fever and spirochetemia separated by short fever-free periods.

The Pathogen

Members of the genus *Borrelia* are motile spirochetes that measure 0.5 μm in diameter and 5 to 40 μm in length. They are aerophilic and require long-chain fatty acids for growth. Louse-borne relapsing fever is caused by *Borrelia recurrentis*. Tick-borne relapsing fever organisms are named after their tick vector and include the closely related species *Borrelia duttonii* (Old World) and *Borrelia hermsii*, *Borrelia turicatae*, and *Borrelia parkeri* (North America).

EPIDEMIOLOGY

Louse-borne epidemic relapsing fever is caused by *B. recurrentis* and is carried from person to person by the human body louse (*Pediculus humanus*). There is no animal reservoir. The spirochete lives in the louse hemolymph; infection is transmitted to humans when the louse is crushed on human skin and infective spirochetes penetrate the skin or mucous membranes. Epidemics have occurred during famines and at wartime when breakdown in sanitation favors the transmission of body lice. Louse-borne disease remains endemic in central and east Africa (Ethiopia, Somalia, Chad, and the Sudan) and in the South American Andes (Bolivia and Peru).

Tick-borne endemic relapsing fever occurs throughout the world and is transmitted to humans by *Ornithodoros* soft ticks. The ticks become infected by feeding on wild rodents (including mice, rats, squirrels, and chipmunks), which serve as natural reservoirs for the organisms. In the United States, relapsing fever is limited to humid, mountainous areas of the West at altitudes of 1500 to 8000 ft, where the tick vector *Ornithodoros hermsii* resides in forests of ponderosa pine and Douglas fir trees. A key diagnostic clue has been a history of sleeping in rodent-infested rustic cabins in western U.S. national parks. In Tanzania, where house infestation with *Ornithodoros* tick vectors can be very high, relapsing fever was identified in 11% of children seen at a clinic with fever.

PATHOBIOLOGY

Borrelia infection begins in the skin at the site of the louse or tick bite and is followed by rapid dissemination of the spirochetes through the blood stream. Spirochetes are visible on Wright-stained peripheral blood smears during the initial febrile episode and during each febrile relapse in most patients. The spirochete burden in blood positively correlates with symptom severity. Clearance of spirochetes from blood is associated with the production of serotype-specific immune sera; anti-*Borrelia* antibodies have been shown in animal models to be the major mechanism of immune clearance of infection.

Relapses are associated with cyclic antigenic variation in the variable major proteins (VMPs), which are the abundant outer membrane proteins of the spirochete that carry the serotype-specific epitopes. Antigenic variation is the consequence of recombination events that occur between VMP genes at silent and expression sites on linear plasmids. A single *B. hermsii* bacterium may produce as many as 40 distinct serotypes. Because spirochetes undergo one or several antigenic phases during infection, no specific or standard procedure has been developed for routine serodiagnosis of relapsing fever.

CLINICAL MANIFESTATIONS

An abrupt onset of fever (temperature >39° C in most patients), headache, myalgia, and shaking chills characterizes the onset of illness. Cough, nausea and vomiting, and fatigue are less frequent complaints. Signs include fever, tachycardia, lethargy or confusion, conjunctival injection, and epistaxis. Hepatosplenomegaly, jaundice, and often a truncal petechial rash are common signs in louse-borne relapsing fever. Neurologic findings may occur, including meningitis, meningoencephalitis, and facial palsy, although these entities are more common with tick-borne relapsing fever. Untreated louse-borne disease lasts 6 days, and relapses occur once after an afebrile period of 9 days. The initial illness of tick-borne relapsing fever lasts about 4 days without antibiotic treatment, with an average of two relapses (each after an average 10-day afebrile period) before the diagnosis is made.

Relapsing fever in pregnancy can cause placental damage and intrauterine growth retardation and results in miscarriage in a third of patients. Neonatal infection by both the tick- and louse-borne forms is accompanied by jaundice, hepatosplenomegaly, and often sepsis and hemorrhage. Fever and hepatosplenomegaly are also common signs in children.

DIAGNOSIS

The diagnosis should be considered in patients with fever who are returning from a stay in cabins in the mountainous and high-elevation areas of the western United States. Only a few patients will remember tick exposure because *O. hermsii* is a night feeder, has a painless bite, and remains attached for only 15 minutes. Internationally, relapsing fever can occur sporadically

FIGURE 330-1. A single spirochete is seen in a Wright-stained thin blood smear from a patient with relapsing fever.

wherever dwellings are infected with *Ornithodoros* ticks, as well as in epidemics with louse-borne disease.

Because the number of organisms in blood is extremely high, the diagnosis is most often made by direct visualization of the organism in a blood smear (Fig. 330-1), although the diagnosis can also be made with polymerase chain reaction and serodiagnostic tests. Spirochetes can be demonstrated in peripheral blood smears taken during febrile episodes in 70% of patients. Additional sensitivity may be gained by examination of a buffy coat preparation of peripheral blood. Because of their characteristic locomotion, spirochetes can be readily detected by direct visualization of thick blood films under low-power microscopy. Culture of the organism requires a special medium and is not practical in a clinical laboratory setting. The white blood cell count is generally normal, but platelet counts of less than 50,000/mm³ occur in up to 90% of cases of louse-borne disease. The prothrombin and activated partial thromboplastin times are often prolonged. In louse-borne disease, elevations in liver function test results (serum transaminases and bilirubin) and blood urea nitrogen are common. Urinalysis may reveal proteinuria and microscopic hematuria. Examination of cerebrospinal fluid may show a lymphocytic pleocytosis, and spirochetes may be directly visualized.

TREATMENT   Rx

Borrelia is generally quite sensitive to antibiotics, which has led to recommendations for single-dose treatments. Although this may be sufficient, especially for louse-borne disease, recent reports suggest that silent, residual infections occur and may best be addressed by longer treatments. For tick-borne relapsing infection, treatment duration should extend for 7 days to reduce the risk for persistent infection. Tetracycline, doxycycline, and erythromycin are all effective antibiotics. Erythromycin should be used in pregnant women and children younger than 7 years (in whom tetracyclines can stain the permanent teeth). Penicillin treatment has been reported to clear the spirochetemia more slowly than tetracycline does.

The Jarisch-Herxheimer reaction (typically characterized by a rise in body temperature of 1° C, rigors, a rise in blood pressure followed by a fall, and transient leukopenia) occurs 2 to 3 hours after treatment in many patients with louse-borne disease, less commonly in tick-borne disease, and should be anticipated and managed supportively. Death as a result of shock from the Jarisch-Herxheimer reaction occurs rarely. The Jarisch-Herxheimer reaction has been associated with accelerated phagocytosis of spirochetes by neutrophils and transient elevations in tumor necrosis factor-α (TNF-α), interleukin-6 (IL-6), IL-8, and IL-10. In small numbers of patients with louse-borne relapsing fever, anti–TNF-α antibodies have been effective in prevention.

PREVENTION

Prevention of louse-borne relapsing fever hinges on improving hygienic conditions, delousing affected areas, and antibiotic treatment of patients and close contacts. Tick-borne relapsing fever can be prevented by reducing the risk of contact with rodents and ticks, including repair of structural flaws in cabins and other residences so that rodents cannot nest in or around them, as well as spraying infested indoor environments.

PROGNOSIS

Epidemics of louse-borne relapsing fever have been reported, with mortality rates approaching 40%; as much as 5% of the mortality is related to Jarisch-Herxheimer reactions with treatment. Mortality from tick-borne disease is less than 5%. Autopsies of patients with louse-borne disease have documented intracranial hemorrhage, brain edema, bronchopneumonia, hepatic necrosis, and splenic infarcts.

SUGGESTED READINGS

Balicer RD, Mimouni D, Bar-Zeev Y, et al. Post exposure prophylaxis of tick-borne relapsing fever. *Eur J Clin Microbiol Infect Dis.* 2010;29:253-258. *In an endemic area, a 5-day course of doxycycline reduces the risk of clinical disease from 38 to 3%.*

Larsson C, Andersson M, Bergstrom S. Current issues in relapsing fever. *Curr Opin Infect Dis.* 2009;22:443-449. *Discusses advances in diagnostics, molecular biology, and host-pathogen interactions.*

331

LEPTOSPIROSIS

ALBERT I. KO

DEFINITION

Leptospirosis, which is a major zoonotic health problem in developing countries, has now been recognized as an emerging infectious disease in developed countries. Infection with *Leptospira* spirochetes occurs during contact with animal reservoirs or an environment contaminated with their urine. The clinical course of leptospirosis ranges from a mild acute febrile illness to life-threatening manifestations such as Weil's disease, which consists of the triad of jaundice, acute renal failure, and bleeding. Leptospirosis has also been recognized as an important cause of pulmonary hemorrhage syndrome worldwide.

The Pathogen

The etiologic agent, which can be identified by darkfield microscopy or silver staining procedures, is a motile spirochete 6 to 20 μm in length and 0.1 μm in diameter (Fig. 331-1). Leptospires are obligate aerobes whose relatively large genome (two chromosomes of approximately 4.3 megabase and 350 kilobase) reflects its ability to adapt to external and host environments. *Leptospira* are classified into 20 species and genomospecies, of which 9 (*L. interrogans, L. kirschneri, L. noguchii, L. weilii, L. borgspetersenii, L. santarosai, L. alexanderi, L. alstonii,* and *L. kmetyi*) are pathogenic and 5 (*L. wolffii, L. inadai, L. fanei, L. broomii,* and *L. licerasiae*) are considered intermediately pathogenic. Serologic classification provides more useful information because serogroups and serovars, of which there are more than 25 and 250, respectively, are associated with specific animal reservoirs and vary with respect to their ability to cause severe disease in humans.

EPIDEMIOLOGY

Leptospirosis has a worldwide distribution because of the broad spectrum of animal reservoirs that support persistent renal carriage of pathogenic *Leptospira* spp, including domestic and wild rodents, dogs, pigs, cattle, and sheep. Leptospires colonize the renal tubules, are excreted in urine, and survive for weeks to months in the environment. Transmission to humans occurs when leptospires penetrate the skin or mucous membranes during contact with contaminated water, soil, or vegetation. Abrasions in the skin facilitate entry of the pathogen. Direct contact with urine and tissues is an important mode of transmission in risk groups such as abattoir workers and veterinarians. Ingestion of contaminated food, inhalation of aerosolized droplets, or swallowing of contaminated water, as occurred during a 1998 outbreak among triathletes, occasionally causes infection. Humans are accidental hosts and do not serve as reservoirs because sufficient concentrations of viable organisms

are not excreted in urine. Rare human-to-human transmission is associated with transplacental infection and breast-feeding.

Leptospirosis is a major public health problem in developing countries, especially in tropical areas, where it is an endemic disease among subsistence farmers, sharecroppers, and livestock herders. Furthermore, it is the cause of large epidemics in urban slums, where inadequate sanitation favors rodent-borne transmission. Although leptospirosis has traditionally been a sporadic occupation-related disease in developed countries, it has emerged to become a health problem associated with travel, water sports, adventure racing, and recreation (white water rafting, swimming). Outbreaks frequently follow natural disasters, heavy seasonal rainfall, and flooding, as seen during the aftermath of hurricanes in the Caribbean and monsoons in Mumbai. Leptospirosis may also be an under-recognized problem in U.S. inner cities inasmuch as sporadic cases have been reported in this setting.

PATHOBIOLOGY

The development of leptospirosis and disease progression are determined by the virulence characteristics of the infecting strain, the dose of the infecting inoculum, and host susceptibility factors. Leptospires disseminate rapidly to all tissues shortly after infection by means of direct tissue penetration and hematogenous spread. The pathogen is resistant to the alternative pathway of complement activation and evades the innate host immune response during the early stages of infection. Symptoms develop 5 to 14 days after exposure, although the incubation period may vary from 2 to 30 days. Leptospires are cleared from the blood stream primarily by agglutinating antibodies, whose titers rise at the end of the early-phase "leptospiremic" illness, although more recent studies have shown that infection also induces an acquired cell-mediated response. The late-phase immunopathogenic process is responsible for the severe manifestations of the disease. *Leptospira* lipopolysaccharide and lipopeptides are potent stimulators of pro-inflammatory cytokines such as tumor necrosis factor-α, and these cytokines produce a septic shock–like picture. Leptospirosis activates the coagulation cascade. A recent study identified disseminated intravascular coagulation (DIC) (Chapter 178) in approximately 50% of hospitalized patients. However, this DIC is usually a milder and less prominent manifestation in leptospirosis than that observed in gram-negative sepsis. Damage to the vascular endothelium, which is a hallmark of severe leptospirosis, causes capillary leakage, hemorrhage, and in a subset of cases, vasculitis. The pronounced disturbances in hepatic and renal function are believed to be due to the toxic effects of products released from killed organisms because pathologic examination of tissues reveals mild inflammatory cell infiltrates and sparse intact leptospires. Although the immune response eventually eliminates the pathogen, leptospires may persist for prolonged periods in immunoprivileged sites, such as the anterior chamber of the eye and the renal tubules, and then may be shed in urine weeks after resolution of the illness.

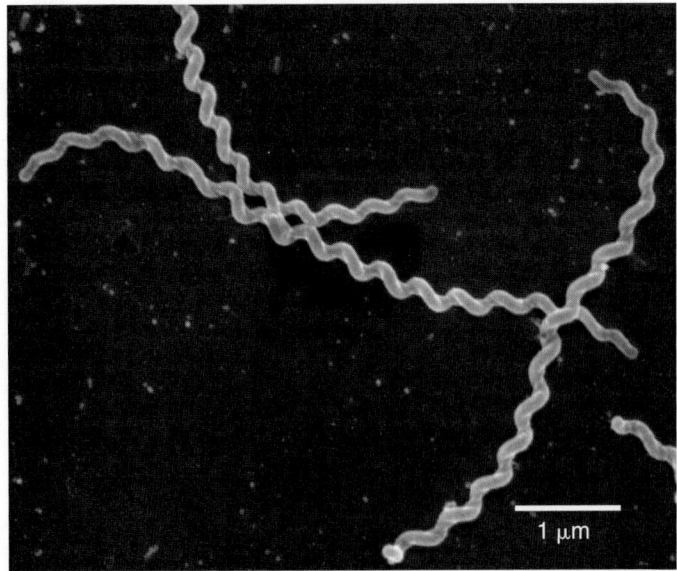

FIGURE 331-1. Scanning electron micrograph of *Leptospira interrogans* serovar *copenhageni.* Original magnification, 17,000; bar = 1 μm.

FIGURE 331-2. Conjunctival suffusion in a patient with Weil's disease. Conjunctival suffusion, a characteristic sign of leptospirosis, is best seen along the right upper palpebral border, above the subconjunctival hemorrhage. (Courtesy of Antonio Seguro and Paulo Marotto, Hospital Emílio Ribas and Universidade de São Paulo.)

CLINICAL MANIFESTATIONS

The clinical findings in early-phase leptospirosis (initial 3 to 7 days of illness) are nonspecific. The onset of high fever (temperature of 38 to 40° C), myalgia, and headache (retro-orbital and frontal) may be abrupt and accompanied by symptoms of nausea, vomiting, abdominal pain, diarrhea, cough, and photophobia. Muscle tenderness is pronounced, especially in the calves and lumbar region; if tenderness involves the abdominal wall musculature, it can mimic the symptoms of an acute abdomen. Rash, which occurs in 10 to 20% of patients, has erythematous macular, papular, urticarial, or purpuric components distributed in a truncal or pretibial ("Fort Bragg fever") pattern. Hepatomegaly, splenomegaly, and lymphadenopathy are less common (<20%) findings. Conjunctival suffusion, which is a characteristic manifestation seen in about 30% of patients, develops toward the end of early-phase illness and involves hyperemia of the conjunctival vessels along the palpebral fissures and chemosis (Fig. 331-2).

A minority (5 to 15%) of patients progress to severe late-phase disease. Jaundice is a poor prognostic sign because acute renal failure and hemorrhage are frequently associated complications (Weil's disease). Anicteric leptospirosis tends to be a milder late-phase finding characterized by prolonged fever and aseptic meningitis. Life-threatening complications are hypotension, hemorrhage, and renal and respiratory failure.

Leptospirosis causes nonoliguric, hypokalemic renal insufficiency, with impaired proximal sodium reabsorption, increased distal sodium delivery, and potassium wasting. As volume loss progresses, oliguric renal insufficiency develops as a result of prerenal azotemia and acute tubular necrosis. Acute renal failure occurs in up to 40 to 60% of patients with severe leptospirosis.

Severe thrombocytopenia and anemia secondary to hemolysis or blood loss are observed in up to 30% of patients. The prothrombin and partial thromboplastin times are normal or mildly elevated. Massive spontaneous gastrointestinal bleeding and pulmonary hemorrhage syndrome are major causes of death. Acute lung injury is a prominent feature of pulmonary hemorrhage syndrome but can occur in the absence of documented bleeding.

Cardiac involvement in the form of electrocardiographic (ECG) changes and myocarditis (Chapter 60) may be overlooked because overt pulmonary hemorrhage and hepatorenal manifestations tend to dominate the clinical picture in seriously ill patients. However, a recent autopsy study of 24 patients who had died of leptospirosis noted myocarditis in 96%, endocardial inflammation in 50%, and pericardial hemorrhage and inflammation in 12 and 29% of cases, respectively. Minor ECG changes have been seen in more than half of all patients. Conduction system abnormalities, such as first-degree atrioventricular block, represent the most common change attributable to myocarditis. Fatal myocarditis has been reported. Other late-phase findings include diffuse or focal interstitial pneumonitis and pneumonia, pancreatitis, and rhabdomyolysis.

Aseptic meningitis, which is the most frequent neurologic manifestation, is characterized by cerebrospinal fluid pleocytosis with early neutrophilic and late mononuclear cell predominance. Leptospirosis has also been reported to cause encephalitis, cerebral hemorrhage and arteritis (moyamoya disease), transverse myelitis, and cranial (Bell's palsy) and peripheral neuropathies.

DIAGNOSIS

Few clinical or laboratory findings differentiate early-phase leptospirosis from other causes of an acute febrile illness associated with myalgias and headache. Conjunctival suffusion is a highly specific, but insensitive clinical finding. The white blood cell count may be mildly elevated or normal in early-phase illness.

Severe leptospirosis is often recognized by the classic manifestations of Weil's disease, but severe complications may occur in anicteric disease. Furthermore, aseptic meningitis and uveitis may develop in patients with icteric leptospirosis, manifestations classically associated with anicteric disease.

Laboratory confirmation of leptospirosis is based on the presence of a four-fold rise in antibody titer in the microagglutination test (MAT) or isolation of pathogenic leptospires from a normally sterile site. However, these standard diagnostic methods provide only retrospective confirmation of the disease. MAT requires acute- and convalescent-phase sera and is performed routinely in few reference laboratories worldwide. A positive MAT titer of ≥1:100 from a single acute-phase sample provides suggestive evidence of leptospirosis but must be interpreted with caution in areas of high endemic transmission. Isolation of *Leptospira* requires specific media (Ellinghausen-McCullough-Johnson-Harris or Fletcher medium), and more than 4 weeks may be needed to identify a positive culture. Commercial anti–whole *Leptospira* immunoglobulin M detection kits in enzyme-linked immunosorbent assay or rapid formats are used to provide presumptive confirmation of leptospirosis. However, sensitivity is low (39 to 72%) during acute-phase illness. Polymerase chain reaction–based diagnostic methods have been developed, but their use has been limited to reference laboratory settings.

Differential Diagnosis

Leptospirosis is frequently confused with other causes of acute fever. Its diagnosis is particularly problematic in regions where dengue (Chapter 389) or malaria (Chapter 353) are endemic diseases. Severe leptospirosis must be differentiated from other causes of acute jaundice, renal and respiratory failure, and hemorrhage, such as viral hepatitis (Chapter 150); typhoid fever (Chapter 316); rickettsial disease (Chapter 335); hantavirus-associated hemorrhagic fever–renal syndrome (Chapter 389) and other viral causes of hemorrhagic fever; gram-negative sepsis; endocarditis; and autoimmune disorders. Icteric leptospirosis is associated with elevated serum conjugated bilirubin concentrations and can be differentiated from viral hepatitis by the finding of elevated serum creatine phosphokinase and mild elevations (<400 U/L) in transaminases. The finding of moderate to severe hypokalemia is useful in distinguishing leptospirosis from other infectious causes of acute renal failure. Leptospirosis-associated pulmonary hemorrhage syndrome is difficult to differentiate from the pulmonary manifestations caused by viral hemorrhagic fevers. The presence of massive pulmonary bleeding may increase suspicion for leptospirosis as the underlying cause because this finding is less frequently observed in patients with dengue hemorrhagic fever and hantaviral pulmonary syndrome.

TREATMENT   Rx

Antimicrobial therapy is efficacious for early- and severe late-phase leptospirosis. Mild leptospirosis is treated with oral doxycycline (100 mg twice a day) or ampicillin (500 mg every 6 hours) or amoxicillin (500 mg every 8 hours). Azithromycin (1 g followed by 500 mg once a day for 2 days) is not inferior to and is better tolerated than doxycycline but is more expensive and less readily available. **1** Severe leptospirosis is treated with intravenous penicillin (1.5 million units every 6 hours). Intravenous ceftriaxone (1 g once a day) **2** and cefotaxime (1 g every 6 hours) have equivalent efficacy as penicillin for severe leptospirosis; parenteral doxycycline (100 mg every 12 hours) is a satisfactory alternative. **3**

Other antimicrobial agents may have potential therapeutic use, although at present their efficacy is unproven. *Leptospira* organisms are susceptible in vitro to chloramphenicol and to quinolone and macrolide agents. The duration of antimicrobial therapy is usually 7 days. Although patients require monitoring for Jarisch-Herxheimer reactions during initiation of antimicrobial therapy, this complication is less frequently observed than with other spirochetal infections.

Reducing mortality from severe leptospirosis requires prompt triage of high-risk patients and aggressive supportive care for hypotension, acute renal and lung injury, and hemorrhage. Patients with nonoliguric hypokalemic renal insufficiency have a better overall prognosis and can be treated by volume and potassium repletion. Timely initiation of dialysis is critical to prevent mortality from oliguric renal insufficiency. Continuous hemofiltration is more effective than peritoneal dialysis in treating infection-associated acute renal failure. To date there is no evidence to indicate the use of pulse glucocorticosteroid and desmopressin in the treatment of severe leptospirosis. **4**

PREVENTION

Prevention of leptospirosis is based on controlling animal reservoirs, interrupting transmission routes, and preventing disease in humans. Control measures that target defined animal populations, such as dogs, pigs, and cattle, are highly effective. Immunization of domestic animals and livestock may reduce carriage and transmission to humans. Chemical pesticides and environmental control of the habitats of domestic rodent reservoirs are important, but difficult to implement, especially in urban slum settings. Control of sylvatic reservoirs is often not feasible. When possible, environmental sources of transmission can be decontaminated with hypochlorite solution and isolated. Protective clothing such as gloves and boots reduces the risk for occupational exposure. Although infection after exposure to human urine has not been documented, precautions need to be taken when handling patients' secretions.

Doxycycline chemoprophylaxis (200 mg orally per week) may be efficacious in preventing clinical disease but does not reduce *Leptospira* seroconversion when used either as postexposure prophylaxis (e.g., in indigenous populations after a flood) or as pre-exposure prophylaxis (e.g., in indigenous populations or deployed soldiers).**5** Doxycycline (100 mg orally twice a day for 3 to 7 days) or amoxicillin is used as chemoprophylaxis in situations where exposure to the pathogen has been documented (e.g., laboratory accident–related exposures); however, the efficacy of these regimens has not been evaluated. Bacterin-based vaccines have been used for high-risk groups in several countries and in mass immunization campaigns in Cuba and China; at present, however, the effectiveness and safety of these vaccines are uncertain.

PROGNOSIS

Although leptospirosis is usually a self-limited illness, mortality is high in patients with severe disease manifestations. Case-fatality rates in patients with Weil's disease and pulmonary hemorrhage syndrome are 5 to 40% and higher than 50%, respectively. Prognostic predictors for death are older age (>40 years), oliguria, respiratory insufficiency, pulmonary hemorrhage, cardiac arrhythmias, and altered mental status. Follow-up of patients has found that hepatic and renal function typically returns to baseline levels within 1 month and 6 months, respectively, after acute illness. However, unilateral or bilateral uveitis characterized by iritis, iridocyclitis, and chorioretinitis may develop up to 18 months after systemic illness and persist for years.

1. Phimda K, Hoontrakul S, Suttinont C, et al. Doxycycline versus azithromycin for treatment of leptospirosis and scrub typhus. *Antimicrob Agents Chemother.* 2007;51:3259-3263.
2. Panaphut T, Domrongkitchaiporn S, Vibhagool A, et al. Ceftriaxone compared with sodium penicillin G for treatment of severe leptospirosis. *Clin Infect Dis.* 2003;36:1507-1513.
3. Suputtamongkol Y, Niwattayakul K, Suttinont C, et al. An open, randomized, controlled trial of penicillin, doxycycline, and cefotaxime for patients with severe leptospirosis. *Clin Infect Dis.* 2004;39:1417-1424.
4. Niwattayakul K, Kaewtasi S, Chueasuwanchai S, et al. An open randomized controlled trial of desmopressin and pulse dexamethasone as adjunct therapy in patients with pulmonary involvement associated with severe leptospirosis. *Clin Microbiol Infect.* 2010;16:1207-1212.
5. Brett-Major DM, Lipnick RJ. Antibiotic prophylaxis for leptospirosis. *Cochrane Database Syst Rev.* 2009;3:CD007342.

SUGGESTED READINGS

Daher EF, Lima RS, Silva Júnior GB, et al. Clinical presentation of leptospirosis: a retrospective study of 201 patients in a metropolitan city of Brazil. *Braz J Infect Dis.* 2010;14:3-10. *The mean age was 39 years, 80% were male, and the common manifestations were fever (97%), jaundice (95%), myalgia (93%), headache (75%), vomiting (72%), and dehydration (64%), with hemorrhage in 36% and death in 15%.*
Katz AR, Buchholz AE, Hinson K, et al. Leptospirosis in Hawaii, USA, 1999–2008. *Emerg Infect Dis.* 2011;17:221-226. *An average of 20 cases are confirmed per year, including recreational exposures and occupational exposures.*
Marchiori E, Lourenço S, Setúbal S, et al. Clinical and imaging manifestations of hemorrhagic pulmonary leptospirosis: a state-of-the-art review. *Lung.* 2011;189:1-9. *Review of this severe complication.*
Stern EJ, Galloway R, Shadomy SV, et al. Outbreak of leptospirosis among adventure race participants in Florida, 2005. *Clin Infect Dis.* 2010;50:843-849. *Instructive study of a multistate outbreak investigation among adventure racers.*
Toyokawa T, Ohnishi M, Koizumi N. Diagnosis of acute leptospirosis. *Expert Rev Anti Infect Ther.* 2011;9:111-121. *Emphasizes PCR.*

TUBERCULOSIS

JERROLD J. ELLNER

DEFINITION

Tuberculosis (TB) is a chronic necrotizing granulomatous disease caused by the acid-fast bacillus (AFB) *Mycobacterium tuberculosis* or the closely related species *Mycobacterium africanum* and *Mycobacterium bovis*. The most common site of disease is the lung, and the most common extrapulmonary sites are the lymph nodes, pleura, bones, and joints. TB is spread from person to person by the inhalation of infectious droplet nuclei aerosolized by patients with pulmonary TB (PTB). TB is a major cause of morbidity and mortality worldwide, but chiefly in resource-limited settings, and has eluded public health measures aimed at its control. The human immunodeficiency virus (HIV) pandemic has led to a resurgence of TB, and the global public health problem of TB has been compounded by increasing drug-resistant disease.

The Pathogen

TB is caused by infection with any of three members of the *M. tuberculosis* complex—*M. tuberculosis*, *M. africanum*, or *M bovis*. The complex also includes the nonpathogenic organisms *Mycobacterium microti* and *Mycobacterium canetti*. The causative organism is a slender, nonmotile, non–spore-forming, non–toxin-producing bacillus that may be beaded and is approximately 2 to 4 μm in length. It is a slow-growing (doubling time of 18 to 24 hours) facultative aerobe that can persist intracellularly for prolonged periods. The organism is identified in clinical specimens as an "acid-fast bacillus." The basis for "acid-fastness" is the waxy coat of the organism, which is composed of mycolic acid and other complex lipopolysaccharides. The organism takes up stain poorly but can be stained with carbol fuchsin by either alkalinization (Kinyoun) or heat (Ziehl-Neelsen) methods. The coat of *M. tuberculosis* precludes decolorization of the stain with a mixture of acid and alcohol. Virulent *M. tuberculosis* may clump or form "cords" in liquid culture.

DNA sequencing of *M. tuberculosis* and other scientific advances have promoted basic understanding of the metabolism and virulence of the organism, its immunodominant antigens, and its capacity to survive adverse conditions and persist intracellularly (Fig. 332-1). These advances have been translated into lead candidates for protective vaccines and targets for drug development. Clinical isolates of *M. tuberculosis* differ in their virulence in experimental models, potential for transmission in humans, and interaction with the host (immunopathology, induction of host cytokines, delayed-type hypersensitivity [DTH]). In the hypervirulent *Beijing* strain family, these differences have been ascribed to overexpression of a phenolic glycolipid that inhibits innate immunity.

A variety of typing systems have been applied to study the lineage of *M. tuberculosis*. Genomic deletion analysis shows six main phylogeographic lineages, each associated with a specific human population. The families differ in geographic distribution. It is not yet clear whether they also differ in their potential for transmission and pathogenesis. Strain typing can be performed by several techniques, such as restriction fragment length polymorphism (RFLP) of the insertional element IS 6110 or spoligotyping. Determining the DNA fingerprint of the causative organism is particularly useful in outbreak investigations. The finding that multiple cases of TB constitute a cluster and are caused by the same strain suggests that they may be epidemiologically linked. Identifying case clusters is important because it suggests recent transmission, possibly in the context of an outbreak.

TB caused by *M. africanum* is clinically identical to that caused by *M. tuberculosis*, and biochemical distinction between the organisms, though feasible, is therefore not generally useful. *M. bovis* has greater than 95% DNA homology with *M. tuberculosis* and can cause disease in humans, cattle, deer, badgers, and other animals. Most strains are resistant to the antituberculosis agent pyrazinamide (PZA). Therefore, the finding that an isolate that appears to be *M. tuberculosis* is monoresistant to PZA raises the possibility that it is, in fact, *M. bovis*, a distinction that can be confirmed only in specialized laboratories.

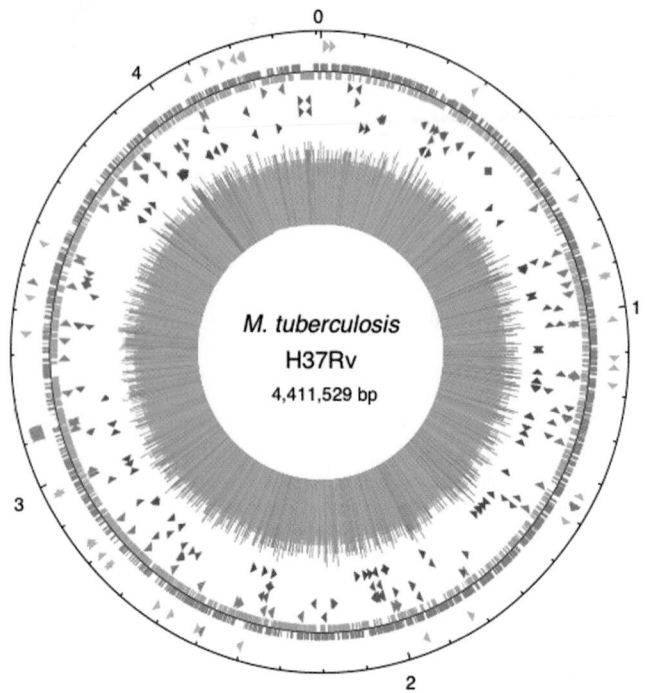

FIGURE 332-1. Circular map of the chromosome of *M. tuberculosis H37Rv*. The outer circle shows the scale in megabases, with 0 representing the origin of replication. The first ring from the exterior denotes the positions of stable RNA genes (tRNAs are *blue*; others are *pink*) and the direct repeat region (*pink cube*), the second ring inward shows the coding sequence by strand (clockwise, *dark green*; anticlockwise, *light green*), the third ring depicts repetitive DNA (insertion sequences, *orange*; 13E12 REP family, *dark pink*; prophage, *blue*), the fourth ring shows the positions of the PPE family members (*green*), the fifth ring shows the PE family members (*purple*, excluding PGRS), and the sixth ring shows the positions of the PGRS sequences (*dark red*). The histogram (center) represents G + C content, with <65% G + C in *yellow* and >65% G + C in *red*. The figure was generated with software from DNASTAR. (Reprinted from Cole ST, Brosch R, Parkhill JH, et al. Deciphering the biology of mycobacteria and tuberculosis from the complete genome sequence. *Nature.* 1998;393: 537-544, with permission.)

The main route of transmission of *M. tuberculosis* is person to person through respiratory aerosols generated by coughing. Bacilli in small droplet nuclei (1 to 5 μm in diameter) remain suspended in air for long periods and, once inhaled, can reach the airways, where one to five organisms are sufficient to cause infection. Laryngeal involvement often renders the patient highly infectious with the possibility of transmission by phonation. Direct cutaneous inoculation ("prosector's wart") does occur, but direct transcutaneous inoculation from infected secretions is rare. *M. bovis* can be transmitted by the gastrointestinal route, usually through the ingestion of contaminated milk.

EPIDEMIOLOGY

In 2009 there were an estimated 9.4 million new cases of TB and 1.7 million deaths as a result of TB; 95% of the cases and 99% of the deaths occurred in resource-limited settings. Fifty-five percent of cases of TB occurred in Asia and 30% in Africa. The largest number of cases was in India and China. Worldwide, TB occurs more commonly in males than females, and the prevalence of disease peaks in young adults. HIV infection has a profound effect on the epidemiology of TB by accelerating the natural history of disease and promoting progression from infection to active TB. There are an estimated 1.1 million HIV-infected persons with TB worldwide, 80% of whom reside in sub-Saharan Africa. As a result, the highest case rates of TB are found in sub-Saharan Africa. TB is a leading cause of death in HIV-infected individuals.

In the United States in 2008, the incidence of TB was 4.2 per 100,000, with 12,904 cases reported. The age-specific prevalence of TB in the United States is skewed toward older adults; the case rate was 6.4 per 100,000 in adults older than 65 years versus 3.4 to 5.1 in 15- to 64-year-olds. Fifty-nine percent of cases occurred in the foreign born, most of whom emigrated with existing *M. tuberculosis* infection from areas endemic for TB. Asians had the highest incidence of TB (25.6/100,000). The countries of origin with the highest prevalence were Mexico, the Philippines, Vietnam, India, and China.

California, Texas, New York, and Florida accounted for 49% of cases, and the prevalence is highest in inner-city areas. Approximately 10% of TB patients in the United States are infected with HIV. Overall, the prevalence of latent tuberculosis infection (LTBI) (defined as a positive tuberculin skin test [TST] or interferon-γ release assay [IGRA] and no active disease) is approximately 4%, and TB disease is more common in this group (12.9/1000 person years). Other conditions that increase the risk for TB are shown in Table 332-1. Smoking and alcoholism also confer an increased risk for TB, though smaller than the conditions listed.

TB caused by drug-resistant organisms is a particular and emerging threat to public health. Multidrug-resistant (MDR) TB (caused by organisms resistant to isoniazid [INH] and rifampin [RIF]) and extensively drug resistant (XDR) TB (MDR plus resistance to fluoroquinolones [FQs] and a second-line injectable—kanamycin, amikacin, or capreomycin) are much more difficult and expensive to treat and in some cases may be incurable. Resistant disease is more common in re-treatment cases of TB. An estimated 500,000 new cases of MDR TB occur annually, and 5 to 10% of these new cases are XDR. Twenty-seven countries account for 85% of the cases of MDR TB, with most occurring in India, China, and the Russian Federation. In the United States, MDR TB was found in 1.0% of new cases of TB, 76.7% of them foreign born, and in 4.2% of re-treatment cases, 88.2% of whom were foreign born.

PATHOBIOLOGY

Typically, the chain of transmission of TB begins with an infectious case of PTB. Infectiousness of a patient is determined by sputum smear status (3 to 4+ AFB), cough strength and frequency, the presence of cavitary lung disease, and the characteristics of the physical space occupied by the source (ventilation and air recirculation). However, not all strongly AFB smear–positive patients with PTB are equally infectious, and there may be high transmitters. Recent studies, in fact, show that only a third of strongly sputum smear–positive persons with PTB generate aerosols that contain viable organisms.

In both low- and high-prevalence countries, exposure often occurs in the household. Even in this setting, where exposure may be intense and protracted, only half of close contacts become infected. In contrast, in outbreaks in residential shelters, hospitals, and prisons, *M. tuberculosis* infection or disease has been documented after brief exposure. Important variables that may explain differences in transmission include virulence of the organism, innate immunity, and susceptibility of the exposed populations (e.g., HIV infected).

Occasionally, primary TB may be associated with minor clinical manifestations as described later. Two to 13 weeks after primary infection, specific adaptive immunity develops and limits bacterial replication. In this time interval, pleural TB may also occur. Infection is usually recognized by conversion of the TST from negative to positive or the development of a positive IGRA. Primary infection is accompanied by occult dissemination of *M. tuberculosis*, and host factors have a great impact on whether progressive primary TB develops, a condition that is most likely in infants younger than 4 years, who are at risk for TB meningitis and miliary TB, and in those with comorbid conditions. In approximately 40% of HIV-infected persons exposed to individuals with infectious TB, active TB will develop and occur in a compressed time frame (within 120 days). In otherwise normal hosts, there is an approximately 2 to 5% risk of primary infection progressing within the first 2 years to PTB. The risk may be higher if exposure to the index case is particularly intense. Granulomas are the focus of infection and the hallmark of primary TB infection and pleural effusion. Recent evidence suggests that granulomas, long thought to be a key element of protective immunity, may be responsible for local spread of the initial infection. The primary focus heals with fibrosis and possibly calcification. Pleural TB will also resolve without treatment, although there is an increased risk for reactivation.

Most (>95%) infected persons thereafter enter a period of clinical latency. During this period, latency is maintained by the active immune system. Evidence for such latency is the increased risk for reactivation TB once immunosuppression supervenes. In HIV-infected individuals, this risk may approach 5 to 10% per year. In addition, bacterial replication occurs during latency as evidenced by the fact that treatment of latent infection with INH and other agents active only in the growth cycle of replication markedly decreases the risk for reactivation. During the period of clinical latency, the TST and IGRA remain positive in most cases. In some there may, however, be reversion of the TST to negative. It is not clear whether this represents waning of the immune response to the tuberculous focus or a diminished number of replicating organisms.

TABLE 332-1 RISK FACTORS FOR TUBERCULOSIS

RISK FACTOR	RISK FOR RECENT INFECTION*	RISK FOR PROGRESSION OF INFECTION TO DISEASE	TST CUT POINT	TB CASES/1000 PERSON YEARS (TST⁺)	RELATIVE RISK— TST UNKNOWN
Household contact of person with PTB	X		≥5 mm	12.9	
Solid organ transplant recipients		X	≥5 mm		20-74
Immunosuppressive treatment (anti-TNF, prednisone ≥15 mg/day for ≥1 mo)		X	≥5 mm		8-30
Fibrotic lesions on chest radiograph consistent with prior TB		X	≥5 mm	2-13.6	
HIV infection	X	X	≥5 mm	35-162	20-37
Foreign born; injecting drug users; TST-positive children, adolescents, young adults	X		≥10mm		
Residents or workers in hospitals, homeless shelters, correctional facilities, nursing homes, residences for the HIV infected	X		≥10 mm		
Underweight (≥15%)		X	≥10 mm	2.6	
Silicosis				68	30
Diabetes mellitus (particularly insulin dependent or poorly controlled)					2.0-4.1
Renal failure/hemodialysis					10-25.3
Gastrectomy					2-5
Jejunoileal bypass					27-63
Carcinoma of the head and neck, lung cancer, lymphoma, leukemia					16
No risk factors			≥15mm		

*Recent infection per se increases the risk for progressing from infection to disease (12.9 cases per 1000 person years in the first year vs. 1.6 per 1000 person years in the subsequent 7 years).
HIV = human immunodeficiency virus; PTB = pulmonary tuberculosis; TB = tuberculosis; TNF = tumor necrosis factor; TST = tuberculin skin test.

Delayed activation (termed *reactivation*) of TB may follow an overt immunosuppressive event or the development of comorbid conditions or occur without clear antecedent. Predisposing medical risk factors are considered in Table 332-1. Reactivation of TB in a host with preexisting immunity leads to a vigorous inflammatory response and, in the case of pulmonary disease, to the development of caseating granulomas and, ultimately, cavitary lung disease. Immunologically, reactivation TB is associated with transient systemic immunosuppression (and sometimes TST reversion) caused by two pro-inflammatory but immunosuppressive cytokines, transforming growth factor-β and interleukin-10. These cytokines are overproduced by activated circulating monocytes, regulatory T cells, or both.

The lung is the site of most cases of reactivation TB. The hallmark of the pathology is granuloma formation with caseation necrosis and multinucleated Langerhans giant cells. The caseous material contains AFBs. *M. tuberculosis* multiplies exuberantly in the liquid caseum. Immunologically, expectorated sputum contains cytokines and both upregulators and downregulators of the immune and inflammatory response, the latter being dominant. Bronchoalveolar lavage shows a lymphocytic alveolitis with an influx of immature macrophages, apparently representing monocytes attracted from blood. In sum, there is an active but downregulated immune response concomitant with bacterial replication. As a consequence of the inflammation, extensive apoptosis occurs and may lead to the deletion of *M. tuberculosis*-responsive T cells, a factor that may play a role in the requirement for a long duration of therapy and in the relapses that may represent reinfection TB. In HIV-infected persons with advanced immunosuppression, granulomas may be poorly formed or absent. There is infiltration with foamy epithelioid cells, which are actually macrophages laden with AFBs. Caseation may or may not be present, but there may be extensive inflammation and necrosis.

Extrapulmonary TB can involve any organ. Persistence of organisms in areas that are relatively well oxygenated has been cited to explain the more frequent sites of reactivation, such as the apices of the lung, cortices of the kidney, and vertebral bodies.

Several forms of extrapulmonary TB have a shared pathogenesis: discharge of a contiguous tuberculous focus into a serosal cavity, a brisk inflammatory reaction based on previous DTH, fever, frequently negative smears of exudative fluid for AFBs, and sometimes a transiently negative TST. The focus that discharges may be a long-standing focus or one seeded during recent dissemination during primary infection. This basic scenario occurs in pleural TB, TB pericarditis, TB meningitis (the parameningeal focus is called a "Rich focus"), TB peritonitis, and TB arthritis.

Pleural TB represents an in situ DTH reaction with activation of T_H1 helper T cells, abundant cytokines, including interferon-γ and tumor necrosis factor-α, and apoptosis. In non–HIV-infected individuals, organisms are sparse, which may be why self-cure of pleural TB can take place. However, in the absence of chemotherapy for TB, there is a high risk for recurrence of TB, usually as PTB on the side contralateral to the effusion.

In addition to reactivation of a latent focus, reinfection with *M. tuberculosis* may occur and progress to disease. Reinfection is more likely to occur if the host is immunosuppressed or there is repeated or intense exposure.

CLINICAL MANIFESTATIONS

Primary Tuberculosis

Most cases of primary TB are asymptomatic and diagnosed by conversion of the TST. There may be fever, shortness of breath, nonproductive cough, and occasionally erythema nodosum. Crepitations and focal wheezes may be present. Chest radiographs show small patchy opacities in the midlung fields, often with unilateral hilar lymphadenopathy. Upper or middle lobe collapse as a result of bronchial compression by enlarged nodes or transient pleural effusion may also be seen. This regresses without specific therapy because of the development of an adaptive immune response. During the subsequent period of clinical latency, evidence of the primary infection may be found as a small calcified parenchymal scar in the midlung fields (Ghon complex), sometimes associated with similar findings in the draining hilar nodes (Ranke complex) (Fig. 332-2A). Small scars caused by arrested lesions in the apices of the lung are called a Simon focus. Pleural TB may be a manifestation of primary or reactivation TB and is discussed later.

Progressive Primary Tuberculosis

Failure to develop adaptive immunity is most common in young children, the elderly and the immunocompromised. Progressive primary TB manifested as TB meningitis, miliary TB, or PTB may develop in this scenario. These syndromes are indistinguishable clinically, regardless of whether they are a manifestation of primary progressive or delayed reactivation TB, and are described subsequently.

Reactivation Tuberculosis

The terms *reactivation TB* and *postprimary TB* are used interchangeably to connote that primary TB is followed by a variable period of clinical latency, after which TB develops and occurs in the setting of DTH/adaptive

FIGURE 332-2. A, Ghon complex. B, Moderately advanced pulmonary tuberculosis. C, Far advanced pulmonary tuberculosis. D, Pulmonary and extrapulmonary tuberculosis. (Radiographs provided courtesy of Thomas M. Daniel, MD.)

immunity, which contributes importantly to the pathogenesis and clinical manifestations.

PTB is the most common form of reactivation TB. The typical findings consist of the insidious onset of a productive cough, night sweats, anorexia, and weight loss. Fever is present in approximately half of those affected. Patients may be asymptomatic and the diagnosis suggested by a chest radiograph obtained for other reasons. The sputum may be purulent, blood streaked, or frankly bloody. Pleuritic chest pain may occur when there is subpleural inflammation. Dyspnea is not a hallmark of PTB, in part because thrombosis of vessels limits the perfusion of inflamed areas, so hypoxemia is not a prominent clinical feature. Physical examination may show dullness to percussion, low-pitched amphoric (hollow sounding) breath sounds, and occasionally crepitations that may be post-tussive. Chest radiographs often reveal more disease than suggested by physical examination (see Fig. 332-2B and C). Typically, lesions are found in the apical and posterior segments of the upper lobes and the superior (dorsal) segment of the lower lobe. There is a progression from patchy opacities and consolidation to cavitation reflective of caseation, liquefaction, and rupture into bronchi. Intrabronchial spread may lead to disease in multiple areas, including the other lung ("TB bronchopneumonia"). There may also be involvement of the larynx and middle ear. Early cavities are thin walled. Ten percent of all cavities have an air-fluid level. There may be an associated pleural effusion or, with rupture of cavities into the air space, rarely pyopneumothorax. If the disease is minimal, it may best be seen on apical lordotic chest radiographs or on computed tomography (CT). Rarely, chest radiographs are normal and the accompanying symptoms and positive sputum smears may be the result of endobronchial lesions or rupture of a tuberculous node into bronchi. With healing, fibrosis and contraction obliterate small cavities, although large cavities may persist and even become the eventual nidus for an aspergilloma.

In immunocompromised persons, the opacities may be located in the mid and lower lung fields and be manifested as poorly resolving lobar or segmental pneumonitis, atelectasis, nodules, and cavities. Early in the course of HIV infection when the CD4$^+$ count exceeds 200/μL, PTB may be typical in its manifestation. At lower CD4$^+$ counts, mid and lower lung abnormalities are more common. At a CD4$^+$ count below 100/μL, the findings may be quite atypical, with prominent hilar and mediastinal adenopathy, pleural disease, interstitial or miliary opacities, or any combination of these manifestations. This picture resembles primary TB and, in fact, may represent progressive primary TB or reinfection disease. Chest radiographs are normal in up to 20% of persons with culture-confirmed TB, sometimes in the presence of a smear that contains AFBs. In this CD4 strata, disseminated and extrapulmonary disease is the rule, with or without concurrent PTB.

FIGURE 332-3. Miliary tuberculosis in a 70-year-old man. **A,** A posteroanterior chest radiograph shows evenly distributed, discrete, uniformly millet-sized nodular opacities in both lungs. **B,** High-resolution computed tomography (1.0-mm section thickness) at the level of the right upper lobar bronchus shows uniformly sized small nodules randomly distributed throughout both lungs. Note the subpleural and subfissural nodules (*arrows*). (From Jeong YJ, Lee KS. Pulmonary tuberculosis: up-to-date imaging and management. *AJR Am J Roentgenol.* 2008;191:834-844.)

Reinfection Tuberculosis

Reinfection TB is clinically indistinguishable from other forms. A shift in the drug susceptibility profile, a documented change in the DNA fingerprint, or occurrence in an outbreak setting may be the only evidence supporting the diagnosis of reinfection TB.

Extrapulmonary Tuberculosis

Approximately 20% of cases of TB in non–HIV-infected populations are extrapulmonary. In areas endemic for TB, extrapulmonary TB often occurs concurrently with PTB and is more common in children and young adults, in whom it represents progressive primary infection. By contrast, in low-prevalence areas, isolated extrapulmonary TB is more common and there is a shift to the elderly that represents reactivation TB. HIV infection is associated with a higher frequency of extrapulmonary disease, including the more serious forms disseminated TB and TB meningitis.

Pleural Tuberculosis

Pleural TB occurs by direct extension when a subpleural caseous focus discharges into the pleural space or through hematogenous seeding. There may be concurrent PTB. Its peak occurrence is 3 to 6 months after primary infection. The typical manifestation is the abrupt onset of fever, pleuritic chest pain, and cough. Occasionally, there is an insidious manifestation consisting of fever, weight loss, and malaise. If the pleural effusion is large enough, shortness of breath may be seen. Physical examination shows dullness to percussion and decreased breath sounds. Above the area of dullness there may be true egophony. Chest radiographs typically show unilateral pleural effusion, more frequently in the right hemithorax. Bilateral disease occurs in 10% of cases. Pleural effusions may be medium sized, large, or uncommonly massive.

Miliary Tuberculosis

Miliary TB usually has an insidious manifestation consisting of fever, weight loss, night sweats, and little in the way of localizing symptoms or signs. There may be concurrent TB meningitis with associated symptoms. Physical examination may show choroidal tubercles (pathognomonic raised white-yellow plaques on funduscopic examination, present in 15% of cases), lymphadenopathy, and hepatomegaly. Chest radiographs may show multiple bilateral small opacities, termed *miliary infiltrates* because of their resemblance to millet seeds. The findings on initial chest radiographs are often subtle and may be clear-cut only in retrospect after 3 months of follow-up. Performance of CT or high-resolution CT is useful because of its increased sensitivity (Fig. 332-3). A variant of miliary TB is "disseminated areactive TB," as may occur in HIV-infected patients or those treated with tumor necrosis factor inhibitors. In this entity, chest radiographic findings may be even more minimal. In the HIV infected with advanced immunodeficiency, blood cultures are positive for *M. tuberculosis* in 20 to 40% of patients and may be the only manifestation of TB.

Tuberculous Meningitis

TB meningitis is usually characterized by less than 2 weeks of fever, headache, and meningismus. There may be depressed levels of consciousness, diplopia,

and rarely, hemiparesis. Physical examination shows a stiff neck and, occasionally, cranial neuropathy (VI, III, IV, VII in order of frequency) and long-tract signs. Chest radiographs may be consistent with PTB or miliary TB. CT of the head may show contrast enhancement over the basilar meninges, hypodense areas consistent with infarcts, hydrocephalus, and sometimes focal inflammatory lesions (tuberculomas).

Tuberculous Lymphadenitis

Lymphadenitis may be the sole manifestation of TB or, more frequently, particularly in the HIV infected, may accompany PTB. Patients with isolated lymph node disease may be afebrile. The supraclavicular and posterior cervical lymph nodes are most frequently involved. This is in contrast to scrofula from atypical mycobacteria or *M. bovis* and is often seen in children, in whom submandibular and high anterior cervical adenopathy predominates. The lymphadenitis is not usually painful, and aspiration of the lymph node with the finding of AFBs is an excellent approach to establish the diagnosis.

Tuberculous Pericarditis

The usual manifestation of TB pericarditis is chronic but may occasionally be subacute with fever, night sweats, chest pain, shortness of breath, pedal edema, and other signs of right heart failure. Physical examination shows signs of pericardial disease, right-sided heart failure, and tamponade (in about 10%). Pericardial aspiration and biopsy are the diagnostic procedures of choice. When tamponade is present, a pericardial window can be both diagnostic and therapeutic.

Tuberculous Peritonitis

TB peritonitis may be accompanied by abdominal pain and fever, at times mimicking an acute abdomen. Alternatively, there may be an insidious manifestation consisting of abdominal pain, swelling, night sweats, and weight loss. The clinical syndrome is caused by discharge of tuberculous lymph nodes into the peritoneal space. Exudative ascites is usually present unless TB is superimposed on preexisting transudative ascites, as in alcoholic liver disease. On physical examination the abdomen has been described as "doughy" because matted loops of bowel may be palpable. A variant of this syndrome is perhaps best termed *abdominal TB*. In this case the abdominal pain is subacute, the associated findings on physical examination less striking, and ascites less prominent or absent. The best method for diagnosis when ascites is present is laparoscopically guided peritoneal biopsy. In areas endemic for TB and HIV, the finding of intra-abdominal lymphadenopathy on abdominal ultrasound or CT is often used to support the diagnosis of abdominal TB.

Gastrointestinal Tuberculosis

Patients with gastrointestinal TB have fever, abdominal pain, and gastrointestinal bleeding or obstruction. Roentgenograms of the small bowel and abdominal CT show involvement of the terminal ileum, similar to Crohn's disease. The diagnosis is made on clinical suspicion in areas endemic for TB and HIV or by the finding of TB elsewhere. Occasionally, intraluminal biopsy of the terminal ileum or other involved sites is used to establish the diagnosis.

Renal Tuberculosis

There may be few symptoms and signs associated with renal TB, although occasionally dysuria, hematuria, and flank pain are present. The diagnosis is often suggested by the finding of sterile pyuria or hematuria as initial abnormalities that trigger evaluation. Physical examination is usually unremarkable. Intravenous pyelography or CT shows cortical scarring, occasionally with mass or cavitary lesions, papillary necrosis with calyceal and ureteral dilation, or "beading" of the ureter because of ureteral strictures (see Fig. 332-2D).

Vertebral Osteomyelitis

The initial site of disease is the subchondral region of the anterior portion of the vertebral body. The lower thoracic and lumbar vertebrae are involved most commonly. The disc space is initially spared but becomes involved late with spread to adjacent vertebrae. Paravertebral "cold abscesses" may dissect through tissue planes. Patients have back and sometimes radicular pain. Occasionally and more often with cervical disease, there may be weakness of the lower extremities and incontinence of stool and urine. Physical examination may show a gibbus deformity caused by anterior compression fractures or paraparesis. Radiographs of the spine, as well as CT and magnetic resonance imaging, may show abnormalities in adjacent vertebrae with anterior compression (Fig. 332-2D). Cold abscesses may be appreciated as well.

Other Forms of Extrapulmonary Tuberculosis

TB of the bone or joints may be manifested subacutely as a combination of synovitis and osteomyelitis. The joints involved may have sustained previous trauma. TB of the female genital tract may result in pelvic pain, menorrhagia, vaginal discharge, or infertility. Males may have an epididymal mass, sometimes seen in patients with miliary TB. TB can cause granulomatous uveitis.

DIAGNOSIS

Infection with *M. tuberculosis*

The diagnosis of LTBI is one of exclusion based on the finding of DTH and the absence of active TB. The TST has been used widely and there is strong epidemiologic evidence supporting its interpretation. Tuberculin purified protein derivative (PPD) derived from autoclaved culture filtrates of *M. tuberculosis* is used to elicit DTH. The response elicited by PPD is nonspecific because of broad cross-reactivity among tuberculous and nontuberculous mycobacteria and other organisms as well. The TST is performed by injecting 5 tuberculin units of PPD in 0.1 mL intradermally. The reaction is assessed as induration after 48 to 72 hours. Problems with the TST are legend. It is the only bioassay used in clinical medicine, and there is no quality control of the application or reading of the TST. The sensitivity of the TST is less in immunosuppressed patients, such as those with HIV infection, and also less in the presence of active TB. The TST may revert to negative over time, and it may be boosted by the application of PPD. This can result in a "pseudoconversion" that does not represent new infection with *M. tuberculosis*. Perhaps the greatest limitation of the TST is its nonspecificity. There has been uncertainty in its interpretation, particularly in the setting of previous vaccination with *M. bovis* bacille Calmette-Guérin (BCG). BCG administered once at birth has little effect on the TST beyond the first year. By 10 years of age, only 1% of positive TSTs can be ascribed to previous BCG administration.

The TST remains of value in the diagnosis of LTBI in at-risk individuals (see Table 332-1) who are candidates for treatment (preventive therapy). Interpretation of the TST is based on a "sliding scale" that takes into account an individual's a priori risk for *M. tuberculosis* infection and the risk for progressing to disease, if infected (Table 332-1). This, in effect, modifies the sensitivity and specificity of the TST. It should be noted that routine testing is not recommended for low-risk populations; however, testing may be performed because of employment. Certain populations should undergo annual testing, including staff or individuals living or working in congregate settings (incarcerated, homeless, HIV infected, correctional facility staff), injection drug users, and others at risk because of sociodemographic factors. For individuals who will undergo an annual TST, a true baseline should be established by two-step skin testing. After the initial negative TST, the test is repeated in 1 to 3 weeks (there is no need to repeat the test if the first TST is positive). An increased reaction size on the second TST is defined as boosting and may be due to previous infection with nontuberculous mycobacteria

or *M. tuberculosis* or vaccination with BCG. TST conversion from negative to positive is the best indicator of intervening new infection with *M. tuberculosis* and is defined as an increase in reaction size of 6 mm or greater from less than 10 mm to 10 mm or greater. It also may be of value to perform a two-step TST on individuals older than 60 years and therefore at risk for TST reversion.

In HIV infection, the TST may be negative before the administration of antiretroviral therapy (ART) and convert to positive with treatment. For this reason it is recommended that the TST be repeated in TST-negative HIV-infected persons once their CD4$^+$ count reaches 200/μL and annually thereafter.

The sensitivity of the TST is decreased in individuals with TB, more so in certain forms of extrapulmonary TB. Though insensitive for the diagnosis of active TB, the TST has another application in low-prevalence areas. If the differential diagnosis of a clinical condition includes TB, establishment of previous *M. tuberculosis* infection increases the likelihood that the clinical findings represent TB. The TST is of particular value in the evaluation of smear-negative patients with pulmonary disease suggestive of PTB and in patients suspected of having extrapulmonary TB. Confirmatory findings such as positive culture or histology or response to therapy are necessary to establish the diagnosis of TB.

IGRAs have also been approved for the diagnosis of LTBI, and the CDC considers them interchangeable with the TST. The main advantage of IGRAs is specificity because the antigens used to stimulate the production of interferon-γ are relatively restricted to *M. tuberculosis* and not present in BCG and most nontuberculous mycobacteria. IGRAs also require only a single patient visit. The disadvantages of IGRAs are expense, technical requirements, and controversy over test sensitivity in certain situations such as HIV infection and in household contacts of patients with PTB. The main indication for performing an IGRA, therefore, is to diagnose LTBI in a person who had received BCG vaccination beyond the first year of age. There are several other situations in which IGRAs may be useful. One would be confirmation of a positive TST. Another might be HIV infection. Because treatment of LTBI is effective in TST-positive HIV-infected persons and the risk for progression of infection is inordinately high in such individuals, it is important to perform tests with high negative predictive value. Therefore, both a TST and IGRA should be performed in HIV-infected persons and others at high risk of progression from infectious diseases or poor outcome. If either is positive, the individual would become a candidate for treatment of LTBI.

Active Tuberculosis

In countries with a high TB burden, the diagnosis of TB is often based on clinical symptoms and sputum microscopy. Clinical diagnosis without the benefit of culture confirmation or radiography is the norm in endemic countries where access to diagnostics is limited. The diagnosis is also made on clinical grounds alone when smears are negative and suspicion for TB is high. Cultures, if available, require several weeks to months, and the decision to begin therapy must be made promptly. Clinical diagnosis is particularly important in HIV-infected persons because of the risk for rapid progression of the TB if left untreated and in those with forms of TB that are paucibacillary (pediatric, meningeal, miliary, abdominal, pleural, pericardial). The diagnosis of miliary, abdominal, pleural, and pericardial TB may be confirmed by the finding of AFBs in biopsied tissue or by culture. In the absence of bacteriologic confirmation, either because cultures are negative or because they are unavailable, the final diagnosis often relies on response to therapy or establishment of an alternative diagnosis. It should be noted that the empirical approach, taken of necessity in resource-limited settings, leads to overdiagnosis and overtreatment of TB, which expends TB program resources and delays treatment of other infections. It is therefore preferable to attempt to establish a definite diagnosis based on demonstration of *M. tuberculosis* by smears, cultures, or nucleic acid amplification tests of infected secretions or tissue specimens.

Sputum microscopy is the standard approach to the diagnosis of PTB. A smear requires 1000 to 10,000 bacilli per mL to be read as positive. Both hot and cold carbol fuchsin methods (Ziehl-Neelsen and Kinyoun) are used extensively. The use of fluorochrome stains such as auramine-rhodamine allows more rapid screening of sputum smears. Three specimens, preferably early morning samples, should be examined to establish the diagnosis. Yield is higher in the presence of cavitary lung disease. Approximately half of individuals with PTB are AFB sputum smear negative, and this proportion is higher in the HIV infected. The quantity of AFBs present in the sputum smear is a measure of the infectiousness of patients with PTB, and on this basis a second important role as a tool to monitor the potential for transmission and response to therapy has evolved for the sputum smear.

HIV-infected persons with PTB carry a particular risk for transmission to health care workers and have been documented as sources of nosocomial outbreaks. Therefore, in the United States, depending on the prevalence of TB, HIV-infected persons with pulmonary symptoms may be placed into respiratory isolation until infectious TB can be reasonably excluded by three negative sputum smears for AFB on specimens separated by at least 8 hours.

The diagnosis of pediatric TB has always been problematic. Children do not produce sputum readily, and TB is often noncavitary, extrapulmonary, or both. Sputum samples may not be readily obtained from infants and children. Options in this case include sputum induction and gastric aspiration. The sensitivity of AFB smears of gastric aspirates and induced sputum is 25 to 30%. Therefore, the diagnosis often is based on clinical and epidemiologic features as well as response to therapy.

Bronchoscopy with bronchoalveolar lavage or transbronchial biopsy is another option for the diagnosis of TB and is useful in all severely ill individuals in whom the diagnosis of TB or an alternative infection must be made quickly if treatment is to have an impact on patient outcome.

AFB smears should be performed on normally sterile fluid obtained from all patients suspected of having TB. The yield of smears from pleural fluid, pericardial fluid, ascitic fluid, and cerebrospinal fluid (CSF) is low in patients with TB but may be higher in those with HIV coinfection, particularly if immunodeficiency is advanced. In TB meningitis, CSF may clot spontaneously and AFB stains of the clot have increased yield. Rapid diagnosis of some forms of extrapulmonary TB may be made by biopsy of tissue (pleural, pericardial, peritoneal, synovial, terminal ileum); the presence of granulomas, particularly if necrotizing, virtually confirms the diagnosis. Necrotizing granulomas are seen in TB and in fungal diseases (particularly histoplasmosis, blastomycosis, coccidioidomycosis, and sporotrichosis). AFBs may also be seen in tissue histology and *M. tuberculosis* cultured from the specimen.

The diagnosis of miliary TB can be suggested by CT of the chest and confirmed by transbronchial lung biopsy (highest yield), as well as biopsy of the liver, bone marrow, or abnormal lymph nodes. If TB meningitis is suspected and the patient is immunosuppressed, it is particularly important to exclude cryptococcal meningitis by performing a cryptococcal polysaccharide antigen test, as well as an India ink preparation on CSF sediment.

The diagnosis of TB from specimens of normally sterile fluid can be difficult and is increased by culturing relatively large volumes. In addition, the yield of biopsy and culture of tissue (pleura, pericardium) is additive. There are particular diagnostic features for various forms of extrapulmonary TB. In TB meningitis, the initial CSF examination may show neutrophil predominance, but this evolves into a lymphocytic meningitis (100 to 500 cells/µL) with high protein and depressed glucose. TB of the pleura, pericardium, and peritoneum is associated with an exudative effusion, often with a lymphocyte predominance. In the words of Maxwell Finland, "The more lymphocytes the more likely it is TB." Low glucose may be found in 20% of TB effusions but limits the differential diagnosis considerably. For example, malignancy, empyema, and rheumatoid arthritis are the other causes of pleural effusion with low glucose. Pericardial fluid in patients with TB pericarditis may be bloody. Eosinophilic meningitis and chylous pleural effusions or ascites may also be seen in TB.

Currently, the "gold standard" for the diagnosis of TB is culture on solid (Löwenstein-Jensen) or in liquid (BACTEC MGIT 960 system) media. The MGIT system, which has replaced BACTEC, is nonradiometric and based on oxygen quenching in the presence of replicating mycobacteria. When compared with solid media, culture with liquid media is more sensitive and growth is more rapid (1 to 3 weeks vs. 3 to 8 weeks for solid media). Once an isolate is available, drug susceptibility testing should be performed to guide therapy. This takes an additional 2 to 4 weeks on solid media, although INH and RIF susceptibility results are available in several days when the molecular line probe assay described later is used. Liquid medium can be inoculated with smear-positive specimens for direct drug susceptibility testing, which also accelerates the process. Once mycobacterial growth occurs, speciation is possible within hours with commercially available DNA probes. Nuclear acid amplification tests are approved and commercially available for use in TB diagnostics. Their sensitivity is somewhat higher than that of AFB smears and their specificity is excellent. Expense precludes routine use of such tests, however.

There has been renewed commitment to develop rapid diagnostics for the detection of *M. tuberculosis* that have a sensitivity and specificity better than

smear and approaching that of culture. As an example, the Xpert MTB-RIF was developed by Cepheid and recently approved for use in Europe. Through in situ DNA amplification reaction, this test allows a specific diagnosis of TB and determination of susceptibility to RIF within 90 minutes. After minimal processing, sputum is added to a cartridge. Gene amplification is done with primers based on the *rpoB* gene, which encodes the target of RIF, and resistance-conferring mutations are detected. This method is capable of establishing the diagnosis of TB in 97% of patients with PTB, including 99% of AFB sputum smear–positive and 90% of smear-negative individuals, thus rivaling the sensitivity of culture. It does not require molecular expertise by the technician and is not subject to amplicon (DNA) contamination because it is a closed system. There are numerous other candidate new diagnostics in various phases of development, mostly based on gene amplification, detection of bacterial constituents and antibodies to them, and host immune and inflammatory responses.

The development of new diagnostics also targets rapid determination of drug susceptibility. The Xpert MTB-RIF test described earlier is promising in this regard. The commercially available molecular line probe assay (Hain Genotype MTBDR plus) has been approved in Europe and is recommended by the World Health Organization. This assay is based on electrophoresis of bacterial constituents and probing for mutations in the targets of INH and RIF. The assay requires that the sputum smear be positive and that the technician be trained in molecular methods, and the results are available in several days. As noted earlier, it is also useful for rapidly establishing drug susceptibility once cultures are positive.

TREATMENT

Comprehensive reviews of TB treatment have been published and provide complete information on drugs for TB, monitoring of therapy, management of adverse events, and treatment of pregnant women, children, and other special populations:

- *http://www.cdc.gov/mmwr/preview/mmwrhtml/rr5211a1.htm* (treatment)
- *http://www.cdc.gov/mmwr/preview/mmwrhtml/rr5804a1.htm* (treatment and prevention in HIV-infected persons)

Treatment of TB is both a clinical and a public health issue. The goals are to cure the patient and to minimize transmission. For that reason, the treating physician has the obligation to ensure that treatment is completed with good adherence to medications. Because of the declining number of TB cases in the United States, with subsequent decline in expertise in TB management, treatment is more likely to occur in a public health clinic than in the private sector. The cornerstone of TB treatment is multidrug therapy. This is necessary because *M. tuberculosis* undergoes spontaneous mutation to drug resistance at a frequency such that most patients with cavitary lung disease—and therefore a high burden of organisms—are likely to harbor resistant mutants.

For the treatment of TB caused by drug-susceptible organisms, there is an intensive phase of therapy for the first 2 months aimed at the rapidly dividing and metabolizing organisms and usually resulting in sterilization of sputum in those with PTB. This is followed by a 4- to 6-month continuation phase that kills the slowly metabolizing, persisting organisms. The five first-line antituberculosis drugs, INH, RIF, ethambutol (EMB), PZA, and streptomycin (SM), form the foundation of chemotherapy for TB. The precepts of therapy have been largely defined by controlled clinical trials. Standard short-course therapy for PTB requires a 2-month intensive phase of four drugs (INH, RIF, EMB, and PZA), followed by a 4-month continuation phase with INH and RIF.

The use of intermittent dosing regimens increases the feasibility of directly observed therapy but is controversial. Recent papers from Hong Kong and the United States have shown, in fact, that intermittent regimens may be slightly less effective than daily 5/7 regimens (5 weekdays observed, 2 weekend days self-administered).▮ For patients with extensive cavitary disease and the severely immunosuppressed, daily therapy should be administered throughout the entire course. For HIV-infected persons with TB who are not severely immunosuppressed, treatment should be daily during the intensive phase and at least three times weekly during the continuation phase. Non–HIV-infected persons without extensive cavitary disease can be treated with intermittent regimens throughout. Originally, EMB was perceived to be a "place holder" should the isolate prove to be resistant to INH, and the recommendation was to eliminate its use once drug susceptibility test results were available. There is recent evidence that EMB may be important because of its synergistic or additive activity with other "first-line" drugs, thereby providing an argument against its premature discontinuation before a full 2 months of therapy has been received.

The problem of nonadherence has led to the directive to provide directly observed therapy. The addition of PZA to the intensive phase allows for the so-called short-course chemotherapy; if PZA is not tolerated, comparable outcomes can be obtained with 9 months of INH-RIF. Treatment of drug-susceptible TB with this standard regimen can be expected to cure approximately 90 to 95% of cases. Routine monitoring of liver function test results is not recommended unless there is preexisting liver disease. Patients should return to the clinic promptly with any signs of drug toxicity, particularly those of early hepatotoxicity (nausea, malaise, anorexia, upper abdominal discomfort). Visits should be scheduled monthly and include clinical assessment and sputum examinations. For those with PTB, sputum cultures are continued until two consecutive cultures are negative. About 20% of patients with cavitary PTB remain sputum culture positive after 2 months of therapy. In uncomplicated PTB, defervescence is expected within 2 weeks, and there should be weight gain and diminution of cough and chest pain. A positive sputum culture at 3 months or failure to improve on chest radiographs suggests nonadherence with therapy, drug-resistant TB, or an alternative or complicating diagnosis. Positive sputum culture at 4 months is defined as treatment failure.

Extrapulmonary TB is usually associated with a smaller bacterial burden than is the case with PTB and can be treated with standard short-course regimens of 6 to 9 months' duration. However, because of the serious ramifications of treatment failure, more prolonged treatment of at least 9 to 12 months is recommended for miliary, meningeal, and skeletal TB. Adjunctive surgical débridement and stabilization may be necessary for skeletal TB. Adjunctive corticosteroids are indicated for TB pericarditis and severe pleurisy, as well as extensive PTB with clinical toxicity or respiratory failure. In TB meningitis, dexamethasone has been shown to improve survival but has not had an impact on the proportion surviving with severe neurologic sequelae. Ventricular shunting may be necessary to relieve hydrocephalus.

HIV-TB coinfection creates additional management issues. Fortunately, the response to treatment of TB is comparable to that in HIV-uninfected individuals, except for higher early mortality. Intermittent regimens have a tendency to lead to RIF resistance; therefore, daily administration of drugs is recommended in the intensive phase, and drugs should be administered no less than three times weekly in the continuation phase. The administration of co-trimoxazole prophylaxis is associated with improved survival.[2] A recent study demonstrated that integration of the treatment of TB and HIV rather than sequential treatment of first TB and then HIV is associated with a 56% reduction in mortality.[3] The results of two randomized controlled trials indicate a survival benefit to starting ART within the first 2 weeks if CD4 <200/mm^3; most of the benefit may be in those with CD4 <50 mm^3.

Early initiation of ART also incurs a risk for paradoxical reaction, a form of immune reconstitution inflammatory syndrome (IRIS) (Chapter 402). TB-IRIS is more likely to occur when the CD4$^+$ count is low, the viral load is high, and the interval between starting TB drugs and ART is short. Immune reconstitution is associated with inflammation and transient exacerbation of disease mimicking progression of TB. There may, for example, be fever, lymphadenitis, and pleural or worsening parenchymal disease, including consolidation and nodular opacities on chest radiographs. In about a third of dually infected patients, IRIS will develop within the first 2 months of treatment and often within the first 2 to 3 weeks of starting ART. TB-IRIS is not usually an important cause of morbidity or mortality and can be managed with supportive care. More problematic is IRIS associated with respiratory failure or neurologic involvement. Initiation of ART in HIV-infected persons may also be associated with "unmasking TB," which occurs within 3 months. This may be due to a missed diagnosis of TB in screening, the development of inflammation at sites of mycobacterial replication in tissue, or progression of latent infection consequent to ART. Unmasking TB is common in countries endemic for TB (5 to 10% but about 25% in South Africa) and associated with morbidity, mortality, and risk for nosocomial transmission.

In general, TB does not affect the response of HIV to ART. A major issue, however, is the interactions between rifamycins that induce CYP3A hepatic microsomal enzymes and protease inhibitors and some non-nucleoside reverse transcriptase inhibitors. RIF can be used safely in efavirenz-based regimens, which are well tolerated and effective for the treatment of persons coinfected with TB and HIV. Where available and affordable, rifabutin can be substituted for RIF because it is less active as an inducer of microsomal enzymes and can be used with protease inhibitors.

Management of TB-HIV coinfection may be complicated for the clinician. For example, a new fever may be due to drug reaction, TB-IRIS, drug resistance, or a complicating opportunistic infection.

Drug-resistant TB is more difficult to cure and in some instances may be incurable. General issues concerning the management of drug-resistant TB are listed in Table 332-2. A major problem, however, is the lack of information on drug susceptibility at the time of initiation of treatment. In resource-limited settings, drug susceptibility testing may not be available at all. Drug resistance is more likely in retreatment cases, so standardized retreatment regimens are administered. The risk for drug resistance is greater if the initial regimen was not administered in a directly observed therapy program. For patients who relapse, did not receive directly observed therapy, were not treated with an RIF-containing regimen, were known or presumed to have irregular treatment, or have severe disease, an expanded regimen should be started, for example, INH, RIF, and PZA plus an injectable (SM if not previously used) and an FQ, with or without an additional oral agent (ethionamide, para-aminosalicylic acid

[PAS], or cycloserine). Ideally, the retreatment regimen should contain at least three drugs to which the isolate is likely to be susceptible. In resource-poor environments, SM alone is often added to INH, RIF, EMB, and PZA. Although most retreatment cases remain drug susceptible, about 25% do not respond adequately to the standard regimen. It has therefore become clear that drug susceptibility testing should be performed for all patients being retreated to ensure success of treatment and to prevent the acquisition of additional resistance.

Monoresistance to INH or SM has little effect on the outcome of TB treatment. INH-resistant TB can be treated with RIF, PZA, and EMB for 6 months. Ofloxacin may be added for extensive or refractory disease. RIF-resistant TB can be treated with 12 to 18 months of INH, EMB, ofloxacin, and PZA (plus an injectable for the first 2 months if there is extensive disease). The acquisition of additional drug resistance is more likely if the initial isolate was resistant to one drug (6%) or more than one drug (14%) versus being pan-susceptible (0.8%).

MDR TB represents a problem of a different order of magnitude. Not only is cure difficult and extremely expensive, but unrecognized MDR TB can also lead to nosocomial outbreaks and rapid and high rates of fatality in the HIV infected. The World Health Organization has recommended a "DOTS-PLUS" strategy for the management of MDR TB in resource-limited settings. An empirical regimen is started based on the predominant drug susceptibility testing profile in the local setting. Unfortunately, this strategy may promote the acquisition of additional drug resistance and even the development of XDR TB if the MDR isolate is resistant to one or more drugs in the empirical regimen. There is no substitute for performing drug susceptibility testing that includes all first-line and available "second-line" drugs. MDR TB is not a homogeneous entity. Frequently, the first diagnosis of MDR TB occurs in the setting of residual susceptibility to most other drugs. However, after repeated treatments, the isolate usually acquires additional drug resistance and, regardless of whether it fulfills the definition, is essentially XDR.

The cornerstone of treatment of MDR TB is the administration of at least four drugs to which the isolate is susceptible (see Table 332-2). Typically, the regimen will include first-line drugs with retained activity, an FQ, an injectable (amikacin, kanamycin, or capreomycin), and a second-line drug if disease is extensive (ethionamide, cycloserine, PAS). The duration of treatment is set at 12 to 18 months (12 to 15 months after sterilization of sputum). Residual susceptibility to FQ treatment and to capreomycin has been shown to be determinants of treatment outcome. Surgical resection is a consideration if the disease is localized, sputum remains culture positive, medical therapy is not tolerated, or massive hemoptysis is present. Cure rates of 60 to 80% can be expected if therapy is targeted to drug susceptibility test results and MDR organisms remain sensitive to enough chemotherapeutic drugs that a reasonable regimen can be established.

The definition of XDR TB requires that an organism be MDR with additional resistance to an FQ plus at least one of three injectables (amikacin, kanamycin, capreomycin). The outcome of treatment of XDR TB has been variable. The best reported results have been obtained in Peru with a comprehensive approach that included therapeutic regimens that were tailored according to drug susceptibility testing. Effective regimens included cycloserine, capreomycin, and PAS. Moxifloxacin may be active even if the isolate is resistant to first-generation FQs. Adjunctive surgery should be considered.

The emergence of drug resistance has emphasized the need for new drugs and new drug regimens. A drug regimen that shortens the course of TB would lessen the emergence of drug resistance because adherence would increase and the administration of direct observed therapy would be simplified. Once MDR TB develops and particularly in the setting of XDR TB, new drugs are necessary to improve efficacy and shorten treatment.

There are promising developments with existing classes of drugs, as well as with as new classes about to enter or already in clinical trials. Rifapentine, a rifamycin with a longer half-life than RIF, is effective when administered to non–HIV-infected TB patients once weekly in the continuation phase. The new FQs moxifloxacin and gatifloxacin have increased activity against *M. tuberculosis* and are being studied in 4-month regimens. There is early evidence that isolates resistant to first-generation FQs may retain susceptibility to moxifloxacin. TMC 207 is a diarylquinoline specific for *M. tuberculosis* ATP synthase. TMC 207 is therefore unlikely to be used to treat pneumonias and other infections and will be reserved for TB, which will slow the emergence of drug resistance. When TMC 207 is used to treat MDR TB, it accelerates sputum clearance of organisms and increases the proportion of patients who sterilize their sputum, very promising evidence of activity.[4] Another approach of considerable interest is the combination of meropenem and clavulanate, a β-lactam and a β-lactamase inhibitor. This combination has activity against XDR TB organisms. Because the drugs are in clinical use for other indications, the time required for development as a TB indication will be considerably shorter. Linezolid has promising early bactericidal activity and may be useful to treat or prevent drug-resistant TB. PA-824 and OPC-67683 are nitroimidazole derivatives that are active against slowly replicating bacilli. Also in development are SQ-109 (ethylenediamine), an ethambutol derivative, and PNU-100480 (an oxazolidinone more active than linezolid).

TABLE 332-2	GUIDELINES FOR THE MANAGEMENT OF TUBERCULOSIS CAUSED BY DRUG-RESISTANT ORGANISMS

Do not add a single drug to a failing regimen.

When starting or modifying therapy, add three previously unused drugs (one an injectable) to which there is likely to be susceptibility.

In multidrug-resistant tuberculosis (MDR TB), when there is resistance to additional first-line drugs, treat with 4 to 6 drugs.

Patients with MDR TB have the highest priority for directly observed therapy because treatment failure may be associated with extensively drug-resistant TB.

Intermittent therapy should not be used (except for injectables after 2-3 mo).

Do not use drugs to which the *M. tuberculosis* isolate is resistant. Low-level resistance to isoniazid may be an exception.

There is cross-resistance among rifamycins but not between streptomycin and other aminoglycosides.

Drug susceptibility testing for pyrazinamide is complex technically and not performed in most laboratories. Monoresistance to pyrazinamide suggests *M. bovis*.

Moxifloxacin may be active in some cases resistant to first-generation fluoroquinolones.

PREVENTION

The issues surrounding prevention are presented in a comprehensive statement published in 2000, *http://www.cdc.gov/mmwr/preview/mmwrhtml/rr4906a1.htm*, and prevention in HIV-infected persons is presented at the website *http://www.cdc.gov/mmwr/preview/mmwrhtml/rr5804a1.htm*.

The approach taken in a low-prevalence setting such as the United States is to target tuberculin skin testing to those at high risk for recent *M. tuberculosis* infection and to those with comorbid conditions that predispose to progression from infection to disease (see Table 332-1). In either category, a positive TST becomes an indication for treatment of LTBI.

LTBI can be treated with INH for 9 months, thereby decreasing the lifetime risk for development of TB by approximately 75 to 90%, depending on the level of adherence to treatment. Pyridoxine should be administered to prevent INH-induced peripheral neuropathy. Monitoring of liver function is indicated in older individuals (the risk for hepatotoxicity increases beyond the age of 35 years) and in those with significant alcohol intake or underlying liver disease (or both). INH should be discontinued if symptoms develop (see Treatment) or hepatic transaminase levels rise to more than three to five times the upper limit of normal. Alternative regimens for the treatment of LTBI are RIF for 4 months or INH and RIF for 3 months. In HIV-infected persons, treatment of LTBI confers short-term efficacy (about 1 year), but this may be extended if ART is administered. In a low-resource setting in the HIV infected, the absence of any cough, any fever, and night sweats for 3 of the preceding 4 weeks has a negative predictive value of 97% and may obviate the need for chest radiography if it is not routinely available. Furthermore, a recent preliminary report suggests that treatment for 3 years confers a survival advantage. Immunosuppression decreases the sensitivity of the diagnosis of LTBI in HIV-infected persons. This creates a quandary because efficacy of treatment has been established only for those with a positive TST. Unfortunately, treatment of LTBI has not been applied broadly. In fact, it is estimated that less than 1% of those who could benefit actually receive appropriate therapy. This is in part due to the concern that if screening is inadequate, patients with active TB will be treated with a single drug and thereby acquire drug resistance. INH can be administered safely if there is no history of cough, fever, or night sweats in the previous 4 weeks.

There are no data on how to treat LTBI caused by a known or probably drug-resistant isolate. PZA plus EMB or ofloxacin has been used after known exposure to MDR TB susceptible to the combination, but gastrointestinal intolerance is very common. Studies of linezolid are planned in this population.

Secondary preventive therapy after completion of TB treatment is indicated in HIV-infected persons in the setting of intense exposure to *M. tuberculosis*. Data demonstrating efficacy of secondary prevention largely result from studies of adults in Congo and gold miners in South Africa.

Tracing of household contacts is a critical element of TB programs. The household is a major site of TB transmission, particularly in an area of low endemicity, so treatment of TST converters is an important strategy for elimination of TB. It is essential that transmission be limited in hospitals and other settings in which infectious PTB patients may co-mingle with susceptible hosts. The risk of transmission to health care workers should be ascertained annually. The finding of excessive risk for new TB infection should lead to focused measures for reducing transmission. All TB suspects should be placed in respiratory isolation in negative-pressure rooms with at least six air exchanges per hour and high-efficiency particulate air (HEPA) filtration or ultraviolet irradiation. N-95 personnel respirator devices that are fit-tested are necessary for individuals entering areas with a known high risk for exposure.

BCG vaccine is widely used and relatively safe except in the setting of immunosuppression. Unfortunately, efficacy has been variable by age and by latitude. A meta-analysis indicated an overall efficacy of 50%. It is approximately 80% effective in preventing the severe forms of TB in childhood, miliary TB, and TB meningitis. However, its failure to prevent adult TB, particularly at low latitudes, which include the most endemic areas, means that BCG vaccine does not have an impact on the public health problem of TB. The development of a more effective protective vaccine has been hampered by the absence of good animal models and the lack of correlates of protective immunity in humans. The issue is further compounded by the natural history of TB such that large, lengthy, and expensive trials may be needed to establish protective efficacy. Nonetheless, several vaccine candidates have been developed and their potential efficacy supported by preclinical studies in animal models. Two of the 12 currently in clinical trials are MVA85A, a recombinant modified vaccinia virus expressing the 85A antigen, a major secretory product of *M. tuberculosis*, and Mtb72f, a combination of two immunogenic antigens, Mtb 32a and Mtb 39a, in two adjuvants, ASO2a and ASO1B.

PROGNOSIS

In the prechemotherapeutic era, minimal PTB stabilized in about 50% of cases. Pleural TB also self-cured with a risk for reactivation as noted previously. With treatment, the prognosis of patients with TB depends on the extent of PTB, the sites of extrapulmonary TB, drug susceptibility of the isolate, and the presence of HIV infection and other comorbid conditions. With extensive PTB, respiratory failure may supervene with a poor prognosis. There is also increased risk for serious, sometimes lethal hemoptysis and pneumothorax. Miliary TB is associated with a high case-fatality rate, in part related to delays in diagnosis. TB meningitis is associated with serious neurologic residua, as well as high mortality. MDR TB and XDR TB are accompanied by high rates of treatment failure, morbidity, and mortality. TB in HIV-infected persons is associated with high early mortality that is poorly characterized. In the absence of ART, there is increased risk for other opportunistic infections and progression of HIV disease. The addition of ART, however, results in the morbidities associated with the concurrent administration of TB and HIV medications and with TB-IRIS.

1. Chang KC, Leung CC, Wing WW, et al. Dosing schedules of 6-month regimens and relapses for pulmonary tuberculosis. *Am J Respir Crit Care Med.* 2006;174:1153-1158.
2. Nunn AJ, Mwaba P, Chintu C, et al. Role of co-trimoxazole prophylaxis in reducing mortality in HIV infected adults being treated for tuberculosis: randomised clinical trial. *BMJ.* 2008;337:215-217.
3. Abdool Karim SS, Naidoo K, Grobler A, et al. Timing of initiation of antiretroviral drugs during tuberculosis therapy. *N Engl J Med.* 2010;362:697-706.
4. Diacon AH, Pym A, Grobusch M, et al. The diarylquinoline TMC 207 for multidrug resistant tuberculosis. *N Engl J Med.* 2009;360:2397-2405.

SUGGESTED READINGS

Cain KP, McCarthy KD, Heilig CM, et al. An algorithm for tuberculosis screening and diagnosis in people with HIV infection. *N Engl J Med.* 2010;361:707-716. *Symptomatic screening has high negative predictive value for the exclusion of TB in patients infected with HIV. Important advance that should allow wider implementation of preventive therapy.*

Gandhi NR, Nunn P, Dheda K, et al. Multidrug-resistant and extensively drug-resistant tuberculosis: a threat to global control of tuberculosis. *Lancet.* 2010;375:1830-1843. *Review.*

Harari A, Rozot V, Enders FB, et al. Dominant TNF-α(+) *Mycobacterium tuberculosis*–specific CD4(+) T cell responses discriminate between latent infection and active disease. *Nat Med.* 2011;17:372-376. *A new tool for the rapid diagnosis of active tuberculosis.*

Horsburgh CR Jr, Rubin EJ. Clinical practice. Latent tuberculosis infection in the United States. *N Engl J Med*. 2011;364:1441-1448. *Case-based review.*

Nathanson E, Nunn P, Uplekar M, et al. MDR tuberculosis—critical steps for prevention and control. *N Engl J Med*. 2010;363:1050-1058. *Review.*

Smith BM, Schwartzman K, Bartlett G, et al. Adverse events associated with treatment of latent tuberculosis in the general population. *CMAJ*. 2011;183:E173-179. *The rate of hospitalization for adverse effects was 0.5%.*

333

THE NONTUBERCULOUS MYCOBACTERIA

STEVEN M. HOLLAND

DEFINITION

Nontuberculous mycobacteria generally include the growing number of mycobacteria other than *Mycobacterium tuberculosis* and its close relatives (Chapter 332) and *Mycobacterium leprae* (Chapter 334). Other names that have been used include *atypical mycobacteria, mycobacteria other than tuberculosis,* and *environmental mycobacteria.* The number of nontuberculous mycobacteria is growing rapidly as a result of the advent of DNA sequence typing for determining criteria for speciation. Accordingly, the number of species of nontuberculous mycobacteria has increased to almost 150 and will continue to increase for the near future.

The Pathogens

Identification of any mycobacterium requires that the appropriate tests be thought of ahead of time and be performed because routine microbiologic testing does not identify mycobacteria. Nontuberculous mycobacteria are typically first detected on acid-fast smears of sputum or other body fluids. When levels of organisms are high, mycobacteria may be seen on Gram stain as gram-positive beaded rods, but this finding is unreliable. The first step in identification is to request the appropriate smear (acid-fast or fluorochrome) and culture. Nontuberculous mycobacteria are broadly differentiated into rapidly growing (<7 days) and slowly growing (>7 days) forms. *M. tuberculosis,* by contrast, typically takes 2 or more weeks to grow. Formation of pigment in light (photochromogens) or dark (scotochromogens) and lack of pigment (nonchromogens) have also been used to help categorize nontuberculous mycobacteria. Current diagnostics use biochemical, nucleic acid, or cell wall composition on high-performance liquid chromatography for speciation (Table 333-1). For purposes of diagnosis, prognosis, and therapy, identification of nontuberculous mycobacteria should be taken to the species level.

EPIDEMIOLOGY

As a group, the nontuberculous mycobacteria are ubiquitous in soil and water and are often found in certain animals, but they rarely cause disease in humans. There are no known instances of human-to-human transmission of nontuberculous mycobacteria. Because these infections are not reported to health agencies and their identification is sometimes problematic, reliable data on incidence and prevalence are lacking. In the United States, however, isolates of nontuberculous mycobacteria have exceeded those for *M. tuberculosis* for many years. In patients with cystic fibrosis (Chapter 89), for example, rates of clinical nontuberculous mycobacterial infection range from 3 to 15%, but even more patients harbor the organism. However, differentiating active disease from commensal harboring of the organism remains problematic. Other patient groups, such as those with bronchiectasis, also have elevated rates of nontuberculous mycobacterial infection, but the rates are undefined. The bulk of nontuberculous mycobacterial disease in North America is due to *Mycobacterium kansasii, Mycobacterium avium* complex (MAC), and *Mycobacterium abscessus.*

PATHOBIOLOGY

Because exposure is essentially universal and disease is rare, normal host defenses against nontuberculous mycobacteria must be highly effective.

TABLE 333-1	COMMON NONTUBERCULOUS MYCOBACTERIA
ORGANISM	**DISEASE**
RAPIDLY GROWING NONTUBERCULOUS MYCOBACTERIA	
M. abscessus	Lung, disseminated, lymph node
M. chelonae	Skin
M. fortuitum	Line infections, lung
M. smegmatis	Almost never associated with disease
SLOWLY GROWING NONTUBERCULOUS MYCOBACTERIA	
M. avium complex	Lung, disseminated, lymph node
M. kansasii	Lung
M. marinum	Skin, tendons (fish tank granuloma)
M. xenopi	Lung
M. simiae	Lung
M. szulgai	Lung
M. malmoense	Lung
M. scrofulaceum	Lymph node
M. haemophilum	Disseminated, skin
M. genavense	Disseminated
M. ulcerans	Skin (Buruli ulcer; toxin producing)
M. neoarum	Disseminated
M. celatum	Disseminated
M. gordonae	Almost never causes disease
M. terrae complex	Disseminated

Therefore, otherwise healthy individuals in whom disease develops may have specific susceptibility factors that permit these infections to become established, multiply, and cause disease.

With the advent of human immunodeficiency virus (HIV) infection, CD4+ T lymphocytes have been identified as key effectors against nontuberculous mycobacteria. Much of the genetic basis of susceptibility to disseminated nontuberculous mycobacterial infection outside HIV infection has been found to be due to specific mutations in the interferon-γ (IFN-γ)/interleukin-12 (IL-12) synthesis and response pathways. However, only about 50% of disseminated cases unassociated with HIV infection have a genetic diagnosis, and genetic causes of predisposition to nontuberculous mycobacterial lung disease are still very few.

Mycobacteria are typically phagocytosed by macrophages, which respond with the production of IL-12, a heterodimer composed of p35 and p40 moieties that together constitute IL-12p70 (Fig. 333-1). IL-12 activates T lymphocytes and natural killer cells through binding to its receptor (composed of IL-12Rβ1 and IL-12Rβ2/IL-23R) and results in phosphorylation of STAT4 (signal transducer and activator of transcription 4). IL-12 stimulation leads to secretion of IFN-γ, which activates neutrophils and macrophages to produce reactive oxidants and increase major histocompatibility complex and Fc receptors. IFN-γ signals through its receptor (composed of IFN-γR1 and IFN-γR2), thereby leading to phosphorylation of STAT1, which in turn regulates IFN-γ–responsive genes such as those for IL-12 and tumor necrosis factor-α (TNF-α). Therefore, the positive feedback loop between IFN-γ and IL-12/IL-23 is pivotal in the immune response to mycobacteria and other intracellular infections. The advent of potent TNF-α inhibitors, such as infliximab, adalimumab, certolizumab, and etanercept (Chapter 35), has provided the ability to neutralize this critical cytokine, which has occasionally resulted in mycobacterial and fungal infections.

CLINICAL MANIFESTATIONS

Disseminated Disease

Disseminated nontuberculous mycobacterial disease secondary to MAC infection used to occur commonly in the setting of advanced acquired immunodeficiency syndrome but is now uncommon in North America because of MAC prophylaxis and improved treatment of HIV infection. The portal of entry was the bowel, with spread to bone marrow and the blood stream. Rapidly growing mycobacteria such as *Mycobacterium fortuitum* sometimes infect deep indwelling lines. The severe disseminated infection seen with immune defects is typically associated with malaise, fever, and weight loss, and it is often accompanied by organomegaly and lymphadenopathy. Disseminated (two or more organ) involvement in a child without an underlying iatrogenic cause should prompt an investigation of the

FIGURE 333-1. Schematization of the critical cytokine interactions between infected macrophages and T and natural killer lymphocytes. Organisms (MYCO) infect macrophages, which release heterodimeric interleukin-12 (IL-12). This acts on the IL-12/23 receptor complex and leads to the production of homodimeric interferon-γ (IFN-γ). IFN-γ acts on its receptor to stimulate the production of tumor necrosis factor-α (TNF-α) and kill intracellular organisms such as mycobacteria, salmonellae, and some fungi. Homotrimeric TNF-α acts on its own receptor and also contributes to killing of intracellular organisms. Both IFN-γ and TNF-α lead to upregulation of IL-12. TNF-α–blocking antibodies work either by blocking the ligand (infliximab, adalimumab, certolizumab) or by providing soluble receptor (etanercept). Mutations in both chains of IFN-γR, IL-12p40, and IL-12Rβ1 and signal elements for IFN-γR and TNF-αR have been identified through their predisposition to mycobacterial infections.

IFN-γ/IL-12 pathway. Nontuberculous mycobacterial osteomyelitis is especially common with dominant negative mutations in IFN-γR1. A male with conical or peg teeth or an abnormal hair pattern and disseminated nontuberculous mycobacterial infection should be evaluated for defects in the pathway that activates nuclear factor κB. Some patients with disseminated, rapidly growing infections (predominantly *M. abscessus*) have high-titer autoantibodies to IFN-γ.

Pulmonary Disease

Lung disease caused by nontuberculous mycobacteria is by far the most common form of the infection in North America. Predisposing factors include underlying lung disease, such as bronchiectasis (Chapter 90), pneumoconiosis (Chapter 93), chronic obstructive pulmonary disease (Chapter 88), primary ciliary dyskinesia, and cystic fibrosis. The manifestations of *M. kansasii* infection can be very similar to those of tuberculosis (Chapter 332) and consist of hemoptysis, chest pain, and cavitary lung disease. MAC infection most commonly occurs in women in their sixth or seventh decade who have had months to years of nagging intermittent cough and fatigue, with or without sputum production or chest pain. Bronchiectasis and nontuberculous mycobacterial infection often coexist and progress in tandem, thus making causality difficult to determine. When compared with male smokers with upper lobe cavitary disease, who tend to carry the very same single strain of MAC indefinitely, nonsmoking females with nodular bronchiectasis tend to have several strains simultaneously and change them over the course of their disease process. Patients with pulmonary alveolar proteinosis (Chapter 91) are prone to pulmonary nontuberculous mycobacterial and nocardial infections. Esophageal motility disorders, such as achalasia (Chapter 140), have been associated with pulmonary disease, especially that caused by rapidly growing nontuberculous mycobacteria such as *M. abscessus.*

Cervical Lymph Nodes

Isolated cervical lymphadenopathy, most frequently caused by MAC, is the most common form of nontuberculous mycobacterial infection in young children in North America. The organism is generally MAC, but other nontuberculous mycobacteria can also cause disease. The cervical swelling is often firm and relatively painless with a paucity of systemic signs. Because the differential diagnosis of painless adenopathy includes malignancy, many of these infections are inadvertently diagnosed at biopsy. Local fistulas usually resolve completely with resection or antibiotic therapy, or both.

Skin and Soft Tissue Disease

Mycobacterium marinum causes skin infections, usually papules or ulcers, associated with water exposure and is known as "fish tank granuloma." Numerous outbreaks of skin infections caused by rapidly growing mycobacteria (especially *M. abscessus, M. fortuitum,* and *Mycobacterium chelonae*) have been due to skin contamination from instruments used for surgical procedures (especially cosmetic surgery), injections, and other procedures.

These infections are typically accompanied by painful, erythematous, draining subcutaneous nodules, usually without associated fever or systemic symptoms.

DIAGNOSIS

With the continued decline in cases of tuberculosis, nontuberculous mycobacteria are now the most common mycobacteria isolated from humans in North America. The conventional tuberculin skin test (purified protein derivative [PPD]) evokes a cell-mediated response to secreted mycobacterial antigens. Unfortunately, the PPD test does not differentiate well between nontuberculous mycobacterial and tuberculosis infection, although large PPD reactions (>15 mm) more commonly signify tuberculosis. With the progressive decline in active tuberculosis in the United States, nontuberculous mycobacteria are likely to account for significant proportions of PPD reactivity. Newer IFN-γ release assays (IGRAs) incubate blood with relatively tuberculosis-specific recombinant proteins and elicit T-cell secretion of IFN-γ, thereby helping clarify whether PPD reactivity is due to tuberculosis.

Isolation of nontuberculous mycobacteria from blood specimens is clear evidence of disease. However, because the slow-growing nontuberculous mycobacteria typically do not grow well in routine blood culture media, the diagnosis must be suspected. Isolation of nontuberculous mycobacteria from a biopsy specimen is strong evidence of infection, but cases of laboratory contamination do occur. Identification of organisms on stained sections of biopsy material confirms the authenticity of the culture. Some unusual nontuberculous mycobacteria require lower incubation temperatures or special additives for growth.

The radiographic appearance of nontuberculous mycobacterial disease in the lung ranges from normal to nodules, bronchiectasis, air space disease, and extensive cavity formation, similar to that seen in tuberculosis (Fig. 333-2). Isolation of nontuberculous mycobacteria from respiratory samples presents special problems in both sensitivity and specificity. *Mycobacterium gordonae* is often recovered from respiratory samples and is almost never thought to be a real pathogen. Many patients, especially those with bronchiectasis, will occasionally have nontuberculous mycobacteria recovered from sputum culture without such mycobacteria being seen on smear. Specific criteria for definitive diagnosis of nontuberculous mycobacterial lung disease exist for MAC, *M. abscessus,* and *M. kansasii,* but they are probably good guidelines for other nontuberculous mycobacteria as well. A positive diagnosis requires that two of three sputum samples grow nontuberculous mycobacteria, regardless of smear findings; a positive bronchoscopic alveolar sample, regardless of smear findings; or a biopsy specimen of pulmonary parenchyma with granulomatous inflammation or mycobacteria found on section and nontuberculous mycobacteria on culture.

Once isolated, identification of nontuberculous mycobacteria is important because it will determine the broad class of antimycobacterial therapy to be used. Many laboratories now use DNA probes to identify MAC, *M. gordonae,* and *M. kansasii.* Drug susceptibility testing is of limited and largely unproven

FIGURE 333-2. Chest computed tomography in a patient with severe pulmonary *Mycobacterium abscessus* infection. Arrows indicate bronchiectasis. Note the extensive left upper lobe destruction and diffuse pleural reaction. In addition, the left lung is smaller than the right as a result of extensive loss of lung parenchyma.

value, although clarithromycin susceptibility testing for MAC and rifampin susceptibility testing for *M. kansasii* are indicated. Initial isolates of MAC that have not been exposed to macrolides are almost always susceptible to macrolides. Any nontuberculous mycobacteria that have resisted a course of antimicrobials should probably be tested for antibiotic susceptibility as well.

PREVENTION

Prophylaxis of MAC disease in patients infected with HIV is started when the CD4+ T-lymphocyte count is less than 50 cells/μL. Azithromycin, 1200 mg weekly, clarithromycin, 1000 mg daily, and rifabutin, 300 mg daily, are effective.

TREATMENT   Rx

It is rarely an emergency to initiate treatment of nontuberculous mycobacterial infections, which are relatively slow-growing, chronic infections that evolve over a period of weeks to years, not hours to days. Therefore, empirical therapy is not usually needed, and identification of the species is advisable before starting complex, often poorly tolerated, and potentially toxic regimens. Similar to the case with tuberculosis, single-drug therapy is almost always associated with the emergence of antimicrobial resistance and is strongly discouraged.

MAC infection frequently requires complex multidrug therapy, the foundation of which is a macrolide (clarithromycin or azithromycin), ethambutol, and a rifamycin (rifampin or rifabutin). For disseminated nontuberculous mycobacterial disease in HIV-infected patients, the use of rifamycins poses special problems of drug interactions with protease inhibitors. For pulmonary MAC disease, three-times-weekly administration of drugs has been used successfully. The duration of therapy is prolonged, generally for 12 months after culture conversion and typically for a total of at least 18 months. Other drugs with activity against MAC include aminoglycosides, fluoroquinolones, and clofazimine.

M. kansasii lung disease is similar to tuberculosis in many ways and is also effectively treated with isoniazid (300 mg/day), rifampin (600 mg/day), and ethambutol (15 mg/kg/day). Treatment should continue until cultures have been negative for at least 1 year. Other drugs with very high activity against *M. kansasii* include clarithromycin, fluoroquinolones, and aminoglycosides.

Rapidly growing mycobacteria pose special therapeutic problems. Extrapulmonary disease in an immunocompetent host is usually due to inoculation (e.g., surgery, injection, trauma) or line infection and is often treated successfully with a macrolide and another drug (based on in vitro susceptibility), along with removal of the offending focus. By comparison, pulmonary disease, especially that caused by *M. abscessus*, is extremely difficult to cure, although repeated courses of treatment are usually effective in reducing the infectious burden and symptoms. Therapy generally includes a macrolide along with an intravenous agent such as amikacin, a carbapenem, cefoxitin, or tigecycline. Other oral agents used according to in vitro susceptibility testing and tolerance include fluoroquinolones, doxycycline, and linezolid.

Treatment of the other nontuberculous mycobacteria is less well defined, but macrolides and aminoglycosides are usually effective, with other agents added as indicated. Expert consultation is strongly encouraged for difficult or unusual nontuberculous mycobacterial infections.

PROGNOSIS

The effect of nontuberculous mycobacterial infection on longevity is closely tied to the underlying condition (e.g., IFN-γ/IL-12 pathway defect, cystic fibrosis). With no or inadequate treatment, symptoms are intrusive, and the infections can lead to fatal complications, including overwhelming infection or severe lung destruction.

SUGGESTED READINGS

Al Houqani M, Jamieson F, Chedore P, et al. Isolation prevalence of pulmonary nontuberculous mycobacteria in Ontario in 2007. *Can Respir J.* 2011;18:19-24. *Documents increasing prevalence, predominatly of Mycobacterium avium.*

Alvarez-Uria G. Lung disease caused by nontuberculous mycobacteria. *Curr Opin Pulm Med.* 2010;16:251-256. *Review of the pathogenesis and treatment of the heterogeneous group of nontuberculous mycobacteria that involve the lungs.*

Esteban J, Ortiz-Perez A. Current treatment of atypical mycobacteriosis. *Expert Opin Pharmacother.* 2009;10:2787-2799. *Current treatment schemes for the most commonly isolated atypical mycobacteria and the increasing problem of resistance.*

Kim RD, Greenberg DE, Ehrmantraut ME, et al. Pulmonary nontuberculous mycobacterial disease: prospective study of a distinct preexisting syndrome. *Am J Respir Crit Care Med.* 2008;178:1066-1074. *Large prospective study of pulmonary MAC infection.*

334

LEPROSY (HANSEN'S DISEASE)

JOEL D. ERNST

DEFINITION

Leprosy (Hansen's disease) is a chronic infection caused by *Mycobacterium leprae,* an acid-fast, slowly growing bacterium that cannot yet be cultured in vitro. Leprosy is found worldwide, although seven countries of high prevalence currently account for more than 80% of reported cases. The primary manifestations of infection with *M. leprae* occur in the skin and peripheral nerves. The skin lesions of leprosy are classically hypopigmented, hypoesthetic or anesthetic, and nonpruritic. Peripheral nerves can be damaged by direct infection with *M. leprae* or by the immune response to the infection; the result is loss of sensation and motor function. Additional morbidity is due to the peripheral nerve dysfunction, including painless traumatic and burn injuries, secondary bacterial infections, and muscle atrophy and contractures. Leprosy per se is not a cause of death, but the debility associated with leprosy contributes to the severity of poverty and the likelihood of death from malnutrition or other infections. Despite the low transmissibility of *M. leprae* and the ability of multiple-drug therapy to cure leprosy, it remains a stigmatized disease that can pose a challenge to diagnosis and therapy.

The Pathogen

M. leprae is an acid-fast bacillus that contains a mycolic acid–rich cell wall and a single membrane. Despite nearly 150 years of effort, *M. leprae* remains uncultivatable in vitro. For biochemical and structural characterization, *M. leprae* can be grown in large quantities in nine-banded armadillos (*Dasypus novemcinctus*), and inoculation of the footpads of athymic mice allows semiquantitation of viable bacilli.

The genome of *M. leprae* consists of 3,268,203 base pairs (bp), compared with the *Mycobacterium tuberculosis* genome of 4,411,529 bp, and the number of expressed genes of *M. leprae* is approximately 60% fewer than that of *M. tuberculosis*. Because *M. leprae* and *M. tuberculosis* probably evolved from a common mycobacterial ancestor, *M. leprae* appears to have lost approximately 2000 genes since this divergence, leaving it dependent on specialized ecologic niches for its survival. Among the genes lacking in *M. leprae* are those of the *mbt* complex, whose products are involved in bacterial acquisition of iron. *M. leprae* also lacks many of the genes for lipid biosynthesis and modification that are characteristic of *M. tuberculosis*. The genome sequence has also allowed a directed approach to identification of 16 "strains" of *M. leprae* from geographically diverse sources.

Leprosy is found worldwide, although endemic leprosy is absent from northern Europe, where it was present in epidemic form as recently as the 19th century. The global prevalence of leprosy is about 213,000 known cases, and the current incidence is about 250,000. By definition of the World Health Organization (WHO) Strategic Plan for the Elimination of Leprosy, a newly diagnosed patient who has been treated with multidrug therapy is removed from the prevalence registry, which explains the lower prevalence than incidence of this chronic infection. Since initiation of the WHO Strategic Plan (whose goal is to eliminate leprosy as a public health problem, that is, a prevalence of <1 in 10,000 in all regions), an estimated 14 million people have been cured of leprosy.

The success of multidrug therapy notwithstanding, leprosy remains a public health problem in four countries in Africa, two in Southeast Asia (India and Nepal), and one in the Americas (Brazil). India and Brazil currently have the largest number of cases. Although domestic transmission of leprosy is extremely rare in the United States, 137 cases of leprosy were diagnosed in 2006, including cases in immigrants from India, Brazil, the Philippines, the Dominican Republic, and Mexico. Because leprosy is not highly transmissible, it is not considered a disease of travelers other than immigrants.

The inability to culture *M. leprae* in vitro has been a major hindrance to understanding of the modes of transmission and reservoirs of the organism. Observational studies reveal a low frequency of leprosy in casual travelers or temporary residents of high-incidence regions, thus indicating that *M. leprae* is not highly transmissible. Even in areas of high incidence, clusters of leprosy are rare outside families or others with prolonged close contact. It is believed that transmission of *M. leprae* commonly occurs through the respiratory route because nasal secretions of people with lepromatous leprosy may contain 10^7 viable bacilli per milliliter. In addition, transmission of *M. leprae* is thought to occur through contact with contaminated soil, although soil has not been found to be a reservoir for the bacilli.

PATHOBIOLOGY

Immunology

There is an inverse correlation between the number of lymphocytes and the number of acid-fast bacteria present in skin lesions. "Tuberculoid" lesions have abundant lymphocytes, well-formed granulomas, and few bacteria (hence this form of leprosy is also termed paucibacillary). In contrast, "lepromatous" lesions have very few lymphocytes, poorly organized or no granulomas, and large numbers of bacteria (also termed multibacillary leprosy). Between these polar extremes are intermediate forms that represent a continuum of the histopathologic and bacteriologic findings, termed borderline tuberculoid, borderline, and borderline lepromatous (Fig. 334-1). In addition to correlating with the number of bacteria in individual lesions, the polar forms of leprosy correlate with the total number of skin lesions in an individual patient: tuberculoid leprosy exhibits few (fewer than five) lesions, whereas lepromatous leprosy is characterized by multiple lesions (five or more, up to hundreds).

Leprosy provides a paradigm for the effect of the cellular immune response to a bacterial pathogen on the clinical manifestations of the infection. Individuals in whom a T helper 1 (T_H1) immune response (characterized by antigen-specific T cells that produce interferon-γ, lymphotoxin [LTA], or interleukin [IL]-2 and no IL-4 or IL-5) develops to *M. leprae* exhibit few skin lesions and few bacteria within the lesions (paucibacillary leprosy). In contrast, people in whom a T_H2 immune response develops (T cells that produce little interferon-γ, lymphotoxin, or IL-2 but produce IL-4, IL-5, and IL-13)

have larger numbers of skin lesions and large numbers of bacteria within their lesions (multibacillary leprosy). The primary determinant of the differential immune response to *M. leprae* is incompletely understood, although substantial evidence indicates that host genetic polymorphisms contribute to the likelihood of paucibacillary versus multibacillary leprosy.

Pathogenesis of Nerve Damage

Peripheral nerve damage, the most important consequence of infection with *M. leprae*, occurs in all forms of leprosy and underlies the complications of the infection. *M. leprae* invades Schwann cells, the glial cells of peripheral nerves. Schwann cells form a functional unit with peripheral nerve axons and are surrounded by laminin-2, a neural-specific extracellular matrix protein. The G domain of laminin-2 can bind simultaneously to *M. leprae* and to the Schwann cell laminin receptor α-dystroglycan, which promotes binding of *M. leprae* to Schwann cells by use of laminin-2 as a bridging molecule. Laminin-2 interacts with two distinct molecules on the surface of *M. leprae*, a 21-kD protein and phenolic glycolipid-1 (PGL-1); either can mediate internalization by Schwann cells. Once *M. leprae* is bound and internalized by Schwann cells, it can cause direct demyelination of peripheral nerves in the absence of an immune response, apparently by signaling through ErbB2 and Erk1/2. *M. leprae*–mediated demyelination occurs without early cell death or toxicity, although Schwann cells and neurons can die by apoptosis later after infection. In addition, dead *M. leprae* or PGL-1 shed from live or dying *M. leprae* can mediate peripheral nerve demyelination and may contribute to the ongoing nerve damage that can follow initiation of chemotherapy. In addition to PGL-1–mediated demyelination, an *M. leprae* 19-kD lipoprotein can mediate Schwann cell apoptosis in vitro, and apoptotic Schwann cells can be found in human leprosy lesions. These mechanisms are probably responsible for the nerve damage in multibacillary leprosy.

In addition to direct damage to peripheral nerves by *M. leprae*, the immune response in leprosy also contributes to nerve damage, especially in paucibacillary (tuberculoid) leprosy, in which the bacteria or PGL-1 or both are present in insufficient quantity to cause widespread nerve damage, and in reversal reactions, in which inflammation is particularly prominent. Several distinct immunologic mechanisms probably contribute to the nerve damage in leprosy. Pro-inflammatory cytokines such as tumor necrosis factor-α (TNF-α), IL-1β, and interferon-γ are especially prominent in lesions during reversal reactions, when irreversible nerve damage can occur. Because these molecules can contribute to inflammatory tissue damage and can induce apoptosis of Schwann cells in vitro, it is likely that these mediators play an active role in nerve damage. Reversal reactions are also characterized by an increase in the number of CD4⁺ T lymphocytes in lesions, and at least some of these CD4⁺ cells exhibit a cytotoxic phenotype and kill *M. leprae*–infected Schwann cells through antigen- and major histocompatibility complex class II–dependent secretion of cytotoxic granule contents. Whether these mechanisms of nerve damage occur in chronic tuberculoid leprosy is not established, but similar cytokines and T lymphocytes are found in tuberculoid lesions.

Genetics

Cases of leprosy cluster in families, partly because of shared environments and similar exposure but also probably because of genetic determinants of susceptibility. Genetic loci whose allelic variants are related to altered susceptibility to infection with *M. leprae* include *NRAMP1*, *TNF*, *TLR1*, *FCN2*, *LTA*, *NOD2*, and *RIPK2*. NRAMP1, NOD2, RIPK2, and TNF are expressed by macrophages, and quantitative or temporal differences in their expression may account for differences in innate susceptibility to infection. TLR1 and ficolin-2 are pattern recognition molecules that recognize bacterial

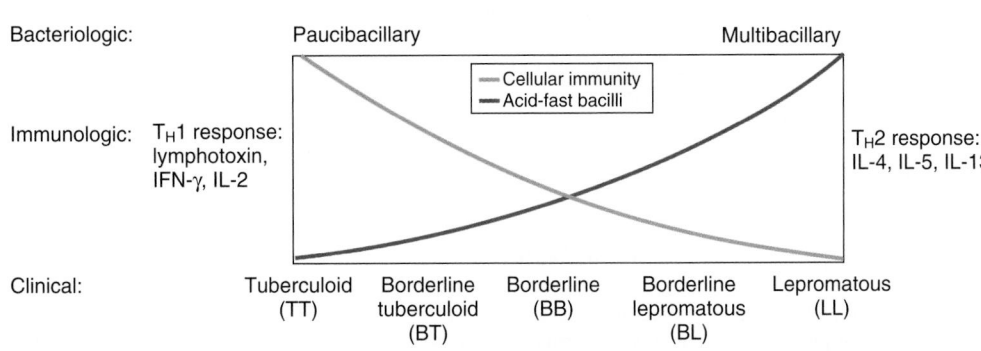

FIGURE 334-1. Bacteriologic, immunologic, and clinical spectrum of leprosy. Tuberculoid (paucibacillary) leprosy is characterized by a T_H1 immune response and few or no detectable bacilli in biopsy specimens of skin lesions or smears of skin slits. At the opposite pole of the spectrum, lepromatous (multibacillary) leprosy is accompanied by a T_H2 immune response, numerous skin lesions, and numerous acid-fast bacilli on skin biopsy specimens or smears. The intermediate forms can be classified according to their resemblance to tuberculoid or lepromatous leprosy. IFN = interferon; IL = interleukin.

FIGURE 334-2. Tuberculoid leprosy. A single large lesion with irregular, raised, erythematous borders and a depressed, hypopigmented center is shown. (From Hansen's disease [leprosy]. In: James WD, Berger TG, Elston DM, eds. *Andrews' Diseases of the Skin*, 10th ed. Philadelphia: Elsevier; 2006.)

FIGURE 334-3. Lepromatous leprosy. Numerous papules and nodules are apparent. Lepromatous macules have ill-defined borders, with normal sensation usually maintained. (From Hansen's disease [leprosy]. In: James WD, Berger TG, Elston DM, eds. *Andrews' Diseases of the Skin,* 10th ed. Philadelphia: Elsevier; 2006.)

lipopeptides and polysaccharides, respectively, whereas NOD2 and its downstream kinase RIPK2 are involved in responses to bacterial peptidoglycan. Genes with polymorphisms associated with a predisposition to distinct clinical forms of leprosy (i.e., lepromatous vs. tuberculoid) include HLA-DRB1*1501 and HLA-DRB1*1502, NRAMP1, TNF, IL-10, and TAP2.

CLINICAL MANIFESTATIONS

The most common manifestations of leprosy involve the skin and peripheral nerves and are determined by the polarity of the disease: paucibacillary (tuberculoid) or multibacillary (lepromatous). The onset of leprosy is usually insidious. Depending on the form of leprosy, numbness may be an initial complaint or finding, and skin lesions may become apparent only months or years later. The classification of leprosy as tuberculoid, lepromatous, or one of the borderline forms is based on the combination of clinical examination, the number of bacteria seen on skin slit smears or skin biopsy specimens, and the histologic appearance. Because the nature of the potential complications and the specific course of chemotherapy are determined by the form of leprosy, accurate diagnosis and classification are essential.

Tuberculoid Leprosy

Tuberculoid leprosy is characterized by the presence of fewer than five skin lesions, which are typically hypopigmented or erythematous macules with raised erythematous borders and an atrophic center (Fig. 334-2). The skin lesions in tuberculoid leprosy are usually hypoesthetic or anesthetic; when multiple lesions are present, their distribution is asymmetrical. The skin lesions may be large and are most commonly found on the face, trunk, or extremities; however, they are not found in the axillae, groin, or perineum or on the scalp, presumably because of the preference of *M. leprae* for lower temperatures.

Local peripheral nerve involvement is common in tuberculoid leprosy and is asymmetrical. In addition to hypoesthesia or anesthesia of the skin lesions, nerve involvement in tuberculoid leprosy is manifested as enlargement or tenderness (or both) of the peripheral nerves that serve the region of the skin lesions. Superficial nerves such as the ulnar, superficial peroneal, or greater auricular nerves may be visibly enlarged, depending on the location of the skin lesions. Functional complications of nerve involvement, such as muscle atrophy and contractures, may be present at the time of diagnosis of tuberculoid leprosy. Tuberculoid leprosy is a stable form; it does not convert to borderline or lepromatous forms.

Lepromatous Leprosy

Lepromatous leprosy is characterized by multiple skin lesions that are smaller than those observed in tuberculoid leprosy (Fig. 334-3). Although the sites of skin lesions are similar to those of tuberculoid leprosy, the multiple lesions of lepromatous leprosy are often symmetrically distributed. Lepromatous macules may have poorly defined borders and no loss of sensation; local nerve enlargement is not characteristic. In addition to macules, lepromatous skin lesions may be nodules or plaques, or they may diffusely infiltrate the skin, especially on the face (which may cause loss of eyebrows and "leonine facies").

Nerve involvement in lepromatous leprosy is characteristically symmetrical and exhibits a stocking-glove distribution, unrelated to the location of skin lesions. Peripheral nerve involvement may initially be manifested as loss of temperature sensation, followed by loss of light touch, pain, and deep pressure sense. In addition, dysesthesia is common. Motor complications, including muscle weakness and atrophy of the muscles of the hands, feet, and face, develop in the absence of effective antileprosy chemotherapy. Involvement of the facial nerve may result in corneal exposure, ulceration, and blindness. People with lepromatous leprosy may also have prominent rhinorrhea as a result of nasal mucosal involvement, and they may shed large numbers of *M. leprae* in their nasal secretions—one of the major sources of bacilli for transmission to other individuals. Like tuberculoid leprosy, lepromatous leprosy is stable; conversion to other forms does not occur.

Borderline Forms of Leprosy

Borderline tuberculoid leprosy is characterized by skin lesions similar to those of tuberculoid leprosy, but they are more numerous and may be accompanied by satellite lesions around large lesions. In borderline leprosy, skin lesions are numerous but remain asymmetrical. The lesions are usually plaques rather than macules and exhibit satellite lesions. Nerve involvement in borderline leprosy is manifested as thickening or tenderness of local nerves, but the skin lesions retain sensation. Borderline lepromatous leprosy is characterized by numerous symmetrical small macules, papules, plaques, and nodules but not the diffuse skin infiltration found in full-blown lepromatous leprosy. Unlike tuberculoid and lepromatous leprosy, the borderline forms are unstable and progress to the lepromatous form over time unless effective treatment is provided. Reactional states, including both reversal reactions and downgrading reactions, occur in people with borderline forms of leprosy.

Reactional States

People with leprosy who may otherwise avoid care may exhibit acute reactional symptoms and signs. Physicians in developed countries may encounter patients with reactional states in acute care settings.

Type 1 reactions, which are mediated by cellular immune responses to *M. leprae* antigens in skin lesions and nerves, occur in people with borderline tuberculoid, borderline, and borderline lepromatous leprosy. Type 1 reactions are frequently accompanied by worsening of peripheral nerve manifestations and may result in permanent nerve damage; they should be considered medical emergencies. Reversal reactions, which are type 1 reactions that occur after initiation of chemotherapy for leprosy or human immunodeficiency virus (HIV) infection, are associated with enhanced T_H1 immune responses that develop in people with a large burden of *M. leprae*; they are most severe in those with borderline lepromatous leprosy. Downgrading reactions occur in association with the transition of borderline disease toward the lepromatous form. Although the immune mechanisms that underlie reversal reactions and downgrading reactions are believed to be distinct, their clinical manifestations are indistinguishable. Type 1 reactions may have an acute or insidious onset, and they are characterized by inflammation of preexisting skin and nerve lesions. Skin lesions, which become erythematous and edematous, may also become tender and thereby resemble cellulitis, but type 1 reactions are not accompanied by fever or other systemic symptoms or signs. Increased expression of TNF has been found in lesions during type 1 reactions and may contribute to the clinical and functional consequences. Moreover, type 1 reactions have been reported when TNF antagonist therapy has been withdrawn after diagnosis of borderline lepromatous leprosy.

Type 2 reactions, also known as erythema nodosum leprosum (ENL), occur in people with borderline lepromatous and lepromatous leprosy; they may be mediated by immune complexes rather than cellular immune responses. Type 2 reactions, which occur most often after initiation of antileprosy chemotherapy or during pregnancy, are generally accompanied by fever and arthralgias. Additional signs of systemic inflammatory disease may appear, including hepatosplenomegaly, lymphadenopathy, arthritis, nephritis, keratitis, and iritis. The skin lesions of ENL resemble those of classic erythema nodosum (Chapter 448), with widely distributed erythematous dermal and subcutaneous nodules whose location is unrelated to the leprosy lesions. Biopsy of ENL lesions shows leukocytoclastic vasculitis.

Leprosy and Human Immunodeficiency Virus
CD4+ T-cell-mediated immunity is essential for control of *M. leprae,* and the extent of T_H1 immunity determines whether an individual will have tuberculoid or lepromatous leprosy. However, coinfection with HIV and depletion of CD4+ T lymphocytes does not affect the rate of progression of leprosy, nor does it cause conversion of tuberculoid leprosy to the lepromatous form. In contrast, type 1 reversal reactions may accompany immune reconstitution subsequent to initiation of effective combination antiretroviral therapy for HIV infection. The manifestations of these reversal reactions are similar to those observed in people who are not infected with HIV.

DIAGNOSIS
The diagnosis of leprosy should be considered in any patient with skin and peripheral nerve manifestations, especially those who have lived in countries where leprosy is endemic. Although leprosy is a chronic infection, its acute complications require prompt diagnosis and therapy to prevent irreversible peripheral nerve damage. It is also important to classify a patient's disease as tuberculoid, lepromatous, or one of the specific borderline forms because correct classification is necessary for selecting optimal therapy and anticipating potential reactional states. Because *M. leprae* cannot be cultured in vitro and there is currently no reliable serologic test or other diagnostic biomarker for leprosy, diagnosis and classification of leprosy depend on the combination of clinical examination, histopathologic evaluation, and acid-fast staining of skin slit or biopsy specimens.

Clinical Examination
Examination of an individual with possible or confirmed leprosy must include evaluation and documentation of the number, location, and characteristics of skin lesions. In addition to descriptions of the skin lesions, accurate classification of leprosy depends on whether the lesions are distributed symmetrically and whether they are hypoesthetic or anesthetic. The examination must also include a search for enlarged and tender peripheral nerves; for the presence of sensory deficits (especially temperature sensation and pain) and skin ulcerations; and for the nature and distribution of motor deficits, muscle atrophy, and contractures. Because some medications used for the treatment of leprosy are contraindicated in pregnancy, women of childbearing age should be evaluated for pregnancy.

Skin Smears and Biopsies
In developing countries, classification of multibacillary or paucibacillary leprosy is made by the combination of clinical examination findings and bacterial counts as determined on acid-fast–stained smears made from skin slits of lesions and skin from cool areas of the body, such as the earlobes. In developed countries, skin biopsies are usually performed instead of skin slits. Skin specimens should be obtained from the active borders of lesions and should include subcutaneous tissue. On hematoxylin-eosin staining, tuberculoid leprosy is characterized by granulomas with giant cells, aggregates of epithelioid macrophages that are neither vacuolated nor foamy, and lymphocytes at the periphery. Although granulomas may be found in other skin diseases, selective destruction of nerve trunks and perineural fibrosis are specific features of leprosy. Acid-fast stains (preferably done with the Fite procedure) show rare or undetectable bacilli in tuberculoid leprosy. Lesions of lepromatous leprosy show poorly organized granulomas without giant cells or lymphocytes; macrophages are foamy and lipid laden. Acid-fast staining of lepromatous leprosy lesions reveals abundant bacilli that usually appear in large clumps ("globi"). The borderline forms of leprosy exhibit less well organized granulomas, with fewer giant cells and lymphocytes but more foamy macrophages and acid-fast bacilli as the spectrum varies from borderline tuberculoid to borderline lepromatous.

Specialized immunohistochemistry stains, such as for CD4+ T lymphocytes or cytokine expression, are useful in research studies but are not currently used for the diagnosis or classification of leprosy. Polymerase chain reaction amplification of *M. leprae* genomic DNA from skin slits or skin biopsy specimens has not yet contributed to enhanced sensitivity or specificity of diagnosis or classification.

Diagnosis of Reactional States
The diagnosis of type 1 reactions is based on clinical findings in a patient with borderline tuberculoid, borderline, or borderline lepromatous leprosy and acute inflammation of preexisting skin lesions, with or without worsening of nerve lesions. Type 1 reactions are not accompanied by systemic findings such as fever or arthritis. At highest risk for type 1 reactions are patients who have recently initiated antileprosy chemotherapy, although type 1 reactions can occur spontaneously. Diagnosis of a type 2 reaction (ENL) is also based on clinical findings of new erythematous subcutaneous or dermal nodules in a patient with borderline lepromatous or lepromatous leprosy. There are currently no diagnostic tests or biomarkers for ENL, and skin biopsy will not distinguish ENL from classic erythema nodosum.

TREATMENT   Rx

Agents to Treat Leprosy
The first-line antimicrobial agents for leprosy are dapsone and rifampin. Clofazimine, minocycline, certain fluoroquinolones, and clarithromycin are also useful in specific contexts, including drug intolerance or resistance.

Dapsone is inexpensive and well tolerated, has a long serum half-life (~28 hours), and is safe for use during pregnancy. Glucose-6-phosphate dehydrogenase (G6PD)–deficient individuals (Chapter 164) are susceptible to dapsone-induced methemoglobinemia and hemolysis, and all patients should be screened for G6PD deficiency before starting dapsone. Patients with mild G6PD deficiency (the African type, caused by mutations that lead to instability of the enzyme) can begin dapsone at 25 mg/day but require close monitoring for anemia. Dapsone can also cause bone marrow suppression and profound neutropenia. Other rare adverse effects of dapsone include hepatitis, cholestatic jaundice, and a syndrome characterized by exfoliative dermatitis, generalized lymphadenopathy, fever, and hepatosplenomegaly.

Rifampin, the most bactericidal drug against *M. leprae,* is well absorbed after oral administration and has a serum half-life of approximately 3 hours. Rifampin should never be used as monotherapy because resistance can develop with single point mutations in its target, RNA polymerase II. Because rifampin is bactericidal and rapid release of components from dead bacteria can have pro-inflammatory effects, some experts withhold rifampin during reversal reactions. Adverse effects of rifampin include maculopapular rash, hepatotoxicity, an influenza-like syndrome (most frequent with intermittent therapy), and orange discoloration of tears, urine, saliva, and sweat. Thrombocytopenia occurs occasionally but is not usually severe. Rifampin also induces metabolism and decreases serum concentrations of other drugs, including antiretroviral protease inhibitors and non-nucleoside reverse transcriptase inhibitors, methadone, and oral contraceptives. Rifampin decreases serum concentrations of dapsone, but this effect is not clinically significant with a dapsone dose of 100 mg/day.

Clofazimine is a lipophilic dye that is bacteriostatic against *M. leprae*. It has a very long (~70 days) half-life and appears to have anti-inflammatory activity as well as direct bacteriostatic activity. Because of its anti-inflammatory activity, clofazimine is useful in the treatment of type 1 reactional states. Clofazimine is generally well tolerated; its major side effect is discoloration of the skin, which occurs in nearly all clofazimine-treated patients. The skin discoloration can range from reddish tan to bluish black and can be blotchy, but it is reversible within 6 to 12 months of discontinuation of the drug. In chronic reactional patients maintained with high doses of clofazimine (200 to 300 mg/day), enteropathy with crampy abdominal pain, mild nausea or diarrhea (or both), and even bowel obstruction can develop.

Regimens to Treat Leprosy

Chemotherapy for leprosy involves the use of multiple drugs to optimize the rate of cure and to prevent emergence of drug resistance. The regimen currently recommended in the United States for paucibacillary leprosy consists of dapsone, 100 mg, and rifampin, 600 mg, both given daily for 12 months. The recommended regimen for multibacillary leprosy is dapsone, 100 mg, plus rifampin, 600 mg, and clofazimine, 50 mg, each given daily for 24 months (available at *http://www.hrsa.gov/hansens/clinical/regimens.htm*). In resource-limited countries, where the burden of leprosy is highest, the WHO regimen for paucibacillary leprosy is dapsone, 100 mg daily, plus rifampin, 600 mg once a month, for 6 months. The WHO regimen for multibacillary leprosy is dapsone, 100 mg daily, plus rifampin, 600 mg once a month, plus clofazimine, 50 mg daily, plus an additional dose of clofazimine, 300 mg once a month (available at *http://www.who.int/lep/resources/pubs/en/index.html*). The monthly doses of rifampin and clofazimine should be administered under supervision.

Response to Therapy

Response to effective therapy for leprosy is seen clinically as flattening and resolution of the papules, nodules, or plaques, with or without improvement in nerve function. Clinical improvement may begin within the first months of therapy, but resolution of skin lesions is often delayed as long as 1 to 2 years after completion of therapy. Quantitation of the bacillary load to assess response to treatment is cumbersome, semiquantitative, and not recommended.

Patients who have been adequately treated may experience worsening of nerve and skin symptoms, perhaps because of a late reversal reaction or relapsed leprosy. If skin specimens do not reveal acid-fast organisms, a therapeutic trial of corticosteroids, which will ameliorate the symptoms of reversal reactions but not those of relapsed leprosy, can help make the distinction and assist in choosing subsequent therapy. Patients who experience relapse after treatment of paucibacillary disease should be treated for multibacillary disease because the most likely cause of relapse is previous multibacillary disease that was misclassified. Patients with multibacillary disease who relapse should be retreated with a regimen containing dapsone and rifampin, with the addition of at least two drugs that were not used in the initial treatment regimen, unless susceptibility testing is available and confirms that the organisms remain susceptible to dapsone and rifampin. The choices among additional drugs include minocycline, moxifloxacin, and clarithromycin. Relapsed multibacillary patients may benefit from lifelong maintenance therapy after completing 2 years of a salvage regimen. Because susceptibility testing cannot be performed with in vitro assays, the mouse footpad assay has been used, but it is becoming less available. The alternative approach to determination of susceptibility by sequencing the targets of dapsone and rifampin (*folP1* and *rpoB*, respectively) offers promise.

Treatment of Reactional States

Type 1 reactions may develop before, during, or years after completion of antileprosy chemotherapy. Type 1 reactions that involve worsening of nerve symptoms and findings are medical emergencies because permanent nerve damage can occur. Type 1 reactions usually respond to prednisone at a daily dose of 60 to 80 mg, which can be tapered slowly once symptoms are controlled. Type 1 reactions can also respond to high-dose clofazimine (200 to 300 mg/day), although reactions with worsening nerve symptoms should be treated initially with prednisone. Patients who have type 1 reactions that occur before or during antileprosy chemotherapy and whose reactions include nerve involvement should have rifampin withheld until the worsened nerve symptoms resolve because release of pro-inflammatory components from dying bacteria may contribute to inflammation and nerve damage. Dapsone and clofazimine should be continued during treatment of type 1 reactions.

The treatment of choice for severe type 2 reactions (ENL) is thalidomide, except in pregnant or potentially pregnant women. Thalidomide requires that patients and the prescribing physician be enrolled in the System for Thalidomide Education and Prescribing Safety (STEPS) program to avoid the drug's teratogenic effects. The mechanism of action of thalidomide is incompletely understood but is likely to include inhibition of TNF. The dose of thalidomide for ENL varies, depending on the severity of the reaction. In patients with ENL and high fever, frank arthritis, and large subcutaneous plaques, up to 100 mg four times daily may be required to achieve a clinical response. Once a clinical response is achieved, the dose of thalidomide may be tapered to a maintenance dose of 50 to 100 mg given once daily at night (because

thalidomide is sedating). For milder cases of ENL, 50 to 100 mg per night may be sufficient to achieve and to maintain control. ENL in women of child-bearing age and thalidomide-unresponsive cases may respond to corticosteroids. Antileprosy chemotherapy, including rifampin, should be continued in patients with ENL.

Other Therapy

Nerve damage in leprosy, which can result in muscle atrophy, contractures, and autoamputation, is the major cause of debility. Supportive care, reconstructive surgery, physical and occupational therapy, and rehabilitation can be extremely valuable in allowing patients to achieve and to maintain optimal function.

PREVENTION

There is currently no effective specific vaccine for leprosy, but several trials have observed a partial protective effect of bacille Calmette-Guérin vaccination. It is likely that improved understanding of transmission of *M. leprae* will be generated by the use of DNA-based strain typing, so better preventive measures are likely to become available in the near future.

PROGNOSIS

Multidrug chemotherapy cures a high proportion of people with paucibacillary and multibacillary leprosy. The currently recommended regimens provide high rates of response, with relapse rates of approximately 0.1% per year in paucibacillary cases and up to 5% per year in multibacillary cases. Some cases of paucibacillary leprosy may enter remission or even self-cure, but all cases of multibacillary leprosy are progressive. Because of its efficacy and low toxicity, multidrug chemotherapy should be used in all people in whom leprosy is diagnosed to minimize long-term morbidity.

SUGGESTED READINGS

Awofeso N. Leprosy control, public health paradigms and stigma. *Aust N Z J Public Health.* 2011; 35:9-11. *Brief review.*

Modlin RL. The innate immune response in leprosy. *Curr Opin Immunol.* 2010;22:48-54. *Review including potential for therapeutic targets.*

Truman RW, Singh P, Sharma R, et al. Probable zoonotic leprosy in the southern United States. *N Engl J Med.* 2011;364:1626-1633. *Wild armadillos in the southern U.S. harbor the same strain of* M. leprae *as southern patients with leprosy and may be spreading leprosy in this area.*

335

RICKETTSIAL INFECTIONS

DIDIER RAOULT

DEFINITION

Rickettsioses are emerging infectious diseases. Because of better diagnostic tools and changes in tick exposure, many new rickettsial diseases have been described in the past 20 years. Three families of diseases are grouped under this name: rickettsioses, ehrlichioses and anaplasmoses, and Q fever.

The Pathogens

The agents of rickettsial diseases (formerly grouped in the order Rickettsiales) are small gram-negative bacteria that grow within eukaryotic cells. They have never been grown in axenic media thus far and for culture require living hosts such as cell cultures, embryonated eggs, or susceptible animals. With the exception of *Rickettsia prowazekii*, the agent of epidemic typhus, these bacteria infect humans incidentally and are mainly animal pathogens. On the basis of molecular phylogeny, the bacteria causing rickettsial diseases have been reclassified into three phyla (Table 335-1).

Because of their difficult growth in vitro, the main diagnostic tool for rickettsioses is serology. Serologic evaluation is frequently hampered by late positivity and cross-reactivity. The development of direct staining in blood

TABLE 335-1 GENETIC CLASSIFICATION OF RICKETTSIALES

	GENUS	GROUP	SPECIES	SUBSPECIES	FIRST YEAR OF ISOLATION OR DISCOVERY
Rickettsiae	Rickettsia	Typhus	R. prowazekii		1916
			R. typhi		1920
		Spotted fever	R. conorii	conorii	1932
				israeli	1974
				caspia	1991
				indica	2001
			R. rickettsii		1919
			R. sibirica	sibirica	1946
				mongolotimonae	1996
			R. slovaca		1997
			R. honei		1991
			R. japonica		1992
			R. parkeri		2003
			R. massiliae		2006
			R. monacencis		2007
			R. heilongjiangensis		1998
			R. aeschlimannii		2001
			R. helvetica		2000
			R. australis		1950
			R. felis		2001
			R. akari		1946
			R. raoultii		2008
	Orientia	Scrub typhus	O. tsutsugamushi		1920
Ehrlichiae	Ehrlichia		E. chaffeensis		1991
			E. ewingii		1999
			E. canis		1996
	Anaplasma		A. phagocytophilum		1992
	Neorickettsia		N. sennetsu		1957
	Wolbachia		W. pipientis		2001
Coxiellae	Coxiella		C. burnetii		1931

smears or skin biopsy samples as well as polymerase chain reaction (PCR) amplification of DNA in blood samples or biopsy specimens has considerably helped identification at the species level and led to the description of emerging pathogens.

RICKETTSIOSES (DISEASES CAUSED BY *RICKETTSIA* SPECIES AND *ORIENTIA TSUTSUGAMUSHI*)

DEFINITION

Rickettsia spp are small gram-negative bacteria that multiply free in the cytoplasm of their host cells. The target cells in humans are endothelial cells or monocytes, and vasculitis is the most prominent clinical manifestation. These bacteria invade cells by phagocytosis and escape the phagosome vacuole.

The genome of *Rickettsia* is small, between 1.1 and 1.6 Mb; some have plasmids and potential for conjugation. These bacteria have a family of outer membrane proteins of the surface cell antigen family, including rOmpA (lacking in typhus group) and rOmpB. These proteins are major antigens that help identify the rickettsial species, and their encoding genes are used for amplification and sequencing for diagnostic or taxonomic purposes. Among rickettsiae, two subgroups, the typhus group and the spotted fever group, were identified on the basis of growth conditions and antigenicity. A specific group antigen, determined to be lipopolysaccharide, has been identified. The optimal growth temperature is 37° C for the typhus group and 32° to 35° C for the spotted fever group. The complete genome sequencing of *R. prowazekii* (from the typhus group) showed that it is mainly a subset of *Rickettsia conorii* (a member of the spotted fever group).

Tick-Borne Rickettsioses
ROCKY MOUNTAIN SPOTTED FEVER

EPIDEMIOLOGY

Rocky Mountain spotted fever (RMSF), the most severe of the rickettsioses, is caused by *Rickettsia rickettsii* (Table 335-2). It is the major tick-transmitted rickettsiosis (Chapter 367) recognized in America, with *Rickettsia africae* in the West Indies, *Rickettsia parkeri* in the southern states of the United States, and, perhaps, *Rickettsia amblyommii*. It was described first in the 19th century in the western United States. RMSF is prevalent in at least 44 states in the United States (Fig. 335-1) and in Central and South America (Argentina, Brazil, Colombia, Costa Rica, Mexico, and Panama).

Rickettsia is transmitted transovarially to tick progeny from one generation to the next. The infecting ticks are mainly *Dermacentor andersoni* (a wood tick) in the western United States; *Dermacentor variabilis* (the American dog tick) in the East, the Midwest, and the South; and *Rhipicephalus sanguineus* in Arizona. In Central and South America, *Amblyomma cajennense* is the major vector. Humans are infected through infected saliva after a tick bite. The duration of attachment is critical in any tick-borne rickettsiosis, and transmission is unlikely when the tick feeds for less than 20 hours. The tick bite is painless and frequently unnoticed. Rarely, an eschar at the site of the tick bite is observed in RMSF. The epidemiology of RMSF undergoes largely unexplained yearly variations. This temporal repartition is determined by tick activity and human encounter. More than 500 cases occur each year, and more than 90% are reported from April to September. The disease is more prevalent in children younger than 10 years. A recent increase has been reported, but the current

TABLE 335-2 RICKETTSIAL DISEASES IN HUMAN BEINGS

DISEASE	ORGANISM	ARTHROPOD HOST	GEOGRAPHIC AREA	RASH	ESCHAR TACHE NOIRE	REGIONAL LYMPH NODE	HIGH FEVER	FATALITY RATE
TICK-TRANSMITTED SPOTTED FEVERS								
Rocky Mountain spotted fever	R. rickettsii	Dermacentor andersoni Dermacentor variabilis Rhipicephalus sanguineus Amblyomma cajennense	America (North, Central, and South)	Yes, may be purpuric	Very rare	No	Yes	High
Mediterranean spotted fever, Astrakhan fever, Israeli spotted fever	R. conorii	Rhipicephalus sanguineus	Mediterranean, India, Caspian Sea, Africa	Yes, papular; may be purpuric	Yes	No	Yes	Moderate
African tick bite fever	R. africae	Amblyomma hebraeum Amblyomma variegatum	Sub-Saharan Africa, West Indies	Yes, half of cases may be vesicular	Yes (frequently multiple)	Yes	No	Low
Queensland tick typhus	R. australis	Ixodes holocyclus	Eastern Australia	Yes, may be vesicular	Yes	?	Yes	Moderate
Siberian tick typhus	R. sibirica	Dermacentor nuttallii	Siberia, China, Mongolia	Yes	Yes	No	Yes	Low
Scalp eschar, neck lymphadenopathy after tick bite (SENLAT)	R. slovaca or R. raoultii	Dermacentor marginatus Dermacentor reticulatus	Europe, Pakistan	Very rare	Yes, may be erythematous	Yes (painful)	No	Low
Lymphangitis-associated rickettsiosis (LAR)	R. sibirica mongolotimonae	Hyalomma asiaticum	Mongolia, Africa, Europe	Yes	Yes	Yes	Yes	Low
Unnamed	R. aeschlimannii	Hyalomma sp	Mediterranean, Africa	Yes	Yes	Yes	Yes	Unknown
Flinders Island spotted fever	R. honei	Ixodes granulosus	Flinders Island, eastern Australia	Yes	Yes	Yes	Yes	Low
Japanese spotted fever	R. japonica	Ixodes ricinus	Japan, Korea (China?)	Yes	Yes	No	Yes	Low
Unnamed	R. parkeri	Amblyomma maculatum	America	Yes	Yes	No	Yes	
Unnamed	R. helvetica	Ixodes ricinus	Europe, Asia	No	Yes	No	No	
	R. massiliae	Rhipicephalus sanguineus	Europe, United States	Yes	Yes	No	Yes	Unknown
	R. monacencis	Ixodes ricinus	Europe	Yes	Yes	No	Yes	Unknown
FLEA-TRANSMITTED DISEASES								
Murine typhus	R. typhi	Xenopsylla cheopis Ctenocephalides felis	Worldwide	Yes	No	No	Yes	Low
Flea-borne spotted fever	R. felis	Ctenocephalides felis	Worldwide	Sometimes	Sometimes	Unknown	Yes	Unknown
LOUSE-TRANSMITTED DISEASE								
Epidemic typhus	R. prowazekii	Pediculus humanus corporis Amblyomma ticks (?)	Worldwide	Yes	No	No	Yes	High
American sylvatic typhus	R. prowazekii	Flying squirrel ectoparasites	United States	Yes	No	No	Yes	Low
Brill-Zinsser disease (relapse of epidemic typhus)	R. prowazekii		Worldwide	Yes, could lack	No	No	No	Low
MITE-TRANSMITTED DISEASE								
Rickettsialpox	R. akari	Liponyssoides sanguineus	Worldwide	Yes, vesicular	Yes	Yes	Yes	Low
Scrub typhus	Orientia tsutsugamushi	Leptotrombidium sp (chiggers)	Central and eastern Asia, Australia	Yes	Yes	Yes	Yes	High, may relapse

diagnostic tools do not allow discrimination between RMSF and other rickettsioses.

CLINICAL MANIFESTATIONS

Two to 14 days after the tick bite, fever and headaches appear. The fever is high (temperature >102° F) and associated with nonspecific symptoms, including malaise, myalgias, nausea, vomiting, anorexia, and diarrhea. At this stage, RMSF is not frequently diagnosed, but during the "tick season," patients with high fever who live in or have a history of travel to an endemic location and, possibly, a history of tick bite should be considered as possibly having RMSF.

The most characteristic feature is a rash. However, the classic triad of fever, headache, and rash is present in only 44% of confirmed cases. Rash is found in 14% of cases on the first day of disease and in less than 50% in the first 3 days. The rash is macular; it appears first on the ankles and wrists and then generalizes. Spots are 1 to 5 mm in diameter and can evolve from pink to purpuric. A rash can appear later or even not at all; Rocky Mountain "spotless" fever represented 34% of cases in a series from the Centers for Disease

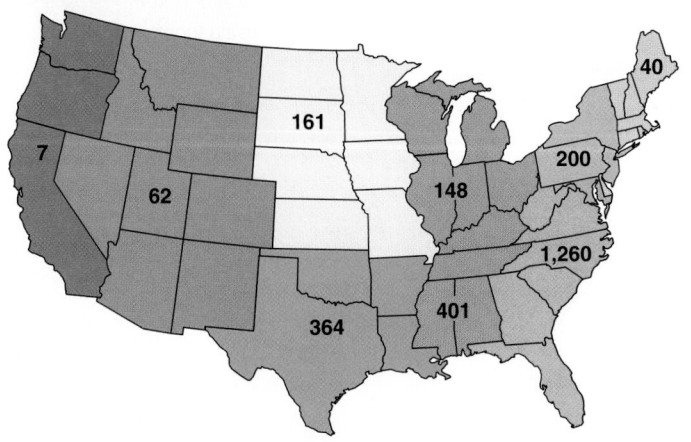

FIGURE 335-1. Number of reported cases of Rocky Mountain spotted fever by region, 1994 to 1998.

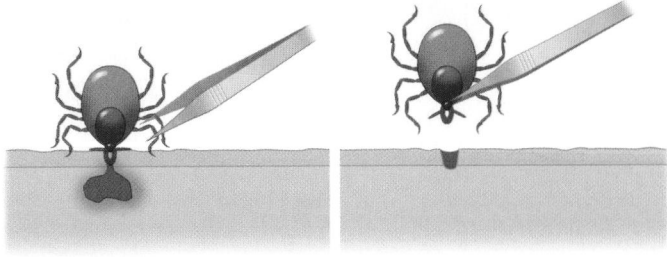

FIGURE 335-2. Tick removal technique.

Control and Prevention (CDC). Involvement of the palms and soles theoretically differentiates the typhus diseases (in which it is absent) from the spotted fevers.

Untreated patients worsen progressively. The disease is associated in various degrees with general manifestations related to vascular inflammation and increased vascular permeability and with multiple organ involvement that can lead to multiple organ dysfunction syndrome (MODS). In severe forms, patients suffer from edema, hypovolemia, hypoalbuminemia, and hypotension leading to shock. In very severe cases, necrosis and gangrene of the extremities occur. In some instances, noncardiogenic pulmonary edema develops; pulmonary involvement leading to respiratory distress can cause death. Renal failure can result either from hypovolemia and shock and be reversible or from acute tubular necrosis and require hemodialysis. The usual neurologic symptoms are confusion, lethargy, and stupor. In severe cases, delirium, coma, and seizures are observed. Cerebrospinal fluid (CSF) sampling exhibits meningitis in a third of cases; in general, a few monocyte cells (10 to 100) are observed, along with increased protein but normal glucose levels. Heart involvement can cause arrhythmia. Liver involvement is manifested as an increase in transaminases in a third of patients and jaundice in 8%. Jaundice can also reflect hemolysis. Intestinal tract involvement is manifested as abdominal pain, diarrhea, vomiting, and severe bleeding (upper gastrointestinal hemorrhage can cause death). Ocular involvement consists of conjunctivitis and retinal abnormalities, including hemorrhages, papilledema, and arterial occlusion.

The blood cell count shows a normal number of white blood cells but often immature myeloid cells. Thrombocytopenia is observed in 30 to 50% of cases and may be marked in severe cases. Anemia develops in 30% of patients. Coagulopathy with decreases in clotting factors (including fibrinogen) and prolonged coagulation times may contribute to bleeding; albuminemia may be low and proteins of the acute phase response increased (C-reactive protein, ferritin, fibrinogen). Hyponatremia and hypocalcemia may be noted and correlate with severity, as with an increase in creatininemia. Increased concentrations of serum enzymes such as aminotransferases (aspartate [AST] and alanine [ALT] aminotransferase), lactate dehydrogenase (LDH), and creatine kinase usually reflect the severity of organ involvement, including the lung, heart, and liver and multifocal rhabdomyolysis.

DIAGNOSIS

The diagnosis of RMSF should be based on clinical and epidemiologic findings and lead to early use of doxycycline. The most important clue is unexplained fever in a patient with a history of tick exposure in an endemic area. When a rash is present, RMSF should be suspected and the patient treated accordingly unless another cause is demonstrated. The differential diagnosis includes other rickettsioses (such as those caused by *R. parkeri* in southeastern states), meningococcemia, enterovirus infections, typhoid, leptospirosis, ehrlichiosis, gonococcemia, toxic shock syndrome, syphilis, rubella, measles, and the Kawasaki syndrome. Drug hypersensitivity, especially after antimicrobial use for febrile illness, is sometimes confused with RMSF.

The main diagnostic test relies on serology, and treatment should never be delayed to obtain diagnostic confirmation. Criteria for laboratory confirmation include a fourfold or greater change in antibody titer determined by

serology (measured by immunofluorescence assay [IFA], complement fixation, or latex agglutination) and direct detection of the bacterium by demonstration of specific antigens by immunodetection, genomic amplification by PCR, or culture. A biopsy specimen of a skin lesion is the best sample for this purpose. Culture of *Rickettsia* takes 3 to 7 days and is restricted to specialized laboratories. It is performed on cell lines such as Vero, L929, or HEL cells. Immunodetection by IFA or immunohistochemistry is sensitive and specific. It can be performed with frozen or fixed and paraffin-embedded material and allows retrospective diagnosis. PCR amplification and identification give promising results in rickettsioses in general but have not been properly evaluated for diagnosis of RMSF. Skin biopsy and direct detection in removed ticks yield the best results because blood contains inhibitors and only few copies of rickettsial DNA.

Two serum samples should be tested (early and convalescent). The early serum is usually negative because patients seroconvert between the 7th and 15th days. IFA is highly sensitive and specific. A cutoff value of 1/64 for total immunoglobulin and 1/32 for IgM antibodies is required for diagnosis. The latex agglutination cutoff is 1/64 or 1/128. Cross-reactive antibodies have been reported with infections caused by other rickettsioses, *Ehrlichia*, *Bartonella*, *Legionella*, and *Proteus*. False-positives, including IgM, may be observed when rheumatoid factor is present in serum and in patients with viral infection generating nonspecific B-lymphocyte proliferation (cytomegalovirus, Epstein-Barr virus). Complement fixation (which lacks sensitivity) and the Weil-Felix test (using antibodies that cross-react with *Proteus* strains) should not be used.

TREATMENT Rx

The prognosis for patients with RMSF depends on the timing of antimicrobial treatment. Doxycycline saves patients with RMSF. The recommended dose is 100 mg two times a day, and treatment should be continued for at least 3 days after the fever resolves. Oral treatment is effective, but in patients with gastric intolerance or coma, the intravenous route is advised. Several antimicrobials are effective in vitro against *R. rickettsii*, including fluoroquinolones, rifampin, and new macrolide antimicrobials (but not erythromycin), but lack of clinical experience precludes their use for RMSF. β-Lactam antimicrobials, aminoglycosides, and cotrimoxazole are not effective.

Severely ill patients should be treated in intensive care units and fluid administration carefully monitored. Mechanical ventilation is used in case of respiratory distress, hemodialysis in patients with renal insufficiency, and antiseizure drugs in patients with seizures. Anemia and coagulation abnormalities may also be corrected. For patients with gangrene of the extremities, amputation may be necessary. Glucocorticoids have not proved useful.

PREVENTION

Prevention is based on avoidance of tick bites (Chapter 367) by use of repellents, protective garments, or both. To discourage tick attachment, repellents containing permethrin can be sprayed on boots and clothing and will last for several days. Repellents containing DEET (N,N-diethyl-m-toluamide) can be applied to the skin but will last only a few hours before reapplication is necessary. It is also useful to check for ticks after exposure. Careful examination of the scalp, groin, and axillae is recommended. The tick can be removed by forceps, and the skin should be disinfected (Fig. 335-2).

PROGNOSIS

The evolution of RMSF depends strongly on the timing of diagnosis and antimicrobial treatment. The current fatality rate is 2.4% on the basis of a 4-year national survey in the United States (27 deaths were attributable to

FIGURE 335-3. Geographic distribution of tick-borne rickettsioses.

RMSF during this period). This rate is currently lowering, but this may result from reporting of confounding rickettsial diseases. No significant difference in outcome was observed between blacks and whites, but the case-fatality rate was highest in people older than 70 years (9%). Patients with glucose-6-phosphate dehydrogenase (G6PD) deficiency were more susceptible to severe infection. Chloramphenicol was associated with a poorer outcome than treatment with doxycycline. Recovery from RMSF is usually complete, but neurologic sequelae can remain, and amputation of extremities may be necessary after gangrene.

OTHER TICK-BORNE RICKETTSIOSES

EPIDEMIOLOGY

Like other tick-transmitted diseases (Chapter 367), rickettsioses have a limited geographic distribution that is determined mainly by the tick vector ecology (Fig. 335-3). *R. parkeri* has recently been identified in the United States and South America. *R. conorii* is found in Europe around the Mediterranean and Caspian seas (*caspia* subspecies); *Rickettsia slovaca, Rickettsia raoultii,* and possibly *Rickettsia helvetica* in western and central Europe; and *Rickettsia sibirica mongolotimonae* in France and Greece. Elsewhere, a number of specific agents of rickettsial disease have been identified (see Table 335-2).

CLINICAL MANIFESTATIONS

R. conorii comprises different but closely related subspecies. Many names are given to the infection caused by *R. conorii*: Mediterranean spotted fever (MSF), boutonneuse fever, Marseilles fever, Kenya tick typhus (caused by the subspecies *R. conorii conorii*), Astrakhan fever (caused by *R. conorii caspia*), Israeli spotted fever (caused by *R. conorii israeli*), and Indian tick typhus (caused by *R. conorii indica*). *R. conorii* is closely related to *R. rickettsii,* with which it shares many common antigens that generate cross-reactive antibodies. MSF resembles RMSF but has several specificities. The spontaneous evolution is milder, but a fatality rate of 1.5 to 2.5% in hospitalized patients is still observed. A malignant form of the disease that includes purpuric rash, shock, and MODS has been described in alcoholic, diabetic, human immunodeficiency virus (HIV)–infected, and old or debilitated patients. The typical clinical manifestation is that of a patient with fever, a rash, and a tache noire (i.e., a black eschar at the site of the tick bite). A tache noire is found in 50 to 80% of cases. Multiple lesions do not occur because the dog tick vector, *R. sanguineus,* seldom bites humans. The rash is frequently clearly papular, which led to one of the names of the disease, boutonneuse

fever. Israeli tick bite fever and Astrakhan fever appear to be milder than typical MSF, and tache noire is usually lacking.

R. africae, which causes African tick bite fever, may be responsible for most of the rickettsioses worldwide. It is extremely common in travelers visiting southern Africa. It is transmitted by African ticks, *Amblyomma hebraeum* and *Amblyomma africanum.* These ticks are often infected; as many as 60% can harbor *R. africae.* They usually feed on ungulates but attack human beings in groups and cause a high prevalence of infection in rural Africa (60% of tested patients exhibit antibodies) and in travelers. The tick attacks typically generate clusters of cases in Safari tourists. The disease differs from MSF in that it is much milder, fever is frequently absent, a rash is observed in only half the patients, and the rash may be vesicular (which has never been reported in confirmed MSF). Moreover, several taches noires are frequently observed. They are prevalently found on the lower limbs and often associated with draining lymphadenopathy in the groin.

Japanese spotted fever (caused by *Rickettsia japonica*) and Siberian tick typhus (caused by *R. sibirica*) resemble MSF. Infections caused by *R. sibirica mongolitimonae* resemble MSF but in some cases exhibit specific clinical features, including a tache noire, groin lymphadenopathy, and lymphangitis joining these two lesions. The disease has recently been named lymphangitis-associated rickettsiosis. *Rickettsia australis* (Queensland tick typhus) and *Rickettsia honei* (Flinders Island spotted fever) cause diseases resembling MSF, but their rash can be vesicular.

R. slovaca and *R. raoultii* cause a disease apparently common in Europe named scalp eschar and neck lymphadenopathy transmitted by ticks (Hungary, Germany, France, Spain). Its tick vectors, *Dermacentor marginatus* and *Dermacentor reticulatus,* preferentially bite in cold months and bite the scalp because they prefer hairy prey. In contrast to other tick-borne rickettsioses, the disease is more prevalent in children and women. It is rarely exanthematic; the typical clinical picture consists of an erythematous skin lesion at the site of the tick bite on the scalp that ranges from 2 to 8 cm in diameter and a draining neck lymphadenopathy (which may be painful). Rarely, patients may exhibit fever and a rash. Deep postinfectious asthenia and residual alopecia at the site of the tick bite can be observed. The occurrence of this rickettsiosis without rash may stimulate research on other new rickettsial diseases with only localized manifestations.

DIAGNOSIS

The diagnosis of other tick-borne rickettsioses is similar to that of RMSF, mainly by serology (IFA; see earlier). An exception is *R. slovaca* infection, in which the serologic response is weak, possibly because of its lack of general infection; in this case, PCR of a skin lesion sample by a swab or a lymph node aspirate is the best solution. In *R. africae* infection, the serologic response occurs later than in RMSF and MSF, and late serum samples are therefore recommended.

TREATMENT Rx

Doxycycline (100 mg twice daily for adults or 4.4 mg/kg body weight per day in two divided doses for children under 45.4 kg [100 lb]) is the drug of choice for treatment. A single day of therapy usually suffices, but in adults with more severe disease, it should be administered until the patient is afebrile for 24 hours. In pregnant women, josamycin, a macrolide antimicrobial, has proved efficient at a dose of 3 g daily for 7 days for MSF; quinolones and newer macrolide antimicrobials give results comparable to those of doxycycline but with longer regimens.

Flea-Transmitted Diseases

Fleas (Chapter 367) can harbor two rickettsial species: *Rickettsia typhi*, the agent of murine typhus; and *Rickettsia felis*, the agent of flea-borne spotted fever. Both rickettsiae can be transmitted transovarially in the flea. Vectors are *Xenopsylla cheopis* and *Pulex irritans* but also *Ctenocephalides felis*, a cat flea. Rats, cats, opossums, and dogs can propagate infected fleas. These reservoirs and vectors are distributed worldwide, and thus these diseases have a global distribution. Fleas can be infected by both species at the same time.

MURINE TYPHUS

DEFINITION

Fleas are usually infected by *R. typhi* when feeding on apparently healthy rats that have blood-borne infection. Humans and other mammals are infected through autoinoculation by scratching a fleabite that is contaminated with feces from an infected flea. Murine typhus, because of its cycle, is more prevalent in hot and humid areas, when rats proliferate.

EPIDEMIOLOGY

In the United States, 50 to 100 cases are reported yearly, mainly in southern California and southern Texas. In California, a transmission cycle involving opossums and cat fleas has been demonstrated. Murine typhus is extremely common in Southeast Asia and North Africa and is a common cause of fever in travelers.

CLINICAL MANIFESTATIONS

On the basis of studies of infected volunteers, the incubation period is generally 8 to 16 days. The disease begins with abrupt fever, nausea, vomiting, myalgias, arthralgias, and headache. A rash is observed in 40 to 50% of patients about 6 days after the onset. It is detected even less frequently in patients with dark skin. The rash begins as pink maculae that can evolve to be maculopapular. It is often discrete, starting in the axilla; it generalizes to the trunk but does not usually involve the face, palms, and soles. In severe cases, it can become purpuric. The most frequently involved organ is the lung. A third of patients have a cough, and in a fourth, a nonspecific interstitial pneumonia develops that is sometimes associated with a pleural effusion. In severe forms, respiratory failure occurs. In patients with severe disease, neurologic symptoms range from confusion and stupor to coma and seizures. Cerebral hemorrhages may occur. Digestive involvement can be manifested as vomiting, abdominal pain, jaundice, and, in severe cases, hematemesis.

The white blood cell count shows leukopenia and then leukocytosis. Thrombocytopenia can be noted as well as anemia, specifically when hemolysis is observed (frequently in patients with G6PD deficiency). A moderate increase in serum liver enzymes is common. In patients with severe disease, hyponatremia and hypoalbuminemia are observed.

DIAGNOSIS

The diagnosis of murine typhus is based mainly on serology (IFA) with titers similar to those of RMSF. On serologic evaluation, *R. typhi* cross-reacts with *R. prowazekii*; it can be differentiated either by comparing titers (two dilutions or more if IgG and IgM titers are discriminative) or by cross-adsorption. In this technique, the serum is absorbed with either antigen and then retested, and the causative agent is that removing antibodies to both bacteria. Skin biopsies and blood samples for culture and PCR may be valuable.

TREATMENT Rx

Treatment is the same as that for RMSF.

PROGNOSIS

The prognosis is usually favorable, but 10% of patients require intensive care and 1% die. Older patients and those with G6PD deficiency (Chapter 164) or chronic debilitating conditions are at higher risk.

FLEA-BORNE SPOTTED FEVER CAUSED BY *RICKETTSIA FELIS*

R. felis is mainly transmitted transovarially. Its genome comprises one or two plasmids, one being apparently conjugative. This is a new, incompletely defined disease. The bacterium is found in fleas in the Americas, Asia, Europe, Africa, and New Zealand. Isolated cases have been reported from Texas, Mexico, Brazil, France, and Germany. Reported cases all exhibited fever, a rash in six of seven cases, and inoculation eschar in some cases. The diagnosis can be based on serologic evaluation using specific *R. felis* antigen or PCR of blood or skin biopsy samples. Treatment has not been established, but the bacterium is highly susceptible to doxycycline and resistant to erythromycin.

Louse and Mite Infections

EPIDEMIC LOUSE-BORNE TYPHUS

EPIDEMIOLOGY

The human body louse (Chapter 367) lives in clothes and multiplies rapidly when cold weather and lack of hygiene allow it to. The body louse transmits three bacterial diseases: trench fever (caused by *Bartonella quintana*), relapsing fever (caused by *Borrelia recurrentis*), and exanthematic typhus (caused by *R. prowazekii*). The name *typhus* is derived from the Greek *tuphos*, which describes the neurologic condition associated with this disease and with typhoid. The body louse is prevalent during war, in poor countries, and in the homeless population of rich countries, including the United States and Europe. A 100,000-person outbreak of typhus was reported during the civil war in Burundi in 1997, and cases were reported in Russia, Peru, the United States, Algeria, and France in the 1990s. Louse-transmitted diseases killed more people than weapons did during central and eastern European wars in the 19th and 20th centuries.

The epidemiology of *R. prowazekii* is mainly related to humans as reservoirs and lice as vectors. In the United States, the eastern flying squirrel (*Glaucomys volans volans*) is also a reservoir, and its fleas, lice, and mites can be infected.

R. prowazekii has also been found in *Amblyomma* ticks, but their role is not known. The louse is infected when feeding on blood, which it does five times a day. *R. prowazekii* multiplies in the gut of the louse and is released in feces; after a few days, it destroys intestinal epithelium, which causes bright red blood to spread from the gut (typhus was also named the red louse disease). The patient is usually contaminated by infected feces (in which *R. prowazekii* survives for weeks), through aerosols, or by skin autoinoculation after scratching. Patients who recover from typhus may harbor the bacterium in a dormant form and suffer relapses under stressful conditions years later; this relapsing form is called Brill-Zinsser disease. During the relapse, a bacteremia occurs that may allow the start of a new outbreak if lice bite the patient.

CLINICAL MANIFESTATIONS

Typhus begins abruptly with fever, headaches, and myalgias, which may have led to the crouched posture termed sutama in the largest recent outbreak in Burundi. Cough and neurologic signs (stupor, confusion, or coma) are common. A rash is observed in 20 to 80% of patients, depending on the population studied; it is probably commonly underobserved on dark skin. It generally starts in the axilla and then spreads. The rash is usually macular but can be papular or purpuric in severe cases. In some cases, diarrhea and jaundice are reported. Splenomegaly is infrequently found. In severe cases, shock occurs and the fatality rate is 20 to 30%. Leukopenia, thrombocytopenia, and anemia as well as an increase in serum hepatic enzymes may be noted.

Sylvatic typhus in the United States is caused by an *R. prowazekii* variant and is a milder disease. The most prominent clinical features are neurologic. Few cases have been described, and nearly all occurred in areas where the eastern flying squirrel is found, east of the Mississippi.

Brill-Zinsser disease is difficult to diagnose because rash is rare and recent exposure to lice can be lacking. Interviewing the patient may reveal prior exposure to lice, associated or not with a diagnosis of typhus in previous years. The disease is mild and the prognosis is good.

DIAGNOSIS

The diagnosis of typhus should be considered when grouped cases of high fever with confusion are observed in patients exposed to lice. The most common diagnostic error is to attribute the findings to typhoid, which can have fatal consequences because the antimicrobials typically prescribed for that condition (β-lactams, cotrimoxazole, and quinolones) are ineffective treatment of typhus. In tropical countries, typhus is frequently confused with malaria, hemorrhagic fever, and dengue. In people with lice, it can be confused with trench fever and relapsing fever, but treatment for both can be prescribed.

The diagnosis of typhus should be clinical because the fatality rate is high and the treatment safe and efficient. Any outbreak of unexplained fever in unhygienic environments may suggest typhus, including outbreaks during civil wars (such as in Algeria, Rwanda, and Burundi), during social collapses (such as in Russia and Ukraine), in jails (such as in Rwanda and Burundi), and in chronically poor and cold countries. The diagnosis is based mainly on serology, in which there is cross-reaction with *R. typhi* (see earlier). When the investigation is performed under difficult field conditions, a drop of blood applied on filter paper and sent to a reference laboratory is valuable for serologic testing. Culture and PCR are helpful and can be performed with a skin biopsy sample or blood. Lice are good diagnostic tools because they can be tested even when dry and can be sent in closed containers without specific temperature conditions.

TREATMENT   Rx

Treatment of typhus is extremely simple, cheap, and effective; 200 mg of doxycycline orally in two divided doses is life-saving. Comatose patients should be treated parenterally. In allergic patients, chloramphenicol is the only known alternative, prescribed at a dose of 2 g/day for 10 days. There is no current vaccination, and the fight against lice is the major prevention strategy. Because lice are fragile, changing and boiling clothes are efficient. When this is not possible, insecticide (primarily permethrin) or ivermectin orally should be used.

SCRUB TYPHUS *(ORIENTIA TSUTSUGAMUSHI)*

EPIDEMIOLOGY

Scrub typhus is transmitted by the bite of trombiculid mite (Chapter 367) larvae infected by *O. tsutsugamushi*. These mites, also named chiggers, are vertically infected through their mother. Scrub typhus distribution is limited to a triangle extending between northern Japan, eastern Australia, and eastern Russia and includes the Far East, China, and the Indian subcontinent. All together, 1 billion people may be exposed. Seasonality is determined by the emergence of larvae. It is one of the three most common causes of prolonged fever in rural Asia; in temperate zones, it occurs mainly in autumn and to a lesser extent in spring. *O. tsutsugamushi* species have a wide heterogenicity that may allow the definition of several species, but a single species is currently recognized with many serotypes. The more frequent are Kato, Karp, Gilliam, and Kawasaki.

CLINICAL MANIFESTATIONS

The disease occurs in patients exposed to rural or urban foci of scrub typhus after a delay of 10 or more days. The onset is usually sudden and includes fever, headache, and myalgias. Attentive examination may reveal an inoculation eschar at the site of the mite bite and tender draining lymph nodes. Generalized lymphadenopathy and rash may be observed. The symptoms vary according to organ involvement. Neuromeningeal symptoms are relatively common. Severe forms can be manifested as septic shock. Abortion commonly occurs in pregnant women.

Leukopenia, thrombocytopenia, and increased levels of hepatic enzymes can occur. Evolution depends on the hosts and strains, and the fatality rate ranges from 0 to 30%. Scrub typhus is not more severe in HIV-infected patients, and surprisingly, HIV suppressive factors appear to be produced during infection. Relapses may occur in this disease.

DIAGNOSIS

Diagnosis may be difficult. Because the clinical features are frequently not specific, epidemiologic factors are critical. A diagnosis of infectious mononucleosis has erroneously been made in patients with scrub typhus. The bacterium can be detected by culture (in cells or mice) or by PCR in blood and biopsy specimens. The serologic technique first used was agglutination of *Proteus mirabilis* serotype OXK in the Weil-Felix reaction. This test lacks sensitivity and specificity and should be replaced by IFA or enzyme-linked immunosorbent assay tests using the three or four major serotypes.

TREATMENT   Rx

Chloramphenicol was the mainstay of treatment for many years, but now doxycycline is recommended. Single-day treatment with doxycycline is followed by relapses, and even repeated treatment for 2 days at a 7-day interval does not prevent all relapses. Hence, the currently recommended regimen is doxycycline, 100 mg orally twice a day, for 7 days. Cases resistant to doxycycline have been reported, and rifampin (600 mg orally daily) is a reasonable alternative. Quinolones should be avoided. Prophylaxis is based on the use of repellents.

RICKETTSIALPOX *(RICKETTSIA AKARI)*

EPIDEMIOLOGY

Rickettsialpox was first described in New York City, where it is still prevalent, by a general practitioner in 1946. *R. akari*, the causal agent, is transmitted by the bite of the mouse mite *(Liponyssoides sanguineus)*. Its prevalence is probably underestimated; an active search revealed 13 cases in a New York hospital in the 1980s. Cases have been reported in Arizona, Utah, and Ohio. After the terrorist attacks of 9/11/01, cases of black skin eschars were investigated as possible anthrax in New York but were in fact rickettsialpox. High seroprevalence was reported among intravenous drug users in Baltimore. Cases have also been reported from Russia, Ukraine, Slovenia, and Korea.

CLINICAL MANIFESTATIONS

Ten days after the mite bite, the beginning of the illness is marked by fever, headache, and myalgia. Careful examination reveals an inoculation eschar and a draining lymphadenopathy that could be mistaken for cutaneous anthrax. Two to 6 days later, a rash appears and comprises 5 to 40 macular, then papular and vesicular spots. This aspect led to the name of the disease. It is frequently mistaken for chickenpox. The disease is usually mild.

DIAGNOSIS

The diagnosis can be made by serologic testing with IFA. Specific antigens react with high titer, but antibodies to other *Rickettsia* may be detected. The diagnosis may also be made on skin specimens by culture, immunodetection, or PCR.

TREATMENT   Rx

Doxycycline is highly efficient in these patients. Prevention is based on the control of mice.

⬤ EHRLICHIOSES AND ANAPLASMOSES

DEFINITION

The index case of modern ehrlichiosis was reported in the United States in 1987. The patient died of fever, presumably acquired after a tick bite in Arkansas, despite receiving chloramphenicol. The patient had several initially confusing diagnostic features; on blood smears, morulae in polymorphonuclear (PMN) cells were seen, and antibodies to *Ehrlichia canis*, a pathogen of dogs but not humans, were detected. He was then thought to have *Ehrlichia chaffeensis*, but this bacterium infects monocytes, not PMN cells. A diagnosis of *Anaplasma phagocytophilum* infection (or human granulocytic ehrlichiosis [HGE]) was considered, but the tick vector of this disease is absent in Arkansas. The most likely diagnosis is currently believed to be infection with *Ehrlichia ewingii*, an agent transmitted by *Amblyomma americanum* that is prevalent in Arkansas, infects PMN cells, and cross-reacts with *E. canis*, although it typically affects immunocompromised hosts. This case illustrates the progress in knowledge on ehrlichioses and how difficult it is to conclude the etiology of an atypical infection definitively on the basis of serology alone.

All *Ehrlichia* pathogenic for humans except *E. ewingii* can be cultured. The ehrlichiae have been reclassified into four genera, mainly on the basis of 16S ribosomal RNA–derived phylogenetic analysis. Two are the tick-associated genera *Ehrlichia* and *Anaplasma* (*A. phagocytophilum*, or the HGE agent that was formerly named *Ehrlichia phagocytophila*). One is a helminth-associated genus, *Neorickettsia*, including *Neorickettsia sennetsu* (formerly *Rickettsia sennetsu*, then *Ehrlichia sennetsu*). The fourth is *Wolbachia pipientis*, a bacterium associated with arthropods (insects, crustaceans, and acarids) and helminth worms (mainly filaria). These organisms elicit cross-reactive antibodies.

Ehrlichiae multiply exclusively in vacuoles of their eukaryotic cell host, where they form clusters known as morulae. The vacuoles are derived from phagosomes and help the organism escape bactericidal lysosomal fusion. In humans, ehrlichiae are associated with monocytes (*E. chaffeensis, E. canis, N. sennetsu*) or PMN cells (*A. phagocytophilum, E. ewingii*).

Ehrlichioses can be acquired through tick bites, by ingestion of nematodes through contaminated water or animals (fish, snails), or as a consequence of filariasis.

American Human Monocytic Ehrlichiosis (*Ehrlichia chaffeensis*)

EPIDEMIOLOGY

Human monocytic ehrlichiosis (HME) is caused by *E. chaffeensis*. This organism has been isolated or identified by PCR mainly in the United States, in the southeastern, south central, and mid-Atlantic states and California (Table 335-3). In the United States, *A. americanum* (Lone Star tick) is the vector (Chapter 367) and the white-tailed deer is the main mammalian reservoir. Immature ticks are infected by blood while feeding on persistently bacteremic reservoirs. *E. chaffeensis* is transmitted transstadially in the tick and infects its next host (deer or human) during its next blood meal. The disease epidemiology reflects the tick habitat and activity, with most cases being contracted in the southern United States, in rural areas, and from April to September. In highly endemic areas, the incidence can reach 100 cases per 100,000 inhabitants. The severity is age dependent, which may explain the lower incidence reported in children. Males are more often affected than females, with a sex ratio of 4:1.

CLINICAL MANIFESTATIONS

The incubation lasts for 7 to 10 days after an identified tick exposure in 80% of cases. Patients have fever, headache, malaise, nausea, and anorexia.

TABLE 335-3	EHRLICHIOSES AND ANAPLASMOSES		
DISEASE	**AGENT**	**VECTOR**	**GEOGRAPHIC REPARTITION**
American monocytic ehrlichiosis	*Ehrlichia chaffeensis*	*Amblyomma americanum*	South central, southeastern, mid-Atlantic coastal states
Human granulocytic ehrlichiosis	*Anaplasma phagocytophilum*	*Ixodes ricinus*	Europe, China
		Ixodes scapularis	Northeast, upper Midwest, northern California
E. ewingii	*Ehrlichia ewingii*	*Amblyomma americanum*	South central, southeastern, mid-Atlantic coastal states
Japanese monocytic ehrlichiosis	*Neorickettsia sennetsu*	Helminth of the gray mullet?	Japan
E. canis	*Ehrlichia canis*	*Rhipicephalus sanguineus*	Venezuela

Untreated patients worsen and may require intensive care. Digestive tract involvement consisting of nausea, vomiting, diarrhea, and abdominal pain is common. Central nervous system infection is manifested in many forms from confusion to coma. A rash is observed in a third of cases and lymphadenopathy in a fourth. In severe forms, sepsis syndrome and MODS may occur.

The white blood cell count typically shows leukopenia, caused by both lymphopenia and neutropenia. Thrombocytopenia is also frequently noticed; anemia may appear later. Coagulopathy may be observed in severe forms. Increases in serum enzymes, including AST, ALT, and LDH, may reflect organ involvement, as does creatininemia. CSF examination in patients with neurologic symptoms reveals pleocytosis and increased protein levels. Cells may be monocytic or PMN. The prognosis depends on early antimicrobial treatment, but the fatality rate is still high at 2.5%. In persons coinfected with HIV, it may be most severe; in one series, 6 of 13 patients died.

DIAGNOSIS

The diagnosis of HME should be considered in patients with a history of tick exposure and unexplained fever. HME resembles RMSF, but rash is less frequent. Later in the disease, it can be misdiagnosed as anything that causes severe sepsis.

Leukopenia associated with thrombocytopenia and an increase in liver enzyme levels may establish the etiology. Careful examination of blood and CSF smears may help identify typical morulae. Treatment should be started in any suspected case. The diagnosis can be confirmed by culture in specialized laboratories using a canine cell line, DH82. However, PCR is more practical; confirmatory PCR using a second target gene is useful. Most cases are currently diagnosed serologically by a fourfold or greater increase in antibody titer or by seroconversion. The reference technique is IFA. A single titer of 25 is indicative of the diagnosis. There are cross-reactive antibodies among *Ehrlichia* species and with *A. phagocytophilum*. Western blotting may be valuable to distinguish among these bacteria.

TREATMENT Rx

Doxycycline (100 mg twice daily for adults) is the drug of choice for patients with ehrlichiosis. The optimal duration of therapy has not been established, but current regimens recommend continuation of treatment for at least 3 days after the fever subsides and until evidence of clinical improvement, for a minimum total course of 5 to 7 days. Severe or complicated disease may require longer treatment courses. Because tetracyclines are contraindicated in pregnancy, rifampin has been used successfully in a limited number of pregnant women with documented HME.

Human Granulocytic Ehrlichiosis (*Anaplasma phagocytophilum*)

EPIDEMIOLOGY

The first human case of *A. phagocytophilum* infection was recognized in 1990. The disease is found in America, Asia, and Europe (Fig. 335-4). It is transmitted by *Ixodes scapularis* (eastern North America), *Ixodes pacificus* (western North America), *Ixodes ricinus* (Europe), and *Ixodes persulcatus* (Asia), the vectors of Lyme disease (Chapter 329), and its epidemiology is similar. Coinfection with the two diseases may occur. The temporal distribution of the disease parallels that of nymph tick activity, with two peaks in spring and autumn. Ticks are born free of *Ehrlichia* and are infected while feeding on bacteremic small mammals. Deer play a major role as hosts of adult ticks and reservoirs. In highly endemic areas, the incidence can reach 50 per 100,000 inhabitants per year. The mean age of diagnosed patients is high, and males are more frequently infected than females, with a sex ratio of 3:1.

CLINICAL MANIFESTATIONS

The incubation time is usually between 7 and 10 days, and 80% of patients report a history of tick exposure. Many infections may be asymptomatic or too mild to require a diagnostic procedure. The disease frequently begins abruptly, with fever, headache, malaise, and myalgias that may be particularly severe. Rash is found in less than 10% of cases. Visceral involvement may be observed and includes digestive symptoms such as nausea, vomiting, and diarrhea. Neurologic symptoms may include confusion, meningitis, and meningoencephalitis.

The evolution of the disease is favorable in most cases, even without specific therapy, but the disease may evolve to septic shock in some patients. Patients with underlying diseases are more at risk of dying. Most deaths are the consequence of *Ehrlichia*-induced immunosuppression, and patients may experience invasive aspergillosis, candidiasis, cryptococcosis, and herpes esophagitis.

DIAGNOSIS

Laboratory findings consist of the association of thrombocytopenia and leukopenia (lymphopenia or neutropenia). An increase in serum transaminases is also frequent. The diagnosis can be made by careful examination of blood smears for morulae within PMN cells. Culture from blood is possible in appropriate cells (HL-60), and PCR is useful as for HME. Most cases are diagnosed by serologic testing with IFA, which is comparable to that in HME (see earlier).

TREATMENT   Rx

Treatment is also similar to that of HME except that *A. phagocytophilum* is susceptible to fluoroquinolones in vitro, but these drugs have not been tested in patients.

Ehrlichia ewingii

Canine granulocytic ehrlichiosis, reported in the United States in 1972, is caused by *E. ewingii*. This bacterium was characterized by amplification and sequencing of the 16S ribosomal RNA gene. The vector of *E. ewingii* is *A. americanum* (Chapter 367), which also transmits *E. chaffeensis*. Among 60 cases of ehrlichiosis in Missouri in 1999, 4 were caused by *E. ewingii*; 4 other cases have been reported since by the CDC. The disease was prevalent in immunocompromised hosts (seven of eight) coinfected with HIV or receiving immunosuppressive drugs. Patients who report tick exposure are noted to have fever, thrombocytopenia, leukopenia, and various symptoms, including meningitis. Morulae may be seen on blood smears in PMN cells. The evolution in reported cases was good; patients responded dramatically to doxycycline. Patients have antibodies to *E. chaffeensis*, and PCR has been shown to be useful when it is applied to blood samples. This diagnosis should be considered when ehrlichiosis is suspected in immunocompromised patients exposed to *A. americanum* ticks.

Ehrlichia canis

Canine monocytic ehrlichiosis was reported first in Algeria in the 1930s. It is caused by *E. canis* and transmitted by the dog tick *R. sanguineus* (Chapter 367). This tick is found worldwide and is prevalent in temperate and hot areas. In 1996, a single case of infection was reported in an asymptomatic man from Venezuela who owned an infected dog. Recently, cases have been reported in patients in South America.

Wolbachia Species

Wolbachia bacteria are endosymbionts of arthropods and nematodes. They were known to be present in filarial worms, but it was later shown that they may play a role in human disease. These bacteria manipulate the fertility of their host. Eradication of *Wolbachia* in filariae may lead to infertility and stop the microfilariae from spreading. This effect was demonstrated by field treatment with doxycycline in patients with onchocerciasis. The patients improved when treated with this drug, which is effective on *Wolbachia* and subsequently on the worm's fertility but not on the worm itself. In 2001, it was shown that the adverse reactions observed after treatment of lymphatic filariasis may be caused by the release of *Wolbachia* from destroyed worms. Some authors suggested that eradicating *Wolbachia* before the anthelmintic prescription would avoid these reactions. For some reason, *Loa loa* (Chapter 366) do not harbor *Wolbachia*, and the genome of *Wolbachia* integrated in the *Brugia malayi* genome makes it inaccessible to therapy.

⬤ Q FEVER

DEFINITION

Q fever is a worldwide zoonosis caused by *Coxiella burnetii*. The name Q fever is derived from "query" to emphasize the surprising aspect of the disease first described in Queensland, Australia, in 1935 by Derrick. The infection in humans is variable in its severity, clinical expression, and natural course (i.e., acute or chronic). It is considered by the CDC to be a potential agent of bioterrorism. Ungulates and pets are the major sources of human infection.

The Pathogen

C. burnetii is a gram-negative bacterium that naturally infects its host's monocytes. It multiplies in an acidic vacuole. Strains are heterogeneous genetically and antigenically and are associated with acute infections of variable severity. *C. burnetii* in vitro generates a deleted, avirulent mutant also named phase II.

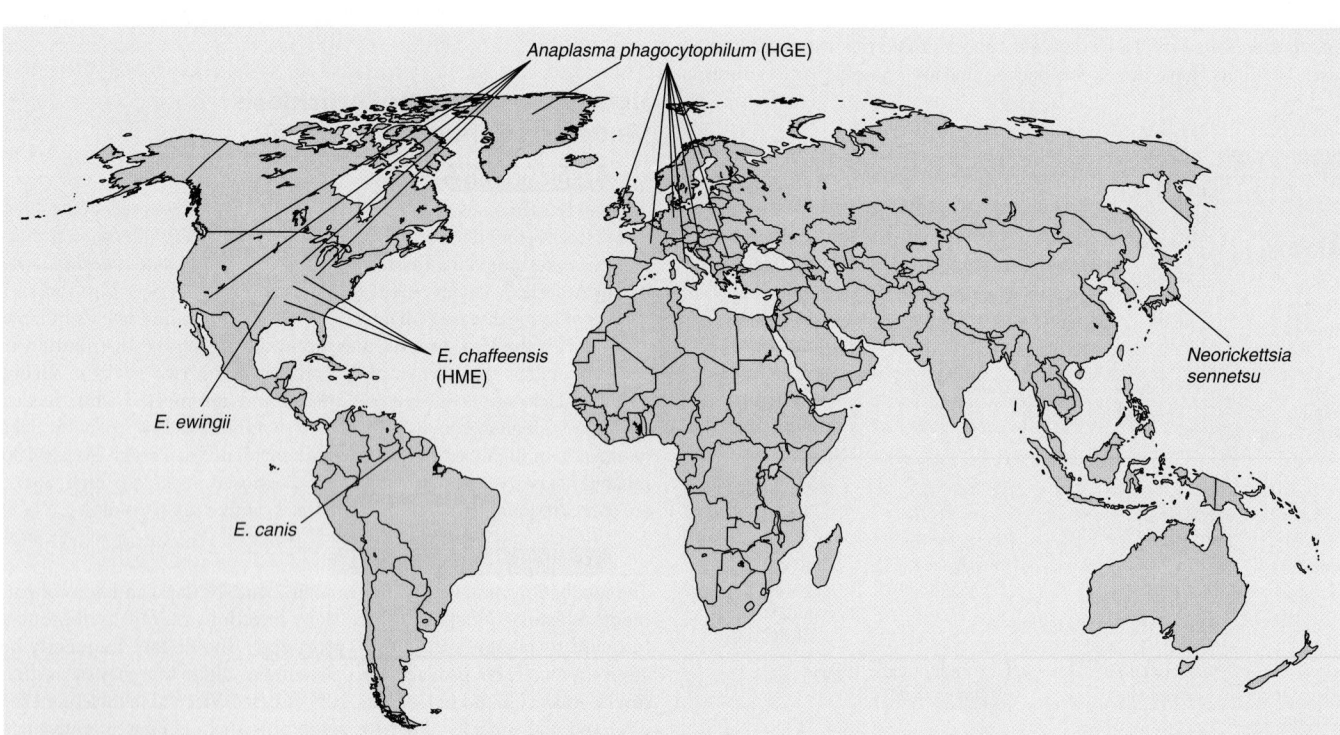

FIGURE 335-4. Geographic distribution of ehrlichioses. HGE = human granulocytic ehrlichiosis; HME = human monocytic ehrlichiosis.

This mutant exhibits diagnostic antigens that are useful because they are more reactive during acute infection.

C. burnetii is incompletely eliminated after acute infection. In immunocompromised hosts and patients with cardiac valve lesions, C. burnetii continues to multiply despite high levels of antibodies and causes chronic infection. Control of the disease in acute Q fever is associated with the formation of a granuloma.

EPIDEMIOLOGY

C. burnetii infects a wide range of animals, including mammals, birds, and ticks. Ungulates and pets (cats and dogs) are the most common source of the disease. Mammals are infected through aerosols and may shed Coxiella in feces, urine, milk, and birth products. Humans are usually infected by aerosols or less frequently by exposure to milk products. Interhuman infections through sexual intercourse, during delivery, or by blood transfusion have been reported. Coxiella survives in the environment and can be spread far by the wind. In the past few years, major outbreaks were related to sheep and goats. The disease is partly seasonal and related to lambing time. The current geographic repartition is largely unknown. Males have more severe disease but are not more often exposed to Q fever, and middle-aged people are more frequently affected and hospitalized. The number of reported cases recently increased dramatically in Europe and Asia. Many American soldiers were infected in Iraq.

CLINICAL MANIFESTATIONS

After contamination by C. burnetii, 60% of patients seroconvert without apparent disease, 38% experience a self-limited disease, and only 2% require diagnostic evaluation. Months to years after the primary infection, a chronic infection associated with an immunocompromised situation, a cardiac valve lesion, or a vascular prosthesis or aneurysm develops in 0.2 to 0.5% of patients.

Patients with diagnosed acute infection may have a variety of symptoms (Table 335-4). Isolated prolonged fever was observed in 14% of more than 1000 patients. Pneumonia was found in 37% and was the only symptom in 17%. This percentage may vary according to the place of study and reach 90% of diagnosed cases. Some cases may be associated with respiratory distress. Hepatitis is found in 60% of patients and is the sole manifestation in 40%. The association of fever and a moderate increase in transaminases is an important clue. Some hepatitides, specifically in middle-aged men, are associated with an inflammatory syndrome and autoantibodies and may be resistant to antimicrobial treatment. Liver biopsy, when it is performed, exhibits granulomas that may be typified by a lipid vacuole and surrounded by a fibrinoid ring in the form of a doughnut. Less frequently, in 1.5% of cases, patients exhibit a rash. Patients can have specific neurologic manifestations such as meningitis, encephalitis, meningoencephalitis, or peripheral neuropathy. In 1 to 2% of cases, patients have cardiovascular manifestations, such as pericarditis or more rarely myocarditis.

Evolution is usually favorable even without treatment, except in special hosts. In pregnant women, symptomatic or not, Q fever compromises the pregnancy. When infected during the first trimester, the patient usually aborts spontaneously. When the patient is infected later, the disease can result in fetal death or prematurity, or the outcome may be normal. Chronic uterine infection may develop in half the patients infected during pregnancy, and they may later experience multiple spontaneous abortions. Thirty percent to 50% of patients with heart valve or vascular lesions may experience chronic endocarditis within 2 years. This evolution is not prevented by regular treatment.

Patients with Q fever endocarditis have a chronic infection with low-grade fever, progressive degradation of valve function, and progressive heart failure. Fever is intermittent, and vegetations are frequently absent on cardiac echocardiography. Endocarditis is therefore not frequently considered in the initial differential diagnosis. If it is not diagnosed, the disease progressively worsens, and emboli (mainly cerebral) as well as renal insufficiency, splenomegaly, and hepatomegaly may be observed. Digital clubbing may also be seen. The main clue to the diagnosis in a patient with a valvulopathy is unexplained sickness (unexplained fatigue, weight loss, fever), a biologic abnormality (leukopenia, increased erythrocyte sedimentation rate, thrombocytopenia, increase in hepatic enzymes), or rapid degradation of a prosthetic valve. Chronic osteomyelitis, hepatitis, and infection of an aneurysm and vascular prosthesis have been reported.

Leukopenia may be observed; thrombocytopenia is frequent, as are increases in hepatic enzymes. Circulating anticoagulant associated with antiphospholipid antibodies may be observed (Chapter 177), as may anti–smooth muscle antibodies. During endocarditis, antinuclear antibodies, microhematuria, and rheumatoid factor are frequently found.

DIAGNOSIS

The diagnosis is based mainly on serology (see Table 335-4). Direct detection by culture and PCR or immunochemistry in valve, liver, or blood samples is also useful, but serologic evaluation by IFA is the best method. Two antigens (phase I and phase II) can be tested. Acute Q fever is diagnosed when seroconversion or a fourfold increase is obtained with phase II antigen. A single serum test exhibiting IgG antibodies of 200 or greater and IgM of 50 or greater against phase II is also diagnostic. During chronic Q fever, antibodies are at higher titer and directed against both phase I and phase II. IgG against phase I at a titer of 800 or 1600 is diagnostic of chronic infection, as is IgA at 100 or greater. Serology is useful for follow-up of patients with acute Q fever and underlying disease and those with treated chronic Q fever.

TABLE 335-4	SITUATIONS THAT SHOULD PROMPT SEROLOGIC TESTING FOR Q FEVER

ACUTE Q FEVER (PHASE II ANTIGEN AND IgG ≥ 200 AND IgM ≥ 50)

Fever in a patient in contact with ungulates
Unexplained prolonged fever (>7 days)
Granulomatous hepatitis
Fever and thrombocytopenia
Meningoencephalitis
Myocarditis
Erythema nodosum
Fever during pregnancy
Fever in a patient in contact with a parturient pet
Unexplained atypical pneumonia
Fever and an increase in transaminases (2-5 times the normal level)
Aseptic meningitis
Guillain-Barré syndrome
Pericarditis
Spontaneous abortion

CHRONIC Q FEVER (PHASE I ANTIGEN AND IgG ≥ 800 AND IgA ≥ 100)

Blood culture–negative endocarditis
Patient with a valvulopathy and unexplained
    Fever
    Weight loss
    Fatigue
    Increased erythrocyte sedimentation rate
    Increased transaminases
    Thrombocytopenia
Patient with unusually rapid degradation of a prosthetic valve
Fever in a patient with a vascular aneurysm or prosthesis
Aseptic osteomyelitis
Chronic pericarditis
Multiple spontaneous abortions

TREATMENT   Rx

Treatment is easy during acute Q fever. Doxycycline is the most efficient antimicrobial, and it should be prescribed for 2 weeks. Some patients with hepatitis do not respond well because of an excessive immune response. They rapidly improve with a short course of glucocorticoids. In pregnant women, cotrimoxazole during the entire pregnancy may decrease the chance of an unfavorable outcome. As for endocarditis, bactericidal treatment is necessary. In vitro, antimicrobial efficacy is impaired by the low pH of the vacuole in which C. burnetii resides. Hydroxychloroquine increases the pH of this vacuole and restores the bactericidal effect of doxycycline. In patients with endocarditis, the recommended treatment is a combination of doxycycline (200 mg daily) and hydroxychloroquine (600 mg/day, then adjusted to reach a 1-mg/mL plasma concentration). This regimen is prescribed for 18 to 36 months according to serologic results. We recently observed that a more rapid favorable outcome was obtained with doxycycline serum levels higher than 5 µg/mL. Some strains may be resistant to doxycycline, and new macrolides may be an alternative. The major problem with this treatment is photosensitivity; sun exposure should be avoided. An alternative treatment is a combination of doxycycline and ofloxacin for 3 years or more.

PREVENTION

Prevention is based on veterinary control in animals. A vaccine is currently available in Australia.

SUGGESTED READING

Openshaw JJ, Swerdlow DL, Krebs JW, et al. Rocky mountain spotted fever in the United Satates, 2000-2007: interpreting contemporary increases in incidence. *Am J Trop Med Hyg.* 2010;83:174-182. *Review noting a 0.3% case-fatality rate.*

ZOONOSES

STUART LEVIN

DEFINITION

Zoonoses are classically, though not without controversy, defined as infections or diseases naturally transmitted between humans and vertebrate animals. There are approximately 1400 human pathogens, of which about 800 species are zoonotic. Of the approximate 180 emerging or reemerging pathogens in the past 3 decades, 130 are known to be zoonotic, with a disproportionate number of the new zoonoses being caused by RNA viruses. As a recent editorial states, this is a microbial world that humans are barely allowed to live in, and nothing microbes do or become should surprise us. We have little ability to predict how an emerging zoonotic pathogen will act. Most zoonotic pathogens, like rabies, enter a human and cause disease, but in these cases, humans are dead-end hosts and are unlikely to transmit the disease to others. Less commonly, pathogens such as human immunodeficiency virus (HIV) or recombinant swine H1N1 enter the human population with great difficulty but are then successfully transmitted to cause global epidemics solely from human-to-human transfer. The recent emphasis on emerging infections, which are predominantly zoonoses, and the potential for new pandemics markedly enhance the need for human medicine to be integrated with veterinary medicine and veterinary research.

EPIDEMIOLOGY

During the course of evolution, humans have sought the company of vertebrates for many reasons, including their companionship as pets. The more than 100 million dogs and cats in the United States facilitate the transmission of more than 250 different infectious species and cause more than 1 million bite injuries each year.

Almost all arthropod-transmitted infectious agents acquired from vertebrates in the United States are due to either ticks or mosquitoes. Ticks are the more common villain, and Lyme disease is the most common arthropod-transmitted infectious disease in the United States. Not all arthropod-transmitted diseases are zoonotic. For instance, arthropod-transmitted infections such as West Nile fever, *Schistosoma japonicum*, and *Trypanosoma rhodesiense* are zoonoses, whereas *Schistosoma mansoni*, *Trypanosoma gambiense*, *Wuchereria bancrofti*, *Onchocerca volvulus*, and vivax malaria are not; these non-zoonoses cause more than a billion infections per year, are transferred from human to human, and do not depend on vertebrate reservoirs. Human infestations with ectoparasites are not considered zoonoses.

The risk of contracting a zoonosis is increased by direct animal contact; in meat handlers, poachers, hunters, exotic animal smugglers, and international travelers; by exposure to and inhalation of infectious air particles; by insect bites, contact with previously infected human blood products, and contact with and ingestion of infectious agents transmitted by animal-contaminated water; and by insufficiently cooked meat, eggs, dairy products, and fish. Raw shellfish, which are the "garbage filters" of the ocean, can transmit at least 25 different infectious or toxic diseases to humans, but shellfish are invertebrates, and such diseases are not zoonoses. Ticks can introduce more than one pathogen while feeding; Lyme disease, ehrlichiosis, and babesiosis can all be transmitted by a single tick bite. Threats from mosquito bites include

St. Louis encephalitis and West Nile virus. Patrons of petting zoos, pet owners, farmers, hunters, laboratory researchers, cave explorers, hikers, and veterinarians, among others, are at higher risk for a zoonosis than is the general population. Infectious agents transmitted by these routes from animal sources essentially include members of all microbial classes: viruses and prions, bacteria and rickettsia, fungi, helminths, and protozoa. Immunocompromised hosts, such as splenectomized patients, transplant recipients, patients with acquired immunodeficiency syndrome (AIDS), and pregnant women and their fetuses, are at higher risk for clinical disease when exposed to these various infectious agents. Chagas' disease, a protozoal infection, is a zoonosis in South America but is not endemic to the United States; however, immigration from Latin America has led to an estimated 300,000 persons with *Trypanosoma cruzi* infection, usually subclinical, in the United States and the potential for transmission of the infection through blood or organ donations. *Leishmania donovani* is almost always a small-animal reservoir zoonosis, but in India, it has set up shop with just human-to-human insect transfer.

As the world shrinks, warms, flattens, and remains in conflict, new infectious diseases seem inevitable, and previously rare ones are seen in unexpected places (Table 336-1) because of global warming, human intrusion into previously underexplored or never-explored sites, world travel, deforestation, and the increasing threat of biologic terrorism or warfare. Increasing urbanization, intermingling of humans and domestic animals, and lack of adequate sanitation can dramatically increase the incidence and severity of epidemic infectious disease.

CLINICAL MANIFESTATIONS

Zoonoses can manifest as a variety of clinical syndromes, including respiratory disease (Table 336-2), central nervous system disease (Table 336-3), and rash or skin lesions (Table 336-4). Other zoonotic clinical syndromes may present as sepsis, polyarthritis, jaundice, acute renal failure, endocarditis, or diarrhea (Table 336-5).

Emerging zoonotic infectious diseases include Nipah virus and Hendra virus encephalitis, *Hantavirus* pneumonia and *Hantavirus* fever with renal failure, the coronavirus that causes severe acute respiratory syndrome (SARS), West Nile encephalitis (which spread coast to coast in the United States over 3 years and is now apparently a permanent resident), monkeypox (an outbreak in the upper Midwest was caused by pet prairie dogs), *Leishmania mexicana* in Texas, and at least 8 to 10 newly identified tick-borne rickettsial spotted fevers worldwide, including the flea-borne *Rickettsia felis* in California. Avian or "bird flu" (H5N1), SARS, monkeypox, H1N1 (swine) influenza, and West Nile fever have recently exposed the fragility of our world village. Nevertheless, exotic zoonoses remain a less frequent cause of fever in travelers than the well-known, ordinary gastrointestinal and pulmonary pathogens.

DIAGNOSIS

Non–animal-associated environment- or travel-related infectious diseases can be confused with zoonoses. The vast majority of clinical diseases caused by *Legionella pneumophila*, *Entamoeba histolytica*, *Giardia lamblia*, *Burkholderia pseudomallei*, *Chromobacterium violaceum*, *Aeromonas hydrophila*, and airborne fungi such as *Blastomyces dermatitidis*, *Coccidioides immitis*, and *Histoplasma capsulatum* are acquired through environmental exposure and are only rarely related to animal hosts. *Sporothrix schenckii*, almost always an environmentally acquired pathogen stemming from vegetation-related injuries, has also been transmitted from cats with draining cutaneous ulcers to owners and animal handlers. Histoplasmosis has been acquired by explorers (spelunkers) in caves contaminated by bat guano. Other noninfectious toxin-induced diseases acquired from animals and insects, such as tick paralysis and the fish toxin illnesses, do not represent zoonoses.

Unfortunately, some descriptive disease titles can be misleading to clinicians and interfere with reaching the correct diagnosis. The transmission of tick-borne Rocky Mountain spotted fever actually occurs much more commonly in the southeastern United States than in the Rocky Mountains and has even occurred in the middle of New York City. Urban New York City continues to be a major source of rickettsialpox, where it was first described 60 years ago. Vegetarians and other strict non–pork-eating persons have been seriously infected with the pig tapeworm *Taenia solium* as a result of fecal contamination of food from infected human food-handlers.

Until recently, human influenza A was not well recognized as a zoonosis; however, interspecies spread and mixing of swine, avian (H5N1 virus), and human influenza viruses can occur in unique geographic areas, such

TABLE 336-1 NEWER ZOONOSES IN THE UNITED STATES (EMERGING INFECTIONS)

DISEASE*	INFECTIOUS AGENT	CLINICAL FINDINGS	VECTOR/ACQUISITION
Ehrlichiosis, monocytic	*Ehrlichia chaffeensis*	Fever, myalgia, leukopenia, monocyte inclusions not often seen, maculopapular rash in a minority	*Amblyomma* (Lone Star) tick bite
Human granulocytic anaplasmosis (HGE)	*Anaplasma phagocytophilium*	Fever, myalgia, leukopenia, granulocyte inclusions often seen on blood smear	*Ixodes* (deer) tick bite
"Flu syndrome"	*Ehrlichia ewingii*	Immunocompromised host—fever, myalgia	*Amblyomma*
Cat-scratch disease	*Bartonella* spp (there are 8 identified zoonotic *Bartonella* spp)	Cervical lymphadenopathy in normal hosts and cutaneous and hepatic angiomatosis in AIDS patients	Cat scratch or bite
Hemorrhagic diarrhea	Enterohemorrhagic *Escherichia coli* O157:H7 (other species)	Rectal bleeding, dysentery, hemolytic-uremic syndrome	Contaminated, undercooked meat
Hantavirus pulmonary syndrome	*Hantavirus*—Sin Nombre	Noncardiac pulmonary edema, elevated hematocrit	Fomites of wild rodents
Cryptosporidium diarrhea	*Cryptosporidium parvum*	Prolonged watery diarrhea	Contaminated water—cattle and sheep
Dysentery	*Campylobacter jejuni*	Dysentery, reactive arthritis, Guillain-Barré syndrome	Contaminated chicken
Pyogenic skin ulcer	*Capnocytophaga canimorsus*	Sepsis, skin infection	Dog bites
West Nile fever encephalitis	West Nile virus	Encephalitis, myelitis, Guillain-Barré syndrome	Mosquito bite, birds
SARS	Coronavirus	Severe lower respiratory tract infection	Masked palm civet (presumed)
Cutaneous leishmaniasis	*Leishmania mexicana*	Skin nodules and ulcers	Wood rat

*See table of contents and index to locate a more detailed discussion of each disease.
AIDS = acquired immunodeficiency syndrome; SARS = severe acute respiratory syndrome.

TABLE 336-2 RESPIRATORY TRACT ZOONOSES

DISEASE*	MICROORGANISM†	CLINICAL FINDINGS	RESERVOIR AND/OR VECTOR
Psittacosis‡	*Chlamydophila psittaci*	Pneumonia, often severe	Aerosols from parrots, ducks, turkeys
Q fever	*Coxiella burnetii*	Pneumonia, hepatitis, myocarditis	Airborne from soil contaminated by sheep, goats, and cats, particularly if parturient
Tularemia	*Francisella tularensis*	Cutaneous ulcer and regional node, pneumonia and hilar node; pleural effusion	Rabbit contact (winter) and tick bites
Plague	*Yersinia pestis*	Inguinal nodes, bubonic plague (basilar pneumonia develops in 10%); hilar node enlargement	Fleas from prairie dogs, rock squirrels, rats
Hantavirus syndrome	*Hantavirus*	Upper respiratory to lower respiratory to adult respiratory distress syndrome (ARDS) to death	Deer mouse fomites: urine, feces, saliva
Rhodococcus pneumonia	*Rhodococcus equi*	Pneumonia often cavitates in those with AIDS and other immunosuppressed patients	Horse manure, soil
Mycoplasma arginini pneumonia	*Mycoplasma arginini*	Pneumonia, sepsis, neutropenia	Sheep, goats
Foot-and-mouth disease	*Aphthovirus*	Nonspecific upper respiratory tract infection, oral vesicles	Cloven-footed mammals
Whooping cough	*Bordetella bronchiseptica*	Pneumonia, bronchitis, whooping cough	Dogs
Histoplasmosis	*Histoplasma capsulatum*	Pneumonia or fever of unknown origin	Bats
Anthrax	*Bacillus anthracis*	Mediastinal widening with CT scan; pneumonia often absent	Herbivore mammals
Glanders	*Burkholderia mallei*	Pneumonia, erosive tracheobronchitis	Horses, mules

*See table of contents and index to locate a more detailed discussion of each disease.
†Because of the fastidious nature of some organisms, the rapid development of diagnostic tools, and the risk some agents pose to laboratory workers, a clinical microbiologist should be consulted if these agents are considered in a patient's differential diagnosis.
‡Occurs in more than 1000 animal species.
AIDS = acquired immunodeficiency syndrome; CT = computed tomography.

as southern China or Mexico (2009 novel H1N1 virus), where dense concentrations of ducks, pigs, and people cohabit. Viral incubation of the three influenza species in the pig, with a reassortment of antigens and subsequent spread of virulent "new" influenza strains to humans, can lead to massive influenza pandemics that in sheer numbers (billions) surpass any past epidemics of smallpox or plague. Initially, HIV-1 and HIV-2 were transmitted as simian immunodeficiency viruses from chimpanzees and mangabey primates, respectively, to humans. As with influenza, the subsequent 33 million (and counting) cases of HIV no longer require an animal reservoir for continuing transmission. Because these pandemics of AIDS and influenza now spread human to human without the help of the initiating animal host, the World Health Organization no longer considers them zoonoses.

Leprosy, an illness of biblical notoriety transmitted from human to human, is endemic in at least three animal species, including the armadillo. This animal has rarely been implicated in the transmission of leprosy to humans in the United States.

Despite the large number of zoonoses described, clinicians evaluating an individual patient usually need to consider only a limited number of historical details to arrive at an appropriate differential diagnosis:

1. A history of direct contact with animals or animal products, animal bites, arthropod exposure, and food ingestion may offer clues to the correct cause.
2. The patient's travel history must be considered because a number of zoonoses are still quite limited in geographic distribution.
3. Occupational and recreational high-risk activities must be ascertained.

TABLE 336-3 CENTRAL NERVOUS SYSTEM ZOONOSES

DISEASE*	ORGANISM	CLINICAL FINDINGS	ACQUISITION
Listeriosis	Listeria monocytogenes	Purulent meningitis during pregnancy, in patients older than 65 yr, in neonates, and in immunosuppressed	Unpasteurized cheese and other dairy products; cattle, goats
Leptospirosis	Leptospira interrogans	Aseptic meningitis, hepatorenal syndrome	Asymptomatic dogs, cattle; common water source
Herpes B encephalitis	Cercopithecine herpesvirus (herpes B virus)	Diffuse, progressive encephalitis	Macaca monkey bites or scratches
Lyme disease	Borrelia burgdorferi	Lymphocytic meningitis, motor-sensory neuropathy, facial palsy	Tick bite
Lymphocytic choriomeningitis	Lymphocytic choriomeningitis virus	Lymphocytic meningitis, occasionally with pneumonia	Inhalation of mouse secretions: urine, feces, saliva
Mosquito-borne encephalitis (U.S.)	Eastern, western equine, St. Louis, California encephalitis; West Nile virus	Diffuse encephalitis, least severe; California encephalitis, most severe; eastern equine encephalitis, myelitis, meningitis	Mosquito-borne from horses, birds
Rabies encephalitis	Rabies virus	Encephalitis; almost always fatal	Bites from dogs, skunks, bats, raccoons, foxes
Toxoplasmosis	Toxoplasma gondii	Multiple brain masses in AIDS patient	Cat feces or ingestion of undercooked lamb or pork
Cerebral cysticercosis	Taenia solium	Epilepsy, CNS cysts, eosinophilic meningitis, hydrocephalus	Fecal-oral; contamination of food with pork tapeworm eggs
New-variant Creutzfeldt-Jakob disease	Prion (proteinaceous infectious particle)	Dementia, ataxia, myoclonus	Beef from cattle fed scraps from contaminated sheep carcasses
Nipah virus	Paramyxovirus	Acute encephalitis, death	Pig contact
Hendra virus	Paramyxovirus	Pneumonitis, encephalitis	Horses, fruit bats

*See table of contents and index to locate a more detailed discussion of each disease.
AIDS = acquired immunodeficiency syndrome; CNS = central nervous system.

TABLE 336-4 ZOONOSES CAUSING RASH OR SKIN NODULE-ULCER

DISEASE*	MICROORGANISM†	CLINICAL FINDINGS	RESERVOIR AND/OR VECTOR
Ehrlichiosis (monocytic)	Ehrlichia chaffeensis	Macular rash (seen in < ⅓ of patients) with a central distribution; prevalent in south-central U.S.	Tick bite
Leptospirosis	Leptospira interrogans	Central macular rash in 20%, with occasional enanthem, conjunctival suffusion, hepatorenal syndrome	Urine-contaminated water; dogs, cattle
Lyme disease	Borrelia burgdorferi	Erythema migrans; 20% have multiple lesions	Mouse reservoir—tick bite
Rocky Mountain spotted fever	Rickettsia rickettsii	Acral or peripheral distribution of maculopapular to hemorrhagic rash to gangrenous lesions—no eschar	Tick bite
Typhus (epidemic)	Rickettsia prowazekii	Macular rash with a central distribution (can be hemorrhagic)	Flying squirrel fleas or fomites
Cat-scratch disease	Bartonella spp	Bacillary angiomatosis, peliosis hepatis in HIV patients, cervical adenopathy, subacute bacterial endocarditis, fever of unknown origin	Cat scratch or bite
Tularemia	Francisella tularensis	Ulcer and node, typhoidal syndrome, pneumonia	Rabbit contact and tick bite
Anthrax	Bacillus anthracis	Painless, edematous, nonpurulent ulcer that becomes black and necrotic over days; mediastinitis	Herbivore animal products, including animal hides
Rickettsialpox (spotted fever Rickettsia)	Rickettsia akari, Rickettsia conorii, Rickettsia africae (8 others found on all continents)	Fever, rash, eschar (multiple), tache noire (R. africae, often multiple)	Mouse mite, tick
Monkeypox	Orthopoxvirus	Multiple maculopustular lesions with lymphadenopathy	Prairie dog (U.S.), African rodents
Erysipeloid	Erysipelothrix rhusiopathiae	Red, tender, swollen finger; subacute bacterial endocarditis	Skin pricked while cleaning fish, domestic meat animals
Seal finger	?	Tender, swollen fingertip	Seal bite?

*See table of contents and index to locate a more detailed discussion of each disease.
†Because of the fastidious nature of some organisms, the rapid development of diagnostic tools, and the risk some agents pose to laboratory workers, a clinical microbiologist should be consulted if these agents are considered in a patient's differential diagnosis.

4. The patient's clinical manifestations (course and organ involvement) are used to focus on the most likely cause (see Tables 336-2 through 336-5).
5. Though neither specific nor sensitive, the inoculation nodule (eschar, tache noire, chancre, necrotic ulcer), with or without fever, rash, or local lymphadenopathy, is the only general clue from the physical examination that might alert the physician to a zoonosis when the history does not.
6. Significant unilateral hilar adenopathy in the presence of acute pneumonia can be a clue to anthrax, plague, or tularemia.

TREATMENT Rx

The approach to treatment of the various zoonoses is presented in their respective chapters.

PREVENTION

Guidelines have been published to help prevent nosocomial transmission of zoonotic diseases. Preventive measures to decrease infection in compromised

TABLE 336-5 OTHER ZOONOTIC CLINICAL SYNDROMES

DISEASE*	ORGANISM
Sepsis syndrome	*Streptococcus suis, Capnocytophaga canimorsus, Yersinia enterocolitica, Pasteurella multocida, Rickettsia rickettsii, Streptobacillus moniliformis, Rickettsia conorii, Leptospira icterohaemorrhagiae*
Polyarthritis	*Streptobacillus moniliformis, Borrelia burgdorferi, Spirillum minus, Brucella* spp, alpha virus—six groups (Ross River, Sindbis, Mayaro, chikungunya, o'nyong-nyong, igbo-ora)
Jaundice	*Coxiella burnetii, Leptospira icterohaemorrhagiae,* yellow fever (sylvatic), hepatitis E, echinococcosis, *Fasciola hepatica*
Renal failure (acute)	*Leptospira, Hantavirus, Rickettsia rickettsii, Rickettsia conorii, Escherichia coli* O157
Endocarditis	*Bartonella, Coxiella burnetii, Erysipelothrix rhusiopathiae, Brucella, Streptococcus suis, Listeria monocytogenes, Chlamydia psittaci*
Diarrhea	*Salmonella, Campylobacter jejuni,* Shiga toxin–positive *E. coli, Giardia intestinalis,* cryptosporidia, *Yersinia pseudotuberculosis, Yersinia enterocolitica*

*See table of contents and index to locate a more detailed discussion of each disease.

TABLE 336-6 HIGHLY FATAL ZOONOSES

DISEASE*	FATALITY RATE (%)
Creutzfeldt-Jakob disease (new variant)	100
Rabies	100
Anthrax, inhalational	80-90
Herpes simiae	50-75[+]
Ebola virus	70
Eastern equine encephalitis	50-70
Hantavirus pulmonary syndrome (U.S.)	60[+]
H5N1 influenza	15-50
Yellow fever (sylvatic)	20-50[§]
Lassa fever	15-25[§]
Plague	50-80[+]
Rocky Mountain spotted fever	20-60[+]
East African sleeping sickness	20-30[+]
Anthrax, cutaneous	20[+]
Tularemia, pneumonic	30-60[+]
Tularemia, cutaneous	2-10
Visceral leishmaniasis	5-25[+]
Louse-borne relapsing fever	5-40[+]

*See table of contents and index to locate a more detailed discussion of each disease.
[+]If untreated.
[‡]Case mortality of hospitalized patients.
[§]If jaundiced.

hosts include the routine immunization of pets, neutering of pets, use of caution when handling pet fomites, rigorous handwashing practices, and avoidance of ingesting undercooked meat, fish, shellfish, and eggs.

Isolation is recommended for anthrax, Andes *Hantavirus* disease, herpes B, monkeypox, Q fever, rabies, plague, SARS, influenza, and the hemorrhagic fever illnesses caused by Argentine, Bolivian, Crimean-Congo, Ebola, Lassa, and Marburg viruses.

PROGNOSIS

The prognosis of zoonoses varies widely, but a number of these disease have very high case-fatality rates (Table 336-6).

SUGGESTED READINGS

Akritidis N. Parasitic, fungal and prion zoonoses: an expanding universe of candidates for human disease. *Clin Microbiol Infect.* 2011;17:331-335. *Review.*

Altizer S, Bartel R, Han BA. Animal migration and infectious disease risk. *Science.* 2011;331:296-302. *Review.*

Christou L. The global burden of bacterial and viral zoonotic infections. *Clin Microbiol Infect.* 2011; 17:326-330. *Review.*

337

ACTINOMYCOSIS

ITZHAK BROOK

DEFINITION

Actinomycosis is an uncommon, subacute to chronic bacterial infection that induces both suppurative and granulomatous inflammation. Localized swelling with suppuration, abscess formation, tissue fibrosis, and draining sinuses characterize this disease. The infection spreads contiguously and often forms draining sinuses that extrude characteristic but not pathognomonic "sulfur granules." Infections of the oral and cervicofacial regions are most common, but any site in the body can be infected, including the thoracic region, the abdominopelvic region, and the central nervous system (CNS). Musculoskeletal or disseminated disease is rare but does occur.

The Pathogen

Actinomycetes of the genera *Actinomyces, Propionibacterium,* and *Bifidobacterium* act as the principal pathogens. However, 98 to 99% of actinomycoses are caused by non–spore-forming anaerobic or microaerophilic bacterial species of the genus *Actinomyces,* family Actinomycetaceae, order Actinomycetales. Of the 30 *Actinomyces* species, 8 may cause disease in humans: the strictly anaerobic *A. israelii, A. gerencseriae* (formerly known as *A. israelii* serotype II), *A. odontolyticus, A. naeslundii, A. meyeri, A. viscosus, A. pyogenes,* and *A. georgiae. A. israelii* is the most common species causing human disease. *Propionibacterium propionicum* (formerly known as *Arachnia propionica*) and *Bifidobacterium dentium* (formerly known as *Actinomyces eriksonii*) are also associated with clinically indistinguishable infection. The organisms are filamentous, branching, gram-positive, pleomorphic, non–spore-forming, non–acid-fast anaerobic or microaerophilic bacilli. *Actinomyces* organisms are fastidious bacteria that require enriched culture media; 6 to 10% ambient CO_2 may aid in their growth, which takes 3 to 10 days or more in culture. Most actinomycotic infections are polymicrobial and involve other aerobic and anaerobic bacteria. The most common co-isolates depend on the infection site and are *Actinobacillus actinomycetemcomitans, Aggregatibacter aphrophilus, Eikenella corrodens, Bacteroides, Fusobacterium, Capnocytophaga,* aerobic and anaerobic streptococci, *Staphylococcus,* and Enterobacteriaceae.

EPIDEMIOLOGY

Actinomyces species are members of the endogenous mucous membrane flora in the oral cavity, lower gastrointestinal tract, bronchi, and female genital tract. No external environmental reservoir, such as soil or straw, has been documented, nor has person-to-person transmission of pathogenic *Actinomyces* species been demonstrated. Although infection can occur in all age groups, it is rarely seen in children or patients older than 60 years. Most cases are encountered in individuals in the middle decades of life. A male-to-female infection ratio of 3:1 is reported in most series. The explanation for this ratio is the higher prevalence of poor oral hygiene and oral trauma in men. The annual reported incidence in the United States is fewer than 100 cases. However, because of the fastidious nature of the organism, many cases are undiagnosed, and the true incidence is probably much higher.

PATHOBIOLOGY

Actinomyces species are agents of low pathogenicity and require mucosal barrier disruption to cause disease. Actinomycosis usually occurs in immunocompetent persons but may afflict those with diminished host defenses. Oral and cervicofacial diseases are commonly associated with dental caries and extractions, gingivitis and gingival trauma, infection in erupting secondary teeth, chronic tonsillitis, otitis or mastoiditis, diabetes mellitus, immunosuppression, malnutrition, and local tissue damage caused by surgery, neoplastic disease, or irradiation. Pulmonary infections generally arise after aspiration of oropharyngeal or gastrointestinal secretions. Gastrointestinal infection frequently follows loss of mucosal integrity, such as with surgery, appendicitis, diverticulitis, trauma, or foreign bodies. The use of intrauterine contraceptive devices (IUDs) increases risk for the development of actinomycosis of the female genital tract. Other predisposing factors are steroid use, immunosuppression, and human immunodeficiency virus infection.

Other bacterial species that are frequently copathogens with *Actinomyces* species may assist in the spread of infection by inhibiting host defenses and reducing local oxygen tension. Once the organism is established locally, it may spread progressively to surrounding tissues. The infection tends to spread without regard for anatomic barriers, including fascial planes and lymphatic channels. The end result is a chronic, indurated, suppurative infection (usually with draining sinuses and fibrosis, especially in pelvic and abdominal infection). The fibrotic walls of the mass before suppuration are "wooden" in nature and may be confused with a neoplasm. Hematogenous spread can be fulminant but is rare.

Actinomyces species grow in microscopic or macroscopic clusters of tangled filaments surrounded by neutrophils. Plasma cells and multinucleated giant cells are often observed with lesions, as are large macrophages with foamy cytoplasm around purulent centers. When visible, these clusters are pale yellow and exude through sinus tracks; they are called sulfur granules (originally called drusen). These granules (1 to 2 mm in diameter) are made of aggregates of organisms and contain calcium phosphate. A central purulent loculation surrounds the granules. Their centers have a basophilic staining property, with eosinophilic rays terminating in pear-shaped "clubs." One to six granules can be present per loculation, and up to 50 loculations can be present in a lesion. Multicenter giant cells can be seen as well.

CLINICAL MANIFESTATIONS

Cervicofacial

Cervicofacial infection is the most common manifestation of actinomycosis (Fig. 337-1). This infection is generally odontogenic in origin and evolves as a chronic or subacute painless or painful soft tissue swelling or mass involving the submandibular or paramandibular region. However, the submental and retromandibular spaces, temporomandibular joint, and cheek can be involved. The swelling may have a ligneous consistency caused by tissue fibrosis. Depending on the composition of the concomitant synergistic flora, the onset of actinomycosis may be acute, subacute, or chronic. When *Staphylococcus aureus* or β-hemolytic streptococci are involved, an acute painful abscess or a phlegmatous cellulitis may be the initial manifestation. The chronic form of the disease is the most common form and is characterized by painless infiltration and bluish or reddish induration that generally progress to form multiple abscesses and draining sinus tracks discharging pus

that may contain sulfur granules in up to 25% of instances. Periapical infection, trismus, fever, pain, and leukocytosis may be present. The infection can extend to the carotid artery, tongue, sinuses, ears, mastoid, orbit, salivary glands, pharynx, masseter muscle, thyroid, larynx, trachea, or thorax. Bone (most commonly the mandible) may be invaded from the adjacent soft tissue and result in periostitis or osteomyelitis. Cervical spine or cranial bone infection may lead to subdural empyema and invasion of the CNS. The differential diagnosis includes tuberculosis (scrofula), fungal infections, nocardiosis, suppurative infections by other organisms, and neoplasms.

Thoracic

Thoracic actinomycosis is an indolent, slowly progressive process involving the pulmonary parenchyma and pleural space. This form accounts for 15 to 30% of actinomycosis cases and is caused by aspiration of infective material from the oropharynx as well as rarely after esophageal perforation, by extension into the mediastinum from the neck, by spread from an abdominal site, or by hematogenous spread to the lung. Infection can spread from a pneumonic focus across lung fissures to involve the pleura and the chest wall, with eventual fistula formation and drainage containing sulfur granules (Fig. 337-2). The mediastinum, pericardium, and myocardium can also rarely be affected. Granules are seldom present in sputum. The incidence of this complication, as well as the destruction of thoracic vertebrae and adjacent ribs, has declined in the antimicrobial era.

The complaints of patients with thoracic actinomycosis are nonspecific. The most common are chest pain, productive cough, dyspnea, weight loss, and fever. Anemia, mild leukocytosis, and elevated sedimentation rate are relatively common. There is often a history of underlying lung disease, and patients are rarely initially seen in an early stage of infection. The pulmonary lesion is either a mass lesion or pneumonitis and may resemble tuberculosis,

FIGURE 337-2. Thoracic computed tomography scan of a 43-year-old woman with pulmonary actinomycosis. There is consolidation of the lung with pleural thickening adjacent to the parenchymal disease (**A**). Abscess extended into the left breast and inferiorly to the costophrenic sulcus, to the retroperitoneum, and into the lateral abdominal wall (**B**, *arrow*).

FIGURE 337-1. Actinomycosis of the jaw, observed at Letterman General Hospital, San Francisco, Calif., in a sergeant who had punctured the floor of his mouth while picking his teeth. (Office of Medical History, Office of the Surgeon General, U.S. Army.)

especially when cavity formation occurs, or blastomycosis, which may destroy ribs posteriorly but rarely forms sinuses. Nocardiosis, bronchogenic carcinoma, cryptococcosis, aspiration pneumonia, pulmonary infection, and lymphoma can also mimic thoracic actinomycosis. Pleural thickening, effusion, or emphysema is common.

Abdominal

Abdominal actinomycosis is a chronic, localized inflammatory process that can occur weeks, months, or years after the integrity of the gastrointestinal mucosa is breached by surgery or trauma. Acute appendicitis with perforation, perforated colonic diverticulitis, and emergency surgery for trauma to the lower intestinal tract are among the predisposing factors. Extension from the thorax or pelvis or through hematogenous dissemination can also occur. The ileocecal region is involved most frequently (usually after appendicitis with perforation) with the formation of a mass lesion. The infection extends slowly to contiguous organs, especially the liver, and may involve retroperitoneal tissues, the spine, or the abdominal wall. Hepatic, renal, or splenic dissemination is an uncommon complication. Persistent draining sinuses may form, and those involving the perianal region can simulate Crohn's disease (Chapter 143) or tuberculosis. The extensive fibrosis of actinomycotic lesions, recognized by the examiner as a mass, often suggests tumor. A frequent finding on computed tomography (CT) is an infiltrative mass with dense inhomogeneous contrast medium enhancement. Constitutional symptoms and signs are nonspecific, the most common being fever, diarrhea or constipation, weight loss, nausea, vomiting, pain, and sensation of a mass.

Pelvic

Pelvic infection is observed in patients with prolonged use of IUDs, usually for longer than 2 years. Pelvic actinomycosis may also occur from extension of intestinal infection, commonly from indolent ileocecal disease. Manifestations of infection may range from a chronic vaginal discharge to pelvic inflammatory disease with tubo-ovarian abscesses or pseudomalignant masses. Patients generally have abnormal vaginal bleeding or discharge, abdominal or pelvic pain, menorrhagia, fever, and weight loss.

Endometritis is the earlier form of the infection, followed by tubo-ovarian abscesses. Extension to the uterus, bladder, rectal area, abdominal wall, peritoneum, pelvic bones, thorax, and systemic circulation can also occur.

Central Nervous System

Infections of the CNS are very rare and generally manifested as single or multiple encapsulated brain abscesses that appear as ring-enhancing lesions with a thick wall that may be irregular or nodular on contrast-enhanced CT scans. There are no features that readily distinguish actinomycosis from other causes of brain abscesses. Rarely, solid nodular or mass lesions termed actinomycetomas or actinomycotic granulomas are found. Headache and focal neurologic signs are the most common finding. Most actinomycotic infections of the CNS are seeded hematogenously from a distant primary site, but direct extension of cervicofacial disease also occurs. Sinus formation is not a characteristic of CNS disease. The rare meningitis caused by *Actinomyces* is chronic and basilar in location, and the cerebrospinal fluid pleocytosis is usually lymphocytic. Thus, it may be misdiagnosed as tuberculous meningitis. Extension to the cranial epidural or subdural space and spinal epidural space can also occur from adjacent foci.

DIAGNOSIS

Appropriate microbiologic and pathologic studies are essential for diagnosis. A high index of suspicion should be communicated to the microbiology laboratory, along with material from draining sinuses, from deep-needle aspiration, or from biopsy specimens. CT or ultrasound needle aspiration can be used to obtain a biopsy specimen. It is important to avoid contamination of the specimen by "normal flora" and administration of antimicrobial therapy before a specimen is obtained. Anaerobic culture is required, and no selective media are available to restrict overgrowth of the slow-growing *Actinomyces* by associated microflora. The presence, in pus or tissue specimens, of non–acid-fast, gram-positive organisms with filamentous branching is suggestive of the diagnosis. The characteristic morphologic features of sulfur granules within are helpful. In tissue sections stained with hematoxylin-eosin, sulfur granules are round or oval basophilic masses with a radiating arrangement of eosinophilic terminal clubs. However, *Actinomyces* species are infrequently visible in sections stained with hematoxylin-eosin; visualization is facilitated by special stains such as Gomori methenamine silver, *p*-aminosalicylic acid, McCallen-Goodpasture, and Brown-Brenn. Multiple biopsy sections from different tissue levels are recommended to improve the histopathologic diagnosis. The granules must be distinguished from similar structures that are sometimes produced in infections caused by *Nocardia, Monosporium, Cephalosporium, Staphylococcus* (botryomycosis), and others. *Actinomyces* and *Arachnia* can generally be differentiated from other gram-positive anaerobes by means of their growth rate (slow), by catalase production (negative, except for *A. viscosus*), and by gas-liquid chromatographic detection of the acetic, lactic, and succinic acids produced in peptone-yeast-glucose broth. Direct fluorescent antibody conjugates and immunofluorescence testing can be used but are not readily available to clinical microbiology laboratories.

Imaging methods such as conventional radiography, CT, and magnetic resonance imaging do not provide a specific diagnosis but allow more accurate definition of the dimensions and extension of the infection.

TREATMENT ℞

Prolonged antimicrobial therapy (i.e., 6 to 12 months) has typically been recommended for patients with all clinical forms of actinomycosis to prevent disease recrudescence. However, individualization of courses of therapy is recommended because the duration of treatment depends on the initial burden of disease, the site of infection, and the clinical and radiologic response. Adequate drainage is indicated if abscesses are present.

Penicillin G is the drug of choice for treatment of an infection caused by any of the *Actinomyces*. It is given in high dosage during a prolonged period because the infection has a tendency to recur. Most deep-seated infections can be expected to respond to intravenous penicillin G, 18 to 24 million units/day given for 2 to 6 weeks, followed by an oral phenoxypenicillin in a dosage of 2 to 4 g/day. A few additional weeks of oral penicillin therapy may suffice for uncomplicated cervicofacial disease; complicated cases and extensive pulmonary or abdominal disease may require treatment for 12 to 18 months. Little evidence exists of acquired resistance to penicillin G by *Actinomyces* during prolonged therapy. The combination of a penicillin (i.e., amoxicillin, piperacillin) and a β-lactamase inhibitor (i.e., clavulanate, tazobactam) offers the advantage of coverage against penicillin-resistant aerobic and anaerobic copathogens. Alternative first-line antibiotics include tetracycline, erythromycin, cephalexin, oxacillin, and clindamycin. Ceftriaxone, imipenem, and fluoroquinolones have also been used successfully. Metronidazole, aminoglycosides, and antifungal drugs are not effective. In vitro antimicrobial susceptibility testing of *Actinomyces* is difficult, and the results may not be predictive of antimicrobial effect in vivo.

The need to use combination antimicrobial therapy to attack microorganisms that are isolated in association with *Actinomyces* has not been established. However, because many of these organisms are known pathogens, treatment is usually appropriate, especially with lower abdominal infections. Surgical removal of infected tissue may also be necessary in some cases, especially if extensive necrotic tissue or fistulas are present, if malignant disease cannot be excluded, and if large abscesses cannot be drained by percutaneous aspiration. When well-defined IUD-related symptoms and Papanicolaou smears demonstrate *Actinomyces* by specific fluorescent-labeled antibody, the IUD should be removed. Antimicrobial administration for a 2-week period may be indicated. More serious infections require prolonged therapy.

PROGNOSIS

The availability of antimicrobial treatment has greatly improved the prognosis for all forms of actinomycosis. At present, cure rates are high, and neither deformity nor death is common.

SUGGESTED READINGS

Choi MH, Hong DG, Seong WJ, et al. Pelvic actinomycosis confirmed after surgery: single center experience. *Arch Gynecol Obstet.* 2010;281:651-656. *Review of 16 cases, 12 related to intrauterine contraceptive devices.*

Song JU, Park HY, Jeon K, et al. Treatment of thoracic actinomycosis: a retrospective analysis of 40 patients. *Ann Thorac Med.* 2010;5:80-85. *Review of medical and surgical therapy.*

Sullivan DC, Chapman SW. Bacteria that masquerade as fungi: actinomycosis/nocardia. *Proc Am Thorac Soc.* 2010;7:216-221. *Review of lung, bone and joint, soft tissue, and central nervous system manifestations.*

338

NOCARDIOSIS

FREDERICK S. SOUTHWICK

DEFINITION

Nocardiosis refers to infections caused by *Nocardia* species. *Nocardia* most commonly causes pneumonia but can also infect the central nervous system (CNS) and skin. Less commonly, this organism can disseminate throughout the body. These infections usually occur in patients with defective immunity.

The Pathogen

Nocardia species are thin, aerobic, gram-positive bacilli that form branching filaments. The bacteria stain irregularly and appear beaded on Gram stain. The speciation of *Nocardia* has been problematic. The original classification was based on the ability to use specific nutrients and to decompose substrates such as adenine, casein, urea, gelatin, and xanthine. However, gene sequencing and DNA-DNA hybridization have now defined the true taxonomy. The species called *Nocardia asteroides* was previously reported to be the most common cause of human disease. However, the majority of these bacteria were misidentified by today's standards. The number of species causing human disease is large and includes *Nocardia abscessus, Nocardia brevicatena/paucivorans* complex, *Nocardia nova* complex, *Nocardia transvalensis* complex, *Nocardia farcinica, Nocardia cyriacigeorgica, Nocardia otitidis-caviarum, Nocardia veterana, Nocardia brasiliensis,* and *Nocardia pseudobrasiliensis.*

EPIDEMIOLOGY

Nocardia species are ubiquitous and originate primarily in soil. Despite being found throughout the environment, they rarely cause symptomatic infection in humans. Because nocardiosis is not a reportable disease, its frequency is unknown. However, the annual incidence is estimated to be 0.4 cases per 100,000 persons. The risk of symptomatic *Nocardia* infection is greatly increased in individuals who are immunocompromised (incidence estimated to be >1000-fold higher), including patients receiving immunosuppressive agents following bone marrow or solid organ transplants and patients with acquired immunodeficiency syndrome (AIDS). Corticosteroids are the most frequent immunosuppressants associated with nocardiosis; however, cases have also been reported in patients receiving anti–tumor necrosis factor-α antibody (infliximab) and other immunosuppressants. It is important to keep in mind that trimethoprim-sulfamethoxazole prophylaxis does not always protect against *Nocardia.* Other risk groups include patients with cancer, Cushing's disease, chronic granulomatous disease, and dysgammaglobulinemia. Patients with chronic pulmonary disorders, particularly alveolar proteinosis, are also more susceptible to this infection. In approximately one third of patients with nocardiosis, no predisposing condition can be identified.

PATHOBIOLOGY

Most *Nocardia* species gain entry to the host via the respiratory tract or, less commonly, by skin inoculation. Invading bacteria elicit a neutrophil response that inhibits but does not kill the organism. The bacteria are phagocytosed by neutrophils and macrophages and become enclosed in a membrane-bound phagolysosome. In this closed environment, neutrophils and macrophages are able to kill many species of bacteria by synthesizing superoxide and hydrogen peroxide. However, *Nocardia* are able to survive in this hostile environment by producing superoxide dismutase, an enzyme that inactivates these toxic oxygen byproducts. In addition, *Nocardia* species produce a mycolic acid called cord factor that inhibits the fusion of lysosomes with the phagolysosomal compartment, preventing toxic proteases and other antibacterial products from reaching the intracellular bacteria. In addition to neutrophils and macrophages, cell-mediated and humoral immunity plays a role in protecting the host against *Nocardia* invasion, explaining the wide range of immunocompromised patients at increased risk for contracting nocardiosis.

CLINICAL MANIFESTATIONS

Nocardiosis has no pathognomonic characteristics, and delays in diagnosis are common. Failure of a pulmonary or skin infection to respond to conventional antibiotic therapy should raise the possibility of a *Nocardia* species infection. Nocardiosis should always be considered in an immunocompromised patient.

Pulmonary Nocardiosis

Approximately two thirds of patients with nocardiosis present with pulmonary infection. Pulmonary disease is usually subacute in onset, mimicking a fungal or mycobacterial infection, and it is most commonly misdiagnosed as tuberculosis. The most common complaints are a persistent cough producing purulent sputum, fever, anorexia, and weight loss. Less commonly, patients may report pleuritic chest pain and dyspnea. Hemoptysis is rare, but it can develop in patients with large cavitary lesions. An acute onset of pneumonia has occasionally been reported in immunocompromised hosts.

Central Nervous System Infection

Approximately 5% of patients with a *Nocardia* infection have CNS involvement. Multilocular brain abscess is the most common CNS manifestation and is usually the consequence of transient bacterial dissemination from the lung. Lesions can occur in any region of the brain, and symptoms depend on location. Headache is the usual initial complaint and is frequently localized to the site of the abscess. Patients may also present with neurologic deficits as well as seizures. In AIDS patients, brain abscess is often accompanied by an abnormal chest x-ray, whereas in other patients, such abnormalities are not always present. The combined findings of a lung nodule on chest x-ray and a ring-enhancing CNS lesion are often mistaken for metastatic lung carcinoma. Other diagnoses that should be considered when an immunocompromised host presents with both lung and CNS foci are disseminated aspergillosis and toxoplasmosis. Meningitis is a less common CNS manifestation and is often associated with brain abscess (40% of meningitis cases). Cerebrospinal fluid cultures are often negative, and patients fail to fully respond to empirical antibiotic therapy.

Cutaneous Infection

Skin infection is usually caused by *N. brasiliensis* and usually follows a break in the skin that is contaminated by soil. Cutaneous disease has been reported in association with trauma, postoperative wounds, insect bites, thorn bush scratches, or even a cat scratch. Initially, a pustule or a moderately erythematous, nonfluctuant nodule develops at the site of inoculation. Erythema can extend along the lymphatic system and is associated with tender lymphadenopathy. This form of cutaneous infection has been termed *lymphocutaneous* or *sporotrichoid* disease. Similar skin manifestations are seen with cat-scratch disease, tularemia, *Mycobacterium marinum* infection, and sporotrichosis. In an immunocompromised host, disseminated infection may manifest as multiple erythematous, raised nodules, which is an ominous finding. In tropical regions of South and Central America, *Nocardia* species can cause ulcerations and large tumor-like lesions called mycetomas that are usually found on the lower legs.

DIAGNOSIS

Radiology

In pulmonary disease, chest x-ray findings are variable, with pulmonary nodules or mass lesions seen most often (Fig. 338-1). Less frequently, consolidation, cavitary lesions with air-fluid levels, interstitial infiltrates, and pleural effusions are found. Chest computed tomography (CT) often demonstrates areas of low attenuation within consolidations, multiple nodules, and extension of the infection to the chest wall. AIDS patients are more likely to have multiple pulmonary nodules, cavitary lesions, and upper lobe infiltrates. In some patients, particularly those with normal immune function, the infiltrate may resolve. However, the patient may present with brain abscess several months later as a consequence of transient dissemination. In CNS infection, CT or magnetic resonance imaging with contrast usually demonstrates one or more ring-enhancing lesions (Fig. 338-2). *Nocardia* brain abscess is more commonly multiloculated, but otherwise, the radiologic findings are similar to those of brain abscess caused by other bacteria. Positron emission tomography is not helpful in differentiating *Nocardia* brain abscess from tumor because both demonstrate increased uptake.

Histopathology

Invasive procedures are generally required for specific diagnosis. For pulmonary infection, bronchoscopy with transbronchial biopsy or skinny needle

FIGURE 338-1. Chest computed tomography showing a peripheral nodular lung lesion *(arrow)* caused by *Nocardia* infection.

FIGURE 338-2. Multiple gadolinium-enhanced brain lesions *(arrows)* caused by *Nocardia* infection.

biopsy is recommended. For brain abscess, CT-guided needle aspirate is the diagnostic procedure of choice. Histopathology usually reveals an acute inflammatory response with a predominance of neutrophils. Micronodular abscesses with minimal capsular formation are usually found. Gram stain or Brown-Brenn stains reveal gram-positive beaded, branching forms. The morphology is identical to *Actinomyces;* however, the high lipid content of its cell wall often renders *Nocardia* modified acid-fast positive, whereas *Actinomyces* species are modified acid-fast negative. Acid fastness may be variable when staining *Nocardia* colonies from cultures, however, and it is unreliable for direct clinical samples.

Culture

Isolation of the organism on culture provides a definitive diagnosis for needle aspirate samples from brain abscess and a presumptive diagnosis when grown from respiratory and cutaneous samples. *Nocardia* species grow best under aerobic conditions with 5 to 10% carbon dioxide. Because the organisms grow slowly on blood agar, taking 3 to 5 days to form colonies, other organisms can overgrow. When *Nocardia* is suspected, the clinical laboratory should be notified to ensure the use of selective media and prolonged incubation. 16S Ribosomal RNA gene sequencing allows the rapid speciation of isolates. Increasing numbers of *Nocardia* have been shown to be resistant to sulfonamides. Therefore, antibiotic susceptibility testing should always be performed to guide the choice of treatment.

Sulfonamides remain the treatment of choice for pulmonary and cutaneous disease. Trimethoprim-sulfamethoxazole given orally at a dose of 160/800 mg (one double-strength tablet) three times a day is the most common adult regimen. When patients with disseminated and/or CNS *Nocardia* are treated with sulfonamides alone, survival is less than 50%. One of the most common species to cause disseminated diseases, *N. farcinica*, is also one of the most common *Nocardia* species to be resistant to sulfonamides. In these more serious conditions, combination therapy is generally recommended, and the exact regimen is guided by antibiotic susceptibility testing. One recommended empirical regimen is trimethoprim-sulfamethoxazole at the doses stated earlier, amikacin (10 mg/kg/day in divided doses), and either ceftriaxone (2 g twice daily) or imipenem (500 mg every 6 hours). In a retrospective study, patients failing trimethoprim-sulfamethoxazole treatment responded to imipenem with or without amikacin. Linezolid 600 mg twice a day has been used successfully in a small number of CNS infections. However, prolonged therapy with this agent can lead to bone marrow toxicity and warrants weekly monitoring of the peripheral cell counts. Recently, the newer fluoroquinolones moxifloxacin and gatifloxacin (400 mg/day orally for both agents) were shown to have activity against several strains of *Nocardia,* including *N. farcinica* and *N. brasiliensis*, and these agents may be useful in patients who cannot tolerate sulfonamides; however, relapse has been reported. Minocycline (100 mg orally twice daily) and amoxicillin/clavulanate (875/125 mg orally twice daily) are other potentially effective alternative treatments for *Nocardia*. Because of the intracellular nature of *Nocardia* and the slow rates of bacterial growth, antibiotic treatment for 6 to 12 months in an immunocompromised host and 4 to 6 months in a normal host is usually required to prevent relapse.

For patients with brain abscess or subcutaneous abscesses, surgical drainage is required for cure, in addition to antibiotics.

The overall mortality for nocardiosis is approximately 25%. In otherwise healthy individuals, pulmonary nocardiosis has a better prognosis (15% mortality). The survival rate is worse in patients with bacteremia, acute infection (symptoms for <3 weeks), disseminated disease involving two or more noncontiguous organs, and meningitis and in those receiving corticosteroids or cytotoxic agents.

SUGGESTED READINGS

Ameen M, Arenas R, Vasquez del Mercado E, et al. Efficacy of imipenem therapy for *Nocardia* actinomycetomas refractory to sulfonamides. *J Am Acad Dermatol*. 2010;62:239-246. *Retrospective study of eight patients with Nocardia soft tissue and bone infections refractory to sulfonamides who responded to imipenem with or without amikacin.*

Decroos FC, Garg P, Reddy AK, et al. Optimizing diagnosis and management of *Nocardia* keratitis, scleritis, and endophthalmitis: 11-year microbial and clinical overview. *Ophthalmology*. 2011. [Epub ahead of print.] *Review of 111 cases of keratitis, 11 cases of scleritis, and 16 cases of endophthalmitis, with a medical response rate of 82% to amikacin therapy for keratitis but a lower rate for scleritis and endophthalmitis.*

Minero MV, Marin M, Cercenado E, et al. Nocardiosis at the turn of the century. *Medicine (Baltimore)*. 2009;88:250-261. *Comprehensive series of cases from a single hospital that, compared with reviews of individual case reports, more accurately reflects the organ distribution of Nocardia infection and the common clinical manifestations, treatment, and outcome.*

339

SYSTEMIC ANTIFUNGAL AGENTS

DAVID A. STEVENS

Methods for in vitro susceptibility testing are available as standardized tools. A variety of assays are available for therapeutic drug monitoring of serum and other body fluids. As more common mutations inducing resistance are uncovered, it becomes possible to develop molecular screening methods that can detect the resistance genes in clinical isolates, in advance of susceptibility test results.

AMPHOTERICIN B–BASED PREPARATIONS

Mechanism of Action

Amphotericin B is a lipophilic molecule that exerts its antifungal effect by insertion into the fungal cytoplasmic membrane. Amphotericin B causes membrane permeability to increase. Loss of intracellular molecules impairs fungal viability. The onset of action is rapid. Amphotericin B also has effects on oxidation that may enhance antifungal activity.

Spectrum of Activity and Mechanisms of Resistance

Amphotericin B is active against most fungi, and its spectrum of activity is not influenced by the choice of formulation. When resistance occurs, it is generally attributed to reductions in ergosterol biosynthesis and the synthesis of alternative sterols that lessen the ability of amphotericin B to interact with the fungal membrane. Primary resistance is common for *Aspergillus terreus* and for *Scedosporium* and *Trichosporon* species. Among the *Candida* species, primary resistance is noted at meaningful frequencies most often for *Candida lusitaniae*. Development of resistance in isolates of normally susceptible species is uncommon. In some studies, the principal pharmacodynamic driver of in vivo response has been the ratio of the peak serum concentration to the minimal inhibitory concentration (MIC).

Available Formulations

There are four commercially available amphotericin B formulations: amphotericin B deoxycholate (ABD) and three lipid-associated formulations— amphotericin B colloidal dispersion (ABCD), amphotericin B lipid complex, and liposomal amphotericin B. All formulations must be infused in 5% dextrose with no electrolytes added. Infusion bottles need not be protected from light. In attempts to produce less expensive lipid-associated formulations, some reports have advocated mixing ABD with a parenteral fat emulsion. Although less nephrotoxicity has been observed in adults given this preparation at a dose of 1 mg/kg/day compared with infusions of ABD in 5% dextrose, no advantage was found in children. Serum amphotericin B concentrations were also lower with the fat emulsion, raising the possibility that amphotericin B was simply aggregating in the fat emulsion, but the cloudiness could not be perceived in the milky-looking lipid. Use of such preparations should be reserved for investigational settings.

Amphotericin B Deoxycholate

Formulation

ABD for intravenous use is a colloidal suspension. If a filter with a 0.22-μm pore diameter is placed in the infusion line, considerable drug is removed by the filter. The addition of electrolyte aggregates the colloids, so the solution becomes cloudy. ABD is available from several generic manufacturers, and significant differences in the formulations have been reported, which may account in part for the intersubject variation in toxicities observed.

Pharmacology

Most of the drug leaves the circulation promptly, with only a small percentage being excreted in urine or bile. Amphotericin B is stored in the liver and other organs; the drug appears to re-enter the circulation slowly. Blood levels are uninfluenced by hepatic or renal failure. Hemodialysis does not alter blood levels, except in an occasional patient with lipemic plasma who may be losing drug owing to its adherence to the dialysis membrane. Concentrations of amphotericin B in fluid from inflamed areas, such as pleura, peritoneum, joint, vitreous humor, and aqueous humor, are roughly two thirds of the nadir serum level. Amphotericin B penetrates poorly into either normal or inflamed meninges, saliva, bronchial secretions, brain, pancreas, muscle, bone, vitreous humor, and normal amniotic fluid. Urine concentrations are similar to serum concentrations. Peak serum concentrations with conventional intravenous doses are roughly 0.5 to 2.0 μg/mL; these concentrations fall rapidly and then slowly approach a plateau of roughly 0.2 to 0.5 μg/mL. The initial half-life is about 24 hours; the β-phase half-life is roughly 15 days. Serum concentrations can be detected for at least 7 weeks after the end of therapy, presumably reflecting release from cell membranes. The drug also has complex immunomodulatory properties that are potentially of clinical significance.

Nephrotoxicity

ABD causes a dose-dependent decrease in the glomerular filtration rate. The direct vasoconstrictive effect of amphotericin B on afferent renal arterioles results in reduced glomerular and renal tubular blood flow. Other effects on the kidney include potassium, magnesium, and bicarbonate wasting and decreased erythropoietin production. Loss of renal function is due to the destruction of renal tubular cells, disruption of tubular basement membrane, and loss of functioning nephron units. Saline loading, such as the infusion of 1 L saline before ABD, has been associated with reduced nephrotoxicity in some studies. Potassium wasting often requires supplemental oral or intravenous potassium. Renal tubular acidosis from bicarbonate wasting rarely requires base replacement, but other drugs and diseases that promote acidosis may act synergistically.

Azotemia caused by amphotericin B is often worse in patients taking other nephrotoxic drugs. Hypotension, intravascular volume depletion, and other preexisting renal disease all magnify the management problems associated with amphotericin B–induced azotemia. These toxicities are lessened by use of the lipid-associated formulations of amphotericin B.

Early in the course of therapy with ABD, azotemia may increase rapidly; it often improves a little and then stabilizes after several days. Adults with no other renal disease have an average serum creatinine level of 2 to 3 mg/dL at therapeutic doses, and therapy should not be withheld unless azotemia exceeds this level. Attempting to give ABD to an adult without causing azotemia usually leads to inadequate therapy.

Other Chronic Toxicity

Nausea, anorexia, and vomiting are common. Phlebitis occurs if peripheral vein catheters are used. Normocytic normochromic anemia occurs gradually. The hematocrit rarely falls below 20 to 25% unless other causes of anemia are present. Rarely, thrombocytopenia, modest leukopenia, arrhythmias, coagulopathy, hemorrhagic enteritis, tinnitus, vertigo, encephalopathy, seizures, hemolysis, or dysesthesia of the soles of the feet may be observed.

Acute Reactions

About 30 to 45 minutes after beginning the first few ABD infusions, chills, fever, and tachypnea may occur, peak in 15 to 30 minutes, and then slowly abate over 2 to 4 hours. A patient with underlying cardiac or pulmonary disease may have hypoxemia. These reactions are less common in young children or in patients receiving corticosteroids. Subsequent infusions of the same dose cause progressively milder reactions. Premedication with acetaminophen or the addition of hydrocortisone 25 to 50 mg to the infusion solution can diminish the reaction. Meperidine given early in a chill shortens the rigors but may induce nausea or emesis. Concern about this kind of reaction in an unstable patient had led some physicians to use a test dose of 1 mg given over a 15-minute period to assess the subsequent reaction over 1 hour before deciding whether to administer a full therapeutic dose. Patients with rapidly progressive mycoses should receive a full therapeutic dose within 24 hours. These reactions should not be mistaken for anaphylaxis or considered a contraindication to further amphotericin B. True allergic reactions are extremely rare.

Administration

ABD is infused over a 2- to 4-hour interval. Infusions 1 hour in duration generally appear to be safe for persons who have tolerated slower infusions. Rapid infusion in patients with severely compromised renal function may lead to acute, marked hyperkalemia and ventricular fibrillation.

Patients receiving a stable daily dose can be changed to a double dose on alternate days to reduce the frequency of infusion-associated toxicity, particularly anorexia, and to make outpatient therapy more convenient. Doses above 1.5 mg/kg are generally not given on this schedule because the toxicity of such infusions is not well described. Continuous infusion of amphotericin B with doses up to 2.0 mg/kg/24 hours is another approach (based on limited data) to reducing toxicity, but this is not consistent with the observation that the principal pharmacodynamic driver of efficacy for amphotericin B is peak drug concentration.

Dosage

Daily ABD doses of 0.3 mg/kg often suffice for esophageal candidiasis. A dose of 0.5 mg/kg is appropriate for blastomycosis, disseminated histoplasmosis, and extracutaneous sporotrichosis. Patients with cryptococcal meningitis are generally given doses of 0.6 to 0.8 mg/kg; those with coccidioidomycosis may require doses of 1 mg/kg. Patients with mucormycosis or invasive aspergillosis are given daily doses of 1 to 1.5 mg/kg until improvement is clearly present. Doses of 0.5 to 1.0 mg/kg are often used in neutropenic patients receiving empirical amphotericin B. Local instillation of amphotericin B into cerebrospinal fluid (CSF), joints, or pleura is rarely indicated. One exception is coccidioidal meningitis, which is treated with intrathecal ABD because it may produce superior results to systemic azole therapy, particularly in the long term, although with far greater toxicity. Intraocular administration for fungal endophthalmitis is occasionally used; doses of 10 μg appear to avoid retinal toxicity. Corneal baths with 1 mg/mL in sterile water are useful for fungal keratitis but are irritating.

Lipid-Associated Formulations of Amphotericin B
Pharmacology and Toxicity

The three lipid-associated formulations have quite different pharmacokinetic patterns. When compared on the basis of equal dosages (mg/kg), the lipid-associated formulations produce tissue amphotericin B concentrations that range from 90% lower to 500% higher than those seen with ABD, with the most consistent relative reduction seen in the kidney. The lipid-associated formulations are typically given at doses that are 3- to 12-fold higher than those used for ABD. All three formulations generally require higher doses in experimental animals to achieve the same therapeutic effect as ABD.

These higher but equipotent doses are notably better tolerated than ABD, with reductions in both the frequency and the severity of acute infusion-related reactions and chronic nephrotoxicity. An exception is ABCD, which generally induces acute infusion-related reactions similar to those for ABD.

Randomized clinical trials comparing ABD as therapy for a defined mycosis are limited to demonstrations that liposomal amphotericin B has a similar efficacy for cryptococcal meningitis and a greater efficacy for histoplasmosis. Randomized comparisons with ABD in persistently neutropenic and febrile cancer patients consistently demonstrate a better tolerability profile, but little data on differential antifungal effect. The aggregate open-label data on efficacy rates for the lipid-associated formulations are similar to those for ABD. Although the lipid-associated formulations are notably more costly than ABD, the purchase cost of the compound must be balanced against the morbidity of ABD-related nephrotoxicity and the financial costs of monitoring, treating, and managing it.

⬤ FLUCYTOSINE
Formulation and Pharmacology

Flucytosine (5-fluorocytosine) is the fluorine analogue of a normal body constituent, cytosine. Flucytosine is marketed as 250- and 500-mg capsules. Absorption from the gastrointestinal tract is rapid and complete, and approximately 90% is excreted unchanged in the urine. CSF concentrations are approximately 74% of simultaneous serum concentrations; the drug also penetrates well into aqueous humor, joints, bronchial secretions, peritoneal fluid, brain, bile, and bone, and it is readily cleared by hemodialysis and peritoneal dialysis.

The half-life of the drug in the serum of patients with normal renal function is 3 to 5 hours and is longer in newborns. Abnormal hepatic function has no influence, but decreased renal function prolongs the half-life.

Mechanisms of Action and Resistance

Isolates of *Candida* species are usually susceptible, as are most isolates of *Cryptococcus neoformans*. Flucytosine is often active against isolates of *Aspergillus* species and against the melanin-pigmented molds that cause chromoblastomycosis. The mechanism of antifungal action appears to be deamination to 5-fluorouracil and then conversion through several steps to 5-fluorodeoxyuridylic acid monophosphate, a noncompetitive inhibitor of thymidylate synthetase, which interferes with DNA synthesis, or conversion to 5-fluouridine triphosphate, which is incorporated into RNA and causes aberrant transcription. In some studies, the principal pharmacodynamic driver of response was the proportion of time the blood level exceeded the MIC. Resistance may be due to loss of the cytosine permease that permits flucytosine to cross the fungal cell membrane or loss of any of the enzymes that lead to its conversion into forms that interfere with DNA or RNA synthesis.

Administration and Dosage

Flucytosine is administered orally, 100 to 150 mg/kg/day, in four divided doses. As an approximation, the total daily dose should be reduced to 75 mg/kg with a creatinine clearance of 26 to 50 mL/minute and to 37 mg/kg when the creatinine clearance is 13 to 25 mL/minute. Ideally, the blood level should be measured in azotemic patients 2 hours after the last dose and immediately before the next dose. These values should range between 10 and 100 µg/mL. Patients requiring hemodialysis can be given a single postdialysis dose of 37.5 mg/kg. Further doses are adjusted by blood level.

Flucytosine given alone to patients with normal renal, hematologic, and gastrointestinal function is infrequently associated with adverse effects, including rash, diarrhea, and hepatic dysfunction. In the presence of azotemia (such as that caused by concomitant amphotericin B), leukopenia, thrombocytopenia, and enterocolitis may appear. These complications seem to be far more frequent among patients whose flucytosine blood levels attain, and especially if they exceed, 100 to 125 µg/mL. Patients receiving flucytosine whose renal function is changing should have their serum flucytosine concentrations determined twice a week, and the leukocyte count, platelet count, alkaline phosphatase, and aminotransferase levels should be measured at a similar frequency. Patients in whom loose stools or dull abdominal pain suddenly develops or who have laboratory evidence consistent with flucytosine toxicity should have their flucytosine blood levels determined, and consideration should be given to withholding the drug until the situation is clarified. Patients with bone marrow and gastrointestinal toxicity from flucytosine often tolerate the drug at a reduced dosage. Uncommonly, vomiting, bowel perforation, confusion, hallucinations, headache, sedation, and euphoria have been reported. Flucytosine is contraindicated in pregnancy.

Conversion of flucytosine to 5-fluorouracil within the human body occurs to a sufficient degree to possibly account for the drug's toxicity to bone marrow and the gastrointestinal tract. It is likely that the drug is secreted into the gut, where flucytosine becomes deaminated by intestinal bacteria and is reabsorbed as 5-fluorouracil.

Flucytosine has a beneficial effect in patients with cryptococcosis, candidiasis, and chromoblastomycosis. It is not the drug of choice for any infection, however, because its clinical efficacy in the first two mycoses is inferior to that of amphotericin B, primary drug resistance is not uncommon in *Candida* infection, and secondary drug resistance is common in cryptococcosis and chromoblastomycosis.

Flucytosine and amphotericin B are at least additive in their effects in vitro and in mice. Flucytosine permits a lower dose of amphotericin B to be used to achieve the same therapeutic effect, and amphotericin B prevents the emergence of secondary drug resistance. The same advantages have been confirmed in two large multicenter studies of cryptococcal meningitis.

Flucytosine therapy is more difficult to manage in patients with diminished bone marrow reserve. Intravenous flucytosine is no longer available in the United States, but it is used at the same dosage as the capsule formulation.

Flucytosine resistance has occurred, albeit uncommonly, during combination therapy. Use of combination therapy in such patients incurs the risk of toxicity without evidence that flucytosine adds to the therapeutic effect. In most laboratories, a MIC of 20 µg/mL or less is considered susceptible.

⬤ AZOLE ANTIFUNGAL AGENTS
Mechanism of Action

The azole ring confers antifungal activity on a variety of synthetic organic compounds.

N-substitution of imidazoles has created a family of drugs called triazoles that have the same mechanism of action as imidazoles, a similar or broader spectrum of activity, and less effect on human sterol synthesis. Both imidazoles and triazoles inhibit C-14α demethylation of lanosterol in fungi; this leads to reduced concentrations of ergosterol, which is essential for a normal fungal cytoplasmic membrane. In some studies, the principal pharmacodynamic driver for response to the triazole antifungal agents has been the ratio of total drug exposure (area under the curve) to the MIC. Because of their interaction with the cytochrome P-450 (CYP) system and, in some cases, the P-glycoprotein pumps, the azoles as a class have a significant number of drug-drug interactions, only some of which are covered here. In any patient in whom azole therapy is contemplated, package inserts for the drug should be consulted to determine which of the patient's other medications could result in a significant drug-drug interaction.

Newer triazoles have properties that make them preferable to ketoconazole. These include not only less hormonal inhibition but also better distribution into body fluids, both parenteral and oral formulations, less hepatotoxicity, and a broader spectrum. Some have fewer drug interactions. Resistance to azoles in previously susceptible species is emerging. Resistance mechanisms include increased drug efflux and altered or increased C-14α demethylase. It has been speculated that some of the common mutations in this demethylase in *Aspergillus* isolates from certain geographic areas, resulting in resistance, may have arisen owing to the widespread agricultural use of azole fungicides. All agents in this class have the potential for embryotoxicity and teratogenicity and should be avoided during pregnancy.

Ketoconazole
Formulations and Pharmacology

Ketoconazole is available in tablet form. It is metabolized in the liver and excreted as inactive drug in bile and, to a small extent, urine. The drug is not removed significantly by hemodialysis or peritoneal dialysis. Decreased renal or hepatic function does not alter plasma drug levels. The initial half-life is approximately 2 hours, with a β-phase half-life of about 9 hours commencing 8 to 12 hours after ingestion.

Oral absorption of ketoconazole differs among individuals. Serious gastrointestinal disease may lead to low blood levels. Inhibitors of gastric acid secretion should not be given to patients taking ketoconazole because blood levels of the latter drug are drastically reduced. The drinking of citrus fruit juices or cola beverages with ketoconazole improves absorption in hypochlorhydric patients. Patients who need antacids should take them 1 to 2 hours after ketoconazole. Rifampin causes substantial lowering of ketoconazole blood levels, by CYP enzyme induction. The levels of other co-administered drugs may be raised owing to CYP enzyme blockade. Cyclosporine blood levels should be monitored during ketoconazole therapy because they usually increase. Penetration into CSF is poor, even in the presence of inflammation. Low concentrations are found in vaginal secretions, saliva, and breast milk, but penetration into inflamed joints is better.

Uses

The main advantage of ketoconazole is its lower cost compared with triazoles. When used at a daily dose of 400 mg, the drug is effective in chronic mucocutaneous candidiasis, coccidioidomycosis, and paracoccidioidomycosis, but fluconazole or itraconazole is preferred. Some patients with chromoblastomycosis, histoplasmosis, blastomycosis, or cutaneous sporotrichosis respond to ketoconazole, as do patients with dermatophytosis, but itraconazole is preferred. Therapy is continued for 6 to 12 months or longer, if the response is slow, to prevent relapse. Improvement may not be evident for weeks to months. Although the dose can be advanced to 600 or 800 mg/day in patients who are not responding to therapy, there is more evidence of increased toxicity than increased efficacy. In coccidioidal meningitis, ketoconazole requires doses exceeding 400 mg/day and has limited efficacy. Aspergillosis does not respond to ketoconazole; additionally, the subsequent use of amphotericin B may be antagonized.

Adverse Effects

The most frequent toxic effects are anorexia, nausea, and vomiting. Dividing doses greater than 400 mg/day is not recommended because hormonal suppression is prolonged. Ketoconazole causes a dose-dependent depression in the serum testosterone- and adrenocorticotropic hormone–stimulated cortisol response. The effect of doses of 800 to 1200 mg/day is profound enough to have prompted trials in the treatment of Cushing's syndrome and prostate cancer. Hypertension is seen in a few of these high-dose patients, in association with increased mineralocorticoid precursors. Gynecomastia, oligospermia, and menstrual irregularities may also be seen during prolonged therapy. Allergic rash and pruritus have been noted.

Perhaps the gravest complication is hepatitis. Fortunately, this complication is estimated to occur in only 1 in 15,000 exposed individuals. A slight, asymptomatic elevation of transaminase levels occurs in 5 to 15% and is generally transient. Ketoconazole-associated hepatitis begins as anorexia, malaise, nausea, and vomiting. Eighty percent of cases occur within the first 3 months. Progression can be swift. If hepatotoxicity is suspected, serum transaminase and alkaline phosphatase levels should be measured. Some authorities have recommended that liver function be measured periodically. This procedure does not protect a patient who has a rapid onset of hepatitis in the interval between tests, but it does require that all patients with abnormalities be contacted to inquire about symptoms and to arrange for repeat testing.

Itraconazole

Formulations and Pharmacology

Itraconazole (Sporanox) is marketed as a capsule and as an oral suspension in cyclodextrin (an oligosaccharide ring). The ring entraps the hydrophobic, water-insoluble drug, thus making it soluble; it is then released either at the lipid membrane of the enterocyte after oral administration or directly into tissues after intravenous administration. The solution can be delivered through a nasogastric tube in intubated patients, and it makes the dosing of infants and small children more convenient. Oral absorption of the capsule is significantly enhanced by food, whereas absorption of the solution is best on an empty stomach. Co-administration of a cola beverage with itraconazole capsules increases absorption. Peak levels with either preparation are achieved 4 to 6 hours after a dose. Steady state is achieved only after 13 to 15 days, at which time the β-elimination half-life is about 19 to 22 hours. Absorption of the capsule is markedly depressed in bone marrow transplant recipients, probably because of hypochlorhydria, mucositis, and

graft-versus-host intestinal changes, and in patients with acquired immunodeficiency syndrome (AIDS) because of enteritis, but this problem can be alleviated by using the solution.

For deep mycoses, an initial itraconazole dose of 200 mg three times a day is recommended for the first 3 days to quickly achieve high serum and tissue levels. Hydroxyitraconazole, a metabolite of itraconazole, appears in the blood in amounts roughly twice that of the parent drug; it has antifungal activity and pharmacokinetics similar to those of the parent compound.

Bioassays of itraconazole give much higher concentrations than does measurement by high-pressure liquid chromatography; the difference depends on the susceptibility of the bioassay organism to hydroxyitraconazole. Concentrations of itraconazole in tissue, pus, and bronchial secretions are generally higher than those in plasma, but CSF concentrations are usually unmeasurable, even in patients with meningitis. Ocular levels are low. Saliva concentrations persist for 8 hours after administration of the solution and may be beneficial in treating oral disease or eradicating oral colonization. The drug is metabolized in the liver and excreted in feces as metabolites. Of the cyclodextrin liquid administered, less than 0.5% is absorbed. No significant amount of bioactive itraconazole appears in urine. Plasma concentrations do not increase in patients with renal insufficiency or decrease with hemodialysis. The half-life is prolonged in those with cirrhosis.

Adverse Effects

The most common adverse effect is dose-related nausea and abdominal discomfort, but symptoms rarely necessitate stopping therapy. Dividing the dose and administering the drug twice daily can improve tolerance and raise blood levels. Hypokalemia and edema may occur at doses of 400 mg/day or higher. Allergic rash is seen occasionally. Itraconazole is rarely hepatotoxic. Diarrhea, nausea, and other gastrointestinal complaints are more frequent with the solution. A negative inotropic effect is rarely seen.

Drug Interactions

Blood levels are reduced by about half in patients taking drugs that decrease gastric acidity. Rifampin, rifabutin, isoniazid, phenytoin, carbamazepine, and phenobarbital decrease itraconazole blood levels. Itraconazole decreases rifampin blood levels and increases blood levels of some antihistamines, potentially causing polymorphic ventricular tachycardia (torsades de pointes), as well as increasing levels of warfarin, benzodiazepines, hepatic hydroxymethylglutaryl–coenzyme A reductase cholesterol-lowering agents, dihydropyridine calcium-channel blockers, digoxin, quinidine, cyclosporine, tacrolimus, methylprednisolone, human immunodeficiency virus (HIV) protease inhibitors (ritonavir, indinavir), and vinca alkaloids (vincristine, vinblastine).

Uses

Itraconazole is useful for the treatment of invasive aspergillosis, allergic bronchopulmonary aspergillosis,[1] blastomycosis, histoplasmosis, meningeal and nonmeningeal coccidioidomycosis, paracoccidioidomycosis, sporotrichosis, phaeohyphomycosis, mucosal candidiasis, ringworm (including onychomycosis), and tinea versicolor. Itraconazole is also useful for the prevention of relapse in AIDS patients with disseminated histoplasmosis. Itraconazole may be useful for prophylaxis against fungal infections during neutropenia and as empirical therapy for febrile episodes in neutropenia.

Fluconazole

Formulations and Pharmacology

Fluconazole is currently available in tablets, as a powder for oral suspension, and as an intravenous formulation. Fluconazole is well absorbed from the gastrointestinal tract. Of the oral dose, 60 to 75% appears unchanged in the urine. Oral absorption is not decreased in patients with AIDS or patients taking H$_2$-blocking agents.

Concentrations of fluconazole in CSF are approximately 70% of simultaneous blood levels, whether or not the meninges are inflamed, and the drug penetrates into the brain. Penetration into saliva, sputum, urine, and other body fluids is also excellent.

The half-life in patients with normal renal function is 27 to 34 hours; it increases to 59 and 98 hours in groups with creatinine clearances of 35 and 14 mL/minute, respectively. The normal dose should be reduced to 50% when the creatinine clearance is reduced to 50 mL/minute and to 25% when the creatinine clearance is below 20 mL/minute. A loading dose of twice the daily dose is recommended. Patients receiving hemodialysis should have one daily dose after each session.

Drug Interactions

Fluconazole can cause significant increases in the blood level of phenytoin, glipizide, glyburide, tolbutamide, warfarin, rifabutin, or cyclosporine. Rifampin lowers fluconazole blood levels by about one fourth.

Adverse Effects

Adverse effects are uncommon. Even with chronic therapy, including doses exceeding 400 mg/day, headache, hair loss, and anorexia were the most common symptoms; 10% of patients had rises in aspartate aminotransferase levels. Alopecia is reversible, in some cases, even when the drug is continued at lower doses. Neurotoxicity has been described after heroic doses of 2000 mg/day. Rarely, anaphylaxis after the first dose or Stevens-Johnson syndrome has been observed.

Indications

Candidiasis

Provided the infection is not caused by fluconazole-resistant *Candida*, fluconazole is effective for the treatment of oropharyngeal and esophageal candidiasis. A single dose of 150 mg is approximately as effective as topical treatment of vulvovaginal candidiasis. Patients with candidemia who are not neutropenic or otherwise seriously immunosuppressed respond as well to intravenous fluconazole therapy as to amphotericin B. A study comparing fluconazole with a combination of fluconazole plus amphotericin as initial therapy of candidemia found that the combination might produce more rapid clearance of the blood stream. In a few patients with *Candida* endocarditis, long-term fluconazole therapy has been used to prevent relapse after amphotericin B therapy. For immunosuppressed patients and for rapidly progressing or severely ill patients with deep candidiasis, amphotericin B or caspofungin is preferred.

Cryptococcal Meningitis

Many authorities recommend amphotericin B or amphotericin B plus flucytosine for at least the first 2 weeks to treat cryptococcal meningitis. Therapy can then be changed to fluconazole 400 mg/day for 2 months if the patient is clinically stable. The propensity of AIDS patients to relapse has led to lifelong maintenance therapy with fluconazole 200 mg/day. Itraconazole capsules are inferior to fluconazole for maintenance therapy. Relapse because of fluconazole resistance is rare. Fluconazole is effective for the eradication of genitourinary foci. For patients without AIDS, fluconazole is useful for those who have completed a course of amphotericin B and seem to be at high risk for relapse.

Other Mycoses

Fluconazole is useful for coccidioidal meningitis and for disseminated nonmeningeal coccidioidomycosis, but a direct comparison with itraconazole found a trend favoring itraconazole owing to its superior efficacy for skeletal infections. The two drugs were similarly efficacious for soft tissue and pulmonary infections. Cutaneous sporotrichosis, ringworm, histoplasmosis, and blastomycosis may respond to fluconazole, but the results are inferior to those with itraconazole.

Prophylaxis in Neutropenic Patients

Fluconazole decreases the incidence of death from deep mycoses in bone marrow transplant recipients. All the protection afforded seems to be related to deep candidiasis. In a long-term follow-up of one study, bone marrow transplant recipients who received at least 75 days of fluconazole prophylaxis also had improved survival. Use of this drug for prophylaxis may result in shifts to less susceptible species.

Prophylaxis in Patients with AIDS

Fluconazole has reduced the incidence of oral and vulvovaginal candidiasis and cryptococcosis in patients with advanced HIV infection, but it has negligible effects on other mycoses. Cost, lack of effect on survival, and the possibility of azole resistance have led the advisory committee of the Infectious Diseases Society of America to recommend against fluconazole prophylaxis in AIDS patients.

Voriconazole

Formulations and Pharmacology

Voriconazole is marketed as a tablet and as a solution in sulfobutyl ether β-cyclodextrin for intravenous administration. Voriconazole is cleared by hepatic metabolism, with less than 2% of the dose excreted unchanged in the urine. Voriconazole exhibits nonlinear pharmacokinetics owing to saturation of the clearance pathways at higher doses. The principal enzyme involved in clearance is hepatic CYP2C19. This enzyme has significant genetic polymorphisms that affect the metabolism of this drug. Despite these differences in metabolism, the achieved plasma levels overlap, and an initial dose adjustment based on genotype or racial group is not necessary. Different studies have suggested that favorable outcomes correlate with serum concentrations greater than 1 to 2 µg/mL, and therapeutic drug monitoring with dose adjustments as necessary is recommended.

Standard loading doses followed by maintenance doses that are 50% of normal are recommended for individuals with mild to moderate hepatic cirrhosis. Dosage adjustments are not required for renal dysfunction, and voriconazole is not significantly cleared by hemodialysis. Because of nephrotoxicity from the cyclodextrin, the intravenous formulation should not be used in patients with a creatinine clearance less than 50 mL/minute.

Drug Interactions

Voriconazole has many drug interactions. Rifampin, carbamazepine, and long-acting barbiturates induce the hepatic enzymes responsible for the clearance of voriconazole and reduce voriconazole levels. Voriconazole and either rifabutin or phenytoin reciprocally alter their clearance. Sirolimus levels are increased dramatically. Reduction in the clearance of pimozide, quinidine, and some antihistamines may be sufficient to place the patient at risk for QTc prolongation. Reduction in the clearance of ergot alkaloids could lead to chronic ergot poisoning. Cyclosporine, tacrolimus, warfarin, oral coumarins, lipid-lowering statin agents, benzodiazepines, calcium-channel blockers, sulfonylureas, and vinca alkaloids can be co-administered, but the dosage of these drugs may need to be reduced, and clinical or laboratory monitoring is suggested. Voriconazole significantly reduces the rate of clearance of omeprazole. Other interactions are possible, and any CYP inhibitors, blockers, or inducers could have an interaction with voriconazole.

Adverse Effects

The most frequently reported adverse event is a transient, reversible visual disturbance beginning approximately 30 minutes after a dose. Patients should be advised to avoid activities that require keen visual acuity while experiencing visual changes. Hallucinations and confusion have also been reported, associated with higher blood levels. Liver enzyme abnormalities also appear to correlate with higher blood levels. Photosensitivity can be severe and has been associated with skin cancers in rare instances. Prolongation of the QT interval and tachyarrhythmias have been noted in patients with pro-arrhythmic factors, such as electrolyte abnormalities.

Indications

Aspergillosis

Voriconazole was licensed for the treatment of invasive aspergillosis on the basis of a randomized, unblinded comparative trial in which patients were randomized to receive initial therapy with either voriconazole or ABD. Following the initial randomization, patients could be switched to other licensed therapies, as dictated by clinical events. After 12 weeks, 53% of the patients randomized to voriconazole, but only 32% of those randomized to ABD, had a successful outcome.

Other Mycoses

Voriconazole is also licensed for the treatment of invasive fusariosis and scedosporiosis, based on high response rates for these diseases. The drug is efficacious in esophageal candidiasis, invasive candidiasis, and refractory candidiasis. Although the drug has appeal for use in prophylaxis, there has been concern about breakthrough zygomycoses with long-term use.

Posaconazole

Formulations and Pharmacology

Posaconazole is available only as an oral suspension. Absorption is maximized by dividing the daily dose into four administrations, each with fatty food. Clearance is primarily by fecal excretion, with only 13% excreted via renal clearance. Hepatic metabolism via uridine diphosphate glucuronidation plays only a small role in clearance, and CYP-mediated oxidation does not occur. The dose is 800 mg/day for treatment of deep mycoses, although 600 mg has been used successfully for prophylaxis, and 200 mg has been used for mucosal candidiasis. At steady state, 800 mg/day produces a C_{max} (peak concentration) of 4.2 µg/mL. Blood levels appear to be rather unpredictable, and outcomes in the treatment of aspergillosis correlate with levels. Therapeutic drug monitoring is advisable, and levels greater than 0.7 µg/mL have been recommended for prophylaxis. Dosage adjustment is not needed for hepatic or renal failure or hemodialysis.

Drug Interactions

Although posaconazole has fewer interactions than itraconazole and voriconazole, there are many significant ones, including increased levels of calcium-channel blockers, cyclosporine, sirolimus, tacrolimus, quinidine, rifampicin, and benzodiazepines. Posaconazole levels are reduced by cimetidine, carbamazepine, efavirenz, and rifampin.

Adverse Effects

The paucity of side effects is similar to that of fluconazole. Gastrointestinal symptoms and headache are occasionally seen. Electrolyte abnormalities should be rectified before therapy to avoid arrhythmias.

Indications

Posaconazole appears to possess a very broad spectrum of activity against molds, including many zygomycetes, a unique property among azoles. The main interest in the drug has been as prophylaxis and for salvage therapy of refractory mycoses. Efficacy in preventing opportunistic mycoses has been shown in the highest-risk patients, transplant patients with graft-versus-host disease, and those with hematologic malignancies and neutropenia.[3,4] Impressive results in salvage have been demonstrated in aspergillosis and coccidioidomycosis. Superficial candidiasis is also responsive.

● ECHINOCANDIN ANTIFUNGAL AGENTS

General Features

The echinocandin antifungal agents act by inhibiting the synthesis of 1,3-β-D-glucan in the fungal cell wall. In studies, the principal pharmacodynamic driver of in vivo response has been the ratio of the peak concentration to the MIC. There are now three licensed echinocandins: caspofungin, micafungin, and anidulafungin. These agents are similar to one another, having very few drug interactions, an admirably low adverse event rate, and essentially identical antifungal spectra. Of the three drugs, caspofungin has the broadest array of approved indications and the most clinical data. Micafungin has the most detailed data on its use in neonates and children. Anidulafungin appears to have somewhat fewer drug-drug interactions. All are cyclic lipopeptides that must be given intravenously.

They are fungicidal against all *Candida* species, including isolates resistant to other agents. Reduced activity against isolates of *Candida parapsilosis* and *Candida guilliermondii* and a paradoxical effect whereby high concentrations permit growth in vitro have been noted in a minority of *Candida* isolates and do not appear to be clinically relevant. All are active against *Aspergillus* species, but activity is limited to growing and dividing hyphal elements. Their activity against other fungi is variable.

Caspofungin
Formulations and Pharmacology

Caspofungin is marketed for intravenous infusion. The clearance of caspofungin is through a combination of spontaneous chemical degradation, hydrolysis, and N-acetylation. Dose adjustments are not required for impaired renal function or hemodialysis. The clearance of caspofungin is modestly reduced in subjects with moderate hepatic insufficiency, and a reduction of the usual daily dose is recommended. Penetration into infected tissues appears to be good.

Drug Interactions

Caspofungin has few meaningful drug interactions. Cyclosporine co-administration increases caspofungin exposure and has been associated with increased hepatic transaminase levels, so concomitant use requires caution. Caspofungin reduces tacrolimus exposure by approximately 20%, and dosage adjustments may be required. Rifampin reduces caspofungin blood levels by approximately 30%, so the daily dosage of caspofungin should be increased from 50 mg to 70 mg if these drugs are co-administered. Likewise, limited data on other inducers of drug clearance (efavirenz, nevirapine, phenytoin, dexamethasone, carbamazepine) suggest that reduced caspofungin levels are possible and that increasing the daily dose to 70 mg should be considered.

Adverse Effects

Overall, the adverse reactions with caspofungin have been infrequent and minor. Symptoms possibly related to histamine release during rapid infusion have been reported.

Indications

Caspofungin is indicated for the treatment of invasive candidiasis[5] and esophageal candidiasis. Caspofungin is also indicated for invasive aspergillosis in patients who are refractory to or intolerant of other therapies. With its activity against these two major opportunistic pathogens, the use of caspofungin for empirical therapy in high-risk situations is logical and is supported by clinical trials.

Micafungin

Micafungin has an in vitro spectrum and properties similar to caspofungin. It is similarly cidal for *Candida* species and noncidal in vitro for *Aspergillus*.

Formulations and Pharmacology

The drug is light sensitive. After an intravenous infusion, the terminal half-life is about 15 hours. A 50-mg dose produces a C_{max} of 3.4 µg/mL. Metabolism appears to be mostly through fecal excretion; less than 1% is excreted in the urine. The drug appears to penetrate particularly well into the lungs, liver, kidneys, and gastric mucosa. No adjustment for hepatic or renal insufficiency is needed.

Drug Interactions

Micafungin has fewer drug interactions than caspofungin. There is no interaction with cyclosporine or rifampin.

Adverse Effects

Micafungin has an excellent safety profile. Histamine release, resulting most prominently in erythema over the body, can be avoided by slow infusion.

Indications

Efficacy is good in invasive candidiasis, similar to that of amphotericin or caspofungin.[6] In clinical dose-finding studies against *Candida* esophagitis, doses of 75 to 150 mg/day were particularly effective. A trial of prophylaxis in neutropenic patients with hematopoietic stem cell transplant showed efficacy at 50 mg/day.[7] Limited experience suggests comparable activity to caspofungin against aspergillosis.

Anidulafungin
Formulations and Pharmacology

Anidulafungin is slowly degraded by the chemical opening of its ring structure. A 100-mg dose produces a C_{max} of 8.6 µg/mL at a T_{max} (time of peak concentration) of 6 to 7 hours. The half-life is 30 to 40 hours. Dose adjustments are not required for renal or hepatic insufficiency.

Drug Interactions

Anidulafungin has no meaningful CYP enzyme interactions. It is not an inducer, inhibitor, or substrate and has no interaction with drugs cleared by these pathways or drugs that induce these pathways.

Adverse Effects

Histamine-mediated symptoms (e.g., rash, urticaria, flushing, pruritus, dyspnea, hypotension) have been noted on occasion, but they are infrequent when the rate of infusion does not exceed 1.1 mg/minute. Other adverse reactions to anidulafungin have generally been infrequent and minor.

Indications

Anidulafungin is indicated for the treatment of invasive candidiasis and esophageal candidiasis. Randomized trials indicate that anidulafungin is at least as efficacious as fluconazole.[8] Inefficacy against *C. parapsilosis* may be of greatest concern with this echinocandin.

● OTHER AGENTS

Combinations of antifungal agents are increasingly being used in an effort to improve the appalling response rates in some diseases and to combine drugs with different mechanisms of action. Although synergy in vitro may be relatively easy to demonstrate, there are few examples of synergy in animal model studies. In patients, the costs are high, and the side effects are likely to be increased. The clinical advantages of the amphotericin-flucytosine combination in cryptococcosis have yet to be documented definitively in other situations.

Immunomodulators, particularly cytokines, hold promise, but insufficient clinical data exist to determine where and how these drugs might be used. Granulocyte-macrophage colony-stimulating factor was shown to be effective in one trial when given prophylactically during induction therapy of high-risk leukemia patients.

Therapy of the various forms of tinea and of onychomycosis with systemic agents is discussed in Chapter 446. Although *Pneumocystis jirovecii* (formerly *Pneumocystis carinii*) is now classified among the fungi, the drugs used to treat it are principally used to treat parasitic infections (Chapter 349).

1. Stevens DA, Schwartz HJ, Lee JY, et al. A randomized trial of itraconazole in allergic bronchopulmonary aspergillosis. *N Engl J Med*. 2000;342:756-762.
2. Herbrecht R, Denning DW, Patterson TF, et al. Voriconazole versus amphotericin B for primary therapy of invasive aspergillosis. *N Engl J Med*. 2002;347:408-415.
3. Ullmann AJ, Lipton JH, Vesole DH, et al. Posaconazole or fluconazole for prophylaxis in severe graft-versus-host disease. *N Engl J Med*. 2007;356:335-347.
4. Cornely OA, Maertens J, Winston DJ, et al. Posaconazole vs. fluconazole or itraconazole prophylaxis in patients with neutropenia. *N Engl J Med*. 2007;356:348-359.
5. Mora-Duarte J, Betts R, Rotstein R, et al. Caspofungin Invasive Candidiasis Study Group. Comparison of caspofungin and amphotericin B for invasive candidiasis. *N Engl J Med*. 2002;347:2020-2029.
6. Kuse ER, Chetchotisakd P, da Cunha CA, et al. Micafungin versus liposomal amphotericin B for candidaemia and invasive candidosis: a phase III randomised double-blind trial. *Lancet*. 2007;369:1519-1527.
7. van Burik JA, Ratanatharathorn V, Stepan DE, et al. Micafungin versus fluconazole for prophylaxis against invasive fungal infections during neutropenia in patients undergoing hematopoietic stem cell transplantation. *Clin Infect Dis*. 2004;39:1407-1416.
8. Reboli AC, Rotstein C, Pappas PG, et al. Anidulafungin versus fluconazole for invasive candidiasis. *N Engl J Med*. 2007;356:2472-2482.

SUGGESTED READINGS

Almyroudis NG, Segal BH. Antifungal prophylaxis and therapy in patients with hematological malignancies and hematopoietic stem cell transplant recipients. *Expert Rev Anti Infect Ther*. 2010;8:1451-1466. *Review*.
Limper AH, Knox KS, Sarosi GA, et al. An official American Thoracic Society statement: treatment of fungal infections in adult pulmonary and critical care patients. *Am J Respir Crit Care Med*. 2011;183:96-128. *Consensus guidelines*.
Muñoz P, Guinea J, Rojas L, et al. New antifungal agents for the treatment of candidaemia. *Int J Antimicrob Agents*. 2010;2:S63-S69. *Review*.
Riddell J 4th, Comer GM, Kauffman CA. Treatment of endogenous fungal endophthalmitis: focus on new antifungal agents. *Clin Infect Dis*. 2011;52:648-653. *Review*.
Ziakas PD, Kourbeti IS, Voulgarelis M, et al. Effectiveness of systemic antifungal prophylaxis in patients with neutropenia after chemotherapy: a meta-analysis of randomized controlled trials. *Clin Ther*. 2010;32:2316-2336. *Systemic antifungal prophylaxis is associated with a reduction in proven fungal infections and mortality attributed to these infections in patients with neutropenia after chemotherapy*.

340

HISTOPLASMOSIS

CAROL A. KAUFFMAN

DEFINITION

Histoplasmosis is the most common endemic mycosis in the United States. Most infections are self-limited, but the organism has the ability to cause acute and chronic pulmonary infections and disseminated infection.

The Pathogen

Histoplasma capsulatum var *capsulatum* is a thermally dimorphic fungus. In the environment and at temperatures lower than 35° C, it exists as a mold that produces conidia, both tuberculate macroconidia, which are helpful for identification purposes in the laboratory, and microconidia, which are the infectious form. In tissues and at 35 to 37° C, *H. capsulatum* transforms into tiny 2- to 4-μm oval yeasts that reproduce by budding and parasitize macrophages. African histoplasmosis is caused by a different subspecies, *H. capsulatum* var *duboisii*, and has different disease manifestations.

EPIDEMIOLOGY

Histoplasmosis, though found worldwide, is primarily a disease of North and Central America. *H. capsulatum* is endemic in the Mississippi and Ohio River valleys, with extension into the St. Lawrence basin; microfoci exist in discrete isolated areas in several eastern states. Soil, caves, and abandoned buildings containing high concentrations of bird or bat guano support luxuriant growth of the organism. Every year, hundreds of thousands of individuals who live in areas endemic for *H. capsulatum* are infected. Most cases are sporadic and the exact source of exposure is unknown. Point source outbreaks that have included as few as 4 persons and as many as 100,000 have been well described in association with disruption of soil; cleaning attics, bridges, or barns; tearing down old structures laden with guano; and spelunking.

PATHOBIOLOGY

After inhalation of microconidia into the alveoli, a localized pulmonary infection ensues. Neutrophils and macrophages phagocytize the organism, now in the yeast phase; the organism is able to survive and travels within macrophages to the hilar and mediastinal lymph nodes and throughout the reticuloendothelial system by hematogenous dissemination. Such dissemination probably occurs in most persons who are infected and in normal hosts is associated with no symptoms. After several weeks, T cells specifically sensitized by *H. capsulatum* antigens activate macrophages, which are then able to kill the intracellular fungi. Histoplasmosis is a classic example of the pivotal importance of the cell-mediated immune system in containing intracellular pathogens.

The extent of disease is determined by both the number of conidia inhaled and the immune response of the host. A small inoculum can cause severe pulmonary infection or progress to acute symptomatic disseminated histoplasmosis in immunosuppressed patients. Conversely, severe life-threatening pulmonary infection may develop in a healthy individual if a large number of conidia are inhaled, as might occur during the demolition of old buildings or while spelunking in a heavily infested cave.

Reinfection can occur in persons who previously had histoplasmosis but is uncommon and almost always occurs in the setting of heavy exposure. Reactivation of latent infection takes place in patients who have deficient cell-mediated immunity, as evidenced by the occurrence of histoplasmosis in immunosuppressed persons who grew up in the endemic area but have not been back in that area for years.

CLINICAL MANIFESTATIONS

Acute Pulmonary Histoplasmosis

Infection is asymptomatic in most people infected with *H. capsulatum*. Those who do have symptomatic pulmonary infection usually have a self-limited illness that begins several weeks after exposure and is characterized by fever, chills, fatigue, nonproductive cough, anterior chest discomfort, and myalgias. A patchy lobar or multilobar nodular infiltrate is noted on chest radiographs.

The differential diagnosis of acute pulmonary histoplasmosis includes pneumonia from *Blastomyces dermatitidis*, *Mycoplasma pneumoniae*, *Legionella* sp, and *Chlamydia pneumoniae*. When enlarged hilar or mediastinal lymph nodes are present, histoplasmosis should be strongly considered. The most difficult to differentiate is acute pulmonary blastomycosis (Chapter 342) because the endemic areas overlap, a comparable history of outdoor activities is often obtained, and radiographs show similar findings.

In patients who have experienced heavy exposure to *H. capsulatum* and in those who are immunosuppressed, acute pulmonary histoplasmosis can be life-threatening. High spiking fevers, chills, prostration, dyspnea, and cough are prominent. Chest radiographs show diffuse reticulonodular pulmonary infiltrates, and respiratory failure can occur rapidly.

Chronic Pulmonary Histoplasmosis

Chronic cavitary pulmonary histoplasmosis is a progressive, often fatal form of histoplasmosis that develops almost exclusively in older patients who have chronic obstructive pulmonary disease. Symptoms include fever, fatigue, anorexia, weight loss, cough productive of purulent sputum, and hemoptysis. On chest radiography the usual findings are unilateral or bilateral upper lobe infiltrates with multiple cavities and extensive fibrosis in the lower lobes. Chronic pulmonary histoplasmosis mimics tuberculosis, other fungal pneumonias (especially blastomycosis and sporotrichosis), and nontuberculous mycobacterial infections with regard to symptoms, signs, and radiographic findings.

Complications of Pulmonary Histoplasmosis

The mediastinal and hilar lymph nodes frequently calcify as the infection resolves; years later they can erode into bronchi and cause hemoptysis and expectoration of broncholiths. Granulomatous mediastinitis is an uncommon syndrome characterized by continuing inflammation and necrosis in the mediastinal lymph nodes. The enlarged nodes are readily apparent on chest radiographs, and computed tomography (CT) shows central necrosis and, in some cases, impingement on adjacent structures, including the esophagus, airways, and blood vessels. Although the symptoms usually resolve without treatment, obstructive syndromes can be severe and the nodes can persist for years.

Fibrosing mediastinitis is a rare complication of histoplasmosis in which the host responds to the infection with an inappropriate excessive fibrotic response. Obstruction of the airways, superior vena cava, or the pulmonary arteries and veins can occur with resultant progressive right heart failure and respiratory insufficiency. Bilateral obstruction of the pulmonary vasculature is less common than unilateral involvement and carries a worse prognosis. Mediastinal widening is seen on chest radiographs, and CT and angiography define the extent of invasion and obstruction of mediastinal structures.

Pericarditis is a manifestation of a local inflammatory reaction to adjacent histoplasmosis. Patients respond promptly to anti-inflammatory medications without antifungal therapy. Hemodynamic compromise, though unusual, requires drainage of pericardial fluid; only rarely has progression to constrictive pericarditis been documented.

Disseminated Histoplasmosis

Symptomatic disseminated histoplasmosis occurs mostly in immunosuppressed patients. Patients with acquired immunodeficiency syndrome (AIDS) and CD4$^+$ counts lower than 150/μL, infants, and those who have a hematologic malignancy, have received an organ transplant, or are taking corticosteroids or tumor necrosis factor antagonists are at greatest risk for acute disseminated histoplasmosis. Symptoms and signs include chills, fever, anorexia, weight loss, hypotension, dyspnea, hepatosplenomegaly, and skin and mucous membrane lesions. Pancytopenia, diffuse pulmonary infiltrates on chest radiography and CT, findings of disseminated intravascular coagulation, and acute respiratory failure are common. This syndrome is indistinguishable from sepsis of any bacterial or viral cause. In AIDS patients, the differential diagnosis includes cytomegalovirus, disseminated *Mycobacterium avium* complex infection, and tuberculosis.

Chronic progressive disseminated histoplasmosis is a fatal form of histoplasmosis that occurs mostly in middle-aged to elderly men who have no known immunosuppressive illness. The illness is characterized by fever, night sweats, weight loss, anorexia, and fatigue. Patients appear chronically ill, hepatosplenomegaly and mucocutaneous ulcerations are common, and adrenal insufficiency can develop. An increased erythrocyte sedimentation rate, elevated alkaline phosphatase, pancytopenia, and diffuse reticulonodular infiltrates on chest radiography and CT are typical. Patients with this form of histoplasmosis often have fever of unknown origin. Miliary tuberculosis, lymphoma, and sarcoidosis must be excluded.

Involvement of almost every organ system has been reported with disseminated infection. Adrenal insufficiency must be sought in any patient who has unexplained hypotension, hyponatremia, and hyperkalemia. Abdominal CT shows markedly enlarged adrenal glands. Central nervous system involvement is manifested either as meningitis or as focal lesions seen on magnetic resonance imaging and is more common in patients with AIDS. Skin lesions, also more common in patients with AIDS, can be papular, pustular, or ulcerated. *Histoplasma* endocarditis is a rare form of disseminated infection.

DIAGNOSIS

The definitive diagnostic test for histoplasmosis is growth of the organism in culture. Unfortunately, *H. capsulatum* may take as long as 6 weeks to grow in vitro. Tissue samples, bronchoalveolar lavage fluid, sputum, and blood are appropriate for culture. For patients who have evidence of dissemination, blood cultures are best performed with the lysis-centrifugation (Isolator tube) system; bone marrow and liver biopsy material often yield *H. capsulatum* in the setting of dissemination. If pulmonary histoplasmosis is a diagnostic consideration, the laboratory should be informed so that a special medium that decreases the growth of commensal fungi can be used for the culture of pulmonary samples. As soon as growth of a mold has been detected, highly specific DNA probes for *H. capsulatum* allow rapid identification of the organism.

If the patient is acutely ill, tissue biopsy should be performed to search for the distinctive 2- to 4-μm oval yeasts with single buds, which allows a tentative diagnosis to be made as quickly as possible. Routine tissue stains do not show the tiny yeasts; biopsy material must be stained with methenamine silver or periodic acid–Schiff stains. In patients with disseminated disease, bone marrow, liver, skin, and mucocutaneous lesions usually reveal many organisms. The organisms can also be seen within neutrophils in peripheral blood smears from patients with acute disseminated infection. In patients with chronic pulmonary histoplasmosis or granulomatous mediastinitis, biopsy of the lung or lymph nodes may reveal the organism.

Serology plays an important role in the diagnosis of some forms of histoplasmosis. Complement fixation (CF) assays that use two different antigens, mycelial and yeast, and immunodiffusion (ID) tests are available. The ID test is more specific than the CF test, but CF tests are more sensitive. Antibody assays can remain positive at low titer for years after the infection. Serology is helpful in diagnosing acute pulmonary histoplasmosis when a four-fold rise in CF titer, a CF titer higher than 1:32, or the appearance of an M precipitin band by ID assay is found. These tests are also useful in patients with chronic forms of pulmonary or disseminated histoplasmosis, but they are rarely helpful in immunosuppressed patients, who often cannot mount an antibody response. Because serologic tests are not definitive in patients with mediastinal lymphadenopathy, the results should always be confirmed by tissue biopsy. An enzyme immunoassay for *H. capsulatum* polysaccharide antigen in urine and serum is extremely helpful in patients with disseminated infection and in those with acute pulmonary histoplasmosis. The sensitivity for antigen detection is higher in urine than in serum. Almost 75% of patients who have experienced heavy exposure and demonstrate diffuse pulmonary infiltrates and more than 90% of patients who have disseminated histoplasmosis will have a positive urinary antigen test. However, the assay is not useful for patients who have chronic cavitary histoplasmosis, granulomatous mediastinitis, or fibrosing mediastinitis. False-positive reactions have been noted commonly with blastomycosis, paracoccidioidomycosis, and penicilliosis and occasionally with acute coccidioidomycosis. Antigen levels usually become undetectable with successful therapy.

TREATMENT   Rx

Guidelines for the treatment of histoplasmosis have been published by the Infectious Diseases Society of America (IDSA). Itraconazole is the drug of choice for mild to moderate histoplasmosis, and lipid formulations of amphotericin B should be used as initial therapy for severe, life-threatening infections. Fluconazole is less active and should be considered a second-line agent, and ketoconazole has become a second-line agent because of increased toxicity in comparison to itraconazole. There is only limited anecdotal experience using voriconazole or posaconazole, although both appear to be effective therapy. The echinocandins are not effective for histoplasmosis.

For all patients who are treated with itraconazole, serum levels should be determined when a steady state has been reached after 2 weeks of therapy to ensure adequate absorption. Serum concentrations should be greater than 1 μg/mL.

Pulmonary Histoplasmosis

Treatment is not usually given for acute pulmonary histoplasmosis; many times the diagnosis is not made until after the symptoms have resolved. However, if the patient remains symptomatic after 4 weeks, therapy with itraconazole, 200 mg once or twice daily for 6 to 12 weeks, should be given. All patients who have severe pulmonary histoplasmosis and all immunosuppressed patients should be treated with an antifungal agent. Lipid formulation amphotericin B, 3 to 5 mg/kg daily, is recommended for several weeks until a response is noted, at which time therapy can be changed to oral itraconazole, 200 mg three times daily for 3 days and then 200 mg twice daily. A short course of methylprednisolone is recommended in the IDSA guidelines for patients in whom respiratory distress develops in association with acute pulmonary histoplasmosis.

Antifungal therapy should be given to all patients with chronic pulmonary histoplasmosis. Itraconazole, 200 mg twice daily for 12 to 24 months, is recommended. A trial of itraconazole for 6 to 12 weeks is often given to patients with symptomatic granulomatous mediastinitis, although there are no data proving such therapy to be effective. Surgical resection of nodes causing obstructive symptoms may be beneficial. Antifungal therapy offers no benefit for patients with fibrosing mediastinitis. However, because of the inexorable downhill course of this illness, a several-month course of itraconazole is frequently tried. Surgery is not indicated and carries a high operative mortality rate. Intravascular stents have been used successfully in patients who have vascular obstruction.

Disseminated Histoplasmosis

All patients with symptomatic disseminated histoplasmosis should receive antifungal therapy. Patients who have only mild to moderate symptoms with acute disseminated disease and most patients with chronic progressive disseminated histoplasmosis can be treated with itraconazole, 200 mg twice daily after a loading dose of 200 mg three times daily for 3 days. A total of 12 months of therapy is generally adequate, but for those with chronic progressive disease, the duration of treatment may need to be longer.

Patients who have moderately severe to severe disseminated histoplasmosis should be treated with liposomal amphotericin B, 3 mg/kg daily.[1] Therapy can be changed to itraconazole after the patient has responded to therapy, generally in a few weeks. Therapy should continue for a total of 12 months. For those who are immunosuppressed, therapy with itraconazole, 200 mg daily, should continue until the immunosuppression resolves. For AIDS patients, suppressive therapy can be safely stopped in those who have had a year of therapy, are receiving antiretroviral therapy, and have CD4$^+$ counts greater than 150 cells/μL.[2]

Prevention of histoplasmosis is difficult because exposure can occur without the person's knowledge in highly endemic areas. Persons who are immunosuppressed should be advised to avoid demolition areas, spelunking, and cleaning of farm buildings or attics. A randomized, blinded, placebo-controlled trial in AIDS patients found that itraconazole, 200 mg daily, was effective in preventing infection.[3] Recommendations are to use prophylaxis only for patients whose CD4$^+$ counts are lower than 150/μL and who live in a highly endemic area with a rate of histoplasmosis that is greater than 10 cases per 100 patient years. There are no recommendations for prophylaxis for other immunosuppressed patients.

PROGNOSIS

Acute pulmonary histoplasmosis is usually a self-limited disease. Patients who require treatment generally respond promptly to antifungal agents. However, the response of patients with chronic cavitary pulmonary histoplasmosis is often poor, primarily because of their severe underlying pulmonary disease. Mediastinal fibrosis has a poor prognosis, but intravascular stenting has led to improvement in many patients. Patients with disseminated histoplasmosis, even those with advanced AIDS, usually respond promptly to antifungal therapy; most deaths in immunosuppressed patients occur when the diagnosis is delayed. Older patients with chronic progressive disseminated histoplasmosis have a slower, but usually complete response to therapy.

Grade A

1. Johnson PC, Wheat LJ, Cloud GA, et al. Safety and efficacy of liposomal amphotericin B compared with conventional amphotericin B for induction therapy of histoplasmosis in patients with AIDS. *Ann Intern Med.* 2002;137:105-109.
2. Goldman M, Zackin R, Fichtenbaum CJ, et al. Safety of discontinuation of maintenance therapy for disseminated histoplasmosis after immunologic response to antiretroviral therapy. *Clin Infect Dis.* 2004;38:1485-1489.
3. McKinsey DS, Wheat LJ, Cloud GA, et al. Itraconazole prophylaxis for fungal infections in patients with advanced human immunodeficiency virus infection: randomized, placebo-controlled, double-blind study. *Clin Infect Dis.* 1999;28:1049-1056.

SUGGESTED READINGS

Buitrago MJ, Bernal-Martinez L, Castelli MV, et al. Histoplasmosis and paracoccidioidomycosis in a non-endemic area: a review of cases and diagnosis. *J Travel Med.* 2011;18:26-33. *Culture had a 73% sensitivity but PCR was more rapid and sensitive.*

Hage CA, Bowyer S, Tarvin SE, et al. Recognition, diagnosis, and treatment of histoplasmosis complicating tumor necrosis factor blocker therapy. *Clin Infect Dis.* 2010;50:85-92. *Deals with the evolving issue of diagnosis and treatment of histoplasmosis in patients who are receiving therapy with tumor necrosis factor antagonists.*

Kauffman CA. Histoplasmosis. *Clin Chest Med.* 2009;30:217-225. *Extensive review of the clinical and laboratory aspects of histoplasmosis.*

Knox KS, Hage CA. Histoplasmosis. *Proc Am Thorac Soc.* 2010;7:169-172. *Review of the most prevalent endemic fungal infection in North America.*

Wheat LJ, Freifeld AG, Kleiman MJ, et al. Clinical practice guidelines for the management of patients with histoplasmosis: 2007 update by the Infectious Diseases Society of America. *Clin Infect Dis.* 2007;45:807-827. *Outlines the current management of histoplasmosis and gives evidence ratings for all treatment recommendations.*

341

COCCIDIOIDOMYCOSIS

JOHN N. GALGIANI

DEFINITION

Coccidioidomycosis is a systemic fungal infection caused by *Coccidioides* species endemic to some deserts of the Western Hemisphere (Table 341-1).

The Pathogen

Coccidioides immitis and *Coccidioides posadasii* are dimorphic fungi classified as Ascomycetes by ribosomal gene homology. In their vegetative state, mycelia with true septations mature to produce arthroconidia, single cells approximately 2 to 5 μm in diameter. After infection, an arthroconidium enlarges to a spherule up to 75 μm in diameter and undergoes internal septation to produce scores of endospores. When the spherules rupture, packets of endospores are released and produce more spherules in infected tissue or revert to mycelia if removed from the body.

EPIDEMIOLOGY

Coccidioides organisms can be recovered from the soil of the low deserts of Arizona; the Central Valley of California; parts of other states, including New Mexico and Texas; and parts of Central and South America. Endemic regions follow the climatologic Sonoran life zone, which is characterized by modest rainfall, mild winters, and low humidity. Mycelia bloom beneath the surface during periods of rain, and arthroconidia develop as the earth dries. Rates of infection are highest during dry months and are accentuated when soil is disturbed by windstorms or construction equipment. Exposure to contaminated bales of cotton or other fomites can result in infection beyond the endemic regions, but this is rare. Person-to-person transmission of pulmonary infection has not been reported, and isolation precautions are unnecessary. *Coccidioides* species are listed by the Centers for Disease Control and Prevention as select agents that could be used for bioterrorism.

Incidence and Prevalence

In general, the annual risk for infection within the most strongly endemic areas is 3%, resulting in approximately 150,000 new infections. Reported infections within endemic areas is increasing. For example, from 2000 to 2010, reported infections increased more than five-fold in Arizona. With unusually intense exposure, such as at archaeology sites or during military

TABLE 341-1	COCCIDIOIDOMYCOSIS: CLINICAL CHARACTERISTICS AND TREATMENT	
CHARACTERISTIC	**DESCRIPTION**
Causative fungi	*Coccidioides immitis* and *Coccidioides posadasii*
Primary geographic distribution	Lower Sonoran deserts of the Western Hemisphere, including parts of Arizona, California, and New Mexico; western Texas; parts of Central and South America
Primary route of acquisition	Respiratory (inhalation of arthroconidia)
Principal site of disease	Lungs most common; spread to skin, bones, meninges, and other viscera uncommon but serious
Opportunistic infection in compromised hosts	Diffuse pneumonia and widespread infections common in patients with T-lymphocyte defects or during high-dose corticosteroid therapy
Drug of choice for most patients	No antifungal is required for uncomplicated pneumonia; fluconazole or itraconazole for progressive forms of infection
Alternative therapy	Amphotericin B (especially with diffuse pneumonia or rapidly progressive infections), voriconazole, posaconazole

maneuvers within endemic regions, infections can develop in the majority of persons exposed for only a matter of days. More than 60% of new infections are likely to occur in Arizona because of the rapid growth of populations in the Phoenix and Tucson areas.

PATHOBIOLOGY

Inhaling as few as a single arthroconidium to the level of the terminal bronchiole initiates virtually all coccidioidal infections. Fungal proliferation engenders both granulomatous inflammation, which is associated with intact spherules, and acute inflammation, including eosinophils, which is associated with spherule rupture. Focal pneumonia is often associated with ipsilateral hilar adenopathy; less frequently, infection enlarges the paratracheal, supraclavicular, and cervical nodes. Lesions occurring elsewhere are the result of hematogenous dissemination, and most become apparent within 2 years of the initial infection. Although progressive dissemination occurs in less than 1% of infections, as many as 8% of persons with self-limited infection manifest asymptomatic chorioretinal scars, suggesting that subclinical hematogenous spread may be frequent. Within weeks after infection, durable T-cell immunity normally arrests fungal proliferation, which allows the inflammation to resolve and prevents reinfection in the future. Mutations of receptors for interferon-γ and interleukin-12 have been associated with disseminated infections. However, control of the infection may occur without sterilizing lesions, and reactivation of the dormant infection is possible, even many years later, in patients whose cell-mediated immunity becomes deficient.

CLINICAL MANIFESTATIONS

At least two thirds of infections are asymptomatic and are detected only by finding dermal hypersensitivity to coccidioidal antigens. Those who become ill usually experience self-limited pulmonary syndromes. However, complications or progressive forms of infection that display a broad variety of manifestations and pose difficult management problems develop in a few patients.

Primary Pulmonary Infections

Symptoms develop within 5 to 21 days after exposure. For residents of or recent visitors to southern Arizona, coccidioidomycosis accounts for approximately one third of cases of community-acquired pneumonia. Fever, weight loss, fatigue, dry cough, and pleuritic chest pain are common but nonspecific complaints. Arthralgia of multiple joints without significant effusion is also frequent and is referred to as "desert rheumatism." Occasionally, skin manifestations develop, including a short-lived nonpruritic maculopapular rash, erythema multiforme, or erythema nodosum. These arthritic and dermatologic manifestations are mediated by circulating immune complexes or other immunologic phenomena rather than by fungal dissemination. Radiographs of the chest may show no abnormalities or may demonstrate pulmonary infiltrates, either segmental or lobar. Hilar adenopathy is often a distinctive finding. Peripneumonic pleural effusions may occur and generally resolve without intervention, although cultures of pleural biopsies usually yield *Coccidioides* species. Eosinophilia may be a prominent finding in differential leukocyte counts of peripheral blood, and the erythrocyte sedimentation rate is generally elevated. Symptoms may persist for several weeks before improvement is clearly under way, and the illness, especially lassitude, may persist for months.

The primary pulmonary process produces a variety of sequelae. The most frequent is the development of a pulmonary nodule (Fig. 341-1), typically measuring 1 to 4 cm and lying within 5 cm of the hilum. Despite their harmless nature, coccidioidal nodules may cause concern because of their similarity to a malignant mass. Positron emission tomography scans are typically positive. For these reasons, management usually requires percutaneous needle aspiration or resection. Another consequence of pulmonary coccidioidomycosis is cavitation of the infiltrate, which occurs in approximately 5% of cases of pneumonia. Most cavities are solitary and thin walled and reside in an upper lobe, close to the pleura. Occasionally, they produce pain, hemoptysis, or adjacent infiltrates. Cavities may acquire mycetomas from either *Coccidioides* species or some other colonizing mold. Infrequently, a cavity ruptures and forms a pyopneumothorax. This is usually the first symptom of coccidioidal infection and typically occurs in otherwise healthy young men. An air-fluid level in the pleural space, detectable by roentgenography, often helps differentiate this problem from a spontaneous pneumothorax. Surgical resection of the cavity is the preferred treatment of this complication. The least common pulmonary complication is persistent fibrocavitary infection that progresses to involvement of both lungs.

FIGURE 341-1. Coccidioidomycosis. **A**, Benign nodule secondary to coccidioidomycosis *(arrows)*. **B**, Computed tomography scan of the nodule shown in **A** *(arrows)*.

Extrapulmonary Dissemination

Coccidioidomycosis in immunosuppressed patients, such as solid organ recipients, those with acquired immunodeficiency syndrome (AIDS) or lymphoma, and women during their third trimester of pregnancy, usually results in dissemination beyond the lungs. Mutations of the genes for gamma-interferon or the IL-12 receptors also predispose persons to dissemination. However, disseminated infection also occurs in some patients who have no underlying disease and do not manifest heightened susceptibility to other infections. The most common locations for disseminated lesions are the skin (cutaneous papules or subcutaneous abscesses); joints (especially the knee); bones, including the vertebrae; and basilar meninges. Such infections may produce one or many lesions and are frequently subacute or chronic in their manifestation. In broadly immunosuppressed patients, coccidioidal infections may be more fulminant, with fungemia detectable in blood cultures and diffuse reticulonodular embolic pulmonary infiltrates. Although the kidneys and the urinary bladder are rarely involved, *Coccidioides* may be recovered from concentrated specimens of urine, usually because of focal dissemination to the prostate. In contrast to histoplasmosis, the gastrointestinal tract is rarely involved in coccidioidomycosis.

DIAGNOSIS

The diagnosis is firmly established by recovering *Coccidioides* species from clinical specimens. On direct examination of respiratory specimens or tissue, spherules appear as large structures with refractile walls and internal organization; they are also seen on hematoxylin-eosin, silver, or periodic acid–Schiff stains of histologic preparations. Gram stain does not detect spherules. In culture, mycelial growth is often evident within the first week of incubation, and DNA probing with commercially available kits allows rapid species identification. Recovery of *Coccidioides* species from patients with only scant respiratory secretions associated with the initial pneumonia and from the cerebrospinal fluid of patients with meningitis may be difficult.

A presumptive diagnosis of coccidioidal infection is often based on the detection of specific antibodies in serum. Within the first weeks of the initial infection, a precipitin-type antibody is detected, usually by immunodiffusion techniques. Later, complement fixation (CF)–type antibodies generally appear. However, these tests may be falsely negative as often as half the time in patients with early infections. When reported quantitatively, concentrations of CF antibodies are usually highest in the most extensive infections and decrease in patients whose infections are controlled. An important means of diagnosing coccidioidal meningitis is the detection of CF antibodies in cerebrospinal fluid, along with other abnormalities such as leukocytosis, elevated protein concentration, or low glucose concentration. Coccidioidal antigens are sometimes found in the urine or serum of patients with widespread infection.

TREATMENT   Rx

The role of antifungal therapy for primary uncomplicated infections is controversial because clinical trials have not been performed to determine whether treatment either shortens the course of symptoms or diminishes the chance of complications. However, the value of treatment is clear for patients with progressive illness. Because many coccidioidal infections are chronic in nature, initial treatment often consists of oral azole antifungal agents, such as fluconazole and itraconazole. Responses to these two drugs are similar, but itraconazole is preferred in patients with skeletal infections.**1** Doses of these azoles are 400 mg/day or higher, and treatment is usually continued for a year or more. Satisfactory responses are obtained in approximately two thirds of patients. Fluconazole is effective therapy for coccidioidal meningitis and has greatly reduced the number of patients treated with intrathecal amphotericin B. Unfortunately, cessation of azole therapy is often followed by a recurrence of symptoms, especially in those with coccidioidal meningitis. Therefore, many patients need protracted or even lifelong therapy to control disease activity. Newer azole antifungals (voriconazole, posaconazole) are also effective and are sometimes useful for refractory infections. Amphotericin B remains a rational choice when treatment with azole antifungals has failed. Daily doses range from 0.4 to 1 mg/kg, and cumulative therapy ranges from 0.5 to 3 g. Occasionally, in a patient with rapid disease progression, amphotericin B may produce a more rapid therapeutic response and is therefore the preferred initial therapy. Delivery of amphotericin B in liposomes or lipid complexes is also effective and is generally less toxic than amphotericin B suspended with deoxycholate. In addition to antifungal agents, surgical removal of necrotic tissue is often essential to control the damage from specific lesions.

PROGNOSIS

After resolution of the initial infection, most patients maintain lifelong immunity, and infections after re-exposure are rare. However, cessation of symptoms is frequently accomplished without eradicating *Coccidioides* completely, and recurrence of the original infection many years after the original episode is a well-recognized risk of intercurrent profound immunosuppression. For patients in whom the initial infection cannot be resolved, the disease typically follows a protracted course. Although infection is more often debilitating than fatal, fulminant respiratory failure can occur, and if untreated, coccidioidal meningitis is nearly always fatal within 2 years.

1. Galgiani JN, Catanzaro A, Cloud GA, et al. Comparison of oral fluconazole and itraconazole for progressive nonmeningeal coccidioidomycosis: a randomized, double-blind trial. Mycoses Study Group. *Ann Intern Med.* 2000;133:676-686.

SUGGESTED READINGS

Adam RD, Elliott SP, Taljanovic MS. The spectrum and presentation of disseminated coccidioidomycosis. *Am J Med.* 2009; 122:770-777. *Retrospective analysis of 150 cases with extrapulmonary and nonmeningeal disease at a single medical center in an endemic region.*
Ampel NM. New perspectives on coccidioidomycosis. *Proc Am Thorac Soc.* 2010;7:181-185. *Most cases are completely asymptomatic, but approximately 40% present as a pulmonary process that may be difficult to distinguish from a community-acquired pneumonia.*
Borchers AT, Gershwin ME. The immune response in coccidioidomycosis. *Autoimmun Rev.* 2010;10:94-102. *Review showing that even the 60% of patients who are asymptomatic have immune responses.*
Galgiani JN, Ampel NM, Blair JE, et al. Coccidioidomycosis. *Clin Infect Dis.* 2005;41:1217-1223. *Revised consensus statement regarding current therapy for coccidioidomycosis, accessible at http://www.idsociety.org.*
Vinh DC, Masannat F, Dzioba RB, et al. Refractory disseminated coccidioidomycosis and mycobacteriosis in interferon-gamma receptor 1 deficiency. *Clin Infect Dis.* 2009;49:e62-e65. *Description of the first of several genetic mutations responsible for severe coccidioidal infection. Thus far, all have been associated with interferon-γ/interleukin-12 expression.*

342

BLASTOMYCOSIS

CAROL A. KAUFFMAN

DEFINITION

Blastomycosis (North American blastomycosis) is an endemic mycosis that primarily causes infection of the lungs and skin and, less commonly, infection of the osteoarticular and genitourinary systems.

The Pathogen

Blastomyces dermatitidis is a thermally dimorphic fungus. In the environment in the mold phase, the organism produces conidia, which when aerosolized and inhaled cause infection. At 37° C on culture media and in tissues, the organism is a yeast that is 5 to 20 μm in diameter, has a thick refractile cell wall, and produces single broad-based buds.

EPIDEMIOLOGY

B. dermatitidis exists in many diverse geographic areas worldwide, but most cases of blastomycosis are reported from the south central and north central regions of the United States and the Canadian provinces surrounding the Great Lakes. The natural niche of *B. dermatitidis* is thought to be soil and decaying vegetation, especially in areas associated with rivers and lakes. Although most cases occur sporadically, several well-described outbreaks have occurred in association with activities along waterways. The typical patient in whom blastomycosis develops is a middle-aged man who has an outdoor occupation or hobby. The association of blastomycosis developing in both hunters and their dogs is well known in endemic areas.

PATHOBIOLOGY

After the inhalation of conidia, *B. dermatitidis* transforms into the yeast phase and causes pulmonary infection. Although many patients manifest only pulmonary symptoms, others have cutaneous lesions in the absence of other organ involvement or have disseminated infection. It is likely that most patients have asymptomatic hematogenous dissemination after the initial pulmonary infection. Thus, cutaneous lesions should be viewed as a manifestation of hematogenous spread of the organism. Except in rare instances, blastomycosis is not acquired by inoculation. Cellular immunity involving T lymphocytes and macrophages is an important component of the host response to infection with *B. dermatitidis*, but neutrophils also play a role. Most patients with blastomycosis are healthy hosts. Patients who are immunosuppressed are more likely to have severe disease. Infection in an immunosuppressed host can occur after new exposure to *B. dermatitidis* or from reactivation of a latent focus of infection acquired years earlier.

CLINICAL MANIFESTATIONS

Pulmonary

Most patients with acute pulmonary blastomycosis are asymptomatic or are thought to have community-acquired pneumonia. Patients with acute pneumonia have fever, malaise, a nonproductive cough, and a pulmonary infiltrate that shows lobar or multilobar patchy or nodular infiltrates on chest radiographs. Development of skin lesions is a strong clue for blastomycosis. Chronic pulmonary blastomycosis must be differentiated from tuberculosis, other fungal infections, and lung cancer. Fever, night sweats, weight loss, fatigue, cough, sputum production, hemoptysis, and dyspnea are commonly noted. On chest radiograph the lesions are cavitary, nodular, fibrotic, or mass-like in appearance. Hilar and mediastinal lymphadenopathy and pleural effusions are not commonly seen. Overwhelming pulmonary disease with acute respiratory distress syndrome occurs infrequently and has a high mortality rate. Whether this is due to inhalation of a large number of conidia or to an exuberant host response is not known.

Disseminated Infection

Cutaneous lesions are the most common manifestation of disseminated blastomycosis. The lesions are usually well-circumscribed, painless papules, nodules, or plaques that become verrucous and develop multiple punctate draining areas in the center. Cutaneous lesions, sometimes single but more often multiple, are most common on the face and extremities but can appear anywhere. The skin lesions of blastomycosis clinically mimic those associated with nontuberculous mycobacteria, other fungal infections, mycosis fungoides, and bromide use. An uncommon manifestation, seen more often in immunocompromised patients, is the appearance of hundreds of pustular lesions that readily reveal the organism when aspirated.

Another manifestation of disseminated blastomycosis is osteoarticular involvement. Osteomyelitis can be associated with contiguous skin lesions or can appear at sites distant from cutaneous lesions. It is helpful to obtain a bone scan in all patients with disseminated blastomycosis because of the propensity of the organism to infect bone. Genitourinary involvement may be asymptomatic or be associated with signs of prostatism and the presence of a nodule on digital examination. Infrequently occurring findings include laryngeal and oropharyngeal nodules; ocular lesions; central nervous system (CNS) involvement, either meningitis or intracerebral mass lesions; and dissemination to the liver, spleen, and lymph nodes.

DIAGNOSIS

The definitive diagnostic test for blastomycosis is growth of the organism from an aspirate, tissue biopsy specimen, sputum, or body fluid. Urine obtained before and after prostatic massage should be sent for fungal culture in those with disseminated blastomycosis. The mold phase takes several weeks to grow at room temperature. Once growth has occurred, the organism can be rapidly identified as *B. dermatitidis* with highly specific and sensitive DNA probes. Histopathologic examination of cutaneous or pulmonary lesions, cytologic examination of sputum, bronchoalveolar lavage fluid, or other tissue fluids, and calcofluor fluorescent staining of sputum or purulent material from pustular lesions should be performed to look for the distinctive large, thick-walled yeast with a single broad-based bud. Identification of characteristic organisms allows a tentative diagnosis of blastomycosis and initiation of antifungal therapy before culture results are known. Serologic assays for blastomycosis are neither sensitive nor specific. A urine enzyme immunoassay for *Blastomyces* cell wall antigens may prove to be useful for diagnosis, but more experience is required to define the role of this assay in disseminated and pulmonary blastomycosis.

TREATMENT   Rx

Guidelines for the treatment of blastomycosis have been published by the Infectious Diseases Society of America (IDSA). With the exception of patients who have acute pulmonary blastomycosis that has totally resolved before the diagnosis is established, all patients with blastomycosis should be treated with an antifungal agent. Patients who have mild to moderate pulmonary or disseminated blastomycosis should be treated with itraconazole, 200 mg once or twice daily. The length of treatment is 6 to 12 months to achieve mycologic cure and prevent relapse. Fluconazole is not as effective as itraconazole. However, if the patient is unable to take itraconazole, fluconazole can be used, but the dosage should be 400 to 800 mg daily for 6 to 12 months. Anecdotal case reports describe success with voriconazole; there are no reports of treatment of blastomycosis with posaconazole. The echinocandins are not active against *B. dermatitidis* and should not be used.

Patients who have severe pulmonary or disseminated blastomycosis, all patients with CNS infection, and most immunosuppressed patients should be treated initially with amphotericin B, preferably a lipid formulation. The dosage is 3 to 5 mg/kg daily, except for CNS infection, for which 5 mg/kg daily should be used. Some physicians prescribe corticosteroids for patients with acute respiratory distress syndrome associated with blastomycosis, but this remains controversial and was not recommended in the IDSA guidelines. After clinical improvement has occurred, usually within several weeks, therapy can be changed to itraconazole, 200 mg twice daily for a total of at least 12 months of therapy.

PROGNOSIS

The prognosis for patients with pulmonary or disseminated blastomycosis treated with itraconazole is excellent; more than 90% are cured. If relapse does occur, a second course of itraconazole is usually successful. Most reported deaths occur in patients with overwhelming pneumonia and acute respiratory distress syndrome.

SUGGESTED READINGS

Bariola JR, Hage CA, Durkin M, et al. Detection of *Blastomyces dermatitidis* antigen in patients with newly diagnosed blastomycosis. *Diagn Microbiol Infect Dis.* 2011;69:187-191. *A sensitive and specific tool for timely diagnosis.*

Bariola JR, Perry P, Pappas PG, et al. Blastomycosis of the central nervous system: a multicenter review of diagnosis and treatment in the modern era. *Clin Infect Dis.* 2010;50:797-804. *Discusses the clinical findings and, most importantly, the approach to treatment of this uncommon, but serious complication of blastomycosis.*

Carlos WG, Rose AS, Wheat LJ, et al. Blastomycosis in Indiana: digging up more cases. *Chest.* 2010;138:1377-1382. *Review of 59 cases, including 34 patients between 2005 and 2008 when major highway projects were underway.*

Chapman SW, Dismukes WE, Proia LA, et al. Clinical practice guidelines for the management of blastomycosis: 2008 update by the Infectious Diseases Society of America. *Clin Infect Dis.* 2008; 46:1801-1812. *Outlines the current management of blastomycosis and gives evidence ratings for all treatment recommendations.*

Smith JA, Kauffman CA. Blastomycosis. *Proc Am Thorac Soc.* 2010;7:173-180. *Review emphasizing the utility of the 2008 treatment guidelines.*

343

PARACOCCIDIOIDOMYCOSIS

CAROL A. KAUFFMAN

DEFINITION

Paracoccidioidomycosis (South American blastomycosis) is a subacute to chronic mycosis that is endemic in Central and South America. The disease is characterized primarily by pulmonary, mucous membrane, and cutaneous lesions, but disseminated disease also occurs.

The Pathogen

Paracoccidioides brasiliensis is a thermally dimorphic fungus. In the environment and at temperatures below 35° C, the organism is a mold that produces conidia, the infectious form. In tissues and at 37° C in vitro, the organism assumes the yeast form with multiple narrow-based daughter cells attached to the mother cell.

EPIDEMIOLOGY

P. brasiliensis exists only in humid areas of Central and South America. More than 80% of cases are from Brazil. The presumed ecologic niche is in soil, but the exact conditions that favor growth of the organism have not been elucidated. The disease is most prevalent in middle-aged to elderly men from rural areas. The reason for the sexual imbalance (male-to-female ratio of 14:1) is possibly related to the inhibitory effects of estrogens on growth of the organism rather than solely environmental exposure. Although the disease classically develops later in life, it is likely that initial exposure occurs in childhood. Cases seen in areas outside Central and South America have all been linked to previous residence in the endemic area.

PATHOBIOLOGY

Paracoccidioidomycosis develops after the inhalation of aerosolized conidia encountered in the environment. Once in the alveoli, the mycelial phase converts to the yeast phase. The infection may remain localized to the lungs, although it is likely that asymptomatic hematogenous dissemination occurs during most infections. In most patients, manifestations of disease do not develop at the time of the initial infection. The primary host defense mechanism against *P. brasiliensis* appears to be cell-mediated immunity, but neutrophils also play a role in host defense. The histopathologic picture includes both neutrophilic and granulomatous responses. There have been increasing reports of paracoccidioidomycosis in patients infected with human immunodeficiency virus (HIV) and in other immunosuppressed patients; in these patients there is widespread dissemination, and histopathology shows poorly formed granulomas. Reactivation of latent infection acquired years earlier is the presumed pathogenesis of most cases of the chronic adult form of paracoccidioidomycosis and cases that appear years after the patient has left the endemic area.

CLINICAL MANIFESTATIONS

Acute-Subacute (Juvenile) Paracoccidioidomycosis

The acute-subacute form of paracoccidioidomycosis occurs in less than 10% of patients. It is a disease of the reticuloendothelial system with widespread dissemination to the liver, spleen, lymph nodes, and bone marrow. Patients younger than 30 years typically have this form of paracoccidioidomycosis; however, older adults, especially those who are immunosuppressed, can also manifest this type of rapidly progressive disease. In patients with HIV infection, rapid progression occurs with multiple cutaneous lesions, lymphadenopathy, hepatosplenomegaly, and severe pulmonary involvement with hypoxemia.

Chronic (Adult) Paracoccidioidomycosis

Chronic paracoccidioidomycosis is seen in more than 90% of patients, most of whom are older men. The disease progresses slowly over a period of years. Pulmonary involvement is prominent and clinically mimics tuberculosis and other chronic fungal pneumonias. Radiographically, nodular, interstitial, or cavitary lesions are seen but differ from those of tuberculosis and histoplasmosis in that the infiltrates tend to be in the middle and lower lung fields rather than the apices. Most patients with the adult form of paracoccidioidomycosis also have ulcerative or nodular mucous membrane lesions, primarily in the anterior nares and oral cavity. Cutaneous lesions, particularly on the face, are also common and may be papular, nodular, ulcerative, or plaquelike. The mucocutaneous lesions must be differentiated from mucocutaneous leishmaniasis and squamous cell carcinoma. Adrenal involvement has been reported in more than 90% of cases at autopsy, but adrenal insufficiency is only noted in about half.

DIAGNOSIS

Definitive diagnosis of paracoccidioidomycosis is established by growth of *P. brasiliensis* in culture. The organism may take as long as 4 weeks to grow. For seriously ill patients, direct examination of body fluids, sputum, or purulent material treated with KOH or calcofluor fluorescent stain or histopathologic examination of tissue biopsy samples can provide a presumptive diagnosis while awaiting culture results. The characteristic appearance of *P. brasiliensis* consists of thick-walled yeast cells that have multiple small, circumferentially attached, narrow-based budding daughter yeast cells—a distinctive morphologic picture likened to a ship's steering wheel.

A variety of immunodiffusion assays, enzyme immunoassays, and complement fixation assays are available in endemic areas, but sensitivity and specificity vary greatly. The immunodiffusion assay appears to be most useful. An assay for circulating cell wall antigens of *P. brasiliensis* has also been developed in endemic areas, but its role has not been established.

TREATMENT Rx

The drug of choice for the treatment of paracoccidioidomycosis is itraconazole (200 mg daily for 6 to 12 months). Ketoconazole at a dosage of 200 to 400 mg daily for 1 year is effective and certainly less expensive than itraconazole, but the incidence of side effects is greater and relapses occur more frequently than with itraconazole. Fluconazole is less effective and should not be used unless no other agent is available. Voriconazole has been shown to be as effective as itraconazole in a randomized open-label pilot study, and there are scattered reports of the successful use of posaconazole as salvage therapy. Sulfonamides have been used for years to treat paracoccidioidomycosis and are clearly the most inexpensive form of treatment. In some areas of Brazil they are the agent of choice for mild to moderate disease; however, relapse rates are higher than with the azoles. Amphotericin B is effective but rarely required, except in immunosuppressed patients with life-threatening disseminated disease. Most HIV-infected patients with paracoccidioidomycosis have been treated with amphotericin B as initial therapy, followed by lifelong suppressive therapy with either itraconazole or trimethoprimsulfamethoxazole. The latter is preferred in patients with acquired immunodeficiency syndrome because it also prevents infections with *Pneumocystis jiroveci* and *Toxoplasma gondii*.

PROGNOSIS

Patients with paracoccidioidomycosis have an excellent response to antifungal therapy, although HIV-infected patients respond less well. Patients who have extensive pulmonary involvement at the time of diagnosis are at risk for progressive fibrosis despite antifungal therapy.

SUGGESTED READINGS

de Freitas RM, Prado R, do Prado FL, et al. Pulmonary paracoccidioidomycosis: radiology and clinical-epidemiological evaluation. *Rev Soc Bras Med Trop.* 2010;43:651-665. *Review of 44 cases, about half of whom had radiographic abnormalities and were more likely to have pulmonary symptoms.*

Laties AM, Fraunfelder FT, Tomaszewski K, et al. Long-term visual safety of voriconazole in adult patients with paracoccidioidomycosis. *Clin Ther.* 2010;32:2207-2217. *Voriconazole was safe long-term.*

Morejon KM, Machado AA, Martinez R. Paracoccidioidomycosis in patients infected with and not infected with human immunodeficiency virus: a case-control study. *Am J Trop Med Hyg.* 2009;80:359-366. *Shows that patients who have paracoccidioidomycosis and are also infected with HIV are younger, more likely to live in urban areas, and more likely than non–HIV-infected patients to have rapidly progressive infection. The initial response to antifungal therapy was similar, but relapse rates and overall mortality were greater in the HIV-infected cohort.*

Nucci M, Colombo A, Queiroz-Telles F. Paracoccidioidomycosis. *Curr Fung Infect Rep.* 2009;3:15-20. *Up-to-date overview of paracoccidioidomycosis.*

344

CRYPTOCOCCOSIS

CAROL A. KAUFFMAN

DEFINITION

Cryptococcosis occurs most often in persons who are immunosuppressed, especially those infected with human immunodeficiency virus (HIV). Meningitis is the most common clinical manifestation, but pulmonary and other organ involvement occur as well.

The Pathogen

Cryptococcus neoformans is a yeast in both the environment and tissues. In tissues, the organism is enveloped by a large polysaccharide capsule that is a major virulence factor. In the environment, *C. neoformans* yeast cells are smaller and less encapsulated and thus more easily aerosolized and inhaled. There are two varieties of the species, *C. neoformans* var *neoformans* and *C. neoformans* var *grubii*; both are pathogenic and cause similar disease manifestations. Most laboratories do not differentiate these varieties. *C. neoformans* var. *neoformans* accounts for most cases of human disease throughout the world.

Cryptococcus gattii is now a separate species distinct from *C. neoformans* and more often infects normal hosts than patients with HIV. It is more restricted in the environment and found mostly in the subtropical and tropical areas of Australia and Southeast Asia, where the ecologic niche is the eucalyptus tree. The epidemiology of *C. gattii* is evolving with its emergence in the past decade in British Columbia and the Pacific Northwest region of the United States. *C. gattii* will not be discussed further.

EPIDEMIOLOGY

C. neoformans has been linked to pigeons; the birds do not become infected, but rather the organism grows luxuriantly in dried pigeon excreta because of its high nitrogen content.

Before highly active antiretroviral therapy (HAART), cryptococcosis occurred in 5 to 10% of patients with acquired immunodeficiency syndrome (AIDS). Patients at highest risk were those with fewer than 50 CD4$^+$ cells/μL. Though less commonly seen now in Europe and North America, cryptococcosis remains extremely common in AIDS patients in Africa, where it is estimated that the prevalence among HIV-infected patients is as high as 30%. In the non-AIDS population, cryptococcosis is a frequent opportunistic infection in patients who have received an organ transplant, have been treated with corticosteroids, or have diabetes mellitus, renal failure, liver dysfunction, or chronic pulmonary disease. For some patients, the only risk factor appears to be older age. In every reported series, separate from those dealing only with HIV infection, approximately 20% of patients have no known underlying illness.

PATHOBIOLOGY

The organism is inhaled from the environment and causes pulmonary infection initially. The primary host defense at this stage is complement-dependent macrophage and neutrophil phagocytosis and killing. Natural killer cells also have the ability to kill the organism. Ultimately, however, T-cell immunity is the most important host determinant in limiting the replication of *C.*

neoformans. In most normal hosts, the infection remains localized to the lungs and does not cause symptomatic infection. It is likely that a few organisms exist as walled-off subpleural granulomas in many who have had pulmonary infection. If the host becomes immunosuppressed, the organism can then reactivate and disseminate to other sites. *C. neoformans* is clearly neurotropic, and the primary disease manifestation is meningoencephalitis. However, dissemination to many organs is likely, especially in those with deficient T-cell immunity.

Virulence factors for *C. neoformans* include the capsule, which requires opsonization for efficient phagocytosis, and the production of melanin, which has been shown to occur in vivo and enables the organism to resist intracellular killing. Both these factors may help explain the virulence of the organism once it has reached the central nervous system (CNS). Antibody and complement levels are low in the brain, and thus phagocytosis of the organism is minimal. Brain tissue provides high concentrations of substrates, such as catecholamines, for the phenol oxidase enzyme systems of *C. neoformans* that produce melanin, thereby aiding survival of the organism.

CLINICAL MANIFESTATIONS
Central Nervous System Infection

The most common manifestation of cryptococcosis is CNS infection. The typical picture is subacute to chronic meningoencephalitis. Patients usually have increasingly severe headaches over a period of several weeks. Other symptoms and signs include nuchal rigidity, lethargy, personality changes, confusion, visual abnormalities (photophobia, diplopia, decreased visual acuity, papilledema, extraocular nerve palsies), and nausea and vomiting. Less commonly, hearing loss, ataxia, and seizures occur. Fever is present in only approximately half the patients. Elderly persons with cryptococcal meningitis may have just dementia, without other neurologic findings. AIDS patients often have subtle CNS symptoms but usually have fever and other constitutional symptoms and rapidly manifest signs of dissemination.

Pulmonary Infection

In non–HIV-infected patients, the most common underlying risk factor for pulmonary cryptococcal infection is chronic obstructive pulmonary disease, followed by corticosteroid use and receipt of a solid organ transplant. *C. neoformans* may merely be an airway colonizer in some patients; in others, symptomatic infection, mostly manifested by fever, cough, and dyspnea, requires treatment with an antifungal agent. The typical lesion noted with pulmonary cryptococcosis is a pleural-based nodular lesion. However, patchy pneumonitis, multiple nodular lesions, cavitary lesions, masslike lesions, and diffuse pulmonary infiltrates have all been noted with pulmonary cryptococcosis. Patients with advanced HIV infection are likely to have diffuse infiltrates that can progress rapidly to acute respiratory insufficiency. All immunosuppressed patients who have pulmonary cryptococcosis and all patients with any CNS symptoms should undergo lumbar puncture to be certain that meningitis is not present. Whether normal hosts with isolated pulmonary cryptococcosis and negative serum antigen tests require lumbar puncture is controversial. The most conservative approach is to perform lumbar puncture in all patients who have pulmonary cryptococcal infection.

Involvement of Other Organs

C. neoformans has been reported to infect most organs during the course of disseminated infection, especially in AIDS patients. Skin lesions are a prominent clue to dissemination. Papules that resemble molluscum contagiosum or an acneiform rash, nodules, ulcers, plaques, draining sinuses, and cellulitis have all been reported. Focal involvement can occur in the prostate and other organs of the genitourinary tract, in osteoarticular structures, in the breast, and in the eye, larynx, and other head and neck structures. The prostate, in particular, has been noted as a sanctuary from which persisting organisms can later disseminate.

DIAGNOSIS

The diagnosis of cryptococcosis is established when the yeast is grown in culture. Appropriate specimens for culture include cerebrospinal fluid (CSF), blood, sputum, material from skin lesions, and other body fluids or tissues that appear to be infected. The organism grows in several days on most standard agar media. Most automated blood culture systems allow rapid growth of *C. neoformans.* Visualization of the capsule and performance of a few simple tests differentiate *C. neoformans* from other yeasts. Tissue biopsy shows the 5- to 10-μm yeast surrounded by the capsule. Definitive diagnosis

of cryptococcosis can be made by mucicarmine staining, which selectively stains the polysaccharide capsule a deep rose color. In CSF or other body fluids, an India ink preparation allows visualization of the budding yeast cells surrounded by the large capsule, but it is not currently done by many laboratories.

The latex agglutination assay for cryptococcal polysaccharide antigen (CRAG) is a highly sensitive and specific diagnostic test. CRAG is positive in CSF in almost 100% and in serum in about 75% of patients who have meningitis. In AIDS patients, serum CRAG is almost always positive and is an excellent screening tool; titers in both CSF and serum are exceptionally high because of the enormous burden of organisms. In non-AIDS patients who have nonmeningeal, pulmonary cryptococcosis, the CRAG assay is positive in only 25 to 50% of cases. False-positive results with the CRAG assay are uncommon, are generally low in titer, and are more likely with serum than with CSF. Patients with *Trichosporon asahii* infection can have a positive CRAG test because of cross-reacting antigens shared by both fungi.

The CSF of patients with cryptococcal meningitis typically has an increased number of white blood cells (but rarely >500/μL), a predominance of lymphocytes (although neutrophils are sometimes prominent early in the course), elevated protein, and decreased glucose. AIDS patients most often have normal or only mildly abnormal findings as a result of their markedly defective immune response. Despite normal CSF findings with regard to cells, protein, and glucose, every AIDS patient with a headache must have a CRAG test, India ink preparation, and culture performed on CSF. It is extremely important that an opening pressure be obtained when lumbar puncture is performed. Especially in AIDS patients, extremely high intracranial pressure (>350 mm H_2O) has been associated with poor outcomes and must be aggressively lowered.

All patients with cryptococcal meningitis should undergo computed tomography or magnetic resonance imaging of the brain to look for mass lesions and to assess ventricular size. Obstructive hydrocephalus is uncommon but requires a shunting procedure to decrease the pressure. More commonly, the increased intracranial pressure with cryptococcal infection is associated with normal-sized ventricles and is due to blockage at the arachnoid villi or increased brain edema (or both), perhaps related to the osmotic effect of the polysaccharide capsule. Different methods for reducing pressure are used in this situation.

TREATMENT

Guidelines for the treatment of cryptococcal infection have been published by the Infectious Diseases Society of America (IDSA).

Central Nervous System Infection

Early multicenter randomized trials in non-AIDS patients showed superiority of the combination of amphotericin B and flucytosine for 6 weeks over amphotericin B alone for 10 weeks. Subsequent randomized trials in the azole era have been performed only in the AIDS population. They have confirmed the benefit of flucytosine added to amphotericin B for induction therapy and have shown that initial therapy with fluconazole alone or with amphotericin B alone is not as effective as therapy with amphotericin B and flucytosine.[1] The combination of amphotericin B and flucytosine has been shown to be the most rapidly fungicidal regimen.[1] Regimens using amphotericin B with fluconazole or flucytosine with fluconazole[2] are less effective, but reasonable alternatives when the preferred regimen of amphotericin B plus flucytosine is not available.

Current recommendations for AIDS patients are to give induction therapy with intravenous amphotericin B deoxycholate, 0.7 to 1 mg/kg daily, combined with oral flucytosine, 100 mg/kg daily given in four divided doses for at least 2 weeks, followed by consolidation therapy with oral fluconazole, 400 mg daily for a minimum of 8 weeks, and then suppressive therapy with fluconazole, 200 mg daily. Lipid formulations of amphotericin B at daily dosages of 3 to 5 mg/kg should be used for patients who have preexisting renal insufficiency and those at risk for nephrotoxicity, including all transplant recipients. For patients who have undergone 12 months of antifungal therapy, who have CD4+ counts higher than 100/μL, and whose HIV viral load is undetectable on antiretroviral therapy, the suppressive therapy can be stopped.[3] Suppressive therapy with fluconazole for transplant recipients is recommended for 6 to 12 months. The IDSA guideline recommendations for non–HIV-infected, nontransplant recipients are to treat with amphotericin B deoxycholate, 0.7 to 1.0 mg/kg daily, plus flucytosine, 100 mg/kg daily, in four divided doses for at least 4 weeks for induction therapy, followed by consolidation therapy with fluconazole, 400 mg daily for 8 weeks, and suppressive therapy with fluconazole, 200 mg daily for 6 to 12 months. Many physicians use lipid formulations of amphotericin B, 3 to 5 mg/kg daily, in this population, many of whom are older and have underlying medical illnesses.

There are only a few case reports on the use of voriconazole and posaconazole for salvage treatment of cryptococcal meningitis. The echinocandins are not active against *C. neoformans* and should not be used.

A significant observation from the AIDS treatment trials was the role of increased intracranial pressure as a cause of early death from cryptococcal meningitis. An aggressive approach to the diagnosis and treatment of increased intracranial pressure in both AIDS and non-AIDS patients is mandatory and should include daily lumbar puncture or placement of a temporary lumbar drain or ventriculostomy until the opening pressure remains lower than 190 mm H_2O. Treatment with corticosteroids, acetazolamide, or mannitol has not proved efficacious in this setting.

Another issue that has emerged is the development of immune reconstitution inflammatory syndrome (IRIS), which can occur in patients with AIDS who are receiving effective antiretroviral therapy that increases the $CD4^+$ count (Chapter 402). Symptoms of meningitis reappear and are due to the inflammatory response and not a relapse of disease. IRIS can also occur in transplant recipients in whom immunosuppressive therapy is decreased rapidly. Generally, no specific therapy is needed for mild IRIS, but sometimes corticosteroids are needed if increased intracranial pressure occurs.

Pulmonary and Other Nonmeningeal Infections

Treatment of nonmeningeal cryptococcosis depends on the severity of the infection. Many patients with isolated pulmonary or other focal infections are not severely ill, and oral fluconazole, 400 mg daily for 6 to 12 months, is recommended. For patients who are severely ill, therapy is the same as noted earlier for CNS infection.

PROGNOSIS

The outcome for both AIDS and non-AIDS patients with cryptococcal meningitis has improved markedly in the developed world, However, in Africa the mortality from cryptococcal meningitis in AIDS patients approaches 100% in some areas because of lack of access to specific therapy. Dementia, which usually occurs in older patients, hearing loss, and visual loss may not be reversed even though mycologic cure is achieved.

1. Brouwer AE, Rajanuwong A, Chierakul W, et al. Combination antifungal therapies for HIV-associated cryptococcal meningitis: a randomised trial. *Lancet*. 2004;363:1764-1767.
2. Nussbaum JC, Jackson A, Namarika D, et al. Combination flucytosine and high-dose fluconazole compared with fluconazole monotherapy for the treatment of cryptococcal meningitis: a randomized trial in Malawi. *Clin Infect Dis*. 2010;50:338-344.
3. Vibhagool A, Sungkanuparph S, Mootsikapun P, et al. Discontinuation of secondary prophylaxis for cryptococcal meningitis in human immunodeficiency virus–infected patients treated with highly active antiretroviral therapy: a prospective, multicenter, randomized study. *Clin Infect Dis*. 2003;36:1329-1331.

SUGGESTED READINGS

Baddley JW, Schain DC, Gupte AA, et al. Transmission of *Cryptococcus neoformans* by organ transplantation. *Clin Infect Dis*. 2011;52:e94-e98. *Three case reports.*

Brizendine KD, Pappas PG. Cryptococcal meningitis: current approaches to management in patients with and without AIDS. *Curr Infect Dis Rep*. 2010;12:299-305. *Combination antifungal therapy with a lipid formulation of amphotericin B plus flucytosine is generally indicated.*

Goldman JD, Vollmer ME, Luks AM. Cryptococcosis in the immunocompetent patient. *Respir Care*. 2010;55:1499-1503. *Review.*

Pappas PG, Chetchotisakd P, Larsen RA, et al. A phase II randomized trial of amphotericin B alone or combined with fluconazole in the treatment of HIV-associated cryptococcal meningitis. *Clin Infect Dis*. 2009;48:1775-1783. *Recent trial assessing the efficacy of treatment with amphotericin B and fluconazole, of most interest for countries that do not have flucytosine available for use.*

Perfect JR, Dismukes WE, Dromer F, et al. Clinical practice guidelines for the management of cryptococcal disease: 2009 update by the Infectious Disease Society of America. *Clin Infect Dis*. 2010;50:291-322. *Outlines the current management of cryptococcosis and gives evidence ratings for all treatment recommendations.*

Tunkel AR. Clinical trial report: treatment of cryptococcal meningitis in the developing world. *Curr Infect Dis Rep*. 2010;12:234-236. *Brief review.*

345

SPOROTRICHOSIS

CAROL A. KAUFFMAN

DEFINITION

Sporotrichosis is a subacute or chronic infection that is usually localized to cutaneous and lymphocutaneous structures, but pulmonary, osteoarticular, and disseminated infection can occur in patients who have certain underlying diseases.

The Pathogen

Sporothrix schenckii is a thermally dimorphic fungus. In the environment at temperatures lower than 35 to 37° C, the organism is a mold and produces conidia, the infectious form. In tissues and at 35 to 37° C, *S. schenckii* transforms into the yeast phase; the yeasts are 4 to 6 μm in diameter; are cigar shaped, round, or oval; and reproduce by budding.

EPIDEMIOLOGY

S. schenckii is found worldwide in climates ranging from temperate to tropical. The organism exists in a variety of environmental niches, including soil, sphagnum moss, hay, decaying wood, and other vegetation. Infection is seen almost entirely in persons whose vocation, avocation, or living condition brings them into contact with the organism in the environment. Landscaping activities, gardening, farming, and motor vehicle accidents have been associated with sporotrichosis. Most cases of sporotrichosis are sporadic, but outbreaks have been described. Inhalation of *S. schenckii* conidia occurs less commonly and results in pulmonary and, rarely, disseminated sporotrichosis.

PATHOBIOLOGY

Infection is almost always acquired by inoculation of conidia and remains localized to the immediate and contiguous cutaneous, subcutaneous, and lymphatic structures. Some strains of *S. schenckii* grow poorly at temperatures higher than 35° C; these strains usually cause fixed cutaneous lesions without lymphatic spread. The typical host response to infection with *S. schenckii* is a mixed neutrophilic and granulomatous reaction. Antibody is not protective; T lymphocytes are important in containing the infection. In individuals who have underlying illnesses, including alcoholism, diabetes mellitus, and chronic obstructive pulmonary disease, *S. schenckii* is more likely to involve osteoarticular structures and the lungs. Widespread dissemination develops in persons infected with human immunodeficiency virus (HIV) but is a distinctly unusual event in normal hosts.

CLINICAL MANIFESTATIONS

Lymphocutaneous

Days to weeks after inoculation of *S. schenckii* conidia, a papular lesion develops at the inoculation site; the lesion becomes nodular and often ulcerates (Fig. 345-1). Drainage is not grossly purulent, and the lesion is not terribly painful. Similar lesions occur along the lymphatic channels proximal to the primary lesion. Verrucous or ulcerative fixed cutaneous lesions do not exhibit lymphatic extension. The differential diagnosis of lymphocutaneous sporotrichosis includes *Nocardia* infections (Chapter 338), particularly *Nocardia brasiliensis*; atypical mycobacterial infections (Chapter 333), especially *Mycobacterium marinum*; *Leishmania brasiliensis* infections (Chapter 356); and tularemia (Chapter 319).

Visceral and Osteoarticular

Pulmonary sporotrichosis occurs most often in middle-aged men who have chronic pulmonary disease and abuse alcohol. Fever, night sweats, weight loss, fatigue, dyspnea, cough, purulent sputum, and hemoptysis are common. Chest radiographs show unilateral or bilateral upper lobe cavities with variable amounts of fibrosis and nodular lesions. The disease mimics reactivation tuberculosis in many aspects. Osteoarticular sporotrichosis is found most often in middle-aged men and occurs more frequently in alcoholics. Infection

FIGURE 345-1. Lymphocutaneous sporotrichosis with a papular lesion at the inoculation site that becomes nodular and often ulcerates. (From CID, Dr. Watanakunakorn, University of Chicago Press.)

may involve one or multiple joints; the joints most commonly affected are the knee, elbow, wrist, and ankle joints. Isolated bursitis, tenosynovitis, and nerve entrapment syndromes have been reported. Osteoarticular infection can follow local inoculation, but most patients probably have had hematogenous spread. Isolated case reports document sporotrichosis involving the pericardium, eye, perirectal tissues, larynx, breast, epididymis, spleen, liver, bone marrow, lymph nodes, and meninges. Disseminated sporotrichosis, manifested as widespread ulcerative cutaneous lesions with or without visceral involvement, is uncommon; most cases have been reported in patients with advanced HIV infection.

DIAGNOSIS

Growth of *S. schenckii* from culture of material aspirated from a lesion, a tissue biopsy specimen, sputum, or body fluid is the most effective method of establishing the diagnosis of sporotrichosis. Growth of the mold phase of the organism is usually evident within a few days. Histopathologic examination of biopsy material shows a mixed granulomatous and pyogenic process; however, the organisms are often present in small numbers and are frequently not visualized. Serology is not useful in the diagnosis of sporotrichosis.

TREATMENT Rx

Because sporotrichosis is usually a localized subacute to chronic infection, oral antifungal agents are preferred; amphotericin B is reserved for severe visceral infections. Guidelines for the management of sporotrichosis have been published by the Infectious Diseases Society of America. Itraconazole is the drug of choice for lymphocutaneous sporotrichosis. The usual dosage is 200 mg daily, and treatment should continue for several weeks after all lesions have disappeared, generally for a total of 3 to 6 months. Saturated solution of potassium iodide (SSKI) has been used to treat sporotrichosis for almost a century. The initial dose is 5 to 10 drops three times daily in water or juice, with the dose increasing over a period of several weeks to a maximum of 40 to 50 drops three times daily. SSKI has many side effects, including salivary gland swelling, metallic taste, rash, and fever; the only advantage is that it is inexpensive. Fluconazole is less effective than itraconazole but for occasional patients can be used at a dosage of 400 to 800 mg daily. Voriconazole is not active against *S. schenckii*, and there is no reported clinical experience with posaconazole. Terbinafine appears to be effective for sporotrichosis at a dosage of 500 mg twice daily, but few patients have been treated with this agent to date. Local hyperthermia, induced by a variety of different warming devices or baths, has been shown to be effective in some patients with fixed cutaneous lesions.

Osteoarticular and pulmonary sporotrichosis is usually treated with itraconazole, 200 mg twice daily for 1 to 2 years. Other azoles are less effective, and SSKI is ineffective. In a seriously ill patient with pulmonary sporotrichosis, 3 to 5 mg/kg of amphotericin B daily, preferably a lipid formulation, should be used as initial therapy. After the patient has shown improvement, therapy can be changed to itraconazole. Amphotericin B is the drug of choice for disseminated sporotrichosis. Therapy can be changed to itraconazole, 200 mg twice daily, once the patient has stabilized. Patients with acquired immunodeficiency syndrome and disseminated sporotrichosis should remain on lifelong maintenance therapy with itraconazole, 200 mg daily.

PROGNOSIS

The prognosis for patients with cutaneous and lymphocutaneous sporotrichosis is excellent. Almost all patients are cured with one course of therapy; relapses occur in only a small proportion of patients. Extracutaneous forms of sporotrichosis do not respond well to therapy, partly because of delays in diagnosis and partly because of the underlying diseases that are frequently found in those who have extracutaneous sporotrichosis. The outcome of disseminated sporotrichosis in patients with HIV infection has been especially poor.

SUGGESTED READINGS

Kauffman CA, Bustamante B, Chapman SW, et al. Clinical practice guidelines for the management of sporotrichosis: 2007 update by the Infectious Diseases Society of America. *Clin Infect Dis.* 2007;45:1255-1265. *Outlines the current management of sporotrichosis and gives evidence ratings for all treatment recommendations.*

Quintella LP, Passos SR, do Vale AC, et al. Histopathology of cutaneous sporotrichosis in Rio de Janeiro: a series of 119 consecutive cases. *J Cutan Pathol.* 2011;38:25-32. *Granulomas were suppurative in about 85% of cases and caseous in 45%.*

346

CANDIDIASIS

CAROL A. KAUFFMAN

DEFINITION

Candidiasis encompasses a wide variety of clinical syndromes caused by yeasts of the genus *Candida*. Of the species that cause infection in humans, *Candida albicans* is the most common; *Candida glabrata, Candida parapsilosis,* and *Candida tropicalis* are responsible for most of the remaining infections. Organisms such as *Candida krusei, Candida lusitaniae,* and *Candida guilliermondii* are less common causes of infection.

The Pathogen

Candida species are 2- to 6-μm yeast-like organisms that reproduce by budding. Most species, with the exception of *C. glabrata*, form pseudohyphae (elongated buds that remain attached to the mother cell) and hyphae in tissues.

Candida species cause a wide spectrum of diseases ranging in severity from localized mucous membrane infection to life-threatening disseminated disease. The major determinant of the severity of infection is the host's immune response. Local infections are often related to overgrowth of *Candida* as a result of changes in the normal flora. Invasive infections that remain within an organ system, such as urinary tract infections, usually occur because of local anatomic abnormalities. In an immunosuppressed host, especially a patient with neutropenia, widespread visceral dissemination is common.

EPIDEMIOLOGY

Candida species are part of the normal human flora of the gastrointestinal and genitourinary tracts and skin. As colonizers, *Candida* species do not cause infection unless there is a defect in host defense mechanisms or unless exogenous factors, such as antibiotic use, have upset the ecology of the normal flora. *C. albicans* is the species most commonly found colonizing humans; *C. glabrata* is the second most common species, and *C. tropicalis, C. parapsilosis,* and others are found less often. The species of *Candida* colonizing patients change during hospitalization and with the use of antifungal agents. *C. glabrata*, a species that is increasingly resistant to fluconazole, and *C. krusei*, which is intrinsically resistant to fluconazole, are associated with increased use of this agent in the hospital setting.

Though uncommon, acquisition of *Candida* from health care workers or from environmental sources has been noted. The *Candida* species most often associated with transmission from contaminated fluids or devices, especially central intravenous catheters, has been *C. parapsilosis*. This species is also the most frequent colonizer of the hands of health care workers.

Candidiasis is the most common opportunistic fungal infection as a result of both the organisms' ubiquity and the increasing number of patients with risk factors for infection with these organisms. The classic immunosuppressed host at risk for serious *Candida* infections was a neutropenic patient with a hematologic malignancy who had received cytotoxic agents and corticosteroids. Increasingly, however, candidiasis is seen in patients in intensive care units (ICUs). Risk factors for the development of serious *Candida* infections in ICU patients include the use of broad-spectrum antimicrobials, indwelling central venous catheters, previous surgical procedures, renal failure, parenteral nutrition, and high Acute Physiology and Chronic Health Evaluation (APACHE) score. Certain ICU populations, especially very low birthweight neonates and burn victims, are at even higher risk for *Candida* infection than is the typical ICU patient.

The acquired immunodeficiency syndrome (AIDS) epidemic has led to a marked increase in *Candida* infections. However, in contrast to candidiasis in the hospital setting, the primary manifestation of *Candida* infection in AIDS patients is mucocutaneous infection, especially oropharyngeal candidiasis. The development of mucosal *Candida* infection is related to deficient T-cell immunity as reflected by a low CD4$^+$ lymphocyte count. With appropriate antiretroviral therapy, oropharyngeal candidiasis has become an uncommon opportunistic infection; it is now seen almost exclusively in patients with advanced human immunodeficiency virus (HIV) infection that is untreated or has become refractory to therapy.

FIGURE 346-1. Thrush.

PATHOBIOLOGY

The usual mode of infection with *Candida* is egress from its normal niche into the blood stream or other tissues; the source is usually the gastrointestinal tract, but the skin and genitourinary tract are other sources. The primary host defense in response to this event is phagocytosis and killing by neutrophils, monocytes, and macrophages. Phagocytosis is enhanced in the presence of specific anti-*Candida* antibody and complement. Several different mechanisms are operative within neutrophils and macrophages that allow the killing of yeasts. Thus, patients who are neutropenic, especially those with chemotherapy-induced disruption of the gut mucosa, are at great risk for invasion with *Candida* species. Once *Candida* gains access to the blood stream, widespread hematogenous dissemination is the rule. Biopsy of many different organs usually shows multiple microabscesses composed of neutrophils (in a host who has these cells), budding yeasts, and often pseudohyphae or hyphae. Over time, the lesions show a mixed neutrophilic and granulomatous response.

T-cell immunity is also an important host defense against infection with *Candida*. T-cell immunity controls *Candida* at mucosal surfaces. In contrast to those with neutropenia, patients with deficient T-cell immunity are at risk for persistent and recurrent mucocutaneous candidiasis, but invasive infection rarely develops.

CLINICAL MANIFESTATIONS

Mucocutaneous Candidiasis
Oropharyngeal Candidiasis
Local mucous membrane and cutaneous lesions are the most common forms of *Candida* infection. Oropharyngeal candidiasis, or thrush (Chapter 433), can be due to either local factors or T-cell dysfunction. Local factors include the use of broad-spectrum antimicrobials or inhaled corticosteroids, xerostomia, and radiation treatment of the head and neck. Denture stomatitis occurs frequently in persons who wear full upper dentures, especially those who do not remove their dentures at night.

Thrush secondary to T-cell dysfunction is most commonly seen in patients with HIV infection (Chapter 397) and is the most frequent opportunistic infection noted in patients with AIDS. The appearance of thrush in a previously healthy individual with no known risk factors should immediately raise suspicion of HIV infection.

Thrush manifests with white plaques on the buccal mucosa, palate, oropharynx, or tongue (Fig. 346-1). Scraping the lesions with a tongue depressor reveals an erythematous, nonulcerated mucosa under the plaques. Denture stomatitis almost always manifests as a painful erythematous palate without plaques. Angular cheilitis, or perlèche, which is the presence of painful cracks at the corners of the mouth, can occur with or without thrush.

Esophagitis
Esophagitis may accompany oropharyngeal candidiasis or may occur independently of lesions in the oropharynx (Chapter 140). The development of *Candida* esophagitis is almost always related to immune dysfunction and not simply to local factors. *Candida* esophagitis occurs in AIDS patients with low CD4 counts, patients with leukemia, and others taking immunosuppressive agents. The classic symptom of *Candida* esophagitis is odynophagia localized to a discrete substernal area. The differential diagnosis includes ulcerations due to herpes simplex or cytomegalovirus and, in AIDS patients, idiopathic ulcers.

Vulvovaginitis
Candida vulvovaginitis is a common infection in women of childbearing age and is the most frequent mucocutaneous manifestation of *Candida* infection. Risk factors include conditions associated with increased estrogen levels, such as the use of oral contraceptives and pregnancy, diabetes mellitus, therapy with corticosteroids or broad-spectrum antimicrobials, and HIV infection. Symptoms include vaginal discomfort, discharge, and vulvar pruritus. The discharge is usually curd-like, but it can also be thin and watery. The labia are erythematous and swollen, and the vaginal walls show erythema and white plaques. Although most women have only a few episodes throughout their lives, a minority have frequent recurrences; in most of these patients, no discrete risk factor is found, and the cause is presumed to be local immune dysregulation.

Cutaneous Candidiasis
Candida infection of the skin (Chapter 444) occurs mostly in the intertriginous areas or under a large pannus or pendulous breasts. The lesions are erythematous, pruritic, and frequently pustular; have a distinct border; and are almost always associated with smaller satellite lesions. The presence of satellite lesions helps distinguish candidiasis from tinea cruris or corporis. *Candida* onychomycosis results in thickened, opaque, and onycholytic nails. *Candida* can also cause paronychia, especially in those whose occupation involves frequent immersion of the hands in water.

Chronic Mucocutaneous Candidiasis
This uncommon syndrome usually begins in childhood and is characterized by recalcitrant and relapsing thrush, vaginitis, onychomycosis, and hyperkeratotic skin lesions on the face, scalp, and hands. It is thought to be due to a specific defect in the T-cell response to *Candida* antigens. Some patients have associated endocrinopathies such as hypoparathyroidism, hypothyroidism, and hypoadrenalism.

Disseminated Infections
Candidemia
The most common manifestation of disseminated *Candida* infection is candidemia. However, candidemia merely implies the presence of *Candida* in blood; it does not define the extent of visceral involvement. *Candida* obtained from a blood culture should never be considered a contaminant and should always prompt a search for the probable source and the extent of infection. Risk factors for candidemia include broad-spectrum antimicrobial therapy, central intravenous catheters, parenteral nutrition, renal failure, surgical procedures involving the gastrointestinal tract, neutropenia, and corticosteroid therapy. The attributable mortality from candidemia approaches 40%; overall mortality is higher in the elderly and neonates.

Although candidemia is the most obvious manifestation of serious infection with *Candida* species, septic shock can also occur, along with invasion

FIGURE 346-2. Skin lesions in invasive candidiasis.

FIGURE 346-3. Retinal involvement.

FIGURE 346-4. Computed tomography of a patient with chronic disseminated candidiasis (hepatosplenic candidiasis). Note the distinctive punched-out lesions in the liver.

of multiple viscera, in the absence of positive blood cultures. The clinical picture of disseminated candidiasis is indistinguishable from that of bacterial infection. The histologic picture characteristic of disseminated candidiasis consists of multiple microabscesses in many organs. The eyes, kidneys, liver, spleen, and brain are the most commonly involved sites, but virtually all organs have been noted to have microabscesses caused by *Candida*. Clinical clues to the diagnosis of disseminated candidiasis include the appearance of the skin and retinal lesions. The nonpainful, nonpruritic skin lesions are papular to pustular and surrounded by a zone of erythema (Fig. 346-2). The eye lesions appear as distinctive white exudates in the retina (Fig. 346-3); with extension into the vitreous body, the retina becomes obscured.

Endocarditis

Candida endocarditis is an uncommon and often fatal complication of candidemia. It occurs most often in intravenous drug users, patients who have prosthetic cardiac valves, and those with central venous catheters in place. Blood cultures are usually persistently positive, and echocardiography reveals large vegetations that can readily embolize to major vessels.

Chronic Disseminated (Hepatosplenic) Candidiasis

This syndrome almost always occurs in leukemic patients who have had an episode of neutropenia. After the neutrophil count returns to normal, fevers that are often quite high, right upper quadrant tenderness, and nausea develop. The alkaline phosphatase level is generally elevated, and distinctive punched-out lesions are seen in the liver, spleen, and sometimes the kidneys on computed tomography (Fig. 346-4). Biopsy of these lesions shows microabscesses that contain budding yeasts.

Focal Invasive Infections

These forms of candidiasis result from local inoculation, contiguous spread, or hematogenous spread. Hematogenous spread, which often goes undetected, is probably the most common pathogenetic mechanism.

Urinary Tract Infections

Candiduria is a frequent finding in hospitalized patients and is related to factors such as diabetes mellitus, broad-spectrum antimicrobial treatment, indwelling urinary devices, and genitourinary tract structural abnormalities. Most patients with candiduria have only bladder colonization and not infection. Urinary tract infection with *Candida* species can arise by two mechanisms. Patients with candidemia can develop multiple microabscesses secondary to hematogenous spread to the kidneys. Other patients, who have the risk factors noted earlier, can develop cystitis or ascending infection with pyelonephritis. Patients with cystitis or pyelonephritis have symptoms indistinguishable from those of bacterial infections. A fungus ball composed of fungal hyphae can develop at any level of the collecting system and lead to obstruction, with subsequent infection.

Osteoarticular Infections

Osteoarticular infections arise secondary to hematogenous seeding or exogenous inoculation during intra-articular injection, a surgical procedure, or trauma. Vertebral osteomyelitis is probably the most common manifestation of osteoarticular candidiasis. The symptoms of back pain and fever may occur many weeks after an episode of fungemia. A unique triad of face, scalp, and upper chest folliculitis; endophthalmitis; and sternoclavicular or costochondral septic arthritis is reportedly due to *C. albicans* in drug users who inject brown heroin intravenously.

Endophthalmitis

Exogenous endophthalmitis occurs secondary to trauma or ophthalmic surgery. Most often, the procedure involved is cataract extraction, with or without lens implantation, and the most common infecting species is *C. parapsilosis*. Primary infection occurs in the anterior chamber, but ultimately the posterior chamber is also involved. Endogenous *Candida* endophthalmitis results from hematogenous seeding of the choroid and retina and is one of the most serious complications of candidemia. Characteristic white lesions are visible in the retina, and with progression of the infection, vitritis occurs; the risk for loss of vision is quite high.

Peritonitis

Candida peritonitis can follow bowel surgery or perforation. Symptoms are the same as those noted in bacterial peritonitis. Usually, this type of infection is polymicrobial, and abscess formation is common. In patients maintained on continuous ambulatory peritoneal dialysis, *Candida* peritonitis generally develops as a late infection after previous episodes of bacterial peritonitis. A cloudy dialysate, abdominal pain, and fever are typically noted.

Meningitis

Acute *Candida* meningitis occurs as part of disseminated infection, especially in low-birthweight neonates. Chronic meningitis, an uncommon manifestation of candidiasis, resembles cryptococcal or tuberculous meningitis with regard to symptoms and cerebrospinal fluid findings.

DIAGNOSIS

The diagnosis of mucocutaneous candidiasis is often made clinically. Culture is rarely indicated. Confirmation can be sought by scraping the lesions and performing either a potassium hydroxide preparation or a Gram stain to look for budding yeasts and pseudohyphae (Chapter 444). Pseudohyphae are not always noted and are never seen in infection with *C. glabrata*. In cases in which the disease is recurrent or unresponsive to standard therapy, lesions should be cultured to establish whether a more resistant species, such as *C. glabrata* or *C. krusei*, is the causative agent. In the event of suspected esophagitis, endoscopy should be performed; biopsy of the plaque-like lesions or ulcerations shows mucosal invasion with budding yeasts and pseudohyphae.

The diagnosis of invasive or disseminated candidiasis is more difficult. Evidence of dissemination is usually sought by culturing blood or other sterile body sites. The automated blood culture systems used by most hospitals are as sensitive as the lysis-centrifugation system for growing *Candida* from blood. However, no system is sensitive enough for clinicians to rely on blood cultures to establish the diagnosis of invasive candidiasis in all cases or to rule out candidiasis as a diagnostic possibility. In addition, 1 to 4 days is required for growth to occur; in a desperately ill patient, this delay is problematic.

The tips of intravenous catheters that have been removed should be sent for culture. However, no studies have evaluated the number of yeasts that is indicative of infection, and many physicians accept the growth of any yeast as affirming infection that requires treatment. Because osteomyelitis and other focal forms of candidiasis are generally indistinguishable from bacterial infection, biopsy should be performed for histopathologic and culture studies.

In a seriously ill patient suspected of having candidiasis, the development of pustular skin lesions or typical retinal lesions can be helpful. Budding yeasts typical of *Candida* species should be sought by smearing material from a pustule on a slide and staining it with Gram stain or by performing a biopsy of a lesion and staining the tissue section with a silver stain. All patients who are candidemic or suspected of having disseminated *Candida* infection should undergo a dilated ophthalmologic examination, preferably by an ophthalmologist, to look for typical retinal lesions.

Imaging studies are invaluable for certain forms of candidiasis, especially chronic disseminated candidiasis, and they can be of major help in defining the extent of infection in other types of *Candida* infection, such as osteoarticular and urinary tract infections and endocarditis.

The serum β-D-glucan assay, which detects a component of the cell wall of many different fungi, may prove beneficial in the diagnosis of invasive fungal infections, including candidiasis; however, more experience is needed to verify this test's usefulness.

TREATMENT   (Rx)

Guidelines for treatment of the various forms of candidiasis were recently published by the Infectious Diseases Society of America (IDSA). Mucocutaneous disease is obviously treated in a much different fashion than disseminated life-threatening infection. Because diagnostic tests are not sensitive, empirical therapy is indicated in some circumstances, and for patients at the highest risk for *Candida* infection, antifungal prophylaxis can decrease that risk.

Mucocutaneous Infections

Most mucocutaneous infections should initially be treated with local creams, solutions, troches, or suspensions. For thrush, clotrimazole troches (10 mg four or five times daily) are preferred to nystatin suspension (commonly given as "swish and swallow" four times daily). Patients with AIDS may not respond to local therapy, especially when their CD4 counts are low; in this situation, oral fluconazole 100 mg daily, or itraconazole solution 200 mg daily, should be used. Posaconazole is as effective as fluconazole but more expensive.[1] For vaginitis, a variety of creams and vaginal tablets (miconazole, clotrimazole, and others) are effective, but many women prefer to take a single 150-mg fluconazole tablet orally. Recurrent vaginitis is a more complicated therapeutic issue and often requires chronic suppressive therapy with fluconazole. Esophagitis should always be treated with a systemically absorbed agent; the usual treatment is fluconazole 200 mg/day for 14 days.

In patients with advanced AIDS and low CD4 counts, who are often taking fluconazole to prevent recurrent candidiasis, fluconazole-refractory disease may develop. For these patients, increasing the dosage of fluconazole or switching to itraconazole suspension, oral voriconazole, or posaconazole should be effective. If oral tablets and solutions are no longer effective, intravenous amphotericin B, caspofungin, anidulafungin, and micafungin are alternative agents that can be used. Patients with the syndrome of chronic mucocutaneous candidiasis require lifelong suppressive therapy with oral azole agents.

Candidemia and Invasive Candidiasis

All patients with candidemia should be treated with an antifungal agent, including patients who have only one blood culture that yields *Candida* and those with a vascular catheter tip that yields *Candida*. The rationale for this recommendation is related to the high rate of metastatic foci in major organs associated with hematogenously disseminated candidiasis. Randomized controlled trials have shown the effectiveness of the following antifungal agents for the treatment of candidemia: fluconazole 400 or 800 mg/day; the three echinocandins—caspofungin 50 mg/day, anidulafungin 100 mg/day, and micafungin 100 mg/day; voriconazole 3 mg/kg twice daily; amphotericin B 0.7 mg/kg/day; and a lipid formulation of amphotericin B 3 to 5 mg/kg/day.[2-6] The IDSA guidelines recommend fluconazole for patients who are not severely ill and have not had recent azole exposure, and an echinocandin for severely ill patients and those who have had recent azole exposure. Patients who have stabilized clinically and are found to have an isolate, such as *C. albicans*, that is likely to be susceptible to fluconazole can be transitioned to fluconazole from an echinocandin. Voriconazole is recommended for step-down therapy rather than initial therapy, and amphotericin B formulations are used infrequently, except for patients who are neutropenic and for neonates. All vascular catheters should be removed, because removal has been shown to help clear *Candida* from blood more quickly. Repeated blood cultures should be obtained to ascertain that the fungemia has resolved, and treatment should continue for 2 weeks after the date of the first negative blood culture.

Because diagnostic tests are not sensitive, seriously ill patients who could have invasive candidiasis may need to be treated before culture confirmation. This approach is used frequently in neutropenic patients, whose outcomes are poor if disseminated fungal infection goes untreated. Several different antifungal agents can be used empirically, including a lipid formulation of amphotericin B, caspofungin, or voriconazole[7-9]; these agents have activity against filamentous fungi as well as *Candida* species. Empirical therapy has also been used in ICU patients. A placebo-controlled, randomized trial failed to show a benefit with empirical therapy; however, there were acknowledged problems with the chosen end point, and the rate of candidemia was too low to allow a proper evaluation of empirical therapy with fluconazole.[10] The IDSA guidelines recommend that empirical therapy be reserved for febrile, critically ill patients who have risk factors for invasive candidiasis; the decision to treat should be based on clinical assessment of risk, serologic markers for invasive candidiasis, and culture data from nonsterile sites. The agents recommended are either fluconazole or an echinocandin, with the caveats noted earlier for treating patients with documented candidemia.

Endocarditis should be treated with a lipid formulation of amphotericin B, with or without flucytosine. Echinocandins are an acceptable alternative. Infected valves should be replaced. In a few patients for whom valve replacement was not an option, lifelong suppression with fluconazole appeared to be effective.

Chronic disseminated candidiasis generally requires months of therapy for cure. Most patients begin therapy with a lipid formulation of amphotericin B and are then switched to fluconazole and treated until the lesions disappear on computed tomography scanning.

Focal Invasive Infections

Treatment of focal infections depends on the organ system involved. Perhaps the simplest to treat are urinary tract infections. Most patients with candiduria are not infected but merely colonized; removing the selective pressure of antimicrobials and indwelling catheters eliminates candiduria in many of these patients. For those who have infection, oral fluconazole at a dosage of 200 mg/day for 2 weeks is recommended. Bladder irrigation with amphotericin B should not be used because it eradicates only bladder colonization, requires that a catheter be placed in the bladder, and is associated with a high recurrence rate. None of the newer antifungal agents has a role in the treatment of urinary tract infections.

Osteoarticular infections require months of therapy; amphotericin B or an echinocandin can be given initially, followed by long-term therapy with an azole. Peritonitis associated with chronic ambulatory peritoneal dialysis can be treated with amphotericin B, fluconazole, or an echinocandin, depending on the species of *Candida* causing infection. Intraperitoneal administration of amphotericin B can be extremely irritating and should not be attempted. The dialysis catheter should be removed. Meningitis should be treated initially with amphotericin B and flucytosine; patients with more chronic disease can be switched to fluconazole for a longer duration of therapy.

Treatment of *Candida* eye infections varies with the extent of ocular involvement. Lesions discovered early at the stage of choroidal or retinal involvement might be treated effectively with systemic antifungal agents (amphotericin B, an echinocandin, fluconazole, or voriconazole) alone, but there are no data that prove this. Many physicians prefer to use an agent, such as voriconazole or fluconazole, that achieves higher concentrations in the eye. Lesions extending into the vitreous body require more aggressive therapy. The best results have been obtained with pars plana vitrectomy, which also provides material for culture; injection of amphotericin B or voriconazole into the vitreous; and a systemic antifungal agent such as fluconazole, voriconazole, or amphotericin B. Clearly, management must be individualized and performed in concert with an ophthalmologist experienced in the treatment of this infection. Treatment of endophthalmitis associated with an intraocular lens implant requires removal of the implant, vitrectomy, and local amphotericin B injections, as well as therapy with fluconazole or voriconazole.

PREVENTION

For certain populations at the highest risk for invasive fungal infection, prophylactic antifungal agents can prevent infection. The populations for whom prophylaxis is recommended include stem cell transplant recipients, patients with acute leukemia who are undergoing induction chemotherapy, high-risk liver transplant recipients, and pancreas and small bowel transplant recipients; in these groups, a variety of different agents are effective. In the ICU population, prophylaxis with fluconazole can be effective, but it is recommended only in units that have a high rate of invasive candidiasis, and only in those patients at the highest risk for infection. Restricting the use of prophylaxis is essential to prevent the widespread use of azoles, with subsequent selection of resistant species.

PROGNOSIS

The prognosis for patients with mucocutaneous infections is excellent. The prognosis for focal invasive infections depends on the organ involved and the patient's immune status. For example, whereas pyelonephritis may respond well to antifungal therapy, endocarditis and meningitis are more difficult to treat and have poor outcomes. Invasive candidiasis has a high mortality rate. Early treatment with an effective antifungal agent is extremely important for a favorable outcome.

Grade A

1. Vazquez JA, Skiest DJ, Nieto L, et al. A multicenter randomized trial evaluating posaconazole versus fluconazole for the treatment of oropharyngeal candidiasis in subjects with HIV/AIDS. *Clin Infect Dis.* 2006;42:1179-1186.
2. Mora-Duarte J, Betts R, Rotstein C, et al. Comparison of caspofungin and amphotericin B for invasive candidiasis. *N Engl J Med.* 2002;347:2020-2029.
3. Kuse ER, Chetchotisakd P, da Cunha CA, et al. Micafungin versus liposomal amphotericin B for candidaemia and invasive candidosis: a phase III randomised double-blind trial. *Lancet.* 2007;369:1519-1527.
4. Reboli AC, Rotstein C, Pappas PG, et al. Anidulafungin versus fluconazole for invasive candidiasis. *N Engl J Med.* 2007;356:2472-2482.
5. Pappas PG, Rotstein CM, Betts RF, et al. Micafungin versus caspofungin for treatment of candidemia and other forms of invasive candidiasis. *Clin Infect Dis.* 2007;45:883-893.
6. Kullberg BJ, Sobel JD, Ruhnke M, et al. Voriconazole versus a regimen of amphotericin B followed by fluconazole for candidaemia in non-neutropenic patients: a randomised non-inferiority trial. *Lancet.* 2005;366:1435-1442.
7. Walsh TJ, Finberg RW, Arndt C, et al. Liposomal amphotericin B for empirical therapy in patients with persistent fever and neutropenia. *N Engl J Med.* 1999;340:764-771.
8. Walsh TJ, Teppler H, Donowitz GR, et al. Caspofungin versus liposomal amphotericin B for empirical antifungal therapy in patients with persistent fever and neutropenia. *N Engl J Med.* 2004;351:1391-1402.
9. Walsh TJ, Pappas P, Winston DJ, et al. Voriconazole compared with liposomal amphotericin B for empirical antifungal therapy in patients with neutropenia and persistent fever. *N Engl J Med.* 2002;346:225-234.
10. Schuster MG, Edwards JE Jr, Sobel JD, et al. Empirical fluconazole versus placebo for intensive care unit patients: a randomized trial. *Ann Intern Med.* 2008;149:83-90.

SUGGESTED READINGS

Avni T, Leibovici L, Paul M. PCR diagnosis of invasive candidiasis: systematic review and meta-analysis. *J Clin Microbiol.* 2011;49:665-670. *The pooled sensitivity for the diagnosis of candidemia was 95% with a specificity of 92%, whereas blood cultures had a sensitivity of only 38%.*
Bassetti M, Mikulska M, Viscoli C. Bench-to-bedside review: therapeutic management of invasive candidiasis in the intensive care unit. *Crit Care.* 2010;14:244. *Review including prophylactic, empirical, and pre-emptive treatment strategies in patients at high risk of candidemia.*
Muñoz P, Guinea J, Rojas L, et al. New antifungal agents for the treatment of candidaemia. *Int J Antimicrob Agents.* 2010;2:S63-S69. *Review.*
Pappas PG, Kauffman CA, Andes D, et al. Clinical practice guidelines for the management of candidiasis: 2009 update by the Infectious Diseases Society of America. *Clin Infect Dis.* 2009;48:503-535. *Outlines the current management of candidiasis, with evidence ratings for all treatment recommendations.*
Summers PR. Topical therapy for mucosal yeast infections. *Curr Probl Dermatol.* 2011;40:48-57. *Approach to vulvovaginal and oral candidiasis.*

347

ASPERGILLOSIS

THOMAS J. WALSH AND DAVID A. STEVENS

DEFINITION

Aspergillosis is defined as infection with one or more species of the genus *Aspergillus*. Sporelike structures called conidia are aerosolized from the mold form of the organism growing in the environment. When conidia reach tissue, they germinate to form invasive filaments called hyphae.

The Pathogens

The most common species infecting humans are *Aspergillus fumigatus*, *Aspergillus flavus*, *Aspergillus terreus*, and *Aspergillus niger*. The species are usually identified in culture by the characteristic microscopic features of their hyphae and the structures producing conidia. When some species are not readily identifiable, they may be reported by the clinical laboratory as "*Aspergillus* species or *Aspergillus* sp." Molecular methods are increasingly being used for identification. *A. fumigatus* may be reported as "*A. fumigatus* species complex." Some species within the *A. fumigatus* complex may be particularly drug resistant. *A. terreus* is frequently resistant to amphotericin B. Aspergilli within tissue appear as dichotomously branched (Y-shaped) septate hyphae. *Scedosporium* spp and *Fusarium* spp may also produce septate hyphae in tissue. The presence of septa and dichotomous branching differentiates *Aspergillus* spp from the Mucorales, which are the causative organisms of mucormycosis (Chapter 348).

EPIDEMIOLOGY

Aspergillus spp are ubiquitous organisms in the external environment, including soil, decaying matter, and air, and can grow at temperatures as high as 40 to 50° C. Aspergilli are easily isolated from houses, particularly from basements, crawl spaces, bedding, humidifiers, ventilation ducts, potted plants, dust, condiments (e.g., pepper), and marijuana samples. Aspergilli cause abortion in cattle and are important pathogens of marine organisms, insects, and domesticated and wild birds. Aflatoxin, which is one of the most potent carcinogens known, is produced by strains of *A. flavus* at ambient temperature on stored grain, spices, and nuts. Food-borne ingestion of preformed aflatoxin may cause hepatic necrosis or hepatocellular carcinoma (Chapter 202) in animals and humans.

Aspergillus spp may be acquired from airborne conidia in inpatient and outpatient settings. Nosocomial aspergillosis is associated with building renovation, new construction, unfiltered air, contaminated ventilation systems, and fireproofing materials. Hospital water, which may become aerosolized during activities such as showering, is a newly described potential source of aspergilli. As human pathogens, *Aspergillus* spp may cause acute invasive disease, chronic infection, or allergic symptoms. A classification of aspergillosis is presented in Table 347-1.

Acute invasive aspergillosis develops in immunocompromised patient populations, particularly those with hematologic malignancies, hematopoietic stem cell transplantation (HSCT), severe aplastic anemia, primary immunodeficiencies, and solid organ transplantation, especially heart, lung, and liver transplants. Persistent neutropenia, use of corticosteroids and other immunosuppressive agents, graft-versus-host disease, and cytomegalovirus disease are the most frequently observed risk factors. The mortality associated with acute invasive aspergillosis varies from as high as 100% with central nervous system (CNS) infection to approximately 65% with pulmonary infection in HSCT recipients. Early recognition of the clinical manifestations followed by prompt initiation of antifungal therapy may improve the ominous prognosis of patients with acute invasive aspergillosis.

CLINICAL MANIFESTATIONS

Invasive Aspergillosis

The classic clinical manifestations of *invasive pulmonary aspergillosis* (IPA) in immunocompromised hosts are fever and focal pulmonary infiltrates, nodules, or wedge-shaped densities resembling infarcts (see Table 347-1). Cough, pleuritic pain, and hemoptysis may also be present. Focal pulmonary infiltrates may progress to a cavity on recovery from neutropenia. Pulmonary

TABLE 347-1 CLASSIFICATION OF ASPERGILLOSIS	
CATEGORY	**SPECIFIC FORMS OF ASPERGILLOSIS**
Acute invasive aspergillosis	Invasive pulmonary aspergillosis
	Empyema
	Tracheobronchial infection
	Extrapulmonary aspergillosis
	Acute sinusitis
	Focal rhinitis
	Cerebral, cerebellar, or brain stem
	infarction
	Endophthalmitis
	Osteomyelitis
	Epidural abscess
	Cardiac aspergillosis
	Myocarditis
	Endocarditis
	Pericarditis
	Gastrointestinal aspergillosis
	Renal infection
	Cutaneous lesions (nodules, ulcers)
	Disseminated aspergillosis
Chronic aspergillosis	Aspergilloma
	Chronic necrotizing pulmonary aspergillosis
	Chronic cavitary pulmonary aspergillosis
	Aspergillus otomycosis
Allergic forms of aspergillosis	Allergic bronchopulmonary aspergillosis
	Extrinsic allergic alveolitis
	Allergic *Aspergillus* sinusitis

FIGURE 347-1. Tomogram of pulmonary aspergillomas *(arrows)*.

infiltrates may also be manifested as bronchopneumonia in an immunosuppressed patient. The pulmonary pathology in all these entities is hemorrhagic infarction caused by the organism's capacity to invade blood vessel walls (angioinvasion). These processes lead to the formation of a necrotic center surrounded by a ring of hemorrhage and edema, which correlates radiographically with a "halo sign" surrounding the nodular density. Concomitant pleural effusion may develop and represents *Aspergillus* empyema. Tracheobronchial aspergillosis in immunocompromised patients is manifested as ulcerative, pseudomembranous, or plaquelike large-airway disease that may presage pulmonary parenchymal invasion.

Acute Aspergillus sinusitis may occur concomitantly or independently of IPA. Although symptoms may include fever, localized pressure, and pain, they may be absent in severely immunocompromised patients. Eschars on the nasal septum and turbinates may be observed by speculum examination or endoscopy. Acute *Aspergillus* sinusitis of the ethmoid and sphenoid sinuses may progress to cavernous sinus thrombosis with symptoms referable to cranial nerves III, IV, V_1, V_2, and VI. *A. flavus* has a high propensity for causing acute sinusitis.

The tissue targets of *extrapulmonary* and *disseminated aspergillosis* most commonly include the CNS, where abscesses and infarcts are characteristic. Patients with CNS aspergillosis suffer from focal paresis, cranial nerve deficits, and seizures. The glucose level in cerebrospinal fluid (CSF) is usually normal, and cultures of CSF are negative. Other extrapulmonary manifestations include endophthalmitis, myocardial infarction, gastrointestinal disease, renal infarction, cutaneous lesions, and Budd-Chiari syndrome. Esophageal ulcers and mesenteric thrombosis may produce gastrointestinal bleeding. Renal infection may cause flank pain and hematuria.

Aspergillus endocarditis usually begins as an isolated infection in intravenous drug users or following cardiac valvular surgery. *Aspergillus* endocarditis is most commonly manifested as major arterial emboli. Blood cultures, which are seldom positive, may be delayed in growth by as much as 14 to 21 days. Diagnosis is difficult, and despite valve replacement and antifungal therapy, mortality approaches 100%. *Aspergillus pericarditis* may arise from contiguous pulmonary lesions or from transmural invasion from an endocardial infection.

Locally invasive aspergillosis is usually manifested in immunocompromised patients as cutaneous ulcers, focal rhinitis, osteomyelitis, and septic arthritis. Cutaneous ulcers have been associated with the use of contaminated adhesive tape and arm boards. Blood-borne infection in illicit intravenous drug users may result in foci of dissemination in the brain, lung, kidney, and bone. Keratitis, endophthalmitis, and infection of burn wounds may develop as a result of traumatic inoculation in otherwise immunocompetent patients.

Chronic Pulmonary Aspergillosis

Aspergilloma appears on chest radiographs as a ball in a cavity. The fungus ball consists of matted hyphae and debris in a preformed cavity from previous pulmonary tuberculosis, histoplasmosis, or fibrocystic sarcoidosis (Fig. 347-1). Symptomatic patients exhibit cough, hemoptysis, dyspnea, weight loss, fatigue, chest pain, or fever. Sputum culture is typically positive for *Aspergillus* spp. Pleural aspergillosis may complicate surgical resection of an aspergilloma or develop spontaneously as a bronchopleural fistula or concomitantly with tuberculosis.

As a stage in the repair process of infarcted lung tissue in neutropenic patients, one or more apparent "aspergillomas" may develop in consolidated lesions during recovery from neutropenia. These apparent aspergillomas do not develop in preexisting cavities. Instead, they create a radiographic "air-crescent sign," or Monod sign, during their formation.

Chronic necrotizing pulmonary aspergillosis (CNPA) and *chronic cavitary pulmonary aspergillosis* (CCPA) occur in patients with underlying chronic lung disease, chronic immunosuppression, such as that due to prolonged use of systemic corticosteroids, or both. CNPA characteristically causes slowly progressive inflammatory destruction of lung tissue superimposed on chronic lung disease. The clinical manifestations of worsening pulmonary function, cough, and dyspnea in CNPA may be indistinguishable from those of concomitant primary chronic respiratory disease.

CCPA is defined as the presence of multiple *Aspergillus*-related cavities, which may or may not contain an aspergilloma. Patients with CCPA may have genetically mediated deficits in innate host defenses. Occurring in association with symptoms of cough, hemoptysis, and dyspnea, the progressive cavities of CCPA tend to coalesce and result in the loss of functional lung tissue.

Aspergillus otomycosis is a chronic infection that usually involves the external auditory canal and causes symptoms of pain, pruritus, hypoacusis, and otic discharge in patients with impaired mucocutaneous immunity, such as those with chronic eczema, hypogammaglobulinemia, diabetes mellitus, human immunodeficiency virus infection, and conditions requiring the administration of corticosteroids. *Aspergillus* may involve the middle ear and extend into the mastoid sinus if the tympanic membrane has been perforated.

Allergic Forms of Aspergillosis

Allergic bronchopulmonary aspergillosis (ABPA) develops most frequently in patients with a history of chronic asthma or cystic fibrosis. Occurring in genetically susceptible patients exposed to specific *Aspergillus* antigens, ABPA is characterized by episodic airway obstruction, fever, eosinophilia, positive sputum cultures, mucous plugs containing hyphae, the presence of grossly visible brown flecks in sputum (hyphae), transient infiltrates, parallel "tramline" or ring markings on chest radiographs, proximal bronchiectasis, upper lobe contraction, and elevated levels of total immunoglobulin E (IgE). Eosinophilia may be present in blood, sputum, and lung tissue. Mucous plugs contribute to development of pulmonary infiltrates, atelectasis, and peribronchial inflammation. The parallel or ring markings are caused by thickened ectatic bronchi, whereas the upper lobe changes are due to progressive apical fibrosis. The pulmonary infiltrates in ABPA may be nonsegmental and transient in association with eosinophilia and asthma; alternatively, they may be segmental and associated with bronchial

Neutropenia

| Halo sign | Air space consolidation | Air-crescent sign |
| D 0–5 | D 5–10 | D 10–20 |

FIGURE 347-2. Evolution of the radiographic appearance of invasive aspergillosis in an immunocompromised host. D = days after the lesion is first noted.

obstruction by mucous plugs, in which case asthma and eosinophilia may be absent.

Extrinsic allergic alveolitis is an unusual allergic form of *Aspergillus* lung disease that has most frequently been associated with *Aspergillus clavatus* in malt workers. A hypersensitivity pneumonitis with dyspnea and fever develops approximately 4 hours after exposure. Diffuse reticulonodular interstitial infiltrates may be present at the time of symptoms. Patients have IgG precipitins and cell-mediated immune reactions against *Aspergillus* antigens. Granulomas are present in lung tissue. In contrast to ABPA, eosinophilia is not a feature of *Aspergillus* extrinsic allergic alveolitis.

Allergic Aspergillus sinusitis (AAS) is a noninvasive form of sinus disease that typically occurs in patients with asthma, nasal polyps, sinus opacification, and eosinophilia. Sinus aspiration yields mucinous material containing eosinophils, Charcot-Leyden crystals, and hyphal elements. AAS and ABPA may coexist in some patients. Advanced forms of AAS may be accompanied by proptosis and optic neuropathy and thus necessitate prompt surgical intervention.

DIAGNOSIS

Invasive Aspergillosis

Diagnosis of IPA and disseminated aspergillosis is difficult. None of the aforementioned clinical manifestations are diagnostic of invasive aspergillosis. Advances in computed tomography have revealed characteristic features of nodules, halo signs, wedge-shaped infiltrates, and air-crescent signs in immunocompromised patients with IPA (Fig. 347-2). However, infections caused by *Fusarium* spp, *Scedosporium* spp, the Mucorales, and *Pseudomonas aeruginosa* may be radiologically indistinguishable from IPA. Microbiologic confirmation, when possible, is important to differentiate aspergillosis from other filamentous fungal infections. Bronchoalveolar lavage (BAL), percutaneous needle aspiration, video-assisted thoracoscopic biopsy, and if necessary, open lung biopsy are standard procedures for establishing a microbiologic diagnosis of invasive aspergillosis. Specimens obtained from these procedures may demonstrate dichotomously branching septate hyphae by direct microscopy or may grow *Aspergillus* species in culture. Each of these procedures is associated with false-negative results, as well as with complications. Conversely, detection of *Aspergillus* by direct examination or culture of tissue from an immunocompromised host with pulmonary nodules or well-circumscribed infiltrates carries a high probability of diagnosis of invasive aspergillosis.

Galactomannan, which is a heteropolysaccharide of the *Aspergillus* cell wall, is a useful biomarker that is released into the circulation and alveolar spaces during IPA. Detection of galactomannan by enzyme immunoassay (EIA) in serum or BAL above certain thresholds is strong microbiologic evidence of a diagnosis of invasive aspergillosis in immunocompromised patients with characteristic clinical manifestations. Nonetheless, false-positive results have been reported in patients who have received piperacillin-tazobactam or amoxicillin-clavulanate, in instances in which Plasma-Lyte was used for BAL, and in other deeply invasive mycoses such as blastomycosis and histoplasmosis. Serum galactomannan may be falsely negative in patients receiving antifungal prophylaxis or empirical therapy.

$(1\rightarrow3)$-β-D-Glucan is another *Aspergillus* cell wall polysaccharide that is detected in serum during invasive disease. The sensitivity of the *Limulus* spectrophotometric assay for detection of $(1\rightarrow3)$-β-D-glucan in patients with invasive aspergillosis appears to be comparable to that of the galactomannan EIA. However, because $(1\rightarrow3)$-β-D-glucan is also present in the cell wall of other medically important fungi, including *Candida* spp, the specificity of $(1\rightarrow3)$-β-D-glucan for *Aspergillus* spp is less than that of galactomannan.

Even though molecular diagnostic tools such as quantitative polymerase chain reaction (PCR) for the diagnosis of invasive aspergillosis are promising, they also remain investigational for this infection. Ultimately, the combined use of improved diagnostic imaging, microscopy, culture methodology, cell wall biomarkers, and possibly PCR in conjunction with careful bedside assessment of risk factors and clinical manifestations will improve the diagnosis of invasive aspergillosis and lead to early initiation of therapy.

Diagnosis of locally invasive extrapulmonary aspergillosis causing mucocutaneous lesions, osteomyelitis, and septic arthritis is best accomplished with biopsy, direct microscopy, and culture. A diagnosis of *Aspergillus* keratitis is established by careful culture of corneal lesions by an ophthalmologist.

Allergic Forms of Aspergillosis

The diagnosis of ABPA is based on the presence of a combination of clinical, biologic, and radiologic criteria (Fig. 347-3). Consensus criteria for establishing a diagnosis of ABPA differ depending on the presence of cystic fibrosis. For patients with ABPA without cystic fibrosis (Chapter 89), the criteria for ABPA include asthma, an immediate cutaneous reaction to *A. fumigatus* antigen, a total serum IgE concentration greater than 1000 ng/mL, elevated *A. fumigatus*–specific serum IgE levels, precipitating serum antibodies to *A. fumigatus*, central bronchiectasis, peripheral blood eosinophilia, and characteristic pulmonary infiltrates. The latter two features (eosinophilia and pulmonary infiltrates) are considered nonessential because they may be present only during the acute phase of ABPA.

In patients with cystic fibrosis, distinguishing between ABPA and an episode of clinical deterioration with colonization by *Aspergillus* spp is challenging. The current criteria of the Cystic Fibrosis Foundation help define ABPA in this setting: clinical deterioration (coughing, wheezing, increased sputum production, exercise intolerance, and decrease in pulmonary function), immediate hypersensitivity to *A. fumigatus* (positive skin test or IgE response), total serum IgE concentration greater than 1000 kIU/L, precipitating antibodies to *A. fumigatus*, and abnormal findings on chest radiography (infiltrate, mucous plugs, or unexplained changes in comparison to previous chest radiograph).

A biphasic skin test response may assist in the diagnosis. A scratch test with *Aspergillus* antigens produces an immediate wheal and flare reaction that is mediated by IgE and blocked by antihistamines but not by corticosteroids. An intracutaneous test with the antigens produces a later (6 to 8 hours) reaction that is mediated by IgG and complement and blocked by corticosteroids.

FIGURE 347-3. Allergic bronchopulmonary aspergillosis in a patient with a long history of asthma. Chest radiographs showed multilobar infiltrates. Computed tomography shows areas of tubular (**A**, *arrows*) and cystic (**A**, *arrowhead*) bronchiectasis, predominantly in the upper lobes, and bilateral mucous plugging (**B**, *arrows*) with mediastinal and hilar lymphadenopathy. (Reproduced with permission from Chen T, Hollingsworth H. Allergic bronchopulmonary aspergillosis [images in Clinical Medicine]. *N Engl J Med.* 2008;359:e7.)

An occupational history of exposure is critical for the diagnosis of *extrinsic allergic alveolitis.* A typical history of recurrent episodes developing within 24 hours after the inhalation of conidial antigens in an agricultural environment in conjunction with a negative scratch test, a positive intradermal test, and granulomas with immunoglobulins and complement in tissue is diagnostically consistent with *Aspergillus* extrinsic allergic alveolitis.

Recurrent sinusitis in a patient with asthma, nasal polyps, eosinophilia, sinus opacification, and a sinus aspirate yielding mucinous material containing eosinophils, Charcot-Leyden crystals, and hyphal elements establishes a diagnosis of AAS.

TREATMENT   Rx

Invasive Aspergillosis

The foundation of treatment of invasive aspergillosis consists of (1) antifungal medical therapy, (2) reversal of immunosuppression, and when appropriate, (3) surgical resection of infected lesions. Dosages of antifungals are listed in Table 347-2. Voriconazole is recommended in most patients for the primary treatment of invasive aspergillosis, including pulmonary, disseminated, and extrapulmonary isolated infection. This recommendation is based on a randomized controlled trial in which voriconazole was found to be superior to deoxycholate amphotericin B as primary treatment of invasive aspergillosis.▉ However, not all patients are candidates to receive voriconazole, including those with substantially elevated hepatic transaminases, hepatic

TABLE 347-2 ANTIFUNGAL THERAPY FOR INVASIVE ASPERGILLOSIS*

FIRST-LINE TREATMENT IN ADULTS†

Drug of choice:	
Voriconazole	IV therapy: 6 mg/kg q12h for 2 doses, then 4 mg/kg q12h
	Oral therapy: 200 mg or 4 mg/kg bid
Alternative (see text for conditions):	
Liposomal amphotericin B	3-5 mg/kg IV daily

SECOND-LINE OR SALVAGE TREATMENT IN ADULTS†

Amphotericin B lipid complex	5 mg/kg IV daily, *or*
Caspofungin	70 mg IV daily for the first dose, then 50 mg IV daily, *or*
Posaconazole	200 mg PO qid or 400 mg PO bid, *or*
Itraconazole	400 mg PO (capsules) daily (in either 1 or 2 doses) or 2.5 mg/kg PO (solution) bid

*Refer to package insert for dose modification of antifungal agents in patients with liver disease or renal impairment.

†The duration of antifungal therapy depends on the therapeutic response of documented lesions, the burden of disease, and host immunocompetence. Guidelines from the Infectious Diseases Society of America recommend at least 6 to 12 weeks for invasive pulmonary aspergillosis. Patients who are immunosuppressed continue treatment throughout the period of immunosuppression and until resolution of the lesions. In patients with previously diagnosed invasive aspergillosis, antifungal therapy should be continued or reinitiated during subsequent periods of immunosuppression (e.g., chemotherapy, stem cell transplantation, graft-versus-host disease) to prevent recrudescence. (See Walsh TJ, Anaissie EJ, Denning DW, et al. Treatment of aspergillosis: clinical practice guidelines of the Infectious Diseases Society of America (IDSA). *Clin Infect Dis.* 2008;46:327-360.)

dysfunction, and a history of hypersensitivity to or intolerance of voriconazole. Such patients should receive liposomal amphotericin B (L-AmB) as primary therapy. This recommendation is based on a randomized trial in which comparable efficacy of approximately 70% was demonstrated with L-AmB dosages of 3 and 10 mg/kg/day in patients predominantly with hematologic malignancies.▉ L-AmB is also indicated as primary therapy for patients in whom there is a suspicion or documentation of concurrent mucormycosis.

Second-line or salvage antifungal therapy is indicated for patients who are intolerant of primary therapy or whose infection is unresponsive to primary therapy. Among the antifungal agents used in this setting are a lipid formulation of amphotericin B, posaconazole, itraconazole, or an echinocandin (caspofungin is the only agent licensed for this indication). For patients who are already receiving voriconazole, a change in class to a lipid formulation, addition of an echinocandin, and use of another azole are possibilities. Such decisions are complicated and warrant infectious disease consultation with consideration of pharmacokinetic and host factors.

Reversal of immunosuppression is a critical factor in the successful management of invasive aspergillosis. Recovery from neutropenia and a decrease in the daily dosage or discontinuation of corticosteroids, when feasible, are two of the most important methods of improving host response. Depending on the protocol used, granulocyte transfusions may stabilize *Aspergillus* lesions until recovery from neutropenia. Granulocyte colony-stimulating factor (G-CSF) and granulocyte-macrophage colony-stimulating factor (GM-CSF) may accelerate recovery from neutropenia. The role of GM-CSF, G-CSF, or interferon-γ in immunocompromised non-neutropenic patients with invasive aspergillosis remains to be defined further.

Surgical management of infected lesions is an important adjunctive component of primary therapy for several forms of invasive aspergillosis: endocarditis, pericarditis, osteomyelitis, epidural abscess, infected vascular catheters and prosthetic devices, and skin and soft tissue infection. Surgical management is also important for several conditions associated with IPA: recurrent hemoptysis from a single cavitary lesion, invasion of a pulmonary lesion into the chest wall, and pulmonary lesions contiguous with great vessels or the pericardium. *Aspergillus* empyema requires closed chest tube drainage and possibly débridement of the infected pleural cavity. Débridement of sinus aspergillosis, particularly when the ethmoid and frontal sinuses are infected, may prevent extension into the orbit or into the cavernous sinus. Surgical resection of selected lesions of the CNS may be indicated for establishing a diagnosis, reducing increased intracranial pressure, or protecting critical neural centers. Location of the CNS lesions and neurologic sequelae after resection are critical factors in the neurosurgical management of aspergillosis.

Local infusion of antifungal agents, particularly intravitreal therapy for endophthalmitis or nephrostomy irrigation for renal disease, provides high concentrations to compartments that may not be reached by systemic therapy. Topical irrigation with voriconazole, amphotericin B, or if available, pimaricin is an important adjunct to the management of *Aspergillus* keratitis.

Chronic Aspergillosis

Medical therapy has shown limited benefit in treatment of aspergilloma; however, some patients may benefit from extended use of an antifungal triazole. Lifelong commitment to an antifungal triazole should be balanced against the natural history of approximately 10% of aspergillomas resolving spontaneously. By comparison, medical therapy with itraconazole or voriconazole is the standard of treatment of CCPA. Patients with CCPA typically achieve improvement in symptoms and stabilization or improvement in radiologic changes. Patients with CNPA also receive an antifungal triazole; however, assessment of response is more difficult as a result of the underlying chronic lung disease. The role of surgical resection in patients with a solitary aspergilloma or CCPA is limited because of the development of a bronchopleural fistula, *Aspergillus* infection of the pleural space, and potentially further worsening of already compromised pulmonary function. However, surgical resection may have a more important role in treating patients with recurrent and severe hemoptysis, in whom the benefits of removing the cavity usually outweigh the known risks. Bronchial artery embolization and transthoracic direct intracavitary instillation of antifungal agents for aspergilloma have only transient benefits but substantial risk.

Topical irrigating solutions of boric or acetic acid or an antifungal azole cream may be effective in treating *Aspergillus* otomycosis. Voriconazole, posaconazole, or itraconazole may be necessary for refractory cases or perforated tympanic membranes.

Allergic Forms of Aspergillosis

APBA is treated with a combination of corticosteroids and itraconazole. Corticosteroid therapy is the mainstay of treatment of ABPA. However, chronic administration of corticosteroids causes severe immunosuppression and multisystem metabolic abnormalities. Addition of itraconazole reduces organism burden, attenuates the antigenic stimulus for destructive bronchial inflammation, and provides a corticosteroid-sparing effect. Intermittent use of corticosteroids or substantially raising the dose in patients receiving chronic therapy can produce rapid resolution of marked symptomatic episodes or deteriorating forced expiratory volume in 1 second (FEV$_1$).

Extrinsic allergic alveolitis is best managed by removing patients from the allergenic environment. An accurate occupational history is critical for this intervention.

AAS is treated by endoscopic drainage to relieve obstruction by tenacious mucin. Itraconazole, nasal corticosteroids, and systemic corticosteroids, alone or in combination, may be beneficial in some patients with AAS. Caution is warranted with the chronic use of systemic or nasal corticosteroids. Itraconazole may have a corticosteroid-sparing effect.

Combination Antifungal Therapy

Combinations of polyenes, triazoles, and echinocandins are being explored. Therapy should be continued after the lesions are resolving, cultures are negative, and reversible underlying predispositions have abated. Reinstating therapy in patients who have previously responded should be considered if immunosuppression is reinstituted or neutropenia recurs.

PREVENTION

Several strategies may be used for the prevention of invasive aspergillosis in immunocompromised patients: primary prophylaxis, empirical therapy, and secondary prophylaxis. Posaconazole is used for the prophylaxis of invasive aspergillosis in patients with hematologic malignancies and in HSCT recipients. Voriconazole and itraconazole are also used for this indication, but with less evidence. Empirical antifungal therapy provides early treatment of persistently febrile immunocompromised patients and systemic prophylaxis for high-risk hosts with or without pulmonary infiltrates. L-AmB, caspofungin, and voriconazole have been used for this strategy. Secondary prophylaxis of invasive aspergillosis with voriconazole is used in patients with a history of previous aspergillosis who are scheduled for a subsequent cycle of immunosuppression that may increase the risk for recurrence.

Reduction of exposure to airborne conidia, such as by high-efficiency particular air (HEPA) filtration of hospital air, avoiding activities that increase conidial aerosols (room maintenance, dust exposure, and contaminated material, e.g., potted plants), and providing clean water distribution systems, may reduce the acquisition of *Aspergillus* by immunosuppressed or neutropenic patients.

For patients with allergic forms of aspergillosis, the use of corticosteroids and itraconazole, alone or in combination, may prevent debilitating exacerbations. The toxicity associated with chronic administration of prednisone warrants strategies for intermittent administration of prednisone or corticosteroid-sparing use of itraconazole.

PROGNOSIS

Untreated invasive aspergillosis is associated with severe morbidity and high mortality in immunocompromised patients. The prognosis is improved by early initiation of antifungal therapy, reversal of immunosuppression, and successful treatment of the underlying primary disease. For patients with chronic aspergillosis, multidisciplinary specialized supportive care may improve outcome and quality of life.

Grade **A**

1. Herbrecht R, Denning DW, Patterson TF, et al. Voriconazole versus amphotericin B for primary therapy of invasive aspergillosis. *N Engl J Med.* 2002;347:408-415.
2. Cornely OA, Maertens J, Bresnik M, et al. Liposomal amphotericin B as initial therapy for invasive mold infection: a randomized trial comparing a high-loading dose regimen with standard dosing (AmBiLoad trial). *Clin Infect Dis.* 2007;44:1289-1297.

SUGGESTED READINGS

Hage CA, Knox KS, Davis TE, et al. Antigen detection in bronchoalveolar lavage fluid for diagnosis of fungal pneumonia. *Curr Opin Pulm Med.* 2011;17:167-171. *A recommended approach for the diagnosis of aspergillosis.*

Patterson K, Strek ME. Allergic bronchopulmonary aspergillosis. *Proc Am Thorac Soc.* 2010;7:237-244. *Review emphasizing its consideration in difficult-to-control asthma or cystic fibrosis.*

Segal BH. Aspergillosis. *N Engl J Med.* 2009;360:1870-1884. *Succinct review of pathogenesis, clinical manifestations, diagnosis, and treatment.*

Sherif R, Segal BH. Pulmonary aspergillosis: clinical presentation, diagnostic tests, management and complications. *Curr Opin Pulm Med.* 2010;16:242-250. *Comprehensive review.*

348

MUCORMYCOSIS

DIMITRIOS P. KONTOYIANNIS

DEFINITION

Mucormycosis describes infections caused by fungi belonging to the order Mucorales. Zygomycosis, an alternative term used to describe these life-threatening infections, has become less accurate because of a recent taxonomic reclassification (using molecular methods) that abolished Zygomycetes as a class (and placed the order Mucorales in the subphylum Mucormycotina). Mucorales organisms typically cause aggressive, acute-onset, frequently fatal angioinvasive infections, especially in immunosuppressed hosts.

EPIDEMIOLOGY AND RISK FACTORS

Mucorales fungi are distributed worldwide and found in decaying organic substrates. The true incidence of mucormycosis is not known and probably underestimated because of difficulties in antemortem diagnosis. In a recent review of more than 900 reported cases, the most common microbiologically confirmed infecting members of the order Mucorales were *Rhizopus* (47%), *Mucor* (18%), *Cunninghamella bertholletiae* (7%), *Apophysomyces elegans* (5%), *Absidia* (5%), *Saksenaea* (5%), and *Rhizomucor pusillus* (4%). Some Mucorales fungi causing infection have unique geographic distributions. The thermophilic fungi *Saksenaea vasiformis* and *A. elegans* are typically isolated in regions with warmer climates; clinical infection with these organisms has shown similar geographic distributions. Additionally, infections may vary seasonally, with the majority of infections occurring in late August to November. Moreover, major natural disasters have been associated with infections by infrequently isolated species, such as *Syncephalastrum racemosum* in areas affected by hurricane Katrina and wound infections caused by *A. elegans* in victims of the 2004 Indian Ocean tsunami.

The classic risk factors for mucormycosis include hematologic malignancy, hematopoietic stem cell or solid organ transplantation, poorly controlled diabetes mellitus, chronic acidemia, prematurity, iron overload, profound chronic debilitation, trauma, burns, and intravenous drug use. Nosocomial cutaneous infections can develop in surgical wound and at intravenous catheter insertion sites. Finally, breakthrough mucormycosis has increasingly been observed in patients with leukemia and recipients of hematopoietic stem cell transplants administered *Aspergillus*-active drugs such as voriconazole (which has no anti-Mucorales activity). This association has been a topic of debate.

PATHOBIOLOGY

Mucorales species are saprophytic, rapidly growing fungi. Angioinvasive growth results in infarction and necrosis of surrounding tissue and is the hallmark of mucormycosis. The major modes of transmission are inhalation, ingestion, and cutaneous inoculation, with inhalation of spores from environmental sources being the most common. Cutaneous or percutaneous transmission occurs with traumatic disruption of skin barriers, and it is the most important mode of transmission in immunocompetent hosts. Gastrointestinal acquisition, which is less common, has occurred in patients repeatedly ingesting non-nutritional substances (pica) containing spores during severe malnutrition and in individuals ingesting contaminated herbal/homeopathic products.

Host immunity in healthy individuals prevents the germination of fungal spores unless the inoculum is heavy. To establish invasive infection, the spores must overcome both innate and adaptive immune responses to germinate into hyphae. Defects in phagocytic activity caused by insufficient numbers (i.e., neutropenia) and functional defects caused by glucocorticoids, hyperglycemia, or acidosis allow unimpeded proliferation of fungi because of the absence of coordinated, effective host responses. Mucormycosis is often disseminated in severely immunosuppressed patients, with high mortality rates. However, lymphopenia may not be as critical in patients as evidenced by the rarity of mucormycosis in patients with acquired immunodeficiency syndrome.

Free iron is an essential component of the pathogenesis of mucormycosis as suggested by the unique predisposition of patients with iron overload (Chapter 219) to such infections. These patients often receive the iron chelator deferoxamine. Both iron overload and use of deferoxamine (which is also used to treat aluminum overload in dialysis recipients) are risk factors for angioinvasive mucormycosis. *Rhizopus oryzae* can use deferoxamine as a xenosiderophore to form a ferrioxamine complex and thereby obtain more iron for its use. The newer iron chelator agents (e.g., deferasirox) are not associated with increased risk for mucormycosis; on the contrary, in preclinical models, deferasirox has exhibited direct fungicidal effects against Mucorales via iron starvation.

Historically, poorly controlled diabetes mellitus (types 1 and 2) has been a major predisposing factor (Chapters 236 and 237) that has been reported in 36 to 88% of all cases of mucormycosis. In particular, diabetic patients with ketoacidosis are susceptible to mucormycosis. Normal human serum cannot support the growth of *R. oryzae*, whereas serum from diabetic patients can. Acidosis disrupts the inhibitory activity of serum by attenuating the ability of transferrin to bind iron from the fungus. In addition, phagocytic cell dysfunction occurs in diabetic patients with ketoacidosis and may play a role in pathogenesis.

CLINICAL MANIFESTATIONS

The clinical manifestations of mucormycosis depend on the host's underlying immune and medical condition. Hence, pulmonary mucormycosis is most common in neutropenic or corticosteroid-treated patients (e.g., hematopoietic stem cell and solid organ transplant recipients). In contrast, rhino-orbital or rhinocerebral mucormycosis is the characteristic finding in patients with diabetic ketoacidosis. Finally, cutaneous mucormycosis in both immunocompetent and immunocompromised hosts is typically seen following the breakdown of skin integrity or after subcutaneous tissue injuries. Infectious syndromes associated with Mucorales are grouped according to clinical manifestation into one of six categories: (1) rhinocerebral, (2) pulmonary, (3) cutaneous, (4) gastrointestinal, (5) disseminated, and (6) unusual manifestations.

Rhinocerebral Mucormycosis

Rhinocerebral mucormycosis describes an infection originating in the paranasal sinuses after the inhalation of Mucorales spores and extending to the orbit (sino-orbital) or brain (rhinocerebral), particularly in patients with diabetic ketoacidosis or those with profound neutropenia. Early signs and symptoms of sinus invasion by rhinocerebral mucormycosis may be indistinguishable from common causes of sinusitis. Common symptoms include sinus pain, congestion, headache, mouth pain, otologic symptoms, and hypo-osmia/anosmia. Involved tissues become red, then violaceous, and finally black with thrombosis and tissue necrosis. Necrotic eschars of the nasal cavity and turbinates, facial lesions, and exophytic or necrotic lesions of the hard palate are signs of extensive, rapidly progressing infection. A painful black eschar on the palate or nasal mucosa is a "classic," yet late sign. Absence of this finding does not rule out rhinocerebral infection because necrotic nasal or palatal lesions occur in only 50% of patients within 3 days of the onset of infection. Extension into the periorbital region is not uncommon at initial evaluation. Signs and symptoms of periorbital and orbital involvement include periorbital swelling, preseptal or orbital cellulitis (or both), proptosis, chemosis, blurred vision or rapidly progressing external ophthalmoplegia, diplopia, eyelid gangrene, retinal detachment, and endophthalmitis. In addition, patients with extensive rhino-orbital or rhinocerebral disease may have trigeminal or other cranial nerve palsy, which is consistent with the frequent histologic findings of perineural invasion. Infection can progress rapidly through the cavernous sinuses into the central nervous system and result in cavernous sinus and internal carotid artery thrombosis. A bloody nasal discharge may be the only sign that the infection has invaded through the nasal turbinates into the brain. Patients with advanced infection may have multiple cranial neuropathies, altered consciousness, or both; bone destruction; retinal artery, internal carotid artery, cavernous, and less often, sagittal sinus thrombosis; frontal lobe necrosis; epidural and subdural abscesses; and basilar artery aneurysm.

Plain films and cerebrospinal fluid findings lack sensitivity in diagnosing rhinocerebral mucormycosis. Computed tomography (CT) and magnetic resonance imaging (MRI) are more useful for revealing soft tissue involvement around the nerve sheaths and bone destruction. CT frequently shows mucosal thickening, air-fluid levels, and bone erosion. Orbital thickening may be detected earlier with MRI than with CT. Findings in the orbits on CT and MRI may be unremarkable during the initial stages of mucormycosis, thus highlighting the importance of serial imaging in monitoring disease progression. Extraorbital muscle thickening is often the first sign of orbital involvement and should prompt empirical antifungal therapy followed by surgical exploration or biopsy.

Accurate diagnosis and prompt medical and surgical intervention are critical because of rapid progression of the infection. Definitive diagnosis of necrotic lesions by biopsy and rapid histologic assessment of frozen sections should be performed as soon as possible because it has a direct impact on outcome. In a review of 929 patients with documented mucormycosis, the mortality rate was 62% in those with rhinocerebral mucormycosis, 24% in those with sino-orbital involvement, and 16% in those with isolated sinus disease. Isolated sinusitis is curable with timely surgical intervention and systemic antifungal therapy.

Pulmonary Mucormycosis

The clinical manifestations of pulmonary mucormycosis are indistinguishable from those of invasive pulmonary aspergillosis (Chapter 347). Patients may have fever refractory to broad-spectrum antibiotics, nonproductive cough, and progressive dyspnea. Less commonly, pleuritic chest pain, hemoptysis, and pleural effusion are seen. If the major pulmonary blood vessels are invaded by hyphae, massive, potentially fatal hemoptysis can occur. Pulmonary mucormycosis can progress and invade adjacent organs by traversing tissue planes, including the diaphragm, chest wall, and pleura (Fig. 348-1). Clues for distinguishing pulmonary mucormycosis from invasive pulmonary aspergillosis include the presence of pansinusitis, a history of prophylaxis with antifungals against *Aspergillus* but not Mucorales (e.g., voriconazole, echinocandins), and possibly, continual absence of detectable *Aspergillus* galactomannan antigen in serum. In rare circumstances, pulmonary mucormycosis can be manifested as an endobronchial or tracheal lesion with a less fulminant course, especially in diabetics. Endobronchial mucormycosis may cause airway obstruction or erosion of major pulmonary blood vessels and fatal hemoptysis. In more immunocompetent hosts, pulmonary mucormycosis may be characterized by more atypical, slowly progressing forms. Like *Aspergillus* species, Mucorales fungi can form mycetomas in preexisting lung cavities and cause slowly necrotizing pneumonia and hypersensitivity syndromes. *Rhizopus* species have also been implicated in allergic alveolitis in farm workers or sawmill workers (wood trimmer's disease).

Because the first-line antifungal typically used for aspergillosis is voriconazole, which lacks activity against Mucorales, timely diagnosis of pulmonary mucormycosis is critical; delay in appropriate antifungal therapy (e.g., amphotericin B) rapidly worsens outcome.

Skin and Soft Tissue Mucormycosis

Cutaneous mucormycosis typically starts as erythema and skin induration at a puncture site and progresses to necrosis with a black eschar. Cutaneous

FIGURE 348-1. Extensive, progressive pulmonary mucormycosis in a young patient with acute myelogenous leukemia and prolonged severe neutropenia. Pneumonia is multifocal with areas of cavitation. Characteristic extension of the infection across tissue planes to the trachea (producing a fistula) and mediastinum (**A**) and adjacent thoracic spine (**B**) are shown by CT and MRI, respectively. The histopathologic characteristics of profound necrosis and hemorrhage (**C**) and pauciseptate, broad-based, ribbon-like Mucorales (**D**) are also shown.

infections can quickly extend into the deep fascia and muscle layers. Necrotizing fasciitis is rare and has a poor prognosis. Neutropenic patients in particular are susceptible to lymphatic and blood vessel invasion, infarction, and necrosis with eventual dissemination. Skin lesions in patients with suspected mucormycosis should raise concern about disseminated disease. Because the differential diagnosis of necrotic skin lesions is broad, especially in neutropenic patients, biopsy specimens should be obtained from the center of a lesion down to subcutaneous fat. Excision and wide débridement of cutaneous lesions coupled with systemic antifungal therapy and, on occasion, hyperbaric oxygen therapy can further reduce mortality rates.

Gastrointestinal Mucormycosis

Primary gastrointestinal mucormycosis is rare and can be manifested as necrotizing enterocolitis and involve any part of the alimentary system with mortality rates higher than 85%. It occurs primarily in malnourished patients and premature infants, in whom the stomach is the most commonly affected site, followed by the colon and ileum. The liver, spleen, and pancreas can also be involved. Physicians have described liver abscesses following the ingestion of herbal products contaminated by *Mucor indicus*. Fungi can invade the bowel wall and blood vessels and result in bowel perforation, peritonitis, and massive gastrointestinal hemorrhage. In neutropenic patients, seeding of the gastrointestinal tract is probably more common than previously thought inasmuch as 75% of cases of gastrointestinal mucormycosis are diagnosed postmortem. Symptoms and signs of gastrointestinal mucormycosis include fever, abdominal distention, nausea, vomiting, abdominal pain, diarrhea, melena, hematemesis, hematochezia, and masslike appendiceal and ileal lesions.

Disseminated Mucormycosis

Disseminated mucormycosis is rarely apparent antemortem. Severely immunosuppressed patients and those receiving deferoxamine are at highest risk. Symptoms vary depending on the site of dissemination and the degree of vascular infarction of the affected organs. The most common organ source of dissemination is the lung, and the most common site of spread is the brain. Diagnosis of disseminated mucormycosis is challenging and requires a high level of suspicion because the infection may be manifested as an unexpected

acute vascular event. Biopsy of suspected sites is critical because of the low yield of blood cultures and suboptimal recovery of the fungus from respiratory specimens. Without appropriate timely treatment, virtually all patients with disseminated mucormycosis die.

Rare Clinical Manifestations of Mucormycosis

Mucormycosis has protean manifestations that can involve any organ. Authors have reported isolated cases of tracheal, mediastinal, bone, heart, kidney, external auditory canal, and corneal involvement. Renal mucormycosis can occur in patients with intravenous drug abuse or those receiving corticosteroids. Cerebral mucormycosis, often manifested as brain abscess involving the basal ganglia and occurring in conjunction with infective endocarditis, has typically been observed in patients using illicit intravenous drugs. In all cases of device-related mucormycosis, prompt removal of the device and several weeks of systemic antifungal therapy are essential for resolution of the infection.

DIAGNOSIS

The clinical signs and symptoms of mucormycosis are nonspecific. Therefore, a high level of suspicion in susceptible patient populations is of paramount importance. Biopsy analysis and culture from sterile sites remain critical. Tissue swabs and cultures of sputum, sinus secretions, and bronchoalveolar lavage fluid are not usually diagnostic. Fungal contamination of clinical specimens and therefore growth in culture may not represent clinically significant invasive disease. However, the value of Mucorales-positive cultures (especially repetitive cultures) as an important indication of infection in immunocompromised patients is quite high. The site of infection has a major impact on the yield of histopathologic diagnosis (e.g., the ease of accessibility of sinuses).

Histopathology

Histopathologic examination of infected tissue typically shows characteristic broad (3 to 25 μm in diameter), thin-walled, primarily aseptate hyphae, focal bulbous dilation, and nondichotomous irregular branching at occasional right angles accompanying tissue necrosis and fungal angioinvasion (see Fig. 348-1). Perineural invasion is found in 90% of tissues containing nerves.

Culture

Blood cultures are rarely positive for these pathogens despite their angioinvasive nature, even when fungal hyphae are seen on histopathologic analysis. Recovery of Mucorales from tissue can be improved by mincing (not homogenizing) tissue specimens and using culture techniques that simulate in vivo fungal growth. Data on the antifungal susceptibility of Mucorales spp are limited, and minimal inhibitory concentration (MIC) testing is rarely available outside research laboratories. The correlation between clinical responses and MIC values is uncertain. Mucorales organisms are resistant to many antifungals, including flucytosine, ketoconazole, fluconazole, voriconazole, and the echinocandins, whereas they have variable susceptibility to itraconazole.

The importance of early differentiation of Mucorales from more common opportunistic molds such as *Aspergillus* spp has generated considerable interest in the development of culture- or histopathology-independent diagnostic tests such as detection of specific antigens or nucleic acids with polymerase chain reaction or in situ hybridization techniques. Molecular techniques for detecting Mucorales are few, not widely available, and investigational. This is an important unmet need for the management of mucormycosis.

TREATMENT Rx

Successful treatment of mucormycosis relies on a multifaceted approach that includes (1) aggressive attempts at diagnosis and rapid initiation of effective antifungal therapy, (2) extensive surgical débridement, and (3) rapid control of any underlying medical conditions.

Early diagnosis is critical to patients' outcome. Small focal lesions should be surgically resected before they progress to involve critical structures or distal organs. Patients often have indolent clinical findings until extensive invasion or dissemination of the infection takes place.

Antifungal Therapy

Delayed administration of systemic antifungal therapy increases the risk for death. No prospective controlled studies on the treatment of primary mucormycosis have been performed. Most of the knowledge about the activity of currently used antifungals comes from small case series, anecdotal reports, and animal models of infection. Therefore, the optimal treatment approach is uncertain. Most of the clinical experience has been with amphotericin B (AMB). Previously, the recommended antifungal therapy for mucormycosis included AMB deoxycholate at the maximum tolerated dosage, usually 1.0 to 1.5 mg/kg/day. Unfortunately, regular AMB had nephrotoxic and systemic toxic effects, which led to the development of lipid formulations of AMB (liposomal AMB, AMB lipid complex, AMB colloidal dispersion). These agents are less nephrotoxic than regular AMB and can be given at high doses (5 to 10 mg/kg/day). Lipid formulations of AMB are considered the drugs of choice for mucormycosis. Furthermore, use of percutaneous or aerosolized AMB in conjunction with concomitant systemic therapy has been successful in selected patients with pulmonary cavitary mucormycosis. Topical therapy with AMB, as well as other polyenes (natamycin), may be effective against primary cutaneous and ocular mucormycosis. Treatment of mucormycosis with AMB-based combinations has been successful in small retrospective case series. In particular, a benefit was suggested for an echinocandin–liposomal AMB combination in 41 diabetic patients with rhino-orbital mucormycosis over the use of amphotericin B lipid complex or liposomal AMB alone. This benefit was most pronounced in patients with cerebral involvement.

Although azoles have traditionally been inactive against Mucorales, the new broad-spectrum triazole posaconazole has demonstrated promising activity. In an open-label study evaluating posaconazole as salvage therapy (800 mg/day) in 24 patients with refractory mucormycosis, the agent's overall success rate was 70%. Furthermore, posaconazole was well tolerated. Similarly, a retrospective survey of posaconazole-based salvage therapy in 91 patients with refractory mucormycosis indicated an overall success rate of 61%. Determining whether posaconazole alone or combined with a lipid formulation of AMB or another agent (e.g., deferasirox) is of value requires further study. Posaconazole has limitations: absorption of the oral suspension is suboptimal in patients with mucositis, severe diarrhea, acid suppression therapy, or poor oral intake. In addition, steady-state plasma concentrations of posaconazole are not reached until around 1 week of therapy.

The duration of antifungal therapy should be determined on an individual basis. Near normalization of radiographic imaging, negative follow-up biopsy specimens and cultures from the affected site, and recovery from immunosuppression are important indicators for stopping antifungal therapy.

Surgery

Surgical débridement of cutaneous lesions is crucial and must be done without delay because of the aggressive nature of mucormycosis. A coordinated effort among all subspecialties involved (surgery, infectious diseases, head and neck, ophthalmology, pathology, clinical microbiology, and plastic surgery) is crucial, and the internist can play a vital role in coordinating this effort.

Repeated removal of necrotic tissue or aggressive surgical measures such as enucleation of the eye may be required for control of the infection. Decisions regarding the extent of débridement are often made at the bedside. CT or MRI before surgery and intraoperative frozen section analysis help determine the extent of tissue and tissue margin involvement. Low platelet counts must be corrected with transfusions before surgical intervention. Unfortunately, bleeding problems can limit surgical options. Surgery in conjunction with systemic antifungal therapy has resulted in significantly improved survival rates.

Management of Comorbid Conditions and Adjunctive Treatments

Rapid correction of underlying conditions, such as control of hyperglycemia, reversal of ketoacidosis, rapid tapering of glucocorticoid therapy, and discontinuation of deferoxamine-based treatment, influences outcomes. Hyperbaric oxygen therapy is a beneficial adjunctive therapy for mucormycosis, particularly in diabetic patients with rhinocerebral disease. Specifically, the increased oxygen pressure achieved seems to improve neutrophil activity and oxidative killing of polyene antifungals. Furthermore, high concentrations of oxygen can inhibit the growth of Zygomycetes in vitro and improve the rate of wound healing by increasing the release of tissue growth factors. However, this treatment has not been studied vigorously to determine its general efficacy and cannot be routinely recommended. In neutropenic patients, granulocyte-macrophage colony-stimulating factor or granulocyte transfusions may be beneficial until granulocyte recovery occurs, but this approach has yet to be studied sufficiently in patients with mucormycosis. Finally, the new iron chelator deferasirox could act as an adjunctive antifungal agent based on preclinical studies and very limited human experience in patients with refractory mucormycosis.

SUGGESTED READINGS

Dan M. Mucormycosis of the head and neck. *Curr Infect Dis Rep.* 2011;13:123-131. *The mortality rate of rhinocerebral mucormycosis has remained 30 to 70% despite aggressive therapy, surgical excision of necrotic tissue, and lipid formulations of amphotericin B.*

Mallis A, Mastronikolis SN, Naxakis SS, et al. Rhinocerebral mucormycosis: an update. *Eur Rev Med Pharmacol Sci.* 2010;14:987-992. *Review.*

Spellberg B, Ibrahim AS. Recent advances in the treatment of mucormycosis. *Curr Infect Dis Rep.* 2010;12:423-429. *Posaconazole may be useful as salvage therapy but is not recommended as primary therapy.*

Spellberg B, Walsh TJ, Kontoyiannis DP, et al. Recent advances in the management of mucormycosis: from bench to bedside. *Clin Infect Dis.* 2009;48:1743-1751. *Review of recent therapeutic advances to improve the outcome of mucormycosis.*

349

PNEUMOCYSTIS PNEUMONIA

JOSEPH A. KOVACS

DEFINITION

Pneumocystis jirovecii is a fungus that causes pneumonia almost exclusively in immunodeficient patients. During the 1960s and 1970s, *Pneumocystis* pneumonia (PCP) was seen with increasing frequency in immunodeficient patients, especially those receiving immunosuppressive chemotherapy. In the early 1980s, an epidemic of PCP in previously healthy adults heralded the onset of the HIV/AIDS epidemic; in the United States and in many other parts of the world, PCP has been the most common life-threatening opportunistic infection in this population. Although the frequency of PCP decreased in HIV-infected patients first in association with the widespread use of anti-*Pneumocystis* prophylaxis and later with the introduction of effective combination antiretroviral therapy, it continues to be seen with regularity in HIV-infected and other immunodeficient patients.

The Pathogen

Pneumocystis, which was long thought to be a protozoan, has now been definitively classified as an ascomycete fungus, based primarily on molecular studies demonstrating that a large number of genes have a high level of homology to other fungi rather than to protozoa. Molecular as well as antigenic studies have further demonstrated that the genus *Pneumocystis* includes a group of closely related organisms that appear to be unique species, each of which can infect only a single host species. This has led to the application of new species names to a group of organisms that were previously called *Pneumocystis carinii*, although this approach has not been universally accepted among investigators in the field. *P. carinii* is reserved for a species that infects rats, and the organism infecting humans has been renamed *P. jirovecii*. Despite the name change, the acronym PCP continues to be used to designate the disease in humans.

Pneumocystis species show a strict host specificity: attempts to transmit, for example, rat or human *Pneumocystis* to mice have been unsuccessful. Molecular evolutionary studies suggest that *Pneumocystis* species co-evolved with their hosts, with rat and mouse *Pneumocystis* diverging an estimated 33 million years ago, similar to the time rat and mouse species diverged.

Studies of *Pneumocystis* have been substantially hampered by an inability to grow any species in culture for a sustained period. Thus, the life cycle of *Pneumocystis* is unknown, although putative life cycles based on morphologic studies have been proposed; there is accumulating evidence supporting a sexual phase in the life cycle. There are two easily recognized forms of the organism: trophic forms ($\approx$2 to 6 μm in diameter) and cysts ($\approx$6 to 8 μm in diameter), which can contain up to eight intracystic bodies; additional intermediate forms are also seen. Trophic forms, which have an amorphous shape, are estimated to outnumber cysts, which are spherical, by approximately 10:1 in an infected lung. β-1,3-Glucan is found in the cyst form only, where it contributes to the rigidity of the cell wall. The estimated genome size is 8 million base pairs. The most abundant surface protein of *Pneumocystis*, the major surface glycoprotein, is found on both cysts and trophic forms and is encoded by a multicopy gene family, only one of which is expressed in a given organism; this provides *Pneumocystis* with the potential for antigenic variability. Although, to date, only a single *Pneumocystis* species has been found that infects humans, recently developed molecular typing techniques have demonstrated a high level of diversity among human *Pneumocystis* isolates.

EPIDEMIOLOGY

Pneumocystis has a worldwide distribution. Serologic studies show a high prevalence of anti-*Pneumocystis* antibodies in all populations studied to date. In America and Europe, serologic studies have demonstrated that most humans develop antibodies to *Pneumocystis* by an early age, suggesting that this is a ubiquitous organism. In support of this, an autopsy study in infants younger than 1 year with no major underlying medical problems identified *Pneumocystis* infection in lung tissue by polymerase chain reaction (PCR) in 100% of cases.

Animal studies have demonstrated that *Pneumocystis* is transmitted by the respiratory route. Human infection is presumably transmitted in the same manner. There is no evidence that water or fomites play a role in transmission. A small number of animal studies and very limited human data suggest that transmission can occur transplacentally, although the clinical relevance is unknown.

Given the strict host specificity of *Pneumocystis*, the source of organisms infecting humans is presumably other humans, by either direct or indirect exposure. There is no evidence that *Pneumocystis* is a zoonosis. PCR-based studies have identified *Pneumocystis* DNA in environmental sources such as apple orchards; however, there are currently no data indicating that such sources play an important role in transmission. *Pneumocystis* infection is likely acquired from apparently healthy humans, in whom subclinical infection (either asymptomatic or minimally symptomatic) must be quite common to allow such rapid and broad dissemination. The high frequency of detection in infants suggests an important role in transmission.

Although infection with *Pneumocystis* is widespread, in immunocompetent hosts it does not appear to cause significant disease. Clinically significant PCP occurs exclusively in patients with severe levels of immunodeficiency that are usually associated with a high risk for other opportunistic pathogens. Populations at risk include those with congenital immunodeficiencies (Chapter 258), especially severe combined immunodeficiency (SCID) and hyper-IgM syndrome; patients with HIV infection (Chapter 392) and human T-lymphotropic virus-1–associated lymphoma (Chapter 386); patients receiving chemotherapy for the treatment of malignancies, especially lymphoma; transplant patients receiving immunosuppressive therapy; and patients being treated with prolonged courses of immunosuppressive drugs (Chapter 34), especially corticosteroids, for inflammatory diseases such as

Wegener's granulomatosis or systemic lupus erythematosus. Among patients with HIV infection, the best predictor of the risk of developing PCP is the CD4 count: patients with CD4 counts less than 200 cells/mm³, and especially those with CD4 counts less than 100 cells/mm³, are at greatest risk. Patients with a prior history of PCP and those with unexplained fever, weight loss, or thrush are also at increased risk. Among other patient populations, laboratory parameters are not as useful in quantifying risk, although non-HIV patients with CD4 counts less than 200 cells/mm³ may be at increased risk. Additional information on risk is provided in the section on prophylaxis.

For many years, development of PCP was thought to result from a reactivation of latent infection by organisms that remained viable following infection at an early age, similar to tuberculosis. However, recent molecular epidemiologic studies based on the detection of mutations in the dihydropteroate synthase (DHPS) gene of *Pneumocystis*, as well as single-nucleotide polymorphism and restriction fragment length polymorphism analysis of isolates from outbreaks of PCP in renal transplant patients, have provided convincing evidence that the infecting strain is often recently acquired. Molecular studies have further documented that in the majority of patients with PCP, more than one strain can be identified in respiratory samples. In patients who develop recurrent PCP, this recurrence can be due to relapse, especially for early recurrences, or to reinfection with a novel strain. Recurrent PCP occurs almost exclusively in HIV-infected patients, in whom the risk was greater than 50% early in the AIDS epidemic, before the availability of highly active antiretroviral therapy (HAART) and the broad use of anti-*Pneumocystis* prophylaxis.

PATHOBIOLOGY

Animal studies have provided important insights into the pathogenesis of *Pneumocystis* infection. Exposure for as little as 1 day to a *Pneumocystis*-infected animal results in transmission of infection. In healthy animals, an adaptive immune response develops by approximately 5 to 6 weeks, which leads to control and clearance before the organism burden produces symptoms. CD4 cells are critical to this control, although other populations, including B cells and macrophages, also play important roles. In immunodeficient animal models, inability to control *Pneumocystis* replication leads to severe pneumonia by 2 to 3 months. Limited human data suggest a similar time course. Host inflammatory responses appear to play a critical role in the development of pulmonary symptoms. This may account for the development of symptoms of PCP in patients in whom corticosteroids are being tapered, as well as the exacerbation of hypoxia that develops approximately 4 days after the initiation of anti-*Pneumocystis* therapy (in the absence of concomitant corticosteroid therapy).

The lung pathology in patients with PCP is characteristic. Staining with hematoxylin-eosin demonstrates an acellular, foamy, eosinophilic, intra-alveolar exudate associated with mild interstitial inflammation (Fig. 349-1). With disease progression, hyaline membrane formation and interstitial as well as intraluminal fibrosis develop. Although methenamine silver stain highlights cysts scattered throughout the eosinophilic exudate, based on Giemsa staining of thin sections as well as electron micrographs, this exudate is composed almost entirely of *Pneumocystis* organisms. Atypical pathology, including noncaseating granulomas and intrapulmonary cystic changes, can also be seen.

CLINICAL MANIFESTATIONS

In non-immunosuppressed humans, no well-defined clinical syndrome is associated with *Pneumocystis* infection. *Pneumocystis* has been identified in infants by PCR and may be associated with a mild respiratory syndrome, but a postulated association with sudden infant death syndrome has not been supported by data from well-controlled studies. *Pneumocystis* has been detected by PCR in pulmonary samples from patients with chronic obstructive pulmonary disease (COPD), but what role, if any, it plays in the development or progression of COPD (Chapter 88) remains to be elucidated.

Pneumonia is the primary clinical manifestation of *Pneumocystis* infection in immunosuppressed patients. PCP typically presents with a fever, nonproductive cough, and shortness of breath that initially occurs only on exertion but, without therapy, inevitably progresses to dyspnea at rest. Only one or two of these symptoms may be present initially. Development of symptoms may be insidious, over the course of a few weeks, as is common in patients with HIV infection; a more rapid onset, over the course of only a few days, is more common in non-AIDS patients. Purulent sputum production is unusual, and chills and chest pain occur in a minority of patients. Patients with HIV infection may present with other manifestations of immunodeficiency, including weight loss and thrush.

FIGURE 349-1. Histopathology of the lung of a patient who died from *Pneumocystis* pneumonia (PCP). **A,** The hematoxylin-eosin–stained section shows the characteristic acellular, eosinophilic, intra-alveolar exudate that is typical of PCP. **B,** Methenamine silver staining of lung tissue from the same patient demonstrates black-staining cysts scattered throughout the intra-alveolar exudates.

In non-AIDS patients, corticosteroids are a common risk factor. Clinical manifestations may develop as corticosteroids are being tapered, which presumably represents the unmasking of an inflammatory response to the infection as immunosuppression is decreased.

Rarely, extrapulmonary disease can involve the skin, eye (choroiditis), central nervous system, bone marrow, thyroid, spleen, liver, gastrointestinal tract, lymph node, or multiple organs in disseminated disease. Extrapulmonary disease can occur with or without concurrent pneumonia. Use of aerosol pentamidine for prophylaxis has been associated with an increased risk of extrapulmonary disease in HIV-infected patients, but even in that circumstance, it remains extremely rare. Symptoms are related to the specific site involved and may be nonspecific; diagnosis is often made at autopsy.

DIAGNOSIS

Given the nonspecific symptoms, especially early in the disease process, clinicians must have a high index of suspicion for PCP even in patients not known to be immunosuppressed; many patients with HIV infection are unaware of their status until they present with an opportunistic infection. Knowledge of the most recent CD4 count is helpful in assessing HIV-infected patients because PCP is rare in those whose CD4 counts are above 200 cells/mm^3.

Physical examination and routine laboratory tests are usually not helpful in making the diagnosis because many pulmonary processes, both infectious and noninfectious, can present in a similar manner. Moreover, even though patients may be tachypneic and appear to be in respiratory distress, those presenting early in the disease course may have an entirely normal lung examination. Lymphopenia is common but is a manifestation of the underlying disease rather than PCP. Lactate dehydrogenase levels may be elevated but have poor specificity.

The initial evaluation should include a chest radiograph and assessment of arterial oxygenation, either by blood gas measurement or by pulse oximetry. The chest radiograph typically shows perihilar or diffuse bilateral interstitial infiltrates that progress to a diffuse alveolar pattern (Fig. 349-2). However, PCP has been associated with unilateral disease, focal disease, consolidation, nodules, cavities, pneumothorax, and, rarely, pleural effusions. In up to 30% of patients with HIV infection, the chest radiograph appears normal; in this situation, a computed tomography (CT) scan of the chest, especially high-resolution CT, is invariably abnormal, usually showing a patchy or diffuse ground-glass pattern (see Fig. 349-2).

Arterial oxygenation at rest is often abnormal, although in 30% or more of cases it is within normal limits. Exercise testing induces desaturation and an increase in the alveolar-arterial oxygen (A-a O$_2$) gradient in the majority of patients with PCP, even those with normal oxygenation at rest or a normal chest radiograph. An abnormal resting diffusing capacity is also common. However, although many of these tests have a high sensitivity for PCP, their specificity is poor because other respiratory processes show similar abnormalities. Gallium scans were frequently performed early in the AIDS epidemic, but they are no longer used owing to low specificity and the 2-day delay in diagnosis inherent with this test.

Serologic tests are not helpful in diagnosing PCP. Although antibody titers against recombinant *Pneumocystis* proteins such as major surface glycoprotein may be increased in patients with PCP, such tests have not shown utility for diagnosis in individual patients. Decreased plasma *S*-adenosyl methionine and increased serum β-D-glucan levels have been proposed as diagnostic tests, but to date, there are inadequate data from well-conducted trials to support their use.

Because *Pneumocystis* cannot be cultured, a definitive diagnosis of PCP requires detection of the organism in a pulmonary sample. This can be accomplished by any number of colorimetric or immunologic stains or by molecular techniques. Until the development of anti-*Pneumocystis* monoclonal antibodies in the 1980s, colorimetric stains were routinely used, and they continue to be used at many centers owing to cost considerations. Such stains include Gomori methenamine silver, toluidine blue O, Gram-Weigert, and cresylecht violet, which stain the cyst wall of *Pneumocystis*, as well as Giemsa-type stains, including Diff-Quik, which can stain both trophic forms, the more abundant form of the organism, and intracystic bodies within cysts, but not the cyst wall. *Pneumocystis* can also be detected by calcofluor white, Papanicolaou, periodic acid–Schiff, and, rarely, Gram stain. None of the colorimetric stains are specific for *Pneumocystis*. Cyst wall stains such as Gomori methenamine silver and toluidine blue O can stain other fungi, and Giemsa-type stains also stain background cells and cellular debris. The latter requires substantial expertise for correct interpretation.

Immunofluorescent assays using anti-*Pneumocystis* monoclonal antibodies provide a number of advantages over colorimetric stains. They are specific for *Pneumocystis* and do not show cross-reactivity with other organisms, including fungi; they can be performed and interpreted rapidly; and they have increased sensitivity, especially when examining induced sputum samples (Fig. 349-3).

Molecular techniques, primarily PCR-based assays, have been extensively evaluated for diagnosing PCP. PCR assays are 10- to 100-fold more sensitive than stains for the detection of *Pneumocystis*; this may allow diagnosis using samples such as oral washes, which have a lower organism burden than induced sputum or bronchoalveolar lavage (BAL). This increased sensitivity, however, is associated with decreased specificity, because it allows the detection of organisms in patients ultimately shown not to have PCP. The latter situation presumably reflects colonization or subclinical infection that does not require specific anti-*Pneumocystis* therapy. PCR-based assays are currently not broadly used because of limited availability and the lack of a commercial product with Food and Drug Administration approval.

As detection methods for *Pneumocystis* improved, there was a parallel improvement in sample acquisition. Before the AIDS epidemic, open lung biopsy was required for diagnosis. During the 1980s, bronchoscopy, initially with brushings and biopsy, and subsequently with BAL, was shown to have a greater than 90% sensitivity for diagnosing PCP; BAL continues to be the primary diagnostic modality at many centers today. Although expectorated sputum has a low diagnostic yield, induced sputum, especially when combined with immunofluorescent staining, can have a sensitivity approaching 90%, although in many centers the diagnostic yield is much lower, likely due in part to variability in the methods used for induction and processing. Ideally, sputum induction should be the first step in diagnosis, followed by

FIGURE 349-2. Chest radiographs (A, C, E) and corresponding computed tomography (CT) scans (B, D, F) from three HIV patients diagnosed with laboratory-confirmed *Pneumocystis* pneumonia. Patient 1 presented with no symptoms; had minimal abnormalities on an incidental chest x-ray (A), suggesting an interstitial process; and had focal infiltrates on CT (B). Patient 2 presented with fever and weight loss but no shortness of breath. Pulse oximetry demonstrated 99% saturation at rest, with a decrease to 89% with exercise. Chest x-ray (C) showed bilateral lower lobe infiltrates, and CT (D) showed bilateral lower lobe interstitial infiltrates with patches of ground-glass attenuation. Patient 3 presented with a 2-week history of fever, night sweats, shortness of breath, and weakness. His PaO$_2$ at diagnosis was 67 mm Hg, and his (A-a)O$_2$ gradient was 53 mm Hg. Chest x-ray (E) showed bilateral mid and lower lung field infiltrates, and CT (F) showed bilateral infiltrates with lower lung consolidation.

bronchoscopy with BAL (Fig. 349-4). Bronchoscopic or open lung biopsy is only rarely needed to make the diagnosis.

The differential diagnosis of pulmonary infiltrates in immunosuppressed patients is very broad and includes infections such as adenovirus, cytomegalovirus, tuberculosis, cryptococcosis, histoplasmosis, aspergillosis, and toxoplasmosis, as well as noninfectious processes such as tumor, congestive heart failure, pulmonary emboli, radiation- and chemotherapy-induced pneumonitis, and, especially in HIV-infected patients, nonspecific interstitial pneumonitis and Kaposi's sarcoma.

TREATMENT   Rx

Specific anti-*Pneumocystis* therapy should be initiated promptly when the diagnosis is suspected in a potentially susceptible patient. Dosing regimens with documented efficacy are listed in Table 349-1. Although there are no controlled studies defining the optimal duration of therapy, HIV-infected patients should be treated for 21 days, and non-HIV patients for 14 days. If the patient has moderate to severe disease (PaO$_2$ <70 mm Hg or A-a O$_2$ gradient >35 mm Hg), concomitant corticosteroid therapy should be administered. The diagnosis should be definitively confirmed by sputum induction or

FIGURE 349-3. Immunofluorescent detection of *Pneumocystis* using a direct fluorescent antibody test to examine an induced sputum sample. **A,** Low power (100× original) allows visualization of multiple clusters or organisms staining bright green. **B,** Under high power (400× original), individual organisms can be seen within a single cluster.

FIGURE 349-4. Algorithm for the evaluation of patients with suspected *Pneumocystis* pneumonia (PCP). CT = computed tomography; HIV = human immunodeficiency virus.

bronchoscopy as soon as possible; however, delaying such confirmation for a few days after the initiation of therapy will not decrease the diagnostic yield because organisms can be detected in clinical samples for more than 3 weeks after the initiation of therapy. Empirical therapy in the absence of a confirmed diagnosis runs the risk of delaying appropriate therapy for another infection, giving inappropriate therapy with known toxicities, and performing a definitive procedure such as bronchoscopy when the patient is failing therapy and consequently has more severe pulmonary compromise.

The treatment of choice for PCP or extrapulmonary disease, regardless of severity, is trimethoprim-sulfamethoxazole, which combines inhibitors of two enzymes in the folate synthetic pathway of *Pneumocystis*: sulfamethoxazole, an inhibitor of DHPS, and trimethoprim, an inhibitor of dihydrofolate

TABLE 349-1 DRUG REGIMENS FOR THE TREATMENT OF *PNEUMOCYSTIS* PNEUMONIA

INDICATION	REGIMEN PREFERENCE	DRUG	ROUTE	DOSE*	COMMENTS
Mild PCP: PaO_2 >70 mm Hg or (A-a)O_2 gradient <35 mm Hg	Preferred	TMP-SMX	PO	2 double-strength (160 TMP + 800 SMX) tablets tid	
	Alternative	Trimethoprim + Dapsone	PO PO	5 mg/kg tid (15 mg/kg/day) 100 mg/day	If possible, test for G6PD deficiency before use
	Alternative	Clindamycin + Primaquine	PO PO	450 mg qid or 600 mg tid 30 mg/day (base)	If possible, test for G6PD deficiency before use
	Alternative	Atovaquone	PO	750 mg bid with food	
Moderate to severe PCP: PaO_2 <70 mm Hg or (A-a)O_2 gradient >35 mm Hg†	Preferred	TMP-SMX	IV†	TMP 5 mg/kg and SMX 25 mg/kg	May switch to oral therapy following clinical improvement
	Alternative	Pentamidine	IV	3-4 mg/kg/day	Infuse over >60 min
	Alternative	Clindamycin +	IV	600 mg q6h or 900 mg q8h	May switch to oral therapy following clinical improvement
		Primaquine	PO	30 mg/day (base)	No parenteral formulation is available
Adjunctive therapy for moderate to severe PCP: PaO_2 <70 mm Hg or (A-a)O_2 gradient >35 mm Hg	Preferred	Prednisone	PO	40 mg bid on days 1-5; 40 mg/day on days 6-10; 20 mg/day on days 11-21	Begin as early as possible and within 72 hr; efficacy has not been demonstrated if started later
	Preferred	Methylprednisolone	IV	30 mg bid on days 1-5; 30 mg/day on days 6-10; 15 mg/day on days 11-21	Use if parenteral therapy is necessary

*HIV-infected patients should receive 21 days of therapy; non–HIV-infected patients should receive 14 days of therapy.
†Moderate PCP ([A-a]O_2 gradient 35-45 mm Hg) can be treated with an oral regimen.
(A-a)O_2 gradient = alveolar-arterial oxygen gradient; G6PD = glucose-6-phosphate dehydrogenase; PaO_2 = arterial partial pressure of oxygen; PCP = *Pneumocystis* pneumonia; SMX = sulfamethoxazole; TMP = trimethoprim.

reductase (DHFR). Trimethoprim-sulfamethoxazole is available in both oral and intravenous formulations. Oral therapy should be reserved for patients with mild to moderate disease in whom poor absorption is not a concern. Outpatient therapy should be reserved for patients with mild to moderate disease who will reliably return for follow-up.

The efficacy of trimethoprim-sulfamethoxazole for both the treatment and the prevention of PCP was first demonstrated in a pediatric cancer population in the 1970s; it has been the first-line therapy since then, when the only alternative was pentamidine. The high incidence of PCP during the early years of the AIDS epidemic led to the identification of a number of new agents with anti-*Pneumocystis* activity, and these were extensively evaluated in randomized controlled trials, primarily in HIV-infected patients. In patients with mild to moderate disease (A-a O_2 gradient <45 mm Hg), trimethoprim-sulfamethoxazole has superior efficacy compared with atovaquone and similar efficacy compared with trimethoprim-dapsone and clindamycin-primaquine. In patients with moderate to severe disease (A-a O_2 gradient >30 mm Hg), it showed superior efficacy to trimetrexate, a potent inhibitor of *Pneumocystis* DHFR that is approved for the treatment of PCP but is no longer commercially available. In smaller, lower-powered studies, trimethoprim-sulfamethoxazole and pentamidine showed similar efficacy.

The major toxicities associated with trimethoprim-sulfamethoxazole include fever, rash, neutropenia, thrombocytopenia, nausea, vomiting, and transaminase elevations. Hyperkalemia and crystalluria have also been reported, and hyponatremia is seen primarily in association with intravenous administration. Toxicities usually appear after the first week of therapy. Toxicities are much more common in HIV-infected patients, occurring in about 50 to 60%; 15 to 35% of these patients discontinue therapy because of these adverse events. Although folinic acid can decrease the toxicities associated with some DHFR inhibitors such as pyrimethamine, it should not be administered with trimethoprim-sulfamethoxazole; in one placebo-controlled trial, it did not decrease side effects but was associated with an increased risk of therapeutic failure and death.

Alternative regimens for patients with mild to moderate disease include trimethoprim-dapsone, clindamycin-primaquine, and atovaquone. Like sulfamethoxazole, dapsone is an inhibitor of *Pneumocystis* DHPS. Adverse reactions to trimethoprim-dapsone include rash, fever, nausea and vomiting, transaminase elevations, methemoglobinemia, anemia, and mild hyperkalemia. Approximately 20 to 30% of patients with adverse reactions to trimethoprim-sulfamethoxazole experience adverse reactions to trimethoprim-dapsone. Toxicities associated with clindamycin-primaquine include fever, rash, diarrhea, anemia, neutropenia, transaminase elevations, and methemoglobinemia. For both dapsone and primaquine and, to a lesser extent, sulfamethoxazole, glucose-6-phosphate dehydrogenase deficiency (Chapter 164) can increase the risk of hemolytic anemia and methemoglobinemia. In a randomized trial comparing trimethoprim-sulfamethoxazole, trimethoprim-dapsone, and

clindamycin-primaquine in 181 HIV-infected patients with mild to moderate disease, response rates and toxicities were similar among the three arms, with an overall therapeutic failure rate of 9% by day 21 and a dose-limiting toxicity rate of 31%. Serious transaminase elevations were more common in the trimethoprim-sulfamethoxazole group, and serious hematologic toxicities were more common in the clindamycin-primaquine group.

Atovaquone is a hydroxynaphthoquinone with activity against *Toxoplasma* and malaria as well as *Pneumocystis*. Atovaquone (tablet formulation) was less effective than trimethoprim-sulfamethoxazole in a randomized trial in HIV-infected patients with mild to moderate disease and showed a trend toward lesser efficacy when compared with pentamidine in another study. Low serum atovaquone levels as well as preexisting diarrhea were associated with therapeutic failure. The current formulation is a suspension that has approximately 50% greater bioavailability than the tablet formulation, which may result in improved responses. Atovaquone should be taken with food because this increases its bioavailability, and it should be avoided in patients with potentially decreased gastrointestinal absorption (e.g., diarrhea). Toxicities of atovaquone include rash, fever, transaminase elevations, nausea, vomiting, diarrhea, neutropenia, and anemia.

Therapeutic alternatives to trimethoprim-sulfamethoxazole for patients with disease requiring parenteral therapy are limited to clindamycin-primaquine (but only clindamycin is available for intravenous administration) and pentamidine. Caspofungin and other echinocandins, which are β-1,3-glucan synthase inhibitors, cannot be recommended because there have been no clinical trials documenting their efficacy; β-1,3-glucan is present in the cyst but not in the trophic form of the organism.

Pentamidine was the first drug demonstrated to have anti-*Pneumocystis* activity. Available data suggest that trimethoprim-sulfamethoxazole and pentamidine have similar efficacy; trimethoprim-sulfamethoxazole is the preferred regimen because the toxicities associated with pentamidine are more frequent and potentially more severe. Intravenous pentamidine was originally associated with severe hypotension, but a slow (>1 hour) infusion is usually well tolerated. Intramuscular administration is associated with a high frequency of sterile abscesses at the injection site. Toxicities associated with pentamidine, which occur in about 50 to 60% of patients and frequently result in discontinuation of the drug, include nephrotoxicity, hypoglycemia, hyperglycemia, fever, neutropenia, thrombocytopenia, hypotension, hyperkalemia, transaminase elevations, and pancreatitis. Hypoglycemia may be life-threatening and may precede the development of hyperglycemia; hyperglycemia may be irreversible. Torsades de pointes (Chapter 65) has also rarely been reported.

Adjunctive Corticosteroid Therapy

Initiation of specific anti-*Pneumocystis* therapy is associated with a deterioration in oxygenation after approximately 3 to 4 days; this likely results from a host inflammatory response to organisms damaged by therapy. Randomized controlled trials have demonstrated that the early addition of corticosteroids to specific anti-*Pneumocystis* therapy in HIV-infected patients can prevent this deterioration and improve survival, without a significant increase in opportunistic complications other than localized herpes simplex infection. In the largest such study, corticosteroid therapy was associated with a 50% decrease in respiratory failure and mortality; this benefit was limited to patients with moderate to severe disease (E-Fig. 349-1). For HIV-infected patients, corticosteroids and specific anti-*Pneumocystis* therapy should be started at the same time; the addition of corticosteroids after 72 hours has shown no benefit, although it is reasonable to add them if patients exhibit deterioration after this time. Although the optimal regimen has not been defined by controlled trials, the tapering regimen from the largest study is most commonly used (see Table 349-1).

Data from controlled trials examining the benefit of corticosteroids are not available for non-HIV patients, who are often already taking corticosteroids, possibly at tapering doses, at the time of PCP diagnosis. One retrospective analysis of 31 such patients suggested that increasing corticosteroids to a prednisone equivalent of 60 mg/day or more was associated with clinical benefit. It is reasonable to administer corticosteroids to non-HIV patients with moderate or severe disease using the same regimen as for HIV-infected patients; for patients already taking corticosteroids at lower doses, the dosage can be increased to those levels.

Initiation of Antiretroviral Therapy

Given that many patients with HIV infection who are diagnosed with PCP are not receiving antiretroviral therapy, an important issue is how soon to start HAART after a diagnosis of PCP. Retrospective and prospective studies have suggested that, in general, it is safe to initiate HAART while patients are being treated for PCP, and early HAART may be associated with an improved outcome. In a randomized trial that examined early versus late initiation of HAART in patients with acute opportunistic infections, 63% of whom had PCP, the early initiation arm (HAART started a median of 12 days after starting therapy for the opportunistic infection) had a decreased rate of AIDS progression or death. Similar findings for tuberculosis in developing countries have emphasized the benefit of early initiation of HAART.

Major concerns about initiating HAART include the risk of adverse drug reactions, which may be confused with adverse reactions to anti-PCP therapy; the risk of overlapping toxicities, which may complicate management; and the risk of immune reconstitution. There are several reports describing apparent immune reconstitution syndrome (Chapter 402), which can be life-threatening, in patients who started HAART soon after being diagnosed with PCP. Thus, many clinicians initiate HAART during or immediately after completion of anti-*Pneumocystis* therapy, assuming the patient has shown clinical improvement, is able to tolerate oral medications, and accepts the commitment to lifelong therapy. However, the parameters for such an approach are difficult to precisely define. Patients who start HAART early should be closely monitored for a recurrence of symptoms that may represent immune reconstitution.

Treatment Failure

The optimal approach to the management of patients who are failing therapy has not been well defined. In patients with progressive respiratory deterioration, it is critical that the diagnosis of PCP be confirmed rather than presumptive and that other concurrent processes (e.g., other infections, congestive heart failure, pulmonary emboli) have been ruled out; bronchoscopy should be considered to facilitate these determinations. Parenteral therapy should be used to eliminate absorption concerns, and corticosteroid medications should be added if this has not already been done. Because patients who will ultimately respond can show clinical deterioration at 3 to 4 days, as noted earlier, it is reasonable to wait 5 to 8 days before considering a change in drug therapy.

Only trimethoprim-sulfamethoxazole and pentamidine are available in parenteral formulations. Parenteral clindamycin is available, but primaquine is available only as a tablet. No randomized trials have examined the relative efficacy of these agents in patients who are failing therapy. For patients who have not received trimethoprim-sulfamethoxazole, this should be the first choice as an alternative agent, assuming the patient did not have a life-threatening adverse reaction previously. Rapid desensitization (similar to penicillin desensitization), ideally in consultation with an allergy specialist, can be considered in patients with prior adverse reactions; however, patients with a history of Stevens-Johnson syndrome or toxic epidermal necrolysis should not be rechallenged. Although meta-analyses have found that clindamycin-primaquine is superior to pentamidine in patients failing a first-line regimen, there are potential biases in such analyses (e.g., severity of illness may have affected the choice of salvage regimen). There are no data to recommend switching to an alternative agent rather than adding an alternative agent (if toxicity is not an issue); both approaches have been used.

Resistance

Although *Pneumocystis* cannot be cultured, molecular studies have identified mutations in genes that are the targets of anti-*Pneumocystis* therapy, and

these mutations appear to represent the development of resistance by *Pneumocystis* to these agents. The best-characterized mutations have been identified in the DHPS gene of *Pneumocystis*, which is the target of sulfamethoxazole and dapsone. Two mutations at the active site of this enzyme, which can occur either individually or together, have been identified with greater frequency in patients receiving trimethoprim-sulfamethoxazole or dapsone for prophylaxis; in vitro studies suggest that these mutations confer resistance. The clinical relevance of these mutations remains uncertain; some studies have found worse outcomes in patients with these mutations, but others have found no such association. Most patients in whom these mutations were identified retrospectively were successfully treated with sulfa-containing drugs. In contrast to DHPS, there are very limited reports suggesting that the DHFR gene of *Pneumocystis*, which is the target of trimethoprim and pyrimethamine, has developed potential drug-resistant mutations.

Atovaquone presumably binds to the mitochondrial BC_1 complex of *Pneumocystis* and thus inhibits electron transport. Multiple mutations have been identified in the cytochrome B gene of *Pneumocystis*, which presumably represent resistance in patients receiving atovaquone for prophylaxis; these mutations have not, however, been associated with clinical outcome.

Because the presence of these mutations has not been definitively associated with worsening prognosis, clinical decisions should not be based on their identification. Methods for detecting these mutations are not readily available, and their presence should remain a research tool until their clinical relevance can be better defined.

PREVENTION

Although *Pneumocystis* is transmitted by the airborne route, the organism appears to be ubiquitous, making avoidance of exposure difficult. In animal models, it takes 2 to 3 months following exposure to develop a heavy infection. If the pattern of growth is similar in humans, clinical symptoms would develop only months after exposure to a source that is likely unknown. Currently, respiratory isolation of patients with active PCP is not required, although it is reasonable to avoid having a susceptible patient share a room with a PCP patient. Recent outbreaks in renal transplant patients strongly suggest a common source of infection; a better understanding of the patterns of transmission in these settings may lead to improved guidelines for preventing the spread of infection.

A major advance in the management of patients at risk for the development of PCP was the demonstration that trimethoprim-sulfamethoxazole was highly effective in preventing the disease in a susceptible pediatric population. Subsequent studies, primarily in HIV-infected patients, demonstrated that additional drug regimens were also effective. This has led to the broad use of anti-*Pneumocystis* prophylaxis in a wide range of susceptible populations.

Two important issues in administering prophylaxis are identifying populations at risk and defining the period of risk during which prophylaxis should be provided. AIDS patients are at especially high risk; before the use of prophylaxis or HAART, the lifetime incidence of PCP in this population was estimated at 60 to 80%. The most recent CD4 count is a validated surrogate marker for HIV-infected patients: patients with CD4 counts below 200 cells/mm³ are at substantially increased risk for developing PCP, and prophylaxis is recommended for this group. Although 10 to 15% of patients who develop PCP have higher CD4 counts, the incidence is very low in this population, given the large number of patients who fall in this category. Patients with CD4 counts greater than 200 cells/mm³ but a CD4 percentage of less than 14% or a history of an AIDS-defining illness are also candidates for prophylaxis. For pediatric patients with HIV infection, in whom the normal CD4 count changes with age, guidelines are based on age. Prophylaxis is recommended for children older than 6 years with CD4 counts below 200 cells/mm³ or 15%, for children between 1 and 5 years old with CD4 counts below 500 cells/mm³ or 15%, and for all children younger than 12 months.

Before the availability of HAART, once patients with HIV infection initiated prophylaxis, they were committed to continuing it for life because immunologic decline was irreversible. With HAART, however, control of HIV replication leads to an increase in the CD4 count, which is associated with a concomitant decrease in the risk of developing PCP. Multiple studies have shown that once the CD4 count has been above 200 cells/mm³ for at least 3 months (ideally in the setting of controlled HIV replication), prophylaxis can be safely discontinued because the risk of developing PCP is no greater than in patients whose CD4 counts never fell below 200 cells/mm³. In most of these studies, the median CD4 count was greater than 300 cells/mm³, and HIV viral loads were below detection limits in the majority of

TABLE 349-2 DRUG REGIMENS FOR THE PREVENTION OF *PNEUMOCYSTIS* PNEUMONIA

REGIMEN PREFERENCE	DRUG	ROUTE	DOSE	COMMENTS
Preferred	TMP-SMX	PO	1 double-strength tablet (160 mg TMP + 800 mg SMX) or 1 single-strength tablet (80 mg TMP + 400 mg SMX) daily	Also active in preventing toxoplasmosis
Alternative	TMP-SMX	PO	1 double-strength tablet (160 mg TMP + 800 mg SMX) 3 times/wk	Also active in preventing toxoplasmosis
Alternative	Dapsone	PO	100 mg/day or 50 mg bid	Test for G6PD deficiency before use
Alternative	Dapsone +	PO	50 mg/day	Also active in preventing toxoplasmosis
	Pyrimethamine +	PO	50 mg once weekly	
	Leucovorin	PO	25 mg once weekly	Should be administered with pyrimethamine to minimize toxicity
Alternative	Atovaquone	PO	1500 mg/day with food	Likely active in preventing toxoplasmosis
Alternative	Pentamidine	Aerosol	300 mg via Respirgard II nebulizer once monthly	Not active in preventing toxoplasmosis

Patients receiving pyrimethamine-sulfadiazine and atovaquone therapy for toxoplasmosis do not appear to need additional prophylaxis for PCP; patients receiving clindamycin-pyrimethamine therapy for toxoplasmosis need additional prophylaxis for PCP.

G6PD = glucose-6-phosphate dehydrogenase; SMX = sulfamethoxazole; TMP = trimethoprim.

patients. Recent uncontrolled studies have suggested that prophylaxis can also be safely discontinued in patients with CD4 counts between 100 and 200 cells/mm^3 who have virologically suppressed HIV, but specific criteria for discontinuation (e.g., duration of viral suppression) were not defined in these studies.

Among non–HIV-infected patients, the CD4 count is not routinely measured, and it has not been shown to have the same predictive value for the development of PCP as in HIV-infected patients; however, CD4 counts below 200 cells/mm^3 do appear to increase their susceptibility. Recommendations for PCP prophylaxis in these populations are based on clinical parameters, including empirical identification of periods of risk and estimation of levels of immunosuppression. Very broad prophylaxis has not been implemented because of the side effects associated with these regimens; for example, there is concern that trimethoprim-sulfamethoxazole might cause bone marrow suppression that would interfere with engraftment or cause nephrotoxicity that would damage a transplanted kidney.

Risk factors for non–HIV-infected patients include underlying disease, use of immunosuppressive drugs, radiation therapy, graft-versus-host disease, and concomitant cytomegalovirus infection (Chapter 384). Patients with malignancies, especially hematologic malignancies, but increasingly solid tumors as well, are at risk for PCP primarily owing to the therapies they receive; the incidence can range from 1 to 43% in the absence of prophylaxis and is highly dependent on the intensity and duration of immunosuppression. In the absence of prophylaxis, the risk of developing PCP in transplant patients, whether hematopoietic stem cell or solid organ transplants, is reportedly about 5 to 15%, although lung and heart-lung transplant patients appear to have a higher incidence (up to 43%). Among patients with collagen vascular disease, the reported risk is less than 2% without prophylaxis, although patients with Wegener's granulomatosis (Chapter 278) reportedly have a risk up to 12%, presumably because of the use of more immunosuppressive treatment regimens. The current risk of developing PCP in non-HIV populations is difficult to quantify because of the widespread use of prophylaxis and because immunosuppressive regimens are evolving.

To facilitate the management of prophylaxis in at-risk populations, a number of guidelines have been developed by expert panels who have made recommendations based on the strength of the available data. HIV guidelines have already been summarized. For allogeneic stem cell transplant recipients, prophylaxis is recommended from the time of engraftment to at least 6 months after transplantation, and longer for patients who continue receiving immunosuppressive therapy or who have chronic graft-versus-host disease. For autologous stem cell transplant recipients, who have a lower risk of PCP, prophylaxis for 3 to 6 months should be considered if the degree of immunosuppression is substantial owing to underlying disease or therapy (e.g., patients with leukemia or lymphoma receiving intensive conditioning or immunosuppressive therapy).

For solid organ transplant patients, prophylaxis has not been universally adopted; it has been used primarily in centers with a known incidence greater than 3%. Guidelines recommend the administration of prophylaxis for 3 to 12 months in renal transplant patients and for longer periods, up to lifelong, in heart, lung, liver, and intestine transplant recipients. As noted earlier, a number of outbreaks of PCP have recently been reported in renal transplant centers, and many of those patients developed disease more than 1 year after transplantation. Changes in immunosuppressive therapy may have contributed to this apparent increase in incidence, given that some of these centers had seen very few cases in prior years.

For patients with inflammatory bowel disease (Chapter 143), who appear to be at increased risk as newer immunosuppressive agents are used, data are limited; however, consensus-based guidelines recommend prophylaxis for patients receiving triple immunomodulators that include either a calcineurin inhibitor or an anti–tumor necrosis factor agent. No consensus was reached for less intensive regimens. For patients with connective tissue disorders or vasculitis, there are currently no consensus guidelines.

Corticosteroid therapy (Chapter 34) is a well-described risk factor in non–HIV-infected patients, with approximately 90% of patients receiving such therapy before developing PCP in some studies. Higher dose and longer duration increase the risk. Not all patients who receive corticosteroids are at risk, however; for instance, asthmatics receiving corticosteroid therapy are at low risk. Although there are no consensus guidelines on the use of prophylaxis for patients receiving corticosteroids, one reasonable approach is to provide prophylaxis to patients with an underlying immunosuppressive or inflammatory disease who receive at least 20 mg of prednisone or equivalent for longer than 1 month. Other immunosuppressive agents (Chapter 34), such as calcineurin inhibitors, sirolimus, tumor necrosis factor antagonists, and rituximab, also appear to increase the risk of developing PCP, primarily in the patient populations noted earlier.

Trimethoprim-sulfamethoxazole is the first-line agent for prophylaxis in all populations (Table 349-2). Alternatives include dapsone alone or combined with pyrimethamine plus leucovorin, atovaquone, and aerosol pentamidine administered by the Respirgard II nebulizer. In a randomized trial of HIV-infected patients comparing trimethoprim-sulfamethoxazole with dapsone and aerosol pentamidine, no significant differences were seen on an intent-to-treat basis, but the lowest failure rates were seen while patients were receiving trimethoprim-sulfamethoxazole. Conversely, trimethoprim-sulfamethoxazole was superior to aerosol pentamidine in another randomized study. In other large randomized trials in HIV-infected patients, the following regimens showed similar efficacy: atovaquone suspension and dapsone, atovaquone suspension and aerosol pentamidine, and dapsone-pyrimethamine and aerosol pentamidine. No randomized trials of these regimens have been conducted in non–HIV-infected populations, but clinical experience suggests that they are effective in these populations as well.

Although the combination of sulfadoxine and pyrimethamine is also efficacious, it is contraindicated in patients with sulfonamide allergies. Moreover, because Stevens-Johnson syndrome and other potentially life-threatening cutaneous reactions are more common with this combination than with trimethoprim-sulfamethoxazole, and because its long half-life results in slow clearance after the drug is discontinued, sulfadoxine plus pyrimethamine should probably not be used in sulfa-tolerant patients if trimethoprim-sulfamethoxazole is available.

HIV-infected patients with a prior history of a mild sulfa allergy (e.g., mild rash, excluding those with prior Stevens-Johnson syndrome or toxic epidermal necrolysis) can often be safely rechallenged with trimethoprim-sulfamethoxazole. Randomized trials have demonstrated that dose escalation over a 6- to 13-day period is associated with better tolerance than direct rechallenge with full-dose trimethoprim-sulfamethoxazole, and that up to 75% of patients can continue to receive trimethoprim-sulfamethoxazole for at least 6 months.[1,2]

PROGNOSIS

Mortality for untreated PCP approaches 100%. With therapy, the survival rate for HIV-infected patients with confirmed PCP is 80 to 90%; a poorer survival rate of 50 to 60% has been reported in patients without HIV infection. Risk factors for death in HIV-infected patients include greater hypoxia, older age, recurrent episodes of PCP, low hemoglobin, and presence of comorbid conditions. Although mortality for patients admitted to an intensive care unit is high, survival for HIV-infected patients has improved in recent years, approaching 50%.

Visit expertconsult.com for e-expanded chapter

1. Leoung GS, Stanford JF, Giordano MF, et al. Trimethoprim-sulfamethoxazole (TMP-SMZ) dose escalation versus direct rechallenge for *Pneumocystis carinii* pneumonia prophylaxis in human immunodeficiency virus-infected patients with previous adverse reaction to TMP-SMZ. *J Infect Dis.* 2001;184:992-997.
2. Para MF, Finkelstein D, Becker S, et al. Reduced toxicity with gradual initiation of trimethoprim-sulfamethoxazole as primary prophylaxis for *Pneumocystis carinii* pneumonia: AIDS Clinical Trials Group 268. *J Acquir Immune Defic Syndr.* 2000;24:337-343.

SUGGESTED READINGS

Beck JM, Cushion MT. *Pneumocystis* workshop: 10th anniversary summary. *Eukaryot Cell.* 2009;8:446-460. *Provides a summary of current research presented at a conference focusing on Pneumocystis.*

Eitner F, Hauser IA, Rettkowski O, et al. Risk factors for *Pneumocystis jirovecii* pneumonia (PcP) in renal transplant recipients. *Nephrol Dial Transplant.* 2011. [Epub ahead of print.] *Patients treated with intensified immunosuppression were at highest risk, and the overall case-fatality rate was 27%.*

Kelley CF, Checkley W, Mannino DM, et al. Trends in hospitalizations for AIDS-associated *Pneumocystis jirovecii* pneumonia in the United States (1986 to 2005). *Chest.* 2009;136:190-197. *Reports the frequency and outcome of hospitalized HIV-infected patients with PCP.*

Opportunistic Infections Project Team of the Collaboration of Observation HIV Epidemiological Research in Europe (COHERE), Mocroft A, Reiss P, et al. Is it safe to discontinue primary *Pneumocystis jiroveci* pneumonia prophylaxis in patients with virologically suppressed HIV infection and a CD4 cell count <200 cells/microL? *Clin Infect Dis.* 2010;51:611-619. *Suggests that discontinuation of prophylaxis may be safe in patients with CD4 counts of 101 to 200 cells/μL and suppressed viral load.*

Zolopa A, Andersen J, Powderly W, et al. Early antiretroviral therapy reduces AIDS progression/death in individuals with acute opportunistic infections: a multicenter randomized strategy trial. *PLoS One.* 2009;4:e5575. *Demonstrates a decrease in AIDS progression and death in patients with an acute opportunistic infection (63% with PCP) who initiated HAART therapy soon after diagnosis of the opportunistic infection.*

MYCETOMA

DIMITRIOS P. KONTOYIANNIS

DEFINITION

Mycetoma (a tumor produced by fungi) was first described in 1842 in the Madura district of India, hence the terms "Madura foot," "maduromycosis," and "maduromycetoma." Mycetoma is a chronic, slowly progressive infection of diverse etiology that starts in subcutaneous tissue and spreads across tissue planes to contiguous structures. The offending organism is inoculated into subcutaneous tissue by trauma that typically involves soil contaminated with pathogens. The hallmarks of mycetoma are the presence of "grains" that consist of colonies of the infectious organism and chronically draining sinus tracts. (The term *pulmonary mycetoma* is used inappropriately to describe the fungus balls typically caused by *Aspergillus* species that colonize a preexisting lung cavity; the term *aspergilloma* [Chapter 347] is more appropriate for this

entity, the pathogenesis of which is distinctly different from that of true mycetoma.)

The Pathogens

Two groups of soil-inhabiting pathogens, each of which accounts for approximately 50% of cases, cause mycetoma: (1) filamentous aerobic actinomycetes (Chapter 337), hence the term *actinomycetoma*, and (2) a wide range of saprophytic soil and woody plant fungi, hence the term *eumycetoma*.

A variety of *Nocardia* species (e.g., *Nocardia brasiliensis, Nocardia asteroides*), *Actinomadura* species (e.g., *Actinomadura pelletieri, Actinomadura madurae*), and *Streptomyces* species (e.g., *Streptomyces somaliensis*) have been reported to cause actinomycetoma. Even more numerous are the agents that cause eumycetoma, such as *Madurella* species, probably the most prevalent mycetoma-causing fungal species worldwide (e.g., *Madurella mycetomatis* causes 70% of all cases of eumycetoma), as well as *Fusarium* species, *Acremonium* species, *Pseudallescheria boydii, Exophiala* species, and *Curvularia* species. There is controversy about whether the various dermatophytes and *Aspergillus* species can cause mycetoma. Eumycetoma is often further characterized on the basis of the color of the grains; specifically, white to yellow grain mycetomas (white piedra) are typically caused by hyalohyphomycetes (e.g., *P. boydii, Fusarium* species, *Acremonium* species), and black grain eumycetomas (black piedra) are caused by *Madurella* species and other less common fungi. However, the geographic distribution of the fungi that cause black grain eumycetoma is variable.

EPIDEMIOLOGY

Although mycetoma has a broad worldwide distribution, it occurs primarily in the tropical and, to a lesser extent, the temperate zones. More specifically, the infection is quite prevalent in India, Mexico, Central America, South America, the Middle East, and especially sub-Saharan Africa (the "mycetoma belt"); Sudan in particular has a high burden of mycetoma. Indigenously acquired mycetoma is sporadic in North America and Europe. However, the globalization of tourism and the increase in immigration from countries with a high endemicity of mycetoma to Western countries necessitates awareness of this entity, even in the developed world.

The relative frequency of actinomycetoma and eumycetoma differs among geographic areas, with eumycetoma being more common in India and Africa and actinomycetoma more common in Latin America. Furthermore, the causative agents of mycetoma differ in their geographic distribution, as shown in Figure 350-1. The recent development of molecular typing procedures such as polymerase chain reaction and restriction fragment length polymorphism holds promise in expanding our knowledge on the environmental sources and pathogenesis of some agents of eumycetoma such as *M. mycetomatis*.

PATHOGENESIS

Local trauma (e.g., wood splinters) introduces a mycetoma-causing organism into the skin and subcutaneous tissue and initiates a chain of events that lead to chronic, suppurative granulomatous inflammation, tumefaction, formation of multiple fistulous tracts and sinuses, deep abscesses, fibrosis and scar formation, and extension to adjacent connective tissue across the lines of least resistance (fascia) and ultimately to bones, muscles, nerves, and tendon sheaths, thereby leading to gross anatomic distortion of the affected site. In addition, a chronic suppurative granuloma featuring reactive fibrosis and grains (sclerotia), which is a matrix consisting of vegetative aggregates of the etiologic agents and host-derived inflammatory response, is characteristic of mycetoma in histologic sections. This infection is not contagious, however. There may be differences in host susceptibility inasmuch as some affected persons have impaired or delayed hypersensitivity reactions. However mycetoma does not appear to be more common in immunocompromised hosts.

CLINICAL MANIFESTATIONS AND NATURAL HISTORY

The clinical manifestations and natural history of mycetoma are variable and, to some degree, related to the pathogenic agent involved. For example, the progression of eumycetoma tends to be slower than that of actinomycetoma. In addition, eumycetoma lesions tend to be more confined and have less inflammation and fewer granulomas and fistulas but more fibrosis than actinomycetoma lesions do. Furthermore, male mycetoma patients predominate over female patients (5:1), and the disease is typically seen in rural areas and in persons susceptible to local trauma and contamination from soil (e.g., thorns). Hence, farmers, gardeners, wood cutters, herders, and people who work outside while barefoot are more susceptible to this infection. Not

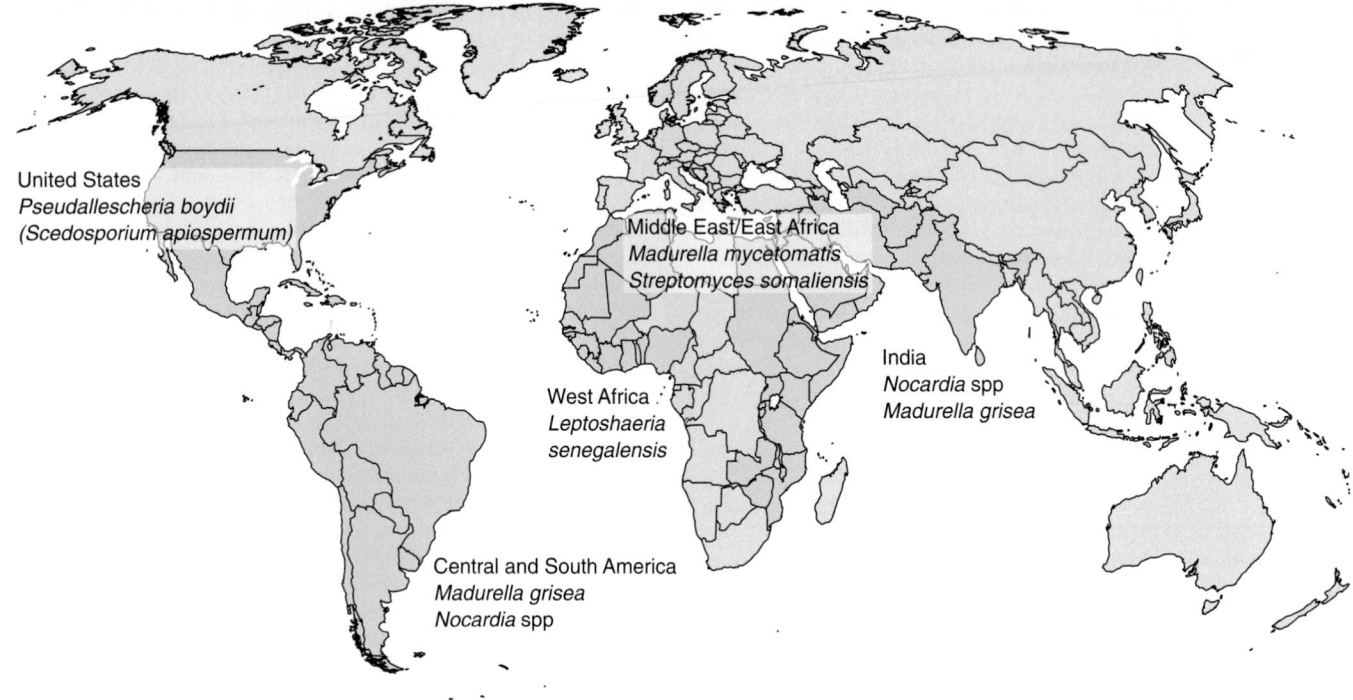

FIGURE 350-1. Predominant agents of mycetoma according to region.

FIGURE 350-2. Madura foot. A 40-year-old farmer from rural Venezuela with a 10-year history of foot edema and slowly progressive deformity following an injury caused by being struck by a hammer exhibited chronic crusted plaques, multiple confluent tender abscesses with fistulization, and release of black grains. The range of motion of the patient's ankle and foot joints was limited, but the joints were not painful. (Courtesy Dr. M. Mendoza, Instituto De Biomedicina, Laboratorio de Micología, San Jose Caracas, Venezuela.)

surprisingly, the foot is the most common site involved in mycetoma (Fig. 350-2), but any other part of the body, such as the hands, thighs, torso, and back of the head, may become involved. Location is typically solitary. Painless nodular or papular swelling (or both) is the most common early manifestation of mycetoma, which is followed by a slow evolution to painless, fixed woody induration. This infection typically runs a chronic, relentless course, sometimes spanning several decades. It is characterized by recurring, vicious cycles of suppuration, draining sinuses, bacterial superinfection, and scar formation. Old sinuses may close up, but new ones may occur, and satellite lesions may be seen. Constitutional symptoms are surprisingly rare. In particular, the presence of fever indicates bacterial superinfection. Bone involvement mimicking clinically chronic osteomyelitis with osteolytic cavitary bone lesions, periosteal reaction or sclerosis (seen on radiographs, computed tomography [CT], or magnetic resonance imaging [MRI]), and osteoporosis may occur; such involvement can be substantial. However, pathologic fractures are rare. In addition, because nerves are relatively spared from involvement, neuropathic manifestations are uncommon. Inexorable limb deformity and misuse because of destruction of deeper tissues may be seen in chronic, refractory, and advanced cases. Finally, because mycetoma does not spread

hematogenously, visceral dissemination is not seen. However, because lymphatic spread may occur (typical incidence of 1 to 3% but more common with actinomycetoma and especially after surgery), regional lymphadenitis may develop.

DIAGNOSIS

Mycetoma, especially in its advanced forms, has rather characteristic findings. The classic triad of painless soft tissue swelling, draining sinus tracts, and extrusion of grains facilitates diagnosis with a high degree of accuracy, especially in endemic areas. For instance, the macroscopic and microscopic appearance of grains in pus-filled draining sinuses frequently allows presumptive diagnosis of the offending pathogen. However, basing the diagnosis on the presence of grains in tissue may be difficult because these grains might be composed of dead organisms. Furthermore, the grains may be contaminated by surface bacteria or fungi. Therefore, a deep tissue biopsy specimen is ideal for staining with hematoxylin and eosin, and appropriate selective bacterial and fungal cultures and stains are preferable for primary detection. Alternatively, aspiration of grains from unopened sinus tracts might provide material for culture.

The culture should be maintained for several weeks because some of the causative agents of mycetoma (e.g., *Nocardia* and *Streptomyces* spp) are slow growing and might take 4 to 6 weeks for growth. Histopathology differentiates eumycetoma from actinomycetoma; however, the multitude of fungi causing eumycetoma necessitates culture identification as agents of eumycetoma might respond differently to antifungal agents. Similarly, cross-reactivity, lack of standardization, and the many agents causing eumycetoma limit the practical value of serologic evaluation.

Differential Diagnosis

The specific manifestations of mycetoma are sometimes confused with those of other rare entities. For example, mycetoma must occasionally be distinguished from chronic cutaneous fungal infections such as sporotrichosis (mycetomatous lymphatic sporotrichosis) and dermatophytic mycetoma. The latter infection, which is typically seen in Africans and sometimes called pseudomycetoma, is a painless granulomatous induration of the skin and subcutaneous tissues caused by ringworm that may be associated with grains consisting of fungi. However, unlike mycetoma, dermatophytic mycetoma is confined to the skin and subcutaneous tissue and does not spread to fasciae or bone. Similarly, chronic severe botryomycosis (typically caused by gram-positive cocci) with purulent exudates, grains, and draining sinus tracts may be confused with mycetoma; however, the presence of visceral dissemination supports a diagnosis of (severe) botryomycosis. Actinomycosis, which is caused by endogenous microaerophilic actinomycetes (part of the normal mucosal flora), also has a propensity for grains and the formation of draining sinus tracts, but unlike mycetoma, its location (neck, chest, pelvis) is rather characteristic. In addition, differentiation between mycetomas with bone involvement and chronic osteomyelitis or osseous tumors may be difficult. Ultrasonography has been used to reliably differentiate mycetoma from either tumor or osteomyelitis. The dot-in-circles sign seen on MRI (tiny hypodense foci, believed to be grains, within hyperintense spherical lesions, believed to be granulomas scattered by areas of fibrosis) might provide an early and specific diagnostic clue for mycetoma. Finally, in cases of mycetoma without draining sinus tracts, benign or malignant skin tumors, chronic granulomatous lesions (e.g., thorn granuloma, cutaneous tuberculosis), chromomycosis, and verrucous leishmaniasis are diagnoses that should be excluded. Unfortunately, delay in specific diagnosis by many months or even years is not uncommon, even in highly endemic areas.

prevent it should be made. Prompt recognition for early curative chemotherapy or surgery (or both) could lead to a better outcome of this difficult-to-manage, chronic infection.

SUGGESTED READINGS

Abd El-Bagi ME, Fahal AH. Mycetoma revisited. Incidence of various radiological signs. *Saudi Med J.* 2009;30:529-533. *A retrospective study of 516 randomly selected mycetoma patients in Sudan to describe the associated radiologic signs.*

Ameen M, Arenas R. Developments in the management of mycetomas. *Clin Exp Dermatol.* 2009;34:1-7. *Review.*

van de Sande WW, Fahal AH, Bakker-Woudenberg IA, et al. *Madurella mycetomatis* is not susceptible to the echinocandin class of antifungal agents. *Antimicrob Agents Chemother.* 2010;54:2738-2740. *Madurella mycetomatis, which typically is treated surgically and with high doses of ketoconazole, was resistant to caspofungin, anidulafungin, and micafungin.*

TREATMENT Rx

Therapy for mycetoma should be individualized. Optimal management has not been well defined, however, because the literature consists of rather heterogeneous and uncontrolled small studies. No single agent is effective against all causative agents of mycetoma. Hence, successful treatment necessitates a reliable diagnosis, differentiation between actinomycetoma and eumycetoma, assessment of the extent of the lesion, and identification of the causative agent. Specifically, the degree of tissue invasion, especially bone involvement (as determined by radiology studies), the site affected, and the specific etiologic diagnosis determine the type and intensity of therapy. Recent studies indicate that MRI and CT (more sensitive, particularly for mycetoma involving bone) are especially useful in "staging" the disease.

In general, in view of the refractoriness of eumycetoma to medical therapy, surgery plays a more prominent role. In contrast, with the satisfactory response of actinomycetoma to medical therapy (success rate of up to 90%) and recognized risk for lymphatic spread following surgery, chronic antibiotic administration is the mainstay of actinomycetoma management.

For actinomycetoma, treatment consists primarily of chronic antibiotic therapy (for at least 9 to 12 months) in conjunction with limited debulking surgery in selected cases; combination therapy designed for potential synergy is preferred. A variety of drugs (trimethoprim-sulfamethoxazole, tetracyclines, dapsone, streptomycin) have been used in different sequences and combinations according to the specific cause of actinomycetoma. Parenteral streptomycin is usually reserved for patients who do not respond to oral therapy. Responses to these drugs tend to occur slowly (within at least 1 month). In addition, relapse is not uncommon, and multiple cycles of therapy may be needed for chronically recurrent disease. Side effects and compliance issues after prolonged administration of antibiotics are common problems.

For eumycetoma, however, medical therapy has produced mixed results. The best results were obtained with prolonged (9 to 12 months) use of oral imidazoles (e.g., 200 to 400 mg/day of ketoconazole or itraconazole). The experience using newer triazoles (e.g., itraconazole, voriconazole, or posaconazole) or the allylamine terbinafine, though encouraging, is not as extensive. Posaconazole or voriconazole might prove to be especially useful for the treatment of eumycetoma caused by *P. boydii*, a fungus that is not susceptible to either ketoconazole or itraconazole. Also, intravenous amphotericin B and its lipid formulations have been used for refractory cases with rather disappointing results. Such results are not surprising because most eumycetoma-causing agents (e.g., *P. boydii*) are resistant to amphotericin B in vitro.

The need for and extent of surgery for mycetoma depend on the etiologic agent and, more important, the extent of the lesion. Early wide-margin surgery for early localized lesions is curative. Major disfiguring or mutilating surgery (e.g., amputation) is reserved for very advanced or refractory cases. Furthermore, primary reliance on surgery could result in recurrence or even spreading of the disease because of incomplete excision.

PROGNOSIS

The prognosis for mycetoma depends on the site and degree of tissue involvement (e.g., worse with involvement of the back because of poor healing or in the presence of bone destruction) and, more important, the timeliness of diagnosis and monitoring of recurrence and extension to other tissues, especially bone. CT and MRI are important modalities for early detection of bone involvement.

PREVENTION

Finally, because mycetoma represents a significant, yet frequently ignored socioeconomic burden for tropical and subtropical countries, every effort to

351

DEMATIACEOUS FUNGAL INFECTIONS

PETER G. PAPPAS

DEFINITION

Dematiaceous fungi represent a large group of fungal organisms characterized by the presence of abundant melanin in the cell wall, which gives rise to a brown-black coloration on artificial culture media. A related term, *phaeohyphomycosis*, refers broadly to infection by these pigmented fungi. The two terms are often used interchangeably, but when dematiaceous fungi are reviewed, three distinct clinical conditions are encountered: eumycetoma (e.g., Madura foot) (Chapter 350), chromomycosis (also known as chromoblastomycosis), and phaeohyphomycosis. This chapter focuses on the latter two entities.

The Pathogens

More than 100 dematiaceous fungi causing colonization or disease have been isolated from humans. The more common organisms and their related conditions are listed in Table 351-1. The taxonomy of the dematiaceous fungi is somewhat confusing because these agents belong to different classes, including Hyphomycetes, Ascomycetes, Basidiomycetes, Coelomycetes, and

TABLE 351-1 DEMATIACEOUS FUNGI AND ASSOCIATED CONDITIONS

CLINICAL CONDITION	COMMON ETIOLOGIC AGENTS
Chromomycosis	*Fonsecaea pedrosoi* *Cladophialophora carrionii* *Phialophora verrucosa*
Cutaneous or subcutaneous condition	*Exophiala jeanselmei* *Wangiella dermatitidis* *Phialophora* sp *Bipolaris* sp *Alternaria* sp
Sinusitis	*Bipolaris* sp *Curvularia* sp *Exserohilum* sp *Alternaria* sp
Central nervous system	*Cladophialophora bantiana* *Ochroconis gallopava* *Ramichloridium mackenziei*
Disseminated	*Wangiella dermatitidis* *Exophiala jeanselmei* *Bipolaris* sp *Ochroconis gallopava* *Phialophora* sp *Scedosporium prolificans*

Zygomycetes. The most common agents of phaeohyphomycosis include species in the following genera: *Bipolaris, Curvularia, Exophiala, Cladophialophora, Alternaria, Exserohilum, Ochroconis, Wangiella, Phialophora, Scedosporium,* and *Phaeoacromonium.* These agents are ubiquitous saprophytes of soil and decaying matter, and some are important plant pathogens. In tissue, these organisms exist as yeastlike cells, septated hyphae, or a combination of yeast and hyphae. Many have a histologic appearance similar to *Aspergillus* and *Fusarium* species, but they may be distinguished on the basis of positive melanin staining with the Fontana-Masson procedure.

Chromomycosis is a chronic skin and soft tissue infection that is observed most frequently in the tropics. Virtually all cases of chromomycosis are caused by three organisms: *Fonsecaea pedrosoi, Cladophialophora carrionii,* and *Phialophora verrucosa.* The distinctive histologic appearance is characterized by the presence of thick-walled, dark brown bodies known as *sclerotic cells* or *copper pennies,* which represent individual organisms and may be seen in clusters or as single cells. The etiologic fungi are indistinguishable on histologic examination of tissue.

EPIDEMIOLOGY AND PATHOBIOLOGY

The agents of chromomycosis and phaeohyphomycosis are found worldwide. Although there is no unique endemic area for most of these infections, some observations are relevant. Allergic fungal sinusitis associated with dematiaceous fungi appears to be more common in the southern portion of the United States. Chronic infections of the lower extremities are more commonly seen in men and in tropical areas. Chromomycosis is more prevalent in rural populations in the tropics and is hyperendemic in certain geographic areas such as Madagascar, where most infections are caused by *C. carrionii.*

Most cutaneous infections occur as a result of minor skin trauma and direct inoculation of the organism. In the nosocomial setting, infection from contaminated intravascular catheters and intravenous fluids has been reported. Other risk factors include intravenous drug abuse, chronic sinusitis, freshwater immersion, and chronic corticosteroid therapy.

In the developed world, phaeohyphomycosis is an important emerging fungal infection, particularly in immunocompromised patients such as solid organ and hematopoietic stem cell transplant recipients, patients with prolonged neutropenia, and other chronically immunocompromised individuals. Phaeohyphomycosis is reported in patients infected with human immunodeficiency virus but is far less common than other opportunistic fungal infections. Extracutaneous invasive disease occurs in otherwise normal patients but is much less common.

CLINICAL MANIFESTATIONS

Chromomycosis is manifested as a cutaneous or subcutaneous lesion that may range in size from a small papule to a large plaque. Single or multiple lesions may be seen, and ulceration may occur. Lesions may remain unchanged in size and consistency for months or years, although most tend to progress in the absence of specific therapy. Chronic lesions may become dry and crusted with a raised border, which may be smooth or irregular. Multiple lesions can coalesce to form larger plaques in which central scarring develops. Occasionally, lesions assume a verrucous, warty appearance. The differential diagnosis includes other fungal infections such as blastomycosis (Chapter 342), coccidioidomycosis (Chapter 341), sporotrichosis (Chapter 345), histoplasmosis (Chapter 340), and paracoccidioidomycosis (Chapter 343). Nocardiosis and cutaneous mycobacteriosis can also mimic the lesions of chromomycosis. Cutaneous lesions usually remain confined to one anatomic site, although nodular lymphangitis and autoinoculation resulting in multifocal cutaneous disease may occur. Common complications include local disfigurement because of scarring and extensive tissue involvement. Disseminated disease involving visceral organs may occur but is rare.

Phaeohyphomycosis is associated with several well-described clinical syndromes. *Superficial* infection is characterized by tinea nigra and black piedra. Tinea nigra is a darkening of the skin caused by growth of *Phaeoannellomyces werneckii* in the stratum corneum. Black piedra is associated with the development of focal thickening on the hair shaft and results from colonization of the shaft by *Piedraia hortae. Cutaneous* phaeohyphomycosis involves deeper skin structures and results in dermatomycosis and onychomycosis; it is frequently due to agents such as *Scytalidium* and *Phyllosticta* species.

Subcutaneous phaeohyphomycosis is relatively common and may be confused with chromomycosis. Patients have discrete subcutaneous nodules or cysts that result from direct inoculation or penetrating trauma. The most common organisms are *Exophiala jeanselmei, Wangiella dermatitidis,* and *Phia-*

lophora spp. *Mycotic keratitis* as a result of infection with *Curvularia, Exophiala,* and *Exserohilum* species has occurred after corneal trauma or surgery.

Foreign body–related infections are seen in patients undergoing chronic ambulatory peritoneal dialysis in whom fungal peritonitis develops, in patients with indwelling intravenous catheters, and rarely with other devices such as breast implants.

Fungal sinusitis is commonly associated with dematiaceous fungi and can be manifested as allergic fungal sinusitis, a fungus ball (eumycetoma) in a sinus cavity, and invasive fungal sinusitis associated with extension into bone, soft tissue, and the central nervous system. This latter manifestation is indistinguishable from rhinocerebral zygomycosis or invasive *Aspergillus* sinusitis. *Bipolaris, Curvularia,* and *Alternaria* species are the most common organisms causing invasive fungal sinusitis.

Systemic phaeohyphomycosis may result from direct extension from a colonized area or dissemination from a distant source. Most patients with systemic disease have significant underlying immunosuppression, and the organisms have a proclivity for involvement of the brain, lungs, endocardium, and other visceral organs. Among patients with primary central nervous system disease, *Cladophialophora bantiana, Ochroconis gallopava,* and *Ramichloridium mackenziei* are the most common etiologic agents, and the majority of them occur in younger patients with no known underlying immunodeficiency.

DIAGNOSIS

The diagnosis of phaeohyphomycosis is suggested by direct examination of a clinical specimen treated with a 10% potassium hydroxide preparation or special stains to demonstrate pigmentation in the cell walls of these organisms. For patients with chromomycosis, the finding of sclerotic bodies or copper pennies on skin biopsy is characteristic, and special stains are usually unnecessary. For patients with other forms of phaeohyphomycosis, the Fontana-Masson stain is useful for distinguishing organisms with significant melanin content. Culture remains the "gold standard" by which a specific etiologic diagnosis is established, and the identity of the organism is largely based on colony and microscopic morphology. Serologic studies and molecular diagnostics are not generally available for these organisms.

TREATMENT   Rx

In many instances, surgical excision of a cutaneous or subcutaneous lesion is curative, although antifungal therapy is usually given in conjunction with surgery. Only limited clinical studies have assessed the efficacy of antifungal therapy for these conditions. Historically, 5-flucytosine (5-FC, 150 mg/kg/day) has been advocated for the oral treatment of chromomycosis based on moderate in vitro activity and clinical experience. Because of limited availability, the need for prolonged therapy, and the necessity of monitoring serum levels, 5-FC is uncommonly used for this purpose. Amphotericin B has only modest in vitro activity against most of the dematiaceous fungi and is most often reserved for patients with life-threatening or disseminated disease. The triazoles, including itraconazole (200 mg orally twice daily), voriconazole (200 mg orally twice daily), and posaconazole (400 mg orally twice daily), demonstrate the best in vitro activity, although clinical studies with these agents are limited. Among the triazoles, posaconazole offers the most potential in the clinical setting based on scattered reports from patients with central nervous system infection, but comparative clinical data are not available because of the relative rarity of these infections. Terbinafine (500 mg orally twice daily) has also been used successfully for the treatment of chromomycosis and is an effective alternative to azole therapy. The length of therapy with any of the oral antifungal agents for dematiaceous fungal infections is unclear, but treatment should probably be continued for at least 6 months or until 1 month after the resolution of all signs and symptoms of disease.

SUGGESTED READINGS

Derber C, Elam K, Bearman G. Invasive sinonasal disease due to dematiaceous fungi in immunocompromised individuals: case report and review of the literature. *Int J Infect Dis.* 2010;3:e329-e332. *Successful outcomes were associated with surgical debridement, aggressive antifungal use, and a reduction of immunosuppression, but 50% of cases were fatal.*

Queiroz-Telles F, Esterre P, Perez-Blanco M, et al. Chromoblastomycosis: an overview of clinical manifestations, diagnosis and treatment. *Med Mycol.* 2009;47:3-15. *Very nice clinical review of chromomycosis in Brazil.*

Revankar SG, Sutton DA. Melanized fungi in human disease. *Clin Microbiol Rev.* 2010;23:884-928. *Spectrum of disease includes local infection, pneumonia, brain abscess, and disseminated infection.*

Taj-Aldeen SJ, Almaslamani M, Alkhalf A, et al. Cerebral phaeohyphomycosis due to *Rhinocladiella mackenziei* (formerly *Ramichloridium mackenziei*): a taxonomic update and review of the literature. *Med Mycol.* 2010;48:546-556. *The disease appears to be nearly uniformly fatal.*

352

ANTIPARASITIC THERAPY

RICHARD D. PEARSON

Several factors, including the development of the global economy, international travel, and immigration, have drawn attention to the importance of parasitic diseases worldwide. A number of effective drugs are available to treat them. This chapter provides an overview of antiparasitic chemotherapy based on taxonomic relationships. Generalizations emerge from this approach that help in organizing an otherwise vast amount of information.

In considering chemotherapy, it is helpful to classify parasitic infections into those caused by helminths, multicellular worms with complex internal structures, and protozoa, single-celled organisms that multiply by cell division. Helminths are further divided into nematodes, or roundworms, which can be grouped into those that live in the gastrointestinal tract and those found elsewhere in the body, and platyhelminths, or flat worms, which are subdivided into cestodes, or tapeworms, and trematodes, or flukes.

The protozoa can be grouped into those that reside under anaerobic conditions in the gastrointestinal tract or vagina and those that live aerobically in the body. The most prevalent systemic protozoan infections are attributable to members of the Apicomplexa, which cause malaria, babesiosis, and toxoplasmosis, and the Kinetoplastida, which are responsible for Chagas' disease, human African trypanosomiasis (sleeping sickness), and leishmaniasis.

Many of the medications used to treat parasitic diseases are not well known by physicians practicing in the United States. They are the focus of this chapter. Some drugs with activity against parasites are also used for the treatment of bacterial or fungal infections and are discussed elsewhere (Chapters 295 and 339). Detailed descriptions of antiparasitic drugs are available in textbooks of infectious diseases and tropical medicine. An excellent compilation of therapeutic recommendations for parasitic diseases is available in tabular form in *The Medical Letter on Drugs and Therapeutics*, "Drugs for Parasitic Infections" (available at *www.medicalletter.org*). A number of antiparasitic drugs are readily available in the United States, whereas others can be obtained from the manufacturer, special pharmacies, or the Centers for Disease Control and Prevention (CDC) Drug Service. Many are approved by the Food and Drug Administration (FDA), but some are available only on an investigational basis.

⬤ TREATMENT OF HELMINTHS

Intestinal Roundworms (Nematodes)

Soil-transmitted intestinal roundworms (Chapter 365) are among the world's most prevalent parasites, and there are good therapeutic options for them.**1** They are found in impoverished areas where sanitation is poor. *Ascaris lumbricoides*, the hookworms *Ancylostoma duodenale* and *Necator americanus*, and *Trichuris trichiura* each infect more than a billion people worldwide. Many residents of these areas harbor more than one soil-transmitted pathogen. Though frequently subclinical, infections can cause malnutrition, iron deficiency anemia, decreased growth, and poor performance in school or at work. *Strongyloides stercoralis* is less prevalent, but unique among common intestinal roundworms in its ability to produce autoinfection and persist for decades. Disseminated hyperinfection can occur in persons concurrently infected with human T-cell lymphotropic virus type 1 (HTLV-1), receiving corticosteroids, or immunocompromised by neoplasm, malnutrition, or other conditions. *Enterobius vermicularis*, the pinworm, infects children and occasionally adults worldwide.

Albendazole has a broad spectrum of activity against intestinal roundworms. It is active against *A. lumbricoides*, the hookworms, and *T. trichiura*. Administered as a single 400-mg dose, it has been used successfully in mass treatment programs in developing areas. However, reinfection is common and treatment is often repeated at 3- to 4-month intervals. Daily doses of albendazole for 3 days are recommended for those with heavy *T. trichiura* infection. Twice-daily doses of albendazole, 400 mg for 7 days, are used as an alternative to ivermectin for the treatment of *S. stercoralis* infections. Failures can occur with either drug, and they are often used together for longer periods to treat those with disseminated infection. Albendazole is effective against the pinworm *Enterobius vermicularis* in a single dose that is repeated in 2 weeks. It is used for cutaneous larva migrans, which is caused by

migrating stages of *Ancylostoma braziliense* and other intestinal helminths of animals. It is the drug of choice for trichinosis, and it is an alternative for the treatment of *Trichostrongylus* species and *Capillaria philippinensis*.

Mebendazole, administered twice daily at a dosage of 100 mg orally for 3 days, has a similar spectrum of activity as albendazole against *A. lumbricoides*, hookworms, and *T. trichiura*. In this regimen it is more effective than a single dose of albendazole and is considered the treatment of choice for *T. trichiura*. A single 500-mg dose of mebendazole has been used in mass treatment programs. It is effective in treating pinworm when given at 100 mg orally in one dose followed by a second dose after 2 weeks. It is an alternative to albendazole for the treatment of trichinosis. Mebendazole is poorly absorbed and not effective against *S. stercoralis*.

Pyrantel pamoate is a relatively safe, poorly absorbed drug with activity against *A. lumbricoides*, hookworms, and pinworms, but it is not effective against *T. trichiura* or *S. stercoralis*. When used for pinworms, it is administered as an oral suspension at a dose of 11 mg/kg (to a maximum of 1 g), which is repeated after 2 weeks.

Ivermectin at an oral dose of 200 μg/kg daily for 2 days is considered the treatment of choice for *S. stercoralis*. It is also effective against cutaneous larva migrans and *A. lumbricoides*, but not hookworms. It is considered an alternative to mebendazole for the treatment of *T. trichiura*. Albendazole, mebendazole, pyrantel pamoate, and ivermectin replaced a number of older anthelmintics that were more toxic, such as piperazine and thiabendazole, or less effective for the treatment of intestinal roundworms.

Systemic Roundworms (Nematodes)

Diethylcarbamazine is the drug of choice for filarial infections (Chapter 366) caused by *Wuchereria bancrofti*, *Brugia malayi*, *Brugia timori*, and *Loa loa*, as well as for persons with tropical pulmonary eosinophilia. It promotes the host's killing of microfilariae of these species and also damages or kills the adult worms. Inflammatory side effects are common and due in part to the release of lipopolysaccharide from endosymbiotic *Wolbachia* bacteria within dying filaria. *Wolbachia* is necessary for filarial development, and it is a potential drug target. Long-term therapy with doxycycline has been shown to result in their elimination and decreased microfilariae. In heavy *L. loa* infections, encephalopathy may result following treatment with diethylcarbamazine. Apheresis or treatment with albendazole is used first to reduce the microfilarial burden in those heavily infected. Diethylcarbamazine can be used prophylactically for *L. loa*. Ivermectin has activity against the microfilariae of *W. bancrofti*, *Brugia* species, and *L. loa*, but it does not kill adult worms and is not recommended for these diseases.

Ivermectin is the treatment of choice for onchocerciasis.**2** It is administered as a single dose of 150 μg/kg. It does not kill adult *Onchocerca volvulus*, but it decreases ova production and reduces microfilariae in the skin and eyes. Retreatment is usually necessary at 6- to 12-month intervals. Profits from the use of ivermectin for treatment of the dog heartworm *Dirofilaria immitis* have permitted the manufacturer to provide the drug free to persons with onchocerciasis in developing areas. Diethylcarbamazine should not be used for onchocerciasis. It kills the microfilariae of *O. volvulus* rapidly but can result in severe ocular and systemic inflammatory responses, known as the Mazzotti reaction. Ivermectin is associated with less rapid killing and less severe reactions.

Tapeworms (Cestodes)

Praziquantel has a broad spectrum of activity against tapeworms (Chapter 362) and flukes. It is the drug of choice for adult tapeworms in the human intestinal tract. It is effective against *Taenia solium* (pork tapeworm), *Taenia saginata* (beef), *Diphyllobothrium latum* (fish), and *Hymenolepis nana* (dwarf tapeworm) when administered as a single dose. Niclosamide, which is not absorbed, is an effective alternative for the treatment of *T. saginata* and *D. latum*. It also kills adult *T. solium*, but disintegration of the worm and release of viable ova into the intestinal lumen raise the theoretical possibility of autoinfection. In the case of *H. nana*, a dose of nitazoxanide, 500 mg daily for 3 days, provides an alternative to praziquantel. It also has activity against *T. saginata* and potentially other tapeworm species.

Neurocysticercosis caused by the larval or tissue phase of *T. solium* is a major cause of seizures and other central nervous system (CNS) abnormalities in residents of and immigrants from endemic areas in Latin America and elsewhere. Symptoms can result from the physical presence of cysticerci, but the inflammation elicited by the release of antigens from dying cysticerci is often more important. Both albendazole and praziquantel are capable of killing cysticerci in the brain; albendazole is the drug of choice for pharmacokinetic reasons. Their use depends on the clinical syndrome. Corticosteroids are administered concurrently—and sometimes alone—to reduce the inflammatory response and the increase in intracranial pressure associated with it. Albendazole is administered for 8 to 30 days at 400 mg twice a day. Praziquantel is administered at 100 mg/kg in three divided doses the first day and then at 50 mg/kg in three divided doses for 29 days. The concurrent use of corticosteroids increases the serum level of albendazole but decreases that of praziquantel. Neither albendazole nor praziquantel should be used if cysticerci are present in the eye or spinal cord because the release of antigens can trigger a locally destructive inflammatory reaction.

Albendazole is the drug of choice for persons with echinococcosis. Administered at a dose of 400 mg twice daily for adults, generally for 1 to 6 months, albendazole can cure approximately a third of persons with uncomplicated *Echinococcus granulosus* liver cysts. Albendazole is also administered before ultrasound-guided percutaneous aspiration-injection-reaspiration (PAIR) of cysts or surgical approaches to prevent seeding of the peritoneum should the cyst's contents spill. Finally, albendazole is used for suppression of inoperable *E. granulosus* and *Echinococcus multilocularis* disease.

Flukes (Trematodes)

Praziquantel is the drug of choice for the treatment of all forms of schistosomiasis (Chapter 363), as well as intestinal, lung, and liver flukes (Chapter 364), with the exception of the liver fluke *Fasciola hepatica*. For schistosomiasis, two or three doses are given in 1 day depending on the species. The flukes are treated with three doses on 1 or 2 days, depending on the species. Oxamniquine is an alternative for *Schistosoma mansoni*, but it is more toxic and less effective. Higher doses of oxamniquine are recommended for *S. mansoni* infections acquired in areas of Egypt or equatorial Africa where the parasite is less susceptible. Either praziquantel or albendazole can be used to treat the liver fluke *Clonorchis sinensis*. *F. hepatica* responds to the veterinary agent triclabendazole. Bithionol, which is more toxic, and nitazoxanide are alternatives.

Drugs Used for Helminthic Infections

Albendazole is poorly soluble in water, but it is well absorbed when administered with a fatty meal. It undergoes rapid first-pass metabolism in the liver to albendazole sulfoxide, which has excellent anthelmintic activity. The serum half-life of albendazole sulfoxide is 8 to 9 hours. Elimination of albendazole sulfoxide and other metabolites is achieved primarily through the kidney. Albendazole binds to tubulin in susceptible parasites, inhibits microtubule assembly, and decreases glucose absorption. It does not affect human tubulin. It also inhibits fumarate reductase in helminths. Concurrent administration of dexamethasone, which is frequently given to prevent cerebral edema in persons with neurocysticercosis, increases serum levels by approximately 50%. The cerebrospinal fluid (CSF) concentration of albendazole is 40% of that in serum.

Albendazole is generally well tolerated when given as a single dose for the treatment of intestinal nematode infections, although gastrointestinal discomfort may develop or patients may experience migration of adult *A. lumbricoides* from the nose or mouth or in stool. Albendazole is contraindicated in persons with cysticerci in the eye or spinal cord, and corticosteroids are administered concurrently in those being treated for neurocysticercosis. High-dose, prolonged therapy with albendazole, such as that recommended for echinococcal disease, can be complicated by alopecia, bone marrow suppression, which is usually reversible after discontinuation of use of the drug, or hepatocellular injury. Albendazole is embryotoxic in animals and contraindicated during pregnancy.

Mebendazole is only slightly soluble in water and is relatively poorly absorbed from the gastrointestinal tract. This is advantageous for the treatment of intestinal parasites but limits its effectiveness against tissue-dwelling helminths. Absorbed drug is metabolized in the liver and excreted in urine. Mebendazole selectively binds to helminthic tubulin, blocks its assembly into microtubules, and inhibits glucose uptake, thereby leading to depletion of glycogen stores and ultimately death of the parasite. It is relatively well tolerated in the doses used to treat intestinal helminths. Transient abdominal pain and diarrhea occur in a small number of recipients. Mebendazole is contraindicated during pregnancy.

Ivermectin is a macrocyclic lactone produced by *Streptomyces avermitilis*. It has a broad spectrum of activity against helminths and arthropods, including *Sarcoptes scabiei*, the cause of scabies. It is well absorbed after oral administration. Ivermectin is highly protein bound, has a serum half-life of 12 hours, and accumulates in adipose tissue and the liver. It is subject to enterohepatic recirculation and ultimately eliminated in stool. Ivermectin activates the opening of gated chloride channels in susceptible helminths and arthropods. The result is an influx of chloride ions and paralysis of the pharyngeal pumping mechanism of helminths. Ivermectin is generally well tolerated in humans, although inflammatory reactions can result in response to antigens released from dying parasites.

Diethylcarbamazine, a piperazine derivative, is well absorbed orally and has a half-life of 8 hours. The parent drug and its metabolites are excreted through the kidney. Although the mechanism of action is uncertain, the piperazine moiety may result in paralysis of sensitive helminths. Diethylcarbamazine also alters the surface membranes of sensitive microfilariae, thereby resulting in destruction by the host's immune system. Side effects include those caused by the drug and those that result from release of the parasite's antigens and lipopolysaccharide from filaria-harbored, endosymbiotic *Wolbachia*. Adverse effects include nausea, vomiting, anorexia, headache, malaise, weakness, arthralgias, and rarely, acute psychotic reactions. In patients with lymphatic filariasis, localized swelling or nodules may develop along the lymphatics during treatment, or transient lymphedema or hydrocele formation may occur.

Praziquantel is well absorbed after oral administration. It undergoes extensive first-pass metabolism, and the metabolites, which are inactive, are excreted in urine. Praziquantel is approximately 80% protein bound, with a serum half-life of 4 to 6 hours. It is rapidly taken up by susceptible cestodes and trematodes. In the case of schistosomes, praziquantel damages the tegument, which results in intense vacuolation and increased permeability to calcium. Adult schistosomes are paralyzed and translocated to the liver through the portal circulation. Sequestered antigens are exposed on their surface, thereby permitting binding of antibodies and phagocytes and immune destruction. Praziquantel is an alternative to albendazole for the treatment of neurocysticercosis. The concurrent administration of corticosteroids, which are necessary to decrease inflammation and edema in the brain, reduces the serum concentration of praziquantel. Its concentration in CSF is approximately 15 to 20% of that in serum.

Praziquantel is frequently associated with mild, transient side effects, including headaches, lassitude, dizziness, nausea, vomiting, and abdominal discomfort, but they are seldom severe enough to interrupt therapy. Untoward reactions attributed to release of the parasite's antigens have been reported in patients treated for schistosomiasis and pulmonary paragonimiasis. Increased intracranial pressure resulting from release of cysticercal antigens is a potentially life-threatening consequence in patients receiving praziquantel for neurocysticercosis. Corticosteroids should be administered concurrently. Praziquantel is contraindicated in persons with cysticerci in the eye or spinal cord.

● TREATMENT OF PROTOZOAL DISEASES

Intestinal and Vaginal Protozoa

Several major luminal pathogens, *Entamoeba histolytica* (Chapter 360), *Giardia lamblia* (Chapter 359), and *Trichomonas vaginalis* (Chapter 361), live in anaerobic conditions in the intestine or vagina and are susceptible to metronidazole and tinidazole. The latter has favorable pharmacodynamics and is generally better tolerated. Because neither metronidazole nor tinidazole reliably eradicates cysts of *E. histolytica*, either paromomycin or iodoquinol, which are active in the lumen of the bowel, is administered as well. Either one of these drugs or diloxanide furoate can be used alone to treat persons with asymptomatic cyst excretion.

Giardiasis can also be treated with nitazoxanide. It is well tolerated, and an oral formulation is available for children. Nitazoxanide is the only drug available for the treatment of cryptosporidiosis (Chapter 358). It is effective in immunocompetent persons, but not usually in those with acquired immunodeficiency syndrome (AIDS). Trimethoprim-sulfamethoxazole, which inhibits successive steps in the folic acid pathway, is the drug of choice for *Cystoisospora* (*Isospora*) *belli* and *Cyclospora cayetanensis*. Ciprofloxacin, a fluoroquinolone antibiotic, is an alternative. Tetracycline is the treatment of choice for *Balantidium coli*; metronidazole and iodoquinol are alternatives. Finally, albendazole is effective in the treatment of intestinal and disseminated microsporidiosis caused by *Encephalitozoon* (*Septata*) *intestinalis* and some, but not all other microsporidial species that cause disease in persons with AIDS.

Metronidazole, a nitroimidazole, is rapidly absorbed after oral administration and has a half-life of 8 hours. More than half of each dose is metabolized in the liver. The metabolites and remaining parent drug are excreted in urine.

Metronidazole is activated by reduction of its 5-nitro group through a sequence of intermediate steps involving microbial electron transport proteins of low redox potential. It is concentrated in susceptible anaerobic organisms and serves as an electron sink. Nausea, vomiting, diarrhea, and a metallic taste are often associated with the use of metronidazole. They are less common with the lower doses recommended for the treatment of giardiasis than with the higher doses used for amebiasis. Other untoward effects include headache, dizziness, vertigo, and numbness. Potentially severe disulfiram-like reactions occur in patients who ingest alcohol while taking metronidazole.

Tinidazole, another 5-nitroimidazole, has a similar mechanism of action and spectrum of activity as metronidazole, but more favorable pharmacodynamics, and is generally better tolerated. It has been used widely around the world for the treatment of giardiasis, intestinal amebiasis, and trichomoniasis. In comparison to metronidazole, it has a longer half-life, a shorter and less complicated dosing regimen, and fewer gastrointestinal side effects. It, too, can cause severe disulfiram-like reactions after alcohol ingestion.

Nitazoxanide, a 5-nitrothiazole salicylamide derivative, has a broad spectrum of activity against protozoa and helminths. It is formulated as a liquid for use in children. Nitazoxanide is well absorbed orally and hydrolyzed to its active metabolite tizoxanide, which undergoes conjugation to tizoxanide glucuronide. The parent compound is not detectable in serum. Maximum concentrations of the metabolites are observed in 1 to 4 hours. They are excreted in urine and bile. Tizoxanide is highly protein bound. Although its mechanism of action is uncertain, tizoxanide inhibits pyruvate:ferredoxin oxidoreductase–dependent electron transport reactions essential for the metabolism of susceptible anaerobic organisms. It is very well tolerated in children and adults.

Malaria: Prophylaxis and Treatment

As discussed in this section, a number of drugs are available for the prophylaxis and treatment of malaria. Most act against *Plasmodium* stages within erythrocytes. Only primaquine kills *Plasmodium vivax* and *Plasmodium ovale* hypnozoites in the liver. The antimalarial drug of choice depends on the geographic site visited and the *Plasmodium* species encountered (Chapter 353). Antimicrobial resistance is now widespread among *Plasmodium falciparum* isolates and well documented in *P. vivax* from some regions. Country-specific recommendations for prophylaxis and treatment are provided by the CDC at *www.cdc.gov/travel/* and in "CDC Health Information for International Travel 2010." Major recent additions to the therapeutic armamentarium in the United States include the fixed drug combination of artemether plus lumefantrine (Coartem), which is used for the oral treatment of acute malaria acquired in areas with chloroquine-resistant *P. falciparum*,[3] and artesunate for intravenous administration in those with severe malaria who cannot take oral medications and for whom quinidine is contraindicated or not available. Artesunate can be obtained from the CDC on an emergency basis as an investigational new drug.

Chloroquine, a 4-aminoquinoline, has a bitter taste but is well absorbed from the gastrointestinal tract. Its half-life, which varies among persons, averages 4 days, thus permitting once-weekly administration for prophylaxis. Chloroquine is concentrated in the hemoglobin-containing digestive vesicles of asexual intraerythrocytic parasites. It inhibits the parasite's heme polymerase that incorporates ferriprotoporphyrin type IX complexes, which are potentially toxic to the parasite, into insoluble, nontoxic, crystalline hemozoin. Chloroquine-resistant strains of *P. falciparum* actively transport chloroquine out of the intraparasitic compartment. Although this action can be blocked by calcium-channel inhibitors in vitro, chloroquine resistance has not been effectively reversed in humans. Hydroxychloroquine (Plaquenil), which is used for rheumatologic diseases, is also effective against chloroquine-sensitive *Plasmodium* species.

Chloroquine is generally well tolerated when used at the doses recommended for the prophylaxis and treatment of malaria. Side effects include headache, nausea, vomiting, blurred vision, dizziness, and fatigue. Some Africans and African Americans experience pruritus, which responds to antihistamines. Rare side effects include depigmentation of hair, exacerbation of psoriasis, blood dyscrasias, seizures, neuropsychiatric effects, and reactions in persons with porphyria. Retinal damage has occurred in persons receiving chloroquine at high doses for the treatment of rheumatologic disorders, but it has not been documented as a problem in those taking it weekly over a period of many years for malaria prophylaxis. Cardiopulmonary collapse and death have occurred after accidental overdose and in adults attempting suicide. As little as 5 g of chloroquine can be fatal unless treatment is initiated

with mechanical respiration, diazepam to control seizures, and blood pressure support.

Doxycycline taken daily provides effective prophylaxis against all *Plasmodium* species. It is begun 1 to 2 days before departure and continued during the time of exposure and for 4 weeks after leaving the malaria-endemic area. Doxycycline or tetracycline is also often administered with quinine for the treatment of acute chloroquine-resistant malaria, but neither drug acts rapidly enough to be used alone for treatment. Doxycycline is generally well tolerated, although it can cause gastrointestinal symptoms and "pill" esophagitis. To avoid the latter, it should be taken with a full glass of water, and the recipient should remain upright for an hour or more after ingestion. Other potential side effects include photosensitivity dermatitis, *Candida albicans* vaginitis, and antibiotic-associated colitis. Finally, tetracyclines should not be used in children younger than 8 years or during pregnancy.

Atovaquone plus **proguanil** (Malarone; adult tablets contain 250 mg of atovaquone and 100 mg of proguanil) is used for prophylaxis in areas with chloroquine-resistant *P. falciparum* and other *Plasmodium* species. Atovaquone is a highly lipophilic compound with low aqueous solubility. Administration with food enhances its absorption two-fold. Plasma concentrations do not increase proportionally with dose. Atovaquone is highly protein bound with a half-life exceeding 60 hours. It undergoes extensive enterohepatic cycling and is eventually excreted unchanged in feces. Atovaquone selectively inhibits electron transport in the mitochondria of susceptible *Plasmodium* species at the level of the cytochrome bc_1 complex, which results in collapse of mitochondrial membrane potential. It also affects pyrimidine biosynthesis, which is obligatorily coupled to electron transport in *Plasmodium*. Resistance develops rapidly when atovaquone is used alone to treat malaria. Atovaquone is generally well tolerated but can cause nausea, vomiting, diarrhea, rash, and pruritus.

Proguanil is absorbed slowly after oral administration. Its serum level falls to zero within 24 hours, so it must be administered daily. Its triazine metabolite, cycloguanil, inhibits dihydrofolate reductase in susceptible *Plasmodium* species. Resistance is well documented when proguanil is used alone. Proguanil also acts synergistically with atovaquone to collapse mitochondrial membrane potential in susceptible *Plasmodium* species.

The combination of atovaquone and proguanil (Malarone) is considered the best tolerated of the options for prevention of chloroquine-resistant malaria, but the most expensive. It is begun 1 to 2 days before departure and continued during the time of exposure and for 7 days thereafter. Higher doses are administered over a period of 3 days to treat acute, uncomplicated malaria. Potential side effects include abdominal pain, nausea, vomiting, diarrhea, headache, pruritus, and rash. Asymptomatic, transient elevations in liver enzymes have been observed with treatment doses.

Mefloquine, a quinoline methanol compound derived from quinine, was once used widely for the prophylaxis and occasionally treatment of chloroquine-resistant *P. falciparum* malaria. Concern about neuropsychiatric and other toxicities and the availability of better-tolerated alternatives have limited its use in recent years. Mefloquine is available for oral administration only. Slowly and incompletely absorbed, it is 99% protein bound. It has a variable half-life ranging from 6 to 23 days with a mean of approximately 14 days. It is metabolized and excreted slowly through bile and feces.

Considerable attention has been paid to the untoward effects of mefloquine. It is reasonably well tolerated in most recipients, although it can cause nausea, dizziness, vivid dreams, fatigue, and lassitude. Less common, but of substantial concern are neuropsychiatric reactions, including anxiety, depression, and acute psychosis. It can also cause seizures. Mefloquine is therefore contraindicated in persons with a history of epilepsy or psychiatric disorders. It can also depress atrioventricular conduction and should not be used in persons taking β-blockers for cardiac indications. It has antibacterial activity and can inactivate the live oral typhoid vaccine (*Salmonella typhi* Ty21a) if administered concurrently. Rare side effects include exfoliative erythroderma, agranulocytosis, and paresthesias. Mefloquine is not approved by the U.S. FDA for use during pregnancy or in children weighing less than 15 kg, but it has been used in situations in which potential benefits were judged to outweigh the risks.

Primaquine, an 8-aminoquinoline, eradicates the hepatic hypnozoite stage of *P. vivax* and *P. ovale* and is used at the end of treatment or for prophylaxis with other drugs to prevent late relapse in persons who are or may be infected with these *Plasmodium* species. It is also effective when used daily for prophylaxis for all *Plasmodium* species. It is begun 1 or 2 days before exposure and continued during and for 7 days after the traveler leaves the endemic area.

Primaquine is well absorbed orally and rapidly converted to carboxyprimaquine, which has a half-life of approximately 7 days. Primaquine is generally well tolerated, although some recipients experience abdominal cramps, epigastric distress, and nausea. The major concern is hemolysis in persons with glucose-6-phosphate dehydrogenase (G6PD) deficiency (Chapter 164). The G6PD status of the recipient should be determined before it is administered. Rarely, primaquine causes neutropenia, methemoglobinemia, hypertension, or arrhythmias. Primaquine is contraindicated during pregnancy and in breast-feeding mothers because life-threatening hemolysis may occur if the fetus or baby is deficient in G6PD. Travelers should be warned not to give the drug to fellow travelers who have not been screened for G6PD deficiency.

Quinine sulfate, a cinchona alkaloid, is the oldest of the antimalarials. It has a very bitter taste. It is rapidly absorbed after oral administration and has a half-life of 16 to 18 hours in persons with malaria. Quinine has the poorest therapeutic-to-toxicity ratio of any antimalarial drug. The side effects, known collectively as cinchonism, include tinnitus, decreased hearing, headache, nausea, vomiting, dysphoria, and visual disturbances. They are dose related and reversible. Quinine has also been associated with severe hypoglycemia in persons with heavy *P. falciparum* infection as a result of the utilization of glucose by the parasites and release of insulin from the pancreas. Hypoglycemia can be prevented or treated by the intravenous administration of glucose. Rare complications with quinine include massive hemolysis in patients with heavy *P. falciparum* infection resulting in hemoglobinuria and renal failure (blackwater fever), cutaneous hypersensitivity reactions, agranulocytosis, and hepatitis. Quinine can cause respiratory paralysis in persons with myasthenia gravis. It stimulates uterine contractions and can produce abortions, but it has saved the lives of many pregnant women with *P. falciparum* malaria. Quinine dihydrochloride given intravenously can cause myocardial depression, peripheral vascular collapse, respiratory depression, and potentially death.

Quinidine gluconate, the stereoisomer of quinine, is recommended for the intravenous treatment of patients with acute malaria who cannot take quinine or other antimalarials orally. Quinidine gluconate was once widely used for the treatment of ventricular ectopy, but it has been replaced by newer antiarrhythmic agents, which has decreased its availability in many hospitals. Side effects include prolongation of the QT interval, arrhythmias, and hypotension, particularly if it is infused too rapidly. Persons receiving intravenous quinidine should be monitored in an intensive care setting, and therapy should be switched to an oral antimalarial medication as soon as possible.

Artemether, artesunate, and other artemisinin derivates are sesquiterpene lactones derived from the wormwood plant *Artemisia annua*, from which qinghaosu, the Chinese herbal medication for malaria, is also derived. They are endoperoxide-containing compounds. In the presence of intraparasitic iron, they are converted into free radicals and other intermediates that alkylate specific malarial proteins and act rapidly to kill intraerythrocytic parasites. They have been used widely around the world for the treatment of acute malaria caused by chloroquine-resistant *P. falciparum*, as well as other *Plasmodium* species. The artemisinins are usually administered with a second antimalarial drug that has a different mechanism of action and longer half-life to prevent the development of resistance. The route of administration with artemisinins varies; some are well absorbed orally, whereas others are administered intravenously, intramuscularly, or by suppository. Their short half-lives preclude their use for prophylaxis. Adverse effects in humans are infrequent and usually mild. Neurologic toxicity and cerebellar dysfunction have been observed in dogs receiving chronic, high-dose therapy.

Artemether plus lumefantrine (Coartem), a fixed drug combination, was recently approved by the FDA for oral use in the United States. In addition, intravenous artesunate is available from the CDC as an investigational new drug for the treatment of acute malaria in persons who cannot take quinidine gluconate or in situations in which it is not available. Side effects with Coartem include headache, dizziness, anorexia, and weakness. Rare hypersensitivity reactions include urticaria, angioedema, and bullous eruptions. Lumefantrine inhibits CYP206 and can reduce the metabolism of medications that prolong the QT interval, so care must be taken in reviewing the recipient's medication list.

Toxoplasmosis and Babesiosis

Toxoplasma gondii (Chapter 357) and *Babesia* species (Chapter 361) are other important pathogens of the phylum Apicomplexa. Pyrimethamine and sulfadiazine are recommended for the treatment of toxoplasmosis. They inhibit sequential steps in the folic acid metabolic pathway. Pyrimethamine preferentially inhibits dihydrofolate reductase in susceptible parasites. It is well absorbed orally. The major side effect is macrocytic anemia, which can be prevented by the concurrent administration of leucovorin. Sulfonamides reduce the activity of dihydropteroate synthetase and the binding of *p*-aminobenzoic acid to it. In ocular toxoplasmosis with macular involvement, corticosteroids are indicated along with anti-*Toxoplasma* therapy to minimize the local inflammatory response. Clindamycin plus pyrimethamine and atovaquone plus pyrimethamine are therapeutic options in sulfonamide-intolerant patients. For prophylaxis in persons with AIDS and CD4+ counts less than 100, options include daily trimethoprim-sulfamethoxazole, pyrimethamine plus dapsone, pyrimethamine plus atovaquone, or atovaquone alone. Spiramycin, a macrolide, is used for the treatment of toxoplasmosis during pregnancy. Two therapeutic regimens are available for babesiosis. The greatest experience has been with the combination of clindamycin plus quinine, but side effects are common. Atovaquone plus azithromycin is effective and better tolerated (Chapter 361).

CHAGAS' DISEASE, AFRICAN TRYPANOSOMIASIS, AND LEISHMANIASIS

The trypanosomes *Trypanosoma cruzi*, the cause of Chagas' disease, and *Trypanosoma brucei rhodesiense* and *Trypanosoma brucei gambiense*, the cause of human African trypanosomiasis (sleeping sickness), pose difficult therapeutic challenges. Nifurtimox and benznidazole orally are the only drugs available to treat *T. cruzi* (Chapter 355). Benznidazole has been used widely in endemic areas in Latin America and nifurtimox in the United States. They lower mortality and shorten the duration of acute Chagas' disease. Treatment is also recommended for asymptomatic children and younger adults with recent or indeterminate-stage *T. cruzi* infection. The percentage of those who are parasitologically cured has been debated. Neither benznidazole nor nifurtimox can reverse the manifestations of chronic Chagas' disease. Side effects are common with both drugs and increase in frequency and severity with age. Benznidazole is associated with allergic dermatitis, peripheral neuropathy, insomnia, and gastrointestinal symptoms, including anorexia and weight loss. Nifurtimox causes anorexia, nausea, vomiting, weight loss, headache, dizziness or vertigo, paresthesias, weakness, and polyneuropathy.

Suramin, pentamidine, eflornithine, and melarsoprol are used for the treatment of human African trypanosomiasis (Chapter 354). Suramin is recommended for the hemolymphatic stage of *T. brucei rhodesiense* infection, and melarsoprol is used in those with CNS involvement. Both drugs are associated with potentially severe side effects. Eflornithine, which is much better tolerated, is effective against both the hemolymphatic and CNS stages of *T. brucei gambiense* infection. It does not have activity against *T. brucei rhodesiense*. Unfortunately, eflornithine is costly and not available in many endemic areas, and supplies are limited. When eflornithine is not available, pentamidine, which has substantial untoward effects, is used for the hemolymphatic stage of *T. brucei gambiense* infection, with suramin being used as an alternative, and melarsoprol is used for CNS disease.

Liposomal amphotericin B (AmBisome) is the only drug approved for the treatment of visceral leishmaniasis (Chapter 356) in the United States. Amphotericin B deoxycholate is also effective. Liposomes deliver amphotericin to macrophages and are theoretically attractive because leishmaniae reside within them. Liposomal amphotericin is also better tolerated than the parent drug. Other lipid-associated amphotericin B preparations appear to be effective, but they have been less extensively studied and are not FDA approved for this indication. For many years two pentavalent antimony drugs, stibogluconate sodium and meglumine antimoniate, were used to treat visceral leishmaniasis, but resistance is now common among *Leishmania donovani* isolates in India, and therapeutic failures occur in other areas. Side effects increase with age and include gastrointestinal complaints, pancreatitis, myalgias, headache, malaise, elevated liver enzyme levels, and occasionally, bone marrow suppression. Nonspecific ST-T wave changes are common. Sudden death has been reported in persons receiving more than the recommended dose. Miltefosine, a phosphocholine analogue that was developed as an antineoplastic drug, has been used effectively for antimony-resistant visceral leishmaniasis in India and is being studied in other areas. It is the only antileishmanial drug that can be administered orally. There is concern that resistance will develop. Miltefosine is relatively well tolerated, but nausea, vomiting, and motion sickness occur, particularly at higher doses. Elevations in liver enzymes, blood urea nitrogen, and creatinine occur but usually resolve with continuation of the drug. Miltefosine is contraindicated during pregnancy. Intravenously administered paromomycin has also been reported to be effective against antimony-resistant visceral leishmaniasis in India.

Treatment of cutaneous leishmaniasis depends on the size and location of the skin lesion or lesions, the infecting *Leishmania* species, and its propensity to cause mucosal disease. Consensus is lacking regarding optimal therapy. Stibogluconate sodium and meglumine antimoniate have been used widely. Miltefosine has been reported to be effective in limited studies and has the advantage of oral administration. Paromomycin has been used topically with methylbenzethonium chloride in soft white paraffin for the treatment of cutaneous leishmaniasis caused by *Leishmania major* and other species not associated with mucosal disease. The imidazole antifungals ketoconazole, itraconazole, and fluconazole vary in their activity against different *Leishmania* species but have been reported to be effective in some trials. Liposomal amphotericin B, amphotericin B deoxycholate, and pentamidine are effective, but more toxic alternatives. Other options include immunotherapy, cryotherapy, and local application of heat. Mucosal leishmaniasis is less responsive than cutaneous leishmaniasis to treatment, and relapses are common. Therapeutic options include stibogluconate sodium, meglumine antimoniate, amphotericin B, and miltefosine.

1. Keiser J, Utzinger J. Efficacy of current drugs against soil transmitted helminth infections: systematic review and meta-analysis. *JAMA.* 2008;299:1937-1948.
2. Basanez MG, Pion SD, Boakes E, et al. Effect of single-dose ivermectin on *Onchocerca volvulus*: a systematic review and meta-analysis. *Lancet Infect Dis.* 2008;8:310-322.
3. Saraga I, Diallo A, Kone M, et al. A randomized trial of artesunate-mefloquine versus artemether-lumefantrine for treatment of uncomplicated *Plasmodium falciparum* malaria in Mali. *Am J Trop Med Hyg.* 2008;79:655-661.

SUGGESTED READINGS

Artemether-lumefantrine (Coartem) for the treatment of malaria. *Med Lett Drugs Ther.* 2009;51:75-76. *The efficacy and toxicity of artemether-lumefantrine (Coartem) for the treatment of acute chloroquine-resistant malaria caused by* Plasmodium falciparum *and other* Plasmodium *species were reviewed after approval by the U.S. Food and Drug Administration.*
Botros S, El-Lakkany N, Seif el-Din SH, et al. Comparative efficacy and bioavailability of different praziquantel brands. *Exp Parasitol.* 2011;127:515-521. *Bioavailability varied substantially enough to affect dosing.*
Centers for Disease Control and Prevention. CDC Health Information for International Travel 2012. Atlanta: U.S. Department of Health and Human Services, Public Health Service, 2011. http://www.cdc.gov/travel. *The "yellow book" is a guide to the practice of travel medicine and the authoritative source of U.S. government recommendations for immunizations and prophylaxis for foreign travel. It is a comprehensive resource for the practitioner and public for finding answers to questions before travel, during travel, or after travel.*
Drugs for parasitic diseases. *Med Lett Drugs Ther.* (www.medicalletter.org.) 2010. *This is an excellent tabular compilation of consensus recommendations for the treatment of parasitic diseases. Key articles are referenced in footnotes.*
Endara P, Vaca M, Chico ME, et al. Long-term periodic anthelmintic treatments are associated with increased allergen skin reactivity. *Clin Exp Allergy.* 2010;40:1669-1677. *The prevalence of allergen skin test reactivity was two-fold higher in children living in treated communities.*

353

MALARIA

PHILIP J. ROSENTHAL AND MOSES R. KAMYA

DEFINITION

Malaria is caused by infection with protozoan parasites of the genus *Plasmodium,* all of which are transmitted by bites of infected anopheline mosquitoes. Malaria is typically characterized by an acute febrile illness, with parasites infecting large numbers of erythrocytes, and classically entails recurrent episodes of fever and chills. It was first described thousands of years ago and is named on the basis of the belief that it was caused by the bad air of the marshes surrounding Rome. Malaria is common, causing hundreds of millions of illnesses each year throughout most of the tropics. Severe disease can occur, primarily with *Plasmodium falciparum* infection, with the acute development of serious organ dysfunction or when chronic and repeated infection

leads to severe anemia. Falciparum malaria kills about 1 million people each year, mostly children in sub-Saharan Africa.

The Pathogen

P. falciparum is responsible for most episodes of severe malaria. It is endemic in most malarious areas and is by far the predominant species in Africa. *Plasmodium vivax* is about as common as *P. falciparum,* except in Africa, but causes severe disease much less commonly. However, studies suggest that severe illness associated with *P. vivax* infection is more common than had previously been appreciated. *Plasmodium ovale* and *Plasmodium malariae* are much less common causes of disease and generally do not cause severe illness. It was recently shown that a fifth parasite causing human infections is *Plasmodium knowlesi,* a parasite of macaque monkeys that is a fairly common zoonosis in parts of Southeast Asia and has been responsible for malarial illnesses, including severe disease, in individuals exposed to macaque-biting vectors in forested areas.

EPIDEMIOLOGY

Malaria in Endemic Countries

Malaria is the most important parasitic disease of humans, causing hundreds of millions of illnesses and approximately a million deaths each year. The disease is endemic in most of the tropics, including many parts of South and Central America, Africa, the Middle East, the Indian subcontinent, Southeast Asia, and Oceania. Transmission, morbidity, and mortality are greatest in Africa, where infection with *P. falciparum* predominates. In most other endemic areas, disease caused by both *P. falciparum* and *P. vivax* is common. In highly endemic areas, the group at greatest risk is young children, who suffer most episodes of disease and the most deaths. A second high-risk group is pregnant women, with high risks of maternal and fetal morbidity from falciparum malaria, including many deaths secondary to low birthweight. In highly endemic areas, in addition to extensive mortality, malaria exerts a massive toll through adverse effects on child development, contributions to school and work absenteeism, and, overall, billions of dollars in lost income among the poorest citizens of the poorest countries of the world. In areas of developing countries with lower levels of malaria transmission, malaria can be epidemic, with intermittent increases in transmission that cause major morbidity in relatively nonimmune populations.

Malaria in Travelers

Malaria is also common in travelers of any age from nonendemic areas to the tropics and may be manifested in those who have returned to nonendemic areas up to many months after travel. Indeed, malaria is the most common documented cause of febrile illness in travelers returning from the tropics to developed countries. Malaria is also rarely transmitted in areas considered nonendemic, including the United States, when imported parasites are transmitted by local anopheline mosquitoes, by blood products, or through congenital spread of infection.

Malaria Transmission

Malaria is transmitted by multiple species of mosquitoes of the genus *Anopheles,* which vary in geographic distribution, ecologic preferences, and susceptibility to mosquito control measures. Anopheline mosquitoes bite at night, and so personal mosquito control measures focus on avoidance of mosquito bites overnight. Levels of malaria transmission in endemic areas vary greatly, from areas where residents experience only rare infectious bites to regions of Africa where individuals may receive hundreds of infectious bites each year.

Recent Changes in the Epidemiology of Malaria

A major effort to eradicate malaria after World War II led to elimination of the disease in many areas, including the United States and Europe, but eventually failed to control the disease in most of the tropics. During the ensuing decades, improvements in malaria control were few, and malarial morbidity worsened in many areas, driven by the loss of enthusiasm for vector control, increasing resistance of mosquitoes to insecticides, and, in particular, resistance of parasites to commonly used antimalarial drugs. Some 50 years later, a new large effort to control and eventually to eradicate malaria has been initiated. Key control measures include indoor residual spraying of insecticides, distribution of insecticide-impregnated bed nets, prompt provision of effective drugs to those with malaria, and targeted intermittent use of drugs to prevent infection in high-risk groups. Recent efforts have led to documented decreases in levels of malarial morbidity and mortality in some areas, notably parts of Africa, Asia, and Oceania with relatively low levels of transmission intensity. It is of great interest to learn whether recent advances due to intensified control efforts can bring significant improvements to those parts of the world most afflicted with malaria, in particular, highly endemic regions of Africa and Asia.

Malaria and Human Immunodeficiency Virus Infection

Malaria does not differ as markedly between those with human immunodeficiency virus (HIV) infection and others as is the case with typical opportunistic infections. However, several interactions between malaria and HIV infection have been established. First, HIV infection appears to disrupt the acquired immune response to malaria and thereby increases incidence and severity of malaria. Second, acute malaria elevates HIV viral load and so may increase the risk of HIV transmission. Third, HIV infection may be associated with reduced efficacy of antimalarial treatment, especially in the setting of severe immune suppression. Fourth, therapies for each infection may have an impact on the other, leading to unanticipated effects on drug efficacy or toxicity. Fifth, routine interventions for HIV infection may affect the incidence of malaria; notably, daily trimethoprim-sulfamethoxazole, a routine regimen in HIV-infected patients, offers partial protection against malaria. As both HIV infection and malaria are common in many areas, in particular sub-Saharan Africa, even modest associations are important. Thus, malaria coinfection in HIV-infected individuals may be an important factor in promoting the spread of HIV infection in Africa.

PATHOBIOLOGY
Parasite Life Cycle

Malaria is transmitted by the bite of infected female anopheline mosquitoes. During feeding, mosquitoes inject sporozoites, which circulate to the liver and infect hepatocytes, causing asymptomatic liver infection (Fig. 353-1). Merozoites are subsequently released from the liver, and they rapidly infect erythrocytes to begin the asexual erythrocytic stage of infection that is responsible for human disease. Multiple rounds of erythrocytic development, with production of merozoites that invade additional erythrocytes, lead to large numbers of circulating parasites and clinical illness. Each erythrocytic cycle lasts approximately 24 hours for *P. knowlesi*; 48 hours for *P. falciparum, P. vivax,* and *P. ovale*; and 72 hours for *P. malariae*. Some erythrocytic parasites also develop into sexual gametocytes, which are taken up by mosquitoes. In the mosquito, gametocytes mature to gametes, and after fusion of male and female gametes to produce zygotes, parasites develop into ookinetes, oocysts, and then salivary gland sporozoites that are infectious for humans, allowing completion of the life cycle and infection of others. *P. vivax* and *P. ovale* also cause a chronic liver infection, in which hypnozoites persist in hepatocytes in a dormant state not eradicated by most therapies for acute disease and subsequently can progress to erythrocytic infection and a relapse of clinical illness.

Pathogenic Features of Malaria Parasites

The most common clinical feature of malaria is fever. Fever coincides with rupture of large numbers of schizont-infected erythrocytes at the completion of the erythrocytic cycle and with high circulating levels of tumor necrosis factor-α. Severe falciparum malaria is associated with very high levels of tumor necrosis factor-α and other inflammatory cytokines, but the specific roles of cytokines in pathogenesis are not well understood. *P. falciparum* infects erythrocytes of all ages, so it is capable of routinely causing high parasitemias, with infection of more than 1% of erythrocytes and more than 10^5 infected erythrocytes per microliter of blood. Non-falciparum parasites infect smaller numbers of erythrocytes, limiting the extent of infection and morbidity. Non-falciparum parasites are more likely to cause highly synchronous infections, leading if untreated to regular cycles of fever every 48 (*P. vivax* and *P. ovale*) or 72 (*P. malariae*) hours, often with minimal symptoms between fever episodes.

The contribution of parasite virulence determinants to the severity of malaria is poorly understood. A key biologic feature of *P. falciparum* infection is the ability of parasites to mediate the adherence of infected erythrocytes to a number of ligands on endothelial cells. By this mechanism, erythrocytes infected with the more mature stages of erythrocytic parasites do not circulate but rather adhere within small blood vessels in the brain and other organs. This phenomenon, termed cytoadherence, allows parasites to avoid passing through the spleen, where abnormal erythrocytes would be cleared. Cytoadherence is also likely to play a major role in mediating severe manifestations of falciparum malaria, with local inflammatory changes mediated by large numbers of adherent parasites leading to organ dysfunction. In

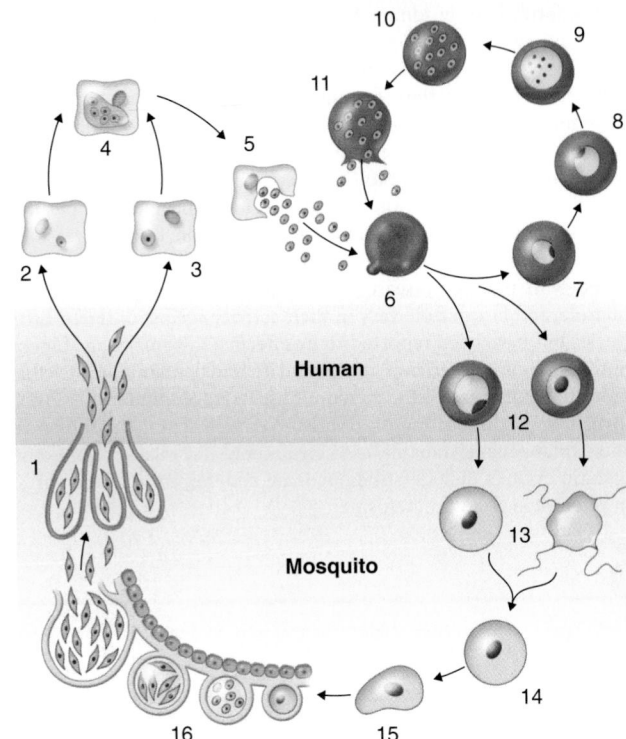

FIGURE 353-1. Life cycle of the malaria parasite. The *upper* and *lower* halves of the diagram indicate the human and anopheline mosquito parts of the cycle, respectively. Sporozoites from the salivary gland of a female *Anopheles* mosquito are injected under the skin (1). They then travel through the blood stream to the liver (2) and mature within hepatocytes to become tissue schizonts (4). Up to 30,000 parasites are then released into the blood stream as merozoites (5) and produce symptomatic infection as they invade and destroy red blood cells. However, in *Plasmodium vivax* and *Plasmodium ovale* infection, some parasites remain dormant in the liver as hypnozoites (3), which can later develop to tissue schizonts and merozoites, leading to relapse. Once within the blood stream, merozoites (5) invade erythrocytes (6) and mature to the ring (7, 8), trophozoite (9), and schizont (10) asexual stages. Mature schizonts lyse their host erythrocytes and release the next generation of merozoites (11), which invade previously uninfected cells. Some erythrocytic parasites differentiate to sexual forms (male and female gametocytes) (12). When taken up by a mosquito, the gametocytes mature to male and female gametes (13), fuse to form zygotes (14), and then develop into ookinetes that invade the gut of the mosquito (15) and develop into oocysts (16). Mature oocysts produce sporozoites, which migrate to the salivary gland of the mosquito (1) to allow another human infection. (From Krogstad DJ: Blood and tissue protozoa. In: Schaechter M, Medoff G, Eisenstein BI, eds. *Mechanisms of Microbial Diseases*, 2nd ed. Baltimore: Williams & Wilkins; 1993:600.)

particular, falciparum malaria can progress to cerebral malaria, including coma; noncardiogenic pulmonary edema, including severe respiratory compromise; and renal failure, severe anemia, acidosis, hypoglycemia, and other syndromes of organ dysfunction. Pregnancy selects for a subset of *P. falciparum* strains that specifically bind to ligands in the placenta. Pregnant women in endemic areas, in particular those in their first pregnancy who lack antibodies specific for placenta-binding parasites, are at high risk of morbidity, including anemia, from high parasite loads in the placenta and of poor fetal outcomes, including intrauterine growth retardation, spontaneous abortion, and low birthweight.

A common cause of death from falciparum malaria, in particular in children in endemic areas, is severe anemia. Anemia is caused by destruction of infected and uninfected erythrocytes, decreased hematopoiesis, and bleeding. In many endemic areas, most asymptomatic young children are infected with *P. falciparum*, with chronic infection contributing to chronic anemia. Other factors contributing to anemia are nutritional deficits and intestinal roundworm infections. With frequent malarial infections and chronic anemia, children are ill-equipped to manage acute worsening of the anemia due to acute malarial illness. With limited access to health care, children often present for medical care late in the course of illness if at all, and many deaths result.

P. falciparum parasites use antigenic variation to evade the host immune response. The principal protein that mediates the cytoadherence of infected erythrocytes to endothelial cells, *P. falciparum* erythrocyte membrane protein-1 (PfEMP-1), is transported to the erythrocyte surface and is a target of host immune responses that limit infection. The PfEMP-1 family comprises about 60 proteins, but only one PfEMP-1 variant is expressed on the surface of infected erythrocytes at a time. During the course of an infection, parasites frequently vary the expression of PfEMP-1s to stymie host responses. This factor and the high variability in sequence of many PfEMP-1 molecules present a broad repertoire of antigens and probably help explain the slow acquisition of protective antimalarial immunity. Antigenic variation and other aspects of immunologic diversity are poorly understood for non-falciparum malaria parasites, but each species appears capable of repeated infections.

Plasmodial parasites other than *P. falciparum* do not cause cytoadherence of infected erythrocytes, infect lower numbers of erythrocytes, and are much less commonly responsible for complicated and severe disease. However, recent reports suggest that *P. vivax* can cause severe disease, in particular respiratory compromise, more commonly than has previously been appreciated. *P. vivax* is also particularly prone to cause splenic rupture, although this complication can be seen with all malarial species. *P. malariae* most commonly causes a mild febrile illness, but chronic or repeated infection has been associated with an immune complex–mediated glomerulonephritis with nephrotic syndrome (Chapter 123). Recent reports indicate that *P. knowlesi* can cause severe illness, including deaths. The short (24-hour) erythrocytic cycle of *P. knowlesi*, which allows more rapid replication of these parasites compared with others, may partly explain the propensity of this zoonotic parasite to cause severe illness.

Host Immunity and Genetics

The nature of human immune responses to malaria remains poorly characterized, but protective responses require multiple infections and apparently humoral and cell-mediated responses. Where falciparum malaria is common, disease occurs primarily in children. After some protection during the first few months of life, probably due to protective effects of maternal antiplasmodial antibodies and fetal hemoglobin, young children are infected frequently, suffer repeated febrile malaria illnesses, and are at high risk of severe disease. With repeated episodes of malaria, children develop partial immunity. Immunity develops gradually, with some protection against severe malaria after only a few infections, increasing protection against symptomatic illness in children, and eventually strong protection against infection. Thus, in highly endemic areas, young children experience frequent episodes of malaria, especially at about age 6 months to 5 years; older children are frequently infected but uncommonly symptomatic, and adults experience identifiable malarial parasitemia only uncommonly. However, antimalarial immunity is not complete; malaria can occur in individuals of any age. In addition, immunity requires boosting by repeated infections, and so adults are at increased risk of disease if they return to a highly endemic site after an extended stay in a nonendemic area.

A number of human genetic polymorphisms offer protection against malaria. The best characterized is sickle hemoglobin (Chapter 166). Hemoglobin S heterozygotes are partially protected against severe falciparum malaria, leading to a balanced polymorphism in which the survival advantage of the polymorphism allows persistence of sickle cell disease in homozygotes. Other erythrocyte polymorphisms that also are likely to offer protection against malaria include hemoglobin C and E, thalassemias (Chapter 165), glucose-6-phosphate dehydrogenase deficiency (Chapter 164), and ovalocytosis (Chapter 164). The Duffy antigen, an erythrocyte chemokine receptor of uncertain function, is the principal receptor on human erythrocytes for attachment and subsequent invasion of *P. vivax*. Most Africans lack the erythrocyte Duffy antigen, explaining the nearly complete absence of vivax malaria in most of Africa.

CLINICAL MANIFESTATIONS

Uncomplicated Malaria

Most malarial episodes, even with *P. falciparum* infection, are uncomplicated. The incubation period after an infectious bite is usually 10 to 14 days for *P. falciparum* and about 2 weeks for other species, but this can be much longer, especially in non-falciparum malaria and in individuals with prior immunity. The hallmark of malaria is fever, often with a nonspecific influenza-like prodrome including headache and fatigue, followed by a classic malarial paroxysm including chills, high fever, and then sweats. Patients may be remarkably well between febrile episodes. Fevers are typically irregular early in the illness but without therapy may become regular, with 48-hour (*P. vivax* and *P. ovale*) or 72-hour (*P. malariae*) cycles, especially with non-falciparum disease. Headache, malaise, myalgias, arthralgias, rigors, confusion, cough, chest pain, abdominal pain, anorexia, nausea, vomiting, and diarrhea are common.

Seizures are often simple febrile convulsions, especially in young children, but they also may represent evidence of severe neurologic disease. Physical findings may be absent or include signs of anemia, jaundice, splenomegaly, and mild hepatomegaly. Rash and lymphadenopathy are not typical in malaria and thus suggestive of another cause of fever. Laboratory studies commonly show anemia, thrombocytopenia, and liver and renal function abnormalities.

Severe Falciparum Malaria

Severe malaria can be defined as presentation with signs of severe illness or organ dysfunction (including prostration, impaired consciousness, convulsions, respiratory distress, shock, acidosis, severe anemia, excessive bleeding, hypoglycemia, jaundice, hemoglobinuria, and renal impairment) or a high parasite load (generally peripheral parasitemia >5% or >200,000 parasites/μL). Cerebral malaria, the most common severe complication in children, is generally defined as altered consciousness in the setting of falciparum malaria. Seizures are common, and deep coma, abnormal posturing, focal neurologic findings, and abnormal respiratory patterns can be seen. Mortality is 15 to 25%, with about 10% with persistence of neurologic sequelae, but many patients do remarkably well with appropriate therapy.

Severe anemia is a common presentation, particularly in young children. Transfusions are avoided when possible but play a key role in management of those with severe compromise. Respiratory failure is caused by noncardiogenic pulmonary edema and is more common in adults than in children. Mechanical ventilation can be life-saving, if available. Acute renal failure is also more common in adults and generally due to hypoperfusion and acute tubular necrosis; hemofiltration and hemodialysis are valuable, if available. Blackwater fever, including intravascular hemolysis and hemoglobinuria, has an uncertain etiology but can be caused by quinine. Hepatic dysfunction, including jaundice, can be seen; jaundice may also be due to hemolysis. Splenic enlargement is common, and splenic rupture can be seen. Hypoglycemia is common because of glucose consumption by parasites, increased demand, impaired gluconeogenesis, and quinine-induced insulin secretion; blood glucose levels should be observed closely, with replacement as needed. Metabolic acidosis due to lactic acidosis and other factors is common; the value of specific therapies for acidosis or aggressive fluid resuscitation is uncertain. Electrolyte derangements can be seen. Coagulopathy, caused by consumption of clotting factors, and marked thrombocytopenia, due to increased platelet turnover, can lead to significant bleeding. Bacterial infection and sepsis can coexist with malaria; presumptive use of antibiotics is warranted when signs of sepsis are seen.

Complications of Non-Falciparum Malaria

The large majority of infections with non-falciparum parasites are uncomplicated both in endemic areas and in nonimmune travelers. Nonetheless, *P. vivax* infection is common in many areas, and studies from a number of sites in Asia and Oceania have shown that it makes up about a quarter of children hospitalized with severe malaria, with a mortality of about 1%. Important features of severe vivax malaria include severe anemia and respiratory distress. All malarias, but in particular *P. vivax* infection, can be complicated by splenic rupture. Chronic malaria infections can be complicated by hyperreactive malarial splenomegaly, with massive splenomegaly and findings of hypersplenism. Chronic infections can also lead to the nephrotic syndrome, particularly with *P. malariae* infection.

DIAGNOSIS

Clinical Features

In individuals with febrile illness and malaria risk, it is essential to make a diagnosis promptly and also important to distinguish the different species that infect humans as management differs according to the infecting species. Malaria is the most common cause of febrile illness in many areas, and with limited diagnostic capabilities, it is frequently diagnosed based only on presentation with a febrile illness. However, formal diagnosis is preferred. In travelers returning from endemic areas with fever, historical details can aid in the diagnosis. Malaria is most likely in individuals who failed to use measures to prevent infection and in travelers to the most highly endemic areas, such as rural sub-Saharan Africa. Falciparum malaria generally has a fairly short incubation period in nonimmune individuals and so presents within 1 to 2 months of return in more than 90% of travelers. Infection with the other malarial species can present a number of months and uncommonly more than a year after exposure.

Blood Smears

The standard means of diagnosis in malaria-endemic areas is by thick blood smear. In this procedure, a drop of blood is allowed to dry on a slide, erythrocytes are lysed, and parasites are then stained with Giemsa. Parasites are easily identified by trained microscopists, and parasite density can be estimated on the basis of counts relative to those of leukocytes. However, thick blood smears do not allow consideration of erythrocyte morphology, which is helpful in species diagnosis, and are difficult for those with limited training. Giemsa-stained thin blood smears offer an improved means of characterizing parasite morphology, but the process is much less efficient than for thick smears. Thus, thick smears are the standard means of diagnosis in highly endemic areas, and thin smears are preferred where malaria is uncommon and where laboratory personnel have ample time to examine multiple microscopic fields. It is important to distinguish infecting species of malaria parasites. In *P. falciparum* infection, generally only ring-form asexual parasites are seen. Trophozoites of *P. vivax* and *P. ovale* are present in enlarged (and ovoid in the case of *P. ovale*) erythrocytes that contain inclusions known as Schüffner's dots. Intraerythrocytic *P. malariae* and *P. knowlesi* trophozoites are often elongate in shape. Sexual stage gametocytes (which have a characteristic oblong shape in *P. falciparum*) are also seen on blood smears; most treatments do not eradicate gametocytes, so persistence of these forms for a few weeks is not a sign of treatment failure.

Antigen Detection

An important new means of malaria diagnosis is antigen detection. Multiple simple tests are now available, incorporating colorimetric detection of one or two antigens in an assay that requires limited training and only a few minutes. The most used assays in Africa use histidine-rich protein-2, a protein that is abundant and long-lived but expressed only by *P. falciparum*. Other assays identify plasmodial lactate dehydrogenase and aldolase, which are produced by all human malarial species. Some tests use two antigens to separately identify *P. falciparum* and all-species plasmodial infection. Rapid diagnostic tests have recently become a standard component of many malaria control programs. One test is approved in the United States. However, with many different tests available around the world, standardization is not optimal, and the specific role of rapid antigen tests for the diagnosis of malaria in different epidemiologic settings is not yet established.

Other Diagnostic Tests

Serologic tests are available to identify prior malaria infection, but responses develop slowly and persist for an extended period, so these tests have limited clinical value, unless it is helpful to diagnose the cause of a febrile illness retrospectively in an individual without prior history of malaria. Malaria parasites can be identified readily with polymerase chain reaction (PCR) using primers encoding genus- and species-specific sequences. These tests are convenient for research purposes as they can be conducted on DNA extracted from blood spotted onto filter paper in field settings. PCR is more sensitive than other diagnostic modalities. It is not practical for routine diagnosis because of the time required to complete an assay, the uncertain significance of a positive test result in endemic areas where low-level parasitemia may be common and clinically insignificant, and the cost and logistical requirements of the procedure in developing countries.

TREATMENT **Rx**

The treatment of falciparum malaria has been challenged by drug resistance for many years and has changed dramatically recently, with recommendations for artemisinin-based combination therapy in nearly all countries endemic for falciparum malaria (Table 353-1). Non-falciparum malaria is still generally treated with chloroquine, although chloroquine resistance is increasing in *P. vivax*.

Chloroquine and Other Aminoquinolines

Chloroquine has been widely used to treat malaria for more than 60 years. It remains the treatment of choice for non-falciparum malaria and falciparum malaria in the few areas where resistance has not been seen (primarily Central America and the Caribbean) and is generally rapidly effective and well tolerated. For *P. vivax* and *P. ovale* infections, primaquine must also be given to eradicate dormant liver forms and thereby prevent subsequent relapse. Chloroquine remains effective as weekly chemoprophylaxis to prevent malaria in areas without resistance. Amodiaquine and piperaquine probably share mechanisms of action with chloroquine, but they are routinely active against chloroquine-resistant parasites because of increased potency compared with

chloroquine and some differences in mechanisms of resistance. Monotherapy with either drug is discouraged, but each is now a component of a leading artemisinin-based combination therapy (Table 353-2). Amodiaquine is somewhat less well tolerated than other aminoquinolines. It is generally safe with short-term use but can cause rare serious toxicities, including hepatic and bone marrow toxicity, especially with chronic use, and so it is not recommended for chemoprophylaxis. Piperaquine was well tolerated during extensive use in China a few decades ago; although resistance was reportedly common in China, it does not appear to be a problem at present.

Mefloquine, Halofantrine, and Lumefantrine

Mefloquine offers effective therapy and chemoprophylaxis for most chloroquine-resistant strains of *P. falciparum* and for other species. Resistance to mefloquine is uncommon but has been seen in parts of Southeast Asia. Mefloquine is now used to treat falciparum malaria in combination with artesunate and is one of three drugs recommended for chemoprophylaxis against *P. falciparum* by the Centers for Disease Control and Prevention (CDC). Tolerability of chemoprophylactic and especially treatment doses of

---

TABLE 353-1 TREATMENT OF MALARIA*

CHLOROQUINE-RESISTANT *P. FALCIPARUM*, RESISTANT *P. VIVAX*, OR SPECIES UNIDENTIFIED

Uncomplicated Disease

Coartem (artemether 20 mg, lumefantrine 120 mg)	4 tablets orally twice daily for 3 days
or	
Malarone (atovaquone 250 mg, proguanil 100 mg)	4 tablets daily for 3 days
or	
Quinine	650 mg quinine sulfate 3 times daily for 3-7 days
plus	
Doxycycline	100 mg twice daily for 7 days
or plus	
Clindamycin	600 mg twice daily for 7 days
or	
Mefloquine	1250 mg (15 mg/kg) once or 750 mg followed by 500 mg in 6-8 hr; can also be given as a single 1250-mg dose, although less well tolerated

Complicated *P. Falciparum* Malaria or Unable to Tolerate Oral Medications[†]

IV artesunate[‡]	2.4 mg/kg every 12 hr on day 1, then daily for 2 additional days
or	
IV quinidine gluconate[§]	10 mg/kg over 1 to 2 hr, then 0.02 mg/kg/min *or* 15 mg/kg over 4 hr, then 7.5 mg/kg over 4 hr every 8 hr
or	
IV quinine dihydrochloride[§,¶]	20 mg/kg over 4 hr, then 10 mg/kg every 8 hr
or	
IM artemether[¶]	3.2 mg/kg IM, then 1.6 mg/kg/day

CHLOROQUINE-SUSCEPTIBLE *P. FALCIPARUM* AND OTHER SPECIES

Chloroquine phosphate	1 g, followed by 500 mg at 6, 24, and 48 hr *or* 1 g at 0 and 24 hr, then 0.5 g at 48 hr
plus (for *P. vivax* and *P. ovale* only)	
Primaquine[§]	30-mg base (52.6 mg primaquine phosphate) daily for 14 days

*Dosages refer to salts unless indicated and are for adults. For pediatric dosing and full CDC recommendations, see http://www.cdc.gov/malaria/pdf/treatmenttable.pdf. For the CDC malaria hotline, call 770-488-7788.

[†]IV regimens should be given until the patient can tolerate oral agents, then followed by a course of oral therapy (doxycycline, clindamycin, or full treatment courses of other drugs, as listed) when patients can tolerate this.

[‡]Available in the United States on an investigational basis through the CDC (phone 770-488-7788 or 770-488-7100).

[§]Cardiac monitoring should be in place during IV administration of quinidine or quinine.

[¶]Not available in the United States.

[§]Use primaquine only after demonstrating normal levels of glucose-6-phosphate dehydrogenase.

TABLE 353-2 RECOMMENDATIONS FOR THE TREATMENT OF FALCIPARUM MALARIA IN DEVELOPING COUNTRIES*

REGIMEN	NOTES
Artemether-lumefantrine (Coartem, Riamet)	First-line therapy in many countries; FDA approved
Artesunate-amodiaquine (ASAQ)	First-line therapy in many African countries; efficacy limited by resistance to amodiaquine in many areas
Artesunate-mefloquine	Standard therapy in parts of Southeast Asia
Artesunate-sulfadoxine-pyrimethamine	Efficacy low compared with other regimens in most areas
Dihydroartemisinin-piperaquine	Newer regimen; highly effective in studies in Asia and Africa
Amodiaquine-sulfadoxine-pyrimethamine	Recommended as an interim option when efficacy established and newer regimens are not available

*Recommendations modified from World Health Organization. *Guidelines for the Treatment of Malaria.* Geneva: World Health Organization; 2010. ISBN 9789241547925.

mefloquine is often limited by neurologic and gastrointestinal toxicity. Halofantrine is an effective drug, but its use is limited by uncommon but dangerous cardiac rhythm disturbances. Lumefantrine is a related drug that does not share this toxicity and offers effective therapy in combination with artemether as Coartem.

Quinine and Quinidine

Quinine has been used to treat malaria for hundreds of years. It offers rapid action against all species, with limited known resistance except in Southeast Asia, where failures against falciparum malaria are fairly common. Quinine can be used to treat uncomplicated malaria, but gastrointestinal and other nonspecific toxicities lead to difficulty in tolerating a full 7-day treatment course. This problem is circumvented by combining a 3-day course of quinine with other agents. For severe disease, intravenous quinine or, in the United States, intravenous quinidine has been standard therapy for many years; therapy should be accompanied by cardiac monitoring because of cardiac toxicities of the drugs.

Primaquine

Primaquine is the only available drug to eradicate dormant liver forms of *P. vivax* and *P. ovale* that are not cleared by other drugs and can lead to relapses after therapy with chloroquine and other agents. Primaquine is also an alternative agent for chemoprophylaxis against *P. falciparum* and other species. Primaquine use is limited principally by hemolysis or methemoglobinemia (Chapter 161) in individuals with deficiency in glucose-6-phosphate dehydrogenase (Chapter 164). Testing for deficiency should ideally be performed before use of the drug.

Inhibitors of Folate Metabolism

Inhibitors of two parasite enzymes involved in folate metabolism, dihydrofolate reductase and dihydropteroate synthase, are used in fixed-dose combination regimens for the treatment and prevention of malaria. For treatment, sulfadoxine-pyrimethamine (Fansidar) was heavily used to treat uncomplicated falciparum malaria, but resistance has increased markedly in most endemic areas. The dihydrofolate reductase inhibitor proguanil is combined with atovaquone in Malarone (see later). For chemoprophylaxis, sulfadoxine-pyrimethamine is no longer recommended because of drug resistance and rare life-threatening dermatologic toxicities. However, less frequent dosing in intermittent preventive therapy regimens has been well tolerated and has decreased malaria in high-risk African groups, in particular, pregnant women and young children. Daily trimethoprim-sulfamethoxazole, a common prophylactic to prevent opportunistic infections in individuals with HIV infection, has offered some protection against malaria in Africa.

Artemisinins

Artemisinin, the active component of an herbal medicine from China, and a number of analogues offer rapid elimination of circulating malaria parasites and also activity against gametocytes to limit disease transmission. The drugs are all short-acting, leading to frequent recrudescences of infection after short-course monotherapy. For this reason and to prevent selection of resistance, artemisinins are now used in combination with longer acting drugs to treat malaria in 3-day regimens. A number of these combinations have become the standard therapies for falciparum malaria in most endemic countries (see Table 353-2). Leading regimens are artemether-lumefantrine, artesunate-amodiaquine, artesunate-mefloquine, and dihydroartemisinin-piperaquine.[1-5] Of these, artemether-lumefantrine is most widely advocated, is now approved in the United States, includes a partner drug that has never been available as

monotherapy, but requires twice-daily therapy. The other regimens offer once-daily therapy but have potential problems with resistance to partner drugs. Resistance to artemisinins is a recent concern, with evidence for prolonged times to parasite clearance in Southeast Asia suggestive of diminished drug responsiveness of *P. falciparum*.[6] Artemisinins also have an increasing role for the treatment of severe malaria. Intravenous artesunate has been shown to be superior to quinine for the treatment of severe malaria in a mostly adult population in Asia.[7] Most recent evidence clearly supports the superiority of parenteral artesunate over quinine for the treatment of severe malaria in both adults and children and in different regions of the world.[8] For settings with limited infrastructure, intramuscular artemether and intrarectal artesunate have also shown good efficacy. Intravenous artesunate should now be considered the first-line therapy for severe malaria in the United States, where it is available from the CDC. Artemisinins are generally very well tolerated, with minimal toxicity.

Atovaquone-Proguanil (Malarone)

This fixed-dose combination of a dihydrofolate reductase inhibitor and atovaquone, which has a unique antimalarial mechanism, has excellent efficacy against most *P. falciparum* infections. It is approved for both treatment and chemoprophylaxis of falciparum malaria and other species in the United States, where it is now widely used for both indications. Malarone offers excellent efficacy with minimal toxicity. Adverse effects may include gastrointestinal symptoms, elevations in liver enzymes, headache, and rash. Widespread use in developing countries is limited by high cost and concerns about resistance, as resistance to each component drug is readily selected.

Antibiotics

A number of antibacterials are slow-acting antimalarials. Tetracyclines and clindamycin should not be used alone to treat malaria but are combined with quinine to allow a shorter duration of therapy with that drug. In addition, doxycycline is effective in chemoprophylaxis of most falciparum malaria and is recommended for this purpose by the CDC, in particular for travelers to regions of Southeast Asia with high-level resistance to other drugs. Macrolides also have antimalarial activity and are currently under study for treatment and prophylaxis.

Treatment of Severe Malaria

Severe malaria is a medical emergency and requires parenteral therapy. With appropriate prompt therapy and supportive care, rapid recoveries may be seen even in very ill individuals. As noted before, standard therapy for severe malaria has been intravenous quinine or quinidine, with continuous cardiac monitoring if possible. However, intravenous artesunate showed superior efficacy and decreased toxicity[7-9] and although it is not yet available in most endemic areas, this is likely to become the worldwide standard to treat severe malaria. In the United States, intravenous quinidine is not available in all hospitals, and intravenous artesunate must be obtained from the CDC; treatment should be with whichever treatment is most rapidly available. Appropriate care of severe malaria includes close nursing care; maintenance of fluids and electrolytes, including glucose; respiratory and hemodynamic support; and consideration of blood transfusions, anticonvulsants, antibiotics for bacterial infections, and hemodialysis or hemofiltration. Aggressive fluid resuscitation, blood transfusion for moderate anemia, exchange transfusion, and specific treatment of acidosis are of uncertain value. After the acute illness, parenteral quinine, quinidine, or artesunate should be followed with oral longer acting drugs, typically doxycycline, clindamycin, Malarone, mefloquine, or a full course of an oral artemisinin-based combination therapy.

PREVENTION

Recent years have been marked by a dramatic increase in interest and investment in the control of malaria. Key malaria control interventions in malaria-endemic regions are control of mosquito vectors by indoor residual spraying of insecticides; personal protection against mosquito bites with insecticide-impregnated bed nets; routine use of artemisinin-based combination therapies, which offer prompt control of malaria infections and activity against gametocytes to limit transmission to mosquitoes; and selected use of intermittent preventive therapies to decrease malarial incidence in high-risk groups. No vaccine to prevent malaria is yet available, but extensive research on potential vaccines including multiple clinical trials is under way. A fully protective malaria vaccine is not expected in the near future, but vaccines that offer significant decreases in malarial incidence for children and other high-risk groups in endemic areas may be available soon.

Preventive Measures for Travelers to Malaria-Endemic Regions

It is important for nonimmune travelers (Chapter 294) to endemic areas to be protected against potentially lethal malaria. Travelers should decrease exposure to night-biting anopheline mosquitoes by use of insecticide repellants

TABLE 353-3 CHEMOPROPHYLAXIS OF MALARIA*

AREAS WITH CHLOROQUINE-RESISTANT *P. FALCIPARUM*	
Malarone	1 tablet (250 mg artesunate/100 mg proguanil) daily
Mefloquine	250 mg weekly
Doxycycline	100 mg daily
Primaquine[†]	30 mg daily during exposure (chemoprophylaxis) or 30 mg daily for 14 days (terminal prophylaxis against *P. vivax* and *P. ovale*)

AREAS WITHOUT CHLOROQUINE-RESISTANT *P. FALCIPARUM*	
Chloroquine phosphate	500 mg weekly

*Recommendations may change on the basis of drug resistance patterns. For additional details and pediatric dosing, see CDC guidelines (*http://www.cdc.gov*) or call 770-488-7788 or 770-488-7100. Begin 1 to 2 weeks before travel for mefloquine and 2 days before for doxycycline, Malarone, and primaquine; continue for 4 weeks after leaving the endemic area (1 week for Malarone; 2 weeks for primaquine). All doses refer to salts unless indicated.
[†]Use primaquine only after demonstrating normal levels of glucose-6-phosphate dehydrogenase.

and sleeping in rooms that are screened or equipped with insecticide-impregnated bed nets. Standard advice for travelers to endemic areas is also to use low doses of preventive drugs chosen on the basis of the resistance profile of the particular region. Chloroquine is still recommended for malaria endemic regions of Central America and the Caribbean. For nearly all other areas, the CDC recommends use of daily Malarone, weekly mefloquine, or daily doxycycline; details of dosing vary, but it is important to continue therapy after return from travel to eliminate parasites as they emerge from the liver (Table 353-3). For areas with high risk of vivax malaria, some authorities recommend a full treatment course of primaquine after travel to eliminate dormant liver stages. For all chemoprophylaxis, it is important to appreciate that no mosquito avoidance methods or drug regimens are fully protective, and so consideration of malaria as a cause of fever in returned travelers is essential (Chapter 294).

PROGNOSIS

Patients with malaria due to *P. vivax*, *P. ovale*, or *P. malariae* generally respond well to chloroquine and make an uneventful recovery. Chloroquine-resistance is increasing with *P. vivax* from many areas; failures of initial treatment are usually not dangerous but should be followed by treatment with another regimen, such as an artemisinin-based combination therapy, Malarone, or mefloquine. Falciparum malaria also generally responds well to prompt therapy as long as the disease is not overly advanced at presentation. The mortality rate in uncomplicated falciparum malaria is about 0.1%. Key contributing factors to most deaths from falciparum malaria are probably delay between the appearance of symptoms and presentation for definitive therapy and the use of suboptimal therapies. Presentation with high-level parasitemia (>200,000 parasites/μL or >5% parasitemia) or signs of severe malaria are predictive of poor outcome. However, with aggressive support, even individuals with severe disease can often experience complete recoveries.

1. Mutabingwa TK, Anthony D, Heller A, et al. Amodiaquine alone, amodiaquine+sulfadoxine-pyrimethamine, amodiaquine+artesunate, and artemether-lumefantrine for outpatient treatment of malaria in Tanzanian children: a four-arm randomised effectiveness trial. *Lancet*. 2005;365:1474-1480.
2. Smithuis F, Kyaw MK, Phe O, et al. Efficacy and effectiveness of dihydroartemisinin-piperaquine versus artesunate-mefloquine in falciparum malaria: an open-label randomised comparison. *Lancet*. 2006;367:2075-2085.
3. Dorsey G, Staedke S, Clark TD, et al. Combination therapy for uncomplicated falciparum malaria in Ugandan children: a randomized trial. *JAMA*. 2007;297:2210-2219.
4. Ratcliff A, Siswantoro H, Kenangalem E, et al. Two fixed-dose artemisinin combinations for drug-resistant falciparum and vivax malaria in Papua, Indonesia: an open-label randomised comparison. *Lancet*. 2007;369:757-765.
5. Zongo I, Dorsey G, Rouamba N, et al. Randomized comparison of amodiaquine plus sulfadoxine-pyrimethamine, artemether-lumefantrine, and dihydroartemisinin-piperaquine for the treatment of uncomplicated *Plasmodium falciparum* malaria in Burkina Faso. *Clin Infect Dis*. 2007;45:1453-1461.
6. Dondorp AM, Nosten F, Yi P, et al. Artemisinin resistance in *Plasmodium falciparum* malaria. *N Engl J Med*. 2009;361:455-467.
7. Dondorp A, Nosten F, Stepniewska K, et al. Artesunate versus quinine for treatment of severe falciparum malaria: a randomised trial. *Lancet*. 2005;366:717-725.
8. Sinclair D, Donegan S, Lalloo DG. Artesunate versus quinine for treating severe malaria. *Cochrane Database Syst Rev* 2011;3:CD005967.
9. Dondorp AM, Fanello CI, Hendriksen IC, et al. Artesunate versus quinine in the treatment of severe falciparum malaria in African children (AQUAMAT): an open-label, randomised trial. *Lancet*. 2010;376:1647-1657.

SUGGESTED READINGS

Freedman DO. Malaria prevention in short-term travelers. *N Engl J Med*. 2008;359:603-612. *A comprehensive review.*

Kappe SHI, Vaughan AM, Boddey JA, Cowman AF. That was then but this is now: malaria research in the time of an eradication agenda. *Science*. 2010;328:862-866. *Recent advances in malaria parasite biology and the implications for intervention targets for eradication.*

Lin JT, Juliano JJ, Wongsrichanalai C. Drug-resistant malaria: the era of ACT. *Curr Infect Dis Rep*. 2010;12:165-173. *Review.*

Taylor SM, Molyneux ME, Simel DL, et al. Does this patient have malaria? *JAMA*. 2010;304:2048-2056. *Case-based review.*

Wellems TE, Hayton K, Fairhurst RM. The impact of malaria parasitism: from corpuscles to communities. *J Clin Invest*. 2009;119:2496-2505. *Genetic and genomic insights into evolutionary adaptations of malaria, processes of parasite transmission and infection, and the challenges of malaria control.*

354

AFRICAN SLEEPING SICKNESS

WILLIAM A. PETRI, JR.

DEFINITION

Human African trypanosomiasis (HAT), commonly known as sleeping sickness, is a vector-borne parasitic disease transmitted to humans and animals by the bite of the tsetse fly (genus *Glossina*). Infection is caused by protozoa of the genus *Trypanosoma* and species *brucei*. In humans, there are two forms of illness caused by two distinct subspecies that are morphologically identical but differ in their geographic range and clinical presentations. *Trypanosoma brucei gambiense* is typically found in west and central Africa and *Trypanosoma brucei rhodesiense* in east Africa. *T. b. gambiense* has a more chronic course, and *T. b. rhodesiense* causes a rapid disease course; both have late stages marked by meningoencephalitis, resulting in coma and death if untreated. There is a third subspecies, *Trypanosoma brucei brucei*, known to cause chronic infection called nagana in cattle; however, humans are not susceptible to this organism.

The Pathogen

As an extracellular microbe, the parasite must evade immune clearance to establish a persistent infection. The surface of the blood stream form of the trypanosome is covered by a dense, homogeneous coat of variant surface glycoproteins (VSGs). VSGs are immunodominant, whereas invariant antigens, such as nutrient receptors, are protected from host antibody recognition by strict localization to a membrane subdomain hidden at the base of the flagellum. Each individual trypanosome expresses only one VSG at a time but possesses more than 1000 different silent copies of the VSG gene, and switching to a new VSG occurs at a frequency of about 1×10^{-6} parasites. Hence, the trypanosomes expressing a given VSG will eventually be cleared by the host antibody response, but any individual trypanosome that has switched to a new VSG will evade immune clearance, resulting in a new peak of parasitemia. Recombination between VSG alleles ensures a virtually limitless repertoire of new VSGs; therefore, antibody-mediated parasite eradication is impossible.

EPIDEMIOLOGY

Although considered one of the "neglected tropical diseases," HAT is relatively less of a problem now than it has been in the prior century, in part because of cyclic epidemics in the past as well as recent increases in public health efforts for control. However, it remains a looming threat to an estimated 60 million people living in tsetse fly–inhabited areas among 36 countries of sub-Saharan Africa and causes significant morbidity, accounting for 1.5 million disability-adjusted life years in Africa as a whole.

The causative organism was first identified during the latter half of the 19th century, roughly corresponding to the first of three epidemics occurring during the past century. The first epidemic occurred in the Congo basin and Uganda between 1896 and 1906, driven in part by various natural disasters that decimated populations of livestock and regional droughts as well as changes in population distribution influenced by colonialism. The second epidemic occurred in numerous endemic countries in the 1920s; control was achieved after major efforts to systematically screen and treat individuals, followed by extensive vector control programs, including bush clearing and insecticide spraying. These acts were nearly successful in halting transmission by the 1960s; however, the independence of many African nations around this time hindered the sustainability of prevention and control programs. The incidence began to rise by the 1970s and surged a decade later, leading to the third epidemic of this century. However, in the past 15 years, increased access to at-risk populations for diagnosis and treatment has led to a 68% reduction in the incidence of reported cases.

Despite increased surveillance efforts during the past 15 years, there are still at-risk areas that lack active monitoring programs, and many people are thought to die of HAT without an accurate diagnosis. The World Health Organization recently reported an annual incidence of 12,000 cases in 2007, a dramatic decrease from the estimated incidence of 300,000 cases a decade ago. It is estimated that 300,000 to 500,000 people are infected, contributing to approximately 100,000 deaths each year. More than 90% of reported cases are due to *T. b. gambiense*, the majority being from the Democratic Republic of the Congo.

The geographic distribution includes areas where the vector, parasite, reservoir hosts, and human hosts cohabit (Fig. 354-1). In general, these include focal areas on the African continent within 15° North and 15° South latitude, with a predilection for rural areas. Humans at greatest risk for infection are those who rely on animal husbandry, agriculture, fishing, and hunting for their livelihoods. Often, disease is concentrated among foci of rural areas, having significant socioeconomic impact on affected villages. With a few exceptions, this infection is never found in urban areas. There have been fewer than 50 cases reported annually outside of Africa, usually the result of travel by North Americans or Europeans to African game reserves.

T. b. gambiense is transmitted by tsetse flies from the *Glossina palpalis* group, which are typically found along riverbanks among wooded areas in the more tropical regions of central and west Africa. The reservoir hosts for *T. b. gambiense* and the focus of public health campaigns are mainly humans. Because of this, *T. b. gambiense* is not generally considered a zoonotic disease; the role of the animal reservoir for this organism remains undetermined, although natural infections have been reported in domestic animals such as dogs, sheep, cattle, and pigs.

T. b. rhodesiense is transmitted by tsetse flies belonging to the *Glossina morsitans* group, which are commonly found among woodland and savannah areas of east and central Africa. *T. b. rhodesiense* is a zoonotic disease with numerous wild and domestic species of animals acting as reservoirs. With this infection, the animal reservoir serves an important role in the cycle, sustaining parasite transmission and human infections. Domestic species, especially cattle, have the potential to drive outbreaks and, not surprisingly, have served as the focus of successful prevention campaigns.

PATHOBIOLOGY

After the bite of a tsetse fly carrying metacyclic trypomastigotes, a local reaction (chancre) may form at the inoculation site. This symptom is seen with *T. b. rhodesiense* infection and is more frequently observed in travelers but is rarely seen with *T. b. gambiense* infection. Parasites subsequently disseminate into the blood and lymphatic systems in what is considered stage I of the disease. Spread of the parasites into the central nervous system (CNS) defines stage II of the disease, which is invariably fatal if untreated. The parasite appears to remain extracellular throughout the course of infection.

Peaks and waves of parasitemia occur during stage I disease and result in the classic symptom of intermittent fever. These bouts of fever correspond to a type 1 inflammatory response (Chapter 47), in which classically activated macrophages produce high levels of tumor necrosis factor and nitric oxide. This helps in the control of parasitemia but also contributes to tissue damage. Type 2 inflammatory responses with high interleukin-10 production may subsequently occur, which limit tumor necrosis factor and nitric oxide production once initial parasitemia has been controlled. Antibody responses are directed to VSGs and other trypanosome antigens (e.g., antigens from lysed parasites), but autoantibodies are also produced. Generalized febrile episodes are observed together with lymphadenopathy and myocardial and pericardial inflammation. Cardiac involvement is typically more severe with *T. b. rhodesiense* infection. Anemia, thrombocytopenia, disseminated intravascular coagulation, and renal disease may also be observed.

In stage II of the disease, parasites cross the blood-brain barrier and invade the CNS. Acute meningoencephalitis develops, with a variety of inflammatory cells infiltrating the brain, including macrophages, lymphocytes, plasma cells, Mott cells, and morular cells. These inflammatory cells are found in the meninges, which become thickened, as well as in the perivascular spaces and neuropil. Edema, hemorrhage, and granulomatous lesions are often present; thrombosis and neuronal degeneration may also be observed.

CLINICAL MANIFESTATIONS

The clinical manifestations of HAT differ on the basis of the infecting organism. *T. b. gambiense* is more of a chronic disease, with an estimated average duration of 3 years; infection with *T. b. rhodesiense* progresses much more rapidly, leading to coma and death within weeks to months. However, infection with *T. b. gambiense* has been known to cause rapid decline. Other similarities exist, including an early hemolymphatic stage (stage I) and a late stage characterized by prominent CNS disease including meningoencephalitis (stage II).

West African Sleeping Sickness

Infection starts after the bite of a fly infected with *T. b. gambiense*. At the site of inoculation, a painful, indurated, and erythematous trypanosomal chancre may develop 1 to 2 weeks after the bite and resolves spontaneously after several weeks. On occasion, the chancre may ulcerate. However, these features are rarely seen at the time of clinical presentation and sometimes are not known to have occurred on history; thus, many develop disseminated disease without awareness of a localized infection.

The hemolymphatic stage, when parasites disseminate throughout the body, may not be manifested clinically until weeks or months after the initial bite. Typical symptoms include intermittent spiking fevers, occasionally accompanied by headaches and malaise. These features may persist for weeks or months because of the cyclic nature of parasitemia and antibody production against the various antigens sequentially expressed by the parasite.

Lymphadenopathy (Chapter 171) is a common finding in West African sleeping sickness. Whereas regional lymphadenopathy may develop after the initial bite, generalized lymphadenopathy around the head and neck is often found as chronic illness develops. Enlargement of nodes in the posterior cervical triangle, commonly known as Winterbottom's sign, is the classic finding; but other cervical and supraclavicular nodes may also be involved. Affected nodes are discrete, movable, rubbery nodes that are nontender to palpation; over time, they may become more indurated because of fibrosis.

Other symptoms reported include pruritus, occasionally accompanied by rash, arthralgias, and periarticular swelling as well as by transient edema of the extremities and face. Less common symptoms include features consistent with neuroendocrine dysfunction: loss of libido and impotence, amenorrhea

T.b.gambiense

T.b.rhodesiense

■ Countries reporting no cases
□ Countries reporting under 100 cases
■ Countries reporting between 100 & 1,000 cases
■ Countries reporting more than 1,000 cases

FIGURE 354-1. Map of human African trypanosomiasis. These 36 sub-Saharan African countries are considered endemic for HAT. *Shaded areas* represent the reported incidence from 1997 to 2006. The *black line* roughly represents the dividing line for the two parasites, although some overlap may already occur.

and infertility, alopecia, and gynecomastia. Signs of disease include hepatomegaly and splenomegaly, cardiac dysfunction including tachycardia, electrocardiographic abnormalities like prolonged QTc intervals and repolarization changes, and, less commonly, pericarditis or myocarditis. Hemolytic anemia and derangements in liver function test results may occur.

Months or even years after the initial infection, stage II disease develops and is characterized by headaches, daytime somnolence, and neuropsychiatric features. Behavioral changes, including irritability, confusion, inability to concentrate, and lassitude, are among the first signs of CNS disease; psychosis has also been described. Neurologic findings are numerous and include a variety of motor and sensory disturbances, including extrapyramidal features, dysesthesias, and visual impairment. Disruption of the normal circadian rhythm has allowed its common name of sleeping sickness and is manifested by daytime somnolence and nocturnal irritability. Late-stage disease is marked by cerebral edema and meningoencephalitis. Progressively, a loss of neurologic function can lead to paralysis, and many may succumb to aspiration pneumonias or malnutrition; otherwise, coma leads to death in the absence of treatment.

East African Sleeping Sickness

In comparison to Gambian sleeping sickness, East African sleeping sickness is more rapidly progressive. The infective bite is more frequently associated with the development of a chancre, although some studies report this in only 20% of patients. An incubation period lasting days to weeks is needed before symptoms are demonstrated. Initial symptoms include severe intermittent fevers that may resemble those found with malaria infection. Lymphadenopathy is not as common with this infecting organism; Winterbottom's sign is typically absent. Skin changes are more prominent, and rashes in the early stage of infection are particularly common in expatriates with the infection. In addition, cardiac manifestations are more commonly and clinically relevant; tachycardia, arrhythmias, myocarditis, and congestive heart failure have been documented and may be severe enough to cause death before the development of severe CNS disease. Hematologic abnormalities include anemia, thrombocytopenia, and disseminated intravascular coagulation. CNS disease mirrors that of West African sleeping sickness, but the onset occurs earlier and the rate of deterioration is more rapid. Death may ensue after weeks or months without treatment.

DIAGNOSIS

Epidemiologic clues and clinical findings may together suggest the diagnosis of HAT, but definitive diagnosis relies on demonstration of the parasite. In the early stage of disease, light microscopy and Giemsa stain may be employed to visualize the highly motile parasites directly from fresh specimens of fluid expressed from chancres or lymph node aspirates. Peripheral blood smears, including Giemsa-stained thick and thin smears and bone marrow aspirates, have been successful. Blood smears have increased sensitivity when they are performed during stage I disease, when parasitemia is high (Fig. 354-2); the threshold for visualization of parasites by thick smear is approximately 5000 parasites/mL. Performance is superior with *T. b. rhodesiense* infection, given the higher parasite load. If the initial smear analysis is negative, subsequent examinations should be pursued. Concentration techniques including buffy coat analysis should be employed when technically feasible. Culture of any of these fluids may yield higher sensitivity than smear preparations.

Cerebrospinal fluid (CSF) must also be analyzed to determine the most appropriate treatment. Abnormalities in CSF analysis often start with increased cell counts and progress to include an elevated opening pressure and total protein levels with an increased polyclonal IgM. Stage II disease is

defined by the presence of more than 5 white blood cells/μL, the presence of trypanosomes, or an elevated total protein count (>370 mg/L) in the CSF. Newer diagnostic methods including polymerase chain reaction analysis of CSF and a latex-agglutination test for CSF IgM hold promise but require validation to determine outcomes after treatment of patients with positive test results.

Serology tests are also available for diagnosis of *T. b. gambiense* infection. The card agglutination test for trypanosomiasis with *T. b. gambiense* (CATT) is commonly used by screening programs; the sensitivity ranges from 87 to 98%, depending on the population under study, and the specificity may be as high as 95%. There are no serology tests available for *T. b. rhodesiense* infection.

Allocation of resources to this neglected tropical disease in recent years has allowed slow but exciting progress in the field of HAT diagnostics. The genomes of *T. brucei* species have been mapped, and molecular assays have been developed that can distinguish between species of HAT with a single polymerase chain reaction test. Novel uses of mass spectrometry have been developed that employ proteomic signature analysis to identify specific fingerprints of HAT with the host. In contrast to these highly technical and expensive methods, other tests suitable for the field are being validated, including the dot-ELISA test, which would be able to provide information on stage of disease.

TREATMENT

There are very few drugs for treatment of HAT, and those that are commonly used are quite toxic (Table 354-1). Treatment is dependent on the infecting organism and the stage of disease. For stage I disease with *T. b. gambiense* infection, pentamidine is the drug of choice. The standard regimen consists of daily parenteral administration for 1 week; however, studies are ongoing to determine the efficacy of shortening therapy to three doses.

Suramin is also used for stage I disease with *T. b. rhodesiense*. This medication is complex to mix and to administer. The drug must be administered in a slow intravenous infusion periodically during 3 weeks. Although anaphylaxis is rare (approximately 1 : 20,000 patients), a test dose is recommended before full treatment is initiated. There are a number of side effects that require close monitoring, the most important being nephrotoxicity. Urinalysis is recommended before each dose, and the drug should be discontinued if proteinuria persists and casts are seen in the urine sediment.

Melarsoprol is a highly effective but impressively toxic drug used for stage II disease with either organism. The side effects are numerous, but the most important is the life-threatening encephalopathy that may develop from the arsenic (highly fatal) or as an inflammatory reaction. Concomitant steroid use is helpful in reducing the risk of encephalopathy and mortality without compromising the efficacy of melarsoprol. Gradual increase in the first round of treatment between 2 and 3.6 mg/kg in divided doses three times daily during 3 days has also been shown to reduce the risks of encephalopathy. Melarsoprol has been replaced by eflornithine for *T. b. gambiense* infection but remains the only agent available for the treatment of stage II *T. b. rhodesiense* infection.

Developed more than 20 years ago, eflornithine is the newest agent and drug of choice for treatment of stage II disease with *T. b. gambiense*. Unfortunately, it is not effective as monotherapy for *T. b. rhodesiense* because of reduced susceptibility of this organism to the drug. Eflornithine requires frequent intravenous administration, and up to 40% of patients may report some adverse effects. The drug is much more tolerable than its predecessor melarsoprol and is associated with a reduced mortality, comparatively.

PREVENTION

To date, there is no vaccine against HAT. The mainstays of prevention include active case finding with early treatment and vector control. Given the nature of each infection, active case surveillance is more suitable for infection with *T. b. gambiense*, whereas vector control is more effective for prevention of infection with *T. b. rhodesiense*. The goal of active case finding is to identify infected individuals who may still be in the asymptomatic stage or early stage. This approach, which is more suited for disease from *T. b. gambiense*, typically consists of a screening examination for lymphadenopathy followed by a CATT test. If results are positive for both, the patient should undergo further evaluation with lymph node aspirate and blood testing. If trypanosomes are found, the patient should be treated. Vector control measures include tsetse fly traps and insecticide-impregnated screens; the traps are easily maintained by locals, whereas the screens require regular re-treatment and thus are more labor intensive and costly to maintain. Mass spraying, once a successful

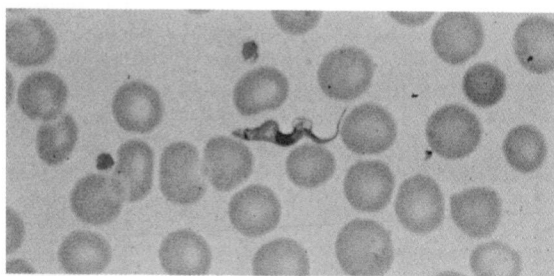

FIGURE 354-2. *Trypanosoma rhodesiense* in peripheral blood. It has a nucleus, posterior kinetoplast, undulating membrane, and flagellum (×1500).

TABLE 354-1 DRUGS USED TO TREAT HUMAN AFRICAN TRYPANOSOMIASIS

DRUG	CLASS	STAGE	ROUTE	ADULT DOSE	ADVERSE EFFECTS
TRYPANOSOMA BRUCEI GAMBIENSE					
Pentamidine	Aromatic diamidine	I	Intramuscular or intravenous	4 mg/kg daily for 7 days	Pain, gastrointestinal symptoms, hypoglycemia or hyperglycemia, electrolyte abnormalities, leukopenia, thrombocytopenia
Eflornithine	Ornithine carboxylase inhibitor	II	Intravenous	100 mg/kg every 6 hr for 14 days	Gastrointestinal symptoms, bone marrow toxicity, seizures
Melarsoprol (alternative option)	Trivalent arsenical	II	Intravenous	2.2 mg/kg daily for 10 days (maximum daily dose is 180 mg)	Encephalopathic syndromes, peripheral neuropathy, paralysis, cardiac dysrhythmias, gastrointestinal symptoms, rash, pruritus, thrombophlebitis
TRYPANOSOMA BRUCEI RHODESIENSE					
Suramin	Polysulfonated naphthylamine derivative of urea	I	Intravenous	1 g IV on days 1, 3, 7, 14, and 21 (after test dose of 100-200 mg)	Anaphylaxis, nephrotoxicity, fever, rash, pruritus, arthralgias, reversible peripheral neuropathy and bone marrow toxicity
Melarsoprol	Trivalent arsenical	II	Intravenous	1.2 mg/kg every 8 hr for 3 consecutive days each week for 3 weeks (maximum daily dose is 180 mg)	Encephalopathic syndromes, peripheral neuropathy, paralysis, cardiac dysrhythmias, gastrointestinal symptoms, rash, pruritus, thrombophlebitis

method until the 1960s, is no longer practiced. However, if an epidemic does occur, ground or aerial spraying combined with disruption of the animal reservoir's habitat may be the most effective in achieving rapid vector control.

Travelers to endemic areas should be aware of this disease and should employ basic protective measures. Protective clothing of at least medium weight should be worn; neutral colors are most effective, as flies are attracted to bright and dark colors. Tsetse flies are attracted to moving vehicles but rest in the shade or bushes. Although use of insect repellant is prudent for other vector-borne illnesses that may be endemic in these areas, it has not been proven to substantially reduce the risk of tsetse fly bites. There is no recommended chemoprophylaxis for travelers.

SUGGESTED READINGS

Brun R, Blum J, Chappuis F, et al. Human African trypanosomiasis. *Lancet*. 2010;375:148-159. *Comprehensive review.*

Frearson JA, Brand S, McElroy SP, et al. N-Myristoyltransferase inhibitors as new leads to treat sleeping sickness. *Nature*. 2010;464:728-732. *Novel and promising approach to therapy based on inhibition of glycosylphosphatidylinositol synthesis.*

355

CHAGAS' DISEASE

LOUIS V. KIRCHHOFF

DEFINITION

Chagas' disease, or American trypanosomiasis, is caused by the protozoan parasite *Trypanosoma cruzi*. The terms *Chagas' disease*, *American trypanosomiasis*, and *T. cruzi infection* are synonyms.

The Pathogen

Several dozen species are included in the genus *Trypanosoma*, but only the African trypanosome *Trypanosoma brucei* (subspecies *T.b. gambiense* [West African] and *T.b. rhodesiense* [East African]) (Chapter 354) and the American trypanosome *T. cruzi* cause disease in humans. Many species of triatomine insects, also called kissing bugs, act as vectors for *T. cruzi*, and many species of wild and domestic mammals, as well as humans, are involved in the complex life cycle of this fascinating organism. The vectors become infected by ingesting blood from mammals that have parasites in their blood stream. The parasites then multiply in the gut of the insects and are ultimately discharged in the feces of the vector. Transmission to a new mammalian host occurs when parasite-laden vector feces contact vulnerable surfaces such as the mucosae of the mouth or nose, the conjunctivae, or breaks in the skin. Once in contact with tissues of the new host, the contaminating parasites enter local cells, multiply intracellularly, and as parasitized cells rupture, are released into the lymphatics and blood stream. The circulating organisms enter new cells at distant sites and in this manner maintain an endless process of asynchronous multiplication. The life cycle is completed as parasites are swept up in blood meals taken by vectors. In addition to vector-borne transmission, *T. cruzi* can be transmitted by blood or organs donated by infected persons, from mother to unborn child, by the ingestion of contaminated food or drink, and in laboratory accidents.

EPIDEMIOLOGY

Epizootiology of *T. cruzi*

The triatomine vectors that transmit *T. cruzi* are found in the Americas from southern Argentina through the southern half of the United States. The parasite has been isolated from more than 100 species of domestic and wild mammals, which for the most part probably become infected when they eat infected vectors. Armadillos, wood rats, raccoons, and opossums are typical wild mammalian reservoirs, and these and other species that harbor *T. cruzi* can be found in large numbers in the southern and western parts of the United States.

Typically, humans acquire *T. cruzi* infection when they live in houses in enzootic areas where the sylvatic cycle of transmission is active. The process begins when vector species adaptable to living in human dwellings take up residence in niches in the primitive wood, mud, and stone houses that are typical in many regions of Latin America. These vectors become domiciliary and they then take blood meals, mostly at night, from the humans who occupy the dwellings that they have invaded, as well as from domestic animals that sleep there, particularly dogs. Thus, Chagas' disease is primarily a public health problem among poor people who live in rural areas.

Epidemiology of Chagas' Disease in Latin America

Chagas' disease is a zoonosis that is endemic in Mexico and all countries of Central and South America. None of the Caribbean islands are endemic. In 2006 the Pan American Health Organization estimated that 8 million people are chronically infected with *T. cruzi* and that up to 14,000 deaths result from Chagas' disease annually. Since 1991 a major international vector control program in the southern cone countries of South America (Chile, Argentina, Paraguay, Brazil, Bolivia, and Uruguay) has achieved a marked reduction in transmission of *T. cruzi* through housing improvement, education of people at risk for acquiring the infection, and spraying of residual insecticides. Substantial reductions in prevalence rates in school-aged children and in blood donors constitute clear evidence of the success of the program. Uruguay, Chile, and Brazil were certified as being free of vector transmission in 1997, 1999, and 2006, respectively. Marked reduction in transmission has been achieved in Argentina as well. Similar programs have been initiated in Central

America and the Andean countries. In parallel with the vector control programs, donor screening has been implemented throughout almost the entire endemic range, and with the notable exception of Mexico, transmission of *T. cruzi* by transfusion has largely been eliminated.

Epidemiology of Chagas' Disease in the United States

As noted, the sylvatic cycle of *T. cruzi* exists in much of the southern and western regions of the United States, but only six cases of autochthonous transmission have been reported: three in Texas and one each in Tennessee, Louisiana, and California. Moreover, the nationwide blood donor screening that started in January 2007, in which more than 35 million units have been tested, has uncovered only a small number of *T. cruzi*–infected donors, who appear to have acquired the infection autochthonously. In the past 30 years only about 15 laboratory-acquired and imported cases of acute Chagas' disease have been reported to the Centers for Disease Control and Prevention (CDC). None of the latter infections occurred in tourists returning to the United States, but three such instances have been reported in Europe. Thus, acute Chagas' disease is extremely rare in the United States.

Census data indicate that including illegal and legal immigrants, 23 million persons born in countries endemic for Chagas' disease currently live in the United States. Roughly 17 million of these individuals are from Mexico, where the overall prevalence of *T. cruzi* infection is thought to range from 0.5% to 1.0%. Moreover, more than half of the non-Mexican immigrants have come from Central America, a region where the prevalence of *T. cruzi* infection is relatively high. A recent estimate puts the number of *T. cruzi*–infected persons currently living in the United States at 300,000. Several studies done before blood donor screening began in 2007 identified *T. cruzi*–infected persons in the donor pool, and seven instances of transmission by transfusion in the United States and Canada were described.

When the Ortho *T. cruzi* ELISA (enzyme-linked immunosorbent assay) Test System (Ortho-Clinical Diagnostics, Raritan, NJ) received approval by the Food and Drug Administration (FDA) in late 2006, shortly thereafter nearly universal screening began. To date, more than 35 million units have been screened and roughly 1200 *T. cruzi*–infected donors have been identified and permanently deferred from donation. The confirmed rate of *T. cruzi* infection in donors is about 1 in 29,000. With the goal of reducing the enormous cost of universal screening ($100 to $200 million per year), a selective screening protocol based on previous negative test results is being implemented in some regions.

The transplantation in the United States of organs from three persons with undiagnosed chronic *T. cruzi* infection resulted in acute Chagas' disease in five recipients, one of whom died of the infection. To date, no instances of congenital transmission of *T. cruzi* here have been reported.

PATHOBIOLOGY

In acute Chagas' disease, an inflammatory lesion, called a chagoma, may appear at the site of entry of the parasites. Local histologic changes include intracellular parasitism of muscle and other subcutaneous tissues, lymphocytic infiltration, interstitial edema, and hyperplasia of lymph nodes that drain the area. As the parasites spread systemically through the lymphatics and blood stream, muscles, including the myocardium, are the most heavily parasitized tissues, but the organisms can invade essentially any tissue. Myocarditis may develop in association with focal areas of infected cardiomyocytes, inflammation, and necrosis. The characteristic pseudocysts seen in sections of *T. cruzi*–infected tissues are actually host cells filled with multiplying forms of the parasite (Fig. 355-1). In some patients parasites can be seen in cerebrospinal fluid (CSF).

In persons with chronic Chagas' disease, the heart is the organ most commonly affected. Hearts obtained at autopsy from patients who died of Chagas' cardiomyopathy usually have a global appearance reflecting biventricular enlargement and thinning of ventricular walls (Fig. 355-2). Mural thrombi are frequently present, and an apical aneurysm of the left ventricle is typical with advanced disease. At the cellular level, the process that underlies these gross pathologic abnormalities is a chronic inflammation with mononuclear cell infiltration, diffuse interstitial fibrosis, and atrophy of myocardial cells. The chronic inflammation affects the conduction system as well and causes a variety of rhythm disturbances, including atrial bradyarrhythmias and fibrillation; premature ventricular contractions; bundle branch blocks, often of the right bundle; ventricular tachycardia; and third-degree atrioventricular block. Parasites are rarely seen in diseased tissues by conventional histologic methods, but several studies using polymerase chain reaction (PCR) assays found a correlation between the intensity of inflammation and the presence

FIGURE 355-1. *T. cruzi* **in cardiac muscle of a child who died of acute Chagas' myocarditis.** An infected myocyte containing several dozen *T. cruzi* amastigotes is in the center of the field (hematoxylin-eosin staining, ×900).

FIGURE 355-2. Chest radiograph of a patient from Bolivia with chronic *T. cruzi* infection, rhythm disturbances, and cardiomyopathy. Pacemaker wires can be seen in the area of the left ventricle.

of parasites. Evidence accumulated to date implicates the persistence of parasites and the resulting chronic inflammation in affected tissues—rather than autoimmune mechanisms—as the basis for the pathogenesis in patients with chronic *T. cruzi* infection.

The dilation and hypertrophy observed on gross examination of the esophagus or colon of a patient with chronic Chagas' disease of the digestive tract (megadisease) is striking. Focal inflammatory lesions with lymphocytic infiltration are seen on microscopic examination of affected tissues. In addition, the number of neurons in the myenteric plexus is reduced, and periganglion and intraganglion fibrosis with Schwann cell proliferation and lymphocytosis is present. In most patients the clinical consequences of this parasympathetic denervation are limited to the esophagus or colon (or to both), but the ureters, biliary tree, and other hollow viscera can be affected as well.

CLINICAL MANIFESTATIONS

Acute Chagas' Disease

Acute Chagas' disease is usually an illness of children but can occur at any age. Symptoms are typically mild and nonspecific. When the parasite has entered through a break in the skin or the site of a vector's puncture, as noted, a chagoma may appear with local lymphadenopathy. The Romaña sign, the classic finding in acute Chagas' disease, consists of painless edema of the palpebrae and periocular tissues and may appear when the conjunctiva is the portal of entry. These initial local signs can be followed by fever, malaise, anorexia, and edema of the face and lower extremities. Generalized lymphadenopathy and hepatosplenomegaly may also be present. Severe myocarditis may develop as well, and most deaths are due to the resulting congestive heart failure. Meningoencephalitis is a rare complication. In untreated patients the acute illness resolves spontaneously over a period of 6 to 8 weeks as the patient enters the indeterminate phase of Chagas' disease, which is characterized by subpatent parasitemia, absence of associated signs and symptoms, and easily detectable antibodies to *T. cruzi*.

Chronic Chagas' Cardiopathy

As noted, in only 10 to 30% of persons chronically infected with *T. cruzi* does clinically manifested disease develop, which most often involves rhythm disturbances or cardiomyopathy. Symptoms of cardiac Chagas' disease can develop insidiously years and often decades after the initial infection. Clinical findings reflect the rhythm disturbances, congestive heart failure, and thromboembolism that characterize the illness. Dizziness, syncope, and even seizures can result from a wide variety of arrhythmias. The cardiomyopathy often leads to biventricular failure, and right-sided heart failure can predominate in patients with advanced disease. A validated risk score assessment tool has been developed to gauge prognosis. Chronic Chagas' disease is an independent risk factor for stroke.

Chronic Gastrointestinal Chagas' Disease (Megadisease)

The esophagus and colon are the segments of the gastrointestinal tract most commonly affected in persons with chronic *T. cruzi* infection. In patients with megaesophagus, the symptoms are similar to those of idiopathic achalasia (Chapter 140) and may include cough, dysphagia, odynophagia, and regurgitation. Hypersalivation and consequent salivary gland hypertrophy develop in some patients with advanced esophageal dysfunction. Aspiration can occur, especially during sleep, and in untreated patients, repeated episodes of aspiration pneumonitis are common. Weight loss and even cachexia in patients with severe megaesophagus can combine with pneumonitis to cause death. Patients with chagasic megacolon suffer from intermittent abdominal pain and chronic constipation and in advanced cases can go for several weeks between bowel movements. Rarely, acute obstruction, occasionally with volvulus, can lead to perforation, septicemia, and death.

Immunosuppression and Transplantation in Patients Infected with *T. cruzi*

When persons with chronic carriage of *T. cruzi* become immunosuppressed, reactivation of the infection can occur, sometimes with an intensity that is atypical of acute Chagas' disease in immunocompetent persons. The overall incidence of reactivation in immunosuppressed persons who harbor the parasite chronically is not known. Reactivation after renal transplantation has been reported, and in two of the patients described the central nervous system was involved. The consensus view is that Chagas' disease should not be a contraindication to kidney transplantation. In *T. cruzi*–infected patients who do undergo the procedure, periodic monitoring for signs and symptoms of acute Chagas' disease should nonetheless be carried out, including careful neurologic evaluation, and parasitologic tests for the parasite should be done when acute illnesses occur postoperatively.

Reactivation of *T. cruzi* infection can also occur in persons coinfected with the parasite and human immunodeficiency virus (HIV). Dozens of such patients have been described, one of whom was a immigrant from El Salvador living in the United States. It is striking that in many of these patients *T. cruzi* brain abscesses developed, which do not occur in immunocompetent patients with chronic Chagas' disease. It has been shown that HIV viral loads increase in the context of reactivated acute Chagas' disease. Calculations based on the overlapping epidemiologies of HIV and *T. cruzi* infections in the endemic countries suggest that the incidence of reactivation of the latter in coinfected persons is quite low.

DIAGNOSIS

Acute Chagas' Disease

The first step in considering the diagnosis of acute Chagas' disease is establishing that a person is at risk for *T. cruzi* infection. Risk factors include recent residence or blood transfusion in an endemic area, birth to a mother with geographic- or transfusion-associated risk in the case of a newborn, or a laboratory accident involving the parasite. Definitive diagnosis of acute Chagas' disease can be made only by detecting parasites. Serologic assays for

T. cruzi–specific IgM are not accurate enough to justify their use. In immunocompetent persons suspected of having acute Chagas' disease, the most productive approach is examination of wet preparations of anticoagulated blood or buffy coat for the highly motile blood stream parasites. They can be seen in Giemsa-stained smears as well. In infected immunocompromised patients, moreover, parasites can sometimes be found in other specimens such as lymph node aspirates, biopsy specimens of skin lesions, bone marrow, endomyocardial tissue, CSF, and pericardial fluid.

When these direct methods fail to detect organisms in an at-risk person, samples should be tested with a PCR assay (see later). PCR assays have been shown to be more sensitive than the direct methods described earlier for detecting *T. cruzi*. Another method is to culture blood or other samples in specialized liquid medium, but the usefulness of this approach is limited by low sensitivity (50 to 70% for hemoculture) and by the fact that cultures take a minimum of 2 weeks before turning positive. In newborns whose blood is negative both by direct examination and in a PCR assay right after birth, serologic evaluation for *T. cruzi*–specific IgG should be performed 6 to 9 months later, by which time maternal antibodies will have disappeared.

Chronic Chagas' Disease

Chronic *T. cruzi* infection is usually diagnosed by detecting IgG antibodies that specifically bind to the parasite's antigens, and in almost all instances isolation of the organism is not necessary. More than 30 serologic assays for diagnosing Chagas' disease are currently available commercially in endemic countries, where they are used widely for testing clinical specimens and screening blood donors. Even though these tests usually have good sensitivity and reasonable specificity, false-positive reactions do occur, typically with specimens from people who have other infectious diseases or autoimmune conditions. The World Health Organization has recommended that testing be done with two assays based on different formats. A number of assays based on recombinant antigens are available commercially or are in development and may offer improved diagnostic accuracy. A Clinical Laboratories Improvement Act (CLIA)-approved radioimmune precipitation assay (Chagas RIPA) is used for confirmatory testing of donor samples that are positive in the screening tests.

Since the publication in 1989 of two reports describing the use of PCR tests to detect *T. cruzi*, well over 100 articles dealing with this approach have appeared. In human studies the sensitivity of the PCR assays ranged from 44.7 to 100%, with most being higher than 90%. It is generally accepted that the level of sensitivity of these assays is not high enough to justify their use for confirmatory testing of serologically positive donor samples. In contrast, PCR assays may be useful in persons who have borderline serologic results, in patients suspected of having congenital or acute Chagas' disease in whom parasites are not detected microscopically, and in infected patients who have received specific treatment. In all such persons, because of the sensitivity issue, only positive PCR results can be taken as being truly indicative of infection status.

TREATMENT ℞

Antiparasitic Drugs (also see Chapter 352)

The two drugs currently available for treating Chagas' disease are unsatisfactory, and the need for a parasitologically curative drug regimen is the most important current challenge in Chagas' disease research. Nifurtimox (Lampit, Bayer 2502, Leverkusen, Germany) is a nitrofuran derivative that has been used for more than 3 decades. Nifurtimox reduces symptoms and decreases mortality in patients with acute Chagas' disease, approximately 70% of whom are cured parasitologically. Nifurtimox also can cure a substantial portion of children in the indeterminate phase, but unfortunately, cure rates may be less than 10% in adults with long-standing chronic *T. cruzi* infection.

Disadvantages of nifurtimox include its long course of treatment and occasionally bothersome side effects, including gastrointestinal complaints such as anorexia, nausea, vomiting, weight loss, and abdominal pain. Patients taking the drug may also have neurologic symptoms such as insomnia, restlessness, paresthesias, twitching, polyneuritis, and even seizures. For adults, the recommended oral dosage is 8 to 10 mg/kg body weight per day. For adolescents, the dose is 12.5 to 15 mg/kg/day, and for children 1 to 10 years of age, it is 15 to 20 mg/kg/day. The drug should be given each day in four divided doses, and treatment should be continued for 90 to 120 days. Nifurtimox can be obtained from the CDC Drug Service (404-639-3670).

The second drug for treating *T. cruzi* infection is the nitroimidazole derivative benznidazole (Rochagan, Radinil, Roche 7-1051; LAFEPE, Pernambuco, Brazil). Cure rates are similar or perhaps a bit higher than those achieved with nifurtimox. A cure rate higher than 90% in babies with congenital infection has been observed with benznidazole. Side effects can include rash, peripheral neuropathy, and granulocytopenia. Benznidazole is considered the drug of choice by most Latin American experts. The recommended oral dosage of benznidazole is 5 to 10 mg/kg body weight per day for children and 5 mg/kg body weight per day for adults, in both cases for 60 days.

There is broad agreement among experts that treatment is indicated in all patients with acute or congenital infections, as well as in chronically infected children up to 18 years old. This recommendation is supported by several studies showing that a majority of such patients can be cured parasitologically. By extension, it would be reasonable to treat anyone 18 years or older known to have acquired *T. cruzi* infection within the last 17 years. There is also broad agreement that persons with advanced symptomatic *T. cruzi* infection should not be given specific treatment. The remaining question, then, is whether adults with long-standing indeterminate-phase infections, who by far constitute the largest group of *T. cruzi*–infected persons, should be treated. This is a thorny question because the burden of taking a full course of either drug can be substantial and also because parasitologic cure rates are so low.

Importantly, there is no clear evidence from randomized controlled trials that therapy with either drug delays the onset of symptoms or the progression of pathology or reduces mortality in adults with chronic *T. cruzi* infection. In 2006 a panel of experts convened at the CDC recommended that adults 19 to 50 years old in the indeterminate phase or with mild symptoms be offered treatment. A large randomized trial (the BENEFIT multicenter trial) designed to assess the clinical and parasitologic efficacy of benznidazole in patients with Chagas' disease 18 to 75 years old without advanced disease is being conducted in Colombia, Bolivia, Brazil, and Argentina. Initial findings will not be available until 2012. An additional important question is whether specific treatment given before pregnancy will reduce the probability of subsequent congenital transmission. To date, only one limited study has addressed this issue, and the findings suggest a protective effect.

Management of Symptomatic Chagas' Disease

An algorithm for the evaluation of persons with newly diagnosed Chagas' disease has been developed (Fig. 355-3). *T. cruzi*–infected patients in whom symptomatic cardiac or gastrointestinal disease develops should be referred

aQRS interval of 0.10 to 0.11 seconds in adults. Criteria based on the *Minnesota Code Manual of Electrocardiographic Findings* with modifications from Maguire et al. Different criteria may be required for ECGs in children.

FIGURE 355-3. Algorithm for baseline evaluation of a patient with newly diagnosed chronic *T. cruzi* infection. (From Bern C, Montgomery SP, Herwaldt BL, et al. Evaluation and treatment of Chagas disease in the United States: a systematic review. *JAMA.* 2007;298:2171-2181.)

to appropriate subspecialists. Beyond the possible use of nifurtimox or benznidazole, treatment of acute and chronic Chagas' disease is symptomatic. In patients with symptomatic chronic Chagas' cardiac disease, treatment should be directed at managing symptoms with the anticoagulants and cardiotropic drugs used in patients with cardiomyopathy of other cause. Pacemakers are useful in patients with ominous arrhythmias. Studies of the usefulness of autologous bone marrow cells in improving heart function in patients with Chagas' cardiomyopathy are under way.

Heart transplantation (Chapter 82) is an option in patients with end-stage Chagas' cardiac disease, and more than 150 such patients have undergone the procedure in Brazil and the United States. As is the case with other *T. cruzi*–infected patients who are immunosuppressed, reactivation is a risk but is manageable. The usefulness and side effects of long-term prophylaxis for reactivation with either benznidazole or nifurtimox in *T. cruzi*–infected patients after heart transplantation have not been evaluated. The long-term survival of Chagas' patients with heart transplants appears to be longer than that in patients undergoing cardiac transplantation for other reasons, probably because the lesions of *T. cruzi*–associated pathology affect mostly the heart.

Chagas' megaesophagus should be treated as normally done for idiopathic achalasia (Chapter 140), which usually responds to balloon dilation of the lower esophageal sphincter when symptoms are mild. Surgical treatment may be required in patients who do not respond to repeated attempts at balloon dilation. Laparoscopic myotomy is being used with increasing frequency to treat Chagas' megaesophagus, as is the case with achalasia. Injection of botulinum toxin into the lower esophageal sphincter is being evaluated as an alternative to myotomy.

Chagas' megacolon in its early stage can be treated with a high fiber diets and occasional laxatives or enemas. Fecal impaction requiring manual disimpaction can occur, and toxic megacolon requires surgery. In patients with advanced megacolon, volvulus (Chapter 144) can develop when an enlarged and lengthened sigmoid colon twists and folds on itself; volvulus causes a constellation of symptoms and in many cases requires immediate surgery. Even if the symptoms associated with volvulus are resolved without operative intervention, however, surgical treatment is usually ultimately necessary because the volvulus tends to recur. Several surgical procedures are used to treat advanced Chagas' megacolon, all of which include resection of the sigmoid and removal of part of the rectum.

PREVENTION

Reducing human contact with triatomine vectors through education of at-risk persons, housing improvement, and spraying of residual insecticides in endemic countries has resulted in reduction or elimination of vector transmission of *T. cruzi* in a major part of the endemic range, and progress in this regard is expected to continue. Serologic screening of donated blood has essentially eliminated transfusion-related transmission of the parasite. Outbreaks of acute Chagas' disease through oral transmission can be avoided by the implementation of better food safety standards. Drug treatment of *T. cruzi*–infected women before pregnancy may reduce the likelihood of congenital transmission, but this issue needs further study. No protocols have been defined and validated for preventing reactivation of *T. cruzi* infection in chronically infected persons who are immunosuppressed iatrogenically or by HIV. A treatment regimen that reliably results in parasitologic cure is needed to prevent the onset or progression of chronic symptomatic Chagas' disease.

PROGNOSIS

The prognosis for patients with acute Chagas' disease is generally excellent because most acutely infected persons have only mild symptoms that resolve spontaneously, even without specific treatment. The occasional patient who has symptomatic acute Chagas' myocarditis should generally do well if treated early. In persons with chronic *T. cruzi* infection, the lifetime risk for the development of related cardiac or gastrointestinal dysfunction is only 10 to 30%. A validated risk score assessment tool has been developed to gauge prognosis. It has not been determined in randomized controlled trials whether this rate of progression to clinical disease or overall mortality is significantly affected by treatment with nifurtimox or benznidazole.

 Visit expertconsult.com for e-expanded chapter

SUGGESTED READINGS

Biolo A, Ribeiro AL, Clausell N. Chagas cardiomyopathy—where do we stand after a hundred years? *Prog Cardiovasc Dis.* 2010;52:300-316. *Review of the main clinical aspects of Chagas' cardiomyopathy and future challenges in control, diagnosis, and management.*

Issa VS, Amaral AF, Cruz FD, et al. Beta-blocker therapy and mortality of patients with Chagas cardiomyopathy: a subanalysis of the REMADHE prospective trial. *Circ Heart Fail.* 2010;3:82-88. *In a subanalysis, Chagas patients had at least as much benefit as other patients with heart failure.*
Lescure FX, Le Loup G, Freilij H, et al. Chagas disease: changes in knowledge and management. *Lancet Infect Dis.* 2010;10:556-570. *Comprehensive review.*
Maya JD, Orellana M, Ferreira J, et al. Chagas disease: Present status of pathogenic mechanisms and chemotherapy. *Biol Res.* 2010;43:323-331. *Review including data on the benefits of aspirin in a mouse model.*
Rassi A Jr, Rassi A, Marin-Neto JA. Chagas disease. *Lancet.* 2010;375:1388-1402. *Review.*

356

LEISHMANIASIS

SIMON L. CROFT AND PIERRE A. BUFFET

DEFINITION

Leishmaniasis is caused by protozoan parasites of the genus *Leishmania* that are transmitted between mammalian hosts by female phlebotomine sandflies. The disease has a number of clinical manifestations ranging in severity from self-curing, limited cutaneous lesions to disseminated, potentially fatal visceral disease. The parasite exists as an extracellular flagellated form, the promastigote, in the sandfly gut and as an intracellular form, the amastigote, that survives and multiplies in a phagolysosomal compartment of macrophages in the mammalian host.

This disease complex is caused by 17 species of *Leishmania*, which are widely distributed in Europe, Asia, Africa, and South and Central America. The characteristics of the main *Leishmania* species are summarized in Table 356-1. There are an estimated 1.5 to 2.0 million new cases each year, with up to 70,000 deaths, although this is probably an underestimate because leishmaniasis is a reportable disease in only 40 of the 88 countries in which it is known to occur. Many *Leishmania* infections are either asymptomatic or misdiagnosed.

Because leishmaniasis is a disease complex, clinical aspects are considered under separate sections for visceral leishmaniasis (VL) and cutaneous leishmaniasis (CL).

EPIDEMIOLOGY

Infection is established in the mammalian host following a bite of the female sandfly belonging to either *Phlebotomus* spp in Europe, Asia, and Africa or *Lutzomyia* spp in the Americas. Different species of sandfly are associated with transmission of different *Leishmania* species. Most species that cause CL have a zoonotic (acquired from a vertebrate animal) transmission cycle, with the exception of *Leishmania tropica*, which is sometimes anthroponotic (transmitted from a human being). VL is either anthroponotic (in the case of *Leishmania donovani*) or zoonotic (in the case of *Leishmania infantum*). The predominant mammalian hosts (the reservoirs) are associated with different *Leishmania* species in diverse ecosystems (Fig. 356-1).

VL is caused by either *L. donovani* or *L. infantum* (which is identical to *Leishmania chagasi* in South America). These species have different geographic distributions, with the highest incidence found in the poorest communities in six countries (Bangladesh, Nepal, India, Sudan, Ethiopia, Brazil), and it is potentially fatal if untreated. An estimated 1 in 5 to 1 in 50 infections are asymptomatic, depending on the parasite species and host immunity. Since 2005 there has been a regional program to eliminate VL (reducing annual incidence to <1 per 10,000) in the Indian subcontinent.

CL, which undergoes self-cure in more than 90% of patients within 3 to 18 months, is widely distributed, but its prevalence is difficult to estimate because of underreporting. Prevalence is associated with age, possibly related to the acquisition of immunity and risk factors, including the presence of domestic animals in some cases or rodent hosts. Ecologic conditions for sandflies, including shaded and humid habitats in crevices and mammal burrows, have been identified.

Urbanization and deforestation have resulted in changing patterns of disease, with transmission occurring in peridomestic cycles. Other forms of transmission, such as via intravenous needles shared by drug users, have been reported in Spain.

TABLE 356-1 CHARACTERISTICS OF THE MAIN *LEISHMANIA* SPECIES

LEISHMANIA SPP	*LEISHMANIA* SUBGENUS	DISTRIBUTION: OLD WORLD	DISTRIBUTION: NEW WORLD	PRIMARY FORM	SECONDARY FORMS	ANTHROPONOTIC: AREAS OF TRANSMISSION	ZOONOTIC: RESERVOIR	ALTERNATIVE NAME
L. donovani	*Leishmania*	Indian subcontinent E. Africa		VL	PKDL CL, ML OIVL	Indian subcontinent E. Africa		Kala-azar
L. infantum (*L. chagasi*)	*Leishmania*	Europe Asia	S. & C. America	VL	CL, ML OIVL		Canid	
L. major	*Leishmania*	Asia N. & E. Africa Europe		CL			Rodent	
L. tropica	*Leishmania*	Asia Europe		CL	Recidivans	Syria Afghanistan	Rodent	Aleppo boil
L. aethiopica	*Leishmania*	Ethiopia		CL	DCL		Hyrax	
L. mexicana	*Leishmania*		C. America	CL			Rodent	Chiclero's ulcer
L. amazonensis	*Leishmania*		C. & S. America	CL	DCL		Rodent	
L. braziliensis	*Viannia*		S. America	CL ML	DissCL Lymph		Rodent, marsupial	ML-espundia
L. panamensis	*Viannia*		C. & S. America	CL	ML Lymph		Edentate rodent	Ulcera de bejuco
L. guyanensis	*Viannia*		S. America	CL	ML Lymph		Rodent, edentates	Pian bois
L. peruviana	*Viannia*		S. America	CL			Canids	Uta

CL = cutaneous leishmaniasis; DCL = diffuse cutaneous leishmaniasis; DissCL = disseminated cutaneous leishmaniasis; Lymph = nodular lymphangitis; ML = mucosal leishmaniasis; OIVL = opportunistic infection with VL in HIV-infected patients; PKDL = Post–kala-azar dermal leishmaniasis; VL = visceral leishmaniasis.

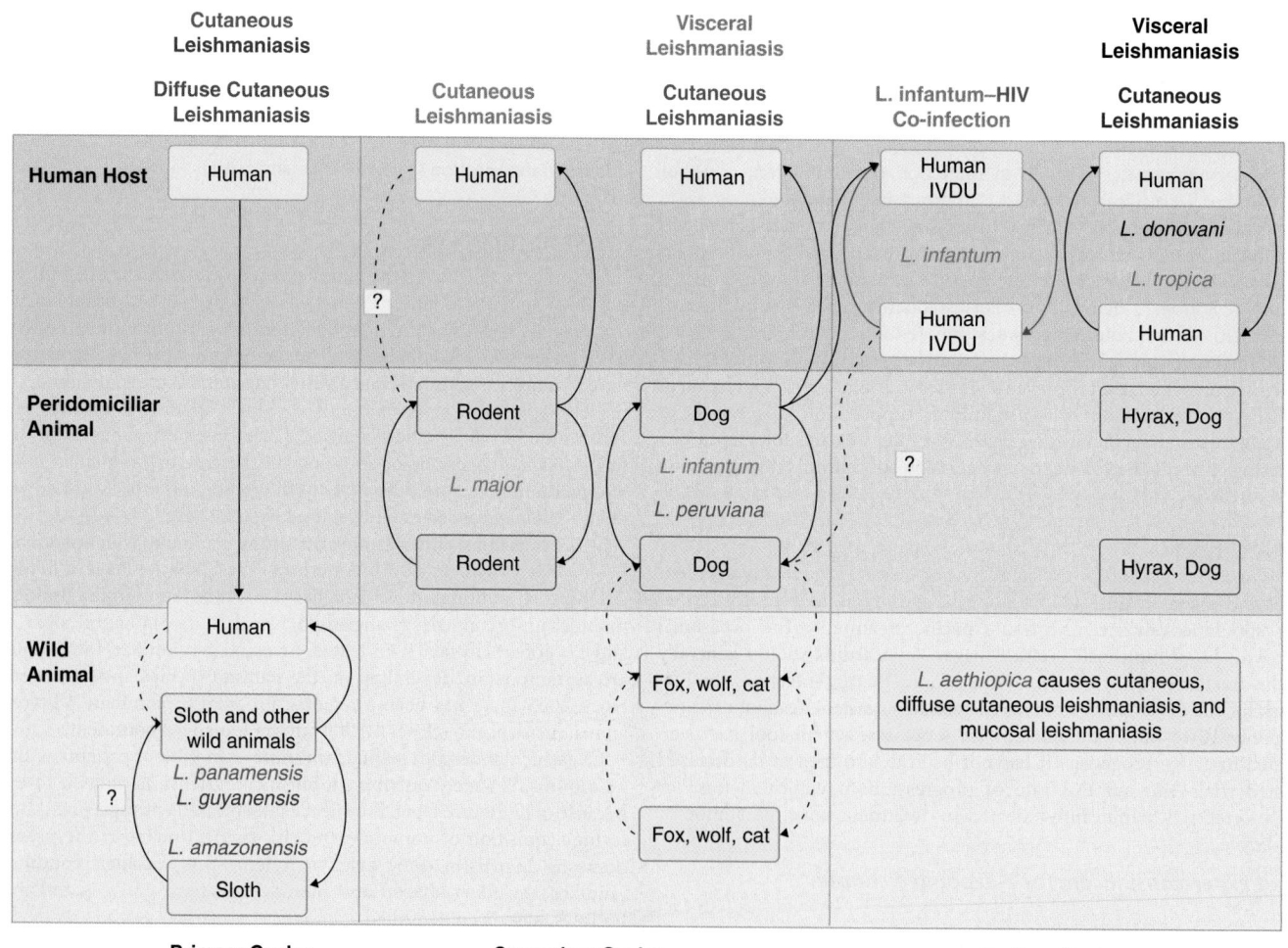

FIGURE 356-1. Old World and New World zoonotic and anthroponotic life cycles of the main species of *Leishmania*. Leishmaniasis is often referred to as a "disease complex" because different forms of disease can be caused by the same parasite species and similar forms of disease can be caused by different parasite species. IVDU = intravenous drug use.

PATHOBIOLOGY

The infection is initially established in the skin after the inoculation of infective metacyclic promastigotes by the sandfly. These infective forms have a glycoprotein coat (a lipophosphoglycan) that enables them to resist complement and attach to and invade host cells. Peptides in sandfly saliva (e.g., maxadilan) cause vasodilation and erythema and help establish infection in the dermal layer of the skin. Early responses to infection involve neutrophil infiltration and invasion of resident macrophages. Progress of the disease depends on the parasite species and host responses. For both VL and CL, disease progression depends on maintenance of a parasite-specific immunosuppressive state. Host cell macrophages are in a deactivated state, but cure follows when macrophages become activated and kill the parasites, which are sensitive to nitric oxide and oxygen radicals in the phagolysosomal compartment. Resolution of disease following the activation of macrophages is mediated by a T-helper cell T_H1 response after interaction between antigen-presenting cells (e.g., dendritic cells) with $CD4^+$ and $CD8^+$ T cells and subsequent secretion of pro-inflammatory cytokines (e.g., interleukin-1 [IL-12], interferon-γ, tumor necrosis factor-α). However, in clinical forms such as active VL or diffuse CL, a T_H2 cell response predominates whereby down-regulation of macrophage activity follows the production of cytokines such as IL-4, IL-10, IL-13, and transforming growth factor-β. This profile has been defined in experimental models, mainly inbred mice, and ongoing clinical studies generally support the notion of a similar profile in human infection.

In patients with VL, the absence of a T-cell–specific immune response to leishmanial antigens is associated with uncontrolled progression of infection. This is related to elevated levels of IL-10 and decreased production of interferon-γ. Genetic susceptibility to *L. donovani* in Sudan has been associated with a solute carrier family (formerly NRAMP1) that regulates macrophage activation and with a polymorphism in the IL-4 gene. In localized simple CL, patients show a T_H1-type response and a delayed-type hypersensitivity (DTH) response. DTH is frequently measured by a Montenegro skin test, which can also be used in epidemiologic prevalence studies. Chronic infections show a T_H2-type response, most predominantly in patients with diffuse CL, in whom there is complete anergy to leishmania antigen and no DTH response. Patients with mucosal leishmaniasis (ML) have both T_H1 and T_H2 cell responses and a strong DTH response.

⬤ VISCERAL LEISHMANIASIS

CLINICAL MANIFESTATIONS

The onset of VL, often referred to as kala-azar when caused by *L. donovani*, occurs weeks to months after the initial infection. Clinical signs and symptoms do not distinguish VL from hyperreactive malarial splenomegaly or other infectious or hematologic conditions. Anemia, leukopenia, thrombocytopenia, systemic inflammation, or polyclonal hypergammaglobulinemia, either isolated or combined, suggests but does not confirm the diagnosis. Parasitologic tests are therefore indispensable before making a therapeutic decision.

DIAGNOSIS

Parasitology

Microscopic visualization of amastigotes in samples from the lymph nodes, bone marrow, liver, spleen, or other organs is usually the first step. Because spleen aspiration causes life-threatening complications in approximately 0.1% of patients, it should be performed only in trained facilities and only if other, lower-risk methods cannot be used. It is still used in the field because of the higher cost, logistic constraints, and lower sensitivity of bone marrow aspiration. Polymerase chain reaction (PCR) is more sensitive than microscopic examination and has become the first-line test in several referral hospitals and research centers. Quantitative PCR with validated thresholds allows accurate diagnosis with venous blood samples, thereby avoiding bone marrow aspiration.

Serology

Serologic tests based on indirect fluorescent antibody (IFA), enzyme-linked immunosorbent assay (ELISA), or Western blot display high performance but require equipment that is poorly adapted to field settings. The field-friendly direct agglutination test (DAT) and immunochromatography using the rK39 antigen have high diagnostic accuracy and can be used in peripheral health centers. Whatever the serologic test used, specific antibodies remain detectable for several years after cure or asymptomatic infection.

Antigen Detection Tests

A latex agglutination test that detects a heat-stable, low-molecular-weight carbohydrate antigen in the urine of patients with VL showed good specificity but low to moderate sensitivity in East Africa and the Indian subcontinent. Further optimization is expected.

Complex Manifestations of Visceral Leishmaniasis

Visceral Leishmaniasis–Human Immunodeficiency Virus Coinfection

Although the clinical manifestations in VL patients infected with human immunodeficiency virus (HIV) without severe immunosuppression are similar to those in immunocompetent patients, atypical clinical features can be found in patients with low $CD4^+$ T-cell counts (<200/μL). In the latter group, physicians may order investigations for VL even in the absence of classic signs (e.g., lack of splenomegaly). A substantial proportion of HIV-VL–coinfected patients may have other opportunistic infections that complicate the clinical diagnosis. The parasitic load is usually higher and parasites may be found in unusual sites, especially in severely immunosuppressed patients. Therefore, the sensitivity of microscopic examination, culture, or PCR of blood (plain blood or buffy coat) or bone marrow aspirates is higher than that in immunocompetent VL patients. *Leishmania* parasites can occasionally be found in biopsy samples from the skin, gastrointestinal tract, or lungs. Limited data have also shown high sensitivity of the latex agglutination test in the urine of HIV-VL–coinfected patients. In contrast, the sensitivity of serologic tests is decreased in coinfected patients, although study results are equivocal and depend on several factors such as the test's format, region of endemicity, and level of immunosuppression. For example, the DAT has shown high sensitivity in Ethiopia. Increased sensitivity can be achieved by using a sequential combination of different serologic tests.

Post–Kala-azar Dermal Leishmaniasis

After successful treatment of visceral disease, a proportion of patients progress to disseminated cutaneous disease. This is reported in up to 20% of patients in Sudan and 0.5% in India. Studies in India have shown that smears are more likely to show amastigotes if taken from nodular lesions rather than papular or macular lesions. Serologic tests such as the DAT, ELISA, and rK39 immunochromatography are of limited value because a positive finding may be the result of persistent antibodies following the past episode of VL. Nevertheless, serology can be helpful when a previous history of VL is uncertain.

TREATMENT   Rx

General Principles

The clinical response to antileishmanial agents depends on the clinical form and the infecting species or even the subspecies (zymodeme). Many antileishmanial agents are either toxic, expensive, or difficult to administer in field conditions. No single satisfactory option for treating most of the clinical forms or species has been validated. Although therapeutic decisions and follow-up have become relatively simple for the treatment of VL in nonendemic countries—based on the powerful, well-tolerated agent liposomal amphotericin B—more complexity persists for the treatment of VL in endemic countries and for CL or ML everywhere.

Visceral Leishmaniasis in Immunocompetent Patients
Single-Agent Therapies

Pentamidine is efficient in treating VL only when high doses (more than seven injections of 4 mg/kg) are used. These are toxic, and pentamidine is no longer used for the treatment of VL. Lower doses (fewer than four injections of 4 mg/kg) induce much less adverse events and are still used for the secondary prophylaxis of VL in HIV-infected patients and in those with CL caused by *Leishmania guyanensis* or *Leishmania panamensis*.

Pentavalent antimonials (sodium stibogluconate, meglumine antimoniate) are still prescribed as first-intention drugs in many areas. In the Indian subcontinent (mainly in northern Bihar), *L. donovani* is resistant to pentavalent antimonials. Their efficacy has decreased from 90% to less than 40% over the past 40 years. In other VL foci, failure rates of initial treatment do not exceed 10% as long as the dosage is respected (20 mg of pentavalent antimony per kilogram per day for 28 days). In an endemic country, mortality in treated patients may exceed 10%, with toxicity positively correlating with age. Pentavalent antimonials are contraindicated in patients with heart, kidney, or liver disease or advanced age and in pregnant women. Generic formulations have demonstrated activity and tolerance identical to that of sodium stibogluconate.

Miltefosine is an alkyl phosphocholine. The oral form (2.5 mg/kg/day for 28 days) is very effective for VL in India. In Ethiopian patients with VL (28% with HIV infection), there was significantly higher mortality with sodium stibogluconate (generic) than with miltefosine (9.7 vs. 2.1%) despite the lower parasitologic efficacy of miltefosine (92.1 vs. 99.3%). Miltefosine is contraindicated in pregnant women or those who may become pregnant. Because of persistent levels of the drug, contraceptive measures must be observed for months after therapy.

Paromomycin (aminosidine sulfate) (15 mg/kg in sulfate form equivalent to 11 mg of base per kilogram intramuscularly for 21 days) is highly effective in India, where it has been available since 2006. In East Africa, its efficacy is lower. Similar to the situation with miltefosine, the longevity of the product would probably be better preserved in combination than as a single-agent therapy.

Amphotericin B (cumulative dose of 7 to 15 mg/kg) cures more than 98% of patients in India, whereas treatment of visceral infection with *L. infantum/chagasi* requires at least 14 mg/kg.

Liposomal amphotericin B achieves very high cure rates in India with lower cumulative doses than needed with the deoxycholate formulation. In preliminary studies in East Africa, the doses of liposomal amphotericin B required to cure VL (about 30 mg/kg cumulatively) are markedly higher than those used in India. Liposomal amphotericin B is associated with less infusion-related fever and chills, less renal toxicity, and a reduction in the number of infusions and length of hospitalization. The better renal tolerance of liposomal amphotericin B is especially beneficial in patients with renal failure or a kidney graft and in those with an increase in serum creatinine during amphotericin B deoxycholate therapy. Liposomal amphotericin B is the antileishmanial agent with the best benefit-risk ratio. It is now the first-line option in most nonendemic countries, both in children and in adults. The very high cost of liposomal amphotericin B has been reduced for use in endemic countries, but wider implementation would be greatly facilitated by a much more drastic reduction. A single infusion of liposomal amphotericin B at a dose of 10 mg/kg of body weight was recently reported not to be inferior to and less expensive than conventional treatment with amphotericin B deoxycholate. In this study, conducted in India, 304 of 304 (100%) patients with VL in the liposomal therapy group and 106 of 108 (98%) in the conventional therapy group had apparent cure responses at day 30. Cure rates at 6 months were similar: 95.7% with liposomal therapy and 96.3% with conventional therapy.**1**

Combinations/Coadministration

To limit extension of the resistance to pentavalent antimonials and prevent the emergence of resistance to paromomycin or miltefosine, shorter courses of therapy are being investigated. Because only miltefosine may be administered orally, this approach is based at least partly on products administered parenterally. Combinations of amphotericin with oral miltefosine and intramuscular paramonomycin can achieve high cure rates with 7 to 10-day courses of therapy.**2** A single infusion of liposomal amphotericin B followed by oral miltefosine has been highly effective in India, but confirmation studies are required here and elsewhere.

Visceral Leishmaniasis in Immunodeficient Patients
Leishmania infantum–HIV Coinfection

As with other major opportunistic infections during HIV infection, treatment may be subdivided into initial course and secondary prophylaxis. With initial treatment, the efficacy of meglumine antimoniate and that of amphotericin B are almost similar. The severe adverse effects of antimony derivatives are more common in this context. Doses of liposomal amphotericin B administered to immunodeficient patients are higher (30 to 40 mg/kg in cumulative dose) than those administered to immunocompetent patients. When therapeutic immunosuppression may not be reduced or optimization of highly active antiretroviral therapy is not possible, secondary prophylaxis is often proposed. Amphotericin B lipid complex moderately reduces the frequency of recurrences. Discontinuous administration of liposomal amphotericin B is generally used, but a progressive reduction in its efficacy has been reported, though apparently not associated with decreased parasitic sensitivity in vitro. Miltefosine is another option, especially if the reduction in parasitic load is backed up by quantitative PCR with a validated threshold (low residual load probably being associated with a lower risk for resistance). Administration of pentamidine once or twice a month is another potentially interesting option because drug levels persist for weeks or months after a single administration. Pancreatic tolerance should be monitored closely.

Leishmania donovani–HIV Coinfection

Patients should benefit from effective antiretroviral treatment. The experience with *L. infantum*–HIV coinfection is in part transposable. The potential risk for the emergence of resistance to antileishmanial agents is still more significant in this context because *L. donovani* (but not *L. infantum*) can be transmitted from human to human. Important clinical research is ongoing in East Africa.

CUTANEOUS LEISHMANIASIS
CLINICAL MANIFESTATIONS

Although the signs and symptoms of CL vary considerably (Fig. 356-2)—from pure nodular lesions to developing ulceration through dry crusty lesions and squamous plaques—there are some fairly constant features. First, firm infiltration is almost constant (the exception being the initial macule of post–kala-azar dermal leishmaniasis). Second, the evolution is subacute, which is a useful criterion in practice. A lesion reaching its maximum size in less than a week is most likely not due to CL. Finally, except in patients with very numerous satellite papulopustules, the lesion or lesions are sharply defined. Colonization of the CL ulceration with bacteria may give the lesion a purulent appearance, whereas patent superinfection adds an erythematous ring distinctly overflowing the infiltrated edge of the ulceration and making a usually cold and painless lesion feel hot and painful. Several dermatologic conditions such as staphylococcal or streptococcal infection, mycobacterial ulcer, leprosy, fungal infection, cancer, sarcoidosis, and tropical ulcer mimic CL or ML lesions (Fig. 356-2). Because treatment is costly, diagnostic confirmation is necessary.

DIAGNOSIS
Parasitology

Scraping, fine-needle aspiration, or biopsy of lesions provides appropriate samples in which amastigotes can be identified (Fig. 356-3). Scraping should be performed at both the center and edges of the lesion with a curved scalpel blade. Local anesthesia considerably reduces patients' discomfort and increases sensitivity. Using an adrenaline-containing local anesthetic (contraindicated for lesions on extremities) or pinching the lesion between the thumb and finger until blanching appears helps obtain a bloodless scraping, thus optimizing microscopic examination. The 2- to 4-mm skin fragment obtained by punch biopsy provides abundant material, which facilitates the search for scarce parasites and for an alternative diagnosis by culture (e.g., mycobacteria, fungi), as well as histopathologic examination. Culture of a biopsy sample requires homogenization in saline or culture medium under sterile conditions.

The material obtained by any of these methods can be used for microscopic examination, culture, and PCR. Microscopic examination of Giemsastained material is the most widely available method. Culture of the parasite in specific media (such as fetal calf serum–supplemented Schneider or Novy-Nicolle-McNeal media) allows identification, characterization, and storage of the isolate. Detection of parasitic nucleic acids by molecular diagnosis (mainly PCR) increases sensitivity and allows identification of the *Leishmania* species. This is particularly useful in regions (e.g., New World) where several *Leishmania* species—with various clinical outcomes and responses to treatment—coexist. Both culture and molecular-based diagnosis require substantial laboratory infrastructure and technical expertise.

Serology

Serologic diagnosis is of limited use for CL because of low sensitivity and variable specificity. The leishmanin (or Montenegro) skin test (LST) evaluates the cell-mediated response against *Leishmania* spp. The LST requires culture and fixation of—preferentially—local species of *Leishmania* and therefore lacks standardization. The production of commercial formulations of the LST lacks sustainability. Like serologic tests, the LST does not distinguish between past and present infections.

COMPLEX MANIFESTATIONS OF CUTANEOUS LEISHMANIASIS
Mucosal Leishmaniasis

A proportion of CL infections (about 1 to 10% in Brazil and Peru) caused by *Leishmania braziliensis* or *L. guyanensis* progress to a metastatic infection of the mucosa of the oral/nasal cavity or larynx, often 1 to 5 years after healing of the initial simple cutaneous lesion. Immunopathology results in extensive destruction of local tissue. Allergic rhinitis, paracoccidioidomycosis or other deep mycosis, cancrum oris, leprosy, and sarcoidosis may mimic the lesions of ML. Positive serology (e.g., IFA, ELISA) or LST indicate possible ML. Parasites are scarce in mucosal lesions. Therefore, a search for parasites in mucosal samples—obtained by scraping or biopsy—by microscopic examination or by culture lacks sensitivity. PCR has proved to be the most sensitive approach to confirm ML.

FIGURE 356-2. **Clinical features of cutaneous leishmaniasis (CL). A,** Typical forms of CL. **A1,** Papular-nodular. **A2,** Squamous. **A3,** Crusty. **A4,** Ulcerated. **A5,** Superinfected lesions. **B,** Atypical forms of CL and mucosal leishmaniasis. **B1,** Multiple papules on the face (*L. infantum,* Balearic islands). **B2,** Nodular lymphangitis (*L. braziliensis,* Brazil). **B3,** Multiple lesions with numerous peripheral papules (*L. major,* Tunisia). **B4,** Initial spread to the nasal mucosa (anterior septum, *L. braziliensis,* Bolivia). **B5,** Infiltration and ulceration of the tonsils (*L. infantum,* France). **C,** Clinical manifestations that are not CL. **C1,** Multiple papules (late secondary syphilis) (Chapter 327). **C2,** Nodular lymphangitis (sporotrichosis) (Chapter 345). **C3,** Single crusty ulceration (*Mycobacterium ulcerans* infection) (Chapter 333). **C4,** Ulcerated acute *Staphylococcus aureus* infection (Chapter 296). **C5,** Ulcerated nodule keratoacanthoma (Chapter 210).

FIGURE 356-3. Amastigotes of *Leishmania major* in scrapings from a skin ulcer.

Diffuse Cutaneous Leishmaniasis

Patients with diffuse CL have an anergic response to *Leishmania* antigens, and nonulcerative nodules, loaded with parasites, disseminate from the initial site of infection to multiple sites on the patient's body. There is no self-cure and treatment is difficult. This form of the disease is found in South America and East Africa, often associated with *Leishmania amazonensis* and *Leishmania aethiopica* infection.

Recidivans Cutaneous Leishmaniasis

Recidivans CL is characterized by the development of lesions containing granulomatous tissue. The lesions often take many years to heal and may arise years after healing of a simple localized lesion. New ulcers and papules may form over the edge of the old scar. Infections are normally associated with *L. tropica* infection and are difficult to treat.

TREATMENT   Rx

The clinical consequences of CL are dermatologic; concomitant visceral impairment is exceptional. The intensity of the discomfort, related to one or several oozing or unsightly lesions, and the impact of atrophic, hypopigmented or hyperpigmented scars depend on the lesions' topography. In the New World, mucosal impairment may affect up to 10 to 15% of patients in some countries (Bolivia, Peru). The risk for metastasis (initially nasal and then affecting the entire otorhinolaryngeal zone) has strongly influenced therapeutic decisions. Systemic treatment of any New World CL has been recommended, but recent data indicate that a different strategy may perhaps be considered, at least in foci where this complication is infrequent (Central America, northern part of the Amazon basin). Inadequate surgical excision and pentavalent antimonials or systemic pentamidine administered in excessive doses or without sufficient follow-up may paradoxically be a major risk for patients with CL. Decisions should therefore be based on a careful analysis of the benefit-risk ratio of any therapeutic intervention. Analysis of the number, size, and topography of the lesions, the clinical signs of spread (cutaneous, mucous, or lymphatic), and the predictable cosmetic or functional impact helps in estimating the benefit-risk ratio.

Oral therapy with relatively nontoxic drugs (ketoconazole, fluconazole, itraconazole, miltefosine) would be the simplest option, and oral miltefosine monotherapy has been successful in Brazil.**3** Local therapy with intralesional injections of pentavalent antimonials (with or without cryotherapy), photodynamic therapy, and thermotherapy are therefore attractive options to avoid potentially toxic, expensive, or impractical systemic schedules. However, implementation of these methods is hampered by logistic constraints and requires skilled health care providers. An efficient topical ointment would resolve most of these issues, but no efficient formulation is widely available. Several formulations of topical paromomycin have been tested with variable results. Recently, an ointment containing paromomycin and gentamicin has shown efficacy with acceptable local tolerance in patients with CL caused by *L. major*. Tentative algorithms for accurate therapeutic decisions in patients with Old World or New World CL are proposed in E-Figures 356-1 and 356-2, respectively.

PREVENTION

There are no modern vaccines for human disease and no prophylactic drug regimens. Leishmanization, or inoculating people with live virulent parasites to cause a local limited lesion and provide protection, has been used for CL

(e.g., in Iran) but is not recommended by the World Health Organization. Sandflies are sensitive to most insecticides, and transmission has been controlled with malaria eradication campaigns and residual spraying in houses. Insecticide-impregnated bed nets and dog collars (to prevent transmission of zoonotic CL) have been investigated.

PROGNOSIS

Most untreated patients with established disease ultimately die. VL has an excellent prognosis with less than a 2% death rate in patients treated soon enough with liposomal amphotericin B. Mortality increases when bleeding (mainly from the digestive tract or lung) or secondary bacterial infection occurs, usually after prolonged untreated evolution. Post-therapeutic relapse is very frequent in HIV-coinfected patients with low initial or persistently low CD4$^+$ counts. In immunosuppressed patients, VL is rarely the direct cause of death but may give rise to complex therapeutic situations. A proportion of *L. donovani*–infected patients experience post–kala-azar dermal leishmaniasis weeks to years after the initial episode. CL caused by *L. braziliensis* may metastasize to the nose and other mucous membranes with variable frequency in different areas. CL caused by *L. tropica* often relapses (recidivans CL). A small proportion of patients infected with *L. amazonensis* and *L. aethiopica* experience diffuse CL. Even when treated, most CL lesions leave disfiguring, hypotrophic, hypopigmented, or hyperpigmented scars.

 Grade A ─────────────────────────────────○

1. Sundar S, Chakravarty J, Agarwal D, et al. Single-dose liposomal amphotericin B for visceral leishmaniasis in India. *N Engl J Med.* 2010;362:504-512.
2. Sundar S, Sinha PK, Rai M, et al. Comparison of short-course multidrug treatment with standard therapy for visceral leishmaniasis in India: an open-label, non-inferiority, randomised controlled trial. *Lancet.* 2011;377:477-486.
3. Chrusciak-Talhari A, Dietze R, Chrusciak Talhari C, et al. Randomized controlled clinical trial to access efficacy and safety of miltefosine in the treatment of cutaneous leishmaniasis caused by *Leishmania* (Viannia) *guyanensis* in Manaus, Brazil. *Am J Trop Med Hyg.* 2011;84:255-260.

SUGGESTED READINGS

Goto H, Lindoso JA. Current diagnosis and treatment of cutaneous and mucocutaneous leishmaniasis. *Expert Rev Anti Infect Ther.* 2010;8:419-433. *Comprehensive review.*
Van Griensven J, Balasegaram M, Meheus F, et al. Combination therapy for visceral leishmaniasis. *Lancet Infect Dis.* 2010;10:184-194. *Combination therapy in attempts to increase treatment efficacy and tolerance, reduce treatment duration and cost, and limit the emergence of drug resistance.*

357

TOXOPLASMOSIS

JOSE G. MONTOYA

DEFINITION

The intracellular parasite *Toxoplasma gondii* is the etiologic agent of toxoplasmosis. The term *toxoplasmosis* is reserved for the disease process in which symptoms and signs are present, whereas *Toxoplasma infection* best describes the asymptomatic presence of the parasite. Toxoplasmosis may result in significant morbidity and mortality of the fetus, newborn, and immunocompromised patient. In addition, *T. gondii* can also be responsible for chorioretinitis, lymphadenopathy, myositis, myocarditis, and hepatitis in immunocompetent patients. A more aggressive form of congenital toxoplasmosis and toxoplasmosis in the adult appears to occur in certain geographic locales in South America, where pneumonia, fever of unknown origin, brain abscesses, and death have been reported in HIV-negative and apparently healthy individuals. Epidemiologic studies have established the role of novel risk factors for the acquisition of the acute infection, including the ingestion of untreated water, oysters, mussels, or clams.

The Pathogen

T. gondii is a protozoan parasite with a high capacity for host cell invasion due to a motile invasive form (tachyzoite or trophozoite) characterized by an evolutionarily unique apical complex and a mechanism of actin-based motility.

T. gondii maintains a highly clonal population structure in North America and Europe that consists of three main lineages: types I, II, and III. This relatively low genetic diversity comes as a surprise given the fact that the parasite has the capacity to infect any warm-blooded animal. It has a sexual life cycle that takes place in the intestine of cats. In North America and Europe, type II strains are most commonly associated with human toxoplasmosis, both in congenital infections and in immunocompromised patients. However, it appears that the type I strain has been reported more frequently in North America than in Europe. In South America, *Toxoplasma* strains appear to be genetically more diverse, with many different genotypes described mainly in Brazil and French Guiana. These atypical South American strains, initially called exotic strains, belong to several haplogroups that are endemic to South America and have been found to be associated with more severe clinical manifestations; physicians need to entertain this possibility in their ill patients who are from or were traveling in these endemic areas.

In nature, the parasite exists in several forms, including the tachyzoite (Fig. 357-1A), the oocyst that contains sporozoites (Fig. 357-1B), the tissue cyst that contains bradyzoites (Fig. 357-1C), and macrogametes and microgametes. The tachyzoite is the rapidly proliferating form of the parasite responsible for the clinical manifestations of toxoplasmosis observed in the setting of the acute infection or reactivation of a latent infection. The tissue cyst is the slower metabolic form of the parasite responsible for chronic infection and for its transmission through meat consumption in humans and animals. Tissue cysts persist in tissues for the life of the host and cannot be eradicated by drugs. Tissue cysts vary in shape and size from younger ones that contain only a few bradyzoites to older tissue cysts that may contain several thousand bradyzoites and may reach more than 100 µm in size. The central nervous system (CNS), eye, and skeletal, smooth, and heart muscles appear to be the most common sites of tissue cyst formation (i.e., latent infection). Oocysts are shed by domestic and feral animals belonging to the Felidae family, and they are primarily responsible for the worldwide and large-scale spread of the parasite among different populations of other animals and humans. Cats shed oocysts after they ingest any of the infectious forms of the parasite: tachyzoites, tissue cysts, and oocysts. As many as 10 million oocysts may be shed in the feces of an infected animal in a single day for periods varying from 7 to 20 days. Oocysts may remain viable for as long as 18 months in moist soil; this results in an environmental reservoir from which incidental hosts may be infected.

EPIDEMIOLOGY

The prevalence of *T. gondii* infection varies significantly according to geographic locale and the socioeconomic status of the population. It can be as low as 7% in England and as high as 80% in the Central African Republic. Seroprevalence increases with age because of increasing length of exposure with age, and it is inversely associated with socioeconomic status because of the strong influence of hygienic and alimentary habits in the transmission of the parasite. The overall age-adjusted seroprevalence of *T. gondii* infection in the United States has been recently reported at 11%, but it may be higher in certain geographic areas or socioeconomic groups. The seroprevalence of the parasite has declined during the past 30 years in the United States and several other countries but appears to be stable or increasing in certain geographic locales, such as in the tropics (e.g., South America).

Humans and non-felid animals are incidental hosts and become infected primarily by the ingestion of infected meat containing tissue cysts or of contaminated food, water, or soil containing oocysts. They can also become infected during gestation by vertical transmission of the parasite from the mother to her offspring. In addition, humans can become infected through organ transplantation and, more rarely, in the setting of laboratory accidents. Ingestion of raw or undercooked meat contaminated with tissue cysts is probably one of the major routes of transmission in humans. Ingestion of untreated water, food, or soil contaminated with oocysts is another significant route of infection with the parasite. Untreated water has been found to be the source of large epidemics of toxoplasmosis in Canada and Brazil.

A study reported the main risk factors for *T. gondii* infection in the United States: eating raw ground beef; eating rare lamb; eating locally produced cured, dried, or smoked meat; working with meat; drinking unpasteurized goat's milk; having three or more kittens. In this study, eating raw oysters, clams, or mussels was also identified as a novel risk factor. Untreated water as a potential vehicle for the transmission of *T. gondii* has been established in several large epidemiologic studies and was found to have a trend toward increased risk for acute infection in the United States.

FIGURE 357-1. *Toxoplasma gondii* **exists in nature primarily in three forms. A,** Tachyzoites are bow or banana shaped, measure 2 to 3 µm wide and 5 to 7 µm long, and can be stained with Wright-Giemsa stain. **B,** Oocysts isolated from cat's feces are subspherical to spherical and measure 10 × 12 µm in diameter. **C,** Tissue cyst observed in human myocardial tissue stained with hematoxylin and eosin. Tissue cysts vary in shape and size and may reach more than 100 µm.

In up to 50% of individuals acutely infected with *T. gondii*, it is not possible to identify the presence of a known risk factor for their acute infection. Thus, attempting to establish whether a patient is at risk for toxoplasmosis solely on the basis of the epidemiologic history is a futile task. Patients may have been infected with *T. gondii* even if they have not owned or been in contact with cats, have not eaten undercooked meat or shellfish, and have not ingested untreated water.

The seroprevalence of *T. gondii* infection in immunocompromised patients reflects the seroprevalence of the particular population from which they come. Latent *T. gondii* infection can reactivate in these patients, particularly in those with the acquired immunodeficiency syndrome (AIDS) and in hematopoietic stem cell transplant (HSCT), bone marrow transplant (BMT), and liver transplant patients. In these patients, it is important to establish whether they have been infected with the parasite before their transplant procedure because serologic testing after transplantation is unreliable. Approximately 30% of AIDS patients who are infected with *T. gondii* will develop toxoplasmosis by reactivation of their chronic infection if their CD4 count falls below 200 cells/μL and they are not taking anti-*Toxoplasma* primary prophylaxis. The advent of highly active antiretroviral therapy, in addition to the use of primary anti-*Toxoplasma* prophylaxis, has clearly contributed to the decline in the incidence of toxoplasmosis in AIDS patients. Among HSCT or BMT patients, those recipients who are *Toxoplasma* seropositive before transplantation, receive an allogeneic graft, and develop graft-versus-host disease (GVHD) have the highest risk of reactivation.

For solid organ transplants, the highest risk for toxoplasmosis is observed when an allograft from a *Toxoplasma*-seropositive donor (D$^+$) is transplanted into a seronegative recipient (R$^-$). In D$^+$/R$^-$ patients, there is a 25% risk for development of potentially life-threatening toxoplasmosis if effective anti-*Toxoplasma* prophylaxis is not instituted. It is highly advised that the *Toxoplasma* serologic status of the donor and the recipient be established before transplantation. Serologic test results are not reliable in the post-transplantation period, and they may significantly vary without any clinical relevance.

Transmission of *T. gondii* to the fetus can occur during pregnancy when a woman acquires her primary infection during gestation. The incidence of seroconversion for pregnant women in the United States has been estimated at 0.27%. The overall rate of transmission of the parasite (prevalence of congenital toxoplasmosis) in seroconverting women has been estimated between 50 and 60% before spiramycin was instituted as an attempt to decrease vertical transmission and 25 to 30% thereafter. The transmission rate increases with the gestational age at which maternal infection is acquired. In women who have been treated for toxoplasmosis during gestation, it can be as low as 4.5% during the first trimester, 31.7% during the second trimester, and as high as 63% during the third trimester. The likelihood of severe disease is inversely proportional to the gestational age at which maternal infection was acquired. Although objective data are lacking on the prevalence of congenital toxoplasmosis in the United States, it has been estimated that among the approximately 4.2 million live births per year, congenital *T. gondii* infection occurs in 500 to 5000 newborns.

Congenital transmission in women who were infected before conception has only rarely been reported in immunosuppressed patients, in those who were acutely infected shortly before conception (i.e., within 3 months of conception), and in those who have been reinfected with a more virulent strain.

PATHOBIOLOGY

Pathogenesis

After oral infection with tissue cysts (e.g., contaminated meat) or oocysts (e.g., contaminated soil or water or food), the wall of both infectious forms is disrupted by the digestive juices of the gastrointestinal tract. Bradyzoites (from cysts) and sporozoites (from oocysts) are released and converted to the tachyzoite form. Tachyzoites have the capacity to infect contiguous cells or distant tissues by hematogenous or lymphatic spread. Tachyzoites appear to actively and rapidly migrate across epithelial cells and may traffic to distant sites while they are extracellular (acute infection). Their histologic hallmark is necrosis surrounded by inflammation.

In immunocompetent individuals, the immune system controls the proliferation of the tachyzoite and induces its conversion to bradyzoites, facilitating the final formation of tissue cysts (chronic infection). Tissue cysts persist for the life of the host, and *T. gondii* can be isolated from tissues of individuals who have died without symptoms of toxoplasmosis.

It appears that the activation of well-orchestrated immune responses is required for the successful resistance against *T. gondii*. Innate, humoral, and

cellular immune responses likely to be involved in preventing the uncontrolled proliferation of tachyzoites include activation of the monocyte-macrophage system, dendritic cells, natural killer cells, and αβ and γδ T cells; *T. gondii*–specific and cytotoxic CD4$^+$ and CD8$^+$ T cells; and interferon-γ, interleukin-12, tumor necrosis factor-α, interleukin-10 and other cytokines, transforming growth factor-β, costimulatory molecules (e.g., CD28, CD40 ligand), and, to a lesser degree, immunoglobulins.

In immunocompromised patients previously infected with *T. gondii*, decreased T-cell-mediated immune responses can facilitate the reactivation of their infection (i.e., conversion of bradyzoites in their tissue cysts into rapidly proliferating tachyzoites). Toxoplasmosis in this setting is 100% lethal if untreated.

Pathology

Most of the data on the pathology of toxoplasmosis come from studies of congenitally infected babies and immunosuppressed patients. CNS lesions of patients with toxoplasmosis are characterized by significant necrosis and surrounding inflammation. In congenitally infected cases, necrotic areas may calcify and lead to typical radiographic findings suggestive but not diagnostic of toxoplasmosis. Hydrocephalus may result from obstruction of the aqueduct of Sylvius or foramen of Monro. Tachyzoites and tissue cysts may be visualized near necrotic foci, near or in glial nodules, in perivascular regions, and in cerebral tissue uninvolved by inflammatory changes.

Formation of multiple brain abscesses is relatively common in patients with AIDS. In the areas around the abscesses, edema, vasculitis, hemorrhage, and cerebral infarction secondary to vascular involvement may also be present. Important associated features in toxoplasmic encephalitis are arteritis, perivascular cuffing, and astrocytosis. A "diffuse form" of toxoplasmic encephalitis has been described with histopathologic findings of widespread microglial nodules without abscess formation in the gray matter of the cerebrum, cerebellum, and brain stem.

Pulmonary involvement by *T. gondii* in the immunodeficient patient can lead to interstitial pneumonitis, necrotizing pneumonitis, consolidation, pleural effusion or empyema, or all of these. Chorioretinitis in AIDS patients is characterized by segmental panophthalmitis and areas of coagulative necrosis associated with tissue cysts and tachyzoites.

Toxoplasmic lymphadenitis in immunocompetent individuals may result in patterns of findings that are often diagnostic of the disease: a reactive follicular hyperplasia; irregular clusters of epithelioid histiocytes encroaching on and blurring the margins of the germinal centers; and focal distention of sinuses with monocytoid cells.

CLINICAL MANIFESTATIONS

Toxoplasmosis should be entertained in the differential diagnosis of several clinical syndromes in immunocompetent, congenitally infected, and immunocompromised patients (Table 357-1). Symptoms result from the primary infection or reactivation of the parasite due to T-cell-mediated immunodeficiency. Primary infection can be asymptomatic in a significant number of individuals, and conventional risk factors for the acute infection may not be present in a particular patient. Thus, the possibility of acute toxoplasmosis or *T. gondii* infection should not be ruled out because of the absence of epidemiologic risk factors (e.g., exposure to cats or undercooked meat) or symptoms in a given patient. For this reason, if the goal is to detect each case of primary *T. gondii* infection in a population of patients (e.g., pregnant women), only systematic and universal screening methods can achieve such an objective; testing of only symptomatic patients or those with conventional epidemiologic risk factors will miss a significant number of acute cases.

Severity of toxoplasmosis due to primary infection or reactivation in a given patient or population may be influenced by the infecting strain (e.g., type I strain), inoculum, infectious form (e.g., oocyst vs. cyst), or genetics of the host (e.g., presence of HLA-DQ3). During the past decade, it has become clear that patients infected in certain geographic locales (e.g., South America) have more aggressive clinical presentations, including a more severe primary infection and disease due to reactivation. These observations need to be entertained on seeing ill travelers returning from the endemic areas or patients who were born in these areas and in whom toxoplasmosis by reactivation has been included in their differential diagnosis.

Lymphadenopathy due to toxoplasmosis may be completely asymptomatic or be accompanied by other symptoms, such as fever (temperature as high as 104° F), headache, general malaise, and fatigue. It can be localized or generalized. A solitary, occipital, and painlessly enlarged lymph node can be the sole manifestation of toxoplasmosis in a child, pregnant woman, or adult.

TABLE 357-1	CLINICAL MANIFESTATIONS OF TOXOPLASMOSIS IN HUMANS	
CLINICAL CATEGORIES	**CLINICAL MANIFESTATIONS AND SYNDROMES**
Primary infection Immunocompetent individuals and pregnant women	Most patients are asymptomatic. However, in ~10% of patients, the following symptoms or syndromes, alone or in various combinations, have been reported: fever, lymphadenopathy, headache, myalgias, arthralgias, sore throat, stiff neck, nausea, abdominal pain, anorexia, rash, confusion, earache, eye pain, general malaise, fatigue. Chorioretinitis resulting in blurred vision, eye pain, decreased visual acuity, floaters, scotoma, photophobia, or epiphora Hepatitis; myositis; myocarditis Disseminated disease, pneumonia, and even death have been observed in immunocompetent individuals infected with *T. gondii* in Latin America.
Congenital toxoplasmosis Fetus	Fetal death; ultrasound study can be normal or reveal hydrocephalus, brain or hepatic calcifications, splenomegaly, ascites, pericarditis.
Newborn	Newborn can be entirely normal, have a nonspecific illness, or have an abnormal physical examination including chorioretinitis, strabismus, blindness, seizures, encephalitis, abnormal cephalic perimeter (microcephaly or hydrocephalus), psychomotor or mental retardation, hepatosplenomegaly, pneumonitis, diarrhea, hypothermia, jaundice, petechiae, rash. Intracranial calcifications can be present in brain imaging studies.
Children and adults	Children can continue to suffer the chronic sequelae of the congenital disease. However, children and adults may become symptomatic for the first time during this phase of their lives, primarily in the form of reactivation of the congenitally acquired chorioretinitis.
Chronic infection	Asymptomatic. However, some investigators have proposed a role of chronic infection in individuals with traffic accidents or schizophrenia. Chorioretinitis can occur as a reactivation of congenital or postnatally acquired disease in otherwise immunocompetent individuals.
Reactivation of chronic infection in immunocompromised patients	Multiple brain abscesses, diffuse encephalitis, chorioretinitis, fever of unknown origin, pneumonia, myocarditis, hepatosplenomegaly, lymphadenopathy, rash

FIGURE 357-2. The morphology of the retinal lesions on funduscopic examination believed to be characteristic of toxoplasmic retinochoroiditis. An active whitish infiltrate is usually attached to the darkly pigmented border of an older scar.

However, more generalized cervical, axillary, and abdominal lymphadenopathy has also been reported. Lymph nodes are usually 1 to 3 cm in size, non-suppurative, and nontender on palpation. They usually regress within 12 weeks, but a mild relapse of the lymphadenopathy has been observed between months 3 and 6. Recurrence of toxoplasmic lymphadenopathy beyond the sixth month is extremely rare.

Ocular disease due to *T. gondii* can be asymptomatic or symptomatic and can be the result of congenital or postnatally acquired infection. In both settings (congenitally and postnatally acquired), toxoplasmic chorioretinitis can be discovered at the time of the diagnosis of the infection or as a reactivation of the subsequent latent infection months to years later. Up to 17% of patients acutely infected with the parasite in Brazil and in a Canadian outbreak of toxoplasmosis presented with concurrent symptomatic toxoplasmic chorioretinitis at the time their acute infection was diagnosed. Similar cases have been described in Europe and the United States. Symptomatic ocular disease primarily consists of a retinochoroiditis that can result in blurred vision, eye pain, decreased visual acuity, floaters, scotoma, photophobia, or epiphora. The morphology of the retinal lesions on funduscopic examination is thought to be characteristic of toxoplasmosis. An active whitish infiltrate is usually attached to the darkly pigmented border of an older scar (Fig. 357-2). However, retinal lesions tend to be less typical in older or immunocompromised patients.

Other less common but well-documented syndromes have been associated with the acute infection, including hepatitis, myositis, myocarditis, and skin lesions. More aggressive disease including pneumonia, brain abscesses, and death has been observed in immunocompetent patients in South America.

Primary infection can be observed in solid transplant patients when an allograft from a seropositive donor is transplanted into a seronegative recipient (D$^+$/R$^-$). Disseminated and localized toxoplasmosis has been reported in this setting, including myocarditis, pneumonia, and encephalitis.

Congenital disease can be asymptomatic in the fetus, newborn, child, or adult. However, most of the infected offspring will eventually develop signs and symptoms of toxoplasmosis (see Table 357-1). The classic triad of chorioretinitis, hydrocephalus (Fig. 357-3A and B), and brain calcifications is highly suggestive of toxoplasmosis and is primarily seen in babies whose mothers have not been treated against the parasite during gestation. Eye examination by an experienced pediatric ophthalmologist may reveal active or inactive toxoplasmic chorioretinitis. New lesions have been reported in up to 30% of congenitally infected children observed up until 11 years of age.

Chronic infection is believed to be asymptomatic. However, several investigators have recently suggested the possibility that chronic infection may play a role in the predisposition of infected individuals to have a higher frequency of traffic accidents or schizophrenia.

Reactivation of the chronic infection is usually observed in patients with significant impairment of their T-cell-mediated immunity. Toxoplasmosis by reactivation can cause brain abscesses, diffuse encephalitis, chorioretinitis, fever of unknown origin, pneumonia, myocarditis, hepatosplenomegaly, lymphadenopathy, and rash. Although multiple brain abscesses (Fig. 357-3C) are commonly described in patients with toxoplasmic encephalitis, diffuse encephalitis without space-occupying lesions by magnetic resonance imaging has been reported with a very high mortality. Fever with pneumonia can be the sole manifestation of toxoplasmosis in immunocompromised patients, including HSCT and solid organ transplants. Toxoplasmic pneumonitis can present with cough, dyspnea, hypoxia, and diffuse bilateral or localized infiltrates. Fever alone has frequently been described in patients with allogeneic HSCT and liver transplant patients. Reactivation in heart tissue causing congestive heart failure, arrhythmias, and pericarditis has been described.

DIAGNOSIS

Laboratory methods for the diagnosis of *T. gondii* infection and toxoplasmosis include serologic tests, the polymerase chain reaction (PCR), histologic and cytologic examination of tissue and body fluids, and attempts to isolate the parasite (Table 357-2).

The diagnosis of acute or latent *T. gondii* infection can be accomplished by serologic testing. Serologic tests can establish whether a patient is acutely or chronically infected regardless of the presence or absence of symptoms. Available serologic tools include methods to detect *T. gondii*–specific IgG-,

FIGURE 357-3. Radiologic manifestations of central nervous system toxoplasmosis. **A,** Fetal ultrasound of a fetus congenitally infected with *T. gondii* in the United States reveals hydrocephalus. **B,** Computed tomography scan of the brain of a newborn congenitally infected with *T. gondii* in the United States reveals hydrocephalus and calcifications. **C,** Magnetic resonance image of the brain of an AIDS patient revealing multiple ring-enhancing brain lesions.

TABLE 357-2 LABORATORY METHODS FOR THE DIAGNOSIS OF *T. GONDII* INFECTION AND TOXOPLASMOSIS* IN HUMANS

METHOD	CLINICAL INTERPRETATION
Serologic tests	
IgG	A positive test result establishes that the patient has been infected with *T. gondii*. However, a negative test result can be seen in patients infected within 4 weeks before serum sampling or in patients unable to produce IgG (e.g., immunocompromised hosts).
IgM	A positive test result suggests but is not necessarily diagnostic of an acute infection. Sera with positive IgM test results should be sent to a reference laboratory for confirmatory testing. Positive IgM test results can be seen in chronically infected patients because of persistence of the IgM response or false-positive results observed in certain commercial kits.
Confirmatory testing for positive IgM test results	IgG avidity test; differential agglutination (AC/HS); IgA, IgE performed at a reference laboratory.[†] At PAMF, a high IgG avidity test result[‡] or a nonacute AC/HS test result indicates that the patient has been infected for more than 4 months (avidity) or 12 months (AC/HS).
Polymerase chain reaction (PCR)	B1 and AF487550 genes are the most commonly used targets for amplification. PCR test can be performed in any body fluid, including peripheral blood, cerebrospinal fluid, bronchoalveolar lavage fluid, vitreous fluid, aqueous humor, peritoneal fluid, pleural fluid, and ascitic fluid. PCR can also be performed in any tissue. A positive test result in any body fluid establishes that the patient has either primary or reactivated toxoplasmosis. However, a positive PCR test result in tissue is more difficult to interpret because it does not differentiate toxoplasmosis from a latent infection. Although DNA extraction is more cumbersome, it can be attempted in paraffin-embedded tissue.
Direct visualization of the parasite	Identification of tachyzoites in any body fluid or tissue is diagnostic of toxoplasmosis due to primary infection or reactivation of a chronic infection. Tachyzoites can be identified by hematoxylin and eosin or cytologic studies but are better visualized with Wright-Giemsa and immunoperoxidase stains. Identification of cysts by hematoxylin and eosin or immunoperoxidase stains confirms the presence of *T. gondii* in the host but does not necessarily establish that the patient has toxoplasmosis. However, a strong inflammatory response surrounding the cysts is highly suggestive of toxoplasmosis, possibly explaining the patient's symptoms.
Attempts to isolate the parasite	A positive isolation study in any body fluid establishes the diagnosis of toxoplasmosis. Isolation of *T. gondii* in cell cultures or peritoneal cavity of mice can be attempted at reference laboratories. These studies can be important in trying to establish a correlation between the genetics of the parasite and its clinical manifestations.
Histology of the lymph node	Classic histologic triad is considered diagnostic: follicular hyperplasia, epithelioid histiocytes impinging on the margins of the germinal centers, and monocytoid cells focally distending sinus walls.

*T. gondii infection = asymptomatic presence of the parasite. Toxoplasmosis = active symptoms and signs are present.
[†]For example, Palo Alto Medical Foundation Toxoplasma Serology Laboratory (PAMF-TSL), Palo Alto, Calif; *www.pamf.org/serology*; 650-853-4828; toxolab@pamf.org.
[‡]The window of exclusion for acute infection varies for different avidity kits (usually between 3 and 5 months).

IgM-, IgA-, IgE-, and IgG-based avidity and differential agglutination (AC/HS).

With the use of commercial kits for the detection of IgG and IgM, most hospital-based or commercial laboratories can reliably diagnose the absence of *T. gondii* infection (negative IgG/negative IgM) and the chronic infection (positive IgG/negative IgM). However, the diagnosis of acute infection is more challenging. A positive IgM test result is observed during the acute infection, but it may remain positive for months to years in certain individuals without any apparent clinical relevance. In addition, commercial IgM kits have been designed to be extremely sensitive so that an acute infection will be rarely missed; as a consequence, their specificity is somewhat sacrificed. Of patients who are found to be IgM positive at hospital-based or commercial laboratories, 60% are found to be chronically infected when their serum is tested at the national reference laboratory for the study and diagnosis of toxoplasmosis in the United States (Palo Alto Medical Foundation

Toxoplasma Serology Laboratory [PAMF-TSL], Palo Alto, Calif; *www.pamf.org/serology*; 650-853-4828; toxolab@pamf.org). At PAMF-TSL, a battery of confirmatory tests (avidity, differential agglutination, IgA, IgE) are performed in addition to the "gold standard" dye test for IgG and the "double" sandwich capture enzyme-linked immunosorbent assay (ELISA) for IgM. These tests are used in various combinations, depending on the clinical scenario of each patient and the questions of the treating physician. For an appropriate interpretation of the serologic test results obtained at PAMF-TSL, it is also crucial to have relevant clinical information available for the medical consultants (for instance, low positive IgG and positive IgM test results with a high IgG avidity test result will mean no risk of congenital toxoplasmosis for a 16-week pregnant woman, but the same results can be highly supportive of the diagnosis of toxoplasmic encephalitis for an AIDS patient with multiple brain lesions). At PAMF-TSL, three interpretations can be given to final serologic test results: (1) acute, results are consistent with a recently acquired infection; (2) chronic, consistent with an infection acquired in the distant past; and (3) equivocal, cannot exclude a recently acquired infection; an earlier or subsequent sample is required to attempt to establish whether the infection is acute or chronic. For serologic test results consistent with an acute infection, an attempt is made by the medical consultants at PAMF-TSL to establish the approximate date that the infection was acquired.

The definitive diagnosis of toxoplasmosis (due to primary infection or reactivation of a chronic infection) requires the identification of tachyzoites in tissues or body fluids or the amplification of parasite DNA in any body fluid (see Table 357-2). Tachyzoites can be visualized in histologic sections stained with hematoxylin and eosin or in cytologic preparations without any specific staining, but they are better visualized with Wright-Giemsa (see Fig. 357-1A) and immunoperoxidase stains. Real-time PCR has become a useful method for the diagnosis of toxoplasmosis, and it is the diagnostic tool of choice for toxoplasmic encephalitis in immunocompromised patients (assuming the lumbar puncture is deemed safe and feasible) and for the prenatal diagnosis of congenital toxoplasmosis. Isolation of the parasite in any body fluid is also diagnostic of toxoplasmosis and can be attempted at reference laboratories. The diagnosis of toxoplasmosis can be supported by the use of serologic tools, demonstration of cysts in tissues (see Fig. 357-1C) surrounded by an inflammatory response, and attempts to isolate the parasite (see Table 357-2); in cases of toxoplasmic lymphadenitis, histologic features can be diagnostic.

Immunocompetent Patients, Pregnant Women, and Patients with Lymphadenopathy

The first diagnostic goal in these patients is to establish whether they have ever been infected with *T. gondii*. If *T. gondii*–specific IgG and IgM test results are negative, the possibility that the patient's symptoms are due to the parasite can be ruled out. During pregnancy, these results confirm that the mother has not been exposed to *T. gondii* but that she is at risk, if exposed, to acquire the primary infection during pregnancy and therefore can potentially transmit *T. gondii* to her offspring. In attempting to determine whether the patient is infected with *T. gondii*, it is important to perform both IgG and IgM tests because during the first 4 weeks of the acute infection, the IgG can still be negative while the IgM will be positive. In these cases, seroconversion can be diagnosed by having a new positive IgG test result in a subsequent serum sample. In rare instances, infected patients may be IgG negative because of their incapacity to produce IgG.

If the patient is found to be IgG positive, the next goal is to determine whether the patient is having an acute infection or has been chronically infected (e.g., >6 months). If the IgG titer is low (e.g., a dye test at PAMF-TSL ≤512) and the IgM test result is negative, the patient has been infected for at least 6 months. With these results, a patient whose symptoms or lymphadenopathy had a date of onset within 6 months of serum sampling will be considered unlikely to have toxoplasmosis. For a pregnant woman whose serum was obtained within 6 months of gestation, they will mean that her infection was acquired before conception and that the risk for congenital toxoplasmosis is essentially zero.

If the patient is found to have a positive IgM test result confirmed to be indicative of a recently acquired infection at a reference laboratory (e.g., PAMF-TSL) and the onset of symptoms or lymphadenopathy falls within the time predicted by the serologic test results for the acquisition of *T. gondii*, the patient will be diagnosed as having acute toxoplasmosis. For a pregnant woman, if the predicted time for when the infection was acquired falls within her gestational age, she will be diagnosed with toxoplasmosis during pregnancy and at risk for transmitting the parasite to her baby.

In patients with lymphadenopathy, the histologic examination of the lymph node tissue obtained by excisional biopsy can be diagnostic or pathognomonic of toxoplasmic lymphadenitis (see earlier under Pathology).

Prenatal and Postnatal Diagnosis of Congenital Toxoplasmosis

Once the diagnosis of acute toxoplasmosis or *T. gondii* infection has been confirmed or is highly suspected in the mother, the next step is to attempt to establish whether her offspring has been infected. Consultation with reference centers for the study and diagnosis of congenital toxoplasmosis is highly recommended.

Ultrasound abnormalities can be consistent with or suggestive of congenital toxoplasmosis (see Fig. 357-3A), but they are not diagnostic. The method of choice for the prenatal diagnosis of congenital toxoplasmosis is a PCR in amniotic fluid obtained at 18 weeks of gestation. Attempts to diagnose

congenital toxoplasmosis from amniotic fluid obtained before 18 weeks of gestation should be avoided because the studies reported to date have included only pregnant women whose gestational age was 18 weeks or more. In addition, false-negative results have been reported in women whose amniocentesis was performed before 18 weeks of gestation. The overall sensitivity of the amniotic fluid PCR has been reported between 64 and 92% and is highly dependent of the gestational age at which the mother acquired the infection.

In the newborn, congenital toxoplasmosis can be confirmed by positive *T. gondii*–specific serologic test results or PCR. Samples for serology should be obtained in the peripheral blood of the baby. Cord blood should be avoided because of the high rate of maternal blood contamination. However, there is still a small degree of maternal blood contamination in newborn blood obtained by peripheral venipuncture, during the first 5 days of life for IgM antibodies and the first 10 days of life for IgA antibodies. A positive IgM immunosorbent agglutination assay (after 5 days of life) or IgA ELISA (after 10 days) is diagnostic of congenital disease. Congenitally infected babies can be positive for both; positive for either one, but negative for the other test; or negative for both. A positive *T. gondii*–specific IgM in cerebrospinal fluid (CSF) is diagnostic of congenital disease, but testing of the CSF by PCR rather than for IgM is strongly recommended because of the higher sensitivity of the PCR test. The diagnosis can also be made by a positive PCR in peripheral blood, CSF, or urine. The CSF of infected infants may exhibit very high levels of protein (e.g., 1000 mg/dL) and eosinophilia in addition to lymphocytosis. Brain imaging studies may reveal calcifications or hydrocephalus; computed tomography scan is superior to ultrasound examination in the detection of these CNS abnormalities (see Fig. 357-3B).

Ocular Disease

Serologic and PCR testing can be helpful in the diagnosis of toxoplasmic chorioretinitis. An IgG-negative/IgM-negative patient is unlikely to have ocular disease due to toxoplasmosis. However, patients should be tested at reference laboratories (e.g., PAMF-TSL) because their *T. gondii*–specific IgG can be present but at very low levels such that only a gold standard method like the dye test can detect it. In patients with eye lesions typical of toxoplasmic chorioretinitis (see Fig. 357-2), a positive IgG test result at a relatively low titer (e.g., a dye test at PAMF-TSL ≤512) and a negative IgM test result are diagnostic of ocular disease due to the parasite reactivation. If the serologic test reveals a positive IgM result and confirmatory testing at PAMF-TSL establishes the diagnosis of an acute infection in patients 1 year of age or older, the eye disease is most likely the result of eye involvement in the setting of a recent and postnatally acquired infection.

In patients with atypically appearing lesions or in whom the response to anti-*Toxoplasma* drugs is slow or absent, a *T. gondii*–specific immune load (aqueous humor) or PCR in ocular fluids (vitreous fluid is preferable to aqueous humor because of probable higher sensitivity, but it is riskier to obtain) should be considered.

Immunocompromised Patients

It appears that acute infection rarely occurs in immunocompromised patients. However, life-threatening disease can occur when the patient's latent infection is reactivated by AIDS, HSCT, or other diseases characterized by severe T-cell deficiency.

Toxoplasmosis can also develop when *T. gondii* is transmitted from a seropositive donor to a seronegative recipient through an infected allograft (e.g., heart). Therefore, to establish the risk for toxoplasmosis and to have a high index of suspicion when patients develop illnesses suggestive of toxoplasmosis, all immunocompromised patients should be tested for *T. gondii*–specific IgG as soon as they have been diagnosed with the underlying disease or it has been established that they will be subsequently immunosuppressed. In addition, serologic testing may not be reliable when immunosuppression is advanced or severe. Post-transplantation serologic test results for IgG antibodies may remain positive or may rise, decrease, or even become negative. Thus, pretransplantation *Toxoplasma* serologic studies are critical for interpretation of subsequent test results and clinical evaluation. Solid organ donors should also be tested for *T. gondii*–specific IgG as their allograft has the potential to transmit the parasite to the transplanted patient (e.g., heart, heart-lung, kidney, kidney-pancreas, liver, liver-pancreas).

In AIDS patients suspected of having toxoplasmic encephalitis, the presence of multiple brain-occupying and ring-enhancing lesions (see Fig. 357-3C), a CD4 count below 200 cells/μL, and a positive *T. gondii*–specific IgG, the response to anti-*Toxoplasma*–specific treatment is considered an additional "diagnostic" indicator of toxoplasmic encephalitis. In these patients, invasive diagnostic tests (e.g., lumbar puncture, brain biopsy) are considered unnecessary unless they do not respond to treatment within a 7- to 10-day period. This diagnostic paradigm should not be applied to other populations of immunosuppressed patients (e.g., transplant patients) because their differential diagnosis often includes other pathogens, such as invasive mold infections. In those patients, examination of the CSF by PCR or brain biopsy should be attempted at the outset of the illness.

The definitive diagnosis of toxoplasmosis in immunosuppressed patients relies on PCR, direct visualization of the parasite, and attempts for isolation of the organism (see Table 357-2). PCR testing is the diagnostic method of choice for immunosuppressed patients at risk for toxoplasmosis who develop unexplained fever, pneumonia, brain lesions, or other compatible syndromes (e.g., in whole blood, bronchoalveolar lavage fluid, CSF, or other fluids as clinically indicated). PCR can be performed in any body fluid or tissue. Attempts to identify the tachyzoite or tissue cyst in tissues should be enhanced with the use of the *T. gondii*–specific immunoperoxidase stain. CSF examination by PCR or brain biopsy should be initially considered in AIDS patients who have a low likelihood of having toxoplasmic encephalitis, such as those who have a single lesion by magnetic resonance imaging examination, have tested seronegative for *T. gondii* infection, have a CD4 count of more than 200 cells/µL, or who are not responding to an appropriate anti-*Toxoplasma* regimen.

TREATMENT Rx

Principles of antiparasitic therapy are discussed in Chapter 352. Treatment of toxoplasmosis is indicated for immunocompetent patients with acute infection in the setting of myocarditis, myositis, hepatitis, pneumonia, brain lesions or skin lesions, and lymphadenopathy accompanied by severe or persisting symptoms. Treatment is indicated as well for patients with active chorioretinitis due to primary infection or reactivation of a latent infection (Table 357-3). In immunocompetent patients, treatment is prescribed for 3 to 4 weeks or until symptoms have subsided, whichever is longer. For toxoplasmic lymphadenitis, co-trimoxazole (48 mg/kg/day divided into two doses for 1 month) increased the cure rate to 65% compared with a 13% resolution rate with placebo.[1] Treatment is also often recommended for all pregnant women suspected of having or diagnosed with primary infection during gestation (Table 357-4) in an attempt to prevent transmission of the parasite to the fetus (spiramycin) or, if congenital infection has occurred, to start treatment of the fetus in utero (pyrimethamine, sulfadiazine, an folinic acid). During pregnancy, treatment regimens are prescribed for the duration of the gestation. There is worldwide controversy about the efficacy of spiramycin to decrease the incidence of congenital toxoplasmosis. There are no definitive studies proving or disproving its efficacy. However, until the results of such studies become available, the use of spiramycin is still recommended in the United States for pregnant women who have been definitively diagnosed to have or are highly suspected of having acute acquired infection during gestation. In addition, newborns and infants diagnosed with or suspected of having congenital toxoplasmosis should also be treated during their first year of life (see Table 357-4).

Treatment, at higher doses, is urgently indicated for all immunocompromised patients with toxoplasmosis due to reactivation of their latent infection or primary infection acquired by natural exposure to the parasite or solid organ transplantation (see Table 357-3). If untreated, toxoplasmosis in these patients has a very high morbidity and mortality.

PREVENTION
Primary Infection

Because approximately 50% of patients may inadvertently become infected with the parasite without having a recognized risk factor for acute infection, only systematic serologic testing can establish whether a patient has been exposed to *T. gondii*. Thus, each pregnant woman and immunocompromised patient should be screened for *T. gondii*–specific IgG and IgM regardless of their epidemiologic history. Seronegative pregnant women and immunocompromised individuals should be counseled on how to maximize their prevention efforts to avoid infection with *T. gondii* (E-Table 357-1). In addition, seronegative pregnant women should be tested serially during gestation in an attempt to diagnose seroconversion at the earliest time possible. In some countries, such as France, seronegative pregnant women are mandated by law

TABLE 357-3 TREATMENT REGIMENS FOR PATIENTS WITH ACUTE OR PRIMARY TOXOPLASMOSIS AND IMMUNOCOMPROMISED PATIENTS WITH TOXOPLASMOSIS DUE TO REACTIVATION*

	IMMUNOCOMPETENT PATIENTS WITH ACUTE INFECTION[†]	IMMUNOCOMPROMISED PATIENTS
Pyrimethamine (PO)	50 mg every 12 hr for 2 days, followed by 25 to 50 mg daily	200 mg loading dose, followed by 50 mg/day (<60 kg) to 75 mg/day (>60 kg)
Folinic acid[‡] (PO)	10-20 mg daily (during and 1 week after therapy with pyrimethamine)	10 to 20 mg daily (up to 50 mg/day)
plus Sulfadiazine (PO)	75 mg/kg (first dose), followed by 50 mg/kg every 12 hr (maximum 4 g/day)	1000 mg (<60 kg) to 1500 mg (>60 kg) every 6 hr
or Clindamycin (PO or IV)	300 mg every 6 hr	600 mg every 6 hr (up to 1200 mg every 6 hr)
or Atovaquone (PO)	1500 mg orally twice daily	1500 mg orally twice daily
Trimethoprim-sulfamethoxazole (PO or IV)	10 mg/kg/day (trimethoprim component) in two or three doses	10 mg/kg/day (trimethoprim component) in two or three doses (doses as high as 15-20 mg/kg/day have been used)
Pyrimethamine and folinic acid	Same doses as above	Same doses as above
plus Clarithromycin (PO)	500 mg every 12 hr	500 mg every 12 hr
or Dapsone (PO)	100 mg/day	100 mg/day
or Azithromycin (PO)	900 to 1200 mg/day	900 to 1200 mg/day

*Preferred regimens: pyrimethamine, sulfadiazine, and folinic acid or trimethoprim-sulfamethoxazole. Assistance is available for the diagnosis and management of patients with toxoplasmosis at the Palo Alto Medical Foundation Toxoplasma Serology Laboratory (PAMF-TSL), Palo Alto, Calif; www.pamf.org/serology; 650-853-4828; toxolab@pamf.org.
[†]Particularly in the setting of myocarditis, myositis, hepatitis, pneumonia, brain or skin lesions, and lymphadenopathy accompanied by severe or persisting symptoms. Also indicated for those with active ocular disease due to primary infection or reactivation.
[‡]Folinic acid = leucovorin; folic acid must not be used as a substitute for folinic acid.
After the successful use of a combination regimen during the acute or primary therapy phase, the same agents at half-dose are usually used for maintenance or secondary prophylaxis.

to be tested every month for *T. gondii*–specific IgG and IgM. Women who seroconvert are offered spiramycin (if infected before 18 weeks of gestation) or pyrimethamine, sulfadiazine, and folinic acid (if infected after 18 weeks) and PCR testing in amniotic fluid. Mothers whose amniotic fluid is found to be positive by PCR or those in whom fetal ultrasound study is highly suggestive of congenital toxoplasmosis are offered pyrimethamine, sulfadiazine, and folinic acid. Although infection often occurs in the absence of known risk factors for the acute infection, educational interventions to avoid exposure to the parasite have been shown to be effective in decreasing the incidence of seroconversion during gestation.

The majority of epidemiologic studies worldwide have recognized contaminated and undercooked meat as one of the main risk factors for the transmission of the parasite. This appears to be the case in Europe, North America, and Latin America. Tissue cysts in meat are rendered nonviable by γ-irradiation (0.4 kGy), heating throughout to 67° C, or freezing to −20° C for 24 hours and then thawing. Cured, dried, or smoked meat has been associated with the acute infection and should not be considered *Toxoplasma* free. Soil exposure and soil-related activities have been reported to play a more prominent role in transmission in certain geographic areas, such as Latin America.

In seronegative recipients of a solid organ from a seropositive donor, trimethoprim-sulfamethoxazole (TMP-SMZ) for at least 6 months or pyrimethamine for at least 6 weeks has been reported to be effective in the prevention of primary infection in the newly immunosuppressed patient.

TABLE 357-4	TREATMENT REGIMENS FOR PREGNANT WOMEN WHO HAVE LIKELY ACQUIRED *T. GONDII* INFECTION DURING GESTATION AND INFANTS SUSPECTED OF HAVING OR CONFIRMED TO HAVE CONGENITAL TOXOPLASMOSIS	
	DURING PREGNANCY	**IN CONGENITAL DISEASE**
Spiramycin (oral)	Recommended for pregnant women suspected of having or confirmed to have acquired the infection before 18 weeks of gestation. Spiramycin should be administered until delivery in those with negative amniotic fluid PCR test results and normal follow-up ultrasound studies or low suspicion of fetal infection. Spiramycin is not teratogenic, and it is available in the United States only through the Investigational New Drug (IND) process at the Food and Drug Administration (301-796-1600). Prior medical consultation is required.* Dosage: 1 g (3 million units) every 8 hr (for a total of 3 g or 9 million units per day)	Not recommended during pregnancy if the fetus has been documented to be or suspected to have been infected. In the setting of fetal infection, pyrimethamine, sulfadiazine, and folinic acid should be instituted (see below)
Pyrimethamine (oral) plus sulfadiazine (oral) plus folinic acid† (oral)	Recommended for women ≥18 weeks of gestation in whom it is suspected or confirmed that the acute infection has been acquired at or after 18 weeks of gestation or who have a positive amniotic fluid PCR test result or an abnormal ultrasound study suggestive of congenital toxoplasmosis. Pyrimethamine is teratogenic and should not be used during pregnancy before week 18 (in some centers in Europe, it is used as early as week 14). Sulfadiazine should not be used alone. Dosages: Pyrimethamine: 50 mg every 12 hr for 2 days followed by 50 mg daily Sulfadiazine: 75 mg/kg (first dose) followed by 50 mg/kg every 12 hr (maximum 4 g/day) Folinic acid† (leucovorin): 10-20 mg daily (during and for 1 week after pyrimethamine therapy)	**Infant** (treatment regimen is usually recommended for 1 year): Pyrimethamine: 1 mg/kg every 12 hr for 2 days; followed by 1 mg/kg/day for 2 or 6 months; followed by 1 mg/kg/day every Monday, Wednesday, Friday Sulfadiazine: 50 mg/kg every 12 hr Folinic acid† (leucovorin): 10 mg three times weekly Prednisone (if CSF protein ≥1 g/dL or severe chorioretinitis): 0.5 mg/kg every 12 hr (until CSF protein <1 g/dL or resolution of severe chorioretinitis) **Older children with active disease** (usually 1-2 weeks beyond resolution of clinical manifestations): Pyrimethamine: 1 mg/kg every 12 hr (maximum 50 mg) for 2 days followed by 1 mg/kg/day (maximum 25 mg) Sulfadiazine: 75 mg/kg (first dose) followed by 50 mg/kg every 12 hr Folinic acid† (leucovorin): 10-20 mg three times weekly Prednisone (severe chorioretinitis): 1 mg/kg/day, divided bid, maximum 40 mg/day, rapid taper

*Palo Alto Medical Foundation Toxoplasma Serology Laboratory (PAMF-TSL), Palo Alto, Calif; *www.pamf.org/serology*; 650-853-4828; toxolab@pamf.org; or U.S. (Chicago) National Collaborative Treatment Trial Study (NCCTS), 773-834-4152.
†Folic acid should not be used as a substitute for folinic acid.

Reactivation of Latent Infection in Immunocompromised Patients and Those with Ocular Disease

Drugs used to prevent reactivation of the latent infection in immunosuppressed hosts include TMP-SMZ (e.g., single-strength or 80 mg TMP and 400 mg SMZ, 1 tablet per day) and atovaquone (1500 mg/day). Dapsone-pyrimethamine and sulfadoxine-pyrimethamine have been also reported to be effective, but their use appears to be limited because of potential hematologic toxicity.

Prophylaxis against reactivation of latent infection has been successful in AIDS patients dually infected with *T. gondii* (*Toxoplasma* IgG seropositive) and whose CD4+ T-cell counts are below 200 cells/μL. For prophylactic purposes, TMP-SMZ should probably not be used below a minimum dose of 160 mg and 800 mg orally twice a day on a thrice-weekly regimen. In AIDS patients, 100 mg of dapsone plus 50 mg of pyrimethamine orally twice weekly or atovaquone (1500 mg/day) has also been effective in preventing toxoplasmic encephalitis. Findings in these studies have been extrapolated to non-AIDS immunosuppressed patients because of the absence of data in this population of patients.

Toxoplasma-seropositive recipients of an allogeneic HSCT (Chapter 181) who develop GVHD represent a unique challenge. Reactivation of toxoplasmosis can be manifested by a nonspecific illness (e.g., fever or pneumonia) and be life-threatening. The disease is often not recognized. Atovaquone prophylaxis has been proposed as an alternative regimen in these patients given the potential bone marrow toxicity of TMP-SMZ. Some investigators have proposed a preemptive strategy in which *Toxoplasma*-seropositive patients who receive an allogeneic HSCT are monitored on a routine basis (e.g., weekly for the first 100 days) with *T. gondii* PCR. Those found positive would receive preemptive prophylaxis with TMP-SMZ or atovaquone.

Discontinuation of prophylaxis against toxoplasmic encephalitis has proved safe in AIDS patients receiving highly active antiretroviral therapy who demonstrate an increase in their CD4+ T-cell counts to at least 200 cells/μL and whose viral load has been undetectable for at least 6 months.

In patients with ocular toxoplasmosis who experience frequent relapses (e.g., more than two episodes per year), TMP-SMZ for at least 1 year has been shown to be effective in the prevention of their recurrences.

PROGNOSIS

The primary infection has a wide spectrum of manifestations in humans, from asymptomatic in most individuals to pneumonia or life-threatening if it is acquired in certain areas of the world. Primary infection can also be fatal in the fetus and in immunocompromised individuals. Early diagnosis and treatment can make a significant difference in the prognosis of these patients.

It is not clear at this time whether chronic infection in immunocompetent individuals is clinically irrelevant. Several investigators have proposed that latent infection with the parasite may play a significant role in mental illness (e.g., schizophrenia) or in the propensity of the infected individual to incur motor vehicle accidents. Immunocompetent patients can reactivate chronic infection in their retina, and the prognosis is influenced by the proximity of the lesions to the macula, involvement of one or both eyes, and number of relapses. It is believed that treatment can slow the progression of these lesions and expedite their healing.

Reactivation of latent infection in immunosuppressed individuals with significant defects in their T-cell–mediated immunity, if untreated, is 100% fatal.

 Visit expertconsult.com for e-expanded chapter

Grade **A**

1. Alavi SM, Alavi L. Treatment of toxoplasmic lymphadenitis with co-trimoxazole: double-blind, randomized clinical trial. *Int J Infect Dis.* 2010;3:e67-e69.

SUGGESTED READINGS

Berrebi A, Assouline C, Bessieres M-H, et al. Long-term outcome of children with congenital toxoplasmosis. *Am J Obstet Gynecol.* 2010;203:552.e1-6. *A 20-year prospective study of the long-term outcome of children with toxoplasmosis infection acquired in utero.*

Magi B, Migliorini L. Western blotting for the diagnosis of congenital toxoplasmosis. *New Microbiol.* 2011;34:93-95. *Detects cases missed by serology.*

Neves ES, Bicudo LN, Curi AL, et al. Acute acquired toxoplasmosis: clinical-laboratorial aspects and ophthalmologic evaluation in a cohort of immunocompetent patients. *Mem Inst Oswaldo Cruz.* 2009;104:393-396. *The most frequent findings were lymphadenopathy (95%), headache (70%), fever (68%), and weight loss (62%); hepatosplenomegaly and elevated transaminase levels were seen in 20 to 30% of cases.*

Wakefield D, Cunningham ET Jr, Pavesio C, et al. Controversies in ocular toxoplasmosis. *Ocul Immunol Inflamm.* 2011;19:2-9. *Review.*

358

CRYPTOSPORIDIOSIS

ALDO A. M. LIMA AND RICHARD L. GUERRANT

DEFINITION

Cryptosporidiosis is the clinical disease caused by protozoal parasites of the genus *Cryptosporidium*. The *Cryptosporidium* species considered important as human pathogens are *Cryptosporidium hominis, Cryptosporidium parvum, Cryptosporidium meleagridis, Cryptosporidium felis, Cryptosporidium canis,* and the *Cryptosporidium* rabbit genotype. *C. parvum* and *C. hominis* are considered the major human pathogens.

The Pathogen

Cryptosporidium spp belong to the protozoal phylum Apicomplexa (sporozoans), which features apical polar rings, micronemes, and subpellicular microtubules, structures responsible for penetration into host cells; the order Eucoccidiorida (Eucoccidiida); and the suborder Eimeriorina (Eimeriina), based on merogony and independent development of male and female gametocytes within vertebrate host. The family Cryptosporidiidae has a hidden sporocyst and undergoes monoxenous completion of its cycle in one host, where it can cause predominantly intestinal, cloacal, and gastric infections.

EPIDEMIOLOGY

The life cycle begins with ingestion of *Cryptosporidium* oocysts (2 to 5 μm) by the vertebrate host, with subsequent excystation within the lumen of the small intestine to release four sporozoites (Fig. 358-1). The sporozoites attach to and enter the host's epithelial cells to form intracellular but extracytoplasmic parasitophorous vacuoles, where they develop into trophozoites and subsequently type 1 meronts (schizonts). By asexual nuclear division they multiply and release six to eight type 1 merozoites that invade neighboring host cells and develop into type 2 meronts, or trophozoites, to complete the asexual reproductive cycle. Type 2 meronts undergo two nuclear divisions and release four type 2 merozoites that can infect the host's cells and further develop into male (microgamont) or female (macrogamete) forms. Microgametes released from the microgamont can penetrate the macrogametes to form zygotes. Approximately 20% of the zygotes develop into thin-walled autoinfectious oocysts; some 80% become thick-walled oocysts, which are excreted in stool.

Cryptosporidium oocysts have at least five characteristics that make this organism a common problem and potential risk for person-to-person spread and for waterborne and food-borne disease outbreaks. First, *Cryptosporidium* oocysts are resistant to many chemical disinfectants such as chlorine. Second, the organism is highly infectious, with the median *C. parvum* infectious dose being 132 or fewer oocysts. Third, the size of the oocysts, 2 to 5 μm, allows them to pass through most conventional filters, even those capable of removing some particles smaller than 1 μm. Fourth, the monoxenous life cycle allows infectious oocysts to be excreted in large numbers in feces, which can easily spread. Fifth, the organism is associated with geographic, seasonal, and socioeconomic differences in the distribution of *Cryptosporidium* spp.

Cryptosporidiosis is seasonal and related to precipitation and temperature fluctuations worldwide. Excystation of *C. parvum* increases in water temperatures up to 46° C (natural sunlight for 12 hours). Two waterborne outbreaks brought cryptosporidiosis to public health attention. In January 1989, an increased number of cases of cryptosporidiosis were reported in Swindon and Oxfordshire, United Kingdom, with a peak reached in March. Mapping of the addresses of early cases showed associations with water supplies. In late February the water authority detected *Cryptosporidium* oocysts in samples from the water that supplied the affected areas and in the treated water. Contamination of the raw Thames River water used at three water treatment plants was found, with evidence of pollution by farm effluent. This outbreak resulted in 516 cases and thus ignited public interest and led to an official inquiry. The second outbreak occurred in early spring 1993 in Milwaukee, Wisconsin, and was the largest documented outbreak of waterborne disease ever in the United States, with an estimated 403,000 people having acute watery diarrhea and potentially 112 deaths. Findings from this outbreak suggested that *Cryptosporidium* oocysts passed through the filtration system of one of the city's water treatment plants. Again, this suggested that the water quality standards and detection methods for *Cryptosporidium* were inadequate. Swimming pool contamination, especially toddler pools, is often associated with accidental fecal contamination. Food-borne outbreaks have also been reported in association with contaminated apple cider, unpasteurized milk, chicken salad, vegetables, raw produce, and shellfish.

The prevalence of cryptosporidiosis varies by geographic region, with the highest rates seen in developing countries. Most cases of cryptosporidiosis occur in young children, thus suggesting that host's immune response plays a key role in susceptibility. Furthermore, cryptosporidiosis in individuals infected with human immunodeficiency virus (HIV) and in those with acquired immunodeficiency syndrome (AIDS) is persistent and occasionally life-threatening and may involve infections of the hepatobiliary and respiratory tracts, in addition to the entire gastrointestinal tract. Only effective antiretroviral therapy with restoration of immune function controls this devastating disease. The prevalence of cryptosporidiosis in patients with HIV/AIDS varies from 23% in those with CD4$^+$ cell counts greater than 1000/μL to 46% in those with CD4$^+$ cell counts less than 100/μL.

PATHOBIOLOGY

Oocysts of *Cryptosporidium* spp excyst in the upper part of the small bowel and release infective sporozoites that invade the mucosal epithelium and occasionally Peyer's patch M cells, often to the terminal ileum and colon. In immunocompromised patients the organisms can be found throughout the gut, biliary tract, pancreas, and respiratory tract. As noted earlier, trophozoites undergo asexual reproduction by merogony to form type 1 and then type 2 meronts. Sporozoites and merozoites are internalized via similar invasion machinery and actin reorganization. Entry into the host's cell occurs within 30 seconds and is dependent on the parasite's actinomyosin cytoskeleton to enter host-derived bimembrane parasitophorous vacuoles in a unique intracellular, but extracytoplasmic niche. Dense polymerized actin forms at the base fusion of the host-parasite bimembranes. Invasion of cells of the host leads to displacement of the microvillous border, villous atrophy, blunting and crypt cell hyperplasia, and marked infiltration by lymphocytes, plasma cells, and some neutrophils into the lamina propria, with apoptosis of infected cells and significant alteration in intestinal permeability, as measured by mannitol and lactulose markers. This noninvasive functional test shows both reduced absorptive area and disrupted barrier function, which is even more severe in patients with HIV/AIDS. Upregulation of nuclear factor κB and the pro-inflammatory cascade causes secretory and mildly inflammatory diarrhea. Pro-inflammatory cytokines, such as tumor necrosis factor-α, interleukin-1β (IL-1β), IL-8, and lactoferrin, are significantly increased in murine and human infections. IL-1β and IL-8 both upregulate cyclooxygenase-2, which results in prostaglandin synthesis in the epithelial cells and production of substance P by the inflammatory cells; these products together decrease net sodium absorption and increase net chloride secretion, which causes the secretory diarrhea often seen with this infection.

Both innate and adaptive immune responses are associated with immunity to cryptosporidiosis. Two chemokines, CXCL-10 and perhaps CXCL-8, are initially implicated in the attraction of pro-inflammatory cells. Activation of the immune system involves early stimulation by IL-15, which may be important for initial clearance of the parasite. CD4$^+$ T cells and interferon-γ play important roles in the eventual immune defense against this infection, probably more so than B cells or CD8$^+$ cells.

CLINICAL MANIFESTATIONS

Cryptosporidiosis is a cosmopolitan, self-limited infection in immunocompetent hosts that affects all age groups and both sexes. In developing

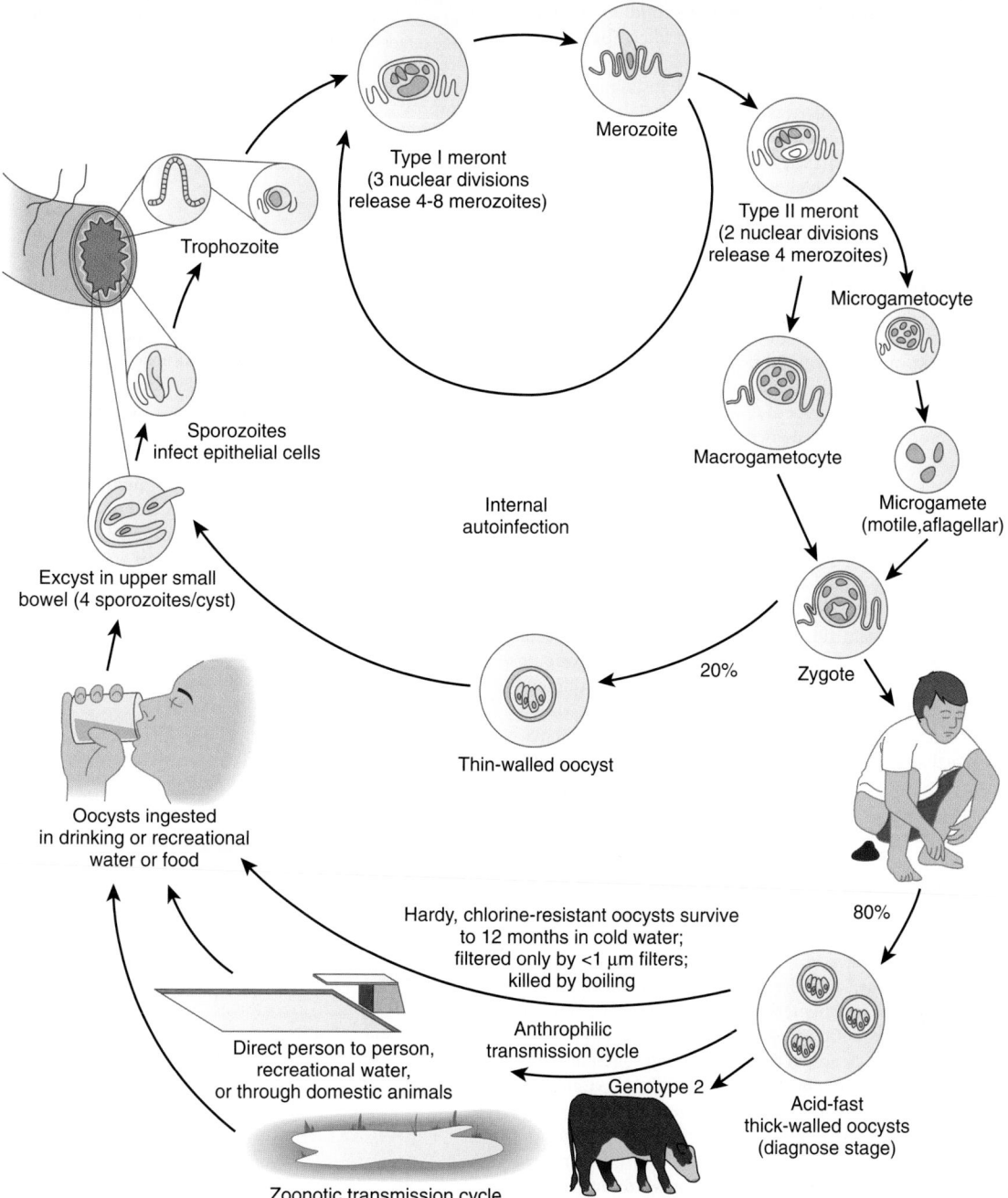

FIGURE 358-1. Life cycle of *Cryptosporidium* spp. (Redrawn with permission from Kosek M, Alcantara C, Lima AAM, et al. Cryptosporidiosis: an update. *Lancet Infect Dis.* 2001;1:262-269.)

countries, the disease occurs most frequently in children younger than 5 years because of high rates of fecal-oral exposure and the development of partial immunity in older children and adults. In developed countries the disease occurs at all ages and most cases are associated with small waterborne outbreaks, frequently with contamination of recreational water. Travelers from developed countries are more often adults. The incubation period is approximately 1 week, with a range of 1 to 30 days. The diarrhea can have a sudden onset, frequently with voluminous watery stools, abdominal pain, nausea or vomiting, bloating, malaise, fatigue and weight loss, occasional pyrexia, and a long-term impact on physical activity, school performance, and development of cognitive function, especially in young children at risk in developing countries. Rarely, respiratory infection and cough have been reported. In normal hosts the disease usually lasts 2 to 3 weeks but sometimes for more than a month. Oocyst shedding typically lasts 1 to 2 weeks but can occur for up to 2 months. Patients with T-cell immune deficiency, such as those with hematologic malignancies (particularly children), primary T-cell deficiencies (severe combined immunodeficiency [SCID] and CD40 ligand deficiency), and HIV/AIDS, are at high risk for the development of more severe disease and have an increased risk for death.

Immunocompetent Host

Data on the natural history of cryptosporidiosis in immunocompetent hosts have been obtained mostly from developed countries, and such data are derived from waterborne outbreaks, patients seeking medical assistance, travelers, animal workers, children in daycare, and their contacts. Most patients in outbreaks and travelers are adults and usually have diarrhea with a median duration of 14 days and a range of 1 to 100 days. The duration and severity of diarrhea appear to be similar for *C. parvum* and *C. hominis*. Recurrence of diarrhea is common and occurs in 30 to 41% of patients. Reports from the United Kingdom describe abdominal pain (96%), vomiting (65%), fever (59%), and bloody diarrhea (11%). The clinical manifestations in 285 people surveyed with a confirmed laboratory diagnosis of *Cryptosporidium* infection in the massive outbreak in Milwaukee showed a median duration of 9 days (range, 1 to 55 days), with watery diarrhea in 93%, abdominal cramps in 84%, fever in 57%, and vomiting in 48%.

Childhood Cryptosporidiosis in Developing Countries

In developing countries, cryptosporidiosis is associated with persistent diarrhea, increased overall burden of diarrhea, risk for malnutrition, and infant mortality. A nested case-control study from a cohort of children in Brazil showed that children younger than 1 year with cryptosporidiosis had subsequent increased diarrheal burdens and growth shortfalls. These findings have been extended in a shantytown in Peru, where cryptosporidiosis is associated with growth faltering and stunting. This was even true for children with asymptomatic infections, which are even more common in endemic areas. The long-term impact of childhood diarrhea and cryptosporidiosis was also evaluated in a cohort study in Brazil in which it was shown that children with more diarrhea morbidity or cryptosporidiosis early in life (0 to 2 years) had reduced fitness and impaired cognitive function at 6 to 9 years of age. Several studies have now shown that oocysts are shed longer and the number of oocysts is higher with *C. hominis* than with *C. parvum* infection. In Brazil, a birth cohort study demonstrated that children with *C. hominis* infection had higher fecal lactoferrin and delayed growth in comparison to those with *C. parvum* infections. Diarrhea, nausea, vomiting, and general malaise were more frequently associated with *C. hominis* infection in a longitudinal study of children in Peru. Subtype family analysis of *C. hominis* (Ia, Ib, Id, and Ie) also showed that Ib was more commonly associated with nausea, vomiting, and general malaise.

Immunocompromised Hosts

Low CD4$^+$ lymphocyte counts in HIV-infected patients are associated with severe cryptosporidial diarrhea. For example, patients with CD4$^+$ counts higher than 180/mm^3 usually have transient or self-limited disease, whereas those with CD4$^+$ counts lower than 50/mm^3 often have severe disease with more than 2 L of stool per day. The introduction of highly active antiretroviral therapy (HAART) heralded reduced rates of cryptosporidiosis in patients with HIV/AIDS. HAART may also directly inhibit sporozoite development and invasion in the host's cells. Patients with other immune disorders such as T-cell immune deficiency (SCID and CD40 ligand deficiency) or hematologic malignancies, particularly children, are at higher risk for more severe, prolonged, or extensive disease, with infection occasionally extending to the gallbladder, pancreatic duct, and even the bronchial tree. Several complications in these patients have been described, including pancreatitis, cholecystitis, sclerosing cholangitis, papillitis, and terminal bile duct stenosis with subsequent biliary cirrhosis.

DIAGNOSIS

The clinical manifestations and physical examination findings in patients with cryptosporidiosis are not unique, and the differential diagnosis should include other causes of infectious gastroenteritis, such as *Giardia, Cyclospora, Isospora,* microsporidia, *E. coli* pathotypes (enteropathogenic [EPEC], enteroaggregative [EAEC], diffusely adherent [DAEC], enterohemorrhagic [EHEC], enteroinvasive [EIEC], and enterotoxigenic [ETEC]), *Campylobacter, Salmonella, Shigella,* rotavirus, norovirus, and others. Definitive diagnosis of *Cryptosporidium* enteric infection is made by stool examination. Up to three fecal samples with fixation and concentration before permanent staining may increase detection rates. Oocysts are stained with the acid-fast stain, modified Ziehl-Nielsen stain, fluorescence staining with auramine-phenol, or immunofluorescent stains. Acid-fast staining requires around 500,000 oocysts per gram for detection in formed stools, whereas immunofluorescence is at least 10 times more sensitive, and commercially available enzyme-linked immunoassays have a sensitivity and specificity approaching 100% for *Cryptosporidium*. Polymerase chain reaction testing can detect as few as 50 to 500 oocysts per milliliter of liquid stool and can be used to differentiate *Cryptosporidium* species and genotypes.

TREATMENT   Rx

Nitazoxanide has emerged as the only promising candidate for treating cryptosporidiosis, is licensed in the United States for treating cryptosporidiosis in nonimmunodeficient children and adults, and has reportedly reduced the duration of diarrhea and oocyst shedding in several double-blind, placebo-controlled clinical trials. A clinical trial in Egypt in adults (500 mg twice daily for 3 days) and children (200 mg for 4- to 11-year-olds and 100 mg for 1- to 3-year-olds, twice daily for 3 days) with cryptosporidiosis showed that 80% exhibited resolution of diarrhea versus 41% of the placebo group. A second clinical trial of a 3-day course of treatment showed resolution of symptoms at 4 days in 96% of the patients receiving nitazoxanide tablets (500 mg twice daily for 3 days) versus only 41% of those receiving placebo tablets.**2**

Prevention and treatment of cryptosporidiosis in immunocompromised patients have been reviewed recently, and there was no evidence of a

reduction in the duration or frequency of diarrhea with nitazoxanide. However, nitazoxanide did result in significantly greater oocyst clearance than did placebo in all children. In patients with HIV/AIDS, HAART has emerged as the most important therapy to prevent and reduce the severity and frequency of cryptosporidiosis. Oral rehydration therapy or intravenous fluid replacement for more severe disease is key to preventing dehydration and risk for immediate death.

PREVENTION

Prevention of person-to-person spread should be achieved with personal hygiene guidelines such as frequent handwashing after using or cleaning the toilet, changing diapers, and caring for a person with diarrhea. It is recommended that people with cryptosporidiosis be excluded from the workplace setting until 48 hours after the last diarrheal episode. Handwashing facilities should be available and used at farms to facilitate personal hygiene. Because most outbreaks of cryptosporidiosis are linked to oocysts in source water, routine survey of treated water for this parasite is key to preventing major spread of this disease. Optimization of multibarrier approaches, including chemical treatment and water filtration and treatment systems, is highly recommended. Ultraviolet irradiation and ozone are effective in inactivating *Cryptosporidium* and *Giardia* cysts in water and may prove useful in controlling the transmission of waterborne protozoa.

Grade A

1. Rossignol JF, Ayoub A, Ayers MS. Treatment of diarrhea caused by *Cryptosporidium parvum*: a prospective randomized, double-blind, placebo-controlled study of nitazoxanide. *J Infect Dis.* 2001;184:103-106.
2. Rossignol JF, Kabil SM, Younis AM, et al. Double-blind placebo controlled study of nitazoxanide in the treatment of cryptosporidial diarrhea in 90 immunocompetent adults and adolescents from the Nile delta of Egypt. *Clin Gastroenterol Hepatol.* 2006;4:320-324.

SUGGESTED READINGS

Borad A, Ward H. Human immune responses in cryptosporidiosis. *Future Mircrobiol.* 2010;5:507-519. *Review of recent advances and future prospects in understanding the human immune responses to* Cryptosporidium *infection.*

Chalmers RM, Davies AP. Minireview: clinical cryptosporidiosis. *Exp Parasitol.* 2010;124:138-146. *A comprehensive review.*

Jagai JS, Castronovo DA, Monchak J, et al. Seasonality of cryptosporidiosis: a meta-analysis approach. *Environ Res.* 2009;109:465-478. *An interesting study on the association of cryptosporidiosis with rain precipitation and temperature fluctuations worldwide.*

Karanis P, Kourenti C, Smith H. Waterborne transmission of protozoan parasites: a worldwide review of outbreaks and lessons learnt. *J Water Health.* 2007;5:1-38. *A comprehensive review.*

Rossignol JF. *Cryptosporidium* and *Giardia*: treatment options and prospects for new drugs. *Exp Parasitol.* 2010;124:45-53. *A comprehensive review.*

359

GIARDIASIS

THEODORE E. NASH AND DAVID R. HILL

DEFINITION

Giardia lamblia (*Giardia duodenalis, Giardia intestinalis*) is a ubiquitous protozoan parasite of humans and other mammals that resides in the small intestine. It is the most common parasitic infection of the gastrointestinal tract in the United States as well as worldwide and is responsible for outbreaks of diarrhea and sporadic endemic disease.

The Pathogen

Giardia has a simple life cycle. The trophozoite, which is 9 to 21 μm long, 5 to 15 μm wide, and 2 to 4 μm thick (Fig. 359-1), resides in the small intestine and is responsible for manifestations of disease. It has four pairs of flagella, two equal functioning nuclei, and a ventral sucking disc by which it may adhere to intestinal epithelial cells. The dorsal surface is pear shaped and bilaterally symmetrical, with the two highly characteristic nuclei best

FIGURE 359-1. Giardia lamblia. This scanning electron micrograph reveals some of the external ultrastructural details displayed by a flagellated *G. lamblia* protozoan parasite.

FIGURE 359-2. Iron hematoxylin stain of *Giardia lamblia* cysts from stool.

visualized after staining. In the lower small intestine, the trophozoite develops into an environmentally resistant cyst. Detection of soluble cyst wall proteins in the feces forms the basis of most stool antigen assays.

Excreted cysts are mature and infectious. They are oval and about 8 to 12 μm in length and 7 to 10 μm in width (Fig. 359-2). After ingestion and exposure to acid and proteases in the stomach and intestines, they excyst in the small intestine, yielding two trophozoites from each cyst, which quickly divide again. Trophozoites double in number every 6 hours for the fastest growing isolates.

A number of morphologically identical but genetically distinct *Giardia* infect humans and animals. There is no agreed on nomenclature. Initially separated into groups, these are now referred to as assemblages or genotypes. Humans and some animals are infected with either assemblage A or B. These two assemblages are genetically and biologically diverse and may be two separate species.

Giardia is well adapted to its existence as a parasite. It has two equal functioning nuclei and lacks mitochondria and peroxisomes. It has a simplified metabolism and is dependent on the host for nutrients such as purines, pyrimidines, cysteine, and cholesterol. The WB isolate, assemblage A, has a compact genome (11.7 Mb) with unusually short promoters. The parasite's rigid cytoskeleton is composed of unique families of structural proteins and carbohydrates.

Giardia is the only bowel-dwelling parasite that undergoes antigenic variation. Only one of a family of about 250 variant-specific proteins (VSPs) is expressed on the surface of the trophozoite at a time. Both immune and biologic selection of trophozoites that express specific VSPs occurs in humans

and animals with giardiasis. Expressed VSPs must be compatible with the host's intestinal environment and are probably not recognized by the host's immune system because antibodies to VSPs are inhibitory or cytotoxic. The mechanisms involved in antigenic variation are incompletely understood, but they do not involve gene movement and appear to be controlled post-transcriptionally. Whereas all VSPs are transcribed, all but one of the transcripts are eliminated by RNA interference–based mechanisms, resulting in expression of a single VSP surface protein. Exactly how selection and switching occur is unclear.

EPIDEMIOLOGY

Giardia is among the most common parasitic infections of humans; it is highly infectious, and cysts are frequently excreted in large numbers (as high as 10^7 cysts per gram of feces), especially in young children. Cysts can survive for months in cold water, are relatively resistant to chlorination, but are intolerant of desiccation and heat in comparison to *Cryptosporidia* and helminth ova. Between 10 and 100 cysts is sufficient to establish infection. Consequently, ingestion of water or food that contains small levels of contamination can result in infection. Approximately 20,000 infections are reported annually in the United States, but because of underreporting, actual infections are estimated at between 100,000 and 2.5 million cases per year.

Infections are most common in young children and are more frequent in summer and fall months. Giardiasis is acquired after ingestion of contaminated water or food or through person-to-person contact. In past decades, large outbreaks in high-income countries such as the United States occurred after ingestion of contaminated drinking water obtained from surface sources such as reservoirs, lakes, and mountain streams. However, with improved water treatment measures, ingestion of contaminated recreational water from pools or lakes is now a more common source of outbreaks and sporadic infection. Backpackers who ingest untreated surface water remain at risk of infection.

Although outbreaks from contaminated food or infected food handlers are well described, they are not often documented. Worldwide, person-to-person transmission may be the most frequent mode of infection and is the primary way children are infected in daycare centers, where historically prevalence has been as high as 50%. Person-to-person spread occurs among family members with infected children and following sexual practices that lead to fecal-oral contact. In low-income, highly endemic regions, almost all children are infected by 2 to 3 years of age. Although partial immunity can develop in previously exposed adults, reinfection of children after treatment is common in highly endemic regions. Longer-term travel, particularly to south Asia, increases the risk of giardiasis. For the returned traveler with persistent diarrhea, giardiasis should be ruled out.

The understanding of immunity in humans is based mostly on animal models that have limited applicability to human infection and disease. In addition, some of the findings are conflicting. In the classic human experimental infections reported by Rendtorff and colleagues in the 1950s, self-cure occurred in about 84% of the persons. In a more recent experimental human challenge study, in which the infecting parasite was well characterized and the inoculum known, rechallenge with the same isolate after treatment resulted in brief, asymptomatic infections in two persons, suggesting development of partial immunity. Humans with hypogammaglobulinemia are susceptible to *Giardia* and have more severe disease that is resistant to treatment. Studies in animals support a major role of intestinal antibodies (particularly IgA) in protective immunity and an essential role of T-cell immunity in the control of *G. lamblia* infection.

Giardia infections are neither more severe nor more common in most other immunosuppressed states and in persons with selective IgA deficiency. Even though most human immunodeficiency virus–infected patients respond to usual treatment, a subset develop recurrent or repeated infections that are difficult to treat.

PATHOBIOLOGY

Giardia infections involve complex interactions between host and parasite. The two assemblages (A and B) that infect humans are composed of genetically distinguishable isolates, which may vary in infectivity, antigenicity, and virulence. They express different sets of VSPs. In addition, human hosts vary in susceptibility to infection and disease and in the response or tolerance to infection. Pathogenic mechanisms need to explain the varied clinical manifestations, as well as the contrasting situation in which there are high rates of infection and disease seen in water-borne outbreaks of giardiasis, compared with the large number of asymptomatic infections in children in low-income regions. In addition, infection with *Giardia* can lead to malabsorption, weight loss, and nutritional deficiencies in some settings and little effect on nutritional parameters in other settings.

Giardia is strictly an intraluminal parasite that adheres to the epithelium by way of an adhesive or sucking disc. Invasion of the epithelium either does not occur or is rare. The number of trophozoites in the intestine can be so large that adherent organisms cover much of the epithelial surface. This could disrupt the epithelial brush border and contribute to disaccharidase deficiency seen in some patients. A number of studies demonstrate direct epithelial cell barrier dysfunction in vitro and in vivo in humans. Exactly how this occurs is not known. There is no evidence of production of a classic enterotoxin, although it is possible that secreted or surface proteins may be injurious to cells. Of patients with persistent giardiasis after treatment, 47% exhibited inflammation on small bowel biopsy specimens, supporting the view that chronic inflammatory responses contribute to disease at least in this subset.

CLINICAL MANIFESTATIONS

The clinical manifestations, course, and duration of *Giardia* infections are variable. Infections may be self-limited or persistent, asymptomatic or symptomatic. In general, patients are not as sick as those with bacterial diarrheas. Acute disease manifestations occur commonly in travelers and in outbreaks and are characterized by diarrhea, nausea, vomiting, anorexia, dehydration, flatulence, eructation, foul-smelling stools, distention, abdominal cramping, and weight loss. Malabsorption is more commonly seen in chronic infection. Fever is uncommon. Blood, mucus, and polymorphonuclear cells in the stool, which are not usual features of small bowel infections, should suggest an alternative or additional diagnosis. Dehydration, although uncommon, may be severe and require hospitalization; hospitalization for giardiasis has occurred in the United States with a frequency similar to that for shigellosis. On occasion, nausea and vomiting will predominate and suggest other causes.

In experimental infections using inoculated cysts, presence of cysts in the stool occurred 6 to 15 days (mean, 9 days) after inoculation. In more recent experimental infections, *Giardia* antigen was detected 1 day before cyst excretion. In one well-documented food-borne outbreak, 74% became ill, with an incubation period of 2 to 19 days and peak symptoms at 5 to 6 days. Symptoms continued for a median of 18 days.

Acute symptoms can resolve, wax and wane, or settle into a chronic phase, which can be prolonged and last weeks to months. Long-lasting symptoms should suggest a search for the parasite. Lactose deficiency is common and can persist for some weeks after treatment, and it needs to be distinguished in symptomatic patients from relapse or reinfection. In extreme cases, malabsorption and weight loss are severe and mimic sprue. Infants and children are particularly susceptible to infection and disease, which can result in growth failure that is reversed on successful treatment.

A typical scenario is a mildly to moderately ill person who complains of an increased number of urgent loose stools, with flatus, cramping, anorexia, and weight loss. There may be periods when the person feels better only to relapse and become noticeably worse. After days to several weeks, the individual will seek medical help. Similar to other causes of infectious diarrheas, symptoms can continue after successful treatment and evolve into irritable bowel syndrome. Uncommonly, *Giardia* is found in biliary and pancreatic ducts and can cause cholecystitis and pancreatitis. Arthritis, uveitis, and urticaria are rarely attributed to *Giardia* infections, but it is unclear if the infection is causative.

Disease and symptoms caused by *Giardia* in children in low-income regions are variably present despite almost universal infection by the age of 3 years and frequent reinfection with prevalence rates that are commonly above 20%. Although there are convincing studies showing detrimental growth and nutritional effects in some populations, other studies show little or no effects. The reasons for these disparate results may be due to differences in the populations, such as prior exposures, maternal factors, and diet, or variability in the organism, including the genetics of the isolate (e.g., assemblage type) and properties of the expressed VSP. In contrast, *Giardia*-naïve visitors frequently develop symptomatic giardiasis while visiting or working in highly endemic regions, in contrast to a mostly asymptomatic population, suggesting that the endemic population has developed an accommodation to the disease.

DIAGNOSIS

The diagnosis of giardiasis is based on detection of cysts, trophozoites, or, more recently, parasite-specific antigens in fecal samples. Polymerase chain reaction analysis for *Giardia* detection in stool is experimental but has been useful to determine assemblage. Because excretion of cysts may be variable or in low concentrations, a single examination for ova and parasites is only 50 to 80% sensitive, and two or three examinations may be necessary. Antigen detection by direct immunofluorescence microscopy increases the sensitivity of a single examination to more than 90%. Stool antigen tests are generally sensitive (>90%), specific (close to 100%), and relatively inexpensive and do not require a trained microscopist. Examination of small intestine biopsy specimens or intestinal contents for trophozoites was the previous "gold standard" for diagnosis but is now uncommonly needed to establish or to confirm the diagnosis. In low-intensity infections, all testing methods can be falsely negative and require repeated testing.

The laboratory findings are nonspecific. Vital signs are generally normal or the patient may have a low-grade fever. The white blood cell count and liver function test results are usually normal. Electrolyte disturbances can be present if diarrhea and vomiting are severe. Lactose deficiency can occur along with other signs or symptoms of small bowel dysfunction. White blood cells, lactoferrin, blood, and mucus are not found in the stool. Immunoglobulin levels are usually normal but abnormally low or absent in susceptible hypogammaglobulinemic individuals.

TREATMENT   Rx

Details of antiparasitic therapy in general are provided in Chapter 352. Tinidazole (Tindamax), a Food and Drug Administration (FDA)–approved nitroimidazole drug similar to metronidazole (Flagyl), is the treatment of choice; other nitroimidazoles (e.g., ornidazole and secnidazole) not approved in the United States are also effective. Tinidazole is given as a single dose, and compared with metronidazole, it has fewer side effects and greater efficacy. In adults, the dose is 2 g orally; in children, the dose is 50 mg/kg as a single dose with a maximum of 2 g. Metronidazole has been used to treat giardiasis for decades but has never been approved by the FDA for this indication; it requires multiple dosing at 250 mg orally three times a day for 5 to 7 days for adults and 15 mg/kg/day in three divided doses for 5 to 7 days for children. Gastrointestinal side effects of metronidazole are relatively common, and alcohol should not be taken concomitantly because of the possibility of a disulfiram reaction with both drugs. Albendazole (400 mg/day for 5 days) is as effective as metronidazole and has fewer side effects.[1] Nitazoxanide[2] is a drug with broad activity against protozoa, helminths, and bacteria and is FDA approved for the treatment of giardiasis. It is given at a dose of 100 mg orally every 12 hours for 3 days for children aged 12 to 47 months, 200 mg orally every 12 hours for 3 days for children 4 to 11 years of age, and 500 mg orally every 12 hours for 3 days for persons older than 12 years. Because it is available in a liquid suspension as well as in a 500-mg tablet, it is advantageous for the treatment of younger children. It should be given with food. Most of the side effects are gastrointestinal symptoms and headache.

Paromomycin, a nonabsorbable aminoglycoside, has activity against *Giardia* and has been used in pregnant women to avoid the theoretical fetal adverse events of nitroimidazoles, particularly during the first trimester. It is given to adults at 500 mg three times a day for 5 to 10 days and to children at 25 to 35 mg/kg/day orally in three divided doses for 5 to 10 days. Albendazole is not approved by the FDA but has activity against *Giardia*. It is usually given at 15 mg/kg/day with a maximum dose of 400 mg for 5 to 7 days. Quinacrine and furazolidone (FDA approved but not usually available) are also active against *Giardia* but should be reserved for use in particular situations.

Patients usually experience relief of symptoms on treatment. Failure of treatment is frequently heralded by a return of symptoms days to weeks after cessation of therapy and requires either re-treatment with an alternative class of drug or an increased dosing of the initial therapy. Clinically resistant cases usually respond to combination treatment; quinacrine and metronidazole have been most effective, with metronidazole plus albendazole also showing efficacy.

PREVENTION

Infection is prevented by scrupulous personal hygiene, proper disposal of sewage, removal of cysts from water supplies, or killing of cysts in potentially contaminated water or food. Cysts are relatively labile and are susceptible to heating and filtration with small water volume filters of 0.2 to 1 μm. Heating (bringing water to a boil) is preferred because other pathogens found in feces are also inactivated. Cysts are susceptible to bleach (chlorine) and iodine, but killing is dependent on turbidity, pH, and temperature of the water as well as on the concentration and physical state of the halogen. Four drops of 5.25% bleach to 1 liter for 1 hour at room temperature is sufficient for killing. At lower temperatures, inactivation may not be complete.

1. Solaymani-Mohammadi S, Genkinger JM, Loffredo CA, et al. A meta-analysis of the effectiveness of albendazole compared with metronidazole as treatments for infections with *Giardia duodenalis*. *PLoS Negl Trop Dis*. 2010;4:e682.
2. Rossignol JF, Ayoub A, Ayers MS. Treatment of diarrhea caused by *Giardia intestinalis* and *Entamoeba histolytica* or *E. dispar*: a randomized, double-blind, placebo-controlled study of nitazoxanide. *J Infect Dis*. 2001;184:381-384.

SUGGESTED READINGS

de Boer RF, Ott A, Kesztyüs B, et al. Improved detection of five major gastrointestinal pathogens by use of a molecular screening approach. *J Clin Microbiol*. 2010;48:4140-4146. *Molecular screening markedly improves detection rates and decreases time to reporting preliminary results.*

Feng Y, Xiao L. Zoonotic potential and molecular epidemiology of *Giardia* species and giardiasis. *Clin Microbiol Rev*. 2011;24:110-140. *Detailed review.*

Lalle M. Giardiasis in the post genomic era: treatment, drug resistance and novel therapeutic perspectives. *Infect Disord Drug Targets*. 2010;10:283-294. *Practical review of limitations of current drugs and potential for future drugs.*

360

AMEBIASIS

WILLIAM A. PETRI, Jr. AND RASHIDUL HAQUE

DEFINITION

Amebiasis is due to infection with the enteric protozoan parasite *Entamoeba histolytica*. Amebiasis can cause asymptomatic colonization, diarrhea, dysentery, and colitis, as well as spread extraintestinally to cause liver and rarely brain abscess (Fig. 360-1).

The Pathogen

E. histolytica has a low infectious dose (<100 organisms), is resistant to chlorine, and is environmentally stable. These properties make it a threat to food and water supplies, as the recent municipal water outbreak of amebic liver abscess in Tbilisi, Georgia, demonstrated. Its tissue-destructive properties are the reason for the parasite being named *histolytica*.

EPIDEMIOLOGY

Most *E. histolytica* infections occur in the developing world, including the Indian subcontinent, Southeast Asia, sub-Saharan Africa, and Central and South America, as a result of fecal-oral transmission. A national serologic survey in Mexico demonstrated antibody to *E. histolytica* in 8.4% of the population. In an urban slum of Fortaleza, Brazil, 25% of the population tested carried antibody to *E. histolytica*, and the prevalence in children 6 to 14 years of age was 40%. In Dhaka, Bangladesh, where diarrheal diseases are the leading cause of childhood death, the annual incidence of *E. histolytica* infection in a cohort of preschool children was 40%. The annual incidence of amebic liver abscess was 21 cases per 100,000 inhabitants in Hue City, Vietnam. The best current estimate by the World Health Organization is that *E. histolytica* infection results in 34 to 50 million symptomatic cases each year worldwide and as many as 100,000 deaths.

In the United States, amebiasis is the third most common parasitic infection after giardiasis and cryptosporidiosis (1.2 cases/100,000 U.S. population). Most cases in industrialized countries occur in travelers to and immigrants from endemic regions, as well as in institutionalized individuals. In returning travelers, diarrhea is the predominant reason for a patient to visit a physician, and amebiasis is the second most common cause of diarrhea in returning travelers. Previously reported high rates of *E. histolytica* infection in homosexual men in the United States actually reflect a high prevalence of *Entamoeba dispar* infection in this population. In contrast, in Asia, amebiasis is more frequently an initial symptom of human immunodeficiency virus (HIV) infection and acquired immunodeficiency syndrome because of the

common risk for acquisition of both HIV infection and amebiasis via the sexual practices of men who have sex with men. The typical patient with an amebic liver abscess in the United States is a 20- to 40-year-old Hispanic male immigrant. Several groups are at increased risk for severe amebiasis, including the very young or old, malnourished persons, pregnant women, and patients treated with corticosteroids.

PATHOBIOLOGY

Killing of host cells is required for invasion of the intestine by the parasite. The process of host cell destruction has been experimentally separated into sequential steps of adherence, contact-dependent cytotoxicity, followed finally by phagocytosis of the host cell corpse. The initial contact of parasite to host is mediated by the parasite's galactose and N-acetyl-D-galactosamine (Gal/GalNAc)-specific lectin, which binds to carbohydrate determinants on the host's intestinal epithelium. Human cells die by apoptosis induced by *E. histolytica*, a process that requires attachment of the Gal/GalNAc lectin to a host cell's receptor, as well as the parasite's acid intracellular vesicles, which may serve as delivery vehicles for an amebic pore-forming protein. *E. histolytica* initiates apoptosis in host cells by directly activating the host cell's distal apoptotic machinery: caspase 3 is activated within minutes of *E. histolytica* adherence, a caspase 3 inhibitor blocks *E. histolytica* killing, and caspase 3–deficient or bcl-2–overexpressing mice are resistant to amebic infection. Recognition and ingestion of the apoptotic host's corpse are required for colonic infection by the parasite, and multiple ligands and receptors are involved, including the Gal/GalNAc lectin, a phosphatidylserine receptor, serine-rich *E. histolytica* protein, and collectins. After ingestion of the corpse of the host cell, additional parasitic factors participate in invasion into the intestinal mucosa. For example, *E. histolytica* encodes at least 44 cysteine proteinase genes that have been implicated in degradation of colonic mucin glycoproteins; digestion of extracellular matrix, hemoglobin, and villin; and inactivation of interleukin-18 (IL-18).

The innate immune response to amebic infection includes activation of the alternative complement pathway, with C3a and C5a recruiting neutrophils to the site of infection but with amebae resisting killing by the membrane attack complex via the Gal/GalNAc lectin. In the murine model of intestinal amebiasis, innate resistance is conferred by nonhematopoietic cells, thus suggesting importance of the epithelial production of cytokines such as tumor necrosis factor-α (TNF-α), IL-1α, IL-6, IL-8, growth related oncogene alpha (GROα), and granulocyte-macrophage colony-stimulating factor. Neutrophils are the earliest innate cellular immune response (within 1 to 2 days) for both intestinal and hepatic amebiasis. Depletion of neutrophils with anti–Gr-1 neutralizing antibody in a murine model results in exacerbated amebic hepatic and intestinal disease. Macrophages and T lymphocytes are also recruited by day 3 of an infection. Macrophages acquire amebicidal activity after in vitro stimulation with interferon-γ (IFN-γ), TNF-α, or colony-stimulating factor-1. Natural killer cells may be important in part as a source of IFN-γ, as well as infiltrating mast cells for their ability to contribute to the innate immune response via the production of IL-6 and TNF-α.

The acquired immune response reflects the opposing roles of IL-4 and IFN-γ in persistence and clearance of amebic infection, respectively. Inbred mice of the CBA strain are susceptible to intestinal amebiasis and develop a rapid T$_H$2 phenotypic immune response, and this response is deleterious in so far as inhibition of IL-4 can convert the response to a healing IFN-γ response. Effective acquired immunity in humans is associated with both a systemic IFN-γ and a mucosal IgA response directed at the Gal/GalNAc lectin. Children with mucosal IgA against the Gal/GalNAc lectin were found to have 86% fewer new *E. histolytica* infections in the following year. Similarly, the risk for amebiasis was 50% lower in children who were in the 50th percentile and above for the production of IFN-γ by peripheral blood mononuclear cells stimulated with soluble amebic antigen. In contrast, there is an association between higher TNF-α production and *E. histolytica* diarrhea, thus indicating that there is a fine line between a pro-inflammatory cellular immune response that is protective and one that is disease enhancing.

CLINICAL MANIFESTATIONS

Asymptomatic Intraluminal Amebiasis

The asymptomatic cyst-passing carrier state is the most common type of amebic infection. All *Entamoeba moshkovskii* and *E. dispar* infections and as many as 80% of *E. histolytica* infections are asymptomatic. Asymptomatically infected individuals represent a risk to the community because they are a source of new infections and a risk to themselves because 1 in 10 to 20 colonized individuals progress to symptomatic infection. The host has a bearing

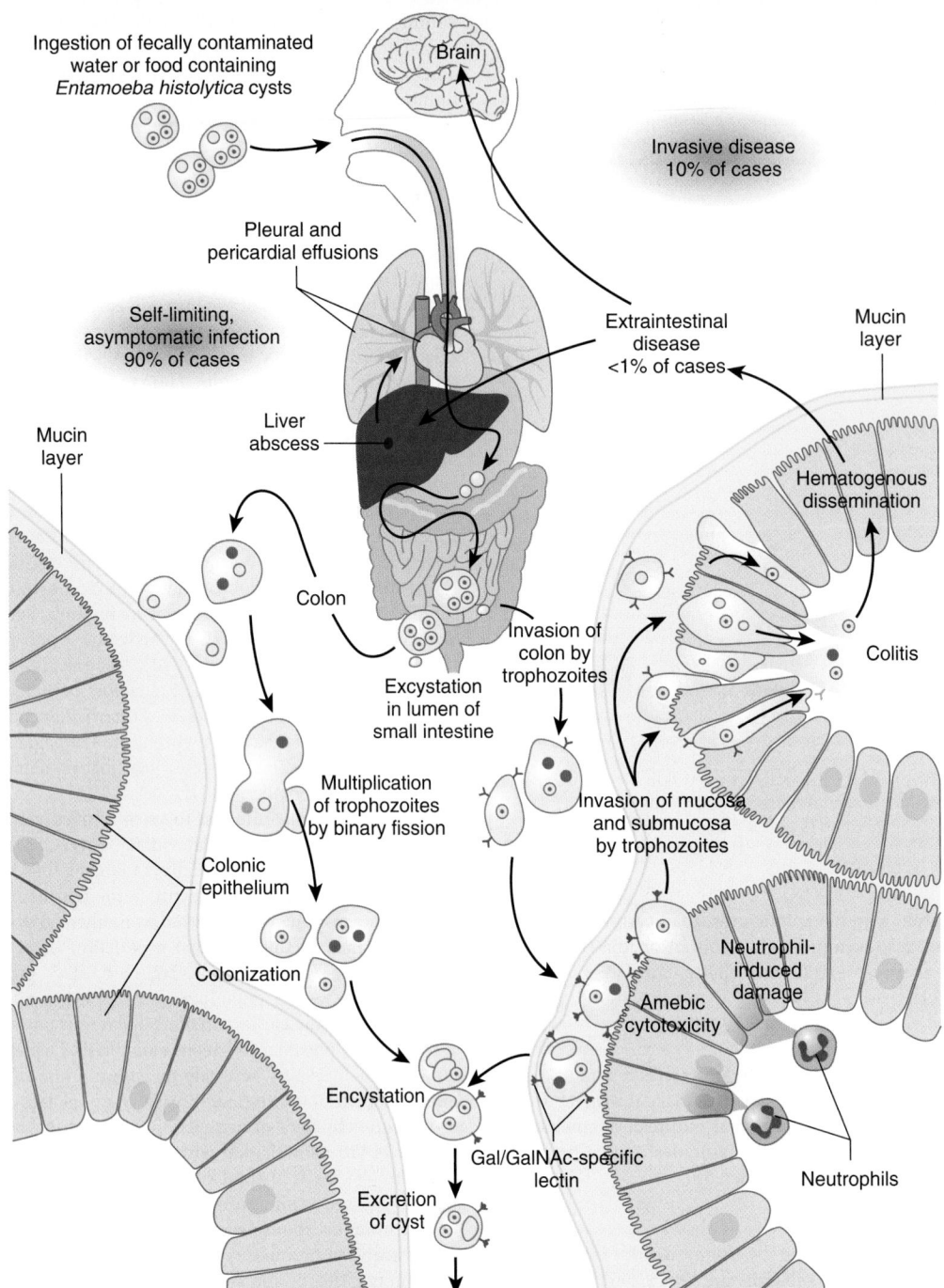

FIGURE 360-1. Life cycle of *Entamoeba histolytica*. Infection is normally initiated by the ingestion of fecally contaminated water or food containing *E. histolytica* cysts. The infective cyst form of the parasite survives passage through the stomach and small intestine. Excystation occurs in the bowel lumen, where motile and potentially invasive trophozoites are formed. In most infections, the trophozoites aggregate in the intestinal mucin layer and form new cysts, which results in a self-limited and asymptomatic infection. In some cases, however, adherence to and lysis of the colonic epithelium, mediated by the galactose and N-acetyl-D-galactosamine (Gal/GalNAc)-specific lectin, initiates invasion of the colon by trophozoites. Neutrophils responding to the invasion contribute to cellular protection at the site of invasion. Once the intestinal epithelium is invaded, extraintestinal spread to the peritoneum, liver, and other sites may follow. Factors controlling invasion, as opposed to encystation, probably include parasitic "quorum sensing" signaled by the Gal/GalNAc-specific lectin, interactions of amebae with the bacterial flora of the intestine, and innate and acquired immune responses of the host. (Redrawn with permission from Haque R, Huston CD, Hughes M, et al. Current concepts: amebiasis. *N Engl J Med.* 2003;348:1565-1573).

on whether infection is asymptomatic in that children heterozygous for the HLA class II DQB1*0601/DRB1*1501 haplotype have been found to be protected from symptomatic infection with amebiasis. In addition, certain genotypes of *E. histolytica* appear to be associated with the propensity for colonization as opposed to invasion.

Amebic Diarrhea

Amebic diarrhea without dysentery is the most common amebic disease. It is defined as diarrhea in an *E. histolytica*–infected individual (there is no requirement for the presence of mucus or visible or microscopic blood in stool for the diagnosis of amebic diarrhea). In one community-based study of a cohort of preschool children in Bangladesh, the annual incidence of

amebic infection, diarrhea, and dysentery was 45%, 9%, and 3%, respectively. The mean duration of amebic diarrhea was 3 days in one study. It causes approximately 2% of cases of diarrhea severe enough to warrant hospital evaluation in developing countries such as Bangladesh.

Amebic Dysentery or Colitis

Diarrhea with mucus or visible or microscopic blood in a patient with *E. histolytica* infection is the definition of amebic dysentery or colitis. Approximately 15 to 33% of patients with *E. histolytica* diarrhea also have amebic dysentery. The onset of symptoms is typically gradual over a period of 3 or 4 weeks after infection, with abdominal tenderness and increasingly severe diarrhea being the primary complaints. Patients with bacterial causes of

FIGURE 360-2. Endoscopic and pathologic features of intestinal amebiasis. **A,** Colonoscopic appearance of intestinal amebiasis. **B,** Colonic ulcers averaging 1 to 2 mm in diameter on gross pathologic examination. **C,** Cross section of a flask-shaped colonic ulcer (hematoxylin-eosin stain, magnification ×20). **D,** Inflammatory response to intestinal invasion by *Entamoeba histolytica* (hematoxylin-eosin stain, magnification ×100). **E** and **F,** *E. histolytica* cysts in a saline preparation (magnification ×1000). **G,** Iodine-stained cyst from stool (magnification ×1000). **H,** *E. histolytica* trophozoite with an ingested erythrocyte in a saline preparation from stool (magnification ×1000). **I,** Trophozoite from stool stained with trichrome (magnification ×1000). (**B-D,** From the slide collection of the late Dr. Harrison Juniper.) (From Haque R, Huston CD, Hughes M, et al. Current concepts: amebiasis. *N Engl J Med.* 2003;348:1565-1573.)

dysentery usually have only 1 to 2 days of symptoms. Surprisingly, fever is present in only a minority of patients with amebic colitis. In young children, intussusception, perforation, peritonitis, or necrotizing colitis may develop rapidly (Fig. 360-2). Unusual manifestations of amebic colitis include toxic megacolon (0.5% of cases, usually requiring surgical intervention) and ameboma (granulation tissue in the colonic lumen mimicking colon cancer in appearance).

Amebic Liver Abscess

Amebic liver abscess is 10 times as common in men as in women and is unusual in children. The typical patient with an amebic liver abscess in the United States is an immigrant from an endemic area, a man aged 20 to 40 years with fever, right upper quadrant pain, leukocytosis, abnormal serum transaminase and alkaline phosphatase levels, and a defect seen on hepatic imaging studies. Most patients have 2 to 4 weeks of prior fever, cough, and abdominal pain in the right upper quadrant or epigastrium. Involvement of the diaphragmatic surface of the liver may lead to right-sided pleural pain or referred shoulder pain and an elevated right hemidiaphragm seen on chest radiography (Fig. 360-3). Hepatomegaly with point tenderness over the liver, below the ribs, or in the intercostal spaces is a typical finding.

If a space-filling defect in the liver is observed, the differential diagnosis includes (1) amebiasis (most common in mean with a history of travel or residence in a developing country), (2) pyogenic or bacterial abscess (particularly suspected in women, patients with cholecystitis, the elderly, individuals with diabetes, and patients with jaundice), (3) echinococcal abscess (which would be an incidental finding because echinococcal abscess should not cause pain or fever), and (4) cancer. Most patients with amebic liver

abscess will have detectable circulating antigen in serum, as well as serum antiamebic antibodies.

In children, abdominal pain is reported infrequently with amebic liver abscess. More commonly, high fever, abdominal distention, irritability, and tachypnea are noted. Some of these children are admitted to the hospital with fever of unknown origin. Hepatomegaly occurs frequently, but elicitation of hepatic tenderness is not well documented. In one report, four of five children younger than 5 years died of amebic liver abscess because the diagnosis was not suspected.

Unusual extraintestinal manifestations of amebiasis include direct extension of the liver abscess to the pleura or pericardium and brain abscess. Death usually results from rupture of the liver abscess into the peritoneum, thorax, or pericardium, but it may also be caused by extensive hepatic damage and liver failure.

Other Extraintestinal Infections

Thoracic amebiasis is the most common type of extra-abdominal amebiasis after liver abscess and occurs in about 10% of patients with amebic liver abscess. It develops via direct extension from the liver. Pericardial amebiasis is the next most common form of extraintestinal involvement and may result from rupture of a liver abscess in the left lobe of the liver into the pericardium or from extension of the right-sided pleural amebiasis. Cerebral amebic abscesses have been found in about 0.5 to 5% of patients with amebic liver abscess. In one series of 18 patients with proven cerebral amebiasis, findings on the initial neurologic examination were normal in 13. Other foci of infection are rare, but amebic rectovesical fistula formation and involvement of the pharynx, heart, aorta, and scapula have been reported. Cutaneous infection may arise from trophozoites emerging from the rectum.

FIGURE 360-3. Radiographic and pathologic features of extraintestinal amebiasis. **A,** Left posteroanterior and right lateral chest radiographs in a patient with amebic liver abscess. The findings include an elevated right hemidiaphragm and evidence of atelectasis. **B,** Luminal narrowing revealed by barium enema examination in a patient with an ameboma. **C,** Two abscesses in the right lobe and one abscess in the left lobe of a patient with amebic liver abscess. **D,** Abdominal computed tomography showing one abscess in the right lobe and one abscess in the left lobe in a patient with amebic liver abscess. (From Haque R, Huston CD, Hughes M, et al. Current concepts: amebiasis. *N Engl J Med.* 2003;348:1565-1573.)

TABLE 360-1   SENSITIVITY OF TESTS FOR DIAGNOSIS OF AMEBIASIS

TEST	COLITIS	LIVER ABSCESS
Microscopy: stool	25-60%	10-40%
Stool antigen detection	80%	≈40%
Serum antigen detection	65%	>95%
Microscopy: abscess fluid	N/A	≤20%
Real-time PCR	>95%	>95%
Serologic testing (indirect hemagglutination)		
Acute	70%	70-80%
Convalescent	>90%	>90%

N/A = not available; PCR = polymerase chain reaction.
Adapted from Haque R, Huston CD, Hughes M, et al. Current concepts: amebiasis. *N Engl J Med.* 2003;348:1565-1573.

DIAGNOSIS

Diagnosis of amebiasis is best accomplished by the combination of serology and identification of the parasite in feces or at extraintestinal sites of invasion (such as pus from a liver abscess). Examination of stool for ova and parasites should *not* be used to diagnose amebiasis (Table 360-1). The most sensitive diagnostic approach is the combined use of *E. histolytica*–specific antigen detection or polymerase chain reaction plus serology.

TREATMENT (also see Chapter 352)   Rx

Therapy for invasive infection differs from that for noninvasive infection, which may be treated with paromomycin (Table 360-2). Invasive infections require treatment with nitroimidazoles, particularly metronidazole, tinidazole, secnidazole, or ornidazole. For amebic colitis, tinidazole reduces treatment failure rates and adverse effects compared with metronidazole.**1** In the rare case of fulminant amebic colitis, it is prudent to add broad-spectrum antibiotics to treat intestinal bacteria that may spill into the peritoneum. Parasites persist in up to half of the patients who are treated with a nitroimidazole, so treatment should be followed with paromomycin or the second-line agent diloxanide furoate to cure luminal infection. Drainage of a liver abscess should be considered in patients who do not show a clinical response to drug therapy within 5 to 7 days or those with a high risk for rupture of the abscess, as defined by a cavity with a diameter of greater than 5 cm or by the presence of lesions in the left lobe. Percutaneous needle aspiration or catheter drainage is the procedure of choice for drainage of a liver abscess. Surgical intervention is occasionally required for drainage of a liver abscess, acute abdomen, gastrointestinal bleeding, or toxic megacolon.

TABLE 360-2   DRUG THERAPY FOR TREATMENT OF AMEBIASIS

DRUG	ADULT DOSAGE	SIDE EFFECTS
AMEBIC LIVER ABSCESS		
Metronidazole	750 mg PO tid × 10 days	Primarily GI side effects: anorexia, nausea, vomiting, diarrhea, abdominal discomfort, or unpleasant metallic taste. Disulfiram-like intolerance reaction to alcoholic beverages. Neurotoxicity, including seizures, peripheral neuropathy, dizziness, confusion, irritability
or Tinidazole	2 g PO once daily × 5 days	Primarily GI side effects and disulfiram-like intolerance reaction to alcoholic beverages as for metronidazole
Followed by a luminal agent Paromomycin	30 mg/kg/day PO in 3 divided doses per day × 5-10 days	Primarily GI side effects: diarrhea, GI upset
or Diloxanide furoate	500 mg PO tid × 10 days	Primarily GI side effects: flatulence, nausea, vomiting. Pruritus, urticaria
AMEBIC COLITIS		
Metronidazole	750 mg PO tid × 5-10 days	Same as for amebic liver abscess
Plus a luminal agent (same as for amebic liver abscess)		
ASYMPTOMATIC INTESTINAL COLONIZATION		
Treatment with a luminal agent as for amebic liver abscess		

GI = gastrointestinal.
Adapted from Haque R, Huston CD, Hughes M, et al. Current concepts: amebiasis. *N Engl J Med.* 2003;348:1565-1573.

ORGANISM	DISEASE	EPIDEMIOLOGY	DIAGNOSIS	CLINICAL COURSE	THERAPY
Naegleria fowleri	Primary amebic encephalitis	Warm freshwater exposure	CSF wet mount for ameba, PCR	Death within 1-2 weeks of onset	Amphotericin B
Acanthamoeba spp	Keratitis	Corneal trauma, usually from contact lens	Corneal scraping for amebae and cysts	Subacute	Polyhexamethylene biguanide, chlorhexidine, propamidine, hexamidine
Acanthamoeba spp	Granulomatous amebic encephalitis	Immunodeficient (organ transplants, HIV/AIDS)	Biopsy of brain or skin abscess—IFA or PCR	Subacute	Combination therapy with pentamidine, fluconazole, or itraconazole. Flucytosine, sulfadiazine
Balamuthia mandrillaris	Granulomatous amebic encephalitis	Immunodeficient but also immunocompetent	Biopsy of brain	Subacute	Combination therapy with flucytosine, pentamidine, fluconazole, and sulfadiazine plus either azithromycin or clarithromycin
Sappinia	Amebic encephalitis	Single patient was not immunodeficient			Azithromycin, pentamidine, itraconazole, flucytosine

AIDS = acquired immunodeficiency syndrome; HIV = human immunodeficiency virus; IFA = indirect fluorescent antibody; PCR = polymerase chain reaction.
Adapted from Visvesvara GS, Moura H, Schuster FL. Pathogenic and opportunistic free-living amoebae: *Acanthamoeba* spp, *Balamuthia mandrillaris*, *Naegleria fowleri*, and *Sappinia diploidea. FEMS Immunol Med Microbiol.* 2007;50:1-26.

PREVENTION

The feasibility of prevention by vaccination with the parasite's Gal/GalNAc lectin is supported by substantial data from human, animal model, and in vitro studies. This vaccine is in the late stages of preclinical development for the prevention of amebiasis in infants and children in the developing world. Provision of sanitation and clean water and safe sexual practices to prevent fecal-oral transmission are of great importance but not universally effective because of the low infectious dose and chlorine resistance of the cyst.

PROGNOSIS

Therapy for amebiasis is highly effective and drug resistance is not reported.

FREE-LIVING AMEBAE

Rare infections of the central nervous system can be seen with infection by free-living amebae of the genera *Naegleria, Balamuthia, Acanthamoeba,* and *Sappinia. Naegleria fowleri* is the agent of primary amebic meningoencephalitis, which occurs in previously healthy children and young adults who have swum in fresh water 2 to 5 days before the onset of meningoencephalitis. Cerebrospinal fluid (CSF) has a polymorphonuclear predominance, and motile amebae can be seen in a wet mount of CSF. The disease is relentlessly progressive to death in most patients. In one case of successful treatment, a combination of intrathecal and intravenous amphotericin B and miconazole and oral rifampin was used. *Acanthamoeba* can cause keratitis in individuals with corneal injuries (usually from contact lens use), as well as granulomatous amebic encephalitis in the immunocompromised. Granulomatous amebic encephalitis can also be caused by *Balamuthia* and *Sappinia*; it is usually associated with focal neurologic findings and has a subacute course (Table 360-3).

1. Gonzales ML, Dans LF, Martinez EG. Antiamoebic drugs for treating amoebic colitis. *Cochrane Database Syst Rev.* 2009;2:CD006085.

SUGGESTED READINGS

Duggal P, Guo X, Haque R, et al. Leptin mediates mucosal immunity to *Entamoeba histolytica* infection in children. *J Clin Invest.* 2010;121:1191-1198. *A common polymorphism in the receptor for leptin has a major influence on susceptibility of children to amebiasis.*

Mortimer L, Chadee K. The immunopathogenesis of *Entamoeba histolytica. Exp Parasitol.* 2010;126:366-380. *New insights into host-parasite interactions and mechanisms of conversion from a harmless enteric commensal to pathogenic parasite.*

Peterson KM, Shu J, Duggal P, et al. The role of TNF-α in susceptibility to amebiasis. *Am J Trop Med Hyg.* 2010;82:620-625. *Demonstration that an over-robust immune response to amebiasis may be deleterious.*

Teixeira JE, Heron BT, Huston CD. C1q- and collectin-dependent phagocytosis of apoptotic host cells by the intestinal protozoan *Entamoeba histolytica. J Infect Dis.* 2008;198:1062-1070. *Study of the cell biology of corpse ingestion by amebae.*

361

BABESIOSIS AND OTHER PROTOZOAN DISEASES

SAM R. TELFORD III AND PETER J. KRAUSE

BABESIOSIS

Babesiosis is a tick-borne malaria-like disease caused by sporozoan parasites of the genus *Babesia*.

EPIDEMIOLOGY

Three epidemiologic patterns are apparent. The first involves the rodent-maintained *Babesia microti*, which is a species complex distributed across the Holarctic. More than 1000 cases of *B. microti* babesiosis have been reported from the northeastern part of the United States and upper Midwestern states, where Lyme disease is endemic. The vector is the same as that for Lyme disease (Chapter 329), the deer tick (*Ixodes dammini*, also known as the northern population of *Ixodes scapularis*), and indeed, concurrent infection may be common. Immune-intact as well as immunocompromised individuals are at risk. In addition, cases of *B. microti* babesiosis have been reported from Germany, Japan, and Taiwan; the vector has not been definitively identified. The second pattern is represented by fewer than 40 cases of babesiosis caused by *Babesia divergens* or closely related species (e.g., "*Babesia venatorum*" or EU1) that have been reported from Europe; all have occurred in splenectomized patients residing in sites where European castor bean ticks (*Ixodes ricinus*) and deer are common. The third pattern of babesiosis involves sporadic cases caused by diverse *Babesia* spp.

Almost all *Babesia* spp are transmitted by ixodid ticks. Although the known zoonotic tick vectors (*I. dammini, I. ricinus*) have marked seasonal periods of activity (May to August) and the majority of reported cases are acquired during these times, babesiosis may be diagnosed at any time of the year. Cases of perinatal transmission have at times been reported outside the typical months of risk. In addition, there have been 70 confirmed reports of transfusion-acquired babesiosis, but the actual number of cases is thought to be much greater. Babesiosis is currently the most commonly reported transfusion-transmitted infection in the United States and may occur year-round. The number of such cases is increasing, including those ending in death. Screening of blood donations for *Babesia* spp is not done other than by targeted questions about a history of previous *Babesia* infection.

PATHOBIOLOGY

The pathophysiology of *Babesia* infection is directly related to the development of parasitemia. In hamsters infected by inoculation of a human-derived *B. microti* strain, intravascular and extravascular hemolysis develops as the parasitemia rises and results in profound anemia; the hematocrit may fall to 20%. During this acute phase of disease, there is extramedullary hematopoiesis and hyperplasia of the splenic red pulp. Livers of infected hamsters contain hypertrophied Kupffer cells, many with ingested parasitized erythrocytes but little hemoglobin breakdown products. The proximal convoluted tubules of the kidneys contain abundant hemosiderin, an observation consistent with the occurrence of marked intravascular hemolysis.

Excessive production of pro-inflammatory cytokines seems to explain the most common symptoms best, which include fever, sweats, chills, headache, myalgia, and nausea. Administration of recombinant tumor necrosis factor (TNF) to human volunteers induces most of the symptoms of babesiosis and malaria. Such symptoms are not seen when the erythrocyte lysis is due to noninfectious causes, which suggests that the release of merozoites serves as a trigger for the pro-inflammatory cascade. Elevated serum concentrations of TNF, as well as interferon-γ (IFN-γ), interleukin-2 (IL-2), IL-6, E-selectin, vascular cell adhesion molecule-1, and intracellular cell adhesion molecule-1, are detected during the acute phase of human *B. microti* infection and return to baseline 1 month after resolution of infection.

Severe illness caused by infection with *Babesia* almost always occurs in people who are immunosuppressed and includes a complex array of metabolic abnormalities and organ dysfunction. Pulmonary disease is the most common complication in people experiencing severe *Babesia* infection, with up to 20% of patients suffering from noncardiogenic pulmonary edema. Pro-inflammatory cytokines appear to mediate the pulmonary complications of *Babesia* infection at least partly. TNF and IFN-γ mRNA is upregulated in the lungs of *B. duncani* ("WA-1")–infected mice, whereas TNF-knockout mice are less likely to die of fulminating *B. duncani* infection than are those with an intact TNF response. It is also likely that lung and other end-organ pathology is mediated, at least in part, by vascular stasis, which has been described in the lungs of hamsters and mice infected with *B. duncani*.

CLINICAL MANIFESTATIONS

About a quarter of *B. microti* infections in adults and half of those in children are subclinical. This estimate is derived from an epidemiologic study that determined the frequency of people who seroconverted over the course of the summer transmission season but reported no illness, coupled with a careful accounting of symptomatic cases. Most people experience a mild to moderate illness lasting about a week. There is a gradual onset of malaise, anorexia, fatigue, fever (temperature as high as 40° C), drenching sweats, and myalgia. Nausea, headache, shaking chills, emotional lability, depression, hemoglobinuria, and hyperesthesia have also been reported. Findings on physical examination consist of fever, pallor, splenomegaly, and hepatomegaly. Laboratory abnormalities include anemia, thrombocytopenia, and leukopenia. Parasitemia generally ranges from barely detectable on blood smear to 5% in previously healthy people but may reach 85% in asplenic and other immunocompromised patients. Lactate dehydrogenase, bilirubin, and transaminase levels may be elevated in more severe cases. Persistent relapsing illness may occur in highly immunocompromised people who fail to clear the infection for months or more than 1 year despite multiple courses of antibiotics. The case-fatality rate for *B. microti* babesiosis has been estimated to be 3 to 5% but may be as high as 20% in immunocompromised hosts. Severe babesiosis usually occurs only in people with asplenia, malignancy, coinfection with human immunodeficiency virus (HIV), immunosuppressive treatment, or age older than 50 years.

Cases of babesiosis caused by species other than *B. microti* tend to be severe, at least in part because they are reported primarily in immunocompromised patients. Virtually all European patients experiencing *B. divergens* infection have been splenectomized and about a third of the patients died. In these patients there was an acute onset of illness with hemoglobinuria, a persistent nonperiodic high fever (temperature of 40 to 41° C), shaking chills, intense sweats, headaches, and myalgia, as well as lumbar and abdominal pain. Vomiting and diarrhea have been reported. Pulmonary, renal, or liver failure may develop rapidly. In fatal cases, patients become comatose with multiorgan failure. *B. duncani*– and *B. divergens*–like infections have also often been reported in immunocompromised hosts with a similarly severe course of illness.

DIAGNOSIS

The diagnosis of babesiosis is based on epidemiologic and clinical findings and confirmed by laboratory testing. Given clinical findings consistent with

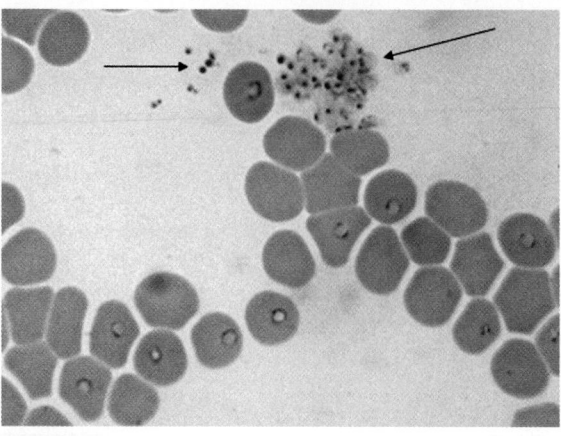

FIGURE 361-1. *Babesia microti* in a human living on Nantucket Island. A predominance of ring forms with a cluster of extraerythrocytic parasites *(arrows)* free in plasma is seen.

babesiosis, the diagnosis may be confirmed by examination of a Giemsa-stained thin blood smear for the presence of parasites within erythrocytes. In an immunocompromised patient, parasitemias are likely to exceed one infected cell per oil immersion field and thus are detected quickly. For *B. microti* babesiosis (Fig. 361-1), examination of a slide for 10 minutes or as many fields as needed to tally 200 leukocytes (that are not infected but serve as a marker for effort) and repeated smears performed twice a day may be required. Standard Romanowsky stains (Giemsa, Wright) using malaria protocols are optimal. Artifactual inclusions are limited mainly to stain precipitates (which can be determined by their presence in the plasma spaces between cells), Howell-Jolly or Heinz bodies (Chapter 160), or platelets superimposed on erythrocytes (which always have a light-colored halo when visualized this way). *Babesia* spp have clearly defined chromatin with a lighter-colored cytoplasm (Fig. 361-2A). They may be mistaken for early malarial trophozoites. Neither malarial nor babesial rings have hemozoin (malarial pigment), so this is not a good feature to distinguish between the two. Paired piriform parasites, arranged in a "v," are very suggestive of *B. divergens* or *B. divergens*–like infection (Fig. 361-2B). "Rings" of all sizes may be seen in all species. Multiple parasites may frequently be seen in single erythrocytes, as well as clumps of extracellular parasites. Tetrad forms (Fig. 361-2C) and "Maltese cross" forms (Fig. 361-2D) are diagnostic but are rarely seen in *B. microti* babesiosis; they seem to be more common with *B. duncani* or CA-type infections.

PCR assays are an important adjunct to blood smears in laboratories with expertise in molecular biology. PCR is usually more sensitive than blood smears in cases in which parasitemias are very sparse. Real-time PCR assays performed in house would provide confirmation nearly as quickly as microscopy with the added advantage of increased sensitivity. As with many molecular diagnostic assays, use of PCR for *Babesia* (either conventional or real time quantitative) is limited by false-positives, validation of experimental assays, and insurance reimbursement. PCR sequencing, performed by collaborating research laboratories, is extremely valuable in retrospectively identifying the species of *Babesia* when the identity is not clear.

Serologic testing is useful for confirming *B. microti* infection. The indirect immunofluorescence test using antigen from infected hamster red cells is sensitive and specific and is currently the serologic method of choice. Analysis of paired acute and convalescent serum samples is most useful for confirmation of *B. microti* infection. The presence of parasite-specific IgM may indicate that the patient has an acute infection even in the absence of readily demonstrable parasitemia. Serology is not generally useful for *B. divergens* babesiosis given its fulminant natural history. Because parasitemia occurs before an antibody response, treatment needs to be initiated immediately based on clinical suspicion and initial laboratory results.

The known vectors for human babesiosis are ticks that also transmit the agents of Lyme disease, human granulocytic anaplasmosis, and tick-borne encephalitis virus. Thus, coinfections should be considered in all patients with babesiosis. Acute illness in patients coinfected with Lyme disease and babesiosis is more severe and more persistent than in patients experiencing Lyme disease alone.

FIGURE 361-2. Diagnosis of *Babesia* infection. **A,** Typical thin-film field demonstrating ring forms of *Babesia microti* with a vacuole or "whitish" cytoplasm demarcated by a dark-staining, defined chromatin. **B,** *Divergens*-like ("MO-1") with robust rings. The accole form and paired piriform parasites are marked by *arrows*. **C,** Tetrad forms of *B. microti*. **D,** "MO-1," classic Maltese cross. (Microscope slide from a human case of "MO-1" kindly provided by Dr. J. F. Beattie, Department of Pathology, The Medical Center, Bowling Green, KY.)

TREATMENT   Rx

Therapy for mild to moderate *B. microti* infection should consist of the combination of atovaquone (750 mg orally twice daily for 7 to 10 days) and azithromycin (500- to 1000-mg initial dose followed by 250 mg orally daily for 7 to 10 days; for immunocompromised hosts, the dosage is 600 to 1000 mg orally daily for 7 to 10 days). A prospective randomized trial■ demonstrated that patients treated with atovaquone and azithromycin cleared parasitemia as effectively as did those receiving clindamycin and quinine and with fewer side effects. For severe babesiosis, a 7- to 10-day course of the combination of quinine (650 mg orally every 8 hours) and clindamycin (either 300 to 600 mg every 6 hours intravenously or 600 mg orally every 8 hours) should be used. The pediatric regimen is quinine, 8 mg/kg given every 8 hours orally (maximum of 650 mg per dose), and clindamycin, 7 to 10 mg/kg given every 6 to 8 hours (maximum of 600 mg per dose).

Treatment may occasionally fail in high-risk patients or in those who must discontinue quinine because of side effects, such as severe tinnitus and gastrointestinal distress. Multiple courses of treatment over a prolonged duration may be required to clear parasitemia in immunocompromised patients; combination therapy should be used. Combination therapy should be used sequentially beginning with clindamycin and quinine and then atovaquone and azithromycin, until an effective combination is identified. If these fail, treatment should include two or more of the following antimicrobials: artemisinin, atovaquone, azithromycin, clindamycin, doxycycline, Malarone, pentamidine, quinine, and trimethoprim-sulfamethoxazole. Once an effective combination is identified, it should be continued for at least 6 weeks and 2 weeks beyond the time when *Babesia* can no longer be visualized on blood smear.

Exchange transfusion should be considered in severely ill patients with parasitemias in excess of 10%, evidence of severe hemolysis, or organ failure. In particularly severe babesiosis cases, partial or complete blood exchange transfusion (2 to 3 blood volumes) should be undertaken, in addition to treatment with clindamycin and quinine.

PREVENTION

Prevention depends on reducing the risk for tick bites. Immunocompromised individuals should be especially careful to use personal protection and may even consider avoiding highly endemic sites such as coastal New England and Long Island during May through July, when risk is the greatest. Use of repellants such as DEET or application of permethrin to clothing will greatly reduce tick attachment. Such products should be applied to shoes, socks, and trouser cuffs. Wearing light-colored long pants and tucking the cuffs into socks will also help prevent ticks from gaining access to attachment sites. Daily examination for attached ticks should be performed; the best way to do this is to feel for new bumps on a soapy body in the shower. Any attached ticks should be promptly removed by simple traction, which is best accomplished with the use of tweezers. As with the agent of Lyme disease, ticks must be attached for at least 36 to 48 hours before a sufficient inoculum of *Babesia* sporozoites is delivered.

● MISCELLANEOUS PROTOZOA

Diarrhea and other lower gastrointestinal signs and symptoms may be caused by diverse protozoa. The gastrointestinal and urogenital tracts may contain representatives of the four major groupings of protozoa (amebae, sporozoa, flagellates, and ciliates). Specific clinical diagnosis is not possible; expert clinical parasitology support is required to determine whether an agent that has been detected in a stool sample is a pathogenic species. Identification is necessary because treatment options differ depending on the agent. With the exception of *Trichomonas vaginalis* infection (sexually transmitted), all of the enteric protozoa are acquired by the ingestion of food or materials contaminated by human feces. Given this shared mode of transmission ("fecal-oral"), demonstrating the presence of any of these protozoa within a stool sample from a patient is justification for an intensified search for those that are recognized as clinically significant pathogens (*Entamoeba histolytica*, *Giardia lamblia/intestinalis*, *Cyclospora cayetanensis*, *Cystoisospora belli*, and *Cryptosporidium parvum/hominis*). Other protozoa, many of which morphologically resemble true pathogens, are commonly detected within the stools of patients with lower gastrointestinal disturbances, but support for their role as etiologic agents is weak.

Cryptosporidiosis (Chapter 358), giardiasis (Chapter 359), and amebiasis (Chapter 360), are discussed in separate chapters. Trichomoniasis and coccidian enteritis are discussed in the following section because they are relatively common infections.

Trichomoniasis

EPIDEMIOLOGY

T. vaginalis is among the most prevalent of all pathogenic protozoa and perhaps the most common sexually transmitted infection globally with the exception of viral and chlamydial agents. As many as 30% of female college students and 40% of pregnant Nigerian women were found to be infected. The highest incidence of infection occurs in women with multiple sexual partners and those with other sexually transmitted diseases (Chapter 293). *T. vaginalis* can also be passed from infected mothers to their newborn daughters, but it is seldom symptomatic in girls before menarche. The parasite is able to survive for some time in moist environments, and nonvenereal transmission, though uncommon, can occur. Trichomoniasis, like other sexually transmitted diseases, may increase the likelihood of transmission of HIV.

PATHOBIOLOGY

T. vaginalis, known colloquially as a "flagellate," is classified in the phylum Metamonada and class Parabasalia, along with another human pathogen, *Dientamoeba fragilis* (previously thought to be an ameba). The 10- to 15-μm-long trophozoites multiply by longitudinal binary fission on the epithelial surface of the vagina or urethra, as well as in vaginal or urethral secretions, and are thereby transmitted by sexual intercourse. No cyst form is known, and the trophozoites are easily killed by drying.

CLINICAL MANIFESTATIONS

Trichomoniasis is one of three common causes of vaginitis or vaginosis (along with bacterial vaginosis and vulvovaginal candidiasis). It is characterized by a thin gray to yellowish green frothy discharge, vulvovaginal erythema, ectocervical erythema or "strawberry cervix" observable mainly by colposcopy, pH higher than 4.5, increased presence of polymorphonuclear leukocytes, and a positive whiff test, in which a foul fishy odor is intensified with the addition of potassium hydroxide. The incubation period for trichomoniasis is 5 to 28 days. In addition to a frothy discharge, vaginitis can be accompanied by vulvovaginal irritation, dyspareunia, abdominal pain, and dysuria. Symptoms may worsen during menstruation. Population-based studies indicate that as many as half of *T. vaginalis* infections in women and the majority in men are asymptomatic. *T. vaginalis* can frequently be isolated from the male partners of infected women and can produce symptomatic urethritis. Urethral discharge is generally scant in these cases. Rarely, *T. vaginalis* is associated with epididymitis, superficial penile ulcerations that are usually located under the prepuce, or prostatitis.

DIAGNOSIS

In women, vaginal and urethral secretions should be examined. *T. vaginalis* is seen in wet mounts of vaginal secretions in approximately 60% of infected women, thus confirming the diagnosis. Live *T. vaginalis* has a twitching or tumbling motion in wet mounts, and polymorphonuclear leukocytes are usually present. Direct immunofluorescent antibody staining is more sensitive than wet mounts, but technically more difficult. Culture is an even more sensitive method of diagnosis and commercial kits for culture are available, but the results are not available for 3 to 7 days. *T. vaginalis* is occasionally identified in Papanicolaou-stained smears; Giemsa stain may also be used (Fig. 361-3). PCR-based assays of vaginal specimens have been sensitive and specific in preliminary studies. For men, a wet mount of material from a platinum loop scraping of the anterior urethra reveals the organism in approximately half of infected individuals. Prostatic massage before collecting urine for *Trichomonas* culture is a more sensitive diagnostic approach. *T. vaginalis* is not found in the gastrointestinal tract, and the presence of trichomonads in wet fecal mounts or stained fixed fecal smears (iron hematoxylin or trichrome) most likely represents the commensal *Pentatrichomonas* (formerly *Trichomonas*) *hominis*. Serologic studies lack sensitivity and specificity.

TREATMENT (ALSO SEE CHAPTER 352) ℞

Tinidazole, a single 2-g oral dose or 500 mg daily for 7 days in adults, or metronidazole, as either a single 2-g oral dose or 500 mg twice daily for 7 days, is the treatment of choice. Tinidazole is the better tolerated of the two. Single-dose therapy (metronidazole or tinidazole) ensures patient compliance but can produce nausea and a metallic taste, particularly with metronidazole. Both tinidazole and metronidazole have a disulfiram-like effect, and patients who consume alcohol within 24 hours of taking metronidazole or 72 hours of tinidazole may experience severe nausea, vomiting, and flushing. Use of tinidazole and metronidazole is relatively contraindicated during pregnancy given the lack of well-controlled studies involving pregnant subjects. Treatment failures with metronidazole are uncommon but well documented. Some result from reinfection and others from poor compliance, but some are caused by metronidazole-resistant parasites. A repeated course of metronidazole (500 mg twice a day orally for 7 days or 2 g orally for 5 days) may be tried.

FIGURE 361-3. *Trichomonas vaginalis.* A Giemsa-stained smear of cultivated trophozoites is seen on bright-field microscopy (×630). The scale bar is 15 μm.

Alternatively, tinidazole, 2 g orally for 5 days, has been effective in treating a subset of persons with metronidazole-resistant isolates. If patients remain refractory to appropriate treatment, sensitivity to metronidazole can be tested by the Centers for Disease Control and Prevention (available at *www.dpd.cdc. gov/dpdx/HTML/DiagnosticProcedures.htm*).

PREVENTION

Condoms (male or female) reduce the risk of acquiring trichomoniasis. Sexual partners should be treated concurrently to prevent reinfection because nearly 20% of male partners also become infected.

PROGNOSIS

Rare complications include pelvic inflammatory disease. Infection during gestation may lead to fetal growth retardation. There is no natural or acquired immunity, so reinfection may be common.

Coccidian Enteritis

EPIDEMIOLOGY

At least two of the coccidia, *C. cayetanensis* (an eimeriid) and *C. belli* (a sarcocystid), are causative agents of enteritis in humans. These parasites are acquired by ingesting food or water contaminated with feces. The infective oocyst stage is moderately resistant to environmental degradation and may remain viable for weeks. *C. cayetanensis* may have both an animal and a human reservoir, but *C. belli* is thought to be an anthroponosis. Cyclosporiasis is a cause of gastroenteritis in tropical and subtropical areas, with Peru, Mexico, Haiti, the Caribbean countries, and Nepal commonly reporting such cases. Since 1990, at least 11 food-borne outbreaks affecting approximately 3600 persons have been documented in the United States and Canada in those who have eaten contaminated raspberries, fresh basil, snow peas, or mesclun. Cyclosporiasis is occasionally diagnosed in returning international travelers.

PATHOBIOLOGY

Oocysts are passed in feces and must sporulate for at least a day (*C. belli*) or 5 to 11 days (*C. cayetanensis*) before attaining infectivity. Sporozoites are liberated in the small bowel and penetrate enterocytes (for *C. cayetanensis*, mainly the jejunum). *C. cayetanensis* appears to have a complicated developmental cycle, with at least two merogonic cycles in the bowel leading to the formation of gametes. The gametes fuse within enterocyte cytoplasm, and an oocyst wall is deposited around the zygote. The sexual cycle begins about a week after infection, with oocysts sloughing into the bowel lumen and subsequently out of the body via feces. Biopsy samples from infected patients demonstrate mononuclear and eosinophilic infiltrates in the lamina propria, as well as alterations in the morphology of villi.

FIGURE 361-4. Diagnosis of coccidian enteritis. **A,** *Cyclospora cayetanensis* seen on formalin-fixed human feces via bright-field microscopy (×1000) with a green contrast filter. The organism is unsporulated. Note the doublet of yeast cells in the lower right of the photomicrograph. The scale bar is 10 μm. **B,** *Cystoisospora belli* seen by bright-field microscopy (×400) on formalin-fixed human feces. The organism is partially sporulated. The scale bar is 15 μm.

TABLE 361-1 OTHER ENTERIC PROTOZOA

ORGANISM	EPIDEMIOLOGY	MANIFESTATIONS	THERAPY*
Balantidium coli	Primarily an infection of animals, especially pigs, but also affects humans	Asymptomatic or mild and self-resolving; occasionally more severe with abdominal pain, blood, and mucus in stool	Tetracycline (500 mg qid for 10 days). Alternative: metronidazole (750 mg tid for 5 days) or iodoquinol (650 mg tid for 20 days)
Blastocystis hominis	Probably worldwide, including North America; often found concomitantly with *Giardia lamblia*	Pathogenicity is debated	The need for treatment is debated, but symptomatic improvement has been reported with metronidazole (750 mg tid for 10 days), iodoquinol (650 mg tid for 20 days), or trimethoprim-sulfamethoxazole (1 double-strength tablet bid for 7 days)
Dientamoeba fragilis	Worldwide distribution; frequently found concomitantly with the pinworm *Enterobius*	Often asymptomatic; diarrhea reported	Paromomycin (25-35 mg/kg body weight per day in 3 doses for 7 days), tetracycline (500 mg qid for 10 days), metronidazole (500-750 mg tid for 10 days), or iodoquinol (650 mg tid for 20 days)
Microsporidia† (*Enterocytozoon bieneusi* and *Encephalitozoon intestinalis*)	Apparent worldwide distribution	AIDS patients with persistent diarrhea and wasting; self-limited cases in immunocompetent persons	Oral fumagillin (20 mg three times daily for 14 days) has been effective for *E. bieneusi*, but it has been associated with thrombocytopenia. Albendazole (400 mg bid for 21 days) has been effective for *E. intestinalis*. Treatment with HAART may lead to clinical response in HIV-infected patients with microsporidial diarrhea
Sarcocystis species	Common pathogens of animals, rare in humans; acquired by ingesting contaminated beef or pork	Often asymptomatic; nausea, vomiting, abdominal pain, and diarrhea may occur; eosinophilic necrotizing enteritis has been reported	No specific therapy

*Recommendations are based on "Drugs for Parasitic Infections" (*Med Lett Drugs Ther*. 2004;46:1-12. www.medicalletter.org). The dosages and durations are for adults.
†Associated with persistent, severe diarrhea in persons with AIDS.
AIDS = acquired immunodeficiency syndrome; HAART = highly active antiretroviral therapy; HIV = human immunodeficiency virus.

CLINICAL MANIFESTATIONS

After an incubation period of approximately 1 week, either agent produces watery diarrhea, nausea, vomiting, abdominal pain, myalgia, anorexia, and fatigue. The illness is usually self-limited, but symptoms can be prolonged (10 to 12 weeks) and be associated with steatorrhea, flatulence, and substantial weight loss in persons who are immunocompromised, especially those with acquired immunodeficiency syndrome (AIDS). Infections may also be asymptomatic.

DIAGNOSIS

The diagnosis is confirmed by identifying coccidia in stool samples stained with modified acid-fast or modified safranin preparations or by phase contrast microscopy or bright-field microscopy (using iodine as a contrast medium) of wet mounts (Fig. 361-4). *C. cayetanensis* and *C. belli* may be sensitively detected by fluorescent microscopy of wet mounts. PCR assays are specific and can be sensitive, depending on the mode of DNA extraction, but they are available only in research settings.

TREATMENT Rx

Rehydration is important, as it is for any severe diarrheal disease. Both infections may respond to treatment with 160 mg trimethoprim and 800 mg sulfamethoxazole taken twice daily for 7 to 10 days. HIV-infected patients may require an increased intensive dosing frequency of four times daily for 10 days. Chronic suppressive therapy with 160 mg trimethoprim/800 mg sulfamethoxazole three times weekly is often necessary thereafter in HIV-infected patients. The widespread use of Bactrim prophylaxis for *Pneumocystis* has reduced the incidence of coccidial diarrhea in patients infected with HIV.

PREVENTION

At the community level, preventing the contamination of water and food (mainly vegetables and fruits) by animal or human feces reduces the risk of transmission. Washing vegetables and fruits in water will reduce the potential inoculum but does not eliminate all risk.

PROGNOSIS

Reactive arthritis, Guillain-Barré syndrome, Reiter's syndrome, cholecystitis, and cholangitis have been reported as complications of either form of coccidiosis, mainly in patients with AIDS. Otherwise, treatment appears to eradicate the organism. Whether reinfection may occur is not known. Reports of extraintestinal infection with *C. belli* and *C. cayetanensis* suggest the possibility of reinvasion of the bowel with ensuing recrudescence of signs and symptoms.

Other Enteric Protozoans

A number of other protozoa transmitted by fecal-oral contamination have been associated with enteric disease (Table 361-1). Some reside in the lumen of the bowel, and others invade and multiply within enterocytes. Enteric protozoa should be considered in the differential diagnosis of patients with persistent diarrhea and abdominal symptoms, particularly those with a history of recent international travel. A clinical diagnosis is rarely possible; laboratory tests, mainly for ova and parasites in stool, establish the diagnosis. Expert microscopists are required because these parasites may be confused with fecal debris. Pathogenic protozoa must also be differentiated from commensals such as *Entamoeba coli*, *Endolimax nana*, *Iodamoeba bütschlii*, *Pentatrichomonas hominis*, and *Chilomastix mesnili*. Therapy includes administration of the appropriate antiprotozoal drug and rehydration, as listed in Table 361-1 (also see Chapter 352).

 Visit expertconsult.com for e-expanded chapter

Grade A

1. Krause PJ, Lepore T, Sikand VK, et al. Atovaquone and azithromycin for the treatment of babesiosis. *N Engl J Med.* 2000;343:1454-1458.

SUGGESTED READINGS

Leiby DA. Transfusion-transmitted *Babesia* spp: bull's-eye on *Babesia microti*. *Clin Microbiol Rev.* 2011;24:14-28. *About 2 or 3 cases occur each year, with about a 15 to 20% case fatality rate, and no effective screening mechanism exists.*

Schwebke JR, Desmond RA. A randomized controlled trial of partner notification methods for prevention of trichomoniasis in women. *Sex Transm Dis.* 2010;37:392-396. *Notification and recommended treatment reduced recurrence from about 12 to 15% to about 6%.*

Stark D, Barratt JL, van Hal S, et al. Clinical significance of enteric protozoa in the immunosuppressed human population. *Clin Microbiol Rev.* 2009;22:634-650. *Comprehensive review of enteric protozoa as opportunistic infections.*

Vannier E, Gewurz BE, Krause PJ. Human babesiosis. *Infect Dis Clin North Am.* 2008;22:469-488. *Review.*

Warren CA. Cyclosporiasis: an update. *Curr Infect Dis Rep.* 2009;11:108-112. *Excellent recent review of cyclosporiasis.*

Wormser GP, Prasad A, Neuhaus E, et al. Emergence of resistance to azithromycin-atovaquone in immunocompromised patients with *Babesia microti* infection. *Clin Infect Dis.* 2010;50:381-386. *Suggests reducing the level of immunosuppression when possible.*

362

CESTODES

A. CLINTON WHITE, JR., AND ENRICO BRUNETTI

DEFINITION
The Pathogens

Cestode parasites are members of the animal kingdom, subphylum Cestoda. The organisms are characterized by several life cycle stages, which typically develop in distinct hosts. The adult stage is the tapeworm, which is acquired by ingestion of uncooked tissues harboring larval forms. After ingestion, the larvae excyst and the scolex attaches to the intestines. Segments, termed *proglottids,* develop at the base of the scolex and are displaced from the scolex by new proglottids to form a chain or tapeworm. The host in which the tapeworm develops is termed the *definitive host.* The proglottids contain male and female sexual organs and produce large numbers of ova. The proglottids

or their ova are shed in stools. Humans are the definitive hosts for a number of different tapeworms, including the *Taenia* species, *Diphyllobothrium* species, and *Hymenolepis nana*. Humans can also be an accidental host for the dog and cat tapeworms of the genus *Dipylidium* (Table 362-1).

The intermediate hosts harbor the larval form of the parasite. Infection follows ingestion of the ova. Under the influence of gastric and intestinal fluids, the ova hatch, releasing the invasive larvae (oncospheres), which migrate to tissues, forming tissue forms. The forms in tissue vary between organisms and may include the cysticercus (a bladder containing a single invaginated scolex), the coenurus (a bladder with multiple scolices), the hydatid (a cystic structure with a germinal layer, which forms numerous protoscolices), or the plerocercoid (a solid form seen in *Spirometra* species). Humans can harbor the intermediate forms of *Taenia solium* (cysticercosis), *Echinococcus granulosus* group (cystic hydatid disease), *Echinococcus multilocularis* (alveolar hydatid disease), and rarely other organisms (Table 362-2). Humans can serve as both the definitive host and an intermediate host for two species, *T. solium* and *H. nana*. In the case of *T. solium*, humans are the obligate host for the tapeworm stage (pork tapeworm) but can also harbor the cystic form (cysticercosis). In the case of *H. nana*, both stages typically develop in a single person, with the cysticercoid form in the intestinal wall and the tapeworm in the lumen.

● INTESTINAL TAPEWORM INFECTIONS
Diphyllobothrium species (Fish Tapeworm)

Diphyllobothrium tapeworms are large segmented parasites that are acquired by ingestion of undercooked or pickled freshwater fish dishes (sushi, sashimi, ceviche, carpaccio, gefilte fish). The tapeworms develop within a few weeks and can live for more than 10 years.

EPIDEMIOLOGY AND PATHOBIOLOGY

Diphyllobothrium species are found worldwide, including foci in Europe, North and South America, and Asia. Perhaps 20 million people are thought to be infected worldwide. Major foci include Russia, Japan, and South America. Disease was formerly highly endemic in Scandinavia, where it is now rarely diagnosed.

In most cases, infection has little impact on the host. However, one species, *Diphyllobothrium latum*, contains vitamin B_{12} receptors on the surface of the tapeworm, which can out-compete the host, leading to vitamin B_{12} deficiency (Chapter 167). This manifestation has been described only in Scandinavia.

CLINICAL MANIFESTATIONS AND DIAGNOSIS

In most of those infected, *Diphyllobothrium* species produce few or no symptoms. Some may complain of gastrointestinal symptoms (abdominal discomfort, nausea, weight loss). The main clinical manifestation is the observation of proglottids being passed in stool. Pernicious anemia with symptoms of anemia or peripheral neuropathy may develop with *D. latum* infection. The diagnosis depends on observation of the characteristic operculated eggs in stool.

TREATMENT AND PREVENTION   Rx

A single oral dose of praziquantel (5 to 10 mg/kg) is usually adequate for therapy (Table 362-3). Niclosamide can be used as an alternative (2 g [adults] or 50 mg/kg [children] in a single dose chewed and swallowed), but it is not available in the United States. Parasites in fish can be killed by cooking (>56° C, >5 minutes) or freezing (−20° C, 24 hours). Infected fish may also be identified by inspection.

Hymenolepis nana

Hymenolepis nana is the human dwarf tapeworm. *Hymenolepis diminuta*, a rat tapeworm, can also cause human infection.

EPIDEMIOLOGY AND PATHOBIOLOGY

H. nana is widely prevalent worldwide, with estimates of 50 to 75 million people infected. Infection follows ingestion of ova. The larvae are released, invade, and develop into cysticercoid forms in the intestinal villi. After a few days, the cysticercoids mature, invade the lumen, and are transformed into a scolex, forming small tapeworms (up to 5 cm long), which begin producing eggs within 2 to 3 weeks. Autoinfection either in the intestines or by the fecal-oral route can lead to heavy infection.

TABLE 362-1 COMMON HUMAN TAPEWORM INFECTIONS

ORGANISM	INTERMEDIATE HOST	COMMON NAME	CLINICAL PRESENTATION	TREATMENT
Diphyllobothrium spp	Fish	Fish tapeworm	Passing segments, pernicious anemia	Praziquantel, niclosamide
Hymenolepis nana	Humans	Dwarf tapeworm	Asymptomatic, diarrhea	Praziquantel, niclosamide
Taenia saginata	Cattle	Beef tapeworm	Asymptomatic, passing segments	Praziquantel, niclosamide
Taenia asiatica	Pigs	Asian tapeworm	Asymptomatic, passing worms	Praziquantel, niclosamide
Taenia solium	Pigs	Pork tapeworm	Asymptomatic, passing segments	Praziquantel, niclosamide
Dipylidium caninum	Fleas	Dog tapeworm	Passing segments	Praziquantel, niclosamide

TABLE 362-2 HUMAN LARVAL CESTODE INFECTIONS

ORGANISM	COMMON NAME	ORGANS INVOLVED
Taenia solium	Cysticercosis	Brain, spinal fluid, eye, muscle
Echinococcus granulosus group	Cystic hydatid disease	Liver, lung, other
Echinococcus multilocularis	Alveolar hydatid disease	Liver
Taenia multiceps, Taenia spp	Coenurosis	Brain, eyes
Spirometra species	Sparganosis	Subcutaneous tissue, viscera

TABLE 362-3 THERAPY FOR INTESTINAL TAPEWORM INFECTIONS

	PRAZIQUANTEL	NICLOSAMIDE	NITAZOXANIDE
Dosage Adults	5-10 mg/kg for all age groups (25 mg/kg for *Hymenolepis nana*)	2 g (4 tablets)	500 mg
Children >34 kg		1.5 g (3 tablets)	200 mg
Children 11-34 kg		1 g (2 tablets)	100 mg
Administration	Taken as a single dose	Taken as a single dose; tablets must be chewed and swallowed	Taken twice a day for 3 days
Side effects	Mild but frequent, including dizziness, myalgias, nausea, vomiting, diarrhea, abdominal pain	Nausea, vomiting, abdominal pain, diarrhea, drowsiness, dizziness, headache, pruritus	
Pregnancy		No known mutagenic effects; considered safe if indicated	

CLINICAL MANIFESTATIONS AND DIAGNOSIS

Most infections are asymptomatic. However, some children may be infected by hundreds or thousands of worms, which can cause abdominal pain, loose stools, diarrhea, and malabsorption. Diagnosis depends on observation of the characteristic eggs in stool. More than one specimen may be required.

TREATMENT AND PREVENTION ℞

Praziquantel (15 to 25 mg/kg as a single oral dose) is usually effective in treating *H. nana* infection, but it may need to be repeated in heavy infection (see Table 362-3). Nitazoxanide (100 mg by mouth twice daily for 3 days for children 1 to 3 years of age, 200 mg by mouth twice daily for 3 days for children 4 to 11 years of age, and 500 mg by mouth twice daily for 3 days for older children) is a reasonable alternative therapy; efficacy is about 75 to 82%. Niclosamide can be used as an alternative. Transmission is by the fecal-oral route and could be prevented by improved hygiene. Mass chemotherapy has been used to control infection in some populations.

Dipylidium caninum

Dipylidium caninum is a common tapeworm of dogs and cats. Dogs are infected by ingestion of fleas, which carry the cysticercoid form in their body cavities. The tapeworms can also develop in children who have ingested the fleas. It is widespread worldwide, but human infections are unusual.

CLINICAL MANIFESTATIONS AND DIAGNOSIS

Infection may be asymptomatic. In some cases, the motile proglottids may be noted in stool. The proglottids are similar in size and shape to rice grains. Diagnosis depends on identification of the ova in stool or identification of the proglottids.

TREATMENT AND PREVENTION ℞

There are no controlled trials of treatment for *Dipylidium* infection, but infection is likely to respond to regimens used for other tapeworms (see Table 362-3). The main measure for prevention is treatment of pets for fleas and tapeworms.

Taenia saginata

Taeniasis refers to infection with the tapeworm form of one of three *Taenia* species. *Taenia solium* and *Taenia asiatica* are acquired from ingestion of undercooked pork. *Taenia saginata*, called the beef tapeworm, is a common intestinal infection worldwide. Cattle are the intermediate hosts, harboring the tissue cysticerci in their muscle. Humans are the obligate definitive host, harboring the tapeworm form.

EPIDEMIOLOGY AND PATHOBIOLOGY

T. saginata is common worldwide in areas where cattle are raised and human fecal material contaminates the pastures. Approximately 45 to 60 million people are thought to be infected. It is found on most continents. Very high rates (>20% of the population) have been noted in east Africa, Bali, and Tibet. It is also endemic in the Middle East, the Americas, and Europe. *T. saginata* is also common in other parts of Asia, but many of the epidemiologic studies did not differentiate *T. saginata* from *T. asiatica*.

T. saginata tapeworms are acquired by ingestion of undercooked beef. The scolex attaches to the intestinal wall, and proglottids form at the base of the scolex. The proglottids gradually enlarge as they are displaced from the scolex by newer proglottids. The chain of proglottids can reach a length of up to 30 feet. The terminal proglottids are shed periodically in the stool. Terminal proglottids are typically off-white, 2 to 3 cm long, 0.5 to 1 cm wide, and 1 to 2 mm thick.

CLINICAL MANIFESTATIONS AND DIAGNOSIS

Mild symptoms (e.g., nausea, abdominal discomfort, anorexia, and pruritus) may be noted. The motile proglottids may cause discomfort as they exit the anus or may be noted in stool.

Ova may be noted in stool. The ova are 40 μm in diameter, surrounded by brown radial striations, and the embryos have six hooks. However, the ova of the three *Taenia* species are morphologically indistinguishable. The proglottids can be distinguished from those of *T. solium* by counting the number of uterine branches (≥14 branches suggests *T. saginata*). However, the proglottids of *T. saginata* cannot be readily distinguished from *T. asiatica*.

TREATMENT, PREVENTION, AND PROGNOSIS Ⓡ

Taeniasis can be treated with praziquantel in a single dose (see Table 362-3). Single doses of niclosamide are also effective. Nitazoxanide has also been used for *T. saginata*. Taeniasis can be prevented by inspection of beef. Also, cooking to 56° C for 5 minutes or freezing at −20° C for 7 to 10 days destroys the infective larvae. Only minor symptoms are noted and are eventually self-limited with or without treatment.

Taenia asiatica

T. asiatica is a cause of taeniasis in Asia, termed *Asian taeniasis*. Infection is acquired by ingestion of undercooked pork. Pigs are infected by ingestion of the ova from tapeworm carriers. *T. asiatica* has been widely described in China, Taiwan, Korea, Indonesia, and Southeast Asia. The clinical manifestations, diagnosis, treatment, and prevention of *T. asiatica* infection are similar to those noted for *T. saginata* infection.

Taenia solium

T. solium, also known as the pork tapeworm, can cause both tapeworm infection and larval infection termed *cysticercosis*. *T. solium* tapeworm infections are caused by ingestion of infected undercooked pork. The scolex evaginates and attaches to the intestines, forming proglottids. The proglottids gradually mature as they are separated from the scolex by new proglottids. The adult worms are often 10 to 20 feet long. Within the mature proglottids, thousands of microscopic ova develop. The ova are either excreted into the stool or shed with the proglottids. By contrast, ingestion of the ova results in development of larval infection, termed cysticercosis (see later). Thus, the tapeworm carrier poses risk of self-infection as well as infection to other people.

EPIDEMIOLOGY AND PATHOBIOLOGY

T. solium is common worldwide in areas where pigs are raised and where pigs have access to human fecal material. Only a few million people are thought to harbor the tapeworm form. Pork tapeworm infection is highly endemic in Latin America, sub-Saharan Africa, south Asia, and Southeast Asia.

T. solium tapeworms are acquired by ingestion of undercooked pork. The scolex attaches to the intestinal wall and proglottids form at the base of the scolex. The proglottids gradually enlarge as they are displaced from the scolex by newer proglottids. The terminal proglottids are shed periodically in the stool. Terminal proglottids are typically off-white, 2 cm long, 0.5 to 1 cm wide, and 1 to 2 mm thick.

CLINICAL MANIFESTATIONS AND DIAGNOSIS

Mild symptoms (e.g., nausea, abdominal discomfort, anorexia, and pruritus) may be noted. The proglottids may be noted in stool. Diagnosis is made by the finding of ova in stool. The ova are 40 μm in diameter, surrounded by brown radial striations, and embryos have six hooks and are morphologically indistinguishable from the other *Taenia* species. The proglottids can be distinguished from those of *T. saginata* and *T. asiatica* by counting the number of uterine branches (<14 branches suggests *T. solium*).

TREATMENT AND PREVENTION   Ⓡ

Taeniasis can be treated with praziquantel in a single dose. Single doses of niclosamide are also effective. Taeniasis can be prevented by inspection of pork. Also, cooking to 56° C for 5 minutes or freezing at −20° C for 7 to 10 days destroys the infective larvae. Current control measures include mass chemotherapy for entire populations with praziquantel. Comprehensive control programs include mass chemotherapy to eliminate tapeworm carriers, treatment of porcine cysticercosis with drugs such as oxfendazole, and improved hygiene to limit access of pigs to human fecal material.

⬤ TISSUE CESTODE (CYST) INFECTION
Taenia solium (Cysticercosis)

DEFINITION

T. solium is the cause of human larval infection termed cysticercosis. The normal hosts for the larval (cysticercus) forms are pigs. When ingested by pigs, the ova hatch, releasing the invasive larvae (termed *oncospheres*), which invade the intestines, migrate to tissues (especially muscle), and mature into cysticercus forms within the tissues. The cysticercus consists of a thick translucent bladder containing an invaginated scolex, which is poised to form a tapeworm after being ingested by a human host. The ova are also infectious to people, including the tapeworm carrier. The sticky ova attach to the hands of the tapeworm carrier and are transmitted by the oral route to the carrier or close contacts. After ingestion, the ova can migrate to tissues and form cysts (cysticercosis). The presence of cysticerci in the central nervous system is termed *neurocysticercosis*. Neurocysticercosis includes cysticerci in the brain parenchyma (parenchymal neurocysticercosis) and cysticerci in the ventricles, subarachnoid space, spine, and eye (extraparenchymal neurocysticercosis).

EPIDEMIOLOGY

Cysticercosis is found in all regions of the world where pigs are raised with access to human fecal material. Some estimate that 60 million people are infected with *T. solium* cysticerci. However, exact data on incidence and prevalence are available from only a limited number of studies because of the requirement for neuroimaging studies to make a diagnosis. In the 19th century, infection was highly endemic in Europe. However, with improving standards of living, local transmission is now limited to a few rural areas in southern and eastern Europe. Cysticercosis is widespread in rural areas of Latin America. High prevalence rates have been documented in parts of Mexico, Guatemala, Honduras, Ecuador, Peru, Brazil, and Bolivia. In endemic villages, more than 10% of the population may have abnormalities on neuroimaging studies consistent with neurocysticercosis. Studies have highlighted the importance of cysticercosis in sub-Saharan Africa. Cysticercosis is widespread in India, Nepal, Southeast Asia, and parts of China. In India, neurocysticercosis most commonly presents with single enhancing lesions, which are the main lesion associated with seizure disorders in that country. In the United States, approximately 2000 cases are diagnosed each year. Most cases are in immigrants from pig-raising villages in Mexico and Latin America. However, there are also imported cases from Asia and a few locally acquired infections.

PATHOBIOLOGY

For cysticercosis, the pathogenesis and pathophysiology vary with the location of the cysticerci and the host inflammatory response. Cysticerci in the brain parenchyma initially suppress the host inflammatory response. After an incubation period, estimated to be several years, the cysticerci lose the ability to suppress the host inflammatory response, leading to parenchymal inflammation, which typically is manifested by seizures. The cysticerci induce a granulomatous response, which gradually degrades the parasites. In some cases, the lesions resolve. However, in others, degradation leads to formation of calcified granulomas. These calcified lesions intermittently become inflamed (as evidenced by edema or contrast enhancement on magnetic resonance imaging [MRI] scan) and may cause recurrent seizures during a period of years. In some cases, cysticerci develop within the ventricles of the brain and can mechanically cause obstructive hydrocephalus. Cysticerci in the subarachnoid space may cause a chronic arachnoiditis, which can be manifested by vasculitis and stroke, communicating hydrocephalus, basilar meningitis, and, in some cases, mass effect. Cysticerci can also develop in the spine (manifested as radiculitis), eye, subcutaneous tissue, and muscle.

CLINICAL MANIFESTATIONS

The clinical manifestations vary with the location of the cysticerci and the associated host response (Fig. 362-1). All forms of disease may be associated with headaches. In general, parenchymal cysticerci are associated with seizures, whereas ventricular and subarachnoid cysticercosis is associated with hydrocephalus.

SINGLE ENHANCING LESION. A single enhancing lesion is the most common manifestation of cysticercosis in India and the United States. Patients typically present with seizures, which can be focal or focal with secondary generalization. Many will have a single seizure or a few seizures during the period when the cysticercus is degenerating, but it is eventually self-limited in most cases. However, a few go on to develop calcified lesions, which are a risk factor for recurrent seizures.

MULTIPLE PARENCHYMAL CYSTICERCI. In patients with multiple lesions, the main presentation is with seizures, associated with parenchymal inflammation. In contrast to those with single lesions, seizures are more likely to recur.

CALCIFIED LESIONS. Many patients do not present until after they have calcified lesions. Patients with calcified lesions may develop recurrent seizures during a period of years.

FIGURE 362-1. Human neurocysticercosis can be classified on the basis of neuroimaging studies. **A,** Multiple cystic lesions. **B,** Single enhancing lesion. **C,** Multiple calcifications. **D,** Intraventricular cysticerci. **E,** Subarachnoid cysticerci. **F,** Diffuse infection with cerebral edema, termed cysticercal encephalitis. **G,** Ocular cysticerci. **H,** Diffuse muscle calcifications. (Reprinted from Garcia HH, Del Brutto OH. Neurocysticercosis: updated concepts about an old disease. *Lancet Neurol.* 2005;4:653-661.)

VENTRICULAR CYSTICERCI. The cysticerci typically are manifested by obstructive hydrocephalus. The patient may present with headache, nausea and vomiting, dizziness, altered mental status, or papilledema with altered vision. This is a medical emergency and can be fatal if it is not treated.

SUBARACHNOID CYSTICERCI. Cysticerci in the basilar cisterns are often accompanied by cysticerci in other locations, including parenchymal cysticerci or calcifications, ventricular cysticerci, and spinal or ocular cysticerci; patients may present with disease attributable to cysticerci at these sites. Cysticerci in the basilar cisterns are particularly prone to cause arachnoiditis. Manifestations of arachnoiditis may include vascular involvement (large- or small-vessel strokes), meningeal signs, or communicating hydrocephalus (headaches, nausea, vomiting, dizziness, and altered mental status).

DIAGNOSIS

The major clinical manifestations of neurocysticercosis (e.g., seizures and hydrocephalus) are not specific, and it is difficult to identify the parasites. The main tools used to diagnose neurocysticercosis are neuroimaging studies. Computed tomography (CT) scans are sensitive for identification of parenchymal calcifications, which appear as 2- to 5-mm nodules. CT may also reveal parenchymal cysticerci or obstructive hydrocephalus. MRI scans are more sensitive for identification of the cysticerci, especially in the subarachnoid space and ventricles. The cysticerci are typically round, 1 to 2 cm in diameter. The cyst fluid is usually isodense with spinal fluid. In uninflamed cysticerci, the walls may not be visible. However, most cases demonstrate enhancement of the cyst walls or surrounding tissues and associated edema. In some cases, the scolex may be visible as a 1- to 2-mm solid nodule, cylinder, or spiral on the side of the cystic lesions. Serologic tests are useful to confirm the diagnosis. Assays using crude antigen, including enzyme-linked immunosorbent assay, are associated with poor sensitivity and specificity. An immunoblot assay using semipurified membrane glycoproteins is highly specific for the diagnosis. The sensitivity is excellent in cases with extraparenchymal or multiple parenchymal cysticerci. However, the sensitivity is poor in those with single enhancing lesions or just calcifications. Antigen detection assays are sensitive and more specific for viable cases but are currently unavailable in the United States.

TREATMENT Rx

Treatment varies with the clinical manifestations and form of infection. Seizures should be treated with antiepileptic drugs (Chapter 410). Phenytoin and carbamazepine are typically used and can control the seizures. Newer antiepileptic drugs may be more effective. There are no viable parasites in those with just calcified lesions, so the main measure is to control symptoms (e.g., antiepileptic drugs for those with seizures). In patients presenting with hydrocephalus, surgery to reestablish cerebrospinal fluid flow is the critical initial step in management. The role of antiparasitic drugs (Chapter 352) varies with the form of infection. Randomized controlled trials have demonstrated more rapid resolution of parenchymal cystic lesions with fewer generalized seizures in those treated with corticosteroids and albendazole (15 mg/kg/day in two daily doses) compared with those treated with placebo.[1,2] Praziquantel (50 to 100 mg/kg/day in three daily doses) can be used as an alternative. A number of clinical trials in subjects with single enhancing lesions have demonstrated a slightly more rapid radiologic resolution and fewer seizures in those treated with steroids or antiparasitic drugs. However, the effects are not dramatically different from spontaneous resolution and were not significant in one meta-analysis.[1] For patients with cysticerci in the ventricles, management usually involves removal of the cysticerci, which can be best achieved by neuroendoscopy. However, the main alternative approach is placement of a ventriculoperitoneal shunt. Chronic steroids or antiparasitic drugs may decrease the rate of shunt failure, which usually results from clogging of the shunts by the cysticerci or proteinaceous debris. There are no controlled trials on the management of cysticercosis in those with subarachnoid cysticercosis. However, expert opinion supports treatment of subarachnoid cysticercosis with prolonged courses of antiparasitic drugs (e.g., albendazole for >28 days) and chronic anti-inflammatory medications (e.g., prednisone, 1 mg/kg/day). Methotrexate can be used as a steroid-sparing agent. Patients with hydrocephalus should be treated by cerebrospinal fluid diversion (e.g., ventriculoperitoneal shunting). Before treatment with antiparasitic drugs, patients should undergo a funduscopic examination. Intraocular parasites may develop brisk inflammatory responses after treatment with antiparasitic drugs. Because this inflammation could lead to blindness, most authorities recommend extraction of the parasites before antiparasitic therapy. However, there are also reports of treatment of intraocular parasites with antiparasitic drugs.

PROGNOSIS

The prognosis varies significantly between the different forms of neurocysticercosis. Parenchymal enhancing lesions and parenchymal cystic lesions will eventually resolve, but this may take months to years. Patients who have or develop calcifications are at high risk for recurrent seizures lifelong. Patients with ventricular or subarachnoid disease are at high risk for morbidity and mortality. However, a recent case series noted no deaths with optimal management.

Cystic Hydatid Disease (*Echinococcus granulosus* group)

DEFINITION

Cystic echinococcosis (CE), also called cystic hydatidosis, is caused by the larval stage of cestodes of the *Echinococcus granulosus* group of parasites. All of these parasites were initially thought to be caused by a single species, *E. granulosus*. However, molecular studies demonstrate that *E. granulosus* comprises a number of different species and genotypes. In humans, the clinical manifestations range from asymptomatic infection to severe, potentially fatal disease.

Echinococcal cysts consist of a periparasitic host tissue (pericyst or adventitia), which encompasses the larval endocyst, and the endocyst itself. The endocyst has an outer, acellular laminated layer and an inner, or germinative, layer that gives rise to brood capsules and protoscolices. The cyst is filled with clear fluid, numerous brood capsules, and protoscolices. Some cysts may also harbor daughter cysts of variable size. The protoscolices convert to tapeworms in the canine definitive hosts but can also form new cysts when released in mammalian tissues.

EPIDEMIOLOGY

E. granulosus species occur on all continents and in circumpolar, temperate, subtropical, and tropical zones. The highest prevalence of the parasite is found in parts of Eurasia, Africa, Australia, and South America. Within the endemic zones, the prevalence of the parasites varies from sporadic to high, but only a few countries can be regarded as being free of *E. granulosus*.

It is difficult to determine the true incidence of CE because of the slow rate of growth and variable clinical presentation. Most epidemiologic reports are based on hospital- and surgery-based surveys that greatly underestimate the actual rates of infection, especially in low socioeconomic groups with limited access to diagnosis and treatment.

Since the mid-1980s, however, mass community-based surveys using portable ultrasound scanners have been conducted in many remote, rural areas of the world. The sensitivity and specificity of ultrasound have been shown to be superior to those of serology in prevalence surveys. These studies showed the real burden of disease, uncovering population infection rates of up to 6.6%.

E. granulosus exists as a complex of species and strains that differ in a variety of criteria that may have an impact on the epidemiology, pathology, and control of CE. To date, 10 distinct genotypes (G1 to G10) have been identified. Some distinct species have been identified (*Echinococcus equinus, Echinococcus ortleppi*). The great majority of *E. granulosus* isolates from human patients thus far have been of the sheep genotype (G1).

CLINICAL MANIFESTATIONS

The presentation of human CE is protean. Patients seek medical attention when a large cyst has some mechanical effect on organ function or rupture of a cyst causes acute hypersensitivity reactions. The cyst is often diagnosed incidentally during ultrasound examination, chest radiography, or body scanning performed for other clinical reasons. The liver is the most frequent location of echinococcal cysts, representing approximately 70% of cases. The lungs are the second most common location. However, CE can occasionally occur in virtually any other organ.

Common symptoms are upper abdominal discomfort and pain, poor appetite, and a mass in the abdomen. Physical findings are hepatomegaly, a palpable mass on the surface of the liver or other organs, and abdominal distention. Other manifestations include jaundice, colic-like pains, portal hypertension, ascites, and compression of the inferior vena cava. If cysts in the lung rupture into the bronchi, symptoms may include intense cough, a salty taste in the mouth, or vomiting of hydatid material and cystic membranes. Patients may present with a chest mass, chest pain, chronic cough, pneumothorax, eosinophilic pneumonitis, pleural effusion, parasitic lung embolism, hemoptysis, or biliptysis. Cysts in the heart can cause a cardiac mass, pericardial effusion, and embolism. Cysts in the breast must be differentiated from neoplasms. Cysts located in the spine and in the brain can cause serious neurologic symptoms, including paralysis and seizures.

DIAGNOSIS

The diagnosis of CE is based on imaging methods and on serology, but serology has only a confirmatory role. Routine laboratory tests are nonspecific. Cyst rupture into the biliary tree may cause elevation of alkaline phosphatase, sometimes in association with hyperamylasemia and eosinophilia (up to 60%). Otherwise, eosinophilia is low grade or absent.

Imaging

Modern imaging tools (ultrasound, CT, and, to a lesser extent, MRI) are central to the diagnosis and clinical management of CE. Ultrasound is the procedure of choice for diagnosis of asymptomatic CE. Ultrasound is also useful for longitudinal studies, such as monitoring the response of cysts to treatment and recording cyst growth rate. In 2003, the World Health Organization (WHO) Informal Working Group on Echinococcosis proposed a standardized ultrasound classification (Fig. 362-2). This classification defines six cyst stages that are assigned to three clinical groups. The active group comprises developing cysts, which may be unilocular (CE1) or multivesicular with daughter cysts (class CE2) and are usually found to be viable. The transitional group (class CE3) contains cysts that are usually starting to degenerate. There are two types of CE3: the "water lily sign" for floating membranes, which is now known as subclass CE3a; and predominantly solid cysts with daughter cysts, or subclass CE3b. This subdivision is based on their

different response to percutaneous treatment (see later) and albendazole, which is generally good for CE3a and poor for CE3b. A study using nuclear magnetic resonance spectroscopy has found that CE3a and CE3b may have different metabolic characteristics. The inactive group (classes CE4 and CE5) exhibits involution and signs of solidification of cyst content with increasing degrees of calcification and is nearly always found to be nonviable.

CT scanning has the advantage of inspecting any organ, detecting smaller cysts located outside the liver, locating cysts precisely, and sometimes differentiating parasitic from nonparasitic cysts. MRI may have some advantages over CT scanning in the evaluation of postsurgical residual lesions, recurrences, and selected extrahepatic infections, such as cardiac infections. Plain radiographs are used for cysts in the lungs, bone, and muscle and for detection of calcified cysts.

Serology

Serologic tests are useful for confirmation of presumptive imaging diagnoses. However, many tests are available, and they are not standardized. Their sensitivity varies with the location of the cysts. Hepatic cysts are more likely to elicit an immune response than are pulmonary, brain, or splenic cysts. Serologic test results are usually positive when the endocyst is detached (CE3a) and in active (CE2) and transitional (CE3b) stages. Serologic test results are generally negative in patients with inactive cysts (CE4 and CE5). Titers tend to slowly decrease when a cyst becomes inactive (CE4, CE5) and after radical surgery. Titers may remain positive after conservative surgery in which the antigen source (the germinal layer) is not completely removed. Antibody titers usually increase immediately after medical or percutaneous treatments because of the mobilization of the antigen following disruption of cyst integrity.

Other Diagnostic Procedures

Fine-needle aspiration biopsy of the cyst performed under ultrasonographic guidance, with a transhepatic approach, under anthelmintic coverage, is useful for differentiation of CE, malignant neoplasms, abscesses, and nonparasitic cysts. The procedure must be carried out in the presence of an anesthesiologist ready to manage the rare but possible anaphylactic reaction.

TREATMENT

The appropriate treatment depends on factors of the individual patient, the characteristics of the cyst, the therapeutic resources available, and the physician's preference. There are few randomized clinical trials evaluating treatment options, so a low level of evidence supports one therapeutic modality over another.

Surgery

Surgery has long been the only option in the treatment of CE. However, in the past two decades, medical treatment, percutaneous procedures, and a

FIGURE 362-2. WHO Informal Working Group on Echinococcosis standardized ultrasound classification of cystic echinococcosis. CL lesions are cystic lesions lacking a distinct wall and may have other diagnoses. CE1 lesions are cystic lesions with a visible wall that may demonstrate protoscolices ("hydatid sand"). CE2 lesions include internal septation. CE3 lesions may be detached from the wall or have daughter cysts with internal thickening. CE4 lesions are heterogeneous lesions with degeneration. CE5 lesions show thick calcification.

"watch and wait" approach have been successfully introduced and replaced surgery as the treatment of choice in selected cases. Surgery remains the main therapy in complicated cysts (i.e., rupture, biliary fistula, compression of vital structures, superinfection, hemorrhage), cysts at high risk of rupture, or large cysts with many daughter vesicles that are not suitable for percutaneous treatments. Surgery can be performed as an open procedure, with either radical and conservative techniques, or laparoscopically, but there are controversies as to the safest and most effective technique and in which cases it should be applied. In all cases, perioperative albendazole prophylaxis, from 1 week before surgery until 4 weeks postoperatively, is recommended as a cautionary measure to minimize the risk of fluid spillage and consequent secondary echinococcosis from seeding of protoscolices in the abdominal cavity. Some authorities treat with praziquantel as well.

Percutaneous Treatments

Percutaneous techniques provide an alternative to surgery and benzimidazole derivatives. These treatment modalities aim either to destroy the germinal layer with scolicidal agents or to evacuate the entire endocyst. The most popular method aimed at destroying the germinal layer is PAIR (puncture, aspiration, injection of a scolicidal agent, and reaspiration). Many modified catheterization techniques are used to evacuate the endocyst and are generally reserved for cysts that are difficult to drain or tend to relapse after PAIR, such as multivesiculated cysts or cysts with predominantly solid content and daughter cysts. A growing number of articles have reported its safety in treating abdominal, especially liver, echinococcal cysts. More than 4000 cysts have been punctured, for either diagnostic or therapeutic purposes, and 16 cases of anaphylactic shock (two of them lethal) have been reported. Prophylactic administration of albendazole for at least 30 days after puncture is a cautionary measure that should always accompany PAIR. PAIR is generally successful at inducing permanent solidification in CE1 and CE3a cysts. A few reports with long-term follow-up indicate that multivesicular cysts (i.e., CE2 and CE3b) tend to relapse repeatedly after PAIR.

Chemotherapy

Albendazole (Chapter 352) is the antiparasitic drug of choice for CE. It is administered orally at a dosage of 10 to 15 mg/kg/day; administration should be continuous without treatment interruptions. However, the optimal dosage and optimal duration of treatment with albendazole have not been formally assessed, and data from the small clinical trials generally fail to take into account the cyst's characteristics. A recent systematic review on the effect of albendazole showed that the efficacy of the drug may have been overstated in previous retrospective, nonrandomized studies. Albendazole induces solidification in small and medium-sized CE1 and CE3a cysts, whereas it has generally little effect on giant (diameter > 10 cm) CE1 and CE3a cysts. It has no effect on most cases of CE2 and CE3b cysts.

Adverse effects of benzimidazoles (Chapter 352) include hepatotoxicity, leukopenia, thrombocytopenia, and alopecia. Increases in aminotransferases may be due to drug-related efficacy or real drug-related toxicity. Whereas teratogenic risks are theoretical, it is nonetheless good practice to avoid use during pregnancy when possible and to delay treatment until after delivery unless it is absolutely necessary.

Watch and Wait

Inactive liver cysts that are free of complications, such as compression on neighboring organs, are increasingly monitored without being treated. Prospective studies need to be carried out to confirm the safety of this option.

Follow-up

Follow-up is crucial to evaluate the efficacy of treatment. Long-term follow-up, generally more than 5 years, is required to evaluate local recurrences, which have been reported up to 10 years after apparently successful treatment. When the combination of imaging and serology is inconclusive, fine-needle aspiration should be performed to ascertain the viability of the cyst contents.

Alveolar Hydatid Disease (*Echinococcus multilocularis*)

Alveolar hydatid disease is caused by the tissue forms of *Echinococcus multilocularis*. In tissues, typically the liver, *E. multilocularis* grows as a budding mass rather than as a large cystic lesion. The tissues resemble lung tissues, hence the name "alveolar." The normal definitive hosts are canines, including wolves and foxes. The normal intermediate hosts are rodents. Humans are accidentally infected by contact with soil containing the ova.

EPIDEMIOLOGY

E. multilocularis is endemic in arctic and alpine areas of the Northern Hemisphere. It is highly endemic in western China, Tibet, and central Asia. In recent years, *E. multilocularis* has emerged as an important problem in Alpine areas of central Europe and adjacent forested areas.

CLINICAL MANIFESTATIONS AND DIAGNOSIS

Human *E. multilocularis* infection almost invariably involves the liver, in which it is manifested as a tumor-like mass that gradually expands during decades. The main symptoms are liver discomfort and swelling. Diagnosis is by demonstration of a characteristic mass on imaging studies, with the etiology confirmed by serologic tests.

TREATMENT

Surgery remains the mainstay of treatment of *E. multilocularis*. When feasible, all infected tissues should be removed. Apparently curative therapy should be followed by a 2-year course of albendazole to decrease the risk of relapse. In some cases, resection is feasible only when it is accompanied by liver transplantation. In cases that are not amenable to surgical resection, prolonged courses of albendazole can suppress growth of the lesion.

Other Larval Cestode Infections

Sparganosis is caused by infection with the larval (plerocercoid) stage of *Spirometra mansonoides*. Infection is acquired by ingestion or application of infected meat (frogs, birds, fish) or exposure of skin to infected flesh (e.g., poultices of infected tissues). After infection, plerocercoids develop in the tissues, typically presenting as subcutaneous or central nervous system nodules or occasionally larva migrans symptoms. Treatment usually involves removal of the nodule.

Coenurosis is a rare larval cestode infection caused by human infection with the larval stage of the dog tapeworms *Taenia multiceps* and *Taenia serialis*. In the tissue, the larva forms a cystic lesion containing multiple scolices (the coenurus). The cystic lesion is usually single and most frequently identified in brain, eye, or soft tissues. Treatment usually involves removal.

Echinococcus oligarthus and *Echinococcus vogeli* have been associated with polycystic hydatid disease in northern South America. *Taenia crassiceps* has been identified in the eye and in tissues of compromised hosts. *Hymenolepis*-like organisms have also been identified in tissues of AIDS patients.

1. Del Brutto OH, Roos KL, Coffey CS, et al. Meta-analysis: cysticidal drugs for neurocysticercosis: albendazole and praziquantel. *Ann Intern Med.* 2006;145:43-51.
2. Garcia HH, Pretell EJ, Gilman RH, et al. A trial of antiparasitic treatment to reduce the rate of seizures due to cerebral cysticercosis. *N Engl J Med.* 2004;350:249-258.

SUGGESTED READINGS

Brunetti E, Junghanss T. Update on cystic hydatid disease. *Curr Opin Infect Dis.* 2009;22:497-502. *Recent review of cystic hydatid disease.*

Brunetti E, Kern P, Vuitton DA. Expert consensus for the diagnosis and treatment of cystic and alveolar echinococcosis in humans. *Acta Trop.* 2010;114:1-16. *Recent expert consensus on diagnosis and management of cystic and alveolar hydatid disease.*

Rangel-Castilla L, Serpa JA, Gopinath SP, et al. Contemporary neurosurgical approaches to neurocysticercosis. *Am J Trop Med Hyg.* 2009;80:373-378. *A review of neurosurgical management of neurocysticercosis.*

Serpa JA, Graviss EA, Kass JS, et al. Neurocysticercosis in Houston, Texas: an update. *Medicine (Baltimore).* 2011;90:81-86. *Review of 111 patients, including 93 Hispanic immigrants.*

Singh G, Rajshekhar V, Murthy JM, et al. A diagnostic and therapeutic scheme for a solitary cysticercus granuloma. *Neurology.* 2010;75:2236-2245. *A practical approach.*

363

SCHISTOSOMIASIS (BILHARZIASIS)

EDGAR M. CARVALHO AND ALDO A. M. LIMA

DEFINITION

Schistosomiasis is one of the most important parasitic diseases of humans and is a global public health problem in the developing world. The disease is caused by trematodes of the genus *Schistosoma*, and it is estimated that 300 million people are infected, another 600 million are at high risk for infection, and 20 million have debilitating disease. Mortality from schistosomiasis is estimated at 280,000 deaths per year and the burden of disease at 1.7 million disability-adjusted life years lost per year.

The Pathogen

Five major species of *Schistosoma* affect humans: *S. mansoni*, *S. haematobium*, *S. japonicum*, *S. intercalatum*, and *S. mekongi*. The sequencing of the *S. mansoni* genome was recently reported. Other *Schistosoma* species that occasionally infect humans include *S. bovis*, *S. mattheei*, and some avian schistosomes. These species differ biologically from one another and in their geographic distribution and the type of disease that they produce. The schistosomes are digenetic parasitic trematodes (Fig. 363-1). Although they are morphologically distinct, the species of *Schistosoma* that infect humans share some common factors. The large male (0.6 to 2.2 cm × 2 to 4 mm) has a ventral gynecophoric canal in which the female (1.2 to 2.6 cm × 1 to 2 mm) is held during copulation.

EPIDEMIOLOGY

Schistosomiasis occurs mainly in rural agricultural and periurban areas. *S. mansoni* is found in 55 countries, including the Arabian peninsula, Egypt, Libya, Sudan, most countries in sub-Saharan Africa, Brazil, Suriname, and Venezuela. *S. haematobium* is endemic in 53 countries in the Middle East and most of the African continent, including the island of Madagascar and Mauritius. *S. japonicum* is endemic in China, Indonesia, and the Philippines; it has also been reported from Thailand. *S. intercalatum* has been reported from 10 countries in Africa. *S. mekongi* is found in Cambodia and Laos.

The endemicity of schistosomiasis depends on the urban disposal of urine (*S. haematobium*) and feces (*S. mansoni*, *S. japonicum*, *S. intercalatum*, *S. mekongi*), the presence of suitable snail hosts, and human exposure to cercariae. The freshwater snail intermediate hosts are *Biomphalaria* spp in Africa and *Biomphalaria glabrata* (*Australorbis*) and *Tropicarbis* in South America and the West Indies. In some cases, the endemicity of schistosomiasis may be maintained by animal reservoirs. Such is the case with *S. japonicum*, which

FIGURE 363-1. Schistosome life cycle.

infects dogs and cows. Rodents, monkeys, and baboons have been found infected in nature, but the role of these animals as reservoirs does not seem to be epidemiologically important.

Etiology and Life Cycle

Adult worms live in the mesenteric veins (*S. mansoni*, *S. japonicum*, *S. mekongi*, and *S. intercalatum*) or in the venous plexus around the lower ends of the ureters and the urinary bladder (*S. haematobium*). In these sites, they start their sexual reproduction by releasing eggs. Once deposited in the host, eggs may stay in the mesenteric vein, be trapped in the intestines, escape to the intestinal lumen, and migrate by portal blood to the liver (*S. mansoni*, *S. japonicum*). Eggs of *S. haematobium* may be trapped in the intestines and bladder and may escape to the intestinal or bladder lumen. After being excreted with feces or urine into fresh water, the eggs hatch and release ciliated motile miracidia that penetrate into the snail intermediate host. Following asexual multiplication in the snail, the development of cercariae, the infective forms for humans, takes 4 to 7 weeks. After leaving the snails, the cercariae can survive in fresh water for almost 72 hours. When penetration of the skin in the human host occurs, the cercariae lose their tails and change into schistosomula. Schistosomula migrate to the lungs and, in about 6 weeks, mature to adult worms and descend to their final habitat. Viable eggs can be seen in excretions (i.e., stool or urine) 5 to 9 weeks after cercarial penetration. The lifespan of the worms ranges from 5 to 10 years.

PATHOBIOLOGY

The pathogenesis of acute human schistosomiasis is mainly related to egg deposition and liberation of antigens of adult worms and eggs. A strong inflammatory response characterized by high levels of pro-inflammatory cytokines such as interleukin (IL)–1, IL-6, and tumor necrosis factor-α (TNF-α) and circulating immune complexes participate in the pathogenesis of the acute phase of the disease.

In chronic schistosomiasis, tissue injury is mediated by egg-induced granulomas and the subsequent appearance of fibrosis. Because the habitat of *S. mansoni*, *S. japonicum*, *S. mekongi*, and *S. intercalatum* worms is the mesenteric blood vessels, the intestines are involved primarily, and egg embolism results in secondary involvement of the liver. Host genetics, immunologic response, and parasite load measured by egg count in the stool are associated with a greater chance for hepatosplenic involvement. IL-4 and IL-13 have been associated with granuloma formation and liver fibrosis. Enzymes and antigens released from eggs sensitize host lymphocytes, which migrate to areas of egg deposition and recruit other cell types, such as macrophages, eosinophils, and fibroblasts. The size of these granulomas and the resulting fibrosis lead to most of the chronic fibro-obstructive lesions in schistosomiasis. In the liver, the granulomas result in perisinusoidal obstruction of portal blood flow, portal hypertension, splenomegaly, esophageal varices, and portosystemic collateral circulation. Liver cell perfusion is not reduced; consequently, liver function test results remain normal for a long time.

In schistosome-infected populations, the intensity of infection increases during the first 2 decades of life as children accumulate worms and then declines. The susceptibility of younger children to infection is even more evident when intensities of reinfection are studied after the elimination of existing worms by chemotherapy. Although there is a decrease in exposure with age, the lower intensities of infection in older individuals are due in part to acquired resistance. Both T_H1 (interferon-γ) and T_H2 types of immune response, mediated by IgE, may participate in resistance to reinfection. In the *S. haematobium*–infected population, IgE increases progressively with age, and IgE antibodies directed against adult worm antigens are associated with subsequent low intensities of reinfection. Similar associations between high IgE levels or a high IgE/IgG4 ratio and resistance to reinfection have been found among Brazilian and Kenyan subjects exposed to *S. mansoni*. Evidence that a T_H1-type immune response may also be involved in the protection against *S. mansoni* comes from immunologic studies in subjects who are highly exposed to contaminated water but have negative stool examination results. In these subjects, there is evidence of higher interferon-γ production in response to *S. mansoni* membrane extract. The existence of a major codominant gene, called *SM1*, that controls the intensity of infection by *S. mansoni* has been demonstrated. The localization of *SM1* on chromosome 5q31-q33, close to several genes involved in regulation of the immune response, including those for colony-stimulating factor-1 receptor, granulocyte-macrophage colony-stimulating factor, IL-3, IL-4, IL-5, IL-13, and immune regulatory factor-1 and a locus regulating IgE levels, indicates that genetic factors are probably critical to susceptibility and resistance to schistosome infection.

Because modulation of the immune response is a characteristic of chronic schistosomiasis, *S. mansoni* infection has modified the clinical course of autoimmune and inflammatory diseases in experimental models and in humans. *S. mansoni* infection attenuates the clinical manifestations of type 1 diabetes and experimental autoimmune encephalitis in mice. In humans, *S. mansoni* attenuates the clinical manifestations of asthma and is inversely associated with the development of myelopathy related to human T-cell leukemia virus type 1 (HTLV-1) infection. *S. mansoni* infection may impair immunologic response to vaccines and change manifestations of other infectious diseases.

CLINICAL MANIFESTATIONS

Clinical manifestations of schistosomiasis are divided into schistosome dermatitis, acute schistosomiasis, and chronic schistosomiasis. Schistosome dermatitis, or swimmer's itch, is seen mainly when avian cercariae penetrate the skin and are destroyed. It is uncommon, but recognition of this clinical entity is gradually expanding. Schistosome dermatitis is a sensitization phenomenon occurring in previously exposed persons. The cercariae evoke an acute inflammatory response with edema, early infiltration of neutrophils and lymphocytes, and later invasion of eosinophils. A pruritic papular rash occurs within 24 hours after the penetration of cercariae and reaches maximal intensity in 2 to 3 days.

Acute schistosomiasis occurs usually 20 to 50 days after primary exposure. Although asymptomatic in endemic areas, acute schistosomiasis is becoming a frequent and major clinical problem in nonimmune individuals from urban regions who are exposed for the first time to a heavy infection in an endemic area. The clinical syndrome (i.e., fever, chills, liver and spleen enlargement, and marked eosinophilia) originally described for *S. japonicum* infection, and still common for this species, is increasingly being diagnosed in Brazil in individuals with *S. mansoni* infection. Malaise, diarrhea, weight loss, cough, dyspnea, chest pain, restrictive respiratory insufficiency, and pericarditis are important findings in this phase. High levels of TNF-α and circulating immune complexes are found in the patient's serum in this phase of illness, and they correlate with the presence of abdominal pain, diarrhea, and weight loss and with respiratory and pericardial manifestations, respectively. Acute disease is not observed in individuals living in endemic areas of schistosomiasis because of the downmodulation of the immune response by antigens or idiotypes transferred from mother to child.

In chronic schistosomiasis, abdominal pain, irregular bowel movements, and blood in the stool are the main symptoms of intestinal involvement. Colonic polyposis may occur, especially in Egypt.

Hepatosplenic involvement is the most important cause of morbidity with *S. mansoni* and *S. japonicum* infection. Patients may remain asymptomatic until the manifestation of hepatic fibrosis and portal hypertension develops. Hepatic fibrosis is caused by a granulomatous reaction to *Schistosoma* eggs that have been carried to the liver. Hepatic fibrosis in *S. mansoni* infection has been associated with the intensity of infection and the patient's genetic background and immunologic response. Although the severity of infection is clearly linked with liver disease, the immune response, collagen deposition, and genetic factors potentiate disease in some individuals with only moderate infections or inhibit disease in others with heavy infections.

Hematemesis from bleeding esophageal or gastric varices may occur. In such cases, anemia and decreasing levels of serum albumin are observed. A few patients have severe hepatosplenic disease with decompensated liver disease. Jaundice, ascites, and liver failure are then observed. Concomitant infection by *Salmonella* species and, less extensively, other gram-negative bacteria with *S. mansoni* or *S. haematobium* leads to a picture of prolonged fever, hepatosplenomegaly, and mild leukocytosis with eosinophilia. Coinfection with *S. mansoni* and hepatitis C virus is associated with a greater chance of chronic hepatitis. Glomerulonephritis, infantilism, and hypersplenism are other complications associated with hepatosplenic schistosomiasis. The finding of pulmonary hypertension is increasing with the use of more advanced diagnostic technology. Pulmonary hypertension has been detected in 10.7% of patients with liver fibrosis. In countries endemic for *S. mansoni*, up to 30% of the cases of pulmonary hypertension are due to schistosomiasis. In hospitalized adult patients with *S. japonicum* infection, cerebral schistosomiasis occurs in 1.7 to 4.3%. It may occur as early as 6 weeks after infection, and the most common sign is focal jacksonian epilepsy. Signs and symptoms of generalized encephalitis may occasionally be found. In *S. mansoni* infection, neurologic involvement is rare and mainly characterized by transverse myelitis. An association between *S. mansoni* or *S. haematobium* and human immunodeficiency virus (HIV) infection has been documented in areas where both infectious agents are found. Although the immune response of

patients with schistosomiasis is altered by HIV, it has not been reported to be associated with any clear changes in the degree of infection or severity of manifestations of schistosomiasis.

In *S. haematobium* infection, the main organ system involved is the urinary tract. The acute granulomatous response to parasite eggs in the early stages causes urinary tract disease, such as urethral ulceration and bladder polyposis. In chronic disease, usually in older patients, granulomas at the lower end of the ureters obstruct urinary flow and may cause hydroureter and hydronephrosis. Bladder fibrosis and calcification are also seen in this phase. Up to 70% of infected individuals have hematuria, dysuria, or urinary frequency. Urine examination reveals proteinuria and hematuria. Radiologic findings include hydronephrosis, hydroureter, ureteral strictures, dilation or distortion, ureteral calcifications, ureterolithiasis, calcified bladder, polyps, reduction in bladder capacity, irregular contraction of the bladder wall, and dilated bladder because of bladder neck fibrosis. An increased incidence of squamous cell carcinoma of the bladder (Chapter 203) has been reported in endemic areas of *S. haematobium* infection, but the mechanism of carcinogenesis is unknown. *S. haematobium* eggs have occasionally been found in the lungs, with subsequent focal pulmonary arteritis and pulmonary hypertension.

DIAGNOSIS

A definitive diagnosis of schistosomiasis can be made only by finding schistosome eggs in feces, urine, or a biopsy specimen, usually from the rectum (Table 363-1). A history of contact with contaminated water and appropriate clinical manifestations are important steps in establishing the diagnosis. Because schistosome eggs may be few, concentration by sedimentation should be performed. All eggs from feces, urine, or tissues should be examined under high power to determine their viability by visualizing the activity of cilia of the excretory flame cells of the enclosed miracidium. Dead eggs may persist for a long time after successful therapy or natural death of the

TABLE 363-1 DIAGNOSIS OF SCHISTOSOMIASIS

SCHISTOSOME	EGGS	DIAGNOSIS
S. haematobium	Mainly found in urine but may be found in stools or rectal biopsy specimens Eggs: 143 × 50 μm; spindle shaped: rounded anterior, conical posterior, tapering to a terminal delicate spine	Obtain urine sample at midday (when eggs are excreted); more than one sample may be needed Examine urine directly or by filtering 10 mL of urine through a Nuclepore membrane Rectal biopsy in suspected cases with normal urine Serologic testing to diagnose early or light infection
S. mansoni	Eggs: 155 × 66 μm; oval with lateral, long spine	Examine stool for eggs Use the Kato-Katz thick smear method for quantification purposes Rectal biopsy or serologic testing to diagnose stool-negative cases, particularly in lightly infected patients
S. japonicum	Found in stool; eggs: 89 × 67 μm; oval or rounded with a lateral, short, sometimes curved spine	Examine stool for eggs Kato-Katz thick smear (for quantitative assessment) Rectal biopsy for those with light infections, especially with less common manifestations (i.e., cerebral schistosomiasis)
S. mekongi	Found in stool; eggs: 60 × 32 μm; smaller than eggs of *S. japonicum*	Examine stool for eggs
S. intercalatum	Found in stool; eggs: 180 × 65 μm; terminal spine	Examine stool for eggs

worms. The presence of only dead eggs does not necessarily require treatment. Because the intensity of infection is associated with morbidity, quantitative techniques are recommended. For *S. mansoni* and *S. japonicum*, the Kato-Katz thick smear method is used. Rectal biopsy may be used for those with light infection. In patients with chronic *S. mansoni* and *S. japonicum* infection and liver disease, the diagnosis is sometimes made by documentation of eggs in liver specimens. Ultrasonography allows determination of the degree of liver fibrosis. *S. mekongi* and *S. intercalatum* infection is diagnosed by examination of the stool for eggs.

Urine examination for *S. haematobium* eggs can be performed by direct or concentration methods. Samples should be obtained at midday, when excretion of eggs is maximal. Rectal biopsy may be performed in patients with light infection and negative urine results. After *S. haematobium* infection is diagnosed, assessment of urinary tract disease by ultrasonography is recommended. Because of an increased incidence of carcinoma of the bladder, cancer surveillance should be performed in patients with *S. haematobium* infection (Chapter 203).

Several serologic tests for detection of IgM, IgG, and IgA antibodies to *Schistosoma* antigens are available. Serologic tests are important in the diagnosis of acute infection because the symptoms are not specific and the finding of eggs in stool may reflect chronic infection.

Quantification of circulating antigens in serum and urine is an alternative for the diagnosis of schistosome infection. However, the sensitivity of the method decreases in patients with light infection (<100 eggs per gram of feces). This test has also been used to monitor the efficacy of antischistosome chemotherapy. A significant decrease in antigen levels or negativity of the test is observed as early as 10 days after therapy.

TREATMENT   **Rx**

Chemotherapy is by far the major method for control and cure of schistosomiasis. Three compounds are in use—metrifonate, oxamniquine, and praziquantel—and all three are included in the World Health Organization's list of essential drugs. Praziquantel, a pyrazinoisoquinoline derivative, is the drug of choice for the treatment of schistosomiasis for four reasons: high efficacy against all schistosome species and against cestodes, lack of serious short-term and long-term side effects, administration as a single oral dose, and competitive cost.

The standard recommended treatment consists of a single dose of praziquantel, 40 mg/kg, for *S. mansoni, S. haematobium*, and *S. intercalatum* infection. In *S. japonicum* infection, a total dose of 60 mg/kg is recommended, split into two or three doses in a single day. Although no significant difference was found in the overall cure rates between single-dose (40 mg/kg) and double treatment (40 mg/kg with 2-week interval) regimens of praziquantel for *S. haematobium*, the effect of double treatment resulted in significant reduction in infection intensity and microhematuria, which may have an impact on reducing subtle morbidity.**1** *S. mekongi* may require two treatments at 60 mg/kg body weight. With these dosages of praziquantel, recorded cure rates are 75 to 85% for *S. haematobium*, 63 to 85% for *S. mansoni*, 80 to 90% for *S. japonicum*, 89% for *S. intercalatum*, and 60 to 80% for double infections with *S. mansoni* and *S. haematobium*. A decrease in the efficacy of praziquantel has been observed in patients coinfected with HTLV-1.

Praziquantel is well tolerated and effective in patients of all ages and for different clinical forms of schistosomiasis, including advanced hepatosplenic cases *(S. mansoni),* cerebral schistosomiasis *(S. japonicum),* and neurologic syndromes *(S. mansoni* and *S. haematobium),* possibly in association with corticosteroids. However, praziquantel has low prophylactic effect, which reduces its efficacy in areas of high transmission. There have been several reports of persistent schistosome egg shedding after treatment, thus posing concern about the emergence of drug resistance.

The effects of praziquantel on schistosomes can be summarized under three headings: muscle contraction, tegumental damage (i.e., vacuolization and blebbing), and metabolic alterations (i.e., decreased glucose uptake, lactate excretion, and glycogen content). Schistosome calcium ion channels are so far the only molecular targets of praziquantel action identified. The drug may also interfere with adenosine uptake, which is relevant because schistosomes are unable to synthesize purines de novo. Several drugs (e.g., phenytoin, rifampin, azole antifungals) decrease plasma concentrations of praziquantel because they inhibit cytochrome P-450 pathway 3A4. Chloroquine and cimetidine also decrease praziquantel bioavailability. Praziquantel's activity also depends on the patient's immune system. Several studies have reported that praziquantel induces the exposure of worm surface antigens that may function as targets for immune responses.

The most common side effects observed with praziquantel or oxamniquine are related to the gastrointestinal tract: abdominal pain or discomfort, nausea,

vomiting, anorexia, and diarrhea. These symptoms can be observed in up to 50% of patients but are usually well tolerated. Other side effects are related to the central nervous system (e.g., headache, dizziness, drowsiness) and the skin (e.g., pruritus, eruptions) or may be nonspecific (e.g., fever, fatigue). In general, the cumulative experience from a large number of studies allows the conclusion that praziquantel is an extremely well tolerated drug that requires minimal medical supervision and is therefore particularly suitable for mass chemotherapy programs. Although a reduction in the intensity of infection and morbidity has been documented after mass chemotherapy, provision of clean water, use of molluscicides, and adequate sanitation should also be implemented to control the disease.

Grade A

1. Sacko M, Magnussen P, Traoré M, et al. The effect of single dose versus two doses of praziquantel on *Schistosoma haematobium* infection and pathology among school-aged children in Mali. *Parasitology.* 2009;136:1851-1857.

SUGGESTED READINGS

Bergquist R, Tanner M. Controlling schistosomiasis in Southeast Asia: a tale of two countries. *Adv Parasitol.* 2010;72:109-144. *Review of remarkable progress in China and good progress in the Philippines.*

Berriman M, Haas BJ, LoVerde PT. The genome of the blood fluke *Schistosoma mansoni. Nature.* 2009;460:352-358. *The sequencing of the S. mansoni genome is a landmark event.*

Clerinx J, Van Gompel A. Schistosomiasis in travelers and migrants. *Travel Med Infect Dis.* 2011;9:6-24. *Review noting the differences in the two groups.*

Danso-Appiah A, Utzinger J, Liu J, et al. Drugs for treating urinary schistosomiasis. *Cochrane Database Syst Rev.* 2008;3:CD000053. *A review of the treatment options and newer drugs for urinary schistosomiasis.*

dos Santos Fernandes CJ, Jardim CV, Hovnanian A, et al. Survival in schistosomiasis-associated pulmonary arterial hypertension. *J Am Coll Cardiol.* 2010;56:715-720. *Compared with patients with idiopathic pulmonary hypertension, patients with schistosomiasis-associated pulmonary arterial hypertension are less likely to respond to vasodilators but have a similar survival.*

Dömling A, Khoury K. Praziquantel and schistosomiasis. *ChemMedChem.* 2010;5:1420-1434. *Comprehensive review.*

King CH. Toward the elimination of schistosomiasis. *N Engl J Med.* 2009;360:106-109. *Why mass treatment with praziquantel has not stopped transmission.*

364

LIVER, INTESTINAL, AND LUNG FLUKE INFECTIONS

EDUARDO GOTUZZO

THE PATHOGENS

Flukes belong to the phylum Platyhelminthes and class Trematoda. The major flukes of medical importance are discussed in this chapter; they belong to the families Fasciolidae, Opisthorchiidae, Heterophyidae, Echinostomatidae, and Troglotrematidae. Approximately 135 million people worldwide are infected with these flukes. With the exception of schistosomes, all flat worms of clinical significance are hermaphroditic. Blood flukes, or schistosomes, are discussed in Chapter 363. The epidemiology, clinical manifestations, diagnosis, and treatment are summarized in Table 364-1.

Liver Flukes
FASCIOLIASIS

Fascioliasis is a zoonosis caused by *Fasciola hepatica* (adult: 30 by 13 mm) or *Fasciola gigantica* (adult: 75 by 20 mm). The most common natural hosts are sheep, cattle, and goats.

EPIDEMIOLOGY

The infection is distributed globally. The highlands of Peru, Bolivia, Ecuador, Egypt, and Vietnam are the most affected regions in the world. Prevalence

TABLE 364-1 CLINICAL MANIFESTATIONS, DIAGNOSIS, AND TREATMENT OF LIVER, INTESTINAL, AND LUNG FLUKE INFECTIONS IN HUMANS

FLUKE, NUMBER OF PEOPLE INFECTED, AND GEOGRAPHIC DISTRIBUTION	CLINICAL MANIFESTATIONS ACUTE AND CHRONIC PHASES	DIAGNOSIS*	TREATMENT†
LIVER FLUKES			
Fasciola spp 17 million Cosmopolitan	‡Hepatomegaly, eosinophilia, fever, abdominal pain, metastatic-like lesions on liver CT §Biliary obstruction, gallstones, fibrosis, cholangitis	Serology (Fas2 ELISA) Eggs in stool	TCZ
Opisthorchis spp 11.2 million Asia	‡Fever, malaise, arthralgia, lymphadenopathy, and rash §Jaundice, cholangitis, cholangiocarcinoma	Serology Eggs in stool	PZQ
Clonorchis spp 35 million Asia	‡Fever, rash, malaise, and RUQ discomfort §Choledocholithiasis, cholangitis, cholecystitis, liver abscess, and possible cholangiocarcinoma	Serology Eggs in stool	PZQ
INTESTINAL FLUKES			
Fasciolopsis buski and others¶ 50 million Asia and North Africa	Small bowel inflammation, ulceration, mucus secretion, protein-losing enteropathy, malabsorption	Eggs in stool	PZQ
LUNG FLUKE			
Paragonimus spp 22 million Asia, Americas, Africa	‡Abdominal pain, pleuritic pain, cough, eosinophilia §Hemoptysis, cough, chronic pleural effusions, pulmonary cysts, abscess	Serology Eggs in sputum or stool	PZQ or TCZ

*For egg morphology and size, refer to text in the section Diagnosis.
†For drug regimens, refer to text in the section Treatment.
‡Acute.
§Chronic. For chronic infection, a sedimentation technique is preferred (suggested technique: rapid sedimentation technique or Kato-Katz technique).
¶Diagnosis and treatment also apply for other intestinal flukes.
CT = computed tomography; ELISA = enzyme-linked immunosorbent assay; PZQ = praziquantel; RUQ = right upper quadrant; TCZ = triclabendazole.

rates higher than 60% have been reported in Peru and Bolivia. Estimates of the number of people infected in some countries are 830,000 in Egypt, 742,000 in Peru, 360,000 in Bolivia, 37,000 in Yemen, 20,000 in Ecuador, and 10,000 in Iran. It has been estimated that between 2.4 and 17 million people are infected worldwide.

The life cycle begins when the parasite's eggs in stool are deposited in water; miracidia appear, develop, and hatch in 9 to 14 days and invade many species of freshwater snails (*Lymnaea* spp), in which they multiply as sporozoites, rediae, and cercariae during a period of 4 to 7 weeks. They then leave as free-swimming cercaria that subsequently attach to watercress, water lettuce, alfalfa, mint, parsley, or khat. The main source of infection is consumption of raw vegetables or water contaminated with metacercariae. Women have a higher incidence of the disease, with more severe infections and complications than seen in men.

PATHOBIOLOGY AND CLINICAL MANIFESTATIONS

After consumption of contaminated vegetables, the larvae excyst in the duodenum and then migrate through the bowel wall to the liver through the peritoneal cavity. In 4 weeks, they reach the liver, penetrate Glisson's capsule, and cause inflammation and pain. During their migration through the liver, the ongoing inflammatory process is accompanied by intense hemorrhage manifested as subcapsular hematoma. Computed tomography (CT), magnetic resonance imaging, or ultrasonography can detect these initial lesions. Furthermore, migration of the parasite leaves a trail or track that can be observed in histologic sections or by imaging (CT). The flukes sometimes die and leave cavities filled with necrotic debris that are eventually replaced by scar tissue and then become calcified. After 3 to 5 months of migration along the liver, the juvenile larvae finally reach the bile ducts. During this invasive, migratory or acute phase the clinical manifestations are prolonged fever, hepatomegaly, abdominal pain, and eosinophilia. Multiple hypodense lesions are seen on CT, similar to metastases, but they change in position, attenuation, and shape in time because the parasites are still migrating. Acute fascioliasis is clinically similar to acute cholecystitis but with the addition of significant eosinophilia. It can occur in travelers with acute subcapsular hematoma or metastatic-like lesions seen on CT of the liver. Hyperbilirubinemia is notably absent in this phase. Other manifestations are anorexia, weight loss, nausea, vomiting, cough, diarrhea, urticaria, lymphadenopathy, and arthralgias. Occasionally, the juvenile larvae reach other ectopic or extrahepatic locations, such as subcutaneous tissue, the pancreas, the eye, the brain, and the stomach wall, among others. In endemic areas, the acute phase manifestation can be superimposed on chronic infection.

Arrival of the parasite in the bile ducts marks the beginning of the chronic phase. Mature flukes consume hepatocytes and duct epithelium and reside for years in the hepatic and common bile ducts and sometimes in the gallbladder. In this chronic phase, the liver contains large dilated, thick-walled, and calcareous bile ducts with yellowish brown bile. The bile ducts have a thickened hyperplastic wall with marked fibrosis. Symptoms usually reflect biliary obstruction with colicky pain in the right upper quadrant and epigastric area. Eosinophilia is absent in half of the chronic cases. Bacterial superinfection of these cysts and consequent cholangitis can develop. Other complications are hemobilia and liver fibrosis. Alkaline phosphatase is commonly elevated because of biliary obstruction, which sometimes requires surgical intervention. On imaging, the initial lesions may be strongly confused with hepatic metastases. Other findings on CT are hepatomegaly, tracklike hypodense lesions in subcapsular locations, multiple hypodense nodular areas (abscess-like lesions), or low-density, serpiginous, tortuous, tunnel-like branching lesions ranging from 2 to 10 mm. CT can also show subcapsular hematoma, enhancement of Glisson's capsule, necrotic granuloma, and cystic calcifications. After maturation, the adult flukes start laying eggs, which are passed from the sphincter of Oddi to the intestines and evacuated to the environment along with stool. Adult parasites can live in the bile ducts for many years, up to 13. In endemic populations, chronic infection has been reported as mildly symptomatic, whereas in travelers or temporary residents, it has been reported to cause biliary obstruction, with adult parasites being seen on endoscopic retrograde cholangiopancreatography (ERCP).

CLONORCHIASIS AND OPISTHORCHIASIS

Clonorchiasis is the disease caused by *Clonorchis sinensis*, also called the Chinese or oriental liver fluke (adult: 10 to 25 mm by 3 to 5 mm). Opisthorchiasis is caused by *Opisthorchis viverrini* (adult: 5 mm to 10 mm by 1 mm to 2 mm) and *Opisthorchis felineus* (adult: 7 to 12 mm by 2 to 3 mm). The most common natural hosts are dogs, cats, pigs, and some small wild mammals.

EPIDEMIOLOGY

The global estimate of the number of people infected is 46.2 million: 35 million with *C. sinensis* (15 million in China), 10 million with *O. viverrini* (8 million in Thailand and 2 million in the Lao People's Democratic Republic), and 1.2 million with *O. felineus*. There are 601 million and 79.8 million people at risk for infection with *Clonorchis* and *Opisthorchis*, respectively. Both infections are endemic in the Far East, Southeast Asia, and Eastern Europe. *C. sinensis* is endemic in northeast China, southern Korea, Japan, Taiwan, northern Vietnam, and the far eastern part of Russia, whereas *O. viverrini* is endemic in Laos, Thailand, Vietnam, and Cambodia. *O. felineus* infection is prevalent in Russia, Ukraine, and Kazakhstan.

The life cycle starts when the adult worm deposits fully developed eggs, which are then passed to the environment through feces. They hatch in water and the miracidia infect their first intermediate host, a freshwater snail (*Bithynia* spp or *Parafossarulus* spp), where they transform into sporocysts, rediae, and cercariae. Cercariae are released from the snail and then penetrate freshwater fish, which are the second intermediate host (*Cyclocheilichthys* spp, *Puntius* spp, *Hampala dispa*); the cercariae encyst as metacercariae in the muscles or under the scales. In general, the infection is acquired by eating raw or uncooked cyprinoid fish products in rural areas or dishes such as koi-pla. The metacercariae pass through the stomach and reach the small intestine unharmed. Then, through the ampulla of Vater, they reach the bile ducts, where they mature into adult worms within 4 weeks and deposit yellow, operculated eggs. The parasites may live for up to 45 years in a human host.

PATHOBIOLOGY AND CLINICAL MANIFESTATIONS

Clonorchiasis as an acute infection caused by *C. sinensis* is usually asymptomatic, but some patients may have fever, rash, malaise, and right upper quadrant abdominal discomfort. Chronic infections may be manifested as recurrent pyogenic cholangitis, cholecystitis, obstructive jaundice, hepatomegaly, cholecystitis, multiple hepatic tumors, cholelithiasis, pancreatitis, and cholangiocarcinoma.

Opisthorchiasis as an acute infection caused by *O. viverrini* can cause right upper quadrant abdominal pain, flatulence, fatigue, and a hot sensation over the abdomen. In the chronic phase, mild hepatomegaly occurs, mainly in more heavily infected patients (egg counts >10,000 per gram). Jaundice and splenomegaly are not observed. Intrahepatic duct stones and recurrent suppurative cholangitis are common manifestations of opisthorchiasis. Whenever jaundice and ascending cholangitis are detected, fluke-related cholangiocarcinoma should be suspected.

In opisthorchiasis caused by *O. felineus*, infestation usually follows the consumption of raw, slightly salted, and frozen fish ("stroganina"), and acute symptoms occur 2 to 4 weeks later, including high-grade fever, nausea, vomiting, abdominal pain, malaise, arthralgias, lymphadenopathy, and rash. Peripheral eosinophilia is a common finding, especially during the initial 2 to 6 weeks of the infection, together with raised liver enzyme levels. In chronic infection, the eosinophilia is usually milder. Patients may have suppurative cholangitis and liver abscesses because of biliary obstruction. Ultrasonography or CT demonstrates the pathologic changes in the liver, including intrahepatic duct dilation and periductal changes.

The pathologic and clinical consequences of these flukes are related to the intensity and duration of cumulative infestations. In general, they cause inflammation around the biliary tree, severe hyperplasia of epithelial cells, metaplasia of mucin-producing cells in the mucosa, and progressive periductal fibrosis. There are clear associations between *O. viverrini* infection and cholangiocarcinoma. Several *N*-nitroso compounds and their precursors occur at low levels in fermented food, such as preserved mud fish paste (*pla ra*), a condiment that is a ubiquitous component of the cuisine of northeastern Thailand and Laos.

Intestinal Flukes

The most common human intestinal trematode is *Fasciolopsis buski* (adult: 20 to 75 mm by 8 to 20 mm). It is found mainly in the central and southeast parts of Asia. *F. buski* is a common parasite in pigs. Others are *Heterophyes heterophyes* (adult: 1 to 2 mm in length), *Metagonimus yokogawai* (adult: 1 to 2.5 mm by 0.4 to 0.75 mm), and *Echinostoma* species (adult: 6.5 by 1 to 2 mm).

EPIDEMIOLOGY

More than 50 species of intestinal trematodes from the Far East, Middle East, and North Africa have been reported to cause human infection. *H. heterophyes* can also be found in the Nile delta region of Egypt. An estimated 40 to 50 million people are infected with one or several species of intestinal flukes. Their life cycles are similar. The adult worm, attached to the intestinal wall of humans, produces eggs that are passed in feces. The eggs reach water, and miracidia develop and penetrate the first intermediate host—snails. During

the course of 6 to 7 weeks inside the host snails, they develop into sporocysts, rediae, and cercariae. The cercariae leave the snails to encyst in the second intermediate host, which can be freshwater snails, fish, tadpoles, or vegetables. Humans are infected by the ingestion of raw stems, leaves (especially bamboo shoots), watercress, or water chestnuts with encysted metacercariae. In the human duodenum, the metacercariae attach to the walls and become adult worms in approximately 3 months.

PATHOBIOLOGY AND CLINICAL MANIFESTATIONS

Despite the fact the majority of intestinal fluke infections are asymptomatic, they may cause inflammation, ulceration, and mucus secretion at the site of attachment, particularly in the duodenum and jejunum. In fact, gastrointestinal hemorrhage, perforation, and abscesses have been observed. In heavy infection, intestinal obstruction, protein-losing enteropathy, malabsorption, impaired vitamin B_{12} absorption, hypoalbuminemia, and anasarca have been reported. The adult worm causes traumatic, toxic, and obstructive damage to the intestinal mucosa. Some cases have been diagnosed by direct visualization of the adult parasite via esophagogastroduodenoscopy.

Pulmonary Flukes

Paragonimiasis is a zoonosis caused by *Paragonimus* spp (adult size: 10 by 5 mm). Reservoir hosts include felids, canids, viverrids, mustelids, some rodents, and pigs. At least 10 species of *Paragonimus* are known to cause human disease; of these, *Paragonimus westermani* is the most common.

EPIDEMIOLOGY

An estimated 22 million people are infected worldwide with *Paragonimus* spp, and 293 million are at risk. Human paragonimiasis is distributed mainly in Southeast Asia, Japan, Korea, China, and the Philippines, where *P. westermani* is the main species. In other areas of low endemicity, other species have been reported, such as *Paragonimus mexicanus* in Latin America, *Paragonimus kellicotti* in North America, *Paragonimus heterotremus* in India, and *Paragonimus africanus* and *Paragonimus uterobilateralis* in West Africa. The life cycle starts when the eggs are excreted unembryonated in sputum, or alternatively they can be swallowed and passed in stool. In the external environment the eggs become embryonated, and miracidia hatch, seek the first intermediate host, a snail (families Pleuroceridae and Thiaridae), and penetrate its soft tissues. Within the snail, asexual reproduction occurs for several weeks with transformation into sporocysts, rediae, and cercariae; the last emerge from the snail and invade the second intermediate host, a crustacean such as a crab or crayfish, where they encyst and become metacercariae. This is the infective stage for the mammalian host. Human infection occurs by eating inadequately cooked or pickled crab or crayfish that harbor metacercariae of the parasite. The metacercariae excyst in the duodenum, penetrate the intestinal wall, and migrate through the peritoneal cavity toward the lungs. During migration through the peritoneum and diaphragm, the inflammatory process causes abdominal pain and dry cough. When invading the lungs, they become encapsulated and develop into adults. Infections may persist for 20 years in humans.

PATHOBIOLOGY AND CLINICAL MANIFESTATIONS

Paragonimiasis typically results from the consumption of raw or improperly cooked crustaceans, especially crabs. Recently, in the United States some autochthonous cases have been reported in the Midwest in people who consumed raw crayfish while camping during the summer. Most of the infected people are asymptomatic and have subclinical disease. During the first month of infection, abdominal pain may represent the juvenile larvae migrating through the abdominal cavity before reaching the lungs. Irritation of the diaphragm or pleura may cause dry cough. Fever, chest pain, fatigue, and urticaria may follow, as well as eosinophilia. Pleural effusions may be seen at this stage, with significant eosinophilia noted on analysis of pleural fluid, which can be the first clue to the diagnosis. In fact, pleural manifestations predominate early in the disease process, whereas lesions of the pulmonary parenchyma predominate later in the course of disease. Moreover, pneumothorax and mild eosinophilia may occur only 1 month after the initiation of infection. The migrating worms may cause bronchiectasis, interstitial pneumonitis, transient hemorrhage, or bronchopneumonia. Again, pulmonary lesions and eosinophilia raise the possibility of paragonimiasis. Cough and recurrent hemoptysis are common clinical findings in this phase. The chronic stage occurs when the worms are paired in a cyst in the pulmonary parenchyma. Eggs are produced 6 weeks after infection, and if there is communication with the bronchial tree, eggs may be seen in a sputum sample under microscopy, or they can be swallowed and passed with stool. The rusty discoloration of sputum is caused by the presence of the tan- to brown-pigmented *Paragonimus* eggs; the sputa of these patients have been classically described as resembling "iron filings." Charcot-Leyden crystals can be seen.

Peripheral blood eosinophilia and elevated total serum IgE levels are observed in approximately 80% of patients. Common findings on CT are pleural effusion, hydropneumothorax, pulmonary nodules or consolidation of air spaces, and cysts. The most common ectopic form is cerebral paragonimiasis, which is manifested as eosinophilic meningitis or meningoencephalitis, brain tumor, or just residual calcifications from a past infection.

Management of Liver, Intestinal, and Lung Fluke Infections

DIAGNOSIS

In general, transmission of food-borne trematodiases is restricted geographically, and their distribution is one of the most important factors in suspecting this diagnosis. In the appropriate clinical setting, laboratory and imaging data can add information to narrow the differential diagnosis. Acute fluke infections require a high level of suspicion. Serologic tests, direct visualization of the migrating larvae, or empirical therapy with a significant clinical response (including reduction of eosinophilia) are major criteria to confirm the diagnosis. In the chronic phase, the diagnosis is usually made by visualization of the eggs in stool or, in the case of *Paragonimus*, in sputum. A sedimentation technique must be performed on a series of at least three stool specimens from alternate days or even weeks. Some of the sedimentation or concentration parasitologic techniques used for these infections include the Lumbreras rapid sedimentation technique, the Kato-Katz technique, and the ether-formalin concentration technique. Immunodiagnostics is an excellent tool, particularly for patients who do not have demonstrable eggs in clinical specimens.

If acute fascioliasis is strongly suspected, serology would be the next step. Cathepsin L1–based antibody enzyme-linked immunosorbent assay (ELISA) has a sensitivity of 92% and a specificity of 84%. If negative, the diagnosis is unlikely. If serology is not available, CT of the liver can visualize the characteristic tracklike lesions. However, because the parasitic lesions are very similar to metastases, liver biopsy may be necessary. If serology or CT is not available, a trial of triclabendazole with clinical (including eosinophilia) resolution is the major criterion for diagnosis. In chronic fascioliasis, the Lumbreras rapid sedimentation technique is the method of choice to detect the eggs in stool. At least three stool examinations are preferred. If negative, serology can be helpful. Ultrasonography and CT have low sensitivity in this phase. ERCP usually finds the adult parasites in the bile duct when performed for other reasons. Nonetheless, ERCP can be useful to eliminate the adult parasites causing biliary obstruction.

In opisthorchiasis, serology or stool examinations can be performed to approach the diagnosis. The Ov-CP-1–based ELISA has a sensitivity of 95% and a specificity of 96%. For *C. sinensis*, ELISA has a sensitivity between 81.3 and 96% and a specificity between 92.6 and 96.2%. For detection of eggs and to measure the intensity of infection, the Kato-Katz technique is preferred. Intestinal fluke eggs can be detected by performing a sedimentation stool technique, preferably in consecutive stool samples.

For paragonimiasis, an immunoblot assay performed with a crude antigen extract of *P. westermani* has been in use at the Centers for Disease Control and Prevention; the sensitivity of the test is 96%, and its specificity is 99%. This would be the ideal first step to confirm the diagnosis. In the acute phase, the precise location of the migrating larva is unknown and a biopsy may not necessarily target the parasite. When serology is negative (or not available), a trial of praziquantel or triclabendazole with a positive clinical response in 48 to 72 hours is a major criterion for diagnosis. In the chronic phase, several sputum samples have to be examined by a sedimentation technique to increase sensitivity. Stool examinations are complementary because the eggs can be swallowed by the host and then passed through stool. If a pulmonary cyst contains adult parasites with eggs but they do not have communication to the main bronchi, serology is indicated to confirm the diagnosis. If not available, biopsy is warranted.

Under the light microscope, the morphologic characteristics and size of the eggs may be sufficient to identify the specific fluke. For *Fasciola*, the egg

is large, ellipsoid, and oval with an indistinct operculum and thin shell. The *F. hepatica* egg measures 120 to 150 μm by 63 to 90 μm, the *F. gigantica* egg measures 160 to 190 μm by 70 to 90 μm, and the *F. buski* egg measures 130 to 159 μm by 78 to 98 μm. *Opisthorchis* eggs are elongated with an operculum on the anterior end and a pointed terminal "knob" on the posterior end (26 to 30 μm by 11 to 15 μm). *C. sinensis* eggs (27 to 35 μm by 11 to 20 μm) are small, ovoid, or elongated with broad rounded posterior ends, a convex operculum resting on "shoulders," and a small "knob" on the posterior ends. *H. heterophyes* and *M. yokogawai* eggs are similar in size, 26 to 30 μm by 15 to 17 μm. *Echinostoma* eggs are brownish and operculated and measure 83 to 116 μm by 58 to 69 μm. *Paragonimus* eggs measure 68 to 118 μm by 39 to 67 μm, are reddish brown and ovoid or elongated, and have a thick shell; the operculum is slightly flattened and fits into the shoulder area of the shell, and the posterior end is thickened. The egg is often asymmetrical, with one side slightly flattened.

TREATMENT Rx

The general principles and details of antiparasitic therapy are provided in Chapter 352. For fascioliasis, 10 mg/kg of triclabendazole once or twice has a cure rate higher than 90%, and it is the treatment of choice.[1] Cure is achieved if stool examinations remain negative for at least 3 months. Serology can usually take more than a year to resolve. In treatment of the chronic phase, the dead parasites can occasionally cause biliary obstruction, which may need surgical consultation. For *O. viverrini*, a single dose of praziquantel (40 to 50 mg/kg) has a cure rate of 91 to 97%. For clonorchiasis, the recommended dose of praziquantel is 25 mg/kg three times for 1 day (total dose of 75 mg/kg), which has a cure rate of 83 to 85%. For intestinal flukes, praziquantel, 25 mg/kg by mouth three times a day for 1 day, is recommended. For paragonimiasis, praziquantel, 25 mg/kg by mouth three times a day for 3 days, or triclabendazole, 10 mg/kg by mouth once or twice, is highly effective.[2] For ectopic cases, surgery may be necessary. In follow-up, negative stool examinations in the ensuing weeks can confirm cure. However, because the rate of reinfection is high in subjects from endemic areas, a suddenly positive stool examination is highly suggestive of a new infection rather than failure to respond to treatment.

PREVENTION

Prevention of infection with these flukes depends on several factors, including recognizing their geographic distribution and avoiding the consumption of raw vegetables, fish, crayfish, or contaminated water in endemic areas. Proper medical advice must be given to individuals traveling or planning to reside in endemic areas, not only to prevent fluke infection but also to inform them about the risk for coinfection with other parasites. Control of these flukes in animals is impractical because of wild animal reservoirs. However, control of human infections is challenging because it involves changing long-established cultural, dietary, and sanitary habits. Massive chemotherapy in highly endemic populations may reduce the infection in humans and in selected animals.

Grade A

1. Hien TT, Truong NT, Minh NH, et al. A randomized controlled pilot study of artesunate versus triclabendazole for human fascioliasis in central Vietnam. *Am J Trop Med Hyg.* 2008;78:388-392.
2. Calvopiña M, Guderian RH, Paredes W, et al. Comparison of two single-day regimens of triclabendazole for the treatment of human pulmonary paragonimiasis. *Trans R Soc Trop Med Hyg.* 2003;97:451-454.

SUGGESTED READINGS

Centers for Disease Control and Prevention (CDC). Human paragonimiasis after eating raw or undercooked crayfish—Missouri, July 2006–September 2010. *MMWR Morb Mortal Wkly Rep.* 2010;59:1573-1576. *An outbreak with fever, cough, pleural effusion, and eosinophilia.*
Fried B, Abruzzi A. Food-borne trematode infections of humans in the United States of America. *Parasitol Res.* 2010;106:1263-1280. *Review.*
Smout MJ, Sripa B, Laha T, et al. Infection with the carcinogenic human liver fluke, *Opisthorchis viverrini*. *Mol Biosyst.* 2011;7:1367-1375. *Review emphasizing its role in cholangiocarcinoma.*
Sripa B, Kaewkes, S, Intapan PM, et al. Food-borne trematodiases in Southeast Asia: epidemiology, pathology, clinical manifestation and control. *Adv Parasitol.* 2010;72:305-350. *Review.*

365

INTESTINAL NEMATODE INFECTIONS

DAVID J. DIEMERT

DEFINITION

Nematodes are nonsegmented roundworms that belong to the phylum Nematoda. Most species are free-living in soil or water but a few parasitize humans. These infections are some of the most prevalent and affect millions worldwide. Nematodes are complex multicellular organisms with specialized organs that include a protective outer coating or cuticle, a complete and functional gastrointestinal tract, and muscular, nervous, and reproductive systems.

Nematodes of medical importance can be divided into those that primarily affect the gastrointestinal tract, where adult worms become established and cause disease, and those that affect other tissues and organ systems. The former group is covered in this chapter and includes the roundworm *Ascaris lumbricoides*, the hookworms (*Ancylostoma duodenale*, *Necator americanus*), the pinworm *Enterobius vermicularis*, the whipworm *Trichuris trichiura*, and the threadworm *Strongyloides stercoralis*. Zoonotic intestinal nematodes such as *Trichostrongylus* and *Anisakis* also occasionally infect and cause disease in the gastrointestinal tract of humans. Nematodes that invade and cause disease primarily in tissues outside the gastrointestinal tract include those that cause lymphatic filariasis (*Wuchereria bancrofti*, *Brugia malayi*, and *Brugia timori*), *Onchocerca volvulus*, *Loa loa*, the guinea worm *Dracunculus medinensis*, *Trichinella spiralis*, and *Angiostrongylus* species.

Nematodes that infect humans vary from several millimeters to more than a meter in length and can often survive for months to years within their host. With the exception of *S. stercoralis* and *Capillaria philippinensis*, adult worms cannot replicate within the host. Instead, eggs or larvae are produced after the mating of sexually mature adult worms.

Nematode infections are rarely acutely fatal; they more commonly result in chronic morbidity such as iron deficiency anemia caused by hookworm infection or elephantiasis caused by lymphatic filariasis. For most nematodes, the severity of the clinical manifestations of infection are proportional to the worm burden in a given host; although light infections with only a few worms are usually asymptomatic, pathologic features appear with heavier worm burdens.

Nematode infections are highly prevalent in the temperate and tropical regions of Africa, Asia, and Latin America. They are transmitted by the oral ingestion of embryonated eggs or by penetration of infective larvae through the skin, either by direct contact with contaminated soil or by blood-feeding arthropod vectors. The prevalence of nematode infections is highest in areas with poor sanitation, where the environment is contaminated by human waste, or in climates that are conducive to survival of the insect vector.

In communities located in endemic areas, the distribution of infections is overdispersed such that most individuals harbor low numbers of worms whereas a minority have relatively high worm burdens and contribute disproportionally to both transmission and morbidity.

ASCARIASIS

The Pathogen

A. lumbricoides, also known as roundworm, is acquired by the oral ingestion of embryonated eggs. After the egg's protective outer shell is dissolved by gastric acid, larvae are released into the small intestine, where they penetrate the intestinal wall; migrate to the liver and then the pulmonary vasculature, where they break into the alveolar spaces; and ascend the bronchial tree and are swallowed to re-enter the small intestine, where they develop into adult, egg-laying worms (if female) approximately 9 to 11 weeks after egg ingestion. Adult worms (Fig. 365-1) are the largest intestinal nematodes and range in length between 15 and 50 cm and can survive in the host for approximately 18 months. A female adult *Ascaris* worm produces approximately 240,000 eggs per day, which are passed in feces. Fertilized unembryonated eggs require warm, moist, shady soil for embryonation to occur, after which they become infective (Fig. 365-2). Eggs in the environment are extremely hardy and resistant to extreme temperatures and desiccation.

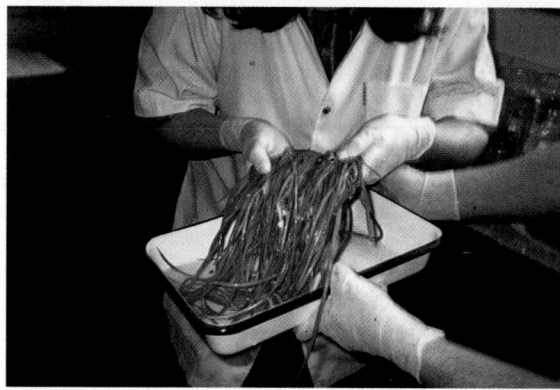

FIGURE 365-1. Mass of adult *Ascaris lumbricoides* worms recovered from a child after the administration of mebendazole. (Reproduced with permission from Dickson Despommier.)

FIGURE 365-2. Fertilized, unembryonated egg of *Ascaris lumbricoides*. (Reproduced with permission from Dickson Despommier.)

EPIDEMIOLOGY

A. lumbricoides is the most prevalent nematode infection worldwide, with approximately a billion people chronically infected. Infection is common in sub-Saharan Africa, south and Southeast Asia, and Latin America, especially in rural areas of high population density with inadequate sanitation or treatment of sewage and where untreated human feces are used as fertilizer. Climate is also an important determinant of disease in that warm temperature and adequate moisture are required for embryonation of eggs in the soil. In endemic areas, the prevalence and intensity of infection with *A. lumbricoides* increase dramatically during the first 2 to 3 years of life; it remains high between the ages of 4 and 15 years and then declines during adulthood.

CLINICAL MANIFESTATIONS

Infection with *A. lumbricoides* is most commonly asymptomatic. Clinical manifestations are usually associated with heavy worm burdens and can be classified into those associated with larval migration through the lungs and into acute and chronic manifestations resulting from parasitism of the gastrointestinal tract by adult worms.

When migrating through the lungs, *Ascaris* larvae can induce an intense reaction that is due to both the physical disruption that their migration causes and the dramatic inflammatory hypersensitivity response to secreted antigens. This phenomenon is more common in areas in which transmission is seasonal, such as on the Arabian peninsula, where outbreaks of pneumonitis typically follow the rainy season because of resumption of transmission. Symptoms may last for 2 to 3 weeks and include a sudden onset of wheezing, dyspnea, paroxysmal nonproductive cough, and high fever. Respiratory symptoms may coincide with or be preceded by urticarial rash, angioedema, abdominal pain, and vomiting. These symptoms are usually self-limited and resolve spontaneously.

With moderate or heavy infestations, intestinal signs and symptoms can result from obstruction caused by a mass of worms in the small intestine or migration of worms to unusual sites such as the biliary tree, pancreatic duct, or appendix. Intestinal obstruction is more common in young children because of their smaller lumen size and is characterized by colicky abdominal pain and vomiting that may progress to signs of perforation. Hepatobiliary and pancreatic ascariasis is more common in adults, presumably because their biliary tree is large enough to accommodate a migrating worm. Chronic intestinal infection can also have more insidious effects, especially in children, including decreased protein and fat absorption, deficiencies of vitamin A and C, and lactose intolerance, which in turn lead to stunted growth and impaired cognitive development.

DIAGNOSIS

The diagnosis of ascariasis is usually made by microscopic examination of a sample of feces for characteristic thick-shelled *A. lumbricoides* eggs. Pulmonary ascariasis cannot be diagnosed on the basis of identification of ova in feces because adult worms have not yet matured and begun producing eggs; instead, larvae, as well as eosinophils or Charcot-Leyden crystals (formed from the breakdown of eosinophils), may be visualized on microscopic examination of sputum. Pulmonary disease is also usually marked by peripheral eosinophilia and transient infiltrates on chest radiographs. The diagnosis of intestinal or biliary obstruction caused by *A. lumbricoides* relies increasingly on radiologic evaluation with ultrasound or endoscopic retrograde cholangiopancreatography (ERCP).

TREATMENT   Rx

Intestinal ascariasis is usually treated with a single oral dose of albendazole (Table 365-1). Alternatives include mebendazole or pyrantel pamoate. No specific treatment is recommended for pulmonary ascariasis because the condition is self-limited. In severe cases of biliary obstruction, such as those with cholangitis, ERCP with or without resection of the ampulla of Vater has proved highly successful and may reduce the need for surgical intervention.

PREVENTION

The major means of preventing *Ascaris* infection is improvement of hygiene and proper disposal of human waste. In endemic communities where this is not feasible, control efforts center on regular (at least annual) mass administration of an anthelmintic medication such as albendazole or mebendazole.

● HOOKWORM

The Pathogen

Hookworm infection in humans is due almost exclusively to two species: *N. americanus* and *A. duodenale*. Humans may also be incidentally infected by the zoonotic hookworms *Ancylostoma caninum*, *Ancylostoma braziliensis*, *Bunostomum phlebotomum*, and *Uncinaria stenocephala*, which can cause self-limited dermatologic lesions in the form of cutaneous larva migrans (Fig. 365-3). Additionally, *Ancylostoma ceylanicum*, normally a hookworm infecting cats, has been reported to cause intestinal hookworm disease in humans, especially in Asia, whereas *A. caninum* has been implicated as a cause of eosinophilic enteritis in Australia.

Infection occurs when exposed skin comes in contact with infective filariform larvae in contaminated soil or grass. Larvae are able to penetrate the skin, enter the afferent circulation, and migrate to the pulmonary vasculature, where they break into the alveolar spaces, ascend the bronchial tree to the trachea, and are swallowed into the gastrointestinal tract. Larvae undergo two molts to mature into adult worms approximately 5 to 9 weeks after skin penetration. Adult hookworms reside in the lumen of the upper part of the small intestine, where they attach to the mucosa by means of cutting teeth in the case of *A. duodenale* or a rounded cutting plate in the case of *N. americanus*. After mating in the host intestinal tract, each female adult worm produces thousands of eggs per day, which then exit the body in feces; *A. duodenale* female worms lay approximately 28,000 eggs daily, whereas the output from *N. americanus* worms is considerably less, averaging around 10,000 a day. Hookworm eggs hatch in warm, moist soil and give rise to larvae that can infect another host. Humans are the only major definitive host for these two parasites, and there are no intermediate or reservoir hosts. *A. duodenale* survives on average for 1 year in the human intestine, whereas *N. americanus* generally lives for 3 to 5 years.

EPIDEMIOLOGY

More than 500 million people are infected with hookworms worldwide. *N. americanus* is the most widespread hookworm globally, whereas *A. duodenale*

TABLE 365-1   TREATMENT OF INTESTINAL NEMATODES

NEMATODE	TREATMENT
Ascaris lumbricoides	Albendazole, 400 mg once. Alternative: mebendazole, 100 mg bid for 3 days
Hookworm	Albendazole, 400 mg once. Alternatives: mebendazole, 500 mg once or 100 mg bid for 3 days, or pyrantel pamoate, 11 mg/kg for 3 days with the maximum daily dose not to exceed 1 g
Trichuris trichiura	Mebendazole, 100 mg bid, or albendazole, 400 mg daily, for 3 days
Enterobius vermicularis	Pyrantel pamoate, 11 mg/kg once, with a second dose 2 wk later; maximum dose of 1 g. Alternatives: mebendazole, 100 mg once, or albendazole, 400 mg once, repeated in 2 wk
Strongyloides stercoralis	Uncomplicated infection: ivermectin, 200 μg/kg daily for 2 days.* Alternative: albendazole, 400 mg daily for 7 days
Trichostrongylus spp	Pyrantel pamoate, 11 mg/kg once; maximum dose of 1 g. Alternatives: albendazole, 400 mg once, or mebendazole, 100 mg bid for 3 days
Capillaria philippinensis	Albendazole, 400 mg daily for 10 days. Alternative: mebendazole, 200 mg bid for 20 days

*Treatment may need to be extended in immunocompromised patients with disseminated disease.

FIGURE 365-3. Typical lesion of cutaneous larva migrans. An erythematous, serpiginous track caused by intradermal migration of a dog (*Ancylostoma caninum*) or cat (*Ancylostoma braziliense*) hookworm larva is apparent. (Reproduced with permission from Gregory L. Zalar.)

is more geographically restricted in distribution. The highest prevalence of infection occurs in rural areas of tropical and less developed countries, where environmental and socioeconomic conditions favor transmission. Climate is an important determinant of hookworm transmission, with adequate moisture and warm temperature being essential for larval development in soil. An equally important determinant of infection is poverty and inadequate sanitation and supply of clean water. In endemic areas, prevalence increases with age in young children and reaches a plateau by around 10 years of age, whereas the intensity of infection rises at a slower rate during childhood, reaches a plateau by around 20 years, and then increases again in the elderly. Whether such age dependency reflects differences in exposure, acquired immunity, or a combination of both is controversial.

Although cutaneous larva migrans is found throughout the tropics, in the United States it is diagnosed primarily in tourists who have recently returned from a vacation to a tropical beach destination, especially in the Caribbean, Brazil, Mexico, and Southeast Asia. Occasionally, autochthonous cases (originating where found) have been reported in the United States, usually from southeastern coastal states such as Florida and South Carolina. Most commonly, cutaneous larva migrans occurs when exposed skin comes in contact with the larval stages of the dog or cat hookworm *A. caninum* or *A. braziliense*, respectively, present in moist soil or sand (especially on beaches) contaminated with animal feces. Other animal hookworms such as *U. stenocephala* and *B. phlebotomum* are less common causes.

PATHOBIOLOGY

The major pathology of hookworm infection is due to the associated gastrointestinal blood loss and the resulting iron deficiency anemia. Hookworms attach to the intestinal mucosa and secrete enzymes that enable them to invade submucosal tissues and ingest villous tissue and blood. Hemoglobinases within the hookworm's digestive canal enable degradation of human hemoglobin for use as an essential nutrient source. The amount of blood loss is directly related to the total worm burden. *A. duodenale* causes more blood loss than *N. americanus* does, with each *N. americanus* worm producing a daily blood loss of 0.03 to 0.1 mL and the corresponding figure for *A. duodenale* being between 0.15 and 0.26 mL.

CLINICAL MANIFESTATIONS

The clinical features of hookworm infection can be separated into acute manifestations associated with larval migration through the skin and other tissues and acute and chronic manifestations resulting from parasitism of the gastrointestinal tract by adult worms. Repeated exposure to hookworm larvae can result in a hypersensitivity reaction known as "ground itch," a pruritic local erythematous and papular rash that appears most commonly on the hands and feet. In contrast, when zoonotic hookworm larvae penetrate the skin to produce cutaneous larva migrans, most commonly on the feet, thighs, and buttocks, they are unable to complete their life cycle in the human host and eventually die after causing a typical clinical syndrome of intensely pruritic erythematous linear tracks with a serpiginous appearance (see Fig. 365-3). Tracks appear after an incubation period of a few days, can be single or multiple, and advance by millimeters to a few centimeters each day. Vesiculobullous or papular lesions may develop along the tracks, as can secondary bacterial infection as a result of scratching. Lesions usually heal spontaneously within weeks to months after the larvae die in the skin.

Migration of hookworm larvae through the lungs may induce mild and transient pulmonary symptoms consisting of a dry cough, sore throat, wheezing, and low-grade fever. Acute symptomatic disease may also result from the oral ingestion of *A. duodenale* larvae, referred to as the Wakana syndrome, which is characterized by nausea, vomiting, pharyngeal irritation, cough, dyspnea, and hoarseness.

Abdominal symptoms and signs caused by hookworm infection are rare. Instead, the manifestations of hookworm disease occur when blood loss via infection exceeds the nutritional reserves of the host and results in iron deficiency anemia. Usually only moderate- and high-intensity (≥2000 eggs per gram of feces) hookworm infections in the gastrointestinal tract produce clinical manifestations, which resemble those of iron deficiency anemia secondary to other causes (Chapter 162). In addition, the protein losses associated with heavy hookworm infection can result in hypoproteinemia and anasarca. The anemia and protein malnutrition that result from chronic intestinal parasitism cause long-term impairments in childhood physical, intellectual, and cognitive development. As iron deficiency anemia develops and worsens, an infected individual may have weakness, palpitations, fainting, dizziness, dyspnea, mental apathy, and headache. Uncommonly, there may be constipation or diarrhea with occult blood in the stool or frank melena, especially in children; there may also be an urge to eat soil (pica). Overwhelming hookworm infection may cause listlessness, coma, and even death, especially in infants. Because children and women of reproductive age have reduced iron reserves, they are at particular risk with hookworm disease. The severe iron deficiency anemia that may arise from hookworm disease during pregnancy can result in adverse consequences for the mother, her unborn fetus, and the neonate.

DIAGNOSIS

The diagnosis of hookworm infection is made primarily by microscopic identification of characteristic eggs in the stool. The eggs of *N. americanus* and *A. duodenale* cannot be distinguished because both are colorless and have a single thin hyaline shell with blunted ends; they range in size from 55 to 75 μm by 36 to 40 μm. Egg concentration techniques, such as the formalin–ethyl acetate sedimentation method, can be used to detect even light infections, although a direct wet mount examination is adequate for detecting moderate to heavy infections. In addition, eosinophilia is a common finding with persistent infection and also during larval migration through the lungs.

TREATMENT

A single oral dose of albendazole, 400 mg, is the recommended treatment of intestinal hookworm infection (see Table 365-1).[1] Alternatives include mebendazole and pyrantel pamoate. For cutaneous larva migrans, although the disease is self-limited and will resolve spontaneously within weeks to a few months, treatment with a single dose of ivermectin will lead to rapid resolution of the symptoms and skin manifestations. Albendazole is an alternative treatment of cutaneous larva migrans.

PREVENTION

The ideal method for preventing hookworm infection is improvement in hygiene and proper disposal of human waste. In endemic communities where this is not feasible, control of disease centers on the regular (at least annual) mass administration of an anthelmintic medication such as albendazole or mebendazole. For cutaneous larva migrans, tourists should be advised to wear shoes or sandals when walking to and on beaches and to avoid beaches frequented by stray cats and dogs.

TRICHURIASIS

The Pathogen

Infection with *T. trichiura*, also known as whipworm, does not have a tissue migratory phase like *A. lumbricoides* and hookworm, and its entire life cycle in the host is limited to the gastrointestinal tract. After embryonated eggs are ingested orally, larvae are released into the small intestine where they undergo a series of molts before being carried passively to the transverse and descending colon. The narrow anterior end of adult worms embeds in the columnar epithelium, with the posterior portion protruding into the lumen, thereby allowing eggs to be released into feces, which are then passed into the environment where they must embryonate in warm, moist soil to complete the life cycle. Adult worms can measure up to 50 mm in length and can survive in the host for approximately 1.5 to 2 years. The period between ingestion of eggs and detection of eggs in feces is about 90 days.

EPIDEMIOLOGY

Like the other soil-transmitted helminths, trichuriasis is most common in poor, mostly rural areas of the tropics and subtropics where disposal of human waste is inadequate. The estimated prevalence worldwide is 800 million. Children are more frequently infected than adults and more likely to have higher worm burdens. Humans are the only host for this parasite.

CLINICAL MANIFESTATIONS

The majority of *T. trichiura* infections are asymptomatic. Most disease is seen in children because the majority of heavy infections (>10,000 eggs per gram of feces) occur in this age group. Heavy infections can be accompanied by acute dysentery or chronic colitis resembling inflammatory bowel disease and result in abdominal pain and diarrhea. The chronic mucosal inflammation and edema of the colon and rectum can lead to protracted tenesmus and resulting rectal prolapse. Chronic *Trichuris* colitis can also lead to malnutrition, impaired growth, and anemia.

DIAGNOSIS

Infection is diagnosed by identification of the typical barrel-shaped eggs with bipolar plugs in direct or concentrated smears of fecal specimens.

TREATMENT

Although *T. trichiura* responds less effectively than *A. lumbricoides* or hookworm to treatment with albendazole or mebendazole, a 3-day course of one of these two benzimidazole drugs is the recommended therapy, as listed in Table 365-1. The addition of ivermectin (200 μg/kg) to either drug increases the response rate significantly.[2]

ENTEROBIASIS

The Pathogen

E. vermicularis, or pinworm, is transmitted by the fecal-oral route. Embryonated eggs on fingernails, bed clothing, or bedding are ingested and hatch in the upper part of the small intestine, where they develop into adults before taking residence in the large intestine. Adult worms measuring between 2 and

5 mm live freely in the lumen of the colon, where they mate. Gravid female worms migrate nightly out of the rectum and deposit large numbers of eggs (11,000 per worm) on the perianal and perineal areas. The eggs rapidly embryonate within 6 hours after being laid. If they are still on the skin, infective larvae are released that can migrate back through the anus into the rectum (retroinfection). In infected females, larvae may also migrate into the genital tract and establish an ectopic infection.

EPIDEMIOLOGY

E. vermicularis is the most prevalent nematode infection found in temperate climes, but it is also found worldwide. Transmission is especially frequent in primary schools and daycare centers where children are in close contact. Up to a quarter of all children worldwide are estimated to be infected with pinworm.

CLINICAL MANIFESTATIONS

Although most pinworm infections are asymptomatic, perianal pruritus is the most common symptom and is caused by an allergic response to worm proteins. The pruritus can be intense and result in chronic sleep deprivation. Rarely, *E. vermicularis* may cause appendicitis, and when hatched larvae migrate into the female genital tract, vulvovaginitis, salpingitis, or peritonitis may develop.

DIAGNOSIS

Pinworm infection is diagnosed by identifying eggs on a piece of cellophane tape applied to the perianal region immediately after waking and before bathing. Characteristic *E. vermicularis* eggs are oval and slightly flattened on one side. It is unusual to find eggs in feces or adult worms in the perianal area. Repeated examination may be necessary.

TREATMENT   Rx

Pinworm infection is treated with a single dose of pyrantel pamoate, mebendazole, or albendazole, which must be repeated 2 weeks later because the drugs do not kill eggs or developing larvae (see Table 365-1). Given the high rate of transmission, all household members and individuals in close contact with the patient (e.g., other children attending the same daycare center) should be treated as well. Bedding and underclothes should be thoroughly washed with hot water to remove and kill the eggs.

⬤ STRONGYLOIDIASIS

The Pathogen

S. stercoralis, or threadworm, infection is endemic in warm climates worldwide, including parts of the United States. Infection occurs when exposed skin comes in contact with free-living filariform larvae living in contaminated soil. After penetrating the skin, larvae enter the afferent circulation and travel to the pulmonary vasculature, where they rupture into the alveolar spaces, ascend the respiratory tree, and are swallowed into the gastrointestinal tract. Further development into adult worms occurs in the upper part of the small intestine, where parasites live embedded in the columnar epithelium. Unlike most nematodes, *S. stercoralis* reproduces by parthenogenesis, with no apparent parasitic male worm present in human infection. Female worms begin laying eggs within 25 to 30 days after infection. The embryonated eggs hatch rapidly in the lumen of the small intestine and release rhabditiform larvae that migrate to the colon and are passed in feces. Alternatively, larvae may directly penetrate the colonic mucosa or perianal skin after migrating out of the anus and enter the circulation directly, a mechanism known as autoinfection. This phenomenon can lead to maintenance of parasitism in the host for decades.

Infective filariform larvae develop in the soil by direct transformation from rhabditiform larvae or indirectly from eggs produced by free-living adult worms that have developed from rhabditiform larvae in warm, moist, sandy soil.

A less common type of strongyloidiasis, called swollen belly syndrome, has been attributed to infection with *Strongyloides fuelleborni* in infants living in sub-Saharan Africa and Papua New Guinea.

EPIDEMIOLOGY

S. stercoralis infection is endemic in the tropical and subtropical regions of sub-Saharan Africa, Asia, Latin America, and areas of eastern and southern Europe, with a worldwide prevalence of between 30 and 100 million. In the United States, infection is diagnosed most frequently in immigrants, commonly from Southeast Asia, although strongyloidiasis is still endemic in parts of rural Appalachia.

PATHOBIOLOGY

In immunologically competent individuals, infection is usually asymptomatic or is associated with mild gastrointestinal symptoms. The main complications of infection with this parasite, however, occur in individuals with cell-mediated immunodeficiency such as those chronically taking corticosteroids, renal transplant recipients, patients with Hodgkin's disease and other lymphomas, leukemic patients, and those infected with human T-cell lymphotropic virus type 1. In these individuals, the autoinfection cycle of the *S. stercoralis* life cycle can become amplified and lead to a hyperinfection syndrome with a large increase in the total worm load in the infected person. Hyperinfection can lead to life-threatening dissemination of larvae and adult worms to aberrant sites such as the brain, pancreas, and kidneys. For unknown reasons, advanced acquired immunodeficiency syndrome has not been associated with hyperinfection syndrome or with disseminated strongyloidiasis. Disseminated strongyloidiasis is frequently accompanied by bacterial sepsis, probably as a result of translocation of enteric organisms carried by migrating larvae.

CLINICAL MANIFESTATIONS

As mentioned previously, most *S. stercoralis* infections, especially in immunocompetent hosts, are asymptomatic or, at most, associated with mild gastrointestinal manifestations such as abdominal pain, bloating, and watery diarrhea. Gastrointestinal bleeding, manifested by hematochezia or melena, occurs in less than 20% of those infected. Rare causes of morbidity related to intestinal *S. stercoralis* infection are small bowel obstruction, paralytic ileus, and a malabsorption syndrome (especially in children).

During the migratory phase of larvae through the lungs, symptoms are rare in immunocompetent patients, although infection may be accompanied by peripheral eosinophilia. However, pulmonary signs and symptoms in immunocompromised persons with hyperinfection syndrome can be severe and resemble those of adult respiratory distress syndrome with an acute onset of dyspnea, productive cough, and hemoptysis accompanied by fever, tachypnea, and hypoxemia.

Migration of filariform larvae from the anus can lead to a dermatologic manifestation known as larva currens, which is characterized by serpiginous erythematous maculopapular tracks and occasionally urticarial lesions on the skin of the buttocks, upper aspect of the thighs, and lower part of the abdomen.

Autoinfection leading to exceptionally high worm loads (i.e., hyperinfection) and disseminated strongyloidiasis can occur in persons with deficient cell-mediated immunity. Because *S. stercoralis* may persist and the person may remain asymptomatic for decades after exposure, it is important to remember that a change in immune status associated with conditions such as the administration of immunosuppressive drugs following solid organ transplantation may result in hyperinfection syndrome even though the infection was previously asymptomatic. Massive increases in the number of *Strongyloides* larvae because of hyperinfection can be manifested as acute enteritis with severe diarrhea and ulcerative disease of the small and large intestine. During disseminated infection, larvae and sometimes adult worms penetrate the intestinal mucosa, migrate to aberrant sites, including the central nervous system, and result in metastatic abscesses and gram-negative meningitis as a result of the enteric bacteria carried by the migrating parasites. Less common complications of disseminated disease include glomerulonephritis and minimal-change nephrotic syndrome, acute respiratory distress syndrome, and alveolar hemorrhage. Mortality from hyperinfection and disseminated disease can be high, although early diagnosis and prompt initiation of treatment are associated with improved outcomes.

Infants with swollen belly syndrome caused by *S. fuelleborni* are often seen acutely with abdominal ascites that is not accompanied by diarrhea or fever. The ascites is due to gastrointestinal protein loss; it can be significant enough to cause respiratory impairment and is associated with a high rate of mortality.

DIAGNOSIS

Definitive diagnosis of *S. stercoralis* infection relies on microscopic identification of larvae in feces or other fluids (such as sputum) or tissues. Detection of filariform larvae in feces implies active autoinfection. Intestinal strongyloidiasis can be diagnosed by identification of larvae in direct smears of freshly passed stool, although the sensitivity of examining a single fecal sample is as low as 30%. Sensitivity can be increased by examining multiple fecal specimens, by using concentration techniques, and by plating feces on an agar plate and inspecting for tracks of colonies created by bacteria being dragged by migrating larvae. Incubating stool mixed with bone charcoal can also enhance recovery (the Harada-Mori culture technique).

Hyperinfection syndrome and disseminated strongyloidiasis can be diagnosed by detection of filariform larvae in duodenal fluid obtained by endoscopy, in sputum, or in bronchoalveolar lavage specimens. Larvae have also been recovered from cerebrospinal fluid, urine, peritoneal washings, skin, and the brains of immunocompromised persons.

Fluctuating eosinophilia is common with uncomplicated intestinal strongyloidiasis, especially during the pulmonary migration phase of initial infection. However, eosinophilia may be absent in patients with hyperinfection and dissemination. In fact, those with hyperinfection and eosinophilia appear to have a better prognosis than do those without eosinophilia.

Serologic diagnosis using an enzyme-linked immunosorbent assay (ELISA) that detects antibodies to filariform larval antigens is both sensitive and specific, even in immunocompromised hosts with disseminated strongyloidiasis.

TREATMENT Rx

Uncomplicated intestinal strongyloidiasis can be treated effectively with ivermectin (200 µg/kg body weight daily for 2 days), with cure rates in excess of 90%. Albendazole is an alternative treatment (see Table 365-1). Decreases in serologic antibody titer and eosinophilia indicate a treatment response in the absence of continued exposure. After 6 months, antibody titers should fall significantly.

In immunocompromised patients with hyperinfection or disseminated disease, daily treatment should be extended. Some experts recommend continuing treatment until 2 weeks after fecal examinations have become negative (i.e., for one autoinfection cycle). For severely ill patients who are unable to tolerate oral therapy, parenteral veterinary and enema ivermectin preparations have been used. Combination therapy with ivermectin and albendazole may also be used to treat disseminated strongyloidiasis, but data on whether this improves prognosis over monotherapy are lacking.

PREVENTION

In endemic areas, the risk for infection can be reduced by minimizing skin contact with contaminated soil, although elimination of this infection will occur only with improvements in sanitation and treatment of human waste. To prevent hyperinfection in individuals already infected, diagnosis should be attempted before the onset of immunosuppression if possible, such as before organ transplantation or cancer chemotherapy. Anyone who has resided in or traveled to an endemic area should undergo screening for asymptomatic infection, preferably by ELISA or, if not possible, by examination of at least three fecal samples for the presence of larvae. Patients with positive screening test results should be treated empirically with ivermectin. Individuals with negative screening test results but unexplained eosinophilia and a history of exposure should also be considered for empirical treatment. In those undergoing hematopoietic stem cell transplantation, documentation of cure with at least three consecutive negative fecal examinations is recommended before proceeding with transplantation.

UNCOMMON INTESTINAL NEMATODIASES

Humans may serve as accidental hosts for several nematodes that ordinarily parasitize the intestines of other mammals.

Trichostrongylus

Human infection with several different species of the genus *Trichostrongylus* has been reported in Iran, the Far East, and Australia. Humans are incidentally infected when larvae are ingested with leafy vegetables that have been contaminated with soil containing the feces of herbivorous animals. *Trichostrongylus* worms are similar to hookworms in their morphology, appearance of their eggs on fecal examination, and the pathology that they induce. Heavy infections may be accompanied by diarrhea and anemia. Drugs recommended for treatment are pyrantel pamoate, albendazole, or mebendazole (see Table 365-1).

Anisakiasis

Anisakiasis results from ingestion of the larvae of nematodes that normally infect sea mammals such as dolphins, whales, and seals. Larvae of the genera *Anisakis*, *Phocanema*, and *Pseudoterranova* infect the flesh of a number of saltwater fish species as intermediate hosts. Consumption of raw or undercooked fish, often in the form of sushi or sashimi, results in release of the infective larvae into the stomach, followed by invasion of the stomach or duodenal wall, which causes upper abdominal pain that can sometimes be intense. Anisakid worms cannot further develop in humans and die within a few days; an eosinophilic granulomatous reaction is provoked that may mimic a gastric tumor. Diagnosis and treatment are accomplished by endoscopic removal of the parasite. Infection is prevented by cooking or freezing seafood before consumption. Of note, salting, smoking, and marinating fish do not kill anisakid larvae.

Capillaria philippinensis

C. philippinensis can cause a serious intestinal infection that has been reported primarily in the Philippines and Thailand, although it has also been observed in Japan, Taiwan, Korea, and Egypt. Adult worms resemble those of *T. spiralis*, although biologically they mimic *S. stercoralis* in that they have an autoinfectious cycle of reproduction in which larvae can develop into adult worms within the host. Even though the life cycle is not completely known, this nematode probably parasitizes waterfowl that feed on fish and crustaceans, which serve as intermediate hosts. Humans become infected by eating raw or undercooked infected shrimp or fish. Adult worms travel to the mucosal crypts of the small intestine, where they deposit living larvae, sometimes resulting in overwhelming infection. Clinical disease consists of severe diarrhea associated with anorexia, vomiting, and weight loss. Mortality rates as high as 10% have been reported, with death resulting from severe malabsorption and protein-losing enteropathy. Diagnosis depends on finding eggs or larvae in feces. The treatment of choice is albendazole or mebendazole (see Table 365-1).

Other Intestinal Nematode Infections

Several nematodes that normally parasitize the intestine of nonhuman primates very rarely infect the human gastrointestinal tract. *Oesophagostomum bifurcum* infections have been reported from Africa, Asia, and South America and result from the oral ingestion of infective larvae. Adult worms can result in the formation of nodules in the intestinal wall that may be manifested as abdominal masses. Finally, infection with *Ternidens diminutus* has been reported to result in colonic ulcerations and nodular lesions in people living in southern Africa.

1. Keiser J, Utzinger J. Efficacy of current drugs against soil-transmitted helminth infections: systematic review and meta-analysis. *JAMA.* 2008;299:1937-1948.
2. Knopp S, Mohammed KA, Speich B, et al. Albendazole and mebendazole administered alone or in combination with ivermectin against *Trichuris trichiura*: a randomized controlled trial. *Clin Infect Dis.* 2010;51:1420-1428.

SUGGESTED READINGS

Alam S, Mustafa G, Rahman S, et al. Comparative study on presentation of biliary ascariasis with dead and living worms. *Saudi J Gastroenterol.* 2010;16:203-206. *Biliary ascariasis with dead worms is more dangerous because it is associated with choledocholithiasis, hepatolithiasis, liver abscess, and cirrhosis.*

Dold C, Holland CV. Ascaris and ascariasis. *Microbes Infect.* 2011. [Epub ahead of print.] *Review from a public health perspective.*

Marcos LA, Terashima A, Canales M, et al. Update on strongyloidiasis in the immunocompromised host. *Curr Infect Dis Rep.* 2011;13:35-46. *Review.*

366

TISSUE NEMATODE INFECTIONS

DAVID J. DIEMERT

The tissue nematodes can be broadly divided into those that normally infect animals but can incidentally infect humans and those for which humans serve as the principal host (the filariases). Several zoonotic nematodes, such as *Toxocara canis*, *Trichinella spiralis*, and *Angiostrongylus cantonensis*, can infect humans through accidental oral ingestion of helminth eggs or larvae but are unable to complete their life cycle in the host. Clinical manifestations are primarily due to the aberrant migration of larvae through various tissues.

TOXOCARIASIS

DEFINITION

Accidental ingestion of embryonated eggs of the dog roundworm *Toxocara canis*, or less frequently of the cat roundworm *Toxocara cati*, can lead to the clinical syndromes of visceral larva migrans and ocular larva migrans. Symptoms are caused by the aberrant migration of larvae through the body, invading organs to cause serious disease and even death.

EPIDEMIOLOGY

Toxocara infections in animals are ubiquitous in their distribution throughout the world and are more common in younger animals than in adults. In humans, children are most frequently infected, probably because they are more likely to ingest soil contaminated with feces of dogs and cats, such as when playing in sandboxes or playgrounds. Although robust epidemiologic data are lacking, recent evidence suggests that this infection may be one of the most common helminthic diseases in North America and Europe, particularly in inner-city urban areas. Visceral larva migrans occurs most commonly in children younger than 5 years, whereas ocular larva migrans typically affects older children between the ages of 5 and 10 years.

PATHOBIOLOGY

The life cycle of *Toxocara* in its normal animal host resembles that of *Ascaris* in humans; larvae penetrate the intestinal wall after being released into the lumen from ingested eggs, migrate through the vasculature to the lungs, enter into the alveolar space, and ascend the bronchial tree until they are swallowed back into the gastrointestinal tract, where they develop into adult worms that can produce eggs. However, when embryonated *Toxocara* eggs are ingested by humans, the released larvae migrate throughout the body (most commonly the lungs, the liver, the central nervous system [CNS], and occasionally the eyes) but cannot develop into adult worms. Ultimately, the larvae die, inducing significant immediate-type and delayed-type hypersensitivity reactions that result in eosinophilic granuloma formation. Visceral larva migrans and ocular larva migrans seem to be mutually exclusive, suggesting that different *Toxocara* strains may have different tissue tropisms. Alternatively, visceral larva migrans may result from repeated infections, whereas ocular larva migrans may be a manifestation of infection in children who have not been previously sensitized.

CLINICAL MANIFESTATIONS

Most *Toxocara* infections in humans are asymptomatic. Visceral larva migrans is characterized by low-grade fever, pulmonary symptoms including cough and wheeze, and less frequently hepatosplenomegaly accompanied by right upper quadrant pain. Symptoms have a gradual onset and resolve during 4 to 8 weeks. Myocarditis, nephritis, and CNS disease are less common. CNS involvement can result in seizures, encephalopathy, neuropsychiatric symptoms, or an eosinophilic meningoencephalitis. A more subtle syndrome referred to as covert toxocariasis has been described that may result from less dramatic migration of larvae through organs. For example, *T. canis* has been suggested as an environmental risk factor for asthma in inner-city populations.

Ocular larva migrans typically presents as unilateral visual impairment that is sometimes accompanied by strabismus. The degree of vision loss is dependent on the particular ocular structure involved, and permanent blindness can occur. Ocular larva migrans involving the retina can be difficult to distinguish from other causes of focal intraretinal lesions, such as retinoblastoma or tuberculosis.

DIAGNOSIS

Toxocariasis can be presumed on the basis of a compatible clinical presentation and history of exposure to dogs or cats. Eosinophilia and hypergammaglobulinemia may be present. Serologic diagnosis by an enzyme-linked immunosorbent assay (ELISA) that employs antigens secreted by second-stage larvae to measure anti-*Toxocara* antibodies may be informative. Although establishment of sensitivity and specificity is difficult because of the inability to make a definitive parasitologic diagnosis, it is estimated that when a titer cutoff of 1 : 32 is used, the sensitivity of the ELISA is 78% for visceral larva migrans but lower for ocular larva migrans; specificity for both syndromes is greater than 90%. Biopsy of tissues to document the presence of larvae is not recommended because of its low sensitivity.

Computed tomography and fluorescein angiography may be helpful in the diagnosis of ocular larva migrans, especially to differentiate it from retinoblastoma and other causes of intraocular space-occupying lesions. Anti-*Toxocara* antibodies can be detected in aqueous and vitreous humor fluid, and elevated levels relative to serum are suggestive of ocular larva migrans.

TREATMENT   Rx

Albendazole (400 mg given twice daily for 5 days) is the treatment of choice for toxocariasis (Table 366-1). Mebendazole is not recommended because of its poor oral bioavailability. In patients with severe pulmonary, cardiac, or neurologic involvement, corticosteroids may be used to reduce symptoms and to shorten the duration of the illness. Ocular larva migrans is treated by vitrectomy, albendazole, or corticosteroids.
See also Chapter 352.

PREVENTION

Visceral larva migrans and ocular larva migrans may be prevented by periodic treatment of dogs and cats with anthelmintics, cleaning up after pets and properly disposing of their feces, covering sandboxes, washing hands after playing with dogs or cats, and keeping children from playing in places where pets have defecated.

TABLE 366-1	TREATMENT OF TISSUE NEMATODE INFECTIONS
NEMATODE INFECTION	**TREATMENT**
Toxocariasis	Albendazole, 400 mg twice daily for 5 days
Trichinellosis	Albendazole, 400 mg twice daily for 8-14 days*
Angiostrongyliasis	Treatment with albendazole or mebendazole is controversial but may relieve symptoms.
Gnathostomiasis	Surgical removal Alternatives: albendazole, 400 mg daily for 3 weeks; ivermectin, 200 µg/kg/day for 2 days
Lymphatic filariasis	Diethylcarbamazine, 6 mg/kg/day divided in 3 doses for 12 days† Alternative: doxycycline, 100-200 mg/day for 4-8 weeks
Onchocerciasis	Ivermectin, 150 µg/kg once, repeated every 6-12 months until resolution of symptoms
Loiasis	Diethylcarbamazine, 6 mg/kg/day divided in 3 doses for 12-21 days†,‡
Mansonella perstans	Doxycycline, 200 mg/day for 6 weeks
Mansonella ozzardi	Ivermectin, 200 µg/kg once
Mansonella streptocerca	Diethylcarbamazine, 6 mg/kg/day divided in 3 doses for 12 days Alternative: ivermectin, 150 µg/kg once
Dracunculiasis	Extraction of the adult worm

*Treatment is effective only if it is initiated during the intestinal phase of infection.
†Start at a dose of 50 mg on the first day, 50 mg three times/day on the second, 100 mg three times/day on the third, and then 6 mg/kg/day on day 4 onward.
‡Repeated treatment after 6 months is often necessary if symptoms and eosinophilia persist.

BAYLISASCARIASIS

Baylisascariasis is a rare zoonosis caused by infection with the ascarid *Baylisascaris procyonis*, which is primarily a nematode parasite of raccoons and other small carnivores. In North America, infection is most commonly associated with contact with raccoons or environments contaminated with their feces and occurs predominantly in infants and young children who ingest the embryonated eggs while playing with soil. Clinically, disease is manifested as neural larva migrans because of the larval invasion of the CNS after release from ingested eggs in the gastrointestinal tract. Characteristic findings include fever and altered mental status accompanied by focal neurologic deficits and seizures; examination of the cerebrospinal fluid (CSF) reveals eosinophilic meningitis. *B. procyonis* has also been associated with ocular larva migrans, usually in otherwise healthy adults. Infection can be fatal or result in significant permanent neurologic or visual impairment. Once neural larva migrans is present, response to treatment with anthelmintics is poor, although corticosteroids may be helpful. Successful use of photocoagulation in ocular larva migrans has been reported. Prophylactic albendazole (25 mg/kg/day for 20 days) started within days of an exposure may prevent clinical disease.

TRICHINELLOSIS

DEFINITION

Trichinella normally infects a range of mammalian hosts, with the domestic pig serving as the most important reservoir worldwide. Humans are infected on eating raw or undercooked pork or other meats of domestic or wild animals that are contaminated with larvae that are encysted in muscle tissue. Although larvae develop into adults in the human intestinal tract, mate, and produce offspring larvae, clinical disease is characterized not so much by the intestinal infection as by the newborn larvae that penetrate through the intestinal wall and disseminate throughout the body.

EPIDEMIOLOGY

Several different species of *Trichinella* can cause disease in humans, although *Trichinella spiralis* is the most important etiologic agent. *T. spiralis* is enzootic throughout the world in omnivorous and carnivorous wild animals, including bears, boars, and rats. *Trichinella nativa* affects predominantly carnivores (e.g., walruses, polar bears, and seals) living in the Arctic and subarctic regions of North America, Europe, and Asia. *Trichinella* is introduced into domestic animal populations, usually pigs or horses, by giving them unprocessed feed containing meat scraps of infected animals, most commonly rats. Because of regulations banning this practice in the United States, Canada, and the European Union, human infection by consumption of undercooked or smoked pork products or beef contaminated with the encysted larvae has been virtually eliminated, although it still occurs throughout the rest of the world. Instead, ingestion of the flesh of poorly cooked wild game, especially bear or boar meat, is now the most common source of infection in these places. An important source of infection with *T. nativa* in Alaskan and Canadian Arctic native populations is eating of uncooked walrus meat.

PATHOBIOLOGY

Infection with *Trichinella* is initiated by ingestion of striated muscle containing encysted infective larvae. Larvae are released from muscle tissue by digestive enzymes in the stomach and then migrate to the upper two thirds of the small intestine, where they rapidly develop into sexually mature adult worms after only 2 days. Adults live embedded in the columnar epithelium, where they grow to a length of 3 mm (females) or 1.5 mm (males). Females begin producing newborn larvae within 5 days of mating. Adult worms remain viable for an additional 3 to 5 weeks, after which acquired immunity develops that leads to their expulsion from the host.

Newborn larvae possess a sword-like stylet in their oral cavity that permits them to penetrate the lamina propria and enter the lymphatic and blood vessels of the host, allowing them to be distributed throughout the body. Larvae enter all types of cells, where they usually die, with the exception of striated skeletal and cardiac muscle cells. Unique among nematodes, mature *Trichinella* larvae have an intracellular phase, developing and transforming muscle cells into "nurse cells" that support the growth and development of the larvae (Fig. 366-1). In nurse cells, parasite larvae can survive for decades. Although nurse cells do not result in any disease in most mammals, they can induce an eosinophilic granulomatous reaction in humans that may result in significant tissue damage and dysfunction.

FIGURE 366-1. Nurse cell in muscle tissue containing a larva of *Trichinella spiralis*. (Courtesy of Dr. I. Kagan, Centers for Disease Control and Prevention.)

CLINICAL MANIFESTATIONS

Clinical disease in humans can be divided into an initial intestinal phase followed by a systemic or muscle phase. The initial phase of infection that occurs within days after ingestion of larvae may be associated with mild gastrointestinal signs and symptoms such as diarrhea, abdominal pain, and vomiting. This phase is self-limited and usually resolves spontaneously within 10 days.

The systemic dissemination of *Trichinella* larvae can result in myocardial damage, pulmonary infiltration, and focal neurologic damage caused by migrating larvae, although usually only in the most heavily infected persons. This systemic phase of infection usually begins 2 to 3 weeks after ingestion of infective larvae and may persist for several weeks. Clinical manifestations typically include fever, periorbital or facial edema, a diffuse inflammatory myositis (Chapter 429) that is characterized by myalgias and muscle tenderness, and petechial hemorrhages most easily observed in the subungual skin and conjunctivae. Larval invasion of the myocardium can lead to myocarditis (Chapter 60) that may result in heart failure or arrhythmias.

As with most nematodes, the severity of symptoms is related to the total worm burden. Because adult worms are incapable of reproducing within the host, the number of encysted larvae ingested is the most important determinant of the number of larvae that invade muscle and other tissues.

DIAGNOSIS

A diagnosis of trichinellosis should be suspected in individuals with a compatible clinical presentation, a history of eating raw or undercooked meat, eosinophilia, and increased muscle enzymes such as creatine kinase and lactate dehydrogenase. Definitive diagnosis depends on visualization of nurse cells in a muscle biopsy specimen or detection of *Trichinella*-specific DNA by the polymerase chain reaction (PCR) technique, although this tool is not widely available. Findings on muscle biopsy may be normal even in heavily infected patients because of sampling error. Detection of anti-*Trichinella* antibodies can be very useful in making a diagnosis; ELISA is the most commonly used method. Antibodies can usually be detected as early as 12 days after initial infection.

TREATMENT   Rx

If patients present during the intestinal phase of infection, albendazole is recommended at a dosage of 400 mg given twice daily for 8 to 14 days to kill the adult worms and thus to prevent release of more newborn larvae (see Table 366-1). Although it is not known if albendazole is effective against newborn larvae, administration of this drug during the systemic phase of infection could potentially worsen symptoms by exacerbating the host inflammatory response to dying larvae. Treatment of severe systemic disease, including myocarditis and neurologic disease, should be directed toward reducing inflammation, most commonly with corticosteroids. Symptomatic treatment with antipyretics and analgesics should also be considered.

See also Chapter 352.

PREVENTION

Trichinella infection is prevented by thoroughly cooking meat products to kill the encysted larvae. Freezing meat solid at −20° C for at least 3 days will kill *T. spiralis* but not all other species of *Trichinella*. Of note, curing and smoking techniques do not reliably kill this nematode.

ANGIOSTRONGYLIASIS

DEFINITION

Angiostrongylus cantonensis and *Angiostrongylus costaricensis* are nematodes that normally infect rodents, primarily rats. The adult worms of *A. cantonensis*, or rat lungworm, inhabit the pulmonary arteries of rodents; larvae are produced that migrate to the pharynx, are swallowed, and then are passed in the feces. Mollusks such as snails, slugs, and prawns serve as intermediate hosts until they are ingested by definitive hosts. Released larvae migrate to the brain, where they develop into immature adult worms before traveling to the pulmonary vasculature to become sexually mature adults. Humans are incidentally infected after eating poorly cooked or raw intermediate mollusk hosts; larvae can migrate to the CNS but cannot develop further. Fresh vegetables may also serve as a vehicle of human infection if they are contaminated with parts of mollusks containing infective larvae. The life cycle of *A. costaricensis* is similar except that the adult worms reside in the arterioles of the small intestine and release eggs and larvae into the intestinal tissue, causing an intense eosinophilic granulomatous reaction.

EPIDEMIOLOGY

Human infections with *A. cantonensis* occur mainly in Southeast Asia and the South Pacific and less frequently in Africa and the Caribbean. Abdominal angiostrongyliasis due to *A. costaricensis* has been reported in Costa Rica, mostly in young children.

CLINICAL MANIFESTATIONS

In human cases of *A. cantonensis* infection, ingested larvae penetrate the intestinal wall and migrate to the brain, the meninges, and less commonly the spinal cord and eye. Fever, severe headache, meningismus, nausea, vomiting, seizures, and focal neurologic deficits may develop. As opposed to *A. cantonensis*, the larvae of *A. costaricensis* can develop into sexually mature adult worms in the local lymphatics and mesenteric arterioles of humans after penetrating the intestinal wall. Clinically, *A. costaricensis* infection can mimic appendicitis with right-sided abdominal pain, vomiting, and fever. Less frequently, gastrointestinal bleeding may occur.

DIAGNOSIS

Diagnosis of *A. cantonensis* infection is based on a history of ingestion of potentially contaminated food, the presence of peripheral eosinophilia, and detection of eosinophils and rarely larvae in the CSF. In neither meningeal nor intestinal angiostrongyliasis are larvae or eggs found in the feces, although both may be seen in specimens removed at surgery.

TREATMENT AND PREVENTION

Most patients infected with either species of *Angiostrongylus* recover completely after approximately 2 weeks. The use of anthelmintics (Chapter 352) is controversial, with only a few reports of benefit with albendazole or mebendazole, usually administered in combination with analgesics and corticosteroids to relieve symptoms. Periodic removal of CSF can relieve symptoms of raised intracranial pressure caused by infection with *A. cantonensis*. Proper cooking of food and washing of vegetables can prevent this infection.

GNATHOSTOMIASIS

Gnathostoma spinigerum is an intestinal nematode of dogs and cats; intermediate hosts include tiny crustaceans (copepods), amphibians, fish, and birds. Accidental human infection occurs throughout the Far East, Thailand, and parts of Mexico on eating of raw or undercooked invertebrate hosts harboring larvae in their tissues. Larvae are released in the intestine and subsequently migrate through the body but are unable to complete their normal life cycle in humans. The most common clinical presentation is migrating painful and pruritic subcutaneous swellings. Eosinophilic meningitis and ocular larva migrans may also occur, with potentially devastating results, including paralysis, subarachnoid hemorrhage, and permanent visual loss. Peripheral eosinophilia, often high, is usually present; with meningitis, eosinophils are also present in the CSF. There is no commercially available serologic test for this infection. Surgical removal is both diagnostic and curative. Alternatively, either a 3-week course of albendazole or a 2-day course of ivermectin (200 µg/kg/day) is recommended (see Table 366-1). The infection may be prevented by thoroughly cooking fish.

FILARIASES

DEFINITION

The filariases are a group of arthropod-borne nematode infections that are endemic mostly in tropical areas of the world. Instead of residing in the intestine, mature adult filarial worms characteristically live in the lymphatics or in connective tissue (Table 366-2). Eight filarial species infect humans: *Wuchereria bancrofti*, *Brugia malayi*, *Onchocerca volvulus*, *Brugia timori*, *Loa loa*, *Mansonella streptocerca*, *Mansonella perstans*, and *Mansonella ozzardi*. The first three are the most common filariases worldwide. Although not usually fatal, these infections can result in significant disability and disfigurement, such as irreversible limb lymphedema in the case of *W. bancrofti* and *B. malayi* or blindness in the case of *O. volvulus*. Most of the filariases require prolonged exposure for disease to be manifested and are therefore uncommon in short-term travelers to endemic areas. The one exception is loiasis, which can occur in returned travelers and expatriates who have spent extended periods in endemic regions.

For all of the filarial nematodes, infection begins with the bite of an infected arthropod vector that deposits infective larvae called microfilariae into the skin or blood. During several months, microfilariae mature into adult worms capable of mating to produce more microfilariae that can be ingested by another arthropod vector to complete the life cycle. Adult worms can survive for 5 to 17 years in the human host; microfilariae live for between 5 months and 5 years. For most of the filarial nematodes except *B. malayi* and *M. perstans*, humans are the only definitive host.

Clinical manifestations of infection are varied and are caused by either the adult worm or the migrating microfilariae. Severity of disease is in most cases directly proportional to the worm burden harbored by an individual, with relatively light infections commonly being asymptomatic. For several of the filariases, the host inflammatory response to infection becomes apparent only on the death of the adult worm or microfilariae. This may be triggered by exposure to filarial antigens that were previously hidden from the immune system or by release of bacterial endosymbionts of the genus *Wolbachia* that live inside several of the filariae and that are critical to the viability and fertility of the worm. *Wolbachia* are of the order Rickettsiales and are found in the

TABLE 366-2 FILARIAL PARASITES OF HUMANS

SPECIES	DISTRIBUTION	VECTOR	PRIMARY LOCATION	Microfilariae PERIODICITY	PRESENCE OF SHEATH
Wuchereria bancrofti	Tropics worldwide	Mosquitoes	Blood	Nocturnal, subperiodic	+
Brugia malayi	India, Southeast Asia	Mosquitoes	Blood	Nocturnal, subperiodic	+
Brugia timori	Indonesia	Mosquitoes	Blood	Nocturnal	+
Onchocerca volvulus	Africa, Central and South America	*Simulium* blackflies	Skin, eye	None or minimal	−
Loa loa	West and central Africa	*Chrysops* flies	Blood	Diurnal	+
Mansonella perstans	Africa, South America, Caribbean	Midges	Blood	None	−
Mansonella ozzardi	Central and South America, Caribbean	Midges, *Simulium* blackflies	Blood	None	−
Mansonella streptocerca	West and central Africa	Midges	Skin	None	−

hypodermis of adults worms and in oocysts, embryos, and microfilariae; they play an essential role in worm fertility and survival.

Diagnosis of filarial infections usually depends on the microscopic examination of either blood or skin specimens for characteristic microfilariae (see Table 366-2). Microfilariae of the different filarial species measure between 170 and 320 μm in length and can be distinguished on the basis of the tissue source of the specimen, the presence or absence of a sheath, and the arrangement of nuclei in the tail. For some filarial species, microfilariae are present in the blood only during certain periods of the day to coincide with biting habits of the arthropod vector, which must be taken into account in timing blood sampling for diagnosis based on microscopy. Serology is not very useful in endemic areas because a positive result does not distinguish between previous and current infection, and there is considerable antigenic cross-reactivity between the filariae and other nematodes. Detection of antifilarial antibodies may, however, be useful in returned long-term travelers or expatriates who are not originally from endemic areas but are suspected of having a filarial infection.

Diethylcarbamazine (DEC), ivermectin, and albendazole are the principal antifilarial drugs, although they have varying efficacies against the different filarial species (see Table 366-1). DEC is macrofilaricidal (active against the adult worm) for *W. bancrofti*, *Brugia* species, and *L. loa*, although prolonged or repeated courses are required for this effect. More commonly, the goal is to suppress microfilaria production by adult female worms, which can be achieved by single doses of antifilarial drugs administered alone or in combination annually or biannually. Reduction of microfilariae in the blood or skin can in some cases ameliorate symptoms or prevent progression of disease as well as interrupt the transmission cycle. Recently, evidence has emerged that targeting the *Wolbachia* endosymbionts of some filarial species with extended courses of antibiotics such as doxycycline can be macrofilaricidal.

Lymphatic Filariasis

DEFINITION

The three etiologic agents of lymphatic filariasis, *W. bancrofti*, *B. malayi*, and *B. timori*, are transmitted to humans through the bite of an infected mosquito. Microfilariae deposited at the bite wound subsequently migrate through the subcutaneous tissue to the lymphatic system, where adult worms develop after approximately 4 to 12 months. The worms reside coiled in lymph nodes and may extend into afferent lymph vessels and surrounding subcutaneous tissue. The lymphatics of the lower and upper extremities and male genitalia are most commonly affected. After mating, females, which measure between 4 and 10 cm in length, twice the length of males, release more than 10,000 microfilariae a day that migrate into the blood stream until ingestion by mosquito intermediate hosts taking a blood meal. In most endemic areas, microfilariae are present in the peripheral blood only at night, when mosquito vectors are most likely to bite. Adult filariae live between 5 and 8 years within the host, although infections lasting for decades have been reported.

EPIDEMIOLOGY

An estimated 120 million people are affected by lymphatic filariasis worldwide; most cases are caused by *W. bancrofti*, and only approximately 10 to 20 million are due to *B. malayi*. *B. timori* is of minor importance, being restricted to southeastern Indonesia. *W. bancrofti* is widely distributed in the tropics, especially in Southeast Asia, the Indian subcontinent, Africa, South America, the Caribbean, and the South Pacific. The major vectors of bancroftian filariasis are *Culex* mosquitoes in urban areas, anopheline mosquitoes in rural areas of Africa, and *Aedes* species in the Pacific. Humans are the only definitive host for *W. bancrofti*.

B. malayi, on the other hand, can be zoonotic, with both monkey and feline species serving as reservoir hosts. Brugian filariasis is found primarily in India, Malaysia, and other restricted areas in Southeast Asia. Zoonotic strains of *B. malayi* are transmitted to humans by *Mansonia* mosquitoes in Malaysia and Indonesia.

PATHOBIOLOGY

The pathologic process due to filarial infections is primarily due to blockage of lymphatic circulation resulting from damage caused by adult worms. Although the worms themselves do not seem to cause obstruction, they induce a local inflammatory lymphangitis, with cell-mediated, cytokine, and humoral components leading to hypertrophy of the vessel walls. It was initially thought that only dead or dying worms induced such an inflammatory response, but more recent evidence suggests that changes to the lymphatic architecture are induced even by living worms.

The initial inflammatory response leads to endothelial and connective tissue proliferation and vessel dilation, which reduces normal lymphatic function and results in lymphedema that is initially reversible. However, worm death results in a granulomatous reaction to released worm and *Wolbachia* antigens. The infiltration of giant cells as well as plasma cells, eosinophils, and neutrophils can completely occlude the lumen of the lymphatic vessel. Over time, fibrosis and obstruction of lymph flow result in irreversible edema and enlargement of the affected limb or body part. Although recanalization and collateralization of lymph vessels may occur, lymphatic function remains compromised.

CLINICAL MANIFESTATIONS

The clinical manifestations of lymphatic filariasis cover a wide spectrum from asymptomatic infection to severe chronic lymphatic obstruction accompanied by lymphedema (referred to as elephantiasis). Other common clinical outcomes include acute episodic lymphadenitis (also called filarial fever) and tropical pulmonary eosinophilia. Most infected individuals living in endemic regions are clinically asymptomatic, although microfilariae can be observed in their blood. Despite the absence of a significant inflammatory response, these individuals may nevertheless exhibit dilation of the affected lymphatics on ultrasound, which is thought necessary to precede the onset of clinically apparent disease.

For unknown reasons, newly exposed individuals may develop acute inflammatory reactions that can rapidly progress to chronic or irreversible changes compared with those born in endemic areas. Severe episodes of lymphadenitis, often with genital involvement, may lead to the relatively rapid development of lymphedema and elephantiasis within a year of arrival. Findings usually resolve quickly if the individual is promptly removed from the endemic area. Microfilariae are usually not detected in these patients.

Acute Lymphadenitis

Acute episodes of retrograde lymphadenitis occur most commonly in adolescents in endemic areas, often in response to a dying adult worm. Painful, erythematous enlargement of an affected lymph node, most commonly inguinal, precedes the onset of lymphangitis and is accompanied by fever and chills. Episodes usually last for about a week, frequently recur, and can be incapacitating. Defervescence is abrupt and associated with desquamation of the overlying skin. In men, inguinal lymphadenitis can be complicated by epididymitis and orchitis. Patients with filarial fevers may be microfilaremic but often are not.

Elephantiasis

Repeated episodes of lymphadenitis eventually lead to dilation of the lymphatic vessels, resulting in chronic lymphedema during the course of months to years (Fig. 366-2), with the prevalence of chronic manifestations increasing with age in affected communities. The extremities, breasts, and genitalia are most commonly affected, although with *B. malayi* infection, usually only the lower parts of the legs are involved. The edema is initially pitting in nature, but the subcutaneous tissue eventually loses its elasticity, resulting in woody edema with thickening of subcutaneous tissue and hyperkeratosis. Secondary

FIGURE 366-2. Elephantiasis, or chronic lymphedema due to infection with *Wuchereria bancrofti*. (Courtesy of the Centers for Disease Control and Prevention.)

bacterial or fungal infection is now recognized to occur more frequently than previously acknowledged and may contribute significantly to the chronic pathologic process of elephantiasis.

In bancroftian filariasis, development of hydrocele is a common manifestation of chronic filariasis in men and can sometimes become massive and debilitating; lymphedema of the vulva is less commonly seen in women. Involvement of the retroperitoneal lymphatics can lead to their rupture to produce intermittent chyluria or chylocele.

Tropical Pulmonary Eosinophilia

Tropical pulmonary eosinophilia develops in a small minority of individuals with filarial infections. The syndrome is most commonly seen in young men living in southern India, although it also occurs in Pakistan, Sri Lanka, Southeast Asia, and Brazil. Characteristic clinical findings include nocturnal paroxysmal cough, wheeze, and low-grade fever that is accompanied by weight loss and prominent peripheral eosinophilia. Levels of both total IgE and antifilarial antibodies are typically high. Chest radiographs generally show diffuse interstitial infiltrates or mottled opacities in the middle and lower lung fields. Without treatment, chronic restrictive lung disease may develop.

DIAGNOSIS

Definitive diagnosis usually relies on microscopic examination of a Giemsa-stained blood sample for microfilariae. Although thick blood smears are relatively insensitive except in cases of high microfilaremia, concentration or filtering techniques can increase diagnostic yield. In the latter case, blood is passed through a 3- to 5-μm pore size membrane filter that is then stained with Giemsa and examined under a microscope. Characteristic microfilariae are 250 to 320 μm in length. Collection of blood should be timed according to the known periodicity of the microfilariae.

Blood can also be assayed by a highly sensitive and specific commercially available rapid immunochromatographic card test that detects circulating *W. bancrofti* antigen (there is no equivalent test for *Brugia* infections). This test has the advantage of not requiring nocturnal collection of blood because it detects antigen of the adult worm and not microfilariae. PCR methods have also been developed to detect filarial antigens in blood, although these are not widely available. Serologic detection of antifilarial antibodies is of limited value because of extensive antigenic cross-reactivity with other nematodes. Furthermore, actively infected individuals cannot be distinguished from those previously infected, and those merely exposed but not infected may also have positive serologic test results.

Ultrasound examination of the lymphatic vessels of the spermatic cord of men can be used to visualize the "filarial dance sign," which is pathognomonic for a nest of filarial parasites.

Individuals with elephantiasis may be amicrofilaremic. Diagnosis therefore depends on a compatible clinical history and physical examination in the context of the appropriate epidemiology, and it may be supported by a positive antigen test result or, in men, by a suggestive scrotal ultrasonogram.

TREATMENT ℞

Management of lymphatic filariasis differs according to whether disease control or curative treatment of an individual patient is the aim. In endemic areas, annual mass drug administration of entire susceptible populations with a combination of two antifilarial drugs has been instituted to break the transmission cycle by reducing the number of microfilariae in the blood available to biting mosquitoes. These programs use different combinations of single-dose DEC, ivermectin, and albendazole, administered once a year. DEC is administered with albendazole except in areas where onchocerciasis or loiasis is also found, in which case ivermectin plus albendazole is used.

It is recommended that all individuals with active infection by a lymphatic filarial parasite, whether symptomatic or asymptomatic, be treated with an antifilarial medication (see Table 366-1). The treatment of choice is DEC (6 mg/kg/day in three divided doses for 12 days). In the United States, DEC is available only through the Centers for Disease Control and Prevention (CDC) drug service (http://www.cdc.gov/ncidod/srp/drugs/drug-service.html). For patients with high levels of microfilariae in the blood, treatment can be started at a low dose of 50 mg daily and scaled up during the first 3 days to reduce side effects of treatment such as fever, headache, dizziness, nausea, vomiting, transient rashes, myalgias, and arthralgias. These normally resolve after a few days of treatment and can be treated with antipyretics, antihistamines, and, if symptoms are severe, corticosteroids.

DEC is both microfilaricidal and partially macrofilaricidal. In individuals who will not be returning to endemic areas, repeated treatments with DEC are often attempted to kill the adult worms instead of just reducing the levels of microfilariae in the blood. Typically, courses of DEC are repeated every 6 to 12 months. Although the adult worm burden is reduced in most treated individuals, all parasites are eliminated in less than a quarter. In men with dancing live adult worms visible by ultrasound in the scrotal lymphatics, serial studies may be performed to monitor the effects of therapy.

Unfortunately, lymphedema due to lymphatic filariasis is usually not reversible with DEC treatment, except in the very early stages. Nevertheless, several management modalities can be employed to limit the chronic sequelae of lymphatic filariasis. Critical among these is the prevention of secondary bacterial and fungal infection through meticulous hygiene and prompt treatment of suspected infections with antimicrobials. Limb elevation, physiotherapy, and use of elastic stockings may slow the worsening of lymphedema. Surgery is usually not indicated except for cases of hydrocele.

Interestingly, treatment directed against the *Wolbachia* endosymbiont has recently been shown to be effective in killing adult *W. bancrofti* and *Brugia* worms. Doxycycline, 100 or 200 mg daily for 4 to 8 weeks, has been shown to reduce female worm fertility with a resulting suppression of microfilaremia for up to a year and to reduce the number of live adult worms.[1] Given the duration of treatment, these regimens are obviously not ideal for disease control programs in endemic countries.

DEC is highly effective in the treatment of tropical pulmonary eosinophilia. Treatment with 6 mg/kg/day for 14 to 21 days results in resolution of symptoms within a week, although relapse may occur even after an interval of years. See also Chapter 352.

PREVENTION

Annual mass treatment with single doses of two antifilarial drugs can significantly reduce the prevalence of infection within a community. In some areas, DEC-fortified table salt has been used to reduce the levels of microfilaremia in affected communities to interrupt the transmission cycle. Vector control through use of insecticide-treated bed nets and residual indoor spraying of insecticides may have some efficacy.

Onchocerciasis

DEFINITION

Onchocerciasis, or river blindness, caused by the nematode *Onchocerca volvulus*, is transmitted to humans by *Simulium* species blackflies. Infective microfilariae develop into male and female adult worms during several months and live for 8 to 10 years coiled within subcutaneous fibrous nodules (onchocercomas). Adult females measure between 20 and 70 cm in length and remain confined to the nodules; males are only 3 to 5 cm long and freely migrate through the subcutaneous tissues. Mature female worms produce about 700 microfilariae per day, which leave the nodule to migrate primarily through the skin and ocular tissues. Microfilariae can survive within the host for approximately 3 to 5 years unless they are ingested by a blackfly taking a blood meal.

EPIDEMIOLOGY

Onchocerciasis is endemic in 30 countries, predominantly in equatorial Africa, with small foci in six Latin American countries (Guatemala, southern Mexico, Venezuela, Brazil, Colombia, and Ecuador) and in Yemen. More than 17 million people are estimated to be infected, 500,000 of whom have significant visual impairment and 270,000 of whom are blind. More than 99% of cases occur in sub-Saharan Africa, with Nigeria being the most highly endemic country. Because *Simulium* blackflies require fast-flowing, well-oxygenated water for egg laying and reproduction, onchocerciasis is concentrated around streams and rivers, often in the most fertile farming areas. In communities bordering such waterways in endemic areas, up to 50% of the population can be affected.

Blindness caused by *O. volvulus* results in significant morbidity, long-term disability, and reduced economic productivity. In addition, onchocerciasis has been associated with a reduced life expectancy of at least 10 years compared with uninfected individuals in the same area, an effect that appears to be independent of the blindness that develops.

PATHOBIOLOGY

The pathologic changes of onchocerciasis are primarily due to an inflammatory reaction elicited by microfilariae. The skin, eyes, and lymph nodes are most affected. Adult worms contained in nodules are relatively isolated from the host immune response. Tissue damage results mainly from a cell-mediated immune response to dying microfilariae, which becomes more pronounced as infection persists. The degree of tissue damage is directly related to the intensity of infection as well as the magnitude of the host response. Sclerosing keratitis, the major cause of blindness, is caused by a lymphocytic inflammatory reaction to dying intraocular microfilariae that appears to be dependent on T helper cell type 2 (T_H2) cytokines. With time, neovascularization and scarring of the cornea lead to corneal opacification and eventual blindness. In the skin, similar immune responses result in pruritus and angioedema. Ongoing low-grade inflammation in the skin eventually leads to loss of elasticity and atrophy. Chronic inflammatory changes and fibrosis are also seen in lymph nodes.

Like the nematodes responsible for lymphatic filariasis, *O. volvulus* adult worms contain endosymbiotic *Wolbachia* bacteria that are obligatory for the development, survival, and fertility of these worms. Pro-inflammatory *Wolbachia* proteins released by dying microfilariae may be responsible for a significant amount of the immunopathologic process associated with onchocerciasis. For example, an endotoxin-like *Wolbachia* product has been shown to interact with the innate immune system through a Toll-like receptor 4–mediated mechanism.

CLINICAL MANIFESTATIONS

Onchodermatitis

Onchocerciasis commonly presents with a diffuse papular dermatitis that is intensely pruritic. In heavily infected individuals in endemic areas, the pruritus is intractable, leading to scratching and excoriation to the point of bleeding and even suicide. Hypersensitivity reactions, scabies, insect bites, and atopic or contact dermatitis should be considered in the differential diagnosis of the acute papular dermatitis seen with onchocerciasis. The skin of affected areas becomes edematous and thickened, losing its elasticity and taking on an orange-peel texture. A lichenified dermatitis (referred to as sowdah) may occur; it consists of an intensely pruritic eruption limited to one extremity, usually a leg, with hyperpigmented papules and plaques accompanied by edema of the entire limb. Over time, the skin will atrophy and fine wrinkles appear, especially over the buttocks. Pruritus is uncommon at this point. Areas of depigmentation may occur most commonly over the shins, a phenomenon called leopard skin.

Subcutaneous Nodules

Subcutaneous onchocercomas containing adult worms are most often palpable over bone prominences. In Africa, the nodules are most commonly found over the hips and lower limbs; in Latin America, they are often located on the head and upper part of the body. Nodules usually measure between 0.5 and 3 cm in diameter and are freely mobile. In lightly infected individuals, such as expatriates, nodules are usually not detectable.

Ocular Lesions

Initial ocular involvement is characterized by conjunctivitis, excess tearing, and photophobia in response to dying microfilariae. At this time, the corneal disease consists of a punctate keratitis or snowflake corneal opacities. During 20 to 30 years, this leads to sclerosing keratitis, neovascularization, and corneal opacification. The anterior chamber of the eye may also be involved, with iritis, iridocyclitis, and secondary glaucoma. Posterior ocular disease can be manifested as chorioretinitis, optic neuritis, and optic atrophy.

Lymphadenopathy

Lymphadenopathy is frequently found in the inguinal and femoral areas in Africa and in the head and neck in Latin America. Advanced disease in the inguinal region can result in the so-called hanging groin, with elongated atrophic skin containing nontender and fibrotic lymph nodes.

DIAGNOSIS

Definitive diagnosis has traditionally been made by observing motile microfilariae released from superficial skin snips. Microfilariae of *O. volvulus* do not have a sheath and measure 200 to 300 μm in length. To take a skin snip, a thin piece of skin overlying a bone prominence that has been tented up with a needle is sliced with a scalpel blade, or a corneal-scleral punch instrument is used to obtain a small piece of skin without drawing blood. Avoidance of blood contamination is critical so as to avoid confusion with blood-borne microfilariae in cases in which patients are coinfected with other filariases. Typically, six snips are taken, one from over each scapula, iliac crest, and lateral aspect of each calf, and then incubated with warm physiologic saline and examined microscopically for motile microfilariae after at least 30 minutes of incubation, although longer periods of up to 24 hours may be

necessary. Newer techniques include PCR amplification of filarial DNA directly from skin snips that are far more sensitive than direct visualization. With ocular disease, free microfilariae may be visible by slit lamp examination in the anterior chamber or aqueous humor.

Subcutaneous nodules can be sampled or examined by ultrasound to demonstrate the presence of adult worms. Serologic tests are usually positive for antifilarial antibodies but are not specific because of extensive antigenic cross-reactivity with other nematodes. Eosinophilia is a common but inconsistent finding.

In the past, the Mazzotti test was used to diagnose onchocerciasis. In this test, a challenge dose of DEC was administered to patients suspected of having onchocerciasis; with *O. volvulus* infection, an intense pruritic skin reaction would develop within hours. However, in patients with high-intensity infections, the Mazzotti reaction could be severe and even worsen ocular disease, resulting in permanent visual loss. Therefore, this test is no longer recommended, although some instead suggest the application of a small amount of DEC to the skin to provoke a localized Mazzotti reaction.

TREATMENT   Rx

Ivermectin is the treatment of choice for onchocerciasis (see Table 366-1). Administration of a single dose of ivermectin (150 μg/kg) is effective in ameliorating ocular and dermatologic disease by destroying microfilariae and suppressing their release from female worms. Because ivermectin is not active against the encapsulated adult worms, treatment must be repeated every 6 to 12 months, probably for at least 10 years in those without further exposure. For unknown reasons, pruritus in lightly infected expatriates may require more aggressive and frequent treatment for the first 2 years. Within 24 hours of treatment with ivermectin, fever and pruritus may occur in reaction to the dying microfilariae or released *Wolbachia* antigens, especially in those with high pretreatment levels of microfilariae. Use of ivermectin in areas where *L. loa* (see later) is co-endemic should be undertaken with caution as treatment may precipitate severe reactions including encephalopathy in those with high microfilaremia. DEC should never be used for treatment of onchocerciasis because of frequent unacceptable reactions to dying microfilariae ranging from urticaria and angioedema to hypotension and death. Although the drug suramin (available from the CDC drug service) is active against adult *O. volvulus* worms, because of its excessive toxicity and potentially life-threatening effects, it is used only in rare situations. Surgical removal of palpable nodules has been successful in resolving the infection in some areas, notably in Central America.

Doxycycline, 100 mg/day administered for 4 to 6 weeks, followed by single-dose ivermectin, has been shown to deplete *Wolbachia* endosymbionts from adult worms and to suppress *O. volvulus* embryogenesis and production of microfilariae for up to 18 months. Some experts now recommend this regimen for patients with onchocerciasis who have left an endemic area and will not be re-exposed.

See also Chapter 352.

PREVENTION

Regular mass administration of ivermectin to affected communities forms the core of the global eradication strategy for onchocerciasis. Implementation of this program has been made easier because the drug is donated by the manufacturer. In addition to benefiting infected individuals, mass drug administration reduces the microfilariae available to vectors and thus interrupts the transmission cycle. For travelers to endemic areas, use of insect repellent may be beneficial.

Loiasis

DEFINITION

Loiasis is caused by infection with the filarial nematode *Loa loa,* otherwise known as the African eye worm. *L. loa* are transmitted by flies of the genus *Chrysops* during a blood meal. Adult worms develop during a period of 1 to 4 years and live for up to 17 years. They migrate freely in the subcutaneous tissue, including the subconjunctiva or sclera of the eye. Adult females measure between 50 and 70 mm in length; males are shorter, measuring between 25 and 35 mm. After mating, females release microfilariae into the blood. *L. loa* microfilariae exhibit a diurnal periodicity coinciding with the feeding habits of *Chrysops,* with microfilaremia peaking around noon.

EPIDEMIOLOGY

Loiasis is endemic in the rain forest regions of central and west Africa. Although accurate numbers are not available, loiasis appears to be most prevalent in Gabon, Cameroon, the Democratic Republic of the Congo, Nigeria, and the Central African Republic. More so than other filarial infections, loiasis seems to require a shorter period of exposure and can be seen in returning travelers or expatriates who have spent extended periods in Africa.

PATHOBIOLOGY

Neither adult *L. loa* worms nor microfilariae have any direct pathologic effects. In a subset of infected individuals, a hypersensitivity response, termed a *Calabar swelling*, develops to secretions from adult worms or released microfilariae, resulting in recurrent localized angioedema that often precedes the migrating worm. Interestingly, this reaction is more commonly observed in visitors to endemic areas rather than in native residents. These patients have very high serum levels of IgE antibodies and eosinophilia. Unlike other filariae, *L. loa* does not contain *Wolbachia* endosymbionts.

CLINICAL MANIFESTATIONS

Most individuals with loiasis are asymptomatic despite being microfilaremic. Clinical manifestations of infection are more common in long-term visitors to endemic areas than in people native to the regions. Recurrent Calabar swellings are the most common finding in these individuals, who are not usually microfilaremic. They are nonerythematous swellings measuring 5 to 20 cm in diameter that typically occur on the extremities and the face and last for a few days. The onset is often preceded by pruritus and pain. On occasion, adult worms may migrate across the subconjunctiva or sclera of the eye in both groups of patients, causing severe pain and inflammation (Fig. 366-3). Rare complications of infection include nephropathy and encephalitis, the latter usually developing in patients with high levels of microfilariae after receiving DEC or ivermectin treatment for other filarial infections. Endomyocardial fibrosis resulting from eosinophilic infiltration of the myocardium has been reported in association with loiasis.

DIAGNOSIS

Definitive diagnosis depends on microscopic examination of a Giemsa- or Wright-stained blood film for characteristic sheathed microfilariae. Blood should be collected between 10 AM and 2 PM because of the diurnal periodicity of the microfilariae. Because individuals who are not native to endemic areas are usually not microfilaremic, diagnosis relies on a compatible history, clinical findings, peripheral eosinophilia, and elevated antifilarial antibody levels. Adult worms can sometimes be surgically removed while migrating across the eye or through subcutaneous tissues. Calabar swellings must be distinguished from onchocercomas and other causes of angioedema.

TREATMENT   Rx

DEC (6 mg/kg/day for 12 to 21 days) is active against both adult *L. loa* worms and microfilariae (see Table 366-1). Treatment is usually increased from a dose of 50 mg/day on the first day to the full dose on the fourth day to minimize the likelihood of treatment-associated complications, the most serious of which are glomerulonephritis and a potentially fatal encephalopathy. Treatment-associated complications are more common with high pretreatment microfilarial levels and result from host allergic reactions to dying microfilariae. Antihistamines and corticosteroids may be employed to reduce allergic side effects. Alternatively, apheresis can be used to remove circulating microfilariae before initiation of DEC in these individuals. Albendazole, which is microfilaricidal but has no activity against adult worms, has also been used to reduce microfilaria levels before treatment with DEC. Repeated courses of DEC may be necessary in about half of patients before clinical manifestations completely resolve. Persistent or increasing eosinophilia or levels of antifilarial antibodies 6 months after treatment should also prompt re-evaluation for repeated treatment. Adult worms in the eye should be surgically removed.

Ivermectin is microfilaricidal but has no macrofilaricidal effect and may cause toxic encephalopathy in individuals with high microfilaria levels. In areas where onchocerciasis is co-endemic, this infection should be ruled out before the initiation of DEC for loiasis to prevent toxicity from dying *O. volvulus* microfilariae.

See also Chapter 352.

PREVENTION

Weekly chemoprophylaxis with DEC administered as a 300-mg dose is effective in preventing loiasis in long-term residents of endemic areas.

FIGURE 366-3. Adult *Loa loa* worm migrating across the eye *(arrow)*.

Less Common Filarial Infections

MANSONELLA PERSTANS

M. perstans infection occurs throughout central Africa, in northeastern South America, and in parts of the Caribbean. Microfilariae are transmitted by midges and develop into adult worms that live in serous body cavities, such as the pleural, pericardial, and peritoneal spaces, as well as in mesenteric and retroperitoneal tissues. Most infections are asymptomatic, although painless conjunctival nodules with eyelid edema have been reported. Transient angioedema and Calabar-like swellings, fever, headache, arthralgias, and neurologic manifestations may also occur. Microfilariae do not exhibit periodicity and can be observed on stained blood films. Eosinophilia is common. *M. perstans* harbor *Wolbachia* endosymbionts, and treatment with doxycycline, 200 mg/day for 6 weeks, has been shown to be highly effective in suppressing microfilaremia for up to 3 years, suggesting that the treatment is macrofilaricidal.[2]

MANSONELLA OZZARDI

Infections with *M. ozzardi* occur only in Central and South America and parts of the Caribbean, especially Haiti. Vectors include *Simulium* blackflies and midges. Adult worms locate to the peritoneal and thoracic cavities or the lymphatics; microfilariae circulate in the blood without periodicity. Infection usually results in asymptomatic eosinophilia, although arthritis and allergic symptoms such as urticaria and lymphadenopathy may occur. Administration of ivermectin as a single dose of 200 µg/kg has been reported to provide long-term suppression of microfilaremia and improvement of symptoms. Neither DEC nor the benzimidazoles are effective.

MANSONELLA STREPTOCERCA

M. streptocerca is endemic in the tropical forest zone of west and central Africa and is transmitted by biting midges. Similar to *O. volvulus*, adult worms live in the subcutaneous tissues, as do microfilariae. In contrast to onchocerciasis, however, microfilariae do not invade the eye. Infection is usually asymptomatic, although a pruritic dermatitis with depigmentation similar to onchodermatitis can affect the trunk and upper extremities. Associated axillary or inguinal adenopathy is common. Microfilariae have characteristic hooked tails and can be visualized in skin snips. In areas where onchocerciasis is co-endemic, skin specimens must be stained to differentiate *M. streptocerca* from *O. volvulus*. DEC is microfilaricidal and macrofilaricidal and is given as 6 mg/kg/day for 12 days. Ivermectin is effective against microfilariae but not adult worms.

ZOONOTIC FILARIAL INFECTIONS

A rare accidental filarial infection of humans with the dog heartworm *Dirofilaria immitis* occurs worldwide. Transmitted by mosquitoes, *D. immitis* microfilariae cannot reach maturity in humans but embolize to the lung after dying in the right ventricle. Most infections are asymptomatic, but some people experience cough, chest pain, and hemoptysis consistent with lung infarction. Chest radiographs demonstrate typical coin lesions that may be mistaken for carcinoma. Other animal filariae, including *Dirofilaria repens* of dogs and *Dirofilaria tenuis* of raccoons, can infect humans and result in subcutaneous nodules that may be migratory. Eosinophilia and antifilarial antibodies are not usually present in zoonotic filarial infections. Surgical removal of lesions is both diagnostic and curative.

DRACUNCULIASIS

Dracunculiasis is a disfiguring disease caused by the nematode *Dracunculus medinensis,* also known as the guinea worm. Although previously found in India, Pakistan, and Latin America, it is now endemic in only four countries in sub-Saharan Africa (Sudan, Ghana, Mali, and Ethiopia) because of concerted efforts at eradication. Currently, fewer than 5000 cases are thought to exist, with the largest concentration being in southern Sudan. Transmission to humans occurs through ingestion of tiny crustacean intermediate hosts called copepods that harbor infective larvae. Released larvae penetrate the intestinal wall and migrate to the subcutaneous tissues, where they develop into adult worms. After approximately a year, female worms induce vesicular skin lesions, usually on the lower extremities, that eventually ulcerate. On direct contact with fresh water, the female worm releases thousands of motile larvae that can then complete the transmission cycle by infecting copepods in the water. Adult worms can measure up to a meter in length. Fever and allergic symptoms, including wheezing and urticaria, may precede rupture of the blister or occur with attempts to extract the worm. Secondary bacterial infection of the skin lesions is frequent. Although not usually fatal, dracunculiasis can result in significant disability.

Traditionally, emerging worms are extracted by slowly winding a few centimeters of the parasite on a stick each day, taking care not to break it. Surgical removal can also be attempted but may exacerbate allergic symptoms. There is no effective chemotherapy for this infection. Prevention efforts have been highly successful in breaking the transmission cycle and have led to eradication of the parasite from many countries. Strategies include filtering of drinking water through finely woven cloth, education of infected individuals not to enter fresh water, treatment of water sources with larvicides, and provision of safe drinking water from wells.

Visit expertconsult.com for e-expanded chapter

1. Taylor MJ, Makunde WH, McGarry HF, et al. Macrofilaricidal activity after doxycycline treatment of *Wuchereria bancrofti*: a double-blind, randomised placebo-controlled trial. *Lancet.* 2005;365: 2116-2121.
2. Coulibaly YI, Dembele B, Diallo AA, et al. A randomized trial of doxycycline for *Mansonella perstans* infection. *N Engl J Med.* 2009;361:1448-1458.

SUGGESTED READINGS

Cupp EW, Sauerbrey M, Richards F. Elimination of human onchocerciasis: history of progress and current feasibility using ivermectin (Mectizan) monotherapy. *Acta Trop.* 2011. [Epub ahead of print.] *Documents the remarkable success of the campaign, which is on track to eliminate the disease in the Americas by 2015 and may eliminate it in parts of Africa.*

Glatz K, Danka J, Kucsera I, et al. Human trichinellosis in Hungary from 1965 to 2009. *Parasite.* 2010;17:193-198. *Backyard pigs and hunted wild boars are the two main sources.*

Padgett JJ, Jacobsen KH. Loiasis: African eye worm. *Trans R Soc Trop Med Hyg.* 2008;102:983-989. *A thorough review of Loa loa infection.*

Rubinsky-Elefant G, Hirata CE, Yamamoto JH, et al. Human toxocariasis: diagnosis, worldwide seroprevalences and clinical expression of the systemic and ocular forms. *Ann Trop Med Parasitol.* 2010;104:3-23. *Review of the current laboratory diagnosis, epidemiology, and clinical features.*

Taylor MJ, Hoerauf A, Bockarie M. Lymphatic filariasis and onchocerciasis. *Lancet.* 2010;376:1175-1185. *Review.*

367

ARTHROPODS AND LEECHES

DIRK M. ELSTON

ARTHROPODS

The Pathogens

Arthropods are invertebrates characterized by an exoskeleton and jointed legs. They commonly act as disease vectors or may cause human injury by means of the direct toxic effects of their venom or through an immune response to their antigens (Tables 367-1 to 367-4). Immediate reactions to

TABLE 367-1	MEDICALLY IMPORTANT ARTHROPODS
Arachnida	
Acari—mites, ticks	
Araneida—spiders	
Scorpionida	
Pentastomida—tongue worms	
Chilopoda—centipedes	
Diplopoda—millipedes	
Crustacea	
Copepoda—*Cyclops, Diaptomus*	
Decapoda—shrimp, lobster, crayfish, crab	
Insecta	
Anoplura—lice	
Coleoptera—beetles	
Diptera—mosquitoes, blackflies, midges, horseflies, deer flies, greenheads, tsetse flies, stable flies, sand flies, houseflies, bluebottle flies	
Hemiptera—bedbugs, reduviids	
Hymenoptera—ants, bees, wasps	
Lepidoptera—moths, caterpillars	
Siphonaptera—fleas	

TABLE 367-2	ARTHROPOD VECTORS
DISEASE	**VECTOR**
African trypanosomiasis	Tsetse flies
American trypanosomiasis	Triatome bugs
Arboviridae	*Culex* mosquitoes
Babesiosis	*Ixodes scapularis* (deer tick)
Bartonellosis	Fleas, lice, sand flies
Dengue	*Aedes* mosquitoes
Endemic typhus	*Ctenocephalides felis* and *Xenopsylla cheopis* (fleas)
Filariasis	Anopheline and *Aedes* mosquitoes
Human anaplasmosis	*Ixodes scapularis*
Human monocytic ehrlichiosis	*Amblyomma americanum* (Lone Star tick)
Leishmaniasis	Sand flies
Lyme disease	*Ixodes scapularis*
Malaria	Anopheline mosquitoes
Onchocerciasis	*Simulium* flies
Plague	*Xenopsylla cheopis* and *Pulex irritans* (human flea)
Rickettsialpox	*Liponyssoides sanguineus* (house mouse mite)
Rocky Mountain spotted fever	*Dermacentor variabilis* (dog tick) *Dermacentor andersoni* (wood tick) *Amblyomma americanum*
Tick paralysis	*Dermacentor andersoni* *Dermacentor variabilis*
Tick-borne relapsing fever	*Ornithodoros* genus (soft tick)
Trypanosomiasis	Tsetse fly, hemipterids
Tularemia	*Amblyomma americanum* *Dermacentor andersoni* *Dermacentor variabilis* *Chrysops* deer flies Horseflies
Typhus	*Pediculus humanus* (lice)
Typhus, endemic	Fleas
Typhus, scrub	Chigger mites
Viral encephalitis	*Aedes* mosquitoes
West Nile fever	*Culex* mosquitoes
Yellow fever	*Aedes* mosquitoes

stings may be related to histamine, serotonin, formic acid, or kinins contained within the venom. Delayed reactions to bites and stings generally represent a host response to proteinaceous allergens contained within venom or saliva.

Whereas many diseases are spread by a single vector, others have multiple potential vectors. For example, tularemia is commonly acquired from ticks or handling of infected carcasses, but it may also be spread by deer flies and horseflies. Rickettsiae are spread by both ticks and fleas. The vector may influence manifestations of the disease. For example, *Bartonella* transmitted by a flea may produce bacillary angiomatosis, whereas the same organism transmitted by a louse is much more likely to be manifested as endocarditis. Disease manifestations may also reflect the underlying immune status of the host, previous sensitization, or associated comorbidities. For example, hypersensitivity reactions to insect stings are more common in those with an atopic diathesis, and anaphylaxis may be a manifestation of underlying mastocytosis. Exaggerated bite reactions (Fig. 367-1) may be a manifestation of an underlying lymphoproliferative disease.

Scabies

DEFINITION

Human scabies is caused by the mite *Sarcoptes scabiei* var *hominis*, an obligate human pathogen, belonging to the class Arachnida, subclass Acari, order Astigmata, and family Sarcoptidae. Animal mange or scab is caused by related *Sarcoptes* or *Psoroptes* mites. These zoonotic mites can produce transient symptoms in exposed humans but are rarely capable of producing sustained infestation. *S. scabiei* var *hominis* is round to oval with a small anterior portion, dorsal spines, and hairlike projections on the rudimentary legs.

PATHOBIOLOGY

After mating on the skin surface, the female mite begins to burrow and lay eggs at a rate of one to three per day. The eggs mature and hatch during 3 to 4 days. The larvae pass through protonymph and tritonymph stages before molting into adults. The entire life cycle ranges between 30 and 60 days. All stages of the mite are capable of penetrating the stratum corneum through secretion of enzymes. In immunosuppressed individuals, mite populations may reach staggering proportions within thick, white, highly infectious crusts.

In immunocompetent patients, scabies mites induce a strong host response characterized by a superficial and deep perivascular inflammatory infiltrate composed of lymphocytes, histiocytes, and eosinophils. There is marked production of interleukin (IL)–6 resulting in proliferation of keratinocytes, activation of T_H1 CD4$^+$ cells causing production of IL-2, and activation of T_H2 CD4$^+$ cells causing production of IL-4. Disease manifestations relate to the complex balance of the immune response.

CLINICAL MANIFESTATIONS

Immunocompetent adults present with severe pruritus and a symmetrical erythematous papulovesicular eruption. There is a predilection for involvement of the interdigital web spaces, the wrists (Fig. 367-2), the anterior

FIGURE 367-1. Exaggerated arthropod bite response in a patient with chronic lymphocytic leukemia.

TABLE 367-3	MEDICALLY IMPORTANT MITES
FAMILY	
Acaridae	Commonly found in grain, flour, and other foods
Cheyletidae	Walking dandruff in dogs, cats, and rabbits
Demodicidae	Human hair follicle mites
Dermanyssidae	Bird and rodent mites
Glycyphagidae	Associated with food, animals, and leaf litter
Psoroptidae	Scab mites
Pyemotidae	Grain and straw mites
Sarcoptidae	Scabies mites
Trombiculidae	Chigger or harvest mites

TABLE 367-4	CAUSES OF DIRECT TOXIC INJURY BY ARTHROPODS AND LEECHES	
ORGANISM	**TYPE OF INJURY**	**DISTRIBUTION AND POPULATION AFFECTED**
Australian funnel web spiders (*Hadronyche* and *Atrax*)	Neurotoxin producing tingling around the mouth, muscle twitching, nausea, vomiting, profuse sweating, coma, myocardial injury	Australians
Blister beetles	Bullous reactions	Widely distributed but more common in hot climates
Brazilian wandering spider (*Phoneutria* spiders)	Neurotoxin resulting in paralysis	Brazilians
Brown *Loxosceles* spiders	Dermonecrotic reactions	Contact through attics and woodpiles
Centipedes	Neurotoxin that may produce pain, paresthesia, erythema, edema, and profuse bleeding; rarely, coronary ischemia, rhabdomyolysis, proteinuria, and renal failure	Most toxic species in Asia
Hymenopterids	Anaphylactic reactions	Wide distribution
Leeches	Bleeding	Fresh water exposure
Lepidopterids	Rash, ophthalmia nodosa, keratoconjunctivitis	Wide distribution
Lonomia caterpillars	Fatal bleeding diathesis	Brazil
Millipedes	Chemical burns	Most toxic species in Australia and Africa
Pacific funnel web spider (*Tegenaria agrestis*)	Dermonecrotic reactions	Basements in the Pacific Northwest
Scorpions	Mild systemic symptoms, sometimes severe in children;	
Centuroides sculpturatus	severe cardiac toxicity	Southwestern United States
Buthid scorpions		Asia, Africa, and Latin America
Tarantulas	Contact urticaria and ophthalmia nodosa	Hot climates
Widow spiders (*Latrodectus*)	Neurotoxin mimicking acute abdomen	Contact through outhouses and woodpiles

FIGURE 367-2. Scabies infestation in children commonly presents with burrows (shown here between the thenar and hypothenar eminences), papulovesicles, and crusts involving the wrists and flexures.

FIGURE 367-3. Scabies preparation demonstrating an adult mite, ova, and feces.

axillary folds, the periumbilical skin, the areolae in women, and the penis and scrotum in men. In infants, the face and scalp are commonly involved. Crusted scabies in immunosuppressed individuals presents with silver to white crusts involving any portion of the body but with a predilection for the hands and ears. In elderly patients, the manifestations may be subtle, with mild pruritus and prurigo-like papules on the trunk and extremities. In patients with human T-lymphotropic virus type 1 infection, scabies often presents with linear hyperkeratotic lesions on the dorsal hands and feet.

The most pathognomonic findings are burrows and genital nodules. The burrow is a short serpiginous gray to white keratotic line measuring 1 to 4 mm in length. Burrows are most common on the hands and feet, particularly on the finger web spaces, the thenar and hypothenar eminences, and the wrists. Genital nodules may involve the glans, scrotum, or labia majora. A history of itch in other family members or sexual partners is highly suggestive of the diagnosis.

DIAGNOSIS

The diagnosis is established by identification of the female mite, ova, or feces in a scraping from a burrow (Fig. 367-3). When the diagnosis is missed initially, it may ultimately be made by transmission to other patients and health care providers. This is particularly true in the case of crusted scabies, when hundreds of individuals may become infested. A high degree of suspicion is required in immunosuppressed and elderly patients, in whom the manifestations may be mild and atypical. Scabies may mimic bullous pemphigoid and Langerhans cell histiocytosis, both clinically and histologically.

TREATMENT   Rx

Commonly employed topical agents include permethrin 5% and precipitated sulfur 2 to 10% in petrolatum. Lindane (gamma benzene hexachloride) 1% was widely used in the past, and topical agents used worldwide include benzyl benzoate 10 to 25%, monosulfiram 5 to 25%, malathion 0.5%, and esdepallethrin 0.63%. Crotamiton 10% has relatively weak antiscabetic activity but is sometimes used for its antipruritic effect. Oral ivermectin has also been used at a single dose of 200 μg/kg (about 12 mg for an average adult).

Proper application of any topical must include the umbilicus, the genitalia, under the nails, and the skin up to the edge of all body orifices. Fomites are important in the spread of crusted scabies, with hospital linens being of particular concern. Caregivers involved in bathing or lifting, sexual partners, and family members are at high risk of infection and should be treated at the same time as the patient regardless of symptoms. It has been estimated that 15 to 20 minutes of close contact with an infected individual is required for transfer of the mites from one person to another. Clothes and bed linens should be machine washed at 60° C, followed by heated drying.

Other Mites

Mites are ubiquitous in the environment and are a frequent cause of dermatitis. The most common medically important mites are listed in Table 367-3.

The majority of mites are free-living, but thousands of species are obligate parasites of animals or plants. Like ticks, mites mature through various life stages. Typically, there is a single six-legged larval stage, followed by several nymphal stages and an adult stage. Both nymphs and adults typically have eight legs. Whereas most mites lay eggs, the spiny rat mite (*Laelaps echidninus*) is viviparous, and the straw itch mite (*Pyemotes tritici*) protects its young internally throughout their life cycle until they emerge as sexually mature adults. Manifestations of mite infestations are protean and include papular, vesicular, urticarial, and morbilliform eruptions. Chigger mites most often affect the lower legs, the edges of underwear, and the genitalia. Summer penile syndrome is a manifestation of chigger mite infestation. It presents with tender to itchy papules of the glans and scrotum and may mimic scabies infestation. Chigger (Trombiculid) mites in Asia are vectors for scrub typhus; house mouse mites in New York City transmit rickettsialpox. The presence of an eschar at the site of the bite suggests rickettsial disease.

The primary treatment is to identify and remove the source of infestation. Many mite-induced rashes represent a "bite and run" injury and can be treated with topical corticosteroids or camphor and menthol lotion for symptomatic relief. Other mites remain attached by a feeding tube and can be removed by scraping or tape stripping of the affected skin. Mite identification can be helpful in establishing the most likely source of the infestation.

Ticks

Ticks are important disease vectors, and *Dermacentor* ticks can cause fatal tick paralysis in children. Tick paralysis presents as progressive ascending paralysis. As the tick attaches to the scalp, it frequently goes unnoticed, and death occurs in more than 10% of affected children. Nodular lesions are commonly pseudolymphomatous histologically.

Rickettsial illnesses typically present with fever and a headache, and treatment with a tetracycline should never be withheld because of absence of a rash. Any delay in the initiation of antibiotic therapy may prove fatal, and empirical treatment should never be delayed until confirmatory test results are available. Doxycycline is generally recommended in both adults and children.

Rickettsial diseases, including Rocky Mountain spotted fever, continue to emerge in much of the world, especially in South America. Recently recognized rickettsial pathogens include *Rickettsia parkeri*. Most of these agents produce milder syndromes similar to Rocky Mountain spotted fever.

Exclusion of animal hosts from recreational areas can be helpful in control of tick-borne illness. Oral agents, including avermectin-laced feed corn, can be used to kill ticks that feed on deer. Removal of leaf debris leads to a reduction in tick numbers through dehydration of adults and ova. Permethrin, a pyrethroid insecticide, is widely marketed as a topical acaricide to be applied to clothing. It is stable through several wash cycles. Some North African *Hyalomma* ticks have demonstrated high-level resistance, and permethrin may produce a pheromone-like attachment response in these ticks. Resistance in North American ticks can be esterase based or related to sodium channel gene mutations, and permethrin resistance has been linked to outbreaks of bovine babesiosis and anaplasmosis.

A veterinarian should be consulted concerning control of ticks in pets and livestock. Topical fipronil is commonly used in dogs. Collars can be impregnated with amitraz and pyriproxyfen, and oral agents are also available.

Antibiotic prophylaxis after tick bites is justified only in the case of endemic disease vectors that are heavily engorged. In some cases, the risk-to-benefit ratio may weigh in favor of prophylactic treatment. If the dose is sufficient and the antibiotic is given at the appropriate time, prophylaxis can prevent tick-borne disease. In the case of Rocky Mountain spotted fever, single-dose prophylaxis should be avoided as it may only delay the onset of clinical symptoms when it is administered too early in the course of incubation. If the decision is made to administer a prophylactic antibiotic, a full 10-day course of therapy is preferable to single-dose prophylaxis. A controlled trial comparing 10 days of oral doxycycline (with or without intravenous ceftriaxone) with 20 days of oral doxycycline for the treatment of early Lyme disease found a similar response rate in all three treatment groups.

Spiders

Toxic spiders are found worldwide. The most feared include the funnel web spiders of Australia and *Phoneutria* wandering spiders in Brazil, which can be fatal. In North America, brown recluse spiders can produce a severe dermonecrotic reaction, but most spider bites result only in a mild local cutaneous reaction.

Black and brown widow spiders have a worldwide distribution. *Latrodectus mactans* is the most common black widow spider in North America. *Latrodectus curacavienis* is common in South America and *Latrodectus tredecimguttatus* in Europe. Both black (*Latrodectus indistinctus*) and brown (*Latrodectus geometricus*) widow spiders are found in Africa and Madagascar; Australia and New Zealand have red-black spiders (*Latrodectus mactans hasselti*).

Widow spiders are commonly encountered in woodpiles, and bites commonly involve the hand. Latrotoxins act by increasing intracellular calcium concentrations, depolarizing neurons, and stimulating uncontrolled release of neurotransmitters. Divalent cation–dependent tetramers of α-latrotoxin produce membrane pores in mammalian cells. Symptoms include local pain as well as systemic symptoms suggestive of an acute surgical abdomen. Both benzodiazepines and intravenous calcium gluconate have been used to treat associated tetany. Antivenin can produce rapid relief of unresponsive tetany and priapism.

Brown *Loxosceles* spiders are found throughout the world; the most famous is the brown recluse spider, *Loxosceles reclusa* (Fig. 367-4). The resulting necrosis can be severe (Fig. 367-5), but most bites do not result in skin necrosis, and those of related spiders, including *Loxosceles rufescens, Loxosceles deserta,* and *Loxosceles arizonica,* are even milder. Brown recluse spiders are most common in the south central United States, from Tennessee and Missouri to Oklahoma and Texas. They are quite shy, and bites are uncommon. Most skin reactions diagnosed as "brown recluse bites" represent furuncles or pyoderma gangrenosum. The diagnosis can be confirmed by an enzyme immunoassay or a passive hemagglutination inhibition test.

Sphingomyelinase D is the major toxin in brown recluse venom, and hyaluronidase allows the eschars to spread in a gravity-dependent fashion. Systemic reactions include disseminated intravascular coagulation and Coombs'-positive hemolytic anemia, but these reactions are rare as well. Most bites can be treated with rest, ice, and elevation. Intradermal injection of polyclonal anti-*Loxosceles* Fab fragments or antivenin may reduce the ultimate size of the necrotic area but is not readily available. Studies with dapsone, colchicine, hyperbaric oxygen, and prednisone have generally been disappointing. Dapsone produces hemolysis, especially in individuals who have inherited glucose-6-phosphate dehydrogenase deficiency (Chapter 164). On the basis of limited animal data and anecdotal human data, intralesional triamcinolone appears to be appropriate for patients with rapidly expanding areas of necrosis.

Tegenaria agrestis is found in basements in the Pacific Northwest. In Europe, it exists as a rural spider; *Tegenaria gigantea* and *Tegenaria domestica* are more likely to be found in homes. Most reactions are mild, although some dermonecrotic reactions have been attributed to these spiders. Australian *Hadronyche* and *Atrax* spiders can produce severe pain and bleeding. Severe myocardial injury has been reported. Tarantulas can cause contact urticaria and ophthalmia nodosa related to hairs that become embedded in the cornea.

Scorpions

Local and systemic symptoms of scorpion stings are typically out of proportion to cutaneous signs. *Centruroides sculpturatus* produces somewhat more severe envenomation in the American Southwest, but the most dangerous

Buthid scorpions are not found in the United States. Most fatalities involve children younger than 10 years. Toxic Buthid scorpions occur in Asia, Africa, and Latin America. Prazosin reverses the autonomic storm characteristic of the Indian red scorpion (*Mesobuthus tamulus*) and is superior to antivenin.

Tongue Worm (Pentastomiasis)

Pentastomiasis is a zoonotic infestation that sometimes affects humans. The pentastomids *Armillifer* and *Linguatula* are wormlike arthropods endemic to Asia and Africa. They commonly infest the respiratory tracts of birds, reptiles, and small mammals. In humans, severe inflammation associated with the infestation can result in coughing, hemoptysis, lacrimation, coryza, and facial edema. Rarely, asphyxiation has been reported. This syndrome is known as halzoun or marrara, meaning suffocation.

Centipedes and Millipedes

Centipedes have powerful jaws that inject a neurotoxic venom. Centipede bites may produce pain, paresthesia, erythema, edema, and profuse bleeding. Rarely, bites have been associated with coronary ischemia, rhabdomyolysis, proteinuria, and renal failure. Millipedes do not bite but cause arcuate chemical burns by a caustic substance that they secrete when threatened. They may be found in line-dried clothing, and the resulting burns may mimic child abuse.

Crustaceans as a Source of Infection

Copepods are tiny aquatic crustaceans that serve as the intermediate hosts for nematodes including the guinea worm *Dracunculus medinensis* and the sushi worm *Gnathostoma spinigerum*. They may also transmit the cestodes *Spirometra mansonoides* and *Diphyllobothrium latum.*

Pediculosis

Pediculosis is the result of infestation by sucking lice of the phylum Arthropoda, class Insecta, order Phthiraptera, suborder Anoplura, family Pediculidae or family Pthiridae. Three types of lice infest humans: *Pediculus humanus*

FIGURE 367-4. Brown recluse spiders are characterized by a dorsal violin-case pattern.

FIGURE 367-5. Dermonecrotic reactions from brown recluse spiders can be severe, but most are mild conditions. Furuncles or pyoderma gangrenosum are commonly misdiagnosed as brown recluse bites. (Image courtesy of Larry Becker, MD.)

capitis (the head louse), *Pediculus humanus humanus* (the body louse), and *Pthirus pubis* (the crab louse).

Head Lice

EPIDEMIOLOGY

Head lice affect 6 to 12 million people per year in the United States alone. Worldwide, much of the human population is affected, with highest prevalence among children between the ages of 3 and 12 years. Transmission occurs by means of direct contact or close contact of hats and scarves.

DIAGNOSIS

Head louse infestation should be suspected in any child with scalp pruritus and cervical adenopathy. Visual inspection can demonstrate nits, especially in the retroauricular area. Small bites and crusts of blood are common on the scalp.

TREATMENT   Rx

Combinations of pyrethrins and piperonyl butoxide are available over-the-counter and have commonly been used before the patient seeks treatment from a physician. Pyrethrins are naturally occurring neurotoxins derived from chrysanthemums. Piperonyl butoxide prevents pyrethroid catabolism, producing a synergistic effect.

Permethrin is a synthetic pyrethroid that acts in a similar manner by inhibiting sodium transport in neurons and causing paralysis of the lice. Permethrin is also available over-the-counter. Permethrin is pregnancy category B and is often used in pregnant patients, but recent data suggest a possible association with childhood leukemia.

Lindane is an organochloride compound that is still available by prescription. Central nervous system toxicity appears rare but together with environmental concerns resulted in banning of the product in California. Malathion is a prescription organophosphate that acts by interfering with acetylcholinesterase. In the United States, it is marketed in a flammable vehicle that contributes substantially to its efficacy. There is relatively little resistance to this agent, but the trend is away from the use of neurotoxins in children and toward agents that kill lice by occlusion of the respiratory spiracles. One such agent (Ulesfia lotion) uses benzyl alcohol to stun the spiracle open and allow occlusion. A recently reported multicenter trial for difficult-to-treat head lice infestation in children showed that oral ivermectin (400 μg/kg), given twice at a 7-day interval, had superior efficacy compared with topical 0.5% malathion lotion, suggesting that it could be an alternative treatment.

Body Lice

EPIDEMIOLOGY

Body louse infestation is common in refugee situations, during war, and among the homeless in urban areas. In this setting, lice act as a vector for *Bartonella* endocarditis. Worldwide, body lice are important vectors for epidemic typhus, louse-borne relapsing fever, and trench fever.

CLINICAL MANIFESTATIONS

Early infestation produces a widespread dermatitis that may mimic atopic dermatitis, allergic contact dermatitis, or a viral exanthem. In patients with widespread excoriations, the most likely differential diagnosis is scabies. The diagnosis is made by finding bluish maculae ceruleae (Fig. 367-6), prompting a search for body lice or nits in the seams of clothing.

TREATMENT   Rx

Washing and hot drying of clothing or ironing will kill lice. Permethrin has also been used on clothing.

Crab Lice

PATHOBIOLOGY

Crab louse infestation is spread as a sexually transmitted disease. Roughly 30% of patients will have another concurrent sexually transmitted disease, and adolescents with pubic lice are twice as likely as uninfested adolescents to have chlamydial or gonorrheal infection.

FIGURE 367-6. Maculae ceruleae are bluish red spots that represent sites where body lice have fed.

CLINICAL MANIFESTATIONS

Patients present with intense itching, and both lice and nits may be found on pubic hairs as well as on the hair of the chest, abdomen, and legs. Pubic lice may occasionally cause scalp infestation in patients with thick curly hair. They may also infest the eyelashes. Maculae ceruleae may be present as in body louse infestation. These are bluish gray macules at the sites of louse bites. Underwear will commonly be stained by minute droplets of blood.

TREATMENT   Rx

Treatment is by means of shaving or with topical agents used to treat head lice. Oral ivermectin has also been used as for scabies at a single dose of 200 μg/kg.

Beetle-Related Dermatitis

Blister beetles (order Coleoptera) are widespread throughout the world and include members of the families Meloidae and Staphylinidae. Members of the family Oedemeridae are classified as "false" blister beetles but can produce similar skin manifestations. Cantharidin accumulates during the larval stages of the beetle and gives it protection from predatory birds. When threatened, the beetles protect themselves by exuding a cantharidin-containing liquid. Contact with blister beetles results in vesicles and bullae. "Nairobi eye," or rove beetle dermatitis, in northern Kenya is caused by *Paederus eximius*. Rove beetles were implicated in a recent epidemic of pustular eruption among U.S. forces in Pakistan. Treatment for all manifestations of blister beetles is largely symptomatic.

Fleas

Fleas (order Siphonaptera) are ubiquitous among pets and wild animals. They serve as vectors for endemic typhus, bubonic plague, brucellosis, melioidosis, and erysipeloid. The most common flea on dogs is the cat flea, *Ctenocephalides felis*. *Pulex irritans*, the human flea, can be found on dogs and became a major plague vector during the great epidemics. Flea bites cluster on the lower legs and present as intensely pruritic papulovesicles. Tungiasis is caused by the jigger or sand flea, *Tunga penetrans*. It typically presents with a necrotic pustule adjacent to the great toenail.

A veterinarian should be consulted about agents for flea control, including lufenuron and fipronil. Beach areas should restrict pets to prevent infestation.

Flies

Mosquitoes and other flies belong to the order Diptera and represent major disease vectors. *Anopheles* mosquitoes bite mostly at night and are the major vectors of malaria. They also transmit filariasis. *Aedes* mosquitoes bite during the day and transmit dengue, viral encephalitis, yellow fever, and filariasis.

FIGURE 367-7. Bedbugs are red-brown and about the size of small ticks.

FIGURE 367-8. Bedbug bites are often arranged in a characteristic "breakfast, lunch, and dinner" pattern.

Culex mosquitoes bite at night and transmit West Nile encephalitis, filariasis, and viral encephalitis. *Culex* mosquitoes also bite at dusk or early evening. Many arthropod diseases have a principal vector but can also be spread by alternative vectors; for example, whereas *Culex* mosquitoes are the major vector for West Nile fever in the United States, *Aedes* and *Anopheles* species can also spread the disease. *Simulium* flies (blackflies, humpback flies, buffalo gnats, turkey gnats) transmit onchocerciasis. *Lutzomyia* and *Phlebotomus* sand flies transmit leishmaniasis, *Bartonella bacilliformis*, and sandfly fever. Biting midges (punkies, gnats, no-see-ums) are small enough to pass through screens and cause papulovesicular and nodular reactions in sensitive individuals. Tabanid flies include the horseflies, deer flies, and greenheads. As a group, they are large and colorful and deliver painful bites. *Chrysops* deer flies transmit loiasis in Africa and tularemia in the United States. *Glossina* tsetse flies transmit trypanosomiasis.

Furuncular myiasis caused by the botfly is common in Latin America. *Dermatobia hominis* glues its eggs to a mosquito, which serves as an intermediate vector. *Cordylobia anthropophaga*, the mango fly, tumbu fly, putzi fly, or skin maggot fly, is native to Africa and lays its eggs on drying clothing. It produces plaque-type myiasis with many maggots. *Cochliomyia hominivorax*, the screwworm, lays its eggs on wounds or mucous membranes. Screwworms are feared because they leave necrotic flesh and continue to travel through viable tissue. Sarcophagid flies deposit their living larvae on the hosts, where they produce a type of larva migrans. Myiasis is treated by means of mechanical removal with tweezers or by incision of the wound. Covering the embedded larvae with an occlusive substance, such as surgical lubricant, petrolatum, or bacon, encourages them to move upward, facilitating removal.

Prevention of vector-borne disease requires control of standing water, use of screening and mosquito netting, and personal protection with repellents. Screening impregnated with pyrethroids is more effective than untreated screening. Secondary prevention includes malaria chemoprophylaxis and early treatment of illness. Other interventions include insecticidal sprays and gas-powered mosquito traps. Most types of mosquito traps generate carbon dioxide and use chemical attractants such as octenol and butanone. Some *Culex* mosquitoes are repelled by octenol.

N,N-Diethyl-3-methylbenzamide (DEET) remains the most widely used insect repellent, although picaridin is widely used in Europe and is gaining market share in the United States. DEET has a long safety record but can occasionally cause bullous dermatitis, anaphylaxis, or toxic encephalopathy. The American Academy of Pediatrics recommends slow-release products below 30% concentration. A soybean oil–based product (Bite Blocker for Kids) is available for those who wish to avoid chemical repellents. Whereas neem oil products perform reasonably well against various mosquitoes, citronella has limited efficacy.

Hemiptera: True Bugs

Bedbugs have become pandemic and are increasingly recognized in suburban homes, in hotels, and, especially, on college campuses. They are reddish brown and about the size of small ticks (Fig. 367-7). The wings are vestigial. *Cimex lectularius* and *Cimex hemipterus* (the tropical bedbug) parasitize birds and bats, who introduce them into buildings. They also spread readily by luggage. The characteristic skin lesions are a string of bites termed breakfast, lunch, and dinner (Fig. 367-8).

Triatome reduviids are important vectors for American trypanosomiasis (Chagas' disease). Their wings overlap and are sclerotic proximally. The striped abdomen is visible lateral to the wings. Unilateral eyelid swelling (Romaña's sign) is caused by a conjunctival reaction to the bite and to triatome feces infected with trypanosomes.

Hymenoptera Stings

Hymenoptera include membranous winged insects such as wasps, bees, and fire ants. They all result in painful stings and present a potential for anaphylactic reactions. Unexpected stings occur frequently; therefore, allergic individuals must always carry a source of epinephrine, such as an EpiPen auto-injector. Bees are eviscerated during the sting, and the venom gland continues to inject additional venom. Therefore, bee stingers should be removed as rapidly as possible, with little concern for the exact method of removal. Venom immunotherapy can improve quality of life. Rush immunotherapy (a method for rapidly desensitizing patients to allergens) should be performed for those with severe reactions. Omalizumab has been used in conjunction with immunotherapy, but its exact role remains to be determined.

Lepidopterids

Moths and caterpillars may have toxic hairs that may contain histamine, kinins, plasminogen activators, and other proteinaceous toxins. The reactions are usually toxic rather than allergic in nature. Clinical manifestations include pain, erythema, swelling, and hemorrhage. Systemic reactions may include renal failure. *Lonomia* caterpillars may cause a fatal bleeding diathesis with intracranial hemorrhage. Ocular reactions to hairs include ophthalmia nodosa, keratoconjunctivitis, subconjunctival nodules, iritis, and vitreoretinal involvement. Children who ingest caterpillars may develop edema of the lips, tongue, and buccal mucosa. Esophageal and tracheobronchial involvement occurs less commonly.

Delusions of Parasitosis

These patients present with an unshakable belief that they are infested. It is difficult to help them. A careful evaluation should exclude formications secondary to cocaine addiction and pruritus related to systemic diseases such as renal failure and hyperthyroidism. Whereas delusions of parasitosis have traditionally been treated with pimozide, newer atypical antipsychotic agents such as olanzapine and risperidone are better tolerated and reduce the need for electrocardiographic monitoring of drug-induced cardiotoxicity.

⬤ LEECHES AND OTHER ANNELIDS

Leeches occur in fresh water and may be associated with *Pseudomonas* or *Aeromonas* wound infections. Leeches contain anticoagulants, and the attachment sites may bleed freely when the leech is removed. More serious coagulation disorders with massive bleeding have been reported. Saturated salt solutions have been used to facilitate leech removal but do not reduce the risk of infection.

1. Chosidow O, Giraudeau B, Cottrell J, et al. Oral ivermectin versus malathion lotion for difficult-to-treat head lice. *N Engl J Med*. 2010;362:896-905.

SUGGESTED READINGS

Graham J, Stockley K, Goldman RD. Tick-borne illnesses: a CME update. *Pediatr Emerg Care.* 2011;27:141-147. *Clinical review.*

Hayes EB. Looking the other way: preventing vector-borne disease among travelers to the United States. *Travel Med Infect Dis.* 2010;8:277-284. *Review.*

Růžek D, Dobler G, Mantke OD. Tick-borne encephalitis: pathogenesis and clinical implications. *Travel Med Infect Dis.* 2010:8:223-232. *Review.*

368

ANTIVIRAL THERAPY (NON-HIV)

JOHN H. BEIGEL

Although some viral infections are self-limited, others can cause significant morbidity and mortality. Effective therapy is available for many of these infections. Emerging viral diseases such as coronavirus and influenza, concern about viral agents of bioterrorism, and treatment of chronic viral diseases such as hepatitis B and hepatitis C have reinvigorated the search for new antiviral agents. This chapter reviews currently available antiviral agents for the treatment of infections caused by viruses other than human immunodeficiency virus (HIV). Not all agents discussed are presently licensed in all countries.

● MECHANISM OF ACTION

Currently available agents can be classified into those that directly inhibit viral replication at the cellular level (antivirals), those that modify the host response to infection (immunomodulators), and those that directly inactivate viral infectivity (antibodies, virucides, or microbicides). Antiviral agents can be further classified into two general mechanisms. First—and most numerous—are nucleic acid analogues that inhibit viral DNA or RNA synthesis by competing with endogenous nucleic acids for incorporation into the viral genome by viral DNA polymerase or RNA transcriptases. The second mechanism is inhibition of the functions of other essential viral enzymes or proteins, including those responsible for attachment to or release from cells. For example, the principal antivirals for influenza viruses inhibit viral proteins responsible for either uncoating (M2 protein) or release and spread (neuraminidase).

Antiviral strategies that are not covered in this chapter include local destructive measures that destroy both host tissues and virus simultaneously, such as cryotherapy, laser, and podophyllin treatment of warts. Although effective, such measures are useful only for discrete or localized mucocutaneous infections.

● ANTIVIRALS FOR HERPESVIRUS INFECTIONS

Acyclovir and Valacyclovir

Acyclovir, which is an acyclic analogue of the nucleoside guanosine, is converted to its active form through initial monophosphorylation by a virus-encoded thymidine kinase (TK). Although normal human cells possess TK, the affinity of acyclovir for viral TK is approximately 200 times greater than for human TK. The monophosphate then undergoes two additional host cell enzyme-mediated phosphorylations to acyclovir triphosphate (acycloguanosine triphosphate), which preferentially inhibits viral DNA polymerase, competitively and through chain termination. The higher concentrations of the activated form in infected cells and its affinity for viral polymerases result in low toxicity to normal host cells.

Valacyclovir is the L-valyl ester prodrug of acyclovir. Addition of the L-valyl ester fosters greater oral absorption, after which valacyclovir is converted to acyclovir; the prodrug provides three to five times greater bioavailability than oral acyclovir.

Clinical Uses

Acyclovir and valacyclovir are used principally to treat infections caused by herpes simplex virus (HSV; Chapter 382) and varicella-zoster virus (VZV; Chapter 383). Depending on country, acyclovir is available in a topical

ointment and cream, oral capsules, and intravenous and ophthalmic formulations. Valacyclovir is available only as an oral capsule.

Oral acyclovir or valacyclovir decreases the duration of symptoms by approximately 50% and reduces the duration of viral shedding by about 90% in initial episodes of genital herpes. Two or 3 days of therapy appears to be sufficient for recurrent genital herpes. Chronic suppression is highly effective in reducing clinical and viral recurrences, and valacyclovir reduces the risk of transmission of genital HSV between heterosexual partners by 48%.◼ For herpes labialis (cold sores), 1 day of therapy with oral valacyclovir improves time to healing and reduces pain, whereas acyclovir ointment has no consistent clinical benefit.

Parenteral acyclovir is indicated for the initial treatment of mucosal or cutaneous HSV infection in immunocompromised patients, neonatal HSV infections, and disseminated or organ-invasive infections in immunocompetent patients. A subsequent switch to oral valacyclovir is possible in some circumstances. High-dose parenteral acyclovir is the therapy of choice for treatment of HSV encephalitis.

Acyclovir is also effective treatment of VZV infections, although higher doses are needed than for mucosal HSV infections (see Table 368-1). In adults treated within 24 hours of the development of a varicella rash, acyclovir decreases the severity of disease and number of lesions, but oral valacyclovir may be more effective than oral acyclovir. Intravenous acyclovir is warranted for initial treatment of varicella and zoster in immunocompromised hosts. Both acyclovir chemoprophylaxis and valacyclovir chemoprophylaxis reduce the incidence of recurrent HSV in recipients of stem cell and solid organ transplants, but valacyclovir is superior for prevention of cytomegalovirus (CMV) disease.

Toxicity

Acyclovir and valacyclovir have excellent safety profiles and are generally well tolerated. Common side effects include nausea, vomiting, and headaches. Major adverse effects include renal dysfunction and central nervous system (CNS) toxicity. Dehydration and preexisting renal dysfunction predispose to the development of renal impairment. Neurologic side effects include tremor, myoclonus, confusion, lethargy, agitation, and hallucination. Renal dysfunction predisposes to the development of neurotoxicity. Neutropenia and other signs of bone marrow toxicity have also been reported rarely.

Antiviral Resistance

Despite widespread use of acyclovir, the development of HSV resistance in immunocompetent subjects is uncommon (prevalence <1%). However, antiviral resistance is higher in immunocompromised subjects, including those with HIV infection (prevalence of 5%) or bone marrow transplants (prevalence of up to 30%). Drug-resistant, refractory VZV infections can occur in highly immunocompromised patients. Intravenous foscarnet or cidofovir may be effective for infections caused by acyclovir-resistant viruses.

Penciclovir and Famciclovir

Penciclovir is an acyclic guanine analogue that unlike acyclovir is not an obligate chain terminator and may be incorporated into DNA. Penciclovir is phosphorylated by viral TK to penciclovir monophosphate, which is then converted to penciclovir triphosphate. Penciclovir demonstrates in vitro activity against VZV and HSV comparable to that of acyclovir. The bioavailability of penciclovir after oral administration is less than 2%. In contrast, famciclovir is an oral prodrug that is deacetylated and oxidized in the liver to form penciclovir; the bioavailability of penciclovir averages 77% after administration of famciclovir.

Clinical Uses

Penciclovir and famciclovir are used to treat HSV and VZV infections. Penciclovir is available as a topical cream and in some countries as an intravenous formulation. Famciclovir is available as a capsule.

Frequent applications of topical penciclovir reduce herpes labialis pain and lesions by about 1 day. Famciclovir is approved for the treatment of recurrent HSV labialis and genital infections and for herpes zoster, for which it is as effective as valacyclovir. It is also as effective as acyclovir when it is used to treat initial genital HSV infection.

Toxicity

Penciclovir is well tolerated as a topical cream; the majority of adverse reactions are local irritation and mild erythema. Adverse effects of oral famciclovir include headache, dizziness, nausea, and diarrhea.

TABLE 368-1 ANTIVIRALS FOR HERPESVIRUS INFECTIONS

VIRAL INFECTION	DRUG	ROUTE	USUAL ADULT DOSAGE
HERPES SIMPLEX VIRUS			
Genital herpes			
First episode	Acyclovir	PO	400 mg tid or 200 mg 5 times/day for 7-10 days
	Famciclovir	PO	250 mg tid for 7-10 days
	Valacyclovir	PO	1 g bid for 7-10 days
Recurrent	Acyclovir	PO	800 mg tid for 2 days, or 400 mg tid or 200 mg 5 times/day for 5 days
	Famciclovir	PO	1000 mg bid for 2 doses
	Valacyclovir	PO	500 mg bid for 3 days or 1 g/day for 5 days
Suppression	Acyclovir	PO	400 mg bid or 200 mg tid
	Famciclovir	PO	250 mg bid
	Valacyclovir	PO	500 mg/day or 1 g/day (10 or more episodes/year)
Orolabial herpes	Penciclovir 1%	Topical	Apply cream every 2 hr while awake for 4 days
	Acyclovir 5%	Topical	Apply cream 5 times/day for 4 days
	Docosanol 10%	Topical	Apply cream 5 times/day until healing
	Valacyclovir	PO	2 g q12h × 2 doses
	Acyclovir	PO	400 mg 5 times/day for 5 days
	Famciclovir	PO	1500 mg single dose
Mucocutaneous disease	Acyclovir	IV	5 mg/kg/8 hr for 7-14 days
	Acyclovir	PO	400 mg 5 times/day for 7-14 days
	Valacyclovir	PO	500 mg or 1 g bid for 7-10 days
Encephalitis	Acyclovir	IV	10 mg/kg/8 hr for 10 days
Neonatal	Acyclovir	IV	10-20 mg/kg/8 hr for 14-21 days
Keratoconjunctivitis	Trifluridine	Topical	1 drop of 1% solution q2h up to 9 drops/day
	Vidarabine	Topical	½-inch ribbon of 3% ointment 5 times daily
Acyclovir-resistant HSV	Foscarnet	IV	40 mg/kg q8-12 h until healed.
CYTOMEGALOVIRUS			
CMV retinitis	Ganciclovir	IV	Induction: 5 mg/kg/12 hr for 14-21 days (maintenance: 5 mg/kg/day)
	Valganciclovir	PO	Induction: 900 mg bid for 21 days (maintenance: 900 mg/day)
	Cidofovir	IV	5 mg/kg once weekly × 2, then every other week (maintenance: 5 mg/kg q2wk)
	Foscarnet	IV	60 mg/kg/8 hr or 90 mg/kg q12h for 14-21 days (maintenance: 90-120 mg/kg daily)
	Fomivirsen	Intravitreal	330 μg q2wk × 2, then q4wk (maintenance: 330 μg every month)
HIV infection, CMV colitis or esophagitis	Ganciclovir	IV	5 mg/kg/12 hr for 14-28 days (until symptoms resolved)
Prophylaxis (transplantation)	Ganciclovir	IV	5 mg/kg/12 hr for 7-14 days, then 5 mg/kg IV once a day
	Valganciclovir	PO	900 mg qd
Prophylaxis (advanced HIV infection)	Ganciclovir	IV	5 mg/kg daily
VARICELLA-ZOSTER VIRUS			
Varicella	Acyclovir	PO	800 mg qid for 5 days
Varicella in immunocompromised hosts	Acyclovir	IV	10 mg/kg/8 hr for 7-10 days
Herpes zoster in immunocompromised hosts	Acyclovir	IV	10 mg/kg/8 hr for 7-10 days
Herpes zoster in normal hosts	Acyclovir	PO	800 mg 5 times daily for 7-10 days
	Valacyclovir	PO	1 g tid for 7 days
	Famciclovir	PO	500 mg tid for 7 days

TABLE 368-2 MECHANISMS OF EXCRETION AND THRESHOLDS FOR DOSE ADJUSTMENT

	MAJOR ROUTE OF ELIMINATION	THRESHOLD FOR ADJUSTMENT IN RENAL INSUFFICIENCY OR FAILURE	ADJUSTMENT FOR HEPATIC FAILURE	ADJUSTMENT FOR OBESITY
Acyclovir IV	Renal	CrCl < 50 mL/min	No adjustment	Dose by ideal body weight
Acyclovir PO	Renal	CrCl < 25 mL/min	No adjustment	Dose by ideal body weight
Valacyclovir	Renal	CrCl < 50 mL/min	No adjustment	Unknown
Famciclovir	Renal	CrCl < 60 mL/min	No adjustment	Unknown
Foscarnet	Renal	CrCl < 1.4 mL/min/kg	No adjustment	Unknown
Ganciclovir IV	Renal	CrCl < 70 mL/min	No adjustment	Unknown
Valganciclovir	Renal	CrCl < 60 mL/min	No adjustment	Unknown
Cidofovir	Renal	CrCl < 55 mL/min	No adjustment	Unknown

Antiviral Resistance

Penciclovir resistance in HSV has been uncommon in immunocompetent subjects but, like acyclovir resistance, more frequent in immunocompromised hosts (2.1%). Most acyclovir-resistant HSV isolates are cross-resistant to penciclovir.

Ganciclovir and Valganciclovir

Ganciclovir is an acyclic deoxyguanosine analogue with antiviral activity against multiple herpesviruses, including HSV, VZV, CMV (Chapter 384), Epstein-Barr virus (EBV; Chapter 385), and human herpesvirus 8. It is much more active than acyclovir against CMV and EBV.

TABLE 368-3 DRUG-DRUG INTERACTIONS

	COADMINISTERED DRUG	RISKS OR TOXICITIES	POSSIBLE MECHANISM
Acyclovir	Fosphenytoin	Decreased phenytoin plasma concentration	Decreased phenytoin absorption
	Meperidine	Increased risk for CNS stimulation and excitation	Increased meperidine metabolites
	Mycophenolate	Increased plasma concentration of acyclovir	Competition for renal secretion
	Valproic acid	Decreased valproic acid plasma concentration	Decreased valproic acid absorption
	Varicella vaccine	Decreased varicella vaccine effectiveness	Inhibition of VZV
	Zidovudine	Increased lethargy and fatigue	Unknown
Valacyclovir	Mycophenolate	Increased risk for neutropenia	Unknown
Ganciclovir	Didanosine	Increased didanosine toxicity (neuropathy, diarrhea, pancreatitis)	Increased didanosine bioavailability
	Imipenem	Increased risk for CNS toxicity (seizures)	Unknown
	Mycophenolate	Increase in plasma concentration of ganciclovir	Competition for renal secretion
	Probenecid	Increase in plasma concentration of ganciclovir	Competition for renal secretion
	Tacrolimus	Increased risk for nephrotoxicity	Additive nephrotoxicity
	Zidovudine	Increased risk for hematologic toxicity (anemia, neutropenia)	Unknown
Valganciclovir	Probenecid	Increase in plasma concentration of ganciclovir	Competition for renal secretion
	Zidovudine	Increased risk for hematologic toxicity (anemia, neutropenia)	Unknown
Cidofovir	Aminoglycosides	Nephrotoxicity	Additive nephrotoxicity
	Foscarnet	Nephrotoxicity	Additive nephrotoxicity
	Pentamidine	Nephrotoxicity	Additive nephrotoxicity
Foscarnet*	Drugs that prolong QRS	Torsades de pointes	Additive toxicity, prolongation of QRS
	Renal toxic drugs	Nephrotoxicity	Additive nephrotoxicity
Idoxuridine	Boric acid	Eye irritation	Formation of precipitate

*Many classes of drugs have added toxicity when they are administered with foscarnet. Consult a pharmacologist if you are uncertain about possible interactions.

TABLE 368-4 SIGNIFICANT ADVERSE EFFECTS (U.S. FDA BLACK BOX WARNING)

DRUG	BLACK BOX SYNOPSIS
Cidofovir	Renal impairment, including renal failure; prehydrate and use probenecid Neutropenia May be carcinogenic and teratogenic and may cause hypospermia or aspermia
Foscarnet	Nephrotoxicity; prehydrate Seizures related to minerals and electrolyte disturbances
Ganciclovir	Neutropenia, anemia, thrombocytopenia May be carcinogenic and teratogenic and may cause hypospermia or aspermia
Valganciclovir	Neutropenia, anemia, thrombocytopenia May be carcinogenic and teratogenic and may cause hypospermia or aspermia

The bioavailability of oral ganciclovir is less than 10%. After the oral administration of valganciclovir, which is an L-valyl prodrug of ganciclovir, bioavailability of ganciclovir averages 60%.

Clinical Uses

Ganciclovir is available as an oral capsule, a parenteral injection, and an ocular implant; valganciclovir is available only as a tablet. Ganciclovir and valganciclovir are effective for treatment of CMV retinitis, for which they are comparably active. In the absence of immune reconstitution, long-term suppression therapy is necessary.

They are also used for life-threatening CMV diseases in patients with acquired immunodeficiency syndrome (AIDS) and other immunocompromised conditions and for prevention of CMV disease in transplant patients. For immunocompromised patients with organ-invasive CMV infections, intravenous ganciclovir provides clinical response rates of 70 to 90%, although response rates are lower for CMV pneumonitis after stem cell transplantation or CMV encephalitis in patients with AIDS. Oral valganciclovir provides long-term outcomes similar to those of intravenous ganciclovir for the treatment of CMV disease.[2]

Long-term prophylaxis with ganciclovir or valganciclovir reduces the incidence of CMV disease after solid organ and stem cell transplantation, but this therapy has substantial side effects, including bone marrow suppression. These drugs can also be used as preemptive therapy for patients who have CMV viremia or antigenemia. In the prevention of CMV disease, preemptive valganciclovir therapy may be equally effective to chronic valacyclovir prophylaxis.[3] Intravenous ganciclovir is the recommended agent for treatment of herpesvirus B infections, particularly those involving the CNS.

Toxicity

The most common adverse effect with ganciclovir and valganciclovir is bone marrow suppression, particularly neutropenia and thrombocytopenia, which occur in up to 50% of patients given intravenous ganciclovir. Fever, edema, phlebitis, headache, neuropathy, disorientation, nausea, anorexia, rash, and myalgias have also been reported with ganciclovir therapy. Intravitreal ganciclovir implants may cause vitreous hemorrhage and retinal detachment.

Antiviral Resistance

Ganciclovir resistance secondary to mutations in CMV kinase and sometimes DNA polymerase is related to the length of ganciclovir exposure and the degree of immunosuppression. Resistance may be associated with progressive disease during continued ganciclovir use; foscarnet and cidofovir are alternative treatments.[4]

Cidofovir

Cidofovir, which is an acyclic phosphonate derivative of cytosine, is phosphorylated to its active diphosphate form by host cellular enzymes. Cidofovir diphosphate competitively inhibits viral DNA polymerase and viral DNA synthesis. Despite a short serum half-life, the antiviral effects are protracted because of prolonged intracellular concentrations of the phosphorylated metabolite.

Clinical Uses

Cidofovir is commercially available as an intravenous infusion. Investigational uses have included topical gel and intravitreal and intralesional injection.

Intravenous cidofovir is indicated in AIDS patients for CMV retinitis for which ganciclovir or foscarnet therapy is failing. Limited data suggest that intravenous cidofovir may be effective in other CMV infections (pneumonitis, gastroenteritis), acyclovir- or foscarnet-resistant HSV infections, certain forms of human papillomavirus disease, invasive adenoviral infections in transplant recipients, and possibly BK virus infection in renal transplant patients. In addition, in vivo and animal data suggest efficacy of cidofovir against smallpox, vaccinia, and monkeypox infections, although clinical trials are lacking.

Toxicity

Dose-related nephrotoxicity, characterized by increased serum creatinine, proteinuria, and tubular dysfunction, is the main side effect of intravenous cidofovir. Adequate hydration and concomitant oral probenecid reduce the risk. Other common side effects include diarrhea, asthenia, nausea, vomiting, neutropenia, fever, and rash. Iritis, intraocular pressure changes, loss of visual acuity, and uveitis have been reported with intravenous cidofovir. Intravitreal cidofovir is effective but locally toxic.

Antiviral Resistance

Sustained exposure to cidofovir does not easily induce resistance, although resistance has infrequently been described in HSV and CMV.

Foscarnet

Foscarnet is a pyrophosphate analogue that acts as a noncompetitive inhibitor of many viral RNA and DNA polymerases. When a nucleotide is incorporated into a DNA or RNA strand by a polymerase, pyrophosphate is released. Foscarnet directly inhibits viral polymerases without phosphorylation, so TK-deficient acyclovir-resistant HSV and VZV are susceptible to this agent.

Clinical Uses

Foscarnet is as effective as ganciclovir for the treatment of CMV retinitis in patients with AIDS, and combination therapy with ganciclovir may be superior to monotherapy with either agent for recalcitrant retinitis. For extraretinal CMV disease, foscarnet has demonstrated efficacy similar to that of ganciclovir. The choice of agent may be dictated by the side effect profile. Foscarnet is also effective for the treatment of acyclovir-resistant HSV and VZV infections.

Toxicity

Nephrotoxicity with azotemia and proteinuria is dose limiting and occurs in more than a third of patients. A slow infusion rate and saline hydration reduce the risk. Other common side effects include anemia (30 to 50% of patients), granulocytopenia, diarrhea, nausea, vomiting, fever, seizures, paresthesias, headache, and genital ulcers. Marked electrolyte disturbances may develop, including hypophosphatemia, hypocalcemia, hypokalemia, and hypomagnesemia. Foscarnet can prolong the QT interval and be associated with cardiac arrhythmias, including ventricular tachycardia, ventricular fibrillation, and torsades de pointes.

Antiviral Resistance

The development of CMV resistance to foscarnet as a result of mutations in viral DNA polymerase is uncommon, except after prolonged administration. In AIDS patients with retinitis, foscarnet resistance is detectable in 13% of patients at 6 months and in 37% at 12 months.

Fomivirsen

Fomivirsen, which is an antisense oligonucleotide that inhibits CMV replication, is currently available as an intravitreal injection that is effective for both newly diagnosed CMV retinitis and CMV retinitis failing usual therapies, although direct comparisons with other agents are lacking. Intravitreal administration of fomivirsen may cause increased intraocular pressure, iritis, vitreitis, and cataracts in 10 to 20% of patients.

Brivudine

Brivudine, also known as bromovinyldeoxyuridine, is a thymidine analogue that is currently licensed for the treatment of herpes zoster in several European Union countries but not in the United States. Its efficacy is comparable to that of acyclovir, with similar time to crusting and cessation of pain. Common side effects include nausea, vomiting, abdominal discomfort, and anorexia.

Docosanol

Docosanol, which is a 22-carbon saturated fatty alcohol that inhibits intracellular penetration of lipid enveloped viruses, is approved as a cream for the treatment of herpes labialis. Frequent topical applications have shown reductions in time to cessation of pain and healing, but direct comparison to other agents is lacking. Local reaction, rash, and pruritus are common side effects.

Idoxuridine and Trifluorothymidine

Idoxuridine and trifluorothymidine (trifluridine) are thymidine analogues that are phosphorylated by both viral and cellular TKs to active triphosphate derivatives that inhibit both viral and cellular DNA synthesis. The result is antiviral activity but also host cytotoxicity, which prevents safe systemic use.

However, the tolerability of these compounds is adequate for topical use. Both idoxuridine and trifluorothymidine are available as ophthalmic formulations and are licensed for the treatment of herpetic keratitis. In direct comparison, trifluridine appears to be the more efficacious of these compounds. In addition, idoxuridine in dimethyl sulfoxide has been used topically in some countries for treatment of mucosal herpes infections. The most frequent adverse effects with trifluridine are transient burning or stinging on instillation and palpebral edema. Irritation and punctate corneal defects have been reported with idoxuridine.

Vidarabine

Vidarabine, an adenosine analogue, is now available only as an ophthalmic ointment indicated for acute keratoconjunctivitis and recurrent epithelial keratitis secondary to HSV. Its clinical activity appears to be superior to that of idoxuridine. Toxicities of the ointment include conjunctival injection, burning, and irritation.

● ANTIVIRALS FOR INFLUENZA VIRUS INFECTIONS

Adamantanes (Amantadine, Rimantadine)

Amantadine and rimantadine are symmetrical tricyclic amines with activity against many influenza A viruses (Chapter 372). By inhibiting the ion channel function of the M2 protein of influenza A, they interfere with uncoating of the virus and release of the viral genome.

Clinical Uses

Amantadine and rimantadine (Tables 368-5 to 368-7) decrease the length and severity of uncomplicated influenza A virus infection by susceptible strains if they are initiated within the first 2 days after the onset of symptoms, but it is uncertain whether they reduce the risk for complications. Both drugs are formulated for oral administration: capsules for amantadine and tablets for rimantadine as well as pediatric syrups. In recent years, marked increases in antiviral resistance in community isolates have limited the utility of these drugs.

Both rimantadine and amantadine are effective when they are used for prophylaxis against influenza A illness (overall 66% average for rimantadine and 74% for amantadine). In persons who take the drug for prophylaxis, subclinical infections may still develop and elicit immune responses that will protect them when they are exposed to antigenically related viruses.

Amantadine is also used in the treatment of parkinsonism, for drug-induced extrapyramidal reactions, and in the management of multiple sclerosis symptoms.

Toxicity

Amantadine causes CNS side effects in 10 to 30% of healthy young adults who take the standard adult dose of 200 mg/day; the frequency is significantly lower with rimantadine. Neuropsychiatric side effects include anxiety, nervousness, insomnia, and, particularly in the elderly or those with renal insufficiency, hallucinations, confusion, disorientation, and psychosis or coma. Amantadine or less often rimantadine is associated with an increased risk for seizures. Both drugs cause gastrointestinal side effects. Orthostatic hypotension occurs in 1 to 5%. Anticholinergic side effects, including dry mouth, occur in amantadine recipients.

TABLE 368-5	ANTIVIRALS FOR INFLUENZA VIRUS INFECTIONS		
VIRUS	**DRUG**	**ROUTE**	**USUAL ADULT TREATMENT DOSAGE**
Influenza A and B virus	Oseltamivir	PO	75 mg bid for 5 days
	Zanamivir	Inhalation	10 mg bid by inhaler for 5 days
Influenza A virus	Amantadine	PO	100 mg bid or 200 mg qd for 5 days
	Rimantadine	PO	100 mg bid for 5 days

TABLE 368-6 MECHANISMS OF EXCRETION AND THRESHOLDS FOR DOSE ADJUSTMENTS

	MAJOR ROUTE OF ELIMINATION	THRESHOLD FOR ADJUSTMENT IN RENAL INSUFFICIENCY OR FAILURE	ADJUSTMENT FOR HEPATIC FAILURE	SPECIAL ADJUSTMENT FOR THE ELDERLY
Amantadine	Renal	CrCl < 50 mL/min	No adjustment	>65 yr: 100 mg daily
Rimantadine	Hepatic and renal	CrCl < 10 mL/min/1.72 m^2	100 mg daily	100 mg daily
Oseltamivir	Renal	CrCl < 30 mL/min/1.72 m^2	No adjustment	
Zanamivir	Renal	No adjustment	No adjustment	

TABLE 368-7 DRUG-DRUG INTERACTIONS

	COADMINISTERED DRUG	RISKS OR TOXICITIES	POSSIBLE MECHANISM
Amantadine	Anticholinergics	Dry mouth, constipation, decreased urination, sedation, blurred vision	Additive anticholinergic effect
	Benztropine	CNS toxicity (confusion, hallucinations)	Unknown
	Bupropion	Nausea, vomiting, excitation, restlessness, postural hypotension	Unknown
	Triamterene	Incoordination, agitation, visual hallucinations	Decreased amantadine clearance
	Trimethoprim	CNS toxicity (insomnia, confusion)	Decreased amantadine clearance

Antiviral Resistance

Single point mutations in M2 confer high-level resistance to these drugs and make them ineffective. Such resistant variants emerge commonly during treatment and are transmissible. In 2005-2006, the frequency of resistance in influenza A (H3N2) viruses was as high as 92% in the United States. Resistance is also present in some seasonal H1N1 and many H5N1 and pandemic H1N1 viruses.

Neuraminidase Inhibitors (Oseltamivir, Zanamivir, Peramivir)

Zanamivir, oseltamivir, and peramivir are sialic acid analogues that inhibit influenza virus neuraminidases by competitively interacting with the active enzyme site of influenza A and B viruses, including adamantine-resistant strains. Influenza neuraminidase cleaves terminal sialic acid residues and destroys the receptors recognized by viral hemagglutinin. These drugs inhibit this action, which is essential for release of virus from infected cells, prevention of viral aggregates, and spread within the respiratory tract.

Oseltamivir is administered orally as the phosphate prodrug, which is rapidly absorbed and hydrolyzed to the active form oseltamivir carboxylate. The oral bioavailability of zanamivir is poor, and it is currently licensed to be delivered as an orally inhaled powder. Peramivir, an intravenous neuraminidase inhibitor, is not licensed but was previously made available for use under an emergency use authorization, a mechanism by which the U.S. Food and Drug Administration (FDA) allows the use of an unapproved medical product during certain types of emergencies, such as pandemic influenza.

Clinical Uses

Oseltamivir and zanamivir are effective for the treatment and prophylaxis of acute influenza A and B infections. Early treatment in adults decreases the duration and severity of illness and reduces lower respiratory tract complications, antibiotic use, and, with oseltamivir, hospitalizations. In cohort studies, treatment with oseltamivir has been associated with a significant reduction in death (odds ratio, 0.21). Zanamivir is also effective in alleviating symptoms and decreasing the risk for lower respiratory complications. Both zanamivir and oseltamivir are highly effective for the prevention of influenza. Peramivir may be useful in patients who are not responding to either oseltamivir or zanamivir antiviral therapy.

Toxicity

The most common side effects with oseltamivir are nausea and vomiting. It may also be associated with headache, rash, and possibly abnormal transaminases. Zanamivir is generally well tolerated, but bronchospasm (sometimes severe) has been reported primarily in patients with underlying airway disease. The most common side effects of peramivir are nausea, diarrhea, and mild neutropenia.

Antiviral Resistance

Oseltamivir resistance as a result of neuraminidase mutations has been detected during treatment of seasonal influenza, more often in children than

TABLE 368-8 ANTIVIRALS FOR HEPATITIS VIRUS INFECTIONS

VIRAL INFECTION	DRUG	ROUTE	USUAL ADULT DOSAGE
Chronic hepatitis C*	PEG-interferon alfa-2a *or* PEG-interferon alfa-2b	SC	180 µg weekly for 48 wk
	plus ribavirin	SC	1.5 µg/kg weekly for 48 wk
		PO	800-1200 mg/day, depending on weight
Chronic hepatitis B	Interferon alfa-2b	SC, IM	5 MU/day or 10 MU 3 times weekly for 16-24 wk
	PEG-interferon alfa-2a	SC	180 µg weekly for 48 weeks
	Entecavir Naive virus	PO	0.5 mg daily; optimal duration of therapy is unknown
	Lamivudine resistant virus	PO	1 mg daily; optimal duration of therapy is unknown
	Lamivudine	PO	100 mg/day
	Adefovir	PO	10 mg/day
	Telbivudine	PO	600 mg/day

*Genotypes 2 and 3 may tolerate shorter treatment.

in adults and recently in H5N1- and H1N1-infected patients. In the immunocompromised host, and possibly in individuals with H5N1 or H1N1, the development of resistance is associated with treatment failure. Zanamivir retains clinical effectiveness against the most common oseltamivir-resistant variant.◢

● ANTIVIRALS FOR HEPATITIS VIRUS INFECTIONS

Adefovir

Adefovir, an acyclic analogue of adenosine monophosphate, is administered orally as a prodrug, adefovir dipivoxil, which is rapidly converted enzymatically to adefovir in intestinal epithelium.

Clinical Uses

In chronic hepatitis B (Chapter 151), prolonged administration of adefovir is effective in improving histologic abnormalities of the liver, decreasing hepatitis B virus (HBV) DNA levels, and normalizing biochemical (alanine aminotransferase) markers in patients with hepatitis B e antigen (HBeAg)–positive and HBeAg-negative chronic hepatitis B (Tables 368-8 to 368-11). Adefovir has been shown to be effective against chronic hepatitis B resistant to lamivudine. The combination of lamivudine and adefovir may decrease the emergence of resistant virus but does not have additive or synergistic antiviral activity.

TABLE 368-9	MECHANISMS OF EXCRETION AND THRESHOLDS FOR DOSE ADJUSTMENT			
	MAJOR ROUTE OF ELIMINATION	**THRESHOLD FOR ADJUSTMENT IN RENAL INSUFFICIENCY OR FAILURE**	**ADJUSTMENT FOR HEPATIC FAILURE**	**SPECIAL ADJUSTMENT FOR ELDERLY**
Adefovir	Renal	CrCl < 50 mL/min	No adjustment	
Entecavir	Renal	CrCl < 50 mL/min	No adjustment	
Lamivudine	Renal	CrCl < 50 mL/min	No adjustment	
Tenofovir	Renal	CrCl < 50 mL/min	No adjustment	
Ribavirin	Renal	CrCl < 50 mL/min	No adjustment	
PEG-interferon alfa-2a	Renal	CrCl < 50 mL/min	Progressive rise in alanine transaminase	>60 yr: consider reduction
Telbivudine	Renal	CrCl < 50 mL/min	No adjustment	

TABLE 368-10	DRUG-DRUG INTERACTIONS		
	COADMINISTERED DRUG	**RISKS OR TOXICITIES**	**POSSIBLE MECHANISM**
Lamivudine	Ribavirin	Lactic acidosis	Unknown
	Sulfamethoxazole	Increased risk for lamivudine adverse effects	Competition for renal secretion
	Trimethoprim	Increased risk for lamivudine adverse effects	Competition for renal secretion
	Zalcitabine	Increased zalcitabine and lamivudine exposure	Inhibition of phosphorylation
Tenofovir	Atazanavir	Decreased atazanavir concentration or increased tenofovir levels	Unknown
	Didanosine	Increased didanosine plasma concentration and risk for toxicity	Increased didanosine bioavailability
	Lopinavir	Increased tenofovir bioavailability	Unknown
	Ritonavir	Increased tenofovir bioavailability	Unknown
Ribavirin	Nucleoside analogues	Lactic acidosis	Unknown
	Interferon alfa-2b	Worsening mental depression, anger, and hostility	Unknown
Interferon alfa-2	Angiotensin-converting enzyme inhibitors	Hematologic abnormalities (granulocytopenia, thrombocytopenia)	Unknown
	Colchicine	Decreased interferon alfa-2a effectiveness	Unknown
	Theophylline	Theophylline toxicity (nausea, vomiting, palpitations, seizures)	Unknown
	Ribavirin	Worsening mental depression, anger, and hostility	Unknown

TABLE 368-11	SIGNIFICANT ADVERSE EFFECTS (U.S. FDA BLACK BOX WARNING)
DRUG	**BLACK BOX SYNOPSIS**
Adefovir	Severe acute exacerbations of hepatitis B may occur with cessation of therapy Nephrotoxicity may occur in patients at risk for or undergoing renal dysfunction Lactic acidosis and severe hepatomegaly with steatosis
Entecavir	Lactic acidosis and severe hepatomegaly with steatosis; severe acute exacerbations of hepatitis B may occur with cessation of therapy
Lamivudine	Severe acute exacerbations of hepatitis B may occur with cessation of therapy Lactic acidosis and severe hepatomegaly with steatosis
Ribavirin	Monotherapy for hepatitis C is not effective Hemolytic anemia Teratogenic and embryocidal
Interferon alfa	May cause or aggravate neuropsychiatric, autoimmune, ischemic, and infectious disorders
Telbivudine	Severe acute exacerbation of hepatitis B may occur with cessation of therapy Lactic acidosis and severe hepatomegaly with steatosis

Toxicity

The major adverse effect is nephrotoxicity, manifested by increased serum creatinine and sometimes hypophosphatemia, both of which are usually reversible with discontinuation of the drug. Common side effects include asthenia, headache, nausea, vomiting, and diarrhea. In addition, severe exacerbations of hepatitis B have been observed after cessation of therapy.

Antiviral Resistance

Adefovir resistance secondary to point mutations in HBV polymerase develops in about 6% of patients after 3 years of adefovir therapy. Lamivudine generally retains activity against adefovir-resistant variants.

Entecavir

Entecavir, which is a deoxyguanosine nucleoside analogue with specific antiviral activity for hepadnaviruses, is more potent than lamivudine and also retains some activity against lamivudine-resistant HBV variants. It is well absorbed after oral administration, and its prolonged half-life (128 to 149 hours) allows once-daily dosing.

Clinical Uses

Entecavir is approved for the treatment of chronic hepatitis B in adults with evidence of active viral replication and either persistent elevations in serum aminotransferases or histologically active disease. Compared with lamivudine, entecavir is more efficacious in reducing HBV DNA levels and normalizing serum aminotransferases as well as in improving histologic abnormalities.**56** Higher doses and longer durations of therapy are indicated for lamivudine-resistant infections. Entecavir is not recommended in patients who have HIV/HBV coinfection and who are not receiving concurrent highly active antiretroviral therapy because of the risk of resistance to HIV nucleoside reverse transcriptase inhibitors.

Toxicity

Adverse effects reported during entecavir therapy include headache, fatigue, dizziness, nausea, abdominal pain, rhinitis, fever, diarrhea, cough, and myalgia. Lactic acidosis and severe hepatomegaly with steatosis have been reported. Severe exacerbations of hepatitis B have been observed after cessation of therapy.

Antiviral Resistance

Entecavir resistance, caused by specific mutations in HBV polymerase, appears to be uncommon, with no evidence after more than 1 year of drug exposure.

Lamivudine

Lamivudine is a deoxycytidine nucleoside analogue active against retroviruses and hepadnaviruses. The triphosphate inhibits HBV polymerase, and its incorporation into viral DNA results in termination of the DNA chain.

Clinical Uses

Prolonged lamivudine administration to patients with chronic hepatitis B suppresses viral replication, improves histologic abnormalities of the liver, reduces progression of fibrosis, and decreases the risk for late complications, but monotherapy with lamivudine appears to be inferior to monotherapy with interferon for sustained control of HBV replication. Combination therapy with lamivudine and interferon has shown inconsistent benefit compared with either drug alone.

Toxicity

Adverse effects of lamivudine include diarrhea, headache, and elevated liver enzymes. Severe post-treatment exacerbations of hepatitis B, including fatalities, have occurred with discontinuation of lamivudine, more commonly in patients coinfected with HBV and HIV.

Antiviral Resistance

Lamivudine resistance, caused by mutations in HBV polymerase, is common during prolonged treatment of hepatitis B and emerges in about 20% of treated patients annually. Resistance is associated with increases in viral replication and aminotransferases.

Tenofovir

Tenofovir is a nucleotide analogue of adenosine monophosphate. The commercially available agent, tenofovir disoproxil fumarate, is an ester prodrug of tenofovir and gives an effective tenofovir bioavailability of 25%.

Clinical Uses

Treatment with tenofovir is more effective than adefovir in producing histologic improvement and viral suppression in patients with HBeAg-negative or HbeAg-positive chronic hepatitis B.[7] In HBV-HIV coinfection, combination antiretroviral therapy that includes tenofovir leads to significantly reduced HBV DNA levels compared with combination therapy with adefovir.

Toxicity

Tenofovir is generally well tolerated; the most common side effects are nausea, diarrhea, vomiting, and anorexia. Lactic acidosis with hepatic steatosis has been reported, primarily when it is used in combination with other nucleoside analogues. Acute exacerbations of hepatitis B have been reported after discontinuation of tenofovir in patients who are coinfected with HIV and HBV.

Antiviral Resistance

Mutations in HBV polymerase that confer reduced susceptibility to tenofovir occur during prolonged use (>12 months), although the clinical significance of these mutations remains to be defined.

Telbivudine

Telbivudine is a synthetic thymidine nucleoside analogue with activity against HBV, including some lamivudine-resistant variants. The triphosphate form competitively inhibits the HBV DNA polymerase (reverse transcriptase).

Clinical Uses

Telbivudine is used for the treatment of chronic hepatitis B. In comparative trials against lamivudine or adefovir, telbivudine demonstrated greater virologic response at week 52 (60% vs. 40% of subjects HBV DNA negative by polymerase chain reaction analysis).

Toxicity

Common side effects include headache, nausea, and vomiting. Severe acute exacerbations of hepatitis B have been reported in patients who have discontinued anti-HBV therapy. Myopathy, manifested by muscle aches or weakness with increased creatine kinase, has rarely been reported.

Ribavirin

Ribavirin is a purine nucleoside with antiviral activity against some DNA viruses and many RNA viruses, including influenza A and B, parainfluenza, measles, respiratory syncytial virus (RSV), retroviruses, arenaviruses such as Lassa virus, and some hantaviruses.

Clinical Uses

Monotherapy with ribavirin for chronic hepatitis C (Chapter 151) has been shown to decrease serum alanine aminotransferase but not hepatitis C virus RNA levels. However, combination therapy with ribavirin and various interferons, most recently pegylated interferons, is superior to interferon monotherapy, improves viral clearance and liver histologic responses, and reduces complications, including mortality. Ribavirin plus pegylated interferon has become the standard treatment of chronic hepatitis C.

Aerosol administration of ribavirin has been used to treat RSV bronchiolitis and pneumonia in children and to treat influenza A and B infections. Limited benefit has been seen with oral ribavirin in uncomplicated influenza. Aerosol ribavirin combined with intravenous immune globulin, particularly with the anti-RSV monoclonal antibody palivizumab, appears to reduce the mortality of RSV infection in bone marrow transplant and other highly immunocompromised patients.

Systemic ribavirin reduces the mortality associated with Lassa fever and Asian (Korean) hemorrhagic fever with renal syndrome (Chapter 389), although not mortality in patients with hantavirus-associated cardiopulmonary syndrome. It appears to have activity in Congo-Crimean hemorrhagic fever and in Nipah virus infections. Ribavirin is often recommended as treatment of hemorrhagic fevers of unknown etiology or secondary to arenaviruses or bunyaviruses in the event that these viruses are used as biologic weapons.

Toxicity

Aerosol delivery may cause bronchospasm. Systemic ribavirin is frequently associated with hemolytic anemia (in up to 61% in some series) and sometimes with electrolyte abnormalities, including hypocalcemia and hypomagnesemia. Arrhythmias, pruritus, rash, nausea, and myalgia have been reported, as have neurologic side effects, including insomnia and irritability. Ribavirin is gonadotoxic and teratogenic in multiple species.

Emtricitabine

Emtricitabine is an analogue of cytidine. It is currently licensed only for the treatment of HIV infection. However, in a large study of patients with chronic hepatitis B, monotherapy with emtricitabine led to significantly better histologic response (62% vs. 25%) and virologic suppression (54% vs. 2%) at 48 weeks compared with placebo.

Interferons

Interferons are glycoprotein cytokines with a complex array of antiviral, immunomodulating, and antineoplastic properties. Interferons are currently classified as α, β, or γ; the natural sources of these classes, in general, are leukocytes, fibroblasts, and lymphocytes, respectively. Each type of interferon can now be produced through recombinant DNA technology. Although the full mechanism of interferon's action is not defined, interferons generally induce synthesis of new cellular RNA and proteins that mediate antiviral effects through multiple different mechanisms.

Interferons generally require administration daily or several times per week. However, the combination of interferon with polyethylene glycol to form pegylated interferon significantly prolongs absorption, decreases elimination, and provides higher, more sustained plasma levels that enable administration once weekly.

Clinical Uses

In chronic active hepatitis B, treatment with interferon alfa leads to loss of HBV DNA and biochemical and histologic improvement in about 25 to 40% of patients. Administration of PEG-interferon alfa-2a or alfa-2b for 48 weeks converts about 30% of patients to seronegative status after 6 months of treatment. Combination therapy with interferon and lamivudine is not clearly superior to interferon alone.

In contrast to hepatitis B, combination therapy is the mainstay of treatment of hepatitis C. Subcutaneous administration of PEG-interferon alfa-2a plus daily ribavirin for 48 weeks results in a sustained virologic response in about 55% of treated patients, compared with less than a 30% response with interferon monotherapy. Patients with hepatitis C genotype 1 have lower levels of response than do patients with genotype 2 or 3 (46% vs. 76%). Patients with genotypes 2 and 3 may need only 24 weeks of combination therapy. Shorter durations of therapy (14 weeks) have lower sustained virologic response.

Toxicity

Common side effects of interferon administration include influenza-like symptoms (fever, chills, headache, and malaise), but these symptoms usually become less severe with repeated treatments; tolerance develops in most patients within several weeks. Major toxicities have included bone marrow suppression, primarily granulocytopenia, and thrombocytopenia, which are generally reversible when therapy is discontinued. Neuropsychiatric disturbance may be manifested by depression, anxiety, somnolence, confusion, and behavioral disturbance. Other side effects include profound fatigue and anorexia, weight loss, hypothyroidism or hyperthyroidism, alopecia, and cardiotoxicity with arrhythmias and reversible cardiomyopathy.

OTHER ANTIVIRALS

Imiquimod

Imiquimod and the related compound resiquimod are topical immune response modifiers that lack direct antiviral effects. Instead, these agents induce activation of immune cells (monocytes, macrophages, natural killer cells) to produce antiviral cytokines, particularly interferon-α and tumor necrosis factor-α.

Topical imiquimod cream is approved for the treatment of anogenital warts (Chapter 381). In immunocompetent patients, imiquimod leads to complete clearance of warts in 37 to 52% of patients. It may also be beneficial in patients with refractory cutaneous leishmaniasis (Chapter 356) and for molluscum contagiosum (Chapter 380). It is administered as a topical cream three times weekly for a maximum of 16 weeks and is washed off 6 to 10 hours after application.

Side effects are primarily local and include erythema, irritation, tenderness, and, less often, erosion. The side effects usually resolve with cessation of the drug.

Grade A

1. Corey L, Wald A, Patel R, et al. Once-daily valacyclovir to reduce the risk of transmission of genital herpes. *N Engl J Med.* 2004;350:11-20.
2. Asberg A, Humar A, Jardine AG, et al. Long-term outcomes of CMV disease treatment with valganciclovir versus IV ganciclovir in solid organ transplant recipients. *Am J Transplant.* 2009;9: 1205-1213.
3. Reischig T, Jindra P, Hes O, et al. Valacyclovir prophylaxis versus preemptive valganciclovir therapy to prevent cytomegalovirus disease after renal transplantation. *Am J Transplant.* 2008;8:69-77.
4. Kawai N, Ikematsu H, Hirotsu N, et al. Clinical effectiveness of oseltamivir and zanamivir for treatment of influenza A virus subtype H1N1 with the H274Y mutation: a Japanese, multicenter study of the 2007-2008 and 2008-2009 influenza seasons. *Clin Infect Dis.* 2009;49:1828-1835.
5. Shim JH, Suh DJ, Kim KM, et al. Efficacy of entecavir in patients with chronic hepatitis B resistant to both lamivudine and adefovir or to lamivudine alone. *Hepatology.* 2009;50:1064-1071.
6. Kobashi H, Takaguchi K, Ikeda H, et al. Efficacy and safety of entecavir in nucleoside-naive, chronic hepatitis B patients: phase II clinical study in Japan. *J Gastroenterol Hepatol.* 2009;24:255-261.
7. Marcellin P, Heathcote EJ, Buti M, et al. Tenofovir disoproxil fumarate versus adefovir dipivoxil for chronic hepatitis B. *N Engl J Med.* 2008;359:2442-2455.

SUGGESTED READINGS

Lange CM, Sarrazin C, Zeuzem S. Review article: specifically targeted anti-viral therapy for hepatitis C—a new era in therapy. *Aliment Pharmacol Ther.* 2010;32:14-28. *Review.*

Lee VJ, Yap J, Maurer-Stroh S, et al. Investigation of causes of oseltamivir chemophrophylaxis failures during influenza A (H1N1-2009) outbreaks. *J Clin Virol.* 2010;50:104-108. *No evidence of viral resistance.*

Tong MJ, Hsu L, Chang PW, et al. Evaluation of current treatment recommendations for chronic hepatitis B: a 2011 update. *J Gastroenterol Hepatol.* 2011;26:829-835. *Comprehensive review.*

369

THE COMMON COLD

RONALD B. TURNER

DEFINITION

The common cold is an upper respiratory syndrome of rhinorrhea and nasal obstruction, frequently accompanied by sore throat, sneezing, and cough. This viral syndrome is among the most common illnesses of humankind.

The Pathogens

The rhinoviruses cause at least half of all common cold illnesses. The rhinoviruses, which are RNA viruses that infect the respiratory epithelium, have long been known as common cold viruses, but they also are important causes of exacerbations of chronic bronchitis and asthma. More recent data suggest

| | TABLE 369-1 | VIRUSES ASSOCIATED WITH THE COMMON COLD |

VIRUS GROUP	ANTIGENIC TYPES	PERCENTAGE OF CASES
Rhinoviruses	>100	40-50
Coronaviruses	5	10-15
Parainfluenza virus	5	5
Respiratory syncytial virus	2	5
Influenza virus	3	25-30
Adenovirus	47	5-10
Metapneumovirus	2	5
Other viruses: enteroviruses, bocavirus		

From Mandell GL, Bennett JE, Dolin R, eds. *Principles and Practice of Infectious Diseases*, 7th ed. Philadelphia: Churchill Livingstone; 2010:810.

that rhinoviruses may also be associated with bronchiolitis in young children.

The coronaviruses (Chapter 374), parainfluenza viruses (Chapter 371), respiratory syncytial virus (Chapter 370), metapneumoviruses, adenoviruses (Chapter 373), and influenza viruses (Chapter 372) may also cause common cold illnesses (Table 369-1). Bocavirus has recently been associated with the common cold, but these viruses are also frequently isolated from healthy control subjects, so their role as pathogens is uncertain. Bacterial pathogens such as *Bordetella pertussis* (Chapter 321) and group A streptococcus (Chapter 298) are occasionally associated with rhinorrhea, but these illnesses are generally readily distinguished from the common cold.

EPIDEMIOLOGY

The incidence of common colds decreases with age, from at least six episodes per year in young children to approximately two episodes per year in adults. The incidence of illness is higher in adults who have occupational or household exposure to children and in children who are cared for in childcare centers. Common cold illnesses occur year-round in temperate climates but have a substantially increased incidence between the early autumn and late spring. This common cold "season" consists of sequential outbreaks caused by the different respiratory viruses. In tropical climates, colds occur year-round without defined seasonality.

PATHOBIOLOGY

Respiratory pathogens are spread from person to person by direct contact with either infected individuals or contaminated objects in the environment, by large-particle aerosols, or by small-particle aerosols. The rhinoviruses appear to be spread most efficiently by direct contact. Respiratory syncytial virus (Chapter 370) may be spread by either direct contact or large-particle aerosols, and influenza (Chapter 372) may be spread by small-particle aerosols.

Regardless of the route of spread, the common cold syndrome is initiated by infection of the nasal epithelium. Influenza and adenovirus produce obvious damage to the respiratory epithelium. Rhinovirus and respiratory syncytial virus, in contrast, have little or no detectable impact on the epithelium. Regardless of the histopathology, all of these viruses stimulate a nonspecific host inflammatory response that appears to be responsible for many of the symptoms associated with the common cold (Fig. 369-1).

The nasal obstruction of the common cold appears to result primarily from increased nasal blood flow and pooling of blood in the capacitance vessels of the nose. The increase in nasal secretion associated with the common cold may also contribute to the nasal obstruction. Rhinorrhea is primarily a result of increased vascular permeability with leakage of serum into the nasal secretions. Increased mucus production contributes to the secretions during the later stages of the illness.

Multiple factors may play a role in the pathogenesis of cough. Cough may be related to infection of the lower airway, irritation of upper airway receptors with neurologically mediated airway reactivity, or postnasal drip with pharyngeal irritation.

The risk of infection after exposure to the respiratory viruses is primarily dependent on the presence of specific neutralizing antibodies. Antibody responses to the rhinoviruses, adenoviruses, and influenza viruses are

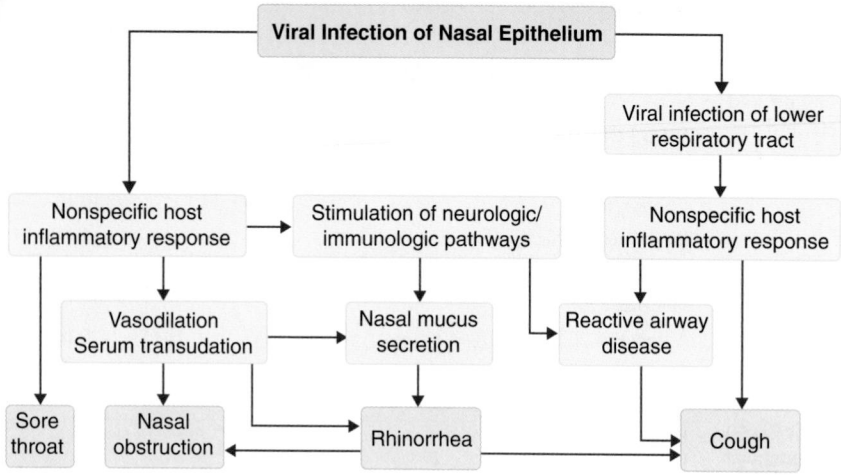

FIGURE 369-1. Proposed pathogenesis of common cold symptoms. (Modified from Richmond D, Hayden FG, Whitley R, eds. *Clinical Virology*, 3rd ed. Washington, DC: ASM Press; 2009:1073.)

protective against subsequent infection. The frequency of infection with these viruses is a result of the large number of distinct serotypes of rhinovirus and adenovirus and the ability of the influenza viruses to behave as though there are multiple virus serotypes by virtue of the rapid mutation of the antigens presented on the surface of the virus. The parainfluenza viruses, respiratory syncytial viruses, and metapneumoviruses do not produce protective immunity, so reinfection is common although preexisting antibody moderates the severity of illness.

Mannose-binding lectin deficiency has been associated with an increased incidence of common colds in young children. Protection by this innate response may become less important as children experience a variety of infections and develop specific immunity. Polymorphisms that enhance inflammatory cytokine responses may be associated with more severe respiratory illness.

CLINICAL MANIFESTATIONS

The incubation of common cold illness is generally short, ranging from 2 to 8 days, although the adenoviruses may have an incubation of as long as 13 days. A sore or scratchy throat is frequently reported as the first manifestation. Sneezing is also a common early symptom. Nasal obstruction and rhinorrhea develop rapidly and, by day 2 or 3 after the onset of illness, are the most bothersome symptoms. Cough generally develops later in the illness and frequently is the most bothersome symptom as the cold resolves. Common cold illnesses generally persist for about 1 week, although about 25% may persist for as long as 2 weeks.

Physical findings are restricted to the upper respiratory tract. Increased nasal secretion may be obvious to the examiner. A change in the color or consistency of nasal secretions is common during the course of the illness and is not indicative of sinusitis or bacterial superinfection.

DIAGNOSIS

The differential diagnosis of the common cold includes noninfectious disorders as well as other upper respiratory tract infections. Allergic rhinitis (Chapter 259) has a symptom complex similar to that of the common cold, although the presence of nasal or conjunctival itching suggests allergic disease. Most patients can reliably differentiate these illnesses.

Sinus involvement is present in uncomplicated cold illnesses, and superimposed bacterial sinusitis (Chapter 434) is difficult to differentiate from an uncomplicated cold. Rhinorrhea that persists without improvement for more than 10 days may suggest the presence of bacterial sinusitis that will respond to antibiotics.

Routine laboratory studies are not helpful for the diagnosis or management of the common cold. Although the viral pathogens associated with the common cold may be detected by culture, antigen detection, polymerase chain reaction, or serologic methods, these studies are of little value unless treatment with an antiviral agent is contemplated.

TREATMENT　Rx

Specific antiviral therapy is generally not useful for the treatment of common cold illnesses. The neuraminidase inhibitors oseltamivir and zanamivir (Chapter 368) have a modest effect on influenza virus infections, but the difficulty of distinguishing influenza from other common cold pathogens

TABLE 369-2	TREATMENTS FOR THE COMMON COLD	
DRUG	**DOSE AND DURATION**	**SIDE EFFECTS**
Topical adrenergic agents: oxymetazoline	2-3 sprays of 0.05% soln every 12 hr as needed for up to 3 days	Rebound nasal congestion with prolonged use Nasal stinging or burning
Oral adrenergic agents: pseudoephedrine	60 mg every 4-6 hr up to 240 mg/day as needed for nasal congestion	Insomnia Agitation
Antihistamines: chlorpheniramine	4 mg orally every 4-6 hr up to 24 mg/day as needed for rhinorrhea or sneezing	Sedation
Anticholinergics: ipratropium bromide	2 sprays per nostril of 0.06% soln every 6-8 hr as needed for rhinorrhea	Nasal dryness

and the need to start treatment early in the illness for maximum benefit are practical limitations to the use of these agents for mild upper respiratory infections. Antibacterial therapy is of no benefit in the treatment of the common cold.

Management of the common cold relies on symptomatic remedies. Treatments for nasal obstruction, rhinorrhea, and sore throat have demonstrated efficacy in adults but are not clearly beneficial in children and are not recommended for children younger than 4 years.

Nasal Congestion

Both topical and oral adrenergic agents (Table 369-2) are effective nasal decongestants. Although direct comparison has not been performed in the common cold, it is generally accepted that topical agents, such as intranasal xylometazoline, are more effective than oral drugs for nasal congestion.[1] Nevertheless, oral pseudoephedrine, 60 mg as a single dose or repeated for 3 to 5 days, is superior to placebo for relief of nasal congestion[2,3] and is safe. A 30-mg dose, however, may be no better than placebo.[4] Prolonged use of the topical adrenergic agents should be avoided to prevent the development of an apparent rebound effect when the drug is discontinued. Systemic absorption of oxymetazoline and xylometazoline has rarely been associated with bradycardia, hypotension, and coma. The antihistamines have no effect on nasal congestion.

Rhinorrhea

The treatment of rhinorrhea is primarily by blockade of cholinergic stimulation of glandular secretion. Intranasal ipratropium bromide reduces rhinorrhea in colds by 22 to 31% compared with placebo, and it can be used as a combined spray with xylometazoline to relieve both rhinorrhea and nasal congestion.[1] The most common side effects of intranasal ipratropium are nasal irritation and bleeding.

The first-generation (sedating) antihistamines reduce rhinorrhea by approximately 25% compared with placebo. The second-generation or "nonsedating" antihistamines have had no effect on common cold symptoms[5] in a limited number of studies. These observations, the absence of histamine in the secretions of most subjects with colds, and the similarity of the response to ipratropium and first-generation antihistamines suggest that any effect of antihistamines on rhinorrhea is related to their anticholinergic rather than their antihistaminic properties. The major side effects associated with the use of the antihistamines are sedation and drying of the eyes, mouth, and nose.

Cough

Cough during colds is produced by several different mechanisms, and treatment should be directed at the most likely underlying cause. If cough is caused by nasal obstruction or postnasal drip, it may respond to treatment with an antihistamine or antihistamine-decongestant combination. If a more persistent cough is the result of virus-induced reactive airway disease or viral infection of the lower airways, patients may benefit from bronchodilator therapy (Chapter 87). Cough that persists after the resolution of other cold symptoms or that persists in association with unremitting rhinorrhea may be due to sinusitis and may respond to antibiotic therapy (Chapter 434). Nonspecific cough suppression with codeine or dextromethorphan hydrobromide has not been demonstrated to be efficacious, and expectorants such as guaifenesin are not effective antitussive agents.

Other Remedies

Many patients have a variety of other symptoms. Nonsteroidal anti-inflammatory agents are effective for headache, ear pain, and muscle and joint pain; however, they do not relieve nasal congestion, rhinorrhea, or cough.[6]

Zinc, which is an inhibitor of rhinovirus 3C protease that is essential for virus replication, does not have a significant antiviral effect and has shown either no or relatively modest effects in reducing the severity of the common cold.[7] This uncertain benefit must also be viewed in light of zinc's side effects; oral zinc lozenges may be associated with sore mouth and occasional nausea, whereas intranasal zinc may cause nasal irritation.

Echinacea has not been shown to be beneficial in reducing symptoms of the common cold in several studies.[8] Given the variation in echinacea products, however, it is possible that echinacea preparations with different phytochemical profiles might be helpful. The accumulating evidence, however, suggests that it is prudent to assume that echinacea has no beneficial effect until positive evidence of a treatment effect is produced.

PREVENTION

Chemoprophylaxis or immunoprophylaxis is generally not available for the common cold. Immunization or chemoprophylaxis against influenza (Chapter 372) may be useful for prevention of colds caused by this pathogen, but influenza is responsible for only a small proportion of all colds. Vitamin C, even in megadoses, is of no benefit.[9] Other nonpharmacologic interventions touted as effective prophylaxis for the common cold but of unproven benefit include zinc, vitamin E, echinacea, ginseng, probiotics, exercise, and handwashing. Handwashing and exercise have undeniable benefits for health in general and can be recommended despite the paucity of evidence specific to common cold prevention. Other interventions, although probably safe, have no demonstrable benefit and simply contribute to the unnecessary health care expenditures related to the common cold.

PROGNOSIS

The common cold generally has little medical significance. However, these illnesses are frequently complicated by otitis media (Chapter 434) or sinusitis (Chapter 434) that may be a direct result of the viral infection or may be due to bacterial superinfection. Exacerbations of asthma (Chapter 87) and chronic bronchitis (Chapter 88) are also important complications of the common cold.

1. Eccles R, Martensson K, Chen SC. Effects of intranasal xylometazoline, alone or in combination with ipratropium, in patients with the common cold. *Curr Med Res Opin.* 2010;26:889-899.
2. Taverner D, Latte J. Nasal decongestants for the common cold. *Cochrane Database Syst Rev.* 2007;24:CD001953.
3. Eccles R, Jawad MS, Jawad SS, et al. Efficacy and safety of single and multiple doses of pseudoephedrine in the treatment of nasal congestion associated with the common cold. *Am J Rhinol.* 2005;19:25-31.
4. Loose I, Winkel M. Clinical, double-blind, placebo-controlled study investigating the combination of acetylsalicylic acid and pseudoephedrine for the symptomatic treatment of nasal congestion associated with the common cold. *Arzneimittelforschung.* 2004;54:513-521.
5. Sutter AI, Lemiengre M, Campbell H, et al. Antihistamines for the common cold. *Cochrane Database Syst Rev.* 2003;3:CD001267.
6. Kim SY, Chang YJ, Cho HM, et al. Non-steroidal anti-inflammatory drugs for the common cold. *Cochrane Database Syst Rev.* 2009;8:CD006362.
7. Marshall I. Zinc for the common cold. *Cochrane Database Syst Rev.* 2006;3:CD001364.
8. Turner RB, Bauer R, Woelkart K, et al. An evaluation of *Echinacea angustifolia* in experimental rhinovirus infections [see comment]. *N Engl J Med.* 2005;353:341-348.
9. Douglas RM, Hemila H, Chalker E, et al. Vitamin C for preventing and treating the common cold. *Cochrane Database Syst Rev.* 2007;18:CD000980.

SUGGESTED READINGS

Meltzer EO, Caballero F, Fromer LM, et al. Treatment of congestion in upper respiratory diseases. *Int J Gen Med.* 2010;3:69-91. *Review.*

Pappas DE, Hendley JO. The common cold and decongestant therapy. *Pediatr Rev.* 2011;32:47-55. *Detailed review and practical guide to therapy.*

370

RESPIRATORY SYNCYTIAL VIRUS

EDWARD E. WALSH

DEFINITION

Respiratory syncytial virus (RSV), which causes yearly winter outbreaks, remains the single most important cause of bronchiolitis and pneumonia in young infants and a common cause of illness in older children and young adults. RSV can cause serious illness in elderly people, adults with underlying cardiopulmonary disease, and the severely immunocompromised.

The Pathogen

RSV is a single-stranded RNA enveloped virus of the family Paramyxoviridae, genus Pneumovirus; it is related to human metapneumovirus. Two major transmembrane glycoproteins (G, attachment protein; F, fusion protein) carry neutralizing epitopes, and two nonstructural proteins (NS1 and NS2) block the antiviral activity of interferon-α, whereas a secreted form of G contains a CX3C chemokine motif that may be important in modulating immune responses to infection. Two major virus groups (A and B), each with four to five subgroups, are distinguishable.

EPIDEMIOLOGY

In the United States, epidemics generally begin in the southern states in late fall, move steadily north, and peak in February and March in colder climates. RSV annually causes approximately 100,000 hospitalizations and accounts for 60% of cases of bronchiolitis and 25% of cases of pneumonia in infants. Mortality is relatively low in U.S. infants, with an estimated 250 deaths annually; however, deaths are more common in underdeveloped countries. About 70% of infants become infected in their first winter and the remainder in the following year. RSV is transmitted principally by direct contact with large-particle fomites of respiratory secretions rather than by small-particle aerosolization.

Approximately 1 to 3% of primary infections result in hospitalization, but lower socioeconomic status, underlying prematurity, congenital cardiac abnormalities, bronchopulmonary dysplasia, and immunosuppression increase the risk for serious disease. Severe disease is associated with specific polymorphisms in the promoter regions of cytokine genes. Hospitalization is most frequent between the ages of 1 and 6 months, with a median age of 2 months. Reinfection occurs frequently throughout life, although subsequent illness is less severe and hospitalization is infrequent, except for persons with underlying cardiac or pulmonary conditions.

Though often not considered in adults, RSV infection is common and may be severe in the elderly. In a British study, RSV accounted for 17% of medically attended respiratory illnesses in persons older than 45 years. In a U.S. study of community-acquired pneumonia in adults (Chapter 97), RSV ranked third behind pneumococcus and influenza. RSV infection is implicated in about 10% of hospitalizations for acute pulmonary symptoms in the winter among community-dwelling elderly persons, a rate similar to that for influenza.

PATHOBIOLOGY

In naturally acquired infection, the virus most commonly enters through the nose or eye and then spreads from the upper to the lower respiratory tract. Pathologic findings include a lymphocytic peribronchiolar infiltration with edema, obstruction, and necrosis. Bronchiolitis, with multiple areas of atelectasis, and pneumonia, with interstitial infiltration of mononuclear cells and alveoli that are filled by edema and necrosis, develop in infected patients. Naturally acquired immunity is incomplete and not lifelong. Repeated infections are common, but severe disease is unusual in adults unless they are immunocompromised.

CLINICAL MANIFESTATIONS

After an incubation period of 2 to 8 days, infants experience upper respiratory symptoms of conjunctival injection, mucopurulent nasal discharge, cough, and low-grade fever. Otitis media occurs commonly, generally in association with bacteria. After several days, lower respiratory tract symptoms appear in 25 to 50% of infants, with cough, wheezing, tachypnea, use of accessory muscle, and cyanosis developing as the disease progresses. Expiratory wheezes, rhonchi, and fine rales are the most common findings on lung examination. Sudden apnea may develop in the youngest infants. Mortality is rare in otherwise healthy infants but can reach 37% in infants with cardiac disorders. Hyperinflation and diffuse interstitial pneumonitis are the most frequent radiographic findings. High-titer virus shedding lasts 7 to 10 days, although immunocompromised infants may excrete virus for a month or longer, even when asymptomatic. Coinfection with other respiratory viruses is not uncommon but is not clinically discernible.

Illness in young adults generally continues for 1 week, typically with upper respiratory symptoms. Many have lower respiratory symptoms, especially wheezing, and may miss work while seeking medical attention. Low-titer virus shedding persists for 3 to 5 days. In elderly persons, RSV attack rates approximate 5% annually; wheezing is more common than with influenza (Chapter 372), whereas a high fever is less common. In frail elderly persons or in patients with underlying chronic obstructive pulmonary disease or heart failure, severe disease can develop. Attack rates in nosocomial nursing home outbreaks average 10 to 15%, with rales and wheezes evident in a third of patients and radiographically confirmed pneumonia in approximately 10%. The precise incidence of bacterial superinfection is unknown but is probably similar to that seen with influenza virus infection.

RSV infection has been documented in up to 10% of bone marrow transplant recipients, patients with acute leukemia, and heart/lung transplant recipients during the winter months. Upper respiratory symptoms frequently lead to lower respiratory tract symptoms.

DIAGNOSIS

In infants, a presumptive diagnosis is suggested by typical symptoms during the epidemic season, but the diagnosis is often not considered in adults. In infants the sensitivity of viral culture is about 75%, and rapid tests that rely on detecting viral antigen in respiratory secretions, such as immunofluorescence or enzyme immunoassay (EIA), have a sensitivity of approximately 80%. Reverse transcription–polymerase chain reaction (RT-PCR) is considerably more sensitive than culture. In immunocompromised adults, RSV antigen is found in only 15% of nasal secretions but in 90% of bronchoalveolar lavage specimens.

In adults, viral culture has a sensitivity of 30%, but RT-PCR detects infection in three quarters of culture-negative cases that would be seropositive with testing of acute and convalescent serum. Immunofluorescence and EIA are not useful in adults. In immunocompromised patients, chest radiographs demonstrate diffuse interstitial and alveolar infiltrates. A useful clinical clue to the presence of RSV is the almost universal presence of radiographically proven sinusitis. The presence of upper respiratory tract symptoms distinguishes this illness from cytomegalovirus pneumonia (Chapter 384).

TREATMENT   Rx

Therapy for hospitalized infants includes hydration, oxygen, bronchodilators, and occasionally specific antiviral medication. The effectiveness of nebulized bronchodilators is variable, but a subset of infants respond. Glucocorticosteroids have not been shown to have benefit. Specific antiviral therapy is limited to inhaled ribavirin (20-mg/mL solution administered by aerosol, typically for 6 hours three times a day for 3 to 5 days). High-dose (2 g at 60 mg/mL), short-duration (2 hours three times daily) treatment is considered equivalent. The majority of infants do not require therapy, but ribavirin treatment appears to benefit infants and children at high risk for serious disease and those who are severely ill. ▪

No placebo-controlled studies of the effect of inhaled ribavirin have been conducted in adults with severe RSV disease, but the evidence accumulated suggests benefit in immunocompromised adults with RSV pneumonia (2 g at 60 mg/mL for 10 days), especially if begun before respiratory failure.

Studies using monoclonal antibody (palivizumab, 15 mg/kg once) combined with inhaled ribavirin suggest benefit in the treatment of RSV pneumonia in immunosuppressed adults, although conclusive randomized studies have not been published. Bacterial superinfection can develop, with *Streptococcus pneumoniae* (Chapter 297) and *Haemophilus influenzae* (Chapter 308) being the most frequent organisms. For such patients, appropriate antimicrobial treatment (Chapter 97) is mandatory.

PREVENTION

Adherence to standard infection control principles (e.g., gloves, gowns, and frequent handwashing) substantially reduces nosocomial spread. A vaccine is not available. Parenteral humanized RSV monoclonal antibody (palivizumab, 15 mg/kg monthly during the RSV season) has demonstrated benefit when administered prophylactically to high-risk infants with underlying cardiopulmonary disease or prematurity in this setting.

PROGNOSIS

RSV infection in severely immunocompromised adults, such as bone marrow transplant recipients (Chapter 181) and those with acute leukemia (Chapter 189) undergoing cytotoxic chemotherapy, carries a 60% mortality rate when pneumonia develops. Risk factors for a poor outcome include the degree of lymphopenia and, in one study, the use of cord blood as a source of allogeneic stem cells (Chapter 181). A link between severe bronchiolitis and the subsequent development of asthma remains unresolved. In otherwise normal hosts the outcome is generally good.

1. Ventre K, Randolph AG. Ribavirin for respiratory syncytial virus infection of the lower respiratory tract in infants and young children. *Cochrane Database Syst Rev.* 2007;1:CD000181.

SUGGESTED READINGS

Centers for Disease Control and Prevention (CDC). Respiratory syncytial virus activity—United States, July 2008–December 2009. *MMWR Morb Mortal Wkly Rep.* 2010;59:230-233. *National data indicate about 180,000 hospitalizations and 14,000 deaths among adults over age 65.*

Welliver RC. Pharmacotherapy of respiratory syncytial virus infection. *Curr Opin Pharmacol.* 2010; 10:289-293. *Review.*

371

PARAINFLUENZA VIRAL DISEASE

GEOFFREY A. WEINBERG AND KATHRYN M. EDWARDS

DEFINITION

Human parainfluenza viruses (hPIVs) are important causes of a wide spectrum of respiratory illnesses. In infants and young children, they produce acute upper and lower respiratory tract infections ranging from the common cold (Chapter 369) and otitis media (Chapter 434) to severe croup, bronchiolitis, and pneumonia (Chapter 97). In older children and adults, hPIV infections are usually limited to the upper respiratory tract (Chapter 96), although immunocompromised individuals may develop fatal respiratory failure.

The Pathogen

The hPIVs are enveloped, single-stranded, nonsegmented RNA viruses that belong to two genera in the family Paramyxoviridae. Members of this family also include respiratory syncytial virus (RSV; Chapter 370), human metapneumovirus (Chapter 369), measles virus (Chapter 375), mumps virus (Chapter 377), Hendra and Nipah viruses, and the animal pathogenic viruses of Newcastle disease, canine distemper, and rinderpest. The hPIV genome encodes six structural proteins. The hemagglutinin-neuraminidase (HN) and fusion (F) proteins, which are exposed on the bilayered lipid envelope surrounding the helical nucleocapsid–RNA complex, mediate both attachment to host sialic acid–containing glycoproteins and penetration of the virus into susceptible mammalian cells. These proteins have retained their antigenic stability for many years, unlike the antigen "drift and shift" of the influenza viruses. The four serotypes of hPIV are called types 1 to 4, including two subgroups (A and B) of type 4 virus.

EPIDEMIOLOGY

The hPIVs are ubiquitous, with a worldwide geographic distribution. Their transmission is principally by large-particle fomites and close person-to-person contact. Parainfluenza virus activity displays both endemic and epidemic patterns, with each serotype favoring different age groups and distinct clinical syndromes but with enough overlap to preclude specific diagnosis based solely on clinical and epidemiologic grounds.

Primary infection with hPIV occurs early in childhood. Among the parainfluenza viruses, type 3 (hPIV-3) generally infects infants first, such that 50 to 67% of infants demonstrate serologic evidence of infection by 1 year of age. Parainfluenza viruses 1 and 2 (hPIV-1 and hPIV-2, respectively) most commonly infect children between 2 and 5 years of age. Parainfluenza virus 4 (hPIV-4) less commonly causes symptomatic respiratory infections.

Until the early 1960s, hPIV-1 caused endemic annual disease in the United States, but for the past several decades, it has been associated with biennial outbreaks in the fall of odd-numbered years. Infections with hPIV-2 largely follow this same curious pattern but occur much less commonly than hPIV-1 infections. Infections with hPIV-3 have remained endemic throughout the year, with peaks in the late spring. The incubation period for all serotypes of hPIV is 3 to 6 days in experimentally infected adults but appears to be 2 to 4 days in natural infections in children.

The hPIVs are second only to RSV as the cause of acute upper and lower respiratory tract infections in young children in the United States. In a population-based study of children younger than 5 years hospitalized with fever or acute respiratory tract infection, 7% had laboratory-confirmed hPIV infection (by cell culture and molecular amplification techniques), compared with 19% with RSV and 6% with influenza A or B virus infections. The hospitalization rate for hPIV infection in children younger than 5 years was 1.02 per 1000 children per year. Extrapolating to the entire U.S. population, these data suggest that approximately 23,000 hPIV annual hospitalizations occur in children younger than 5 years. The rates of emergency department and outpatient health care visits attributable to hPIV infections in young children are 10- to 50-fold greater. Further, immunity to hPIV infection is neither complete nor durable, so older children and adults can exhibit symptomatic infection, sometimes leading to office visits and hospitalization.

CLINICAL MANIFESTATIONS

Primary Infection

Illness associated with primary hPIV infection varies by age and viral serotype. Underlying medical conditions, such as cardiopulmonary compromise and immune disorders, increase the severity of disease. Large cohort and longitudinal family studies have shown that hPIV infections are responsible for about 65% of croup, 20 to 40% of lower respiratory infection, and 20% of upper respiratory infection in young children. The majority of children have experienced primary hPIV infection by the time they enter elementary school. Thus, although hPIV also causes upper respiratory infections in adults, these are reinfections rather than primary infections (see later). In general, hPIV-1 and hPIV-2 are most commonly associated with croup, whereas hPIV-3 infection often presents as undifferentiated febrile illness, bronchiolitis, or pneumonia.

Infection typically begins with upper respiratory signs and symptoms, notably coryza, rhinorrhea, pharyngitis without cervical adenopathy, and low-grade fever. Symptoms, which typically persist for 3 to 5 days, may be unpredictable and can result in sudden respiratory failure. In approximately 15 to 25% of infected children, signs of lower respiratory tract disease develop, usually presenting as croup but sometimes as bronchiolitis or pneumonia, indistinguishable from RSV infection. When croup develops, the child has a raspy, barking cough with notable inspiratory stridor, dyspnea, and respiratory distress. These symptoms, which are generally spasmodic, result from subglottic inflammation and edema. On occasion, severe stridor may develop and make differentiation from epiglottitis caused by *Haemophilus influenzae* type b (Chapter 308) difficult, although epiglottitis is much less common in the United States since universal Hib vaccination became routine in 1990.

Croup is very rare in adults but has been associated with hPIV in isolated case reports. Epiglottitis is seen more often in adults, but it is more commonly associated with staphylococcal or streptococcal infection. Epiglottitis is a medical emergency for patients of all ages and must be distinguished from croup to allow proper therapy, including emergent intubation of the airway (Chapter 437). The differences between these two entities are clearly shown in lateral neck radiographs, on which subglottic edema and narrowing are seen with croup, and swelling of the epiglottis is seen with epiglottitis (Figs. 371-1 and 371-2). Children with bronchiolitis or pneumonia caused by hPIV have cough, rales, and wheezing associated with hypoxia, and their chest radiographs often exhibit air trapping.

FIGURE 371-1. Subglottic edema. Endoscopic view of subglottic edema in viral croup (**A**). Radiologic presentation of subglottic edema in viral croup causing narrowing ("steeple sign") of the tracheal air shadow (**B**) compared with a normal tracheal air shadow (**C**). (From Hammer J. Acquired upper airway obstruction. *Paediatr Respir Rev.* 2004;5:25-33.)

FIGURE 371-2. Epiglottitis. Schematic (**A**) and endoscopic view (**B**) of epiglottitis. The typical lateral neck radiographs of a normal child (**C**) and a child with epiglottitis (**D**; "thumb sign" of swollen epiglottis) are displayed. (From Hammer J. Acquired upper airway obstruction. *Paediatr Respir Rev.* 2004;5:25-33.)

Reinfection

Reinfection with hPIV is less severe and typically causes cold symptoms in normal children and adults. Reinfection with hPIV is estimated to account for 1 to 15% of all acute respiratory illnesses in adults, the majority of whom present with simple upper respiratory tract infections. However, as with RSV, some adults may develop severe disease that requires hospitalization and even ventilatory support. In such patients, fever, cough, dyspnea, and wheezing are common. Radiographic changes, primarily lobar or interstitial infiltrates, are seen in more than 50% of adults hospitalized with hPIV infection.

Elderly and Immunocompromised Patients

Nursing home outbreaks of hPIV infection may include a high incidence of pneumonia, just as hPIV infections often cause severe pneumonia in immunocompromised children and adults. Among healthy elderly residents of long-term care facilities, hPIV infections are as common as infections caused by influenza A virus, influenza B virus, or RSV. In a large study of hematopoietic stem cell transplant recipients, 7% developed hPIV infections, with about 90% of those due to hPIV-3. Although nearly 80% of these cases were community acquired, nosocomial outbreaks occurred even in stem cell transplant units.

Approximately 25% of hPIV-infected stem cell transplant recipients develop lower respiratory disease, mostly in the first 100 days after transplantation, when lymphopenia is most pronounced. The strongest identified risk factors for any hPIV infection and for severe infection in this setting are allogeneic transplantation from unrelated or nonmatched sibling donors and the use of corticosteroids, especially at higher doses. Fever, cough, dyspnea, and sputum production are the most common symptoms. Coinfection, especially with *Aspergillus* (Chapter 347), may occur in hematopoietic stem cell transplant recipients with pneumonia.

DIAGNOSIS

Although hPIV may be suspected on clinical and epidemiologic grounds, specific diagnosis requires isolation of the virus or detection of viral antigen or RNA in respiratory secretions. Reverse transcription–polymerase chain reactions (RT-PCR) are highly sensitive and specific for diagnosis. Alternatively, cultures of monkey kidney or human embryonic kidney cells can be used to grow the virus, with cytopathic effects detected in 5 to 10 days (except for hPIV-4, which requires up to 3 weeks). Rapid direct or indirect immunofluorescence tests are less sensitive than culture but still are used in many clinical laboratories.

Definitive diagnosis of parainfluenza infection in adults, even by RT-PCR, may be more difficult than in children, presumably because less virus is shed by partially immune adults. However, virus can usually be recovered from the nasopharyngeal secretions or bronchoalveolar lavage fluid in hematopoietic stem cell transplant recipients with pneumonia.

TREATMENT Rx

Specific antiviral treatment of hPIV infection is currently unavailable. Aerosolized ribavirin, approved for use in RSV infection, has in vitro activity against hPIV, but studies in immunocompromised children and adults with severe hPIV pneumonia have shown no benefits even when it was administered with concomitant intravenous immune globulin.

For previously healthy children with croup, general comfort, which usually means sitting in the lap of a parent or caregiver, is widely recommended. Humidified air (mist) repeatedly has been shown to have no benefits and actually has associated adverse effects, including anxiety, difficulty with monitoring, and bacterial and fungal contamination of both hot and cold mist humidifiers. Oxygen may be given by holding the end of the tubing near the nose and mouth ("blow-by" oxygen).

Children with mild to moderate croup (i.e., without stridor or significant chest wall indrawing at rest, or with stridor and indrawing but without agitation) may be given oral dexamethasone, 0.6 mg/kg body weight, and observed; if they improve, they may be discharged to home. Children with severe croup (stridor, chest wall indrawing, and agitation) may benefit from blow-by oxygen, inhaled racemic epinephrine (0.05 mL/kg body weight of a 2.25% solution of racemic epinephrine for nebulization, up to a maximum dose of 0.5 mL **1**; if racemic epinephrine is not available, the equivalent effects can be achieved by nebulizing 0.5 mL/kg of 1:1000 L-epinephrine, up to a maximum dose of 5 mL), and dexamethasone. Children should be admitted to the hospital if no significant clinical improvement is seen after several hours of observation and therapy.

Oral dexamethasone is as effective as intramuscular dexamethasone or nebulized budesonide, and it is easier to administer. Corticosteroids decrease the need for hospitalization and return visits,**2** decrease length of stay both in emergency departments and after hospital admission,**2** and decrease the need for intubation for mechanical ventilation. In general, there are no reasons to institute either antibiotic therapy or short-acting bronchodilator therapy in children with croup.

PREVENTION

Clinical trials of live attenuated hPIV vaccines are ongoing. At least one vaccine candidate under study combines hPIV-3 and RSV in an attempt to prevent both of these common infections in young children.

Grade A

1. Bjornson C, Russell KF, Vandermeer B, et al. Nebulized epinephrine for croup in children. *Cochrane Database Syst Rev.* 2011;2:CD006619.
2. Russell KF, Liang Y, O'Gorman K, et al. Glucocorticoids for croup. *Cochrane Database Syst Rev.* 2011;1:CD001955.

SUGGESTED READINGS

Hodson A, Kasliwal M, Streetly M, et al. A parainfluenza-3 outbreak in a SCT unit: sepsis with multiorgan failure and multiple co-pathogens are associated with increased mortality. *Bone Marrow Transplant.* 2011. [Epub ahead of print.] *Despite treatment, the mortality rate was 63% in a transplant unit.*

Schiffer JT, Kirby K, Sandmaier B, et al. Timing and severity of community acquired respiratory virus infections after myeloablative versus non-myeloablative hematopoietic stem cell transplantation. *Haematologica.* 2009;94:1101-1108. *Large retrospective series describing the epidemiology of hPIV and other respiratory virus infections in stem cell transplant recipients.*

Wald EL. Croup: common syndrome and therapy. *Pediatr Ann.* 2010;39:15-21. *Review.*

372

INFLUENZA

FREDERICK G. HAYDEN

DEFINITION

Influenza is an acute febrile respiratory illness that occurs in annual outbreaks of varying severity and commonly in unpredictable worldwide epidemics (pandemics). The causative virus infects the respiratory tract, is highly contagious, and typically produces prominent systemic symptoms early in the illness. Influenza virus infection can produce various clinical syndromes in adults, including nonfebrile common colds, pharyngitis, tracheobronchitis, and pneumonia. Conversely, infections with other respiratory viruses, such as respiratory syncytial virus (Chapter 370) or adenovirus (Chapter 373), may produce influenza-like illness. Influenza A viruses have caused five pandemics of varying severity within the past 120 years (Table 372-1). The pandemic in 1918 to 1919 caused at least 500,000 deaths in the United States and more than 40 million worldwide, whereas the 2009 H1N1 pandemic was associated with substantially less mortality. Seasonal epidemics may cause enormous morbidity, economic loss, and often substantial mortality. Recent epidemics have caused on average more than 24,000 respiratory- and circulatory-related deaths and more than 200,000 hospitalizations in the United States alone.

The Pathogen

Influenza viruses belong to the family Orthomyxoviridae and are divided into three types (A, B, and C) distinguished by their internal and external proteins (Table 372-2). The virion (Fig. 372-1) is a medium-sized, enveloped, pleomorphic particle covered with two types of surface glycoprotein spikes, the trimeric hemagglutinin (H or HA) and the tetrameric, mushroom-shaped neuraminidase (N or NA). The envelope is composed of a lipid bilayer overlying the matrix (M1) protein that surrounds the viral genome consisting of eight segments of single-stranded RNA. Influenza C viruses have seven segments and only a single surface glycoprotein. Whereas influenza B and C viruses are principally human pathogens, influenza A viruses primarily infect aquatic birds and sometimes other animal hosts, including other avians, swine, horses, marine mammals, felids, and dogs. Influenza A viruses are further classified into subtypes on the basis of their HA and NA glycoproteins. Sixteen HA and nine NA subtypes are currently recognized in nature, but only three HAs (H1, H2, and H3) and two NAs (N1 and N2) have been documented thus far in epidemic and pandemic human influenza A viruses. Each strain is identified by type, subtype if influenza A, site, sample number, and year of isolation.

EPIDEMIOLOGY

Antigenic and Genetic Variation

Influenza viruses are unique among the respiratory viruses with regard to their extent of genetic and antigenic variation, epidemic behavior, and frequent association with excess mortality during community outbreaks. The changing antigenicity of the surface glycoproteins largely accounts for repeated influenza epidemics in humans. Antibody to HA neutralizes viral infectivity and is thus the major determinant of immunity. Anti-NA antibody limits viral replication and probably reduces the severity of infection. Variation involves either relatively minor (antigenic drift) or major (antigenic

TABLE 372-1 ANTIGENIC SUBTYPES OF INFLUENZA A VIRUS ASSOCIATED WITH PANDEMIC AND PANDEMIC-LIKE INFLUENZA

YEAR	INTERVAL (YR)	SUBTYPE DESIGNATION	EXTENT OF ANTIGENIC CHANGE IN INDICATED SURFACE PROTEIN*	SEVERITY OF PANDEMIC (MORTALITY)
1889	?42-59	H3N?	H+++N?	Severe
1918	18	H1N1[†]	H+++N+++	Very severe
1957	39	H2N2	H+++N+++	Severe
1968	11	H3N2	H+++N−	Moderate[‡]
1977	9	H1N1	H+++N+++	Negligible[§]
2009	32	H1N1	H++N++	Mild-moderate[§]

*Compared with antecedent or cocirculating virus.
[†]Formerly designated H0N1 (swine virus prototype) or Hsw1N1.
[‡]The population had some immunity to N2 neuraminidase.
[§]The older population was largely immune because of previous infection with earlier circulating, antigenically identical (1977) or related (2009) viruses; those born after 1957 were primarily affected. The impact of the 2009 pandemic virus, based on estimated years of life lost, was comparable to that observed in the 1968 pandemic in the United States.
+ = Minor change; ++ = moderate change; +++ = major change; − = no change.

TABLE 372-2 INFLUENZA VIRUS PROTEINS

DESIGNATION	LOCATION (APPROXIMATE NO. PER VIRION)	FUNCTION	OTHER
Hemagglutinin (HA)	Surface (500)	Cell attachment and penetration; fusion activity	Type-, subtype-, and strain-specific antigens; key antigen in inactivated vaccine
Neuraminidase (NA)	Surface (100)	Virus release and spread; enzymatic activity	Type-, subtype-, and strain-specific antigens; activity linked to risk for pneumonia; site of action of zanamivir, oseltamivir carboxylate
Membrane or M1 matrix	Internal (3000)	Major structural envelope protein; virus assembly	Type-specific antigen
M2	Surface (20-60)	Virus uncoating and assembly; ion channel	Influenza A only; site of action of amantadine/rimantadine
Nucleoprotein (NP)	Internal (1000)	Associated with RNA and polymerase proteins	Type-specific antigen
Polymerase proteins (PB1, PB2, PA)	Internal (30-60)	RNA replication and transcription	Determinant of replication efficiency; probable site of action of ribavirin
NS1	Nonstructural (infected cells)	Regulation of virus replication	Interferon antagonist
NEP	Internal (130-200)	Nuclear export factor	Formerly NS2
PB1-F2	Nonstructural (infected cells)	Proapoptotic factor; proinflammatory effects	Expressed from 1+ reading frame of PB1 of certain viruses

Modified from Lamb RA, King RM. Orthomyxoviridae. In: Fields BN, Knipe DM, Howley PM, eds. *Fields Virology,* 4th ed. Philadelphia: Lippincott Williams & Wilkins; 2001:1487.

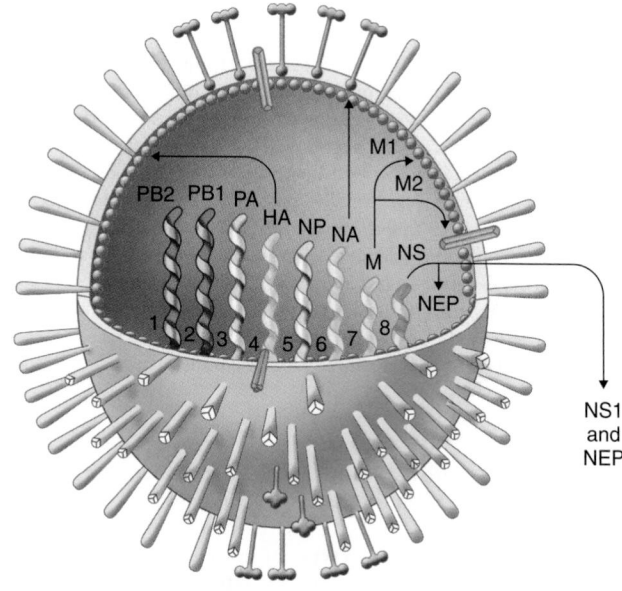

FIGURE 372-1. Diagram of influenza virus structure. Eight segments of viral RNA are contained within the envelope and matrix (M1) shell. Each codes for one or two proteins that form the virus or regulate its intracellular replication. The presumed functions of each are listed in Table 372-2. (Courtesy of Dr. Robert G. Webster.)

shift) changes in antigenicity. Significant antigenic variation is much less frequent with influenza B than with influenza A.

Antigenic drift results from point mutations in the RNA segment that codes for HA, thereby causing amino acid substitutions in at least one of five antigenic sites on HA. Drift can also occur in NA. These mutations occur frequently (every year or every few years) within an influenza A or B virus. For example, the original H3N2 variant, A/Aichi/68, has undergone successive drifts resulting in epidemic strains that include the recent circulation of A/Perth/16/2009–like viruses. Immunologic selection favors transmission of the new variant over the old because of the less frequent presence of antibody to the new virus in the population.

Antigenic shift results from the appearance of an influenza A virus with HA or HA and NA glycoproteins that are new to humans or that reappear after decades of absence. Because of the lack of population immunity, a new strain that is transmissible from person to person can cause pandemic disease (see Table 372-1). The origin of new pandemic strains and the basis for their possible recirculation remain incompletely understood. Avian influenza viruses have served as the reservoir of new genes for human pandemic viruses. Reassortment of gene segments may occur when two influenza

viruses simultaneously infect a single cell, and reassortment events in which human viruses acquired avian genes led to both the 1957 and 1968 pandemic viruses. Because swine can support replication of both human and avian viruses, they have been postulated to serve as a mixing vessel for the generation of new strains or as the host in which avian viruses can adapt to mammals. The 2009 H1N1 pandemic virus arose as a quadruple reassortant, which derived gene segments from Asian and North American swine lineage viruses that harbored genes derived from swine, avian, and human viruses. Frequent intra-subtypic reassortment also occurs among seasonal human influenza A viruses and sometimes leads to new antigenic variants. The 1918 pandemic virus was probably a reassortant composed of both human and swine genes, including those of avian origin that underwent mutational adaptation in a mammalian host, perhaps human or swine, before causing the pandemic.

Zoonotic infections occur from swine, poultry, or rarely other animals. Although most avian influenza viruses do not cause infections directly in humans, human infection by avian subtype H5, H7, and H9 viruses has been well documented. Initially recognized by a cluster of human cases in Hong Kong in 1997, an epizootic of avian H5N1 infections has affected many areas of Asia, the Middle East, Europe, and Africa and continues to cause sporadic human illnesses with high mortality.

Epidemic or Interpandemic Influenza

An *epidemic* is an outbreak of influenza confined to one geographic location. In temperate climates, community epidemics of influenza A virus infection often have a characteristic pattern, typically reaching a sharp peak in 2 or 3 weeks after initial recognition and persisting for 6 to 10 weeks. Increased numbers of schoolchildren with febrile respiratory illness are often the first indication of influenza in a community, soon followed by illnesses in adults and, 1 to 2 weeks later, by increased hospital admission of patients with influenza-related complications. Hospitalization rates in high-risk persons increase two- to five-fold during major epidemics (Table 372-3). School and employment absenteeism increases, as does mortality from pneumonia and underlying conditions, especially in older persons during A/H3N2 epidemics. Epidemics occur almost exclusively during the winter months in temperate areas, but inderlying conditions, activity may occur year-round in the tropics or display other patterns. Outbreaks sometimes occur in tour groups (land or ship) and in facilities during summer months, particularly after the appearance of a drift variant. Regional differences in the time and magnitude of occurrence of influenza outbreaks are common. During epidemics, overall attack rates typically range from 5 to 20% in adults. Attack rates of 40 to 50% are not uncommon in closed populations, such as in hospitals and nursing homes, and in highly susceptible age groups such as children. Two different strains within a single subtype, two different influenza A subtypes, two different influenza B lineages, or both influenza A and B viruses may cocirculate or occur sequentially. In addition, simultaneous outbreaks of influenza A

TABLE 372-3	AGE-SPECIFIC RATES FOR ILLNESS AND MORTALITY DURING URBAN INFLUENZA EPIDEMICS		
AGE (YR)	PHYSICIAN VISITS PER 100	ACUTE RESPIRATORY DISEASE HOSPITALIZATIONS PER 10,000	PNEUMONIA- AND INFLUENZA-RELATED MORTALITY PER 100,000
<5	28	43	3
5-14	14	5	1
15-44	10	8	1
45-54	9	13	10
55-64	10	21	10
≥65	Not stated	73	104

Modified from Glezen WP. Anatomy of an urban influenza epidemic. In: Hannoun C, Kendal AP, Klenk HD, et al, eds. *Options for the Control of Influenza II.* Amsterdam: Elsevier; 1993:12.

virus and respiratory syncytial virus or other respiratory viruses occur. Strains circulating at the end of one season's epidemic are sometimes responsible for the next season's outbreak (the so-called herald wave phenomenon).

Pneumonia- and influenza-related deaths fluctuate annually, with peaks in the winter months in temperate climates. When such deaths exceed the expected threshold, the cause is typically influenza A, but influenza B virus or respiratory syncytial virus can occasionally be responsible. Although mortality is usually greatest during pandemics, substantial mortality occurs in epidemics. During seasonal influenza, more than 85% of pneumonia- and influenza-related deaths occur in persons 65 years of age and older. Mortality risk is especially high in those aged 85 years and older. Other cardiopulmonary and chronic diseases also result in increased mortality after influenza epidemics, so the overall influenza-associated mortality is about two- to fourfold higher than pneumonia- and influenza-related deaths.

Pandemic Influenza

Pandemics of influenza A result from the emergence of a new virus capable of sustained person-to-person transmission and to which the population contains no or limited immunity. The virus spreads worldwide, often circulating outside of the usual influenza season, and usually infects persons of all ages. Preexisting immunity due to prior infection with antigenically related viruses can provide partial protection, as occurred in older adults during the 2009 H1N1 pandemic. Pandemics are associated with high morbidity rates, especially in children, and sometimes notably increased mortality rates in pregnant women and young and middle-aged adults. For example, more than 90% of deaths in the 1918 and 2009 pandemics occurred in persons younger than 65 years.

The pandemics of 1957 and 1968 began in mainland China, but the geographic origin of the 2009 H1N1 pandemic virus is uncertain. The interval between pandemics is variable (10 to 40 years) and unpredictable. The most severe pandemics have been associated with major antigenic alterations in both major surface antigens. Depending on population susceptibility and perhaps changes in the virus, one or more waves, sometimes with increased severity, may occur. As the level of immunity in the population increases, antigenic drift within the subtype may cause repeated epidemics in subsequent years, and excess mortality in younger adults may continue for some years.

PATHOBIOLOGY

Influenza virus infection is transmitted from person to person by virus-containing respiratory secretions. Large- and small-particle aerosols over short distances (1 to 2 meters) both appear to contribute, but transmission by other routes, including fomites, may be possible. Infection by avian viruses also can occur after direct contact with infected birds or their excreta, ingestion of contaminated food, and sometimes inoculation into the conjunctiva. Virtually all levels of cells lining the respiratory tract can support viral replication, although receptors for avian viruses appear to be concentrated on cells in the distal bronchioles, alveoli, and conjunctiva. Once the virus initiates infection of the respiratory tract epithelium, successive cycles of viral replication infect large numbers of cells and result in destruction of respiratory epithelium and sometimes pneumocytes through direct cytopathic effects or apoptosis. Virulence, which is a multigenic characteristic with contributions

from HA, NA, NS, and polymerase proteins (see Table 372-2), varies among strains and is not necessarily linked to transmissibility.

The incubation period, which averages 2 days and varies from about 1 to 4 days, may be somewhat longer in infections caused by avian viruses. The quantity of virus in respiratory tract specimens generally correlates with the severity of illness and levels of host pro-inflammatory cytokine-chemokine responses, findings that support the importance of ongoing viral replication in producing acute illness. Elevated levels of mediators such as interferon-α, interleukin-6, and tumor necrosis factor-α occur in blood and respiratory secretions and probably contribute to systemic symptoms and fever. The duration of viral replication depends on age, immune status, underlying conditions, and viral strain. In seasonal influenza, upper respiratory viral shedding generally continues for 3 to 5 days in adults and often into the second week in young children, and it may persist for weeks to months in immunocompromised hosts. Higher level and more prolonged viral replication occurs in the lower respiratory tract of patients with viral pneumonia, and excessive cytokine-chemokine responses have been found in severe H5N1 infections and pandemic H1N1 infections. Viremia or extrapulmonary dissemination is rarely detected in typical human influenza, but both occur in some patients with avian H5N1 infections, in whom gastrointestinal replication may also occur.

Nasal and bronchial biopsy specimens from persons with uncomplicated influenza reveal desquamation of the ciliated columnar epithelium. Individual cells show shrinkage, pyknotic nuclei, and loss of cilia. In addition, the lungs in fatal influenza may show necrotizing bronchitis, alveolar edema and hemorrhage, hyaline membrane formation, diffuse alveolar damage, and, later, fibrosis and squamous metaplasia. Secondary bacterial infections develop as a result of altered bacterial flora, damage to bronchial epithelium with depressed mucociliary clearance, decreased polymorphonuclear and alveolar macrophage functions, accumulation of alveolar fluid, and suppression of other host immune responses. Bacterial infections were associated with more than 90% of fatal pneumonias in 1918 and about 20 to 40% in 2009. Neutralizing, hemagglutination-inhibiting (HAI), anti-NA, complement-fixing, enzyme-linked immunosorbent assay, and immunofluorescent antibodies begin to develop in the sera of persons with primary influenza virus infection during the second week after infection and reach a peak by 4 weeks. Secretory antibodies develop in the upper respiratory tract and consist predominantly of IgA antibodies. Cell-mediated immune responses develop by 1 week after infection and are considered important for termination of viral replication. Adaptive immunity to influenza appears to be largely subtype specific and durable for a particular strain. Protection against illness caused by human viruses is generally associated with serum HAI titers of 1 : 40 or greater, serum-neutralizing antibody titers of 1 : 8 or greater, or nasal-neutralizing antibody titers of 1 : 4 or greater.

CLINICAL MANIFESTATIONS

Influenza Syndrome

An abrupt onset of feverishness, chilliness, rigors, headache, myalgia, and malaise is characteristic of influenza but occurs in less than two thirds of cases. Systemic symptoms predominate initially, and prostration occurs in more severe cases. Myalgia, arthralgias, malaise, and headache are usually the most troublesome early symptoms, and their severity is related to the level of fever. Ocular symptoms, including photophobia, tearing, burning, and pain on moving the eyes, are sometimes present. Conjunctivitis is characteristic in avian H7 virus infections. Respiratory symptoms, particularly dry cough and nasal discharge, are typical early in the illness but are overshadowed by the systemic symptoms. Nasal obstruction, hoarseness, and sore throat are likewise common. Pandemic H1N1 2009 illness also was notable for nausea, vomiting, and diarrhea in some adults. As systemic illness diminishes, respiratory complaints and findings become more apparent. Cough is the most frequent and troublesome symptom and may be accompanied by substernal discomfort or burning. Cough, lassitude, and malaise may persist for several weeks before full recovery.

Fever is the most important initial physical finding. The temperature usually rises rapidly to a peak of 38° to 40° C within 12 hours of onset, concurrently with systemic symptoms. Fever is usually continuous but may be intermittent, especially if antipyretics are administered. Typically, the duration of fever in adults is about 3 days, but it may persist from only 1 to 5 or more days. Uncommonly, the fever takes a biphasic course. Early in the course of illness, the patient appears toxic, the face is flushed, and the skin is hot and moist. The eyes are watery and reddened. Clear nasal discharge is common. The mucosa of the nose and throat is hyperemic, but exudate is not

TABLE 372-4 PARTICULAR TARGET GROUPS FOR SEASONAL INFLUENZA IMMUNIZATION*

GROUPS AT INCREASED RISK FOR COMPLICATIONS

Persons 50 years and older

Residents of nursing homes and other chronic care facilities

Patients with a chronic pulmonary (including asthma) or cardiac (except hypertension) disorder

Patients with chronic metabolic (including diabetes), renal, hepatic, hematologic (including hemoglobinopathies), or neurologic (including those that compromise respiratory function or increase aspiration risk) disorder

Patients with immunosuppression (including that caused by medications or HIV infection)

Women who will be pregnant or within 2 works post partum during the influenza season

Persons who are morbidly obese (body mass index ≥ 40)

Persons who are American Indians or Alaskan Natives

Children 6 months through 4 years old

Children and teens receiving long-term aspirin

GROUPS IN CONTACT WITH HIGH-RISK PERSONS

Physicians, nurses, and other health care providers, including those in training†

Employees of nursing homes and chronic care and assisted-living facilities

Household contacts (parents including breast-feeding mothers, siblings) and caregivers of at-risk persons, including children 0-5 years old, adults ≥50 years old, and persons with medical conditions associated with risk of severe influenza complications (above)

OTHER GROUPS

Travelers (including to the tropics, large organized groups, or to the Southern Hemisphere in its winter)

Students, dormitory residents

Anyone wishing to reduce their risk for influenza

*Note: Starting with the 2010-2011 season, routine annual immunization is recommended for all persons aged 6 months or older who do not have contraindications. The risk groups for influenza complications have been expanded because of observations from the 2009 influenza pandemic.
†Trivalent inactivated influenza vaccine is recommended for vaccination of household members, health care personnel, and others who have close contact with severely immunosuppressed persons (e.g., patients with hematopoietic stem cell transplants) during those periods in which the immunosuppressed person requires care in a protective environment.
HIV = human immunodeficiency virus.
Modified from Centers for Disease Control and Prevention. Prevention and control of seasonal influenza with vaccines: recommendations of the Advisory Committee on Immunization Practices, 2010. http://www.cdc.gov/mmwr/.htm.

observed. Small, tender cervical lymph nodes are often present. Transient scattered rhonchi or localized areas of rales are found in less than 20% of cases.

The same pattern of illness occurs with any strain of influenza A or B virus. However, illness is more frequent and severe in smokers. In children, maximum temperatures are often higher; cervical adenopathy may be more frequent, and nausea, vomiting, and abdominal pain are more common. Persons at higher risk for influenza-associated complications and hospitalization (Table 372-4) include pregnant women (especially during the second and third trimesters or early postpartum period), morbidly obese patients, and immunosuppressed persons. Older adults, especially the infirm elderly, develop fever, muscle aches, sore throat, and headache less often but have higher rates of altered mental status and pulmonary complications. Immunocompromised hosts may also have an apparently mild initial illness but often progress to severe lower respiratory tract involvement. In sporadic illness attributable to H5N1 virus, upper respiratory complaints are less frequent, diarrhea is more common, and progressive viral pneumonia with high mortality is much more likely. Influenza C virus generally causes sporadic upper respiratory tract illness or febrile bronchitis.

Respiratory Complications

Three pneumonic syndromes have been described—primary influenza viral pneumonia, secondary bacterial pneumonia, and mixed viral and bacterial pneumonia—but their clinical presentations and courses overlap considerably. Influenza A and B virus infections are often associated with other respiratory tract complications, including exacerbations of chronic bronchitis, asthma, or cystic fibrosis; croup and bronchiolitis in young children; and otitis media, sinusitis, and, rarely, parotitis or bacterial tracheitis. Apparently uncomplicated influenza frequently causes tracheobronchitis and is often accompanied by abnormal tracheobronchial clearance, airway hyperactivity, and dysfunction of small airways lasting weeks. A syndrome mimicking

pulmonary embolism with transiently altered perfusion scans has also been described.

Primary influenza viral pneumonia is uncommon during epidemics but accounts for about 20 to 50% of pneumonias during pandemics and has been the principal manifestation of severe pandemic H1N1 or H5N1 illness. It occurs predominantly in persons with underlying pulmonary and cardiac disorders, pregnancy, or immunodeficiency states, although up to 40% of reported cases and almost all patients with H5N1 have no recognized underlying disease. After a typical onset of influenza, there is rapid progression of fever, cough, dyspnea, and even cyanosis. Bilateral pulmonary infiltrates, often consistent with adult respiratory distress syndrome, and hypoxia may evolve rapidly. Gram staining of sputum may show abundant polymorphonuclear leukocytes but scant bacterial flora. Sputum may be bloody. Sputum and endotracheal aspirates usually yield high titers of influenza virus by RNA detection or culture, but upper respiratory samples are sometimes negative.

In patients with classic bacterial superinfection, transient improvement for 1 to 4 days may be followed by recrudescence of fever, increased cough, sputum production, pleuritic chest pain, and a localized area of consolidation; in some patients, fulminant pneumonia develops. Gram staining and culture of sputum most often reveal *Streptococcus pneumoniae* (Chapter 297), *Staphylococcus aureus* (Chapter 296) including community-acquired methicillin-resistant *S. aureus, Haemophilus influenzae* (Chapter 308), or *Streptococcus pyogenes*. Such patients usually respond to specific antibiotic therapy, although staphylococcal infections may be particularly virulent and cause destructive pulmonary lesions. Invasive aspergillosis (Chapter 347) occurs rarely after influenza.

In addition, during an outbreak of influenza, many less distinct syndromes are observed; patients may have viral tracheobronchitis (Chapter 96), milder forms of localized viral pneumonia, or mixed viral and bacterial infection. Many such patients respond to antibiotics. Immunocompromised hosts, including transplant recipients and acute leukemia patients undergoing chemotherapy, may have high rates of pneumonia and mortality after influenza if they are not treated with appropriate antiviral and antimicrobial medications.

Nonrespiratory Complications

Severe influenza, including both pandemic H1N1 and H5N1 disease, may be associated with sepsis syndrome (Chapter 108), acute renal insufficiency (Chapter 122), and multiorgan failure. Lymphopenia and thrombocytopenia are common in severe influenza, and the hemophagocytic syndrome can occur. Myositis with tender leg muscles and elevated serum creatine kinase levels is uncommon, except in children. Rhabdomyolysis (Chapter 115) can be severe, and virus has been recovered rarely from skeletal muscle. Disseminated intravascular coagulation (Chapter 178) develops rarely, as does renal failure related to disseminated intravascular coagulation or myoglobinuria. Reye's syndrome (Chapter 152), which is a well-recognized hepatic and central nervous system complication of influenza A and B virus infections in children and rarely in adults, is associated with salicylate use. Toxic shock syndrome (Chapter 296) caused by respiratory tract infection with toxin-bearing *S. aureus* or *Streptococcus pyogenes* can occur, and outbreaks of meningococcal infection (Chapter 306) have been associated with both influenza A and B virus infections. Myocarditis (Chapter 60) or pericarditis (Chapter 77) occurs uncommonly. Aseptic meningitis (Chapter 420), myelitis, encephalopathy (Chapter 422), and postinfluenzal Guillain-Barré syndrome (Chapter 428) also can develop.

DIAGNOSIS

In an individual case, influenza often cannot be distinguished from infection with a number of other viruses or nonviral pathogens that produce similar clinical manifestations (Chapters 96 and 437). Conversely, when public health authorities report an epidemic of influenza A and B virus infection in a given community and a patient is seen with typical febrile respiratory illness, it is highly likely that these symptoms are caused by an influenza virus infection. In such circumstances, the presence of fever and cough has a positive predictive value of about 80% for laboratory-proven influenza in ambulatory adults. Influenza virus is readily isolated from nasal, sputum, or tracheal secretion specimens in the first 2 or 3 days of illness. Throat samples have lower yield than nasal samples in infections by human viruses but appear to be superior to nasal samples for detection of H5N1 infections. Endotracheal aspirates and bronchoalveolar lavage fluid have higher yields in patients with serious lower respiratory illness. Infectious virus is usually recovered in cell culture within 48 to 72 hours. Immunofluorescence testing of respiratory cells or inoculated cell cultures (shell vials) can reduce time to detection. Commercially available enzyme immunoassays can detect influenza virus antigens rapidly but have limited sensitivity (<20 to 70%) in adults; some do not distinguish between influenza A and B. The limited specificity of some assays makes their predictive value low, especially outside the influenza season. Detection of viral RNA by reverse transcription–polymerase chain reaction, which is more sensitive and specific than viral culture, is the rapid test of choice for serious illness and for suspected pandemic H1N1 or H5N1 illness. Serologic methods are less useful clinically because they require convalescent serum obtained 14 to 21 days after the onset of infection.

PREVENTION

Vaccination

Inactivated influenza vaccines for persons 6 months of age and older, a high-dose inactivated vaccine for persons 65 years of age and older, and a live attenuated, intranasal vaccine for otherwise healthy persons aged 2 to 49 years are currently licensed in the United States. The target groups for seasonal vaccine have continued to expand; beginning with the 2010-2011 season, immunization is recommended for all persons aged 6 months or older in the United States. However, persons at higher risk for influenza-related complications should continue to be a focus of vaccination efforts (see Table 372-4) during the transition to routine annual immunization or if vaccine shortages occur. Racial and ethnic disparities in influenza vaccination rates persist, and rates for other target groups, including health care workers, remain suboptimal. Immunization of health care personnel can be enhanced by improved access and employer recommendations or requirements.

Seasonal vaccine should be given each year in the fall, preferably October or November, before the influenza season. The antigenic composition of seasonal vaccines is reviewed annually so that these trivalent vaccines contain the most recently circulating strains, usually two subtypes of influenza A (H3N2, H1N1) and an influenza B virus. Both vaccine types are grown in eggs, and episodic production problems have sometimes led to shortages of the inactivated vaccine. For the 2010-2011 season, pandemic 2009 virus has been incorporated as the H1N1 component. Alternative vaccines (cell culture grown; oil-in-water adjuvanted) are available in some countries, and various investigational vaccines (mammalian or insect cell produced; vectored and DNA based; and those directed to conserved antigens) are in clinical study. An intradermal vaccine is approved in Europe.

Inactivated vaccines (Chapter 17) given by intramuscular injection provide about 70 to 90% protection against seasonal influenza illness and reduce work absenteeism, use of health care resources, and antibiotics in adults younger than 65 years when the vaccine is well matched to the epidemic strain.[1] Live attenuated vaccines are highly protective against influenza in children but appear less effective in adults compared with inactivated vaccine.[2] Immunogenicity and hence protection rates with inactivated vaccine are often lower in elderly persons, particularly infirm nursing home residents, and in immunosuppressed patients. For example, the effectiveness of influenza vaccine for prevention of medically attended acute respiratory illness among the elderly in nursing homes is estimated to be 20 to 40%. In ambulatory high-risk patients, immunization reduces hospitalizations from pneumonia, influenza,

and cardiovascular disease as well as all-cause mortality during the influenza season. Higher dose inactivated vaccines (four-fold more HA per strain) and those containing oil-in-water adjuvant are more immunogenic in older ambulatory adults,[3] and their comparative effectiveness to standard dose vaccines is under study. Immunization of children appears to reduce respiratory illness in household and community contacts[4] and, in one Japanese study, excess deaths in the elderly. Immunization of health care providers reduces the risk of transmission to patients as well as their own risk of infection. Maternal immunization benefits both mother and child. Persons with malignant disease should receive vaccine between courses of chemotherapy.

Nonadjuvanted, inactivated pandemic 2009 H1N1 vaccines were highly immunogenic in older children and adults after one standard 15-μg HA dose, perhaps in part related to preexisting immunity. Oil-in-water adjuvants (e.g., MF-59, AS03) are immunogenic at lower HA doses. For H5 vaccines, two doses of high HA antigen content or coadministration with an oil-in-water adjuvant appears to be necessary for adequate immunogenicity; the latter is also associated with cross-clade immunogenicity.

With inactivated vaccine, fever and systemic symptoms occur at rates comparable to those of adults given placebo but are more common in young children. Among adults, 25% or more may have mild local reactions at the site of injection. Ocular or respiratory symptoms have occasionally been reported within 24 hours after administration, but these symptoms typically are mild and resolve quickly without specific treatment. Injection site reactions and systemic complaints are more frequent after the high HA content[3] or oil-in-water adjuvanted inactivated vaccines. Intranasal vaccine causes coryza and sore throat in adults. Hypersensitivity reactions to residual egg proteins or other vaccine components occur rarely, and vaccine is contraindicated in persons with chicken egg anaphylactic hypersensitivity unless the patient has been desensitized. Inactivated vaccine does not cause exacerbation of asthma but might rarely be associated with Guillain-Barré syndrome in older adults.

Medications

Inhaled zanamivir and oral oseltamivir appear to be effective for chemoprophylaxis of both influenza A and B virus infections, including postexposure prophylaxis in households (Table 372-5), with each reducing the risk of symptomatic influenza infections by about 60 to 80%.[5,6] Unimmunized persons can be given prophylaxis when an outbreak develops and be given inactivated vaccine simultaneously with cessation of prophylaxis after 14 days. Alternatively, if vaccine is not available or is a poor match or if the patient is highly immunosuppressed, administration may be continued for the duration of the outbreak. When given to patients and staff alike, these drugs may be helpful in managing nosocomial outbreaks.

Rimantadine and amantadine are 70 to 90% effective in preventing influenza A illness caused by susceptible strains. However, the recent global circulation of adamantane-resistant H3N2 and pandemic H1N1 strains has made use of these agents unreliable. Transmission of resistant virus from drug-treated close contacts (households, nursing homes) may cause failure of prophylaxis and has been associated with failure to terminate nursing home outbreaks.

TABLE 372-5	ANTIVIRAL DOSE RECOMMENDATIONS IN ADULTS				
DRUG	ROUTE	TREATMENT	PROPHYLAXIS	DOSE REDUCTIONS	COMMENT
Amantadine	Oral	100 mg bid	100 mg bid	Age >64 yr, Cr_{cl} < 50-80 mL/min	Consider further dose reductions in elderly <70 kg
Rimantadine	Oral	100 mg bid	100 mg bid	Age >64 yr, Cr_{cl} < 10 mL/min or severe hepatic dysfunction	Lower risk of CNS side effects than with amantadine
Oseltamivir	Oral	75 mg bid	75 mg once daily	Cr_{cl} < 30 mL/min	
Zanamivir	Inhaled	10 mg bid	10 mg once daily	Avoid in those with underlying airways disease	Training in use of the inhaler device is important
Peramivir*	Intravenous	600 mg once daily	Not applicable	Cr_{cl} < 50 mL/min	Currently investigational in U.S.
Zanamivir*	Intravenous	600 mg bid	Not applicable	Cr_{cl} < 80 mL/min	Currently investigational in U.S.

*Currently intravenous oseltamivir, peramivir, and zanamivir are in clinical development and are available on a compassionate use/emergency investigational new drug (zanamivir) use basis in the United States. Peramivir is licensed for use in Japan.

The standard duration of treatment in uncomplicated illness is 5 days; a longer duration (e.g., 10 days) should be considered for infections in seriously ill patients, immunosuppressed hosts, or infections caused by novel viruses. Higher doses (e.g., 150 mg twice daily) of oseltamivir have been used in patients with serious lower respiratory illness, immunocompromise, or infections by novel viruses. The duration of prophylaxis depends on the epidemiologic setting; durations of 2 weeks after immunization or 7 to 10 days for postexposure prophylaxis are appropriate. Antiviral prophylaxis may interfere with response to intranasal, live attenuated but not to intramuscular, inactivated vaccine.

CNS = central nervous system; Cr_{cl} = creatinine clearance.

Precautions

Patients hospitalized with human influenza should be managed with standard and droplet precautions. Masks appear to be as effective as respirators in protecting health care workers during seasonal influenza.[7] Patients hospitalized with presumed H5N1 or other novel strains warrant airborne, droplet, and contact precautions, including eye protection. Compliance with masks and hand hygiene also appears to reduce the risk of secondary infections in household contacts.[8]

TREATMENT   Rx

Inhaled zanamivir and oral oseltamivir (see Table 372-5) are active against both influenza A and B viruses. Antiviral treatment is recommended as soon as possible for patients with proven or suspected influenza who manifest severe, complicated, or progressive illness; are hospitalized; or have underlying conditions that increase the risk for complications (Table 372-4), including adults >64 years of age and children <5 years of age (especially those <2 years). Treatment within 2 days of symptom onset may be considered in outpatients with uncomplicated febrile illness. Therapy within 2 days of the onset of febrile illness in ambulatory patients reduces symptoms by 1 to 2 days, time to functional recovery, and risk for lower respiratory complications such as bronchitis and pneumonia.[5] Early oseltamivir therapy also decreases the risk for hospitalization, and even delayed use appears to reduce mortality in hospitalized patients. During therapy, oseltamivir resistance is infrequent but is more common in children and immunocompromised hosts and has developed in H5N1 and pandemic 2009 H1N1 infections owing to a specific mutation (H275Y). Global circulation of oseltamivir-resistant seasonal H1N1 viruses in 2008-2009 highlights the need for ongoing susceptibility monitoring. Zanamivir is inhibitory for most oseltamivir-resistant variants, including those with H275Y. Inhaled zanamivir may be infrequently associated with bronchospasm, sometimes severe, and nebulization of the lactose-containing commercial form is contraindicated in intubated patients. Oseltamivir is associated with nausea, vomiting, rash, and possibly rare neuropsychiatric symptoms.

Oral rimantadine or amantadine shortens the duration of fever and symptoms in uncomplicated influenza A caused by susceptible strains (see Table 372-5). The possible effectiveness of these drugs in preventing or treating the pulmonary complications of influenza is uncertain. Rimantadine carries a lower risk for central nervous system side effects than amantadine does, but both may cause gastrointestinal upset. These agents are ineffective for influenza B infections. Antiviral resistance emerges in 30% or more of treated persons. Circulating H3N2 and pandemic H1N1 as well as increasingly seasonal H1N1 and many H5N1 viruses show high-level resistance to this antiviral class, so these drugs are not recommended for routine use at present.

Symptomatic measures include antipyretics and cough suppressants. Aspirin should not be used, especially in children younger than 16 years, because of its association with Reye's syndrome.

Influenza viral pneumonia, particularly pandemic H1N1 and H5N1 disease, requires intensive respiratory monitoring, often including ventilatory support. Early oseltamivir appears to reduce mortality in such patients.[5] Intravenous formulations of zanamivir and peramivir provide reliable delivery of high drug levels in seriously ill persons and are available for compassionate use in the United States. Oral amantadine or rimantadine combined with a neuraminidase inhibitor is reasonable for susceptible strains. Intravenous ribavirin, aerosolized ribavirin, nebulized zanamivir, and convalescent plasma have been used with uncertain benefit. Systemic corticosteroids have been associated with prolonged viral replication, side effects, and possibly increased mortality. Intensive care unit complications, including ventilator-associated pneumonia, are common. Secondary bacterial pneumonia should be treated with appropriate antibiotics. When studies of sputum do not clearly indicate an infecting bacterium, antibiotics that are effective against the probable pathogens, including methicillin-resistant *S. aureus*, should be used.

PROGNOSIS

The mortality rate from seasonal influenza or pandemic 2009 H1N1 illness has been very low. However, although 90% of seasonal influenza-related deaths occur in persons older than 65 years or at high risk because of comorbid conditions, most pandemic 2009 deaths were in those younger than 65 years. Most patients make a full recovery, but they may require several weeks to return to full function. In patients whose viral pneumonia progresses to respiratory failure, the mortality rate is up to 50% (60% in H5N1) but is reduced by early antiviral therapy and intensive care support.

1. Kwong JC, Maaten S, Upshur RE, et al. The effect of universal influenza immunization on antibiotic prescriptions: an ecological study. *Clin Infect Dis.* 2009;49:750-756.
2. Monto AS, Ohmit SE, Petrie JG, et al. Comparative efficacy of inactivated and live attenuated influenza vaccines. *N Engl J Med.* 2009;361:1260-1267.
3. Falsey AR, Treanor JJ, Tornieporth N, et al. Randomized, double-blind controlled Phase 3 trial comparing the immunogenicity of high-dose and standard-dose influenza vaccine in adults 65 years of age and older. *J Infect Dis.* 2009;200:172-180.
4. Loeb M, Russell ML, Moss L, et al. Effect of influenza vaccination of children on infection rates in Hutterite communities: a randomized trial. *JAMA.* 2010;303:943-950.
5. WHO Guidelines for Pharmacological Management of Pandemic Influenza A (H1N1) 2009 and Other Influenza Viruses, revised February 2010; Part I: Recommendations and Part II: Review of Evidence. http://www.who.int/csr/resources/publications/swineflu/h1n1_use_antivirals_20090820/en/index.html.
6. Khazeni N, Bravata DM, Holty JE, et al. Systematic review: safety and efficacy of extended-duration antiviral chemoprophylaxis against pandemic and seasonal influenza. *Ann Intern Med.* 2009;151:464-473.
7. Loeb M, Dafoe N, Mahony J, et al: Surgical mask vs N95 respirator for preventing influenza among health care workers: a randomized trial. *JAMA.* 2009;302:1865-1871.
8. Cowling BJ, Chan KH, Fang VJ, et al: Facemasks and hand hygiene to prevent influenza transmission in households: a cluster randomized trial. *Ann Intern Med.* 2009;151:437-446.

SUGGESTED READINGS

Center for Infectious Diseases Research & Policy, University of Minnesota website. http://www.cidrap.umn.edu/cidrap/content/influenza/general/index.html. *Daily updated resource site for current events, new publications, and thoughtful commentary related to influenza.*

Centers for Disease Control and Prevention. Prevention and control of influenza with vaccines: recommendations of the Advisory Committee on Immunization Practices. http://www.cdc.gov/mmwr/preview/mmwrhtml/rr5908a1.htm. *Annually updated review of epidemiology and recommendations for immunization.*

Centers for Disease Control and Prevention Influenza website. http://www.cdc.gov/cnidod/diseases/flu/weekly.htm. *Information on surveillance, prevention, detection, and control, with weekly updates.*

Centers for Disease Control and Prevention 2009 H1N1 Influenza website. http://www.cdc.gov/h1n1flu. *Dedicated site for information related to pandemic H1N1.*

Centers for Disease Control and Prevention. Antiviral agents for the treatment and chemoprophylaxis of influenza. Recommendations of the Advisory Committee on Immunization Practices (ACIP). *MMWR Morbid Mortal Wkly Rep.* 2011;60(No. RR-1):1-25. *Updated antiviral guidance and review of dosing, safety, and effectiveness data.* http://www.cdc.gov/mmwr/pdf/rr/rr6001.pdf.

World Health Organization website. http://www.who.int/topics/influenza/en. *A frequently updated, authoritative source with global perspectives.*

373

ADENOVIRUS DISEASES

JOHN J. TREANOR

DEFINITION

The adenoviruses are found in a variety of animal species, including humans, simians, horses, pigs, goats, and dogs. Specific disease syndromes or hosts are often associated with specific adenovirus serotypes (Table 373-1).

The Pathogen

The virus is nonenveloped and has a double-stranded DNA genome. The human adenoviruses are grouped into six subgenera (A to F) on the basis of differences in genome content, pattern of hemagglutination, and ability to cause tumors in experimental animals. In addition, at least 51 distinct serotypes are defined on the basis of neutralization tests. The majority of adenoviruses, like the coxsackieviruses (Chapter 387), use the same cellular receptor called the coxsackievirus-adenovirus receptor. The cell surface marker CD46 has also been identified as a potential receptor for some adenoviruses.

EPIDEMIOLOGY

The adenoviruses can infect and cause disease in a variety of human epithelial tissues, including those of the eye, respiratory tract, gastrointestinal tract, and urinary bladder. Virus may be shed from either the gastrointestinal or respiratory tract for months after acute infection. Most infections in immunologically competent individuals are subclinical.

Many outbreaks of epidemic keratoconjunctivitis have been attributed to contamination of ophthalmologic equipment, such as tonometers. Sterilization of such equipment between patients, good handwashing, segregation of patients, and other infection control procedures are critical in terminating nosocomial outbreaks.

PATHOBIOLOGY

Adenoviruses appear to use multiple mechanisms to circumvent the host's immune response, including inhibition of the antiviral effects of interferons,

TABLE 373-1	ADENOVIRUS SEROTYPES AND ASSOCIATED SYNDROMES	
HOST AND DISEASE CATEGORY	**EPIDEMIOLOGIC FEATURES**	**SEROTYPES**
IMMUNOCOMPETENT HOSTS		
Pharyngoconjunctival fever	Epidemics in schools, families, and military personnel; associated with swimming pools	3, 7
Epidemic keratoconjunctivitis	Sporadic epidemics in schools, families, and industrial sites; may cause nosocomial outbreaks; more common in fall and winter	8, 19, 37
Endemic upper respiratory disease	Seen predominantly in children, families, and daycare settings	1, 2, 5
Acute lower respiratory tract disease	Most common in military recruits, but other healthy adults can also be affected	3, 4, 7, 14, 21
Acute hemorrhagic cystitis	Male preponderance	7, 11, 21, 35
Gastroenteritis	Predominantly in children <2 yr old	40, 41
IMMUNOCOMPROMISED HOSTS		
Transplantation		7, 11, 31, 34, 35
Acquired immunodeficiency syndrome		Multiple, 35, 42-47

downregulation of the expression of human leukocyte antigen molecules on the surface of infected cells, and inhibition of apoptotic cell death. They are capable of establishing persistent asymptomatic infection in some tissues.

CLINICAL MANIFESTATIONS
● DISEASE IN NORMAL HOSTS
Eye Disease
PHARYNGOCONJUNCTIVAL FEVER
The syndrome of pharyngoconjunctival fever is seen predominantly in children and is characterized by bilateral conjunctivitis accompanied by mild pharyngitis without exudate. Fever, myalgias, and malaise may also be present. The eyes are itchy but not painful, with a boggy, hyperemic conjunctiva and watery discharge. Occasionally, the syndrome may be complicated by punctate keratitis.

Pharyngoconjunctival fever is highly contagious (see Table 373-1) and can be spread by contact with the eyes and mouth for 8 to 10 days after the onset of symptoms. The incubation period is 5 to 8 days. The illness is self-limited, with a duration of a few days to as long as 3 weeks. There is no specific therapy.

EPIDEMIC KERATOCONJUNCTIVITIS
In contrast to pharyngoconjunctival fever, epidemic keratoconjunctivitis occurs as unilateral disease in the majority of patients and is not generally accompanied by sore throat, fever, or systemic symptoms. Patients may complain of a mild foreign body sensation with watery tearing but are not in significant discomfort. Physical findings include a swollen eyelid, conjunctival hyperemia with edema and chemosis, and tender preauricular adenopathy. Keratitis eventually develops in about 80% of patients and is usually noted on about the eighth day of illness with the onset of pain, photophobia, lacrimation, and blepharospasm. Visual acuity may be temporarily reduced during the height of illness. Subepithelial corneal infiltrates can be detected in about a third of patients and may take weeks or months to resolve. Some cases of adenoviral conjunctivitis may result in prominent subconjunctival hemorrhage and resemble enteroviral acute hemorrhagic conjunctivitis.

Respiratory Disease
UPPER RESPIRATORY TRACT ILLNESS
Acute pharyngitis is the most common respiratory syndrome attributed to the adenoviruses. Adenoviruses can cause an exudative tonsillitis similar to that caused by group A streptococci (Chapter 298). In children, common associated syndromes include otitis media, coryza, and undifferentiated fever. Overall, adenoviruses are associated with about 7% of acute febrile illnesses in children, with the peak incidence occurring between 6 months and 2 years of age. High secondary attack rates are seen in families or in the daycare setting.

LOWER RESPIRATORY TRACT ILLNESS
Adenoviruses have been etiologically implicated in approximately 10% of childhood pneumonias. Clinical features are nondescript, and findings on chest radiography are similar to those in patients with other forms of viral pneumonia, with the exception that hilar adenopathy is more common in children with adenoviral pneumonia than in those with other forms of viral pneumonia. Mixed bacterial-viral pneumonia is often present and may be suggested by elevations in band forms in peripheral blood.

Adenoviruses can also be responsible for acute, febrile lower respiratory tract disease in healthy adults, seen most commonly in military recruits. The increased incidence in military recruits may be related to the special conditions of fatigue and crowding found in military training. Formerly well controlled by vaccination, adenovirus types 4 and 7 have reemerged as an important cause of acute respiratory illness in recruits after the production of adenovirus vaccine was discontinued in the 1990s. The disease is manifested as an atypical pneumonia syndrome and clinically resembles *Mycoplasma* pneumonia (Chapter 325). Prodromal symptoms of upper respiratory tract infection are reported by most patients, and pharyngitis is often found on initial evaluation. Bacterial superinfection may occur, particularly with *Neisseria meningitidis*. Although the illness is typically mild, more severe disseminated infections and deaths have been reported. Radiographic patterns can include focal infiltrates that resemble acute bacterial pneumonia, as well as large pleural effusions.

Acute, severe lower respiratory tract disease has also been reported in healthy adults in civilian populations in a variety of settings. Nosocomial outbreaks of adenoviral respiratory disease in healthy adults and children in long-term care facilities, psychiatric hospitals, and hospitals have been reported. Recently, outbreaks of severe respiratory disease in normal hosts have been associated with type 14 adenoviruses in the United States and elsewhere.

Because adenoviruses are relatively rare causes of pneumonia in otherwise healthy civilian adults but are frequently shed asymptomatically, isolation of adenovirus from stool or respiratory secretions in normal adults with pulmonary infiltrates should be interpreted with caution.

Urinary Disease: Hemorrhagic Cystitis
Acute hemorrhagic cystitis caused by adenoviruses is seen predominantly in children. The patient complains of gross hematuria and dysuria. The findings may be confused with those of glomerulonephritis, but laboratory tests of renal function remain normal, and fever and hypertension do not occur. Acute hemorrhagic cystitis is generally self-limited.

Gastrointestinal Disease: Gastroenteritis
Although multiple adenovirus serotypes may be shed in stool, only types 40 and 41, referred to as the enteric adenoviruses, have been convincingly associated with acute gastroenteritis. These adenovirus types belong to subgroup F and differ from other adenoviruses in being acid stable and highly restricted in their ability to replicate in conventional cell culture.

Gastroenteritis caused by enteric adenovirus is a disease predominantly of children younger than 2 years. Clinical features include watery diarrhea and vomiting similar to that seen with group A rotavirus infection (Chapter 388). In contrast to gastroenteritis associated with the rotaviruses and astroviruses, adenoviral gastroenteritis has no significant seasonal variability. The frequency of illness is about 5 to 10% of that caused by rotavirus in the same age group. Adenoviruses are rarely causes of acute gastroenteritis in adults.

Other Syndromes Associated with Adenoviruses in Immunocompetent Hosts
Adenoviruses are often isolated in cases of pertussis-like syndrome, but there is no evidence that adenoviruses by themselves are important causes of

whooping cough (Chapter 321). A toxic shock–like manifestation (Chapter 296) of disseminated adenovirus infection in a normal host has been reported. Adenoviruses have occasionally been isolated from cerebrospinal fluid in immunocompetent individuals with meningitis or meningoencephalitis and have been reported to be associated with an acute flaccid paralysis resembling polio (Chapter 423) in children. These viruses have also been implicated in sudden infant death syndrome. Adenoviruses may be detected in mesenteric lymph nodes at the time of surgery for intussusception, and it is postulated that viral infection causes an acute mesenteric lymphadenitis that leads to the development of this condition. Adenoviruses have also been isolated from myocardial biopsy specimens in adults with acute myocarditis (Chapter 60), thus suggesting a role for adenoviruses in its pathogenesis.

● DISEASE IN IMMUNOCOMPROMISED HOSTS

In contrast to infection in normal hosts, infection in immunocompromised subjects tends to be disseminated, with virus being isolated from multiple body sites, including the lung, liver, gastrointestinal tract, and urine. The spectrum of serotypes includes those found in immunocompetent individuals and a markedly increased frequency of higher-numbered serotypes rarely found in immunologically normal subjects (see Table 373-1). Because adenoviruses are often isolated from immunocompromised patients in conjunction with multiple other opportunistic pathogens, it is difficult to ascribe specific clinical syndromes to them. The source of infection may be reactivation of latent virus, but nosocomial infection has also been documented.

Adenovirus infections are reported in 3 to 47% of patients undergoing bone marrow transplantation (Chapter 181), usually in association with respiratory disease, gastrointestinal infection, hepatitis, or cystitis. Hemorrhagic cystitis is common and infrequently progresses to disseminated disease. Disseminated disease, defined as involvement of two or more organ systems, generally in association with viremia, is accompanied by high mortality. Symptomatic disease is more common in children and in those with acute graft-versus-host disease.

Adenovirus infections following solid organ transplantation frequently involve the transplanted organ and may become disseminated. Infection may mimic rejection and can lead to graft loss. Infections are more common in pediatric recipients and may be newly acquired or arise endogenously from the donor organ or the recipient.

Adenoviruses are also frequently isolated from the stool and urine of individuals with acquired immunodeficiency syndrome, particularly patients with relatively low CD4$^+$ lymphocyte counts. The most remarkable aspect of this situation is the isolation of a wide variety of serotypes in these patients (see Table 373-1), including new, higher-numbered serotypes isolated for the first time in such subjects. In addition, antigenically intermediate types have been isolated that possibly reflect recombination events made possible by prolonged viral replication in these hosts.

___ DIAGNOSIS

Adenovirus can be cultured efficiently from conjunctival swabs, respiratory secretions, urine, or stool in as little as 2 days by applying centrifugation culture systems coupled with detection by immunofluorescence. Other widely used methods of directly detecting viral antigen or nucleic acid in clinical specimens include enzyme immunoassays, immunofluorescence tests, and polymerase chain reaction (PCR) techniques. Virus can be detected in the blood of immunocompromised individuals with disseminated disease and in healthy children with primary infections. Assessment of viral load by quantitative PCR techniques may be useful in monitoring the course of disease.

___ PREVENTION

Live adenovirus vaccines administered orally in enteric-coated capsules provide effective protection against serotypes 4 and 7 but are no longer in production. There is an active program to reintroduce these vaccines in the military. Adenovirus vaccines have not been used in civilian populations, partially because of the plethora of additional serotypes causing severe disease in these populations.

TREATMENT   Rx

Conjunctivitis
Therapy is generally supportive. Corticosteroids should be avoided in patients with mild conjunctivitis (Chapter 431) because the symptoms usually recur when these agents are discontinued. In more severe cases of keratitis,

mild topical corticosteroids may be used with cycloplegics as needed for iritis (Chapter 431). Topical antibiotics may be administered to prevent bacterial superinfection. Topical cidofovir may decrease the frequency of severe corneal opacities but is associated with significant local toxicity.

Systemic Infections
No antiviral therapy has been proved to be effective for any systemic adenoviral syndrome. Cidofovir, which is highly active in cell culture, has been used (5 mg/kg intravenously weekly for 2 weeks and then every 2 weeks until three consecutive negative samples are obtained from previously positive sites) to treat disseminated disease in immunosuppressed individuals. The patient should be well hydrated and probenecid (2 g orally 3 hours before the dose and 1 g 2 and 8 hours after the dose) should be given to reduce the risk for renal toxicity. When compared with historical controls, use of cidofovir appears to be associated with decreased mortality, but no controlled trials are available to evaluate its efficacy. The utility of intravenous immunoglobulin for the treatment of adenovirus infection is unclear.

SUGGESTED READINGS

Gray GC, Chorazy ML. Human adenovirus 14a: a new epidemic threat. *J Infect Dis.* 2009;199:1413-1415. *A novel adenovirus strain emerged in the Unites States in 2007 and was associated with severe disease in healthy young persons.*

Hoffman JA. Adenovirus infections in solid organ transplant recipients. *Curr Opin Organ Transplant.* 2009;14:625-633. *Review of epidemiology, diagnosis, and therapy.*

Tebruegge M, Curtis N. Adenovirus infection in the immunocompromised host. *Adv Exp Med Biol.* 2010;659:153-174. *Review of pathobiology and clinical manifestations.*

374

CORONAVIRUSES

LARRY J. ANDERSON AND EILEEN SCHNEIDER

___ DEFINITION

Human coronaviruses were, until 2003, recognized as a frequent cause of common cold symptoms, occasionally a cause of lower respiratory tract disease, but rarely if ever a cause of serious disease. In 2003, a novel coronavirus was introduced into humans from animals as the etiologic agent of the outbreak of severe acute respiratory syndrome (SARS). The SARS outbreak demonstrated that coronaviruses can be serious human pathogens and led to discovery of other novel human coronaviruses as well as multiple novel coronaviruses in bats, the likely reservoir for SARS coronavirus. The novel non-SARS coronaviruses detected in humans have usually been associated with mild respiratory disease, similar to the clinical syndromes associated with the previously described human coronaviruses 229E and OC43.

The Pathogens
Coronaviruses are members of the family Coronaviridae, which includes two genera, coronaviruses and toroviruses. Coronaviruses are single-stranded, positive-sense RNA viruses with a genome of approximately 30 kD, the largest genome among RNA viruses. These viruses were named coronaviruses because by electron microscopy they have club-shaped surface projections that give them a crownlike appearance. The genome encodes four or five structural proteins (a spike protein [S], a small envelope protein [E], a membrane protein [M], a nucleocapsid protein [N], and sometimes a hemagglutinin-esterase protein [HE]), a varying number of open reading frames scattered among the structural genes, and a polyprotein that is processed into multiple (usually 16) nonstructural proteins. These nonstructural proteins participate in virus replication but are not incorporated into the virion. Coronaviruses have also been isolated from a variety of animals and birds and, in their respective species, cause a wide range of respiratory, gastrointestinal, neurologic, and systemic illnesses. The coronaviruses have traditionally been divided into three antigenic groups; human and animal viruses compose groups I and II and avian viruses group III.

The first two human coronaviruses, 229E and OC43, are members of groups I and II, respectively. SARS coronavirus is a distant member of group II, and the two most recent human coronavirus isolates, NL63 and HK1, are members of groups I and II, respectively. Detection of novel coronaviruses in bats has greatly expanded our understanding of diversity among coronaviruses and suggests that additional groups may be needed to classify these viruses.

EPIDEMIOLOGY

The coronaviruses, which are common pathogens of humans, appear to be transmitted through close contact that probably includes contamination of hands from person-to-person contact or from fomites, followed by autoinoculation to the mucosal surfaces of the mouth, nose, or eyes or inhalation of infectious droplets and possibly aerosols. Symptoms occur 2 to 4 days after infection. The non-SARS coronaviruses are detected in patients with acute respiratory illnesses, most often a mild, upper respiratory tract illness (i.e., the common cold), but also in patients with more serious respiratory illnesses including pneumonia, bronchiolitis, and croup. Coronavirus infections are detected early in childhood, and repeated infections can occur throughout life. About 50% of children have antibodies against OC43 by 3 years of age, and about 70% of adults have such antibodies. Up to 75% of children have antibodies against NL63 and 229E by 3.5 years of age. Studies looking for 229E- and OC43-like infections suggest that coronaviruses are associated with about 15% of cases of the common cold and with up to 10% of cases of acute respiratory illnesses in children and adults. Individually, 229E, OC43, HKU1, and NL63 are detected in less than 1% to 4% of cases, and their individual contributions will vary by location and year. Serious illness has been reported in outbreaks among elderly patients in nursing homes. In one outbreak associated with OC43 infection, for example, 23 residents and 24 staff reported influenza-like illness, and three residents died. The non-SARS coronaviruses can be detected throughout the year, but peak detection is often during fall and winter months in temperate climates. A second respiratory viral pathogen can be detected in 20 to 60% of specimens positive for a non-SARS coronavirus.

Most documented SARS coronavirus infections in humans occurred in persons ill with a SARS-like illness during the 2002-2003 global outbreak. It is likely that wild animal markets in Guangdong Province, China, played a key role in amplifying and introducing the virus into humans, but the original source of the outbreak virus has not been determined. Detection of multiple SARS-like and other coronaviruses in bats suggests that they are a rich source of coronaviruses and likely the source of SARS coronavirus. The parent to the outbreak virus has, however, not yet been detected. Although animals were the original source of human infections, global spread of SARS coronavirus occurred through human-to-human transmission and involved droplet, person-to-person, and fomite transmission and, in some instances, probably small-particle aerosol transmission. Most transmission occurred within households, hospitals, or other health care facilities, and little transmission occurred in the community. The fact that most transmission occurred after the patient's illness had become serious and required hospitalization helps explain the importance of transmission in health care settings and the relative lack of transmission in the community.

PATHOBIOLOGY

The human coronaviruses characterized to date, including SARS coronavirus, infect humans through the respiratory tract. The site of virus replication is determined, at least in part, by which cells express the respective receptors. The receptors for antigenic group I human coronaviruses 229E and the recently described NL63 are aminopeptidase N and angiotensin-converting enzyme 2 (ACE2), respectively. The receptors for the two group II human coronaviruses characterized to date, OC43 and the recently described HK1, have not yet been determined, but OC43 may use several cell surface molecules as receptors, including 9-O-acetylated neuraminic acid. The primary receptor for SARS coronavirus is ACE2, but the virus also binds to two C-type lectins expressed on dendritic cells, DC-SIGN and L-SIGN. Aminopeptidase N is expressed in various cells, including respiratory, gastrointestinal, kidney epithelial, and myeloid cells, but 229E is known to infect only respiratory epithelial cells. ACE2 is found in various tissues, including the lung, gastrointestinal tract, heart, and kidneys. The SARS coronavirus has consistently been detected in pneumocytes in the lung and enterocytes in the gastrointestinal tract, and it is occasionally found in other cells, including distal tubular cells in the kidney and macrophages in various tissues. Autopsy studies suggest that infection in the

lung leads initially to diffuse alveolar damage and later may lead to a repair process that includes fibrosis in the alveolar walls. It is not known whether NL63, which also uses ACE2 as its receptor, infects sites other than the respiratory tract.

It is likely that the illness associated with SARS and non-SARS coronavirus infections results from both the cytopathic effect of the virus and the host immune and inflammatory response to the viral infection. How this interplay contributes to disease, however, is not understood. The biphasic course of SARS in some patients, with the onset of severe disease in the second week of illness, and the decrease in the number of lymphocytes suggest a role for the host response and virus-induced immune suppression in the disease process.

CLINICAL MANIFESTATIONS

Non-SARS coronavirus infections are commonly associated with acute respiratory illnesses that are usually mild and consistent with the common cold (Chapter 369) but can also result in the full range of acute respiratory illnesses including pneumonia (Chapter 97), croup (Chapter 437), bronchiolitis (Chapter 92), and bronchitis (Chapter 96). The best studied of the non-SARS coronaviruses, human coronaviruses 229E and OC43, cause respiratory symptoms, such as rhinorrhea, nasal congestion, sore throat, and cough, as well as systemic symptoms, including fever, headache, and malaise, when they are inoculated intranasally in adult volunteers. Symptoms develop 2 to 4 days after inoculation, but about 30% of the volunteers who excrete virus had no associated illness. Symptoms usually persist for about 1 week but sometimes for as long as 3 weeks. Previous infection does not induce high levels of protective immunity. Humans can be reinfected with respiratory coronaviruses throughout life, and human volunteers can be symptomatically reinfected with the same strain of coronavirus 1 year after the first infection. As with other infections, the severity of disease varies among individual patients during the same outbreak and among groups of patients during different outbreaks in the same community. Patients with compromised cardiac, pulmonary, or immune systems are at increased risk of more serious lower respiratory tract illness, and outbreaks of human coronavirus infections in elderly patients in chronic care facilities can cause severe lower respiratory illnesses and deaths.

In contrast to the mild illness associated with 229E and OC43, SARS coronavirus infection nearly always results in a serious illness that requires hospitalization, often in an intensive care unit, and a high fatality rate. Radiologic evidence of pneumonia was seen in nearly all SARS coronavirus–infected persons, and acute respiratory distress syndrome (Chapter 104) requiring admission to an intensive care unit and mechanical ventilation developed in 20% or more of patients. Nearly 10% of outbreak-associated patients died. The death rate was especially high, approaching 50%, in elderly patients and patients with underlying illnesses. The initial clinical manifestation of SARS was often systemic symptoms of fever, malaise, and myalgias from 2 to 10 days (rarely longer than 10 days) after exposure. Several days after the onset of systemic symptoms, lower respiratory tract symptoms of nonproductive cough and shortness of breath were noted. Unlike patients with other respiratory virus infections, the majority of patients never experience upper respiratory tract symptoms such as rhinorrhea, sore throat, or nasal congestion (Table 374-1). As with other infections, the expected signs and symptoms with SARS coronavirus infection may be obscured or not present in elderly patients or patients with underlying chronic illnesses. During the course of their illness, most SARS coronavirus–infected patients had elevated liver enzyme levels and lymphopenia, including a substantial drop in numbers of both CD4$^+$ and CD8$^+$ T cells. SARS coronavirus–infected patients with severe complications also often suffered complications associated with intensive supportive care, such as secondary bacterial infections. A more severe illness with infection has been associated with older age, underlying chronic illness, higher liver enzyme values, lower lymphocyte levels and platelet counts, and higher titers of virus or viral RNA. Asymptomatic or mild illness occurred but was uncommon. In studies of exposed health care workers and patients who did not have a SARS-like illness, less than 1% of those tested had definitive serologic evidence of SARS coronavirus infection (i.e., a positive neutralization test result). In general, children had less severe illness than adults did.

Although most survivors of SARS coronavirus infection appeared to achieve full recovery, as many as 25% had abnormal pulmonary findings, such as ground-glass opacities on chest radiograph or abnormal pulmonary function test results (e.g., decreased diffusing capacity), 6 months or more after their illness.

TABLE 374-1	PERCENTAGE OF SARS CORONAVIRUS–INFECTED PATIENTS WITH SELECTED CLINICAL AND LABORATORY FEATURES OF SARS CORONAVIRUS INFECTION	
	SARS Coronavirus–Infected Patients with Symptoms or Laboratory Findings	
CLINICAL OR LABORATORY FINDING	**AT HOSPITAL ADMISSION**	**SOMETIME DURING THE ILLNESS**
Fever	90-100%	≈100%
Upper respiratory tract symptoms	10-25%	Not available
Cough or shortness of breath	40-75%	Up to 100%
Diarrhea	20-30%	40-70%
Elevated liver function test results	35-90%	70-100%
Pneumonia on chest radiograph	65-90%	90-100%
Lymphopenia*	50-90%	70-95%

*Both CD4+ and CD8+ lymphocyte counts are decreased.
SARS = severe acute respiratory syndrome.

DIAGNOSIS

Because illness is usually mild and there is no effective treatment, the diagnosis of non-SARS coronavirus infection has not been important to management of patients. The diagnosis of SARS coronavirus infection, however, is critical for the management of individual patients and for the public health response to reemergence of SARS.

Non-SARS Coronavirus Infection

Non-SARS coronavirus polymerase chain reaction (PCR) assays, which can be designed to detect both known and novel coronaviruses, are the assays of choice for diagnosis of infection. Most coronavirus PCR assays are type specific, that is, specific to SARS coronavirus, 229E, OC43, HKU1, or NL63 RNA. Coronavirus diagnostic assays have not been generally available and may have to be obtained by special requests from a limited number of sites that perform human coronavirus diagnostics. Presence of the virus can also be inferred by electron microscopy and confirmed by in situ or immunohistologic assays of affected tissues. Positive immunohistologic and in situ hybridization studies document the site of infection and help support a link between the virus and the disease process. A variety of enzyme or fluorescent immunoassays for antibodies have been used successfully to detect infection. Most assays detect IgG antibodies, but virus neutralization antibody assays are more specific. The need to detect a diagnostic rise in antibodies between acute and convalescent serum specimens for non-SARS coronavirus infections means that serologic tests are not helpful for managing the acute care of individual patients, although they are very helpful for epidemiologic studies.

SARS

Three features of SARS cases help guide approach to its diagnosis. First, SARS has occurred only in persons who have some potential exposure, that is, to patients with SARS, to a location with SARS transmission, to a laboratory working on SARS coronavirus, or to a setting where SARS-infected animals might be located (e.g., southern China). Second, nearly 100% of infected patients develop chest radiographic abnormalities by day 10 of their illness. Finally, SARS nearly always developed within 10 days of exposure. Thus, a suspicion of SARS and a diagnostic evaluation can be limited to patients who have a severe lower respiratory tract illness and some potential exposure to SARS within 10 days before the onset of illness.

Laboratory confirmation of SARS coronavirus infection early in the illness proved to be problematic, even with sensitive real-time PCR assays. Unlike in most respiratory viral infections, the highest titer of virus, or viral RNA, was found in clinical specimens from the second week of illness. During the first week of illness, the best way to detect infection is by a sensitive PCR assay or a sensitive enzyme immunoassay for N protein antigen applied to respiratory and serum specimens. During the second week of illness, respiratory and stool specimens are most likely to be positive for viral RNA. Because most populations are negative for SARS coronavirus antibodies, detection of serum SARS coronavirus antibodies is a reliable indicator of infection. Antibodies were sometimes detected early in the second week of illness but at times were not detected until 4 weeks into the illness. Because antibodies persist in serum, a specimen can be collected late without compromising the ability to detect antibodies. Serologic assays, unlike PCR assays, are not confounded by problems with specimen contamination. Because antibodies to SARS coronavirus were rarely present before the 2003 outbreak, a single positive antibody test result from an ill person could be considered diagnostic of an acute SARS coronavirus infection. However, because the reemergence of SARS coronavirus will have substantial public health, social, and economic impact, and because of occasional cross-reacting antibodies induced by other coronaviruses, a neutralization antibody test and repeated testing by a reference laboratory are required to confirm the diagnosis.

TREATMENT

There is no virus-specific treatment of non-SARS coronavirus infections, but the illnesses are mild and usually resolve in a few days to a week. Patients require symptomatic therapy or, uncommonly, management of complications of infection.

Treatment of SARS coronavirus infection is more complex. Currently, no antiviral drug has proved to be effective. With the high death rate, fast pace of the outbreak, and no clinical or in vitro data to guide treatment, a combination of ribavirin, steroids, and various mechanical ventilation and oxygenation regimens was often used to treat SARS patients. Later in the outbreak, in vitro data showed little if any antiviral effect with ribavirin and suggested that interferon alfa, SARS convalescent phase immune globulin, and lopinavir plus ritonavir might be useful. Although many people were treated during the outbreak, lack of control groups makes it impossible to determine which if any therapies were beneficial. If SARS reemerges, it is hoped that in vitro and animal studies can provide clearer guidance for treatment.

PREVENTION

A variety of candidate vaccines have been evaluated in animals, and two have entered clinical trials in humans. Handwashing and other infection control measures (Chapter 372) probably decrease the spread of coronaviruses in the home, health care facilities, and other settings. These strategies focus on reinforcing the need for patients with respiratory illnesses to cover the nose and mouth when coughing or sneezing, to use tissues to contain respiratory secretions, and to wash the hands after contact with respiratory secretions. Staff should use good infection control practices.

Within 4 months of the initiation of the 2003 SARS outbreak, the outbreak was contained and human-to-human transmission stopped without a vaccine or effective antiviral therapy but with thorough implementation of the classic public health tools of case finding, isolation, and contact tracing management. The low risk of SARS transmission early in the illness and the very low rate of asymptomatic infection were key factors to the success of these preventive measures.

The cases of laboratory-acquired SARS coronavirus infection and the subsequent transmission of disease to others after one such case reinforce the importance of strict attention to safe laboratory practices. Because the reemergence of SARS could lead to global spread, the local, national, and global public health and health care communities must be alerted quickly and updated regularly about new cases and the status of transmission.

SUGGESTED READINGS

Peiris JS, Poon LL. Detection of SARS coronavirus. *Methods Mol Biol.* 2011;655:369-382. *Review of a highly accurate PCR protocol.*

www.cdc.gov/ncidod/sars/index.htm. *This website contains background information on SARS and provides comprehensive guidance for the health care and public health communities on approaches to diagnosis and containment of SARS and control of a SARS outbreak.*

www.who.int/cxr/sars/en. *This website contains information on SARS and the global SARS outbreak and global strategies to diagnose and contain SARS and to control a SARS outbreak.*

375

MEASLES

MARTIN WEISSE AND MARK PAPANIA

DEFINITION

Measles (synonyms: rubeola, red measles, hard measles, 7-day measles) is a highly contagious systemic viral disease characterized by generalized maculopapular rash, fever, cough, coryza (rhinitis), and conjunctivitis. The measles virus is a negative-stranded RNA virus of the genus *Morbillivirus*, family Paramyxoviridae, with only one serotype and 23 genotypes.

EPIDEMIOLOGY

In the pre-vaccine era, measles was a nearly universal rite of childhood, affecting almost every child by 15 years of age. As a result of high vaccination coverage, measles has not been endemic in the United States for more than a decade (incidence <1 case/million people). However, a limited number of measles cases occur annually in the United States from the international importation of the virus. Many other countries have eliminated endemic measles, including all countries in the Americas. Unfortunately, measles is still endemic in many developed and developing countries and still causes an estimated 164,000 annual deaths worldwide.

Measles, which is one of the most contagious diseases, infects more than 90% of susceptible people who come into close contact with an infectious patient. The measles virus is transmitted mainly by direct contact with large respiratory droplets, but airborne spread is also possible. Persons with measles are considered infectious from 4 days before the onset of the rash until 4 days after its onset. Immunocompromised patients may shed virus for a prolonged time and should be considered infectious as long as they have catarrhal symptoms.

Measles infection confers lifelong immunity, as does measles vaccination. Maternal measles antibody, which is transferred through the placenta, protects infants of immune mothers during the first months of life. More than 90 to 95% of a population must be immune to sustain interruption of measles transmission.

PATHOBIOLOGY

Measles infection usually occurs through inhalation of infectious droplets into the respiratory epithelium or direct inoculation onto the conjunctiva. The virus attaches to host cells by its hemagglutinin protein, and its fusion protein allows viral entry and facilitates spread between cells. The virus initially replicates in the respiratory epithelial tissues or the adjacent lymph nodes. A primary viremia disseminates the virus to the reticuloendothelial tissues of the tonsils, lungs, gastrointestinal tract, spleen, and distant lymph nodes. Several days later, the onset of prodromal symptoms heralds a secondary viremia that results in further spread of the virus to the skin, viscera, kidney, and bladder. Histologic changes in the skin and mucous membranes consist of epithelial giant cells with surrounding mononuclear infiltrates and edema. Koplik spots, which are inflammatory lesions of the buccal submucous glands, have similar histologic features.

The development of IgM antibody coincides with the appearance of the rash; during the next week, IgG antibodies appear and persist for life. Cell-mediated immunity is also critical for resolution of acute infection. Measles virus infection causes a significant immunosuppression that predisposes infected patients to secondary bacterial and viral infections, which increase the mortality rate of measles. The exact mechanisms of immunosuppression are unknown.

CLINICAL MANIFESTATIONS

The incubation period of measles is usually 8 to 12 days after exposure until the development of the first symptoms. The well-known description of the prodrome of measles is fever associated with cough, coryza, conjunctivitis, and Koplik spots, often accompanied by malaise, myalgia, and headache. Fever increases with the severity of catarrhal symptoms and peaks at the onset of the exanthem; it frequently reaches 40° or 41° C and may persist for 6 days. Koplik spots, an enanthem of small bluish white spots on a red background on the buccal mucosa lateral to the molar teeth (Fig. 375-1), are

FIGURE 375-1. Typical Koplik spots.

FIGURE 375-2. Typical morbilliform eruption of measles, with broad areas of confluent red maculopapular lesions interspersed with islands of normal skin.

pathognomonic for measles. Koplik spots precede the rash by 1 day and are no longer evident 2 days into the rash.

The measles rash (Fig. 375-2) typically arises 2 to 6 days after the onset of the catarrhal symptoms. It begins on the face or behind the ears as individual red macules that blanch with pressure. During 12 to 24 hours, the macules become papular and tend to coalesce. The rash progresses from head to trunk to extremities and maintains the same pattern of progression from macules to coalescing papules. By the fourth day of the rash, the entire body is typically involved, although the hands and feet may be spared. The rash fades in the same head-to-toe order in which it appeared and often peels with a brawny desquamation during the subsequent weeks. In darkly pigmented individuals, the erythema may be difficult to appreciate, and the rash may be better felt than seen.

Important variations in the classic presentation of measles include "modified measles" in patients who have received immune globulin prophylaxis and "mild measles" in previously vaccinated persons. In both variations, any of the classic symptoms may be attenuated or absent. Such cases are extremely difficult to diagnose in the absence of known exposure to measles. Also, immunocompromised patients can have severe measles pneumonia without rash. Measles should be considered in any immunocompromised patient with pneumonia of unknown etiology.

TABLE 375-1 A GUIDE TO THE DIFFERENTIAL DIAGNOSIS OF MEASLES

	CONJUNCTIVITIS	RHINITIS	SORE THROAT	ENANTHEM	LEUKOCYTOSIS	DIAGNOSTIC TESTS AVAILABLE
Measles	++	++	0	+	0	Yes
Rubella	±	0	0	0	0	Yes
Exanthem subitum	0	0	0	0	0	Yes
Enterovirus infection	0	0	±	±	0	Yes
Adenovirus infection	+	+	+	0	0	Yes
Scarlet fever	0	0	++	+	+	Yes
Infectious mononucleosis	0	0	++	+	±	Yes
Drug rash	0	0	0	0	0	No

0 = not usually present or no test available; ± = variable in occurrence; + = present: test available (virus or bacterial culture, serology); ++ = present and severe.
Modified from Brunell PA. Measles. In: Ausiello D, Goldman L, eds. *Cecil Textbook of Medicine*, 23rd ed. Philadelphia: Saunders Elsevier; 2008:2477.

Complications

The most common complications of measles are diarrhea, otitis media, and pneumonia. Diarrhea occurs early in the disease and is probably the result of intestinal measles virus infection. Measles-associated diarrhea significantly contributes to morbidity and mortality in malnourished patients. Pneumonia is the most severe common complication and is responsible for the majority of deaths associated with measles. Measles-associated pneumonia may be a giant cell pneumonitis consistent with direct infection by measles virus or be caused by a secondary bacterial pathogen, most often *Staphylococcus aureus* (Chapter 296) or *Streptococcus pneumoniae* (Chapter 297).

Overall, children younger than 5 years and adults older than 20 years have the highest complication rates. Complication rates do not vary substantially by sex except that pregnant women are at high risk. Measles is especially hazardous during the first trimester, often leading to fetal demise. Later in pregnancy, the rate of prematurity is high, as is maternal pneumonia.

Malnutrition is associated with increased fatality rates, and children with vitamin A deficiency are at high risk for severe keratoconjunctivitis, which can lead to blindness. Immunocompromised patients (e.g., those with human immunodeficiency virus [HIV] infections, with cancer, or receiving chemotherapy or immunosuppressive drugs such as steroids) are at higher risk for severe measles complications. Interstitial pneumonia occurs 1 to 2 weeks after the onset of measles and is the most common cause of measles-related death in immunocompromised patients. Measles inclusion body encephalitis occurs in immunocompromised patients 1 to 6 months after acute measles and is usually fatal.

Postinfectious encephalomyelitis occurs in 1 in 1000 measles cases. Patients present during the 2 weeks after the onset of the rash with headache, recurrence of fever, vomiting, and stiff neck. Up to 25% of patients die, and 33% of survivors suffer neurologic sequelae. Elevated IgG and IgM can be found in cerebrospinal fluid, but measles virus cannot be isolated, thereby suggesting an autoimmune pathologic process. A rare late central nervous system complication of measles is subacute sclerosing panencephalitis (Chapter 378), a degenerative demyelinating disease due to chronic infection. Subacute sclerosing panencephalitis occurs years after the acute measles infection and is almost universally fatal.

DIAGNOSIS

In many countries, measles has become such a rare disease that most physicians have never seen a patient. One key to making the diagnosis is to consider measles in any patient with a generalized maculopapular rash and fever. The index of suspicion should be raised if cough, coryza, and conjunctivitis are present and if measles virus transmission is occurring in the area or if the patient has traveled internationally or had any association with international travelers. Although Koplik spots are pathognomonic, the absence of Koplik spots does not exclude the diagnosis. The lack of vaccination should increase the level of suspicion, but measles can occur despite two documented doses of measles vaccine.

The standard laboratory test for measles is an IgM measles antibody assay on a single serum specimen. However, during the first 3 days of rash, up to 25% of cases may not have IgM; the test can be repeated if the rash and fever persist for 3 days. Acute and convalescent sera to test for a rise in IgG antibody are sometimes useful. Urine, throat swabs, or blood specimens can be sent for viral culture or for detection of viral RNA by reverse transcription–polymerase chain reaction. Genotype sequence analysis aids in tracking the source of the virus, monitoring transmission patterns, and distinguishing a mild case of measles from a vaccine reaction in patients who have recently received measles vaccine.

Differential Diagnosis (Table 375-1)

Other viral infections that may be confused with measles are rubella (Chapter 376), human herpesvirus 6 and 7 infection (Chapter 382), infectious mononucleosis (Chapter 385), and parvovirus B19 infection (erythema infectiosum, Chapter 379). In general, these infections have a milder course. Bacterial infections that may mimic measles include secondary syphilis (Chapter 327), scarlet fever (Chapter 298), streptococcal or staphylococcal toxic shock syndrome (Chapter 447), and leptospirosis (Chapter 331). Drug eruptions (Chapter 448) and Kawasaki disease (Chapter 278) must also be considered. It can be extremely difficult to distinguish measles vaccine reactions, which may include fever and rash, from a mild case of measles. In highly vaccinated populations, measles is rare and clinical symptoms may be attenuated; serologic and virologic assays are critical in distinguishing measles from other diseases and conditions.

TREATMENT

Vitamin A treatment (100,000 IU orally for children 6 to 12 months of age, 200,000 IU orally for children 1 year of age and older) on 2 consecutive days [1] is recommended for children 6 months to 2 years of age who are hospitalized with measles and for any child older than 6 months who has evidence of immune deficiency, clinical evidence of vitamin A deficiency, impaired intestinal absorption, or moderate to severe malnutrition or who comes from communities where vitamin A deficiency is common or measles case-fatality rates are 1% or higher. In these settings, vitamin A can reduce blindness due to severe keratoconjunctivitis and decrease mortality by as much as 50%. For patients with ophthalmologic evidence of vitamin A deficiency, the dose should be repeated once 4 weeks later.

No specific antiviral or other therapies are recommended for measles. Ribavirin, isoprinosine, and interferon alfa have demonstrated modest benefit in small clinical trials, but no controlled trials have been conducted. For most patients, treatment of measles consists of symptomatic therapy with antipyretics and analgesics and encouraging fluids to maintain hydration.

PREVENTION

Vaccination

Live attenuated measles virus vaccines are the best means of preventing measles. Although the vaccine virus strains vary from different manufacturers, all provide equivalent protection. Measles vaccine is typically given as a component of the combination measles-mumps-rubella (MMR) vaccine or the measles-mumps-rubella-varicella (MMRV) vaccine. Measles-containing vaccines can be given at the same time as other live or killed vaccines.

Infants with known or suspected HIV infection also should be vaccinated at 6 months and then again at 9 months if they are at risk of exposure to measles. The first dose of vaccine is given at 9 months of age in countries where transmission is widespread and mortality is high, and it can be given as early as 6 months of age in U.S. infants at high risk of exposure. In the United States, the first dose of measles vaccine is usually given at 12 to 15 months of age (Chapter 17).

376

In the United States, a second dose of measles vaccine is given when a child enrolls in school at 4 to 6 years of age. Many other countries also recommend a routine second dose at various ages or provide a second opportunity for vaccination in mass campaigns to ensure protection. However, a high rate of first-dose coverage should always be the top priority.

Contraindications to measles vaccination include pregnancy, immunodeficiency, leukemia and other immunosuppressive diseases, administration of immunosuppressive drugs such as systemic corticosteroids or antimetabolites, and untreated active tuberculosis. Extreme caution should be used in considering vaccination in patients with severe allergies to gelatin, neomycin, or other vaccine components or a history of thrombocytopenic purpura. Persons with HIV infection should be vaccinated against measles unless they have signs of severe immunosuppression.

Common adverse events after vaccination with measles vaccine include transient fever and mild rash, each of which occurs in roughly 5% of vaccine recipients. More serious adverse events are very rare.

Prevention of Measles Virus Transmission
To prevent transmission of measles, contact should be minimized between persons with suspected or confirmed measles and all persons who might be susceptible to measles; isolation and airborne precautions are indicated for hospitalized patients. When a case of measles is suspected, the local health department should be contacted immediately to assist with measures to prevent virus transmission.

Postexposure Prophylaxis
If susceptible persons 6 months of age or older are identified within 72 hours of exposure to measles, vaccination is recommended (if it is not contraindicated) as it may prevent or alter the course of the disease. Susceptible household contacts of measles cases should be given immune globulin within 6 days of exposure, especially those who have contraindications to measles vaccination, such as pregnancy or immunodeficiency, and those who were not identified within 72 hours of exposure. Immune globulin may prevent measles or result in a less severe case of measles.

PROGNOSIS
In well-nourished populations with access to modern medical care, the case-fatality rate is typically 1 to 3 deaths/1000 cases, but case-fatality rates as high as 20% are seen in some developing countries as a result of malnutrition, limited access to health care, and immunodeficiency. Most measles deaths are associated with pneumonia or encephalitis. Antimicrobial treatment of secondary infections, especially pneumonias, can significantly reduce measles deaths. Vitamin A deficiency is associated with more severe disease, blindness, and increased mortality from respiratory and diarrheal causes, but vitamin A supplementation can reduce the severity of these complications. Patients with HIV infection and other immunocompromising conditions often have more severe cases with higher complication rates and case-fatality rates.

1. Sudfeld CR, Navar AM, Halsey NA. Effectiveness of measles vaccination and vitamin A treatment. *Int J Epidemiol.* 2010;39(Suppl 1):i48-55.

SUGGESTED READINGS

Centers for Disease Control and Prevention (CDC). Global measles mortality, 2000-2008. *MMWR Morb Mortal Wkly Rep.* 2009;58:1321-1326. *Global measles mortality declined by 78%, from an estimated 733,000 deaths in 2000 to 164,000 in 2008.*

Parker Fiebelkorn A, Redd SB, Gallagher K, et al. Measles in the United States during the postelimination era. *J Infect Dis.* 2010;202:1520-1528. *About 60 to 70 cases occur annually in the U.S., with 42% imported from other countries and most of the remainder occurring in U.S. residents who claimed exemptions for personal beliefs.*

Sugerman DE, Barskey AE, Delea MG, et al. Measles outbreak in a highly vaccinated population, San Diego, 2008: role of the intentionally undervaccinated. *Pediatrics.* 2010;125:747-755. *Emphasizes the individual risks and the high public health costs of intentional nonvaccination.*

RUBELLA (GERMAN MEASLES)

SUSAN E. REEF

DEFINITION
Rubella, also known as German measles, is an acute viral illness that usually presents with a generalized maculopapular rash of 1 to 3 days' duration, low-grade or no fever, and associated clinical symptoms such as lymphadenopathy, arthropathy, and conjunctivitis. However, about 20 to 50% of persons infected with rubella may present without a rash or other symptoms.

The Pathogen
Rubella virus is a member of the Togaviridae family and the genus *Rubivirus*. Rubella virus is a single-stranded enveloped RNA with a single antigenic type. It measures 50 to 70 nm in diameter and has two envelope proteins (E1, E2) and a core protein (c). The core protein is surrounded by a single-layer lipoprotein envelope with spikelike projections that contain the two glycoproteins, E1 and E2. Humans are the only known reservoir.

EPIDEMIOLOGY
In the pre-vaccine era, rubella epidemics occurred approximately every 6 to 9 years in the United States. The last major American epidemic, which occurred in 1964-1965, resulted in an estimated 12.5 million cases and approximately 20,000 cases of congenital rubella syndrome. In 1969, live attenuated rubella vaccines were licensed in the United States and were introduced into the routine childhood immunization program. The initial rubella vaccination strategy was to target children from 12 months of age to puberty with a catch-up mass campaign. During the first 8 years of the vaccination program, the reported number of cases of rubella and congenital rubella syndrome decreased by 78% and 66%, respectively. When a rubella resurgence occurred mainly among adolescents and young adults in 1977-1978, however, the rubella vaccination program was modified to include susceptible postpubertal girls, persons in military service, college students, and persons in certain work settings (e.g., health care). In 1979, the RA 27/3 rubella virus vaccine replaced the other rubella virus vaccines (HPV-77 and Cendehill). Since 2003, 16 or fewer cases have been reported annually in the United States, and rubella is no longer endemic in the United States.

Although rubella and congenital rubella syndrome are no longer endemic in the United States, they continue to be of global public health importance. For most countries, the epidemiology of rubella mirrors the epidemiology seen in the United States during the pre-vaccine era, when rubella occurred mainly among children. The number of reported rubella cases globally has decreased from 875,000 in 1999 to about 120,000 in 2009, but the incidence is substantially underestimated because rubella cases in many countries are identified through case-based measles surveillance, which focuses only on the detection of suspected measles cases. The annual number of new cases of congenital rubella syndrome in developing countries is estimated to be 110,000 during nonepidemic years.

During the 1970s and 1980s, the use of rubella-containing vaccine (RCV) was mainly limited to industrialized countries. The number of World Health Organization member countries using RCV in national childhood immunization schedules increased from 83 (43%) in 1996 to 130 (67%) in 2008. As of 2009, rubella control and congenital rubella syndrome prevention or elimination goals have been established in three of six World Health Organization regions (Americas, European, and western Pacific). With the success of the vaccination strategy in the Americas, the number of reported rubella cases decreased from 135,947 in 1998 to a provisional total of 11 in 2009, and only Argentina had endemic rubella virus transmission. The other three World Health Organization regions (i.e., Southeast Asia, eastern Mediterranean, Africa) have not established regional rubella control or congenital rubella syndrome prevention goals.

PATHOBIOLOGY
Rubella
Rubella virus is transmitted through person-to-person spread by droplets shed from the respiratory secretions of infected persons. The first point of

entry is the nasopharynx, where replication occurs and then spreads to the lymph nodes. Subsequent viremia may seed multiple organs, including the placenta. Viremia occurs between 8 and 9 days after exposure and peaks at 10 to 17 days, just before the onset of the rash, which usually occurs 16 to 18 days after exposure. Although individuals with rubella are considered to be only moderately contagious, they may shed virus from 7 days before the onset of the rash to approximately 5 to 7 days or more after its disappearance. Persons with both clinical and subclinical infections are considered contagious.

Congenital Rubella

Rubella virus viremia can infect the placenta of pregnant women, and viral replication can infect all fetal organs. In tissue specimens, infections with rubella virus have diverse effects, ranging from small foci of infected cells in apparently normal tissue to hypoplasia, generalized vasculitis, and cell destruction. The hallmark of fetal infection is chronic infection that persists throughout fetal life, with shedding of virus up to 1 year of age.

Infants with congenital rubella syndrome may shed large quantities of virus from body secretions, particularly from the throat. Rubella virus can be found in the nasopharyngeal secretions of more than 80% of infants during the first month of life. Rubella virus is found in 11% of infected infants between 9 and 12 months of age and in only 3% in the second year of life. Viral shedding by infants with congenital rubella syndrome can result in nosocomial outbreaks, so only individuals immune to rubella virus should be in contact with infants with congenital rubella syndrome or with congenital infection even in the absence of clinical signs of congenital rubella syndrome.

CLINICAL MANIFESTATIONS

Postnatally Acquired Rubella

Acquired rubella, which occurs in 50 to 80% of persons infected with rubella virus, is characterized by a generalized maculopapular rash that usually persists for 1 to 3 days (Fig. 376-1). The rash usually starts on the face and neck and progresses downward. The rash is fainter than the rash of measles (Chapter 375) and does not coalesce. Because of the mildness of the rash, it may be difficult to detect in persons with darker skin. Children usually have few or no prodromal symptoms, so the rash is usually the first sign of illness. However, in older children and adults, a 1- to 5-day prodrome of low-grade fever, malaise, and upper respiratory symptoms often precedes the rash. The incubation period is 14 days, with a range of 12 to 23 days. Lymphadenopathy, particularly occipital and postauricular, may be noted during the second week after exposure.

FIGURE 376-1. Rash of rubella on the skin of a child's back. The distribution is similar to that of measles, but the lesions are less intensely red. (From the Centers for Disease Control and Prevention Public Health Image Library, ID #: 712.)

Rubella disease is usually mild and results in few complications. Arthralgia and arthritis are commonly observed in infected adults, particularly in postpubertal girls. Other less common complications are thrombocytopenia (1 in 3000 rubella cases) and encephalitis (1 in 6000 rubella cases).

Congenital Rubella Syndrome

The most serious consequences of rubella virus infection occur when a woman becomes infected during pregnancy, particularly during the first trimester. Complications can include miscarriage, fetal death, or a live birth with a constellation of congenital defects known as congenital rubella syndrome. The most common defects of congenital rubella syndrome affect the eyes (e.g., cataracts, pigmentary retinopathy, microphthalmos, congenital glaucoma), the ears (e.g., hearing impairment), and the heart (e.g., patent ductus arteriosus, pulmonary arterial stenosis). Other clinical manifestations of congenital rubella syndrome may include microcephaly, developmental delay, and purpura, including dermal erythropoiesis (blueberry muffin syndrome).

Among pregnant women infected with rubella virus during the first 10 weeks of gestation, up to 90% of their live born infants may have congenital rubella syndrome. Among women infected during the first 20 weeks of pregnancy, the rate of congenital rubella syndrome in live born infants is 20%. Infants who are born with rubella virus infection but who do not have any apparent signs or symptoms of congenital rubella syndrome are referred to as infants with congenital rubella infection only.

DIAGNOSIS

Postnatally Acquired Rubella

Because many rash illnesses may mimic rubella virus infection and because 20 to 50% of rubella virus infections may be subclinical, laboratory testing is the only way to confirm the diagnosis. Some illnesses with clinical presentation similar to that of rubella include scarlet fever (Chapter 298), roseola (Chapter 447), fifth disease (Chapter 379), and measles (Chapter 375).

Serologic testing is the most common method of diagnosis of acquired rubella. IgM antibody is generally detectable for up to 6 weeks after the onset of the rash. Because IgM antibodies may not be detectable before day 5 of the rash, serologic testing should be repeated no sooner than then. Diagnosis also can be made on the basis of a significant rise in the IgG antibody titer in paired acute and convalescent specimens. The acute serum specimen should be collected within 7 to 10 days after the onset of the rash, and the convalescent serum specimen should be collected 14 to 21 days after the first specimen.

Rubella virus can be isolated from nasopharynx (i.e., nasal, throat), blood, urine, and cerebrospinal fluid specimens of persons with rubella and congenital rubella syndrome. The most frequently positive results are from throat swabs. Rubella virus can be isolated during the prodromal period and up to 2 weeks after onset of the rash. For viral cultures, specimens should be obtained during the time of maximum virus secretion—up to 4 days after the onset of rash. During the first 4 days after the onset of the rash, rubella RNA detection by reverse transcription–polymerase chain reaction (RT-PCR) is more sensitive than rubella IgM testing.

Diagnosis in Pregnant Women

In the United States, all pregnant women should be screened for rubella IgG antibodies as part of routine prenatal care. Pregnant women who have a positive serologic test result for IgG antibody to rubella virus are considered to be immune if they do not have a recent history of exposure to rubella virus. Susceptible pregnant women should be vaccinated postpartum. Pregnant women exposed to rubella virus should be evaluated for evidence of acute infection by testing for presence of IgM antibodies in sera or a significant rise of IgG antibodies in acute and convalescent sera. Pregnant women with evidence of acute infection should be monitored clinically and evaluated for gestational age at infection to assess the risk of fetal infection.

Congenital Rubella

Diagnosis of congenital rubella syndrome in infants can be confirmed by either serologic or virologic methods. Serum IgM antibodies may be present in an infant with congenital rubella syndrome for up to a year after birth; however, IgM antibody may not be detectable during the first month of life. Thus, infants younger than 1 month and with symptoms consistent with congenital rubella syndrome should be retested at 1 month of age. Congenital rubella syndrome also can be confirmed by documentation of a persistent rubella serum IgG titer beyond the time expected from passive transfer of maternal IgG antibody (i.e., a rubella titer that does not decline at the expected rate of a two-fold dilution per month).

Rubella virus from congenitally infected infants can be isolated most commonly from throat swabs and less commonly from urine and cerebrospinal fluid specimens. Infants with congenital rubella may excrete virus for up to 1 year, but specimens for virus isolation are most likely to be positive if they are obtained within the first 6 months after birth. Rubella virus in infants with congenital rubella syndrome also can be detected by RT-PCR with use of the same specimens as for viral isolation.

TREATMENT   Rx

There is no specific treatment of rubella or congenital rubella syndrome. For persons with rubella, symptomatic treatment may be warranted for clinical manifestations such as arthralgias, myalgias, and fever. Infants with congenital rubella syndrome should be evaluated and treated by specialists for their specific clinical manifestations.

PREVENTION

Passive Immunization

Administration of immune globulin after exposure to rubella virus will not prevent infection or viremia but might modify or suppress symptoms. Therefore, immune globulin is not recommended for routine postexposure prophylaxis of rubella in any circumstance.

Active Immunization

One dose of live attenuated rubella vaccine (RA 27/3, RCV) induces rubella IgG antibody seroconversion in 95% or more of persons. Immunity is considered long term, probably lifelong. RCV is available as a monovalent formulation or in combination with measles-mumps (MMR) and measles-mumps-varicella (MMRV) vaccines (Chapter 17).

In the United States, the routine rubella vaccination policy is to immunize children with the first dose of MMR at 12 to 15 months of age and to provide a second dose at 4 to 6 years of age. The MMRV vaccine also can be given to children up to age 12 years. Persons who were born in 1957 or later (except women of childbearing age who are or could become pregnant) and who do not have a medical contraindication (e.g., pregnancy) should receive at least one dose of MMR unless they have documentation of one dose of live rubella virus vaccine or laboratory evidence of immunity or laboratory confirmation of disease. High-risk groups who should be targeted for vaccination include health care personnel, persons attending post–high school educational facilities, the military, international travelers, and nonpregnant women of childbearing age.

In follow-up studies of more than 2700 susceptible women who were unknowingly pregnant and who received a live attenuated rubella vaccine, none of their infants was born with congenital rubella syndrome. Nevertheless, because of the theoretical risk of congenital rubella syndrome in infants born to pregnant women vaccinated with RCV, the vaccine should not be given to pregnant women, and pregnancy should be avoided for at least 28 days after receipt of vaccine. Receipt of RCV during pregnancy is not generally considered to be an indication for termination of pregnancy.

PROGNOSIS

Because rubella is usually a mild disease, the prognosis is excellent, with complete recovery in almost all persons. Deaths are seen in 0 to 50% of patients who develop rubella encephalitis. The prognosis for infants with congenital rubella syndrome is dependent on their clinical manifestations and access to quality medical care.

SUGGESTED READINGS

Centers for Disease Control and Prevention. Manual for the Surveillance of Vaccine-Preventable Diseases. http://www.cdc.gov/vaccines/pubs/surv-manual/chpt14-rubella.htm. *U.S. guidelines for rubella surveillance, including information to collect in suspected cases, discussion of laboratory testing, and management of outbreaks.*

Centers for Disease Control and Prevention. Progress toward control of rubella and prevention of congenital rubella syndrome—worldwide, 2009. *MMWR Morb Mortal Wkly Rep.* 2010;59:1307-1310. *Review.*

377

MUMPS

JOHN W. GNANN, Jr.

DEFINITION

Mumps is an acute systemic viral infection that occurs most commonly in children, is usually self-limited, and is clinically characterized by nonsuppurative parotitis.

The Pathogen

Mumps virus is a member of the Paramyxoviridae family. Mumps virions are pleomorphic, roughly spherical enveloped particles with an average diameter of 200 nm. Glycoprotein spikes project from the surface of the envelope, which encloses a helical nucleocapsid composed of nucleoproteins and linear, nonsegmented, single-stranded, negative-sense RNA. Humans are the only natural hosts for mumps virus, although infection can be induced experimentally in a variety of mammalian species. In vitro, mumps virus can be cultured in many mammalian cell lines and in embryonated hens' eggs.

EPIDEMIOLOGY

In unvaccinated urban populations, mumps is a disease of school-aged children (5 to 9 years), and more than 90% of individuals have mumps antibodies by 15 years of age. Before the mumps vaccine was released in the United States in 1967, mumps was an endemic disease with a seasonal peak of activity between January and May. The largest number of cases reported in the United States occurred in 1941, when the incidence of mumps was 250 cases per 100,000 population. In 1968, when the mumps vaccine was first entering clinical use, the incidence of mumps was 76 cases per 100,000 population. In 1985, only 2982 cases of mumps were reported, an incidence of 1.1 per 100,000 population, which represents a 98% decline from the number of cases reported in 1967. Epidemiologic studies of mumps epidemics in high schools, colleges, and military units during the 1980s demonstrated that outbreaks were principally due to failure to vaccinate. In 1989, the Centers for Disease Control and Prevention (CDC) Advisory Committee on Immunization Practices issued a recommendation that all children receive a second dose of the measles-mumps-rubella (MMR) vaccine, which reduced the problem of primary vaccine failure. In 2003, the CDC reported only 231 cases of mumps in the United States, the lowest annual total ever recorded. However, a series of outbreaks in the United States and Canada in 2005-2006 reemphasized the potential for mumps virus to cause epidemics even in highly vaccinated populations. In 2006, a total of 6584 cases of mumps were reported, with a national incidence of 2.2 cases per 100,000 population. In a 2006 Midwest outbreak, the highest risk group was persons aged 18 to 24 years (median age, 22 years), many of whom were college students; 7% of cases were unvaccinated, 14% had received only one dose of MMR, 49% had received two doses, and 30% had an unknown vaccination status. In 2009, another mumps outbreak resulted in more than 1500 cases in New York and New Jersey, with the highest rate among boys who were 7 to 18 years old and who attended tradition-observant Jewish schools. Among patients with known vaccination status, 88% had received at least one dose and 75% had received a second dose. Although some cases in recent U.S. outbreaks can be attributed to failure to vaccinate, most represented primary (insufficient initial immune response) or secondary (waning immune response) vaccine failure, thereby suggesting the need either for a mumps vaccine with a longer duration of protection or for a vaccination policy focusing on young adults.

PATHOBIOLOGY

Mumps is highly contagious and can be transmitted experimentally by inoculation of virus onto the nasal or buccal mucosa, thus suggesting that most natural infections result from droplet spread of upper respiratory secretions. The mean incubation period for mumps is 18 days. Primary viral replication takes place in epithelial cells of the upper respiratory tract, followed by spread of virus to regional lymph nodes and subsequent viremia. Because virus can be isolated from saliva for 5 to 7 days before and up to 9 days after the onset of clinical symptoms, an infected individual is potentially able to transmit mumps for a period of about 2 weeks. An estimated 30% of mumps infections

FIGURE 377-1. **Mumps.** Child with submandibular swelling due to mumps parotitis. (From the Centers for Disease Control and Prevention Public Health Image Library, ID #: 4491.)

in children are subclinical or associated only with nonspecific upper respiratory infection symptoms. Transient IgM antibody responses are detected early in the course of mumps infection, followed by the appearance of IgG antibody and cytotoxic T lymphocytes. Mumps-specific IgG can be detected during the first week of acute infection, peaks at 3 to 4 weeks, and persists for decades. Lifelong immunity follows natural infection. Patients who report more than one episode of mumps probably had parotitis of another cause.

CLINICAL MANIFESTATIONS

Parotitis
Mumps usually begins with a short prodromal phase of low-grade fever, malaise, headache, and anorexia. Young children may complain of ear pain initially. The characteristic parotid tenderness and enlargement, in which the earlobe is lifted forward and obscures the angle of the mandible, then develops (Fig. 377-1). The parotid glands are involved most commonly, although other salivary glands may occasionally be enlarged. Parotitis may initially be unilateral, with swelling of the contralateral parotid gland occurring 2 to 3 days later; bilateral parotitis with symptomatic salivary gland involvement eventually develops in 70% of patients. Painful parotid gland enlargement progresses for a period of about 3 days, followed by defervescence and resolution of the parotid pain and swelling within about 7 days. Long-term sequelae of mumps parotitis are uncommon.

Aseptic Meningitis
Symptomatic meningitis occurs in 15% of cases and is the second most common manifestation of mumps. About 50% of patients with mumps parotitis have cerebrospinal fluid (CSF) pleocytosis, but many have no clinical evidence of meningitis. Signs and symptoms of meningeal inflammation (headache, neck stiffness, vomiting, and lethargy) plus high fever usually develop 4 to 5 days after the onset of parotitis, although the meningitis may occasionally precede the parotitis. Indeed, 40 to 50% of all cases of documented mumps meningitis occur in patients who never exhibit clinical parotitis. For unexplained reasons, symptomatic central nervous system (CNS) involvement with mumps is two to three times more common in boys than in girls. Examination of CSF usually reveals normal opening pressure and a mononuclear cell pleocytosis with an average cell count of 450/mm³. Polymorphonuclear leukocyte predominance in CSF may be seen in some patients early during the course of mumps meningitis. CSF protein is generally normal or mildly elevated (<100 mg/dL). Hypoglycorrhachia, which is not usually seen in viral meningitis, may be present in 10 to 30% of patients with mumps meningitis. Mumps virus can be recovered from CSF. Whereas the symptoms of mumps meningitis typically resolve within 7 to 10 days, the CSF abnormalities may persist for up to 5 weeks. Mumps meningitis is generally benign, and significant neurologic complications are rare.

Encephalitis
The spectrum of mumps-induced CNS disease ranges from mild "aseptic" meningitis (which is common) to severe encephalitis (which is rare). Some cases of encephalitis develop concurrently with the parotitis and are thought to result from direct extension of viral infection from the choroid plexus

ependyma into parenchymal neurons. Other cases of mumps encephalitis occur 1 to 2 weeks after the onset of parotitis and may represent a demyelinating postinfectious encephalitis. Clinical findings in mumps encephalitis include obtundation (and less commonly delirium), generalized seizures, and high fever. Other neurologic findings can include focal seizures, aphasia, paresis, and involuntary movements. Recovery from mumps encephalitis is generally complete, although complications such as aqueductal stenosis with hydrocephalus, seizure disorders, and psychomotor retardation have been reported. The overall mortality from mumps encephalitis is 0.5 to 2.3%.

Orchitis
Epididymo-orchitis is rare in young boys with mumps but occurs in 15 to 35% of postpubertal boys with mumps. Orchitis is most often unilateral (bilateral involvement occurs in 17 to 38% of cases) and results from replication of mumps virus in the seminiferous tubules, with resulting lymphocytic infiltration and edema. Orchitis typically develops within 1 week of the onset of parotitis, although orchitis, like mumps meningitis, can develop before or even in the absence of parotitis. Mumps orchitis is characterized by marked testicular swelling and severe pain accompanied by fever, nausea, and headache. The pain and swelling resolve within 5 to 7 days, but residual testicular tenderness can persist for weeks. Testicular atrophy may follow orchitis in 35 to 50% of cases; however, sterility is an uncommon complication, even in men with bilateral orchitis.

Other Manifestations
Mumps can cause inflammation of other glandular tissues, including pancreatitis and thyroiditis. Oophoritis and mastitis have been reported in postpubertal women with mumps. Transient renal function abnormalities are common in mumps, and virus can be isolated readily from urine; significant renal damage is rare, however. Other infrequent manifestations of mumps include sensorineural deafness (either transient or permanent), arthritis, myocarditis, and thrombocytopenia. Maternal mumps infection during the first trimester of pregnancy results in an increased frequency of spontaneous abortions, but no clear association between congenital malformations and maternal mumps has been demonstrated.

DIAGNOSIS
The diagnosis of mumps is usually based on clinical findings in a child with fever and parotitis, particularly if the individual is known to be susceptible and has been exposed to mumps during the preceding 2 to 3 weeks. An atypical clinical presentation (e.g., meningitis or orchitis without parotitis) requires laboratory confirmation. Culturing for mumps virus is definitive but not universally available. Testing of acute and convalescent sera should demonstrate a diagnostic four-fold rise in mumps IgG antibody titer. Alternatively, finding mumps IgM antibody provides good evidence of recent infection. About 30% of patients have an elevated serum amylase level that may be due to parotitis or pancreatitis.

The differential diagnosis of a mumps-like syndrome includes infections caused by other viruses, such as Epstein-Barr virus (Chapter 385), adenovirus (Chapter 373), influenza A virus (Chapter 372), parainfluenza virus (Chapter 371), coxsackievirus (Chapter 387), or lymphocytic choriomeningitis virus. Parotid gland enlargement can also occur in patients with AIDS, particularly children. Bacteria such as *Staphylococcus aureus* can cause suppurative parotitis. Parotid gland enlargement can also be associated with Sjögren's syndrome (Chapter 276), sarcoidosis (Chapter 95), amyloidosis (Chapter 194), thiazide ingestion, iodine sensitivity, tumor, or salivary duct obstruction. Careful examination should distinguish parotitis from lymphadenopathy.

TREATMENT

Management of a patient with mumps consists of conservative measures to provide symptomatic relief, adequate hydration, and nutrition. Treatment of orchitis includes bedrest, scrotal support, analgesics, and ice packs. Patients with significant CNS involvement require hospitalization for observation and supportive care. There is currently no established role for antiviral drugs, corticosteroids, or passive immunotherapy in the treatment of mumps.

PREVENTION
The cornerstone of mumps prevention is active immunization with the live attenuated mumps vaccine. In the United States, mumps vaccine is

administered in combination with the measles and rubella vaccines (MMR) to children at 12 to 15 months of age, with a second dose at 4 to 6 years of age. Efficacy of the mumps vaccine is estimated to be 79 to 95% after two doses. The mumps vaccine is also indicated for susceptible adults.

The Jeryl-Lynn strain of attenuated mumps virus used in the United States since 1967 is a very well tolerated vaccine, although rare instances of fever, parotitis, and possibly aseptic meningitis have been reported after immunization. In recent years, an increased frequency of cases of vaccine-related mumps meningitis has been recognized in other countries. These cases occurred after the administration of an MMR vaccine that contained the Urabe AM9 or Leningrad 3 strains of mumps virus. This problem has not been recognized in the United States, where the Jeryl-Lynn mumps vaccine continues to be used.

Questions about prevention often arise when an individual with no history of mumps (typically an adult man) is exposed to a patient with active mumps. The immune status of the exposed individual can be determined by enzyme-linked immunosorbent assays. The mumps skin test is not a reliable indicator of immune status. Most adults born in the United States before 1957 were naturally infected and are therefore immune. Mumps vaccine can be safely administered to an individual of unknown immune status, although vaccine given to a susceptible individual after exposure to mumps may not provide protection.

For infection control purposes, patients with mumps require both standard precautions and droplet precautions. In the outpatient setting, a patient with suspected mumps should wear a mask and be isolated from other potentially susceptible persons. When a patient with mumps is hospitalized, a private room is required; caregivers should wear masks, and the patient should wear a mask while being transported.

SUGGESTED READINGS

Choi KM. Reemergence of mumps. *Korean J Pediatr.* 2010;53:623-628. *Characteristics of an outbreak in a high-vaccination country.*

Levine H, Ankol OE, Rozhavski V, et al. Sub-optimal prevalence of mumps antibodies in a population based study of young adults in Israel after 20 years of two dose universal vaccination policy. *Vaccine.* 2011;29:2785-2790. *The sub-optimal population seroprevalence despite a universal vaccination policy helps explain periodic outbreaks, especially in crowded settings.*

378

CYTOMEGALOVIRUS, EPSTEIN-BARR VIRUS, AND SLOW VIRUS INFECTIONS OF THE CENTRAL NERVOUS SYSTEM

JOSEPH R. BERGER AND AVINDRA NATH

CYTOMEGALOVIRUS INFECTION

Human cytomegalovirus (CMV) is a ubiquitous herpesvirus that is acquired throughout life (Chapter 384). In children, CMV is an important and relatively common cause of congenital neurologic deficits. In the United States, seroprevalence rates are 40% in adolescents and 60 to 90% in adults. Primary infection is usually asymptomatic in young, healthy adults but may be associated with a transient mononucleosis-like syndrome. CMV results in major neurologic disability in the setting of immunosuppression, particularly in transplant recipients and in persons with acquired immunodeficiency syndrome (AIDS) and hematologic malignant neoplasms. In addition to the retina, CMV may involve the meninges, brain, spinal cord, peripheral nerves, and muscle.

CLINICAL MANIFESTATIONS AND DIAGNOSIS

Cytomegalovirus Encephalitis

CMV encephalitis has several manifestations in patients with AIDS. The most typical is a subacute, diffuse encephalopathy evolving during a period of weeks and characterized by headache, impaired cognition and sensorium, apathy, and social withdrawal. Neurologic examination reveals abnormal mentation and variable motor features, including hyperreflexia, ataxia, and weakness. CMV ventriculitis is characteristically present, and progressive ventricular enlargement may be observed. Other features may suggest brain stem encephalitis, including internuclear ophthalmoplegia, nystagmus, cranial nerve palsies, gaze paresis, ataxia, and quadriparesis. Rarely, CMV infection may be manifested as a cerebral mass lesion. Other findings in these patients include cerebral infarction resulting from CMV vasculitis, acute subarachnoid hemorrhage, and intracerebral hemorrhage. Virtually all patients with CMV encephalitis have systemic CMV infection. CMV myelitis, polyradiculitis, and multifocal neuritis may also occur with CMV encephalitis. Distinctive retinal lesions can often be seen ophthalmoscopically (Chapter 384).

Cerebral imaging studies are of limited sensitivity and low specificity in patients with CMV encephalitis. Ependymal or meningeal enhancement as well as areas of focal infarction or necrosis may be visualized. Progressive ventricular enlargement should suggest CMV ventriculitis. Cerebrospinal fluid (CSF) findings are variable. Most patients have elevated protein levels and a CSF pleocytosis, but leukocytes may be absent and glucose levels may be normal or decreased. A marked pleocytosis with a polymorphonuclear leukocyte preponderance may occur in patients with CMV ventriculo-encephalitis. CMV can rarely be cultured from CSF. CSF polymerase chain reaction (PCR) is the most specific diagnostic method, but the diagnosis is often difficult and relies on a high index of clinical suspicion.

Myelitis

CMV transverse myelitis, which may be seen in both immunocompetent and immunosuppressed patients, is indistinguishable neurologically from other forms of transverse myelitis (Chapters 407 and 419). A severe necrotizing CMV myelitis may occur in the immunosuppressed host, particularly with human immunodeficiency virus (HIV) infection, and is commonly associated with polyradiculitis. Some cases of necrotizing myelitis in the absence of a typical polyradiculitis syndrome have been described, with patients displaying acute or progressive paraplegia and disturbances in urinary and rectal sphincter function. Reflexes are preserved or enhanced in the legs unless concurrent neuropathy is present. A sensory level may be demonstrable. The combination of radicular complaints and a CSF polymorphonuclear pleocytosis may serve as clues to the diagnosis. Serology for CMV may be useful in immunocompetent individuals.

Polyradiculomyelitis

Approximately 25% of patients dying of AIDS have neuromuscular disease from CMV, predominantly localized to the perineurial and epineurial regions. CMV polyradiculomyelitis in HIV-infected patients is manifested subacutely during a period of days to weeks. Initial symptoms of paresthesias or dysesthetic pain localized to the perineum and lower extremities are followed by rapidly progressive paraparesis with hypotonia and diminished or absent lower extremity reflexes. Urinary retention is characteristic, and rectal sphincter incontinence is common. Variable sensory findings are typically overshadowed by weakness. Babinski signs and diminished sensation below a discrete level across the trunk are evidence of an associated myelitis. With time, symptoms progress by ascending to involve the upper limbs and sometimes the cranial nerves. CSF examination generally shows polymorphonuclear pleocytosis, prominent elevation of protein levels, and a low glucose level. Spinal magnetic resonance imaging (MRI) may be normal or show enhancement of the conus medullaris, cauda equina, meninges, and nerve roots. Electrophysiologic studies reveal axonal neuropathy with evidence of acute denervation. Variable slowing of nerve conduction may occur.

The appearance of acute cauda equina syndrome in a patient with AIDS or in a solid organ or bone marrow transplant recipient is suggestive of CMV infection when a polymorphonuclear pleocytosis is present in CSF; however, the syndrome is not pathognomonic. Other conditions that may produce a cauda equina syndrome in AIDS patients include lymphomatous meningitis, syphilis, toxoplasmosis, other herpesvirus infections, and cryptococcal or bacterial meningitis. Progressive multifocal motor and sensory neuropathy that evolves during a period of weeks to months has also been seen in patients with CMV infection. Paresthesia and dysesthesia are quickly followed by prominent motor weakness involving both the upper and lower limbs asymmetrically. Neurogenic atrophy may be prominent. Nerve biopsy reveals necrotizing neuritis with mononuclear and polymorphonuclear infiltrates and cytomegalocytes localized around endoneurial capillaries in the nerve trunks and roots. Some patients may have necrotizing arteritis. PCR for CMV in CSF may be useful in establishing the diagnosis.

TREATMENT   Rx

CMV neurologic complications should be treated with ganciclovir (5 mg/kg intravenously every 12 hours) plus foscarnet (60 mg/kg intravenously every 8 hours or 90 mg/kg intravenously every 12 hours until symptomatic improvement), followed by maintenance therapy with oral valganciclovir (900 mg daily) and intravenous foscarnet (90 to 120 mg/kg intravenously during 2 hours, every 24 hours); however, evidence of efficacy in these conditions is limited chiefly to case reports and small series. Cidofovir is a second-line agent (5 mg/kg by intravenous infusion during 1 hour once a week for 2 consecutive weeks, with saline hydration and probenecid, 2 g orally 3 hours before the dose and 1 g orally at 2 hours and 8 hours after the dose). CMV strains resistant to these agents have emerged, and CMV encephalitis has developed in the presence of maintenance ganciclovir therapy for CMV retinitis. Combination therapy (foscarnet and ganciclovir) or different drugs should be considered in patients already undergoing suppressive monotherapy or in those with persistent CSF pleocytosis. Maintenance therapy, which is the same regimen given every other week, is required unless the patient experiences immune reconstitution, such as after highly active antiretroviral therapy (HAART) in an AIDS patient or discontinuation of immunosuppressive regimens in a transplant or cancer patient.

PROGNOSIS

The prognosis for long-term survival, especially with AIDS, is very poor.

EPSTEIN-BARR VIRUS INFECTION

Epstein-Barr virus (EBV), the cause of infectious mononucleosis (Chapter 385), is distributed worldwide. Individuals in areas of high population density and lower social strata acquire the virus in early childhood. However, seroepidemiologic studies indicate that virtually all persons are infected by EBV by 30 years of age.

Neurologic manifestations occur in 1 to 5% of patients with primary EBV infection and may be the predominant clinical finding. The most common neurologic disorder associated with infectious mononucleosis is meningoencephalitis, which is rare in early childhood and is most often observed in persons between the ages of 15 and 25 years. Its onset may be gradual during a span of several days or be explosive. Fever, headache, mild stiff neck, confusion, lethargy, seizures, and hyperreflexia are the most typical features. On occasion, focal neurologic features, including hemiparesis, focal seizures, and cerebellar and brain stem findings, may be detected. Hyperintense signal abnormalities on T2-weighted and fluid attenuated inversion recovery (FLAIR) cranial MRI are frequently observed but are nondiagnostic. PCR for EBV in CSF may be useful.

Ganciclovir treatment (10 mg/kg/day intravenously for 3 weeks followed by 1000 mg/day orally for another 3 weeks or until the virus is cleared) has been used in some cases but is of unproven value. The prognosis for patients with EBV meningoencephalitis is excellent, with complete resolution anticipated in 1 to 2 weeks.

SLOW VIRUS INFECTIONS OF THE CENTRAL NERVOUS SYSTEM

Human T-Lymphotropic Virus Type 1 and Human Immunodeficiency Virus

These viruses and their neurologic sequelae are considered in Chapters 386 and 401, respectively.

Subacute Sclerosing Panencephalitis

EPIDEMIOLOGY AND PATHOBIOLOGY

Subacute sclerosing panencephalitis (SSPE), which is caused by the measles virus (Chapter 375), usually affects children but can present in young adulthood. Patients generally have a history of measles within the first 2 years of life, and it is speculated that such early host exposure allows the emergence of persistent but defective virus replication because the SSPE virus genome, particularly the matrix gene, differs from wild-type measles. As a result of effective vaccination strategies against measles virus, the incidence of SSPE has decreased markedly.

Gray matter is most prominently involved. The pathologic features of SSPE include gliosis, loss of myelin, and perivascular infiltrates of lymphocytes and plasma cells in white and gray matter. Neuronal cell loss is seen in later stages of the illness. Intranuclear Cowdry type A inclusions containing viral nucleocapsids are identified in neurons and glia.

CLINICAL MANIFESTATIONS AND DIAGNOSIS

SSPE usually begins with cognitive and behavioral changes, and cortical blindness is often an early feature. Progression is associated with motor dysfunction, including prominent myoclonus, choreoathetosis, dystonia, and rigidity. Its course progresses during a period of 1 to 3 years to rigid quadriparesis and a vegetative state, frequently accompanied by autonomic features, such as hyperthermia, excessive sweating, and altered pulse and blood pressure. The condition is more common in rural settings and affects boys more often than girls.

The electroencephalogram reveals periodic complexes with synchronous bursts of two or three high-amplitude slow waves per second, with recurrence at regular intervals of 5 to 8 seconds and a 1 : 1 relationship with myoclonic jerks. Computed tomography (CT) of the brain shows generalized atrophy. CSF protein, glucose, and cell levels are usually normal; CSF is characterized by a high immunoglobulin concentration, oligoclonal bands, and intrathecal synthesis of antibody to measles virus antigens. Serum measles antibody titers are also high. These findings are usually sufficiently characteristic for diagnosis, but measles RNA can be detected in the brain by PCR. Rarely, brain biopsy is needed for definitive diagnosis in atypical cases. Measles virus may also cause subacute encephalitis in an immunocompromised host. The prominence of cognitive and motor dysfunction in these patients resembles that of SSPE, but in the clinical setting, its subacute onset and more rapid evolution and the presence of generalized seizures rather than myoclonus are distinctive. Brain abnormalities include abundant intranuclear inclusions, but inflammation is minimal, and neither serum nor CSF antibody titers against measles virus are high. For this reason, brain biopsy is generally needed for diagnosis.

TREATMENT AND PROGNOSIS   Rx

There is no established, unequivocally effective treatment of SSPE, but arrest of the disease has been reported in some patients with SSPE after long-term treatment with intrathecal interferon alfa or with intrathecal ribavirin. The usual prognosis is progression to coma, brain stem involvement, and death in 2 to 5 years.

Progressive Rubella Panencephalitis

Progressive rubella panencephalitis is a rare disorder resembling SSPE but caused by rubella virus (Chapter 376). It occurs as a complication of congenital rubella syndrome or, more typically, after childhood rubella. With the advent of widespread rubella immunization, this disorder has been nearly eliminated in the United States.

A hiatus of years separates early infection from the onset of neurologic deterioration, which is characterized by behavioral changes, cognitive impairment, cerebellar ataxia, spasticity, and sometimes seizures. Myoclonus is a less prominent feature than it is in SSPE. Serology or isolation of the virus from brain or peripheral blood lymphocytes confirms the cause. There is no effective treatment, and the prognosis is similar to that for SSPE.

Progressive Multifocal Leukoencephalopathy

DEFINITION

This demyelinating disease is associated with infection of oligodendrocytes by JC virus, a papovavirus widely distributed in humans. JC virus exhibits a neurotropism exclusive to glial cells. Progressive multifocal leukoencephalopathy (PML) was the first demyelinating disease to be unequivocally associated with a viral infection.

EPIDEMIOLOGY

Serologic studies indicate that approximately 10% of children have antibody to JC virus by 5 years of age, 40 to 60% have antibody by the age of 10 years, and 80% have antibody by the age of 20 years. Despite the wide dissemination of JC virus infection, PML is rarely observed in the absence of underlying cellular immunosuppression. It is also rarely observed in childhood. Until the AIDS epidemic, PML was most commonly observed in patients with lymphoproliferative disorders (62% of cases) and less commonly with myeloproliferative diseases (7%), carcinomatous diseases (2%), acquired immunodeficiency states (11%), and no underlying disease (6%). Since the

FIGURE 378-1. Pathology of progressive multifocal leukoencephalopathy. **A,** An area of demyelination is seen in the white matter that fails to stain with Luxol fast blue dye. **B,** Immunohistochemical staining with antibody to papovavirus shows brown-staining nuclei in oligodendrocytes, indicative of JC virus infection. **C,** Immunohistochemical staining for glial fibrillary acidic protein shows large bizarre astrocytes. (Courtesy of Dr. Carlos Pardo, Johns Hopkins University, Baltimore.)

inception of the AIDS epidemic, AIDS has been the most common underlying disorder associated with PML. PML develops in up to 4% of AIDS patients. PML also occurs in association with the administration of monoclonal antibodies for diseases that had not previously been associated with it, including natalizumab, an α4β1 and α4β7 integrin inhibitor used in the treatment of multiple sclerosis (Chapter 419) and Crohn's disease (Chapter 143); efalizumab, an anti-CD11a antibody that is effective in the treatment of psoriasis (Chapter 446); rituximab, an anti-CD20 antibody; and mycophenolate mofetil.

PATHOBIOLOGY

The cardinal feature of PML is demyelination, which is typically multifocal but occasionally unifocal (Fig. 378-1). These lesions may occur in any location in the white matter but have a predilection for the parieto-occipital regions. The lesions range in size from 1 mm to several centimeters; larger lesions may reflect the coalescence of multiple smaller lesions. The other histopathologic hallmark of PML is the presence of hyperchromatic, enlarged oligodendroglial nuclei and enlarged bizarre astrocytes with lobulated hyperchromatic nuclei. Electron microscopic examination reveals the JC virions, which are 28 to 45 nm in diameter and appear singly or in dense crystalline arrays in oligodendroglial cells and, less frequently, in reactive astrocytes. Inflammatory infiltrates are typically absent, except in patients who have reconstitution of their immune system, such as HIV-infected patients being treated with HAART, in whom macrophages and lymphocytes may be found.

CLINICAL MANIFESTATIONS

The clinical hallmark of PML is the presence of focal neurologic symptoms and signs associated with radiographic evidence of white matter disease in the absence of a mass effect. The most common initial symptoms include weakness, speech abnormalities, and cognitive disturbances, each seen in approximately 40% of patients. Although it is rare in non-AIDS patients, headache may occur in as many as one third of patients with AIDS. Gait disturbances, sensory loss, and visual impairment all occur in approximately 20 to 30%. Seizures and brain stem symptoms are less common. Signs noted on physical examination parallel the reported symptoms, with weakness, typically a hemiparesis, detected in more than half of patients at initial evaluation. Gait abnormalities, cognitive problems, and language disorders (i.e.,

dysarthria and dysphasia) are observed in about 25% of patients at initial contact. Limb and trunk ataxia, which reflects cerebellar involvement, is detected in as many as 10% of patients but may occasionally result from severe impairment in position sense (i.e., sensory ataxia). Neuro-ophthalmic symptoms occur in 50% of patients with PML and are the initial manifestation in 30 to 45%. The most common visual deficit is homonymous hemianopia or quadrantanopia secondary to lesions of the optic radiations. Cortical blindness is present in as many as 5 to 8% of patients at the time of diagnosis. Other neuro-ophthalmic manifestations include optic agnosia, alexia without agraphia, and ocular motor abnormalities. Sensory disturbances occur with PML but are distinctly less common than impairment of strength or visual function.

DIAGNOSIS

The diagnosis of PML may be strongly suggested by the clinical manifestations and the radiographic imaging. When the clinical manifestations are coupled with a positive JC virus PCR finding in CSF, the diagnosis of PML is virtually certain. Brain biopsy with demonstration of the characteristic histopathologic triad of PML coupled with immunohistochemical or electron microscopic evidence of JC virus remains the "gold standard" for diagnosis.

CT of the brain reveals hypodense lesions of the affected white matter that generally have a "scalloped" appearance because of involvement of the subcortical arcuate fibers lying directly beneath the cortex. Cranial MRI shows a hyperintense lesion on T2-weighted or FLAIR images in the affected regions (Fig. 378-2) and usually shows a hypointense lesion on T1-weighted images. Faint contrast enhancement at the periphery of lesions is seen in approximately 5 to 10% of pathologically confirmed cases of PML with either brain imaging technique, but intense intralesional nodular enhancement may be seen in patients with immune reconstitution. In patients without AIDS, the lesions of PML have a predilection for the parieto-occipital lobes, but the lesions are more often found in the frontal lobes in AIDS patients. Involvement of the basal ganglia, external capsule, and posterior fossa structures (i.e., cerebellum and brain stem) is also seen.

The results of routine analysis of CSF are not diagnostic, but CSF protein may be elevated. CSF PCR for JC virus is of great value in diagnosis; although not always positive, it is highly specific.

FIGURE 378-2. Cranial magnetic resonance images of progressive multifocal leukoencephalopathy. **A,** A T1-weighted image shows a hypointense signal abnormality of the left frontal lobe white matter. **B,** On T2-weighted imaging, the lesion is hyperintense.

TREATMENT   Rx

There is no effective therapy for PML. Although cytosine arabinoside prevents JC virus replication in vitro, a randomized, double-blind trial in which it was administered intrathecally or intravenously in patients with AIDS-associated PML demonstrated no benefit. This lack of efficacy may have been a reflection of inadequate concentrations of the drug at the sites of infection. The antimalarial agent mefloquine has demonstrated efficacy in suppressing viral replication in vitro and is under investigation as a therapy. Spontaneous recovery in untreated patients, especially in patients who have immunologic recovery with HAART or after the removal of an offending immunosuppressive agent, makes it difficult to assess the results of experimental treatments in small or uncontrolled treatment trials.

PROGNOSIS

Previously, PML was regarded as a fatal illness, with survival averaging 3 to 4 months in the typical patient. After the introduction of HAART, approximately 50% of patients with AIDS-associated PML survive for more than 12 months, often with partial or nearly complete clinical and radiographic recovery. Factors associated with a more benign course include the presence of PML as the heralding manifestation of AIDS, high or climbing CD4$^+$ T-lymphocyte counts, contrast enhancement of the lesions on radiographic studies, and any clinical or radiographic evidence of recovery. JC virus–specific T lymphocytes appear to be critical for control of the infection.

SUGGESTED READINGS

Gutierrez J, Issacson RS, Koppel BS. Subacute sclerosing panencephalitis: an update. *Dev Med Child Neurol.* 2010;52:901-907. *Review.*

Silva CA, Oliveira AC, Vilas-Boas L, et al. Neurologic cytomegalovirus complications in patients with AIDS: retrospective review of 13 cases and review of the literature. *Rev Inst Med Trop São Paulo.* 2010;52:305-310. *CMV may present with encephalitis (62% of cases) or polyradiculopathy (54% of cases), with an in-hospital mortality of about 40%.*

White MK, Khalili K. Pathogenesis of progressive multifocal leukoencephalopathy—revisited. *J Infect Dis.* 2011;203:578-586. *Review of both AIDS and PML as complications of immunomodulatory drugs.*

379

PARVOVIRUS

NEAL S. YOUNG

DEFINITION

B19 parvovirus, which was discovered in the mid-1970s by electron microscopic observation of an anomalous precipitin reaction of a normal blood donor's serum (occupying position 19 in plate B), was first linked to human disease by the observation of virus-specific IgM antibody or the virus itself in the sera of sickle cell disease patients suffering transient aplastic crisis (Chapter 166). The common illness caused by the virus was identified later during outbreaks of fifth disease, a highly contagious rash illness of childhood long suspected of having a viral etiology. The ability of parvovirus to persist and to be manifested as an isolated hematologic syndrome was demonstrated by the presence of the virus in fetal liver at autopsy of hydropic newborns and in immunosuppressed patients with chronic pure red cell aplasia (Chapter 168).

The Pathogen

The parvoviruses form small icosahedral capsids of about 25 nm. They have a limited genome of single-stranded DNA. The approximately 5600 nucleotides of B19 parvovirus show remarkably little sequence variation among isolates; two variants, V9 and A6, are of uncertain clinical significance.

The Parvoviridae family contains many pathogenic animal viruses: feline panleukopenia virus, the cause of a fatal agranulocytosis in cats; canine parvovirus, which probably arose from the cat virus as a host range variant in the 1970s to produce a global pandemic and can cause fatal myocarditis in puppies; Aleutian mink virus infection, a model of immune complex disease; and porcine parvovirus, responsible for fetal wastage in pig litters. B19 is the only parvovirus known to be pathogenic in humans.

EPIDEMIOLOGY

B19 infection is global; infectivity rates, inferred from the presence of anti-parvovirus IgG antibody in sera, are similar in the United States, Europe, and Asia, and only isolated populations, Amazonian tribesman and residents of remote islands off the coast of Africa, have escaped exposure. B19 parvovirus infection is common in childhood, and half of 15-year-old adolescents have specific antiparvovirus B19 antibodies. Infection continues throughout adult life, and the great majority of the elderly are seropositive. In temperate climates, most infections occur in the spring, with small epidemics every few years being typical. Transmission is respiratory by droplet spread, and secondary infection rates among household contacts are high. Nosocomial infection can occur, and B19 parvovirus has been transmitted in blood products, especially pooled components such as factor VIII and IX concentrates. Producers of plasma derivatives now voluntarily screen by quantitative measurement of B19 DNA to reduce the risk for iatrogenic transmission. The lack of a lipid envelope and the stable DNA genome make parvoviruses notoriously resistant to heat inactivation and solvent detergents.

PATHOBIOLOGY

The biology of the Parvoviridae makes them especially dependent on helper function from host cells or other viruses. The autonomous parvoviruses propagate in actively dividing cells; the family Parvoviridae includes disease-causing animal parvoviruses. Adeno-associated viruses grow in tissue cultures infected with adenoviruses and herpesviruses and are popular vectors for gene transduction and therapy. B19 is the type member of the

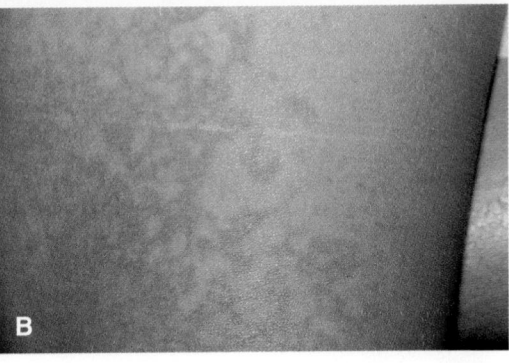

FIGURE 379-1. Erythema infectiosum. In this infection by parvovirus B19, a child will develop prominent erythema of the cheeks, "slapped cheeks" (A), followed by a lacelike erythema on the extremities (B) and buttocks. It is also known as fifth disease.

Erythrovirus genus, which includes very similar simian viruses, all of which are best propagated in the erythroid progenitor cells that are responsible for red blood cell production in the bone marrow. Active replication of virus can be detected by the presence of double-stranded intermediate forms by simple DNA hybridization methods. The transcription map of the erythroviruses differs markedly from that of other Parvoviridae. Only three genes produce proteins of known function. Many antigenic determinants recognized by the host immune system are located in helical loops that form the surface of each capsomere. Most of the capsid is composed of a major structural protein, called VP2, but about 5% of the capsid is a minor structural protein, VP1, which differs from VP2 only by an additional 226 amino acids at the amino terminus; this VP1 unique region is located external to the capsid surface and contains linear epitopes recognized by neutralizing antibodies.

The only known natural host cell of B19 parvovirus is the human erythroid progenitor. The tropism of the virus for an erythroid cell host results from its cellular receptor, globoside, a neutral glycolipid also known as erythrocyte P antigen. Rare individuals with the p phenotype, who congenitally lack globoside on their erythrocytes, are genetically insusceptible to B19 parvovirus infection; they show no serologic evidence of previous infection, and their marrow erythroid progenitors proliferate normally in the presence of high concentrations of virus. Parvovirus kills erythroid progenitors by expression of its nonstructural protein, and it is possible that some cells, such as megakaryocytes, may be lysed by restricted expression of viral proteins in the absence of viral propagation. B19 can be efficiently propagated in tissue culture of primary human hematopoietic cells in which erythropoietic differentiation is stimulated by erythropoietin.

The humoral immune response is dominant in B19 parvovirus infection. Natural antibody production correlates with disappearance of the virus from blood, and the presence of IgG appears to confer lasting protection against a second infection. Parvovirus infection can persist if immunoglobulin production is defective such that antibody fails to neutralize the virus; reactivity of antibodies to the unique amino-terminal region of VP1 is especially important.

CLINICAL MANIFESTATIONS

Fifth Disease

Most B19 parvovirus infections are asymptomatic. The most common manifestation of infection is erythema infectiosum, or fifth disease, a rash illness of childhood characterized by a "slapped cheek" appearance (Fig. 379-1). In volunteers inoculated intranasally with B19, nonspecific influenza-like complaints occurred early along with viremia; the cutaneous eruption a week later corresponded to the appearance of antiviral antibodies. These more specific symptoms of B19 parvovirus infection are secondary to immune complex formation and deposition. Serologic testing generally shows seroconversion, IgM antibody, or the appearance of IgG antibody to parvovirus. The rash of fifth disease may be evanescent, and recurrences can be provoked by sunlight, heat, emotion, or exercise. Fifth disease can be confused with rubella. In adults, the rash is less characteristic and may be difficult to visualize in dark-skinned individuals.

B19 Arthropathy

In contrast to the mild course in children with fifth disease, acute parvovirus infection in adults, particularly middle-aged women, may cause significant arthropathy. Not only arthralgia but also a true inflammatory arthritis occurs in about 50% of older patients, and approximately 15% of new arthritis cases may be the sequelae of B19 parvovirus infection. Symmetrical joint involvement of the hands, ankles, knees, and wrists can resemble rheumatoid

FIGURE 379-2. Bone marrow aspirate of a patient with chronic pure red cell aplasia secondary to persistent B19 parvovirus infection. Mature erythroid precursors are absent, and giant pronormoblasts are typical of B19 infection.

arthritis (Chapter 272), and the test result for rheumatoid factor may be positive. B19 arthropathy usually resolves within a few weeks; joint destruction does not occur. Parvovirus is not the cause of rheumatoid arthritis, but case reports suggest that B19 infection may mimic, precipitate, or worsen a variety of rheumatologic diseases, including juvenile rheumatoid arthritis, systemic lupus erythematosus, and fibromyalgia.

Transient Aplastic Crisis

In persons with underlying hemolysis or a high demand for production of circulating erythrocytes, acute B19 parvovirus infection causes transient aplastic crisis, an abrupt cessation of red blood cell production that exacerbates or, in previously compensated states, provokes severe anemia. Erythropoiesis is temporarily suppressed in all B19 parvovirus infections, but hemoglobin levels ordinarily remain stable because of the long lifespan of erythrocytes. The anemic crises associated with low or absent reticulocytes in hereditary spherocytosis and sickle cell disease are virtually always secondary to B19 parvovirus infection. Parviviremia is present in patients with transient aplastic crisis, and red cell production resumes once antibodies to the virus are produced and the infection is cleared. Transient aplastic crisis is generally a unique event in the patient's life, thus suggesting induction of long-lasting protective immunity. Although it is self-limited, aplastic crisis often requires transfusion and can lead to severe, occasionally fatal anemia that precipitates congestive heart failure and cerebrovascular accidents. Transient aplastic crisis is associated with a pathognomonic bone marrow appearance, absence of maturing erythroid precursors, and the presence of "giant pronormoblasts" (Fig. 379-2) that represent the cytopathic effect of parvovirus infection.

White blood cell and platelet counts may fall modestly during transient aplastic crisis, especially in patients with functioning spleens. Occasional cases of agranulocytosis may be due to B19; thrombocytopenia and pancytopenia have been reported, and B19 can precipitate a benign virus-associated hemophagocytic syndrome.

Persistent Infection

B19 parvovirus persists in the absence of an appropriate host antibody response. Absent specific immunity, there are none of the clinical features of fifth disease but instead a purely hematologic syndrome of pure red cell aplasia. The anemia is severe and requires transfusion; reticulocytes are absent from blood, as are erythroid precursors from marrow. Observation of giant pronormoblasts in the marrow may lead to the diagnosis. There is no antibody to parvovirus in the blood, but the virus can be detected in the circulation, often at extremely high levels (>10^{12} genome copies per milliliter). Failure to produce neutralizing antibodies to B19 parvovirus occurs in patients with congenital immunodeficiency (Nezelof's syndrome), in those with iatrogenic immunodeficiency (chemotherapy or immunosuppressive drugs), or as a result of acquired immunodeficiency secondary to HIV-1. Pure red cell aplasia secondary to parvovirus may be the first manifestation of acquired immunodeficiency syndrome (AIDS).

Hydrops Fetalis

B19 parvovirus infection of the pregnant mother followed by transplacental transmission to the fetus can lead to an adverse outcome, either miscarriage or hydrops fetalis. Parvovirus infects the fetal liver, the site of erythrocyte production during early development. Hydrops is the result of severe anemia as well as perhaps myocarditis, contributing to congestive heart failure. Prospective studies have led to an estimated 30% risk of transplacental infection and 9% risk of fetal loss in women who are exposed to B19 during pregnancy. Infection during the second trimester poses the greatest risk for birth of a hydropic infant; B19 parvovirus probably accounts for 10 to 20% of all cases of nonimmune hydrops fetalis. The risk of spontaneous abortion resulting from first trimester infections has been more difficult to quantitate. The likelihood of an infection increases in epidemic years and correlates with the level of contact of the pregnant woman with children. Although most B19 infections during pregnancy probably do not lead to either loss of the fetus or congenital anomalies, B19 infection is a relatively frequent cause of fetal death. Congenital malformations have not been consistently associated with intrauterine parvovirus infection. However, severe anemia at birth with a bone marrow histology consistent with either constitutional pure red cell aplasia (Diamond-Blackfan anemia) or congenital dyserythropoietic anemia has occurred in infants salvaged by in utero blood transfusions or exchange transfusion at birth.

Other Syndromes

Elevated levels of hepatic transaminases can accompany fifth disease, and parvovirus infection has been associated with severe but self-limited hepatitis in a few children. The presence of B19 genetic sequences in cardiac tissue has led to a diagnosis of parvovirus myocarditis. Serologic and DNA evidence of B19 infection implicated parvovirus in some patients with necrotizing vasculitis, Kawasaki disease, Henoch-Schönlein purpura, and giant cell arteritis. Glove-and-sock syndrome, an exanthem localized to the hands and feet and consisting of edema, erythema, paresthesia, and pruritus, has been linked to B19. Chronic fatigue syndrome may follow parvovirus infection. Meningitis, encephalitis, and a variety of neurologic complications may occur with fifth disease and parvovirus infection.

False-positive results arise when the diagnosis of infection rests on detection of amplified B19 genome by polymerase chain reaction, and furthermore, B19 parvovirus can persist at low levels in normal individuals for many months after infection.

DIAGNOSIS

Because of the difficulty in propagating B19 parvovirus in standard tissue culture, laboratory diagnosis relies on serologic and DNA tests (Table 379-1). Virus-specific antibodies are measured in standardized commercial solid-phase enzyme-labeled immunoassays, generally involving the use of capsid proteins generated in the baculovirus system. "Capture" formats are preferred to detect serum IgM, which is first bound to a solid phase coated with anti–μ-chain antibodies, followed by the addition of viral antigen and an antiviral monoclonal antibody. IgM antibodies are diagnostically positive in almost all cases of fifth disease at initial evaluation and appear within a few days of the onset of transient aplastic crisis, and IgM may persist for months after acute infection. IgG is usually assayed in conventional indirect assays. IgG circulates later than IgM, generally at the end of the first week of illness. Although titers of IgG are generally highest in the year after an acute infection, substantial interindividual variation and the presence of IgG in a large proportion of the population make measurement of IgG less helpful than other tests for diagnosis of parvovirus. DNA assays are required for persistent B19 infection, in which antibody production is absent or minimal. Parvovirus can also be found in the sera of patients with early transient aplastic crisis. Direct hybridization methods are reliable, and they detect clinically relevant viral titers of greater than 10^6 international units (orders of magnitude below levels present in both acute and persistent infection). Gene amplification methods are more sensitive but less reliable because of false-positive results. Virus can be detected in amniotic fluid, and both virus and IgM antibody to B19 are found in umbilical cord blood; the mother's serum will show seroconversion during pregnancy, but maternal IgM may be absent at the onset of hydrops fetalis.

PREVENTION

Effective vaccines exist for animal parvoviruses, and human B19 infection can also probably be prevented. A recombinant immunogen in development for the human virus lacks DNA and is therefore noninfectious; the empty capsids have been engineered to overexpress the highly immunogenic minor structural protein VP1, and a single 2.5-μg dose of empty capsids elicited excellent neutralizing antibody responses in normal volunteers. Vaccination could prevent transient aplastic crisis in patients with sickle cell disease and other hemolytic anemias, pure red cell aplasia in some immunodeficient individuals, and hydrops if seronegative mothers were inoculated early in pregnancy.

TREATMENT   Rx

Most parvovirus infections in normal children and adults do not require specific therapy. Isolation of infected individuals is impractical, with the exception of hospitalized cases. Pure red cell aplasia and the underlying persistent B19 parvovirus infection can be dramatically terminated by discontinuation of immunosuppressive therapy or institution of effective antiretroviral drugs in patients with AIDS. Commercial immunoglobulins are a good source of antibodies to parvovirus, and persistent B19 infection responds to a 5- or 10-day course of IgG at 0.4 g/kg with a prompt decline in serum viral DNA, as measured by hybridization methods, accompanied by reticulocytosis and increased hemoglobin levels. This regimen has been curative in congenital immunodeficiency, but in AIDS, parvovirus often persists at lower levels, and relapses of anemia may require repeated IgG administration. Immunoglobulin therapy can precipitate fifth disease rash and arthralgia. Hydrops fetalis may resolve spontaneously, but intrauterine blood transfusions have been used with apparent success. Chronic arthropathy has been treated symptomatically with anti-inflammatory drugs, and there is not a clear role for the administration of immunoglobulin. As important as recognizing parvovirus infection is avoiding misinterpretation of laboratory studies, such as positive IgG serology or borderline IgM and DNA test results, and misguided maneuvers that delay appropriate alternative treatments.

TABLE 379-1   DIAGNOSIS OF PARVOVIRUS B19

DISEASE	IgM	IgG	B19 DOT BLOT*	B19 PCR
Fifth disease	+++	++	−	+
Polyarthropathy syndrome	++	+	−	+
Transient aplastic crisis	+/−	+/−	++	++
Persistent anemia	+/−	+/−	++	++
Hydrops/congenital infection	+/−	+	+/−	++
Previous infection	−	++	−	+/−

*Sensitivity about 10^6 genome copies per milliliter.
PCR = polymerase chain reaction.

SUGGESTED READINGS

Douvoyiannis M, Litman N, Goldman DL. Neurologic manifestations associated with parvovirus B19 infection. *Clin Infect Dis.* 2009;48:1713-1723. *Review of peripheral and central nervous system manifestations.*

Oiwa H, Shimada T, Hashimoto M, et al. Clinical findings in parvovirus B19 infection in 30 adult patients in Kyoto. *Mod Rheumatol.* 2011;21:24-31. *Initial symptoms were flu-like, but about 85% of patients developed arthralgias and about 80% developed rash.*

380

SMALLPOX, MONKEYPOX, AND OTHER POXVIRUS INFECTIONS

INGER K. DAMON

DEFINITION

Human illness caused by a poxvirus is characterized by a cutaneous manifestation; illness may be localized or systemic, depending on the particular poxvirus and the route of introduction. DNA-based assays, including DNA sequencing, are the most precise methods for identification and differentiation of poxvirus genera, species, strains, and variants. The guanosine plus cytosine content of orthopoxviruses, yatapoxviruses, molluscum contagiosum virus, and parapoxviruses is approximately 33%, 32%, 60%, and 63%, respectively.

The Pathogens

All poxviruses described in this chapter (Table 380-1) belong to the family Poxviridae, subfamily Chordopoxvirinae.

EPIDEMIOLOGY

Recognition of the epidemiologic characteristics of poxvirus diseases is valuable in assessing the potential etiologic agent of a particular suspected poxvirus lesion. Knowledge of zoonotic reservoirs, geographic localizations, and capacity for epidemic transmission is critical for clinical assessment and control measures. All human poxvirus infections are zoonotic in nature, with the exception of molluscum contagiosum and variola, which are solely human pathogens. Parapoxvirus and molluscipoxvirus infections are endemic worldwide; orthopoxvirus and yatapoxvirus infections are geographically restricted, probably by the distribution of competent reservoir hosts. With the exception of variola virus (the causative agent of smallpox, a disease declared eradicated in 1980), none of these diseases is required to be reported to public health systems; furthermore, diagnostics are not widely available, so it is difficult to estimate disease incidence and prevalence with any certainty. In addition to variola virus, both monkeypox and camelpox viruses are considered to be select agents by the U.S. government; they must be reported and appropriately handled if discovered and if samples are maintained in the United States.

Orthopoxvirus

The epidemiology of smallpox, caused by the orthopoxvirus variola, is understood through detailed studies conducted during the end of the eradication campaign. Interhuman transmission of variola virus generally occurred through the inhalation of large airborne respiratory droplets of infectious variola virus. Transmission usually required prolonged face-to-face or other close contact, although airborne transmission over longer distances had been reported. Transmission by fomites or contact with infectious material from the rash also occurred. Aggregate data, collected during the smallpox eradication campaign, suggest a secondary attack rate of 58.4% in unvaccinated close or household contacts and a secondary attack rate of 3.8% in previously vaccinated close or household contacts. Case-fatality rates for variola major varied with the type of disease manifested, but aggregate rates of 10 to 30% in various outbreaks have been recorded. Severity of disease

correlated with rash burden and was also more severe in children and pregnant women. Variola alastrim minor, a variant of variola with a case-fatality rate of less than 1%, has similar human-to-human disease transmission characteristics.

Monkeypox has a more complex epidemiology. The virus is zoonotic, and two genetically discrete virus clades have been described, each with apparent distinct clinical and epidemiologic parameters. Human infections in western and central Africa were first identified in 1970. Investigations in the Congo basin country Zaire, now the Democratic Republic of Congo, demonstrated that human-to-human transmission of monkeypox was less prevalent than that of smallpox. The secondary attack rate in unvaccinated contacts of monkeypox cases was calculated to be 9.3% versus 37 to 88% for smallpox. Previous smallpox vaccination (3 to 19 years previously) appeared to be 85% protective in preventing disease acquisition in contacts and also ameliorated the severity of disease. Overall, the majority of identified cases acquired disease from presumed animal exposure; only 28% of cases were ascribed to person-to-person transmission. A case-fatality rate of approximately 10% was observed in unvaccinated persons, and the majority of fatalities and the most severe disease manifestations were observed in children younger than 5 years. Serosurveys suggested that subclinical infection may have occurred in up to 28% of close contacts of monkeypox patients in some communities; this relatively low rate may contribute to the rarity of sustained generations of human-to-human transmission in household and other close contact situations.

Among primary cases, recent close contact—through hunting, skinning, killing, cooking, or playing with carcasses—was identified with *Cercopithicus, Colobus,* and *Cercocebus* (primate); *Cricetomys* (terrestrial rodent); and *Funisciurus* and *Heliosciurus* (squirrel species). Samples of animals collected in areas of western and central Africa surrounding human cases demonstrated orthopoxvirus and sometimes monkeypox-specific seroprevalence in various members of these species, except in *Cricetomys* species. The prevailing hypothesis was that squirrel species were the probable reservoir of disease.

The disease reemerged in 1996 in the Democratic Republic of Congo, this time with 88% of cases derived from secondary human-to-human contact because of the cessation of routine smallpox vaccination in 1980 after the eradication of smallpox. Mortality was only 1%. Ecologic serosurveys showed orthopoxvirus seroprevalence in terrestrial rodents (*Cricetomys emini*) and in one domestic pig (*Sus scrofa*).

Monkeypox virus was introduced to the United States in 2003 through a consignment of animals from the west African country of Ghana. The virus was identified as belonging to a distinct clade of monkeypox that included previous west African monkeypox isolates as well as isolates derived from earlier outbreaks in primate colonies. The U.S. cases had a less pronounced rash and a less severe illness, with no mortality or human-to-human transmission. These data suggest at least two populations of monkeypox virus.

Cowpox virus is found in Europe and Asia and is maintained in rodents; in Britain, the reservoirs are bank voles and wood mice. Human infection is a zoonosis. The domestic cat is the most common source of human infection, which probably explains the occurrence of cases in children; 26% of 54 cases occurred in children younger than 12 years. Most feline and human cases occur between July and October, with only occasional cases between January and June. No case of bovine cowpox has been detected since 1976. Cowpox virus also is prevalent in European zoos, where cheetahs, lions, anteaters, rhinoceros, elephants, and okapi have occasionally transmitted infection to animal handlers.

Vaccinia is the live virus contained in preparations of the smallpox vaccines used to eradicate smallpox. In the United States, the vaccine is recommended for laboratory workers who use replicative orthopoxviruses and for selected military personnel. Contacts of vaccinees occasionally develop vaccinia infections. The origin of vaccinia is unknown, and no natural host for the virus is known. Vaccinia "variants" have been described, including buffalopox from contact with infected animals in India and vaccinia viruses in cattle handlers in Brazil.

Parapoxvirus

Human infection is an occupational hazard of farm workers, abattoir workers, veterinary surgeons, and students. It is most common in the lambing and calving seasons and among sheep workers.

Factors responsible for ongoing transmission have been attributed both to the environmental stability of orf virus in scab material and to the manifestation of chronic infections in some animals. There is no known latent state for

TABLE 380-1 TAXONOMY OF POXVIRUSES KNOWN TO INFECT HUMANS

GENUS	SPECIES
Orthopoxvirus	Variola virus, vaccinia virus, cowpox virus, monkeypox virus
Parapoxvirus	Orf virus, milker's node virus, bovine papular stomatitis virus, sealpox virus
Yatapoxvirus	Tanapox virus (Yaba-like disease virus), Yaba monkey tumor virus
Molluscipoxvirus	Molluscum contagiosum virus

this or any other poxvirus. Transmission of virus to humans and to animals is through direct contact with lesions or by fomites.

Molluscipoxvirus

Molluscum contagiosum virus occurs worldwide, and increasing reports of the disease have paralleled the number of reported cases of acquired immunodeficiency syndrome (AIDS). Traditional modes of transmission are associated with mild skin trauma such as abrasions, direct contact with a lesion, and fomites (e.g., shared towels) in some cases. However, the disease appears to be sexually transmitted, and genital lesions are more common than lesions elsewhere on the body. Children in daycare or school situations may transmit the disease to other children. Secondary spread of lesions may occur by autoinoculation (excoriation of primary lesions and spread to areas of normal skin) as well as by shaving. No known animal reservoir exists.

Yatapoxvirus

Tanapox virus is restricted to Africa, principally to Kenya and the Democratic Republic of Congo, and probably has a simian reservoir. Direct primate-to-human transmission through a break in skin has rarely been described in animal handlers, but an insect or arthropod intermediary may be involved in the transmission of tanapox virus to humans. No human-to-human transmission has been reported. Yaba monkey tumor virus causes localized infections after contact with infected primate lesions. Little is known about the epidemiology of this virus.

PATHOBIOLOGY

The majority of smallpox infections were initiated by inhalation of respiratory droplets and implantation of virus on the oropharyngeal and respiratory mucosa. No primary localized site of infection was evident if the route of exposure was by inhalation. Disease could also be introduced through suspensions of virus obtained from scabs of patients that were introduced percutaneously and constituted the practice of variolation. In these cases (when skillfully administered), illness was usually less virulent, a localized primary infectious lesion was present, and the asymptomatic incubation period was truncated.

After entry, virus moves to local lymph nodes and then disseminates to the reticuloendothelial system to replicate further. At this time, the individual is asymptomatic. In 10 to 14 days, secondary viremia occurs and heralds the prodrome of symptomatic illness. During this time, virus seeds the oropharynx and epidermis. The absence of a keratinized structure in the mucosa of the oropharynx leads to ulceration and release of virus in saliva; virus replicates in the epidermis to cause the characteristic macular, papular, and vesicular eruptions of smallpox.

In experiments in monkeys, high levels of type I interferons, interleukin-6, and interferon-γ are seen; D-dimers and thrombocytopenia suggest disseminated intravascular coagulation. Apoptosis with loss of T cells in lymphoid organs was also observed. Of note, tumor necrosis factor-α (TNF-α) levels were minimal in the infected animals, with a notable decrease in the expression of genes regulated by nuclear factor κB and TNF-α.

In humans, the viral lesion primarily develops in the epidermis, where the cells of the malpighian layer swell and vacuolate to undergo ballooning degeneration. The cytoplasm continues to enlarge, loss of nuclear material is noted, and coalescence of vacuoles through cell rupture creates reticulating degeneration of the middle and upper layers of the stratum spinosum. In the next stages, the vesicle is formed. High titers of virus are found within the lesions. In mucosal surfaces, the absence of a horny layer allows the necrosis caused by proliferation of virus within the epithelium to create ulcers and leads to liberation of large quantities of virus into the oropharynx. Evaluation of other organs in human smallpox has been done only in select autopsy cases. Mild pathologic changes are seen in the lungs.

CLINICAL MANIFESTATIONS
Orthopoxvirus
Smallpox

Naturally acquired variola virus infection is characterized by fever and a distinctive rash, with several different clinical presentations (Table 380-2). When the disease still existed, an asymptomatic incubation period of 10 to 14 days (range, 7 to 17) was followed by a fever that quickly rose to about 103° F (38° to 40° C), sometimes with dermal petechiae. Associated constitutional symptoms included backache, headache, vomiting, and prostration. Within a day or two after incubation, a systemic rash with a characteristic centrifugal distribution (i.e., lesions present in greater numbers on the oral

TABLE 380-2	WORLD HEALTH ORGANIZATION SMALLPOX TYPES
WHO SMALLPOX TYPE	**CLINICAL DEFINITION**
Variola sine eruptione	Fever, no rash
Modified	Like ordinary, with an accelerated course
Ordinary discrete	Fever, rash; areas of normal skin between pustules, even on the face
Ordinary semiconfluent	Fever, rash; pustules confluent on the face, discrete elsewhere
Ordinary confluent	Fever, rash; pustules confluent on the face and forearms
Flat	Fever, erythema, and edema of the skin; vesicles soft, flat, and bullous
Hemorrhagic, early	Fever (persistent), hemorrhages and petechiae, purpuric rash at illness onset
Hemorrhagic, late	Fever (persistent), rash, hemorrhage into the base of vesicles late in illness

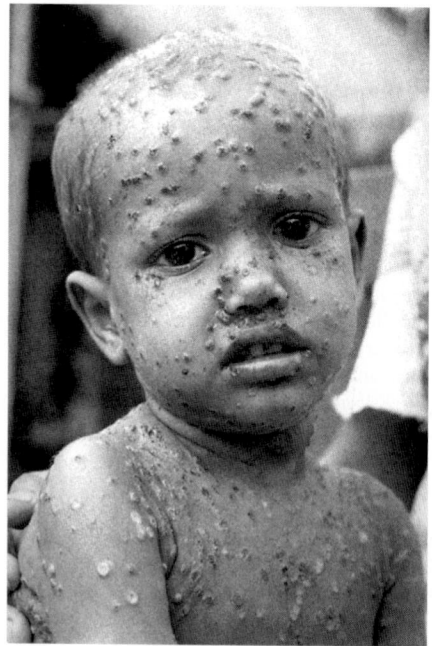

FIGURE 380-1. Pustular lesions of smallpox and beginning of scarring on the face and upper part of the torso. (From the Centers for Disease Control and Prevention Public Health Image Library, ID #: 7055. Photograph by Stan Foster.)

mucosa, face, and extremities than on the trunk) appeared. The fever typically abated as the rash developed. Lesions commonly appeared on the palms and soles. The rash lesions were initially macular and then advanced to the papular stage, at which point they enlarged and progressed to a vesicle by day 4 to 5 and a pustule by day 7. When lesions became pustular, the fever typically returned. Lesions became encrusted and scabbed by day 14 and then sloughed off. Skin lesions in the vesicular and pustular stages were deep seated and in the same stage of development in any one area of the body (Fig. 380-1). The ordinary disease type was subgrouped into three categories based on the extent of rash on the face and the body: confluent, semiconfluent, and discrete. In *ordinary confluent disease*, no area of skin was visible between vesiculopustular rash lesions on the trunk or the face. In *ordinary semiconfluent* and *discrete disease*, patches of normal skin were visible between rash lesions on the trunk and face, respectively. Less severe manifestations (modified smallpox or variola sine eruptione) occurred in both unvaccinated and, more commonly, vaccinated individuals. The mortality rate correlated with the rash burden.

Four main clinical types of variola can be subgrouped according to the World Health Organization (WHO) classification schema: *ordinary smallpox* (≈90% of cases) produced viremia, fever, prostration, and rash, and mortality rates were generally proportional to the extent of rash and ranged as described earlier; *(vaccine) modified smallpox* (5% of cases) produced a mild prodrome with few skin lesions in previously vaccinated people and had a mortality rate well below 10%; *flat smallpox* (≈5% of hospitalized cases) produced slowly developing lesions that were difficult to ascertain because they appeared flush with the (edematous) skin at the vesicular stage, and it was almost always fatal; and *hemorrhagic smallpox* (<1% of cases) induced bleeding into the skin and the mucous membranes and was invariably fatal. A discrete type of the ordinary form, with a typical febrile prodrome and rash, resulted from alastrim variola minor infection. Individuals with this form of disease were not nearly as moribund or "toxemic" as individuals with variola major infection. Previous vaccination was not necessarily protective against the hemorrhagic forms of disease but seemed to be protective against flat forms of disease.

In flat smallpox, illness was heralded by the abrupt onset of fever to 38.3° to 38.9° C and the appearance of the rash after 3 to 4 days. The oral enanthem was often confluent, and sloughing of rectal mucosal membranes was also reported. At the papulovesicular stage of disease, lesions appeared as small indentations (day 6) with hemorrhages in the bases and were surrounded by an erythematous ring. By day 7 or 8, the lesions appeared flat. Bullous lesions that would slough were reported. Fever persisted throughout the disease course, and respiratory complications were often observed by day 7 or 8 of illness. Thrombocytopenia, neutropenia, and lymphocytosis were reported.

In hemorrhagic forms of smallpox, illness began with fever and typical prodromal symptoms; the fever never abated. Early after the onset of fever, petechiae and purpuric rashes became apparent; subconjunctival hemorrhages, hematuria, and vaginal bleeding were also seen. Patients usually died by day 6 of illness, well before any classic vesiculopustular rash was evident. In late hemorrhagic disease, after the onset of fever, typical maculopapular lesions developed, but the fever did not abate. The lesion evolved slowly, and areas of hemorrhage were evident at the base of the lesions. Bleeding occurred in the mucous membranes, thrombocytopenia was profound, and death occurred between days 8 and 10 of illness.

Monkeypox

After an incubation period of 7 to 17 days (mean, 12 days), a prodrome of fever, headache, backache, and fatigue begins. The cutaneous eruption evolves similar to that of smallpox. Lesions evolve in the same stage in any one part of the body from macules, papules, and vesicles to pustules, and then they crust and scar (Fig. 380-2). After resolution of the rash, hypopigmentation is followed by hyperpigmentation of the scarred lesions. Pronounced cervical, postauricular, submandibular, and inguinal lymphadenopathy clinically distinguishes monkeypox from smallpox.

Vaccinia

Multiple-puncture vaccinia virus infection by a bifurcated needle is the current smallpox vaccination regimen used for laboratory personnel working with orthopoxviruses, public health care personnel, and military in the United States. Most commonly, the infection progresses through a standard course of events from vesicle to pustule. However, of all vaccines used today, the smallpox vaccine, which is composed of live, replicative vaccinia virus, has one of the highest rates of adverse events. Major complications include progressive vaccinia, eczema vaccinatum, generalized vaccinia, postvaccinial encephalitis, accidental infection, and carditis.

Progressive vaccinia, which is a rare and often fatal vaccine complication in persons with severe deficiencies in cellular immunity, occurs in about 1 per million vaccines, with a case-fatality rate of about 35%. Progressive vaccinia is characterized by frequently painless growth and spread of the vaccine virus beyond the inoculation site, often leading to necrosis and sometimes metastases to other body sites. The possibility of progressive vaccinia should be considered if the vaccination site lesion continues to progress and expand without apparent healing more than 15 days after vaccination.

Eczema vaccinatum can occur in people with a history of atopic dermatitis (eczema), irrespective of its severity or activity, owing to local spread or dissemination from the primary vaccination site or contact with the unscabbed vaccination site of another person. A localized or generalized papular, vesicular, or pustular rash can develop anywhere on the body or be localized to previous eczematous lesions. Systemic illness with fever, malaise, and lymphadenopathy may occur. In the 1968 national U.S. surveillance of smallpox vaccination, there were 66 cases (no deaths) of eczema vaccinatum among 14.5 million vaccinees (4.6 cases/million) and 60 cases (1 death) among their several million contacts.

Generalized vaccinia describes the vesicular rash that develops after vaccination. Excluding dissemination associated with eczema vaccinatum and progressive vaccinia, it has been extremely rare to document virus in these lesions. True generalized vaccinia is believed to represent the end product of viremic spread of virus, and no predisposing factors have been identified. Generalized vaccinia is estimated to occur in about 242 of every million primary vaccinations.

Postvaccination encephalomyelitis is a rare but serious complication that usually occurs only in primary vaccinees. Patients have variably displayed clinical and diagnostic features suggestive of a postimmunization demyelinating encephalomyelitis or direct viral invasion of the nervous system. This postvaccination reaction typically occurs 11 to 15 days after vaccination. Symptoms include fever, headache, vomiting, confusion, delirium, disorientation, restlessness, drowsiness or lethargy, seizures, and coma. Cerebrospinal fluid can demonstrate elevated pressure but generally has a normal cell count and chemistry profile. The diagnosis is one of exclusion, and no specific tests are available to confirm it.

Accidental infection occurs when virus from the vaccination site is transferred to another site or to another person through intimate skin contact. This complication generally occurs with primary vaccinees rather than revaccinees. Accidental self-inoculation, which most commonly occurs on the face, mouth, lips, or genitalia, is not usually serious and requires no specific treatment. Inoculation of the eye or eyelid is more serious and can be sight threatening if it is not evaluated and treated appropriately (Fig. 380-3). Between 1963 and 1968, ocular vaccinia was observed in 348 persons, including 22 who had evidence of corneal involvement and 11 who experienced permanent defects.

With buffalopox viruses in India and the Cantagalo virus in Brazil, up to 10 lesions have been described on the hands or arms of human handlers; fever, lymphadenopathy, backache, and fatigue are also associated symptoms. Transmission is believed to occur by unprotected contact with active lesions

FIGURE 380-2. Rash of monkeypox of the head (A) and extremities (B) in a 7-year-old girl in central Zaire. (From Peters W, Pasvol G. *Tropical Medicine and Parasitology*, 5th ed. New York: Mosby; 2002:238.)

FIGURE 380-3. Vaccinia autoinoculation of an eye. (From the Centers for Disease Control and Prevention Public Health Image Library, ID #: 3322.)

present on animal teats and udders. Interhuman transmission of buffalopox to family members has been reported to occur through contact.

Cowpox

Cowpox lesions are generally restricted to the hands and face; most patients (72%) have only one lesion. Multiple lesions may be caused by multiple primary inoculations, by autoinoculation, and very infrequently by lymphatic or viremic spread. The cowpox lesion passes through macular, papular, vesicular, and pustular stages before forming a hard black crust. The lesion is generally very painful, and erythema and edema are common at the late vesicular and pustular stages. Patients usually have lymphadenitis, fever, and general malaise. These features are generally severe in children, and absence from school or work is common. About 30% may be hospitalized. Most patients take 6 to 8 weeks to recover, but up to 12 weeks may be required. On occasion, a very severe infection and death may occur, typically in immunosuppressed individuals. Scarring is usually permanent.

Parapoxvirus

Lesions, such as from the orf virus, start as erythematous papules and progress in 1 to 2 weeks to target lesions with a red center surrounded by a white halo and an outer inflamed halo. Lesions then progress to a nodular and then a papillomatous stage, which often has a "weeping" surface. In some patients, lesions may enlarge and persist for weeks before resolving by a crusting stage, which also may persist for weeks. Very large granulomatous lesions may occasionally require surgical removal.

Most patients have only one lesion, but multiple primary lesions may develop. Systemic reaction is relatively uncommon, and the lesion is often not particularly painful. Lymphadenopathy is present in some patients, and lymphangitis is relatively uncommon. Erythema multiforme (Chapter 447) can develop in up to one third of patients.

Molluscum Contagiosum Virus

Molluscum infection occurs when molluscum contagiosum virus comes into contact with nonintact skin. The characteristic lesion begins as a small papule and, when mature, is a discrete, 2- to 5-mm-diameter, smooth, dome-shaped, pearly or flesh-colored nodule that is often umbilicated. A cheesy, off-white or yellowish material is easily expressed from lesions. Most patients have 1 to 20 lesions, but hundreds of lesions may occasionally be present. Because of multiple simultaneous infections or mechanical spread, the lesions may become confluent along the line of a scratch, and satellite lesions are sometimes seen.

In children, molluscum lesions occur mainly on the trunk and proximal ends of the extremities; in adults, lesions tend to occur on the trunk, pubic area, and thighs. In all cases, however, infection can be transmitted to other areas by autoinoculation. In men infected with human immunodeficiency virus (HIV), molluscum lesions can occur along the beard line and result in ocular involvement.

Individual lesions persist for about 2 months, but the disease usually persists for 6 to 9 months. Individuals with impaired cell-mediated immunity, including persons with HIV infection, tend to have more severe and prolonged infection.

Yatapoxvirus

Tanapox infection begins with a short febrile (38° to 39° C) illness that persists for 2 to 4 days and is sometimes accompanied by headache, backache, or prostration. The eruption of a lesion is frequently heralded by pruritus at the site of the outbreak. The lesion appears as a hyperpigmented macule, which often has central elevation and evolves to a papule with palpable induration. About 80% have a solitary nodule, but as many as 10 lesions can occur. Most lesions (72%) occur on the lower extremities, and the fewest occur on the face and areas normally covered by clothing.

Fever and systemic symptoms wane as the lesion erupts. The papule then becomes more "pocklike" but contains no fluid; umbilication or a pseudocrust may develop. Typically, the papule evolves into a firm, deep-seated, elevated nodule. At the end of the first week, the lesion is surrounded by erythema and indurated skin, and regional lymphangitis is common. Lesions then either ulcerate or become larger nodules (up to 2 cm in diameter) within about 2 weeks, after which the local inflammatory response wanes and the lesions began to granulate. Resolution of lesions occurs within 6 weeks. Infection appears to confer lifelong immunity.

DIAGNOSIS

Before its eradication, smallpox was relatively easy to recognize. Chickenpox (Chapter 383) produces a centripetally distributed rash and rarely appears on the palms and soles; in chickenpox, prodromal fever and systemic manifestations are mild, the lesions are superficial in nature, and lesions in different developmental stages may be present in the same area of the body. Other diseases and conditions that could be confused with vesicular-stage smallpox include monkeypox, generalized vaccinia, disseminated herpes zoster or herpes simplex virus infection (Chapters 382 and 383), drug reactions (eruptions), erythema multiforme (Chapter 447), enteroviral infections (Chapter 387), scabies (Chapter 367), insect bites, impetigo (Chapter 447), and molluscum contagiosum. Diseases confused with hemorrhagic smallpox included acute leukemia (Chapter 189), meningococcemia (Chapter 306), and idiopathic thrombocytopenic purpura (Chapter 175). The Centers for Disease Control and Prevention has developed a worksheet for evaluation of patients for potential smallpox (available at *http://www.bt.cdc.gov/agent/smallpox/diagnosis/evalposter.asp*) and an algorithm for assessment of the vesiculopustular stage of rash (available at *http://www.bt.cdc.gov/agent/smallpox/diagnosis/rashtestingprotocol.asp*).

Orthopoxvirus

Viral culture or electron microscopic evaluation of virion particles from clinical rash specimens has been the approach to diagnosis of orthopoxvirus infections. Serologic tests are largely genus specific, detect IgG, and usually cannot differentiate among species, although IgM levels can help differentiate recent orthopoxvirus infection from remote vaccination. Nucleic acid–based tests and polymerase chain reaction (PCR) assays are other options. If the diagnosis of smallpox is being considered, viral culture requires a biosafety level 4 (BSL-4) containment facility that is sanctioned by the WHO to use variola virus.

Parapoxvirus

The differential diagnosis of parapoxvirus lesions can include ecthyma gangrenosum as a result of a *Pseudomonas aeruginosa* infection (Chapter 314), vaccinia or cowpox infection, cutaneous anthrax (Chapter 302), erysipeloid (Chapter 303), tularemia (Chapter 319), and tumor. Farm workers recognize the infection and tend not to seek medical attention for routine cases, so about 45% of reported cases may have no known contact with infected animals, and the clinical diagnosis of such cases may be difficult. With negative-stain electron microscopy, virions with the characteristic morphology of parapoxviruses are usually seen easily in lesion extracts, thereby providing a rapid, certain diagnosis of the genus. The virus can be grown in cell culture, and PCR detection can be performed. Species-specific and species-generic protein-based diagnostics have also been developed for parapoxviruses.

Molluscum Contagiosum Virus

The clinical appearance of molluscum lesions usually is sufficiently characteristic to permit a clinical diagnosis. Brick-shaped virions typically can be seen in large numbers if the cheesy material expressed from the lesion is examined by electron microscopy. The virus has not been cultured in standard tissue culture systems. The characteristic histopathology of these lesions is diagnostic, but PCR methods can also identify molluscum contagiosum.

Yatapoxvirus

The limited geographic distribution of tanapox virus and the patient's travel history help with the diagnosis of tanapox infection. Unique clinical features that differentiate tanapox from other orthopoxvirus infections are the nodular nature of the rash lesion, the paucity of lesions, the benign disease course, and the protracted resolution of the rash. The solid nodular and ulcerated lesions are larger and develop more slowly than those of monkeypox, but they are smaller and develop more rapidly than those of tropical ulcers.

Tanapox virus can be detected by electron microscopy, but the appearance of the virions cannot exclude infection with other morphologically similar brick-shaped poxviruses. Nucleic acid testing or cell line culture can make the definitive diagnosis.

TREATMENT AND PREVENTION

Orthopoxvirus

Vaccination with smallpox vaccine is the mainstay for prevention of orthopoxvirus infection and was the primary method used to eradicate smallpox. Stockpiles of vaccine are available should smallpox recur. In the United States, however, smallpox vaccine is currently recommended only for laboratory personnel who work with infectious orthopoxvirus, certain public health personnel, and certain members of the military. Adverse events are rare with vaccination, but myocarditis or pericarditis was documented in 18 of 230,734 (8 per million) U.S. military primary vaccinees immunized in 2002 and 2003. In recent trials, both an attenuated tissue-cultured smallpox vaccine (LC16m8) and a replication-deficient smallpox vaccine (MVA) were about 95% effective both in newly vaccinated adults and as a booster.[1,2]

Currently, no antiviral drugs are licensed to treat orthopoxvirus or other poxvirus illnesses. Early administration of vaccinia immune globulin (VIG) may reduce the mortality of eczema vaccinatum from 30 to 40% to 7%, and VIG may also be useful for other complications (e.g., progressive vaccinia, severe generalized vaccinia or contact infection) of vaccinia (smallpox) vaccine administration and for other orthopoxvirus infections. However, VIG alone has no clear benefit for treatment of smallpox infection itself.

Antiviral compounds with in vitro and in vivo activity against poxviruses include specifically 5-iodo-2′-deoxyuridine, adenine arabinoside, and trifluorothymidine. Because of their systemic toxicity, these compounds have been used topically for the treatment of orthopoxvirus ocular infections. In vitro, cidofovir is active against cowpox, vaccinia, monkeypox, and variola; in vivo, it protects challenged animals when it is given prophylactically or early in the evolution of disease. Cidofovir has known renal toxicity and is administered with hydration and probenecid. CMX-001 has been effective in treatment of systemic rabbitpox infection in rabbits and was used as part of a multiple-drug regimen to treat a case of progressive vaccinia. The drug ST-246 is effective in animal models of systemic orthopoxvirus infection and has been used as part of a multiple-drug regimen to treat a human case of eczema vaccinatum and a case of progressive vaccinia.

Parapoxvirus

Most workers at risk for parapoxvirus become infected, and reinfection also occurs. The vaccine used to control orf in sheep is fully virulent and has caused human infection. Treatment options are limited; anecdotal reports have described the use of topical cidofovir, and other options may be topical formulations of interferon-modulating compounds such as imiquimod.

Molluscum Contagiosum Virus

Molluscum contagiosum infection is benign and recovery is usually spontaneous, but treatment may be sought for cosmetic reasons, particularly for facial or multiple lesions. Options include cryotherapy, mechanical curettage, and chemical treatments such as podophyllin or podofilox, cantharidin, iodine, and tretinoin. Irritation has been a side effect of many of the chemical treatments. Topical application of a 3% cidofovir antiviral cream or suspension has been reported to be beneficial, as has the use of potentially immune-modulating cimetidine or topical imiquimod therapy. However, no therapy is documented to be beneficial by well-controlled randomized trials.[3] Covering of lesions and the use of proper hand hygiene after contact with lesions should prevent transmission in most situations. For individuals with AIDS and molluscum, highly active antiretroviral therapy with a resulting improvement in the CD4+ cell count appears to be efficacious.

PROGNOSIS

Monkeypox and smallpox both cause human illness, with mortality ranging from 10% to 40%; variola minor variants, however, have mortality rates of less than 1%. Yatapoxvirus infections are self-limited, and the illness resolves in the course of a few weeks. Parapoxvirus infections are manifested chiefly by localized symptoms, and the lesions resolve during a month or so in non-immunocompetent hosts. Molluscum contagiosum infection is benign, usually with a spontaneous recovery, but the infection can persist for months. Variola minor has a mortality rate of less than 1%.

1. Saito T, Fujii T, Kanatani Y, et al. Clinical and immunological response to attenuated tissue-cultured smallpox vaccine LC16m8. *JAMA.* 2009;301:1025-1033.
2. von Krempelhuber A, Vollmar J, Pokorny R, et al. A randomized, double-blind, dose-finding Phase II study to evaluate immunogenicity and safety of the third generation smallpox vaccine candidate IMVAMUNE. *Vaccine.* 2010;28:1209-1216.
3. van der Wouden JC, van der Sande R, van Suijlekom–Smit LW, et al. Interventions for cutaneous molluscum contagiosum. *Cochrane Database Syst Rev.* 2009;4:CD004767.

SUGGESTED READINGS

Moss B. Smallpox vaccines: targets of protective immunity. *Immunol Rev.* 2011;239:8-26. *Comprehensive review.*

Roess AA, Galan A, Kitces E, et al. Novel deer-associated parapoxvirus infection in deer hunters. *N Engl J Med.* 2010;363:2621-2627. *Description of a new human infection.*

381

PAPILLOMAVIRUS

JOHN M. DOUGLAS, Jr.

DEFINITION

Human papillomaviruses (HPVs) are a group of small DNA viruses that cause a variety of benign and malignant lesions of the skin and mucous membranes. The most commonly recognized HPV-associated diseases include warts (Chapter 448) at anogenital sites (condyloma acuminatum), other skin surfaces (common warts or verruca vulgaris), and the plantar surface of the foot (verruca plantaris).

In addition, HPV infection causes squamous intraepithelial lesions of the cervix, also known as cervical intraepithelial neoplasia (CIN), and of other anogenital sites. It is considered the etiologic agent of a variety of anogenital cancers, especially cervical cancer (Chapter 205).

The Pathogen

HPV is a member of the family Papillomaviridae. Like all papillomaviruses, HPV is nonenveloped, measures 55 nm in diameter, and has a double-stranded circular DNA genome of approximately 7900 base pairs enclosed by an icosahedral capsid. The HPV genome contains three functional regions: early genes (E), which are expressed soon after infection and control replication, transcription, and cellular proliferation; late genes (L), which are expressed in later stages of infection and encode the structural capsid proteins; and the long control region, which contains regulatory sequences that control the replication and transcription of early and late genes. Papillomaviruses complete their life cycle only in terminally differentiated epithelial cells and thus are difficult to grow in cell culture. Papillomavirus taxonomy is based on a genotyping system involving the use of DNA sequence relatedness of the gene encoding L1, the major capsid protein, with different types defined as having less than 90% homology.

Papillomaviruses are classified taxonomically by genus (Greek letters) and species (numbered), each containing one or more types. Most HPV types are included in two large genera: alpha (primarily mucosal or genital types) and beta (primarily cutaneous types). Currently, more than 100 types of HPV have been well characterized, approximately 40 of which infect genital skin and mucosa. Of the genital types, approximately 15 are considered high risk because they are associated with high-grade squamous intraepithelial lesions and cervical and other genital tract cancers, whereas others are considered low risk because they are largely associated with genital warts and low-grade squamous intraepithelial lesions.

EPIDEMIOLOGY

HPV infections are primarily transmitted by direct contact of skin or mucous membranes with an infected lesion. Genital HPV infection is typically contracted through sexual intercourse, although nonpenetrative genital contact, oral-genital contact, and manual-genital contact are also possible routes of transmission. In addition, genital HPV infection can be transmitted to the mouth and upper respiratory tract perinatally from infected mothers to newborns. For nongenital HPV infection, personal skin-to-skin contact also plays a primary role, although for plantar warts, fomite transmission from moist surfaces is likely to be an important source of infection. Both genital and nongenital infection can be transmitted to new sites by autoinoculation.

Overall, in the United States, it is estimated that more than 6 million new infections of genital HPV occur annually in sexually active adolescents and adults and that the lifetime risk for infection is 50 to 80%, thus making genital HPV one of the most common sexually transmitted infections. Acquisition of infection begins shortly after sexual debut, with an estimated 40 to 60% incidence of at least one type within 2 years of initiation of sex. Risk factors for infection include variables related to probable exposure (e.g., younger age, increased number of recent and lifetime partners, and number of partners of the sex partners), susceptibility (e.g., lack of circumcision for men), and absence of prevention factors (e.g., lack of consistent condom use or immunization). Most infections are asymptomatic and clear without treatment; only 10% are estimated to persist longer than 2 years. Only such persistently detectable HPV infections are associated with the development of high-grade squamous intraepithelial lesions and cancer. The prevalence of genital HPV infection is estimated to range from 25 to 35% in U.S. women. The prevalence of anogenital warts is estimated to be approximately 1% in the sexually active adult population. Cervical cancer has declined in developed countries since the initiation of cytologic screening programs, although an estimated 11,000 cases and 4000 deaths still occur in the United States annually. However, the disease is a major problem in the developing world, where screening is limited, and it is the second most common cancer in women worldwide, with an estimated 490,000 cases annually.

Nongenital HPV infection is most typically recognized as common and plantar warts, especially in children and adolescents, in whom prevalence rates of 3 to 20% have been reported. All types and manifestations of HPV infection are more common in persons with impaired cell-mediated immunity, such as those infected with human immunodeficiency virus (HIV) or receiving immunosuppressive therapy.

PATHOBIOLOGY

HPV infections cause disease by producing aberrant cell growth. In the case of cutaneous and low-risk genital types, lesions such as warts result from HPV-induced benign proliferation of epidermal layers. For high-risk genital types, precancerous and cancerous lesions result from replacement of the epithelium by undifferentiated cells as a result of HPV-induced interference with normal cellular growth.

Infection begins in the lowest and least well differentiated layer of the epithelium, the basal cells, where exposure is thought to be facilitated by microtrauma. Transcription and protein expression are highly coordinated with the level of cellular differentiation. In the basal layer, the viral genome becomes established in the nucleus as an episome that replicates in tandem with cellular replication, thus maintaining a stable copy number of viral genomes. As basal cells migrate up and differentiate in the superficial layers of the epithelium, full vegetative viral DNA replication and expression of structural proteins occur, with assembly of infectious virions in the most superficial layer of the epithelium, where they are released with the sloughing of dead cells during normal cellular turnover.

On the basis of a variety of epidemiologic and laboratory studies, persistent infection with various high-risk types of genital HPV is firmly established as the cause of squamous cell carcinoma and adenocarcinoma of the cervix (Chapter 205), and HPV 16 plays a causal role in other anogenital and oropharyngeal squamous cell cancers (Chapters 147 and 196). There are also associations of HPV of the genus beta with squamous cell cancer of the skin (Chapter 210). HPV DNA can be detected in more than 99% of cases of cervical cancer, with 70% of cancers being associated with the two most common high-risk types, HPV 16 and 18. The pathogenesis of HPV-induced cancer involves viral integration into the host genome with resulting disruption of the E2 transcription regulatory gene and increased expression of E6 and E7 proteins. These proteins have oncogenic activity and affect cell growth by binding with tumor suppressor proteins, E6 with p53 and E7 with the retinoblastoma tumor suppressor protein, thereby disrupting apoptosis and cell cycle regulation. Although persistent infection with high-risk types is

"necessary" for the development of cervical cancer, it is not considered "sufficient" because cancer does not develop in the majority of infected women. Data support a variety of possible cofactors, including cigarette smoking, prolonged hormonal contraceptive use, multiparity, micronutrient deficiency, and other infections, (i.e., *Chlamydia trachomatis* and herpes simplex virus type 2). In addition, a variety of specific HLA class II alleles have been associated with both increased (e.g., DQB1*0301) and decreased (DRB1*13) risk for cancer, whereas polymorphisms of the p53 gene and the tumor necrosis factor-α promoter region have been associated with increased susceptibility to cancer.

The immune response after initial infection is less robust than for most viral infections; measurable antibody develops in only an estimated 60% of infected individuals, often as long as 6 to 12 months after infection. The limited immune response is probably due to the superficial location of infection in the epithelium and the fact that the capsid proteins are not expressed except in the most well differentiated cells, which are the least accessible to antigen-presenting cells of the immune system. The dynamics of the immune response are quite different after the administration of L1-containing vaccines, with almost 100% seroconversion within several months and antibody levels approximately 10-fold higher than those after natural infection. The high efficacy of these vaccines, which are believed to produce primarily humoral immunity, supports the importance of the antibody response in protection from infection. In contrast, once infection occurs, cellular immunity appears to be critical for clearance of infection on the basis of the experience of persons with impaired cell-mediated immunity, in whom persistent HPV infection and high-grade squamous intraepithelial lesions are more common than in normal hosts.

The histopathologic changes of warts include epithelial papillomatosis and acanthosis, with hyperkeratosis, parakeratosis, and hyperplasia of the parabasal cells. A characteristic feature is the presence in the upper epidermis of koilocytes, or large atypical keratinocytes with irregular, hyperchromatic nuclei surrounded by a perinuclear halo. Squamous intraepithelial lesions are characterized by hyperkeratosis, parakeratosis, and epidermal hyperplasia, with increased mitotic figures in the upper half of the epidermis; koilocytosis is common and often detected cytologically but less prominently than in warts. Several classification systems have been used to classify these lesions and their probable risk for progression based on the proportion of the epithelium replaced by undifferentiated cells. The CIN system grades lesions as CIN 1 (with undifferentiated cells occupying the lower third), CIN 2 (with undifferentiated cells in the lower third to two thirds), and CIN 3/carcinoma in situ (CIS, with undifferentiated cells across the full thickness of the epithelium). A newer classification, the Bethesda system, was originally developed for use with cytology but has increasingly been used for histologic classification; it includes only two categories: low-grade squamous intraepithelial lesions (CIN 1) and high-grade squamous intraepithelial lesions (CIN 2 and CIN 3/CIS).

CLINICAL MANIFESTATIONS

The clinical manifestations of HPV infection vary by anatomic site and viral type. Common warts are exophytic, hyperkeratotic papules that typically occur on the hands but can appear on any skin surface, including the genital skin; they are most commonly caused by HPV types 1, 2, 4, 27, and 57. Plantar warts, which are caused by similar types of HPV, are hyperkeratotic, endophytic, and often very painful. In contrast, flat warts (verruca plana), which are small flat-topped papules that occur more commonly on the face, hands, and legs, are caused by a different group of nongenital HPV types (e.g., types 3, 10, 28, 38, 42, 49, 75, 76).

Epidermodysplasia verruciformis is an uncommon autosomal recessive disease that is usually manifested in childhood as diffuse warts that respond poorly to treatment and typically are caused by HPV types uniquely associated with it (e.g., types 5, 8, 9, 12, 14, 15, 17, 19-25). This syndrome, which is thought to be due to a selective defect in cell-mediated immunity because other opportunistic infections do not occur, is associated with two types of lesions: flat warts caused by the same HPV types as in normal hosts and scaly tinea versicolor–type lesions caused by a large number of unusual types. The latter are associated with the development of squamous cell cancer in sunexposed areas. Similar skin lesions and, rarely, associated skin cancers can develop in other patients with acquired defects in cell-mediated immunity. Other uncommon lesions caused by unique HPV types include butchers' warts (type 7), which are verrucous lesions found on the hands of meat handlers, and focal epithelial hyperplasia, which consists of flat mucosal lesions of the oropharynx (types 13 and 32).

The majority of genital HPV infections do not produce recognized lesions and remain subclinical, detected only by HPV DNA testing. Anogenital warts are papillomatous growths that occur throughout the anogenital skin and mucosa, generally at sites of genital friction. Perianal warts, which are more common in persons with a history of anal intercourse, are often associated with intra-anal warts but can occur without such contact, presumably through autoinoculation. The warts can range from flat or papular lesions to the classic pedunculated, cauliflower-shaped condyloma acuminatum. They are typically caused by low-risk types (>90% are due to HPV 6 or 11), although warts caused by high-risk or multiple types can occur in immunocompromised patients. Warts are typically asymptomatic, noticed either by the patient as a "bump" or inadvertently during a genital examination, although they can cause itching, burning, pain, or, rarely, bleeding or mechanical obstruction of the birth canal in pregnant women. Warts caused by genital types can also rarely occur in the mouth and upper respiratory tract, producing a serious condition known as recurrent respiratory papillomatosis, which can cause hoarseness and even airway compromise.

Squamous intraepithelial lesions are most commonly found on the cervix as a result of screening for cervical cancer precursors by cytology (Pap test) or HPV DNA testing, with confirmation by colposcopy and biopsy. Like warts, they also occur at other anogenital sites, and like cervical lesions, they are categorized either as low-grade or high-grade squamous intraepithelial lesions or as various stages of intraepithelial neoplasia (e.g., vulva—VIN; vagina—VaIN; anus—AIN; penis—PIN). At all sites, low-grade squamous intraepithelial lesions can be caused by either low- or high-risk types, whereas high-grade squamous intraepithelial lesions are primarily due to high-risk types. Most squamous intraepithelial lesions are not visible on mucosal surfaces without the application of 3 to 5% acetic acid and magnification, although they can appear as flat hyperpigmented papules known as bowenoid papulosis on the external genitalia.

DIAGNOSIS

Both cutaneous (Fig. 381-1) and genital (Fig. 381-2) warts generally present an easily recognized clinical picture and can be diagnosed by history and physical examination without laboratory testing. The application of 3 to 5% acetic acid causes whitening of HPV lesions on genital mucosa ("acetowhitening") and may be useful with magnification in women; however, because its sensitivity and specificity have not been defined, it is not recommended for routine use.

The differential diagnosis of cutaneous warts includes seborrheic and solar keratoses, nevi, irritated acrochordons, clavi, and squamous cell carcinoma (Chapters 210 and 448); lichen planus (Chapter 446) can mimic flat warts and calluses of the foot or plantar warts. Genital warts must also be distinguished from the condyloma latum lesions of secondary syphilis (Chapter 327) and molluscum contagiosum (Chapters 380 and 448). Biopsy for histopathologic examination may be helpful for lesions that are atypical or not responsive to therapy, those suggestive of high-grade squamous intraepithelial lesions or cancer (e.g., pigmented, indurated, fixed, bleeding, or ulcerated), or lesions in immunocompromised patients.

The principal approach to the diagnosis of cervical squamous intraepithelial lesions is cytologic screening, with assessment of abnormal results by colposcopy and biopsy for histopathologic examination. In the United States, the Digene Hybrid Capture 2 High-Risk HPV test (QIAGEN, Valencia, Calif) detects any of 13 high-risk types (16, 18, 31, 33, 35, 39, 45, 51, 52, 56, 58, 59, 68), whereas the Cervista HPV HR (Hologic, Inc., Bedford, Mass) detects the same 13 types as well as type 66. Results of both tests are reported as positive for any type or negative. Type-specific results are not available with these tests, but another assay (Cervista 16/18) can specifically identify HPV 16 and 18. HPV DNA testing is approved as an adjunct to cytology, referred to as the DNA Pap or HPV co-test, to enhance the sensitivity of screening in women older than 30 years but is not recommended for younger women. HPV DNA tests are also recommended for triage of women whose Pap test results show atypical squamous cells of undetermined significance, which is an equivocal test result (Chapter 205).

PREVENTION

Primary Prevention

Primary prevention of HPV infection depends on avoidance of contact with infectious lesions and reduction of susceptibility through immunization. For example, the use of footwear in locker rooms may prevent plantar warts. For genital HPV infection, avoidance of sexual contact is the most reliable preventive measure, but correct and consistent condom use can reduce the risk for both HPV infection and the HPV-associated diseases of genital warts, cervical squamous intraepithelial lesions, and cervical cancer. Male circumcision reduces the prevalence of both high-risk and low-risk types of genital HPV infection.[1]

Of greatest importance for prevention are newly licensed vaccines, composed of virus-like particles assembled from the major capsid protein, L1. The quadrivalent vaccine (types 6, 11, 16, and 18) given in three doses during a period of 6 months is highly effective for the prevention of CIN 1

TABLE 381-1 U.S. ADVISORY COMMITTEE ON IMMUNIZATION PRACTICES RECOMMENDATIONS FOR QUADRIVALENT (HPV 6, 11, 16, 18) and BIVALENT (HPV 16, 18) HPV VACCINES

Routine vaccination with quadrivalent or bivalent vaccine recommended in females aged 11-12 years, starting as young as 9 years

Catch-up vaccination recommended in females aged 13-26 years who have not previously received full vaccine series

Quadrivalent HPV vaccine may be given to males aged 9 to 26 years to reduce their likelihood of genital warts

Recommended dosage and schedule: 0.5 mL IM at 0, 2, and 6 months

Schedule modifications: if doses are missed, series does not need to be restarted, but second and third doses should be given as soon as possible

Cervical cancer screening: no change in recommended interval

Special situations: females with genital warts, abnormal Pap test results, or positive HPV test results are unlikely to be infected with all four vaccine types and should be immunized per other recommendations

Pregnant and lactating women: not recommended for use in pregnancy based on lack of data; may be used in lactating women

Immunocompromised persons: no safety concerns because vaccine is noninfectious, but immune response and effectiveness might be reduced

Not recommended for females or males <9 and >26 years

Modified from Markowitz LE, Dunne EF, Saraiya M, et al; Centers for Disease Control and Prevention. Quadrivalent human papillomavirus vaccine. Recommendations of the Advisory Committee on Immunization Practices. *MMWR.* 2007;56:1-24.
Centers for Disease Control and Prevention. FDA licensure of bivalent human papillomavirus vaccine (HPV2, Cervarix) for use in females and updated HPV vaccination recommendations from the Advisory Committee on Immunization Practices. *MMWR Morb Mortal Wkly Rep.* 2010;59:626-629.
Centers for Disease Control and Prevention. FDA licensure of quadrivalent human papillomavirus vaccine (HPV4, Gardasil) for use in males and guidance from the Advisory Committee on Immunization Practices. *MMWR Morb Mortal Wkly Rep.* 2010;59:630-632.

TABLE 381-2 RECOMMENDED TREATMENT OF GENITAL WARTS

Patient applied
   Podophyllotoxin (podofilox) 0.5% solution or gel; to be applied in up to 4 weekly cycles (bid for 3 days, followed by 4 days without treatment)
   Imiquimod 5% cream; to be applied once daily at bedtime 3 times per week for 6-10 hours for up to 16 weeks
   Sinecatechins 15% ointment; to be applied 3 times daily for up to 16 weeks
Provider administered
   Cryotherapy with liquid nitrogen or cryoprobe; to be applied once every 1-2 weeks*
   Podophyllin resin 10-25% in compound tincture of benzoin; to be applied once weekly
   Trichloroacetic or bichloroacetic acid 80-90% solution; to be applied once weekly*
   Office surgery* (excision, electrocautery, curettage)

*Safe for use in pregnancy.
Modified from Workowski KA, Berman SM; Centers for Disease Control and Prevention. Sexually transmitted disease treatment guidelines, 2010. *MMWR Morb Mortal Wkly Rep.* 2010;59(RR-12): 70-74.

TREATMENT   Rx

Management of HPV infection is directed toward diagnosis and treatment of the lesions themselves because there are no virus-specific therapies. Many lesions resolve spontaneously, so the goal of treatment is amelioration or prevention of symptoms or, in the case of high-grade squamous intraepithelial lesions, prevention of progression to cancer. Treatment generally involves destruction of lesions by physical techniques or topically applied or injected cytotoxic agents. Because treatment does not eradicate infection in surrounding tissues, recurrent lesions are common.

Treatment of warts depends on their location and size, the patient's preferences, and the provider's experience. Recommended first-line treatment of common, flat, and plantar warts includes the application of topical salicylic acid and cryotherapy; second-line treatment of recalcitrant lesions includes topical imiquimod (5% cream applied once daily at bedtime three times a week for up to 16 weeks), intralesional bleomycin, pulsed dye laser therapy, and surgical excision.[7] Recommended treatment of genital warts (Table 381-2) includes patient-applied podophyllotoxin (0.5 or 0.15% solution or gel applied twice a day for 3 days, repeated weekly for four cycles), imiquimod, or sinecatechins and provider-administered cryotherapy, podophyllin, trichloroacetic acid, or surgical excision; alternative treatments include intralesional interferon and laser surgery.

For cervical lesions, treatment depends on histologic staging after colposcopy and biopsy and on the clinical context. Because CIN 1 usually regresses spontaneously, conservative management with close follow-up is recommended with either HPV DNA testing every 12 months or cervical cytology every 6 to 12 months. Treatment is generally recommended for all CIN 2/3 lesions, except in adolescents and pregnant women, who have higher rates of spontaneous regression and a greater risk of reproductive tract complications after treatment. Treatment options include a variety of ablative and excisional techniques such as cryosurgery, loop electrosurgical excision procedure, and laser surgery.

PROGNOSIS

Although the natural history of HPV infection is not fully characterized, the large majority of infections and premalignant lesions are self-limited in most immunocompetent patients. Whether infections no longer detectable have been cleared by the immune system or remain latent in the basal layer of the epithelium with the potential for reactivation is not clear, but the higher prevalence of detectable infection in advanced than in early HIV infection supports the possibility of long-term infection. Many if not most clinical lesions resolve spontaneously, presumably as a result of the development of cell-mediated immunity. Spontaneous regression is estimated to occur in 25% of genital warts and more than 50% of common warts in children.

The natural history of CIN has been most intensively studied because of its relationship to cervical cancer, although many questions remain unanswered. Estimates of the likelihood of regression versus the risk of progression to invasive cancer are 60% and 1% for CIN 1, 40% and 5% for CIN 2, and 32% and 12% for CIN 3. Traditionally, the various stages of precursor lesions have been viewed as a biologic continuum, with CIN 1 progressing through higher grades to invasive cancer. However, emerging data indicate that low-grade squamous intraepithelial lesions and high-grade squamous intraepithelial lesions may be distinct processes, in which low-grade lesions

and CIN 2/3 as well as genital warts and VaIN and VIN, caused by any of the four types.[2] A bivalent vaccine (types 16 and 18) provides a high level of protection against CIN but not genital warts.[3] Both vaccines are recommended for the routine immunization of 11- to 12-year-old girls as well as females 13 to 26 years of age; girls 9 to 10 years of age may also be vaccinated at the discretion of the provider (Table 381-1). The vaccines have no therapeutic benefit against existing infection or lesions, and they are most effective if given before initiation of sexual activity. Because they provide protection against only two of the high-risk types associated with cancer, immunized women will continue to need Pap test screening. The quadrivalent vaccine is also recommended in males aged 9 to 26 years, in whom it reduces the likelihood of genital warts. Although men experience fewer HPV-related cancers than women do, the vaccine is likely to be particularly beneficial in preventing AIN in men who have sex with men on the basis of their high incidence of anal cancer. The quadrivalent vaccine is also effective in preventing HPV infection and disease in males.[4]

Secondary Prevention

Screening plus treatment of high-grade cervical squamous intraepithelial lesions is one of the most successful of all cancer prevention strategies. Current guidelines in the United States vary slightly among recommending organizations, but all agree that screening should begin within 3 years of initiation of sexual activity or by the age of 21 years and continue at 1- to 3-year intervals. Women older than 30 years who have had three negative Pap test results can be screened less frequently (e.g., every 2 to 3 years). Because of the higher sensitivity of the DNA Pap test, some groups recommend that women who are negative by both tests be screened no more frequently than every 3 years. Among women older than 30 years, HPV DNA testing appears to be more sensitive than cytology for detection of high-grade lesions and cancer,[5,6] thereby suggesting a potential shift in screening approaches. Assessment by colposcopy and biopsy is recommended for most abnormal results, although women with atypical squamous cells of undetermined significance can be managed safely without colposcopy if an HPV DNA test result is negative.

The value of cytologic screening for anal intraepithelial lesions in HIV-positive men who have sex with men is controversial but not currently recommended because of limited data on the natural history of these precursor lesions, the reliability of screening methods, and the safety and effectiveness of treatment.

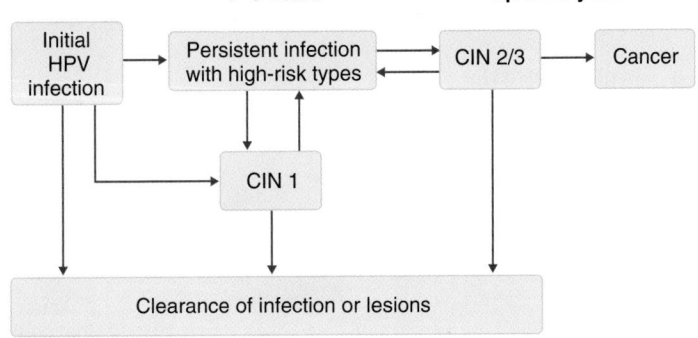

1–5 Years   **Up to 20 years**

Risk factors for infection
- Younger age
- Increasing number of lifetime sex partners
- Lack of circumcision
- Lack of consistent condom use
- Not immunized

Initial HPV infection → Persistent infection with high-risk types ⇄ CIN 2/3 → Cancer

CIN 1

Clearance of infection or lesions

Cofactors for disease progression
- Hormonal exposure (long-term oral contraceptive use)
- Multiparity
- Other STIs (e.g., *Chlamydia trachomatis*, HSV-2)
- Smoking
- Nutritional deficiency
- Host genetics (e.g., polymorphisms in HLA and other genes)
- Deficiency of cell-mediated immunity
- Lack of Pap test screening

FIGURE 381-3. Natural history of genital human papillomavirus (HPV) infection and cervical cancer. CIN = cervical intraepithelial neoplasia; HSV = herpes simplex virus; STIs = sexually transmitted infections.

(CIN 1) represent a usually transient productive infection characterized by the production of capsid protein (and probably infectious virions) and only minor cellular abnormalities, whereas high-grade lesions (CIN 2/3) represent proliferation of immature cells as a result of the activity of oncogenic proteins of high-risk types. In this model (Fig. 381-3), initial infection frequently leads to a transient low-grade squamous intraepithelial lesion and less frequently to persistent infection. Persistent infection can, in turn, lead directly to high-grade squamous intraepithelial lesions within several years of initial infection and can progress to invasive cancer during a period of several decades. The natural history of squamous intraepithelial lesions at other anogenital sites is less well defined, but they may be associated with higher rates of regression.

Immunodeficient patients, such as those with HIV infection, have a lower rate of spontaneous regression of squamous intraepithelial lesions and may have a higher rate of progression to cancer. Whether antiretroviral therapy reduces the risk of progression of HPV-associated lesions in HIV-infected persons is unresolved, but current data indicate that it may reduce incidence of genital warts and progression of CIN but not the risk of high-grade AIN or VIN or of cervical or anal cancer.

Grade A

1. Tobian AAR, Serwadda D, Quinn TC, et al. Male circumcision for the prevention of HSV-2 and HPV infections and syphilis. *N Engl J Med.* 2009;360:1298-1309.
2. Munoz N, Kjaer SK, Sigurdsson K, et al. Impact of human papillomavirus (HPV)-6/11/16/18 vaccine on all HPV-associated genital diseases in young women. *J Nat Cancer Inst.* 2010;102: 325-339.
3. Paavonen J, Salmeron J, Wheeler CM, et al. Efficacy of human papillomavirus (HPV)–16/18 AS04-adjuvanted vaccine against cervical infection and precancer caused by oncogenic HPV types (PATRICIA): final analysis of a double-blind, randomised study in young women. *Lancet.* 2009; 374:301-313.
4. Giuliano AR, Palefsky JM, Goldstone S, et al. Efficacy of quadrivalent HPV vaccine against HPV infection and disease in males. *N Engl J Med.* 2011;364:401-411.
5. Mayrand MH, Duarte-Franco E, Rodrigues I, et al. Human papillomavirus DNA versus Papanicolaou screening tests for cervical cancer. *N Engl J Med.* 2007;357:1579-1588.
6. Ronco G, Giorgi-Rossi P, Carozzi F, et al. Efficacy of human papillomavirus testing for the detection of invasive cervical cancers and cervical intraepithelial neoplasia: a randomised controlled trial. *Lancet Oncol.* 2010;11:249-257.
7. Gibbs S, Harvey I, Sterling JC, et al. Local treatments for cutaneous warts. *Cochrane Database Syst Rev.* 2004;4:CD001781.

SUGGESTED READINGS

Romanowski B. Long term protection against cervical infection with the human papillomavirus: review of currently available vaccines. *Human Vaccines.* 2011;7:161-169. *Review of duration of protection of quadrivalent and bivalent HPV vaccines.*
Roteli-Martins CM, de Carvalho NS, Naud P, et al. Prevalence of human papillomavirus infection and associated risk factors in young women in Brazil, Canada, and the United States: a multicenter cross-sectional study. *Int J Gynecol Pathol.* 2011;30:173-184. *The prevalence of oncogenic strains is about 20% in all three countries and is directly linked to sexual behavior.*
Workowski KA, Berman SM; Centers for Disease Control and Prevention. Sexually transmitted disease treatment guidelines, 2010. *MMWR.* 2010;59(RR-12):70-74. *CDC recommendations for treatment of genital warts.*

382

HERPES SIMPLEX VIRUS INFECTIONS

RICHARD J. WHITLEY

DEFINITION

The Pathogen

Herpes simplex virus (HSV), a member of the family Herpesviridae, has been implicated in human infections since descriptions of cutaneous spreading lesions in ancient Greek times. Scholars of Greek civilization defined *herpes* to mean "to creep or crawl," in reference to the spreading nature of the observed skin lesions. More recently, infection has been defined by the spectrum of illnesses caused by HSV. In 1968, well-defined antigenic and biologic differences were demonstrated between HSV type 1 (HSV-1) and HSV type 2 (HSV-2). Of all the herpesviruses, HSV-1 and HSV-2 are most closely related, with approximately 60% genomic homology. Historically, HSV-1 was more frequently associated with nongenital infection and HSV-2 with genital disease, but these distinctions are much less relevant now. These two viruses can be distinguished most reliably by DNA restriction enzyme analysis, but differences in antigen expression and biologic properties also serve as methods for differentiation.

Inclusion in the family Herpesviridae is based on the structure of the virion (Fig. 382-1). HSV contains double-stranded DNA at its central core, has a molecular weight of approximately 100 million, and encodes at least 80 polypeptides. The DNA core is surrounded by a capsid that consists of 162 capsomers arranged in icosahedral symmetry. The capsid is 100 to 110 nm in diameter. Tightly adherent to the capsid is the tegument, which consists of amorphous material. Loosely surrounding the capsid and tegument is a lipid bilayer envelope derived from host cell membranes. The envelope consists of polyamines, lipids, and glycoproteins. These glycoproteins confer distinctive properties to the virus and provide unique antigens to which the host is capable of responding. Notably, glycoprotein G (gG) provides antigenic specificity to HSV and therefore results in an antibody response that allows distinction between HSV-1 (gG-1) and HSV-2 (gG-2).

EPIDEMIOLOGY

HSV infections occur worldwide and have been reported in both developed and underdeveloped countries. Animal vectors for human HSV infections have not been described, and there is no seasonal variation in the incidence of HSV infections. HSV is transmitted from infected to susceptible individuals during close personal contact, and the virus must come in contact with mucosal surfaces or abraded skin for infection to be initiated. Because approximately a third of the world's population has recurrent HSV infections and because infection is rarely fatal, a large reservoir of HSV exists in the community.

Seroprevalence studies have demonstrated that acquisition of HSV-1 infection is related to socioeconomic factors. Antibodies, which indicate past

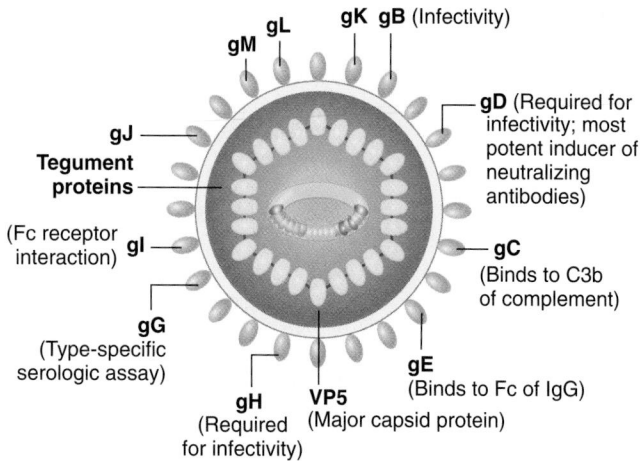

FIGURE 382-1. Schematic diagram of the herpes simplex virion.

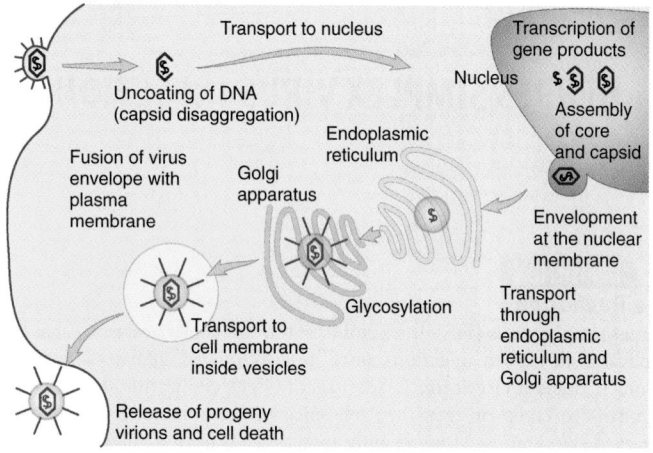

FIGURE 382-2. Schematic diagram of replication of herpes simplex virus.

FIGURE 382-3. Schematic diagram of primary herpes simplex virus infection.

infection, are found early in life among individuals of lower socioeconomic groups, presumably a consequence of crowded living conditions that provide a greater opportunity for direct contact with infected individuals. Antibodies develop in as many as 75 to 90% of individuals from lower socioeconomic populations by the end of the first decade of life. In contrast, only 30 to 40% of persons in the middle and upper socioeconomic groups are seropositive by the middle of the second decade of life.

Because infections with HSV-2 are usually acquired through sexual contact, antibodies to this virus are rarely found until the onset of sexual activity. There is a progressive increase in infection rates with HSV-2 in all populations beginning in adolescence. Overall, about one in five Americans has genital HSV-2 infection. As with HSV-1 infections, the rate of acquisition of HSV-2 infection appears to be related to socioeconomic factors. The number of sexual partners is also an important risk factor for the acquisition of HSV-2. Genital herpes infection has been found to be a risk factor for another sexually transmitted virus, human immunodeficiency virus (HIV; Chapter 394).

Localized, recurrent HSV-2 infection is the most common form of HSV infection during gestation. Transmission of infection to the fetus is most frequently related to shedding of the virus at the time of delivery. The incidence of cervical shedding in pregnant women with asymptomatic HSV infection is approximately 1%. Most infants in whom neonatal disease develops are born to women who are completely asymptomatic for genital HSV infection at the time of delivery and who have neither a past history of genital herpes nor a sexual partner reporting a genital vesicular rash. These women account for 60 to 80% of all women whose children acquire neonatal HSV infection.

PATHOBIOLOGY

Replication of HSV is a multistep process (Fig. 382-2). After the onset of infection, DNA is uncoated and transported to the nucleus of the host cell. This step is followed by transcription of immediate-early genes, which encode the regulatory proteins, and is followed by the expression of proteins encoded

by early and then late genes. These proteins include enzymes necessary for viral replication and structural proteins.

Assembly of the viral core and capsid takes place within the nucleus. Envelopment at the nuclear membrane and transport out of the nucleus occur through the endoplasmic reticulum and the Golgi apparatus. Glycosylation of the viral membrane occurs in the Golgi apparatus. Mature virions are transported to the outer membrane of the host cell inside vesicles. Release of progeny virus is accompanied by cell death. Replication for all herpesviruses is considered inefficient, with a high ratio of noninfectious to infectious viral particles.

A critical factor for transmission of HSV, regardless of virus type, is intimate contact between a person who is shedding virus and a susceptible host. With inoculation onto skin or mucous membranes, HSV replicates in epithelial cells; the incubation period is 4 to 6 days (Fig. 382-3). As replication continues, cell lysis and local inflammation ensue and result in the characteristic vesicles on an erythematous base. Regional lymphatics and lymph nodes become involved as a result of draining of infected secretions from the area of viral replication. Viremia and visceral dissemination may develop, depending on the immunologic competence of the host. In all hosts, the virus generally ascends peripheral sensory nerves to reach the dorsal root ganglia. Replication of HSV within neural tissue is followed by spread of the virus to other mucosal and skin surfaces by means of peripheral sensory nerves. HSV replicates further in epithelial cells and reproduces the lesions of the initial infection until infection is contained through host immune responses.

The histopathologic changes induced by HSV replication are similar in both primary and recurrent infection. Changes induced by viral infection include ballooning of infected cells and the appearance of condensed chromatin within the nuclei of cells, followed by subsequent degeneration of cellular nuclei. Cells lose intact plasma membranes and form multinucleated giant cells. They may also demonstrate intranuclear inclusions known as Cowdry type A bodies, which are suggestive but not diagnostic of HSV infection. With cell lysis, clear vesicular fluid containing large quantities of virus accumulates between the epidermis and dermal layer. The dermis reveals an intense inflammatory response, more so with primary infection than with recurrent disease. As healing progresses, the clear vesicular fluid becomes pustular with the recruitment of inflammatory cells. The pustule then forms a scab; scarring is uncommon.

Vascular changes in the area of infection include perivascular cuffing and hemorrhagic necrosis. These changes are particularly prominent when organs other than skin are involved, as is the case with herpes simplex encephalitis or disseminated neonatal HSV infection. Local lymphatics can show evidence of infection with intrusion of inflammatory cells because of draining of infected secretions from the area of viral replication. As host defenses are mounted, an influx of mononuclear cells can be detected in infected tissue.

A unique characteristic of all herpesviruses is their ability to establish latent infection, to persist in an apparently inactive state for varying amounts of time, and then to be reactivated (Fig. 382-4). The latent viral genome may be either extrachromosomal or integrated into host cell DNA, depending on the virus.

Dorsal root ganglia

Latent viral genome (may be integrated or extrachromosomal)

Stimulus for reactivation (stress, UV light, etc.)

Viral replication

Transport along peripheral sensory nerves

Replication in the epithelium with the production of vesicles

FIGURE 382-4. Schematic diagram of herpes simplex virus latency and reactivation. UV = ultraviolet.

FIGURE 382-5. Herpes labialis, classic grouped blisters.

Latency is established when HSV reaches the dorsal root ganglia after retrograde transmission through sensory nerve pathways. Latent virus may be reactivated and enter a replicative cycle at any point in time. Reactivation of latent virus is a well-recognized biologic phenomenon but not one that is understood from a molecular standpoint. Stimuli associated with the reactivation of latent HSV have included stress, menstruation, and exposure to ultraviolet light. Precisely how these factors interact at the level of the ganglia remains to be defined. Reactivation may be clinically asymptomatic, or it may produce life-threatening disease.

CLINICAL MANIFESTATIONS

Gingivostomatitis

Gingivostomatitis (usually caused by HSV-1) occurs most frequently in children younger than 5 years. Illness is characterized by fever, sore throat, pharyngeal edema, and erythema, followed by the development of vesicular or ulcerative lesions on the oral and pharyngeal mucosa. Recurrent HSV-1 infections of the oropharynx are most frequently manifested as herpes simplex labialis (cold sores) and usually appear on the vermilion border of the lip (Fig. 382-5). Recurrences are triggered by fever, stress, and exposure to ultraviolet light as well as by other factors. Intraoral lesions as a manifestation of recurrent disease are uncommon.

Genital Herpes

Genital herpes is most frequently caused by HSV-2. However, an increasing percentage is being caused by HSV-1. Indeed, among all new primary cases in young adults, approximately 50% are caused by HSV-1. Primary infection in women usually involves the vulva, vagina, and cervix. In men, initial infection is most often associated with lesions on the glans penis, prepuce, or penile shaft. In individuals of either gender, primary disease is associated with fever, malaise, anorexia, and bilateral inguinal adenopathy. Women frequently have dysuria and urinary retention as a result of urethral involvement. Aseptic meningitis develops in as many as 10% of individuals with primary infection. Sacral radiculomyelitis may occur in both men and women and results in neuralgias, urinary retention, or obstipation. Complete healing of primary infection may take several weeks. The first episode of genital infection is less severe in individuals who have previously had HSV-1 infections at other sites. Antibodies to HSV-1 appear to ameliorate the expression of HSV-2 clinical disease, although this effect is controversial.

Recurrent genital infections in either men or women can be particularly distressing. The frequency of recurrence varies significantly from one individual to another. Of note, viral DNA can be detected by polymerase chain reaction (PCR) in genital secretions three- to four-fold more frequently than symptomatic recurrences. Furthermore, recurrences detected by PCR can occur frequently during 24 hours and persist for brief periods. A third of infected individuals have virtually no or few clinical recurrences, a third have approximately three recurrences per year, and another third have more than three per year. Several seroepidemiologic studies have found that between 25 and 65% of individuals in the United States have antibodies to HSV-2 and that seroprevalence is correlated with the number of sexual partners.

Herpetic Keratitis

Herpes simplex keratitis is usually caused by HSV-1 and is accompanied by conjunctivitis in many cases. It is considered the most common infectious cause of blindness in the United States. The characteristic lesions of HSV keratoconjunctivitis are dendritic ulcers best detected by fluorescein staining. Deep stromal involvement has also been reported and may result in visual impairment.

Other Cutaneous Manifestations

HSV infections can occur at any skin site. Common among health care workers are lesions on abraded skin or the fingers, known as herpetic whitlow. Similarly, in wrestlers, disseminated cutaneous lesions known as herpes gladiatorum may develop as a result of physical contact.

HERPES SIMPLEX VIRUS INFECTIONS IN IMMUNOCOMPROMISED HOSTS

HSV infections in immunocompromised hosts, including patients with acquired immunodeficiency syndrome, are usually due to reactivation of latent infection and are clinically more severe, may be progressive, and require a longer time to heal. Manifestations of HSV infections in this population of patients include pneumonitis, esophagitis, hepatitis, colitis, and disseminated cutaneous disease. Individuals suffering from HIV infection may have extensive perineal or orofacial ulcerations. HSV infections are also noted to be of increased severity in individuals with extensive burns.

DIAGNOSIS

Definitive diagnosis of HSV infection requires isolation of virus. Swabs of clinical specimens or other body fluids can be inoculated into susceptible cell lines and observed for the development of characteristic cytopathic effects. This technique is useful for the diagnosis of HSV-1 and HSV-2 infection because of their short replicative cycles.

In the absence of diagnostic virology facilities, cytologic examination of cells scraped from a clinical lesion may be useful in making a presumptive diagnosis of HSV infection. Material obtained from scraping the base of a lesion should be smeared on a glass slide and promptly fixed in cold ethanol. The slide can be stained according to the methods of Papanicolaou, Giemsa, or Wright. The presence of intranuclear inclusions and multinucleated giant cells is indicative but not diagnostic of HSV infection. This method has a sensitivity of only 60 to 70% and should not be the sole diagnostic method used.

DNA amplification by PCR has gained greater acceptance for routine diagnostic purposes. DNA amplification has become the diagnostic method of choice in assessing cerebrospinal fluid (CSF) specimens for evidence of HSV infection of the central nervous system. Furthermore, PCR has significantly improved sensitivity for confirmation of HSV as the cause of lip and genital herpes infection.

In addition to new tests for viral DNA, type-specific serologic assays are commercially available. These tests are based on differences in HSV-1 and HSV-2 gG.

TREATMENT

For *immunocompromised* patients, such as patients with cancer or receiving immunosuppressive drugs, with mucocutaneous infections or for patients with herpes encephalitis, intravenous acyclovir (5 mg/kg every 8 hours for 5 to 7 days) is the treatment of choice.**1** Caution must be exercised when acyclovir is used intravenously because it may crystallize in the renal tubules when it is given too rapidly or to dehydrated patients. Valacyclovir (500 to 1000 mg two or three times daily) and famciclovir (250 to 500 mg three times daily), depending on severity, are equally efficacious**2** and have improved pharmacokinetics as demonstrated by improved biodistribution and less frequent dosing compared with oral acyclovir. Thus, they should preferentially be used for the treatment of non–life-threatening HSV infection. For life-threatening disease, only intravenous medications should be given. Immunocompromised individuals with non–life-threatening mucocutaneous HSV infections may be given oral acyclovir (400 mg two or three times daily for 7 to 10 days), valacyclovir (500 to 1000 mg once or twice daily for 3 to 5 days), or famciclovir (250 to 500 mg three times daily for 7 days or 1000 mg twice daily for 1 day).

In *immunocompetent* hosts with mucocutaneous infections, oral acyclovir (200 mg five times daily for 5 days) reduces lesions and speeds recovery. Oral valacyclovir (1 g/day for 5 days or 500 mg twice daily for 3 days) and oral famciclovir (1 g twice daily for 1 day) are equally effective. **3-5** In general, recurrent episodes are not as responsive to treatment as first episodes are. Topical acyclovir is not as reliable as oral acyclovir and is not recommended.

HSV has been used for experimental gene therapy. By removal of the $\gamma_1 34.5$ gene, both neurovirulence and the propensity to establish latency are ablated. These engineered viruses are being experimentally tested in patients with glioblastoma multiforme and colorectal metastases to liver.

PREVENTION

Some patients with particularly disabling oral recurrences, genital recurrences, or aseptic meningitis triggered by genital recurrences are candidates for chronic suppressive therapy. Potential regimens include oral acyclovir 400 mg twice daily, oral valacyclovir 1 g/day, and oral famciclovir 250 mg twice daily. Such regimens are approved by the Food and Drug Administration for genital herpes but not for herpes labialis.

At present, experimental vaccines for HSV-1 and HSV-2 remain under investigation. Acyclovir, valacyclovir, and famciclovir are given to recipients of solid organ and bone marrow transplants in the immediate post-transplantation period in an effort to prevent reactivation of latent disease at the doses noted before. Valacyclovir (500 mg daily) decreases person-to-person transmission of HSV-2.

HERPES SIMPLEX ENCEPHALITIS

Herpes simplex encephalitis is characterized by hemorrhagic necrosis of the temporal lobe (Chapter 422). Disease begins unilaterally and spreads to the contralateral temporal lobe (Fig. 382-6). It is the most common cause of focal, sporadic encephalitis in the United States today and occurs in approximately 1 in 150,000 individuals. Most cases are caused by HSV-1. The actual pathogenesis of herpes simplex encephalitis requires further clarification, although it has been speculated that primary or recurrent virus can reach the temporal lobe by ascending neural pathways, such as the trigeminal tracts or the olfactory nerves.

CLINICAL MANIFESTATIONS AND DIAGNOSIS

Clinical manifestations of herpes simplex encephalitis include headache, fever, altered consciousness, and abnormalities in speech and behavior, findings characteristic of temporal lobe involvement. Focal seizures also may occur. CSF findings in these patients are variable but usually consist of a pleocytosis with both polymorphonuclear leukocytes and monocytes present. The protein concentration is characteristically elevated, and the glucose level is usually normal. Magnetic resonance imaging can suggest the diagnosis by demonstrating edema of either temporal lobe. Diagnosis can be confirmed by PCR detection of HSV DNA in the CSF by experienced laboratories.

FIGURE 382-6. Hemorrhagic necrosis in herpes simplex encephalitis.

TREATMENT AND PROGNOSIS

Mortality and morbidity are high, even with appropriate acyclovir antiviral therapy. At present, the mortality rate is approximately 30% 1 year after treatment. In addition, approximately 50% of survivors have moderate or severe neurologic impairment.

● NEONATAL HERPES SIMPLEX VIRUS INFECTION

Neonatal HSV infection is estimated to occur in approximately 1 in 3500 deliveries in the United States each year. Approximately 70% of cases are caused by HSV-2 and usually result from contact of the fetus with infected maternal genital secretions at the time of delivery. Manifestations of neonatal HSV infection can be divided into three categories: skin, eye, and mouth disease; encephalitis; and disseminated infection. As the name implies, skin, eye, and mouth disease consists of cutaneous lesions and does not involve other organ systems. Involvement of the central nervous system may occur with encephalitis or disseminated infection and generally results in diffuse encephalitis. CSF assay characteristically reveals elevated protein levels and mononuclear pleocytosis. Disseminated infection involves multiple organ systems and can cause disseminated intravascular coagulation, hemorrhagic pneumonitis, encephalitis, and cutaneous lesions. Diagnosis is difficult in the absence of skin lesions, which occurs in as many as 36% of cases. The mortality rate for each disease classification varies from zero for skin, eye, and mouth disease to 5% for encephalitis and 25% for neonates with disseminated infection, even with appropriate antiviral treatment. In addition to the high mortality associated with these infections, morbidity is significant in that children with encephalitis or disseminated disease develop normally in only 40% of cases, even with appropriate antiviral therapy (acyclovir, 10 mg/kg every 8 hours for 14 days for skin, eye, and mouth infections and 21 days for central nervous system or disseminated disease).

1. Watts DH, Brown ZA, Money D, et al. A double-blind, randomized, placebo-controlled trial of acyclovir in late pregnancy for the reduction of herpes simplex virus shedding and cesarean delivery. *Am J Obstet Gynecol.* 2003;188:836-843.
2. Glenny AM, Fernandez Mauleffinch LM, Pavitt S, et al. Interventions for the prevention and treatment of herpes simplex virus in patients being treated for cancer. *Cochrane Database Syst Rev.* 2009;1:CD006706.
3. Cernik C, Gallina K, Brodell RT, et al. Treatment of herpes simplex infections. *Arch Intern Med.* 2008;168:1137-1144.
4. Abudalu M, Tyring S, Koltun W, et al. Single-day, patient-initiated famciclovir therapy versus 3-day valacyclovir regimen for recurrent genital herpes: a randomized, double-blind, comparative trial. *Clin Infect Dis.* 2008;47:651-658.
5. Corey L, Wald A, Patel R, et al. Once daily valacyclovir to reduce the risk of transmission of genital herpes. *N Engl J Med.* 2004;350:11-20.

SUGGESTED READINGS

Centers for Disease Control and Prevention. Seroprevalence of herpes simplex virus type 2 among persons aged 14-49 years—United States, 2005-2008. *MMWR Morb Mortal Wkly Rep.* 2010;59: 456-459. *Seroprevalence is 16%.*
Corey L, Wald A. Maternal and neonatal herpes simplex virus infections. *N Engl J Med.* 2009;361:1376-1385. *Review.*
Gardella C, Brown Z. Prevention of neonatal herpes. *BJOG.* 2011;118:187-192. *Review of maternal treatment and neonatal risks.*
Patel R, Alderson S, Geretti A, et al. European guideline for the management of genital herpes, 2010. *Int J STD AIDS.* 2011;22:1-10. *Review including consensus guidelines.*

383

VARICELLA-ZOSTER VIRUS (CHICKENPOX, SHINGLES)

JEFFREY COHEN

DEFINITION

Primary infection with varicella-zoster virus (VZV) results in the rash of varicella (chickenpox). The virus establishes a latent infection in the nervous system and can reactivate later in life to cause zoster (shingles).

The Pathogen

VZV is a member of the alphaherpesvirus family and has a DNA core surrounded by a nucleocapsid, which is in turn surrounded by a viral envelope that is studded with glycoproteins. Antibody to viral glycoproteins is important for neutralizing the virus's infectivity and for protecting against primary infection. The virus encodes a thymidine kinase, which phosphorylates acyclovir, which in turn inhibits viral DNA replication by inhibiting the VZV DNA polymerase.

EPIDEMIOLOGY

Before the advent of an effective vaccine, more than 95% of children in temperate climates were infected with VZV. By comparison, infection is usually delayed until adulthood in tropical climates. Varicella usually occurs in children younger than 5 years. Zoster is less common in tropical areas, probably because of a delay in acquisition of varicella. Varicella is more common in the winter and spring, whereas zoster has no seasonal predilection.

Primary varicella infection can occur after exposure to either chickenpox or zoster. The virus is spread by droplets and aerosols from patients or by contact with vesicular lesions. Persons are infectious beginning about 2 days before the rash appears and continuing until all lesions have crusted. Although 60 to 90% of susceptible household contacts develop varicella, only 20 to 30% of susceptible persons exposed to zoster become infected. More than 95% of primary infections result in the symptoms of varicella, and second episodes of varicella are rare. Varicella is more severe in persons with impaired cellular immunity, including patients with acquired immunodeficiency syndrome (AIDS) and infants whose mothers present with varicella 5 days before to 2 days after delivery.

About 30% of persons who have had varicella will develop zoster. The risk of zoster rises with increasing age (especially 50 years of age and older) and with increasing impairment of cellular immunity. For example, men with AIDS have a 20-fold higher risk for development of zoster than that of age-matched controls. Less than 5% of persons have a second episode of zoster, but recurrent zoster is more common in persons with impaired cellular immunity.

PATHOBIOLOGY

Varicella is transmitted by the respiratory route. The virus is thought to infect epithelial cells and lymphocytes in the oropharynx and upper respiratory tract or in the conjunctiva, and then infected lymphocytes subsequently spread the virus throughout the body. The virus then enters the skin through endothelial cells in blood vessels and spreads to epithelial cells, where it causes the vesicular rash of varicella. Lesions initially are vesicular but become pustular after the infiltration of inflammatory cells. Later the lesions break open and dry to form crusts that usually heal without scarring. During primary infection, neurons in cranial nerve ganglia and dorsal root ganglia become latently infected with the virus.

If VZV-specific cellular immunity declines, the virus can reactivate from a ganglion, travel down the axon, and replicate in epithelial cells to cause dermatomal zoster. In highly immunocompromised persons, high-grade viremia during reactivation causes disseminated zoster.

Antibodies, which usually are present at the time varicella presents clinically, persist for life. Antibody is important for protection against varicella, as evidenced by the ability of varicella immune globulin to attenuate the disease. Cytotoxic T cells are present within 2 to 3 days after the onset of varicella and limit its severity. Varicella is more severe in persons with impaired cellular immunity but not in patients with hypogammaglobulinemia. Cellular immunity, not antibody, is required to prevent reactivation of virus and zoster.

CLINICAL MANIFESTATIONS

Varicella

Varicella begins with fever and malaise followed 1 to 2 days later by a disseminated, pruritic, vesicular rash (Fig. 383-1). The usual incubation period for varicella is 2 weeks (range, 10 to 21 days) after exposure to an infected person. The lesions begin as papules that become vesicles, followed by pustules and then crusts. Lesions appear on the head and then spread to the trunk and then to the extremities; the mucosa can also be involved. There are typically 200 to 500 lesions in different stages on the skin. New lesions occur for up to 5 days in normal hosts, and crusting is complete within 2 weeks.

The most common complication of varicella is bacterial superinfection of skin lesions. Group A streptococcus (Chapter 298) or *Staphylococcus aureus* (Chapter 296) infections can cause cellulitis, bacteremia, and necrotizing

FIGURE 383-1. Child with varicella. (Courtesy of Centers for Disease Control and Prevention.)

FIGURE 383-2. Dermatomal zoster. (Courtesy of Centers for Disease Control and Prevention.)

fasciitis. Other complications include cerebellar ataxia, viral pneumonitis, hepatitis, and thrombocytopenia. Less frequent complications include viral meningitis, encephalitis, vasculopathy (which presents as a stroke), disseminated intravascular coagulopathy (Chapter 178), and Reye's syndrome (more common in children receiving aspirin). Complications involving the lungs and liver are more common in children with impaired cellular immunity including those receiving systemic steroids, children with chronic pulmonary or skin disease, adults, and pregnant women during the third trimester. The fetal varicella syndrome, which occurs in fetuses infected during the first trimester, is characterized by atrophy of limbs with scarring of skin, chorioretinitis or cataracts, and central nervous system abnormalities. Patients with AIDS and moderately reduced CD4 cell counts may develop recurrent varicella lesions in the absence of new exposures, and patients with CD4 cell counts below 200/mm^3 may develop progressive varicella with new lesions occurring for at least 1 month or chronic verrucous lesions.

Zoster

In healthy persons, zoster presents with localized pain and increased sensation for 1 to 3 days before the development of a dermatomal vesicular rash that does not cross the midline (Fig. 383-2). Zoster most frequently presents in the dermatomes innervated by trigeminal or thoracic ganglia. The rash is usually accompanied by itching, tingling, or pain. The lesions evolve from vesicles to pustules, and crusting is usually complete by 10 days. In normal hosts, a few lesions may develop outside of the dermatome owing to low-grade viremia. Some patients with zoster sine herpete never develop a rash. In persons with very impaired cellular immunity, reactivation is often associated with high-grade viremia with dissemination to large areas of the skin and involvement of multiple organs.

A dreaded complication of zoster is postherpetic neuralgia (Chapter 29) with pain persisting for at least 1 month after the rash has resolved. Patients may have allodynia (sensation of pain after nonpainful stimuli), paresthesias, dysesthesias, or severe neuropathic pain. Postherpetic neuralgia is more common in persons older than 50 years. Other complications of zoster include bacterial superinfection; ocular disease, involving any of the structures of the eye, due to reactivation in the ophthalmic branch of the trigeminal ganglia; facial palsy caused by reactivation in the VII cranial nerve; Ramsay Hunt syndrome, with pain and vesicles in the ear, numbness of the anterior tongue, and ipsilateral facial palsy due to reactivation in the geniculate ganglion of the VII cranial nerve; motor neuropathy; and meningitis. Zoster vasculopathy, occurring at the time of zoster or a few months later, can present with stroke due to inflammation of the cerebral arteries.

Progressive outer retinal necrosis, with few inflammatory ocular cells, occurs when VZV reactivates in the eye of severely immunocompromised persons, including patients with AIDS and low CD4 cell counts. In contrast, acute retinal necrosis with a marked inflammatory response occurs when the virus reactivates in otherwise healthy persons. Patients with AIDS or recipients of hematopoietic stem cell transplants can have pancreatitis, hepatitis, and pneumonitis in the absence of or preceding a rash.

DIAGNOSIS

Most cases of varicella and zoster are diagnosed on the basis of their clinical presentation. A disseminated vesicular rash with lesions in various stages of evolution is usually sufficient for a diagnosis of varicella. The differential diagnosis includes impetigo (Chapter 449), enterovirus infections (Chapter 387), herpes simplex (Chapter 382), Stevens-Johnson syndrome (Chapter 448), and guttate psoriasis (Chapter 446). A dermatomal vesicular rash that does not cross the midline in a patient with a prior history of pain in the area is usually diagnostic of zoster. Herpes simplex is the most common disease that resembles zoster.

When the diagnosis of varicella or zoster must be confirmed definitively, polymerase chain reaction (PCR) for VZV from vesicular fluid is the most sensitive and specific test. PCR for VZV in the blood can be useful for diagnosis of visceral zoster in highly immunocompromised persons before the onset of rash. PCR for VZV in the cerebrospinal fluid and intrathecal synthesis of VZV-specific antibody is useful for diagnosis of VZV neurologic diseases. Culture is less sensitive than PCR because the virus is very labile. Direct fluorescent antibody testing of vesicle fluid is rapid and sensitive. Detection of multinucleated giant cells (Tzanck smear) is less specific because lesions of herpes simplex virus have a similar appearance. Biopsy specimens show eosinophilic intranuclear inclusion bodies and multinucleate giant cells.

Serology for VZV is useful to determine the need for postexposure prophylaxis in persons who are at high risk for disease after exposure to varicella or zoster. Enzyme-linked immunosorbent assay tests are less sensitive than latex agglutination assays and may not detect antibodies in vaccinees.

TREATMENT   Rx

Varicella

Symptomatic treatment includes acetaminophen for fever and lotion or baths for pruritus. Although acyclovir is licensed for the treatment of varicella, the drug is not recommended for otherwise healthy children because it only modestly decreases symptoms by about 1 day.**1** Acyclovir reduces visceral dissemination in immunocompromised persons, in whom intravenous acyclovir (500 mg/m^2 every 8 hours for children, 10 mg/kg every 8 hours for adults) is recommended for 7 to 10 days or until all lesions have crusted. Oral acyclovir (20 mg/kg four times daily for children or 800 mg five times daily for adults) given within 24 hours after the onset of rash reduces the duration of symptoms and is recommended for treatment of adolescents, adults, newborns whose mothers developed varicella near the time of delivery, immunocompromised persons, children with chronic pulmonary or skin disease, and persons with complications of varicella. Acyclovir also should be considered for household contacts of persons with varicella or for pregnant women in the third trimester; these patients often have more severe disease. Although acyclovir is the only drug approved for treatment of varicella, more expensive medications (e.g., oral valacyclovir, 1 g three times daily, or famciclovir, 500 mg three times daily) result in higher antiviral drug levels than does oral acyclovir and can be used in nonpregnant adolescents and adults.

Zoster

Acyclovir, valacyclovir, and famciclovir (for 7 days at the same doses as for varicella) are licensed for the treatment of zoster. Oral valacyclovir and famciclovir result in higher levels of antiviral activity than oral acyclovir does.

Although therapy should be started within 3 days of the rash, therapy may still be of benefit if new lesions continue to occur after this time. Because patients younger than 50 years usually have little pain associated with zoster, antiviral therapy is not used in these patients unless they have moderate to severe pain or disease involving the eye. Antiviral drugs (see earlier) reduce the duration of lesions and zoster-associated pain but not the incidence of postherpetic neuralgia.**2** In severely immunocompromised persons, intravenous acyclovir (7 to 10 days or until all lesions have crusted) reduces the risk of visceral dissemination. Oral valacyclovir or famciclovir may be used in persons who are less severely immunocompromised.

Corticosteroids (e.g., prednisone, 60 mg/day and tapered over 21 days) in combination with acyclovir reduce acute pain and improve the quality of life in persons older than 50 years but do not reduce the risk of postherpetic neuralgia.**3** Patients with moderate to severe pain often require narcotics.

Treatment of postherpetic neuralgia is challenging. In addition to long-acting narcotics (Chapter 29) for persons with severe pain, gabapentin (initiated at a dose of 300 mg at bedtime and titrated to a maximum dose of 1200 mg three times daily) or pregabalin (initiated at a dose of 75 mg at bedtime and titrated to a maximum dose of 300 mg twice daily) may reduce pain.

Treatment of VZV Complications and Acyclovir-Resistant VZV

Intravenous acyclovir is recommended for persons with acute retinal necrosis. Corticosteroids (e.g., prednisone, 1 mg/kg/day for 3 to 5 days) and intravenous acyclovir (10 to 15 mg/kg every 8 hours for 14 days) are recommended for nonimmunocompromised persons with VZV vasculopathy. Zoster involving the eye should be evaluated by an ophthalmologist to assess the potential value of topical or intraocular therapy, such as the need to reduce intraocular pressure to treat possible glaucoma or to use mydriatics to prevent synechiae.

Acyclovir-resistant VZV infections are rare and are limited almost exclusively to patients with AIDS or recipients of transplants. Foscarnet (40 mg/kg every 8 hours) for 2 weeks or until all lesions have crusted is the treatment of choice for acyclovir-resistant VZV.

PREVENTION

Varicella

Patients with varicella or zoster are considered infectious until all lesions have completely crusted. Airborne and contact precautions are recommended for varicella, whereas only contact precautions are necessary for immunocompetent persons with localized zoster.

The live attenuated varicella vaccine is recommended for children aged 1 to 12 years and for persons 13 years of age and older without immunity to the virus. The vaccine is 75 to 90% effective in protection against symptomatic varicella and more than 95% effective in protecting against severe disease.**4** Two doses of vaccine are given subcutaneously. The varicella vaccine is also given as part of a combined measles, mumps, rubella vaccine (MMRV) for children 1 to 12 years of age in the United States. The rate of disease due to varicella declined by 85% in the United States during the first 10 years after the vaccine was licensed.

The most common complications of varicella vaccination are pain at the injection site, fever, and a mild rash within 2 weeks after vaccination. The rash is usually localized to areas of vaccination and is often papular; in some healthy persons, the rash can be disseminated, although there are fewer lesions and symptoms are much less severe than with wild-type virus. In persons with severely impaired cellular immunity, rash is more common, can be extensive, and may be accompanied by organ dysfunction. The varicella vaccine establishes latency and can cause shingles, although this complication occurs less commonly with vaccine virus than with wild-type virus. The vaccine strain of varicella has been transmitted to third parties only by vaccinees who developed a rash. Varicella vaccine is contraindicated in pregnant women and persons receiving high-dose immunosuppressive therapy (e.g., ≥ 2 mg/kg of prednisone daily) or with hematologic malignant neoplasms. Vaccination should be considered for human immunodeficiency virus (HIV)–infected children with age-specific CD4$^+$ T cells of 15% or more and adolescents and adults with CD4$^+$ T cell counts of 200 cells/mm^3 or higher. Serologic testing to verify immunity is not recommended for health care workers who have received two doses of vaccine because the currently available commercial antibody assays are not sensitive enough to detect protective levels of antibody.

Zoster

Zoster vaccine is recommended for persons 60 years of age or older. This vaccine is similar to the varicella vaccine, except that the titer of virus is ~14-fold higher. The vaccine is about 50% protective in preventing zoster and 66% effective in preventing postherpetic neuralgia.[5] Although the vaccine's efficacy to prevent zoster declines in persons older than 70 years, efficacy to prevent postherpetic neuralgia does not decline. Transient pain and erythema at the injection site are not uncommon, but serious complications attributable to the vaccine have not been reported. The vaccine is contraindicated in persons with hematologic malignant neoplasms, AIDS, or HIV infection with CD4 count of 200/mm^3 or lower and in persons receiving high-dose immunosuppressive therapy (e.g., ≥20 mg of prednisone daily) or anti–tumor necrosis factor-α therapy.

Postexposure Prophylaxis

In persons exposed to varicella, three options are available. Varicella vaccine is preferred if exposure occurred within the prior 3 days and the patient is not immunocompromised.[6] Vaccine is estimated to be 70 to 90% effective in healthy persons. VariZIG (formerly available as varicella immune globulin) prevents or attenuates varicella in 90% of susceptible persons if it is given within 4 days of exposure. VariZIG (given intramuscularly at 125 units/10 kg body weight, up to a maximum of 625 units) is indicated for susceptible persons at risk of severe varicella (e.g., pregnant women, preterm infants, neonates whose mothers have varicella between 5 days before and 2 days after delivery, immunocompromised persons) and for persons in close contact with patients with varicella or zoster. VariZIG has no effect in the treatment of zoster.

Oral acyclovir (40 to 80 mg/kg for 1 week beginning 7 to 9 days after exposure) is estimated to be 80 to 85% effective as postexposure prophylaxis. It is often used when the exposure occurred too long ago for vaccination or VariZIG.

PROGNOSIS

Before vaccination, about 100 children died of varicella each year in the United States. Now, only eight varicella-related deaths were reported during an 18-month period from 2003 to 2004.

Additional agents including nortriptyline (initiated at a dose of 25 mg at bedtime and titrated to a maximum dose of 150 mg daily), carbamazepine, lidocaine patches, topical capsaicin (which itself causes pain that is not tolerated in up to one third of patients), regional nerve blocks, acupuncture, and transcutaneous nerve stimulation have been effective in some patients.

1. Klassen TP, Hartling L, Wiebe N, et al. Acyclovir for treating varicella in otherwise healthy children and adolescents. *Cochrane Database Syst Rev.* 2005;4:CD002980.
2. Li Q, Chen N, Yang J, et al. Antiviral treatment for preventing postherpetic neuralgia. *Cochrane Database Syst Rev.* 2009;2:CD006866.
3. He L, Zhang D, Zhou M. Corticosteroids for preventing postherpetic neuralgia. *Cochrane Database Syst Rev.* 2008;1:CD005582.
4. Marin M, Güris D, Chaves SS, et al. Prevention of varicella: recommendations of the Advisory Committee on Immunization Practices (ACIP). *MMWR Recomm Rep.* 2007;56:1-40.
5. Tseng HF, Smith N, Harpaz R, et al. Herpes zoster vaccine in older adults and the risk of subsequent herpes zoster disease. *JAMA.* 2011;305:160-166.
6. Macartney K, McIntyre P. Vaccines for post-exposure prophylaxis against varicella (chickenpox) in children and adults. *Cochrane Database Syst Rev.* 2008;3:CD001833.

SUGGESTED READINGS

Donahue JG, Kieke BA, Gargiullo PM, et al. Herpes zoster and exposure to the varicella zoster virus in an era of varicella vaccination. *Am J Public Health.* 2010;100:1116-1122. *Found no relation between exposure to varicella and the development of zoster.*

Harpaz R, Ortega-Sanchez IR, Seward JF, et al. Prevention of herpes zoster: recommendations of the Advisory Committee on Immunization Practices (ACIP). *MMWR Recomm Rep.* 2008;57:1-30. *Recommendations for use of the zoster vaccine.*

Paster Z, Morris CM. Treatment of the localized pain of postherapeutic neuralgia. *Postgrad Med.* 2010;122:91-107. *Practical review.*

Whitley RJ. A 70-year-old woman with shingles: review of herpes zoster. *JAMA.* 2009;302:73-80. *Case-based review.*

Whitley RJ, Volpi A, McKendrick M, et al. Management of herpes zoster and post-herpetic neuralgia now and in the future. *J Clin Virol.* 2010;48:S20-S28. *Review.*

384

CYTOMEGALOVIRUS

W. LAWRENCE DREW

DEFINITION

Cytomegalovirus (CMV) is a member of the herpesvirus family and shares, with the other members, the ability to establish a long-lived latent infection. Most of the clinical disease caused by this virus results from reactivation of latent virus in immune-impaired patients, although primary infection in such patients and in antibody-negative fetuses can also be devastating.

The Pathogen

CMV has a linear, double-stranded DNA genome with about 250,000 base pairs that encode about 160 proteins. On microscopic examination, the hallmark of CMV infection is a large (cytomegalic), 25- to 35-μm cell containing a large central, basophilic intranuclear inclusion (Fig. 384-1), referred to as an owl's eye.

EPIDEMIOLOGY

Multiple mechanisms account for the spread of this virus, including vertical (in utero, during vaginal delivery, and by breast milk) and horizontal (saliva, genital, urine) contact. These routes of transmission lead, collectively, to a 15 to 20% seroprevalence by 15 years of age in developed countries, with a higher seroprevalence in lower socioeconomic settings. From that age on, there is a steady upward trend of 1 to 2% per year that is due in part to sexual transmission. As a result, approximately 50% of the general population of the United States is antibody positive by 35 years of age, and a 1% per year rate of increase occurs thereafter. In underdeveloped countries, up to 90% of persons may be seropositive by 2 years of age. Presumably, crowded living conditions permit spread of the virus through close contact with body fluids. Two additional mechanisms of transmission are blood transfusion and organ transplantation. A final important epidemiologic fact is that reinfection with a different strain of CMV may occur in a CMV-seropositive person, especially those who are immunocompromised, pregnant, or sexually promiscuous.

PATHOBIOLOGY

In fully immunocompetent individuals, CMV rarely causes clinically evident end-organ disease. When immune mechanisms are deficient, especially those mediated by CD4$^+$ and CD8$^+$ lymphocytes, latent virus replicates and causes both direct and indirect effects. Examples of direct virally mediated diseases are necrotizing CMV retinitis and esophagitis. In contrast, CMV pneumonitis is frequently manifested as subtle histologic alterations accompanied by limited viral replication, thus suggesting that immune-mediated injury may be the primary pathologic mechanism. Such injury may result from the upregulation and release of cytokines, including tumor necrosis factor-α, interferon-γ, and interleukin-2. Immune-mediated tissue injury may also be

FIGURE 384-1. Cytomegalovirus (CMV) pneumonia. A lung biopsy specimen was stained with hematoxylin and eosin and magnified 250-fold. The inset shows a CMV "owl's eye" inclusion.

effected by CD8+ cytotoxic T lymphocytes directed against CMV-infected target cells. The clinical manifestations of CMV infection, including meningoencephalitis, retinitis, enteritis, vasculitis, pneumonitis, myocarditis, lymphadenitis, hepatitis, adrenalitis, and pancreatitis, reflect the range of cell types that CMV is capable of infecting.

The immune response to CMV infection involves both the humoral and cell-mediated arms, but the CD8+ cytotoxic T-cell response appears to be the most important. The CMV envelope glycoproteins that participate in viral entry are gB, gH/gL, and gCII. Humoral immunity directed at gB has been detected in convalescent phase sera and has been shown to block viral entry, cell to cell transmission, and syncytium formation in CMV-infected cells.

Fundamental to the pathogenesis of CMV is latency, or persistence of the viral genome in host cells without evidence of productive viral replication. It is thought that monocytes and bone marrow progenitor cells are sites of human CMV latency. Reactivation from the latent state has classically been associated with immunosuppression. Exposure to a rich milieu of cytokines and growth factors results in the activation of signal transduction pathways, generation of increased levels of intracellular transcription factors, and production of viable virus.

CLINICAL MANIFESTATIONS

Congenital and Neonatal Infection

In the United States each year, approximately 40,000 infants are born excreting CMV, and about 4000 of these newborns show clinical evidence of congenital disease, such as microcephaly, intracerebral calcification, hepatosplenomegaly, and rash. Ninety percent of these clinically infected newborns will survive, but most will have unilateral or bilateral hearing loss or mental retardation (or both). Mothers of most infants with these stigmata had a primary infection during pregnancy.

Infection in Immunocompetent Persons

Virtually all CMV infections occurring in immunocompetent persons are asymptomatic. In some patients, a clinical illness resembling infectious mononucleosis may develop (Chapter 385), but with minimal pharyngitis and lymphadenopathy. Atypical lymphocytosis develops in these patients, similar to Epstein-Barr virus infection, but they have a negative heterophil antibody test result. CMV reactivation is common (33%) in critically ill immunocompetent patients, in whom it is associated with prolonged hospitalization and mortality, but whether it causes these effects is unclear.

Infection in Transplant Recipients

When a CMV-seronegative recipient receives a solid organ from a CMV-seropositive donor, the resulting illnesses include the "CMV syndrome," characterized by fever, neutropenia, atypical lymphocytes, and often hepatosplenomegaly. CMV disease may also develop in the transplanted organ. For example, CMV hepatitis in liver transplant recipients is associated with fever, hyperbilirubinemia, and elevated liver enzymes; liver failure may ensue and necessitate retransplantation.

CMV pneumonia may occur after solid organ transplantation but is most common after stem cell transplantation. Fever, nonproductive cough, and dyspnea can progress rapidly. The diagnosis is suggested by interstitial to nodular infiltrates rather than by alveolar densities on chest radiographs. In contrast to solid organ transplantation, CMV disease after stem cell transplantation usually results from reactivation of latent CMV in a seropositive recipient rather than from a new, primary infection.

CMV may cause disease throughout the gastrointestinal tract. Colitis, which is a common syndrome in transplant recipients, is manifested as diarrhea, weight loss, and fever. It is characterized by diffuse submucosal hemorrhages and ulcerations.

Infection in Patients with Acquired Immunodeficiency Syndrome

In the era before highly active antiretroviral therapy, CMV retinitis occurred in approximately a third of patients with acquired immunodeficiency syndrome (AIDS), most often in those with CD4 counts below 50/mm³. It usually begins unilaterally with visual blurring, floaters, decreased acuity, and loss of visual fields and progresses to blindness if it is untreated. Retinal examination reveals apparent hemorrhages and exudates (Fig. 384-2). CMV colitis is similar to that seen in transplant recipients, but esophagitis is also common and characterized by distal ulceration, which may be single but extensive. CMV neurologic disease occurs in multiple forms, including encephalitis and a polyradiculopathy/myelitis syndrome.

FIGURE 384-2. Cytomegalovirus retinitis as seen by direct ophthalmoscopic examination.

DIAGNOSIS

Culture

Historically, culture has been regarded as the "gold standard" for detection of CMV infection, but false-negative culture results do occur. Furthermore, CMV may require at least 4 to 6 weeks for detection. More rapid culture results may be achieved by centrifuging specimens in a shell vial seeded with diploid fibroblast cells and examining them after 1 to 2 days of incubation by immunofluorescence. Interpretation of cultures positive for CMV may be difficult, particularly in immunosuppressed patients. For example, CMV may be present in saliva or urine in up to 60 to 90% of transplant recipients or patients with AIDS. Recovery from these sites, however, does not prove that CMV is the cause of a patient's pneumonia or fever. Cytologic and histologic abnormalities are not sensitive measures of CMV infection, but they are specific and more indicative of CMV disease than is culture of virus from the tissue.

CMV Antigen or Nucleic Acid Detection

Identification of CMV in blood has greater diagnostic utility, but an assay for antigenemia or CMV DNA, not blood culture, should be used. Monoclonal antibodies can detect and count CMV antigens directly in peripheral blood leukocytes (antigenemia) (Fig. 384-3) with a high sensitivity. Assays of viral DNA by polymerase chain reaction or hybrid capture are also more sensitive than culture and at least comparable to antigenemia assays. These quantitative assays may be particularly useful for early detection of CMV disease and for monitoring of therapy.

Serology

Seroconversion is an excellent marker for primary CMV infection, but rises in IgG titers, even four-fold or greater, are not diagnostic of newly acquired infection. CMV-specific IgM antibody develops during primary infection but may reappear during reactivation of latent CMV. The presence of IgG antibody is a sensitive marker of past infection and is used to screen transplant recipients and donors as well as certain blood product recipients and donors.

PREVENTION

A nonviable CMV vaccine, containing the gB antigen, decreases primary infection in young women by 50%,[1] but a strategy for use of this or any vaccine has yet to be developed.

Because CMV is transmitted by exchange of secretions or excretions, infection can be diminished by reducing exposure to body fluids. For example, both vaginal and anal intercourse, which are bidirectional risks for transmission, can be diminished by "safe sex." Similarly, limiting the contact of seronegative pregnant women with the secretions and excretions of preschool children can decrease primary infection and, in turn, congenital disease.

The risk of acquiring CMV disease can be reduced in seronegative, immunosuppressed patients through the use of blood products or organ grafts from CMV-seronegative donors. Valganciclovir and ganciclovir provide effective prophylaxis in solid organ transplantation.[2] Prophylaxis is uncommon for stem cell transplant recipients; instead, these patients are monitored weekly

FIGURE 384-3. Peripheral blood leukocytes stained with monoclonal antibody to cytomegalovirus pp65 antigen by the immunoperoxidase technique (magnification ×500).

(from day 10 to day 100 after transplantation) for CMV DNA or antigenemia, and antiviral therapy is introduced preemptively if seroconversion occurs. Thus, active infection is not prevented, but end-organ disease is avoided.

TREATMENT   Rx

Oral valganciclovir, IV ganciclovir, IV ganciclovir followed by oral valganciclovir, IV foscarnet, IV cidofovir, and the ganciclovir intraocular implant coupled with valganciclovir are all effective treatments of CMV retinitis.[3,4]

Ganciclovir (dihydroxypropoxymethylguanosine [DHPG], Cytovene) is given intravenously, 5 mg/kg two times daily during initial induction (2 to 3 weeks); maintenance therapy consists of 5 mg/kg once daily (Chapter 368). The oral form of ganciclovir is given at a dose of 3 g/day for maintenance treatment, but it has been largely replaced by valganciclovir, which achieves levels comparable to intravenous ganciclovir at 5 mg/kg when it is given orally in a 900-mg dose. Initial response in retinitis (improvement or stabilization of vision or ophthalmoscopic appearance) occurs in approximately 75% of patients treated with ganciclovir alone. CMV retinitis can also be treated locally by implantation of a sustained-release device, but this approach should be accompanied by an oral drug to treat and to prevent extraocular end-organ disease. Ganciclovir together with CMV hyperimmune globulin may reduce the mortality of CMV pneumonia after stem cell transplantation from approximately 85% to 40%. CMV gastrointestinal disease should be treated with ganciclovir therapy. Ganciclovir resistance may occur as a result of mutations in the phosphorylating gene (*UL97*) or in the DNA polymerase gene (*UL54*). Granulocyte colony-stimulating factor may be needed to offset neutropenia.

Foscarnet, or phosphonoformic acid, blocks the pyrophosphate-binding site of viral DNA polymerase, thereby preventing cleavage of pyrophosphate from deoxyadenosine triphosphate. The recommended initial therapy with foscarnet is 60 mg/kg intravenously every 8 hours or 90 mg/kg every 12 hours. The maintenance dose ranges from 90 to 120 mg/kg daily. Adverse effects include renal impairment, anemia, hypocalcemia (especially ionized calcium), hypomagnesemia, and hypophosphatemia. Resistance to foscarnet can develop because of mutations in DNA polymerase. Toxicity and the absence of an oral formulation usually make foscarnet a second choice for treatment of CMV, but it is used in combination with ganciclovir for infections such as central nervous system disease or for treatment of ganciclovir-resistant virus.

Cidofovir, or 3-hydroxy-2-phosphonomethoxypropyl cytosine (HPMPC), appears to the cell as a nucleotide and does not require phosphorylation by virus-encoded enzyme. It is therefore active against ganciclovir-resistant CMV strains that have resistance mutations only in *UL97*, the phosphorylating gene. When polymerase, *UL54*, mutations occur in ganciclovir-treated patients, cross-resistance to cidofovir is frequent. These resistance mutations also occur in patients treated with cidofovir de novo. The drug has an extremely long half-life that permits intravenous administration as infrequently as every 2 weeks during maintenance treatment.

Cidofovir is nephrotoxic, especially to the proximal renal tubule, but this side effect can be diminished by prehydration and concomitant probenecid therapy. Cidofovir toxicities make it a second- or third-line agent for CMV.

PROGNOSIS

In immunocompetent patients, the mononucleosis-like CMV syndrome resolves spontaneously. Infections in immunocompromised patients are much more serious and may result in failure of a transplanted solid organ. For CMV pneumonia, death occurs even with antiviral therapy, especially after stem cell transplantation. In AIDS patients, CMV infection generally resolves when CD4 counts exceed 100/mm³, but it is a grave prognostic sign if counts do not recover to those levels.

 Grade A   ————————————————◯

1. Pass RF, Zhang C, Evans A, et al. Vaccine prevention of maternal cytomegalovirus infection. *N Engl J Med.* 2009;360:1191-1199.
2. Hodson EM, Craig JC, Strippoli GF. Antiviral medications for preventing cytomegalovirus disease in solid organ transplant recipients. *Cochrane Database Syst Rev.* 2008;2:CD003774.
3. Martin DF, Sierra-Madero J, Walmsley S, et al. A controlled trial of valganciclovir as induction therapy for cytomegalovirus retinitis. *N Engl J Med.* 2002;346:1119-1126.
4. Studies of Ocular Complications of AIDS Research Group. The ganciclovir implant plus oral ganciclovir versus parenteral cidofovir for the treatment of cytomegalovirus retinitis in patients with acquired immunodeficiency syndrome: The Ganciclovir Cidofovir Cytomegalovirus Retinitis Trial. *Am J Ophthalmol.* 2001;131:457-467.

SUGGESTED READINGS

Boeckh M, Geballe AP. Cytomegalovirus: pathogen, paradigm, and puzzle. *J Clin Invest.* 2011;121:1673-1680. *Recent review of mechanisms of persistence and pathogenesis of cytomegalovirus in various human illnesses.*

Cannon MJ, Schmid DS, Hyde TB. Review of cytomegalovirus seroprevalence and demographic characteristics associated with infection. *Rev Med Virol.* 2010;20:202-213. *The seroprevalence among women of reproductive age ranges from 45 to 100%.*

Eid AJ, Razonable RR. New developments in the management of cytomegalovirus infection after solid organ transplantation. *Drugs.* 2010;70:765-781. *Review.*

Palmer SM, Limaye AP, Banks M, et al. Extended valganciclovir prophylaxis to prevent cytomegalovirus after lung transplantation: a randomized, controlled trial. *Ann Intern Med.* 2010;152:761-769. *Shows benefit of extending prophylaxis to 12 months.*

Peled Y, Yogev Y, Oron G, et al. Suggested algorithm for cytomegalovirus surveillance in low-risk pregnancies. *J Matern Fetal Neonatal Med.* 2011. [Epub ahead of print.] *Description of a successful algorithm to guide evaluation and therapy.*

 385

EPSTEIN-BARR VIRUS INFECTION

ROBERT T. SCHOOLEY

DEFINITION

Epstein-Barr virus (EBV), a member of the gamma human herpesvirus family, is the etiologic agent of infectious mononucleosis. In addition, the etiologic role of EBV in the pathogenesis of a number of neoplastic syndromes is increasingly becoming apparent.

EPIDEMIOLOGY

Ubiquitous in the human population, EBV is found in 90 to 95% of adults throughout the world. As in the case of other herpesviruses, infection with EBV is lifelong. The virus resides in B lymphocytes and is intermittently shed asymptomatically in oropharyngeal secretions, which accounts for the bulk of its transmission in the human population. The virus is not highly contagious; it is usually acquired during early childhood through sharing of saliva-bearing fomites or during adolescence through kissing, although it can be acquired in any decade of life. Thus, for example, EBV-seronegative platonic roommates of patients with acute infectious mononucleosis in college dormitory settings are not at higher risk than others in the college population for acquiring the virus. In addition to oropharyngeal spread, the virus can be transmitted by blood transfusion or through organ donation.

Most childhood EBV infections are clinically silent, but infection of adolescents and adults results in the clinical syndrome of infectious mononucleosis between 25 and 70% of the time, depending on the setting. The incidence of infectious mononucleosis is highest in the 15- to 24-year-old age group. Incidence rates in men and women are equal, but the peak incidence occurs 2 years earlier in women than in men. Incidence rates are lower in lower socioeconomic populations, in whom the likelihood of acquisition is greater in childhood than in adolescence.

PATHOBIOLOGY

EBV enters B lymphocytes through the CD21 molecule (also known as the C3d receptor) on the surface of B cells or nasopharyngeal epithelial cells.

Major histocompatibility complex class II molecules serve as secondary receptors on B cells. Once inside the cell, the virus expresses a series of nuclear proteins (called Epstein-Barr nuclear antigens [EBNAs]), which in turn activate EBV-encoded latent membrane proteins and other gene products responsible for the regulation of B-cell growth. This sequence of events leads to transformation or immortalization of B cells, which is the phenotypic hallmark of B-cell infection. EBV-transformed B cells proliferate vigorously both in vivo and in vitro and maintain EBV DNA within progeny cell nuclei in an episomal state. During acute EBV infection, up to 20% of peripheral blood B cells express EBNA.

The host response to acute EBV infection consists of a vigorous and coordinated cellular and humoral immune response. The humoral immune response includes IgM and IgG antibodies directed at the viral capsid antigen (VCA) and to EBNA, as well as antibodies to antigens on the surface of sheep red blood cells. Sheep red blood cell–directed antibodies, termed *heterophile antibodies*, are useful diagnostically and are present in up to 90% of patients, although they are not always demonstrable at initial evaluation. These antibodies are probably an epiphenomenon in host defense and are not cross-reactive with any known viral antigens.

The cellular immune response includes both natural killer (NK) and EBV-specific CD4$^+$ and CD8$^+$ T lymphocytes. Expansion of the CD8$^+$ subset of T lymphocytes during acute EBV infection includes a subset of large, activated cells that appear on standard peripheral blood smears as "atypical" lymphocytes. This vigorous cellular immune response is associated with an outpouring of cytokines, including tumor necrosis factor, interleukin-1, and interleukin-6, which are probably responsible for many of the symptoms and signs of infectious mononucleosis. Over a period of 4 to 6 weeks after initial evaluation in most patients, immune response mechanisms gain control of the EBV-driven B-cell proliferation and the virus enters into a lifelong period of symbiosis with the host. The virus is shed asymptomatically approximately 15% of the time in the oropharyngeal fluids of healthy human immunodeficiency virus type 1 (HIV-1)-seronegative adolescents and adults. The shedding rate increases significantly in patients with defects in cellular immunity, such as those that occur with HIV-1 infection or immunosuppression associated with organ allografts.

CLINICAL MANIFESTATIONS

Most cases of acute EBV infection are clinically silent. The syndrome of infectious mononucleosis consists of the clinical triad of fever, sore throat, and lymphadenopathy, in association with an atypical lymphocytosis and the transient appearance of heterophile antibodies. Epidemiologic studies indicate that the incubation period between exposure and the onset of symptoms is generally 30 to 50 days. The onset of symptoms may be abrupt, or it may be heralded by a several-day nonspecific prodrome of malaise and low-grade fever. Although the classic syndrome includes fever, sore throat, and adenopathy, the findings may be dominated by only one or any combination of these symptoms. Other common clinical manifestations include headache, malaise, and anorexia. On physical examination, patients are usually febrile. Pharyngeal erythema, tonsillar enlargement, and cervical adenopathy are generally present. Mild periorbital edema may also be observed. Abdominal findings may include splenomegaly, hepatomegaly, or both. Although most patients will have mild splenomegaly at some point in their illness, splenic enlargement is usually maximal in the second or third week of illness and might not be detectable at initial evaluation. Adenopathy may be observed in noncervical regions, but it is usually much less prominent than in the cervical regions. Approximately 5% of patients will exhibit a rash that may be macular, scarlatiniform, or urticarial. If patients with acute EBV infection are given ampicillin or its derivatives, a pruritic maculopapular eruption will develop in 90 to 100% of them. Patients with an ampicillin-induced rash during acute EBV infection generally tolerate the drug and other penicillin products when administered later in life.

DIAGNOSIS

Because the clinical manifestations of acute EBV infection vary from patient to patient and other organisms may cause similar clinical syndromes, laboratory tools are required to confirm an etiologic diagnosis. Heterophile antibodies to sheep red blood cells are classically used to diagnosis EBV-induced infectious mononucleosis. Though ultimately demonstrable in approximately 90% of symptomatic acute EBV infections, these antibodies are present in only about two thirds of patients at initial encounter. If antibodies are negative at the outset and clinical suspicion is high, repeated testing in the second or third week of the illness is warranted. Although EBV-specific antibodies

remain the "gold standard" for the diagnosis of acute EBV infection, if heterophile antibodies are demonstrated in a straightforward case of infectious mononucleosis, it is not generally necessary to order EBV-specific serologic studies. IgM antibodies to the EBV capsid antigen (VCA) are the most useful serologic study for the diagnosis of acute EBV infection. Relatively high titers of IgG antibodies to VCA persist for life after initial infection and are not useful in making the diagnosis of acute EBV infection. Antibodies to EBNA are slower to arise than those to capsid antigens, and acute infection may be diagnosed by demonstration of seroconversion to this antigen. If the diagnosis is based on the emergence of antibodies to EBNA, both tests should be performed in the same laboratory.

Among pathogens causing clinical syndromes that can be mistaken for acute EBV infection, cytomegalovirus (Chapter 384) is the most frequent. Patients with cytomegalovirus infection are less likely to have an acute onset of illness, and pharyngitis is less frequently a prominent manifestation of the illness. *Toxoplasma gondii* (Chapter 357) infection can also cause a nonspecific febrile illness that can be confused with infectious mononucleosis. Streptococcal pharyngitis (Chapter 298) and primary herpes stomatitis (Chapter 382) may occasionally cause symptoms that are mistaken for acute EBV infection. None of these syndromes are associated with heterophile antibodies or with other serologic evidence of acute EBV infection. The differential diagnosis is generally made by serologic studies directed at these organisms or by culture. Nonetheless, physicians should be cognizant that organisms such as group A β-hemolytic streptococci and herpes simplex virus are also common in the human population and may be demonstrated in people whose symptoms are nonetheless due to acute EBV infection.

PREVENTION AND TREATMENT   Rx

Because the virus is usually transmitted by asymptomatic oral shedders and is so common in the human population, epidemiologic interventions to prevent spread are not practical. No vaccine has yet been developed. The clinical course is generally self-limited and does not usually require specific therapeutic intervention beyond the use of aspirin or acetaminophen for antipyresis and mild pain relief, except in the presence of specific complications, such as when lymphadenopathy threatens the airway or in certain cases of autoimmune hemolytic anemia (Chapter 163) or thrombocytopenia (Chapter 175). Short courses of corticosteroids, which have been used to hasten symptomatic recovery in patients in whom the symptoms are severe or refractory,[1] should not be used routinely and should consist of no more than a 10- to 14-day tapering course that begins at a dose equivalent of 0.5 mg/kg of prednisone. Although EBV replication can be inhibited in vitro or in vivo by acyclovir and related antiviral agents, the symptoms of infectious mononucleosis are primarily driven by the immune response to the virus and follow the time of maximal viral replication. Antiviral agents have not been demonstrated to accelerate the resolution of symptoms significantly or to prevent complications of the disease.

PROGNOSIS

Most patients recover uneventfully from the acute symptoms and signs of infectious mononucleosis over a 2- to 3-week period, although many patients may have a variable period of malaise and fatigue that can last for another 3 to 4 weeks. Some patients, however, experience fatigue and difficulty concentrating for up to 6 months after diagnosis. Symptoms often wax and wane and can be extremely troublesome. Reassurance is usually the best approach to these patients. There is less evidence that corticosteroids are of benefit in this setting. Recovery may be less straightforward in patients with certain specific complications of acute EBV infection (outlined in the next section). Death from infectious mononucleosis is rare. When it does occur, it is most frequently associated with neurologic complications of the illness, splenic rupture, or X-linked lymphoproliferative syndrome (discussed later).

Complications

Although most patients recover spontaneously from acute EBV infection, a number of complications may arise. In some patients, these complications dominate the clinical findings, and seroconversion to EBV may be the only evidence of acute EBV infection. Mild hepatomegaly can occur in acute infectious mononucleosis, and biochemical evidence of hepatitis is to be expected in virtually every acute infection. More severe hepatic complications are uncommon.

The most serious complication of acute EBV infection arises in individuals with X-linked lymphoproliferative syndrome, which occurs in males with mutations in the signaling lymphocyte activation molecule (SLAM)-associated protein (SAP) that regulates T and NK cells. These otherwise healthy individuals have severe clinical symptoms, a large lymphocytosis consisting of T and B cells, and severe hepatitis. If patients survive the acute infection, the syndrome may evolve into progressive agammaglobulinemia or lymphoma in the following months.

Patients with acute EBV infection should be specifically warned about splenic rupture, a complication attributable to splenomegaly (Chapter 171) and associated stretching of the splenic capsule that occurs most frequently in the second or third week of the illness, when other symptoms of the disease are abating. Rupture is generally accompanied by trauma but can occasionally occur without an obvious antecedent event. Patients should be counseled against activities that might result in abdominal trauma for 6 to 8 weeks after the onset of symptoms. Left upper quadrant pain, especially pain radiating to the subscapular region, should raise this diagnostic consideration. As with other complications of acute EBV infection, splenic rupture may occur occasionally in patients without other prominent clinical manifestations of acute EBV infection.

Other hematologic complications of acute EBV infection include autoimmune hemolytic anemia (Chapter 163), thrombocytopenia (Chapter 175), and neutropenia (Chapter 170). These complications usually arise from a combination of self-reactive antibodies and hypersplenism and are generally self-limited and resolve with resolution of the illness. Corticosteroids may be of benefit in more severe cases of autoimmune hemolytic anemia or thrombocytopenia.

Neurologic complications during acute EBV infection can rarely cause clinical manifestations that are similar to those seen with herpes simplex encephalitis (Chapter 422). Although these patients have a much better prognosis than do patients with herpes simplex encephalitis, they should receive parenteral acyclovir (10 mg/kg every 8 hours). Other neurologic complications include aseptic meningitis (Chapter 420), cerebellitis, mononeuritis multiplex (Chapter 428), Bell's palsy (Chapter 428), Guillain-Barré syndrome (Chapter 428), and transverse myelitis (Chapter 407). These complications may be clinically dramatic but are usually self-limited and associated with full recovery in 85% of patients without specific antiviral therapy. Renal, cardiac, pulmonary, and skeletal muscle complications are rare.

OTHER CLINICAL MANIFESTATIONS

In addition to infectious mononucleosis, EBV is also associated with neoplasia and lymphoproliferative disorders, which are seen most frequently in patients with defects in cellular immunity but are not restricted to such patients.

Post-transplantation Lymphoproliferative Disease

EBV-driven B-cell proliferation that is insufficiently regulated in the presence of prolonged periods of severe T-cell immunodeficiency may result in a B-cell polyclonal proliferation that is initially similar to that seen in acute infectious mononucleosis. Though most frequently occurring in the setting of organ transplantation, especially when patients are immunosuppressed with agents directed specifically at T lymphocytes, such as anti-CD3 antibodies or cyclosporine, this syndrome can be seen in other conditions with similar levels and durations of immunodeficiency, such as HIV-1 infection. Patients with this disorder, termed *post-transplantation lymphoproliferative disease* (PTLD), often initially have fever, adenopathy, and splenomegaly. Intestinal B-cell proliferation is also common. If the immunodeficiency persists, these disorders often proceed from a polyclonal stage, which can be reversed with restoration of immunity, to a monoclonal or oligoclonal stage that is progressive despite restoration of cellular immunodeficiency. Elevated plasma levels of EBV DNA are associated with an increased risk for PTLD, but their predictive value is less well established after solid organ transplantation than after bone marrow transplantation. These tumors are becoming less common as allograft-associated immunosuppression is better targeted and less intense.

The diagnosis is not generally difficult to make in the appropriate clinical setting and can be made histopathologically. Successful management depends on the extent to which the immunosuppressive condition can be reversed before the evolution of restricted clonality. Therapy for PTLD with rituximab (375 mg/m² weekly for 4 weeks) is used in some centers. PTLD may be less frequent in patients who have received acyclovir or ganciclovir after

transplantation, but these agents are less useful once the syndrome develops. Surgery or radiation therapy, or both, are also used.

Burkitt's Lymphoma

EBV is the cause of African Burkitt's lymphoma (Chapter 191), which is composed of small, noncleaved B cells and, unless aggressively treated, is rapidly fatal. This aggressive B-cell lymphoma with a predilection for the head and neck is endemic in equatorial Africa and is geographically linked to *Plasmodium falciparum* malaria. EBV DNA is readily demonstrable in tumor biopsy specimens, and high titers of antibodies to EBV structural antigens are found in plasma. Sporadic cases of abdominal B-cell lymphomas with a histologic appearance compatible with Burkitt's lymphoma are also observed but are associated with EBV only about 25% of the time. The tumor is likewise seen in patients with HIV-1 infection, but it is not as clearly associated with advanced immunodeficiency as are other complications of HIV-1 infection. The tumor is often quite responsive to combination chemotherapy with or without radiation therapy (Chapter 191).

Hodgkin's Lymphoma

EBV is associated with a subset of Hodgkin's lymphomas (Chapter 192), especially the lymphocyte-depleted and mixed-cellularity histologic subtypes. EBV DNA and proteins are detected in the Reed-Sternberg cells that are characteristic of Hodgkin's lymphoma. Therapy for EBV-associated Hodgkin's lymphoma is directed at the tumor (Chapter 192), not at EBV.

Central Nervous System Lymphoma

EBV is associated with central nervous system (CNS) lymphoma (Chapter 191). This tumor was most frequently observed in the post-transplantation setting before the HIV epidemic but is now the most frequent CNS neoplasm in HIV-1–infected individuals. The major differential diagnostic challenge is with *T. gondii* infection (Chapter 357). Although a tissue-based diagnosis is definitive, noninvasive neurodiagnostic approaches coupled with the demonstration of EBV DNA in cerebrospinal fluid by polymerase chain reaction can strongly support the diagnosis of lymphoma over that of *T. gondii* infection. Radiation therapy may be used but is generally only palliative.

Nasopharyngeal Carcinoma

EBV has been associated with certain cases of nasopharyngeal carcinoma (Chapter 196), a tumor that is rare in Western countries but is much more frequent in southern China and in the Inuit population of Alaska. EBV-associated cases are usually less histologically differentiated than the sporadic forms of nasopharyngeal carcinoma. EBV DNA is demonstrable in tumor tissue, and high titers of IgA and IgG antibodies to the EBV capsid antigens are found in plasma. The prognosis for this tumor is poor, although it is often treated with radiation therapy (Chapter 196).

Other Epstein-Barr Virus–Associated Neoplasms

EBV collaborates with another human gamma herpesvirus, human herpesvirus-8, to cause primary effusion lymphoma in the HIV-1–infected population. These aggressive tumors occur in body cavities such as the pleural, peritoneal, and pericardial spaces. EBV DNA may also be found in the moderate to slowly progressive destructive midline facial angiocentric tumors of T- and NK-cell phenotypes; this neoplasm is clinically manifested as a syndrome that was previously known as lethal midline granuloma (Chapter 191). EBV also plays a key role in the pathogenesis of an angiocentric EBV-associated B-cell tumor that is clinically manifested as lymphomatoid granulomatosis (Chapter 278).

Oral Hairy Leukoplakia

EBV infection can cause a corrugated or "hairy" plaquelike lesion that extends around the lateral aspects of the tongue. Oral hairy leukoplakia is most often observed in patients with chronic forms of cellular immunodeficiency, especially those with HIV-1 infection and CD4⁺ cell counts lower than 200/mm³. It is most often clinically confused with mucocutaneous candidiasis (Chapter 346) but can be differentiated because its distribution is restricted to the lateral surface of the tongue and, unlike thrush, does not involve the buccal mucosa, palate, or pharynx and is not readily removed by superficial scraping. Biopsy specimens demonstrate a characteristic histopathologic pattern, as well as the presence of EBV antigens and DNA within squamous epithelial cells. Although the lesions may be cosmetically troublesome, they are not generally painful. In HIV-1–associated oral hairy leukoplakia, the lesions resolve with successful antiretroviral chemotherapy. If the immunosuppression cannot be reversed, oral hairy leukoplakia usually responds to weekly local treatment with podophyllin resin (25%), with or without topical acyclovir cream (5%),**2** and to oral valacyclovir (1 g every 8 hours for 1 month).

Chronic Active Epstein-Barr Virus Infection

Infrequent patients with no apparent defect in cellular immunity may have chronic EBV infection associated with persistent or intermittent hepatitis, interstitial pulmonary disease, or both. These rare patients with bona fide organ system disease should not be confused with patients who have chronic fatigue syndrome. This nonspecific clinical syndrome, seen most frequently in young and middle-aged women, is characterized by malaise and difficulty concentrating but lacks objective physical findings. Although an etiologic or contributing role for EBV had been posited in the past, there is no convincing evidence that the virus plays a role in this condition.

1. Candy B, Hotopf M. Steroids for symptom control in infectious mononucleosis. *Cochrane Database Syst Rev.* 2006;3:CD004402.
2. Moura MD, Guimarães TR, Fonseca LM, et al. A random clinical trial study to assess the efficiency of topical applications of podophyllin resin (25%) versus podophyllin resin (25%) together with acyclovir cream (5%) in the treatment of oral hairy leukoplakia. *Oral Surg Oral Med Oral Pathol Oral Radiol Endod.* 2007;103:64-71.

SUGGESTED READINGS

Dinardo CD, Tsai DE. Treatment advances in posttransplant lymphoproliferative disease. *Curr Opin Hematol.* 2010;17:368-374. *Reviews treatment options, including reduction in immunosuppression, rituximab, and chemotherapy.*
Luzuriaga K, Sullivan JL. Infectious mononucleosis. *N Engl J Med.* 2010;362:1993-2000. *Comprehensive review.*
Odumade OA, Hogquist KA, Balfour HH Jr. Progress and problems in understanding and managing primary Epstein-Barr virus infections. *Clin Microbiol Rev.* 2011;24:193-209. *Overview.*

386

RETROVIRUSES OTHER THAN HUMAN IMMUNODEFICIENCY VIRUS

WILLIAM A. BLATTNER

DEFINITION

There are now four members of the human T-lymphotropic virus (HTLV) family: HTLV-1, discovered in 1979; HTLV-2, discovered in 1982; and HTLV-3 and HTLV-4, discovered in 2005. HTLV-1 has been causally linked to adult T-cell leukemia/lymphoma (ATL) and to several chronic degenerative conditions, most notably HTLV-1–associated myelopathy/tropical spastic paraparesis (HAM/TSP), whereas disease associated with HTLV-2 is rare, and no disease associations have been established with HTLV-3 or HTLV-4.

The Pathogens

Within the taxa of RNA reverse transcribing viruses, the HTLV viruses, along with bovine leukemia virus, are classified in the subfamily Retroviridae within the genus Deltaretrovirus (formerly termed *oncovirus*). The oncogenic properties of these viruses and their molecular structure distinguish them from the human immunodeficiency retroviruses HIV-1 and HIV-2 (Chapter 394), which are members of the genus Lentivirus. Both deltaretroviruses and lentiviruses are capable of prolonged asymptomatic infection. In vitro, however, HIV-1 and HIV-2 have cytopathic effects on human T cells, whereas HTLV-1 and HTLV-2 are capable of transforming T cells into immortalized cell lines. The HTLVs are diploid single-stranded RNA viruses that replicate through cDNA, a proviral intermediate, by reverse transcriptase, a viral enzyme.

EPIDEMIOLOGY

HTLV-1 is widely disseminated worldwide and is estimated to infect 10 to 25 million persons, with the aggressive T-cell malignant neoplasm ATL developing in 2 to 6% and chronic inflammatory diseases, mainly HAM/TSP, developing in another 1 to 5% in their lifetime. Similar to HIV, molecular epidemiology suggests that the four major subtypes of HTLV identified in humans arose from separate interspecies transmission from simians to humans. The recent discovery of HTLV-3 and HTLV-4 was made in Cameroon, where closely related viruses in nonhuman primates led to discovery in humans with exposure as bush meat hunters. Related to such interspecies transmission, there are three major lineages of HTLV-1: Melanesian (Papua New Guinea, Melanesia, and Australian aborigines), central African, and cosmopolitan groups. Within the cosmopolitan group are four subtypes: A, transcontinental; B, Japanese; C, West African; and D, North African. The virus from Melanesia differs molecularly from the Japanese and African strains by 5 to 10%, the result of independent evolution of the virus in these populations separated for tens of thousands of years. The stability of HTLV-1 in comparison to HIV-1 reflects the observation that HTLV favors viral expansion through proliferation of proviral DNA-harboring cells rather than infection of new cells by cell-free virions. The HTLV subtypes differ phylogenetically by approximately 30 to 40% among each other.

HTLV-1 is not universally present in all human populations but rather clusters geographically: southern Japan; Melanesia; Australia, in aboriginal peoples; West Africa and, by the slave trade from Africa, the Caribbean and the United States in African Americans; southern India; and the Mashhad region of Iran. In the United States, HTLV-1 infection is often found in persons who migrate from these regions. HTLV-2 is found in Native American people throughout North, Central, and South America and in West Africa. Most HTLV-2 infections in the United States and Europe occur in injection drug users, in whom the virus is spread by needle sharing and other injection practices. Initial isolations of HTLV-3 and HTLV-4 are from Cameroon, but their extent in West Africa is not yet known.

Routes of Transmission

HTLV, like HIV-1, is transmitted sexually, perinatally, and by transfusion or injection drug use (Table 386-1).

Sexual Transmission

Sexual transmission of HTLV-1 from male to female and from female to male as well as from male to male has been documented. HTLV-1 transmission is cell associated and appears to be at least an order of magnitude less infectious than HIV-1. Coincidental infection with other sexually transmitted diseases,

TABLE 386-1	TRANSMISSION OF HTLV-1 AND HTLV-2	
MODE OF TRANSMISSION	**HTLV-1**	**HTLV-2**
MOTHER TO INFANT		
Transplacental	Yes	Not known
Breast milk	Yes	Probable
SEXUAL		
Male to female	Yes	Yes
Female to male	Yes	Yes
Male to male	Yes	Not known
PARENTERAL		
Blood transfusion	Yes	Yes
Intravenous drug use	Yes	Yes
COFACTORS		
Ulcerative genital lesions	Yes	Not known
Cellular transfusion products	Yes	Yes
Sharing of "works"*	Yes	Yes
ELEVATED VIRUS LOAD		
Mother to infant	Yes	Not known
Heterosexual	Yes	Not known

*Intravenous paraphernalia, such as needles.

particularly those associated with ulcerative and inflammatory genital lesions, amplifies the risk of transmission. For HTLV-1, elevated viral load is linked to heightened transmission. In regions endemic for the virus, there is a characteristic age-dependent rise in HTLV-1 seroprevalence. This increase first becomes evident in the adolescent years; it is steeper in women than in men and continues in women after 40 years of age, whereas rates in men plateau around the age of 40 years. This pattern reflects more efficient male to female transmission. For HTLV-2, the rates for both genders are equal, thus suggesting that there may be differences in the kinetics of transmission between the two viruses.

Perinatal Transmission

For HTLV-1, transmission through breast-feeding is more efficient than in utero or perinatal transmission. On average, 20% of infants breast-fed by HTLV-1–positive mothers seroconvert to HTLV-1, whereas only 1 to 2% of bottle-fed infants of HTLV-1–positive mothers become infected. In contrast, in utero and perinatal transmission accounts for virtually all HIV-1 transmission in the West, and breast-feeding accounts for an additional 15 to 20% of infant HIV infection in Africa. This difference may reflect the fact that maternal antibody to HTLV-1 transmitted across the placenta appears to neutralize perinatal HTLV-1 but not the highly mutable HIV-1. HTLV-2 is detectable in breast milk and, similar to HTLV-1, accounts for many childhood infections.

Transfusion and Injection Drug Use

Parenteral transmission, through either transfusion or injection drug use, is a major source of HTLV infection. Among blood donors in the United States, more than half of HTLV infections are due to HTLV-2. Among injection drug users, most infections are due to HTLV-2, and HTLV-2 is more efficiently transmitted by this route than HTLV-1 is.

Both HTLV-1 and HTLV-2 are transmitted in association with cellular components through a "virologic synapse," unlike HIV-1, which is transmitted by cells, plasma, or plasma products. Approximately 50% of the recipients of HTLV-1/HTLV-2–positive blood seroconvert, compared with more than 95% for HIV-1.

The only documented illness linked to HTLV-1 or HTLV-2 transfusion-associated transmission is the HTLV-associated demyelinating neurologic syndrome HAM/TSP. Leukemia has not been associated with transfusion of HTLV-positive blood. Among U.S. blood donors who are confirmed to be HTLV positive (slightly less than half are HTLV-1 positive and the others are HTLV-2 positive), the major risk factors are intravenous drug use, birthplace in an area in the Caribbean or Japan endemic for the virus, and sexual contact with a person with this profile.

Coinfection with HTLV-1 and HIV-1 appears to increase the progression to acquired immunodeficiency syndrome (AIDS) through unexplained mechanisms, possibly related to the cell-proliferative effects of HTLV-1 on HIV-1–infected T cells. Such a relationship has not been shown for HTLV-2. Other modes of transmission involving "casual contact" are not a source of infection. Health care and laboratory workers who experience a needlestick or skin or mucous membrane exposure in the absence of protective barriers have little or no risk for infection but should be monitored.

PATHOBIOLOGY

Virology

The HTLV viruses, which are single-stranded RNA viruses that contain a diploid genome, replicate through a DNA intermediary that integrates into the genome of the target T cell as a provirus, thereby resulting in lifelong infection. HTLV-1 is approximately 100 nm in diameter and has a thin, electron-dense outer envelope and an electron-dense, roughly spherical core. The total provirus genome contains 9032 nucleotides with two identical sequences termed *long terminal repeats* (LTRs) at the 5′ and 3′ ends of the genome, which contain regulatory elements that control virus expression and virion production. The retroviral structural genes (*gag* and *pol*) code for large overlapping polyproteins that are later processed into functional peptide products by virally encoded protease and cellular proteases. The encoding genes of the virus are *gag* (group-specific antigen), *pol* (polymerase/integrase/protease), and *env* (envelope), and it has a series of regulatory genes, *tax* and *rex*, and several smaller gene products that regulate infection and virus expression. A newly discovered viral gene is the basic leucine zipper factor (*HBZ*) gene, encoded by the minus strand of the HTLV-1 provirus and transcribed from the 3′ LTR. Tax protein plays a central role in enhancing the transcription of viral and cellular gene products that promote viral replication and transformation of human T lymphocytes. Through binding to the LTR, Tax promotes transcriptional activation of the viral genome, and by binding to key regulatory proteins of the cell, it promotes cell activation and disease pathogenesis. Through binding to regulatory enhancers of the cell and through abrogation of key suppressor genes, Tax not only promotes cellular growth but also appears to have an impact on pathogenesis of the disease (see later). Rex stabilizes viral mRNA, essential for export of full-length Gag/Pol and single-spliced Env mRNA from the nucleus to the cytoplasm. HBZ inhibits the Tax-mediated activation of viral gene transcription through the 5′ LTR and promotes the proliferation of infected cells.

Viral Life Cycle

The life cycle of the HTLVs involves attachment, membrane fusion, and reverse transcription from an RNA template to a circular DNA provirus that is transported to the cell nucleus and integrated into the host genome. Both cell-free transmission and cell to cell transmission of HTLV-1 have been documented, with a cell to cell viral synapse involved in cell to cell transmission. Once the cell is infected, viral expansion is primarily achieved through proliferation of proviral DNA–harboring cells rather than through repeated cycles of cell to cell infection. Glut-1, the major vertebrate glucose transporter, is the cellular receptor for HTLV-1 attachment to the cell. Given the ubiquity of this receptor, the cellular trophism of HTLV-1 for CD4$^+$ cells and HTLV-2 for CD8$^+$ cells appears to involve postinfection transcriptional mechanisms; in contrast, HIV targets CD4$^+$ cells through direct binding with a cell-specific receptor. After uptake and uncoating, viral RNA is transcribed by reverse transcriptase, an RNA-dependent DNA polymerase complexed to the RNA in the core of the virus particle, into double-stranded DNA. This double-stranded viral DNA is integrated into the host cell nucleus by the virally encoded integrase, which results in lifelong cell infection. The viral LTR elements are essential for integration and regulation of viral genome expression with regulation from both Tax and HBZ.

Pathogenesis of Adult T-Cell Leukemia

HTLV-1 is integrally involved in the pathogenesis of ATL through a multistage process that includes clonal integration of virus (sometimes including partial viral sequences that always include *tax*) into active cellular gene sequences. Interestingly, HBZ is always present in ATL, and its quantification may be a useful marker for monitoring of the response to treatment. The clonal pattern of integration indicates that ATL is derived from a single transformed tumor cell that evolved from a virus infection *before* transformation rather than afterward as a passenger virus. Tax is an oncoprotein that interacts with numerous cellular proteins to reprogram cellular processes to alter transcription, cell cycle regulation, DNA repair, and apoptosis, thereby allowing cells with potential carcinogenic mutations to survive and to escape cell death.

In some healthy carriers, T-cell polyclonal and oligoclonal proliferations develop that can later progress to malignant transformation or may disappear spontaneously. Morphologically distinct "flower cells" (Fig. 386-1B), which represent T cells with deeply lobulated nuclei resembling ATL leukemic cells, are seen on peripheral blood smears of healthy carriers, and increased numbers are detected in persons with higher HTLV viral loads.

Pathogenesis of Myelopathy/Spastic Paraparesis

Viral overproduction, as measured by high viral loads, appears to result from defective host immune responses characterized by very high levels of cytotoxic T cells. Local pathologic changes in neuronal tissue may result from immune-mediated damage caused by misdirected responses to molecular mimics of viral proteins or by local damage due to cytokine-induced damage of neuronal tissue as HTLV-1 cells infiltrate the perivascular space and the neurons of the central nervous system (CNS), particularly the spinal cord.

ADULT T-CELL LEUKEMIA/LYMPHOMA

EPIDEMIOLOGY AND PATHOBIOLOGY

The cumulative lifetime incidence of adult T-cell leukemia/lymphoma (ATL) in persons infected with HTLV-1 is between 2 and 6%, so about 2500 to 5000 cases per year occur in the approximately 10 to 25 million infected persons worldwide. About 30 cases develop in the United States annually. Although rates of HTLV-1 infection in adults are much higher in women, the equal male to female rates of ATL suggest that early life exposure is associated with the greatest risk for subsequent disease. In areas endemic for HTLV-1, such as southern Japan and the Caribbean Islands, ATL accounts for half or more

FIGURE 386-1. Photomicrographs demonstrating the morphologic features of leukemic cells observed in different subtypes of adult T-cell leukemia/lymphoma (ATL). **A** and **B,** Polylobulated morphology of the acute type, with the highly characteristic "flower cell" shown in **B. C,** Typical cleaved cell seen in chronic-type ATL. **D,** Typical morphology of smoldering ATL. (Courtesy of K. Yamaguchi and K. Takatsuki.)

TABLE 386-2   HTLV-ASSOCIATED DISEASES

DIAGNOSIS	NATURE OF SYNDROME	STRENGTH OF ASSOCIATION
HTLV-1–ASSOCIATED DISEASES		
Adult T-cell leukemia/lymphoma	Aggressive lymphoproliferative malignant disease of mature T lymphocytes	Strong
HTLV-associated myelopathy/tropical spastic paraparesis (HAM/TSP)	Chronic progressive demyelinating syndrome of long motor tracts of spinal cord	Strong
Polymyositis	Degenerative inflammatory syndrome of skeletal muscles	Probable
Sporadic inclusion body myositis	Recently described HTLV-associated inflammatory muscle disease	Possible
Infective dermatitis	Chronic generalized eczema in adults and children; potential for pre-leukemia and immunodeficiency	Strong
Uveitis	Inflammatory infiltration of the uvea of the eye	Strong
Sjögren's syndrome/ keratoconjunctivitis sicca	Loss of tear production and dry eyes and dry mouth	Probable
Pulmonary lymphocyte alveolitis/ cryptogenic fibrosing alveolitis	Pulmonary infiltrate involving T lymphocytosis in lungs of patients with HAM/TSP and HTLV uveitis	Possible
HTLV-associated arthritis	Large-joint polyarthropathy; rheumatoid factor positive, with HTLV-1–positive cells infiltrating the synovia	Probable
Immunodeficiency	Subclinical (e.g., decreased PPD response) or clinical (e.g., association with clinical tuberculosis and poor response to therapy for symptomatic strongyloidiasis)	Probable
Miscellaneous clinical conditions	Case reports of small cell lung cancer with monoclonal HTLV-1 integration and invasive cervical cancer	Uncertain
HTLV-2–ASSOCIATED DISEASES		
HTLV-associated myelopathy	Increased numbers of cases among blood donors	Definite but rare

PPD = purified protein derivative.

of adult lymphoid malignant neoplasms. In one series of pediatric cases of ATL, four of the eight patients shared a homozygous deletion in the p16 gene locus, and deletion of exons 7 and 8 of p53 was detected in another child, thereby suggesting that a genetic predisposition interacts with viral infection to accelerate disease progression.

CLINICAL MANIFESTATIONS

The most common disease caused by HTLV-1 is ATL, a type of T/natural killer–cell lymphoma in the new World Health Organization classification (Table 386-2). ATL is a high-grade lymphoma (Chapter 191), usually of large, medium, or pleiotropic morphology (or combined morphology) and advanced clinical stage, and it is associated with a poor prognosis.

The acute form of ATL, accounting for about 55% of cases, is characterized by an aggressive, mature T-cell lymphoma that presents with a high white blood cell count, hypercalcemia, and cutaneous involvement. Lymphoma type (about 20% of cases) shares all features of acute ATL except for peripheral blood involvement. Other cases resemble T-prolymphocytic leukemia and are termed *chronic ATL* (about 20% of cases). Smoldering ATL (about 5%) may clinically resemble mycosis fungoides/Sézary syndrome, with cutaneous involvement manifested as erythema or as infiltrative plaques or tumors. A long prodrome of signs (e.g., cutaneous rashes) and symptoms (e.g., fevers) is sometimes noted in chronic and smoldering ATL before transformation to an acute or lymphoma-type ATL that is rapidly fatal.

DIAGNOSIS

The diagnosis should be considered in an adult with mature T-cell lymphoma and hypercalcemia or cutaneous involvement (or both) with characteristic flower cells (Fig. 386-1B), particularly if the individual is from a known risk group or endemic region. The diagnosis is established by testing of serum for HTLV-1 antibodies. HTLV-1 and HTLV-2 are routinely detected through blood bank screening assays and confirmed by Western blotting. Polymerase chain reaction (PCR) can detect infection and distinguish the type of virus. The cytologically distinct flower cell, a sine qua non of HTLV-1–associated leukemia (see Fig. 386-1), is also seen in apparently healthy carriers and may presage the risk for future ATL. Occasional cases with characteristic clinical features are antibody negative but provirus positive as detected by PCR in blood cells or in biopsy specimens.

TREATMENT Rx

Watchful waiting is an option for patients with smoldering or chronic ATL, but conventional chemotherapy (Chapter 191), including prednisone with or without cyclophosphamide, is sometimes used in the chronic form. More aggressive therapy is associated with altered immunity and high rates of opportunistic infection.

The acute and lymphoma types of ATL are aggressive high-grade lymphomas whose initial response rates to standard regimens (Chapter 191) are 66%, including a 32% complete response rate. However, responses are of short duration, with relapses occurring in weeks to months, often involving the CNS. Novel therapies with denileukin diftitox (interleukin-2–diphtheria toxin conjugate) that target the high-affinity interleukin-2 receptor on ATL cells are in clinical trials. Recent reports suggest a therapeutic role for allogeneic hematopoietic stem cell transplantation (Chapter 181), with a reported 3-year overall survival rate of 73% and progression-free survival of 67%, with disappearance of detectable virus in a majority of patients.

PROGNOSIS

Smoldering ATL has a relatively good prognosis, with a 5-year survival rate of 70%. The chronic subtype has a 5-year survival rate of 20%. For the aggressive forms of acute and lymphoma-type ATL, median disease-free survival is 0.6 years, with an overall survival of 0.8 years. Significant negative prognostic factors include poor performance status at diagnosis, older age, advanced stage, hypercalcemia, and elevated serum lactate dehydrogenase levels. Death usually results from rapid growth of tumor cells, hypercalcemia, bacterial sepsis, and opportunistic and other infectious complications.

HTLV-ASSOCIATED MYELOPATHY/TROPICAL SPASTIC PARAPARESIS

EPIDEMIOLOGY AND PATHOBIOLOGY

HTLV-1 causes an inflammatory neurologic syndrome known as HAM/TSP. The lifetime incidence is approximately half the rate for ATL, with approximately 1 to 2% of carriers affected. HAM/TSP is approximately two times more likely to develop in females. The majority of adult cases occur in the 30- to 50-year age group, but cases have occurred in children as young as 3 years. These patterns suggest that the latency period for HAM/TSP is shorter than that for ATL and that both early-life and adult exposure causes disease. More than a dozen HAM/TSP cases associated with HTLV-2 have been reported, but the occurrence is infrequent compared with HTLV-1 carriers.

The pathogenesis results from trafficking of infected T cells in the perivascular areas and parenchyma of the spinal cord, where they cause astrocytosis. Ongoing inflammation of spinal gray and white matter results in a progressive and preferential demyelination and degeneration of the lateral and posterior columns, followed over time by loss of myelin and axons in the anterior columns.

CLINICAL MANIFESTATIONS

Symptoms include stiff gait, spasticity, lower extremity weakness, back pain, urinary incontinence and impotence, and (rarely) ataxia. The presenting symptom is stiff gait that progresses (usually slowly) to increasing spasticity and weakness, with incontinence and impotence developing later. In contrast

to classic multiple sclerosis (Chapter 419), HAM/TSP is characterized by a generally slow and progressive course, absence of waxing and waning symptoms, and demyelination of long motor neurons rather than the CNS. However, some cases are acutely progressive, especially those associated with transfusion of HTLV-1–positive blood. It is not uncommon for other manifestations of HTLV-1–associated "autoimmune" disease to present coincident with the neurologic syndrome (see later).

DIAGNOSIS

The diagnosis is suspected in patients with unexplained CNS disease and loss of pyramidal tract functions and is confirmed by testing of sera for HTLV-1 antibodies. Oligoclonal immunoglobulin bands in the cerebrospinal fluid (CSF) of patients with HAM/TSP react to HTLV-1 antigens, and the CSF to serum ratio of HTLV-1 antibodies is greater than 1. PCR detection of HTLV-1 antigen in the CSF is also diagnostic. Spinal cord lesions often appear hyperintense on T2-weighted magnetic resonance imaging.

TREATMENT Rx

Corticosteroids (intravenous methylprednisolone 1.5 g for 3 consecutive days in the first week, 2 consecutive days in the second week, 1 day in the third week, and then monthly for 6 months; an alternative is oral prednisone, 1 mg/kg/day in tapering doses for 2 to 4 months) reduce symptoms in approximately 40% of cases, especially in early disease or patients with rapid progression. Interferon alfa (3 MU three times per week) can improve neurologic symptoms. Pentoxifylline (400 to 1200 mg daily) decreases tumor necrosis factor-α and interferon-γ levels and has improved motor disability, especially spasticity, in uncontrolled trials. Cyclophosphamide also benefits some patients. Spasticity can be treated with tizanidine (2 to 12 mg daily) and botulinum toxin injection (100 to 400 IU every 4 to 6 months). Urinary incontinence is treated with oxybutynin (5 to 30 mg daily), imipramine (10 to 75 mg daily), or doxazosin mesylate (1 to 6 mg daily), and urinary retention is treated with bethanechol (10 to 50 mg daily). Treatment with danazol (100 to 400 mg daily in two divided doses) has resulted in improvement in urinary and fecal incontinence but not in the underlying neurologic deficit. Clinical trials are under way with Hu-Mik-(Beta)1, a genetically engineered antibody that blocks the action of interleukin-15 with the goal of blunting the autoimmune response that results in HAM/TSP.

PROGNOSIS

The prognosis of HAM/TSP is poor, with inexorable progression of neurologic deterioration.

OTHER HTLV-ASSOCIATED CONDITIONS

HAM/TSP is the prototype for a series of immune-mediated syndromes characterized by a high viral load, immune activation, and an indirect pathogenic mechanism produced by virally induced perturbations in immune function. Examples include skeletal muscle polymyositis, sporadic inclusion body myositis, uveitis (30 to 40% of cases in areas endemic for HTLV), large-joint arthropathy, pulmonary lymphocyte alveolitis/cryptogenic fibrosing alveolitis, Sjögren's syndrome/keratoconjunctivitis sicca, and infective dermatitis, which is a pediatric syndrome characterized by inability to clear saprophytic skin infections (see Table 386-2). Carriers of HTLV-1 also have elevated rates of invasive cervical cancer, tuberculosis, parasitic infestations (e.g., strongyloidiasis), scabies, and refractory generalized eczema associated with infective dermatitis. One prospective study of HTLV-2–positive drug users showed an excess of asthma-related deaths and an increased frequency of skin and soft tissue infections.

PREVENTION

Patients often seek medical attention when confronted with a positive HTLV test result based on blood bank screening. Confirmation with Western blot or PCR is needed. Confirmed positive patients must be told that complications related to HTLV-1 infection are rare and that HTLV-2 is hardly ever responsible for clinical disease. Second, it should be emphasized that these viruses are not easily transmitted. Third, the patient should be clearly counseled concerning the distinction between HTLV and HIV because the greatest fear that patients may experience is that they have the "AIDS virus." Other guidelines for prevention include the following:

- Blood for donation should be screened before transfusion, and positive donors should be deferred from donating.

- HTLV-1/HTLV-2–positive mothers should be discouraged from breast-feeding to prevent mother to infant transmission (except in particular settings, such as in the tropics, where diarrheal disease in non–breast-fed infants presents a high risk for morbidity and mortality).
- Condoms should be used by discordant couples, but given the relatively low frequency of sexual transmission per sexual encounter, couples who desire a pregnancy could time unprotected sexual intercourse to coincide with periods of maximal fertility. Such decisions, however, require careful discussion between the physician and the patient.

Postexposure prophylaxis with zidovudine is not recommended because the efficacy of such prophylaxis for HTLV infection has not been established. Vaccines containing whole virus and recombinant HTLV-1 envelope antigens have successfully prevented HTLV-1 infection in monkeys and in a rabbit model. However, a vaccine for humans is unlikely to be a high priority because of the relatively low incidence of clinical disease.

SUGGESTED READINGS

Bittencourt AL, de Oliveira Mde F. Cutaneous manifestations associated with HTLV-1 infection. *Int J Dermatol.* 2010;49:1099-1110. *Review.*

Iwanaga M, Watanabe T, Utsunomiya A, et al. Human T-cell leukemia virus type 1 (HTLV-1) proviral load and disease progression in asymptomatic HTLV-1 carriers: a nationwide prospective study in Japan. *Blood.* 2010;116:1211-1219. *Among 1218 HTLV-1 carriers observed prospectively for 6 years, 14 progressed to ATL, and high baseline viral load was a risk factor.*

Suzumiya J, Ohshima K, Tamura K, et al. The International Prognostic Index predicts outcome in aggressive adult T-cell leukemia/lymphoma: analysis of 126 patients from the International Peripheral T-Cell Lymphoma Project. *Ann Oncol.* 2009;20:715-721. *Update on risk factors and prognosis in the context of current therapy.*

TABLE 387-1 CLASSIFICATION OF HUMAN ENTEROVIRUSES

TRADITIONAL CLASSIFICATION

Species	Serotypes*
Polioviruses (PV)	1-3
Group A coxsackieviruses (CAV)	1-22, 24
Group B coxsackieviruses (CBV)	1-6
Echoviruses (E)	1-7, 9, 11-21, 24-27, 29-33
Enteroviruses (EV)	68-71

REVISED CLASSIFICATION

Species†	Serotypes‡
Human enterovirus A	CAV2-8, 10, 12, 14, 16 EV71, 76, *90, 91*
Human enterovirus B	CAV9 CBV1-6 E1-7, 9, 11-21, 24-27, 29-33 EV69, 73-75, 77, 78, *79-88, 100, 101*
Human enterovirus C	PV1-3 CAV1, 11, 13, 17, 19-22, 24
Human enterovirus D	EV 68, 70

*CAV23, E8, E10, E22, E23, E28, and EV72 have been reclassified.
†Polioviruses have been merged into human enterovirus C.
‡Serotypes in bold italics represent those not yet recognized by the International Committee on Taxonomy of Viruses.

387

ENTEROVIRUSES

JOSÉ R. ROMERO

DEFINITION

The enteroviruses belong to the genus Enterovirus in the family Picornaviridae. The original taxonomic classification of the enteroviruses was initially based on disease manifestations in humans and animal models but was later based on patterns of replication in cell culture, as well as physicochemical characteristics. According to this scheme, the traditional classification recognized five species within the genus: polioviruses, group A coxsackieviruses, group B coxsackieviruses, enteroviruses, and numbered enteroviruses (Table 387-1). With the advent of molecular virology, the classification is now based on phylogenetic analysis of the nucleic acid sequence of VP1, the major enteroviral capsid protein. This molecular methodology expanded the number of recognized species from 64 to more than 100.

The Pathogens

Enteroviruses are small (30 nm in diameter), nonenveloped, icosahedral-shaped viruses. The viral capsid is composed of four viral proteins (VP1 to VP4). The enteroviruses possess an approximately 7.4-kilobase (kb) positive-sense single-stranded RNA genome. The 5′ end of the genome is covalently linked to a small protein, VPg. The genome is organized into a long (≈740 nucleotides) 5′ noncoding region that precedes a single continuous open reading frame measuring approximately 6630 nucleotides. The open reading frame, which is followed by a short 3′ noncoding region and a terminal polyadenylated tail, yields a single large polyprotein that is post-translationally modified to produce four capsid proteins and seven nonstructural proteins.

The 5′ and 3′ noncoding regions participate in replication of the viral genome. Determinants of neurovirulence have been identified within the 5′ noncoding region of polioviruses.

EPIDEMIOLOGY

Worldwide, an estimated 1 billion or more enteroviral infections occur annually. In the United States, about 30 to 50 million annual infections result in approximately 10 to 15 million symptomatic cases.

TABLE 387-2 MOST COMMON ENTEROVIRUS SEROTYPES SUBMITTED BY STATE AND LOCAL PUBLIC HEALTH LABORATORIES TO THE CDC, 1970-2005

ENTEROVIRUS SEROTYPE	PERCENTAGE
Echovirus 9	11.8
Echovirus 11	11.4
Echovirus 30	10.1
Coxsackievirus B5	8.7
Echovirus 6	6.1
Coxsackievirus B2	5.2
Coxsackievirus A9	4.8
Echovirus 4	4.6
Coxsackievirus B4	4.2
Echovirus 7	4.0
Coxsackievirus B3	3.9
Echovirus 18	2.7
Coxsackievirus B1	2.3
Echovirus 3	1.9
Echovirus 5	1.8
Total	83.5

From Centers for Disease Control and Prevention (CDC). Enterovirus surveillance—United States, 1970-2005. *MMWR Surveill Summ.* 2006;55(8):1-20.

Humans are the only known reservoir for enteroviruses. Enteroviral infections are seasonal, and the majority of infections occur during the summer and early autumn in temperate regions. For example, more than 80% of infections occur in the United States from June through October. In tropical and subtropical regions, infections continue year-round, with an increased incidence during the rainy season.

Globally, the dominant circulating enterovirus serotypes may vary annually by geographic region. In the United States, 15 serotypes accounted for about 85% of all isolates reported (Table 387-2).

More than 80% of infections occur in individuals younger than 20 years, with the highest incidence in infants and children 4 years and younger. Nearly 45% of all infections occur in infants younger than 1 year. Among household members of infected children, clinical or serologic evidence of secondary infection can be seen in more than 50% of susceptible individuals. A male preponderance is noted in persons younger than 20 years (male-to-female ratio of 1.4), but not in older individuals.

Community-wide as well as localized outbreaks have been reported in neonatal units, nurseries, daycare centers, schools, camps, and sports teams. The enteroviruses have also occasionally been associated with pandemics, as occurred with acute hemorrhagic conjunctivitis caused by enterovirus 70 and group A coxsackievirus 24.

The use of live attenuated poliovirus vaccines has led to the problem of vaccine-derived polioviruses (VDPVs) as a result of the excretion of neurorevertant vaccine (Sabin) strains from immunodeficient individuals or as a result of natural recombination between Sabin strains of poliovirus and members of the human enterovirus C species. VDPVs that can circulate in the environment with evidence of person-to-person transmission have been termed circulating vaccine-derived polioviruses (cVDPVs). A third group of VDPVs, designated ambiguous VDPVs, are clinical isolates from individuals without known immunodeficiency or sewage isolates whose ultimate source is unknown. Similar to wild-type poliovirus, cVDPVs can cause acute flaccid paralysis in unimmunized or incompletely immunized individuals. Outbreaks of cVDPV disease have been reported in Cambodia, China, the Dominican Republic, Egypt, Haiti, Indonesia, Madagascar, Myanmar, Nigeria, and the Philippines. As a result of effective antipolio immunization programs, wild-type polioviruses remain endemic only in India, Afghanistan, Pakistan, and Nigeria, where they are periodically introduced into neighboring countries.

PATHOBIOLOGY

The polioviruses and the majority of the nonpolio enteroviruses are transmitted via a fecal-oral route. Notable exceptions include group A coxsackievirus 21, which is spread via the respiratory route, and enterovirus 70, which may spread via contaminated fomites or ocular and respiratory secretions. Evidence also supports transplacental transmission.

Ingestion of the enteroviruses results in infection of cells of the pharynx and, because the virus is acid resistant, the lower gastrointestinal tract. Initial viral replication, which is thought to occur in the mucosal tissues of the nasopharynx and intestinal tract (i.e., tonsils and Peyer's patches), leads to seeding of the deep cervical and mesenteric lymph nodes. Further replication at these sites results in a minor viremia with seeding of multiple organs, including the liver, lungs, heart, and central nervous system (CNS). Viral replication at these sites causes many of the clinical manifestations of infection and is followed by a major viremia that may infect the CNS if it was spared during the initial viremia. The virus is cleared by type-specific neutralizing antibodies directed at the capsid proteins by day 7 to 10 after infection. IgA antibodies appear in the respiratory and gastrointestinal tracts 2 to 4 weeks after infection.

The host humoral immune response appears to be pivotal in the prevention and eradication of enteroviral infections. Congenital or acquired B-cell immunodeficiencies may result in prolonged or chronic infection, and the interferons, natural killer cells, and gamma or delta T cells may play roles in regulating the host T-cell response.

Histopathologic findings in patients who are dying of poliomyelitis (Chapter 423) reveal neuronal necrosis in association with mononuclear and polymorphonuclear infiltrates that are initially perivascular in distribution but are later found diffusely within the gray matter of the anterior horns of the spinal cord, the reticular formation of the hindbrain, the vestibular nuclei, and the roof nuclei of the cerebellum. In nonpolio enterovirus CNS infections in immunocompetent hosts, findings include edema of the meninges and cerebral parenchyma, with microscopic perivascular lymphocytic infiltration, increased numbers of oligodendrocytes, and focal areas of necrosis and hemorrhage. In cases of enteroviral myocarditis (Chapter 60), a mononuclear cell inflammation is associated with widespread myocardial necrosis followed by fibrosis, which may be focal but results in myocardial damage.

CLINICAL MANIFESTATIONS

The incubation period for enterovirus infections is generally 3 to 6 days. Depending on serotype and the age of the patient, as many 90% of infected individuals may have subclinical infections. The enteroviruses are responsible for a wide array of clinical syndromes affecting nearly every organ system, and no enterovirus serotype is uniquely associated with a single disease or clinical syndrome (Table 387-3).

TABLE 387-3 CLINICAL MANIFESTATIONS OF NONPOLIO ENTEROVIRUS INFECTIONS*

CLINICAL SYNDROME	GROUP A COXSACKIEVIRUSES[†]	GROUP B COXSACKIEVIRUSES	ECHOVIRUSES[‡]	ENTEROVIRUSES
Asymptomatic infection	All serotypes	All serotypes	All serotypes	All serotypes
Undifferentiated febrile illness ("summer grippe") with or without respiratory symptoms	All serotypes	All serotypes	All serotypes	68, 70, 71
Aseptic meningitis (often associated with an exanthem)	1, 2, 3, 4, 5, 6, 7, 8, 9, 10, 11, 14, 16, 17, 18, 22, 24	1, 2, 3, 4, 5, 6	1, 2, 3, 4, 5, 6, 7, 8, 9, 10, 11, 12, 14, 16, 17, 18, 19, 20, 21, 25, 30, 31, 33	70, 71
Encephalitis	2, 4, 5, 6, 7, 9, 10, 16	1, 2, 3, 4, 5	2, 3, 4, 6, 7, 9, 11, 14, 17, 18, 19, 25, 30, 33	70, 71
Paralytic disease (poliomyelitis-like)	4, 5, 6, 7, 9, 10, 11, 14, 16, 21, 24	1, 2, 3, 4, 5, 6	1, 2, 4, 6, 7, 9, 11, 14, 16, 17, 18, 19, 30	68, 70, 71
Myopericarditis	1, 2, 4, 5, 7, 8, 9, 14, 16	1, 2, 3, 4, 5, 6	1, 2, 3, 4, 6, 7, 8, 9, 11, 14, 16, 17, 19, 25, 30	
Pleurodynia	1, 2, 4, 6, 9, 10, 16	1, 2, 3, 4, 5, 6	1, 2, 3, 6, 7, 8, 9, 11, 12, 14, 16, 19, 25, 30	
Herpangina	1, 2, 3, 4, 5, 6, 7, 8, 9, 10, 16, 22	1, 2, 3, 4, 5	6, 9, 11, 16, 17, [22], 25	71
Hand-foot-and-mouth disease	4, 5, 7, 9, 10, 16	2, 5	7	71
Exanthems	2, 4, 5, 6, 7, 9, 10, 16	1, 2, 3, 4, 5	2, 4, 5, 6, 9, 11, 16, 18, 25	71
Common cold	2, 10, 21, 24	1, 2, 3, 4, 5	2, 4, 8, 9, 11, 20, 25	
Lower respiratory tract infections (bronchiolitis, pneumonia)	7, 9, 16	1, 2, 3, 4, 5	4, 8, 9, 11, 12, 14, 19, 20, 21, 25, 30	68, 71
Acute hemorrhagic conjunctivitis[§]	24			70
Generalized disease of the newborn	3, 9, 16	1, 2, 3, 4, 5	3, 4, 6, 7, 9, 11, 12, 14, 17, 18, 19, 20, 21, 30	

*A great many enterovirus serotypes have been implicated in most of these syndromes, at least in sporadic cases. The serotypes listed are those that have been clearly or frequently implicated. Serotypes with a strong association are underlined.
[†]Because isolation of many of the group A coxsackieviruses requires suckling mouse inoculation, they are likely to be underreported as causes of illness.
[‡]Conjunctivitis without hemorrhage is frequently seen in association with other manifestations in patients infected with many group A and group B coxsackieviruses and echoviruses, especially coxsackieviruses A9, A16, and B1 to B5 and echoviruses 2, 7, 9, 11, 16, and 30.
From Modlin JR. Enterovirus. *Cecil Textbook of Medicine*, 23rd ed. Philadelphia, PA: WB Saunders; 2008, with minor changes.

The most frequent enteroviral syndrome, seen in about 50 to 80% of cases, is febrile illness, which occurs most commonly in infants, toddlers, and young children. The onset of illness is abrupt, with fever, poor appetite, lethargy, irritability, emesis, diarrhea, and upper respiratory tract symptoms. Physical findings are minimal and consist of mild pharyngeal and conjunctival injection and lymphadenopathy. Exanthems may be present in about 25% of cases.

DIAGNOSIS

Nucleic acid amplification techniques (e.g., reverse transcription–polymerase chain reaction [RT-PCR] and nucleic acid–based sequence amplification) are the preferred methods for detecting and identifying all enteroviruses. Multiple studies have documented that nucleic acid amplification techniques are more sensitive than cell culture for the detection of enteroviruses in cerebrospinal fluid (CSF). RT-PCR can detect enteroviruses in CSF, blood, tissue, stool, and other body fluids within hours, and the results can shorten hospitalizations, decrease the use of antibiotics, and reduce health care costs.

Serologic testing is now of limited use, although a four-fold change in antibody titer to a specific serotype of enterovirus in paired acute and convalescent sera can establish the diagnosis. Viral cultures are not recommended because of their limited sensitivity, prolonged positivity even after the related clinical syndrome may have resolved, and the several days required for viral detection.

TREATMENT AND PROGNOSIS Rx

Nonspecific febrile enteroviral infections generally resolve in less than 5 days without sequelae. Because of concern for possible occult bacterial infection, however, significant numbers of young infants and children are hospitalized for evaluation and empirical therapy. Following infection, virus may be shed into the nasopharynx for 2 to 6 weeks and in feces for several months.

⬤ SPECIFIC CLINICAL SYNDROMES
Central Nervous System Infections
ACUTE FLACCID PARALYSIS

CLINICAL MANIFESTATIONS AND DIAGNOSIS

During poliovirus epidemics, 90 to 95% of infections are subclinical. In another 4 to 8% of patients, infection results in fever, fatigue, headache, anorexia, myalgia, and sore throat, which resolve in 2 to 3 days. Paralytic polio (Chapter 423) develops in less than 1 to 2% of infected individuals.

Acute flaccid paralysis is also seen with other enteroviruses, including group A coxsackievirus 7, enterovirus 70, and enterovirus 71. With the exception of enterovirus 71, the paralysis associated with nonpolio enteroviruses tends to be milder, and fever is not present at the time of onset of the paralysis. The upper extremities and face are more commonly involved. Sensory pathways remain intact.

CSF may reveal a mild lymphocytic pleocytosis (<100 cells/mm³) in association with mildly increased protein and a normal glucose concentration. Neuroimaging is not generally useful, but increased signal may be seen on T2-weighted magnetic resonance imaging (MRI) in the anterior horn regions in patients with acute flaccid paralysis caused by poliovirus and nonpolio enteroviruses.

TREATMENT AND PROGNOSIS Rx

No specific therapy exists. Efforts should focus on monitoring for the development of respiratory failure or airway compromise, as well as control of pain associated with muscle spasms.

The mortality associated with spinal poliomyelitis is about 5%. Before modern methods of respiratory and cardiovascular support, mortality rates higher than 50% were common in patients with bulbar or medullary poliomyelitis. The ultimate outcome of the paralysis is highly variable and can range from complete resolution to lifelong persistence. The greatest gains in recovery of strength occur during the first 6 months. Paralytic limbs become atrophic, thereby leading to skeletal deformities. Patients with nonpolio enteroviruses usually have a more rapid recovery and less atrophy than do those with classic polio.

A syndrome of postpoliomyelitis muscular atrophy, which may be seen in up to 25% of individuals 2 to 3 decades after recovery from paralytic disease, is characterized by the gradual development of weakness, pain, and atrophy. Possible mechanisms include aging and neuronal dropout in compromised neuromuscular connections or reactivation/ongoing poliovirus infection.

MENINGITIS

The enteroviruses, especially echoviruses and group B coxsackieviruses, are the dominant cause of viral meningitis (Chapter 420) in all ages.

CLINICAL MANIFESTATIONS AND DIAGNOSIS

The clinical picture varies with age. The predominant symptoms of meningitis in neonates are nonspecific fever, irritability, lethargy, and poor feeding, often with a full fontanelle and a generalized rash. In neonates with meningoencephalitis, clinical findings may consist of fever, lethargy, seizures, full fontanelle, and focal neurologic abnormalities. Hepatitis, myocarditis, or pneumonitis, singly or in combination, may be present in severe cases.

In older infants and children, an abrupt onset of fever is the most frequent initial symptom. The fever may persist for 1 to 5 days and may exhibit a biphasic pattern. Irritability or lethargy is common. Other nonspecific symptoms include poor feeding, vomiting, diarrhea, and rash. Headache is present in nearly all children old enough to report it. Rash, malaise, sore throat, abdominal pain, and myalgia are common, and photophobia may be reported. Seizures occur in less than 5% of cases. Examination may reveal a full fontanelle. Signs of meningeal irritation (i.e., nuchal rigidity, Brudzinski's and Kernig's signs) occur in less than 10% of infants younger than 3 months and increase with age.

In adolescents and adults, headache is nearly always present and severe enough to require narcotic analgesics for control. Some patients report temporary relief of headache following lumbar puncture. Fever is not universal, but photophobia, signs of meningeal irritation, nausea, emesis, and neck stiffness occur in more than two thirds of patients. Myalgia is reported in 20 to 90% of patients. Less frequent findings include rash and abdominal pain.

CSF analysis generally reveals a mild to moderate pleocytosis (<500 cells/mm³). However, some patients have no cells and others may have several thousand. The protein concentration may be increased. Although the glucose concentration is generally normal, hypoglycorrhachia may occur, particularly in association with group B coxsackievirus meningitis. Neuroimaging in cases of meningitis is generally unrevealing. Nucleic acid amplification testing can detect enteroviruses in CSF. The serotypes most frequently identified from CSF specimens are, in descending order, enterovirus 9, enterovirus 11, enterovirus 30, group B coxsackievirus 5, enterovirus 6, group B coxsackievirus 2, group A coxsackievirus 9, enterovirus 4, group B coxsackievirus 4, enterovirus 7, enterovirus 18, enterovirus 5, and enterovirus 13.

TREATMENT AND PROGNOSIS

Treatment is supportive, with control of fever and pain. Hospitalization may not be necessary in adolescents and adults who appear well if a bacterial cause can be confidently excluded. In children or infants or when bacterial infection cannot be confidently excluded in adults, hospitalization and initial empirical antimicrobial therapy are advisable (Chapter 420) while awaiting the results of bacterial cultures of blood and CSF. Intravenous fluids may be required to prevent dehydration. Control of headache pain may require narcotic analgesics. Uncommon complications in all ages include coma, increased intracranial pressure, and inappropriate secretion of antidiuretic hormone.

The overwhelming majority of patients recover fully. The duration of illness in infants and children is generally less than 1 week. In adults, full recovery may take up to 3 weeks.

ENCEPHALITIS

The enteroviruses are responsible for up to 20% of identifiable causes of viral encephalitis (Chapter 422). In the single largest report of enterovirus-related encephalitis, 73% of confirmed cases occurred in individuals younger than 20 years, including about 40% of cases in patients younger than 10 years.

CLINICAL MANIFESTATIONS AND DIAGNOSIS

The onset of neurologic findings may be abrupt or be preceded by fever, headache, malaise, myalgia, upper respiratory symptoms, rash, nausea, emesis, and diarrhea. Somnolence, lethargy, and altered consciousness are common. Patients may exhibit irritability, changes in personality, or hallucinations. Generalized or focal seizures occur in up to 30% of patients, and a minority of patients may progress to coma. Neck stiffness and ataxia are frequent physical findings. Focal neurologic findings such as hemiplegia, hemichorea, and paresthesias are reported in nearly 30% of patients. The focal nature of the seizures and abnormal neurologic findings may be reminiscent of herpes simplex virus encephalitis (Chapter 382).

Among enteroviral encephalitides, enterovirus 71 is uniquely associated with severe brain stem encephalitis (rhombencephalitis), primarily in children. The initial manifestation may be a prodrome of either hand-foot-and-mouth disease or herpangina, which is followed by myoclonus that may be associated with ataxia, tremors, or cranial nerve abnormalities and a rapid onset of neurogenic pulmonary edema, shock, coma, and apnea.

Evaluation of CSF may reveal mild to moderate pleocytosis (<500 cells/mm³), but the CSF white cell count may be normal. The protein concentration may be increased and may be the sole abnormality. The glucose concentration is generally normal. Enteroviruses may frequently be detectable by nucleic acid amplification testing of CSF.

TREATMENT AND PROGNOSIS

Management is supportive, with monitoring for the development of respiratory failure or airway compromise. Nearly 50% of patients require intensive care. In patients with focal neurologic findings, empirical acyclovir (10 to 15 mg/kg every 8 hours) is warranted until herpes simplex virus is excluded.

The median duration of hospitalization is less than 1 week, and mortality is below 10%. For severe enterovirus 71 rhombencephalitis, however, mortality may approach 70%. Long-term sequelae following rhombencephalitis include myoclonus, abducens nerve palsy, facial diplegia, ataxia, dysarthria, internuclear ophthalmoplegia, and central apnea.

Myopericarditis

The enteroviruses—predominantly group B coxsackieviruses—are responsible for approximately a third of cases of acute myocarditis (Chapter 60). The majority of cases occur in young adults.

CLINICAL MANIFESTATIONS AND DIAGNOSIS

An upper respiratory tract infection may precede the onset of cardiac symptoms by 1 to 2 weeks. Fever may be present, and common initial symptoms include dyspnea, chest pain, and fatigue. Physical examination may reveal a gallop rhythm or a pericardial friction rub.

Cardiomegaly may be seen on the chest radiograph. Electrocardiographic findings vary and include low-voltage QRS complexes, ST segment depression, T wave inversion, pathologic Q waves, ventricular arrhythmias, and heart block. Echocardiographic findings include a decreased ejection fraction, ventricular dilation, or pericardial effusion. Blood troponin levels are frequently elevated. Cardiac MRI may help localize areas of myocarditis. Myocardial biopsy is recommended in selected patients who have refractory heart failure or suspected giant cell myocarditis (Chapter 60); enterovirus can be detected by nucleic acid amplification tests.

TREATMENT AND PROGNOSIS

Supportive treatment includes bedrest and management of heart failure (Chapter 59), arrhythmias (Chapters 64 and 65), and pericarditis with or without pericardial effusion (Chapter 77). Immunosuppressive therapy is not generally recommended (Chapter 60). In approximately a third of patients with acute myocarditis, chronic dilated cardiomyopathy develops. In patients with pericarditis, recurrent pericardial effusions or chronic constrictive pericarditis may develop in the future.

Exanthems and Enanthems

Enterovirus infections may result in a wide spectrum of febrile exanthems and enanthems, including macular, papular, maculopapular, morbilliform, rubelliform, vesicular, urticarial, papulopustular, and scarlatiniform types. Exanthems are more commonly observed in children 15 years or younger. Any serotype is capable of causing several different rashes. With the exception of group A coxsackievirus 16, no serotype is associated with a unique rash. Echovirus 9 and group A coxsackievirus 9 can cause petechial or purpuric rashes reminiscent of meningococcemia (Chapter 306).

Hand-Foot-and-Mouth Disease and Herpangina

Hand-foot-and-mouth disease is typically associated with group A coxsackievirus 16, but other group A coxsackieviruses and enterovirus 71 may also cause this syndrome. Herpangina is most commonly caused by the group A

coxsackieviruses but has also been associated with group B coxsackieviruses, echoviruses, and numbered enteroviruses.

CLINICAL MANIFESTATIONS AND DIAGNOSIS

Hand-foot-and-mouth disease begins with low-grade fever, malaise, anorexia, and oral soreness. In 1 to 2 days, oral macules appear and then rapidly vesiculate and ulcerate. Oral lesions are typically distributed on the buccal mucosa and tongue, but they may also occur on the palate, uvula, anterior pillars, and gums. In approximately two thirds of patients, the enanthem is accompanied by an exanthem, with tender 3- to 7-mm vesicles on the dorsum of the hands and feet, frequently involving the palms and soles. Lesions may appear on the buttocks but tend not to be vesicular.

Herpangina begins with high fever, particularly in young patients. Additional findings include sore throat, mild cervical lymphadenopathy, sialorrhea, anorexia, dysphagia, abdominal pain, and emesis. Examination of the mouth and throat reveals 1- to 2-mm papulovesicular, grayish white lesions with an areola of erythema, primarily located on the anterior pillars of the tonsillar fauces. The soft palate, uvula, and tonsils may also be involved. Rarely, the posterior buccal surfaces and dorsal tip of the tongue may be involved. Over a period of 2 to 3 days, the lesions increase to 3 to 4 mm in size. On average, five lesions are present.

TREATMENT AND PROGNOSIS

Hand-foot-and-mouth disease usually resolves in less than 1 week and herpangina generally resolves in 10 days, both typically uneventfully, without the need for hospitalization, and without sequelae. Infants and young children may require hospitalization for administration of parenteral fluids.

Acute Hemorrhagic Conjunctivitis

Acute hemorrhagic conjunctivitis is associated with enterovirus 70 and group A coxsackievirus 24. The illnesses caused by the two serotypes are indistinguishable from each other. However, acute hemorrhagic conjunctivitis caused by group A coxsackievirus 24 may be more commonly accompanied by upper respiratory and systemic symptoms and may be associated with less severe conjunctival hemorrhage. High secondary attack rates within households are common. Other enteroviruses can cause acute conjunctivitis or keratoconjunctivitis but generally without hemorrhagic manifestations.

CLINICAL MANIFESTATIONS

An incubation period of about 1 to 2 days precedes the rapid onset of palpebral swelling associated with lacrimation, photophobia, blurring of vision, and severe ocular pain. The hallmark subconjunctival hemorrhages vary in size from petechiae to large blotches. Although transient keratitis occurs frequently, it seldom results in subepithelial opacities. Preauricular adenopathy is common, but fever is not. An ocular mucopurulent discharge may occasionally be present.

TREATMENT AND PROGNOSIS

Management is supportive. The illness usually persists for 1 to 2 weeks, but complete recovery is generally the rule. A transient lumbar radiculomyelopathy and acute flaccid paralysis–like illness may develop in some patients.

Respiratory Tract Syndromes

The enteroviruses may cause upper and lower respiratory tract syndromes, alone or accompanying other syndromes. As determined by nucleic acid amplification testing, enteroviruses are responsible for up to 15% of upper respiratory tract syndromes. They also cause 18% of lower respiratory tract syndromes in hospitalized children and 25% of hospitalizations in patients with acute wheezing.

CLINICAL MANIFESTATIONS AND DIAGNOSIS

The enterovirus "summer cold" (Chapter 369) consists of nasal congestion, rhinorrhea, and sneezing. Malaise and cough may be present. Fever and sore throat are typically absent or minimal.

Pharyngitis, tonsillitis, or pharyngotonsillitis begins abruptly with fever and sore throat. The nasopharynx, tonsils, uvula, and soft palate demonstrate erythema and inflammation. Petechiae may be present, and cervical lymphadenitis is common.

Enteroviral pneumonias begin gradually with coryza, anorexia, and low-grade fever. A nonproductive cough, tachypnea, retractions, nasal flaring, and wheezing may be present. In severe cases, cyanosis may develop. The chest radiograph may demonstrate perihilar infiltrates, patchy consolidation, air trapping, and atelectasis.

TREATMENT AND PROGNOSIS   Rx

Treatment is supportive and consists of control of fever and pain. In older children and adults, hospitalization is not usually required. Resolution occurs in 7 days or less.

Myositis
PLEURODYNIA

The group B coxsackieviruses are the usual cause of sporadic and epidemic pleurodynia, but the syndrome may also be caused by other enteroviruses.

CLINICAL MANIFESTATIONS AND DIAGNOSIS

The onset of illness is abrupt in approximately 75% of patients. In the remainder, the onset of pleuritic chest pain is preceded by a prodrome of headache, malaise, anorexia, and vague myalgia lasting up to 10 days. Pain may be referred to the lower ribs or the sternum, and it can radiate to the shoulders, neck, or scapula. Pain is exacerbated by deep breathing, coughing, sneezing, or movement. During paroxysms, patients tend to be tachypneic and to have shallow breathing. Additional findings can include abdominal pain, headache, cough, anorexia, nausea, vomiting, and diarrhea. Fever may be biphasic.

Physical examination does not generally reveal muscle tenderness, obvious myositis, or muscle swelling. A pleural friction rub may be present in 25% of patients. The chest radiograph is typically normal.

TREATMENT AND PROGNOSIS   Rx

Treatment is supportive, with an emphasis on nonsteroidal analgesics (e.g., ibuprofen, 200 to 400 mg per dose every 4 to 6 hours) or hydrocodone (5 to 10 mg four times per day) alone or in combination with acetaminophen to control pain. The symptoms may persist for 1 to 14 days (mean of 3.5 days) and resolve without sequelae, although recurrent symptoms may occur in 25% of patients.

INFLAMMATORY MYOSITIS

Multiple enteroviral serotypes are associated with focal or generalized myositis. In patients with B-cell immunodeficiencies, a dermatomyositis-like syndrome may develop.

CLINICAL MANIFESTATIONS AND DIAGNOSIS

Nonspecific findings include fever and chills. Involved muscles may be weak, tender, and edematous. Chemical evidence of myositis may be evidenced by elevated serum levels of creatine kinase, myoglobinemia, and myoglobinuria.

TREATMENT AND PROGNOSIS   Rx

Treatment is supportive. With the exception of patients with B-cell immunodeficiencies, recovery is complete and rapid.

Enterovirus Infections in Special Populations
PATIENTS WITH B-CELL IMMUNODEFICIENCIES

Nonpolio enteroviruses and polioviruses may result in chronic or prolonged infections in patients with congenital or acquired B-cell immunodeficiencies (Chapter 258), such as those with X-linked agammaglobulinemia, hyper-IgM syndrome, severe combined immunodeficiency syndrome, or common variable immunodeficiency, or in patients who are receiving chemotherapy or immunomodulatory therapies or undergoing bone marrow or solid organ transplantation.

CLINICAL MANIFESTATIONS AND DIAGNOSIS

Meningoencephalitis, pulmonary infections, and severe gastroenteritis can occur. The initial symptoms may consist of only persistent headaches and lethargy. As the disease progresses, additional neurologic findings develop and may include ataxia, loss of cognitive skills and memory, dementia, emotional lability, paresthesias, weakness, dysarthria, and seizures. Non-CNS manifestations include dermatomyositis-like syndrome, edema, exanthems, and hepatitis. CSF demonstrates a persistently elevated protein concentration and pleocytosis. Enterovirus is detectable in CSF by viral culture or RT-PCR.

TREATMENT AND PROGNOSIS   Rx

Children with humoral immunodeficiency (Chapter 258) should receive life-long immunoglobulin replacement therapy in an attempt to prevent chronic infection. However, chronic meningoencephalitis develops in some patients and is usually ultimately fatal.

PREVENTION

Handwashing is the primary method for the prevention of enteroviral infections. Only poliovirus infections (Chapter 423) are preventable through vaccination.

SUGGESTED READINGS

Centers for Disease Control and Prevention (CDC). Nonpolio enterovirus and human parechovirus surveillance—United States, 2006-2008. *MMWR Morb Mortal Wkly Rep.* 2010;59:1577-1580. *Coxsackievirus B1, echovirus 6, echovirus 9, echovirus 18, and coxsackievirus A9 account for more than 50% of enteroviral infections.*

Rhoades RE, Tabor-Godwin JM, Tsueng G, et al. Enterovirus infections of the central nervous system. *Virology.* 2011;411:288-305. *Review of pathophysiology, clinical aspects, and treatment.*

388

ROTAVIRUSES, NOROVIRUSES, AND OTHER GASTROINTESTINAL VIRUSES

MANUEL A. FRANCO AND HARRY B. GREENBERG

DEFINITION

Viruses are the agents of acute infectious gastroenteritis, a syndrome of vomiting, watery diarrhea, or both that begins abruptly in otherwise healthy persons. Two distinct viruses account for the majority of cases. Rotaviruses are the principal agent of sporadic, severe gastroenteritis in young children and are responsible for the death of approximately 1600 children daily worldwide, mainly in developing countries (Fig. 388-1). Noroviruses are the principal agent of epidemic infectious gastroenteritis in both infants and adults. For example, outbreaks of gastroenteritis in closed settings, such as cruise ships and nursing homes, are a typical manifestation of norovirus infections. However, noroviruses are also a common cause of sporadic, severe gastroenteritis in young children.

The Pathogens
Noroviruses

Noroviruses, which are one of the five genera of the Caliciviridae family, are nonenveloped, icosahedral viruses with a relatively small, positive-sense, single-stranded RNA genome. The norovirus genus is further classified into five genogroups (GI to GV), only three of which (GI, GII, and GIV) are known to infect humans. GIII and GV viruses infect bovines and mice, respectively, and to date these animal viruses have not been shown to infect humans. Viruses in each genogroup are further divided into genotypes (more

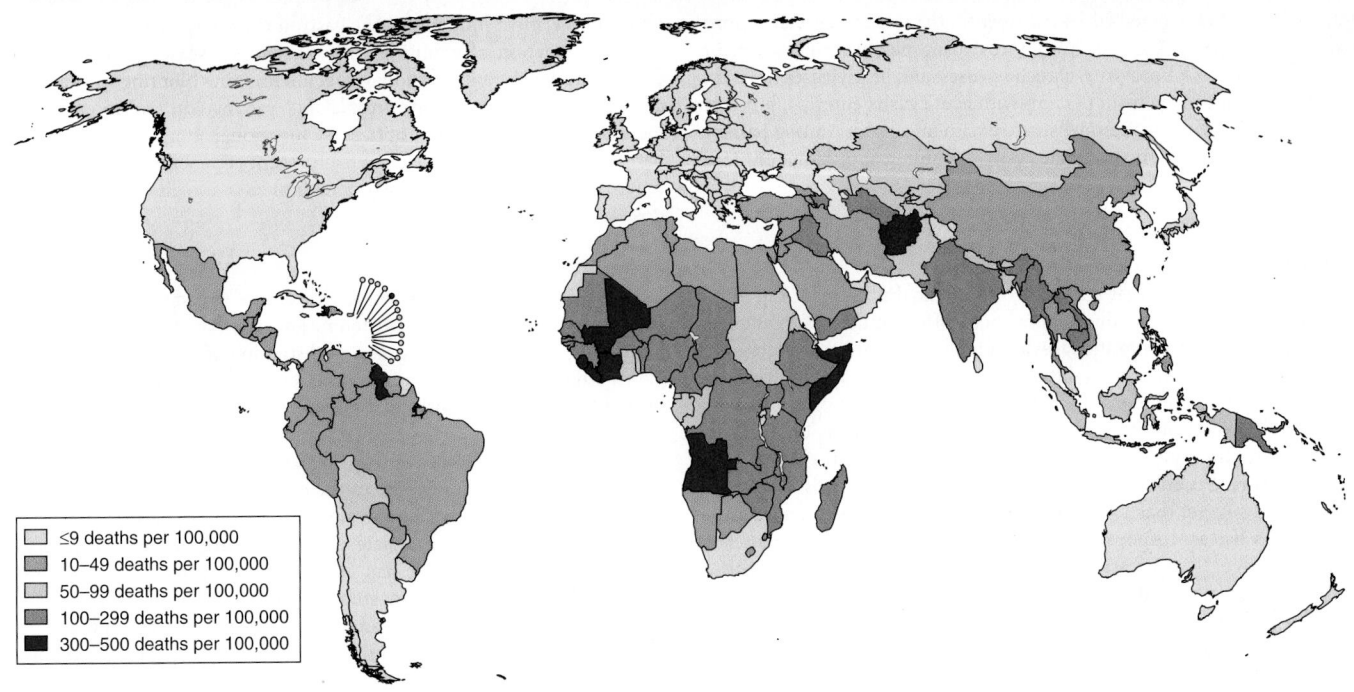

FIGURE 388-1. Mortality rate associated with rotavirus disease worldwide. (Based on World Health Organization data and modified with permission from Danchin MH, Bines JE. Defeating rotavirus? The global recommendation for rotavirus vaccination. *N Engl J Med.* 2009;361:1919-1921.)

Legend:
- ≤9 deaths per 100,000
- 10–49 deaths per 100,000
- 50–99 deaths per 100,000
- 100–299 deaths per 100,000
- 300–500 deaths per 100,000

TABLE 388-1 EPIDEMIOLOGIC AND CLINICAL FEATURES OF NOROVIRUS AND ROTAVIRUS

	NOROVIRUS	ROTAVIRUS	ASTROVIRUS
Epidemics	Occurs year-round; outbreaks tend to peak in cold weather	Year-round in equatorial countries; winter peak in others	Winter epidemics in children and endemic year-round
Key driver of epidemics	Antigenic drift strains promoted by population-based immunologic pressure	Size of the susceptible birth cohort	Unknown
Transmission	Fecal-oral, water, and food-borne outbreaks	Fecal-oral	Fecal-oral
Severity of diarrhea in children	Generally mild but can be severe	Most severe	Milder than rotavirus or noroviruses
Reservoir	Humans are the only known reservoir of noroviruses that infect humans	Mostly humans, but rotaviruses from farm animals and pets (especially in developing countries) infect humans	Humans are the only known reservoir of astroviruses that infect humans
Prevention	Viral protein 1-based vaccine in development	Several vaccines available	No vaccine in development
Age predisposition	All ages	Children <5 years; disease transmission in older family contacts is low (<25%)	Generally children, but adults may also get disease

VLP = Norwalk virus (NV) virus-like particles.

than 25 have been described) and subgroups. Norwalk virus is a prototype genogroup I genotype 1 (GI.1) virus. The norovirus genome is approximately 7.7 kilobases in size and consists of three open reading frames, the first of which encodes the nonstructural proteins that are essential for virus replication. The second open reading frame encodes the major capsid protein, viral protein 1 (VP1). When it is expressed as a recombinant protein, 180 molecules of VP1 autoassemble into virus-like particles that are critical to the study of noroviral epidemiology and immunity. Human noroviruses have not yet been adapted to cell culture, so diagnosis generally depends on amplification of virus genes by the polymerase chain reaction (PCR; see later).

Rotavirus

Rotaviruses, which belong to the family Reoviridae, are large, icosahedral, nonenveloped viruses with a segmented, double-stranded RNA genome and a triple-layered protein coat. Rotaviruses are classified into groups A through G on the basis of the presence of cross-reactive antigenic epitopes and their overall genetic relatedness. Group A rotaviruses are the principal enteric pathogen of humans and many other species. Group B viruses have been identified sporadically in outbreaks of adult diarrheal illness in China and more recently in studies of children with sporadic gastroenteritis, principally in India. Group C rotaviruses are relatively infrequently associated with diarrheal disease in humans and animals around the world. Groups D through G rotaviruses have been isolated only from animals, primarily avian species.

Rotaviruses are 100-nm particles that have three concentric layers of proteins: the core is composed of VP1, VP2, and VP3 and the segmented, double-stranded RNA genome; the intermediate layer is formed by VP6, the most abundant and antigenic structural viral protein; and the external layer is composed of VP7 and VP4. The genome is composed of 11 segments of double-stranded RNA that together are approximately 18 kilobases and encode six structural and six nonstructural proteins. As is the case among virtually all other RNA viruses, the rotavirus RNA polymerase is error prone and, along with selective pressure such as the evolution of immunity, drives viral diversity. For rotaviruses, gene reassortment, which is the mixing of gene segments from different parental viruses in cells coinfected by two or more strains, and rearrangement of the viral genome also contribute to genetic diversity. Reassortment of gene segments between animal and human rotavirus strains also occurs in natural settings, especially in less developed countries.

Other Agents

Other viral agents that cause human acute infectious gastroenteritis that is difficult to distinguish from disease caused by rotaviruses and noroviruses include the sapovirus (like norovirus, a member of the Caliciviridae family), enteric adenoviruses (Chapter 373) belonging to types 40 and 41, and astroviruses (Table 388-1). The frequency of detection (by PCR assays) of these viruses in individuals with acute gastroenteritis depends on the setting, but they are almost always detected less frequently than rotaviruses and noroviruses. Coronaviruses (Chapter 374), toroviruses, picobirnaviruses, picornavirus (Chapter 387), bocavirus, parechoviruses, and pestiviruses have also been isolated occasionally from persons with acute gastroenteritis, but their roles as causative agents of enteric disease remain uncertain. Among patients with acute gastroenteritis, no etiologic agent is found in approximately 25 to 50% of cases.

EPIDEMIOLOGY

Norovirus

Over time, noroviruses appear to undergo antigenic drift in response to the acquisition of immunity in the general population, much like influenza viruses. At present, gastroenteritis cases around the world are most frequently caused by the GII.4 norovirus strain, but new strains generally evolve every 2 to 4 years owing to antigenic drift. Outbreaks frequently take place in settings of close human contact, such as military establishments, cruise ships, nursing homes, and schools, especially in cold and dry weather (see Table 388-1). Viral spread is enhanced by the very high level of infectivity of noroviruses, as data suggest that 1 to 10 particles constitute an infectious dose.

Noroviruses also are responsible for about 12% of sporadic gastroenteritis in children younger than 5 years in both developed and developing countries. Overall, it is estimated that noroviruses annually cause 900,000 outpatient visits and 64,000 hospitalizations among children in developed countries as well as up to 200,000 deaths of children younger than 5 years in developing countries.

Rotavirus

The incidence of rotaviral disease is similar in children in both developed and developing countries, suggesting that measures such as access to clean water will not replace the need for an effective vaccine. Before the introduction of an effective vaccine, rotavirus was estimated to be responsible for about 600,000 annual deaths worldwide. In developed countries, rotavirus rarely is fatal; but before the introduction of vaccines in the United States, it resulted in hospitalization for rotavirus-mediated gastroenteritis in about 1 in 75 children by 5 years of age.

In the temperate zones of the world, rotaviral infection occurs primarily during epidemic peaks in the cooler months of the year (see Table 388-1). This pattern is not seen, however, in countries within 10 degrees of the equator, where infection occurs in an endemic fashion year-round. Before the introduction of rotavirus vaccination, a yearly wave of rotaviral illness spread across the United States and Europe following peculiar spatiotemporal patterns. In the United States, this pattern of spread has been correlated with variation in birth rates, thereby suggesting that the number of babies experiencing their first infection is one of the primary drivers of rotavirus epidemics. The high birth rates in developing countries may also influence the differential epidemiologic distribution of rotaviruses. Antibodies against the outer capsid proteins are the basis of serotypic classification of rotaviruses into G (glycoprotein, VP7) and P (protease-sensitive, VP4) serotypes. For technical reasons, P serotyping reagents are infrequently available, and classification is based on the P genotype (provided in brackets). Worldwide, most human infections are caused by five types of group A rotavirus; P[8] G1 is by far the most common (approximately 53% of strains), followed by P[8]G3, P[4]G2, P[8]G9, and P[8]G4. In some developing areas like India, Brazil, and Africa, P[6]G9, G5, and G8 rotaviruses, respectively, are most frequently encountered. Some human rotavirus strains may have arisen after reassortment with bovine or porcine rotaviruses. A high prevalence of G12 viruses has recently been observed in several countries, thereby suggesting that this serotype may be an emerging rotavirus strain.

PATHOBIOLOGY

Norovirus

Histo-blood group antigens (HBGAs) are the receptors for noroviruses and determine susceptibility to disease in a strain-specific manner. The HBGAs are complex carbohydrate oligosaccharides linked to proteins or lipids that are expressed on the mucosal epithelia of the digestive tract. All three major families of HBGA, the ABO, Lewis, and secretor families, are involved in binding noroviruses. The secretor status of a person is controlled by the fucosyltransferase 2 (*FUT2*) gene. Secretor-negative individuals are specifically resistant to infection with the Norwalk virus (GI.1) and some GII viruses.

Although norovirus RNA has been detected in the blood stream of up to 15% of patients with norovirus gastroenteritis, the site of primary viral

replication is most probably in the gastrointestinal tract. Consistent with the strong association of vomiting with norovirus disease, gastric emptying is delayed. Proximal jejunal biopsy specimens show blunting of the villi with crypt cell hyperplasia and cytoplasmic vacuolation, sometimes with an increase in epithelial cell apoptosis. A functional alteration of the epithelial barrier is likely to occur. Unknown at present is the effectiveness and persistence of immunity in the context of natural infection, in which the infectious dose is generally quite low.

Rotavirus

Rotaviruses replicate in the villus tip cells of the small bowel, where the pathologic process includes shortening and atrophy of the villi, mononuclear infiltration in the lamina propria, and distention of the cisternae of the endoplasmic reticulum. However, the severity of clinical disease is not directly related to the extent of intestinal disease; rather, it is related to levels of viral RNA in stool.

During the initial phases of the disease, altered intestinal secretion, motility, and permeability contribute to the pathophysiologic mechanism of diarrhea. Later in the course of disease, malabsorption can occur. Rotaviral NSP4 is a viral enterotoxin that mediates, at least in part, the early secretory components of the diarrhea. It has also been postulated that viral infection increases intestinal motility by stimulating the enteric nervous system, possibly through NSP4. Whether and to what degree the enterotoxic effect of NSP4 is clinically relevant in children or other animal species remains to be determined. Infected individuals have a short period of viremia, but its clinical consequences are unclear other than correlating with the level of fever.

Rotavirus serum IgA levels measured shortly after natural infection in children generally correlate with intestinal IgA levels and appear to correlate with protection. One explanation for recurrent rotavirus (and norovirus) infections is that protection from reinfection is mediated by intestinal IgA, which is not long-lasting in humans. Another explanation is that protection is dependent on neutralizing antibodies to one or both of the highly variable outer rotaviral proteins. However, a monovalent P[8]G1 vaccine induces significant protection against strains with different serotypes, thereby supporting the conclusion that protective immunity to rotavirus infection is, in part, heterotypic.

CLINICAL MANIFESTATIONS

Norovirus

The clinical manifestations of norovirus infection are variable and depend in part on the age of the individual infected. About one third of infections are asymptomatic, but symptoms include diarrhea, nausea, vomiting, abdominal cramps, fever, and malaise that generally persist for 2 to 3 days. In children younger than 11 years, disease typically begins with the sudden onset of vomiting and can last 4 to 6 days. Virus can be shed in low titers for up to 8 weeks from otherwise healthy individuals and for more than a year in patients with severe immunodeficiency syndromes. In neonates and premature infants, vomiting often is not a symptom, and infection has been associated with necrotizing enterocolitis. To support the diagnosis of norovirus outbreaks, the following four criteria have been proposed: (1) vomiting in more than half of affected persons; (2) mean (or median) incubation period of 24 to 48 hours; (3) mean (or median) duration of illness of 12 to 60 hours; and (4) absence of bacterial pathogens in stool culture.

Rotavirus

Rotavirus diarrhea and dehydration tend to be more severe than illness caused by the other childhood enteric pathogens. Rotavirus diarrhea is watery, persists for approximately 5 days, is often preceded by the sudden onset of vomiting, and is frequently accompanied by fever and dehydration. The incubation period of rotavirus is estimated to be less than 48 hours. Viral excretion in feces persists for 10 days in the majority of children and rarely can persist for up to 57 days. Excretion times are longer on examination by sensitive PCR-based assays rather than solid-phase immunoassay. By the age of 5 years, virtually all children have acquired immunity to rotavirus, and severe disease after this age is uncommon.

DIAGNOSIS

Norovirus

Reverse transcription–PCR (RT-PCR) is currently the procedure of choice to detect norovirus in clinical specimens, in food, and in water. Although enzyme-linked immunosorbent assays (ELISAs) to detect noroviruses are available in Europe, their sensitivity is genotype dependent, and diagnostic specificity and sensitivity vary on the basis of the diversity of the circulating strains in the population. Moreover, these immunoassays are not easily adaptable for detection of new strains. Norovirus RNA is detected by RT-PCR in stool samples of up to 16% of healthy individuals, a finding that complicates the diagnosis of norovirus gastroenteritis. Although the relationship between disease symptoms and viral load has not been fully established, a quantitative real-time RT-PCR has been proposed to establish a relative threshold of positivity for attributing disease to norovirus.

Rotavirus

Before the introduction of the rotavirus vaccine in developed countries, well above 50% of the moderate to severe diarrheal episodes in young children during the rotavirus "season" were due to rotavirus. In tropical countries, the presence of other enteric pathogens and the absence of seasonal occurrence of rotaviral disease make it more difficult to determine which diarrheal episodes are caused by rotavirus without a diagnostic assay. Numerous ELISAs for rotavirus are commercially available, and these are generally sensitive, specific, and easy to use under most conditions. PCR has increased sensitivity for detection of rotavirus and has permitted easy typing of viruses. With PCR-based methods, however, up to 29% of healthy children younger than 1 year may be rotavirus positive, so it is difficult to associate the detection of the virus with gastroenteritis. Thus, ELISA or quantitative RT-PCR (using a threshold level as for norovirus) is preferable for diagnosis of rotavirus gastroenteritis.

PREVENTION

Norovirus

The development of a norovirus vaccine for humans is a challenge owing to the great degree of antigenic heterogeneity among circulating strains, the propensity of noroviruses to undergo antigenic drift, and the lack of known correlates of protection. High percentage alcohol-based sanitizers (99.5% ethanol) and 10% povidone-iodine antiseptics are superior to other alcohol-based sanitizers at reducing norovirus contamination. Simple household antimicrobial hand soap and handwashing with tap water also decrease viral contamination.

Rotavirus

Rotavirus vaccines have been based on two different approaches. One type of vaccine uses a mixture of reassortant viruses, each part human rotavirus and part animal rotavirus, to provide attenuation.[1,2] Another approach uses a single attenuated human virus.[3,4] Neither type of vaccine prevents subsequent rotavirus infection or mild illness, but both types prevent severe illness.

The first vaccine (Rotashield, Wyeth-Lederle), which used a mixed rhesus-human rotavirus, was effective and licensed for use in the United States, but it was subsequently withdrawn from the market because of its association with intussusception. Subsequently, two second-generation vaccines were shown in large studies to be safe without detectable risk of intussusception, effective, and cost-effective in developed and developing countries. RotaTeq (Merck) is a modified pentavalent vaccine made of bovine and human virus. Rotarix (GlaxoSmithKline) is a monovalent attenuated human virus vaccine.

Protection rates in developed and middle-income countries for each vaccine are similar, varying from 70 to 80% against any rotavirus disease to 90 to 100% against severe gastroenteritis.[1-4] These two vaccines may be only about 50% efficacious against severe diseases in the poorest developing countries.[5] However, even with the reduced effectiveness, the two licensed vaccines are still cost-effective. The World Health Organization now recommends the routine use of these vaccines.

TREATMENT Rx

Because both norovirus and rotavirus disease resolves within days without treatment, the basic therapeutic goal is to prevent acute dehydration. The recommended oral rehydration salts solution, which now has an osmolarity of 331 mmol/L, is as effective as higher osmolarity solutions.[6] After rehydration, rapid age-appropriate refeeding is recommended. Rotavirus disease induces self-limited intestinal lactase deficiency, but lactose-containing products, particularly maternal milk, should not be withheld.

Passive oral immunotherapy with diverse preparations of immunoglobulins can shorten the duration of rotavirus infection but probably is economically feasible only for immunodeficient patients or low-birthweight infants. *Lactobacillus*, a bacterium present in yogurt, is safe and, in limited studies, appears

moderately effective for treatment of acute rotavirus gastroenteritis. Nonetheless, different preparations of lactobacilli vary greatly in dose of bacteria, and a general recommendation on their use has not been issued. Several studies in developing countries have shown that zinc supplementation (10 mg/day for infants younger than 6 months and 20 mg/day for older children) is useful for the treatment and prevention of diarrhea, but further studies are needed to determine whether treatment will be useful in all developing and developed countries.

At present, no pharmacologic treatment of rotavirus or norovirus diarrhea is recommended. Racecadotril (4.5 mg/kg per day), an enkephalinase inhibitor that acts on the enteric nervous system, has been shown to be useful as an adjunct to treat rotaviral diarrhea in several small studies. Ondansetron (0.15 mg/kg per day), a serotonin antagonist, is effective in reducing the emesis from gastroenteritis during the phase of oral rehydration. In several small studies, nitazoxanide (15 mg/kg per day) was helpful in the treatment of rotavirus gastroenteritis. More studies are needed before any of these various preparations can be generally recommended for treatment of rotavirus diarrhea.

1. Vesikari T, Matson DO, Dennehy P, et al. Safety and efficacy of a pentavalent human-bovine (WC3) reassortant rotavirus vaccine. *N Engl J Med.* 2006;354:23-33.
2. Vesikari T, Karvonen A, Prymula R, et al. Efficacy of human rotavirus vaccine against rotavirus gastroenteritis during the first 2 years of life in European infants: randomised, double-blind controlled study. *Lancet.* 2007;370:1757-1763.
3. Ruiz-Palacios GM, Pérez-Schael I, Velázquez FR, et al. Safety and efficacy of an attenuated vaccine against severe rotavirus gastroenteritis. *N Engl J Med.* 2006;354:11-22.
4. Linhares AC, Velázquez FR, Pérez-Schael I, et al. Efficacy and safety of an oral live attenuated human rotavirus vaccine against rotavirus gastroenteritis during the first 2 years of life in Latin American infants: a randomised, double-blind, placebo-controlled phase III study. *Lancet.* 2008;371:1181-1189.
5. Madhi SA, Cunliffe NA, Steele D, et al. Effect of human rotavirus vaccine on severe diarrhea in African infants. *N Engl J Med.* 2010;362:289-298.
6. CHOICE Study Group. Multicenter, randomized, double-blind clinical trial to evaluate the efficacy and safety of a reduced osmolarity oral rehydration salts solution in children with acute watery diarrhea. *Pediatrics.* 2001;107:613-618.

SUGGESTED READINGS

Anderson EJ, Rupp A, Shulman ST, et al. Impact of rotavirus vaccination on hospital-acquired rotavirus gastroenteritis in children. *Pediatrics.* 2011;127:e264-e270. *Vaccination programs have reduced cases by >60%.*

Glass RI, Parashar UD, Estes MK. Norovirus gastroenteritis. *N Engl J Med.* 2009;361:1776-1785. *Review of clinical manifestations and diagnosis and therapy.*

Managing acute gastroenteritis among children. http://www.cdc.gov/mmwr/preview/mmwrhtml/rr5216a1.htm. *A review on the treatment of gastroenteritis in children performed by a CDC team.*

Wilhelm CM, Hanna SL, Welch CA, et al. Viral gastroenteritis in Charleston, West Virginia, in 2007: from birth to 99 years of age. *Infect Control Hosp Epidemiol.* 2010;31:816-821. *Norovirus was responsible for 77% of cases and rotavirus for 14%.*

389

VIRAL HEMORRHAGIC FEVERS

DANIEL G. BAUSCH

DEFINITION

Viral hemorrhagic fever is an acute systemic illness classically involving fever, a constellation of initially nonspecific signs and symptoms, and a propensity for bleeding and shock. It may be caused by more than 25 different viruses from four taxonomic families, Filoviridae, Arenaviridae, Bunyaviridae, and Flaviviridae (Table 389-1), although not every virus in these families causes the syndrome. Hemorrhagic fever viruses are often named after the site of the first recognized case. All are single-stranded RNA viruses with small genomes (10 to 19 kilobases). The individual viruses have negative, positive, or ambisense polarities, depending on the specific virus. Pathogenicity varies widely

TABLE 389-1   PRINCIPAL VIRUSES CAUSING HEMORRHAGIC FEVER

VIRUS	DISEASE	PRINCIPAL RESERVOIR/ VECTOR	GEOGRAPHIC DISTRIBUTION OF DISEASE	ANNUAL CASES	DISEASE TO INFECTION RATIO	HUMAN TO HUMAN TRANSMISSIBILITY	CASE-FATALITY
FILOVIRIDAE							
Ebola	Ebola HF	Fruit bat (Egyptian fruit bat or *Rousettus aegyptiacus*, perhaps others)	Sub-Saharan Africa, Philippines	—[1]	1:1	High	25-85%, depending on species[2]
Marburg	Marburg HF	Fruit bat (Egyptian fruit bat or *Rousettus aegyptiacus*, perhaps others)	Sub-Saharan Africa	—[1]	1:1	High	25-85%
ARENAVIRIDAE[3]							
Old World							
Lassa	Lassa fever	Rodent (multimammate rat or *Mastomys natalensis*)	West Africa	30,000-50,000	1:5-10	Moderate	5-50%
Lujo[4]	Lujo HF	Unknown; presumed rodent	Zambia	Unknown	Unknown	Moderate to high	80%
New World							
Junin	Argentine HF	Rodent (corn mouse or *Calomys musculinus*)	Argentine Pampas	<50	1:1.5	Low	15-30%
Machupo	Bolivian HF	Rodent (large vesper mouse or *Calomys callosus*)	Beni department, Bolivia	<50	1:1.5	Moderate	15-30%
Guanarito	Venezuelan HF	Rodent (cane mouse or *Zygodontomys brevicauda*)	Portuguesa State, Venezuela	<50	1:1.5	Low	30-40%
Sabiá[5]	Brazilian HF	Unknown; presumed rodent	Rural area near São Paulo, Brazil?	—[5]	1:1.5	Low?	33%
Chapare[6]	Chapare HF	Unknown; presumed rodent	Cochabamba, Bolivia	Unknown	Unknown	Unknown	Unknown
BUNYAVIRIDAE							
Old World Hantaviruses							
Hantaan, Seoul, Puumala, Dobrava-Belgrade, others	HF with renal syndrome	Rodent (Hantaan: striped field mouse or *Apodemus agrarius*; Seoul: Norway rat or *Rattus norvegicus*; Puumala: bank vole or *Clethrionomys glareolus*; Dobrava-Belgrade: yellow-necked field mouse or *Apodemus flavicollis*)	Hantaan: northeast Asia Seoul: urban areas worldwide Puumala and Dobrava-Belgrade: Europe	50,000-150,000	Hantaan: 1:1.5 Others: 1:20	None	<1-50%, depending on specific virus

New World Hantaviruses

Disease	Reservoir/vector	Geographic distribution	Ratio inapparent:apparent	Estimated cases/yr	Person-to-person transmission	Case-fatality rate
Sin nombre, Andes, Laguna negra, others / Hantavirus pulmonary syndrome	Rodent (sin nombre: deer mouse or *Peromyscus maniculatus*; Andes: long-tailed rat or *Oligoryzomys longicaudatus*; Laguna negra: vesper mouse or *Calomys laucha*)	Sin nombre: North America, Andes; Laguna negra: Southern South America	Sin nombre: 1 : 1; Others up to 1 : 20	50,000-150,000	None except for Andes virus	<1-50%, depending on specific virus
Rift Valley fever	Domestic livestock/mosquitoes (*Aedes* and others)	Sub-Saharan Africa, Saudi Arabia, Yemen[7]	1 : 100	100-100,000[8]	None	50%
Crimean-Congo HF	Wild and domestic vertebrates/tick (primarily *Hyalomma* species)	Africa, Balkans, southern Russia, Middle East, India, Pakistan, Afghanistan, western China	1 : 1-2	~500	High	15-30%
FLAVIVIRIDAE						
Yellow fever	Monkey/mosquito (*Aedes aegypti*, other *Aedes* and *Haemagogus* spp)	Sub-Saharan Africa, South America up to Panama	1 : 2-20	5000-200,000[8]	No	20-50%
Dengue	Human/mosquito (*Aedes aegypti* and *albopictus*)	Tropics and subtropics worldwide	1 : 10-100, depending on age, previous infection, genetic background, and infecting serotype	Dengue HF: 100,000-200,000[8]	None	Untreated: 10-15% Treated: <1%
Kyasanur Forest disease	Vertebrate (rodents, bats, birds, monkeys, others)/tick (*Haemaphysalis* species and others)	Karnataka State, India; Yunnan Province, China; Saudi Arabia[9]	Unknown	~500	Not reported, but laboratory infections have occurred	3-5%
Omsk HF	Rodent/ticks (primarily *Dermacentor* and *Ixodes* species)	Western Siberia	Unknown	100-200	Not reported	1-3%

[1] Although some endemic transmission of the filoviruses (Ebola > Marburg) and Rift Valley fever virus occurs, these viruses have most often been associated with outbreaks. Filovirus outbreaks are typically fewer than 100 cases and have never been more than 500.
[2] Five species or subtypes of Ebola virus with varying associated case-fatality ratios are recognized: Ebola Zaire, 85; Ebola Sudan, 55; Ebola Bundibugyo, 25%; Ebola Cote d'Ivoire, 0% (only one recognized case); Ebola Reston, 0% (not pathogenic to humans). All are endemic to sub-Saharan Africa, with the exception of Ebola Reston virus, which is found in the Philippines.
[3] In addition to the arenaviruses listed in the table, Flexal and Tacaribe viruses have caused human disease as a result of laboratory accidents. Another arenavirus, Whitewater Arroyo, has been noted in sick persons in California, but its role as a pathogen has not been clearly established.
[4] Discovered in 2008 in an outbreak of five cases (four of them fatal) in South Africa. The index case came to South Africa from Zambia.
[5] Discovered in 1990. Only three cases (one fatal) of Sabiá virus infection have been noted, two of them from laboratory accidents.
[6] Discovered in 2003 from a "small outbreak" in Cochabamba, Bolivia. Blood was obtained from one fatal case and Chapare virus isolated, but few other details from the outbreak have been reported.
[7] Although Rift Valley fever virus can be found throughout sub-Saharan Africa, large outbreaks usually occur in East Africa.
[8] Based on estimates from the World Health Organization. Significant underreporting occurs. Incidence may fluctuate widely, depending on epidemic activity.
[9] Numerous variants of Kyasanur Forest disease virus have been identified, including Nanjianyin virus in Yunnan Province, China, and Alkhurma virus (also spelled Alkhurma in some publications) in Saudi Arabia and Egypt.
HF = hemorrhagic fever.

by the specific virus and sometimes among strains of the same virus. Many of the hemorrhagic fever viruses have been placed on the Centers for Disease Control and Prevention select agents list of pathogens that pose a potential bioterrorism threat (Chapter 20).

EPIDEMIOLOGY

Maintenance in Nature and Transmission to Humans

With the exception of dengue virus, for which humans can now be considered the reservoir, hemorrhagic fever viruses are zoonotic, maintained in nature in mammalian reservoirs (see Table 389-1). The viruses may be transmitted to humans through direct contact with the reservoir or, in the case of the flaviviruses and most of the bunyaviruses, by an arthropod vector. Although viral hemorrhagic fever can be found worldwide, the endemic area of any given hemorrhagic fever virus is restricted by the distribution of its natural reservoir or arthropod vector. With the exception of dengue, human infection is generally rare, and humans are dead-end hosts who play no role in the natural maintenance of the viruses. The infectious dose for most hemorrhagic fever viruses appears to be low, sometimes on the order of just a few virions.

Bat-Borne Viruses

The filoviruses (from the Latin *filo*, "thread," referring to their filamentous shape), Marburg and Ebola, are perhaps the most feared of all hemorrhagic fever viruses. Fruit bats appear to be the filovirus reservoir, with transmission to humans likely from exposure to infected bat excreta or saliva. Nonhuman primates, especially gorillas and chimpanzees, and other wild animals may become infected, presumably from similar bat exposure, and transmit filoviruses to humans through contact with blood and body fluids of these animals, usually in association with hunting. Nonhuman primates are also dead-end hosts who develop severe and usually fatal disease, similar to that seen in humans, and are likely to be easier prey for hunters. Because hemorrhagic fever viruses are rapidly inactivated by heating, infection probably occurs by exposure during butchering and preparation. Ebola Reston virus has been isolated from pigs in the Philippines, presumably from exposure to bats.

Rodent-Borne Viruses

Arenaviruses (from the Latin *arena*, "sand," referring to their sandy appearance on electron microscopy) are divided into two groups: the Old World (or lymphocytic choriomeningitis/Lassa) complex and the New World (or Tacaribe) complex. Lassa virus and the recently discovered Lujo virus are found in Africa, whereas Junin, Machupo, Guanarito, Sabiá, and Chapare viruses are found in South America. Although there may be subtle differences among the syndromes produced by the New World arenaviruses, they are usually grouped simply as the South American hemorrhagic fevers.

The genus Hantavirus of the Bunyaviridae family is similarly divided into Old and New World groups. The Old World hantaviruses, such as Hantaan, Seoul, and Puumala, among many others, cause hemorrhagic fevers with prominent renal involvement across Europe and Asia. New World hantaviruses, such as sin nombre and Andes, among many others, cause a viral hemorrhagic fever named hantavirus pulmonary syndrome, sometimes also called hantavirus cardiopulmonary syndrome to emphasize the significant cardiogenic component of this disease.

Arenaviruses and hantaviruses are maintained in nature through chronic asymptomatic infection in rodents of the Muridae family, with a strict pairing between the specific virus and rodent species. Transmission between rodents may be by vertical or horizontal transmission or both, depending on the specific virus. Transmission to humans occurs through exposure to rodent excreta, either from aerosols produced when rodents urinate or by direct inoculation to the mucous membranes. The relative importance of these modes of transmission is unknown. Secondary aerosol generation is notoriously inefficient, so disturbing shed urine is a less likely mechanism of infection. In West Africa, Lassa virus is sometimes contracted when rodents are trapped and prepared for consumption or, more rarely, through a rodent bite. Experimental data suggest that humans may be infected with arenaviruses by the oral route.

The rodents that transmit Lassa, Machupo, and many of the Old World hantaviruses commonly invade the peridomestic environment, thereby putting housewives, children, and others who spend time at home at risk. In contrast, the reservoirs for Junin, Guanarito, and most of the New World hantaviruses typically inhabit agricultural fields, wood lots, or other rural habitats, thereby putting outdoor workers, campers, and hikers at risk.

Mosquito-Borne Viruses

Rift Valley fever virus is maintained in domestic livestock, such as cattle, buffalo, sheep, goats, and camels, in which it often provokes spontaneous abortion. The virus may be transmitted to humans by direct exposure to these animals, especially during parturition, or by mosquitoes. Farmers, abattoir workers, and veterinarians are at particular risk.

Yellow fever virus is maintained in a cycle between monkeys and forest canopy mosquitoes. Sporadic cases occur when humans are bitten by these mosquitoes. Larger outbreaks occur when humans bring the virus back to more settled environments, where the urban mosquito *Aedes aegypti* can spread the virus directly between humans. *Ae. aegypti,* which typically lay eggs in artificial containers around the home and bite during the day, become infective a few weeks after feeding on a viremic monkey or human. Sanitation and mosquito control measures have virtually eliminated urban yellow fever in the Americas, but urban outbreaks continue to occur in Africa.

Although nonhuman primates are also a reservoir for sylvatic strains of dengue, the virus is now largely maintained in humans, with a regular transmission cycle akin to urban yellow fever. Despite the presence of dengue virus in the tropics worldwide, less than 10% of infected persons develop hemorrhagic fever, primarily children between the ages of 4 and 12 years.

Tick-Borne Viruses

Kyasanur Forest disease and Crimean-Congo and Omsk hemorrhagic fever viruses are maintained in small mammals, such as rodents, hares, and hedgehogs, among which the viruses are spread by ticks. Humans are infected either by tick bites or by exposure to contaminated blood or excreta of the reservoir animals. Ticks also spread Crimean-Congo hemorrhagic fever virus to large mammals, including cattle and other domestic livestock, whose transient and asymptomatic viremia puts farmers, abattoir workers, and veterinarians at risk.

Human to Human Transmission

Secondary human to human transmission occurs with many of the hemorrhagic fever viruses, but tertiary transmission is unusual and often associated with milder disease. Secondary attack rates for hemorrhagic fever viruses are generally low (15 to 20% for Ebola Zaire virus), probably because transmission between humans requires direct contact with contaminated blood or body fluids. Human to human infection probably usually occurs through oral or mucous membrane exposure, most often in the context of providing care to a sick family member (community) or patient (nosocomial transmission). Large outbreaks are almost always fueled by nosocomial transmission, usually in resource-poor regions. Funeral rituals that entail the touching of the corpse before burial have also played a significant role in transmission of the filoviruses. Infection through fomites cannot be excluded.

With the exception of hantaviruses and some of the flaviviruses, infectivity generally parallels the clinical state. Persons are generally most infectious late in the course of severe disease, especially when bleeding. Transmission during the incubation period or from asymptomatic persons is negligible.

PATHOBIOLOGY

Microvascular instability and impaired hemostasis are the hallmarks of viral hemorrhagic fever. Although the pathophysiologic mechanism varies with the specific virus, mortality usually results not directly from exsanguination but rather when an intense inflammatory process akin to septic shock results in insufficient effective circulating intravascular volume that leads to hypotension, cellular dysfunction, and multiorgan system failure. In fact, external bleeding is seen in a minority of all cases. Cardiac inotropy may be directly or indirectly inhibited, especially in Lassa fever.

After inoculation, virus first replicates in dendritic cells and other local tissues, with subsequent migration to regional lymph nodes and then dissemination through the lymph and blood monocytes to a broad range of tissues and organs, including the liver, spleen, lymph nodes, adrenal glands, lungs, and endothelium. Migration of tissue macrophages results in secondary infection of permissive parenchymal cells.

The interaction of virus with immune cells, especially macrophages and endothelial cells, results in cell activation and the unleashing of an inflammatory and vasoactive process consistent with the systemic inflammatory response syndrome. Although lymphocytes remain free of infection, they may be destroyed in massive numbers during the course of illness through apoptosis, as seen in other forms of septic shock. The synthesis of cell surface tissue factor triggers the extrinsic coagulation pathway. Impaired hemostasis

TABLE 389-2 PATHOBIOLOGIC AND CLINICAL ASPECTS OF VIRAL HEMORRHAGIC FEVERS

DISEASE	INCUBATION PERIOD (DAYS)	ONSET	BLEEDING	RASH	JAUNDICE	HEART	LUNG	KIDNEY	CNS	EYE
FILOVIRIDAE										
Ebola HF	3-21	Abrupt	++	+++	+	++?	+	+	+	+
Marburg HF	3-21	Abrupt	++	+++	+	++?	+	+	+	+
ARENAVIRIDAE										
Lassa fever and Lujo HF[1]	5-16	Gradual	+	++	0	++	+	0	+	0
South American HFs[1]	7-14	Gradual	+++	0	0	++	+	0	+++	0
BUNYAVIRIDAE										
HF with renal syndrome	9-35	Abrupt	+++	0	0	++	+	+++	+	0
Hantavirus pulmonary syndrome	7-35	Gradual	0 (except for Andes virus infection)	0	0	+++	+++	+	+	0
Rift Valley fever[2]	2-5	Abrupt	+++	+	++	+?	0	+	++	++
Crimean-Congo HF	3-12	Abrupt	+++	0	++	+?	+	0	+	0
FLAVIVIRIDAE										
Yellow fever	3-6	Abrupt	+++	0	+++	++	+	++	++	0
Dengue HF	3-15	Abrupt	++	+++	+	++	+	0	+	0
Kyasanur Forest disease	3-8	Abrupt	++	0	0	+	++	0	+++	+
Omsk HF	3-8	Abrupt	++	0	0	+	++	0	+++	+

[1]Data are insufficient to distinguish between the syndromes produced by the various Old and New World arenaviruses.
[2]Hemorrhagic fever, encephalitis, and retinitis may be seen in Rift Valley fever independently of each other.
CNS = central nervous system; HF = hemorrhagic fever; 0 = sign not typically noted/organ not typically affected; + = sign occasionally noted/organ occasionally affected; ++ = sign commonly noted/organ commonly affected; +++ = sign characteristic/organ involvement severe.

may entail endothelial cell, platelet, or coagulation factor dysfunction. Disseminated intravascular coagulopathy (DIC) is frequently noted, especially with Ebola, Marburg, and Crimean-Congo hemorrhagic fever virus infections.

Tissue damage may be mediated through direct necrosis of infected cells or indirectly through apoptosis of immune cells. The most affected organs vary with the virus (Table 389-2). For example, renal tubular necrosis and retroperitoneal edema are seen in hemorrhagic fevers with renal syndrome, whereas interstitial pneumonitis and myocardial depression are the hallmarks of hantavirus pulmonary syndrome. The liver is particularly affected in yellow fever, with fatty degeneration, coagulative midzonal necrosis of hepatocytes, and the presence of Councilman bodies. The brain and meninges are particularly affected in Kyasanur Forest disease and Omsk hemorrhagic fever and often in the South American hemorrhagic fevers as well. Reticuloendothelial proliferation is seen in Kyasanur Forest disease, with marked erythrophagocytosis in the spleen.

With the exception of disease caused by the hantaviruses and some of the flaviviruses, the pathogenesis of viral hemorrhagic fever appears to be unchecked viremia, with most fatal cases failing to mount a significant antibody response. Inflammatory cell infiltrates are usually mild. In some viral hemorrhagic fevers, such as Ebola, virus replication and dissemination are facilitated by virus-induced suppression of the host adaptive immune response.

In contrast to this process, hantavirus, yellow fever virus, and dengue virus are usually cleared from the blood before the most severe phase of the disease. The host immune response is thought to play a detrimental role. The unique process of antibody-mediated immune enhancement, in which secondary infection with a different dengue virus serotype is more severe than the primary one, may play a role in the pathogenesis of dengue hemorrhagic fever.

CLINICAL MANIFESTATIONS

Viral hemorrhagic fever is seen in both genders and all age groups, with a spectrum from relatively mild or even asymptomatic infection to severe vascular permeability resulting in shock, multiorgan system failure, and death. Although the clinical presentation may differ for each viral hemorrhagic fever as it progresses, the limited data do not permit clear distinctions in most cases, especially in the early phases of disease. Dengue and Rift Valley fever viruses cause a range of syndromes, including rash and central nervous

system involvement (Chapters 390 and 391). Hemorrhagic fever occurs in a minority of infections with these viruses.

Most patients present with nonspecific signs and symptoms difficult to distinguish from a host of other febrile illnesses (see Table 389-2). Illness typically begins with fever and constitutional symptoms, including general malaise, anorexia, headache, chest or retrosternal pain, sore throat, myalgia, arthralgia, lumbosacral pain, and dizziness. Relative bradycardia and orthostatic hypotension may be noted. The pharynx may be erythemic or, less frequently, exudative, especially in Lassa fever, and incorrectly lead to a diagnosis of streptococcal pharyngitis. Gastrointestinal signs and symptoms readily ensue, including nausea, vomiting, epigastric and abdominal pain, abdominal tenderness (especially over the liver in filovirus infection), and diarrhea. Bleeding, including from the gastrointestinal tract, may be profuse in some viral hemorrhagic fevers, especially with Crimean-Congo hemorrhagic fever, Ebola (Fig. 389-1), and Marburg viruses. Significant internal bleeding from the gastrointestinal tract may occur even in the absence of external hemorrhage.

Viral hemorrhagic fever has sometimes been mistaken for acute appendicitis (Chapter 144) or other abdominal emergencies. A dry cough, sometimes accompanied by a few scattered rales on auscultation, is common, but prominent pulmonary symptoms are uncommon early in the course of the disease, except with hantavirus pulmonary syndrome. Conjunctival injection or hemorrhage is frequent but is not accompanied by itching, discharge, or rhinitis (Fig. 389-2). Various forms of rash, including morbilliform, maculopapular, petechial, and ecchymotic, may be seen. A maculopapular rash on the torso or face may be one early and relatively specific although insensitive indicator of Ebola or Marburg hemorrhagic fever. Rash almost always occurs in fair-skinned persons with Lassa fever but, for unclear reasons, rarely in blacks.

In severe cases, patients progress to vascular instability, which may be manifested by conjunctival injection and hemorrhage, facial flushing, edema, bleeding, hypotension, shock, and proteinuria. Swelling in the face and neck is sometimes seen in Lassa fever and is relatively specific to this disease (see Fig. 389-2). The likelihood of clinically discernible hemorrhage varies with the infecting virus, but it is seen in a minority of cases and almost never in the first few days of illness. Hematemesis, melena, hematochezia, metrorrhagia, petechiae, purpura, epistaxis, and bleeding from the gums and venipuncture sites may develop, but hemoptysis and hematuria are infrequent. Large ecchymoses are characteristic of Crimean-Congo hemorrhagic fever.

FIGURE 389-1. Bleeding in a patient with Ebola hemorrhagic fever. (From Bausch DG. Viral hemorrhagic fevers. In: Schlossberg D, ed. *Clinical Infectious Disease.* New York: Cambridge University Press; 2008.)

FIGURE 389-2. Subconjunctival hemorrhage and facial swelling in a boy with Lassa fever in Sierra Leone.

TABLE 389-3	INDICATED CLINICAL LABORATORY TESTS AND CHARACTERISTIC FINDINGS IN PATIENTS WITH VIRAL HEMORRHAGIC FEVER
TEST	**CHARACTERISTIC FINDINGS AND COMMENTS**
Leukocyte count	Early: moderate leukopenia, sometimes with atypical lymphocytes (except for the VHFs caused by hantaviruses, in which early leukocytosis is typical) Later: leukocytosis with left shift
Hemoglobin and hematocrit	Hemoconcentration (especially noted in hantavirus pulmonary syndrome)
Platelet count	Mild to moderate thrombocytopenia
Electrolytes	Sodium, potassium, and acid-base perturbations, depending on fluid balance and stage of disease
Lactate	A level >4 mmol/L (36 mg/dL) may indicate persistent hypoperfusion and sepsis
BUN/creatinine	Renal failure may occur late in disease
AST, ALT, amylase	Increased, usually AST > ALT
Coagulation studies (PT, PTT, fibrinogen, fibrin split products, platelets, D-dimer)	DIC common except in hantavirus pulmonary syndrome
Urinalysis	Proteinuria common
Blood culture	Useful early to exclude VHF and later to evaluate for secondary bacterial infection
Stool culture	Useful to exclude VHF (in favor of hemorrhagic bacillary dysentery)
Thick and thin smears or other assay for malaria	Negative in VHF unless coinfection with malaria
Febrile agglutinins or other assay for *Salmonella typhi*	Negative in VHF unless coinfection with *S. typhi*

ALT = alanine aminotransferase; AST = aspartate aminotransferase; BUN = blood urea nitrogen; DIC = disseminated intravascular coagulation; PT = prothrombin time; PTT = partial thromboplastin time; VHF = viral hemorrhagic fever.

the most severe manifestations, including hemorrhage, shock, renal failure, and meningoencephalitis. Distinct phases of disease and recovery are classically described for hemorrhagic fever with renal syndrome (prodrome, hypotension, oliguria, diuresis) and yellow fever (infection, intoxication, recovery), although not seen in all cases. The initial manifestations for hantavirus pulmonary syndrome may be mild and nonspecific, but the disease may progress to require mechanical ventilation and pressor support within 24 hours; sinus bradycardia and ventricular tachycardia or fibrillation may occur. Encephalitis and retinitis may develop in Rift Valley fever independently of the presence or absence of viral hemorrhagic fever.

A variety of clinical laboratory findings are seen (Table 389-3) but are nonspecific. Radiographic and electrocardiographic findings also are generally nonspecific and usually correlate with the physical examination. Bilateral noncardiogenic interstitial pulmonary edema consistent with the adult respiratory distress syndrome (ARDS) is the hallmark of hantavirus pulmonary syndrome, although chest radiographs may be normal early in the disease even when the patients complain of shortness of breath. Only about 30% of patients with hantavirus pulmonary syndrome have radiographic evidence of pulmonary edema on initial evaluation, although it develops in virtually all persons within 48 hours.

DIAGNOSIS

The nonspecific presentation of most viral hemorrhagic fevers makes them extremely difficult to diagnose clinically, especially early in the course of the disease, when hemorrhage is usually absent. The differential diagnosis includes a broad array of febrile illnesses that may vary by geographic region (Table 389-4). A diagnosis of viral hemorrhagic fever should be considered in patients with a clinically compatible syndrome who, within 3 weeks before disease onset, traveled in areas where a viral hemorrhagic fever is known or suspected to be endemic, had potential direct contact with blood or body fluids of a person or animal with viral hemorrhagic fever during the acute illness, had contact with live or recently killed wild animals (especially nonhuman primates), recently arrived from an area where a viral hemorrhagic

Central nervous system manifestations, including disorientation, tremor, gait anomalies, convulsions, and hiccups, may be noted in end-stage disease, especially in Kyasanur Forest disease, Omsk hemorrhagic fever, and the South American hemorrhagic fevers, particularly Argentine hemorrhagic fever. Nevertheless, the cerebrospinal fluid findings are usually normal, with the exception of patients who have meningoencephalitis due to Kyasanur Forest disease and Omsk hemorrhagic fever, in which an elevated protein level is common. Renal insufficiency or failure is common, especially in hemorrhagic fever with renal syndrome. Pregnant women often present with spontaneous abortion and vaginal bleeding. Maternal and fetal mortality may approach 100% in the third trimester. With the exception of yellow fever, jaundice is not typical.

Biphasic illnesses are classically noted for the flavivirus hemorrhagic fevers, in which a quiescent period of days (yellow fever and dengue) to weeks (Kyasanur Forest disease and Omsk hemorrhagic fever) is followed by

TABLE 389-4 DIFFERENTIAL DIAGNOSIS OF VIRAL HEMORRHAGIC FEVER

DISEASE	DISTINGUISHING CHARACTERISTICS AND COMMENTS
PARASITES	
Malaria (Chapter 353)	Classically shows paroxysms of fever and chills; hemorrhagic manifestations less common; malaria smears or rapid test result usually positive; responds to antimalarials
Amebiasis (Chapter 360)	Hemorrhagic manifestations other than bloody diarrhea generally not seen; amebic trophozoites identified in the stool; responds to antiparasitics
Giardiasis (Chapter 359)	Diagnostic findings in stool; responds to antiparasitic medications
African trypanosomiasis (acute phase) (Chapter 354)	Acute stages may mimic VHF if neurologic syndrome not prominent
BACTERIA	
Typhoid fever (Chapter 316)	Hemorrhagic manifestations other than bloody diarrhea generally not seen; responds to antibiotics
Bacillary dysentery (including shigellosis, campylobacteriosis, salmonellosis, and enterohemorrhagic *Escherichia coli* and others) (Chapter 291)	Hemorrhagic manifestations other than bloody diarrhea generally not seen; responds to antibiotics
Meningococcemia (Chapter 306)	Bacterial-induced DIC may mimic the bleeding diathesis of VHF; large ecchymoses typical of meningococcemia are unusual in the VHFs except for Crimean-Congo HF; may respond to antibiotics
Staphylococcemia (Chapter 296)	Bacterial-induced DIC may mimic the bleeding diathesis of VHF; may respond to antibiotics
Septicemic plague (Chapter 320)	Bacterial-induced DIC may mimic the bleeding diathesis of VHF; large ecchymoses typical of plague are unusual in the VHFs except for Crimean-Congo HF; may respond to antibiotics
Streptococcal pharyngitis (Chapter 298)	May mimic the exudative pharyngitis sometimes seen in Lassa fever
Tularemia (Chapter 319)	Ulceroglandular and pneumonic forms more common; responds to antibiotics
Acute abdominal emergencies (Chapter 144)	Appendicitis and peritonitis
Pyelonephritis and post-streptococcal glomerulonephritis (Chapters 123 and 292)	May mimic HF with renal syndrome
Anthrax (inhalation or gastrointestinal) (Chapter 302)	Prominent pulmonary manifestations in inhalational form; may respond to antibiotics
Psittacosis (Chapter 326)	Pulmonary symptoms often not present until late in the illness; responds to antibiotics
VIRUSES	
Influenza (Chapter 372)	Prominent respiratory component to clinical presentation; no hemorrhagic manifestations; influenza rapid test result may be positive; may respond to anti-influenza drugs
Arbovirus infection (including dengue and West Nile fever) (Chapters 390 and 391)	Encephalitis unusual but when present may mimic the VHFs with significant neurologic involvement (Kyasanur Forest disease, Omsk HF); usually less severe than VHF; hemorrhage not reported
Viral hepatitis (including hepatitis A, hepatitis B, hepatitis E, Epstein-Barr, and cytomegalovirus) (Chapter 150)	Jaundice atypical in HF except yellow fever; test results for hepatitis antigens positive
Measles (Chapter 375)	Rash may mimic that seen in early stages of some VHFs; prominence of coryza and upper respiratory symptoms in measles should help differentiate; vaccine preventable
Rubella (Chapter 376)	Rash may mimic that seen in early stages of some VHFs; usually a mild disease; vaccine preventable
Hemorrhagic or flat smallpox (Chapter 380)	Diffuse hemorrhagic or macular lesions; in contrast to the VHFs, the rash may involve the oral mucosa, palms, and soles; smallpox in the wild has been eradicated
Alphavirus infection (including chikungunya and o'nyong-nyong) (Chapter 390)	Joint pain often prominent
SPIROCHETES, RICKETTSIA, EHRLICHIA, AND COXIELLA	
Relapsing fever (Chapter 330)	Recurrent fevers and influenza-like symptoms, with direct neurologic involvement and splenomegaly; spirochetes visible in blood while febrile; responds to antibiotics
Leptospirosis (Chapter 331)	Jaundice, renal failure, and myocarditis in severe cases; responds to antibiotics
Spotted fever group rickettsioses (including Rocky Mountain spotted fever, boutonneuse fever, African tick bite fever) (Chapter 335)	Necrotic lesion (eschar) at site of tick bite in some forms; responds to antibiotics
Typhus-group rickettsioses (including murine- and louse-borne typhus) (Chapter 335)	History of exposure to lice; interstitial pneumonia on a chest radiograph; responds to antibiotics
Q fever (Chapter 335)	Pneumonia may be prominent; responds to antibiotics
Ehrlichiosis (Chapter 335)	Responds to antibiotics
NONINFECTIOUS CAUSES	
Idiopathic and thrombotic thrombocytopenic purpura (ITP/TTP) (Chapter 175)	Presentation usually less acute than VHF; may have prominent neurologic symptoms in TTP; coagulation factors normal and DIC absent; often respond to corticosteroids (ITP) or plasma exchange (TTP)
Acute glaucoma (Chapter 431)	May mimic the acute ocular manifestations of Rift Valley fever
Leukemia (Chapter 189)	May resemble the leukemoid reaction occasionally seen in HF with renal syndrome

DIC = disseminated intravascular coagulopathy; HF = hemorrhagic fever; VHF = viral hemorrhagic fever.

fever is endemic, worked in a laboratory or animal facility where hemorrhagic fever viruses are handled, or had sexual relations with someone recovering from a viral hemorrhagic fever in the last 3 months. Acts of bioterrorism (Chapter 20) must be considered if clusters of cases are seen in the absence of such risk factors. ARDS or other respiratory compromise in a person living in an endemic area for New World hantaviruses should prompt consideration of hantavirus pulmonary syndrome. Risk of tick infection, including physical examination for an eschar, should be assessed if a tick-borne viral hemorrhagic fever is suspected. However, most viral hemorrhagic fevers are rare even in persons possessing one of the risk factors, so alternative diagnoses should always be aggressively sought, especially malaria and typhoid fever in areas where they are endemic. All confirmed cases of viral hemorrhagic fever should be reported immediately to local, state, and federal health authorities.

Laboratory Testing

No commercial assays are available except for the serologic diagnosis of dengue and hantavirus pulmonary syndrome. Specialized testing can be arranged through the U.S. Centers for Disease Control and Prevention (001-404-639-1115). The enzyme-linked immunosorbent assay is the mainstay of diagnosis, with sensitivities and specificities usually above 90%. Immunofluorescent antibody tests are not as routinely sensitive or specific. Serologic diagnosis of flavivirus infection is often complicated by cross-reactions. Reverse transcription–polymerase chain reaction (RT-PCR) is also useful, although careful attention must be paid to the potential for false-positive results due to laboratory contamination. The most definitive test is viral culture, but the time to diagnosis (2 to 10 days for the virus to grow, depending on the specific virus and titer in the test sample), variability, and need for high containment facilities render this technique more of a confirmatory test and research tool.

TREATMENT   Rx

Patients with viral hemorrhagic fever should generally be treated in intensive care units or the highest level of care available. A broad range of clinical laboratory parameters should be monitored (see Table 389-3).

General Supportive Measures

Severe microvascular instability, often complicated by vomiting, diarrhea, and decreased fluid intake, normally requires aggressive fluid replacement. However, overaggressive and unmonitored rehydration may lead to significant third-spacing and pulmonary edema, especially in hantavirus pulmonary syndrome. Because of the risk of bleeding at intravascular insertion sites, hemodynamic status should be monitored by blood pressure cuff and other noninvasive means.

Fluid and blood pressure management is as for septic shock (Chapter 108). Crystalloids (lactated Ringer's solution or normal saline) and, if necessary, vasopressors (Chapter 108) should be infused to maintain central venous pressure between 8 and 12 mm Hg or mean arterial blood pressure above 65 mm Hg.**1** Early use of vasopressors, especially dopamine and norepinephrine, may diminish the risk of fluid overload, and dobutamine should be added if these measures and blood transfusion fail to maintain the target blood pressure and adequate organ perfusion (Chapter 108). Extrapolating from data on septic shock, transfusions, preferably with packed red blood cells, should be used to maintain a hematocrit above 30% while avoiding volume overload.

Electrolyte values should be monitored closely. Vomiting and diarrhea frequently result in hypokalemia, so potassium supplementation may be needed (Chapter 119).

The possibility of DIC (Chapter 178) should be assessed and treatment (see Table 178-2) implemented in patients with consistent laboratory parameters (see Table 389-3) *and* active bleeding. Transfusion of platelet concentrate (1 to 2 units/10 kg) should be considered when the platelet count is less than 50,000/μL in a bleeding patient or less than 20,000/μL without bleeding. The platelet count should generally rise by at least 2000/μL per unit of platelets transfused, although a lesser response may occur if there is ongoing DIC and platelet consumption. Impaired platelet aggregation may promote hemorrhage in some viral hemorrhagic fevers, especially Lassa fever, even when platelet counts are not drastically low. Transfusion of fresh-frozen plasma (FFP; 15 to 20 mL/kg) should be considered when bleeding is present and fibrinogen levels are less than 100 mg/dL. Fibrinogen concentrates (total dose, 2 to 3 g) or cryoprecipitates (1 unit/10 kg) may be administered instead of FFP, although FFP has the theoretical advantage of containing all coagulation factors and inhibitors deficient in DIC but no activated coagulation factors. Vitamin K (10 mg on 2 consecutive days) may be given, especially if underlying malnutrition or liver disease is suspected.

With the exception of hantavirus pulmonary syndrome, impaired gas exchange is not typically a prominent feature of viral hemorrhagic fever, especially in the absence of iatrogenic pulmonary edema. Intubation and mechanical ventilation (Chapter 105) should be avoided because of the risk of barotrauma and pleural-pulmonary hemorrhage, except in hantavirus pulmonary syndrome, in which patients should be immediately covered with appropriate broad-spectrum antibacterial or antiparasitic therapy, with specific consideration of antimalarial agents for malaria (Chapter 353) and doxycycline for tick-borne rickettsial diseases, until a diagnosis of viral hemorrhagic fever can be confirmed (see Table 389-4). If patients have persistent or new fever after about 2 weeks of illness, secondary bacterial infection should be suspected.

Acetaminophen (500 to 1000 mg every 4 to 6 hours), tramadol (50 to 100 mg every 4 to 6 hours), opiates (see Table 29-4), or other analgesics should be used as needed for pain control. Salicylates and nonsteroidal anti-inflammatory drugs should not be used, and intramuscular and subcutaneous injections should be avoided because of the risk of bleeding. Prophylactic therapy for stress ulcers with H2-receptor antagonists (e.g., ranitidine, 50 mg intravenously every 8 hours; see Table 140-1) is appropriate.

Seizures sometimes occur in late-stage viral hemorrhagic fever but can usually be managed with benzodiazepines or phenytoin (Chapter 410). The use of sedatives and neuromuscular blocking agents should be minimized, but haloperidol (0.5 to 5 mg, two or three times daily) or a benzodiazepine (e.g., lorazepam, 1 to 10 mg orally daily in two or three divided doses) may be used.

Uterine evacuation appears to lower maternal mortality and should be seriously considered, although only with extreme caution to avoid nosocomial transmission of hemorrhagic fever viruses. Peritoneal dialysis and hemodialysis are often used in patients with hemorrhagic fever with renal syndrome without major complications, but there is little published experience in other viral hemorrhagic fevers.

Antiviral Therapy

Intravenous ribavirin (a loading dose of 30 mg/kg, maximum 2 g; followed by 15 mg/kg, maximum 1 g, every 6 hours for 4 days; followed by 7.5 mg/kg, maximum 500 mg, every 8 hours for another 6 days) for 10 days decreases mortality in severe Lassa fever from 55% to 5% when it is begun within the first 6 days of illness,**2** although it is not approved by the Food and Drug Administration for this indication. The drug should be diluted in 150 mL of 0.9% saline and infused slowly, with the dose diminished in persons with a creatinine clearance of less than 50 mL/min (Chapter 368).

Ribavirin reduces mortality in hemorrhagic fever with renal syndrome if it is administered within 4 days of onset.**3** It also appears to be efficacious in the South American hemorrhagic fevers and Crimean-Congo hemorrhagic fever, although randomized trials have not been performed for these diseases. There are no published data on the clinical efficacy of ribavirin for Rift Valley fever, although the drug has in vitro activity against the virus. Ribavirin is not efficacious in Ebola or Marburg hemorrhagic fevers. Until more data are available, ribavirin should not be used for dengue and yellow fever virus infections.

Convalescent Immune Plasma

Transfusion of appropriately titered convalescent plasma within the first 8 days of illness reduces the case-fatality of Argentine hemorrhagic fever from 15 to 30% to less than 1%.**4** However, this therapy has been associated with a convalescent phase neurologic syndrome characterized by fever, cerebellar signs, and cranial nerve palsies in 10% of treated patients. Convalescent plasma also has been used in Lassa fever. Immune plasma also appears to be efficacious for Crimean-Congo hemorrhagic fever and Rift Valley fever, although there are no controlled data, but it should not be used for Ebola and Marburg hemorrhagic fevers.

Immune Modulators

Immune modulators have not shown conclusive benefit in the viral hemorrhagic fevers. Intravenous corticosteroids (e.g., hydrocortisone, 200 to 300 mg/day divided into three or four doses for 7 days) should not be administered unless adrenal insufficiency is demonstrated, target blood pressure is not maintained despite adequate fluid repletion and vasopressors, or (in conjunction with mannitol) cerebral edema is suspected.

Activated protein C (24 μg/kg/hr constant infusion) is efficacious for some patients with septic shock (Chapter 108) and reduces mortality in Ebola virus–infected monkeys but is still experimental for viral hemorrhagic fever in humans. An experimental recombinant inhibitor of the tissue factor/factor VIIa coagulation pathway (rNAPc2) also decreases mortality in Ebola virus–infected monkeys and has completed a phase I trial in humans.

PREVENTION

Infection control of the hemorrhagic fever viruses relies on classic public health principles of isolation of infected persons. All patients with a clinically compatible syndrome should be presumed infectious and kept isolated until a specific diagnosis is made. If it is available, a negative airflow room is prudent, but hermetically sealed isolation chambers are not required. Access to the patient should be limited to a small number of designated staff and family members with specific instructions and training on infection control guidelines and the use of personal protective equipment. Insecticide-treated bed nets and room screens should be used in open-air settings to prevent transmission of arthropod-borne viruses.

Personal Protection and Nursing Precautions

Although specific viral hemorrhagic fever isolation precautions (surgical mask, double gloves, gown, protective apron, face shield, and shoe covers) are advised for added security, routine strict barrier nursing is protective in most cases. Positive airway pressure masks and other small-particle aerosol precautions should be used in performing procedures that may generate aerosols, such as endotracheal intubation.

Items that were in direct contact with a patient with viral hemorrhagic fever should be decontaminated with household bleach. A 1 : 100 (1%) solution of ordinary 5% chlorine bleach should be used for reusable items, and a 1 : 10 (10%) solution for disinfection of excreta, corpses, and items to be discarded.

Contact Tracing

The early nonspecific presentation of the viral hemorrhagic fevers poses a serious challenge to effective epidemiologic surveillance. Fortunately, the low secondary attack rates afford a measure of reassurance even when cases go unrecognized as long as proper barrier nursing is maintained. Furthermore, because mild cases, which may be still more difficult to recognize, are usually not very infectious, missed or delayed diagnosis of these patients is unlikely to pose a problem from an infection control standpoint.

Persons with unprotected direct contact with a patient during the symptomatic phase of a person to person communicable hemorrhagic fever virus should be monitored daily for evidence of disease for the duration of the longest possible incubation period starting after their last contact (see Table 389-2). Contacts should check their temperature daily and record the results in a log. Despite the lack of evidence for transmission during the incubation period, it is usually recommended that exposed persons avoid close contact or activities with household members that might result in exposure to body fluids, such as sex, kissing, and sharing of utensils. Hospitalization or other confinement of asymptomatic persons is not warranted, but persons who develop fever or other signs and symptoms suggestive of viral hemorrhagic fever should immediately be isolated until the diagnosis can be excluded.

Reservoir and Vector Control

Avoiding contact with bats, primarily by avoiding entry into caves and mines in endemic areas, is a key prevention measure for Ebola and Marburg viruses. Personal protective equipment may be indicated for miners and other persons who work in these environments. Humans should also avoid exposure to fresh blood, body fluids, or meat of wild animals, especially nonhuman primates.

For rodent-borne viruses whose reservoirs often colonize human dwellings, prevention is best accomplished by improving "village hygiene," such as eliminating unprotected storage of garbage and foodstuffs and plugging holes that allow rodents to enter homes. Prevention of the mosquito-borne hemorrhagic fever viruses hinges on controlling *Aedes* mosquitoes in and around the home, primarily by elimination of clean standing water containers that serve as larval habitats and by use of screened windows and doors, insecticide-treated bed nets, protective clothing, mosquito repellent, and aerosol bomb insecticides in enclosed spaces. Analogous measures can help protect against tick bites.

Vaccines

The only widely licensed, validated, and available vaccine for a viral hemorrhagic fever is the yellow fever 17D (YF-17D) live attenuated vaccine. The vaccine is highly efficacious; a single 0.5-mL injection confers protection in more than 95% of recipients within 10 days. Immunity is probably lifelong, although revaccination is recommended every 10 years and required by International Health Regulations published by the World Health Organization. Hence, confirmed previous vaccination with YF-17D should strongly suggest a diagnosis other than yellow fever unless the patient was immunocompromised at the time of vaccination (see later).

YF-17D is indicated for persons 9 months of age and older who are traveling to or living in areas with risk of yellow fever transmission. The overall safety profile of YF-17D is excellent, with mild adverse events (low-grade fever, headache, myalgia) occurring in 10 to 30% of cases. However, severe and fatal vaccine-associated neurotropic and viscerotropic disease has been increasingly reported in the last decade, especially in persons older than 60 years, in whom the actual risk of exposure must be carefully weighed. YF-17D is contraindicated in persons allergic to eggs or chicken, breast-feeding women, and immunocompromised persons. Physicians are advised to consult state and federal health departments when considering vaccination of persons with relative contraindications.

A live attenuated vaccine called Candid #1 decreases the morbidity and mortality of Argentine hemorrhagic fever and may also protect against Bolivian hemorrhagic fever, although it does not appear to cross-protect against Guanarito or Sabiá viruses or any of the Old World arenaviruses.[5] The

vaccine is not approved in the United States, however, and supplies are insufficient even in Argentina, the sole country in which the vaccine is produced.

A formalin-inactivated vaccine for Rift Valley fever (TSI-GSD-200) is efficacious in humans but is not widely available and requires yearly boosters. It is sometimes available for high-risk groups, such as veterinarians working in endemic areas and laboratory workers. A number of other Rift Valley fever vaccines are in development. Vaccines for Kyasanur Forest disease and hemorrhagic fever with renal syndrome are available in India and northeast Asia, respectively, but their efficacy has not been extensively evaluated, and they are not generally licensed or available outside these regions. The vaccine for hemorrhagic fever with renal syndrome is based on hantaviruses found in Asia and is unlikely to protect against the viruses that commonly cause this disease in Europe. A mouse brain–derived vaccine for Omsk hemorrhagic fever has been used for those at risk of environmental exposure but is not widely available.

A number of experimental approaches also show promise; a live recombinant vesicular stomatitis virus vector engineered to express the key immunogenic proteins of the hemorrhagic fever viruses has shown protective immunity in animal models for Ebola, Marburg, and Lassa virus infection. Furthermore, these vaccines also are effective when they are given by the nasal or oral route. A DNA plasmid vaccine for Ebola hemorrhagic fever has been shown to be safe and immunogenic in a phase I trial, as has a recombinant vaccine for dengue fever.

Postexposure Prophylaxis

Postexposure prophylaxis with oral ribavirin (loading dose of 35 mg/kg, maximum 2.5 g; followed by 15 mg/kg, maximum 1 g, three times daily for 10 days) may be considered for persons with distinct and direct unprotected contact with blood or body fluids from a person with a confirmed infection with arenaviruses, Crimean-Congo hemorrhagic fever virus, and perhaps Rift Valley fever virus, although there are no data on efficacy, dose, or duration of administration of the drug for this purpose. Persons who are exposed to an arenavirus and who develop manifestations of viral hemorrhagic fever should be immediately converted to intravenous ribavirin. Convalescent plasma is as efficacious as postexposure prophylaxis for Argentine hemorrhagic fever. Various experimental therapies show potential promise as postexposure prophylaxis for the filoviruses. Prophylaxis should never be given if the only exposure was during the incubation period.

PROGNOSIS

The clinical course of viral hemorrhagic fever unfolds quite rapidly. In fatal cases, death usually occurs within 7 to 10 days after the onset of hemorrhagic fever symptoms in filovirus infection and in about 2 weeks with the arenaviruses and some of the other viruses. Common indicators of a poor prognosis include shock, bleeding, neurologic manifestations, high levels of viremia, elevated levels of aspartate aminotransferase (>150 IU/L), and pregnancy, especially during the third trimester. However, mild and even asymptomatic cases have been reported even for what are considered the most virulent viral hemorrhagic fevers. Reasons for this heterogeneity are largely unknown.

Viremia clears rapidly in survivors of viral hemorrhagic fever, who can be discharged without concern of subsequent transmission at home. However, clearance of virus may be delayed for weeks to months from a few immunologically protected sites, such as the kidney, chambers of the eye, and gonads. Sexual transmission can occur months after recovery from acute disease, especially with Ebola, Marburg, and Lassa viruses.

Persons who survive viral hemorrhagic fever usually suffer no obvious long-term sequelae. Notable exceptions include deafness in up to 30% of patients after Lassa fever and sometimes after Venezuelan hemorrhagic fever and optic retinopathy with vision loss in Rift Valley fever. Convalescence may be prolonged, especially for Ebola and Marburg hemorrhagic fevers, with the potential for persistent myalgia, arthralgia, anorexia, weight loss, alopecia, pancreatitis, uveitis, and orchitis up to a year after infection. The psychological effects of viral hemorrhagic fever may also be significant, with some patients experiencing depression or post-traumatic stress.

Clinical management during convalescence includes the use of warm packs, acetaminophen, nonsteroidal anti-inflammatory drugs, cosmetics, hair growth stimulants, anxiolytics, antidepressants, nutritional supplements, and nutritional and psychological counseling as indicated. Uveitis in patients recovering from Ebola hemorrhagic fever responds to topical steroids and atropine. Because of the risk of sexual transmission during convalescence, abstinence or condom use is recommended for 3 months after acute illness. Similarly, breast-feeding should be avoided during convalescence unless there is no other way to support the baby. Transmission through toilet facilities or eye secretions has not been noted, but simple precautions to avoid contact with these potentially infected body fluids are prudent, including separate toilet facilities, if possible, and regular handwashing.

1. Levy MM, Dellinger RP, Townsend SR, et al. The Surviving Sepsis Campaign: results of an international guideline–based performance improvement program targeting severe sepsis. *Crit Care Med.* 2010;38:367-374.
2. McCormick JB, King IJ, Webb PA, et al. Lassa fever. Effective therapy with ribavirin. *N Engl J Med.* 1986;314:20-26.
3. Huggins JW, Hsiang CM, Cosgriff TM, et al. Prospective, double-blind, concurrent, placebo-controlled clinical trial of intravenous ribavirin therapy of hemorrhagic fever with renal syndrome. *J Infect Dis.* 1991;164:1119-1127.
4. Maiztegui JI, Fernández NJ, de Damilano AJ. Efficacy of immune plasma in treatment of Argentine hemorrhagic fever and association between treatment and a late neurological syndrome. *Lancet.* 1979;2:1216-1217.
5. Maiztegui JI, McKee KT Jr, Barrera Oro JG, et al. Protective efficacy of a live attenuated vaccine against Argentine hemorrhagic fever. *J Infect Dis.*1998;177:277-283.

SUGGESTED READINGS

Bausch DG, Hadi CM, Khan SH, et al. Review of the literature and proposed guidelines for the use of oral ribavirin as postexposure prophylaxis for Lassa fever. *Clin Infect Dis.* 2010;51:1435-1441. *Comprehensive review and detailed guidelines.*

Feldmann H, Geisbert TW. Ebola haemorrhagic fever. *Lancet.* 2011;377:849-862. *Review.*

Moraz ML, Kunz S. Pathogenesis of arenavirus hemorrhagic fevers. *Expert Rev Anti Infect Ther.* 2011;9:49-59. *Review.*

Růžek D, Yakimenko VV, Karan LS, et al. Omsk haemorrhagic fever. *Lancet.* 2010;376:2014-2113. *Review.*

Simpson SQ, Spikes L, Patel S, et al. Hantavirus pulmonary syndrome. *Infect Dis Clin North Am.* 2010;24:159-173. *Comprehensive review.*

390

ARBOVIRUSES CAUSING FEVER AND RASH SYNDROMES

STANLEY J. NAIDES

COLORADO TICK FEVER

DEFINITION

Colorado tick fever (mountain fever, American mountain fever) is an acute, often self-limited, typically biphasic febrile illness that is common in the Rocky Mountain areas, the Sierra Nevada and Wasatch ranges, and the Black Hills mountain areas. The virus is transmitted through the bite of the hard-shelled tick *Dermacentor andersoni* (Rocky Mountain wood tick), and the disease's range corresponds to the vector's range. Other coltiviruses, such as the Salmon River, Eyach, Banna, Beijing, and Gansu viruses, have also been implicated in human disease.

The Pathogen

The causative agent, Colorado tick fever virus, is a member of the genus Coltivirus, family Reoviridae. Coltiviruses have a genome consisting of 12 double-stranded RNA segments. Colorado tick fever virus is the prototype member.

EPIDEMIOLOGY

D. andersoni is found at elevations of 4000 to 10,000 ft. Seasonal temperatures tend to influence the range, with the vector being found at higher elevations in warmer seasons and at lower elevations in colder seasons. Human exposure usually occurs during outdoor recreational activities in these areas. Occasional exposure occurs in nonendemic areas from ticks exported out of the endemic region in clothes, hiking equipment, or baggage. Infections generally take place between March and September, when the adult tick is most plentiful. Ticks are most abundant in south-facing dry and rocky slope habitats that favor small rodents (e.g., chipmunks, ground squirrels, marmosets), with underbrush cover, burrows, and humidity for the ticks. Colorado tick fever virus is found in nymphal and adult ticks that overwinter on the rodent host, in which viremia persists for weeks to months. In the endemic area, as many as 14% of *D. andersoni* ticks carry Colorado tick fever virus. Humans are an incidental host. Fewer than 50 cases have been reported annually in Colorado beginning in 1992. The actual number of cases is probably significantly larger and includes subclinical, mild, and unreported cases.

The geographic range of Colorado tick fever may be larger than the well-recognized endemic mountain areas. Serologically confirmed cases in California have been attributed to the Colorado tick fever–related virus S1-14-03, which is transmitted by *Dermacentor variabilis* (American dog tick). Salmon River virus causes a Colorado tick fever–like illness in rafters on the Salmon River in Idaho. Another similar virus, Eyach virus, has been implicated in neurologic illness in France and Germany and has been isolated from the deer ticks *Ixodes ricinus* and *Ixodes ventalloi*.

PATHOBIOLOGY

Colorado tick fever virus replicates in CD34$^+$ stem cells in bone marrow and leads to mild to moderate leukopenia and thrombocytopenia. The virus also replicates in committed erythrocyte precursors and may be detected in circulating erythrocytes up to 4 weeks after infection.

CLINICAL MANIFESTATIONS

Patients report a tick bite or exposure in 90% of cases, but there is no notable local reaction to the tick bite. After a mean incubation of 3 to 4 days (range, 0 to 14 days), sudden-onset fever develops in association with malaise, chills, myalgia, weakness, headache, photophobia, retro-orbital pain, and cutaneous hyperesthesia. Conjunctival and oropharyngeal injection, palatal enanthem, lymphadenopathy, and splenomegaly may be present. The absence of prominent respiratory and gastrointestinal symptoms helps exclude other febrile illnesses. A petechial or maculopapular exanthem, found in 15% of patients, may be confused with the rash of Rocky Mountain spotted fever (Chapter 335). The illness has a "saddleback" fever pattern consisting of resolution of the initial fever within 1 week and recrudescence after a 2- to 3-day hiatus. A third fever episode may occur.

Leukopenia develops 5 to 6 days after onset of the illness. Mild thrombocytopenia and anemia may occur.

Myocarditis, pneumonitis, hepatitis, orchitis, and epididymitis may complicate adult infection, and aseptic meningitis or encephalitis may occur in up to 10% of childhood infections.

DIAGNOSIS

Clinical diagnosis is confirmed by demonstration of the Colorado tick fever viral genome or specific acute phase IgM antibody. The viral genome may be detected up to 6 weeks after infection by nucleic acid–based methods such as reverse transcription–polymerase chain reaction (RT-PCR) on blood or stored blood clots. Virions in circulating erythrocytes may be detected by immunofluorescent antibody labeling. Anti–Colorado tick fever virus IgM antibody is detected by antibody capture enzyme-linked immunosorbent assay (ELISA) or complement fixation. Neutralization assays using Vero or BHK-21 cells have been helpful.

Differentiating Colorado tick fever from Rocky Mountain spotted fever (Chapter 335) may be difficult before the appearance of the typical rash of the latter. However, Rocky Mountain spotted fever does not have a saddleback fever pattern and is 20 times less common than Colorado tick fever in the western endemic area.

TREATMENT

Treatment is supportive. Aspirin is contraindicated to avoid complicating thrombocytopenia.

PROGNOSIS

Extreme weakness and malaise may persist for weeks to months after final resolution of the fever. Older patients have a prolonged recovery. Seventy percent of patients older than 30 years may still have fatigue 3 weeks after the fever, whereas children and adolescents may recover completely within a week. Rare instances of maternal-fetal transmission have been reported. Full recovery eventually occurs, except when the disease course is complicated by neurologic insult. Patients should refrain from donating blood for 6 months.

DENGUE

DEFINITION

Dengue is an acute febrile illness characterized by severe muscle and joint pain, rash, malaise, and lymphadenopathy. The severity of the musculo-skeletal complaints gave rise to the sobriquet *breakbone fever*. Dengue occurs in the tropical and subtropical climes of the Caribbean, Central and South America, Asia, and Africa. The mosquito range extends into the southeastern part of the United States, where dengue reemerged in the 1980s. After World War II, a spreading global pandemic has been associated with erosion of mosquito control programs, human populations that have spread into rural settings, accelerated population movement as a result of travel by airplane, and large areas that have experienced deterioration in public health infra-structure. Approximately 40% of the world's population lives in endemic areas; tens of millions of individuals are infected annually.

The Pathogen

Dengue virus is a member of the Flaviviridae family, which consists of single-stranded RNA viruses with a lipid envelope approximately 50 nm in diame-ter. There are four serotypes of dengue: DEN-1, DEN-2, DEN-3, and DEN-4. No cross-protection is seen among the serotypes, so dengue can develop after infection with another serotype. Infection with a second serotype places the individual at risk for the development of hemorrhagic fever (Chapter 389).

EPIDEMIOLOGY

Dengue is transmitted to humans by the bite of female *Aedes aegypti* and *Aedes albopictus* mosquitoes. *A. albopictus* has become the dominant pest mosquito in many urban centers. Members of the two mosquito species acquire dengue virus by biting humans, typically during the day. Zoonotic life cycles involving nonhuman primates (i.e., chimpanzees, gibbons, and macaques) and canopy-dwelling forest *Aedes* species have been demon-strated in western Africa and Malaysia. The mosquitoes nest in stagnant water around human dwellings; they are not typically encountered in the forest. In the human host, dengue virus may reach a titer of greater than 10^8 median infectious doses per milliliter. The mosquito becomes infected when taking its meal from a viremic host. The virus continues replication in the midgut epithelium and salivary glands of female mosquitoes, which remain infectious for life. Within 8 to 12 days of the initial infection, the mosquito's salivary glands become infected and virus is shed with saliva during the next blood meal. A given mosquito may infect multiple indi-viduals, especially in view of its skittishness during feeding—slight move-ment of the host interrupts its meal, after which it returns to the original or another host.

The incubation period is typically 4 to 7 days but may range from 3 to 14 days. During outbreaks in the southeastern United States and Puerto Rico, the risk for infection may be as high as 79% in naïve hosts, and clinical disease may develop in up to 20%. Immunity against the infecting serotype is prob-ably lifelong, but individuals remain susceptible to the remaining serotypes. Peak transmission occurs after increased rainfall, when rainwater collected in household containers allows expansion of mosquito populations. Epidemics tend to occur in 3- to 5-year cycles, but interepidemic cases occur regularly.

Dengue is a particular risk to visitors to the tropics and is a leading cause of pediatric morbidity and mortality in endemic areas. Globalization and climate change have contributed to expansion of the geographic range. Dengue accounts for approximately 2% of the febrile illnesses in travelers returning to the United States.

PATHOBIOLOGY

Dengue hemorrhagic fever (Chapter 389) and dengue shock syndrome are forms of dengue reinfection characterized by capillary leakage and hemor-rhage. Previous infection with an alternative serotype allows antibody to the previously encountered serotype to combine with the newly infecting sero-type. Although the first exposed serotype antibody is not neutralizing, it does allow enhanced antibody-mediated macrophage uptake, thereby leading to macrophage activation and increasing viral replication and viral load. Excre-tion of vasoactive inflammatory mediators by macrophages results in vascular leakage; severe vascular leak causes shock. Endothelial cell swelling and peri-vascular edema may occur. Rarely, dengue shock syndrome may occur with primary infection. Variation in a strain's ability to generate enhancing

antibody, as well as differences in virulence, may account for differences in clinical behavior.

CLINICAL MANIFESTATIONS

Dengue infection is often subclinical. When symptomatic, dengue may be manifested as classic dengue, dengue hemorrhagic fever, or dengue shock syndrome. Patients may also have mild illness characterized by nonspecific fever, anorexia, and headache.

Classic dengue, which typically occurs in nonindigenous older children and adults, is characterized by sudden-onset fever, severe frontal headache, retro-orbital pain, myalgia, and in many cases, nausea, vomiting, rash, lymph-adenopathy, and arthralgia. Patients may experience generalized weakness, altered taste, rigors, and cutaneous hyperesthesia. Classic dengue is self-limited, but some patients progress to dengue hemorrhagic fever or dengue shock syndrome, which is characterized by capillary leakage, hypotension, narrowed pulse pressure, and shock. Dengue in pregnancy may be severe.

Physical examination demonstrates fever, relative bradycardia, scleral injection, ocular pressure tenderness, and pharyngeal injection. A transient macular rash appears on days 1 or 2 of illness. On days 2 and 3 of illness, fever and other symptoms may improve. The fever is typically, but not consistently biphasic. After a hiatus of typically 2 days, fever and other symptoms recru-desce, though less severely. Generalized, nontender lymphadenopathy of the posterior cervical, epitrochlear, and inguinal regions may develop. Rash also recurs and appears as 2- to 5-mm speckles of pallor surrounded by erythema and occasionally accompanied by burning dysesthesia of the palms and soles. The rash may desquamate.

DIAGNOSIS

An adequate travel history and knowledge of occurrence of disease in the community can lead to consideration of dengue in the differential diagnosis. Viremia is of adequate intensity in infections with DEN-1, DEN-2, and DEN-3 to allow viral isolation. Viremia in DEN-4 infections is often less intense and more difficult to detect through inoculation of mosquito cells in vitro. Specific IgM antibody appears 3 to 5 days after infection. IgG antibody appears 9 to 10 days after infection. Cross-reactivity with other flaviviruses prevents serotype-specific diagnosis. Neutralization testing with hemagglutin-ation inhibition is more specific, and complement fixation testing for IgG in paired sera is helpful. PCR-based assays are available.

Leukopenia develops by the second day of fever, reaches 2000 to 4000 cells/mL by day 4 or 5, and is associated with granulocytopenia. In dengue hemorrhagic fever, thrombocytopenia of less than 100,000 cells/mL and a prolonged prothrombin time are characteristic. Mild to moderate proteinuria and a few casts may be detected. Aspartate transaminase levels may be increased.

TREATMENT AND PROGNOSIS ℞

Classic dengue resolves abruptly in 5 to 7 days, but fatigue and depression may linger for weeks; survival is uniform. The prognosis of patients with dengue hemorrhagic fever (Chapter 389) and dengue shock syndrome depends on early diagnosis and the introduction of supportive measures. Treatment is supportive and consists of antipyretics and analgesics. Initial resuscitation of patients with shock syndrome (Chapter 108) with crystalloid and colloidal solutions is indicated in those with moderately severe dengue shock syndrome. Fresh-frozen plasma and blood products are used as necessary.

WEST NILE FEVER VIRUS

DEFINITION

West Nile fever is an acute febrile illness associated with malaise, rash, head-ache, myalgia, and lymphadenopathy. Infection involves a bird-mosquito-human cycle. Viremia develops in all varieties of birds. Bats, cats, chipmunks, domestic rabbits, horses, skunks, squirrels, dogs, sheep, llamas, and alpacas may be infected.

The Pathogen

West Nile fever virus, which is the most widely distributed flavivirus, is trans-mitted by a variety of mosquito species. The mosquito vector varies: *Culex univittatus*, *Culex pipiens*, and *Culex molestus* in the Middle East and Africa; *Mansonia metallicus* in Uganda; and *Culex tritaeniorhynchus* in Asia. After introduction into the New York City area in 1999, *C. pipiens* became the most important vector in the United States. Other mosquito species may carry the virus.

EPIDEMIOLOGY

Viral transmission involves mosquitoes and wild birds, with mammals, including humans, being incidental end-stage hosts. In endemic areas, more than 60% of young adults have antibodies, thus suggesting a high prevalence of inapparent or undifferentiated febrile illness in children. There is no gender predominance.

Between 0.5 and 1% of infected individuals experience a more severe illness. Incubation is typically 3 to 14 days but may be as short as 1 day.

West Nile virus emerged in the United States in New York and has spread throughout the continental United States, Canada, Mexico, the Caribbean, and Central and South America. In America, birds of the Corvidae family (e.g., crows, jackdaws, ravens) are often infected, and recognition of increased death in crow populations continues to serve as a sentinel for the presence of West Nile virus. In addition to mosquito transmission, the virus has been transmitted by a transplanted organ, via blood transfusion, transplacentally, and in the laboratory.

Zika virus, a flavivirus related to dengue and West Nile virus, has emerged in Africa, Asia, and the Yap Islands of the southwestern Pacific. It causes outbreaks of fever, rash, arthralgia, and conjunctivitis.

PATHOBIOLOGY

West Nile virus grows in a variety of cells in vitro and produces cytopathic effects in *A. albopictus* cells. Individuals in whom encephalitis develops show evidence of diffuse brain inflammation and neuronal degeneration, with virus detected early in multiple sites. The virus probably replicates in skin dendritic cells, which then migrate to local lymph nodes and initiate the innate immune response.

CLINICAL MANIFESTATIONS

Approximately 80% of infections are asymptomatic, and most of the remaining infections are mild and manifested by fever, malaise, headache, nausea, anorexia, generalized lymphadenopathy, and myalgia. Aseptic meningitis or encephalitis (Chapter 391) may occur in the elderly and, less commonly, in the very young. Severe neurologic disease, including meningitis, myelitis, encephalitis, and flaccid paralysis of the limbs and respiratory muscles, can develop. Like Colorado tick fever and dengue, West Nile fever may be biphasic. Nonpruritic, maculopapular, or roseolar rash occurs on the chest, back, and arms in half the patients, beginning during or with resolution of the fever. The rash persists for up to 1 week and then resolves with desquamation. Patients may experience vomiting, diarrhea, abdominal pain, and pharyngitis. Anterior myelitis or hepatitis may also occur. Disease is usually milder in children than in adults.

DIAGNOSIS

West Nile virus may be isolated from up to 77% of patients with West Nile fever on the first day of illness, but viral isolation is less common in patients with encephalitis (Chapter 391). Low-titer viremia may persist for the first 5 days of illness. Tests for virus-specific antibody using ELISA or immunofluorescence are available. RT-PCR may detect viral RNA in human samples and in avian and insect specimens.

TREATMENT   Rx

Treatment is supportive. The clinical value of antiviral agents is unknown. Infection is controlled by the endogenous development of neutralizing antibodies to protein E, the viral envelope protein.

PROGNOSIS

Illness generally persists 3 to 6 days before rapid recovery. The prognosis is excellent, but mortality rates of 10% or higher occur in patients with encephalitis (Chapter 391).

⬤ PHLEBOTOMUS FEVER

DEFINITION

Phlebotomus fever (i.e., sandfly fever, pappataci, and 3-day fever) is an acute, mild, self-limited febrile illness transmitted through the bite of *Phlebotomus* flies.

The Pathogen

Phlebotomus fever viruses are members of the genus Phlebovirus, family Bunyaviridae. The latter consists of a group of single-stranded RNA viruses that are 80 to 120 nm in diameter, possess a lipid envelope, and have three segments in the genome. A related virus, the Toscana virus hosted by *Phlebotomus perniciosus*, causes a similar illness in central Italy, Cyprus, Spain, and Portugal. Punique virus, a related virus, has been found in blood pools in Sicily.

EPIDEMIOLOGY

The virus's distribution parallels the distribution of *Phlebotomus* flies found throughout the Mediterranean basin, Middle East, and western India and Pakistan. In Central America, *Lutzomyia* fly species may transmit the virus. These tiny sandflies pass through mosquito netting to feed in the early evenings. Virus is maintained by transovarial and trans-stadial transmission. During outbreaks, humans may serve as a reservoir. Human infection is more common in rural areas during the summer months. The incubation period is 2 to 6 days. Sandflies spread by hopping, thus limiting their travel range. Use of insect sprays locally is effective in decreasing risk.

CLINICAL MANIFESTATIONS

Sandfly fever virus causes an acute febrile illness associated with malaise, headache, photophobia, ocular pain, altered taste, myalgia, and arthralgia. The myalgias may be localized to specific regions (e.g., the chest) and simulate regional syndromes such as pleurodynia. A macular or urticarial rash may appear. Examination may show relative bradycardia after the first day, conjunctival injection, mild papilledema, or small palatal vesicles. Fever lasts 2 to 4 days and then subsides. Weakness and malaise may persist during convalescence. About 15% of patients experience recrudescence in 2 to 12 weeks. Aseptic meningitis may occur with mild cerebrospinal fluid pleocytosis. Peripheral leukopenia and lymphopenia may be present early in the illness. However, leukopenia may be delayed in some patients until the third day of illness, and a rebound relative lymphocytosis may be encountered.

DIAGNOSIS

The diagnosis of phlebotomus fever is confirmed by isolation of virus after intracerebral inoculation of suckling mice, detection of the viral genome by RT-PCR, or detection of specific IgM antibody by ELISA.

TREATMENT AND PROGNOSIS   Rx

Treatment is supportive, and recovery is complete. Ribavirin (Chapter 368) has been proposed as a therapeutic option.

⬤ RIFT VALLEY FEVER

Rift Valley fever, which is an acute-onset, febrile illness, is often associated with epizootic waves of spontaneous abortion in livestock.

DEFINITION

The Rift Valley fever virus is a member of the family Bunyaviridae, genus Phlebovirus, but unlike other members of the genus, it is transmitted by *Aedes* mosquitoes.

EPIDEMIOLOGY

Rift Valley fever occurs throughout most of Africa, with the majority of epizootic outbreaks occurring in eastern and southern Africa. Rift Valley fever was documented in Saudi Arabia and Yemen in 2000. The principal initial vectors are probably the *Aedes* species associated with flooding. Shallow pools along rivers and streams play an important role as mosquito breeding sites. Feeding on nearby livestock allows a local epizootic outbreak and amplification of the virus in local mosquito populations, including *C. pipiens* in Egypt and *Culex theileri* in eastern Africa.

Hemorrhagic fever in humans is typically seen 1 to 2 weeks after a wave of abortion in livestock. Initial human cases usually occur in those who have close contact with livestock. The virus is highly transmissible through aerosolization. Although the risk for severe human infection is less than 1%, the extensive exposure associated with outbreaks can lead to significant morbidity and mortality. For example, in the 1977-1978 Egyptian outbreak associated with movement of camels from Sudan, an estimated 200,000 people were infected, with 600 deaths. Zinga virus, isolated in central Africa and Madagascar and shown to be responsible for mild human illness, is a strain of Rift Valley fever virus.

PATHOBIOLOGY

Rift Valley fever virus grows well in a variety of cell cultures and has cytopathic effects. After infection by a mosquito bite, virus is transported through the lymphatics to regional lymph nodes, where replication allows amplification of the input inoculum and development of viremia with systemic spread. Viral replication in liver, spleen, lymph node, adrenal, lung, and kidney tissues is highly cytopathic. In severe cases, hepatic necrosis and, rarely, focal brain necrosis may occur. Encephalitis is not associated with viremia, thus suggesting that this sequela is immune mediated rather than a direct viral effect. Inflammatory cell infiltration is associated with focal necrosis in the brain. Spontaneous abortion is common in livestock, but fetal loss in humans is not clearly correlated with viral infection.

CLINICAL MANIFESTATIONS

Most human infections are mild, with an abrupt onset of fever, chills, malaise, and arthralgia following a 2- to 6-day incubation. Despite the development of neutralizing antibodies, however, about 1 to 2% of infections progress to more severe disease, including a severe hemorrhagic fever associated with hepatic necrosis and disseminated intravascular coagulopathy. Recovery is complicated by retinal vasculitis or encephalitis, which occurs in less than 0.5% of patients 1 to 4 weeks after recovery and is associated with recurrent fever. In severe cases, focal brain necrosis and encephalitis may lead to hallucinations, stupor, coma, and death.

DIAGNOSIS

Intense viremia allows detection of virus by quantitative real-time RT-PCR. Specific IgM and IgG are detectable by ELISA applied to acute and convalescent (after 1 to 2 weeks) paired sera.

TREATMENT, PREVENTION, AND PROGNOSIS   **Rx**

Treatment is supportive. Ribavirin (Chapter 368) has been proposed as a therapeutic option but exhibits limited penetration of the blood-brain barrier. In endemic areas, vaccination of livestock is the most effective preventive measure.

The prognosis is good in the absence of retinitis or encephalitis. A high viral load at initial evaluation is a prognostic indicator for a poor outcome.

● CHIKUNGUNYA FEVER

DEFINITION

Chikungunya fever is a febrile arthritis that occurs in sporadic cases and in epidemics.

The Pathogen

Chikungunya, an enveloped, single-stranded RNA virus 60 to 70 nm in diameter, is a member of the family Togaviridae, genus Alphavirus. Chikungunya virus is transmitted by mosquitoes, principally *Aedes* species, but also by *Mansonia africana* and other genera. Known animal reservoirs are monkeys, baboons, and in Senegal, *Scotophilus* bat species. During outbreaks, humans are the major reservoir.

EPIDEMIOLOGY

Chikungunya, which is endemic in sub-Sahara Africa, India, the Philippines, and Southeast Asia, spread in 2005 to the Seychelles, Mauritius, and Mayotte Islands with a genotype better adapted to *A. albopictus*. This genotype then spread to India, where the outbreak continues with millions being affected. In 2007, an outbreak occurred in Italy. Outbreaks typically develop after heavy rains. In urban settings, outbreaks are explosive. In endemic areas, seroprevalence rates may be as high as 90%, thus suggesting that time required for loss of herd immunity is the reason for the prolonged absence of cases in a region after an outbreak. Globalization may contribute to increasing propensity for spread. An outbreak in Malaysia from 1998 to 1999 was attributed to migrant workers from endemic areas. After inoculation, the incubation period is typically 2 to 3 days but ranges from 1 to 12 days.

PATHOBIOLOGY

Intense viremia develops within 48 hours of the mosquito bite and wanes 2 to 3 days later. Onset of hemagglutination inhibition and neutralizing antibodies clears the viremia. Superficial capillaries in rash-involved skin demonstrate erythrocyte extravasation and perivascular cuffing. The virus adsorbs to human platelets and causes them to aggregate. Synovitis probably results from direct chikungunya viral infection of synovium.

CLINICAL MANIFESTATIONS

Chikungunya fever is characterized by an explosive onset of fever and severe arthralgia. Constitutional symptoms, fever to 40° C, rigors, headache, photophobia, retro-orbital pain, conjunctival injection, pharyngitis, anorexia, nausea, vomiting, abdominal pain, tense lymphadenopathy, and myalgia are common. A maculopapular rash located on the torso, extremities, and occasionally the face, palms, and soles occurs in most patients 1 to 10 days after onset of the illness. Appearance of the rash is often associated temporally with initial defervescence; the rash may recur with fever and may be pruritic. Isolated petechiae and mucosal bleeding may occur, but significant hemorrhage is rare. Desquamation may take place when the rash resolves. The initial acute illness may last 2 to 3 days (range, 1 to 7 days). Fever may recrudesce after a 1- to 2-day hiatus. The polyarthralgia is migratory and predominantly affects the small joints of the hands, wrists, feet, and ankles, with less prominent involvement of the large joints. Previously injured joints may be more severely affected. Stiffness and swelling may occur, but large effusions are uncommon. Synovial fluid shows decreased viscosity with poor mucin clot and 2000 to 5000 white blood cells per milliliter. Symptoms, including arthralgia, arthritis, and tenosynovitis, may persist for months. Maternal-fetal transmission may result in severe neonatal infection.

DIAGNOSIS

Chikungunya fever must be differentiated from dengue and o'nyong-nyong fever. Chikungunya virus may be isolated from blood during the initial 2 to 4 days of illness. In some patients, viral antigen may be detected in acute sera by hemagglutination assay as a result of the intensity of the viremia. Commercially available real time RT-PCR assays on acute phase serum may be used to confirm the diagnosis. Specific IgM antibody may be detected for 6 months or longer. Hemagglutination inhibition and neutralization antibodies develop as the viremia is cleared. Complement fixation antibodies are positive by the third week and slowly decrease over the subsequent year.

TREATMENT AND PROGNOSIS   **Rx**

Treatment is supportive. Nonsteroidal anti-inflammatory agents are useful. During the acute arthritis, range-of-motion exercises lessen the stiffness. In most cases, mild joint symptoms may persist for months. Destructive arthropathy is rare and may be associated with low-titer rheumatoid factor, thus suggesting an unrelated, underlying inflammatory arthritis. Approximately 10% of patients have joint symptoms 1 year after infection. In children, arthralgia and arthritis are milder and briefer in duration.

● O'NYONG-NYONG FEVER

DEFINITION

O'nyong-nyong means "joint breaker" in the Acholi dialect of northwestern Uganda, where o'nyong-nyong fever first appeared in February 1959.

The Pathogen

O'nyong-nyong fever is clinically similar to chikungunya fever, and the viruses share antigenic similarity. O'nyong-nyong virus is also a member of the family Togaviridae, genus Alphavirus.

EPIDEMIOLOGY

Within 2 years of its appearance in 1959, the o'nyong-nyong fever virus spread through Uganda and eastern Africa and affected 2 million people. Serologically determined attack rates ranged from 50 to 60%, with case rates of 9 to 78%. Disease spread at a rate of 2 to 3 km daily. After the epidemic, the virus was not detected again until it was isolated from *Anopheles funestus* mosquitoes in Kenya in 1978. *Anopheles gambiae* also serves as a vector. Serologic surveys suggested that o'nyong-nyong virus is endogenous, but cases were not detected again until 1996-1997, during an outbreak in south central Uganda. An outbreak in western Côte d'Ivoire occurred in 2003. The nonhuman vertebrate reservoir for o'nyong-nyong virus is not known. The incubation period lasts at least 8 days. O'nyong-nyong fever virus vectors include *A. funestus, A. gambiae,* and other species.

Igbo-ora (meaning "the disease that breaks your wings") virus is a variant of o'nyong-nyong, with 98.5% homology between the two at the genomic level. Igbo-ora is serologically similar to the chikungunya and o'nyong-nyong viruses. In 1984, an epidemic of fever, rash, arthralgia, and myalgia occurred in four villages on the Ivory Coast. The virus was isolated from *A. funestus* and *A. gambiae* mosquitoes and from affected individuals.

PATHOBIOLOGY

Little is known about the pathobiology of o'nyong-nyong fever.

CLINICAL MANIFESTATIONS

Illness begins with a sudden onset of polyarthralgia and polyarthritis. Between 4 and 7 days later, rash begins with improvement in joint symptoms. The rash is uniform in nature, begins on the face, and then spreads to the torso and extremities and occasionally to the palms. The rash lasts 4 to 7 days before fading. Fever is not prominent, but postcervical lymphadenopathy may be marked. Arthralgia is incapacitating in most patients for up to a week, but residual joint pain may persist for months.

DIAGNOSIS

O'nyong-nyong fever is difficult to differentiate from chikungunya fever and may also be mistaken for measles. Specific hemagglutination inhibition and complement fixation tests are available. Mouse antisera raised against chikungunya virus react equally well with o'nyong-nyong virus, but o'nyong-nyong antisera do not react well with chikungunya virus. O'nyong-nyong–specific RT-PCR is available in reference laboratories.

TREATMENT AND PROGNOSIS

Treatment is symptomatic. Although residual joint pain often persists, there do not appear to be any long-term sequelae.

MAYARO FEVER

DEFINITION

Mayaro fever is an acute febrile illness characterized by fever, rash, arthralgia, and arthritis. Mayaro virus was first recognized in Trinidad in 1954. It has caused recorded outbreaks in Bolivia and Brazil and is endemic in the rain forest region where Bolivia, Brazil, and Peru share borders. Mayaro virus has a monkey reservoir and is transmitted to humans by *Haemagogus* mosquitoes dwelling in the tropical rain forest canopy.

The Pathogen
Mayaro virus is a member of the family Togaviridae, genus Alphavirus.

EPIDEMIOLOGY

Mayaro virus was responsible for an outbreak in Belterra, Brazil, in 1988. Eight hundred of 4000 exposed latex gatherers became infected, with a clinical attack rate of 80%. Cases of imported Mayaro virus infection have been documented in the United States after travel from the endemic Brazil-Bolivia-Peru interborder region. Mayaro virus has been isolated from a bird in Louisiana, thus raising the specter of emergence of Mayaro virus in North America.

PATHOBIOLOGY

Viremia occurs during the first 1 to 2 days of illness.

CLINICAL MANIFESTATIONS

Illness is characterized by a sudden onset of fever, headache, dizziness, chills, and arthralgia in the small joints of the hands and feet. About 20% of patients have joint swelling. Unilateral inguinal lymphadenopathy is seen occasionally. Leukopenia is common. Fever resolves after 2 to 5 days, but a maculopapular rash then develops on the trunk and extremities of about two thirds of patients and lasts about 3 days.

DIAGNOSIS

Mayaro virus may be isolated from blood by growth in Vero or C6/36 cells. RT-PCR with ELISA is available. A specific IgM is also available as an antibody capture ELISA.

TREATMENT AND PROGNOSIS

Recovery is complete, although some patients have persistent arthralgia 2 months later.

ROSS RIVER FEVER VIRUS (EPIDEMIC FEBRILE POLYARTHRITIS)

Ross River fever virus causes an acute-onset, febrile illness characterized by rash and arthralgia. Ross River virus is a member of the family Togaviridae, genus Alphavirus.

EPIDEMIOLOGY

Epidemics of fever and rash have been observed in Australia since 1928. Isolation of Ross River virus from mosquitoes, its serologic association with epidemic polyarthritis, and isolation of the virus from epidemic polyarthritis patients in Australia confirmed Ross River virus as the etiologic agent of epidemic polyarthritis. Seroprevalence has been observed in endogenous populations in Papua New Guinea, western New Guinea, the Bismarck Archipelago, Rossel Island, and the Solomon Islands. An outbreak in the Fiji Islands affected more than 40,000 individuals in 1979 to 1980. A similar epidemic occurred in the Cook Islands early in 1980. Antibodies to Ross River virus are not found in individuals west of Weber's line, a hypothetic line separating the Australian geographic zone from the Asiatic zone. Endemic cases and epidemics occur in tropical and temperate regions in Australia. Queensland and New South Wales have a particularly high annual incidence associated with higher rainfall. High rainfall usually precedes epidemic periods, with cases subsequently occurring from spring through fall. Seroprevalence may reach just 6 to 15% in temperate coastal zones but is 27 to 39% in the plains of the Murray Valley river system. In Queensland, annual rates of disease range from 31.5 to 288.3 per 100,000 person years. From 1992 to 2006, 55,000 cases of Ross River virus infection were reported in Australia.

Aedes vigilax is the major vector on the eastern coast of Australia and *Aedes camptorhynchus* in the salt marshes of southern Australia. *Culex annulirostris* is a freshwater breeding vector. Other Australian *Aedes* species and *Mansonia uniformis* may also serve as vectors. In outbreaks on the Pacific islands, *Aedes polynesiensis, A. aegypti, A. vigilax,* and *C. annulirostris* may have contributed to transmission. Domestic animals, rodents, and marsupials may serve as intermediate hosts. Virus may persist in *Aedes* mosquitoes.

Most infected individuals become symptomatic. Although male and female infection rates are similar, there is a predominance of women among infected individuals. Children have a case attack rate ratio lower than that of adults. The incubation period is 7 to 11 days.

Barmah Forest virus, another alphavirus found in Australia in 1986, may be manifested in a fashion similar to epidemic febrile polyarthritis. The number of cases reported annually has been increasing since its initial discovery.

PATHOBIOLOGY

Ross River viral antigen may be detected in monocytes and macrophages early in infection, but intact virus is not identifiable by electron microscopy or cell culture. Dermal vessels show mild perivascular mononuclear cell infiltrates, mostly T lymphocytic, in erythematous and purpuric areas. Vessels in purpuric areas also show erythrocyte extravasation. Antigen can be demonstrated in epithelial cells in erythematous or purpuric skin and in the perivascular zone in erythematous skin. However, viral antigens have not been found in normal skin. Synovium undergoes lining cell hypertrophy and sublining vascular proliferation and mononuclear cell infiltration. Viral RNA can be identified by RT-PCR. Synovial fluid cell counts range from 1500 to 13,800 cells/mL and consist of monocytes, vacuolated macrophages, and a few neutrophils. Animal models of infection indicate that Ross River virus targets bone, joint, and skeletal muscle and elicits an inflammatory response mediated by the innate immune system.

CLINICAL MANIFESTATIONS

Arthralgia typically occurs abruptly, followed in 1 to 2 days by a macular, papular, or maculopapular rash that may be pruritic. Three fourths of patients have severe, incapacitating arthralgia in an asymmetrical and migratory distribution. Commonly affected joints are the metacarpophalangeal joints, finger interphalangeal joints, wrists, knees, and ankles. The shoulder, elbow, toe, spine, hip, and temporomandibular joints may also be affected. Arthralgias are worse in the morning and after periods of inactivity. A third of patients have synovitis. Polyarticular swelling and tenosynovitis are common. Up to a third of patients have paresthesias or palm or sole pain. Classic carpal tunnel syndrome may occur.

In some individuals, rash may precede or follow the joint symptoms by 11 or 15 days, respectively. Occasionally, vesicles, papules, or petechiae are seen. The trunk and extremities are typically involved, but the palms, soles, and face may also be affected. The rash resolves by fading to a brownish discoloration or by desquamation. Fever tends to be mild to moderate and lasts 1 to 3 days. Headache, nausea, and myalgia are common. Mild photophobia, respiratory symptoms, and lymphadenopathy may occur.

DIAGNOSIS

In the Australian epidemics before 1979, patients were antibody positive at the time of initial evaluation. However, in the Pacific island epidemics of 1979 to 1980, patients remained viremic and serologically negative for up to a week after the onset of symptoms. Virus in serum is stable for up to a month at 0 to −10° C. Current testing in Australia is performed with an indirect ELISA. The presence of specific IgM or evidence of seroconversion to IgG positivity supports a recent infection.

TREATMENT AND PROGNOSIS   Rx

Treatment is supportive. Nonsteroidal anti-inflammatory drugs provide relief of joint pain. Half of all patients return to activities of daily living within 4 weeks despite residual polyarthralgia. Joint symptoms may recur, but episodes gradually resolve. In some patients, joint symptoms may persist for up to 3 years. Mild exercise tends to improve the joint symptoms.

● SINDBIS

Sindbis virus causes a sudden-onset, febrile illness associated with arthralgia and rash. It is known as Ockelbo disease in Sweden, Pogosta disease in Finland, and Karelian fever in the Karelian Isthmus of Russia. *Aedes*, *Culex*, and *Culiseta* mosquitoes transmit the virus to humans, with birds serving as intermediate hosts. Sindbis virus is the prototype alphavirus used for molecular virology studies of its genus.

EPIDEMIOLOGY

The virus was first isolated from *Culex* mosquitoes in the Egyptian village of Sindbis in 1952. Outbreaks frequently occur in the forested areas of Sweden, Finland, and the Karelian Isthmus, but sporadic cases and small outbreaks have occurred in Uganda, South Africa, Zimbabwe, central Africa, and Australia. Individuals involved in outdoor activities or occupations are at greatest risk.

PATHOBIOLOGY

Skin lesions show perivascular hemorrhage, lymphocytic infiltrates, edema, and areas of necrosis. Virus has been isolated from skin lesions. Antiviral IgM may persist for years, thus raising the possibility that Sindbis virus arthritis is associated with viral persistence and a direct viral effect on the synovium. Autophagy, an evolutionarily conserved intracellular mechanism for recycling cytoplasmic material to lysozymes for degradation during times of stress, may be disrupted in neurons by Sindbis virus infection, thereby leading to programmed cell death or apoptosis.

CLINICAL MANIFESTATIONS

Arthralgia and rash are the initial symptoms, although one may precede the other by a few days. Arthralgia and arthritis involve the small joints of the hands and feet, wrists, elbows, ankles, and knees. Occasionally, arthralgia affects the spine. Tendinitis is common and often involves the Achilles and hand extensor tendons. Fever, if present, tends to be mild to moderate. Constitutional symptoms, headache, fatigue, malaise, nausea, vomiting, pharyngitis, and paresthesias may be present but are not usually severe. Macular rash typically begins on the torso and then involves the arms, legs, palms, soles, and occasionally the head. Macules evolve to papules that have a tendency to vesiculate. Vesiculation is prominent on pressure points, including the palms and soles. As the eruption fades, a brownish discoloration is left. Vesicles on the palms and soles may become hemorrhagic. Rash may recur during convalescence.

DIAGNOSIS

Specific IgM detected by enzyme immunoassay supports a diagnosis of Sindbis virus infection. IgM titers may wane over a period of 3 to 4 years.

TREATMENT AND PROGNOSIS   Rx

Treatment is supportive. Nonerosive chronic arthropathy is common in Sweden and Finland, with up to half of all patients having joint symptoms 2.5 years after infection. In a few cases, symptoms may persist for up to 6 years.

SUGGESTED READINGS

Gibney KB, Fischer M, Prince HE, et al. Chikungunya fever in the United States: a fifteen year review of cases. *Clin Infect Dis.* 2011;52:e121-e126. *Review of 109 U.S. cases, all in adult travelers.*
Weaver SC, Reisen WK. Present and future arboviral threats. *Antiviral Res.* 2010;85:328-345. *Review, including the changing epidemiology with global warming.*

391

ARBOVIRUSES AFFECTING THE CENTRAL NERVOUS SYSTEM

THOMAS P. BLECK

Arboviruses, which are also termed *arthropod-borne viruses*, can affect the central nervous system (CNS). These viruses share a number of clinical and epidemiologic similarities and have an RNA genome, but they do not form a formal virologic taxonomic group. Arboviruses generally have avian or small mammalian reservoirs and are transmitted to humans and other large mammals incidentally when an infected mosquito or other arthropod obtains a blood meal.

EPIDEMIOLOGY

Most human disease is subclinical; a few patients have a brief febrile illness resembling influenza, and a small percentage, usually at the extremes of age, suffer meningitis or encephalitis. The diseases (Table 391-1) reflect the quotidian and seasonal characteristics of their insect vectors. Other viruses of the same genera cause hemorrhagic fever (Chapter 389), and other less frequently encountered arboviruses are also capable of producing encephalitis.

Many of these agents cause notifiable disease in the United States: St. Louis, West Nile, Powassan, eastern equine, western equine, and the California serogroup encephalitis viruses. Case definitions and additional information are available at *http://www.cdc.gov/ncidod/dvbid/arbor/index.htm*.

The diseases described here are zoonoses (Chapter 336), that is, illnesses caused by viruses transmitted from animals to humans. They are more prevalent in the tropics and subtropics and are usually localized because of ecologic restrictions on their transmission.

PATHOBIOLOGY

Two pathologic processes are common to the arboviral encephalitides: neuronal and glial damage mediated by intracellular viral infection; and migration of immunologically active cells into the perivascular space and brain parenchyma. Endothelial cell swelling and proliferation, destruction of myelin sheaths in deep white matter areas, and vasculitis are present in some arboviral encephalitides.

After a bite by an infected arthropod, viral replication occurs in local tissues and regional lymph nodes. Viremia, which seeds extraneural tissues, occurs and persists, depending on the extent of replication in extraneural sites, the rate of viral clearance by the reticuloendothelial system, and the appearance of humoral antibodies. The sites of extraneural infection vary among the viruses. Many alphaviruses and flaviviruses involve striated muscle and endothelium, whereas Venezuelan encephalitis virus is associated with

TABLE 391-1 ARTHROPOD-BORNE VIRUSES ASSOCIATED WITH HUMAN ENCEPHALITIS

VIRUS	INSECT VECTOR	COMMON VERTEBRATE HOSTS	GEOGRAPHIC DISTRIBUTION
TOGAVIRIDAE			
Alphaviruses	Mosquitoes		
Eastern equine encephalitis	*Culiseta* spp, *Aedes* spp, *Coquillettidia* spp		Eastern United States and Gulf Coast, Caribbean region, South America
Western equine encephalitis	*Culiseta* spp, *Culex* spp		Western United States, Canada
Venezuelan equine encephalitis	*Aedes* spp, *Culex* spp, *Psorophora* spp, and *Mansonia* spp		South America, Central America, Florida and southwestern United States
FLAVIVIRIDAE			
Japanese serocluster	Mosquitoes		
Japanese encephalitis	*Culex* and *Aedes* spp		East and Southeast Asia, India, Australia
West Nile encephalitis	*Aedes* spp, *Culex* spp, and others		Africa, Middle East, North America
St. Louis encephalitis	*Culex* spp		Western Hemisphere
Murray Valley encephalitis	*Culex* spp		Australia
Tick-borne encephalitis complex			
Central European encephalitis	*Ixodes* spp	Goats, sheep	Europe, Russia
Russian spring-summer encephalitis	*Ixodes* spp		Europe, northern and central Asia
Kyasanur Forest disease	*Haemaphysalis spinigera*	Rodents, insectivores	India
Omsk hemorrhagic fever	*Dermacentor reticulatus*	Rodents	Central Asia
Powassan	*Ixodes* spp	Squirrels, groundhogs	North America, Russia
Louping ill	*Ixodes ricinus*	Small mammals, sheep, birds	British Isles
Langat	*Ixodes* spp	Rodents	Malaysia, Thailand, parts of former Soviet Union
BUNYAVIRIDAE			
California encephalitis	*Aedes melanimon, Aedes dorsalis*	Rodents, rabbits	California
La Crosse encephalitis	*Aedes triseriatus*	Chipmunks, squirrels	Eastern and Midwestern United States

TABLE 391-2 FEATURES OF ARBOVIRAL ENCEPHALITIDES IMPORTANT IN THE UNITED STATES

	EASTERN EQUINE ENCEPHALITIS	WESTERN EQUINE ENCEPHALITIS	VENEZUELAN EQUINE ENCEPHALITIS	WEST NILE ENCEPHALITIS	ST. LOUIS ENCEPHALITIS	CALIFORNIA SEROGROUP ENCEPHALITIS
Annual U.S. cases of symptomatic disease	10	0-2 cases, mostly infants and children	Rare, mostly children	Up to 3000, mostly >40 yr	0-2000, mostly >50 yr	10-50, mostly children
Time of year	Late summer, early fall	Early and mid summer	Summer	Summer, fall	Mid to late summer	July-September
Case-fatality rate	50-70%, highest in children <15 yr and adults >55 yr	3-5% in children	35% in children, <10% in older persons	14-19%, 30% in adults >70 yr	9% overall; 0% <20 yr, 30% >65 yr	<1%
Residual damage	30-50%, especially in children	33% in infants	Frequent in children	50%, more frequent in elderly	Frequent in elderly	Probably rare
Cerebrospinal fluid findings (cells/μL)	500-2000 cells, predominantly neutrophils	<500 cells, predominantly lymphocytes	<500 cells, predominantly lymphocytes	<500 cells, predominantly lymphocytes	<500 cells, predominantly lymphocytes	<500 cells, predominantly lymphocytes

myeloid and lymphoid tissue invasion. During viremia, the neural parenchyma may be invaded, but the mode of penetration of virus across the blood-brain barrier is not completely understood. Possible mechanisms include passive movement of virus across vascular membranes and viral replication in the cerebral capillary endothelium. Factors increasing vascular permeability promote nervous system invasion. In experimental animal infection, flaviviruses enter the CNS through the olfactory epithelium.

The immature brain is more susceptible to damage by western equine, Venezuelan equine, and California serogroup encephalitis viruses (Table 391-2). St. Louis encephalitis and West Nile encephalitis principally affect the elderly, whereas Japanese encephalitis and eastern equine encephalitis have a bimodal incidence and strike both children and elderly persons. In endemic areas, immunity accumulated with increasing age may reduce the incidence of disease in older persons for some viruses; however, the reasons for the increased severity of illness with other viruses remain unknown.

CLINICAL MANIFESTATIONS

Clinical symptoms and signs vary among the viral causes (see later), although all share common signs and symptoms of encephalitis (Chapter 422).

DIAGNOSIS

Diagnosis depends on a careful history that includes exposure to vertebrate animals and arthropod vectors, age, season, and travel, including the geographic site of exposure. Laboratory confirmation of infection is essential. The virus may be isolated from acute phase serum or whole blood in laboratory animals or in tissue culture. Neutralization, complement fixation (CF), hemagglutination inhibition (HI), fluorescent antibody, and enzyme-linked immunosorbent assay (ELISA) of acute and 3-week convalescent sera can also produce the correct diagnosis. Antigen detection and IgM capture ELISA often permit diagnosis on initial evaluation and within a week of the onset of illness in most cases. Sensitive nucleic amplification assays using reverse transcription–polymerase chain reaction (RT-PCR) are under development for a number of the arboviruses and may lead to earlier diagnosis.

Differential Diagnosis

The most important initial consideration is to differentiate arboviral encephalitides from other acute CNS infections, including infections other than encephalitis (Chapters 420 and 421), treatable causes of encephalitis (Chapter 422), and paraneoplastic and autoimmune encephalitis (Chapters 420 and 422). The early prodrome resembles influenza (Chapter 372).

Bacterial meningitis (Chapter 420; especially early or partially treated), infective bacterial endocarditis (Chapter 76), brain abscess (Chapter 421), subdural empyema (Chapter 421), and cerebral thrombophlebitis may mimic viral encephalitis, and the cerebrospinal fluid (CSF) profile is sometimes similar. Other infections that occasionally cause meningoencephalitis that may resemble arthropod-borne viral encephalitis include tuberculosis (Chapter 332), cryptococcosis (Chapter 344), histoplasmosis (Chapter 340), coccidioidomycosis (Chapter 341), Rocky Mountain spotted fever (Chapter 335), leptospirosis (Chapter 331), falciparum malaria (Chapter 353), trichinosis (Chapter 365), *Naegleria* meningitis (Chapter 420), typhoid fever (Chapter 316), Lyme disease (Chapter 329), and *Mycoplasma* pneumonia (Chapter 325).

Acute meningoencephalitis may result from infections with other viruses, including herpesviruses (Chapter 382), human immunodeficiency virus (Chapter 394), mumps virus (Chapter 377), enteroviruses (Chapter 387), lymphocytic choriomeningitis virus (Chapter 420), rabies (Chapter 422), influenza (Chapter 372), and the exanthematous viral infections of childhood (Chapters 375 and 376). The exposure history, the presence of similar disease in the community, and the summer-fall occurrence are principal clues to an arboviral etiology. Enteroviruses (Chapter 387) also cause summer-fall outbreaks, but the predominant syndrome is aseptic meningitis, and the concomitant occurrence of rash or pleurodynia is a helpful clue. Herpes simplex encephalitis (Chapter 422) presents an important diagnostic challenge because effective therapy is available and should be started quickly. The presence of localizing neurologic signs, localizing findings on computed tomography (CT) or magnetic resonance imaging (MRI), and detection of herpes simplex DNA in CSF by PCR help distinguish herpes simplex encephalitis from the arboviral encephalitides.

Noninfectious diseases of the CNS such as stroke (Chapter 414) may rarely be confused with viral encephalitis. Subarachnoid hemorrhage (Chapter 415) produces meningismus, fever, headache, and neurologic signs that mimic an infectious etiology. Metabolic encephalopathies occasionally have features suggesting infectious encephalitis. Neoplastic or granulomatous diseases involving the CNS and a variety of diseases of uncertain etiology (Behçet's disease [Chapter 278], Reye's syndrome, acute multiple sclerosis [Chapter 419], and systemic lupus erythematosus [Chapter 274]) must be considered in the differential diagnosis as well.

PREVENTION

Control can be achieved by interruption of the cycle, including vaccination of reservoir animals, vector control, and education on vector avoidance. Practical measures include wearing long-sleeved clothing, using insect repellents, limiting outdoor activities during peak mosquito season, and eliminating standing pools of water. Vaccines are currently available for Japanese encephalitis.

TREATMENT   Rx

Treatment is symptomatic and may include bedrest, antipyretics, and analgesics. Early empirical treatment of herpes simplex encephalitis (Chapter 382) may be appropriate while the diagnostic evaluation to document arboviral encephalitis proceeds.

● EASTERN EQUINE ENCEPHALITIS

EPIDEMIOLOGY

Human disease is relatively rare, with fewer than 10 cases occurring each year in the Gulf Coast and Atlantic states, usually in association with an equine epizootic involving 100 to 300 animals. Outbreaks generally occur during the late summer and early fall. The occurrence of equine cases or outbreaks of fatal encephalitis in penned exotic birds precedes the appearance of human cases by several weeks or more. Epizootics of eastern equine encephalitis have been reported in the Caribbean (Hispaniola) and South America.

In temperate areas, eastern equine encephalitis virus circulates between wild birds and *Culiseta melanura* mosquitoes in a freshwater swamp habitat. Equine epizootics and associated human cases result from extension of the transmission cycle to involve *Aedes* and *Coquillettidia* mosquitoes, which feed on horses and humans.

PATHOBIOLOGY

The brain is grossly edematous and congested, and the inflammatory response is predominantly polymorphonuclear. The areas most affected are the basal ganglia, thalamus, hippocampus, and frontal and occipital cortices. Focal vasculitis, endothelial cell swelling, intravenous and arteriolar thrombus formation, demyelination, necrosis, neuronolysis, and neuronophagia are prominent.

CLINICAL MANIFESTATIONS

Onset is abrupt, with high fever, vomiting, and somnolence. Stupor, coma, myoclonus, and generalized convulsions appear within 24 hours to as long as 10 days later. Autonomic disturbances (sialorrhea) may be prominent, and respiratory difficulty and cyanosis are frequent. In children, facial, periorbital, or generalized edema may be present.

A striking peripheral leukocytosis with immature neutrophils occurs frequently in patients with eastern equine encephalitis. CSF examination reveals 500 to 2000 white blood cells/µL (predominantly neutrophils). As the total cell count falls, neutrophils may persist as a significant fraction. Red blood cells may be present, protein concentration is elevated, and the glucose level is normal.

DIAGNOSIS

Brain CT and MRI are frequently abnormal and reveal lesions in the basal ganglia, thalami, and brain stem. The virus can rarely be isolated from blood or CSF. Serologic diagnosis by demonstration of a rise in antibody titer in appropriately timed paired sera is the most practical and available test. Because of the rapid course of the clinical disease, sera should be obtained at 2- to 3-day intervals during the acute phase of illness.

PREVENTION

An experimental formalin-inactivated chick embryo cell culture vaccine is used to protect laboratory and field workers. Reduction of mosquito populations by appropriate use of insecticides may be effective in threatened or established outbreaks.

TREATMENT   Rx

Treatment is supportive. Control of fever, intracranial pressure, seizures, fluid and electrolyte disturbances, and the airway is critical. Although attempts at immunologic therapy have been reported, no controlled data are available.

PROGNOSIS

The case-fatality rate is 50 to 70%. Mortality, like incidence, is highest in children younger than 15 years and in persons older than 55 years, with no gender predilection. Death usually occurs during the first week; in surviving patients, recovery begins during the second week and may progress rapidly. Good functional recovery is associated with a long prodromal course and absence of coma. Residual damage, found in 30 to 50% of patients, is often severe, especially in children, and is characterized by mental retardation, spastic paralysis, and radiographic evidence of brain atrophy.

● WESTERN EQUINE ENCEPHALITIS

EPIDEMIOLOGY

Few cases of western equine encephalitis have been reported in the past decade; the most recent epidemic occurred in Colorado in 1987. Epidemics occur in early or mid summer and may follow heavy snow melt or flooding, conditions favorable for breeding of mosquitoes. Cases of encephalitis in equines often precede the appearance of human disease. The illness principally affects residents of rural communities, and the incidence is higher in males than in females.

The ratio of inapparent to apparent infection is also age dependent and ranges from about 1 : 1 in infants younger than 1 year, to 58 : 1 in children 1 to 4 years old, to more than 1000 : 1 in persons older than 14 years. Western equine encephalitis virus also occurs in South America. Equine epizootics in Argentina have been associated with human cases.

Western equine encephalitis virus circulates between wild birds and *Culex tarsalis* mosquitoes. *C. tarsalis* is responsible for infection of humans and equines, which have low or undetectable viremia and do not perpetuate the chain of transmission. In temperate areas, transmission ceases during the winter months.

PATHOBIOLOGY

Pathologic examination of the brains of infants reveals massive parenchymal destruction; children dying months or years after the acute insult often have large cystic lesions in many areas of the brain. In older children and adults, acute western equine encephalitis is characterized by focal necrosis and perivascular cuffing, predominantly in the basal ganglia and thalami but also in deep cerebral white matter.

CLINICAL MANIFESTATIONS

The disease usually begins with an influenza-like illness consisting of fever, headache, malaise, and myalgia lasting 1 to 4 days. Somnolence, lethargy, photophobia, vomiting, and neck stiffness may follow; neurologic involvement may rapidly progress to stupor, coma, and seizures. Pareses, cranial nerve deficits, tremors, and abnormal reflexes may be present. In fatal cases, patients die 1 to 2 days after coma develops. Congenital infections have been documented and result in severe and progressive neurologic deterioration.

Leukocytosis and a shift to the left are common. The CSF contains fewer than 500 white blood cells/μL (at first polymorphonuclear, then mononuclear) and an elevated protein concentration (usually 90 to 110 mg/dL).

DIAGNOSIS

Viral isolation from blood or CSF is almost never successful. Diagnosis is achieved by demonstration of a rise in HI, fluorescent antibody, CF, ELISA, or neutralizing antibody titers in appropriately timed (10 to 14 days apart) paired sera. Demonstration of IgM antibodies in serum or CSF by ELISA provides a presumptive diagnosis.

PREVENTION

An experimental formalin-inactivated vaccine grown in chick embryo cell culture has been used to protect laboratory workers but is not indicated for others. In threatened or ongoing epidemics, residents should be advised to use protective clothing, insect repellents, and window screens and to restrict outdoor activity in the early morning, late afternoon, and evening (times of greatest mosquito activity). Public health measures include spraying insecticides aimed at the adult *C. tarsalis* vector.

TREATMENT

There is no specific therapy for western equine encephalitis. Supportive therapy is similar to that discussed earlier for eastern equine encephalitis.

PROGNOSIS

Western equine encephalitis is most severe in infants and young children. The case-fatality rate is between 3 and 5%. Survivors generally experience sudden and rapid recovery. However, about a third of surviving infants suffer mental retardation, cerebellar damage, choreoathetosis, and spastic paralysis. Children with protracted illnesses in whom convulsions develop during the acute stage are more likely to suffer long-term neurologic sequelae. Adults may have a prolonged convalescent syndrome, but objective residua are rare.

⬤ VENEZUELAN EQUINE ENCEPHALITIS

Six antigenic subtypes of Venezuelan equine encephalitis virus (I to VI) with several antigenic variants of subtypes I and III are recognized serologically. Subtypes IAB and IC are responsible for epidemics involving humans and equines. In Florida, subtype II is enzootic and produces sporadic human disease. Methods of transmitting Venezuelan equine encephalitis virus as a biologic warfare agent were developed in the 1960s; an epidemic of Venezuelan equine encephalitis, especially if humans and horses become ill simultaneously, could represent an attack rather than naturally occurring illness.

EPIDEMIOLOGY

Before 1973, large equine epizootics occurred at 5- to 10-year intervals in Venezuela, Colombia, Ecuador, and Peru and involved many thousands of animals with mortality rates as high as 40%. Associated human morbidity was also great (up to 32,000 clinical cases). The disease was quiescent for several years but has reemerged in the past decade. The last major outbreak occurred in Venezuela and Colombia in 1995, with more than 85,000 human cases. Laboratory infections are common in unvaccinated persons working with the virus or infected animals.

A large variety of mosquito vectors, including species of the genera *Aedes, Psorophora,* and *Mansonia,* transmit subtypes IAB and IC during epizootic epidemics. Equines are the principal viremic hosts. Virus may be present in the pharyngeal excretions of human patients; contact or aerosol person to person spread, although possible, is not epidemiologically important.

The other members of the Venezuelan equine encephalitis viral complex, including subtype II in Florida, have enzootic transmission cycles involving *Culex* mosquitoes and small forest rodents and marsupials. Human disease is sporadic and relatively uncommon.

PATHOBIOLOGY

Pathologic changes in the CNS include edema, congestion, meningeal and perivascular inflammation, intracerebral hemorrhage, neuronal degeneration, and vasculitis. In addition, hepatocellular degeneration and necrosis, widespread lymphoid depletion and follicular necrosis, and interstitial pneumonitis are frequent. Congenitally infected fetuses demonstrate massive and widespread necrosis of brain tissue, hemorrhage, and resorption of brain material resulting in hydranencephaly.

CLINICAL MANIFESTATIONS

The predominant syndrome is a self-limited influenza-like illness; encephalitis develops in only about 4% of infected persons, principally children younger than 15 years. Subclinical infections are rare.

After an incubation period of 2 to 5 days, there is a sudden onset of fever, chills, malaise, and headache, followed by myalgias, nausea, vomiting, and occasionally diarrhea. Physical examination reveals fever, tachycardia, conjunctival injection, and, in some cases, nonexudative pharyngitis. The acute illness generally subsides in 4 to 6 days, and convalescent symptoms may last up to 3 weeks. A biphasic course has sometimes been noted; acute symptoms can reappear after a brief remission, within a week after initial onset.

When it occurs, severe encephalitis is characterized by meningeal signs, seizures, tremor, stupor, coma, spastic paralysis, abnormal reflexes, cranial nerve palsies, and central respiratory failure. Residual neurologic damage occurs in severe cases. Infections of pregnant women acquired during the first and second trimester may result in fetal encephalitis and death.

The peripheral leukocyte count is often low, with a decrease in both lymphocytes and neutrophils, or normal with relative lymphopenia. In patients with CNS signs, the CSF contains up to 500 cells/μL, predominantly lymphocytes. Serum lactate dehydrogenase and aspartate aminotransferase concentrations may be elevated.

DIAGNOSIS

In contrast to the other arboviral encephalitides, Venezuelan equine encephalitis virus can be isolated from blood or from throat swabs or washings during the first 3 or 4 days of illness. Serodiagnosis is usually more practical and is achieved by testing appropriately timed paired sera by HI, CF, ELISA, neutralization, or IgM immunoassay.

PREVENTION

An experimental live attenuated vaccine made from subtype IAB is used for adult laboratory personnel. It provides solid immunity to subtypes IAB and IC but incomplete protection against heterologous Venezuelan equine encephalitis viruses. Epidemics and epizootics can be prevented by effective vaccination of equines. Spraying insecticides to reduce adult (infective) mosquito populations is the only means of immediate control in the face of an ongoing epidemic. Individual protection against mosquitoes is advised.

TREATMENT

No specific therapy is available, and treatment of encephalitis cases is supportive.

PROGNOSIS

The case-fatality rate in children 5 years or younger with encephalitis is approximately 35%, but it is less than 10% in older persons.

⬤ JAPANESE ENCEPHALITIS

EPIDEMIOLOGY

Japanese encephalitis virus causes epizootics of clinical encephalitis in equines. The disease occurs throughout Asia, including Japan, the Korean peninsula, Taiwan, the People's Republic of China, Okinawa, Vietnam, the Philippines, Burma, Malaysia, Bangladesh, east and south India, Sri Lanka, Thailand, and Indonesia. More than 30,000 clinical cases occur annually, about one third of which are fatal. Japanese encephalitis is a summertime disease in temperate areas but occurs sporadically year-round in the tropics. Epidemics are most frequent at the northern fringe of the tropical zone. It is a predominantly rural disease, and the incidence in males is often higher than in females. In hyperendemic areas, more than 70% of adult populations surveyed have antibodies, and children younger than 15 years are principally affected by the disease. In areas without a high prevalence of background immunity (e.g., northern India), however, all age groups are affected. In Japan, where schoolchildren have been protected by vaccination campaigns targeted at this age group, encephalitis has become prominent in the elderly. The ratio of clinically inapparent to apparent infection is higher than 500 : 1 in children and decreases with age; in Korea, the ratio in American servicemen was estimated at 25 : 1.

PATHOBIOLOGY

Neuropathologic changes and the distribution of lesions are similar to those described for St. Louis encephalitis (see later).

CLINICAL MANIFESTATIONS

Manifestations of Japanese encephalitis include abrupt fever, headache, and gastrointestinal symptoms. Meningeal irritation develops within 24 hours and is followed on the second or third day by the appearance of irritability, impaired consciousness, seizures (especially in children), muscle rigidity, parkinsonian findings, ataxia, coarse tremor, involuntary movements, cranial nerve deficits, paresis, hyperactive deep tendon reflexes, and pathologic reflexes. Weight loss and dehydration are often striking findings. In mild cases, fever subsides after the first week, and neurologic signs resolve by the end of the second week after onset. In severe cases, hyperpyrexia, progressive neurologic dysfunction, and coma result in death, usually between the seventh and tenth days. About 25% of patients undergo a prolonged recovery, with permanent sequelae often remaining. The occurrence of such sequelae correlates with severity of the acute stage of illness, and young children are most susceptible. Cardiorespiratory complications are frequent during the acute stage in these patients. A poor prognosis is associated with protracted high fever, frequent or prolonged seizures, high protein content in CSF, Babinski signs, and early respiratory depression. Fetal death from transplacental Japanese encephalitis infection has been reported.

DIAGNOSIS

Moderate peripheral leukocytosis and neutrophilia occur early in the disease. Pleocytosis (predominantly lymphocytic), protein elevation, and normal glucose concentration in CSF are usual findings.

MRI in Japanese encephalitis reveals edema in the basal ganglia, thalami, and focal area of the cerebral cortex; evidence of hemorrhage in these areas may likewise be present. Enhancement may also be noted in the meninges, brain stem, and spinal cord.

Virus is rarely isolated from blood. Virus is also rarely recovered from the CSF of patients who live but may be recovered from the CSF of a third of patients who die. HI and neutralizing antibodies appear during the first week, and CF antibodies appear during the second week. Cross-reactions with other flaviviruses make serodiagnosis difficult. Specific IgM antibodies in serum or CSF are detectable by immunoassays in more than three fourths of patients at the time of hospital admission.

PREVENTION

The inactivated, partially purified mouse brain vaccines produced in Japan are safe and effective in preschool- and school-aged children.[1] A vaccine produced in Japan is available to U.S. citizens traveling to high-risk areas. However, generalized urticaria and angioedema may occur in 0.3% of recipients, and anecdotal cases of encephalomyelitis have been reported; as a result, the precise indications for vaccination of travelers are unclear. Because two or three doses of the inactivated vaccine are used and approximately 1 month is required to confer protection, vaccination is not a practical measure in the event of an ongoing epidemic. Two Japanese encephalitis (JE) vaccines are licensed in the United States. An inactivated mouse brain–derived vaccine (JE-MB) was licensed to prevent Japanese encephalitis in persons older than 1 year, but it is not currently in production. The remaining stores of JE-MB are reserved for children. A newer inactivated Vero cell culture–derived vaccine (JE-VC; ICS1, or IXIARO) is licensed for use in persons older than

17 years[2] and has recently been shown to be safe in children. Reduction of vector mosquito populations by the application of insecticides may help abort outbreaks. Immunization of swine is an ancillary control strategy.

TREATMENT Rx

Treatment is supportive (see Eastern Equine Encephalitis). A randomized trial of interferon alfa showed no benefit.

PROGNOSIS

The case-fatality rate is probably about 25%. Sequelae such as mental impairment, emotional lability, choreoathetosis, tremor, parkinsonism, autonomic disturbances, paralysis, and psychiatric disturbances have been reported in up to 75% of patients.

WEST NILE FEVER AND ENCEPHALITIS

Before 1996, the predominant clinical manifestation of West Nile virus was a brief influenza-like illness, sometimes with a rash (Chapter 390) but infrequently with neurologic manifestations. Epidemics since then in Romania, Israel, and North America have added meningitis, meningoencephalitis, and myelitis to the list of disorders attributable to the virus. Sequence analyses of various isolates of the virus indicate two lineages. The first includes viruses from North America, Europe, Israel, western Africa, India, Russia, and Australia; the second includes viruses from sub-Saharan Africa and Madagascar.

EPIDEMIOLOGY

See Chapter 390. The incidence of neuroinvasive West Nile disease varies in different parts of the United States but can be seen nearly everywhere (Fig. 391-1).

CLINICAL MANIFESTATIONS

The majority of infected people are asymptomatic. Fever develops in about 20%, and CNS manifestations are seen in less than 1%, although this percentage is higher in the elderly (Chapter 390). In those in whom clinical manifestations develop, an incubation period of 1 to 6 days is followed by the abrupt onset of symptoms, usually without a prodrome. The temperature rises quickly to 38.3° to 40.0° C, with rigors in a third of patients. Symptoms include drowsiness, severe frontal headache, ocular pain, myalgia, and pain in the abdomen and back. A small number of patients have dryness of the throat, anorexia, and nausea. Cough is common. Examination shows facial flushing, conjunctival injection, and coating of the tongue. Generalized lymphadenopathy had been a prominent feature in past epidemics but is no longer commonly reported. The spleen and liver are occasionally slightly enlarged. The temperature curve may be biphasic. A pale roseolar maculopapular rash, predominantly on the trunk and upper part of the arms, may appear from the second to fifth day but is now less common as well; it may be evanescent (several hours) or persist until defervescence, and it does not desquamate. Vesicular lesions occur rarely. The illness lasts 3 to 5 days in 80% of patients.

In the past decade, the incidence of CNS disease has increased in several epidemics, apparently because of a true increase in the invasiveness and neurovirulence of the virus. The virus causes a syndrome resembling poliomyelitis (Chapter 423), with prominent lower motor neuron dysfunction (acute flaccid paralysis with asymmetrical weakness and decreased deep tendon reflexes but preserved sensory function), which may be seen independently or with signs of meningoencephalitis. In some patients, prolonged, possibly permanent ventilatory failure requiring mechanical ventilation develops. A parkinsonian syndrome has also been noted, but it generally remits after months. Some patients may have seizures, cranial nerve involvement, ataxia, tremors, or myoclonus. Acute inflammatory polyneuropathy (e.g., Guillain-Barré syndrome; Chapter 428) has also been reported. Other rare complications include myocarditis, pancreatitis, and hepatitis. Convalescence is often prolonged, lasting several weeks with prominent symptoms of fatigue. Lymph node enlargement requires several months to regress. Laboratory findings often include leukocytosis, whereas 10 to 15% of patients have leukopenia.

DIAGNOSIS

CSF examination may reveal a lymphocytic pleocytosis (<1800 cells/μL) with some increase in protein but a normal glucose concentration. Although

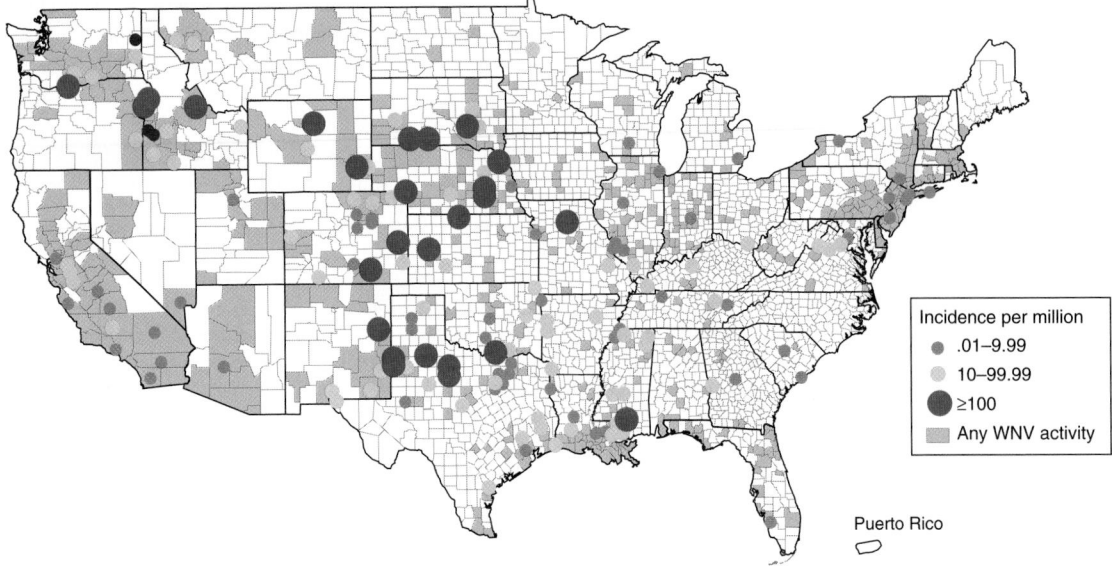

FIGURE 391-1. Incidence of human neuroinvasive West Nile disease in 2009. (Available at http://www.cdc.gov/ncidod/dvbid/westnile/images/2009BL_300410.jpg. Accessed May 27, 2010.)

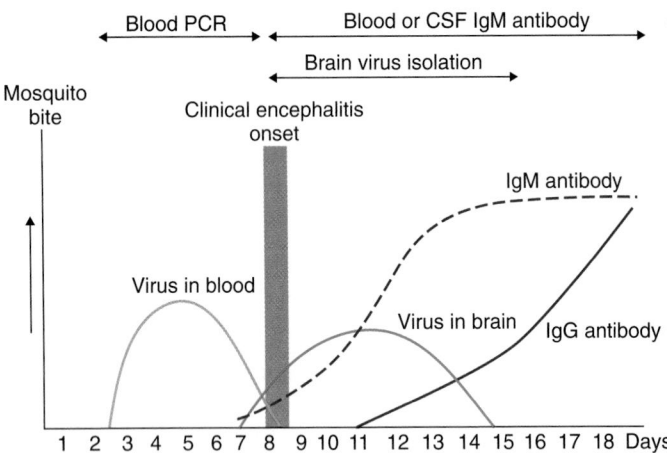

FIGURE 391-2. Typical time course for development of West Nile virus in blood and brain and occurrence of IgG and IgM antibodies in humans after West Nile virus infection. CSF = cerebrospinal fluid; PCR = polymerase chain reaction. (Reproduced from Davis LE, Beckham JD, Tyler KL. North American encephalitic arboviruses. *Neurol Clin.* 2008;26: 727-757.)

West Nile virus may be isolated from the blood of three fourths of patients with West Nile fever on the first day of illness (Chapter 390), patients with West Nile encephalitis appear less likely to be viremic, and isolation of virus from CSF is infrequent. Viral RNA is detected in CSF by RT-PCR in about 50% of cases (Fig. 391-2). IgM antibody capture immunoassay, which is the test of choice, is more sensitive than RT-PCR. IgM antibodies may remain detectable for up to 500 days after infection, so their presence should suggest acute infection only with compatible clinical manifestations. In some situations, cross-reactions with other flaviviruses, particularly St. Louis encephalitis virus, may complicate the interpretation of IgM immunoassays.

TREATMENT ℞

Treatment is symptomatic and similar to that suggested for eastern equine encephalitis. Patients may require prolonged mechanical ventilation for either the polio-like syndrome or Guillain-Barré syndrome. The Guillain-Barré syndrome seen in West Nile patients does not appear to respond to plasma exchange. A large trial of intravenous immune globulin is under way. Ribavirin has activity against West Nile virus, but its clinical utility is unknown.

PROGNOSIS

The overall case-fatality rate is 4 to 14%, but it is higher in the elderly. Risk factors for death include more severe weakness or coma,

immunocompromise, and failure to produce virus-specific IgM. The prognosis for neurologic recovery is generally good; most U.S. patients regain physical and mental function by 1 year, but about half the patients in some series still report difficulties 1 year after the illness.

ST. LOUIS ENCEPHALITIS

ETIOLOGY

St. Louis encephalitis virus, a member of the family Flaviviridae, shares close antigenic relationships with Japanese encephalitis, Murray Valley encephalitis, and West Nile viruses and is related to yellow fever (Chapter 389) and dengue (Chapter 390) viruses. Strains associated with *Culex pipiens*–borne epidemics in the eastern United States are distinct from endemic strains transmitted by *C. tarsalis* in the western states.

EPIDEMIOLOGY

The virus is present in all parts of the Western Hemisphere, but epidemics occur only in North America and some Caribbean islands. During epidemic years, the virus has been responsible for up to 80% of all reported cases of encephalitis of known etiology in the United States. Epidemics of up to 2000 cases have taken place, mainly in urban-suburban localities of the Ohio-Mississippi River basin and in eastern and central Texas and Florida. Small outbreaks have also occurred in the western United States. Epidemics generally take place between July and September but may arise later in the year in warm areas such as Florida. Previous exposure and immunity to dengue may provide a degree of cross-protection against clinical St. Louis encephalitis. The ratio of inapparent to apparent infection is 800 : 1 in children up to 9 years of age, 400 : 1 in persons aged 10 to 49 years, and 85 : 1 in persons older than 60 years.

In most of the eastern United States, St. Louis encephalitis virus circulates between wild birds and *C. pipiens* mosquitoes, which breed in polluted water. In Florida and in parts of the Caribbean, *Culex nigripalpus* is the principal vector. The cycle in the western United States also involves wild birds, but the vector is *C. tarsalis*, also that of western equine encephalitis. Because of the similar ecology of St. Louis encephalitis and western equine encephalitis viruses in the West, mixed outbreaks occur, mostly in rural, agricultural areas.

Above-average summer temperatures and conditions such as deficient rainfall, which create stagnant pools suitable for *C. pipiens* breeding, are associated with epidemics in the eastern United States. St. Louis encephalitis in the western states is favored by warm spring temperatures, heavy snow melt, and flooding.

PATHOBIOLOGY

Pathologic changes in fatal cases are limited to microscopic findings. Leptomeningitis is characterized by lymphocytic inflammation. Parenchymal changes consist of lymphocytic perivascular cuffing, cellular nodule formation, and neuronal degeneration.

CLINICAL MANIFESTATIONS

Three clinical syndromes are recognized: febrile headache, aseptic meningitis, and encephalitis. After an incubation period of 4 to 21 days, a variable period of nonspecific symptoms, including fever (temperature of 38° to 41° C), headache, malaise, drowsiness, myalgia, and sore throat, may be followed by an acute or subacute onset of meningeal or encephalitic signs, or both. Nausea, vomiting, and photophobia are common.

Neurologic abnormalities occur in up to 25% of patients. Extrapyramidal abnormalities and altered consciousness are the most significant findings. Other findings include meningismus, cranial nerve deficits (particularly the facial nerve), abnormal reflexes, tremors, myoclonic twitching, nystagmus, and ataxia. Motor abnormalities are infrequent, and sensory changes are extremely uncommon. Seizures occur in 10% of patients and are a poor prognostic sign, as is a persistent high temperature of 40° to 41° C. Signs of markedly increased intracranial pressure are unusual. A Guillain-Barré–like syndrome (Chapter 428) has occasionally been associated with St. Louis encephalitis, both as an acute manifestation and during the convalescent period.

In uncomplicated cases of St. Louis encephalitis, a moderate peripheral neutrophilic leukocytosis and shift to the left are noted. CSF pressure is elevated, protein level is mildly elevated, and glucose concentration is normal; a pleocytosis of up to 500 cells/μL is present, with an early neutrophilia predominance changing to lymphocytes within days. Serum creatine kinase, aspartate aminotransferase, and aldolase levels are frequently elevated. The electroencephalogram typically shows polymorphic delta activity, most prominently in the frontal and temporal regions; electrographic seizures are common. CT scans are normal, but MRI may show edema involving deep structures such as the substantia nigra. Hypo-osmolality, presumably as a result of the syndrome of inappropriate antidiuretic hormone secretion (Chapter 232), is noted in a third of patients.

Genitourinary tract symptoms (urgency, frequency, incontinence, and retention), microscopic hematuria, pyuria, proteinuria, and elevated blood urea nitrogen are frequent. St. Louis encephalitis viral antigen in cells of the urinary sediment has been detected by fluorescent techniques, and virus-like particles have been detected in urine by immunoelectron microscopy.

DIAGNOSIS

St. Louis encephalitis virus is rarely isolated from blood or CSF obtained during the acute phase of illness. Serologic diagnosis is achieved by demonstration of changing antibody titers; the HI, fluorescent, ELISA, and neutralizing tests demonstrate antibody within the first week after onset, and titers rise during the ensuing 2 weeks. CF antibodies appear 10 to 20 days after onset. Rapid, early diagnosis is possible by detection of IgM antibodies by ELISA in serum and CSF. Serologic cross-reactions may occur in persons with previous exposure to dengue, West Nile, and other related flaviviruses. RT-PCR provides a more specific diagnosis, but its sensitivity is uncertain.

PREVENTION

No vaccine is available for St. Louis encephalitis. Surveillance of viral activity in vectors and avian hosts is used to define the risk for human infection and to initiate vector control efforts. In an established outbreak, avoidance of mosquito bites and spraying to reduce infected adult mosquitoes are the only effective means of control.

TREATMENT   Rx

Treatment is supportive.

PROGNOSIS

A convalescent syndrome characterized by weakness, fatigue, nervousness, tremulousness, sleeplessness, irritability, depression, difficulty concentrating, and headaches occurs in 30 to 50% of older persons and clears in 80% of them within 3 years. The overall case-fatality rate is approximately 9%. Mortality is negligible in persons younger than 20 years but rises steeply after 55 years to approximately 30% in patients older than 65 years. Approximately 50% of the deaths occur during the first week, and 80% occur within 2 weeks after onset.

MURRAY VALLEY ENCEPHALITIS AND ROCIO ENCEPHALITIS

Murray Valley encephalitis and Rocio encephalitis, which are similar to Japanese encephalitis in their pathogenesis and clinical features, are caused by closely related flaviviruses. Murray Valley encephalitis has occurred in small epidemics in the Murray and Darling River valleys of Victoria and New South Wales, Australia. The virus is endemic in northern Australia and New Guinea, where it is maintained in a bird-mosquito cycle. Rocio encephalitis has caused epidemics of 1000 or more cases in São Paulo State, Brazil.

TICK-BORNE ENCEPHALITIS

PATHOGENS

A complex of six antigenically related tick-borne flaviviruses cause encephalitis: Powassan, tick-borne encephalitis, louping ill, Kyasanur Forest disease, Omsk hemorrhagic fever, and Langat viruses. The predominant syndrome is hemorrhagic fever (Chapter 389), but meningoencephalitis may be a component of the disease spectrum. Two subtypes of tick-borne encephalitis virus (central European encephalitis and Russian spring-summer encephalitis) are distinguished by serologic tests, are ecologically distinct, and differ in virulence for humans. Powassan and louping ill viruses are rare causes of encephalitis in North America and the British Isles, respectively. These viruses are easily distinguished serologically from mosquito-borne flaviviruses but induce cross-reactions within the complex.

EPIDEMIOLOGY

Tick-borne encephalitis occurs in Europe (including eastern Europe and Ukraine), southern Scandinavia, and far eastern Russia during the summer months, which corresponds to peak tick vector populations. Several hundred to more than 2000 cases are reported annually, with morbidity rates of up to 20 per 100,000 inhabitants. Adults older than 20 years are mainly affected, and persons frequenting wooded areas that are heavily tick infested are at highest risk. In Europe, the disease is relatively mild (case-fatality rate of 1 to 2%), but in the Far East, it is severe (20 to 25%).

The vector of tick-borne encephalitis is *Ixodes ricinus* in Europe and *Ixodes persulcatus* in the Far East. The tick vector also serves as a reservoir for the virus. Larval ticks parasitize small rodents, which serve as amplifying viremic hosts during the spring and summer. Large vertebrates (goats, sheep, cattle) are hosts for nymphal and adult ticks. Outbreaks have occurred in families or groups of individuals ingesting unpasteurized milk or cheese from goats or sheep.

CLINICAL MANIFESTATIONS

Inapparent infections are common. Symptomatic tick-borne encephalitis in Europe typically (but not invariably) has a biphasic course beginning 7 to 14 days after exposure with an influenza-like illness that lasts 1 week, followed by a period of clinical remission for several days and then an abrupt onset of aseptic meningitis or meningoencephalitis. The meningoencephalitis is usually benign, although severe paralytic illness, myelitis, myeloradiculitis, and bulbar forms may occur.

In the Far East, tick-borne encephalitis begins suddenly with fever, headache, and gastrointestinal symptoms, followed rapidly by the appearance of depressed sensorium, coma, convulsions, and paralysis. Bulbar paralysis and cervical myelitis are frequent findings. In fatal cases, death occurs in the first week after onset. Aseptic meningitis and milder forms of encephalitis also occur. Chronic forms of tick-borne encephalitis have been described, with active clinical and pathologic abnormalities present a year or more after onset.

DIAGNOSIS

Brain MRI in patients with tick-borne encephalitis shows evidence of edema in the basal ganglia, thalami, and brain stem in about 20% of cases. MRI of the spinal cord may show anterior horn cell lesions corresponding to lower motor neuron weakness on examination.

Isolation of virus from blood is also possible during the early phase of illness. Serologic diagnosis is achieved by the HI, CF, neutralization, or ELISA techniques.

PREVENTION

In eastern Europe and the former Soviet Union, vaccines are used in high-risk groups (forestry and agricultural workers, military personnel). In Austria, immunization of the general population has resulted in a marked decline in incidence. Avoidance of tick exposure by wearing of protective clothing and use of repellents may be recommended in areas of high tick-borne encephalitis activity.

PROGNOSIS

In European tick-borne encephalitis, convalescence is often prolonged, and residual paralysis may follow in severe cases. In the Far East, survivors frequently have residual paralysis, especially lower motor neuron paralysis of the upper extremities or shoulder girdle as a result of spinal cord involvement.

Louping III Encephalitis

Louping ill causes encephalitis in sheep (rarely in cattle, horses, and swine) in Scotland, northern England, and Ireland. Sporadic human cases have been recognized. Louping ill virus is maintained in nature by *I. ricinus* ticks and a variety of hosts, including small mammals, ground-dwelling birds (grouse), and probably sheep. The clinical features of louping ill resemble the European form of tick-borne encephalitis.

Powassan Virus Encephalitis

Powassan virus encephalitis has been documented in a small number of cases in the northeastern United States and eastern Canada. The virus is not associated with animal disease. The transmission cycle of Powassan virus involves *Ixodes cookei, Ixodes marxi,* and possibly other tick species along with mammals, particularly rodents and carnivores. Powassan encephalitis is characterized by fever and nonspecific symptoms, followed by encephalitic signs, which are frequently severe. Peripheral blood and CSF changes are similar to those described for other forms of flaviviral encephalitis. The case-fatality rate is about 50%, and residual paralysis may persist in survivors.

● CALIFORNIA SEROGROUP ENCEPHALITIS

At least four members of the California serogroup of the Bunyaviridae family (Bunyavirus genus)—La Crosse, California encephalitis, Jamestown Canyon, and snowshoe hare viruses—cause encephalitis. California encephalitis virus occurs in the western United States (California, New Mexico, Utah, Texas) and has been implicated in only three human cases. In contrast, La Crosse virus, distributed more widely in the eastern half of the United States and southern Canada, is a major human pathogen. Jamestown Canyon and snowshoe hare viruses have also been implicated in sporadic cases of human encephalitis in the north central United States and Canada. California serogroup viruses have been implicated in human disease in China and the former Soviet Union.

EPIDEMIOLOGY

California serogroup encephalitis occurs as an endemic rather than an epidemic disease, with individual or small clusters of cases scattered across affected areas. Seventy to 115 cases are reported each year, generally between July and September, with a peak incidence in August. The virus primarily affects persons younger than 15 years living in rural and suburban areas characterized by deciduous hardwood forests. It is most prevalent in the north central states, where it is responsible for as many as 20% of cases of acute CNS infection in children. Focal "hot spots" (communities, even backyards) of recurrent summertime viral activity are recognized. The ratio of inapparent to apparent infection has been estimated variably at between 26 : 1 and 157 : 1.

The vector of La Crosse virus is *Aedes triseriatus,* which breeds both in forest tree holes and in artificial containers, notably discarded tires. This vector also serves as a reservoir for La Crosse virus. Wild rodents (squirrels, chipmunks) contribute to the cycle of transmission as viremic hosts. Humans acquire the disease by being bitten by an infected mosquito. *Aedes communis, Aedes stimulans, A. triseriatus,* and possibly anopheline mosquitoes are involved in transmitting Jamestown Canyon virus, and deer are the principal vertebrate hosts.

PATHOBIOLOGY

Histopathologic features in the CNS are qualitatively similar to those of other viral encephalitides. However, absence of inflammatory lesions in the cerebellum, medulla, and spinal cord may be a distinguishing feature of La Crosse infection.

CLINICAL MANIFESTATIONS

The clinical spectrum of California serogroup virus infection includes nonspecific febrile illness, aseptic meningitis, and meningoencephalitis. The disease begins with fever, headache, sore throat, and gastrointestinal symptoms. In mild cases, CNS signs appear on the third day after onset and subside within 7 to 8 days. In the more severe form, neurologic signs appear within 24 to 48 hours of onset, usually in the form of generalized seizures, elevated intracranial pressure, and altered consciousness, and persist longer. Encephalitis may be severe in the acute stage, but the disease is almost always self-limited; death is extremely rare.

The peripheral white blood cell count is elevated, with a predominance of polymorphonuclear cells and a shift to the left. CSF contains up to 500 lymphocytes/μL; the protein level is normal or mildly elevated, and the glucose concentration is normal. The electroencephalogram reveals generalized slowing in the delta and theta range; focal delta wave activity related to cortical destruction and focal seizures are also common findings.

DIAGNOSIS

In contrast to the other arboviral encephalitides, brain MRI in patients with California serogroup encephalitides may show lesions involving the temporal lobe in a pattern similar to that of herpes simplex encephalitis. The virus cannot be recovered from blood or CSF obtained during the acute phase. Diagnosis is best achieved by counterimmunoelectrophoresis, HI, CF, fluorescent, ELISA, and neutralization tests for antibody in paired acute and convalescent sera. The most practical, sensitive, and reliable methods are the HI test with La Crosse viral antigen and IgM antibody capture ELISA. Viral RNA can be detected in CSF or brain tissue by RT-PCR, although the sensitivity of the test remains to be determined.

PREVENTION

There is no vaccine for California encephalitis, although research involving DNA-based vaccines appears promising. Vector control methods are of uncertain usefulness in this disease. In defined hot spots of recurrent viral activity, breeding sites for *A. triseriatus* should be eliminated, particularly by draining or eliminating standing water (e.g., discarded tires or birdbaths) and filling holes in trees. Parents should protect children by limiting exposure and using mosquito repellents.

PROGNOSIS

The case-fatality rate is less than 1%. The risk for permanent neuropsychiatric sequelae is unclear, but hemiparesis and persistent seizure disorders have been reported.

1. Schiøler KL, Samuel M, Wai KL. Vaccines for preventing Japanese encephalitis. *Cochrane Database Syst Rev.* 2007;3:CD004263.

2. Tauber E, Kollaritsch H, Von Sonnenburg F, et al. Randomized, double-blind, placebo-controlled phase 3 trial of the safety and tolerability of IC 51, an inactivated Japanese encephalitis vaccine. *J Infect Dis.* 2008;198:493-499.

SUGGESTED READINGS

Fischer M, Lindsey N, Staples JE, et al. Centers for Disease Control and Prevention (CDC). Japanese encephalitis vaccines: recommendations of the Advisory Committee on Immunization Practices (ACIP). *MMWR Recomm Rep.* 2010;59(RR-1):1-27. *Current discussion of options for Japanese encephalitis immunization.*

Gao X, Nasci R, Liang G. The neglected arboviral infections in mainland China. *PLoS Negl Trop Dis.* 2010;4:e624. *Review of infections that may affect travelers.*

Lindsey NP, Staples JE, Lehman JA, et al. Centers for Disease Control and Prevention (CDC). Surveillance for human West Nile virus disease—United States, 1999-2008. *MMWR Surveill Summ.* 2010;59:1-17. *Summary of the epidemiology.*

Murray KO, Walker C, Gould E. The virology, epidemiology, and clinical impact of West Nile virus: a decade of advancements in research since its introduction into the Western Hemisphere. *Epidemiol Infect.* 2011;139:807-817. *Review of virology, history, epidemiology, clinical features, and sequelae.*

XXIV

HIV AND THE ACQUIRED IMMUNODEFICIENCY SYNDROME

392

EPIDEMIOLOGY OF HUMAN IMMUNODEFICIENCY VIRUS INFECTION AND ACQUIRED IMMUNODEFICIENCY SYNDROME

THOMAS C. QUINN

HISTORICAL PERSPECTIVE

Twenty-five years after initial recognition of acquired immunodeficiency syndrome (AIDS) in the United States, the disease has become epidemic in every country of the world. Initially reported as a disease primarily affecting homosexual men, AIDS was rapidly identified in many other risk groups, and it became evident that it was caused by an infectious agent transmitted through sexual activities, parentally through blood transfusions and injecting drug use, and perinatally from mother to infant. Early investigations in the 1980s demonstrated that the etiologic agent of AIDS was human immunodeficiency virus (HIV), which existed in two types, HIV-1 and HIV-2. After the development of diagnostic assays for HIV antibody, it became possible to track and monitor the escalating spread of HIV throughout the world, definitively define the modes and probabilities of transmission, and study the natural history of HIV infection. Within years of its recognition, HIV disseminated rapidly throughout the world, caused a massive epidemic, and became one of the leading causes of death worldwide. Efforts at prevention and treatment with antiretroviral drugs have tempered the spread and decreased the fatality rate in some countries, but in developing countries where the social, demographic, cultural, and economic impact of the AIDS epidemic has been the greatest, these gains were initially too limited and too slow to reverse the escalating trend of the epidemic. More recently, with the increased availability of antiretroviral drugs in many countries, the annual rate of increase in HIV infections may have peaked and mortality has declined.

GLOBAL STATISTICS

By January 2010, approximately 75 million people had become infected with HIV since the beginning of the epidemic in 1981. Of these individuals, more than 40 million people had already died of AIDS, and it became ranked as one of the leading causes of death throughout the world. According to estimates by the Joint United Nations Program on HIV/AIDS (UNAIDS), 33.4 million people were living with HIV by December 2008 (Fig. 392-1; Table 392-1). In 2008 alone, 2.7 million people became newly infected, half of whom were young individuals between the ages of 15 and 24 years. The continuing rise in the population of people living with HIV infection reflects the combined effects of continued high rates of HIV infection and the beneficial impact of antiretroviral therapy (ART) resulting in fewer deaths.

The latest epidemiologic data indicate that globally, the spread of HIV appears to have peaked in 1996, when 3.5 million new HIV infections occurred. In 2008 the estimated number of new HIV infections was approximately 30% lower than at the epidemic's peak 12 years earlier. The epidemic appears to have stabilized in most regions, although prevalence continues to increase in Western Europe, central Asia, and other parts of Asia because of the high rates of HIV infection. Sub-Saharan Africa remains the most heavily affected region and accounted for 71% of all new HIV infections in 2008.

Nearly 90% of all new infections occurred in developing countries; 50% occurred in women; and the major mode of transmission was heterosexual transmission, although infections continue to spread at high rates among men who have sex with men (MSM). Resurgence of the epidemic among MSM in high-income countries is increasingly well documented. Differences are apparent in all regions, with some national epidemics continuing to expand even as the overall regional incidence of HIV infection stabilizes. Epidemic patterns have been changing over time. In eastern and central Asia, epidemics that were once characterized primarily by transmission among injecting drug users (IDUs) are now increasingly being characterized by significant sexual transmission, whereas in parts of Asia, epidemics are increasingly becoming characterized by significant transmission among heterosexual couples. Perinatal transmission also continues to occur in developing countries, where

access to antiretroviral drugs to prevent mother-to-infant transmission is limited. In 2008, 430,000 children became newly infected, and 25 million children have been orphaned by the premature deaths of their parents from AIDS. In 2008, 2.0 million people died of AIDS, including 280,000 children.

From these epidemiologic trends it is projected that within the next 8 years an additional 25 million people could become infected with HIV in 126 low- and middle-income countries, which have the most concentrated or generalized epidemics, unless the world succeeds in mounting a drastically expanded global prevention and treatment effort. It is anticipated that more than 40% of these new infections will occur in Asia, the Pacific, and Eastern Europe, although it is apparent that the epidemic will continue to devastate nearly all countries of the African continent. During the next decade, without full access to treatment and care in many countries, millions of individuals will join the ranks of the more than 40 million people who have already died of AIDS.

DEMOGRAPHIC, SOCIAL, AND ECONOMIC IMPACT OF HIV AND AIDS

AIDS is the leading cause of death in sub-Saharan Africa and the fourth largest killer worldwide. The average life expectancy in sub-Saharan Africa is now 47 years; it would have been 62 years without AIDS (Fig. 392-2). Life expectancy at birth in Botswana has dropped to a level not seen in that country since the 1950s. Even in Haiti, life expectancy is nearly 6 years less than it would have been in the absence of AIDS. In Asia, Cambodia has experienced a reduction in life expectancy of 4 years. Current HIV prevalence levels merely hint at the greater lifetime probability of AIDS developing. In Lesotho, it is estimated that a person who is 15 years old has a 74% chance of being infected with HIV by his or her 50th birthday.

According to one report, AIDS is expected to cause a decline in life expectancy in 51 countries over the next 20 years. Seven nations in sub-Saharan Africa now have life expectancies of less than 40 years, and this number will increase by 11 countries over the next 7 years. The declining life expectancies will soon reach levels that have not existed since the 19th century. In Zimbabwe and South Africa, the infant mortality rate is higher than it was in 1990. Five African nations will experience more deaths than births by 2010, with a resultant decrease in population. Life expectancy will drop to just 27 years in Botswana and Mozambique in the next 8 years, and Swaziland will have an estimated life expectancy of 33. In Zimbabwe, Zambia, and Namibia, the expected lifespan will be 34 years. In contrast, the overall life expectancy in an African nation without AIDS would be 70 years by 2010.

THE GLOBAL RESPONSE

At a 2001 special session of the United Nations General Assembly on AIDS, 189 nations agreed that AIDS was a national and international security issue of the highest priority. The Global Fund for AIDS, Tuberculosis, and Malaria raised funds from private donations and industrialized countries to help support access to care and treatment within developing countries. This initiative was complemented by the U.S. government's Emergency Plan for AIDS Relief (PEPFAR), now committed over a 10-year period through the Bush and Obama administrations to provide treatment and care for HIV-infected individuals, as well as additional resources for enhancing prevention efforts to prevent further transmission. As of December 2008, approximately 4 million people in low- and middle-income countries were receiving ART—a 10-fold increase over a period of 5 years (Fig. 392-3). ART coverage rose from 7% in 2003 to 42% in 2008, with especially high coverage achieved in eastern and southern Africa (48%). Even though the rapid expansion of access to ART is helping lower AIDS-related death rates in multiple countries and regions, it is also contributing to increases in HIV prevalence. Scale-up in sub-Saharan Africa has been the most dramatic, with an increase from 100,000 people receiving treatment in 2003 to more than 3 million in December 2008. Sixty-three percent of all people now receiving treatment in low- and middle-income countries are living in sub-Saharan Africa, as compared with 25% in late 2003.

Effective prevention of mother-to-child transmission depends on the simultaneous support of several strategies that work synergistically to reduce the odds that an infant will become infected as a result of exposure to the mother's virus. In ideal conditions, provision of antiretroviral prophylaxis and replacement feeding or continued antiretroviral treatment with breastfeeding can reduce transmission from an estimated 30 to 35% with no intervention to 1 to 2%. Unfortunately, most countries have not yet reached all

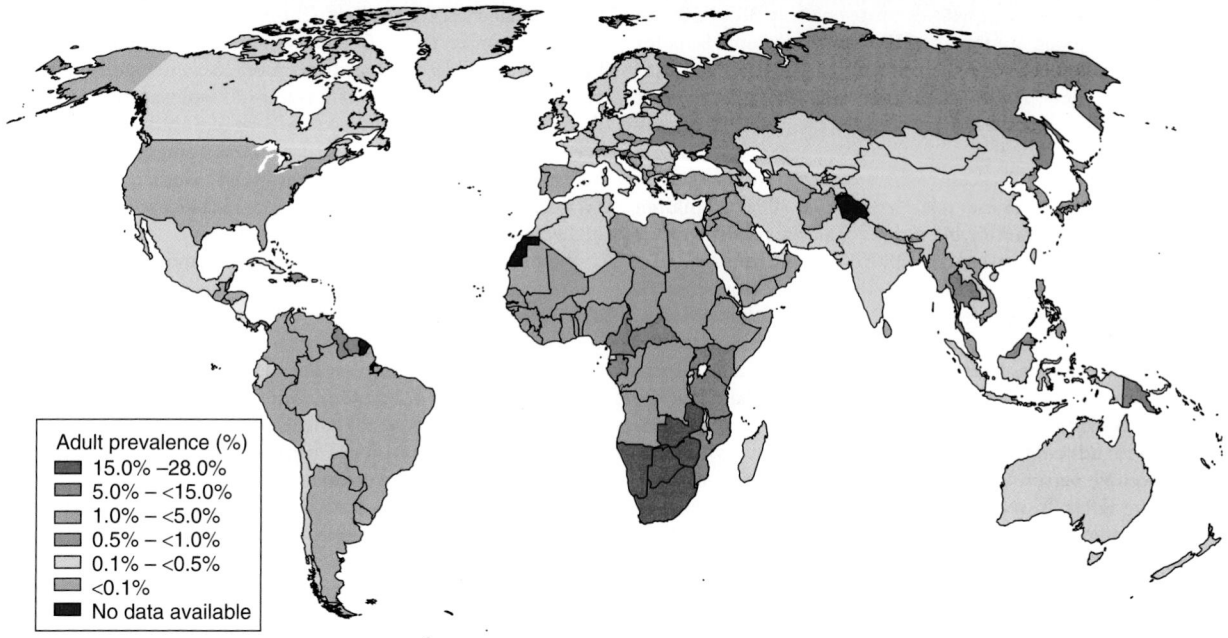

Adult prevalence (%)
- 15.0% –28.0%
- 5.0% – <15.0%
- 1.0% – <5.0%
- 0.5% – <1.0%
- 0.1% – <0.5%
- <0.1%
- No data available

FIGURE 392-1. A total of 33.4 million people (31.1 to 38.5 million) were living with HIV infection in 2008. The adult prevalence of HIV infection is shown by country. (Data from UNAIDS.)

TABLE 392-1 REGIONAL HIV AND AIDS STATISTICS AND FEATURES AT THE END OF 2008

REGION	ADULTS AND CHILDREN LIVING WITH HIV/AIDS	ADULTS AND CHILDREN NEWLY INFECTED WITH HIV	ADULT PREVALENCE RATE*	MAIN MODES OF TRANSMISSION FOR ADULTS LIVING WITH HIV/AIDS
Sub-Saharan Africa	22,400,000	1,900,000	5.2%	Hetero
North Africa and Middle East	310,000	35,000	0.2%	Hetero, IDU
South and Southeast Asia	3,800,000	280,000	0.3%	Hetero, IDU
East Asia and Pacific	850,000	75,000	0.1%	IDU, Hetero, MSM
Oceania	59,000	3,900	0.3%	MSM, Hetero
Latin America	2,000,000	170,000	0.6%	MSM, IDU, Hetero
Caribbean	240,000	20,000	1.0%	Hetero, MSM
Eastern Europe and central Asia	1,500,000	110,000	0.7%	IDU, Hetero, MSM
Western Europe	850,000	30,000	0.3%	MSM, IDU, Hetero
North America	1,400,000	55,600	0.4%	MSM, IDU, Hetero
Total	33,400,000	2,700,000	0.8%	

*The proportion of adults (15 to 49 years of age) living with HIV infection or AIDS in 2008 using 2008 population numbers.
Hetero = heterosexual transmission; IDU = transmission through injecting drug use; MSM = sexual transmission among men who have sex with men.

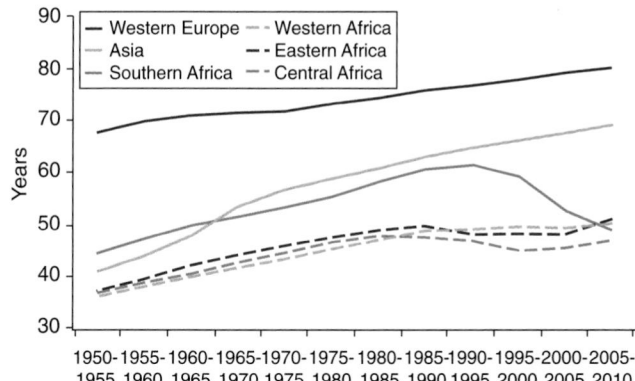

FIGURE 392-2. Impact of AIDS on life expectancy in six regions between 1950 and projected to 2010. (From the United Nations Population Division, 2004. World Population Prospects: the 2004 Revision Database.)

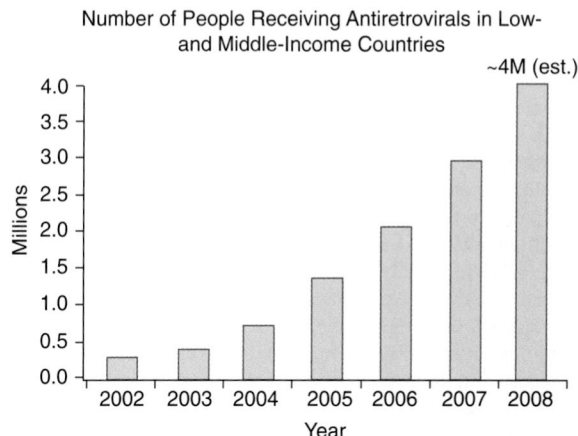

FIGURE 392-3. Estimated number of people receiving antiretroviral therapy in low- and middle-income countries from 2002 through 2008. (Data from World Health Organization and UNAIDS.)

pregnant women with these services, with estimates of only 30 to 50% of HIV-infected mothers receiving appropriate HIV care and prophylaxis for mother-to-child transmission. Despite these limitations, it has been estimated that nearly 200,000 new HIV infections have been averted in the past decade because of provision of antiretroviral prophylaxis during pregnancy and to newborn infants.

Unfortunately, not all have equal access to therapy, even within countries with middle to high prevalence. For example, an estimated 800,000 children younger than 15 years now require ART, but only 200,000 are receiving treatment. Children account for approximately 14% of AIDS deaths. Nearly 90% of children infected with HIV are African. The median proportion of HIV-infected children receiving treatment is just 25% in sub-Saharan Africa. Similarly, less than 40% of HIV-infected pregnant women in low- and middle-income countries are benefiting from antiretroviral prophylaxis despite success in certain countries such as Botswana, Brazil, and Thailand and the virtual elimination of pediatric HIV disease in the industrialized world. Likewise, in Eastern Europe and central Asia, injecting drug use accounts for more than 70% of HIV-positive persons. However, only 25% of treatment recipients in this region are IDUs. In years to come, additional resources will be required to reach the additional millions of HIV-infected people who require treatment with antiretroviral drugs, especially in light of recent recommendations to expand access to all HIV-infected adults who have a CD4$^+$ count of less than 350/mm^3 based on the finding that early (versus standard) initiation of ART reduces mortality and incident tuberculosis.∎

● REGIONAL EPIDEMICS

HIV and AIDS in Sub-Saharan Africa

Sub-Saharan Africa represents the epicenter of the global HIV/AIDS pandemic (see Table 392-1). Studies in the late 1990s and early 2000s support the theory that HIV originated in Africa and that humans probably became infected sometime in the mid-20th century from a similar, related retrovirus in chimpanzees and sooty mangabey monkeys. For years, the infection remained limited to remote rural regions of Africa, but with urbanization, infected individuals migrated to major urban centers, where transmission was amplified and HIV spread to thousands of individuals within a relatively short period.

Most HIV transmissions in sub-Saharan Africa occur through sexual intercourse, with unsafe blood transfusions and unsafe injections accounting for a smaller fraction. Although sexual behavior is the most important factor influencing the spread of HIV in Africa, that behavior varies greatly across cultures, age groups, socioeconomic class, and gender. The interplay of multiple factors, biologic and behavioral, determines the spread of HIV. One study of four African cities (Cotonou, Kisumu, Ndola, and Yaounde) revealed that the most common behavioral and biologic factors in those cities with the highest HIV prevalence were young age at a woman's first sexual intercourse, young age at first marriage, age difference between spouses, the presence of herpes simplex type 2 infection and trichomoniasis, and lack of male circumcision. There is substantial evidence that sexually transmitted diseases (STDs) enhance the risk for sexual transmission of HIV, that the level of the HIV viral load in an individual enhances the probability of infectiousness, and that male circumcision is associated with a reduced risk for transmission. Although the complex interplay of factors makes it difficult to estimate the probable growth of the epidemic within the region, evidence from the past 25 years demonstrates that HIV can spread rapidly and widely from very low-prevalence levels.

Sub-Saharan Africa remains the worst affected region in the world for HIV infection. A little more than a 10th of the world's population lives in sub-Saharan Africa, but it is home to 64% of all people infected with HIV in the world. In 2008 an estimated 1.9 million people living in sub-Saharan Africa became newly infected with HIV, thus bringing the total number of people infected with HIV to 22.4 million. Sub-Saharan Africa accounted for 72% of all the world's AIDS-related deaths in 2008. Even though the rate of new HIV infections in sub-Saharan Africa has slowly declined, with the number of new infections in 2008 being approximately 25% lower than at the epidemic's peak in the region in 1995, the number of people infected with HIV has slightly increased in 2008, in part because of the increased longevity stemming from improved access to treatment.

Seventy-five percent of all women infected with HIV live in sub-Saharan Africa. In Côte d'Ivoire, home to the most serious epidemic in West Africa, HIV prevalence in females (6.4%) was more than twice as high as that in males (2.9%). In sub-Saharan Africa as a whole, women account for 60% of the estimated HIV infections. The risk of becoming infected is especially disproportionate for girls and young women. In Kenya, young women between 15 and 19 are three times more likely to be infected than their male counterparts, whereas 20- to 24-year-old women are 5.5 times more likely than men in their age cohort to be living with HIV infection. Among people aged 15 to 24 in Tanzania, females are four times more likely than males to be living with HIV. In the nine countries of southern Africa most affected by HIV, the prevalence in young women 15 to 24 was on average three times higher than that in men of the same age.

Women's vulnerability to HIV in sub-Saharan Africa stems not only from their greater physiologic susceptibility to heterosexual transmission but also from the severe social, legal, and economic disadvantages that they often confront. HIV prevalence generally tends to peak at a younger age for women than for men. The very young are often at extremely high risk for infection through mother-to-child transmission.

A third of all AIDS deaths globally occurred in sub-Saharan Africa in 2008. As noted earlier, access to ART has increased more than 10-fold since the end of 2003, and more than 3 million people now receive treatment. Unfortunately, progress is uneven, with coverage reaching or exceeding 50% in some countries (Botswana, Namibia, and Uganda) but remaining below 20% in most others.

Although some countries in sub-Saharan Africa such as Kenya, Uganda, and Zimbabwe have shown recent declines in HIV prevalence, there is no evidence of any decline in southern Africa, including the Republic of South Africa, Botswana, Namibia, and Swaziland, where exceptionally high infection levels continue. Southern Africa remains the area most heavily affected by the epidemic. The nine countries with the highest HIV prevalence worldwide are all located in this subregion, with each of these countries experiencing adult HIV prevalence greater than 10%; prevalence is as high as 26% in Swaziland, 24% in Botswana, and 23% in Lesotho. South Africa is home to the world's largest population of people living with HIV (5.7 million). In Swaziland, the national adult HIV prevalence is estimated to be 33.4%. HIV prevalence in pregnant women attending antenatal clinics rose from 4% in 1992 to 43% in 2004. In the Republic of South Africa, an estimated 5.5 million people were living with HIV in 2005. An estimated 18.8% of adults (15 to 49 years old) were living with HIV in 2005. Almost one in three pregnant women attending public antenatal clinics was infected with HIV. Although South Africa's HIV prevention efforts have not made a significant impact on the epidemic, there has been considerable progress on the treatment front as noted earlier. South Africa accounts for a large percentage of the treatment scale-up in sub-Saharan Africa, but as of 2006, nearly 80% of the 1 million South Africans in need of ART were still without treatment.

In Botswana, the national adult HIV prevalence was 24.1% in 2005. More than a third of pregnant women attending antenatal clinics and close to 50% of women 30 to 34 years of age were infected with HIV. The prevalence in pregnant women has generally remained at 34 to 37% since 2001. Similarly, Lesotho has a national adult HIV prevalence of 23.2%, with 27% documented in women attending antenatal clinics. A third of pregnant women 25 to 34 years of age were infected. In Namibia, the prevalence of HIV infection is 19.6% in all adults, with an HIV prevalence of 42% in antenatal clinics in selected areas. In neighboring Mozambique, Malawi, and Zambia, HIV prevalence has been documented to be between 16 and 17%. There is wide geographic variation, however, with HIV infection rates in pregnant women ranging from less than 10% in some places to as high as 30% in others.

In the countries of eastern Africa, HIV prevalence has either decreased or remained stable in the past several years. In Uganda, which saw a steep decline in HIV prevalence during the mid and late 1990s, adult HIV prevalence was estimated to be 6.7% in 2005. However, trends in 2006 suggest that HIV prevalence may be increasing in selected areas, in part because of a decrease in mortality with access to ART but potentially also because of increasing incident rates as a result of decreasing condom use and an increased percentage of multiple partners. In neighboring Kenya, Eritrea, Tanzania, Burundi, and Rwanda, the HIV epidemic has been stable in recent years, with prevalence rates ranging from 2% in Eritrea to 7% in Kenya, Tanzania, Burundi, and Rwanda. In Ethiopia, HIV prevalence has stabilized in urban areas but appears to be increasing in more distant rural areas, where access to treatment and care is more limited.

Western Africa is less severely affected than other parts of sub-Saharan Africa, with national adult HIV prevalence rates of 2% in several countries. The highest rate in the region is in Côte d'Ivoire: 7.1%. In Nigeria, infection levels vary radically across the country from 2.6% in the southwest to 6.1% in the north central zones. HIV continues to spread rapidly among female sex workers and their clients, as well as in the general population. In some urban populations, more than 10% of adults are infected and the annual incidence is as high as 3%.

As of December 2008, 44% of adults and children in need of ART in the region were estimated to be receiving such services. ART coverage is notably higher in eastern and southern Africa (48%) than in western and central Africa (30%). Treatment coverage for adults (44%) remains higher than that for children (35%). Children's access to ART is especially limited in western and central Africa.

AIDS-related deaths have fallen by 29% in Kenya, and a study in Uganda found that timely initiation of ART and cotrimoxazole prophylaxis reduced mortality by 95% and produced a 93% reduction in HIV-related orphans. In Botswana, where ART coverage exceeds 80%, the estimated annual number of AIDS-related deaths declined by more than half. More than 50% of all people in need of treatment are still not receiving such services.

AIDS is now the leading cause of death and years of productive life lost throughout the continent. Excess deaths attributable to HIV are highest in the 25- to 34-year-old group, usually a group with low mortality. Nearly 90% of deaths in this age group are in excess of background rates and were attributable to HIV. Because AIDS deaths are concentrated in childhood and young adult age groups, their effects are substantial, with life expectancy reduced by more than 20 years in several countries. Demographic projections have estimated that population growth will decline more rapidly than expected and that the size of the African population in 2015 will be smaller than it would have been without AIDS. HIV or AIDS cases will put an increasing strain on health care systems, which are already overburdened, and on individual households that are trying to manage with limited economic resources. Care and support for children orphaned by AIDS will become a growing concern throughout the region.

HIV and AIDS in Asia and the Pacific

After sub-Saharan Africa, Asia and the Pacific, home to 60% of the world's population, have the second largest number of HIV-infected individuals in the world, estimated at 4.7 million. In 2008, 360,000 adults and children became newly infected, in part because of growth of the HIV epidemic in China, India, and several other countries in Southeast Asia. With the exception of Thailand, national HIV prevalence levels remain comparatively low in most countries of Asia and the Pacific, with HIV prevalence being less than 1%, to some extent being due to their large population base. Thus, because of the region's large population, Asia's comparatively low HIV prevalence translates into a substantial portion of the global HIV burden. India's national adult HIV prevalence rate of 0.3% offers little indication of the serious situation facing the country. An estimated 2.4 million people were living with HIV at the end of 2008—one of the highest figures in the world after South Africa.

Throughout the region, injecting drug use remains one of the most prominent modes of transmission of HIV. More than 50% of IDUs have already acquired HIV in Malaysia, Myanmar, Nepal, Thailand, Indonesia, Manipur, and southern China. Very high rates of needle sharing have been documented among users in Bangladesh and Vietnam, along with evidence that a considerable proportion of sex workers in Vietnam also inject drugs. More recently, the epidemic in many parts of Asia is steadily expanding into lower-risk populations through transmission to the sexual partners of the most at risk. In China, where the epidemic was previously driven by transmission through injecting drug use, heterosexual transmission has become the predominant mode of HIV transmission.

China, with a fifth of the world's population, has also witnessed a dramatic escalation of the HIV epidemic in the past decade. A total of 700,000 Chinese individuals are estimated to be living with HIV. The HIV epidemic is particularly severe among IDUs, who account for almost half (44%) of all HIV infections. To compound the tragedy of the epidemic in China, reports from Henan province in central China demonstrate that tens of thousands and possibly more rural villagers became infected by selling their blood to collecting centers that did not follow basic blood donation safety procedures. It has been estimated that 150,000 people have been infected through these practices. There are new signs of heterosexually transmitted HIV epidemics in at least three provinces—Guangdong, Guangxi, and Yunnan. Several other factors highlight the swift escalation of HIV infection in China. STDs quadrupled between 1997 and 2002, thus suggesting that unprotected sex with nonmonogamous partners is increasing in China. There is massive population mobility. Approximately 100 million Chinese are temporarily or permanently away from their registered addresses, and increasing socioeconomic disparities add to the likelihood of the spread of HIV.

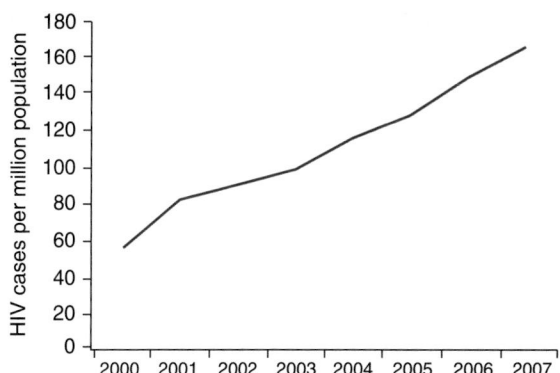

FIGURE 392-4. HIV cases per million population in Eastern Europe by year of notification, 2000 to 2007. *Note*: Data from the Russian Federation are not included. (Data from UNAIDS 2008.)

Indonesia, the world's fourth most populous country, is another example of how quickly the AIDS epidemic can emerge. After more than 10 years of negligible HIV prevalence, the infection rate in IDUs, sex workers, and blood donors in some regions is rapidly increasing. Papua New Guinea has also reported the highest HIV infection rates among the Pacific Island countries and territories. Even though the Philippines has maintained a low HIV prevalence, higher rates of STDs among Filipino sex workers, their clients, and MSM indicate low levels of condom use and the potential for rapid spread of HIV.

In some countries of Southeast Asia where HIV prevalence rose rapidly in the 1990s, strong prevention programs have limited the spread, most notably in Thailand, Cambodia, and Myanmar. Furthermore, the increased access to ART has coincided with a drastic drop in AIDS-related deaths. Despite these advances, AIDS is still a leading cause of death in Thailand, and 1.4% of the country's 63.6 million people are infected with HIV. Although STDs and heterosexual transmission have declined as a result of the government's prevention programs, HIV continues to spread rapidly among IDUs and MSM.

Treatment scale-up in Asia has been mixed. As of December 2008, 37% of those in Asia needing ART were receiving it, lower than the global average (42%) for all low- and middle-income countries. This, however, represents a seven-fold increase in access to treatment in 5 years.

HIV and AIDS in Eastern Europe and Central Asia

The HIV epidemic has increased faster in Eastern Europe and central Asia between 2000 and 2009 than in any other area of the world (Fig. 392-4). In 2008 there were an estimated 1.5 million people living with HIV, a 20-fold increase in less than a decade. In recent years, the Russian Federation has experienced an exceptionally steep rise in reported HIV infections, 90% of which have been attributed to injecting drug use. It is estimated that nearly 1% of the young people in Eastern Europe and central Asia are injecting drugs, which places these individuals and their sex partners at high risk for becoming infected with HIV. In countries such as Azerbaijan, Georgia, Tajikistan, and Uzbekistan, HIV has experienced explosive growth. Similar explosive high rates of HIV are being documented in IDUs and heterosexuals at risk for STDs in other countries of the Commonwealth of Independent States, in the Baltic states, and in Romania.

In Estonia, Latvia, and Lithuania, major HIV outbreaks are also occurring in selected populations, such as prison inmates. In one prison in Lithuania, 15% of the inmates were HIV positive, thus confirming the role of prisons in the spread of HIV in many countries of the region. The concentration of large numbers of young people in overcrowded prisons or juvenile justice facilities, often marked by an abundance of drugs but a scarcity of HIV information, clean needles, or condoms, provides fertile ground for the rapid spread of HIV among inmates and, on their eventual release, into the wider population.

Initially driven by injecting drug use in young people, heterosexual transmission of HIV has become a prominent mode of spread in Belarus and Ukraine. With an estimated adult HIV prevalence rate of 1.6%, Ukraine is one of the most severely affected countries in the region. Three fourths of HIV infections in Ukraine are related to injecting drug use, with a prevalence ranging from 38.5 to 50.3% in IDUs, but the proportion of sexually transmitted infection is increasing. Although many of these infections may occur in sex partners of IDUs, the trend may also indicate spread into the wider population of these countries. In the Russian Federation in the Ukraine, up to 30%

of female IDUs are also involved in commercial sex work. In Odessa, 67% of sex workers who inject drugs were HIV positive. The public health efforts to stem the tide of the epidemic in these countries are limited and, in some cases, nonexistent. In contrast, HIV prevalence remains low in Poland, the Czech Republic, Hungary, and Slovenia, where well-designed national HIV/AIDS programs are in operation.

A number of countries in the region have expanded access to ART, although treatment coverage remains relatively low. By December 2008, only 22% of adults in need of therapy were receiving it—a level much less than the global average. IDUs, the population most at risk for HIV in eastern Europe and central Asia, are often least likely to receive ART when they are medically eligible. If effective interventions are not implemented in the more severely affected countries, it is likely that the situation will become dramatically worse over the next 5 years.

HIV and AIDS in Latin America and the Caribbean
An estimated 2.25 million adults and children are living with HIV in Latin America and the Caribbean. Twelve countries in this region have an estimated HIV prevalence of 1% or greater in pregnant women. In several Caribbean countries, adult HIV prevalence rates are surpassed only by the rates experienced in sub-Saharan Africa, which makes this region the second most affected in the world. Haiti and the Bahamas remain the worst affected, with an estimated national prevalence higher than 2.2% in Haiti and a prevalence of 3.3% in the Bahamas. AIDS is the leading cause of death in some countries of the Caribbean basin. In Haiti, the Bahamas, and Guyana, the number of deaths in 15- to 34-year-olds is 2.5 times higher than it would have been in the absence of AIDS.

Homosexual and heterosexual transmission continues to be the major mode of transmission throughout the region, although there is evidence that spread of HIV is increasing through sharing of infected drug equipment. Population mobility, spurred by high rates of unemployment and poverty, is emerging as a significant factor in the epidemic's growth in this region. Central America's geographic position also makes it an important transit zone for people moving between the rest of the region and North American countries. Appropriately, protecting vulnerable populations on the move, including adolescent girls and young women, is now the focus of a regional prevention program in Central America. In Mexico, adult HIV prevalence in the wider population is still well under 1%, but prevalence rates are higher in specific population groups—6% in IDUs and 15% in MSM. There is significant overlap between IDUs and MSM, especially in Brazil and the southern Latin American countries, where injecting drug use is a growing social phenomenon. Injecting drug use is also a major route of HIV transmission in Argentina, Chile, and Uruguay.

Despite many constraints, the region has made progress in the provision of treatment and care. By reducing HIV-related morbidity through treatment, Brazil's treatment and care program is estimated to have avoided 234,000 hospitalizations in a 4-year period, thereby demonstrating a cost-effective approach to care. Argentina, Costa Rica, Uruguay, and Cuba now guarantee free and universal access to drugs through the public sector, and sharp reductions have recently been secured in Honduras and Panama. Treatment coverage has risen from 10% of those in need in 2004 to 54% in 2008. Similarly, pediatric antiretroviral coverage in the Caribbean was high (55%) in comparison to the global average for children of 38%. Consistent with the evolving guidelines of HIV treatment, a growing number of people living with HIV in Latin America are starting treatment earlier at CD4+ cell counts of 350 or lower rather than waiting until the count drops below 200. Earlier initiation of therapy offers the possibility that medical outcomes in the region may improve further still and reduce the population-level viral load, which might result in lower transmission rates.

HIV and AIDS in Western Europe
More than 850,000 HIV-infected individuals reside in Western Europe, with trends similar to those witnessed in the United States, Australia, and New Zealand. Longer survival of people infected with HIV has led to a steady increase in the number of people living with the virus in high-income countries. In a multicountry study in Europe, Australia, and Canada, mortality rates in people living with HIV in the first 5 years after infection now approach those in the non–HIV-infected population, although excess mortality in HIV-infected people increases with the duration of infection. In the United Kingdom, half of all people living with HIV are receiving ART, with no appreciable increase in the number of patients with virologic failure or resistance to the drugs.

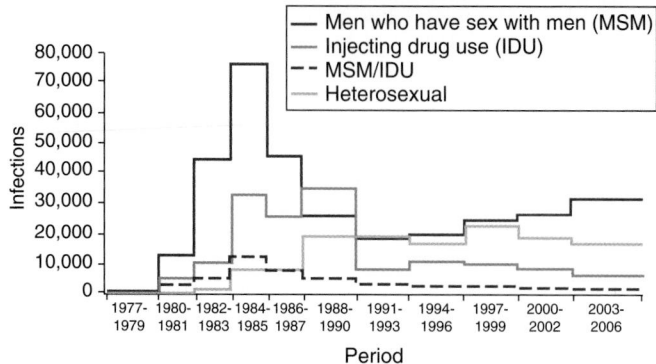

FIGURE 392-5. Estimated new HIV infections by transmission category for the United States, 1977 to 2006. Tick marks denote the beginning and end of a year. The model specifies periods within which the number of HIV infections was assumed to be approximately constant. (Data from Centers for Disease Control and Prevention and Hall HI, Song R, Rhodes P, et al. Estimation of HIV incidence in the United States. *JAMA.* 2008;300:520-529.)

The HIV epidemic in Western Europe is a result of a multitude of epidemics that differ in their timing, scale, and effects on populations. A larger proportion of new HIV diagnoses in Western European countries occur through heterosexual intercourse. More than half of the new HIV infections in the United Kingdom in 2008 resulted from heterosexual sex, as compared with 33% in 1998. In Ireland, a similar trend is visible, with numbers of heterosexually transmitted HIV infection increasing four-fold between 1998 and 2001. Unsafe sex between men remains an important factor for spread in most European countries, particularly in the United Kingdom, Germany, the Netherlands, and Spain. Injecting drug use remains a major mode of transmission in Spain, France, and Portugal, but like other countries in Europe, about a fourth of all HIV infections are now heterosexually transmitted. Most data from high-income countries demonstrate that the epidemic has shifted to the poor and marginalized sections of society. Underscoring the need for renewed prevention efforts, especially in young people, are findings of increases in high-risk behavior, less frequent condom use, and higher rates of STDs in several countries. In the United Kingdom, for example, rates of gonorrhea, syphilis, and chlamydial infections have more than doubled since 1995, and increases have been found in other Western European countries as well.

HIV and AIDS in the United States
By 2009, more people than ever were living in the United States with HIV—1.2 million (see Table 392-1). Nationally, the adult HIV prevalence was estimated to be 0.6%. This increase reflects mixed results in the U.S. effort to combat its epidemic. More people infected with HIV are living longer because of ART, but unfortunately, the early gains made in prevention have not been sustained (Fig. 392-5). The number of newly recorded HIV cases in 33 states with confidential name-based reporting has varied only slightly since the late 1990s. In 2006, the annual incidence of HIV infection was estimated at 56,300, which was approximately 40% higher than previously estimated. Half of all HIV infections diagnosed in men, women, and children in 2008 were in MSM, a rise from previous years.

Another aspect of the U.S. epidemic is that more women are being infected with HIV through unprotected heterosexual exposure and injecting drug use. Overall, nearly 20% of new HIV infections are attributable to injecting drug use. The main risk factor for women who acquire HIV during sex is the risk behavior of their male partners, such as injecting drug use, commercial sex, or sex with other men. As in Latin America, women living in impoverished and marginal circumstances appear to be at disproportionate risk for HIV infection. In North Carolina, HIV-positive women were considerably more likely to be unemployed, requiring public assistance, and exchanging sex for money and gifts.

As the U.S. epidemic evolves, it is becoming more an epidemic of African Americans and other minorities. African Americans make up 12% of the U.S. population but account for 45% of new HIV diagnoses. Hispanics represent 14% of the population but account for 18% of new HIV diagnoses. Among African Americans and Hispanics, most men infected with HIV were exposed during sex with other men (49% and 59%, respectively), whereas most women with HIV become infected heterosexually (78% and 73%, respectively). African American women are more than 10 times more likely to be infected with HIV than white women are. AIDS continues to be the leading cause of death in African American women aged 25 to 34 years and ranks in the top three causes of death in African American men aged 25 to 54 years. African Americans are about half as likely to receive ART as other population groups, and twice as many African Americans as whites die of AIDS. In the United States, the challenge of slowing the rate of new HIV infections overlaps with the need to provide diagnosis, treatment, and care services more equitably. The number of AIDS-related deaths was 69% lower than in 1994. However, further declines in mortality will require greater success in encouraging timely diagnosis of HIV infection. An estimated 21% of people living with HIV are unaware of their HIV status. Moreover, in 36% of people in whom HIV was diagnosed, AIDS was diagnosed within 12 months. With the aim of increasing the percentage of people who receive a timely diagnosis of HIV, the Centers for Disease Control and Prevention recommends routine voluntary HIV testing in all health care settings unless the patient opts not to be tested.

With an epidemic that is nearly into its third decade, complacency has increased, and prevention efforts have dwindled as a result of declining mortality. Multiple studies illustrate that prevention efforts are not reaching the large number of at-risk individuals who engage in unsafe sex. Increased rates of sexually transmitted infections among MSM have been documented in the United States, Australia, Great Britain, Canada, and other developed countries. Rates of gonorrhea, syphilis, and chlamydia have more than doubled in the past 5 years among MSM in selected U.S. and European cities. Renewed efforts to enhance prevention efforts, particularly in HIV care clinics, are being echoed throughout all these countries.

1. Severe P, Juste MAJ, Ambroise A, et al. Early versus standard antiretroviral therapy for HIV-infected adults in Haiti. *N Engl J Med.* 2010;363:257-265.

SUGGESTED READINGS

Cambiano V, Rodger AJ, Phillips AN. "Test-and-treat": the end of the HIV epidemic? *Curr Opin Infect Dis.* 2011;24:19-26. *Discusses the impact of test-and-treat on the future risk of HIV transmission.*

El-Sadr WM, Mayer KH, Hodder SL. AIDS in America—forgotten but not gone. *N Engl J Med.* 2010;362:967-970. *The prevalence of HIV infection within some U.S. populations now rivals that in some sub-Saharan countries.*

Hall HI, Song R, Rhodes P, et al. Estimation of HIV incidence in the United States. *JAMA.* 2008;300:520-529. *Revision of the number of people newly infected in the United States to a level higher than previously estimated.*

Lawn SD, Harries AD, Wood R. Strategies to reduce early morbidity and mortality in adults receiving antiretroviral therapy in resource-limited settings. *Curr Opin HIV AIDS.* 2010;5:18-26. *Strategies to reduce disease burden in light of fundamental need for much earlier HIV diagnosis and initiation of antiretroviral therapy.*

WHO, UN Children's Fund, UNAIDS. Towards Universal Access: Scaling Up Priority HIV/AIDS Interventions in the Health Sector. Geneva, Switzerland: World Health Organization; 2009. *An extensive report on the scale-up of antiretroviral drugs and prevention initiatives worldwide.*

393

IMMUNOPATHOGENESIS OF HUMAN IMMUNODEFICIENCY VIRUS INFECTION

JOEL N. BLANKSON AND ROBERT F. SILICIANO

Human immunodeficiency virus type 1 (HIV-1) infection results in a progressive state of immune system dysregulation that ultimately leads to the acquired immunodeficiency syndrome (AIDS), a syndrome characterized by a profound depletion of CD4$^+$ T lymphocytes and the inability to control infections by opportunistic pathogens that do not cause disease in individuals with a normal immune system. Despite almost 30 years of research on this condition, the basic pathogenic mechanisms are still incompletely understood. This chapter reviews current understanding of the mechanisms involved in HIV-1 immunopathogenesis.

PRIMARY INFECTION

The natural history of HIV-1 infection is illustrated in Figure 393-1. During acute HIV-1 infection, massive viral replication occurs in CD4$^+$ T

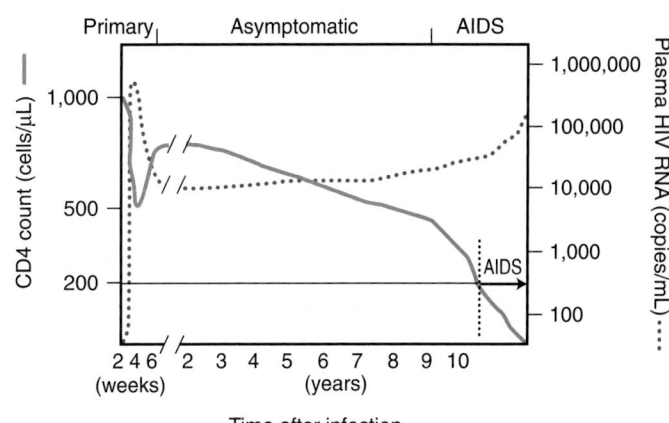

FIGURE 393-1. Natural history of HIV-1 infection. CD4 counts and viral load are shown in the three phases of infection.

lymphocytes in the absence of an adaptive immune response. CD4$^+$ T cells in the gut-associated lymphoid tissue and other mucosal sites express high levels of the HIV coreceptor CCR5 and are thus particularly prone to infection and depletion by the commonly transmitted R5 variants of HIV-1. In animal models, it has been shown that approximately 30% of memory CD4$^+$ T cells are infected and depleted by 4 days after infection. This is in contrast to chronic infection, in which less than 1% of all CD4$^+$ T cells are infected at any given time. As a result of this massive early infection, levels of virion-associated HIV RNA of more than 1 million copies/mL are typically seen in plasma within 2 weeks of infection, and patients tend to experience a constellation of signs and symptoms known as the *acute retroviral syndrome*. There can be significant declines in peripheral CD4$^+$ T-cell counts in primary infection resulting in opportunistic infections. Within several weeks, the development of an effective HIV-1–specific cytolytic T-lymphocyte response results in the partial control of viral replication, and peak viral loads fall and reach a steady state known as the *set point*. The magnitude of the set point viral load during the second asymptomatic phase of the infection reflects a dynamic equilibrium between viral replication and the HIV-1–specific immune response. This set point determines the rate of progression to the final phase, clinical AIDS. The median set point is approximately 30,000 HIV-1 RNA copies per milliliter, and most patients who have this level of viremia will develop AIDS in a 5- to 10-year period if they are left untreated. Patients with much higher set point viral loads will tend to be rapid progressors who develop AIDS much more quickly; patients with much lower viral loads tend to be long-term nonprogressors.

HIV-1–SPECIFIC IMMUNITY

The host mounts a vigorous immune response after HIV-1 infection. The virus is thought to activate plasmacytoid dendritic cells through Toll-like receptors, resulting in the secretion of type I interferons and other inflammatory cytokines. Whereas type I interferons have direct antiviral properties and enhance the HIV-1–specific immune response, excessive secretion may play a key role in pathogenic immune activation of CD4$^+$ and CD8$^+$ T cells (Fig. 393-2). Natural killer (NK) cells are important effector cells in the innate immune response that become activated when infection of target cells by HIV-1 or other viruses results in the downregulation of HLA molecules. Patients expressing certain NK receptor alleles are more likely to become long-term nonprogressors, suggesting that these cells may play a protective role possibly by controlling early HIV-1 replication, leading to the development of an effective adaptive immune response. Myeloid dendritic cells play a key role in the presentation of HIV-1 antigens to HIV-1–specific CD4$^+$ and CD8$^+$ T cells, which results in the initiation of the adaptive immune response. They express CD4 molecules and have been shown to bind HIV-1. It is thought that in the process of presenting antigen, these cells may inadvertently transmit HIV-1 to clusters of activated CD4$^+$ T cells.

The role of the humoral response in HIV-1 infection is not clear. HIV-1–specific antibodies, which are used to diagnose HIV-1 infection, do not develop until after peak viremia occurs. There is thus a window period in primary HIV-1 infection during which viremia is present in the absence of detectable antibodies. A subset of the antibodies that eventually appear are capable of preventing infection by blocking the interaction of the HIV-1 envelope protein gp120 with CD4 and coreceptor proteins on the surface of

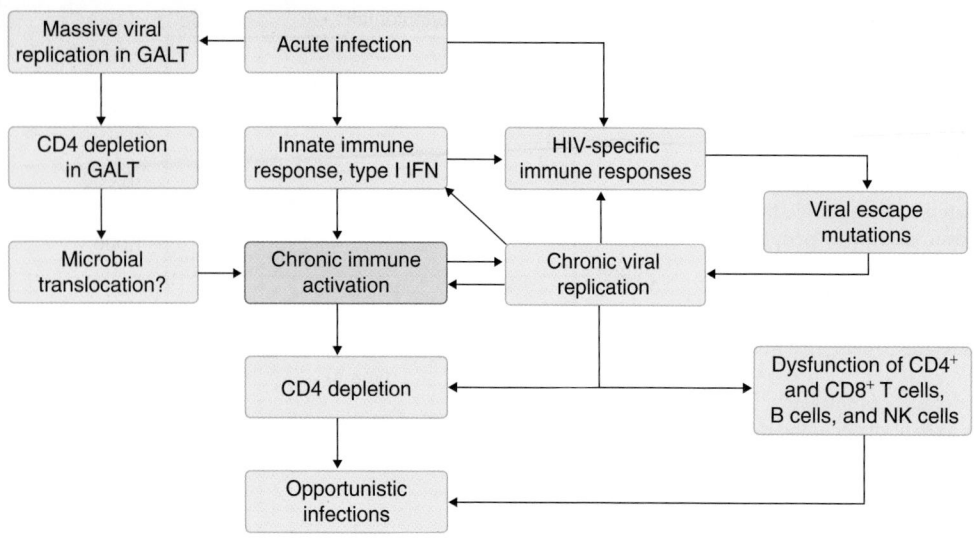

FIGURE 393-2. Parameters involved in chronic immune activation and CD4⁺ T-cell depletion. GALT = gut-associated lymphoid tissue; IFN = interferons; NK = natural killer.

target cells. These so-called neutralizing antibodies are present at relatively low titers and have limited access to the critical regions of gp120. Whereas they can exert significant selective pressure on the virus, immunologic escape is common, and the bulk of evidence suggests that these antibodies do not play a major role in the control of viral replication in most long-term nonprogressors.

The selective depletion of CD4⁺ T cells is the main reason that HIV-1 infection results in such profound immunosuppression; these so-called helper T cells play a major role in every facet of the adaptive immune response. The ability of HIV-1–specific CD4⁺ T cells to proliferate and to secrete key cytokines such as interleukin-2 is lost shortly after primary infection, setting up the entire HIV-1–specific response for failure.

CD8⁺ T cells contribute to the control of HIV-1 infection by the direct lysis of infected cells and by the secretion of soluble factors like macrophage inflammatory protein 1β that bind to chemokine receptors, thereby preventing HIV-1 entry into target cells. However, the HIV-1–specific CD8⁺ T-cell response that partially controls HIV-1 replication after peak viremia in primary infection does not achieve sterilizing immunity, partly because of a reservoir of latent virus in resting memory CD4⁺ T cells that develops shortly after infection. These quiescent cells probably do not make HIV-1 proteins and thus are not recognized by cytolytic T lymphocytes. Furthermore, the cytolytic T-lymphocyte response in patients with progressive disease is of poor quality with limited proliferative capacity. Most important, the low fidelity of HIV-1 reverse transcriptase results in the development of mutations with each round of replication. Mutations that lead to escape from cytolytic T-lymphocyte responses have an advantage and are thus rapidly selected for.

THE EFFECT OF HIV-1 REPLICATION ON THE IMMUNE SYSTEM

Whereas the HIV-1–specific immune response helps limit the rate of viral replication, sterilizing immunity is never achieved and the virus has a negative impact on the immune system. Continuous viral replication results in chronic immune activation (see Fig. 393-2). The mechanism is not understood. The chronic immune response to the virus may lead to nonspecific inflammation, and microbial translocation resulting from the depletion of CD4⁺ T cells in the gut-associated lymphoid tissue may also be important. Whatever the mechanism, immune activation appears to drive the depletion of CD4⁺ T cells. The level of immune activation markers on CD4⁺ and CD8⁺ T cells correlates better with the rate of CD4 decline than does the magnitude of the viral load in untreated patients.

Increased levels of activation markers are seen on NK cells, B cells, CD4⁺ T cells, and CD8⁺ T cells. Activation is accompanied by an increase in the turnover rate of these cells. The function of NK cells is compromised, which may predispose to the poor control of other viruses. B-cell defects result in hypergammaglobulinemia and the production of autoantibodies. Poor antibody responses to vaccines are also seen as CD4⁺ T cells decline.

Studies of viral dynamics make it clear that most productively infected cells live only a short time (~1 day) before succumbing to viral cytopathic effects

or host cytolytic T lymphocytes or NK cells. Although the loss of infected CD4⁺ T cells contributes to CD4 depletion, there is marked depletion of CD4⁺ T cells even though at any given time during chronic infection only 1% or less of these cells are infected. Thus, it is currently thought that chronic immune activation leading to the death of noninfected CD4⁺ T cells is the principle mechanism for CD4 depletion. Support for this idea comes from studies of the closely related simian immunodeficiency virus that replicates in natural simian hosts without causing immune activation or CD4 depletion. In addition to the quantitative loss of CD4⁺ T cells in HIV-1 infection, marked skewing of the CD4 T-cell repertoire is seen, and there is a diminished qualitative memory response to recall antigens long before the CD4⁺ T-cell count drops to 200 cells/μL. The chronic activation and high turnover rate of these cells eventually result in the progressive CD4 decline that is characteristic of HIV-1 infection.

There is evidence of immune exhaustion for both CD4⁺ and CD8⁺ T cells, and there is decline in the qualitative features of the CD8⁺ T-cell response to other chronic viruses such as cytomegalovirus and Epstein-Barr virus. This may be the result of anergy or depletion of the CD4⁺ T cells that are needed to sustain functional CD8⁺ T-cell responses.

CLINICAL CONSEQUENCES OF HIV INFECTION

Clinical immunodeficiency is associated with the late stages of HIV-1 infection, when profound CD4⁺ T-cell depletion has occurred. However, some level of immunodeficiency may be present shortly after infection because of qualitative changes in the immune response related to ongoing viral replication. As a result, patients are more susceptible to infections like *Mycobacterium tuberculosis* infection before the CD4 count reaches the 200 cells/μL threshold that defines AIDS. Patients are also much more susceptible to malignant neoplasms such as non-Hodgkin's lymphoma at any CD4⁺ T-cell count. Other opportunistic infections arise at fairly predictable CD4⁺ T-cell counts. *Pneumocystis jiroveci* infections occur at CD4 counts of lower than 200 cells/μL, *Cryptococcus neoformans* and *Toxoplasma gondii* infections occur at CD4 counts of lower than 100 cells/μL, and *Mycobacterium avium* complex and cytomegalovirus infections occur at CD4 counts below 50 cells/μL. Whereas these infections are a consequence of diminished cellular immunity, there is also a marked increase in invasive pneumococcal infections in HIV-1–infected patients, possibly due to defects in humoral immunity.

The Response to Antiretroviral Therapy

Treatment with selected combinations of antiretroviral drugs, which is known as highly active antiretroviral therapy (HAART), suppresses viral replication to below the limits of detection of current commercial assays (50 copies of HIV-1 RNA per milliliter of plasma). Current evidence suggests that HAART produces a complete or nearly complete arrest in viral replication in adherent patients, but trace amounts of viremia persist because of stable viral reservoirs, including the latent reservoir in resting CD4⁺ T cells. This suppression of viral replication is usually accompanied by a substantial increase in CD4⁺ T-cell counts. The initial rise in CD4⁺ T-cell counts occurs mostly as a consequence of migration of cells from lymph nodes (where 98%

of all CD4 T cells reside) to the peripheral blood as inflammation diminishes in lymphoid tissue. Subsequently, there is an increase in the production of memory CD4$^+$ T cells in most individuals. Naive T cell production is also sometimes seen at lower levels. Clinical studies have shown that patients who experience significant immune reconstitution can safely discontinue prophylactic therapy for opportunistic infections. However, it is not clear whether patients who maintain undetectable viral loads while receiving HAART yet do not achieve significant CD4 T-cell immune reconstitution are still at risk for opportunistic infections. Two large studies have shown that although the use of interleukin-2 treatment in conjunction with HAART will cause a significant increase in CD4$^+$ T-cell counts in these patients, the enhanced immune reconstitution is not associated with any clinical benefit.

Just as a decline is seen in the functional CD4$^+$ T-cell response shortly after primary infection, there is a qualitative improvement in CD4$^+$ T-cell function shortly after HAART is initiated. In some cases, there are exaggerated immune responses to opportunistic infections leading to the immune reconstitution inflammatory syndrome (IRIS; Chapter 402), particularly when there is rapid control of viral replication after the initiation of HAART. IRIS usually presents as a paradoxical worsening of a disease process a few weeks after HAART is started and can occur even before there are significant changes in the absolute CD4$^+$ T-cell counts. IRIS has been reported for virtually all known opportunistic infections, and in some cases it can occur in response to previously unrecognized infections. There have not been clinical trials looking at treatment of this condition, but nonsteroidal anti-inflammatory drugs and corticosteroids have been routinely used with varying degrees of success (Chapter 402).

SUGGESTED READINGS

Hersperger AR, Migueles SA, Betts MR, et al. Qualitative features of the HIV-specific CD8+ T-cell response associated with immunologic control. *Curr Opin HIV AIDS.* 2011;6:169-173. *Detailed analysis of the role of HIV-specific CD8 T-cell in long-term noprogressors.*

Moir S, Fauci AS. B cells in HIV-1 infection and disease. *Nat Rev Immunol.* 2009;4:235-245. *An analysis of B cell dysfunction in HIV-1 infection.*

Muller M, Wandel S, Colebunders R, et al. Immune reconstitution inflammatory syndrome in patients starting antiretroviral therapy for HIV infection: a systematic review and meta-analysis. *Lancet Infect Dis.* 2010;10:251-261. *Detailed review of the immune reconstitution inflammatory syndrome.*

O'Connell KA, Bailey JR, Blankson JN. Elucidating the elite: mechanisms of control on HIV-1 infection. *Trends Pharmacol Sci.* 2009;12:631-637. *An analysis of the immunologic mechanisms seen in patients who maintain undetectable viral loads without antiretroviral therapy.*

FIGURE 394-1. Transmission electron micrograph of HIV-1. Virions are shown at all stages of morphogenesis: early *(A)* and late *(B)* budding forms and cell-free mature virions *(C and D)* with condensed central cores. Virion diameter is approximately 110 nm.

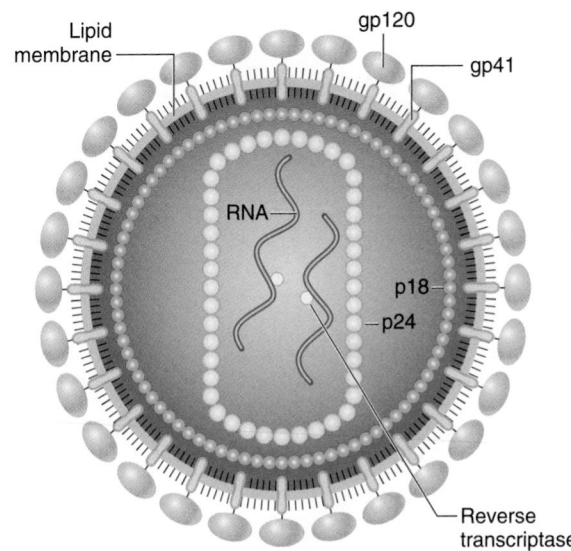

FIGURE 394-2. Structure of HIV-1. (Adapted from Gallo RC. The AIDS virus. *Sci Am.* 1987;256:46-56. Copyright © 1987 by Scientific American, Inc., and George V. Klein.)

BIOLOGY OF HUMAN IMMUNODEFICIENCY VIRUSES

GEORGE M. SHAW

DISCOVERY OF HUMAN IMMUNODEFICIENCY VIRUSES

Identification of human immunodeficiency virus type 1 (HIV-1) as the causative agent of acquired immunodeficiency syndrome (AIDS) just 3 years after the clinical syndrome was initially described represents a remarkable scientific achievement that had its roots in earlier discoveries of animal and human retroviruses. The selective loss of CD4$^+$ helper T lymphocytes in patients with AIDS implicated an agent with T-lymphocyte tropism. HIV-1 had this property, and as expected for an etiologic agent, the virus was shown to be invariably present in subjects with AIDS and to reproduce the hallmark of the disease in tissue culture: destruction of T lymphocytes.

HUMAN IMMUNODEFICIENCY VIRUS TYPE 1

General Biologic Properties

Soon after its discovery, HIV-1 was shown to be biologically, structurally, and genetically distinct from human T-lymphotropic virus type 1 (HTLV-1) and

type 2 (HTLV-2) and more like members of the lentivirus subfamily of retroviruses. Unlike the leukemia viruses, which lead to immortalization of lymphocytes in vitro and in vivo, HIV-1 produces pronounced cytopathic properties in lymphocytes and causes syncytia formation and cell death. Morphologically, HIV-1 differs from HTLV-1 and other type C oncogenic retroviruses in exhibiting a dense, cylindrical core surrounded by a lipid envelope typical of lentiviruses (Fig. 394-1).

The structural organization of HIV-1 is shown diagrammatically in Figure 394-2. Like all retroviruses, HIV-1 is a single-stranded, plus-sense RNA virus. The RNA-dependent DNA polymerase, or reverse transcriptase, is packaged within the virion core and is responsible for replicating the single-stranded RNA genome through a double-stranded DNA intermediate that serves as the precursor molecule for proviral integration within the host cell genome. The major structural core proteins of HIV-1 are the p24 capsid protein and the p18 matrix protein. Surrounding the viral core protein structures is a bilayered lipid envelope that is derived from the outer limiting membrane of the host cell as the virus buds from the cell surface during replication. Studding this outer viral membrane are the envelope glycoproteins gp120 and gp41, which are encoded by virus-specific genes and are responsible for cell attachment and entry.

The life cycle of HIV-1 is shown diagrammatically in Figure 394-3. Features of this life cycle distinguish retroviruses from all other viruses. The cell-free virion first attaches to the target cell through a specific interaction between the viral envelope and the host's cell membrane. The specificity of this interaction between virus and cell results from a high-affinity interaction between the viral gp120 envelope glycoprotein and the target cell–associated

A

B

C

FIGURE 394-3. Different representations of the HIV-1 life cycle. **A**, *Thick arrows* denote amplification of viral products that may occur in the latter half of the replication cycle. **B**, Pictorial overview of the virus life cycle outlined in **A**. **C**, Major transformations of retroviral genetic information during the life cycle. A_n = poly(A) tract; Cap = 5′-methyl-G nucleotide; CHO = glycosylation site; LTR = long terminal repeat; P = phosphorylation site; Psi = viral packaging signal sequence; S_A = splice acceptor site; S_D = splice donor site. (From Varmus H, Brown P. Retroviruses. In: Berg DE, Howe MM, eds. *Mobile DNA*. Washington, DC: American Society for Microbiology; 1989:53.)

CD4 molecule and leads to a conformational change in gp120 and subsequent interaction with a member of the cellular chemokine receptor family (CCR5 or CXCR4). These highly specific interactions among gp120, CD4, and CCR5/CXCR4 culminate in fusion of the viral and cellular membranes and internalization of the nucleoprotein-viral complex. Reverse transcription

catalyzed by viral reverse transcriptase generates a double-stranded DNA copy of the viral RNA within the nucleoprotein complex, and this copy migrates to the nucleus, where covalent integration of viral DNA into host chromosomes leads to formation of the provirus. Subsequent expression of viral DNA is controlled by a combination of viral and host cellular proteins that interact with viral DNA and RNA regulatory elements. Transcribed viral mRNA is translated into viral proteins, and new virions are assembled at the cell surface, where genomic-length viral RNA, reverse transcriptase, structural and regulatory proteins, and envelope glycoproteins are assembled. Importantly, most of the steps in the HIV-1 life cycle can now be inhibited by antiretroviral drugs, which when used in combination, result in sustained clinical benefit. However, because the HIV-1 provirus is covalently integrated within the host cell's chromosomes, it can persist in a transcriptionally silent or latent state in unactivated memory CD4+ T lymphocytes for years, only to resume productive replication should therapy be discontinued. Thus, HIV-1 latency is a viral feature that has stood in the way of curative therapy.

Molecular Structure and Function of HIV-1

The genomic organization of HIV-1 is shown diagrammatically in Figure 394-4. The HIV-1 genome, like other retroviral genomes, is diploid and consists of two identical viral RNA molecules assembled in a hydrogen-bonded 70S complex. These genomic subunits are plus strands of viral RNA in that they have the same chemical polarity as the mRNA from which the viral products are translated. Like eukaryotic mRNA, the genomic viral RNA contains a 5′-methyl-G nucleotide, a poly(A) tract of 100 to 200 nucleotides at its 3′ end, and a number of methylated(A) residues. Host cell–derived tRNA incorporated within the virion is base-paired over a stretch of 18 nucleotides to the primer-binding site of the genomic viral RNA near its 5′ terminus and serves to prime the synthesis of minus-strand DNA during the initial stages of viral replication after infection.

The HIV-1 genome is bounded by long terminal repeat (LTR) elements and contains genes encoding the structural and enzymatic proteins (gag, pol, and env) found in all other replication-competent retroviruses. In addition to these genes, HIV-1 contains genes encoding other viral functions unique to this family of viruses that are responsible for their biologic behavior. The LTR sequences of HIV-1 direct and regulate expression of the viral genome (Fig. 394-5).

The *gag* gene encodes a precursor protein (p55) of 55 kD that is cleaved into four smaller products with the linear order NH₂-p18-p24-p9-p7-COOH. These proteins constitute the core protein structure of the virus and subserve nucleic acid– and lipid membrane–binding functions. The gag proteins of HIV-1, like those of other retroviruses, are synthesized as a polyprotein precursor that is subsequently cleaved during the viral maturation process. This facilitates assembly of the different components of the viral core structure into a three-dimensional configuration that when cleaved by a specific virus-derived protease, acquires the specialized functions characteristic of the mature virion. The polymerase gene products are translated from the same genomic RNA message as the gag proteins but in a different, overlapping reading frame as a result of ribosomal frame shifting. The *pol* gene encodes three proteins that are cleaved from a larger precursor polypeptide. These genes include NH₂-protease (p13)-reverse transcriptase (p66/p51)-integrase (p31)-COOH. The HIV-1 protease plays a critical role in viral biology in that it acts specifically to cleave gag and pol precursor polypeptides into functionally active proteins. The reverse transcriptase of HIV-1 is a magnesium-requiring, RNA-dependent DNA polymerase responsible for replicating the RNA viral genome. The integrase protein is required for proviral integration into the host cell's genome.

The envelope gene *(env)* encodes a glycosylated polypeptide precursor (gp160) that is cleaved to form the exterior envelope glycoprotein (gp120) and the transmembrane glycoprotein (gp41), the latter of which anchors the envelope complex to the viral surface. The gp120/gp41 heterodimer exists as a trimeric spike complex on the virion surface and must serve two separate but essential functions: (1) mediation of viral binding and entry into cells and (2) avoidance of neutralization by virus-specific antibodies. The former task is accomplished by sequential gp120 binding to cell-associated CD4 followed by a chemokine receptor, which triggers a gp41-mediated fusion event. The latter function results from a combination of carbohydrate cloaking of the exposed viral env surface, mutation of exposed env epitopes, and masking of conserved env receptor surfaces by conformational or energetic barriers to antibody binding.

Within the HIV-1 genome, additional genes serve important viral functions and distinguish HIV-1 from oncogenic retroviruses. They include the

FIGURE 394-4. Genomic organization of HIV-1. LTR = long terminal repeat.

FIGURE 394-5. Regulatory regions in the long terminal repeat (LTR) of HIV-1. Deletion mutant studies of the LTR have identified at least five regions for gene expression, including the TATA box and promotor, where RNA polymerase binds and transcription is initiated (+1); a negative regulatory element (NRE) located between nucleotides −340 and −185, deletion of which increases the level of gene expression directed by the viral LTR; enhancer elements (NFκB and Sp-1) located between nucleotides −137 and −17; and a *trans*-acting responsive region (TAR) located between nucleotides +1 and +80, which represents the putative binding region for regulatory factors responsible for tat-mediated transcriptional activation.

vif, vpr, and *vpu* genes located between *pol* and *env*; the *nef* gene located 3′ to *env* and extending into the U3 region of the viral LTR; and the *tat* and *rev* genes, both of which exist as bipartite coding exons in the central and 3′ end of the virus. The *tat* gene encodes a 14-kD protein that upregulates HIV-1 expression at transcriptional and post-transcriptional levels and is thus essential for HIV-1 replication. The target sequence for *tat*-mediated upregulation of HIV-1 expression is the *trans*-acting responsive region (TAR) of the LTR, which interacts with cellular factors to bind and activate TAR (see Fig. 394-5). The *rev* gene encodes a 20-kD protein that is required for transport of unspliced and singly spliced viral mRNA from the nucleus to the cytoplasm. In the absence of *rev*, gag and env mRNA transcripts become multiply spliced and gag and env proteins are not made. The *vif* gene encodes a protein product of 23 kD that suppresses the antiretroviral cellular enzyme apolipoprotein B mRNA-editing enzyme-catalytic polypeptide-like 3G (APO-BEC3G), thereby enabling the production of infectious virions. The *vpr* gene encodes a protein of 15 kD that induces G_2/M cell cycle arrest, thereby enhancing viral production. The *vpu* gene encodes a 16-kD protein that is involved in virus assembly and release. The *nef* gene encodes a 27-kD protein that facilitates viral pathogenesis by downregulating cell surface–bound CD4, altering T-cell activation, and interfering with major histocompatibility complex (MHC) antigen presentation.

In summary, HIV-1 encodes the usual structural and enzymatic proteins typical of other replication-competent retroviruses, including gag, pol, and env, but it also encodes a group of at least six regulatory or auxiliary proteins (vif, vpr, vpu, tat, rev, and nef) whose activities are critically important in regulating the life cycle and pathogenesis of the virus.

Cell Tropism
The hallmark of AIDS is selective depletion of CD4+ helper-inducer T lymphocytes. This defect is believed to result largely from the selective tropism of HIV-1 for this population of cells based on the high affinity of the viral gp120 envelope protein for the CD4 molecule. CD4 normally serves as a ligand for MHC type II interactions, but in HIV-1 infection, it is used as the primary receptor molecule for HIV-1 targeting. This has been shown conclusively by studies demonstrating (1) direct complexing of gp120 and CD4 during viral infection, (2) inhibition of viral attachment and infection by anti-CD4 monoclonal antibodies that prevent gp120 binding, and (3) the ability of recombinant CD4 to confer susceptibility to HIV-1 infection to transfected human cells that normally do not express CD4.

CD4 expression alone is not sufficient to mediate HIV-1 entry. Coreceptors essential for viral entry include members of the chemokine receptor family, which are G protein–coupled receptors for pro-inflammatory chemokines. They include CCR5, which normally responds to the chemokines RANTES, MIP-1α, and MIP-1β, and CXCR4, which normally binds SDF-1. CCR5 and CXCR4 are differentially expressed on normal human cells that serve as targets of HIV-1 infection and are importantly involved in the cellular and tissue tropism of HIV-1 and in viral transmission and pathogenesis.

FIGURE 394-6. Natural history model for HIV-1 infection. Viremia denotes cell-free virus in plasma, p24 Ag denotes circulating viral p24 antigen in plasma, and anti-p24 and anti-gp160 correspond to antibodies to viral core and envelope proteins.

A variety of cell types other than helper-inducer T lymphocytes are known to express CD4 on their surface and are capable of replicating HIV-1. Such cells include tissue macrophages, Langerhans cells in skin, and microglial and multinucleated giant cells in the central nervous system (CNS). These cells generally express smaller amounts of CD4 on their cell surface, but in each case they express one or more coreceptor molecules. Infection of such cells is believed to play a role in the pathogenesis of AIDS. Other cell types, including neurons, glial cells, gastrointestinal epithelial cells, and kidney epithelium, can support HIV-1 infection, but the pathophysiologic significance of such findings in regard to viral pathogenesis in vivo is uncertain.

Viral Pathogenesis
Lentiviral (*lenti* = slow) diseases are typically characterized by prolonged periods of restricted viral gene expression, clinical latency, and lifelong persistence of virus in the face of substantial host immune responses and effective suppressive antiretroviral drug therapy. From cohort studies of individuals infected with HIV-1 before the era of highly active antiretroviral therapy (HAART), it was estimated that AIDS will develop in 26 to 36% of infected individuals within 7 years of infection and that lesser signs of immune dysfunction will develop in an additional 40%. This protracted clinical course suggested that expression of the HIV-1 genome in vivo is downregulated with respect to in vitro infection of lymphocytes by HIV-1, which is characterized by explosive lytic viral infection.

However, clinical quiescence can be misleading, and Figure 394-6 depicts the natural history of HIV-1 infection in humans to be one of continuous viral replication and progressive lymphocyte destruction. Initial infection with HIV-1 frequently causes an acute viral syndrome with protean manifestations

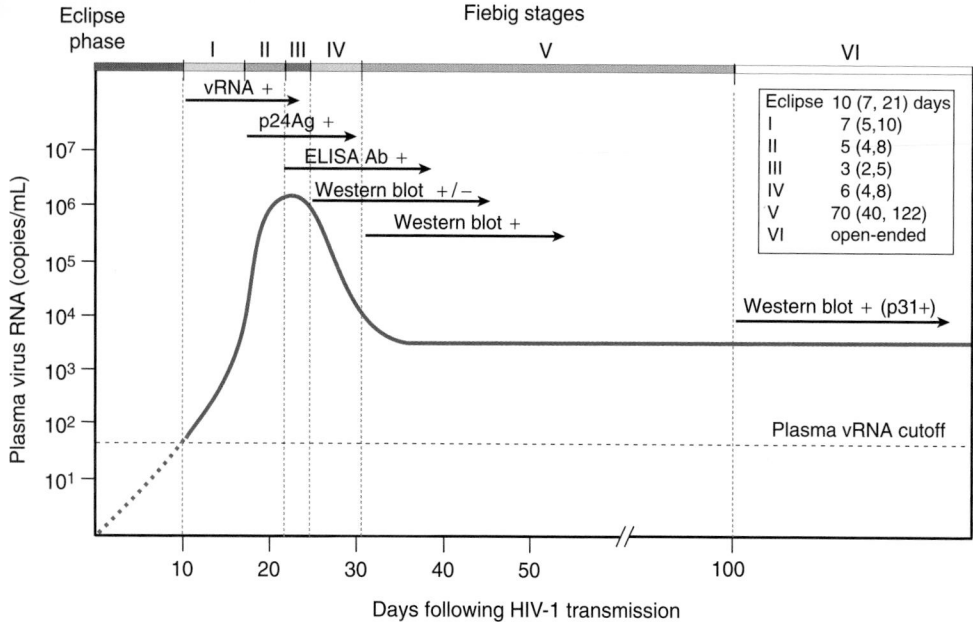

FIGURE 394-7. Laboratory markers and clinical staging of acute and early HIV-1 infection. HIV-1 transmission is followed by an orderly appearance of viral markers and host antibodies in plasma. The average duration (with 95% confidence intervals in parentheses) of each clinicopathologic stage is depicted in the *boxed inset*. (Adapted from Fiebig EW, Wright DJ, Rawal BD, et al. Dynamics of HIV viremia and antibody seroconversion in plasma donors: implications for diagnosis and staging of primary HIV infection. *AIDS.* 2003;17:1871-1879.)

but typically characterized by fever, lymphadenopathy, pharyngitis, and rash. Other symptoms and signs that may occur with acute HIV-1 infection include myalgia, arthralgia, leukopenia, thrombocytopenia, nausea, diarrhea, headache, and encephalopathy. During this primary phase of infection, CD4+ lymphocytes in blood may be normal or transiently diminished, but CD4+ lymphocytes in gut-associated lymphoreticular tissue and in lymph nodes become widely infected and rapidly depleted, thereby leading to a long-lasting quantitative and qualitative loss of CD4+ helper T-cell function. Regardless of the presence or absence of discernible clinical symptoms during primary infection, the emergence of viral and host immune markers of infection occurs in an orderly process (Fig. 394-7). Immediately following viral transmission, there is an eclipse phase during which virus replicates in mucosal tissues, draining lymphatics, and gut-associated lymphoid tissue but neither virus nor viral-specific antibodies are detectable in plasma. This is followed by an exponential rise in viral RNA (Fiebig stage I) and viral RNA and p24 antigen (Fiebig stage II) in plasma while viral antibodies are still not detectable. Peak plasma viremia titers typically reach 10^6 to 10^8 virions/mL. Clinically, Fiebig stages I and II are important because patients are highly infectious, oftentimes symptomatic, and commonly seek medical attention, but rapid antibody tests are negative. To diagnose acute HIV-1 infection, clinicians must thus have a high index of clinical suspicion and specify HIV-1 RNA tests in addition to antibody tests. The typical "window" period during which a patient is HIV-1 antibody negative but plasma virus positive is about 12 days but ranges from 9 to 18 days. This antibody-negative, plasma viral RNA–positive period generally begins about 7 to 21 days after transmission and persists for as long as 2 weeks before HIV-1–specific antibodies are first detectable by sensitive recombinant protein-based enzyme-linked immunosorbent assay (ELISA). Confirmation of HIV-1 infection based on the appearance of antibodies to multiple viral proteins on Western immunoblot generally follows within a week or two. In rare instances, antibody seroconversion has been reported to occur as long as 3 or even 6 months after a presumed date of infection. After peak viremia, HIV-1 replication is downregulated by host defense mechanisms with resolution of the acute proinflammatory infectious state, although viral replication is not altogether abrogated. Even during the clinically quiescent stages of infection, substantial viral replication takes place and leads to progressive CD4+ cell destruction. This serves as the rationale for clinical studies examining the risk-benefit ratio of antiviral therapy initiated at the earliest stages of infection, a question that has still not been answered.

The precise biologic mechanisms responsible for the cytopathic effects and immunosuppressive properties of HIV-1 in vivo are unknown. Molecularly cloned HIV-1 proviral DNA, transfected into human cells, has been shown in cell culture experiments to contain all the necessary information to generate infectious and cytopathic virus. Expression of HIV-1 proteins in activated lymphocytes leads to cell cycle arrest in G₂ and cell death within approximately 2 days. HIV-1 alone exerts direct cytopathic activity against CD4+

lymphocytes in vitro and in vivo. Expression of only the HIV-1 envelope on lymphocytes is sufficient to induce fusion of cells with normal uninfected CD4+ bystander cells, thus suggesting that syncytium formation mediated by gp120-CD4 interaction may contribute to cell loss in vivo. Other mechanisms of CD4+ cell loss may also be operative. Cell-free HIV-1 gp120 envelope protein adsorbs to CD4+ cells and may serve as an antigen for mediating antibody-dependent cell-mediated cytotoxicity and, when processed by antigen-presenting cells, be a target for direct T-cell cytotoxicity. In the CNS of infected individuals, in which the predominant cell types infected with HIV-1 are cells of the monocyte-macrophage lineage, additional mechanisms of cellular and organ dysfunction are involved. These mechanisms are believed to include the elaboration of cytotoxic factors from infected cells and interference with neurotropic factors leading to the clinically recognized AIDS dementia complex (Chapter 401).

Despite uncertainties regarding the precise mechanisms of CD4+ lymphocyte destruction and immune dysfunction, the relationship between HIV-1 expression (as reflected by the plasma viral load) and disease outcome is clear. Outcome measures of death or AIDS-defining illness are related to plasma viral load at a set point beginning about 6 months after infection, and effective antiretroviral therapy that reduces viral load improves clinical outcome. It was the introduction of HAART that illuminated the extraordinary dynamics of ongoing viral replication and infected cell turnover in chronic HIV-1 infection that drive HIV-1 pathogenesis and made the case for earlier treatment intervention. Such therapy combined with a kinetic analysis of plasma virus decay curves revealed a lifespan of HIV-1 in plasma of less than 6 hours, a lifespan of activated, virus-producing CD4+ lymphocytes in lymphoreticular tissue of less than 1.2 days, and a virus production rate as high as 10 billion HIV-1 particles per day released into the circulation. Steady-state plasma viral load measurements in patients directly reflect this extraordinary, incessant reiteration of the HIV-1 life cycle: cellular infection, viral production, cell death, de novo infection of cells by newly released virus, and so on. It is not surprising that clinical outcome as measured by time to diagnosis of AIDS or time to death from AIDS is significantly related to the steady-state plasma viral load, although other factors, including activated T-cell levels, are also prognostically important. With the advent of HAART, viral replication in vivo can be all but eliminated for prolonged periods lasting months and years. However, the toxicities of therapy are cumulative, and residual latently infected CD4+ memory T lymphocytes (with a lifespan measured in years) remain an insurmountable obstacle to cure of infection.

Host immune and immunogenetic factors contribute to partial containment of HIV-1 replication in vivo. Neutralizing antibodies, antibody-dependent cell-mediated cytotoxicity, antibody-dependent complement-mediated cytotoxicity, MHC-restricted virus-specific cytotoxic T-lymphocyte-mediated cytotoxicity, and natural killer cell–mediated cytotoxicity all have activity against HIV-1 in vitro and may play a role in the downmodulation of viral replication. The most convincing evidence for a significant role of cytotoxic

T cells in viral containment comes from human studies in which virus escape mutants have been detected and from primate studies in which plasma viral loads increased dramatically after elimination of CD8$^+$ cells by the administration of monoclonal antibody. However, CD8$^+$, or killer, T cells lose their ability to combat HIV-1 infection over time despite their persistence in large numbers in the body of an infected patient. This "T-cell exhaustion" may be due to the enhanced activity of a T-cell receptor protein, programmed death 1 (PD-1), whose ligand (PD-L1) is located on antigen-presenting cells. This interaction diminishes the capacity of these T cells to be activated, most likely reflecting a normal pathway for dampening immune responses to prevent the consequences of uncontrolled cytotoxicity.

Genetic variability is a hallmark of HIV-1. Variability of the HIV-1 genome is characteristic of retroviruses because reverse transcription of viral RNA into proviral DNA and transcription of proviral DNA into genomic viral RNA are not subject to cellular proofreading mechanisms. The rate of nucleotide misincorporation by the viral reverse transcriptase is on the order of 10^{-4} per nucleotide per replication cycle. Because the HIV-1 genome is 10^4 nucleotides long, this high rate of nucleotide misincorporation means that virus strains that infect patients or that are isolated from patients must be described as a "quasispecies" composed of populations of viruses with highly related, but distinct viral genomes. Such variation in the HIV-1 genome leads to viral resistance to reverse transcriptase, protease, and entry inhibitors and to escape from the cellular and humoral arms of the adaptive immune system. Genetic variability can also lead to other biologic changes in the virus over time, including altered cellular tropism. Patients in whom predominant viral strains develop that use the CXCR4 coreceptor, for example, generally have an accelerated decline in CD4$^+$ cell counts and a less favorable clinical prognosis. On a population level, the variability in HIV-1 can be recognized in the phylogenetic relationships among circulating viral strains (Fig. 394-8). HIV-1 viruses are composed of four distinct groups: M, N, O, and P. Group M is responsible for more than 99% of infections worldwide. Groups N, O, and P are largely restricted to west-central Africa. It is believed that HIV-1 groups M, N, O, and P represent separate introductions of virus into the human population from African primates sometime early in the 20th century, most likely as a consequence of direct blood exposure. Group M viruses can be further subdivided by phylogeny into subtypes A through K. Although these phylogenetic distinctions allow molecular epidemiologic tracking of HIV-1 at a population level, there is little evidence to suggest that the various virus groups and subtypes differ in any clinically meaningful manner. All are pathogenic in humans.

HUMAN IMMUNODEFICIENCY VIRUS TYPE 2

After the discovery of HIV-1 as the cause of the global AIDS pandemic, patients in West Africa with AIDS-like symptoms were identified whose serum antibodies reacted not with HIV-1 but with a distantly related lentivirus isolated from captive rhesus macaques in U.S. primate centers and from wild-living sooty mangabey monkeys in West Africa. These latter two simian viruses were found to be genetically indistinguishable, and it thus became apparent that the new West African AIDS-like illness in humans had originated from zoonotic transmission of a virus from sooty mangabey monkeys (SIVsmm). The new human virus was designated HIV-2 to distinguish it from HIV-1. An extensive survey of African primate species for other related lentiviruses then led to the identification of phylogenetically distinct but related lentiviruses in approximately 40 African primate species (see Fig. 394-8).

Though originally restricted geographically to western Africa, HIV-2 has been identified in patients in Europe, the United States, South America, and India. HIV-2 is approximately 40 to 50% similar to HIV-1 in overall nucleotide sequence homology. There are two major differences in the genomic organization of HIV-1 and HIV-2. The *vpu* gene of HIV-1 is not present in HIV-2, and HIV-2 contains an additional gene, *vpx*, in its central region that is not present in HIV-1. Vpx is an 18-kD protein involved in nuclear transport of the HIV-2 preintegration complex in nondividing cells. Antigenically, HIV-2 and HIV-1 are distinct, with the greatest cross-reactivity in structural proteins and the least in envelope proteins. Licensed ELISA tests to detect HIV-1 infection include HIV-2 antigens as well.

Like HIV-1, HIV-2 selectively infects CD4$^+$ cells. Although HIV-2 has the potential to cause profound immunodeficiency and an AIDS syndrome indistinguishable from that caused by HIV-1, evidence suggests that it is less virulent than HIV-1 and causes disease in a smaller fraction of individuals and over a more protracted period. Moreover, transmissibility of HIV-2 is less than that of HIV-1, and as a consequence, the prevalence of HIV-2 is declining.

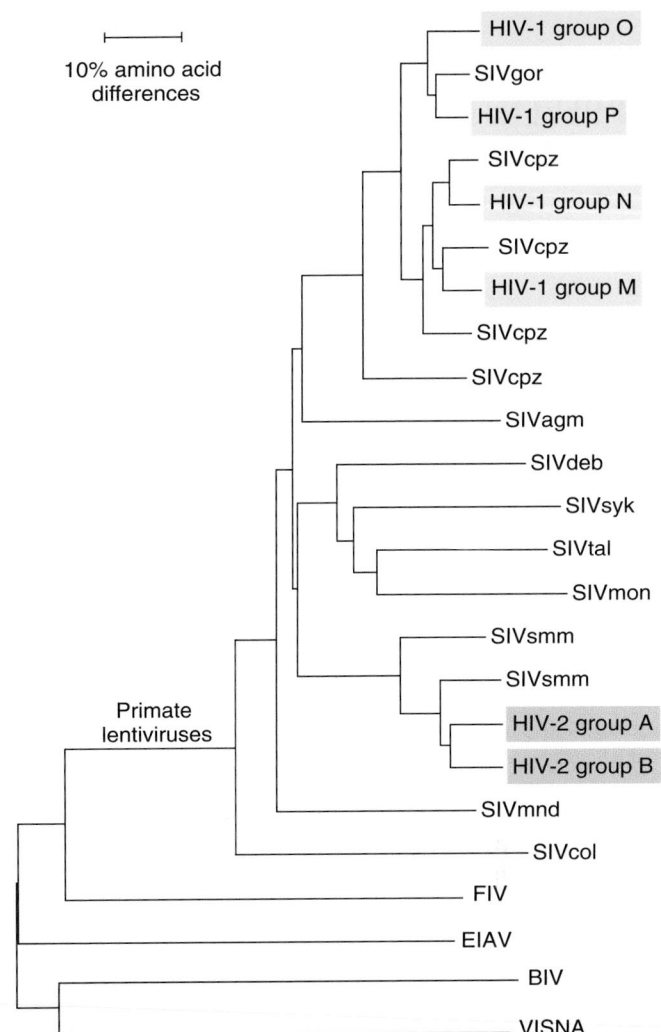

10% amino acid differences

Primate lentiviruses

HIV-1 group O
SIVgor
HIV-1 group P
SIVcpz
HIV-1 group N
SIVcpz
HIV-1 group M
SIVcpz
SIVcpz
SIVagm
SIVdeb
SIVsyk
SIVtal
SIVmon
SIVsmm
SIVsmm
HIV-2 group A
HIV-2 group B
SIVmnd
SIVcol
FIV
EIAV
BIV
VISNA

FIGURE 394-8. Phylogenetic relationships among HIV-1, HIV-2, and other lentiviruses inferred from pol protein sequences. Sequences from the HIV-1 pandemic group M ("main" group) and the less widely distributed HIV-1 group N cluster with chimpanzee viruses SIVcpz. HIV-1 groups O and P cluster with gorilla viruses SIVgor. HIV-2 groups A and B cluster with sooty mangabey viruses SIVsmm. More divergent primate lentiviruses (SIVagm = African green monkey; SIVdeb = De Brazza's monkey; SIVsyk = Sykes monkey; SIVtal = Talapoin monkey; SIVmon = Mona monkey; SIVmnd = Mandrill monkey; SIVcol = Colobus monkey) and lower vertebrate lentiviruses (FIV = feline immunodeficiency virus; EIAV = equine infectious anemia virus; BIV = bovine immunodeficiency virus; VISNA = visna virus from sheep) are also represented. Horizontal branch lengths are drawn to scale and can be used to infer the percent difference in pol protein sequences between the different viral lineages.

The discovery of two distinct types of human immunodeficiency viruses (HIV-1 and HIV-2) having closely related counterparts in African primates (SIVcpz in chimpanzees and SIVsmm in sooty mangabeys) suggested a cross-species (zoonotic) origin for HIV-1 and HIV-2. This conclusion has been confirmed by molecular epidemiologic studies that have unequivocally identified the chimpanzee subspecies *Pan troglodytes troglodytes* in west-central Africa as the source of the HIV-1 pandemic (HIV-1 group M) and the sooty mangabey (*Cercocebus atys*) in western Africa as the source of HIV-2. A recent intriguing finding is that the closest relatives to HIV-1 groups O and P are viruses that naturally infect gorillas, thus raising the possibility that this second great ape species represents a natural reservoir for HIV-1.

SUGGESTED READINGS

Coiras N, Lopez-Huertas, Perez-Olmeda M, et al. Understanding HIV-1 latency provides clues for the eradication of long-term reservoirs. *Nat Rev Microbiol.* 2009;7:798-812. *Review of the molecular mechanisms involved in establishment of HIV-1 latency, cellular reservoirs, and future perspectives on targeting viral persistence.*

Haase AT. Targeting early infection to prevent HIV-1 mucosal transmission. *Nature.* 2010;464:217-223. *Potential viral vulnerabilities at the mucosal portal of entry in the earliest stages of infection.*

International HIV Controllers Study. The major genetic determinants of HIV-1 control affect HLA class I peptide presentation. *Science.* 2010;330:1551-1557. *Review of polymorphisms that increase or reduce the likelihood of durable control of HIV infection.*

McMichael AJ, Borrow P, Tomaras GD, et al. The immune response during acute HIV-1 infection: clues for vaccine development. *Nat Rev Immunol.* 2010;10:11-23. *Review of the early host and viral factors that determine the outcome of HIV infection.*

395

PREVENTION OF HUMAN IMMUNODEFICIENCY VIRUS INFECTION

CARLOS DEL RIO

Prevention of infection with human immunodeficiency virus (HIV) requires a thorough understanding of the epidemiology of HIV infection and knowledge of the science of human behavior. Only then can science-based prevention strategies be designed and implemented. HIV has been identified in virtually every body fluid and tissue, including blood, semen, vaginal secretions, saliva, tears, breast milk, cerebrospinal fluid, amniotic fluid, urine, and fluid obtained from bronchoalveolar lavage. In most instances, the virus resides in lymphocytes present within body fluids; therefore, any fluid that contains lymphocytes could theoretically be implicated in spread of the virus. Nonetheless, HIV transmission occurs primarily through exposure to blood, semen, vaginal secretions, and breast milk. HIV has also been transmitted through transplanted organs, including kidney, liver, heart, pancreas, and bone.

The advent of antiretroviral therapy has resulted in new challenges in the field of HIV prevention, and concern about reports of an upsurge in sexually transmitted infections in people known to be infected with HIV has resulted in guidelines for the incorporation of HIV prevention into the medical care of HIV-infected persons.

● MODES OF HIV TRANSMISSION AND PREVENTION

Sexual Transmission

The primary mode of HIV transmission throughout the world is sexual contact. However, the geographic distribution of cases attributable to homosexual or heterosexual transmission varies markedly. In the United States, most sexually transmitted cases reported have occurred through male homosexual activity, and heterosexual transmission accounts for a smaller, albeit growing proportion of cases. In contrast, heterosexual transmission is the leading mode of transmission worldwide and is the primary mode of disease acquisition in Africa. Like other sexually transmitted diseases (STDs) (Chapter 293), HIV spreads bidirectionally and appears to be more efficiently transmitted from male to female. Sexual transmission of HIV is relatively inefficient, but behavioral and biologic factors influence the likelihood of HIV transmission in a given sexual encounter. In particular, the coexistence of an STD (most notably the presence of genital ulcerative disease) greatly increases the infectiousness as well as the susceptibility of the individual. In a study conducted in Rakai, Uganda, there were no cases of transmission between heterosexual serodiscordant couples when the infected partner had a serum HIV RNA level of less than 1500 copies/mL. The risk for acquisition of HIV per coital act has been estimated to be 5 per 10,000 for insertive unprotected penile-vaginal intercourse to 50 per 10,000 for receptive unprotected anal intercourse. However, the risk is not stable and varies depending on the stage of infection. It is highest in early HIV infection and in advanced infection, thus suggesting that the HIV viral load of the index partner is the strongest predictor of the risk for transmission, with risk being greater when the viral load is higher.

Prevention

Abstinence is the only absolute way of preventing sexual acquisition of HIV infection. Persons who have been engaged in a mutually monogamous relationship since the mid-1970s are at extremely low risk of acquiring disease; however, assurance that both partners have remained "faithful" is sometimes difficult to confirm. Strategies for the prevention of sexual transmission of HIV have focused on reducing unsafe sexual behavior, encouraging condom use, and treating STDs.

In situations in which a decision to engage in sexual activity has been made and the HIV status of the partner is positive, unknown, or in doubt, safe sexual practices ("safe sex") should be implemented (Table 395-1). Mutual masturbation is considered "safe," assuming that it is nontraumatic and not followed by the ingestion of body fluids such as semen or vaginal secretions.

TABLE 395-1	SAFE AND UNSAFE SEXUAL PRACTICES IN ORDER OF "SURENESS" OF SAFETY
SAFE	
Abstinence	
Monogamous relationship with a confirmed seronegative partner	
Manual sex (manual masturbation)	
Kissing	
Intercourse with a latex condom	
UNSAFE	
Intercourse with a "natural skin" condom	
Intercourse with a latex condom lubricated with petroleum-based products	
Unprotected oral-genital sex	
Unprotected vaginal intercourse	
Unprotected anal intercourse	

The probability of HIV transmission through saliva during oral-oral and oral-genital contact is extremely low but not zero. Condom use is the most effective means of preventing HIV infection in individuals who engage in oral, vaginal, or anal intercourse. Consistent use of latex condoms has been shown to be effective in preventing of HIV transmission at both an individual and population level. Multiple epidemiologic studies of heterosexual couples in which one partner is HIV positive and the other is HIV negative indicate that correct and consistent use of condoms can significantly reduce transmission of HIV and other STDs.

To be effective, however, the condom should be made of latex and must be used properly. Natural skin condoms should not be used because they do not prevent transmission of HIV. Petroleum-based lubricants enhance the likelihood of rupture of latex condoms and should be avoided. If needed, water-based lubricants such as K-Y jelly should be used.

Both partners should be knowledgeable about the correct use of condoms. Discussions regarding condom use should occur before the need arises, and ideally, condom placement should be practiced in advance. A new condom should be used for each act of intercourse, and each condom should be used only one time. The effectiveness of condoms in preventing heterosexual transmission of HIV has been estimated to be 87%, but it may be as low as 60% or as high as 96%. Many factors can affect the effectiveness of condoms in reducing the risk for transmission of HIV, such as condom breakage, leakage, and slippage. The effectiveness of condoms during anal intercourse is probably lower because the frequency of condom breakage and slippage may be considerably higher than during vaginal intercourse. Thus, although condom use during intercourse is considered "safer" sex, it is not absolutely safe.

Three randomized clinical trials have demonstrated a protective benefit of male circumcision, with the risk for acquisition of HIV infection through heterosexual intercourse decreasing by approximately 60%.[1-3] This benefit has not been confirmed for men who have sex with men.

Antiretroviral therapy may influence infectivity and the subsequent risk for transmission through sexual contact. Emerging data seem to suggest that the risk for transmission of HIV from a patient receiving highly active antiretroviral therapy (HAART) with a viral load below the limit of detection of the current assays (<50 copies/mL) is exceedingly low. However, even in the presence of suppression of HIV RNA in plasma, proviral DNA has been detected in the seminal cells of infected men and genital secretions of women. Thus, any protective effect of antiretrovirals on sexual transmission of HIV is not absolute, and current antiretroviral therapy does not render an individual completely noninfectious. Ongoing studies are also looking at the prospect of using antiretrovirals for prevention of HIV when administered prophylactically to HIV-uninfected, but at-risk individuals (pre-exposure prophylaxis). In a randomized trial, daily administration of co-formulated tenofovir plus emtricitabine to men who have sex with men decreased the risk of HIV infection by 44%.[4] Similarly, a tenofovir-containing vaginal gel led to a 39% reduction in the risk of HIV infection among women.[5] In addition, antiretrovirals can be given after exposure to prevent HIV acquisition (postexposure prophylaxis). In 2005 the Centers for Disease Control and Prevention (CDC) published guidelines for antiretroviral postexposure prophylaxis after sexual, injection drug use, and other nonoccupational exposures to HIV (see Suggested Readings). In these guidelines it is recommended that persons seeking care 72 hours or sooner after nonoccupational exposure to the blood, genital secretions, or other potentially infected body fluids of a person known to have HIV infection be offered a 28-day course of antiretroviral therapy. In contrast, acyclovir was not shown to be effective for the prevention of HIV transmission.[6]

HIV Transmission in Intravenous Drug Users

The primary mode of HIV transmission in intravenous drug users (IVDUs) is sharing of contaminated needles and syringes. Sharing of injection paraphernalia ("works") is commonplace among IVDUs and is reinforced by the cultural, economic, and legal environment in the IVDU community. The risk for transmission of HIV is highest in IVDUs who share needles and use drugs that are injected more often, such as cocaine. HIV is frequently transmitted from IVDUs to their sexual partners through heterosexual and homosexual activity, and ultimately, the virus may be transmitted to their children through perinatal exposure. Many cases of heterosexual transmission, including transmission from prostitutes, are associated with intravenous drug use.

Prevention

The primary mode of preventing HIV transmission in IVDUs is to stop the use of intravenous drugs in the first place. Education programs that are culturally sensitive and geared to young audiences have the best chance of preventing drug use. Access to treatment centers is the best approach for individuals already using intravenous drugs. However, approximately 80% of active drug users in the United States are not in substance abuse treatment because of either choice or the unavailability of treatment centers. For IVDUs who do not wish to seek treatment or who are unable to gain access to treatment, the most effective way to prevent HIV infection is to avoid sharing needles and works. Where works are in short supply, needles and syringes should be cleaned after each use, preferably with readily accessible virucidal cleansers such as chlorine bleach (diluted 1:10). Some communities have adopted programs that provide free needles and syringes for IVDUs, and there is strong evidence that these programs, when implemented properly, are effective in reducing HIV transmission and do not result in increased drug use among participants. As with sexual transmission, preliminary data from Vancouver, Canada, suggest that voluntary HIV testing followed by antiretroviral therapy may decrease transmission of HIV among drug users. The efficacy of many community programs is limited, however, by cultural barriers, including lack of trust, fear of prosecution, misconceptions regarding the prevalence of HIV infection within the local drug-using population, and the use of ineffective language in delivering anti-HIV messages by program staff. When combined with the relative paucity of intravenous drug treatment resources, HIV education among IVDUs that ultimately results in behavioral changes remains a challenging HIV prevention goal.

Transmission of HIV through Blood Products and Other Tissues

HIV has been transmitted through the transfusion of single-donor blood and blood products, including whole blood, fresh-frozen plasma, packed red blood cells, cryoprecipitate, clotting factors, and platelets. Confidential donor exclusion, as well as the institution of HIV antibody screening in 1985, followed by additional testing for antibodies to HIV-2 and p24 antigen in 1996 and nucleic acid testing in 2002, has reduced the risk for HIV infection through the transfusion of blood or blood products to approximately 1 in 2,135,000.

Transmission of HIV by liver, heart, kidney, pancreas, bone, and possibly skin transplantation has been reported. In contrast, relatively avascular tissues such as corneas and processed tissues have not been associated with transmission.

Prevention

The institution of HIV antibody testing of donated blood and blood products in 1985 has had the most dramatic effect on lowering the incidence of transfusion-related transmission. When combined with voluntary self-deferral and nucleic acid testing, the blood supply has become relatively free of HIV. The effectiveness of self-deferral is limited, however, by social pressures. Self-deferral programs are most effective when free, voluntary testing centers are readily available elsewhere in the community and when blood drives encourage potential donors to come to donation centers by themselves and not in groups. Heat inactivation processes for cryoprecipitate and clotting factor concentrates have virtually eliminated transmission of HIV through use of these products. Other products, such as immune globulin preparations and hepatitis B vaccines, are produced by methods that inactivate HIV and have never been associated with transmission of HIV.

Organ and tissue donors should be evaluated and serologically screened in a manner similar to blood donors. In addition, donations of semen and

TABLE 395-2	SUMMARY OF UNIVERSAL PRECAUTIONS

Specimens, including blood, blood products, and body fluids, obtained from all patients should be considered hazardous and potentially infected with transmissible agents.

Handwashing should be performed before and after patient contact, after removing gloves, and immediately if hands are grossly contaminated with blood.

Gloves should be worn when hands are likely to come in contact with blood or body fluids.

Gowns, protective eyewear, and masks should be worn when splashing, splattering, or aerosolization of blood or body fluids is likely to occur.

Sharp objects ("sharps") should be handled with great care and disposed of in impervious receptacles.

Needles should never be manipulated, bent, broken, or recapped.

Blood spills should be handled by initial absorption of the spill with disposable towels, cleaning the area with soap and water, followed by disinfecting the area with a 1:10 solution of household bleach.

Contaminated reusable equipment should be decontaminated by heat sterilization or, when heat is impractical, with a mycobactericidal cleanser.

Pocket masks or mechanical ventilation devices should be available in areas where cardiopulmonary resuscitation procedures are likely.

Health care workers with open lesions or weeping dermatitis should avoid direct patient contact and should not handle contaminated equipment.

Private rooms are not required for routine care; select circumstances, however, such as the presence of a concomitant transmissible opportunistic disease, may warrant respiratory, enteric, or contact isolation.

bone from a living donor may be quarantined until subsequent testing has definitively ruled out the possibility of delayed seroconversion in the donor.

Transmission of HIV to Health Care Workers

Transmission of HIV in the health care delivery setting has been the subject of intense investigation throughout the course of the epidemic. The percentage of health care workers with AIDS who have "no identified risk" for HIV infection has remained low (<10%) and has not increased over time despite the dramatic increase in the number of AIDS cases and concomitant exposure of health care workers to patients with HIV disease. More importantly, detailed studies examining the risk associated with specific exposures, such as needlestick injuries and mucous membrane exposure, have demonstrated very low risk for acquisition of disease in the workplace. More than 3628 health care workers have been prospectively examined in carefully designed surveillance studies at 10 high-incidence medical centers. The overall risk for seroconversion after a percutaneous needlestick from a known HIV-positive source is 0.3% per exposure. A retrospective study conducted by the CDC found that the risk for transmission of HIV to health care workers is increased when the device causing the injury is visibly contaminated with blood, when the device has been used for insertion into a vein or artery, when the device causes a deep injury, or when the source patient dies within 2 months after the exposure. Although exposure of mucous membranes to HIV-positive blood has resulted in seroconversion in at least five health care workers, the risk for transmission is estimated to be 0.09%. No transmission has occurred after exposure to body fluids other than blood or fluids heavily contaminated with blood. Although the potential for HIV transmission to health care providers clearly exists, the risk for infection is inherently low and can be further minimized by following routine precautions to prevent transmission.

Prevention

In August 1987, the CDC published guidelines recommending that the principles of "universal precautions" be incorporated into health care settings to minimize exposure of health care workers to blood and body fluids that may be infected with blood-borne pathogens such as HIV. The guidelines, updated in June 2001 and in September 2005 (available at *http://www. aidsinfo.nih.gov/guidelines/*), remain the principal mode of HIV prevention among health care workers today. "Universal precautions" are based on the premise that any patient may be infected with blood-borne infectious agents and it may be difficult, if not impossible, to differentiate those with infection from their uninfected counterparts. All specimens containing blood or blood-tinged fluids obtained from *any* patient should be considered hazardous and handled as such (Table 395-2). The use of universal precautions helps minimize the transmission of many transmissible diseases in addition to HIV.

Handwashing is the cornerstone of universal precautions, as it is with all infection control practices. Gloves should be worn when spillage of blood or body fluids is likely. Gloves should *never* be washed and should be changed

TABLE 395-3 CDC RECOMMENDATIONS FOR POSTEXPOSURE PROPHYLAXIS (PEP) FOR PERCUTANEOUS AND MUCOUS MEMBRANE EXPOSURE TO HIV

EXPOSURE TYPE	HIV POSITIVE, CLASS 1*	HIV POSITIVE, CLASS 2†	HIV STATUS OR SOURCE UNKNOWN	HIV NEGATIVE
Percutaneous exposure: less severe (e.g., solid needlestick)	Recommend basic 2-drug PEP‡	Recommend expanded ≥3-drug PEP	No PEP, but should consider 2-drug PEP if source has risk factors for HIV	No PEP
Percutaneous exposure: more severe (e.g., large-bore hollow needlestick)	Recommend expanded 3-drug PEP‡	Recommend expanded ≥3-drug PEP	No PEP, but should consider 2-drug PEP if source has risk factors for HIV	No PEP
Mucous membrane exposure: small volume (e.g., few droplets)§	Consider basic 2-drug PEP	Recommend basic 2-drug PEP	Generally no PEP warranted	No PEP
Mucous membrane exposure: large volume (e.g., major blood splash or prolonged contact)	Recommend basic 2-drug PEP	Recommend expanded ≥3-drug PEP	Generally no PEP warranted, but should consider 2-drug PEP if source has risk factors for HIV	No PEP

*Asymptomatic patient with HIV infection, low viral load (<1500 copies/mL). If drug resistance is suspected, obtain expert consultation regarding the choice of antiretroviral regimen. PEP should not be delayed while awaiting consultation.
†Symptomatic patient with HIV, high viral load (>1500 copies/mL), AIDS, or acute seroconversion syndrome.
‡Basic PEP refers to dual-nucleoside therapy (e.g., zidovudine plus lamivudine); expanded PEP includes dual nucleosides combined with a potent protease inhibitor (such as lopinavir-ritonavir). PEP should be discontinued if the source patient is later determined to be HIV negative.
§Body fluids considered to be potentially infectious include blood, blood products, cerebrospinal fluid, amniotic fluid, menstrual discharge, inflammatory exudates, pleural fluid, peritoneal fluid, pericardial fluid, and any fluid visibly contaminated with blood. All other fluids are considered noninfectious.
Consider PEP indicates that PEP is optional and should be individualized for each situation based on the nature of the exposure and the opinion of the exposed health care worker and the treating clinician.
Adapted from Henderson D, Gerberding J. Occupational and nonoccupational exposure management. In: Dolin R, Masur H, Saag M, eds. *AIDS Therapy*, 2nd ed. New York, NY: Churchill-Livingstone; 2003:327-346; and Panlilio AL, Cardo DM, Grohskopf LA, et al. Updated U.S. Public Health Service guidelines for the management of occupational exposures to HIV and recommendations for postexposure prophylaxis. *MMWR Recomm Rep.* 2005;54(RR-9):1-17.

after soiling or after gross contamination, with handwashing immediately after the gloves are removed. Handwashing may be performed with soap and water or with the use of commercially available alcohol-based cleansing gels. Gowns, protective eyewear, and masks are not usually needed except in circumstances in which splattering or splashing of blood-containing fluids is likely to occur. Masks should always be worn in situations in which eyewear is required. Reusable equipment should be cleaned of visible organic material, placed in an impervious bag, and returned to central supply for decontamination. Although heat is the single best decontamination method, chemical agents that possess mycobactericidal activity are effective against hepatitis B virus and HIV and are acceptable alternatives when heat inactivation is impractical. Blood spills should be cleaned with appropriate caution. After putting on gloves and using other appropriate barrier precautions, excess blood should be removed with absorbent material (e.g., paper towels) and the area then cleaned with soap and water and disinfected with a 1:10 solution of sodium hypochlorite (i.e., household bleach) and water. Health care workers with denuded skin, open lesions, or active dermatitis should avoid direct patient contact and should not process contaminated equipment or materials. Private rooms are not generally required for patients known to be infected with HIV unless a concomitant opportunistic disease is present that requires respiratory, enteric, or contact isolation. Food service should be provided as usual on reusable dishware.

Because *all* blood and body fluids should be handled as though potentially hazardous and *all* patients presumed to be infected, it makes little sense to identify infected patients or their specimens with "blood and body fluid" labels. The use of such labels on known infected patients implies that unlabeled specimens or specimens from patients of unknown status are less hazardous and may be handled with less care. Studies have shown that more than half of specimens containing antibodies to hepatitis B surface antigen or HIV went to the laboratory unlabeled.

Handling of sharp instruments ("sharps") represents the greatest risk for transmission of HIV to health care workers. Although injuries from sharps cannot be eliminated entirely, the number of exposures can be reduced substantially by adhering to guidelines put forth in universal precautions. Before a sharp instrument is used, thought should be given to where the instrument will be disposed after use. Impervious containers should be readily available in all patient care areas and identified by the health care worker *before* the use of sharps. These containers should be checked frequently and should not be allowed to overfill. Used needles should never be manipulated, bent, broken, or recapped. Recapping of needles is the single most common activity that results in needlestick injuries. Technologic developments that do not rely on health care worker compliance such as self-sheathing needles have also been important in decreasing the risk for needlestick injury.

Even in the best of circumstances, accidental mucous membrane and percutaneous exposure to blood from HIV-infected patients does occur. Each institution and health care facility should adopt procedures for managing such exposure based on guidelines published by the CDC (see Suggested

Readings). The essential elements of management after needlestick or mucous membrane exposure include defining the type of exposure, appropriately evaluating the donor (patient) and recipient (health care worker) at the time of exposure, and providing follow-up of the health care worker for at least 1 year after exposure.

Proposed definitions of the types of exposure are summarized in Table 395-3. Health care workers with any type of parenteral exposure should be counseled and evaluated for possible acquisition of HIV and should receive routine prophylaxis against hepatitis B virus. The source patient (donor) should be evaluated for HIV infection; if the donor's HIV status is unknown, the donor should be informed about the incident and encouraged to allow voluntary, confidential screening of blood for HIV and hepatitis B antibody. If a patient refuses or cannot give consent, that patient should be considered to be infected. In cases in which exposure to HIV is documented or presumed to have occurred, the health care worker should be evaluated serologically for the presence of HIV as soon as possible after the exposure (baseline) and again at 6 weeks, 12 weeks, 24 weeks, and 1 year after the exposure to determine whether transmission of HIV has occurred. The health care worker should report any acute illnesses that occur during the follow-up period, especially during the first 6 to 12 weeks after exposure. Exposed workers should follow the recommended guidelines for preventing HIV transmission, including using safe sexual practices; refraining from blood, semen, and organ donation; and avoiding breast-feeding. If the source patient is seronegative for HIV and has no clinical manifestations of HIV disease, no further follow-up of the exposed health care workers is necessary, although some workers prefer follow-up for their own peace of mind. Serologic testing should be made available to all health care workers who are concerned about potential on-the-job exposure.

For occupational exposure to HIV among health care workers, the CDC recommended the use of zidovudine for postexposure prophylaxis in 1990. This recommendation was further supported by a case-control study in which it was shown that the risk for HIV seroconversion after occupational exposure was decreased by approximately 81% with the use of zidovudine. Subsequent recommendations have incorporated the newer antiretroviral drugs, as well as risk stratification for the type of exposure, in the management of occupational exposure to HIV. The current CDC recommendations are different, depending on the type of exposure and the clinical status of the source patient. For less severe exposures (e.g., a solid needle or a superficial injury), two nucleosides/nucleotides are recommended (e.g., tenofovir and emtricitabine). For more severe exposures (e.g., large-bore hollow needle, deep puncture, visible blood in the device, or a needle used in a patient's artery or vein), a regimen that includes three antiretrovirals is recommended (e.g., zidovudine, lamivudine. and lopinavir/ritonavir). Postexposure prophylaxis should be initiated as soon as possible, preferably within hours of exposure, and administered for 4 weeks.

The U.S. Public Health Service has established a National Clinicians' Post-Exposure Prophylaxis Hotline (PEPline) to provide expert consultation about the management of health care workers with potential HIV exposure. The PEPline can be accessed at 1-888-448-4911 or through the Internet at *http://www.ucsf.edu/hivcntr/Hotlines/PEPline*.

Transmission from Infected Health Care Workers to Their Patients

Transmission of HIV from a health care worker to patients has been documented in two instances: in a dental practice in Florida and from an orthopedic surgeon in France. The Florida cluster of cases was reported in July 1990. Six patients are believed to have acquired infection from the dentist based on the absence of other risk factors in the patients and the high degree of homology between the virus isolated from the dentist and those isolated from the patients. Although each patient underwent an invasive procedure in the dental office, the precise mode of transmission remains unknown. Aside from these two instances, investigation of 22,759 patients treated by 53 other HIV-infected health care workers has not identified other episodes of transmission of HIV from health care worker to patient.

PREVENTION INTERVENTIONS FOR HIV-POSITIVE INDIVIDUALS

Increases in high-risk sex practices and STDs among HIV-infected individuals have prompted considerable concern over increased risk for transmission of HIV infection and have led to initiatives to increase STD screening and risk reduction measures in the HIV-infected population. The available evidence indicates that risk reduction counseling is effective, and improved attention to risk reduction counseling in the HIV medical care setting is needed. CDC 2006 STD treatment guidelines recommend that all patients with newly diagnosed HIV infection undergo screening for gonorrhea, chlamydial infection, hepatitis B and C virus infection, and syphilis. Screening for curable STDs (gonorrhea, chlamydial infection, and syphilis) should be performed at least annually in sexually active patients. The CDC, Health Resources and Services Administration, National Institutes of Health, and Infectious Diseases Society of America have also published joint recommendations for incorporating HIV prevention into the HIV medical care setting. These guidelines reflect four basic priorities: (1) screening for risky behavior and STDs, (2) providing general and tailored risk reduction messages to patients, (3) when indicated, referring patients for additional risk reduction services and other services that may affect risk reduction (e.g., substance abuse treatment), and (4) ensuring that patients are provided with partner counseling and referral services.

VACCINE DEVELOPMENT

Education and modification of behavior are the only means of preventing transmission of HIV currently available. During the past years, significant effort has been directed toward the development of an effective vaccine against HIV. Although substantial progress has been achieved, several obstacles remain. Despite enormous advances in understanding the immunopathogenesis of HIV infection, the precise mechanism of protective immunity remains unknown. Without such knowledge, it is difficult to develop vaccines that ensure targeting the appropriate arm of the immune system that confers long-term protective immunity. Another obstacle is the lack of correlation of data from animal models to the potential protective effects of vaccines in humans. Although vaccine research has been continuing for many years, the results from phase IIB and phase III clinical trials have thus far been disappointing, and it was only recently that the results of a phase III efficacy trial showed a modest 30% protection. Over the next few years new trials with novel candidate HIV vaccines will be taking place around the world.

1. Auvert B, Taljaard D, Lagarde E, et al. Randomized, controlled intervention trial of male circumcision for reduction of HIV infection risk: the ANRS 1265 trial. *PLoS Med.* 2005;2:1-11.
2. Bailey RC, Moses S, Parker CB, et al. Male circumcision for HIV prevention in young men in Kisumu, Kenya: a randomized controlled trial. *Lancet.* 2007;369:643-656.
3. Gray RH, Kigozi G, Serwadda D, et al. Male circumcision for HIV prevention in men in Rakai, Uganda: a randomised trial. *Lancet.* 2007;369:657-666.
4. Grant RM, Lama JR, Anderson PL, et al. Preexposure chemoprophylaxis for HIV prevention in men who have sex with men. *N Engl J Med.* 2010;363:2587-2599.
5. Abdool Karim Q, Abdool Karim SS, Frohlich JA, et al. Effectiveness and safety of tenofovir gel, an antiretroviral microbicide, for the prevention of HIV infection in women. *Science.* 2010;329:1168-1174.
6. Celum C, Wald A, Lingappa JR, et al. Acyclovir and transmission of HIV-1 from persons infected with HIV-1 and HSV-2. *N Engl J Med.* 2010;362:427-439.

SUGGESTED READINGS

Centers for Disease Control and Prevention (CDC). Interim guidance: preexposure prophylaxis for the prevention of HIV infection in men who have sex with men. *MMWR Morb Mortal Wkly Rep.* 2011;60:65-68. *Review of the potential benefits.*

Dieffenbach CW, Fauci AS. Universal voluntary testing and treatment for prevention of HIV transmission. *JAMA.* 2009;301:2380-2382. *Important editorial that suggests as a prevention strategy the expansion of testing and treatment of all HIV-infected individuals.*

Doherty T, Sanders D, Goga A, et al. Implications of the new WHO guidelines on HIV and infant feeding for child survival in South Africa. *Bull World Health Organ.* 2011;89:62-67. *Review of guidelines and "call to action" for the implementation of national or subnational programs.*

Donnell D, Baeten JM, Kiarie J, et al. Heterosexual HIV-1 transmission after initiation of antiretroviral therapy: a prospective cohort analysis. *Lancet.* 2010;375:2092-2098. *Provision of ART to HIV-1 infected patients can be effective for reducing population-wide HIV-1 transmission.*

Long EF, Brandeau ML, Owens DK. The cost-effectiveness and population outcomes of expanded HIV screening and antiretroviral treatment in the United States. *Ann Intern Med.* 2010;153:778-789. *Expanding HIV screening and treatment is cost effective but not sufficient by itself to markedly reduce the U.S. HIV epidemic.*

Pirrone V, Thakkar-Rivera N, Jacobson JM, et al. Combinatorial approaches to the prevention and treatment of HIV-1 infection. *Antimicrob Agents Chemother.* 2011;55:1831-1842. *Review.*

396

TREATMENT OF HUMAN IMMUNODEFICIENCY VIRUS INFECTION AND ACQUIRED IMMUNODEFICIENCY SYNDROME

HENRY MASUR, LETHA HEALEY, AND COLLEEN HADIGAN

When the first cases of acquired immunodeficiency syndrome (AIDS) were recognized in the United States in the late 1970s, strategies for management of the patient focused on prompt diagnosis and treatment of opportunistic infections. Clinicians recognized that this strategy improved survival only modestly, but until the causative virus was discovered and antiretroviral drugs were developed, this was the best that could be accomplished. In that era, the median time to death after the first AIDS-defining opportunistic process was about 9 months, and very few patients survived more than 2 years after their initial opportunistic disease.

By the mid-1980s, clinicians began to recognize that chemoprophylaxis against the most common and severe opportunistic infections could be beneficial. Trimethoprim-sulfamethoxazole (TMP-SMX) to prevent *Pneumocystis jirovecii* pneumonia (PCP) and toxoplasmosis and rifabutin or clarithromycin or azithromycin to prevent *Mycobacterium avium* complex disease became the standard of care and provided a modest benefit in terms of prolonged AIDS-free survival.

With the licensing of zidovudine in 1987, treatment of the underlying retroviral cause of immunosuppression became possible for the first time. Monotherapy with nucleosides (zidovudine, didanosine, zalcitabine, stavudine, and lamivudine) in that era slowed the immunologic decline caused by human immunodeficiency virus (HIV), reduced the number of HIV-related opportunistic infections, and prolonged survival by months or a few years. The development of more potent antiretroviral agents in the mid-1990s and the opportunity to use drug combinations of agents with different mechanisms of action led to regimens that provided more potent and durable virologic and immunologic effects and better clinical benefit. These regimens were a major advance in the management of patients infected with HIV who had access to medical care and who were capable of taking and willing to take these drugs.

The development of multiple categories of antiretroviral drugs is one of the most gratifying testaments to the ability of biomedical science to recognize a new syndrome, to identify the novel causative agent, to develop active antiretroviral drugs, and to carry out rapidly clinical trials that demonstrated the benefits and toxicities of these new drug regimens. The evolution of this therapy also demonstrated how difficult it is to operationalize therapy in the developed or the developing world and underlined the importance of collaboration among basic science, clinical medicine, and social science if benefit is to be delivered to the full range of infected persons.

Whereas some current combination antiretroviral therapies are available as single pills or as convenient once-daily or twice-daily regimens, taking these drugs has been no small challenge for patients in every social and economic stratum. For many patients who can tolerate and adhere to these regimens, the quality and duration of survival have improved dramatically. However, both patients and clinicians must recognize that all regimens have some adverse effects. As these drugs are evaluated in larger and larger populations, in diverse groups of patients, and during increasing periods, those toxicities are becoming better defined. Although some of these toxicities can be mitigated by screening for predisposing viral or host phenotypes or genotypes, toxicities can still be treatment limiting and occasionally fatal.

As patients who have access to care and who can adhere to treatment regimens have survived longer with potent, combination antiretroviral regimens, causes of morbidity and mortality have evolved. Liver, kidney, cardiovascular, and metabolic diseases have become more prominent causes of morbidity and mortality compared with AIDS-defining opportunistic infections and malignant neoplasms. Current evidence suggests that chronic inflammation, induced by persistent HIV replication, plays an important role in producing this end-organ damage, suggesting that the concept of "HIV-associated" processes needs to be reconsidered.

Guidelines from various professional societies around the world review current data and make recommendations.[1,2] When prospective, randomized, adequately powered clinical trials have been performed, recommendations can be made with more certainty than when data are derived from nonrandomized cohort studies or from other observational databases. Recommendations have evolved during the past 20 years as more drugs have been developed and as more studies have been published. For some populations, such as those with CD4 counts below 200 cells/mm^3, there is consensus that treatment is indicated because all clinical trials have supported such intervention. For patients with CD4 counts above 200 cells/mm^3, there is more debate because prospective randomized trials either have not been done or are not as convincing.[3]

A plausible argument can be made for starting antiretroviral therapy when HIV infection is first recognized, regardless of how high CD4$^+$ T-lymphocyte cell counts are, and continuing therapy for life,[3,4] even in developing countries.[5] Such an approach has the potential to provide clinical benefit to the individual patient, to reduce sexual transmission to HIV-uninfected partners, and to have long-term economic benefit. Proponents of this approach consider the benefits of early intervention to outweigh the known and as yet unknown toxicities of long-term antiretroviral therapy. A plausible argument can also be made that given this lack of knowledge of the long-term consequences of chronic antiretroviral therapy and uncertainty about the benefits at CD4$^+$ T-lymphocyte counts above 350 cells/mm^3, drug regimens should not be started until patients reach a CD4$^+$ T-lymphocyte cell threshold at which therapeutic intervention is documented by randomized prospective studies to be associated with improved survival and tolerable toxicity.

Until there are randomized, prospective trials assessing the long-term benefits of early versus late therapy for patients with CD4$^+$ T-lymphocyte cell counts above 350 cells/mm^3 and for patients with CD4$^+$ T-lymphocyte counts above 500 cells/mm^3, uncertainty about the best strategies will continue because published observational cohort studies are not as scientifically convincing as randomized prospective trials.

In 2011, there are more than two dozen licensed antiretroviral agents in six mechanistic categories. The challenge for clinicians and public health authorities in the developed and developing world is to define the best strategies to optimize clinical outcome in each geographic area and to determine how best to operationalize those strategies given the resources that are available.

Treatment of HIV and AIDS can be organized into four major areas: antiretroviral therapy, prophylaxis for opportunistic infections, treatment of HIV-related infections, and management of noninfectious complications related to HIV infection or antiretroviral therapy. These treatments need to be used with the goal of minimizing or preventing HIV-related complications and producing as little disruption as possible in the patient's lifestyle. With currently available therapies, patients with access to care who can adhere to recommended regimens can live for longer and longer times with very low risk for HIV-related complications.

● ANTIRETROVIRAL THERAPY

Clinicians and patients must be clear about the goals of antiretroviral therapy. Current therapies cannot eradicate the virus because pools of latently infected CD4$^+$ T-lymphocyte cells are established soon after acute infection and have a long half-life. When HIV-infected patients have stopped antiretroviral therapy, even after many years of combination regimens and viral loads below 50 copies/mL, their viremia invariably rebounds to pretherapy levels within days or weeks of drug termination. Thus, a measured undetectable plasma viral RNA level does not indicate that the virus has been eliminated from the body. Virus may be present in plasma at levels below the detection capability of the laboratory assay and in body compartments other than blood, such as lymphoid tissue or the central nervous system (CNS). Provirus may be present in a variety of cells that can act as reservoirs for HIV, such as memory T cells. Thus, once therapy is initiated, treatment should be continued without interruption, except for serious toxicities or concurrent conditions that preclude oral therapy.

The realistic goal of antiretroviral therapy is to reduce HIV-associated morbidity and to prolong survival. The success of regimens is currently monitored by surrogate markers; reduction in the viral load in plasma to levels below 50 copies/mL and increase in CD4$^+$ T-lymphocyte cell counts to levels in the normal range are considered likely to correlate with long-term disease-free survival.

For most patients, antiretroviral therapy can reliably reduce viral loads to levels below 50 copies/mL when the circulating virus is susceptible to available drugs. When viral loads are reduced to low levels, further immune decline is usually prevented, and immune function is usually improved substantially both in the period immediately after initiation of therapy and then more slowly during subsequent months and years. Whereas most patients with effective virologic suppression will demonstrate improvement in CD4 count, a few patients will not show such benefit, for reasons that are usually not clear.

Patients may be identified during acute infection (within a few days to 6 months after acquisition of infection); or they may be identified when CD4 counts are relatively high, before they are highly susceptible to AIDS-defining complications (>200 cells/mm^3); or they may be identified when they meet the definition of AIDS (CD4 count < 200 cells/mm^3), when they are highly susceptible to AIDS-defining conditions. A case can be made for treating each of these groups of patients with antiretroviral therapy, although there is universal, long-standing agreement based on solid data only for the groups who have CD4 counts below 200/mm^3 or who have had an AIDS-defining condition.

As public health efforts expand testing for patients who engage in high-risk activities and offer "opt out" testing at medical and nonmedical venues, more and more patients are being identified early in the course of HIV infection, when they are asymptomatic and their CD4$^+$ T-lymphocyte cell counts are relatively high. Consensus about the benefits of treating such patients with antiretroviral therapy will develop as more prospective data are accumulated about patients' outcomes with such an approach.

A substantial number of patients still come to medical attention only when they develop opportunistic infections such as PCP, toxoplasmosis, cryptococcal meningitis, or cytomegalovirus (CMV) retinitis, times when their CD4$^+$ T-lymphocyte cell counts are characteristically low. These patients either have ignored the possibility of HIV infection due to high-risk activities or have not accessed early voluntary testing. There is virtually universal agreement that these patients should receive antiretroviral therapy, although there is debate as to the precise timing of such therapy in relation to treatment of their opportunistic process.

As antiretroviral regimens have become less toxic and more convenient, there is enhanced enthusiasm for initiation of antiretroviral therapy early as soon as HIV infection is recognized. However, antiretroviral therapy is not likely to be effective unless the patient is committed and able to adhere to the antiretroviral regimen and the clinician is skilled at managing the regimen. Studies have shown, as is intuitively obvious, that the likelihood of achieving a durable virologic response (i.e., plasma viral load below the limit of detection of the assay system used) depends on adherence. There is a direct relationship between missing doses of the antiretroviral therapy regimen and the development of HIV drug resistance. If a patient is not fully invested in taking the drugs regularly or is unable to adhere because of psychiatric, social, economic, or medical issues, initiation of antiretroviral therapy may not be indicated. Active drug and alcohol abuse, mental illness including depression, concomitant medical problems, poor clinician-patient relationship, history of drug toxicity, and fear of drug toxicity can be strong predictors of poor adherence. Directly observed therapy can be a successful strategy to improve adherence, but this approach is not practical in most settings.

Successful management of HIV therapy also requires an experienced clinician. In the 1980s, there was considerable emphasis on "mainstreaming" HIV-infected patients (i.e., encouraging general internists, family practitioners, and a variety of other primary care providers to care for patients with HIV infection). Since that era, management has become dramatically more complex. Studies show that clinicians with experience (regardless of their formal training or certification) are more likely to follow current standards and guidelines than are clinicians with less experience. When it is feasible, patients should be managed by clinicians who have considerable experience and the capacity to keep abreast of the rapidly evolving field.

HIV has an extremely high mutation rate. Resistance to therapeutic agents can emerge rapidly, especially when viral loads are high, adherence is suboptimal, or resistance exists at baseline to one or more agents being used for therapy. Resistance to reverse transcriptase inhibitors is associated with amino acid substitutions in the reverse transcriptase enzyme. Resistance to protease inhibitors is associated with amino acid substitutions in the protease enzyme. Clinically important resistance can occasionally occur in untreated patients as a result of spontaneous mutations. For some drugs, a single mutation can produce clinically important resistance. For other drugs, significant resistance occurs only if several mutations take place. Most clinically important resistance, however, is a result of selective pressure from antiretroviral therapy. This resistance can be assessed by genotypic and phenotypic assays.

Resistance can emerge rapidly; for example, with nevirapine monotherapy, resistance can emerge within the first few days of treatment. Resistance can even emerge after a single dose of nevirapine because of the long half-life of this compound, which essentially exposes the patient to many days of monotherapy. Early experience with zidovudine showed that zidovudine resistance emerged during the initial 6 to 12 months of therapy. Current recommendations for therapy emphasize the use of combination regimens that include at least two and ideally three potent agents so that viral replication is maximally inhibited and mutation rates conferring resistance occur infrequently. This is best measured by consistent plasma HIV RNA (viral load) values below the level of detection with use of commercially available assays.

Thus, the goal of antiretroviral therapy is reduction of HIV infection–associated morbidity and mortality, best accomplished by maximal inhibition of HIV replication. Inhibition of viral replication should prevent HIV-related immunologic decline and promote immune reconstitution as well as bring about reduction in HIV infection–associated inflammation and its complications. Effective therapy should also reduce HIV transmission from the patient to sexual partners. Development of an effective program for individual patients requires considerable knowledge and commitment for both the health care provider and the patient.

When to Initiate Antiretroviral Therapy

All patients being considered for antiretroviral therapy need a careful evaluation by history, physical examination, and laboratory assessment including virologic and immunologic status (HIV viral load and CD4+ T-lymphocyte cell count), clinical status (presence of AIDS-related opportunistic infections or tumors), and presence of comorbidities. The resistance pattern of the virus should be measured because drug resistance is increasingly prevalent in most communities. More assays are being developed to help predict the efficacy and safety of particular drugs, for instance, the presence of HLA B*5701 allele in the patient if abacavir therapy is being considered, and CCR5 coreceptor status of the virus if maraviroc is being considered.

Current guidelines for initiation of therapy are summarized in Tables 396-1 to 396-3. Patients with acute HIV infection (i.e., those in the process of seroconverting) and patients who have seroconverted in the previous 6 months should be considered for early therapy. About 40 to 90% of acutely infected patients experience symptomatic illnesses, and if the patient or health care provider considers the possibility that the symptoms might have been related to high-risk behavior, HIV infection can potentially be identified by serologic and virologic assays. In theory, early therapy should reduce the viral load in lymphoid tissue during the period before an effective host immune response is initiated and subsequently lead to lower viral loads and higher CD4+ T-lymphocyte cell counts. The long-term clinical benefit of treating acute or early HIV infection has not been shown conclusively, however, and the potential benefits of treating acute HIV infection must be weighed against the disadvantages of toxicity, cost, and inconvenience. Many clinicians would offer at least 2 to 6 months of this therapy in an effort to

TABLE 396-1	CONDITIONS FAVORING MORE RAPID INITIATION OF ANTIRETROVIRAL THERAPY

Pregnancy
AIDS-defining conditions
Acute opportunistic infections
Lower CD4 counts (e.g., <200 cells/mm^3)
Rapidly declining CD4 counts (e.g., >100 cells/mm^3 decrease per year)
Higher viral loads (e.g., >100,000 copies/mL)
HIV-associated nephropathy
Hepatitis B virus (HBV) coinfection when treatment for HBV is indicated

Modified from Panel on Antiretroviral Guidelines for Adults and Adolescents. Guidelines for the use of antiretroviral agents in HIV-1–infected adults and adolescents. Department of Health and Human Services. Jan. 10, 2011. http://www.aidsinfo.nih.gov/ContentFiles/AdultandAdolescentGL.pdf.

TABLE 396-2	WHEN TO INITIATE ANTIRETROVIRAL THERAPY IN TREATMENT-NAIVE PATIENTS

ART should be initiated in all patients with a history of an AIDS-defining illness or with a CD4 count of <350 cells/mm^3.
ART is also recommended for patients with CD4 counts between 350 and 500 cells/mm^3.
ART should also be initiated, regardless of CD4 count, in patients with the following conditions: HIVAN and HBV coinfection when treatment of HBV is indicated.
A combination ARV drug regimen is also recommended for pregnant women who do not meet criteria for treatment, with the goal to prevent perinatal transmission.
For patients with CD4 counts >500 cells/mm^3, 50% of the panel members favor starting ART; the other 50% of members view treatment as optional in this setting.
Patients initiating ART should be willing and able to commit to lifelong treatment and should understand the benefits and risks of therapy and the importance of adherence.
Patients may choose to postpone therapy, and providers, on a case-by-case basis, may elect to defer therapy based on clinical and/or psychosocial factors.

HIVAN = HIV-associated nephropathy.
Modified from Panel on Antiretroviral Guidelines for Adults and Adolescents. Guidelines for the use of antiretroviral agents in HIV-1–infected adults and adolescents. Department of Health and Human Services. Jan. 10, 2011. http://www.aidsinfo.nih.gov/ContentFiles/AdultandAdolescentGL.pdf.

reduce viral replication in lymphoid tissue and to produce a lower plasma HIV viral load. It is often difficult to stop such therapy when both the patient and the clinician witness the rapid fall in plasma viral load and the rebound in CD4+ T-lymphocyte cell count. There is no consensus about the benefits of continuing such therapy lifelong.

For patients with chronic HIV infection, the decision to initiate therapy is influenced by data that demonstrate clinical benefits for patients with comparable clinical and laboratory findings. Observational studies provide some important clues about the risk for progression of patients to AIDS-defining complications. Figure 396-1 demonstrates the natural history of the interaction of HIV infection and CD4+ T-lymphocyte cell count and their effect on the patient's outcome during a 3-year follow-up of untreated patients in the Multicenter AIDS Cohort Study. This figure indicates that the CD4+ T-lymphocyte cell count and plasma HIV viral load influence the 3-year risk for progression to AIDS.

These data by themselves do not prove which patients would respond to therapy or which patients would respond best. These data do provide information about the magnitude of potential benefit in terms of AIDS-defining events. Contemporary understanding of the pathogenesis of HIV infection emphasizes the importance of non–AIDS-defining events that were not measured in this study and does not take into account potential benefits, such as reduced HIV transmission.

In terms of assessing patients in specific CD4+ T-lymphocyte cell strata, chronically infected patients with CD4+ T-lymphocyte cell counts of less than 200 cells/mm^3 are at high risk for development of opportunistic diseases, non–AIDS-defining morbidity, and death. These patients have been shown by clinical end point studies to benefit from antiretroviral therapy in terms of longer survival and delayed disease progression. For patients with CD4+ T-lymphocyte cell counts of more than 200 cells/mm^3, there have been few prospective clinical end point studies to show conclusively when therapy should be initiated. A randomized trial in Haiti evaluated patients randomized to receive therapy when their CD4+ T-lymphocyte cell counts were 200

TABLE 396-3 WHAT ANTIRETROVIRAL REGIMEN TO CHOOSE FOR INITIAL THERAPY

PREFERRED REGIMENS	COMMENTS
NNRTI-based regimen EFV/TDF/FTC	EFV should not be used during the first trimester of pregnancy or in women trying to conceive or not using effective and consistent contraception.
PI-based regimens (in alphabetical order) ATV/r + TDF/FTC DRV/r (once daily) + TDF/FTC INSTI-based regimen RAL + TDF/FTC Preferred regimen for pregnant women LPV/r (twice daily) + ZDV/3TC	ATV/r should not be used in patients who require >20 mg omeprazole equivalent per day.

ALTERNATIVE REGIMENS	COMMENTS
NNRTI-based regimens (in alphabetical order) EFV + (ABC or ZDV)/3TC NVP + ZDV/3TC PI-based regimens (in alphabetical order) ATV/r + (ABC or ZDV)/3TC FPV/r (once or twice daily) + either [(ABC or ZDV)/3TC] or TDF/FTC LPV/r (once or twice daily) + either [(ABC or ZDV)/3TC] or TDF/FTC	NVP Should not be used in patients with moderate to severe hepatic impairment (Child-Pugh B or C) Should not be used in women with pre-ARV CD4 >250 cells/mm³ or men with pre-ARV CD4 >400 cells/mm³ ABC Should not be used in patients who test positive for HLA-B*5701 Use with caution in patients with high risk of cardiovascular disease or with pretreatment HIV RNA >100,000 copies/mL Once-daily LPV/r is not recommended in pregnant women.

ACCEPTABLE REGIMENS

SQV/r + TDF/FTC
NVP

ABC = abacavir; ATV = atazanavir; 3TC = lamivudine; ddI = didanosine; DRV = darunavir; EFV = efavirenz; FPV = fosamprenavir; FTC = emtricitabine; LPV = lopinavir; NVP = nevirapine; RAL = raltegravir; r = low dose ritonavir; SQV = saquinavir; TDF = tenofovir; ZDV = zidovudine. The following combinations in the recommended list are available as fixed-dose combination formulations: ABC/3TC, EFV/TDF/FTC, LPV/r, TDF/FTC, and ZDV/3TC. INSTI = integrase strand transfer inhibitor; NNRTI = non-nucleoside reverse transcriptase inhibitor; NRTI = nucleos(t)ide reverse transcriptase inhibitor; PI = protease inhibitor. Modified from Panel on Antiretroviral Guidelines for Adults and Adolescents. Guidelines for the use of antiretroviral agents in HIV-1–infected adults and adolescents. Department of Health and Human Services. Jan. 10, 2011;1-161. http://www.aidsinfo.nih.gov/ContentFiles/AdultandAdolescentGL.pdf.

to 350 cells/mm³ rather than less than 200 cells/mm³; patients deferring therapy had a higher mortality and a higher rate of tuberculosis. Other observational studies support the benefit of treating these patients with antiretroviral therapy. Given the cumulative data, most clinicians are convinced that all patients with CD4⁺ T-lymphocyte cell counts below 350 cells/mm³ should be treated.

For patients with CD4⁺ T-lymphocyte cell counts between 350 and 500 cells/mm³, there are no randomized trials using current regimens to provide guidance about when to start therapy. Data from two cohort studies suggest that there is a declining risk of AIDS or death for subjects who start antiretroviral therapy at CD4⁺ T-lymphocyte cell counts above 350 cells/mm³ compared with those who start therapy later. Whereas these studies have relatively few end point events and cohort studies can be confounded by unrecognized biases, the weight of these trials plus the concern about end-organ damage from sustained HIV viral replication has led to recommendations in current guidelines that patients with CD4⁺ T-lymphocyte cell counts of 350 to 500 cells/mm³ should be treated.

For patients with CD4⁺ T-lymphocyte cell counts above 500 cells/mm³, there are also no prospective randomized trials. Data from one cohort study suggest that deferring therapy until patients' CD4⁺ T-lymphocyte cell counts fall below 500 cells/mm³ is associated with increased mortality. These data were not confirmed in another cohort study. Given the fact that no harm could be identified with earlier intervention, at least to date, some experts endorse treatment of all HIV-infected patients, regardless of CD4⁺ T-lymphocyte cell count. Other experts, however, would not endorse treatment of patients with CD4⁺ T-lymphocyte cell counts above 500 cells/mm³.

In addition to CD4⁺ T-lymphocyte cell count, there are a number of conditions that should favor rapid initiation of therapy. These include acute opportunistic infection, rapid decline in CD4⁺ T-lymphocyte cell count (>100 cells/year), and high viral load (>100,000 copies/mL) (see Table 396-1).

Current guidelines also recommend that therapy be started regardless of CD4⁺ T-lymphocyte cell counts in patients who have AIDS-defining diseases, HIV-associated nephropathy, pregnancy, or hepatitis B that will be treated (see Tables 396-1 and 396-2). Some experts would favor starting therapy in all patients with hepatitis C virus coinfection to slow progression of liver disease or cardiovascular disease. Whereas some antiretroviral agents may enhance the likelihood of cardiovascular disease, often by producing a more atherogenic lipid profile, some clinicians would favor initiation of therapy with drugs that are least likely to have cardiovascular effects. Uncontrolled HIV replication has also been associated with neurocognitive decline. Some studies have, additionally, shown neurocognitive improvement when antiretroviral therapy is initiated. Thus, there may be some neurocognitive advantage to initiation of antiretroviral therapy as either prevention of or therapy for the CNS process. There are also data indicating that age is related to treatment-related immune reconstitution. Therefore, initiation of therapy at an "early" age may be associated with more favorable immune response

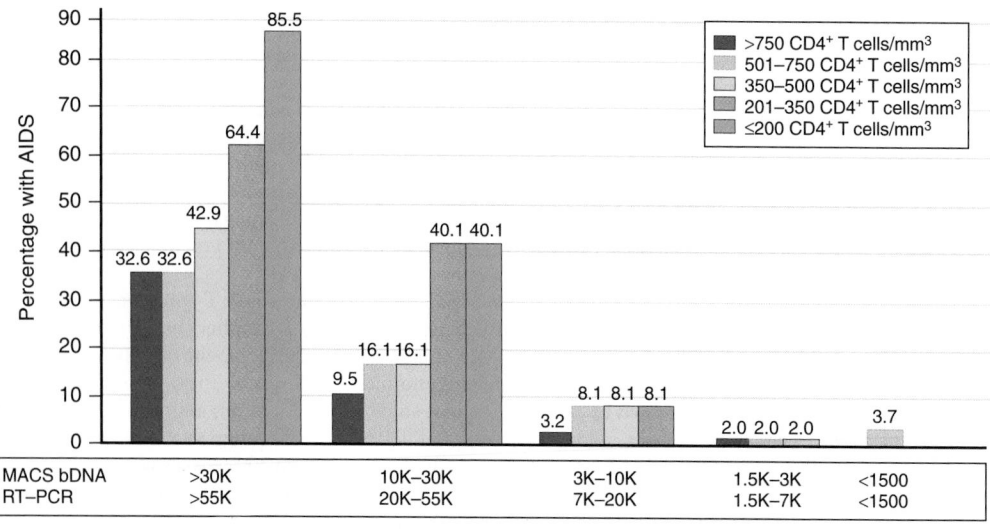

MACS bDNA RT–PCR	>30K >55K	10K–30K 20K–55K	3K–10K 7K–20K	1.5K–3K 1.5K–7K	<1500 <1500

Plasma viral load (copies/mL)

FIGURE 396-1. Likelihood for development of AIDS within 3 years. MACS = Multicenter AIDS Cohort Study; RT-PCR = reverse transcription–polymerase chain reaction.

than initiation of therapy "later," and age would thus be a factor in deciding when to initiate therapy.

HIV-infected patients with acute opportunistic infections deserve special focus in terms of when to start antiretroviral therapy. When antiretroviral therapy–naive patients develop an opportunistic infection, there has been considerable debate about the optimal time to initiate antiretroviral therapy. The advantages of immediate initiation of antiretroviral therapy include augmentation of immune response and reduction in likelihood that other HIV infection–associated complications will occur. There have been well-publicized cases, however, in which the augmented immune response has caused life-threatening exacerbations of the primary opportunistic process or of a previously unrecognized process (immune reconstitution syndrome [Chapter 402]), although the frequency of such cases has been unclear. A major argument against starting therapy has been that patients may not be dedicated to adherence when they leave the hospital. There are also concerns that toxicities of the antiretroviral agents may be confused with toxicities due to the drugs used to treat the acute infection and that drug interactions might interfere with the efficacy or safety of the drugs used to treat the opportunistic infection or the drugs used for antiretroviral therapy. Although it is difficult to generalize because not all opportunistic infections behave uniformly during immune reconstitution, retrospective and prospective studies do support the benefits of early versus deferred initiation of antiretroviral therapy. What the optimal time frame for initiation is (i.e., after how many days of opportunistic infection therapy or after how much clinical improvement) and what specific exceptions should be made for specific opportunistic infections and specific geographic areas remain to be determined.

What Antiretroviral Regimen to Initiate

More than 20 unique antiretroviral drugs in six mechanistic classes are currently approved by the U.S. Food and Drug Administration for sale in the United States. Some of these drugs are available in combination formulations of two or three agents in the United States (e.g., zidovudine plus lamivudine, lamivudine plus abacavir, zidovudine plus lamivudine plus abacavir, emtricitabine plus tenofovir, emtricitabine plus tenofovir plus efavirenz, and lopinavir plus ritonavir). Some of the drugs are also available in liquid formulations.

The regimen that is initiated should be potent enough to suppress the viral load below the level of assay detection for a prolonged period. This goal currently requires a combination regimen that optimally includes two nucleoside reverse transcriptase inhibitors plus either efavirenz or a ritonavir-boosted protease inhibitor.

Table 396-3 shows regimens recommended by the U.S. Department of Health and Human Services guidelines. Such recommendations are updated regularly as new data become available.

It is notable that the list of preferred regimens has changed during the past few years as more drugs have been developed and as trials have been published that demonstrated enhanced efficacy or improved safety with new regimens. Drugs that were popular a decade ago, such as nelfinavir, indinavir, didanosine, and stavudine, are seldom used currently, and zalcitabine and delavirdine are no longer marketed in the United States. Even drugs such as zidovudine, lamivudine, and lopinavir, which have benefited many patients, are no longer preferred agents, although they continue to have a role in certain patients. The field continues to evolve rapidly as trials are completed and analyzed.

Which regimen a health care provider should choose for an individual patient depends on a variety of factors. The regimen should be compatible with a patient's lifestyle. Adherence is more likely with regimens that can be taken once or twice per day than with those that are taken more often. Comorbid conditions such as cardiovascular disease, chemical dependency, liver disease, psychiatric disease, renal disease, and tuberculosis are relevant, as is pregnancy or the potential for the patient to become pregnant. For instance, ritonavir-based regimens that enhance atherogenic lipid profiles might be less desirable in patients with cardiovascular disease, and tenofovir might be less desirable in patients with renal or metabolic bone disease. Drug interactions are major considerations that should be carefully considered; ritonavir has multiple interactions that make it a poor choice in patients receiving rifampin for tuberculosis, for instance, or certain antiseizure regimens. Pregnancy would preclude the use of efavirenz during at least the first trimester because of evidence of this drug's teratogenicity. HLA B*5701 and coreceptor tropism results would influence the safety or efficacy of abacavir and maraviroc, respectively.

Drugs must be acceptable to the patient; if the patient cannot swallow certain sized pills, if the taste is unacceptable, or if the patient is convinced

that the drugs will produce unacceptable toxicity, the patient is not likely to be adherent and to achieve the virologic results that would produce long disease-free survival.

Planned interruptions (structured or strategic treatment interruptions) of antiretroviral therapy have been considered by some patients and health care providers to reduce the lifestyle burden of taking medications, to reduce medication-related toxicity, to decrease cost, or to improve immune control of HIV infection. These approaches are no longer recommended because of adverse immunologic and clinical events after interruption of treatment.

Immune-based therapies have been investigated in an attempt to augment immunity against HIV-associated infections and tumors. Interleukin-2, given subcutaneously 5 days every 2 months for several cycles, has been shown to increase $CD4^+$ T-lymphocyte cell counts in a substantial fraction of patients. However, in long-term controlled, randomized studies, these increases in $CD4^+$ T-lymphocyte cell counts did not correlate with improved prognosis in conjunction with standard antiretroviral therapy.

Changing an Unsuccessful Antiretroviral Regimen

The initial antiretroviral therapy regimen may need to be changed because of toxicity, drug availability, cost, preference of the patient, lack of efficacy, or comorbid conditions. The initial decision to start therapy and considerations to change a regimen are important because of the limited number of antiretroviral agents that can be used in subsequent regimens. A long-term strategy needs to be developed for each patient, with a focus on what approach might be available if the current regimen fails. If the patient is unlikely to be adherent to the new regimen, the best long-term strategy may be a drug holiday, with deferral of a new regimen until the patient is ready to be adherent. Similarly, if a patient's viral load were detectable but less than 5000 copies/mL and the $CD4^+$ T-lymphocyte cell count were stable and greater than 200 to 350 cells/mm^3, it might be reasonable to consider maintaining the current regimen rather than switching to a more complex regimen that would expose the patient to other previously untried classes of drugs, although many experts would be reluctant to allow even that degree of viral replication to persist.

Lack of efficacy can be defined in a variety of ways: failure to meet the virologic milestones (in a treatment-naive patient, the HIV RNA level should be below 400 copies/mL by 24 weeks and below 50 copies/mL by 48 weeks after starting of therapy); $CD4^+$ T-lymphocyte cell counts that either fail to increase or decline; and clinical deterioration. Not all of these outcomes will benefit from a change in treatment. Changing the regimen may not alter the outcome of patients who have deteriorated clinically or failed to increase their $CD4^+$ T-lymphocyte cell count despite virologic suppression. Moreover, virologic suppression must be carefully defined. Small and intermittent virologic breakthroughs of 50 to 200 copies/mL are not necessarily indications to change the regimen, that is, they are not necessarily a harbinger of poor immunologic or clinical response.

In terms of their implications for therapy, each of these aspects of failure must be interpreted in context. A patient with a high initial viral load (e.g., >1 million copies/mL) whose viral loads are declining might be recommended to remain on a regimen if the viral load is still declining at 6 months. Similarly, a patient who started a regimen when the $CD4^+$ T-lymphocyte cell count was low and in whom an opportunistic infection developed at a time when the HIV viral load was below the level of assay detection might be unlikely to benefit from a different antiretroviral therapy regimen. Decisions about changing therapies must also consider what treatment options are feasible in view of previous drug exposure, viral resistance, drug tolerability, and drug availability.

There are many reasons for treatment to fail. Poor adherence of the patient is probably the most common cause, and clinicians may find it especially difficult to identify this factor. Altered drug pharmacokinetics resulting from abnormal absorption or metabolism of the drug may also be a factor. Drug interactions with licensed drugs or "alternative" medicines may be relevant. The patient may have acquired a drug-resistant virus on initial infection, or the patient's virus may have become resistant during therapy. These causes of regimen failure must be investigated carefully to maximize the likelihood that the next regimen will succeed.

After a regimen has failed, the new regimen should include at least two and ideally three agents proven to be currently active by the results of resistance testing obtained while the patient was taking the failing regimen. Both phenotypic and genotypic resistance assays can provide useful information if the assay is performed while the patient is receiving the failing regimen. There is no definitive guideline regarding which assay is more useful. Some agents (i.e., the nucleoside inhibitors lamivudine and emtricitabine) may confer partial antiviral activity for other drugs (e.g., zidovudine) despite predicted drug resistance on genotypic and phenotypic testing. In general, adding a single new agent to a failing regimen is not recommended because of the risk for development of rapid resistance. Newer agents have demonstrated potent activity against virus shown to be resistant to multiple agents and can be considered for inclusion in a new regimen for a patient determined to have failed prior regimens. Tipranavir, darunavir, maraviroc, etravirine, enfuvirtide, and raltegravir are examples of newer agents that show promise in combination regimens for patients with highly resistant virus.

Potential Complications of Antiretroviral Regimens

Like any medication, each antiretroviral agent is associated with toxicities. Some are class specific, such as mitochondrial toxicities with nucleoside analogues or rash and CNS dysfunction with non-nucleoside reverse transcriptase inhibitors. Others are drug specific, such as urolithiasis and interstitial nephritis with indinavir, diarrhea with nelfinavir, or a characteristic hypersensitivity reaction with abacavir.

Certain toxicities deserve special mention. Chronic compensated hyperlactatemia occurs during treatment with nucleoside and nucleotide reverse transcriptase inhibitors (NRTIs). As fewer patients are receiving ddI, d4T, or ddC, this complication is likely to become less common. In rare cases, decompensated lactic acidosis (Chapter 120) accompanied by hepatic steatosis and hepatomegaly can occur and is associated with high mortality. Risk factors for this potentially fatal syndrome include female gender, obesity, late-stage pregnancy or the postpartum period, and use of didanosine and stavudine. The lactic acidosis syndrome often presents as nonspecific gastrointestinal symptoms, including nausea, abdominal pain, vomiting, diarrhea, weakness, myalgias, paresthesias, and hepatomegaly. Hepatic enzymes may be normal or only slightly elevated. Elevated lactate levels may be associated with an anion gap, elevated creatine kinase and lactate dehydrogenase, and an enlarged fatty liver on computed tomography. Therapy consists of supportive measures and discontinuation of all nucleoside analogue drugs. Bicarbonate infusions and hemodialysis may be helpful. There is growing evidence that most patients can be successfully restarted on a new antiretroviral therapy regimen.

Mitochondrial dysfunction in association with NRTIs may be accompanied by several complications, including peripheral neuropathy, cardiomyopathy, myopathy, pancreatitis, and lipoatrophy. Although antiretroviral drug toxicity can contribute to these conditions, it is possible that HIV itself or opportunistic infections, or both, may also play an etiologic role. As tenofovir and emtricitabine are replacing nucleosides that have had greater risk of mitochondrial toxicity, it is expected that mitochondrial complications will become less frequent.

HIV infection and antiretroviral therapies have been associated with body fat abnormalities or lipodystrophy. Loss of peripheral fat or lipoatrophy, most notable in the face and extremities, as well as abnormal accumulation of abdominal and dorsocervical fat may be seen, each alone or in combination. Lipoatrophy has been most closely linked to NRTIs in association with mitochondrial toxicity. Although causality has not been established, lipid accumulation may be a consequence of protease inhibitors, more so than of NRTIs. It remains unknown whether fat distribution abnormalities represent various manifestations of a single pathologic process, but increasingly they seem to represent distinct entities or toxicities of antiretroviral therapy. When fat maldistribution occurs, it can be disfiguring and distressing. There is growing evidence that switching antiretroviral therapy to regimens with less mitochondrial toxicity (e.g., switching from stavudine-, didanosine-, or zidovudine-containing regimens to tenofovir or nucleoside-sparing regimens) can result in improvements in lipoatrophy during a period of many months or years. Strategies to restore physiologic growth hormone levels can reduce abdominal visceral fat and improve lipid profile, but these benefits do not appear to persist after withdrawal of growth hormone therapies.

Before the advent of antiretroviral therapy, HIV infection was associated with reduced high-density lipoprotein cholesterol and elevated triglyceride levels. Antiretroviral therapy, in particular most protease inhibitors, is associated with elevated total serum cholesterol and fasting triglyceride levels (Chapter 213). Evidence is mounting that these atherogenic lipid profiles are important factors contributing to the accelerated atherosclerosis manifested as increased risk for cardiovascular and cerebrovascular disease independent of other recognized risk factors, such as age, tobacco use, and family history. Most clinicians monitor and treat these lipid abnormalities as they would manage abnormalities in an HIV-uninfected patient. When lipid management programs (Chapter 213) are implemented, however, careful consideration must be given to drug interactions, especially interactions between protease inhibitors and β-hydroxy-β-methylglutaryl–coenzyme A reductase inhibitors (statins). Replacement of the offending agent with an alternative antiretroviral (using atazanavir or atazanavir-ritonavir in place of alternative protease inhibitors, or nevirapine instead of efavirenz) may be effective in reducing the lipid elevations.

Elevations in lipids alone do not appear to account for all the excess risk for cardiovascular disease observed in HIV-infected patients. Other factors, possibly related to drug toxicity or chronic inflammation, are probably implicated. For example, insulin resistance and diabetes are increasingly identified in HIV-infected patients, in particular in patients treated with antiretroviral therapy. As with hyperlipidemia, the use of certain protease inhibitors is linked to impaired insulin sensitivity. However, the risk of diabetes has been associated with some NRTIs. The combination of insulin resistance, hyperlipidemia, and abnormal fat distribution represents many of the components of metabolic syndrome (Chapter 237), a condition known to be associated with increased risk for diabetes and cardiovascular disease. Therefore, accelerated atherosclerosis may be due in part to this combination of factors as well as to traditional risk factors as indicated earlier.

Hepatotoxicity is an important complication of antiretroviral therapy. Serum transaminase elevations have been reported with all licensed protease inhibitors and non-NRTIs and have been associated with nucleoside agents as well. In some patients, the transaminase elevations are mild and unassociated with symptoms. In other cases, symptomatic hepatitis or associated hepatic steatosis with or without lactic acidosis requires cessation of the drug. Among the non-NRTIs, nevirapine has the greatest potential for causing symptomatic hepatitis. Manifestations often include fever, rash, and eosinophilia and usually occur within 12 weeks of initiation of therapy. Protease inhibitor–associated liver enzyme abnormalities can occur at any juncture during therapy. Ritonavir-containing regimens are particularly likely to be associated with hepatic toxicity. Hepatitis C, hepatitis B, alcohol, elevated baseline liver function test results, and other hepatotoxic drugs are risk factors for the development of protease inhibitor–associated liver toxicity. Preliminary results from the use of integrase inhibitors and CCR5 antagonists suggest that hepatotoxicity is relatively uncommon with these agents.

Decreased bone mineral density and avascular necrosis are complications of HIV infection that appear to be associated with HIV and antiretroviral therapy. Evidence indicates that fractures may be increased in patients with HIV infection. Avascular necrosis of the hips and other joints appears to be a separate and distinct syndrome, possibly associated with previous steroid use. There are few data to guide the development of preventive or therapeutic strategies for these bone disorders.

Nephrotoxicity is an emerging concern for patients receiving long-term tenofovir therapy.

● PREVENTION OF HIV-ASSOCIATED OPPORTUNISTIC INFECTIONS

Patients with HIV infection and severe immunodeficiency develop characteristic and predictable opportunistic infections. Because the period of susceptibility to opportunistic infections in patients with HIV infection can be measured by CD4$^+$ T-lymphocyte cell counts, a strategy of chemoprophylaxis is particularly attractive for patients whose immunity has not been restored with antiretroviral therapy or immunomodulating therapies.

Chemoprophylaxis regimens are available for most treatable HIV-associated opportunistic infections. Table 396-4 and E-Table 396-1 summarize regimens that are recommended for primary and secondary chemoprophylaxis. Table 396-4 and E-Table 396-1 summarize the CD4$^+$ T-lymphocyte cell counts at which chemoprophylaxis should be implemented. Chemoprophylaxis for various pathogens should be started when the CD4$^+$ T-lymphocyte cell count declines to specific levels (depending on the pathogen) to prevent an initial episode of disease (primary prophylaxis). This prophylaxis can be stopped if immunity is augmented by antiretroviral therapy (Table 396-5) but must be restarted if immunity again declines below designated thresholds. Similarly, if an opportunistic infection develops, suppressive therapy (secondary prophylaxis) is indicated for life for most opportunistic infections unless immunity is restored by antiretroviral therapy.

The regimens recommended in Table 396-4 and E-Table 396-1 have been shown to prevent primary and subsequent occurrence of disease. The use of these regimens improves survival of the patient in several instances (PCP, *M. avium* complex disease, and *M. tuberculosis* infection) and decreases the patient's morbidity.

TABLE 396-4 PROPHYLAXIS TO PREVENT FIRST EPISODE OF HIV-RELATED OPPORTUNISTIC DISEASE

PATHOGEN	INDICATION	FIRST CHOICE	ALTERNATIVE
Pneumocystis pneumonia (PCP)	CD4$^+$ count <200 cells/mm^3 or oropharyngeal candidiasis CD4$^+$ <14% or history of AIDS-defining illness CD4$^+$ count >200 but <250 cells/mm^3 if monitoring CD4$^+$ count every 1-3 months is not possible	Trimethoprim-sulfamethoxazole (TMP-SMX) 1 double-strength PO daily; *or* 1 single-strength daily	TMP-SMX 1 double-strength PO 3 times weekly; *or* Dapsone 100 mg PO daily or 50 mg PO bid; *or* Dapsone 50 mg PO daily + pyrimethamine 50 mg PO weekly + leucovorin 25 mg PO weekly; *or* Aerosolized pentamidine 300 mg via Respirgard II nebulizer every month; *or* Atovaquone 1500 mg PO daily; *or* Atovaquone 1500 mg + pyrimethamine 25 mg + leucovorin 10 mg PO daily
Toxoplasma gondii encephalitis	*Toxoplasma* IgG–positive patients with CD4$^+$ count <100 cells/mm^3 Seronegative patients receiving PCP prophylaxis not active against toxoplasmosis should have *Toxoplasma* serology retested if CD4$^+$ count declines to <100 cells/mm^3. Prophylaxis should be initiated if seroconversion occurred.	TMP-SMX, 1 double-strength PO daily	TMP-SMX 1 double-strength PO 3 times weekly; *or* TMP-SMX 1 single-strength PO daily; Dapsone 50 mg PO daily + pyrimethamine 50 mg PO weekly + leucovorin 25 mg PO weekly; *or* (Dapsone 200 mg + pyrimethamine 75 mg + leucovorin 25 mg) PO weekly; (Atovaquone 1500 mg ± pyrimethamine 25 mg + leucovorin 10 mg) PO daily
Mycobacterium tuberculosis infection (TB) (treatment of latent TB infection or LTBI)	(+) diagnostic test for LTBI, no evidence of active TB, and no prior history of treatment for active or latent TB (−) diagnostic test for LTBI, but close contact with a person with infectious pulmonary TB and no evidence of active TB A history of untreated or inadequately treated healed TB (i.e., old fibrotic lesions) regardless of diagnostic tests for LTBI and no evidence of active TB	Isoniazid (INH) 300 mg PO daily or 900 mg PO twice weekly for 9 months—both plus pyridoxine 50 mg PO daily; *or* For persons exposed to drug-resistant TB, selection of drugs after consultation with public health authorities	Rifampin (RIF) 600 mg PO daily × 4 months; *or* Rifabutin (RFB) (dose adjusted based on concomitant antiretroviral therapy) × 4 months
Disseminated *Mycobacterium avium* complex (MAC) disease	CD4$^+$ count <50 cells/mm^3—after ruling out active MAC infection	Azithromycin 1200 mg PO once weekly; *or* Clarithromycin 500 mg PO bid; *or* Azithromycin 600 mg PO twice weekly	RFB 300 mg PO daily (dosage adjustment based on drug-drug interactions with antiretroviral therapy); rule out active TB before starting RFB
Streptococcus pneumoniae infection	CD4$^+$ count >200 cells/mm^3 and no receipt of pneumococcal vaccine in the past 5 years CD4$^+$ count <200 cells/mm^3—vaccination can be offered In patients who received polysaccharide pneumococcal vaccination (PPV) when CD4$^+$ count <200 cells/mm^3 but has increased to >200 cells/mm^3 in response to antiretroviral therapy	23-valent PPV 0.5 mL IM × 1 Revaccination every 5 years may be considered	
Influenza A and B virus infection	All HIV-infected patients	Inactivated influenza vaccine 0.5 mL IM annually	
Histoplasma capsulatum infection	CD4$^+$ count ≤150 cells/mm^3 and at high risk because of occupational exposure or live in a community with a hyperendemic rate of histoplasmosis (>10 cases/100 patient-years)	Itraconazole 200 mg PO daily	
Coccidioidomycosis	Positive IgM or IgG serologic test result in a patient from a disease-endemic area; and CD4$^+$ count <250 cells/mm^3	Fluconazole 400 mg PO daily Itraconazole 200 mg PO bid	
Varicella-zoster virus (VZV) infection	*Pre-exposure prevention:* Patients with CD4$^+$ count ≥200 cells/mm^3 who have not been vaccinated, have no history of varicella or herpes zoster, or who are seronegative for VZV Note: Routine VZV serologic testing in HIV-infected adults is not recommended. *Postexposure—close contact with a person who has active varicella or herpes zoster:* For susceptible patients (those who have no history of vaccination or of either condition, or are known to be VZV seronegative)	*Pre-exposure prevention:* Primary varicella vaccination (Varivax), 2 doses (0.5 mL SC) administered 3 months apart If vaccination results in disease because of vaccine virus, treatment with acyclovir is recommended. *Postexposure therapy:* Varicella-zoster immune globulin (VariZIG) 125 IU per 10 kg (maximum of 625 IU) IM, administered within 96 hours after exposure to a person with active varicella or herpes zoster Note: As of June 2007, VariZIG can be obtained only under a treatment IND (1-800-843-7477, FFF Enterprises).	VZV-susceptible household contacts of susceptible HIV-infected persons should be vaccinated to prevent potential transmission of VZV to their HIV-infected contacts. *Alternative postexposure therapy:* Postexposure varicella vaccine (Varivax) 0.5 mL SC × 2 doses, 3 months apart if CD4$^+$ count >200 cells/mm^3; *or* Preemptive acyclovir 800 mg PO 5×/day for 5 days These two alternatives have not been studied in the HIV population.

TABLE 396-4 PROPHYLAXIS TO PREVENT FIRST EPISODE OF HIV-RELATED OPPORTUNISTIC DISEASE—cont'd

PATHOGEN	INDICATION	FIRST CHOICE	ALTERNATIVE
Human papillomavirus (HPV) infection	Women aged 15-26 yr	HPV quadrivalent vaccine 0.5 mL IM months 0, 2, and 6	
Hepatitis A virus (HAV) infection	HAV-susceptible patients with chronic liver disease, or who are injection-drug users, or men who have sex with men. Certain specialists might delay vaccination until CD4$^+$ count >200 cells/mm^3.	Hepatitis A vaccine 1 mL IM × 2 doses—at 0 and 6-12 months IgG antibody response should be assessed 1 month after vaccination; nonresponders should be revaccinated	
Hepatitis B virus (HBV) infection	All HIV patients without evidence of prior exposure to HBV should be vaccinated with HBV vaccine, including patients with CD4$^+$ count <200 cells/mm^3. _Patients with isolated anti-HBc:_ (consider screening for HBV DNA before vaccination to rule out occult chronic HBV infection) _Vaccine nonresponders:_ Defined as anti-HBs <10 IU/mL 1 month after a vaccination series For patients with low CD4$^+$ count at the time of first vaccination series, certain specialists might delay revaccination until after a sustained increase in CD4$^+$ count with antiretroviral therapy.	Hepatitis B vaccine IM (Engerix-B 20 µg/mL or Recombivax HB 10 µg/mL) at 0, 1, and 6 months Anti-HBs should be obtained 1 month after completion of the vaccine series. Revaccinate with a second vaccine series.	Some experts recommend vaccinating with 40-µg doses of either vaccine. Some experts recommend revaccinating with 40-µg doses of either vaccine.

Modified From Centers for Disease Control and Prevention. Guidelines for Prevention and treatment of opportunistic infections in HIV-infected adults and adolescents. Recommendations from CDC, the National Institutes of Health, and the HIV Medicine Association of the Infectious Disease Society of America. _MMWR Morb Mortal Wkly Rep._ 2009;58(RR-4).

TABLE 396-5 CRITERIA FOR DISCONTINUING AND RESTARTING OPPORTUNISTIC INFECTION PROPHYLAXIS FOR ADULTS AND ADOLESCENTS WITH HUMAN IMMUNODEFICIENCY VIRUS INFECTION

OPPORTUNISTIC INFECTION	CRITERIA FOR DISCONTINUING PRIMARY PROPHYLAXIS	CRITERIA FOR RESTARTING PRIMARY PROPHYLAXIS	CRITERIA FOR DISCONTINUING SECONDARY PROPHYLAXIS/ CHRONIC MAINTENANCE THERAPY	CRITERIA FOR RESTARTING SECONDARY PROPHYLAXIS/ CHRONIC MAINTENANCE
Pneumocystis pneumonia (PCP)	CD4$^+$ count >200 cells/mm^3 for >3 months in response to antiretroviral therapy (ART)	CD4$^+$ count <200 cells/mm^3	CD4$^+$ count increased from <200 cells/mm^3 to >200 cells/mm^3 for ≥3 months in response to ART If PCP is diagnosed when CD4$^+$ count >200 cells/mm^3, prophylaxis should probably be continued for life regardless of CD4$^+$ count rise in response to ART.	CD4$^+$ count <200 cells/mm^3, or if PCP recurred at a CD4$^+$ count >200 cells/mm^3
Toxoplasma gondii encephalitis (TE)	CD4$^+$ count >200 cells/mm^3 for >3 months in response to ART	CD4$^+$ count <100-200 cells/mm^3	Successfully completed initial therapy, remain asymptomatic of signs and symptoms of TE, and CD4$^+$ count >200 cells/mm^3 for >6 months in response to ART	CD4$^+$ count <200 cells/mm^3
Microsporidiosis	Not applicable	Not applicable	No signs and symptoms of non-ocular microsporidiosis and CD4$^+$ count >200 cells/mm^3 for >6 months in response to ART Patients with ocular microsporidiosis should be on therapy indefinitely regardless of CD4$^+$ count.	No recommendation
Disseminated _Mycobacterium avium_ complex (MAC) disease	CD4$^+$ count >100 cells/mm^3 for ≥3 months in response to ART	CD4$^+$ count <50 cells/mm^3	If fulfill the following criteria Completed ≥12 months therapy, and No signs and symptoms of MAC, and Have sustained (≥6 months) CD4$^+$ count >100 cells/mm^3 in response to ART	CD4$^+$ count <100 cells/mm^3
Bartonellosis	Not applicable	Not applicable	If fulfill the following criteria Received 3-4 months of treatment CD4$^+$ count >200 cells/mm^3 for ≥6 months Certain specialists would discontinue therapy only if _Bartonella_ titers have also decreased by four-fold.	No recommendation
Mucosal candidiasis	Not applicable	Not applicable	If used, reasonable to discontinue when CD4$^+$ count >200 cells/mm^3	No recommendation

TABLE 396-5 CRITERIA FOR DISCONTINUING AND RESTARTING OPPORTUNISTIC INFECTION PROPHYLAXIS FOR ADULTS AND ADOLESCENTS WITH HUMAN IMMUNODEFICIENCY VIRUS INFECTION—cont'd

OPPORTUNISTIC INFECTION	CRITERIA FOR DISCONTINUING PRIMARY PROPHYLAXIS	CRITERIA FOR RESTARTING PRIMARY PROPHYLAXIS	CRITERIA FOR DISCONTINUING SECONDARY PROPHYLAXIS/ CHRONIC MAINTENANCE THERAPY	CRITERIA FOR RESTARTING SECONDARY PROPHYLAXIS/ CHRONIC MAINTENANCE
Cryptococcal meningitis	Not applicable	Not applicable	If fulfill the following criteria Completed course of initial therapy Remain asymptomatic of cryptococcosis CD4$^+$ count ≥200 cells/mm^3 for >6 months in response to ART Certain specialists would perform a lumbar puncture to determine if cerebrospinal fluid is culture and antigen negative before stopping therapy.	CD4$^+$ count <200 cells/mm^3
Histoplasma capsulatum infection	If used, CD4$^+$ count >150 cells/mm^3 for 6 months on ART	For patients at high risk for acquiring histoplasmosis, restart at CD4$^+$ count ≤150 cells/mm^3.	If fulfill the following criteria Received itraconazole for ≥1 year Negative blood cultures CD4$^+$ count >150 cells/mm^3 for ≥6 months in response to ART Serum *Histoplasma* antigen <2 units	CD4$^+$ count ≤150 cells/mm^3
Coccidioidomycosis	If used, CD4$^+$ count ≥250 cells/mm^3 for ≥6 months	If used, restart at CD4$^+$ count <250 cells/mm^3	**Only for patients with focal coccidioidal pneumonia:** Clinically responded to ≥12 months of antifungal therapy CD4$^+$ count >250 cells/mm^3 Receiving ART Suppressive therapy should be continued indefinitely, even with increase in CD4$^+$ count on ART for patients with diffuse pulmonary, disseminated, or meningeal diseases.	No recommendation
Cytomegalovirus retinitis	Not applicable	Not applicable	CD4$^+$ count >100 cells/mm^3 for >3-6 months in response to ART. Therapy should be discontinued only after consultation with an ophthalmologist, taking into account magnitude and duration of CD4$^+$ count increase, anatomic location of the lesions, vision in the contralateral eye, and the feasibility of regular ophthalmologic monitoring. Routine (every 3 months) ophthalmologic follow-up is recommended for early detection of relapse or immune restoration uveitis.	CD4$^+$ count <100 cells/mm^3
Isospora belli infection	Not applicable	Not applicable	Sustained increase in CD4$^+$ count to >200 cells/mm^3 for >6 months in response to ART and without evidence of *I. belli* infection	No recommendation

Modified From Centers for Disease Control and Prevention. Guidelines for Prevention and treatment of opportunistic infections in HIV-infected adults and adolescents. Recommendations from CDC, the National Institutes of Health, and the HIV Medicine Association of the Infectious Disease Society of America. *MMWR Morb Mortal Wkly Rep.* 2009;58(RR-4).

Several caveats about the use of chemoprophylaxis are worth noting, however. First, some opportunistic infections occur at CD4$^+$ T-lymphocyte cell counts above the recommended thresholds for starting chemoprophylaxis. Of PCP cases, 5 to 10% occur at CD4$^+$ T-lymphocyte cell counts above 200 cells/mm^3. In some instances, clinical information, such as the development of oral candidiasis or substantial weight loss, may provide additional clues that the patient is clinically more immunosuppressed than the laboratory parameters would predict. A high viral load (e.g., >100,000 copies/mL) may also suggest that earlier institution of chemoprophylaxis is warranted.

Second, patients may be unable to tolerate certain chemoprophylactic agents. TMP-SMX is often associated with intractable pruritus or rash and cannot be used by many patients with HIV infection.

Third, no chemoprophylactic regimen is completely effective. Some regimens fail because of poor adherence, but some fail because of poor host immune response or pathogen resistance. Prescribing a chemoprophylactic regimen does not guarantee that the targeted disease will never develop.

Finally, a decision to use a chemoprophylactic agent depends on the balance between its benefit in terms of efficacy and its disadvantages in terms of toxicity, inconvenience, drug interactions, ecologic effects (e.g., effects on producing resistance in targeted and bystander organisms), and cost. Some effective drugs, such as fluconazole for *Candida* and *Cryptococcus* and valganciclovir for CMV, are generally not recommended because their disadvantages were judged to outweigh their benefits.

TMP-SMX is the agent of choice for prevention of PCP. This drug should be started when the CD4$^+$ T-lymphocyte cell count decreases to 200 cells/mm^3, when oral candidiasis develops (regardless of the CD4$^+$ T-lymphocyte cell count), or when the patient has had a previous episode of PCP. Prophylaxis should be continued until the CD4$^+$ T-lymphocyte cell count increases to more than 200 cells/mm^3 for a period of at least 3 months as a result of antiretroviral therapy. Several regimens of TMP-SMX are effective; one double-strength tablet per day, one single-strength tablet per day, and one double-strength tablet three times weekly are all recommended. The daily regimens have proven to be moderately more effective than the three-times-per-week regimen. TMP-SMX can be associated with a variety of toxicities, including rash, fever, pruritus, nausea, vomiting, nephritis, hyperkalemia, and aseptic meningitis. For reasons that have not been well delineated, rash occurs at an unusually high frequency in HIV-infected patients who take TMP-SMX. Lower-dose regimens (e.g., a single-strength rather than a double-strength tablet or three times weekly rather than daily) seem to be better tolerated. Gradual dose escalation may also improve the tolerability of TMP-SMX prophylaxis. Evidence of enzyme mutations in *Pneumocystis*, which probably confers sulfonamide resistance, raises the ominous possibility that this useful prophylactic and therapeutic agent may lose the impressive efficacy that it has enjoyed to date. The clinical relevance of this mutation is not certain.

Alternatives to TMP-SMX for the chemoprophylaxis of PCP include dapsone, dapsone-pyrimethamine, sulfadiazine-pyrimethamine, atovaquone, and aerosolized pentamidine. These regimens are not as effective as TMP-SMX in preventing PCP. In addition, TMP-SMX provides protection against toxoplasmosis, bacterial pneumonia, and enteric infections. None of the alternative regimens provides protection against all these pathogens, and all have associated toxicities.

Chemoprophylaxis against toxoplasmosis should be offered to patients with CD4$^+$ T-lymphocyte cell counts below 100 cells/mm^3 with positive *Toxoplasma* serology (IgG) and should be continued until the CD4$^+$ T-lymphocyte cell count increases to more than 200 cells/mm^3 for at least 3 months after treatment with antiretroviral therapy. The preferred treatment is TMP-SMX (one double-strength tablet daily), but alternative regimens are dapsone plus pyrimethamine (with or without folinic acid) daily or atovaquone administered daily. For patients intolerant of TMP-SMX therapy, recommended alternatives for both PCP and toxoplasmosis prophylaxis include dapsone plus pyrimethamine plus leucovorin or atovaquone with or without leucovorin plus pyrimethamine.

Clarithromycin or azithromycin is the chemoprophylactic agent of choice for *M. avium* complex disease in HIV-infected patients with CD4$^+$ T-lymphocyte cell counts below 50 cells/mm^3. Each of these agents is more effective than placebo, and each is preferred to rifabutin because rifabutin is less effective and associated with multiple complex drug interactions. Clarithromycin and azithromycin provide additional protection against bacterial pneumonia. These drugs are relatively well tolerated; however, the weekly regimen of azithromycin can be associated with considerable nausea. Azithromycin causes fewer drug interactions than clarithromycin does and is preferred by some clinicians when multiple other drugs metabolized by the cytochrome P-450 system are being used.

Prophylaxis for *M. tuberculosis* infection is an important aspect of the management of HIV-infected patients, especially in communities in which tuberculosis is common. Purified protein derivative (PPD) or interferon-γ release assay screening for all patients with newly diagnosed HIV infection and regular screening thereafter are important for identification of subclinically infected patients because HIV-infected individuals have such a high likelihood for reactivation of latent tuberculosis. Latently infected patients (defined as a PPD reaction ≥5 mm for this population of patients) or patients recently exposed to active tuberculosis should be treated with one of the recommended regimens, with careful attention to the toxicities and interactions of the regimen chosen.

Immunization is an important component of preventive therapy for HIV-infected patients. Vaccination with pneumococcal vaccine is generally recommended for all HIV-infected patients with CD4$^+$ T-lymphocyte cell count above 200 cells/mm^3 unless they have received a prior dose within the past 5 years, as clinical trials have demonstrated a lower risk of pneumococcal bacteremia after vaccination. Revaccination can be considered in patients who received initial immunization when their CD4$^+$ T-lymphocyte cell count was below 200 cells/mm^3 but have subsequently experienced a rise in CD4$^+$ T-lymphocyte cells to above 200 as a result of antiretroviral therapy. HIV-infected patients who do not have evidence of prior exposure to hepatitis A or B or have high risk of acquiring these infections or concomitant hepatitis C should be vaccinated with the appropriate hepatitis A or B vaccine. It is generally recommended that hepatitis B surface antibody testing be conducted 1 month after the third and final dose of the vaccine is administered to document an appropriate response. Some experts would recommend either repeating the entire hepatitis B vaccination series (single or double doses) or administering a single booster dose in patients who fail to develop hepatitis B surface antibody after completion of the usual three-dose series.

Primary chemoprophylaxis for fungal or herpesvirus diseases is not currently recommended in the United States. Primary prophylaxis may be effective, but the benefits are currently thought to be outweighed in the United States and western Europe by the effects of prophylaxis on pathogen resistance and by the toxicity and cost of drugs that target diseases that are usually readily treatable.

MANAGEMENT OF HIV-ASSOCIATED OPPORTUNISTIC INFECTIONS

Minimizing the effect of acute opportunistic infections on the lifestyle and survival of patients depends on prompt recognition of such diseases and expeditious institution of appropriate therapy. Patients and health care providers need to be familiar with the signs and symptoms of HIV-associated opportunistic infections and neoplasms so that diseases can be treated early, before manifestations are severe.

The manifestations of HIV-related opportunistic infections often differ from manifestations in other populations of patients. PCP, for instance, is usually much less acute in patients with HIV infection than in those receiving high-dose corticosteroids or antineoplastic chemotherapy. CMV disease is associated with retinitis or colitis most often in patients with HIV disease and only rarely with pneumonitis; in contrast, organ transplant recipients almost always manifest pneumonitis, and retinitis rarely develops. *M. avium* complex disease is common in patients with HIV infection but rare in patients with most other causes of immunosuppression. Similarly, therapy for various opportunistic infections may also differ. Certain drugs may not be tolerated as well by HIV-infected patients as by other immunosuppressed patients; the unusually high incidence of rash associated with TMP-SMX is a good example of this phenomenon. Drug regimens need to be continued for longer periods; unless the immune competence can be augmented substantially by antiretroviral therapy, the likelihood of recurrence for most HIV-associated infections is so high that lifelong suppressive or maintenance therapy (e.g., secondary prophylaxis) must be maintained. Drug-drug interactions are often important considerations, especially if patients are receiving antiretroviral therapy; rifampin, rifabutin, and fluconazole are examples of drugs that may have clinically important drug interactions with antiretroviral agents that could require dose modifications of either the antiretroviral agent or the drug used to treat the opportunistic infection. HIV-infected patients frequently have multiple concurrent opportunistic infections. Patients are often being treated or receiving prophylaxis for multiple infections simultaneously, thereby leading to potential additive toxicities or drug interactions. Finally, HIV-infected patients are administered multiple courses of antimicrobial agents, often for prolonged periods. These patients have the potential for the development of drug-resistant pathogens themselves, and they are exposed to drug-resistant pathogens in clinics, hospitals, and other group settings. They are at high risk for disease caused by drug-resistant pathogens, such as *M. tuberculosis*, *P. jirovecii*, *Streptococcus pneumoniae*, and *Candida*. All of these issues support the concept that optimal management should emphasize identification of the specific organism causing a specific syndrome because the range of possible etiologic agents is broad and the adverse consequences of unnecessary drugs are magnified in patients with HIV infection compared with many other populations.

The manifestations and treatment of specific opportunistic and nonopportunistic pathogens are discussed in other chapters. Additional chapters detail pulmonary disease (Chapter 398), skin disorders (Chapter 399), hematologic problems (Chapter 400), gastrointestinal disease (Chapter 397), and neurologic disorders (Chapter 401). Several additional syndromes deserve particular mention.

Fever is a common finding in patients with HIV infection. As noted earlier, patients with HIV infection are susceptible to a wide range of processes that can cause fever, including opportunistic and nonopportunistic infections, neoplasms, and drug toxicities. The CD4$^+$ T-lymphocyte cell count is a valuable indicator of the likelihood for opportunistic pathogens. At high CD4$^+$ T-lymphocyte cell counts (e.g., >300 cells/mm^3), the evaluation should probably be similar to that for HIV-uninfected healthy individuals, although patients do have enhanced predisposition to certain processes, notably pneumococcal disease, tuberculosis, and specific neoplasms such as lymphoma and Kaposi's sarcoma.

Fever and Wasting

Early in the HIV epidemic, patients often sought care for fever of several weeks' or months' duration, associated with considerable weight loss. This is less common in the era of effective antiretroviral therapy, but it still occurs in the United States and western Europe and is especially common in emerging countries. Many of the opportunistic infections associated with HIV infection can cause this syndrome. In some patients, chronic cough, chronic diarrhea, abnormal liver function test results, and other focal findings can lead to a directed evaluation. Some patients have no focal or localizing findings. In such patients, methodical evaluation is required with specific attention to the possibility of pulmonary or disseminated tuberculosis, disseminated *M. avium* complex or fungal disease, lymphoma, and endocrine abnormalities such as adrenal insufficiency. Diagnostic evaluations that merit special consideration include mycobacterial blood cultures and serum cryptococcal and *Histoplasma* antigen testing. Extensive imaging procedures should be considered before empirical therapy is initiated.

Retinitis

Ocular manifestations are one of the most common complications of HIV infection. When patients have visual complaints, it is important to determine the anatomic location of the lesion (e.g., cornea, choroid, retina, cranial nerve, or occipital lobe) to establish the appropriate diagnostic and therapeutic approach.

CMV retinitis is the most common vision-threatening lesion. Patients almost universally have positive serum anti-CMV IgG levels and CD4$^+$ T-lymphocyte cell counts below 50 cells/mm^3. CMV causes irreversible necrosis of the retina, although treatment can restore some vision as edema of the retina subsides. Untreated, CMV retinitis causes progressive loss of vision in both eyes.

The diagnosis of CMV retinitis can be made during routine retinal examination (dilated indirect ophthalmoscopy) performed by an experienced ophthalmologist. Examination with a direct ophthalmoscope evaluates just 10% of the total retinal area; disease can be excluded only by a full funduscopic evaluation. Polymerase chain reaction (PCR) of the aqueous or vitreous can be used to document CMV, as can retinal biopsy, but such procedures are almost never used given the characteristic clinical findings. In patients with CMV retinitis, CMV disease may also be present or eventually develop in other anatomic locations, such as the colon or CNS.

The goal of therapy for CMV retinitis is to arrest progression of the disease, to prevent further spread of infection, and to preserve visual function. Therapy with one of the recommended modalities (e.g., oral valganciclovir, intravenous ganciclovir or foscarnet, or an ocular implant plus oral valganciclovir) is usually effective; maintenance therapy is necessary lifelong unless antiretroviral therapy leads to substantial immunologic reconstitution. If such reconstitution occurs, immune reconstitution syndrome (Chapter 402) can cause substantial ocular disease.

Other pathogens can also cause retinitis. Varicella-zoster virus (VZV) can cause acute retinal necrosis (CD4$^+$ T-lymphocyte cell count >50 cells/mm^3) or progressive outer retinal necrosis (CD4$^+$ T-lymphocyte cell count <50 cells/mm^3). The former often responds to acyclovir; the latter usually does not. Toxoplasmosis can likewise cause retinitis. Experienced ophthalmologists can generally distinguish *Toxoplasma* retinochoroiditis from CMV or VZV disease or from disease caused by herpes simplex virus, mycobacteria, or fungi. However, such diagnoses can be difficult to establish solely on the basis of funduscopic examination.

Central Nervous System Mass Lesions

In the era before antiretroviral therapy, focal brain lesions developed in 10% of patients, and the majority of such patients came to attention when their CD4$^+$ T-lymphocyte cell counts were less than 100 cells/mm^3. Initial signs and symptoms range from focal deficits (hemiparesis, aphasia, diplopia, seizures) to generalized weakness or altered mental status. Neuroimaging is important to confirm the clinical diagnosis of a mass lesion and to distinguish among general diagnostic categories (e.g., bacterial brain abscess, tumor, opportunistic infection, or progressive multifocal leukoencephalopathy). Neuroimaging does not, however, provide a microbiologic diagnosis. Positron emission tomography with radiolabeled glucose to measure tissue metabolism or single-photon emission computed tomography to measure metabolically linked cerebral blood flow appears to be useful to distinguish tumors (e.g., lymphoma) from infections (e.g., toxoplasmosis).

The majority of focal contrast-enhancing brain lesions in HIV-infected patients are caused by cerebral toxoplasmosis or primary CNS lymphoma. On magnetic resonance imaging or computed tomography, these lesions are often associated with surrounding edema. Although primary CNS lymphoma typically involves solitary brain lesions and cerebral toxoplasmosis is more commonly associated with multiple lesions, these diagnoses cannot be distinguished solely by neuroradiographic parameters.

Toxoplasmosis almost always is a result of reactivation of previously acquired disease in patients with CD4$^+$ T-lymphocyte cell counts below 50 cells/mm^3. Almost all patients have positive serum IgG antibodies against *Toxoplasma* if serology is performed by a reference laboratory. The diagnosis of toxoplasmosis is usually established by either response to empirical therapy

or brain biopsy. Cerebrospinal fluid (CSF) examination is rarely helpful in establishing toxoplasmosis as the diagnosis.

The majority of patients with cerebral toxoplasmosis (65 to 90%) respond rapidly to standard two-drug anti-*Toxoplasma* therapy with pyrimethamine (200 mg orally once, followed by 50 to 75 mg daily) plus either sulfadiazine (1 to 1.5 g orally every 6 hours) or clindamycin (600 mg orally or intravenously every 6 hours). Clinical improvement is generally seen within several days, and neuroradiographic improvement occurs within 2 to 3 weeks. Failure to reach these milestones should suggest other diagnoses, such as lymphoma. Patients who respond should be treated for a minimum of 6 weeks after resolution or stabilization of the clinical and radiologic abnormalities. Lifelong suppressive therapy is necessary to prevent recurrences (80% recurred in the pre–antiretroviral therapy era without secondary prophylaxis), unless the patient responds immunologically to antiretroviral therapy.

Primary CNS lymphoma and generalized lymphoma both occur in patients who are usually naive to antiretroviral therapy and commonly have less than 100 cells/mm^3. Both diseases progress rapidly, with high morbidity and mortality. HIV-associated primary CNS lymphoma occurs most often in patients with CD4$^+$ T-lymphocyte cell counts of 100 cells/mm^3 or lower. Epstein-Barr viral DNA can be detected by PCR in the CSF of most but not all patients.

Most authorities recommend treatment of primary CNS lymphoma with combination chemotherapy. Lesions are highly responsive to irradiation, but radiation therapy is associated with considerable morbidity and a dismal long-term prognosis.

Progressive multifocal leukoencephalopathy involves white matter lesions and is generally clinically distinct from the manifestations of toxoplasmosis or lymphoma. Patients usually have subacute limb weakness, sensory loss, gait difficulties, cognitive impairment, or any combination of these findings. Magnetic resonance imaging shows predominantly white matter lesions with no contrast enhancement or mass effect. JC viral DNA can be demonstrated by PCR examination of CSF.

The prognosis for progressive multifocal leukoencephalopathy is dismal; most patients die within 4 months unless they have a robust immunologic response to antiretroviral therapy. No specific therapy has been shown to be effective for progressive multifocal leukoencephalopathy.

Diarrhea

Chronic diarrhea is a common problem for patients with HIV infection and CD4$^+$ T-lymphocyte cell counts below 100 to 200 cells/mm^3. Bacteria, viruses, and protozoa are often identified, as is *Clostridium difficile* colitis. See Chapter 397 for detailed information.

Parasitic and Fungal Infections Acquired Outside the United States

In patients who live in emerging countries or those who have traveled to such areas, latent infections may reactivate once they return to the United States or emigrate there. Leishmaniasis, Chagas' disease, and malaria are examples of parasitic diseases that can be more frequent and more severe in patients with HIV infection than in those without HIV infection. *Leishmania*, for example, can reactivate years after residence in an endemic area such as the Mediterranean basin or Brazil and be associated with fever, cytopenia, and hepatosplenomegaly. Therapy with liposomal amphotericin B or pentavalent antimony is effective, although treatment may have to be lifelong unless immunity is reconstituted with highly active antiretroviral therapy. Similarly, *Trypanosoma cruzi* can be manifested as a focal cerebral mass lesion or lesions years after residence in an endemic area; therapy with benznidazole or nifurtimox has been used successfully.

⬤ IMMUNE RECONSTITUTION SYNDROMES

When patients with HIV infection initiate antiretroviral therapy, their augmented immune response may produce clinical syndromes that seem to represent immunologic or inflammatory reactions rather than disease progression from proliferating organisms. Within days, weeks, or months after antiretroviral therapy is started and sometimes before the CD4$^+$ T-lymphocyte cell count has risen, patients may manifest such a syndrome. Immune reconstitution inflammatory syndrome in HIV/AIDS is discussed in detail in Chapter 402.

⬤ MANAGEMENT OF HIV-ASSOCIATED NEOPLASMS

Therapy for HIV-associated lymphoma, Kaposi's sarcoma, human papillomavirus (HPV)–associated neoplasms, and other malignant processes such as primary effusion cell lymphoma and multicentric Castleman's disease is detailed in Chapter 400. Early in the HIV epidemic, there was little optimism that these neoplastic processes could be treated successfully. More recent studies, however, suggest that even for HIV-associated lymphoma, rates of remission and long-term survival are improving. In treatment of HIV-associated neoplasms, particular attention to antiretroviral regimens, drug toxicities, drug interactions, and chemoprophylaxis for HIV-associated opportunistic infections is required if the prognosis is to be optimized.

For patients treated successfully with long-term antiretroviral therapy, there is growing evidence that other tumors (i.e., tumors that are not AIDS defining) are becoming increasingly frequent. Lung cancer, hepatoma, Hodgkin's disease, and rectal carcinoma are examples of tumors that are occurring with increased frequency; the frequency may well be related both to HIV-related immunosuppression and to cofactors such as tobacco, alcohol, and HPV.

● PREGNANCY AND HIV INFECTION

All pregnant women should be offered antiretroviral therapy after the first trimester to minimize transmission of virus to the fetus. The choice of drugs and the timing of initiation of therapy should be influenced by the pregnancy.

Most antiretroviral drugs are safe in pregnant women, to the extent they have been studied. Many of the toxicities caused by antiretroviral agents may contribute to parallel complications of pregnancy, however (e.g., the hyperglycemia associated with protease inhibitors may exacerbate pregnancy-associated diabetes). There are specific concerns about the use of nucleosides during pregnancy, especially stavudine and didanosine, in view of their association with hepatic steatosis and lactic acidosis in several pregnant women. There is also particular concern about the use of efavirenz because of teratogenicity studies in animals and anecdotal human reports. Antiretroviral regimens must be chosen carefully and monitored.

Grade **A**

1. Panel on Antiretroviral Guidelines for Adults and Adolescents. *Guidelines for the use of antiretroviral agents in HIV-1–infected adults and adolescents.* Department of Health and Human Services. Jan. 10, 2011. http://www.aidsinfo.nih.gov/ContentFiles/AdultandAdolescentGL.pdf.
2. Centers for Disease Control and Prevention. Guidelines for Prevention and treatment of opportunistic infections in HIV-infected adults and adolescents. Recommendations from CDC, the National Institutes of Health, and the HIV Medicine Association of the Infectious Disease Society of America. *MMWR Morb Mortal Wkly Rep.* 2009;58(RR-4).
3. When To Start Consortium, Sterne JA, May M, Costagliola D, et al. Timing of initiation of antiretroviral therapy in AIDS-free HIV-1–infected patients: a collaborative analysis of 18 HIV cohort studies. *Lancet.* 2009;373:1314-1316.
4. Kitahata MM, Gange SJ, Abraham AG, et al. Effect of early versus deferred antiretroviral therapy for HIV on survival. *N Engl J Med.* 2009;360:1815-1826.
5. Severe P, Juste MA, Ambroise A, et al. Early versus standard antiretroviral therapy for HIV-infected adults in Haiti. *N Engl J Med.* 2010;363:257-265.

SUGGESTED READINGS

Abdool Karim SS, Naidoo K, Grobler A, et al. Timing of initiation of antiretroviral drugs during tuberculosis therapy. *N Engl J Med.* 2010;362:697-706. *An important study related to the timing of antiretroviral therapy when patients in South Africa present with TB and HIV coinfection.*

Deeks SG, Gange SJ, Kitahata MM, et al. Trends in multidrug treatment failure and subsequent mortality among antiretroviral therapy–experienced patients with HIV infection in North America. *Clin Infect Dis.* 2009;49:1582-1590. *A study on the outcomes for patients being treated with antiretroviral therapy despite prior failures.*

Li JZ, Paredes R, Ribaudo HJ, et al. Low-frequency HIV-1 drug resistance mutations and risk of NNRTI-based antiretroviral treatment failure: a systematic review and pooled analysis. *JAMA.* 2011;305:1327-1335. *Review.*

Pirrone V, Thakkar-Rivera N, Jacobson JM, et al. Combinatorial approaches to the prevention and treatment of HIV-1 infection. *Antimicrob Agents Chemother.* 2011;55:1831-1842. *Review of existing and developing combination therapies.*

Rerks-Ngarm S, Pitisuttithum P, Nitayaphan S, et al. Vaccination with ALVAC and AIDSVAX to prevent HIV-1 infection in Thailand. *N Engl J Med.* 2009;361:2209-2220. *The first major trial to support the concept that vaccines could have a beneficial effect in terms of reducing HIV transmission, but clearly a support of concept, not yet a tool for widespread use.*

The HIV-CAUSAL Collaboration. When to initiate combined antiretroviral therapy to reduce mortality and AIDS-defining illness in HIV-infected persons in developed countries: an observational study. *Ann Intern Med.* 2011;154:509-515. *AIDS-free survival but not overall mortality improves when cART is initiated at a threshold CD4 count of 0.500 cells/µL rather than 200 cells/µL.*

Thompson MA, Aberg JA, Cahn P, et al. Antiretroviral treatment of adult HIV infection: 2010 recommendations of the International AIDS Society-USA panel. *JAMA.* 2010;304:321-333. *Consensus guidelines.*

Volberding PA, Deeks SG. Antiretroviral therapy and management of HIV infection. *Lancet.* 2010;376:49-62. *Review.*

397

GASTROINTESTINAL MANIFESTATIONS OF HIV AND AIDS

TAMSIN A. KNOX AND CHRISTINE WANKE

● INTRODUCTION

Gastrointestinal (GI) diseases were among the leading causes of morbidity and mortality in persons infected with human immunodeficiency virus (HIV) before the advent of highly active antiretroviral therapy (HAART) in 1996. Profound wasting and chronic diarrhea are still manifestations of end-stage acquired immunodeficiency syndrome (AIDS) in persons not receiving or resistant to antiretroviral therapy (ART). However, the common GI problems found today in persons receiving effective ART have shifted away from the enteric and hepatobiliary infections associated with low CD4$^+$ counts. Current GI issues are mainly due to side effects of antiretroviral medications, to nutritional and metabolic disorders associated with chronic HIV disease and therapy, and to liver disease from coinfection with hepatitis B virus (HBV) and hepatitis C virus (HCV).

The degree of immunosuppression, measured by the CD4$^+$ count, is the most important determinant of the likelihood of a GI illness, the type of disease, and its severity. The more profound the CD4$^+$ count suppression, the more likely a GI disease will be present.

The route of transmission of HIV may affect GI function; men who have sex with men (MSM) have higher rates of diarrhea and Kaposi's sarcoma than do those who acquired HIV from intravenous drug use (IVDU). Alcohol abuse or IVDU predisposes to liver disease. Regional exposures may increase the risk for disease. In resource-limited settings, lack of ART, increased exposure to pathogens, lack of clean water, poverty, and hunger are associated with increased prevalence and severity of GI disease. In contrast, nutritional and metabolic diseases such as obesity, metabolic syndrome, and fatty liver are seen in HIV populations with high caloric and fat intake and lack of exercise. All treatment recommendations are summarized in Table 397-1.

● GASTROINTESTINAL DISEASES FOUND WITH CD4$^+$ COUNTS GREATER THAN 200 TO 500 CELLS/µL

The GI diseases discussed in this section may also be seen with more advanced HIV infection.

Side Effects of Medications

Adverse effects of medications are frequently seen in the course of HIV treatment and may be due to ART or to the medications required for treatment or prevention of opportunistic infections. Gastric effects, including nausea, vomiting, loss of appetite, and dyspepsia, may occur as a symptom of the HIV infection itself or in response to ART regimens, particularly those with zidovudine, didanosine, ritonavir, amprenavir, or indinavir. Hypersensitivity reactions to ART, such as occurs in persons with the HLA-B5701 haplotype who take abacavir, may also be manifested as fever, abdominal pain, and rash. Didanosine, stavudine, and pentamidine may cause acute pancreatitis.

Lactic acidosis is a life-threatening condition caused by mitochondrial toxicity from nucleoside reverse transcriptase inhibitors (NRTIs), particularly stavudine, didanosine, and zidovudine. Early discontinuation of NRTIs and supportive care are key to recovery, but the syndrome may be difficult to diagnose because of nonspecific findings such as fatigue, nausea, muscle aches, weight loss, or abdominal pain. Blood lactate levels are usually greater than 5 mmol/mL. Nevirapine has been associated with liver toxicity when used in individuals with CD4$^+$ counts higher than 400 cells/µL. One of the most common adverse effects of atazanavir has been asymptomatic elevation in indirect bilirubin. Some ART agents have also been associated with the development of significant elevations in triglycerides, to levels above 1000 mg/dL, and the development of pancreatitis.

Although all antiretrovirals have been associated with diarrhea, nelfinavir is particularly known to cause a secretory form of diarrhea. Intestinal

TABLE 397-1 RELATIONSHIP OF GASTROINTESTINAL DISEASES TO CD4+ COUNTS IN HIV-INFECTED PATIENTS

CD4+ COUNT	SYSTEM	SYMPTOMS AND DISEASES	TREATMENT
>200-500 cells/μL	Gastrointestinal and pancreas	**Nausea, vomiting, abdominal pain**	
		Side effects of medications	Changes in antiretroviral regimen
		Pancreatitis	Lipid-lowering agents, low-fat diet, no alcohol
		Diarrhea	Treat specific pathogens, if present
			Antimotility agents and fiber
	Nutritional and metabolic	**Lactic acidosis**	Stop nucleoside reverse transcriptase inhibitors
		Stavudine, didanosine, zidovudine	
		Changes in body shape	
		Obesity	Diet, exercise
		Metabolic syndrome	Diet, exercise, lipid-lowering agents, insulin-sensitizing agents
		Visceral obesity	hGH/GHRH in clinical trials
	Liver	**Liver function abnormalities, cirrhosis**	
		Chronic hepatitis with HCV	Pegylated interferon and ribavirin
		Chronic HBV infection	Nucleosides/tides for HBV infection
		Hepatotoxicity	Stop implicated antiretrovirals
	Oral lesions (≈400-500 cells/μL)	**Plaques, pain**	
		Oral thrush	Clotrimazole troche, nystatin, oral azoles
		Hairy leukoplakia	Acyclovir
		Herpes simplex-1	Acyclovir, famciclovir, valacyclovir
		Idiopathic ulcers	Corticosteroids, thalidomide (men)
		Gingivitis	Topical chlorhexidine, oral metronidazole
		Kaposi's sarcoma	Radiation, intralesional injection, systemic chemotherapy
	Anorectal lesions	**Anorectal pain, mass, discharge, tenesmus**	
		Anal fissure, fistula, or perirectal abscess	Local care, surgery
		Foreign body in rectum	Endoscopic or surgical removal
		Sexually transmitted disease	
		Gonorrhea, *Chlamydia trachomatis*, syphilis	Specific antibiotic therapy
		Herpes simplex infection	Acyclovir, famciclovir, valacyclovir
		Condyloma	Podophyllin, surgical excision, or ablation
		Anal cancer	Surgery, chemoradiation therapy
<200 cells/μL	Esophagus	**Dysphagia, odynophagia**	
	<200 cells/μL	*Candida*	Fluconazole, itraconazole, (voriconazole)
	<50 cells/μL	CMV	Ganciclovir
		Idiopathic ulcers	Oral corticosteroids, thalidomide (men)
		HSV	Acyclovir, famciclovir, valaciclovir
<100 cells/μL	Intestine	**Diarrhea**	
		Bacterial, viral, or protozoal infection	Treat specific pathogens
		AIDS enteropathy	Antimotility agents, nutritional support, ART
		Abdominal pain, fever	
		CMV	Treat specific pathogens
		Mycobacterium tuberculosis, MAC, *Histoplasma*	Surgery if perforation or dead bowel
		Cryptosporidium	
	Malignancy	**GI bleeding, weight loss, or abdominal pain**	
		Kaposi's sarcoma	As above
		Lymphoma	Systemic chemotherapy
<50 cells/μL	Wasting	**Weight loss**	
		Increased metabolic demands (infection, HIV)	Treat HIV and underlying infections
		Decreased oral intake	Appetite stimulants
		Malabsorption	Anabolic steroids, hGH
	Hepatobiliary	**Hepatomegaly, elevated liver function test results**	
		Opportunistic infections—MAC, fungal	Consider liver biopsy
		Lymphoma	
		Jaundice, RUQ pain, elevated liver function test results	
		AIDS cholangiopathy	ERCP and sphincterotomy
		Acalculous cholecystitis	Laparoscopic cholecystectomy

AIDS = acquired immunodeficiency syndrome; ART = antiretroviral therapy; CMV = cytomegalovirus; ERCP = endoscopic retrograde cholangiopancreatography; GHRH = growth hormone–releasing hormone; GI = gastrointestinal; HBV = hepatitis B virus; HCV = hepatitis C virus; hGH = human growth hormone; HIV = human immunodeficiency syndrome; HSV = herpes simplex virus; MAC = *Mycobacterium avium* complex; RUQ = right upper quadrant.

pathogens should be sought in stool examinations despite a normal CD4+ count or low HIV load.

Nutritional and Metabolic Disorders

With the advent of effective ART and the conversion of HIV to a chronic, manageable disease, overnutrition and obesity have become frequent complications of HIV infection. Lifestyle factors and poor dietary choices may help promote the development of overweight/obesity, but some weight gain and increases in visceral fat may be related to the use of specific ART agents. HIV-associated lipodystrophy syndrome, which was recognized after the introduction of effective triple ART regimens, is a complex of four distinct components: visceral fat accumulation, subcutaneous fat atrophy,

atherogenic lipid profiles, and glucose intolerance. The pathogenesis remains unclear, but nutritional intake probably contributes to all components except fat atrophy. Chronic inflammation caused by long-term HIV infection and selected antiretrovirals has been implicated as well, particularly the protease inhibitors. Host factors (genetics) also probably play a role in producing these syndromes. The co-occurrence of visceral fat accumulation, atherogenic lipid profiles, and glucose intolerance defines metabolic syndrome, diagnosis of which requires three of the following factors: high triglyceride levels, low high-density lipoprotein levels, hypertension, elevated waist circumference, and glucose intolerance. The prevalence of metabolic syndrome has increased dramatically in HIV-infected individuals, and there is concern that it may contribute to the increased risk for cardiovascular disease in persons infected with HIV.

Liver Disease

Liver disease is now the second leading cause of death in those with HIV infection because of the prevalence of coinfection with chronic viral hepatitis (Chapter 151). Coinfection with HCV is present in approximately 25%, depending on the HIV transmission category: 50 to 90% of IVDUs and hemophiliacs, 10 to 20% of heterosexuals, and 5 to 10% of MSM. Chronic HBV infection, defined by the presence of hepatitis B surface antigen (HBsAg), is found in approximately 10% of persons with HIV, and some have more than one viral coinfection. Hepatic fibrosis progresses more rapidly in HIV-infected individuals and leads to cirrhosis, decompensated liver disease, or hepatic failure (Chapter 157). This may be further accelerated by alcohol use, steatosis, or fatty liver disease and by hepatotoxicity from ART. Coinfection with HCV or HBV increases the risk for death by four- to six-fold over HIV infection alone. Mortality from liver disease increases as CD4$^+$ cells decline, more markedly with CD4$^+$ counts lower than 100 cells/μL. Early diagnosis and treatment of HCV and HBV may arrest or slow the progression of hepatic fibrosis and reduce the hepatotoxicity associated with antiretroviral treatment.

All persons with HIV infection should be screened for coinfection with HBV and HCV. A positive serologic test for HBsAg indicates chronic HBV infection and should be followed by tests for HBV DNA and hepatitis B e antigen. Those without chronic HBV infection and with no protective antibody to HBV surface antigen (negative anti-HBs) should be vaccinated against HBV. If treatment of hepatitis B is to be initiated in the absence of ART, a dual regimen of telbivudine and adefovir is appropriate because these agents will not select for HIV resistance. A positive test for HCV antibody should prompt testing for HCV RNA, which determines whether chronic HCV infection is present. Noninvasive markers of hepatic fibrosis, serum biomarkers, and hepatic elastography (to measure hepatic stiffness) are being developed to replace liver biopsy. The prevalence of hepatocellular carcinoma (HCC) (Chapter 202) is increased in those with HIV coinfection; it is found at a younger age and is more aggressive in HIV-infected patients. Regular 6-month screening for HCC by serum α-fetoprotein levels and ultrasound imaging of the liver in persons with cirrhosis may help identify lesions earlier.

Randomized clinical trials have shown that anti-HCV therapy can induce a sustained virologic response (SVR), that is, undetectable levels of HCV RNA measured 6 months after the end of treatment. However, SVR rates are approximately 60 to 80% of those achieved in persons with HCV monoinfection. Pegylated interferon alfa given for 48 weeks with ribavirin■ is associated with significant side effects, including anemia, bone marrow suppression, weight loss, flulike symptoms, and depression. To avoid drug interactions, neither didanosine (lactic acidosis) nor zidovudine (anemia) should be given with ribavirin.

Hepatotoxicity from ART occurs in up to 12% of patients started on a new ART regimen. Risk factors for hepatotoxicity include chronic HCV or HBV infection, female sex, and the use of ritonavir or nevirapine in the regimen. Effective ART has been associated with reduced hepatic inflammation, less progression of hepatic fibrosis, and decreased mortality from liver disease.

Oral Lesions

New oral lesions should raise suspicion for HIV disease. The lesions may be unsightly but asymptomatic or cause discomfort and difficulty eating. Thrush appears as white plaques, usually on the buccal mucosa. Oral hairy leukoplakia, which is associated with Epstein-Barr virus, consists of raised shaggy, dirty white patches on the sides of the tongue but is not premalignant.

Oral ulcers are caused by infection with herpes simplex virus type 1 (HSV-1) and tend to be more severe and persistent than ulcers in immunocompetent hosts. Idiopathic ulcers, similar to those found in the esophagus, are found in patients with advanced HIV disease. These deep, necrotic ulcers are most commonly found on the buccal and pharyngeal mucosa. They respond to systemic corticosteroids or thalidomide. Gingivitis and periodontal disease appear as linear or diffuse erythema of the gums. With declining CD4$^+$ counts, it may progress to necrotizing gingivitis with pain and hemorrhage. There is increasing concern that these bacterial diseases may contribute to systemic inflammation and more rapid progression of HIV disease.

Kaposi's sarcoma (Chapter 400), a multicentric malignancy of endothelial cells caused by human herpesvirus 8 infection, is more common in MSM with HIV infection in the United States but is also prevalent in Africa. Oral lesions are found in half of persons with other sites of Kaposi's sarcoma and appear on the palate or gums as raised reddish or bluish nodules.

Anorectal Diseases

Anorectal disorders in HIV-infected individuals are more prevalent in MSM. Anal fissures, fistulas, abscesses, and foreign objects may be found on anal examination as a consequence of receptive anal intercourse or manipulation. Proctitis caused by gonorrhea (Neisseria gonorrhoeae) (Chapter 307) is characterized by mucopurulent discharge from the anus, tenesmus, and bleeding. Chlamydia trachomatis infection (Chapter 326) also causes proctitis and inguinal lymphadenopathy. Cultures and swabs of the discharge are diagnostic.

Primary syphilis (Chapter 327) is manifested as an anal chancre or ulcer that may be tender because of its location. Secondary syphilis appears 2 to 6 months later as condylomata lata, or warty masses around the anus. Perianal, shallow painful ulcers caused by HSV (Chapter 382) evolve as the initial vesicles rupture. These ulcerations may be cultured for HSV, or scrapings will show viral inclusions. Patients may have concurrent herpes proctitis.

Anal condylomata or warts are caused by infection with human papillomavirus (HPV) (Chapter 381) and appear as white, pink, or gray painless lesions around the anus and in the anal canal. HPV types 16 and 18 are associated with the development of dysplasia and squamous cell cancer of the anus, which is manifested as bleeding or a mass. The prevalence of anal dysplasia may be as high as 50% in HIV-positive MSM, and the incidence of anal cancer has increased more than six-fold in the past 2 decades. Screening via anal cytology is being pioneered for high-risk individuals.

● GASTROINTESTINAL DISEASES MORE COMMONLY SEEN WITH CD4$^+$ COUNTS LESS THAN 200 CELLS/μL

GI illness increases in prevalence and severity as the CD4$^+$ count declines. With marked immunosuppression, there may be multiple concurrent infections. Although specific antimicrobial therapy may control the infection, HAART is the most effective therapy.

Esophageal Diseases

Candidal esophagitis (Chapter 346) is the most common esophageal infection in HIV-infected individuals. The combination of oral thrush and dysphagia has a positive predictive value of 90% for esophageal candidiasis. If the symptoms do not resolve with treatment in 7 days, endoscopy is indicated. Cytomegalovirus (CMV) (Chapter 384) and idiopathic esophageal ulcerations may appear when the CD4$^+$ count falls below 50 cells/μL. Odynophagia, or severe pain on swallowing, is the initial symptom. Endoscopy shows large ulcerations with elevated margins, and CMV inclusions are seen in biopsy samples. HSV infections are much less common and appear as confluent shallow ulcerations in the esophagus. Idiopathic ulceration is diagnosed by the absence of viral inclusions on biopsy specimens.

Diarrhea

Diarrhea remains a common illness in HIV-infected individuals, even in the era of effective ART. Infections of the small intestine are accompanied by large-volume watery diarrhea. Colonic disease may be manifested as bloody, inflammatory, or small-volume diarrhea and tenesmus. Routine bacterial pathogens, including Salmonella, Campylobacter, and Shigella, have all been documented to cause diarrhea in HIV-infected patients. Enteroaggregative Escherichia coli has been identified as a cause of persistent diarrhea in HIV-infected individuals. The use of multiple antibiotics in HIV-infected patients has led to the frequent occurrence of Clostridium difficile colitis. Mycobacterial infections with either Mycobacterium tuberculosis or atypical mycobacteria, most commonly Mycobacterium avium complex (MAC), may infiltrate the small bowel in HIV-infected patients. Although M. tuberculosis infection occurs with exposure in individuals with moderate CD4$^+$ cell depletion, disseminated MAC disease occurs only in individuals with CD4$^+$ counts lower than 50 cells/μL.

Most often, viral diarrheas are similar in manifestation to those in the general population, pathogens are not routinely identified in the clinical setting, and disease is self-limited. However, CMV may cause disease throughout the length of the GI tract in HIV-infected patients with CD4$^+$ counts lower than 50 cells/μL. In the small bowel, CMV may cause a watery diarrhea and, in the colon, a colitis with blood and signs of inflammation on endoscopy. Biopsy with identification of virus in tissue is required to make the diagnosis of CMV enteric disease.

Parasitic causes of diarrhea are common in HIV-infected individuals. Opportunistic parasitic pathogens include *Cryptosporidium parvum*, the microsporidial organisms *Enterocytozoon bieneusi* and *Encephalitozoon intestinalis*, and *Cyclospora cayetanensis*. Persistent diarrhea caused by cryptosporidiosis (Chapter 358) occurs when the CD4$^+$ count is less than 200 cells/μL, and the most effective control of this pathogen is treatment of HIV.

Pathogens are not found in up to half of cases of diarrhea in HIV-infected patients, even after a full diagnostic evaluation. This condition has been called *AIDS enteropathy* and is associated with chronic diarrhea, malnutrition, and wasting. It is possible that some of the chronic diarrhea is caused by pathogens that are not yet recognized or by noninfectious causes such as lymphoma. It is also likely that some of these pathogen-negative diarrheas are caused by HIV itself, which may infect the enterocyte, as well as lymphoid tissue within the gut.

Malignancy

Kaposi's sarcoma (Chapter 400) may develop at any location in the GI tract. Kaposi's lesions appear endoscopically as raised reddish nodules that may bleed spontaneously. Non-Hodgkin's lymphomas may involve any portion of the GI tract, as well as the liver, and are manifested as bleeding, obstruction, weight loss, or abdominal pain.

Wasting

Wasting in HIV-infected individuals is defined by the World Health Organization as a body mass index of less than 18.5 kg/m^2. Weight loss and wasting are still seen in patients with treated HIV infection, and even modest weight loss of 3% or greater increases mortality.

In uncontrolled HIV infection, multiple factors contribute to wasting. Caloric requirements are increased by the metabolic demands of HIV replication, concurrent opportunistic infections, and fever. Oral intake may be poor because of nausea, anorexia, dysphagia, odynophagia, or chronic diarrhea or as a result of food insecurity, depression, or dementia. Weight loss is exacerbated by malabsorption of nutrients from small intestinal or pancreatic disease. HIV-infected persons may not be able to increase caloric intake to overcome the loss of nutrients in stool and meet the metabolic demands of their illness. Targeted approaches to wasting and weight loss include treatment of HIV or opportunistic infections, frequent small meals, and use of appetite stimulants (megestrol acetate, dronabinol), anabolic steroids (testosterone, oxandrolone, nandrolone), or recombinant human growth hormone, as indicated. With control of HIV replication, nutritional status and weight generally improve, although they may not return to premorbid levels if the wasting was severe.

Hepatobiliary Disease

Hepatobiliary disease is associated with very low CD4$^+$ counts, often less than 20 cells/μL. Evaluation of abnormalities in liver function should initially exclude HBV and HCV infection and drug-induced hepatotoxicity, particularly that involving antiretroviral or sulfa-containing medications. The presence of hepatomegaly suggests an infiltrative process such as MAC or fungal infection or lymphoma. Alkaline phosphatase is disproportionately elevated. Liver imaging often does not show a localized lesion but determines whether biliary dilation is present, a finding suggestive of extrahepatic disease. Liver biopsy with special stains and cultures may be definitive.

In contrast, the presence of right upper quadrant pain with or without jaundice indicates biliary tract disease (Chapter 158). AIDS cholangiopathy includes a sclerosing cholangitis–like process with diffuse biliary strictures and dilations and papillary stenosis with narrowing of the distal common bile duct at the entrance to the duodenum. In papillary stenosis, the common bile duct is dilated proximal to the stenosis. Acalculous cholecystitis may also be seen. These changes are caused by infection of the biliary tree with *Cryptosporidium*, microsporidia, *Isospora belli*, or CMV in the setting of profound immunosuppression. Endoscopic retrograde cholangiopancreatography can be performed to establish the diagnosis, obtain brushings for examination, and treat papillary stenosis by sphincterotomy. Treatment of the specific organism seldom eradicates infection because of the degree of immunosuppression. However, treatment with ART can result in marked improvements in biliary findings.

● APPROACH TO GASTROINTESTINAL DISEASES

The GI tract is host to a myriad of infectious and infiltrative diseases in HIV-infected persons. Even so, routine GI diseases such as diverticulitis, choledocholithiasis, or peptic ulcer disease must be considered, particularly in those treated with ART. The clinician is guided by the symptom complex, as laid out in Table 397-1, to identify the probable organisms or tumors by clinical findings. The CD4$^+$ count influences the likelihood of the type of GI infection. It is important to remember that multiple illnesses may occur simultaneously with HIV infection and that finding one cause of a symptom or complaint may not be sufficient.

With diarrhea, careful stool evaluations should include cultures for *Salmonella*, *Shigella*, and *Campylobacter*; assay for *Clostridium difficile* toxin; and at least three examinations for parasites, including acid-fast stains for MAC and *Cryptosporidium*. If these measures are unrevealing, upper GI endoscopy with biopsy of the small intestine is indicated to diagnose protozoal infections with *Cryptosporidium*, *Isospora belli*, or microsporidia. Signs of colitis are best evaluated by flexible sigmoidoscopy or colonoscopy with biopsy and cultures. Examination and biopsy of the terminal ileum with acid-fast stain is necessary to confirm the diagnosis of pathogens such as *M. tuberculosis* or MAC.

All persons with HIV should be screened for coinfection with HBV and HCV and vaccinated against hepatitis A and B if not immune. Finally, close attention to serial measurement of weight and calculation of the body mass index is crucial to identify those who may have poor outcomes as a result of weight loss or excessive weight gain.

1. Núñez M, Miralles C, Berdún MA, et al. Role of weight-based ribavirin dosing and extended duration of therapy in chronic hepatitis C in HIV-infected patients: the PRESCO trial. *AIDS Res Hum Retroviruses*. 2007;23:972-982.

SUGGESTED READINGS

Cello JP, Day LW. Idiopathic AIDS enteropathy and treatment of gastrointestinal opportunistic pathogens. *Gastroenterology*. 2009;136:1952-1965. *An approach to the evaluation and treatment of diarrhea in HIV-infected patients in the HAART era.*

Huppmann AR, Orenstein JM. Opportunistic disorders of the gastrointestinal tract in the age of highly active antiretroviral therapy. *Hum Pathol*. 2010;41:1777-1787. *The most common were* Candida *(esophagus);* H. pylori *(stomach); and* Cytomegalovirus, Mycobacterium avium *complex, and* Cryptosporidium *(small and large bowel).*

Silva RC, Benati FJ, Pena GP, et al. Molecular characterization of viruses associated with gastrointestinal infection in HIV-positive patients. *Braz J Infect Dis*. 2010;14:549-552. *In HIV-infected patients with diarrhea in Brazil, viral infections (especially CMV) were more common than parasitic infections.*

Stensvold CR, Nielsen SD, Badsberg JH, et al. The prevalence and clinical significance of instestinal parasites in HIV-infected patients in Denmark. *Scand J Infect Dis*. 2011;43:129-135. *Review showing* Entamoeba *were more common than* Isospora *and* Cryptosporidium.

398

PULMONARY MANIFESTATIONS OF HUMAN IMMUNODEFICIENCY VIRUS INFECTION AND ACQUIRED IMMUNODEFICIENCY SYNDROME

LAURENCE HUANG

DEFINITION

Respiratory symptoms are common in individuals infected with human immunodeficiency virus (HIV), and HIV-infected patients are subject to a wide spectrum of pulmonary diseases, both those associated with HIV (Table 398-1) and those not associated with HIV. The spectrum of HIV-associated pulmonary diseases encompasses opportunistic infections, neoplasms, and other pulmonary disorders. Table 398-1 lists the most frequent pulmonary diseases seen in HIV-infected patients in the United States. In other parts of the world, these frequencies may be strikingly different. Although each pulmonary disease has characteristic clinical and radiographic findings, they can vary and often overlap.

TABLE 398-1 HIV-ASSOCIATED PULMONARY DISEASES

Opportunistic Infections

BACTERIAL	MYCOBACTERIAL	FUNGAL	VIRAL/ PARASITIC
Streptococcus pneumoniae	Mycobacterium tuberculosis	Pneumocystis jirovecii*	Cytomegalovirus
Haemophilus species	Mycobacterium kansasii	Cryptococcus neoformans	Influenza
Pseudomonas aeruginosa	Mycobacterium avium complex	Histoplasma capsulatum	Toxoplasma gondii
Staphylococcus aureus		Coccidioides immitis	
Klebsiella pneumoniae		Aspergillus species (esp. fumigatus)	

Neoplasms and Selected Noninfectious Diseases

NEOPLASM	LYMPHOPROLIFERATIVE DISORDERS	MISCELLANEOUS DISORDERS
Kaposi's sarcoma	Nonspecific interstitial pneumonitis	Pulmonary arterial hypertension
Non-Hodgkin's lymphoma	Lymphocytic interstitial pneumonitis	Chronic obstructive pulmonary disease
Lung cancer		Sarcoidosis
		Immune reconstitution syndromes

*The form of *Pneumocystis* that infects humans is *Pneumocystis jirovecii* (formerly *Pneumocystis carinii*).

TABLE 398-2 DIAGNOSTIC APPROACH TO PULMONARY DISEASE IN HIV-INFECTED PERSONS: CLUES

CLINICAL SETTING

Ambulatory: URI > acute bronchitis > bacterial pneumonia > *Pneumocystis* pneumonia
Hospital: bacterial pneumonia > *Pneumocystis* pneumonia > TB > pulmonary KS
Intensive care unit: *Pneumocystis* pneumonia > bacterial pneumonia; non–AIDS associated > AIDS associated conditions

CD4⁺ CELL COUNT (see Table 398-3)
PATIENT BACKGROUND

HIV transmission category: MSM—increased incidence of KS; IDU—increased incidence of bacterial pneumonia, TB
Habits: cigarettes—increased incidence of bacterial bronchitis, bacterial pneumonia, COPD, RB-ILD, bronchogenic carcinoma
Travel and residence: assess risk for endemic fungal diseases, TB

MEDICAL BACKGROUND AND USE OF PROPHYLAXIS

Previous disease: increased incidence of recurrence of bacterial pneumonia, *Pneumocystis* pneumonia, fungal pneumonias
Prophylaxis/maintenance: decreased incidence of disease—*Pneumocystis* pneumonia, fungal pneumonias, TB (if PPD positive or positive interferon-γ release assay)

SYMPTOMS AND SIGNS

Respiratory symptoms: especially cough (productive or nonproductive) and symptom duration
Symptoms suggesting extrapulmonary or disseminated disease
Physical examination of the chest: focal or nonfocal findings
Signs suggesting extrapulmonary or disseminated disease

LABORATORY TESTS

WBC count: elevated or, if normal, elevated relative to baseline—bacterial pneumonia
Serum LDH: elevated—nonspecific but classically seen in *Pneumocystis* pneumonia
Arterial blood gas: nonspecific but useful for prognosis, management decisions (e.g., admission and whether corticosteroids are indicated for *Pneumocystis* pneumonia)

CHEST RADIOGRAPH (see Figs. 398-9 and 398-10)

AIDS = acquired immunodeficiency syndrome; COPD = chronic obstructive pulmonary disease; HIV, human immunodeficiency virus; IDU = injection drug user; KS = Kaposi's sarcoma; LDH = lactate dehydrogenase; MSM = men who have sex with men; PPD = purified protein derivative (in an HIV-infected person, PPD is considered positive if ≥5-mm induration); RB-ILD = respiratory bronchiolitis–interstitial lung disease; TB = tuberculosis; URI = upper respiratory tract infection; WBC = white blood cell.

DIAGNOSIS

Initial Diagnostic Approach

The frequency of HIV-associated opportunistic pneumonias and the need for prompt treatment of these infections often focus the initial diagnostic approach and management on identifying and treating possible infectious causes. However, HIV-infected persons may have HIV-associated neoplasms or other disorders, and the prevalence of these noninfectious conditions may be increasing. In addition, risk factors for HIV infection, such as injection drug use, may also contribute to pulmonary disease (e.g., endocarditis with septic pulmonary emboli). Finally, HIV-infected individuals may have preexisting pulmonary disease (e.g., asthma), or pulmonary disease unrelated to their HIV infection (e.g., pulmonary embolism) may develop and be the cause of their respiratory symptoms. Therefore, in the proper clinical context, clinicians must also consider noninfectious HIV-associated pulmonary diseases and non–HIV-associated disorders before embarking on an exhaustive search for HIV-associated opportunistic infections. This is especially important inasmuch as HIV-infected patients receiving combination antiretroviral therapy are living longer and new associations with traditionally non–HIV-related disorders are increasingly being found.

Clinical Setting

The clinical setting in which the patient is encountered and evaluated has an impact on the relative frequency of the pulmonary diseases seen (Table 398-2). The Pulmonary Complications of HIV Infection Study found that patients seen as outpatients more often had upper respiratory tract infections and acute bronchitis than pneumonia secondary to bacteria or *Pneumocystis jirovecii* (formerly *Pneumocystis carinii*). However, neither of the former conditions typically necessitates hospitalization, whereas a significant number of patients with the latter diseases require hospitalization. The most common pulmonary diseases in hospitalized HIV-infected patients are bacterial pneumonia, followed by *Pneumocystis* pneumonia, both of which are significantly more frequent than the next most common diagnoses: tuberculosis, pulmonary Kaposi's sarcoma (KS), and *Cryptococcus neoformans* pneumonia. The Pulmonary Complications of HIV Infection Study found that the most common pulmonary disease in patients requiring critical care was *Pneumocystis* pneumonia, followed by bacterial pneumonia. Currently, non–acquired immunodeficiency syndrome (AIDS)-associated conditions are often more frequent indications for critical care than are AIDS-associated conditions in HIV-infected persons.

The geographic location may also influence the frequency of different diagnoses. In specific populations or particular geographic regions, mycobacterial and endemic fungal pneumonias become important considerations. Worldwide, tuberculosis is the dominant disease. In endemic areas, diseases caused by *Histoplasma capsulatum* or *Coccidioides immitis* are among the most frequent infections seen.

Laboratory Findings

CD4⁺ Lymphocyte Count

The CD4⁺ cell count is an excellent indicator of an HIV-infected patient's risk for the development of a specific opportunistic infection or a particular neoplasm. Many of the HIV-associated pulmonary diseases become manifested once a patient's CD4⁺ cell count has declined to a certain level, and these diseases only occasionally occur in a patient whose CD4⁺ cell count is above that level (Table 398-3). The exceptions are diseases that can develop in persons without underlying immunodeficiency, such as bacterial pneumonia, tuberculosis, and non-Hodgkin's lymphoma. These diseases can occur at any CD4⁺ cell count in HIV-infected patients. However, their incidence increases as the CD4⁺ cell count declines. One study found that the risk for bacterial pneumonia in HIV-infected subjects with a CD4⁺ cell count of less than 200 cells/μL was more than 5.5 times greater than that in subjects whose CD4⁺ cell count was higher than 500 cells/μL. In addition, as the CD4⁺ cell count declines, the incidence of bacterial pneumonia accompanied by bacteremia (especially *Streptococcus pneumoniae*) and the incidence of *Mycobacterium tuberculosis* infection accompanied by extrapulmonary or disseminated disease increase, features that have important implications for diagnosis.

At CD4⁺ cell counts lower than 200 cells/μL, *Pneumocystis* and *C. neoformans* pneumonias become significant diagnoses to consider. A review from

TABLE 398-3 CD4⁺ CELL COUNT RANGES FOR HIV-ASSOCIATED PULMONARY DISEASES

ANY CD4⁺ CELL COUNT

Bacterial pneumonia (most often *S. pneumoniae*, *Haemophilus* species)
M. tuberculosis pneumonia
Influenza
Non-Hodgkin's lymphoma
Lung cancer
Nonspecific interstitial pneumonitis
Lymphocytic interstitial pneumonitis
Pulmonary arterial hypertension
Chronic obstructive lung disease

CD4⁺ CELL COUNT <200 CELLS/μL

Pneumocystis pneumonia
Cryptococcus neoformans pneumonia

CD4⁺ CELL COUNT <100 CELLS/μL

Bacterial pneumonia caused by *Pseudomonas aeruginosa*
Toxoplasma gondii pneumonia
Pulmonary Kaposi's sarcoma

CD4⁺ CELL COUNT <50 CELLS/μL

Mycobacterium avium complex—usually associated with disseminated disease
Histoplasma capsulatum—usually associated with disseminated disease
Coccidioides immitis—usually associated with disseminated disease
Aspergillus species (most often *Aspergillus fumigatus*) pneumonia
Cytomegalovirus pneumonia—usually associated with disseminated disease

---

the Clinical Center of the National Institutes of Health found that 46 of 49 patients (94%) in whom *Pneumocystis* pneumonia was diagnosed had a CD4⁺ cell count of less than 200 cells/μL. The Multicenter AIDS Cohort Study demonstrated that HIV-infected subjects with a CD4⁺ cell count lower than 200 cells/μL at study entry had nearly a five-fold greater risk for *Pneumocystis* pneumonia than did subjects who had a CD4⁺ cell count higher than 200 cells/μL at entry. Finally, the Pulmonary Complications of HIV Infection Study reported that 95% of 145 cases of *Pneumocystis* pneumonia occurred in subjects whose CD4⁺ cell count was less than 200 cells/μL (median CD4⁺ count, 29 cells/μL).

At CD4⁺ cell counts lower than 100 cells/μL, pneumonias secondary to *Pseudomonas aeruginosa* and *Toxoplasma gondii* and lung involvement by KS are increasingly diagnosed. One study of 64 HIV-infected patients with pulmonary toxoplasmosis diagnosed by bronchoalveolar lavage (BAL) reported a mean CD4⁺ cell count of 40 cells/μL; 82% had a CD4⁺ count of less than 50 cells/μL, and only 4% had a count higher than 200 cells/μL. A series of 168 consecutive HIV-infected patients with pulmonary KS diagnosed by bronchoscopy reported a median CD4⁺ cell count of 19 cells/μL; 68% had a CD4⁺ count lower than 50 cells/μL, and only 4% had a count higher than 200 cells/μL.

Finally, at CD4⁺ cell counts lower than 50 cells/μL, nontuberculous mycobacteria (*Mycobacterium avium* complex), endemic (*H. capsulatum*, *C. immitis*) and nonendemic (*Aspergillus* species) fungi, and cytomegalovirus increasingly become important causes to consider. These diseases are usually accompanied by extrapulmonary or disseminated disease, which can dominate the clinical findings. In many of these cases, the patient may have minimal or no respiratory complaints, and findings on chest radiography are often normal. One review noted respiratory complaints in 53% of HIV-infected patients with disseminated histoplasmosis and normal findings on chest radiography in 43%.

History
Patient Background

A number of important diagnostic clues can be gleaned from a patient's personal and medical background that may help suggest specific diagnoses (see Table 398-2).

Health Habits and Mode of HIV Transmission

A patient's health-related habits and mode of acquiring HIV influence the relative frequency of various HIV-related and non–HIV-related pulmonary diseases. In the United States, HIV-associated KS is seen almost exclusively in men who report having sexual relationships with other men. Bacterial pneumonia and tuberculosis are more common in HIV-infected patients who

are injection drug users than in HIV-infected patients without a history of injection drug use. Furthermore, injection or other illicit drug use can cause a variety of non–HIV-related pulmonary diseases such as endocarditis-associated septic pulmonary emboli, pulmonary talcosis/interstitial lung disease, aspiration pneumonia secondary to respiratory depression, and drug-induced pulmonary edema.

HIV-infected patients who smoke tobacco are at increased risk for a variety of smoking-related respiratory illnesses and diseases. Both bacterial bronchitis and bacterial pneumonia are more common in HIV-infected cigarette smokers than in HIV-infected nonsmokers or former smokers. This is especially the case in persons with a CD4⁺ cell count lower than 200 cells/μL. In addition, HIV-infected patients who report a long history of cigarette use may have manifestations of chronic obstructive pulmonary disease (COPD) or respiratory bronchiolitis/interstitial lung disease as the cause of their symptoms. Emerging evidence suggests that HIV infection itself is associated with an increased risk for lung carcinoma.

Travel and Residence

Travel to or residence in a geographic region that is endemic for fungi such as *C. immitis*, *H. capsulatum*, or *Penicillium marneffei* is a strong determinant of the risk for exposure, infection, and ultimately disease. HIV-infected patients without such a history are unlikely to have been exposed and infected and are therefore unlikely to contract these diseases. Clinicians caring for patients in nonendemic areas would be wise to query their patients for details on their residence and travel history if the findings are suggestive of an endemic fungal infection.

Tuberculosis is more common in certain geographic areas and in certain populations. HIV-infected patients who were born in or have traveled to a country with a high prevalence of tuberculosis and patients who are homeless or previously incarcerated are at higher risk for exposure to *M. tuberculosis*. Patients with a positive purified protein derivative (PPD) tuberculin skin test result (defined as ≥5-mm induration in HIV-infected persons), especially if recent converters, and those with a positive result on an interferon-γ release assay are at increased risk for the development of tuberculosis.

Medical Background and Use of Prophylaxis

Many HIV-related opportunistic infections recur, and the current manifestation may be due to recurrence or relapse of a previous pulmonary disease (see Table 398-2). Bacterial infections are often recurrent, and patients with recurrent episodes of bacterial pneumonia are subject to the development of airway damage or bronchiectasis, which in turn predisposes them to further bacterial infections. Patients with previous *Pneumocystis* pneumonia are at high risk for recurrence, especially if their CD4⁺ cell count remains lower than 200 cells/μL. If the CD4⁺ cell count rises to higher than 200 cells/μL with antiretroviral therapy, prophylaxis against *Pneumocystis* can be safely discontinued in the majority of patients. Similarly, patients with previous cryptococcosis, coccidioidomycosis, or histoplasmosis are at high risk for relapse. Patients with a positive PPD reaction, a positive interferon-γ release assay result, or a chest radiograph with fibrotic lesions consistent with tuberculosis and no evidence of active tuberculosis and no previous history of treatment of latent tuberculosis infection (LTBI) should receive therapy for LTBI; failure to do so places the patient at a high risk for tuberculosis. In HIV-infected patients, adherence to the prescribed prophylaxis regimen lessens the probability of disease, whereas failure to adhere to the regimen frequently results in recurrent or relapsed disease.

Diagnostic Evaluation (see Table 398-2)
Symptoms

All of the HIV-associated pulmonary diseases may be accompanied by cough, dyspnea, or less commonly, pleuritic chest pain, or any combination of these symptoms. However, each pulmonary disease has a characteristic manifestation, and particular aspects of these symptoms may be useful in suggesting a specific diagnosis. For example, most patients with bacterial pneumonia have a cough productive of purulent sputum, whereas most patients with *Pneumocystis* pneumonia have a nonproductive cough. Bacterial pneumonias caused by *S. pneumoniae* and *Haemophilus* species characteristically have an acute onset and symptom duration of 3 to 5 days. In contrast, *Pneumocystis* pneumonia usually has a subacute onset and symptom duration of 2 to 4 weeks. Thus, in an HIV-infected patient with a CD4⁺ count lower than 200 cells/μL (and hence at risk for both pneumonias), the presence of cough productive of purulent sputum with a symptom duration of a few days favors the diagnosis of bacterial pneumonia. In contrast, the absence of purulent sputum with a symptom duration of a few weeks strongly favors the diagnosis of *Pneumocystis* pneumonia.

Constitutional symptoms such as fever, night sweats, and weight loss may suggest the presence of a systemic or disseminated disease. Fever and weight loss may be the sole complaints associated with disseminated mycobacterial or fungal disease, or they may be "B" symptoms associated with non-Hodgkin's lymphoma.

Extrapulmonary symptoms, when present, are often useful in suggesting a specific diagnosis. Although HIV-infected patients can have multiple concurrent illnesses, many of the HIV-associated pulmonary diseases have important extrapulmonary manifestations that account for their nonpulmonary findings. For example, respiratory symptoms and headache in a patient with a CD4$^+$ cell count lower than 200 cells/μL should suggest the possibility of *C. neoformans* pneumonia and meningitis. In fact, although the lungs are the portal of entry for *Cryptococcus*, many patients have no respiratory complaints or have minimally symptomatic pulmonary disease and the diagnosis is suggested only by the presence of extrapulmonary symptoms.

Signs

HIV-infected patients with pneumonia may be febrile, tachycardic, and tachypneic. The presence of systemic hypotension often suggests a fulminant disease process (e.g., bacterial septicemia). Pulse oximetry frequently reveals a decrease in oxygen saturation and also provides an estimate of the severity of the disease. The presence of exercise-induced oxygen desaturation is reported to be a sensitive indicator of *Pneumocystis* pneumonia.

Examination of the lungs may suggest a cause of the respiratory symptoms. Patients with bacterial pneumonia often have focal lung findings suggestive of consolidation or pleural effusion, or both. In contrast, patients with *Pneumocystis* pneumonia most often have normal findings on lung examination and only a minority have inspiratory crackles (usually bilateral). Abnormal findings on lung examination may be the result of a nonpulmonary disease. For example, rales in association with an S$_3$ cardiac gallop and elevated jugular venous pressure suggest a cardiac etiology.

The remainder of the physical examination may also suggest a cause of the respiratory symptoms. Altered mental status in a patient with pulmonary disease whose CD4$^+$ cell count is lower than 200 cells/μL suggests *C. neoformans* with neurologic involvement. A patient with focal neurologic findings and pulmonary disease may have concurrent *T. gondii* encephalitis and pneumonitis. The presence of mucocutaneous KS lesions may point to pulmonary KS. However, the absence of KS lesions on the skin and mucous membranes does not preclude the possibility of significant visceral disease, including the lung. An abdominal examination revealing hepatosplenomegaly suggests either disseminated mycobacterial or fungal disease or non-Hodgkin's lymphoma.

Laboratory Tests

Laboratory tests may provide important clues to the diagnosis of pulmonary disease (see Table 398-2). In general, however, HIV-infected patients typically have a host of laboratory abnormalities that are nonspecific or caused by conditions unrelated to the pulmonary disease. Laboratory tests that may be useful include a complete blood count with a white blood cell count and differential, serum lactate dehydrogenase (LDH), and arterial blood gas (ABG) analysis. These tests also serve as prognostic markers and as baseline values for subsequent measurements. Serial measurements are useful in any patient who fails to exhibit a clinical response or who worsens despite appropriate therapy.

Serum LDH is often elevated in patients with *Pneumocystis* pneumonia. However, it may be elevated with other pulmonary (including bacterial pneumonia and tuberculosis) and nonpulmonary conditions. Despite its diagnostic limitations, the degree of LDH elevation has been shown to correlate with prognosis and response to therapy. Patients with *Pneumocystis* pneumonia and an initially markedly elevated or increasing serum LDH level despite treatment of *Pneumocystis* pneumonia have a poor prognosis. ABG analysis is useful for prognosis, as well as for clinical decisions regarding whether to admit the patient and whether corticosteroids are indicated in those with *Pneumocystis* pneumonia.

Imaging

Chest Radiograph

The chest radiograph is the cornerstone for evaluation of pulmonary diseases in HIV-infected patients. Because each of these diseases has a characteristic

FIGURE 398-1. Chest radiograph of an HIV-infected person, CD4$^+$ cell count higher than 200 cells/μL, revealing left lingular consolidation. Sputum and blood cultures were positive for *Streptococcus pneumoniae*. (Courtesy Laurence Huang, MD, and Chin Tang Huang, MD.)

FIGURE 398-2. Chest radiograph of an HIV-infected person, CD4$^+$ cell count higher than 200 cells/μL, demonstrating a right upper lobe infiltrate with areas of cavitation. Sputum acid-fast bacillus stain was positive, and multiple sputum cultures grew *Mycobacterium tuberculosis*.

radiographic appearance, the radiograph can narrow the diagnostic possibilities and suggest a diagnostic approach.

Bacterial pneumonia is currently the most common pulmonary disease seen in HIV-infected persons at many institutions in the United States. The most frequently identified pathogens are *S. pneumoniae*, *Haemophilus* species, *Staphylococcus aureus*, and *P. aeruginosa*. Classically, chest radiographs of HIV-infected patients with bacterial pneumonia demonstrate focal, segmental, or lobar consolidation, similar to that observed in non–HIV-infected persons (Fig. 398-1). However, this finding may be more frequent in pneumonias caused by *S. pneumoniae* and to a lesser extent *Haemophilus* species than in community-acquired *P. aeruginosa*. The presence of cavitary pneumonia may be more suggestive of *Staphylococcus* or *Pseudomonas* than either *Streptococcus* or *Haemophilus*.

Tuberculosis can be associated with a variety of chest radiographic findings, including upper lung zone infiltrates, often with cavitation (Fig. 398-2), middle or lower lung zone consolidation (or both) mimicking bacterial pneumonia (Fig. 398-3), miliary or nodular disease, and pleural effusions or intrathoracic adenopathy (or both). The frequency with which each of these specific findings is seen is influenced in part by the patient's CD4$^+$ cell count. HIV-infected patients with a CD4$^+$ cell count well higher than 200 cells/μL are more likely to have a radiograph showing upper lung zone infiltrates and cavitation than are patients with a CD4$^+$ count lower than 200 cells/μL. In this latter group, patients are as likely or more likely to have a radiograph demonstrating mid or lower lung zone involvement (or both) or diffuse involvement and are more likely to have associated intrathoracic adenopathy. One study of radiographic findings in HIV-infected patients with tuberculosis found that the proportion of patients with cavitary infiltrates declined significantly as the CD4$^+$ cell count decreased from 400 cells/μL or higher to less than 200 cells/μL whereas the proportion with noncavitary infiltrates and with intrathoracic adenopathy increased significantly as the CD4$^+$ count declined. Thus, the radiographic key to diagnosis of tuberculosis is

FIGURE 398-3. Chest radiograph of an HIV-infected person, CD4+ cell count less than 200 cells/μL, revealing right lower lung zone consolidation with air bronchograms. Sputum culture grew *Mycobacterium tuberculosis* that was resistant to rifampin treatment. In this case, the key to the diagnosis of tuberculosis was knowledge of the patient's CD4+ cell count and an understanding that tuberculosis can be manifested in this manner in such an individual.

FIGURE 398-5. Close-up of the left lung from a chest radiograph of an HIV-infected person, CD4+ cell count less than 200 cells/μL. Two thin-walled cysts *(arrows)* are present as a result of *Pneumocystis* pneumonia.

FIGURE 398-4. Chest radiograph of an HIV-infected person, CD4+ cell count less than 200 cells/μL, demonstrating the characteristic bilateral, reticular-granular opacities of *Pneumocystis* pneumonia. Bronchoscopy with examination of bronchoalveolar lavage fluid revealed *Pneumocystis jirovecii*.

knowledge of the patient's CD4+ cell count and the patterns common at that CD4+ count.

Classically, *Pneumocystis* pneumonia is characterized by bilateral interstitial-reticular or granular opacities (Fig. 398-4). Frequently, the opacities are symmetrical, and they are diffuse when the disease is severe. One large study revealed that 7% of HIV-infected patients with *Pneumocystis* pneumonia had thin-walled cysts (pneumatoceles) (Fig. 398-5) and 4% had honeycomb lesions. Infiltrates were bilateral in 95% and involved the entire lung in 48%. Several reports have described the radiographic findings in patients receiving aerosolized pentamidine prophylaxis; these radiographs characteristically revealed an upper lung zone predominance mimicking mycobacterial disease. However, upper lung zone predominance can also be seen in patients who never received aerosolized pentamidine, and the pattern present (reticular, granular) is more important than the distribution in suggesting the diagnosis of *Pneumocystis* pneumonia.

Although bilateral interstitial-reticular infiltrates are the most common radiographic manifestation (mimicking *Pneumocystis* pneumonia), pulmonary involvement by *Cryptococcus* can also result in an alveolar or nodular pattern, thin-walled cysts or cavities, nodules, masses (Fig. 398-6A and B), intrathoracic adenopathy, and pleural effusions.

Pulmonary KS is characteristically accompanied by bilateral opacities in a central or perihilar distribution (Fig. 398-7). One large study of HIV-infected patients with pulmonary KS diagnosed by bronchoscopy (in which BAL studies were negative for infectious organisms) found that 95% of chest radiographs demonstrated peribronchial cuffing and tram track opacities with (45%) or without (50%) more extensive perihilar coalescent opacities. Small nodules (50%) or nodular opacities (28%) were seen on 78%, Kerley's B lines on 71%, and pleural effusions on 53% of the radiographs.

FIGURES 398-6. A and B, Chest radiograph and chest computed tomography (CT) scan of an HIV-infected person, CD4+ cell count less than 200 cells/μL. A multilobulated noncalcified mass measuring 4.6 × 2.4 cm is present in the left lower lobe with multiple adjacent satellite nodules. Culture from CT-guided transthoracic needle aspiration revealed *Cryptococcus neoformans*.

Chest Computed Tomography

Chest computed tomography (CT) is more sensitive than chest radiography for detecting the presence and defining the characteristics and extent of pulmonary disease. However, CT is unnecessary in most evaluations because the clinical and chest radiographic findings often suggest a single or a few diagnoses to consider primarily. There are a number of specific clinical scenarios in which chest CT may be of particular use in HIV-infected patients. High-resolution CT (HRCT) is extremely useful in patients with clinically suspected *Pneumocystis* pneumonia and normal or unchanged findings on chest radiography. Patients with *Pneumocystis* pneumonia and normal chest radiographic findings have patchy areas of ground-glass opacity on HRCT (Fig. 398-8). Although the presence of ground-glass opacity is nonspecific and

FIGURE 398-7. Chest radiograph of an HIV-infected person, CD4+ cell count less than 100 cells/μL, with the characteristic bilateral, middle, and lower lung zone, predominantly central distribution of abnormalities of pulmonary Kaposi's sarcoma. The patient had no evidence of mucocutaneous Kaposi's sarcoma, and the diagnosis of pulmonary disease was made by bronchoscopy with visualization of characteristic erythematous-violaceous Kaposi's sarcoma lesions throughout the visible airway (see Fig. 398-11).

FIGURE 398-8. Chest high-resolution computed tomography (HRCT) in an HIV-infected person, CD4+ cell count less than 200 cells/μL, whose chest radiograph showed normal findings. Because of clinical suspicion of *Pneumocystis* pneumonia (PCP), the patient underwent HRCT, which demonstrates the characteristic patchy ground-glass opacities of PCP. Induced sputum examination revealed *Pneumocystis jirovecii*.

may be seen with a number of pulmonary disorders, its absence strongly argues against the presence of *Pneumocystis* pneumonia.

Chest CT can also be useful in suggesting a diagnosis in cases in which the chest radiograph reveals multiple pulmonary nodules. A predominance of nodules less than 1 cm in diameter in a centrilobular distribution strongly suggests the presence of an opportunistic infection, whereas a predominance of nodules larger than 1 cm in diameter is suggestive of neoplasm. When the nodules are mostly less than 1 cm in diameter, the presence of intrathoracic adenopathy, especially if low attenuation (another use for CT), indicates that mycobacterial (or fungal) disease is probable. When the nodules are mostly greater than 1 cm in diameter, the finding of associated peribronchovascular thickening inevitably results in a diagnosis of pulmonary KS.

In patients suspected of having disseminated mycobacterial or fungal disease, the chest radiograph may reveal little or no parenchymal lung involvement. However, chest CT may reveal intrathoracic adenopathy, which if low attenuation, strongly suggests these infections. Finally, chest CT is useful in guiding diagnostic procedures such as bronchoscopy, transthoracic needle aspiration (see Fig. 398-6B), and occasionally, surgical procedures.

Pulmonary Function Tests

Pulmonary function testing can be useful in evaluating respiratory complaints in HIV-infected patients. In patients complaining of dry cough or dyspnea (or both) whose findings on chest radiography are normal, spirometry may diagnose airflow obstruction that is often responsive to bronchodilators. It may also reveal a pattern suggestive of COPD, which is increasingly being recognized as a noninfectious complication of HIV infection. Pulmonary function testing in patients with *Pneumocystis* pneumonia frequently reveals a restrictive ventilatory defect with decreased lung volumes and increased airflow. In addition, the diffusing capacity for carbon monoxide

(D_{LCO}) is a sensitive, but nonspecific indicator of *Pneumocystis* pneumonia, and a normal D_{LCO} makes the diagnosis of *Pneumocystis* pneumonia extremely unlikely.

Selected Diagnostic Tests

The approach to the evaluation of HIV-infected patients with suspected pulmonary disease begins with consideration of the spectrum of pulmonary diseases outlined in Table 398-1. After a careful history and physical examination supplemented by selected laboratory tests and a chest radiograph, the goal is to arrive at a probable diagnosis (or at most a few diagnoses) for which specific diagnostic tests can be ordered and appropriate treatment can be initiated (Figs. 398-9 and 398-10). The next sections provide a discussion of selected diagnostic tests (E-Table 398-1).

Blood Cultures

Blood can be obtained for bacterial, fungal, and mycobacterial culture. Because *S. pneumoniae* is the most frequent cause of bacterial pneumonia and because pneumococcal pneumonia is often accompanied by bacteremia in HIV-infected patients (especially those with a CD4+ cell count <200 cells/μL), blood cultures should usually be performed in patients with suspected bacterial pneumonia. When positive, blood cultures are specific for the diagnosis, and in an era of increasing antibiotic resistance, the utility of drug susceptibility testing cannot be overemphasized. Tuberculosis and many of the fungal pneumonias may be manifested as extrapulmonary or disseminated disease with minimal or absent respiratory complaints and normal findings on chest radiography. For this reason, mycobacterial and fungal blood cultures should usually be performed for suspected tuberculous or fungal infection, especially if the CD4+ cell count is lower than 200 cells/μL.

Serology

Serum cryptococcal antigen (sCRAG) is an extremely sensitive test for the presence of cryptococcemia and cryptococcal meningitis, and a negative sCRAG test result virtually rules out the diagnosis of cryptococcal meningitis. However, sCRAG may occasionally be negative in HIV-infected patients who have isolated cryptococcal pneumonia. sCRAG is extremely specific for cryptococcal infection; false-positive test results are rare. Therefore, sCRAG should be determined in all patients with suspected cryptococcal disease, and patients positive for sCRAG should undergo evaluation to determine the extent of disease (i.e., lumbar puncture for possible meningitis), whereas those negative for sCRAG but with respiratory complaints or chest radiographic findings should undergo further pulmonary evaluation (i.e., bronchoscopy with BAL). There appears to be little to no utility in measuring serial sCRAG titers in patients with cryptococcal disease.

Similar to sCRAG, *H. capsulatum* polysaccharide antigen (HPA) is a sensitive test for the presence of disseminated histoplasmosis. However, the HPA test may be negative in patients with mild or localized disease. The antigen, which can be measured in blood and other fluids (including BAL fluid) but is most commonly assayed from urine, should be determined in patients with suspected histoplasmosis. In the proper clinical context, a positive result indicates *H. capsulatum* infection. However, patients with a positive HPA test result should have appropriate material (i.e., blood) sent for fungal culture because fungal pathogens such as *P. marneffei*, *Blastomyces dermatitidis*, and *Paracoccidioides braziliensis* may cause a false-positive result. One important benefit of serial HPA testing is its use in diagnosing relapsed disease; a 2-unit increase is associated with relapsed disease.

Most cases of *T. gondii* encephalitis result from reactivation of latent infection. In studies of central nervous system toxoplasmosis, up to 97% of HIV-infected patients were positive for *Toxoplasma* IgG, with a smaller percentage being positive for *Toxoplasma* IgM. Although a positive *Toxoplasma* IgG finding merely indicates previous infection and cannot itself be taken as proof of acute toxoplasmosis, a negative *Toxoplasma* IgG finding, especially if accompanied by a negative IgM finding, makes the diagnosis of toxoplasmosis unlikely.

Sputum

Most patients with bacterial pneumonia have a productive cough. Current U.S. guidelines recommend that sputum Gram stain and culture be performed in hospitalized patients with suspected bacterial pneumonia and whenever the presence of identified pathogens would alter empirical therapy.

Sputum acid-fast bacillus (AFB) smear and culture are the foundations for the diagnosis of pulmonary tuberculosis and other nontuberculous

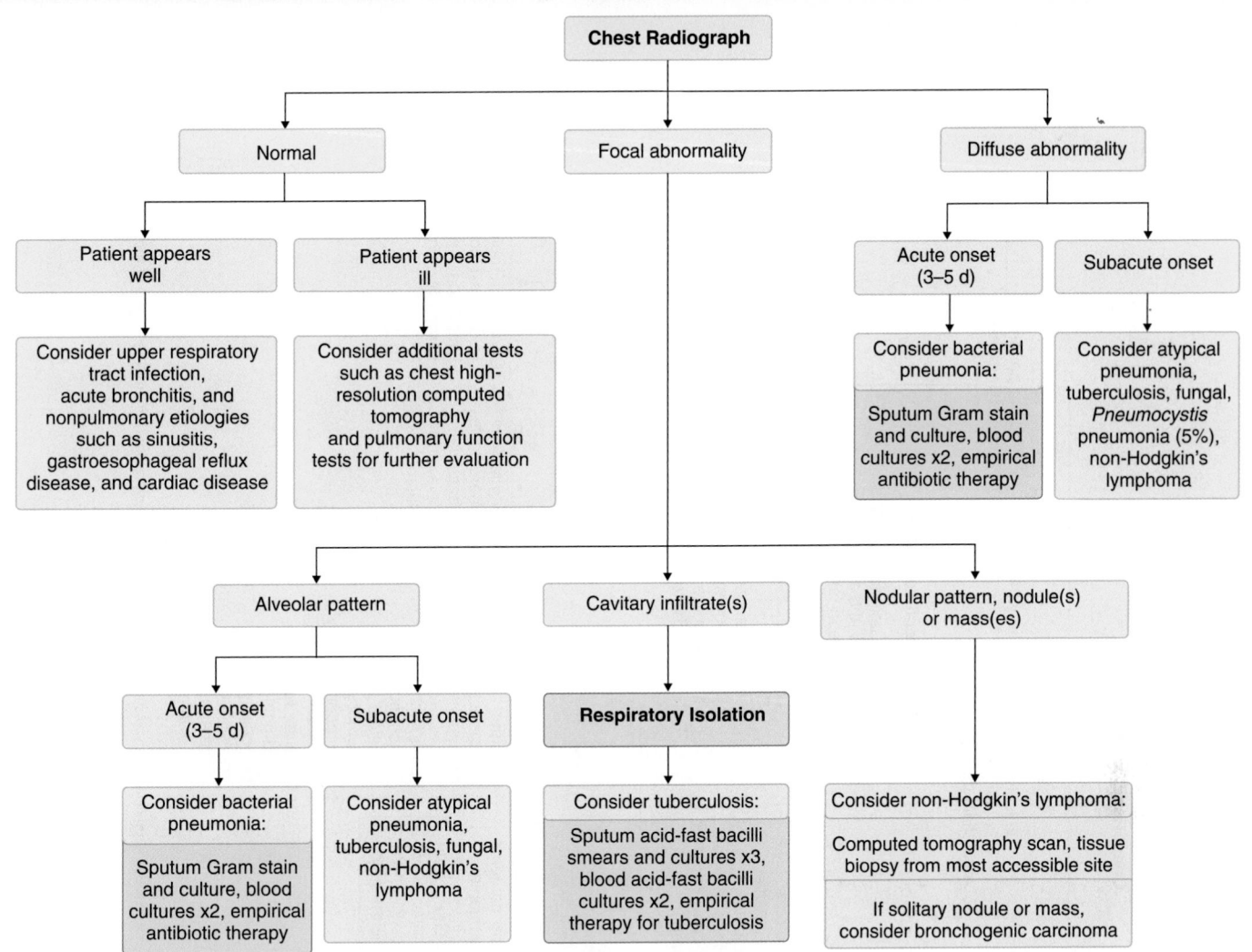

FIGURE 398-9. Diagnostic approach to an HIV-infected patient with suspected pulmonary disease, CD4⁺ cell count greater than 200 cells/μL, according to the predominant chest radiograph findings.

mycobacterial pneumonias. Sputum AFB specimens—either spontaneous or induced—should ideally be obtained on 2 to 3 consecutive days, preferably in the morning. Several studies report that the sensitivity of sputum AFB smear and culture for tuberculosis in HIV-infected patients is similar to that seen in the overall population; other studies report that its sensitivity is lower. The sensitivity of sputum AFB smear for *M. tuberculosis* ranged from 50% to 60% in two large series; in HIV-infected persons with disseminated disease, the sensitivity was significantly higher (90%). In one of these studies, the proportion of patients who were sputum AFB smear positive was no different in those with normal chest radiographic findings and those with abnormal findings. Thus, all patients with suspected tuberculosis, even if the findings on chest radiography are negative, should have two to three sputum specimens sent for AFB smear and culture. Patients with a positive AFB smear must be presumed to have tuberculosis, and appropriate measures must be instituted while awaiting either culture or nucleic acid amplification test results. Patients with negative sputum AFB smear results may still have tuberculosis detected on culture or determined by clinical and radiographic response but are at reasonably low likelihood for transmission, so respiratory isolation (if hospitalized) can be discontinued. A single positive sputum AFB culture result for *M. tuberculosis* is diagnostic of tuberculosis, but the same cannot be said for a sputum specimen positive for a nontuberculous mycobacterium (i.e., *Mycobacterium kansasii, M. avium* complex). In these patients a positive sputum culture can be due to colonization, and determination of when these mycobacteria are causing pulmonary disease relies on a constellation of clinical, radiographic, and microbiologic criteria.

Most patients with *Pneumocystis* pneumonia have a dry, nonproductive cough, and sputum must be induced. Sputum induction should be performed in a properly engineered room to minimize transmission of infectious microorganisms. Sputum induction is a sensitive diagnostic test for *Pneumocystis* pneumonia, with a reported sensitivity ranging from 55% in early studies

to 95% with fluorescent antibody testing. At institutions where sputum induction is performed, the need for bronchoscopy is decreased significantly. In addition, induced sputum has led to the diagnosis of cases of certain bacterial, mycobacterial, fungal, and parasitic pneumonias and suggested the presence of bacterial bronchitis/bronchopneumonia. Polymerase chain reaction–based assays applied to noninvasive respiratory specimens (i.e., oropharyngeal washing or gargle) have been reported to have encouraging results but are typically available only in a research setting. Thus, sputum induction should be the initial diagnostic test for patients with suspected *Pneumocystis* pneumonia at institutions where it is available.

Although experience is limited when compared with that for tuberculosis and *Pneumocystis* pneumonia, sputum examination, culture, or both can occasionally diagnose fungal pneumonias, including *C. neoformans, H. capsulatum*, and *C. immitis*, but not invasive *Aspergillus* disease.

Bronchoscopy

Bronchoscopy is a mainstay in the diagnosis of HIV-associated pulmonary disease. It should be considered for any patient with pulmonary disease whose severity warrants prompt and accurate diagnosis, for patients with suspected pulmonary KS, for patients in whom the diagnosis is unclear despite less invasive diagnostic tests (e.g., sputum), and for those who are failing empirical therapy for a presumed pathogen.

Bronchoscopy with BAL is the "gold standard" diagnostic test for *Pneumocystis* pneumonia. The sensitivity of BAL alone for *Pneumocystis* pneumonia is reported to be 95% or greater. Bronchoscopy with BAL can be performed in patients with suspected *Pneumocystis* pneumonia whose induced sputum examination is negative. There are institutional differences in the sensitivity of BAL, and both BAL and transbronchial biopsy (TBBX) are warranted at institutions where the yield of these two procedures is complementary.

Bronchoscopy is an important modality for diagnosing cryptococcal pneumonia, especially if the disease is limited to the lungs. BAL fluid culture has

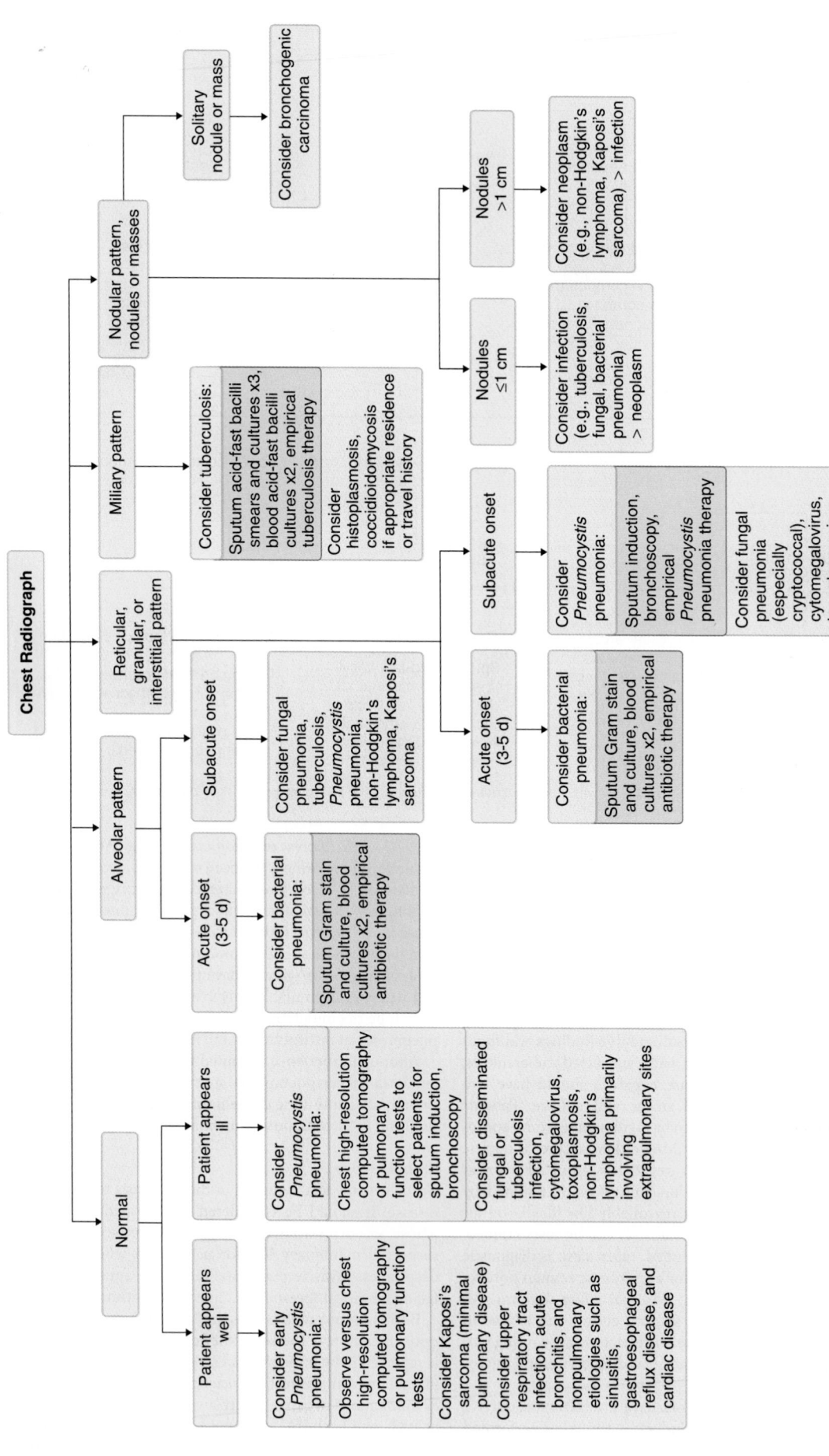

FIGURE 398-10. Diagnostic approach to an HIV-infected patient with suspected pulmonary disease, CD4+ cell count less than 200 cells/μL, according to the predominant chest radiograph findings. Some of the diagnoses listed usually occur when the CD4+ cell count is below 100 cells/μL or even below 50 cells/μL (see Table 398-3).

FIGURE 398-11. Characteristic Kaposi's sarcoma lesions located in the trachea in an HIV-infected person, CD4+ cell count less than 100 cells/µL. Concurrent bronchoalveolar lavage also revealed *Pneumocystis* pneumonia.

been reported to be positive in more than 80% of HIV-infected patients with cryptococcal pneumonia.

Bronchoscopy with a thorough visual inspection of the airways is the procedure of choice for the diagnosis of pulmonary KS. In these patients, neither TBBX nor endobronchial biopsy adds to the yield when the characteristic KS lesions are seen (Fig. 398-11). However, the absence of visible KS lesions does not preclude their presence in more distal airways, nor does it preclude the possibility of parenchymal KS involvement. In these select patients, TBBX can occasionally establish the diagnosis.

Bronchoscopy with BAL may diagnose *M. tuberculosis* (although the diagnostic yield improves with the addition of TBBX), *H. capsulatum*, *C. immitis*, and *T. gondii* pneumonia. Bronchoscopy with TBBX (or other tissue biopsy specimen) is required to establish a definitive diagnosis of *Aspergillus* and cytomegalovirus pneumonia. Similarly, biopsy is an important tool for the diagnosis of pulmonary disease caused by non-Hodgkin's lymphoma and lung cancer.

Other Procedures

Diagnostic thoracentesis should be considered for any HIV-infected patient with evidence of pleural effusion in whom other tests are nondiagnostic or empyema is a concern. In most situations, pleural fluid culture or cytology in the case of non-Hodgkin's lymphoma or lung cancer can establish the diagnosis. However, in patients with pleural effusion and suspected tuberculosis, the diagnostic yield is improved with the addition of pleural biopsy.

CT-guided transthoracic needle aspiration is an important and useful diagnostic procedure for selected patients. HIV-infected patients with focal parenchymal lesions, most often peripheral lung nodules or masses that may be beyond the reach of a bronchoscope, are ideal candidates for CT-guided aspiration. Mediastinoscopy should be considered for patients with a mediastinal mass or adenopathy, or both. Video-assisted thoracoscopic surgery can be an important procedure in selected patients.

Occasionally, despite all these efforts, HIV-infected patients with pulmonary disease may elude definitive diagnosis. In such patients, consideration should be given to open lung biopsy, although the results have been mixed. Even though open lung biopsy often provides important new information, patients who undergo this procedure are frequently already so ill that this new information fails to translate into improved survival.

Complications

Noninfectious Complications

The focus of the evaluation and management of respiratory symptoms in an HIV-infected patient is frequently placed on opportunistic infections and their prompt diagnosis and treatment. However, several noninfectious complications associated with HIV infection warrant discussion.

Kaposi's Sarcoma

The overwhelming majority of HIV-infected patients with KS in the United States are men who have sexual relationships with other men (Chapter 400). Clinically symptomatic pulmonary KS occurs at the lower range of CD4+ cell

counts, but tracheobronchial lesions may be seen in patients with higher CD4+ counts who are undergoing bronchoscopy for other reasons. Most patients with pulmonary KS have mucocutaneous disease.

Pulmonary KS is characterized by nonproductive cough, dyspnea, and occasionally fever. Chest pain and hemoptysis are less frequently noted. Symptoms are usually present for weeks or months but may also progress rapidly in a manner indistinguishable from opportunistic infection. Pulmonary KS is characteristically accompanied by bilateral middle to lower lung zone opacities in a central or perihilar distribution; the presence of isolated upper lung zone opacities should raise suspicion for opportunistic pneumonia. Typical chest radiographic findings include linear densities (bronchial wall thickening), nodules or nodular opacities of varying size, Kerley's B lines, pleural effusions, and intrathoracic adenopathy. Chest CT often demonstrates the characteristic peribronchovascular distribution with associated nodules.

The diagnosis of pulmonary KS is usually established by bronchoscopy. The finding of characteristic endobronchial, reddish purple, flat or slightly raised lesions is sufficient to diagnose pulmonary disease in the proper clinical context (Fig. 398-11). Most patients with chest radiographic findings suggestive of pulmonary KS have endobronchial KS lesions seen below the level of the carina. However, the absence of lesions in the observable airway does not preclude more distal airway disease or parenchymal, pleural, or nodal involvement. When clinical suspicion for pulmonary KS is strong but no endobronchial KS lesions are seen, TBBX should be considered to establish the diagnosis. A significant proportion of patients with pulmonary KS have concurrent opportunistic infection, and patients undergoing evaluation for pulmonary KS should be concomitantly evaluated for opportunistic infection.

Non-Hodgkin's Lymphoma

Most HIV-infected patients with non-Hodgkin's lymphoma have widely disseminated disease and extranodal involvement (Chapter 400). Frequent extranodal sites include the liver, spleen, bone marrow, meninges, and gastrointestinal tract, whereas intrathoracic involvement is seen in a smaller proportion. Occasionally, the lung is the only site involved. Patients with non-Hodgkin's lymphoma can have a wide range of CD4+ counts.

When the lungs are involved, the most common symptoms are cough and dyspnea, with pleuritic chest pain and hemoptysis occurring less frequently. Classic "B" symptoms such as fever, sweats, and weight loss are also common features. The most frequent parenchymal lung findings on chest radiography are multiple nodular opacities or masses, lobar infiltrates, and diffuse interstitial infiltrates. Occasionally, a solitary nodule or mass is seen. Pleural effusions are the most common radiographic abnormality; they are detected in 40 to 70% of cases and may occur in the absence of parenchymal disease. Hilar and mediastinal adenopathy is found in up to 60% of patients.

The diagnosis of non-Hodgkin's lymphoma requires demonstration of malignant lymphocytes on cytology or biopsy specimens. Persons with isolated intrathoracic involvement should undergo bronchoscopy with biopsy or CT-guided transthoracic needle aspiration. Other options include mediastinoscopy, thoracoscopy, and open lung biopsy. For patients with effusions, pleural fluid cytology or biopsy (or both) is often diagnostic.

Lung Cancer

The incidence of lung cancer is higher in HIV-infected persons than in non–HIV-infected persons. Whether this increased incidence is due to HIV infection itself or to potential confounders such as greater rates of tobacco smoking in HIV-infected persons remains somewhat controversial. Most HIV-infected persons in whom lung cancer develops are tobacco smokers. Adenocarcinoma is the most frequently reported type. The clinical and chest radiographic findings, diagnosis, and management of lung cancer in HIV-infected patients are identical to those in immunocompetent patients (Chapter 197). Importantly, HIV infection should not be considered a contraindication to resection but instead be considered an important concurrent underlying medical problem, much the same as one would consider underlying cardiac or pulmonary disease. The median survival in HIV-infected patients with lung cancer is similar to that of age-matched, non–HIV-infected lung cancer patients.

Nonspecific Interstitial Pneumonitis

Nonspecific interstitial pneumonitis (NSIP) has been reported at various frequencies. Because it is a histologic diagnosis, its incidence depends partly on the frequency that biopsy is performed during the diagnostic evaluation.

FIGURE 398-12. Chest high-resolution computed tomography in an HIV-infected person, CD4⁺ cell count less than 200 cells/μL. Lymphocytic interstitial pneumonitis was diagnosed by transbronchial biopsy.

Symptoms of NSIP include dyspnea, nonproductive cough, and fever. These clinical features are indistinguishable from *Pneumocystis* pneumonia. However, NSIP may occur at CD4⁺ cell counts higher than 200 cells/μL, whereas *Pneumocystis* pneumonia rarely does. Chest radiographic findings in patients with NSIP are nonspecific and usually indistinguishable from those of *Pneumocystis* pneumonia, and as with *Pneumocystis* pneumonia, patients with NSIP can have normal radiographic findings. The most common radiographic abnormality seen was a diffuse interstitial pattern. Other abnormalities include pleural effusions, alveolar infiltrates, and nodules. Pulmonary function tests often reveal a mildly decreased diffusing capacity. The diagnosis of NSIP requires histologic confirmation and exclusion of other causes.

Lymphocytic Interstitial Pneumonitis
The most striking feature of HIV-associated lymphocytic interstitial pneumonitis (LIP) is the effect of age on its incidence. LIP has been a frequent AIDS-defining diagnosis in children but is rare in adults. Symptoms of LIP include slowly progressive dyspnea, nonproductive cough, and fever indistinguishable from that caused by opportunistic infection. The chest radiograph is nonspecific in patients with LIP and characteristically shows bilateral reticulonodular "interstitial" infiltrates with lower lung zone predominance. Hilar or mediastinal adenopathy is occasionally seen and can potentially be used to distinguish LIP from *Pneumocystis* pneumonia. Pulmonary function tests often reveal a restrictive ventilatory defect and a decreased diffusing capacity. Chest CT demonstrates small (2 to 4 mm) nodules, frequently in a peribronchovascular distribution, or diffuse areas of ground-glass opacity (Fig. 398-12). The diagnosis of LIP requires histologic confirmation by biopsy.

Pulmonary Arterial Hypertension
Increasingly, pulmonary arterial hypertension (Chapter 68) is being recognized as an HIV-associated condition, although many HIV-infected persons with this condition have concurrent risk factors for pulmonary hypertension (e.g., cigarette smoking resulting in COPD and end-stage liver disease causing portal hypertension). The characteristic clinical manifestation is progressive dyspnea, with nonproductive cough, chest pain, and syncope or near-syncope seen in a minority. Chest radiographic findings include cardiomegaly and prominence of the pulmonary arteries. Most often, a chest radiograph or an electrocardiogram with evidence of right ventricular hypertrophy first suggests the diagnosis of pulmonary hypertension. Patients in whom pulmonary hypertension is diagnosed should undergo an evaluation for secondary causes, including underlying cardiac and pulmonary diseases (e.g., COPD, recurrent pulmonary emboli). In general, treatment of HIV-associated pulmonary arterial hypertension is similar to that in non–HIV-infected persons (Chapter 68), except that concurrent antiretroviral therapy has been used, with varying success.

Chronic Obstructive Pulmonary Disease
COPD (Chapter 88) is emerging as an HIV-associated condition. Early reports suggested that HIV-infected cigarette smokers were at greater risk for the development of emphysema than were HIV-infected nonsmokers or non-immunocompromised cigarette smokers, and large cohort studies support this association. In addition to cigarette smoking, repeated opportunistic pulmonary infections may eventually result in the development of chronic bronchitis and bronchiectasis. The clinical and radiographic findings,

diagnosis, and management of obstructive lung disease in HIV-infected patients are identical to that in immunocompetent patients (Chapter 88), including the use of inhaled corticosteroids, when indicated.

Sarcoidosis
Several cases of sarcoidosis in HIV-infected patients have been reported. In these cases the clinical and radiographic manifestations, diagnosis, and clinical course with corticosteroid therapy were similar to cases of sarcoidosis in non–HIV-infected persons (Chapter 95).

Pulmonary Manifestations of Immune Reconstitution Inflammatory Syndromes
The initiation of combinations of potent antiretroviral medications and the subsequent improvement in immune function have also resulted in several syndromes that have important clinical implications (Chapter 402). Interestingly, in some of the reports, the use of antiretroviral therapy transiently exacerbated the disease, whereas in others, its use was seemingly solely responsible for the reported improvements. Finally, in some cases, the use of antiretroviral therapy has been associated with the development of pulmonary disease that is host mediated.

The transient worsening of clinical symptoms and signs and chest radiographic findings of tuberculosis after the initiation of appropriate antituberculous therapy has been well recognized. These paradoxical reactions are thought to represent an enhanced antituberculous immune response, and they usually resolve with continued therapy alone. HIV-infected patients in whom tuberculosis develops and who receive concurrent antiretroviral and antituberculous therapy appear to have an increased incidence of paradoxical worsening and immune reconstitution inflammatory syndrome. The radiographic findings can consist of new or worsening parenchymal disease, new or worsening intrathoracic lymphadenopathy, and new or worsening pleural effusion. HIV-infected patients with tuberculosis and suspected paradoxical reactions must also be thoroughly evaluated for progressive tuberculosis resulting from drug resistance or patient nonadherence and for the presence of a concurrent, superimposed opportunistic infection.

Similar to tuberculosis, paradoxical reactions in HIV-infected patients have been reported in those receiving concurrent therapy for HIV and opportunistic infection, including important pulmonary pathogens such as *Pneumocystis* and *Cryptococcus*. In some of these cases the manifestations of immune reconstitution are severe and patients require mechanical ventilation for respiratory failure.

The use of antiretroviral therapy, even in the absence of specific chemotherapy, often results in clinical regression and, occasionally, complete resolution of KS lesions (including pulmonary KS). However, case reports also indicate that patients with pulmonary KS may likewise experience a paradoxical worsening as a result of immune reconstitution inflammatory syndrome.

Improved immune function may also play a role in the development of host-mediated pulmonary disease. There are several reports of sarcoidosis or a sarcoidosis-like disease that developed after the initiation of antiretroviral therapy. In addition, hypersensitivity pneumonitis to avian antigen that developed only after the patient's immune function improved with antiretroviral therapy has been described. Diseases in which the host's immune response plays an essential role in pathogenesis can be expected to become more prevalent as more HIV-infected patients receive potent antiretroviral therapy.

SUGGESTED READINGS

Almodovar S, Cicalini S, Petrosillo N, et al. Pulmonary hypertension associated with HIV infection: pulmonary vascular disease: the global perspective. *Chest.* 2010;137(6 Suppl):6S-12S. *Review of screening approaches to HIV-related pulmonary arterial hypertension and mechanistic insights.*

Calligaro G, Meintjes G, Mendelson M. Pulmonary manifestations of the immune reconstitution inflammatory syndrome. *Curr Opin Pulm Med.* 2011;17:180-188. *Tuberculosis, nontuberculous mycobacterial, and* Pneumocystis *infections occur within days to weeks of starting antiretroviral therapy, whereas cryptococcal infection occurs later and with a much higher mortality.*

Kaplan JE, Benson C, Holmes KH, et al. Guidelines for prevention and treatment of opportunistic infections in HIV-infected adults and adolescents: recommendations from CDC, the National Institutes of Health, and the HIV Medicine Association of the Infectious Diseases Society of America. *MMWR Recomm Rep.* 2009;58(RR-4):1-207. *Current U.S. guidelines for the treatment and prevention of opportunistic infections.*

Kovacs JA, Masur H. Evolving health effects of *Pneumocystis*: one hundred years of progress in diagnosis and treatment. *JAMA.* 2009;301:2578-2585. *An excellent review recognizing the 100 years since the discovery of* Pneumocystis *and summarizing our current understanding.*

Morris A, Crothers K, Beck JM, et al. An official ATS workshop report: emerging issues and current controversies in HIV-associated pulmonary diseases. *Proc Am Thorac Soc.* 2011;8:17-26. *Review of noninfectious lung diseases in HIV patients.*

399

SKIN MANIFESTATIONS IN PATIENTS WITH HUMAN IMMUNODEFICIENCY VIRUS INFECTION

TOBY MAURER

From the beginning of the epidemic, skin disease has frequently been the initial feature of infection with human immunodeficiency virus (HIV). Cutaneous manifestations are often predictive of the stage of immunosuppression and long-term prognosis. Morbidity from skin diseases, particularly from opportunistic infections, has decreased with the advent of antiretroviral treatment (ART), although there are still significant dermatologic problems for patients in the post-ART era. Cutaneous manifestations seen in patients with HIV may be categorized as infectious, neoplastic, inflammatory, or related to ART.

INFECTIOUS MANIFESTATIONS

HIV Seroconversion Exanthem

Frequently observed in acute HIV infection is an infectious mononucleosis–like illness that precedes seroconversion by 2 to 6 weeks. The rash is characterized by erythematous macules and papules ranging from 2 mm to a few centimeters, particularly on the upper part of the trunk and face with relative sparing of peripheral regions. It is commonly accompanied by aphthous or penile ulceration, or both. There is evidence that very early after infection, HIV goes to dendritic cells in skin and causes an inflammatory response, which may explain the rash. At this stage the viral load may be very high and is suggestive of acute HIV seroconversion, although the HIV antibody test is likely to be negative.

Viruses

Herpes Zoster

Herpes zoster (Chapter 383) is often observed even at relatively normal CD4$^+$ counts and may therefore be the first feature of HIV infection. The mouth may also be affected. In any patient younger than 50 years with zoster, risk factors for HIV should be explored and consideration given to HIV testing. Zoster infection may be multidermatomal or disseminated even in patients with relatively high CD4$^+$ counts, and if it involves the eye, treatment with intravenous acyclovir should be considered. Antiviral treatment should be started at any time during the disease course (not only within the first 48 hours, as with zoster not associated with HIV). Less severe disease normally responds to standard treatment. There have been a few reports of a verrucous chronic form of zoster occurring in more severely immunosuppressed patients; this form of zoster is usually associated with acyclovir resistance. Zoster has been one of the more commonly reported diseases in patients with immune reconstitution inflammatory syndrome (IRIS) (Chapter 402) and has been noted to appear in the second phase of IRIS, that is, later than the initial 3 months of ART.

Herpes Simplex Virus

Infection with herpes simplex virus (HSV) (Chapter 382) should always be considered in patients with HIV who have mucocutaneous ulcerations (Fig. 399-1), particularly in the anogenital area. Patients with CD4$^+$ counts lower than 200 cells/μL may require higher doses of acyclovir to treat the infection. (See Table 399-1 for skin conditions occurring at CD4$^+$ counts lower than 200 cells/μL in patients not receiving ART.) Patients who fail to respond may have HSV with acyclovir resistance, and alternative agents such as foscarnet or cidofovir may be required. The presence of HSV clinically or subclinically increases the likelihood of transmission of HIV. There also appears to be synergy between HSV and HIV, which may mean faster progression of HIV disease. Daily acyclovir therapy to suppress coinfection with HSV-2 has recently been found not to reduce the risk for transmission of HIV.

Human Papillomavirus

Human papillomavirus infection (Chapter 381) is very common in all stages of HIV infection. Common, flat, genital, and plantar warts are all seen with

FIGURE 399-1. Chronic herpes simplex infection.

TABLE 399-1	SKIN CONDITIONS COMMON IN PATIENTS WITH CD4$^+$ COUNTS LESS THAN 200 CELLS/μL AND NOT RECEIVING ANTIRETROVIRAL THERAPY

Photodermatitis
Psoriasis, difficult to control or involving more than 50% of the body
Pruritic papular eruption associated with HIV infection
Prurigo nodularis
Oral hairy leukoplakia
Molluscum contagiosum
Eosinophilic folliculitis

TABLE 399-2	SKIN CONDITIONS THAT CAN OCCUR AT ANY CD4$^+$ COUNT

Eczema
Xerosis
Tinea/onychomycosis
Kaposi's sarcoma
Warts
Syphilis

increased frequency. Patients with significant immunosuppression may have particularly extensive warts that are recalcitrant to standard treatment. Most patients commencing ART often notice considerable improvement or resolution of the warts. However, some patients receiving ART will not clear their warts despite improvement in the CD4$^+$ count, suppressed viral load, and resolution of all other opportunistic infections. The reasons for this observation remain obscure. Treatment modalities include cryotherapy, surgery, laser, topical salicylic acid preparations, podophyllin, intralesional bleomycin, and contact sensitization immunotherapy. Imiquimod has proved to be a useful modality for genital warts but appears to be less effective in the HIV setting. Anal carcinoma and anal intraepithelial neoplasia are frequent in HIV-infected patients (men and women), and screening anal Papanicolaou smears may be helpful in identifying anal dysplasia.

Molluscum Contagiosum

Molluscum contagiosum is a poxvirus (Chapter 380) that causes a self-limited papular umbilicated eruption commonly seen in children. It is rarer in adults and, when present on the face, persistent, or severe, raises the possibility of HIV coinfection. It tends to occur when the CD4$^+$ count falls below 200 cells/μL. First-line treatment is ART because molluscum contagiosum is invariably cleared with rising CD4$^+$ counts. Ablative treatments such as cryotherapy or curettage will treat individual lesions more expeditiously but can leave scarring; however, without ART the lesions are likely to recur.

Epstein-Barr Virus (Oral Hairy Leukoplakia)

Oral hairy leukoplakia (OHL) is characterized by nonpainful white plaques with a feathered edge, particularly on the lateral border of the tongue. It is associated with Epstein-Barr virus (Chapter 385) and is very rare in immunocompetent hosts. OHL can occur at any CD4$^+$ count and may therefore be the initial feature of HIV infection. (See Table 399-2 for skin diseases not

FIGURE 399-2. Staphylococcal folliculitis.

FIGURE 399-3. Secondary syphilis.

affected by the CD4$^+$ count.) The appearance of OHL was a poor prognostic indicator before ART. There is no specific treatment of OHL, although it tends to resolve when patients are receiving ART. Superinfection with *Candida* spp should be considered if the lesions are painful.

Bacteria
Staphylococcus aureus

Infections with *Staphylococcus aureus* (Chapter 296) are commonly seen in HIV disease. Staphylococcal folliculitis (Fig. 399-2) tends to be more severe or refractory to treatment in HIV-infected patients than in those who are HIV negative. Other cutaneous manifestations of staphylococcal infection include cellulitis, ecthyma (necrotic plaques), or, rarely, botryomycosis. Treatment of folliculitis includes antiseptic washes such as chlorhexidine solution, eradication of nasal carriage with mupirocin ointment, and, occasionally, systemic antibiotics. More severe infections may require intravenous antibiotics. There has been concern that patients infected with HIV are at increased risk for the development of infections, particularly recurrent infections with methicillin-resistant *S. aureus* (MRSA). Rifampicin is often used to clear MRSA, but caution should be used in patients receiving ART because rifampicin is a potent inducer of cytochrome P-450 and will therefore interfere with protease inhibitors. Risk factors for infection, including colonization with *S. aureus*, are being explored.

Bartonella

Bacillary angiomatosis is caused by *Bartonella* species (most commonly *Bartonella henselae* and *Bartonella quintana*) (Chapter 323). Occult infection with *Bartonella* should be considered in any HIV-infected patient with fever of unknown origin. The cutaneous lesions appear as purple papules, nodules, or ulcers in HIV-positive individuals. Clinically, they may resemble lesions of Kaposi's sarcoma (KS) and may also be confused with pyogenic granuloma or cutaneous lymphoma. These lesions should always undergo biopsy with tissue sent for culture. Bacillary angiomatosis responds to antibiotics such as macrolides, which will be needed for at least a 2-month course of treatment. Bacillary angiomatosis can be associated with visceral disease; in particular, the liver and spleen may be affected.

Syphilis

Syphilis (Chapter 327) is frequently seen in patients with HIV infection. Its cutaneous manifestations are protean, and therefore syphilis should be considered in any patient infected with HIV who has a new cutaneous eruption. An example of a secondary syphilis exanthem is shown in Figure 399-3. Primary, secondary, and tertiary forms of syphilis may be manifested clinically as they are in HIV-negative individuals, although atypical findings are not uncommon. Serology is not as reliable in patients with HIV infection, and skin biopsy may be useful in establishing the diagnosis. First-line

treatment is still with penicillin. Azithromycin resistance has been reported. Follow-up titers of syphilis serology should be documented to ensure adequate treatment and central nervous system (CNS) clearance.

Fungi
Candida

Oral candidiasis (Chapter 346) is commonly seen in patients with immunodeficiency, including HIV infection. It is characterized by white, cheesy plaques and papules loosely adherent to the tongue and oropharynx. Topical therapies include clotrimazole troches and nystatin oral suspension. First-line oral treatment is with fluconazole, although there is emerging resistance in *Candida* species, including *Candida albicans*, the most common species associated with thrush. Second-line treatment consists of oral itraconazole, although it is unclear whether pulsed therapy is preferable.

Dermatophytes

The prevalence of dermatophyte infection (Chapter 446) is not higher in HIV-infected patients than in control groups. However, increased severity and variability in the manifestations of dermatophyte infection are seen in HIV coinfection. Tinea corporis and tinea cruris can occur at all stages of immunosuppression and may be treated successfully with topical antidermatophytic preparations such as ketoconazole or terbinafine. Treatment of onychomycosis is systemic therapy with oral antifungals, although onychomycosis recurrence rates have not been studied.

Other Fungi

Cryptococcus neoformans is a yeast that tends to cause clinical problems when patients are profoundly immunosuppressed (CD4$^+$ count <100 cells/µL). It commonly affects the CNS and causes meningitis, but it can affect the skin and give rise to papules indistinguishable from molluscum contagiosum. *Histoplasma capsulatum* and *Penicillium marneffei* may morphologically resemble molluscum. Patients who have had these diseases need long-term suppressive doses of antifungal medications.

Infestations
Scabies

Scabies (Chapter 367) is caused by infestation with the mite *Sarcoptes scabiei* and is commonly seen in HIV-infected individuals. It can be manifested as the classic rash of scabies with burrows affecting the finger and toe webs and widespread excoriated papules with a predilection for the axillae, nipples, and genitalia. It can also appear as crusted scabies with hyperkeratotic plaques that tend not to be pruritic. Combination treatment with a topical agent such as permethrin or benzoyl benzoate and systemic treatment with ivermectin tablets is recommended for crusted scabies. Topical agents may be sufficient for classic scabies. Lindane lotion is often used to treat scabies, but there have been reports of lindane-resistant scabies and neurologic side effects attributed to this treatment.

● TUMORS
Kaposi's Sarcoma

KS is the most common HIV-associated malignancy (Chapter 400), but since the introduction of ART, there has been a significant decrease in its incidence. It is characterized by dusky, purple nodules and plaques with

FIGURE 399-4. Kaposi's sarcoma.

FIGURE 399-5. Eosinophilic folliculitis.

a predilection for the extremities and the oral mucosa (Fig. 399-4). Poor prognostic factors include lymphedema and internal organ involvement. It is caused by human herpesvirus 8, also known as Kaposi's sarcoma–associated virus. The virus may be transmitted vertically, sexually, or casually, and its presence is necessary for the development of KS. First-line treatment consists of ART, with the addition of chemotherapy for aggressive or unresponsive KS.

Malignant Melanoma and Nonmelanoma Skin Cancer

Malignant melanoma (Chapter 210) may develop at an increased incidence in HIV-positive patients. The behavior of melanoma in the ART era is unclear. There appears to be a three-fold increased risk for the development of nonmelanoma skin cancer in patients with HIV disease. The clinical manifestations of squamous cell carcinoma (SCC) and basal cell carcinoma (BCC) do not appear to be any different than those in the uninfected population (Chapter 210). However, in the context of HIV infection, SCC behaves more aggressively and is associated with reduced survival. Management of SCC is surgical excision, whereas curettage and electrodesiccation may be appropriate for BCC lesions on the extremities or trunk. Surgical excision should be the treatment of choice for BCC on the face.

⬤ INFLAMMATORY MANIFESTATIONS

Immune Reconstitution Inflammatory Syndrome

After commencement of ART, a subset of patients experience unmasking of new skin disease or paradoxical worsening of existing dermatologic conditions, attributable to IRIS (also see Chapter 402). The list of skin manifestations of IRIS continues to grow, with the current literature highlighting the emergence of tropical skin diseases, such as leishmaniasis and leprosy, manifested in the context of immune recovery. Increasingly, we are recognizing that common skin eruptions such as acne may be associated with IRIS. *Mycobacterium avium* infection can be associated with cutaneous ulceration and an epidermodysplasia verruciformis–like eruption of warts.

Certain cutaneous diseases are more common in early versus late IRIS, such as herpes zoster. Cutaneous KS can be manifested as organ involvement during IRIS. Eosinophilic folliculitis is one of the more common manifestations of IRIS and can be seen within the first 16 weeks of ART. It may be confused with a drug reaction, but the distribution of urticarial papules on the scalp, neck, face, upper part of the chest, and upper part of the back is a distinguishing factor. HSV disease may be seen 3 to 4 months into treatment and is thought to appear in the later stages of immune reconstitution.

Seborrheic Dermatitis

Seborrheic dermatitis is a common dermatosis in the general population, but it has a strikingly increased prevalence in HIV-infected patients, and its frequency increases with more severe immunosuppression. It appears as orange-red scaly patches affecting the scalp, eyebrows, nose, and cheeks. Seborrheic dermatitis can also affect the central portion of the chest and genitalia. It responds well to a combination of topical antifungals such as econazole or ketoconazole and low-potency corticosteroids. The condition also tends to improve with ART.

Atopic Dermatitis

Atopic dermatitis is common in HIV-infected patients. As with other dermatoses, it improves with ART, but in patients who had a CD4$^+$ nadir of less than 200 cells/μL, it tends to be more persistent, even with ART. Treatment consists of topical steroids and emollients as in the non–HIV-infected population. Topical pimecrolimus and tacrolimus are licensed for the treatment of atopic dermatitis, but their safety has not been demonstrated in patients with HIV infection.

Psoriasis

HIV infection can be associated with severe psoriasis (Chapter 446) as the CD4$^+$ count drops. This observation is paradoxical because psoriasis is thought to be a T-cell-mediated disease but may be explained by immune dysregulation. Topical treatments, systemic retinoids, and ultraviolet phototherapy are all reasonable treatment options. Immunosuppressive agents such as methotrexate and cyclosporine should be avoided if possible. ART invariably reduces the severity of psoriasis.

Papular Pruritic Eruption of HIV

Papular pruritic eruption is commonly seen in Africa and Asia in association with HIV. It should be considered in the differential diagnosis of any widespread itchy dermatosis, but it does appear to be a separate entity. Papular pruritic eruption has a rather nondescript appearance of red excoriated papules on the trunk and limbs. Other itchy skin diseases such as eczema or eosinophilic folliculitis should be considered in the differential diagnosis. Recent evidence has suggested that exaggerated arthropod bite reactions may be the predominant cause. Potent topical corticosteroids and, anecdotally, ART have been of benefit.

Eosinophilic Folliculitis

Eosinophilic folliculitis is characterized by edematous papules and pustules on the face and upper part of the trunk (Fig. 399-5). These lesions are intensely itchy, and skin biopsy is helpful in ruling out other causes of folliculitis. Eosinophilic folliculitis tends to be seen when CD4$^+$ counts are lower than 200 cells/μL and may improve with ART. It can also be seen as a manifestation of IRIS within the first 16 weeks of ART. Treatments such as itraconazole, permethrin, retinoids, and phototherapy are all effective.

Prurigo Nodularis

In patients with prurigo nodularis, symmetrically distributed papules and nodules develop on the limbs and trunk with sparing of the midportion of the back (because of inaccessibility for scratching). It is commonly seen in HIV-infected persons, is sometimes associated with hepatitis C virus coinfection, and may be exacerbated by light. Standard treatment options include emollients, potent topical steroids, and sedating antihistamines such as chlorpheniramine or hydroxyzine. Thalidomide is often effective in recalcitrant cases but requires careful monitoring for peripheral neuropathy, and women of childbearing potential require effective contraception.

FIGURE 399-6. HIV-associated facial lipoatrophy.

TABLE 399-3	MOST COMMON SKIN DISEASES SINCE THE ADVENT OF ANTIRETROVIRALS

Acne
Staphylococcal infections of soft tissue and skin
Erythema nodosum
Eosinophilic folliculitis
Lipodystrophy

METABOLIC MANIFESTATIONS

HIV Lipodystrophy Syndrome

Lipodystrophy syndrome consists of peripheral lipoatrophy, central lipohypertrophy, lipid abnormalities, and insulin resistance. It is likely that it is caused by a number of factors, including ART (Chapter 396) (Table 399-3), although it is unlikely that a single agent is responsible. Cutaneous facial lipoatrophy tends to be the most problematic dermatologic aspect, with significant associated psychological morbidity (Fig. 399-6). Currently, no treatments are effective for lipodystrophy syndrome, although surgical correction with dermal fillers may improve the cosmetic appearance.

1. Celum C, Wald A, Lingappa JR, et al. Acyclovir and transmission of HIV-1 from person infected with HIV-1 and HSV-2. *N Engl J Med.* 2010;362:427-439.

SUGGESTED READINGS

Huang XJ, Li HY, Chen DX, et al. Clinical analysis of skin lesions in 796 Chinese HIV-positive patients. *Acta Derm Venereol.* 2011. [Epub ahead of print.] *With HAART, the prevalence of skin lesions declined from over 80%, primarily infectious etiologies, to about 30%, with nearly half caused by drug eruptions.*
Menon K, Van Voorhees AS, Bebo BF Jr, et al. Psoriasis in patients with HIV infection: from the medical board of the National Psoriasis Foundation. *J Am Acad Dermatol.* 2010;62:291-299. *Issues and treatments for HIV-associated psoriasis are discussed.*
Rodgers S, Leslie KS. Skin infections in HIV-infected individuals in the era of HAART. *Curr Opin Infect Dis.* 2011;24:124-129. *Review including herpes, syphilis, Kaposi's sarcoma, and MRSA infections.*

400

HEMATOLOGY AND ONCOLOGY IN PATIENTS WITH HUMAN IMMUNODEFICIENCY VIRUS INFECTION

PAUL A. VOLBERDING

A wide variety of cancers and hematologic disorders remain important clinical complications of infection with human immunodeficiency virus (HIV) despite advances in HIV suppression with antiretroviral (ARV) drug regimens. Hematologic abnormalities can be caused by HIV infection itself, be a consequence of immune deficiency and related opportunistic infections, or result from side effects of drugs used to manage HIV disease. Acquired immunodeficiency syndrome (AIDS)-defining cancers (ADCs) usually occur in patients with advanced immune deficiency and a second infection in addition to HIV. Recently, reports have described an increased incidence of a widening spectrum of other non–AIDS-defining cancers (NADCs), possibly caused by continued immune activation/inflammation, even in the setting of seemingly successful ARV therapy. Cancers and hematologic disorders have changed with the advent of effective ARV therapy. Study of these clinical problems affords insight into the consequences of immune deficiency and its reversal and highlights the benefits and limitations of ARV treatment.

HIV HEMATOLOGY

Disorders in all major blood cell lines were recognized early in the HIV epidemic. The underlying biology of HIV-associated hematologic disease is complex and often involves multiple lineages and mechanisms of pathogenesis. HIV itself infects cells involved in hematopoiesis or disturbs the bone marrow microenvironment. HIV infection also causes both immune activation and immune deficiency. The former, analogous to inflammation, can cause anemia of chronic disease (also called *anemia of inflammation,* Chapter 161), whereas the dysregulation of lymphocyte subsets can disrupt the balance of cytokines and other factors needed for normal myelopoiesis. The combination of immune activation and dysregulation can also contribute to hypergammaglobulinemia and reticuloendothelial activation and result in accelerated blood cell destruction. The effect of ARV therapy on HIV-associated hematologic disease is similarly complex. ARV drugs, fortunately ones less commonly prescribed today, have well-described direct hematologic toxicities, but their ability to reverse established immune deficiency and to control HIV infection within marrow reduces the incidence and severity of many HIV-associated hematologic disorders.

Red Blood Cell Disorders and Anemia

The prevalence of anemia in HIV-infected patients varies by threshold definition and demographics. Before the advent of effective ARV therapy, estimates ranged as high as 75%.

EPIDEMIOLOGY

Anemia in HIV-infected patients can be caused by many factors (Table 400-1). Those unrelated to HIV infection, such as the hemoglobinopathies, should always be considered in the differential diagnosis, as should those associated with the mode of HIV acquisition, particularly injection drug use.

HIV-associated anemia is usually caused by decreased red blood cell (RBC) production. RBC loss from bleeding or intravascular hemolysis can occur but is less common. Decreased RBC production is seen with chronic inflammation, nutritional deficiencies, erythropoietic defects, and marrow suppression as a result of infection or drug therapy.

Anemia of chronic disease (anemia of chronic inflammation) follows ineffective iron utilization in the setting of an underlying chronic inflammatory process (Chapter 161). Iron studies generally show reductions in serum iron and transferrin concentrations. RBCs are typically normochromic and normocytic. In HIV-infected patients, this anemia presumably reflects the chronic infection of lymphocytes and ongoing immune activation and cytokine dysregulation. Direct HIV infection of precursor hematopoietic cells may also be involved. The frequency and severity of this anemia are often reduced with the use of effective ARV therapy.

Relative or absolute hypogonadism is common in persons with HIV infection and probably contributes to the reduced erythropoietic effect. This anemia may respond to testosterone replacement. Total and free serum levels of testosterone should be measured in HIV-infected men with anemia. The role, if any, of testosterone deficiency in HIV-infected women with anemia is uncertain.

PATHOBIOLOGY

Infections and Malignancies within Marrow

Bone marrow can be infected by a variety of opportunistic pathogens, especially *Mycobacterium avium-intracellulare* and *Mycobacterium tuberculosis.* The causative relationship of such infections to anemia is complicated by the advanced stage of HIV disease in many of these patients, which may itself cause marrow failure. Fortunately, these serious opportunistic infections are much less common in the era of effective ARV but still occur in patients

TABLE 400-1 CAUSES OF ANEMIA IN HIV-INFECTED PATIENTS

CAUSED PREDOMINANTLY BY DECREASED RED BLOOD CELL PRODUCTION

Anemia of chronic disease (anemia of inflammation)
Hypogonadism and decreased erythropoietic effect
Infections and cancers in marrow
   Mycobacterium-avium intracellulare
   Mycobacterium tuberculosis
   Parvovirus B-19
   Bartonella henselae
   Bartonella quintana
   Non-Hodgkin's lymphoma
   Hodgkin's lymphoma
Nutritional deficiency
   Iron deficiency
Drug effects
   Zidovudine
   Trimethoprim-sulfamethoxazole
   Ganciclovir
   Amphotericin
   Cytotoxic chemotherapeutics
   Others

CAUSED PREDOMINANTLY BY ACCELERATED RED BLOOD CELL LOSS

Hypersplenism
   HIV
   Portal hypertension from hepatitis C, hepatitis B with cirrhosis
Hemolysis
   Microangiopathy—thrombotic thrombocytopenic purpura
   Others
   Intravascular hemolysis secondary to oxidative stress in glucose-6-phosphate
     dehydrogenase deficiency and exposure to dapsone and other drugs

unable to access or maintain expert HIV care. The hematologic effects of these infections are reversed with the initiation of ARV therapy and specific treatment of the complicating infection. Chronic parvovirus B19 infection in an HIV-infected patient can cause normocytic anemia as a result of pure red cell aplasia (Chapters 168 and 379). This uncommon cause of HIV-related anemia is rarely seen with effective ARV therapy. It responds to intravenous immunoglobulin that contains parvovirus B19 antibodies. Bacillary angiomatosis, seen with *Bartonella henselae* or *Bartonella quintana* infection (Chapter 323), can also result in anemia. This condition can cause skin lesions resembling those of Kaposi's sarcoma (KS) and responds to antibiotic therapy. HIV-associated cancers, particularly non-Hodgkin's lymphoma (NHL), can involve bone marrow. Extensive marrow replacement by lymphoma may result in anemia or other cytopenias, but it is uncommon.

Nutritional Deficiencies

The presence of severe and complex nutritional deficiencies with extreme wasting is a feature of untreated HIV infection. It was common in the United States before the advent of effective ARV therapy but is now rare. Wasting remains common globally, of course, especially since HIV infection occurs against a backdrop of societal nutritional deficits (Chapter 222). Although severe wasting is less common, many patients have poor diets or other conditions, and deficiencies of vitamins such as folate and B12 should be considered, although they are less common than iron deficiency as a cause of anemia in individuals infected with HIV.

Iron Deficiency

Iron deficiency is not uncommon as a cause of anemia in HIV-infected persons. It is most often seen in women and injection drug users. Submucosal KS lesions are seen frequently in the gastrointestinal tract in advanced stages, although they rarely cause sufficient gastrointestinal blood loss to lead to iron deficiency.

Drug Toxicity

In early ARV development, anemia was often seen as a drug toxicity, particularly with zidovudine (or azidothymidine [AZT]). Stavudine (or d4T) can also cause anemia but is most frequently associated with macrocytosis. Stavudine is seldom used outside resource-limited settings because of serious toxicities, and AZT is also seldom used, again because less toxic drugs are now available. Newer ARV drugs rarely cause anemia.

A variety of drugs used to treat HIV-associated conditions can cause bone marrow suppression with resulting anemia, neutropenia, thrombocytopenia, or any combination of these disorders. Such drugs include trimethoprim-sulfamethoxazole, ganciclovir, amphotericin, and many cytotoxic chemotherapeutic agents. These side effects are very common, especially since the infections for which they are prescribed occur in late-stage HIV infection, which is itself a cause of anemia and other hematologic disorders.

Red Blood Cell Antibodies

HIV infection is associated with polyclonal gammopathy as a result of dysregulation and altered balance of the CD4$^+$ and CD8$^+$ cell populations of T lymphocytes and corresponding B-cell function. RBC autoantibodies are not uncommon in patients with HIV infection and cause a positive direct Coombs antiglobulin test (Chapter 163). This is not usually associated with hemolysis and requires no specific therapy.

CLINICAL MANIFESTATIONS

Anemia from accelerated RBC loss in HIV infection is uncommon. Frank bleeding is rare in HIV-infected patients, except in those with concomitant conditions such as portal hypertension from coincident cirrhosis associated with hepatitis B virus (HBV) or hepatitis C virus (HCV) infection. Hypersplenism, most often also seen with portal hypertension, may lead to anemia and other types of cytopenia. Finally, hemolytic anemia (as well as methemoglobinemia) can occur with microangiopathic disease or as a consequence of oxidative stress from some drugs, particularly dapsone, when used in patients with underlying glucose-6-phosphate dehydrogenase deficiency.

Anemia in HIV-infected persons is associated with accelerated disease progression and shortened survival. This association is seen even after adjusting for baseline CD4$^+$ cell counts and plasma HIV load.

Clinical evaluation of anemia in HIV infection is similar to that in other disease settings (Chapter 161), and both HIV-related and HIV-unrelated causes should be explored. Reversible causes are especially important to identify. Peripheral cell counts, including reticulocytes, are determined, as well as careful review of the peripheral blood smear. Iron studies can help differentiate between anemia of chronic disease and iron deficiency. Underlying malignancies and opportunistic infections must be considered, as should exposure to drugs with potential bone marrow suppression, especially AZT. Bone marrow biopsy is rarely indicated specifically for anemia.

TREATMENT

Potent ARV therapy has changed the frequency and severity of anemia in individuals with HIV infection, although it has not eliminated this problem.
Anemia in HIV is managed according to its etiology. Reversible causes such as iron deficiency or unnecessary exposure to a toxic drug should be addressed, as should bone marrow infections or malignancies. ARV therapy should be started if other indications exist. Replacement therapy with testosterone in the case of hypogonadism should be recommended. RBC transfusion is indicated for the acute onset of severe anemia, especially in a patient with underlying cardiovascular disease. Transfusion carries its own set of risks and should be performed only when other options are limited.
The use of replacement erythropoietin in HIV-infected patients is approved in the United States solely for AZT-associated anemia. It has not been shown to prolong survival and is rarely if ever needed because ARV options not associated with anemia are now so available and preferred by HIV treatment guidelines.

White Blood Cell Disorders

Apart from lymphocytes, the primary pathogenic target of HIV infection, the white blood cell population is relatively spared in HIV disease in comparison to other cell lines. Neutrophils are affected to some degree, whereas eosinophils and monocytes usually remain normal in number and function.

Even though neutropenia is not uncommon, it is rarely severe. Neutropenia in HIV infection is most commonly a manifestation of drug toxicity, although HIV infection within bone marrow might contribute to reduced myelopoiesis. Drugs used to treat or prevent opportunistic infections (such as trimethoprim-sulfamethoxazole) or malignancies are common offenders. Neutrophil function is well preserved in HIV infection, especially in earlier-stage disease. Although mucocutaneous candidal infections are very common in patients with HIV disease, dissemination is extremely rare, even with advanced CD4$^+$ cell depletion. Presumably, preserved neutrophil function prevents these and related infections.

Lymphocyte subset analysis, possible even early in the HIV epidemic, highlights the striking CD4⁺ cell depletion associated with HIV infection, although the mechanism for this loss remains, surprisingly, an active research question. The total lymphocyte count may be decreased in advanced HIV disease but is not a reliable surrogate for actual CD4⁺ cell enumeration. This is unfortunate because the cost of CD4⁺ counts remains an important barrier to effective ARV therapy in many global settings, although new devices for easy testing in the field may overcome this hurdle.

CD8⁺ lymphocytes are activated, not destroyed, in HIV infection. CD8⁺ cell number is relatively preserved until the most advanced disease stage. This cell population is, however, of research interest because CD8⁺ activation may accelerate disease progression.

Immune Thrombocytopenia

HIV infection is associated with thrombocytopenia. Immune thrombocytopenic purpura (ITP), though never common, was more often seen in the early years of the epidemic—in up to 8.7% of individuals with advanced AIDS. Its severity varies, but as with non–HIV-associated autoimmune or idiopathic thrombocytopenic purpura, life-threatening bleeding is uncommon (Chapter 175).

Increased splenic clearance of platelets (sometimes associated with hypersplenism) is the major mechanism of thrombocytopenia in these HIV-infected patients, but whether platelets are coated with nonspecific antibodies from immune activation and polyclonal gammopathy or with specific antiplatelet autoantibodies remains uncertain. Although HIV may directly infect megakaryocytes, accelerated platelet loss appears to be more important than decreased production. Further anecdotal evidence supporting increased platelet destruction is the observation that platelet counts tend to normalize in late HIV disease, presumably because of decreased reticuloendothelial function and hence less platelet clearance.

TREATMENT   Rx

Therapy for HIV-associated ITP (HIV-ITP) resembles that for ITP without HIV infection (Chapter 175), but effective HIV suppression should be established whenever possible before treating the thrombocytopenia per se. Splenectomy is successful in many cases. Splenectomy also results in an increase in peripheral CD4⁺ cell counts. Corticosteroids are likewise effective in treating HIV-ITP, although many fear the use of immunosuppressants in the setting of an acquired immunodeficiency disease. Other treatments with some reported success in HIV-ITP include interferon alfa, danazol, intravenous IgG/RhoGAM, and plasmapheresis.

The advent of effective ARV regimens has reduced the incidence of severe HIV-ITP. HIV-ITP should prompt initiation of ARV therapy if other indications exist. It should otherwise be managed essentially as it is in non–HIV-infected persons, with corticosteroids in a tapering dose as the initial management strategy.

Thrombotic Thrombocytopenic Purpura

Thrombotic thrombocytopenic purpura (TTP), often involving some combination of microangiopathy, renal disease, and neurologic disorders, has been reported to occur at increased frequency in persons with HIV infection. Most of these series, however, are very small, with an uncertain relationship to HIV. Presumably, HIV triggers TTP, as do many other infectious diseases (Chapter 175). Management and outcome in these reports resemble those for TTP in patients without HIV infection. Response to plasma exchange is typically rapid. The effect of effective ARV therapy on this condition—either on its incidence or on its disease course—is unknown.

Thrombosis

Reports of increased deep vein thrombosis in HIV-infected patients are relatively rare, which is perhaps surprising in the setting of a chronic viral infection and persistent elevation in markers of immune activation and inflammation. Reports may reflect the overlap between two relatively common diseases. Deep vein thrombosis in an HIV-infected person should be evaluated and managed as for noninfected patients (Chapter 81).

Bone Marrow in HIV Infection

Numerous reports early in the HIV epidemic identified alterations in bone marrow morphology and suggested ways in which bone marrow biopsy might affect management. These conclusions may require adjustment in the era of effective ARV therapy. In the absence of opportunistic infections or malignancies, bone marrow is not strikingly abnormal. Relative RBC aplasia may be seen in anemic patients, and plasma cell number is often increased, but not usually to a striking degree. The marrow findings may resemble mild cases of myelodysplasia. Marrow has been considered a site for the diagnosis of systemic opportunistic infections but has little added utility over peripheral blood culture. Marrow can be affected by HIV-related malignancies, and biopsy of marrow is commonly performed to stage HIV-related lymphoma. Bone marrow biopsy is not required for the evaluation of KS.

HIV ONCOLOGY

HIV is strongly associated with cancers, but even after 25 years of investigation no direct causal relationship has been established. Most ADCs seem to result from interaction of HIV with a second viral coinfection, especially human herpesvirus 8 (HHV-8). Other causative factors may include defects in "immune surveillance" or activation of the immune system.

In addition to ADCs, persons infected with HIV are at increased risk for the development of a widening spectrum of other malignancies that have not been considered to be AIDS defining. Such NADCs may include anal neoplasms, colorectal cancer, Hodgkin's lymphoma, liver and lung cancer, melanoma, oropharyngeal cancer, leukemia, and renal carcinoma. The association of HIV infection with NADCs is a field of intense interest because this risk appears to increase with the duration of HIV infection. In addition, much interest focuses on the role of a second infection—usually viral—in the pathogenesis of NADCs. These include cancers associated with human papillomavirus (HPV), Epstein-Barr virus (EBV), HCV, HBV, and the recently described Merkel cell virus. HIV-infected men have reduced risk for at least one cancer, that of the prostate gland, itself possibly virally related.

ADCs have been profoundly affected by the common use of effective ARV therapy. The incidence of some has declined sharply, and even advanced-stage KS has regressed after the initiation of ARV therapy. Some cancers are less affected, whereas others, such as cervical cancer—perhaps reflecting a longer period of development—have been less immediately affected by HIV treatment.

Kaposi's Sarcoma

Reports of KS in previously healthy young men heralded the onset of the AIDS epidemic. The striking novelty of this cancer in this population, along with simultaneous reports of previously rare infections, allowed almost immediate recognition of underlying immune impairment.

Before the HIV epidemic, KS was uncommon in the United States. It typically affected very elderly men or recipients of solid organ transplants. In Africa, KS was common in a region overlapping an area with a high incidence of Burkitt's lymphoma. As a result, KS was speculated to arise from immune deficiency, along with intriguing suggestions of genetic, environmental, or hormonal factors explaining the predominance of affected men in all settings.

EPIDEMIOLOGY

In the case of HIV, especially before the use of effective ARV therapy, KS affected a very specific subpopulation in the Western world. Women and children were almost always spared, and men with KS typically reported sexual contact with other men as their probable source of HIV infection. These and other observations fueled early speculation that an agent, sexually transmitted between men, might be involved in the pathogenesis of KS. These predictions have proved true with the identification of a new human herpesvirus, HHV-8, as a causative agent of KS and other malignancies.

In the early HIV epidemic, KS was a common initial manifestation of AIDS and was included as an AIDS-defining condition. In the population of men who have sex with other men (MSM), it was present in nearly 50% of new AIDS cases before the use of effective ARV therapy. In contrast, KS was seen in only 2% of new AIDS cases in women, and most of them reported sexual contact with MSM. KS rarely developed in HIV-infected children in the United States.

PATHOBIOLOGY

The viral etiology of KS, later shown to be due to HHV-8 infection, was suggested by its distinctive epidemiology. HHV-8, a gamma herpesvirus, was discovered after viral gene sequences characteristic of this viral family were found in KS lesions, but not in adjacent normal tissue. HHV-8 infects B lymphocytes, macrophages, and endothelial cells. Lytic and latent forms are

FIGURE 400-1. Kaposi's sarcoma.

seen in KS lesions. The precise mechanism of oncogenesis remains unclear, but it is dramatically accelerated in the setting of HIV coinfection.

HHV-8 is a common infection, although serologic diagnosis remains nonstandardized, with wide variation from study to study. In one multicenter study its prevalence in all U.S. blood donors was estimated to be 3.5%. In HHV-8–endemic areas of sub-Saharan Africa, children are infected by puberty, probably from salivary transmission. In San Francisco, the prevalence of HHV-8 was already high in MSM before the HIV epidemic. In the United States, the higher prevalence in MSM suggests sexual transmission.

Active HHV-8 infection, as opposed to simple seropositivity, is required for the development of KS, and HHV-8 serum titers correlate with KS incidence and disease progression rates. Together, these observations suggest a rationale for HHV-8 therapy to prevent or treat KS. The incidence of KS was reduced in several clinical trials of antiherpes therapy in HIV-infected adults. These studies, however, were very small and not powered to detect this effect, and gamma herpesviruses, including HHV-8, are relatively resistant to antiviral control. Whether such approaches offer promise for prevention or treatment of KS requires further research.

KS results from the proliferation of endothelial cells. At least in its later stages it appears to be a true malignancy and typically shows monoclonality and growth independence. Histologically, KS is characterized by both proliferation of spindle-shaped cells and poorly formed vascular channels, often with extensive RBC extravasation.

CLINICAL MANIFESTATIONS

KS lesions typically involve the visible skin surface (Fig. 400-1), although internal lesions may be seen in essentially any organ. Cutaneous lesions are generally violaceous, occasionally with surrounding ecchymosis. They are nodular and range in size from several millimeters to 2 cm in diameter, although multiple lesions can coalesce into large tumor plaques. Lesions are nonpruritic and painless except in advanced stages. KS lesions can appear simultaneously in widely separated regions rather than as a primary site with metastatic spread. Lesions may appear in clusters, may be symmetrical, and may be somewhat linear and appear to follow skin creases. KS lesions may appear on scars or other sites of previous trauma. Lesions are also common in the oral cavity, where they correlate with gastrointestinal involvement.

KS commonly involves the gastrointestinal tract, and bulky disease can cause obstruction. Frank hemorrhage is uncommon. Pulmonary KS involvement is typically evidenced by reticulonodular, patchy infiltrates on chest radiographs. Pleural effusions, if seen, are often hemorrhagic and frequently cytologically "benign." Advanced KS disease can cause intractable lymphedema, especially common in the lower extremities and head and neck.

TREATMENT Rx

KS lesions are usually quite distinct in appearance, but biopsy confirmation is essential. HHV-8 is invariably present. Bacillary angiomatosis may resemble KS morphologically but is distinguishable histologically.

ARV therapy is currently regarded as the treatment of choice for HIV-associated KS because it is remarkably active. The incidence of KS has fallen precipitously (5- to 10-fold) with wide use of ARV therapy. Moreover, established KS often responds rapidly after initiation of ARV therapy. In one series 90% of patients responded, with complete and durable resolution in 18 of 20 patients. ARV therapy may decrease HHV-8 viremia. Several preliminary reports suggest

an especially active KS response with HIV protease inhibitors. This possibility is being explored in ongoing clinical trials. An immune reconstitution inflammatory syndrome response (Chapter 402) has also been reported in patients with KS after initiation of ARV therapy.

Before the use of effective ARV therapy, KS was treated with a variety of cytotoxic agents. Vinblastine, administered either systemically or intralesionally, was later replaced by paclitaxel, anthracyclines, or etoposide. Monotherapy is generally preferred over more aggressive drug combinations. Biologic agents, including interferon alfa, topical retinoids, and tumor necrosis factor inhibitors, are also active against KS. Radiation therapy may be useful for systematic control of bulky KS plaques causing pain or lymphatic obstruction. Despite the vascular proliferation of KS lesions histologically, experimental angiogenesis inhibitors have not yet proved active in treating KS.

Non-Hodgkin's Lymphoma

NHL (Chapter 191) is the second ADC whose incidence is clearly increased with HIV infection. NHL occurs in two distinct forms in HIV-infected patients: those of peripheral or central nervous system (CNS) origin.

EPIDEMIOLOGY

Peripheral Non-Hodgkin's Lymphoma

HIV-associated peripheral NHL (HIV-NHL) is a B-cell tumor. The malignancy is often of moderate- to high-grade classification. The most common histologic variants are intermediate-grade large cell and high-grade immunoblastic lymphomas. The most common subtype is diffuse large B-cell lymphoma; the second most common is Burkitt's lymphoma. HIV-NHL is often found to be advanced at initial evaluation. Extranodal sites, including the gastrointestinal tract, lungs, and liver, are more common with HIV-NHL than in the absence of HIV infection. NHL arising in the bile duct, in the appendix, or as a solitary parenchymal pulmonary nodule has been reported. Intravascular NHL has also been seen, occasionally in vessels within the CNS.

The epidemiology of peripheral HIV-NHL is more straightforward than that of KS. Both sexes are affected equally, as are HIV-infected children and adolescents. The CD4+ cell count at diagnosis, though variable, is typically only moderately suppressed in HIV-NHL, and ARV therapy has decreased its incidence by only two-fold.

The cause of peripheral HIV-NHL is unknown. Many affected patients, but not all, are EBV positive and the tumors are HHV-8 negative except for primary effusion lymphomas (PELs).

Central Nervous System HIV-NHL

High-grade B-cell NHL can arise within the CNS in HIV-infected patients. This occurs at a much higher rate and is considered diagnostic of AIDS. HIV-related CNS lymphomas frequently exhibit leptomeningeal involvement or are associated with multiple parenchymal lesions, both unusual in the absence of HIV infection. Moreover, CNS lymphoma in HIV-infected individuals is almost always seen in those with strikingly advanced stages of immune deficiency. The median CD4+ cell count in one report, for example, was 12 cells/μL. Given the close relationship between immune deficiency and risk for CNS NHL, it is not surprising that the common use of effective ARV therapy has reduced its incidence by 100-fold.

CLINICAL MANIFESTATIONS

Apart from frequent occurrence in extranodal sites, peripheral HIV-NHL closely resembles the disease in HIV-uninfected individuals. It can be an aggressive tumor with rapid enlargement, pain, and erythema. Nodes are usually asymmetrically affected and have a firm, rubbery consistency on palpation. Any unusual mass or asymmetrical lymphadenopathy in an HIV-infected patient should undergo prompt biopsy. Systemic "B" symptoms (fever, sweats, weight loss) may be present but are neither sensitive nor specific for HIV-NHL.

Peripheral HIV-NHL is typically an aggressive malignancy—unsurprising given its high-grade histology, advanced stage at diagnosis, and underlying immune deficiency. Apart from the inherent risk for opportunistic infections in these patients, the course of the disease is not specifically affected by HIV infection. Progression can occur at local or distant sites, and CNS involvement (distinct from primary CNS HIV-NHL) is seen commonly.

CNS NHL is typically associated with signs and symptoms of a space-occupying mass. Although the specific manifestations depend on the precise location, as well as the size and rate of tumor growth, sensory and motor deficits are common, as are seizures. Headache, fever, and changes in personality are less common than in the frequent differential diagnostic considerations of CNS toxoplasmosis or cryptococcal meningitis. CNS NHL has some predilection for periventricular involvement, as well as involvement of the base of the skull.

DIAGNOSIS

Peripheral HIV-NHL is diagnosed and staged similar to the situation when HIV is not present (Chapter 191). Bone marrow biopsy, thoracic and abdominal imaging, and cerebrospinal fluid (CSF) examination are routine. Conventional histologic examination and immunoassays are used to evaluate specimens, and cell surface markers are determined by flow analysis.

CNS NHL is diagnosed by brain imaging and tissue biopsy and by detecting EBV in CSF. Although a solitary mass is common, several may be seen, especially if magnetic resonance imaging is used, which is more sensitive than computed tomography. Positron emission tomography is also useful. The most common site is deep in the white matter, and periventricular sites are disproportionately involved. CNS toxoplasmosis is more typically multicentric, but imaging alone cannot reliably differentiate most cases. CNS NHL is much more suspect if the patient has no serum *Toxoplasma* antibodies, although many patients with CNS NHL are also *Toxoplasma* antibody positive. Essentially all CNS NHL cases in the HIV setting are EBV positive. Detection of EBV on CSF polymerase chain reaction (PCR) in a patient with advanced-stage HIV and CNS imaging findings typical of CNS NHL has been considered adequate by some to establish this diagnosis, but many still demand tissue confirmation, usually obtained by stereotactic brain biopsy. CSF cytology is relatively insensitive, with 80% of patients showing no malignant cells. Flow analysis of malignant cells is characteristically diagnostic of NHL; essentially all malignant cells are CD20+.

TREATMENT AND PROGNOSIS Rx

HIV-NHL, whether diffuse large B-cell lymphoma or Burkitt's lymphoma, generally requires systemic combination chemotherapy. It is seldom so localized that it benefits from local radiation therapy and does not, itself, respond to ARV therapy as seen with KS. Various regimens have commonly been used. CHOP (cyclophosphamide, hydroxydaunomycin, Oncovin [vincristine], and prednisone) is often used in standard doses. The addition of rituximab to the CHOP regimen does not significantly increase response rates or survival and is associated with an increased risk for bacterial infection.[1] A more aggressive regimen (R-EPOCH and others) based on prolonged chemotherapy infusion has been used with success and is considered the standard regimen by many experts. This regimen includes rituximab, etoposide, vincristine, doxorubicin, cyclophosphamide, and prednisone.

Because of the high risk for CNS relapse, prophylactic administration of methotrexate or cytosine arabinoside is recommended.

The use of ARV therapy in patients with HIV-NHL improves survival. Most practitioners would initiate ARV therapy with chemotherapy because the former difficulties caused by the use of AZT can now be avoided with combinations not associated with hematologic toxicity. In one series, HIV-NHL patients treated with ARV therapy had a median duration of survival of 30 months as compared with only 6.1 months in the group not receiving ARV therapy.

The common use of ARV therapy has decreased the incidence of HIV-NHL by more than two-fold. This is less of a reduction than with KS, however, and HIV-NHL has thus become the most common HIV-related malignancy, even though its absolute prevalence is reduced from that in the era before effective ARV therapy was available.

The aggressive nature of CNS NHL, the relative isolation of the body compartment affected from systemic chemotherapy, and the severe underlying immune deficiency combine to limit survival. Before the common use of ARV therapy, the median duration of survival was measured in weeks. The use of effective ARV therapy has improved this expectation and allows the implementation of more aggressive systemic therapy for CNS NHL, but it remains a serious disease. In one series, the median survival without radiation or ARV therapy was 29 days, whereas six of seven ARV-treated patients were alive 667 days after diagnosis.

Given the severe underlying immune deficiency and the high mortality rate from opportunistic infections in early series, initiation of effective ARV therapy as soon as possible is indicated. Mass lesions can be palliated with combined chemotherapy and brain irradiation, although neurologic impairment is common in longer-term survivors. The use of ARV therapy may allow high-dose systemic chemotherapy alone, particularly high-dose methotrexate with leucovorin rescue. Radiation therapy can be used to control recurrent disease, unfortunately still an expected part of this tumor's disease course.

HHV-8–RELATED LYMPHOPROLIFERATIVE DISEASES

Primary Effusion Lymphoma

PEL is an interesting HIV-related malignancy; it is often grouped with peripheral NHL but is distinct in many respects. PEL was first reported in HIV-infected patients. These lymphomas arise as a malignant, exudative effusion in essentially any body cavity and thus have also been called *body cavity lymphomas*. These cancers are quite rare. Even rarer are solid tumor variants, with only several reported cases.

PEL typically occurs in persons with advanced HIV disease. Like KS, PEL is closely associated with HHV-8 infection. HHV-8 infects B lymphocytes, but the precise mechanism of malignant transformation has not yet been established.

CLINICAL MANIFESTATIONS

PEL has been reported in many body cavities. Pleural and pericardial disease is the most frequent, but peritoneal and synovial sites are also seen. Fever and other "B" symptoms are present in many patients. The diagnosis must be considered in an HIV-infected patient with any localized effusion, and the diagnosis of PEL should prompt HIV testing in a patient not known to be so infected.

The effusion is exudative with a lymphocyte predominance. HHV-8 DNA is found by PCR in essentially all cases.

TREATMENT AND PROGNOSIS Rx

Even though response to chemotherapy is expected, complete resolution is rare. PEL is treated with systemic chemotherapy. Although no large series or controlled trials have been reported, standard doses of CHOP regimens are often used. Some have advocated a more aggressive chemotherapeutic approach, but the rarity of these tumors has not allowed a prospective comparative clinical trial of this strategy. ARV therapy is also typically initiated, analogous to the situation with CNS NHL, but PEL does not, itself, respond to ARV treatment. Effective ARV therapy has decreased the incidence of PEL and prolongs survival, although it remains an aggressive malignancy with a short median duration of survival. Median survival in one series was 6.2 months.

Multicentric Castleman's Disease

Multicentric Castleman's disease (MCD) is a lymphoproliferative disorder associated with overexpression of interleukin-6. MCD in the HIV-infected population is associated with HHV-8 infection. Though "benign," the proliferation is often extensive, with diffuse nodal enlargement, splenomegaly, and "B" symptoms seen in the majority of patients. MCD may have a malignant phenotype and may be associated with KS, HIV-NHL, or PEL.

CLINICAL MANIFESTATIONS

MCD is commonly accompanied by diffuse lymphadenopathy, hepatic and splenic enlargement, and a variety of systemic signs and symptoms. In some series, pulmonary manifestations were common and anemia was also frequent. Lymph node biopsy is essential for diagnosis. Histologic patterns vary, but B cells predominate. EBV studies are not consistently positive, whereas HHV-8 DNA is typically detected. The course may be relapsing and remitting but in some individuals is a highly aggressive disorder that responds poorly to treatment.

TREATMENT AND PROGNOSIS Rx

MCD carries a high risk for the simultaneous or subsequent development of an HIV-related malignancy. Depending in part on the predominant histologic pattern of MCD at biopsy, progression may be toward HIV-NHL or PEL/KS. MCD itself responds to low-dose chemotherapy, such as vinblastine, which may prolong survival but rarely results in prolonged remission. In addition to chemotherapy, other agents such as corticosteroids and antiherpesvirus drugs have provided additional benefit. More promising results have been seen with the use of rituximab, which has been associated with durable response in some patients. The effect of ARV therapy on MCD has been incompletely examined, but such therapy should be initiated.

Plasmablastic Lymphoma

Often associated with HHV-8, this lymphoproliferative disease has been recognized with increasing frequency. These are typically highly aggressive, high–growth fraction tumors with phenotypes that fall in the spectrum between B-cell NHL and plasma cell malignancies. They are frequently seen in the oral cavity. No prospective treatment studies have been reported. Aggressive treatment regimens such as those used for Burkitt's lymphoma are often recommended.

Human Papillomavirus–Associated Anal-Cervical Disease

HPV infection is transmitted sexually and, unsurprisingly, is often seen in combination with HIV, also a sexually transmitted infection. HPV-related cancers are less easily linked to HIV infection given their common occurrence in demographically similar but HIV-uninfected persons and because of their typically prolonged period of development. Both cervical and anal cellular atypia are common in patients dually infected with HIV and HPV, and several reports have found a higher frequency of higher-grade or premalignant atypia in such dually infected populations. Similarly, both cervical and anal cancers have been diagnosed in HIV-infected persons. These cancers are seen more frequently as a result of HIV infection. HPV infection is common in the MSM population (with or without HIV infection), and anal cancer is clearly more common in the MSM community, but at even higher rates in those concurrently infected with HIV. Cervical cancer is also seen in HIV-infected women at a somewhat higher frequency than in non–HIV-infected women. More effective ARV therapy has, however, not led to a declining incidence of these cancers as opposed to those more directly associated with HIV infection, possibly reflecting the very prolonged time that these cancers take to develop from lower grades of cellular atypia.

The association between HPV infection, HIV infection, and cervical and anal cancer may become even more evident as survival is prolonged with effective ARV therapy. Moreover, regardless of any cause-and-effect relationship, it is clear that proliferative changes with a potential for malignant transformation occur frequently in HIV-infected persons. These observations have led to increasingly strong recommendations for regular physical and cytologic examination of cervical and anal tissue in HIV-infected patients. Standard Papanicolaou (PAP) testing has been adapted for anal examination and is increasingly routine. Abnormal PAP cytology should prompt further diagnostic and therapeutic approaches, although proof of improved outcome with specific algorithms remains under investigation. Detection of HPV by molecular techniques is also a promising way to establish risk for disease and may be applied in settings globally where PAP testing is unavailable. The role and prophylactic effect of HPV vaccine have not yet been fully evaluated in HIV-infected persons, but it is generally anticipated to play a major role in the prevention of both cervical and anal cancer as it is made available internationally.

Hepatitis C, Hepatitis B, and Hepatocellular Cancer

HIV infection accelerates the course of disease of both hepatitis B and hepatitis C. Both are associated with an increased risk for hepatocellular cancer (HCC) (Chapter 202). In the case of HCV infection, this risk requires underlying cirrhosis. HCC in an HBV-infected patient can arise without cirrhosis. It is not clear that screening for HCC should be affected by HIV infection because of the relative insensitivity and nonspecific nature of all techniques. Perhaps more importantly, this association should increase interest in ensuring wide use of HBV vaccination at an early age and in developing effective antivirals for HBV and HCV infection. If effective, such antivirals would presumably prove useful in decreasing the risk for malignancy, particularly with the potential curability of each infection.

Cancers in HIV-Infected Persons Not Proved to Be Linked Causally (NADCs)

A wide variety of cancers have been diagnosed in HIV-infected persons. This may, of course, represent the coincidence of common diseases. Such cancers may, in fact, increase in frequency as a larger number of people survive HIV infection for prolonged periods as a result of effective ARV therapy. Moreover, HIV-infected persons may have higher exposure to cancer through smoking or other cancer risk behavior. Some causal relationship may exist, though difficult to prove, and the natural history of cancers may be altered by HIV infection.

Hodgkin's lymphoma (Chapter 192) has most closely been linked to HIV infection, and most of these tumors are EBV positive. Several epidemiologic studies have shown an increased incidence in HIV-infected persons. Other reports suggest an altered histology with less favorable subtypes, including mixed cellularity and lymphocyte depletion seen at higher frequency with an associated impact on outcome. Not all reports show a causative relationship, however, and the management of individual patients is probably not specifically changed in the setting of HIV infection.

The questions surrounding NADCs have generated substantial research interest, particularly as the population of those living with treated HIV infection increases along with their duration of infection. It does appear clear from numerous cohort studies that the incidence and variety of NADCs are increasing in HIV-infected persons. A frequent suggestion is that this may result from continuing inflammation and immune activation in these patients, even with the use of potent ARV therapy, as opposed to those who are not infected with HIV. In addition, many cancers seen in HIV-infected persons but not strictly AIDS defining are associated with a second infection in addition to HIV. Examples include Hodgkin's lymphoma and EBV, esophageal cancer and anal cancer with HPV, and Merkel cell carcinoma with the Merkel virus. Research may be able to clarify the nature of these associations, particularly through use of the large and well-characterized patient cohorts now being monitored in many countries. Pending clarification, physicians treating HIV-infected patients must be increasingly vigilant to prevent, screen, and treat a widening spectrum of cancers and to avoid overconfidence that these diseases are prevented simply by the use of ARV therapy.

FUTURE DIRECTIONS

HIV-related hematologic and malignant diseases were vital indicators of the AIDS epidemic. They remain significant clinical problems, although their severity and frequency have changed, in some cases dramatically, after the widespread use of effective ARV therapy. Research will continue to investigate the relationship between HIV infection and these problems. This research may also be able to elucidate the general relationship between inflammation, immune activation, and immune deficiency and oncogenesis. Because many HIV-related cancers require the participation of a second virus, this work will also provide strong motivation for the development of vaccines and antivirals directed at these pathogens. Such research, if positive, could well benefit an even broader population.

1. Kaplan LD, Lee JY, Ambinder RF, et al. Rituximab does not improve clinical outcome in a randomized phase 3 trial of CHOP with or without rituximab with HIV-associated non-Hodgkin lymphoma: AIDS-Malignancies Consortium Trial 010. *Blood*. 2005;106:1538-1543.

SUGGESTED READINGS

Bower M, Francis N, Newsom-Davis T, et al. The effects of HAART in 254 consecutive patients with AIDS related Kaposi's sarcoma. *AIDS*. 2009;23:1701-1706. *Review of the clinical outcomes of patients with histologically confirmed AIDS-related Kaposi's sarcoma diagnosed since the introduction of highly active antiretroviral therapy (HAART).*

Castillo JJ, Beltran BE, Bibas M, et al. Prognostic factors in patients with HIV-associated peripheral T-cell lymphoma: a multicenter study. *Am J Hematol*. 2011;86:256-261. *HIV-associated PTCL presents predominantly in young men with low CD4(+) counts and high HIV viral loads.*

Collaboration of Observational HIV Epidemiological Research Europe (COHERE) study group. Prognosis of HIV-associated non-Hodgkin lymphoma in patients starting combination antiretroviral therapy. *AIDS*. 2009;23:2029-2037. *Review of examined survival and prognostic factors in patients in whom HIV-associated NHL developed in the era of combination antiretroviral therapy.*

Patel M, Philip V, Fazel F. Human immunodeficiency virus infection and Hodgkin's lymphoma in South Africa: an emerging problem. *Adv Hematol*. 2011;2011:578163. *Review in a region where HAART is rapidly changing the natural history of HIV.*

Shiels M, Cole S, Kirk G, et al. A meta-analysis of the incidence of non-AIDS cancers in HIV-infected individuals. *J Acquir Immune Defic Syndr*. 2009;52:611-622. *Review to estimate summary standardized incidence ratios of non-AIDS cancers among HIV-infected individuals in comparison to general population rates overall and stratified by gender, AIDS, and HAART era.*

Uldrick TS, Whitby D. Update on KSHV epidemiology, Kaposi sarcoma pathogenesis, and treatment of Kaposi sarcoma. *Cancer Lett*. 2011;305:150-162. *Comprehensive review of pathogenesis and treatment for the developed and developing world.*

401

NEUROLOGIC COMPLICATIONS OF HUMAN IMMUNODEFICIENCY VIRUS INFECTION

JOSEPH R. BERGER AND AVINDRA NATH

The neurologic complications of human immunodeficiency virus (HIV) infection can affect any portion of the neuraxis. They can be broadly divided into two large groups: those that are the consequence of HIV infection and those that are secondary in nature and occur chiefly as a result of the associated immunosuppression (Table 401-1). With respect to the former group, some of these disorders, such as acute HIV meningitis, are relatively rare, whereas others, such as HIV-associated neurocognitive disorders (HAND) and HIV-associated peripheral neuropathy, are common. HIV meningitis generally occurs at the time of seroconversion, but other disorders, such as HAND, HIV myelopathy, and HIV peripheral neuropathy, are typically not observed until advanced stages of immunosuppression.

The most common neurologic complications occurring as a secondary consequence of the virus are opportunistic infections. The most frequent of such infections are central nervous system (CNS) toxoplasmosis (Chapter 357), cryptococcosis (Chapter 344), tuberculosis (Chapter 332), cytomegalovirus encephalitis (Chapter 384), JC virus infection that results in progressive multifocal leukoencephalopathy (Chapter 378), and varicella-zoster virus encephalitis or myelitis (Chapter 383). However, many noninfectious complications occur as well. The incidence of primary CNS lymphoma is remarkably high. Unlike non–AIDS-associated primary CNS lymphoma, in which Epstein-Barr virus can be recovered from only 50% of tumors (Chapter 191), all AIDS-related primary CNS lymphomas have been associated with Epstein-Barr virus infection (Chapter 400). A wide variety of toxic and metabolic complications have been observed in HIV-infected patients, including Wernicke's encephalopathy and vitamin B_{12} deficiency. Drugs, particularly antiretroviral agents, have also been associated with neurologic complications. Certain nucleoside analogues (e.g., the "d" drugs didanosine [ddI], dideoxycytidine [ddC], and stavudine [d4T]; see Table 401-5) are frequently associated with peripheral neuropathy. Finally, a wide variety of cerebrovascular disorders have been associated with HIV infection. Thrombotic ischemic stroke in this population has been attributed to an as yet undefined procoagulant tendency. Certain infections seen with increased frequency in patients infected with HIV, such as syphilis, tuberculosis, and cryptococcosis, may be associated with stroke. In addition, CNS vasculitis has occasionally been observed with HIV infection, either from HIV or from an associated varicella-zoster infection.

In recent years, it is being increasingly recognized that in a few weeks or months after initiation of combination antiretroviral therapy (ART), some patients will clinically deteriorate even when there is a robust drop in plasma viral load and recovery of CD4 cell counts. In these patients, the recovery of immune function may result in an inflammatory syndrome termed immune reconstitution inflammatory syndrome (IRIS; Chapter 402). This most often occurs when a patient has an underlying opportunistic infection, in which case the inflammation is targeted to the site of the infection. On occasion, IRIS may occur in the brain without any identifiable opportunistic infection.

Few HIV-infected individuals will escape experiencing one or more of these complications during their lifetime. They are responsible for a significant amount of morbidity and mortality. Not infrequently, more than one neurologic condition coexists in the same patient, which is often a source of confusion because one of the illnesses may be appropriately diagnosed and treated, yet the patient continues to deteriorate. Furthermore, one must also consider that any neurologic abnormalities observed are the consequence of more pedestrian disorders, such as radiculopathy secondary to disc herniation, and are unrelated to the HIV infection. In patients not responding to appropriate therapy for a proven disorder, careful clinical reevaluation is essential.

HIV-ASSOCIATED NEUROCOGNITIVE DISORDERS

DEFINITION

HIV dementia has been referred to by a number of names, including *subacute encephalitis, multinucleated giant cell encephalitis, AIDS dementia complex,* and *HIV-associated neurocognitive disorders (HAND)*.

A spectrum of increasing cognitive impairment has been described in association with HIV infection. An acquired impairment in cognitive function involving two ability domains, with a performance at least 1.0 SD below the mean for norms on standardized neuropsychological tests but no cognitive impairment in everyday function, has been referred to as *asymptomatic neurocognitive impairment*. Patients with mild neurocognitive disorder have a similar disorder on neuropsychological testing but exhibit problems with daily functions. Those with HIV dementia have marked impairment (≥ 2 SD) on at least two domains in neuropsychological testing and marked interference in day-to-day activities because of cognitive impairment. By definition, the diagnosis of HAND requires that there be no delirium and no other etiology to explain the deficit.

EPIDEMIOLOGY

In the pre-ART era, HIV dementia was observed more commonly. Early studies suggested that it was evident in more than 50% of preterminal patients. The Multicenter AIDS Cohort Study found an incidence of 4% coincident with the diagnosis of AIDS, and dementia developed in 7% within 1 year of the development of AIDS and in 14% within 2 years. Other studies have found slightly higher rates. After the introduction of combination ART in 1996, the incidence rate of HIV dementia declined substantially but the prevalence of the disorder increased; this finding may be the result of prolonged survival of affected patients. Studies suggest that the incidence of HAND may be climbing to involve as many as 50% of patients with HIV infection, but most patients have milder forms of cognitive impairment. Risk factors for HAND include low CD4 cell counts, concurrent anemia, extremes of age, and history of substance abuse or addiction. Depression is also a common comorbidity. Congenitally or perinatally infected children may exhibit delayed development. Genetic factors such as *APOE4* and polymorphisms in chemokine monocyte chemotactic protein-1 and tumor necrosis factor receptor have been identified as risk factors for the development of HAND.

PATHOBIOLOGY

HIV enters the brain early after the initial infection. In all likelihood, the virus enters the brain in infected mononuclear cells, although it is possible that it also enters as cell-free virus. HIV can be demonstrated in the brain as early as 2 weeks after infection. The viral infection predominates in invading macrophages in the brain, microglial cells, and multinucleated giant cells, usually in perivascular areas. HIV can also infect astrocytes, and studies suggest that in patients with cognitive impairment, 16 to 19% of astrocytes may be infected. HIV may remain latent for extended periods. Infection of other cell types is a rare event. The brain may thus be an important reservoir for HIV. Certain proteins of the virus, Tat and gp120, have been demonstrated to have a significant pernicious effect on neuronal function and viability either through direct toxic effects on neurons or by stimulation of glial cells, which in turn produce neurotoxic metabolites—cytokines and chemokines. Similarly, the perivascular, HIV-infected inflammatory cells produce a wide variety of chemokines and cytokines that also have similar deleterious effects. Therefore, there appear to be parallel paths, direct viral neurotoxicity and toxicity from inflammatory byproducts that lead to the development of HAND. Drugs of abuse, such as opiates, cocaine, and methamphetamine, can

TABLE 401-1	CLASSIFICATION OF THE NEUROLOGIC COMPLICATIONS OF HIV INFECTION

DIRECT	INDIRECT
Acute meningitis	Opportunistic infections
Chronic meningitis	Neoplasms
Encephalopathy	Toxic/metabolic
Myelopathy	Drug effects
Peripheral neuropathy	Cerebrovascular disease
Myositis/myopathy	

FIGURE 401-1. Histopathology of HIV dementia. **A,** Multinucleated giant cell immunostaining for HIV antigen. **B,** A microglia nodule shows a collection of inflammatory cells. The HIV-infected cells are immunostained for HIV antigen and are brown. **C,** A confocal photomicrograph shows astrocytosis. The astrocytes are stained blue with antibody to glial acidic fibrillary protein (GAFP). The macrophages are immunostained with antibody to CD14 (red). (Courtesy of Carlos Pardo, Johns Hopkins University, Baltimore.) **D,** In neurons immunostained with antibody to amyloid precursor protein, beading of the neuritis suggests interruption of axonal flow. (Courtesy of Chris Zink, Johns Hopkins University, Baltimore.)

stimulate HIV replication in glial cells and synergize with the HIV proteins to cause neurotoxicity and glial cell activation.

On gross examination, the brain typically exhibits cortical atrophy, sulcal widening, and ventricular dilation. Histopathologic examination shows multinucleated giant cells, microglial nodules, white matter pallor, astrogliosis, and perivascular inflammation (Fig. 401-1). The multinucleated giant cell, which is a syncytium of macrophages, has been regarded as the hallmark of infection, but it is not uniformly present in patients with HAND. The pathologic changes are most prominent in the basal ganglia, prefrontal cortex, and hippocampus. Concomitant vacuolar myelopathy is seen in as many as 40% of patients, although it has become less common since the introduction of ART.

CLINICAL MANIFESTATIONS

Most commonly, patients describe impaired memory, poor concentration, impairment of executive function, and difficulty reading. They often find it difficult to recall a passage recently read. Other frequent symptoms include gait problems, depression, and tremors, and patients may appear apathetic and slow or become socially withdrawn. Headaches, fatigue, and sexual dysfunction are frequent. The most commonly observed physical findings are psychomotor slowing with bradyphrenia and impaired rapid repetitive and alternating movements, hyperreflexia, increased tone, facial masking, frontal release signs (snout, glabellar, involuntary grasp), and abnormal ocular motility. The dementia has the features of a subcortical dementia not inconsistent with the relatively marked disease burden observed in dopaminergic basal ganglia. Screening tools for HAND have been proposed (Table 401-2) and a battery of specific neuropsychological tests used (Table 401-3). Staging of the disease along a continuum has been widely adopted (Table 401-4).

DIAGNOSIS

Computed tomography of the head typically shows brain atrophy, but findings may be normal. Central atrophy is generally more pronounced than cortical atrophy. In children, calcification of the basal ganglia is often observed. Similar findings are seen on magnetic resonance imaging. Basal ganglia hyperintensity is seen rarely on T2-weighted images and may resolve during the course of ART. White matter hyperintensities are also commonly detected on T2-weighted images and fluid-attenuated inversion recovery (FLAIR) sequences (Fig. 401-2). These lesions may be discrete and focal or large and confluent. They are generally symmetrically distributed and may be confused with lesions of progressive multifocal leukoencephalopathy (Chapter 378). Unlike progressive multifocal leukoencephalopathy lesions, they are typically not hypointense on T1-weighted sequences.

TREATMENT Rx

Whether ART needs to cross the blood-brain barrier for a better neurocognitive outcome remains uncertain. Higher cerebrospinal fluid (CSF) penetrant ability is associated with lower levels of HIV RNA in the CSF. Prudence dictates that highly CNS penetrant ARTs would best be used, although other factors should be considered (e.g., the drug's pharmacokinetics, protein binding, and

TABLE 401-2	SCREENING TEST FOR HIV-ASSOCIATED NEUROCOGNITIVE DISORDERS	
MAXIMUM SCORE	**SCORE**	
		MEMORY REGISTRATION
		Give 4 words to recall (dog, hat, green, peach), 1 second to say each. Then ask the patient all 4 after you have said them.
4	( )	**ATTENTION**
		Anti-saccadic eye movements: 20 commands _____ errors of 20 trials
		≤3 errors = 4; 4 errors = 3; 5 errors = 2; 6 errors = 1; >6 errors = 0
6	( )	**PSYCHOMOTOR SPEED**
		Ask patient to write the alphabet in uppercase letters horizontally across the page (use the back of this form) and record the time: _____ sec
		≤21 sec = 6; 21.1-24 sec = 5; 24.1-27 sec = 4; 27.1-30 sec = 3; 30.1-33 sec = 2; 33.1-36 sec = 1; >36 sec = 0
4	( )	**MEMORY RECALL**
		Ask for 4 words from Registration above. Give 1 point for each correct. For words not recalled, prompt with a "semantic" clue, as follows: animal (dog); piece of clothing (hat), color (green), fruit (peach). Give ½ point for each correct after prompting.
2	( )	**CONSTRUCTION**
		Copy the cube below; record the time: _____ sec <25 sec = 2; 25-35 sec = 1; 35 sec = 0

TOTAL SCORE: _____ /16

From Power C, Selnes OA, Grim JA, McArthur JC. HIV dementia scale: a rapid screening test. *J Acquir Immune Defic Syndr Hum Retrovirol.* 1995;8:273-278.

TABLE 401-3	NEUROPSYCHOLOGICAL BATTERY PROPOSED FOR EVALUATION OF HIV-ASSOCIATED NEUROCOGNITIVE DISORDERS

Fine motor control
    Grooved pegboard
    Finger tapping

Rapid sequential problem solving
    Trail making A and B
    Digit symbol

Visuospatial problem solving
    Block design

Spontaneity
    Verbal fluency

Visual memory
    Visual reproduction

TABLE 401-4	MEMORIAL SLOAN-KETTERING SCALE FOR HIV-ASSOCIATED NEUROCOGNITIVE DISORDERS
Stage 0 (normal)	Normal mental and motor function
Stage 0.5 (equivocal or subclinical)	Absent, minimal, or equivocal symptoms without impairment of work or capacity to perform activities of daily living
Stage 1 (mild)	Able to perform all but the more demanding aspects of work or activities of daily living
Stage 2 (moderate)	Able to perform all the basic activities of daily self-care but cannot work or maintain the more demanding aspects of daily life
Stage 3 (severe)	Major intellectual incapacity or motor disability with slowing
Stage 4 (end stage)	Nearly vegetative

From Price RW, Brew BJ. The AIDS dementia complex. *J Infect Dis.* 1988;158:1079-1083.

FIGURE 401-2. Magnetic resonance image of the brain in HIV dementia. The FLAIR image shows confluent areas of signal hyperintensity adjacent to ventricles.

TABLE 401-5	CEREBROSPINAL FLUID–PLASMA RATIOS FOR ANTIRETROVIRAL THERAPIES
	CEREBROSPINAL FLUID–PLASMA RATIO
NUCLEOSIDE REVERSE TRANSCRIPTASE INHIBITORS	
Zidovudine (AZT)	0.3-1.35
Stavudine (d4T)	0.16-0.97
Abacavir (ABC)	0.3-0.42
Didanosine (ddI)	0.16-0.19
Lamivudine (3TC)	0.11
Zalcitabine (ddC)	0.09-0.37
Emtricitabine	0.04
NUCLEOTIDE REVERSE TRANSCRIPTASE INHIBITORS	
Tenofovir	<0.05
FUSION INHIBITORS	
Enfuvirtide	NA
NON-NUCLEOSIDE REVERSE TRANSCRIPTASE INHIBITORS	
Nevirapine (NVP)	0.28-0.45
Delavirdine	0.02
Efavirenz	0.01
PROTEASE INHIBITORS	
Indinavir	0.02-0.76
Saquinavir	<0.05
Nelfinavir	<0.05
Ritonavir	<0.05
Amprenavir	<0.05
Lopinavir	<0.05
Atazanavir	0.0021-0.0226
Fosamprenavir	<0.05

Adapted from McArthur JC, Haughey N, Gartner S, et al. Human immunodeficiency virus–associated dementia: an evolving disease. *J Neurovirol.* 2003;9:205-221.

IC_{95}). Newer CCR5 antagonists, maraviroc and vicriviroc, demonstrate good CSF penetration and may be uniquely suited for the treatment of HAND. Table 401-5 provides a list of ARTs with their respective CSF-plasma ratios, which may provide a proxy for CNS penetration. A variety of other therapies have been proposed for the treatment of HAND that chiefly addresses the proposed inflammatory pathway of the pathogenesis of the disorder. To date, none has been established to be effective. The flow chart in Figure 401-3 provides an algorithm for the management of HAND. Careful attention to treatment of comorbidities is also essential.

PROGNOSIS

In the pre-ART era, the life expectancy of patients with HIV dementia was less than 6 months. The institution of effective ART has considerably increased the life expectancy of affected patients, and partial recovery of neurocognitive deficits may be seen.

● HIV MYELOPATHY

A broad spectrum of myelopathies occurs with HIV infection (Table 401-6). HIV causes a distinct myelopathy referred to as *HIV vacuolar myelopathy*. Evident in 20 to 55% of autopsies, this myelopathy is underrecognized clinically. It is characterized by an insidious onset of leg weakness and gait abnormality that usually occurs during the course of advanced HIV infection. Sensory complaints include vague leg discomfort and distal paresthesias. Bowel and bladder dysfunction is frequent. Physical examination reveals spastic paraparesis with lower extremity hyperreflexia, a spastic-ataxic gait,

and impaired sensation with vibratory and position perception disproportionately affected. The sensory loss may be asymmetrical, but the presence of a discrete sensory level should suggest an alternative cause of the myelopathy. Magnetic resonance imaging of the spinal cord is usually normal but may show cord atrophy or hyperintense signal abnormalities within the cord on T2-weighted images. The value of spinal magnetic resonance imaging lies in exclusion of other diagnostic possibilities, particularly structural abnormalities of the cord. Somatosensory evoked potentials generally demonstrate delayed conduction. Although findings on gross examination of the cord and dura are usually normal, histopathologic examination typically reveals loss of myelin with spongy degeneration, axonal preservation, microglial nodules, and multinucleated giant cells involving the lateral and posterior columns of the spinal cord. The pathogenesis of this disorder remains obscure. The clinical and pathologic features are suggestive of vitamin B_{12} deficiency (Chapter 167), but no consistent abnormalities are found in serum levels of vitamin

FIGURE 401-3. Flow chart for the treatment of HIV dementia. ART = antiretroviral therapy; CNS = central nervous system; CSF = cerebrospinal fluid; HIV = human immunodeficiency virus; MRI = magnetic resonance imaging.

TABLE 401-6	SPECTRUM OF MYELOPATHIES IN HIV INFECTION

HIV ASSOCIATED

Vacuolar myelopathy
Acute myelitis
Relapsing remitting encephalomyelitis
Spinal myoclonus

VIRAL

Cytomegalovirus
HTLV-1 and HTLV-2
Varicella-zoster virus
Measles virus
Progressive multifocal leukoencephalopathy

BACTERIAL

Mycobacterium tuberculosis
Treponema pallidum
Pseudomonas cepacia

FUNGAL

Cryptococcus immitis
Aspergillus sp
Nocardia

PARASITIC

Toxoplasma gondii
Schistosoma

MALIGNANCY

Primary CNS lymphoma
Metastatic CNS lymphoma
Other tumors (e.g., glioma)

VASCULAR

Necrotizing vasculitis
Disseminated intravascular coagulation

TOXIC/METABOLIC

Vitamin B_{12} deficiency
Protease inhibitor epidural lipomatosis

CNS = central nervous system; HTLV = human T-lymphotropic virus.

B_{12} or its metabolites, and replacement therapy with cyanocobalamin or S-methyl-L-methionine has not proved to be beneficial. The most effective management appears to be ART coupled with physical therapy.

HIV PERIPHERAL NEUROPATHY

Although a large number of peripheral neuropathies have been described in association with HIV infection, the one most commonly observed is a distal symmetrical sensorimotor peripheral neuropathy that ultimately affects at least a third of all HIV-infected persons. This neuropathy is seen more often in advanced disease. The patient typically complains of "burning feet." Distal paresthesias and numbness are reported, and the pain may be debilitating. Distal vibratory, pinprick, and temperature sensory perceptions are diminished, and the Romberg sign is often present. Ankle jerks are depressed or absent, and mild weakness of the toes with associated atrophy of the intrinsic muscles of the foot is frequently noted. Nerve conduction studies show reduced sensory nerve action potentials and conduction velocities. Nerve conduction amplitudes are reduced disproportionately to the reduction in conduction velocity. Electromyography may demonstrate features consistent with either acute or chronic denervation. Skin biopsy shows a reduction in cutaneous nerve fibers.

A clinically indistinguishable neuropathy may be seen with some of the antiretroviral agents, particularly with ddI, ddC, and d4T. The neuropathy associated with these agents appears to be dose dependent. Other drugs used in treatment of AIDS or its complications, such as hydroxyurea, isoniazid, vincristine, and thalidomide, may also result in a similar peripheral neuropathy. Discontinuation of the use of these drugs should result in improvement in the neuropathic features; however, a phenomenon referred to as *coasting*, in which continued worsening of the neuropathy occurs after discontinuation of the offending agent, may be observed for a period of several months.

Shortly after seroconversion, a demyelinating peripheral neuropathy identical to Guillain-Barré syndrome or chronic inflammatory polyradiculoneuropathy (Chapter 428) may be observed if it progresses for a duration of 3 weeks or more. An autoimmune process is the probable pathogenesis, and these neuropathies respond to therapy routinely used in the treatment of these conditions. In rare instances, mononeuritis multiplex (Chapter 428) may be seen with HIV infection.

HIV MYOPATHY

Several forms of muscle disease occur with HIV infection and, like other neurologic disorders, may be due to HIV or be secondary to other processes. Among the latter are myopathies associated with drugs such as zidovudine and cholesterol-lowering agents, opportunistic infections, neoplastic infiltrates, and vasculopathies. HIV myopathy mirrors the clinical and laboratory findings of classic polymyositis (Chapter 277). It is characterized by a progressive symmetrical weakness of the limb girdle and neck flexor muscles. Fatigue, myalgias, and wasting are observed in up to 50% of affected persons. Muscle enzymes, including creatine kinase and aldolase, are elevated, and the electromyogram shows short, brief, polyphasic unit action potentials. Muscle biopsy reveals myofibrillar necrosis, phagocytosis, variation in fiber size, and regeneration and degeneration typically with endomysial inflammatory infiltrates. This myopathy is rare, with an incidence of less than 1%, and has been observed in any stage of HIV infection. All patients with weakness who are taking a nucleoside reverse transcriptase inhibitor (NRTI) should have blood lactate levels measured because of an association between a recently described neuromuscular weakness syndrome and lactic acidosis in patients taking

NRTIs. The contribution of zidovudine to the genesis of HIV-associated myopathy remains controversial. As in non-HIV polymyositis, corticosteroid therapy is beneficial and can be administered with tolerable side effects.

SUGGESTED READINGS

McArthur JC, Steiner J, Sacktor N, et al. Human immunodeficiency virus-associated neurocognitive disorders: mind the gap. *Ann Neurol.* 2010;67:699-714. *A comprehensive review.*

Robinson-Papp J, Simpson DM. Neuromuscular diseases associated with HIV-1 infection. *Muscle Nerve.* 2009;40:1043-1053. *Comprehensive clinical review of the clinical manifestations and management of neuropathies associated with HIV infection.*

Schouten J, Cinque P, Gisslen M, et al. HIV-1 infection and cognitive impairment in the cART era: a review. *AIDS.* 2011;25:561-575. *Cognitive impairment continues to occur in 15 to 50% of patients.*

Singer EJ, Valdes-Sueiras M, Commins D, et al. Neurologic presentations of AIDS. *Neurol Clin.* 2010;28:253-275. *Review of HIV-associated neurologic syndromes.*

Sonneville R, Ferrand H, Tubach F, et al. Neurological complications of HIV infection in critically ill patients: clinical features and outcomes. *J Infect.* 2011;62:301-308. *Review of 210 patients, 20% of whom were not known to be infected on admission.*

402

IMMUNE RECONSTITUTION INFLAMMATORY SYNDROME IN HIV/AIDS

ROBERT COLEBUNDERS AND MARTYN A. FRENCH

DEFINITION

Treatment of human immunodeficiency virus (HIV) infection with combination antiretroviral therapy (ART) results in the restoration of protective pathogen-specific immune responses and the regression or prevention of opportunistic infections (OIs) and cancers (Chapter 396). However, restoration of an immune response against a pathogen may also result in immunopathology at body sites infected by the pathogen. This has been referred to as *immune restoration disease* (IRD) to differentiate it from immunodeficiency disease, but it is now commonly known as *immune reconstitution inflammatory syndrome* (IRIS) because an inflammatory illness is the most common clinical feature.

Essentially any pathogen that causes an infection as a result of HIV-induced cellular immunodeficiency may be associated with IRIS after ART is commenced. However, the clinical characteristics and severity of IRIS associated with each type of pathogen vary greatly (Table 402-1). For example, IRIS associated with *M. tuberculosis*, cryptococcal, or JC polyomavirus (JCV) infection is manifested differently from an OI caused by these pathogens, and the resulting illness is often severe and may result in death. In contrast, herpes zoster after ART is usually indistinguishable from that occurring before ART, and it is only the timing of onset that suggests that it results from IRIS.

IRIS develops mainly during the first 3 months of ART but occasionally later. Two patterns are recognized. *Paradoxical IRIS* refers to the worsening or atypical manifestation (or both) of an established OI after ART is commenced. In most cases the infection had been treated before ART was initiated, and the immune response appears to be against residual antigens of the pathogen. *Unmasking IRIS* refers to disease that occurs for the first time after ART is commenced and appears to result from an immune response against a subclinical infection by an opportunistic pathogen.

EPIDEMIOLOGY

The reported incidence of IRIS has varied from 8% to greater than 40% in different studies. To some extent, the large variation reflects the lack of universally accepted diagnostic criteria. It also probably reflects differences in risk factors in the populations of patients studied. The most important risk factors for IRIS are a low CD4$^+$ T-cell count when ART is initiated and, in patients in whom paradoxical IRIS develops, disseminated infection and a short time between treatment of the infection and commencement of ART.

TABLE 402-1 EXAMPLES OF IMMUNE RECONSTITUTION INFLAMMATORY SYNDROME

PATHOGEN	NOMENCLATURE	TYPICAL CHARACTERISTICS OF THE DISEASE
Mycobacterium tuberculosis	TB-IRIS	Paradoxical exacerbation of TB
Nontuberculous mycobacteria (NTM)	NTM immune reconstitution syndrome	Mainly lymphadenitis, also pulmonary disease and hepatitis
Bacille Calmette-Guérin (BCG)	BCG-IRIS	Necrotizing regional lymphadenitis
Mycobacterium leprae	Leprosy-related IRIS	Borderline and type 1 reactional state
Cryptococcus neoformans	Cryptococcal-IRIS	Mainly meningitis, also lymphadenitis
Pneumocystis jirovecii	*Pneumocystis*-IRIS	Paradoxical exacerbation of pneumonitis
Cytomegalovirus (CMV)	CMV retinitis after ART or immune recovery uveitis	Acute retinitis after commencing ART or uveitis
JC polyomavirus	Inflammatory PML	Multifocal leukoencephalopathy with inflammatory features
Human herpesvirus 8	KS-IRIS	Rapid progression of existing and/or new KS lesions
Hepatitis B or C virus	Some cases of ART-associated hepatotoxicity	Hepatitis flare and/or liver enzyme elevation
Herpes-zoster virus		Mainly dermatomal or multidermatomal zoster, occasionally myelitis
Molluscum contagiosum virus	Inflammatory molluscum contagiosum	Inflamed molluscum lesions
Pityrosporon sp	Inflammatory seborrheic dermatitis	Abnormally inflamed seborrheic dermatitis

ART = antiretroviral therapy; IRIS = immune reconstitution inflammatory syndrome; KS = Kaposi's sarcoma; PML = progressive multifocal leukoencephalopathy; TB = tuberculosis.

PATHOBIOLOGY

Information about the pathogenesis of IRIS has been obtained mostly by studying patients who experience disease associated with a mycobacterial infection. Both clinicopathologic and immunologic studies have shown an association with a T$_H$1 cellular immune response against mycobacterial antigens, which has been demonstrated by measuring delayed-type hypersensitivity skin test responses or the frequency of circulating antigen-specific T cells that produce interferon-γ (IFN-γ). The immunopathogenesis of IRIS associated with other pathogens is less well understood and appears to vary depending on the provoking pathogen. For example, IRIS associated with JCV infection (inflammatory progressive multifocal leukoencephalopathy [PML]) is characterized by an inflammatory cell infiltrate in affected areas of the brain that is dominated by CD8$^+$ T cells.

CLINICAL MANIFESTATIONS

The clinical manifestations of IRIS are different for each associated pathogen and will therefore be described for each pathogen. Only disease that presents a significant patient management problem will be discussed.

Mycobacterium tuberculosis

M. tuberculosis is the most common pathogen involved in IRIS, with estimates of incidence ranging from 7 to 43% of patients with HIV infection and treated tuberculosis (TB). Most TB-IRIS develops within the first 3 months after the initiation of ART. Patients in whom paradoxical TB-IRIS develops typically give a history of having improved with treatment of TB before initiation of ART. After starting ART, recurrent, worsening, or new clinical or radiologic manifestations of TB develop. Common manifestations include fever, enlargement of lymph nodes, and worsening radiographic pulmonary infiltrates. Tracheal compression by intrathoracic lymph nodes or massive pleural effusions can cause life-threatening dyspnea. Respiratory failure as a result of worsening pulmonary infiltrates and acute respiratory distress syndrome have occasionally been reported. In a prospective case series from South Africa, neurologic TB-IRIS accounted for 12% of cases of paradoxical TB-IRIS. Meningitis, tuberculoma, or both were the most common manifestations. TB-IRIS should be considered as a potential cause of hepatitis, especially in patients with disseminated TB who are being treated with a combination of antituberculosis therapy and ART. Peritonitis secondary to bowel perforation and splenic rupture are other unusual findings. Though usually negative, mycobacterial cultures may be positive, particularly if IRIS occurs early during antituberculosis therapy and in patients with multidrug-resistant TB. Histologic examination often reveals necrotizing granulomas.

High rates of TB have been reported during ART, especially in the initial months of treatment in ART programs in resource-limited settings. This type of TB has been referred to as ART-associated TB because the mechanisms underlying the manifestations of TB after initiating ART are likely to be heterogeneous. Diagnoses of active TB before initiation of ART may be missed because of the inherent insensitivity of TB diagnostics in this patient group and only later be diagnosed during ART. Because ART-induced immune recovery is a time-dependent process and some patients fail to respond immunologically, a proportion of cases may develop as a result of persisting immunodeficiency. Other patients may have active subclinical disease at the time of ART initiation, and progression to symptomatic disease may be accelerated by ART-induced restoration of a cellular immune response against *M. tuberculosis* antigens. Of patients in this latter group, some have exuberant inflammatory clinical features that are consistent with a diagnosis of TB-IRIS.

Nontuberculous Mycobacteria

Atypical manifestations of *Mycobacterium avium* complex (MAC) disease in patients who had commenced zidovudine monotherapy were the first indication that IRIS may be a complication of ART. MAC and other nontuberculous mycobacteria have been associated with IRIS in 3 to 4% of patients who commence combination ART with a CD4$^+$ T-cell count lower than 100/µL. Disease is usually localized, as opposed to the disseminated nontuberculous mycobacterial disease of patients with acquired immunodeficiency syndrome (AIDS), and is most commonly manifested as fever, night sweats, and lymphadenitis. Unmasking disease is most common. Peripheral lymphadenitis may suppurate and sometimes cause chronically discharging fistulas to the skin. Abdominal disease frequently causes pain, which is usually associated with lymphadenitis and occasionally with omental masses, hepatitis, and inflammation of the spleen (Fig. 402-1). Pulmonary and thoracic disease usually causes cough that is sometimes associated with chest pain. Bronchoscopy may reveal endobronchial lesions. Microscopic examination of biopsy material or aspirates from affected tissues often reveals mycobacteria, but these may not be cultured.

In HIV-seropositive children vaccinated with bacille Calmette-Guérin (BCG), a BCG-associated lymphadenitis and abscesses may develop after starting highly active antiretroviral therapy (HAART) (Fig. 402-2).

Leprosy-related IRIS is usually manifested as unmasking of previous subclinical *Mycobacterium leprae* infection, with a borderline and a type I reactional state.

Cryptococci

The proportion of patients with HIV infection and treated cryptococcosis in whom cryptococcosis-IRIS develops ranges from 8 to 42%. The majority represent a recurrence of previously treated cryptococcal meningitis. Inflammatory reactions to quiescent meningeal infection during the first few weeks of ART have also been reported. The time at onset of cryptococcosis-IRIS varies from 4 days after initiation of ART to around 3 years. Central nervous system (CNS) features of cryptococcosis-IRIS include intracranial cryptococcoma or abscesses, spinal cord abscesses, recalcitrant raised intracranial pressure, optic disc swelling, cranial nerve lesions, dysarthria, hemiparesis, and paraparesis. Extracranial manifestations of cryptococcosis-IRIS include lymphadenitis, eye disease, suppurating soft tissue lesions, and pulmonary disease that may include cavitating or nodular lesions.

FIGURE 402-1. *Mycobacterium avium* complex–associated immune reconstitution inflammatory syndrome manifested as necrotizing inflammation in the spleen and abdominal lymph nodes.

FIGURE 402-2. Bacille Calmette-Guérin (BCG)-associated immune reconstitution inflammatory syndrome after antiretroviral therapy for HIV infection in a child who received BCG vaccination shortly after birth. A biopsy specimen from the larger lesion demonstrated necrotizing granulomatous inflammation.

Cerebrospinal fluid (CSF) profiles in paradoxical cryptococcosis-IRIS may show an increased white blood cell count and an increased opening pressure of greater than 25 cm H$_2$O, but these features overlap significantly with those observed in patients with non–IRIS-related relapses of cryptococcal meningitis. The value of determining serum and CSF cryptococcal antigen in patients with cryptococcosis-IRIS is unclear. Direct examination of tissue or fluid samples obtained at the time of IRIS may be negative. In contrast to the unmasking form of cryptococcosis-IRIS, the paradoxical forms are often culture negative.

Pneumocystis jirovecii

Patients who have been treated for *P. jirovecii* pneumonitis (PJP) may experience pulmonary inflammation after ART is commenced. It is usually characterized by fever, cough, dyspnea, chest discomfort, and patchy alveolar infiltrates on the chest radiograph (Fig. 402-3). In some patients organizing pneumonia develops.

JC Polyomavirus

Progressive PML of the brain occurs when cellular immune responses fail to control JCV infection of oligodendrocytes and astrocytes. It is characterized by a paucity of inflammatory cells in brain lesions. ART is the only effective therapy, presumably because it enhances cellular immune responses against JCV antigens. However, ART may also result in a paradoxical worsening of established PML or in unmasking of subclinical JCV infection and

FIGURE 402-3. *Pneumocystis jirovecii*–associated immune reconstitution inflammatory syndrome. *Left,* Before treatment of the *P. jirovecii* infection. *Right,* After treatment of the *P. jirovecii* infection and commencing antiretroviral therapy.

appearance of PML for the first time. These manifestations of PML are often atypical in that imaging studies of the brain demonstrate changes associated with inflammation and brain biopsy specimens demonstrate inflammatory cell infiltrates with a prominence of CD8+ T cells. Between 19 and 23% of cases of PML in HIV-infected patients are due to paradoxical or unmasking IRIS. The median time at onset is 7 weeks, and most cases occur within the first 3 months of ART but very occasionally as late as 26 months after commencing ART. Predictors of PML-IRIS have not been identified.

Human Herpesvirus 8

A prospective study of Kaposi's sarcoma (KS) in patients from Mozambique commencing ART found that paradoxical IRIS developed in 31% of patients with pre-ART KS and that unmasking IRIS developed in 7% of patients without pre-ART KS. Clinical manifestations included an increased number of preexisting skin lesions that sometimes exhibited increased nodularity and ulceration, new skin or mucosal lesions, and lymphedema. Independent risk factors for the development of KS-IRIS were KS before ART, human herpesvirus 8 DNA detectable in plasma, a hematocrit of less than 30%, and a plasma HIV RNA level greater than 5 log$_{10}$ copies/mL.

Some cases of KS-IRIS will resolve without treatment, but chemotherapy is usually necessary. Doxorubicin has been used most often.

Cytomegalovirus

Eye disease is the most common manifestation of IRIS associated with cytomegalovirus (CMV) infection. Retinitis usually develops during the first few weeks of ART as a "paradoxical" worsening of treated retinitis or as a new manifestation of CMV retinitis. Previously treated CMV infection is the most common cause of immune recovery uveitis (IRU), which presumably results from the restoration of an immune response against residual CMV antigens in the eye. The risk for development of CMV-associated IRU is greatest in patients who had a large proportion of the retina affected by CMV infection. It may develop up to 21 months after ART is commenced, and the clinical manifestations vary in severity from a transient vitreitis to persistent uveitis, papillitis, cystoid macular edema, and epiretinal membranes.

Hepatitis B and C Viruses

Hepatotoxicity manifested as elevated serum liver enzyme levels occurs in up to 18% of patients after ART is initiated. Several causes have been defined, but the most important risk factor is concomitant infection with hepatitis B virus (HBV) or hepatitis C virus (HCV). In a prospective study of patients with HIV and HBV infection who commenced ART that was effective against both viruses, 8 of 36 (22%) patients experienced a "flare" of hepatitis that was associated with increased plasma levels of several immune mediators, thus suggesting that it was a manifestation of IRD in the liver. Patients who experienced hepatitis "flares" had higher plasma HBV DNA levels and serum alanine transaminase levels before ART was commenced. There are also data from retrospective studies suggesting that elevated serum enzyme levels after commencement of ART in patients with HIV and HCV infection also reflects IRD in the liver. Severe hepatotoxicity after ART in patients with HIV infection and coinfection with HBV or HCV is uncommon but can occasionally result in liver decompensation and death.

Herpes Simplex Virus

Exacerbation of mucocutaneous herpes simplex virus (HSV) disease may occur after ART is initiated. Sometimes, lesions become hemorrhagic and exhibit tissue necrosis. Rarely, HSV infection of the brain may be unmasked by commencing ART and be manifested as encephalitis.

DIAGNOSIS

Immunologic tests for diagnosing IRIS are currently not available for routine use, although there are data suggesting that whole blood IFN-γ release assays might be of value in predicting and diagnosing TB-IRIS. In the absence of diagnostic tests, IRIS may be established with diagnostic criteria that take into consideration the timing, clinical characteristics, and pathology of the disease, as well as the virologic response to the ART.

TREATMENT

The general approach to the treatment of IRIS is to continue ART and provide antimicrobial therapy for the provoking infection when it is active (usually in unmasking IRIS). Cessation of ART should be considered only in patients with life-threatening disease when all other measures have failed. Anti-inflammatory therapy should not be given routinely but be reserved for patients with severe inflammation, particularly when it is life-threatening. Corticosteroid therapy is used most often, but its effectiveness may vary from one type of IRIS to another. Thus, a randomized controlled trial in South Africa demonstrated that corticosteroids (prednisone 1.5 mg/kg/day for 2 weeks, then 0.75 mg/kg/day for 2 weeks) are a safe and effective treatment option for paradoxical TB-IRIS.**[1]** In contrast, in an analysis of data from previously reported cases of PML-IRIS, it was suggested that corticosteroid therapy is not effective, although it was indicated that only early use of corticosteroid therapy is likely to be effective. There is anecdotal evidence suggesting that corticosteroid therapy can be effective in other types of IRIS, but there are potential risks to using corticosteroid therapy in HIV patients who are very immunodeficient, and it should only be used after weighing all considerations and should be based on evidence from clinical trials if available. Corticosteroid therapy for IRIS affecting the eye should be supervised by an ophthalmologist.

PREVENTION

Given that a low CD4+ T-cell count is a major risk factor for the development of IRIS, commencing ART at a CD4+ T-cell count higher than 350/μL, as recommended by many treatment guidelines, will prevent most cases. However, this is not possible in patients who are seen for the first time with an OI or in many patients from countries with limited resources. Other strategies to prevent paradoxical IRIS are therefore under investigation.

Observations that disseminated OIs and a shorter duration of treatment of the OI are risk factors for IRIS suggest that the pathogen load is an important factor. Therefore, delaying the introduction of ART so that the OI can be fully treated might be beneficial. However, doing so may increase the risk for the development of other OIs or cancers. The results of the AIDS Clinical Trial Group study A5164 provided evidence supporting the introduction of ART at the same time as antimicrobial therapy, particularly in patients with PJP.**[2]** In addition, randomized studies in patients with TB have provided evidence that survival is better in patients who commence ART at the same time as treatment of TB (Starting Antiretroviral Therapy at Three Points in Tuberculosis [SAPIT] study).**[3]** In contrast, commencing ART at the same time as treatment of cryptococcal meningitis has been shown to reduce long-term survival when compared with delaying ART until the meningitis has been treated. It seems probable that IRIS affecting the CNS is more likely than other types of IRIS to result in morbidity and mortality. Therefore, a single approach to this issue may not be possible, and a strategy for commencing antimicrobial therapy and ART may have to be determined for each pathogen or for infections of the CNS.

PROGNOSIS

The prognosis for patients in whom IRIS develops is highly variable because of differences in the extent of the infection by the provoking pathogen, the characteristics of the immunopathology caused by the restored immune response, and the body site affected. Most cases of IRIS are self-limited and outcomes are usually good. However, mortality rates of up to 66% have been reported for cryptococcosis-IRIS. The mortality rate for TB-IRIS is much lower at about 1%, but hospital admissions are common. Mortality and hospitalization rates are particularly high when TB- or cryptococcosis-IRIS affects the CNS. Indeed, involvement of the CNS by any type of IRIS may result in death or permanent neurologic disability. For example, mortality rates of 53% have been reported for paradoxical PML-IRIS and 31% for unmasking PML-IRIS. Furthermore, patients who survive PML-IRIS may have neurologic sequelae, such as hemiparesis or seizures. Patients with lymphadenitis resulting from TB-IRIS and those with meningitis resulting from cryptococcosis-IRIS occasionally undergo recurrent relapses and can become steroid dependent.

Autoimmune Disease and Sarcoidosis

Patients with HIV infection who are receiving ART have an increased susceptibility to some autoimmune diseases, mainly Graves' disease, and sarcoidosis. Although sometimes referred to as types of IRIS, they appear to have a different immunopathogenesis.

1. Meintjes G, Wilkinson RJ, Morroni C, et al. Randomized placebo-controlled trial of prednisone for paradoxical tuberculosis-associated immune reconstitution inflammatory syndrome. *AIDS.* 2010;24:2381-2390.
2. Zolopa A, Andersen J, Powderly W, et al. Early antiretroviral therapy reduces AIDS progression/death in individuals with acute opportunistic infections: a multicenter randomized strategy trial. *PLoS One.* 2009;4:e5575.
3. Abdool Karim SS, Naidoo K, Grobler A, et al. Timing of initiation of antiretroviral drugs during tuberculosis therapy. *N Engl J Med.* 2010;362:697-706.

SUGGESTED READING

Calligaro G, Meintjes G, Mendelson M. Pulmonary manifestations of the immune reconstitution inflammatory syndrome. *Curr Opin Pulm Med.* 2011;17:180-188. *Tuberculosis, nontuberculosis mycobacterial, and Pneumocystis infections occur within days to weeks of starting anti-viral therapy, whereas cryptococcal infections occur later but with a much higher mortality.*

French MA. Immune reconstitution inflammatory syndrome: a reappraisal. *Clin Infect Dis.* 2009;48:101-107. *A contemporary review of IRIS, including discussion of immune reconstitution–associated autoimmune disease and sarcoidosis.*

Martin-Blondel G, Delobel P, Blancher A, et al. Pathogenesis of the immune reconstitution inflammatory syndrome affecting the central nervous system in patients infected with HIV. *Brain.* 2011;134 (Pt 4):928-946. *Review including the nature of the provoking pathogens and the composition and specificity of the evoked immune responses.*

Müller M, Wandel S, Colebunders R, et al. Immune reconstitution inflammatory syndrome in patients starting antiretroviral therapy for HIV infection: a systematic review and meta-analysis. *Lancet Infect Dis.* 2010;10:251-261. *IRIS developed in 16% of all patients, including 38% of patients with cytomegalovirus retinitis, 20% of patients with cryptococcal meningitis, 16% of patients with tuberculosis, and 17% of patients with PML; the overall mortality was 4.5%.*

Sereti I, Rodger AJ, French MA. Biomarkers in immune reconstitution inflammatory syndrome: signals from pathogenesis. *Curr Opin HIV AIDS.* 2010;5:504-510. *Markers such as C-reactive protein may be helpful.*

Smith K, Kuhn L, Coovadia A, et al. Immune reconstitution inflammatory syndrome among HIV-infected South African infants initiating antiretroviral therapy. *AIDS.* 2009;23:1097-1107. *Study describing the incidence, clinical manifestations, and risk factors for IRIS in young children initiating HAART.*

XXV

NEUROLOGY

403

APPROACH TO THE PATIENT WITH NEUROLOGIC DISEASE

ROBERT C. GRIGGS, RALPH F. JÓZEFOWICZ,
AND MICHAEL J. AMINOFF

CLINICAL MANIFESTATIONS

The symptoms of nervous system diseases are a part of everyday experience for most normal people. Slips of the tongue, headaches, backache and other pains, dizziness, lightheadedness, numbness, muscle twitches, jerks, cramps, and tremors all occur in totally healthy persons. Mood swings with feelings of elation and depression, paranoia, and displays of temper are equally a part of the behavior of completely normal people. The rapid increase in information about neurologic diseases coupled with the intense interest of people in all walks of life in medical matters has focused public attention on both common and rare neurologic conditions.

Most older people are concerned that they or their spouse have or are developing Alzheimer's disease or stroke. The almost ubiquitous tremor of the elderly prompts concern about Parkinson's disease. Many younger patients are concerned about multiple sclerosis or brain tumor, and few normal people lack one or more symptoms suggesting the diagnosis of a serious neurologic disease. For most of these and other common diagnoses, the results of imaging and other tests are typically normal when symptoms first appear, and such tests should not be performed to reassure the patient or physician. Moreover, the widespread availability of neurodiagnostic imaging and electrophysiologic, biochemical, and genetic testing has led to the detection of "abnormalities" in many young and most elderly persons. In evaluating a patient's symptoms, it is imperative that a clinical diagnosis be reached without reference to a neurodiagnostic laboratory finding. Patients with disorders such as headache, anxiety, and depression do not usually have abnormal laboratory results. Abnormalities noted on various neurodiagnostic studies are often incidental findings whose treatment may be justified and necessary, but they do not improve the patient's symptoms. Abnormalities detected incidentally that are not accompanied by signs or symptoms may, as for disorders such as hypertension, require aggressive evaluation and treatment, but in general, the adage that it is difficult to improve an asymptomatic patient should be kept in mind. Thus, in elderly patients, few imaging or electrophysiologic studies are interpreted as "normal," but in the absence of specific complaints consistent with the findings, treatment and even further evaluation should reflect an estimate of the specificity and sensitivity of the test as well as the likelihood that the patient will require and benefit from treatment. It is a good rule of thumb that one should never perform (or refer to the result of) a neurodiagnostic procedure without a specific diagnosis or at least a differential diagnosis in mind.

It is important to allow patients to describe any symptoms in their own words. Direct questions are often necessary to fully characterize the problem, but suggested terms or descriptors for symptoms are frequently grasped by a patient unfamiliar with medical terminology and then parroted to subsequent interviewers. The patient's terms should always be used in recording symptoms. Terms such as *lameness, weakness, numbness, heaviness, cramps,* and *tiredness* may each mean pain, weakness, or alteration of sensation to some patients.

DIAGNOSIS
History

In neurologic diagnosis, the history usually indicates the nature of the disease or the diagnosis, whereas the neurologic examination localizes it and quantitates its severity. For many diseases, the history is almost the only avenue to explore. Examples of such disorders include headaches, seizures, developmental disorders, memory disorders, and behavioral diseases. In arriving at a diagnosis, the following points are useful. Consider the entire medical history of the patient. Early life events or long-standing processes such as head or spine trauma, unilateral hearing or visual loss, poor prowess in sports, poor performance in school, spinal curvature, and bone anomalies are easily overlooked but may point to the underlying disease process.

Consider the tempo and duration of the symptoms. Have the symptoms been progressive without remission, or have there been plateaus or periods of return to normal? Cerebral mass lesions (tumor, subdural) tend to have a progressive but fluctuating course; seizures and migraine, an episodic course; and strokes, an abrupt, ictal onset with worsening for 3 to 5 days, followed by partial or complete recovery.

Can one disease account for all of the symptoms and signs? The clinician should formulate a diagnostic opinion in anatomic terms. Is the history suggestive of a single (e.g., stroke or tumor) focus or multiple sites of nervous system involvement (e.g., multiple sclerosis), or is the process a disease of a system (vitamin B_{12} deficiency, myopathy, or polyneuropathy)?

The neurologic history is the most important component of neurologic diagnosis. A careful history frequently determines the cause and allows one to begin localizing the lesions, which aids in establishing whether the disease is diffuse or focal. Symptoms of acute onset suggest a vascular cause or seizure; symptoms that are subacute in onset suggest a mass lesion, such as a tumor or abscess; symptoms that have a waxing and waning course with exacerbations and remissions suggest a demyelinating cause; and symptoms that are chronic and progressive suggest a degenerative disorder.

The history is often the only way of diagnosing neurologic illnesses that typically have normal or nonfocal findings on neurologic examination. These illnesses include many seizure disorders, narcolepsy, migraine and most other headache syndromes, the various causes of dizziness, and most types of dementia. The neurologic history may often provide the first clues that a symptom is psychological in origin. The following are points to consider in obtaining a neurologic history.

- *Carefully identify the chief complaint or problem.* Not only is the chief complaint important in providing the first clue to the physician about the differential diagnosis, but it is also the reason that the patient is seeking medical advice and treatment. If the chief complaint is not properly identified and addressed, the proper diagnosis may be missed and an inappropriate diagnostic work-up may be undertaken. Establishing a diagnosis that does not incorporate the chief complaint frequently focuses attention on a coincidental process irrelevant to the patient's concerns.
- *Listen carefully to the patient for as long as necessary.* A good rule of thumb is to listen initially for at least 5 minutes without interrupting the patient. The patient often volunteers the most important information at the start of the history. During this time, the examiner can also assess mental status, including speech, language, fund of knowledge, and affect, and observe the patient for facial asymmetry, abnormalities in ocular movements, and an increase or a paucity of spontaneous movements as seen with movement disorders.
- *Steer the patient away from discussions of previous diagnostic test results and the opinions of previous caregivers.* Abnormal results of laboratory studies may be incidental to the patient's primary problem or may simply represent a normal variant.
- *Take a careful medical history, medication history, psychiatric history, family history, and social and occupational history.* Many neurologic illnesses are complications of underlying medical disorders or are due to adverse effects of drugs. For example, parkinsonism is a frequent complication of the use of metoclopramide and most neuroleptic agents. A large number of neurologic disorders are hereditary, and a positive family history may establish the diagnosis in many instances. Occupation plays a major role in various neurologic disorders, such as carpal tunnel syndrome (in machine operators and people who use computer keyboards) and peripheral neuropathy (caused by exposure to lead or other toxins).
- *Interview surrogate historians.* Because patients with dementia or altered mental status are generally unable to provide exact details of the history, a family member may need to provide the key details required to make an accurate diagnosis. This situation is especially common with patients who have dementia and certain right hemispheric lesions with various agnosias (lack of awareness of disease) that may interfere with their ability to provide a cogent history. Surrogate historians also provide missing historical details for patients with episodic loss of consciousness, such as syncope and epilepsy.
- *Summarize the history for the patient.* Summarizing the history is an effective way to ensure that all details were covered sufficiently for a tentative diagnosis to be made. Summarizing also allows the physician to fill in historical gaps that may not have been apparent when the history was initially taken. In addition, the patient or surrogate may correct any historical misinformation at this time.
- *End by asking what the patient thinks is wrong.* This question allows the physician to evaluate the patient's concerns about and insight into the

condition. Some patients have a specific diagnosis in mind that spurs them to seek medical attention. Multiple sclerosis, amyotrophic lateral sclerosis, Alzheimer's disease, and brain tumors are diseases that patients often suspect may be the cause of their neurologic symptoms.

Diagnostic Challenges

Two common situations provide special challenges to the diagnostic skills of the physician.

Physical Abuse as a Cause of Neurologic Symptoms

Traumatic injury inflicted by family members or others is usually difficult to detect by the medical history and examination. Physically battered babies, abused children, battered women, and traumatized seniors are often unable or unwilling to complain of this cause or contribution to symptoms. The only method to prevent overlooking of this frequent cause of common problems is systematic consideration of the possibility in every patient and awareness of the often subtle signs that suggest physical trauma: ecchymoses or fractures (often attributed to a logical cause), denial of expected symptoms, failure to keep appointments, and unexplained intensification of neurologic symptoms (headache, dizziness, ringing in the ears, blackouts).

Alcoholism and Drug Abuse

See Chapters 32 and 33. A host of neurologic disorders can be the result of intentional ingestion of toxins (Chapter 110). Patients do not give an accurate account of their use of these agents. Consequently, physical signs and laboratory screening test results that give evidence of drug-related hepatic and other metabolic abnormalities may point to a major underlying problem.

⬤ ACUTE NEUROLOGIC DISORDERS REQUIRING IMMEDIATE DIAGNOSIS AND TREATMENT

Most neurologic diagnoses are arrived at by a careful, thorough history and an appropriately complete examination. However, the tempo of illness and the availability of life-saving treatment that is effective only if it is administered within minutes of first evaluating a patient dictate rapid action in several specific circumstances. Coma (Chapter 411), repetitive seizures (Chapter 410), acute stroke (Chapters 414 and 415), suspected meningitis and encephalitis (Chapters 420 and 422), head and spine trauma (Chapter 406), and acute spinal cord compression are diagnosed by clinical and laboratory assessment, and urgent treatment must be instituted as soon as ventilation and cardiac status are stabilized.

⬤ NEUROLOGIC EXAMINATION

The neurologic examination is always tailored to the clinical setting of the patient. A complete neurologic examination of a child is much different from that of an elderly adult, and the examination of a patient with specific complaints focuses on findings pertinent to that patient. Thus, more detailed testing of cognition is indicated in patients with behavioral or memory disturbance, and more detailed testing of sensation should be performed in patients with complaints of pain, numbness, or weakness.

However, many tests of neurologic function are routinely indicated in all patients because they provide a baseline for future examination and are frequently helpful in detecting unsuspected neurologic disease in apparently normal persons or in patients whose symptoms initially suggest disease outside the nervous system. It is particularly important to perform all routine tests in patients with abnormalities in one sphere of neurologic dysfunction; otherwise, erroneous localization of a lesion or disease process is likely. For deviations from normal to be recognized and quantitated, it is essential for a physician to have extensive experience in the routine assessment of normal persons.

The General Examination

Specific neurologic symptoms or signs should prompt attention to the assessment of general findings. Head circumference should be measured in patients with central nervous system (CNS) or spinal cord disease (normally 55 ± 5 cm in adults). Head enlargement is occasionally a normal, often hereditary variant but should suggest a long-standing anomaly of the brain or spinal cord. The skin should be inspected for cafe au lait maculae, adenoma sebaceum, vascular malformations, lipomas, neurofibromas, and other lesions (Chapter 426). Neck range of motion, straight leg raising, and spinal curvature (scoliosis) should be assessed. Carotid auscultation for bruits is indicated in all older adults; carotid palpation is seldom informative. In patients with bladder, bowel, or leg symptoms, a rectal sphincter examination for tone and ability to contract voluntarily is usually indicated. Limitation of joint

range of motion or painless swelling of joints is often a sign of an unsuspected neurologic lesion.

Neurologic Examination

The various aspects of the detailed neurologic examination are considered in specific symptom and disease sections noted later. The five major divisions of the examination should be assessed in all patients. During a careful medical history, mental status is often adequately assessed: level of consciousness, orientation, memory, language function, affect, and judgment. If any of these functions are abnormal, more detailed testing is needed. Cranial nerve function that should be tested in all patients includes visual acuity (with and without correction); optic fundi; visual fields; pupils (size and reactivity to direct and consensual light); ocular motility; jaw, facial, palatal, neck, and tongue movement; and hearing.

Examination of the motor system (Chapter 429) is essential in all patients because incipient weakness is generally overlooked by the patient. Muscle tone (flaccid, spastic, or rigid), muscle size (atrophy or hypertrophy), and muscle strength can be assessed rapidly. Muscle strength testing should always assess specific functional activities, including the ability to walk on heel and toe, to sit up from a supine position, to rise from a deep knee bend or deep chair, to lift the arms over the head, and to make a tight fist. Gait, stance, and coordination are assessed. The patient should be observed for tremor and other abnormal movements and the muscles inspected for fasciculations.

Sensory testing (Chapter 428) need not be detailed unless there are sensory symptoms. However, vibration perception in the toes and the normality of perception of pain, temperature, and light touch in the hands and feet should be assessed.

Muscle stretch reflexes and plantar responses should always be assessed by evaluating right-left symmetry and disparity between proximal and distal reflexes or arm and leg reflexes. Biceps, triceps, brachioradialis, quadriceps, and ankle reflexes should be quantitated from 1 to 4 (4 = clonus; 3 = spread; 2 = brisk; 1 = hypoactive).

The Comatose Patient

The rapid examination required for a patient with an altered state of consciousness is much different from that of an alert, aware individual (Chapter 411). Many aspects of the neurologic examination cannot be tested: cognitive function, subtleties of sensory perception, specific motor functions, coordination, gait, and stance. Moreover, the muscle stretch reflexes are likely to fluctuate from one moment to the next, and minor asymmetries are much less important than in an awake patient. Instead, attention should focus on examination of the level of consciousness, respiratory pattern, eyelid position and eye movements, pupils, corneal reflexes, optic fundi, and motor responses. Particular elements of the general examination must also be assessed quickly: evidence of cranial and spine trauma, tenderness of the skull to percussion, nuchal rigidity (but not in patients with head or neck trauma), and evidence of physical abuse.

⬤ COMMON COMPLAINTS OF POSSIBLE NEUROLOGIC ORIGIN

Weakness

It is axiomatic that patients typically have motor signs before motor symptoms and, conversely, sensory symptoms before sensory signs. Thus, patients with even severe weakness may not report symptoms of weakness. Somewhat paradoxically, patients who complain of "weakness" often do not have confirmatory findings on examination that document the presence of weakness.

Weakness, when it is actually a symptom of neurologic disease, is frequently caused by diseases of the motor unit (Chapters 418, 429, and 430) and is usually reported by a patient in terms of loss of specific functions, for example, difficulty with tasks such as climbing stairs, rising from a chair, sitting up, lifting objects onto a high shelf, or opening jars. Symptoms may also reflect the consequences of weakness, such as frequent falls or tripping. Such symptoms can be remarkably quantitative. A patient with leg muscle weakness who is falling even as infrequently as once a month almost invariably has severe weakness of the knee extensor muscles and can be shown on examination to have a knee extension lag, an inability to lift the leg fully against gravity and to lock the knee.

The symptom of weakness without findings of weakness on examination is not generally the result of neuromuscular disease but can be a sign of neurologic disease outside the motor unit or, more commonly, a symptom of disease outside the nervous system altogether (Table 403-1).

TABLE 403-1 DISORDERS COMMONLY ACCOMPANIED BY WEAKNESS

Disorders of the motor unit
Upper motor neuron lesions—spasticity
Basal ganglia disorders—rigidity
General medical conditions
    Heart failure
    Respiratory insufficiency
    Renal, hepatic, and other metabolic disease
    Alcoholism and other toxin-related disease
Psychiatric and behavioral disorders
    Depression
    Malingering

Fatigue

The complaints of "fatigue," "tiredness," and "lack of energy" are even less likely than the symptom of weakness to reflect definable neurologic disease. With the exception of neuromuscular junction disorders such as myasthenia gravis, fatigue is rarely a complaint of diseases of the motor unit. Fatigue can be a sign of upper motor neuron disease (corticospinal pathways) and is a common complaint of established multiple sclerosis and other multifocal CNS disease. Similarly, any process that produces bilateral corticospinal tract or extrapyramidal disease can cause fatigue. Examples include motor neuron disease (Chapter 418), spinal cord disease in the cervical cord region (Chapter 407), and Parkinson's disease (Chapter 416). In addition, disorders that impair sleep (Chapter 412) may include fatigue as a complaint.

Fatigue, like weakness, is much more often than not a sign of disease outside the central and peripheral nervous system. Depression and other psychiatric and behavioral disorders (Chapter 404) as well as the medical illnesses associated with a complaint of weakness are all frequent causes of fatigue.

Chronic fatigue syndrome and many cases of fibromyalgia (Chapter 282) have fatigue as a dominant, disabling symptom. These disorders are defined in part by the absence of consistent neurologic findings and lack of demonstrable disease in the nervous system.

Spontaneous Movements

Muscle tremors, jerks, twitches, cramps, and spasms (Chapter 417) are frequent symptoms. The cause of spontaneous movements can reside at any level of the nervous system. In general, movements that occur in an entire limb or in more than one muscle group concurrently are caused by CNS disease. Movements confined to a single muscle are likely to be a reflection of disease of the motor unit (including the motor neurons of the brain stem and spinal cord). When spontaneous movements of a muscle are associated with severe pain, patients often use the term *cramp*. Cramp is a medically defined disorder that reflects the intense contraction of a large group of motor units. Leg cramps are occasionally a sign of an underlying disease of the anterior horn cell, nerve roots, or peripheral nerve; however, cramps are frequent in normal persons and particularly common in older patients, and they are usually benign. When they are severe, cramps can produce such intense muscle contraction that muscle injury is caused and muscle enzyme (e.g., creatine kinase) levels are elevated in blood.

The rare muscle diseases in which an enzyme deficiency interferes with substrate use as fuel for exercise (e.g., McArdle's disease) are often associated with severe, exercise-provoked muscle *contractures*. These contractures are electrically silent on electromyography, in contrast to the intense motor unit activity seen with cramps. Contractures must not be confused with the limitation of joint range of motion resulting from long-standing joint disease or long-standing weakness—also termed contractures.

The intense muscle contractions of *tetany* are frequently painful. Although tetany is usually a reflection of hypocalcemia (Chapter 253), it can occasionally be seen without demonstrable electrolyte disturbance. Tetany results from hyperexcitability of peripheral nerves. Similarly, in the syndrome of *tetanus* produced by a clostridial toxin (Chapter 304), intensely painful, life-threatening muscle contractions arise from hyperexcitable peripheral nerves. A number of toxic disorders, such as strychnine poisoning and black widow spider envenomation, produce similar neurogenic spasms.

Muscle Pain

Acute muscle pain in the absence of abnormal muscle contractions is an extremely common symptom. When such pain occurs after strenuous exercise or in the context of an acute viral illness (e.g., influenza), it probably

TABLE 403-2 CHARACTERISTIC GAIT DISORDERS

SPECIFIC DISORDER	LOCATION OF LESION	CHARACTERISTICS
Spastic gait	Bilateral corticospinal pathways within the thoracic or cervical cord or in the brain	Legs stiff, feet turning inward, "scissoring"
Hemiparetic gait	Unilateral central nervous system, cervical cord, or brain	Affected leg circumducted, foot extended, arm flexed
Sensory ataxia	Posterior columns of the spinal cord or peripheral nerve	Wide-based, high steps; Romberg's sign present
Cerebellar ataxia	Brain stem or cerebellum	Wide-based steps; Romberg's sign absent
Parkinsonian gait	Basal ganglia	Shuffling, small steps
Dystonic gait	Basal ganglia; also corticospinal pathways	Abnormal posture of the arms, head, neck
Gait disorder of the elderly	Multifactorial: bihemispheric disease, spinal cord disease, impaired proprioception, muscle weakness	Stooped posture, wide-based steps; often retropulsion
Steppage gait	Distal muscle weakness	High steps ("steppage")
Waddling gait	Proximal muscle weakness	Both legs circumducted to allow locking of the knees
Antalgic gait	Non-neurologic; reflects disease of joints, bones, or soft tissue	Minimizes pain in the hip, spine, leg
Hysterical gait	Psychiatric or behavioral disorder	Reeling side to side, associated astasia-abasia, bizarre arm and trunk movements

reflects muscle injury. In such patients, the serum creatine kinase level is often raised. It is uncommon for this frequent and essentially normal sign of muscle injury to be associated with weakness or demonstrable ongoing muscle disease. *Chronic* muscle pain is a common symptom but is seldom related to a definable disease of muscle.

Episodic and Intermittent Weakness

The complaint of attacks of severe weakness or paralysis occurring in a patient with baseline normal strength is an uncommon symptom. It is typical of the periodic paralyses and may also be seen with episodic ataxias and myotonic disorders (Chapter 429). All of these disorders are ion channelopathies. These channelopathies (e.g., the calcium channelopathy hypokalemic periodic paralysis) are rare but treatable disorders (Chapter 429). Episodic weakness is also seen in patients with neuromuscular junction disorders, such as myasthenia gravis and the myasthenic syndrome (Chapter 430). On occasion, patients with narcolepsy complain of intermittent paralysis as a reflection of *sleep paralysis* (Chapter 412).

Loss of Balance

Unsteadiness of gait is a common symptom. When it is associated with complaints of dizziness or vertigo (Chapter 436), disease of the labyrinth, the vestibular nerve, the brain stem, or the cerebellum is a probable cause. When unsteadiness and loss of balance are unassociated with dizziness, particularly if the unsteadiness appears to be out of proportion to other symptoms of the patient, a widespread disorder of sensation or motor function is likely.

Abnormal Gait and Posture

The ability to stand and to walk in a well-coordinated, effortless fashion requires the integrity of the entire nervous system. Relatively subtle deficits localized to one part of the central or peripheral nervous system produce characteristic abnormalities (Table 403-2).

Sensory Symptoms

Sensory symptoms can be negative or positive. Negative symptoms represent a loss of sensation, such as a feeling of numbness. Positive symptoms, by contrast, consist of sensory phenomena that occur without normal stimulation of receptors and include paresthesias and dysesthesias. *Paresthesias* may include a feeling of tingling, crawling, itching, compression, tightness, cold, or heat and are sometimes associated with a feeling of heaviness. The term *dysesthesias* is used correctly to refer to abnormal sensations, often tingling, painful, or uncomfortable, that occur after innocuous stimuli, whereas *allodynia* refers to painful perception from a stimulus that is not normally painful. For some patients, it may be difficult to distinguish paresthesias and dysesthesias from pain. *Hypesthesia* and *hypalgesia* denote a loss or impairment of touch or pain sensibility, respectively. By comparison, *hyperesthesia* and *hyperalgesia* indicate a lowered threshold to tactile or painful stimuli, respectively, such that there is increased sensitivity to such stimuli.

With the use of a wisp of cotton, a pin, and a tuning fork, the trunk and extremities are examined for regions of abnormal or absent sensation. Certain instruments are available for quantifying sensory function, such as the computer-assisted sensory examination, which is based on the detection of touch, pressure, vibratory, and thermal sensation thresholds.

Alterations in pain and tactile sensibility can generally be detected by clinical examination. It is important to localize the distribution of any such sensory loss to distinguish between nerve, root, and central dysfunction. Similarly, abnormalities in proprioception can be detected by clinical examination when patients are unable to detect the direction in which a joint is moved. In severe cases, there may be pseudoathetoid movements of the outstretched hands, sensory ataxia, and sometimes postural and action tremors.

Disorders of peripheral nerves commonly lead to sensory disturbances that depend on the population of affected nerve fibers (Chapter 428). Some neuropathies are predominantly large-fiber neuropathies. Appreciation of movement and position is impaired, and paresthesias are common. Examination reveals that vibration, position, and movement sensations are impaired, and movement becomes clumsy and ataxic. Pain and temperature appreciation is relatively preserved. The tendon reflexes are lost early. In other neuropathies, it is the small fibers especially that are affected; spontaneous pain is common and may be burning, lancinating, or aching in quality. Pain and temperature appreciation is disproportionately affected in these neuropathies, and autonomic dysfunction may be present. Examples of small-fiber neuropathies include certain hereditary disorders, Tangier disease, and diabetes. Most sensory neuropathies are characterized by a distal distribution of sensory loss, whereas sensory neuronopathies are characterized by sensory loss that may also involve the trunk and face and tends to be particularly severe. Sensory changes in a radiculopathy conform to a root territory; in cauda equina syndromes, sensory deficits involve multiple roots and may lead to saddle anesthesia and loss of the normal sensation associated with the passage of urine or feces.

Lesions of the *posterolateral columns* of the cord, such as occur in multiple sclerosis (Chapter 419), vitamin B_{12} deficiency (Chapter 425), and cervical spondylosis (Chapter 407), often lead to a feeling of compression in the affected region and to a Lhermitte sign (paresthesias radiating down the back and legs on neck flexion). Examination reveals ipsilateral impairment of vibration and joint position senses, with preservation of pain and temperature appreciation. Conversely, lesions of the *anterolateral region* of the cord (as by cordotomy) or *central* lesions interrupting fibers crossing to join the spinothalamic pathways (as in syringomyelia; Chapter 426) lead to impairment in pain and temperature appreciation with relative preservation of vibration, joint position sense, and light touch. Motor deficits may also be present and help localize the lesion. Upper motor neuron dysfunction

(Chapter 407) from cervical lesions leads to quadriplegia, whereas more caudal lesions lead to paraplegia; lesions below the level of the first lumbar vertebra may simply compress the cauda equina and result in lower motor neuron deficits from a polyradiculopathy as well as impairment of sphincter and sexual function.

● NEUROLOGIC DIAGNOSTIC PROCEDURES

Lumbar Puncture

Sampling of cerebrospinal fluid (CSF) by lumbar puncture is crucial for accurate diagnosis of meningeal infections and carcinomatosis (Fig. 403-1). CSF analysis is also helpful in evaluating patients with central or peripheral nervous system demyelinating disorders and with intracranial hemorrhage, particularly when imaging studies are inconclusive.

The CSF formula often provides an important clue to the pathologic process involved (Table 403-3). An elevated white blood cell count is seen with infections and other inflammatory diseases as well as with carcinomatosis. The differential white blood cell count may point to a specific class of pathogen; polymorphonuclear leukocytes suggest a bacterial process, whereas mononuclear cells suggest a viral, fungal, or immunologic cause. The CSF glucose concentration is typically reduced in bacterial and fungal infections as well as with certain viral infections (e.g., mumps virus) and with sarcoidosis. The CSF protein concentration is elevated in a variety of disorders, including most infections and demyelinating neuropathies.

Specialized tests that can be performed on CSF include oligoclonal bands, a pathologic pattern of bands on CSF electrophoresis that is seen in up to 90% of patients with multiple sclerosis. The bands, which represent monoclonal immunoglobulins that are locally synthesized in the CNS, are not specific for multiple sclerosis and may be seen with other inflammatory and noninflammatory conditions, including systemic lupus erythematosus, human immunodeficiency virus infection, and stroke.

CSF polymerase chain reaction is a rapid, sensitive, and specific test for the diagnosis of herpes simplex encephalitis (Chapter 422), for which it has replaced brain biopsy as the diagnostic procedure of choice. The CSF VDRL (Venereal Disease Research Laboratory) assay is a specific although insensitive test for neurosyphilis (Chapter 327).

FIGURE 403-1. Cerebrospinal fluid examination. **A**, Normal crystal-clear CSF. **B**, Blood in the CSF, which could result from a traumatic (bloody) tap or from subarachnoid hemorrhage. In a traumatic tap, subsequent tubes of CSF are usually less bloody. **C**, Centrifuged CSF in a traumatic tap. The supernatant is nearly clear. **D**, CSF from a patient with subarachnoid hemorrhage. There is blood at the bottom of the tube and the supernatant is yellow (xanthochromic) as a result of breakdown of blood cells in the CSF before the lumbar puncture. (From Forbes CD, Jackson WD. *Color Atlas and Text of Clinical Medicine,* 3rd ed. London: Mosby; 2003, with permission.)

TABLE 403-3	CHARACTERISTIC CEREBROSPINAL FLUID FORMULAS						
	TURBIDITY AND COLOR	**OPENING PRESSURE**	**WBC COUNT**	**DIFFERENTIAL CELLS**	**RBC COUNT**	**PROTEIN**	**GLUCOSE**
Normal	Clear, colorless	70-180 mm H_2O	0-5 cells/μL^3	Mononuclear	0	<60 mg/dL	> ⅔ serum
Bacterial meningitis	Cloudy, straw colored	↑	↑↑	PMNs	0	↑↑	↓
Viral meningitis	Clear or cloudy, colorless	↑	↑	Lymphocytes	0	↑	Normal
Fungal and tuberculous meningitis	Cloudy, straw colored	↑	↑	Lymphocytes	0	↑↑	↓↓
Viral encephalitis	Clear or cloudy, straw colored	Normal to ↑	↑	Lymphocytes	0 (herpes ↑)	Normal to ↑	Normal
Subarachnoid hemorrhage	Cloudy, pink	↑	↑	PMNs and lymphocytes	↑↑	↑	Normal (early); ↓ (late)
Guillain-Barré syndrome	Clear, yellow	Normal to ↑	0-5 cells/μL^3	Mononuclear	0	↑	Normal

PMN = polymorphonuclear leukocyte; RBC = red blood cell; WBC = white blood cell.

FIGURE 403-2. Normal and abnormal electroencephalograms. **A,** The EEG of a normal awake adult. **B,** A 3-Hz spike and wave activity, a pattern seen in absence epilepsy. In each record, channels 1 through 8 and 11 through 18 represent left- and right-sided bipolar electrode placements, respectively. Channels 9 and 10 represent midline bipolar electrode placements, and channels 19 and 20 represent the left and right electro-oculograms (eye movements). Each major horizontal division represents 1 second. **C,** Triphasic slow waves, a pattern seen in hepatic or other metabolic encephalopathies.

A lumbar puncture should not be performed in patients who have an obstructive, noncommunicating hydrocephalus or a focal CNS mass lesion causing raised intracranial pressure because reducing CSF pressure acutely in these settings by lumbar puncture may result in cerebral or cerebellar herniation. Lumbar puncture may be safely performed in patients with a *communicating* hydrocephalus, such as with idiopathic intracranial hypertension (pseudotumor cerebri), and it may even be an effective treatment in selected patients with this condition.

Electroencephalography

Electroencephalography is the recording and measurement of scalp electrical potentials to evaluate baseline brain functioning and paroxysmal brain electrical activity suggestive of a seizure disorder.

Electroencephalography is performed by securing 20 electrodes to the scalp at predetermined locations based on an international system that uses standardized percentages of the head circumference, the "10-20 system." Each electrode is labeled with a letter and a number, the letter identifying the skull region (Fp = frontopolar; F = frontal; P = parietal; C = central; T = temporal; O = occipital) and the number identifying the specific location, with odd numbers representing left-sided electrodes and even numbers right-sided electrodes. These electrodes are then connected in various combinations of pairs to generate voltage potential differences, and the potentials are recorded on a chart recorder.

To delineate the spatial distribution of the changing electrical field for an electroencephalogram (EEG), an orderly arrangement of electrode pairs is used, and each specific arrangement is known as a montage. Montages are generally of two types: *referential,* in which each electrode is connected to a single reference electrode, such as the ear; and *bipolar,* in which electrodes are connected sequentially to one another to form a chain. A standard EEG generally records about 30 minutes of brain activity, both in the awake state and in the first two stages of sleep. Various activating procedures are used during the recording of an EEG, including hyperventilation and photic stimulation. These activating procedures may precipitate seizure discharges in some patients with seizure disorders, thereby increasing the sensitivity of the test.

The amplitudes of scalp electrical potentials are quite low, averaging 30 to 100 μV. They represent a summation of excitatory postsynaptic potentials and inhibitory postsynaptic potentials that are largely generated by the pyramidal cells in layer 4 of the cerebral cortex. Action potentials are of too brief a duration to have an effect on the EEG.

The EEG is analyzed with respect to symmetry between each hemisphere; wave frequency and amplitude; and the presence of spikes (20 to 70 msec) and sharp waves (70 to 200 msec), which may indicate a seizure focus. Electroencephalographic frequencies are divided into four categories as follows: delta: <4 Hz; theta: 4-7 Hz; alpha: 8-13 Hz; beta: >13 Hz.

The normal waking EEG (Fig. 403-2A) in a patient with eyes closed contains rhythms of alpha frequency in the occipital leads and beta frequency in the frontal leads. Normal sleep causes a generalized slowing of electroencephalographic frequencies and an increase in amplitude in each stage of sleep such that stage 4 sleep consists of more than 50% large-amplitude delta rhythms. Electroencephalographic abnormalities are of two types: abnormalities in background rhythm and abnormalities of a paroxysmal nature (Table 403-4).

The major usefulness of electroencephalography is for diagnosis and categorization of a seizure disorder (Fig. 403-2B). EEGs are neither highly sensitive nor completely specific for diagnosis of seizures. Because seizures are paroxysmal events, it is not unusual for an EEG to be normal—or only minimally abnormal—in a patient with epilepsy if it is recorded during an interictal phase (the period between seizures). Only about 50% of patients with seizures show epileptiform activity on the first EEG. Repeating the EEG with provocative maneuvers, such as sleep deprivation, hyperventilation, and photic stimulation, may increase this percentage to 90%. Conversely, about

TABLE 403-4	ELECTROENCEPHALOGRAPHIC ABNORMALITIES
ELECTROENCEPHALOGRAPHIC ABNORMALITY	**CLINICAL CORRELATE**
BACKGROUND RHYTHM ABNORMALITIES	
Generalized slowing	Most metabolic encephalopathies
Triphasic waves	Hepatic, renal, and other metabolic encephalopathies
Focal slowing	Large mass lesions (tumor, large stroke)
Electrocerebral inactivity with lack of response to all stimuli	Brain death
PAROXYSMAL ABNORMALITIES	
3-Hz spike and wave, augmented by hyperventilation	Absence epilepsy
3- to 4-Hz spike and wave in light sleep or with photic stimulation	Primary generalized epilepsy
Central to midtemporal spikes	Benign rolandic epilepsy, other partial epilepsies
Anterior temporal spikes or sharp waves	Simple or complex partial seizures of mesial temporal origin
Hypsarrhythmia (high-voltage chaotic slowing with multifocal spikes)	Infantile spasms (West's syndrome)
Burst suppression	Severe anoxic brain injury, barbiturate coma

TABLE 403-5	NERVE CONDUCTION STUDY ABNORMALITIES
ABNORMALITY	**CLINICAL CORRELATE**
Reduced CMAP amplitude	Axonal neuropathy
Prolonged terminal latency	Demyelinating neuropathy Distal compressive neuropathy
Conduction block	Severe focal compressive neuropathy Severe demyelinating neuropathy
Slowed conduction velocity	Demyelinating neuropathy

CMAP = compound muscle action potential.

lesion is axonal or demyelinating. The NCS is also helpful in diagnosis of compressive mononeuropathies, such as carpal tunnel syndrome, ulnar palsy, peroneal nerve palsy, and tarsal tunnel syndrome.

F Wave and H Reflex

The F wave and H reflex are ways of looking at the conduction characteristics for proximal portions of nerves, including the nerve roots. The F wave is a late CMAP evoked intermittently from a muscle by a *supramaximal* electrical stimulus to the nerve, and it is due to antidromic activation (backfiring) of alpha motor neurons. F waves can be elicited from practically all distal motor nerves. The H reflex is a late CMAP that is evoked regularly from a muscle by a *submaximal* stimulus to a nerve, and it is due to stimulation of Ia afferent fibers (a spinal reflex). The H reflex can be routinely obtained from calf muscles only with stimulation of the tibial nerve in the popliteal fossa.

F waves are helpful in diagnosis of Guillain-Barré syndrome, in which demyelination is often confined to the proximal portions of nerves early in the course of the disease. The H reflex is often absent in patients with acute S1 radiculopathy.

Repetitive Stimulation Study

A repetitive stimulation study is a method of measuring electrical conduction properties at the neuromuscular junction. To perform a repetitive stimulation study, a surface recording electrode is placed over a muscle belly, and the nerve innervating that muscle is electrically stimulated with a supramaximal stimulus at a certain frequency. A series of electrical potentials are then recorded whose amplitude is roughly proportional to the number of muscle fibers that are being activated.

A repetitive stimulation study is helpful in diagnosis of neuromuscular junction disorders, such as myasthenia gravis and myasthenic syndrome (Lambert-Eaton syndrome). In myasthenia gravis, the amplitudes of evoked potentials become progressively smaller with repetitive stimulation in clinically involved muscles. Clinically uninvolved muscles often do not demonstrate this decrement. In myasthenic syndrome, an *increment* is seen in the amplitudes of evoked potentials with rapid repetitive electrical stimulation.

Electromyography

Electromyography (EMG) is the recording and study of insertional, spontaneous, and voluntary electrical activity of muscle. It allows physiologic evaluation of the motor unit, including the anterior horn cell, peripheral nerve, and muscle.

EMG is performed by insertion of a needle electrode into the muscle in question and evaluation of the motor unit action potentials both visually (on the oscilloscope screen) and aurally (over the loudspeaker). Muscles are typically studied at rest and during voluntary contraction. During EMG, the electrical activity of muscle is studied in four settings (Table 403-6): *insertional activity* (occurring within the first second of needle insertion), *spontaneous activity* (electrical activity at rest), *voluntary activity* (electrical activity with muscle contraction), and *recruitment pattern* (change in electrical activity with maximal contraction).

EMG is helpful in evaluation of patients with weakness in that it can help determine whether the weakness is due to anterior horn cell disease, nerve root disease, peripheral neuropathy, or an intrinsic disease of muscle itself (myopathy). EMG can differentiate acute denervation from chronic denervation and may thus give an indication about the time course of the lesion causing the neuropathy. In addition, on the basis of which muscles have an abnormal EMG pattern, it is possible to determine whether the neuropathy is due to a lesion of a nerve root (radiculopathy), the brachial or lumbosacral plexus (plexopathy), an individual peripheral nerve (mononeuropathy), or multiple peripheral nerves (polyneuropathy).

1% of adults and 3.5% of children who are neurologically normal and who never had a seizure have epileptiform activity on an EEG.

The EEG may provide clues to the diagnosis of certain neurologic conditions, including viral encephalitis, prion disorders, and some forms of coma. In each of these situations, the EEG can have specific patterns that suggest a specific neurologic diagnosis. In herpes simplex encephalitis, periodic lateralizing epileptiform discharges emanating from the temporal lobes are frequently present. Triphasic slow waves are common in hepatic encephalopathy (Fig. 403-2C) but are a nonspecific finding. Creutzfeldt-Jakob disease is characterized by the presence of bilateral synchronous repetitive sharp waves. The EEG is also helpful in evaluating comatose patients, in confirming brain death when an apnea test cannot be performed because of cardiac instability, and for staging sleep in polysomnography.

In the past, the EEG was often used to localize neurologic lesions such as stroke, brain tumor, and abscess. With the advent of neuroimaging, EEG is almost never used for these purposes.

Nerve Conduction Study

A nerve conduction study (NCS) is the recording and measurement of the compound nerve and muscle action potentials elicited in response to an electrical stimulus.

To perform a motor NCS, a surface (active) recording electrode is placed over the belly of a distal muscle that is innervated by the nerve in question. A reference electrode is placed distally over the tendon. The nerve is then supramaximally stimulated at a predetermined distance proximal to the active electrode, and the resultant compound motor action potential (CMAP) is recorded. The terminal latency, amplitude, and duration of the evoked potential are measured directly, and the conduction velocity is calculated from the latencies of the evoked potentials with stimulation at two different points; the distance between the two points (conduction distance) is divided by the difference between the corresponding latencies (conduction time) to derive a calculated velocity (conduction velocity = distance ÷ time).

To perform a sensory NCS, the active recording electrode is placed over the portion of the skin innervated by the nerve in question, and a sensory nerve action potential is recorded after electrical stimulation of the nerve, similar to that noted for a motor NCS. NCS abnormalities include reduced amplitudes, prolonged terminal latencies, conduction block, and slowed conduction velocities (Table 403-5).

The NCS is helpful in documenting the existence of a neuropathy, quantifying its severity, and noting its distribution (i.e., whether it is distal, proximal, or diffuse). In addition, the NCS can provide information on the modality involved (i.e., motor versus sensory) and can suggest whether the

EMG is also helpful in differentiation of active (inflammatory) myopathies from chronic myopathies. Active myopathies include dermatomyositis, polymyositis, inclusion body myositis, and some forms of muscular dystrophy, such as Duchenne's dystrophy. Chronic myopathies include the other muscular dystrophies, the congenital myopathies, and some metabolic myopathies. Myotonic dystrophy and myotonia congenita produce characteristic myotonic discharges.

It may take several weeks for a muscle to develop EMG signs of acute denervation after nerve transection. For this reason, EMG performed in the acute setting after nerve injury should be interpreted with caution, and it may need to be repeated at a later date.

Evoked Potentials

Evoked potentials are ways of measuring conduction velocities for sensory pathways in the CNS by means of computerized averaging techniques. Three types of evoked potentials are routinely performed: visual, brain stem auditory, and somatosensory.

Pattern Reversal Visual Evoked Responses

The pattern reversal visual evoked response (PVER) assesses the function of central visual pathways, in particular the optic nerves. To perform this test, EEG electrodes are placed over the occipital regions of the scalp, and the patient is asked to look at the center of a black-and-white checkerboard screen with one eye patched. The color of the checks alternates about twice per second, a process known as pattern reversal. The scalp potentials elicited by approximately 100 such pattern reversals are then recorded and signal averaged by a computer. This signal averaging cancels the random EEG activity and differentially amplifies the evoked potential. A single waveform (P 100) is recorded for each eye, and its latency is measured. Normal latency for the P 100 waveform is approximately 100 msec. A prolonged P 100 latency in one eye, in the absence of ocular disease, implies slowed conduction velocity in the optic nerve and suggests demyelination of that nerve. PVER testing is helpful when multiple sclerosis is suspected clinically and it is necessary to document the presence of a second demyelinating lesion in the CNS that may not be clinically evident (Fig. 403-3).

Brain Stem Auditory Evoked Responses

The brain stem auditory evoked response (BAER) assesses function in the central auditory pathways in the brain stem. EEG electrodes are placed over the vertex and mastoid process, and a series of clicks at a frequency of 5 Hz are delivered to each ear separately for 3 minutes. The scalp potentials elicited by the clicks are then recorded and signal averaged by a computer. This signal averaging cancels the random EEG activity and differentially amplifies the evoked potential. A series of five waves are recorded for each ear, and each wave corresponds to a different point in the central auditory pathway (Table 403-7). The wave latencies for the right and left ears are compared, and a delay in any of the latencies suggests a lesion at that point in the central brain stem auditory pathway. BAER testing is helpful in diagnosis of acoustic schwannoma and other tumors in the cerebellopontine angle.

Somatosensory Evoked Responses

The somatosensory evoked response (SER) assesses conduction in the central somatosensory pathways in the posterior columns of the spinal cord, brain stem, thalamus, and primary sensory cortex in the parietal lobes. To perform SER testing, recording electrodes are placed over Erb's point and the

TABLE 403-6	ELECTROMYOGRAPHIC ABNORMALITIES
ABNORMALITY	**CLINICAL CORRELATE**
INSERTIONAL ACTIVITY	
Prolonged	Acute denervation
	Active (usually inflammatory) myopathy
SPONTANEOUS ACTIVITY	
Fibrillations and positive waves	Acute denervation
	Active (usually inflammatory) myopathy
Fasciculations	Chronic neuropathies
	Motor neuron disease (rare fasciculations may be normal)
Myotonic discharges	Myotonic disorders
	Acid maltase deficiency
VOLUNTARY ACTIVITY	
Neuropathic potentials: large-amplitude, long-duration, polyphasic potentials	Chronic neuropathies and anterior horn cell diseases
Myopathic potentials: small-amplitude, short-duration, polyphasic potentials	Chronic myopathies
	Neuromuscular junction disorders
RECRUITMENT	
Reduced	Chronic neuropathic disorders
Rapid	Chronic myopathies

TABLE 403-7	BRAIN STEM EVOKED RESPONSE WAVE GENERATORS	
WAVE		**LOCATION**
I		Auditory nerve
II		Cochlear nucleus
III		Superior olivary nucleus
IV		Lateral lemniscus
V		Inferior colliculus

FIGURE 403-3. Abnormal pattern reversal visual evoked response in a patient with multiple sclerosis. The prolonged P 100 wave latency with left eye stimulation suggests a conduction defect in the left optic nerve. The top three channels represent right eye stimulation, and the bottom three channels represent left eye stimulation. Each horizontal division represents 20 msec.

TABLE 403-8   STRENGTHS AND WEAKNESSES OF SELECTED IMAGING MODALITIES

MODALITY	STRENGTHS	WEAKNESSES
Computed tomography (CT)	Fast; best test for acute intraparenchymal or subarachnoid hemorrhage and calcification; easy to monitor patients; excellent for bones	Less sensitive to parenchymal lesions than MRI; potential for significant reaction to contrast material; radiation exposure
Conventional angiography	Best imaging modality for aneurysms, vascular malformations, and vasculitis	Invasive and often lengthy; risk of stroke and other complications
Conventional myelography	Good images of nerve roots and small osteophytic lesions; accurate for bony stenosis; useful in patients with contraindications to MRI	Invasive, with risk of complications from lumbar puncture and instillation of contrast material; does not image intramedullary lesions well
CT myelography	Excellent for imaging nerve roots and detecting root compression from degenerative processes	Invasive, with risk of complications from lumbar puncture and instillation of contrast material
Magnetic resonance imaging (MRI)	Noninvasive; no radiation; multiplanar; extremely sensitive, safe contrast agent	Less sensitive than CT for detection of subarachnoid hemorrhage and calcification; less sensitive for bony skull fractures; contraindicated in patients with implanted metallic devices or foreign bodies; the patient must be able to cooperate and tolerate confined space; time-consuming relative to CT
Magnetic resonance angiography (MRA)	Noninvasive; good for screening for extracranial and intracranial vascular disease; may be performed with or without contrast agent	Need cooperative patient; technically demanding; may overestimate the degree of vascular stenosis (noncontrast MRA); cannot image distal vessels optimally without contrast agent; may miss small lesions (e.g., aneurysms)
Positron emission tomography (PET)	Limited role in helping to distinguish radiation necrosis from tumor; sometimes helpful in the diagnosis of Alzheimer's disease and epilepsy	Requires a cyclotron to generate radioisotopes with a short half-life; lower resolution and less available than MRI or CT
Single-photon emission computed tomography (SPECT)	Occasionally useful in epilepsy; sensitive for diffuse pathologic processes; easier to use than PET	Lower resolution than PET, MRI, or CT
Proton magnetic resonance spectroscopy	Localization of seizure focus; may help diagnose and classify dementias, such as Alzheimer's disease; may distinguish brain tumors from other mass lesions; may distinguish radiation necrosis from recurrent tumor	Specificity not yet determined; not routinely available; lower resolution; time-consuming
Ultrasonography	Fast; easy to use; can be performed at the bedside to assess vessel patency	Does not assess the vertebral arteries; less sensitive and specific than MRA; cannot visualize vessels in the upper neck and cranial base
Transcranial Doppler (TCD)	Fast; easy to use; assesses vascular velocities quantitatively; can assess cerebral vasospasm and occluded vessels	Does not provide images of vessels

Reproduced and modified from Hackney D. Radiologic imaging procedures. In: Goldman L, Ausiello D, eds. *Cecil Medicine*, 23rd ed. Philadelphia: Saunders Elsevier; 2008:2623-2627.

cervical spine (for medial or ulnar nerve stimulation), over the popliteal fossa and lumbar spine (for peroneal or tibial nerve stimulation), and over the scalp. A series of 1000 to 2000 electrical shocks at a frequency of 5 Hz are delivered to the median or ulnar nerve (for an upper extremity SER) or to the peroneal or tibial nerve (for a lower extremity SER). The scalp potentials elicited by the electrical shocks are then recorded and signal averaged by a computer. This signal averaging cancels the random EEG activity and differentially amplifies the evoked potential. A series of waves are recorded for each nerve stimulated, with each wave corresponding to a different point in the somatosensory pathways in the spinal cord, brain stem, and cerebral cortex. The wave latencies for the right and left limbs are compared, and a delay in any of the latencies suggests a lesion at that point in the somatosensory pathways.

SER testing, like PVER, is helpful when multiple sclerosis is suspected clinically and it is necessary to document the presence of a second demyelinating lesion in the CNS that may not be clinically evident. SER testing is also useful for monitoring of spinal cord function intraoperatively in patients undergoing spinal surgery.

Electronystagmography

Electronystagmography accurately records eye movements and nystagmus after certain provocative maneuvers. To perform this test, disc electrodes are placed over the bridge of the nose and lateral to each outer canthus, and the electrical leads from these discs are connected to an oscilloscope. Because the cornea is electropositive and the retina is electronegative, these electrodes accurately record lateral eye movements. The patient is first observed for spontaneous nystagmus with the eyes open and closed and then for nystagmus evoked with lateral gaze, for nystagmus induced by hot and cold air instilled in the outer ears (caloric induced), and for positional nystagmus. The last is performed by rotating the patient in a specialized chair. Spontaneous

nystagmus suggests a vestibular pathologic lesion, as does an imbalance in the nystagmus evoked by these maneuvers in the right and left ears.

Imaging

On the basis of the relative advantages and disadvantages of computed tomography (CT), magnetic resonance imaging (MRI), and other neuroimaging modalities, different clinical entities can and should be assessed differently (Table 403-8). In acute ischemic stroke (Chapter 414) without bleeding, CT abnormalities typically appear within 4 to 12 hours and are seen even earlier with larger infarctions and embolic infarctions. CT detects hemorrhagic stroke (Chapter 415) acutely and can estimate its age. CT is also the preferred initial imaging modality for detection of intraparenchymal hemorrhage and subarachnoid hemorrhage, and it often suggests whether an aneurysm is the likely cause. Either CT angiography or magnetic resonance arteriography can display the three-dimensional anatomy of aneurysms with sufficient detail for therapy to be planned, but surgical treatment generally requires pre-procedure catheter arteriography. CT is the first-line method for evaluation of brain trauma and diagnosis of a subdural or epidural hematoma (Chapter 406), usually without requiring intravenous contrast material. However, MRI is better than CT to delineate the anatomy of a subdural hematoma and to estimate the age of the lesion. Many brain tumors are initially recognized on CT scans, but MRI is the preferred modality for detection and characterization of all brain tumors (Chapter 195).

SUGGESTED READINGS

De Luigi AJ, Fitzpatrick KF. Physical examination in radiculopathy. *Phys Med Rehabil Clin N Am.* 2011;22:7-40. *Review.*

Loder E, Cardona L. Evaluation for secondary causes of headache: the role of blood and urine testing. *Headache.* 2011;51:338-345. *Review.*

404

PSYCHIATRIC DISORDERS IN MEDICAL PRACTICE

JEFFREY M. LYNESS

OVERVIEW

Disorders in Psychiatry

Psychiatric disorders, also known as mental illnesses, are extraordinarily common and have a profound impact on well-being and functional status. Collectively, psychiatric disorders account for more aggregate disability than do those involving any other organ system, with depression alone being second only to cardiovascular disorders.

Psychiatric disorders are defined as *disorders of the psyche*, that is, as conditions that affect *thoughts*, *feelings*, or *behaviors*. By definition, such mental disturbances must be sufficient to produce significant *distress* in the patient or *impairment in role or other functioning*. Because the causes and pathogenesis of most psychiatric disorders are incompletely understood, current classification is based on clinical syndromes, which are defined by diagnostic criteria that have high inter-rater reliability because they emphasize discrete reportable or observable symptoms and signs.

Specific Syndromes

Because many *psychiatric disorders* result from the direct influence of neurologic conditions, systemic diseases, or drugs on brain functioning, assessment of any new or worsened psychiatric condition must include evaluation for their potential contributions (Table 404-1). Delirium (Chapter 27) and dementia (Chapter 409), which are *cognitive disorders* that are always the result of one or more neurologic, systemic, or drug causes, are defined by impairment in intellectual functions such as attention, memory, or language. Although cognitive impairment is the hallmark of cognitive disorders, these conditions may also be manifested as alterations in other aspects of mental status, including mood, thought content, thought process, and behavior. If a noncognitive psychiatric syndrome is caused by an identifiable underlying condition, it is known as a *secondary psychiatric disorder* (e.g., depression secondary to hypothyroidism).

The major nonsecondary, noncognitive psychiatric syndromes (Table 404-2) can coexist with multiple syndromes; for example, a patient with severe depression may have depressive, anxiety, and psychotic syndromes simultaneously. Substance use disorders, also known as addictions, are considered in Chapters 32 and 33.

Comorbid Conditions in Psychiatry

It is common for persons who suffer from mental disorders to meet the diagnostic criteria for more than one condition. Although such comorbidity may reflect the limitations of current approaches to diagnosis, psychiatric comorbidity influences the choices or sequence of indicated treatments and may worsen the overall prognosis. Comorbidity with general medical conditions, probably reflecting complex bidirectional causal relationships between physical and mental illnesses, is also common, and such comorbidity often worsens the overall prognosis for both conditions.

Treatments in Psychiatry

Treatments in psychiatry are intended to reduce or eliminate symptoms, thereby improving the patient's distress and dysfunction and averting suicidal behavior. Pharmacotherapy remains an evidence-based mainstay of the treatment of many psychiatric conditions despite the previously underestimated side effects of some drugs. The evidence for a number of forms of psychotherapy, administered in individual, group, or family contexts, supports its use as primary treatment or as co-treatment of many conditions. Other psychosocial interventions, ranging from self-help groups to the use of structured treatment or residential programs, are often important adjuncts to treatment.

TABLE 404-1	IMPORTANT CAUSES OF PSYCHIATRIC SYNDROMES

CENTRAL NERVOUS SYSTEM DISEASES

Trauma
Tumor
Toxins
Seizures
Vascular
Infections
Genetic/congenital malformations
Demyelinating diseases
Neurodegenerative diseases
Hydrocephalus

SYSTEMIC DISEASES

Cardiovascular
Pulmonary
Endocrine
Metabolic
Nutritional
Infections
Cancer

DRUGS (e.g., recreational, prescription, or over-the-counter drugs)

Drug intoxication
Drug withdrawal

TABLE 404-2	IMPORTANT PSYCHIATRIC SYNDROMES AND DISORDERS	
SYNDROME	**MAIN SYMPTOMS AND SIGNS**	**MAY OCCUR AS PART OF THESE DISORDERS**
Cognitive	Deficits in intellectual functions, e.g., level of consciousness, orientation, attention, memory, language, praxis, visuospatial, executive functions	Cognitive disorders Mental retardation (if onset in childhood)
Mood	Depressive: lowered mood, anhedonia, negativistic thoughts, neurovegetative symptoms *or* Manic: elevated or irritable mood, grandiosity, goal-directed hyperactivity with increased energy, pressured speech, decreased sleep need	Cognitive disorders Mood disorders (primary or secondary) Psychotic disorders (schizoaffective disorder)
Anxiety	All include anxious mood and associated physiologic symptoms (e.g., palpitations, tremors, diaphoresis). May include various types of dysfunctional thoughts (e.g., catastrophic fears, obsessions, flashbacks) and behavior (e.g., compulsions, avoidance behavior)	Cognitive disorders Mood disorders (primary or secondary) Psychotic disorders (primary or secondary) Anxiety disorders (primary or secondary)
Psychotic	Impairments in reality testing: delusions, hallucinations, thought process derailments	Cognitive disorders Mood disorders (primary or secondary) Psychotic disorders
Somatoform	Somatoform symptoms: physical symptoms resulting from unconscious psychogenic causes	Mood disorders (primary or secondary) Anxiety disorders (primary or secondary) Somatoform disorders
Personality pathology	Enduring patterns of dysfunctional emotional regulation, thought patterns, interpersonal behavior, impulse regulation	Cognitive disorders (dementia) Change in personality because of general medical condition Personality disorders

Based on categories and criteria from American Psychiatric Association. *Diagnostic and Statistical Manual of Mental Disorders (DSM-IV)*, 4th ed. Washington, DC: American Psychiatric Association; 2000.

Nonpharmacologic evidence-based therapies include electroconvulsive therapy or light therapy for particular forms of major depression, and encouraging data are emerging to support deep brain stimulation for severe depressive or obsessive-compulsive disorders.

Mood Disorders

Mood disorders are categorized as either *unipolar*, characterized by depressive episodes only, or *bipolar*, characterized by manic or hypomanic episodes but typically also including depressive episodes.

● MAJOR DEPRESSIVE DISORDER

DEFINITION

Major depressive disorder is characterized by one or more episodes of idiopathic major depressive syndrome (Table 404-3).

TABLE 404-3 SYMPTOMS/SIGNS OF AN EPISODE OF MAJOR DEPRESSIVE SYNDROME

DIAGNOSTIC CRITERIA (*EACH MUST BE PRESENT PROMINENTLY, MOST OF THE DAY AND NEARLY EVERY DAY FOR A MINIMUM OF 2 CONSECUTIVE WEEKS*)

Depressed mood (may be irritable mood in children and adolescents) *or*
Diminished interest or pleasure *and*
Weight loss or change in appetite (decrease or increase)
Change in sleep (insomnia or hypersomnia)
Psychomotor agitation or retardation
Fatigue or anergia
Feeling of worthlessness or guilt
Diminished concentration or indecisiveness
Recurrent thoughts of death or suicidal ideation, a suicide attempt, or a specific suicide plan

MNEMONIC TO AID RECALL OF DIAGNOSTIC CRITERIA

SIG: E CAPS (*i.e., prescribe energy capsules*) for depressed mood
  Sleep change
  Interests
  Guilt
  Energy
  Concentration
  Appetite/weight
  Psychomotor changes
  Suicide

DEPRESSIVE SYMPTOMS/SIGNS GROUPED CONCEPTUALLY, WITH ADDITIONAL COMMON PHENOMENA

Emotional

Depressed mood, sadness, tearfulness
Irritability (*seen in all ages, perhaps most commonly in children/adolescents and the elderly*)
Anxiety
Loss of interests or pleasure (anhedonia)

Ideational

Worthlessness/lowered self-esteem
Guilt
Hopelessness/nihilism
Helplessness
Thoughts of death, dying, suicide

Somatic/Neurovegetative

Change in appetite/weight
Change in sleep
Anergia
Decreased libido
Trouble concentrating
Diurnal variation in symptoms (*mornings—worst pattern is most characteristic*)

Other

Ruminative thinking (*tendency to dwell on one [negativistic] theme*)
Somatoform symptoms or somatic worry
Psychotic symptoms (*negativistic delusions most characteristic*)—defines the subtype "Major Depression with Psychotic Features"

Based on criteria from American Psychiatric Association. *Diagnostic and Statistical Manual of Mental Disorders (DSM-IV)*, 4th ed. Washington, DC: American Psychiatric Association; 2000.

EPIDEMIOLOGY

In the United States, major depression has a point prevalence of approximately 3 to 5% in males and 8 to 10% in females. Lifetime prevalence is up to 10% in males and 20 to 25% in females. It is difficult to determine the true incidence rates of a new depressive disorder, but new episodes have an annual incidence of approximately 3%. Despite minor variations, similar rates are found in most industrialized nations. Depression accounts for more than twice as much disability in midlife as any other medical condition does, and its overall cumulative burden is greater than that from all but cardiovascular disorders. The economic impact is also enormous, with U.S. estimates of annual costs for depression exceeding $12 billion for treatment, $8 billion for associated morbidity, and $33 billion for lost earnings and work productivity.

PATHOBIOLOGY

Major depression is probably not a single disease entity but rather a heterogeneous group of conditions with multiple pathogenic mechanisms. It is both multifactorial and polygenic: genetic factors account for up to 50% of the risk for depression, but multiple gene loci, most of which are currently unknown, are probably involved in a complex interplay with developmental and environmental influences. Alterations in the brain's noradrenergic and serotonergic systems are present and are most likely related to the efficacy of current antidepressant medications. The hypothalamic-pituitary-adrenal axis is hyperactive in depression, as evidenced by a nonsuppressed response to the dexamethasone suppression test, although this test is too insensitive and nonspecific for clinical use as a diagnostic tool. Neuroimaging studies in subjects with depression show an array of findings, including smaller hippocampal volumes, which are thought to be the result of exposure to elevated cortisol levels, and altered regional cerebral metabolic activity of the frontal-striatal circuitry and anterior cingulate cortex. Cognitive psychology studies have demonstrated dysfunctional patterns of negative thinking, with distorted thoughts about self, the future, and the environment. Poor quality or absence of social relationships and stressful life events, particularly events such as deaths, separations, or functional impairment, are powerfully associated with depression as well.

CLINICAL MANIFESTATIONS

The symptoms of depression (see Table 404-3) may be conceptually grouped as alterations in mood, ideation (i.e., thought content), and somatic/neurovegetative functioning. Importantly, patients with depressive illness may be seen without a depressed mood, albeit by definition they must have loss of interest or pleasure in their usually desired activities. They may also exhibit prominent anxiety, irritability, or somatization. Although mild forms of major depression in the community often remit spontaneously within a few months without medical care, patients may already have had persistent symptoms for months or years before seeking treatment.

DIAGNOSIS

The diagnosis is made clinically by elicitation of findings from the history and mental status examination to determine the presence of major depressive syndrome. The differential diagnosis includes other idiopathic disorders with episodes of major depression, such as bipolar disorder (distinguished by a history of manic episodes) and schizoaffective disorder (distinguished by a history of psychotic episodes in the absence of depression). Major depression may accompany delirium or dementia, and secondary depression also commonly accompanies serious medical illnesses; these comorbid conditions require careful, well-coordinated care.

TREATMENT **Rx**

The three phases of treatment include (1) *acute*, in which treatment is provided to resolve the major depressive episode; (2) *continuation*, in which the acute treatment is continued for at least 4 to 8 months to prevent relapse; and (3) *maintenance*, for those with two to three or more episodes of recurrent depression, for whom treatment is maintained indefinitely to reduce the frequency and severity of future recurrences. Combinations of psychotherapy and medication are used for more complex or severe clinical conditions.

Acute treatment of depression includes focused psychotherapies (Table 404-4), which are more efficacious than usual care and equivalent to medications when used for patients in primary care settings.█ Based on the patient's preference, psychotherapy rather than medications may be the initial treatment of mild to moderate major depression with prominent psychosocial stressors. Involvement of family members for education and support and sometimes for formal family therapy may be an important adjunctive or primary therapeutic approach. These therapies may be administered with decreased frequency during the continuation or maintenance phases of treatment. However, psychotherapies may be difficult to implement and are not likely to help patients with more severe forms of depression, including major depression with psychotic features.

Medications should be used as initial treatment for most patients with more severe forms of major depression. Antidepressant medications (Table 404-5) are also effective for acute, continuation, and maintenance therapy. A recent meta-analysis found that sertraline and escitalopram have the best profiles of efficacy and tolerability whereas mirtazapine and venlafaxine also have strong efficacy in head-to-head comparisons with other antidepressants.[2] Because antidepressant medications typically do not begin to improve symptoms for at least 1 to 2 weeks, with maximal benefit accruing up to at least 6 to 8 weeks, it is crucial to see patients regularly (every 1 to 2 weeks initially) to monitor their clinical status, to provide support and education, and to foster adherence. Antidepressant medications appear to increase the relative risk for suicidal behavior in adolescents and young adults, so careful benefit/risk assessments must be made in such patients. The relative risk for suicidal behavior is not increased by drug treatment in individuals older than 25 years and is substantially lowered in older adults. Electroconvulsive therapy is preferred for the most severe forms of major depression, including major depression with psychotic features, and is also used for depression that is refractory to other forms of treatment.

Optimal care for depression in primary care settings may be enhanced by the use of on-site mental health collaborative care models. However, despite considerable evidence supporting such models,[3] the lack of reimbursement mechanisms has limited their implementation in most communities and clinical settings.

PROGNOSIS

Optimal, guideline-based treatment of major depression results in full remission in at least 80% of patients, and the expectation is that patients with major depression will return to baseline functioning after resolution of the depressive episodes. However, at least 50 to 70% of patients will suffer recurrent episodes, up to 20% may experience chronic major depression, and many more will be in incomplete remission with persistent lower-level symptoms because of a variety of factors, including limited access to care, nonadherence, or insufficiently assertive treatments.

BIPOLAR DISORDER

DEFINITION AND EPIDEMIOLOGY

Bipolar disorder is characterized by recurrent episodes of idiopathic mania. Most persons with bipolar disorder also have recurrent episodes of major depression.

The point prevalence of bipolar disorder is approximately 1%. Males and females are affected equally. The average age at first onset is late adolescence or early adulthood. Childhood onset is possible, but diagnosis may be difficult because of symptomatic overlap with other conditions of childhood, including attention-deficit/hyperactivity disorder. Onset in midlife to late life is also possible, although most persons in whom mania develops in later life have mania secondary to medical conditions or drugs rather than idiopathic bipolar disorder.

PATHOBIOLOGY

Even though the pathogenesis of bipolar disorder remains unclear, genetic factors play a greater role than in unipolar depressive conditions. Heritability has been traced to several specific loci in rare families, but genetic screening is not clinically useful and the gene associations have, to date, revealed no unifying pathophysiologic themes. Most cases of bipolar disorder are polygenic and multifactorial, with nongenetic factors accounting for approximately 50% of the risk for the disorder. Dysregulation of the frontostriatal systems is probably involved in the manifestations of the illness. Though not specific enough to be diagnostic, structural neuroimaging studies show increased ventricular-brain ratios suggestive of parenchymal atrophy. Phase advance of central circadian rhythms can precipitate episodes of mania, so the decreased sleep of persons with incipient mania may produce a vicious cycle in which phase-advanced circadian cycles lead to a further decreased need for sleep, thereby resulting in further phase advancement. Psychosocial stressors also often play a role in precipitating episodes of both mania and depression.

CLINICAL MANIFESTATIONS AND DIAGNOSIS

The symptoms of mania include a distinct period of abnormally and persistently elevated (euphoric) or irritable mood; goal-directed hyperactivity, often for pleasurable activities with poor judgment that leads to long-lasting adverse financial, psychosocial, or medical consequences, such as sprees of spending, sexual activity, or gambling; decreased need for sleep; pressured speech; and distractibility.

As with major depression, the diagnosis is based on findings from the history and examination revealing a pattern of recurrent manic episodes (Table 404-6), which are usually interspersed with major depressive episodes and cannot be explained by general medical conditions, medications, or other substances. Although persons with bipolar disorder may become psychotic while in manic or depressed states, a history of psychotic symptoms in the absence of mania or depression indicates a diagnosis of schizoaffective disorder rather than bipolar disorder. Manic and depressive episodes may also be seen in the course of delirium (Chapter 27) and dementia (Chapter 409), in which case the psychiatric symptoms are accompanied by the cognitive impairment that is the hallmark of the latter conditions.

TREATMENT

The mainstay of treatment of bipolar disorder is mood stabilizer medications to reduce the frequency and severity of recurrent manic and depressive episodes. Traditional mood stabilizers with substantial evidence base to support their use include lithium (typical dose of 600 to 1500 mg/day or higher given in two or three divided doses as needed to achieve plasma levels of 0.6 to 1.2 mEq/L [up to 1.4 mEq/L in acute mania]), valproic acid (typical dose of 500 to 1500 mg/day or higher as tolerated to achieve plasma levels of 50 to 100 µg/mL), and carbamazepine (typical dose of 400 to 1200 mg/day as tolerated to achieve plasma levels of 4 to 12 µg/mL). The combination of lithium plus valproate is superior to valproate alone for prevention of relapses.[4] A number of other anticonvulsants have been tried, but generally with less empirical support for their use, although lamotrigine (starting at 25 mg/day, maximum dose of 200 mg/day, titrated slowly to minimize the risk for Stevens-Johnson syndrome) can be used for prophylaxis against depressive episodes. Even though several second-generation antipsychotic medications have received approval by the Food and Drug Administration for their mood-stabilizing properties, their potential to precipitate metabolic syndrome and, to a lesser extent, tardive dyskinesia should limit their use as *maintenance* medications to patients for whom true mood stabilizers are inefficacious or poorly tolerated. For *acute* episodes of mania, second- or first-generation antipsychotics are more rapidly efficacious than mood stabilizers, with doses similar to their use for acute psychosis (see Table 404-12). For acute treatment of depressive episodes, antidepressants may be required, but they may precipitate mania; therefore, patients should receive therapeutic doses of a mood stabilizer first, and exposure to antidepressant medication should be for the minimum dose and duration required to reach euthymia. Electroconvulsive therapy is useful for refractory mania or depression and for patients with relative contraindications to medications, such as pregnant women. Standard psychotherapeutic approaches for unipolar depression may also be used for bipolar patients during depressive episodes. Ongoing psychotherapy may be important to encourage compliance with maintenance therapies and to help patients manage psychosocial stressors in order to minimize their impact on precipitating acute manic or depressive decompensations.

PROGNOSIS

Although the classically described course of bipolar disorder includes return to baseline functioning between episodes, some patients may experience frequent debilitating episodes (known as "rapid cycling," defined as four or more episodes per year), whereas others may experience a deterioration in overall functioning over time.

TABLE 404-4	TREATMENTS OF DEPRESSION
NAME OF PSYCHOTHERAPY	**APPROACH**
Cognitive psychotherapy	Identify and correct negativistic patterns of thinking
Interpersonal psychotherapy	Identify and work through role transitions or interpersonal losses, conflicts, or deficits
Problem-solving therapy	Identify and prioritize situational problems; plan and implement strategies to deal with top-priority problems
Psychodynamic psychotherapy	Use therapeutic relationship to maximize use of the healthiest defense mechanisms and coping strategies

TABLE 404-5 COMMONLY USED ANTIDEPRESSANT MEDICATIONS

NAME OF CLASS/ SPECIFIC MEDICATION	IMMEDIATE MECHANISM OF ACTION	INITIAL DOSE	TARGET DOSE RANGE*	SIDE EFFECTS	COMMENTS
SSRIs (selective serotonin re-uptake inhibitors)	Inhibit presynaptic re-uptake of serotonin			Nausea, diarrhea, sexual dysfunction, serotonin syndrome	
Citalopram		20 mg qd	20-60 mg qd		Few drug-drug interactions
Escitalopram		10 mg qd	10-20 mg qd		Enantiomer of citalopram
Fluoxetine		20 mg qd	20-40 mg qd (depression), up to 80 mg qd (OCD)		Long half-life; tends to be activating
Paroxetine		20 mg qd	20-50 mg qd	Anticholinergic effects	Tends to be sedating
Sertraline		25-50 mg qd	50-200 mg qd		Few drug-drug interactions
SNRIs (serotonin and norepinephrine re-uptake inhibitors)	Inhibit presynaptic re-uptake of serotonin and norepinephrine			Nausea, diarrhea, serotonin syndrome, sinus tachycardia, mild elevation in blood pressure, tremor	
Duloxetine		30-60 mg qd	30-60 mg qd on a twice-daily schedule, maximum of 120 mg/day		
Venlafaxine		37.5 mg bid	150-375 mg/day on bid schedule		XR form allows once-daily dosing
Desvenlafaxine		50 mg qd	50 mg qd, maximum of 100 mg ER qd		Metabolite of venlafaxine
TCAs (tricyclic antidepressants)	Inhibit presynaptic re-uptake of serotonin and norepinephrine (in varying proportions depending on the specific TCA)			Anticholinergic effects, sedation, orthostatic hypotension, tremor, cardiac conduction delays, ventricular arrhythmias	
Amitriptyline		25-75 mg qhs	150-300 mg qhs		Strongly anticholinergic and sedating; aim for combined amitriptyline/ nortriptyline blood level of 120-250 ng/mL
Desipramine		25-75 mg qd	150-300 mg qd		Aim for blood level of 115-250 ng/mL
Doxepin		25-75 mg qhs	150-300 mg qhs		Strongly sedating
Imipramine		25-75 mg qd	150-300 mg qd		Strongly anticholinergic; aim for combined imipramine/ desipramine blood level of 180-350 ng/mL
Nortriptyline		25-50 mg qhs	50-150 mg qhs		Aim for blood level of 50-150 ng/mL; least anticholinergic of the TCAs
MAOIs (monoamine oxidase inhibitors)	Inhibit monoamine oxidase, the enzyme that catalyzes oxidative metabolism of monoamine neurotransmitters			Need for tyramine-free diet to avoid sympathomimetic (hypertensive) crisis; sedation, anticholinergic effects, tremor, orthostatic hypotension	
Isocarboxazid		10 mg bid	20-60 mg/day in bid-qid dosing		
Phenelzine		15 mg tid	45-90 mg/day in tid or qid dosing		
Selegiline	(selective MAO-B inhibitor)	5 mg bid	5 mg bid	Tyramine-free diet not required	Take with meals
Tranylcypromine		10 mg tid	30-60 mg/day in tid dosing		
Other					
Bupropion	Unknown, although it is a weak inhibitor of presynaptic re-uptake of norepinephrine and dopamine	75-150 mg/day	300-450 mg/day	Activating; risk for seizures reduced by divided dosing and careful dosage titration	Divided dosing required unless using SR or XR forms
Mirtazapine	Antagonist at α_2 and 5-HT$_2$ receptors	15 mg qhs	30-45 mg qhs; maximum of 45 mg qhs	Sedation, hyperphagia	Becomes more stimulating at higher doses
Trazodone	Inhibits presynaptic re-uptake of serotonin; antagonist at 5-HT$_2$ and 5-HT$_3$ receptors	25-50 mg qhs	300-600 mg qhs for depression, 25-100 mg qhs for insomnia	Sedation, priapism	Few sexual side effects

*Target doses in the elderly may be lower.
ER = extended release; 5-HT$_2$ = 5-hydroxytryptamine; OCD = obsessive-compulsive disorder; qhs = at bedtime; SR = sustained release; XR = extended release.

● OTHER MOOD DISORDERS

Although chronic major depression should be the diagnosis in patients with long-lasting major depressive episodes, others may have chronic (≥2 years) lower-level depressive symptoms, known as *dysthymic disorder*, that can be treated with a combination of antidepressant medication and psychotherapy. A significant minority (perhaps 20 to 40%) of such patients will improve substantially with aggressive treatment. Other patients may have "less than major depression" of shorter duration, increasingly being referred to as "subsyndromal" or "subthreshold" depression; growing evidence suggests that broad psychosocial interventions (e.g., bibliotherapy, social activation) may improve outcomes in such patients.

Less severe bipolar spectrum disorders include *bipolar II disorder*, which is characterized by episodes of hypomania (i.e., low-level manic symptoms

TABLE 404-6   SYMPTOMS/SIGNS OF AN EPISODE OF MANIA

DIAGNOSTIC CRITERIA

A distinct period of abnormally, persistently elevated, expansive, or irritable mood lasting ≥1 week *and*

3 or more of the following symptoms/signs (4 or more if the mood abnormality is only irritability):

Inflated self-esteem/grandiosity

Decreased need for sleep

More talkative or pressure to keep talking

Subjective experience of racing thoughts or flight of ideas observed on examination

Distractibility

Increase in goal-directed activity or psychomotor agitation

Excessive involvement in pleasurable activities with high potential for painful consequences

MANIC SYMPTOMS/SIGNS GROUPED CONCEPTUALLY, WITH ADDITIONAL COMMON PHENOMENA

Emotional

Euphoria

Irritability

Labile affect

Ideational

Grandiosity

Somatic/Neurovegetative

Psychomotor agitation

Decreased need for sleep

Distractibility

Other

Goal-directed hyperactivity

Pressured speech

Impaired judgment

Flight of ideas

Psychotic symptoms (may include delusions, hallucinations, or derailment of thought processes such as loose associations)—defines the subtype "mania with psychotic features"

Based on criteria from American Psychiatric Association. *Diagnostic and Statistical Manual of Mental Disorders (DSM-IV)*, 4th ed. Washington, DC: American Psychiatric Association; 2000.

TABLE 404-7   TYPES OF ANXIETY DISORDERS

ANXIETY DISORDER	MAJOR CLINICAL CHARACTERISTICS
Panic disorder	Recurrent unexpected panic attacks, typically with anticipatory anxiety and avoidance behavior
Obsessive-compulsive disorder (OCD)	Recurrent obsessions (distressing thoughts experienced as ego-alien) and compulsions (mental or physical actions in an attempt to neutralize obsessions or in response to rigid rules)
Acute stress disorder and post-traumatic stress disorder (PTSD)	Responses to a severely traumatic event, including re-experiences of the trauma, avoidance behavior, and hyperarousal
Generalized anxiety disorder	Excessive anxiety and worry, not meeting the criteria for other anxiety disorders, lasting ≥6 months
Phobias	
Agoraphobia	Anxiety about or avoidance of places or situations from which escape might be difficult or embarrassing or in which help might not be available in the event of panic symptoms
Social phobia	Anxiety provoked by exposure to social situations, typically with ensuing avoidance behavior; may be generalized (i.e., in response to many interpersonal situations) or specific in response to a particular social situation (e.g., using a public restroom, public speaking)
Specific phobia	Anxiety provoked by exposure to a specific feared object or (nonsocial) situation, typically with ensuing avoidance behavior

Based on categories and criteria from American Psychiatric Association. *Diagnostic and Statistical Manual of Mental Disorders (DSM-IV)*, 4th ed. Washington, DC: American Psychiatric Association; 2000.

without substantial functional impairment and without psychosis) and episodes of major depression. Such patients typically seek care during depressive episodes rather than during hypomania, but antidepressant medication may worsen the manic symptoms. It is therefore imperative to ask about a history of manic or hypomanic symptoms in the evaluation of all patients with depression. *Cyclothymic disorder*, which includes episodes of hypomania and low-level depressive episodes, may be difficult to distinguish from the mood instability seen in "cluster B" personality disorders (see later).

ANXIETY DISORDERS

DEFINITION

The anxiety disorders (Table 404-7) are a group of conditions whose hallmark is idiopathic anxiety, typically accompanied by psychological (i.e., thought content) and somatic symptoms. Anxiety is a common accompanying symptom in many other psychiatric disorders, but the primary anxiety disorders lack the cognitive deficits, depressive or manic symptoms, or psychosis seen in these other disorders.

EPIDEMIOLOGY

Panic disorder and obsessive-compulsive disorder (OCD) each have point prevalence rates of approximately 1 to 2%. The prevalence of acute stress disorder and post-traumatic stress disorder (PTSD) varies widely by population. Generalized anxiety disorder has a prevalence of approximately 2 to 3%, whereas the phobias collectively have a prevalence of 10% in the adult population. Clear data on incidence rates are not available. Most primary anxiety disorders have an age at first onset in late adolescence through the mid-30s. Most anxiety symptoms with new onset in later life are due to mood or cognitive disorders or are secondary to medical illnesses or drugs; true late-onset primary anxiety disorders are often triggered by traumatic or other stressful life events.

PATHOBIOLOGY

Most of the anxiety disorders may be understood as inappropriate triggering of the stress response system, which is commonly referred to as the "fight or

flight" response. However, it is important to recognize that the responses involve a wide range of cognitive, motor, neuroendocrine, and autonomic systems and thus are not limited to manifestations of sympathetic nervous system activity. The central nucleus of the amygdala is believed to play a crucial role in coordinating the anxiety response. The amygdala receives excitatory glutamatergic input from several cortical areas and from the thalamus, thereby allowing it to respond to a wide variety of stimuli, including sensory input from the external world, as well as stressors that are processed and recognized by cortical association areas. The amygdala in turn projects to the many brain regions that subserve the clinical manifestations of the anxiety response, in part through its direct projections to the important centers of monoaminergic systems: dopaminergic neurons of the ventral tegmental area in the midbrain, noradrenergic neurons in the locus caeruleus, and serotonergic neurons in the raphe nuclei.

From a cognitive psychology perspective, the pathogenesis of many anxiety disorders, particularly panic, may be understood as catastrophic misinterpretations of normal somatic sensations. A vulnerable individual may become aware of a normal or minimally abnormal body sensation, which is interpreted as something concerning, thereby leading to sympathetic and other autonomic arousal, which in turn leads to further somatic sensations (e.g., tachycardia, sweating) in what becomes a vicious cycle of thoughts and somatic symptoms. The pathogenesis of acute stress disorder and PTSD may be understood from psychodynamic perspectives as psychological attempts to cope with or master a traumatic life event that is difficult or impossible to "master" and integrate into one's sense of self and the world.

OCD appears to have a pathogenesis distinct from that of the other anxiety disorders. It probably involves altered functioning of the striatofrontal systems, as well as a prominent role of the serotonergic systems. The obsessions and compulsions of OCD may represent inappropriate triggering of neural "scripts" involving thoughts and behaviors that have been analogized to the scripts involved in animal grooming and other complex behavior. Patterns of heritability and symptomatic comorbidity strongly suggest that the pathogenesis of OCD is more closely related to that of movement disorders, such as tic disorders (Chapter 417), than to the other primary anxiety disorders.

CLINICAL MANIFESTATIONS

Most individuals experience one or more somatic symptoms (Table 404-8) that accompany the psychic anxiety, regardless of whether the anxiety is normal or part of a pathologic condition. Such somatic symptoms may be referable to virtually every body organ system.

TABLE 404-8	COMMON SOMATIC MANIFESTATIONS OF ANXIETY

CARDIORESPIRATORY

Palpitations
Chest pain
Dyspnea or sensation of being smothered

GASTROINTESTINAL

Sensation of choking
Dyspepsia
Nausea
Diarrhea
Abdominal bloating or pain

GENITOURINARY

Urinary frequency or urgency

NEUROLOGIC/AUTONOMIC

Diaphoresis
Warm flushes or chills
Dizziness or presyncope
Paresthesias
Tremor
Headache

TABLE 404-9	COMMON TYPES OF OBSESSIONS AND COMPULSIONS IN OBSESSIVE-COMPULSIVE DISORDER

OBSESSIONS

Aggressive (fears of harming self or others, of blurting out obscenities, or of other unwanted aggressive acts; unwanted violent or horrific images)
Contamination (concerns about dirt, germs, body waste or secretions, environmental contaminants, or animals/insects)
Sexual (concerns about unwanted sexual images or impulses)
Hoarding/saving
Religious (scrupulosity) (excessive concerns about sacrilege, blasphemy, right/wrong, morality)
Need for symmetry/exactness
Somatic (excessive concern about illness, body part, or appearance)

COMPULSIONS

Cleaning/washing (excessive or ritualized handwashing, showering, or other grooming)
Checking (checking locks, stove, appliances; checking body in relation to somatic obsessions; checking that did not or will not harm self or others)
Repeating rituals (rereading or rewriting; routine activities such as going through a door or arising from a chair)
Counting
Ordering/arranging
Hoarding/saving

Adapted from Goodman WK, Price LH, Rasmussen SA, et al. The Yale-Brown Obsessive Compulsive Scale. I. Development, use, and reliability. *Arch Gen Psychiatry*. 1989;46:1006-1011.

Many anxiety disorders include acute, discrete periods of symptoms known as *panic attacks*. In a panic attack, the patient experiences a rapid rise in anxiety, fear-related thoughts, and somatic symptoms in the space of a few minutes, known as a crescendo onset. The acute symptoms resolve quickly, typically within an hour or less.

Panic Disorder

Panic disorder consists of *recurrent panic attacks*. Although some panic attacks may be precipitated by situations known to be stressful, at least some attacks must be *unexpected* ("out of the blue"). Patients also exhibit *anticipatory anxiety*, in which they experience ongoing psychic distress by worrying about their next panic attack or the attack's effects (e.g., humiliation if the attack were to happen in public view). In addition, patients manifest *avoidance behavior* by staying away from known triggers or from situations in which having a panic attack might be dangerous (e.g., driving) or particularly distressing (e.g., in public spaces). For many patients, the anticipatory anxiety and avoidance behavior may be more disabling than the panic attacks themselves. Avoidance behavior may overlap with *agoraphobia*, which is defined as a distressing and disabling fear of places or situations from which escape might be difficult or embarrassing or from which help might not be available in the event of a panic attack. Common agoraphobic foci include being outside one's home alone, being on bridges or in tunnels, traveling by vehicle, or being in crowds or lines. Up to 40 to 50% of patients with panic disorder have agoraphobia (termed *panic disorder with agoraphobia*), whereas the others have agoraphobia without panic disorder (termed *agoraphobia without history of panic disorder*).

Obsessive-Compulsive Disorder

Patients with OCD have recurrent *obsessions* or *compulsions* (Table 404-9); the vast majority of patients have both. OCD should not be confused with obsessive-compulsive personality traits or disorder, described later under Personality Disorders. *Obsessions*, not to be confused with obsessing (ruminating) on a topic, are recurrent distressing (ego-dystonic) thoughts that at some point during the course of the disorder are experienced as intrusive and inappropriate (ego-alien). Patients may describe their obsessions in language such as "I don't know where this thought comes from" or "I don't know why I have this thought, I would never actually do such a thing!" However, it is important to recognize that the ego-alien quality of obsessions may not be reported by children with OCD or by those with chronic OCD symptoms; for such patients the thought is merely experienced as distressing. *Compulsions* are recurrent mental or physical actions, typically related to the content of obsessions or to rigid rules that must be obeyed; for example, compulsive handwashing may relate to obsessional thoughts about germs or contamination. Again, most adults, at least early in the course of the disorder, experience the compulsions as intrusive and inappropriate or excessive. Patients with OCD typically attempt to ignore, suppress, or neutralize their obsessions and compulsions, but doing so causes great psychic distress, including anxiety until "giving in" and experiencing the unpleasant thought or performing the

action. OCD patients may spend many hours per day engaged in or attempting to resist their obsessions and compulsions.

Acute Stress Disorder and Post-traumatic Stress Disorder

Acute stress disorder and PTSD are specific manifestations of symptoms referable to an extremely traumatic event. The event by definition must involve exposure to actual or threatened death, serious injury, or destruction of the physical integrity of the patient or others such that the patient's immediate reaction includes intense fear, helplessness, or horror. Formerly, definitions of the traumatic event involved descriptions such as "beyond usual human experience." It is important to recognize that acute stress disorder or PTSD does not develop in all individuals exposed to a common traumatic event (e.g., a natural or man-made disaster)—major depression may develop in some; other anxiety disorders may develop in others; mania, psychosis, or other conditions may develop in a few; and diagnosable psychopathology may never develop at all in some or many. In acute stress disorder, the patient develops a sense of numbing or emotional detachment, a reduction in awareness of the surroundings ("in a daze"), and dissociative symptoms such as derealization, depersonalization, or dissociative amnesia, as well as symptoms similar to those seen in PTSD. However, PTSD symptoms, by definition, persist for more than 1 month after the traumatic event and include three types of clinical phenomena: (1) re-experiencing the trauma (e.g., intrusive memories, dreams, or flashbacks or intense distressing psychological or physiologic responses to reminders of the trauma), (2) avoidance (e.g., avoiding specific reminders of the trauma; more generalized social withdrawal, emotional detachment, or blunting; or a sense of a foreshortened future), and (3) hyperarousal (e.g., insomnia, irritability, difficulty concentrating, or exaggerated startle response). Several PTSD symptoms overlap considerably with those of major depression, which is commonly a comorbid condition and should also be diagnosed when the diagnostic criteria are met.

Generalized Anxiety Disorder

This diagnostic term encompasses a more heterogeneous group of conditions, defined by the presence of clinically significant anxiety and associated somatic symptoms for 6 or more months. Generalized anxiety disorder is not diagnosed if the anxiety is part of a diagnosable anxiety, mood, or other psychiatric disorder; that is, it is superseded in the diagnostic hierarchy by other conditions that produce anxiety.

Phobias

The phobias are a group of conditions defined by the consistent ability of a specific environmental stimulus to elicit a pathologic anxiety response. Exposure to such a stimulus nearly always produces this response, so the patient avoids the stimulus whenever possible or endures the stimulus with considerable distress. In addition to agoraphobia, the other main types of phobias are *social phobia* and *specific phobias* (see Table 404-7).

DIAGNOSIS

Diagnosis of anxiety disorders must rest on consideration of both syndromic and etiologic perspectives. From a syndromic perspective, a careful history and mental status examination are required to determine the pattern of anxiety and associated symptoms and to determine whether the phenomenology fits the pattern for any of the anxiety disorders as described earlier. The history and mental status examination must also assess for the presence of any other psychiatric disorder that might truly be comorbid with the anxiety disorder but might also supersede the anxiety disorder in the diagnostic hierarchy. For example, generalized anxiety may be seen as part of cognitive disorders (delirium or dementia), mood disorders (depressed or manic phases), and psychotic disorders; if the generalized anxiety is present only during the cognitive, mood, or psychotic disorder, a separate diagnosis of generalized anxiety disorder is not warranted. As another example, however, major depression may develop in a patient with long-standing PTSD or OCD symptoms, perhaps partly as a consequence of the social and other disability conferred by the PTSD or OCD; in such cases, both the anxiety disorder and major depression would be diagnosed.

From an etiologic perspective, it is important to determine whether the anxiety disorder is primary (idiopathic) or secondary to a systemic or neurologic condition (see Table 404-1), drug intoxication, or withdrawal state. The evaluation should include laboratory tests, such as a toxic drug screen, as guided by the differential diagnosis that is generated from the clinical evaluation.

TREATMENT   Rx

Considerable empirical evidence from controlled trials demonstrates the efficacy of cognitive-behavioral psychotherapies for most of the anxiety disorders.[5] Such therapies, which use the principles of learning theory to extinguish unhelpful behavior and positively reinforce more functional behavior, help the patient learn to identify and correct the dysfunctional patterns of thinking ("automatic thoughts") that underlie or trigger the cognitive-physiologic cascade of pathologic anxiety responses. Cognitive behavioral therapy may be used as sole therapy, particularly for specific phobias, or in combination with pharmacotherapy. Frequently, cognitive behavioral therapy may be administered as part of family therapy (e.g., to help family members avoid behavior that inadvertently reinforces the patient's obsessions and compulsions) or in group therapy settings.

Although anxiolytic drugs, such as the benzodiazepines (Table 404-10), will usually relieve acute anxiety symptoms, concerns about their long-term efficacy and side effects (e.g., risk for abuse, risk for cognitive impairment or falls) make antidepressant medications the more attractive pharmacologic agents for most anxiety disorders (see Table 404-5). Most classes of antidepressants, with the probable exception of bupropion, are helpful for panic disorder, PTSD, generalized anxiety disorder, and social phobia. For OCD, the only efficacious antidepressants are those with strong activity on the serotonergic system, such as selective serotonin re-uptake inhibitors and also the tricyclic compound clomipramine.

PROGNOSIS

In general, most persons with anxiety disorders, other than transient acute stress disorder or other situation-dependent anxiety states, tend to have a chronic course of waxing and waning symptoms. At one extreme, a small minority of patients ($\approx$5%) with OCD have intermittent episodes alternating with periods of full remission; at the other extreme, up to 15% of OCD patients may have a continuous and progressively worsening course over time. Maintenance therapies should often be used for patients with more chronic anxiety disorders, although evidence to support long-term therapies is not as robust as for mood disorders.

● PSYCHOTIC DISORDERS

Psychotic symptoms, defined as a loss of reality testing, include delusions (fixed false beliefs), hallucinations (false sensory perceptions), and major derailments in thought processes (e.g., loose associations). Psychotic symptoms may be seen in the course of cognitive, secondary, and mood disorders. The psychotic disorders are defined by the presence of psychotic symptoms in the absence of prominent mood disturbance or cognitive deficits at the level seen in delirium or dementia. In general, the diagnosis and care of most patients with psychotic disorders should be conducted in mental health specialty settings, but primary care settings are common points of entry (and re-entry) to care.

Schizophrenia

DEFINITION AND EPIDEMIOLOGY

Schizophrenia, which is the prototypical psychotic disorder, includes acute episodes of psychosis ("positive" symptoms), often accompanied by a decline in overall functioning over time because of "negative symptoms," such as affective flattening, abulia, apathy, and social withdrawal. The point prevalence of schizophrenia is approximately 1%, and its chronic, debilitating course takes a considerable toll on patients, families, and society. Peak onset is in late adolescence to young adulthood, slightly younger for males than females. The annual incidence is approximately 15 per 100,000, but with marked variability across study samples and populations; recent data suggest that the condition is slightly more common in males than in females.

PATHOBIOLOGY

The pathogenesis of schizophrenia remains unknown. Twin studies show that the disease is multifactorial. Genetic factors account for about 50% of the risk, and multiple gene loci appear to be involved. Studies of postmortem brains indicate a nongliotic neuropathologic process with subtle disruptions of cortical cytoarchitecture. It is likely that psychosocial factors and neurodevelopment interact with a nonlocalizable brain "lesion" that is either present at birth or acquired early in life. The dopaminergic mesocortical and mesolimbic pathways are important in the production of psychotic symptoms.

DIAGNOSIS

The diagnosis of schizophrenia is based on the presence of delusions, disorganized speech and behavior, and major impairment in social functioning for

TABLE 404-10   DRUGS FOR ANXIETY AND PANIC

DRUG	TRADE NAME	INITIAL DOSE	TARGET DOSE RANGE*	SIDE EFFECTS	COMMENTS
Benzodiazepines				Sedation, ataxia, risk for falls	Potential for abuse/dependence
Lorazepam	Ativan	0.5 mg bid-qid	2-6 mg/day, tid-qid dosing		Reliable IM absorption
Diazepam	Valium	2-5 mg bid-tid	10-40 mg/day, bid-tid dosing		Long half-life of drug and active metabolites
Triazolam	Halcion	0.125 mg qhs	0.125-0.25 mg qhs	Rebound insomnia	Used as hypnotic
Chlordiazepoxide	Librium	5 mg bid-tid	10-40 mg/day, bid-tid dosing		Long half-life of drug and active metabolites
Temazepam	Restoril	7.5 mg qhs	7.5-30 mg qhs		Used as hypnotic
Alprazolam	Xanax	0.25 mg tid-qid	2-8 mg/day, tid-qid dosing	Possibly greater addictive potential	
Clorazepate	Tranxene	7.5-15 mg bid-tid	15-60 mg/day, bid-tid dosing		
Flurazepam	Dalmane	15-30 mg qhs	15-30 mg qhs	Daytime somnolence	Used as hypnotic
Oxazepam	Serax	10-15 mg tid-qid	10-30 mg tid-qid		
Clonazepam	Klonopin	0.5 mg bid-tid	0.5-5 mg bid-tid		Long duration of action
Zaleplon	Sonata	5-10 mg qhs	5-20 mg qhs		"Nonbenzodiazepine" hypnotic
Zolpidem	Ambien	5-10 mg qhs	5-10 mg qhs		"Nonbenzodiazepine" hypnotic
Eszopiclone	Lunesta	1-2 mg qhs	1-3 mg qhs		"Nonbenzodiazepine" hypnotic
β-Blockers					
Propranolol	Inderal	20 mg bid	Individualize, 40-120 mg/day	Bradycardia, hypotension, potential for mental slowing	Only helps with sympathetically mediated somatic symptoms of anxiety

*Target doses in the elderly may be lower.
qhs = at bedtime.

at least 6 months (Table 404-11). In patients with single schizophrenia-like psychotic episodes of briefer duration, with subsequent return to asymptomatic baseline functioning, *brief psychotic disorder* (<1 month) or *schizophreniform disorder* (1 to 6 months) may be diagnosed.

TABLE 404-11 SYMPTOMS AND SIGNS OF MAJOR PSYCHOTIC DISORDERS

SCHIZOPHRENIA

Delusions
Hallucinations
Disorganized speech (i.e., thought process derailments)
Grossly disorganized or catatonic behavior
Negative symptoms: affective flattening, alogia, avolition
Major impairment in social or occupational functioning
Duration of at least 6 months

SCHIZOAFFECTIVE DISORDER

During the course of illness, at least one episode of schizophrenia-like psychotic symptoms *plus* a mood syndrome (either major depression, mania, or mixed episode) *and*
During the course of illness, at least 2 weeks of schizophrenia-like psychotic symptoms *in the absence of* a mood syndrome

DELUSIONAL DISORDER

Delusions that are nonbizarre (i.e., potentially plausible, such as delusions of being followed, poisoned, infected, loved at a distance, deceived by a spouse or lover, or having a disease)
Not meeting full criteria for an acute episode of schizophrenia
Functioning *not* markedly impaired other than as related to the impact of the delusion (or delusions) and its ramifications

Based on criteria from American Psychiatric Association. *Diagnostic and Statistical Manual of Mental Disorders (DSM-IV)*, 4th ed. Washington, DC: American Psychiatric Association; 2000.

TREATMENT Rx

Antipsychotic medications (Table 404-12), often with adjunctive benzodiazepines, are used to treat acute psychotic episodes, commonly in acute inpatient settings so that the patient can be managed safely until the acute symptoms improve. Although maintenance antipsychotic medications help reduce the severity and frequency of acute psychotic episodes, comprehensive psychosocial rehabilitation programs are required to help patients manage interpersonal and other stressors and to improve overall clinical outcomes. In the past decade, second-generation ("atypical") antipsychotic medications have replaced first-generation antipsychotics because of their greater short-term tolerability and lower rates of extrapyramidal side effects, including tardive dyskinesia, although their efficacy is not generally better than that of first-generation drugs.[6] However, second-generation drugs contribute to the increase in obesity and metabolic syndrome in patients with chronic schizophrenia (Chapter 442). One trial found that oral long-chain ω-3 polyunsaturated fatty acids reduced the rate of onset of psychosis by more than four fifths during a 1-year follow-up of adolescents and young adults with especially high risk profiles for incipient psychosis, but the usefulness of this approach in broader populations remains to be determined.

PROGNOSIS

The prognosis of individuals with schizophrenia may often be poor, with recurrent episodes of psychotic exacerbations superimposed on progressively deteriorating baseline functioning. However, some patients may have preservation of relatively high baseline functioning, and some experience periods of prolonged remission or improvement in functioning. Prominent negative symptoms, younger age at first onset, and enduring psychosocial stressors and family discord all predict poorer outcomes. Although many patients with schizophrenia survive into later life, overall life expectancy is shortened by at least 10 to 15 years because of poor health behavior and self-care, higher rates of medical disorders, including metabolic syndrome, and a lifetime suicide risk of approximately 10%.

TABLE 404-12 COMMONLY USED ANTIPSYCHOTIC MEDICATIONS

DRUG NAME	INITIAL DOSE FOR PSYCHOSIS IN SCHIZOPHRENIA*	TARGET DOSE FOR PSYCHOSIS IN SCHIZOPHRENIA†	SIDE EFFECTS	CHLORPROMAZINE DOSAGE EQUIVALENCE (FIRST-GENERATION DRUGS ONLY)/ OTHER COMMENTS
First-generation drugs			Low-potency drugs: anticholinergic effects, orthostatic hypotension, prolongation of QT interval, cholestatic jaundice High-potency drugs: extrapyramidal side effects (dystonias, akathisia, parkinsonism, neuroleptic malignant syndrome), hyperprolactinemia with galactorrhea	
Chlorpromazine	100 mg qd	300-1000 mg/day, qd-bid dosing		100 mg
Thioridazine	50-100 mg qd	300-800 mg/day, qd-bid dosing	Pigmentary retinopathy at higher doses	100 mg
Thiothixene	2-5 mg qd	5-60 mg/day, qd-bid dosing		5 mg
Trifluoperazine	2-5 mg qd	5-40 mg/day, qd-bid dosing		5 mg
Perphenazine	4-8 mg qd	8-64 mg/day, qd-tid dosing		8 mg
Haloperidol	0.5-2 mg qd	2-10 mg/day (up to 40 mg/day or higher in refractory cases), qd-bid dosing		2 mg; available in depot IM form
Fluphenazine	1-2.5 mg qd	2.5-10 mg/day (up to 40 mg/day in refractory cases), qd-bid dosing		2 mg; available in depot IM form
Second-generation drugs			Metabolic syndrome, risk for stroke and mortality in older patients with dementia, QT prolongation	
Risperidone	0.5-1 mg qd-bid	2-4 mg/day, qd-bid dosing	Extrapyramidal side effects at higher doses	Available in depot IM form
Olanzapine	5 mg qd	5-10 mg qd (up to 20 mg/day in refractory cases)		
Ziprasidone	20 mg bid	20-80 mg bid		
Quetiapine	25-50 mg bid-tid	300-800 mg/day, bid-tid dosing		Extended-release form for qd dosing
Asenapine	5 mg bid	5-10 mg bid		Sublingual form only
Paliperidone	3-6 mg qd	6-12 mg qd		
Iloperidone	1 mg bid	2-12 mg qd		
Aripiprazole	10-15 mg qd	10-30 mg qd		Partial agonist/antagonist at D_2 receptors
Clozapine	12.5 mg qd-bid	300-900 mg/day, qd-bid (titrate dose slowly by 25-50 mg/day every 3-7 days)	Risk for agranulocytosis, requires ongoing monitoring of complete blood count	Efficacy superior to that of other antipsychotics, but hematologic risks and need for monitoring limit its use

*Doses for other indications, such as agitation in delirium or dementia, may be much lower.
†Target doses in the elderly may be lower.

Schizoaffective Disorder

Schizoaffective disorder is a chronic, recurrent disorder with a prevalence slightly lower than that of schizophrenia. It is characterized by episodes of non–mood-associated psychosis and also by mood episodes (manic or depressed) with psychotic features. As a result, the diagnosis of schizoaffective disorder cannot be based on the patient's clinical findings at any one point in time but rather requires knowledge of the overall course. Treatment is symptomatic and involves the use of antipsychotic medications (see Table 404-12), mood stabilizers (see the section on treatment of bipolar disorders), and antidepressant medications (see Table 404-5) to target specific psychotic and mood symptoms. The outcomes of schizoaffective disorder are heterogeneous but on average intermediate between those of schizophrenia and mood disorders.

Delusional Disorder

Delusional disorders are characterized by potentially plausible ("nonbizarre") delusions, such as those regarding marital infidelity, in the absence of a thought process disorder, prominent hallucinations, or the negative symptoms seen in schizophrenia. Delusional disorder has a point prevalence of approximately 0.03% and a lifetime prevalence of 0.05 to 0.1%. The pathogenesis of delusional disorder, like the other the nonschizophrenic primary psychotic disorders, remains largely unknown. It is often only partially responsive to antipsychotic medications (see Table 404-12), but patients' functioning may be largely unimpaired if they are able, with the aid of antipsychotics and psychotherapy, to avoid speaking publicly about their delusions or acting on them.

● SOMATOFORM DISORDERS

Somatoform symptoms (Table 404-13), often broadly referred to as "somatization," resemble the symptoms caused by systemic or neurologic diseases but are thought to arise from unconscious psychogenic causes rather than identifiable physical causes. Somatization may range from normal human experiences (e.g., abdominal cramping in response to an acute stressor), to time-limited episodes, to chronic, disabling conditions.

The prevalence of somatoform disorders varies widely among various populations, in part based on diagnostic ascertainment. Full-fledged somatization disorder may have a lifetime prevalence of 0.2 to 2% in females and less than 0.2% in males. Prevalence estimates for conversion disorder are as low as 0.01% in the general population but may be much higher (1 to 14%)

in medical/surgical inpatients and even higher in neurologic treatment settings.

Although the symptoms of somatoform disorders are not due to identifiable physical disease, they are nonetheless "real" and are just as distressing and baffling to patients as would be similar symptoms produced by physical disease. Somatoform symptoms and disorders must be distinguished from other conditions in which psychological factors lead to manifestations resembling physical disorders. *Factitious disorder* (also known as Munchausen's syndrome) is a mental disorder in which patients consciously produce stigmata of disease (e.g., simulated or artificially induced fever or hypoglycemia) for the unconscious gain of assuming the sick role. *Malingering* is the conscious feigning of illness for conscious gain and is therefore not a mental disorder.

TREATMENT ℞

Management of patients with somatoform disorders is often difficult because physicians must simultaneously maintain an appropriate level of vigilance for undiagnosed physical illness while avoiding unnecessary tools and therapies. Keys to ongoing care include maintaining an ongoing therapeutic alliance, setting regular office visits, conveying empathy for the patient's very real distress without colluding with the patient's belief in an identifiable physical disorder, and assertively treating depression, anxiety, or other comorbid psychopathology. Antidepressant medications may benefit selected patients (e.g., some chronic pain syndromes), even in the absence of comorbid psychiatric disorders.

● PERSONALITY DISORDERS

Personality is defined as the total repertoire of enduring patterns of thinking, feeling, and behaving, including affect and impulse regulation, defense and coping mechanisms, and interpersonal relatedness. Personality and personality disorders are the result of complex interactions among genetic, environmental, and developmental factors. The cumulative point prevalence of all personality disorders in the general adult population is approximately 10 to 15%, with rates as high as 50% in patients receiving care in psychiatric treatment settings.

CLINICAL MANIFESTATIONS AND DIAGNOSIS

A *personality disorder* is diagnosed when personality trait repertoires lead to enduring (if variable) subjective distress or dysfunction in social role performance (Table 404-14). In diagnosing personality disorders, care must be taken to distinguish personality *traits*, which by definition are enduring, from time-limited *states*. Most persons can regress to more primitive personality styles, not characteristic of their baseline personality traits, under the influence of substantial psychosocial stressors, including those posed by significant medical illnesses. For example, a patient who exhibits dependent features only while acutely ill does not have a dependent personality disorder. Similarly, patients with personality disorders are prone to mood, anxiety, eating, and substance abuse disorders, which should be diagnosed and treated assertively.

TABLE 404-13	TYPES OF SOMATOFORM DISORDERS
TYPE	**MAIN CLINICAL MANIFESTATIONS**
Disorders characterized by somatoform symptoms (i.e., physical symptoms due to unconscious psychological factors)	
Somatization disorder	Also known as Briquet's syndrome: chronic recurrent disorder with multiple somatoform symptoms across multiple organ systems, including pain, neurologic, sexual, and other symptoms, beginning before the age of 30 years
Conversion disorder	Neurologic somatoform symptoms (other than pain), e.g., paralysis, blindness, dyscoordination, convulsion-like phenomena, memory or other cognitive complaints
Pain disorder	Pain (may or may not be associated with a physical disorder)
Undifferentiated somatoform disorder	Other somatoform symptoms not meeting criteria for the disorders above
Other types of somatoform disorders	
Hypochondriasis	Inappropriate worry about illness and help seeking (in the absence of somatoform symptoms per se)
Body dysmorphic disorder	Preoccupation with a perceived body defect or deformation ("imagined ugliness"); may have more in common with the obsessions of obsessive-compulsive disorder than with the other somatoform disorders

Based on criteria from American Psychiatric Association. *Diagnostic and Statistical Manual of Mental Disorders (DSM-IV)*, 4th ed. Washington, DC: American Psychiatric Association; 2000.

TREATMENT ℞

In most circumstances the goal is not to alter fundamental personality structure, but rather to help the patient maximize use of personality strengths (e.g., optimal defense and coping mechanisms) while minimizing the harmful effects of emotional dysregulation, dysfunctional defenses, and destructive behavior. Dialectic behavior therapy is an evidence-based, focused psychotherapy that is based on specific cognitive-behavioral techniques and has been demonstrated to reduce self-injurious behavior and suicidality in patients with borderline personality disorder.

Although pharmacotherapy is not the mainstay of treatment of most personality disorders, drugs can be useful in selected patients. Antipsychotic drugs may be used to target escalating paranoia in paranoid personality disorder or for short-term reduction in emotional and impulse regulation with a wide range of (often cluster B, see Table 404-14) personality disorders in times of crisis. For longer-term treatment of emotional dysregulation in borderline and other cluster B personality disorders, mood stabilizers or antidepressants may be used.

TABLE 404-14 PERSONALITY DISORDERS	
TYPE OF PERSONALITY DISORDER	**MAIN IDENTIFYING CHARACTERISTICS**
CLUSTER A: ODD/ECCENTRIC	
Schizoid personality disorder	Detachment from social relationships, restricted emotional expression
Schizotypal personality disorder	Discomfort with close relationships, cognitive or perceptual distortions, eccentric behavior
Paranoid personality disorder	Pervasive distrust and suspiciousness of others' motives as malevolent
CLUSTER B: DRAMATIC/EMOTIONAL	
Borderline personality disorder	Instability of interpersonal relationships and self-image and poorly regulated emotional states and impulse control
Narcissistic personality disorder	Inflated self-esteem, need for admiration from others, and lack of empathy for others
Antisocial personality disorder	Pervasive disregard for and violation of the rights of others, lack of conscience
Histrionic personality disorder	Pervasive excessive emotionality (theatricality) and attention seeking
CLUSTER C: ANXIOUS/FEARFUL	
Avoidant personality disorder	Social inhibition because of feelings of inadequacy and sensitivity to negative views from others
Dependent personality disorder	Submissive and clinging behavior because of excessive need to be taken care of
Obsessive-compulsive personality disorder	Preoccupation with orderliness, perfectionism, and control

Based on criteria from American Psychiatric Association. *Diagnostic and Statistical Manual of Mental Disorders (DSM-IV)*, 4th ed. Washington, DC: American Psychiatric Association; 2000.

SUICIDE AND EVALUATION OF SUICIDALITY

Suicide is a leading cause of death worldwide. Suicide rates in the United States average approximately 11 per 100,000 per year, with considerable variability geographically and demographically. Of all age-, gender-, and race-based demographic groups, the highest suicide rates occur in older white men. Suicide is the 3rd leading cause of death in adolescents and young adults and the 11th leading cause of death in the population overall. Suicide attempts, which outnumber completed suicides by a factor of at least 3:1, lead to considerable morbidity and utilization of health care resources. Persons who attempt suicide represent an overlapping but distinct population from those who die by suicide. Nonetheless, a previous history of a suicide attempt is a powerful risk for subsequent death by suicide. Suicide attempts and verbal threats should always be evaluated carefully and never dismissed as "gestures" or "attention-seeking" behavior.

Suicide is a potentially preventable cause of death, but despite considerable research on risks for suicidal behavior, specific predictions about an individual's behavior cannot be made with certainty. Nonetheless, the linchpin of clinical evaluation is a methodic assessment of risks for suicide (Table 404-15), together with direct questioning of the patient regarding thoughts of death, dying, and suicide; specific plans (in ideation or action) for suicide; and the details of any attempts. Patients at significantly increased risk for suicide should immediately be referred for psychiatric evaluation, with emergency referral if the risk is deemed to be imminent or increasing.

WHEN TO REFER A PATIENT FOR PSYCHIATRIC EVALUATION

Clinical decisions to refer a patient for specialty psychiatric evaluation must be made on an individual basis by taking into account both the patient's clinical findings, including any previous history and immediate needs, and the clinician's own experience and expertise in assessing and managing the disorder (Table 404-16).

TABLE 404-15 SOME IMPORTANT RISKS FOR SUICIDE AND SUICIDE ATTEMPTS
Mental disorder, particularly mood, substance use, psychotic, and personality disorders
Other symptoms of acute psychic distress, particularly hopelessness and panic attacks
Previous history of suicide attempt
Family history of suicide or suicide attempt (and, to a lesser degree, of any mental disorder)
Family violence, including physical or sexual abuse
Access to firearms or other lethal methods
Exposure to suicidal behavior of others (family, peers, public figures)
Social isolation
Interpersonal discord or other psychosocial stressors
Demographic factors, including male gender, non-Hispanic white or American Indian/Alaska Native race, older age

TABLE 404-16 GENERAL CONSIDERATIONS IN DECIDING TO REFER A PATIENT FOR PSYCHIATRIC SPECIALTY CARE
Diagnosis or ongoing care of severe/chronic mental disorders, including bipolar disorder, psychotic disorders such as schizophrenia, and psychotic symptoms in other disorders
Management of more severe forms of other mental disorders (as well as those refractory to treatment), including depression, anxiety disorders, and substance use disorders
Need for safety evaluation or management, including suicidality, homicidality or other aggressivity, or inability to care for self
Diagnostic uncertainty
Psychiatric comorbid conditions complicating diagnosis or treatment, including personality and substance use disorders coexisting with other psychiatric disorders
Psychiatric-medical comorbid conditions complicating diagnosis or treatment, including management of psychiatric disorders during pregnancy
Need for expertise in psychopharmacologic treatment
Need for expertise in other somatic therapies, e.g., electroconvulsive therapy
Need for expertise in psychotherapy or other psychosocial interventions

1. Bortolotti B, Menchetti M, Bellini F, et al. Psychological interventions for major depression in primary care: a meta-analytic review of randomized controlled trials. *Gen Hosp Psychiatry.* 2008;30:293-302.
2. Cipriani A, Furukawa TA, Salanti G, et al. Comparative efficacy and acceptability of 12 new-generation antidepressants: a multiple-treatments meta-analysis. *Lancet.* 2009;373:746-758.
3. Katon WJ, Lin EH, Von Korff M, et al. Collaborative care for patients with depression and chronic illnesses. *N Engl J Med.* 2010;363:2611-2620.
4. BALANCE investigators and collaborators. Lithium plus valproate combination therapy versus monotherapy for relapse in bipolar I disorder (BALANCE): a randomized open-label trial. *Lancet.* 2010;375:385-395.
5. Hofmann SG, Smits JA. Cognitive-behavioral therapy for adult anxiety disorders: a meta-analysis of randomized placebo-controlled trials. *J Clin Psychiatry.* 2008;69:621-632.
6. Kahn RS, Fleischhacker WW, Boter H, et al. Effectiveness of antipsychotic drugs in first-episode schizophrenia and schizophreniform disorder: an open randomised clinical trial. *Lancet.* 2008; 371:1085-1097.

SUGGESTED READINGS

Abramowitz JS, Taylor S, McKay D. Obsessive-compulsive disorder. *Lancet.* 2009;374:491-499. *Review.*

Frye MA. Clinical practice. Bipolar disorder—a focus on depression. *N Engl J Med.* 2011;364:51-59. *Review.*

Leichsenring F, Leibing E, Kruse J, et al. Borderline personality disorder. *Lancet.* 2011;377:74-84. *Review.*

O'Connor EA, Whitlock EP, Beil TL, et al. Screening for depression in adult patients in primary care settings: a systematic evidence review. *Ann Intern Med.* 2009;151:793-803. *Review.*

U.S. Preventive Services Task Force. Screening for depression in adults: U.S. Preventive Services Task Force recommendation statement. *Ann Intern Med.* 2009;151:784-792. *Review.*

van Os J, Kapur S. Schizophrenia. *Lancet.* 2009;374:635-645. *Review.*

Weissman MM, Neria Y, Gameroff MJ, et al. Positive screens for psychiatric disorders in primary care: a long-term follow-up of patients who were not in treatment. *Psychiatr Serv.* 2010;61:151-159. *Emphasizes the high rate of enduring symptoms and use of emergency psychiatric services for untreated patients with positive screening.*

405

HEADACHES AND OTHER HEAD PAIN

KATHLEEN B. DIGRE

DEFINITION

Headache, which is a very common symptom, can be caused by a serious underlying abnormality but is usually a primary headache disorder, such as migraine headache, tension-type headache, cluster headache, and paroxysmal hemicrania.

EPIDEMIOLOGY

About 90% of all adults experience headache at some time in their lives, and more than 75% of children have reported significant headaches by the age of 15 years. In the United States, the cost associated with migraine is almost $17 billion annually in both direct and indirect costs. Patients at most risk for lost days of employment are those with transformed migraine and daily headache.

In large population-based studies, the relative risk of having migraine, tension-type headaches, or cluster headaches increases up to four times if a first-degree relative has the same kind of headaches. Studies of twins, especially identical twins, also show a similar susceptibility.

PATHOBIOLOGY

Headache pain is initiated by primary trigeminal afferents that innervate the blood vessels, mucosa, muscles, and tissues. Fibers from these sources coalesce in the trigeminal ganglion, especially the first division. The trigeminal afferents terminate in the primary sensory nucleus of cranial nerve V and its spinal nucleus, which has several small subnuclei, the most important of which is the subnucleus caudalis. This subnucleus receives afferents from meningeal vessels, dura-sensitive neurons, and even the upper cervical cord and then projects them to the lateral and medial thalamus by way of the spinothalamic tract and to diencephalic and brain stem regions that are involved in the regulation of autonomic functions. Thalamic nociceptive information ascends to the sensory cortex, as well as to other areas of the brain.

Although secondary headaches may stimulate the pathway by way of processes such as inflammation and compression, primary headache disorders occur spontaneously by means of chemical mediators. The sequence of events commences with peripheral activation caused by neurogenic plasma extravasation activated spontaneously or by cortical spreading depression. The trigeminocervical complex, especially the nucleus caudalis, is then activated, and patients can experience allodynia, a condition in which a non-noxious stimulus is sensed as painful.

Aura is defined as a focal visual, sensory, or motor neurologic disturbance that may occur with or without headache. Aura is thought to occur when cortical spreading depression causes depolarization of membranes. Both neurons and glia can cause both constriction and dilation of blood vessels.

Migraine headache clearly has a genetic component. Familial hemiplegic migraine can be caused by mutations in the *CACNA1A* gene, which is located on chromosome 19p13.2-p13.1 and encodes for voltage-gated neuronal calcium channels. Many mutations are found in the *CACNA1A* gene, and other phenotypes include episodic ataxia and epilepsy. Another mutation is on *ATP1A2*, also called the familial hemiplegia migraine 2 (*FHM2*) gene, which is located on chromosome 1q21-q23 and encodes for the sodium-potassium adenosine triphosphatase (Na^+,K^+-ATPase) transport protein. A third genetic locus is the *SCN1A* gene on chromosome 2q24.3, which is a voltage-gated sodium channel. Although there are linkages to many genetic loci for more common forms of migraine, migraine and other headaches probably have multiple gene interactions with environmental factors.

CLINICAL MANIFESTATIONS

Patients with headache may describe the pain as throbbing, bandlike, or aching, but it is invariably moderate to severe and interferes with activities. The pain is frequently unilateral but can be bilateral. Migraine headache is often associated with nausea, vomiting, photophobia, and phonophobia. Other autonomic manifestations that can accompany migraine, cluster, and other headache variants include ptosis, rhinorrhea, Horner's syndrome, and facial edema. Secondary headaches may appear to be similar to tension-type

TABLE 405-1	REASONS FOR FURTHER EVALUATION TO LOOK FOR SECONDARY HEADACHES

Beginning of headaches at an older age without a previous history or a positive family history

Unexplainable and abnormal worsening of previously existing migraines

Dramatic or unusual change in character of the prodrome or the headache previously present

Headaches awakening the patient in the middle of the night (except for a cluster headache)

Headaches much worse when recumbent or with coughing, sneezing, or the Valsalva maneuver

Unusually severe headache of sudden onset ("worst headache of my life")

Focal deficits that do not disappear after the headache is over

Any abnormal neurologic finding on examination

A new headache in a patient with human immunodeficiency virus infection, malignancy, or pregnancy

or migraine headaches, but there may be "red flags" suggesting a secondary rather than a primary headache disorder (Table 405-1).

DIAGNOSIS

Evaluation of an individual's headache is almost entirely based on five elements of the history. The family history helps determine whether a person has a genetic predisposition to headache. The life history of headache determines whether the headache is new or has evolved over the course of a lifetime. The attack history provides the clinical features of the headache or headaches. The medical and psychiatric history determines whether there are comorbid conditions that can cause or worsen the headache. The medication and drug history determines whether the headache could be caused by or worsened by medications or drugs that the person has ingested.

Diagnosis of the type of headache is based on the type of pain, the duration of headache, and accompanying features (Table 405-2). Secondary headaches are usually due to an underlying condition, such as a brain tumor (Chapter 195), increasing intracranial pressure, sinus disease (Chapter 434), or a vascular malformation (Chapter 415); on removing the cause, the headache generally improves. Headaches that occur at a frequency of less than 15 days a month are called episodic, whereas headaches that occur more than 15 days a month are considered chronic.

The diagnostic evaluation for headache depends on the clinical findings. If there is a typical history without any reason for further evaluation and if the findings on neurologic examination are completely normal, no further evaluation is needed. The features of the history that are most likely to predict migraine headache without a secondary disorder include a pulsating quality, duration of 4 to 72 hours, unilateral headache, nausea, and disabling headache. However, if there are atypical features of the history or any abnormality on neurologic examination, further evaluation is indicated. Patients with cluster headache types and headaches of undetermined cause need imaging to exclude secondary causes.

In patients with acute headache, computed tomography (CT) is best for assessing acute hemorrhage as the cause of the headache, whereas magnetic resonance imaging (MRI) is best for assessing most persistent headaches to look for mass lesions, evidence of intracranial hypertension or hypotension, hemosiderin (old hemorrhage), and congenital abnormalities (e.g., Chiari malformation). In individuals older than 60 years with an unexplained new or unusual headache, the erythrocyte sedimentation rate (ESR) needs to be determined to evaluate for giant cell arteritis (Chapter 78). Cerebrospinal fluid (CSF) analysis, including opening pressure, protein, glucose, cells, culture, and cytology, is indicated in patients with suspected intracranial hypertension or meningitis.

TREATMENT

Treatment of acute headache depends on the type and severity of the headache. For mild headaches, simple analgesics such as acetaminophen[1] (500 to 1000 mg), aspirin (250 to 1000 mg)[2] and nonsteroidal anti-inflammatory drugs[3] (NSAIDs) (e.g., ibuprofen, 400 to 800 mg; naproxen sodium, 220 to 500 mg) will suffice. If the migraine headaches are moderate to severe, patients benefit from migraine-specific therapies (Table 405-3) such as triptans (sumatriptan, zolmitriptan, rizatriptan, almotriptan, naratriptan, frovatriptan, and eletriptan), ergotamine (dihydroergotamine, ergotamine tartrate), or iso-methepttene[3] and the combination of naproxen plus sumatriptan is better than either alone[4]

TABLE 405-2 DIFFERENTIAL DIAGNOSIS OF HEADACHE

HEADACHE TYPE	GENETICS	EPIDEMIOLOGY	CHARACTERISTIC FEATURES	LENGTH	ACCOMPANYING SYMPTOMS
Migraine headache	Complex genetics but usually a family history	More frequent in women	Unilateral, bilateral; throbbing; moderate to severe; worsens with activity	Hours to days	Photophobia, phonophobia, nausea and/or vomiting
Tension-type headache	Usually a family history	Equal frequency in men and women	Tight band–like pain; bilateral; pain may be mild to moderate; improves with activity	Hours to days	No nausea or vomiting; small amount of light or sound sensitivity, but not both
Cluster headache	May have a family history	More frequent in men	Unilateral, severe pain in the face	Minutes to hour	Ipsilateral ptosis, miosis, rhinorrhea, eyelid edema, tearing
Paroxysmal hemicrania	Usually no family history	More frequent in women	Unilateral pain in the face	Minutes	Ipsilateral ptosis, miosis, rhinorrhea, eyelid edema, tearing; responds to indomethacin
Hemicrania continua	No family history	More frequent in women	Unilateral, continuous headache with episodic stabbing pains	Continuous	Ipsilateral autonomic features: ptosis, miosis, rhinorrhea, eyelid edema, tearing

TABLE 405-3 ACUTE MIGRAINE-SPECIFIC TRIPTAN MEDICATIONS FOR THE TREATMENT OF MIGRAINE

	SUMATRIPTAN	ZOLMITRIPTAN	NARATRIPTAN	RIZATRIPTAN	ALMOTRIPTAN	FROVATRIPTAN	ELETRIPTAN
Trade Name	Imitrex	Zomig	Amerge	Maxalt	Axert	Frova	Relpax
Forms	SQ, nasal (NS), oral	Oral: tablet/ZMT, NS	Oral	Oral: tablet/MLT	Oral	Oral	Oral
Dose	Oral: 50-100 mg (200 mg/24 hr max.) SQ: 4-6 mg (12 mg/24 hr max.) NS: 5-20 mg (40 mg/24 hr max.)	2.5-5 mg (10 mg/24 hr max.) 5 mg (10 mg/24 hr max.)	1-2.5 mg (5 mg/24 hr max.)	5-10 mg (30 mg/24 hr max.)	6.25-12.5 mg (25 mg/24 hr max.)	2.5 mg (7.5 mg/24 hr max.)	20-40 mg (80 mg/24 hr max.)
Half-life	2-3 hr	3-4 hr	6-8 hr	2-3 hr	3-4 hr	26 hr	4-6 hr
Crosses blood-brain barrier	–	+	+	+	+	+	+
Use with monoamine oxidase inhibitor (MAOI)	–	–	+	–	+	+	–
Good for recurrences	–	–	+	–	–	+	–
Rapid response	SQ, 10-15 min NS, 15-20 min Oral, 30 min	30 min	1-4 hr	30 min	60 min	1-4 hr	20-30 min
Menstrual migraine	+	+	+	+	+	+	+
Other	Now in combination with naproxen (Treximet)			Decrease dose by ½ with propranolol			Do not use with CYP3A4 drugs (ketoconazole and some macrolide antibiotics)

NS = nasal spray; SQ = subcutaneous.

PREVENTION

Preventive medications are recommended when headaches are frequent or severe enough to interfere with quality of life. The choice of medications should be based on the type of headache (migraine, tension type), their side effect profiles, and the patient's comorbid conditions (Table 405-4).[5]

PROGNOSIS

The natural history of headache depends on many factors, including the type of headache, the comorbid conditions that accompany the headache, and the success of treatment. Risk factors for chronic headache include female gender, migraine-type headaches, frequent headaches, obesity, low education and socioeconomic level, overuse of medication, stressful events, and sleep apnea.

● MIGRAINE HEADACHE

DEFINITION

Migraine is an inherited headache disorder that is typically unilateral but sometimes bilateral, moderate to severe, worsened by routine physical activity, associated with nausea and vomiting, and accompanied by photophobia and phonophobia. The headache occurs anytime and persists from 4 to 72 hours. It may occur with an aura (a focal neurologic symptom that may be visual, sensory, or motor) or without an aura. Visual auras may have positive (photopsias) and negative (scotomas) features.

EPIDEMIOLOGY

The prevalence of migraine is 15 to 20% in women and 4 to 7% in men. In children the prevalence may be as high as 17% and is equal in boys and girls. At puberty, the prevalence rises in girls and remains higher throughout their lifespan. The highest prevalence occurs between the ages of 25 and 55. Migraine with aura affects 5% of the adult population, and 90% of auras are visual. Migraine is more prevalent in white persons and in those with a lower socioeconomic status or income.

Comorbid conditions that may be associated with migraine headache include epilepsy, stroke, depression, anxiety, myocardial infarction, patent foramen ovale, Raynaud's syndrome, irritable bowel syndrome, and pain disorders such as fibromyalgia. Menstruation and ovulation may increase the frequency of headache.

PATHOBIOLOGY

The aura of a migraine headache is thought to be due in part to cortical spreading depression, which is associated with a brief reduction in flow followed by hyperemia. These changes do not seem to correlate with the phase of the headache. Pain occurs when trigeminal afferents of the dura are stimulated.

TABLE 405-4 PREVENTIVE MEDICATIONS FOR HEADACHE

DRUG	RATIONAL USE	DOSAGE	SIDE EFFECTS	CONTRAINDICATIONS/ CAUTION	LEVEL OF EVIDENCE
β-Blockers: e.g., propranolol, nadolol, timolol	Migraine, anyone with elevated blood pressure	20-80 mg; may increase	Lethargy, depression	Asthma, low blood pressure	A
Calcium-channel antagonists: verapamil, amlodipine	Cluster headache, elevated blood pressure	Verapamil, 120 to 480 mg/day	Low blood pressure		B
Nonsteroidal anti-inflammatory drugs: naproxen sodium, ibuprofen	Migraine, tension-type, and menstrual migraine	Naproxen, 200-600 mg/day; ibuprofen, 600-800 mg bid-tid	Gastrointestinal	Ulcers, sensitivity, allergy	A
Indomethacin	Paroxysmal hemicrania, hemicrania continua	25 mg tid	Gastrointestinal	Ulcers	A
Tricyclic antidepressants: amitriptyline, nortriptyline, imipramine	Migraine, tension-type headache, anyone with poor sleep	10-25 mg qhs	Dry mouth, orthostatic hypotension	Sensitivity	A—amitriptyline
Anticonvulsants: topiramate valproate	Migraine, cluster headache	Topiramate, 25-50 mg bid; valproate, 250-500 mg bid	Topiramate: weight loss, kidney stones, intra-ocular hypertension Valproate: weight gain	Pregnancy	A

CLINICAL MANIFESTATIONS

Migraine headache often begins with a prodrome, which may persist for hours to days, when patients note difficulty concentrating or fatigue without headache. An aura may or may not occur but is generally present before the headache begins. The headache may be unilateral or bilateral, throbbing, moderate to severe, and worsened with activity. Accompanying clinical features include nausea, vomiting, and sensitivity to light and sound. Other clinical features include neck pain, occasionally dizziness, osmophobia, and difficulty thinking.

The migraine aura is generally visual but can be sensory or can include aphasia or vertigo. Migraine aura without headache begins with a neurologic disturbance, such as a visual phenomenon, but without a subsequent headache.

DIAGNOSIS

The diagnosis of migraine is based on the history. The differential diagnosis includes tension-type headache, but most moderate to severe headaches are migraine. In patients with a history suggestive of a secondary headache, further evaluation with MRI should be considered (see Table 405-2). However, if the headache is typical of migraine and the findings on neurologic examination are normal, no further studies are needed.

TREATMENT   Rx

Treatment of migraine is divided into treatment of the acute headache and prevention of subsequent migraine attacks. Acute treatment is most effectively accomplished with migraine-specific stepped care: a nonspecific analgesic agent, combination analgesic therapy, opioids, and aggressive migraine-specific therapy (see Table 405-3). For example, *mild attacks* can generally be treated successfully with over-the-counter analgesics such as acetaminophen (suggested dose, 650 to 1000 mg[1]) or NSAIDs (aspirin, 900 to 1000 mg[2]; ibuprofen, 1000 to 1200 mg; naproxen, 500 to 825 mg; or ketoprofen, 75 mg). During pregnancy, mild to moderate attacks can be treated with acetaminophen. Moderate headaches may respond to the combination of acetaminophen, isometheptene mucate (a mild vasoconstrictor, 65 mg), and dichloralphenazone (a mild sedative, 100 mg). Antinausea agents include prochlorperazine (10 to 25 mg) and metoclopramide (2.5 to 10 mg).

Stratification of care, including tailoring the treatment according to the type of headache, results in fewer days of disability and use of medications.[6] Which migraine-specific drug will work for any individual patient depends on the patient. It is important to avoid overuse of analgesic and other medications because overuse can cause chronic daily headache in susceptible individuals. Prompt treatment improves the outcome of headache when compared with late treatment. Contraindications to use of the triptans (Table 405-3) include uncontrolled hypertension, clinical evidence of ischemic heart disease, and Prinzmetal's angina.

Opioids such as *N*-acetyl-*p*-aminophenol (APAP) with codeine, or butorphanol, benefit some patients, but meperidine is not effective. Oral opiates should not be used for chronic recurrent, primary headaches, although sometimes opiates (e.g., acetaminophen, 325 mg, with codeine, 30 mg) are the only option during pregnancy or in patients with severe vascular disease. When opiates are used, caution is required, and the associated risks of rebound headache and dependency must be recognized by both the patient and physician. Barbiturates (e.g. APAP, caffeine, and butalbital or aspirin) have not been efficacious in controlled trials but may be helpful in individual patients in whom other migraine-specific drugs cannot be used.

For *moderate to severe attacks*, options include dihydroergotamine (1 to 2 mg intranasally); oral, intranasal, or subcutaneous administration of sumatriptan (25 to 100 mg orally, 20 mg intranasally, or 4 to 6 mg subcutaneously); or sumatriptan-like drugs (e.g., naratriptan, 2.5 mg; zolmitriptan, 5 mg; rizatriptan, 10 mg; eletriptan, 40 mg; frovatriptan, 2.5 mg; or almotriptan, 12.5 mg).[7] Ergotamine (2 mg sublingually or 1 to 2 mg orally), when given early in the migraine attack, can be effective if the associated nausea and peripheral vasoconstriction are tolerable. Telcagepant (300 mg), a calcitonin gene–related peptide antagonist, may be as effective as zolmitriptan (5 mg), with fewer side effects.[8]

For *very severe attacks*, dihydroergotamine (1 mg subcutaneously or 0.5 to 1 mg intravenously) is usually effective but generally requires an antiemetic (e.g., promethazine, 25 mg) before intravenous use. Intramuscular injections of ketorolac (60 mg) or prochlorperazine (10 to 25 mg) may be helpful. For patients who are nonresponsive or have contraindications to vasoactive abortive agents, 10 mg of intravenous prochlorperazine (10 mg delivered over a 5-minute period) is another alternative.[9]

PREVENTION

Preventive treatment (see Table 405-4) is often recommended when the headaches interfere with activities on 3 or more days per month, the headaches are severe or prolonged, or migraine is complicated by events such as cerebral infarction. Prophylactic options include β-adrenergic blockers, calcium-channel antagonists, NSAIDs, tricyclic antidepressants, and anticonvulsants. Other alternatives include the serotonergic drug cyproheptadine (4 to 20 mg) or the monoamine oxidase inhibitor phenelzine (30 to 60 mg). Acupuncture and biofeedback have been used successfully.[10] OnabotulinumtoxinA injection is also effective for prophylaxis.[11]

PROGNOSIS

The prognosis for patients with migraine is variable. In many patients, headaches decrease in severity with age, but migraine aura without headache becomes more frequent with older age. Modification of inciting factors such as avoiding dietary triggers (tyramine, phenylethylamine, ethanol), ameliorating or preventing insomnia, and averting environmental triggers (light, sound, odor) may improve outcome. Migraines may become chronic, defined as more than 15 days per month, especially when associated with obesity and low socioeconomic status.

TENSION-TYPE HEADACHE

DEFINITION

Tension-type headache is defined as a holocranial headache without nausea or vomiting. Patients may have either photophobia or phonophobia but not both, and the headache does not worsen with activity.

EPIDEMIOLOGY

The 1-year prevalence is 14 to 93 per 100,000 individuals for episodic tension-type headache and 8.1 per 100,000 for chronic tension-type headache. Tension-type headaches are more common in women than in men, regardless of age, race, and educational level. Tension-type headaches are more common in Western countries and less frequent in Asian countries, and they are more common in white persons than in African Americans.

PATHOBIOLOGY

The pathophysiology of tension-type headache is less well understood than that of the other types of headache. Myofascial tenderness is increased, especially in chronic tension-type headache. Genetic factors are uncertain. Migraine and tension-type headache often coexist. Although tension-type headaches are not due to emotion or muscle contraction, triggers of a tension-type headache are similar to those associated with migraine: stress, fatigue, and lack of sleep. Comorbid conditions in patients with tension-type headache include depression and anxiety in more than 50% of individuals.

CLINICAL MANIFESTATIONS

Tension-type headaches are usually mild to moderate in severity, and most individuals do not seek care. Tension-type headache can be episodic, occurring less than 15 days per month, or chronic, occurring more than 15 days per month. In many patients headaches remain episodic, but about 25% progress to chronic headache. Of the patients with chronic tension-type headache, about a quarter to a third continue as chronic, half can improve to episodic, and in about a quarter medication overuse headache can develop. Episodic tension-type headaches can last minutes, hours, or days.

DIAGNOSIS

Headaches that can be misdiagnosed as tension-type headache include migraine, hemicrania continua, new daily persistent headache, and headaches caused by brain tumors, elevated or low intracranial pressure, or giant cell arteritis. A careful history is the best way to distinguish other types of headaches.

TREATMENT   (Rx)

Episodic tension-type headaches are generally treated successfully[12] with acetaminophen (650 to 1000 mg) or NSAIDs (aspirin, 900 to 1000 mg; naproxen, 250 to 500 mg; ibuprofen, 200 to 800 mg; or ketoprofen, 12.5 to 75 mg). However, analgesic use for more than 3 days per week can worsen headaches.

PREVENTION

Chronic tension-type headaches may benefit from prophylactic treatment with amitriptyline (starting with 10 mg at bedtime and increased slowly up to 100 mg until the patient improves or intolerable side effects develop), nortriptyline (25 to 100 mg each evening), doxepin (25 to 75 mg/day), maprotiline (10 to 25/mg/day), or fluoxetine (10 to 20 mg/day). Muscle relaxants, physical therapy, and acupuncture are also useful.[13]

PROGNOSIS

Tension-type headache has a variable prognosis. Adolescents with tension-type headache and two or more psychiatric factors (e.g., depression and anxiety) have a worse prognosis.

⬤ CLUSTER HEADACHE AND OTHER TRIGEMINAL AUTONOMIC CEPHALALGIAS

DEFINITION

Trigeminal autonomic cephalalgias, including cluster headaches, are unilateral headaches associated with ipsilateral autonomic features. Other trigeminal autonomic cephalalgias include paroxysmal hemicrania, which is characterized by bouts of headache that persist for 5 to 30 minutes, is generally unilateral, and usually occurs in women; they typically respond to indomethacin. Hemicrania continua, another indomethacin-responsive headache that is seen in both men and women, is characterized by continuous unilateral pain and mild associated autonomic features; it is frequently observed in conjunction with chronic daily headache but not with trigeminal autonomic cephalalgia. Short unilateral neuralgiform headache with conjunctival injection and tearing is a rare trigeminal autonomic cephalalgia that occurs in men, and the individual headache attack persists for only a very short time.

EPIDEMIOLOGY

Cluster headache occurs in 56 to 401 per 100,000 persons and is more frequent in men (3:1 to 7:1). Attacks usually begin between 20 and 30 years of age. Paroxysmal hemicrania occurs in 56 to 381 per 100,000 persons; it affects women more often (2:1) and can begin at any age but usually commences at 34 to 41 years. Short unilateral neuralgiform headache with conjunctival injection and tearing is rare, with a slight male preponderance (2:1).

PATHOBIOLOGY

There appears to be a genetic predisposition for cluster headache. Imaging studies such as positron emission tomography and functional MRI show inferior posterior hypothalamic activation at the onset of cluster headache and other trigeminal autonomic cephalalgias. In addition, the trigeminovascular complex and the cranial autonomic system are activated. The pathophysiology of hemicrania continua is unknown, and there is debate whether it is associated with hypothalamic involvement or whether it resembles migraine.

CLINICAL MANIFESTATIONS

Cluster headaches are almost always unilateral, rarely bilateral, and have characteristic ipsilateral autonomic features, commonly including lacrimation and conjunctival injection and sometimes including nasal congestion, rhinorrhea, ptosis, miosis, flushing, and eyelid edema (Table 405-5). The location of the pain is usually behind or above the eye or in the temple, but other areas of pain can include the forehead, cheek, teeth, or jaw. The pain reaches its maximum intensity in about 9 minutes and tends to end abruptly. Attacks occur one to eight times a day and are usually described as "boring" or "stabbing" excruciating pain that persists for 15 minutes to 2 hours. Migraine symptoms may coexist, including unilateral photophobia, phonophobia, and rarely, an aura. Unlike migraine patients, who usually try to rest, patients with cluster headaches pace and are unable to sit or lie down. Cluster headaches, when precipitated by alcohol, histamine, or nitroglycerin, have a daily periodicity and may also have a seasonal periodicity. For example, episodic cluster headache may occur annually or every 2 years, often in the same season each time. Chronic cluster headache may occur without a remission.

Paroxysmal hemicrania is pain of short duration, usually 2 to 30 minutes, and occurs unilaterally around the eye, temple, or maxillary region, sometimes precipitated by head movements. Autonomic features similar to cluster headache can occur. The usual attack rate is up to 40 episodes each day. Bouts of pain may be episodic, separated by a remission, but most patients have daily chronic paroxysmal hemicrania without a remission.

Short unilateral neuralgiform headache with conjunctival injection and tearing attacks are unilateral and consistently on the same side. Although the pain is excruciating, the attack is brief, usually seconds; most patients are free of pain between attacks, although a dull ache can be present. Associated autonomic features include ipsilateral conjunctival injection and tearing.

DIAGNOSIS

The diagnostic criteria for *cluster headache* include severe unilateral orbital, supraorbital, or temporal pain persisting for 15 to 180 minutes with at least one of the following: ipsilateral conjunctival injection or lacrimation, nasal congestion or rhinorrhea, eyelid edema, forehead and facial sweating, miosis with or without ptosis, and restlessness or agitation. Attacks occur between once and as often as eight times each day. There is no other cause of the disorder.

Paroxysmal hemicrania is defined by unilateral pain persisting for 2 to 30 minutes, about 5 times each day, with one or more autonomic features such as conjunctival injection, nasal congestion, eyelid edema, forehead and facial sweating, and miosis or ptosis (or both). Complete prevention may be achieved with indomethacin.

Hemicrania continua is a unilateral headache that occurs daily and continuously without pain-free periods; its intensity is moderate with exacerbations of severe pain. During the exacerbations, at least one autonomic feature is present and is ipsilateral to the pain: conjunctival redness, lacrimation, nasal congestion, ptosis, or miosis.

Short unilateral neuralgiform headache with conjunctival injection and tearing is diagnosed by unilateral orbital, supraorbital, temporal stabbing pain persisting for 5 to 240 seconds at a frequency of 3 to 200 per day. It is associated with conjunctival injection and tearing.

TABLE 405-5   DISTINGUISHING CHARACTERISTICS OF THE TRIGEMINAL AUTONOMIC CEPHALALGIAS

CHARACTERISTIC	CLUSTER	PAROXYSMAL HEMICRANIA	HEMICRANIA CONTINUA	SHORT UNILATERAL NEURALGIFORM HEADACHE WITH CONJUNCTIVAL INJECTION AND TEARING
Sex—F:M	1:3-7	2:1	2:1	1:2
Unilateral	+	+	+	+
Attack frequency	1-8/day	1-40/day		3-200/day
Attack duration	15-80 min	2-30 min	Continuous with episodic exacerbations	5-240 sec
Autonomic features	+	+	+ with exacerbations	+
Indomethacin effect	−	+++	+++	−
Acute treatment at onset	Oxygen, sumatriptan SQ, DHE nasal spray; sumatriptan or zolmitriptan nasal spray (A level evidence)	None	None	None
Preventive medications	Verapamil, lithium, corticosteroids, anticonvulsants (A level)	Indomethacin (A level)	Indomethacin (A level)	Lamotrigine, topiramate, gabapentin (B level)

DHE = dihydroergotamine.

An imaging procedure such as MRI is indicated for all patients with cluster headaches or the other trigeminal autonomic cephalalgias because they can be caused by a primary lesion such as an infection (Chapters 420 through 422), vascular malformation (Chapter 415), or neoplasm, especially a pituitary tumor (Chapter 195). Other possibilities in the differential diagnosis include migraine, hypnic headache (rare, short-lasting headaches exclusively during sleep in the elderly), and trigeminal neuralgia.

TREATMENT ℞

Because the course of the headache is brief, oral medications take too long to work to be effective. The use of 100% oxygen at 7 to 10 L/min for 15 to 30 minutes benefits some patients.[14] Sumatriptan or zolmitriptan nasal spray or sumatriptan subcutaneously (4 to 6 mg) can be helpful. Dihydroergotamine can be helpful when given nasally, intramuscularly, or even intravenously. Refractory cases may respond to occipital nerve stimulation. Short unilateral neuralgiform headache with conjunctival injection and tearing attacks is so short that there are no medications to treat it acutely.

PREVENTION

Preventive medications should be started at the beginning of a cluster bout. Verapamil, 240 to 480 mg, is the drug of choice. Lithium (300 mg twice daily) is another alternative. Corticosteroids (e.g., prednisone, 40 mg/day, or dexamethasone, 4 mg twice daily for 2 weeks) act rapidly to prevent cluster headache and can be used acutely while other preventive medications are started. Valproic acid (500 to 1500 mg/day in divided doses), topiramate (50 to 100 mg/day), melatonin (4 mg at bedtime), and gabapentin (300 mg three times daily) are sometimes beneficial. Surgical approaches, including occipital nerve stimulators, hypothalamic stimulation, and destructive procedures, are sometimes necessary for this disabling headache.

Paroxysmal hemicrania and hemicrania continua respond to daily indomethacin (25 to 50 mg three times daily). If the patient cannot tolerate indomethacin, calcium-channel blockers (e.g., verapamil, 240 to 480 mg/day) may be helpful. Preventive treatment of short unilateral neuralgiform headache with conjunctival injection and tearing includes lamotrigine (100 to 400 mg/day), topiramate (50 to 100 mg), gabapentin (300 to 900 mg), or intravenous lidocaine (starting at 2 mg/min with cardiac monitoring).

PROGNOSIS

Cluster headache is often a lifelong problem, but remissions may persist for longer periods as the patient ages. The other trigeminal autonomic cephalalgias are probably lifelong; nevertheless, symptomatic treatment combined with preventive medications is helpful.

● CHRONIC DAILY HEADACHE

DEFINITION

Though not a specific disorder, chronic daily headache, defined as a headache that is present on more than 15 days per month, is challenging for both patients and physicians. These headaches may be chronic migraine, chronic tension-type headache, new daily persistent headache, or chronic cluster headache, with or without overuse of medications.

EPIDEMIOLOGY

About 4 to 5% of the population suffers from chronic daily headache, most commonly chronic tension type. Trigger factors such as a previous infection, mild head injury, or stressful life event can be present in 40 to 60% of patients with new daily persistent headache. Risk factors for chronic daily headache include medication overuse, history of migraine headache, depression, female gender, obesity, snoring, stressful life events, and low educational level.

PATHOBIOLOGY

The pathophysiology of chronic daily headache is probably related to migraine, with both central and peripheral abnormalities. Once migraine has been prolonged and headache occurs on a daily basis, allodynia, a sense that a usually nonpainful stimulus is becoming painful, often develops. Central sensitization associated with painful structures around the head increases.

CLINICAL MANIFESTATIONS

New daily persistent headache is characterized by daily occurrence and an unrelenting course. It is generally bilateral, nonpulsating, mild to moderate, and associated with no more than one of the following: photophobia, phonophobia, or nausea. Severe nausea or vomiting is rare. New daily persistent headache can be disabling.

Chronic daily headache is often associated with profound psychiatric comorbidity, especially depression and anxiety, and psychiatric comorbidity predicts intractability.

Use of an opiate for more than 8 days per month, especially in men, use of barbiturates for more than 5 days per month, especially in women, or use of triptans for more than 10 to 14 days per month can often lead to chronic migraine headache or at least worsening of headaches.

DIAGNOSIS

Diagnosis of chronic daily headache is based on the history. It is important to identify the underlying type of primary chronic daily headache: chronic migraine, chronic tension-type headache, new daily persistent headache, or hemicrania continua. Of note is that headaches of less than 4 hours' duration can also be chronic and daily: cluster headache; paroxysmal hemicrania; hypnic headaches, occurring every night, usually in the elderly; and episodic stabbing headache. It is most important to exclude secondary headaches, including post-traumatic headache, headaches associated with vascular disorders (e.g., giant cell arteritis, arteriovenous malformations, carotid and vertebral artery dissections), and headaches associated with nonvascular disorders (e.g., intracranial hypertension, intracranial hypotension, infections). MRI and laboratory studies (e.g., ESR in an elderly individual) are commonly recommended. Lumbar puncture to assess intracranial pressure may also be indicated in selected patients.

TREATMENT ℞

The most common cause of chronic daily headache is overuse of medications, so patients must be weaned off the overused symptomatic medication. Treatment of underlying depression, anxiety, and pain may also be helpful. Occasionally, hospital admission is necessary to break the headache cycle. Acute migraine–specific treatments (see earlier), especially intravenous dihydroergotamine (0.5 to 2 mg), are helpful in terminating migrainous attacks.

PREVENTION

Medications that are helpful in preventing chronic daily headache include tricyclic antidepressants, selective serotonin re-uptake inhibitors if patients are depressed, anticonvulsants, β-blockers, and calcium-channel blockers (see Tables 405-3 and 405-4). For hemicrania continua, indomethacin (25 to 50 mg three times daily) is the preferred treatment.

PROGNOSIS

The prognosis depends on the underlying headache diagnosis. If medication overuse is the cause but the patient is successfully detoxified, about 75% of patients improve when treated with preventive medications. Treatment may fail if the diagnosis is incorrect or because of continued overuse of medications, overuse of caffeine, lack of sleep, dietary or other life triggers, hormonal factors, or psychiatric factors.

SINUS HEADACHE

Rhinosinusitis (Chapter 434) is characterized by inflammation or infection of the nasal mucosa and sinuses. The sinuses themselves are relatively insensate, but ducts, turbinates, and ostia are the painful structures.

Headaches attributed to rhinosinusitis are frontal headaches with pain in the face, ears, or teeth. The onset of pain is simultaneous with the rhinosinusitis, and the headache and face pain resolve within 7 days after successful treatment. The diagnosis requires imaging (see Fig. 434-4) and clinical evidence that support the diagnosis of acute or chronic rhinosinusitis, and most headaches that are initially thought to result from sinus disease are found to be migraine or tension-type headache.

Treatment of acute sinusitis (Chapter 434) should resolve the headache. If it does not, an underlying primary headache disorder is likely.

SECONDARY CAUSES OF HEADACHES
Temporal (Giant Cell) Arteritis

Temporal arteritis (Chapter 279) is an inflammatory process seen mainly in elderly individuals. Headache is one of the most common features. Its incidence is approximately 12 per 100,000 and increases with age to 51 per 100,000 in individuals over 80 years of age. It affects women more often than men (3:1) and is more common in white individuals, especially those of Scandinavian and British descent. It is associated with polymyalgia rheumatica.

The headache has no specific feature, but the pain is usually continuous, generalized, and occasionally throbbing. The temples are generally painful, and patients complain of pain when performing certain activities of daily living, such as chewing food or combing their hair. Transient monocular blindness and diplopia can occur.

Elevation of the ESR and C-reactive protein occurs almost invariably. The diagnosis is made by finding giant cells in a temporal artery biopsy specimen. Immediate treatment with corticosteroids, sometimes before the biopsy result is available, is necessary in doses between 40 and 80 mg daily, with the dose then titrated downward while monitoring the ESR. Used early enough, corticosteroids generally prevent the complications of temporal arteritis, including blindness. The disorder can be long lasting.

Intracranial Hypertension

Intracranial hypertension can be primary and idiopathic in obese women of childbearing age. Secondary intracranial hypertension can be seen with cerebral venous thrombosis (Chapters 414 and 421), masses in the brain (Chapter 195), hydrocephalus, or other intracranial processes.

Idiopathic increased intracranial pressure occurs in 20 per 100,000 individuals (15 to 55 years of age) who are obese. Women are affected more frequently than men. Onset is usually in young adulthood. The cause of the increased pressure is either poor CSF absorption, as is thought to be the problem in idiopathic intracranial hypertension, venous hypertension, as is seen in venous thrombosis, or a mass that causes an increase in pressure.

CLINICAL MANIFESTATIONS

Idiopathic intracranial hypertension is characterized by headache in more than 90% of individuals, about 90% of whom are obese. Other symptoms include pulsatile tinnitus, transient visual obscurations, and double vision.

On examination, papilledema (see Fig. 431-27) may be found. The remainder of the general and neurologic examination is usually normal in patients with idiopathic intracranial hypertension, but abnormalities on examination may point to a secondary cause, such as underlying venous sinus thrombosis (Chapter 414), ischemic stroke, central nervous system infection (Chapter 420), or brain tumor (Chapter 195). Although some individuals have idiopathic intracranial hypertension for years, the condition can be self-limited. In about a third of patients, permanent visual sequelae related to the effect of papilledema develop.

DIAGNOSIS

The diagnosis of intracranial pressure is made by the presence of clinical features, as well as by signs such as papilledema (see Fig. 431-27). MRI is necessary to exclude secondary causes of increased intracranial pressure. MR or CT venography is often needed to exclude venous sinus thrombosis (Chapter 414). Lumbar puncture must be performed unless patients have a contraindication such as an intracranial mass lesion, and CSF pressure should be measured. The diagnosis can be made if the pressure is elevated (CSF > 200 mm H_2O), but the fluid itself is normal. Visual fields must be examined formally because visual acuity is not affected until late in the course of the disorder.

> **TREATMENT AND PROGNOSIS** Rx
>
> Although no controlled trials of treatment of intracranial hypertension have been conducted, acetazolamide in doses of 500 to 1000 mg/day appears to be useful for the treatment of idiopathic intracranial hypertension. Any underlying secondary cause should also be treated. Weight loss may be beneficial in obese subjects. The prognosis of patients with idiopathic intracranial hypertension is good with treatment, but up to a third of inadequately treated patients can experience permanent loss of visual fields or visual acuity.

Intracranial Hypotension

Intracranial hypotension causes a headache that is characteristically better when the patient is supine and worse when the patient is upright. It can be primary (spontaneous) or secondary to another underlying cause, most commonly a previous lumbar puncture.

Intracranial hypotension was once considered rare, but modern imaging techniques suggest an incidence of about 5 per 100,000 per year.

PATHOBIOLOGY

The cause of primary intracranial hypotension is thought to be a small leak or tear in the dura, usually in the lumbar region around cystic structures called Tarlov's cysts. The cause of intracranial hypotension may not be not the tear itself, but low epidural venous pressure that assists in development of the lower pressure and hence the leak.

CLINICAL MANIFESTATIONS

Intracranial hypotension is characterized clinically by a positional headache. The location of the pain is variable, and the most constant characteristic is the orthostatic change in the pain. Double vision can develop if hindbrain herniation occurs.

DIAGNOSIS

The diagnosis of intracranial hypotension is made by MRI showing pachymeningeal enhancement and thickening, along with herniation of the hindbrain. Lumbar puncture may also show low (<50 mm H_2O) CSF pressure. The differential diagnosis includes chronic daily headache, migraine, or a secondary headache. The diagnosis is confirmed if a CSF leak is demonstrated by isotope studies or CT myelography.

> **TREATMENT AND PROGNOSIS** Rx
>
> Treatment of CSF leaks includes bedrest, caffeine, and fluids. For post–dural puncture headache, an epidural blood patch improves the symptoms.[15] Surgical repair is rarely required. With treatment, the symptoms and MRI findings should resolve completely.

Trigeminal Neuralgia

Trigeminal neuralgia is a distinct, excruciatingly painful condition provoked by sensory stimuli in the distribution of the trigeminal nerve. Trigeminal neuralgia occurs in 4 per 100,000 individuals, most commonly in persons between 50 and 70 years of age and in women slightly more than in men (1.5:1).

In younger individuals, multiple sclerosis (Chapter 419) can be associated with the condition. In older individuals, an ectatic artery in the vertebrobasilar system can cause the syndrome. The trigeminal nerve root entry zone is thought to be the site of pathology. Either demyelination or compression of this region increases the firing of trigeminal afferents. When a specific cause can be defined, the term "symptomatic trigeminal neuralgia" is often used.

Trigeminal neuralgia pain is characteristically sharp, shooting, and electric shock–like in the distribution of the trigeminal nerve: cheek (V2), chin or lower teeth (V3), and around the eye (V1). A combination of V2 and V3 is the most common. The paroxysms are brief—seconds to up to 2 minutes. Some patients have a dull and continuous interictal pain, whereas most have only staccato-like volleys of pain. Pain is usually triggered by stimuli such as touching the face, brushing the teeth, air moving across the face, or masticating food. Once a volley of pain is triggered, there is usually a refractory period in which pain will not occur.

DIAGNOSIS

Diagnostic criteria include paroxysmal attacks of pain persisting for a second to 2 minutes and affecting one or more divisions of the trigeminal nerve. To make the diagnosis, the pain must be intensely sharp, stabbing, or precipitated by a trigger. Each attack is stereotypical, and there are usually no other neurologic defects. Idiopathic trigeminal neuralgia by definition has no causative lesion, whereas symptomatic trigeminal neuralgia has a cause, such as vascular compression of the trigeminal nerve root exit zone. The differential diagnosis includes trigeminal autonomic cephalgia, which has autonomic accompaniments that are not associated with trigeminal neuralgia. Atypical facial pain and Tolosa-Hunt syndrome, an inflammatory syndrome of the anterior cavernous sinus, are also included in the differential.

TREATMENT   Rx

Trigeminal neuralgia is treated with medications or surgery. Carbamazepine (400 to 1200 mg) is considered the first-line agent for the neuralgia.**16** Phenytoin (200 to 300 mg), baclofen (40 to 80 mg), clonazepam (2 to 6 mg), valproic acid (500 to 1500 mg), lamotrigine (100 to 400 mg), gabapentin (900 to 1800 mg), oxcarbazepine (300 to 1800 mg), and topiramate (50 to 200 mg) are also used. Surgical treatments include microvascular decompression, which may alleviate the symptoms and preserve sensory function. Other treatments include partial destruction of the trigeminal nerve with heat (radio frequency lesions) or with glycerol (chemical destruction).

PROGNOSIS

Patients with trigeminal neuralgia can have spontaneous or medication-induced remissions. Microvascular decompression is often curative.

Glossopharyngeal Neuralgia

Less common than trigeminal neuralgia, glossopharyngeal neuralgia is unilateral pain in the distribution of the glossopharyngeal and vagal nerves in the ear, jaw, throat, and tongue. The cause is thought to be compression of the glossopharyngeal nerve by blood vessels, tumor, aneurysm, or infection. The pains are paroxysmal and persist for less than seconds to 2 minutes, but patients can experience 30 to 40 attacks in a day. Like trigeminal neuralgia, the pain is triggered by chewing, swallowing, or talking. Pharmacologic therapy is similar to that for trigeminal neuralgia. Rarely, surgical therapy and microvascular decompression are required.

1. Prior MJ, Codispoti JR, Fu M. A randomized, placebo-controlled trial of acetaminophen for treatment of migraine headache. *Headache.* 2010;5:819-833.
2. Kirthi V, Derry S, Moore RA, et al. Aspirin with or without an antiemetic for acute migraine headaches in adults. *Cochrane Database Syst Rev.* 2010;4:CD008041.
3. Evers S, Afra J, Frese A, et al. EFNS guideline on the drug treatment of migraine—revised report of an EFNS task force. *Eur J Neurol.* 2009;16:968-981.
4. Brandes JL, Kudrow D, Stark SR, et al. Sumatriptan-naproxen for acute treatment of migraine: a randomized trial. *JAMA.* 2007;297:1443-1454.
5. Silberstein SD: Preventive migraine treatment. *Neurol Clin.* 2009;27:429-443.

6. Lipton RB, Stewart WF, Stone AM, et al. Disability in Strategies of Care Study Group. Stratified care vs step care strategies for migraine: the Disability in Strategies of Care (DISC) Study: a randomized trial. *JAMA.* 2000;284:2599-2605.
7. Bigal ME, Krymchantowsky AV, Ho T. Migraine in the triptan era: progresses achieved, lessons learned and future developments. *Arq Neuropsiquiatr.* 2009;67(2B):559-569.
8. Ho TW, Ferrari MD, Dodick DW, et al. Efficacy and tolerability of MK-0974 (telcagepant), a new oral antagonist of calcitonin gene–related peptide receptor, compared with zolmitriptan for acute migraine: a randomized, controlled, parallel-treatment trial. *Lancet.* 2008;372:2115-2123.
9. Kostic MA, Gutierrez FJ, Rieg TS, et al. A prospective, randomized trial of intravenous prochlorperazine versus subcutaneous sumatriptan in acute migraine therapy in the emergency department. *Ann Emerg Med.* 2010;56:1-6.
10. Linde K, Allais G, Brinkhaus B, et al. Acupuncture for migraine prophylaxis. *Cochrane Database Syst Rev.* 2009;1:CD001218.
11. Dodick DW, Turkel CC, DeGryse RE, et al. OnabotulinumtoxinA for treatment of chronic migraine: pooled results from the double-blind, randomized, placebo-controlled phases of the PREEMPT clinical program. *Headache.* 2010;50:921-936.
12. Fumal A, Schoenen J. Tension-type headache: current research and clinical management. *Lancet Neurol.* 2008;7:70-83.
13. Linde K, Allais G, Brinkhaus B, et al. Acupuncture for tension-type headache. *Cochrane Database Syst Rev.* 2009;1:CD007587.
14. Bennett MH, French C, Schnabel A, et al. Normobaric and hyperbaric oxygen therapy for migraine and cluster headache. *Cochrane Database Syst Rev.* 2008;3:CD005219.
15. Boonmak P, Boonmak S. Epidural blood patching for preventing and treating post–dural puncture headache. *Cochrane Database Syst Rev.* 2010;1:CD001791.
16. Gronseth G, Cruccu G, Alksne J, et al. Practice parameter: the diagnostic evaluation and treatment of trigeminal neuralgia (an evidence-based review): report of the Quality Standards Subcommittee of the American Academy of Neurology and the European Federation of Neurological Societies. *Neurology.* 2008;71:1183-1190.

SUGGESTED READINGS

Garza I, Schwedt TJ. Diagnosis and management of chronic daily headache. *Semin Neurol.* 2010;30:154-166. *Review.*
Halker RB, Hastriter EV, Dodick DW. Chronic daily headache: an evidence-based and systematic approach to a challenging problem. *Neurology.* 2011;76:S37-S43. *Review.*
Ju YE, Schwedt TJ. Abrupt-onset severe headaches. *Semin Neurol.* 2010;30:192-200. *Emphasizes serious causes, including subarachnoid hemorrhage, intracranial aneurysm, cervical artery dissection, and cerebral venous sinus thrombosis.*
Leone M, Bussone G. Pathophysiology of trigeminal autonomic cephalalgias. *Lancet Neurol.* 2009;8:755-764. *Review.*
Mathew PG, Garza I. Headache. *Semin Neurol.* 2011;31:5-17. *Review.*

406

TRAUMATIC BRAIN INJURY AND SPINAL CORD INJURY

GEOFFREY S. F. LING

EPIDEMIOLOGY

Traumatic brain injury and traumatic spinal cord injury are all too common preventable diseases. Traumatic brain injury is the leading cause of traumatic death and disability (Chapter 112). Approximately 1.4 million cases per year result directly in about 52,000 deaths in the United States annually—almost a third of all injury-related deaths. The majority of traumatic brain injuries are due to falls (Chapters 24), motor vehicle accidents, and assaults. An additional approximately 11,000 cases of severe spinal cord injury occur each year in the United States, primarily the result of motor vehicle accidents, falls, sports-related injuries, and work-related accidents (Chapter 112). The majority of patients with traumatic brain and spinal cord injuries are young adult men.

During the past 20 years, the marked improvement in overall mortality associated with traumatic brain and spinal cord injuries can largely be ascribed to improved care in intensive care units, early aggressive neurosurgical intervention, and prevention of long-term conditions such as deep vein thrombosis and decubitus ulcers. The almost 5.5 million survivors of traumatic brain and spinal cord injuries in the United States often require extended rehabilitation. Because the majority of these patients are young and otherwise in good physical health at the time of injury, many need chronic care for decades. Even minor injury can lead to major disability; approximately 75% of patients who are classified as having mild to moderate traumatic brain injury continue to have residual symptoms months later, and many of these patients are unable to return to gainful employment.

PATHOBIOLOGY

Traumatic injury to the central nervous system has two phases. The first, neuronal injury, is a direct result of the initiating traumatic event. The second or late phase, which is caused by multiple neuropathologic processes, can continue for days to weeks after the initial insult.

Primary Injury Phase

The primary injury phase is immediate, and its damage, which can cause death almost instantaneously, is often complete by the time that medical care can be instituted. In closed compartment injury to the head or spine, the direct impact of neuronal tissue against the bony vault and shearing of neurovascular structures result in wounding. Because the neuronal structures reside in a fluid-filled compartment, these structures often lag behind the bony structure as it moves during sudden stopping of the body in motion. Thus, the structures will strike both anteriorly and posteriorly against the inner bony table, and a coup-contrecoup lesion will result. If a rotational component is present, the structures will torque, twist, and shear, thereby causing diffuse axonal injury. Motor vehicle accidents are particularly injurious because of the sudden deceleration. In penetrating lesions, the moving projectile will tear neural, vascular, and support structures as it traverses through the brain or spinal cord. If the projectile is moving at high velocity, such as a bullet, the vacuum created by its wake will give rise to tissue cavitation. The temporary cavity, which will ultimately collapse, may be many-fold larger than that of the projectile itself; the transient expansion of surrounding tissue will be sufficient to cause substantial irreversible damage.

Secondary Injury Phase

The delayed secondary phase of injury, which begins quickly after the primary phase and can continue for a prolonged period, involves both neurons and glia. Most neurologic injury is thought to be related to this secondary injury, when "neuron suicide" is caused by processes such as hypoxia, ischemia, and inflammation and the effects of free radicals, excitatory amino acids, and certain ions (e.g., calcium).

The injured brain is more susceptible to hypoxic-ischemic states. The most commonly affected areas are the hippocampus and "watershed" areas. It has been hypothesized that delayed neurologic compromise can be attributed to delayed ischemia.

Diffuse microvascular damage is due to early loss of cerebral vascular autoregulation and loss of integrity of the blood-brain barrier, with resulting endothelial changes such as the formation of intraluminal microvilli. Although the clinical significance of this injury is uncertain, it may play a role in the development of cerebral edema.

Diffuse axonal injury, which consists of shearing of axons in cerebral white matter, causes neurologic deficits such as nonfocal encephalopathy. The consequences of this type of injury can be delayed for up to 12 hours after the initial trauma.

CLINICAL MANIFESTATIONS

Traumatic Brain Injury

The signs and symptoms of traumatic brain injury vary with its severity. Patients suffering from mild traumatic brain injury often experience headache, difficulty concentrating, anxiety, and disrupted sleep; findings on clinical examination are normal, but detailed neuropsychological testing may reveal mild cognitive abnormalities. With moderate traumatic brain injury, patients may have an abnormal sensorium, motor and sensory involvement, and impaired language; the results of neurologic examination will be abnormal. In very severe traumatic brain injury, patients are comatose; at best, they may exhibit some eye opening and decorticate or decerebrate posturing to stimulation.

Focal injuries cause neurologic deficits related to the site of impact. The orbitofrontal and anterior temporal lobes are most commonly affected. Extreme vigilance is needed to recognize the development of delayed hematomas and edema, which can be manifested days later.

Traumatic brain injury may be accompanied by a transient increase in systemic arterial pressure. Apnea or cerebral dysfunction may develop. Depending on the degree of injury, spontaneous resolution may be delayed, and laceration of the microvasculature will exacerbate this injury.

Traumatic Spinal Cord Injury

Spinal Cord Syndromes

There are three main spinal cord syndromes: Brown-Séquard, central cord, and anterior cord syndrome. In Brown-Séquard syndrome, the deficits are referable to a lesion of a lateral half of the cord; findings consist of loss of ipsilateral motor, touch, proprioception, and vibration sensation as well as contralateral pain and temperature sensation. Central cord or "man in a barrel" syndrome is manifested as bilateral loss of motor function involving the upper extremities but sparing the lower extremities. Proximal weakness is greater than distal weakness. Pain and temperature sensation is generally reduced, whereas proprioception and vibration are usually spared. Anterior cord syndrome is manifested by deficits referable to bilateral anterior and lateral spinal cord columns or funiculi. There is loss of touch, pain, and temperature sensation and motor function below the level of the lesion, but the posterior column functions of proprioception and vibratory sensation remain intact.

Spinal Shock

After acute traumatic spinal cord injury, patients may suffer from spinal shock, or temporary loss of spinal reflexes below the level of injury. Clinically, there is loss of deep tendon reflexes, the bulbocavernosus reflex, and the anal wink. In high cervical injuries, the lower reflexes (bulbocavernosus and anal wink) may be preserved. Some patients demonstrate the Schiff-Sherrington phenomenon, in which reflexes are affected above the level of injury. Loss of autonomic reflexes can lead to neurogenic shock, ileus, and urinary retention.

DIAGNOSIS

Traumatic Brain Injury

The Glasgow Coma Scale score (Table 406-1) should be calculated promptly, and a detailed neurologic examination should be performed to determine the extent of injury and the severity of impairment. Important clinical signs of occult injury may be revealed on a general physical examination. For example, a scalp laceration should be palpated for evidence of an underlying skull fracture. Periorbital ecchymosis ("raccoon eyes") and postauricular ecchymosis ("Battle's sign") are concerning for a basal skull fracture. A clear or blood-tinged watery discharge from the nose or ear may be a cerebrospinal fluid leak.

Intracranial bleeding caused by traumatic brain injury includes subdural hematoma, epidural hematoma, intraparenchymal hemorrhage, contusion, and traumatic subarachnoid hemorrhage (Chapter 415). The most common is subdural hematoma, which is the basis of approximately 50% of admissions for head injury. Epidural hematoma accounts for about 3%. An associated skull fracture, especially at the temporoparietal junction, increases the incidence of epidural hematoma, usually by disrupting the middle meningeal artery.

Imaging

A computed tomography (CT) scan without contrast should be obtained as soon as possible after the initial clinical assessment. The need for neuroimaging is best determined by use of the Glasgow Coma Scale score and a validated clinical prediction instrument such as the Canadian CT Head Rule (Table 406-2). In any patient thought to have suffered a head injury, the

TABLE 406-1 GLASGOW COMA SCALE SCORE

BEST EYE RESPONSE	BEST VERBAL RESPONSE	BEST MOTOR RESPONSE
1 = No eye opening	1 = No verbal response	1 = No motor response
2 = Eye opening to pain	2 = Incomprehensible sounds	2 = Extension to pain
3 = Eye opening to verbal command	3 = Inappropriate words	3 = Flexion to pain
4 = Eyes open spontaneously	4 = Confused	4 = Withdrawal from pain
	5 = Oriented	5 = Localizing pain
		6 = Obeys commands

To calculate the score, sum the numbers from each of the three columns.

TABLE 406-2 DECISION RULES TO DETERMINE INDICATIONS FOR CT SCAN IN PATIENTS WITH MINOR HEAD INJURY

STUDY	POPULATION OF PATIENTS	INDICATIONS FOR CT SCAN	Reported Validity (%)*	
			SENSITIVITY	SPECIFICITY
Canadian CT Head Rule[†]	GCS score of 13-15, loss of consciousness, no neurologic deficit, age ≥16 yr	High-risk patients: GCS score <15 at 2 hr after injury, suspected skull fracture, any sign of basal skull fracture, vomiting (≥2 times), age ≥65 yr[‡] Medium-risk patients: retrograde amnesia >30 min, dangerous mechanism (pedestrian vs. motor vehicle, ejection from motor vehicle, fall from height >1 m or 5 stairs)[§]	100	24.5
New Orleans Criteria[¶]	GCS score of 15, loss of consciousness, no neurologic deficit, no seizure, no anticoagulation, age >3 yr	Headache, vomiting, seizure, intoxication, short-term memory deficit, age ≥ 60 yr, or injury above the clavicles	98.4	49.6

*Validity for identification of patients with traumatic CT findings.
[†]Stiell IG, Wells GA, Vandemheen K, et al. The Canadian CT Head Rule for patients with minor head injury. *Lancet.* 2001;357:1391-1396.
[‡]High-risk patients in whom a CT scan is mandatory.
[§]Medium-risk patients in whom a CT scan is recommended but close clinical observation is an alternative.
[¶]Haydel MJ, Preston CA, Mills TJ, et al. Indications for computed tomography in patients with minor head injury. *N Engl J Med.* 2000;343:100-105.
CT = computed tomography; GCS = Glasgow Coma Scale.

TABLE 406-3 AMERICAN ACADEMY OF NEUROLOGY: DIAGNOSIS AND MANAGEMENT OF CONCUSSION

GRADE 1 (MILD)*	GRADE 2 (MODERATE)[†]	GRADE 3 (SEVERE)[‡]
Remove from duty/ work/play	Remove from duty for the rest of the day	Take to the emergency department
Examine immediately and at 5-minute intervals	Examine frequently for signs of CNS deterioration Physician's neurologic examination as soon as possible (within 24 hours)	Neurologic evaluation, including appropriate neuroimaging
May return to duty/work if clear within 15 minutes	Return to duty after 1 full asymptomatic week (after being cleared by the physician)	Consider hospital admission

GRADE OF CONCUSSION	RETURN TO PLAY/WORK
Grade 1 (first)	15 minutes
Grade 1 (second)	1 week
Grade 2 (first)	1 week
Grade 2 (second)	2 weeks
Grade 3 (first) (brief loss of consciousness)	1 week
Grade 3 (first) (long loss of consciousness)	2 weeks
Grade 3 (second)	1 month
Grade 3 (third)	Consult a neurologist

*Mild: transient confusion, no loss of consciousness, symptoms associated with concussion (such as amnesia) or mental status changes lasting less than 15 minutes.
[†]Moderate: transient confusion, no loss of consciousness, symptoms lasting longer than 15 minutes.
[‡]Severe: any loss of consciousness.

FIGURE 406-1. Subdural hematoma.

FIGURE 406-2. Epidural hematoma.

severity of the concussion should be assessed (Table 406-3). A subdural hematoma (Fig. 406-1) is blood that accumulates above the brain but below the dura; on CT imaging, it appears as a crescentic or concave opacity overlying the brain. An epidural hematoma (Fig. 406-2) is blood that accumulates below the skull but above the dura; it appears as a convex or lenticular opacity on CT imaging. Skull fractures are best diagnosed with the use of CT bone windows.

Traumatic Spinal Cord Injury

A detailed neurologic examination is needed to identify the level of the injury and the severity of any deficits as well as to document the degree of neurologic dysfunction at the earliest time possible. The level of the injury is the lowest spinal cord segment with intact motor and sensory function. Normal neurologic findings in patients with a clear sensorium obviate the need for

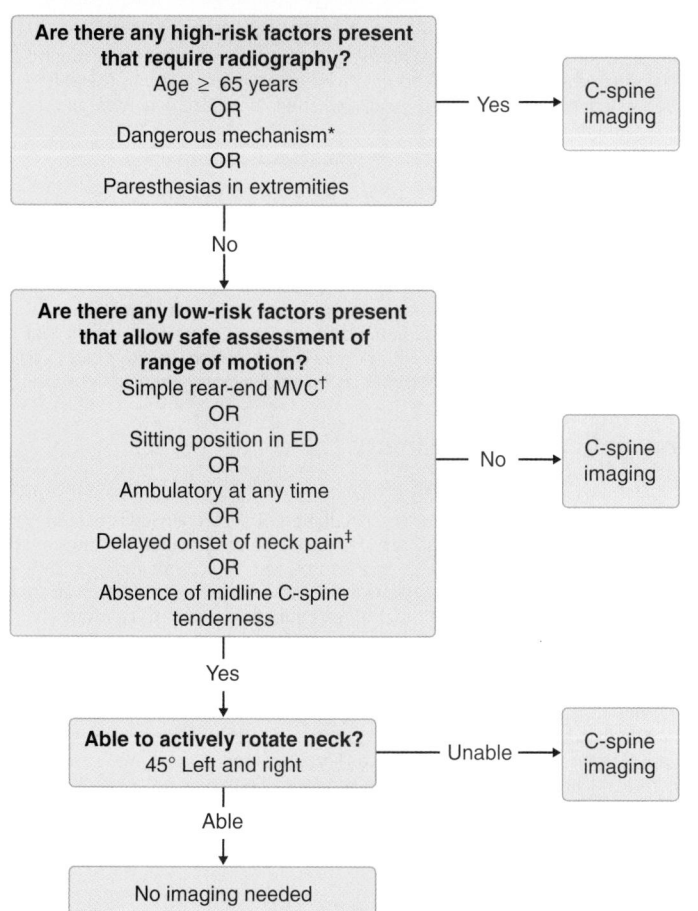

Are there any high-risk factors present that require radiography?
Age ≥ 65 years
OR
Dangerous mechanism*
OR
Paresthesias in extremities

—Yes→ C-spine imaging

—No→

Are there any low-risk factors present that allow safe assessment of range of motion?
Simple rear-end MVC†
OR
Sitting position in ED
OR
Ambulatory at any time
OR
Delayed onset of neck pain‡
OR
Absence of midline C-spine tenderness

—No→ C-spine imaging

—Yes→

Able to actively rotate neck?
45° Left and right

—Unable→ C-spine imaging

Able

No imaging needed

Canadian C-Spine Rule should not be used if:
• Nontrauma case
• GCS < 15
• Unstable vital signs
• Age < 16 years
• Acute paralysis
• Known vertebral disease
• Previous C-spine surgery

*Dangerous mechanism:
• Fall from elevation ≥ 3 ft/5 stairs
• Axial load to head (e.g., diving)
• MVC high speed (>100 km/hr), rollover, ejection
• Motorized recreational vehicles
• Bicycle struck or collision

†Simple rear-end MVC excludes:
• Pushed onto incoming traffic
• Hit by bus/large truck
• Rollover
• Hit by high-speed vehicle

‡Delayed:
• i.e., not immediate onset of neck pain

FIGURE 406-3. Canadian C-Spine Rule. For alert (Glasgow Come Scale ≥ 15) and stable trauma patients in whom cervical spine injury is a concern. ED = emergency department; GCS = Glasgow Coma Scale (see Table 406-1); MVC = motor vehicle collision. (Modified from Stiell IG, Clement CM, McKnight RD, et al. Comparative validation of the Canadian C-Spine Rule and the NEXUS low-risk criteria in alert and stable patients. *N Engl J Med.* 2003;349:2510-2518; and Stiell IG, Wells GA, Vandemheen KL, et al. The Canadian C-Spine Rule for radiography in alert and stable trauma patients. *JAMA.* 2001; 286:1841-1848).

imaging studies. However, any complaints of pain over the spine, numbness, tingling, or weakness should raise suspicion of spinal cord injury. In particular, a complaint of "burning hands" suggests traumatic spinal cord injury.

The time of injury should be recorded as accurately as possible. The prognosis for neurologic improvement is better if the lesion is incomplete as opposed to complete. During the acute period, serial examinations must be performed frequently.

If spinal cord injury is suspected, the patient should be appropriately immobilized, such as with a rigid collar and back board. In patients who are able to cooperate with a neurologic examination, are not intoxicated, and do not have painful distracting injuries (such as a femoral fracture, which would interfere with the leg motor and sensory examination), normal neurologic findings effectively rule out cervical spine disease.

Imaging
In patients in whom a cervical injury cannot be excluded, the radiologic evaluation should begin with plain radiographs of the bony spine, with further neuroimaging of any abnormalities that are found. In patients who are alert and stable, the Canadian C-Spine Rule (Fig. 406-3) can be used to reduce unnecessary imaging without any adverse effect on patients' outcomes.**1** Bony vertebrae should be examined with CT and the spinal cord with magnetic resonance imaging. Intervertebral and paravertebral soft tissues are best studied with magnetic resonance imaging. A chest radiograph is usually indicated to provide images of the lower cervical and thoracic vertebrae; the presence of a pleural effusion in the setting of a possible thoracic spine injury suggests a hemothorax.

Ligamentous Injury Versus Spinal Cord Injury
If plain radiographs of the cervical spine are normal but the patient still complains of neck pain, a ligamentous injury should be considered. Ligamentous injury can be evaluated by flexion-extension radiographs of the cervical spine. If pain prevents an adequate study, patients should be kept in a rigid cervical collar for 3 to 5 days until the pain and muscle spasm resolve. If studies at that time are normal, the patient will no longer require the collar. Conversely, abnormal results warrant surgical evaluation to determine whether further immobilization or surgical correction is necessary.

TREATMENT ℞

The immediate goals of therapy are to arrest ongoing injury, to preserve and if possible to restore neurologic function, and to avoid secondary medical complications. To achieve these goals, an organized team approach is essential. Despite major research efforts, current clinical treatment is largely confined to supportive measures: maintaining perfusion pressure, minimizing intracompartment hypertension (e.g., increased intracranial pressure [ICP]), and indirectly treating edema.

Traumatic Brain Injury
Initial Management
It is crucial that prehospital providers optimize perfusion and oxygenation because the duration and severity of hypoxia and hypotension in this critical early period have dramatic consequences on clinical outcome. Treatment begins with immediate attention to airway and cardiopulmonary function, early identification of the potential for traumatic brain injury, and minimization of secondary insults such as hypoxia and ischemia.

Patients with mild or moderate traumatic brain injury often have returned to normal or are rapidly recovering by the time that they reach an emergency department. The critical element is the duration of amnesia or loss of consciousness (see Table 406-3). Longer periods of abnormal sensorium are associated with higher grades of concussion, and higher grades of concussion necessitate longer periods of convalescence.

Severe Traumatic Brain Injury
Patients with Glasgow Coma Scale scores of 8 or lower are considered to have severe traumatic brain injury. With this level of impaired consciousness, even with an intact gag reflex, patients are unable to protect the airway adequately. Intubation should be performed with either an endotracheal or a nasotracheal tube, depending on clinical circumstances. The patient should be in a rigid neck collar with the head elevated 30 degrees. The neck collar is used not only to protect the cervical spine until appropriate imaging can be performed but also to keep the head midline to avoid compromising venous drainage.

If intracranial hypertension is suspected, a 30-mL intravenous dose of 23% hypertonic saline through a central venous catheter **2** may be better than mannitol (intravenously at a dose of 0.5 to 1.0 g/kg) to reduce it. Continuous infusion of 3% hypertonic saline through a central venous catheter may be started at a rate of 75 to 100 mL/hr with the goal of a serum sodium level of 150 to 155 mM/L to maintain ICP below 20 mm Hg. Intravenous steroids are of no benefit acutely and increase mortality at 2 weeks after the injury.[3] Hyperventilation may also be tried but has the potential to exacerbate ischemia; if it is used, the goal should be hyperventilation to a PCO_2 of 34 to 36 mm Hg. Induced hypothermia reduces ICP in patients with traumatic brain injury. However, its use is not currently recommended,[4] and a large study found no benefit and potential harm in children.[5]

In addition to ICP control, cerebral perfusion must be maintained. The goal is to maintain cerebral perfusion pressure, which is the difference between mean arterial pressure and ICP, higher than 60 mm Hg. Volume resuscitation is the first therapeutic intervention, with the aim of achieving euvolemia or only slight hypervolemia to a central venous pressure (CVP) goal of 4 to 6 mm Hg. For fluid resuscitation, saline is preferred to albumin.[6] Furthermore, for treatment of elevated ICP, an osmolar gradient between the systemic vasculature and the brain is needed. Thus, intravenous hyperosmolar solutions may be used, including normal saline and hypertonic saline (e.g., 3% sodium solutions). The initial goal is 310 mOsm or a serum sodium level of 150 to 155 mM/L. If a cerebral perfusion pressure above 60 mm Hg cannot be achieved with intravenous fluids alone, vasoactive pharmacologic agents such as norepinephrine (beginning at 2 µg/min by continuous intravenous infusion) and phenylephrine (100 µg/min) may be required. Invasive hemodynamic monitoring with an arterial pressure line and CVP catheter may be needed.

Types of Injury

Certain lesions require prompt surgical intervention, whereas others do not. Penetrating wounds, intracerebral hemorrhage with a mass effect (including subdural and epidural blood), and bone injury (such as a displaced fracture and vertebral subluxation) require emergency surgical evaluation for intervention. However, focal, hypoxic-anoxic, diffuse axonal, and diffuse microvascular injuries do not warrant surgical intervention; treatment remains primarily with the critical care clinician. Skull fractures and intracranial hemorrhages require neurosurgical evaluation. In general, if a fracture is displaced more than the thickness of the skull, it needs to be elevated.

If a surgical lesion is not identified, the patient should be admitted to an intensive care unit. If the patient is still at a Glasgow Coma Scale score of 8 or lower, an ICP-monitoring device should be used. An intraventricular catheter provides the most reliable data. It is also a treatment option because it allows drainage of cerebrospinal fluid. However, a subdural bolt and fiberoptic catheter are less invasive alternatives.

Pharmacologic Coma and Surgical Decompression

If ICP remains poorly controlled after the aforementioned efforts, pharmacologic coma or surgical decompression is considered. The postulated effect of pharmacologic coma on ICP is through reduction of cerebral metabolism. If the decision to use pharmacologic coma is made, pentobarbital can be administered at a loading dose of 5 mg/kg intravenously, followed by an infusion of 1 to 3 mg/kg/hr. Another option is propofol (loading dose of 2 mg/kg intravenously, followed by an infusion of up to 100 µg/kg/hr). Continuous electroencephalographic monitoring is helpful because the target response is burst suppression. Barbiturates and propofol are myocardial depressants, so aggressive cardiovascular management is often necessary to achieve the desired cerebral perfusion pressure. Recalcitrant elevated ICP despite these interventions is an ominous sign; serious consideration should be given to frontal or temporal lobe decompression and hemicraniectomy.

Complications

If the patient is agitated, an evaluation should be made to determine whether the patient is in pain or poorly tolerating mechanical ventilation. If pain is a concern, a narcotic analgesic such as fentanyl (50 to 100 µg intravenously) or morphine (1 to 2 mg intravenously) should be administered. Because these agents are easily reversed by naloxone, periodic reassessment of neurologic status can be performed. If agitation alone is the issue, haloperidol (0.5 to 2 mg intravenously), a nonsedating agent that still maintains the ability for a neurologic examination to be performed, should be considered.

The PO_2 level should be maintained at approximately 100 mm Hg. Phenytoin (loading dose of 1000 mg intravenously followed by a maintenance dose of 300 mg/day intravenously) reduces seizures during the first week after traumatic brain injury, but its later usefulness is less clear. Fever greatly increases cerebral metabolism; antipyretic interventions such as acetaminophen and cooling blankets should be used as needed. Gastric stress ulcers may be prevented with H_2-antagonists such as ranitidine (50 mg intravenously four times daily) or proton pump inhibitors such as omeprazole (20 mg/day orally). Low-dose heparin (5000 units subcutaneously twice daily) or a low-molecular-weight heparin such as enoxaparin (40 mg/day subcutaneously) and pneumatic stockings should be instituted to avoid deep vein thrombosis. A nasogastric or orogastric tube should be placed for nutrition. Feeding should be initiated as soon as practical, usually on the second day after injury. Because cerebral edema is a concern, hyperosmotic feeding should be instituted. If ileus is present, total parenteral nutrition (TPN; Chapter 224) should be given.

After the first 6 to 12 hours, effort should be made to reduce hyperventilation. Otherwise, the metabolic compensation to chronic hyperventilation negates the ameliorative effects of the respiratory alkalosis.

Regular neurologic examinations and monitoring of ICP and cerebral perfusion pressure are useful to guide ongoing therapy. In general, the peak period of cerebral edema is 48 to 96 hours after traumatic brain injury. Thereafter, cerebral edema spontaneously resolves, often in association with clinical improvement.

Recovery

Recovering patients may experience "postconcussive syndrome," which is primarily manifested as headache. Other symptoms may include difficulty concentrating, changes in appetite, sleep abnormalities, and irritability. In general, postconcussive syndrome lasts a few weeks after injury, but it can persist beyond a year or more. Therapies are based on the patient's symptoms. For headache, nonsteroidal anti-inflammatory agents (such as ibuprofen at an oral dose of 400 to 600 mg), migraine drugs (such as sumatriptan at an oral dose of 25 to 50 mg), and biofeedback may be considered. For cognitive dysfunction, neuropsychological testing may be helpful in determining appropriate intervention.

Traumatic Spinal Cord Injury

Initial Management

Emergency management of traumatic injury to the spinal cord begins with the basics of airway, breathing, and circulation. A secure airway is essential. For patients suffering from high cervical lesions, spontaneous ventilation will be lost. Cervical lesions below C5 may also be associated with impaired ventilatory capability. If there is any concern that the airway or ventilatory effort is compromised, emergency intubation is required. In a patient in whom the cervical spine has not been imaged, the preferred method is nasotracheal intubation under fiberoptic guidance. Other approaches are nasotracheal (blind) or orotracheal intubation, provided that in-line traction is applied.

Other immediate concerns are bleeding and circulation. Hypotension (systolic blood pressure < 90 mm Hg) may be due to either neurogenic shock or hypovolemia and should be avoided. For neurogenic shock, vasopressive pharmacologic agents such as phenylephrine (beginning as a continuous intravenous infusion at 100 µg/min with titration to clinical effect) may be needed. If tachycardia is present, hypovolemia is more likely, so fluid resuscitation would be more appropriate.

Targeted Therapy

If closed compartment spinal cord injury is identified, immediate pharmacologic therapy with methylprednisolone may be instituted,[7] but treatment must be started within 8 hours of injury. The initial dose is an intravenous bolus of 30 mg/kg administered during 15 minutes, followed 45 minutes later by a continuous infusion of 5.4 mg/kg/hr for 23 hours; longer durations of therapy are significantly more toxic. The utility of methylprednisolone in penetrating traumatic spinal cord injury has not been demonstrated, and it should not be used.

At this time, the decision for surgical intervention should be based on the stability of the anterior, middle, and posterior vertebral columns. The anterior column consists of the anterior half of the vertebral body and the vertebral disc. The middle column is the posterior half of the body and the disc. The posterior column is composed of the arch, facets, and ligaments. In general, if two of the three columns are damaged, surgical stabilization is needed. If immediate surgery is not indicated, the patient should be admitted to the intensive care unit for further management.

Acute and Subacute Management

Patients with severe spinal cord injuries require close cardiovascular and ventilatory care, supportive care for bladder and bowel function, approaches to avoid pressure ulcers (Chapter 24), and general measures similar to those used for patients with traumatic brain injury.

Neurogenic Shock and Dysautonomia

After traumatic spinal cord injury, patients are at risk for neurogenic shock and dysautonomia. Lesions of the cervical and thoracic spine disrupt the descending sympathetic pathways to the intermediolateral cell column of the thoracolumbar spinal cord, thereby leading to peripheral vasodilation and hypotension. If the lesion is at T3 or above, sympathetic tone to the heart is compromised. In this setting, hypotension is accompanied by bradycardia, thus producing the neurogenic shock triad of bradycardia, hypotension, and peripheral vasodilation.

Initial therapy for dysautonomia should be fluid administration to restore an adequate circulating volume with a target CVP of 4 to 6 mm Hg. A hematocrit of 30 is optimal for perfusion of the central nervous system, so blood can be used if the patient is anemic. If blood is not required, either colloid (e.g., albumin solutions) or crystalloid (e.g., normal saline) may be used. If there is a suspicion of cardiac or pulmonary disease, a pulmonary artery catheter may be needed briefly to assess fluid status and the relationship between pulmonary pressure and CVP.

Once adequate circulating volume has been achieved, hypotension should be managed with vasopressive agents such as phenylephrine (see earlier), norepinephrine (see earlier), or dopamine (beginning at 1 µg/kg/min by continuous intravenous infusion; Chapter 106), with the goal of a mean arterial pressure of 85 to 90 mm Hg that should be maintained for 7 days after injury. Symptomatic bradycardia can be treated with atropine (1 mg intravenously).

Ventilatory Compromise

An injury at C5 or higher results in diaphragmatic denervation and requires complete ventilatory assistance. Proper management requires endotracheal or nasotracheal intubation and mechanical ventilation, with an appropriate tidal volume (6 to 10 mL/kg), an FIO_2 to achieve a PO_2 between 80 and 100 mm Hg, and a rate to give a PCO_2 of 40 mm Hg. Positive end-expiratory pressure should also be given to minimize atelectasis (Chapter 105). If the patient does not show signs of ventilatory recovery within 2 weeks of intubation, a tracheostomy should be considered.

Lesions below C5 may also be associated with inadequate spontaneous ventilation. Midcervical lesions may be associated with intact but compromised diaphragm function. If this is suspected, a "sniff" test under fluoroscopy can be performed to determine whether both hemidiaphragms are functioning properly. If they are not, intubation or tracheostomy with volume-controlled ventilation may be needed. If function is intact, pressure support ventilation may be sufficient (Chapter 105) to achieve an appropriate tidal volume.

Cervical lesions at C6 and below spare the phrenic nerves but may disrupt innervation of the intercostal muscles. The primary finding is decreased cough and an inability to increase ventilation when needed, thereby leading to atelectasis and pneumonia; assisted elimination of tracheal secretions is essential.

Thromboembolic Disease

Thromboembolic disease (Chapters 81 and 98) is a leading cause of morbidity and mortality after traumatic spinal cord injury. Prolonged immobility of the lower extremities leads to deep vein thrombosis in up to 70% of spinal cord–injured patients. Patients should receive prophylaxis with heparin alone or in combination with intermittent compression devices (e.g., pneumatic stockings) or graduated compression stockings. Anticoagulation therapy with warfarin to a therapeutic goal of an international normalized ratio of 2 to 3 should begin during rehabilitation. An inferior vena cava filter may be placed if anticoagulation and mechanical therapies are contraindicated.

Visceral Function

The abdominal wall musculature is innervated by T7 to T12. The stomach, small bowel, liver, pancreas, and proximal two thirds of the colon receive innervation from T5 to L2. Spinal cord injury at these levels or above may impair visceral function. For ileus, a nasogastric tube should be placed to decompress the stomach. Parenteral nutrition should be started as soon as possible. Enteral feeding should be delayed until gastrointestinal motility returns, usually within 2 to 3 weeks. In comparison with conservative bowel management, transanal irrigation improves constipation, fecal incontinence, and symptom-related quality of life in patients with spinal cord injuries.[8]

Stress-induced peptic ulcer disease occurs in nearly a third of patients without prophylaxis. An H_2-receptor antagonist such as ranitidine (50 mg intravenously four times daily) or a proton pump inhibitor such as omeprazole (20 mg/day orally) reduces the incidence of ulcers.

Bladder tone may be lost because of spinal shock. A Foley catheter should be placed for a minimum of 5 to 7 days to drain the bladder and to evaluate volume and renal status. After spinal shock has resolved, autonomic dysreflexia may occur as a result of bladder distention. Clinical signs such as sweating, skin flushing, and hypertension may be present. Clinical examination with palpation and percussion will reveal a distended bladder, which can be treated by bladder training or intermittent catheterization.

Nutrition

Until enteral feeding can begin, parenteral nutrition should be used. Ideally, TPN should be started. However, if TPN is not possible, peripheral parenteral nutrition should be used until TPN (Chapter 224) can begin. Energy expenditures of 19 kcal/kg/day for high cervical injuries to 35.8 kcal/kg/day for injuries at T10 and below have been reported. A calorie level of 80% of the Harris-Benedict prediction should be used for quadriplegic patients. The full Harris-Benedict predicted amount should be used in patients with thoracic spine injuries and below.

Other Therapy

Patients with traumatic spinal cord injury have a propensity for the development of decubitus ulcers and pressure sores (Chapter 24). Mechanical kinetic beds, regular log rolling (every 2 hours), and padded orthotics are useful in minimizing this complication. Orthotics, physical therapy, and occupational therapy (for cervical cord injury) are also important to minimize contractures and to begin the rehabilitation process.

PROGNOSIS

Traumatic Brain Injury

The most useful prognostic indicator after traumatic brain injury is the neurologic examination at initial evaluation. For patients with severe traumatic brain injury, the initial Glasgow Coma Scale score is the most reliable

TABLE 406-4 AMERICAN SPINAL INJURY ASSOCIATION IMPAIRMENT SCALE

GRADE	INJURY TYPE	DEFINITION	LIKELIHOOD OF RECOVERY*
A	Complete	No motor or sensory function below the lesion	15.5% (cervical) and 7% (thoracic)
B	Incomplete	Sensory but no motor function	47%
C	Incomplete	Some motor strength (<3)	84%
D	Incomplete	Motor strength > 3	84%
E	None	Sensory and motor function normal	100%

*Data from Coleman WP, Geisler FH. Injury severity as primary predictor of outcome in acute spinal cord injury: retrospective results from a large multicenter clinical trial. *Spine J.* 2004;4:373-378.

prognostic indicator. The lower the initial Glasgow Coma Scale score, the less likely a patient will have meaningful neurologic or functional recovery. After traumatic brain injury, 40% of patients with a score of 8 have a good recovery versus only 7% when the score is 3. Furthermore, only 27% of patients with a score of 3 survive versus 88% of patients with a score of 8. Patients in whom the Glasgow Coma Scale score remains the same or worsens during a period of 6 hours do worse clinically than those whose score improves. Further prognostic stratification at 24 hours can be based on pupillary responses, motor responses, and age (see Chapter 411).

A subsequent head injury before full recovery from even a mild traumatic brain injury may occasionally result in "second impact syndrome," which can worsen the clinical outcome. When seen (mostly in children and adolescents), coma develops rapidly after the second injury, often within minutes. There is decreased autoregulation, diffuse cerebral edema, and intracranial hypertension. Second impact syndrome is associated with high mortality.

Traumatic Spinal Cord Injury

For traumatic spinal cord injury, the completeness of the injury is the most useful predictor (Table 406-4). A grade "A" or complete motor and sensory deficit below the lesion has a poor prognosis. If such a lesion persists for 24 hours, there is little likelihood of meaningful recovery. On the other hand, even severe partial injuries have a higher probability of recovery.

1. Stiell IG, Clement CM, Grimshaw J, et al. Implementation of the Canadian C-Spine Rule: prospective 12 centre cluster randomised trial. *BMJ.* 2009;339:b4146.
2. Wakai A, Roberts I, Schierhout G. Mannitol for acute traumatic brain injury. *Cochrane Database Syst Rev.* 2007;1:CD001049.
3. CRASH Trial Collaborators. Final results of MRC CRASH, a randomized placebo-controlled trial of intravenous corticosteroid in adults with head injury—outcomes at six months. *Lancet.* 2005;365:1957-1959.
4. Sydenham E, Roberts I, Alderson P. Hypothermia for traumatic head injury. *Cochrane Database Syst Rev.* 2009;2:CD001048.
5. Hutchison JS, Ward RE, Lacroix J, et al. Hypothermia therapy after traumatic brain injury in children. *N Engl J Med.* 2008;358:2447-2456.
6. SAFE Study Investigators. Saline or albumin for fluid resuscitation in patients with traumatic brain injury. *N Engl J Med.* 2007;357:874-884.
7. Bracken MB, Shepard MJ, Holford TR, et al. Administration of methylprednisolone for 24 or 48 hours or tirilazad mesylate for 48 hours in the treatment of acute spinal cord injury. Results of the Third National Acute Spinal Cord Injury Randomized Controlled Trial. National Acute Spinal Cord Injury Study. *JAMA.* 1997;277:1597-1604.
8. Christensen P, Bazzocchi G, Coggrave M, et al. A randomized, controlled trial of transanal irrigation versus conservative bowel management in spinal cord–injured patients. *Gastroenterology.* 2006; 131:738-747.

SUGGESTED READINGS

Gupta R, Bathen ME, Smith JS, et al. Advances in the management of spinal cord injury. *J Am Acad Orthop Surg.* 2010;18:210-222. *Review.*
Husson EC, Ribbers GM, Willemse-van Son AH, et al. Prognosis of six-month functioning after moderate to severe traumatic brain injury: a systematic review of prospective cohort studies. *J Rehabil Med.* 2010;42:425-436. *Glasgow Coma Scale score, midline shift, and subdural hematoma predicted outcome.*
van Middendorp JJ, Hosman AJ, Donders AR, et al. A clinical prediction rule for ambulation outcomes after traumatic spinal cord injury: a longitudinal cohort study. *Lancet.* 2011;377:1004-1010. *Age, motor scores of the quadriceps femoris (L3) and gastrocsoleus (S1) muscles, and light touch sensation of dermatomes L3 and S1 distinguished independent walkers with excellent predictive accuracy.*

407

MECHANICAL AND OTHER LESIONS OF THE SPINE, NERVE ROOTS, AND SPINAL CORD

RICHARD L. BARBANO

DEFINITION

Disorders of the spine, nerve roots, and spinal cord together are frequent reasons for a patient to visit a physician. Many of these disorders either initially or eventually involve more than one element of the vertebra–spinal cord–nerve root unit, so there is much overlap in the pathobiology and clinical manifestations of these diseases.

The spine consists of 30 vertebrae: 7 cervical (C), 12 thoracic (T), 5 lumbar (L), 5 sacral (S), and the coccyx (Fig. 407-1). The ring shape of the bony vertebrae forms a protective circle around the spinal cord while leaving ample room to allow the cord to move within this canal during flexion and

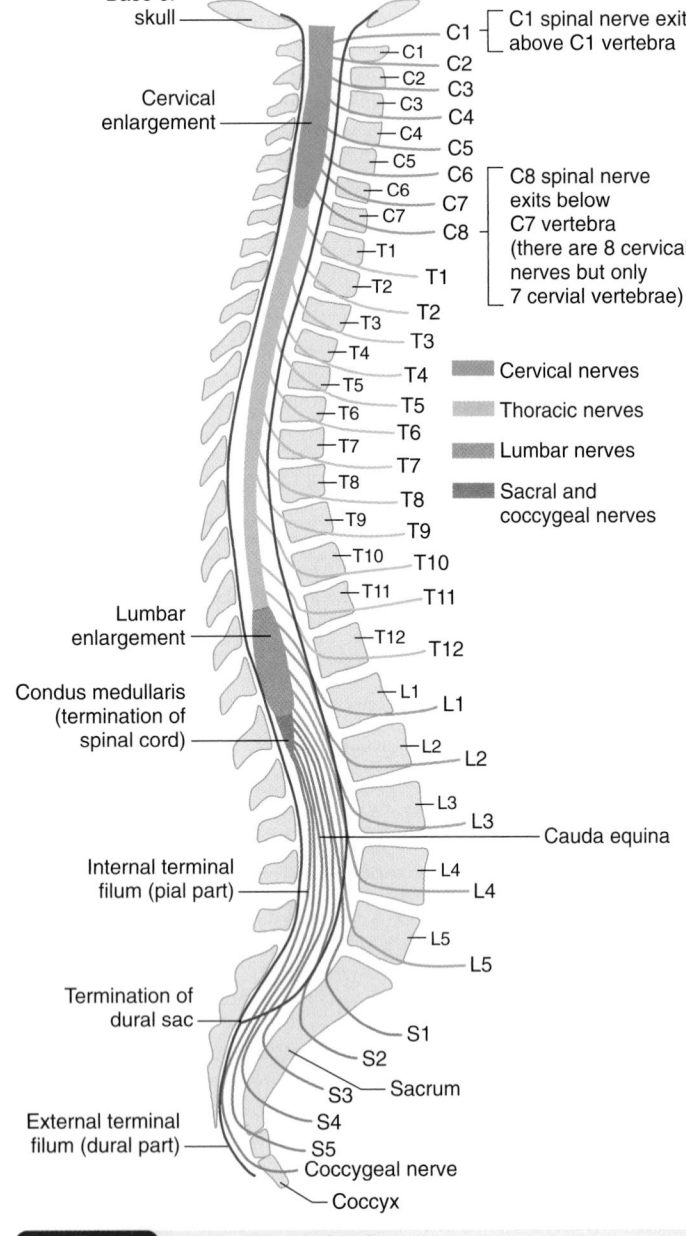

FIGURE 407-1. Anatomy of the spinal cord.

*Labels in figure:*

Base of skull — C1 spinal nerve exits above C1 vertebra

C1, C2, C3, C4, C5, C6, C7, C8

Cervical enlargement

C8 spinal nerve exits below C7 vertebra (there are 8 cervical nerves but only 7 cervial vertebrae)

T1–T12

■ Cervical nerves
■ Thoracic nerves
■ Lumbar nerves
■ Sacral and coccygeal nerves

Lumbar enlargement

Condus medullaris (termination of spinal cord)

L1–L5

Cauda equina

Internal terminal filum (pial part)

Termination of dural sac

S1, S2, S3, S4, S5 — Sacrum

External terminal filum (dural part)

Coccygeal nerve

Coccyx

extension of the spine. The vertebral bodies help bear the compressive weight of the body and provide the surface area to support the intervertebral discs, which act to cushion the axial force along the spine. The overlapping facet joints and multiple sets of longitudinal ligaments give the spine stability during its many ranges of motion. The posteriorly placed foramina allow the exit of spinal nerves.

The spinal cord consists of 31 spinal segments, with one more cervical cord segment (8) than vertebrae; each gives rise to a bilateral pair of spinal nerves. Spinal nerves C1 to C7 exit the canal above their corresponding vertebral body, the C8 nerve exits below the C7 vertebra, and subsequent inferior nerves also exit below the numbered vertebrae. The spinal segments of the cord itself, however, lie progressively superior to the vertebrae, so that the end of the spinal cord, the conus medullaris, in adults is approximately adjacent to the L1 vertebra. The more caudal spinal nerves travel as the cauda equina in the subarachnoid space within the spinal canal before exiting their respective foramina. The spinal cord does not have a uniform diameter; the cervical and lumbar segments are wider compared with the thoracic and lower sacral areas because the increased motor and sensory neurons supplying the arms and legs enlarge the cord.

Spinal nerves are formed by the joining of the anterior and posterior spinal roots, which directly exit and enter the spinal cord. The anterior root derives from axons of the anterior horn cells and lateral columns, and it serves motor and autonomic efferent pathways; the posterior root mostly derives from the axons from the dorsal root ganglion and carries afferent sensory signals (Fig. 407-2). The sensory root is twice the thickness of the motor root and lies in a more anterior and inferior location as it crosses the foramen.

CLINICAL MANIFESTATIONS

Disorders of the spinal nerve root produce signs and symptoms referable to the corresponding dermatome or myotome. By far the most frequent complaint is localized neck or back pain, but compromise of the nerve roots or spinal cord will cause symptoms such as abnormal or painful sensations (paresthesias or dysesthesias), loss of sensation, weakness, and autonomic dysfunction (most commonly bladder or bowel incontinence).

When it affects a myotome (the group of muscles served by motor neurons of a spinal cord segment; Fig. 407-3), the motor deficit associated with a spinal root disorder is of the *lower motor neuron* type. Typical findings are weakness, hypotonia, depressed or absent reflexes, and, if the syndrome has persisted for at least several weeks, atrophy with or without fasciculations. Sensation at the root level is diminished or absent for all modalities, but sensation below the affected root level is intact.

Conversely, disorders of the spinal cord produce a "level" below which sensation is abnormal and motor deficits are of the *upper motor neuron* type, with weakness without atrophy (unless complicated by disuse), hypertonia, and increased reflexes. At the level of a spinal cord lesion, the motor deficits can be of the lower motor neuron type as the anterior horn cell bodies or exiting fibers are affected; below this level, an upper motor neuron syndrome will predominate. With strokes (Chapter 414) and other central nervous system disorders (Chapter 195), the full upper motor neuron syndrome may not be present in the acute phase of cord injury and can take time to appear.

DIAGNOSIS

The clinical history can help localize the patient's symptoms, especially complaints of pain and sensory alterations that may exist in the absence of objective sensory loss on probing with light touch, pinprick, and vibration stimuli. The neurologic examination should include evaluation of the sensory, motor (Table 407-1), and reflex (Table 407-2) functions. Careful side-to-side comparisons can help assess subtle deficits. For example, elderly patients often have decreased or absent ankle jerks, so contralateral comparison is necessary. However, all muscles receive innervation from more than one root/spinal cord level, and all roots send fibers to multiple muscles. The clinical implication of this anatomic pattern is that individual muscles are rarely profoundly weak, and patients rarely report isolated muscle weakness in single root involvement syndromes. Likewise, overlap of the sensory dermatomes (see Fig. 407-3) explains why sharp demarcations in the sensory examination rarely occur.

DISORDERS OF THE SPINE
Neck and Back Pain

DEFINITION

Most neck and back pain is *mechanical*, that is, theoretically emanating from the spine's structural elements, which are the vertebrae, discs, ligaments,

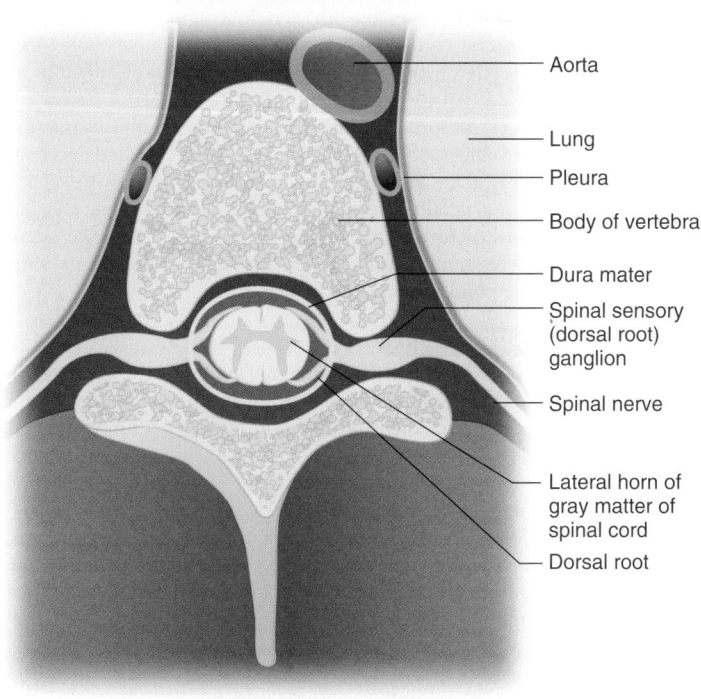

- Aorta
- Lung
- Pleura
- Body of vertebra
- Dura mater
- Spinal sensory (dorsal root) ganglion
- Spinal nerve
- Lateral horn of gray matter of spinal cord
- Dorsal root

FIGURE 407-2. Anatomy of the spinal cord: section through a thoracic vertebra.

tendons, and muscles. The location of pain is either *axial*, which means it is located along the spine itself, or *referred*; the term *perceived pain* is sometimes used when the pain from a spinal lesion is felt elsewhere by the patient, whereas *referred pain* is often used to describe pain caused by nonspinal structures that is experienced by the patient in the spinal area. If the pain follows a dermatomal (nerve root) distribution, it is referred to as *radicular pain*, which is likely to involve the nerve root.

EPIDEMIOLOGY

Neck and back pain is a frequent reason for visits to a primary care physician. Low back pain is more common than neck pain, but both are common. The thoracic spine, possibly because of rib attachments and limited range of motion, is an uncommon location for back pain.

In the general population, the incidence of self-reported neck pain is 213 per 1000; the 12-month prevalence of any pain is typically between 30 and 50%, and pain severe enough to limit activity is between 1.7 and 11.5%. The prevalence is higher among women. Risk factors for neck pain include inherited factors, poor psychological health, and tobacco use; the presence of disc degeneration is not a significant factor.

More than 70% of people will experience low back pain significant enough to inhibit their participation in daily activities at some time in their life. The highest prevalence is in the 45- to 64-year age group. There is less of a gender difference than with neck pain, although tobacco use is an associated risk factor. Physical work–related factors, such as heavy lifting, prolonged sitting, and repetitive twisting, increase risk; prospective studies show that psychosocial issues, such as work monotony and job dissatisfaction, also are major predisposing factors.

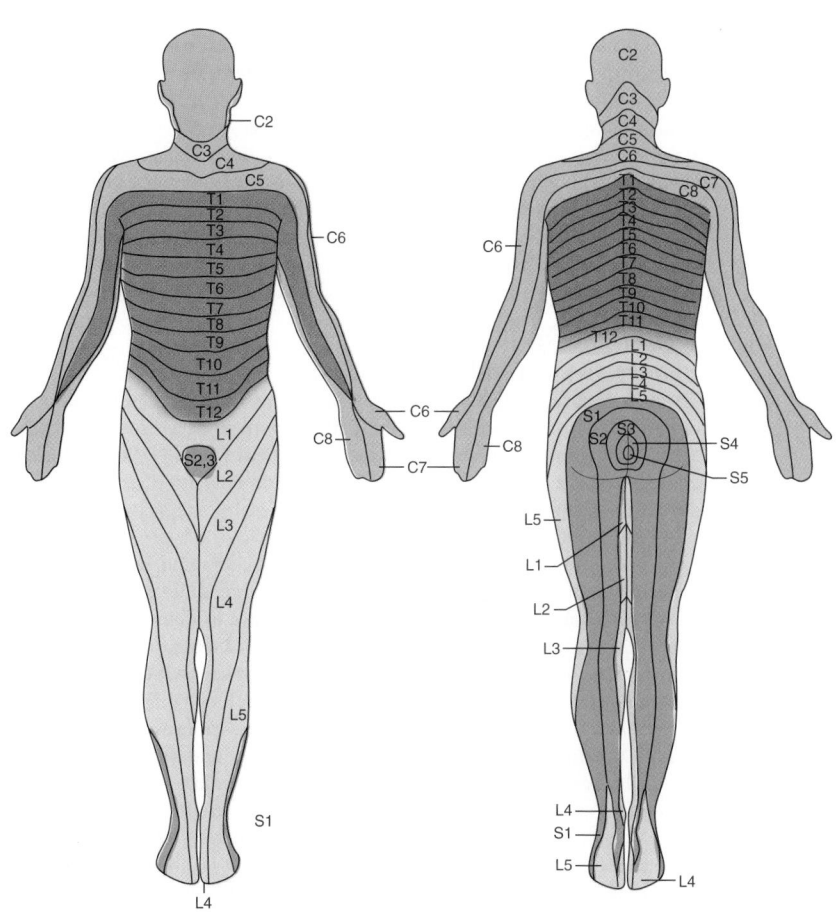

Levels of principal dermatomes

C5	Clavicles
C5,6,7	Lateral parts of upper limbs
C8, T1	Medial sides of upper limbs
C6	Thumb
C6,7,8	Hand
C8	Ring and little fingers
T4	Level of nipples
T10	Level of umbilicus
T12	Inguinal or groin regions
L1,2,3,4	Anterior and inner surfaces of lower limbs
L4,5 S1	Foot
L4	Medial side of great toe
S1,2, L5	Posterior and outer surfaces of lower limbs
S1	Lateral margin of foot and little toe
S2,3,4	Perineum

FIGURE 407-3. Schematic demarcation of levels of principal dermatomes shown as distinct segments. There is actually considerable overlap between any two adjacent dermatomes.

TABLE 407-1 ESSENTIAL MUSCLE TESTING

ROOT	MUSCLES	ACTION/TESTING
ARM		
C5	Deltoid	Abducts arm
	Infraspinatus	Externally rotates arm with elbow flexed
C6	Brachioradialis	Flexes elbow (along with biceps [C5-6])
C7	Triceps	Extends elbow
	Extensor digitorum	Extends fingers
C8	Flexor digitorum	Flexes fingers (both superficialis and profundus)
	Flexor pollicis longus	Flexes distal phalanx of thumb
T1	Interossei	Spread fingers
LEG		
L1-2	Iliacus	Flexes hip
L2-3	Adductor magnus	Adducts thigh (as part of adductor group)
L3-4	Quadriceps	Extends knee
L4	Tibialis anterior	Dorsiflexes foot
L5	Extensor hallucis longus	Great toe extension
	Extensor digitorum longus	Toe extension
S1	Hamstrings	Flex knee
	Flexor hallucis longus	Flexes great toe (along with S2)

TABLE 407-2 ESSENTIAL REFLEX EXAMINATION

REFLEX	EFFECT	ROOT/IMPLICATION
Jaw jerk	Jaw closes with tap on slightly opened jaw	Cranial nerve V; implies lesion above cervical cord
Biceps	Tap tendon: elbow flexion	C5-6; musculocutaneous nerve
Brachioradialis	Tap tendon over distal radius with elbow flexed and mid pronation: elbow flexion	C5-6; radial nerve
Triceps	Tap tendon: elbow extension	C6 < C7
Finger flexion	Tap partially flexed fingertips: finger flexion	C6-T1; when hyperactive, may imply lesion above midcervical spinal cord
Patella	Tap patella: quadriceps contraction (knee extension)	L2-4
Achilles	Tap Achilles tendon: foot plantar flexion	S1-2
Babinski	Scratch sole: great toe flexion	Great toe extension implies lesion of cord (or brain) above L4
Anal wink	Scratch perineum: external anal sphincter contraction	Absence of contraction implies S2-4 lesion

PATHOBIOLOGY

Although the popular impression is that the disc is the source of most spine pain, it is estimated that disc disease such as protrusion accounts for only 5% of all low back problems. Degenerative changes are a much more common cause of both acute and chronic spine pain. There is a genetic predisposition to intervertebral disc degeneration, with heritability estimates in the range of 34 to 61%.

Degenerative changes can result in *spondylosis,* a condition that includes degenerative disc disease with bulging and occasionally herniation. The condition is often accompanied by the formation of osteophytes, ligamentous hypertrophy, and sometimes facet fracture and vertebral subluxation. Spondylosis, which is a consequence of age-related disc disease, is exemplified by the fact that almost everybody has at least anterior osteophytes by the age of 40 years, and it is not necessarily painful. Spondylosis probably starts with age-related disc desiccation and loss of elasticity of the annulus fibrosus. Tension of the longitudinal ligaments results in the formation of hypertrophic osteophytes. Compromise of microvascular supply may also contribute. Eventually, the facet joints can ride over one another, thereby leading to instability, the formation of more osteophytes, and inflammation of the synovial joints. If there is fracture of the pars interarticularis, the term *spondylolysis*

is used. Further instability between the intervertebral segments leads to *spondylolisthesis,* in which one vertebral body shifts sagittally in relation to its adjacent vertebra. Spondylolisthesis is graded by the amount of shift as measured with flexion and extension lateral spine films.

Whiplash, an acute flexion-extension injury of the cervical spine, is common after motor vehicle accidents and other situations of rapid deceleration. Although specific acute and chronic manifestations are controversial, the acute syndrome is generally accepted to be a result of mechanical irritation of pain-sensitive structures in the cervical spine with or without nerve root injury. More severe trauma can cause fracture and vertebral instability, both of which require rapid surgical evaluation.

CLINICAL MANIFESTATIONS

Acute neck pain and low back pain are commonly limited to the axial region, although radicular signs and symptoms can occur in the presence of nerve root irritation. The most common radicular pain occurs in the distribution of a dermatome. Other radicular signs and symptoms can include dysesthesias or sensory loss in the affected dermatome, decreased strength in muscles of the affected myotome, and decreased reflex. Cranial nerve findings, diffuse weakness throughout a limb or in more than one limb, hemisensory symptoms, autonomic symptoms, and increased reflexes are not manifestations of spine disease and should prompt more extensive evaluation for other conditions that affect the brain or brain stem. Bowel and bladder symptoms should prompt urgent evaluation of a cauda equina or myelopathy syndrome (see later).

Acute spine problems can also cause referred or perceived pain at sites other than their anatomic source. For example, mechanical low back pain may include aching in the buttocks or thigh, most often posteriorly and occasionally the hip region but rarely below the knee. More commonly, however, the term *referred pain* denotes the situation in which other structures, usually internal organs, refer pain to the spine or back. Areas of referred pain usually share the same embryologic origin and, during development, the same sensory pathways. Differentiation of referred pain from localized back pain depends on the history and examination. Mechanical pain is often exacerbated by movement, such as twisting, bending, extension, or flexion, whereas referred pain tends to be independent of such activities.

Chronic spine disorders lead to chronic back pain directly and as a secondary complication. For example, chronic degenerative arthropathy can lead to degenerative lumbar scoliosis with secondary involvement of neural structures. Back pain and radiculopathy are the most prominent symptoms, present in upward of 80% of patients, but symptoms of neurogenic claudication also develop in about 50% of patients.

DIAGNOSIS

History and Clinical Examination

The history and examination are essential for the initial evaluation and triage of patients with neck and back pain. Patients with so-called red flags (Table 407-3) merit special attention, as does any patient who awakens from sleep because of pain or has pain that is constant and unchanged by position, is unremitting and progressive, or is accompanied by any systemic signs or symptoms.

As part of the history in the setting of acute neck trauma, well-established screening protocols such as the Canadian C-Spine Rule and the NEXUS Low-Risk Criteria (Fig. 407-4) are validated ways to detect cervical spine fracture and to direct appropriate radiographic evaluation. In such a setting, a computed tomographic (CT) scan of the cervical spine would be the imaging test of choice.

On clinical examination, inspection should assess evidence of trauma, muscle wasting, fasciculations, erythema, rashes, and scars. Palpation is directed to areas of point tenderness during evaluation for more diffusely tender regions, muscle spasm, and masses. If light percussion of the spinous process evokes significant pain, a focal process, such as fracture, malignant neoplasm (Chapter 195), or infection (Chapter 421), should be considered because such a finding is unusual in typical mechanical spine pain. Finally, the active and passive range of motion for flexion, extension, rotation, and tilt should be noted. Many provocative tests have been described for the evaluation of neck and back pain, but few have undergone formal evaluation of their diagnostic accuracy. For neck pain, contralateral rotation of the neck with extension of the arm and fingers (Video 407-1) suggests cervical root involvement, particularly in combination with other provocative tests, such as the Spurling maneuver, in which the patient's head is rotated 45 degrees to the contralateral side with the neck in slight extension to minimize the

TABLE 407-3 "RED FLAGS" IN THE EVALUATION OF SPINE PAIN

Recent significant trauma or minor trauma at age >50 years
Unexplained weight loss
Unexplained fever
Immunosuppression
History of cancer
History of prior local surgery
Systemic disorder, bone or arthritic disorder
Intravenous drug use
Prolonged use of corticosteroids or osteoporosis
Age >70 years
Focal neurologic deficit with progressive symptoms
Duration >6 weeks
Thoracic spine pain

Modified from Davis PC, Wippold FJ, Brunberg JA, et al. ACR Appropriateness Criteria on low back pain. *J Am Coll Radiol.* 2009;6:401-407.

The NEXUS Low Risk Criteria (NLC) Algorithm for screening of neck injuries

- No posterior midline cervical spine tenderness—Midline posterior bony cervical-spine tenderness is present if the patient reports pain on palpation of the posterior midline neck from the nuchal ridge to the prominence of the first thoracic vertebrae, or if the patient evinces pain with direct palpation of any cervical spinous process.
- No evidence of intoxication—Patients should be considered intoxicated if they have either of the following: a recent history provided by the patient, or an observer of intoxication or intoxicating ingestion, or evidence of intoxication on physical examination such as an odor of alcohol, slurred speech, ataxia, dysmetria, or other cerebellar findings, or any behavior consistent with intoxication. Patients may also be considered to be intoxicated if tests of bodily secretions are positive for alcohol or drugs that affect level of alertness.
- A normal level of alertness—An altered level of alertness can include the following: a Glasgow Coma Scale score of 14 or less; disorientation to person, place, time, or events; an inability to remember three objects at five minutes; a delayed or inappropriate response to external stimuli; or other findings.
- No focal neurological deficit—A focal neurological deficit is any focal neurological finding on motor or sensory examination.
- No painful distracting injuries—No precise definition of painful distracting injury is possible. This category includes any condition thought by the clinician to be producing pain sufficient to distract the patient from a second (neck) injury. Such injuries may include, but are not limited to, any long-bone fracture; a visceral injury requiring surgical consultation; a large laceration, degloving injury, or crush injury; large burns; or any other injury causing acute functional impairment. Physicians may also classify any injury as distracting if it is thought to have the potential to impair the patient's ability to appreciate other injuries.

FIGURE 407-4. The NEXUS Low-Risk Criteria (NLC) algorithm for screening of neck injuries. (Reproduced from Hoffman JR, Mower WR, Wolfson AB, et al. Validity of a set of clinical criteria to rule out injury to the cervical spine in patients with blunt trauma. National Emergency X-Radiography Utilization Study Group. *N Engl J Med.* 2000;343:94-99.)

foraminal opening. Downward pressure on the top of the head by the examiner will reproduce arm dysesthesias (Video 407-2). Provocative tests also can diminish symptoms. For example, in the cervical distraction test, the examiner's hands are placed under the jaw and occiput; gentle upward pulling of the head will temporarily reduce or alleviate the symptoms (Video 407-3).

For low back pain, the straight leg raise (Video 407-4) has sensitivity of 0.85 to 0.91 but a specificity of only 0.26 to 0.52 for the diagnosis of sciatica due to a herniated disc. The crossed straight leg raise test (Video 407-5) has a lower sensitivity of 0.23 to 0.34 but a much higher specificity of 0.86 to 0.90. The seated straight leg raise (Video 407-6) can be used for confirmation of root irritation as the spine-leg angle is increased to 90 degrees. A negative result of the seated straight leg raise in the setting of a positive result of the straight leg raise suggests the possibility of a nonorganic component, although a mechanical alteration of the root exit zone in this position should also be considered.

Ancillary Testing

For neck pain (Fig. 407-5), plain radiography and CT scanning, which are the mainstays of cervical spine imaging, allow adequate view of the bony structures. Magnetic resonance imaging (MRI) has largely replaced myelography, which is still used occasionally to provide information about the spinal cord and nerve roots. However, magnetic resonance abnormalities are common and can have a high false-positive rate; for example, 12 to 17% of patients younger than 30 years and 86 to 89% of patients 60 years of age have disc degeneration as evidenced by loss of signal intensity, disc protrusion, narrowing of the disc space, or foraminal stenosis. Cervical discography also has a high false-positive rate and cannot be recommended as a diagnostic test in the assessment of neck pain.

Uncomplicated acute low back pain, with or without radiculopathy, is generally self-limited, and imaging studies are unnecessary unless any of the red flags (see Table 407-3) are present.█ For trauma, osteoporosis, or patients older than 70 years, plain radiography *may* suffice if the results are normal and no other abnormalities are present. Otherwise, with few exceptions, MRI is the test of choice given its superiority in evaluating soft tissue structures and its lack of radiation exposure. Care must be taken, however, to ensure correlation with the clinical syndrome because 28% of asymptomatic volunteers with a mean age of 42 years have herniated discs, 52% have bulging discs, and 14% have annular tears. The percentage of imaging abnormalities increases even more in asymptomatic volunteers older than 60 years; 57% have significantly abnormal scans, with 36% showing herniated discs and close to 98% showing disc degeneration. Abnormalities of the Modic end plate, anterolisthesis, and disc extrusion are more strongly associated with low back pain than is disc degeneration without end plate changes. Situations in which alternative imaging should be considered include spondylosis and stress fracture, for which bone scintigraphy with single-photon emission computed tomography is more sensitive than MRI. CT can also be useful when MRI is contraindicated or to evaluate scoliosis, bone graft integrity, surgical fusion, and instrumentation. For back and neck pain that persists for 6 weeks, electrodiagnostic testing can demonstrate compromise of spinal root function but is not usually helpful in axial spine pain without neurologic symptoms.

Differential Diagnosis

Mechanical or idiopathic pain explains up to 97% of cases of neck pain (Table 407-4) and low back pain (Table 407-5); the remaining 3% is nonmechanical in origin and includes referred pain and other conditions. Acute mechanical neck pain is most often caused by a neck strain, a herniated nucleus pulposus, or whiplash; for pain of insidious onset, osteoarthritis and myelopathy are the leading causes. For back pain, muscle strain and a herniated nucleus pulposus are acute causes; insidious causes include osteoarthritis, spinal stenosis, spondylolisthesis, and scoliosis. Queries regarding the red flags will identify serious and nonmechanical causes of neck and back pain (Table 407-6).

Abdominal and pelvic structures can refer pain *to* the low back (referred pain). Abdominal aortic aneurysms (Chapter 78) can present with a mid to low back ache that may radiate to the hips or anterior thighs. Cholecystitis (Chapter 158) can cause pain in the midthoracic area; pancreatic disease (Chapter 146) can cause pain in the L1 region; and diverticulitis (Chapter 144) in the left lower quadrant can cause diffuse low back pain. Genitourinary disorders (Chapter 128) can cause colicky referred pain to the flanks and costovertebral angle. Bladder disorders (Chapter 125) may occasionally refer pain to the sacral area, as can prostate problems (Chapter 131). Pelvic disorders in women that can cause referred low back pain include endometriosis (Chapter 244), ectopic pregnancy, and pelvic inflammatory disease (Chapters 307 and 326). Most of these disorders have additional signs and symptoms to aid in the diagnosis.

Myocardial ischemia (Chapter 71) can be associated with anterior neck pain, although less commonly than with left arm or jaw pain. Arterial dissections (Chapter 78) are more commonly associated with neck pain; for example, up to 20% of patients with carotid dissections complain of anterolateral pain, and about 80% of patients with vertebral dissections have posterior or occipital pain. Patients with arterial dissections frequently but not necessarily have signs and symptoms of stroke (Chapter 414). Disorders of the esophagus (Chapter 140) and mass lesions of the throat (Chapters 196 and 437) can also present as neck pain.

Acute spine pain can precede the rash in herpes zoster (Chapter 383) or can be seen in the vaso-occlusive crisis of sickle cell anemia (Chapter 166).

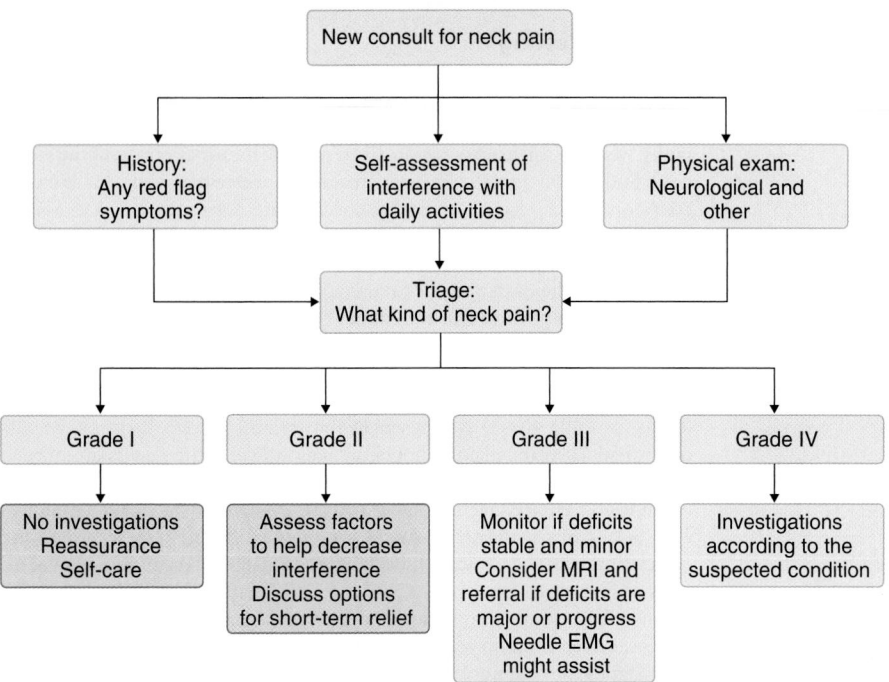

FIGURE 407-5. Approach to new-onset neck pain. (Modified from Guzman J, Haldeman S, Carroll LJ, et al. Clinical practice implications of the Bone and Joint Decade 2000-2010 Task Force on Neck Pain and Its Associated Disorders. From concepts and findings to recommendations. *Spine.* 2008;33:S199-S213.)

TABLE 407-4 MECHANICAL NECK PAIN

	NECK STRAIN	HERNIATED NUCLEUS PULPOSUS	OSTEOARTHRITIS	MYELOPATHY	WHIPLASH
Age (yr)	20-40	30-50	>50	>60	30-40
Pain location	Neck	Arm	Neck	Arm/leg	Neck
Onset	Acute	Acute	Insidious	Insidious	Acute
Flexion	+	+	−	−	+
Extension	−	+/−	+	+	+
Plain radiography	−	−	+	+	−

+ = present; − = absent.
From Borenstein DG, Wiesel SW, Boden SD. *Neck Pain: Medical Diagnosis and Comprehensive Management.* Philadelphia: WB Saunders; 1996.

TABLE 407-5 MECHANICAL LOW BACK PAIN

	MUSCLE STRAIN	HERNIATED NUCLEUS PULPOSUS	OSTEOARTHRITIS	SPINAL STENOSIS	SPONDYLOLISTHESIS	SCOLIOSIS
Age (yr)	20-40	30-50	>50	>60	20	30
Pain pattern location	Back (unilateral)	Back (unilateral)	Back (unilateral)	Leg (bilateral)	Back	Back
Onset	Acute	Acute (prior episodes)	Insidious	Insidious	Insidious	Insidious
Standing	↑	↓	↑	↑	↑	↑
Sitting	↓	↑	↓	↓	↓	↓
Bending	↑	↑	↓	↓	↑	↑
Straight leg	−	+	−	+ (stress)	−	−
Plain radiography	−	−	+	+	+	+

From Borenstein DG, Wiesel SW, Boden SD. *Low Back Pain: Medical Diagnosis and Comprehensive Management,* 2nd ed. Philadelphia: WB Saunders; 1995.

Infections of the disc (Chapter 421) cause sharp back pain worsened by movement. Arachnoiditis (Chapter 420), an inflammatory process of the arachnoid space, can cause diffuse, chronic back pain, often after the introduction of foreign substances or manipulation of the intrathecal space. Finally, 20 to 50% of patients with depression (Chapter 404) will complain of back pain that often is diffuse and described in emotionally laden terms. Complaints of low back pain are also common in malingering patients.

TREATMENT Rx

Treatment options vary according to the severity of pain, presence of radicular signs or symptoms, and any underlying disease. *Acute nontraumatic neck pain* is common and usually benign. Beneficial treatments include nonsteroidal anti-inflammatory drugs (NSAIDs, e.g., ibuprofen 600 mg three times daily for 2 weeks), exercise, and physical therapy. The low risk of myocardial

TABLE 407-6 DIFFERENTIAL DIAGNOSIS OF ORGANIC CAUSES OF LOW BACK PAIN*		
MECHANICAL LOW BACK OR LEG PAIN (97%)†	**NONMECHANICAL SPINAL CONDITIONS (~1%)‡**	**VISCERAL DISEASE (2%)**
Lumbar strain, sprain (70%)§	Neoplasia (0.7%)	Disease of pelvic organs
Degenerative processes of discs and facets, usually age related (10%)	Multiple myeloma	Prostatitis
	Metastatic carcinoma	Endometriosis
Herniated disc (4%)	Lymphoma and leukemia	Chronic pelvic inflammatory disease
Spinal stenosis (3%)	Spinal cord tumors	Renal disease
Osteoporotic compression fracture (4%)	Retroperitoneal tumors	Nephrolithiasis
Spondylolisthesis (2%)	Primary vertebral tumors	Pyelonephritis
Traumatic fracture (<1%)	Infection (0.1%)	Perinephric abscess
Congenital disease (<1%)	Osteomyelitis	Aortic aneurysm
Severe kyphosis	Septic discitis	Gastrointestinal disease
Severe scoliosis	Paraspinous abscess	Pancreatitis
Transitional vertebrae	Epidural or subdural abscess	Cholecystitis
Spondylolysis‖	Shingles	Penetrating ulcer
Internal disc disruption or discogenic low back pain¶	Inflammatory arthritis (often associated with HLA-B27) (0.3%)	Cardiac or pericardial disease
Presumed instability**	Ankylosing spondylitis	Pulmonary or pleural disease
Other structural anomalies	Rheumatoid arthritis	
	Psoriatic spondylitis	
	Reiter's syndrome	
	Inflammatory bowel disease	
	Arachnoiditis	
	Scheuermann's disease (osteochondrosis)	
	Paget's disease of bone	

*Values in parentheses indicate the estimated percentages of patients with these conditions among all adult patients with low back pain in primary care, excluding nonorganic causes such as conversion reaction, psychosis, litigation-related disorders, malingering, and substance abuse. Diagnoses in italics are often associated with neurogenic leg pain. Percentages may vary substantially according to demographic characteristics or referral patterns in a practice. For example, spinal stenosis and osteoporosis will be more common in geriatric patients, spinal infections in injection drug users, and so forth.
†The term *mechanical* is used to designate an anatomic or functional abnormality without an underlying malignant, neoplastic, or inflammatory disease. Approximately 2% of cases of mechanical low back pain or leg pain are accounted for by spondylolysis, internal disc disruption, or discogenic low back pain and presumed instability.
‡Scheuermann's disease and Paget's disease of bone probably account for less than 0.1% of nonmechanical spinal conditions.
§Strain and sprain are nonspecific terms with no pathoanatomic confirmation. Idiopathic low back pain may be a preferable term.
‖Spondylolysis is as common in asymptomatic persons as in those with low back pain, and its role in causing low back pain remains ambiguous.
¶Internal disc disruption is diagnosed by provocative discography (injection of contrast material into a degenerated disc, with assessment of pain at the time of injection). However, discography often causes pain in symptomatic adults, and the condition of many patients with positive discograms improves spontaneously. The clinical importance and appropriate management of this condition remain unclear. Discogenic low back pain is used more or less synonymously with internal disc disruption.
**Presumed instability is loosely defined as more than 10 degrees of angulation or 4 mm of vertical displacement on lateral flexion and extension radiographs. However, the diagnostic criteria, natural history, and surgical indications remain controversial.
From Deyo RA, Weinstein JN. Low back pain. *N Engl J Med.* 2001;344:363-370.

infarction or upper gastrointestinal bleed from NSAIDs must be weighed against pain relief and the relative benignity of the condition. Chiropractic manipulation is of benefit but has the rare complication of posterior circulation stroke from arterial dissection, especially in patients younger than 45 years. Low-level laser therapy[3] and acupuncture[4] are also of short-term benefit. Cervical collars and traction are not of established benefit. Even in the absence of radicular pain, surgical intervention for neck pain is indicated in cases of vertebral instability, such as caused by fracture or dislocation. Surgery, including fusion, may be needed for stabilization after surgery for lesions such as tumors, infections, or hemorrhages. For neck pain that is accompanied by signs or symptoms of radiculopathy, surgery should be considered but is not usually the initial therapy (see later). If a cervical spine lesion is causing spinal cord compression, emergent evaluation for possible surgery is indicated (see later).

Because *acute low back pain* is generally benign, invasive therapy should be avoided in the first 3 months. Conservative treatment includes NSAIDs (e.g., ibuprofen 600 mg three times daily as needed) and controlled physical activity; strict bed rest for longer than 2 days is no better than restricted physical activity.[5] Other options include local heat and massage. Spinal manipulation, exercise therapy, yoga, acupuncture, and cognitive-behavioral therapy are moderately effective.[6]

For *persistent, nonradicular low back pain*, exercise and cognitive-behavioral therapy are recommended. Prolotherapy, in which a mild irritant is injected into a tendon or ligament to increase blood flow and to promote healing, and facet joint injections can be helpful, but intradiscal steroid injections and percutaneous intradiscal radiofrequency thermocoagulation are not effective.[7] When persistent nonradicular low back pain is accompanied by associated degenerative spine changes, surgical fusion is of benefit but not superior to interdisciplinary rehabilitation.

Surgery is indicated for spine instability, progressive neurologic deficits, or severe radicular pain that persists for more than 3 months despite conservative therapy,[8] especially in patients with spinal stenosis and herniated discs. When degenerative changes lead to lumbar scoliosis with or without neurologic signs, decompressive surgery with or without fusion appears effective for at least 5 years for the majority of patients. In more focal disorders, surgery to remove disc material pressure from pain-sensitive structures can be considered; techniques include open, laser, and microdiskectomy approaches, with little evidence to favor one option over the other.

PROGNOSIS

Between 50 and 85% of patients who have neck pain that persists for more than 1 day report recurrence of symptoms in 1- and 5-year follow-up. Patients younger than 45 years have less recurrence, and patients aged 45 to 59 years have the highest risk. Prior neck injury or pain, coexistent low back pain, and self-perceived poor general health are risk factors for recurrence.

Mechanical spine pain, even with radicular symptoms, resolves without specific intervention within 30 days in many patients and within 3 months in 90% of patients. Recurrence is frequent, however, especially in patients with spondylosis, because the underlying process persists and further degeneration of the spinal elements can be expected.

Long-term disability is more common with obesity, low education level, tobacco use, high levels of pain at the onset, tendency to somatization, job dissatisfaction, lack of availability of light-duty employment, and need to perform significant lifting at work. The strongest factors affecting outcome are psychological, especially worrying, fear avoidance, anger, and frustration.

Spinal Stenosis

DEFINITION

Spinal stenosis, which is a narrowing of the spinal canal, results in compression of neural structures in the cervical and lumbar regions, where the diameter of the spinal cord is largest. Signs and symptoms of spinal stenosis are referable to these levels. In the lumbar region, L4-5 is the most common level of stenosis, followed by L3-4 and L5-S1.

EPIDEMIOLOGY

The annual incidence of spinal stenosis in the United States is about 1 to 2 per l00,000 for the cervical region and 5 per 100,000 for the lumbar region. Spinal stenosis often coexists in the cervical and lumbar regions, and the incidence is higher in patients with more complex degenerative anatomy.

PATHOBIOLOGY

Primary spinal stenosis is due to a congenital narrowing of the spinal canal. Causes of secondary stenosis include chronic degenerative conditions, such as spondylosis and thickening of the ligamenta flava and longitudinale posterius neoplasia, osteomyelitis, and rheumatoid arthritis. In patients receiving corticosteroids long term, epidural lipomatosis is a cause predominantly at the thoracic level.

In spinal stenosis, myelopathy results from compression of the veins that drain the canal, thereby leading to capillary stasis and edema, which result in further compromise of the spinal cord. If the anterior spinal artery is also occluded intermittently or chronically, ischemic gliosis develops. The cord itself can be compressing, and dynamic injury can occur during flexion and extension, especially in chronic degenerative conditions associated with thickening and buckling of the ligamentum flavum. Superimposed trauma, such as severe flexion-extension from whiplash injury or falls, can cause the central cord syndrome (see later, Disorders of the Spinal Cord).

CLINICAL MANIFESTATIONS

Cervical stenosis, which usually results from spondylosis (cervical spondylotic myelopathy) and degenerative spine changes superimposed on congenital stenosis, can be manifested in a number of ways. At the C5-8 level, both the cord and roots are involved, and patients develop lower motor neuron findings in the arms and upper motor neuron signs in the legs; the result is the slow onset of painless atrophy of the weakened hand muscles, accompanied by gait abnormalities. Above the C5 level, the arms may become numb and clumsy, but there is little atrophy. Gait problems are frequently described as leg stiffness, heaviness, or incoordination, and patients may complain of falls or fear of falling, difficulty walking on uneven surfaces, and needing to watch where they are walking. In general, neck pain is not as prominent a complaint as is low back pain in lumbar spinal stenosis, but radicular pain occurs in about one third of patients. On examination, a Lhermitte sign, which is a shocklike tingling traveling down the spine with neck flexion or less commonly with extension, may be elicited. Sensation to pinprick examination will often be decreased in the hands, but this finding may be patchy and not well demarcated. Increased muscle tone will predominate in the legs, and reflexes will likely be increased; the Babinski sign is often present. The stance and gait may be wide based, with slow, short steps. A Romberg sign may be present.

Lumbar spinal stenosis can present with intermittent or persistent signs and symptoms referable to both cord and roots; axial neck or back pain is almost always present. The pain can also radiate in a pseudoradicular pattern from the lumbar region into the gluteal region, groin, and one or both upper legs, but pain rarely radiates distal to the knee unless spinal root involvement occurs. Lumbar neurogenic claudication is perhaps the most specific; symptoms are precipitated by compressive effects on the spinal cord and exiting roots and are characterized by increasing leg paresthesias and weakness as the patient remains standing and gravity pulls the lumbar cord enlargement into the narrowed spinal segment. As opposed to vascular claudication (Chapter 79), symptoms occur even at rest and can be relieved only by bending at the waist or sitting; the patient will characteristically report improved ability to walk if bent at the waist. Other features that suggest neurogenic claudication rather than vascular claudication include back pain, paresthesias, numbness, weakness, and prolonged presence of symptoms after changing of position (seconds to 1 to 2 minutes in vascular claudication but 2 to 20 minutes in neurogenic claudication).

DIAGNOSIS

MRI can localize and quantify the severity of the stenosis. The normal diameter of the lumbar canal is approximately 22 to 25 mm, relative lumbar stenosis is 10 to 12 mm diameter, and a diameter of less than 10 mm is considered absolute stenosis. MRI also can identify any comorbid spinal disease, such as degenerative changes and spondylolisthesis. However, CT myelography, which provides the details needed for surgical treatment, is another alternative. Electromyography (EMG) is not generally useful in the diagnosis of spinal stenosis except in assessment of comorbid conditions, such as localized radiculopathy, which might be important for surgical planning, as well as for detection of other potentially significant disorders, such as polyneuropathy.

The differential diagnosis of lumbar spinal stenosis includes vascular claudication from peripheral vascular disease (Chapter 79) and abdominal aortic aneurysm (Chapter 78). The symptoms of vascular claudication are activity dependent, unlike the positional dependency of the spinal stenosis. Other conditions that can mimic lumbar stenosis include radiculopathy or disc prolapse, polyneuropathy, tethered cord, and spina bifida. Because cervical stenosis can cause both arm and leg symptoms, the differential diagnosis also includes multiple sclerosis (Chapter 419), syringomyelia (Chapter 426), Arnold-Chiari malformation (Chapter 426), cerebrovascular disease (Chapters 414 and 415), normal-pressure hydrocephalus (Chapter 195), and motor neuron disorders (Chapter 418).

TREATMENT   Rx

Spinal stenosis is not necessarily an indication for surgery. Conservative therapy with NSAIDs (e.g., ibuprofen or acetaminophen 600 mg three times daily or acetaminophen 650 mg every 6 hours as needed), muscle relaxants, physical therapy, and a hard cervical collar can help many patients. However, surgery should be considered in patients with severe symptoms and signs of progressive myelopathy. Decompressive laminectomy, with or without fusion, is superior to nonsurgical therapy for improvement of pain and function for at least a year in patients with lumbar spinal stenosis.[9]

PROGNOSIS

Because spinal stenosis is usually degenerative, it is a slowly progressive condition. After symptoms develop and the condition is affecting quality of life, decompressive surgery should be considered. Because the underlying condition itself is progressive, however, surgery is not a permanent cure, and symptoms often recur.

● DISORDERS OF THE NERVE ROOTS

DEFINITION

Disorders of the nerve root, termed radiculopathy, lead to symptoms referable to a dermatome or myotome. Either the ventral (anterior, motor) or posterior (dorsal, sensory) root can be involved independently or after they join to form the spinal nerve. Symptoms will follow the anatomic location. Because the root must traverse the vertebral foramen, it is prone to disorders of the spine at these locations. *Sciatica*, which is a commonly used but poorly defined term, often connotes low back pain with radiation into the ipsilateral leg, thereby implying pain radiating along the sciatic nerve, which anatomically contains fibers originating in the L4-S2 roots. The *cauda equina syndrome* results from disease involving the roots of the lower lumbar and sacral spinal cord levels as they traverse inside the spinal canal on their way to exit below their respective vertebral bodies.

PATHOBIOLOGY

Irritation of the spinal sensory nerve root or dorsal root ganglion causes symptoms referable to that dermatome. Spontaneous dysesthesias are hypothesized to result from ectopic discharges from the injured nerve; sensitization of the injured nerve leads to tactile evoked dysesthesias in the same distribution. Mechanical compression of the nerve contributes to the syndrome. In addition, inflammatory cytokines leak from the nucleus pulposus into the epidural space, where they result in endoneurial edema and pain. The pro-inflammatory cytokine tumor necrosis factor-α is a likely main contributor. Rupture of the nucleus pulposus releases phospholipase A_2, which also plays an important role in the inflammatory process. The inflammatory process itself can cause pain even in the absence of frank root compression.

The nerve root exits through the intervertebral foramen, where it is subject to compression and injury. The proximal portion of the nerve root has a small region of decreased vascular supply, where it is especially prone to edema, which can exacerbate the effect of the original injury. Treatment of this edema is one of the potential therapeutic effects of corticosteroid injections. The S1 root is the most susceptible to injury at the foramen because it is the largest diameter spinal nerve and exits through the narrowest lumbar foramen. In addition, because it is traveling inferiorly from the S1 spinal cord level to pass out of the foramen under the S1 vertebral body, it passes through the superior, most narrow part of the foramen. The superior location of the sensory root on these nerves may account for the early predominance of sensory symptoms versus motor symptoms.

CLINICAL MANIFESTATIONS

The symptoms of radiculopathy depend on the affected root. Root involvement is likely if pain radiates beyond the shoulder or the knee. In the thoracic region, root involvement often produces symptoms that "wrap around" the trunk. Radicular pain is often worsened by activities that increase intraspinal pressure, such as coughing, sneezing, straining, and other Valsalva maneuvers. The characteristics of the pain vary, but when they are exacerbated by such provocation, they are often described as sharp, shooting, electrical, and tingling. When reporting the symptoms, patients may point to or rub the distal dermatome where they are experiencing the discomfort (perceived pain). Patients also may report specific positions that increase or decrease pain; for example, sitting will often worsen the pain of acute lumbar disc herniation, and neck extension can produce radiating pain in cervical disc herniation or other processes that narrow the foramen.

It is uncommon for patients to spontaneously note anesthesia, but they often note dysesthesias in radiculopathy, even in the absence of spine pain. The localization of these dysesthesias often follows the dermatome but also may be described diffusely by the patient. Likewise, complaints of weakness may be difficult to isolate to a particular muscle; however, exceptions exist, such as when the patient complains of a weak grip or a foot drop.

On examination, side-by-side strength testing of specific muscles (see Table 401-1) can help identify slight weakness. Slight weakness may also be identified by evaluating for pronator drift in the arms or asking patients to walk on their toes, walk on their heels, and do shallow knee bends on each leg independently. Sensory examination should test all potential root distributions; pinprick is often sufficient, and it is helpful to ask the patient to report any abnormalities, not just frank hypesthesia. Hyperreflexia in the arms is not expected in a spinal nerve disorder and, if unexplained, should be further investigated for an injury to the spinal cord or brain (Chapter 406). Patients who are older than 65 years or who have a peripheral neuropathy (Chapter 428) might have reduced or even absent ankle jerks.

The cauda equina syndrome is manifested as unilateral or bilateral leg weakness, saddle anesthesia, urinary dysfunction with hesitancy or retention, and, less commonly, bowel dysfunction. Depending on the cause, it is frequently accompanied by low back pain. The syndrome can be accompanied by severe sciatica, which can be unilateral or bilateral but also involve perineal pain. The weakness of the legs, which may be asymmetrical, is of the lower motor neuron type. The major causes of the cauda equina syndrome include lumbar disc herniation, neoplasm, and lumbar spinal stenosis.

DIAGNOSIS

The history and physical examination are similar to the evaluation of neck and back pain (see earlier), with special emphasis on finding evidence of nerve root involvement.

The patient should be queried about bowel and bladder dysfunction. Frank incontinence needs to be investigated for either the cauda equina syndrome or a myelopathy. If the patient has any loss of perineal sensation, such as might be noted during or after voiding or bowel movement, the examination should test perianal sensation, anal sphincter tone, and anal wink reflex. Because the cauda equina syndrome involves nerve roots, reflexes should be normal or decreased; hyperactive reflexes or a Babinski sign would indicate a myelopathy (see later).

Ancillary Testing

Imaging to evaluate a potential radiculopathy is similar to the evaluation for neck and back pain (see earlier). EMG can localize radicular abnormalities and their severity as well as assess possible comorbid neurologic diseases, such as diffuse peripheral or entrapment neuropathies. EMG electrodiagnostic localization can be extremely helpful in determining whether a finding on MRI is truly associated with neurologic impairment, and it has a high sensitivity and specificity for identification of acute and chronic denervation when the motor (anterior) aspect of the root is involved. However, EMG is less sensitive (about 30 to 70%) if only the sensory (posterior) limb of the root is involved by the lesion. MRI with its high sensitivity and EMG with its high specificity should be considered complementary tests.

Differential Diagnosis

Many mechanical processes can injure the spinal nerve root (see earlier, Neck and Back Pain), and most of the causes of spine pain can cause root disorders. Spinal cord compression may accompany radiculopathy.

In addition to conditions that can affect the nerve root as it leaves the spinal column, intra-column abnormalities below the level of the conus medullaris can affect the lumbar and sacral roots before they exit, thereby resulting in the cauda equina syndrome. Most commonly, the cauda equina syndrome is caused by extrinsic compression of the caudal sac by a mass, such as a large and centrally herniated lumbar disc, metastatic tumor, abscess, or epidural hematoma, but arachnoiditis or chronic meningitis must be considered.

Disorders of the brachial or lumbosacral plexus can cause pain radiating down a limb in a radicular or polyradicular pattern. Painful peripheral neuropathies (Chapter 428) can also resemble a radiculopathy. Non-neurologic disorders, such as fibromyalgia (Chapter 282) and polymyalgia rheumatica (Chapter 279), can cause axial pain that mimics a radiculopathy. Cervical radiculopathy also can be mimicked by acromioclavicular joint arthropathy, shoulder bursitis, and the shoulder impingement syndrome; lumbar radiculopathy can be mimicked by hip arthritis, trochanteric bursitis, iliotibial band syndrome, and hamstring tendinitis (Chapter 264).

TREATMENT   Rx

Acute neck and back pain, even with radicular symptoms, is usually self-limited and resolves. If radiculopathy is associated with an underlying non-structural lesion, such as infection or tumor, treatment should be directed toward that underlying lesion (see also later, Metastatic Spinal Cord Compression). If symptoms or neurologic dysfunction progresses or persists for more than 6 weeks, interventional options should be considered.

In *cervical radiculopathy,* either foraminal or epidural corticosteroid injection may be of benefit.[10] A series of injections, usually between one and three, provides short-term relief of radicular symptoms, with an acceptable adverse event profile. Although minor events, such as increased neck pain, headache, and vasovagal reactions, are relatively frequent (5 to 20%), serious events, such as epidural hematoma or abscess, are uncommon (<1%). In cervical spondylopathy with radiculopathy, surgery provides more rapid pain relief than does physiotherapy but little additional benefit in the long term.[11] Anterior cervical discectomy, with or without fusion, is beneficial.[3] Cervical anterior discectomy and arthroplasty result in a lower risk of postoperative dysphagia compared with discectomy and fusion,[12] but more complicated surgeries are not of established benefit.

In *lumbar radiculopathy,* transforaminal epidural steroid injections provide short-term symptom relief,[13] but there are no clear guidelines on how many injections or on the indications for continuing the series. Chemonucleolysis of a lumbar disc is moderately superior to placebo but inferior to surgery.

For symptomatic radiculopathy associated with a herniated disc, either open surgical discectomy or microdiskectomy is superior to nonsurgical therapy for at least 3 months.[8] If the condition is isolated to a single disc and no significant degenerative changes are present, longer periods of benefit are more likely. Systematic reviews suggest that conservative discectomy allows a quicker return to work and has less long-term back pain than does more aggressive surgery, but with the downside of an increased risk of recurrent disc herniation. Video 407-7 demonstrates a right L4-5 hemilaminectomy with removal of a herniated disc fragment. The presurgical magnetic resonance images show the position and extent of the disc herniation.

DISORDERS OF THE SPINAL CORD

DEFINITION AND GENERAL OVERVIEW

A disorder of the spinal cord itself is termed a myelopathy. A myelopathy can be intramedullary, as the result of a disorder intrinsic to the cord, or extramedullary, as the result of an abnormality that is extrinsic to the cord but compressing it.

EPIDEMIOLOGY AND PATHOBIOLOGY

Spinal cord disorders can be caused by a wide range of conditions (Table 407-7).

The functional elements of the spinal cord (Fig. 407-6) include descending tracts largely to motor and autonomic neurons, motor neurons, autonomic neurons, and sensory ascending tracts. The anterior horn cell motor neuron is the cell body for the axon that will become the anterior nerve root and continue directly to innervate the muscle. The cell bodies for the primary sensory neurons reside in the dorsal root ganglion outside the spinal cord itself.

CLINICAL MANIFESTATIONS

The clinical manifestations of myelopathy result from the spinal level of the lesion. The majority of signs will be bilateral, but asymmetry, or even unilaterality, does not exclude a spinal cord lesion.

In general, the three major functions affected are motor, sensory, and autonomic, especially bowel, bladder, and erectile function. If anterior horn cells are involved at the lesion level, the corresponding myotome will exhibit lower motor neuron function (hypotonic weakness), and reflexes may be decreased at that level. Below the lesion, however, patients will have hypertonic weakness that can progress to spastic paralysis, hyperreflexion, and Babinski sign. Sensation will be decreased from the level of the lesion and distally. Because increased tone and spasticity often develop over time, they may not be dramatic at the initial clinical presentation. If the posterior columns are compromised, patients may lose joint position sense and develop ataxia, especially

of gait. If the posterior columns of the cervical cord are impaired, patients may have *pseudoathetosis* of the fingers, manifested as unconscious athetotic movements of the fingers of the outstretched arm when the eyes are closed.

The *anterior cord syndrome* is manifested as lower motor neuron weakness at the level of the lesion (anterior horn); upper motor neuron weakness and spasticity below the lesion (corticospinal tracts); autonomic dysfunction below the level of the lesion (lateral horn), most often bowel and bladder dysfunction; and loss of pain and temperature sensation below the level of the lesion (spinothalamic tract). Vibration and joint position sense remain intact (posterior columns). The major causes of this syndrome are vascular, such as an anterior spinal artery, or an anteriorly impinging mass lesion, such as disc or vertebral body mass.

The *central cord syndrome* is manifested as lower motor neuron signs and symptoms at the level of the lesion (anterior horn cells) and upper motor neuron signs and symptoms below the lesion (corticospinal tracts), urinary retention, and a band of loss of temperature and pain sensation at the level of the lesion (anterior white commissure decussation of these fibers). In the midcervical level, this syndrome is typical of syringomyelia (Chapter 426). Other major causes include intramedullary tumors (Chapter 195) and post-traumatic cervical injury (Chapter 406) in patients with disc herniation or preexisting cervical spondylosis.

The *posterior cord syndrome* is manifested as complaints of imbalance, especially in the dark or with eyes closed, and an examination notable for ataxia, presence of Romberg sign, and loss of vibration sense and proprioception below the level of the lesion (posterior columns), with preservation of pain and temperature sensation. Patients are seldom weak. Posterior compression may be caused by spondylotic disease, but other major causes include deficiencies of vitamin B_{12} or vitamin E (Chapters 225 and 425), syphilis (Chapter 327), AIDS-associated vacuolar myelopathy (Chapter 401), and nitrous oxide inhalation (Chapter 425).

The *Brown-Séquard (cord hemisection) syndrome* combines features of these syndromes. At the level of the lesion, patients exhibit *ipsilateral* lower motor weakness (anterior horn) and loss of all sensation (posterior root entry zone). Below the level of the lesion, patients have *ipsilateral* upper motor weakness and spasticity (corticospinal tract) and *ipsilateral* loss of vibration sense and proprioception (posterior columns), with *contralateral* loss of pain and temperature (spinothalamic tract, the fibers of which have crossed from the opposite side through the anterior white commissure). The Brown-Séquard syndrome is often caused by trauma (Chapter 406) or eccentric compression.

TABLE 407-7   CAUSES OF MYELOPATHY

Trauma/compression	Neoplastic
Direct ± vertebral spine disease	Metastatic cord compression
Spondylotic myelopathy/stenosis	Spinal tumors
Post-traumatic syrinx	Paraneoplastic
Arachnoid cyst	Infectious
Vascular	Epidural abscess
Cord infarction	Syphilis
Dural arteriovenous malformation	Lyme disease
Inflammatory/autoimmune	Tuberculosis
Multiple sclerosis	HIV infection
Devic's disease	Tropical spastic paraparesis
Acute disseminating encephalomyelitis	Herpes zoster
Adrenomyeloneuropathy	Toxic/metabolic
Systemic lupus erythematosus	Post-radiation myelopathy
Sjögren's syndrome	Vitamin B_{12} deficiency
Mixed connective tissue disease	Vitamin E deficiency
Postinfectious/postvaccination	Heroin
Arachnoiditis	Epidural lipomatosis
	Congenital/hereditary
	Chiari malformation
	Syringomyelia

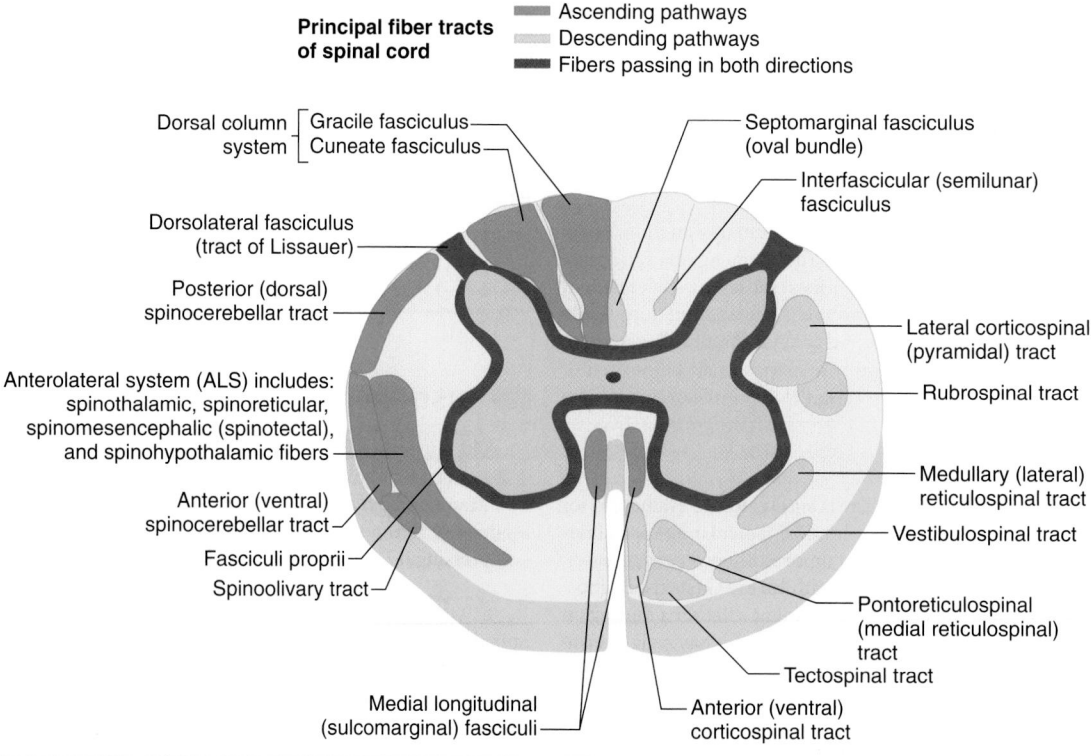

Principal fiber tracts of spinal cord

- Ascending pathways
- Descending pathways
- Fibers passing in both directions

Dorsal column system [Gracile fasciculus — Cuneate fasciculus]

Septomarginal fasciculus (oval bundle)

Interfascicular (semilunar) fasciculus

Dorsolateral fasciculus (tract of Lissauer)

Posterior (dorsal) spinocerebellar tract

Lateral corticospinal (pyramidal) tract

Rubrospinal tract

Anterolateral system (ALS) includes: spinothalamic, spinoreticular, spinomesencephalic (spinotectal), and spinohypothalamic fibers

Medullary (lateral) reticulospinal tract

Vestibulospinal tract

Anterior (ventral) spinocerebellar tract

Fasciculi proprii

Spinoolivary tract

Pontoreticulospinal (medial reticulospinal) tract

Tectospinal tract

Anterior (ventral) corticospinal tract

Medial longitudinal (sulcomarginal) fasciculi

FIGURE 407-6. Principal fiber tracts of spinal cord.

The *conus medullaris syndrome* refers to dysfunction of the distal-most tapered portion of the spinal cord, which anatomically lies at approximately the T12-L1 vertebral spine level. The arms are normal; weakness in the legs is variable but often symmetrical when it is present. The main signs and symptoms are sexual dysfunction, loss of bowel and bladder control, and perianal anesthesia with loss of the anal wink reflex. The major causes are disc herniation, lumbar stenosis, and neoplasm.

DIAGNOSIS

Symptoms of bilateral involvement of the arms or legs suggest a myelopathy, although bilateral leg involvement can be seen in lumbar spinal stenosis and the cauda equina syndrome. Complaints of leg stiffness or incoordination suggest spasticity from myelopathy. Other symptoms include a recent change in bowel or bladder function, erectile dysfunction, imbalance (especially in the dark or with eyes closed), and catching of feet when walking. These central symptoms can also reflect lesions of the brain stem and higher, so the patient should be queried about cortical and brain stem symptoms (e.g., cognitive function, vision, facial strength, sensation, and swallowing). Focal back pain supports a myelopathy.

Examination for a potential myelopathy must include an evaluation of anal tone and perineal sensation. The patient should be examined in a gown to allow inspection of the spine as well as the overlying skin. A *sensory level,* which represents a point where distal (inferior) sensation is altered, should also be sought, but a spinal cord lesion rarely causes a sharp line of sensory demarcation. Joint position sense can be diminished if the posterior columns are involved. A tandem gait will assess possible gait ataxia. Finally, the patient should be examined for distal hypertonicity, if not frank spasticity, by assessment for hyperreflexia and Babinski signs. *In acute spinal cord lesions, however, a state of "spinal shock" can cause hyporeflexia or even a flaccid paralysis.*

Ancillary Testing

MRI is the test of choice because it provides anatomic detail of the spine and subarachnoid space as well as the spinal cord. MRI may also show evidence of demyelinating or metastatic disease. Plain films are not adequate to evaluate the spinal cord. If the MRI is normal, lumbar puncture is sometimes useful for evaluation of conditions that resemble myelopathy: Guillain-Barré syndrome (Chapter 428), infectious or carcinomatous meningitis (Chapter 420), arachnoiditis, and transverse myelitis.

Differential Diagnosis

The many causes of myelopathy (see Table 407-7) can typically occur at any spinal level, but certain conditions predominate at specific spinal levels.

Any lesion that has an upper *cervical* location must be evaluated for disorders of the craniocervical junction, especially disorders that can produce atlantoaxial instability, such as rheumatoid arthritis (Chapter 272); after trauma, cervical or odontoid fracture must be excluded. Disorders at the base of the skull, such as Chiari I and other congenital malformations (Chapter 426), can sometimes affect the upper cervical cord. Syringomyelia (Chapter 426), which may or may not be associated with Chiari malformation, also has a predilection for the cervical cord.

The *thoracic* cord is relatively protected from all but direct trauma, but it is the most common site for metastatic cord compression. Transverse myelitis is most commonly thoracic, and the thoracic cord also is particularly vulnerable to a watershed ischemic myelopathy due to severe hypotension. Epidural lipomatosis often is most symptomatic at the thoracic level.

The *lumbar-conus* region is the most common site for disc herniations. In addition, ependymomas are relatively more common in this region, as are metastases from more caudal locations and compression from arachnoiditis.

The rapidity of onset helps in diagnosis. *Acute or relatively acute myelopathy* suggests vascular causes, trauma, demyelinating lesions, or sudden decompensation of a preexisting lesion, such as a pathologic fracture. In a young person, with no other comorbid illnesses, a demyelinating illness, such as multiple sclerosis (Chapter 419) or acute disseminated encephalomyelitis (Chapter 422), is suggested; other central nervous system lesions separated in space with white matter signal abnormalities on MRI would increase the likelihood of this diagnosis. In older persons or patients with known vascular risk factors, hypotension, or an onset in the immediate postoperative period, a spinal cord infarction is possible. Sudden, sharp back pain suggests mechanical disorders (e.g., pathologic fracture, sudden worsening spondylolisthesis) or spinal cord infarction, whereas demyelinating lesions are often painless. Myelopathy developing *subacutely,* especially accompanied by back pain, can be caused by metastatic disease (Chapter 195) and abscesses (Chapter

421). Both of these conditions must be evaluated and treated as true emergencies to prevent permanent paralysis. *Subacute* or *chronic* myelopathies include vitamin B_{12} deficiency (Chapter 425), although nitrous oxide inhalation may cause an acute expression of the disorder; syringomyelia (Chapter 426); and more slowly growing tumors, such as meningiomas (Chapter 195), lipomas, and neurofibromas (Chapter 426).

In the setting of known malignant disease or unexplained weight loss, metastatic cord compression (Chapter 195) must be considered. Weight loss, back pain, and fever can be seen in infection (Chapter 421) and occasionally spondyloarthropathies (Chapter 273). Infectious causes also include tropical spastic paraparesis (HTLV-1, Chapter 386). Syphilis (Chapter 327) is the cause of tabes dorsalis; patients may have other signs and symptoms, such as lancinating pains, ataxia, depressed leg reflexes, and Argyll Robertson pupils. Myelopathies that follow an infectious illness include acute disseminated encephalomyelitis and progressive necrotizing myelopathy. Transverse myelitis can follow viral infections, such as herpes zoster (Chapter 383). Myelopathy accompanied by evidence of multifocal cortical dysfunction would likely be multiple sclerosis or acute disseminated encephalomyelitis (Chapter 419). An accompanied peripheral neuropathy is seen in vitamin B_{12} deficiency myelopathy (Chapter 425), which tends to cause gait ataxia. Rheumatoid arthritis (Chapter 272) causes progressive loss of cartilage and bone destruction, potentially leading to atlantoaxial instability and cervical subluxation. Other systemic illnesses, such as systemic lupus erythematosus (Chapter 274), Behçet's syndrome (Chapter 278), and sarcoidosis (Chapter 95), can also cause myelopathies. In patients with exogenous or endogenous hypercortisolemia (Chapter 234), epidural deposition of unencapsulated fat can cause epidural lipomatosis that compresses the spinal column. Patients with a distant history of trauma might be evaluated for post-traumatic syringomyelia. Patients with a history of lumbar puncture, surgery, or intrathecal injections can develop arachnoiditis.

Younger patients are more likely to be symptomatic from congenital disorders, ankylosing spondylitis, or multiple sclerosis. In patients older than 55 years, cervical spondylytic myelopathy is the most common cause of myelopathic symptoms.

TREATMENT AND PROGNOSIS   Rx

Acute traumatic spinal cord lesions are treated with high-dose steroids (Chapter 34). Steroids should also be used in cord compression from metastatic tumors (Chapter 195). Steroids are also frequently used in transverse myelitis, although no controlled trials have been performed.

Patients with spinal cord lesions must be assessed emergently for any potential complications. With high cervical spine lesions, paresis or paralysis of the diaphragm and respiratory depression can occur. Although not emergent, higher cervical or medulla extension of inflammatory myelopathies can cause distressing hiccups and nausea. In lesions at the thoracic level or above, interruption of the lateral column autonomic pathways can lead to autonomic instability, including altered blood pressure responses. At almost any level, but especially at the conus and cauda equina, acute urinary retention may require catheterization. Long-term complications of spinal cord injury include osteoporosis (Chapter 251), orthostatic hypotension (Chapters 50 and 62), and chronic neuropathic pain (Chapter 428), all of which may require specific therapy. Other aspects of treatment and prognosis depend on the specific cause.

Specific Causes of Myelopathy
VASCULAR MYELOPATHIES

The central nervous system tissue of the spinal cord is as intolerant of ischemia as the brain is. Vascular myelopathy occurs when there is loss of blood flow to the spinal cord, whether it is acute or chronic and whether the cause is ischemic or hemorrhagic.

The blood supply to the spinal cord comes from the anterior and posterior spinal arteries that run longitudinally along the length of the spinal cord (Fig. 407-7). The paired posterior spinal arteries are derived in their most rostral origin as branches of the vertebral arteries at the level of the medulla and then run inferiorly along the posterolateral surface of the spinal cord. Along their course, they are fed by a series of small arteries that enter the spinal canal through the intervertebral foramina. Inside the canal, they anastomose extensively to provide redundancy. The anterior spinal artery is formed superiorly when branches of the vertebral artery join to form a single anterior spinal artery, which then runs down the midline of the anterior surface of the spinal

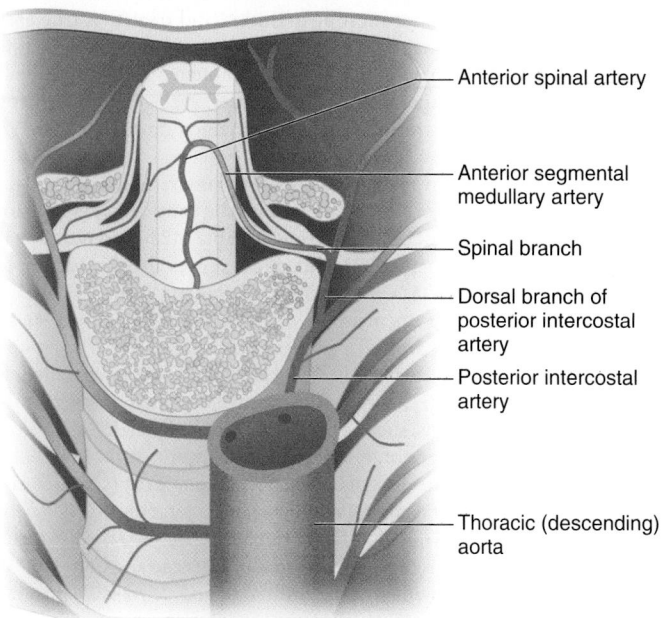

FIGURE 407-7. Blood supply of the spinal cord: section through thoracic level, antero-superior view.

Labels on figure:
- Anterior spinal artery
- Anterior segmental medullary artery
- Spinal branch
- Dorsal branch of posterior intercostal artery
- Posterior intercostal artery
- Thoracic (descending) aorta

cord. It also receives feeders along its length, but not to the same extent as the posterior segmental branches do. A large anterior radicular artery at C5-6 supplies the cervical enlargement. The main caudal anterior blood supply, however, is from the large artery of Adamkiewicz that enters the spinal canal between the cord levels of T9 and L2 and serves as the main blood supply to the anterior spinal artery, which supplies the lumbar enlargement, the lower thoracic cord, and the conus medullaris.

Compromise of the microvascular supply to the cord underlies the gliotic changes in many slowly progressive myelopathies, such as spondylotic myelopathy. Ischemic causes include general hypotension, atherosclerotic disease, embolic events, vasculitis, and vascular steal; hemorrhagic events usually result from rupture of abnormal vascular malformations.

Severe global hypotension or aortic dissection or surgery can cause ischemic myelopathy, especially in watershed areas of the spinal cord, notably the thoracic region. Atherosclerosis, especially of the artery of Adamkiewicz, can lead to ischemic infarction of the cord by either decreased perfusion or thromboembolic events. Ischemia has also been reported to be a result of compression of the anterior spinal artery by a centrally herniated T12-L1 disc.

Embolic events and local thrombosis can occur in pregnancy and sickle cell disease (Chapter 166). During decompression sickness (Chapter 94), nitrogen bubbles cause microvascular emboli and ischemia. Vasculitis affecting the spinal cord is rare, but granulomatous angiitis of the central nervous system and polyarteritis nodosa (Chapter 278) can lead to infarction.

Spinal dural arteriovenous fistulas are the most common type of vascular malformation of the spinal cord. Arteriovenous malformations are most common in the thoracic cord, especially in patients older than 30 years. Vascular malformations can cause myelopathy by being mass lesions that compress local structures, by interfering with normal venous drainage, by diverting blood as part of a vascular steal with exercise of muscles that compete for blood flow, or by hemorrhage.

Spinal cord hemorrhage, which is rare, can occur intramedullary in the cord itself or in subarachnoid, subdural, or epidural locations. Intramedullary hemorrhage is most often caused by trauma, although bleeding can also occur into a tumor or from an intramedullary vascular malformation. Bleeding from a malformation that enters the subarachnoid space can cause back pain and headache. Epidural hematomas, which cause extramedullary cord compression, can occur as a complication of surgery, myelography, or lumbar puncture, particularly in patients with bleeding diatheses.

CLINICAL MANIFESTATIONS

Occlusion of the artery of Adamkiewicz usually presents with signs of thoracic watershed ischemia—paraplegia with relative sparing of the sacral roots. Infarction in the anterior spinal artery distribution results in dysfunction of

the anterior two thirds of the cord, including the anterior horns, the spinothalamic tracts, and the corticospinal tracts; patients usually present with acute paraparesis and impaired bowel and bladder function. Sharp and sometimes circumferential pain at the level of the infarct is often described. Below the level of the lesion, temperature and pain sensation are lost, but vibration and position sense (posterior columns) are preserved.

Infarction of the posterior arteries is less common because of their better collateral circulation. Clinical manifestations, which are less dramatic, include loss of vibratory and position sense, ataxia, gait coordination problems, and Romberg sign; reflexes may be depressed at the level of the infarction.

The central cord vasculature syndrome is similar clinically to a traumatic central cord syndrome (Chapter 406). It may occur as a watershed lesion between the territories of the anterior and posterior spinal circulation and is most common in the cervical cord in older patients with preexisting cervical spondylotic disease.

Vascular malformations most often have a chronic progressive clinical course. Pain is common. Arteriovenous fistulas, commonly in the thoracic cord, present as progressive paraplegia. Patients may have exacerbations of symptoms with exercise and certain postures, and sudden worsening usually indicates hemorrhage.

DIAGNOSIS

Vascular malformations are initially evaluated by MRI, which also can assess the health of the surrounding tissue. When the vascular malformation is connected to the dura (arteriovenous fistula), myelography can occasionally detect lesions that are not seen or are poorly defined by MRI. If embolization or surgery is being considered, spinal angiography is needed to identify feeding and draining vessels, although the test carries a small risk of infarction. Intramedullary arteriovenous malformations are more commonly found in the cervical and thoracic levels and may require angiography to be visualized.

TREATMENT AND PROGNOSIS

Prognosis for most cases of spinal cord infarct is poor unless blood flow is restored rapidly. Treatment options are limited and include reversal of the cause of ischemia, for example, by correcting hypotension (Chapter 106) or treating for emergent sickle crisis (Chapter 166).

Arteriovenous fistulas are treated by occluding the shunt with embolization or surgery. Successful treatment may arrest and occasionally improve symptoms. Patients with suspected epidural hematomas (Chapter 406) require emergency treatment and surgery if there is progressive neurologic dysfunction.

INFLAMMATORY AND METABOLIC MYELOPATHIES

Transverse myelitis, multiple sclerosis, and other demyelinating diseases are considered in Chapter 419. Metabolic myelopathies can be caused by vitamin B$_{12}$, vitamin E, and copper deficiencies (Chapter 225).

Acute disseminated encephalomyelitis is mostly a monophasic disorder of demyelination of the spinal cord and brain. If it is isolated to the spinal cord, it might best be termed transverse myelitis. Parainfectious or postvaccination causes account for at least 75% of cases. Postvaccination acute disseminated encephalomyelitis is associated with measles-mumps-rubella vaccinations and diphtheria-tetanus-polio vaccinations as well as with vaccinations for influenza, hepatitis B, pertussis, and Japanese B encephalitis.

Connective tissue diseases can infrequently be a cause of myelopathy. Systemic lupus erythematosus (Chapter 274), with or without antiphospholipid antibody, can include myelitis in 1 to 3% of patients. Sjögren's syndrome (Chapter 276), Behçet's syndrome (Chapter 278), sarcoidosis (Chapter 95), ankylosing spondylitis (Chapter 273), mixed connective tissue disease (Chapter 278), and systemic sclerosis (Chapter 275) can be associated with inflammatory myelitis.

Human T lymphotropic virus type 1 (HTLV-1)–associated myelopathy/tropical spastic paraparesis (Chapter 386) is a chronic progressive myelopathy that causes leg weakness, spasticity, loss of vibratory sense, and bladder dysfunction. More than 90% of infected people remain asymptomatic, with transformation to a symptomatic condition thought to be largely related to the host's inflammatory response. Other neurologic dysfunctions associated with HTLV-1 infection include mild cognitive impairment, sensory neuropathy, and erectile dysfunction. There is no effective therapy.

DIAGNOSIS

In general, diagnosis of the inflammatory myelopathies is based on the clinical examination. MRI often shows a high T2 signal focal enlargement of the cord.

TREATMENT AND SECONDARY PREVENTION Rx

Intravenous corticosteroid infusions (e.g., methylprednisolone, 1 g intravenously daily for 5 days) are usually the mainstay for treatment of acute attacks of inflammatory myelopathies.

In patients who do not respond to corticosteroids, plasma exchange is effective in the acute treatment of central nervous system demyelinating disorders; about 60% of patients show improvement at 6 months. Factors predicting improvement are initiation of treatment within 15 days of the onset of symptoms and evidence of early improvement.

METASTATIC SPINAL CORD COMPRESSION

When metastatic cancer invades the spine or epidural space, the resultant destruction and growth compress the spinal cord and lead to a myelopathy. The prevalence of metastatic spinal cord compression may be as high as 5% in patients with cancer, depending on the type of malignant neoplasm and its tendency to metastasize to bone. Prostate (Chapter 207), breast (Chapter 204), and lung (Chapter 197) cancers each account for approximately 15 to 20% of cases, and non-Hodgkin's lymphoma (Chapter 191), renal cell cancer (Chapter 203), and multiple myeloma (Chapter 193) account for about 5 to 10% each.

Most metastatic disease causes compression as a result of an extradural lesion, although a smaller number of metastatic lesions can be intradural-extramedullary disease. Intramedullary metastases are rare. Symptoms can be caused by direct compression of the cord and roots in the epidural space as the result of direct extension from hematogenous metastasis to the vertebral body. However, some tumors, such as lymphomas, may grow through the intervertebral foramen without causing significant bone destruction; the accompanying edema can compromise the local vasculature and cause ischemic damage in addition to direct compression. Vertebral destruction can make the spine unstable and cause pathologic fractures, which can lead to cord and root damage.

CLINICAL MANIFESTATIONS

About 90% of patients present with pain that is classically worse on lying down and increases with the Valsalva maneuver. If the nerve root is involved, the pain will have a radicular component; if there is bone collapse, pain can be made worse by movement. Muscle weakness is present in 35 to 75% of patients at the time of diagnosis; sensory deficits are present in 50 to 70% of patients and autonomic dysfunction in 50 to 60% of patients. The range of signs will depend on the level of compression.

DIAGNOSIS

Spinal cord compression, which must be suspected when any patient with cancer complains of spine pain even in the absence of neurologic signs or symptoms, is a neurologic emergency. MRI is the test of choice because plain films, which might recognize bone metastases and vertebral collapse, will miss soft tissue tumors that are in the epidural space and yield no information about the spinal cord itself. Conventional myelography should be used if MRI cannot be performed because of availability or the presence of metallic implants in the patient. Because up to 35% of patients have more than one site of metastasis, care should be taken to image the entire spine by MRI, myelography, or isotope bone scanning.

Differential Diagnosis

For extradural lesions, the differential diagnosis includes lipomas, fibromas, meningiomas, and chordomas as well as vascular malformations and abscesses. Intradural-extramedullary lesions include neurofibromas (Chapter 426), neurinomas, meningiomas, vascular malformations, and, less often, metastases. Arachnoid cysts, although benign, can cause compression through pressure effect. Finally, intramedullary lesions that can present as myelopathy and must be considered in the differential of metastatic cord compression include intramedullary vascular malformations, ependymomas, astrocytomas, and syringomyelia.

TREATMENT Rx

Prompt initiation of corticosteroids (e.g., dexamethasone, loading dose of 10-16 mg followed by tapering over 10 to 14 days) and radiation therapy are the mainstays of initial therapy. Surgical decompressive surgery plus radiation therapy is better than radiation therapy alone for maintaining ambulation 15 in patients who have a radioinsensitive tumor, have displacement of the spinal cord on MRI, have a single site of cord compression, and have not been totally paraplegic for more than 48 hours.

PROGNOSIS

Metastatic spinal cord compression usually occurs in the setting of metastases to multiple locations, and the expected survival prognosis is generally less than 6 months. Prognosis is improved in patients with malignant neoplasms that are sensitive to steroid therapy (especially lymphoma and leukemia) or are radiosensitive (e.g., multiple myeloma, small cell lung cancer). Patients who are ambulatory at the time of diagnosis, have a single site of compression, and had a less rapid onset of symptoms also generally have a better prognosis.

Grade **A**

1. Chou R, Fu R, Carrino JA, et al. Imaging strategies for low-back pain: systemic review and meta-analysis. *Lancet.* 2009;373:463-472.
2. Gross A, Miller J, D'Sylva J, et al. Manipulation or mobilization for neck pain. *Cochrane Database Syst Rev.* 2010;5:CD004249.
3. Chow RT, Johnson MI, Lopes-Martins RA, et al. Efficacy of low-level laser therapy in the management of neck pain: a systematic review and meta-analysis of randomised placebo or active-treatment controlled trials. *Lancet.* 2009;374:1897-1908.
4. Vas J, Perea-Milla E, Mendez C, et al. Efficacy and safety of acupuncture for chronic uncomplicated neck pain: a randomized controlled trial. *Pain.* 2006;126:245-255.
5. Hagen KB, Jamtvedt G, Hilde G, et al. The updated Cochrane review of bed rest for low back pain and sciatica. *Spine.* 2005;30:542-546.
6. Chou R, Huffman LH, American Pain Society, American College of Physicians. Nonpharmacologic therapies for acute and chronic low back pain: a review of the evidence for an American Pain Society/American College of Physicians clinical practice guideline. *Ann Intern Med.* 2007;147:492-504.
7. Chou R, Atlas SJ, Stanos SP, et al. Nonsurgical interventional therapies for low back pain. A review of the evidence for an American Pain Society Clinical Practice Guideline. *Spine.* 2009;34:1078-1093.
8. Peul WC, van Houwelingen HC, van den Hout WB, et al. Surgery versus prolonged conservative treatment for sciatica. *N Engl J Med.* 2007;356:2245-2256.
9. Weinstein JN, Tosteson TD, Lurie JD, et al. Surgical versus nonsurgical therapy for lumbar spinal stenosis. *N Engl J Med.* 2008;358:794-810.
10. Benyamin R, Singh V, Parr AT, et al. Systemic review of the effectiveness of cervical epidurals in the management of chronic neck pain. *Pain Physician.* 2009;12:137-157.
11. Nikolaidis I, Fouyas IP, Sandercock PA, et al. Surgery for cervical radiculopathy or myelopathy. *Cochrane Database Syst Rev.* 2010;1:CD001466.
12. McAfee P, Cappuccino A, Cunningham B, et al. Lower incidence of dysphagia with cervical arthroplasty compared with ACDF in a prospective randomized clinical trial. *J Spinal Disord Tech.* 2010;23:1-8.
13. Roberts ST, Willick SE, Rho ME, et al. Efficacy of lumbar transforaminal epidural steroid injections: a systematic review. *Phys Med Rehabil.* 2009;1:657-658.
14. Weinshenker BG, O'Brien PC, Patterson TM, et al. A randomized trial of plasma exchange in acute central nervous system inflammatory demyelinating disease. *Ann Neurol.* 1999;46:878-886.
15. Patchell RA, Tibbs PA, Regine WF, et al. Direct decompressive surgical resection in the treatment of spinal cord compression caused by metastatic cancer: a randomized trial. *Lancet.* 2005;366:643-648.

SUGGESTED READINGS

Chou R, Qaseem A, Owens DK, et al; for the Clinical Guidelines Committee of the American College of Physicians. Diagnostic imaging for low back pain: advice for high-value health care from the American College of Physicians. *Ann Intern Med.* 2011;154:181-189. *Clinical guidelines.*

Chou R, Shekelle P. Will this patient develop persistent disabling low back pain? *JAMA.* 2010;303:1295-1302. *Review of the risk factors associated with the development of chronic pain.*

Deyo RA, Mirza SK, Martin BI, et al. Trends, major medical complications, and charges associated with surgery for lumbar spinal stenosis in older adults. *JAMA.* 2010;303:1259-1265. *Complications increase with the invasiveness of surgery.*

Graber J, Nolan C. Myelopathies in patients with cancer. *Arch Neurol.* 2010;67:298-304. *Review of the diagnosis and treatment.*

Klineberg E. Cervical spondylitis myelopathy: a review of the evidence. *Orthop Clin North Am.* 2010;41:193-202. *A review of clinical trial data, including current controversies.*

408

REGIONAL CEREBRAL DYSFUNCTION: HIGHER MENTAL FUNCTIONS

DAVID S. KNOPMAN

DEFINITION

Higher mental function is at the core of what defines competent, independent individuals. Impairment of higher mental function can be broadly classified into four categories. Mental retardation is a form of cognitive impairment that is present from infancy. Acquired forms of cognitive impairment are delirium, dementia, and focal cognitive disorders. Delirium (Chapter 27) is defined by its acute or subacute onset and coexistent alterations in alertness. Dementia (Chapter 409) represents an acquired cognitive impairment that is usually gradual in onset and not associated with alterations in alertness. Focal cognitive disorders involve only one aspect of cognition: memory, language, visuospatial cognition, or executive cognitive functioning, each of which is supported by a different cerebral region.

For the majority of patients in a non-neurology practice, a global description such as "normal mental function" or "cognitively impaired" will suffice. "Cognitive impairment" then becomes a diagnosis that subsumes all forms of altered higher mental function regardless of which domains are affected or how severely they are affected.

CLINICAL MANIFESTATIONS AND DIAGNOSIS

An informal conversation with a patient lacks sensitivity for detecting cognitive impairment. If cognitive impairment is suspected from the patient's history, formal assessments such as the Mini-Cog Test (see Table 26-4) should be performed. Bedside evaluations of orientation, memory, language, reasoning, and visuospatial function can be used to derive an overall view of cognitive function but do not automatically translate into diagnoses because alertness, cooperation, education, native language, sensorimotor function, and mood must be taken into account. Although scores on bedside mental status examinations correlate strongly with severity and prognosis, they provide only rough guides to cognitive ability and cannot localize a cognitive deficit anatomically in the brain. If cognitive dysfunction is discovered in the course of the bedside examination, further exploration of individual cognitive domains must be undertaken.

● MEMORY FUNCTION AND AMNESIC DISORDERS

DEFINITION

Human memory operates over a wide time range, from seconds to decades, and with quantities of information ranging from a single word to a lifetime's experience. Each neural system that achieves this monumental dynamic range has its own brain localization (Table 408-1).

Declarative memory describes the type of learning and retrieval of facts and information that occur with conscious attention and intent; examples include remembering conversations, events, and intentions. Declarative memory has semantic and episodic components. Semantic memory refers to the brain's storehouse of knowledge, words, and facts. Episodic memory refers to learning and recall of specific events. Retention of information for more than a few seconds, in the face of exposure to additional facts, details, or events, requires declarative episodic memory to store and organize the information suitable for later recall. It is this declarative, episodic memory system that is assessed as "memory" in the clinical setting. Anterograde amnesia is the clinical manifestation of disturbances in declarative episodic memory. "Anterograde" refers to failure to learn and hence recall new information on an ongoing basis. Most disorders of memory also exhibit retrograde amnesia, a disturbance of the ability to retrieve information from the past.

Immediate recall of information with zero delay and zero intervening information is a very short-term declarative memory function. Immediate memory is capable of storing an image of an auditory message in exact form, but only a small amount and for a short period. The fidelity of immediate memory recall accuracy drops off dramatically over seconds, particularly if intervening sensory stimuli attract attention. A comparable system exists in the visual modality in that the memory acts like a photograph that fades rapidly. From a clinical perspective, immediate memory is separate from declarative episodic memory. Immediate recall is generally used as a marker of attention and alertness and not memory per se. Loss of immediate recall is not usually indicative of memory loss.

PATHOBIOLOGY

The hippocampal formations are the anatomic structures of importance for the declarative episodic memory system. The hippocampal formations are imaged well with magnetic resonance imaging (MRI) (Fig. 408-1). The principal input to the hippocampus comes through the entorhinal cortex from multimodal association areas in the frontal, parietal, and temporal neocortex. A second important input is a cholinergic pathway that originates in the septum of the medial-orbital frontal lobe. There are two principal output circuits of the hippocampal formations. One is via the subiculum back to multimodal association areas. The other hippocampal efferent pathway projects via the fornix to the mammillary bodies. The projection from the mammillary bodies passes through the medial thalamus to the ventral anterior nucleus of the thalamus, then to the posterior cingulate, and then back to the entorhinal cortex. The hippocampal circuit is believed to facilitate the formation of memory in association neocortices. The hippocampus does not store a particular learned fact, but rather it enables the appropriate region in a multimodal association cortical region to do so.

Lesions in one hippocampal formation will not generally have as devastating an impact on episodic memory as bilateral lesions will. However, in older people who may have subclinical bilateral hippocampal pathology, a unilateral lesion, particularly in the dominant hemisphere, may produce a dense

TABLE 408-1	**DESCRIPTION OF MEMORY SYSTEMS**					
TYPE OF MEMORY FUNCTION	**REGIONAL LOCALIZATION**	**LEARNING EFFICIENCY**	**TIME SPAN UNTIL EFFECTIVE RETRIEVAL**	**CAPACITY**	**CLINICAL TESTING TECHNIQUES**	**EXAMPLES IN DAILY LIFE**
Declarative episodic memory	Hippocampus, medial thalamus	Single exposure	Decades	Very large, with rehearsal and elaboration	Recall of 3-4 words after 5 minutes	Recall of recent events and conversations
Declarative semantic memory	Temporal-parietal association cortices	Capable of single exposure; enhanced with repetition	Decades	Very large, perhaps limitless	Confrontation naming, general knowledge	Vocabulary, knowledge of life events from remote past
Attention span, "immediate memory"	Primary auditory or visual cortex	Single exposure only	Seconds	Very small: 7 ± 2 digits (auditory)	Digit span	Dialing a telephone number after hearing it or reading it
Working memory	Lateral frontal cortex	Single exposure only	Seconds	Small	Digits backward	Supporting many mental activities, such as mental arithmetic, abstract reasoning
Procedural memory	Basal ganglia, probably association neocortices	Requires extensive training	Decades	Moderate	Experimental laboratory methods only	Retention of motor skills, e.g., riding a bicycle or typing

FIGURE 408-1. Magnetic resonance images of a normal brain. **Upper left,** Midsagittal view; **upper right,** left lateral view; **lower left,** axial view through the head of the caudate and body of the thalamus; **lower right,** coronal view through the mammillary bodies, with a magnified view of the medial temporal lobe. at = anterior temporal; c = caudate nucleus; e = entorhinal cortex; h = hippocampus; hf = hippocampal formation; ip = inferior parietal cortex; it = inferior temporal; lpf = lateral prefrontal cortex; mf = medial frontal cortex; of = orbital frontal cortex; pif = posterior inferior frontal cortex (Broca's area); pst = posterior superior temporal; pv = primary visual cortex (area 17); s = subiculum; t = temporal; va = visual association cortex (areas 18 and 19). (Courtesy Maria Shiung and Clifford Jack, MD.)

anterograde amnesia. Lesions in the columns of the fornix, mammillary bodies, and medial thalamus have also been linked to anterograde amnesia.

CLINICAL MANIFESTATIONS

Patients with anterograde amnesia have poor or no recollection of events, conversations, or observations. Family members report that patients repeat themselves in conversation or re-ask the same questions over the course of a few minutes to hours. Patients will generally forget important events and conversations, even when they were fully engaged in them. They will lose track of the date and time of day. They will forget appointments, even with reminders. Generally, patients with anterograde amnesia will fail to encode most events and happenings around them. The consequences of such memory failure are usually more evident to the family and acquaintances of patients with the disorder than they are to the patients themselves. Anosognosia (lack of awareness) for the deficit of anterograde amnesia is very common, though not universal. Patients who most vehemently complain of memory loss are often suffering from depression rather than focal cognitive dysfunction.

Because some degree of forgetting is ubiquitous in human experience, it is challenging to distinguish between "everyday" forgetting and forgetting that is pathologic. All adults occasionally misplace important items, overlook an appointment, or forget some part of a conversation. In cognitively normal individuals, distraction, preoccupation, inattention, exhaustion, sleep deprivation, or other major life stressors inevitably produce some instances of excess forgetting. Pathologic forgetting as a result of a brain disorder produces a much greater degree of forgetting than occurs in the course of normal daily life, but there is no formulaic description of the boundary at which normal forgetting ends and pathologic forgetting begins.

DIAGNOSIS

The diagnosis of anterograde amnesia begins with a complaint of memory impairment from the patient or from someone close to the patient. Testing of memory can be performed at the bedside in alert patients. The patient is asked to learn three or four words and recall them after 1 or 2 minutes. A patient with severe anterograde amnesia will recall none or at most one of the words, whereas individuals with normal memory can recall all of the words or all but one.

In patients with questionable memory difficulties, assessment by an experienced neuropsychologist is often a necessary part of the evaluation.

Standardized tests of memory have greater precision and reliability and involve the use of lengthier material to be remembered and a longer delay between learning and recall.

Determining the Cause

Alzheimer's disease is the most common disorder in which anterograde amnesia occurs (Chapter 409). In Alzheimer's disease, anterograde amnesia is usually the dominant cognitive symptom, particularly early in the illness. Hippocampal atrophy is common (see Fig. 409-3). Anterograde amnesia also occurs in other dementing illnesses, such as vascular dementia and dementia with Lewy bodies.

Strokes can damage regions involved in episodic memory. Occlusion of the medial temporal branch of the posterior cerebral artery causes infarction of the hippocampus. Infarction in the territory of penetrating branches of the tip of the basilar artery causes bilateral medial thalamic infarcts.

Anterograde amnesia may be a major residual deficit after herpes simplex encephalitis (Chapter 382). Herpes simplex encephalitis has a predilection for damaging structures at the base of the cerebral hemispheres; frequently, the temporal lobes are severely damaged. Korsakoff's syndrome, the residual of the encephalopathy of thiamine deficiency (Chapter 425), is characterized by profound anterograde amnesia. Hemorrhagic necrosis of the mammillary bodies occurs in Korsakoff's syndrome. Survivors of closed head injuries (Chapter 406) may have anterograde amnesia because the medial temporal lobes are vulnerable to trauma as a result of their close proximity to the temporal bone. Survivors of an episode of anoxic-ischemic encephalopathy may also have dense anterograde amnesia. The pyramidal neurons of the CA1 region of the hippocampus are particularly vulnerable to hypoxic injury.

The syndrome of transient global amnesia involves anterograde amnesia, but the duration of the amnesia is a matter of 6 to 12 hours rather than the weeks or months seen in post-traumatic amnesia or the permanent deficits in patients with Alzheimer's disease or Korsakoff's syndrome. Transient global amnesia generally affects middle-aged or elderly individuals. Its cause is not known, although it is not usually due to typical cerebrovascular disease or epilepsy. Electroencephalography is typically not specifically abnormal, but diffusion-weighed MRI often shows distinctive abnormalities of the hippocampus a day or more after the onset of transient global amnesia.

● THE APHASIAS

DEFINITION

Aphasia is a disorder of language at the conceptual level. Aphasics may have difficulty producing language, comprehending language, or both.

PATHOBIOLOGY

In more than 99% of right-handed individuals, language is localized to the left hemisphere. In left-handed individuals, language is also predominantly localized to the left hemisphere, although varying degrees of bilateral or rarely right hemispheric dominance may be seen. The hemisphere involved in language is referred to as the dominant hemisphere. Anatomic differences in the temporal and parietal lobes of the dominant hemisphere versus the other hemisphere also reflect its specialization for language.

In clinical practice, lesions in the dominant hemisphere's auditory association areas cause receptive language dysfunction. The critical regions are located in the superior temporal lobes adjacent to the primary auditory cortex and in the adjacent supramarginal and angular gyri of the inferior parietal lobule, an area known as Wernicke's area. Lesions in the dominant hemisphere's lateral inferior posterior frontal lobes, often referred to as Broca's area, result in expressive language deficits. Loss of access to one's vocabulary for either understanding spoken language or expressing oneself results from lesions in any portion of the region of the dominant hemisphere around the sylvian fissure, including the lateral posterior inferior frontal lobe, the inferior parietal lobule, and the superior and middle temporal gyri. Coronal and axial MRI scans give a detailed view of the critical language regions (see Fig. 408-1).

CLINICAL MANIFESTATIONS

The language comprehension difficulties in persons with aphasia must be distinguished from hearing disorders (Chapter 436), and the motor speech dysfunction in aphasia must be distinguished from dysarthria. Errors of articulation in persons with aphasia reflect altered conceptual selection of what is to be said. In aphasia, mispronunciation of a sound within one word may be followed by perfect pronunciation of the same sound in a different word. In dysarthria, by comparison, the errors in articulation or phonation are consistent.

Aphasia has three principal components: impaired verbal comprehension, disordered verbal expression, and impaired naming. Disorders of reading, writing, and sentence repetition are additional elements of the aphasia syndrome. The disordered verbal comprehension may range from profound to mild. When profound, patients are unable to grasp the meaning of single words. In milder forms of disordered comprehension, patients may be able to follow one-step, but not two- or three-step commands. Usually, the comprehension difficulty involves both spoken and written language, but each can be affected separately. Anomia, which is an inability to produce names of people or objects, is common in almost all aphasic syndromes.

In expressive aphasic syndromes, written material and spoken speech are most often affected in parallel. Speech is labored in the expressive aphasias, and it lacks the normal melody and variation in intonation that characterize normal speaking. Melody and intonation are referred to as the prosody of speech. Speech is often grammatically impoverished. The number of words per utterance is greatly reduced, thus giving the speech a choppy, staccato character. These features are referred to as speech apraxia. Nonfluency is a related term that describes the reduced number of words and the terseness of verbal output. In some aphasic syndromes, speech is often degraded by anomia and paraphasic errors (word or syllable substitutions), even when fluency, melody, and intonation are preserved.

Specific Aphasic Syndromes

Specific, common aphasic syndromes exhibit various combinations of receptive and expressive difficulty (Table 408-2).

WERNICKE'S APHASIA

In Wernicke's aphasia, verbal comprehension of both written and verbal language is severely impaired. Patients with Wernicke's aphasia have difficulty understanding the meaning of individual words and may not be able to follow any command consisting of greater than one step. Their speech is fluent but marred by paraphasia and anomia. Wernicke's aphasics tend to lack awareness of the extent of their communicative difficulties and are often unaware that the words they are uttering are fundamentally incorrect. The location that typically causes Wernicke's aphasia is the dominant posterior superior temporal lobe or inferior supramarginal gyrus (see Fig. 408-1).

BROCA'S APHASIA

Broca's aphasia is a syndrome in which expressive language is prominently affected. Patients with Broca's aphasia have nonfluent, labored speech. The location of the lesion that typically causes Broca's aphasia is the dominant posterior inferior frontal lobe (see Fig. 408-1). Patients with Broca's aphasia have largely preserved comprehension and, as a result, are acutely aware of their difficulties and become frustrated with them. Depression is common in Broca's aphasics.

GLOBAL APHASIA

Global aphasia occurs when both expressive and receptive problems are present. Global aphasia often appears acutely after a major infarction, hemorrhage, or traumatic brain injury involving the dominant hemisphere.

ANOMIA

Anomia is at the milder end of the spectrum of language disorders. Some anomic aphasics also have difficulty with sentence repetition, even in the presence of relatively preserved comprehension and verbal expressive abilities. There is some controversy whether this latter syndrome, called conduction aphasia, represents a disconnection between the perisylvian centers for comprehension and expression or whether it represents a lesion in the cortical auditory areas involved in immediate auditory memory.

IDEOMOTOR APRAXIA

Ideomotor apraxia is a disorder at the interface between comprehension and execution of facial or limb motor actions. Patients with ideomotor apraxia have no paresis of the face or limb musculature and are able to carry out simple tasks, but they are unable to execute more complex tasks or commands. For example, in a woman who is able to name a comb and use her right hand to point to parts of her body, ideomotor apraxia can be demonstrated if she is unable to indicate through her actions how she would use the comb.

DIAGNOSIS

The diagnosis of aphasia is made by listening to the patient speak and by examining comprehension, naming ability, reading, and writing in a standardized fashion. Frequently, the diagnosis of aphasia is made during attempts to obtain a history from the patient. It is helpful to prompt patients to speak about a neutral topic, such as what they had for their last meal or what they did the previous day. Listening to their spontaneous speech allows the examiner to characterize its fluency, grammatical form, articulation, melody, and intonation, as well as difficulty finding words, the presence of paraphasias, and the overall information content.

Comprehension should be examined formally by asking the patient to perform tasks that range from one to at least three steps. Naming can be tested by asking the patient to name a series of common objects, such as the parts of the hand and arm (e.g., thumb, palm, knuckles, wrist, elbow). In general, the more commonly a word is used in the language, the easier it will be to name, whereas infrequent words are harder for aphasics. Reading and writing should also be tested.

Portions of the dominant perisylvian cerebral cortex may be damaged by infarction (Chapters 414 and 415), hemorrhage, and other space-occupying brain lesions such as neoplasms (Chapter 195) and abscesses (Chapter 421). Aphasia secondary to stroke has an abrupt onset, usually with some subsequent improvement. Recovery from aphasia after a stroke may occur as ischemic zones around an infarction eventually regain function. Regions remote from the infarction may also be synaptically depressed acutely after a stroke ("diaschisis") but eventually regain function. Finally, regions in the nondominant hemisphere may become more active over the course of recovery. Aphasia that has a gradual and slowly progressive onset occurs in the degenerative dementia syndromes of progressive aphasia and semantic dementia (Chapter 409).

TREATMENT   Rx

Speech therapy may be helpful for patients in the first few months after a brain injury that causes aphasia.

TABLE 408-2	MAJOR APHASIC SYNDROMES				
APHASIA SYNDROME	REGIONAL LOCALIZATION	SPONTANEOUS SPEECH ABNORMALITIES	AUDITORY COMPREHENSION	CONFRONTATION NAMING	SENTENCE REPETITION
Broca's aphasia	Lateral inferior frontal lobe	Nonfluent, labored, agrammatic	Preserved	Poor	Poor
Wernicke's aphasia	Posterior superior temporal-parietal supramarginal gyrus	Fluent, many paraphasic errors, very little information content	Very impaired	Poor	Poor
Global aphasia	Major portions of the frontoparietal operculum and superior temporal lobe	Nonfluent or virtually absent	Very impaired	Poor	Poor
Anomic aphasia	Small lesion somewhere in the perisylvian region	Fluent, may contain some paraphasias	Normal or mildly impaired	Poor to moderately impaired	Preserved or impaired

CORTICAL DISORDERS OF VISUAL FUNCTION AND HEMISPATIAL NEGLECT

DEFINITIONS

Cortical disorders of vision and spatial cognition are caused by lesions in the occipitoinferotemporal or occipitoposteroparietal lobes. The principal disorders of cortical visual functioning are alexia (impaired reading), object agnosia (impaired recognition of visual forms), and prosopagnosia (impaired face recognition). The principal disorders of spatial cognition are simultanagnosia (impaired integration of complex visual scenes), dressing apraxia, and visual hemispatial neglect (lack of awareness of the personal or extrapersonal hemispace). Diagnosis of a cortical visual disorder requires integrity of primary visual function from the cornea to the lateral geniculate nuclei.

PATHOBIOLOGY

Higher visual function is localized to a network centered in the occipital lobe and includes the inferior temporal and posterior parietal lobes (see Fig. 408-1). From area 17, processing of visual information passes to visual association areas 18 and 19. From there it proceeds in several directions. Disorders of higher visual function can be related to a ventral or to a dorsal pathway. The ventral pathway from the visual centers to the medial temporal lobe links visual information to meaning ("What is the object?"). The dorsal visual processing pathway, which links the visual centers to the parietal lobes, is concerned with locating objects in space and determining spatial relationships among objects in order to grasp a complete visual scene ("Where is the object?"). Cortical control of the extraocular muscles in the parietal lobes is an integral part of the process whereby the eyes are directed to various elements of a visual scene so that the individual elements are synthesized into a coherent ensemble.

Alexia occurs as a result of lesions in the ventral pathway of the dominant hemisphere. Object agnosia may also occur with lesions, usually bilateral, in the ventral pathway. Simultanagnosia, dressing apraxia, and hemispatial neglect are syndromes caused by lesions in the dorsal pathway. Simultanagnosia usually requires bilateral posterior parietal lesions. Dressing apraxia and hemispatial neglect arise from unilateral lesions, most often in the nondominant hemisphere. Cortical blindness is a consequence of bilateral occipitoparietal pathology.

CLINICAL MANIFESTATIONS

Alexia may occur as an isolated deficit, or it may occur in the context of other evidence of aphasia. Patients may be able to recognize individual letters but are unable to recognize a string of letters as a word. In pure alexia, auditory comprehension of words and sentences is preserved. Patients with object agnosia may be unable to identify objects visually, but they will be able to recognize the object based on its characteristic sound or how it feels to touch. In simultanagnosia, patients may be able to identify small objects easily if they happen to appear within the narrow viewing area at the center of their visual field. At the same time, such patients will fail to grasp the bigger visual picture. They may appear to be functionally blind. This clinical picture is referred to as Balint's syndrome.

Patients with cortical disorders usually have difficulty with visuoconstructional tasks such as copying figures or drawing simple objects such as a flower, a house, or a clock. Dressing apraxia represents a deficit of practical significance in which patients are unable to comprehend the orientation of articles such as a shirt or a blouse and to manipulate them.

The most severe form of a cortical disorder of visuospatial processing is cortical blindness. In this condition, in which the anterior visual pathways can be reasonably believed to be intact, patients appear functionally blind. On occasion, they also exhibit anosognosia for the blindness and claim that they can see. This latter condition is referred to as Anton's syndrome.

Hemispatial neglect occurs in the setting of acute strokes involving the nondominant perisylvian region. Even when there is no hemianopia as measured by single visual stimuli, presentation of double simultaneous stimuli to the patient reveals unawareness in the nondominant field. Hemispatial neglect can be demonstrated at the bedside with a task such as drawing a clock. A patient with hemispatial neglect will fail to place the numbers on the nondominant side (i.e., the left side in a right-handed person). Patients with hemispatial neglect may sometimes deny that their paretic limb belongs to them.

DIAGNOSIS

Information about visual functioning can be obtained from the history. The patient or the patient's informant may report that the patient cannot read, cannot read a clock, or cannot find objects when asked to get something off a table or out of a cupboard. There is often a history of motor vehicle accidents in which the patient failed to see another vehicle, the curb, or the side of a garage. Patients may report difficulty recognizing people's faces, even though they are able to recognize them by their voices or by other cues.

Bedside tests that screen for visuospatial deficits include either copying a simple geometric design or drawing an object. Intersecting pentagons and a cube are objects used clinically. Clock drawing is a brief, but informative exercise. Reading of words or commands and naming of objects can be done at the bedside as well. Face recognition is more difficult to assess at the bedside. Formal testing of visuospatial function in the neuropsychology laboratory involves the use of specially designed instruments to characterize visual processing.

The etiology of lesions that cause deficits in cortical vision and spatial cognition ranges from focal cerebrovascular disease, neoplasms, infectious processes, and brain trauma to neurodegenerative disorders. When a stroke causes a disorder of cortical visuospatial processing or hemispatial neglect, it is usually abrupt in onset. Space-occupying brain lesions such as neoplasms or brain abscesses that cause cortical visual disorders do so on a subacute basis. Disordered visuospatial function may also appear insidiously when caused by the degenerative disorder posterior cortical atrophy.

EXECUTIVE COGNITIVE DYSFUNCTION AND CONTROL OF PERSONAL BEHAVIOR

DEFINITIONS

Integrative abilities that are broadly referred to as executive cognitive function include mental agility, abstract reasoning, and problem solving. Executive cognitive function represents processes that support mental flexibility, adaptability, focus, and tenacity. Control of personal actions and regulation of interpersonal relationships are also closely related to executive cognitive dysfunction. The term "comportment" denotes how a person behaves, particularly toward other people.

PATHOBIOLOGY

The anatomic basis of executive cognitive function and comportment is a network of brain regions anchored by the prefrontal and anterior temporal lobe neocortex (see Fig. 408-1). These regions receive input from multiple cortical and subcortical regions. The caudate nucleus is the site of a major frontal lobe efferent pathway. The medial thalamus is a major afferent source to the frontal lobes. The anterior temporal lobes are also part of the same integrative circuitry as the prefrontal regions. Lesions in the lateral prefrontal regions are associated with slowing of cognitive processing, difficulty with set shifting (switching from one idea or task to another), difficulty initiating tasks, and loss of mental flexibility. The frontal and anterior temporal lobes are involved in the modulation of personal behavior and interpersonal relationships. Patients with lesions in the medial prefrontal lobes are often apathetic and lack initiative. Patients with lesions in the orbital frontal or right anterior temporal lobe may exhibit disinhibition, impulsivity, and a striking loss of ability to interpret or predict the feelings of others.

Traumatic brain injury (Chapter 406) is a common cause of frontal lobe and anterior temporal damage. The orbital frontal, frontal polar, and anterior temporal regions are particularly vulnerable to contusions because of their proximity to the skull. Patients with traumatic brain injuries may also suffer diffuse white matter damage as a result of shear injuries. Disconnection of the frontal and anterior temporal lobes from other parts of the brain can produce executive cognitive dysfunction and altered control of personal behavior.

CLINICAL MANIFESTATIONS

Executive cognitive functioning and control and regulation of behavior are usually affected concurrently. Patients with executive dysfunction are deficient in goal-oriented behavior; they lose the ability to predict the consequences of their actions or words. Patients with executive dysfunction also exhibit poor mental agility and inflexibility in their thinking and control of their actions. They are easily distracted and exhibit a tendency to perseverate, in which the answer to a prior question is repeated in response to subsequent questions. They are disinhibited; as a consequence, when asked to recall a specific event, they may glibly answer with a fabrication, a phenomenon referred to as confabulation.

Patients with lateral prefrontal pathology exhibit poor performance on tests of abstract reasoning and mental agility. In a test such as verbal similarities, they tend to be very concrete and narrowly focused. They become easily distracted and are slow in performing tasks that require sustained attention. Because of their mental rigidity and difficulty in set shifting, they do poorly on tests that require the ability to vary their response strategies, such as verbal fluency tests.

Patients with medial frontal lesions are often profoundly apathetic and lack initiative and motivation. They may be laconic and completely unable to express emotion, whether it be anger, sadness, or elation. They tend to be indifferent to their surroundings, a state referred to as "abulia." The majority of patients with substantial prefrontal or anterior temporal lobe pathology lack insight into the extent of their inappropriate behavior.

In contrast, other patients with altered comportment exhibit different manifestations of dysregulation of personal actions and interpersonal behavior. These alterations may include difficulty controlling impulsivity, poor social graces manifested as rude behavior or caustic comments, a disregard for the feelings of others (loss of empathy), and a general failure to understand what constitutes acceptable behavior in a particular social context. If the underlying disease is progressive, gross alterations in table manners and loss of interest in maintaining personal hygiene may appear. Inappropriate sexual behavior may occur. Patients with prominent disease of the frontal lobes may also exhibit hyperorality, which is a compulsion to put nonfood objects into their mouths. Hyperorality can be life-threatening, depending on the substance ingested.

DIAGNOSIS

The clinical history is essential for documenting the characteristic changes in personality, behavior, and interpersonal relationships. The history must almost always be obtained from an informant who knows the patient well because the patient may assert that there are no problems.

Mental status examination is an integral part of the diagnosis of an executive cognitive disorder. Simply interacting with the patient may be quite revealing. The patient may exhibit abulia, disinhibition, socially inappropriate behavior, or easy distractibility. Tests of executive cognitive function that are suitable for bedside use include verbal similarities and differences, the digits backward test, reciting the months of the year backward, or spelling a word backward. Verbal fluency, which is a very useful test of mental flexibility and set shifting, is tested by asking patients to produce as many words as they can that begin with a particular letter of the alphabet in 60 seconds. Frequently, a patient with a frontal lesion will quickly produce two or three words and then stop.

Bedside testing of executive cognitive dysfunction provides only a superficial view of the cognitive domain. Assessment in the neuropsychology laboratory gives a more refined estimate of the degree of executive dysfunction.

Space-occupying lesions of the frontal lobes such as neoplasms or brain abscesses can lead to the cognitive and behavioral syndromes of frontal lobe dysfunction. With these diseases, executive cognitive dysfunction and alteration of control of personal behavior develop over a period of weeks.

Neurodegenerative diseases such as frontotemporal lobar degeneration (Chapter 409) are associated with dysfunction and brain loss in the prefrontal (see Fig. 409-4) and anterior temporal lobes. These disorders may produce the entire spectrum of executive cognitive dysfunction and altered control of personal behavior over a period of a year or longer.

Some diseases that do not directly damage the frontal or anterior temporal neocortex may cause executive cognitive dysfunction and alteration of control of personal behavior because of the interconnectedness of the frontal and anterior temporal lobes with other cortical and subcortical regions. Multiple sclerosis (Chapter 419), a disorder of white matter pathways, may cause abnormalities in cognition and behavior of the frontal type. Similarly, Huntington's disease (Chapter 417) and progressive supranuclear palsy, which affect the caudate nuclei, may also resemble a frontal cognitive and behavioral syndrome and result in executive cognitive dysfunction and alterations in comportment.

TREATMENT   Rx

Cognitive-behavioral therapies offer modest, but definite benefit for patients with aphasia and for those with mild attention deficits and mild memory deficits caused by brain injury.

SUGGESTED READINGS

Bartsch T, Deuschl G. Transient global amnesia: functional anatomy and clinical implications. *Lancet Neurol.* 2010;9:205-214. *Review.*

Budson AE. Understanding memory dysfunction. *Neurologist.* 2009;15:71-79. *Clinically oriented review of memory disorders.*

Mahoney CJ, Rohrer JD, Omar R, et al. Neuroanatomical profiles of personality change in frontotemporal lobar degeneration. *Br J Psychiatry.* 2011;198:365-372. *Personality change in FTLD can be correlated with changes in regional gray matter.*

409

ALZHEIMER'S DISEASE AND OTHER DEMENTIAS

DAVID S. KNOPMAN

DEMENTIA

DEFINITION

Dementia, which is a disorder of cognition, interferes with daily functioning and results in loss of independence (Table 409-1). The majority of dementias are of gradual onset, are progressive in course, and occur in persons with previously normal cognition. However, none of these features are necessary aspects of the definition of dementia. Some dementias, such as those caused by an acute neurologic illness secondary to stroke, encephalitis, or head trauma, may begin abruptly and then remain static for long periods. Conversely, a small subset of dementias, such as Creutzfeldt-Jakob disease (Chapter 424), have a rapid onset and a course that can run for less than a year. Dementia may also occur in persons with developmental disabilities and long-standing cognitive deficits.

EPIDEMIOLOGY

The prevalence and incidence of dementia increase with advancing age. Dementia is uncommon before 50 years of age. In individuals older than 65 years, the prevalence of dementia of all types is about 7%. In the age range of 65 to 69 years, the prevalence of dementia is only 1 to 2%, but it increases to 20 to 25% in the 85- to 89-year age range and continues to rise steadily thereafter. The incidence of new cases of dementia is about 1 per 100 per year at the age of 70 years and rises to about 2 to 3 new cases per 100 per year by about the age of 80 years. Incidence rates continue to rise into the ninth and tenth decades of life. With the dramatic increase in longevity in North America, the societal burden of dementia has risen substantially.

In absolute numbers, far more women than men have dementia because women live longer. However, men and women have an equal age-adjusted risk for the development of dementia. There are no racial or ethnic differences in the risk for dementia.

TABLE 409-1   DEFINITION OF DEMENTIA

Based on evidence from the history and mental status examination, a disorder characterized by the presence of at least two of the following:
    Impairment in learning and retaining new or recently acquired information (impairment in episodic declarative memory)
    Impairment in handling complex tasks and reasoning abilities (impairment in executive cognitive functions)
    Impaired visuospatial ability and geographic orientation
    Impaired language functions

The cognitive disturbance significantly interferes with work, usual social activities, or relationships with others

The cognitive disturbance and the consequences for daily functioning represent a significant decline from a previous level of functioning

The cognitive disturbance does not occur exclusively during the course of delirium (which includes reversibility as a criterion)

The disturbance is not better accounted for by a major psychiatric diagnosis

PATHOBIOLOGY

Dementia is the culmination of dysfunction in the cerebral hemispheres, especially the association cortices, hippocampal formations, their supporting subcortical nuclear structures such as the caudate nuclei and thalamus, and their white matter interconnections (see Fig. 408-1). Specific diseases that cause dementia do so by affecting particular parts of the cerebral cortex, subcortical nuclei, or the underlying white matter pathways linking different cortical regions.

CLINICAL MANIFESTATIONS

Any of the major domains of cognition—declarative episodic memory, executive cognitive functioning, visuospatial function, or language—may be affected in dementia (Chapter 408). Because Alzheimer's disease is the most common dementia, anterograde amnesia is typically present first and most intensely in the majority of dementia patients. In other dementing illnesses, deficits in the other cognitive domains may be dominant. A pervasive and nearly invariant aspect of dementia is a loss of insight (anosognosia) into the extent of one's cognitive and functional losses.

Neuropsychiatric symptoms are also common in dementia. Apathy and loss of initiative are almost always present. Depression and anxiety are frequent, as are irritability, paranoia, delusional thinking, and hallucinations. Daily functioning of patients with dementia is compromised. In early dementia, difficulty is likely to be present in management of finances and medications, independent travel, preparation of meals, and keeping of appointments. In more advanced disease, difficulty becomes evident in basic activities of daily living, such as bathing, dressing, toileting, and feeding oneself. Dementias secondary to cerebrovascular or Lewy body disease are often associated with specific abnormalities in strength, coordination, gait, or balance. Alzheimer's disease, the most common dementia, typically has no associated motor abnormalities.

DIAGNOSIS

Clinical Examination

Dementia is strictly a clinical diagnosis based on evidence of cognitive dysfunction in both the history and the mental status examination. The key elements of the history flow from the definition of dementia: What is the evidence for impairment in one or more domains of cognition? What is the evidence that daily functioning is affected? The mental status examination is necessary to establish that alertness is preserved (i.e., the patient does not have delirium; Chapter 27) and to determine what specific areas of cognition

exhibit directly observable impairment. For diagnosis of the syndrome of dementia, no laboratory test supersedes the clinical history and the mental status examination. Laboratory testing is critical, however, to determine the cause of the dementia.

Bedside testing of mental status is based on the principles of cognitive neurology (Chapters 27 and 408). For moderate or severe dementia to be distinguished from normal cognitive states, a bedside mental status examination such as the Mini-Cog test (Table 26-4) is accurate. However, for mild dementia, bedside mental status examinations lack sensitivity (i.e., they fail to diagnose some cases of mild dementia). For patients with suspected mild dementia, neuropsychometric testing is a useful adjunct to the bedside examination. The neurologic examination is also important for evaluation of signs of specific causes of dementia, including signs of cerebrovascular disease (e.g., hemiparesis; Chapter 413) and signs of extrapyramidal disease (e.g., rigidity, bradykinesia, resting tremor; Chapter 416).

Differential Diagnosis

Dementia must be distinguished from other disorders of cognition (Fig. 409-1). Delirium (Chapter 27) also affects cognition directly; key features distinguishing it from dementia include impaired arousal and attention. Delirium is almost always of sudden onset, whereas the majority of cases of dementia are of gradual onset.

Primary psychiatric diseases (Chapter 404) such as major depression, bipolar disorder, and schizophrenia may also impair cognition. In dementia, however, the impairment in cognition is typically equivalent to or more pervasive than the changes in mood and behavior.

The principal diseases that cause dementia are three neurodegenerative diseases—Alzheimer's disease, Lewy body disease, and frontotemporal lobar degeneration—and cerebrovascular disease (Fig. 409-2). The neurodegenerative diseases that cause dementia are typically slow and insidious in onset and inexorably progressive. Dementia secondary to cerebrovascular disease may be of either sudden or gradual onset.

Many much less common secondary causes account for less than 2% of all dementias. Drug intoxication (Chapter 33), metabolic disorders (Chapter 425), central nervous system infections (Chapters 420 and 422), and brain structural lesions (Chapter 195) are typically subacute in onset; if they are diagnosed and treated early, the cognitive deficits improve or resolve completely. A number of medications such as sedatives, pain medications, corticosteroids, digoxin, and others cause mental confusion, particularly but not always at toxic levels (Chapter 110). Metabolic disorders that may also cause subacute confusion and produce a cognitive disorder include hypothyroidism or hyperthyroidism (Chapter 233), vitamin B_{12} deficiency

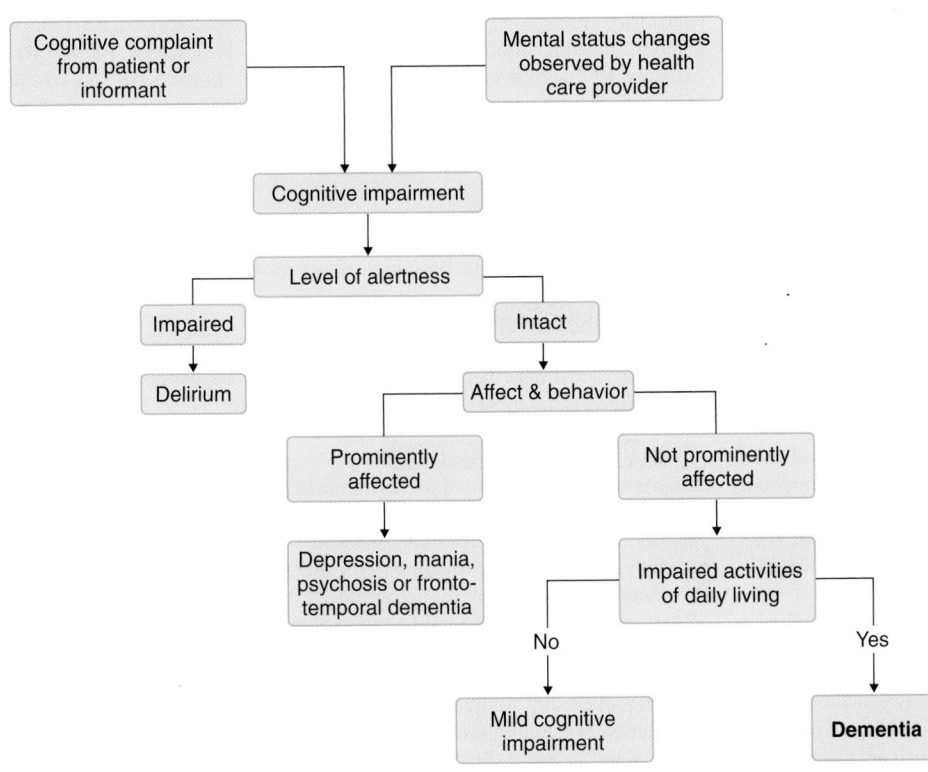

FIGURE 409-1. Flow diagram to establish the diagnosis of dementia.

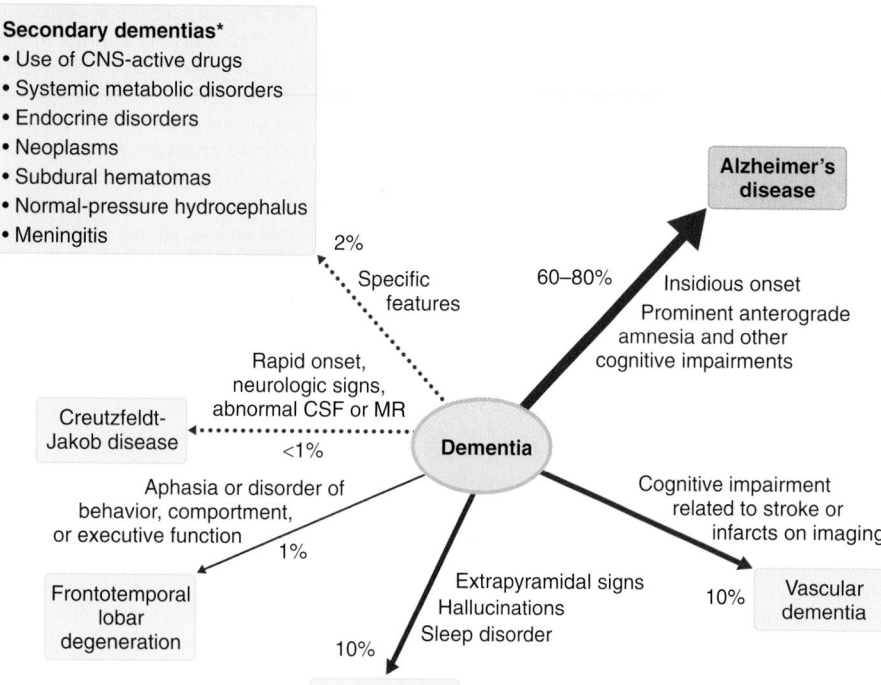

Secondary dementias*
- Use of CNS-active drugs
- Systemic metabolic disorders
- Endocrine disorders
- Neoplasms
- Subdural hematomas
- Normal-pressure hydrocephalus
- Meningitis

Alzheimer's disease — 60–80% — Insidious onset, Prominent anterograde amnesia and other cognitive impairments

2% — Specific features

Rapid onset, neurologic signs, abnormal CSF or MR — <1% — Creutzfeldt-Jakob disease

Dementia

Aphasia or disorder of behavior, comportment, or executive function — 1% — Frontotemporal lobar degeneration

Extrapyramidal signs, Hallucinations, Sleep disorder — 10% — Dementia with Lewy bodies

Cognitive impairment related to stroke or infarcts on imaging — 10% — Vascular dementia

FIGURE 409-2. Flow diagram for the differential diagnosis of dementia. The percentage contributions of various diagnoses are approximate. *The list of secondary causes of dementia is not exhaustive. CNS = central nervous system; CSF = cerebrospinal fluid; MR = magnetic resonance imaging.

(Chapter 425), chronic liver disease (Chapter 156), chronic renal failure (Chapter 132), and hypocalcemia or hypercalcemia (Chapter 253). Chronic viral infections of the brain, especially human immunodeficiency virus infection, frequently cause dementia (Chapter 401). Chronic meningitides in the differential diagnosis of dementia include cryptococcal meningitis (Chapter 344), tuberculous meningitis (Chapter 332), and tertiary syphilis (Chapter 327). Finally, structural lesions of the brain, including primary and metastatic tumors (Chapter 195), chronic subdural hematomas (Chapter 406), and normal-pressure hydrocephalus (Chapter 195), can cause a syndrome resembling dementia that consists of a subacute or slowly progressive decline in cognition with few or no other neurologic symptoms or signs.

PROGNOSIS

Except for the secondary causes of dementia and the rare dementing illnesses caused by single episodes of brain injury, such as severe head trauma or anoxic encephalopathy, dementia is a condition that invariably leads to worsening of cognition and function. Almost all dementia patients progress from mild stages to severe dementia during the course of several years, if they do not die prematurely. The rate of cognitive decline is variable among individuals and, of course, also varies with the specific disease. In general, dementia can be said to decrease life expectancy by half compared with the life expectancy of nondemented individuals.

End-of-Life Care

The terminal stage and end-of-life care issues (Chapter 3) associated with the common dementias are usually similar. Dementia itself does not directly cause death, but it is strongly linked to reduced survival. Patients with dementia typically die of the same illnesses that affect debilitated individuals, such as sepsis, pneumonia, pulmonary embolism, or heart disease.

Most patients with dementia experience their terminal illnesses in hospitals or extended care facilities. Given the inexorably progressive nature of most dementing illnesses and their likelihood of producing severe and completely disabling cognitive and functional impairment, it is widely accepted that patients with end-stage dementia should receive conservative care. Feeding tubes and ventilatory support should not generally be considered.

● MILD COGNITIVE IMPAIRMENT

DEFINITION

Mild cognitive impairment represents the transition between the state of normal cognition and dementia. Patients with mild cognitive impairment have abnormalities in a specific aspect of cognition to such an extent that it

TABLE 409-2 DIAGNOSTIC CRITERIA FOR AMNESIC MILD COGNITIVE IMPAIRMENT

The presence of a new memory complaint, preferably corroborated by an informant
Objective evidence of an impairment in episodic declarative memory (for age)
Normal general cognitive functions
No substantial interference with work, usual social activities, or other activities of daily living
No dementia

is clearly different from normal performance but does not interfere with daily functioning to any appreciable degree. More than one domain of cognition may be affected. The amnesic form of mild cognitive impairment, in which declarative episodic memory is impaired, is the most common. Alterations in attention, concentration, and mental agility may also be seen (Table 409-2). The term "cognitively impaired, not demented" includes patients whose mild cognitive impairment may progress to dementia but also encompasses anyone who is neither cognitively normal nor demented, such as individuals with stable, lifelong cognitive impairment.

EPIDEMIOLOGY

The prevalence and incidence of mild cognitive impairment are about the same as those of dementia. Both increase with advancing age.

PATHOBIOLOGY

Mild cognitive impairment is a risk state for the subsequent development of dementia. Alzheimer's disease, followed by cerebrovascular disease and Lewy body disease, is the most common underlying cause.

CLINICAL MANIFESTATIONS

Patients with mild cognitive impairment may have more insight into their emerging cognitive difficulties than do patients with dementia. Hence, some patients with mild cognitive impairment may themselves seek medical consultation because of concern about their memory or their thinking. They or their family members may report a milder extent of many of the symptoms of dementia. Patients with mild cognitive impairment forget recent events and conversations or have trouble with mental flexibility, multitasking, problem solving, or completing mentally challenging activities at the speed that they once did. Mental status testing will sometimes corroborate the complaints, but neuropsychometric testing may be needed to document impairment. Other patients with mild cognitive impairment may have virtually no insight into their memory loss, but the impairment is diagnosed after family members force the patient to undergo an evaluation.

DIAGNOSIS

When mild cognitive impairment is suspected, the principal alternative diagnosis is that the person is cognitively intact or that the person has dementia. The diagnosis of normal function should be straightforward when the patient and family have no complaints of cognitive impairment and the patient scores normally on bedside cognitive testing. However, a number of circumstances may cloud the issue, including very low or very high levels of prior educational and occupational achievement, instances in which English (or whatever the dominant language is) was a second language, severe hearing loss or blindness, and major alterations in mood or major motor disabilities that interfere with daily functioning. In such circumstances, the history of cognitive difficulty and the examination of cognitive status may be so confounded by these other phenomena that distinguishing between normal cognitive function and mild cognitive impairment is challenging. Conversely, distinguishing between mild cognitive impairment and dementia may be straightforward when daily functioning is obviously impaired. In other circumstances, it may be difficult to ascertain whether a person is functioning fully independently or not. For example, many older people reside in assisted living facilities that provide services such as cooking and housekeeping. In such individuals with few daily responsibilities, it is difficult to determine whether they are functionally impaired.

TREATMENT   Rx

As of 2011, no treatments have been approved for mild cognitive impairment, although a randomized trial demonstrated that donepezil therapy, 10 mg/day, significantly reduced the rate of development of dementia secondary to Alzheimer's disease at 1 year but not at 3 years.[1] Physical activity appears to provide a modest slowing of cognitive decline.[2]

PROGNOSIS

Mild cognitive impairment should be viewed as a risk state for the subsequent development of dementia. With use of the definition of amnesic mild cognitive impairment in Table 409-2, the rate of evolution from mild cognitive impairment to dementia is 15% per year.

● ALZHEIMER'S DISEASE

DEFINITION

Alzheimer's disease is defined as a dementing illness in which anterograde amnesia is a dominant symptom (Table 409-3). The clinical diagnosis implies that the causative pathologic process is of the Alzheimer type, whereas the pathologic diagnosis rests on the findings of characteristic histopathologic features.

EPIDEMIOLOGY

Between 60 and 80% of all dementing illness is due to Alzheimer's disease. Among all individuals older than 65 years, the prevalence of Alzheimer's disease is estimated to be about 5%. As with dementia in general, the prevalence doubles in every 5-year interval after 65 years of age, and the incidence continues to rise into the 10th and 11th decades of life. Men and women may

TABLE 409-3	DIAGNOSTIC CRITERIA FOR THE ANTEROGRADE AMNESIC SYNDROME OF ALZHEIMER'S DISEASE

Dementia (as defined in Table 409-1) with:
   Major impairment in learning and retaining new information and at least one other domain of cognitive impairment:
      Impairment in handling complex tasks and reasoning abilities (impairment in executive cognitive functions)
      Impaired visuospatial ability and geographic orientation
      Impaired language functions

The cognitive disturbance is of insidious onset and is progressive, based on evidence from the history or serial cognitive examinations

The cognitive disturbance is not better accounted for by a systemic disease or another brain disease

be equally affected, although on an absolute basis, far more women have prevalent Alzheimer's disease because women live longer than men do. There are no ethnic or racial differences in the predilection for Alzheimer's disease.

Risk Factors

Established risk factors for Alzheimer's disease include advancing age and a family history. Putative risk factors include diabetes mellitus, hypertension, cardiovascular disease, and head trauma; evidence for and against each of these four conditions is inconclusive, but the consensus is that at least diabetes and hypertension may play a role in the pathogenesis of Alzheimer's disease. Low educational achievement is also a consistent risk factor, but most experts believe that educational level is a proxy for some other factor, such as socioeconomic status or the early childhood medical and psychosocial environment. Protective factors have also been proposed, but their status is much debated.

PATHOBIOLOGY

The histopathologic diagnosis of Alzheimer's disease is based on the joint presence of a substantial cerebral burden of neuritic plaques and neurofibrillary tangles. Neuritic plaques consist of a core of aggregated β-amyloid peptide surrounded by degenerating neurites, which are fragments of axons and dendrites. β-Amyloid contains 39 to 42 amino acids and is proteolytically derived from a larger protein, the amyloid precursor protein. Neurofibrillary tangles are intracellular aggregations of an excessively phosphorylated form of the microtubule-associated protein tau. Neurofibrillary tangles, which are self-aggregates of tau, are thought to represent a nonspecific response to a cellular injury, which in Alzheimer's disease is triggered by β-amyloid. The altered tau protein self-aggregates and forms neurofibrillary tangles. In a low-powered microscopic section of frontal, temporal, or parietal cortex, at least six neuritic plaques and neurofibrillary tangles should be visible for the diagnosis of Alzheimer's disease to be made.

Pathophysiology

The progression of changes of β-amyloidosis follows a roughly predictable pattern in Alzheimer's disease. Positron emission tomographic imaging with ligands that bind to β-amyloid shows that β-amyloid begins to accumulate in the neocortex as long as 20 years before dementia occurs. Soluble aggregates of β-amyloid in oligomeric (consisting of a small number of monomers) forms may be the key pathogenic molecules that eventually induce neuronal injury. By the time that clinical dementia due to Alzheimer's disease is present, large numbers of β-amyloid peptide–containing deposits invariably are found in neuritic plaques in the neocortex. Neuritic plaques represent the end-stage of the Alzheimer process. Because β-amyloidosis begins well before clinical symptoms appear and probably reaches a plateau in terms of abundance, the amount of β-amyloidosis does not closely mirror the severity of dementia in Alzheimer's disease.

The regional extent of neurofibrillary tangles in Alzheimer's disease also follows a remarkably predictable pattern. The location of the earliest accumulation of neurofibrillary tangles is in the entorhinal cortex and hippocampus. At the time that clinical symptoms develop, neurofibrillary tangles are found in association neocortices of the frontal, parietal, and temporal lobes. It is only in the most severe and final stages that neurofibrillary tangles are found in the occipital lobes and primary motor and sensory cortices. The location of neurofibrillary tangles corresponds faithfully to the clinical evolution of specific symptoms and severity of Alzheimer's disease. In mild cognitive impairment, the earliest clinical manifestation of Alzheimer's disease, the most intense burden of neurofibrillary tangles is in the entorhinal cortex and hippocampi, precisely the regions that are involved in declarative episodic memory. Hippocampal atrophy is characteristic, and reductions in hippocampal volumes may be observed on magnetic resonance imaging (MRI; Fig. 409-3). Involvement of the association neocortices with neurofibrillary tangles represents the histopathologic correlate of the progression to dementia. Quantitative MRI in patients with mild cognitive impairment who later progress to dementia shows increasing atrophy of key cortical association areas, such as the lateral temporal lobes, inferior parietal lobes, posterior cingulate cortex, and lateral frontal lobes. Reflecting the spread to association neocortex, language functions, visuospatial functions, and executive cognitive functions typically become impaired some time after declarative episodic memory dysfunction occurs.

The most consistent neurotransmitter deficit in Alzheimer's disease is in cholinergic neurotransmission. The cells of origin of hippocampal and neocortical cholinergic projections are located in the septum, diagonal band, and

FIGURE 409-3. Serial coronal images from MRI of a patient with Alzheimer's disease. The scan on the *left* was performed when the patient was clinically normal. The scan on the *right* was performed 11 years later when the patient was demented. Hippocampal atrophy has increased dramatically from the first to the subsequent scan. (Courtesy of Maria Shiung and Clifford Jack.)

nucleus basalis. Neurofibrillary tangles accumulate in the neurons in these regions as Alzheimer's disease develops, but there is also neurochemical evidence that these neurons are stressed much earlier in the disease.

Genetics

The overwhelming majority of Alzheimer's disease is due to sporadic (not genetic) disease. However, in a very small number of instances, Alzheimer's disease occurs as an autosomal dominant disease. The three known genes involved in autosomal dominant Alzheimer's disease all are directly involved in the production of β-amyloid peptide. The first is the amyloid precursor protein (*APP*) gene, located on chromosome 21q21.3. Eighteen known mutations in this gene lead to excess production of β-amyloid and are reliably associated with a very early onset (20 to 50 years of age) of Alzheimer's disease. Another line of evidence implicating the *APP* gene in Alzheimer's disease is the invariable appearance of the pathologic process of Alzheimer's disease in individuals with Down syndrome (trisomy 21; Chapter 40), who have an extra copy of the *APP* gene as a result of the trisomy.

The other two genes associated with autosomal dominant Alzheimer's disease are the presenilin 1 and 2 genes, located on chromosomes 14q24.3 and 1q31.42. A large number of presenilin 1 mutations account for the majority of autosomal dominant Alzheimer's disease. Both genes code for a similar protein known as presenilin. Presenilin is involved in degradation of the APP molecule at the gamma cleavage site. It is believed that the Alzheimer's disease–causing mutations in presenilin 1 and 2 lead to a "toxic gain of function" that produces excess β-amyloid peptide. The presenilin mutations are also associated with early-onset (40 to 60 years of age) Alzheimer's disease.

Studies of the familial aggregation of Alzheimer's disease have shown that later-onset disease also displays genetic risks, but only one gene has been definitively linked to later-onset Alzheimer's disease. That gene, located on chromosome 19q13.2, encodes apolipoprotein E (apo E), a protein involved in lipid transport. In humans, three allelic variants of apolipoprotein gene (*APOE*) are determined by differences in the amino acids cysteine and arginine at positions 112 and 158 of the 299–amino acid protein. One of the allelic variants, with arginine at both positions, designated the ε4 variant, is strongly associated with a 14-fold increased risk for Alzheimer's disease in homozygotes and a 3-fold increase in heterozygotes. In many series, almost 50% of Alzheimer's disease patients but only about 25% of nondemented controls have at least one copy of the *APOE* ε4 allele. The presence of an *APOE* ε4 allele does not always cause Alzheimer's disease in that the disease never develops in some carriers of the genotype. The mechanism by which the *APOE* ε4 allele predisposes to Alzheimer's disease is not established, but the tertiary structure of the APOE protein with arginine at positions 112 and 158 may lead to impaired binding to β-amyloid, which in turn reduces the clearance of β-amyloid from cells.

CLINICAL MANIFESTATIONS

The early course of Alzheimer's disease is dominated by difficulties with anterograde amnesia. Some of the usual complaints include forgetting recent events and conversations, misplacing items, problems with keeping track of the date, getting lost in familiar surroundings, and problems with remembering to complete tasks. The frequency and severity of the memory lapses progress from occasional difficulty to more pervasive and consistent failure.

In mild Alzheimer's disease, declarative episodic memory function may be lost. Familiarity and access to previous knowledge may allow patients to function in their usual daily routines as long as nothing out of the ordinary is required of them. They may still retain the ability to prepare simple meals and to take walks in their neighborhood without getting lost. However, even in mild Alzheimer's disease, medication-taking errors and difficulty managing money or balancing a checkbook are likely to occur. Traveling to unfamiliar places often accentuates confusion. Changes in personality commonly accompany the cognitive losses. Apathy, loss of initiative, and loss of interest in previous hobbies and pastimes are ubiquitous in early Alzheimer's disease.

As the disease progresses, the ability to perform necessary daily tasks becomes more and more difficult to the point that the patient will need assistance preparing meals, paying bills, taking transportation, and keeping house. As the disease moves into the severe stages, assistance and supervision in basic activities such as bathing, dressing, toileting, and eating become necessary.

In the terminal stages of the disease, all communicative abilities may be lost. Mobility may still be preserved until late in the disease. Alzheimer's disease patients commonly die of illnesses that strike other debilitated elderly individuals, such as sepsis, pneumonia, and congestive heart failure.

The duration of the course of clinical Alzheimer's disease is long but variable. The time from mild dementia to death may be as short as 2 to 3 years or may be well over a decade. For patients in whom mild dementia is diagnosed, about 10% per year reach the stage of severe dementia.

Rarely, Alzheimer's disease is associated with prominent symptoms in cognitive domains other than memory. The most common of the atypical syndromes is one in which profound visuospatial deficits occur without the typical severe anterograde amnesia. This syndrome is referred to as posterior cortical atrophy.

DIAGNOSIS

The diagnosis of Alzheimer's disease, like that of dementia itself, is largely a clinical one based on the history and examination. The key elements in the history are a gradual onset and insidious progression of cognitive impairment, especially anterograde amnesia. The mental status examination should demonstrate impairment in short-term memory and other cognitive deficits. Alzheimer's disease should be thought of as a diagnosis of inclusion: if the history and examination are compatible with Alzheimer's disease and if certain exclusions can be verified, the diagnosis can be made with confidence.

No laboratory tests can confirm the diagnosis of Alzheimer's disease with sufficient sensitivity and specificity. For example, the presence of the *APOE* ε4 allele increases diagnostic accuracy only marginally after consideration of the history and physical examination. Findings on MRI, such as a decreased hippocampal volume, are useful when atrophy is present, but hippocampal atrophy is neither sensitive nor specific enough to be useful in diagnosis. Positron emission tomography with fluorodeoxyglucose or with newer amyloid-binding agents has yet to deliver the necessary precision or predictive abilities to warrant use in routine practice.

Differential Diagnosis

A number of other conditions that bear similarity to Alzheimer's disease must be excluded on clinical or laboratory grounds (see Fig. 409-2). One is dementia with Lewy bodies, which is suggested by the presence of parkinsonism, prominent visual hallucinations, and a specific sleep disorder. At autopsy, the pathologic processes of Lewy body disease and Alzheimer's disease often coexist, thus suggesting that the diagnoses overlap. Frontotemporal lobar degeneration is suggested by prominent behavioral and personality changes or by prominent language difficulties early in the course. Hippocampal sclerosis has unique neuropathologic findings but is virtually impossible to distinguish from Alzheimer's disease by clinical features. Other neurodegenerative conditions in the differential diagnosis of Alzheimer's disease include Huntington's disease (Chapter 417), progressive supranuclear palsy, corticobasal degeneration, amyotrophic lateral sclerosis (Chapter 418), and Wilson's disease (Chapter 218); however, these diseases invariably have prominent motor manifestations early in their course.

It is particularly challenging to distinguish dementia caused by cerebrovascular disease from Alzheimer's disease (see later). The fact that Alzheimer's disease and cerebrovascular disease often coexist requires clinicians to consider both simultaneously.

PREVENTION AND TREATMENT   Rx

There are no established preventive therapies. Although a healthy diet, physical exercise, and stimulating cognitive leisure activities are sensible, they have not been shown to protect against Alzheimer's disease. Except in patients who have folate or vitamin B_{12} deficiency, vitamin B supplementation is not effective in slowing cognitive decline.[3] Treatment of diabetes (Chapters 236 and 237) and hypertension (Chapter 67) is beneficial for other reasons, but it is not clear that such treatment alters the course of Alzheimer's disease.

Once Alzheimer's disease becomes symptomatic, support for family caregivers is a critical intervention that cannot be overemphasized. Support groups through the Alzheimer's Association (available at *www.alz.org*) can benefit families coping with the disease.

Important safety issues include supervision of medications, supervision of finances, and close scrutiny of motor vehicle operation. Operation of other potentially dangerous tools, firearms, appliances, and equipment should also be carefully monitored or avoided. Patients with Alzheimer's disease often wander and can become lost long distances from home. Identification of patients can prevent tragic occurrences (*www.alz.org/Media/newsreleases/2003/033003wandering.asp*).

Evidence-Based Treatments

Two classes of drugs are approved for the treatment of Alzheimer's disease: cholinesterase inhibitors and memantine, a glutamate receptor antagonist. The rationale for the use of cholinomimetic drugs (donepezil, 5 or 10 mg/day; galantamine, 16 or 24 mg/day; or rivastigmine, 6 to 12 mg/day) is the reduced levels of cholinergic markers in the neocortex of patients dying of Alzheimer's disease. All three agents delay the progression of symptoms to a statistically significant but clinically marginal extent at 6 to 12 months in patients with mild to moderate Alzheimer's disease, but not at 3 years.[1,4,5] Furthermore, there is no compelling evidence that they alter its biologic progression. Individual patients often do not show any clear benefits of treatment.

Memantine, which is a low- to moderate-affinity, uncompetitive *N*-methyl-D-aspartate receptor antagonist that acts on glutamate neurotransmission, also delays the progression of functional decline at a dose of 10 mg twice per day.[6] It is not clear why modulation of glutamate neurotransmission is beneficial in Alzheimer's disease, and studies of memantine in patients with mild to moderate Alzheimer's disease have not yet been published.

One study of patients with moderately severe Alzheimer's disease showed that vitamin E was effective in delaying progression, but recent studies showed no benefit in subjects with mild cognitive impairment.[1] By comparison, donepezil appears to be beneficial for severe as well as for mild disease,[7] although it has not been proven useful for the agitation that may accompany Alzheimer's disease.[8]

PROGNOSIS

Alzheimer's disease is inevitably progressive, and severe cognitive impairment and complete dependence on others develop in virtually all patients, unless they die prematurely. Alzheimer's disease also contributes to premature death; the mortality rate in patients with Alzheimer's disease is about 10% per year. In patients with advanced dementia, the 6-month mortality is about 55%; pneumonia, fever, and eating problems are associated with poor prognosis.

FUTURE DIRECTIONS

Intensive research on the pathogenesis of Alzheimer's disease is elucidating information on production and degradation of the β-amyloid molecule and mechanisms of induction of tau aggregation. Research is also focusing on the development of biomarkers, cerebrospinal fluid (CSF) markers, and imaging techniques for the early diagnosis of Alzheimer's disease. A number of therapeutic agents are also being studied.

TABLE 409-4	DIAGNOSTIC CRITERIA FOR THE SYNDROME OF DEMENTIA CAUSED BY CEREBROVASCULAR DISEASE (VASCULAR DEMENTIA)

Dementia as defined in Table 409-1

Clinically important cerebrovascular disease is demonstrable by *either* of the following:

    Onset of the cognitive disturbance *or* dramatic worsening of an existing disturbance that occurred within 3 months of a stroke, where stroke is defined as a focal neurologic deficit of acute onset in which the symptoms and signs persist for more than 24 hours

    Neuroimaging evidence of bilateral brain infarctions rostral to but including the thalamus

⬤ VASCULAR DEMENTIA

DEFINITION

Vascular dementia is a dementing illness in which the underlying cause is cerebral infarction. For a cognitive disorder to be attributed to cerebrovascular disease from a neuropathologic perspective, there must be sufficient cerebral infarction in locations known to be responsible for the cognitive deficits in the absence of other neurodegenerative neuropathologic changes (Table 409-4). When cerebrovascular disease produces cognitive impairment that is not severe enough to meet the criteria for dementia, it is referred to as vascular cognitive impairment.

EPIDEMIOLOGY

In clinical studies, as many as 20% of dementia patients have cerebrovascular disease. Like Alzheimer's disease, it is less common in patients younger than 65 years and increases steadily thereafter. In neuropathologic studies, about 25% of all cases of dementia have some vascular component. Roughly half that number are relatively pure vascular dementia; the remainder consists of vascular disease mixed with Alzheimer's disease. Men and women are equally affected.

Risk Factors

Risk factors for vascular dementia include cardiovascular disease, diabetes, and hypertension. There are no known protective factors other than treatment of these risk factors. Populations with high rates of generalized vascular disease should have higher rates of vascular dementia, but competing mortality from cardiovascular disease may obscure part of the relationship. In the first year after a stroke, the risk for development of dementia is about 9-fold higher than the rate in persons without a stroke; the risk remains about 2-fold higher in subsequent years.

PATHOBIOLOGY

The majority of vascular disease causing cognitive impairment is due to atherosclerosis. One mechanism is through large infarctions, such as those secondary to occlusive disease in major cerebral vessels, including the carotid arteries and the anterior, middle, and posterior cerebral arteries (Chapter 413). A second mechanism of infarction is at the arteriolar level, with lacunar infarctions in the thalamus, basal ganglia, and subcortical white matter. Both these processes can be detected by brain MRI. Infarcts in the hippocampal formations, medial thalamus, caudate nuclei, and parietal association areas are highly likely to produce cognitive impairment but not necessarily dementia. Microinfarcts, which are small zones of infarction that are not visible to the naked eye but can be observed with light microscopy, may also contribute to the dementia. The simultaneous presence of Alzheimer's disease is common in vascular dementia.

There are other uncommon causes of vascular dementia. Cerebral autosomal dominant arteriopathy with subcortical infarcts and leukoencephalopathy (CADASIL) is a very rare inherited disease that usually becomes clinically evident between the ages of 30 and 50 years and causes severe white matter disease, headaches, and dementia. The cause of CADASIL is mutations in the *notch3* gene on chromosome 19q12. Cerebral amyloid angiopathy, a β-amyloidosis in which the β-amyloid peptide accumulates in the media of small to medium-sized arteries in the leptomeninges and superficial cortex, causes cerebral hemorrhages that may lead to dementia if it occurs in sufficient number and in critical locations. Cerebral amyloid angiopathy is also seen in Alzheimer's disease, but its hemorrhagic manifestations may occur in individuals with little evidence of Alzheimer's disease clinically and modest evidence pathologically. Cerebral vasculitis (Chapter 278) is a very rare cause of dementia.

CLINICAL MANIFESTATIONS

The spectrum of cognitive changes in patients with cerebrovascular disease is broad. The more common cognitive syndromes in cerebrovascular disease include mild cognitive impairment, a dementia with prominent anterograde amnesia, and a dementia with prominent changes in personality and executive function. Some patients with vascular cognitive impairment without dementia may have deficits in only one domain (Chapter 408). A number of aphasia syndromes are a result of cerebral infarction or hemorrhage in the perisylvian regions of the dominant hemisphere. Infarction or hemorrhage in the occipitotemporal or occipitoparietal regions may produce one of the disorders of visual cognition, such as alexia or visual agnosia. Infarcts in the caudate nuclei, particularly if they are bilateral, may produce a cognitive syndrome that includes both amnesia and disordered executive function, thus mimicking dementia. Large infarcts in the right parietal lobe can also produce dementia. Infarcts in the medial thalami or in the hippocampal formations can produce isolated amnesia.

The evolution of symptoms in vascular dementia does not follow a stereotypical pattern. In some, the dementia syndrome may remain static. In others, new strokes may lead to substantial declines in cognition and function. Some patients with vascular dementia may experience a gradually declining illness. Patients with vascular cognitive impairment without dementia or vascular dementia may also have other neurologic signs typical of patients with cerebrovascular disease, such as hemiparesis, hemianopia, hemisensory changes, or cranial nerve abnormalities.

DIAGNOSIS

The diagnosis of vascular dementia is based on the neurologic history and examination. Brain imaging, preferably with MRI, is essential to establish the presence of infarcts. The cardinal diagnostic features of vascular dementia are that (1) the cognitive disorder should have begun within 3 months of a clinical stroke event and (2) there should be multiple, bilateral infarcts in the cerebral hemispheres visible on brain imaging studies. A temporal link between the onset or worsening of cognitive impairment and a stroke is important in demonstrating that cerebrovascular disease is etiologically relevant to the cognitive impairment. Brain imaging of infarcts in the cerebral cortex, basal ganglia, thalamus, and cerebral white matter has obvious value for establishment of cerebrovascular disease. In contrast to actual infarcts on imaging, the presence of white matter hyperintensities without infarcts on brain MRI is much less specific.

The accuracy of the clinical diagnosis of vascular dementia is generally lower than that of Alzheimer's disease. The combination of (1) a temporal relationship between dementia and a stroke and (2) imaging evidence of bilateral infarcts is diagnostically specific for vascular dementia but is insensitive. Broader diagnostic criteria (see Table 409-4) are more sensitive but less specific. The usual alternative diagnosis is Alzheimer's disease, and there is typically no way to be certain whether and how much Alzheimer's disease is simultaneously present.

PREVENTION AND TREATMENT **Rx**

Some cases of vascular dementia should be preventable. With early, lifelong aggressive treatment of diabetes (Chapters 236 and 237), hypertension (Chapter 67), and hyperlipidemia (Chapter 213), the number of cerebral infarcts should be reduced, with a corresponding reduction in the number of cases of vascular dementia. Evidence for this link comes from large-scale studies in which the treatment of hypertension reduced the frequency of strokes and incident dementia. Once vascular dementia develops, cholinesterase inhibitors have shown some benefit,[9] but the major goal is to prevent future strokes.

PROGNOSIS

Patients with vascular dementia can often be expected to have severe cardiovascular disease and a greater likelihood of future strokes and cardiac ischemic events. Survival of patients with vascular dementia is poorer than that of patients with Alzheimer's disease.

TABLE 409-5	DIAGNOSTIC CRITERIA FOR THE DEMENTIA SYNDROME ASSOCIATED WITH LEWY BODY PATHOLOGY

Dementia as defined in Table 409-1

The cognitive disturbance is of insidious onset and is progressive, based on evidence from the history or serial cognitive examination

The presence of at least two of the following:
 Parkinsonism (rigidity, resting tremor, bradykinesia, postural instability, parkinsonian gait disorder)
 Prominent, fully formed visual hallucinations
 Substantial fluctuations in alertness or cognition
 Rapid eye movement sleep behavior disorder (see Chapter 412)
 Severe worsening of parkinsonism by antipsychotic drugs

The disturbance is not better accounted for by a systemic disease or another brain disease

DEMENTIA WITH LEWY BODIES

DEFINITION

Dementia with Lewy bodies is a multifaceted dementing disorder in which the underlying pathologic process includes Lewy bodies in limbic and cortical structures (Table 409-5). Some clinicians make a distinction between patients in whom parkinsonism preceded the cognitive disorder and those in whom the cognitive disorder occurred either simultaneously with or before the movement disorder. This distinction may be somewhat useful in clinical practice, but there are few clinical or neuropathologic differences based on different sequences of signs and symptoms. The diagnosis of dementia with Lewy bodies is similar in principle to diagnosis of both dementia and Parkinson's disease (Chapter 416) in the same individual, but dementia with Lewy bodies is a term with broader connotations because of other features (hallucinations, fluctuations, and sleep disorder) that may be more apparent than the movement disorder.

EPIDEMIOLOGY

Dementia with Lewy bodies is about a quarter as common as Alzheimer's disease. Lewy body disease becomes more common with advancing age, and the prevalence of dementia with Lewy bodies increases with advancing age as well. As with the other dementias, there are no known ethnic or racial differences, but dementia with Lewy bodies may be more common in men. There are no known risk factors for dementia with Lewy bodies. Dementia develops in up to 30% of patients with Parkinson's disease, and advancing age is the major risk factor.

PATHOBIOLOGY

The pathology of dementia with Lewy bodies is a mixture of Lewy body disease and Alzheimer's disease. In general, the more intense the Lewy body disease, the less abundant the Alzheimer disease. Lewy bodies, which are intraneuronal inclusions that contain α-synuclein, are found in the nucleus basalis, pars compacta of the substantia nigra, locus caeruleus, other brain stem structures, amygdala, cingulate gyrus, and neocortex. The earliest locations of Lewy bodies are the brain stem, where they affect nuclei involved in sleep and arousal, and the substantia nigra, the locus caeruleus, and cranial nerve nuclei IX and X. Typically, the nucleus basalis, transentorhinal cortex, cingulate gyrus, and neocortex become involved later.

In Lewy body disease, the α-synuclein protein becomes misfolded and aggregates intraneuronally. Mutations in the α-synuclein gene have been seen in a few families with autosomal dominant Parkinson's disease, but most cases of dementia with Lewy bodies are sporadic.

CLINICAL MANIFESTATIONS

The clinical manifestations of dementia with Lewy bodies include four major abnormalities: the cognitive disorder, the neuropsychiatric disorder, the motor disorder, and the disorder of sleep and wakefulness. The cognitive disorder may differ from Alzheimer's disease, although there is considerable overlap. In a typical patient with dementia with Lewy bodies, visuospatial deficits, impaired concentration, and impaired attention dominate the picture. In some patients, the deficits in executive functions may be similar to what is seen in frontotemporal lobar degeneration. Anterograde amnesia is usually present but milder than in Alzheimer's disease. Language deficits are not prominent. The neuropsychiatric manifestations of dementia with

Lewy bodies, including prominent apathy, loss of initiative, and depression, may be more disabling than the cognitive symptoms. The motor manifestations include bradykinesia, gait disturbances, postural disturbances, and rigidity. Rest tremor is less common in dementia with Lewy bodies in patients in whom the cognitive disorder appears before the parkinsonism. Visual hallucinations, fluctuations in alertness, and REM sleep disorders are part of a broader disorder of the regulation of sleep and wakefulness. Visual hallucinations are often graphic, detailed, and bizarre, perhaps because the sleep phenomenon of dreaming intrudes into wakefulness. Patients with dementia with Lewy bodies have large fluctuations in their alertness and arousal from day to day.

REM sleep behavior disorder (Chapter 412) is a parasomnia in which patients exhibit dream enactment behavior, often with violent, threatening overtones. Patients typically relate that they feel as though they are being chased by something or someone. Their behavior, while they are asleep, consists of excessive talking, calling out or shouting, and thrashing about, often to the point of striking a bed partner or falling out of bed. The REM sleep behavior disorder may precede the development of Parkinson's disease and dementia with Lewy bodies by years.

DIAGNOSIS

The diagnosis of dementia with Lewy bodies is based on clinical information that corroborates the presence of abnormalities in cognition, motor function, neuropsychiatric behavior, and regulation of sleep and wakefulness. Formal neuropsychological testing is often helpful in evaluating memory, executive function, and visuospatial function in a detailed manner. Neuroimaging has only a limited role in the diagnosis of dementia with Lewy bodies.

Differential Diagnosis

Other disorders that must be considered in patients with dementia and a movement disorder include progressive supranuclear palsy (Chapter 417), which can resemble dementia with Lewy bodies in terms of both the dementia and the motor disorder. In progressive supranuclear palsy, patients are much less likely to have disorders of arousal and typically have other distinctive signs and symptoms, including the characteristic supranuclear gaze palsy and other brain stem findings. The corticobasal degenerations, which are members of the family of frontotemporal lobar dementias (see later), may also produce a movement disorder and dementia. Huntington's disease (Chapter 417) is associated with dementia and a movement disorder, but the movement disorder of Huntington's disease includes prominent chorea and athetosis, neither of which is present in dementia with Lewy bodies.

Normal-pressure hydrocephalus (Chapter 195) is a rare disorder typically characterized by the triad of a gait disorder, dementia, and urinary incontinence. Normal-pressure hydrocephalus can be suspected when computed tomography or MRI shows ventricular enlargement that is out of proportion to the amount of sulcal widening. Predicting a favorable response to ventriculoperitoneal shunting in suspected normal-pressure hydrocephalus has proved to be difficult. Imaging studies that measure CSF flow through the aqueduct of Sylvius or that measure flow of radiolabeled CSF with radionuclide cisternography have not been useful. Clinical response to the removal of a high volume (e.g., 30 mL) of CSF through lumbar puncture is sometimes used to select patients for surgery, although its positive and negative predictive value is unclear. Normal-pressure hydrocephalus is very rare relative to dementia with Lewy bodies and Alzheimer's disease.

TREATMENT ℞

Management of patients with dementia with Lewy bodies is challenging because of the simultaneous appearance of a cognitive disorder, a neuropsychiatric disorder, a motor disorder, and a sleep and wakefulness disorder. Treatment of the motor disorder is accomplished with antiparkinsonian drugs such as levodopa and dopaminergic agonists (Chapter 416). Treatment with these agents should be instituted for dementia with Lewy bodies if there are prominent gait or balance problems that threaten safety and interfere with independence. These medications may worsen hallucinations and exacerbate confusional states, but this concern should not preclude a treatment trial if the motor symptoms pose safety risks or interfere with independence. Cholinesterase inhibitors, which do not exacerbate parkinsonian symptoms, have a beneficial effect on neuropsychiatric symptoms but not clearly on the cognitive disorder.[10]

Hallucinations and agitation impair quality of life for the patient and family and often require treatment. Some antipsychotic agents that might otherwise control these symptoms dramatically exacerbate the parkinsonism in dementia with Lewy bodies. Atypical antipsychotics are usually recommended, but there is insufficient experience from controlled clinical trials. Many movement disorder specialists prefer to use quetiapine in doses of 25 to 200 mg/day or clozapine at 6.25 to 50 mg/day because these agents appear to have the lowest rate of extrapyramidal side effects. However, it is not possible to make any strong statements about the relative efficacy of atypical antipsychotics in treating the hallucinations in dementia with Lewy bodies, especially in view of the possibility that atypical antipsychotic agents may be associated with higher than expected mortality.

The REM sleep behavior disorder (Chapter 412) can be disabling, but there are no controlled clinical trials to inform treatment. Some sleep disorder specialists typically use either melatonin, 3 to 12 mg, or clonazepam, 0.5 to 2 mg, at bedtime.

Treatment of depressive symptoms may substantially improve a patient's functioning. Use of one of the newer generation of antidepressants, such as sertraline in a dose of 25 to 100 mg/day or citalopram in a dose of 10 to 20 mg/day, may be beneficial and does not necessarily interfere with management of the other symptoms (Chapter 404).

PROGNOSIS

As opposed to patients with Alzheimer's disease, some studies show that patients with dementia with Lewy bodies have a more rapidly progressive course and poorer survival. As a result of the combination of manifestations, patients with dementia with Lewy bodies may become disabled sooner in their course.

FUTURE DIRECTIONS

Because the REM sleep behavior disorder often precedes the development of dementia with Lewy bodies, early diagnosis offers an opportunity for early intervention. Progress in understanding of the production and degradation of α-synuclein may lead to more specific therapies.

FRONTOTEMPORAL LOBAR DEGENERATION

DEFINITION

The frontotemporal lobar degenerations are a group of neurodegenerative disorders with distinctive clinical manifestations and a predilection for the prefrontal and anterior temporal neocortices. The most common clinical syndrome is a disorder of behavior and personal relationships (comportment) with a loss of executive functions (Table 409-6). This syndrome is referred to as behavior-variant frontotemporal dementia. Other syndromes in the clinical spectrum of frontotemporal lobar degeneration involve different aspects of language or motor dysfunction of the limbs.

EPIDEMIOLOGY

Unlike Alzheimer's disease, the frontotemporal lobar degenerations have a peak age at onset in the 50- to 70-year range, and the incidence declines after the age of 70 years. In patients with dementia who are younger than 70 years, frontotemporal lobar degeneration makes up 10 to 20% of cases. However,

TABLE 409-6	DIAGNOSTIC CRITERIA FOR FRONTOTEMPORAL DEMENTIA

Based on evidence from the history and mental status examination, a disorder characterized by the early *and* predominant presence of *either* of the following:
    Decline in regulation of personal or social interpersonal conduct (as characterized by loss of empathy for the feelings of others; socially inappropriate behavior that is rude, caustic, irresponsible, or sexually explicit; mental rigidity; impulsivity typically with poor judgment; inflexibility in interpersonal relationships or emotional blunting; apathy; disregard for personal hygiene and grooming; deviations in previous dietary preferences or habits; binge eating)
    Impairment in mental agility, reasoning, or handling of complex tasks out of proportion to impairment in the domains of declarative episodic memory or visuospatial abilities

The cognitive or behavioral disturbances are of gradual onset and are progressive, based on evidence from the history or serial cognitive examination

The cognitive disturbance significantly interferes with work, usual social activities, or relationships with others

The cognitive disturbance and the changes in daily functioning represent a significant decline from a previous level of functioning

Not occurring exclusively during the course of delirium

The disturbance is not better accounted for by a major psychiatric diagnosis, a systemic disease, or another brain disease across the entire age spectrum, the frontotemporal lobar degenerations are much less common than Alzheimer's disease, dementia with Lewy bodies, or vascular dementia. Both men and women are affected equally. There are no known risk factors for the frontotemporal lobar degenerations except a family history.

PATHOBIOLOGY

The clinical syndrome in frontotemporal lobar degeneration is determined by the lobar location of the pathologic process. Right prefrontal or anterior temporal disease and brain atrophy produce behavioral syndromes like frontotemporal dementia. Left frontal involvement tends to produce progressive nonfluent aphasia. Predominant left anterior temporal lobe involvement may produce semantic dementia.

On histopathologic grounds, patients with frontotemporal lobar degeneration can be divided into three groups: those whose inclusions contain the microtubule-associated protein tau; those whose inclusions contain the TAR DNA-binding protein 43 (TDP-43); and those whose inclusions contain the fused in sarcoma (FUS) protein, another nucleic acid–binding protein. Each type includes both genetically determined and sporadic forms.

Among the tau-positive varieties are Pick's disease, in which intracellular tau-positive inclusions known as Pick bodies are seen. Several other pathologic tau-positive subtypes occur, including progressive supranuclear palsy, corticobasal degeneration, and the disorder associated with mutations in the tau gene. Nearly 50 mutations in the tau gene on chromosome 17q21 are associated with autosomal dominant frontotemporal lobar degeneration syndromes, each with a slightly different clinical and neuropathologic phenotype. The most common is a proline to leucine mutation at codon 301, located in exon 10. The tau gene undergoes alternative splicing, resulting in six isoforms of the tau protein. Pathologic mutations appear to disrupt splicing of alternative isoforms of tau protein, which in turn adversely affects the binding of tau to microtubules in neurons. Reduced binding of tau to microtubules is deleterious to microtubule function and neuronal integrity.

The TDP-43–positive frontotemporal lobar degenerations are almost equally common. Immunostaining shows that there are distinctive TDP-43–containing inclusions. Mutations in the granulin (*GRN*) gene, also located on chromosome 17q21, cause familial, autosomal dominant forms of frontotemporal lobar degeneration with TDP-43–positive inclusions. Nearly 70 different mutations in the granulin gene are linked to frontotemporal lobar degenerations. All of the mutations lead to premature degradation of the messenger RNA, a process termed haploinsufficiency. Granulin mutation carriers have an abnormally low amount of the protein progranulin. The normal function of granulin in the brain is unclear, and the pathophysiologic basis for dementia in persons with granulin gene mutations is unknown. The link between alterations in TDP-43 and *GRN* mutations is also unknown at this time.

Frontotemporal lobar degenerations that are FUS positive are much less common. At this time, all FUS-positive cases have had the behavioral variant of frontotemporal dementia.

CLINICAL MANIFESTATIONS

The clinical manifestations of the syndrome of frontotemporal dementia begin insidiously. Apathy, loss of initiative, and flattening of affect are common early symptoms. As the disease progresses, the entire spectrum of behavioral changes associated with dysfunction of the frontal and anterior temporal lobes appears. On cognitive assessments, patients may have preserved memory functions, but they typically have difficulty with tests of executive cognitive function. When frontotemporal dementia progresses to moderate or severe stages, the behavioral changes remain prominent, but the disease becomes more difficult to distinguish from other dementias such as Alzheimer's disease. The neuropathology of behavior-variant frontotemporal dementia may be either tau positive or TDP-43 positive.

In some patients with frontotemporal lobar degeneration, signs and symptoms of motor neuron disease develop, such as weakness, atrophy, and fasciculation in the limbs or the bulbar musculature (Chapter 418). In other patients with frontotemporal lobar degeneration, asymmetrical limb apraxia develops that is part of the corticobasal syndrome. Features of progressive supranuclear palsy may also appear in patients with behavior-variant frontotemporal dementia.

Frontotemporal lobar degeneration can be manifested as a progressive nonfluent aphasia in which patients experience a feeling of hesitancy in selecting words in their speech, a problem that may be difficult for others to appreciate at first. Anomia is an early sign. Gradually, the patient's speech becomes laconic and labored. Eventually, a nonfluent, apractic, agrammatic speech develops. In other cognitive domains, progressive nonfluent aphasics as well as progressive anomic aphasics often have no deficits. As the diseases progress, however, a pervasive cognitive disorder develops in some patients. Other progressive nonfluent aphasics may eventually become virtually mute, even though they may appear to have preserved memory and visuospatial functions. Patients with progressive nonfluent aphasia often have tau-positive neuropathologic findings.

Semantic dementia is a disorder that involves dissolution of the meaning of words or objects. A patient with semantic dementia may also become unable to access knowledge about objects (object agnosia) and people's faces (prosopagnosia). The most striking demonstration of the deficit in semantic dementia is when a patient can produce the name of an object—a watch, for example—but then cannot say what a watch is for when asked. Often, patients with semantic dementia have preservation of the ability to learn a list of words, even if their knowledge of the meaning of the words is diminished. Patients with semantic dementia usually have TDP-43–positive neuropathologic findings.

DIAGNOSIS

Frontotemporal lobar degeneration must first be suspected on clinical grounds, based on the appearance of one of the distinctive clinical syndromes such as frontotemporal dementia (see Table 409-6) or one of the aphasic subtypes. Neuropsychological testing can also aid in the diagnosis by detecting abnormalities in executive function and verifying that memory function is preserved, as it often is. For all of the frontotemporal lobar degeneration syndromes, MRI showing focal atrophy of the frontal (Fig. 409-4) or temporal lobes is highly likely to be diagnostic. Imaging with fluorodeoxyglucose-enhanced positron emission tomography can also be useful when the clinical diagnosis is uncertain and MRI is nondiagnostic.

FIGURE 409-4. Parasagittal image from MRI of a patient with frontotemporal dementia *(left)*. Atrophy of the frontal lobes is dramatic compared with the brain of a normal individual *(right)*. (Courtesy of Maria Shiung and Clifford Jack.)

There is no symptomatic therapy specifically for frontotemporal lobar degeneration. In patients with agitation, paranoia, delusions, or obsessive behavior, atypical antipsychotics (e.g., quetiapine, 25 to 200 mg/day) are used, but no controlled clinical trials are available. There are no preventive treatments of frontotemporal lobar degeneration.

PROGNOSIS

Specific frontotemporal lobar degeneration syndromes have dramatic differences in their clinical course and outcome. In patients with motor neuron signs and symptoms, the prognosis is usually poor, with survival of only about 2 years from the time of diagnosis. Patients with semantic dementia and progressive nonfluent aphasia have much more protracted and gradual trajectories; survival for more than 10 years is not uncommon. Frontotemporal dementia itself can also exhibit a more protracted course.

FUTURE DIRECTIONS

Drugs that delay or prevent the pathologic consequences of tau protein dysfunction could be of great value for many patients with frontotemporal lobar degeneration.

 Grade

1. Petersen RC, Thomas RG, Grundman M, et al. Vitamin E and donepezil for the treatment of mild cognitive impairment. *N Engl J Med.* 2005;352:2379-2388.
2. Lautenschlager NT, Cox KL, Flicker L, et al. Effect of physical activity on cognitive function in older adults at risk for Alzheimer disease: a randomized trial. *JAMA.* 2008;300:1027-1037.
3. Aisen PS, Schneider LS, Sano M, et al. High-dose B vitamin supplementation and cognitive decline in Alzheimer disease: a randomized controlled trial. *JAMA.* 2008;300:1774-1783.
4. Courtney C, Farrell D, Gray R, et al; AD2000 Collaborative Group. Long-term donepezil treatment in 565 patients with Alzheimer's disease (AD2000): randomised double-blind trial. *Lancet.* 2004;363:2105-2115.
5. Raina P, Santaguida P, Ismaila A, et al. Effectiveness of cholinesterase inhibitors and memantine for treating dementia: evidence review for a clinical practice guideline. *Ann Intern Med.* 2008;148:379-397.
6. Reisberg B, Doody R, Stöffler A, et al. Memantine in moderate-to-severe Alzheimer's disease. *N Engl J Med.* 2003;348:1333-1341.
7. Winblad B, Kilander L, Eriksson S, et al. Donepezil in patients with severe Alzheimer's disease: double-blind, parallel-group, placebo-controlled study. *Lancet.* 2006;367:1057-1065.
8. Howard RJ, Juszczak E, Ballard CG, et al. Donepezil for the treatment of agitation in Alzheimer's disease. *N Engl J Med.* 2007;357:1382-1389.
9. Erkinjuntti T, Kurz A, Gauthier S, et al. Efficacy of galantamine in probable vascular dementia and Alzheimer's disease combined with cerebrovascular disease: a randomised trial. *Lancet.* 2002;359:1283-1290.
10. McKeith IG, Del Ser T, Spano P, et al. Efficacy of rivastigmine in dementia with Lewy bodies: a randomised, double-blind, placebo-controlled international study. *Lancet.* 2000;356:2031-2036.

SUGGESTED READINGS

Arvanitakis Z. Update on frontotemporal dementia. *Neurologist.* 2010;16:16-22. *Review.*
Ballard C, Gauthier S, Corbett A, et al. Alzheimer's disease. *Lancet.* 2011;377:1019-1031. *Review.*
Mayeux R. Clinical practice. Early Alzheimer's disease. *N Engl J Med.* 2010;362:2194-2201. *Review.*
Plassman BL, Williams JW Jr, Burke JR, et al. Factors associated with risk for and possible prevention of cognitive decline in later life. *Ann Intern Med.* 2010;153:182-193. *Review.*
Querfurth HW, LaFerla FM. Alzheimer's disease. *N Engl J Med.* 2010;362:329-344. *Review.*
Yaffe K, Weston A, Graff-Radford NR, et al. Association of plasma beta-amyloid level and cognitive reserve with subsequent cognitive decline. *JAMA.* 2011;305:261-266. *A low plasma beta-amyloid level is associated with greater cognitive decline in non-demented elderly, especially those with low cognitive reserve.*

410

THE EPILEPSIES

SAMUEL WIEBE

DEFINITION

A *seizure* is defined by transient focal or generalized signs or symptoms due to abnormal excessive or synchronous neuronal activity in the brain. *Focal seizures*, which originate within neuronal networks limited to one cerebral hemisphere, produce signs and symptoms corresponding to the specific region of the brain that is affected by the seizure. *Generalized seizures* rapidly affect extensive neuronal networks on both cerebral hemispheres, and their signs and symptoms are consistent with substantial involvement of both sides of the brain.

Seizures are not synonymous with epilepsy. The epilepsies should be distinguished from situations in which acute brain insults (e.g., infections, trauma, intoxication, metabolic disturbances) cause one or more seizures without a resulting chronic seizure tendency. *Acute symptomatic seizures,* or *provoked seizures*, constitute about 40% of all incident cases of nonfebrile seizures, typically respond to treatment of the provoking factor, and do not require long-term treatment with antiepileptic drugs.

The *epilepsies* are a group of conditions in which an underlying neurologic disorder results in a chronic tendency to have recurrent, unprovoked seizures. Under these circumstances, *the occurrence of two or more seizures establishes the diagnosis of epilepsy.* The causes, types, and clinical expression of the epilepsies are numerous and varied. However, some of the epilepsies conform into identifiable *epileptic syndromes*, which consist of clusters of clinical and electroencephalographic (EEG) features that have specific causes, respond to particular treatments, and may have specific prognostic implications.

EPIDEMIOLOGY

Incidence and Prevalence

Seizures are common in the general population, and about 1 in 10 people will experience a seizure in their lifetime. Most of these seizures are provoked by acute events and are not related to epilepsy. The overall annual incidence of acute symptomatic seizures, excluding febrile seizures, in developed countries is about 39 per 100,000 people. The incidence is higher in men and follows a bimodal age distribution. Incidence is at its highest peak in the first year of life (up to 300 per 100,000), reaches a nadir of 15 per 100,000 in the third and fourth decades of life, and rises again to 123 per 100,000 after 75 years of age. These differences are attributable to the high incidence of acute symptomatic seizures associated with metabolic, infectious, and encephalopathic causes during the neonatal period, and of cerebrovascular and degenerative diseases in elderly people.

The *epilepsies* are common and affect humans of any age. After headache, the epilepsies are the most frequent chronic neurologic condition seen in general practice worldwide. In developed countries, the prevalence of active epilepsy ranges from 5 to 7 per 1000 people, and the annual incidence ranges from 35 to 52 per 100,000, varying by age. The incidence of epilepsy peaks in children younger than 5 years at 60 to 70 per 100,000, decreases throughout adolescence to 30 per 100,000 in early adulthood, and rises again after the sixth decade, reaching a peak of 150 to 200 per 100,000 people older than 75 years. Overall, the incidence and prevalence of the epilepsies are higher in developing countries, largely owing to a higher frequency of perinatal insults, trauma, and infectious disorders of the brain and to suboptimal treatment. In these countries, the median prevalence of active epilepsy is 12.5 per 1000 (range, 5 to 57 per 1000), and the annual incidence ranges from 78 to 190 per 100,000. Furthermore, the patterns of age-specific incidence are quite different in developing countries, where incidence peaks in young adults, not in elderly people.

Risk Factors

Among all age groups, the top five risk factors for developing *acute symptomatic seizures* are head trauma (16%), stroke (16%), infectious disorders (15%), toxic-metabolic disorders (15%), and drug and alcohol withdrawal (14%) (Table 410-1).

The risk factors for developing *epilepsy* differ in adults and children. In childhood, excluding inherited epilepsies, the risk is increased by febrile seizures, head trauma, infections of the brain, mental retardation, cerebral palsy, and attention-deficit hyperactivity disorder. Perinatal insults do not carry an increased risk for epilepsy unless they are accompanied by mental retardation or cerebral palsy.

In adults, risk factors for developing *epilepsy* can be identified in only one third of patients, in whom head trauma, brain infections, stroke, and Alzheimer's disease are the most common. The risk of developing epilepsy is increased more than 500-fold by a history of a military head injury, 30-fold by a severe civilian head injury (Chapter 406), 20-fold each by stroke (Chapter 414) and brain infections (Chapters 420 and 422), and 10-fold each for Alzheimer's disease (Chapter 409), migraine headache (Chapter 405), and hypertension.

In Latin America, the most frequently identified risk factor is brain infection. In endemic areas, neurocysticercosis (Chapter 362) accounts for about 10% of all newly diagnosed cases of epilepsy.

Pathobiology

Pathogenesis

The pathologic substrates and mechanisms underpinning initiation and propagation differ for focal and generalized seizures. In focal seizures, an aggregate of cortical or subcortical neurons develop high-frequency bursts of sodium-dependent action potentials caused by a shift in calcium conductance, thereby resulting in the typical EEG spike discharge (Fig. 410-1). Spread of bursting activity to other neurons is normally prevented by surrounding inhibitory mechanisms, such as hyperpolarization and inhibitory interneurons. When a sufficient number of neurons are engaged in sustained bursting, further excitatory phenomena ensue, including the increased release of excitatory neurotransmitters owing to presynaptic accumulation of Ca^{2+},

depolarization of surrounding neurons owing to increased extracellular K^+, and further neuronal activation caused by depolarization-induced activation of N-methyl-D-aspartate (NMDA) receptors. As excitation increases and inhibition decreases, additional neurons are recruited regionally and distantly, thereby resulting in seizure propagation. The mechanisms by which neurons develop a tendency toward anomalous bursting activity include alterations in neurotransmitters, membrane receptors, ion channels, second-messenger systems, and gene expression of various proteins.

Considerably less is known about the basic mechanisms underlying generalized seizures, which depend prominently on thalamocortical circuits. In absence seizures, the classic generalized spike-and-wave discharges seen on EEG (Fig. 410-2) are related to alterations in oscillatory rhythms generated by circuits that connect the thalamus and cortex and that involve T-type Ca^{2+} channels, which are located in the reticular nucleus of the thalamus. In generalized convulsive seizures, cortical neurons exhibit prolonged depolarization during the tonic phase, followed by rhythmic depolarization and repolarization during the clonic phase. Activation of NMDA receptors increases calcium Ca^{2+} influx, thereby leading to further neuronal excitation. The initiation and modulation of generalized convulsive seizures involve cholinergic, noradrenergic, serotonergic, and histaminergic afferents from the brain stem and basal forebrain structures, which modulate excitability of hemispheric motor mechanisms.

Genetics

Only 15% of patients have one or more first-degree relatives who also suffer from epilepsy, and of those, about 75% have just one affected relative. However, the risk is still higher in first-degree relatives of patients with epilepsy than in the general population. In a large population-based study, the cumulative incidence of epilepsy to age 20 years was 2.5-fold higher in siblings and 3.4-fold higher in offspring of patients with epilepsy.

The genetic aspects of epilepsy can be categorized in three large groups: *Conditions in which epilepsy forms part of a mendelian disorder* include over 200 rare conditions, which encompass neurocutaneous disorders (Chapter 426), neurodegenerative disorders, inherited malformations of cortical development (Chapter 426), and inherited metabolic disorders. For example, genes have been identified in progressive myoclonic epilepsies (e.g., Unverricht-Lundborg disease, Lafora's disease, and the neuronal ceroid lipofuscinosis), X-linked myoclonic epilepsy with mental retardation, and cortical malformation syndromes, such as polymicrogyria, pachygyria, and periventricular nodular heterotopia.

TABLE 410-1	COMMON CAUSES OF ACUTE SYMPTOMATIC (PROVOKED) SEIZURES

METABOLIC

Hypernatremia, hyponatremia, hypocalcemia, hypoxia, hypoglycemia, nonketotic hyperosmolar hyperglycemia, renal failure

DRUG INDUCED

Theophylline, meperidine, tricyclic antidepressants, ephedra, gingko, phenothiazines, quinolones, β-lactams, isoniazid, antihistamines, cyclosporine, interferons, tacrolimus, cocaine, lithium, amphetamines

DRUG WITHDRAWAL

Alcohol, benzodiazepines, barbiturates

ENDOCRINE

Hyperthyroidism, hypothyroidism, peripartum

OTHER SYSTEMIC CONDITIONS

Sickle cell crisis, hypertensive encephalopathy, systemic lupus erythematosus, polyarteritis, eclampsia, high fever

CENTRAL NERVOUS SYSTEM DISORDERS

Trauma, stroke, intracerebral hemorrhage, encephalitis, abscess, bacterial meningitis

FIGURE 410-1. Selected electroencephalogram channels showing a typical right anterior temporal spike, the archetypal interictal footprint of temporal lobe epilepsy. The patient had right hippocampal sclerosis.

FIGURE 410-2. Electroencephalogram pattern of 3-Hz generalized spike and wave, the characteristic correlate of generalized absence seizures. This episode lasting 6 seconds had no discernible clinical manifestations.

Epilepsies that can be directly explained by simple mendelian inheritance are rare and account for only about 1% of all epilepsy cases. More than a dozen genes have been identified in the following eight autosomal dominant epilepsy syndromes, of which all but two encode voltage-gated or ligand-gated ion channels. Benign familial neonatal seizures are associated with mutations in the potassium-channel genes *KCNQ2* and *KCNQ3*. Benign familial neonatal-infantile seizures are associated with mutations in the sodium-channel *SCN2A*. Generalized epilepsy with febrile seizures plus is associated with mutations in the genes for sodium-channel subunits *SCN1A*, *SCN1B*, and *SCN2A* and the *GABRG2* subunit of the GABA$_A$ receptor. Childhood absence epilepsy with febrile seizures is associated with mutations in the *GABRG2* subunit of the GABA$_A$ receptor. Autosomal dominant juvenile myoclonic epilepsy has been associated with a mutation in the *GABRA1* subunit of the GABA$_A$ receptor and in *EFHC1*, which regulates calcium currents. Autosomal dominant idiopathic generalized epilepsy is associated with mutations in the chloride-channel gene *CLCN2*. In autosomal dominant nocturnal frontal lobe epilepsy, mutations have been found in the genes encoding nicotinic acetylcholine receptor subunits *CHRNA4* and *CHRNB2*. In autosomal dominant partial epilepsy with auditory features, mutations have been found in the *LGI1* gene, which appears to be involved in development of the central nervous system (CNS).

In some patients, the epilepsy is associated with *"complex" disease genes*. In this large group, which constitutes about 50% of all patients with epilepsy, multiple genes with individually small but additive effects act in combination with environmental factors to produce an increased risk for epilepsy.

CLINICAL MANIFESTATIONS

The clinical expression of seizures varies widely depending on the type of seizure and the areas of the brain that are involved by the epileptic activity. Accurate identification of the specific types of seizures determines the syndrome and dictates the type of drug that the patient should receive.

Focal Seizures

Focal seizures originate within neuronal networks limited to one area of one cerebral hemisphere and produce signs and symptoms corresponding to the function subserved by the area of cerebral cortex engaged by the seizure (Table 410-2). Focal seizures are now subclassified according to their clinical expression; if consciousness or awareness is predominantly impaired, they are referred to as dyscognitive seizures. For example, patients who formerly were classified as having simple partial seizures now are classified as having focal seizures with preserved consciousness.

An *aura* consists of sensory, autonomic, or psychic symptoms that are experienced at the start of an observable seizure. The aura is a focal seizure itself, and it is often missed because patients and clinicians focus on the more dramatic dyscognitive or convulsive seizure that follows. Careful inquiry about the occurrence of an aura is of crucial importance for three reasons. First, it points to a focal as opposed to a generalized onset, thereby implying an underlying focal structural or functional brain abnormality (e.g., a tumor) that requires further investigation. Second, focal seizures have important implications for therapy and for prognosis (see later). Third, the nature of the symptoms points to the area of the brain that gives rise to the seizure and that could be a target for surgical treatment.

The neuronal discharge causing the focal seizure may remain confined to the region where it began (as an aura or more objective focal event), or it may spread to involve additional brain areas. Thus, a focal seizure originating in the cortical area that represents sensation of the hand (rolandic area) may begin with contralateral hand tingling and then progress to involve additional cortical regions ipsilaterally, producing more extensive sensory symptoms as well as clonic motor signs. Seizures of rolandic origin in particular exhibit a peculiar type of propagation, in which the seizure activity "marches" from hand to arm to leg area ipsilaterally, a process referred to as a jacksonian march. After the clonic motor activity ends, patients are often weak; a postictal or Todd's paralysis may last hours or even a day or two, with gradual resolution. The seizure may also propagate to distant ipsilateral or contralateral regions along known anatomic pathways.

In dyscognitive seizures, seizure propagation sufficiently involves limbic and bilateral structures to cause alteration of consciousness. Focal seizures originating from any region can become dyscognitive seizures, and unilateral focal seizures can progress to involve bilateral brain areas and cause a convulsive seizure. Such convulsive seizures usually take the form of generalized tonic-clonic events rather than another type of generalized seizure (Table 410-3).

The evolution of the focal clinical seizure reflects the evolution of the EEG changes, which in turn reflects the pathophysiology of the process. A

TABLE 410-2 CLINICAL MANIFESTATIONS OF DIFFERENT TYPES OF FOCAL SEIZURES AND AREAS OF THE BRAIN INVOLVED

SEIZURE TYPE	AREAS OF BRAIN INVOLVED	CLINICAL EXPRESSION
Somatosensory	Postcentral rolandic; parietal	Contralateral intermittent or prolonged tingling, numbness, sense of movement, desire to move, heat, cold, electric shock. Sensation may spread to other body segments.
	Parietal	Contralateral agnosia of a limb, phantom limb, distortion of size or position of body part
	Second sensory; supplementary sensory-motor	Ipsilateral or bilateral facial, truncal or limb tingling, numbness, or pain. Often involve lips, tongue, fingertips, feet
Motor	Precentral rolandic	Contralateral regional clonic jerking, usually rhythmic, may spread to other body segments in jacksonian motor march. Often accompanied by sensory symptoms in same area
	Supplementary sensory-motor	Bilateral tonic contraction of limbs causing postural changes, may exhibit classic fencing posture, may have speech arrest or vocalization
	Frontal	Contralateral head and eye version, salivation, speech arrest or vocalization; may be combined with other motor signs (as above) depending on seizure spread
Auditory	Heschl's gyrus—auditory cortex in superior temporal lobe	Bilateral or contralateral buzzing, drumming, single tones, muffled sounds
Olfactory	Orbitofrontal; mesial temporal cortex	Often described as unpleasant odor
Gustatory	Parietal; rolandic operculum; insula; temporal lobe	Often unpleasant taste, acidic, metallic, salty, sweet, smoky
Vertiginous	Occipitotemporal-parietal junction; frontal lobe	Sensation of body displacement in various directions
Visual	Occipital	Contralateral static, moving, or flashing colored or uncolored lights, shapes, or spots. Contralateral or bilateral, partial or complete loss of vision.
	Temporal; occipitotemporal-parietal junction	Formed visual scenes, faces, people, objects, animals
Limbic	Limbic structures: amygdala, hippocampus, cingulum, olfactory cortex, hypothalamus	Autonomic: abdominal rising sensation, nausea, borborygmi, flushing, pallor, piloerection, perspiration, heart rate changes, chest pain, shortness of breath, cephalic sensation, lightheadedness, genital sensation, orgasm Psychic: déjà vu, jamais vu, depersonalization, derealization, dreamlike state, forced memory or forced thinking, fear, elation, sadness, sexual pleasure, hallucinations or illusions of visual, auditory, or olfactory nature
Dyscognitive	Usually bilateral involvement of limbic structures (see above)	Previously known as "complex partial seizures," characterized by a predominant alteration of consciousness or awareness. The current definition requires involvement of at least two of five components of cognition: perception, attention, emotion, memory, and executive function.

Note: Focal seizures may evolve into bilateral convulsive seizures.

TABLE 410-3 GENERALIZED SEIZURES: CLASSIFICATION AND CLINICAL EXPRESSION

SEIZURE TYPE	SUBTYPE	CLINICAL EXPRESSION
Absence	Typical	Abrupt cessation of activities, with motionless, blank stare and loss of awareness lasting about10 seconds. The attack ends suddenly, and patient resumes normal activities immediately.
	Atypical	Longer duration than typical absence, often accompanied by myoclonic, tonic, atonic, and autonomic features as well as automatisms
	With myoclonias	Absence with myoclonic components of variable intensity
Myoclonic	Myoclonic	Sudden, brief (<100 msec), shocklike, involuntary, single or multiple contractions of muscle groups of various locations
	Myoclonic Atonic	A sequence consisting of a myoclonic followed by an atonic phase
	Myoclonic Tonic	A sequence consisting of a myoclonic followed by a tonic phase
Tonic		Sustained increase in muscle contraction lasting a few seconds to minutes
Clonic		Prolonged, regularly repetitive contractions involving the same muscle groups at a rate of 2-3 cycles per second
Atonic		Sudden loss or diminution of muscle tone lasting 1-2 seconds, involving head, trunk, jaw or limb musculature
Tonic-clonic		A sequence consisting of a tonic followed by a clonic phase

simultaneous rhythmic, localized discharge (often in the 4- to 7-Hz range) becomes higher in amplitude and lower in frequency as the seizure continues (Fig. 410-3). Some seizures that begin in the association cortex (e.g., frontal or parietal lobes) have bizarre or extremely brief clinical manifestations, without postictal deficits, and create diagnostic challenges. The stereotyped nature of the clinical events, with the identification of EEG changes if present, may be the only way to make an appropriate diagnosis. The diagnosis can be even more challenging if the seizure spreads to different cortical regions during different seizure episodes, thereby producing variable constellations of clinical findings at different times.

Focal seizures with or without dyscognitive features can also occur as a series of single events without intervening normal behavior, thereby resulting in focal status epilepticus. Focal status epilepticus with dyscognitive seizures is characterized by prolonged confused behavior. EEG findings may be normal in a focal seizure without altered awareness, even in patients with status epilepticus, but the diagnosis is usually evident from the clinical features. In status epilepticus of focal dyscognitive seizures, EEG recordings show continuous abnormalities that are not of the same nature as seen in single seizures in that individual. The most common are a slow background

with superimposed rhythmic high-amplitude sharp waves or repetitive rhythmic seizure discharges (Fig. 410-4). This type of status epilepticus is most frequent with frontal lobe seizures but can occur in temporal lobe seizures as well. The factors that precipitate status epilepticus are not well defined, nor are the implications for treatment or prognosis.

Nonconvulsive status epilepticus consists of a state of confusion or impaired mental status in patients with various neurologic diagnoses (i.e., trauma, stroke) in the acute intensive care unit setting. It also denotes a condition that can occur de novo in older adults without a precipitating cause and that is characterized by prolonged confusional episodes, which are caused by generalized slow spike-and-wave status epilepticus. Clinical suspicion should prompt an EEG study, which is essential for diagnosis (Fig. 410-5).

Generalized Seizures

Generalized seizures rapidly affect both cerebral hemispheres, and their clinical expression is consistent with substantial involvement of both sides of the brain (see Table 410-3). *Convulsive seizures,* which are also referred to as grand mal seizures, consist of excessive, abnormal muscle contractions that may be sustained or interrupted, and usually are a combination of tonic and

FIGURE 410-3. Right temporal lobe dyscognitive seizure in a patient with right hippocampal sclerosis. The focal onset is characteristic, with 4-Hz rhythmic waves in the right anterior temporal region.

FIGURE 410-4. Focal, right hemisphere nonconvulsive status epilepticus in a comatose patient with a large right hemisphere infarct.

FIGURE 410-5. Generalized nonconvulsive status epilepticus in an older adult presenting with a prolonged episode of confusion and catatonic behavior.

clonic phases (generalized tonic-clonic seizures). This type of seizure may involve both hemispheres at the onset or may result from propagation of a focal seizure. These dramatic seizures often frighten witnesses and cause severe disruption of social interaction and development. They may begin with a "cry" as a result of abrupt air movement across the glottis from sudden tonic muscle contraction. The patient becomes diffusely stiff, usually with limb and body extension. Breathing is suspended, cyanosis occurs, and urinary incontinence is common. After 15 to 45 seconds, the tonic activity gives way to clonic, rhythmic, sometimes asymmetrical jerking of all four extremities. The rhythmic contractions gradually become slower in frequency until the event stops; the patient is apneic, comatose, and diaphoretic, but breathing with stridor and gasping begins within 60 seconds. Patients who have generalized tonic-clonic seizures in public often prompt bystanders to initiate resuscitation efforts, although such patients begin spontaneous respiration within 1 minute or so. Postictal stupor persists for a variable length of time. The patient generally sleeps for 2 to 8 hours and then complains of severe headache, sore muscles, a bitten tongue, and the inability to concentrate for a day or more. After generalized tonic-clonic seizures, some individuals have severe memory loss that gradually improves, sometimes over a period of weeks. Generalized tonic-clonic seizures also are a common expression of many metabolic, toxic, traumatic, or ischemic insults (see Table 410-1), but these provoked seizures do not qualify for the diagnosis of epilepsy.

Absence seizures, or petit mal seizures, are the second most common type of generalized seizure. Patients experience an abrupt onset and termination of a momentary lapse of awareness. Patients have no perception of any aspect of the event and may or may not realize that some time was lost, although individuals often lose their train of thought. Because consciousness is abruptly lost and immediately regained, there is neither an aura nor residual postictal symptoms. These seizures begin in childhood, and school teachers are often the first to notice them. Absence seizures may be accompanied by brief eye blinking or myoclonic movements (see Table 410-3), particularly if the event, as judged by EEG, extends beyond 10 seconds. These seizures can occur many times a day but are not associated with progressive neurologic disease. They can also occur in a more continuous form as nonconvulsive status epilepticus with resultant confusion (see Fig. 410-5).

Some patients with extensive bilateral brain disease have a variation of absence seizures, known as *atypical absence.* The event is similar in terms of loss of contact, but there is more motor, autonomic, or automatic activity, and the EEG demonstrates discharges that are slower than the 3-Hz spike and wave of typical absence seizures.

Myoclonic seizures consist of brief episodes of sudden motor contraction (see Table 410-3), which can be focal, with one arm involved, or bilateral and massive, with involvement of both upper extremities and the trunk. Consciousness is preserved but can be difficult to evaluate because of the brevity of these seizures. Myoclonic seizures form part of three main clinical constellations: juvenile myoclonic epilepsy, which starts in childhood or adolescence and often persists into adulthood; epilepsy with various combinations of absence and myoclonic seizures; and epilepsy in the setting of degenerative or inherited syndromes with bilateral cerebral involvement and abnormal cerebral function. Myoclonic seizures most commonly occur in the morning after awakening and often increase in frequency to culminate in a generalized tonic-clonic seizure.

Atonic and tonic seizures are brief but extremely disabling motor events that are characterized by a sudden increase or decrease in muscle tone. The result is falls and injuries with variable impairment of awareness. Such seizures frequently begin in children with diffuse CNS disease and multiple types of seizures, but they persist during adulthood.

DIAGNOSIS

The basic diagnosis of seizures is established by the clinical history. Although EEG, imaging, and laboratory studies are commonly required to determine the type of epilepsy, epilepsy syndrome, site of origin of focal seizures, and occurrence of nonepileptic seizures, the answer to the basic question of whether the patient's episodes are seizures or not rests almost entirely on a careful clinical history. Because epilepsy is defined as the occurrence of two or more unprovoked seizures, this diagnosis is also established by history.

Differential Diagnosis

The first question facing clinicians is whether the episodes under consideration are indeed seizures. The diverse clinical expression of seizures entails a large differential diagnosis among conditions that produce episodic neurologic dysfunction (Table 410-4). Common conditions resembling seizures include syncope (Chapters 50 and 62), transient ischemic attacks (Chapter 414), migraine (Chapter 405), movement disorders (Chapter 417), and psychogenic nonepileptic seizures (see Table 410-4).

A number of historical elements dramatically change the likelihood of this diagnosis. Three essential elements help determine whether an episode is a seizure (Table 410-5) and distinguish seizures from other causes of temporary loss of consciousness, especially syncope (Chapters 50 and 62):

1. The clinical context, including medical and family history, and circumstances under which the episode occurred
2. Specific triggers or provoking factors
3. A detailed clinical description that entails four components:
   - What is the first symptom or sign (presence and type of aura, evidence of focal seizure at onset)?

TABLE 410-4 DISORDERS RESEMBLING SEIZURES

VASCULAR AND PERFUSION DISORDERS

Migraine, syncope, transient ischemic attack, transient global amnesia, arrhythmia/hypoperfusion

PSYCHIATRIC DISORDERS

Psychogenic nonepileptic seizures, panic disorder, dissociative disorder

MOVEMENT DISORDERS

Tics, paroxysmal dystonia, paroxysmal choreoathetosis, paroxysmal ataxia

SLEEP DISORDERS

Night terrors, sleep walking, sleep myoclonus, narcolepsy/cataplexy, rapid eye movement sleep intrusions

METABOLIC DISTURBANCES

Alcoholic blackouts, delirium tremens, hypoglycemia, hallucinogenic drugs

OTHER

Breath-holding spells, paroxysmal vertigo, migraine with recurrent abdominal pain and cyclic vomiting

TABLE 410-5 CLINICAL FEATURES THAT HELP DISTINGUISH A GENERALIZED TONIC CLONIC SEIZURE FROM SYNCOPE

	SEIZURE	SYNCOPE
Clinical context and circumstances	Neurologic or systemic conditions that predispose to seizures, family history of seizures. Mental fatigue, sleep deprivation, alcohol use or withdrawal, systemic illness	Cardiovascular disorders, dehydration, anemia. Family history of syncope
Triggers	Usually none (unless reflex epilepsy)	Orthostatic hypotension, venipuncture, painful and noxious stimuli, emotional stress, micturition, Valsalva maneuver
Clinical features		
Onset	No warning unless there is an aura. Abrupt loss of consciousness, generalized stiffening, and fall. Occurs in any position	Tiredness, nausea, diaphoresis, tunneling of vision. Loss of consciousness over few seconds and fall. Occurs usually standing
Course	Prominent tonic phase then clonic movements lasting about 1 minute, cyanosis, labored breathing, may bite tongue or cheeks, sometimes urinary incontinence	Usually loss of tone, pallor, multifocal myoclonic jerks lasting less than 15 seconds, sometimes urinary incontinence, usually no tongue or cheek biting
Offset	Postical sleepiness and confusion lasting up to hours, headache, myalgia	Rapid recovery over seconds to less than few minutes, no confusion, headache or myalgia. May have fatigue

- How does it evolve after onset (what happens during the seizure proper, what are the signs or symptoms, how long does it last)?
- How does it end (gradually or abruptly)?
- Are there any neurologic deficits after the seizure ends?

Because patients have limited or no recall, the history from others is crucial. Observers can contribute important information about the patient's activity, responses, and appearance, including changes in color, diaphoresis, respirations, vocalization, and muscle tone. This information is often essential to characterize the type of seizure and to distinguish seizures from conditions that resemble seizures.

Migraine (Chapter 405) and focal seizures not only resemble each other but also coexist as comorbid conditions. Features that favor a diagnosis of seizures over classic migraine include an inconsistent occurrence of headache during the event, a brief duration, and the occurrence of more severe seizures. Myoclonus (Chapter 417) occurs in a variety of settings (e.g., metabolic encephalopathies) without any association with epilepsy or the EEG changes seen in myoclonic epilepsy.

Frontal lobe seizures arise predominantly during sleep and can have dramatic motor expression. They can be confused with nonepileptic psychogenic seizures, sleep disorders (Chapter 412), or movement disorders (Chapters 416 and 417). Video EEG monitoring may be necessary for diagnosis.

Patients with panic attacks (Chapter 404) can experience events that mimic focal seizures with autonomic and psychic features. However, panic attacks usually have a longer duration, do not progress to more severe seizures, and can be linked to specific circumstances. Nevertheless, focal seizures with limbic symptoms are often misdiagnosed as panic attacks.

Psychogenic nonepileptic seizures are behaviors that resemble seizures and are often part of a conversion reaction (Chapter 404) precipitated by underlying psychological distress. Psychogenic seizures can be difficult to diagnose because they can mimic almost any type of seizure, and they often coexist with epilepsy in the same patient. An erroneous diagnosis of nonepileptic seizures poses a risk for inappropriate discontinuation of medication, with resulting status epilepticus. Conversely, an erroneous diagnosis of seizures can result in iatrogenic illness owing to unnecessary therapy, excessive sedation, and cardiorespiratory depression. Features suggesting nonepileptic seizures include variable clinical manifestations across episodes, frequent and prolonged episodes, lack of response to antiseizure medication, out-of-phase upper and lower body movements, prominent pelvic thrusting, and lack of rigidity. Secondary gain is usually evident, and there is often a history of sexual abuse. Nevertheless, the peculiarities of these attacks may require continuous video EEG monitoring for diagnosis.

Diagnostic Investigations

A detailed history, EEG recordings, and magnetic resonance imaging (MRI), can lead to a definitive diagnosis of epilepsy and its cause in up to 50% of patients. In other patients, the information is insufficient or inconsistent, but the physiologic and CNS abnormalities surrounding the actual event allow it to be placed provisionally into a specific diagnostic category in about another 30% of patients. Continuous video-EEG monitoring in an inpatient epilepsy unit can increase diagnostic sensitivity.

Single Seizures

Acute symptomatic seizures (see Table 410-1) are the known consequence of an acute condition, and investigations should be directed at the possible cause of these seizures. When no known cause is readily apparent, the seizures are considered to be *unprovoked*. The evaluation of patients who present with a first unprovoked seizure includes either brain computed tomography (CT) or MRI, which reveals a possible cause in about 10% of patients. An EEG obtained after the seizure will demonstrate abnormalities with prognostic significance in 20 to 25% of these patients. Blood tests (including levels of serum electrolytes, glucose, calcium, and magnesium; tests of liver and kidney function; a complete blood cell count; and screening for suspected toxins) will reveal abnormalities in up to 15% of these patients but are often nonspecific. Lumbar puncture is indicated if CNS infections are suspected and in all patients infected with human immunodeficiency virus (HIV), even in the absence of clinical findings suggestive of infection.

Epilepsy

Electroencephalogram

The EEG is the keystone investigation in all patients with seizures and epilepsy. Between seizures, the EEG can assess overall brain function and the type, location, and amount of epileptiform (spike) discharges. The EEG is crucial in determining the epilepsy syndrome and choosing appropriate anti-epileptic drugs. In focal epilepsies, the EEG often demonstrates focal slowing and spike discharges in the area of abnormality.

The EEG can establish the definitive diagnosis of epilepsy if electrical changes consistent with a seizure are recorded during a clinical seizure. However, the EEG may fail to demonstrate electrical changes during a typical clinical seizure if the seizure focus is too small (at least 6 cm² of cortical involvement is needed to create an EEG epileptiform change), the seizure focus is deep or in the mesial or inferior surfaces of the brain, or the event in question may not be an epileptic seizure. The EEG is always abnormal during generalized convulsive and absence seizures.

The initial EEG is normal in up to 60% of people with known epilepsy. However, epileptiform abnormalities occur in more than 80% of individuals with focal epilepsy if three or more interictal EEG studies are performed. In generalized epilepsies, interictal epileptiform discharges are more common and are easier to capture in the EEG (see Fig. 410-2).

The type of abnormality points to the epileptic syndrome. For example, the EEG can show hypsarrhythmia in West's syndrome (see later), or the classic 3-Hz generalized spike wave in generalized epilepsies with absence seizures (see Table 410-3; see Fig. 410-2).

In some circumstances, it is imperative to record seizures, such as in the evaluation of patients for epilepsy surgery and when the diagnosis of seizures is in question. Continuous video EEG monitoring for prolonged periods has made it possible to capture these events. Continuous EEG is also used in comatose patients in the intensive care unit setting when nonconvulsive seizure or status epilepticus is suspected.

Magnetoencephalography

Magnetoencephalography measures the small magnetic fields that are generated by electrical activity in the brain and approximates their location using mathematical models. Its use is largely restricted to the evaluation of patients for epilepsy surgery, in whom it is used for mapping interictal discharges and the localization of brain function when superimposed on brain MRI.

Imaging Studies

Brain MRI, which can demonstrate lesions in most patients whose epilepsy is associated with a structural cause, should be performed in essentially all patients with new-onset seizures. The use of fluid-attenuated inversion recovery (FLAIR) sequences increases the sensitivity to detect abnormalities of cortical development as well as hippocampal sclerosis, which point to the need for chronic anticonvulsant therapy or possible surgical treatment. Functional imaging procedures such as positron emission tomography (PET) for analysis of metabolism and single-photon emission computed tomography (SPECT) for determination of blood flow are also used to help localize areas of the brain to be targeted with epilepsy surgery.

Epileptic Syndromes and Constellations

Epileptic syndromes include 27 age-related syndromes, of which all but 6 begin or occur in infancy and childhood (Table 410-6). In addition, specific clinical constellations represent diagnostically meaningful forms of epilepsy, with specific implications for treatment, especially surgery, and also categorize for structural-metabolic causes, epilepsies of unknown cause, and conditions characterized by seizures that are not a form of epilepsy (e.g., febrile seizures). The diagnosis of epileptic syndromes and constellations is based on the types of seizures, the setting in which seizures occur, the patient's neurologic and cognitive status, age at onset, family history, and results of diagnostic studies, including EEG and MRI. The selection of specific drug and surgical treatment depends on the types of seizures present (see Table 410-8, later). The need for lifelong treatment, the risk for genetic transmission, the likelihood of concurrent neurologic diseases, the risk for comorbid conditions, and the long-term prognosis are critical factors that can be addressed only with knowledge of the specific epileptic syndrome or constellation.

Some Specific Seizure Syndromes and Constellations
Neonatal and Infantile Epilepsy Syndromes

Benign neonatal convulsions occur in previously healthy newborns on about day 5 as focal or generalized tonic seizures. Mutations in two potassium channel genes (*KCNQ2, KCNQ3*) have been associated with this syndrome. Potassium-channel regulation may be age dependent and therefore account for the age-related appearance of the seizures. The EEG shows rhythmic slow-wave activity or spiking with seizures. The seizures are refractory to

TABLE 410-6	EPILEPTIC SYNDROMES AND CONSTELLATIONS ACCORDING TO THE NEW INTERNATIONAL CLASSIFICATION

BY AGE AT ONSET

Neonatal Period
Benign familial neonatal epilepsy
Early myoclonic encephalopathy
Ohtahara's syndrome

Infancy
Epilepsy of infancy with migrating partial seizures
West's syndrome
Myoclonic epilepsy in infancy
Benign infantile epilepsy
Benign familial infantile epilepsy
Dravet's syndrome
Myoclonic encephalopathy in nonprogressive disorders

Childhood
Febrile seizures plus (can start in infancy)
Panayiotopoulos' syndrome
Epilepsy with myoclonic atonic (previously astatic) seizures
Benign epilepsy with centrotemporal spikes
Autosomal-dominant nocturnal frontal lobe epilepsy
Late-onset childhood occipital epilepsy
Epilepsy with myoclonic absences
Lennox-Gastaut syndrome
Epileptic encephalopathy with continuous spike and wave during sleep
Landau-Kleffner syndrome
Childhood absence epilepsy

Adolescence-Adult
Juvenile absence epilepsy
Juvenile myoclonic epilepsy
Epilepsy with generalized tonic-clonic seizures alone
Progressive myoclonus epilepsies
Autosomal dominant partial epilepsy with auditory features
Other familial temporal lobe epilepsies

LESS SPECIFIC AGE RELATIONSHIP

Familial focal epilepsy with variable foci (childhood to adult)
Reflex epilepsies

DISTINCTIVE CONSTELLATIONS

Mesial temporal lobe epilepsy with hippocampal sclerosis
Rasmussen's syndrome
Gelastic seizures with hypothalamic hamartoma
Hemiconvulsion-hemiplegia-epilepsy

---

treatment, are recurrent over a brief interval, and disappear within a month. About 90% of such infants subsequently have normal development, whereas 10% have subsequent seizures.

Generalized epilepsy with febrile seizures plus is a syndrome that consists of febrile seizures in combination with other nonfebrile types of seizures, including myoclonic, absence, atonic, tonic-clonic, and focal seizures. Mutations in at least four different voltage-gated ion channel and GABA receptors genes have been identified.

Dravet's syndrome (severe myoclonic epilepsy of infancy) starts in the first year of life with myoclonic seizures plus other seizure types, including absence, atonic, and focal. In this devastating syndrome, the seizures are resistant to treatment and are accompanied by developmental and cognitive decline. Mutations in the *SCN1A* sodium channel have been identified.

West's syndrome comprises a triad of epileptic spasms, developmental arrest, and an EEG pattern called hypsarrhythmia (a markedly abnormal EEG pattern with high-amplitude slowing and superimposed multifocal spikes, polyspikes, and spike and slow-wave complexes). It appears before the age of 12 months and ceases by 5 years of age, often to be replaced by other epilepsy syndromes such as Lennox-Gastaut syndrome. Tuberous sclerosis (Chapter 426) and hypoxia are among the common causes, but a cause may not be found. Associated abnormalities often include developmental delay, porencephaly, atrophic lesions, calcifications, and agenesis of the corpus callosum.

Childhood Epilepsy Syndromes

Childhood absence epilepsy begins before age 12 years, and its onset peaks at age 5 to 7 years, with a strong genetic tendency. It is more common in girls than boys and is characterized by very frequent daily absence seizures (up to hundreds per day), rarely with other types of generalized seizures. It occurs in the setting of otherwise normal brain structure and function, and it is self-limited in about 40% of cases. The seizures are accompanied by a characteristic 3-Hz spike-and-wave EEG discharge, which appears in short bursts between seizures and in continuous runs during seizures. Remission usually occurs before the age of 12 years, but generalized tonic-clonic seizures occasionally may develop in adolescence.

Lennox-Gastaut syndrome is one of the most severe childhood epilepsies. It starts before age 8 years (peak from 3 to 5 years) and is characterized by a triad of mental retardation, multiple types of generalized seizures (atypical absence, generalized tonic-clonic, tonic, atonic), focal seizures that are highly resistant to treatment, and a typical EEG pattern of slow spike and wave (slower than the typical 3 Hz associated with absence seizures) and bursts of fast rhythms at 10 to 12 Hz during sleep. It often follows the resolution of West's syndrome.

Benign epilepsy with centrotemporal spikes (*benign rolandic epilepsy*) starts between 3 and 13 years of age and is characterized by almost exclusively nocturnal focal motor or sensory seizures that have a facial or oral onset and often evolve to convulsive seizures. Nearly 50% of cases have a family history of epilepsy, but most patients have no known brain abnormality. The EEG shows spiking in the centrotemporal region. In some cases, the disorder may not require treatment because it usually remits spontaneously.

Adolescence and Adult Epilepsy Syndromes and Constellations

Juvenile myoclonic epilepsy usually starts in the second decade with generalized tonic-clonic and myoclonic seizures. Mutations in GABA receptors, including *GABRG1*, can be found. Seizures typically occur in the morning, immediately after awakening. The seizures are especially linked to sleep deprivation and tend to appear in college students. A proportion of these patients have had absence seizures as well. The EEG typically shows fast (4 to 6 Hz) generalized spike and wave. Lifetime treatment is generally needed.

Mesial temporal lobe epilepsy with hippocampal sclerosis is the most common epilepsy to produce focal dyscognitive seizures in adults. It is characterized by recurrent focal limbic seizures (see Table 410-2), with and without impaired awareness, that originate in mesial temporal and limbic structures. Up to 70% of patients have a risk factor, such as lengthy and complicated seizures before the age of 4 years, frequently associated with fever or with encephalitis, meningitis, or trauma. However, the characteristic seizures generally begin some years later. Most cases are sporadic, but there are familial forms of mesial temporal lobe epilepsy.

Various components of the mesial temporal limbic network (including the hippocampus, entorhinal cortex, amygdala, neocortical areas of the frontal and temporal lobes, and dorsal medial thalamus) are probably involved in the pathogenesis of these seizures. Mesial temporal sclerosis, also called hippocampal sclerosis, is characterized by neuronal loss and gliosis, mostly in the CA1 and CA3 regions of the hippocampus, with mossy fiber reorganization that is seen as sprouting of neuropeptide Y and dynorphin interneurons into the inner third of the dentate molecular layer. Whether hippocampal sclerosis is the cause or the result of seizures (or both) is not known. The seizures of mesial temporal lobe epilepsy often begin at 5 to 15 years of age. Seizures are typically dyscognitive with limbic symptoms; they begin with an aura of a rising epigastric sensation or a feeling of déjà vu, followed by oral and alimentary automatisms and later by contralateral arm dystonia and ipsilateral arm automatisms. The seizures are lengthy (lasting several minutes), rarely generalize, and typically occur three to five times a month. Auras without subsequent seizures are common. Hippocampal atrophy and increased hippocampal signal are best seen on T2-weighted and FLAIR coronal MRI sequences, and widespread interictal hypometabolism is seen in the temporal lobe on PET. Material-specific (verbal or visual) memory impairment corresponds to primary involvement of the dominant or nondominant hippocampus. EEG recordings show temporal lobe spikes interictally as well as rhythmic 4- to 7-Hz discharges over the appropriate temporal lobe during seizures.

Seizures with Less Specific Age Relationship

Reflex seizures are triggered reliably by specific simple (e.g., flashing lights) or elaborate (e.g., reading) stimuli. The mechanisms are diverse and may involve cortical and brain stem pathways, cortical dysregulation of extracellular calcium concentrations, and an imbalance between excitatory and inhibitory neurotransmitters. Visual-sensitive seizures (triggered by light or visual patterns) are the most common type of reflex seizures. They occur most commonly in females, and their incidence peaks around puberty, when they represent up to 10% of all new cases of epilepsy. Other triggers of reflex seizures include specific thoughts, actions, reading, tactile stimuli, adopting certain positions, eating, listening to music, startle, and contact with hot water. The triggered seizures can be myoclonic, convulsive, atonic, or focal, depending on the triggering stimulus. Avoiding the offending stimulus is crucial to avoid seizures, emphasizing the importance of careful questioning about seizure triggers in patients with epilepsy.

TREATMENT

The treatment of seizures and epilepsy is guided by accurate knowledge of the type of seizure and epileptic syndrome, the probability of recurrent seizures, the likelihood and severity of psychosocial or physical consequences with further seizures, and whether the benefit from treatment substantially outweighs the risks for side effects. It is important to identify and correct any environmental, physiologic, or lifestyle factors, such as sleep deprivation and irregular sleep habits, that can lower the seizure threshold and trigger seizures in patients with epilepsy.

Single Unprovoked Seizures

The decision to treat single unprovoked seizures depends on the likelihood of recurrence according to prognostic variables (see Prognosis) and on the individual patient's profile and preference. A meta-analysis demonstrated that antiepileptic drug treatment after a first seizure reduces the absolute risk of having a second seizure in the short-term by 33%, corresponding to a number needed to treat (NNT) of 3.[1] However, at least two randomized trials have shown that treatment of the first seizure with antiepileptic drugs does not prevent the development of epilepsy in the long term.[1,2] Therefore, the decision to treat the first seizure should be individualized based on the patient's preference, the risk for and impact of recurrent seizures (e.g., driving and employment), and the risk for medication side effects.

Acute Symptomatic (Provoked) Seizures

Seizures that are provoked by specific exposures are usually self-limited and not associated with an enduring seizure tendency, so the primary therapeutic consideration should be identification and treatment of the underlying disorder (see Table 410-1). If antiepileptic drugs are needed to treat seizures acutely, they usually can be discontinued after the patient has recovered from the primary illness. Some acute conditions like stroke (Chapter 414), brain infections (Chapters 420 and 422), and trauma (Chapter 406) can produce both acute symptomatic seizures and an enduring seizure tendency, so it would seem logical to use long-term antiepileptic drug treatment. To date, however, randomized controlled trials have not been able to demonstrate that antiepileptic drugs prevent the development of epilepsy in these conditions, so long-term therapy is not recommended unless epilepsy develops.

Epilepsy Syndromes with a Favorable Course

In syndromes such as benign epilepsy of childhood with centrotemporal spikes and some types of childhood occipital epilepsy, seizures are mild, infrequent, or exclusively nocturnal, and they remit spontaneously, thereby making treatment generally unnecessary. In selected cases, treatment may be desirable to prevent recurrences and to help alleviate parental concerns. In such cases, drug treatment is usually limited to 1 to 2 years regardless of interictal EEG abnormalities, which can persist long after seizures have remitted. The recommended antiepileptic drugs are those used in focal epilepsy in children, including oxcarbazepine, carbamazepine, valproate, gabapentin, lamotrigine, and topiramate (Table 410-7). Some patients with reflex seizures may require antiseizure medication, which should be chosen according to seizure type (Table 410-8).

Choice of Antiepileptic Drugs

The ultimate goal of treatment is to obtain complete freedom from seizures without side effects. Some of the newer antiepileptic drugs (see Table 410-7) are better tolerated and have better pharmacokinetics than older drugs, but there is no robust evidence to support superior efficacy of one drug over another.[3,4] The choice of medication depends on the type of seizure, thereby making a correct diagnosis crucial, and the medication's side effects, cost, and ease of use. Specific drugs are effective for specific types of seizures, and some drugs can worsen other types of seizures. Knowledge of individual drugs as they relate to age, sex, comorbid conditions, drug interactions, sedation, tolerance, mood, and withdrawal is critical in the drug selection process (see Table 410-8).[5,6] For example, ethosuximide and valproic acid are more effective than lamotrigine for the treatment of childhood absence epilepsy.[7]

Drugs that cause enzyme induction (e.g., carbamazepine, phenytoin, phenobarbital, oxcarbazepine, topiramate) or inhibition (e.g., valproic acid) can be difficult to manage when additional medications, such as oral contraceptives, are used for independent conditions. For these settings and in elderly patients, gabapentin and levetiracetam are particularly useful because they have no appreciable drug interactions.

TABLE 410-7　CHARACTERISTICS OF MAJOR ANTIEPILEPTIC DRUGS

NAME	TOTAL MILLIGRAMS PER DAY (USUAL SCHEDULE)	THERAPEUTIC RANGE (μG/mL)	PROMINENT SIDE EFFECTS	OTHER EFFECTS	OTHER ISSUES
Carbamazepine	400-1600 (bid)	4-12	Diplopia, fatigue, hyponatremia	Mood stabilizer	Enzyme inducer
Ethosuximide	750-1250 (qd, bid)	40-100	Ataxia, lethargy	Skin rash, bone marrow suppression	
Gabapentin	600-6000 (tid, qid)	2-12	Fatigue	Treatment of pain	No drug interactions
Lamotrigine	100-600 (bid)	4-18	Insomnia, headache, tremor, anxiety	Mood stabilizer	Risk for Stevens-Johnson syndrome; slow start-up
Levetiracetam	500-3000 (bid)	3-63	Mood change, irritability, lethargy		No drug interactions
Oxcarbazepine	300-2400 (tid)	6-40	Diplopia, hyponatremia, sedation	Mood stabilizer	
Phenobarbital	60-240 (hs)	15-40	Fatigue, depression, sedation	Joint pain	Enzyme inducer
Phenytoin	200-600 (bid)	10-20	Fatigue, hirsutism, gingival hypertrophy	Treatment of some pain	Enzyme inducer
Topiramate	50-600 (bid)	2-12	Anorexia, weight loss, kidney stones, speech disturbance, distal paresthesias	Headache prophylaxis, mood stabilizer	Enzyme inducer
Valproate	500-6000 (tid)	50-100	Weight gain, hair loss, tremor	Headache prophylaxis, mood stabilizer	Enzyme inhibitor, parkinsonian effects in elderly patients
Zonisamide	100-600 (hs)	10-40	Anorexia, kidney stones, dizziness, distal paresthesias	Mood stabilizer	

TABLE 410-8　ANTIEPILEPTIC DRUG SELECTION BY SEIZURE TYPE

SEIZURE TYPE	COMMONLY USED (ALPHABETICAL ORDER)	LESS COMMONLY USED (ALPHABETICAL ORDER)	Effectiveness (Grade A Recommendation)*	
			NEW-ONSET SEIZURES	REFRACTORY SEIZURES
Focal seizures with or without dyscognitive features or evolution to convulsions	Carbamazepine (CBZ) Gabapentin (GBP) Lamotrigine (LTG) Levetiracetam (LEV) Oxcarbazepine (OXC) Phenytoin (PHT) Tiagabine (TIAG) Topiramate (TPM) Valproate (VPA) Zonisamide (ZNS)	Acetazolamide (ACZ) Clonazepam (CLN) Clorazepate (CLZ) Phenobarbital (PB) Primidone (PRM) Felbamate (FBM)	CBZ* GBP* LTG* OXC* PB* PHT* TPM* VPA*	CBZ† GBP* LAM* LEV* OXC* PB† PHT† TIAG* TPM* VPA† ZNS*
Generalized convulsive seizures (tonic-clonic seizures, tonic seizures, atonic seizures)	Carbamazepine Lamotrigine Levetiracetam Oxcarbazepine Phenytoin Topiramate Valproate Zonisamide	Acetazolamide Clonazepam Clorazepate Felbamate Phenobarbital Primidone	CBZ† LEV* LTG* PHT† VPA*	CBZ† LAM* LEV* PHT† TPM* VPA*
Absence seizures	Ethosuximide (ETH) Lamotrigine Valproate Topiramate	Acetazolamide Clonazepam Phenobarbital Primidone	ETH* LTG* VPA*	
Myoclonic seizures	Clonazepam Valproate Zonisamide Levetiracetam	Phenobarbital	VPA†	LEV

*Supported by class I evidence (American Academy of Neurology).
†Often the "standard" of comparison, without evidence of effectiveness by randomized controlled trials.

In patients with newly diagnosed focal epilepsy, the underlying cause influences the response to antiepileptic drugs. The likelihood of achieving seizure freedom is higher for patients with vascular malformations, stroke, and tumors (63 to 78%), and lower for patients with hippocampal sclerosis and malformations of cortical development (40 to 50%). Among patients presenting with a new diagnosis of epilepsy, about 65% achieve seizure remission on antiepileptic drug treatment. Of these patients, about 45 to 50% achieve seizure remission with the first antiepileptic drug, 10 to 15% with the second, 1% with the third, and 3% with a combination of two or more antiepileptic drugs. Because the likelihood of achieving subsequent seizure remission is small if two drug trials fail, the 35% or so of patients who fail adequate trials of two antiepileptic drugs are considered to be *drug resistant*. In these patients, other forms of treatment, including surgery, should be considered. The first consideration in managing apparently drug-resistant patients is to ensure that the diagnosis is correct and the antiepileptic drug is appropriate. Other common issues include poor adherence to antiepileptic drugs, sleep deprivation, alcohol use, fatigue, emotional stress, systemic illnesses, use of concurrent medications, and nonepileptic seizures. After addressing these factors, patients who remain drug resistant should be considered potential candidates for surgical therapy.

Surgical Treatment

Surgical treatment entails resection or disconnection of the cerebral region that contains the seizure focus. Removal of an epileptogenic region requires accurate identification of the region as well as documentation of a lack of functional consequences after its removal. Video EEG monitoring with seizure recording from scalp electrodes, MRI protocols with special attention to areas commonly associated with refractory seizures (e.g., the medial temporal and frontal lobes), and functional neuroimaging, including PET and SPECT, are used to make the assessment. In temporal lobe epilepsy, neuropsychological evaluation is essential to localize dysfunction and to establish the level of function in the region considered for resection. EEG localization of the region of seizure onset and mapping of brain function may require the surgical implantation of intracranial electrodes for recording and for stimulating cortical tissue. These procedures are performed by multidisciplinary teams in specialized epilepsy centers.

Epilepsy surgery interventions that have been subjected to rigorous randomized trials include temporal lobe resection compared with medical therapy for mesial temporal lobe epilepsy, comparison of different amounts of temporal lobe resection, different intensities of vagus nerve stimulation, and thalamic stimulation compared with medical therapy. The most dramatic surgical effect is seen for temporal lobe resection compared with medical therapy. In one series, 58% of surgical patients and only 8% of medical patients became seizure free (NNT of 2 at 1 year).[8] As a result, patients with drug-resistant temporal lobe epilepsy should be evaluated for epilepsy surgery. Nonrandomized studies demonstrate enduring freedom from seizures at 10 years or more after hemispheric disconnection (61%), temporal lobe resection (64%), parieto-occipital resection (46%), and frontal lobe resection (27%). Palliative surgical procedures, such as callosotomy and multiple subpial transections, have lower success rates and are used when surgical resection of the seizure focus is not possible. Promising surgical therapies for epilepsy include radiosurgery and various types of electrical stimulation of the brain.

Status Epilepticus

Status epilepticus is a medical emergency in which seizures occur continuously or repeatedly without intervening resumption of consciousness for 30 minutes. However, even 5 minutes of generalized tonic-clonic seizures cause hypoxia, lactic acidosis, muscle breakdown, and neuronal damage. Most episodes of status epilepticus are caused by an acute brain insult in people without underlying epilepsy, so a cause should be sought promptly. After securing the airway and stabilizing cardiovascular function, immediate intervention with parenteral agents is needed to stop the seizures. Intravenous lorazepam (0.1 mg/kg given at 2 mg per minute) is the emergent treatment of choice, followed by intravenous phenytoin (15 mg/kg at a rate of 50 mg per minute) or fosphenytoin (15-20 mg/kg at a rate of 150 mg per minute) to provide a more long-lasting effect. If seizures continue for 10 to 15 minutes, options include phenobarbital (20 mg/kg intravenously) or continuous intravenous midazolam (0.1 to 2 mg/kg/hour), pentobarbital (0.5 to 3 mg/kg/hour), or propofol (2 to 4 mg/kg/hour), most appropriately in an intensive care setting. In refractory cases, general anesthesia for 24 hours is used.

Considerations in Women

Changes in hormone levels during the menstrual cycle may aggravate seizures perimenstrually in some women (i.e., catamenial epilepsy). The administration of oral contraceptives (Chapter 246), Depo-Provera, or acetazolamide (250 to 500 mg per day) may reduce perimenstrual seizures. Enzyme-inducing antiepileptic drugs (see Table 410-7) that reduce estrogen levels by enhancing its metabolism require patients to be treated with higher doses of estrogen or alternative methods of contraception.

Pregnancy poses challenges with regard to seizure control, teratogenesis, and outcomes of pregnancy. Nevertheless, pregnancy itself has no consistent effect on the frequency of seizures, and more than 90% of pregnancies in women with epilepsy are safe and successful. Freedom from seizures for at least 9 months preceding pregnancy is associated with a high probability of freedom from seizures during the pregnancy. Serum levels of lamotrigine, phenytoin, carbamazepine, levetiracetam, and oxcarbazepine may change during pregnancy and should be monitored. To reduce the risk for major congenital malformations, the use of valproate should be avoided if seizure control permits it. Similarly, polytherapy and high doses of antiepileptic drugs should be avoided, if possible, but antiepileptic drugs should not be discontinued. There is no increased risk for cesarean section or premature contractions, and epilepsy itself does not increase the risk for cognitive impairment in the child. Supplementation with at least 0.4 mg of folic acid daily should be given before conception and during pregnancy to reduce the risk for neural tube defects.

Discontinuing Antiepileptic Drugs

About 60% of patients have seizures that are easy to control with antiepileptic drugs. Medications may be slowly tapered over 4 to 6 months in patients who have remained free of seizures for 2 years or longer, have had few seizures before treatment started, and who have a normal neurologic examination and EEG. However, the increased absolute risk for recurrent seizures after withdrawal of medication is about 20% (number needed to harm of 5). The consequences of a recurrent seizure, the costs and side effects of drugs, and aspects such as personal preferences influence the decision to withdraw antiepileptic drugs in patients who have been free of seizures.

PROGNOSIS

The prognosis is favorable in the majority of patients who experience either unprovoked seizures or one of the epilepsies.

Prognosis after Febrile Seizures

Febrile seizures are common and usually consist of generalized tonic-clonic seizures. They are provoked by fever and therefore are not considered epilepsy. The seizures begin after 6 months of age and stop before 6 years of age. Usually, febrile seizures are left untreated because the prognosis is benign. When febrile seizures occur in the setting of a neurologic abnormality or are prolonged or complicated, the risk for later epilepsy is increased.

Prognosis after a Single Unprovoked Seizure

The risk of experiencing recurrent seizures after a first unprovoked seizure ranges from 21 to 69% at 2 years and from 34 to 70% at 5 years. The risk is lower in the general population than in hospital-based studies (36% at 1 year and 45% at 2 years). The probability of a relapse decreases with time; about 50% of recurrences occur within 6 months of the initial seizure, and 76 to 96% occur within 2 years. The two most consistent predictors of recurrence are the presence of a neurologic cause for the seizure, which is often uncovered on brain MRI or by the neurologic examination and history, and an epileptiform or slow EEG. The 2-year risk for recurrence is lowest for patients without an identified neurologic cause and with a normal EEG (about 25%), intermediate for patients with an identified neurologic cause or without a cause but with an abnormal EEG (48%), and highest for those with a neurologic cause and an abnormal EEG (about 65%). The risk rises dramatically if more than one seizure has occurred; after a second unprovoked seizure, the risk for a third seizure is 73%, and after a third seizure, the risk for a fourth seizure is 76%.

Prognosis of Epilepsy

The natural history of untreated epilepsy, mostly in developing countries, shows that 30 to 40% of patients obtain 5- to 10-year remissions without treatment. In developed countries, where treatment is generally started after two unprovoked seizures have occurred, the likelihood of 5-year remission is about 60% when patients are followed for 10 years, and about 70% when patients are followed for 20 years. The rate of 5-year remission in children is about 75%.

Conversely, the duration of active epilepsy before achieving control is one of the most powerful predictors of remission. If seizures remain uncontrolled during the first year after diagnosis, the chance of ever achieving control is only 60%. If the period of uncontrolled seizures extends to 4 years, the chance of ever achieving control is only 10%. The presence of multiple seizure types and frequent generalized tonic-clonic seizures is associated with a lower likelihood of remission. Less than 40% of patients with newly diagnosed mesial temporal lobe epilepsy will be controlled with medications, although familial cases are more easily managed medically.

Patients with epilepsy are at risk for poor psychosocial outcomes, depression, and increased mortality. The risk for death is two to three times higher in epilepsy than in the general population, and it can be up to six times higher in patients with frequent generalized convulsions and drug-resistant epilepsy. The major causes of death are underlying conditions such as stroke and pneumonia. Sudden unexpected death in epilepsy occurs in 1 per 1000 patient years and is particularly devastating because it affects young individuals with frequent, uncontrolled seizures.

1. Wiebe S, Téllez-Zenteno JF, Shapiro M. An evidence-based approach to the first seizure. *Epilepsia.* 2008;49(suppl 1):50-57.
2. Marson A, Jacoby A, Johnson A, et al. Immediate versus deferred antiepileptic drug treatment for early epilepsy and single seizures: a randomised controlled trial. *Lancet.* 2005;365:2007-2013.
3. Marson AG, Al-Kharusi AM, Alwaidh M, et al. The SANAD study of effectiveness of carbamazepine, gabapentin, lamotrigine, oxcarbazepine, or topiramate for treatment of partial epilepsy: an unblinded randomised controlled trial. *Lancet.* 2007;369:1000-1015.
4. Marson AG, Al-Kharusi AM, Alwaidh M, et al. The SANAD study of effectiveness of valproate, lamotrigine, or topiramate for generalised and unclassifiable epilepsy: an unblinded randomised controlled trial. *Lancet.* 2007;369:1016-1026.
5. French JA, Kanner AM, Bautista J, et al. Efficacy and tolerability of the new antiepileptic drugs I: treatment of new onset epilepsy. Report of the Therapeutics and Technology Assessment Subcommittee and Quality Standards Subcommittee of the American Academy of Neurology and the American Epilepsy Society. *Neurology.* 2004;62:1252-1260.
6. French JA, Kanner AM, Bautista J, et al. Efficacy and tolerability of the new antiepileptic drugs II: treatment of refractory epilepsy. Report of the Therapeutics and Technology Assessment

Subcommittee and Quality Standards Subcommittee of the American Academy of Neurology and the American Epilepsy Society. *Neurology*. 2004;62:1261-1273.

7. Glauser TA, Cnaan A, Shinnar S, et al. Ethosuximide, valproic acid, and lamotrigine in childhood absence epilepsy. *N Engl J Med*. 2010;362:790-799.

8. Wiebe S, Blume WT, Girvin JP, et al. A randomized, controlled trial of surgery for temporal-lobe epilepsy. *N Engl J Med*. 2001;345:311-318.

SUGGESTED READINGS

Chong DJ, Bazil CW. Update on anticonvulsant drugs. *Curr Neurol Neurosci Rep*. 2010;10:308-318. *Review*.

Christensen J, Pedersen MG, Pedersen CB, et al. Long-term risk of epilepsy after traumatic brain injury in children and young adults: a population-based cohort-study. *Lancet*. 2009;373:1105-1110. *The risk for epilepsy is significantly increased after skull fracture (2-fold), mild traumatic brain injury (2.2-fold), or severe brain injury (7.4-fold).*

Geerts A, Arts WF, Stroink H, et al. Course and outcome of childhood epilepsy: a 15-year follow-up of the Dutch Study of Epilepsy in Childhood. *Epilepsia*. 2010;51:1189-1197. *Epilepsy remains active in about 30% of patients and becomes intractable in approximately 10%.*

Kahane P, Depaulis A. Deep brain stimulation in epilepsy: what is next? *Curr Opin Neurol*. 2010;23:177-182. *Review*.

Martindale JL, Goldstein JN, Pallin DJ. Emergency department seizure epidemiology. *Emerg Med Clin North Am*. 2011;29:15-27. *Review*.

Noe KH. Seizures: diagnosis and management in the outpatient setting. *Semin Neurol*. 2011;31:54-64. *Practical review*.

411

COMA, VEGETATIVE STATE, AND BRAIN DEATH

JAMES L. BERNAT

Assessment and treatment of a comatose patient are among the most challenging and critical activities in clinical medicine. Physicians must systematically and rapidly identify the cause of coma while simultaneously supporting vital systems and reversing the pathologic process. For example, resuscitation from cardiac arrest (Chapter 63) is successful only if the brain is not irreversibly damaged by a hypoxic-ischemic injury that can cause a vegetative state or brain death.

Coma, stupor, the vegetative state, and the minimally conscious state are disorders of consciousness (Table 411-1) that must be differentiated from brain death and locked-in syndrome. Human consciousness has two measurable clinical dimensions that correspond to two distinct brain neuronal systems: (1) wakefulness, which is the organism's arousal and readiness to respond to internal or external stimuli and which is provided by the reticular system of the rostral brain stem and its thalamic and forebrain ascending projections, and (2) awareness of self and environment, which is provided by a diffuse parallel network of thalamocortical and corticocortical circuits. Wakefulness is a prerequisite for awareness, but as exemplified by patients in a vegetative state, awareness may be lost despite maintained wakefulness.

Consciousness is usually considered a global brain function. Focal cerebral hemispheric lesions (Chapters 403 and 413) may disturb fragments of consciousness and produce disturbances such as aphasia, apraxia, or agnosia. Although language, praxis, and gnosis are elements of normal consciousness, their selective loss does not usually result in a diminution of the quantity of consciousness, so these focal syndromes are not classified as disorders of consciousness.

COMA

Coma is a pathologic state of eyes-closed unresponsiveness in which the patient has neither awareness nor wakefulness and from which the patient cannot be aroused to awareness or wakefulness by vigorous stimuli. Stupor is a similar disorder in which stimuli can temporarily arouse the patient to limited responsiveness but, in the absence of stimuli, the patient returns to an unresponsive state. Sleep, by contrast, is a normal state of active cyclic unconsciousness from which subjects can be fully and persistently aroused to full normal consciousness.

Coma is not a univocal state; it has levels of depth depending on the degree of reflex response to stimulation. Disorders of consciousness comprise a continuum from the mildest state of lethargy to the deepest stage of coma. Obtundation is a nonspecific term that describes any degree of altered consciousness without stipulating its depth.

EPIDEMIOLOGY

The frequencies of the various causes of coma vary widely depending on the setting. In most settings, however, post-traumatic, metabolic, anoxic, and toxic causes are the most common (Table 411-2).

PATHOBIOLOGY

Wakefulness is provided by a network of neurons and their connections in the central tegmentum of the pons and midbrain (reticular system) that receives input at each level as it ascends into the central basal forebrain, thalamus, and cerebral cortex. Damage to this neuronal network by trauma, ischemia, hypoxia, edema, or metabolic or toxic insults leads to coma because the ascending arousal mechanism is disturbed.

Awareness of self and environment requires not only wakefulness but also normal functioning of massive parallel reverberating neuronal circuits between the thalamus and multiple cortical regions to provide an integrated and unified experience. These structures and their connections can be damaged by the same pathologic conditions that affect the arousal system, but thalamic and cortical neurons are more susceptible to damage because of their higher metabolic demands. A given global brain insult, such as systemic hypoxia and ischemia suffered during cardiac arrest, can selectively damage the cortical and thalamic neurons necessary for awareness while largely sparing the phylogenetically older and less metabolically demanding neurons of the arousal network of the reticular system. This selective damage can result in the vegetative state, which is characterized by wakefulness without awareness.

Coma can be caused by (1) structural damage as a result of brain trauma, edema, inflammation, ischemia, or mass lesions or (2) diffuse metabolic and toxic effects on brain neurons. Structural lesions can affect the arousal neuronal network of the brain stem and basal forebrain directly through local neuronal damage or indirectly by downward or lateral pressure or displacement that causes local ischemia. Metabolic and toxic encephalopathies diffusely affect all brain neurons, particularly the metabolically sensitive cortical and thalamic neurons.

Structural lesions that cause coma typically produce clinically recognizable syndromes of cerebral "herniation" in which intracranial pressure shifts produce caudal displacement and ischemia of the midbrain and medial temporal lobe through the tentorial incisura and induces dysfunction of cranial nerves, breathing, and motor systems. Central transtentorial herniation from slowly expanding axial lesions is uncommon; more common is uncal herniation from rapidly expanding and laterally placed lesions that trap the ipsilateral oculomotor nerve against the uncus of the temporal lobe. Lateral displacement of brain structures can supplement or exceed downward displacement. The ascending arousal system can also be damaged directly by primary brain stem catastrophes such as pontomesencephalic hemorrhage or infarction or indirectly by downward-directed pressure waves produced by hemispheric mass lesions such as from brain trauma (Chapter 406) or supratentorial neoplasms (Chapter 195), abscesses (Chapter 421), hemorrhages (Chapter 415) or large infarctions (Chapter 414).

Metabolic encephalopathies disturb the neuronal microenvironment by altering the precise metabolic conditions necessary for normal neuronal excitability. Disturbances in the neuronal milieu can be caused by alterations in blood flow, oxygen delivery, glucose concentration, temperature, electrolyte concentrations, and intracranial pressure, as well as by meningitis, seizures, and organ failure. The depth of the resulting alteration of consciousness depends on the severity of the metabolic disturbance: mild metabolic encephalopathies can cause slowness or lethargy, whereas severe metabolic encephalopathies can produce deep coma. The rapidity of onset is of particular importance. A sudden drop in the serum sodium concentration (Chapter 118) may result in coma and seizures, whereas a slow decline to an equivalent level may not. Toxic encephalopathies can be caused by poisoning with exogenous agents such as depressant drugs or by endogenous toxins resulting, for example, from renal or hepatic failure and produce the same continuum of severity. Acute meningeal inflammation, caused most commonly by bacterial meningitis, induces coma by a combination of inflammatory and vascular changes.

TABLE 411-1 COMPARISON OF DISORDERS OF CONSCIOUSNESS*

	AWARENESS	WAKEFULNESS	BRAIN STEM/ RESPIRATORY	MOTOR	EEG	EVOKED POTENTIALS	PET/FMRI	COMMENT
Brain death	Absent	Absent	Absent	Absent	ECS	Absent	Absent cortical metabolism	Legally dead in most jurisdictions
Coma	Absent	Absent	Depressed, variable	Reflex or posturing	Polymorphic delta, burst suppression	BAER variable; cortical ERPs often absent	Resting <50%	Prognosis variable
Vegetative state	Absent	Present, intact sleep-wake cycles	Intact	Reflex, nonpurposeful	Delta, theta, or ECS	BAER preserved; cortical ERPs variable	Resting <50%; primary areas stimulatable	Prognosis variable
Minimally conscious state	Intact but poorly responsive	Intact	Intact	Variable with purposeful movements	Nonspecific slowing	BAER preserved; cortical ERPs often preserved	Reduced; secondary areas also stimulatable	Prognosis variable
Locked-in syndrome	Intact but communication difficult	Intact	Intact breathing; often brain stem signs	Quadriplegia, pseudobulbar palsy	Usually normal	BAER variable; cortical ERPs normal	Normal or nearly normal	Not a disorder of consciousness

*The table lists typical findings, which are not necessarily present in all patients.
BAER = brain stem auditory evoked response; ECS = electrocerebral silence; EEG = encephalography; ERP = event-related potential; fMRI = functional magnetic resonance imaging; PET = positron emission tomography.
From Bernat JL. *Ethical Issues in Neurology*, 3rd ed. Philadelphia: Lippincott Williams & Wilkins; 2008:292.

TABLE 411-2 CAUSES OF STUPOR AND COMA

Traumatic brain injury*
  Contusion
  Intracerebral, epidural, subdural, or subarachnoid hemorrhage
  Raised intracranial pressure
Neoplasms and other mass lesions
Infections
  Meningitis
  Encephalitis
  Brain abscess or empyema
  Sepsis or other infection, especially in the elderly or a demented patient*
Cerebrovascular disease
  Subarachnoid hemorrhage
  Infarction in the brain stem or cerebellum or large hemispheric infarction
  Hemorrhage in the brain stem or cerebellum or large hemispheric hemorrhage
  Vasculitis, disseminated intravascular coagulation, thrombotic thrombocytopenic purpura
Seizures
  Status epilepticus
  Spike-wave stupor
  Postictal state
Metabolic encephalopathies*
  Hypoglycemia, hyperglycemia
  Hypercalcemia
  Hyponatremia, hypernatremia
  Hypoxemia, including anoxia after cardiac arrest
  Acidosis
  Organ system failure: hepatic, renal, pulmonary, cardiac
  Endocrinopathy, e.g., myxedema coma
Toxic encephalopathies
  Drug intoxications*: alcohol, barbiturates, benzodiazepines, opioids, stimulants, salicylates, anticonvulsants, anticholinergics, psychotropic drugs, or others
  Poisoning: carbon monoxide, industrial toxins
Other encephalopathies
  Hypertensive encephalopathy
  Acute hydrocephalus
  Pituitary apoplexy
Other
  Conversion, malingering, catatonia

*Most common causes.

TABLE 411-3 FOUR SCORE COMA ASSESSMENT SCALE*

EYE RESPONSE

E4 = Eyelids open or unopened, tracking or blinking to command
E3 = Eyelids open but not tracking
E2 = Eyelids closed but open to pain
E1 = Eyelids remain closed with pain stimuli

MOTOR RESPONSE

M4 = Thumbs up, fist, or peace sign
M3 = Localizing to pain
M2 = Flexion response to pain
M1 = Extension response to pain
M0 = No response to pain or generalized myoclonic status epilepticus

BRAIN STEM REFLEXES

B4 = Pupillary and corneal reflexes present
B3 = One pupil dilated and unreactive to light
B2 = Pupillary or corneal reflexes absent
B1 = Pupillary and corneal reflexes absent
B0 = Absent pupillary, corneal, or cough reflexes

RESPIRATION

R4 = Regular breathing pattern
R3 = Cheyne-Stokes breathing pattern
R2 = Irregular breathing pattern
R1 = Triggers or breathes above the ventilator rate
R0 = Apnea or breathes at the ventilator rate

*For nontraumatic coma and other disorders of consciousness.
From Wijdicks EFM. *The Comatose Patient*. New York: Oxford University Press; 2008:72a.

especially useful because it elicits primitive reflex mechanisms to protect the airway. Many painful stimuli should be avoided as unnecessary and cruel, but a sternal rub with fingers or knuckles is acceptable. Responses can be graded as voluntary movement, withdrawal, reflex posturing, and none.

Coma assessment scales are useful to describe the depth of coma, serially assess changes, and by correlation to outcomes, provide a prognosis. The widely used Glasgow Coma Scale (see Table 406-1) was devised to assess patients with traumatic brain injury. The FOUR Score scale is more useful for all causes of coma because it more accurately assesses brain stem function and quantifies awareness (Table 411-3).

DIAGNOSIS

The diagnosis of coma requires a rapid history, physical and neurologic examination (Table 411-4), laboratory tests, and neuroimaging studies, during which patient's vital functions must be supported. Immediate attention should be paid to whether the patient has signs of meningitis (e.g., fever, nuchal rigidity) or head trauma (Chapter 406) or focal findings suggestive of

CLINICAL MANIFESTATIONS

A comatose patient is unresponsive and cannot be aroused to awareness or wakefulness. The level of consciousness can be assessed by loudly speaking the patient's name directly in the ear. Patients should be asked to look up and down to test for locked-in syndrome, in which vertical eye movements may be the only remaining voluntary movement. Noxious stimuli can be applied to elicit responses. Tickling the nasal hairs with a cotton-tipped swab is a mass, lesion, bleeding, or ischemic injury. If signs of meningitis are present, a lumbar puncture should be performed without the delay of obtaining brain imaging if no marked focal signs (e.g., hemiparesis) are present. Brain computed tomography (CT) should be performed urgently in nearly every patient in coma.

The relevant history includes eyewitness accounts of any preceding headache, vomiting, confusional state, prescription and street drug use, alcohol consumption, diabetes, fever, head trauma, seizure activity, and medical illnesses, especially atrial fibrillation. The rate at which neurologic function declined can be especially helpful. On the general physical examination, assessment of vital signs, otoscopy, optic funduscopy, and inspection for head trauma, nuchal rigidity, and needle tracks can provide key findings.

TABLE 411-4	SOME INITIAL CLINICAL CLUES TO THE DIAGNOSIS OF STUPOR AND COMA

STRUCTURAL CAUSES

History
  Abrupt onset of unconsciousness
  Sudden headache
  Vomiting
Examination
  Focal neurologic signs (hemiparesis, posturing, asymmetrical reflexes)
  Abnormal pupillary light reflexes

METABOLIC OR TOXIC CAUSES

History
  Gradual onset of unconsciousness
  Preceding confusional state
  Seizures
  Known cognitive impairment
  Taking insulin or street drugs
Examination
  Absence of focal neurologic signs
  Presence of frontal release signs
  Intact pupillary light reflexes
  Tremor, asterixis, or multifocal myoclonus
  Evidence of systemic infection
  Needle tracks

MENINGITIS

History
  Worsening headache
  Neck stiffness and pain
  Fever, chills
  Progressive stupor and coma
Examination
  Fever, rigors
  Nuchal rigidity and signs of meningeal inflammation

Oximetry and a finger stick blood glucose assessment should be performed immediately. Emergency laboratory testing should generally include a complete blood count, serum electrolytes, a blood glucose level, tests of renal and liver function, coagulation tests, thyroid function tests, arterial blood gas analysis, a blood alcohol concentration, a urine drug screen, and an electrocardiogram.

The neurologic examination focuses on five systems whose careful assessment can distinguish structural from metabolic causes of coma and delineate the functional brain level caused by the pathologic process: the respiratory rate and pattern; the pupils' size, shape, and reactivity; eye movements and vestibulo-ocular reflexes; and motor responses to stimuli (Table 411-5).

The respiratory rate and pattern should be observed for 30 to 60 seconds. The earliest abnormalities seen in patients with altered consciousness are yawning, sighing, and posthyperventilation apnea, which occurs especially in those with metabolic encephalopathies. Stuporous patients should be asked to take five deep breaths and then be observed for the duration of subsequent apnea, which is normally less than 5 seconds. Cheyne-Stokes respiration (Chapter 86) is a periodic form of breathing whose amplitude forms a sine wave, with 5- to 45-second periods of apnea punctuating periods of hyperpnea; it is seen in the metabolic encephalopathies, especially those caused by heart failure, and during sleep. Central neurogenic hyperventilation, which is continuous hyperpnea and tachypnea that produces a pure respiratory alkalosis, occurs with lesions of the rostral brain stem tegmentum at the midbrain level; rapid, deep breathing (Kussmaul) that is compensating for a severe metabolic acidosis (Chapter 236) can look similar. Apneustic breathing, which is characterized by a prolonged inspiratory pause, is seen with pontine lesions. Ataxic breathing is an irregular and agonal sign of medullary failure.

Pupillary size and reactivity to a bright light stimulus can be assessed to evaluate the integrity of the optic and oculomotor nerves, the midbrain, and the sympathetic nerves. The reactivity of the pupils to light is an important sign that discriminates structural coma from metabolic-toxic coma. The pupils remain reactive through varying depths of metabolic-toxic coma, often until apnea ensues, whereas pupillary reflexes are lost earlier in structural coma that is caused by transtentorial herniation. The pupils are small, equal, and reactive in patients with metabolic encephalopathies. When the oculomotor nerve or the midbrain is involved, the ipsilateral pupil becomes unreactive to light because of damage to the parasympathetic pupilloconstrictors and dilates because of unopposed sympathetic pupillodilators. When herniation proceeds further, the brain stem sympathetic tracts are also damaged, so the pupil returns to midposition and becomes unreactive to light or dark. Lesions that affect only the pons and not the midbrain, such as pontine hemorrhage or infarction, can cause pinpoint pupils whose intact reaction to light can be seen with a magnifying glass. Preexisting disease (e.g., diabetes) or locally applied eye medications can also impair pupillary reflexes.

TABLE 411-5	BRAIN FUNCTIONAL LEVELS DETERMINED BY FINDINGS IN FIVE CLINICAL SYSTEMS

FUNCTIONAL LEVEL	CONSCIOUSNESS	RESPIRATION	PUPILS	VESTIBULO-OCULAR REFLEXES	MOTOR RESPONSES
CENTRAL TRANSTENTORIAL HERNIATION					
High diencephalic	Light stupor	Eupnea, yawning, posthyperventilation apnea	Small, reactive	Loss of checking component	Paratonia, grasp
Low diencephalic	Deep stupor	Cheyne-Stokes	Small, reactive	Loss of checking component	Decorticate posturing
Midbrain	Coma	Central neurogenic hyperventilation	Midposition, fixed	Loss of medial rectus function	Decerebrate posturing
Upper pons	Coma	Central neurogenic hyperventilation	Midposition, fixed	Loss of medial rectus function	Decerebrate posturing
Lower pons	Coma	Ataxic	Midposition, fixed	Absent	Flaccid
Medulla	Coma	Apnea	Midposition, fixed	Absent	Flaccid
UNCAL TRANSTENTORIAL HERNIATION					
Early third nerve	Unreliable	Normal	Ipsilateral dilated, fixed	Normal	Contralateral hemiparesis
Late third nerve	Coma	Cheyne-Stokes or central neurogenic hyperventilation	Ipsilateral dilated, fixed; contralateral dilated, fixed	Medial rectus dysfunction	Ipsilateral hemiparesis and contralateral decerebrate posturing
Midbrain-pons	Coma	Central neurogenic hyperventilation or ataxic	Midposition, fixed	Absent	Bilateral decerebrate posturing

Spontaneous eye movements may have localizing value. Conjugate horizontal eye deviation points to the side of brain lesions rostral to the brain stem (usually in the cerebral hemisphere) but to the side opposite brain stem lesions. Tonic downward eye deviation suggests acute lesions of the thalamus or dorsal midbrain. Tonic upward eye deviation is unusual but is seen in patients with hypoxic-ischemic lesions. Ocular bobbing with a rapid downward movement followed by a slow return upward suggests a pontine lesion. Reverse ocular bobbing with a slow downward and rapid upward movement ("ocular dipping") has poor localizing value but may be seen after hypoxic-ischemic insults and metabolic disorders. "Ping-Pong" gaze with alternating conjugate horizontal eye movements is nonspecific, but a slower and otherwise similar disorder, called periodic alternating gaze, is seen in those with portosystemic encephalopathy (Chapter 157). Ocular skew deviation, in which one eye is higher than the other on primary gaze, suggests a brain stem lesion.

The vestibulo-ocular reflex assesses brain stem and cerebral hemispheric function by reflexively inducing eye movements. First, the external auditory canal should be inspected to exclude perforation of the tympanic membrane and obstruction by cerumen. Ice water is then injected into the canal (10 mL for usual assessment but 50 mL for assessment of brain death), and the induced reflex eye movements are observed (see Table 411-5). In patients with normal consciousness, such as in psychogenic coma, marked horizontal nystagmus is produced. In those with stupor at a diencephalic level, such as from metabolic encephalopathy, the fast component of nystagmus is suppressed, so the patient responds with full tonic conjugate eye movements toward the injected ear. With lesions of the oculomotor or abducens nerves or lesions of the midbrain or pons, ophthalmoplegia of localizing value is observed. In brain death or total brain stem failure, no response is observed. The vestibulo-ocular reflexes may be ablated after treatment with ototoxic antibiotics.

Motor responses are observed after noxious stimulation, particularly nasal tickle, sternal rub, and ice water irrigation of the external auditory canal. In light coma from metabolic encephalopathy, symmetrical paratonia and grasp reflexes may be present. At lower functional levels of structural coma, limb posturing is often observed. Limb posturing is a unilateral or bilateral, stereotyped, tonic brain stem reflex movement induced by stimulation, especially noxious stimuli. Decorticate posturing, in which the arm is flexed and the ipsilateral leg is extended, suggests a midbrain functional level. Decerebrate posturing, in which both the arm and the ipsilateral leg are extended, suggests a pontine functional level. When the entire brain stem is destroyed, as in brain death, all limbs remain flaccid during stimulation. Metabolic-toxic encephalopathies usually produce symmetrical motor signs, whereas structural causes of coma frequently produce asymmetrical motor signs. Hypoglycemia and acute hyponatremia are exceptions in which aphasia, gaze paresis, and hemiparesis may be seen. Myoclonic seizures with continuous or intermittent rhythmic clonic movements frequently develop in patients who have suffered hypoxic-ischemic neuronal damage during cardiopulmonary arrest. Progression to myoclonic status epilepticus is a bad prognostic sign.

After the neurologic examination, screening laboratory tests, brain CT, and lumbar puncture have been accomplished, a tentative diagnosis can be made in most patients. If focal signs are present despite normal findings on CT, consideration should be given to an acute stoke involving the posterior circulation (Chapter 414). Brain CT angiography or magnetic resonance imaging (MRI) can clarify the diagnosis. If lateralizing signs are absent, metabolic and toxic causes are most likely. An electroencephalogram (EEG) is useful in patients in whom nonconvulsive seizure activity may be causing stupor or coma.

TREATMENT Rx

Management of coma requires simultaneous diagnostic, supportive, and treatment measures (Table 411-6). Specific treatments, which depend on the causative diagnosis, include urgent attention to any head trauma (Chapter 406). Emergency stabilization of respiration and circulation and control of seizures are critical for all patients. In patients without focal findings or obvious meningitis, 50% dextrose (25 g intravenously), thiamine (50 mg intravenously), naloxone (0.4 to 2.0 mg intravenously), and flumazenil (0.2 mg intravenously) should be administered during the diagnostic assessment. If fever, nuchal rigidity, or leukocytosis is present, the patient should be treated presumptively for bacterial meningitis (Chapter 420) with intravenous antibiotics before neuroimaging and lumbar puncture.

Elevated intracranial pressure must be lowered urgently. Treatments include hyperventilation by bag or ventilator, intravenous hyperosmolar

agents (Chapter 112) such as mannitol, and intravenous glucocorticoid drugs for patients with vasogenic edema from brain tumors (Chapter 195), abscesses (Chapter 421), or bacterial meningitis (Chapter 420). Intravenous barbiturate or benzodiazepine therapy remains of uncertain benefit. Therapeutically induced hypothermia for several days improves outcomes in patients who are in coma after diffuse hypoxic-ischemic neuronal damage caused by cardiac arrest.[1]

PROGNOSIS

The prognosis is highly variable and depends on the cause, stage, degree of structural brain damage, and potential reversibility. Prediction rules for recovery apply only to a specific cause. The prognosis after traumatic brain injury is predicted by the Glasgow Coma Score (see Table 406-1). In patients who have survived cardiopulmonary arrest and resuscitation and in whom toxic and metabolic factors (e.g., sedation, neuromuscular blockade, hypothermia, organ failure, and shock) are not an issue, the likelihood for recovery of awareness is less than 1% if the following are present:

Day 1: presence of myoclonic status epilepticus

Days 1 to 3: bilateral absence of the N20 response of the somatosensory evoked potential

Days 1 to 3: serum neuron-specific enolase concentration higher than 33 μg/L

Day 3: absent pupillary or corneal reflexes; extensor or absent motor responses

If the patient remains comatose on day 3 without these findings and without a contribution from a potentially reversible metabolic or toxic encephalopathy, the probability of recovery of awareness is below 10% if there is no withdrawal response to painful stimuli and below 40% if the patient withdraws to painful stimuli but lacks spontaneous eye opening.

THE VEGETATIVE STATE

The vegetative state is a disorder of consciousness in which wakefulness is retained but awareness of self and environment is entirely absent, to the extent that it can be tested clinically. The vegetative state may be a transient stage during spontaneous recovery from coma to awareness, or it may be a chronic, unchanging state. Adjectives such as "persistent" or "permanent" should be avoided because they generate confusion by confounding the diagnosis and prognosis.

EPIDEMIOLOGY AND PATHOBIOLOGY

The vegetative state is caused by diffuse or multifocal brain lesions that disconnect the polymodal cerebral cortices from the thalami but spare the brain stem and hypothalamus. The prevalence of a transient vegetative state after brain injury is unknown. The prevalence of the chronic vegetative state is 19 per million.

Causative lesions can be located bilaterally in the thalami, diffusely in the cerebral cortex, or diffusely in the white matter that connects the thalami to the cortex. Two clinical disorders are most commonly responsible: diffuse hypoxic-ischemic neuronal damage to the thalami and cortex suffered during cardiopulmonary arrest and diffuse axonal injury from a traumatic injury

TABLE 411-6	EMERGENCY MANAGEMENT OF COMATOSE PATIENTS

1. Ensure oxygenation
2. Maintain the circulation
3. Administer 50% dextrose, 25 g IV, and control glucose
4. Lower raised intracranial pressure
5. Stop seizures with lorazepam, 1.0-2.0 mg IV
6. Search for and treat infections
7. Restore acid-base and electrolyte balance
8. Normalize body temperature
9. Administer thiamine, 50 mg IV, and multivitamins
10. Consider administration of opioid antagonists (naloxone, 0.4-2.0 mg IV)
11. Consider administration of benzodiazepine antagonists (flumazenil, 0.2 mg IV)
12. Control agitation
13. Protect the eyes
14. Consider inducing therapeutic hypothermia for diffuse hypoxic-ischemic causes

Modified from Posner JB, Saper CB, Schiff ND, et al. *Plum and Posner's Diagnosis of Stupor and Coma*, 4th ed. New York: Oxford University Press; 2007:311.

TABLE 411-7	DIAGNOSIS OF THE VEGETATIVE STATE

I. Absence of:
   Awareness of self or environment
   Purposeful or voluntary behavioral response to all stimuli
   Language comprehension or expression

II. Presence of:
   Intermittent wakefulness manifested by the presence of sleep-wake cycles
   Autonomic functions
   Cranial nerve and spinal reflexes

III. Potential behavioral repertoire:
   Breathe spontaneously
   Spontaneous roving eye movements
   Utter sounds but no words
   Grimace to pain, make facial expressions
   Yawn, make chewing jaw movements, swallow saliva
   Move limbs nonpurposefully, arch back, decorticate limb posturing
   Flexion withdrawal from noxious stimuli
   Move head or eyes briefly toward sound or movement
   Auditory startle

TABLE 411-8	DIAGNOSIS OF THE MINIMALLY CONSCIOUS STATE

Globally impaired responsiveness

Limited but discernable evidence of awareness of self and environment as demonstrated by the presence of one or more of the following behaviors that occur in a contingent relationship to relevant environmental stimuli and are not simply reflexive movements:
   Follow simple commands
   Gesture yes/no answers
   Make intelligible vocalizations or gestures in direct response to a question's linguistic content
   Reach for objects that demonstrates a clear relationship between object location and direction of reach
   Touch and hold objects in a manner that accommodates the size and shape of the object
   Sustain visual pursuit to moving stimuli
   Smile or cry appropriately to linguistic or visual content of emotional but not to affectively neutral topics or stimuli

caused by a torque force. These two disorders have different pathologies: hypoxic-ischemic injury affects cortical, thalamic, and cerebellar neurons, whereas diffuse axonal injury shears the axons at the gray matter–white matter junction in the cortex.

CLINICAL MANIFESTATIONS AND DIAGNOSIS

The clinical features of the vegetative state (Table 411-7) are dominated by what patients do. A careful neurologic examination must be performed to search for any evidence of awareness because up to 40% of patients in whom a vegetative state is initially diagnosed are actually in a minimally conscious state (see later).

The vegetative state is a clinical syndrome with a spectrum of severity. The typical patient has diffuse slow-wave activity on the EEG, but the most severely affected patients have isoelectric EEGs. As determined by functional neuroimaging studies, an occasional patient with a clinically diagnosed vegetative state can perform ideational tasks on command, with evidence on functional MRI that they possess awareness. Such functional neuroimaging tests are not yet part of routine clinical practice but may become standard clinical assessment tools for patients who are suspected to be in a vegetative state.

TREATMENT AND PROGNOSIS Rx

No treatments reverse or improve the vegetative state. The aggressiveness of medical treatment of patients in the vegetative state should ideally be guided by their previously stated wishes. Patients require the same medical and nursing care, physical therapy, and nutritional needs as patients in coma. Patients should be referred to specialized neurorehabilitation units when possible. Patients who are in a vegetative state from nontraumatic causes and who do not regain awareness within 3 months of the insult have less than a 1% chance of experiencing significant neurologic recovery. After traumatic brain injury, the prognosis cannot be estimated with a similar degree of certainty until after 1 year, although functional neuroimaging is a promising approach to identify patients who are destined to recover awareness.

THE MINIMALLY CONSCIOUS STATE

The minimally conscious state (Table 411-8) is a disorder of altered consciousness characterized by a profound lack of responsiveness but partial or intermittent evidence of awareness of self and environment. Patients may typically have suffered less severe injuries than patients in the vegetative state. The minimally conscious state is much more common than the vegetative state, from which it must be distinguished. When compared with patients in the vegetative state, patients in the minimally conscious state are more likely to respond to environmental and sensory stimuli, to stimulant medications such as levodopa or dopamine agonists (which stimulate thalamic dopaminergic neurons and are prescribed in the same dose ranges as for the treatment of Parkinson's disease, Chapter 416), and perhaps to deep brain electrical stimulation of the intralaminar thalamic nuclei. Patients in the minimally conscious state require the same specialized neurorehabilitation

services as those in the vegetative state. There are no good prognostic data for the minimally conscious state other than for recovery after traumatic brain injury (Chapter 406).

THE LOCKED-IN SYNDROME

The locked-in syndrome, a state of profound paralysis, is not a disorder of consciousness but may be mistaken for one. In its classic form, it is produced when a large infarction or hemorrhage in the pontine tegmentum and base produces quadriplegia, pseudobulbar palsy, and paralysis of horizontal eye movements. Once the acute encephalopathy resolves, locked-in patients usually remain awake and alert, breathe spontaneously, and have normal consciousness and cognition, to the extent that they can be tested accurately. Inexperienced examiners may incorrectly diagnose locked-in patients as being comatose because of their profound paralysis, pinpoint pupils, and seeming unresponsiveness. A similar state of profound, global paralysis with intact cognition can be produced by advanced amyotrophic lateral sclerosis (Chapter 418), Guillain-Barré syndrome (Chapter 428), or critical illness polyneuropathy (Chapter 428).

Locked-in patients can be taught to communicate with voluntary vertical eye movements and eyelid movements, which are typically their only retained volitional movements because they are controlled rostral to the pons. Most affected patients die within a few months, but some otherwise healthy young patients who have become locked in as a result of basilar artery occlusion have survived for many years; occasional patients may recover function to become independent. Computerized systems can help patients communicate.

BRAIN DEATH

Brain death is the term popularly applied to the determination of human death based on tests that show irreversible cessation of all clinical brain functions. Once illness or injury has destroyed the brain or rendered its clinical functions irreversibly lost, a human being is dead. Brain death is a medically and legally accepted determination of human death throughout North America, Europe, Australia, most of the developed world, and much of the undeveloped world. Brain-dead patients serve as ideal multiorgan donors.

EPIDEMIOLOGY AND PATHOBIOLOGY

Most cases of brain death result from massive traumatic brain injury (Chapter 406), intracranial hemorrhage (Chapter 415), meningitis (Chapter 420), or diffuse hypoxic-ischemic neuronal damage secondary to cardiac arrest (Chapter 63) or asphyxia. Marked cerebral edema from the primary injury or illness produces severe intracranial hypertension. When intracranial pressure exceeds mean arterial blood pressure (or systolic blood pressure in some cases), intracranial blood flow ceases and widespread ischemic death of brain neurons ensues. Syndromes of transtentorial herniation commonly occur.

CLINICAL MANIFESTATIONS AND DIAGNOSIS

Brain-dead patients have no brain functions measurable at the bedside. The diagnosis should be suspected in any patient who is deeply comatose,

TABLE 411-9 TESTS FOR BRAIN DEATH

I. Preconditions showing irreversibility: all necessary
- Presence of a structural brain lesion sufficient to produce all the clinical signs
- Absence of reversible significant toxic or metabolic encephalopathy:
   No depressant drug intoxication
   No neuromuscular blockade (use electroneurography if uncertain)
   No severe hypothermia
   No severe hypotension
- Sequential repeated testing or one test followed by a confirmatory blood flow test

II. Signs showing complete cessation of all clinical brain functions: all necessary
- Coma: No spontaneous movements, no response to any stimuli, and no reflex movements integrated by the brain
- Apnea: No breathing or respiratory effort when the $P_{ACO_2} \geq 60$ mm Hg while protecting the P_{AO_2}
- Brain stem areflexia: all necessary
   Absent pupillary light and dark reflexes
   Absent corneal touch reflexes
   Absent facial movement to noxious stimuli
   Absent vestibulo-ocular reflexes tested by caloric irrigation of the external auditory canal with 50 mL of ice water
   Absent pharyngeal and tracheal reflexes to endotracheal tube suctioning

III. Confirmatory tests: optional but desirable; neuroimaging preferred
- Neuroimaging that shows complete absence of intracranial blood flow; one test
   Intravenous radionuclide angiography
   Transcranial Doppler ultrasound
   Computed tomographic angiography
   Magnetic resonance angiography or diffusion
   Single-photon emission computed tomography
- Electrophysiologic testing (use only if intracranial pressure is not elevated)
   Electroencephalography + brain stem auditory evoked responses + somatosensory evoked responses: all isoelectric

is unresponsive to stimuli, has absent pupillary light reflexes, and is completely ventilator dependent. The diagnosis requires a comprehensive evaluation (Table 411-9) that demonstrates both total loss of brain functions and its irreversibility as documented by at least two sequential examinations performed by an experienced physician or one examination followed by a neuroimaging test to confirm the complete absence of intracranial blood flow.

TREATMENT   Rx

There is no treatment. Once the diagnosis has been made, the patient is declared dead. If the family has agreed to allow the deceased patient to serve as an organ donor, the ventilator is reattached following the apnea test, and the patient is moved to the surgical suite. If the patient is not an organ donor, the ventilator is not reattached, and all lines and monitors are discontinued. Physicians should be knowledgeable about local laws that may restrict making the diagnosis in patients belonging to certain religious groups that do not accept brain death as human death.

1. Holzer M, Bernard SA, Hachimi-Idrissi S, et al. Hypothermia for neuroprotection after cardiac arrest: systematic review and individual patient data meta-analysis. *Crit Care Med.* 2005;33:414-418.

SUGGESTED READINGS

Bernat JL. Chronic consciousness disorders. *Annu Rev Med.* 2009;60:381-392. *Reviews vegetative and minimally conscious states.*

Holzer M. Targeted temperature management for comatose survivors of cardiac arrest. *N Engl J Med.* 2010;363:1256-1264. *Review the technique, outcomes, and adverse effects of therapeutic hypothermia to protect the brain of cardiac arrest survivors.*

Wijdicks EFM, Varelas PN, Gronset GS, et al. Practice parameter update: determining brain death in adults: report of the Quality Standards Subcommittee of the American Academy of Neurology. *Neurology.* 2010;74:1911-1918. *Clinical and laboratory approach to diagnosing brain death.*

Wu O, Batista LM, Lima FO, et al. Predicting clinical outcome in comatose cardiac arrest patients using early noncontrast computed tomography. *Stroke.* 2011;42:985-992. *Median Hounsfield units in the whole brain and the ratio in the putamen compared with the posterior limb of the internal capsule predict poor outcome.*

412

DISORDERS OF SLEEP

MARK W. MAHOWALD

DEFINITION

Wake-sleep complaints are second only to complaints of pain as the reason that patients seek medical attention. Undiagnosed and untreated wake-sleep complaints extract an enormous toll at the personal level in terms of misery and at the societal level in socioeconomic consequences. Knowledge of sleep and its disorders has expanded rapidly over the past half century, particularly with the discovery that sleep is far more than the passive absence of wakefulness. Sleep is an active brain process that includes two divergent states: non–rapid eye movement (NREM) and rapid eye movement (REM) sleep. A complex array of neurotransmitters, neuropeptides, and circulating humoral sleep-promoting factors interact with multiple areas of the central nervous system to determine wakefulness, REM sleep, and NREM sleep.

PATHOBIOLOGY

Wakefulness is controlled by the reticular activating system of the rostral brain stem, which projects to the thalamus and cortex. Inhibition of these projections, which is modulated by neurons in the pons and midbrain, results in sleep. REM sleep, during which most dreaming occurs, is generated within the tegmentum of the pons with modulation from the norepinephrine- and serotonin-containing neurons of the locus caeruleus and the dorsal raphe nucleus. Electrical events generated in the pontine reticular formation (i.e., ponto-geniculo-occipital [PGO] waves) are propagated through the oculomotor and visual system during REM sleep simultaneously with REMs. PGO waves are suppressed by norepinephrine, and the serotonin neuronal systems suppress PGO waves and REM; cholinergic neurons are stimulatory. PGO input can induce an action potential in neurons below their usual threshold. Such PGO-facilitated activity in the visual system may play a role in the random imagery of dreaming.

Hypocretins (orexins) are sleep modulatory neuropeptides made in the lateral hypothalamus with projections to the locus caeruleus and dorsal raphe, as well as to the thalamus, where they modulate the release of excitatory (glutamate) and inhibitory (γ-aminobutyric acid) neurotransmitters. Disruption of this system induces narcolepsy in animals, and hypocretin neurotransmission is deficient in most narcoleptic patients.

Stage of Sleep

Sleep stages in humans are defined electroencephalographically and behaviorally (Table 412-1). Sleep includes NREM and REM sleep. NREM sleep can be divided into four stages. In *stage I NREM sleep*, patients are drowsy and may maintain some environmental awareness. The electroencephalogram (EEG) loses its alpha rhythm (8 to 13 Hz) and develops theta (3 to 7 Hz) activity; vertex potentials (i.e., negative deflections recorded from the midline) occur, especially in response to sensory stimuli. Slow lateral eye movements take place, and spontaneous motor activity, as monitored by electromyography (EMG), is diminished. Stage I represents about 5% of normal sleep time.

Stage II NREM sleep is characterized by sleep spindles (12 to 14 Hz), vertex sharp waves, and K complexes (i.e., biphasic, high-voltage slow waves often followed by sleep spindles). Slow lateral eye movements may persist. EMG activity is further reduced. Stage II NREM sleep represents 50 to 60% of sleep and increases with age.

Stages III and IV NREM sleep are characterized by slow or delta waves (<4 Hz) and are therefore called delta sleep or deep sleep. If 20 to 50% of the EEG is delta activity, the patient is in stage III sleep; if delta activity is 50% or greater, the sleep event is called stage IV. Deep sleep constitutes 10 to 20% of sleep time (less with advancing age). EMG activity is diminished. Eye movements are not seen, and ventilation is regular.

In REM sleep, the EEG resembles that of waking, with low-voltage, mixed frequencies. Abrupt REMs and irregular ventilation and heart rate are present. Penile tumescence occurs, and muscle tone is depressed because of suppression of activity in all somatic muscles except the diaphragm. REM

TABLE 412-1 STAGES OF SLEEP

SLEEP STAGE	EEG	EYE MOVEMENTS	EMG ACTIVITY	IMAGERY
Wakefulness	Alpha and beta activity (low voltage, fast)	Random, rapid	Active, spontaneous	Vivid, external
Non-REM sleep (NREM)				
Stage I (drowsiness)	Theta activity	Slow, rolling	Attenuated, episodic	Dulled
Stage II (light sleep)	Sleep spindles, K complexes	Slow or absent	Attenuated	Nonvivid
Stage III and IV (slow wave sleep)	Delta activity	Absent	Attenuated	
REM sleep	Low amplitude, irregular	Abrupt, rapid eye movements	Absent	Vivid, bizarre

EEG = electroencephalogram; EMG = electromyogram; REM = rapid eye movement.

TABLE 412-2 CAUSES OF HYPERSOMNIA (EXCESSIVE DAYTIME SLEEPINESS*)

Sleep deprivation

Obstructive sleep apnea (Chapter 100)

Narcolepsy

Circadian rhythm disorders
  Shift work sleep disorder
  Jet lag
  Advanced and delayed sleep phase syndrome

Restless legs syndrome (may be associated with extreme daytime sleepiness but is always manifested as insomnia)

Drug use

Syndromes associated with subjective sleepiness but usually without true, verifiable sleepiness by objective testing
  Depression
  Chronic pain
  Insomnia

*Excessive daytime sleepiness is usually confirmed by objective testing.

TABLE 412-3 EPWORTH SLEEPINESS SCALE

How likely are you to doze off or fall asleep in the following situations, in contrast to just feeling tired? This refers to your usual way of life in recent time. Even if you have not done some of these things recently, try to work out how they would have affected you. Use the following scale to choose the most appropriate number for each situation.

0 = would never doze
1 = slight chance of dozing
2 = moderate chance of dozing
3 = high chance of dozing

SITUATION	CHANCE OF DOZING
Sitting and reading	_____
Watching TV	_____
Sitting and inactive in a public place (theater or meeting)	_____
As a passenger in a car for an hour without a break	_____
Lying down to rest in the afternoon when circumstances permit	_____
Sitting and talking to someone	_____
Sitting quietly after lunch (without alcohol)	_____
In a car, while stopped for a few minutes in traffic	_____
Total	_____

From Johns MW. A new method for measuring daytime sleepiness: the Epworth Sleepiness Scale. *Sleep.* 1991;14:540-545.

sleep occupies 20 to 25% of sleep time. Dreaming occurs during all stages of NREM sleep and during REM sleep.

There is some evidence that procedural (i.e., motor learning such as typing) and declarative (i.e., episodic learning such as recalling places or events) memory consolidation occurs during REM sleep. REM sleep time increases after task training. After episodic learning, memory consolidation is accomplished during slow wave sleep by rapid reactivation of the hippocampal neurons previously activated by the place or event to be remembered. Alternatively, it has been hypothesized that dream sleep functions as a random stimulator of the cortex to remove weak memories and thus permit only stronger memories to be retained.

CLINICAL MANIFESTATIONS

Most sleep complaints fall into four categories: hypersomnia (excessive daytime sleepiness), insomnia (trouble falling or staying asleep), circadian rhythm (biologic clock) disorders, and parasomnias (complex behavior arising during the sleep period).

Hypersomnia is typically manifested as the tendency to fall asleep in inappropriate or undesirable settings such as at work, while talking with others, or while driving. Sleepiness from any cause can result in impaired sustained attention, with adverse, occasionally disastrous socioeconomic consequences in the classroom, in the workplace, or on the highways. The most common cause of hypersomnia is volitional sleep deprivation for social or economic reasons. Volitional sleep deprivation can usually be diagnosed by the history or sleep diary. Nonvolitional sleep deprivation–related sleepiness is almost always due to an underlying sleep disorder, most commonly either obstructive sleep apnea or narcolepsy (Table 412-2).

DIAGNOSIS
Subjective
Sleep Diaries and Sleepiness Scales

Sleep diaries kept for a period of 2 or 3 weeks may reveal valuable information about a patient's subjective perception of wakefulness and sleep. One useful scale is the Epworth Sleepiness Scale (Table 412-3), which is frequently used as a screening tool for identifying excessive daytime sleepiness and generally correlates with other measures of sleep propensity. A score higher than 11

suggests a high probability of a sleep problem. This scale may be limited by its lack of sensitivity in that there may be a striking discrepancy between self-perceived sleepiness and the physiologic sleepiness that can be documented by formal sleep studies.

Objective
Polysomnography

Polysomnography (Chapter 100) determines states of sleep and wakefulness by recording eye movements, submental EMG activity, and the EEG. If sleep-disordered breathing is suspected, additional monitoring such as oral/nasal airflow, chest/abdominal movement, hemoglobin oxygen saturation, and transcutaneous or end-tidal CO_2 is used. A full EEG helps evaluate disorders of arousal, REM sleep behavior disorder, and nocturnal seizures.

Multiple Sleep Latency Test

The multiple sleep latency test, which assesses the tendency to fall asleep during normal waking hours, consists of five 20-minute nap opportunities at 2-hour intervals. An all-night polysomnograph is generally performed the night before to determine the quality and quantity of the preceding night's sleep. Normal, fully rested adults do not usually fall asleep in less than 10 minutes and uncommonly display REM sleep during daytime naps. Patients with narcolepsy typically fall asleep in 5 minutes or less and often display REM sleep during at least two of the daytime naps. This test is not generally performed in patients with obstructive sleep apnea because an explanation for the hypersomnia should have been identified by the preceding all-night polysomnograph.

Actigraphy

Analysis of sleep diaries may be insufficient to verify a tentative diagnosis in patients with reported insomnia or suspected abnormalities in the wake-sleep cycle. In such cases, definitive objective data may be obtained by actigraphy, in which a small, wrist-mounted device records activity plotted against time—usually over a period of 1 to 3 weeks. There is direct correlation between the rest/activity recorded by the actigraph and the wake-sleep pattern as determined by polysomnography.

● SPECIFIC SLEEP DISORDERS
Obstructive Sleep Apnea

Obstructive sleep apnea (Chapter 100), which is the most common medical disorder causing hypersomnia, affects more than 2% of adult women and 4% of adult men. It is seen primarily in overweight people who are loud snorers, but it may also occur in children and thin individuals.

Obstructive sleep apnea is characterized by collapse of the upper airway during sleep. This upper airway collapse may be associated with a fall in the blood oxygen level and results in repetitive arousal (up to 100 per hour of sleep) to re-establish upper airway airflow. These brief arousals are not perceived by the individual but result in excessive daytime sleepiness. Obstructive sleep apnea is described in detail in Chapter 100.

Narcolepsy

EPIDEMIOLOGY AND PATHOBIOLOGY

Narcolepsy affects 1 in 2000 individuals. It has a clear genetic component, with more than 90% of affected individuals carrying the HLA-DR2/DQ1 (under current nomenclature, HLA-DR15 and HLA-DQ6) gene, which is found in less than 30% of the general population. Despite a genetic component, the risk in a first-degree relative is only 1 to 2%, but this risk represents a 10- to 40-fold increase over that in the general population. Thus, the genetic component is neither necessary nor sufficient to cause narcolepsy.

Hypocretin-1 is an excitatory neuropeptide found in a very circumscribed group of neurons confined to the hypothalamic region. Patients with narcolepsy have lost hypocretin cells, possibly by an immune-mediated phenomenon.

CLINICAL MANIFESTATIONS

Narcolepsy is characterized by the tendency to fall asleep inappropriately during the daytime, particularly during sedentary or nonstimulating activities, despite having obtained an adequate amount of sleep the preceding night. Other symptoms of narcolepsy include (1) cataplexy (sudden brief spells of muscle weakness), often triggered by emotionally laden events; (2) hypnagogic (occurring at sleep onset) or hypnopompic (occurring at sleep offset) hallucinations; (3) sleep paralysis (awakening to find the entire body paralyzed—with the exception of being able to breathe and move the eyes); (4) automatic behavior; and (5) disrupted nighttime sleep.

Patients with narcolepsy do not sleep more per 24 hours than non-narcoleptics do; instead, they are unable to maintain the normal boundaries of wakefulness, NREM sleep, and REM sleep. The automatic behavior (driving past the desired freeway exit, putting clothing into the refrigerator) represents an admixture of wakefulness and NREM sleep, with enough wakefulness to perform complex behavior but not enough for conscious awareness of the behavior. Sleep paralysis and cataplexy represent the simultaneous occurrence of REM sleep–related muscle paralysis and wakefulness. If the paralysis intrudes into wakefulness, the result is cataplexy; if it persists into wakefulness from a period of REM sleep, sleep paralysis results. The waking hallucinations represent the release of sleep-related dreaming into wakefulness, and the disrupted nighttime sleep is a manifestation of the "state boundary dyscontrol" aspect of narcolepsy. Sleep paralysis and hypnagogic/hypnopompic hallucinations, but not cataplexy, are often experienced by people who do not have narcolepsy—particularly in the setting of sleep deprivation.

DIAGNOSIS

Sleep laboratory evaluation of patients with narcolepsy includes polysomnography and the multiple sleep latency test. Results of the all-night polysomnograph will usually be unremarkable. The multiple sleep latency test will demonstrate objective hypersomnolence, and REM sleep may be present during the daytime naps.

Levels of hypocretin-1 are undetectable in the cerebrospinal fluid (CSF) of most patients with narcolepsy who experience cataplexy and are HLA-DQB1*0602 positive. Absent CSF hypocretin-1 levels are not found in any conditions that could be confused clinically with narcolepsy, thus suggesting that CSF hypocretin determinations could be of value in the diagnosis of narcolepsy in difficult cases.

TABLE 412-4 CLASSIFICATION OF ADULT INSOMNIA

PRIMARY INSOMNIA

Idiopathic insomnia—Insomnia arising in infancy or childhood with a persistent, unremitting course

Psychophysiologic insomnia—Insomnia caused by a maladaptive conditioned response in which the patient learns to associate the bed environment with heightened arousal rather than sleep; its onset is often associated with an event causing acute insomnia, with the sleep disturbance persisting despite resolution of the precipitating factor

Paradoxical insomnia (sleep-state misperception)—Insomnia characterized by a marked mismatch between the patient's description of sleep duration and objective polysomnographic findings

SECONDARY INSOMNIA

Adjustment insomnia—Insomnia associated with active psychosocial stressors

Inadequate sleep hygiene—Insomnia associated with lifestyle habits that impair sleep

Insomnia caused by a psychiatric disorder—Insomnia secondary to an active psychiatric disorder, such as anxiety or depression

Insomnia caused by a medical condition—Insomnia secondary to a condition such as restless legs syndrome, chronic pain, nocturnal cough or dyspnea, or hot flashes

Insomnia caused by a drug or substance—Insomnia secondary to consumption or discontinuation of medications, drugs of abuse, alcohol, or caffeine

Reproduced with permission from *The New England Journal of Medicine*. Silber M. Clinical practice. Chronic insomnia. *N Engl J Med*. 2005;353:803-810.

TREATMENT **Rx**

Stimulant medications such as methylphenidate (e.g., 10 to 60 mg/day), methamphetamine (e.g., 20 to 60 mg/day), dextroamphetamine (e.g., 5 to 60 mg/day), and modafinil (e.g., 100 to 400 mg/day) are generally effective and well tolerated. Sodium oxybate (20 to 40 mg/kg per night in divided doses), alone or combined with modafinil, can reduce sleep disruption significantly. However, responses to these medications are variable among individuals, and clinical judgment is needed to titrate to an effective dose. Dependency, tolerance, or abuse of stimulant medications is uncommon in patients with narcolepsy, and there is no indication for "drug holidays." Cataplexy is often controlled by tricyclic antidepressants (e.g., imipramine, 25 to 50 mg at bedtime), selective serotonin re-uptake inhibitors (e.g., fluoxetine, 10 to 20 mg/day), or selective norepinephrine re-uptake inhibitors (e.g., venlafaxine, 25 to 37.5 mg/day). γ-Hydroxybutyrate (20 to 40 mg/kg per night in divided doses) has been used in difficult cases.

Insomnia

Insomnia (Table 412-4) is defined not simply by total sleep time but rather by difficulty in initiation and maintenance of sleep, poor quality of sleep, and a insufficient duration of sleep, such that functioning in the awake state is impaired.

EPIDEMIOLOGY

Insomnia, the most prevalent sleep complaint, affects up to 10 to 20% of the adult population and is second only to the complaint of pain as a reason to seek medical attention.

PATHOBIOLOGY

There is growing evidence that some insomniacs may be in a constant state of hyperarousal because many are actually less sleepy during the day than normal subjects are as measured by objective daytime nap studies, and some also have increased 24-hour metabolic activity.

Many people with insomnia have identifiable psychiatric or psychological problems, and untreated insomnia is a risk factor for the future development of psychiatric problems such as depression (Chapter 404) or substance abuse (Chapter 33). Importantly, the relationship between insomnia and psychiatric conditions is bidirectional: depression may cause insomnia, and insomnia may cause depression.

CLINICAL MANIFESTATIONS

Patients with insomnia complain of an inability to sleep long enough or well enough to awaken feeling rested or restored despite having an adequate amount of time to devote to sleep. Sleep deprivation as a result of inadequate time to devote to sleep is not insomnia. Many patients complain of

TABLE 412-5   COGNITIVE BEHAVIORAL THERAPY FOR INSOMNIA

STIMULUS-CONTROL THERAPY

Go to bed only when sleepy
Use the bedroom only for sleeping and sex
Go to another room when unable to sleep in 15 to 20 minutes, read or engage in other quiet activities, and return to bed only when sleepy; repeat if necessary
Have a regular wake time regardless of the duration of sleep
Avoid daytime napping

SLEEP-RESTRICTION THERAPY

Reduce time in bed to the estimated total sleep time (minimum, 5 hr)
Increase time in bed by 15 minutes every week when the estimated sleep efficiency (ratio of time asleep to time in bed) is at least 90%

RELAXATION THERAPY

Physical component: progressive muscle relaxation, biofeedback
Mental component: imagery training, meditation, hypnosis

COGNITIVE THERAPY

Education to alter faulty beliefs and attitudes about sleep, such as that a minimum of 8 hours of sleep per night is required for health

SLEEP-HYGIENE EDUCATION

Correct extrinsic factors affecting sleep, such as environmental disruption (pets or snoring bed partner); bedroom temperature; fixation on the bedside clock; use of alcohol, nicotine, or caffeine; lack of exercise or exercise too close to bedtime

Reproduced with permission from *The New England Journal of Medicine*. Silber M. Clinical practice. Chronic insomnia. *N Engl J Med*. 2005;353:803-810.

nonrestorative sleep. Daytime consequences include feeling tired or fatigued or having trouble concentrating. True excessive daytime sleepiness (inappropriate or uncontrollable sleep episodes during the day) is extremely rare in insomniacs.

DIAGNOSIS

Insomnia is a clinical diagnosis. Sleep diaries and actigraphy may be very helpful in difficult cases. Formal sleep studies are rarely indicated unless there is reason to suspect a coexisting sleep disorder such as obstructive sleep apnea.

TREATMENT   Rx

Behavioral therapy for insomnia (Table 412-5) can be quite effective but may be very time-consuming.**1** Over-the-counter sleep aids are of little, if any benefit.

Although medications used to treat depression are often prescribed to treat insomnia, there is very little evidence that they are effective in the treatment of insomnia not associated with depression. Nevertheless, if patients with insomnia are physiologically hyperaroused, a case may be made for chronic administration of sedative-hypnotic agents.**2** Three classes of medications are approved for the treatment of insomnia: the benzodiazepines (e.g., temazepam, 15 to 30 mg at bedtime; triazolam, 1.25 to 2.5 mg at bedtime; or estazolam, 1 to 2 mg at bedtime), the newer, nonbenzodiazepines (e.g., zolpidem, 5 to 10 mg at bedtime; zolpidem controlled release, 6.25 to 12.5 mg at bedtime; zaleplon, 5 to 10 mg at bedtime; or eszopiclone, 1 to 3 mg at bedtime), and a melatonin agonist (ramelteon, 8 mg at bedtime). Combined behavioral and pharmacologic treatments are often effective. Benzodiazepines may be administered safely and effectively for longer than 3 weeks. Tolerance, abuse, and dependency can be associated with chronic benzodiazepine administration in patients with well-documented sleep disorders, but the incidence of these complications is relatively low. Melatonin is normally secreted by the pineal gland (Chapter 230) in synchronization with the light-dark cycle. Its effect on sleep is variable, and its efficacy in treating insomnia has been disappointing.

Restless Legs Syndrome

Restless legs syndrome, which is one of the most common causes of severe insomnia, is a neurologic sensory/movement disorder that affects 5 to 15% of the general population. It is described in detail in Chapter 417.

Disorders of Circadian Rhythm

DEFINITION

Most living creatures follow a relentless and pervasive daily rhythm of activity and rest that is ultimately linked to the geophysical light-dark cycle. Plants, animals, and even unicellular organisms show daily variations in metabolic activity, locomotion, feeding, and many other functions. The importance of the light-dark cycle on the human biologic clock is underscored by the fact that only a third of totally blind humans will be entrained to the environment, a third will have a 24-hour cycle that is out of phase with the environment, and the remaining third have a free-running pattern that is longer than 24 hours.

EPIDEMIOLOGY

In the absence of blindness, the etiology of primary circadian dysrhythmias is unknown. There is good evidence that genetic factors contribute in some cases.

PATHOBIOLOGY

The function of the biologic clock is to promote wakefulness. Normally, maximal wakefulness occurs during daylight hours. For reasons that are not understood, the biologic clocks of people with circadian dysrhythmias are inexorably out of synchronization with the environment, thus making it difficult or impossible to adjust to demands of the environment.

Exposure to bright light has a potent effect on the biologic clock, and exposure at strategic times during the wake-sleep cycle results in a change in the underlying rhythm. For example, evening light exposure may delay the clock, whereas morning light exposure may advance it.

CLINICAL MANIFESTATIONS AND DIAGNOSIS

The primary symptom of disorders of circadian rhythm is an inability to sleep during the desired sleep time. Once asleep, there is no abnormality of sleep per se, only an abnormality of the timing of sleep. The result is often a complaint of insomnia if sleep is attempted during the "wake" cycle of the clock or a complaint of sleepiness if wakefulness is attempted during the clock's sleep period. Wake-sleep schedule disorders fall into two categories: (1) primary malfunction of the biologic clock per se and (2) secondary malfunction as a result of environmental effects on the underlying clock. The primary disorders may be difficult to diagnose because they typically masquerade as other sleep, medical, or psychiatric disorders, such as hypersomnia, insomnia, substance (sedative-hypnotic or stimulant) abuse, or psychiatric conditions.

The diagnosis is made by the history. Most people, if asked what their wake-sleep pattern would be if they had 3 weeks of vacation without any constraints on their wake-sleep activities (meals, work, school, family activities), can provide an accurate estimate of their inherent wake-sleep pattern. Sleep diaries and actigraphy may be helpful in difficult cases. The secondary disorders (such as jet lag and shift work) are usually immediately apparent on simple questioning of the patient.

TREATMENT

The mainstays of treatment of the primary circadian dysrhythmias are chronotherapy, phototherapy, and pharmacologic therapy.

Chronotherapy

In chronotherapy, the desirable total sleep time is determined by sleep logs during a "free-running" period. The patient then delays or advances the onset of sleep by a few hours every day and sleeps only the predetermined number of hours until the onset of sleep occurs at the desired time, at which point the patient attempts to maintain that time. This method requires several days of free time and can be difficult if sleeping quarters cannot be kept dark and quiet during the several day sleeps required.

Phototherapy

The timing and duration of phototherapy depend on the diagnosis and individual response. The patient sits at a prescribed distance from a bright light that furnishes an illuminance of greater than 2500 lux at that distance. The effect of light on human rhythms varies with the intensity, wavelength, timing, and duration of exposure. This intervention can be performed at home, with the timing of light exposure individualized for a given patient's complaint. Light exposure in the morning will advance the clock, whereas evening exposure will delay the clock. Once the desired sleep period time has been achieved, continued light exposure must be maintained.

Pharmacologic Therapy

The administration of melatonin, 3 mg 4 to 5 hours before the desired time of sleep onset, may assist in advancing the timing of the biologic clock.

JET LAG, SHIFT WORK, AND PERSISTENT PRIMARY CIRCADIAN DYSRHYTHMIAS

The best way to manage jet lag is to assume the wake-sleep pattern of the destination site immediately. Sedative-hypnotic medication may reduce the sleep-onset insomnia associated with jet lag. Jet lag usually resolves at a rate of 1 day per time zone change.

Management of shift work may be difficult; options include stimulant medications and exposure to bright light at night or sedative-hypnotic medication and protection of the sleep environment during the day (or both). The biologic clocks of night shift workers virtually never completely adjust to the night shift because the drive home in the morning resets the clock every day and workers tend to sleep at conventional times during nights off.

Treatment with medications is justified in patients who have persistent symptoms despite chronotherapy and phototherapy. For example, modafinil, 100 to 200 mg during the night shift, is effective for the excessive sleepiness and loss of attention associated with shift work sleep disorder. Caffeine has modest benefits[3] but is no better than napping, bright light, or modafinil.[3] The administration of 3 mg of melatonin 4 to 5 hours before the desired onset of sleep may be of benefit, especially in individuals who travel across five or more time zones, particularly in an eastward direction.[4]

DELAYED SLEEP SYNDROME

In delayed sleep phase syndrome, the patient falls asleep late and rises late. There is a striking inability to fall asleep at an earlier, more desirable time. This syndrome may be manifested as either sleep-onset insomnia or daytime hypersomnia, particularly in the morning. Delayed sleep phase syndrome is the most common of the primary circadian dysrhythmias and may, in part, be the consequence of societal increases in opportunities for nighttime activity. Combinations of chronotherapy, phototherapy, and medications may be effective in "resetting" the clock, as for circadian dysrhythmias. Unfortunately, the treatment regimen must be maintained, or the clock will again become delayed.

ADVANCED SLEEP PHASE SYNDROME

Individuals suffering from advanced sleep phase syndrome fall asleep early and awaken earlier than desired. They are unable to remain awake until the desired time; they fall asleep in the early evening and awaken in the very early hours of the morning. This syndrome may be manifested as hypersomnia, particularly in the evening, or sleep maintenance insomnia. Patients complain of interruption of evening activities by their sleepiness. They may avoid evening social activities for fear of the intrusive sleepiness. The undesirable early morning awakenings in this condition may lead to a misdiagnosis of depression. Exposure to bright light in the evening may delay the clock to a more acceptable pattern.

OTHER ABNORMALITIES OF CIRCADIAN RHYTHM

Other, less common circadian dysrhythmias include a "non–24-hour wake-sleep pattern" in which the wake-sleep period is longer than 24 hours and sleep begins at a later time each cycle, as well as an "irregular wake-sleep pattern" characterized by a completely chaotic and unpredictable wake-sleep pattern.

Parasomnias

Parasomnias are defined as unpleasant or undesirable behavioral or experiential phenomena occurring predominantly or exclusively during sleep. Initially attributed to psychiatric disease, it is now clear that parasomnias are the manifestation of a wide variety of completely different conditions, most of which are diagnosable and treatable. The common parasomnias are examples of "dissociated sleep states," which represent the simultaneous admixture of wakefulness with either NREM sleep (disorders of arousal such as confusional arousal, sleepwalking, or sleep terrors) or REM sleep (REM sleep behavior disorder). The parasomnias, like narcolepsy, support the concept that wake and sleep are not mutually exclusive states and that sleep is not necessarily a global brain phenomenon.

Isolated, often bizarre sleep-related events may be experienced by perfectly normal individuals, and most do not warrant further extensive or expensive evaluation. However, serious attention should be paid to complaints of sleep-related behavior that is potentially violent or injurious. In these cases, formal sleep studies using a full EEG montage with continuous audiovisual monitoring is indicated to establish a correct diagnosis and treatment plan.

DISORDERS OF AROUSAL

Disorders of arousal tend to arise from NREM sleep and usually occur in the first third of the sleep cycle and rarely during naps. They are common in childhood and usually decrease in frequency with increasing age.

Disorders of arousal may be triggered by febrile illness, prior sleep deprivation, physical activity, emotional stress, or medications. They are not caused by significant underlying psychiatric problems.

Clinical manifestations vary across a broad spectrum ranging from confusional arousal to somnambulism (sleepwalking) to sleep terrors. Some patients perform more specialized behavior, such as sleep-related eating and sleep-related sexual activity, without conscious awareness. Such behavior may have forensic implications.

TREATMENT

Most disorders of arousal, such as simple sleepwalking or sleep terrors, require no treatment other than reassurance of their benign nature. If the behavior is bothersome or potentially injurious, medical management with benzodiazepines (e.g., clonazepam, 0.5 to 1.0 mg 30 minutes before bedtime) or tricyclic antidepressant medications (e.g., imipramine, 25 to 50 mg 30 minutes before bedtime) or behavioral treatment in the form of self-taught relaxation exercises is often effective.

RAPID EYE MOVEMENT SLEEP BEHAVIOR DISORDER

The most common and best-studied REM sleep parasomnia is the REM sleep behavior disorder.

EPIDEMIOLOGY AND PATHOBIOLOGY

REM sleep behavior disorder predominantly affects males (about 90%) and usually begins after the age of 50 years. Acute REM sleep behavior disorder is often due to undesirable side effects of prescribed medications, most commonly antidepressant medications and particularly the selective serotonin re-uptake inhibitors. Chronic REM sleep behavior disorder, which may be preceded by a lengthy prodrome of REM sleep behavior disorder, can be idiopathic or associated with neurodegenerative disorders, particularly the synucleinopathies (Parkinson's disease, multiple system atrophy, or dementia with Lewy bodies), in which it may be the first symptom and precede other manifestations of the underlying process by more than 10 years (Chapter 416). There is also a higher incidence of REM sleep behavior disorder in patients with narcolepsy, in whom this tendency may be aggravated by the tricyclic antidepressants or selective serotonin re-uptake inhibitors prescribed to treat cataplexy.

CLINICAL MANIFESTATIONS

In these patients, somatic muscle atonia—one of the defining features of REM sleep—is absent, thereby permitting the acting out of dream mentation, often with violent or injurious results. The initial complaint is vigorous sleep behavior usually accompanying vivid dreams. Such behavior may result in repeated injury, including ecchymoses, lacerations, and fractures.

DIAGNOSIS

The diagnosis may be suspected by the clinical history, but formal sleep studies are indicated. Patients with REM sleep behavior disorder will demonstrate increased EMG activity during REM sleep, thus confirming the clinical suspicion.

TREATMENT

The benzodiazepine clonazepam (0.5 to 2.0 mg 30 minutes before bedtime) is a highly effective treatment of REM sleep behavior disorder, with a sustained response rate of nearly 90%, although its mechanism of action is unknown. Melatonin, 6 to 12 mg at bedtime, may also be effective.

1. Schutte-Rodin S, Broch L, Buysse D, et al. Clinical guideline for the evaluation and management of chronic insomnia in adults. *J Clin Sleep Med.* 2008;4:487-504.
2. Drugs for insomnia. *Med Lett.* 2009;7:23-26.
3. Ker K, Edwards PJ, Felix LM, et al. Caffeine for the prevention of injuries and errors in shift workers. *Cochrane Database Syst Rev.* 2010;5:CD008508.
4. Herxheimer A, Petrie KJ. Melatonin for the prevention and treatment of jet lag. *Cochrane Database Syst Rev.* 2002;2:CD001520.

SUGGESTED READINGS

Cao M. Advances in narcolepsy. *Med Clin North Am.* 2010;94:541-555. *Review.*
Centers for Disease Control and Prevention (CDC). Unhealthy sleep-related behaviors—12 States, 2009. *MMWR Morb Mortal Wkly Rep.* 2011;60:233-238. *In the prior 30 days, about 48% of people snored, 38% unintentionally fell asleep during the day, and about 5% nodded off or fell asleep while driving.*
Sack RL. Clinical practice. Jet lag. *N Engl J Med.* 2010;362:440-744. *Case-based review recommending short-acting sleep medications and consideration of oral melatonin.*
Sullivan SS. Insomnia pharmacology. *Med Clin North Am.* 2010;94:563-580. *Review.*
Trenkwalder C, Paulus W. Restless leg syndrome: pathophysiology, clinical presentation and management. *Nat Rev Neurol.* 2010;6:337-346. *Review emphasizing the use of dopaminergic agents.*

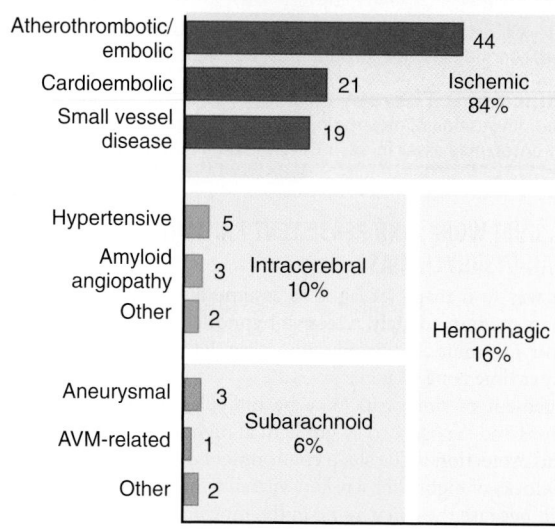

FIGURE 413-1. Classification of cerebrovascular disease. AVM = arteriovenous malformation.

413

APPROACH TO CEREBROVASCULAR DISEASES

JUSTIN A. ZIVIN

DEFINITION

Stroke is the generally preferred term for a group of diseases that are of abrupt onset and cause neurologic damage (Fig. 413-1). Approximately 85% of strokes are caused by a sudden onset of inadequacy of blood flow to some or all of the brain (Chapter 414). The remaining strokes are divided between hemorrhage (Chapter 415) into brain tissue (parenchymatous hemorrhage) and hemorrhage into the spaces surrounding the brain, most frequently the subarachnoid space. A commonly used synonym for stroke was *cerebrovascular accident*, but this term has lost favor because strokes are not really accidents. Well-established prophylactic and acute therapies are now available, and diagnostic tools have improved markedly. Management of stroke has become much more rational and successful.

EPIDEMIOLOGY

Stroke is the second leading cause of mortality worldwide and the third most common cause of death in the industrialized world (after heart disease and all types of cancer combined). It is the most common cause of adult disability in the United States. In China and Japan, stroke is the most frequent cause of death.

In the United States, the annual incidence and death rate for stroke declined steadily for most of the 20th century. In more recent years, however, the rate of decline has slowed and the incidence of stroke may be increasing. About 750,000 new strokes reach medical attention per year in the United States, and strokes cause about 150,000 deaths annually. At any given time there are about 3 million stroke survivors in the United States. Incidence rates in Western European countries are slightly higher than those in the United States, and several Eastern European countries, China, and Japan have much higher rates based at least partly on smoking and on environmental and dietary factors.

The rate of stroke approximately doubles with each decade after the age of 55. Blacks and Hispanics have about twice the risk as whites, and men have about a 40% higher incidence of stroke than women do. Hypertension increases the risk by four-fold, smoking nearly doubles the risk, and diabetes increases the risk two- to six-fold. Carotid stenosis and atrial fibrillation are perhaps the strongest risk factors. Other factors that increase risk include obesity, hypercholesterolemia, physical inactivity, alcohol abuse, hyperhomocysteinemia, drug abuse, and use of oral contraceptive agents.

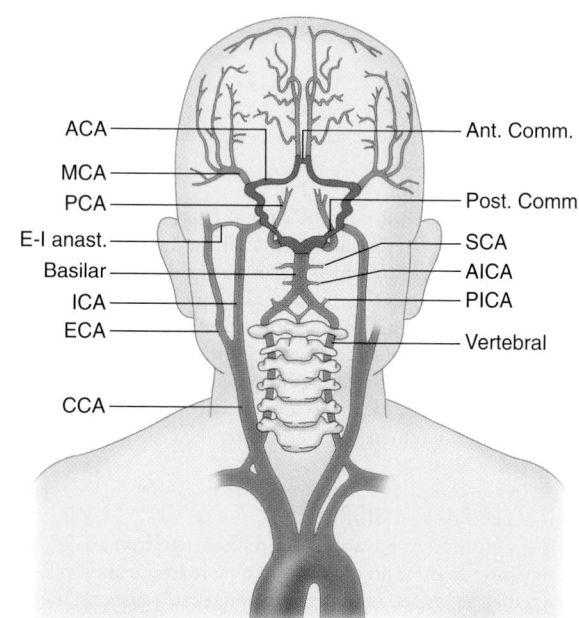

FIGURE 413-2. Extracranial and intracranial arterial supply to the brain. Vessels forming the circle of Willis are highlighted. ACA = anterior cerebral artery; AICA = anterior inferior cerebellar artery; Ant. Comm. = anterior communicating artery; CCA = common carotid artery; ECA = external carotid artery; E-I anast. = extracranial-intracranial anastomosis; ICA = internal carotid artery; MCA = middle cerebral artery; PCA = posterior cerebral artery; PICA = posterior inferior cerebellar artery; Post. Comm. = posterior communicating artery; SCA = superior cerebellar artery. (Modified from Lord R. *Surgery of Occlusive Cerebrovascular Disease.* St. Louis, MO: CV Mosby; 1986.)

PATHOBIOLOGY

Cerebrovascular Anatomy

Strokes are usually caused by abnormalities in the cerebral circulation. Anatomic variations are frequent, however, and the territory receiving its blood supply from a given artery is not entirely predictable; as a result, stroke syndromes may not correlate well with the location of the vascular injury. Appropriate imaging studies are needed to provide detailed information about each individual patient. In many situations, noninvasive imaging is adequate. For vascular anomalies such as stenosis, malformations, and aneurysms, angiography is crucial for diagnosis because an understanding of the anatomy is necessary to develop treatment plans.

Four major arteries supply the brain: the bilaterally paired internal carotid and vertebral arteries (Fig. 413-2). The left common carotid artery arises directly from the aortic arch, but the right originates from branches of the aorta. The right common carotid artery is a branch of the innominate artery, and the left and right vertebral arteries originate from the subclavian arteries.

Internal Carotid Arteries

In most individuals, each common carotid artery bifurcates into an internal and external carotid artery just below the angle of the jaw and approximately at the level of the thyroid cartilage. The internal carotid artery (ICA) enters the skull through the foramen lacerum and travels a short distance within the petrous portion of the temporal bone. It then enters the cavernous sinus before penetrating the dura and ascends above the clinoid processes to divide into the anterior cerebral artery (ACA) and middle cerebral artery (MCA). The portion of the ICA that lies between the cavernous sinus and the supra-clinoid process forms an S shape and is sometimes termed the *carotid siphon*. The ICA gives off its first important branches at the supraclinoid level: the ophthalmic, posterior communicating, and anterior choroidal arteries, usually in that order. In some cases, the ophthalmic artery arises from the ICA within the cavernous sinus.

External Carotid Arteries

Branches of the external carotid artery sometimes form anastomoses that provide collateral circulation to the ICA. These branches include the facial artery and the superficial temporal artery. Both vessels may anastomose with the supratrochlear branches of the ophthalmic artery. In instances of ICA occlusion below the level of the ophthalmic branch, the facial and superficial temporal arteries sometimes supply blood through the ophthalmic branch to the distal ICA.

Vertebral-Basilar Arteries

Anatomic variation is considerably more common in the vertebral artery system than in the ICA. The paired vertebral arteries usually arise from the subclavian arteries, but their origins may be more proximal on the aortic arch, or they may form a common branch of the thyrocervical trunk. The vertebral arteries generally enter the foramina of the sixth cervical vertebra or, much less commonly, the fourth, fifth, or seventh vertebral foramina. The vertebral arteries ascend through the transverse foramina and exit at C1, where they turn nearly 90 degrees posteriorly to pass behind the atlantoaxial joint before penetrating the dura and entering the cranial cavity through the foramen magnum. The portion of the vertebral artery that loops behind the atlanto-axial joint is prone to mechanical deformation, and excessive rotation of the head may cause arterial narrowing and reduction of blood flow to the ipsilateral vertebral artery.

Intracranially, the vertebral arteries are lateral to the medulla oblongata and then course ventrally and medially, where they unite rostrally at the medullopontine junction to form the basilar artery. The basilar artery ultimately bifurcates at the pontomesencephalic junction to form the posterior cerebral arteries (PCAs).

In a few individuals, the right or left vertebral arteries terminate before reaching the basilar artery, which is consequently supplied, proximally, by a single vertebral artery. The vertebral arteries usually have medial branches that turn caudally and unite to form the anterior spinal artery, as well as lateral branches supplying the dorsolateral medulla and posterior cerebellum, called the *posterior inferior cerebellar arteries*.

Circle of Willis

The circle of Willis, which is at the base of the brain, is formed by the union of the right and left ACAs via the anterior communicating artery, the MCAs, and the PCAs via the posterior communicating arteries. Anomalies of the circle of Willis occur frequently; in large autopsy series of normal individuals, more than half show an incomplete circle of Willis. The most common sites for these abnormalities, which are usually manifested as hypoplasia or absence, are the posterior communicating arteries and the ACAs.

Anterior Cerebral Arteries

The ACAs travel medially above the optic chiasm and pass rostrally toward the interhemispheric fissure, where they arch caudally to lie just dorsal to the corpus callosum. In a small fraction of normal individuals, the A1 segment of the ACA (the portion between the origin at the MCA and the first major branch, the anterior communicating artery) is hypoplastic or absent, which leaves its distal portion to be supplied by the opposite ACA via the anterior communicating artery. Branches of the ACA normally supply the frontal poles, the superior surfaces of the cerebral hemispheres where their distal branches anastomose with those of the MCA, and all of the medial surfaces of both cerebral hemispheres with the exception of the calcarine cortex (Figs. 413-3 and 413-4). Cortical areas served by the ACA include the motor and

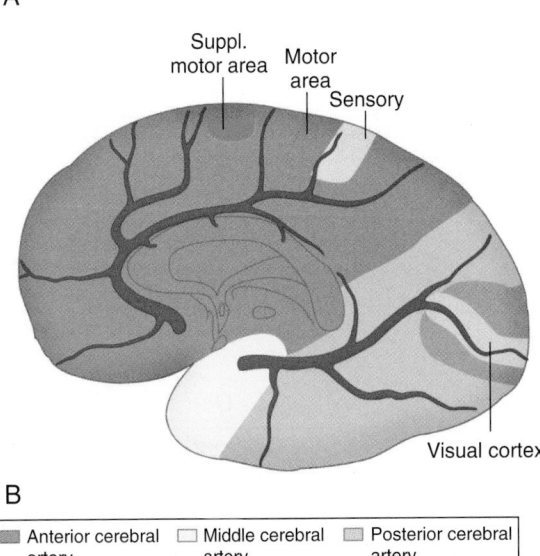

| Anterior cerebral artery | Middle cerebral artery | Posterior cerebral artery |

FIGURE 413-3. Surface cerebral arterial anatomy. Lateral (**A**) and medial (**B**) views of the cerebral hemisphere show the surface distributions of the anterior, middle, and posterior cerebral arteries.

sensory cortex of the legs and feet, the supplementary motor cortex, and the paracentral lobule.

The A1 and A2 segments (the portions between the anterior communicating artery and the genu of the corpus callosum) give off many small branches that penetrate the anterior perforated substance of the brain. These small penetrating branches include all of the anterior and some of the medial lenticulostriate arteries. Usually, there is a dominant medial striate vessel called the *recurrent artery of Heubner*, which commonly arises from the A1 segment of the ACA. This artery penetrates the perforated substance of the brain and, along with the other small perforators, supplies the anterior and inferior portions of the anterior limb of the internal capsule, the anterior and inferior head of the caudate nucleus, the anterior globus pallidus and putamen, the anterior hypothalamus, the olfactory bulbs and tracts, and the uncinate fasciculus.

Anterior Choroidal Artery

The anterior choroidal artery arises from the supraclinoid portion of the ICA in most people. It travels caudally and medially over the optic tract, to which it provides a few small branches, and enters the brain via the choroidal fissure. Many important brain structures receive blood flow from the anterior choroidal artery, including portions of the anterior hippocampus, uncus, amygdala, globus pallidus, tail of the caudate nucleus, lateral thalamus, geniculate body, and a large portion of the most inferior, posterior limb of the internal capsule.

Middle Cerebral Artery

The MCA provides flow to most of the lateral surface of the cerebral hemispheres and is the vessel most frequently involved in ischemic stroke. As the

Anterior cerebral artery	Thalamogeniculate arteries	Middle cerebral artery
Recurrent artery of Heubner	Anterior choroidal artery	
Lenticulostriate arteries	Posterior cerebral artery	

FIGURE 413-4. Arterial supply of the deep brain structures. **A,** Sagittal view of the brain showing the computed tomographic (CT) planes through which views **B, C,** and **D** were taken. **B,** CT plane through the head of the caudate nucleus (HC), putamen (P), amygdala (A), tail of the caudate nucleus (TC), hypothalamus, temporal lobe, midbrain, and cerebellum. **C,** CT plane through the frontal horn of the lateral ventricle (FLV), head of the caudate nucleus (HC), anterior and posterior limbs of the internal capsule (AIC, PIC), putamen (P), globus pallidus (GP), thalamus (T), optic radiations (OR), and posterior horn of the lateral ventricle (PLV). **D,** CT plane through the centrum semiovale. (Modified from De Armond S, Fusco MM, Dewey MM. *Structure of the Human Brain, a Photographic Atlas,* 3rd ed. New York: Oxford University Press; 1989, with permission.)

main MCA trunk passes laterally toward the sylvian fissure, it gives rise to some of the medial and all of the lateral lenticulostriate arteries. These arteries supply the putamen, the head and body of the caudate nucleus, the lateral globus pallidus, the anterior limb of the internal capsule, and the superior portion of the posterior limb of the internal capsule. The MCA extends into the sylvian fissure, where it branches into several smaller arteries grouped into a superior division, which feeds the cortical surface above the fissure, and an inferior division, which supplies the cortical surface of the temporal lobe. The territory of the MCA includes the major motor and sensory areas of the cortex, the areas for contraversive eye and head movement, the optic radiations, the auditory sensory cortex, and in the dominant hemisphere, the motor and sensory areas for language.

Posterior Cerebral Arteries

Blood flow to both PCAs is derived in most people from the basilar artery and infrequently from the ICA. Sometimes the ICA is the origin of one PCA and the other PCA originates from the basilar artery. The PCAs pass dorsal to the third cranial nerves and across the cerebral peduncles and then ascend upward along the medial edge of the tentorium, where they branch into anterior and posterior divisions. The anterior division supplies the inferior surface of the temporal lobe, where its terminal branches form an anastomosis with branches of the MCA. The posterior division supplies the occipital lobe, where its terminal branches anastomose with the ACA and the MCA.

In its most proximal course along the base of the brain, the PCA gives off several groups of penetrating arteries commonly called the *thalamogeniculate,* the *thalamoperforating,* and the *posterior choroidal* arteries. The red nucleus, the substantia nigra, medial portions of the cerebral peduncles, the nuclei of the thalamus, the hippocampus, and the posterior hypothalamus receive blood from these penetrating branches.

Brain Stem Blood Supply

The ventral medial portion of the brain stem receives its blood supply from short paramedian vessels, the ventrolateral region receives its blood from short circumferential branches of the vertebral or basilar arteries, and long circumferential branches supply the dorsolateral brain stem and cerebellum (Fig. 413-5). These vessels include the posterior inferior cerebellar arteries, which arise from the vertebral arteries, and the anterior inferior and superior cerebellar arteries, which arise from the basilar artery.

The pyramids, the inferior olives and medial lemnisci, the medial longitudinal fasciculi, and the emerging fibers of the hypoglossal nerve derive blood from the vertebral arteries. Longer branches from the vertebral arteries and posterior ICAs supply the spinothalamic tracts, the vestibular nuclei, the sensory nuclei of the fifth cranial nerve, the descending fibers of the sympathetic nervous system, the restiform body, and the emerging fibers of the vagus and glossopharyngeal nerves. The most cephalad and dorsal segment of the medulla includes the vestibular and cochlear nuclei, which along with the posterior portion of the cerebellum, receive flow from the posterior inferior cerebellar artery.

The basilar artery gives rise to perforating branches as it spans the ventral midline pons and midbrain. These short perpendicular branches distribute blood to the paramedian structures, including the corticospinal tracts, the pontine reticular nuclei, the medial lemnisci, the medial longitudinal fasciculi, and the pontine reticular nuclei. The anterior ICA feeds blood to the lateral pons, including the emerging seventh and eighth cranial nerves, the trigeminal nerve root, the vestibular and cochlear nuclei, and the spinothalamic tracts. It also branches to the most dorsal and lateral of these structures on its dorsal course toward the cerebellum.

At the midbrain level, the basilar artery lies in the midline in the interpeduncular fossa. Short branches pass laterally and dorsally on both sides to supply the cerebral peduncles, the emerging fibers of the third nerve, medial portions of the red nuclei, the medial longitudinal fasciculus, the oculomotor nuclei, and the midbrain reticulum. The superior cerebellar arteries contribute to the dorsal midbrain supply, including that of the colliculi and the superior portion of the cerebellum on each side.

Venous Drainage

The veins in the brain, in contrast to those in many other parts of the body, often do not accompany the arteries. Cortical veins drain into the superior sagittal sinus, which runs between the cerebral hemispheres. Deeper structures drain into the inferior sagittal sinus and great cerebral vein (of Galen), which join at the straight sinus (Fig. 413-6). The straight sinus runs along the attachment of the falx cerebri and tentorium to join with the superior sagittal sinus at the torcular Herophili, from which the two transverse sinuses arise. Each transverse sinus passes laterally toward the petrosal bone to become the sigmoid sinus, which exits the skull into the internal jugular vein. Each cavernous sinus communicates with its contralateral twin and surrounds the ipsilateral carotid artery. Both drain into the petrosal sinuses, which drain into the sigmoid sinus.

Normal Physiology
Cerebral Metabolism and Blood Flow

Although the brain is normally about 2% of body weight in humans, it is supplied with approximately 14% of the resting cardiac output. The energy demands to support normal brain activity in conscious humans are equal, on a per-weight basis, to the demands of the most metabolically active tissues, such as the heart and kidney. Aerobic glucose metabolism in a normal, conscious human brain consumes an average of 140 μmol of oxygen and 24 μmol of glucose per 100 g of brain tissue each minute. Normal brain activities, such as thinking or sleeping, do not alter total blood flow, glucose use, or oxygen uptake in the brain, but they do change the patterns of blood supply and energy use in specific brain areas.

The brain extracts approximately 10% of available blood glucose in a single pass, yet only 80% of this glucose is used to generate energy. About 10 to 15% of the glucose is metabolized to lactate, which may be lost to the circulation; the remainder is used for the synthesis of neurotransmitters, fats, and to a

FIGURE 413-5. Brain stem blood supply. **A,** Cross section of the medulla oblongata at the level of the hypoglossal nuclei (cranial nerve XII). Short branches of the vertebral and anterior spinal arteries supply the medulla. Longer circumferential branches, including the posterior inferior cerebellar artery, supply the lateral portions of the medulla. **B,** Cross section of the midpons region. The medial portion receives blood supply from short, perforating basilar artery branches. More laterally, the blood supply comes from lateral basilar artery branches.

FIGURE 413-6. Venous drainage of intracranial structures. CS = cavernous sinus; CV = cortical veins; GV = great vein of Galen; ICV = internal cerebral vein; IJ = internal jugular vein; ISS = inferior sagittal sinus; LS = lateral sinus; PS = petrosal sinus; SS = sigmoid sinus; *SS = straight sinus; SSS = superior sagittal sinus; TH = torcular Herophili; TS = transverse sinus. (From Gates P, Barnett HJ, Mohr JP, et al, eds. Stroke: *Pathophysiology, Diagnosis and Management.* New York, NY: Churchill Livingstone; 1986.)

small degree, proteins. Each mole of glucose metabolized by the brain through glycolysis and the mitochondrial respiratory chain yields approximately 30 mol of adenosine triphosphate (ATP) instead of the theoretical maximum of 38 mol.

In contrast to most other tissues, the brain stores little glucose, glycogen, or high-energy phosphates (ATP, phosphocreatine) but instead relies on continuous, well-regulated blood flow to satisfy its needs for energy. Cerebral blood flow (CBF) averages 50 mL/100 g of brain tissue per minute in a normal, conscious human. In the absence of this flow, the brain has sufficient high-energy stores to support its metabolic needs for only a few minutes. The vascular reserves of oxygen and glucose are small, as illustrated by the fact that all changes in synaptic activity, whether related to thinking, talking, or

directing muscular activity, are tightly coupled, temporally and anatomically, to an almost instantaneous increase in local CBF. The mechanisms responsible for this coupling of blood flow to metabolic activity have not been fully elucidated, but the relationship is well established, under normal conditions, and provides a basis for the use of imaging methods to assess regional brain activity. Regional CBF can be precisely quantified with positron emission tomography. Other less invasive techniques such as magnetic resonance imaging and single-photon emission computed tomography provide qualitative measurements of local CBF. The brain's functional activities result in a frequently and rapidly changing pattern of regional metabolic and blood flow values that reflect moment-to-moment changes in activity. On a larger scale, the low stores and high metabolic rate of the brain are responsible for the rapid loss of consciousness and subsequent irreversible damage that accompany loss of the critical energy sources of the brain, glucose and oxygen.

The coupling of CBF to regional synaptic and metabolic activity is only one of several mechanisms known to regulate normal CBF. Another is alteration of carbon dioxide. Hypercapnia dilates and hypocapnia constricts cerebral resistance vessels such that CBF shows a linear relationship to $PaCO_2$ within the normal range. This physiologic response to $PaCO_2$ can be exploited clinically to treat cerebral herniation. Increases in intracranial pressure (ICP) in the absence of adequate intracranial volume may force the hemispheres through the tentorium or the cerebellum through the foramen magnum. Mechanical hyperventilation to a $PaCO_2$ of 20 to 25 mm Hg reduces CBF by approximately 40 to 45% and normal adult cerebral blood volume from 50 to approximately 35 mL. Though seemingly small, this reduction sometimes suffices to retard the progression of herniation and is the fastest way to reduce ICP. The response is short-lived, however, and brain and blood HCO_3^- and H^+ ions controlling blood vessel tone re-equilibrate within 30 to 60 minutes. More definitive therapy must be initiated quickly.

A complex system of neural pathways also helps control CBF. Some of these pathways participate in autoregulation, a process that maintains CBF at a constant level despite fluctuations in arterial blood pressure over a fairly wide range (Fig. 413-7). Autoregulation has upper and lower limits; at a mean arterial pressure greater than about 150 mm Hg, blood flow increases and capillary pressure rises, whereas at a mean arterial pressure of less than 50 mm Hg, CBF falls. In patients with chronic hypertension, the upper and lower autoregulatory limits are shifted toward higher systemic pressure. Consequently, a rapid therapeutic reduction in blood pressure to levels that would be normal in most people carries the risk of further lowering CBF in hypertensive patients who have ongoing cerebral ischemia. Long-term treatment with antihypertensive agents readjusts the autoregulatory curve toward more normal values. Conversely, excessive reduction of blood pressure in

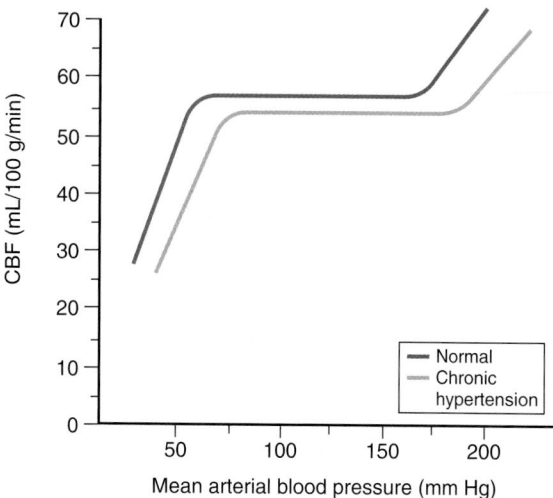

FIGURE 413-7. Autoregulatory cerebral blood flow (CBF) response to changes in mean arterial pressure in normotensive and chronically hypertensive people. Note the shift of the curve toward higher mean pressure with chronic hypertension.

previously normal patients to a mean arterial pressure of less than approximately 50 mm Hg inevitably leads to loss of autoregulation, possible expansion of an ischemic zone, or production of global cerebral ischemia. These injuries are seen in patients who are treated too aggressively with antihypertensive agents in the immediate aftermath of a stroke and in patients who are anesthetized during surgical procedures.

Blood-Brain Barrier

The brain's extracellular ionic and molecular environment is tightly regulated. Small changes in extracellular concentrations of Na^+, K^+, and Ca^{2+} ions or neurotransmitters, including glutamate, acetylcholine, and norepinephrine, alter neuronal function. Intracellular communication within the brain, perhaps its most important basic function, depends on a carefully controlled extracellular space. The blood-brain barrier (BBB), which has evolved to protect this milieu, is composed of unique endothelial cells that lack the usual transendothelial channels and closely abut one another in tight junctions. This anatomy protects the brain against the fluctuating composition of blood and reduces the entry of potentially toxic compounds. A negative consequence is that the BBB prevents the entry of polar molecules into the brain, thus limiting the utility of many drugs, small molecules, and proteins, which cannot gain entry into the brain by the oral or intravenous routes.

The entry of nutrients and egress of metabolic waste across the BBB can occur by simple diffusion, facilitated transport, or active transport. Lipid-soluble compounds can diffuse rapidly across endothelial cell membranes, whereas some polar compounds can be transported by special carrier molecules that are driven either by concentration gradients (facilitated transport) or through the expenditure of energy (active transport). Gas molecules, such as oxygen and carbon dioxide, freely diffuse across plasma membranes and rapidly equilibrate between blood and brain. Glucose, a highly polar molecule, enters the brain on a special glucose transporter. The rate of brain glucose transport is normally two to three times faster than the metabolism of glucose, but because glucose uptake depends so highly on its blood concentration, a reduction in blood glucose level to a third of normal, caused by either ischemia or hypoglycemia, may compromise normal brain energy metabolism.

● CEREBRAL ISCHEMIA

Inadequate delivery of oxygen or glucose to the brain initiates a cascade of events that ultimately result in infarction. The severity of the insult, defined by the degree and duration of reduced blood flow, hypoxia, or hypoglycemia, determines whether the brain suffers only temporary dysfunction, such as a transient ischemic attack; irreversible injury to only a few of the most vulnerable neurons (selective necrosis); or cerebral infarction, in which damage occurs to extensive areas involving all cell types (pan-necrosis).

Types of Cerebral Hypoxia-Ischemia

Cerebral hypoxia-ischemia can be divided into focal ischemia caused by vascular occlusion, global ischemia as a result of complete cardiovascular failure, and diffuse hypoperfusion-hypoxia produced by respiratory disease or severely reduced blood pressure.

Focal Ischemia

Focal cerebral ischemia results most frequently from embolic or thrombotic occlusion of extracranial or intracranial blood vessels and the resulting reduction in blood flow within the related vascular territory. Blood flow to the central zone of the ischemic vascular bed is usually severely reduced but rarely reaches zero because of partial supply from collateral blood vessels. The best treatment option for this intensely ischemic region is acute restoration of blood flow. A transition zone may be present between the normally perfused tissue and the more ischemic central core. This rim of moderately deprived tissue has been called the *ischemic penumbra*. It is thought that brain cells in the penumbra remain viable for a longer time than do cells in the ischemic core. This marginally viable tissue may die if inadequate blood flow persists but may be salvaged by restoring flow or, possibly, by neuroprotective therapeutic agents. The size and duration of the penumbra are unknown in any individual patient and poorly defined by current diagnostic techniques. In more recent years, salvage of the penumbra with neuroprotective agents has been the subject of intense basic and clinical research.

Cerebral ischemia sufficient to cause clinical signs or symptoms, if severe, can produce irreversible injury to highly vulnerable neurons in 5 minutes. Progressively longer durations of ischemia increase the probability of permanent damage. If cerebral ischemia persists for more than about 6 hours, infarction of part or all of the involved vascular territory is completed, and the only strategies for therapy entail rehabilitation, such as treatment with neurotrophic factors or neural transplantation. Whether clinical evidence of permanent brain injury from ischemia is detectable depends on the location of the brain tissue involved.

Global Ischemia

Global cerebral ischemia results from cardiac asystole or ventricular fibrillation that reduces the blood flow rate to zero throughout the brain and body. Global ischemia for more than 5 to 10 minutes is generally incompatible with full recovery of consciousness in normothermic humans. If blood flow is restored in time to prevent cardiac death, selective ischemic necrosis usually involves the most vulnerable neurons in the CA1 pyramidal neurons of the hippocampus, the cerebellar Purkinje cells, and the pyramidal neurons in neocortical layers 3, 5, and 6. Anything that prevents adequate oxygen or glucose supply to the brain, such as hypoxemia, carbon monoxide poisoning, and severe and prolonged hypoglycemia, can also produce such injury. Cardiac resuscitation or other causes of prolonged hypotension may cause cerebral infarction, particularly in border zones that lie between the terminal branches of major arterial supplies, often termed *watershed zones*.

Diffuse Hypoxia

Diffuse cerebral hypoxia initially causes cerebral dysfunction but not irreversible brain injury. Individuals with cerebral hypoxia from high altitude, pulmonary disease, or severe anemia can exhibit confusion, cognitive impairment, and lethargy. The onset of coma heralds permanent brain damage. With acute changes in Pao_2 from normal to less than 40 mm Hg or a decrease in the hemoglobin concentration to less than 7 g/dL, compensatory increases in CBF become inadequate, and clinical signs and symptoms of cerebral hypoxia develop. A slower onset of reduced oxygenation, such as caused by moving to high elevations or the gradual development of anemia, permits compensation by a variety of mechanisms; if the hypoxia increases, however, the compensation ultimately fails.

Neuropathology of Cerebral Ischemia

Four general classes of histopathologic damage can occur. Cerebral infarction caused by focal vascular occlusion is characterized by destruction of all cellular elements: neurons, glia, and endothelial cells (pan-necrosis). Cerebral infarcts are initially grossly pale (anemic) or hemorrhagic (showing gross petechial bleeding). Later, necrotic tissue is removed and replaced by a glial scar or a cavity. Transient arrest of the cerebral circulation (global ischemia) can cause selective *ischemic necrosis* of highly vulnerable neurons. Using conventional stains, histologic change begins to outline the margins between living and dying neurons and glia within a few hours, although the full extent of damage may not be evident for several days. The neurologic functionality of the cells is irreversibly lost within the first 6 hours. Newer imaging techniques can reveal abnormal cell function much more rapidly than conventional histology can.

Cerebral *autolysis* is observed most frequently in brain-dead patients who are maintained on mechanical ventilators for more than a few days; it reflects enzymatic autodigestion of brain tissue. *Demyelination* of the central hemispheric white matter is usually a consequence of carbon monoxide poisoning or other prolonged periods of moderately severe hypoxemia or cerebral hypoperfusion. Development of these lesions may take several days, and the onset of neurologic dysfunction may be delayed. Patients may have a lucid interval after such an injury and subsequently manifest neurologic symptoms. Within these lesions, nerve cell axons are demyelinated, and oligodendroglial cells die.

Ischemic Cascade

In severe ischemia, energy-rich compounds become depleted within minutes. As energy-dependent membrane pumps fail, neuronal and glial cell membranes depolarize and allow the influx of Ca^{2+} ions. Elevated intracellular Ca^{2+} and other second messengers activate lipases and proteases, which release membrane-bound free fatty acids that denature proteins. Depolarization of presynaptic terminals releases abnormally high concentrations of excitatory neurotransmitters, such as glutamate, which may elevate metabolic demand at a time when energy supplies are inadequate and thus exacerbate the injury. If blood flow is restored within 5 minutes and there are no other complicating factors such as hyperglycemia, these events are completely reversible. As the duration of ischemia increases, selectively vulnerable neurons die first; if the ischemia persists for hours or longer, cerebral infarction develops. Prompt restoration of blood flow permits full functional recovery and maintenance of tissue integrity. Tissues with partial depletion of ATP and impaired calcium homeostasis may benefit from pharmacologic therapies that reduce calcium movement through voltage- and neurotransmitter-dependent ion channels. Many other neuroprotective strategies have also been shown to be effective in animal models, including prevention of the detrimental actions of excitatory neurotransmitters, inhibition of many biochemical pathways leading to cell death, and therapies that may delay the denaturation of proteins. Thus far, however, none of these therapies has proved useful in clinical trials in stroke patients.

Leukocytes

More recently, the role of leukocytes in ischemic damage has been recognized. Two proposed mechanisms of injury are (1) microvascular occlusion from direct mechanical obstruction and damage to the endothelium and (2) infiltration into central nervous system tissue and cellular cytotoxic injury. The white blood cell–mediated damage may be irreversible even if blood flow is restored.

White blood cells require considerable deformation to pass through capillaries. When activated by chemotactic substances during ischemia, their cytoplasmic stiffness increases, and they adhere to capillary endothelium. Under conditions of reduced perfusion pressure, white blood cells may obstruct the microcirculation. This leukocyte capillary plugging may be the major cause of the *no-reflow phenomenon*, which is defined as incomplete restoration of normal blood flow after a period of ischemia. Areas of parenchyma that might be viable when blood flow returns are inadequately reperfused. This phenomenon was a laboratory curiosity until the advent of thrombolytic therapy; it may now be a cause of apparent stroke in evolution or the development of increased neurologic deficits after apparently successful thrombolysis.

Leukocytes may potentiate injury by toxic damage to vascular endothelium and by transendothelial migration to the parenchyma. Release of leukocyte granule contents, which include reactive oxygen metabolites and membrane phospholipases, can injure the endothelium and is usually responsible for the removal of necrotic tissue after irreversible damage. The resultant effects include increased endothelial permeability, interstitial edema, expansion and injury of individual cells (endothelial, glial, and neuronal), vasoconstriction, and generation of substances that induce further leukocyte adhesion.

Anoxic Encephalopathy

In industrialized countries, out-of-hospital cardiac arrest (Chapter 63) occurs in 0.04 to 0.13% of the total population per year. Only a minority of these patients will survive the arrest and be discharged with a good neurologic outcome, in part because of the risk for anoxic encephalopathy. If brain stem function is preserved but the cerebral hemispheres are destroyed, the patient enters a persistent vegetative state (Chapter 411).

CEREBRAL HEMORRHAGE

Bleeding into the subarachnoid space from a ruptured aneurysm or other vascular malformation produces a chemical (sterile) meningitis and can induce vasospasm, particularly in the vessels constituting the circle of Willis. If the vasospasm is sufficiently severe, it can result in cerebral infarction and death.

Intraparenchymal hemorrhage may be relatively benign. Bleeding into a region of previous infarction, called *hemorrhagic transformation*, causes no additional functional loss. Primary parenchymatous hemorrhage damages tissue in several ways, however. If a large vessel ruptures, the amount of bleeding into the brain can be severe. The portion of the vascular distribution distal to the site of rupture is no longer supplied with blood, and infarction results. At the site of rupture, bleeding into the brain may cause traumatic injury to the exposed tissue, and blood or its breakdown products in the parenchyma damage brain tissue. In addition, the extravascular blood in the brain parenchyma increases total brain volume, and the edema, which forms rapidly in and around the site of bleeding, increases the intracranial contents. Because cranial capacity is fixed, ICP increases rapidly, and cerebral herniation may occur.

The biochemical pathology caused by exposure of brain tissue to blood has not been established. Hypertension is closely associated with intracerebral hemorrhage. Research suggests that the matrix metalloproteinases in vessel walls are activated, thereby leading to degradation of vascular tissue with subsequent bleeding.

CEREBRAL EDEMA

A pathologic increase in the water content of brain tissue (edema) eventually develops in all types of ischemic and hemorrhagic stroke. Brain swelling and raised ICP relate proportionally to the volume of accumulated water; in some instances, edema can cause neurologic deterioration and death by herniation syndromes.

The intracranial space contains the brain, which weighs approximately 1400 g, about 75 mL of blood, and approximately 75 mL of cerebrospinal fluid (CSF). An increase in the volume of any of these contents must be accompanied by a decrease in another component because the intracranial cavity is of relatively fixed size and surrounded by bone. Normally, the brain's tissue volume is constant, whereas intracranial blood and CSF vary reciprocally to maintain normal ICP. A variety of mechanisms can compensate for increased intracranial contents to a limited extent, including displacement of CSF into other cranial compartments, reduction of venous blood volume, reduction of normal cerebral interstitial fluid, and chronic cerebral atrophy. If there is a rapid increase in extravascular blood, reduced venous outflow, blockage or resorption of CSF, or cerebral edema, ICP increases markedly.

Brain edema is categorized on the basis of pathophysiologic and anatomic criteria as intracellular or interstitial. Intracellular edema, also called *cytotoxic edema*, develops as energy-dependent membrane ion pumps fail; as a result, Na^+ and other osmoles enter the cell and draw water in from the interstitial and vascular compartments. This process can begin within a few hours after the onset of ischemia. Cell swelling occurs predominantly in astrocytes, but neurons, oligodendroglial cells, and endothelial cells are also involved.

Interstitial edema, also called *vasogenic edema*, occurs later than the intracellular form. Damage to endothelial cells of the BBB allows macromolecules, such as plasma proteins, to enter the cerebral interstitial space accompanied by osmotically bound water. Interstitial edema after cerebral infarction progressively worsens for about 3 days after a stroke. Fluid accumulation within the vicinity of damaged endothelial cells and the zone of infarction can raise the local water content of brain by 10%. The osmolality of ischemic brain increases from 310 to approximately 350 mOsm. The intracellular accumulation of water increases from a normal value of approximately 79 to 81% of brain weight.

If the cerebral circulation is re-established before permanent brain injury develops, the intracellular edema resolves without permanent sequelae. A large increase in the brain's volume can, however, lead to transtentorial herniation of the cerebral hemispheres or to cerebellar herniation. These syndromes can result in irreversible global ischemia of the hemispheres or crushing of the brain stem, loss of cerebral control of the circulation, and death from respiratory arrest. The edema-induced increase in ICP usually reaches a maximum about 3 days after the onset of a stroke. If a patient has a large stroke and survives after the third day, the patient is unlikely to die as a result of that stroke.

SUGGESTED READINGS

Butcher K, Emery D. Acute stroke imaging. Part I: fundamentals. *Can J Neurol Sci.* 2010;37:4-16. *Review.*

Gorelick PB, Ruland S. Cerebral vascular disease. *Dis Mon.* 2010;56:39-100. *Review.*

Thompson AM, Hu T, Eshelbrenner CL, et al. Antihypertensive treatment and secondary prevention of cardiovascular disease events among persons without hypertension: a meta-analysis. *JAMA.* 2011;305:913-922. *Antihypertensive medications decrease the risk of stroke even in people without hypertension.*

414

ISCHEMIC CEREBROVASCULAR DISEASE

JUSTIN A. ZIVIN

DEFINITION

Ischemic stroke is caused by insufficient blood flow to part or all of the brain. *Focal stroke* is defined as an infarction in a part of the brain as the result of reduced blood flow in an artery that supplies that part of the brain. During the early phases of a stroke, when acute therapy is potentially beneficial, it is impossible to predict whether an individual patient will recover because the treatment is effective only if given before it is known whether the symptoms will resolve spontaneously.

The important distinction between a transient ischemic attack (TIA) and a stroke is whether the ischemia has caused brain infarction, a difference that may not be possible to distinguish within the first few hours after the onset of symptoms but commonly becomes apparent retrospectively. With a stroke, symptoms usually persist for more than 24 hours, but clinical deficits that persist for more that 1 to 2 hours commonly are associated with permanent brain damage, often demonstrable by computed tomography (CT) or magnetic resonance imaging (MRI), despite complete recovery. Many events that were defined as TIAs in the era before neuroimaging were actually infarcts. By comparison, the symptoms of TIAs usually do not persist for more than 1 to 2 hours and do not cause permanent damage on neuroimaging studies. Patients with TIAs are at considerably increased risk of having a stroke within hours to days after a TIA.

Ischemic strokes are differentiated from hemorrhagic strokes (Chapter 415) by the lack of extravasated blood in the brain parenchyma. There are two main classifications of ischemic stroke. *Thrombosis* and *embolism,* which are caused by arterial occlusion with either a thrombus that forms locally at the site of an atherosclerotic plaque or an embolic clot, are responsible for 65% of all strokes. Emboli are produced when a piece of a larger clot breaks off from a mural thrombus in the heart or a more proximal artery and lodges downstream at a point where the diameter of the vessel has decreased in size so that the clot can no longer pass through the arterial lumen. It is often impossible to distinguish a thrombus from an embolus by imaging methods or histopathologic material, so the two processes are classified together. *Small vessel strokes,* commonly called *lacunes,* are caused by occlusion of small arterioles and account for about 20% of strokes. The histologic lesion in blood vessels in these strokes is classically called lipohyalinosis, which does not help in identifying the cause of these strokes. Some of these strokes are caused by local vascular abnormalities, but others are almost certainly caused by small emboli. The other 15% or so of strokes are caused by hemorrhage (Chapter 415).

EPIDEMIOLOGY

Hypertension is the most important risk factor for ischemic and hemorrhagic stroke (Chapter 67). The incidence of stroke increases directly in relation to the degree of elevation of systolic and diastolic arterial blood pressure above threshold values. More important, there has been conclusive evidence for more than 30 years that control of hypertension prevents strokes. Meta-analyses of randomized controlled trials confirm an approximate 30 to 40% reduction in stroke risk with lowering of blood pressure.

Approximately 7 to 10% of men and 5 to 7% of women older than 65 years have asymptomatic carotid stenosis of greater than 50%. Epidemiologic studies suggest that the rate of unheralded stroke ipsilateral to a stenosis is about 1 to 2% annually.

Nonvalvular atrial fibrillation (Chapter 64) carries a 3 to 5% annual risk for stroke, with the risk becoming even higher in the presence of advanced age, previous TIA or stroke, hypertension, impaired left ventricular function, and diabetes mellitus.

In epidemiologic studies, the risk for stroke in smokers is almost double that in nonsmokers, but the risk becomes essentially identical to that of nonsmokers by 2 to 5 years after quitting. The relative risk for stroke is two to six times greater for patients with insulin-dependent diabetes (Chapter 236). Patients with sickle cell disease (Chapter 166) have a markedly increased risk for stroke. Hyperlipidemia also increases the risk for stroke, and reduction of low-density lipoprotein (LDL) cholesterol levels with statins reduces this risk. Some evidence suggests that abdominal obesity in men and obesity and weight gain in women are independent risk factors for stroke. Weight reduction in overweight people is recommended, but weight loss has not been proved to reduce the risk for stroke.

Epidemiologic studies have found that consumption of fruits and vegetables is associated with a lower risk for stroke, but no randomized trials have proved the value of changing dietary habits. Heavy alcohol consumption may be a risk factor for ischemic and hemorrhagic stroke.

Postmenopausal hormone replacement therapy has been shown to increase the risk for stroke. The absolute risk for stroke remains low, however, in otherwise healthy, low-risk patients. Meta-analysis suggests an increase in the relative risk for stroke in women taking oral contraceptives, but the absolute risk for stroke is small. Women who smoke, are hypertensive or diabetic, have migraine headaches, or have previously suffered thromboembolic events may be at increased risk for stroke when taking oral contraceptives.

PATHOBIOLOGY

The precise signs and symptoms of ischemic stroke depend primarily on the region deprived of blood flow. The tempo with which deficits develop has important clinical implications.

Pattern of Development of Strokes

Shortly after the onset of vascular occlusion, it is common for symptoms and signs to fluctuate and either to improve or to deteriorate, often rapidly. Some patients may be in denial and anticipate that their symptoms will resolve, thereby resulting in delay in seeking medical care until sufficient time has elapsed that acute therapy is useless.

If the symptoms resolve completely in 1 or 2 hours, the patient has had a TIA. The basis for this resolution is unclear. Possibilities include dissolution of an embolus with subsequent restoration of normal regional blood flow, decrease in vasospasm, and improvement in perfusion secondary to increased collateral flow.

Ischemic episodes that ultimately develop into infarction often fluctuate for several hours after onset. Early in the course it is impossible to predict what will happen. Recovery may stop suddenly, and deficits may plateau or increase. Persistence of any neurologic deficit beyond 2 hours, even if the patient subsequently recovers fully, is nearly always accompanied by some degree of tissue destruction.

Hours to days after the abnormality becomes stable, increased neurologic deficits may develop, a deterioration termed *stroke in evolution.* Probable reasons include reperfusion injury, clot extension, or a new stroke in the same vascular distribution. Compromised cardiac output and systemic hypotension resulting from myocardial ischemia, cardiac arrhythmias, or heart failure may also contribute in some cases. Patients may appear to have stroke in evolution because of systemic disorders, such as electrolyte imbalances or glucose abnormalities that initially appear to be exacerbations of a stroke but are really comorbid problems that do not cause extension of the infarct. Cerebral edema may increase neurologic deterioration in large strokes by causing herniation syndromes. Secondary bleeding into an infarct can occur; ordinarily, this process does not increase neurologic deficits unless the blood extends into an area outside the initial boundaries of the infarction or causes a mass effect and increased intracranial pressure. The term *stroke in evolution* describes a clinical picture rather than a specific pathologic process.

Common Causes and Pathogenesis of Stroke

Atherosclerosis

Atherosclerosis (Chapter 70) is the most common disorder that leads to stroke. Atherosclerotic plaques are thought to cause stroke in three ways: (1) mural thrombosis forms at the site of an atherosclerotic lesion, and the clot obstructs the artery at that location; (2) ulceration or rupture of a plaque leads to formation of a clot and distal embolization; and (3) hemorrhage into a plaque obstructs the artery. The clinical manifestations of a stroke depend on the rate of occlusion. If occlusion occurs slowly, there may be time for collateral blood supply to develop, and a stroke is avoided. If the occlusion is abrupt, a stroke ensues, and the degree of damage depends on the extent of collateral supply that is available to the territory of the brain supplied by the occluded vessel. If collateral supply is marginal, just enough blood may pass through the stenotic region to maintain minimally adequate blood flow. In these circumstances, neurologic function may become critically dependent on changes in blood pressure, and small decreases can cause a stroke or recurrent TIAs.

More frequently, a platelet-fibrin thrombus forms on the roughened surface of an atherosclerotic plaque. The thrombus can break off and float distally in the blood stream, eventually becoming lodged in a distal, smaller branch; this process is termed *artery-to-artery embolization*. These embolic occlusions are more likely to be symptomatic because the more distal end vessels have no collateral supply. The amount of territory that is deprived of blood is smaller, however, and symptoms are usually less severe than with occlusion of the main stem of a vessel. The most common locations for an intravascular thrombus to form are the base of the aorta, the bifurcation of the common carotid artery, or the point at which the vertebral arteries originate from the subclavian arteries.

Emboli of Cardiac Origin

Emboli originating from the heart may lodge in any part of the body; however, because about 20% of the normal cardiac output goes to the brain, it is a common site of cardioembolism. Thrombus formation and release of emboli from the heart are promoted by arrhythmias and by structural abnormalities of the valves and chambers. The frequency of the various types of stroke produced by cardioembolism can only be estimated. Although some strokes are clearly embolic in origin, and others are unquestionably thrombotic, it is generally impossible to distinguish them pathologically. There is no diagnostic test to prove that a thrombus or embolus is of cardiac origin.

Mural Thrombi

Myocardial infarction may produce a region of dyskinetic myocardium that predisposes to the formation of mural thrombi (Chapter 73). Anterior wall myocardial infarction is associated with the highest frequency of thromboembolic stroke. Cardiomyopathies (Chapter 60), such as those caused by alcohol abuse or viral infections, also produce dyskinesia that promotes mural thrombi and can result in cerebral embolization, as can any cause of severe heart failure (Chapter 59). In some instances, a cardiac mural thrombus may release numerous pieces that produce a shower of emboli and cause several simultaneous strokes at various locations in the brain.

Valvular Heart Disease

Rheumatic heart disease (Chapter 298), which is now rare in industrialized countries, is associated with systemic emboli, especially in patients who have mitral stenosis (Chapter 75). Acute or subacute infectious endocarditis (Chapter 76) produces vegetations on heart valves, and these vegetations can embolize to the cerebral circulation. Endocarditis caused by staphylococci, fungi, or yeast is often extensive enough to occlude large intracranial arteries. Infective endocarditis is associated with other forms of cerebrovascular disease, including intracerebral hemorrhage, subarachnoid hemorrhage, and mycotic aneurysm (Chapter 415). Strokes can occur during the acute phases of the disease, and the combination of fever, a new murmur, and petechiae should prompt collection of blood for culture and consideration of empirical treatment with antibiotics. Anticoagulants may increase the risk for intracerebral hemorrhage in patients with bacterial endocarditis.

Nonbacterial endocarditis (Chapter 60), which is usually associated with various types of cancer, can also give rise to vegetations that produce cerebral embolization and cause focal strokes or diffuse encephalopathy, sometimes in the form of disseminated intravascular coagulopathy. Systemic lupus erythematosus (Chapter 274) is associated with atypical verrucous (Libman-Sacks) endocarditis in which friable vegetations form on the leaflets of any of the heart valves and can rarely produce cerebral embolization.

In patients with prosthetic heart valves, the incidence of stroke is 1 to 5% per year despite oral anticoagulation (Chapter 75). Mechanical valves have a higher risk than biologic valves. Many studies have suggested that anticoagulants reduce but do not completely eliminate cerebral embolization in these patients.

Arrhythmias

Atrial fibrillation, independent of the presence or absence of valvular disease, is a proven cause of embolic stroke and increases the relative risk, compared with age-matched controls, to about 5% per year (Chapter 64). Approximately 15% of all ischemic strokes are associated with nonvalvular atrial fibrillation. Most patients with atrial fibrillation never have a stroke, however. The strokes are often large and disabling, but minor strokes, silent strokes, and TIAs can occur. Most ischemic strokes in patients with atrial fibrillation are due to embolism from left atrial mural thrombi. The risk for atrial fibrillation–associated strokes is increased in patients who have chronic hypertension. The risk for embolic stroke is highest shortly after the development of atrial fibrillation, but embolism can also accompany cardioversion to normal sinus rhythm regardless of whether the conversion is spontaneous, induced by medication, or electrical.

Paradoxical Emboli

Embolic occlusion of intracranial vessels can be of venous origin. The embolic material gains access to the arterial circulation through various cardiac defects, such as a patent foramen ovale, atrial septal defect (Chapter 69), or arteriovenous malformation. When venous emboli enter the heart, a right-to-left shunt allows the emboli to enter the arterial circulation. A patent foramen ovale has been detected in 40% of patients with acute ischemic stroke of uncertain origin, and it is often assumed that paradoxical embolization is the cause of the stroke. Patients with an atrial septal aneurysm and a patent foramen ovale are at highest risk.

CLINICAL MANIFESTATIONS

The clinical manifestations are summarized in Table 414-1.

Internal Carotid Artery

The common carotid artery bifurcation, at the origin of the internal carotid artery (ICA), is the most frequent site of atherosclerotic lesions of the cerebral vasculature. Occlusion of the ICA is often clinically silent if the circle of Willis is complete. It is often impossible to distinguish ICA occlusion from similar damage to the middle cerebral artery (MCA) on clinical examination (see later). Because the ophthalmic artery originates from the ICA, however, TIAs of the ICA may be manifested as transient monocular blindness (also called *amaurosis fugax*). Severe stenosis of the ICA, particularly if bilateral, can cause hypoperfusion of the cerebral hemispheres and symptoms in border zones between the MCA and other major vascular territories (watershed areas), especially if superimposed on generalized hypoperfusion secondary to severe hypotension.

Anterior Cerebral Artery

Isolated occlusion of the anterior cerebral artery (ACA), which is relatively rare in comparison to strokes in other major branches of the circle of Willis, accounts for about 2% of all cerebral infarcts. The principal symptoms associated with occlusion of an ACA distal to the anterior communicating artery are upper motor neuron weakness and cortical sensory deficits (neglect) in the contralateral leg. Other manifestations of ACA occlusion can include urinary incontinence, generalized depression of psychomotor activity (abulia), and transcortical motor aphasia manifested as loss of verbal fluency with preserved ability to repeat. Bilateral occlusion may occur because the origins of the two ACAs are separated by only a short stretch of anterior communicating artery, and there are frequent anomalies in which both ACAs originate from a common source. Bilateral damage usually causes a patient to be mute, with severe mood disturbances and long-lasting incontinence from bilateral damage to the frontal lobes.

Middle Cerebral Artery

Strokes in the distribution of the MCA are the most common type of focal stroke, and such strokes cause approximately two thirds of all infarcts. Occlusion of the stem of the MCA often results in massive, devastating infarction of much of the hemisphere. Edema during the first 3 to 4 days may lead to

TABLE 414-1   CLINICAL MANIFESTATIONS OF ISCHEMIC STROKE

OCCLUDED BLOOD VESSEL	CLINICAL MANIFESTATIONS
ICA	Ipsilateral blindness (variable) MCA syndrome (see below)
MCA	Contralateral hemiparesis, sensory loss (arm, face worst) Expressive aphasia (dominant) or anosognosia and spatial disorientation (nondominant) Contralateral inferior quadrantanopsia
ACA	Contralateral hemiparesis, sensory loss (worst in leg)
PCA	Contralateral homonymous hemianopia or superior quadrantanopia Memory impairment
Basilar apex	Bilateral blindness Amnesia
Basilar artery	Contralateral hemiparesis, sensory loss Ipsilateral bulbar or cerebellar signs
Vertebral artery or PICA	Ipsilateral loss of facial sensation, ataxia, contralateral hemiparesis, sensory loss
Superior cerebellar artery	Gait ataxia, nausea, dizziness, headache progressing to ipsilateral hemiataxia, dysarthria, gaze paresis, contralateral hemiparesis, somnolence

ACA = anterior cerebral artery; ICA = internal carotid artery; MCA = middle cerebral artery; PCA = posterior cerebral artery; PICA = posterior inferior cerebellar artery.

severely increased intracranial pressure and herniation. The classic picture of occlusion of the MCA stem is contralateral weakness and sensory loss in the face and arm (with relative sparing of the leg) and homonymous hemianopia on the side of the weakness; initially, there may be depressed consciousness and deviation of gaze toward the side of the lesion. There is little chance of substantial recovery. In right-handed people, occlusion of the left MCA produces global aphasia in which the patient can neither understand the speech of others nor produce meaningful speech. In the nondominant hemisphere, unilateral neglect, anosognosia (unawareness of the deficit), and spatial disorientation occur.

Occlusion of branches of the MCA produces partial syndromes. An embolus to the MCA frequently lodges in one of its two main divisions. Occlusion of the superior division can cause dense sensorimotor deficits in the contralateral face and arm without initial impairment of alertness. Later, some neurologic function may recover, and the aphasia may decrease. Strokes of the inferior division in the dominant hemisphere characteristically produce receptive aphasia of the Wernicke type (severe loss of speech comprehension with preserved spoken and written language). Damage to either hemisphere can result in contralateral loss of integrated sensation, such as perception of shapes (stereognosis). Occlusion of more distal branches causes less clinical damage.

Posterior Cerebral Artery

In about three fourths of people, both posterior cerebral arteries (PCAs) arise from the basilar artery; in most others, one PCA arises from the basilar artery and the other arises from the ICA. In a few individuals, both PCAs originate from the ICAs. As a consequence, the syndromes associated with occlusion of the PCA are highly variable. Strokes of the perforating branches most frequently cause complete contralateral hemianesthesia with loss of all sensation and complete hemianopia on that side. Macular (central) vision may be spared because of collateral blood supply from the MCA. Difficulty reading (dyslexia) and performing calculations (dyscalculia) may occur. Recovery is often good, but the initial numbness may be replaced by paresthesias or excruciating pain; this Dejerine-Roussy syndrome is caused by damage to the thalamus. Involvement of the subthalamic nucleus may produce hemiballismus, with wild flinging movements of the limbs on one side of the body. Distal branch occlusions of the PCA cause partial syndromes; occlusion of the terminal branch can produce a variety of incomplete visual field deficits, although the loss is characteristically congruous (superimposable) in both visual fields.

Vertebral and Basilar Arteries

Characteristic of occlusion of the blood supply to the brain stem are "crossed syndromes" (i.e., contralateral loss of strength and selected contralateral and ipsilateral sensory symptoms below the level of the lesion, in addition to ipsilateral motor and sensory deficits localized to the level of the lesion). Weber's syndrome is caused by a mesencephalic lesion that produces an ipsilateral third cranial nerve palsy resulting from damage to the oculomotor nerve as well as contralateral weakness.

The vertebral arteries are the principal blood supply for the medulla. The posterior inferior cerebellar artery is usually a branch of the vertebral artery. The consequences of occlusion of the posterior inferior cerebellar artery are variable, but lateral medullary infarction (Wallenberg's syndrome) is classically produced. In about 80% of cases, occlusion of the vertebral artery causes lateral medullary syndrome, which consists of severe vertigo, nausea, vomiting, nystagmus, ipsilateral ataxia (of the cerebellar type), and ipsilateral Horner's syndrome (ptosis, miosis, and decreased sweating). The syndrome also includes ipsilateral loss of facial pain and temperature sensation and contralateral loss of these sensory modalities in the trunk and limb. Partial syndromes are the rule; a complete lateral medullary syndrome is rare, so it is often misdiagnosed.

The basilar artery supplies most of the brain stem, and occlusion of this artery produces a variety of syndromes. Obstruction of the basilar artery trunk is often fatal because the main motor and sensory pathways between the cerebral hemispheres and the remainder of the body are compact and travel through the brain stem. The findings in occlusion of the basilar artery consist of a combination of bilateral sensory and motor long-tract signs, cerebellar dysfunction, and cranial nerve abnormalities: paralysis or weakness of all extremities and the bulbar muscles, impaired vision with various visual field defects, bilateral cerebellar ataxia, and a variety of sensory disturbances ranging from normal to total anesthesia. Coma may occur, or the locked-in syndrome may develop in which consciousness is preserved but the victims are unable to move anything voluntarily except their eyes or eyelids. It is possible to communicate with these patients and demonstrate normal mental status by codes involving eye movements.

Occlusion of the various branches of the basilar artery produces a large variety of syndromes. Because the pathways are so closely spaced in the brain stem, even small brain infarctions can cause substantial motor and sensory deficits. The characteristic findings are crossed syndromes with motor and sensory dissociation, unless the findings are bilateral. Distinguishing mild vertebrobasilar ischemia from the common causes of dizziness is occasionally difficult (Chapters 50 and 62), but ischemia is rarely a cause of isolated vertigo in the absence of other brain stem signs or symptoms.

DIAGNOSIS

The history gives initial clues about the site and severity of a stroke, and the physical examination helps refine a hypothesis on the location of the lesion. Based on this information, definitive laboratory testing can proceed efficiently.

History

As the name implies, stroke ordinarily starts at a clearly identifiable time. The most important aspect of the history, which must be elicited from a patient or accompanying observers if a stroke is suspected, is the time of onset of symptoms. If abnormalities began within the preceding 3 hours, the patient should be managed as an acute emergency, and thrombolytic therapy may be indicated. Patients may be confused, anxious, or aphasic, and they may not remember the duration of symptoms. It may be necessary to try to associate the onset of symptoms with events that the patient or accompanying persons can identify accurately. Did the patient wake up with symptoms? In this case the symptoms must be assumed, in terms of considering acute treatment, to have started at the time that the patient was last known to be in a premorbid state—usually at the time of going to sleep. Was the patient watching television, and if so, what program was it? Consultation with the program guide can be used to assign a time of onset. Was an ambulance called, and if so, what time was the patient first examined by paramedics? This information is usually available in the ambulance records.

TIAs may not be distinguishable from a stroke during the early phases, but TIAs usually resolve within the first hour or two. Rapid progression of deficits or the presence of headache occurs more often in patients with intracerebral hemorrhage (Chapter 415). Although intracerebral hemorrhage is responsible for only about 15% of strokes, hemorrhages generally produce more severe symptoms that cannot be denied. By comparison, patients with minor strokes or predominantly sensory symptoms are often in a state of denial and do not seek medical care until long after vessel occlusion. Because ischemic strokes are nearly always painless, they do not awaken patients from sleep and are frequently discovered at the time of normal awakening in the morning. There is some diurnal variation in the onset of stroke, with a peak in the late morning.

Physical Examination

The neurologic examination (Chapter 403) is a cost-effective method for initiating a diagnostic evaluation, and it often helps localize the site of the lesion. The cardiovascular examination (Chapter 50) should focus on measurement of arterial blood pressure, including measurement in both arms to evaluate the possibility of aortic dissection (Chapter 78) or vascular abnormalities that result in reduced blood flow to the brain when the arms are exercised (subclavian steal). The greatest risk factor for stroke is preexisting hypertension. In many patients, transient hypertension develops in the immediate aftermath of a stroke, however, so it is important to determine whether a patient has had sustained hypertension (Chapter 67). Extremely elevated blood pressure at initial evaluation can lead to heart failure, which may have to be managed urgently. If hypertension is a transient manifestation of acute stroke, aggressive reduction may cause hypotension and enlarge the infarct. The pulse may reveal arrhythmias, such as atrial fibrillation, that can result in cerebral embolism. Cardiac murmurs may suggest valvular lesions (Chapter 75) that can cause cerebral embolism. Bruits of the carotid arteries can be produced by atherosclerotic disease of the arteries, and such disease is associated with embolic and thrombotic strokes. Evidence of peripheral vascular disease (Chapter 79) may be a reflection of generalized atherosclerosis.

Ophthalmoscopic visualization of retinal cholesterol or platelet-fibrin emboli suggests more proximal atherosclerotic disease. Examination of the retinal vessels may also reveal signs of chronic hypertension or diabetes (arteriovenous crossing defects or retinal hemorrhages; Chapter 431).

The neurologic examination usually suggests the location and size of the stroke. If the patient's mental status is depressed, bilateral cerebral lesions or a brain stem lesion is suggested. Multiple smaller strokes may lead to dementia. Speech is commonly affected, with various aphasic patterns suggesting the site of the lesion. Testing of strength, sensation, and deep tendon reflexes provides information about the patterns of the deficits and suggests the site of the vascular lesion. Plantar stimulation (Babinski's sign), which is a classic finding in patients with damage to the long tracts, indicates upper motor neuron damage caused by stroke. However, during the early phases of a large stroke, reflexes may be depressed rather than hyperactive.

Laboratory Examination
Hematologic Tests

A complete hemogram, including a platelet count, is essential to evaluate for polycythemia (Chapter 169), thrombocytosis, bacterial endocarditis (Chapter 76), and severe anemia. An erythrocyte sedimentation rate is also a useful screening test because it may be elevated in patients with hypercoagulable states (Chapter 179) and is markedly elevated in patients with giant cell arteritis (Chapter 279). A blood glucose level must be checked because hyperglycemia and hypoglycemia can produce focal and global neurologic deficits, sometimes mimicking stroke. Diabetes (Chapter 236) increases the risk for stroke, and stroke may be the initial symptom of diabetes. A prothrombin time and partial thromboplastin time should be obtained in patients who may have received anticoagulants before the onset of stroke to determine whether they have been taking their medications or the anticoagulation is excessive.

Although moderate hyperlipidemia is not a proven risk factor, extremely high lipid levels are strongly associated with stroke. Antiphospholipid antibodies are elevated in some patients with immune-related diseases. Measurement of protein C, protein S, antithrombin III, blood viscosity, and platelet function (Chapter 179) and tests for homocystinuria, collagen vascular diseases (Chapter 264), amyloidosis (Chapter 194), and syphilis (Chapter 327) should be performed in selected cases.

Cardiovascular Testing

Patients with acute myocardial infarction or a new or chronic atrial arrhythmia may have suffered an embolic stroke. A standard electrocardiogram and rhythm strip should be obtained at initial evaluation to determine whether acute myocardial ischemia or arrhythmia is present. Echocardiography is indicated urgently only in patients with a history of cardiac disease and an abnormal electrocardiogram; if no cause for the stroke is identified, however, particularly if the patient is relatively young, echocardiography is generally indicated.

Noninvasive Brain Imaging

Brain imaging (Chapter 403), which is essential to verify causes of focal neurologic dysfunction, can generally distinguish ischemic stroke from other diseases. The most important disorders to differentiate from acute ischemic stroke are intracerebral hemorrhage (Chapter 415), subarachnoid hemorrhage (Chapter 415), and brain tumors (Chapter 195).

CT is the standard initial imaging study (Fig. 414-1). Non–contrast-enhanced imaging usually detects intracerebral hemorrhage. Signals indicating tissue hypodensity, particularly in the region of the brain appropriate to the neurologic deficits, and loss of the distinction between gray and white matter are often observed 3 to 24 hours after the onset of stroke. These findings cannot predict the size of the infarction, however, and noncontrast CT findings may be normal for 3 to 24 hours after an ischemic stroke. The hypodensity typically becomes progressively more apparent over the first 3 to 24 hours and is usually readily detectable by 24 hours in patients with large infarcts. Small ischemic strokes in the brain stem can produce major neurologic dysfunction and may not be detected by CT. Contrast enhancement of CT scans seldom improves detection of acute stroke, but it may distinguish ischemic lesions from some types of neoplasms.

FIGURE 414-1. Computed tomographic imaging. **A,** A computed tomography (CT) scan of a patient with a left hemisphere infarction 6 to 24 hours after the onset of symptoms shows a hypodense area in the basal ganglia region and compression of the frontal horn of the lateral ventricle. **B,** A CT scan shows the chronic infarction 1 year later; atrophy and loss of tissue volume are visible. (Courtesy of Gregory W. Albers, Stanford University, Stanford, Calif.)

FIGURE 414-2. Magnetic resonance imaging showing early ischemic changes obtained 6 hours after the onset of right-sided weakness in a patient with an occluded left internal carotid artery. (Courtesy of Gregory W. Albers, Stanford University, Stanford, Calif.)

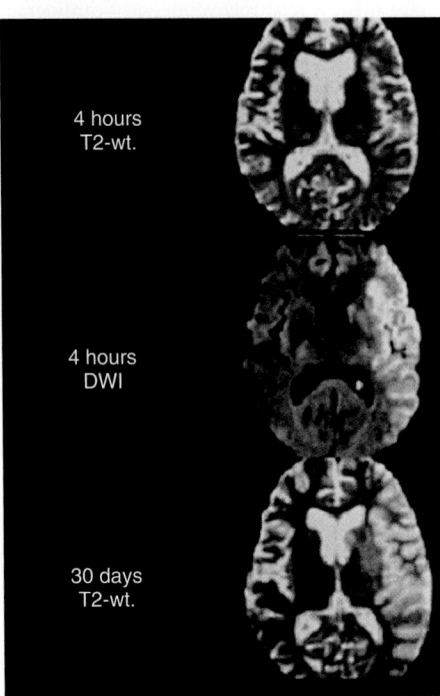

4 hours
T2-wt.

4 hours
DWI

30 days
T2-wt.

FIGURE 414-3. Magnetic resonance imaging (MRI) showing possible advantages of diffusion-weighted imaging (DWI) relative to conventional MRI at early times after vascular occlusion. *Top,* Conventional T2-weighted MRI 4 hours after symptom onset that appears normal. *Middle,* At the same time, a DWI scan shows abnormalities in the left hemisphere. *Bottom,* Repeat T2-weighted MRI 1 month later showed an infarction in the same location as the initial DWI scan. (Courtesy of Gregory W. Albers, Stanford University, Stanford, Calif.)

CT is currently the only imaging method useful for deciding whether to administer thrombolytic therapy. Detection of hemorrhage in areas of infarction is important because it precludes thrombolytic therapy. Small hemorrhages may be detected by CT scanning during the first few hours but may not have clinical importance. Hemorrhages become more evident with time and appear on repeat scans hours to weeks after infarction. Whether this apparent increase in the detection of hemorrhage is due to a progressive increase in the size of the initial hemorrhage or to alterations in the extravasated blood is not known.

MRI is more sensitive than CT for detecting early ischemia (Fig. 414-2). MRI sequences can identify tissue or blood flow abnormalities within minutes after the onset of ischemia (Fig. 414-3). These early indicators of

tissue injury are qualitative and have not been shown to predict the ultimate volume of the lesion or whether the tissue damage is irreversible. MRI cannot be used in patients who have ferromagnetic materials within their bodies, is often impossible to use in critically ill patients, and renders the patient inaccessible for several minutes. No MRI sequences successfully distinguish ischemia from hemorrhage, especially during the early phases of injury, when decisions regarding whether thrombolysis should be administered are needed. CT remains the imaging procedure of choice for acute patient management.

Lumbar Puncture

Lumbar puncture is no longer performed routinely in the evaluation of a patient with stroke because CT detects intracerebral hemorrhage more reliably (Chapter 403). CT can also usually identify blood in the subarachnoid space, although lumbar puncture is more sensitive for this purpose and can give some indication about when the bleeding occurred (Chapter 415). After subarachnoid hemorrhage, erythrocytes hemolyze. As hemoglobin is metabolized, cerebrospinal fluid becomes xanthochromic. Lumbar puncture is required to determine whether a patient has neurosyphilis (Chapter 327), although screening blood testing should be conducted first. Lumbar puncture is also occasionally indicated if there is concern that a patient may have bacterial meningitis (Chapter 420).

Noninvasive Cerebrovascular Examination

Ultrasonography provides an estimate of luminal diameter and the direction and speed of blood flow. B-mode ultrasonography, which produces real-time images of the carotid vessels, and range-gated pulsed Doppler, which is guided visually by the B-mode image, can detect increased blood velocity through a stenotic lumen. The combination of the location of the Doppler frequency signal and the B-mode image provides a noninvasive method for analyzing the condition of the extracranial circulation. Limitations of the technique include (1) access to only the portion of the carotid circulation that lies between the clavicles and the mandible (in approximately 10% of patients, the carotid bifurcation lies above the angle of the jaw, thus making ultrasonography difficult or impossible); (2) absorption of sound waves by calcium within a mural plaque, a process that may "shadow" and obscure a plaque on a distal vessel wall; and (3) echolucency of acute thrombi, which can be indistinguishable from flowing blood. The direction and velocity of blood flow in the intracranial blood vessels originating from the circle of Willis can be examined with low-frequency pulsed transcranial Doppler. Although these methods are useful screening techniques with essentially no risk to the patient, the "gold standard" for defining the status of the cerebral vasculature remains cerebral angiography. Moreover, ultrasound technique is critically dependent on the training and skill of the technician; there is considerable variation among different laboratories, and the clinician must confirm new or suspicious findings with repeat examinations or other tests.

CT and magnetic resonance (MR) angiography can visualize the larger cerebral vessels and detect abnormalities such as stenosis, aneurysms, or arteriovenous malformations. These methods lack sensitivity for small lesions, however, and the degree of stenosis tends to be exaggerated.

Cerebral Angiography

Cerebral angiography is reserved for patients who are suspected to have a surgically correctable lesion. Arterial vessels are displayed initially, and delayed images can outline the venous system. Patients commonly receive anticoagulants during the procedure. The images give high-quality resolution of the vessels but do not provide quantitative information about blood flow. This method is the only one that has been proved useful for selecting patients who can benefit from carotid endarterectomy.

Angiography, particularly in patients with abnormal vasculature, can itself cause stroke and result in permanent neurologic deficits or death. The rate of injury varies in different surveys but is about 0.5% in good facilities. Angiography requires exposure to ionizing radiation, may be associated with adverse reactions to the contrast material, and involves a fluid load that poses a risk to patients with severe cardiac disease.

Other Techniques

Single-photon emission computed tomography provides only qualitative blood flow rates. Positron emission tomography quantitatively measures blood flow or brain metabolism. CT and MRI methods for measurement of cerebral blood flow and metabolism are in development. None of these techniques has yet been shown to be useful for the management of stroke patients (Chapter 403).

Differential Diagnosis

The characteristic feature of ischemic stroke is the abrupt, painless onset of a neurologic deficit. Blood supply is lost in the distribution of a terminal vessel, and loss of function begins within seconds. The brain does not have pain receptors in its parenchyma, so the symptoms are painless unless the dura mater, which does have pain fibers, is stretched or irritated. One type of stroke that can evolve slowly is subdural hematoma (Chapter 415), which may be distinguishable from ischemic stroke because a hematoma produces deficits more slowly. Focal symptoms and signs of tumors (Chapter 195) of various types typically evolve over a period of weeks or longer, except in uncommon cases in which a tumor erodes a vessel and causes bleeding or crushes it and causes infarction. TIAs cannot initially be distinguished from strokes, but they generally resolve within the first 1 or 2 hours.

Other neurologic disorders can be manifested as an abrupt onset of neurologic abnormalities. Migraine (Chapter 405) with or without aura may simulate stroke or TIA because of its associated hemiparesis or other focal deficits. Migraine is primarily an exquisitely painful, throbbing, unilateral headache that sometimes has an aura (symptoms preceding the headache) of scintillating scotomas (flashing lights). Complicated migraine (migraine accompanied by focal deficits) can rarely evolve into a true ischemic stroke, probably because of the decreased blood flow that often accompanies migraine.

Seizures (Chapter 410) can be confused with TIAs. Many seizures produce tonic (sustained) or clonic (rapid) motor activity or positive sensory phenomena. Strokes and TIAs produce weakness and sensory loss without involuntary motor activity. Seizures can sometimes be associated with these negative symptoms, particularly in the postictal state after (unobserved) seizures. The patient generally returns to the premorbid state after a seizure, however. Serial observations usually permit the differentiation of stroke from seizure, but early differentiation may be difficult and require laboratory testing, particularly an electroencephalogram. In a few patients with stroke, especially with emboli, a seizure occurs at the onset of the stroke.

Hyperglycemia and hypoglycemia can cause focal neurologic deficits. Most patients have a history of diabetes, and the glucose abnormality is substantial at the time of focal neurologic deficits.

Hemorrhagic stroke (Chapter 415) cannot generally be definitively distinguished from ischemic stroke on the basis of the history or clinical examination. Primary hemorrhages are often severe at onset and may result in headache and rapidly evolving deficits. Ischemic strokes are normally painless and characterized by a fixed deficit or a stuttering onset followed by rapid waxing and waning fluctuations. Headaches can occur in conjunction with many ischemic strokes, however, and the only way to distinguish infarct from hemorrhage definitively is with a CT scan.

Brief global cerebral anoxia causes syncope without any permanent sequelae. Prolonged diffuse ischemia, by contrast, can have devastating consequences. The most common causes are cardiac asystole or other forms of overwhelming cardiopulmonary failure. Aortic dissection (Chapter 78), global hypoxia, or carbon monoxide poisoning (Chapter 94) can cause a similar picture. Clinically, these disorders result in unconsciousness. If ischemia persists for more than 4 to 5 minutes, patients often remain in a coma, sometimes evolving into the vegetative state, in which brain stem functions are preserved but the patient has no higher cortical function (Chapter 411). If patients do not regain consciousness within 2 or 3 days, the prognosis for return of independent function is poor. Prompt and aggressive effort to restore cardiovascular circulation is most important. Clinical trials have shown that induced hypothermia within minutes to hours improves outcome in adults who remain comatose after initial resuscitation from out-of-hospital ventricular fibrillation cardiac arrest.**1**

In young patients, hypoxia caused by near-drowning in cold water may result in resistance to prolonged hypoxic-ischemic damage. Therapeutic hypothermia has not yet been proved useful in adults with stroke.

TREATMENT   **Rx**

Acute Stroke

Thrombolytic therapy is the only safe and effective method for acute management of ischemic stroke of typical cause (i.e., atherosclerotic and embolic stroke). Meta-analyses provide support for the efficacy and safety of thrombolysis if patients are treated within 4.5 hours after the onset of

---

symptoms,**2,3** with about a one third increase in the likelihood of a favorable neurologic outcome, directly attributable to the drug, despite the minimal risk for hemorrhage. Obstacles to thrombolytic treatment include the need to redesign and implement acute stroke care systems, delay of patients in reaching medical facilities, and insufficient expertise in the use of thrombolysis by many physicians. Telemedicine approaches, whereby physicians can communicate through audio, video, and digital imaging with consultants at referral institutions, can improve the evidence-based use of acute thrombolytic therapy.**4**

The recommended therapy with intravenous tissue plasminogen activator (t-PA) requires adherence to relatively stringent eligibility criteria (Table 414-2 and Fig. 414-4). Therapy must be started within 4.5 hours after the onset of stroke. Before initiating therapy, a non–contrast-enhanced CT scan should be obtained to exclude patients with intracranial hemorrhage. Blood pressure limits are a maximum of 185 mm Hg systolic or 110 mm Hg diastolic. If blood pressure exceeds these limits, it should be lowered with an antihypertensive drug such as labetalol before initiating t-PA. In addition, patients who have had major surgery or serious trauma within the preceding 2 weeks or evidence of gastrointestinal bleeding should not be treated. The recommended dose of intravenous t-PA is 0.9 mg/kg to a maximum of 90 mg, administered as a 10% initial bolus with the remainder given over a 60-minute period.

Treatment should begin as soon as possible, and even patients with mild strokes or rapidly resolving deficits probably merit treatment. Patients with severe strokes, as evidenced by major clinical deficits or early signs of a large infarct by CT scan, do not fare well regardless of whether they are treated. Treatment 3 to 6 hours after the onset of ischemic stroke is not currently recommended, although one study of intra-arterial prourokinase given 3 to 6 hours after the onset of an ischemic stroke showed benefit from such therapy. Streptokinase is not of benefit. Intra-arterial t-PA has been used in patients who are not candidates for intravenous t-PA, but there are no controlled studies of this form of treatment.

Acute anticoagulation with various forms of heparin or warfarin is of no benefit in patients with ischemic stroke. Patients with stroke in evolution, in which deficits increase over the first day after the onset of the stroke, commonly receive anticoagulants, but there is no strong evidence that such therapy is effective. Vital signs and neurologic status should be monitored. After the acute stroke has stabilized and begun to improve, hypertension must be treated.

Blood pressure is often transiently elevated in the initial hours after a stroke and should not be rapidly lowered except as a prelude to t-PA therapy (see earlier). Many stroke patients have markedly elevated blood pressures, even in the absence of a history of hypertension. Until multiple ongoing trials are completed, a reasonable acute blood pressure goal is less than 180 mm Hg systolic in patients who have an intracerebral hemorrhage or are eligible for thrombolysis (<220 mm Hg otherwise), then a goal of 160/100 mm Hg after 24 hours.

If a patient has suffered an acute myocardial infarction, the preferred therapy is primary angioplasty (Chapter 74). It is uncertain what dose of t-PA should be administered if a patient simultaneously has a stroke and myocardial infarction. If a patient is a candidate for coronary artery bypass graft surgery and is found to have surgically correctable carotid stenosis, the more urgent procedure should generally be performed first.

There is an increased risk for pulmonary embolism and deep vein thrombosis in patients with ischemic stroke, particularly those with neurologic deficits that produce immobility. In these patients, prophylactic low-dose subcutaneous heparin or low-molecular-weight heparin (Chapter 37) is recommended unless there are other contraindications to anticoagulation. The use of graduated compression stockings does not significantly reduce deep vein thrombosis after stroke but results in adverse skin effects.**5**

⬤ UNUSUAL CAUSES OF STROKE

Atrial Myxoma

Atrial myxomas (Chapter 60) are the most common type of primary cardiac tumor and are found in about 0.05% of autopsies of young adults with ischemic strokes or TIAs. Nonspecific constitutional symptoms are frequent, and less than half of myxomas produce emboli. When these tumors do produce emboli, the danger period usually lasts days to weeks. Metastasis can rarely cause cerebral aneurysms. Other primary and metastatic cardiac tumors can embolize neoplastic tissue or thrombus.

Vasculitis

Vasculitis (Chapters 274, 278, and 279) can produce focal or multifocal cerebral ischemia by means of inflammation and necrosis of extracranial or intracranial blood vessels. Segmental inflammation of cerebral blood vessels is associated with cerebral ischemia acutely at the site of involvement.

Vasculitis of the central nervous system (CNS) is often manifested as cognitive disturbances, headache, and seizures. Because the vascular damage is commonly diffuse, these nonfocal neurologic abnormalities occur more

TABLE 414-2 TISSUE PLASMINOGEN ACTIVATOR THERAPY FOR ACUTE ISCHEMIC STROKE

Clinical manifestation—focal neurologic deficits

Patient selection

    Therapy must be started within 3 hr of the onset of acute ischemic stroke symptoms

    A baseline CT scan must be obtained before initiation of therapy

Contraindications

    Evidence of intracranial hemorrhage on pretreatment evaluation

    Suspicion of subarachnoid hemorrhage

    Recent intracranial surgery, serious head trauma, or previous stroke

    History of intracranial hemorrhage

    Uncontrolled hypertension at the time of treatment—≥185 mm Hg systolic or >110 diastolic—that cannot be reduced with acute antihypertensive therapy

    Seizure at stroke onset

    Active internal bleeding

    Intracranial neoplasm, AVM, or aneurysm

    Known bleeding diathesis, including but not limited to

        Oral anticoagulation with a prothrombin time >15 sec

        Heparin administration within the preceding 48 hr and an elevated activated partial thromboplastin time at initial evaluation

        Platelet count <100,000/mm^3

Warnings

    Patients with a severe neurologic deficit (NIH Stroke Scale >22) at initial evaluation have an increased risk for ICH

    Patients with major early infarct signs on CT (edema or mass effect) are probably >3 hr since vessel occlusion

Dosing information for acute ischemic stroke

    0.9 mg/kg to a maximal dose of ≤90 mg

    10% of the total dose administered as an intravenous bolus over a 1-min period

    90% of the remainder infused continuously over a 60-min period

Follow-up

    Monitor vital signs and neurologic status

    Maintain blood pressure at ≤185/≤110 mm Hg

    No anticoagulant or antiplatelet therapy for 24 hr

AVM = arteriovenous malformation; CT = computed tomography; ICH = intracranial hemorrhage; NIH = National Institutes of Health.

Modified from package insert for Activase, Genentech, Inc., South San Francisco, Calif.

---

frequently with vasculitis than with focal ischemic disorders. The diagnosis is often difficult to make because the signs and symptoms are frequently nonspecific. The angiographic appearance of a beadlike segmental narrowing of cerebral blood vessels, when present, is virtually diagnostic, but cerebral angiograms are often normal in histologically proven cases. Definitive diagnosis requires the demonstration of characteristic inflammatory histopathology in leptomeningeal or cortical biopsy specimens. Because of the segmental and highly focal nature of the inflammatory process, the histopathology may go undetected at biopsy despite a positive angiogram.

Primary CNS vasculitis, Behçet's disease (Chapter 278), Takayasu's arteritis (Chapters 78 and 278), and temporal arteritis (Chapter 279) are notable for their infrequent involvement of the peripheral nervous system. By contrast, hypersensitivity and systemic necrotizing vasculitides frequently produce polyneuropathies. Primary CNS arteritis (Chapter 278), giant cell arteritis (Chapter 279), and vasculitis associated with certain CNS infections may be manifested initially or solely as neurologic abnormalities.

Primary arteritis of the CNS causes headache and other encephalopathy-like symptoms in young or middle-aged individuals. The course is usually insidiously progressive but may wax and wane for periods of several months. A few of these patients initially have a strokelike episode.

Giant cell arteritis (Chapter 279) can affect any medium or large artery in the body. When it is present in the cerebral vasculature, it is called *temporal arteritis* and is characterized by panarteritis, including intimal proliferation, destruction of the internal elastic lamina, and thickening of the media. Luminal obstruction is caused by edema, thickening of the intima, and thrombosis. A prominent inflammatory infiltrate consisting of mononuclear cells, giant cells, and eosinophils with granuloma formation is present with active disease. Giant cell arteritis is the most common angiitis causing ischemic stroke. Temporal arteritis predominantly affects patients older than 55 years. Symptoms include fever, malaise, weight loss, and headache. In many patients, constitutional symptoms consistent with polymyalgia rheumatica may coexist, including jaw, neck, and facial pain and morning stiffness. Pain over the temporal arteries and an erythrocyte sedimentation rate greater than 50 mm/hour are frequently present. Biopsy of the superficial temporal artery provides a definitive diagnosis; because of the segmental nature of the

vasculitis, however, serial sections must be examined or the characteristic histology may be missed. The diagnosis is important to establish because early initiation of corticosteroid therapy (e.g., prednisone, 60 mg/day) may decrease the risk for acute ischemic blindness or stroke (Chapter 279). This treatment can be started shortly before performing the biopsy.

Takayasu's arteritis, also called *pulseless disease* (Chapters 78 and 278), is a chronic, idiopathic inflammatory disorder, primarily of young women. It affects mainly the aortic arch, the large brachiocephalic arteries, and the abdominal aorta. Mononuclear infiltrates and fibrous proliferation produce progressive narrowing of the lumen of these vessels and thus reduced flow into the upper extremities and cerebral ischemia. Although initially diagnosed in Japanese families, it has been recognized in Western countries.

Fibromuscular dysplasia is a segmental vasculopathy of unknown etiology (Chapters 78 and 127). Its frequency in large angiographic series is less than 1%. Bilateral extracranial involvement of the ICA is common, but abnormalities of the intracranial carotid or vertebrobasilar artery are rare. Dysplasia of the arterial wall may involve the intima, media, or adventitia. This disorder, which may also affect the renal arteries and is associated with hypertension, can lead to aneurysm formation and cervicocephalic arterial dissection. The diagnosis is made by cerebral angiography. Little information on treatment is available; angioplasty and stenting to open the narrowed lumen are unproven experimental procedures.

Other types of vasculitis are unusual causes of stroke. Such diseases include Wegener's granulomatosis (Chapter 278); sarcoidosis (Chapter 95); bacterial, fungal, and viral infections; meningovascular syphilis (Chapter 327); and lymphomatoid angioendotheliomatosis.

Hemoglobinopathies

In sickle cell anemia (Chapter 166), irreversible sickling results in increased blood viscosity, microvascular sludging, and brain infarction. Sickle cell disease also causes hyperplasia of fibrous tissue and muscle cells of the vascular intima, thereby leading to stenosis and occlusion of some medium to large cerebral arteries.

Estimates of the incidence of stroke vary but are generally reported to be 8 to 17% in patients with hemoglobin SS and about 2% in individuals with hemoglobin SA. The mean age at first stroke is about 8 years in people with hemoglobin SS. Ischemic stroke occurs more frequently in children. In adults, hemorrhagic strokes are more common.

Hyperviscosity Syndrome

Cerebral blood flow decreases with increasing blood viscosity. Blood viscosity increases with increasing levels of red and white blood cells, platelets, and plasma proteins. A hyperviscosity syndrome can occur when any of these blood components is markedly increased and produce focal or multifocal neurologic dysfunction, including headache, encephalopathy, and seizures. Common causes of hyperviscosity include polycythemia vera (Chapter 169) and paraproteinemias (Chapter 193) secondary to macroglobulinemia or multiple myeloma.

Coagulation Disorders
Hereditary

Four circulating proteins that inhibit coagulation are protein C, protein S, antithrombin III, and factor V (Chapters 81 and 179). Deficiencies of these proteins rarely cause arterial strokes but more frequently cause venous thrombosis. Deficiencies of proteins C and S are dominantly inherited. Homozygotes have serious, frequently fatal clotting abnormalities at birth, whereas heterozygotes may show no signs of hypercoagulability. Because of incomplete penetrance, the occurrence of thrombosis and stroke in adults is extremely rare; testing for these abnormalities should be undertaken only in unusual cases. Antithrombin III is vitamin K independent and synthesized in the liver. Deficiency should be suspected in young patients with a history of recurrent deep vein thrombosis or pulmonary embolism, especially if there is a similar family history. Inheritance is autosomal dominant with incomplete penetrance. Arterial stroke is rare.

Acquired

Cancer and pregnancy, including the postpartum period, are associated with hypercoagulable states that predispose to arterial and venous thrombosis (Chapters 81, 179, and 187). Although a variety of clotting abnormalities may be present, no tests have been devised to detect patients at risk for stroke. No treatments have been proved useful for strokes associated with these conditions.

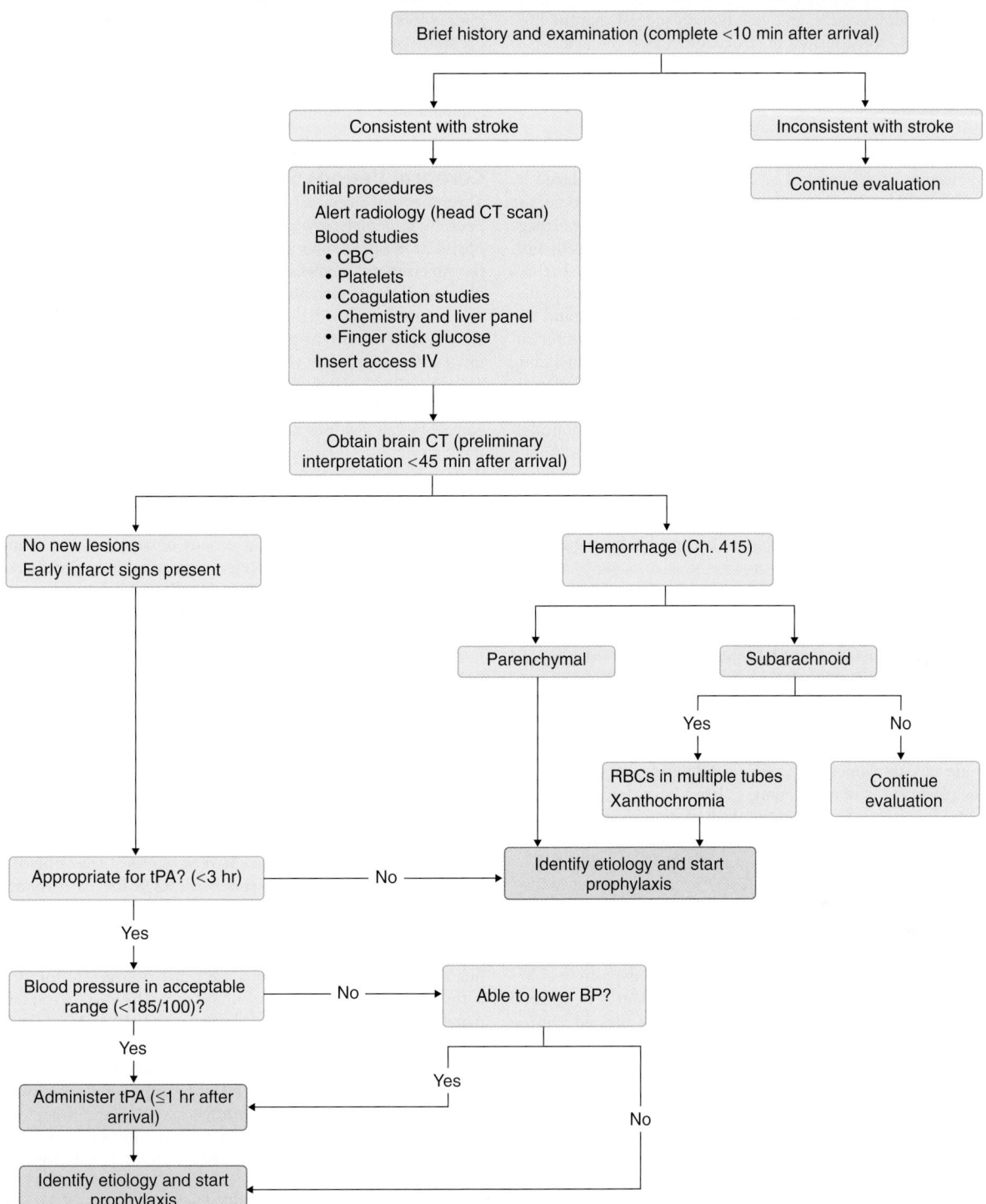

FIGURE 414-4. Algorithm for the emergency evaluation of a patient with suspected stroke. BP = blood pressure; CBC = complete blood count; CT = computed tomography; RBCs = red blood cells; tPA = tissue plasminogen activator.

Antiphospholipid Antibodies

The antiphospholipid antibody syndrome is associated with cerebral arterial and venous infarction, particularly in young adults (Chapter 179). There is no clear relationship between the levels of these antibodies and the risk for stroke. Other laboratory abnormalities include a prolonged activated partial thromboplastin time, biologic false-positive Venereal Disease Research Laboratory results, thrombocytopenia, and a positive antinuclear antibody test. There is an association with atypical migraine, TIA, and ischemic encephalopathy. The reason for the relationship between the antibodies and cerebral thrombosis is unknown.

Drug-Related Causes of Stroke

Numerous legal and illicit drugs have been associated with stroke (Chapter 33). Even the process of drug administration may cause a stroke. Intravenous

drug abuse may lead to septicemia and diseases that cause strokes, such as bacterial endocarditis and mycotic aneurysms. Particles of adulterants can be trapped by pulmonary arterioles and cause local arteritis and later arteriovenous shunts that are thought to allow the microemboli to reach the brain. Paradoxical embolization is also possible through structural cardiac defects or arteriovenous malformations.

Some of the drugs that are associated with stroke are potent vasoconstrictors and may initiate cerebral vasospasm. In other instances, cerebral vasculitis is associated with either immune responses to the primary drug or hypersensitivity to contaminating adulterants.

Over-the-counter common cold remedies and nasal decongestants containing sympathomimetic amines, such as ephedrine, phenylpropanolamine, and fenoxazoline, have been associated with ischemic stroke, although hemorrhages are more common (Chapter 415). These drugs are often used in high doses as appetite suppressants, and case reports suggest that the high doses are especially likely to be related to stroke, often after the first use of these products. Herbs taken as dietary supplements may also include sympathomimetics (e.g., ephedra, also known as *ma huang*) that have been associated with stroke (Chapter 38).

Cervical Artery Dissection

Spontaneous dissection of the cervical or cerebral arteries is produced by subintimal dissection of blood with subsequent longitudinal extension of the intramural hematoma between its layers for various distances. Hemorrhage into the intima can cause luminal stenosis and obstruction, whereas hemorrhage into the media or adventitia produces a pseudoaneurysm that can rupture. Most dissections are spontaneous, but this process is also associated with trauma, including whiplash and other neck-stretching injuries, and chiropractic cervical manipulation. Some cases are associated with fibromuscular dysplasia and others with a variety of inherited conditions, including Ehlers-Danlos and Marfan syndromes (Chapter 268) and tuberous sclerosis (Chapter 426). Recognition of dissection is sometimes difficult, and the physician must probe carefully for recent injuries to the neck. Cerebral angiography can occasionally show a double lumen, although a tapered lumen leading to an obstruction is more common. MRI with attention to vessel cross section may show a crescent-shaped hyperintense mass adjacent to a flow void. Some patients with this condition have been treated by thrombolysis or anticoagulation and surgical repair, but no therapy has been proved to be useful in randomized trials.

Homocystinuria

Homocystinuria (Chapter 216) is associated with a variety of disorders, including dislocated ocular lenses, bone deformities, mental retardation, and accelerated atherosclerosis of large and medium-sized arteries. Strokes commonly occur before 20 years of age. Detection of homocystine in urine is the diagnostic test of choice. Individuals with modest increases in serum homocystine levels may also have an increased risk for stroke. Treatment with a diet low in methionine and supplements of cysteine and pyridoxine (vitamin B_6) can decrease the plasma level of methionine. Folate administration may also be helpful because it is necessary for methylation of homocystine. Vitamin therapy has not been proved to reduce the risk for stroke in patients with homocystinuria, however.

Fat Embolism

Fat embolism (Chapter 98) is mostly a complication of long bone trauma (Chapter 112), intramedullary manipulation during orthopedic procedures, contusions of soft tissues, and severe trauma to large fat deposits. Strokes typically occur several days after the trauma. Clinical features of cerebral embolization depend on the sites within the brain that are affected. Diffuse embolization can produce encephalopathy or seizures, but more discrete lesions can cause focal neurologic deficits. The condition is probably underdiagnosed clinically and at autopsy. Peripheral features that suggest the diagnosis include petechiae and fat emboli visible on ophthalmoscopic examination. Laboratory abnormalities include hypoxemia, anemia, lipuria, and disorders of blood coagulation. The chest radiograph commonly shows bilateral fluffy infiltrates.

Air Embolism

Air embolism can occur with a variety of surgical procedures, particularly cardiac surgery, and as a complication of neurosurgical procedures performed with the patient in the sitting position. Trauma can produce pneumothorax, and air may enter the pulmonary vein and subsequently lodge in the brain. Extended underwater dives and too rapid an ascent can cause the air in the blood to come out of solution and form bubbles that can be pumped into the cerebral circulation (caisson disease). Arterial gas embolism can cause disturbances in cortical function, including seizures and focal deficits. Segmental areas of pallor may be observed on the tongue, marbling of the skin may be seen, and air emboli can be detected on funduscopic examination. When caused by rapid decompression, barotrauma is treated in a decompression chamber.

Moyamoya

Moyamoya disease is a chronic, noninflammatory occlusive vasculopathy of unknown etiology. It is a rare condition that is most common among the Japanese. It has a bimodal age distribution, with peaks in the first and fourth decades. Diagnostic criteria include stenosis or occlusion involving the bifurcation of the ICA and proximal portions of the ACA and MCA, the presence of unusual netlike ("puff of smoke") collateral arteries arising from the circle of Willis, and bilateral occurrence. In adults, the clinical manifestation is usually hemorrhages. Moyamoya is diagnosed by cerebral angiography. No treatment has been proved effective.

Cerebral Venous Sinus Thrombosis

Thrombosis of a cerebral venous sinus may be manifested as headache, focal neurologic deficits, seizures, altered mental status, and papilledema. With obstruction of the superior sagittal sinus, veins draining into the sinus from the superior and medial surfaces of both cerebral convexities are commonly obstructed; in its early stages, the condition can result in bilateral weakness and sensory changes in the legs. The presence of bilateral leg weakness should alert the clinician to the possibility of sinus thrombosis. Seizures occur more often with venous than with arterial occlusion. The most dangerous form of venous disease arises when the superior sagittal sinus is occluded, but obstruction of a transverse sinus or one of the major veins over the cerebral convexity can also produce major damage. These venous occlusions occur most commonly in association with coagulopathies, often in the puerperal period, or in patients with disseminated cancer. The transverse sinus can be occluded as a consequence of inner ear infections, a condition called *otitic hydrocephalus*.

The differential diagnosis of venous obstruction can include an arterial stroke, but the findings more often suggest a diffuse process, such as herpes simplex encephalitis or meningitis. The diagnosis depends on the recognition of impaired venous flow, which can be suspected on routine CT or MRI and confirmed by CT or MR angiography; conventional angiography is rarely needed. Unfractionated dose-adjusted heparin (see Table 81-4 in Chapter 81) and perhaps low-molecular-weight heparin may be safe and effective for cerebral venous sinus thrombosis during the acute phase, even in the presence of hemorrhagic infarction caused by the sinus thrombosis. Oral warfarin anticoagulation is generally continued for 3 to 6 months with the usual target international normalized ratio of 2.0 to 3.0.

Rare Genetic Causes

More than 50 genetic disorders have stroke as at least one of their features, but the prevalence of these abnormalities is low, so strokes produced by monogenetic anomalies are relatively rare. Cerebral autosomal dominant arteriopathy with small subcortical infarcts and leukoencephalopathy (CADASIL) is characterized by recurrent strokes resulting in multiple deep infarcts and dementia, without the usual risk factors for stroke. It has an autosomal dominant pattern of inheritance. The mean age at onset is approximately 40 years, and dementia ensues within 10 to 15 years. Migraine with aura often precedes the strokes by several years. The responsible gene on chromosome 19 results in mutations of the Notch3 receptor protein. As is true of all these genetic causes of stroke, treatment is symptomatic. Antenatal diagnosis is possible in these disorders.

Fabry's disease (angiokeratoma corporis diffusum) (Chapter 215) is an X-linked disease that causes a reduction in α-galactosidase A enzyme activity. Patients have diseases of the skin, eyes, and kidneys as well as frequent neurologic complications that result from either vascular occlusion or, infrequently, intracerebral hemorrhage related to the accumulation of glycolipids in small and medium-sized arteries. The gene encoding this enzyme is located at Xq22. Enzyme replacement therapy is of benefit (Chapter 215).

Neurofibromatosis (Chapter 426) is associated with strokes as a result of occlusion of the internal carotid arteries or the proximal part of the anterior cerebral circulation. Histologically, arterial lesions consist of hyperplasia of the intimal layer with fragmentation and reduplication of the elastic layer. Cerebral aneurysms can also occur. The diagnosis of type I neurofibromatosis is usually based on clinical findings. *DNA-based testing* of the *NF1* gene is available clinically but is infrequently needed for diagnosis.

Marfan syndrome (Chapter 268), which is an autosomal dominant disorder of the fibrillin gene on chromosome 15, affects the skeletal, ocular, cardiovascular, and central nervous systems. Expression is highly variable, and only one system may be involved. Involvement of large arteries, such as the aorta and carotid arteries, is common and may cause death. The most life-threatening problem is dissection of these arteries. Pathologically, the disease results from defective fibrillin, which is an important component of connective tissue.

PREVENTION AND TREATMENT OF STROKE AND TRANSIENT ISCHEMIC ATTACK

Primary Prevention

Risk factors for stroke fall into two general categories, nonmodifiable and modifiable (Table 414-3). Within the modifiable group are risk factors that are well documented and others that are not. Blood pressure control (Chapter 67) is the most important primary prevention strategy. It is especially important in patients with diabetes, in whom tight control of hypertension with angiotensin-converting enzyme inhibitors substantially reduces the incidence of stroke. Statins are recommended in patients who meet the criteria for treating hyperlipidemia (Chapter 213), in whom they reduce the risk of stroke proportionately to the reductions in the LDL cholesterol levels.[6] Statins also reduce the risk for stroke in patients with an elevated C-reactive protein level even when the LDL level is less than 130 mg/dL.[7] Smoking cessation (Chapter 31) is routinely recommended, but there are no prospective randomized trials to prove that cessation of smoking reduces the risk for stroke. Anticoagulation markedly reduces the risk for stroke in patients with atrial fibrillation (Chapter 64), and blood transfusion is the usual treatment to prevent strokes in patients with sickle cell disease (Chapter 166).

Prophylactic Carotid Interventions

In asymptomatic patients, ipsilateral carotid endarterectomy benefits patients who have a 60% or greater reduction in diameter of the artery without ulceration, provided that the perioperative complication rate is less than 3%,[8] a rate that requires a skilled surgeon. Carotid artery angioplasty and stent placement are not as efficacious as operative endarterectomy, mainly because of their higher risk for stroke.[9]

Secondary Prevention in Patients with Previous Stroke or Transient Ischemic Attack

All the risk factor reductions that are recommended for primary prevention are also recommended in patients who have suffered a previous stroke or TIA and have no contraindication. In addition, specific medical and surgical therapies should be considered.

Medications

Aspirin and other antiplatelet agents reduce the odds of nonfatal stroke by 31% when used in patients with known vascular disease (Chapter 37). All patients who have sustained a stroke and have no contraindication should receive an antiplatelet agent to reduce the risk for recurrent stroke. The optimal dose of aspirin has not yet been established, and doses of 50 to 1300 mg/day have been used. Clopidogrel, 75 mg/day, instead of or in addition to aspirin appears to be no better than aspirin alone[10] but is substantially more expensive. The addition of dipyridamole to aspirin can benefit high-risk patients with prior cerebral ischemia.[11] Warfarin anticoagulation is not superior to antiplatelet agents in preventing recurrent strokes, except in patients with atrial fibrillation or another cardiac source of emboli, because of its risks for cerebral hemorrhage.[12] In patients with previous cerebrovascular disease or high-risk conditions, aggressive cholesterol reduction with 40 mg of simvastatin or 80 mg of atorvastatin reduces the rate of stroke by 25% or more.[13]

Surgery

Carotid endarterectomy reduces the cumulative risk for any ipsilateral stroke at 2 years from 26 to 9% in patients with a 70 to 99% symptomatic (i.e., previous TIA or nondisabling stroke) internal carotid stenosis and from 22 to 16% at 5 years in patients with a 50 to 70% symptomatic stenosis. Patients with less than a 50% symptomatic stenosis do better with medical management alone. In patients with advanced occlusive disease of the carotid arterial system, extracranial-intracranial bypass is no better than medical therapy.[14]

Devices

Carotid artery stents can restore patency to stenotic arteries with an efficacy and safety comparable to that of open endarterectomy in experienced centers. Intra-arterial clots can also be extracted under radiologic guidance with a corkscrew-like device inserted into the common or internal carotid artery for occlusion of the anterior circulation or into the subclavian artery for occlusion of the posterior circulation and then advanced to remove clot located in medium or large intracranial vessels (ICA, MCA, vertebral artery, basilar artery, PCA, or ACA). Using proximal balloon occlusion to arrest flow, the corkscrew device can grab and hold the clot as it is extracted from the patient's artery. Currently, however, outcomes appear to be better with endarterectomy than with stenting, suggesting that stenting should be reserved for selected situations.[9,15]

TABLE 414-3 WELL-DOCUMENTED MODIFIABLE RISK FACTORS FOR STROKE

FACTOR	PREVALENCE (%)	RELATIVE RISK	RISK REDUCTION WITH TREATMENT
Hypertension (by age group)			38%
50 yr	20	4	
60 yr	30	3	
70 yr	40	2	
80 yr	55	1.4	
90 yr	60	1	
Smoking	25	1.8	50% within 1 yr, baseline after 5 yr
Diabetes	20	1.8-6	Reduction of stroke risk in hypertensive diabetics with blood pressure control No demonstrated benefit in stroke reduction with tight glycemic control
Asymptomatic carotid stenosis	2-8	2	50%
Hyperlipidemia			20-30% with statins in patients with known coronary disease
Adults <35 yr	8-9	1.8	
Men >55 yr	25	2.6	
Women >65 yr	40		
Atrial fibrillation (nonvalvular)			68% warfarin 21% aspirin
50-59 yr	0.5	4	
60-69 yr	1.8	2.6	
70-79 yr	4.8	3.3	
80-89 yr	8.8	4.5	

Modified from Goldstein LB, Adams R, Becker K, et al. Primary prevention of ischemic stroke. *Stroke.* 2001;32:280-299.

PROGNOSIS AND REHABILITATION

Patients who receive care in specialized, acute stroke units are less likely to die, more likely to go home, and more likely to be independent 3 months later. In most clinical trials, about 15% of patients with ischemic stroke die within the first 3 months. Immediate causes of death include herniation because of brain swelling or neurologic dysfunction directly related to the stroke. Deaths that occur days after stroke and are not directly related to neurologic dysfunction are commonly produced by pulmonary embolism or pneumonia. Most large population studies report that about 20% of patients who survive a stroke require long-term institutionalization and that 33 to 50% of the others are left with substantial disability. Stroke is the most common cause of adult disability in the United States. Most functional recovery takes place during the first month, but some continued slow improvement is possible for 1 year. The most common long-term cause of death in patients with stroke is myocardial infarction.

1. Hypothermia after Cardiac Arrest Study Group. Mild therapeutic hypothermia to improve the neurologic outcome after cardiac arrest. *N Engl J Med.* 2002;346:549-556.
2. Hacke W, Kaste M, Bluhmki E, et al. Thrombolysis with alteplase 3 to 4.5 hours after acute ischemic stroke. *N Engl J Med.* 2008;359:1317-1329.
3. Lees KR, Bluhmki E, von Kummer R, et al. Time to treatment with intravenous alteplase and outcome in stroke: an updated pooled analysis of ECASS, ATLANTIS, NINDS, and EPITHET trials. *Lancet.* 2010;375:1695-1703.
4. Schwamm LH, Holloway RG, Amarenco P, et al. A review of the evidence for the use of telemedicine within stroke systems of care: a scientific statement from the American Heart Association/American Stroke Association. *Stroke.* 2009;40:2616-2634.
5. Dennis M, Sandercock PA, Reid J, et al, for the CLOTS Trials Collaboration. Effectiveness of thigh-length graduated compression stockings to reduce the risk of deep vein thrombosis after stroke (CLOTS trial 1): a multicentre, randomised controlled trial. *Lancet.* 2009;373:1958-1965.
6. De Caterina R, Scarano M, Marfisi R, et al. Cholesterol-lowering interventions and stroke: insights from a meta-analysis of randomized controlled trials. *J Am Coll Cardiol.* 2010;55:198-211.
7. Everett BM, Glynn RJ, MacFadyen JG, et al. Rosuvastatin in the prevention of stroke among men and women with elevated levels of C-reactive protein. Justification for the Use of Statins in Prevention: an Intervention Trial Evaluating Rosuvastatin (JUPITER). *Circulation.* 2010;121:143-150.

8. MRC Asymptomatic Carotid Surgery Trial (ACST) Collaborative Group. Prevention of disabling and fatal strokes by successful carotid endarterectomy in patients without recent neurological symptoms: randomised controlled trial. *Lancet.* 2004;363:1491-1502.

9. Murad MH, Shahrour A, Shah ND, et al. A systematic review and meta-analysis of randomized trials of carotid endarterectomy vs stenting. *J Vasc Surg.* 2011;53:792-797.

10. Bhatt DL, Fox KA, Hacke W, et al. Clopidogrel and aspirin versus aspirin alone for the prevention of atherothrombotic events. *N Engl J Med.* 2006;354:1706-1717.

11. The ESPRIT Study Group. Aspirin plus dipyridamole versus aspirin alone after cerebral ischaemia of arterial origin (ESPRIT): randomised controlled trial. *Lancet.* 2006;367:1665-1673.

12. Chimowitz MI, Lynn MJ, Howlett-Smith H, et al. Comparison of warfarin and aspirin for symptomatic intracranial arterial stenosis. *N Engl J Med.* 2005;352:1305-1316.

13. The Stroke Prevention by Aggressive Reduction in Cholesterol Levels (SPARCL) investigators. High-dose atorvastatin after stroke or transient ischemic attack. *N Engl J Med.* 2006;355:549-559.

14. Fluri F, Engelter S, Lyrer P. Extracranial-intracranial arterial bypass surgery for occlusive carotid artery disease. *Cochrane Database Syst Rev.* 2010;2:CD005953.

15. International Carotid Stenting Study investigators. Carotid artery stenting compared with endarterectomy in patients with symptomatic carotid stenosis (International Carotid Stenting Study): an interim analysis of a randomised controlled trial. *Lancet.* 2010;375:985-997.

SUGGESTED READINGS

Gorelick PB, Ruland S. Cerebral vascular disease. *Dis Mon.* 2010;56:39-100. *Detailed review.*

Ifejika-Jones NL, Harun N, Mohammed-Rajput NA, et al. Thrombolysis with intravenous tissue plasminogen activator predicts a favorable discharge disposition in patients with acute ischemic stroke. *Stroke.* 2011;42:700-704. *Patients who receive intravenous recombinant tissue plasminogen activator are more likely to be discharged directly home.*

O'Kelly CJ, Butcher KS, Marchak BE, et al. Carotid revascularization: an update. *Can J Neurol Sci.* 2010;37:320-335. *Review of indications, methods, and timing of interventions.*

Xian Y, Holloway RG, Chan PS, et al. Association between stroke center hospitalization for acute ischemic stroke and mortality. *JAMA.* 2011;305:373-380. *Admission to a designated stroke center is associated with modestly lower mortality and more frequent use of thrombolytic therapy.*

415

HEMORRHAGIC CEREBROVASCULAR DISEASE

JUSTIN A. ZIVIN

Approximately 15% of all strokes are due to intracranial hemorrhage. Hemorrhagic stroke can be diffuse (i.e., bleeding into the subarachnoid or intraventricular spaces) or focal (i.e., intraparenchymal hemorrhage). About two thirds of intracranial bleeding cases are predominantly subarachnoid hemorrhages, whereas about one third are intracerebral hemorrhages. Subarachnoid hemorrhage is usually caused by rupture of vessels on or near the surface of the brain or ventricles (e.g., aneurysms, vascular malformations), with bleeding mainly into the cerebrospinal fluid (CSF) spaces. Intracerebral hemorrhage is most frequently caused by the rupture of arteries that are within the brain substance (e.g., hypertensive hemorrhage, vascular malformations) but do not extend to the CSF spaces. Both types of hemorrhagic stroke have high mortality rates, depending on subtype and location. Prevention is the mainstay of management because there are no sufficiently efficacious therapies for hemorrhage-induced cerebral injury.

⬤ SUBARACHNOID HEMORRHAGE

EPIDEMIOLOGY

In the United States, about 30,000 new cases of subarachnoid hemorrhage occur each year and predominantly involve young adults. Both genders are equally affected, and the rate may be twice as high in African Americans as in whites. Rupture of aneurysms is by far the most common cause of nontraumatic subarachnoid hemorrhage. Advances in diagnostic imaging have improved the detection of intracranial aneurysms, but most cases are not discovered until after rupture.

Risk factors include cigarette smoking, binge drinking, illicit drugs, phenylpropanolamine, and other sympathomimetic agents. Although hypertension is well established as a risk factor for ischemic stroke, the relationship of nonmalignant hypertension to subarachnoid hemorrhage is less well documented; the decline in hypertension in the general population has not been accompanied by a decrease in the incidence rate of subarachnoid hemorrhage.

PATHOBIOLOGY

The principal causes of subarachnoid hemorrhage are aneurysms and arteriovenous malformations (AVMs), but trauma can also cause subarachnoid bleeding (Chapter 406). Rare causes of subarachnoid hemorrhage include vasculitis, central nervous system neoplasms (Chapter 195), and hematologic disorders such as hemophilia, disseminated intravascular coagulopathy, and thrombocytopenic purpura.

CLINICAL MANIFESTATIONS

The classic symptom of a subarachnoid hemorrhage is a very rapidly developing, severe headache, typically called the "worst headache of my life," that is sometimes accompanied by a stiff neck. Aneurysms may generate prodromal signs and symptoms as they gradually expand or cause sentinel (warning) leaks that produce focal or generalized head pain. Such sentinel headaches are frequently severe, and they may be accompanied by nausea or vomiting and may cause meningeal irritation.

Arterial blood pressure is often elevated, and body temperature usually increases, particularly during the first few days after bleeding as subarachnoid blood products produce chemical meningitis. Transient alterations in mental status occur in nearly half the patients, particularly if intracranial pressure exceeds cerebral mean arterial pressure. Patients can remain in coma for several days, depending on the location of the aneurysm and the amount of bleeding.

Acute subarachnoid hemorrhage causes meningeal irritation; nuchal rigidity and photophobia can require several hours to develop. Ophthalmoscopic observation reveals well-circumscribed, bright red, preretinal hemorrhages, known as subhyaloid hemorrhages and thought to be a result of increased intracranial pressure, raised retinal venous pressure, and dissection of blood along the optic nerve sheath. Focal neurologic dysfunction is not usually a prominent feature unless an aneurysm compresses surrounding brain structures, a jet of blood dissects directly into a clinically eloquent brain region, or vasospasm subsequently develops.

DIAGNOSIS

Laboratory Findings

A complete blood cell count, including platelets, should be obtained, and clotting times should be determined to assess whether the patient has an infection or clotting abnormalities. Blood should also be sent for electrolyte analysis to serve as a baseline for detecting later complications.

Imaging

The patient should then be sent immediately for emergency computed tomography (CT). A scan performed within 24 hours of onset generally reveals an area of high signal attenuation consistent with hemorrhage; if blood is present in the subarachnoid space, it is seen within the basal cisterns in more than 90% of patients. By 48 hours after onset, the sensitivity of CT declines to about 75%. Conventional magnetic resonance imaging (MRI) sequences (T1- or T2-weighted scans) are less sensitive than CT scans.

The location of subarachnoid hemorrhage by CT suggests the source of bleeding. High signal attenuation in the basal cisterns, sylvian fissure, or intrahemispheric fissure often indicates rupture of a saccular aneurysm, whereas higher concentrations of blood over the convexities or within the superficial parenchyma of the brain are more consistent with rupture of an AVM or a mycotic aneurysm. A large amount of blood in the subarachnoid space increases the likelihood of subsequent vasospasm. A contrast-enhanced CT scan may aid in the identification of an AVM and some large aneurysms.

An electrocardiogram should be performed to detect peaked or inverted T waves and increased U waves. These abnormalities and subsequent arrhythmias have been attributed to multifocal myocardial necrosis caused by elevated levels of circulating catecholamines.

If the CT findings are normal but the index of suspicion remains high for subarachnoid hemorrhage, a lumbar puncture is usually diagnostic. A traumatic lumbar puncture (i.e., penetration of the needle into a small blood vessel of the venous plexus on the anterior wall of the spinal canal) produces a declining number of red blood cells in subsequent tubes, whereas subarachnoid hemorrhage produces a relatively constant number of red blood cells in each tube. In the presence of bloody fluid, one of the CSF samples should be centrifuged immediately and the supernate examined for the presence of hematin or xanthochromia by visual inspection. Red blood cells in CSF begin to lyse within a few hours, and the centrifuged supernate then appears pink. Later (about 10 hours), as the hemoglobin is converted to bilirubin, the fluid becomes slightly yellow. Opening CSF pressure is generally elevated and may remain so for many days. CSF samples obtained within the first day may show a white blood cell count consistent with the normal circulating white cell–to–red cell ratio (about 1:1000). Chemical meningitis is produced by the presence of blood or breakdown products within the subarachnoid space, and CSF samples contain increased numbers of polymorphonuclear and mononuclear cells relative to red blood cells. The CSF glucose concentration is usually normal shortly after the onset of bleeding, but as chemical meningitis develops, the glucose level may decline, rarely to less than 40 mg/dL. After a subarachnoid hemorrhage, the protein content of CSF is generally elevated, consistent with contamination by blood (the usual ratio is 1 mg/dL of protein for every 1000 red blood cells).

Cerebral angiography remains the definitive study to identify the source of subarachnoid hemorrhage. When the diagnosis of aneurysmal subarachnoid hemorrhage seems highly probable, the timing and need for a cerebral angiogram should be determined by surgical considerations. If doubt exists, angiography should be performed with minimal delay. Because many patients have multiple cerebral aneurysms, the carotid and vertebral artery systems should be examined angiographically. The initial cerebral angiogram fails to detect the source of bleeding in about 20% of patients; such patients are thought to have a fairly good prognosis, with only a 1 to 2% annual risk for recurrent hemorrhage. Failure to detect the bleeding source can be due to obliteration of the aneurysm because of clot or may be due to the small size of the ruptured aneurysm. A superficial venous angioma, a spinal cord aneurysm, or a spinal AVM also will not be seen on a cerebral angiogram. The presence of back pain or neurologic signs localized to the spinal cord at onset should prompt a search for a spinal source of hemorrhage. If the initial angiogram is negative and no other clues to the bleeding site can be found, repeat cerebral angiography is usually performed within a few weeks; MRI or CT with and without contrast may also be helpful.

TREATMENT ℞

Treatment of Complications

If a patient does not die immediately after a subarachnoid hemorrhage, a number of neurologic complications can occur. Some result from blood in the subarachnoid space, and other concerns include rebleeding from the same aneurysm, cerebral vasospasm and its ischemic consequences, hydrocephalus caused by blockage of CSF outflow pathways, and seizures. Non-neurologic complications include cardiac and electrolyte abnormalities.

Rebleeding

If an aneurysm is not repaired promptly, it can rupture again. A new headache or neurologic worsening suggests repeat rupture, which can be diagnosed only if a repeat CT scan or lumbar puncture shows the presence of new blood in the subarachnoid space. Approximately 30% of patients with aneurysmal subarachnoid hemorrhage rebleed during the first month, and the incidence is highest during the first 2 weeks after the initial episode. Patients with unrepaired aneurysms who survive their initial bleeding for more than 1 month have a 2 to 3% annual risk for rebleeding. Infusion of factor VII can reduce the growth of the hemorrhage but does not improve outcomes. **[1]**

Vasospasm

A common cause of death and disability in patients with aneurysmal subarachnoid hemorrhage is cerebral vasospasm. The vessels at the base of the brain become narrowed, thereby reducing blood flow; if the vasospasm is severe, it can produce infarction of the brain distal to the site of the spasm. The vessels that go into spasm are often different from the artery that was responsible for the initial bleeding. Vasospasm has been reported in up to 75% of patients after subarachnoid hemorrhage, and delayed neurologic deficits develop in as many as 30% of patients with vasospasm. The onset of vasospasm is typically between days 3 and 14 after bleeding, but this complication can develop as late as 3 weeks after subarachnoid hemorrhage. The arteries of the circle of Willis and their major branches are the usual initial site of spasm, with more distal arteries becoming involved later. The amount and location of blood detected within the basal cisterns on CT correlate with the incidence and location of vasospasm. The pathogenesis of cerebral vasospasm is unknown.

Cerebral angiography, which is the best established method to diagnose vasospasm, shows narrowing of the dye column. However, other methods such as transcranial Doppler ultrasonography and magnetic resonance angiography are increasingly being used. Transcranial Doppler has high specificity, but its sensitivity is not as good as that of angiography.

Hydrocephalus

Acute hydrocephalus occurs in up to two thirds of patients within 3 days after subarachnoid hemorrhage. Hydrocephalus is caused by obstruction of

CSF outflow pathways at the level of the fourth ventricle and the pacchionian granulations lining the venous sinuses. Increasing age, a history of hypertension, intraventricular hemorrhage, focal neurologic findings, a decreased level of consciousness, and hyponatremia are associated with risk for the development of hydrocephalus. Chronic ventricular enlargement occurs in as many as 60% of patients within 1 month after subarachnoid hemorrhage and is often asymptomatic. Several forms of treatment have been advocated for the management of hydrocephalus, including repeated lumbar puncture and shunt placement, but their value has not been proved.

Seizures

Seizures may occur shortly after subarachnoid hemorrhage in 15 to 90% of patients. Seizures are thought to be caused by cortical damage from bleeding into the neocortex or from ischemic necrosis related to vasospasm. The development of persistent epilepsy is unusual. Prophylactic anticonvulsant therapy has not been useful.

Non-neurologic Complications

Cardiac complications occur as a consequence of subarachnoid hemorrhage. In the acute phases of subarachnoid hemorrhage, electrocardiographic patterns can mimic acute myocardial infarction (Chapter 73). A pattern of deep inverted T waves across the pericardium is classic. Appropriate biomarker assays and repeat electrocardiograms are needed to document true myocardial damage.

Hyponatremia (Chapter 118) is the most common electrolyte abnormality after subarachnoid hemorrhage. Sodium loss, which is typically mild, may occur in up to 25% of patients. The natriuresis has been attributed to inappropriate levels of antidiuretic hormone (Chapter 232), but this hypothesis has not been proved. Hyponatremia can itself result in a decreased level of consciousness and seizures, but it is often impossible to distinguish the effects of hyponatremia from the other possible causes of these neurologic abnormalities.

● SPECIFIC CAUSES AND THEIR TREATMENT AND PROGNOSIS
Saccular Aneurysms

DEFINITION AND EPIDEMIOLOGY

Saccular or "berry" aneurysms, which account for 80 to 90% of all intracranial aneurysms, are thin-walled outpouchings that protrude from the arteries of the circle of Willis or its major branches; 85% are located at branching points (Fig. 415-1). Because of the local weakness and degeneration of the media, the intima bulges outward and is covered only by the adventitia. A saccular aneurysm may be an incidental finding on a scan or may be detected at autopsy in patients who die of other diseases; in symptomatic cases, however, the sack gradually enlarges and ultimately ruptures.

Saccular aneurysms are rarely detected in children, and the incidence of subarachnoid hemorrhage increases with age; therefore, it seems clear that congenital wall defects develop into aneurysms only after some time. Congenital defects in the muscle and elastic tissue of the arterial media are observed at autopsy in up to 80% of normal vessels of the circle of Willis. It is postulated that these defects gradually degenerate over time as they are exposed to pulsatile arterial blood pressure. Multiple aneurysms are found in about 15% of people with at least one aneurysm. Because the incidence of aneurysmal subarachnoid hemorrhage is approximately 1 in 10,000, it is evident that most saccular aneurysms do not rupture.

PATHOBIOLOGY

Approximately 10 to 20% of patients with known aneurysms have a family history. Diseases that are associated with intracranial saccular aneurysms include polycystic kidney disease (Chapter 129), Marfan and Ehlers-Danlos syndromes (Chapter 268), fibromuscular dysplasia (Chapter 78), pseudoxanthoma elasticum (Chapter 268), systemic lupus erythematosus (Chapter 274), and sickle cell anemia (Chapter 166). Screening of other family members is often recommended when two or more members of a family have aneurysms.

TREATMENT ℞

Primary Prevention of Bleeding

Because the natural history of aneurysms may be highly variable and the risk-to-benefit ratio for the various invasive techniques is unknown, expectant waiting may sometimes be the best option. However, an aneurysm may rupture without warning, and the uncertainty is unacceptable to some patients and physicians. Medical therapies may delay the time of rupture but cannot repair the lesion.

Treatment of Aneurysms that Have Bled
Medical Treatment

Medical management of a ruptured aneurysm aims to reduce the risk for rebleeding and cerebral vasospasm and prevent other medical complications before and after surgical intervention. The only form of medical therapy that has been useful in treating subarachnoid hemorrhage patients is the voltage-regulated calcium-channel antagonist nimodipine. Although it does not reduce the frequency of vasospasm, nimodipine (60 mg orally every 4 hours for 21 days) lowers the incidence of cerebral infarction by about one third.

General support consisting of bed rest, analgesics for headache, and gentle sedation as needed is provided to quiet the patient. Stool softeners can minimize straining. Hypertension should be treated appropriately but not aggressively (Chapter 67) because elevated blood pressure may represent a normal compensatory mechanism, particularly in a chronically hypertensive patient, and excessive reduction may cause extension of the infarct. There is no conclusive evidence that modification of blood pressure in patients with acute subarachnoid hemorrhage is of benefit. Antifibrinolytic drugs, including tranexamic acid and ε-aminocaproic acid, may reduce rebleeding, but any such benefit is outweighed by an increased incidence of infarction.

Interventional Therapies

The objectives of interventional procedures are to exclude the aneurysm from the circulation or relieve pressure on adjacent brain tissue caused by expansion of the sack. The optimal timing of these therapies is uncertain, but many surgeons recommend treatment as soon as possible after the subarachnoid hemorrhage.

An electrical current applied to a detachable coil threaded into an aneurysm by means of percutaneous angiography causes the surrounding blood to clot. The coil is detached and left in place, and the catheter is then removed. This approach is more effective than surgical clipping for achieving disability-free survival in patients who have had ruptured aneurysms.[2] With very large aneurysms, for which use of a coil is not possible, wrapping the sack with various types of material to prevent it from rupturing or growing is sometimes performed. Indirect procedures include various methods of occluding the feeding artery; if there is sufficient collateral supply, the risk for infarction may be less than that of spontaneous rupture of the aneurysm with subsequent extensive subarachnoid hemorrhage.

Middle cerebral artery — Ophthalmic artery
— Anterior cerebral artery
— Anterior communicating artery
— Internal carotid artery
— Posterior communicating artery
— Anterior choroidal artery
— Superior cerebellar artery
— Basilar artery
— Internal auditory artery
— Anterior inferior cerebellar artery
— Posterior inferior cerebellar artery
Posterior cerebral artery — Anterior spinal artery — Vertebral artery

FIGURE 415-1. Saccular aneurysms. Saccular or berry aneurysms typically develop at the bifurcations of arteries on the undersurface of the brain.

PROGNOSIS

Mortality and morbidity rates differ among studies. About 12% of subarachnoid hemorrhage victims die before reaching medical attention. By 30 days, approximately 50% die, but 30-day survivors generally survive for at least a year. An equally high mortality rate accompanies each episode of rebleeding. Approximately 25% of survivors have persistent neurologic deficits.

Fusiform Aneurysms

Fusiform aneurysms are so named because they are elongated dilations (i.e., ectasia) of large arteries associated with atherosclerosis. These aneurysms typically develop in the basilar artery but also may affect the internal, middle, and anterior cerebral arteries of individuals with widespread arteriosclerosis and hypertension. These aneurysms may progressively dilate and become tortuous, thereby producing neurologic dysfunction, most frequently by compressing surrounding structures. Thrombi may form in them and embolize distally to cause ischemic strokes. Typically, ectatic aneurysms of the basilar artery compress cranial nerves and cause facial pain (V), hemifacial spasm (VII), and hearing loss with vertigo (VIII). Fusiform aneurysms may mimic pituitary and suprasellar mass lesions or cerebellopontine angle tumors. Fusiform aneurysms rarely rupture; if they do, they are difficult to treat surgically because their shape and stiff walls generally preclude easy surgical clipping, and total occlusion is usually required.

Mycotic Aneurysms

Infected emboli, usually originating on an infected heart valve (Chapter 76), may lodge in a distal branch of a cerebral artery and cause small areas of infarction or microabscesses. In arteries that do not rupture immediately, focal arteritis and mycotic aneurysms, also known as septic aneurysms, may develop. Mycotic aneurysms are frequently multiple and can be found distally in the cerebral arteries. Rates of rupture of these aneurysms may be as high as 10%. Such lesions may be detected by noninvasive imaging studies, but the definitive test is contrast-enhanced angiography, for which the indications are controversial. Aside from treatment of the underlying infection, other treatments are not established.

Vascular Malformations

EPIDEMIOLOGY

About 1% of all strokes and 10% of intracerebral hemorrhages are caused by vascular malformations. The prevalence of AVM is approximately 0.5%, and the annual incidence of hemorrhage is between 1 and 3 cases per 100,000 people. Familial cases occur but are rare.

PATHOBIOLOGY

Conventional classifications of cerebrovascular malformations are based on the histologic appearance of the vessels and the intervening neural parenchyma. The most frequent type of vascular malformation is an AVM, which has a core of dysplastic vessels (i.e., nidus), feeding arteries, and draining veins. In the nidus, arteries connect directly to veins without intervening capillaries to produce a low-resistance, high-flow shunt that ultimately dilates feeding arteries and thickens the walls of the draining veins. The classic arteriographic appearance includes an early draining vein. Ordinarily, there is no intervening neural tissue in the nidus. The nidus is the usual site of hemorrhage in an AVM.

The next most common lesions are cavernous malformations (i.e., cavernous angiomas or hemangiomas), which are composed of small-caliber sinusoidal vascular channels that are commonly thrombosed. The low flow rate through these vessels makes them difficult to detect by angiography, and they are unlikely to hemorrhage; these malformations also do not contain neural tissue. Cavernous AVMs are often associated with venous malformations, which are composed of small veins separated by normal parenchyma. Smaller venous channels drain into a dilated venous trunk that ultimately drains into a large vein and sinus in the brain. The classic angiographic appearance is a caput medusae in the late venous phase. These anomalies are readily detected by CT, but they rarely hemorrhage.

A cerebral varix is a single dilated vein that seldom causes clinical symptoms. Telangiectasis, also called capillary malformation, is a cluster of enlarged capillaries surrounded by normal parenchyma. These lesions are too small to be detected by conventional imaging methods and are usually noted as petechiae that are found incidentally at autopsy; these benign lesions rarely hemorrhage.

CLINICAL MANIFESTATIONS

Although increasing numbers of probably asymptomatic vascular malformations are being diagnosed by brain imaging as part of the evaluation of nonspecific headaches, about 50% of AVMs are manifested as intracranial hemorrhage, a lower proportion initially present as seizures, and the remainder cause progressive neurologic disability as the first symptom. Hemorrhage, which is the most feared complication of an AVM, has an associated mortality rate of 10 to 15%. The mortality and morbidity rates associated with AVMs are somewhat less than for aneurysms. The initial hemorrhage tends to occur during the second through fourth decades, and hypertension before the hemorrhage is uncommon. The risk for acute rebleeding averages approximately 6 to 7%. In the next 5 years, the rate is about 2% per year, and it is 1 to 2% per year thereafter. If this rebleeding rate is maintained for life, a young individual who has a hemorrhagic AVM faces a 50 to 60% chance of an incapacitating or fatal subsequent hemorrhage during a normal lifespan.

AVMs can bleed into the subarachnoid space, the brain parenchyma, or the ventricular system. Focal neurologic abnormalities depend on the severity of the bleeding and the location of brain parenchyma that has been affected. The frequency of cerebral vasospasm after hemorrhage from an AVM is less than that for aneurysmal bleeding.

Approximately 30% of patients who have an AVM are initially evaluated for seizures, which often have a focal onset. Focal neurologic deficits independent of seizures can develop, possibly caused by vascular thrombosis and perhaps by shunting of blood through arteriovenous fistulas away from normal brain tissue.

DIAGNOSIS

If a hemorrhage has occurred, unenhanced CT scanning may show evidence of bleeding in an unusual location for primary intracerebral hemorrhage or a ruptured aneurysm. Contrast-enhanced CT scans may demonstrate marked enhancement of the feeding arteries and draining veins. MRI with signal void on T1- or T2-weighted images can also establish the diagnosis. Angiography remains the definitive test to identify the AVM and delineate its size, gross morphology, feeding arteries, and draining veins. Because AVMs are occasionally multiple and may be associated with saccular aneurysms, four-vessel angiography is indicated even if an AVM is found by unilateral carotid injection. Extracranial or contralateral arteries occasionally supply intracranial AVMs and should be considered in the angiographic evaluation.

TREATMENT   Rx

There is uncertainty regarding the prognosis of unruptured AVMs as a result of their various locations, sizes, and morphology. Because the safety and efficacy of the various procedures for treating AVMs have not been established, there are no guiding therapeutic principles.

Conservative treatment is often recommended for unruptured AVMs manifested as seizures or headache, especially in patients older than 55 to 60 years. This approach emphasizes control of hypertension, avoidance of anticoagulants, and use of anticonvulsants to control seizures.

If an AVM has ruptured and the patient has recovered from the initial hemorrhage, the two goals of interventional therapy are to remove the AVM completely and to avoid deterioration of neurologic dysfunction. Removal can be curative, but it is important to eliminate residual abnormal vessels, which may produce hemorrhages, especially if reduction of outflow increases perfusion pressure within the remaining anomalous vasculature. However, it is particularly dangerous to perform these procedures in critical neurologic areas, such as in or near the speech centers.

Therapeutic options include surgical resection of the AVM, embolization of the feeding arteries, and radiation-induced thrombosis. In some cases, combinations of these treatments are used. Selective embolization of the lesion through the transfemoral angiographic approach is commonly the initial procedure, with the goal of reducing blood flow through the AVM. Embolization may be performed in stages to reduce the size of the lesion sequentially, but endovascular treatment seldom obliterates an AVM. A risk for embolization is that embolic material may escape from the AVM and occlude normal vessels.

Stereotactic radiosurgery can eliminate an AVM but is satisfactory only for small lesions. The therapeutic effect of this technique is delayed because the abnormal vessels shrink gradually after the procedure.

Direct surgical intervention involves the use of microsurgical techniques. If the AVM is large, the procedures are often performed in stages to reduce blood flow in an adjacent region and make subsequent surgery easier. Surgery is considered successful if the postoperative angiogram shows no residual AVM. However, long-term occlusion rates are unknown, and recanalization with recurrent hemorrhage is possible.

TABLE 415-1 CAUSES, MEANS OF DIAGNOSIS, AND CHARACTERISTICS OF INTRACEREBRAL HEMORRHAGES

CAUSES	PRIMARY MEANS OF DIAGNOSIS	CHARACTERISTICS
Hypertension	Clinical history	Rupture of small arterioles related to degenerative changes induced by uncontrolled hypertension
Amyloid angiopathy	Clinical history	Rupture of small and medium-sized arteries with deposition of β-amyloid protein; manifested as lobar hemorrhages in people older than 70 years
Arteriovenous malformation	MRI or angiogram	Rupture of abnormal small vessels connecting arteries and veins
Intracranial aneurysm	MRI or angiogram	Rupture of a saccular dilation from a medium-sized artery; usually associated with subarachnoid hemorrhage
Cavernous angioma	MRI or angiogram	Rupture of abnormal capillary-like vessels with intermingled connective tissue
Venous angioma	MRI or angiogram	Rupture of an abnormal dilation of venules
Venous sinus thrombosis	MRI or angiogram	Result of hemorrhagic venous infarction
Intracranial neoplasm	MRI or angiogram	Result of necrosis and bleeding within hypervascular neoplasms
Coagulopathy	Clinical history	Most commonly associated with the use of anticoagulants or thrombolytics
Vasculitis	Serologic and cerebrospinal fluid markers, brain biopsy	Rupture of small or medium-sized arteries with inflammation and degeneration
Cocaine or alcohol abuse	Clinical history	Underlying vascular abnormalities may be present
Hemorrhagic transformation	CT	Hemorrhage in the region of cerebral infarction as a result of ischemic damage to the blood-brain barrier

CT = computed tomography; MRI = magnetic resonance imaging.
Modified from Qureshi AI, Tuhrim S, Broderick JP, et al. Spontaneous intracerebral hemorrhage. *N Engl J Med.* 2001;344:1450-1460.

● PRIMARY INTRACEREBRAL HEMORRHAGE

DEFINITION

Primary nontraumatic intracerebral hemorrhage (i.e., hemorrhage that does not result from ischemic injury) occurs predominantly as a consequence of chronic, poorly controlled hypertension (Chapter 67). Less frequently, a ruptured vascular malformation or amyloid angiopathy is responsible. Intracerebral hemorrhage can also be caused by a bleeding diathesis and certain drugs of abuse (Table 415-1).

EPIDEMIOLOGY

In the United States, primary intracerebral hemorrhage is responsible for 10 to 15% of strokes and about 80% of all intracranial hemorrhages. The average annual incidence in the United States is approximately 50,000. Intracerebral hemorrhage has the highest mortality rate of all subtypes of stroke, and almost 60% of affected patients die within the first year. The risk for primary intracerebral hemorrhage in blacks is about 40% higher than in whites. Worldwide, the incidence of intracerebral hemorrhage ranges from 10 to 40 per 1 million people, with the rate in Japan being at the top end of this range. Age-adjusted rates for men are about 50% higher than those for women. As with ischemic stroke, the incidence appears to be declining in the industrialized world, concurrent with the decline in hypertension.

PATHOBIOLOGY

Primary intracerebral hemorrhage typically consists of a large, confluent area of blood that clots (Fig. 415-2). Most bleeding occurs at or near bifurcations

FIGURE 415-2. Pathology specimen showing a large basal ganglia parenchymal hemorrhage in the left hemisphere. (Courtesy of Gregory W. Albers, Stanford University, Stanford, Calif.)

of arteries with prominent degeneration of the media and smooth muscle. Several weeks later, the blood is slowly removed by phagocytosis, and after several months, only a small, collapsed cavity lined by hemosiderin-containing macrophages may remain. Rupture into the ventricles with bleeding into the subarachnoid space commonly occurs with large hemorrhages. Edematous parenchyma rapidly develops around the clot. Although hemorrhage may destroy brain tissue locally, histologic examination suggests that displacement of normal brain tissue and dissection of blood along fiber tracts account for much of the pathology. Viable and salvageable neural tissue may exist in the vicinity of the hematoma.

The most important risk factor for intracerebral hemorrhage is hypertension, particularly in people who are younger than 55 years, smokers, and poorly compliant with antihypertensive medications. Excessive chronic alcohol consumption also increases the risk for intracerebral hemorrhage. A less well established risk factor is a low serum cholesterol concentration (<160 mg/dL).

Hypertension is associated with hemorrhage in various locations throughout the brain, especially in the external capsule–putamen, internal capsule–thalamus, central pons, and cerebellum (Fig. 415-3). A smaller number of hemorrhages occur in the subcortical white matter, especially in the frontal, temporal, and occipital lobes.

Evidence, especially from serial CT scans, shows that hematomas expand for many hours after the onset of bleeding in many patients. Bleeding may cease when the lesion grows to a size sufficient to produce increased tissue pressure with consequent tamponade.

Amyloid (congophilic) angiopathy is a pathologic diagnosis that is more frequently made in people older than 55 years. This condition, which is unrelated to generalized amyloidosis and is occasionally hereditary, commonly produces multiple, small hemorrhages. It often appears in the brains of patients with Alzheimer's disease (Chapter 409) and has been associated with nonhypertensive hemorrhage in unusual lobar locations in the cerebral hemispheres. Amyloid deposits, chemically similar to those in Alzheimer's plaques, are seen in the media and adventitia of small and medium-sized arteries.

Anticoagulation, thrombolysis, and various hematologic abnormalities (Chapters 175 to 178) are associated with intracerebral hemorrhages. Warfarin anticoagulation to conventional intensities (i.e., international normalized ratio of 2.0 to 3.0) has been associated with a risk for intracranial hemorrhage of approximately 1% per year in many stroke-prone patients (Chapter 37). This rate is about 7 to 10 times greater than the risk in similar patients who have not undergone anticoagulation. On average, when such hemorrhages occur, the fatality rate is about 60%. Predictors are advanced age, previous ischemic stroke, hypertension, and the intensity of anticoagulation.

The most feared complication of thrombolytic therapy for acute myocardial infarction (Chapter 73) or ischemic stroke (Chapter 414) is intracerebral hemorrhage. When tissue plasminogen activator (t-PA) is administered within 3 hours after the onset of stroke symptoms, the intracerebral hemorrhage rate is 6.5%, compared with 0.5% in placebo patients; 50% of the patients who sustain these hemorrhages die. However, the overall benefit of t-PA therapy in appropriate patients persists because the increased risk for hemorrhage is more than counterbalanced by the improvement in ischemic strokes (Chapter 414).

Cerebral hemorrhages also occur in patients with leukemia (Chapter 189), polycythemia vera (Chapter 169), thrombocytopenia (Chapter 175),

FIGURE 415-3. Typical sites and sources of intracerebral hemorrhage. Intracerebral hemorrhages most commonly involve the cerebral lobes and originate from penetrating cortical branches of the anterior, middle, or posterior cerebral arteries (A); the basal ganglia and originate from ascending lenticulostriate branches of the middle cerebral artery (B); the thalamus and originate from ascending thalamogeniculate branches of the posterior cerebral artery (C); the pons and originate from paramedian branches of the basilar artery (D); and the cerebellum and originate from penetrating branches of the posterior inferior, anterior inferior, or superior cerebellar arteries (E). (From Qureshi AI, Tuhrim S, Broderick JP, et al. Spontaneous intracerebral hemorrhage. *N Engl J Med.* 2001;344:1450-1460.)

hemophilia (Chapter 177) and other clotting abnormalities, infectious and noninfectious vasculitis, intracranial neoplasms, and venous thrombosis. In addition, intracerebral hemorrhage can occur in patients who abuse various sympathomimetic agents and cocaine (Chapter 33).

CLINICAL MANIFESTATIONS

Neck stiffness, seizures, diastolic blood pressure higher than 110 mm Hg, vomiting, and headache increase the likelihood of a hemorrhagic stroke rather than an ischemic stroke. Otherwise, however, the neurologic abnormalities caused by intracerebral hemorrhage do not differ from those caused by ischemic strokes (Chapter 414) because destruction of neural tissue is the basis of the neurologic dysfunction caused by both entities. The signs and symptoms are related to the location of the lesion. Because the site of intracerebral hemorrhage often differs from that of ischemic strokes, characteristic patterns of neurologic loss may be more frequently associated with intracerebral hemorrhage than with ischemic strokes (Table 415-2). Hemorrhages may grow as the bleeding continues, whereas ischemic lesions usually do not change in size after vascular occlusion; as a result, hemorrhages characteristically cause progressively increasing loss of neurologic function until a plateau is reached, whereas ischemic strokes may fluctuate or remain static after the early phases of the stroke. Subsequent deterioration in the level of consciousness after an intracerebral hemorrhage occurs in about one fourth of patients who are initially alert.

Intracranial hemorrhages in each of the four typical locations produce characteristic findings. Patients with massive *putaminal hemorrhages* become lethargic or comatose within minutes to hours after onset and concurrently experience contralateral weakness (including the face) with contralateral hemianopia and gaze paresis (i.e., eyes deviated toward the side of the hemorrhage). *Cerebellar hemorrhages* initially spare the brain stem, and consciousness is generally preserved in the early stages. Occipital headache may be the first symptom. The usual findings are unsteady gait, ataxia, nausea, and vomiting, which is often severe and repetitive. A variety of eye movement abnormalities may be present. Weakness is not prominent at onset, but with progression and brain stem compression, focal or bilateral weakness and coma develop, often rapidly. Further deterioration can result from herniation of cerebellar tissue downward through the foramen magnum or upward across the tentorium; hydrocephalus may be caused by obstruction of CSF flow. With continued bleeding or tissue swelling, severe brain stem damage ensues and causes rapid demise of the patient. Less frequent are *thalamic*

TABLE 415-2 CLINICAL FEATURES OF COMMON HYPERTENSIVE HEMORRHAGES

	Site of Hemorrhage			
CLINICAL FEATURES	**PUTAMINAL**	**THALAMIC**	**PONTINE**	**CEREBELLAR**
Unconsciousness	Later	Later	Early	Late
Hemiparesis	Yes	Yes	Quadriparesis	Late
Sensory change	Yes	Yes	Yes	Late
Hemianopia	Yes	Yes	No	No
Pupils				
Size	Normal	Small	Small	Normal
Reaction	Yes	Yes or no	Yes or no	Yes
Gaze paresis side	Contralateral, sometimes ipsilateral	Contralateral	Ipsilateral	Ipsilateral
Response to calorics	Yes	Yes	No	Yes or no
Downward eye deviation	Yes	No	No	
Ocular bobbing	No	No	Sometimes	Sometimes
Gait loss	No	No	Yes	Yes
Vomiting	Occasional	Occasional	Often	Severe

hemorrhages, which cause patients to lose consciousness relatively rapidly; those who survive often experience contralateral hemiparesis, sensory deficits, and homonymous hemianopia. *Pontine hemorrhage* was once thought to produce coma invariably, but modern imaging detects smaller hemorrhages that are not fatal. Patients with severe pontine hemorrhages become comatose, usually with very small but detectable reactive pupils. Oculovestibular responses are often lost early, vomiting can occur at onset, and these patients generally have quadriplegia and bilateral extensor posturing. Patients may be "locked-in" (Chapter 411).

Lobar hemorrhages, which are more characteristic of amyloid angiopathy than hypertension, usually originate at the junctions between gray and white matter in the cerebral hemispheres. Such hemorrhages account for about one third of intracerebral hemorrhages and are approximately as common as putaminal hemorrhages. The clinical manifestation depends on the location of the hemorrhage. Most patients are elderly because amyloid angiopathy and hypertension are relatively frequent in this age group. Nonspecific symptoms, including headache, nausea, and vomiting, probably occur with about the same frequency but with less intensity than with deep, hypertensive hemorrhages. Coma and seizures are uncommon, possibly because most of these hemorrhages are comparatively small and located in subcortical white matter.

DIAGNOSIS

Intracerebral hemorrhage often cannot be distinguished from other types of stroke based on clinical findings alone. The test of choice for making the diagnosis is a non–contrast-enhanced CT scan (Fig. 415-4) that shows areas of hemorrhage as zones of increased density, which may or may not have associated regions of decreased density indicating infarction. Primary parenchymal hemorrhages typically display homogeneous areas of increased density and a mass effect (i.e., shift of normal tissue from its usual location), whereas hemorrhagic infarctions are characterized by areas of increased density (i.e., blood) interspersed with areas of decreased density (i.e., infarction).

MRI findings depend on the precise imaging sequence and the age of the hemorrhage. The sensitivity and specificity of MRI for the diagnosis of hemorrhage, particularly in the presence of infarction, are unknown. MRI is able to detect small lesions, particularly in the posterior fossa, better than CT, but how much of the lesion is hemorrhage or hypoperfusion is uncertain. Cerebral angiography is not needed for the acute evaluation of hemorrhages, but it is commonly used later to identify a suspected aneurysm or AVM that may be considered for intervention.

FIGURE 415-4. Intracerebral hemorrhage. A computed tomographic scan shows a parenchymal hemorrhage involving the left thalamus and posterior internal capsule. (Courtesy of Gregory W. Albers, Stanford University, Stanford, CA.)

TREATMENT   Rx

General Measures
The usual medical management of acute parenchymal hemorrhage has been supportive, with initial care directed at maintenance of the airway, oxygenation, nutrition, and prevention and treatment of secondary complications. Optimal blood pressure treatment is uncertain, although the general guidelines for excessive hypertension and reduction of cerebral perfusion apply as for ischemic strokes (Chapter 414). There is no accepted protocol for the management of increased intracranial pressure; osmotherapy, hyperventilation, and neuromuscular paralysis rarely are beneficial. Fluid management should maintain euvolemia; fluid restriction or volume expansion is not of proven value. Seizures are particularly harmful in critically ill patients and are treated despite lack of data from randomized trials. Maintenance of normal body temperature is theoretically desirable because fever may accelerate tissue destruction.

Medical Therapy
Intravenous administration of recombinant factor VIIa within 4 hours after onset reduces the volume of hemorrhage and surrounding cerebral edema, as measured by CT, but does not improve clinical outcomes. ■ Larger trials of this promising therapy are in progress. Small clinical trials of corticosteroids, glycerol, and hemodilution have not demonstrated benefit, and corticosteroids may increase the risk for infectious complications.

Surgical Therapy
The goal of surgical treatment of intracerebral hemorrhage is to remove as much blood clot as possible as quickly as possible. Ideally, surgery should remove the underlying cause, such as an AVM, and prevent hydrocephalus. Early surgical intervention to evacuate intracerebral hematomas within 24 hours is no better than medical therapy. ■ However, patients who have cerebellar hemorrhages and are deteriorating because of brain stem compression and hydrocephalus caused by ventricular obstruction are still recommended by some for removal of the clot or amputation of part of the cerebellum, although no proof exists to support this approach.

PROGNOSIS

In recent series, the 30-day case-fatality rate averaged 30 to 50%. Most early deaths result from the direct neurologic consequences of the hemorrhage; the severity of bleeding (e.g., size, extension into ventricles) and level of neurologic function are the best predictors of poor outcomes. Supratentorial hemorrhages smaller than 30 mL rarely lead to death unless they are located in the thalamus. The long-term prognosis for various degrees of recovery is similar or better than that of cerebral infarctions of comparable severity. The risk for recurrent intracerebral hemorrhage has not been well studied, but the risk for at least one rebleeding episode may be as high as 25% over the next several years. The risk for intracerebral hemorrhage can be reduced by appropriate treatment. Control of mild to moderate hypertension decreases the risk for hemorrhagic stroke by one third to one half (Chapter 67).

HYPERTENSIVE ENCEPHALOPATHY

DEFINITION

Hypertensive encephalopathy is usually defined as malignant hypertension associated with central nervous system abnormalities (Chapter 67). Malignant hypertension is commonly defined as sustained, elevated arterial blood pressure, with diastolic levels of 130 mm Hg or greater and systolic pressure in excess of 200 mm Hg. Abnormal funduscopic findings include papilledema, retinal linear hemorrhages, or extravascular cotton-wool exudates. Hypertensive encephalopathy is classically characterized by rapidly evolving severe hypertension associated with headache, nausea, vomiting, visual disturbances, seizures, confusion, stupor, and ultimately coma. Focal neurologic signs are common.

PATHOBIOLOGY

The pathogenesis of hypertensive encephalopathy remains unclear. Pathologic findings include purpura in the brain, retinal hemorrhages, papilledema, and fibrinoid arteriolar lesions of the glomeruli. Diffuse fibrinoid necrosis and thrombotic occlusion of arterioles cause microinfarctions and petechial hemorrhages, and these changes lead to distal ischemia. Ring hemorrhage around a thrombosed precapillary is the characteristic microscopic lesion of hypertensive encephalopathy. Multiple, compacted petechiae can resemble a hematoma.

CLINICAL MANIFESTATIONS AND DIAGNOSIS

Hypertensive encephalopathy is associated with hypertension of any cause and can occur in patients of any age. Severe headache is the most frequent manifestation. Nausea, vomiting, impaired vision, and dizziness are common. Confusion, stupor, and coma with generalized seizures may develop. Retinal changes characteristic of severe hypertension are common and often include hemorrhages or papilledema, but arteriolar narrowing may be the only abnormality. Because there are no pathognomonic findings in this disorder, it is a diagnosis of exclusion.

Uremic encephalopathy also occurs in patients with renal failure (Chapter 132). Uremia can cause altered mental status and seizures, and differentiation from hypertensive encephalopathy may be difficult. However, uremia is usually accompanied by metabolic acidosis or water intoxication, which may differentiate it from hypertensive encephalopathy, and correction of the uremia by dialysis may help clarify the picture.

Other complications of hypertension to be considered in the differential diagnosis of hypertensive encephalopathy include hemorrhagic and ischemic strokes. Focal neurologic signs predominate in these other conditions, whereas mental status changes are characteristic of hypertensive encephalopathy. Increased intracranial pressure from obstructive hydrocephalus (Chapter 195), brain tumor (Chapter 195), or subdural hematoma (Chapter 406) can elevate blood pressure and slow the pulse, but encephalopathy and markedly elevated blood pressure are absent.

TREATMENT   Rx

Therapy should be initiated immediately, but the rate of decrease in blood pressure should be controlled to avoid hypotension (Chapter 67). Seizures can usually be stopped with intravenous diazepam (10 mg); in eclamptic patients (Chapter 247), fosphenytoin (15 to 20 mg phenytoin equivalent per kilogram

intravenously) or magnesium sulfate (4 g intramuscularly every 4 hours as needed) are often used, particularly because they may not depress the respiratory drive of the fetus as much as some other drugs. Prompt delivery of the fetus may be quite helpful.

Grade A

1. Mayer SA, Brun NC, Begtrup K, et al. Efficacy and safety of recombinant activated factor VII for acute intracerebral hemorrhage. *N Engl J Med.* 2008;358:2127-2137.
2. Molyneux AJ, Kerr RS, Birks J, et al. Risk of recurrent subarachnoid haemorrhage, death, or dependence and standardised mortality ratios after clipping or coiling of an intracranial aneurysm in the International Subarachnoid Aneurysm Trial (ISAT): long-term follow-up. *Lancet Neurol.* 2009;8:427-433.
3. Mendelow AD, Gregson BA, Fernandes HM, et al. Early surgery versus initial conservative treatment in patients with spontaneous supratentorial intracerebral haematomas in the International Surgical Trial in Intracerebral Haemorrhage (STITCH): a randomised trial. *Lancet.* 2005;365:387-397.

SUGGESTED READINGS

Runchey S, McGee S. Does this patient have a hemorrhagic stroke? Clinical findings distinguishing hemorrhagic stroke from ischemic stroke. *JAMA.* 2010;303:2280-2286. *Neck stiffness, seizures, diastolic blood pressure >110 mm Hg, vomiting, and headache increase the likelihood of a hemorrhagic stroke rather than an ischemic stroke, but neuroimaging is required for reliable diagnosis.*
Smith SD, Eskey CJ. Hemorrhagic stroke. *Radiol Clin North Am.* 2011;49:27-45. *Review of imaging options.*

416

PARKINSONISM

ANTHONY E. LANG

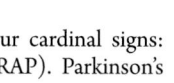

Parkinsonism is a clinical syndrome that consists of four cardinal signs: tremor, rigidity, akinesia, and postural disturbances (TRAP). Parkinson's disease is a common cause of the TRAP syndrome, but there are numerous other causes (Table 416-1).

PARKINSON'S DISEASE

EPIDEMIOLOGY

Parkinson's disease, which is the second most common neurodegenerative disorder after Alzheimer's disease, occurs in approximately 1 in 1000 in the general population and in 1% of persons older than 65 years. Men are affected slightly more often than women (3:2).

PATHOBIOLOGY

The cause of Parkinson's disease is believed to be a variable combination of poorly understood genetic and environmental factors. Both autosomal dominant and recessive genes can cause classic Parkinson's disease. The protein α-synuclein, which is the chief constituent of the hallmark cytoplasmic inclusion, the Lewy body (Chapter 409), is critical in the pathogenesis of Parkinson's disease. Abnormal aggregation of the protein, either from mutations in the α-synuclein gene or as a result of excessive production of the normal protein because of gene duplications or triplications, is associated with varying disease phenotypes. Other defined genetic abnormalities may be associated with classic later-onset Parkinson's disease, including *LRRK2*, which is currently the most common cause of autosomal dominantly inherited Parkinson's disease, or with early-onset parkinsonism, typically found in the autosomal recessive forms associated with *parkin*, *DJ-1*, and *PINK1*. Other genes in which mutations may increase the risk for development of Parkinson's disease include the glucocerebrosidase gene (*GBA*).

Although monogenetic forms of Parkinson's disease are uncommon, knowing that parkin is an E-3 ubiquitin protein ligase has implicated the ubiquitin proteasome system in the pathogenesis of Parkinson's disease. Proteasome inhibitors, which may be present in the environment, are being studied for their potential to cause parkinsonism in animals. Such findings support the "environmental hypothesis" of sporadic Parkinson's disease, similar to the discovery that the selective neurotoxin 1-methyl-4-phenyl-1,2,3,6-tetrahydropyridine (MPTP) is oxidized to the active toxin MPP^+, which is a selective inhibitor of complex I of the mitochondrial electron transport chain. This knowledge, combined with recognition of the importance of dopamine (see later), has implicated oxidative stress in the pathogenesis of Parkinson's disease. Other proposed pathogenetic factors include mitochondrial dysfunction, protein misfolding or aggregation, excitotoxicity, and inflammation.

Pathology

Many of the features of Parkinson's disease are due to loss of dopamine in the neostriatum (especially the putamen) secondary to loss of pigmented dopaminergic neurons in the substantia nigra pars compacta (SNc) of the midbrain. Approximately 60% of these dopaminergic neurons will have degenerated before clinical features of the disease develop.

In addition to the prominent degenerative changes in the SNc (cell loss, gliosis, abnormal deposition of aggregated α-synuclein as Lewy bodies and Lewy neurites), pathologic changes are also evident in other brain stem nuclei, in cortical regions, and in peripheral autonomic neurons. Indeed, it has been suggested that Parkinson's disease may begin in the lower brain stem and the olfactory system, where it causes early loss of the sense of smell and only later involves the substantia nigra. Independent of the order of involvement, it is likely that the widespread extranigral neurodegenerative changes account for the many symptoms that do not respond to dopamine replacement and that become increasingly problematic as the disease progresses.

CLINICAL MANIFESTATIONS

Typically, the symptoms begin in one limb. This asymmetry often persists into later stages of the disease.

Motor Symptoms
Tremor

The classic "resting tremor" of Parkinson's disease has characteristic clinical features. The tremor has a frequency of 4 to 6 cycles per second, typically with a "pill-rolling" character when it involves the hand. It is generally present with the limb in complete repose and typically subsides when the limb moves and takes up a new position, although the tremor may reemerge ("reemergent tremor") within a short time after maintaining the new position (Video 416-1). Because resting tremor diminishes or subsides with action, it may not be disabling but can be embarrassing and may be associated with aching or fatigue of the affected limb. Resting tremor is usually accentuated by stress (e.g., by asking the patient to perform mental calculations). It is also characteristically present in the upper limbs while walking. A higher-frequency (e.g., 7 to 10 Hz) postural and kinetic tremor is also common in patients with various causes of parkinsonism.

Rigidity

Rigidity is a form of increased muscle tone appreciated best on slow passive movements. It may be characterized as "cogwheel" when a tremor is superimposed or as "lead pipe" when it is not. Rigidity is "activated" or accentuated on examination by asking the patient to move the limb opposite the one being tested. Patients may complain of stiffness, but the rigidity is not usually disabling.

Akinesia

Akinesia or bradykinesia comprises a variety of disturbances in movement, including slowness, reduced amplitude, fatiguing, and interruptions in ongoing movement. This disabling aspect of parkinsonism interferes with all voluntary activities and accounts for many of the well-known features of parkinsonism: lack of facial expression with reduced blinking (hypomimia or masked facies—the "reptilian stare"), soft monotonous speech (hypophonia), impaired swallowing resulting in drooling (sialorrhea), small handwriting (micrographia), reduced arm swing while walking, shortened stride and shuffling gait, difficulty arising from a low chair, and problems turning over in bed. Arrest in ongoing movement ("motor block") can interfere with a variety of activities, but it is best appreciated as freezing of gait (Video 416-2). Bradykinesia is evident on inspection and elicited by testing rapid repetitive and alternating movements: finger tapping, opening

and the closing the fist, pronating and supinating the wrist, and toe and heel tapping.

Postural Disturbances

Postural disturbances include a flexed posture in the limbs and trunk (stooped, simian posture), as well as postural instability resulting in imbalance and falls. Patients may complain of being unable to stop themselves from going forward (propulsion) or backward (retropulsion). Clinical assessment of postural instability includes the "pull test," in which the examiner abruptly pulls the patient off balance while being ready to catch the patient in the event of a fall.

Other Symptoms

In addition to the motor features of parkinsonism, a variety of non–motor-related features are extremely common and include pain and other sensory disturbances; dysautonomic complaints, such as urinary urgency and frequency; orthostatic faintness; constipation; male erectile dysfunction; sleep abnormalities, including rapid eye movement behavioral disorder (Chapter 412); anxiety; fatigue; depression; and cognitive disturbances, including dementia. As the disease progresses, more resistant features develop, including "axial" motor disturbances (speech and swallowing abnormalities, freezing, and postural instability), as well as neurobehavioral and cognitive dysfunction.

TABLE 416-1 DIFFERENTIAL DIAGNOSIS OF PARKINSONISM

PARKINSON'S DISEASE

Sporadic
Genetic
    Autosomal dominant (e.g., α-synuclein gene mutations, duplications, triplications; *LRRK2* mutations)
    Autosomal recessive (e.g., *parkin, DJ-1, PINK-1*)

SECONDARY PARKINSONISM

Neurodegenerative diseases (sporadic or genetic)
    Progressive supranuclear palsy* (Videos 416-3 through 416-6)
    Multiple system atrophy* (Videos 416-7 through 416-9)
    Corticobasal degeneration* (Videos 416-10 and 416-11)
    Dementia with Lewy bodies*
    Alzheimer's disease*
    ALS-parkinsonism-dementia complex of Guam
    Huntington's disease
    Rapid-onset dystonia-parkinsonism
    Pallidopyramidal degeneration (including PARK9 and PARK15)
    Neuroacanthocytosis
    Spinocerebellar ataxias (e.g., SCA-3, SCA-2)
    Wilson's disease
    Pantothenate kinase–associated neurodegeneration (Hallervorden-Spatz syndrome)
    Neuroferritinopathy
    Calcification of the basal ganglia (Fahr's disease)
    Dopa-responsive dystonia (not a degenerative disorder)
Drugs*
    Neuroleptics, metoclopramide, prochlorperazine, tetrabenazine, reserpine, cinnarizine, flunarizine, α-methyldopa, lithium
Toxic
    MPTP, manganese (including illicit use of ephedrone), carbon monoxide, mercury
Infectious
    Encephalitis lethargica
    Other encephalitis, including HIV associated
    Subacute sclerosing panencephalitis
    Creutzfeldt-Jakob disease
Vascular*
    Atherosclerosis
    Amyloid angiopathy
Neoplastic
    Brain tumor
    Other mass lesions
Normal-pressure hydrocephalus*
Head trauma
Multiple sclerosis

*See Table 416-4 for additional details.
ALS = amyotrophic lateral sclerosis; HIV = human immunodeficiency virus; MPTP = 1-methyl-4-phenyl-1,2,3,6-tetrahydropyridine.
Adapted from Cloutier M, Lang AE. Movement disorders: an overview. In: Factor SA, Lang AE, Weiner WJ, eds. *Drug Induced Movement Disorders*. Malden, Mass: Blackwell; 2005:3-19.

TABLE 416-2 PROBLEMS IN LATE-STAGE PARKINSON'S DISEASE

PROBLEM	SYMPTOMS
LATER TREATMENT-RESISTANT SYMPTOMS	
Motor	Dysarthria
	Dysphagia
	Freezing of gait (on-period freezing)
	Postural instability with falls
Non–motor related*	Dysautonomia, weight loss
	Sensory symptoms, including pain (some may be responsive to levodopa)
	Changes in mood or behavior (depression, anxiety), sleep disturbances (excessive daytime sleepiness often caused by or aggravated by dopaminergic medication)
	Rapid eye movement sleep behavior disorder (may develop before parkinsonism)
	Fatigue
	Cognitive dysfunction and dementia
RELATED TO TREATMENT AND DISEASE	
Motor fluctuations	Wearing off of drug effect (predictable end-of-dose deterioration, morning akinesia), increased latency to benefit ("delayed-on"), dose failures ("no-on")
	On-off phenomenon, more rapid and unpredictable fluctuations
	Concomitant fluctuations of non–motor-related symptoms that may be as disabling as motor symptoms (or more so)
Dyskinesias (abnormal involuntary movements)	Peak-dose dyskinesias: chorea, athetosis, and less often, more prolonged dystonia, typically worse on the initially affected side (Video 416-12)
	Diphasic dyskinesia ("beginning-of-dose" and "end-of-dose" dyskinesias): mixtures of choreoathetosis, ballism, dystonia, alternating movements (especially in the legs)
	Off-period dystonia: most often involving the legs and feet (including morning foot dystonia)
Psychiatric disturbances	Vivid dreams and nightmares
	Visual hallucinations with a clear sensorium
	Hallucinations with confusion
	Mania, hypersexuality, problem gambling, dopaminergic drug addiction
	Paranoid psychosis

Adapted from Lang AE, Lozano AM. Parkinson's disease—second of two parts. *N Engl J Med.* 1998;339:1130-1143.

Complications

In addition to the manifestations of the disease itself, complications of drug therapy include motor- and non–motor-related fluctuations and psychiatric or behavioral disturbances. Thus, in the later stages of the disease, the clinical picture often fluctuates from hour to hour and even from minute to minute; accordingly, patients exhibit a mixtures of the classic features of parkinsonism, which may improve considerably in response to medication, symptoms that persist despite the peak benefit of medication, and symptoms that occur as a complication of dopaminergic medication (Table 416-2).

DIAGNOSIS

Testing for monogenetic forms of Parkinson's disease (e.g., parkin) is becoming available, but guidelines for its use have not yet been developed. Given the classic clinical manifestations, the diagnostic evaluation focuses largely on ways to exclude other causes of parkinsonism (Table 416-3). Young-onset patients should have Wilson's disease excluded by determination of 24-hour urine copper and serum ceruloplasmin and by slit lamp examination (Chapter 218). Findings on magnetic resonance imaging are generally normal in Parkinson's disease, but it is indicated to exclude other diagnoses (Table 416-4). Positron emission tomography, which can assess the presynaptic and postsynaptic sides of the nigrostriatal dopamine system, is useful for research, but the most common ligand, $[^{18}F]$fluorodopa, does not reliably distinguish Parkinson's disease from many other neurodegenerative diseases that mimic it. The same

TABLE 416-3 CLINICAL CLUES TO AN ALTERNATIVE (NON-PARKINSON'S DISEASE) CAUSE OF PARKINSONIAN SIGNS AND SYMPTOMS

Extraocular movements—e.g., nystagmus, limitation of vertical gaze, especially with slowing of downward saccadic eye movements (see Video 416-4)

Early and prominent dysarthria/dysphagia

Prominent or early abnormal neck postures: flexion or extension (see Video 416-8)

Ataxia—limb, gait (impaired tandem gait)

Lower body distribution with relative sparing of upper limb function

Early postural instability/falls/freezing (see Video 416-3)

Dysautonomia (early/prominent), prominent hypotensive response to dopaminergic medication

Pyramidal tract signs—very brisk reflexes, clonus, extensor plantar responses

Peripheral nerve dysfunction—loss of reflexes, distal sensory loss, weakness

Apraxia/cortical sensory changes

Early severe dementia

Poor response to levodopa

limitations apply to evaluation of the dopamine transporter by single-photon emission computed tomography. The finding of increased echogenicity in the SNc of the midbrain on transcranial ultrasound may be more specific in diagnosing Parkinson's disease, but the data are not conclusive.

For evidence-based recommendations on investigation of parkinsonism, see the article by Suchowersky and colleagues in Additional Suggested Readings.

TREATMENT   Rx

Treatment of Parkinson's disease is directed at slowing its progression ("neuroprotective" or "disease-modifying" treatments); improving symptoms, typically by restoring dopaminergic tone medically or by correcting basal ganglia neurophysiology surgically ("symptomatic"); or attempting to restore or regenerate the damaged neurons ("neurorestorative" or "neuroregenerative" therapy).

Medical Treatment

To date, no medical treatment (Table 425-5) has been proved to modify the progressive course of Parkinson's disease. The selective monoamine oxidase B (MAO-B) inhibitors selegiline and rasagiline **1** may exert disease-modifying effects, and the potential effects of agents such as coenzyme Q_{10}, creatine, the calcium-channel blocker isradipine, the pro-urate agent inosine, and the dopamine agonist pramipexole are currently under study.

Early treatment in a patient with little or no disability may entail only education, psychological support, encouragement to remain active and become involved in an exercise program, and ongoing follow-up. There is some evidence that early treatment, even when patients are only mildly symptomatic, may preserve quality of life. A treatment philosophy that still requires evidence-based support involves the early initiation of symptomatic therapy to bolster the brain's compensatory mechanisms that have begun to fail as the physical symptoms of parkinsonism become manifested.

When symptoms begin to interfere with function, mildly effective drugs such as an MAO-B inhibitor, amantadine, and anticholinergics (the latter predominantly for tremor in younger patients) may provide adequate benefit (see Table 425-5). When symptoms are more pronounced or inadequately controlled with these approaches, dopaminergic therapy should be introduced. In patients younger than 65 years who are cognitively intact and lack other major medical problems, initial therapy with a dopamine agonist may delay the development of motor complications.**2** However, these drugs result in more excessive sleepiness, leg edema, "impulse control disorders" (such as pathologic gambling, hypersexuality, binge eating, and shopping), and hallucinations than levodopa does. If a full dose of a dopamine agonist does not provide adequate clinical benefit or has intolerable side effects, levodopa should be initiated. In older patients, in those with cognitive dysfunction (more prone to hallucinations with dopamine agonists), and in circumstances that require more rapid improvement of pronounced disability, levodopa should be the initial drug used.

Alleviating Symptoms

Levodopa is the most effective treatment of Parkinson's disease, but it is associated with a variety of side effects (see Table 416-2). For the first year or

TABLE 416-4 DISEASES THAT MUST BE DISTINGUISHED FROM PARKINSON'S DISEASE

DIAGNOSIS	IMPORTANT DISTINGUISHING CLINICAL FEATURES	RESPONSE TO LEVODOPA/COMMENTS (INCLUDING IMAGING)
Multiple system atrophy (MSA) (includes striatonigral degeneration, sporadic olivopontocerebellar atrophy, and Shy-Drager syndrome)	Early dysautonomia (including orthostatic hypotension and sexual impotence) and bladder dysfunction (with autonomic and nonautonomic components) Cerebellar dysfunction	Good response initially evident in 20% and sustained partial response in ≈15% Dyskinesias or motor fluctuations possible; cranial dystonia may be prominent (see Video 416-7) Patient is wheelchair bound despite response to levodopa (early loss of postural reflexes, with or without ataxia) MRI (including diffusion-weighted imaging and gradient-echo sequences) often shows diagnostic changes in the striatum in MSA-P and "hot cross bun sign" in the pons and hyperintensity in middle cerebellar peduncles in MSA-C
MSA-P = a predominant parkinsonian manifestation	Pyramidal tract signs Stimulus-sensitive myoclonus of the hands and face	
MSA-C = a predominant cerebellar manifestation (mixed features are common)	Extreme forward neck flexion (anterocollis) Mottled, cold hands Inspiratory stridor (see Video 416-9) Prominent dysarthria	
Progressive supranuclear palsy	Supranuclear vertical ophthalmoplegia (see Video 416-4) Other oculomotor and eyelid disturbances (see Video 416-6) Axial rigidity greater than limb rigidity Early falls, speech and swallowing disturbances Nuchal extension Cognitive or behavioral changes Possibly a higher incidence of hypertension than in Parkinson's disease and other neurodegenerative causes of parkinsonism	Good response rarely evident; benefit only for classic parkinsonian features such as limb rigidity, bradykinesia, and rare examples of tremor at rest MRI often demonstrates profound midbrain atrophy ("hummingbird sign" on a midline sagittal view)
Corticobasal (cortical-basal ganglionic) degeneration	Apraxia, cortical sensory loss, alien-limb phenomenon (see Video 416-10) Pronounced asymmetrical rigidity Limb dystonia Stimulus-sensitive myoclonus (see Video 416-11) Aphasia (progressive nonfluent aphasia) Cognitive dysfunction (frontotemporal dementia)	Usually negligible MRI may show pronounced asymmetrical cortical atrophy
Vascular parkinsonism	"Lower-half" parkinsonism with gait disturbances predominating, often with minimal or much milder upper body involvement Additional neurologic deficits (e.g., pyramidal tract signs, pseudobulbar palsy)	Usually poor but some respond well Imaging demonstrates multiple infarcts involving the basal ganglia and subcortical white matter
Dementia with Lewy bodies	Early dementia (cognitive profile somewhat different from that of Alzheimer's disease) Spontaneous hallucinations, fluctuating cognitive status, falls, orthostatic hypotension, RBD Pronounced sensitivity to the extrapyramidal side effects of neuroleptic drugs Parkinsonism may be similar to typical Parkinson's disease, although rigidity may be more prominent than bradykinesia or tremor	Motor features may respond well; psychiatric side effects of dopaminergic drugs are typically dose limiting
Alzheimer's disease	Early dementia (memory loss, apraxia, aphasia) Tremor uncommon Spontaneous hallucinations less common than in dementia with Lewy bodies	Poor
Normal-pressure hydrocephalus	"Lower-half" parkinsonism ("gait apraxia") Urinary complaints (frequency, urgency, incontinence) Cognitive disturbances	Generally poor Imaging demonstrates ventriculomegaly out of proportion to cortical atrophy
Drug-induced parkinsonism	All the classic features of parkinsonism (tremor may be less common than in Parkinson's disease) Usually symmetrical signs and symptoms Other drug-induced movement disorders (e.g., tardive dyskinesia with neuroleptics)	Usually poor because of ongoing dopamine receptor blockade; may aggravate movements of tardive dyskinesia

MRI = magnetic resonance imaging; RBD = rapid eye movement sleep behavior disorder.
Adapted from Lang AE, Lozano AM. Parkinson's disease—first of two parts. *N Engl J Med.* 1998;339:1044-1053.

more the benefit of levodopa lasts throughout the day with little symptomatic variability. However, in time the duration of benefit declines, with worsening of symptoms the first thing in the morning (morning akinesia) and for a variable time before scheduled daytime doses (wearing-off/end-of-dose akinesia). Within 2 to 5 years of initiating treatment, up to 50% of patients may also experience involuntary movements (chorea, athetosis, dystonia), most often at the peak action of the medication. These complications, which are generally more prominent and occur earlier in patients with an onset of disease at a younger age, reflect the short half-life of levodopa combined with the underlying progressive loss of presynaptic dopamine neurons and result in nonphysiologic "pulsatile" stimulation of striatal dopamine receptors, which then induces "neuroplastic" changes in postsynaptic striatal neurons. Initially, these complications rarely cause major disability.

Although initiating therapy with a dopamine agonist rather than levodopa may be associated with a delay in the onset of these motor problems, the clinical benefit is generally less than with levodopa, and all patients eventually require the addition of levodopa to control symptoms. No data support delaying treatment with levodopa, and some data suggest that levodopa could have a neuroprotective effect.[3] Even as Parkinson's disease progresses, most of the classic features continue to respond after 20 or more years of treatment.

TABLE 416-5 DRUGS FOR PARKINSON'S DISEASE

CLASS	DRUG	USUAL STARTING DOSE	USUAL FINAL DOSAGE	IMPORTANT ADVERSE EFFECTS	COMMENTS	INDICATIONS
Anticholinergic	Many (e.g., benztropine, trihexyphenidyl)	Benztropine or trihexyphenidyl, 1-2 mg 2-3 times per day	Varied	Peripheral effects, e.g., dry mouth, blurred vision, constipation, difficulty with urination Central effects, e.g., confusion, memory problems, hallucinations	Relatively contraindicated in the elderly and contraindicated in patients with cognitive disturbances	Early treatment of tremor
Miscellaneous	Amantadine	100 mg once per day	100 mg 2 or 3 times per day	Confusion, visual hallucinations; livedo reticularis, swelling of the ankles; dose reduction or drug withdrawal necessary in patients with renal failure	Previously considered a dopaminergic drug, now thought to act primarily through NMDA antagonist effects	Early treatment; later for dyskinesias
	Memantine	5 mg once daily	10 mg twice daily	Confusion, fatigue, dizziness, headache	NMDA antagonist	Possibly effective for cognitive dysfunction in PDD
Dopamine precursor	Levodopa given with peripheral dopa decarboxylase inhibitor (DDCI) (carbidopa [in 4:1 and 10:1 ratios] or benserazide [4:1]*)	50 (levodopa)/12.5 (DDCI) mg (4:1 preparation) 3 times per day (with meals to reduce nausea and vomiting)	Varied; begin with 3-times-daily schedule (controlled-release levodopa-carbidopa may be given twice daily at first); late in the disease patients may require multiple doses per day (sometimes > 2 g/day). Initially give with meals to reduce GI upset; later avoid meals to improve absorption and reliability of response	Peripheral and central dopaminergic side effects Peripheral: nausea, vomiting, and orthostatic hypotension Central: motor fluctuations, dyskinesias, psychiatric disturbances	Peripheral side effects often controlled by additional carbidopa or the peripheral dopamine receptor blocker domperidone* Controlled-release formulations often less bioavailable with less reliable absorption (more "dose failures" later on)	Formulations: immediate release—for early and later treatment Controlled-release (with carbidopa [4:1] or benserazide [4:1]*)—for predictable motor fluctuations (wearing off) and nighttime akinesia Stalevo (with carbidopa and entacapone)—for wearing off Parcopa (orally disintegrating tablets for faster absorption)—for patients with problematic long latency to benefit with individual doses Duodopa* (used with a pump for duodenal infusions)—for problematic motor fluctuations
Dopamine agonists Ergot derived	Bromocriptine	1.25 mg 3 times per day with meals	30-40 mg/day	Peripheral and central dopaminergic side effects; pedal edema, excessive daytime sleepiness Pleuropulmonary reaction, retroperitoneal fibrosis, erythromelalgia Impulse control disorders probably equally common with all dopamine agonists	Peripheral side effects often well controlled with domperidone* Rare pulmonary, retroperitoneal, and skin effects possibly caused by ergot derivation (drug withdrawal usually required)	Early and adjunctive therapy
	Pergolide	0.05 mg once per day × 2 days, increasing slowly thereafter	3-5 mg/day	As for bromocriptine; cardiac valvulopathy	As for bromocriptine	Not the first agonist because it causes restrictive cardiac valve disease
	Cabergoline*	0.5-1 mg once per day	2-6 mg/day	As for pergolide	As for pergolide	As for pergolide, although advantage of a long half-life may outweigh this concern
	Lisuride*	0.1-0.2 mg 1-3 times per day	2-5 mg/day	As for bromocriptine	As for bromocriptine	Uncertain whether cardiac valve abnormalities occur Parenteral formulations allow chronic infusion (pump) therapy

Class	Drug	Starting Dose	Usual Dose Range	Adverse Effects	Indications/Comments	Additional Comments
Non–ergot derived	Ropinirole	0.25 mg 3 times per day	Up to 24 mg/day in 3 divided doses; Once daily extended/prolonged-release formulation available	Peripheral and central dopaminergic side effects similar to those of ergot-derived dopamine agonists, with the probable exceptions of pleuropulmonary reaction, retroperitoneal fibrosis, erythromelalgia, and cardiac valvulopathy	Effective as first-line and adjunctive therapy; dopamine D_3 agonist effects may contribute to efficacy	De novo therapy shown to be associated with less motor complications than with levodopa; Implications of less progressive loss of dopamine terminal function on imaging uncertain
	Pramipexole	0.125 mg 3 times per day	Up to 4.5 mg/day in 3 divided doses; Once daily extended/prolonged-release formulation available	As for ropinirole	As for ropinirole, possibly greater "D_3-preferring" effects—may account for antidepressant effect	As for ropinirole
	Rotigotine*	4.5 mg/day (10 cm²)	Transdermal patch (4.5-27.0 mg/day; 10-60 cm²)	As for ropinirole; Additional adverse effects related to skin patch application (dermatitis)	May be effective for both first-line and adjunctive therapy	Limited availability because of problems with patch formulation
	Apomorphine	3-5 mg SC injection	Parenteral agent given as needed or as continuous infusion	Peripheral and central dopaminergic side effects; Local skin reactions, including nodule formation	Concomitant antiemetic (eg, domperidone,* trimethobenzamide) needed	Late-stage problematic motor fluctuations; Long-term use of infusions may reduce dyskinesias, as well as motor fluctuations
Monoamine oxidase B inhibitors	Selegiline	5 mg once per day	5 mg 2 times per day	Dopaminergic effects of other drugs possibly accentuated, insomnia, confusion	Last dose given at midday to avoid insomnia	Early mild disease; Some controversial evidence suggesting disease-modifying effects; Predictable motor fluctuations (wearing off)
	Zydis selegiline	1.25 mg once per day	1.25 or 2.5 mg/day (wafer formulation)	As for selegiline	As for selegiline; Absorbed from the buccal mucosa, thereby avoiding first-pass hepatic metabolism and methamphetamine metabolite of selegiline	As for selegiline
	Rasagiline	1 mg once per day	1-2 mg once per day	As for selegiline		Possible disease-modifying effects; As for selegiline
Catechol O-methyltransferase (COMT) inhibitors	Tolcapone	100 mg 3 times per day	100 or 200 mg 3 times per day (at 6-hr intervals)	Effects of levodopa accentuated; Diarrhea in approximately 5% of patients; Hepatotoxicity	Dose of levodopa may have to be reduced by as much as 25%; diarrhea (sometimes explosive) typically forces discontinuation; Ongoing monitoring of liver function tests required (second-line COMT inhibitor)	Motor fluctuations, especially wearing off (probably more effective than entacapone)
	Entacapone	200 mg with each dose of levodopa	200 mg 4-10 times per day (given with doses of levodopa)	Effects of levodopa accentuated	As for tolcapone; diarrhea possibly less frequent; Liver function monitoring unnecessary	As for tolcapone; Available in a combination tablet with levodopa/carbidopa (Stalevo)

TABLE 416-5   DRUGS FOR PARKINSON'S DISEASE—cont'd

CLASS	DRUG	USUAL STARTING DOSE	USUAL FINAL DOSAGE	IMPORTANT ADVERSE EFFECTS	COMMENTS	INDICATIONS
Atypical neuroleptics	Clozapine	12.5 mg hs	Wide range (6.25-150 mg/day), usually <75 mg/day	Agranulocytosis, sedation, hypotension, sialorrhea	Very low risk of worsening parkinsonism; agranulocytosis rare (<1%) and reversible if discovered early (requires regular monitoring of complete blood count)	Drug-induced psychosis Other "off-label" indications include drug-resistant tremor and possibly levodopa-induced dyskinesias
	Quetiapine	12.5-25 mg hs	25-150 mg/day	Sedation May worsen parkinsonism	Probably less effective than clozapine	Drug-induced psychosis
Acetylcholinesterase inhibitors	Donepezil	5 mg once per day	5-10 mg/day	Peripheral cholinergic side effects: nausea, vomiting, diarrhea Increased tremor, worsening of other Parkinson's features		Dementia Possibly effective for psychotic symptoms
	Rivastigmine	1.5 mg twice per day	3-12 mg/day	As for donepezil	Patch formulation available for transdermal administration—tolerability may be improved over oral formulation	As for donepezil

*Unavailable in the United States.

GI = gastrointestinal; NMDA = N-methyl-D-aspartate, PDD = Parkinson's disease dementia.

For evidence-based treatment recommendations, see Suchowersky O, Gronseth G, Perlmutter J, et al. Practice parameter: neuroprotective strategies and alternative therapies for Parkinson disease (an evidence-based review): report of the Quality Standards Subcommittee of the American Academy of Neurology. *Neurology.* 2006;66:976-982; Pahwa R, Factor SA, Lyons KE, et al. Practice parameter: treatment of Parkinson disease with motor fluctuations and dyskinesia (an evidence-based review): report of the Quality Standards Subcommittee of the American Academy of Neurology. *Neurology.* 2006;66:983-995; and Miyasaki JM, Shannon K, Voon V, et al. Practice parameter: evaluation and treatment of depression, psychosis, and dementia in Parkinson disease (an evidence-based review): report of the Quality Standards Subcommittee of the American Academy of Neurology. *Neurology.* 2006;66:996-1002.

It is not clear that delaying motor complications in the first 5 years of treatment by the initial use of a dopamine agonist improves long-term outcome or quality of life; indeed, clinical status, including the incidence of motor complications, may be no different after 10 years of treatment in those initiating therapy with a dopamine agonist and those starting with levodopa.[4]

There is no clear advantage to starting a controlled-release rather than an immediate-release preparation of levodopa or combining levodopa with a catechol *O*-methyltransferase [COMT] inhibitor. The motor fluctuations that develop during levodopa therapy are managed by a number of approaches (see Table 416-5), including increasing the frequency of the dose, using a controlled-release preparation, prolonging the action by blocking metabolism (MAO-B or COMT inhibition), or adding a dopamine agonist. For example, adding rasagiline or entacapone to levodopa provides significant incremental benefits. Dyskinesias improve when doses of dopaminergic medications are reduced, but the parkinsonism often increases to an intolerable level. Amantadine may improve the dyskinesias without worsening the parkinsonism.

Medical management of Parkinson's disease often includes a variety of other agents, for example, drugs directed at the treatment of orthostatic hypotension, depression (Chapter 404), anxiety (Chapter 404), urinary frequency and urgency (Chapters 25 and 125), and male erectile dysfunction (Chapter 242). Management of late-stage Parkinson's disease requires skill in polypharmacy and an understanding of the complicated benefit-risk ratios of the many drugs needed.

Surgical Treatment

Surgical therapy, which involves deep brain stimulation of the subthalamic nucleus, improves the symptoms of Parkinson's disease[5] and permits lower doses of antiparkinson medications to be used, whereas deep brain stimulation of the internal segment of the globus pallidus may provide a less consistent and durable response. Nevertheless, a randomized trial comparing these two approaches found no differences in outcome at 24 months.[6] Bilateral deep brain stimulation of the subthalamic nucleus or globus pallidus is more effective (71%) than medical therapy (32%); it also improves self-reported quality of life despite the adverse events associated with the procedure.[5,7] Thalamic deep brain stimulation is of limited utility because it is effective only for tremor. The best predictor of a good response to deep brain stimulation of the subthalamic nucleus is the patient's ongoing clinical response to levodopa. Apart from tremor, which may be resistant to the highest tolerable dose of levodopa, symptoms that are resistant to the peak effect of levodopa (e.g., dysarthria, postural instability with falls) also fail to respond to deep brain stimulation. The typical good candidate for deep brain stimulation of the subthalamic nucleus is an otherwise healthy, relatively young, cognitively intact, and psychiatrically stable patient who still responds well to levodopa but is suffering from disabling motor fluctuations and dyskinesias.

Double-blind randomized trials of transplantation of fetal substantia nigra into the striatum have not only failed to show significant efficacy but have also been associated with the side effect of transplant-induced off-medication dyskinesias. Postmortem assessments in a small number of patients surviving for more than 10 years following fetal transplants have shown Lewy bodies in the transplanted dopamine neurons, thus suggesting that the pathology can be "transmitted" to neurons placed in the diseased host. Double-blind randomized trials of bilateral intraputamenal infusion of glial-derived neurotrophic factor and gene therapy with AAV-neurturin failed to confirm the benefits found in unblinded studies.

OTHER CAUSES OF PARKINSONISM

The numerous causes of parkinsonism (see Table 416-1) are sometimes termed "akinetic-rigid syndrome," "Parkinson's syndrome," "atypical parkinsonism," or even "Parkinson-plus syndrome" to emphasize that these patients commonly demonstrate additional clinical features indicative of the more widespread and particularly more severe pathologic involvement of areas beyond the dopaminergic SNc. These other parkinsonism conditions are generally associated with "postsynaptic" changes that result in a poor or unsustained response to levodopa, and this unresponsiveness serves as one of the most important of several clues that the parkinsonism features are caused by conditions other than Parkinson's disease (see Table 416-4) (i.e., "parkinsonism minus" a levodopa response; see Table 416-3).

1. Olanow CW, Rascol O, Hauser R, et al. A double-blind, delayed start trial of rasagiline in Parkinson's disease. *N Engl J Med.* 2009;361:1268-1278.
2. Parkinson Study Group CALM Cohort Investigators. Long-term effect of initiating pramipexole vs levodopa in early Parkinson disease. *Arch Neurol.* 2009;66:563-570.
3. Fahn S, Shoulson I, Kieburtz K, et al. Levodopa and the progression of Parkinson's disease. *N Engl J Med.* 2004;351:2498-2508.
4. Katzenschlager R, Head J, Schrag A, et al. Parkinson's Disease Research Group of the United Kingdom. Fourteen-year final report of the randomized PDRG-UK trial comparing three initial treatments in PD. *Neurology.* 2008;71:474-480.
5. Deuschl G, Schade-Brittinger C, Krack P, et al. A randomized trial of deep-brain stimulation for Parkinson's disease. *N Engl J Med.* 2006;355:896-908.
6. Follett KA, Weaver FM, Stern M, et al. Pallidal versus subthalamic deep brain stimulation for Parkinson's disease. *N Engl J Med.* 2010;362:2077-2091.
7. Weaver FM, Follett K, Stern M, et al. Bilateral deep brain stimulation vs best medical therapy for patients with advanced Parkinson disease: a randomized controlled trial. *JAMA.* 2009;301: 63-73.

SUGGESTED READINGS

Benabid AL, Chabardes S, Mitrofanis J, et al. Deep brain stimulation of the subthalamic nucleus for the treatment of Parkinson's disease. *Lancet Neurol.* 2009;8:67-81. *An excellent review.*
Brooks DJ. Imaging approaches to Parkinson disease. *J Nucl Med.* 2010;51:596-609. *Overview of positron emission tomography and single-photon emission computed tomography.*
International Parkinson Disease Genomics Consortium. Imputation of sequence variants for indentification of genetic risks for Parkinson's disease: a meta-analysis of genome-wide association studies. *Lancet.* 2011;377:641-649. *Eleven loci were associated with risk for Parkinson's disease.*
Lang AE. When and how should treatment be started in Parkinson disease? *Neurology.* 2009;72:S39-S43. *A practical overview.*
Lees AJ, Hardy J, Revesz T. Parkinson's disease. *Lancet.* 2009;13:2055-2066. *Review.*

417

OTHER MOVEMENT DISORDERS

ANTHONY E. LANG

PROGNOSIS

Parkinson's disease progresses inexorably over a period of many years; the speed and course of progression vary considerably from patient to patient. Some patients maintain an excellent response to treatment and seem to change very little over prolonged follow-up, but most note increasing disability, with the development of many symptoms that are poorly responsive to medications. Factors such as poor postural stability, falls, dysarthria, dysphagia, dysautonomia, excessive daytime sleepiness, and dementia contribute to the disability and increased mortality.

FUTURE DIRECTIONS

Gene therapies directed at either modifying neurotransmitter function or inducing neuroregeneration and other cell-based therapies are under development. Future treatments must also address the widespread, multisystemic nature of the disease, especially symptoms that are unrelated to nigrostriatal dopamine deficiency and that fail to respond to current therapies.

DEFINITION

Movement disorders are first divided into hypokinetic and hyperkinetic categories. *Hypokinetic disorders,* which are characterized by akinesia, bradykinesia, and rigidity, are parkinsonian syndromes and are discussed elsewhere (Chapter 416). The common *hyperkinetic movement* disorders (Table 417-1) are defined by their specific clinical phenomena.

CLINICAL MANIFESTATIONS AND DIAGNOSTIC APPROACH

The traditional approach to a neurologic symptom is first to address localization within the nervous system (i.e., "Where is the lesion?"), followed by an evaluation of the origin ("What is the lesion?"). The neurologic examination is critical in determining the localization of the lesion, and generally the history, including the nature of onset and the progression of the symptoms, determines the most likely diagnosis. However, when a movement disorder is the predominant problem, the approach is somewhat different. The pathophysiology of most movement disorders is complex and often poorly understood. Many of these disorders are the result of dysfunction of different

TABLE 417-1 HYPERKINETIC MOVEMENT DISORDERS
Tremor
Chorea
Ballism
Dystonia
Athetosis
Tics
Myoclonus
Startle
Stereotypies
Miscellaneous

circuits in the brain, and it is often impossible to ascertain a specific anatomic localization. Instead, an accurate appreciation of the clinical phenomena is the first important step in evaluating these patients. The clinician must observe and examine the patient to define the type of movement disorder that best describes the clinical picture. This accurate characterization then allows the generation of a differential diagnosis for the specific movement disorder. The age and nature of onset, the distribution, the progression of symptoms, a family history of similar or related symptoms, and the presence of systemic signs then help to determine the most likely explanation for that movement disorder.

TREMOR

Tremor, which is a rhythmic, sinusoidal movement of a body part, is caused by regular, either synchronous or alternating, contractions of reciprocally innervated muscles. Tremors are classified based on whether they occur at rest (weight fully supported against gravity) or in action. Resting tremors are typically seen in Parkinson's disease and other parkinsonism syndromes (see Table 416-1 in Chapter 416). Action tremors are further divided into postural, kinetic, or intention tremors. A *postural tremor* is seen with the maintenance of a posture against gravity (e.g., when the arms are outstretched in front of the body). A *kinetic tremor* is seen with a voluntary movement of the limb (e.g., a tremor in an upper limb when performing the finger-to-nose test). An *intention tremor* increases in amplitude on approaching a target.

CLINICAL MANIFESTATIONS

Most action tremors (Table 417-2) combine postural and kinetic components. All tremors worsen with stress, including performing an affected activity in public. Initially, a tremor may be evident only when one attempts fine, dextrous tasks such as threading a needle, soldering, or using a screwdriver. More severe tremors interfere with activities such as handwriting, fastening buttons, shaving, eating soup with a spoon, or drinking from a cup. Patients often adapt or use compensatory measures, such as switching an activity to a less affected hand (e.g., shaving with the nondominant hand), using two hands to drink, drinking only from an incompletely filled glass or cup, or completely avoiding more challenging feeding activities in public. Severe action and intention tremors can cause handwriting to become completely illegible and can result in dependence on others for care.

Head tremors, which may be side to side, up and down, or mixed, are rarely disabling but are often a source of embarrassment. Tremor of the larynx, which causes the voice to quaver, is best appreciated by asking the patient to sustain a note. Action tremor of the lower limbs is assessed by having the patient hold the foot up to a target (e.g., the examiner's hand) and then perform a heel-knee-shin test.

Most upper limb action tremors affect many activities to a similar extent. Less commonly, tremors can affect a single task in isolation (*task-specific tremors*), the most common being a primary writing tremor. *Orthostatic tremor* is apparent in the legs and in antigravity muscles only when the patient is standing in one spot and subsides during walking or leaning against a wall; these patients commonly complain of a tremendous sense of insecurity while standing and a fear of falling. Electrophysiologic assessment demonstrates a very characteristic high-frequency tremor (14 to 16 Hz).

Enhanced Physiologic Tremor

A 7- to 12-Hz tremor is found in everyone on electrophysiologic recording. This physiologic tremor is enhanced and may become symptomatic in a

TABLE 417-2 DIFFERENTIAL DIAGNOSIS OF TREMOR AND RHYTHMIC MOVEMENT DISORDERS
ENHANCED PHYSIOLOGIC TREMOR
Metabolic disorders
Hyperthyroidism
Hyperparathyroidism
Hypoglycemia
Pheochromocytoma
Drugs
Caffeine
Theophylline
Amphetamines
Lithium
Valproic acid
Antidepressants
Amiodarone
β-Agonists
Others
Withdrawal of drugs
Benzodiazepines
Alcohol
Others
Fever, sepsis
Anxiety, stress, fatigue
PRIMARY OR IDIOPATHIC TREMOR
Essential tremor
Task-specific tremor
Orthostatic tremor
Idiopathic palatal tremor
TREMOR ASSOCIATED WITH CENTRAL NERVOUS SYSTEM DISEASES
Tremor with parkinsonian syndromes
Idiopathic Parkinson's disease
Multiple system atrophy
Progressive supranuclear palsy
Corticobasal degeneration
Neuroleptic-induced parkinsonism
Wilson's disease
Multiple sclerosis
Fragile X premutation-tremor/ataxia syndrome
Stroke
Arteriovenous malformation
Tumor
Head trauma
Midbrain tremor (Holmes' tremor)
TREMOR ASSOCIATED WITH PERIPHERAL NEUROPATHIES
PSYCHOGENIC TREMOR
OTHER RHYTHMIC MOVEMENT DISORDERS
Rhythmic movements in dystonia ("dystonic tremor")
Rhythmic myoclonus (including "myoclonic tremor")
Asterixis
Clonus
Epilepsia partialis continua
Hereditary chin quivering
Spasmus nutans
Head bobbing with hydrocephalus
Nystagmus

Adapted from Cloutier M, Lang AE. Movement disorders: an overview. In: Factor SA, Lang AE, Weiner WJ, eds. *Drug Induced Movement Disorders.* Malden, Mass: Blackwell; 2005:3-19.

variety of circumstances, including fatigue, anxiety, and excitement. This same tremor may be accentuated by drugs and systemic processes.

Essential Tremor

Essential tremor affects up to 5% of the general population after the age of 60 years. Essential tremor is often inherited in an autosomal dominant fashion, with the phenotype showing genetic heterogeneity from at least three different genes, most recently *LINGO1*, as well as environmental influences. Recent pathology studies have demonstrated microscopic abnormalities of cerebellar Purkinje cells. The age of onset may be as early as the first or second decade of life, but senile tremor may be delayed until the mid-60s. Patients first become aware of a mild postural and action tremor in the hands, which is indistinguishable from an enhanced physiologic tremor and may result in little functional impairment for many years until it gradually interferes with activities. Older patients with large-amplitude, lower-frequency tremors can have a resting component that is often misdiagnosed as Parkinson's disease (see Table 416-1 in Chapter 416). (Video 417-1).

TREATMENT   Rx

Treatment of essential tremor does not influence the course of the illness and therefore is justified only when the tremor interferes with function. At least 50% of patients note improvement or complete amelioration of tremor following the ingestion of a small amount of ethanol.

First-line drug treatment includes trials of a noncardioselective β-adrenergic blocker (e.g., propranolol, ≤320 mg/day) or primidone (starting in a low dose of 25 to 62.5 mg at night and increasing to 500 to 750 mg/day).◼ Other drugs that have been shown to be effective in double-blind crossover trials include gabapentin (1200 to 1800 mg/day), topiramate (≤400 mg/day), and alprazolam (0.125 to 3 mg/day),◼ but many patients remain resistant to all drugs. If disability is substantial, thalamic deep brain stimulation or thalamotomy can be of major benefit, but a few patients suffer permanent neurologic sequelae owing to intracranial hemorrhage or other postoperative complications.

● CHOREA

Chorea (Table 417-3) consists of irregular, random, brief, flowing movements that often flit from one body part to another in an unpredictable and purposeless sequence. Patients may incorporate choreiform movements into a voluntary movement to mask them. The severity varies from the appearance of being slightly fidgety or restless, to striking, continuous movements involving the whole body. Many patients with chorea seem unaware of their movements, whereas others can be very troubled and disabled.

Huntington's Disease

DEFINITION AND EPIDEMIOLOGY

Huntington's disease is a fully penetrant autosomal dominant neurodegenerative disorder caused by an expanded trinucleotide (CAG) repeat in the gene for the protein *huntingtin*. The prevalence is approximately 10 per 100,000.

PATHOBIOLOGY

Huntington's disease is characterized neuropathologically by neuronal loss accompanied by intraneuronal inclusions and gliosis, especially in the caudate nucleus and putamen (the striatum) and the cerebral cortex. Understanding how these changes result from the expanded polyglutamine tract in the mutated huntingtin protein is the goal of current research.

CLINICAL MANIFESTATIONS

Symptoms typically begin between the ages of 30 and 55 years, but 5 to 10% of patients have an onset before the age of 20 years (juvenile Huntington's disease), and a few patients begin to have symptoms quite late in life. Symptoms include a combination of a movement disorder, psychiatric disturbances, and cognitive dysfunction. Early on, the movement disorder is predominantly chorea, but parkinsonism and dystonia develop later (Video 417-2). Some patients, especially those with juvenile onset, have a more rapidly progressive akinetic-rigid and dystonic form (the Westphal variant). Psychiatric manifestations, which are universal but widely variable, include personality changes, impulsiveness, aggressive behavior, depression, and paranoid psychosis. These psychiatric symptoms may precede the motor manifestations, and psychotropic drug therapy may be incorrectly blamed for the subsequent development of the movement disorder. Cognitive changes result in progressive "subcortical dementia" with disturbed attention, concentration, judgment, and problem-solving that differs from the typical "cortical dementia" of Alzheimer's disease. Oculomotor dysfunction, most often manifested by difficulties with refixating the gaze and a resulting tendency to use blinks and head thrusts, is another common feature.

DIAGNOSIS

The diagnosis is confirmed by genetic testing. Normal alleles of the *IT15* gene have fewer than 30 CAG repeats, whereas 40 or more repeats invariably result in clinical illness. An earlier age of onset correlates with larger numbers of CAG repeats.

TABLE 417-3   DIFFERENTIAL DIAGNOSIS OF CHOREA

GENETIC DISORDERS

Benign hereditary chorea
Huntington's disease
Huntington-like conditions
Neuroferritinopathy
Neuroacanthocytosis including McLeod's syndrome
Dentatorubropallidoluysian atrophy
Wilson's disease
Neurodegeneration with Brain Iron Accumulation 1 (NBIA 1) (previously Hallervorden Spatz disease)
Spinocerebellar ataxias
Ataxia-telangiectasia
Ataxia-oculomotor apraxia type 1
Tuberous sclerosis

INFECTIONS/PARAINFECTIOUS CAUSES

Sydenham's chorea
Acquired immunodeficiency syndrome (including complications)
Encephalitis and postencephalitic disorders
Creutzfeldt-Jakob disease

DRUGS

Levodopa
Dopaminergic agonists used for Parkinson's disease
Amphetamines
Anticholinergics
Anticonvulsants (especially phenytoin)
Neuroleptics
Tricyclic antidepressants
Selective serotonin reuptake inhibitors (occasionally)
Oral contraceptives (typically in patients with a prior history of Sydenham's chorea)
Antihistaminics

ENDOCRINOLOGIC/METABOLIC CONDITIONS

Hyperthyroidism
Hypoparathyroidism
Chorea gravidarum
Acquired hepatolenticular degeneration

IMMUNOLOGIC DISORDERS

Systemic lupus erythematosus
Antiphospholipid syndrome
Henoch-Schönlein purpura

VASCULAR DISORDERS

Stroke
Hemorrhage
Arteriovenous malformation
Polycythemia rubra vera

OTHER CONDITIONS

Cerebral palsy
Kernicterus
Head trauma
Cardiopulmonary bypass with hypothermia
Neoplastic and paraneoplastic syndromes
Paroxysmal dyskinesias

Adapted from Cloutier M, Lang AE. Movement disorders: an overview. In: Factor SA, Lang AE, Weiner WJ, eds. *Drug Induced Movement Disorders.* Malden, Mass: Blackwell; 2005:3-19.

TREATMENT AND PROGNOSIS

Current care for patients with Huntington's disease involves a multidisciplinary team of clinical geneticists, neurologists, psychiatrists, psychologists, social workers, occupational and physical therapists, speech therapists, nutritionists, and nurses. Genetic counseling for patients and family members is critical. Chorea may be extremely responsive to drugs that reduce central dopamine activity, especially tetrabenazine, starting at 12.5 mg two or three times daily and gradually increasing to up to 200 mg per day.◼ Other potential agents include haloperidol (3 to 30 mg/day), pimozide (0.5 to 10 mg/day), fluphenazine (0.5 to 20 mg/day), and reserpine (0.75 to 5 mg/day). These agents should be reserved for patients with disabling chorea because they may be associated with increased parkinsonism, postural instability, depression, sedation, and other adverse effects. Unfortunately, physical function may not improve significantly even when the chorea is controlled. Psychiatric symptoms (e.g., anxiety, psychosis, depression) can be managed effectively with the same strategies as in other psychiatric diseases (Chapter 404). The disease progresses to institutionalization and death over the course of approximately 15 years.

Other Choreas

Most of the non-neurodegenerative causes of chorea (see Table 417-3) can be excluded by a careful history (including a detailed drug history) and a focused set of investigations, including, in appropriate circumstances, wet preparation of peripheral blood for acanthocytes, immunologic studies (including anticardiolipin antibodies), endocrine assessment (hyperthyroidism, pregnancy), and neuroimaging. *Sydenham's chorea*, which is a late component of rheumatic fever (Chapter 298), is presumably the result of immunologic cross-reactivity between the causative group A β-hemolytic streptococcus and the basal ganglia. This disorder is infrequently seen in North America but is more common in developing countries. Sydenham's chorea usually affects children and young adults, and it is more common in girls before puberty. Adults with a past history of Sydenham's chorea in childhood may develop chorea during pregnancy or in response to taking oral contraceptive agents or estrogen preparations. Drugs that can cause chorea should be withdrawn if possible.

Ballism

Ballism, which is considered an extreme form of chorea, involves large-amplitude, random, often violent flinging movements of the proximal limbs (Table 417-4). It is most often a consequence of an acute cerebral insult, such as a stroke, and it usually involves one side of the body, particularly the arm, hence the term *hemiballism* (Video 417-3). When a causative lesion can be demonstrated, it typically involves the region of the subthalamic nucleus or the striatum. When the condition is caused by a stroke, movements usually subside spontaneously over days to weeks, although they may persist indefinitely in some patients. Treatment often requires the use of medication that antagonizes the effects of dopamine in the brain, including dopamine receptor blockers (neuroleptics such as haloperidol, 3 to 30 mg/day) or dopamine depleters (e.g., tetrabenazine, 50 to 200 mg/day). Functional neurosurgery (e.g., pallidotomy, deep brain stimulation) can be considered in patients with refractory, persistent symptoms.

● DYSTONIA

DEFINITION AND PATHOBIOLOGY

In *dystonia*, sustained muscle contractions result in twisting and repetitive movements and abnormal postures. Dystonia can be classified according to its origin (Table 417-5). *Primary dystonia* includes syndromes in which the only phenotypic expressions are dystonia and tremor. These diseases can be hereditary or sporadic. *Dystonia-plus* is characterized by a combination of dystonia with other neurologic signs resulting from a known or presumed genetic defect without an underlying progressive neurodegenerative process; *dopa-responsive dystonia* and *myoclonus dystonia* are examples of such diseases. *Secondary dystonias* are the result of acquired injury to the central nervous system. *Heredodegenerative dystonias* include a large number of genetic as well as idiopathic neurodegenerative diseases.

CLINICAL MANIFESTATIONS

Common forms of dystonia include eyelid closure (blepharospasm), jaw opening or closing (oromandibular dystonia), pulling or turning of the neck

in any one or combination of directions (cervical dystonia: rotatory torticollis, laterocollis, retrocollis, anterocollis), hyperadduction and less often excessive abduction of the vocal cords (laryngeal dystonia or spasmodic dysphonia), abnormal posturing and tightness of the hand while writing or using the hand for other tasks (writer's cramp, manual dystonia), abnormal posturing of the trunk or pelvis (axial dystonia), or abnormal posturing of the lower limb, including plantar flexion and inversion of the foot (Videos 417-4 through 417-7). The movements are often slow and sustained, although they may also be rapid (*dystonic spasms*). Slower, sinuous writhing dystonic movements, particularly present in the distal limbs, are referred to as *athetosis*. Dystonia is often made worse by activity (*action dystonia*), and a unique aspect of dystonia is that only selected acts may be affected, with complete sparing of all other activities in the same limb (*task-specific dystonia*, including *writer's cramp* and *musician's cramp*) (Video 417-8). In some patients, dystonia remains isolated and action specific over many years, whereas in others, it progresses to involve adjacent muscles (*overflow dystonia*) and may eventually be present at rest, in which case joint contractures may result. Another common feature of dystonia is its transient improvement with the use of a sensory trick (*geste antagoniste*), such as lightly touching the chin to relieve severe cervical dystonia or the lid to relieve disabling blepharospasm (Video 417-9). Patients with dystonia, independent of cause, often have additional postural and action tremors, phenotypically similar to essential tremor. Some patients also demonstrate more irregular, coarse, lower-frequency rhythmic movements called *dystonic tremor*.

Dystonia is often classified according to the site of involvement: focal, only one body part (e.g., blepharospasm, cervical dystonia, writer's cramp); segmental, two or more contiguous body parts; multifocal, two or more noncontiguous body parts; generalized, legs and other body areas; and hemidystonia, unilateral (generally a causative focal brain lesion is found most often involving the putamen).

DIAGNOSIS AND PROGNOSIS

For diagnostic and prognostic purposes, dystonia also may be distinguished by age of onset as childhood-onset, adolescent-onset, or adult-onset dystonia. The younger the age of onset, the more likely that a cause can be defined. Conversely, isolated dystonia beginning in adult life is most often an idiopathic disorder; further investigations are typically unrewarding and are usually not indicated. Likewise, independent of the cause, dystonia beginning in childhood commonly progresses to segmental or generalized involvement, whereas adult-onset dystonia usually remains focal or segmental.

Specific Dystonias
PRIMARY (IDIOPATHIC) DYSTONIAS

Primary dystonia accounts for up to 90% of patients with a pure dystonic syndrome. To date, no consistent neuropathologic changes have been found in the small numbers of brains affected by primary dystonia that have been studied.

When symptoms begin in *childhood*, a definable genetic cause is often identified, the most common being DYT1 resulting from the autosomal dominant inheritance of a GAG deletion in the *torsin A* gene (*Oppenheim's dystonia*). This disorder is more common in persons of Ashkenazi Jewish descent. The dystonia often begins in the first decade of life and can progress to severe disability, although the spectrum of disease, even within the same family, can be quite varied, and penetrance is relatively low (~40%) (Video 417-10). Genetic testing is available but is recommended only when the age of onset in the patient or another affected family member is less than 26 years. Increasing numbers of other genetic forms of primary dystonia, most recently *THAP1* for DYT6, are being defined, but genetic testing is not yet available for most of them.

ADULT-ONSET IDIOPATHIC DYSTONIA

Adult-onset idiopathic dystonia is the most common type of dystonia seen in general neurologic practice. The dystonia typically begins in the face, neck, or arm and may remain focal and nonprogressive or spread only to contiguous muscles after many years. The cause of this disorder is not known, although a positive family history may be noted if multiple family members can be examined.

DYSTONIA-PLUS

Dopa-responsive dystonia, which usually results in dystonia beginning in the first decade of life, most often in the lower limbs, sometimes can be mistaken for hereditary spastic paraplegia or cerebral palsy. Most patients with

TABLE 417-5 CLASSIFICATION AND CAUSES OF DYSTONIA

PRIMARY DYSTONIAS (PRIMARY TORSION DYSTONIA)	HEREDODEGENERATIVE DYSTONIAS

Familial (several genetic causes and types)
Sporadic, usually adult onset, focal, or segmental
	X-linked
	  Lubag disease
	  Deafness-dystonia-optic atrophy (Mohr-Tranebjaerg) syndrome
	  Pelizaeus-Merzbacher disease
	  Lesch-Nyhan syndrome

DYSTONIA-PLUS	Autosomal dominant Rapid-onset dystonia-parkinsonism

Dystonia with parkinsonism
  Dopa-responsive dystonia
  Dopamine agonist–responsive dystonia (e.g., aromatic acid decarboxylase deficiency)
Myoclonus dystonia
	Juvenile parkinsonism (e.g., from mutations in the parkin gene)
	  Huntington's disease
	  Machado-Joseph disease (SCA3) and other SCAs
	  Dentatorubropallidoluysian atrophy

SECONDARY DYSTONIAS	Autosomal recessive
	  Wilson's disease
	  Niemann-Pick disease type C

Perinatal cerebral injury
  Athetoid cerebral palsy
  Delayed-onset dystonia
  Pachygyria
  Kernicterus
	GM1 gangliosidosis
	  GM2 gangliosidosis
	  Metachromatic leukodystrophy
	  Homocystinuria
	  Glutaric acidemia

Encephalitis
  Reye's syndrome
  Subacute sclerosing leukoencephalopathy
  Wasp sting
  Creutzfeldt-Jakob disease
  Human immunodeficiency virus infection
	Triose-phosphate isomerase deficiency
	  Hartnup's disease
	  Ataxia-telangiectasia
	  Neurodegeneration with Brain Iron Accumulation (NBIA 1) (previously Hallervorden Spatz disease)
	  Juvenile neuronal ceroid lipofuscinosis

Head trauma
Thalamotomy
Brain stem lesion
Primary antiphospholipid syndrome
Stroke
Arteriovenous malformation
Hypoxia
	Neuroacanthocytosis
	  Intranuclear hyaline inclusion disease
	  Hereditary spastic paraplegia with dystonia
	Probably autosomal recessive
	  Familial basal ganglia calcifications (also dominantly inherited)
	  Progressive pallidal degeneration
	  Rett's syndrome

Brain tumor
Multiple sclerosis
Central pontine myelinolysis
Cervical cord injury
Peripheral injury
Drugs
Toxins
Hypoparathyroidism
Psychogenic conditions
	Mitochondrial
	  Leigh's disease
	  Leber's disease
	  Other mitochondrial cytopathies
	Sporadic, with parkinsonism
	  Parkinson's disease
	  Progressive supranuclear palsy
	  Multiple system atrophy
	  Corticobasal degeneration

Adapted from Cloutier M, Lang AE. Movement disorders: an overview. In: Factor SA, Lang AE, Weiner WJ, eds. *Drug Induced Movement Disorders*. Malden, Mass: Blackwell; 2005:3-19.

dopa-responsive dystonia have a mutation in the *GCH1* gene, which results in reduced production of dopamine. Approximately 75% of patients have notable worsening of dystonia as the day progresses (*diurnal variation*). Exercise often aggravates the dystonia. Patients commonly demonstrate some degree of bradykinesia (especially in the legs) and postural instability. Rare adult-onset disease may result in a pure parkinsonian phenotype. Dopa-responsive dystonia should be considered in all children with dystonia. Symptoms are exquisitely sensitive to low doses of levodopa (typically as little as 50 mg/day of levodopa), and this treatment allows patients to live a normal life without the usual complications seen in Parkinson's disease (Chapter 416).

Myoclonus dystonia, which usually begins within the first decade of life, combines dystonia with separate multifocal myoclonic jerks. Myoclonus dystonia is genetically heterogeneous; the most common definable cause is a mutation in the *e-sarcoglycan* gene. The dystonia in these patients most often involves the neck or upper limbs, is mild, and is often overlooked. The disorder can also include psychopathology, such as obsessive-compulsive behavior. A characteristic feature of this disorder is the marked ameliorative effect of ethanol on both the myoclonus and the dystonia, a feature that sometimes results in alcohol abuse.

OTHER DYSTONIAS

Dystonia may be a symptom of many diseases. The nature and extent of the investigations undertaken depend on such factors as age of onset, clues provided on the history, and additional neurologic or systemic features on examination. *Wilson's disease* (Chapter 218) is an important consideration in the diagnosis of dystonia beginning in children and young adults.

Some patients with dystonia, chorea, or a mixture of the two ("choreoathetosis") have intermittent symptoms (*paroxysmal dyskinesias*) and may be normal between episodes. The duration of symptoms can be as brief as a few seconds to a few minutes or persist for several hours. Symptoms triggered by sudden movement, which are termed *kinesigenic*, are typically brief; prolonged episodes are commonly triggered by exercise, stress, fatigue, caffeine, or alcohol. These paroxysmal dyskinesias may be genetically determined, idiopathic, the manifestation of another disorder (e.g., head injury, brain tumor, or stroke), or even psychologically based.

TREATMENT Rx

Ideally, treatment is directed at the underlying cause, such as dopa-responsive dystonia, which is treated with levodopa (usually up to 300 mg per day) or Wilson's disease (Chapter 218). Unfortunately, cause-specific treatment usually is not possible, so a variety of symptomatic treatments may be tried, often unsuccessfully, in an attempt to reduce disability.

Focal injections of botulinum toxin are now usually the first choice for treatment of focal and segmental dystonias.[3] This approach can improve the condition of patients with cranial (blepharospasm, oromandibular dystonia) and cervical dystonia. Patients with task-specific limb dystonias (e.g., writer's cramp) often benefit less because weakness of the treated muscles, which is the most common side effect of this therapy, can impair other important upper limb functions.

Young patients in particular can tolerate and benefit from high doses of anticholinergic drugs such as trihexyphenidyl (6 to 40 mg/day, but sometimes as much as 100 mg/day). Muscle relaxants, including benzodiazepines (diazepam, 5 to as much as 100 mg/day) and baclofen (40 to 120 mg/day), may provide some benefit. Dopamine-depleting (e.g., tetrabenazine, 50 to 200 mg/

day) and dopamine-blocking (e.g., haloperidol, 3 to 30 mg/day) agents are occasionally helpful (more often effective in tardive dystonia than in other types). Neurosurgical treatments, particularly deep brain stimulation of the internal segment of the globus pallidus, can be considered in medically refractory, disabling dystonia, especially in patients with idiopathic dystonia (e.g., DYT1, adult-onset cervical dystonia).

TICS

EPIDEMIOLOGY AND PATHOBIOLOGY

Tics are repetitive, stereotyped movements (motor tics) or vocalizations (vocal tics). Transient tics are extremely common in childhood, and simple tics may begin in childhood and persist throughout adult life. Most tics (Table 417-6) are primary or idiopathic and have no identifiable cause. Secondary tics are caused by a defined underlying brain disease or environmental factor.

CLINICAL MANIFESTATIONS

Tics vary in terms of complexity, from abrupt, brief, meaningless movements or sounds (*simple motor tics* such as eye blinking, nose wrinkling, or head jerking; *simple vocal-phonic tics* such as sniffing, throat clearing, or grunting) to more sustained, more deliberate, almost meaningful gestures or utterances (*complex motor tics* such as touching, hand shaking, and jumping; *complex vocal tics* such as echolalia [repeating others], palilalia [repeating oneself],

TABLE 417-6	ETIOLOGIC CLASSIFICATION OF TICS

PRIMARY OR IDIOPATHIC TICS

Transient motor or phonic tics
Chronic motor or phonic tics
Adult-onset tics
Tourette's syndrome

SECONDARY TICS

Genetic disorders
  Neuroacanthocytosis
  Huntington's disease
  Neurodegeneration with Brain Iron Accumulation 1 (NBIA 1) (previously
    Hallervorden Spatz disease)
  Idiopathic dystonia*
  Tuberous sclerosis*
Chromosomal disorders
Infections
  Sydenham's chorea
  PANDAS†
  Encephalitis and postencephalitic disorders
  Creutzfeldt-Jakob disease
  Neurosyphilis
Drugs
  Methylphenidate
  Amphetamines
  Cocaine
  Levodopa
  Carbamazepine
  Phenytoin
  Phenobarbital
  Lamotrigine
  Neuroleptics
Developmental disorders
  Mental retardation
  Pervasive developmental disorders/autism
Other causes
  Head trauma
  Stroke
  Carbon monoxide poisoning
  Cardiopulmonary bypass with hypothermia

RELATED DISORDERS

Mannerisms, stereotypies
Compulsions
Self-injurious behavior

*Tics have been described with these conditions but may simply be coincidental.
†Pediatric autoimmune neuropsychiatric disorders associated with streptococcal infections. The existence of this disorder remains somewhat controversial.
Adapted from Cloutier M, Lang AE. Movement disorders: an overview. In: Factor SA, Lang AE, Weiner WJ, eds. *Drug Induced Movement Disorders.* Malden, Mass: Blackwell; 2005:3-19.

and coprolalia [uttering profanities]). The frequency of the tics in an individual patient varies markedly over minutes, hours, days, weeks, and years.

DIAGNOSIS

Various characteristics help to differentiate tics from other abnormal movements. Tics are often described by patients as being "semivoluntary" in response to an inner, irresistible urge. Premonitory sensory symptoms occasionally precede the tic, generally in the same general anatomic area as the tic itself. Relief is often associated with the production of the tic. Tics can be partially or completely voluntarily suppressed for variable periods, but often at the expense of mounting inner tension and psychological discomfort. Performing the tic or sometimes even substituting another more acceptable behavior for the socially inappropriate tic alleviates the tension. Many patients report that some tics occur in response to a typical urge, whereas the same or different tics may be unexpected and totally involuntary.

Tourette's Syndrome

EPIDEMIOLOGY AND PATHOBIOLOGY

The exact relationship between childhood tics and Gilles de la Tourette's syndrome remains uncertain. Tourette's syndrome is a common disorder, with prevalence estimates varying from 10 to 700 per 100,000. There is a male preponderance of 3:1 for the classic syndrome, but female patients manifest obsessive-compulsive features more often than tics. A functional mutation in the *HDC* gene encoding L-histidine decarboxylase can result in Tourette's syndrome, thereby suggesting a role for histaminic neurotransmission in its pathogenesis (Video 417-11).

CLINICAL MANIFESTATIONS AND DIAGNOSIS

The criteria for this disorder include the presence of multiple motor and at least one vocal tic beginning before the age of 21 years (typically between ages 2 and 10 years) and lasting for more than 1 year, waxing and waning symptoms over time (new tics replacing old ones; previous tics sometimes recurring years after they had originally resolved), and the absence of other explanatory medical conditions. Involuntary swearing (coprolalia), a highly publicized feature of the syndrome, is present in fewer than 10% of patients and is usually manifested by aborted forms such as "fu" and "shi." Patients commonly exhibit a variety of comorbid disorders including obsessive-compulsive disorder, attention-deficit disorder (with or without hyperactivity), impulse control problems, and other behavioral disturbances.

TREATMENT

Most patients who fulfill diagnostic criteria for Tourette's syndrome have mild symptoms that do not require treatment; education, reassurance, behavioral therapy, [5] and follow-up are often sufficient. When tics (isolated or as part of Tourette's syndrome) interfere with social and physical function, low-dose clonazepam (0.5 to 4 mg/day) may be effective. Clonidine (0.05 to 0.5 mg/day) is variably effective in controlling tics and may be useful for impulse control and symptoms of attention-deficit/hyperactivity disorder (ADHD); alternatively, guanfacine (0.5 to 4 mg/day) can be used. The most effective treatments for disabling tics are the dopamine receptor blockers such as risperidone (0.5 to 16 mg/day), haloperidol (0.5 to 20 mg/day), pimozide (0.5 to 10 mg/day), fluphenazine (0.5 to 20 mg/day), and aripiprazole (5 to 15 mg/day), but caution is required in view of the potential for important side effects, including tardive dyskinesia, with long-term use. An alternative without this complication is the dopamine depleter tetrabenazine (50 to 200 mg/day dopamine). Injected botulinum toxin may be effective for simple motor tics of the face and neck and may also reduce the urge to perform the tic. Comorbid ADHD can be treated safely with stimulant therapy (e.g., methylphenidate, 2.5 to 60 mg/day) without a significant risk for increasing the severity of tics. Obsessive-compulsive symptoms may respond well to selective serotonin reuptake inhibitors (e.g., clomipramine, 25 to 250 mg/day; paroxetine, 10 to 60 mg/day; or citalopram, 10 to 40 mg/day). Behavioral disorders, which remain a major therapeutic challenge, may require a variety of psychotherapeutic or behavioral modification approaches. Promising preliminary reports of deep brain stimulation require confirmation in controlled clinical trials.

PROGNOSIS

The natural history of Tourette's syndrome is to stabilize and often improve in adolescence. Approximately 50% of patients have a complete or partial remission at this time.

TABLE 417-7 CLASSIFICATION AND CAUSES OF MYOCLONUS

PHYSIOLOGIC MYOCLONUS

Sleep myoclonus
Anxiety-induced myoclonus
Exercise-induced myoclonus
Hiccups
Benign infantile myoclonus during feeding

ESSENTIAL MYOCLONUS

Essential myoclonus*
   Hereditary
   Sporadic
Myoclonus dystonia*

EPILEPTIC MYOCLONUS

Fragments of epilepsy
   Isolated epileptic myoclonic jerks
   Photosensitive myoclonus
   Myoclonic absences
   Epilepsia partialis continua
   Idiopathic stimulus-sensitive myoclonus
Childhood myoclonic epilepsies
   Infantile spasms
   Lennox-Gastaut syndrome
   Cryptogenic myoclonus epilepsy
   Juvenile myoclonic epilepsy of Janz
Benign familial myoclonic epilepsy
Baltic myoclonus (Unverricht-Lundborg)

SYMPTOMATIC MYOCLONUS

Storage disease
   Lafora body disease
   Lipidoses
   Neuronal ceroid lipofuscinosis
   Sialidosis
Spinocerebellar degeneration
   Friedreich's ataxia
   Ataxia-telangiectasia
   Other spinocerebellar degenerations
Basal ganglia degenerations
   Wilson's disease
   Idiopathic torsion dystonia
   Neurodegeneration with Brain Iron Accumulation 1 (NBIA 1)
      (Hallervorden-Spatz disease)
   Progressive supranuclear palsy
   Corticobasal degeneration
   Parkinson's disease
   Multiple system atrophy
   Huntington's disease
   Dentatorubropallidoluysian atrophy

Mitochondrial cytopathies
Dementias
   Alzheimer's disease
   Creutzfeldt-Jakob disease
   Dementia with Lewy bodies
Viral encephalopathies
   Subacute sclerosing panencephalitis
   Encephalitis lethargica
   Herpes simplex encephalitis
   Arbovirus encephalitis
   Human immunodeficiency virus infection
   Postinfectious encephalitis
Metabolic disorders
   Hepatic failure
   Renal failure
   Dialysis dysequilibrium syndrome
   Hyponatremia
   Hypoglycemia
   Nonketotic hyperglycemia
   Infantile myoclonic encephalopathy
   Multiple carboxylase deficiency
   Biotin deficiency
Toxins
   Bismuth
   Heavy-metal poisoning
   Methylbromide, dichlorodiphenyltrichloroethane (DDT)
   Drugs (multiple)
Physical encephalopathies
   Posthypoxic myoclonus (Lance-Adams)
   Post-traumatic status
   Heat stroke
   Electric shock
   Decompression injury
Focal central nervous system damage
   Stroke
   Post-thalamotomy status
   Tumor
   Trauma
   Spinal cord lesions
Paraneoplastic syndromes
Psychogenic myoclonus

*Probably represents the same entity.
Adapted from Cloutier M, Lang AE. Movement disorders: an overview. In: Factor SA, Lang AE, Weiner WJ, eds. *Drug Induced Movement Disorders*. Malden, Mass: Blackwell; 2005:3-19.

MYOCLONUS

DEFINITION

Myoclonus (or myoclonic jerks) consists of sudden, brief, shocklike, involuntary movements that result from both active muscle contraction (positive myoclonic jerks) and brief inhibition of ongoing muscle activity (negative myoclonic jerks). The most common form of negative myoclonic jerk is *asterixis*.

PATHOBIOLOGY

Myoclonus generally arises in the central nervous system, although rare peripheral causes are described, and it is distinct from abnormal muscle activity associated with peripheral nervous system diseases, such as fasciculations or myokymia. Myoclonus can be classified according to origin (Table 417-7), including physiologic, essential, epileptic, and symptomatic forms. Physiologic myoclonus, such as hypnic (sleep) jerks and hiccups, occurs in normal healthy subjects. Patients with essential myoclonus, which may be sporadic or inherited, often have additional postural tremor or dystonia, and this disorder is probably the same as what is now referred to as *myoclonus dystonia* (see Dystonias, earlier). Epileptic myoclonus arises in the context of seizures (Chapter 410), including many inherited generalized epileptic syndromes and the progressive myoclonic epilepsies. Symptomatic myoclonus occurs in association with a large number of encephalopathic states.

CLINICAL MANIFESTATIONS AND DIAGNOSIS

Myoclonic jerks are very short, typically lasting less then 150 milliseconds. Myoclonus can be spontaneous, action induced, or reflex (induced by various sensory stimuli), or a combination. Spontaneous myoclonus occurs at rest, without any provocation. Action myoclonus occurs during purposeful movement and is often very disabling owing to its interference with volitional activity. Reflex myoclonus can be triggered by visual, auditory, or somesthetic stimuli. The distribution of myoclonus may be focal, segmental, multifocal, or generalized. When myoclonus involves more than one body area, the movements may be synchronous or asynchronous. Myoclonus can be intermittent or repetitive, and it sometimes is rhythmic (e.g., usually originating in the brain stem or spinal cord). *Palatal myoclonus*, recently redesignated as *palatal tremor*, is a rhythmic movement disorder originating in the brain stem and involving the soft palate as well as the eyes, facial muscles, neck, and limbs; it is commonly the result of a focal lesion (e.g., stroke, demyelination) in the connections between the dentate nucleus of the cerebellum and the inferior olives of the medulla (*symptomatic palatal tremor*).

DIAGNOSIS

Myoclonus can be classified according to the anatomic site of origin, usually with the assistance of detailed electrophysiologic assessments. These sites may be cortical, subcortical (e.g., thalamus; lower brain stem [reticular myoclonus]), or spinal (two types: spinal segmental and propriospinal).

TREATMENT

Management of myoclonus, when possible, should be directed specifically at the underlying cause. Drug treatment includes a variety of anticonvulsant medications, most notably clonazepam (1.5 to 15 mg/day), valproic acid (10 to 15 mg/kg/day), carbamazepine (600 to 1200 mg/day), and levetiracetam (1000 to 4000 mg/day). Postanoxic action myoclonus (the Lance-Adams syndrome) in some patients who survive severe cerebral anoxia may also respond to 5-hydroxytryptophan (400 to 2800 mg/day) given with carbidopa (75 to 300 mg/day). Acetazolamide (250 to 1000 mg/day) may be useful for patients with action myoclonus.

HYPEREXPLEXIA

A disorder related to myoclonus, known as *hyperexplexia,* manifests as excessive response to startle. It may be inherited (startle disease, most often caused by a mutation in the α_1-subunit of the glycine receptor gene). Some patients demonstrate only generalized body jerking or an exaggerated startle response that habituates poorly after repeated stimuli. Others also experience disabling stiffness in response to sudden unexpected stimuli such as loud sound. The disorder responds well to clonazepam (1.5 to 15 mg/day) therapy.

OTHER MOVEMENT DISORDERS
Drug-Induced Movement Disorders

All the movements listed in Table 417-1 can be induced by medications. Neuroleptic drugs, which block postsynaptic dopamine receptors, particularly the D2 subtype, can result in a variety of movement disorder syndromes, including acute dystonic reactions, akathisia, drug-induced parkinsonism (including "the rabbit syndrome" with perinasal and perioral rest tremor), the neuroleptic malignant syndrome, and a variety of later-onset, often persistent, movements referred to as *tardive dyskinesia.*

ACUTE DYSTONIC REACTIONS

Acute dystonic reactions are most often seen in young patients who are receiving potent antipsychotic agents (e.g., young male patients receiving high doses of haloperidol for acute psychosis), but they also occur in patients receiving dopamine receptor blockers, including metoclopramide as antiemetic therapy. Symptoms range from overt dystonic postures of the face and neck, to involuntary prolonged deviation of the eyes (oculogyric crises), to simple slurring of speech and difficulty coordinating the tongue. Symptoms often vary from moment to moment and can increase with anxiety and improve with relaxation or reassurance. Acute dystonic reactions are self-limited and respond rapidly to a parenteral injection of an anticholinergic drug such as benztropine (2 mg intravenously followed by 2 mg three times daily orally for a variable duration depending on neuroleptic use) or an antihistaminic such as diphenhydramine (50 mg intravenously followed by oral benztropine).

AKATHISIA

Akathisia refers to a sense of restlessness and a need to move. Typically, the patient performs a variety of purposeful or semipurposeful, often complex, movements in response to an uncomfortable subjective restlessness, including pacing when standing, marching in place, rocking, shifting weight, moving legs when sitting, picking at clothing or hair, rubbing body parts with hands, and other similar movements. Akathisia is most often a side effect of medications, especially neuroleptic drugs and selective serotonin reuptake inhibitors (Chapter 404). Symptoms occur in a dose-related fashion and usually resolve on drug withdrawal. Akathisia is a common reason for psychiatric patients to comply poorly with their medications; management includes adjustment of the dose or type of antipsychotic agent and trials of β-blockers (e.g., propranolol, 80 mg/day) or antiparkinson agents, such as anticholinergics (e.g., benztropine (6 mg/day) or amantadine (200 to 300 mg/day). Rare patients experience a very disabling and persistent form referred to as *tardive akathisia.* Akathisia is also sometimes seen in patients with Parkinson's disease.

NEUROLEPTIC MALIGNANT SYNDROME

The *neuroleptic malignant syndrome* (Chapters 440 and 442) is an uncommon but severe, sometimes fatal, complication of neuroleptic therapy. Patients usually manifest a combination of features including fever, marked rigidity, changes in level of arousal, and autonomic instability. Laboratory abnormalities include a marked increase in the serum creatine kinase level and the blood leukocyte count. Management involves early recognition, withdrawal of the causative agent, systemic supportive therapy, a dopamine agonist (most experience has been with the older agent bromocriptine, ≤60 mg/day), and, when necessary, dantrolene sodium (50 to 600 mg/day orally or ≤10 mg/kg/day intravenously) to reduce muscle contraction.

TARDIVE DYSKINESIA
EPIDEMIOLOGY AND PATHOBIOLOGY

The term *tardive dyskinesia* encompasses a wide variety of abnormal movements caused by chronic neuroleptic therapy. The cumulative 5-year incidence rate in patients taking classic neuroleptics is approximately 25%, and the incidence may continue to increase almost linearly beyond that point. The propensity to develop tardive dyskinesia on newer atypical neuroleptics appears to be much lower (Video 417-12).

CLINICAL MANIFESTATIONS

Tardive dyskinesia generally begins after a minimum of 6 weeks of treatment. One of the most common forms involves the lower facial muscles and has been given a variety of names, including *orobuccolinguomasticatory dyskinesia.* The movements generally include repetitive chewing and smacking movements with the tongue either protruding between the lips (fly-catching movements) or pushing into the cheek (bonbon sign). Although the movements are somewhat choreic, they are not as random as true chorea. The more stereotypical, repetitive nature of the movements, involving not only face but also the limbs (e.g., piano playing movements of the fingers, rocking or thrusting of the pelvis), has encouraged the more recent term *tardive stereotypies.* Many patients with classic orofacial tardive dyskinesia seem unaware of the presence of the movements and are not disabled by them, but others are embarrassed or otherwise impaired.

Tardive akathisia and tardive dystonia are less common but particularly disabling subtypes of tardive dyskinesia. Rarer forms include tardive tics (tourettism), tardive tremor, tardive myoclonus, and even tardive oral or genital pain.

TREATMENT AND PROGNOSIS

Treatment is often unsatisfactory, but the dopamine depleter tetrabenazine (50 to 200 mg/day) can be very effective. Prevention is the most important consideration. The physician must regularly reassess the need for ongoing neuroleptic therapy, consider switching to an atypical agent when possible (particularly quetiapine and clozapine; Chapter 404), and routinely evaluate the patient for the presence of early subtle clinical features, such as mild pursing of the lips or rolling movements of the tongue in the mouth. Unfortunately, tardive dyskinesia may persist for many years despite withdrawal of neuroleptic treatment in up to 50% of patients. Several atypical neuroleptics, such as risperidone and olanzapine, nevertheless block dopamine D2 receptors sufficiently to cause drug-induced parkinsonism and tardive dyskinesias.

Restless Legs Syndrome
EPIDEMIOLOGY

Restless legs syndrome (Chapter 412) is now recognized as an extremely common disorder affecting between 3 and 29% of the general population. Women are affected more frequently than men. Although the incidence increases with age, it can also affect children, in whom it may be confused with "growing pains" or ADHD.

PATHOBIOLOGY

Restless legs syndrome is most often primary or idiopathic, in which case it is frequently inherited in an autosomal dominant fashion. Five genetic loci associated with restless legs syndrome by recent genome-wide studies are variants in MEIS1, BTBD9, MAP2K5/LBXCOR1, and PTPRD. Restless legs syndrome also may be secondary to other causes, including peripheral neuropathy, uremia, pregnancy, and iron deficiency, and it may occur more commonly than by chance in some neurodegenerative disorders such as Parkinson's disease. The pathophysiology of restless legs syndrome is uncertain, but central iron dysregulation may somehow alter central dopamine. Serum ferritin levels are often low, even in the presence of normal values of hemoglobin, hematocrit, iron, and iron-binding capacity.

CLINICAL MANIFESTATIONS AND DIAGNOSIS

In restless legs syndrome, as in akathisia, movements occur because of the subjective need to move. However, unlike in akathisia, the patient typically complains of a variety of sensory disturbances in the legs, including pins and needles, creeping or crawling sensations, aching, itching, stabbing, heaviness, tension, burning, or coldness. Occasionally, similar symptoms are appreciated in the upper limbs. These symptoms are usually experienced during periods of prolonged inactivity, especially with recumbency in the evening, and are often associated with insomnia (Chapter 412). The discomfort appears particularly during the transition from wake to sleep in the evening and often follows a circadian pattern, peaking between midnight and 4 A.M. Symptoms are typically relieved only by movement or stimulation of the legs; although these maneuvers are effective while they are being performed, the discomfort usually returns as soon as the individual becomes inactive or returns to bed to try to sleep. Patients often have significant problems with immobility during long automobile drives or plane flights.

In approximately 80% of patients, this condition is associated with another movement disorder, periodic leg movements in sleep, sometimes inappropriately called nocturnal myoclonus. These periodic, slow, sustained (1 to 2 seconds) movements range from synchronous or asynchronous dorsiflexion of the toes and feet to triple flexion of one or both legs. In 15% of patients, more rapid myoclonic movements or slower, prolonged dystonic-like movements of the feet and legs are present while patients are awake. In the absence of evidence of a secondary cause of restless legs syndrome, the only useful routine test is a serum ferritin level.

TREATMENT Rx

Dopamine agonists (e.g., pramipexole, 0.125 to 1.5 mg at bedtime) and ropinirole (1 to 4 mg at bedtime) are the treatments of choice in moderate to severe restless legs syndrome and can be very effective.[6] Levodopa preparations (100 to 300 mg of levodopa at bedtime; consider controlled-release preparation) are also effective but are more often associated with disabling rebound symptoms early in the morning or during the day (augmentation). A new nondopaminergic agent, XP13512, is also effective, but is not yet approved in the United States.[7] Patients with milder symptoms may respond to gabapentin (300 to 2400 mg/day). Opiate agonists (e.g., oxycodone, 5 mg at bedtime; codeine, 30 mg at bedtime; propoxyphene, 65 mg or N-100 mg at bedtime) and less often benzodiazepines (e.g., clonazepam, 0.5 to 2 mg at bedtime) may also be effective. Tolerance or loss of original benefit may occur with all these treatments. Iron replacement is indicated in patients with reduced serum ferritin levels (325 mg ferrous sulfate two to three times per day for 3 to 4 months until ferritin levels exceed 50 mg/L and iron saturations surpass 20%).

Painful Legs and Moving Toes

Another uncommon but well-defined movement disorder of the lower limbs has been termed *painful legs and moving toes*. Patients typically complain of a deep pulling or searing pain in the lower limbs, associated with continuous involuntary wriggling or writhing of the toes. Occasionally, the ankle and less commonly more proximal muscles of the legs are involved. Rarely, a similar problem is seen in the upper limbs as well. Various treatments have been tried without much benefit to the pain, which is typically the major concern of the patient.

Other Abnormal Movements

Numerous abnormal movements are caused by dysfunction of the peripheral nerves (e.g., fasciculations, myokymia); these movements are usually easily separated from the movement disorders described earlier. *Hemifacial spasm* is a common disorder in which irregular clonic and tonic movements involve the muscles innervated by the facial nerve, usually owing to compression of the seventh nerve as it exits the brain stem, most often by a normal small artery or vein and less often by a mass lesion or inflammatory process. Eyelid twitching is usually the first symptom, followed at variable intervals by lower facial muscle involvement. A magnetic resonance image with careful assessment of the posterior fossa is necessary to exclude secondary causes. Treatment usually involves injections of botulinum toxin into selected facial muscles, although surgical decompression can be curative (Video 417-13).

Hereditary Cerebellar Ataxias and Spastic Paraplegias
CEREBELLAR ATAXIAS

The hereditary cerebellar ataxias, which may begin in childhood or adulthood, can progress at widely varying rates. These ataxias are divided into early-onset ataxias, which are usually inherited as autosomal recessive disorders, and adult-onset ataxias, which are usually autosomal dominant. A small number are X-linked. Because most of these ataxias are untreatable, it is important to recognize the rare causes of treatable or preventable progressive ataxias.

Friedreich's Ataxia

EPIDEMIOLOGY AND PATHOBIOLOGY

The most common progressive inherited ataxia in children is Friedreich's ataxia. Friedreich's ataxia is a trinucleotide-repeat disorder that affects the central and peripheral nervous systems, the heart, and many other organs. Friedreich's ataxia is an autosomal recessive disorder with no anticipation. It has an estimated carrier frequency in the population of about 1 in 100 and a resulting disease prevalence of about 1 per 50,000.

The normal length of the GAA repeat on the long arm of chromosome 9 (9q13-q21) is 10 to 21 copies, but expansion in individuals with Friedreich's ataxia results in 200 to 900 copies and disrupts the expression of the protein frataxin. GAA unstable expansion, which occurs on an intron, leads to gene silencing rather than to the production of an abnormal protein. Higher numbers of copies correlate with more severe neurologic deficits. Frataxin appears to be critical for iron export and mitochondrial function. Because accumulation of mitochondrial iron affects the production of oxygen radicals, loss of frataxin may lead to oxidative mitochondrial damage. The pathology of Friedreich's ataxia includes spinal cord atrophy, which often is evident on magnetic resonance imaging, with loss of neurons in Clarke's columns and the dorsal root ganglia. Degeneration occurs in spinocerebellar tracts, pyramidal tracts, dorsal column tracts, and peripheral nerves, with minor cell loss in the brain stem and cerebellum. Cardiomyopathy is associated with ventricular hypertrophy and chronic interstitial myocardial fibrosis.

CLINICAL MANIFESTATIONS AND DIAGNOSIS

Typical Friedreich's ataxia first presents clinically during puberty with progressive ataxia, loss of lower extremity deep tendon reflexes, and extensor plantar responses (i.e., Babinski's signs). Other common clinical features include nystagmus, dysarthria, stocking-glove sensory loss, and weakness in the lower extremities. Patients frequently have kyphosis, scoliosis, and pes cavus. Interstitial myocardial disease may cause a typical hypertrophic cardiomyopathy (Chapter 60). A small number of patients have a later onset and less severely progressive course.

The diagnosis is made by genetic testing for the trinucleotide repeat expansion, which usually is present on at least one allele. Point mutations are sometimes present in the other allele and are more difficult to detect. Potentially treatable conditions with similar clinical manifestations include vitamin B_{12} deficiency (Chapter 225), abetalipoproteinemia (Chapter 142), and a selective defect in vitamin E absorption (Chapter 225).

TREATMENT AND PROGNOSIS

Treatment consists of supportive measures. A randomized trial using idebenone showed no benefit. The disorder is progressive, and patients usually are wheelchair bound by their mid-20s. The average age at death is 37 years, and the major cause of death is hypertrophic cardiomyopathy (Chapter 60).

Other Spinocerebellar Ataxias

The hereditary spinocerebellar ataxias are routinely classified by their specific molecular diagnosis. At least 10 autosomal recessive and nearly 30 autosomal dominant cerebellar ataxias have been identified. Clinical features, ethnic origin, and family history may suggest an autosomal recessive, autosomal dominant, or X-linked inheritance and often narrow the search for the genetic mutation. As the molecular pathogenesis of many of the hereditary ataxias is unraveled, the current numerical classification, which largely reflects the chronology of the identification of causative mutations, is likely to be replaced by a more pathophysiologic approach. Spinocerebellar ataxias 1, 2, 3, 6, 7, and 17 are caused by trinucleotide expansions in or adjacent to a protein-coding region of a gene. These expansions result in polyglutamine expansions in the protein product, which likely results in a toxic gain of function in a manner analogous to the pathogenesis of Huntington's disease.

CLINICAL MANIFESTATIONS AND DIAGNOSIS

The predominant clinical features of the spinocerebellar ataxias are ataxia and dysarthria. Other cerebellar signs include titubation, dysdiadochokinesia, and dysmetria. With increasing ataxia, patients can become wheelchair bound. Additional clinical signs include ophthalmoplegia, dementia, optic atrophy, retinal pigmentary degeneration, deafness, dysphagia, and peripheral neuropathy. Extrapyramidal features include masked facies, cogwheel rigidity, dystonia, athetosis, and chorea. Levodopa-responsive parkinsonism (Chapter 416) may be seen in some patients, particularly in spinocerebellar ataxia 2 and spinocerebellar ataxia 3. Pyramidal dysfunction includes spastic limbs, especially legs; hyperreflexia; and Babinski's response. Diagnosis is based on genetic testing.

TREATMENT AND PROGNOSIS

No treatment is currently available. The spinocerebellar ataxias are progressive, with worsening gait, hand coordination, speech, and eye movements, but with preserved mental function. Pneumonia is a common cause of death.

HEREDITARY SPASTIC PARAPLEGIAS

Hereditary spastic paraplegia, also known as Strümpell's disease, can be an autosomal dominant disorder (70 to 80%), an autosomal recessive disorder, or an X-linked disorder. The prevalence of hereditary spastic paraplegia is about 1 per 10,000 in the population. At least 14 loci have been identified for autosomal dominant hereditary spastic paraplegias; 15 loci for autosomal recessive hereditary spastic paraplegias; and 3 loci for X-linked hereditary spastic paraplegias. The autosomal dominant spastic gait genes include *SPG4*, which encodes for spastin, and the less common *SPG3A* (atlastin) and *SPG31* (*REEP1*) genes.

At autopsy, patients with hereditary spastic paraplegia have axonal degeneration of the pyramidal tracts and dorsal column tracts with lesser involvement of the spinocerebellar tracts. The neurons of origin are intact. The peripheral nervous system is unaffected.

CLINICAL MANIFESTATIONS

Patients with hereditary spastic paraplegia have a progressive gait disturbance with spasticity of lower extremities, hyperreflexia, clonus, and extensor plantar responses. Cranial nerves, speech, swallowing, and upper extremities remain normal. Although patients can experience weakness of their lower extremities, spasticity is usually the disabling component. The progressively increased leg spasticity results in tripping and an inability to run. Strength is generally preserved, and pain is infrequent. Sensation is normal. Pure hereditary spastic paraplegia is limited to symptoms and signs of spasticity, whereas complex or complicated hereditary spastic paraplegia includes additional neurologic or other abnormalities. Other clinical features include pes cavus (30 to 50%), decreased vibratory sensation, and urinary frequency, urgency, and hesitancy.

DIAGNOSIS

Hereditary spastic paraplegia is diagnosed when patients meet clinical criteria and when other causes of spasticity are excluded. Magnetic resonance imaging may show spinal cord atrophy, but cerebrospinal fluid analysis and nerve conduction studies are normal. The differential diagnosis includes other genetic conditions, spinal cord disease from structural lesions, multiple sclerosis, and vitamin deficiencies or retroviral infections (Table 417-8). Even a positive family history does not obviate the need to exclude potentially treatable alternative diagnoses.

TREATMENT AND PROGNOSIS

No specific treatment is available. Symptomatic therapy is aimed at decreasing disability and preventing complications, such as contractures. Antispastic agents, such as oral baclofen (usually 10 to 20 mg three times daily), improve spasticity but should be used with caution because they may worsen weakness. Some reports suggested an improved therapeutic response to intrathecal baclofen, but no controlled trials have addressed this issue. Preliminary data also raise the possible utility of injected botulinum neurotoxin type A injections for improving spasticity. Most patients become nonambulatory between 60 and 70 years of age. Patients with complicated hereditary spastic paraplegia often have other disabling features.

TABLE 417-8   DIFFERENTIAL DIAGNOSIS OF HEREDITARY SPASTIC PARAPLEGIAS

Hereditary
    Dopa-responsive dystonia
    Spinocerebellar ataxias
    Adult-onset adrenoleukodystrophy

Structural lesions of the spinal cord
Cervical spondylosis

Tumor
Arteriovenous malformation

Syringomyelia
Multiple sclerosis

Primary lateral sclerosis
Vitamin B$_{12}$ deficiency

Copper deficiency

Infections
    Human immunodeficiency virus
    Human T-lymphotropic virus type 1
    Tertiary syphilis

1. Zesiewicz TA, Elble R, Louis ED, et al. Practice parameter: therapies for essential tremor—report of the quality standards subcommittee of the American Academy of Neurology. *Neurology.* 2005;64:2008-2020.
2. Mestre T, Ferreira J, Coelho MM, et al. Therapeutic interventions for symptomatic treatment in Huntington's disease. *Cochrane Database Syst Rev.* 2009;8(3):CD006456.
3. Jankovic J, Esquenazi A, Fehlings D, et al. Evidence-based review of patient-reported outcomes with botulinum toxin type A. *Clin Neuropharmacol.* 2004;27:234-244.
4. Mueller J, Skogseid IM, Benecke R, et al. Pallidal deep brain stimulation improves quality of life in segmental and generalized dystonia: results from a prospective, randomized sham-controlled trial. *Mov Disord.* 2008;23:131-134.
5. Piacentini J, Woods DW, Scahill L, et al. Behavior therapy for children with Tourette disorder: a randomized controlled trial. *JAMA.* 2010;303:1929-1937.
6. Trenkwalder C, Hening WA, Montagna P, et al. Treatment of restless legs syndrome. *Mov Disord.* 2008;23:2267-2302.
7. Kushida CA, Becker PM, Ellenbogen AL, et al. Randomized, double-blind, placebo-controlled study of XP13512/GSK1838262 in patients with RLS. *Neurology.* 2009;72:439-446.

SUGGESTED READINGS

Abdo WF, van de Warrenburg BP, Burn DJ, et al. The clinical approach to movement disorders. *Nat Rev Neurol.* 2010;6:29-37. *Review.*
Gasser T, Finsterer J, Baets J, et al. EFNS guidelines on the molecular diagnosis of ataxias and spastic paraplegias. *Eur J Neurol.* 2010;17:179-188. *Current approach to identifying the specific mutation.*
Kurlan R. Tourette's Syndrome. *N Engl J Med.* 2010;363:2332-2338. *Review.*
Müller U. The monogenic primary dystonias. *Brain.* 2009;132:2005-2025. *Thorough review.*
Ostrem JL, Racine CA, Glass GA, et al. Subthalamic nucleus deep brain stimulation in primary cervical dystonia. *Neurology.* 2011;76:870-878. *Deep brain stimulation improved dystonia.*
Poon LH, Kang GA, Lee AJ. Role of tetrabenazine for Huntington's disease-associated chorea. *Ann Pharmacother.* 2010;44:1080-1089. *Review of benefits and side effects.*
Thevathasan W, Gregory R. Deep brain stimulation for movement disorders. *Pract Neurol.* 2010;10:16-26. *Review.*

418

AMYOTROPHIC LATERAL SCLEROSIS AND OTHER MOTOR NEURON DISEASES

PAMELA J. SHAW

DEFINITION

The motor neuron diseases (Table 418-1) are a heterogeneous group of disorders in which selective loss of function of upper motor neurons, lower motor neurons, or both results in impairment of the nervous system's control of voluntary movement. The most common acquired motor neuron disease, amyotrophic lateral sclerosis (ALS), is a combined upper and lower motor neuron disorder. The features of lower motor neuron involvement are muscle wasting, fasciculations, and flaccid weakness, with normal or depressed tendon reflexes. Upper motor neuron dysfunction may cause increased muscle tone, clonus, weakness in the pyramidal distribution, and extensor plantar responses. Recent advances in the molecular genetics of hereditary motor neuron diseases have improved their classification and enhanced the careful diagnosis that is essential for genetic counseling, guidance, treatment, and advising patients about prognosis.

AMYOTROPHIC LATERAL SCLEROSIS

EPIDEMIOLOGY

ALS is a neurodegenerative disorder that causes progressive injury and cell death of lower motor neurons in the brain stem and spinal cord, as well as upper motor neurons in the motor cortex. ALS has an incidence of about 2 per 100,000 and a prevalence of 6 to 8 per 100,000. The global incidence is fairly uniform, with the exception of a few high-incidence foci such as the Western Pacific island of Guam. The disease affects predominantly middle-aged and elderly individuals, with a mean age at onset of 55 to 60 years, although younger individuals can also be affected. Increasing age, male sex (male-to-female ratio ≈1.6:1), and genetic susceptibility are the only proven risk factors, although ongoing research is assessing the effects of athleticism/physical exercise and other potential environmental risk factors. Approximately 90% of cases of ALS occur sporadically, but 5 to 10% are familial, usually with an autosomal dominant mode of inheritance.

PATHOBIOLOGY

The process of neuronal degeneration in ALS is complex. The subtype of disease caused by *SOD1* mutations accounts for 20% of familial ALS cases and 2% of ALS overall. Mutant *SOD1* appears to trigger a complex interplay of multiple pathogenic processes, including oxidative stress, protein aggregation, mitochondrial dysfunction, excitotoxicity, and impaired axonal transport. Non-neuronal cells in the vicinity of motor neurons may contribute importantly to neuronal injury. Genetically engineered mouse models of *SOD1*-related ALS have shown that normal astrocytes can protect motor neurons expressing mutant *SOD1* and that removing the expression of mutant *SOD1* from microglia or astrocytes has a significant effect in slowing the progression of disease in these murine models. Astrocytes expressing mutant *SOD1* exert toxic effects on neighboring motor neurons through as yet undefined mechanisms.

Familial motor neuron disease has been linked to mutations in *SOD1*, alsin, senataxin, angiogenin, VAPB, dynactin, TDP-43, and FUS/TLS, with a suggestion that defective RNA processing may play a key role in the pathogenesis of ALS. In the sporadic disease, associations have been reported with alterations in at least eight other genes.

Pathology

At autopsy, the gross pathologic features of ALS consist of atrophy of the cerebral precentral gyrus, as well as sclerosis and pallor of the corticospinal tracts of the spinal cord. Thinning of the hypoglossal nerves and ventral spinal roots may be observed, and muscle atrophy is obvious. Microscopically, ALS patients will typically have lost 50% of their spinal motor neurons and have

TABLE 418-1	CLASSIFICATION OF THE MAJOR MOTOR NEURON DISEASES

COMBINED UPPER AND LOWER MOTOR NEURON DISORDERS

Amyotrophic lateral sclerosis
   Familial adult onset
   Familial juvenile onset
   Sporadic
   ALS-plus syndromes
      ALS with frontotemporal dementia
      Western Pacific ALS–parkinsonism-dementia complex

UPPER MOTOR NEURON DISORDERS

Primary lateral sclerosis
Hereditary spastic paraplegias
Neurolathyrism
Konzo

LOWER MOTOR NEURON DISORDERS

Hereditary
   Spinal muscular atrophies (SMAs)
      Proximal autosomal recessive SMA (associated with *SMN* mutations) types I to IV
      Other forms of SMA not associated with *SMN* mutations
   Distal spinal muscular atrophies/hereditary motor neuronopathies
      Kennedy's disease (X-linked spinobulbar neuronopathy)
      Hexosaminidase deficiency (GM2 gangliosidosis)
Acquired
   Monomelic focal and segmental spinal muscular atrophies
   Multifocal motor neuropathies
   Acute motor axonal neuropathy (AMAN)
   Postpolio syndrome
   Postirradiation syndrome
Infective disorders
   Acute poliomyelitis
   West Nile fever
   Other viral infections, e.g., enterovirus 71 and rabies virus
   Human immunodeficiency virus–associated motor neuron disorder
   Lyme disease
   Creutzfeldt-Jacob disease (amyotrophic forms)

DISORDERS OF THE BULBAR MOTOR SYSTEM

Kennedy's disease (X-linked bulbospinal neuronopathy)
Brown-Vialetto-Van Laere syndrome
Fazio-Londe disease

TOXIC DISORDERS OF THE MOTOR NEURON

Neurolathyrism
Konzo
Heavy metal toxicity (lead, mercury)
Western Pacific ALS–parkinsonism-dementia complex
Postirradiation motor neuron injury

DISORDERS OF MOTOR NEURON OVERACTIVITY

Neuromyotonia
Stiff person syndrome

MISCELLANEOUS MOTOR NEURON DISORDERS

Endocrinopathies, e.g., hyperthyroidism, hyperparathyroidism, hypoglycemia
Copper deficiency syndrome
Benign cramp-fasciculation syndrome

diffuse astrocytic gliosis in the spinal gray matter. By comparison, motor neurons in Onuf's nucleus in the sacral spinal cord, which innervate the pelvic floor muscles, and the motor nuclei of cranial nerves III, IV, and VI, which control eye movements, are relatively preserved. A cardinal feature in residual motor neurons is the presence of ubiquitinated proteinaceous inclusions, which may be compact or skeinlike. TDP-43 has recently been recognized as a major protein constituent of these aggregates. In the motor cortex, there is variable loss of upper motor neurons and astrocytic gliosis. In the descending corticospinal tracts, axonal loss, myelin pallor, and gliosis are seen. The atrophied skeletal muscle shows clusters of angular atrophic fibers and fiber-type grouping, which results from serial denervation and reinnervation. The selectivity of the disease process for the motor system is now recognized to be relative, and involvement of extramotor parts of the central nervous system can be found, especially in the sensory and spinocerebellar pathways, substantia nigra neurons, and dentate granule cells in the hippocampus.

CLINICAL MANIFESTATIONS

ALS is characterized by a combination of upper and lower motor neuron degeneration. Lower motor neuron degeneration causes weakness, atrophy, and fasciculation of the limb and bulbar musculature. Features of upper motor neuron dysfunction include the incongruous presence of active or brisk tendon reflexes in a wasted limb, increased muscle tone, and sometimes the presence of Babinski's sign. Upper motor neuron bulbar disease causes pseudobulbar palsy, with emotional lability, a brisk jaw jerk, slowing of repetitive tongue movements, and strained effortful speech. Fatigue and weight loss are also common symptoms. With end-stage disease, most patients will have features of upper and lower motor neuron dysfunction affecting all four limbs and the bulbar musculature.

In approximately 75% of patients, the disease starts distally, focally, and asymmetrically in the upper limb, lower limb (Video 418-1), or bulbar territories, followed by progressive spread of injury in an anatomically logical progression to contiguous groups of motor neurons. Affected individuals may notice weakness, wasting or clumsiness of one hand, or unilateral footdrop. Muscle cramps may precede other clinical features, and fasciculations are most noticeable in the large proximal limb muscles. In the upper limbs, the thenar and intrinsic hand muscles tend to be severely affected, whereas the triceps and finger flexors are relatively spared until late in the disease. In the lower limbs, the pattern of weakness is often in a pyramidal distribution (flexors weaker than extensors), with early weakness of hip flexion and ankle dorsiflexion and severe involvement of the distal muscles.

Bulbar symptoms, which are the initial feature in approximately 25% of patients, are especially common in elderly women with ALS (Video 418-2). The first problem is usually slurring of speech, initially apparent only when the individual is tired. Patients often have a mixed spastic/flaccid dysarthria, in which speech develops a tight, strangled quality because of the upper motor neuron component, with a superimposed nasal quality as a result of the flaccid lower motor neuron weakness of the palate and nasopharynx. In patients with bulbar disease, examination often reveals weakness of the facial muscles; a spastic, weak, wasted, and fasciculating tongue; and a brisk jaw jerk. Dysphagia, initially more pronounced for liquids than for solids, usually follows the dysarthria within a few weeks or months (Video 418-3). Complications include weight loss and prolonged and arduous meal times with frequent episodes of coughing, drooling of saliva, and aspiration pneumonia.

Respiratory muscle weakness is rarely the initial feature of ALS. More commonly, respiratory muscle weakness develops insidiously and causes dyspnea and orthopnea. Diaphragmatic weakness may be apparent from the paradoxical movement of the abdominal wall during inspiration and a marked decline in forced vital capacity in the supine position. Symptoms of nocturnal carbon dioxide retention may develop, including morning headaches, anorexia, and daytime somnolence.

Neck muscle weakness, which is common later in the course of disease, causes difficulty holding the head upright (dropped head syndrome). Eye movements tend to be spared even in advanced disease, thereby permitting limited communication by movements of the eyes. Similarly, the strength of the pelvic floor muscles is relatively preserved, so patients with ALS usually remain continent throughout the course of the disease.

Overt features of frontotemporal dementia (Chapter 409), with progressive deterioration in personality and behavior, will develop in approximately 5% of patients with ALS. Cognitive dysfunction may precede, follow, or coincide with the features of motor dysfunction. Up to 50% of ALS patients without overt dementia may show more subtle features of frontal lobe dysfunction.

About 5 to 10% of ALS patients have the progressive muscular atrophy variant with clinical features reflecting only degeneration of lower motor neuron groups in the spinal cord. In primary lateral sclerosis, patients have pure upper motor neuron degeneration. Although severe spastic spinobulbar paresis ultimately develops in these patients, the duration of survival is commonly 10 to 15 years after the onset of symptoms. The progressive bulbar palsy variant usually progresses to involve the limbs, although limb signs may not be present initially.

Several ALS variants follow a more segmental pattern than is typical in ALS. Up to 10% of patients with ALS have flail arm syndrome, which is more common in men and is associated with a longer median survival than seen in

those with typical ALS. A similar focal manifestation in the lower limbs, flail leg syndrome, is another recognized variant.

DIAGNOSIS

The diagnosis of ALS is essentially clinical, and there is no specific diagnostic test. Diagnosis requires evidence of *lower motor neuron degeneration* by clinical, electrophysiologic (Chapter 403), or neuropathologic examination; upper motor neuron degeneration by clinical examination; and progressive spread of symptoms or signs within a region or to other regions, as determined by the history or examination. The diagnosis also requires the absence of other disease processes as determined by electrophysiologic testing, neuroimaging, and if performed, biopsy. Generally accepted criteria (Table 418-2) classify patients as having definite, probable, or possible ALS. However, a number of other conditions may mimic ALS (Table 418-3), and about 8% of patients in whom ALS is initially diagnosed have other lower motor neuron syndromes such as multifocal motor neuropathy with conduction block, Kennedy's disease, or mixed spinal cord and root compression. Conversely, 10 to 15% of patients in whom ALS is ultimately diagnosed may first undergo inappropriate surgery for presumed spinal cord or root compression abnormalities.

Blood tests that may be helpful in distinguishing ALS from mimic syndromes (see Table 418-3) include a complete blood count and serum calcium level, thyroid function tests, serum protein electrophoresis, Venereal Disease Research Laboratory test, creatine kinase level, inflammatory markers (erythrocyte sedimentation rate and C-reactive protein), and levels of anti-GM1 ganglioside and anti–myelin-associated glycoprotein (MAG) antibodies. Further testing, which is guided by the patient's clinical findings, might include acetylcholine receptor antibody; mutation screening in patients with familial disease, suspected Kennedy's disease, or spinal muscular atrophy (SMA); heavy metal screening; urinary porphyrins; serum hexosaminidase A and B levels; *Borrelia* titers; and testing for human immunodeficiency virus.

Typical features of ALS on electromyography (EMG) include evidence of active denervation (i.e., positive sharp waves, fibrillation, and fasciculation potentials) and chronic denervation, as evidenced by large motor unit potentials that cannot be explained by a single nerve, root, or plexus lesion. Neuroimaging of the brain and spinal cord is often needed to exclude structural pathology.

Baseline respiratory function tests should be performed on all patients. Muscle biopsy is indicated only in rare or atypical cases, when diagnostic uncertainty persists.

TABLE 418-2 REVISED EL ESCORIAL DIAGNOSTIC CRITERIA FOR AMYOTROPHIC LATERAL SCLEROSIS

The diagnosis of ALS requires:
[A:1] Evidence of LMN degeneration by clinical, electrophysiologic, or neuropathologic examination
[A:2] Evidence of UMN degeneration by clinical examination and
[A:3] Progressive spread of symptoms or signs within a region or to other regions, as determined by history or examination

Together with the absence of:
[B:1] Electrophysiologic and pathologic evidence of another disease that might explain the signs of LMN and/or UMN degeneration and
[B:2] Neuroimaging evidence of other disease processes that might explain the observed clinical and electrophysiologic signs

Levels of diagnostic certainty:
Definite ALS
- UMN signs and LMN signs in 3 regions

Probable ALS
- UMN signs and LMN signs in 2 regions with UMN signs rostral to LMN signs

Probable ALS—laboratory supported
- UMN signs in 1 or more regions *and* LMN signs defined by EMG in at least 2 regions

Possible ALS
- UMN signs and LMN signs in 1 region (together) or
- UMN signs in 2 or more regions
- UMN and LMN signs in 2 regions with *no* UMN signs rostral to LMN signs

UMN signs: clonus, Babinski's sign, absent abdominal reflexes, hypertonia, loss of dexterity.
LMN signs: atrophy, weakness. If only fasciculation, search with EMG for active denervation.
Regions reflect segmental motor neuron pools: bulbar, cervical, thoracic, and lumbosacral.
EMG = electromyography; LMN = lower motor neuron; UMN = upper motor neuron.

TABLE 418-3 DISORDERS THAT CAN MIMIC AMYOTROPHIC LATERAL SCLEROSIS/MOTOR NEURON DISEASE

FORM OF MOTOR NEURON DISEASE	MIMIC SYNDROMES	CLINICAL CLUES
Progressive muscular atrophy (PMA)/LMN-predominant phenotype	Multifocal motor neuropathy	Weakness out of proportion to wasting. Neurophysiology identifies conduction block. Anti-GM1 antibodies may be raised
	Kennedy's disease	Gynecomastia, distal sensory features, perioral fasciculation, indolent progression
	Spinal muscular atrophy	SMA can be adult onset. Pure LMN syndrome. Slower progression than PMA. Probably no family history
	Chronic idiopathic demyelinating polyneuropathy	Electrophysiology identifies peripheral nerve demyelination
	Benign cramp-fasciculation syndrome	Predominantly middle-aged men. Largely calf involvement. Failure to progress. No active denervation on EMG
	Postpolio syndrome	Pure LMN syndrome. Past history of an illness compatible with poliomyelitis. Indolent progression
	Lead poisoning	Extramotor clinical features, e.g., constipation, nail and buccal signs
	Acute motor axonal neuropathy (AMAN—a Guillain-Barré syndrome variant)	Acute onset, with progression ceasing after a few weeks. Nerve conduction studies show features of motor axonopathy
	Hereditary motor neuropathies	Pure LMN syndrome. Family history, clinical signs indicating chronicity, slower rate of progression
	Porphyria	Extramotor clinical features, family history, episodic exacerbations
	Compressive focal motor neuropathies	Pure motor disorders can result from compression of the deep palmar branch of the ulnar nerve and posterior interosseous branch of the radial nerve. Failure to extend beyond territory of one nerve. Electrophysiology with or without imaging helpful
Amyotrophic lateral sclerosis	Multilevel spinal cord and root compression by discs, osteophytes, or tumor	Sensory symptoms and pain are common. UMN signs often caudal to LMN signs
	Thyrotoxicosis	Systemic symptoms and signs
	Combined peripheral neuropathy and cervical myelopathy	MRI of the spine and electrophysiology will differentiate
	Inclusion body myositis	Rarer than ALS. Characteristic pattern of weakness with early involvement of the long finger flexors and quadriceps
	Paraneoplastic syndromes, especially lymphoma	History of malignancy or systemic features
	Sjögren's syndrome	Non–motor-related symptoms
	Radiation myelopathy	History of radiotherapy
	Structural lesions of the bulbar region, e.g., tumor of the tongue base	Pain, failure of features to extend outside the bulbar territory
Primary lateral sclerosis	Hereditary spastic paraplegia	Family history. Symptoms rarely extend beyond the lower limb territory. Prominent bladder dysfunction
	Multiple sclerosis	Non–motor-related symptoms and signs, e.g., eye, bladder, cerebellar, and sensory involvement
	Spinal cord compression by disc or tumor	Pain and sensory involvement usually present

ALS = amyotrophic lateral sclerosis; EMG = electromyography; LMN = lower motor neuron; MRI = magnetic resonance imaging; SMA = spinal muscular atrophy; UMN = upper motor neuron.

TREATMENT AND PROGNOSIS   Rx

ALS is best managed in specialized centers that offer multidisciplinary care. Teams typically include a neurologist, nurse specialist, occupational therapist, physical therapist, speech and language therapist, and dietitian. During the course of the disease, patients frequently require referral for placement of a gastrostomy tube and to provide respiratory support.

No therapy currently has a dramatic effect in slowing the progression of ALS. Riluzole, which is a sodium-channel blocker whose primary mechanism of action is to reduce excitotoxicity through inhibition of presynaptic glutamate release, prolongs survival by approximately 3 months when given at 50 mg twice daily.[1] It may cause fatigue, nausea, and dizziness, but these effects are frequently transient. Liver function tests should be performed at baseline and monthly for the first 3 months of therapy.

Management must focus on symptoms and preservation of independence and quality of life. In patients with progressive bulbar problems, optimal positioning, attention to food and fluid consistency, and protective swallowing techniques are helpful. If weight loss continues, high-calorie nutritional supplements are added between meals. Placement of a gastrostomy tube via endoscopy or under radiologic guidance is recommended in patients in whom dehydration, weight loss of 10 to 15%, frequent distressing choking episodes, prolonged and tiring mealtimes, or aspiration pneumonia develops. Tube placement is higher risk in patients with respiratory insufficiency. Tubes should ideally be placed before the patient's forced vital capacity falls below 50% of expected.

Respiratory muscle weakness, which can develop insidiously during the course of ALS, causes breathlessness, orthopnea, daytime somnolence, morning headaches, and interrupted sleep. Management must emphasize detection and prevention of aspiration pneumonia, assistance in clearing of secretions by providing a suction machine, use of a mucolytic agent such as carbocysteine (in a dose of up to 750 mg three times daily), adoption of a semiupright position for sleep, and aggressive antibiotic therapy for bronchitis (Chapter 96) or pneumonia (Chapter 97). A small dose of sublingual lorazepam (0.5 to 1 mg) may be useful if the dyspnea is accompanied by extreme anxiety; opiate therapy (such as morphine, diamorphine, or fentanyl; see Table 29-4) may be given orally, transdermally, or by subcutaneous infusion to relieve respiratory distress during the later stages of the disease.

As respiratory function worsens, noninvasive ventilation can alleviate symptoms of chronic hypoventilation, significantly improve quality of life, and prolong survival,[2] especially in patients with orthopnea, daytime hypercapnia, and nocturnal oxygen desaturation. Full 24-hour ventilation via a tracheostomy is an option that is chosen uncommonly by fully informed patients. Palliative care teams and hospices can contribute substantially to the care of ALS patients in the later stages of the disease. In the absence of ventilatory support, ALS patients will almost always die in their sleep from hypercapnic coma. In the terminal phases (Chapter 3), the aim of treatment is to ensure comfort by prescribing opiates and anxiolytic medications as required to alleviate discomfort or distress.

PROGNOSIS

Clinical features associated with a worse prognosis include older age at onset of symptoms, early compromise of respiratory function, bulbar symptoms, and more rapid need for medical attention. The mean duration from the onset of symptoms to death in patients with sporadic ALS ranges from 27 to 43 months. The average 5-year survival rate is 25%, and approximately 5% of patients will survive for more than 10 years. The usual cause of death is respiratory failure, which may be accompanied by bronchopneumonia.

● SPINAL MUSCULAR ATROPHIES

DEFINITION

The term *spinal muscular atrophy* encompasses a group of pure lower motor neuron disorders that cause progressive, symmetrical muscle weakness and wasting. Because the bulbar musculature may be affected, an alternative term, "hereditary motor neuronopathy," has been proposed. The time of onset is variable and ranges from in utero to adult life.

EPIDEMIOLOGY AND PATHOBIOLOGY

The most common type of SMA is caused by mutations in the survival motor neuron (*SMN*) gene and is inherited as an autosomal recessive disorder. The estimated carrier frequency of an *SMN* mutation is 1 in 50. Type 1 SMA (Werdnig-Hoffmann disease) has an incidence of 1 in 8000 births. SMA is divided into subtypes I to IV according to age at onset and severity of the phenotype.

The human *SMN* gene on chromosome 5q13 exists in two forms with 5–base pair differences between *SMN1* and its centromeric homologue *SMN2*. A change in exon 7 of *SMN2* leads to skipping of exon 7, and as a result, 80% of the protein encoded by *SMN2* is truncated and nonfunctional rather than full length. The majority of patients with SMA have homozygous absence of *SMN1* exon 7, but *SMN1* may be replaced by a copy of *SMN2* during DNA replication by a process known as gene conversion. An individual may have one to four copies of *SMN2*, with a proportional increase in the amount of full-length SMN protein. A molecular basis for the wide variation in the phenotypic severity of SMA, which can range from in utero onset (SMA type I) to adult onset (SMA type IV), is the number of copies of *SMN2* and the SMN protein levels, although other disease-modifying factors have also been implicated.

The SMN protein oligomerizes and associates with other proteins to form the SMN complex, which in turn has an important role in the assembly of spliceosomal small nuclear ribonucleoproteins that have a function in pre-mRNA splicing in the nucleus. These cellular processes are ubiquitous, so either the clinical features of SMA may be caused by a particular susceptibility of lower motor neurons to defects in RNA processing or SMN may have functions that are specific to the motor neuron, including axonal transport of mRNA molecules essential for the health of the distal axon.

At autopsy, patients with SMA have atrophic spinal cords with loss of α-motor neurons and evidence of motor neuron degeneration and gliosis. The ventral roots are atrophic, and muscle atrophy is apparent with microscopic evidence of denervation and reinnervation.

CLINICAL MANIFESTATIONS

Type I SMA (Werdnig-Hoffman disease) is characterized by severe generalized muscle weakness and hypotonia at birth or by the age of 6 months; affected children never sit or walk. Type II is an intermediate form with an onset of muscle weakness before the age of 18 months; patients can sit but are never able to walk unaided. Type III SMA (Wohlfart-Kugelberg-Welander disease) appears after 18 months of age; patients acquire the ability to stand and walk but often become wheelchair dependent in adolescence or adult life, although life expectancy is normal. Patients with type IV SMA have an onset of muscle weakness in adult life.

DIAGNOSIS

The diagnosis of SMA caused by changes in *SMN* can be made by genetic testing in a patient with appropriate clinical signs and symptoms. Ninety-five percent of affected individuals have *SMN* deletions. Prenatal diagnosis is available. Electrophysiology and muscle biopsy reveal evidence of denervation.

Other disorders that may be manifested in infancy or childhood as hypotonia and a pattern of weakness similar to *SMN*-related SMA can be distinguished by associated clinical features, such as early respiratory distress or vocal cord paralysis or an atypical distribution of motor features, such as upper limb– or lower limb–predominant or scapuloperoneal involvement. The etiologic relationship of these disorders to classic SMA can be clarified by testing for *SMN* mutations.

It is important to distinguish SMA type I from infantile botulism, which can have a similar initial clinical picture. EMG with high-frequency repetitive nerve stimulation shows a decrement in botulism, and testing for the presence of botulinum toxin can confirm the diagnosis. SMA II and SMA III can be distinguished from chronic inflammatory demyelinating polyneuropathy (Chapter 428) by the presence of normal cerebrospinal fluid protein and normal nerve conduction studies in SMA. Patients with SMA III can have clinical features that are similar to those of the hereditary motor and sensory neuropathies, but it can be distinguished by neurophysiologic assessment and genetic testing.

SPINOBULBAR MUSCULAR ATROPHY/ KENNEDY'S DISEASE

EPIDEMIOLOGY

Kennedy's disease, or spinobulbar muscular atrophy (SBMA), is an X-linked degenerative disorder of the lower motor neurons. Though rare, it is important not to miss the diagnosis because of the genetic implications for the family and a more benign course than occurs with ALS. The diagnosis should be considered in any male patient with a pure lower motor neuron disorder, particularly when the disease course is relatively indolent, gynecomastia is present, or there is evidence of a mild accompanying sensory neuropathy.

PATHOBIOLOGY

SBMA is a trinucleotide repeat disorder in which a CAG expansion encodes for a polyglutamine tract in the first exon of the androgen receptor gene on chromosome Xq11-12. The androgen receptor, which contains three functional domains, is transported to the nucleus, where it binds to DNA and acts as a transcription factor. Expansion of the polyglutamine tract results in reduced target gene transactivation, and neurodegeneration occurs when the polyglutamine tract reaches a critical length of approximately 40 repeats. The neurodegeneration in patients with SBMA is considered to result from a ligand-dependent, toxic gain of function of the mutant androgen receptor protein. Complete loss of its function, as seen in testicular feminization syndrome (Chapter 241), does not lead to motor neuron degeneration. The toxicity has not been fully characterized, but protein aggregation, impairment of protein degradation pathways, disruption of gene transcription, impairment of axonal transport, and neurotrophic factor signaling may all contribute.

Pathologic examination reveals mild spinal cord atrophy, with ventral horn gliosis and loss of α-motor neurons. Misfolding of the polyglutamine (Q)-expanded protein leads to the formation of nuclear inclusions that contain the amino-terminal epitopes of the mutant androgen receptor within motor neurons and certain non-neuronal tissues.

CLINICAL MANIFESTATIONS AND DIAGNOSIS

The mean age at onset of SBMA is 30 years, with a range of 15 to 60 years, and the severity of the disease and its age at onset correlate with the size of the repeat expansion. Initial symptoms consist of hand tremors, fasciculations, and muscle cramps, followed by progressive weakness and atrophy of the limb and bulbar muscles. Limb muscle weakness tends to be proximal and predominantly involves the lower limbs. There are no clinical signs of upper motor neuron dysfunction. Weakness of the lower facial and tongue muscles causes dysarthria, and jaw weakness may cause the mouth to hang open. The presence of perioral fasciculations with quivering of the chin is a characteristic feature. Pharyngeal involvement can cause dysphagia, and respiratory muscle weakness causes breathlessness. Mild distal sensory loss is frequently present in the lower limbs. Features of mild androgen insensitivity with gynecomastia, testicular atrophy, and erectile dysfunction will often be apparent. Heterozygous female carriers of SBMA may show mild clinical manifestations of the disease.

EMG and muscle biopsy, which are often performed because the creatine kinase level tends to be elevated, reveal evidence of chronic denervation. Genetic screening for the CAG repeat expansion in exon 1 of the androgen receptor gene is diagnostic.

TREATMENT AND PROGNOSIS

Current therapy consists of supportive care. The course of the disease is slowly progressive in comparison to ALS and is compatible with normal life expectancy, although a proportion of patients may die of respiratory failure. Patients may become wheelchair dependent over a period of 2 to 3 decades, but some remain ambulatory until late in life.

Grade A

1. Miller RG, Mitchell JD, Lyon M, et al. Riluzole for amyotrophic lateral sclerosis (ALS)/motor neuron disease (MND). *Cochrane Database Syst Rev.* 2007;24:CD001447.
2. Bourke SC, Tomlinson M, Williams TL, et al. Effects of non-invasive ventilation on survival and quality of life in patients with amyotrophic lateral sclerosis: a randomized controlled trial. *Lancet Neurol.* 2006;5:140-147.
3. Bosboom WM, Vrancken AF, van den Berg LH, et al. Drug treatment for spinal muscular atrophy types II and III. *Cochrane Database Syst Rev.* 2009;1:CD006282.

SUGGESTED READINGS

Bede P, Oliver D, Stodart J, et al. Palliative care in amyotrophic lateral sclerosis: a review of current international guidelines and initiatives. *J Neurol Neurosurg Psychiatry.* 2011;82:413-418. *Highlights the importance of early palliative care for ALS patients and existing national differences in the availability of such care.*
Douglass CP, Kandler RH, Shaw PJ, et al. An evaluation of the neurophysiological criteria used in the diagnosis of motor neuron disease. *J Neurol Neurosurg Psychiatry.* 2010;81:646-649. *Highlights the usefulness of the new Awaji-shima neurophysiologic criteria in allowing earlier diagnosis of ALS.*
Kiernan MC, Vucic S, Cheah BC, et al. Amyotrophic lateral sclerosis. *Lancet.* 2011;377:942-955. *Comprehensive review.*

419

MULTIPLE SCLEROSIS AND DEMYELINATING CONDITIONS OF THE CENTRAL NERVOUS SYSTEM

PETER A. CALABRESI

The disorders of myelin encompass a wide range of diseases in which either myelin is not formed in a normal fashion (dysmyelinating disease) or normally formed myelin is destroyed or not maintained appropriately (demyelinating disease) (Table 419-1). Dysmyelinating diseases are uncommon and include an array of leukodystrophies that have a genetic basis. Demyelinating diseases are much more common and include multiple sclerosis (MS), which represents more than 95% of all types of disorders of central nervous system (CNS) myelin.

Some disorders of myelin actually have a distinct pathogenesis in which the disruption of myelin is secondary. Further, in many of the diseases of myelin, the axon degenerates as a result of loss of trophic support from loss of myelin or because of increased susceptibility to injury in the absence of myelin. This observation has led to the recent hypothesis that axonal loss is the underlying substrate for permanent disability in MS, adrenoleukodystrophy, and perhaps other diseases of myelin.

MULTIPLE SCLEROSIS

DEFINITION

MS is a disease characterized by multifocal areas of demyelination in the brain and spinal cord, with associated inflammatory cell infiltrates, reactive gliosis, and axonal degeneration. It typically presents in young adults with episodic neurologic dysfunction. Although the exact origin of MS remains enigmatic, evidence suggests that it is an immune-mediated attack on myelin, with

---

TABLE 419-1	DISEASES OF MYELIN

IDIOPATHIC

Recurrent or chronic progressive demyelination (multiple sclerosis and its variants)
Monophasic demyelination (may be the first clinical episode of multiple sclerosis)
Optic neuritis
Acute transverse myelitis
Acute disseminated encephalomyelitis; acute hemorrhagic leukoencephalopathy

VIRAL INFECTIONS

Progressive multifocal leukoencephalopathy
Subacute sclerosing panencephalitis (Chapters 375 and 378)

NUTRITIONAL AND METABOLIC DISORDERS (Chapter 425)

Combined systems disease (vitamin B_{12} deficiency)
Copper deficiency (dorsal columns and subacute optic neuropathy)
Demyelination of the corpus callosum (Marchiafava-Bignami disease)
Central pontine myelinolysis

ANOXIC-ISCHEMIC SEQUELAE (Chapter 411)

Delayed postanoxic cerebral demyelination
Progressive subcortical ischemic encephalopathy

LEUKODYSTROPHIES PRIMARILY AFFECTING CENTRAL NERVOUS SYSTEM MYELIN

Adrenoleukodystrophy (Schilder's disease)
Pelizaeus-Merzbacher disease (sudanophilic leukodystrophies)
Spongy degeneration
Vanishing white matter disease
Others (Alexander's disease, Canavan's disease)
Leukodystrophies of the central and peripheral nervous system
Metachromatic leukodystrophy
Globoid cell leukodystrophy (Krabbe's disease)

---

secondary disruption of axons leading to progressive disability over time in most afflicted patients.

EPIDEMIOLOGY

The annual incidence of MS varies by location and ranges between 1.5 and 11 per 100,000 people. MS is second only to trauma as the most common cause of neurologic disability in young adults. More recent studies suggest that the incidence rate has increased, in part because of better recognition of more cases at an earlier stage. The prevalence is estimated at 350,000 to 400,000 in the United States and more than 1,000,000 worldwide, but these numbers may be underestimates owing to incomplete recognition of the disease even in developed countries.

MS occurs 2- to 2.5-fold more frequently in women than in men, a sex predilection that is common in autoimmune diseases. The disease most often presents in the third to fourth decades of life, but with an incidence age range from postpubertal teenagers to persons in their 50s. Rare cases occur in infants or in patients in their 60s, but extreme caution is warranted in these situations to exclude alternative processes. In many of the late-onset cases, symptoms were present in younger years and were attributed to other causes.

MS is most common in people of Northern European descent, and whites acquire multiple sclerosis at nearly twice the rate of African Americans in the United States. In many areas of the world, MS is more prevalent in temperate latitudes (approaching 1 in 500 in some locations) and becomes less common toward the equator (1 in 20,000 or rare case reports only in some locations), perhaps explained, in part, by migration patterns of people with the same gene pools. However, the absence of complete genetic penetrance in monozygotic twin studies suggests an environmental component to the disease. Indeed, an outbreak of MS was documented on the Faroe Islands following World War II, and numerous other clusters have been reported, although an environmental trigger has not been identified.

Several studies have linked cigarette smoking with risk for MS. High levels of vitamin D and early exposure to excessive sunlight (sunburns) have been linked with lower risk for MS, possibly related to the beneficial effects of cholecalciferol on regulating immune cell responses.

PATHOBIOLOGY AND GENETICS

Monozygotic twins with MS show a concordance rate of between 15 and 50%, compared with only 3 to 5% concordance in dizygotic twins, consistent with a strong but incomplete role for genes in causing MS. The lifetime risk for MS is increased to 2 to 4% in individuals with a first-degree relative with

MS, compared with the general population risk of 0.1%. In addition, between 10 and 20% of patients with MS have a first-degree relative with another autoimmune disease, commonly rheumatoid arthritis, systemic lupus erythematosus, or autoimmune thyroid disease. Hashimoto's disease and Crohn's disease also may be more common in patients with MS. Genetic modeling of the disease strongly argues against a single MS gene and suggests that many different genes predispose to MS and account for its many phenotypes. Linkage and association studies have identified the human leukocyte antigen (HLA) or major histocompatibility complex (MHC) region on chromosome 6 as one genetic determinant for MS. The MHC class II region, involved in presentation of antigen to $CD4^+$ T cells, is the most strongly associated locus. The HLA-DR2 allele and, more specifically, the molecular haplotype HLA-DRB*1501 allele have repeatedly been implicated. Two single nucleotide polymorphisms in the interleukin-2 (IL-2) receptor α gene and the IL-7 receptor gene also appear to be associated with a higher risk for MS. Other loci of interest on other chromosomes, including chromosome 1, continue to be investigated, but the associations appear less strong.

Pathology

Pathologically, most cases are characterized by multifocal areas of demyelination and gross gliotic scar in the brain and spinal cord. Classic locations of these lesions, called *plaques,* are the optic nerves, periventricular white matter, deep white matter, juxtacortical white matter, corpus callosum, cerebellar peduncles, and dorsolateral spinal cord. However, there may be a bias toward recognition of lesions in white matter because of the relative ease of detecting demyelination and inflammation in white compared with gray matter. Indeed, more recent pathologic studies have confirmed demyelination, neuritic damage, and atrophy in the cortex and deep gray matter. At the microscopic level, one usually sees multiple areas of perivenular inflammatory cell infiltrates with extravasation into the surrounding tissue parenchyma. In the acute active plaque, CD4 helper T (T_H) cells are prominent in the perivenular areas. Proinflammatory cytokines released from T_H1 (interferon-γ [IFN-γ]) and T_H17 (IL-17) cells are thought to mediate damage. Increasingly large numbers of CD8 cytotoxic T cells have been documented in brain tissue, especially in the parenchyma, and these cells may mediate direct damage to axons through release of proteases such as granzyme B. Most parenchymal inflammatory cells are $CD68^+$ macrophages and microglia. In addition to the influx of circulating immune cells, prominent astroglial activation and even oligodendrocyte precursor cell proliferation occur in response to injury. Over time, the inflammation becomes less prominent in the center of the plaque, but a chronic active rim of inflammation with microglial activation exists at a well-demarcated border between abnormal and normal unharmed myelin. This characteristic of MS is seldom seen in other disorders of myelin. Although oligodendrocytes may survive, proliferate, and result in partial remyelination (shadow plaques) in some early cases, this process is hardly ever complete in MS. Over time, remyelination is less successful, and oligodendrocyte progenitor cells appear unable to differentiate into mature myelinating oligodendrocytes.

The number of damaged axons correlates with the extent of inflammation. Further, axonal damage and even neuronal apoptosis are seen in the cortex. Atrophy of both the brain and spinal cord, which occurs more rapidly in MS than in normal aging, reflects loss of both myelin and axons.

No consistent microbial cause has been discerned from careful examination of MS tissues for known infectious pathogens. Differential expression of human herpesvirus type 6, which is acquired by most people in childhood, has been noted in oligodendrocytes of patients with MS, but whether this virus is a cofactor in demyelination or just a bystander remains unclear. Evidence suggests the possibility that the earliest event in MS may be an insult to the oligodendrocytes, with subsequent activation of resident immune cells and secondary recruitment of other immune cells only at later stages.

Some pathologists believe that four distinct subtypes of MS can be discerned, in which the pathologic characteristics are consistent in every lesion, thereby allowing classification of patients with differing pathologic categories rather than just describing evolution of lesions over time. Type I lesions are characterized by typical perivenular inflammatory infiltrates consisting mainly of T cells, with early preservation of oligodendrocytes. Type II lesions are similar to type I but have an additional humoral component with immunoglobulin G (IgG) deposition and complement activation. Type III lesions are distinguished by not being based around venules and by prominent loss of myelin-associated glycoprotein, with evidence for oligodendrocyte apoptosis. Type IV lesions have inflammatory infiltrates more similar to types I

TABLE 419-2	CONDITIONS THAT CAN BE MISTAKEN FOR MULTIPLE SCLEROSIS AND OTHER DISEASES OF MYELIN

VASCULAR DISEASE

Small-vessel cerebrovascular disease
Vasculitides
Arteriovenous malformation
CADASIL
Antiphospholipid antibody syndrome

STRUCTURAL LESIONS

Craniocervical junction, posterior fossa, or spinal tumors
Cervical spondylosis or disc herniation
Chiari malformation or syrinx

DEGENERATIVE DISEASES

Hereditary myelopathy
Spinocerebellar degeneration

INFECTIONS

HTLV-1 infection
HIV myelopathy or HIV-related cerebritis
Neuroborreliosis (e.g., Lyme disease)
JC virus/progressive multifocal leukoencephalopathy
Neurosyphilis

OTHER INFLAMMATORY CONDITIONS

Systemic lupus erythematosus
Sjögren's syndrome
Sarcoidosis

MONOFOCAL OR MONOPHASIC DEMYELINATING SYNDROMES

Transverse myelitis
Optic neuritis
Neuromyelitis optica/Devic's disease
Acute disseminated encephalomyelitis

OTHER CONDITIONS

Hashimoto's thyroiditis with or without encephalopathy
Nonspecific MRI abnormalities related to migraine, aging, or trauma

CADASIL = cerebral autosomal dominant arteriopathy with subcortical infarcts and leukoencephalopathy; HIV = human immunodeficiency virus; HTLV = human T-cell lymphotropic virus; MRI = magnetic resonance imaging.

and II but also have oligodendrocyte loss as in type III. These varying pathologic features may begin to explain clinical subtypes of the disease.

Pathogenesis

It remains possible that the autoimmune hypothesis is wrong and that the inflammation observed in MS is secondary to an as yet uncharacterized primary degenerative process. Proponents of this theory cite evidence from pathologic features of hyperacute cases, in which the oligodendrocytes appear to die before any systemic immune response occurs, as well as recent data revealing neuronal and axonal death or demyelination in the absence of inflammation.

Macrophages and microglia, which make up the majority of cells within the parenchymal infiltrate in chronic MS plaques, are potent antigen-presenting cells and express HLA and costimulatory molecules. Activated macrophages and microglia also have effector functions, including release of cytokines that are partly (IL-6, tumor necrosis factor-α) or completely distinct from the T cells (IL-1β, IL-12, and IL-23). In high concentrations, these cytokines may damage oligodendrocytes and neurons and activate T cells.

CLINICAL MANIFESTATIONS
Presenting Symptoms

MS, which can present in many ways across a broad age range, may initially masquerade as a variety of different illnesses (Table 419-2; see Table 419-1). In a classic presentation, a young white person, more often a woman, will have the acute to subacute onset of impaired vision or sensation. Fatigue, depression, bladder urgency, weakness, impaired balance, and impaired coordination are also common symptoms. The often remarkably mild nature of the first symptoms often dissuades the patient from seeking medical attention or is insufficiently impressive to stimulate the physician to order diagnostic tests. Furthermore, patients may initially have few objective neurologic findings, especially between attacks.

Paresthesias of a limb that are circumferential and do not follow a dermatome suggest a spinal cord lesion; these symptoms often manifest distally and then ascend to involve more proximal parts of the limb, spread to the contralateral limb, or progress from a leg to an arm. Similarly, bandlike sensations around a limb or the torso also suggest a myelopathic process.

Incomplete transverse myelitis is a focal (partial) spinal cord syndrome that is usually inflammatory and does not follow vascular territories. It is a common presentation of MS.

Lhermitte's symptom, an electrical sensation moving down the spine into the limbs on flexion of the neck, is characteristic of cervical myelitis from any cause, including MS. Frank loss of sensation is less common as an early symptom or sign but is seen in more advanced cases. Burning, electrical, or deep aching sensations are also common in MS.

Sensory Abnormalities

On examination, the most common sensory findings are loss of vibration perception, most prominent in the feet, and incomplete spinal cord levels to pin prick or vibration, which are often more notable in a graded fashion rather than at a distinct level. Such sensory levels may be asymmetrical and differ by sensory modality because of isolated demyelination in the dorsal columns compared with the spinothalamic tracts. Patchy or seemingly nonanatomic focal areas of impaired sensation can occur, and some patients describe bizarre sensations such as water dripping or bugs crawling on an area of the body.

Visual Effects

Optic neuritis (Chapter 432) is a classic presenting syndrome, typically with visual symptoms in one eye. In optic neuritis, patients often complain of pain over the lateral eyebrow and worsening on lateral eye movement. The visual impairment may be described as looking through frosted glass or a veil. The scotoma or area of greatest loss can often be mapped in a centrocecal distribution (central focal point to the blind spot laterally), which in mild cases may be evident only as desaturation to red color using the head of a pin. More severe cases may result in total loss of light perception. In most acute cases of optic neuritis, the inflammation is retrobulbar (behind the disc), so no immediate changes are visible on the optic disc, thereby leading to the aphorism "the patient sees nothing, and the doctor sees nothing." However, there should be a relative afferent papillary defect (Marcus-Gunn pupil; Chapter 432) with paradoxical dilation of the affected eye to direct light on swinging a flashlight from the unaffected eye in which consensual constriction was induced. In cases of bilateral optic neuritis (new or old), this abnormality may not be seen. Patients usually spontaneously recover substantial vision after weeks to months. Later, the optic disc may become pale, especially in the temporal region, a finding reflecting damage to the axons following inflammation and demyelination, even with recovery of normal visual acuity. Patients often have more subtle chronic visual impairment for colors, low contrast visual acuity, and contrast sensitivity. Visual testing using low contrast letter acuity charts commonly reveals substantial visual loss after clinical optic neuritis.

Visual impairment from impaired tracking of eye movements owing to brain stem or cerebellar disease most commonly occurs in the setting of an acute lesion affecting the medial longitudinal fasciculus, which is the neurologic pathway that yokes the eyes together on lateral saccades. Patients may experience frank diplopia or just blurred vision, especially when they look off to one side rapidly, such as when looking over one's shoulder while driving. The neurologic sign of this problem is called *internuclear ophthalmoplegia* (Chapter 432) and manifests as slowed or absent adduction of one eye with abducting nystagmus of the other eye. It may occur bilaterally or may exist in milder forms, such that the adduction lag is imperceptible to the human observer. Blurred vision from cerebellar damage with nystagmus is very common in MS and is often worse on extreme lateral or vertical gaze. *Oscillopsia*, the sensation that the environment is moving when it actually is not, is another symptom of impaired cerebellar coordination of the eyes. Saccadic eye movement or loss of smooth pursuit is also common in MS and also can be seen in numerous neurologic conditions or with aging.

Motor Symptoms

The most common motor symptoms of MS are weakness and impaired coordination in a leg, with ascending involvement from distal to proximal and commonly spreading to the contralateral leg or ipsilateral arm. The lesion causing these symptoms is more commonly in the cervical spinal cord rather than the thoracic spinal cord, even when the first sign is partial footdrop. It is likely that axons that must conduct impulses over the longest distance (entire length of the spinal cord) from a site of inflammatory demyelination will become symptomatic before axons delivering signals to closer synapses (adjacent anterior horn cells in the cervical cord). Clinically, the weakness may be severe and may result in an obvious paralysis or be so subtle as to be undetectable. Heat-induced fatigue and weakness, as manifested by focal symptoms (slapping of a foot or dragging a leg) occurring after 15 to 20 minutes of exercise and resolving with rest, are characteristic of early demyelinating disease. The early absence of associated hyperreflexia and plantar extensor responses (Babinski's sign) may make it difficult to document corticospinal tract involvement. Later, in more established MS, classic corticospinal tract signs are often evident and manifest clinically as spastic gait (either hemiparetic or paraparetic), muscle cramps, and clonus (sustained reflex loop), sometimes occurring with positional changes and mistaken for signs of a cerebellar tremor.

Ataxia may occur as a result of impaired delivery of sensory information up the spinal cord or from demyelination of cerebellar pathways in the brain stem or cerebellum. Often, the two are mixed and may be confounded further by visual loss and impaired ability to compensate by fixing on the environment; this combination commonly causes dizziness in crowds, in which fixation may be further obscured. Appendicular dysmetria resulting in tremor on reaching for an object is a common cause of impaired coordination and dexterity. Lower extremity and truncal ataxia may result in a wide-based (drunk) gait. Other movement disorders, such as postural tremor and titubation (head tremor), are much less common in MS. *Myokymia* (wormlike muscle movements) under the skin, especially around the face, however, is fairly common. Pseudoathetosis and parkinsonism can be seen in severe cases.

Organ Dysfunction

Bladder symptoms are extremely common, but often are not volunteered, so specific questions must be asked. A careful bladder history may reveal isolated or mixed patterns of urinary frequency, urgency, incontinence, or retention. Careful delineation of a spastic bladder (detrusor muscle spasm) causing incontinence from an atonic bladder or spasm of the external sphincter (the latter two are causes of retention) leading to overflow incontinence is critical to designing an appropriate therapeutic strategy (Chapter 25). Urinary tract infections (Chapter 292), which are commonly the result of bladder dysfunction, may aggravate the underlying symptoms of MS.

Bowel dysfunction commonly manifests as constipation (Chapter 138), which may be primary (related to spinal cord involvement) or secondary (related to self-induced dehydration to manage urinary frequency or to side effects of anticholinergic drugs). Bowel incontinence secondary to an incompetent anal sphincter is less common and most often occurs as an isolated episode of fecal urgency, sometimes related to dietary change or diarrheal illness.

Sexual dysfunction is also common and underdiscussed in MS. In men, erectile dysfunction is frequent. In women and men, loss of libido and inability to achieve orgasm can occur as a result of medication, loss of sensation, heat-induced worsening of symptoms, physical barriers to intercourse (impaired mucosal moisture, spasticity, and pain), depression, or disorders of body image.

Systemic Symptoms

Fatigue, which is common in MS, may be linked to depression but often occurs independently and can be the most disabling symptom of the disease. A sleep history is important to exclude daytime fatigue resulting from disrupted sleep secondary to pain, cramps, bladder frequency, sleep apnea, periodic limb movements, depression, or disrupted sleep-wake cycles. Daytime fatigue even after a good night of sleep may occur in midafternoon and may be described as being "unplugged" or completely drained. Many patients obtain benefit from a short daytime nap.

Sensitivity to heat, which is a classic symptom of MS, occurs only in some patients. Even minor elevations of the body temperature can dramatically worsen symptoms. Symptoms usually (but not always) improve on cooling. Cooling devices can prevent this phenomenon, but there is no persistent benefit of cooling below normal body temperature. Some patients complain of worsened symptoms in cold weather, likely related to increased dysfunction of already stiff muscles and increased pain.

Pregnancy

Many women with MS successfully have multiple children, and the activity of MS lessens during the course of pregnancy, especially by the third trimester, when the frequency of exacerbations is reduced by approximately two thirds. Relapses are more frequent in the first 6 postpartum months, but no evidence indicates that pregnancy changes the natural history of the disease. Whether breast-feeding alters the course of MS is debated, but it is contraindicated for patients who resume disease-modifying drugs following delivery.

Types of Multiple Sclerosis

The three major clinical types of MS are relapsing remitting, secondary progressive, and primary progressive. Approximately 85 to 90% of patients present with relapsing remitting MS, characterized by acute or subacute episodes of new or worsening old neurologic symptoms that increase in severity, plateau, and then partly or completely remit. Patients may have no detectable residual deficit, or they may accumulate significant permanent disability from an attack. Most patients with relapsing remitting MS convert to secondary progressive MS after 20 to 40 years. This stage of the disease, which is characterized by at least 6 months of progressive worsening without evidence of a relapse, can be diagnosed with confidence only retrospectively. Some patients with secondary progressive MS also have interposed relapses distinct from their periods of progressive worsening, although these episodes become less frequent with time. Primary progressive MS, which is characterized by progressive deterioration from the onset for at least 1 year without a history of distinct relapses, occurs in approximately 10 to 15% of patients. It is more common in middle-aged men and typically has more involvement of the spinal cord and fewer inflammatory brain lesions.

Several other uncommon types of MS also are described. Progressive relapsing MS refers to a fairly uncommon variant of MS (6%), in which a relapse ensues after an initially primary progressive course. Acute progressive MS (Marburg's disease) causes acute or subacute progressive neurologic deterioration leading to severe disability within days to a month in a patient with no prior history of MS. This rare form of the disease may progress to a quadriplegic, obtunded state with death as a result of intercurrent infection, aspiration, or respiratory failure from brain stem involvement.

DIAGNOSIS

The diagnosis of MS rests on demonstrating evidence of at least two inflammatory demyelinating lesions referable to different locations within the CNS, occurring at different times (usually ≥1 month apart), and for which no better explanation exists. Diagnostic criteria allow for the diagnosis to be made on clinical grounds alone as long as appropriate exclusionary testing is performed (Table 419-3). Clinical evidence of a lesion requires objective findings on examination, not just a symptom. Further, repeated episodes of neurologic dysfunction that could be explained based on one lesion (e.g., a cervicomedullary junction lesion causing brain stem, cerebellar, and corticospinal tract dysfunction) is not enough evidence to diagnose MS.

Laboratory Findings
Magnetic Resonance Imaging

No definitive diagnostic laboratory test exists for MS, but magnetic resonance imaging (MRI) of the brain is extremely useful and should be performed in all patients in whom MS is a diagnostic consideration. More than 95% of patients with clinically definite MS have an abnormal brain MRI, and the presence of high-signal, bright lesions is so characteristic of MS that a normal brain MRI should suggest an alternative diagnosis. Brain MRI is also useful in predicting future MS at the time of a clinically isolated demyelinating syndrome. Specific MRI findings allow for confirmation of disease disseminated in time and space (different parts of the brain or spine) as well as fulfilling evidence for dissemination in time (Table 419-4). MS plaques typically appear as high-signal (white) areas on fluid attenuation inversion recovery (FLAIR) T2-weighted images, which allow for the best discrimination of these lesions by suppressing high-signal from cerebrospinal fluid (CSF) in the ventricles (Fig. 419-1). Lesions generally range in size from 2 mm to 2 cm; larger plaques occasionally resemble a tumor. Features of an MRI lesion suggesting MS include an elliptical shape, discrete borders, lack of mass effect, and gadolinium enhancement. Typical locations include the periventricular area (perpendicular to or abutting the walls of the ventricles) (Fig. 419-2), the corpus callosum, the cerebellar peduncles, the brain stem, the

TABLE 419-3	2010 REVISIONS TO THE MCDONALD DIAGNOSTIC CRITERIA FOR MULTIPLE SCLEROSIS
CLINICAL PRESENTATION	**ADDITIONAL DATA NEEDED FOR DIAGNOSIS OF MULTIPLE SCLEROSIS**
Two or more attacks; objective clinical evidence of two or more lesions; or one lesion with a prior attack	None*
Two or more attacks; objective clinical evidence of one lesion	Dissemination in space, demonstrated by: (1) MRI (see Table 419-4), or (2) Two or more MRI-detected lesions consistent with MS plus positive CSF, or (3) Await further clinical attack implicating a different site
One attack; objective clinical evidence of two or more lesions	Dissemination in time, demonstrated by: (1) MRI (see Table 419-4), or (2) Second clinical attack
One attack; objective clinical evidence of one lesion (monosymptomatic presentation; clinically isolated syndrome)	(1) Dissemination in space, demonstrated by: (a) MRI (see Table 419-4), or (b) Two or more MRI-detected lesions consistent with MS plus positive CSF, and (2) Dissemination in time, demonstrated by: (a) MRI (see Table 419-4), or (b) Second clinical attack

*Must rule out other causes (e.g., see Table 419-2).
CSF = cerebrospinal fluid; MRI = magnetic resonance imaging; MS = multiple sclerosis. Adapted with permission from Polman CH, Reingold SC, Banwell B, et al. Diagnostic criteria for multiple sclerosis: 2010 revisions to the McDonald criteria. *Ann Neurol.* 2011;69:292-302.

TABLE 419-4	MAGNETIC RESONANCE IMAGING CRITERIA IN MULTIPLE SCLEROSIS (INTERNATIONAL PANEL RECOMMENDATIONS: 2010)

DISSEMINATION IN TIME

Detection of a new T2 or gadolinium-enhancing lesion if it appears at any time compared with a reference scan*
Simultaneous presence of asymptomatic gadolinium-enhancing and non-enhancing lesions at any time

DISSEMINATION IN SPACE

At least one gadolinium-enhancing lesion in at least 2 of 4 areas:
 Periventricular
 Juxtacortical
 Infratentorial
 Spinal cord

DIAGNOSIS OF PRIMARY PROGRESSIVE MULTIPLE SCLEROSIS

One year of disease progression (retrospectively or prospectively determined) plus two of the following:
 a. Positive brain magnetic resonance imaging (≥1 T2 lesion in at least one characteristic area: periventricular, juxtacortical, or infratentorial)
 b. Positive spinal cord magnetic resonance imaging (two focal T2 lesions)
 c. Positive cerebrospinal fluid (isoelectric focusing evidence of oligoclonal immunoglobulin G bands or increased immunoglobulin G index, or both)

*Caution: Determination that a T2 lesion is indeed new can be challenging. A new T2 lesion must be of sufficient size and location to reflect one that could not have been missed previously for technical reasons of slice orientation, thickness or spacing, tissue contrast, patient motion, or other artifacts. This judgment requires standardized scanning procedures, with emphasis on careful repositioning, as well as input from qualified evaluators experienced in multiple sclerosis imaging. From Polman Ch, Reingold SC, Banwell G, et al. Diagnostic criteria for multiple sclerosis: 2010 revisions to the McDonald criteria. *Ann Neurol.* 2011;49:292-302.

juxtacortical area, and the dorsolateral spinal cord (Fig. 419-3). Cortical and deep gray matter lesions also occur but are less clearly seen on conventional MRI. Gadolinium enhancement, which suggests permeability of the blood-brain barrier, is correlated with new or active inflammation in lesions (Fig. 419-4). Lesions that enhance on a T1-weighted sequence usually have a concomitant lesion in the same location on a T2-weighted image. However,

FIGURE 419-1. Axial fluid attenuation inversion recovery image of the brain from a patient with multiple sclerosis revealing classic multiple periventricular and deep white matter high signal lesions.

FIGURE 419-3. Sagittal T2-weighted image of the brain and cervical spine from a patient with multiple sclerosis. The image shows a high-signal plaque from C3-C5 in the spinal cord.

FIGURE 419-2. Sagittal fluid attenuation inversion recovery image of the brain from a patient with multiple sclerosis revealing classic periventricular lesions radiating outward from the ventricles (arrows).

FIGURE 419-4. Axial T1-weighted image after gadolinium contrast showing an actively inflamed ring-enhancing lesion in a patient with multiple sclerosis.

T2-weighted lesions may form without evident enhancement. Gadolinium enhancement typically persists for 2 to 8 weeks and thus may be missed on intermittent scans. Persistent areas of low signal on T1-weighted images before contrast ("black holes") correlate with pathologic evidence of axonal loss and atrophy (Fig. 419-5).

Cerebrospinal Fluid
Examination of the CSF is useful in many cases but is not mandatory in patients with a typical clinical presentation and MRI evidence of disseminated disease. CSF evaluation includes cell counts, total protein, glucose, oligoclonal bands with a paired serum sample, and an IgG index. The presence of myelin basic protein is not specific for MS because it can be elevated secondary to any disruption of CNS tissue. Oligoclonal bands in the CSF or an elevated IgG index provides evidence for intrathecal production of immunoglobulins, and oligoclonal bands are common in MS but can occur with

infection or other immune-mediated processes; the test lacks specificity for MS and has a sensitivity of only approximately 85 to 90% of patients with clinically definite MS. In clinically isolated demyelinating syndromes (see later), the sensitivity is even lower (~50%).

CSF evaluation is generally recommended if an alternative diagnosis is considered, especially if one suspects an infectious process (e.g., fever, sweats, unusual travel history, tick bite, or rash). CSF analysis may also be useful if clinical or MRI criteria are incomplete to provide confirmation of the diagnosis.

Evoked Potential Tests
Evoked potentials (Chapter 403) may also be useful in some situations to document objective evidence of slowed conduction owing to demyelination in locations different from those recognized clinically. However, visual evoked potentials (VEPs), brain stem auditory evoked potentials, and somatosensory

evoked potentials are less sensitive and less specific for MS than is high-resolution MRI. Multifocal VEPs may be more sensitive than global VEPs in revealing focal areas of abnormal conduction along the optic nerve.

Optical Coherence Tomography

Optical coherence tomography is an office-based device that uses the reflection of infrared light (from an exogenous source directed through the pupil) off the back of the eye to quantify the thickness of retinal tissues, including the retinal nerve fiber layer and macula. This test, which has been widely used in glaucoma, can monitor axonal damage, both in the setting of acute optic neuritis and in detecting subclinical axonal damage (Fig. 419-6). Retinal nerve fiber layer thinning correlates with brain atrophy and may be useful as a surrogate marker of more global neurodegeneration in MS.

Differential Diagnosis

The diagnosis of MS may be so clear that it is recognized by the patient and is readily confirmed by the primary physician or so obscure that even experienced specialists disagree. Many processes (see Table 419-2) can mimic the clinical, radiologic, and CSF findings associated with MS, and there is no "gold standard" diagnostic test that is 100% sensitive and specific for the disease.

FIGURE 419-5. Axial T1-weighted image showing numerous areas of T1 low signal ("black holes"), ventricular enlargement, and diffuse atrophy.

Processes that mimic MS include structural lesions, especially of the base of the brain and of the spinal cord, in which one lesion can cause symptoms referable to many different tracts and at different perceived locations in the body. Chiari malformations with or without syrinx (Chapter 426), disc herniation (Chapter 407), cervical spondylosis, and low-grade tumors (Chapter 195) can produce symptoms of MS both in newly presenting patients and in patients who truly have MS but who also have a second process.

Various infectious diseases can mimic MS. Examples include human T-cell lymphotropic virus types I and II (virally associated myelopathy or tropical spastic paraparesis; Chapter 386), human immunodeficiency virus (neuropathy, myelopathy, cognitive impairment, CNS white matter changes; Chapter 401), neuroborreliosis (Lyme disease; Chapter 329), neurosyphilis (Chapter 327), Epstein-Barr virus (Chapter 385), cytomegalovirus (Chapter 384), herpes simplex virus (Chapter 382), varicella-zoster virus myelitis (Chapter 383), and JC virus (progressive multifocal leukoencephalopathy; Chapter 378).

Other inflammatory diseases that usually involve other parts of the body can concomitantly affect the CNS or rarely present in the CNS. Examples include sarcoidosis (Chapter 95), systemic lupus erythematosus (Chapter 274), Sjögren's syndrome (Chapter 276), and vasculitides (Chapter 278). Ischemic vascular disease secondary to any cause also can resemble MS. Metabolic and nutritional disorders that can mimic MS include vitamin B_{12} deficiency and methylmalonic acidemia (in some cases distinct from cyanocobalamin deficiency). Central pontine myelinolysis (Chapters 118 and 425) secondary to overly rapid correction of sodium is rarely mistaken for MS. Thyroid disease (Chapter 233) may mimic the fatigue of MS and may cause dysesthesias and disorders of the optic nerve and muscles. Nutritional deficiency (Chapter 222) and malabsorption have been associated with demyelination and may mimic MS. Copper deficiency can cause dorsal column pathology, neuropathy, anemia, and optic neuropathy. Vitamin D deficiency (Chapter 252), which is becoming increasingly common, can cause proximal weakness, fatigue, and asthenia, in addition to bone loss.

Monophasic demyelinating syndromes with or without multiple other lesions often, but not always, progress to become MS (see later). Spinocerebellar atrophy and hereditary myelopathy cause slowly progressive disease but do not cause sensory and visual abnormalities.

TREATMENT   Rx

The treatment of MS can be divided into drugs designed to relieve symptoms, drugs designed to modify the course of the disease, and nondrug measures. In addition, numerous drugs can target specific aspects of MS: depression, fatigue, muscle spasticity, pain, insomnia, and bladder, bowel, and sexual dysfunction. Before considering a symptomatic therapy, the

Time from AON onset	− 3 Months	+ 2 Weeks	+ 3.5 Months	+ 8 Months	+ 10 Months
Average RNFL (microns)	108	164	98	99	97
Superior	131	197	131	123	125
Nasal	78	126	74	75	74
Inferior	141	246	118	130	126
Temporal	79	84	69	66	65

FIGURE 419-6. Serial optical coherence tomography (OCT) scans in a patient who developed unilateral optic neuritis. Immediate swelling and increased thickness of the retinal nerve fiber layer (RNFL) thinning can be seen followed by focal thinning, especially in the temporal quadrants, as depicted by the *yellow* and *red* regions. AON = acute optic neuritis.

patient should be educated about the purpose of the drug and its side-effect profile. On learning that these drugs have no long-term impact on disease activity, patients may elect not to use them for relief of symptoms alone. Symptomatic therapies are best started at low doses and frequently require titration to obtain the optimal balance between efficacy and side effects.

Treatment of Specific Symptoms

Depression and emotional lability are common symptoms of MS. In addition to appropriate supportive care and counseling, antidepressant therapy with one of the "activating" serotonergic or noradrenergic drugs (fluoxetine, sertraline, citalopram, escitalopram, venlafaxine, or bupropion) can be of benefit (see Table 404-5 in Chapter 404). If anxiety and panic symptoms predominate, a less activating drug such as paroxetine may be preferable. Patients with concomitant pain or insomnia may benefit more from a sedating antidepressant (amitriptyline, nortriptyline, or trazodone) given at bedtime.

Spasticity can be managed by physical therapy, stretching, and institution of either baclofen (5 to 160 mg in divided doses) or tizanidine (2 to 32 mg in divided doses). Either drug should be started as a single agent at a low dose, generally three to four times a day, but a larger dose at bedtime is often the best tolerated and may target nocturnal symptoms. Decreasing muscle tone can result in weakness. Baclofen should never be discontinued abruptly because of the potential for a severe withdrawal reaction.

Bladder urgency resulting from detrusor muscle spasm can be managed effectively with anticholinergics such as oxybutynin (5 to 20 mg in divided doses) or tolterodine (1 to 4 mg), but these agents can cause temporary urinary retention. Bladder ultrasonography permits accurate bedside assessment of postvoid residual volume to determine whether a patient is retaining excessive amounts of urine. Urinary retention may be improved by removing drugs known to induce it. Primary urinary retention is difficult to treat with drugs, but external sphincter spasm can be treated with α_{1a}-adrenergic receptor blockers such as tamsulosin (0.4 to 0.8 mg) and doxazosin (1 to 8 mg). Bethanechol (10 to 150 mg in divided doses) may be tried for an atonic bladder, but intermittent catheterization is often required. Alternative causes of bladder symptoms such as urinary tract infections, prostatic enlargement, or anatomic changes following pregnancy should be considered and managed separately.

Painful dysesthesias and paroxysmal dystonic spasms may be managed effectively with antiepileptic drugs (gabapentin, 300 to 5400 mg/day in divided doses; pregabalin, 75 to 600 mg/day in divided doses; or carbamazepine, 100 to 2400 mg/day in divided doses) or tricyclic antidepressants (amitriptyline, 10 to 150 mg; or nortriptyline, 10 to 50 mg). Patients with trigeminal neuralgia (Chapter 405) may respond to these drugs or to baclofen, misoprostol, botulinum toxin, or decompression surgery.

Sexual dysfunction in MS is often multifactorial. Patients with erectile dysfunction usually respond well to the phosphodiesterase inhibitors, which enhance penile vasodilation (Chapter 242). Education regarding the use of lubrication, alternative sensory stimulation, and the adverse effect of heat can improve sexual function.

Systemic Treatments

Corticosteroids (e.g., intravenous methylprednisolone, 1 g/day for 3 to 5 days) shorten the duration and severity of symptoms from an acute exacerbation but have no proven effect on long-term disability. Oral corticosteroids used in equivalent dosage are probably equally efficacious and safe. Intravenous immunoglobulin and plasma exchange have been reported occasionally to benefit steroid-refractory patients, but randomized placebo-controlled trials have failed to show consistent benefits, perhaps because only patients with type II disease (humoral component) are likely to respond.

Seven disease-modifying agents have been approved by the U.S. Food and Drug Administration (FDA): IFN-β1b (Betaseron and Extavia), IFN-β1a (Avonex), IFN-β1a (Rebif), glatiramer acetate (Copaxone), natalizumab (Tysabri), and mitoxantrone (Novantrone). The first six agents were approved for relapsing remitting MS, and mitoxantrone is indicated for worsening forms of MS and for secondary progressive MS.

The three IFN-β drugs[1-3] and glatiramer acetate[4] reduce the relapse rate by approximately one third. IFN-β1b (8 million IU, subcutaneously every other day [Betaseron and Extavia]) and IFN-β1a (30 μg intramuscularly weekly [Avonex] or 22 to 44 μg subcutaneously three times a week [Rebif]) appear to have a more rapid onset of action, perhaps based on their dosing regimen, compared with weekly IFN-β1a (30 μg weekly intramuscularly). However, weekly IFN-β1a Avonex is less immunogenic and results in only a 3% incidence of neutralizing antibodies, which reduce efficacy, compared with 20 to 30% for the other IFN-β preparations. The major side effects of IFN-β are a flulike reaction (low-grade fever, chills, and myalgias 6 to 24 hours after the injection), local reactions at the injection site (pain, erythema, and rarely necrosis), and elevated aminotransferase levels (rarely severe hepatitis). These side effects can be managed by initiating the drug slowly and by prophylaxis with

acetaminophen and nonsteroidal anti-inflammatory agents, and they improve in most patients after 3 to 6 months.

Glatiramer acetate is a copolymer of four amino acids designed to mimic myelin basic protein; given as 20 mg/day subcutaneously, it also reduces relapses by about one third and is well tolerated by most patients.[4] Major side effects are local reactions at the injection site, swelling, hives, and a rare, self-limited (15 to 20 minutes) systemic reaction consisting of chest pain, palpitations, and anxiety. No monitoring of blood tests is required for this medication. The effect of glatiramer acetate on MRI T2-weighted and gadolinium-enhancing lesions is less dramatic than for the IFNs (30% reduction) perhaps because its primary effect is not at the blood-brain barrier.

Natalizumab is a monoclonal antibody directed against the α_4-integrin chain of the leukocyte adhesion molecule VLA-4. In a large phase III trial, this drug, at a dose of 300 mg intravenously every 4 weeks, reduced relapses by 68% compared with placebo and reduced gadolinium-enhancing lesions by 92%.[5] However, about 1 per 500 patients develop JC virus brain infection (Chapter 378) after 24 months of exposure, which causes progressive multifocal leukoencephalopathy.

In a randomized study, yearly courses of alemtuzumab (12 or 24 mg daily for 5 consecutive days in year 1 and for 3 days in years 2 and 3), which is a monoclonal antibody that targets CD52 in lymphocytes and monocytes, reduced relapse rates and disability by up to 75% compared with IFN-β1a given three times a week.[6] Serious side effects associated with alemtuzumab include an increased rate of autoimmune thyroid and thrombocytopenic purpura.

Mitoxantrone, which is an anthracenedione antineoplastic agent with potent immunosuppressive activity, has been approved to slow progression of neurologic disability and to reduce the relapse rate in patients with relapsing remitting MS and secondary progressive MS.[7] The recommended dose is a 5- to 12-mg/m^2 intravenous infusion every 3 months. In a phase III randomized, placebo-controlled, multicenter trial of 188 patients, the number of treated relapses was reduced by 67%. Side effects of mitoxantrone include nausea and alopecia. The lifetime use of this drug is limited to 2 to 3 years (or a cumulative dose of 120 to 140 mg/m^2) because of its cardiotoxicity. Heart failure or asymptomatic decreases in left ventricular ejection fraction (LVEF) can occur even after one to four doses, so careful monitoring of LVEF after each dose is mandatory. The risk for leukemia is increased and may be as high as 0.8%. A complete blood count, including platelets, should be done before each course of mitoxantrone therapy, and women of childbearing age should have a pregnancy test and should know the results before each dose, regardless of whether or not they are using birth control. Patients should be made aware that mitoxantrone may impart a blue-green color to the urine for 24 hours after administration. It also may cause bluish discoloration of the sclera. Rituximab (1000 mg intravenously 2 weeks apart every 6 months), which is a monoclonal antibody that depletes B-cell lymphocytes, can significantly reduce inflammatory brain lesions and relapse by about 50% for up to 48 weeks in patients with relapsing remitting MS,[8] but has not been effective in primary progressive MS. A trial of rituximab in primary progressive MS failed to show an effect on progression, although a post hoc analysis suggested that younger patients with enhancing lesions on MRI did have reduced progression after treatment compared with controls.

Fingolimod is a sphingosine-1 phosphate receptor modulator that is given orally once a day at 0.5 mg. Fingolimod reduces relapse rates and the progression of disease compared with placebo[9] and compared with IFN therapy.[10] Fingolimod's side effects include first-dose bradycardia, macular edema, and respiratory infections. Cladribine (2-chlorodeoxyadenosine, 3.5 or 5.25 mg/kg/day) given as a short course once a year reduced the annualized relapse rate by 55% and disease progression by one third compared with placebo in a phase III trial.[11] Both these drugs may have a role in treating MS but also have global immunosuppressive effects that increase the risk for serious infections and possibly other systemic complications.

In a phase 2 trial, treatment with 0.6 mg/day of laquinimod, a novel oral immunomodulatory agent, resulted in a 40% decrease in MR lesions in relapsing-remitting multiple sclerosis at 36 weeks.[12] In another phase II trial, oral fumarate, which also has anti-inflammatory effects, reduced new gadolinium-enhancing lesions by 69%.[13] In a randomized trial, sustained-release fampridine, a potassium-channel blocker at 10 mg twice daily, improved walking in 35% of patients compared with only 8% of patients receiving placebo, leading to its recent approval by the FDA.[14] Teriflunomide is an oral dihydro-orotate dehydrogenase inhibitor that reduced MRI activity in a phase II clinical trial. Other forms of immunosuppression, including methotrexate, azathioprine, mycophenolate mofetil, and cyclophosphamide, also appear to have some efficacy in MS, although no definitive clinical trials have been done with these agents, and none is as yet approved for MS by the FDA.

MS patients are at high risk of developing osteopenia or osteoporosis, so prophylaxis with vitamin D and calcium and treatment with bisphosphonates or other proven approaches should be considered. Patients with suboptimal 25-OH vitamin D levels (<30 ng/mL) on standard 1000 IU cholecalciferol replacement therapy should consider increasing to 2000 to 4000 IU/day or 50,000 IU ergocalciferol every other week or, in some cases, weekly, with appropriate monitoring of vitamin D and calcium levels. If osteoporosis has already been diagnosed, bisphosphonate therapy, such as alendronate (10 mg daily or 70 mg weekly) or similar drug is generally indicated.

Nondrug Approaches to Well-Being

Nonmedical treatment of MS is a critical part of managing the disease. Patients derive benefit from a health care team approach consisting of an experienced MS physician, nurse, social worker, therapist, and counselor, with appropriate referral to other subspecialties as needed. Alternative and complementary therapies (Chapter 38) are commonly used by patients with MS, and the risks and benefits of these approaches must be discussed with the patient.

PROGNOSIS

The average lifespan of patients with MS is about 8 years less than normal, a finding reflecting a bimodal distribution in which many patients live a normal lifespan and a few die at a significantly younger age owing to aggressive disease, severe disability, infection, or suicide. Most patients presenting with relapsing remitting MS convert to secondary progressive MS after 20 to 40 years. Only one third of patients will require use of a wheelchair, but 50% may need assistive devices, and nearly two thirds will have disability that prevents them from working. African Americans and men of all races tend to have a more aggressive course and are more likely to become disabled. Institution of immunomodulating therapy early in the course of the disease may slow progression of disability, but no long-term follow-up data are available to quantify the extent of this benefit.

OTHER DISEASES OF MYELIN

Monofocal and Monophasic Demyelinating Processes

OPTIC NEURITIS AND TRANSVERSE MYELITIS

Optic neuritis (Chapter 432) and transverse myelitis are inflammatory processes that can occur as entities distinct from MS or as part of MS (see earlier). In addition, optic neuritis and transverse myelitis can occur together in the syndrome called *neuromyelitis optica* (Devic's disease).

Optic Neuritis

Optic neuritis (Chapter 432) is an inflammatory disease that usually involves the retrobulbar portion of the optic nerve and sometimes parts of the optic chiasm. Although optic neuritis is most often associated with MS (50 to 75%), it also can be seen as an isolated idiopathic disorder (25 to 50%), as part of neuromyelitis optica, or associated with other inflammatory and infectious diseases such as systemic lupus erythematosus, Sjögren's syndrome, sarcoidosis, Lyme disease, syphilis, and human immunodeficiency virus infection. The pathobiologic features are thought to be similar to those of MS and are characterized by idiopathic inflammatory demyelination followed by secondary axonal injury.

CLINICAL MANIFESTATIONS AND DIAGNOSIS

The clinical presentation, which typically is monocular visual loss with pain over the brow that worsens with lateral eye movement, is similar regardless of whether it presents as part of MS (see the earlier discussion of the visual effects of MS) or not. When it involves the optic nerve head, it is called *papillitis* and, in bilateral cases, can be impossible to differentiate from papilledema. Optic neuritis can also be mimicked by anterior segment, choroidal, or retinal diseases. Optic neuritis is distinguished from optic neuropathy, which is a chronic, generally noninflammatory condition of the optic nerve caused by tobacco or nutritional amblyopia, ischemia, Leber's disease, or other rare hereditary diseases (Chapter 432).

TREATMENT

Among patients with optic neuritis, the 15-year risk of developing MS is 25% in patients without lesions on their baseline brain MRI but 72% in patients with one or more baseline MRI lesions. Treatment with intravenous methylprednisolone as in MS may shorten the duration and severity of the attack, but no definitive evidence indicates that it changes the long-term outcome. Oral prednisone alone, without prior treatment with intravenous methylprednisolone, may increase the risk for recurrent optic neuritis and should be avoided. Data support the use of IFN-β drugs and glatiramer acetate in patients whose optic neuritis is at high risk for conversion to MS (one or more typical brain MRI lesions).

Transverse Myelitis

Transverse myelitis is a rare (~1 in 100,000 people) monophasic inflammatory process of the spinal cord that is usually distinct from MS in that it either involves the entire cross section or is longitudinally extensive along three vertebral body segments rostrocaudally. Transverse myelitis may be idiopathic or associated with inflammatory diseases (systemic lupus erythematosus, Sjögren's syndrome, vasculitis, or MS), infectious diseases, or vascular diseases (antiphospholipid antibody syndrome or dural venous fistula).

CLINICAL MANIFESTATIONS AND DIAGNOSIS

In its fulminant form, transverse myelitis causes complete loss of motor and sensory function below the affected level of the spinal cord and causes concomitant bowel, bladder, and sexual dysfunction. Autonomic involvement can be seen in cervical and high thoracic spine cases. Transverse myelitis may also manifest in an incomplete or partial form, which is more commonly associated with MS.

TREATMENT AND PROGNOSIS

Treatment is usually with methylprednisolone (1000 mg intravenously for 3 to 5 days), followed by specific treatment of any identifiable underlying disease process. The prognosis is worse than in MS in that significant recovery is seen in fewer than 50% of patients, and many patients remain completely paralyzed after the initial attack. Plasma exchange or cyclophosphamide may be considered in steroid-refractory cases.

NEUROMYELITIS OPTICA

Neuromyelitis optica is now recognized as a distinct entity from MS and is characterized by an optic neuritis, often bilateral and temporally associated with a fulminant multilevel transverse myelitis. A specific IgG directed against aquaporin 4 strongly predicts this process. Brain lesions may be seen on MRI and have a predilection for the brain stem. Neuromyelitis optica may be similar to what is called *opticospinal MS* in Japan. There is no proven effective treatment, but patients are usually given anti-inflammatory and immunosuppressive medications. Therapies directed against B cells or humoral factors are being explored. The prognosis is generally poor; most patients develop sustained disabling visual loss and weakness.

ACUTE DISSEMINATED ENCEPHALOMYELITIS

Acute disseminated encephalomyelitis and its hyperacute form, acute necrotizing hemorrhagic encephalopathy, are thought to be forms of monophasic immune-mediated inflammatory demyelination. They differ from MS in that they are typically monophasic, whereas MS is by definition multiphasic or chronically progressive. However, no reliable clinical or pathologic criteria are available to differentiate the two processes, which may represent a continuum. Patients may present with fever, headache, meningeal signs, and altered consciousness, which are exceedingly rare in MS. There is no known effective treatment. Large numbers of patients, especially children, make remarkable recoveries, but the necrotizing form can be severely disabling or fatal.

Leukodystrophies

The leukodystrophies represent a variety of diseases formerly characterized by their common clinical and pathologic characteristics of white matter and, presumably, myelin. Many of these diseases now have a defined biochemical and genetic basis, and some (e.g., Alexander's disease) are no longer considered dysmyelinating diseases.

ADRENOLEUKODYSTROPHY AND ADRENOMYELONEUROPATHY

Adrenoleukodystrophy and adrenomyeloneuropathy, which are caused by impaired ability of the peroxisomes to metabolize very long chain fatty acids, represent different phenotypes resulting from the same X-linked, incompletely recessive genetic defect. Impaired oxidation of very long chain fatty acids results from deficient function of the enzyme lignoceroyl–coenzyme A ligase. The defective gene maps to Xq28 and codes for a peroxisomal membrane protein (ALDP), which is a member of a large family of proteins referred to as the adenosine triphosphate–binding cassette (ABC) transporters, specifically *ABCD1*.

Childhood cerebral adrenoleukodystrophy, which is the most common form of the disorder, represents 45% of all cases; it is seen only in male patients, with an onset at ages 4 to 11 years. Adolescent (5%) and adult (3%) cerebral forms progress at a similar or slower rate compared with the childhood form.

CLINICAL MANIFESTATIONS

Adrenomyeloneuropathy begins in young men as slowly progressive paraparesis with hypogonadism, impotence, sphincter disturbances, variable adrenal insufficiency, and axonal neuropathy affecting mainly the lower extremities. A rare acute inflammatory form with rapid progression and dementia may occur. A similar, but usually milder, disorder can be seen in up to 20% of women who are hemizygous for the disease.

DIAGNOSIS

Diagnosis is established in male patients by finding elevated very long chain fatty acids in the plasma. DNA-based diagnosis in carriers is reliable and is recommended in women because of false-negative results using the plasma assay.

TREATMENT Rx

Treatment is unsatisfactory. A 4:1 mixture of glyceryl trioleate and glyceryl trierucate (i.e., "Lorenzo's oil") normalizes plasma very long chain fatty acids within 4 weeks and has few side effects. Although clinical trials suggested that treatment in presymptomatic patients delayed or prevented the onset of disease, this treatment is ineffective after symptoms have begun, and the disease progresses relentlessly.

PELIZAEUS-MERZBACHER DISEASE

Pelizaeus-Merzbacher disease is an extremely rare, chronic, familial leukodystrophy usually caused by a genetic defect in the myelin proteolipid (PLP; lipophilin) protein gene. In classic Pelizaeus-Merzbacher disease, age at onset varies between 3 months and 9 years, the age at death varies between 6 years and 25 years, and the longest duration of the disease is approximately 24 years. The disease manifests as a slowly progressive myelopathy, often with cerebellar and cognitive involvement. The diagnosis is established by genetic testing for mutations in the *PLP* gene. No specific treatment exists for Pelizaeus-Merzbacher disease.

METACHROMATIC LEUKODYSTROPHY

Metachromatic leukodystrophy usually results from a recessively inherited defect in the lysosomal enzyme arylsulfatase A. Absence of arylsulfatase A results in the accumulation of sulfatide in both central and peripheral myelin and myelin-forming cells; instability of the myelin membranes results in the breakdown of myelin. Metachromatic leukodystrophy is generally divided into four subtypes: congenital, late infantile (most common), juvenile, and adult. It appears in all ethnic groups and has an overall frequency of 1 in 40,000.

The clinical manifestations are variable and may include progressive spastic paraparesis, extrapyramidal signs, seizures, and peripheral neuropathy. Brain MRI usually shows large confluent symmetrical high-signal areas in the cerebral white matter, brain stem, and cerebellum, but a more patchy appearance resembling MS is occasionally seen in adult cases. At present, no satisfactory treatment exists. Some evidence suggests that bone marrow transplantation delays the onset in presymptomatic patients and may slow progression of the disease.

GLOBOID CELL LEUKODYSTROPHY

Globoid cell leukodystrophy is characterized biochemically by accumulation of galactocerebroside in cerebral white matter as a result of deficient galactocerebroside β-galactosidase activity. The disease is transmitted as an autosomal recessive trait and affects infants in the first 2 to 3 months of life, initially manifesting with behavioral changes and failure to achieve developmental milestones. Rare late-onset cases present with progressive motor impairment and, less frequently, visual failure. Neuropathologic examination reveals marked loss of myelin throughout the brain, with the presence of round or oval macrophages and large, irregular, multinucleated cells, termed *globoid cells,* which are filled with galactocerebroside. Accumulation of galactosylsphingosine (psychosine) is thought to cause destruction of oligodendrocytes and marked reduction of myelin formation.

CANAVAN'S DISEASE

Canavan's disease is a fatal, progressive leukodystrophy with an autosomal recessive inheritance, caused by mutations in the gene for aspartoacylase, an enzyme that hydrolyzes *N*-acetylaspartate into L-aspartate and acetate. Aspartoacylase deficiency results in elevated levels of its substrate molecule, *N*-acetylaspartate, brain edema, and dysmyelination. Clinically, the disease manifests with retardation, seizures, and diffuse, symmetrical white matter degeneration in the subcortical areas, with involvement of the globus pallidum on MRI. No treatment is available.

1. The IFN-β Multiple Sclerosis Study Group. Interferon beta-1b is effective in relapsing-remitting multiple sclerosis. I. Clinical results of a multicenter, randomized, double-blind, placebo-controlled trial. *Neurology.* 1993;43:656-661.
2. Jacobs LD, Cookfair DL, Rudick RA, et al. Intramuscular interferon beta-1a for disease progression in relapsing multiple sclerosis: The Multiple Sclerosis Collaborative Research Group (MSCRG). *Ann Neurol.* 1996;39:285-294.
3. PRISMS Study Group (Prevention of Relapses and Disability by Interferon beta-1a Subcutaneously in Multiple Sclerosis). Randomised double-blind placebo-controlled study of interferon beta-1a in relapsing/remitting multiple sclerosis. *Lancet.* 1998;352:1498-1504.
4. Johnson KP, Brooks BR, Cohen JA, et al. Copolymer 1 reduces relapse rate and improves disability in relapsing-remitting multiple sclerosis: results of a phase III multicenter, double-blind placebo-controlled trial. *Neurology.* 1995;45:1268-1276.
5. Polman C, O'Connor PW, Havrdovra E, et al. A randomized, placebo-controlled trial of natalizumab for relapsing multiple sclerosis. *N Engl J Med.* 2006;354:899-910.
6. Coles AJ, Compston DA, Selmaj KW, et al, for the CAMMS223 Trial Investigators. Alemtuzumab vs. interferon beta-1a in early multiple sclerosis. *N Engl J Med.* 2008;359:1786-1801.
7. Hartung H-P, Gonsette R, Konig N, et al. Mitoxantrone in progressive multiple sclerosis: a placebo-controlled, double-blind, randomized, multicentre trial. *Lancet.* 2002;360:2018-2025.
8. Hauser SL, Waubant E, Arnold DL, et al. B-cell depletion with rituximab in relapsing-remitting multiple sclerosis. *N Engl J Med.* 2008;358:676-688.
9. Cohen JA, Barkhof F, Comi G, et al. Oral fingolimod or intramuscular interferon for relapsing multiple sclerosis. *N Engl J Med.* 2010;362:402-416.
10. Kappos L, Radue EW, O'Connor P, et al. A placebo-controlled trial of oral fingolimod in relapsing multiple sclerosis. *N Engl J Med.* 2010;362:387-401.
11. Giovannoni G, Comi G, Cook S, et al. A placebo-controlled trial of oral cladribine for relapsing multiple sclerosis. *N Engl J Med.* 2010;362:416-426.
12. Comi G, Pulizzi A, Rovaris M, et al. Effect of laquinimod on MRI-monitored disease activity in patients with relapsing-remitting multiple sclerosis: a multicentre, randomised, double-blind, placebo-controlled phase IIb study. *Lancet.* 2008;371:2085-2092.
13. Kappos L, Gold R, Miller DH, et al. Efficacy and safety of oral fumarate (240 mg thrice daily but not lower doses) in patients with relapsing-remitting acute multiple sclerosis: a multicentre, randomised, double-blind, placebo-controlled phase IIb study. *Lancet.* 2008;372:1463-1472.
14. Goodman AD, Brown TR, Krupp LG, et al. Sustained-release oral fampridine in multiple sclerosis: a randomised, double-blind, controlled trial. *Lancet.* 2009;373:732-738.

SUGGESTED READINGS

Fancy SP, Kotter MR, Harrington EP, et al. Overcoming remyelination failure in multiple sclerosis and other myelin disorders. *Exp Neurol.* 2010;225:18-23. *Overview of pathobiology.*
Frohman EM, Wingerchuk DM. Transverse myelitis. *N Engl J Med.* 2010;363:564-572. *Clinical review.*
Polman CH, Reingold SC, Banwell B, et al. Diagnostic criteria for multiple sclerosis: 2010 revisions to the McDonald criteria. *Ann Neurol.* 2011;69:292-302. *Review.*
Tremlett H, Zhao Y, Rieckmann P, et al. New perspectives in the natural history of multiple sclerosis. *Neurology.* 2010;74:2004-2015. *Review.*

420

MENINGITIS: BACTERIAL, VIRAL, AND OTHER

MORTON N. SWARTZ AND AVINDRA NATH

BACTERIAL MENINGITIS

DEFINITION

Meningitis is an inflammation of the arachnoid membrane, the pia mater, and the intervening cerebrospinal fluid (CSF). The inflammatory process extends throughout the subarachnoid space around the brain and spinal cord and involves the ventricles. Pyogenic meningitis is usually an acute bacterial infection that evokes a polymorphonuclear response in CSF. By comparison, tuberculous meningitis (Chapter 332) is often subacute and characterized initially by a modest polymorphonuclear pleocytosis that rapidly evolves to lymphocytic predominance.

EPIDEMIOLOGY

The incidence of bacterial meningitis has dropped dramatically in developed countries since the introduction of vaccines against bacterial pathogens such as *Haemophilus influenzae* type b (Chapter 308), *Streptococcus pneumoniae* (Chapter 297), and *Neisseria meningitidis* (Chapter 306). Worldwide, however, bacterial meningitis remains a major cause of mortality and morbidity. Although all human microbes have the potential to cause meningitis, only a few organisms account for most cases of bacterial meningitis.

The clinical setting in which meningitis develops may provide a clue to the specific bacterial cause. *H. influenzae* (Chapter 308) affects primarily children, whereas *S. pneumoniae* (Chapter 297) causes meningitis in adults, especially those older than 50 years with comorbid conditions. Meningococcal meningitis (Chapter 306) most often occurs in outbreaks. In developed countries, *Listeria monocytogenes* (Chapter 301) is emerging as the most common cause of bacterial meningitis, with peak frequencies in the neonatal period and in persons 60 years of age and older. Simultaneous mixed bacterial meningitis is rare but occurs in the setting of neurosurgical procedures, penetrating head injury, head trauma with fracture of the cribriform plate, erosion of the skull or vertebrae by adjacent neoplasm, extension of osteomyelitis, or intraventricular rupture of a cerebral abscess; isolation of anaerobes should strongly suggest the latter two of these situations. Meningitis involving anaerobes may also occur very rarely as a result of an intestinal-meningeal fistula following surgery and radiation therapy for colorectal cancer. In approximately 10% of patients with pyogenic meningitis, the bacterial cause cannot be defined.

Over the past several decades, gram-negative bacillary meningitis has doubled in frequency in adults, a change reflecting more frequent and extensive neurosurgical procedures, as well as other nosocomial factors. *L. monocytogenes* has increased 8- to 10-fold as a cause of bacterial meningitis in large urban general hospitals. *Listeria* infections are most often food-borne via dairy products, processed meats, uncooked vegetables, and precut salads. Although *Listeria* meningitis may occur in immunocompetent individuals, it occurs mostly in organ transplant recipients, patients undergoing hemodialysis, patients receiving corticosteroids or cytotoxic drugs for treatment of cancer or autoimmune diseases, patients with liver disease, alcoholic patients, pregnant women, and neonates. Meningitis caused by coagulase-negative staphylococci, which represents approximately 3% of cases in large urban hospitals, occurs as a complication of neurosurgical procedures and is often caused by methicillin-resistant strains. *Streptococcus viridans, Pseudomonas,* and other gram-negative bacteria are the agents most often associated with meningitis that complicates diagnostic myelography and percutaneous trigeminal rhizotomy.

In large tertiary care hospitals, approximately 40% of cases of bacterial meningitis in adults are of nosocomial origin. The leading causes are gram-negative bacilli (primarily *Escherichia coli* and *Klebsiella*), which account for approximately 40% of nosocomial episodes, as well as various streptococci, *Staphylococcus aureus*, and coagulase-negative staphylococci, each responsible for approximately 10% of nosocomial cases.

Meningococcal disease, including meningitis, may occur sporadically and in cyclic outbreaks. High-risk groups include individuals who live in close quarters such as crowded classrooms, college dormitories, military barracks, or jails. The meningococcal vaccine is about 85% protective. In industrialized countries, serogroups B and C account for the majority of infections. In developing countries, serogroups A and, to a lesser extent, C are dominant. In sub-Saharan Africa, the so-called meningitis belt, recurrent yearly waves of serogroup A meningococcal infections can occur.

Predisposing factors for the development of pneumococcal meningitis include acute otitis media (Chapters 297 and 434), with or without mastoiditis, which is seen in approximately 20% of adult patients. Pneumonia is present in approximately 15% of patients with pneumococcal meningitis, a much higher frequency than in meningitis caused by *H. influenzae* or *N. meningitidis*. Acute pneumococcal sinusitis (Chapter 434) is occasionally the initial focus from which infection spreads to the meninges. A recent or remote major head injury (Chapter 406) precedes approximately 10% of episodes of pneumococcal meningitis, and CSF rhinorrhea (usually caused

by a defect or fracture in the cribriform plate) is present in approximately 5% of patients. Cochlear implants, particularly those that include a positioner, have been implicated in cases of childhood bacterial meningitis, especially episodes resulting from *S. pneumoniae*. Occasionally, meningitis caused by *S. pneumoniae* develops in patients with central nervous system (CNS) shunts. Splenectomy or splenic dysfunction, as in sickle cell anemia (Chapter 166) or in cirrhosis (Chapter 156) with portal hypertension, or other defects in humoral immunity also predispose patients to pneumococcal meningitis. Alcoholism (Chapter 32) is an underlying problem in 10 to 25% of adults with pneumococcal meningitis in urban hospitals. The estimated annual incidence of bacterial meningitis (primarily pneumococcal) in patients infected with human immunodeficiency virus (HIV) is 150-fold higher than in the general population.

S. aureus meningitis is seen most commonly as a complication of a neurosurgical procedure, after penetrating skull trauma, or occasionally secondary to staphylococcal bacteremia and endocarditis. Meningitis attributable to gram-negative bacilli takes one of three forms: neonatal meningitis, meningitis after trauma or neurosurgery, or spontaneous meningitis in adults (e.g., bacteremic *Klebsiella* meningitis in a patient with diabetes mellitus). The most common causes of gram-negative bacillary meningitis in adults are *E. coli* (≈30%) and *Klebsiella-Enterobacter* (≈40%). Meningitis caused by group A streptococci is uncommon but occasionally occurs after acute otitis media, more often in children than in adults. *H. influenzae* type b meningitis in an adult should raise the question of the presence of an underlying anatomic or immunologic defect.

Patients with defects in cell-mediated immunity are susceptible to the development of CNS infections with intracellular organisms such as *L. monocytogenes*. Patients with defective humoral immunity and an inadequate antibody response are particularly vulnerable to meningitis with *S. pneumoniae* and *H. influenzae*. Patients with neutropenia are at higher risk for meningitis with *Pseudomonas aeruginosa* and members of the Enterobacteriaceae family.

PATHOBIOLOGY

Pathology

On gross examination, purulent exudate in the subarachnoid space is most abundant in the cisterns at the base of the brain and over the convexities of the rolandic and sylvian sulci, which are expansions of the subarachnoid space. Although neither the infecting organism nor the inflammatory exudate directly invades cerebral tissue, the subjacent brain becomes congested and edematous. The effectiveness of the pial barrier generally prevents bacterial meningitis from causing a cerebral abscess; when these two processes coexist, the sequence is usually that an initial abscess leaks its contents into the ventricular system and produces secondary meningitis.

The inflammatory exudate can extend around the perivascular spaces to adjacent structures, especially the arteries and veins that carry a layer of pia mater and arachnoid membrane as they enter the brain from the cortical surface. *Cortical thrombophlebitis* results from venous stasis and adjacent meningeal inflammation. Infarction of cerebral tissue may follow. *Involvement of cortical and pial arteries* by peripheral aneurysm formation and vascular occlusion or narrowing (related to spasm, arteritis, or both) of the supraclinoid portion of the internal carotid artery at the base of the brain occurs in approximately 15% of patients with meningitis. The anterior and middle cerebral arteries may have markedly increased intracerebral blood flow velocity (an index of stenosis or arterial spasm) on transcranial Doppler ultrasonography, a finding corresponding to focal cerebral signs. In fulminating cases, particularly meningococcal meningitis, *cerebral edema* may be marked even though the pleocytosis is only moderate. Rarely, temporal lobe herniation through the tentorium develops in such patients and compresses the midbrain, thereby leading to ipsilateral third nerve palsy and contralateral hemiparesis or cerebellar herniation through the foramen magnum with compression of the medulla, which results in apnea, hemodynamic instability, and coma. *Damage to cranial nerves* occurs in areas where dense exudate accumulates around the nerves; the third and sixth cranial nerves are also vulnerable to damage by increased intracranial pressure. *Ventriculitis*, which probably occurs in most cases of bacterial meningitis, rarely progresses to *ventricular empyema*. As the exudates continue to accumulate, obstruction of the flow of CSF may result in *hydrocephalus*. Obstruction of the foramina of Magendie and Luschka at the base of the fourth ventricle results in noncommunicating or obstructive hydrocephalus, whereas obstruction at the level of the arachnoid granulations in the venous sinuses results in communicating hydrocephalus. *Subdural effusions* are sterile transudates that develop over the cerebral cortex and can be demonstrated readily by computed tomography (CT) as low-density areas about the cerebrum; rarely, such effusions become infected and produce subdural empyema.

Pathogenesis

Bacteria may gain access to the meninges by several routes: (1) hematogenous spread from a distant site, (2) direct ingress from the upper respiratory tract or skin through an anatomic defect (e.g., skull fracture, eroding sequestrum, meningocele, sequela of surgery), (3) passage intracranially through venules in the nasopharynx, or (4) spread from a contiguous focus of infection (infection of the paranasal sinuses, leakage of a brain abscess). Bacteremic spread of *H. influenzae*, *N. meningitidis*, and *S. pneumoniae* is probably the most frequent path of infection. Bacteremia is usually initiated by pharyngeal adhesion and colonization by an infecting strain. Adhesion of such strains, as well as of *S. pneumoniae*, to mucosal surfaces is abetted by their capacity to produce proteases that cleave immunoglobulin A, thus inactivating this local antibody defense. Adhesion of *N. meningitidis* to nasopharyngeal cells is affected by fimbriae or pili and promoted by previous damage to ciliated cells such as from smoking or viral infections. Meningococci invade the nasopharyngeal mucosal cells by means of endocytosis and are transported to the abluminal side in membrane-bound vacuoles. *H. influenzae*, in contrast, invades intercellularly by causing separation of the apical tight junctions between columnar epithelial cells. When these meningeal pathogens gain access to the blood stream, their intravascular survival is aided by the presence of polysaccharide capsules that inhibit phagocytosis and confer resistance to complement-mediated bactericidal activity.

The mechanism by which bacteria gain access to the subarachnoid spaces from blood appears to be related to specific adhesion molecules on brain endothelial cells. Once established in any part of the meninges, infection quickly extends throughout the subarachnoid space. Bacterial replication proceeds relatively unhindered because the low CSF levels of immunoglobulin and complement early in meningeal inflammation result in minimal or no opsonic or bactericidal activity and because surface phagocytosis of unopsonized organisms is meager in such a fluid environment. During meningitis, the concentrations of immunoglobulins in CSF increase but still remain relatively low. Secondary bacteremia may follow meningeal infection and may itself contribute to continuing further inoculation of CSF.

Bacterial meningitis following head trauma occurs because of a dural fistula from the nasal cavity, paranasal sinuses, or the middle ear to the subarachnoid space. The most frequent site is at the cribriform plate, where the bone is very thin and the dura is tightly adherent to the bone. Leakage of CSF results in CSF rhinorrhea and loss of smell.

Bacterial components (e.g., pneumococcal cell walls or lipoteichoic acid, *H. influenzae* lipopolysaccharide) are major elicitors of meningeal inflammation by causing release into the subarachnoid space of various pro-inflammatory cytokines such as interleukin-1 and tumor necrosis factor from endothelial and meningeal cells, macrophages, and microglia. Cytokines appear to enhance the passage of leukocytes by inducing several families of adhesion molecules that interact with the corresponding receptors on leukocytes. Cytokines can also increase the binding affinity of a leukocyte selectin, leukocyte adhesion molecule, for its endothelial cell receptor and may thereby further contribute to trafficking of neutrophils into the subarachnoid space.

In bacterial meningitis, neutrophils move into the subarachnoid space but are not able to control the bacterial infection because their phagocytic properties are inefficient as a result of a lack of opsonic and bactericidal activity. Within the subarachnoid space, neutrophils release products such as prostaglandins, matrix metalloproteinases, and free radicals that disrupt the endothelial intercellular tight junctions and the subendothelial basal lamina. The increased local vascular permeability of the blood-brain barrier may cause cerebral edema, which can also be caused by increased CSF pressure as a result of obstruction of CSF outflow because of interstitial inflammation at the level of the arachnoidal villi.

Cerebral blood flow, which depends on mean arterial pressure, appears to be increased in the very early stages of meningitis, but it subsequently decreases, substantially in some patients, in whom it may be responsible for ensuing neurologic injury. Localized regions of marked hypoperfusion, attributable to focal vascular inflammation or thrombosis, can occur in patients with normal blood flow. Impairment of cerebral blood flow autoregulation, as measured by transcranial Doppler ultrasonography of the middle cerebral artery, occurs in the early phase of acute bacterial meningitis and causes cerebral blood flow to correspond directly to mean arterial blood pressure, with attendant hyperperfusion or hypoperfusion of the brain. On recovery, the ability of the cerebral vasculature to maintain a constant level of perfusion despite variations in mean arterial pressure is restored.

CLINICAL MANIFESTATIONS

History

Acute-onset fever, generalized headache, vomiting, and stiff neck are common to many types of meningitis (Table 420-1). Most patients with community-acquired pyogenic meningitis have had an antecedent or accompanying upper respiratory tract infection or nonspecific febrile illness, acute otitis (or mastoiditis), or pneumonia. Myalgia, particularly in patients with meningococcal disease, backache, and generalized weakness are common symptoms. The illness usually progresses rapidly, with the development of confusion, obtundation, and loss of consciousness. Occasionally, the onset may be less acute, with meningeal signs being present for several days to a week.

General Physical Findings

Evidence of meningeal irritation is usually present as evidenced by a stiff neck, Kernig's sign, and Brudzinski's sign. Although the classic triad of fever, stiff neck, and change in mental status is present in only 44% of episodes, a combination of two of four symptoms (headache, fever, stiff neck, and altered mental status) is found in 95% of patients. The findings of meningitis may easily be overlooked in infants, obtunded patients, elderly patients with heart failure or pneumonia, or immunosuppressed individuals, who may have

TABLE 420-1	CHARACTERISTICS OF THE STUDY POPULATION*	
CHARACTERISTIC	**EPISODES OF MENINGITIS** (***N* = 696**)	
Duration of symptoms <24 hr	48%	
Predisposing conditions		
Otitis or sinusitis	25%	
Pneumonia	12%	
Immunocompromise[†]	16%	
Symptoms at initial evaluation		
Headache	87%	
Nausea	74%	
Neck stiffness	83%	
Triad of fever, neck stiffness, and change in mental status	44%	
Focal neurologic deficits	33%	
Aphasia	23%	
Hemiparesis	7%	
Indices of CSF inflammation		
Opening pressure (mm H$_2$O)[‡]	370 ± 130	
White cell count[§]		
Mean (cells/mm^3)	7753 ± 14,736	
<100/mm^3	7%	
100-999/mm^3	14%	
>999/mm^3	78%	
Protein (g/L)	4.9 ± 4.5	
CSF/blood glucose ratio	0.2 ± 0.2	
Positive blood culture[‖]	66%	
Blood tests		
ESR (mm/hr)[¶]	46 ± 37	
C-reactive protein (g/L)**	225 ± 132	
Platelet count (platelets/mm^3)[††]	198,000 ± 100,000	

*The study included 671 patients who had a total of 696 episodes of community-acquired meningitis. Plus-minus values are means ± standard deviation.
[†]Immunocompromise was defined by the use of immunosuppressive drugs, a history of splenectomy, or the presence of diabetes mellitus or alcoholism, as well as patients infected with human immunodeficiency virus.
[‡]CSF pressure was measured in 216 patients.
[§]The CSF leukocyte count was determined in 659 patients; CSF specimens from 14 patients had too many leukocytes for an exact count to be performed.
[‖]Blood culture was performed in 611 patients.
[¶]The ESR was determined in 549 patients.
**C-reactive protein levels were determined in 394 patients.
[††]The thrombocyte count was determined in 653 patients.
CSF = cerebrospinal fluid; ESR = erythrocyte sedimentation rate.
Data from 696 cases reported in van de Beek D, de Gans J, Spanjaard L, et al. Clinical features and prognostic factors in adults with bacterial meningitis. *N Engl J Med.* 2004;351:1849-1859.

meningitis without prominent meningeal signs; in such patients, lethargy should be investigated carefully, meningeal signs should be sought, and examination of CSF is indicated if any doubt exists. In elderly patients, neck stiffness may be difficult to evaluate because of osteoarthritis in the neck or stiffness of neck muscles secondary to basal ganglia disorders. When neck stiffness is caused by meningitis, the neck resists flexion but can be rotated passively from side to side; with cervical spine disease, however, resistance is present in all directions of neck movement. Neck stiffness disappears during coma.

The presence of a petechial or ecchymotic rash (see Fig. 306-3 in Chapter 306) in a patient with meningeal findings almost always indicates meningococcal infection and requires prompt treatment because of the rapidity with which this infection can progress (Chapter 306). Rarely, extensive petechial and ecchymotic lesions occur in meningitis caused by *S. pneumoniae, H. influenzae,* or echovirus type 9. Very rarely, skin lesions almost indistinguishable from those of meningococcal bacteremia occur in patients who have acute *S. aureus* endocarditis (see Fig. 76-1) and who also have meningeal signs and pleocytosis (secondary either to staphylococcal meningitis or to embolic cerebral infarction). Usually, one or two of the lesions in such a patient represent purulent purpura; aspiration of material reveals staphylococci on Gram staining. In the summer, viral aseptic meningitis may produce meningeal signs, macular and petechial skin lesions, and a pleocytosis of several hundred cells, sometimes with neutrophils predominating initially.

Fulminant meningococcal septicemia may cause hemorrhages within the adrenal glands and result in Waterhouse-Friderichsen syndrome (Chapter 234), a condition characterized by the sudden onset of a febrile illness, large petechial hemorrhages in the mucous membranes and skin, cardiovascular collapse, and disseminated intravascular coagulation. In contrast, hyponatremia and the syndrome of inappropriate secretion of antidiuretic hormone may develop in patients with meningitis attributable to *H. influenzae.* A concurrent respiratory tract infection or acute otitis media may be present with either *H. influenzae* or *S. pneumoniae.*

In patients with a basilar skull fracture, the potential for development of a dural fistula and bacterial meningitis is indicated by the presence of CSF rhinorrhea, periorbital ecchymoses, bruising behind the ear (Battle's sign), hemotympanum, or blood in the external auditory canal. Meningitis complicating neurosurgical procedures may be insidious in onset and difficult to distinguish from the altered consciousness and signs of meningeal irritation that are expected in the postoperative period. However, fever or prolonged obtundation is an indication for evaluation of CSF.

Neurologic Findings and Complications

Neurologic complications in patients with inadequately treated bacterial meningitis can be severe and disabling. Cranial nerve abnormalities, involving principally the third, fourth, sixth, or seventh nerve, occur in 5 to 10% of adults with community-acquired meningitis and usually disappear shortly after recovery. Persistent sensorineural hearing loss occurs in 10% of children with bacterial meningitis, and another 16% have transient conductive hearing loss. The most likely sites of involvement in patients with persistent sensorineural deafness appear to be the inner ear (infection or toxic products possibly spreading from the subarachnoid space along the cochlear aqueduct) and the acoustic nerve. In children, permanent hearing impairment is more common after meningitis caused by *S. pneumoniae* than by *H. influenzae* or *N. meningitidis.*

Seizures (focal or generalized; Chapter 410) occur in 20 to 30% of patients and may result from reversible causes (high fever or hypoglycemia in infants, penicillin neurotoxicity when large doses are administered intravenously to patients with renal failure) or, more commonly, from focal cerebral injury related to arterial hypoperfusion and infarction, cortical venous thrombosis, or focal edema and cerebritis. Seizures can occur during the first few days or can appear with associated focal neurologic deficits caused by vascular inflammation some days after onset of the meningitis. In adults with seizures accompanying meningitis, *S. pneumoniae* is more commonly the cause, but alcohol withdrawal is a confounding factor.

Increased CSF pressure, which can be caused by brain swelling or hydrocephalus, is associated with seizures, vomiting, sixth and third nerve dysfunction, abnormal reflexes, reduced consciousness or coma, dilated and poorly reactive pupils, and the Cushing response of decerebrate posturing, hypertension, bradycardia, and irregular respirations. In approximately a fourth of fatal cases of community-acquired meningitis in adults, cerebral edema accompanied by temporal lobe herniation is observed at autopsy.

Papilledema (see Fig. 431-27 in Chapter 431) occurs in less than 1% of patients with bacterial meningitis, even with high CSF pressure, probably because the patient is seen early in the process before changes in the nerve head have occurred. The presence of this sign should indicate the possibility of another associated and independent suppurative intracranial process, such as subdural empyema or brain abscess. Marked central hyperpnea sometimes occurs in patients with severe bacterial meningitis; CSF acidosis, which is principally due to increased lactic acid levels, provides much of the respiratory stimulus.

Focal cerebral signs (principally hemiparesis, dysphasia, visual field defects, and gaze preference) occur in approximately a third of adults with community-acquired bacterial meningitis. These signs may develop because of arterial or venous occlusion. In addition, cerebral blood flow velocity may be decreased in patients with increased intracranial pressure and may lead to temporary or lasting neurologic dysfunction. It is important to distinguish these vascular effects from postictal changes (Todd's paralysis), which usually persist for less than a day. Meningitis may also cause the syndrome of inappropriate secretion of antidiuretic hormone.

DIAGNOSIS

Bacterial meningitis is a medical emergency that requires immediate diagnosis and rapid institution of antimicrobial therapy. Delay in treatment is the most critical factor in determining the morbidity and mortality of patients with bacterial meningitis. The diagnosis of bacterial meningitis is not difficult in a febrile patient with meningeal symptoms and signs developing in the setting of a predisposing illness. The diagnosis may be less obvious in an elderly, obtunded patient with pneumonia or a confused alcoholic patient in impending delirium tremens.

When the diagnosis of bacterial meningitis is entertained, blood cultures should be performed, CSF examined and cultured, and antimicrobial therapy instituted promptly. If a mass lesion (cerebral abscess, subdural empyema) is suspected from the history, clinical setting, or physical findings (papilledema, focal cerebral signs), CT with or without contrast enhancement or magnetic resonance imaging (MRI) should be performed because of the danger of brain herniation with lumbar puncture. Antibiotics can and commonly should be started immediately, even before performing lumbar puncture, because it takes approximately 2 hours for antibiotics to affect CSF cultures. Diagnostic lumbar puncture should not be delayed to perform CT or MRI except in patients who have focal neurologic findings suggestive of a parameningeal collection or other intracranial mass lesions; in such patients, it is critical to initiate antimicrobial therapy for meningitis of unknown origin or brain abscess before CT or MRI is performed. Patients with community-acquired meningitis rarely have important abnormalities detected on CT in the absence of focal neurologic findings.

Laboratory Findings
Cerebrospinal Fluid Examination

Initial CSF pressure is usually moderately elevated (200 to 300 mm H_2O in adults). Striking elevations ($\geq$450 mm H_2O) occur in occasional patients with acute brain swelling complicating meningitis in the absence of an associated mass lesion. Findings on CSF analysis are strikingly abnormal in patients with meningitis, and such findings help suggest the cause even before the results of culture are available (Table 420-2). In patients with skull fractures, CSF rhinorrhea can be distinguished from nasal secretions by the presence of glucose.

Gram-Stained Smear

By the time of hospitalization, most patients with pyogenic meningitis have large numbers ($\geq$10^5/mL) of bacteria in their CSF. Careful examination of the Gram-stained smear of the spun sediment of CSF reveals the etiologic agent in 60 to 80% of cases. In most instances when gram-positive diplococci (or short-chain cocci) are observed on a stained CSF smear, they are pneumococci. In certain clinical settings, it is important to distinguish pneumococci from the relatively penicillin-resistant *Enterococcus,* an occasional cause of nosocomial meningitis, by latex particle agglutination. Rarely, three species may morphologically mimic *Neisseria* in CSF or may suggest a mixed infection with short gram-negative rods and meningococci: *Acinetobacter baumannii, Moraxella* sp, and *Pasteurella multocida.* Culture of CSF reveals the etiologic agent in 80 to 90% of patients with bacterial meningitis if CSF is obtained before or within 1 to 2 hours of the initiation of antibiotics.

TABLE 420-2 COMMON CEREBROSPINAL FLUID FINDINGS IN PATIENTS WITH MENINGITIS

MICROORGANISM	CSF OPENING PRESSURE (cm H$_2$O)	CELL COUNT (CELLS/mm^3)	PROTEIN (mg/dL)	GLUCOSE (mg/dL)
Bacteria*	>20	>1000	>100	<10
Mycobacterium tuberculosis	>20	100-500	>100	10-45
Borrelia burgdorferi	<20	100-500	50-150	10-45
Treponema pallidum	<20	5-500	50-150	10-45
Fungi	<20	5-500	>100	10-45
Viruses	<20	5-500	50-150	Normal

*Group B streptococci, *Escherichia coli*, *Listeria monocytogenes*, *Streptococcus pneumoniae*, *Neisseria meningitidis*, and *Haemophilus influenzae* type b.
CSF = cerebrospinal fluid.
Adapted from Kim KS. Acute bacterial meningitis in infants and children. *Lancet Infect Dis.* 2010;10:32-42.

Special Testing Procedures

Broad-range polymerase chain reaction (PCR), which can be performed on CSF within 1.5 hours, can diagnose bacterial meningitis in patients in whom antimicrobial therapy was begun before lumbar puncture or when cultures are negative and a bacterial origin is still suspected. However, specific real-time PCR for the diagnosis of pneumococcal and meningococcal meningitis is currently available only in the research setting. The sensitivity and specificity of rapid antigen testing by latex agglutination are highest (>90%) for *H. influenzae*, lower for *S. pneumoniae*, and considerably lower for *N. meningitidis*. Gram-stained smears almost invariably show the causative microorganism when the latex agglutination test result is truly positive, so latex agglutination is not used routinely for the diagnosis of bacterial meningitis. However, latex agglutination testing may be very useful when the CSF cell count is abnormal, the Gram stain is negative, and blood and CSF cultures are unrevealing at 48 hours, at which time a stored sample of the initial CSF specimen can be tested. Occasionally, when only rare organisms of ambiguous morphology or Gram-staining properties are seen, latex agglutination may be helpful in providing a more specific diagnosis. Other promising new techniques include a nucleic acid amplification technique, which may be useful in resource-poor settings, and a rapid immunochromatographic test for *S. pneumoniae*.

Cell Count

Cells counts should be determined promptly because the cells will begin to lyse after 90 minutes. The normal CSF white blood cell count is less than 5/mm^3 (all mononuclear). The cell count in untreated meningitis usually ranges between 100 and 10,000/mm^3, with polymorphonuclear leukocytes predominating initially (>80%) and lymphocytes appearing subsequently.

The cell count in *L. monocytogenes* meningitis tends to be lower (median, 585/mm^3) than in other types of community-acquired pyogenic meningitis. Extremely high cell counts (>50,000/mm^3) should raise the possibility of intraventricular rupture of a cerebral abscess. Cell counts as low as 10 to 20/mm^3 may be observed early in bacterial meningitis, particularly that caused by *N. meningitidis* and *H. influenzae*. Occasionally, in granulocytopenic patients or in elderly persons with overwhelming pneumococcal meningitis, CSF may contain very few leukocytes and yet may appear grossly turbid because of the presence of a myriad of organisms and an elevated protein level. Meningitis caused by several bacterial species (*Mycobacterium tuberculosis*, *Borrelia burgdorferi*, *Treponema pallidum*, *Leptospira* sp, *Francisella tularensis*, *Brucella* sp) is characteristically associated with a lymphocytic pleocytosis. With *L. monocytogenes* meningitis in an adult, there is usually a polymorphonuclear response, but lymphocytes may predominate in rare instances.

Glucose

CSF glucose is reduced to values of 40 mg/dL or less (or <50% of the simultaneous blood level) in 50% of patients with bacterial meningitis; this finding can be valuable in distinguishing bacterial meningitis from most viral meningitides or parameningeal infections. However, a normal CSF glucose value does not exclude the diagnosis of bacterial meningitis. The blood glucose level should be determined simultaneously because patients with diabetes mellitus (or those who are receiving intravenous glucose infusions) have an elevated CSF glucose level that can be appreciated only by comparison with the simultaneous blood level; however, it may take 90 to 120 minutes for equilibration to occur after major shifts in the level of glucose in the circulation. The hypoglycorrhachia characteristic of pyogenic meningitis appears to result from interference with normal carrier-facilitated diffusion of glucose and increased utilization of glucose by host cells.

Protein

The level of protein in lumbar CSF is usually elevated to greater than 100 mg/dL, and higher values are more commonly observed in pneumococcal meningitis. Extreme elevations, 1000 mg/dL or greater, may indicate subarachnoid block with obstruction of CSF flow. Values higher than 15 mg/dL in ventricular CSF are considered abnormal. If the lumbar puncture is traumatic, the CSF protein level is corrected by subtracting 1 mg/dL for every 1000 red blood cells.

Other Abnormalities

Elevated levels of lactic acid occur in pyogenic meningitis, but other conditions (cerebral ischemia, metabolism of CSF neutrophils, hypoxia) may also increase CSF lactate concentrations. Although lactate dehydrogenase levels are higher in patients with bacterial meningitis than in patients with viral infections of the CNS, these alterations are not helpful in determining the specific etiologic agent.

Blood and Respiratory Tract Cultures

Bacteremia is demonstrable in approximately 80% of patients with *H. influenzae* meningitis, 50% of patients with pneumococcal meningitis, and 30 to 40% of patients with meningococcal meningitis. Hence, blood cultures should be performed routinely in patients suspected of having bacterial meningitis. Cultures of the upper respiratory tract are not helpful in establishing an etiologic diagnosis.

Determination of serum creatinine and electrolyte levels is important in view of the gravity of the illness, the occurrence of specific abnormalities secondary to the meningitis (syndrome of inappropriate secretion of antidiuretic hormone), and problems with therapy in patients with renal dysfunction (seizures and hyperkalemia with high-dose penicillin therapy). In patients with extensive petechial and purpuric skin lesions, evaluation for coagulopathy is indicated. Elevated serum procalcitonin levels have been used to distinguish bacterial meningitis from that of viral origin, but CSF examination (Gram stain, white blood cell count, glucose, culture) usually provides more direct and specific information.

Radiologic Studies

Because of the frequency with which pyogenic meningitis is associated with primary foci of infection in the chest, nasal sinuses, or mastoid, radiographs of these areas should be taken when clinically indicated at the appropriate time after antimicrobial therapy is begun. Initial head CT or MRI is not indicated in most patients with bacterial meningitis. For example, in patients who undergo head CT or MRI before lumbar puncture for suspected meningitis, only approximately 5% have a mass effect identified on CT. Baseline clinical features associated with abnormal findings on CT include age older than 60 years, history of CNS disease, seizure within the previous week, abnormal level of consciousness, abnormal visual fields, limb drift, and aphasia. In patients without any of these clinical findings, only approximately 1% have a mass effect identified on CT or MRI that would raise concern regarding lumbar puncture.

Specific changes that may be observed on CT or MRI during meningitis include cerebral edema and enlargement of the subarachnoid spaces, contrast enhancement of the leptomeninges and the ependyma, or patchy areas of diminished density as a result of associated cerebritis and necrosis. In patients with meningitis whose clinical status deteriorates or fails to improve, CT or MRI may help demonstrate suspected complications: sterile subdural collections or empyema; ventricular enlargement secondary to communicating or obstructive hydrocephalus; prominent persisting basilar meningitis; extensive areas of cerebral infarction resulting from occlusion of major cerebral arteries, veins, or venous sinuses; or marked ventricular wall enhancement suggesting ventriculitis or ventricular empyema. MRI is superior to CT for visualizing these abnormalities. Rarely, cerebral hemorrhage identifiable on CT may complicate acute bacterial meningitis in adults. In approximately 10% of adults with bacterial meningitis, findings on cranial CT (mastoid or sinus wall defect, eroding retrobulbar mass, pneumocephalus) are indicative of disruption of the dural barrier.

Rarely, paraparesis or tetraparesis resulting from myelitis may complicate bacterial meningitis. In this situation, T2-weighted or short tau inversion recovery (STIR) sequences on MRI can be helpful to exclude spinal cord compression by an extramedullary mass.

Differential Diagnosis

Headache, fever, stiff neck, confusion, vomiting, and pleocytosis are features of meningeal inflammation and are common to many types of meningitis (e.g., bacterial, fungal, viral, chemical) and also to some parameningeal processes. The CSF findings are most helpful in distinguishing among these processes (Chapters 421 and 422). Although a lymphocyte-predominant pleocytosis without hypoglycorrhachia is characteristic of viral (usually enteroviral or herpes simplex virus type 2 [HSV-2]) meningitis or meningoencephalitis (HSV-1), the initial CSF finding may be a polymorphonuclear response (of ≤60%) that quickly becomes mononuclear. HSV-1 encephalitis is suggested by neurologic findings (dysphasia, hemiparesis, olfactory hallucinations, other temporal lobe signs, seizures), abnormalities in the orbitofrontal and medial temporal lobes on MRI, and distinctive electroencephalographic changes in the temporal lobe or lobes. The rash, fever, and headache of Rocky Mountain spotted fever (Chapter 335) may suggest meningococcal infection, but the geographic and seasonal predilections of the former can provide clues. Approximately 10% of patients hospitalized with Rocky Mountain spotted fever have CSF cell counts higher than 100/mm³ (>70% polymorphonuclear), and thus the condition may initially be confused with bacterial meningitis. The rash associated with enteroviral infections typically consists of erythematous macules and papules on the face, neck, and trunk. Acute subarachnoid hemorrhage (Chapter 415) may be confused with bacterial meningitis because of headache, stiff neck, and vomiting. However, subarachnoid hemorrhage usually has a more abrupt onset without a prodromal fever but with evidence of subarachnoid blood on CT or CSF examination. In patients with neuroleptic malignant syndrome (Chapters 417 and 427), fever, generalized rigidity, and a fluctuating level of consciousness with autonomic instability and leukocytosis may develop. The most specific laboratory abnormality in these patients is a markedly elevated creatine kinase level.

In a patient with meningitis but whose CSF does not reveal the etiologic agent on a Gram-stained smear, particularly when the CSF glucose level is normal and the polymorphonuclear pleocytosis is atypical, certain treatable processes that can mimic bacterial meningitis should be considered in the differential diagnosis:

1. *Parameningeal infections.* The presence of infections (chronic ear or nasal accessory sinus infections, lung abscess) predisposing to brain abscess, epidural (cerebral or spinal) abscess, subdural empyema, or pyogenic venous sinus phlebitis should be sought (Chapter 421). Neurologic symptoms may appear in the course of primary bacterial meningitis, but their presence should alert the physician to the need for close scrutiny for the presence of a space-occupying infectious process in the CNS. Neurologic symptoms or findings antedating the onset of meningeal symptoms should suggest the possibility of a parameningeal infection. Isolation of an anaerobic organism should suggest the possibility of intraventricular leakage of a cerebral abscess.
2. *Bacterial endocarditis.* Bacterial meningitis may occur during bacterial endocarditis (Chapter 76) caused by pyogenic organisms such as *S. aureus* and enterococci. In subacute bacterial endocarditis, sterile embolic infarctions of the brain may produce meningeal signs and a pleocytosis consisting of several hundred cells, including polymorphonuclear leukocytes. A history of dental manipulation, fever, and anorexia antedating the meningitis should be sought; careful examination for heart murmurs and peripheral stigmata of endocarditis is indicated.
3. *"Chemical" meningitis.* The clinical and CSF findings (polymorphonuclear pleocytosis and even reduced glucose level) of bacterial meningitis may

be produced by chemically induced inflammation. Acute meningitis after diagnostic lumbar puncture or spinal anesthesia may result from bacterial or chemical contamination of equipment or anesthetic agent. Chemical meningitis, characterized by polymorphonuclear pleocytosis, hypoglycorrhachia, and a latent period of 3 to 24 hours, occurs after 1% of metrizamide myelograms. Endogenous chemical meningitis resulting from material from an epidermoid tumor or a craniopharyngioma leaking into the subarachnoid space can produce polymorphonuclear pleocytosis and hypoglycorrhachia; birefringent material may be seen on polarizing microscopy of the CSF sediment.

Complications

Non-neurologic Complications

Shock

When shock occurs in patients with pyogenic meningitis, it is usually a manifestation of the accompanying intense bacteremia, as in fulminant meningococcemia, rather than a manifestation of the meningitis itself. Management is guided by the principles of septic shock therapy (Chapter 108), with appropriate modifications in patients with heart failure (Chapter 59).

Coagulation Disorders

Coagulopathies (Chapter 177) are frequently associated with the intense bacteremia (usually meningococcal, occasionally pneumococcal) and hypotension that can accompany meningitis. The changes may be mild, such as thrombocytopenia (with or without prolongation of the prothrombin and partial thromboplastin times), or more marked, with clinical evidence of disseminated intravascular coagulation (Chapter 178).

Septic Complications

Endocarditis

In patients with pneumococcal meningitis, particularly those with concomitant bacteremia and pneumonia, acute endocarditis (Chapter 76) can develop, most commonly on the aortic valve. In such patients, febrile relapse and a new cardiac murmur may appear shortly after the completion of antimicrobial therapy for meningitis.

Pyogenic Arthritis

Septic arthritis may result from the bacteremia associated with meningitis caused by *S. pneumoniae*, *N. meningitidis*, or *H. influenzae*.

Prolonged Fever

With appropriate antimicrobial treatment of community-acquired bacterial meningitis, patients become afebrile within 2 to 5 days. Sometimes, however, the fever persists or recurs after an afebrile period. In a patient with persisting headache, obtundation, and cerebral findings, inadequate drug therapy or neurologic sequelae (cortical venous thrombophlebitis, ventriculitis, subdural collections) are important considerations. Re-evaluation of CSF, particularly Gram-stained smear and culture, is essential in these circumstances. Drug-induced fever (Chapters 262 and 288) should be suspected in patients who continue to show clinical improvement in all other respects. Metastatic infection (septic arthritis, purulent pericarditis, thoracic empyema, endocarditis) may be the cause of continuing or recurrent fever. A syndrome, probably immunologic, consisting of fever, arthritis, and pericarditis 3 to 6 days after the initiation of effective antimicrobial therapy for meningococcal meningitis occurs in approximately 10% of patients (Chapter 306).

Recurrent Meningitis

Repeated episodes of bacterial meningitis generally indicate a host defect, either in local anatomy or in antibacterial and immunologic defenses (e.g., recurrent *N. meningitidis* infections in patients with congenital or acquired deficiencies of complement, particularly the late-acting components). Approximately 10% of episodes of pneumococcal meningitis in adults are recurrent meningitis, but only 0.5% of patients with community-acquired meningitis caused by other microorganisms have recurrent attacks. *S. pneumoniae* is the cause of a third of episodes of community-acquired recurrent meningitis; various streptococci, *H. influenzae*, and *N. meningitidis* are the cause of another third of episodes. In contrast, in nosocomial recurrent meningitis, gram-negative bacilli and *S. aureus* are the cause of approximately 60% of episodes. A history of head trauma is much more frequent in patients with recurrent meningitis. Organisms may enter the subarachnoid space directly, through a defect in the cribriform plate (the most common site), in association with the empty sella syndrome, by means of a basilar skull fracture, through an erosive sequestrum of the mastoid, through congenital dermal defects along the craniospinal axis (usually evident before adult life), or as a consequence of penetrating cranial trauma or neurosurgical procedures. The anatomic defect may produce a frank CSF leak (rhinorrhea or, less commonly, otorrhea) or may entrap a vascular cuff of meninges that may subsequently serve as a direct route for organisms to reach the meninges. CSF rhinorrhea may be intermittent, and meningitis may occur months or years after head injury.

Any patient with bacterial meningitis, particularly if the meningitis is recurrent, should be evaluated carefully for congenital or post-traumatic defects. The presence of CSF rhinorrhea should be sought at admission and subsequently (rhinorrhea may clear during active meningitis only to recur when the inflammation has resolved). Clinical clues suggesting the presence of a CSF fistula through the cribriform plate, pericranial air sinuses, or temporal bone include (1) a salty taste in the throat, (2) positionally dependent rhinorrhea (rhinorrhea only in the lateral recumbent or prone position suggests an otic or sphenoid origin), (3) anosmia (cribriform plate leak), and (4) hearing loss or full feeling in the ear, often with a finding of fluid or bubbles behind the tympanic membrane (leakage into the middle ear). Quantitative determination of the glucose and chloride content of nasal secretions and detection of a transferrin band unique to CSF by protein electrophoresis can definitively establish the presence of CSF rhinorrhea.

Recurrent pneumococcal meningitis may develop without apparent predisposing circumstances, and cryptic CSF leaks should be sought actively in such patients by CT of the frontal and mastoid regions and by radioisotope techniques. Radioiodine-labeled albumin is introduced intrathecally, and pledgets of cotton placed in the nares are subsequently examined for the radionuclide. Intrathecal introduction of fluorescein as a visual tracer (under ultraviolet light) can similarly be used to detect active leaks. Surgical closure of CSF fistulas should be performed to prevent further episodes of meningitis. Extracranial approaches through the ethmoidal sinuses can be used to repair cribriform plate or sphenoidal sinus dural defects and avoid the higher morbidity associated with craniotomy.

In most patients with CSF otorrhea and rhinorrhea after an acute head injury, the leak ceases in 1 or 2 weeks. *Persistent rhinorrhea for more than 4 to 6 weeks is an indication for surgical repair.* Prolonged administration of penicillin does not prevent pneumococcal meningitis and may encourage infection with more drug-resistant species.

TREATMENT   Rx

Antimicrobial Agents

Antimicrobial therapy should be initiated promptly in this life-threatening emergency. Subsequent management should be undertaken with close monitoring, often in an intensive care unit. Treatment should be aimed at the most likely causes based on clinical clues, such as the age of the patient, the presence of a petechial or purpuric rash, a recent neurosurgical procedure, and CSF rhinorrhea. However, it is difficult to distinguish among the various causes of bacterial meningitis on clinical grounds alone, although patients with pneumococcal meningitis frequently have altered mental status and progress rapidly to coma, often with recurrent seizures and the rapid development of focal neurologic deficits. If the infecting organism is observed on examination of a Gram-stained smear of the CSF sediment, specific therapy is initiated. If the etiologic agent is not seen on a smear from a patient with suspected bacterial meningitis or if lumbar puncture is delayed because head CT is needed, empirical antimicrobial therapy should be initiated (Table 420-3).

Adequate CSF bactericidal activity, which is critical to cure the meningitis, depends on the ability of the antibiotic to penetrate CSF and to maintain its activity in the purulent exudate, as well as on its metabolism and rate of clearance from CSF. The ability of the antibiotic to penetrate CSF depends on its lipid solubility, protein binding in serum, molecular size, and the status of the blood-CSF barrier. For example, chloramphenicol has very high lipid solubility, whereas β-lactam antibiotics have poor solubility. With the exception of rifampin and chloramphenicol, the commonly used antimicrobial agents do not readily penetrate the normal blood-brain barrier, but the passage of penicillin and other antimicrobial agents is enhanced in the presence of meningeal inflammation (Table 420-4). Antimicrobial drugs should be administered intravenously throughout the treatment period; the dose should not be reduced as the patient improves because normalization of the blood-brain barrier during recovery reduces the achievable CSF drug levels. Bactericidal drugs (penicillin, ampicillin, third-generation cephalosporins) are preferred whenever possible, and CSF levels of antibiotics at least 10 to 20 times the minimal bactericidal concentration are needed for optimal therapy. Some antibiotics are removed from CSF by active transport into blood via the epithelium of the choroid plexus; by comparison, third-generation cephalosporin antibiotics persist in CSF for longer periods. Antimicrobial drugs (first- or second-generation cephalosporins, clindamycin) do not provide effective levels in CSF and should not be used.

Empirical Treatment

Initial treatment of presumed bacterial meningitis when the etiologic agent cannot be identified on a Gram-stained smear of CSF is based on the available clinical clues. In older children and adults, therapy with vancomycin and a third-generation cephalosporin (cefotaxime or ceftriaxone) is recommended (see Table 420-3). In adults older than 50 years and in high-risk groups, ampicillin is also added because of penicillin-resistant pneumococci, the increased frequency of aerobic gram-negative bacilli in nosocomial meningitis and meningitis in immunocompromised patients, and the possibility of *L. monocytogenes*, which is susceptible to ampicillin but not to third-generation cephalosporins. In a penicillin-allergic individual, trimethoprim-sulfamethoxazole is a suitable alternative for *Listeria* meningitis. In special settings, such as nosocomial meningitis associated with neurosurgical procedures or penetrating head trauma, more resistant species such as methicillin-resistant *S. aureus*, coagulase-negative staphylococci, and *P. aeruginosa* may be responsible; in these situations, vancomycin in addition to cefepime is indicated as initial therapy.

Meningitis of Specific Bacterial Cause

Pneumococcal Meningitis

The treatment of choice for pneumococcal meningitis in adults has historically been penicillin, with vancomycin (or chloramphenicol) being a reasonable alternative in patients allergic to penicillin (see later). However, penicillin-resistant pneumococcal strains are found worldwide, including 25% of clinical isolates in the United States. Thus, antimicrobial susceptibilities should be determined for all pneumococcal isolates from CSF, blood, or sterile body fluids (see Table 420-4). Approximately 9% of pneumococcal isolates from patients with meningitis in the United States are resistant to third-generation cephalosporins, with a minimal inhibitory concentration of 2 µg/mL or greater. If the minimal inhibitory concentration for cefotaxime or ceftriaxone (≤1.0 µg/mL) indicates a susceptible isolate, cefotaxime or ceftriaxone would be the drug of choice. If the isolate is highly penicillin resistant or is resistant to 1.0 µg/mL ceftriaxone or cefotaxime, alternative therapy (vancomycin with or without rifampin intravenously) is indicated. Because of the increasingly wide distribution of highly resistant strains, initial therapy (pending susceptibility testing) with cefotaxime (or ceftriaxone) in addition to vancomycin intravenously is recommended. When initial adjunctive therapy with dexamethasone is used (see later) along with vancomycin, it should be borne in mind that vancomycin levels in CSF may be reduced by concomitant corticosteroid use.

Although resistance to chloramphenicol is unusual in pneumococcal isolates from the United States, chloramphenicol has poor bactericidal activity against penicillin-resistant isolates from children with meningitis in South Africa. The relative chloramphenicol resistance of such strains may not be discerned on usual laboratory testing, but it is revealed when the minimum bactericidal concentration is determined. For this reason, vancomycin is preferred over chloramphenicol for the initial treatment of pneumococcal meningitis in a highly penicillin-allergic patient.

The β-lactam antibiotic meropenem is as effective as cefotaxime for meningitis caused by *S. pneumoniae*, *N. meningitidis*, and *H. influenzae* in adults and in children. Cefepime is also similar to ceftriaxone and cefotaxime for infection with *S. pneumoniae*, *N. meningitidis*, and *H. influenzae*, and it has greater activity than these antibiotics against *Enterobacter* sp and *P. aeruginosa* (Table 420-5).

Meningococcal Meningitis

Intravenous administration of penicillin G and ampicillin, in doses used to treat meningitis caused by penicillin-susceptible pneumococci, successfully treats *N. meningitidis* meningitis resulting from susceptible strains. Meningococci resistant to penicillin have occasionally been isolated in Spain (≤50% of strains), South Africa, and Canada but rarely in the United States. Most of these isolates have been only intermediately resistant to penicillin (minimal inhibitory concentration of 0.1 to 1.0 µg/mL), although rare strains have had high-level resistance related to β-lactamase production and require third-generation cephalosporins such as ceftriaxone, which is as effective as the potentially more toxic chloramphenicol.[1] Nevertheless, "meningitis doses" of penicillin or ampicillin may provide CSF levels that are sufficient for infections with some strains of intermediately penicillin-resistant *N. meningitidis*. Usually, a 7-day course of antibiotics is sufficient.

Haemophilus influenzae Meningitis

At present, 25 to 35% of isolates of *H. influenzae* type b in the United States are β-lactamase producers and are ampicillin resistant; cefotaxime or ceftriaxone is the initial therapy of choice (see Table 420-5). Alternatives include cefepime or the combination of chloramphenicol and ampicillin; if the isolate proves susceptible to ampicillin, chloramphenicol may be discontinued. Although more than 50% of isolates are chloramphenicol resistant in some

TABLE 420-3 INITIAL EMPIRICAL THERAPY FOR COMMUNITY-ACQUIRED AND NOSOCOMIAL PURULENT MENINGITIS BASED ON AGE AND CLINICAL SETTING

PREDISPOSITIONS	LIKELY PATHOGENS	PREFERRED ANTIMICROBIALS	ALTERNATIVE ANTIMICROBIALS
Age			
<1 mo	Group B streptococcus, *Escherichia coli*, *Listeria monocytogenes*, *Klebsiella* sp	Ampicillin plus cefotaxime	Ampicillin plus aminoglycoside
1-23 mo	*Streptococcus pneumoniae*, *Neisseria meningitidis*, group B streptococci, *Haemophilus influenzae*, *Escherichia coli*	Vancomycin* plus ceftriaxone or cefotaxime	Meropenem (? plus vancomycin*)
2-50 yr	*Neisseria meningitidis*, *Streptococcus pneumoniae*	Vancomycin* plus ceftriaxone or cefotaxime	Meropenem (? plus vancomycin*)
>50 yr	*Streptococcus pneumoniae*, *Neisseria meningitidis*, *Listeria monocytogenes*	Vancomycin* plus ceftriaxone or cefotaxime plus ampicillin	Vancomycin* plus ceftriaxone or cefotaxime plus trimethoprim-sulfamethoxazole
Impaired immunity	*Listeria monocytogenes*, gram-negative bacilli, *Streptococcus pneumoniae*	Ampicillin plus ceftazidime plus vancomycin*	Trimethoprim-sulfamethoxazole plus meropenem
Cerebrospinal fluid leak or basilar skull fracture	*Streptococcus pneumoniae*, various streptococci, *Haemophilus influenzae*	Vancomycin* plus cefotaxime or ceftriaxone	Vancomycin* plus meropenem
After neurosurgery or penetrating trauma	*Staphylococcus aureus*, coagulase-negative staphylococci, aerobic gram-negative bacilli (including *Pseudomonas aeruginosa*)	Vancomycin* plus cefepime	Vancomycin* plus ceftazidime or vancomycin* plus meropenem
Cerebrospinal fluid shunts (external or internal)	Coagulase-negative staphylococci, *Staphylococcus aureus*, aerobic gram-negative bacilli (including *Pseudomonas aeruginosa*), *Propionibacterium acnes*	Vancomycin* plus cefepime	Vancomycin* plus ceftazidime or vancomycin* plus meropenem

*If dexamethasone is also administered, consideration should be given to the addition of rifampin.
Modified from Tunkel AR, Hartman BJ, Kaplan SL, et al. IDSA practice guidelines for the management of bacterial meningitis. *Clin Infect Dis.* 2004;39:1267-1284.

TABLE 420-4 PERMEABILITY OF ANTIBIOTICS INTO CSF

GOOD CONCENTRATIONS IN CSF WITH AND WITHOUT MENINGITIS	ADEQUATE CONCENTRATIONS IN CSF IN MENINGITIS	FAIR TO POOR CONCENTRATIONS IN CSF IN MENINGITIS
Chloramphenicol	Penicillin	Early cephalosporins
Sulfonamides	Ampicillin	Cephalothin
Cephalosporins	Methicillin	Cefoxitin
Cefotaxime	Oxacillin	Aminoglycosides
Ceftriaxone	Nafcillin	Gentamicin
Ceftazidime	Carbenicillin	Tobramycin
Moxalactam	Ticarcillin	Amikacin
Cefepime	Tetracycline	Clindamycin
Metronidazole	Erythromycin	Benzathine penicillin
Trimethoprim-sulfamethoxazole	Ethambutol	
Isoniazid	Rifampin	
	Vancomycin	
	Meropenem	

CSF = cerebrospinal fluid.
Courtesy Allen Aksamit, Mayo Clinic, Rochester, Minn.

TABLE 420-5 ANTIMICROBIAL THERAPY FOR COMMUNITY-ACQUIRED BACTERIAL MENINGITIS OF KNOWN CAUSE IN ADULTS OR CHILDREN

ORGANISM	PREFERRED ANTIMICROBIAL THERAPY	ALTERNATIVE ANTIMICROBIAL THERAPY
Streptococcus pneumoniae		
Penicillin MIC <0.1 µg/mL	Penicillin G or ampicillin	Cefotaxime, or ceftriaxone, or vancomycin, or chloramphenicol
Penicillin MIC 0.1-1 µg/mL	Ceftriaxone or cefotaxime	Vancomycin,* or meropenem, or cefepime
Penicillin MIC ≥2.0 µg/mL	Vancomycin* (plus cefotaxime or ceftriaxone)	Moxifloxacin or gatifloxacin
Cefotaxime or ceftriaxone MIC ≥1.0 µg/mL	Vancomycin* (plus cefotaxime or ceftriaxone)	Moxifloxacin or gatifloxacin
Neisseria meningitidis		
Penicillin MIC <0.1 µg/mL	Penicillin G or ampicillin	Ceftriaxone, or cefotaxime, or chloramphenicol
Penicillin MIC 0.1-1.0 µg/mL	Ceftriaxone or cefotaxime	Chloramphenicol, or meropenem, or gatifloxacin, or moxifloxacin
Haemophilus influenzae		
β-Lactamase negative	Ampicillin	Ceftriaxone, or cefotaxime, or cefepime, or chloramphenicol
β-Lactamase positive	Ceftriaxone or cefotaxime	Cefepime, or chloramphenicol, or gatifloxacin, or moxifloxacin
Listeria monocytogenes	Ampicillin† or penicillin G†	Trimethoprim-sulfamethoxazole or meropenem
Streptococcus agalactiae (group B streptococci)	Ampicillin† or penicillin G†	Cefotaxime or ceftriaxone

*Addition of rifampin should be considered. Consider intrathecal (or intraventricular vancomycin, 5 to 20 mg/day) if not responding to intravenous therapy.
†Addition of intravenous gentamicin should be considered.
MIC = minimal inhibitory concentration.
From Tunkel AR, Hartman BJ, Kaplan SL, et al. IDSA practice guidelines for the management of bacterial meningitis. *Clin Infect Dis.* 2004;39:1267-1284.

areas of Spain, less than 1% of isolates have been found to be resistant in the United States. A 10-day course of antibiotics is usually sufficient.

Staphylococcal Meningitis

For the treatment of adult meningitis caused by methicillin-susceptible *S. aureus* or in a penicillin-allergic patient, vancomycin is the alternative of choice (Tables 420-6 and 420-7). Because penetration of vancomycin into CSF is limited, adjunctive intrathecal (or intraventricular) therapy with vancomycin (without preservative) is occasionally used when CSF cultures have remained positive after 48 hours of intravenous therapy alone and CSF levels can be monitored. For adult meningitis caused by methicillin-resistant *S. aureus*, intravenous vancomycin (with adjunctive intrathecal vancomycin as needed) is the treatment of choice. In severe or refractory cases, the addition of rifampin is warranted.

Listeria Meningitis

Ampicillin is the drug of choice for *Listeria* meningitis. When combined with gentamicin, it can have a synergistic bactericidal effect. Third-generation cephalosporins and vancomycin are not effective. In patients allergic to

---

TABLE 420-6 THERAPY FOR NOSOCOMIAL MENINGITIS OF KNOWN BACTERIAL CAUSE IN ADULTS

ORGANISM	THERAPY OF CHOICE	ALTERNATIVE THERAPY
Staphylococcus aureus		
Methicillin susceptible	Nafcillin or oxacillin; in difficult cases may add rifampin	Vancomycin or meropenem
Methicillin resistant	Vancomycin; in difficult cases may add rifampin	Linezolid or trimethoprim-sulfamethoxazole
Coagulase negative	Vancomycin; may consider addition of rifampin	Linezolid
Enterococcus sp		
Ampicillin susceptible	Ampicillin plus gentamicin	Vancomycin plus gentamicin
Ampicillin resistant	Vancomycin plus gentamicin	Linezolid
Ampicillin and vancomycin resistant	Linezolid	
Escherichia coli and other	Cefotaxime or ceftazidime	Meropenem or aztreonam or ampicillin or trimethoprim-sulfamethoxazole
Enterobacteriaceae*		
*Pseudomonas aeruginosa**	Cefepime or ceftazidime	Meropenem or aztreonam or ciprofloxacin

*Selection of specific antimicrobial drug should be based on in vitro susceptibility results, with consideration given to the addition of an aminoglycoside (e.g., tobramycin, gentamicin, or amikacin).

TABLE 420-7 DOSES OF ANTIMICROBIAL DRUGS FOR TREATMENT OF BACTERIAL MENINGITIS*

ANTIMICROBIAL DRUG	ADULTS (24-HR DOSE)	INFANTS AND CHILDREN (24-HR DOSE)
β-LACTAMS		
Penicillin G	24 million U, q4h aliquots	300,000 U/kg, q4h aliquots
Ampicillin	12 g, q4h aliquots	300 mg/kg, q4h aliquots
Nafcillin	10-12 g, q4h aliquots	200 mg/kg, q4h aliquots
Oxacillin	10-12 g, q4h aliquots	200 mg/kg, q4h aliquots
Aztreonam (a monobactam)	6-8 g, q6-8h aliquots	
Meropenem (a carbapenem†)	6 g, q8h aliquots	120 mg/kg, q8h aliquots
CEPHALOSPORINS		
Cefotaxime	12 g, q4h aliquots	200-300 mg/kg, q6h aliquots
Ceftriaxone‡	4 g, q12h aliquots	80-100 mg/kg, q12h aliquots
Ceftazidime	6 g, q8h aliquots	150 mg/kg, q8h aliquots
Cefepime	6 g, q6-8h aliquots	150 mg/kg, q8h aliquots
AMINOGLYCOSIDES		
Gentamicin§	5 mg/kg, q8h aliquots	7.5 mg/kg, q8h aliquots
Tobramycin§	5 mg/kg, q8h aliquots	7.5 mg/kg, q8h aliquots
Amikacin§	15 mg/kg, q8h aliquots	20-25 mg/kg, q8h aliquots
FLUOROQUINOLONES		
Ciprofloxacin	800-1200 mg, q8-12h aliquots	—
Gatifloxacin‖	400 mg, q24h dosing	—
Moxifloxacin‖	400 mg, q24h dosing	—
OTHERS		
Chloramphenicol	4-6 g, q6h aliquots	75-100 mg/kg, q6h aliquots
Vancomycin¶	2-3 g, q6-8h aliquots	50-60 mg/kg, q6h aliquots
Rifampin	600 mg, q24h dosing	10-20 mg/kg, q12-24h aliquots
Trimethoprim-sulfamethoxazole**	20 mg/kg, q6h aliquots	20 mg/kg, q6h aliquots
Linezolid	1200 mg, q12h aliquots	30 mg/kg, q8h aliquots

*Dosages are intravenous and for patients with normal renal and hepatic function.
†Use may be associated with seizures, but much less so than with imipenem.
‡Four-gram maximum daily dose.
§Peak and trough serum levels should be monitored.
‖No data are available on the optimal dosage required for bacterial meningitis.
¶Monitoring of trough serum levels is advisable; they should be maintained at concentrations of 15 to 20 μg/mL. If the patient is not responding well, one may need to monitor cerebrospinal fluid levels and, if low, temporarily increase the daily dose accordingly or add adjuvant intrathecal vancomycin (5 to 20 mg), as for the treatment of methicillin-resistant *Staphylococcus aureus* meningitis.
**Dosage based on the trimethoprim component of the combination.

ampicillin, intravenous trimethoprim-sulfamethoxazole may be used, followed by oral trimethoprim alone.

Gram-Negative Bacillary Meningitis

Cefotaxime or ceftriaxone (see Tabless 420-6 and 420-7) is used to treat meningitis known to be caused by susceptible gram-negative bacilli (e.g., *E. coli*, *Klebsiella*, *Proteus*), but they should not be used to treat meningitis caused by less susceptible species such as *P. aeruginosa* and *Acinetobacter*. After identifying the specific pathogen and determining its drug susceptibilities, alterations in antimicrobial therapy may be indicated. Although experience is limited, fluoroquinolones can also be used. If the organism is *P. aeruginosa*, ceftazidime or cefepime is recommended and may be combined with vancomycin (see Tables 420-6 and 420-7).

Zoonotic Meningitis

Uncommonly, systemic or bacteremic zoonotic infections are complicated by bacterial meningitis. *F. tularensis* (Chapter 319) meningitis, a rare complication of tularemia, develops approximately a week after the onset of infection. Illness is acquired from direct (or airborne) contact with wild rabbits or squirrels, with domestic animals, or through tick bites. Tularemia occurs throughout the United States, particularly in the Southeast and Midwest. CSF usually exhibits a lymphocytic pleocytosis (several hundred to 2000 cells/mm³), hypoglycorrhachia, and increased protein concentration. Treatment of adults consists of chloramphenicol (4 g/day intravenously in 6-hour aliquots) in addition to either gentamicin (3 to 5 mg/kg/day intravenously in 8-hour aliquots) or streptomycin (15 mg/kg intramuscularly every 12 hours for 3 days followed by 7.5 mg/kg every 12 hours for the remainder of treatment). The duration of therapy is 14 days or longer.

Brucella meningitis (Chapter 318) is a subacute or chronic process that is often accompanied by other manifestations of neurobrucellosis (encephalitis, polyradiculitis, myelitis). Infection is transmitted to humans in endemic areas (Central and South America, Mediterranean littoral, Arabian peninsula) from the ingestion of unpasteurized milk or cheese or direct contact with domestic animals. Neurobrucellosis occurs in 2 to 5% of patients with brucellosis. CSF findings consist of a lymphocytic pleocytosis (<500 cells/mm³), hypoglycorrhachia, and an elevated protein level, findings that could mistakenly suggest tuberculous meningitis. The diagnosis is based on demonstration of antibody in serum and CSF or by isolation of *Brucella* from blood; the microorganism is isolated from CSF in only a minority of cases. Treatment of adults involves the three-drug combination of doxycycline (200 mg/day), rifampin (600 mg/day), and trimethoprim-sulfamethoxazole (20 mg/kg/day, based on trimethoprim component, in 6-hour aliquots) intravenously for several months, depending on the clinical and CSF responses.

Streptococcus suis is an uncommon cause of meningitis seen in pig breeders, butchers, and abattoir workers in Europe, Canada, and China. *S. suis* meningitis, which is an acute illness with a brisk neutrophilic pleocytosis, is often initially mistaken for pneumococcal meningitis on the basis of Gram stain of CSF. Treatment of adults consists of penicillin (12 to 24 million U/day in 4-hour aliquots) or ampicillin (12 g/day in 4-hour aliquots) intravenously for 10 to 14 days.

Bacillus anthracis (Chapter 302) is a rare cause of meningitis that most often develops as a complication of inhalation anthrax following exposure to aerosols of anthrax spores in the setting of large-scale processing of wool and hides or a bioterrorism attack (Chapter 20). Anthrax meningitis is an acute process characterized by hemorrhagic or serohemorrhagic CSF with a neutrophilic predominance (several thousand cells per cubic millimeter), hypoglycorrhachia, an elevated protein level, and prominent large gram-positive bacilli on stained smear. Treatment of adults initially includes ciprofloxacin (400 mg at 12-hour intervals) in addition to penicillin (24 million U/day in 4-hour aliquots) and chloramphenicol (4 g/day in 6-hour aliquots) intravenously. Whether all drugs are continued (or treatment is narrowed to one or two antimicrobials) and the duration of treatment depend on whether the meningitis is of suspected bioterrorist origin (Chapter 20) or caused by cutaneous anthrax resulting from animal (or animal product) exposure (Chapter 302). Consultation with infectious disease and public health authorities should be sought.

Duration of Therapy

The frequency of CSF examination depends on the clinical course, but examination should be repeated in 24 to 48 hours if there has not been satisfactory improvement or if the causative microorganism is a more resistant gram-negative bacillus or a highly penicillin-resistant (or cephalosporin-resistant) *S. pneumoniae* strain, especially in patients who are receiving adjunctive dexamethasone therapy. Routine "end-of-treatment" CSF examination is unnecessary in most patients with the common types of community-acquired bacterial meningitis. Meningococci are rapidly eliminated from the circulation and CSF with appropriate antimicrobial therapy, which should be continued for 4 to 7 days after the patient becomes afebrile. If the patient has responded well, a follow-up lumbar puncture is not necessary. *H. influenzae* meningitis should be treated for 7 to 10 days. Follow-up CSF examination may be omitted in patients who have responded with rapid clinical resolution of the meningitis. In pneumococcal meningitis, antimicrobial treatment should be continued for 10 to 14 days and follow-up examination of CSF should be performed, particularly when the patient has coexistent mastoiditis. More prolonged therapy is indicated with concomitant parameningeal infection. Meningitis caused by *L. monocytogenes* should be treated for 21 days. Treatment of gram-negative bacillary meningitis with parenteral antimicrobials is prolonged, usually for a minimum of 3 weeks (particularly in patients after a recent neurosurgical procedure) to prevent relapse. Repeated examinations of CSF are necessary both during and at the conclusion of treatment to determine whether bacteriologic cure has been achieved. When treating meningitis resulting from vancomycin-resistant *Enterococcus faecium* with linezolid, an antibiotic that is bacteriostatic, approximately 4 weeks of therapy is indicated.

Other Aspects of Treatment

Adjunctive Corticosteroids

In children, the routine use of dexamethasone administered intravenously (either 0.15 mg/kg every 6 hours for 4 days or 0.4 mg/kg every 12 hours for 2 days), either at the time of or 10 to 20 minutes before initiating antimicrobial therapy (third-generation cephalosporin), has no effect on mortality but reduces the incidence of neurologic sequelae (primarily bilateral sensorineural hearing loss). However, the benefits are seen predominantly in *H. influenzae* type b meningitis, the incidence of which has been sharply reduced by the use of protein-conjugate vaccines. In a randomized double-blind study in adults with community-acquired bacterial meningitis, adjunctive dexamethasone therapy (10 mg every 6 hours intravenously for 4 days) significantly reduced the proportion of patients with an unfavorable neurologic outcome from 25 to 15% or a fatal outcome from 15 to 7%.[2] Adverse events were not increased in those receiving dexamethasone. Notably, the risk for gastrointestinal bleeding was not increased in the dexamethasone-treated group. The beneficial effect of dexamethasone was most evident in the subgroup of patients with pneumococcal meningitis, in whom the rate of unfavorable outcomes was reduced from 52 to 26% and deaths from 34 to 14%. In this trial, adjuvant dexamethasone was not beneficial in patients with meningococcal meningitis, but the number of patients in this subgroup was small. In a study of adolescents and adults with bacterial meningitis in Vietnam, dexamethasone significantly reduced death and disability by approximately 54% at 6 months in patients with confirmed disease but not in those with suspected disease.[3] By comparison, adjunctive corticosteroids were not effective in treating bacterial meningitis in a large trial of predominantly HIV-positive patients in sub-Saharan Africa.[4] Based on these data, adjunctive dexamethasone (0.15 mg/kg every 6 hours for 2 to 4 days, with the initial dose given 10 to 20 minutes before or simultaneously with the initial dose of antimicrobial therapy) is recommended in adults with suspected or demonstrated pneumococcal meningitis and perhaps routinely in all cases of bacterial meningitis,[5] at least in non–HIV-infected patients in high-income countries.[6] Continuation of dexamethasone requires demonstration of gram-positive diplococci on the CSF Gram stain or positive blood or CSF cultures for *S. pneumoniae*. When vancomycin is used for treatment of meningitis resulting from highly cephalosporin-resistant *S. pneumoniae*, as is recommended in the United States, the addition of rifampin should be considered because dexamethasone may reduce the CSF concentration of vancomycin (see Table 420-4).

Elevated Cerebrospinal Fluid Pressure (Brain Swelling)

Occasional patients with acute bacterial meningitis experience marked brain swelling (CSF pressure >450 mm H₂O), which may lead to temporal lobe or cerebellar herniation after lumbar puncture. To decrease the possibility of this complication when the pressure is found to be this high, only a small amount of CSF should be removed for analysis (the amount present in the manometer), and a 20% solution of mannitol (0.25 to 0.5 g/kg) should be infused intravenously over a period of 20 to 30 minutes while monitoring (if possible) for a decline in CSF pressure to a lower level before the spinal needle is removed. Continued control of increased intracranial pressure, if needed thereafter, may be effected with additional mannitol; dexamethasone (10 mg intravenously, followed by 0.15 mg/kg every 6 hours) should be used in patients with brain swelling regardless of the suspected bacteriologic cause of meningitis.

In a stuporous patient or one with respiratory insufficiency and markedly increased intracranial pressure, use of a ventilator to reduce the arterial carbon dioxide pressure to between 25 and 32 mm Hg is reasonable, and the patient's head should be elevated 30 to 45 degrees. Intubation should be performed with minimal stimulation to avoid an appreciable further rise in pressure; pharmacologic aids to intubation are recommended, such as succinylcholine and opioids, with the possible use of adjunctive intravenous lidocaine. Subsequently, transient increases in intracranial pressure associated with hyperactive airway reflexes can be mitigated by intratracheal instillation of lidocaine before vigorous suctioning. With continued marked and fluctuating elevations in intracranial pressure, use of a continuous intracranial monitoring device may be warranted.

Hypotension

Initial hypovolemia or hypotension, if present, should be treated with fluid to prevent significantly decreased cerebral blood flow. Over the next 24 to 48 hours, inappropriate secretion of antidiuretic hormone may contribute to further brain swelling; in such cases, fluid should be restricted to 1200 to 1500 mL daily in adults if possible, although a study in children suggests that routine fluid restriction does not improve outcome and that the resulting decrease in extracellular water may increase the likelihood of hypovolemia and an adverse outcome.

Supportive Care

Patients with acute bacterial meningitis should receive constant nursing attention in an intensive care unit to ensure prompt recognition of seizures and to prevent aspiration. If seizures occur, they should be treated acutely in adults with diazepam (administered slowly intravenously at a dose of 5 to 10 mg) or lorazepam (4 to 8 mg). Maintenance anticonvulsant therapy can be continued thereafter with intravenous phenytoin (Chapter 410) until the medication can be administered orally. Sedation should be avoided because of the danger of respiratory depression and aspiration.

Surgery

Surgical treatment of an accompanying pyogenic focus such as mastoiditis should be undertaken when recovery from the meningitis is as complete as possible but under continuing antibiotic administration. Rarely, the mastoid infection (e.g., Bezold's abscess) is so hyperacute that early drainage may be required after 48 hours or so of antibiotic therapy when the acute meningeal process has subsided somewhat.

PROGNOSIS

Prompt treatment of bacterial meningitis usually results in rapid recovery of neurologic function. Persistent or late-onset obtundation and coma without focal findings suggest brain swelling, subdural effusion, hydrocephalus, loculated ventriculitis, cortical thrombophlebitis, or sagittal sinus thrombosis. The last three conditions are commonly associated with fever and continuing pleocytosis.

The mortality rate for community-acquired bacterial meningitis in adults varies with the etiologic agent and the clinical circumstances. With current antimicrobial therapy, the mortality rate for *H. influenzae* meningitis is less than 5% and that for meningococcal meningitis is approximately 10%. The highest mortality is seen with pneumococcal and *L. monocytogenes* meningitis, for which the rates are approximately 20% and 20 to 30%, respectively.

The mortality rate for gram-negative bacillary meningitis, commonly nosocomial in origin, has been 20 to 30% in adults, but it appears to be decreasing. The mortality rate for recurrent community-acquired meningitis in adults (≈5%) is strikingly lower than the 20% rate for nonrecurrent episodes. Poor prognostic factors include advanced age, the presence of other foci of infection, underlying diseases (leukemia, alcoholism), obtundation, seizures within the first 24 hours, and delay in instituting appropriate therapy.

Residual neurologic damage is seen in 10 to 20% of patients who recover from bacterial meningitis. Approximately 25% of adults considered clinically well recovered (expected to function independently and to resume activities of daily life, including work) from pneumococcal meningitis show neuropsychological abnormalities, mainly loss of cognitive speed, when they are examined 6 to 24 months after hospital discharge. Developmental delay and speech defects are each observed in approximately 5% of children. In infants surviving neonatal meningitis, significant sequelae are much more frequent (15 to 50%).

PREVENTION

Vaccination

Effective vaccines are now available for many subtypes of *H. influenzae* type b (Chapter 308) and many meningococcal (Chapter 306) infections that cause meningitis. Adherence to recommended vaccination (Chapter 17) substantially reduces meningitis from each of these organisms.

Chemoprophylaxis

Prompt prophylaxis of close contacts (individuals who frequently slept and ate in the same household with the patient, girlfriend, or boyfriend) is warranted because up to a third of secondary cases of meningococcal disease develop within 2 to 5 days of illness in the initial case. Only hospital personnel who were in close contact with a patient (mouth-to-mouth resuscitation, initial examination before institution of respiratory precautions) are at special risk. Commonly, rifampin orally is used for prophylaxis: for adults (other than pregnant women), 600 mg twice daily for 2 days; for children, 10 mg/kg twice daily for 2 days. Alternatively, for adults, ciprofloxacin (500 mg),

ofloxacin (400 mg), or azithromycin (500 mg), each given orally as a single dose, may be used. Another choice is ceftriaxone intramuscularly as a single dose in adults (250 mg) or children (125 mg).

Widespread use of *H. influenzae* type b polysaccharide protein-conjugate vaccine in developed countries has largely eliminated the need for chemoprophylaxis of close childhood contacts of patients with *H. influenzae* meningitis or invasive infection. However, prophylaxis would be indicated for unimmunized close household contacts of an index patient (e.g., recent immigrant) younger than 6 years. If two or more cases of invasive *H. influenzae* type b disease occur in children at a daycare center, prophylaxis of other unimmunized attendees is warranted. Rifampin (20 mg/kg orally) once daily for 4 days is recommended for such children.

VIRAL MENINGITIS

DEFINITION

The nonspecific term *aseptic meningitis* describes an inflammatory process involving the meninges, usually accompanied by a mononuclear pleocytosis, without evidence of pyogenic bacterial infection on Gram stain or culture. The definition encompasses various processes that produce similar clinical pictures and inflammatory responses: *viral meningitis, atypical and nonpyogenic bacterial and fungal meningitis, chemically induced meningitis, drug-induced meningitis, neoplastic meningitis, meningeal inflammation caused by adjacent pyogenic infections,* and *meningitis associated with autoimmune hypersensitivity diseases.* Aseptic meningitis, which is usually an acute or subacute process, can be further divided into types by the duration of illness (*chronic versus chronic-intermittent*) and by distinctive cellular responses in CSF (e.g., *eosinophilic meningitis*).

Many of the viruses causing meningitis may also cause infection of the brain parenchyma (encephalitis; Chapter 422) or spinal cord. Sometimes, parenchymatous involvement and meningeal involvement occur simultaneously in the same patient and are referred to as meningoencephalitis and meningomyelitis, respectively.

EPIDEMIOLOGY

Most cases of community-acquired aseptic meningitis are the result of viruses, principally enteroviruses, which account for more than 60% of viral meningitides and for 90% of those for which an etiologic agent is identified (Table 420-8). Enteroviruses are members of the Picornaviridae (small RNA) family, which consists of more than 60 serotypes: 28 echoviruses, 23 group A and 6 group B coxsackieviruses, 4 numbered enteroviruses (68 to 71), and 3 polioviruses. The most common serotypes implicated in viral meningitis from year to year have been echoviruses 4, 6, 9, 11, 16, and 30 (most recently 13 and 33) and coxsackie B serotypes 2 to 5. Currently, poliovirus infections (Chapter 423) are limited to parts of Asia and Africa, although rare cases occur secondary to attenuated vaccine strains.

Many viruses that produce the clinical picture of aseptic meningitis, such as arthropod-borne viruses, HSV-1, enterovirus 71, lymphocytic choriomeningitis virus, mumps virus, HIV-1, cytomegalovirus, and Epstein-Barr virus, can also produce the clinical picture of meningoencephalitis and encephalitis (Chapter 422). In addition, some viruses involve the spinal cord, including the anterior horn cells (poliovirus, West Nile virus) or the dorsal root ganglia (HSV-2).

Enterovirus

An estimated 10 to 15 million clinical enteroviral infections (Chapter 387) occur annually in the United States, and these include an estimated 50,000 to 75,000 cases of enteroviral meningitis. In temperate climates, enteroviral meningitis peaks during the summer and fall, especially in children. Serotypes tend to cycle with varying periodicity, and outbreaks are related to lack of previous exposure to a particular serotype. Serotype-specific protective antibodies develop following infection, so subsequent episodes of enteroviral meningitis are uncommon and are caused by a different serotype.

Humans are the only known reservoir of enteroviruses. Enteroviral infection is spread predominantly by the fecal-oral route and occasionally by the respiratory route.

Herpes Simplex Virus

HSV (Chapter 382) accounts for 1 to 3% of all episodes of aseptic meningitis and occurs most commonly in sexually active adults or adolescents. In individuals with primary genital herpes (HSV-2) infection, up to 36% of women

TABLE 420-8 AGENTS OF VIRAL MENINGITIS

COMMON

Nonarthropod Viruses

Picornavirus (RNA)
    Enterovirus
        Echovirus
        Coxsackie A
        Coxsackie B
        Enterovirus 70, 71
        Poliovirus
Herpes simplex virus type 2 (HSV-2) (DNA)

Arthropod-Borne Viruses (Arboviruses)

Togavirus (alphavirus, RNA)
    Eastern equine encephalitis (EEE)
    Western equine encephalitis (WEE)
    Venezuelan equine encephalitis (VEE)
Flavivirus (RNA)
    St. Louis encephalitis (SLE)
    West Nile virus (WNV)
Bunyavirus (RNA)
    California encephalitis

UNCOMMON

Arenavirus (RNA)
    Lymphocytic choriomeningitis (LCM)
Paramyxovirus (RNA)
    Mumps
Retrovirus (RNA)
    Human immunodeficiency virus (HIV-1)

RARE

Herpesvirus (DNA)
    Herpes simplex virus type 1 (HSV-1)
    Epstein-Barr virus (EBV)
    Cytomegalovirus (CMV)
    Varicella-zoster virus (VZV)
    Human herpesvirus type 6 (HHV-6)
Adenovirus (DNA)
Coltivirus (RNA)
    Colorado tick fever
Bunyavirus (RNA)
    Toscana virus (a Phlebovirus)

and 13% of men have symptoms of aseptic meningitis. Recurrences of genital herpes are common and are sometimes accompanied by aseptic meningitis. More than 80% of cases of benign recurrent aseptic meningitis are caused by HSV-2. In contrast, HSV-1 CNS infection is almost always manifested as encephalitis rather than aseptic meningitis. Herpesviruses may also be reactivated in patients taking immunomodulatory drugs, which are often used to treat autoimmune diseases.

Arboviruses

Although the most common form of CNS infection caused by arboviruses (Chapters 391 and 422) is encephalitis, aseptic meningitis may also occur. These vector-borne viruses are introduced subcutaneously by a mosquito (e.g., West Nile virus), tick (e.g., Colorado tick fever), or sandfly (e.g., Toscana virus). Birds, which are vectors of mosquito-borne arboviruses, may not be obviously sick, although West Nile virus may cause prominent die-offs of corvine species, especially crows and blue jays, which can provide clues to an outbreak affecting humans.

The geographic spread of alphavirus infections (Eastern equine encephalitis, Western equine encephalitis, Venezuela equine encephalitis) in the United States is determined by the range of their individual mosquito vectors. Eastern equine encephalitis occurs sporadically or as focal outbreaks in the summer in the eastern and Gulf coasts, most frequently in children and elderly persons. Western equine encephalitis occurs predominantly in the western states, and Venezuela equine encephalitis is found in Florida. St. Louis encephalitis infections were originally recognized in the Midwest, but sporadic cases and outbreaks have occurred more recently in most parts of the United States; it is the most common arbovirus causing aseptic meningitis in the United States. West Nile virus infections first appeared in the United States in 1999 and now account for approximately 3000 cases of meningitis and another 3000 cases of encephalitis annually.

Mumps

Mumps virus (Chapter 377) was the leading identifiable cause of viral meningitis before widespread immunization in the 1960s. Episodes occurred most frequently in the winter and spring. It is now an uncommon cause of viral meningitis in the United States.

Lymphocytic Choriomeningitis

Lymphocytic choriomeningitis virus is transmitted to humans by rodents through direct contact, through ingestion of animal-contaminated food, or via aerosol or an animal bite. Cases tend to occur in early winter when mice seek shelter in homes. Outbreaks have occurred following exposure to pet or laboratory hamsters. Currently, lymphocytic choriomeningitis virus is infrequently a cause of aseptic meningitis.

PATHOBIOLOGY

The two basic routes for virus to gain access to the CNS are hematogenous (enteroviral infection) or neuronal (HSV infection). Enteroviruses pass through the stomach, where they resist the acid pH, and proceed to the lower gastrointestinal tract. Some virus also undergoes replication in the nasopharynx and spreads to regional lymphatics. After presumably binding to specific enterocyte receptors, the virus breaches the epithelial lining and undergoes primary replication in a permissive cell. From there, the virus progresses to Peyer's patches, where further replication occurs. A minor enterovirus viremia then seeds the CNS, heart, liver, and reticuloendothelial system. Following extensive replication at the latter sites, a major viremia ensues, often accompanying the onset of clinical illness. The mechanism by which enterovirus enters the CNS is presumed to involve crossing the blood-CSF barrier's tight endothelial junctions and then entering CSF, probably at the choroid plexus.

In contrast, HSV infections may reach the CNS via the neuronal route: in HSV-1 encephalitis, from oral sites via the trigeminal and olfactory nerve; in HSV-2 (and the rare HSV-1) aseptic meningitis, by spread from a primary genital lesion and ascent along the sacral nerve roots to the meninges. After subsidence of the primary infection, HSV-1 may remain dormant in the trigeminal or olfactory root ganglia only to reactivate at a later date, enter the temporal lobe, and produce encephalitis. Similarly, HSV-2 may remain latent in the sacral root ganglia until subsequent reactivation causes later episodes of aseptic meningitis.

CLINICAL MANIFESTATIONS

Enteroviral Meningitis

The clinical features of enteroviral meningitis (Chapter 387) in older children and adults often begin abruptly with headache (85 to 100%), fever (80 to 100%), and stiff neck (50 to 80%). In some patients the course is biphasic, with the initial prodromal phase being characterized by low-grade fever and nonspecific symptoms (malaise, sore throat, diarrhea), followed by a second phase at which time the meninges are seeded, with the development of higher fever, nausea, vomiting, myalgia, photophobia, and stiff neck. Other enteroviral syndromes may coexist, particularly pleurodynia or pericarditis resulting from coxsackieviruses. Rash may be a manifestation of infections caused by echoviruses, particularly echovirus type 9, coxsackieviruses A9 and A16, and enterovirus 71; the latter three cause hand-foot-and-mouth disease, which may occur alone or accompany aseptic meningitis. Echovirus 9 epidemics often produce syndromes of exanthem, enanthem (small, grayish white lesions resembling Koplik's spots on the buccal mucosa), and aseptic meningitis, either alone or in combination; a macular and petechial rash in the presence of a meningitic syndrome must be differentiated from meningococcal meningitis.

Neurologic abnormalities affecting the cerebrum are rarely observed because such cases would be defined as encephalitis or meningoencephalitis rather than enteroviral meningitis. In agammaglobulinemic individuals in whom enteroviral CNS infection develops, meningitis may progress to a chronic meningoencephalitis with multiple neurologic features, including headache, seizures, ataxia, weakness, hearing loss, obtundation, and coma.

The clinical course of enteroviral meningitis is benign, even in the minority of patients in whom the onset is acute and even fulminant. Symptoms subside within a week in children but may continue for several weeks in adults.

Herpes Simplex Virus Type 2 Meningitis

Aseptic meningitis is a common complication of primary genital HSV-2 infection (Chapter 382); up to 36% of women and 13% of men have headache (developing over a period of 2 to 3 days), stiff neck, and photophobia. Clinical features of meningitis occur 3 to 12 days after the appearance of genital lesions and usually last for 4 to 7 days. Neurologic complications occur in up to 37% of patients and include dysesthesia or paresthesia in the perineum or sacral area, urinary retention, and constipation; evidence of transverse myelitis with motor weakness in the lower extremities, hyporeflexia, and paraparesis occasionally ensues. Recurrent episodes of HSV-2 meningitis may occur at intervals of months or years in 20% of patients. In recurrent HSV-2 meningitis, fever may develop but is not as prominent as in bacterial or acute enteroviral meningitis. Recurrent vesicular lesions, paresthesia, or dysesthesia in areas of previous genital herpes may or may not precede individual recurrences of meningitis. Between recurrences, CSF findings and clinical manifestations return to normal. In patients who have had neurologic complications with a first episode of HSV-2 meningitis, the findings subside within 6 months.

Mumps Meningitis

Symptomatic CNS disease, principally meningitis or meningoencephalitis, occurs in 1 to 10% of patients with mumps parotitis (Chapter 377), but pleocytosis occurs in more than 50% of patients with mumps, most of whom lack CNS symptoms. When meningitis occurs in patients with mumps, it usually follows parotitis by 4 to 10 days, but it may precede parotitis by up to 1 week. The typical features of viral meningitis (headache, fever, vomiting) are each present in 50 to 100% of patients. Stiff neck (40 to 90%) is common, and abdominal pain (perhaps complicating pancreatitis or oophoritis) or orchitis (in ≤20% of men with mumps) may be present. Other complications of mumps may involve the nervous system (eighth nerve damage, transient facial nerve paralysis, and rarely, fifth nerve palsy) but are usually independent of mumps meningitis or meningoencephalitis. The incubation period for mumps is 18 to 21 days. When mumps meningitis occurs in the absence of clinical parotitis, it is difficult to distinguish it from other forms of viral meningitis.

When meningitis complicates mumps, fever, which had been low grade, rises to 103° F or higher and persists at this level for 3 or 4 days. Most cases are uncomplicated, with approximately a 10-day duration of illness and then complete recovery. However, symptomatic mumps meningitis may persist for more than 14 days in some patients.

Meningitis Caused by Lymphocytic Choriomeningitis Virus

Lymphocytic choriomeningitis virus infections are uncommon, and clinical illness occurs after an incubation period of 1 to 3 weeks. Illness begins with a grippe-like syndrome of fever, rigors, malaise, myalgia, anorexia, and photophobia. Sore throat and arthralgia or arthritis of the digits are noted by some patients. Orchitis or parotitis occurs rarely. This grippe-like illness lasts 1 to 3 weeks in humans, but 15% of patients have a biphasic illness consisting of transient improvement and then recrudescence, 1 to 2 days later, of fever, photophobia, and more prominent headache. Meningeal signs are observed during the second phase. The duration of meningitis caused by lymphocytic choriomeningitis virus, like that of mumps meningitis, tends to be longer than the 7 to 10 days for enteroviral meningitis.

Meningitis Caused by Human Immunodeficiency Virus

Initial infection with HIV-1 (Chapter 392) is symptomatic in 40 to 90% of patients but is frequently overlooked. The interval between exposure and onset of symptoms is 2 to 4 weeks. This acute illness resembles mononucleosis, with fever, malaise, lymphadenopathy, arthralgia, myalgia, anorexia, nausea, headache, and morbilliform rash. A few patients with this initial syndrome have manifestations of aseptic meningitis (headache, photophobia, nausea, vomiting, and stiff neck). Occasionally, encephalopathy or cranial nerve palsies (seventh, eighth, and fifth) develop. Symptoms of the initial HIV-1 aseptic meningitis syndrome last several weeks and then subside. Occasionally, manifestations similar to those of the initial infection may appear later in the course of untreated infection.

DIAGNOSIS

Cerebrospinal Fluid Examination

CSF findings in all types of viral meningitis are similar and consist of a predominantly lymphocytic pleocytosis, usually 50 to 1000/mm³ but occasionally up to several thousand per cubic millimeter, a normal glucose

concentration, and a mildly elevated protein level, usually less than 150 mg/dL. During the first 24 to 48 hours of enteroviral meningitis, a predominance of neutrophils (55 to ≤90%) is observed in approximately 50% of patients; subsequently, the principal cells in CSF change to lymphocytes. Occasionally, no pleocytosis is noted in patients proved by culture or PCR to have early enteroviral meningitis. Rarely, hypoglycorrhachia occurs in meningitis resulting from mumps or lymphocytic choriomeningitis virus or in infants with enterovirus.

Polymerase Chain Reaction versus Culture or Antibody Detection

The recent development of reverse-transcription PCR for enteroviruses can reduce detection time to as little as 5 hours, thereby shortening hospital stay and minimizing the unnecessary use of antimicrobial agents. Its sensitivity in CSF is 85 to 100%, with a specificity of 90 to 100%, depending on the laboratory. The test is available in research settings, large hospitals, and commercial laboratories. By comparison, viral culture of enterovirus from CSF has a sensitivity of only 65 to 75% and takes 4 to 8 days.

HSV-2 can be cultured from CSF in approximately 75% of patients with aseptic meningitis during an initial episode of genital HSV-2 infection, but it is rarely isolated from CSF during meningitis associated with recurrent genital herpes. PCR for HSV-2 DNA is usually positive in the CSF of patients with initial episodes of meningitis and is positive in approximately 80% of patients with benign recurrent meningitis caused by lymphocytic choriomeningitis virus.

The diagnosis can be made retrospectively by demonstrating seroconversion in antibody to gG-2 antigen in HSV-2 meningitis. A four-fold rise in titer to mumps or lymphocytic choriomeningitis virus between acute and convalescent sera is also diagnostic. Serodiagnosis is not practical for sporadic enteroviral meningitis because of the specificity of antibodies to individual serotypes.

Differential Diagnosis

The most important process to distinguish from viral meningitis is bacterial meningitis. A predominance of CSF neutrophils, hypoglycorrhachia, and bacteria on Gram-stained smear or culture indicate bacterial meningitis. An early neutrophilic predominance in CSF combined with a macular and petechial rash in enteroviral meningitis may mimic meningococcemia with meningitis. Occasional bacteria and fungi cause meningitis with a predominantly lymphocytic pleocytosis similar to that of most viral meningitides (Table 420-9). Epidemiologic considerations and clinical findings aid in distinguishing leptospiral, Lyme *Borrelia*, and syphilitic meningitis, whereas hypoglycorrhachia suggests tuberculous and cryptococcal meningitis.

TABLE 420-9	NONVIRAL INFECTIOUS CAUSES OF ASEPTIC MENINGITIS	
UNCOMMON	**RARE**
Bacterial	
Leptospira interrogans serovars	*Mycoplasma pneumoniae*
Borrelia burgdorferi	*Ehrlichia chaffeensis*
Treponema pallidum	*Listeria monocytogenes*
Mycobacterium tuberculosis	*Borrelia recurrentis* and *Borrelia hermsii*
Brucella sp	*Chlamydia psittaci*
Parameningeal infections	Staphylococcal enterotoxin or TSST-1
Subacute bacterial endocarditis	*Rickettsia rickettsii* and *Rickettsia prowazekii*
Partially treated bacterial (pyogenic) meningitis	
Fungal	
Cryptococcus neoformans	*Blastomyces dermatitidis*
Coccidioides immitis	*Sporothrix schenckii*
Histoplasma capsulatum	*Candida* sp
Protozoan	
	Trypanosoma brucei sp
	Toxoplasma gondii
	Acanthamoeba sp

TSST-1 = toxic shock syndrome toxin 1.

PREVENTION AND TREATMENT

The introduction of live attenuated mumps vaccine in the United States reduced mumps from the leading cause of aseptic meningitis and meningo-encephalitis to the point at which it occurs only rarely. Chronic enteroviral meningitis and meningoencephalitis in agammaglobulinemic patients have been controlled by parenteral (even intrathecal) administration of immune globulin.

No approved antiviral chemotherapy is available for enteroviral meningitis. Pleconaril, a drug that prevents attachment of virus to host cells, can produce clinical improvement in agammaglobulinemic patients with chronic enteroviral meningoencephalitis.

Intravenous acyclovir (5 to 10 mg/kg every 8 hours) is used to treat hospitalized, symptomatic patients with HSV-2 meningitis, particularly when the disease is associated with primary genital herpes, although it has not been shown in clinical trials to alter the course of illness. In patients with frequent recurrences of HSV meningitis, it is reasonable to attempt prophylaxis with oral antivirals: valacyclovir (500 mg once daily), famciclovir (250 mg twice daily), or acyclovir (400 mg twice daily).

PROGNOSIS

The course and outcome in patients with enteroviral meningitis are almost always benign, although approximately 1% of patients have subsequent abnormalities, probably reflecting a meningoencephalitic process. Most viral meningitides are self-limited, but some cause chronic or recurrent illness. Persistent meningitis or meningoencephalitis, sometimes fatal, can occur in individuals with hereditary (usually X-linked agammaglobulinemia or common variable immunodeficiency) deficiencies in B-lymphocyte function. HIV-1 may produce a prolonged meningeal inflammation. HSV-2 infection is the most common viral cause of recurrent episodes of aseptic meningitis.

OTHER MENINGITIDES
Nonviral Infectious Causes of Aseptic Meningitis
Categories of aseptic meningitis other than the viral meningitides include nonviral infectious processes (see Table 420-9), noninfectious processes (Table 420-10), chronic meningitides (Table 420-11), recurrent meningitis (Table 420-12), and eosinophilic meningitis (Table 420-13). Nonviral infectious causes are uncommon or rare in comparison to viral or acute suppurative meningitis. Some of the bacterial causes (e.g., *Leptospira* serovars,

TABLE 420-10	NONINFECTIOUS CAUSES OF ASEPTIC MENINGITIS

Drug hypersensitivity

Systemic disease
   Systemic lupus erythematosus
   Familial Mediterranean fever
   Behçet's syndrome
   Wegener's granulomatosis
   Cogan's syndrome
   Sarcoidosis
   Still's disease
   Kawasaki disease
   Lead poisoning

Neoplastic disease
   Metastatic carcinomatous meningitis
   Central nervous system tumors (meningeal gliomatosis, dysgerminomas, ependymomas)
   Tumors that leak inflammatory material into cerebrospinal fluid (squamous cells in epidermoid tumors of the posterior fossa, cholesteatomas)

Inflammatory processes involving central nervous system structures primarily
   Chemical meningitis following myelography (water-soluble nonionic contrast material)
   Continuous spinal and epidural anesthesia, inflammation after neurosurgery
   Granulomatous cerebral vasculitis
   Vogt-Koyanagi-Harada syndrome

B. burgdorferi, *Brucella* sp, *T. pallidum*) produce a lymphocytic pleocytosis; others (partially treated bacterial meningitis, subacute bacterial endocarditis with embolic cerebral infarcts) produce a mixed neutrophilic-mononuclear pleocytosis; and *M. tuberculosis*, though producing a lymphocytic response with developing hypoglycorrhachia, may show a predominantly neutrophilic response in a minority of patients early in the disease. Although patients with *L. monocytogenes* infection usually have neutrophilic pleocytosis, this infection may suggest aseptic meningitis because of its sometimes indolent onset and, occasionally, an early predominantly lymphocytic response in young children. Fungal (e.g., *Cryptococcus neoformans*, *Coccidioides immitis*, *Histoplasma capsulatum*) meningitides are associated with a predominantly mononuclear response, sometimes with a small percentage of eosinophils, particularly in coccidioidal meningitis (Chapter 341). Patients with Rocky Mountain spotted fever (Chapter 335), an acute disease with a macular and petechial rash, may exhibit confusion. When examined, the CSF in

TABLE 420-11	INFECTIOUS CAUSES OF CHRONIC (PERSISTENT) LYMPHOCYTIC MENINGITIS
CAUSATIVE CONDITIONS	**OTHER CSF FINDINGS**
Bacterial	
Mycobacterium tuberculosis	Usually <500 white blood cells/mm³, low glucose, high protein
Borrelia burgdorferi (Lyme disease)	Normal glucose, elevated protein
Treponema pallidum (secondary syphilitic meningitis, tertiary meningovascular syphilis)	Elevated protein; Venereal Disease Research Laboratory positive in CSF and serum
Brucella sp (uncommon)	Often low glucose; elevated protein
Tropheryma whippelii (rare)	Periodic acid–Schiff–positive cells on meningeal biopsy
Partially treated bacterial meningitis	Mixture of PMNs and lymphocytes, bacteria on Gram stain and culture
Parameningeal infections	Lymphocytes or mixed lymphocytic-PMN response, normal glucose
Fungal	
Cryptococcus neoformans	Low glucose, elevated protein, budding yeast on India ink or fungal wet mount, antigen detectable
Coccidioides immitis	Often low glucose, may have 10-20% eosinophils, elevated protein, presence of complement-fixing antibody
Histoplasma capsulatum	Low glucose; complement-fixing antibodies in CSF; antigen detectable in urine, CSF, serum
Blastomyces dermatitidis	Low glucose
Candida sp	Low glucose, may have PMN or lymphocyte predominance, fungal stain may be positive
Aspergillus sp	Lymphocytes or PMNs predominate
Sporothrix schenckii (sporotrichosis)	Low glucose; protein, 200-800 mg/dL
Protozoal	
Toxoplasma gondii	Usually, picture is that of an encephalitis; often in patients with AIDS; pleocytosis is mild (<60 cells/mm³) and protein is mildly elevated
Trypanosoma gambiense or *Trypanosoma rhodesiense*	Meningoencephalitis is stage II of disease, elevated protein and immunoglobulin M, trypanosomes on Giemsa-stained smear
Viral	
Mumps	Rarely, low glucose
Lymphocytic choriomeningitis	Rarely, low glucose
Echovirus (in patients with congenital agammaglobulinemia)	Occasionally, low glucose
HIV-1	Cell counts lower (10-20/mm³) than in acute self-limited meningitis at clinical onset of HIV infection or may develop during course of AIDS

AIDS = acquired immunodeficiency syndrome; CSF = cerebrospinal fluid; HIV = human immunodeficiency virus; PMN = polymorphonuclear leukocyte.

TABLE 420-12 CAUSES OF CHRONIC (RECURRENT) MENINGITIS

Infections
Herpes simplex virus type 2

Leakage of contents from central nervous system tumors (chemical meningitis)
Epidermoid tumors
Craniopharyngiomas
Cholesteatomas

Drug hypersensitivity with repeated use of agent

Inflammatory processes
Behçet's syndrome
Systemic lupus erythematosus
Mollaret's meningitis
Vogt-Koyanagi-Harada syndrome

TABLE 420-13 CAUSES OF EOSINOPHILIC MENINGITIS*

CAUSATIVE CONDITIONS	SOURCE
Parasitic Disease	
Angiostrongylus cantonensis	Ingestion of raw shellfish; Pacific
Taenia solium (cysticercosis)	Fecal-oral transmission of *T. solium* eggs
Gnathostoma spinigerum	Ingestion of raw fish; Japan, Southeast Asia
Baylisascaris procyonis	Accidental ingestion of *B. procyonis* eggs from raccoon feces
Trichinella spiralis (trichinosis)	Ingestion of poorly cooked pork
Schistosoma sp	Exposure of skin to fresh water; Africa, Middle East
Echinococcus granulosus	Contact with infected dogs passing eggs in feces
Toxoplasma gondii	Ingestion of meat containing cysts or food contaminated with oocysts from cat feces
Toxocara canis (visceral larva migrans)	Ingestion of infective eggs from dog feces
Fungal Infections	
Coccidioides immitis	Southwestern United States
Neoplastic Disease	
Lymphoma, leukemia, metastatic carcinoma	
Hypereosinophilic syndrome (myeloproliferative disorder)	
Inflammatory Processes	
Sarcoid	
Drug hypersensitivity	
Presence of foreign body in the central nervous system	

*The percentage of eosinophils varies from as little as 6% to the majority of cells.

approximately 20% of such patients shows a pleocytosis of 10 to 100 or more cells/mm³, with either a neutrophilic or lymphocytic predominance. The clinical picture may suggest either enteroviral or meningococcal disease.

Epidemiologic factors are important in raising suspicion for nonviral aseptic meningitis. Leptospirosis (Chapter 331) may be suggested by a history of recent direct or indirect exposure to animals (e.g., dogs, rodents, dairy cattle) and their urine. Neurobrucellosis (Chapter 318) is suggested by the recent ingestion of unpasteurized cheese from the Mediterranean littoral, Middle East, or Mexico or by work as a veterinarian or in an abattoir. Specific endemic mycoses may be a consideration with residence in the southwestern United States (coccidioidomycosis; Chapter 341) and the Mississippi River valley (histoplasmosis; Chapter 340). The setting of immunosuppression by drugs or illness such as acquired immunodeficiency syndrome would raise the possibility of *C. neoformans* (Chapter 344) or *L. monocytogenes* (Chapter 301). Sexual promiscuity and the macular rash of secondary syphilis could suggest *T. pallidum* (Chapter 327) as the cause in a patient with lymphocytic meningitis.

Noninfectious Causes of Aseptic Meningitis

Noninfectious causes fall into four principal categories (see Table 420-10): drug hypersensitivity; systemic processes such as systemic lupus erythematosus and other collagen-vascular diseases; neoplastic disease, primary or metastatic, infiltrating the leptomeninges; and inflammatory processes primarily involving the CNS. Although a mononuclear cell predominance is found in the CSF in most noninfectious aseptic meningitides, there are several important exceptions. Drug hypersensitivity meningitis usually causes a neutrophilic response, although occasionally mononuclear cells or eosinophils predominate. In systemic lupus erythematosus (Chapter 274), the pleocytosis may be predominantly lymphocytic or neutrophilic (sometimes several thousand per cubic millimeter) with a normal CSF glucose level. Hypoglycorrhachia is a feature of few noninfectious aseptic meningitides and suggests malignant disease or sarcoidosis. Various drugs, most commonly the nonsteroidal anti-inflammatory drugs, have also been implicated in aseptic meningitis.

Chronic (Persistent) Meningitis

Chronic meningitis is defined by the clinical syndrome of headache, stiff neck, altered mental status, nausea and vomiting, evidence of myelopathy or radiculopathy with or without cranial nerve palsies (e.g., III, IV, VI, VII, VIII), and an inflammatory response in the CSF for 4 weeks or longer. Obstruction of CSF flow may produce hydrocephalus and papilledema.

Infectious Causes

Among the more common bacterial causes of chronic meningitis, *M. tuberculosis* (Chapter 332) is the most important to identify because if untreated, it is almost always fatal within 4 to 8 weeks (see Table 420-11). Similarly, parameningeal infections (Chapter 421) must be recognized and treated promptly because surgery is often necessary to provide a specific bacteriologic diagnosis and prevent neurologic residua. Tuberculosis should be suspected in patients with a previous history of a tuberculous illness, a history of recent exposure, HIV infection or another immunosuppressed state, fever and night sweats, sixth cranial nerve palsies, stroke related to arteritis, or lesions on the chest radiograph. The purified protein derivative skin test may be negative in patients with recently acquired or overwhelming disease. Acid-fast smear and culture of concentrated CSF can provide the diagnosis, and PCR can be very helpful. When clinical and CSF findings suggest the diagnosis, treatment (Chapter 332) should be initiated while one awaits the results of culture.

Parameningeal infections (Chapter 421) should be suspected when chronic meningitis with focal neurologic signs develops in the setting of chronic otitis media or sinusitis, pleuropulmonary infection, or right-to-left cardiopulmonary shunting. Contrast-enhanced CT or MRI of the head is important to delineate brain abscess, sinus infection, and epidural or subdural infections.

Meningitis may accompany the skin, mucous membrane, and lymph node features of secondary syphilis (Chapter 327), or it may occur alone. Individual cranial nerves (II to VII) may be involved; visual abnormalities, hearing loss, and facial palsy are most frequent. The fluorescent treponema antibody absorption test or microhemagglutination *T. pallidum* serologic studies are helpful in distinguishing the process from biologic false-positive Venereal Disease Research Laboratory (or rapid plasma reagent) results in serum.

Lyme disease meningitis (Chapter 329) should be suspected on the basis of epidemiologic grounds (geographic location, season, tick exposure) and associated clinical features (erythema chronicum migrans rash, Bell's palsy, radiculopathy). The diagnosis is made by enzyme-linked immunosorbent assay with Western blot confirmation.

Noninfectious Causes

Noninfectious causes of meningitis include malignant disease, chemical meningitis, and primary inflammatory conditions (Table 420-14). Malignant disease may be diagnosed by cytologic examination of large volumes of CSF. Contrast-enhanced MRI may disclose thickening of the meninges and nerve roots, but meningeal biopsy may be required for diagnosis. Chemical meningitis from previous subarachnoid injection may persist, with xanthochromia noted in CSF; meningeal inflammation may be identified on contrast-enhanced CT or MRI.

Meningeal or CNS sarcoid (Chapter 95) may be isolated or occur with other organ involvement, such as pulmonary granulomas, lymphadenopathy, or myopathy. Neurologic findings can include diabetes insipidus and cranial nerve palsies. Wegener's granulomatosis (Chapter 278) may produce

TABLE 420-14	NONINFECTIOUS CAUSES OF CHRONIC (PERSISTENT) LYMPHOCYTIC MENINGITIS
CAUSATIVE CONDITIONS	**OTHER CSF FINDINGS**
Neoplasms	
Metastatic: lung, breast, stomach, pancreas, lymphoma, melanoma, leukemia	Low glucose; elevated protein, cytologic examination; polarizing microscopy; clonal lymphocyte markers
Central nervous system: meningeal gliomatosis, meningeal sarcoma, cerebral dysgerminoma; epidermoid tumors/cysts	
Chemical Inflammation	
Endogenous: epidermoid tumor, craniopharyngioma	Low glucose, elevated protein
Exogenous: recent injection into the subarachnoid space	Low glucose, elevated protein
Primary Inflammatory Processes	
Central nervous system sarcoid	Often low glucose, elevated protein, elevated angiotensin-converting enzyme levels in CSF (and serum)
Wegener's granulomatosis	Elevated protein
Behçet's syndrome	Elevated protein
Isolated granulomatous angiitis of the central nervous system	Elevated protein
Systemic lupus erythematosus	Elevated protein
?Chronic idiopathic benign meningitis	Elevated protein

CSF = cerebrospinal fluid.

TABLE 420-15	CAUSES OF CHRONIC (PERSISTENT) MENINGITIS WITH NEUTROPHIL PREDOMINANCE
UNCOMMON	**OTHER CSF FINDINGS**
Bacterial	
Nocardia asteroides	Low glucose, markedly elevated protein, culture positive
Actinomyces israelii	Low glucose, elevated protein, anaerobic culture positive
Arachnia propionica	Low glucose, elevated protein, anaerobic culture positive
Fungal	
Candida sp	Low glucose, elevated protein, culture positive
Aspergillus sp	Low glucose, elevated protein, enzyme immunoassay or enzyme-linked immunosorbent assay for *Aspergillus* galactomannan
Zygomycetes	Low glucose, elevated protein
Dematiaceous fungi	Low glucose, protein may be markedly elevated
Noninfectious	
Systemic lupus erythematosus	Low glucose, elevated protein
Chemical meningitis	Low glucose, protein may be markedly elevated
VERY RARE	
Bacterial	
Brucella sp	Low glucose, elevated protein
Mycobacterium tuberculosis	Low glucose, elevated protein, polymerase chain reaction positive for *M. tuberculosis* DNA
Fungal	
Pseudoallescheria boydii	Low glucose, protein may be markedly elevated
Coccidioides immitis	Low glucose, elevated protein, presence of complement-fixing antibody
Blastomyces dermatitidis	Low glucose, protein elevated, antigen detection possible in CSF and urine
Histoplasma capsulatum	Low glucose; protein mildly elevated; complement-fixing antibodies in CSF; antigen detectable in CSF, urine, serum

CSF = cerebrospinal fluid.

meningeal inflammation and cranial nerve palsies, often in association with air sinus disease. The diagnosis is suggested by lesions on the chest radiograph, microscopic hematuria, skin lesions, peripheral neuropathy, and serum antineutrophil cytoplasmic antibodies. Aseptic meningitis associated with systemic lupus erythematosus (Chapter 274) may be accompanied by other neurologic manifestations (seizures, encephalopathy, stroke, transverse myelopathy), systemic manifestations (rash, arthritis), and antinuclear and anti-DNA antibodies.

Chronic (Intermittent) Meningitis

In chronic intermittent meningitis, all clinical and CSF abnormalities resolve completely between episodes without antimicrobial therapy (see Table 420-11). Uncommonly, a patient may have several episodes resulting from different viral agents. The major causes of recurrent aseptic meningitis are infections (almost always viral and resulting from HSV-2), endogenous chemical meningitis, drug hypersensitivity with meningitis following each use, and inflammatory and autoimmune diseases.

In HSV-2 recurrent meningitis, lymphocytes predominate, with the cell numbers being approximately 40% higher in the initial episode than in recurrences. Leakage of material from intracranial epidermoid cysts produces 1000 to 5000 cells/mm^3 (≈80% polymorphonuclear leukocytes) initially, with a subsequent mononuclear cell predominance. Occasionally, polarizing microscopy may demonstrate keratin and cholesterol crystals in the CSF of patients with endogenous chemical meningitis. In Behçet's syndrome (Chapter 278), the CSF may have predominantly mononuclear cells or polymorphonuclear leukocytes. Mollaret's meningitis, a syndrome of benign recurrent meningitis usually caused by HSV-2, is initially associated with neutrophils and monocytes in the CSF without hypoglycorrhachia but subsequently transitions to a predominantly lymphocytic pleocytosis. Vogt-Koyanagi-Harada syndrome, a rare uveomeningoencephalitis, consists of recurrent meningitis/meningoencephalitis and anterior or posterior uveitis, followed by vitiligo, poliosis, alopecia, and dysacousia; the CSF cellular response is mononuclear, and an autoimmune origin, directed against a melanocyte antigen, has been suggested.

Chronic Meningitis with Predominantly Neutrophilic Pleocytosis

Chronic persistent neutrophilic meningitis (Table 420-15) is defined by the following combination: (1) clinical features consistent with meningitis; (2) initial CSF examination showing greater than 50% neutrophils, hypoglycorrhachia, and elevated protein concentration; (3) antimicrobial therapy that would be appropriate for the usual causes of bacterial meningitis; (4) negative smears and cultures for bacteria on the initial CSF specimen; and (5) repeated CSF examination 7 days or more after initial analysis showing 50% or greater neutrophils, hypoglycorrhachia, and elevated protein concentration.

Among the bacterial causes (see Table 420-15) are organisms (*Actinomyces israelii* and *Arachnia propionica* [Chapter 337]) that can be isolated by culture only under anaerobic conditions. Coexisting pulmonary lesions may suggest *Nocardia* (Chapter 338) or *M. tuberculosis* (Chapter 332) as the cause, although the initial polymorphonuclear pleocytosis in some cases uncommonly persists much beyond a week before changing to a lymphocytic predominance. *Brucella* (Chapter 318) and endemic invasive mycotic infections would be suggested by epidemiologic considerations. Other fungal causes may be diagnosed, particularly in immunocompromised patients, by antigen testing with enzyme-linked immunosorbent assay (*Aspergillus* sp galactomannan; Chapter 347), or meningeal biopsy may be required.

Occasionally, exogenous chemical meningitis secondary to intrathecal injection of antimicrobials, chemotherapeutic agents, or contrast media may produce persisting pleocytosis and hypoglycorrhachia resulting from sclerosing arachnoiditis well after the inciting medication has been withdrawn. Systemic lupus erythematosus (Chapter 274) can produce a variety of meningitides, including acute lymphocytic or neutrophilic aseptic meningitis, as well as chronic persistent lymphocytic or neutrophilic CSF responses.

Eosinophilic Meningitis

The presence of 5% or greater eosinophils in CSF is uncommon and suggests parasitic disease, certain fungal infections such as coccidioidal or candidal meningitis, neoplastic diseases, or a few inflammatory processes (see Table 420-13). In most cases, eosinophils are mixed with lymphocytes, which predominate; the highest percentage of eosinophils is seen with meningitis caused by migrating larvae of the raccoon ascarid *Baylisascaris procyonis* (Chapter 365) and the rat lung worm *Angiostrongylus cantonensis* (Chapter 365). In fungal meningitides, particularly those resulting from *C. immitis* (Chapter 341), the CSF response is primarily mononuclear with 6 to 20% eosinophils; hypoglycorrhachia may be a feature of *C. immitis* and *Candida* meningitis (Chapter 346) and of neoplastic processes and sarcoid.

Most patients with eosinophilic meningitis, except those with cases resulting from trichinosis (Chapter 365) or drug hypersensitivity, have prolonged symptoms suggesting chronic meningitis. Most patients with meningitis of parasitic or neoplastic origin have evidence of cerebral involvement as well.

1. Nathan N, Borel T, Djibo A, et al. Ceftriaxone as effective as long-acting chloramphenicol in short-course treatment of meningococcal meningitis during epidemics: a randomised non-inferiority study. *Lancet.* 2005;366:308-313.
2. van de Beek D, Farrar JJ, de Gans J, et al. Adjunctive dexamethasone in bacterial meningitis: a meta-analysis of individual patient data. *Lancet Neurol.* 2010;9:254-263
3. Nguyen TH, Tran TH, Thwaites G, et al. Dexamethasone in Vietnamese adolescents and adults with bacterial meningitis. *N Engl J Med.* 2007;357:2431-2440.
4. Scarborough M, Gordon SB, Whitty CJ, et al. Corticosteroids for bacterial meningitis in adults in sub-Saharan Africa. *N Engl J Med.* 2007;357:2441-2450.
5. Vardakas KZ, Matthaiou DK, Falagas ME. Adjunctive dexamethasone therapy for bacterial meningitis in adults: a meta-analysis of randomized controlled trials. *Eur J Neurol.* 2009;16:662-673.
6. Assiri AM, Alasmari FA, Zimmerman VA, et al. Corticosteroid administration and outcome of adolescents and adults with acute bacterial meningitis: a meta-analysis. *Mayo Clin Proc.* 2009;84:403-409.

SUGGESTED READINGS

Edmond K, Clark A, Korcczak VS, et al. Global and regional risk of disabling sequelae from bacterial meningitis: a systematic review and meta-analysis. *Lancet Infect Dis.* 2010;10:317-328. *Review.*
Kallio-Laine K, Seppanen M, Kautiainen H, et al. Recurrent lymphocytic meningitis positive for herpes simplex virus type 2. *Emerg Infect Dis.* 2009;15:1119-1122. *Describes the epidemiology, clinical manifestations, management, and outcome of HSV-2–associated meningitis.*
Sinner SW. Approach to the diagnosis and management of tuberculous meningitis. *Curr Infect Dis Rep.* 2010;12:291-298. *Comprehensive review.*
van de Beek D, Drake JM, Tunkel AR. Nosocomial bacterial meningitis. *N Engl J Med.* 2010;362:146-154. *Review of pathophysiology and treatment.*

421

BRAIN ABSCESS AND PARAMENINGEAL INFECTIONS

AVINDRA NATH AND JOSEPH BERGER

Brain abscess affects the brain's parenchyma directly, whereas parameningeal infections produce suppuration in potential spaces covering the brain and spinal cord (epidural abscess and subdural empyema) or produce occlusion of the contiguous venous sinuses and cerebral veins (cerebral venous sinus thrombosis).

BRAIN ABSCESS

EPIDEMIOLOGY

The frequency of various causes of brain abscess (Table 421-1) in the population has been difficult to ascertain because of wide variations among case series, in part as a result of referral patterns. In addition, case series of children with brain abscesses contain a sizable contingent of cases related to cyanotic

TABLE 421-1 CONDITIONS THAT PREDISPOSE TO THE DEVELOPMENT OF BRAIN ABSCESS

Otogenic
  Otitis media
  Mastoiditis

Dental

Cardiac
  Cyanotic heart disease
  Tetralogy of Fallot
  Patent foramen ovale
  Infective endocarditis

Pulmonary
  Pulmonary arteriovenous fistula
  Lung infection
    Lung abscess
    Bronchiectasis

Esophageal strictures

Cerebral infarcts and tumors

Penetrating and nonpenetrating head injury

Postoperative neurosurgical procedure (trauma and nontrauma related)

Dermal sinus tracts

Sepsis

Immunosuppression

Unknown mechanism

congenital heart disease or otogenic infection. Cryptogenic abscesses account for a greater percentage of cases in more recent series, perhaps related to the presence of a patent foramen ovale. On average, 90% of brain abscesses occur as a consequence of a focus of suppuration elsewhere in the body, with the remainder due to introduction of the infection from head wounds or neurosurgical procedures. Males predominate in virtually all series of brain abscess. Terminally ill patients in whom medical care may be withdrawn may be found to have abscesses at autopsy, but these abscesses are of little clinical importance.

PATHOBIOLOGY

Brain abscesses are collections of purulent material (neutrophils and necrotic tissue) caused by infection with a variety of bacterial, fungal, and parasitic organisms. Infection arising from other sites typically seeds the brain hematogenously. When contiguous to the brain, infection enters the brain by direct extension or by traveling along veins with associated thrombophlebitis of pial veins and sinuses. Within the brain, the infection begins as a cerebritis with perivascular infiltrates and infiltration of neutrophils into the brain parenchyma. With time, the developing abscess is characterized by a purulent exudate that includes necrotic brain tissue as well as viable and necrotic neutrophils. Granulation tissue develops at the interface between necrotic and viable tissue, and eventually, the abscess is walled off by a fibrous capsule. Formation of the capsule depends on the virulence of the organism and the immune status of the individual. More virulent organisms are associated with larger lesions, more necrosis, earlier ependymitis, and more frequent areas of inflammatory escaping outside the collagen capsule. Immunocompromised patients, such as human immunodeficiency virus (HIV)-infected patients with *Toxoplasma* species abscesses, are unable to mount an immune response to form a capsule and hence respond well to antibiotic therapy alone.

CLINICAL MANIFESTATIONS

The clinical picture reflects a triad of the infectious nature of the lesion, focal brain involvement, and an increasing intracranial mass effect (Table 421-2). One or two elements may be absent in a given case, particularly early in the course. Among infectious symptoms, fever is present at onset or early in the course in only about 60% of cases. Neck stiffness is an infrequent complaint, and meningeal signs are elicited in about 30% of cases.

Focal neurologic deficits depend on the site of the lesion, which in turn will be determined by the causal or predisposing condition. In some patients, seizures precede the diagnosis. The early deficits in patients with temporal lobe lesions, which are typically caused by spread of an otogenic abscess, are contralateral homonymous superior quadrantic visual field defects and, if in the dominant hemisphere, aphasia. Motor deficits eventually occur in 40 to 50% of supratentorial abscesses. Cerebellar abscesses, which are often caused

TABLE 421-2	BRAIN ABSCESS: INITIAL FEATURES IN 123 CASES	
Headache		55%
Disturbed consciousness		48%
Fever		58%
Nuchal rigidity		29%
Nausea, vomiting		32%
Seizures		19%
Visual disturbance		15%
Dysarthria		20%
Hemiparesis		48%
Sepsis		17%

by aural-mastoid infections, are characterized by ipsilateral limb ataxia; there may also be abnormal head positioning, forward and away from the side of the lesion, and nystagmus that is slow and coarse on gaze to the side of the abscess and rapid in the opposite direction. Patients with multiple brain abscesses may have multifocal signs or encephalopathy. Patients with *Toxoplasma* species (Chapter 357) brain abscesses often have movement disorders because these abscesses frequently localize to the basal ganglia. In fact, nearly all patients with HIV infection in whom hemiballism or hemichorea is present have *Toxoplasma* species brain abscesses.

Headache is an important initial symptom in 80 to 90% of patients with bacterial abscess but is less frequent (approximately 20%) in patients with fungal abscesses. Symptoms of increased intracranial pressure, such as nausea, depressed level of consciousness, and papilledema, occur less often. The development of headache in a patient with a known chronic anaerobic infection, such as aural-mastoid, paranasal sinus, or pulmonary suppuration, suggests the possibility of brain abscess. Similarly, the development of headache in a child with cyanotic congenital heart disease is often related to a brain abscess. Tetralogy of Fallot (Chapter 69) is the most common congenital heart anomaly associated with brain abscess.

DIAGNOSIS

Examination of the cranium, ears, paranasal sinuses, oral cavity, heart, and lungs may provide important clues to the etiology, as may overt signs of infection at other sites. Cultures of blood and sputum may identify the organism and its antimicrobial sensitivity. In patients with signs of raised intracranial pressure, lumbar puncture may be contraindicated.

Magnetic resonance imaging (MRI) can detect early changes, such as brain edema, and is preferable to computed tomography (CT). In the early cerebritis stage, T2-weighted MRI shows abnormally high signal intensity corresponding to low signal intensity on the T1-weighted images. The fluid-attenuated inversion recovery (FLAIR) sequence provides superior visualization of brain edema. On T1-weighted images, the area of cerebritis that is seen initially as a low-signal-intensity, ill-defined area later progresses to a central cavity with slightly higher signal intensity than cerebrospinal fluid (CSF), surrounded by edema that is slightly hypointense in comparison to brain parenchyma. Later stages of infection show central necrosis and formation of a rim of slightly high signal intensity on T1-weighted images (Fig. 421-1). Gadolinium administration shows a ring-enhancing lesion. Diffusion-weighted imaging helps differentiate abscesses from brain tumors; an abscess cavity demonstrates high signal with decreased apparent diffusion coefficient values, whereas necrotic tumor cavities demonstrate the opposite.

Surgical aspiration or excision of the lesion may be necessary to establish a microbial diagnosis. Gram stain and culture from abscess fluid, with proper handling, have high yield, with or without previous antibiotic therapy. If immediate surgery is planned, antibiotics can be deferred until culture material has been acquired. Multiplex polymerase chain reaction testing is being developed for rapid identification of bacterial organisms and detection of antibiotic resistance genes.

TREATMENT ℞

Brain abscess requires urgent intervention. Because of the risk for cerebral herniation with large lesions, treatment of cerebral edema (intravenous dexamethasone, 16 to 24 mg/day in four divided doses) may be needed even while initiating surgical intervention. Corticosteroids often decrease edema within

FIGURE 421-1. **Brain abscess.** Magnetic resonance imaging with gadolinium shows a multiloculated ring-enhancing lesion caused by *Nocardia* species infection.

FIGURE 421-2. **Brain stem abscess.** Magnetic resonance imaging with gadolinium shows an enhancing lesion in the brain stem caused by *Listeria* species infection.

8 hours but may retard the formation of a capsule around the brain abscess, may suppress the immune response to the infection, and may decrease penetration of antibiotics; hence, they should be used for short periods, usually only until surgical decompression by needle drainage or surgical removal is possible. A trial of nonsurgical treatment may be considered in patients with (1) small lesion size; (2) an already identified pathogen; (3) no symptoms or signs of increased intracranial pressure requiring neurosurgical intervention; (4) a deep or inaccessible lesion; (5) multiple abscesses; (6) a contraindication to surgery (e.g., a bleeding diathesis); (7) a short duration of symptoms, which suggests that the lesion is in the cerebritis stage; and (8) availability of monitoring with MRI. Patients with acquired immunodeficiency syndrome and suspected cerebral toxoplasmosis (Chapter 357) should receive antimicrobial therapy initially. In patients who are suspected of having a brain stem abscess, the possibility of listerial infection (Chapter 301) should be considered (Fig. 421-2), even in the absence of a clear immunodeficiency. Empirical parenteral antibiotics to cover *Listeria* species should be started (Chapter 301).

Successful antibiotic management of brain abscess is based on knowledge of proved or suspected pathogens as well as familiarity with a drug's spectrum of activity and penetration into the central nervous system. When surgery cannot be performed, empirical antibiotic therapy must be initiated even if the organism cannot be isolated from the abscess (Table 421-3).

PROGNOSIS

Before the CT scan era, the mortality of brain abscesses ranged from 40 to 60%, and even with the drastic reduction in mortality in the era of modern neuroimaging, the mortality rate remains about 15%. In post-transplantation patients and those with deep hemispheric or brain stem abscesses, mortality

TABLE 421-3 COMMON PATHOGENS AND EMPIRICAL THERAPY FOR BRAIN ABSCESS

PREDISPOSING CONDITION	COMMON PATHOGENS	ANTIMICROBIAL AGENTS
Dental abscess	Streptococci, *Bacteroides fragilis*	Penicillin + metronidazole
Chronic otitis	*Bacteroides fragilis*; *Pseudomonas, Proteus, Klebsiella* species	Cefotaxime or ceftriaxone + metronidazole; ceftazidime or cefepime for *Pseudomonas* species
Sinusitis	Streptococci; *Haemophilus, Staphylococcus* species	Cefotaxime, ceftriaxone, or nafcillin + metronidazole
Penetrating trauma or postsurgical	*Staphylococcus, Pseudomonas, Enterobacter* species; streptococci	Nafcillin or vancomycin + ceftriaxone or cefotaxime + metronidazole
Bacterial endocarditis or drug use	Mixed flora, streptococci, *Staphylococcus* species	Nafcillin or vancomycin + ceftriaxone or cefotaxime + metronidazole
Congenital heart disease	Streptococci	Cefotaxime or ceftriaxone
Pulmonary infection	*Nocardia* species, *Bacteroides fragilis*, streptococci, mixed flora	Penicillin + metronidazole + trimethoprim-sulfamethoxazole
HIV infection	*Toxoplasma gondii*	Pyrimethamine + sulfadiazine + folinic acid

TABLE 421-4 INITIAL CHARACTERISTICS OF 915 SPINAL EPIDURAL ABSCESSES

STAGE 1	
Back pain	71%
Fever	66%
STAGE 2	
Radicular pain	20%
STAGE 3	
Muscle weakness	26%
Sphincter incontinence	24%
Sensory deficits	13%
STAGE 4	
Paralysis	31%
Quadriplegia	3%

From Reihsaus E, Waldbaur H, Seeling W. Spinal epidural abscess: a meta-analysis of 915 patients. *Neurosurg Rev.* 2000;23:175-204.

rates may exceed 80%. Other factors associated with a poor prognosis include extremes of age, multiple abscesses, and diagnostic delay in the absence of systemic signs of infection. Impaired level of consciousness is a poor prognostic sign even with early hospitalization and rapid diagnosis. Anaerobic and gram-negative organisms and culture-negative cases also have a poor prognosis. Seizure (Chapter 410) is a long-term risk that develops in up to 50% of patients, sometimes after latencies as long as 5 years.

● SPINAL EPIDURAL ABSCESS

DEFINITION

Infection within the epidural space around the spinal cord is an uncommon but readily treatable potential cause of paralysis and death. The epidural space surrounds the dural sac and is limited by the posterior longitudinal ligament anteriorly, the ligamenta flava and the periosteum of the laminae posteriorly, and the pedicles of the spinal column and the intervertebral foramina containing their neural elements laterally. The space communicates with the paravertebral space through the intervertebral foramina. Superiorly, the space is closed at the foramen magnum. Caudally, the space is closed by the sacrococcygeal ligament. The epidural space contains loose areolar connective tissue, semiliquid fat, lymphatics, arteries, an extensive plexus of veins, and the spinal nerve roots.

EPIDEMIOLOGY

Spinal epidural abscesses can result from hematogenous spread of infection; risk factors include intravenous drug use, organ transplantation, chronic steroid use, malignancy, and diabetes. Local infection after acupuncture for back pain or epidural analgesia can also cause epidural abscesses. Cutaneous sites of infection are the most common remote sources, especially in intravenous drug users. Abdominal, respiratory tract, and urinary sources are also common. Osteomyelitis may be a cause of either direct extension or hematogenous spread, particularly when associated with sepsis. Contiguous spread may occur from epidurally placed catheters, psoas abscesses, decubitus ulceration, perinephric and retropharyngeal abscesses, or surgical sites. Minor back trauma has been implicated in causing a paraspinal hematoma, which may subsequently be seeded hematogenously. *Staphylococcus aureus* is the most common organism isolated from spinal epidural abscesses.

PATHOBIOLOGY

Because the dura mater around the cord is adherent to the vertebral column anteriorly, more epidural abscesses lie posteriorly, and because no anatomic barriers separate the spinal segments in the posterior epidural space, such abscesses usually extend over several vertebral segments. Spinal cord dysfunction probably reflects toxic processes secondary to inflammation, as well as venous thrombosis, thrombophlebitis, ischemia secondary to compression of the spinal arteries, and edema.

CLINICAL MANIFESTATIONS

The presence of a risk factor (>80% of patients) in the setting of neurologic deficits or back or radicular pain should suggest a spinal epidural abscess. The clinical manifestations can be divided into four stages (Table 421-4). Back pain (71%), fever (66%), tenderness of the spine with focal percussion (17%), spinal irritation (20%), and headache (3%) are common. Radicular pain can be mistaken for sciatica, a visceral abdominal process, chest wall pain, or cervical disc disease. Clinical signs are often substantially greater than would be predicted from the anatomic extent of pus or granulation tissue.

Unfortunately, the diagnosis often is missed initially. If the condition goes unrecognized at an early stage, the symptoms can evolve, over a period of hours to days, to paralysis below the spinal level of infection.

DIAGNOSIS

The differential diagnosis includes compressive and inflammatory processes involving the spinal cord: transverse myelitis (Chapter 419), herniation of an intervertebral disc (Chapter 407), epidural hemorrhage (Chapter 407), or metastatic tumor (Chapter 195), none of which are associated with evidence of systemic infection. Blood leukocytosis may not be present, but the sedimentation rate is often elevated. Other infectious processes that may produce back or neck pain or tenderness must be excluded: bacterial meningitis (Chapter 420), perinephric abscess, disc space infection (Chapter 407), and bacterial endocarditis (Chapter 76).

Lumbar puncture should be avoided in patients suspected of having a spinal epidural abscess for fear of spreading the infection to the subarachnoid space and causing meningitis. Gadolinium-enhanced MRI (Fig. 421-3) is the method of choice for diagnosis, but MRI findings in patients undergoing epidural analgesia can resemble those of epidural spinal abscess, even when no infection is present.

TREATMENT ®x

Patients with a progressing neurologic deficit should undergo urgent surgical drainage; CT-guided aspiration may be useful, and antibiotics plus percutaneously guided needle aspiration may be as therapeutically effective as antibiotics plus surgery. Unless culture results and sensitivities dictate otherwise, empirical therapy should cover *S. aureus* (nafcillin, 2 g every 6 hours; vancomycin, 1 g every 12 hours for methicillin-resistant strains). Additional gram-negative coverage with a third-generation cephalosporin (e.g.,

FIGURE 421-3. Epidural abscess. **A** and **B**, Magnetic resonance images of the lumbosacral spine show a lesion in the epidural space compressing the thecal sac. (Courtesy of Drs. Martin Pomper and Dima Hammoud, Johns Hopkins University.)

cefotaxime, 2 g every 6 hours, or ceftriaxone, 2 g every 12 hours) or a quinolone (e.g., ciprofloxacin, 400 mg every 12 hours) should be considered for severe disease. Rifampin (300 mg every 12 hours) may be added because of its ability to penetrate the abscess cavity. Intravenous therapy should be continued for 3 to 4 weeks, except in the presence of osteomyelitis (6 to 8 weeks).

PROGNOSIS

The mortality rate associated with spinal epidural abscess is about 15%. Approximately 50% of survivors have residual neurologic deficits. More severe preoperative neurologic deficits and deficits of longer duration are associated with a worse prognosis. In general, patients who develop paralysis that persists for longer than 36 hours do not recover function.

SUBDURAL EMPYEMA

Subdural empyema is an infection in the space between the dura and the arachnoid. It usually results from infected paranasal sinuses and rarely from infected mastoid sinuses by extension of thrombophlebitis from the sinuses into the subdural space. The infection is most commonly unilateral because bilateral spread is prevented by the falx. The empyema may evolve to cause cortical vein thrombosis, cerebral abscesses, or purulent meningitis.

CLINICAL FEATURES AND DIAGNOSIS

The most common symptoms are headache, fever, a neurologic deficit, and a stiff neck. However, subdural empyema may progress and cause signs of raised intracranial pressure, such as vomiting, altered level of consciousness, seizures, and papilledema. A high degree of suspicion is needed to establish the diagnosis early in the course of the illness. In patients with sinusitis (Chapter 434), the symptoms of subdural empyema may be incorrectly attributed to the sinusitis.

MRI with gadolinium enhancement and diffusion-weighted images is particularly useful in visualizing the subdural infection as a crescent-shaped mass with an enhancing rim over the cerebral convexities and below the inner table of the skull. CSF evaluation is useful only if there is accompanying meningitis. In a patient with signs of raised intracranial pressure, lumbar puncture should be avoided because of the risk for herniation.

TREATMENT   Rx

Surgical drainage of the empyema is mandatory. Intravenous antibiotic therapy is also necessary and is based on the organisms isolated at the time of craniotomy.

PROGNOSIS

Mortality rates in most series are about 25%, with severe neurologic sequelae remaining in 20% of survivors. Accompanying venous sinus thrombosis or brain abscess carries a poor prognosis.

VENOUS SINUS THROMBOSIS SECONDARY TO INFECTION

The venous sinus system lacks valves, thereby permitting retrograde propagation of clots or infections that emanate from structures located in the central portion of the face or the middle ear.

Septic Cavernous Sinus Thrombosis

DEFINITION

The cavernous sinuses are the most caudal dural venous chambers at the base of the skull. The paired structures lie on either side of the pituitary fossa immediately above the midline sphenoid sinus. The cavernous sinus encloses the "cavernous portion" of the internal carotid artery as well as the third, fourth, and sixth cranial nerves en route to the apex of the orbit.

EPIDEMIOLOGY AND PATHOBIOLOGY

The infection usually spreads from the paranasal sinuses, dental abscesses, or other infections affecting the orbit or middle third of the face. *S. aureus* is the most common organism. Streptococci, pneumococci, and gram-negative bacilli are less common; anaerobic infection has also been reported. Many cases of idiopathic intracranial hypertension (Chapter 195) are due to thrombosis in the lateral sinuses.

CLINICAL MANIFESTATIONS

Cavernous sinus thrombosis may be manifested as an acute, fulminant disease or have an indolent, subacute manifestation. Fever and other systemic symptoms from sepsis may be present. Clinical symptoms and signs are related to anatomic structures within the cavernous sinuses or drained by them: unilateral periorbital edema, headache, photophobia, proptosis, ophthalmoplegia, pupillary dilation, decreased corneal reflex, and periorbital sensory loss. Obstruction of venous drainage from the retina can result in papilledema, retinal hemorrhages, and visual loss. The infection can spread rapidly (24 to 48 hours) through the intercavernous sinuses to the contralateral cavernous sinus. Thrombus can extend to other dural venous sinuses, adjacent vascular structures, or the brain parenchyma.

DIAGNOSIS

The diagnosis is made on clinical grounds and confirmed by radiographic studies. Radiologic evaluation includes sinus imaging, particularly the sphenoid and ethmoid sinuses. MRI using flow parameters and a magnetic resonance (MR) venogram is very sensitive and may reveal deformity of the cavernous portion of the internal carotid artery, a heterogeneous signal from the abnormal cavernous sinus, and an obvious hyperintense signal of thrombosed vascular sinuses. MRI with intravenous gadolinium can demonstrate venous thrombosis by illustrating a lack of the normal "flow void" within vascular structures. Cranial CT scans are less helpful but may show a subtle increase in the size and enhancement of the thrombosed sinus. MR angiography may demonstrate extrinsic narrowing of the intracavernous portion of the internal carotid artery.

TREATMENT AND PROGNOSIS   Rx

Blood cultures are often negative, so delays in diagnosis are common. Even when the diagnosis is established, empirical antimicrobial treatment may not provide full coverage.

Treatment consists of prompt drainage of infected paranasal sinuses or other identifiable source of infection as well as specific antistaphylococcal agents (Chapter 296). Heparin anticoagulation without a loading dose is sometimes initiated to reduce morbidity from associated brain ischemia, but experience in septic venous thrombosis is limited compared with the more frequent use of anticoagulation in nonseptic venous thromboses. Hemorrhage caused by anticoagulation is rare in this setting. Despite modern therapy, mortality rates remains as high as 44%.

FIGURE 421-4. Lateral sinus thrombosis. Magnetic resonance imaging shows a thrombus in the lateral sinus *(short arrow)* with accompanying mastoiditis *(long arrow)*. (Courtesy of Drs. Martin Pomper and Dima Hammoud, Johns Hopkins University.)

Lateral Sinus Thrombosis

Septic thrombosis of the lateral sinus results from acute or chronic infections of the middle ear.

CLINICAL MANIFESTATIONS AND DIAGNOSIS

Symptoms consist of ear pain and fever followed by headache, nausea, vomiting, loss of hearing, and vertigo, usually evolving over a period of several weeks. Symptoms or signs suggestive of otitis media (Chapter 434), including mastoid swelling, may be seen. Sixth cranial nerve palsies can occur, but other focal neurologic signs are rare. In some patients with nonseptic lateral sinus thrombosis, headache may be the only symptom. Papilledema occurs in 50% of cases, and elevated CSF pressure is present in most, especially with occlusion of the right lateral sinus, which is the major venous conduit from the superior sagittal sinus (Fig. 421-4).

CSF is usually normal, although a parameningeal inflammatory profile (mild pleocytosis, slight elevation in protein level, and a normal glucose level) may be seen. The diagnosis is confirmed by MR venography.

TREATMENT Rx

Treatment includes intravenous antibiotics to cover staphylococci, anaerobes, and gram-negative bacilli such as *Proteus* species and *Escherichia coli* (nafcillin, 2 g every 6 hours, or vancomycin, 1 g every 12 hours; plus cefotaxime, 2 g every 6 hours, or ceftriaxone, 2 g every 12 hours; plus metronidazole, 7.5 mg/kg every 6 hours, or clindamycin, 300 mg every 6 hours; plus ciprofloxacin, 400 mg every 12 hours). Surgical drainage (mastoidectomy or tympanoplasty) may be required to eradicate the nidus of infection and to determine the antibiotic susceptibility of the organism. If the sinus contains pus, it must be opened so that the septic thrombus can be removed. Unless vision is compromised, increased intracranial pressure seldom requires specific treatment such as drainage or placement of a shunt.

PROGNOSIS

Broad intravenous antibiotic coverage and eradication of the perisinus infection, which may require surgical drainage, early in the course of the illness lead to a good prognosis. Neurologic sequelae may include a sixth nerve palsy, ataxia, and hearing loss.

Septic Sagittal Sinus Thrombosis

Although superior sagittal sinus thrombosis is the most common form of venous sinus thrombosis and is frequently associated with the use of oral contraceptives, septic sagittal sinus thrombosis is an uncommon condition that occurs as a consequence of purulent meningitis, infections of the ethmoid or maxillary sinuses spreading through venous channels, compound infected skull fractures, or rarely, neurosurgical wound infections.

CLINICAL MANIFESTATIONS AND DIAGNOSIS

Symptoms are primarily related to the elevated intracranial pressure and can evolve rapidly to stupor and coma. Seizures and hemiparesis may result from cortical infarction. Early recognition and treatment are necessary because septic sagittal sinus thrombosis carries a high mortality rate. The rate of progression, severity of symptoms, and prognosis are all related to the location of thrombosis. Obstruction of the anterior third of the sinus produces less intense symptoms and evolves more slowly.

CSF abnormalities are frequent, including enough red blood cells that the CSF can sometimes be mistaken for a subarachnoid hemorrhage; the opening pressure is increased in proportion to the extent of sagittal sinus involvement. A septic sagittal sinus is best visualized during the venous phase of cerebral angiography or MR venography. The diagnosis can also be made by MRI, which demonstrates an abnormal increase in signal intensity (absent flow void) within the affected venous sinus. Contrast-enhanced CT scanning may reveal a contrast void lying at the junction of the transverse and sagittal sinuses (the region of the torcular); this so-called delta sign is an intraluminal clot surrounded by contrast material.

TREATMENT

Intravenous antibiotics should be directed at organisms recovered from the meningeal process or the meningeal site. *S. aureus* (Chapter 296), β-hemolytic streptococci (Chapter 298), pneumococci (Chapter 297), and gram-negative aerobes such as *Klebsiella* species (Chapter 314) are the most common organisms. Associated paranasal sinusitis should be drained surgically.

PROGNOSIS

If the thrombosis progresses to involve the middle and posterior thirds of the sinus, deterioration progresses rapidly. The prognosis is poor, with a mortality rate of nearly 30%.

NEUROLOGIC COMPLICATIONS OF INFECTIOUS ENDOCARDITIS

Neurologic complications develop in nearly one third of patients with infective endocarditis (Chapter 76), and neurologic manifestations are the initial symptom in 20% of patients with infective endocarditis. In nearly 30% of patients, the neurologic complications occur within 2 weeks after the initiation of treatment. Stroke is the most common manifestation; most strokes are due to cerebral emboli, and others are due to intracerebral hemorrhage. Infective endocarditis should always be considered in a patient with a fever and stroke.

PATHOBIOLOGY

Cerebral embolization occurs as a result of dislodgement or disruption of the cardiac vegetations that frequently cause occlusion of cerebral blood vessels. Emboli occurring before the initiation or completion of treatment with antibiotics may contain microorganisms capable of causing metastatic infections such as abscesses, arteritis, meningitis, or mycotic aneurysms. Most cerebral emboli involve small or moderate-sized blood vessels, and multiple cerebral emboli are common. Intracranial hemorrhage is usually due to rupture of a mycotic aneurysm (Chapter 415), septic erosion of the arterial wall without the formation of an aneurysm, or hemorrhagic transformation of a large cerebral infarct. About 20% of patients with mycotic aneurysms have multiple aneurysms; involvement of the middle cerebral artery and its branches occurs in more than 75% of patients, unlike congenital aneurysms, which occur predominantly in the circle of Willis. Mycotic aneurysms develop as a result of either septic embolization into the vasa vasorum or direct penetration of the microorganism into the wall of the artery. Streptococci and staphylococci account for nearly 90% of all mycotic aneurysms.

CLINICAL MANIFESTATIONS

The nature of the clinical manifestations depends on the underlying pathophysiology. Embolic stroke typically causes the acute onset of a focal neurologic deficit. Seizures may also occur. Multiple microemboli result in an altered or fluctuating level of consciousness not adequately explained by other abnormalities.

Most patients with mycotic aneurysms have a sudden, often fatal subarachnoid or intracerebral hemorrhage without warning signs. Warning signs, if present, include severe localized headache, ischemic events, seizures, and cranial nerve abnormalities. In some patients, mycotic aneurysms may be asymptomatic and resolve with antibiotic therapy. Clinical features of brain abscess and meningitis (Chapter 420) may also be observed in the setting of bacterial endocarditis.

DIAGNOSIS

MRI is the modality of choice for the diagnosis of cerebral infarcts and brain abscesses related to endocarditis, a CT scan is the best test for intracranial hemorrhage, and an MR angiogram is preferred for diagnosing an aneurysm. CSF evaluation is useful if accompanying meningitis or a slow leak from an aneurysm is suspected but not visualized with these imaging tests.

TREATMENT   Rx

Treatment of patients with infective endocarditis and cerebral emboli requires prevention of embolization with appropriate antibiotic therapy and sometimes cardiac surgery (Chapter 76). Anticoagulation is contraindicated in patients with cerebral infarcts and septic emboli because of the high risk for complications from intracerebral bleeding.

Patients with unruptured aneurysms smaller than 7 mm in diameter, proximal aneurysms, multiple aneurysms, ruptured aneurysms without an intracerebral hematoma, and aneurysms for which excision is likely to cause a neurologic deficit can be monitored conservatively with serial MRI and MR angiography. All other aneurysms require surgical excision of the aneurysm and the adjacent septic vessel wall. Patients who cannot undergo surgery may be candidates for endovascular embolization of the aneurysmal vessel.

PROGNOSIS

Mortality rates in patients with infective endocarditis and cerebral emboli range from 30 to 80%. Mortality is high if there is hemorrhagic transformation of the infarct. Mortality in patients with ruptured mycotic aneurysms is 80%, and even patients with unruptured aneurysms have a mortality rate of 30%.

SUGGESTED READINGS

Arlotti M, Grossi P, Pea F, et al. Consensus document on controversial issues for the treatment of infections of the central nervous system: bacterial brain abscesses. *Int J Infect Dis.* 2010;14:S79-S92. *A detailed review with consensus guidelines.*

Johnson MD, Johnson CD. Neurologic presentations of infective endocarditis. *Neurol Clin.* 2010;28:311-321. *Review.*

Tsou TP, Lee PI, Lu CY, et al. Microbiology and epidemiology of brain abscess and subdural empyema in a medical center: a 10 year experience. *J Microbiol Immunol Infect.* 2009;42:405-412. *Review of 151 brain abscesses and 10 subdural empyemas.*

422

ACUTE VIRAL ENCEPHALITIS

ALLEN J. AKSAMIT, JR.

DEFINITION

Encephalitis is an inflammatory process that affects the parenchyma of the brain, usually in a diffuse manner. The term *encephalitis* indicates that the predominant clinical syndrome arises from infection and inflammatory reaction in the parenchyma of the brain rather than in the leptomeninges. When both the leptomeninges and brain parenchyma are involved, the term *meningoencephalitis* is used.

EPIDEMIOLOGY

Viral encephalitis has an estimated incidence of 7 per 100,000 per year. In general, a specific cause is identified in only 10 to 20% of patients in

| TABLE 422-1 | COMMON CAUSES OF ENCEPHALITIS IN THE UNITED STATES |

I. Causes of viral encephalitis
   A. Nonseasonal
     Herpes simplex virus type 1 (herpes simplex encephalitis)
     Herpes simplex virus type 2 (neonatal encephalitis)
   B. Seasonal—summer and fall—arboviruses (arthropod borne)
     West Nile virus
     St. Louis encephalitis virus
     Eastern equine encephalitis virus
     Western equine encephalitis virus
     LaCrosse/California encephalitis virus
   C. Seasonal—non–arthropod borne
     Summer and fall: enteroviruses (including coxsackieviruses, ECHO viruses, polioviruses, and enterovirus 71)
     Winter: influenza virus
   D. Immunosuppressed patients
     Human immunodeficiency virus (chronic HIV encephalitis)
     Varicella-zoster virus (subacute encephalitis)
     JC virus (progressive multifocal leukoencephalopathy)
     Cytomegalovirus (ventriculitis or encephalitis)
     Human herpesvirus 6 (possible subacute encephalitis)
     Epstein-Barr virus (subacute encephalitis)

II. Uncommon causes in the United States
     Lymphotrophic choriomeningitis virus
     Rabies
     Measles (subacute sclerosing panencephalitis)
     Mumps
     Adenovirus
     Herpes B virus (of monkeys)
     Rubella (progressive rubella panencephalitis)

III. Causes outside the United States
     Tick-borne encephalitis virus (Russia, Asia)
     Japanese encephalitis virus (Japan, Southeast Asia, Malaysia)
     Venezuelan equine encephalitis virus (Central and South America)
     Dengue virus (Southern Asia, Africa, South America)
     Rift Valley fever virus (east central Africa)
     Murray Valley encephalitis virus (Australia)
     Powassan fever encephalitis virus (Canada)
     Nipah virus (Malaysia and Bangladesh)

the United States. Many viruses (Table 422-1) are implicated, and testing by serologic or nucleic acid identification (by polymerase chain reaction [PCR]) is required to identify the specific virus. The epidemiology of each virus responsible for central nervous system infection is unique in terms of the types of patients who are at highest risk, geographic distribution, and seasonal occurrence, especially the arboviruses (Chapter 391) and enteroviruses (Chapter 387), which are covered in separate chapters.

In the United States, the most common cause of nonepidemic encephalitis is herpes simplex encephalitis, which is caused by herpes simplex virus type 1 (Chapter 382). The most common epidemic virus in the United States is now West Nile virus (Chapter 391), which is a Flavivirus related to St. Louis encephalitis virus and to its Asian counterpart Japanese encephalitis virus. There is serologic cross-reactivity between St. Louis encephalitis, Japanese encephalitis, and West Nile viruses.

PATHOBIOLOGY

In general, gross pathologic inspection of an encephalitic brain does not reveal purulence visible to the naked eye. If focal purulence is present, *cerebritis* is the more correct term. If frank necrosis and purulence are present, the correct pathologic term is *brain abscess* (Chapter 421). Encephalitis, however, can be associated with substantial necrosis, and patients with severe acute viral encephalitis frequently have microscopic evidence of necrosis. Certain viral encephalitides, such as herpes simplex encephalitis, can be frankly hemorrhagic. Viruses that cause acute encephalitis may often also cause meningitis (Chapter 420). Indeed, patients with encephalitis virtually always have some microscopic inflammatory changes in the leptomeninges. Conversely, patients with viral meningitis will inevitably have some component of microscopic encephalitis. The degree of inflammatory change present in the brain is determined by the individual viral pathogen and by host immune factors, which are responsible for the reaction to the invading virus.

CLINICAL MANIFESTATIONS

The clinical findings in patients with acute viral encephalitis start with a prodrome of fever, malaise, myalgia, and nonspecific symptoms. Nausea, vomiting, diarrhea, cough, sore throat, and rash can precede the neurologic symptoms. Invasion of the nervous system is typically accompanied by headache, photophobia, and altered consciousness, with symptoms progressing over a period of several days. Seizures are also a common heralding symptom. Meningeal signs are variably present and are an unreliable finding in encephalitis.

Focal brain dysfunction is seen with some viruses. For example, West Nile virus (Chapter 391) can cause a brain stem encephalitis with an early onset of coma. Herpes simplex virus (Chapter 382) tends to cause focal cortical neurologic deficits, including hemiparesis, aphasia, and seizures. Limbic system involvement in herpes simplex encephalitis or rabies can lead to prominent behavioral changes at the beginning of the illness before the patient's level of consciousness is depressed. Focal or generalized seizures, which suggest cortical involvement, are particularly common when herpes simplex encephalitis affects the hippocampus and limbic system. Rabies is typically associated with laryngospasm, hydrophobia, and depressed consciousness. Because of spinal cord involvement, West Nile virus, St. Louis encephalitis virus, poliovirus, and rabies virus infections can cause focal or asymmetrical weakness of the lower motor neuron type with areflexia.

DIAGNOSIS

In patients with coma or focal deficits, computed tomography (CT) of the head is typically performed before spinal fluid analysis to exclude a substantial mass effect and to avoid the risk for herniation during lumbar puncture. In patients without focal findings, however, lumbar puncture should be performed immediately to establish the diagnosis and allow early treatment. Opening pressures should be measured because increased intracranial pressure can occur with all forms of viral encephalitis.

Spinal fluid analysis, essential in suspected cases of viral encephalitis, typically reveals an elevated protein level, which usually is less than 120 mg/dL. The cerebrospinal fluid (CSF) glucose level is typically normal and greater than 40% of the coincident serum value, but some patients may rarely have a low CSF glucose level suggestive of a bacterial infection (Chapter 420). The white blood cell count is typically elevated, usually in the range of 10 to 500 cells/mm^3 and generally with a lymphocytic predominance. However, a polymorphonuclear predominance is seen in some cases of West Nile encephalitis and cytomegalovirus ventriculitis.

Serologic or PCR testing on spinal fluid is frequently helpful (Table 422-2). PCR testing has the added advantage of proving direct viral infection within the central nervous system, but serologic testing is more appropriate for West Nile virus encephalitis, which is best confirmed by an IgM antibody response in spinal fluid.

Magnetic resonance imaging (MRI) of the brain is the most sensitive technique for defining abnormalities in patients with viral encephalitis. However, frank viral encephalitis can occur with normal findings on MRI. The specific patterns can suggest the virus responsible; the best example is herpes simplex encephalitis, which has a characteristic pattern involving the mesiotemporal, inferofrontal, and insular cortices, usually unilateral or asymmetrically bilateral.

Differential Diagnosis

A number of nonviral pathogens can cause encephalitis that is clinically and pathologically indistinguishable from viral encephalitis. Examples include *Rickettsia* (Chapter 335), *Borrelia* (Chapter 329), Whipple's disease (Chapter 142), *Toxoplasma* (Chapter 357), and *Acanthamoeba* (Chapter 360). Additionally, autoimmune encephalitides that mimic viral encephalitis include limbic paraneoplastic encephalitis, Hashimoto's encephalopathy associated with autoimmune thyroiditis (Chapter 233), and encephalitis associated with anti–N-methyl-D-aspartate (NMDA) receptor antibodies. In parainfectious encephalitis, a systemic viral infection is associated with a febrile encephalopathy, sometimes with inflammatory spinal fluid but without direct evidence of brain invasion by the organism. Examples of parainfectious encephalitis include infection and encephalopathy associated with influenza virus (Chapter 372), varicella virus (Chapter 383), and Epstein-Barr virus (Chapter 385). Furthermore, manifestations of parainfectious effects by viruses may include severe brain white matter inflammation or demyelination referred to as acute disseminated encephalomyelitis.

TABLE 422-2 SELECTED TESTS FOR VIRAL ENCEPHALITIS

ORGANISM/SYNDROME	TEST	COMMENT
WEST NILE VIRUS		
West Nile encephalitis	IgM in CSF	Diagnostic of CNS invasive disease or acute flaccid paralysis
HERPES SIMPLEX VIRUS TYPE 1		
Herpes simplex encephalitis	PCR in CSF	Sensitive and specific in the acute phase
	CSF–serum antibody ratio	Useful 2 weeks to 3 months after onset
HERPES SIMPLEX VIRUS TYPE 2		
Neonatal encephalitis	PCR in CSF	Confirmatory, high sensitivity
Relapsing meningitis	PCR in CSF	Sensitive and specific in first 3 days of illness
VARICELLA-ZOSTER VIRUS		
Meningoencephalitis	PCR in CSF	Confirmatory when used with clinical and spinal fluid findings; sensitivity unclear
EPSTEIN-BARR VIRUS		
EBV encephalitis	PCR in CSF	Suggests CNS invasion by virus
JC VIRUS		
Progressive multifocal leukoencephalopathy	PCR in CSF	Diagnostic but incompletely (70%) sensitive
CYTOMEGALOVIRUS		
CMV ventriculitis	PCR in CSF	Sensitive and specific

CNS = central nervous system; CSF = cerebrospinal fluid; PCR = polymerase chain reaction.

SELECTED SPECIFIC VIRUSES
Herpes Simplex Encephalitis

EPIDEMIOLOGY

Herpes simplex (Chapter 382) encephalitis, which is second only to West Nile encephalitis as the most common form of nonepidemic encephalitis in the United States, has an annual incidence of two to four cases per million people per year. There is no seasonal or gender predisposition. The encephalitis can strike older children as well as adults, although it is most commonly a disease of adults.

PATHOBIOLOGY

Herpes simplex encephalitis can occur in immunosuppressed or immunocompetent patients. Patients who are deficient in toll-like receptor 3 in the immune system may be selectively vulnerable to herpes simplex encephalitis.

Herpes simplex virus type 1 infects and establishes latency in the majority of the population. Whether herpes simplex encephalitis arises from reactivation of a latent viral infection in the trigeminal ganglion or is a primary nasopharyngeal infection that ascends into the olfactory nervous system is uncertain.

The pathology of herpes simplex encephalitis is a necrotizing, hemorrhagic, inflammatory encephalitis in the mesiotemporal, inferofrontal, and insular cortices, with gray matter being affected more than white matter. When the brain is affected bilaterally, the pathologic features are usually asymmetrical, a pattern that helps distinguish herpes simplex from other forms of limbic encephalitis.

CLINICAL MANIFESTATIONS

The clinical manifestations of herpes simplex encephalitis usually begin with a nonspecific febrile prodrome, which is followed within hours to days by the symptoms of headache, malaise, nausea, and vomiting. A reduced level of consciousness may occur early. Seizures may be the first manifestation of this encephalitis. Focal deficits, especially hemiparesis or aphasia, are common. More specific manifestations of herpes simplex encephalitis are symptoms of limbic system–associated behavioral changes, such as behavioral or emotional lability and inappropriateness. Memory is affected early if consciousness is preserved. As the encephalitis progresses, symptoms of increased intracranial pressure, lethargy, and coma are usual. Focal findings alone in the context of encephalitis are not sufficient to confirm a diagnosis of herpes simplex encephalitis.

DIAGNOSIS

Spinal fluid analysis is a mainstay in the diagnosis of herpes simplex encephalitis. In a patient with focal encephalitis or coma, however, CT of the brain should be performed before spinal fluid analysis to avoid the risk for herniation. Elevation of the protein level and the white blood cell count, with a predominance of lymphocytes, is the most frequent pattern; red blood cells are also commonly seen. The CSF glucose level is usually normal, but it can be less than 50% of the blood glucose level in about 5% of patients.

The best and most accurate test for proof of herpes simplex encephalitis is the presence of herpes simplex virus type 1 DNA amplified by PCR in the spinal fluid. Herpes simplex virus type 1 can be distinguished from herpes simplex virus type 2 by specific primer amplification, applied as part of the PCR analysis. Because herpes simplex type 2 can cause encephalitis in neonates and meningitis in adults, this distinction may affect therapy.

MRI, which is the imaging technique of choice for this form of suspected encephalitis, typically shows characteristic focal involvement with increased T2 and fluid-attenuated inversion recovery (FLAIR) signal in the mesiotemporal lobes (including the amygdala, hippocampus, and uncus), the inferofrontal lobes (cingulate gyrus and orbital frontal cortex), and the insular cortex. The abnormalities seen on MRI are often unilateral but can be bilateral and asymmetrical. Focal MRI abnormalities must be distinguished from brain abscess (Chapter 421), cerebral infarction (Chapter 414), cerebral hemorrhage (Chapter 415), brain tumors (Chapter 195), and paraneoplastic limbic encephalitis(Chapter 197); radiographically detected involvement of the mesiotemporal rather than the lateral temporal areas and involvement of the gray matter rather than the white matter suggest herpes simplex encephalitis as the diagnosis. Early gadolinium contrast enhancement may occur but is not universal.

CT of the head is less sensitive than MRI for detecting mild cases of herpes encephalitis. However, because herpes simplex encephalitis can be hemorrhagic, CT may sometimes identify the hemorrhage more accurately than MRI can.

Electroencephalography is an adjunctive test that can show periodic lateralized epileptiform discharges ipsilateral to the involved temporal lobe. However, the findings are not specific for herpes simplex encephalitis and commonly occur in patients with cerebral infarction (Chapter 414) and occasionally other forms of viral encephalitis.

TREATMENT   Rx

Multicenter prospective trials emphasize that early treatment affects outcome. When suspicion for herpes simplex encephalitis is raised in the acute setting by the presence of focal signs or symptoms, early empirical treatment is recommended even while the diagnostic evaluation is proceeding.

Intravenous acyclovir (30 mg/kg daily given three times per day in divided doses for 14 to 21 days) is the therapy of choice.**1** Some experts have suggested treatment using the same doses for 21 days, but no prospective data show that a longer duration of therapy or higher doses of acyclovir affect neurologic outcomes.

Rabies

Human rabies, which is an encephalitic illness caused by the rabies virus, is usually transmitted by an animal bite. It produces a fatal encephalitis, although the latency between animal bite exposure and occurrence of neurologic symptoms may make the diagnosis unsuspected.

EPIDEMIOLOGY AND PATHOBIOLOGY

Rabies is a rare illness in the United States and developed world. However, initially unsuspected cases have been transmitted via trivial bites by infected bats, which are widely distributed in every state in the United States except Hawaii. Rabies virus variants in bats are now responsible for the majority of recent human cases in the United States and Canada. Raccoon rabies has extended from Florida into Georgia, Alabama, and South Carolina.

Canine rabies is still endemic in much of the developing world, including Africa, Latin America, Eastern Europe, and Asia, and the vast majority of human rabies cases occur as a result of untreated dog bites from endemic

areas. Dog rabies came under control in the United States during the 1950s and was associated with a marked reduction in the number of human cases transmitted by dogs. Much of the dog-related clinical rabies seen in the United States is the result of dog bites that occurred in developing countries, before the patient migrated to the United States. Rare cases of transmission of rabies to transplant organ recipients have occurred recently in the United States.

The presence of Negri bodies (intracytoplasmic viral inclusions) in neurons of the brain stem, cerebellum (especially the Purkinje cells), or hippocampus defines rabies pathologically. These inclusions are often not present, but detection of antigen by immunohistochemical means can aid in the pathologic diagnosis. Because the disorder tends to be a brain stem encephalitis, the cardiovascular, bulbar, and respiratory centers are affected.

CLINICAL MANIFESTATIONS

Clinically, human rabies usually develops 20 to 90 days after a bite, although rarely disease develops after only a few days or after a year or more following bite exposure. Multiple bites and facial bites are associated with shorter incubation times.

Nonspecific prodromal symptoms include fever, chills, malaise, fatigue, insomnia, anorexia, headache, and irritability. In the majority of patients, pain or paresthesias will develop in the limb that was affected by the bite. Following the prodromal illness, an encephalitic form develops in about 80% of patients and causes varied behavior from episodes of agitated arousal to quiet lethargy. Fever is a common accompaniment but not universal at this phase. Disinhibition of brain stem reflexes leads to hydrophobia with laryngospasm and an inability to deal with salivation, swallowing of water, or other oral intake. When the brain stem encephalitis affects the bulbar, cardiovascular, and respiratory centers, autonomic dysfunction, cardiopulmonary complications, and respiratory failure may occur.

Another form of rabies that affects up to a third of patients is known as paralytic rabies. This form of rabies is manifested as acute flaccid paralysis, which may be multifocal and affect the limbs, as well as the bulbar musculature. The weakness can mimic poliomyelitis (Chapter 423) because of its multifocality, and it can be confused with Guillain-Barré syndrome (Chapter 428). Paralytic rabies typically occurs in conjunction with encephalitis.

DIAGNOSIS

Findings on spinal fluid analysis may be abnormal in human rabies. A pleocytosis, usually less than 100 white cells/μL, is found in more than 50% of patients in the first week of illness; the leukocytes are predominantly mononuclear. The protein concentration is commonly mildly elevated, and the glucose level is usually normal.

Imaging of patients with rabies is sometimes useful. MRI may show gray matter involvement and involvement of the brain stem in particular, with increased T2 signal, commonly without enhancement. Spinal cord MRI in patients with paralytic rabies may show increased T2 signal mimicking acute disseminated encephalomyelitis. Involvement of brain gray matter, including the hippocampus and basal ganglia structures, indicates the gray matter predilection and often bilateral involvement of supratentorial structures. However, imaging cannot be relied on to exclude rabies.

Serum antibodies against rabies virus are not usually present in unimmunized patients until the second week of illness, and patients can die before having a detectable serum antibody level. Serum antibodies may also be present in spinal fluid, but their absence is unreliable in excluding the diagnosis. Classically, staining a skin biopsy sample taken from an area near the nape of the neck for rabies antigen in the sensory nerves can confirm the diagnosis of rabies. Alternatively, small amounts of rabies RNA can be detected by PCR testing. Typical specimens to detect virus include saliva, brain tissue, or spinal fluid. A positive result confirms the diagnosis, but the exclusionary value of negative results is unknown.

TREATMENT

After an animal bite, local treatment with antirabies immunoglobulin and systemic treatment with vaccination are typically offered. Rabies postexposure prophylaxis includes local wound cleansing, passive immunization with immunoglobulin, and active immunization with rabies vaccine. Inactivated cell culture rabies vaccines are used for active immunization, and the risk for vaccination-induced acute disseminated encephalomyelitis has been markedly reduced by the use of these vaccines. However, once rabies encephalitis is manifested, it is unclear whether vaccination, though regularly used, has any role in improving outcome. Antiviral therapy and a variety of immunotherapies, including ribavirin and interferon alfa, have been tried in the treatment of rabies, usually without success. Although one patient was reputed to survive with the use of therapeutic coma without vaccination, subsequent reports of patients treated in similar fashion have been associated with a fatal outcome.

Rare Causes of Encephalitis

Lymphocytic choriomeningitis (Chapter 420) virus is a human infection acquired from mice. Typically, humans acquire the infection by contact with food or dust that is contaminated by excreta of the common house mouse. Most commonly, human disease occurs in winter, when the natural host tends to move indoors. It can also be acquired as a consequence of laboratory exposure by human caretakers.

Mumps virus (Chapter 377) is typically acquired by the respiratory route. Infection can occur throughout the year, but the incidence is higher during the spring. Although mumps virus infects both sexes equally, meningoencephalitis develops in males three times more frequently than in females. Vaccination programs in the United States have made mumps encephalitis rare.

TREATMENT   Rx

Effective antiviral therapy does not exist for viral encephalitis, except for herpes simplex encephalitis. However, because of the usual delay in establishing or excluding the diagnosis of herpes simplex encephalitis, patients suspected of having encephalitis should start acyclovir therapy (10 mg/kg intravenously every 8 hours for 2 weeks) even while specific serologic and spinal fluid analyses are being performed to make a specific diagnosis.

Supportive measures for patients with encephalitis typically include intensive care unit monitoring and treatment in the initial phases of the illness. Seizures are common and frequently refractory to antiepileptic drugs; however, the seizures themselves can increase morbidity and mortality, so vigorous treatment attempts are required (Chapter 410).

In patients who are immunosuppressed (see Table 422-1), the spectrum of possible infections is broader and potentially more treatable. Examples include varicella-zoster virus (Chapter 383), with acyclovir administered at doses similar to those used for herpes simplex virus, and cytomegalovirus (Chapter 384), with ganciclovir administered at 5 mg/kg intravenously every 12 hours for 2 weeks or cidofovir administered at 5 mg/kg intravenously weekly for 2 weeks, although some patients require long-term oral valganciclovir (900 mg every 24 hours) or intravenous cidofovir (5 mg/kg every 2 weeks). By comparison, no specific treatments are currently effective for Epstein-Barr virus (Chapter 385) and JC virus (progressive multifocal leukoencephalopathy, Chapter 378).

PROGNOSIS

The prognosis of encephalitis is dependent on the cause. Herpes simplex encephalitis, even with adequate treatment, has a 20% mortality, and the likelihood of major persistent morbidity with seizures or defects in memory and behavior is 35 to 40%. Each of the arboviruses has a different mortality rate, with eastern equine encephalitis virus associated with the highest mortality. LaCrosse encephalitis virus has the lowest mortality and is the most benign. Some forms of encephalitis have specific sequelae, such as sensorineural deafness or hydrocephalus associated with mumps encephalitis.

Grade A

---

1. Whitley RJ, Alford CA, Hirsch MS, et al. Vidarabine versus acyclovir therapy in herpes simplex encephalitis. *N Engl J Med.* 1986;314:144-149.

SUGGESTED READINGS

Centers for Disease Control and Prevention (CDC). Surveillance for human West Nile virus disease—United States, 1999-2008. *MMWR Surveill Summ.* 2010;59(SS-2):1-17. *Review.*

Long SS. Encephalitis diagnosis and management in the real world. *Adv Exp Med Biol.* 2011;697:153-173. *Review of viral, other infectious, and noninfectious causes.*

423

POLIOMYELITIS

ALLEN J. AKSAMIT, JR.

DEFINITION

Poliomyelitis is an acute viral illness that is associated with encephalitic features and acute flaccid paralysis. Enterovirus 71 (Chapter 387) and West Nile virus (Chapter 391) can cause an identical clinical illness.

EPIDEMIOLOGY

The cause of poliomyelitis is the poliovirus, which is serotyped into three subtypes (types 1, 2, and 3) and belongs to the group of enteroviruses in the family Picornaviridae. Most clinical disease is caused by the type 1 strain. Vaccination eliminated polio epidemics in the United States and Europe in the 1960s. The last major polio epidemic in the United States occurred in 1960, with a steady decline in cases subsequently. The last case of wild-virus poliomyelitis in the United States was reported in 1979. However, polio continues to remain a significant illness in unvaccinated areas of the world, particularly in Nigeria, Pakistan, and Afghanistan. In temperate climates, poliovirus infections occur most often in the summer and fall months, but infection occurs throughout the year in tropical areas.

Because of its oral-fecal, host-to-host transmission, poliovirus infection is influenced by standards of hygiene. The greatest risk for transmission occurs in family members and other direct contacts, especially under crowded conditions. The incubation period is about 3 to 6 days, after which virus may be shed into the nasopharynx for 2 to 6 weeks and into feces for several months.

Although poliovirus infects many exposed individuals, the acute flaccid paralysis of poliomyelitis occurs in only 1 to 2% of infected persons. The precise factors that cause dissemination of virus to the nervous system and susceptibility to paralytic disease are unknown. Paralytic disease occurs more commonly in children and young adults.

Historically, in the United States, poliomyelitis occasionally resulted from the live attenuated poliovirus vaccine. The risk for *vaccine-associated poliomyelitis* was about 1 case in 2.4 million doses, with most of the risk occurring with the first dose. About 75% of cases were related to immunocompetent vaccine recipients; about half of these cases occurred in the vaccinated person, most of the remainder occurred in healthy close contacts of vaccine recipients, but about 5% occurred in healthy community contacts who had not been vaccinated recently and had not been in direct contact with vaccine recipients. The remaining 25% or so cases occurred in immunocompromised persons, in whom clinical disease is about 5000-fold more likely to develop than in immunocompetent persons, or in the direct contacts of immunocompromised persons. The live attenuated virus in the vaccine can also mutate to cause *vaccine-derived poliomyelitis*, which can infect unvaccinated persons and lead to clinical polio with an attack rate and severity similar to that of wild-type virus. The inactivated polio vaccine, which is the only vaccine currently in use in the United States since the year 2000, does not cause vaccine-induced polio.

PATHOBIOLOGY

Polioviruses are small (approximately 27 nm), roughly spherical particles with a single-stranded RNA core surrounded by a protein capsid. Poliovirus is an enterovirus that is ingested orally and replicates initially in the lymphatic system of the gastrointestinal tract, especially in Peyer's patches in the small intestine. Spread to the local gastrointestinal lymphatics is followed by systemic viremia, which seeds the nervous system, although the precise mechanism of entry into the nervous system is not well established. The virus can replicate in skeletal muscle, where it may cause the myalgias that often precede weakness. One hypothesis is that the virus is then spread via peripheral motor axons to the spinal cord by retrograde transport, where it selectively replicates in the anterior horn cells. Pathology indicates a disseminated asymmetrical pattern of infection of the anterior horn cells of the spinal cord. Death of anterior horn cells leads to permanent paralysis, but compensation by collateral sprouting from uninfected cells in the same segment of the cord can allow some improvement in functional status and motor recovery.

CLINICAL MANIFESTATIONS

Acute poliomyelitis has two phases. An initial phase coincides with viremia and is associated with fever and headache and sometimes with sore throat; it resolves in 1 to 4 days. The second phase of illness, which usually occurs 7 to 21 days (range, 4 to 30 days) after the initial infection, is associated with abrupt fever, headache, vomiting, and meningismus, presumably as a result of viral infection in the central nervous system. The meningitic symptoms of headache and stiff neck subsequently resolve but are rapidly followed by asymmetrical, multifocal muscle weakness of the lower motor neuron type, sometimes with severe myalgias.

Clinical examination shows weakness affecting muscles in an asymmetrical and multifocal fashion, with a corresponding reduction in muscle stretch reflexes. Sensation is normal, thereby attesting to the selective involvement of the anterior horns of the spinal cord. Neurogenic muscular atrophy rapidly follows in affected muscles. The extent of motor involvement is typically completed within 1 week.

The upper and lower limb, truncal, and respiratory muscles are affected. Muscles innervated by the bulbar (medullary) cranial nerves (9th, 10th, 11th, or 12th) are often involved. The facial nerve can be involved, but the eye muscles are usually spared. Rarely, direct involvement of the brain stem reticular formation can cause an encephalitic illness with coma or cause death by its effects on breathing and cardiovascular control.

DIAGNOSIS

In addition to the typical symptoms and signs, the diagnosis of poliomyelitis is aided by analysis of spinal fluid. Spinal fluid typically shows a pleocytosis with lymphocytic predominance. The spinal fluid protein level is elevated, but the glucose level is normal. Enteroviruses may be cultured from the spinal fluid, but specific viral studies identifying poliovirus and other enteroviruses are best accomplished by polymerase chain reaction (PCR) testing. More specific characterization of the individual virus type can be accomplished by direct sequencing of the genome.

Differential Diagnosis

Other viral causes of encephalomyelitis can mimic poliomyelitis. Enterovirus 71 (Chapter 387) can cause epidemics of fever and acute flaccid paralysis. Coxsackievirus 7 and enterovirus 70 can cause milder paralytic syndromes, usually without fever. West Nile virus (Chapter 391) infection of the central nervous system is also associated with fever and acute flaccid paralysis. Tick-borne encephalitis virus (Chapter 391), native to Russia, may behave similarly. A paralytic form of rabies encephalitis (Chapter 422) can lead to asymmetrical acute flaccid paralysis. Serologic and virologic testing can distinguish these other agents. Testing for West Nile virus detects IgM antibodies against the virus in spinal fluid. Rabies may be tested for by either serology or PCR testing for the rabies virus (Chapter 422).

Ascending or descending paralysis can also be seen in a variety of non-infectious or postinfectious illnesses, such as Guillain-Barré syndrome (Chapter 428) and acute inflammatory myelopathy (Chapter 407). Diphtheria (Chapter 300) can be associated with focal paralytic syndromes.

PREVENTION

Poliomyelitis can be prevented by lifelong immunity induced by either the live attenuated (oral) or killed (inactivated) polio vaccines, which are routinely given to children. Oral polio vaccine is relatively inexpensive, about $0.08 per dose. Short-term shedding of vaccine virus in the stools of recently immunized children leads to passive immunization of close contacts, thereby providing the ability of mass campaigns to interrupt the transmission of wild poliovirus. However, about 1 in every 2.5 million doses of the vaccine can cause *vaccine-associated* poliomyelitis with paralysis in the vaccinated child, in a close contact, or even in another person. Rarely, a strain of poliovirus in the oral polio vaccine may change genetically and circulate to cause *vaccine-derived* poliomyelitis. In endemic countries, this low risk for vaccine-associated polio and vaccine-derived polio is preferable to the much higher risk for polio from wild-type virus without vaccination.

In countries where the risk of disease from wild-type poliovirus is zero, however, programs have shifted to using inactivated polio vaccine. Inactivated polio vaccine, which is about five times as expensive as oral vaccine, produces protective antibodies that prevent the poliovirus from spreading from the intestinal tract to the central nervous system. Unlike oral polio vaccine, it does not prevent the spread of wild poliovirus and cannot contain an epidemic because virus can still multiply inside the intestines and be shed in stool.

In the United States, debate about the efficacy and risks of live attenuated versus killed vaccine ended in 2000 with a policy that exclusively uses the inactivated polio vaccine, which does not lead to vaccine-associated or vaccine-derived polio. Global eradication strategies using live attenuated vaccine now focus especially on Nigeria, India, Afghanistan, and Pakistan, where polio remains endemic.

TREATMENT AND PROGNOSIS Rx

No specific treatment is available for patients affected by poliomyelitis caused by poliovirus. However, supportive therapy, including intensive care treatment to maintain respiratory function and provide cardiovascular support, can stabilize the patient and allow rehabilitation.

Death in patients with poliomyelitis is usually the result of bulbar muscle, respiratory, and cardiovascular impairment. With intensive treatment of respiratory insufficiency, patients can survive the acute paralytic illness. In general, motor improvement begins within a month after the onset of illness. On follow-up, many patients are left with profound neurologic deficits; others may return fully to activities of daily living, but some neurologic residua can usually be found on clinical or electrophysiologic examination.

Postpolio Syndromes

In patients who have had paralytic poliomyelitis, progressive atrophy and weakness can develop after more than 10 to 15 years of stable neurologic function. This syndrome, which is known as postpolio progressive muscular atrophy, is postulated to result from the normal age-related loss of motor neurons from a motor neuron pool already depleted by the viral illness. A second symptom complex in survivors of paralytic polio is characterized by progressive muscle pain, weakness, and fatigue; this "postpolio syndrome," which may affect up to 60% of patients infected during a polio epidemic, is not related to persistent viral infection and is of unknown cause.

SUGGESTED READINGS

Jenkins HE, Aylward RB, Gasasira A, et al. Implications of a circulating vaccine-derived poliovirus in Nigeria. *N Engl J Med*. 2010;362:2360-2369. *The attack rate and severity of disease with vaccine-derived poliovirus in Nigeria was similar to that of wild-type virus.*

Koopman FS, Uegaki K, Gilhus NE, et al. Treatment for postpolio syndrome. *Cochrane Database Syst Rev*. 2011;2:CD007818. *Review of pharmacological and rehabilitative treatments.*

Zangwill KM, Yeh SH, Wong EJ, et al. Paralytic syndromes in children: epidemiology and relationship to vaccination. *Pediatr Neurol*. 2010;42:206-212. *The incidence was 1.4 per 100,000 children per year in California, but no cases were related to polio vaccination.*

424

PRION DISEASES

PATRICK J. BOSQUE

DEFINITION

Prion diseases, which are a group of closely related neurodegenerative conditions of humans and other mammals, are caused by an accumulation of aggregated forms of the prion protein (PrP) in the central nervous system (CNS). These conditions can be transmitted by an infectious agent, the prion, that is composed of misfolded and aggregated PrP. The prion contains no specific nucleic acid. The name Creutzfeldt-Jakob disease (CJD) is applied to most human forms of prion disease, although other names are used for some forms.

EPIDEMIOLOGY

Prion diseases occur worldwide, with an incidence of about one case per million annually in most populations. These conditions can be acquired sporadically, genetically, or infectiously. Sporadic disease accounts for about 90% of cases, and genetic forms account for almost all the remainder. Cases acquired by infection are exceedingly rare in humans and account for less than 1% of cases in most populations. Both dietary and iatrogenic exposure has transmitted prion disease to humans.

Kuru, the first human prion disease recognized to be transmissible, was caused by ceremonial cannibalism in tribes of the Fore language group in the highlands of New Guinea. The last episodes of exposure are thought to have occurred in the late 1950s, but the few cases that have occurred in the past decade indicate an incubation period that approaches 50 years.

Variant CJD is caused by exposure, presumably by the alimentary route, to prions from cattle with bovine spongiform encephalopathy. It first arose in Great Britain in 1994, about 10 years after the first cases of bovine spongiform encephalopathy there. Despite the exposure of millions of people to meat contaminated with bovine spongiform encephalopathy prions, fewer than 200 people worldwide have contracted variant CJD. The incidence of variant CJD has decreased in recent years as the bovine spongiform encephalopathy outbreak in cattle has been contained and the entry of contaminated meat into the food supply restricted.

Most cases of iatrogenic transmission of CJD have involved contaminated cadaveric dura mater allografts, and these have almost all been from a single product, Lyodura, manufactured before May 1987. The other large group of iatrogenic cases occurred in recipients of growth hormone derived from cadaveric pituitaries, before the availability of recombinant growth hormone. Blood and blood products derived from donors with variant CJD have transmitted the illness, but surprisingly, CJD appears not to be transmissible from the blood of persons with the sporadic form of the disease. Contaminated surgical instruments are persuasively documented to have transmitted CJD on only four occasions.

PATHOBIOLOGY

PrP is a cell surface glycoprotein normally produced in the brain and several other tissues in mammals. Its normal function is unknown, but it may play a role in copper metabolism. In prion diseases, an abnormal misfolded and aggregated isoform of PrP, termed PrP^{Sc}, accumulates. Remarkably, PrP^{Sc} is able to recruit the normal form of PrP into the pathologic aggregate. The precise structure of PrP^{Sc} aggregates and the mechanism of prion propagation are incompletely understood, but a basic conceptual model proposes that the normally α-helical regions of PrP directly interact with the β-sheets of PrP^{Sc}, lose their normal structure, and then join the aggregate. At some point, the growing aggregate fractures, thereby creating additional aggregate particles. In this way, aggregates of PrP^{Sc} can propagate as infectious agents.

What precisely initiates sporadic or genetic prion diseases is not known. In infectious forms of prion disease that are transmitted by the alimentary route, prions first replicate in the enteric lymphatic system, including Peyer's patches. From the lymphatic system, prions spread to the CNS via sympathetic nerves in lymphatic tissue. Once in the CNS, prions appear to spread trans-synaptically. As with other neurodegenerative diseases associated with accumulations of aggregated proteins (e.g., β-amyloid in Alzheimer's disease), the mechanism by which the formation PrP^{Sc} causes neuronal dysfunction and death is unknown.

Pathology

Traditionally, prion diseases are recognized by a combination of vacuolization or "spongiosus" of the gray matter, astrocytic gliosis, and loss of neurons. In modern practice, the presence of PrP^{Sc}, demonstrated by immunohistochemical or biochemical techniques, is the pathologic hallmark of these conditions. In some forms of prion disease, PrP^{Sc} will form amyloid plaques, which are dense aggregates of protein linked by intermolecular β-sheets that bind Congo red. However, most commonly the PrP^{Sc} aggregates are smaller and more diffuse.

Genetics

All inherited forms of prion disease are caused by mutations in the PrP coding sequence of the gene *PRNP*. Mutations associated with familial forms of prion disease include more than 20 missense mutations, 2 premature stop mutations, and a series of insertions that code for an additional series of eight amino acids in a region where five of these octapeptide repeats normally occur. Genetic forms of prion disease are transmitted in an autosomal dominant pattern, usually with high but incomplete penetrance. Certain genotypes affect susceptibility to prion disease. Codon 129 of *PRNP* is polymorphic in most populations, with alleles coding for either valine or methionine. Persons who are homozygous (129VV or 129MM) at this allele are overrepresented among victims of sporadic CJD, and all victims of variant CJD (see later) carry 129M on both *PRNP* alleles.

Three distinctive forms of prion disease are associated with certain *PRNP* mutations: Gerstmann-Sträussler-Scheinker syndrome, fatal familial insomnia, and slowly progressive forms of CJD. Gerstmann-Sträussler-Scheinker syndrome is caused by any of several mutations in *PRNP*, the most common of which codes for a substitution of leucine for proline at codon 102 (P102L). Pathologically, there are accumulations of plaques of PrP amyloid in the brain, especially in the cerebellum.

Fatal familial insomnia is caused by a D178N mutation on the same allele as a methionine at the polymorphic codon 129 of *PRNP*. Pathologically, there is neuronal loss and accumulation of PrP^{Sc} in the thalamus. In contrast, the D178N mutation on an allele with valine at codon 129 causes a disease that is indistinguishable from sporadic CJD.

Some *PRNP* mutations cause a slowly progressive dementia. The most common of these mutations are large expansions of the octapeptide repeat region.

CLINICAL MANIFESTATIONS

Sporadic

The most common form of human prion disease is sporadic CJD. Onset is typically in later midlife at an average of about 60 years of age, although onset as young as 17 years and as old as 80 years has been reported. In about 25% of cases, patients or their families report a prodrome of a psychiatric disturbance, such as anxiety, depression, or altered sleep. Cognitive dysfunction is usually the most prominent neurologic sign. Unlike Alzheimer's disease, however, prion disease typically involves other brain systems and causes motor signs (such as ataxia, bradykinesia, or spasticity), vague somatic sensory disturbances, or alterations in visual perception. Myoclonus is a characteristic but not pathognomonic sign. Perhaps the most distinctive feature of prion disease is the pace of its progression. Typically, clear decrements in neurologic function can be observed over a period of weeks.

Genetic

Most genetic forms of prion disease are accompanied by symptoms indistinguishable from the those of the common sporadic syndrome just described. However, the mean age at onset may be somewhat younger.

In Gerstmann-Sträussler-Scheinker syndrome, the clinical signs are prominent ataxia, a slower rate of progression than occurs with sporadic CJD (typically 5 to 6 years from onset to death), and late dementia. Fatal familial insomnia begins with anxiety, depression, and sleep disturbance. Ataxia or other motor signs may also develop early in the disease course. Dementia occurs relatively late in the condition. Very rarely, a sporadic form of CJD will be manifested as a clinical syndrome of sporadic fatal insomnia that is indistinguishable from fatal familial insomnia.

Slowly progressive CJD may have clinical manifestations similar to those of familial Alzheimer's disease (Chapter 409) or resemble Huntington's disease (Chapter 417).

Infectiously Acquired

The extremely rare infectiously acquired forms of prion disease have features that are different from the common sporadic manifestation. The three infectiously transmitted forms of prion disease are variant CJD, kuru, and iatrogenic CJD.

Variant CJD is distinguished clinically from sporadic CJD by a much younger mean age at onset (mean, 26 years; range, 12 to 74 years), the prominence of psychiatric and sensory signs early in the disease, and the later emergence of dementia and motor signs, typically more than 6 months after the first symptoms. Iatrogenic CJD usually resembles sporadic CJD, but a subset of patients may have an ataxic form that clinically and pathologically shares some features with Gerstmann-Sträussler-Scheinker syndrome.

Kuru begins with limb pain followed by cerebellar ataxia and tremor ("kuru" means "shiver" in the Fore language). Overt dementia occurs late in the disease course.

DIAGNOSIS

The diagnosis of prion disease should be considered in patients with relatively rapidly progressive dementia, especially when structural, inflammatory, and more common metabolic, endocrine, and deficiency diseases have been excluded (Table 424-1). If the initial evaluation fails to yield an alternative diagnosis, a number of available tests further support the diagnosis of prion disease. However, prion diseases are rare, and ancillary tests have less than perfect specificity and sensitivity; if they are applied indiscriminately, these

TABLE 424-1 EVALUATION OF RAPIDLY PROGRESSIVE DEMENTIA

Initial screening	**Serum tests:** glucose, sodium, calcium, blood urea nitrogen, creatinine, hepatic aminotransferases, albumin, prothrombin time, TSH, antinuclear antigen, vitamin B_{12}, HIV and syphilis serology **Imaging:** brain MRI **CSF:** glucose, protein, cell counts, VDRL
Test findings supporting a diagnosis of prion disease	**MRI:** T2 hyperintensity in the basal ganglia, sometimes in the cortex **CSF 14-3-3 protein:** elevated levels fairly specific for CJD **EEG:** Periodic sharp wave complexes

CJD = Creutzfeldt-Jakob disease; CSF = cerebrospinal fluid ; EEG = electroencephalography; HIV = human immunodeficiency virus; MRI = magnetic resonance imaging; TSH = thyroid-stimulating hormone; VDRL = Venereal Disease Research Laboratory test.

TABLE 424-2 DIFFERENTIAL DIAGNOSIS OF RAPIDLY PROGRESSIVE DEMENTIA

Neurodegenerative diseases that may mimic CJD	Alzheimer's disease, diffuse Lewy body disease, frontotemporal dementia, corticobasal ganglion degeneration, progressive supranuclear palsy
Some less common treatable diseases that mimic CJD	**Autoimmune:** central nervous system vasculitis, limbic encephalitis, Hashimoto's encephalopathy, anti–voltage-gated potassium channel encephalopathy **Infections:** viral encephalitis, chronic meningitis **Toxicities:** lithium, bismuth, methotrexate **Neoplasms:** primary central nervous system lymphoma, intravascular lymphoma **Structural:** Normal-pressure hydrocephalus

CJD = Creutzfeldt-Jakob disease.

tests will frequently yield false-positive results. The presence of elevated cerebrospinal fluid levels of a protein called 14-3-3 is relatively specific for CJD if inflammatory and ischemic causes of dementia are excluded. An unusual hyperintensity of the deep gray matter (basal ganglia and thalamus) and sometimes the cortical gray matter on certain magnetic resonance imaging sequences (T2-weighted, fluid-attenuated inversion recovery, and diffusion-weighted weighting) occurs in about two thirds of CJD cases. The electroencephalogram in patients with CJD may show a pattern of periodic large-amplitude triphasic complexes.

Most diseases that cause rapidly progressive dementia are, like prion disease, untreatable and relentlessly progressive, for example, atypical Alzheimer's disease and diffuse Lewy body dementia (Table 424-2). However, it is important to exclude rare and at least partially treatable entities that can mimic prion disease, including autoimmune, infectious, toxic, malignant, and structural causes.

Certain diagnosis of prion disease can be made by brain biopsy. Tissue is examined immunohistochemically for the presence of abnormal aggregates of PrP. National or regional specialized prion disease centers, such as the National Prion Disorders Pathology Service Center (available at *http://www.cjdsurveillance.com*) in the United States, can assist pathologists in tissue analysis. In patients with a family history of neurodegenerative disease consistent with prion disease, determining the sequence of the protein-coding region of the prion protein gene can be diagnostic if a mutation is found.

TREATMENT AND PROGNOSIS [Rx]

Prion diseases are incurable, and no treatment significantly improves the course of disease. Most patients with sporadic CJD die within a year of the onset of symptoms. Patients with Gerstmann-Sträussler-Scheinker syndrome and certain other genetic or variant forms of prion disease may live longer. Excellent animal models of prion disease exist, and a number of novel therapeutic approaches are under active investigation. It is worthwhile to consider enrollment in experimental clinical trials if they are available (*http://clinicaltrials.gov*).

PREVENTION

Most cases of prion disease occur sporadically and cannot be prevented. Genetic cases can potentially be prevented through genetic counseling and prenatal testing, although whether such measures are warranted to prevent a disease that may not be manifested until midlife or later is an ethically complex question. Infectiously transmitted cases are currently amenable to preventive measures, including avoidance of surgical transmission as a result of contaminated instruments or tissue grafts and protection of the human food supply from meat products contaminated with bovine spongiform encephalopathy or other ruminant prions. Chronic wasting disease is epidemic among deer and elk in certain regions of the United States, and scrapie, which affects sheep and goats, is endemic at low levels in the United States and many other countries. Neither of these prion diseases has been convincingly linked to human illness, but prudence dictates that humans should avoid eating any prion-infected animal.

SUGGESTED READINGS

Frost B, Diamond MI. Prion-like mechanisms in neurodegenerative diseases. *Nat Rev Neurosci.* 2010;11:155-159. *Propagation of protein misfolding may be a common pathogenetic mechanism in neurodegenerative diseases.*

Geschwind MD, Shu H, Haman A, et al. Rapidly progressive dementia. *Ann Neurol.* 2008;64:97-108. *Summarizes alternative diagnoses found in patients referred to a large center with an initial diagnosis of CJD.*

Mastrianni JA. The genetics of prion diseases. *Genet Med.* 2010;12:187-195. *Review.*

Samson AO, Levitt M. Normal modes of prion proteins: from native to infectious particle. *Biochemistry.* 2011;50:2243-2248. *Review of the conformational biology.*

425

NUTRITIONAL AND ALCOHOL-RELATED NEUROLOGIC DISORDERS

BARBARA S. KOPPEL

An adequate supply of vitamins and minerals is necessary for development and metabolic function of both the central and peripheral nervous systems. Deficiencies of vitamins and minerals can cause a variety of neurologic syndromes (Table 425-1).

Vitamin deficiency (Chapter 225) can be caused by either malnutrition (Chapter 222) or malabsorption (Chapter 142). In malnutrition, it may be difficult to determine the specific vitamin responsible for particular neurologic symptoms and signs because multiple deficiencies are likely to coexist. Malnutrition is the most common cause of vitamin deficiency in economically disadvantaged countries. When adequate food supplies are readily available, malnutrition may be caused by surgery for obesity, unbalanced ("fad") diets, prolonged vomiting or anorexia, excess alcohol consumption, incomplete parenteral nutrition, or a genetic predisposition to malabsorption or dysfunction of transport proteins.

DEFICIENCY OF WATER-SOLUBLE VITAMINS
Thiamine (Vitamin B_1) Deficiency

Thiamine is converted to thiamine pyrophosphate, which serves as a coenzyme in glucose and lipid metabolism and in the synthesis of neurotransmitters from branched-chain amino acids. To avoid deficiency, thiamine must be consumed regularly in adequate amounts.

BERIBERI

In developing countries, the most common manifestation of thiamine deficiency is beriberi, which results in a painful sensorimotor peripheral neuropathy and heart failure ("wet beriberi"). Other causes of thiamine deficiency include consumption of foods in which the vitamin has been inactivated by processing or overcooking or foods that contain thiaminase-producing bacteria (e.g., raw fish). Headache, vomiting, seizures, and cranial nerve dysfunction can develop in babies born to malnourished mothers or fed thiamine-deficient formula.

TABLE 425-1 SUMMARY OF VITAMIN AND MINERAL DEFICIENCIES

VITAMIN AND MINERAL DEFICIENCIES	NEUROLOGIC SYNDROME OR SYNDROMES	SUPPORTING TESTS	TREATMENT	CAUSES (OTHER THAN MALNUTRITION)
A (Retinol)	Blindness from retinal or corneal damage	Visual fields, visual acuity Serum level <30-65 μg/dL	30,000 IU vitamin A daily × 1 wk	Hypothyroidism, diabetes, renal or liver failure
B_1 (thiamine)	Wernicke's encephalopathy: ataxia, nystagmus, ophthalmoparesis, confusion, delirium Korsakoff's syndrome: amnesia, confabulation Beriberi: axonal neuropathy	MRI: symmetrical lesions of midbrain (periaqueductal area), pons, hypothalamus, thalamus, cerebellum MRI: necrosis of mamillary bodies, dorsomedial and anterior thalamus Nerve conduction tests: decreased amplitude Serum thiamine level <20 ng/dL Erythrocyte transketolase	Prevent by 100 mg PO daily before and 1 year after bariatric surgery, 100 mg IV before glucose administration or refeeding Treat Wernicke's encephalopathy with 5 days of thiamine, 100-500 mg IV or IM daily, then PO 100 mg daily Antioxidants (*N*-acetylcysteine)	Alcoholism, bariatric or other major GI surgery, prolonged vomiting, hemodialysis, diuretic treatment of heart failure, cachexia, 5-fluorouracil, other blockers of thiamine phosphate production
B_3 (niacin)	Pellagra: confusion, dementia, weakness, ataxia, spasticity, myoclonus, glossitis, dermatitis, photosensitivity	Erythrocyte NAD, plasma niacin, urinary N1-methylnicotinamide	Nicotinic acid, 50 mg PO tid or 25 mg IV tid; nicotinamide, 50-100 mg IM or PO tid	Alcoholism, corn- or cereal-based diet, Hartnup's syndrome, carcinoid syndrome
B_5 (pantothenic acid)	Dysesthesias, foot paresthesias	Deficient coenzyme A	5 mg PO daily	Severe malnutrition
B_6 (pyridoxine)	Neuropathy, sensory ataxia, depression Infantile pyridoxine-deficient epilepsy	Plasma PLP <27 nmol/L; urinary 4-pyridoxic acid, <3 nmol ↑ Homocysteine after methionine loading challenge ↑ α-AASA in urine, plasma, CSF	50-100 mg PO daily for neuropathy (preventive use if taking B_6 antagonist) 100-200 mg daily for adult epilepsy	Diverticulosis, isoniazid, cycloserine, other antagonists Genetic defects in antiquitin (aldehyde dehydrogenase), pyridoxal synthesis
B_{12} (cobalamin)	Myelopathy with spastic paraparesis and sensory ataxia, peripheral neuropathy, optic neuropathy, memory loss, dementia; indirect contributor to stroke	Blood level <200 pg/mL ↑ Methylmalonic acid >145 nmol/L Intrinsic factor antibodies Schilling test, megaloblastic anemia Delayed somatosensory evoked potentials ↑ Homocysteine, total >12.5 μmol/L	IM B_{12}, 1000 μg daily for 1 week, then weekly for 1 month, then monthly or oral B_{12}, 1000 μg daily, or nasal B_{12}, 500 μg weekly for lifetime if abnormal absorption, 50-100 μg daily if normal absorption	Achlorhydria, gastric or ileal resection, blind loop syndrome, sprue, HIV infection, nitrous oxide anesthesia (especially abuse), fish tapeworm, vegan diet
D (calciferol)	Proximal myopathy, often painful; cognitive impairment Secondary compression of spinal cord, plexus, or peripheral nerves from rickets or osteomalacia	25-(OH) vitamin D_3 level <10 ng/mL in urine Serum calcium ↑ PTH >54 pg/mL Osteopenia/porosis on bone densitometry	Daily supplementation with 400 IU, >50,000 IU 3 times per wk if malabsorption; use blood level or urine calcium excretion to guide (should be >100 mg/day)	Lack of exposure to sunlight, including sunblock protection; chronic antiepileptic drug use
E (tocopherol)	Spinal and cerebellar ataxia, Babinski's sign, ophthalmoplegia, peripheral neuropathy, retinitis pigmentosa	Vitamin E level <2.5 mg/L (normal, 6-15 with normal lipid level) ↑ A-β-lipoprotein levels, antigliadin antibodies Genetic analysis to rule out other spinocerebellar ataxias such as Friedreich's ataxia	Supplement with 6-800 IU, 5-10 mg/kg twice daily, for ataxia of genetic causes, water-soluble 200 mg/kg/day or IM α-tocopherol for malabsorption	Biliary atresia, celiac sprue, Genetic: ↓ α-tocopherol transport protein (8q13), microsomal triglyceride transfer protein
Folate	Dementia, B_{12} deficiency, stroke	↑ Homocysteine, plasma level <2.5 μg/L	1 mg 3 times per day until normal level, then maintenance of 1 mg/day Pregnancy: additional 0.4 mg/day if taking a folate antagonist	Malabsorption or use of antagonist (methotrexate) or antiepileptic medication
K (phytonadione)	Intracranial hemorrhage	INR or PT elevation	IM phytonadione at birth, maternal vitamin K for last month of pregnancy	Medication use that increases metabolism, such as phenytoin
Copper	Myelopathy, neuropathy	Serum Cu <75 μg/dL, ↓ urinary Cu, ceruloplasmin <23 mg/dL MRI: ↑ T2 signal in cervical cord, dorsal column Mutation in *ATP7A* gene (Menkes' disease)	Elemental Cu, 8 mg/day PO week 1, 6 mg/day week 2, 4 mg/day week 3, 2 mg/day ongoing malabsorption Menkes' disease: 250 mg SC bid	Wilson's disease, Menkes' disease, alcoholism, malabsorption, gastric bypass, zinc toxicity
Magnesium	Seizures, encephalopathy	Serum magnesium <1.5 mg/dL, correct for low albumin	Magnesium sulfate IV or PO Avoid magnesium-wasting drugs	Alcoholism, especially beer
Potassium	Muscle weakness, chronic, acute	Serum potassium <3.5 mEq/L, ECG	IV or PO KCl until normalized	Diuretic use, bulimia

AASA = aminoadipic semialdehyde; CSF = cerebrospinal fluid; ECG, electrocardiography; GI = gastrointestinal; INR = international normalized ratio; MRI = magnetic resonance imaging; NAD = nicotinamide adenine dinucleotide; PLP = pyridoxal-5-phosphate (active coenzyme of pyridoxine); PT = prothrombin time; PTH = parathyroid hormone.

WERNICKE'S ENCEPHALOPATHY

Severe short-term thiamine deficiency results in Wernicke's encephalopathy, a syndrome characterized by confusion and other changes in mental status, abnormal eye movements, and ataxia. Wernicke's encephalopathy occurs most commonly in the setting of chronic alcohol abuse, but it can also be seen following bariatric surgery, refeeding after a period of starvation, or after the intravenous administration of glucose without thiamine. The symptoms and signs of Wernicke's encephalopathy reflect dysfunction of brain regions that are dependent on thiamine or have high rates of energy metabolism, where lactate production from anaerobic metabolism causes damage to astrocytes or the blood-brain barrier. These regions include the periaqueductal gray matter of the midbrain, pons, and medulla, as well as the cerebellum, anterior thalamus, mamillary bodies, and rarely, the cerebral cortex and hypothalamus.

The classic triad of mental status changes, ocular abnormalities, and ataxia is present in less than 50% of patients. Changes in mental status range from mild memory impairment or inattention to delirium. Eye movement abnormalities include nystagmus, dysconjugate gaze, and gaze palsies. Ataxia can affect the limbs, trunk, and gait. Patients with Wernicke's encephalopathy can also have autonomic and hypothalamic dysfunction, such as bradycardia and hypothermia, as well as papilledema, optic neuropathy, seizures, and myoclonus. In symptomatic patients, T2-weighted magnetic resonance imaging (MRI) demonstrates increased signal from edema or hemorrhage in affected areas, most often the thalamus.

KORSAKOFF'S SYNDROME

Korsakoff's syndrome becomes apparent in 80% of patients with Wernicke's encephalopathy as the ataxia and eye movement abnormalities improve. Korsakoff's syndrome is characterized by disproportionate retrograde and anterograde episodic amnesia, confabulation or hallucinations, and sometimes apathy. The primary pathologic findings occur in the limbic system, especially the mamillary bodies, amygdala, and anterior thalamus.

The memory deficit, which prevents the learning of new information or the acquisition of new memories, is disproportionately severe in relation to other aspects of the cognitive function. For example, alertness, attention, social interactions, and motor learning are generally well preserved. There may be mild disorientation with respect to time and place, and sometimes apathy and other emotional changes are present. Confabulation, in which the intrusion of errors in response to questions leads to fabrication without the intention of deceiving, is often present spontaneously in the first weeks. Confabulation may be a compensatory mechanism, and it usually lessens over time. Neuropsychological testing often demonstrates emotional changes and mild problems in executive function, which are suggestive of frontal lobe involvement.

> ### TREATMENT   **Rx**
>
> Treatment with thiamine (see Table 425-1) can prevent or treat beriberi and Wernicke's encephalopathy. Korsakoff's syndrome, however, does not respond to replacement of thiamine and must be prevented by timely recognition and treatment of Wernicke's encephalopathy.

Cobalamin (Vitamin B₁₂) Deficiency

Cobalamin deficiency results in combined system disease or subacute combined degeneration, which is a spinal cord syndrome (myelopathy) in which damage to the dorsal (sensory) and lateral (motor) tracts results in impaired position and vibratory sensation and spastic paraparesis.

EPIDEMIOLOGY AND PATHOBIOLOGY

Cobalamin deficiency (Chapters 167 and 225) is most common in individuals older than 60 years because the incidence of atrophic gastritis (Chapter 141) and achlorhydria rises in older individuals who lack the gastric intrinsic factor needed for absorption of vitamin B₁₂. Cobalamin deficiency is rarely due to inadequate dietary intake (e.g., a vegan diet for several years). Nitrous oxide toxicity, from illicit use but not from administration for anesthesia, can cause cobalamin deficiency by inactivating the cobalamin-dependent enzyme methionine synthase, so this anesthetic should be avoided in people with known or suspected cobalamin deficiency. Low vitamin B₁₂ levels have been associated with increased homocysteine levels, but a relationship to vascular disease or vascular-related dementia has not been established.

CLINICAL MANIFESTATIONS

The proprioceptive loss results in sensory ataxia with Romberg's sign (failure to maintain balance with the eyes closed). A peripheral neuropathy with numbness and tingling in the hands and feet is almost always present. Cerebral involvement includes memory loss, changes in personality, and occasional psychosis. Symptoms generally progress slowly, but they may appear especially rapidly after exposure to nitrous oxide anesthesia by individuals with preexisting subclinical cobalamin deficiency.

DIAGNOSIS

Serum vitamin B₁₂ levels are almost always low but can rarely be normal in symptomatic patients. In such cases, serum levels of methylmalonic acid and

homocysteine are useful ancillary tests because these levels are increased in persons with vitamin B₁₂ deficiency as a result of impaired cobalamin-dependent reactions (Chapter 167). Pernicious anemia (Chapter 167) is severe in about 20% of patients. However, both the hematocrit and mean corpuscular volume can be normal because the hematologic effects of cobalamin deficiency can be partially masked by folate supplementation.

Low levels of cobalamin can also be present in many normal people, especially the elderly. Because of the increasing frequency of dementia, peripheral polyneuropathy, and myelopathy with age, a low cobalamin level does not necessarily imply cause and effect. Nonetheless, the triad of dementia, polyneuropathy, and myelopathy is rare. The definitive definition of causality is clinical improvement after cobalamin replacement.

> ### TREATMENT   **Rx**
>
> Treatment usually begins with a subcutaneous or intramuscular injection of 500 to 1000 μg of cobalamin daily for 1 week and then weekly for 1 month. After that time, oral supplementation with 50 to 100 μg daily of cyanocobalamin usually suffices in patients with achlorhydria or other causes of malabsorption; 1000 μg daily should be used in patients with intrinsic factor antibodies. A nasal gel form (500 μg weekly) may also be effective.

PROGNOSIS

Neurologic symptoms, especially paresthesias, typically improve to some extent within 3 months of achieving adequate serum levels. Numbness and areflexia often persist, especially if treatment is delayed. If there is no improvement whatsoever, vitamin B₁₂ deficiency is most likely not responsible for the condition. For example, human immunodeficiency virus–associated myelopathy, which can have a similar clinical manifestation, does not reverse with supplemental vitamin B₁₂ because it is caused by disruption of transmethylation pathways, not low cobalamin levels (see Table 425-1).

Folate Deficiency

Folate is an important coenzyme in the metabolism of nucleic and amino acids. Inborn errors of folate metabolism cause mental retardation and seizures. Although folate deficiency is more likely to produce hematologic abnormalities than neurologic deficits, it is an important risk factor for neural tube defects in babies born to mothers who have insufficient folate intake or use anticonvulsant drugs such as valproate, antituberculosis medications, or folate antagonists such as methotrexate. Women of childbearing age who are taking these medications are now routinely given 0.4 mg of folate daily in addition to the 1 mg contained in prenatal vitamins. Vitamin B₁₂ levels should be checked to avoid ongoing neurologic damage as a result of unrecognized cobalamin deficiency when anemia is treated with folate alone. Folate deficiency is treated with 1 mg three times daily for 1 month followed by 1 mg each day.

Folate deficiency results in increased levels of homocysteine, which is associated with an increased risk for ischemic heart disease and stroke. However, multiple trials of supplementation of folate and B vitamins in patients with elevated homocysteine levels but not with classic homocysteinemia have been uniformly unsuccessful in reducing adverse clinical events.

Pyridoxine (Vitamin B₆) Deficiency

Pyridoxine is a coenzyme in multiple reactions that involve gluconeogenesis, biosynthesis of neurotransmitters, and the metabolism of amino acids, nucleic acids, and lipids. Pyridoxine deficiency can be caused by genetic defects, such as defective antiquitin, that lead to increased utilization of pyridoxine. In adults, low levels of pyridoxine are well tolerated, so symptomatic deficiency is rare. However, symptomatic deficiency can occur in the setting of renal failure or dialysis; cirrhosis; the use of medications such as isoniazid for antitubercular therapy or hydralazine for hypertension without concurrent supplementation; or extreme malnutrition, especially diets consisting predominantly of white rice.

CLINICAL MANIFESTATIONS AND DIAGNOSIS

Prolonged pyridoxine deficiency causes a painful axonal peripheral neuropathy that leads to weakness and sensory ataxia. Some patients may have skin thickening, seborrheic dermatitis, or glossitis, which suggest pellagra. Serum levels of the active form of pyridoxine, pyridoxal 5′-phosphate, and urine levels of the metabolite 4-pyridoxic acid are low. Ancillary tests include nerve conduction studies, which show decreased amplitude, typical of axonal neuropathy. In inherited forms of pyridoxine deficiency, electroencephalography shows generalized 1- to 4-Hz spiked wave discharges and slowing.

Toxicity from excess intake of pyridoxine (>100 mg daily), usually from vitamin supplements, causes a ganglionopathy that is characterized by impaired sensation, sensory ataxia with Romberg's sign, and areflexia.

TREATMENT   Rx

Patients in whom symptoms of pyridoxine deficiency develop or who take pyridoxine antagonists should receive supplemental pyridoxine (50 to 100 mg daily). Children with pyridoxine-dependent epilepsy require lifelong supplementation with 100 mg of pyridoxine daily. For pyridoxine toxicity, simply stopping vitamin intake will usually reverse the damage.

⬤ DEFICIENCY OF FAT-SOLUBLE VITAMINS
Vitamin E (Tocopherol) Deficiency

Although vitamin E is composed of several tocopherols, it is the α form that is biologically active in humans and contained in most foods. Because it is so widely available, deficiency is almost never due to inadequate dietary consumption. Rather, vitamin E deficiency is almost always the result of malabsorption because of such conditions as biliary and pancreatic disease (Chapters 158 and 146), cystic fibrosis (Chapter 89), celiac disease (Chapter 142), Crohn's disease (Chapter 143), extensive small bowel resection, and blind loop syndrome (Chapter 142). In addition, vitamin E deficiency is associated with genetic defects such as those causing hypolipoproteinemia and abetalipoproteinemia, chylomicron retention disease, and ataxia with vitamin E deficiency.

CLINICAL MANIFESTATIONS AND DIAGNOSIS

Neurologic manifestations of vitamin E deficiency include a spinocerebellar syndrome with ataxia, loss of vibration and position senses, hyporeflexia, and extensor plantar responses. Other findings can include ophthalmoplegia, retinopathy, ptosis, and rarely, myopathy.

Serum levels of vitamin E can vary with the serum lipid levels. In extreme hyperlipidemia, such as cholestasis, the ratio of vitamin E to cholesterol will be more reliable than the absolute vitamin E level, which can be normal despite a low ratio.

TREATMENT   Rx

The amount of vitamin E replacement depends on the cause. Malabsorption syndromes require 1000 to 2000 mg daily for infants and 10 to 20 g for adults. Genetic causes can be treated with 5 to 10 g/day. After bariatric surgery, 300 mg daily is recommended. For vitamin E, 1 mg is equivalent to 1.49 IU. Although vitamin E has been advocated to forestall neurodegenerative diseases such as Alzheimer's disease, this role has not been established.[2]

Vitamin D (Calciferol) Deficiency

Vitamin D deficiency results from inadequate exposure to sunlight, dietary insufficiency, or malabsorption because of celiac disease, inflammatory bowel disease, or extensive small bowel resection. The most important consequences of vitamin D deficiency are rickets in children, osteomalacia in adults, and hypocalcemia with secondary hyperparathyroidism. Hypocalcemia, in turn, can cause tetany, encephalopathy, and seizures. A proximal myopathy, worse in the legs than the arms, and cutaneous hyperalgesia have been reported. Inadequate vitamin D levels, present in 44% of Americans older than 65 years, are associated with cognitive dysfunction or dementia. Lower levels of vitamin D are also correlated with the risk for multiple sclerosis (Chapter 419). Individuals who can absorb vitamin D normally require 400 to 600 IU of vitamin D_3 (cholecalciferol) (10 to 15 µg), but persons with malabsorption may need more than twice that amount. The eventual dose should be titrated to produce a serum 25-hydroxyvitamin D level of at least 30 ng/mL.

Vitamin A Deficiency

Vitamin A deficiency, which is most often associated with night blindness, can also impair taste and has rarely been associated with raised intracranial pressure in children. Malabsorption rarely leads to vitamin A deficiency. Vitamin A toxicity, which is occasionally a complication of the use of isotretinoin for acne or excessive consumption of liver in the diet, can cause pseudotumor cerebri with headache and papilledema.

Vitamin K Deficiency

Vitamin K deficiency, which is a rare consequence of malabsorption, is seen more commonly in patients who have compromised liver synthesis or who are receiving warfarin therapy. Vitamin K deficiency causes excessive bleeding and increases the risk for intracerebral hemorrhage (Chapter 415), especially in newborns whose mothers are taking antagonists such as phenytoin. Five milligrams daily is usually adequate supplementation, but the dose may need to be adjusted based on the prothrombin time.

⬤ DEFICIENCY OF MISCELLANEOUS ELEMENTS AND NUTRIENTS
Copper Deficiency

Acquired copper deficiency is rare but may occur in premature or malnourished infants and in patients with malabsorption from celiac disease, cystic fibrosis, or Crohn's disease. It can also occur in patients with nephrotic syndrome and following gastric surgery, especially bariatric surgery. Copper deficiency is also a well-recognized consequence of excessive intake of zinc, usually as a result of the overuse of zinc-containing products, such as denture cream or herbal preparations to treat rhinitis and sinusitis, or because of parenteral overload during hemodialysis.

The most common neurologic complication in persons with copper deficiency is a myelopathy that is clinically very similar to that seen with cobalamin deficiency. The most prominent features are spastic paraparesis and sensory ataxia. A peripheral polyneuropathy of the axonal type is usually present as well. Copper levels, including excreted urinary copper, should be measured in patients who are suspected of having vitamin B_{12} deficiency but fail to respond to treatment with cyanocobalamin. Optic neuropathy, wristdrop, and footdrop have also been reported. Menkes' disease, an X-linked recessive copper deficiency caused by mutations in the *ATP7A* gene needed for absorption, is characterized by severe mental retardation and kinky hair. The diagnosis is made by finding low serum copper levels or changes in the ratio of dopamine to norepinephrine. Large doses of copper histidine (250 mg twice daily until age 1, then daily until age 3) must be delivered subcutaneously, but improvement is variable. Patients survive to adulthood only if copper injections start neonatally.

Wilson's disease (Chapter 218) is an autosomal recessive disorder that results from excessive copper accumulation, primarily in the liver and brain, as a result of failed transport and impaired copper excretion. Ceruloplasmin, the transport protein for copper, is deficient. Neurologic manifestations can include depression, psychosis, dementia, dysarthria, tremor, chorea, and other movement disorders. Accumulation of copper in the liver leads to chronic liver failure. Wilson's disease is treated by copper chelation (Chapter 218) and by minimizing dietary intake.

Other Nutritional Disorders

Biotin deficiency is caused by an autosomal recessive disorder affecting biotinidase. It results in developmental delay, seizures, ataxia, and deafness.

Some epidemics that are manifested as peripheral neuropathy or optic neuropathy, such as Strachan's Jamaican neuropathy and Cuban tobacco-alcohol amblyopia, occur in the setting of malnutrition and respond to replacement of B vitamins or folate. Toxicity from foods should always be suspected in populations that are reliant on a single main source of nutrition, even when the exact cause is not known. Examples include spastic paraparesis or muscle atrophy from overconsumption of legumes in the *Lathyrus* genus, such as chick peas, which contain the neurotoxic glutamate agonist oxalyl-diaminoproprionic acid; konzo, probably from cyanide poisoning (Chapter 110), which is related to improperly prepared cassava in Africa; and amyotrophic lateral sclerosis and Parkinson-dementia complex in Guam, probably caused by cycad toxins in flour.

⬤ ALCOHOL-RELATED DISORDERS

Alcohol (Chapter 32) is responsible for a wide spectrum of neurologic disorders. At one extreme, it can cause irreversible dementia, cerebellar degeneration, optic neuropathy, and peripheral polyneuropathy. Alcohol also causes transient neurologic syndromes such as seizures, tremors, hallucinosis, and delirium tremens. Acute intoxication can range from mild euphoria, to vestibular and cerebellar dysfunction, to coma and death. When alcohol is the main source of calories, it contributes to nutritional deficiency syndromes such as Wernicke-Korsakoff syndrome, beriberi, and pellagra. Alcohol-induced liver toxicity results in hepatic encephalopathy and non-wilsonian hepatolenticular degeneration. Coagulopathy caused by liver disease or suppressed platelet production raises the risk for subdural or intracranial hematoma. Fetal alcohol syndrome reflects the vulnerability of the developing nervous system to the toxic effects of alcohol.

Signs of intoxication correlate with blood alcohol levels: from 50 mg/dL for personality changes; 150 mg/dL for ataxia, vestibular dysfunction, and nystagmus; 300 mg/dL for stupor; 400 mg/dL for coma; and up to 500 mg/dL for respiratory depression or apnea. However, the effects vary greatly, depending on the chronicity of intake and the rate at which high levels develop. Intoxication alone should never be assumed to be the sole cause of a depressed mental state because alcoholics are at increased risk for other causes of coma (Chapter 411).

Specific Clinical Syndromes

Seizures and status epilepticus (Chapter 410) can be a direct consequence of intoxication, withdrawal, hyponatremia (Chapter 118), and hypomagnesemia (Chapter 121) or result from epileptogenic foci from previous head trauma or stroke.

Hepatic encephalopathy can be the result of alcoholic cirrhosis (Chapter 156), especially in patients who have bleeding esophageal varices, and is characterized by irritability alternating with depressed mental status, seizures, tremor, and asterixis.

Dementia develops even when nutrition is well maintained because of alcohol's direct neurotoxic effects. Contributing factors include head injury, status epilepticus, and cerebrovascular disease. Further evidence of alcohol's deleterious effect is cerebral atrophy involving both gray and white matter. The dementia is probably not reversible.

Wernicke's encephalopathy and *Korsakoff syndrome* are described in the section on thiamine.

Marchiafava-Bignami syndrome was first described in postmortem studies of Italian chianti drinkers but can occur in persons who consume any type of alcohol. Acute signs include coma, seizures, hemiparesis, rigidity, and sometimes death. The most severe pathology involves demyelination and necrosis of the corpus callosum. Findings on MRI include increased T2- and diffusion-weighted signals in the corpus callosum, especially the splenium.

Cerebellar degeneration and ataxia result from the alcohol-induced loss of Purkinje cells, mainly in the anterior superior parts of the cerebellar vermis; the cerebellar hemispheres are less affected. As a result, the clinical picture is mainly truncal and gait ataxia, with a wide-based unsteady gait and inability to walk tandem. The arms are much less involved, if affected at all. Intention tremor, nystagmus, and dysarthria are rare. Findings are exacerbated by concurrent thiamine deficiency and Wernicke's encephalopathy.

Optic neuropathy, which occurs with severe chronic alcohol abuse, is manifested as progressive, painless visual loss as a result of damage to the optic nerve fibers. The macular region is most affected. Similar findings, first described in Cuban men who were heavy cigar smokers, have also been attributed to tobacco. However, neither alcohol nor tobacco is apparently directly responsible for the optic nerve damage, so it is more likely that the syndrome results from malnutrition and deficiencies of multiple vitamins, including vitamins A and B.

Peripheral neuropathy (Chapter 428) ("alcoholic neuropathy") is the most common neurologic complication of chronic alcoholism. It is an axonal sensorimotor neuropathy that causes dysfunction of small nerve fibers, thereby leading to distal sensory symptoms such as burning dysesthesias and paresthesias of the soles of the feet. The typical numbness develops in a stocking-glove distribution, with loss of ankle reflexes. Mild distal weakness eventually occurs in some patients. Involvement of the autonomic nervous system frequently causes impotence, as well as urinary or bowel complaints. Although vitamin supplements, especially thiamine and pyridoxine, may lead to some improvement, especially in the painful paresthesias, complete resolution is rare. If abstinence from alcohol is not also achieved, the symptoms persist, thereby implying that a direct toxic effect of alcohol is likely.

Compressive neuropathies, especially of the radial nerve ("Saturday night palsy") and peroneal nerve, occur in individuals who injure peripheral nerves during periods of prolonged pressure on a nerve while obtunded from heavy alcohol consumption. Recovery takes several weeks but is generally complete.

Myopathy occurs in binge drinkers, in whom severe muscle injury with rhabdomyolysis (Chapter 115) can develop, especially in the setting of fasting and prolonged absence of movement. Myoglobinuria can result in kidney damage. Heavy alcohol consumption is also associated with cardiomyopathy (Chapter 60), which can lead to arrhythmias even in the absence of hypokalemia. Chronic alcohol abuse causes a symmetrical proximal weakness (Chapter 429), but it is rarely the only neurologic finding; although weakness can be demonstrated in up to 50% of chronic alcoholics, it is not usually severe enough to prevent walking or standing.

Fetal alcohol syndrome is recognized at birth in infants whose mothers consumed significant amounts of alcohol, especially in the early stages of pregnancy. The characteristic findings are growth retardation, microcephaly, hypotonia, skeletal and cardiac anomalies, and characteristic facial features (micrognathia, small palpebral fissures). Recently, migration defects have been demonstrated by diffusion-weighted MRI and tractography. Exposure of the developing brain to alcohol can also lead to subtle or severe neurocognitive defects and attention deficit disorder, which may not be detected until later in childhood. The teratogenic effects of alcohol are not prevented by adequate amounts of thiamine, folate, and other vitamins.

Grade A

1. Andrès E, Fothergill H, Mecili M. Efficacy of oral cobalamin (vitamin B$_{12}$) therapy. *Expert Opin Pharmacother.* 2010;11:249-256.
2. Isaac MG, Quinn R, Tabet N. Vitamin E for Alzheimer's disease and mild cognitive impairment. *Cochrane Database Syst Rev.* 2008;3:CD002854.

SUGGESTED READINGS

Kopelman MD, Thomson AD, Guerrini I, et al. The Korsakoff syndrome: clinical aspects, psychology and treatment. *Alcohol Alcohol.* 2009;44:148-154. *About 75% of abstinent patients have some recovery.*

Kumar N: Neurologic presentation of nutritional deficiencies. *Neurol Clin.* 2010;28:107-170. *Review.*

Mellion M, Gilchrist JM, De La Monte S. Alcohol-related peripheral neuropathy: nutritional, toxic, or both? *Muscle Nerve.* 2011;43:309-316. *Review suggesting that it is mostly toxic.*

Rudnicki SA. Prevention and treatment of peripheral neuropathy after bariatric surgery. *Curr Treat Options Neurol.* 2010;12:29-36. *Review of vitamin deficiencies, with specific recommendations for testing for and supplementation with vitamins A, C, D, K, E; iron; zinc; selenium; magnesium; and copper.*

426

CONGENITAL, DEVELOPMENTAL, AND NEUROCUTANEOUS DISORDERS

JONATHAN W. MINK

● CONGENITAL DISORDERS
Malformations of Cerebral Cortex

Developmental malformations of the cerebral cortex arise from a wide variety of etiologies, including genetic mutations, intrauterine infections, intrauterine ischemia, and toxic exposures. These malformations are heterogeneous and can result from disrupted neuronal proliferation, migration, or cortical organization. In general, disorders that arise early in development are more severe than those that arise after the basic architecture of the brain has developed. When small areas of the brain are involved, the patient may have minor impairment of neurologic function. When larger areas of the brain are involved, patients often have cognitive deficits and more severe neurologic dysfunction. Epilepsy (Chapter 410), which is the most common manifestation of abnormal cortical development, may occur with or without other neurologic signs or symptoms.

Disorders of Neuronal Proliferation

Neuronal proliferation can be abnormally increased or decreased owing to a variety of mechanisms. These disorders can manifest with megalencephaly or microcephaly, or head size can be normal. Abnormal proliferation can involve specific cell types, thereby resulting in focal or multifocal areas of dysplasia or in the formation of hamartomas (see Tuberous Sclerosis, later).

FOCAL CORTICAL DYSPLASIA WITH BALLOON CELLS

Focal cortical dysplasia is caused by abnormal proliferation of both neurons and glia. Its neuropathology is characterized by the presence of giant dysmorphic neurons and "balloon cells" associated with altered cortical lamination, but some lesions have abnormal cortical layering with ectopic neurons in white matter. Affected patients typically present with partial seizures that are often intractable to medical therapy. These seizures can begin at any age but most commonly present during childhood or adolescence. The type of seizure depends on the anatomic location of the dysplasia. Other neurologic manifestations, such a sensory, motor, or cognitive impairments, depend on the extent of the dysplasia and whether multiple brain regions are affected. The diagnosis of focal cortical dysplasia is usually made with brain magnetic resonance imaging (MRI), which demonstrates focal thickening of a gyrus or alteration of the gray-white matter junction. Management includes medical treatment of seizures, but surgical resection of the epileptic focus may be required for complete remission (Chapter 410).

Disorders of Neuronal Migration

Disorders of neuronal migration typically result in disruption of the normal laminar organization of the cerebral cortex. Defects include impaired initiation of neuronal migration, impaired orderly migration, and impaired termination of migration. All result in abnormal cortical organization and function.

LISSENCEPHALY AND BAND HETEROTOPIA

The lissencephalies (smooth brain) are a group of disorders that are caused by arrested migration of neurons to the cerebral cortex. Lissencephaly genes include *LIS1* (chromosome 17p13.3) and *DCX* (chromosome Xq22), both of which are thought to be involved in the regulation of microtubule organization and function. Individuals with mutations of *LIS1* typically have severe malformations that are most prominent in the posterior cerebrum. More extensive mutations in the region of *LIS1* result in Miller-Dieker syndrome, a condition characterized by lissencephaly and distinctive facial features that include a prominent forehead, midface hypoplasia, low-set and abnormally shaped ears, and a small jaw. Males with *DCX* mutations typically have a severe lissencephaly that is most prominent in the anterior cerebrum. Lissencephaly is typically diagnosed in infancy or early childhood, usually accompanied by microcephaly, severe global developmental delay, cerebral palsy, and intractable epilepsy. Diagnosis of lissencephaly is made by brain MRI that shows a smooth cortex with minimal sulcation. Genetic testing for *LIS1* and *DCX* is available. Management consists of seizure control, genetic counseling, and supportive care.

Band heterotopia (double cortex) is a less severe form of lissencephaly that is usually seen in women with *DCX* mutation. Clinical manifestations of band heterotopia range from mild to severe and include seizures, intellectual disability, and developmental delay. Women with a *DCX* mutation are at risk of having male children with severe lissencephaly. Brain MRI demonstrates a band of gray matter underlying a nearly normal-appearing cerebral cortex. Management consists of seizure control and genetic counseling.

NODULAR HETEROTOPIA

Nodular heterotopias are characterized by nodular ectopic collections of neurons and glia in the subependyma or in the subcortical white matter. The most important form is subependymal nodular heterotopia, a condition characterized by multiple gray matter nodules in the walls of the lateral ventricles bilaterally. This X-linked condition is due to a mutation in *FLNA* (chromosome Xq28), which codes for filamin A, an actin-cross-linking phosphoprotein that is critical for the initiation of migration. As a result of this mutation, many neurons do not migrate out of the subventricular zone. Most affected individuals are heterozygous females. Males are severely affected and often die in infancy. Most affected females present with seizures during childhood or adolescence. Females may be intellectually normal or have mild disability. Individuals with subependymal nodular heterotopia appear to be at increased risk for aortic or carotid dissection and for cardiac valvular abnormalities.

The diagnosis is based on brain MRI, which shows gray matter nodules along the walls of the lateral ventricles. Genetic testing for FLNA is available. Management consists of seizure control and genetic counseling.

Disorders of Cortical Organization

Disorders of cortical organization include conditions such as polymicrogyria and schizencephaly. These disorders are not due to abnormal numbers of neurons or impaired migration but instead include abnormalities of gyration, sulcation, connectivity, or synaptogenesis. The best understood of these disorders are polymicrogyria and schizencephaly.

POLYMICROGYRIA

Polymicrogyria is characterized by regions of complex cortical convolutions with miniature gyri that are fused and superimposed together. Polymicrogyria is caused by failure of cortical organization as a result of in utero injury or genetic mutation; it has been associated with prenatal infections, such as cytomegalovirus, and possible vascular abnormalities, but often it is idiopathic. A single gene, *GPR56* (chromosome 16q13), has been associated with bilateral frontoparietal polymicrogyria. *GPR56* codes for a G protein–coupled receptor that appears to be important for human cerebral cortical development. Clinical manifestations include epilepsy, developmental delay, cerebral palsy, and intellectual disability, depending on the location and extent of the abnormality. The diagnosis of polymicrogyria is made by brain MRI. Clinical management consists of seizure management and supportive therapies.

SCHIZENCEPHALY

Schizencephaly is characterized by infolding of cortical gray matter along a hemispheric cleft near the primary cerebral fissures. It is thought to represent a more extensive injury than what leads to polymicrogyria. In most cases, the cause cannot be determined, but it has been associated with in utero insult. A rare familial form has been described, but no gene has been identified. Clinical features include developmental delay, cerebral palsy, dysarthria, and epilepsy. The clinical abnormalities are more severe with large open-lip schizencephaly and with bilateral lesions than with small unilateral closed-lip schizencephaly. Diagnosis is made by brain MRI. Management consists of seizure control and supportive therapies when indicated.

Malformations of Cerebellum and Brain Stem

Developmental abnormalities of the hindbrain are less well understood than are abnormalities of cerebral cortical development. Two of the better known and important syndromes are Joubert's syndrome and Dandy-Walker malformation.

JOUBERT'S SYNDROME

Joubert's syndrome is characterized by a distinctive pattern of cerebellar and brain stem developmental malformation. Four causative genes (*NPHP1*, *CEP290*, *AHI1*, and *TMEM67* [*MKS3*]) together account for approximately 30% of cases. Clinical features include hypotonia, truncal ataxia, developmental delay, abnormal eye movements, and disordered breathing. The combination of signs and severity can be variable. Some individuals with Joubert's syndrome also have retinal dystrophy, renal disease, ocular colobomas, occipital encephalocele, or hepatic fibrosis. No formal diagnostic criteria exist. The diagnosis is usually based on the combination of hypotonia in infancy with later development of ataxia, intellectual impairment, and abnormal breathing pattern, or abnormal eye movements in combination with a characteristic MRI finding known as the molar tooth sign. The molar tooth sign results from hypoplasia of the cerebellar vermis and accompanying brain stem abnormalities on axial imaging through the junction of the midbrain and pons. Genetic testing is available for the four identified genes. Management is supportive. Caffeine can be helpful for periodic hypoventilation, but some patients require tracheostomy.

DANDY-WALKER MALFORMATION

Dandy-Walker malformation is characterized by cerebellar vermis hypoplasia and cystic dilation of the fourth ventricle. Rare familial cases have been reported, but a genetic basis has not been identified. This heterogeneous disorder is usually accompanied by hypotonia, delayed motor development, and ataxia. Intellectual disability is present in about 50% of affected individuals. In some cases, hydrocephalus requires shunting. Diagnosis is based on characteristic findings on brain MRI. Treatment is supportive, with cerebrospinal fluid (CSF) shunting when indicated.

FIGURE 426-1. Chiari I malformation. A sagittal magnetic resonance image shows low, pointed cerebellar tonsils (i.e., Chiari I malformation, T) that extend to the level of C1 (*black arrow*) and a dilated central canal of the spinal cord (i.e., syringohydromyelia, S). (From Barkovich AJ, Kuzniecky RI. Congenital, Developmental, and Neurocutaneous Disorders. In Goldman L, Ausiello D, eds. *Cecil Textbook of Medicine,* 23rd ed. Philadelphia: Saunders Elsevier; 2008:2790.)

CHIARI MALFORMATIONS

Four types of Chiari malformation have been described. The most common of these are Chiari types I and II. Chiari I malformations are most often diagnosed in adulthood, whereas Chiari II malformations are associated with spina bifida and are usually diagnosed in childhood.

Chiari I malformations are characterized by downward displacement of the cerebellar tonsils through the foramen magnum, often first accompanied by compression of the tonsils. Chiari I is a developmental abnormality that is thought to be congenital in most cases, even though symptoms may not present until adulthood, typically in the third or fourth decade of life. The abnormality is often asymptomatic and discovered only as an incidental finding. However, clinical manifestations can result from compression of neural structures at the cranial-cervical junction or obstruction of CSF flow. Signs and symptoms include headaches that worsen with straining or coughing, lower cranial nerve findings, downbeat nystagmus, ataxia, or long-tract signs. Chiari I malformations are accompanied by syringomyelia (see later) in up to 80% of cases. Diagnosis is made with brain MRI, which shows the cerebellar tonsils extending through the foramen magnum 5 mm or more (Fig. 426-1). Surgical treatment with craniocervical decompression is recommended for symptomatic patients but usually not for asymptomatic individuals or patients whose only symptom is headache.

Chiari II malformations, commonly called Arnold-Chiari malformations, are characterized by descent of the cerebellar tonsils, the inferior vermis, and portions of the cerebellar hemispheres into the spinal canal along with elongation and displacement of the brain stem and fourth ventricle. Chiari II malformations are almost always associated with meningomyelocele and spina bifida. Hydrocephalus requiring shunting occurs in most cases. Brain stem dysfunction may result from intrinsic malformation or from compression of neural structures at the craniocervical junction. Treatment is surgical repair of the myelomeningocele, relief of hydrocephalus, and occasionally, cervical bone decompression. The prognosis depends on the level and extent of the myelomeningocele and on the severity of brain anomalies.

Malformations of Spinal Cord

Tethered Spinal Cord

Tethered spinal cord syndrome is a disorder caused by an anomalous filum terminale that restricts the normal ascent of the conus medullaris and limits the movement of the spinal cord within the spinal column. The result is an abnormal stretching of the spinal cord with neurologic symptoms referable to the lower spinal cord. Tethering may also develop after spinal cord injury. Associated spinal anomalies are common and may include diastematomyelia, spinal lipomas, dermal sinuses, and fibrolipomas of the filum terminale. Symptoms can occur at any age but usually develop during periods of rapid growth in childhood or adolescence. However, tethered spinal cord syndrome may go undiagnosed until adulthood, when sensory and motor problems and loss of bowel and bladder control emerge. Erectile dysfunction may occur in males. Symptoms are typically progressive. Diagnosis is made with MRI, which shows a low conus medullaris (i.e., below the bottom of the L2 vertebral body) or a thickened or fat-containing filum terminale. Diminished pulsations of the spinal cord may also be seen. Treatment consists of surgical release of the tethered cord. With successful surgery, symptoms typically do not progress and may improve.

SYRINGOHYDROMYELIA

Syringohydromyelia is a condition in which the central canal of the spinal cord (hydromyelia) or the substance of the spinal cord (syringomyelia) is expanded by the accumulation of CSF. In many cases, both hydromyelia and syringomyelia are present (syringohydromyelia). The proximate cause of syringes probably is altered flow of CSF with variations in pressure in different parts of the subarachnoid space. The pressure variations create forces that drive CSF into the spinal cord. Possible causes include narrowing of the foramen magnum, Chiari I and II malformations, intramedullary and extramedullary spinal cord tumors, and subarachnoid scarring. Subsequent extension of the cyst may result from rapid changes in intraspinal pressure owing to such events as coughing or sneezing. Symptoms of syringohydromyelia most commonly begin in late adolescence or early adulthood and progress irregularly, with long periods of stability. The classic presentation is asymmetrical weakness and atrophy in the upper extremities, loss of upper limb deep tendon reflexes, and loss of pain and temperature sensation (with preservation of vibration and proprioception) in the neck, arms, and upper part of the trunk. With progression, spasticity and hyperreflexia develop in the lower extremities. Progressive ascending and descending levels of weakness and sensory impairment typically occur over time. The diagnosis is made by spinal MRI (see Fig. 426-1). If syringohydromyelia is identified, it is important to perform a brain MRI to look for associated abnormalities of the craniocervical junction. Occasionally, mild central canal dilation is discovered incidentally in patients without spinal cord symptoms or signs. If no associated cause is found, the prognosis of such incidentally discovered anomalies is generally good. Treatment is directed at the cause, if one can be identified. Syringopleural or syringoperitoneal shunting is sometimes performed with variable benefit.

⬤ DEVELOPMENTAL DISORDERS

Disorders that result from impaired postnatal neurodevelopmental function range from specific disorders such as fragile X syndrome and Rett's syndrome, to complex syndromes such as autism, to nonspecific developmental delay and learning disabilities.

Fragile X Syndrome

Fragile X syndrome is an X-linked trinucleotide repeat disorder that is characterized by nonsyndromic mental retardation in most affected males. The pathogenesis of fragile X syndrome is not well understood. The classic disorder is seen in males with full mutations (>200 repeats) in the *FMR1* gene. Fragile X syndrome may present as only moderate to severe mental retardation, but it is often associated with a prominent forehead, large ears, prominent jaw, and macro-orchidism. Postpubertal males often have poor impulse control, perseveration, and poor eye contact. Up to 25% of affected males have autism. Heterozygous females may be asymptomatic or may have a syndrome similar to what is seen in males, depending on repeat size and random X-inactivation.

Other disorders associated with *FMR1* include the fragile X ataxia syndrome, which is characterized by the late onset, usually after age 50 years, of progressive cerebellar ataxia and intention tremor in individuals who have an *FMR1* premutation (60 to 200 repeats). It occurs equally in males and females. Diagnosis is by molecular genetic testing. Cytogenetic testing for fragile sites is no longer recommended because it is less sensitive and more expensive than molecular testing. Treatment is symptomatic and supportive. Genetic counseling is recommended for affected individuals and their families.

Rett's Syndrome

Rett's syndrome is a neurodevelopmental disorder that occurs in females with mutations in the *MECP2* gene. *MECP2* mutations are generally lethal in male embryos, but Rett's syndrome has been reported in males with XXY karyotype or with somatic mosaicism. *MECP2* is thought to mediate transcriptional silencing of methylated DNA. Most mutations are probably de novo or may reflect germline mosaicism; 99% of cases represent a single occurrence within a family. Affected girls are usually normal at birth and have apparently normal development for the first 6 to 18 months of life. Brain growth decelerates, and development stagnates, followed by rapid regression of language and motor skills. A classic feature of Rett's syndrome is the loss of purposeful hand use and the development of repetitive stereotyped hand movements that usually have the appearance of wringing or clapping. Other features present to variable degree are bruxism, episodic apnea and hyperpnea, seizures, gait disorders, and tremor. Non-neurologic features include growth failure and wasting, bowel dysmotility, scoliosis, osteopenia, and vasomotor changes in the limbs. Diagnosis is by molecular genetic methods. Treatment is symptomatic.

Autism

Autism is a neurodevelopmental syndrome characterized by impaired communication, impaired social interaction, and restricted interests or repetitive behaviors. Fragile X syndrome and tuberous sclerosis are two important entities in which an autistic phenotype can occur and in which autism may be the most prominent feature. Symptoms typically present before 3 years of age and persist into adulthood. Autism is a spectrum ranging from severe, with impairment in all domains, to mild with normal intellect and language but with impaired social interactions and repetitive behaviors or restricted interests. Autism has many causes but in most cases is idiopathic. Epilepsy is common in autism. Diagnosis is based on careful diagnostic interview and examination. When epilepsy is present, treatment with antiepileptic medications is indicated. Behavioral therapy can help individuals learn rules for social interaction and can improve communication. It can also help with problematic behavior. Educational support is important. Medications such as atypical antipsychotics, selective serotonin reuptake inhibitors, and anxiolytics (Chapter 404) can help with aggressive behavior, repetitive behaviors, and anxiety.

⬤ NEUROCUTANEOUS DISORDERS

Neurocutaneous disorders are congenital syndromes characterized by dysplastic and neoplastic lesions primarily involving the nervous system and skin. The more than 40 described syndromes include neurofibromatosis, tuberous sclerosis, Sturge-Weber syndrome, and von Hippel-Lindau disease.

Neurofibromatosis

Neurofibromatosis encompasses a spectrum of syndromes with distinctive neural and cutaneous lesions. The two major forms of neurofibromatosis are genetically and clinically distinct.

NEUROFIBROMATOSIS TYPE 1

Neurofibromatosis type 1, which is the classic disorder described by von Recklinghausen, is an autosomal dominant condition with an incidence of 1 per 2500 to 3000 births. Although it is an autosomal dominant disease, approximately 50% of cases are due to new mutations. Most mutations in *NF1* occur in the parental germline. The *NF1* gene, which is located on chromosome 17q11.2, codes a protein called neurofibromin, which is thought to function as a tumor suppressor by acting as a negative regulator of the Ras signaling pathway. Neurofibromatosis type 1 is characterized by multiple cafe au lait spots, axillary and inguinal freckling, multiple discrete cutaneous neurofibromas (Fig. 426-2), and Lisch nodules (Table 426-1). Subcutaneous neurofibromas may be painful or disfiguring. Learning disabilities are present in at least 50% of individuals. Other manifestations include plexiform neurofibromas, optic nerve and other central nervous system (CNS) gliomas, malignant peripheral nerve sheath tumors, tibial dysplasia, and vasculopathy.

Management of patients depends on the specific manifestations and often requires multidisciplinary collaboration. Most patients with neurofibromatosis type 1 do not require treatment, but all require surveillance (Table 426-2). Subcutaneous, intraspinal, and intracranial tumors can be treated surgically. Optic nerve gliomas may be treated with chemotherapy; both cisplatin and temozolomide have shown some benefit. Radiation is not recommended. Genetic counseling should be provided to all patients and their families.

NEUROFIBROMATOSIS TYPE 2

Neurofibromatosis type 2, which is often referred to as central neurofibromatosis, is an autosomal dominant condition with an incidence of approximately 1 in 25,000 individuals. The *NF2* gene is located on chromosome 22q12.2. Its gene product, merlin, is cytoskeletal protein that is thought to act as a

FIGURE 426-2. Multiple neurofibromas covering the back of a patient with neurofibromatosis type 1.

TABLE 426-1	DIAGNOSTIC CRITERIA FOR NEUROFIBROMATOSIS TYPE 1

Two or more of the following clinical features signify the presence of neurofibromatosis type 1:

- Six or more cafe au lait macules (>0.5 cm at largest diameter in prepubertal individuals or >1.5 cm in individuals past puberty)
- Axillary freckling or freckling in inguinal regions
- Two or more neurofibromas of any type or ≥1 plexiform neurofibroma
- Two or more Lisch nodules (iris hamartomas)
- A distinctive osseous lesion
- A first-degree relative with neurofibromatosis type 1 diagnosed by using the above-listed criteria

TABLE 426-2	RECOMMENDED SURVEILLANCE IN PATIENTS WITH NEUROFIBROMATOSIS TYPE 1

Annual physical examination by a physician who is familiar with the individual and with the disease

Annual ophthalmologic examination in early childhood, less frequent examination in older children and adults

Regular developmental assessment by screening questionnaire (in childhood)

Regular blood pressure monitoring

Other studies only as indicated on the basis of clinically apparent signs or symptoms

Monitoring of those who have abnormalities of the central nervous system, skeletal system, or cardiovascular system by an appropriate specialist

membrane-stabilizing protein. The specific function of merlin is unknown. Neurofibromatosis type 2 is characterized by bilateral vestibular schwannomas, which usually present with symptoms of tinnitus, hearing loss, and imbalance. The age at onset is usually in young adulthood, but some individuals may develop posterior subcapsular lens opacities or mono-neuropathy in childhood. Almost all affected individuals develop bilateral vestibular schwannomas by age 30 years (Table 426-3). Affected individuals may also develop schwannomas of other cranial and peripheral nerves, meningiomas, and, rarely, ependymomas or astrocytomas. Posterior subcapsular lens opacities are the most common ocular abnormality.

Management is dependent on the specific manifestations and complications. In individuals who either have tested positive for known *NF2* mutations or have a family history of neurofibromatosis type 2 and whose genetic status cannot be determined with genetic testing, annual brain MRI is recommended starting between ages 10 and 12 years and continuing until at least age 40 years. Hearing evaluations may be useful in detecting changes in auditory nerve function before changes can be visualized by MRI. Routine complete eye examinations should be part of the care of all individuals.

Bevacizumab, a vascular endothelial growth factor inhibitor (5 mg/kg intravenously every 2 weeks), can improve hearing in some patients with neurofibromatosis type 2 and vestibular schwannomas.◼ Surgical treatment of schwannomas and meningiomas may be indicated to preserve function or to relieve compression of adjacent structures, especially in patients with intramedullary spinal tumors. Genetic counseling should be provided to affected individuals and their families.

TABLE 426-3	DIAGNOSTIC CRITERIA FOR NEUROFIBROMATOSIS TYPE 2

Presence of one or more of the following makes the diagnosis of neurofibromatosis type 2:

- Bilateral vestibular schwannomas
- A first-degree relative with neurofibromatosis type 2, *and*
    Unilateral vestibular schwannoma, *or*
    Any two of: meningioma, schwannoma, glioma, neurofibroma, posterior subcapsular lenticular opacities*
- Unilateral vestibular schwannoma, *and*
    Any two of: meningioma, schwannoma, glioma, neurofibroma, posterior subcapsular lenticular opacities*
- Multiple meningiomas, *and*
    Unilateral vestibular schwannoma, *or*
    Any two of: schwannoma, glioma, neurofibroma, cataract*

*"Any two of" refers to two individual tumors or cataracts.

TABLE 426-4	DIAGNOSTIC CRITERIA FOR TUBEROUS SCLEROSIS COMPLEX

Definite—Two major features or one major feature plus two minor features
Probable—One major feature plus one minor feature
Possible—One major feature or two or more minor features

Major features
    Facial angiofibromas or forehead plaque
    Nontraumatic ungual or periungual fibromas
    More than three hypomelanotic macules (ash leaf spots)
    Shagreen patch (connective tissue nevus)
    Multiple retinal nodular hamartomas
    Cortical tuber
    Subependymal nodule
    Subependymal giant cell astrocytoma
    Cardiac rhabdomyoma, single or multiple
    Lymphangiomyomatosis
    Renal angiomyolipoma
Minor features
    Multiple dental enamel pits
    Hamartomatous rectal polyps
    Bone cysts
    Cerebral white matter radial migration lines
    Gingival fibromas
    Nonrenal hamartoma
    Retinal achromic patch
    "Confetti" skin lesions
    Multiple renal cysts

FIGURE 426-3. Subependymal nodules and multiple cortical tubers in a patient with tuberous sclerosis.

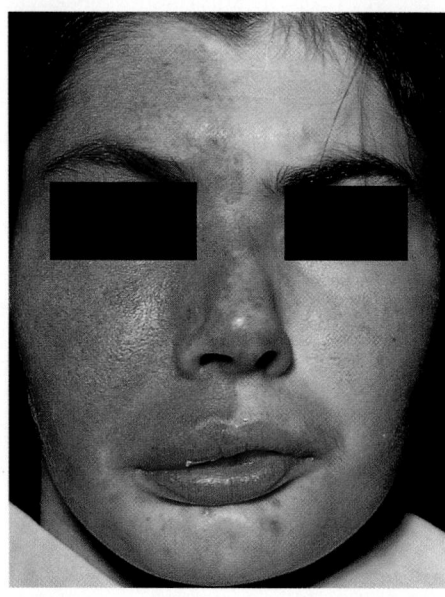

FIGURE 426-4. Sturge-Weber syndrome. This patient has a classic diffuse capillary hemangioma in the distribution of the ophthalmic, nasociliary, and maxillary branches of the trigeminal nerve. The lesion extends backward over the anterior two thirds of the crown of the head. (From Forbes CD, Jackson WD. *Color Atlas and Text of Clinical Medicine*, 2nd ed. London: Mosby; 1996.)

Tuberous Sclerosis

Tuberous sclerosis complex is characterized by abnormalities of the brain, kidney, and heart. Tuberous sclerosis may occur as an autosomal dominant syndrome or result from spontaneous mutation. Two tuberous sclerosis genes have been identified. *TSC1* (chromosome 9q34) codes for a protein called hamartin, a protein that interacts with the product of the *TSC2* gene to inhibit the mammalian target of rapamycin (mTOR). *TSC2* (chromosome 16p13) codes for tuberin, which interacts with hamartin. *TSC2* mutations account for about 60% of individuals with clinical tuberous sclerosis.

The specific findings vary across individuals, and severity ranges from minimal to severe. Skin lesions are seen in almost 100% of affected individuals, but CNS lesions are the leading cause of morbidity and mortality. Epilepsy is seen in as many as 80% of patients with CNS lesions. Intellectual impairment and developmental delay are common, and up to 40% of patients have an autism spectrum disorder. Giant cell astrocytoma is the leading cause of death. Up to 80% of children with tuberous sclerosis have an identifiable renal lesion (Chapter 203) by 10.5 years of age, and renal disease is the second leading cause of early death in individuals with tuberous sclerosis. Cardiac rhabdomyomas, which can occur in up to 50% of patients, are usually present at birth and typically regress over time. Diagnosis of tuberous sclerosis (Table 426-4) is usually clinical and confirmed by identification of calcified or uncalcified hamartomas on imaging studies (Fig. 426-3).

Treatment is directed at complications of the disease, particularly epilepsy (Chapter 410). Neurosurgical intervention may sometimes be indicated for epilepsy and for symptomatic treatment of complications, such as hydrocephalus, which results from midline giant cell tumors. In a small, nonrandomized study, treatment with sirolimus (dosed to achieve blood levels of 1 to 5 ng/mL) for 1 year reduced the size of the angiomyolipomas during the year of treatment. Rapamycin has shown promise in early investigations for treatment of giant cell astrocytomas. Serial brain MRI and renal ultrasound screening may be indicated in some patients because benign tumors of these organs may enlarge rapidly. Genetic counseling is an important part of management.

Sturge-Weber Syndrome

Sturge-Weber syndrome is a sporadic disorder characterized by facial vascular nevi, epilepsy, cognitive impairment, and sometimes hemiparesis, hemianopsia, or glaucoma. The characteristic CNS feature of this disorder is capillary angiomatosis of the pia mater. Cerebral cortical calcifications are generally seen in a pericapillary distribution and are progressive. Most patients with Sturge-Weber syndrome have epilepsy. The diagnosis is usually based on the presence of a facial nevus (Fig. 426-4), which is manifested as a typical portwine stain, and confirmatory imaging on a contrast brain MRI showing leptomeningeal enhancement.

Regular ophthalmologic examination is warranted because of the risk for glaucoma. Treatment is usually aimed at the epilepsy, which can be medically intractable. In patients with intractable epilepsy and infantile-onset hemiplegia, hemispherectomy can improve the seizures and the neurodevelopmental outcome.

Von Hippel-Lindau Disease

Von Hippel-Lindau disease (i.e., CNS angiomatosis) is an autosomal dominant disorder caused by a defective tumor suppressor gene at chromosome 3p25-p26. It is characterized by retinal angiomas, brain (usually cerebellar) and spinal cord hemangioblastomas, renal cell carcinomas, endolymphatic sac tumors, pheochromocytomas, papillary cystadenomas of the epididymis, angiomas of the liver and kidney, and cysts of the pancreas, kidney, liver, and epididymis. Both sexes are affected equally.

Symptoms typically begin during the third or fourth decade. Retinal inflammation with exudate, hemorrhage, and retinal detachment from the retinal angiomas typically precedes the cerebellar complaints, but the order is not constant. The ocular findings are nonspecific, and the retinal detachment may mask the underlying lesion. Headache, vertigo, and vomiting result from cerebellar tumors. Cerebellar signs such as ataxia, dysdiadochokinesis, and dysmetria are common. Rare patients present with symptoms of spinal cord or visceral lesions, or may have hearing loss from tumors of the endolymphatic sac.

Clinical diagnosis is established if the patient has more than one CNS hemangioblastoma, one hemangioblastoma with a visceral manifestation of the disease, or one manifestation of the disease and a known family history. Molecular genetic testing detects mutations in the *VHL* gene in nearly 100% of affected individuals.

For patients with von Hippel-Lindau disease and for those with a disease-causing VHL mutation, surveillance is recommended with annual ophthalmologic examination, annual blood pressure monitoring, measurement of urinary catecholamine metabolites beginning at age 5 years in families with pheochromocytoma, and annual abdominal ultrasound examination beginning at age 16 years with evaluation of suspicious lesions by computed tomography or MRI. Treatment is symptomatic. Retinal detachments and tumors are treated by laser therapy. Large brain tumors (Chapter 195), renal cell carcinomas (Chapter 203), pheochromocytomas (Chapter 235), epididymal tumors (Chapter 206), and endolymphatic sac tumors are treated surgically; smaller CNS tumors may be treated by gamma knife.

1. Plotkin SR, Stemmer-Rachamimov AO, Barker FG 2nd, et al. Hearing improvement after bevacizumab in patients with neurofibromatosis type 2. *N Engl J Med.* 2009;361:358-367.

SUGGESTED READINGS

Evans GR, Lloyd SK, Ramsden RT. Neurofibromatosis type 2. *Adv Otorhinolaryngol.* 2011;70:91-98. *Review emphasizing the role of surgery.*

Ferner RE. The neurofibromatoses. *Pract Neurol.* 2010;10:82-93. *Review.*

Krueger DA, Care MM, Holland K, et al. Everolimus for subependymal giant-call astrocytomas in tuberous sclerosis. *N Eng J Med.* 2010;363:1801-1811. *In a nonrandomized study, oral everolimus decreased the volume of subependymal giant-cell astrocytomas and the frequency of seizures in patients with tuberous sclerosis.*

Nordstrom-O'Brien M, van der Luijt RB, van Rooijen E, et al. Genetic analysis of von Hippel-Lindau disease. *Hum Mutat.* 2010;31:521-537. *Review of mutations and their clinical manifestations.*

427

AUTONOMIC DISORDERS AND THEIR MANAGEMENT

WILLIAM P. CHESHIRE, JR.

The peripheral autonomic nervous system and the central integration of autonomic reflexes maintain homeostasis and modulate the complex physiologic responses at the interface between the internal milieu and the external world. Autonomic activity, which generally occurs below the level of conscious control, regulates cardiovascular, thermal, metabolic, gastrointestinal, urinary, and reproductive functions and coordinates the adaptive response to stress.

Many diseases can involve the autonomic nervous system, which in turn can involve all organ systems. Examples include brain lesions that affect any part of the central autonomic network, disorders that damage peripheral nerve function, and systemic illnesses that impair autonomic responses.

EPIDEMIOLOGY

The most frequently disabling manifestation of autonomic failure is orthostatic hypotension, which increases in prevalence with aging and is associated with a two-fold increased risk for falls, fractures, syncope, transient ischemic attacks, and decreased functional capacity in elderly individuals. The prevalence of orthostatic hypotension is 5 to 20% among all elderly persons, but it rises to 30% in persons older than 75 years and to greater than 50% in frail individuals who live in nursing homes. Neurally mediated syncope (vasodepressor, vasovagal), as well as various situational syncopes that occur in response to emotional distress, micturition, defecation, coughing, carotid sinus stimulation, and other factors, accounts for 1 to 3% of all emergency room visits. The lifetime prevalence of syncope is about 20%. Another common autonomic syndrome is postprandial hypotension, which occurs in 20 to 60% of elderly individuals and increases the risk for mortality by 80%.

Diabetes mellitus (Chapter 236) is the most common cause of autonomic neuropathy in the developed world. Within 10 to 15 years of the onset of diabetes, laboratory evidence of autonomic neuropathy can be detected in about 30% of patients, and symptomatic autonomic failure with orthostatic hypotension can be detected in about 5% of patients. Other autonomic symptoms in diabetics include constipation in 40 to 60% of patients, gastroparesis in 20 to 40%, bladder dysfunction in 30 to 80%, erectile impotence in more than 30% of males, and occasionally, intermittent diarrhea.

Hyperhidrosis involving the palms and soles represents the most common form of essential hyperhidrosis and affects about 1% of the population. Although excessive sweating is usually symptomatic, anhidrosis may go unnoticed unless it interferes with the thermoregulatory response to heat stress. Impaired thermoregulation can cause increased mortality rates during heat waves or in times of heat stress (Chapter 109).

PATHOBIOLOGY

The peripheral autonomic nervous system comprises three main divisions: (1) *sympathetic*, or outflow from the thoracolumbar segments of the spinal cord; (2) *parasympathetic*, or outflow from cranial nerves III, VII, IX, and X and from the sacral spinal segments; and (3) *enteric*, or the ganglionated plexuses intrinsic to the wall of the gut. Disorders of the autonomic nervous system may occur suddenly or evolve gradually. They may affect specific or multiple autonomic pathways depending on their pathogenesis and localization. Orthostatic hypotension, a hallmark of autonomic disorders, results from sympathetic vasomotor denervation, which renders a standing patient unable to constrict the splanchnic and other peripheral vascular beds in response to the pooling of blood volume (500 to 1000 mL) secondary to gravity.

Physiologic effects of sympathetic activation include pupillary dilation, increased heart rate and contractility, increased peripheral vascular resistance, bronchodilation, increased glandular secretions, decreased gastrointestinal motility, increased sweating, decreased function of reproductive organs, and mobilization of energy substrates. The effects of parasympathetic activation include pupillary constriction, lacrimal and salivary secretion, decreased heart rate and contractility, bronchoconstriction, increased gastrointestinal motility, and contraction of the detrusor muscle of the bladder. Sympathetic and parasympathetic responses, though generally antagonistic, are not always equally counterbalanced.

Sympathetic preganglionic neurons, which use acetylcholine as their primary neurotransmitter, originate in the segmentally organized intermediolateral column of the spinal cord and exit via the ventral roots to pass through the white rami communicans and reach the paravertebral sympathetic chain ganglia, which innervate all organs and tissues except those of the abdomen and pelvis. The superior cervical ganglion, for example, innervates cranial structures, and the stellate ganglion innervates the upper limb. Sympathetic preganglionic axons also form the splanchnic nerves, which innervate the celiac, superior mesenteric, and hypogastric ganglia, as well as the adrenal medulla. With the exception of neurons that innervate the sweat glands, which are cholinergic, all other sympathetic postganglionic neurons are adrenergic and use norepinephrine as their primary transmitter.

Preganglionic innervation of parasympathetic neurons is also cholinergic; however, in contrast to their sympathetic counterparts, the major postganglionic parasympathetic neurotransmitter is acetylcholine. Parasympathetic preganglionic fibers originate in the Edinger-Westphal, salivatory, and vagal dorsal motor nuclei in the brain stem. The ciliary, sphenopalatine, otic, submandibular, sublingual, and pelvic ganglia send postganglionic parasympathetic fibers to their target organs. Cranial nerves IX and X, which constitute the afferent limbs of the baroreceptor reflex, relay beat-to-beat information about systemic arterial pressure to the nucleus of the solitary tract.

The gastrointestinal tract contains neural plexuses, the most prominent of which are the myenteric (Auerbach) plexus found between the two layers of the muscularis externa and the submucosal (Meissner) plexus. Disorders of the enteric nervous system mainly affect gastrointestinal motility or sphincter control rather than absorptive or secretory functions.

● BRAIN DISORDERS

Important disease targets involved in central autonomic regulation include the interrelated neuronal cell groups of the hypothalamus, as well as the ventrolateral medulla, nucleus of the solitary tract, parabrachial nucleus, periaqueductal gray matter, amygdala, and insular and prefrontal cortices. Together, these relay systems and integrative centers compose the central autonomic network, which when impaired, fails to activate or modulate sympathetic and parasympathetic tone and neurohumoral responses.

A number of neurodegenerative disorders disrupt the central pathways of autonomic regulation. The most severe form is multiple system atrophy, a sporadic, adult-onset disease in which severe autonomic failure accompanies and occasionally precedes parkinsonism (Shy-Drager syndrome; Chapter 416) or cerebellar ataxia (Chapter 417). In multiple system atrophy, there is degeneration of the striatum, pigmented nuclei, pontine nuclei, inferior olives, cerebellar Purkinje cells, and dorsal vagal and vestibular nuclei. Autonomic dysfunction also occurs in dementia with Lewy bodies (Chapter 409) and, to a lesser degree, in Parkinson's disease, both of which also involve abnormal neuronal accumulation of α-synuclein.

Essential to the integration of behavioral, autonomic, and neuroendocrine responses is the tightly packed, interwoven group of cells that constitute the hypothalamus. Lesions of the anterior hypothalamus may alter thirst perception and sodium regulation. Dysfunction of the magnocellular arginine vasopressin neurons of the supraoptic and supraventricular nuclei can be manifested as decreased secretion of antidiuretic hormone, thereby resulting in diabetes insipidus (Chapter 232) with hypovolemia, or as inappropriately increased secretion of antidiuretic hormone, thereby resulting in hyponatremia. Medial preoptic–anterior hypothalamic dysfunction associated with dysgenesis of the corpus callosum (Shapiro's syndrome) is characterized by episodic hyperhidrosis and hypothermia. Lesions of the posterior hypothalamus can result from hypothermia, Wernicke-Korsakoff syndrome (Chapter 425), acute traumatic brain injury (Chapter 406), multiple sclerosis (Chapter 419), mesodiencephalic hematoma, and toluene toxicity.

Catastrophic neurologic conditions such as subarachnoid hemorrhage, head trauma, status epilepticus, and acute hydrocephalus with increased intracranial pressure can profoundly stimulate sympathetic responses with cardiovascular consequence. Release of the hypothalamus as a result of cortical inhibition is the presumed mechanism. These paroxysmal sympathetic storms (diencephalic syndrome) are characterized by episodic sympathetic hyperactivity with hypertension, tachycardia, hyperventilation, pupillary dilation, flushing, and diaphoresis. Communicating hydrocephalus, structural lesions affecting the medial frontal cortex, and degenerative conditions affecting the frontobasal ganglia can cause urinary incontinence with uninhibited bladder contractions.

Autonomic responses are closely linked to emotional states. Portions of the insular and anterior cingulate cortices mediate the autonomic responses to emotional stress. Because cardioregulatory function is represented within the insular cortex, insular strokes have been associated with destabilization of sympathoregulatory balance and occasional adverse cardiac events. Correlations of electroencephalography and electrocardiography have shown that seizures arising from the mesial temporal lobe may induce ictal tachycardia or, more rarely, bradycardia or asystole.

Lesions of the brain stem may also be manifested as autonomic dysfunction. Damage to the medulla oblongata may give rise to hypertension, orthostatic hypotension, or syncope. Medullary ischemia or compression can cause acute neurogenic hypertension (Cushing's response). Lateral medullary infarction (Wallenberg's syndrome) typically produces ipsilateral Horner's syndrome and occasionally more extensive dysautonomia,

TABLE 427-1	SOME CAUSES OF PERIPHERAL AUTONOMIC NEUROPATHY
Metabolic	Diabetes mellitus
	Alcohol
	Acute intermittent porphyria
	Uremia
Autoimmune	Autoimmune autonomic ganglionopathy
	Guillain-Barré syndrome
	Morvan's syndrome
	Lambert-Eaton myasthenic syndrome
	Chronic inflammatory demyelinating polyradiculoneuropathy
	Sjögren's syndrome
	Systemic lupus erythematosus
	Mixed connective tissue diseases
Paraproteinemic	Amyloidosis
Nutritional	Cyanocobalamin deficiency
	Thiamine deficiency
	Gluten-sensitive neuropathy
Toxic	Heavy metals
	Organic solvents
	Organophosphates
	Vacor
	Acrylamide
Drug induced	Cisplatin
	Vincristine
	Amiodarone
	Metronidazole
	Perhexiline
	Paclitaxel
Infectious	Human immunodeficiency virus
	Leprosy
	Chagas' disease
	Botulism
	Diphtheria
	Lyme disease
Genetic	Hereditary sensory and autonomic neuropathies
	Types I and II
	Type III (familial dysautonomia)
	Type IV (congenital insensitivity to pain)
	Type V
	Fabry's disease
Idiopathic	Adie's syndrome
	Ross' syndrome
	Acute cholinergic neuropathy
	Chronic idiopathic anhidrosis
	Amyotrophic lateral sclerosis

including bradycardia, acute hypertension, supine hypotension, or central hypoventilation.

● SPINAL CORD DISORDERS

Lesions of the spinal cord, whether compressive, demyelinating, vascular, or neoplastic, commonly result in an overactive bladder (Chapter 25) with symptoms of frequency, urgency, and sometimes incontinence. Lesions that involve the sacral cord segments or cauda equina result in an underactive bladder with incomplete emptying, overflow incontinence, sphincter atonia, and sexual dysfunction.

After spinal cord injuries above the level of T5, sprouting of afferent fibers in the thoracolumbar dorsal horns and necrosis of the descending white matter connections to sympathetic preganglionic neurons result in autonomic dysreflexia. In these patients, peripheral sensory stimuli such as bladder distention can induce a reversible state of sympathetic hyperresponsiveness, including hypertension, diaphoresis, flushing, and headache.

● PERIPHERAL GANGLIONOPATHIES AND NEUROPATHIES

Autonomic dysfunction can arise at the level of the autonomic ganglia or peripheral nerves (Table 427-1). Peripheral autonomic nerves are generally small in caliber and unmyelinated or thinly myelinated. Peripheral neuropathies selectively involve small nerve fibers and cause various combinations of sensory, sympathetic, or parasympathetic signs and symptoms.

TABLE 427-2 AUTOIMMUNE AUTONOMIC NEUROPATHIES

CLINICAL SYNDROME	ASSOCIATED AUTOANTIBODY
Autoimmune autonomic ganglionopathy	Anti-GAChR
Guillain-Barré syndrome	Anti-GM$_1$, anti-GM$_3$
Paraneoplastic autonomic neuropathy	ANNA-1 (anti-Hu), PCA-2, CRMP-5
Lambert-Eaton myasthenic syndrome	Anti-VGCC
Morvan's syndrome	Anti-VGKC
Sjögren's syndrome	SSA (anti-Ro), SSB (anti-La)

ANNA-1 = antineuronal nuclear antibody; anti-GAChR = nicotinic ganglionic acetylcholine receptor antibody; anti-GM$_1$, anti-GM$_3$ = antiganglioside antibody; anti-VGCC = P/Q-type voltage-gated calcium-channel antibody; anti-VGKC = voltage-gated potassium-channel antibody; CRMP-5 = collapsin response mediator protein 5; PCA-2 = Purkinje cell cytoplasmic antibody type 2.

Among the peripheral dysautonomias is the syndrome of pure autonomic failure, which is defined as the insidious onset of severe, generalized autonomic failure as the sole clinical feature in the absence of any signs of extrapyramidal, cerebellar, or sensory or motor peripheral nerve dysfunction. Pathologic studies have found Lewy body accumulation in autonomic ganglia, peripheral autonomic nerves, the substantia nigra, and the locus ceruleus.

Diabetic neuropathy involves autonomic nerves early in its course but advances to clinically apparent autonomic neuropathy only in about 14% of patients. The incidence increases with the duration of diabetes and advancing age. In diabetic patients, microvascular ischemia causes progressive peripheral nerve damage, although an autoimmune mechanism may also play a role in a subset of patients. Some patients with otherwise unexplained distal small fiber autonomic neuropathy have impaired fasting glucose. Whether this association reflects an early stage of diabetic neuropathy or a chance association, given the prevalence of glucose intolerance, remains to be determined.

Other syndromes of neurologic autoimmunity (Table 427-2) include Guillain-Barré syndrome, in which antiganglioside antibodies mediate an acute inflammatory demyelinating polyradiculoneuropathy that may be associated with tachycardia, blood pressure lability, and pupillomotor, sudomotor, and vasomotor disturbances (Chapter 428). The syndrome of acute pandysautonomia is typically manifested dramatically over a period of days to weeks as combined sympathetic and parasympathetic failure with gastrointestinal dysmotility and, in contrast to Guillain-Barré syndrome, sparing of the somatic nerves. An antecedent, presumably viral infection is reported in about 50% of cases. The finding of antibodies against the nicotinic acetylcholine receptor in the autonomic ganglia in many of these patients has led to the clinical designation autoimmune autonomic ganglionopathy. Ganglionic acetylcholine receptor antibodies occur in some patients with lung cancer or thymoma. Low levels of these antibodies have also been found in a subset of patients with isolated gastrointestinal dysmotility.

Autoimmune neuromyotonia is characterized by peripheral nerve hyperexcitability, insomnia, fluctuating delirium, and prominent dysautonomia with hyperhidrosis and orthostatic intolerance. Most patients have antibodies to voltage-gated potassium channels.

Paraneoplastic autonomic neuropathies (Chapter 187), which can predate the diagnosis of malignancy, are a rare epiphenomenon of malignancy, most frequently small cell lung carcinoma (Chapter 197), and can also occur in association with ovarian carcinoma (Chapter 205), breast carcinoma (Chapter 204), thymoma, lymphoma (Chapter 191), and other cancers. The most commonly encountered paraneoplastic antibody is antineuronal nuclear antibody type 1 (ANNA-1 or anti-Hu), which binds to a 35- to 40-kD family of neuronal nuclear RNA-binding proteins, including those in autonomic and enteric ganglia. Antibodies against collapsing response mediator proteins (CRMP-5 or anti-CV2) have also been associated with paraneoplastic autonomic neuropathy. Dysautonomia occurs in approximately 10 to 30% of patients with ANNA-1 and in 30% of patients with CRMP-5 seropositivity. Small cell lung cancer (Chapter 197) has been found in more than 80% of patients seropositive for ANNA-1 or CRMP-5.

Hereditary sensory and autonomic neuropathy (HSAN) type I, which is due to a mutation of the gene for serine palmitoyltransferase long-chain base subunit 1, is inherited in an autosomal dominant pattern and is characterized by distal anhidrosis with loss of nociceptive and thermal perception. Mutations in *HSN2* have been linked to HSAN type II, an autosomal

recessive neuropathy that causes distal anhidrosis and sensory loss. Sural nerve biopsy specimens disclose virtual absence of myelinated fibers and decreased numbers of unmyelinated fibers. Autonomic involvement is most prominent in HSAN type III, commonly known as familial dysautonomia, or Riley-Day syndrome. This autosomal recessive disorder, which affects 1 in 3600 live births in parents of Ashkenazi Jewish descent, has been linked to mutations in the I-κB kinase–associated protein gene (*IKBKAP*). Pathologic studies disclose severely depleted sympathetic preganglionic and postganglionic neuronal populations with preservation of parasympathetic neurons. Affected children cry without tears, feed poorly, lack fungiform papillae, have depressed patellar reflexes, and are subject to orthostatic hypotension and autonomic storms.

HSAN type IV, or congenital insensitivity to pain with anhidrosis, is an autosomal recessive disorder that is associated with mental retardation and repeated episodes of fever. HSAN type IV results from mutations in the gene for neurotrophic tyrosine kinase receptor type 1 (*NTRK1*), which is important for inducing neurite outgrowth in embryonic sensory and sympathetic neurons. Peripheral nerve biopsy discloses virtual absence of unmyelinated fibers.

HSAN type V is an autosomal recessive disorder characterized by loss of pain sensation and sudomotor abnormalities.

The age-related decline in baroreflex sensitivity, adrenergic responses to sympathetic activation, parasympathetic control of heart rate, esophageal and gastrointestinal motility, and efficient thermoregulation predisposes the elderly to orthostatic, postprandial, and drug-induced hypotension. Pheochromocytomas (Chapter 235) and carcinoid syndrome (Chapter 240) can also be accompanied by autonomic symptoms, including blood pressure lability.

CLINICAL MANIFESTATIONS

Several common patterns of autonomic dysfunction may be distinguished.

Generalized Autonomic Failure

Early symptoms of adrenergic failure typically include lightheadedness on arising in the morning or following a warm shower, physical exercise, or a large meal. Other common symptoms include male erectile dysfunction, decreased sweating, dry mouth, constipation, and bladder dysfunction. Severe orthostatic hypotension without pulse acceleration, which is the hallmark of severe generalized autonomic failure, may be accompanied by supine and nocturnal hypertension, thus reversing the normal diurnal decrease in blood pressure during sleep.

Acute Autonomic Syndromes

Acute or subacute manifestations of autonomic dysfunction may result from rapidly developing disease or from decompensation of chronic autonomic disease. An abrupt onset of new focal autonomic signs, particularly when accompanied by headache or motor or sensory deficits, should prompt a detailed neurologic assessment for an acute cerebral or spinal syndrome, which may be caused by vascular, traumatic, inflammatory, neoplastic, or infectious diseases.

Chronic Autonomic Syndromes

The clinical spectrum of chronic autonomic neuropathies includes distal small fiber neuropathies with a stocking-and-glove distribution of anhidrosis, often combined with loss of pain and temperature sensibility. Other patients may have orthostatic hypotension and impaired exercise tolerance, with either an increased resting heart rate because of a parasympathetic cardiovagal neuropathy or a fixed heart rate that does not increase adequately in response to physiologic demands as a result of the involvement of sympathetic fibers. Some patients with distal sudomotor neuropathy will complain of spontaneous or gustatory proximal hyperhidrosis with episodic sweating involving the face, head, and upper part of the trunk.

Gastroparesis, which is a common feature of autonomic neuropathies, is characterized by delayed gastric emptying, which may be manifested as early satiety, nausea, anorexia, bloating, and sometimes pain and weight loss. Intestinal dysmotility may cause severe constipation (Chapter 138). In advanced peripheral neuropathies, in ganglionopathies in which involvement is not length dependent, and in central degenerative disorders, the loss of sweating may extend to proximal body regions or globally. Widespread anhidrosis may result in impaired thermoregulatory sweating and the potential for hyperthermia in conditions of heat stress (Chapter 109).

Paroxysmal Dysautonomias

Paroxysmal and episodic autonomic symptoms include postprandial hypotension, which is a reduction in systolic blood pressure of at least 20 mm Hg within 2 hours of the start of a meal, typically one high in carbohydrate content. Postprandial hypotension may occur in elderly individuals with or without orthostatic hypotension.

Dysfunction of the afferent limb of the baroreflex system leads to volatile blood pressure in patients with acute inflammatory demyelinating polyneuropathy and syndromes of baroreflex failure. Additional causes of aberrant activation of autonomic reflexes include epilepsy, diencephalic syndrome, subarachnoid hemorrhage, acute head trauma, pheochromocytoma, intoxication, drug withdrawal, neurally mediated syncope, and panic disorder.

Selective Autonomic Syndromes

Regional autonomic disorders are characterized by focal or system-selective autonomic dysfunction. An example is harlequin syndrome, in which heat stress, exercise, or sudden emotion in a patient with hemifacial cutaneous sympathetic denervation evokes a dramatic facial division in which the denervated half remains pale and dry and the intact half flushes red. Oculosympathetic paresis or Horner's syndrome may also be present. Harlequin syndrome may occur in patients with Holmes-Adie syndrome, which consists of tonic pupils with asymmetrical or absent tendon reflexes, and has been described in patients with Ross' syndrome, a partial dysautonomia consisting of the clinical triad of unilateral or bilateral tonic pupils, tendon hyporeflexia, and segmental body anhidrosis.

Other Specific Syndromes

Baroreflex failure is commonly the result of damage to the carotid sinus baroreceptors or the glossopharyngeal nerves. Similarly, interruption of vagal input from the aortic arch baroreceptors to the nucleus of the solitary tract can impair baroreflex responses. Baroreflex failure also occurs in patients who have undergone surgery or irradiation of the neck. These patients will exhibit severe and labile hypertension with concomitant tachycardia, palpitations, headache, diaphoresis, and emotional lability.

Serotonin syndrome develops within hours or days of the addition of a new serotonergic agent to a drug regimen that already enhances serotonergic neurotransmission, on overdose with a selective serotonin reuptake inhibitor, or from abuse of psychostimulants such as amphetamine, methamphetamine, and 3,4-methylenedioxymetamphetamine (MDMA or "ecstasy"). Manifestations include agitation, hypervigilance, confusion, hyperthermia, increased sweating, fluctuating blood pressure, hyperreflexia, and myoclonus.

Neuroleptic malignant syndrome (Chapters 440 and 442) is a potentially life-threatening hypermetabolic condition that develops within days to weeks in 0.2% of patients who receive drugs that block dopamine 2 receptors. The clinical findings consist of hyperthermia, profuse sweating, muscle rigidity, bradykinesia, and delirium. If the offending medication is not withheld, the syndrome may progress to tachycardia, tachypnea, labile blood pressure, myoclonus, obtundation, and catatonia.

Among the infectious neuropathies, tetanus infection (Chapter 304) causes sympathetic overactivity in a third of patients because of the exotoxin tetanospasmin, which is taken up by peripheral nerve terminals and transported across synaptic junctions to reach the central nervous system. There it binds to gangliosides at presynaptic junctions to disinhibit preganglionic neurons and damages autonomic brain stem nuclei. Sympathetic hyperactivity results in labile or persistent hypertension or hypotension, tachyarrhythmias, peripheral vasoconstriction, fever, and profuse sweating. Diphtheritic neuropathy (Chapter 300) causes bulbar weakness and may be associated with cardiovagal impairment but not usually with orthostatic hypotension.

The acute cholinergic neuropathy of botulism (Chapter 304) occurs along with bulbar and generalized neuromuscular paralysis 12 to 36 hours after the ingestion of food contaminated with the gram-positive anaerobic bacterium *Clostridium botulinum*. Botulinum toxin binds with high affinity to presynaptic receptors of cholinergic nerve terminals and inhibits the release of acetylcholine, thereby blocking neuromuscular and cholinergic autonomic transmission. Autonomic manifestations include anhidrosis, dry eyes, dry mouth, paralytic ileus, gastric dilation, urinary retention, and sometimes orthostatic hypotension with fluctuating blood pressure and vasomotor tone.

Human immunodeficiency virus infection commonly causes autonomic disturbances, particularly in its advanced stages. Manifestations can include orthostatic hypotension, tachycardia, urinary dysfunction, impotence,

TABLE 427-3	SOME COMMONLY PRESCRIBED DRUGS THAT AFFECT SWEATING
Drugs that increase sweating	
Opioids	
Serotonin re-uptake inhibitors	
Anticholinesterases	
Cholinergic agonists	
Drugs that decrease sweating	
M_3 anticholinergics	
Carbonic anhydrase inhibitors	
Tricyclic antidepressants	
Neuroleptics	
Antihistamines	
Central α-adrenergic agonists	
Botulinum toxin	

diarrhea, and cardiac conduction defects. Perivascular mononuclear inflammatory infiltrates and neuronal degeneration in biopsy specimens of sympathetic ganglia suggest an autoimmune pathogenesis.

Chagas' disease (Chapter 355) causes a predominantly parasympathetic neuropathy characterized by megaesophagus, megaduodenum, and megacolon, as well as sympathetic cardiovascular failure with cardiomegaly and conduction defects. The autonomic neuropathy has an autoimmune basis and develops years to decades following primary infection with *Trypanosoma cruzi*.

Leprosy (Chapter 334), one of the most common causes of neuropathy worldwide, frequently causes peripheral autonomic neuropathy as a result of an immune reaction against *Mycobacterium leprae*. Focal anhidrosis occurs in areas of hypopigmented and hypoesthetic skin. Cardiac denervation and orthostatic hypotension have been described.

Toxins known to cause autonomic neuropathy include the rodenticide Vacor, as well as thallium, arsenic, mercury, acrylamide, and organic solvents such as carbon disulfide and hexacarbon. Organophosphate poisoning (Chapter 110) induces miosis and copious secretions. Ergot poisoning from rye contaminated with the fungus *Claviceps purpurea* results in intense vasoconstriction, paresthesia, seizures, and diarrhea. Poisoning with muscarine, which is present in certain poisonous mushrooms (Chapter 110), results in increased salivation, sweating, and lacrimation followed by nausea, abdominal pain, and diarrhea.

Medicinal drugs that may induce an autonomic peripheral neuropathy include cisplatin, vincristine, amiodarone, metronidazole, perhexiline maleate, and paclitaxel. Many drugs are capable of increasing or decreasing sweating (Table 427-3).

Nutritional deficiencies that lead to autonomic dysfunction include alcoholic neuropathy, which is a dying-back neuropathy identical to that of beriberi that is caused by thiamine deficiency (Chapter 425). Distal parts of the vagus nerve are affected early, and orthostatic hypotension may occur in more advanced stages. Subacute combined degeneration from vitamin B_{12} deficiency (Chapter 225) results in axonal degeneration and is occasionally manifested as orthostatic hypotension. Autonomic neuropathy has been described in some cases of celiac disease (Chapter 142).

Amyloidosis (Chapter 194) results from the focal deposition of insoluble fibrillary proteins arranged in β-pleated sheet configurations within the extracellular space of various tissues, which may include the vasculature of peripheral autonomic nerves and sympathetic ganglia. Amyloid neuropathy is typically manifested as a painful distal small fiber sensory and severe autonomic neuropathy. Autonomic dysfunction frequently occurs in primary AL, immunoglobulin light chain–associated disease, and hereditary amyloidosis, but only rarely in reactive or AA amyloidosis.

DIAGNOSIS

Clinical evaluation of autonomic dysfunction begins with a careful history. It is important to distinguish chronic and stable conditions from progressive and episodic phenomena and to recognize the circumstances that provoke or modify symptoms. Orthostatic hypotension, for example, is typically worse in the morning and may be aggravated by prolonged standing, physical exertion, heat, carbohydrate ingestion, or menstruation (Table 427-4).

Bedside Evaluation

The skin examination should assess turgor, pallor, flushing, and acral cyanosis, as well as any asymmetry of sweating, which may be more palpable than

TABLE 427-4	GRADING OF ORTHOSTATIC INTOLERANCE			
	SYMPTOM FREQUENCY	**ACTIVITIES OF DAILY LIVING IN THE UPRIGHT POSTURE**	**STANDING TIME (ON MOST OCCASIONS)**	**ORTHOSTATIC BLOOD PRESSURE**
Grade I	Infrequent orthostatic symptoms developing only under conditions of increased stress*	Unrestricted	>15 min	May or may not be abnormal
Grade II	Intermittent orthostatic symptoms occurring at least weekly	Some limitation	>5 min	Some changes in cardiovascular indices, e.g., oscillations, or decrease in pulse pressure by >50%
Grade III	Frequent orthostatic symptoms occurring on most occasions	Marked limitation	>1 min	Orthostatic hypotension is present >50% of the time, recorded on different days
Grade IV	Orthostatic symptoms are consistently present	Incapacitated and unable to stand without presyncope or syncope developing	<1 min	Orthostatic hypotension is severe and consistently present

*Conditions that increase orthostatic stress include dehydration, deconditioning from prolonged bedrest, physical exertion, heat stress, and medications that lower blood pressure or impair adrenergic function.
Adapted from Low PA, Singer W. Update on management of neurogenic orthostatic hypotension. *Lancet Neurol.* 2008;7:451-458.

visible. Signs of pupillary asymmetry, ptosis, mucosal dryness, distal sensory or reflex changes, bradykinesia, or rigidity should be noted.

Blood pressure and heart rate should be measured with the patient supine and again after standing for 1 to 3 minutes and correlated with symptoms. Orthostatic hypotension is defined as a reduction in systolic blood pressure of at least 20 mm Hg or a reduction in diastolic blood pressure of at least 10 mm Hg, with or without symptoms, within 1 to 3 minutes of assuming an erect posture. Neurogenic orthostatic hypotension is typically sustained with continued standing. Measurements taken immediately on standing can be misleading because some healthy young persons without orthostatic hypotension will exhibit transient hypotension within 30 seconds of standing but then recover. Except in patients treated with β-blockers, orthostatic hypotension without reflex tachycardia is evidence of generalized adrenergic failure. If reflex tachycardia occurs, dehydration or excessive venous pooling should be considered.

Some patients with orthostatic intolerance experience an abnormal increase in heart rate rather than a drop in blood pressure on standing. Postural tachycardia syndrome is defined as an increase in heart rate by more than 30 beats per minute or to consistently greater than 120 beats per minute when standing.

Laboratory Evaluation

Laboratory testing depends on the type and distribution of autonomic dysfunction. Investigations may include a complete blood count, fasting glucose, electrolytes, morning cortisol, thyroid function testing, vitamin B_{12} level, and when appropriate, autoimmune markers. Creatine kinase should be checked in patients with hyperthermia.

In a patient with an autonomic neuropathy, seropositivity for any of the characterized paraneoplastic autoantibodies should prompt a careful search for an underlying malignancy, even if the results of routine imaging studies are normal. Positron emission tomography is more sensitive than computed tomography in detecting small tumor foci. In patients with suspected pheochromocytoma, the most sensitive screening test is the free metanephrine level (Chapter 235).

Pupillary responses to the instillation of dilute pilocarpine, epinephrine, and cocaine can assist in the localization of oculosympathetic and oculoparasympathetic deficits. Lacrimal secretion may be quantified by the Schirmer and rose bengal tests (Chapter 276). Sialography may be useful to quantify salivary flow. Salivary gland biopsy may be necessary to diagnose Sjögren's syndrome, particularly the seronegative form.

Manometry and scintigraphic studies are useful in the diagnosis of disorders of gastrointestinal motility. Urodynamic studies can elaborate patterns of urinary bladder dysfunction. Suspected amyloid may require biopsy (Chapter 193).

Ambulatory blood pressure testing (Chapter 67), usually over a period of 24 hours, is useful to detect patterns of nocturnal hypertension, postprandial hypotension, and the labile hypertension of baroreflex failure. Adrenergic function can be assessed noninvasively by tilt table testing (Chapter 62). Adrenergic failure can also be defined by deficient recovery and overshoot of arterial pressure following 15 seconds of expiration at 40 mm Hg. The Valsalva ratio, defined as the maximum heart rate generated by the Valsalva maneuver divided by the lowest heart rate within 30 seconds of the peak, is a measure of parasympathetic cardiovagal function. A sensitive index of cardiovagal function is the heart rate response to sinusoidal deep breathing, which quantifies respiratory sinus arrhythmia.

TREATMENT ℞

Treatment begins with educating patients about the underlying physiology, helping them avoid exacerbations, and managing their symptoms. In cases of mild dysautonomia, medications may not be needed. Elderly patients may be able to compensate for some of the age-associated decline in autonomic function through regular exercise.

Efforts at treating the underlying cause of an autonomic neuropathy should be pursued. Good control of glucose in patients with diabetes mellitus (Chapters 236 and 237) reduces the rate of complications, including neuropathy. Meticulous foot care can prevent cutaneous and joint trauma, ulceration, and infection of desensitized skin.

Orthostatic Intolerance

The goals of treatment are to increase the time that the patient is able to stand without orthostatic symptoms developing while simultaneously avoiding excessive recumbent hypertension. Mild orthostatic hypotension may respond to conservative measures such as increasing oral hydration (2 to 2.5 L/day), drinking sports beverages, and adding dietary salt or sodium tablets to increase daily salt intake to 10 to 20 g. Prolonged bedrest and medications that could potentially exacerbate orthostatic hypotension should be avoided if possible. Elevating the head of the bed by inserting 4- to 6-inch blocks under the head posts can improve orthostatic tolerance by reducing nocturnal natriuresis and stimulating release of renin.

Water bolus treatment (drinking 16 oz of water) can increase systolic blood pressure by 20 mm Hg for about 2 hours by a sympathetic reflex. Lower extremity resistance strength training combined with education about physical countermaneuvers (leg crossing, squatting, bending forward, or placing one foot on a chair) can help patients increase venous return to the heart and improve orthostatic tolerance by activating leg muscles.**1** Compressive stockings are effective if they are tightly fitting, especially if they provide abdominal compression in addition to leg compression.**2** However, they may be poorly tolerated in warm climates and are cumbersome to apply.

Pharmacologic measures include fludrocortisone (0.1 to 0.4 mg/day) to expand plasma volume, midodrine (5 to 10 mg three times daily) to constrict capacitance vessels,**3** and pyridostigmine (30 to 60 mg two or three times daily) to enhance ganglionic transmission during orthostatic stress.**4** Pyridostigmine has a more modest pressor effect but has the advantage of inducing less supine hypertension.**4** Yohombine (5.4 mg three times daily) improves orthostatic hypotension by engaging residual sympathetic tone.**5** Droxidopa (100 to 600 mg three times daily), an orally active synthetic precursor of norepinephrine, is approved in Japan for the treatment of orthostatic hypotension and is under study in the United States. Nocturnal hypertension may be minimized by avoiding pressor agents within several hours of bedtime, elevating the head of the bed, or having a nighttime snack. In severe cases, bedtime hydralazine (25 mg), nifedipine (10 mg), amlodipine (2.5 to 5 mg), or a nitroglycerin patch (0.1 mg/hr) may be needed.

Postprandial hypotension may be managed by dividing meals to avoid large carbohydrate loads. Caffeine or midodrine with breakfast may be helpful.

Sweating Disorders

Initial therapy for palmar hyperhidrosis begins with tap water iontophoresis, in which a low-level electric current applied to the skin surface blocks sweat ducts at the level of the stratum corneum; for severe cases, endoscopic thoracic sympathotomy is effective. Focal hyperhidrosis, such as gustatory sweating caused by aberrant innervation of the facial sweat glands by regenerating parasympathetic fibers of the facial nerve, responds well to botulinum toxin injections. Generalized hyperhidrosis can be suppressed by oral anticholinergic drugs (e.g., glycopyrrolate, 1 to 2 mg one to three times daily), which tend to be well tolerated because very little crosses the blood-brain barrier; dry mouth is an invariable side effect. Aluminum chloride hexahydrate (20%) in anhydrous ethyl alcohol applied topically to dry skin at bedtime), oral belladonna (0.2 mg 1 to 2 times daily), propantheline (15 mg three times daily), topiramate (beginning at 25 mg twice daily), and clonidine (0.1 mg three times daily orally or by transdermal patch) may also be helpful for hyperhidrosis. Botulinum toxin types A and B, injected intradermally, are effective for axillary hyperhidrosis.

In a patient who is unable to sweat, hyperthermia cannot be prevented by drinking more water. Seeking shade, avoidance of exertion in hot weather, moistening the skin with a wet washcloth, and the use of portable fans can be quite effective. Carbonic acid inhibitors such as topiramate and zonisamide, which can inhibit thermoregulatory sweating, should be avoided if patients experience heat intolerance.

PROGNOSIS

The prognosis depends on the nature of the autonomic disorder. In general, the development of orthostatic hypotension worsens the prognosis.

A diagnosis of multiple system atrophy carries an estimated life expectancy of 7 to 9 years. A patient with pure autonomic failure may have a prolonged and stable clinical course, but it is not unusual for this syndrome to progress years later to a phenotype of multiple system atrophy or dementia with Lewy bodies. Amyloid neuropathy portends a median survival of less than 1 year if orthostatic hypotension is present. Diabetic autonomic neuropathy is associated with an approximately two-fold increased risk for silent myocardial ischemia and overall mortality.

Regional Sympathetic Dysfunction

Regional sympathetic dysfunction may accompany the pain that sometimes follows peripheral nerve injuries. For example, sympathetic activation can occur as a normal physiologic response to any painful state.

Complex regional pain syndrome is characterized by severe, ongoing neuropathic pain that is disproportionate in intensity, duration, and distribution to the expected sequela of limb trauma. In this syndrome, allodynia (pain in response to normally nonpainful stimuli, such as light touch or cold) or hyperalgesia (increased sensitivity to painful stimuli) accompany cutaneous vasomotor or sudomotor abnormalities. The vasomotor changes are manifested as vasodilation with a warm, red or swollen limb or, alternatively, as vasoconstriction with a cold, pale limb. The sudomotor findings range from regional hyperhidrosis to anhidrosis. Regional dystrophic changes, such as dry atrophic skin, sparse or coarse hair, brittle nails, and osteopenia, may also develop. Although sympathetic dysfunction may be pronounced, it does not appear to cause the pain. The mechanisms of pain and sympathetic dysfunction in this condition are incompletely understood and may result from crosstalk among aberrantly regenerated peripheral nerve fibers, expression of new α-adrenergic receptors on sensory nerve fibers and sweat glands, release of substance P and pro-inflammatory peptides at the site of injury, and sensitization of pain-mediating structures at multiple levels within the central nervous system.

Mobilization of the affected limb is of paramount importance in the early treatment of complex regional pain syndrome. A primary goal of analgesic medication or regional anesthesia in early treatment is to facilitate participation in physical therapy. Randomized controlled trials report improvement with the use of bisphosphonates (e.g., alendronate, 40 mg orally or 7.5 mg intravenously daily), steroids (e.g., prednisone, 40 mg daily, or methylprednisolone, 8 mg four times daily initially and then tapered), dimethyl sulfoxide (50% cream one to four times daily), epidural clonidine (300 to 700 μg daily), intrathecal baclofen (25 to 75 μg daily), and epidural spinal cord stimulation. One randomized trial of intravenous immunoglobulin, 0.5 g/kg, found that pain was reduced.[6]

1. Winker R, Barth A, Bidmon D, et al. Endurance exercise training in orthostatic intolerance: a randomized, controlled trial. *Hypertension.* 2005;45:291-298.
2. Podoleanu C, Maggi R, Brignole M, et al. Lower limb and abdominal compression bandages prevent progressive orthostatic hypotension in elderly persons: a randomized single-blind controlled study. *J Am Coll Cardiol.* 2006;58:1425-1432.
3. Kaufmann H, Saadia D, Voustianiouk A. Midodrine in neurally mediated syncope: a double-blind, randomized, crossover study. *Ann Neurol.* 2002;52:342-345.
4. Singer W, Sandroni P, Opfer-Gehrking TL, et al. Pyridostigmine treatment trial in neurogenic orthostatic hypotension. *Arch Neurol.* 2006;63:513-518.
5. Shibao C, Okamoto LE, Gamboa A, et al. Comparative efficacy of yohimbine against pyridostigmine for the treatment of orthostatic hypotension in autonomic failure. *Hypertension.* 2010;56:847-851.
6. Goebel A, Baranowski A, Maurer K, et al. Intravenous immunoglobulin treatment of the complex regional pain syndrome. *Ann Intern Med.* 2010;152:152-158.

SUGGESTED READINGS

Frasson E, Brigo F, Acler M, et al. Botulinum toxin type A vs type B for axillary hyperhidrosis in a case series of patients observed for 6 months. *Arch Dermatol.* 2011;147:122-123. *Data suggesting a benefit.*
Tran de QH, Duong S, Bertini P, et al. Treatment of complex regional pain syndrome: a review of the evidence. *Can J Anaesth.* 2010;57:149-166. *Review of evidence from randomized controlled trials.*

PERIPHERAL NEUROPATHIES

MICHAEL E. SHY

APPROACH TO PERIPHERAL NEUROPATHIES

DEFINITION AND PATHOBIOLOGY

Peripheral neuropathy is a general term for disorders affecting peripheral nerves. The peripheral nervous system consists of motor, sensory, and autonomic neurons that extend outside the central nervous system (CNS) and are ensheathed by Schwann cells or ganglionic satellite cells. The peripheral nervous system includes the dorsal and ventral spinal roots, spinal and cranial nerves, sensory and motor terminals, and part of the autonomic nervous system. Motor neurons extend from their cell body in the ventral horn of the spinal cord to the neuromuscular junctions at the muscle that they innervate. The cell bodies of primary sensory neurons lie outside the spinal cord in the dorsal root ganglia, where they extend peripherally to specialized sensory end organs, including nociceptors, thermoreceptors, and mechanoreceptors. Central projections from dorsal root ganglia enter the spinal cord through the dorsal roots. At each spinal segment, the ventral roots, which carry motor axons, and the dorsal roots, which carry sensory axons, join to form mixed sensorimotor nerves. In the cervical, brachial, and lumbosacral areas, the mixed spinal nerves form plexuses from which arise the major anatomically defined limb nerves. Each mixed nerve is composed of large numbers of myelinated and nonmyelinated nerve fibers of varying diameter. The large myelinated axons include motor neurons and large fiber sensory nerves that mediate position and vibration sense. Small, thinly myelinated and nonmyelinated axons primarily provide nociception and autonomic functions. Preganglionic sympathetic autonomic fibers begin in the intermediolateral column of the spinal cord and synapse in ganglia of the sympathetic trunk. Preganglionic parasympathetic fibers travel long distances from their cell bodies in the brain stem or sacral spinal cord to reach terminal ganglia near the organs that the parasympathetic fibers innervate.

CLINICAL MANIFESTATIONS

Symptoms of peripheral neuropathy include weakness, sensory loss, abnormal balance, and autonomic dysfunction. Weakness is often distal and more severe in the legs than the arms. Deep and superficial muscles that are innervated by the peroneal nerve, such as the tibialis anterior and peroneus brevis and longus muscles, often cause more symptoms than do the plantar flexion muscles innervated by the tibial nerve, such as the gastrocnemius. As a result, tripping on a carpet or curb and ankle sprains are frequent symptoms. In the hands, symptoms typically involve fine movements, such as using buttons or zippers and inserting and turning keys in locks. Cramps, the painful knotting of a muscle, frequently occur with motor or sensorimotor neuropathies.

The sensory symptoms of neuropathy reflect disease of small, thinly myelinated or nonmyelinated fibers subserving pain and temperature, as well as large myelinated fibers subserving position sense. Common symptoms of small fiber sensory neuropathy include feeling as though the feet are "walking on pebbles" or "ice cold" and difficulty determining whether bath water is hot or cold with the foot. Painful dysesthesias, such as feeling as though the feet

FIGURE 428-1. A systematic approach to evaluate neuropathy. The diseases listed are examples of neuropathies associated with specific neurophysiologic and clinical findings. Diabetic distal, predominantly sensory neuropathies are manifested as chronic axonal neuropathies; acute asymmetrical neuropathies can also occur with diabetes. Most neuropathies caused by toxins or by side effects of medication are chronic, symmetrical axonal neuropathies. AIDP, AMAN, and AMSAN are subtypes of Guillain-Barré syndrome. These and other examples are discussed in more detail in the text. AIDP = acute inflammatory demyelinating polyradiculoneuropathy; AMAN = acute motor axonal neuropathy; AMSAN = acute motor and sensory axonal neuropathy; CIDP = chronic inflammatory polyradiculoneuropathy; CIP = chronic illness polyneuropathy; CMT1 = Charcot-Marie-Tooth disease type 1, a genetic disorder; ENMG = electroneuromyography; HIV = human immunodeficiency virus–related neuropathy; α-MAG = anti-myelin-associated glycoprotein; MMN = multifocal motor neuropathy.

are "on fire," "on hot coals," or "stuck with pins," are also associated with small fiber abnormalities. Similar symptoms occur less frequently in the hands because most neuropathies are dependent on the length of the nerves; as a general rule, sensory symptoms begin in the hands when sensory symptoms in the legs have progressed up to the knee. An exception is when the patient also has carpal tunnel syndrome, which is often manifested as pain and tingling in the hands and can awaken patients from sleep. Large fiber sensory loss usually impairs balance, which may be worse at night when vision cannot overcome the loss of proprioception. Loss of proprioception is also frequently length dependent, so a patient may improve balance by lightly touching a wall with the hand to improve proprioceptive input to the brain.

Autonomic symptoms are frequent in neuropathies associated with diabetes or amyloidosis and include urinary retention or incontinence, abnormalities of sweating, constipation alternating with diarrhea, and lightheadedness when standing. Impotence is frequent.

DIAGNOSIS

Systematic Approach to Patients with Peripheral Neuropathy

Evaluation begins with the history and physical examination to demonstrate peripheral nerve disease and proceeds to neurophysiologic testing to characterize whether the process is demyelinating or axonal. Other specific tests are then ordered (Fig. 428-1).

Peripheral neuropathies usually affect both motor and sensory nerves, thereby causing both weakness and sensory loss. However, certain neuropathies are predominantly sensory, such as diabetes, or motor, such as multifocal motor neuropathy (Tables 428-1 and 428-2). Most neuropathies are symmetrical and length dependent. Pronounced asymmetries in symptoms suggest specific disorders, such as mononeuritis multiplex or hereditary neuropathy with liability to pressure palsies. It is also useful to know whether symptoms are acute (<1 month), subacute (<6 months), or chronic (>6 months). For example, Guillain-Barré syndrome develops over a period of days to weeks, whereas chronic inflammatory demyelinating polyneuropathy (CIDP) evolves over months, and inherited neuropathies may develop over years.

Neurologic Examination

Wasting of muscle is prominent in many sensorimotor or motor neuropathies, regardless of whether they are primary axonal or primary demyelinating disorders, because even demyelinating neuropathies are associated with secondary axonal degeneration. Atrophy frequently occurs in muscles of dorsiflexion, such as the tibialis anterior, and in intrinsic hand muscles, such as the first dorsal interosseus. Fasciculations, which appear as small twitches of the muscle, are sometimes present, particularly in axonal neuropathies.

Weakness is often most pronounced in foot dorsiflexion and eversion and in the intrinsic hand muscles. In the lower extremities, weakness usually progresses to the muscles of plantar flexion before more proximal muscles become involved.

TABLE 428-1	PREDOMINANTLY SENSORY NEUROPATHIES		
CLASSIFICATION	**SUBGROUP**	**TYPE**	**FIBERS**
Genetic		HSAN	Large, small
Inflammatory, immune	Monoclonal gammopathy	Anti-MAG (early on)	Mainly large
	Vasculitis	Sjögren's syndrome	Large, small
	Paraneoplastic	Anti-Hu	Large
Metabolic	Diabetic	Distal symmetrical polyneuropathy	Large, small
Infectious	HIV	HIV neuropathy	Small
	Herpes zoster	Focal radiculoneuropathy	Small
	Leprosy	Tuberculoid	Small
Toxic, deficiency	Medications	Vincristine	Small
		Paclitaxel	Large
		Cisplatin	Large
		Thalidomide	Large
		NRTIs	Small
	Toxins	Thallium	Small
		Acrylamide	Large
		Pyridoxine (B$_6$)	Large, small
	Deficiency states	Vitamin B$_1$	Large, small
		Vitamin B$_{12}$	Large
		Vitamin E	Large
Idiopathic	Frequent		Large, small

HIV = human immunodeficiency virus; HSAN = hereditary sensory and autonomic neuropathy; MAG = myelin-associated glycoprotein; NRTIs = nucleoside reverse transcriptase inhibitors.

TABLE 428-2	PREDOMINANTLY MOTOR NEUROPATHIES	
CLASSIFICATION	**SUBGROUP**	**TYPE**
Genetic		HMN
Inflammatory, immune	Guillain-Barré	AMAN
	Multifocal motor neuropathy	MMN
	Critical illness myopathy	CIM
Toxic, deficiency	Medications	Dapsone
	Toxins	Lead (adults)

AMAN = acute motor axonal neuropathy; CIM = critical illness myopathy; HMN = hereditary motor neuropathy; MMN = multifocal motor neuropathy.

Sensory loss is usually in a stocking-glove distribution in both large and small fiber neuropathy. Cold, erythematous, or bluish discolored feet suggest loss of small fiber function. Large fiber sensory loss, or *sensory ataxia*, in the upper extremities can often be detected by an inability of the patient to locate the thumb accurately with the opposite index finger while the eyes are closed or by the presence of a characteristic irregular tremor (pseudoathetosis) of the fingers.

The sensory examination should include vibration, position, and light touch as well as pain and temperature. It is important to determine the degree and extent of sensory loss in addition to the pattern of deficits (symmetrical or asymmetrical; distal or generalized; focal, multifocal, or diffuse).

The complete absence of reflexes early in the course of a neuropathy suggests a demyelinating neuropathy ; for example, the absence of reflexes in early childhood is often the first detectable abnormality in children with inherited demyelinating neuropathies. Alternatively, the absence of ankle reflexes but the presence of normal patellar or upper extremity reflexes is common in "dying back" (length-dependent) axonal neuropathies, both acquired and inherited. Reflexes may be present in small fiber neuropathies.

On gait testing, subtle weakness in the feet can be detected by an inability of the patient to heel walk. Sensory ataxia can be appreciated by a wide-based gait or inability to tandem walk.

Neurologic Testing
Neurophysiology

Electromyography (EMG) and nerve conduction studies can determine whether a neuropathy is primarily demyelinating or axonal and can confirm whether the process is symmetrical or asymmetrical (Chapter 403).

Motor nerve conduction velocities measure conduction over the main body of nerves but not their proximal or distal portion. Distal motor latencies and F wave latencies measure velocities over the distal and proximal portions of the nerves. When slowing is roughly the same over the proximal, distal, and main portion of the nerve, the slowing is said to be uniform. When slowing is multifocal or asymmetrical, either along the same nerve or between different nerves, the slowing is said to be nonuniform. Slowed conduction velocities (to less than 70% of normal) suggest that the neuropathy is primarily demyelinating.

The sensory nerve action potential is a summation of action potentials from individual large-diameter sensory axons. In axonal neuropathies, amplitudes of the compound muscle action potential or sensory nerve action potential are reduced. When there has been a loss of individual sensory axons, amplitudes of the sensory nerve action potential are reduced.

The presence of spontaneous activity on EMG, such as fibrillations or positive sharp waves, suggests that an acute or active process is damaging axons and denervating muscle. The presence of large, polyphasic motor units suggests partial reinnervation of muscle by regenerating axons (i.e., a more chronic process). Recruitment of motor units is also reduced in patients with demyelinating and axonal neuropathies.

Quantitative Sensory Testing

Quantitative sensory testing can assess and quantify vibratory, thermal, or painful sensory function in patients with peripheral neuropathies or other sensory disorders. Although the stimulus is an objective physical event, the response represents a subjective report and requires cooperation from the patient; as a result, this test by itself cannot diagnose sensory neuropathies or sensory loss.

Nerve and Skin Biopsy

Nerve biopsy is occasionally indicated to address specific questions, such as whether vasculitis, tumor, or another infiltrative or metabolic disorder is present. Biopsy of sural nerves is performed just above the ankle. After biopsy, patients lose sensation over the region on the lateral aspect of the foot that is innervated by the sural nerve, and transient painful dysesthesias may develop around the biopsy site. Teased sural nerve fiber analysis can demonstrate segmental demyelination or remyelination, and electron microscopy can demonstrate features of nerve regeneration and identify specific pathologic processes.

Epidermal skin biopsies with quantification of the loss of small epidermal nerve fibers may aid in the diagnosis of sensory neuropathies, particularly in neuropathies that involve a loss of small fibers, such as diabetes mellitus, human immunodeficiency virus (HIV) infection, or chemotherapeutic drugs. Skin biopsies also are increasingly being used to evaluate myelinated sensory nerves.

Laboratory Findings

Evaluation of all patients with suspected neuropathy should include blood glucose and creatinine levels as well as a complete blood count (including red blood cell indices to detect possible macrocytosis). If the history and EMG are consistent with exposure to a toxin or a vitamin-deficiency state,

specific testing is indicated. Most patients should also have vitamin B_{12} level measurement (Chapter 167), rapid plasmin reagent test (Chapter 327), and serum immunofixation electrophoresis for possible monoclonal gammopathy (Chapter 193). In unexplained sensory neuropathies, HIV testing should be considered (Chapter 401). In selected patients, electrodiagnostic studies will suggest the need to test for specific antibodies, such as antibodies reacting to ganglioside GM_1 or myelin-associated glycoprotein (MAG). Genetic testing is most cost-effective when selection of candidate genes is based on the patient's nerve conduction studies, inheritance pattern, and clinical findings.

INHERITED NEUROPATHIES

DEFINITION

Inherited neuropathies are frequently called Charcot-Marie-Tooth (CMT) disease based on the names of the three physicians who initially characterized the disorders in the late 19th century. They are also referred to as hereditary motor and sensory neuropathies, hereditary motor neuropathies, or hereditary sensory and autonomic neuropathies, depending on their clinical manifestation. Autosomal dominant forms are subdivided into demyelinating (CMT1) and dominantly inherited axonal (CMT2) forms based on electrophysiologic and neuropathologic criteria. X-linked (CMTX) and autosomal recessive (CMT4) forms are also seen. Each type of CMT disease is subdivided according to the specific genetic cause of the neuropathy. For example, the most common form of CMT1, termed CMT1A, is caused by a duplication of a fragment of chromosome 17 containing the peripheral myelin protein 22-kD (*PMP22*) gene (see later). Currently, mutations in more than 40 genes have been identified as causes of inherited neuropathies (available at *www.uia.ac.be/CMTMutations/*) (Table 428-3).

EPIDEMIOLOGY

The prevalence of CMT is about 1 in 2500 people, without ethnic predisposition. The 17p11.2 duplication causing CMT1A accounts for 60 to 70% of CMT1 patients, CMT1X for approximately 10 to 20% of CMT cases, CMT1B for less than 5% of patients, and CMT2 for about 20% of cases. The prevalence of hereditary neuropathy with liability to pressure palsies is not known, but about 85% of patients with clinical evidence of this syndrome have a chromosome 17p11.2 deletion.

PATHOBIOLOGY
Pathology

Segmental demyelination, remyelination, and axonal loss are characteristic features of the various demyelinating forms of CMT1. In Dejerine-Sottas neuropathy, the demyelination is more severe. In CMT1, onion bulbs of concentric Schwann cell lamellae are usually present on nerve biopsies, with loss of both small- and-large diameter myelinated fibers and sometimes axons. Focal, sausage-like thickenings of the myelin sheath (tomacula) are characteristic of hereditary neuropathy with liability to pressure palsies (HNPP) but may also be found in other forms of CMT1, particularly CMT1B. In CMT1, disability typically correlates better with secondary axonal degeneration than with demyelination itself, thereby demonstrating the importance of Schwann cell–axonal interactions in demyelinating disease (Fig. 428-2).

Genetics

Mutations in *PMP22* and *MPZ* cause CMT1, and mutations in *GJB1* cause CMT1X. All three genes code for myelin proteins. Mutations in the neurofilament light (*NEFL*), gigaxonin (*GAN*), and *dynactin* genes cause CMT2; all three genes have roles in the axonal cytoskeleton and axonal transport. LITAF/SIMPLE, the myotubulin-related proteins 2 and 13, and RAB7 are involved in intracellular trafficking. MFN2 and ganglioside-induced differentiation-associated protein-1 (GDAP1) are nuclearly encoded mitochondrial proteins.

CLINICAL MANIFESTATIONS

Despite phenotypic variability, the typical clinical course of CMT1 and CMT2 patients includes normal development before weakness, and sensory loss appearing gradually within the first two decades of life. Affected children are often slow runners and have difficulty with activities that require balance (e.g., skating, walking across a log). Ankle-foot orthoses are frequently required by the third decade. Fine movements of the hands for activities such

TABLE 428-3 INHERITED NEUROPATHIES

DISORDER	LOCUS/GENE	INHERITANCE	PROTEIN	MUTATION (FREQUENCY)	TESTING METHOD	TYPE OF TESTING
HEREDITARY MOTOR AND SENSORY NEUROPATHIES						
CMT1A	17p11.2/*PMP22*	AD	Peripheral myelin protein 22	Duplication (98%)	Pulsed-field gel electrophoresis, FISH, Southern blot	Clinical
				Sequence alteration (2%)	Sequencing	
HNPP	17p11.2/*PMP22*	AD	Peripheral myelin protein 22	Deletion (80%)	Pulsed-field gel electrophoresis, FISH, Southern blot	Clinical
				Sequence alteration (20%)	Sequencing	
CMT1B	1q22/*MPZ*	AD	Myelin protein zero	Sequence alteration	Sequencing, mutation scanning, mutation analysis	Clinical
CMT1C	16p13.1-p12.3/*LITAF*	AD	SIMPLE	Sequence alteration		Research
CMT1D	10q21.1-q22.1/*EGR2*	AD	Early growth response protein 2	Sequence alteration	Sequencing, mutation scanning, mutation analysis	Clinical
CMT2A	1p36.2/*MFN2*	AD	Mitofusin 2	Sequence alteration	Direct DNA, linkage analysis	Research
CMT2B	3q21/*RAB7*	AD	Ras-related protein Rab-7	Sequence alteration	Direct DNA, linkage analysis	Research
CMT2C	12q23-24/unknown	AD	Unknown		Direct DNA, linkage analysis	
CMT2D	7p15/*GARS*	AD	Glycyl-tRNA synthetase	Sequence alteration	Direct DNA, linkage analysis	Research
CMT2E	8p21/*NEFL*	AD	Neurofilament triplet L protein	Sequence alteration	Sequencing	Clinical
CMT2F	7q11-21	AD	Heat shock protein 27 (B1)	Sequence alteration	Sequencing	Research
CMT2L	12q24	AD	Heat shock protein 22 (B8)	Sequence alteration	Sequencing	
CMT4A	8q13-q21.1/*GDAP1*	AR	Ganglioside-induced differentiation protein 1	Sequence alteration	Sequencing	Clinical
CMT4B1	11q22/*MTMR2*	AR	Myotubularin-related protein 2	Sequence alteration		Research
CMT4B2	11p15/*CMT4B2*	AR	SET binding factor 2	Sequence alteration		Research
CMT4C	5q32/*KIAA1985*	AR	KIAA1985	Sequence alteration		Research
CMT4D	8q24.3/*NDRG1*	AR	NDRG1 protein	Sequence alteration		Research
CMT4E	10q21.1-q22.1/*EGR2*	AR	Early growth response protein 2	Sequence alteration	Mutation analysis, sequencing	Clinical
CMT4F	19q13.1-q13.2/*PRX*	AR	Periaxin	Sequence alteration	Sequencing	Clinical
CMT4G (HMSN-R)	10q23	AR	Unknown			
CMT4H	12p11.21-q13.11	AR	FRABIN	Sequence alteration	Sequencing	Research
CMT4J	6q21	AR	FIG4	Sequence alteration	Sequencing	Clinical
CMT1X	Xq13.1/*GJB1*	X-linked	Gap junction β1 protein (connexin 32)	Sequence alteration (deletion rare)	Sequencing	Clinical
DI-CMTA	10q24.1-q25.1	AD	Unknown			
DI-CMTB	19p12-p13.2	AD	Dynamin 2	Sequence alteration	Sequencing	Research
DI-CMTC	1p34-p35	AD	Tyrosine tRNA Synthetase	Sequence alteration	Sequencing	Research
Slow-NCV	8p23	AD	ARHGEF10	Sequence alteration	Sequencing	Research
DISTAL HEREDITARY MOTOR NEUROPATHIES						
dHMN I	Unknown	AD	Unknown			Research
dHMN II	12q24.3/unknown	AD	Unknown			Research
dHMN III	1q21-23/unknown	AR	Unknown			Research
dHMN V	7p15/*GARS*	AD	Glycyl-tRNA synthetase	Sequence alteration	Sequencing	Clinical
dHMN VI	Unknown	AR	Unknown			Research
dHMN VII	2q14/unknown	AD	Unknown			Research
dHMN Jerash	9p21.1-p12/unknown	AR	Unknown			Research
ALS4	9q34/unknown	AD	SETX	Sequence alteration		Research
HMN Dynactin	2p13/*DCTN1*	AD	Dynactin	Sequence alteration		Research
HEREDITARY SENSORY AND AUTONOMIC NEUROPATHIES						
HSAN I	9q22.1-q22.3/*SPTLC1*	AD	Serine palmitoyltransferase light chain 1	Sequence alteration	Sequencing	Clinical
HSAN II	Unknown	AR	Unknown			Research
HSAN III (Riley-Day syndrome)	9q31/*IKBKAP*	AR	IκB kinase complex-associated protein	Two mutations account for 99% of affected patients of Ashkenazi Jewish descent	Mutation analysis, quantitative PCR	Clinical
HSAN IV	1q21-q22/*NTRK1*	AR	Tyrosine kinase for nerve growth factor	Sequence alteration		Research

CMT = Charcot-Marie-Tooth disease; FISH = fluorescence in situ hybridization; HNPP = hereditary neuropathy with liability to pressure palsies; dHMN = distal hereditary motor neuropathy; HSAN = hereditary sensory and autonomic neuropathy; PCR = polymerase chain reaction; RFLP = restriction fragment length polymorphism.

FIGURE 428-2. Schematic view of an axon and its myelinating Schwann cell. Proteins mutated in inherited peripheral neuropathies are shown in color at their cellular location. In the *upper part* of the panel, the myelinating Schwann cell has been unraveled to show the nucleus and regions of both compact myelin and noncompact myelin. Cytoskeletal elements within the axon are also illustrated. (From Shy ME, Garbern JY, Kamholz J. Hereditary motor and sensory neuropathies: a biological perspective. *Lancet Neurol.* 2002;1:110-118.)

as turning a key or using buttons and zippers may be impaired, but the hands are rarely as affected as the feet. Most patients remain ambulatory throughout life and have a normal lifespan.

A minority of CMT patients have a more severe phenotype with delayed motor milestones and onset in infancy, termed *Dejerine-Sottas neuropathy*. Especially severe cases are classified as congenital hypomyelination if myelination appears to be disrupted during embryologic development. Many patients have de novo autosomal dominant disorders, and the term *Dejerine-Sottas neuropathy* is currently used primarily to denote severe early-onset clinical phenotypes regardless of the inheritance pattern. Patients with hereditary motor neuropathies sometimes have mild sensory abnormalities, and patients with hereditary sensory and autonomic neuropathies usually have some weakness. The same mutations in the same gene (*GARS*) cause both CMT2D and hereditary motor neuropathy type V.

DIAGNOSIS

Molecular testing, performed after the family history, neurologic examination, and neurophysiologic testing have suggested the probable candidate genes (GeneClinics—available at *www.geneclinics.org*), is the "gold standard" for the diagnosis of inherited neuropathies. Nerve conduction velocity testing can distinguish between demyelinating and axonal neuropathies. Most CMT1 patients, particularly those with CMT1A, have a uniformly slow nerve conduction velocity of about 20 m/second. Asymmetrical slowing, which is characteristic of hereditary neuropathy with liability to pressure palsies, may be found in patients with missense mutations in *PMP22*, *MPZ*, *EGR2*, and *GJB1*. Although CMT2 is characterized by axonal loss and reduced compound muscle action potential or sensory nerve action potential amplitudes, virtually all forms of CMT1 have axonal loss as well as demyelination.

Differential Diagnosis

Inherited neuropathies must be distinguished from acquired neuropathies (see later). Additionally, genetic disorders of the CNS such as hereditary spastic paraplegia (Chapter 417) or leukodystrophies (Chapter 419) may mimic inherited neuropathies by causing length-dependent weakness, sensory loss, and foot deformities such as pes cavus; these patients will frequently have upper motor neuron signs, such as increased reflexes or Babinski's signs, and do not have neurophysiologic evidence of neuropathy.

TREATMENT

There is no specific therapy for the inherited neuropathies, but clinical and genetic counseling and symptomatic and rehabilitative treatment are important. A detailed family history and often examination of family members are required for prognosis and genetic counseling.

Ankle-foot orthoses to correct footdrop may return gait and balance to normal for years. Foot surgery is sometimes offered to correct inverted feet, pes cavus, and hammertoes. Surgery may improve walking, alleviate pain over pressure points, and prevent plantar ulcers. However, foot surgery is generally unnecessary and does not improve weakness and sensory loss.

Ascorbic acid, antagonists to progesterone, and subcutaneous injections of neurotrophin 3 have demonstrated improvement in animal models of CMT1A. However, no medication has yet demonstrated efficacy in patients with CMT1A or any other form of CMT.

INFLAMMATORY AND IMMUNOLOGIC NEUROPATHIES
Guillain-Barré Syndrome

DEFINITION

Guillain-Barré syndrome refers to acquired, inflammatory peripheral neuropathies that have (1) an acute onset, (2) elevated cerebrospinal fluid (CSF) protein levels with low CSF cell counts (cytoalbuminologic dissociation), and (3) a monophasic illness with at least partial recovery. Guillain-Barré syndrome is subdivided into acute inflammatory demyelinating polyneuropathy, acute motor and sensory axonal neuropathy, acute motor axonal neuropathy, and Miller-Fisher syndrome (Table 428-4).

EPIDEMIOLOGY

Acute inflammatory demyelinating polyneuropathy accounts for up to 97% of cases of Guillain-Barré syndrome in North America and Europe. It is a sporadic disorder with an incidence of 0.6 to 1.9 cases per 100,000 people in North America and Europe. Men are more likely to be affected than women (1.4:1). In 60% of cases, acute inflammatory demyelinating polyneuropathy is preceded by a respiratory tract infection (e.g., cytomegalovirus [Chapter 384], Epstein-Barr virus [Chapter 385], or gastroenteritis (*Campylobacter jejuni* [Chapter 311]). Acute motor axonal neuropathy and acute motor and sensory axonal neuropathy are rare in North America and Europe but more frequent in China, Japan, Mexico, Korea, and India.

PATHOBIOLOGY

All forms of Guillain-Barré syndrome probably result from postinfectious molecular mimicry in which nerve antigens are attacked by the immune system because they resemble antigens presented by microbes, in particular, *C. jejuni*. For example, the HS/0:19 serotype of *C. jejuni* is common in northern Chinese patients with Guillain-Barré syndrome and has also been isolated from such patients in other countries. Assays with antiganglioside antibodies, bacterial toxins, and lectins have characterized potential immunogenic regions of diarrhea-associated *C. jejuni* strains. However, it is not clear that molecular mimicry is the cause of acute inflammatory demyelinating polyneuropathy, which is the most common form in the United States and Europe.

CLINICAL MANIFESTATIONS

Weakness, which is the most common initial symptom in both acute inflammatory demyelinating polyneuropathy and acute motor and sensory axonal neuropathy, can be mild, such as difficulty walking, or severe, such as total quadriplegia and respiratory failure. Bilateral weakness of facial muscles (facial diplegia) occurs in about 50% of cases. The most common manifestation is leg weakness that subsequently "ascends" into the arms. Although Guillain-Barré syndrome has been described as an "ascending paralysis," proximal weakness is common, and 5% of cases have isolated cranial nerve involvement that subsequently descends into the limbs. Sensory loss occurs in most patients. The autonomic nervous system is involved in about 65% of patients.

Length-dependent weakness without sensory loss develops in patients with acute motor axonal neuropathy, including cranial nerve involvement in about 25%. Miller-Fisher syndrome consists of the triad of ophthalmoplegia, ataxia, and areflexia. Facial weakness, ptosis, and pupillary abnormalities may be present. Nerve conduction velocities in Miller-Fisher syndrome are generally normal, unlike the case with acute inflammatory demyelinating polyneuropathy.

DIAGNOSIS

The diagnosis of acute inflammatory demyelinating polyneuropathy and acute motor and sensory axonal neuropathy is based on the history, physical examination, and CSF evaluation. Deep tendon reflexes are decreased or absent, and the CSF is abnormal with cytoalbuminologic dissociation. The weakness is symmetrical. The presence of CNS abnormalities should cast doubt on the diagnosis. Acute inflammatory demyelinating polyneuropathy is distinguished from acute motor and sensory axonal neuropathy by nerve conduction studies. In both acute inflammatory demyelinating polyneuropathy and acute motor and sensory axonal neuropathy, the CSF should have fewer than five white blood cells (WBCs)/mL. If the CSF cell count is greater than 50 WBCs/mL, another diagnosis, such as HIV infection (Chapter 401) or Lyme disease (Chapter 329), should be considered. Elevated CSF protein may not be apparent in the first 7 to 10 days of the illness; in up to 10% of cases, CSF protein levels remain normal. Approximately 5% of patients with Guillain-Barré syndrome have Miller-Fisher syndrome, and more than 85% of these patients have polyclonal antibodies that react with the ganglioside GQ_{1b}.

Differential Diagnosis

The differential diagnosis varies in different parts of the world. Historically, poliomyelitis (Chapter 423) was the major cause of acute flaccid quadriparesis. In North America, polio has been eradicated, but other viral illnesses may induce polio-like syndromes: ECHO 70 (Chapter 387), coxsackievirus

TABLE 428-4	INFLAMMATORY AND IMMUNE-RELATED NEUROPATHIES				
DISORDER	**TYPE**	**CLINICAL TRAITS**	**PATHOBIOLOGY**	**TREATMENT***
Guillain-Barré syndrome	AIDP	Acute flaccid weakness, sensory loss	Demyelination, lymphocyte infiltration	Plasma exchange, IVIG
	AMAN/AMSAN	Acute flaccid weakness, no sensory loss in AMAN	Molecular mimicry, association with *Campylobacter jejuni*	? Plasma exchange or IVIG
	Fisher's syndrome	Acute ataxia, ophthalmoparesis and areflexia	Anti-GQ1b antibodies	? Plasma exchange or IVIG
CIDP		Slower onset of weakness, sensory loss	Inflammatory/immune-mediated demyelination	Corticosteroids, plasma exchange, IVIG
Monoclonal gammopathy	IgM	Sensory > motor	Particularly anti-MAG	Immune suppression (Chapter 193)
	IgG	Sensorimotor	Many probably chance associations, osteosclerotic myeloma, solitary plasmacytoma; POEMS may be immune mediated	Treatment of myeloma
Multifocal motor neuropathy		Pure motor	Focal demyelination, antibodies to GM_1 frequent	IVIG

*Typical regimens: IVIG, 0.4 g/kg/day × 5 days for a total of 2 g/kg; may be repeated monthly as needed. Corticosteroids: prednisone, 60 to 80 mg/day for up to 3 months, followed by gradual tapering, depending on the clinical response, with a goal to about 20 mg on an alternate-day regimen.
AIDP = acute idiopathic demyelinating polyneuropathy; AMAN = acute motor axonal neuropathy; AMSAN = acute motor and sensory axonal neuropathy; CIDP = chronic inflammatory polyradiculoneuropathy; IgG = immunoglobulin G; IVIG = intravenous immune globulin; MAG = myelin-associated glycoprotein; POEMS = polyneuropathy, organomegaly, M protein, skin changes.

(Chapter 387), West Nile virus (Chapter 390), and rarely, rabies (Chapter 422). Because these diseases are not demyelinating disorders, they can be distinguished from acute inflammatory demyelinating polyneuropathy by their normal nerve conduction velocity. However, the results of electrodiagnostic studies are similar in both acute motor axonal neuropathy and the polio-like syndromes, thus making distinction between acute motor axonal neuropathy and these syndromes difficult.

Tick paralysis (Chapter 390), caused by a toxin within the tick, can mimic Guillain-Barré syndrome, particularly in children. Usually, removal of the tick is associated with improvement within hours, although progression can occur. Progression is particularly likely in Australia, where the toxin differs from that found in North America.

Botulism (Chapters 304 and 430) rapidly produces a flaccid paralysis. Patients have ophthalmoplegia, bulbar weakness, dry mouth, constipation, and orthostatic hypotension, but sensory symptoms do not develop. Other entities that can mimic Guillain-Barré syndrome are acute spinal cord compression (Chapter 407), acute transverse myelitis (Chapter 419), and vascular myelopathies, all of which are characterized by decreased reflexes before the development of upper motor neuron signs such as increased reflexes. Carcinomatous or lymphomatous meningitis can also cause a rapidly developing quadriparesis, but both are associated with elevated CSF WBC counts.

TREATMENT   Rx

Patients with Guillain-Barré syndrome require hospitalization because of the potential for respiratory compromise. Pulmonary function tests should be performed frequently; a vital capacity of less than 1 L or a negative inspiratory force of less than −70 suggests that ventilator support may be needed in an intensive care unit setting. Autonomic instability and difficulty swallowing also need to be monitored.

Therapies directed at modulating the immune system are effective in Guillain-Barré syndrome. Intravenous immunoglobulin (IVIG) therapy, which is the preferred treatment, is typically given as 2 g/kg divided over 2 to 5 days within the first 2 weeks. Although plasma exchange and IVIG are equally effective,**1** at least in the first 2 weeks, IVIG is often preferred for its convenience unless there are contraindications, such as low serum immunoglobulin A (IgA) levels, renal failure, or severe hypertension.

Plasma exchange, usually four exchanges of 1.5 L of plasma spread over a 10-day period, is also effective.**2** Two plasma exchanges may be sufficient in mild cases, and six exchanges are not superior to four in severely affected patients. This therapy should ideally be administered within the first 2 weeks and not later than 4 weeks from clinical onset.

Ten percent of patients with Guillain-Barré syndrome relapse after initially responding to plasma exchange or IVIG; they usually respond to a second cycle of the previously effective treatment. The combined use of plasma exchange followed by IVIG does not improve the prognosis.**3**

Corticosteroids in different forms (intravenous methylprednisolone, oral prednisolone or prednisone, intramuscular adrenocorticotropic hormone) are not of benefit. Intravenous methylprednisolone (500 mg/day for 5 days) in association with IVIG has a slight initial advantage over IVIG alone but no benefit in terms of long-term disability.

PROGNOSIS

Fifty percent of patients progress to their nadir, or maximal disability, within 2 weeks, 75% within 3 weeks, and more than 90% within 4 weeks of the onset of symptoms. With modern supportive care, acute mortality is about 2%. After a brief period of stabilization, slow spontaneous recovery occurs over a period of weeks or months. Most patients either undergo complete recovery or are left with minor sequelae; about 20% have a persistent disability. The long-term prognosis depends at least in part on the extent of axonal loss. Patients with low compound muscle action potential amplitudes in the upper extremities are more likely to have a poor prognosis.

Patients with acute motor axonal neuropathy will recover after approximately 2 months, but the extent of recovery may be less than in Guillain-Barré syndrome. In general, the prognosis for recovering from Miller-Fisher syndrome is excellent.

Chronic Inflammatory Demyelinating Polyradiculoneuropathy

DEFINITION

CIDP is a chronic acquired demyelinating sensorimotor neuropathy that may be monophasic, relapsing, or progressive. By definition, CIDP develops over at least a 2-month period as opposed to acute inflammatory demyelinating polyneuropathy, which it otherwise resembles.

EPIDEMIOLOGY

CIDP occurs in all age groups, with a mean age range of 30 to 50 years. Women are slightly more likely to be affected than men. Antecedent events are less common than in Guillain-Barré syndrome; they occur in about 30% of patients and include upper respiratory infections, gastrointestinal infections, vaccinations, surgery, and trauma.

PATHOBIOLOGY

CIDP is considered an autoimmune disorder based on pathologic findings in nerve biopsy samples from patients and on findings in animal models such as experimental allergic neuritis, in which a similar disorder follows immunization with peripheral nervous system myelin components and Freund's adjuvant. Nerve biopsy shows macrophage-mediated segmental demyelination, occasional endoneurial lymphocytic T-cell infiltrates, and endoneurial edema. The major histocompatibility complex class I and II antigens are upregulated, and there are often deposits of immunoglobulins and complement split products on the outer Schwann cell membranes or myelin sheaths. CIDP can be passively transferred to animals by patient sera, but no clear autoantigen has been identified.

CLINICAL MANIFESTATIONS

Weakness and sensory loss begin insidiously and progress over a period of months to years. Weakness is commonly proximal as well as distal. Patients can become bedridden. Loss of proprioception from damage to large-diameter sensory nerves may affect balance and result in an action tremor. Deep tendon reflexes are usually absent or markedly decreased. Facial weakness (15%), ptosis or ophthalmoparesis (5%), and papilledema occur occasionally. Variant forms include pure motor, pure sensory, and multifocal disease.

DIAGNOSIS

Diagnosis is based on clinical symptoms and signs, electrodiagnostic studies, and CSF examination. Nonuniform, asymmetrical slowing on nerve conduction studies is characteristic. One portion of a nerve may have different conduction than another. For example, if damage is primarily in the spinal roots, proximal conduction velocities and F wave latencies may be most affected. Compound muscle action potentials are generally reduced because of the concomitant axonal degeneration that occurs with demyelinating neuropathies. However, temporal dispersion and conduction block may also reduce the amplitude of muscle action potential in any demyelinating neuropathy. Sensory nerve conduction is also slow in CIDP, but because sensory nerve action potentials are often not detectable, sensory conduction velocity may be unmeasurable.

CSF results resemble those of acute inflammatory demyelinating polyneuropathy: WBC counts are usually less than 10 cells/mm^3, and protein levels are higher than 60 mg/dL. CSF cell counts higher than 50/mm^3 suggest another diagnosis, such as HIV infection or hematologic malignancy. CSF protein levels may be normal early in the course of CIDP.

Differential Diagnosis

CIDP is distinguished from acute inflammatory demyelinating polyneuropathy by its time course. A similar manifestation can also occur in diabetes, lymphoma, monoclonal gammopathies (see later), and asymmetrical inherited neuropathies (see earlier).

TREATMENT

Corticosteroids are effective in more than two thirds of patients with CIDP. A standard approach is to use oral prednisone (1 mg/kg/day) for 6 to 8 weeks, followed by slow tapering over a 3- to 12-month period to a maintenance level of about 0.1 mg/kg/day. A response to prednisone may take months to occur, and occasional patients may worsen before they respond. As a result, plasma exchange**2** or IVIG**4,5** is often used as initial treatment. Because of the side effects of long-term corticosteroids or the lack of response to them, azathioprine, cyclosporine, cyclophosphamide, methotrexate, mycophenolate mofetil, rituximab, and interferon-α or -β have been used with variable success in uncontrolled reports.

Neuropathy Associated with Monoclonal Gammopathy

DEFINITION

Monoclonal gammopathy refers to the presence in the β-γ region of serum protein electrophoresis of an abnormal spike (variably called a paraprotein, monoclonal protein, or M protein) consisting of immunoglobulins of the same isotype, all produced by a single clone of abnormally proliferating lymphocyte and plasma cells. In some cases, the M protein is part of a malignant lymphoproliferative disease such as multiple myeloma, solitary plasmacytoma (IgG and IgA), Waldenström's macroglobulinemia (IgM) (Chapter 193), lymphoma (Chapter 191), chronic lymphocytic leukemia (IgM) (Chapter 190), primary amyloidosis (Chapter 194), or cryoglobulinemia (Chapter 193). In most instances, however, monoclonal gammopathy is not initially associated with any of these disorders and is classified as a monoclonal gammopathy of uncertain significance (MGUS), although in patients with MGUS, the gammopathy may evolve into a malignant form (Chapter 193).

EPIDEMIOLOGY

Monoclonal gammopathy occurs in up to 8% of patients with peripheral neuropathy of unknown etiology. However, MGUS is frequent, being found in 1% of the population older than 50 years and in 3% older than 70 years, and most subjects with MGUS do not have neuropathy. In some cases, the co-occurrence of neuropathy and M protein may be a coincidence, but in other cases, the M protein is clearly related to the neuropathy.

The prevalence of neuropathy is higher in patients with IgM versus IgG or IgA M proteins. The prevalence of symptomatic neuropathy associated with IgM monoclonal gammopathy in patients older than 50 years is approximately 20 per 100,000. In half of such patients, the M protein reacts either with the HNK1 carbohydrate moiety of MAG or with other glycoproteins (MPZ, PMP22) and glycolipids (sulfoglucuronyl paraglycoside [SGPG] and lactosaminyl paraglycoside [SGLPG]). IgM M proteins associated with neuropathy may also bind to other neural antigens.

In patients with IgG monoclonal gammopathy and neuropathy, the relationship is less clear than with IgM. Although about 10% of patients with multiple myeloma have neuropathy, in most cases, the M protein does not react with a neural antigen, and patients do not improve with immunotherapy (see later). Conversely, approximately 50% of patients with the osteosclerotic form of myeloma have neuropathy, often associated with the non-neurologic manifestations of organomegaly, endocrine abnormalities, and brown, tannish discoloration of the skin. Collectively, the M protein, polyneuropathy, and other features are referred to by the acronym POEMS (Chapter 193). Similarly, about 50% of patients with light-chain amyloidosis have neuropathy.

PATHOBIOLOGY

In patients with IgM M proteins that immunoreact with MAG, nerve biopsies demonstrate segmental demyelination with deposits of M protein and complement. The myelin lamellae are often widened on sural nerve biopsies, but a biopsy is not necessary for diagnosis. High titers (>1:10,000) of anti-MAG IgM antibodies are associated with neuropathy, and intraneural or systemic injection of anti-MAG IgM M proteins causes complement-mediated demyelination of nerves in animals.

CLINICAL MANIFESTATIONS

Most patients with anti-MAG neuropathies are initially seen in their sixth to seventh decade of life with dysesthesias and paresthesias in their legs and unsteadiness while walking because of loss of proprioception. Physical examination shows a length-dependent large fiber sensory neuropathy. Weakness may develop later.

DIAGNOSIS

Nerve conduction velocities are slow (about 25 m/second) with pronounced delays in distal motor latencies, thus prompting the designation *distal acquired demyelinating symmetrical neuropathy* to distinguish the disorder from CIDP.

TREATMENT   **Rx**

Treatment of neuropathies associated with monoclonal gammopathy is similar to that for CIDP (see earlier). However, patients with anti-MAG-related neuropathies do not respond as well to treatment as do patients with CIDP. Anecdotal data support the benefit of rituximab in some patients.

PROGNOSIS

Progression of the neuropathy of monoclonal gammopathy disables about 25% of patients after 10 years and 50% after 15 years. The course of patients with osteosclerotic myeloma and neuropathy depends on the response to treatment of the myeloma. In patients whose myeloma responds to treatment, more than 50% have improvement in neuropathy. In other patients with sensorimotor neuropathies associated with plasma cell dyscrasias, the course is variable, and the M protein may not be related to their neuropathy.

Multifocal Motor Neuropathy and Lewis-Sumner Syndrome

DEFINITION

Multifocal motor neuropathy is characterized by progressive, distal more than proximal, asymmetrical limb weakness, mostly affecting the upper limbs with minimal or no sensory impairment.

EPIDEMIOLOGY

The prevalence of multifocal motor neuropathy is estimated at 2 per 100,000. Men are more frequently affected than women (2.6:1). Initial symptoms develop in 80% between the ages of 20 and 50 years, with a mean age at onset of 40 years. Lewis-Sumner syndrome occurs less frequently than multifocal motor neuropathy.

PATHOBIOLOGY

Multifocal motor neuropathy is considered an autoimmune neuropathy based on its clinical improvement with immunologically based therapies and because of a frequent association with antiglycolipid antibodies. Patients with MMN often have serum antibodies that react with ganglioside GM_1, and these titers decrease during effective treatment. GM_1 is highly represented in neural membranes at the nodes of Ranvier, compact myelin, and the motor end plate at the neuromuscular junction. A blocking effect on mouse distal motor nerve conduction has been induced in vitro by sera from multifocal motor neuropathy patients with and without high anti-GM_1 antibody titers. These data support the presence of serum factors responsible for conduction block in the sera of patients with multifocal motor neuropathy, although these factors are not invariably related to anti-GM_1 antibodies. The Lewis Sumner syndrome, however, is not associated with anti-ganglioside antibodies.

CLINICAL MANIFESTATIONS

The usual pattern is progressive, distal, asymmetrical arm weakness, often in the distribution of a single nerve. In a minority of patients, weakness may start proximally or in the legs. The disease will frequently affect other nerves, occasionally with a crossed distribution (i.e., one arm and the contralateral leg). Asymmetry and predominance of arm weakness may become less evident as the disease progresses. Localized muscle atrophy may be mild or absent in the early stage of the disease but can become prominent later as a result of axonal degeneration.

Fasciculations, cramps, and myokymia occur in patients with multifocal motor neuropathy and those with amyotrophic lateral sclerosis (Chapter 418), making distinction between the two disorders difficult. Marked asymmetry in the degree of clinical findings and electrophysiologic abnormalities between contiguous nerves is suggestive of multifocal motor neuropathy rather than amyotrophic lateral sclerosis. Cranial nerve involvement or respiratory failure as a result of unilateral or bilateral phrenic nerve palsy rarely occurs in multifocal motor neuropathy. The presence of sensory loss suggests Lewis-Sumner syndrome.

DIAGNOSIS

The diagnosis is established by the presence of multifocal, persistent partial conduction blocks on motor but not sensory nerve conduction studies. Lewis-Sumner syndrome has sensory loss as well as weakness, with conduction block in both sensory and motor nerves.

TREATMENT   **Rx**

IVIG (2 g/kg) is the initial treatment of multifocal motor neuropathy, and almost 80% of patients respond within a week. However, improvement is typically brief (3 to 6 weeks), so repeated treatments are required indefinitely. Clinical improvement is often accompanied by a reduction or resolution of the motor conduction block in some nerves, but it does not consistently correlate with a reduction in antiganglioside antibody titers. Patients may eventually become refractory to IVIG, and another agent may be needed, such as rituximab (e.g., 375 mg/m² weekly for four weeks) or azathioprine (2 to 3 mg/kg/day). Plasma exchange and corticosteroids are generally ineffective and have been associated with worsening neuropathy in some patients. Lewis-Sumner syndrome is considered a multifocal variant of CIDP and responds to the same treatments as CIDP.

PARANEOPLASTIC NEUROPATHIES

DEFINITION

Paraneoplastic neuropathies (Chapter 187) are a "remote effect of cancer" not caused by metastatic invasion of neural tissue; radiation therapy or chemotherapy; metabolic, vascular, or hormonal disturbances; or opportunistic infections. It is hypothesized that they are the result of host immune responses to a tumor antigen or antigens that are also present in neural tissues.

EPIDEMIOLOGY

Paraneoplastic syndromes occur in less than 1% of patients with cancer; peripheral neuropathy is only one of the paraneoplastic syndromes. Although more than 25% of patients with cancer have evident neuropathy on neurologic examination, the relationship to malignancy is unclear in most. Paraneoplastic neuropathy may develop before, during, or after the tumor is diagnosed. In certain tumors, neuropathies are distinctive and should prompt a thorough investigation for cancer. Small cell carcinoma of the lung (Chapter 197) is by far the most common underlying neoplasm, followed by carcinoma of the stomach, breast, colon, rectum, ovary, and prostate.

PATHOBIOLOGY

Subacute sensory neuropathy, the most characteristic paraneoplastic neuropathy, results from an immune-mediated ganglionitis that destroys sensory neurons in the dorsal root ganglia. Mononuclear inflammatory infiltrates composed of CD4+ and prominent CD8+ T cells, along with plasma cells, are found in the stroma surrounding the dorsal root ganglion neurons. Other findings include atrophy of the dorsal roots; loss of sensory neurons, which appear to be replaced by a proliferation of satellite cells (Nageotte's nodule); axonal degeneration; and secondary degeneration of the dorsal column of the spinal cord. Inflammatory infiltrates can also be found in peripheral nerves or muscle. Sural nerve biopsies typically reveal only loss of myelinated nerve fibers and are not useful for diagnosis.

CLINICAL MANIFESTATIONS

Subacute sensory neuropathy is characterized by subacute, progressive impairment of all sensory modalities and is associated with severe sensory ataxia and areflexia. Subacute sensory neuropathy may precede the diagnosis of tumor by months or even years.

At onset, patients may have shooting pain and burning sensations. Other symptoms include numbness, tingling, and a progressive sensory loss that may be asymmetrical. Symptoms usually progress rapidly to involve all four limbs, the trunk, and face. Findings may then stabilize, although by this time the patient is often totally disabled. Occasional patients have an indolent course.

Neurologic examination reveals loss of deep tendon reflexes and involvement of all modalities of sensation; large fiber modalities such as vibration and joint position sense are most severely affected. The loss of position sense may lead to severe sensory ataxia with pseudoathetoid movements of the hands and an inability to walk despite normal strength. Cranial nerve involvement may cause sensorineural deafness, loss of taste, and facial numbness. The frequent asymmetrical pattern of symptoms sometimes suggests a radiculopathy or plexopathy.

A paraneoplastic encephalomyelitis characterized by patchy, multifocal neuronal loss in regions of the cerebral hemispheres, the limbic system, the cerebellum, the brain stem, the spinal cord, and autonomic ganglia often develops in patients with subacute sensory neuropathy. Autonomic symptoms include impotence, dry mouth, and constipation.

DIAGNOSIS

The diagnosis is based on recognizing the typical neuropathy in the setting of malignancy. The results of routine laboratory studies are generally normal. The diagnosis is supported by finding serum polyclonal IgG anti-Hu

antibodies, also called antineuronal antibodies type 1, or by indirect immunofluorescence or immunohistochemistry and confirmed by Western blot analysis.

Subacute painful, asymmetrical neuropathy or neuronopathy in an elderly patient should prompt a search for carcinoma of the lung because small cell lung cancer (Chapter 197) accounts for more than 80% of the associated tumors. Subacute sensory neuropathy has also been reported in patients with adenocarcinoma of the lung, breast, ovary, stomach, colon, rectum, and prostate as well as Hodgkin's and non-Hodgkin's lymphoma. In patients with no evidence of cancer, detection of anti-Hu antibodies should prompt a computed tomography study of the chest with special attention to the mediastinal lymph nodes. The use of whole body positron emission tomography with fluorodeoxyglucose has been advocated for early diagnosis in patients with anti-Hu antibodies or clinical suspicion of subacute sensory neuropathy because it may reveal neoplastic adenopathy months before computed tomography or magnetic resonance imaging can detect them.

TREATMENT   Rx

Subacute sensory neuropathy responds poorly to plasma exchange, IVIG, or various immunosuppressant medications, even when such treatment is started early in the course of the disease, possibly before the loss of sensory neurons. Even successful treatment of the tumor rarely induces remission of subacute sensory neuropathy, but the symptoms may stabilize.

Other Neuropathies Possibly Associated with Cancer

SENSORIMOTOR NEUROPATHY

Sensorimotor neuropathy occurs in approximately 25% of patients with all types of tumors. The neuropathy can have an acute or subacute onset, with a progressive or relapsing remitting course. Because no antineuronal antibody has been specifically associated with these neuropathies, their paraneoplastic nature is not established. Severe or relapsing neuropathies often precede the diagnosis of cancer, but the search for malignancy is generally limited to a chest radiograph, stool samples for blood, and routine blood tests. There are no specific treatments of these neuropathies, and their progression does not necessarily correlate with that of the malignancy.

PARANEOPLASTIC VASCULITIS OF NERVES

A nonsystemic vasculitic neuropathy, which may also involve muscle, occurs with various types of tumor, including small cell lung cancer, lymphoma, and carcinoma of the kidney, stomach, and prostate. Neurologic symptoms may develop either before or after the tumor is diagnosed. The neuropathy is subacute and progressive and usually affects older men. Like many paraneoplastic disorders, these neuropathies often do not respond well to treatment, which is similar to that for the vasculitic neuropathies (see later).

VASCULITIC NEUROPATHIES

DEFINITION

Vasculitic neuropathies (Table 428-5) typically present as painful acute or semiacute axonal mononeuritis multiplex. There is acute motor and sensory loss in multiple nerve territories. The number of nerves involved may be extensive enough to make the distinction between a multifocal and diffuse neuropathy difficult. Occasionally, vasculitic neuropathy can present as sensory neuropathy, trigeminal neuropathy, compressive neuropathy, or autonomic neuropathy. Neuropathy can occur in systemic vasculitis associated with other organ systems as well as in nonsystemic vasculitis affecting just nerve and muscle.

EPIDEMIOLOGY

Systemic vasculitic neuropathy is more common than nonsystemic vasculitic neuropathy. Peak ages at onset of both are the fifth to eighth decades, but vasculitis can occur at any age. Neuropathy, particularly mononeuritis multiplex, is common in several forms of systemic vasculitis. Rheumatoid arthritis (Chapter 272) evolves into systemic rheumatoid vasculitis in 5 to 15% of patients, and vasculitic neuropathy will develop in about 50% of these patients. More than 50% of patients with Churg-Strauss syndrome (Chapter 278), 40 to 50% with Wegener's granulomatosis (Chapter 278), 35 to 75% with polyarteritis nodosa (Chapter 278), and most patients with mixed

TABLE 428-5 SYSTEMIC VASCULITIS AND NEUROPATHY

TYPE	SEROLOGY FEATURES	ASSOCIATED FEATURES	USUAL NEUROPATHY TYPE	NEUROPATHY PREVALENCE
Rheumatoid arthritis	RF 80-90%	Arthralgias, arthritis frequent; multiple organs	Mononeuritis multiplex and sensorimotor neuropathy	50% of patients with vasculitis
Churg-Strauss syndrome	c-ANCA < 30% p-ANCA < 50%	Eosinophilia Asthma	Mononeuritis multiplex	20% of patients
Wegener's granulomatosis	c-ANCA 75-90% p-ANCA < 20%	Pulmonary and renal	Mononeuritis multiplex	15% of patients
Polyarteritis nodosa	c- and p-ANCA rare	Multiple organs, 30% hepatitis B	Mononeuritis multiplex	60% of patients
Mixed cryoglobulinemia	No	Hepatitis C, purpura frequent	Mononeuritis multiplex	20-90% of patients
Sjögren's syndrome	α-Ro/SS-A 60%, α-La/SS-B 50%	Dry eyes, dry mouth; women 90%	Sensory	25% of patients
Systemic lupus erythematosus	ANA screen > 90%	Multiorgan	Sensorimotor neuropathy	5-20% of patients

ANA = antinuclear antigen; p- and c-ANCA = perinuclear and cytoplasmic antineutrophil cytoplasmic antibodies; RF = rheumatoid factor; α-Ro/SS-A and α-La/SS-B = antibodies to the Ro/SS-A and La/SS-B antigens.

cryoglobulinemia (Chapter 193) have neuropathy. Patients with Sjögren's syndrome (Chapter 276) are often initially found to have sensory neuropathies. Neuropathies are uncommon in systemic lupus erythematosus.

PATHOBIOLOGY

In patients with mononeuritis multiplex, axonal degeneration develops as a result of nerve ischemia caused by the vasculitic process. Immune-mediated inflammation and necrosis of blood vessel walls occlude the vessel's lumen, thereby resulting in ischemic damage. Small arteries or arterioles (50 to 300 μm) are most commonly affected, particularly those that occur in watershed areas between the distribution of the major nutrient arteries of proximal nerves. True nerve infarcts are rare.

The immune-mediated inflammation is associated with antibody-antigen complexes that are deposited in the wall of the blood vessel. Antibodies also bind directly to endothelial cell antigens. In both circumstances, complement is activated, as evidenced by deposition of membrane attack complex. Chemotactic factors then recruit neutrophils, which release proteolytic enzymes and generate toxic oxygen free radicals.

The sensory neuropathy of Sjögren's syndrome probably results from the infiltration of dorsal root ganglia by cytotoxic T cells. Some patients with systemic vasculitis have symmetrical neuropathies rather than mononeuritis. The pathogenesis of such cases is not defined.

CLINICAL MANIFESTATIONS

Patients typically have a relatively sudden onset of painful, focal or multifocal weakness or sensory loss. These symptoms reflect ischemia anywhere along the length of the nerve or nerves, generally in the lower extremities. Onset usually occurs rapidly (hours to days) as a result of the abrupt, ischemic etiology.

DIAGNOSIS

Nerve biopsy of clinically affected sensory nerves (sural, superficial peroneal, or superficial radial) is often necessary and is justified because therapy may be aggressive and long-term. Superficial peroneal nerve biopsy may be combined with muscle biopsy from the same incision. Pathologic features diagnostic of vasculitis occur in 60% of patients, and less specific features such as multifocal loss of fibers occur in others. Findings diagnostic of vasculitis include destruction of the vessel and inflammation within the vessel wall. Fibrinoid necrosis, vessel wall scarring, recanalization, neovascularization, and hemosiderin are common, but not essential, histopathologic features of vasculitis.

Although nerve biopsy is the gold standard for diagnosis, clinical, serologic, and electrophysiologic findings can suggest the diagnosis. For example, EMG and nerve conduction velocity studies can distinguish between mononeuritis multiplex and symmetrical neuropathy. It is essential to confirm nerve conduction velocity abnormalities in a nerve before biopsy, which is always required before treatment. An acute or subacute onset of asymmetrical weakness or sensory loss in the distribution of individual nerves suggests mononeuritis multiplex, particularly in the setting of a known connective tissue disorder. Systemic symptoms, such as unexplained weight loss and purpura, or constitutional symptoms, such as fever, myalgias, arthralgias, pulmonary disease, abdominal complaints, rashes, or night sweats, suggest systemic vasculitis in a patient with mononeuritis multiplex.

The erythrocyte sedimentation rate is usually elevated in the systemic vasculitides but is normal in nonsystemic cases. Perinuclear and cytoplasmic antineutrophil cytoplasmic antibody (p-ANCA and c-ANCA) suggests Wegener's granulomatosis (Chapter 278) or Churg-Strauss syndrome (Chapter 278). Hepatitis C (Chapter 151) is usually associated with the presence of cryoglobulins. Serum complement levels, extractable nuclear antigen, angiotensin-converting enzyme levels, serum protein electrophoresis, and HIV serology are generally indicated. CSF analysis is not usually helpful in cases of vasculitic neuropathy but may be needed to exclude infectious (e.g., Lyme disease [Chapter 329]) or other inflammatory causes.

Differential Diagnosis

Acute or subacute mononeuritis multiplex may also result from diabetes, sarcoidosis, Lyme disease, and malignant infiltration of nerves. Multifocal motor neuropathy with conduction block and Lewis-Sumner syndrome can resemble vasculitic mononeuritis multiplex. Sensory neuropathies similar to those in Sjögren's syndrome may occur in patients with diabetes, paraneoplastic syndromes associated with anti-Hu antibodies, and pyridoxine deficiency.

TREATMENT   Rx

Systemic Vasculitis

Corticosteroid therapy is used for most vasculitic neuropathies (Chapter 278). Oral prednisone (1 mg/kg) is appropriate for relatively mild cases, but intravenous methylprednisolone (1000 mg/day for 3 to 5 days) may be indicated as initial treatment in severe cases. Daily dosing is commonly used for the first 2 months or longer if the disease remains active. Subsequently, the dose is gradually tapered, with a transition to alternate-day dosing and discontinuation depending on the clinical picture and associated systemic features.

Corticosteroid treatment may be adequate for Churg-Strauss syndrome, but additional medication is generally needed in other forms of systemic vasculitic neuropathy. In most cases of Wegener's granulomatosis and microscopic polyangiitis, combined therapy with glucocorticoids and oral cyclophosphamide (2 mg/kg/day) or weekly oral methotrexate (7.5 mg/week) is used. Azathioprine (2 to 3 mg/kg/day) is also used.

Nonsystemic Vasculitis

Because patients with nonsystemic vasculitic neuropathy may recover spontaneously or have a relatively benign course, low-dose or alternate-day oral prednisone (60 to 80 mg/day) is often adequate therapy. Azathioprine or weekly methotrexate can be used as a glucocorticoid-sparing agent. Doses such as 60 mg of prednisone on alternate days, 2 to 3 mg/kg/day of azathioprine, or 7.5 to 15 mg/week of methotrexate, are reasonable starting doses that can ultimately be tapered if the treatments prove effective.

PROGNOSIS

Most systemic and nonsystemic vasculitis responds to treatment, and patients make at least partial recovery with gradual return of function after a static period. The prognosis of patients with nonsystemic vasculitis is better than that of patients with systemic vasculitis, with fewer episodes of nerve damage; the disease may be monophasic or relapsing remitting over a period of years, and most patients recover the ability to walk.

CRITICAL ILLNESS NEUROPATHY

DEFINITION

Critical illness polyneuropathy is an acute or subacute axonal length-dependent neuropathy that occurs in critically ill patients, not as a direct consequence of their underlying illness. The neuropathy is monophasic and recovers, at least in part, if the patient survives the underlying illness.

EPIDEMIOLOGY

The incidence of critical illness polyneuropathy is uncertain because of variable diagnostic criteria. Moreover, it frequently accompanies critical illness myopathy (Chapter 429), which may be indistinguishable from it. Critical illness polyneuropathy frequently occurs in patients with systemic inflammatory response syndrome (Chapters 106 and 108), a generalized inflammatory host response to severe illness; up to 70% of patients with sepsis have a length-dependent axonal neuropathy.

PATHOBIOLOGY

Nerve biopsies have identified perivascular lymphocytic infiltration, macrophages, and cytokines such as interleukin-1β, interferon-γ, and interleukin-12. Ischemia caused by a sepsis-induced abnormal distribution of capillary blood flow, nutritional deprivation, and hypoglycemia has also been implicated in critical illness polyneuropathy.

CLINICAL MANIFESTATIONS

The typical finding is rapid development of profound limb weakness days to weeks after acquiring a severe illness that necessitated intensive care unit admission and ventilator support. Respiratory muscles are often involved, and inability to wean from the ventilator is a common problem. Elicitable deep tendon reflexes distinguish critical illness polyneuropathy from acute inflammatory demyelinating polyneuropathy. Sensory findings are typically absent, but sensory testing is difficult to perform in severely disabled patients.

DIAGNOSIS

Laboratory studies are rarely helpful. CSF protein is normal, unlike the case with acute inflammatory demyelinating polyneuropathy. A lack of cells also excludes infectious or inflammatory disorders. Creatine kinase levels are normal, unlike critical illness myopathy, in which they may be elevated.

Motor conduction velocities are normal with reduced or absent compound muscle action potential amplitudes. Critical illness polyneuropathy is a predominantly motor disorder, so sensory conduction velocities and sensory nerve action potential amplitudes are normal. Abnormal spontaneous activity from axonal damage may occur within 1 to 3 weeks of onset. The presence of neuropathic and myopathic abnormalities suggests that critical illness polyneuropathy and critical illness myopathy coexist.

Differential Diagnosis

Distinguishing between critical illness myopathy and critical illness polyneuropathy can be difficult. Glucocorticoids and neuromuscular blocking agents predispose to critical illness myopathy (Chapter 429), which occurs in up to 5% of critically ill patients and is also manifested as rapidly progressive weakness of the limbs and diaphragm. Muscle biopsy and special electrical techniques are often needed to diagnose critical illness myopathy. If patients with critical illness myopathy survive their critical illness, their long-term prognosis may be better than that of patients with critical illness polyneuropathy.

Acute inflammatory demyelinating polyneuropathy can mimic critical illness polyneuropathy but can be distinguished by slow nerve conduction velocity and abnormal CSF. Acute motor axonal neuropathy or acute motor and sensory axonal neuropathy may be more difficult to distinguish, particularly if sepsis or another underlying disorder induces an abnormal CSF; nevertheless, the presence of antiganglioside antibodies may help distinguish these disorders from critical illness polyneuropathy. Myasthenia gravis (Chapter 430), botulinum toxin (Chapter 304), acetylcholinesterase inhibitor poisoning (Chapter 110), and other toxins can cause a similar clinical picture.

TREATMENT   Rx

The main treatment is directed at the underlying disease or diseases, such as sepsis. Glucocorticoids and neuromuscular blocking agents should be avoided if possible because both have been associated with critical illness myopathy.

PROGNOSIS

In-hospital mortality has been reported to be as high as 84% in patients with critical illness polyneuropathy, compared with 50% in similarly ill patients without it. Although most patients improve if they survive their underlying illness, up to 10% have persistent severe limb weakness and are ventilator dependent. Most patients have at least some evidence of weakness 2 years after discharge.

DIABETIC AND OTHER METABOLIC NEUROPATHIES

DEFINITION

Diabetic peripheral neuropathies can be separated into two large groups: (1) symmetrical, predominantly sensory or autonomic neuropathies (or both), and (2) asymmetrical mononeuropathies or plexopathies.

EPIDEMIOLOGY

Diabetes (Chapter 236) is the most common cause of neuropathy in the Western world. Diabetic neuropathy occurs in 8 to 70% of patients with diabetes, depending on the criteria used to diagnose neuropathy, and patients with retinopathy or overt albuminuria are more than twice as likely to have neuropathy. Distal symmetrical polyneuropathies are the most common diabetic neuropathy, but distal autonomic neuropathy is also common. For example, impotence develops in 20 to 60% of diabetic men, but widespread autonomic dysfunction develops in less than 5% of diabetic patients.

PATHOBIOLOGY

Distal Symmetrical Polyneuropathy and Autonomic Neuropathy

The pathogenesis of distal symmetrical polyneuropathy and autonomic neuropathy involves both microvascular and metabolic abnormalities, with a causal link between increased blood glucose levels and the development and progression of diabetic neuropathy. The mechanisms by which hyperglycemia causes nerve dysfunction may include activation of the polyol pathway, extensive glycation, altered diacylglycerol and protein kinase activity, and oxidative stress. Evidence from animal models suggests a role for neurotrophic factors, in particular, nerve growth factor, which selectively supports small fiber sensory and sympathetic neurons.

Acute Asymmetrical Neuropathies

The focal nature of these diabetic neuropathies is presumed to result from occlusion of endoneurial arterioles with resultant ischemic damage to the nerve. Changes suggestive of vasculitis are observed in epineurial and perineurial blood vessels in about 50% of cases, and perivascular lymphocytic infiltrates are common.

CLINICAL MANIFESTATIONS

Distal Sensory Polyneuropathy and Autonomic Neuropathy

Distal symmetrical polyneuropathy is typically manifested as insidious symmetrical sensory loss of small (pain and temperature) and large (proprioception) fiber modalities. Paresthesias or painful dysesthesias (e.g., burning or tingling feet) are common, although not invariable. An unsteady gait may be the initial finding. Weakness is usually minimal, even in the distal foot muscles. Ankle reflexes are generally absent, although patellar reflexes may be present. Feet and distal calves are often cold and erythematous. Slow distal proximal progression of sensory symptoms and signs is the rule. By the time that symptoms reach the knees, abnormalities often begin in the hands.

When sensory changes reach the level of the knees, symptoms of autonomic neuropathy often begin: gastroparesis, which may alternate with diarrhea, orthostatic hypotension, anhidrosis, cardiac arrhythmias, and impotence. Autonomic abnormalities can be the most disabling component of diabetic neuropathy.

Acute Asymmetrical Neuropathies

Asymmetrical acute neuropathies cause focal or multifocal symptoms, depending on the peripheral nerve or nerves affected. They are usually accompanied by acute pain in the afflicted region. The pain may be deep and aching or throbbing and lancinating. Most cases of acute focal or multifocal diabetic neuropathy eventually resolve, at least partially. Pain may resolve within a few months, whereas weakness may take a year or more to recover and may persist. Characteristic manifestations include the following:

1. Compressive *mononeuropathies*. Compressive neuropathies, such as carpal tunnel syndrome, occur more frequently in diabetic patients for unclear reasons. It is not known whether the response of carpal tunnel syndrome to treatment is as effective as when these mononeuropathies occur independently of diabetes.

2. Diabetic *lumbosacral radiculoplexus neuropathy*. Patients are frequently elderly with type 2 diabetes (Chapter 237). Asymmetrical pain in the upper part of the thigh is followed by progressive weakness and atrophy of the proximal leg muscles. Progression to the other leg occurs frequently. In about 50% of those affected, autonomic symptoms also develop, including orthostatic, gastrointestinal, and sexual dysfunction. Weakness may progress for up to 6 months. About 50% of patients require a wheelchair for ambulation, and many require opiates for pain. After the nadir, the patient will usually stabilize for several months, followed by progressive improvement. As many as 50% of patients do not regain full ambulation.

3. *Truncal radiculopathy*. An acute, focal onset of pain and sensory loss develop over a region of the trunk. In extreme cases, the abdominal wall muscles may become weak, resembling a hernia. As with diabetic lumbosacral radiculoplexus neuropathy, at least partial improvement will probably occur after a period of months, but the pain is difficult to control.

4. *Cranial neuropathies*: The classic manifestation is an acute oculomotor nerve palsy in which retro-orbital pain is followed by diplopia and ptosis. Pupillary fibers are often spared, distinguishing the disorder from lesions that compress the oculomotor nerve and cause a dilated pupil. Similar findings may occur with the trochlear (fourth nerve) or abducens nerves. Bell's palsy is more frequent and is less likely to involve taste in diabetic patients than in patients without diabetes.

DIAGNOSIS

Distal Sensory Polyneuropathy

The diagnosis of distal symmetrical polyneuropathy is based on identification of a predominantly sensory length-dependent neuropathy in the presence of either type 1 or type 2 diabetes. Neuropathy can develop independently of good control of blood sugar. Clinically similar neuropathies occur in patients with glucose abnormalities that are detectable only by oral glucose tolerance testing. Nerve conduction studies usually show low-amplitude or nondetectable sensory nerve action potential amplitudes; when detectable, sensory conduction may be slightly slow. Compound muscle action potential amplitudes are often reduced. Motor conduction studies are slightly slowed even if there is only minimal motor involvement clinically. Needle EMG in distal muscles typically demonstrates changes characteristic of chronic denervation. Occasional fibrillations and positive sharp waves may also be present.

Acute Asymmetrical Neuropathy

The focal neuropathies tend to occur in older patients with type 2 diabetes. The characteristic syndromes are diagnosed on the basis of their clinical manifestations and association with diabetes. EMG may demonstrate pronounced denervation in affected muscles. Concomitant evidence of distal symmetrical polyneuropathy is often present clinically and by electrophysiologic studies.

TREATMENT   Rx

Distal Symmetrical Polyneuropathy

An important treatment goal in distal symmetrical polyneuropathy is prevention of osteomyelitis and the resultant amputation of toes and feet. Because patients often do not sense injuries to their feet, diligence in foot care is important. Specific treatments to reverse or halt progression of the distal symmetrical polyneuropathy in diabetic patients are not yet available. Current therapy is based on control of hyperglycemia, management of symptoms, and foot care. Careful control of blood glucose (Chapter 236) remains the only treatment proven to delay the onset and slow progression of distal symmetrical polyneuropathy. There is, however, no hemoglobin A$_{1c}$ threshold below which patients avoid risk for neuropathy. For the treatment of pain (Chapter 29), combination therapy of gabapentin (usually starting at about 300 mg three times a day but titrating up to as high as 3600 mg per day) with either

nortriptyline (three times a day, titrated to as high as 100 mg per day or as tolerated)[6] or sustained-release morphine (15 mg twice daily) in low doses is effective when less aggressive treatments fail.[7] Pregabalin is effective at doses of 300 mg to 600 mg daily.[8] Duloxetine at 60 to 120 mg daily is another option.[9]

Acute Asymmetrical Neuropathy

Although acute asymmetrical neuropathy generally improves spontaneously, improvement may take months and remain incomplete. Intravenous corticosteroids, IVIG, or plasma exchange may improve the speed and extent of recovery, but these treatments are not of established benefit. Pain management is similar to that just described. Because the pain in patients with diabetic lumbosacral radiculoplexus neuropathy and truncal radiculopathy is focal, topical therapy may be effective.

INFECTIOUS NEUROPATHIES

Neuropathies Associated with HIV Infection

The peripheral nervous system may be involved in all phases of HIV infection (Chapter 401). The most common peripheral neuropathy is a distal, painful, sensory axonal polyneuropathy that is very similar to the toxic neuropathy caused by nucleoside reverse transcriptase inhibitors (NRTIs), including zidovudine, zalcitabine, didanosine, stavudine, and lamivudine. When an iatrogenic neuropathy is suspected, discontinuation of NRTIs may improve symptoms. Conversely, a neuropathy caused by HIV is likely to stabilize or improve with antiretroviral treatment.

Inflammatory neuropathies such as chronic or acute inflammatory demyelinating polyneuropathy can also occur in the early stages of HIV infection; the CSF cytoalbumin dissociation usually seen with these conditions may not be evident in these patients because of a mild CSF mononuclear pleocytosis. The response of these neuropathies to plasma exchange or IVIG is generally good. In later stages of HIV infection, cytomegalovirus (Chapter 384) may cause either an acute lumbosacral polyradiculopathy as a result of direct invasion of nerve roots or a mononeuritis multiplex through a vasculitic mechanism.

Neuropathies Associated with Herpes Zoster

Varicella-zoster virus (Chapter 383) usually remains latent in cranial or spinal ganglia after resolution of a systemic infection. Reactivation, which tends to occur in elderly persons and immunocompromised patients, causes a vesicular skin eruption accompanied by pruritus and dysesthesias. Herpes zoster normally undergoes spontaneous resolution but is frequently followed by a severe post-herpetic neuralgia, which is defined as pain persisting for more than 6 weeks after the rash appears. Early treatment with oral acyclovir (800 mg, five times daily for 7 days) may reduce both the duration of the acute phase and the chance of post-herpetic neuralgia developing, which is usually treated with symptomatic drugs for neuropathic pain (Chapter 29).

The use of concomitant corticosteroids in addition to acyclovir appears to reduce acute pain without exacerbating viral spread. However, corticosteroids do not appear to reduce the incidence or severity of post-herpetic neuralgia.

Neuropathy Associated with Lyme Disease

Borrelia burgdorferi causes a disease with three stages (Chapter 329). In the first stage, shortly after and in the same area of a tick bite, a nonpruritic rash (erythema migrans) appears and spontaneously disappears after a few weeks. The second stage is frequently associated with neurologic complications such as lymphocytic meningitis and focal and multifocal peripheral and cranial neuropathies; characteristic manifestations are unilateral or bilateral facial palsy and radiculitis. The third stage is associated with severe neurologic complications, including encephalopathy, encephalomyelitis, and a predominantly sensory axonal polyneuropathy. A lymphocytic pleocytosis in CSF and demonstration of *B. burgdorferi* infection in serum or CSF are the main laboratory findings. Treatment is discussed in Chapter 329.

Neuropathy Associated with Leprosy

Leprosy (Chapter 334) is the most common cause of peripheral neuropathy in developing countries, although it is infrequent in the Western world. Leprosy may be manifested in different forms, depending on the host's immune system. Patients with normal cell-mediated immunity are more likely to have a tuberculoid form characterized by hypopigmented skin lesions associated with decreased sensation. In patients with abnormal cell-mediated immunity, the more severe lepromatous form with large disfiguring lesions may develop. A mononeuritis multiplex pattern with prominent superficial sensory loss is the most typical clinical manifestation of leprosy.

If treated early, neuropathies in leprosy can improve significantly. World Health Organization recommendations call for combination therapy that includes dapsone (50 to 100 mg/day or 200 to 250 mg/wk), rifampicin (600 mg monthly), and clofazimine (100 mg/day) (Chapter 334).

Neuropathy Associated with Diphtheria

Although vaccination has made diphtheria (Chapter 300) rare in developed countries, it is still an important cause of subacute neuropathy in developing countries. Some strains of *Corynebacterium diphtheriae* produce a potent neurotoxin that causes palatal weakness, accommodation deficits, and extraocular palsies. This acute manifestation is followed by an ascending paralysis secondary to a demyelinating neuropathy that shares many clinical features with acute inflammatory demyelinating polyneuropathy.

The neuropathy caused by the neurotoxin usually resolves with resolution of the infection. The diphtheria organism can be eradicated by therapy with antibiotics such as erythromycin (2 g/day intravenously divided twice daily for adults) or penicillin (procaine penicillin G, 1.2 million U/day intramuscularly divided twice daily for 14 days). However, the neuropathy, as with other manifestations of the disease, generally requires treatment with diphtheria antitoxin, a hyperimmune antiserum produced in horses. Depending on the severity of the disease, antitoxin is administered intramuscularly or intravenously (80,000 to 120,000 units for extensive disease with a duration of 3 or more days) (Chapter 300).

● TOXIC AND DEFICIENCY SYNDROMES

In Western countries, toxic neuropathies are frequently the side effects of medications rather than a result of environmental exposure. In most cases, iatrogenic neuropathy is manifested as a length-dependent or "dying-back" axonal neuropathy. Treatment requires a correct diagnosis (Table 428-6) and discontinuation of the drug, but improvement is often slow and may take several months.

Compressive Neuropathies

Peripheral nerves are vulnerable to chronic compression in many sites: median nerve compression at the wrist within the carpal tunnel (*carpal tunnel syndrome*), median nerve compression in the upper part of the forearm, ulnar nerve compression in the hand (*cubital tunnel syndrome*), ulnar nerve compression at the elbow or wrist, tibial nerve compression behind the medial malleolus (*tarsal tunnel syndrome*), and peroneal nerve compression over the lateral fibular head.

CARPAL TUNNEL SYNDROME

Entrapment of the median nerve at the wrist reflects the limited space available for the median nerve because of the surrounding bone, joint, ligaments, tendons, and synovium. Repetitive motion of the fingers is an exacerbating element. Other precipitating factors include trauma, osteoarthritis, synovial cysts, myxedema (Chapter 233), and amyloid deposition (Chapter 194). Mild symptoms typically involve paresthesias of the first three digits, often occur overnight, and are relieved by shaking or elevating the hands. In more severe disease, objective sensory loss in the median nerve distribution, weakness of median-innervated muscles such as the abductor pollicis brevis, and

prolongation of nerve conduction across the carpal tunnel (prolonged distal latency) are characteristic. The diagnosis is supported by identification of *Tinel's sign*, in which tapping the carpal tunnel elicits paresthesias in the median nerve distribution, and by paresthesias produced by sustained flexion of the wrist (*Phalen's sign*). Treatment begins with splinting of the wrist in slight dorsiflexion during sleep. Injection of corticosteroids into the carpal tunnel provides temporary benefit. More severe carpal tunnel syndrome is treated surgically by release of the carpal ligament.[10]

Bell's Palsy

Unilateral facial paralysis of acute onset frequently occurs on an idiopathic basis (Bell's palsy). The diagnosis is one of exclusion. Facial nerve palsies also occur in the setting of *herpes zoster oticus* (Chapter 383), in which they are typically associated with otalgia and varicelliform lesions affecting the external ear, ear canal, or tympanic membrane. Facial paralysis of a lower motor neuron type can be caused by carcinomatous meningitis (Chapter 195), sarcoidosis (Chapter 95), Lyme disease (Chapter 329), and HIV infection (Chapter 401).

Primary tumors of the facial nerve can occur with apparently rapidly developing facial paralysis. Facial paralysis can also occur in primary *CNS disease* affecting the pontomedullary junction, such as stroke or multiple sclerosis (Chapter 419).

CLINICAL MANIFESTATIONS AND DIAGNOSIS

Most cases of facial paralysis are idiopathic. Patients typically notice facial paralysis on inspection in the mirror in the morning. Facial paralysis may be heralded or accompanied by pain behind the ear. The severity of paralysis varies widely.

TREATMENT

In a randomized trial, 10 days of oral corticosteroids (prednisolone, 25 mg twice daily for 10 days) administered early in the course increased the return of facial function from 63 to 83% at 3 months in patients with idiopathic Bell's palsy;[11] acyclovir added to prednisone is of uncertain benefit.[11] In severe cases, protection of the cornea from drying and injury is essential.

PROGNOSIS

The prognosis is favorable in most cases, but about 10% of patients achieve little recovery. Aberrant regeneration of the facial nerve can cause synkinesias, such as "jaw winking" (when the eye is closed) or tearing accompanying salivation ("syndrome of crocodile tears").

Trigeminal Neuralgia (Tic Douloureux)

Trigeminal neuralgia and other painful cranial neuralgias are discussed in Chapter 405.

1. Plasma Exchange/Sandoglobulin Guillain-Barré Syndrome Trial Group. Randomised trial of plasma exchange, intravenous immunoglobulin, and combined treatments in Guillain-Barré syndrome. *Lancet.* 1997;349:225-230.
2. Hahn AF, Bolton CF, Pillay N, et al. Plasma-exchange therapy in chronic inflammatory demyelinating polyneuropathy: A double-blind, sham-controlled, cross-over study. *Brain.* 1996;119:1055-1066.
3. Hughes RA, Raphaël JC, Swan AV, et al. Intravenous immunoglobulin for Guillain-Barré syndrome. *Cochrane Database Syst Rev.* 2006;1:CD002063.
4. Mendell JR, Barohn RJ, Freimer ML, et al. Randomized controlled trial of IVIG in untreated chronic inflammatory demyelinating polyradiculoneuropathy. *Neurology.* 2001;56:445-449.
5. Hughes R, Bensa S, Willison H, et al. Randomized controlled trial of intravenous immunoglobulin versus oral prednisolone in chronic inflammatory demyelinating polyradiculoneuropathy. *Ann Neurol.* 2001;50:195-201.
6. Gilron I, Bailey JM, Tu D, et al. Nortriptyline and gabapentin, alone and in combination for neuropathic pain: a double-blind, randomized controlled crossover trial. *Lancet.* 2009;374:1252-1261.
7. Gilron I, Bailey JM, Tu D, et al. Morphine, gabapentin, or their combination for neuropathic pain. *N Engl J Med.* 2005;352:1324-1334.
8. Moore RA, Straube S, Wiffen PJ, et al. Pregabalin for acute and chronic pain in adults. *Cochrane Database Syst Rev.* 2009;3:CD007076.
9. Lunn MP, Hughes RA, Wiffen PJ. Duloxetine for treating painful neuropathy or chronic pain. *Cochrane Database Syst Rev.* 2009;4:CD007115.
10. Jarvik JG, Comstock BA, Kliot M, et al. Surgery versus non-surgical therapy for carpal tunnel syndrome: a randomised parallel-group trial. *Lancet.* 2009;374:1074-1081.
11. Sullivan FM, Swan IR, Donnan PT, et al. Early treatment with prednisolone or acyclovir in Bell's palsy. *N Engl J Med.* 2007;357:1598-1607.

TABLE 428-6 TOXIC AND DEFICIENCY NEUROPATHIES
Associated with antineoplastic agents: vincristine, paclitaxel (Taxol), cisplatin, suramin, thalidomide
Associated with antimicrobials: chloroquine, dapsone, isoniazid, metronidazole, nitrofurantoin
Associated with cardiac medications: amiodarone, perhexiline, hydralazine
Associated with other medications: colchicine, tacrolimus, gold salts, phenytoin, disulfiram (Antabuse), pyridoxine (vitamin B_6)
Associated with heavy metals: lead, arsenic, mercury, thallium
Associated with chemical compounds: acrylamide, carbon disulfide, ethylene glycol, hexacarbons, organophosphate esters, Vacor
Deficiency neuropathies: vitamin B_1 deficiency, vitamin B_{12} deficiency, vitamin E deficiency

SUGGESTED READINGS

Brannagan TH 3rd. Current treatments of chronic immune-mediated demyelinating polyneuropathies. *Muscle Nerve.* 2009;39:563-578. *Review.*

Dworkin RH, O'Connor AB, Audette J, et al. Recommendations for the pharmacological management of neuropathic pain: an overview and literature update. *Mayo Clin Proc.* 2010;84:3-14. *Evidence-based review.*

England JD, Gronseth GS, Franklin G, et al. Practice parameter. Evaluation of distal symmetric polyneuropathy: role of laboratory and genetic testing (an evidence-based review). Report of the American Academy of Neurology, American Association of Neuromuscular and Electrodiagnostic Medicine, and American Academy of Physical Medicine and Rehabilitation. *Neurology.* 2009;72:185-192. *Review.*

Kanji JN, Anglin RE, Hunt DL, et al. Does this patient with diabetes have large-fiber peripheral neuropathy? *JAMA.* 2010;303:1526-1532. *Case-based review emphasizing the value of altered vibration and pressure sensation on the physical examination.*

Schenone A, Nobbio L, Monti Bragadin M, et al. Inherited neuropathies. *Curr Treat Options Neurol.* 2011;13:160-179. *Comprehensive review.*

429

MUSCLE DISEASES

PATRICK F. CHINNERY

DEFINITION

Muscle diseases, or myopathies, are disorders of skeletal muscle structure or function. Myopathies can be primary and occur in isolation, or they can be part of multisystem diseases that involve other organs.

EPIDEMIOLOGY

Many muscle diseases (Table 429-1) are genetically determined, with an autosomal dominant, autosomal recessive, X-linked, or maternal (mitochondrial) inheritance pattern. Precipitating environmental factors of muscle disease include recent infections, foreign travel, medications such as statins that may increase the likelihood of muscle pain, and alcohol abuse (Chapter 425). Exercise tends to precipitate symptoms in patients with metabolic disorders, whereas cold and damp conditions and a high-carbohydrate meal can precipitate weakness in muscle channelopathies. The prevalence of muscle disease, which is estimated to be 1 per 1000 people, includes acute or short-lived disorders (e.g., myositis owing to infectious or toxic causes; see later), or chronic inflammatory and genetic disorders that cause substantial morbidity over decades. Muscle disease can cause premature death owing to neuromuscular weakness and secondary chest infections or to involvement of other organs in multisystem diseases. Cardiac involvement, which is particularly common in muscle diseases, can cause life-threatening dysrhythmias or chronic heart failure.

PATHOBIOLOGY

The basic unit of motor function is the motor unit, which is defined as the anterior horn cell body, its axon, the neuromuscular junction, and all the skeletal muscle fibers innervated by the one axon. The number of muscle fibers innervated by each motor nerve varies, from a few (e.g., in muscles controlling very precise movements, such as extra-ocular muscle) to more than 1000 (e.g., large and powerful but less precise muscles, such as the quadriceps).

Skeletal muscle fibers are multinucleate giant cells that are the principal component of skeletal muscle. Muscle also contains fibrous connective tissue, blood vessels, and blood components, all of which can be involved in muscle disease. The muscle fiber itself contains interdigitated myofibrils that are composed of thick (myosin) and thin (actin, troponin, tropomyosin) filaments. The myofibrils are organized into a functional unit called the sarcomere, which is about 2 mm in length and is bound by the Z disc. Subcellular organelles between the myofibrils include mitochondria, which are the principal energy source, the endoplasmic reticulum, transverse tubules that communicate with the extracellular space, and vacuoles that contain glycogen and lipid. The muscle cell nuclei are found in the periphery, just below the plasma membrane, which is the sarcolemma.

Muscle function (Fig. 429-1) is dependent on a chemical energy source—adenosine triphosphate (ATP), which in the first 30 minutes of sustained activity is produced by the breakdown of muscle glycogen (glycolysis) and after 30 minutes by fatty acid β-oxidation and oxidative phosphorylation within the mitochondria. Muscle contraction is initiated by the release of calcium from the endoplasmic reticulum and transverse tubules into the sarcoplasm. The calcium binds to troponin, which interacts with tropomyosin and results in actin-myosin binding. The conformational change that results from actin-myosin binding moves the thick filaments relative to the thin filaments, and the Z discs are pulled closer together, thereby leading to muscle contraction in an ATP-dependent process.

The structural integrity of the muscle fiber is maintained by a network of interlinking protein fibers within the muscle, including the cytoskeletal scaffolding protein, titin. These fibers are connected to the sarcomere, to the sarcolemma, and then to the extracellular matrix and connective tissue. Dystrophin anchors the sarcomere to the sarcolemma through its interaction with several glycoproteins called sarcoglycans (α, β, γ, δ), dystroglycans (α, β), and syntrophins (α, β1, β2), which form the dystrophin-sarcoglycan complex that links to the extracellular basal lamina. The basal lamina contains several important proteins that, when abnormal, cause clinical disease, including collagen types I or VI, fibronectin, and laminin, which includes merosin and related proteins.

CLINICAL MANIFESTATIONS

Muscle diseases are often present with nonspecific symptoms, including fatigue, muscle pain, and generalized weakness. As a consequence, muscle disease is often overlooked in patients with multisystem diseases, or its symptoms are masked by other neurologic or systemic features.

History

Weakness is usually symmetrical. In the legs, proximal weakness causes difficulties in getting out of low chairs or a bathtub or in climbing stairs. Distal weakness can lead to the "flapping feet" characteristic of a bilateral foot drop or to frequent tripping over small objects, such as uneven paving stones or the curb of the sidewalk. In the arms, proximal weakness leads to difficulties with self-care, including washing, brushing the hair, or feeding. Distal hand weakness leads to problems opening jars or bottles, typing at a computer keyboard, or writing. Weakness of the bulbar muscles can lead to swallowing and speech difficulties, neck weakness can lead to a dropped head, and respiratory muscle weakness can lead to symptoms suggestive of nocturnal hypoventilation or respiratory failure.

Fatigue and exercise intolerance can be the presenting features of primary muscle diseases, but they also are common in many systemic and psychiatric disorders. In the absence of objective clinical signs, these symptoms are unlikely to be caused by muscle pathology.

Muscle pain can be difficult to distinguish from joint pain (Chapter 264) or fibromyalgia (Chapter 282). Diffuse, generalized, and persistent muscle pain is rarely due to muscle disease, and sometimes patients describe muscle stiffness as pain. Proximal muscle pain at rest may suggest an underlying inflammatory myopathy, whereas pain precipitated by exercise may suggest a metabolic myopathy. Pain beginning within the first 30 minutes of exercise suggests a disorder of carbohydrate metabolism; symptoms typically are short lived, and further exercise leads to their resolution (the warm-up phenomenon). Muscle pain developing later during exercise suggests a disorder of fatty acid β-oxidation.

TABLE 429-1	CLASSIFICATION OF MYOPATHIES

HEREDITARY

Muscular dystrophies
Congenital myopathies
Myotonias and channelopathies
Metabolic myopathies
Mitochondrial myopathies

ACQUIRED

Inflammatory myopathies
Endocrine myopathies
Myopathies associated with systemic illness
Drug-induced/toxic myopathies

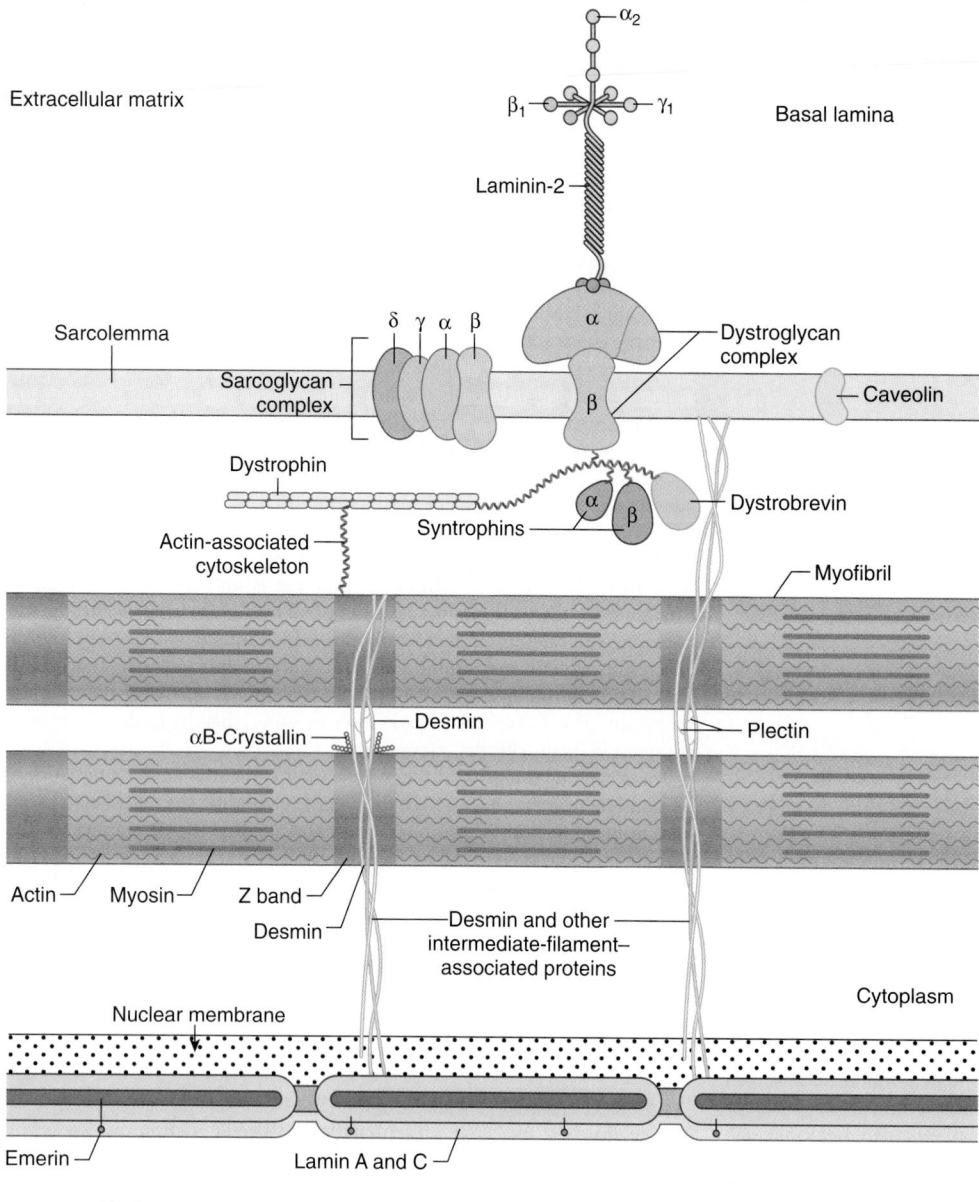

FIGURE 429-1. Muscle structure.

Muscle pain should be distinguished from muscle cramps, which typically affect specific muscles, persist for seconds or minutes, and rarely indicate muscle disease. However, persistent muscle contraction results in contractures, which are particularly seen in the myophosphorylase deficiency of McArdle's disease.

Muscle stiffness, which can be totally subjective and not associated with abnormal muscle fiber contraction, can occur in inflammatory, metabolic, and ion-channel muscle diseases and in nonmuscle diseases such as multiple sclerosis, polymyalgia rheumatica, and connective tissue diseases. Conversely, stiffness associated with weakness or an inability to move the affected muscle suggests myotonia. Myotonia can be painful (paramyotonia), painless, or associated with perceived stiffness if caused by a muscle channelopathy; it can affect limb, facial, or bulbar muscles and lead to persistent limb muscle contraction, eyelid closure, or dysphagia. Patients who describe their hands as "locking" but do not have objective myotonia rarely have a physical explanation for the symptom. Severe acute muscle damage, termed *rhabdomyolysis* (Chapter 115), results in myoglobinuria that presents as dark brown or red urine.

The family history should include questions about muscle diseases as well as systemic illnesses such as heart failure or diabetes that can be the clue to an underlying multisystem mitochondrial disorder.

Physical Examination

A full physical examination is critical to assess for systemic diseases with muscular involvement. The skin also should be evaluated for any signs of systemic disease, including the characteristic heliotrope rash of dermatomyositis (Chapter 277).

The neurologic and motor examinations should help distinguish muscle disease from nerve diseases (Table 429-2). Patients may have facial muscle wasting and weakness, ptosis, or dysmorphic features that lead to an instant diagnosis, such as the characteristic appearance of patients with myotonic dystrophy (Fig. 429-2). Proximal muscle weakness may be evident if patients push themselves up on their thighs or waddle into the consultation room.

Patients should be asked to rise from a low crouched posture and walk on their toes to assess calf muscle weakness or their heels to assess ankle dorsiflexion weakness. The posture should be examined, and the spine should be inspected for evidence of scoliosis. The spine and joints should be moved passively to determine whether there are any contractures, which are usually asymptomatic.

All muscle groups should be inspected for evidence of muscle wasting, hypertrophy, and fasciculation, which is the spontaneous firing of muscle fibers innervated by a single motor unit. Palpation of the large muscles occasionally reveals an unusual texture. The examiner should test for myotonia with both percussion (inability to relax the muscle belly after percussion with a reflex hammer) and grip (inability to relax the fingers from a firm grip).

Muscle strength should be assessed at the bedside (Table 429-3) while distinguishing proximal (limb-girdle), distal (in the legs and arms), axial, neck, orofacial, extraocular, and bulbar muscle weakness. Weakness is usually but not always symmetrical in muscle disease, and specific patterns of weakness can be highly specific for a particular diagnosis.

TABLE 429-2 CLINICAL FINDINGS DIFFERENTIATING MUSCLE FROM NERVE DISEASE

FINDING	MYOPATHY	ANTERIOR HORN CELL DISEASE	PERIPHERAL NEUROPATHY	NEUROMUSCULAR JUNCTION DISEASE
Distribution	Usually proximal, symmetrical	Distal, asymmetrical, and bulbar	Distal, symmetrical	Extraocular, bulbar, proximal limb
Atrophy	Slight early, marked late	Marked early	Moderate	Absent
Fasciculations	Absent	Frequent	Sometimes present	Absent
Reflexes	Lost late	Variable, can be hyperreflexic	Lost early	Normal
Pain	Diffuse in myositis	Absent	Variable, distal when present	Absent
Cramps	Rare	Frequent	Occasional	Absent
Sensory loss	Absent	Absent	Usually present	Absent
Serum creatine kinase	Usually elevated	Occasionally slightly elevated	Normal	Normal

Adapted from Goldman L, Ausiello DA, eds. *Cecil Textbook of Medicine*, 23rd ed. Philadelphia: Elsevier; 2008.

TABLE 429-3 UNITED KINGDOM MEDICAL RESEARCH COUNCIL SCALE

5—Normal power
4—Active movement against gravity and resistance (often subdivided into 4−, 4, and 4+)
3—Active movement against gravity but not against resistance
2—Active movement only possible when gravity has been eliminated
1—Observable muscle contraction, but not capable of initiating movement
0—No contraction

TABLE 429-4 GUIDING PRINCIPLES FOR ASSESSING MUSCLE DISEASES

1. **History**
   Age of onset (most inherited and acquired disorders have a characteristic age of onset)
   Rate of progression (acute suggests an acquired, often inflammatory cause)
   Fluctuating weakness (may indicate a neuromuscular junction disorder, metabolic muscle disease, or a channelopathy)
   Relationship to exercise (may indicate a metabolic myopathy)
   Muscle pain (may indicate inflammatory or metabolic muscle disease)
   Relevant multisystem involvement (may indicate a mitochondrial disorder or myotonic dystrophy)
   Family history (may indicate a genetically determined muscular dystrophy or myopathy)

2. **Pattern of weakness**
   Limb-girdle weakness is relatively nonspecific.
   Inherited disorders often have specific patterns of muscle involvement and are usually symmetrical.
   Fluctuating weakness may indicate a neuromuscular junction disorder, metabolic muscle disease, or a channelopathy.

3. **Testing**
   The serum creatine kinase may be normal.
   Electromyography is often normal in metabolic muscle disease.
   All patients should have an electrocardiogram and echocardiogram to look for cardiomyopathy and/or a conduction defect.
   Muscle magnetic resonance imaging is increasingly being used to guide the muscle biopsy or reveal diagnostic patterns of muscle involvement.
   Some inherited muscle diseases can be diagnosed clinically and confirmed by genetic testing without requiring other investigations (e.g., myotonic dystrophy; Duchenne's, facioscapulohumeral, and Becker's muscular dystrophies)
   Muscle biopsy will reveal the cause in most cases—it identifies specific inflammatory myopathies and muscular dystrophies and often provides diagnostic clues for other muscle and neurogenetic disorders.

FIGURE 429-2. Myotonic dystrophy in a 50-year-old man. His appearance is typical, with facial weakness, atrophy of the temporal muscles and sternomastoids, and frontal baldness, which gives a monklike appearance. (From Forbes CD, Jackson WF. *Color Atlas and Text of Clinical Medicine*, 3rd ed. London: Mosby; 2003.)

DIAGNOSIS

A systematic approach can help guide the diagnosis of muscle diseases (Table 429-4).

Serum Enzymes

The muscle (MM) isoform of creatine kinase (CK) is frequently elevated in patients with muscle disease, although the CK is often normal in metabolic myopathies and in chronic, slowly progressive myopathies. A mild to moderate increase in CK is also seen in patients with acute and subacute neurogenic weakness, including amyotrophic lateral sclerosis (Chapter 418). The degree of CK elevation can be a strong clue for a specific muscle disease in an appropriate clinical context; for example, calf muscle weakness and a very high CK (>1000 I/U) is suggestive of dysferlinopathy, and a CK of more than 20,000 I/U indicates rhabdomyolysis (Chapter 115). Alanine aminotransferase, aspartate aminotransferase, and lactate dehydrogenase levels, which are increased in liver disease (Chapter 148), also can be elevated in muscle disease, but the CK level usually exceeds the upper limit of normal by about ten-fold in muscle disease before these other enzymes can be detected in the plasma.

Neurophysiologic Tests

Nerve conduction studies (see Table 403-5 in Chapter 403), which identify focal or general disturbances of the conduction velocity or amplitude of the nerve impulse, are normal in myopathies. Electromyograms (EMGs) (see Table 403-6 in Chapter 403), together with nerve conduction studies, can distinguish neuropathies and disturbances of the neuromuscular junction from myopathies based on such features as prolonged insertional activity, myotonic discharges, rapid recruitment, and myopathic potentials, which are short amplitude, short duration, and polyphasic. Contractures are electrically silent on EMGs, but muscle cramps are associated with persistent bursts of motor unit activity. EMG changes can be highly focal, particularly in inflammatory myopathies, so the EMG can be normal in patients with muscle disease. Metabolic myopathies also are often associated with a normal EMG.

Imaging

Muscle computed tomography (CT) and magnetic resonance imaging (MRI) can show specific patterns of atrophy and the replacement of muscle with fat in some inherited myopathies. The MRI can also be used to guide the EMG or muscle biopsy if the pathology is patchy or focal, as in inflammatory myopathy. In specific circumstances, functional MRI is used to investigate suspected metabolic muscle disease, especially mitochondrial disorders.

Muscle Biopsy

Muscle biopsy remains a key investigation for patients with suspected muscle disease, although it has been replaced by molecular genetic analysis in patients with typical Duchenne's or Becker's muscular dystrophy. The biopsy can be the final step in discerning whether limb weakness is neurogenic or myopathic. In addition to the overall appearance, the size distribution of muscle fibers, the degree and distribution of atrophic fibers, the presence of necrosis or inflammatory infiltrates, muscle fiber regeneration, and the replacement of muscle with fat and fibrous connective tissue provide important diagnostic clues.

Molecular Genetic Tests

The widespread availability of molecular genetic testing has had a dramatic impact on the investigation of suspected muscle disease. Disorders that can now be diagnosed with a blood test include Becker's muscular dystrophy and several of the channelopathies. However, given the large number of possible genes, a systematic approach to the investigation of suspected muscle disorders is recommended. Furthermore, molecular diagnosis is currently not possible in some patients, and many of the tests are available only in research laboratories or expensive commercial laboratories.

Other Investigations

Routine hematologic and biochemical tests of liver and kidney function (complete blood count, sedimentation rate, and levels of alanine and aminotransferases, creatine kinase, and creatinine) can assess possible systemic involvement. The erythrocyte sedimentation rate and C-reactive protein level are elevated in inflammatory muscle diseases, and antibody studies (antinuclear antibodies, extractable nuclear antigens, rheumatoid factor, and antineutrophil cytoplasmic antibodies) are useful in patients with suspected autoimmune disorders.

In patients with dermatomyositis (Chapter 277), the evaluation should include an appropriate evaluation for a possible underlying paraneoplastic myopathy (Chapter 187). For patients with suspected metabolic muscle disease, useful screening tests include a fasting blood lactate level in patients with suspected mitochondrial myopathy and a blood acylcarnitine analysis in those with suspected fatty acid β-oxidation disorders.

● SPECIFIC MUSCLE DISEASES

Inherited Muscle Diseases

Inherited muscle diseases fall into four main categories: muscular dystrophies (Table 429-5), hereditary myopathies, muscle ion-channel disorders (channelopathies; Table 429-6), and metabolic myopathies (Table 429-7). Some diseases overlap these categories, such as myotonic dystrophy, which includes a characteristic muscular dystrophy, myotonic discharges indicating an ion-channel disorder on EMG, and secondary mitochondrial abnormalities in skeletal muscle suggestive of a metabolic component. Some specific gene defects cause specific phenotypes, now instantly recognizable at the bedside, but other phenotypes are caused by a range of different diseases. A confident clinical diagnosis remains challenging, even in expert hands, so a systematic approach is key to the investigation of these disorders.

Muscular Dystrophies

The term *muscular dystrophy* refers to a pathologic description of muscle fiber degeneration and abnormal muscle regeneration (dystrophy), usually associated with an increase in fat and fibrous connective tissue. From a clinical perspective, muscular dystrophies are a group of genetically determined clinical syndromes with a particular pattern of muscle involvement owing to known or presumed genetic defects. Although the molecular basis of common muscular dystrophies has been defined, new genes are still being identified.

BECKER AND DUCHENNE MUSCULAR DYSTROPHY

Becker and Duchenne muscular dystrophies are both due to mutations in the *DYSTROPHIN* gene, which is located on the X chromosome and determines

TABLE 429-5 MUSCULAR DYSTROPHIES
X-LINKED
Duchenne's/Becker's (dystrophin)
Emery-Dreifuss (emerin)
LIMB-GIRDLE
Thirteen different autosomal dominant (3) and recessive (10) conditions
CONGENITAL
Autosomal Recessive with CNS Involvement
Fukuyama's, Walker-Warburg, muscle-eye-brain
Autosomal Recessive without CNS Involvement
Merosin-deficient, merosin-positive, integrin-deficient, rigid spine syndrome
DISTAL
Autosomal Dominant
Late adult onset
Autosomal Recessive
Early adult onset 1A (Nonaka)
Autosomal Dominant
Early adult onset
OTHER
Autosomal dominant facioscapulohumeral
Autosomal dominant oculopharyngeal
Autosomal dominant myotonic dystrophy
Autosomal dominant myofibrillar myopathy
Autosomal dominant Bethlem myopathy

CNS = central nervous system.

TABLE 429-6 CHANNELOPATHIES AND RELATED DISORDERS	
DISORDER	**PATTERN OF CLINICAL FEATURES**
Thomsen's disease	Myotonia
Becker's disease*	Myotonia and weakness
Paramyotonia congenita	Paramyotonia
Hyperkalemic periodic paralysis	Periodic paralysis with myotonia and paramyotonia
Hypokalemic periodic paralysis	Periodic paralysis
Myotonia fluctuans	Myotonia
Myotonia permanens	Myotonia
Acetazolamide-responsive myotonia	Myotonia
Hypokalemic periodic paralysis	Periodic paralysis
Schwartz-Jampel syndrome (chondrodystrophic myotonia)	Myotonia, dysmorphic
Rippling muscle disease	Muscle mounding/stiffness
Andersen-Tawil syndrome	Periodic paralysis, cardiac arrhythmia, skeletal abnormalities
Brody's disease*	Delayed relaxation, no EMG myotonia
Malignant hyperthermia	Anesthetic-induced delayed relaxation

*Becker's disease, Schwartz-Jampel syndrome, and Brody's disease are autosomal recessive diseases; all other listed diseases have autosomal dominant inheritance.

the amount and structure of the dystrophin protein. Female carriers can develop milder adult-onset disease but can be very difficult to diagnose, especially if there is no family history.

Duchenne's Muscular Dystrophy

Duchenne's muscular dystrophy affects about 1 in 3500 males. About one third of cases arise from a de novo mutation without a family history. Most patients have a frame-shift mutation in the *DYSTROPHIN* gene with a complete loss of the dystrophin protein. The absence of dystrophin disrupts the mechanical link between the sarcomere and the sarcolemma, probably with a calcium leak that leads to muscle cell necrosis.

TABLE 429-7	METABOLIC AND MITOCHONDRIAL MYOPATHIES

GLYCOGEN METABOLISM DEFICIENCIES

Type II: α-1,4-Glucosidase (acid maltase)
Type III: Debranching
Type IV: Branching
Type V: Phosphorylase (McArdle's disease)*
Type VII: Phosphofructokinase (Tarui's disease)*
Type VIII: Phosphorylase B kinase*
Type IX: Phosphoglycerate kinase*
Type X: Phosphoglycerate mutase*
Type XI: Lactate dehydrogenase*

LIPID METABOLISM DEFICIENCIES

Carnitine palmitoyltransferase*
Primary systemic/muscle carnitine deficiency
Secondary carnitine deficiency
β-Oxidation defects
Medications (valproic acid)

PURINE METABOLISM DEFICIENCIES

Myoadenylate deaminase deficiency*

MITOCHONDRIAL MYOPATHIES

Alpers-Huttenlocher syndrome
Chronic progressive external ophthalmoplegia
Kearns-Sayre syndrome
Pearson's syndrome
Mitochondrial encephalomyopathy with lactic acidosis and strokelike episodes (MELAS)
Mitochondrial neurogastrointestinal encephalomyopathy (MNGIE)
Myoclonic epilepsy with ragged-red fibers (MERRF)
Leber's hereditary optic neuropathy
Leigh's syndrome
Infantile myopathy and lactic acidosis

*Deficiency can produce exercise intolerance and myoglobinuria.

CLINICAL MANIFESTATIONS

Duchenne's muscular dystrophy typically presents in young boys between 3 and 5 years of age with delayed motor milestones and proximal muscle weakness. The disorder is relentlessly progressive and causes a cardiomyopathy (Chapter 60) that can result in heart failure and fatal arrhythmias. Mild cognitive impairment is also a feature. By 10 to 12 years of age, most affected individuals are usually confined to a wheelchair. By age 20 years, most patients develop joint contractures and a kyphoscoliosis that lead to respiratory muscle weakness and eventual respiratory failure.

DIAGNOSIS

Affected individuals have a high CK level that is 20- to 100-fold the upper limit of normal from birth. EMG and muscle biopsy are abnormal, with characteristic dystrophic features and reduced size and amount of the protein on immunoblotting studies. However, these investigations are rarely needed to make the diagnosis because the *DYSTROPHIN* gene rearrangement can be detected in blood.

TREATMENT Rx

Management is largely supportive, including physical therapy to prevent contractures, management of the cardiomyopathy using β-blockers and angiotensin-converting enzyme inhibitors (Chapter 59), and noninvasive ventilation in later stages. Prednisolone (0.75 mg/kg/day) prolongs the period of ambulation and other functions in Duchenne's muscular dystrophy.**1** Creatine (30 mg/kg/day and sometimes higher doses) increases muscle strength and lean body mass.**2** Albuterol is of uncertain benefit, and calcium-channel blockers are not beneficial.

PROGNOSIS

Without ventilating support, patients usually die in their late teens to early 20s. With such support, patients often live well into the third or fourth decades before succumbing to pneumonia, cardiac failure, or gastrointestinal complications.

Becker's Muscular Dystrophy

Becker's muscular dystrophy is a milder form of Duchenne's muscular dystrophy due to a non-frame-shift mutation in the *DYSTROPHIN* gene. It has a similar spectrum of findings but a much wider variation in course of progression.

CLINICAL MANIFESTATIONS

Becker's muscular dystrophy typically presents in boys older than 5 years, teenagers, or even adults with proximal weakness and prominent calf hypertrophy. The clinical course is progressive, and cardiac features are frequent.

DIAGNOSIS

The CK is elevated, although not to the same degree as seen in Duchenne's muscular dystrophy. In about two thirds of patients, a mutation in *DYSTROPHIN* can be detected in blood. The muscle biopsy findings resemble Duchenne's muscular dystrophy but are less dramatic. On immunocytochemistry or on immunoblotting of muscle sections, the amount of the dystrophin protein is decreased.

Female carriers of a *DYSTROPHIN* gene mutation can develop mild symptoms with proximal muscle weakness and an elevated CK in adult life. Diagnosis can be difficult in the absence of a family history, and protein abnormalities are often subtle in the muscle biopsy.

TREATMENT AND PROGNOSIS

Management is largely supportive. Corticosteroids are rarely used. Careful cardiac monitoring is essential. Heart transplantation (Chapter 82) has been performed in patients with severe restrictive cardiomyopathy (Chapter 60).

Many patients have a normal lifespan, although some develop respiratory failure in middle age and have a shortened lifespan owing to respiratory complications. Heart failure and arrhythmias occur late in the course of disease.

EMERY-DREIFUSS MUSCULAR DYSTROPHY

Emery-Dreifuss muscular dystrophy is due to mutations in the X-chromosomal gene encoding the nuclear membrane protein emerin.

CLINICAL MANIFESTATIONS AND DIAGNOSIS

Emery-Dreifuss muscular dystrophy is characterized by progressive joint contractures, scapula-peroneal distribution weakness, and cardiomyopathy with a progressive cardiac conduction disorder.

The CK is often elevated but can be normal. The ECG shows conduction delay. The muscle biopsy shows dystrophic changes, and the protein emerin is deficient on muscle cell nuclear membranes.

TREATMENT AND PROGNOSIS

Management is supportive, with physical therapy to reduce contractures and cardiac pacing to prevent sudden death due to the conduction defect. Patients usually live many decades with appropriate supportive care.

FACIOSCAPULOHUMERAL MUSCULAR DYSTROPHY

Facioscapulohumeral muscular dystrophy, which is an autosomal dominant disorder with variable penetrance, affects about 1 person in 20,000 of the population. It is associated with a deletion of chromosome 4q35 in about 95% of patients, although the responsible gene has yet to be identified.

CLINICAL MANIFESTATIONS

The disease has a highly variable penetrance, ranging from severe proximal facial weakness in early childhood to mild, almost asymptomatic distal weakness presenting in late adult life. Some gene carriers never present clinically. The entire range of phenotypes can be seen in the same family. The muscle weakness affects the face, where it causes difficulty with whistling or smiling, and includes periscapular involvement that leads to scapular winging and to weakness of the shoulder girdle, biceps, and triceps. Distal weakness causes a foot drop, and proximal leg weakness is a late feature. Unlike other muscular dystrophies, muscle involvement is often asymmetrical.

DIAGNOSIS

The CK is usually elevated but can be normal. EMG shows myopathic features. Muscle biopsy shows dystrophic changes occasionally with an inflammatory infiltrate.

TREATMENT AND PROGNOSIS   Rx

Clinical management is supportive, and corticosteroids are of no benefit. Cardiac features are not prominent, and respiratory muscle weakness is a late feature. The prognosis is highly variable, depending on the severity and related age of onset. Many patients have a normal lifespan.

LIMB-GIRDLE MUSCULAR DYSTROPHIES

Limb-girdle dystrophies are a diverse group of genetically determined myopathies caused by defects or deficiencies of muscle proteins, often proteins associated with the muscle cell membrane and particularly the dystrophin-sarcoglycan complex. Although it is possible to identify some specific causes at the bedside, muscle biopsy, immunolabeling studies, and genetic studies are often required to make a precise diagnosis. Each form is rare, and management is largely supportive. The prognosis is usually years to decades after diagnosis.

CONGENITAL MUSCULAR DYSTROPHIES

Congenital muscular dystrophies are a group of rare autosomal recessive muscle diseases that present in childhood with hypotonia (floppy infant) and muscle weakness. The main differential diagnosis is spinal muscular atrophy (Chapter 418), although congenital myasthenia gravis (Chapter 430) also should be considered. Affected infants often have joint contractures, which can be severe at birth. Some congenital myopathies have a pure muscle phenotype, with limited disability and survival well into adult life. Others with central nervous system involvement may be fatal in childhood.

Myotonic Dystrophies

Myotonic muscular dystrophies are the most common inherited muscle diseases. The two main genetic causes, DM1 and DM2, are inherited in an autosomal dominant manner. Both forms cause multisystem disease and can be difficult to distinguish from each other. DM1 is due to an abnormal expansion of CTG nucleotide repeats in a protein kinase gene on chromosome 19. DM2 is due to an abnormal tetranucleotide repeat on chromosome 3.

CLINICAL MANIFESTATIONS

Classic myotonic dystrophy can be diagnosed visually owing to characteristic myopathic facies (see Fig. 429-2), frontal balding in males, nasal speech, and high-steppage gait due to the distal myopathy. Additional features include ptosis, proximal weakness of the neck flexor muscles, especially the sternomastoid, and proximal muscle weakness in later stages. Patients show percussion, grip, and eyelid myotonia (inability to open forcibly closed eyelids). Systemic features include premature posterior subcapsular lens cataracts, testicular atrophy, intellectual impairment, impotence, and hypersomnolence mediated by both central and neuromuscular mechanisms. Diabetes mellitus may develop later in the disease, and dysphagia and constipation are common. Progressive cardiac conduction defects lead to sudden death. Women who transmit DM1 have a high risk of having a child with a severe congenital form.

DIAGNOSIS

The CK may be normal or mildly elevated. EMG reveals myopathic features and myotonic discharges. A muscle biopsy, which is rarely required, will reveal myopathic features. Molecular genetic analysis of the DM1 and DM2 loci usually confirms the diagnosis.

TREATMENT   Rx

All patients should have regular electrocardiogram, echocardiogram, respiratory function, and blood glucose level monitoring and undergo sleep studies to detect nocturnal hypoventilation. Management is largely supportive. Physical therapy can help prevent contractures. Cardiac pacing is frequently required. Hypersomnolence can be treated with overnight positive-pressure ventilation and modafinil (200 to 400 mg daily in the morning) for the central component. Diabetes (Chapter 236) and cataracts (Chapter 431) are managed in the standard manner.

Other Inherited Myopathies

CONGENITAL MYOPATHIES

Congenital myopathies are a group of rare inherited muscle diseases that are generally less severe than congenital muscular dystrophies, both clinically and histopathologically. They often have characteristic morphologic features on the muscle biopsy, present at birth with hypotonia and motor delay, and are slowly progressive. Respiratory muscle weakness is common, and patients can present with ventilator failure at birth or insidiously in adult life.

Central core myopathy, which is a rare autosomal dominant congenital myopathy due to mutations in the ryanodine receptor gene, is associated with malignant hyperthermia (Chapters 427, 440, and 442). *Nemaline myopathies* are a group of diseases with characteristic "nemaline rods" apparent in the muscle biopsy. Different genetic forms have been defined, including mutations in the *NEBULIN, TITIN*, and *α-TROPOMYOSIN* genes. *Myotubular myopathy*, which is an X-linked myopathy defined by the presence of central nuclei within muscle fibers, is due to mutations in the *MYOTUBULARIN* gene. Patients typically have ptosis and ophthalmoplegia.

Myofibrillar myopathies are inherited muscle diseases characterized by the presence of desmin fibrils in the muscle biopsy. Other features in the muscle biopsy include the presence of vacuoles with blue rims and the presence of eosinophilic inclusions. Autosomal dominant or sporadic mutations in *ZASP*, a Z-line association protein, *DESMIN, MYOTILIN*, and *AB-CRYSTALLIN* have been identified. The phenotypes overlap, and patients typically present with very slowly progressive distal muscle weakness that cause a foot drop, pes cavus, and proximal weakness. Cardiomyopathy is common in desmin myopathy.

Other distal myopathies include *Welander's myopathy*, an autosomal disorder that presents with finger extensor weakness and appears to be largely restricted to families of Scandinavian origin. *Tibial muscular dystrophy*, which is an autosomal dominant disorder due to mutations in *TITIN*, presents with bilateral foot drop due to tibialis anterior weakness. *Nonaka myopathy*, which is an autosomal recessive disorder due to mutations in *GNE*, affects the post-translational glycosylation of muscle proteins.

Oculopharyngeal muscular dystrophy is an autosomal dominant inherited disorder due to a triplet repeat expansion of the *PABP2* gene. The disorder typically presents in late life (>50 years of age) with dysphagia and marked ptosis without ophthalmoplegia. Mild distal and proximal weakness occurs later in the disease course. Surgical correction of the ptosis often yields excellent results, but the dysphagia can be difficult to manage. Patients often have a normal lifespan.

Ion-Channel Myopathies

Ion-channel myopathies (see Table 429-6) are genetically determined muscle ion-channel disorders, with specific molecular causes but substantial clinical overlap.

CHLORIDE CHANNELOPATHIES

Autosomal dominant (Thomson's) and autosomal recessive (Becker's) myotonia congenita, which are due to a mutation in the muscle chloride-channel gene *CLC1*, present with painless myotonia, muscle hypertrophy, grip and percussion myotonia, and myotonic discharges on EMG. Patients usually complain that their symptoms get worse in cold and damp conditions and improve with exercise (the warm-up phenomenon). There are usually no cardiac complications. The myotonia responds to mexiletine (150 to 200 mg three times a day).[3] Patients usually have a normal lifespan.

SODIUM CHANNELOPATHIES

Mutations in the voltage-gated sodium-channel gene *SCN4A* cause a range of autosomal dominant phenotypes, including hyperkalemic periodic paralysis, paramyotonia congenital (Eulenburg's disease), and potassium-aggravated myotonia. Periodic paralysis is typically precipitated by sustained exercise, which leads to weakness during the rest period, or by a high carbohydrate meal. The attacks can persist for hours, during which patients can be quadriplegic with no tendon reflexes but normal sensation, normal eye movements, and normal respiration. The serum potassium level may be high during attacks. The physical examination is usually normal between attacks, although later in the disease course, some patients develop fixed proximal weakness associated with tubular aggregates on muscle biopsy. Patients with paramyotonia congenita have myotonia that paradoxically improves with exercise, is often painful, and affects the eyelids. For both phenotypes, avoidance of high carbohydrate loads and treatment with dichlorphenamide[4] (50

TABLE 429-8 SECONDARY CAUSES OF PERIODIC PARALYSIS

HYPOKALEMIC

Thyrotoxic
Primary hyperaldosteronism (Conn's syndrome)
Renal tubular acidosis (e.g., Fanconi's syndrome)
Juxtaglomerular apparatus hyperplasia (Bartter's syndrome)
Gastrointestinal potassium wastage
Villous adenoma
Laxative abuse
Pancreatic non–insulin-secreting tumors with diarrhea
Nontropical sprue
Barium intoxication
Potassium-depleting diuretics
Amphotericin B
Licorice
Corticosteroids
Toluene toxicity
p-Aminosalicylic acid
Carbenoxolone

HYPERKALEMIC

Addison's disease
Hypoaldosteronism
Excessive potassium supplementation
Potassium-sparing diuretics
Chronic renal failure

From Goldman L, Ausiello DA, eds. *Cecil Textbook of Medicine,* 23rd ed. Philadelphia: Elsevier; 2008.

to 100 mg twice daily) or acetazolamide (125 to 250 mg three times daily) are effective.

CALCIUM CHANNELOPATHIES

Mutations in the muscle sodium-channel gene *CNA4A* cause hypokalemic periodic paralysis, which is an autosomal dominant disorder that resembles hyperkalemic periodic paralysis, except that the episodes of weakness can persist for up to 24 hours. Avoidance of high carbohydrate loads and treatment with dichlorphenamide[4] (50 to 100 mg twice daily) or acetazolamide (125 to 250 mg three times daily) are effective.

OTHER FORMS OF PERIODIC PARALYSIS AND MUSCLE STIFFNESS

Periodic paralysis can occur secondary to a wide range of metabolic and electrolyte disorders (Table 429-8).

Mutations in *KCNJ2* cause *Andersen-Tawil syndrome,* an autosomal dominant periodic paralysis associated with mild distinctive facial features, including hypertelorism and low-set ears, and a propensity to ventricular dysrhythmias. *Brody's disease,* which is an autosomal recessive disorder due to mutations in the SR calcium ATPase gene, is characterized by exercise-induced muscle stiffness that is electrically silent on EMG. *Rippling muscle disease,* which is due to mutations in the *CAVEOLIN3* gene, is characterized by rippling muscles triggered by exercise or percussion.

Neuromyotonia (Isaacs' syndrome) is an autoimmune disorder associated with voltage-gated potassium-channel antibodies and is part of a spectrum of disorders including limbic encephalitis.

Metabolic Myopathies

Metabolic myopathies are caused by enzyme defects that affect the three principal stages of muscle metabolism: (1) carbohydrate disorders due to a defect of glucose-glycogen metabolism; (2) disorders of fatty acid oxidation; and (3) disorders of mitochondrial oxidative phosphorylation. Symptoms can be mild and develop in adult life but can sometimes cause rhabdomyolysis (see Table 429-7).

DISORDERS OF CARBOHYDRATE METABOLISM

Glucose and glycogen are the primary energy source for immediate muscle contraction, so defects of this metabolic pathway cause muscle pain, cramps, contracture, and weakness within the first 30 minutes of exercise, thereby leading to exercise intolerance and muscle deconditioning. Severe episodes are associated with CK levels higher than 1000 I/U, rhabdomyolysis, and myoglobinuria. Most diseases are autosomal recessive, although phosphoglycerate kinase deficiency is X-linked. The most common is McArdle's disease, and the others are extremely rare.

Mcardle's Disease

McArdle's disease (type IV glycogenosis, myophosphorylase), which typically presents with muscle pain or cramps after short bursts of exercise, leads to contractures and exercise intolerance. Some patients present with recurrent rhabdomyolysis. Persistent exercise beyond about 30 minutes leads to the "second wind" phenomenon, when symptoms subside as fatty acids become the primary source of muscle energy. Clinical examination and the CK can be normal between the attacks, although some patients develop fixed proximal muscle weakness with myopathic features on EMG. Histochemical and enzyme analysis of skeletal muscle confirms the diagnosis. Common founder mutations (e.g., R49X) are often found in blood DNA samples. Graded exercise and 75 g of oral sucrose[5] before exercise may improve symptoms.

Pompe's Disease

Pompe's disease (type II glycogenosis, α-1,4-glucosidase, or acid-maltase deficiency; Chapter 215) can present in childhood with proximal weakness, hypotonia, and a fatal cardiomyopathy, or in adult life with progressive ventilatory failure. The EMG can reveal myotonic discharges. Abnormal glycogen storage is seen in the muscle biopsy. Enzyme replacement therapy has been shown to be effective in children with the severe form.[6] The disorder can be diagnosed by measuring the enzyme activity in leukocytes.

DISORDERS OF FATTY ACID METABOLISM

Fatty acids are the principal source of muscle energy during sustained exercise, especially when the muscle glycogen reserves become exhausted after about 30 minutes of exercise. Fatty acid metabolism involves the transport of fatty acids from the serum into the muscle cell and into mitochondria, where key components of the β-oxidation pathway reside. Both carnitine and carnitine palmitoyltransferase are required to complete this process.

Clinically, disorders of fatty acid metabolism can present with a proximal myopathy, exercise intolerance, muscle pain, and rhabdomyolysis. Cardiomyopathy is an important component of some fatty acid oxidation disorders, and multiorgan metabolic crises, such as hypoketotic hypoglycemia, can occur along with neurologic complications, including a peripheral neuropathy.

Carnitine palmitoyltransferase I deficiency presents in childhood with an encephalopathy and liver failure associated with hypoglycemia and a high blood ammonia during metabolic crises. Despite the similar name, *carnitine palmitoyltransferase II deficiency* presents with muscle pain, exercise intolerance, and myoglobinuria, typically after a long period of fasting or sustained exercise. All standard clinical investigations, including the CK, EMG, and muscle biopsy, can be normal. The measurement of fasting acylcarnitines by tandem mass spectrometry on a dried blood spot is the key to making the diagnosis, and molecular genetic blood tests can detect common mutations in the *CPTII* gene.

Carnitine deficiency can be primary or secondary. Primary carnitine deficiency causes myopathy, cardiomyopathy, and encephalopathy in association with hypoketotic hypoglycemia, although pure muscle presentations have been described. Blood carnitine levels below the laboratory reference range reveal the diagnosis, although prominent fat deposition in muscle is another clue.

Many metabolic myopathies cause a secondary carnitine deficiency, including β-oxidation disorders, disorders of mitochondrial oxidative phosphorylation, and other systemic diseases. The accumulation of lipid within the muscle fibers leads to a lipid storage myopathy. Low carnitine levels can be detected in blood.

TREATMENT ℞

Both primary and secondary carnitine deficiencies respond well to oral carnitine replacement (200 to 400 mg/kg/day in divided doses). Modifying the diet to increase the intake of carbohydrates relative to fat can improve symptoms in carnitine palmitoyltransferase deficiency. Some patients have a multiple acyl-coenzyme A dehydrogenase deficiency (also called trifunctional enzyme deficiency, or glutaric aciduria type II), which responds well to riboflavin (100 mg daily).

DISORDERS OF MITOCHONDRIAL OXIDATIVE PHOSPHORYLATION

Disorders of mitochondrial oxidative phosphorylation (see Table 429-7) are among the most common causes of inherited metabolic disease. They can present with isolated muscle disease, but often they are multisystemic with cardiac involvement, diabetes mellitus, and both central and peripheral neurological features.

Mitochondria are present in every nucleated cell and are the major source of ATP, which is generated by oxidative phosphorylation, which in turn involves five respiratory chain complexes situated on the inner mitochondrial membrane. Mitochondrial dysfunction results in an energy deficit and, if severe, ultimately leads to organ failure. The genetic basis of mitochondrial disorders is complex because mitochondrial proteins have two genetic origins: mitochondrial DNA (mtDNA), which is maternally inherited, and nuclear DNA. Autosomal dominant, recessive, and X-linked nuclear genetic mitochondrial disorders have been described. Mitochondrial DNA disorders affect the structure or amount of the respiratory chain proteins. Both deletions of mtDNA and point mutations of mtDNA are important causes of disease. Nuclear genetic disorders can affect the proteins, the assembly of the respiratory chain, or the maintenance of mtDNA.

CLINICAL MANIFESTATIONS

Mitochondrial diseases should be considered in all patients with a complex, multisystemic myopathy, especially patients with neuromuscular, ocular, and endocrine involvement. The myopathy is often only a minor feature. Although the list of mitochondrial disorders is extensive, they can be divided into defined clinical syndromes, or ill-defined multisystem disorders.

Mitochondrial encephalomyopathy with lactic acidosis and strokelike episodes is usually due to a specific point mutation of mtDNA (m.3243A>G). Patients can have myopathy, cardiomyopathy, encephalopathy, complicated migraine, seizures, encephalopathy, and attacks superficially resembling stroke. Some patients have one or only a few of these features, some have a more limited phenotype with only diabetes and deafness, and some have an isolated cardiomyopathy.

Myoclonic epilepsy with ragged-red fibers presents with a proximal myopathy associated with slowly progressive degenerative ataxia, epilepsy, myoclonus, and peripheral neuropathy; it is usually caused by a point mutation of mtDNA (m.8344A>G).

Leber hereditary optic neuropathy predominantly affects young adult males who have a history of subacute bilateral visual failure affecting both eyes within 2 to 3 months; more than 95% of cases have mtDNA point mutations in m.3460G>A, m.11778G>A, or m.14484T>C.

Chronic progressive external ophthalmoplegia with ptosis and the gradual limitation of eye movements is seen in up to 20% of mitochondrial disorders. About 95% of patients have sporadic mtDNA point mutations or deletions, but the disease can also be inherited as either an autosomal dominant or recessive trait. This disease can occur in isolation, with a proximal myopathy, or with ataxia, diabetes, deafness, and cardiac conduction block (Kearns-Sayre syndrome).

Mitochondrial disorders in children are invariably severe and result in premature death as a result of subacute necrotizing encephalomyopathy (*Leigh's syndrome*), hepatorenal failure (*mtDNA depletion syndromes*), cardiomyopathy, and severe lactic acidosis. Children with *Pearson's syndrome*, caused by the accumulation of mtDNA deletions, typically present with pancytopenia, sideroblastic anemia, and exocrine pancreatic failure. *Primary coenzyme Q10 (ubiquinone) deficiency* is a rare recessive disorder that can present with myoglobinuria and myopathy in childhood, or with ataxia and seizures in adult life.

DIAGNOSIS, TREATMENT, AND PROGNOSIS ◯ Rx

The investigation of suspected mitochondrial disorders involves a systematic screen for multisystem complications, especially diabetes and cardiomyopathy; muscle biopsy to look for histochemical cytochrome *c* oxidase deficiency or biochemical evidence of respiratory chain dysfunction; and molecular genetic tests. Some primary mtDNA defects are not detectable in blood, so skeletal muscle is often required for the genetic tests. For example, the diagnosis of ubiquinone deficiency can be made by measuring coenzyme Q10 in muscle.

Vitamins and cofactors, including thiamine, riboflavin, and ubiquinone (coenzyme Q10), have shown varying degrees of benefit in individual cases. Management is largely supportive, with surveillance and treatment of complications. Prognosis varies depending on the phenotype, ranging from the relatively normal life expectancy with chronic external ophthalmoplegia to a relatively rapid demise with Leigh's syndrome.

TABLE 429-9 TOXIC MYOPATHIES

INFLAMMATORY

Cimetidine
D-Penicillamine
Procainamide
L-Tryptophan
L-Dopa

NONINFLAMMATORY NECROTIZING OR VACUOLAR

Cholesterol-lowering agents
Chloroquine
Colchicine
Emetine
ε-Aminocaproic acid
Labetalol
Cyclosporine and tacrolimus
Isoretinoic acid (vitamin A analogue)
Vincristine
Alcohol

RHABDOMYOLYSIS AND MYOGLOBINURIA

Cholesterol-lowering drugs
Alcohol
Heroin
Amphetamine
Toluene
Cocaine
ε-Aminocaproic acid
Pentazocine
Phencyclidine

MALIGNANT HYPERTHERMIA

Halothane
Ethylene
Diethyl ether
Methoxyflurane
Ethyl chloride
Trichloroethylene
Gallamine
Succinylcholine

MITOCHONDRIAL

Zidovudine

MYOTONIA

2,4-D-Chlorophenoxyacetic acid
Anthracene-9-carboxycyclic acid
Cholesterol-lowering drugs
Chloroquine
Cyclosporine

MYOSIN LOSS

Nondepolarizing neuromuscular blocking agents
Intravenous glucocorticoids

From Goldman L, Ausiello DA, eds. *Cecil Textbook of Medicine*, 23rd ed. Philadelphia: Elsevier; 2008.

OTHER METABOLIC AND TOXIC MYOPATHIES

Myopathy can complicate many metabolic disorders, including hypothyroidism (Chapter 233), Addison's disease (Chapter 234), Conn's syndrome, hyperparathyroidism (Chapter 253), vitamin D deficiency (Chapter 252), and liver and renal failure (Chapters 132 and 157). The myopathy is often subtle, the CK level and EMG are often normal, and the muscle biopsy may be nonspecifically abnormal.

Many drugs cause myopathies (Table 429-9) with proximal muscle weakness, muscle pain, and exercise intolerance. The CK and EMG can be normal, and muscle biopsy findings may be nonspecific. Often the diagnosis is reached only after removal of the toxic agent leads to a resolution of symptoms. Statins can cause muscle pain and, rarely, myoglobinuria.

● INFLAMMATORY MUSCLE DISEASES

Inflammatory myopathies are a heterogeneous group of acquired muscle diseases (Table 429-10). Most patients present with muscle weakness, with or without pain, and exercise intolerance. Most patients have an elevated CK, abnormal EMG, abnormal muscle MRI, and an inflammatory infiltrate on muscle biopsy. However, the inflammatory process can be patchy and missed

TABLE 429-10 IDIOPATHIC INFLAMMATORY MYOPATHIES: CLINICAL AND LABORATORY FEATURES

	SEX	TYPICAL AGE AT ONSET	RASH	PATTERN OF WEAKNESS	CK LEVEL	MUSCLE BIOPSY	RESPONSE TO IMMUNOSUPPRESSIVE THERAPY	COMMON ASSOCIATED CONDITIONS
Dermatomyositis	F > M	Childhood and adult	Yes	Proximal > distal	Increased (up to 50× normal)	Perimysial and perivascular inflammation; CD4+ T cells, B cells; MAC, Ig, C deposition on vessels	Yes	Myocarditis, interstitial lung disease, vasculitis, other connective tissue diseases, malignancy
Polymyositis	F > M	Adult	No	Proximal > distal	Increased (up to 50× normal)	Endomysial inflammation; CD8+ T cells, macros	Yes	Myocarditis, interstitial lung disease, other connective tissue diseases; ? malignancy
Inclusion body myositis	M > F	Elderly (>50 yr)	No	Proximal = distal; predilection for finger/wrist flexors, knee extensors	Increased (<10× normal)	Endomysial inflammation; CD8+ T cells, macros; rimmed vacuoles; amyloid deposits; EM: 15- to 18-nm tubulofilaments	No	Neuropathy

C = complement; CK = creatine kinase; F = female; Ig = immunoglobulin; M = male; MAC = membrane attack complex; macros = macrophages.
From Goldman L, Ausiello DA, eds. *Cecil Textbook of Medicine,* 23rd ed. Philadelphia: Elsevier; 2008.

TABLE 429-11 CLASSIFICATION OF INFLAMMATORY MYOPATHIES

IDIOPATHIC

Polymyositis
Dermatomyositis
Inclusion body myositis
Overlap syndromes with other connective tissue disease (scleroderma, systemic lupus erythematosus, mixed connective tissue disease, Sjögren's syndrome, rheumatoid arthritis, polyarteritis nodosa)
Sarcoidosis and other granulomatous myositis
Behçet's syndrome
Inflammatory myopathies and eosinophilia
   Eosinophilic polymyositis
   Diffuse fasciitis with eosinophilia
Focal myositis
Myositis ossificans

INFECTIOUS

Bacterial: *Staphylococcus aureus*, streptococci, *Escherichia coli*, *Yersinia* sp., *Legionella* sp., gas gangrene (*Clostridium welchii*), leprous myositis, Lyme disease (*Borrelia burgdorferi*)
Viral: acute myositis after influenza or other viral infections (adenovirus, coxsackievirus, echovirus, parainfluenza virus, Epstein-Barr virus, arbovirus, cytomegalovirus), retrovirus-related myopathies (HIV, HTLV-1), hepatitis B and C
Parasitic: trichinosis (*Trichinella spiralis*), toxoplasmosis (*Toxoplasma gondii*), cysticercosis, sarcosporidiosis, trypanosomiasis (*Taenia solium*)
Fungal: *Candida, Cryptococcus,* sporotrichosis, actinomycosis, histoplasmosis

HIV = human immunodeficiency virus; HTLV-1 = human T-lymphotropic virus 1.
From Goldman L, Ausiello DA, eds. *Cecil Textbook of Medicine,* 23rd ed. Philadelphia: Elsevier; 2008.

microorganisms also cause myositis (Table 429-11), which rarely dominates the clinical picture.

1. Manzur AY, Kuntzer T, Pike M, et al. Glucocorticoid corticosteroids for Duchenne muscular dystrophy. *Cochrane Database Syst Rev.* 2008;1:CD003725.
2. Kley RA, Vorgerd M, Tarnopolsky MA, et al. Creatine for treating muscle disorders. *Cochrane Database Syst Rev.* 2007;1:CD004760.
3. Logigian EL, Martens WB, Moxley RT 4th, et al. Mexiletine is an effective antimyotonia treatment in myotonic dystrophy type 1. *Neurology.* 2010;74:1441-1448.
4. Sansone V, Meola G, Links TP, et al. Treatment for periodic paralysis. *Cochrane Database Syst Rev.* 2008;1:CD005045.
5. Vissing J, Haller RG. The effect of oral sucrose on exercise tolerance in patients with McArdle's disease. *N Engl J Med.* 2003;349:2503-2509.
6. van der Ploeg AT, Clemens PR, Corzo D, et al. A randomized study of alglucosidase alfa in late-onset Pompe's disease. *N Engl J Med.* 2010;362:1396-1406.

SUGGESTED READINGS

Dalakas MC. Inflammatory muscle diseases: a critical review on pathogenesis and therapies. *Curr Opin Pharmacol.* 2010;10:346-352. *Review emphasizing dermatomyositis, polymyositis, necrotizing myositis, and inclusion body myositis.*
Rider LG, Miller FW. Deciphering the clinical presentations, pathogenesis, and treatment of the idiopathic inflammatory myopathies. *JAMA.* 2011;305:183-190. *Case-based review.*
Rocha CT, Hoffman EP. Limb-girdle and congenital muscular dystrophies: current diagnostics, management, and emerging technologies. *Curr Neurol Neurosci Rep.* 2010;10:267-276. *Review including the potential usefulness of DNA sequencing technologies and potential new therapies.*
Selcen D. Myofibrillar myopathies. *Neuromuscul Disord.* 2011;21:161-171. *Review.*
Turner C, Hilton-Jones D. The myotonic dystrophies: diagnosis and management. *J Neurol Neurosurg Psychiatry.* 2010;81:358-367. *Review.*

on the EMG and the muscle biopsy. Similarly, a short period of corticosteroid treatment can mask the findings.

Inclusion body myositis is the most common inflammatory myopathy presenting in men older than 50 years. It typically begins insidiously with proximal weakness and then evolves to affect the quadriceps, the long finger flexors in the arms, and the tibialis anterior, where it results in a foot drop. The signs are often asymmetrical. Bulbar and respiratory muscle weakness occur later in the disease course, which is usually refractory to immunomodulatory therapy. No treatment has been proved to influence the disease's slow progression, with significant disability resulting within 5 years.

Polymyositis, Dermatomyositis, and Other Inflammatory Myopathies

Polymyositis and dermatomyositis are covered in Chapter 277. Systemic lupus erythematosus (Chapter 274), mixed connective tissue disease (Chapter 278), Sjögren's syndrome (Chapter 276), and rheumatoid arthritis (Chapter 272) can cause an inflammatory myopathy, as can sarcoidosis (Chapter 95). Systemic viral illnesses frequently cause muscle pain and an elevated CK, which are rarely a major clinical concern. Other

430

DISORDERS OF NEUROMUSCULAR TRANSMISSION

ANGELA VINCENT AND AMELIA EVOLI

DEFINITION

Neuromuscular transmission depends on the release of acetylcholine from synaptic vesicles that are stored in the terminal boutons of the motor nerve axon (Fig. 430-1). Invasion of the motor nerve terminal by the action potential opens voltage-gated calcium channels, resulting in the Ca^{2+}-dependent

FIGURE 430-1. Diagrammatic representation of the neuromuscular junction, indicating the ion channels, receptors, enzymes, and associated proteins that are the most frequent targets for autoimmune diseases *(left)* or mutations in genetic diseases *(right)*. The acetylcholine receptor exists in fetal and adult isoforms as illustrated at *top left*. The replacement of the fetal form by the adult form takes place toward the end of gestation in humans. Voltage-gated sodium channels are located at the bottom of the postsynaptic folds.

release of the vesicular contents into the synaptic space. Acetylcholine binds to the acetylcholine-gated ion channels (acetylcholine receptors [AChRs]) on the postsynaptic membrane, thereby leading to the opening of these channels and a local depolarization, the end plate potential. If the end plate potential exceeds the critical firing threshold, voltage-gated sodium channels (sited at the bottom of the postsynaptic folds) open to generate the muscle action potential that propagates along the muscle fiber and activates muscle contraction. The action of acetylcholine is terminated by its dissociation from the AChRs, which close spontaneously after 1 to 4 milliseconds; hydrolysis of acetylcholine by acetylcholinesterase; and acetylcholine diffusion from the synaptic cleft. Meanwhile, in the motor nerve terminal, the voltage-gated calcium channels close spontaneously, and the resting membrane potential is restored through the transient opening of voltage-gated potassium channels.

The extent to which the amplitude of the end plate potential exceeds the threshold for activation of the voltage-gated sodium channels is called the safety factor. In healthy individuals, the amplitude decreases during repeated activity but does not fall below this threshold; thus, neuromuscular transmission is not compromised. However, if there is a an abnormally low end plate potential amplitude, failure of neuromuscular transmission may occur. Causes include defects in the release of acetylcholine, the postsynaptic response to acetylcholine, or the number or sensitivity of the voltage-gated sodium channels. Morphologic changes to the presynaptic or postsynaptic components or to the basal lamina between them may also influence the efficacy of transmission. Although myasthenia gravis and some neurotoxic envenomations (Chapter 113) are the most common disorders of neuromuscular transmission, a number of conditions have been implicated (Table 430-1).

AUTOIMMUNE DISEASES
Myasthenia Gravis

EPIDEMIOLOGY

Myasthenia is the most common disorder of neuromuscular transmission, with a prevalence of about 15 per 100,000 in Western countries. All races can be affected. It can occur at any age from about year 1 onward, with a small peak in the third decade. It also increasingly is being recognized at later ages, with an annual incidence rising above 5 per 100,000 in individuals older than 70 years, in whom it is important to differentiate from other causes of limb or bulbar muscle weakness.

Myasthenia gravis itself is heterogeneous and can be divided into different subtypes; the relative frequency of these different forms is not known, but relatively mild childhood forms are frequent in some Asian countries.

Neonatal myasthenia gravis, due to the placental transfer of maternal antibodies to the AChR or to the muscle-specific kinase, affects up to one in eight babies born to mothers with myasthenia gravis. Autoimmune myasthenia gravis must be distinguished from congenital myasthenic syndromes, which are caused by gene mutations.

PATHOBIOLOGY
Pathophysiology

Myasthenia gravis is the result of a defect in neuromuscular transmission. The postsynaptic response to acetylcholine, the end plate potential, is reduced so that the threshold for activation of the muscle action potential is not reached. At a severely affected end plate, this deficiency can occur at the initiation of contraction, but it is most common during repetitive activity when the end plate potential naturally declines. This phenomenon, occurring across many end plates within a muscle, is responsible for the decrement in the amplitude of the compound muscle action potential on repetitive nerve stimulation, a finding that is diagnostic of a disorder of neuromuscular transmission.

In myasthenia gravis, the reduced end plate potentials result from loss of functional AChRs on the postsynaptic membrane and also from morphologic damage to the membrane. This damage leads to loss of AChR-containing membrane and to simplification of the postsynaptic folds, which contain the voltage-gated sodium channels. The result is a raised threshold for generation of the action potential, thereby further compromising neuromuscular transmission. In most patients, these changes are caused by antibodies against the AChRs. The pathophysiology in patients without such antibodies, including patients with muscle-specific kinase antibodies, is not well studied.

Like most synapses, the neuromuscular junction is highly regulated. If the nerve is cut, leading to loss of neuromuscular transmission, the muscle responds by upregulating the expression of AChR that revert to a fetal phenotype (see Fig. 430-1). Alternatively, if the activity of the postsynaptic muscle decreases, the motor nerve attempts to compensate. Consequently, in myasthenia gravis, there is some increase in the release of acetylcholine from the motor nerve and an increase in the synthesis of AChRs in the muscle fiber.

Pathogenesis

Myasthenia gravis is an antibody-mediated autoimmune disease that is associated with other autoimmune diseases, most often thyroid disease, and, in younger patients, with an increased incidence of the human leukocyte antigen (HLA)-B8 and -DR3 haplotype that also is associated with several other autoimmune diseases. Anti-AChR antibodies act by three main mechanisms (Fig. 430-2). First, a few antibodies directly inhibit the binding of

TABLE 430-1 DISORDERS OF NEUROMUSCULAR TRANSMISSION

DISEASE	TARGET	PATHOBIOLOGY
AUTOIMMUNE		
Myasthenia gravis	AChRs	Antibodies to AChR in 85% reduce AChR numbers and EPP amplitude
		Antibodies to MuSK in 5-10%—mechanism not clear
Transient neonatal myasthenia	AChRs, MuSK	Maternal antibodies cause transient disease in neonate; not seen commonly if mother receiving treatment
Arthrogryposis	Fetal AChR	Maternal antibodies that inhibit fetal AChR function paralyze baby in utero, leading to joint contractures; very rare cause of arthrogryposis
Lambert-Eaton myasthenic syndrome	VGCCs	Antibodies to VGCC in 90% reduce VGCC numbers and ACh release and EPP amplitude
Acquired neuromyotonia	VGKCs	Antibodies to VGKCs in 40% lead to increased and spontaneous ACh release
GENETIC		
Acetylcholine receptor deficiency	AChR	Recessive mutations in AChR-subunit genes cause reduced AChR expression
Acetylcholine receptor deficiency		Recessive mutations in *RAPSYN* cause reduced anchoring of AChR on the postsynaptic membrane, or in *DOK-7* causing a synaptopathy
AChR kinetic abnormalities	AChR	Dominant or recessive mutations in AChR-subunit genes cause kinetic defects—"slow" and "fast" channel syndromes
Choline acetyltransferase deficiency	Choline acetyltransferase	Recessive mutations in the gene for choline acetyltransferase (*CHAT*) cause reduced ACh release
Acetylcholine esterase deficiency	AChE	Recessive mutations in the collagen tail (*COLQ*) that anchors AChE at the neuromuscular junction cause absence of AChE
Arthrogryposis, multiple pterygium, Escobar's syndrome	Can occur with rapsyn, δ- or γ-subunit AChR mutations	Fetal akinesia
NEUROTOXIC		
Botulism	Presynaptic ACh release	Botulinum toxin gains entry into the presynaptic motor nerve and cleaves proteins involved in ACh release mechanism
Envenomation following bites from snakes, spiders, scorpions, etc.	Varied sites of action	Neurotoxins specific for VGCCs, VGKCs, AChE, AChRs, voltage-gated sodium channels, and other targets are frequent in many animal venoms and generally inhibit function
Drugs and insecticides	Varied sites of action	Muscle relaxants and other drugs
		Many antibiotics and quinine-related drugs can alter neuromuscular transmission at high dose
		Organophosphates block AChE and have complicated acute and chronic actions

AChE = acetylcholinesterase; AChR = acetylcholine receptor; EPP = end plate potential; MuSK = muscle-specific kinase; VGCC = voltage-gated calcium channel; VGKC = voltage-gated potassium channel.

FIGURE 430-2. Mechanisms of loss of the acetylcholine receptor (AChR) at the neuromuscular junction. Antibodies can act (A) by directly blocking ACh binding or ion channel function; (B) by cross-linking the AChRs in the membrane, thereby leading to increased internalization and degradation; or (C) by complement-dependent lysis of the AChR-containing postsynaptic membrane. In myasthenia gravis, complement-dependent lysis is likely to be the most important mechanism overall. Interestingly, there is no evidence of complement-dependent mechanisms in either the Lambert-Eaton myasthenic syndrome or acquired neuromyotonia, in which cross-linking of the respective ion channels with increased internalization seems to be the main mechanism.

acetylcholine to the AChR and cause a pharmacologic-like blockade of function. Second, because of their divalence, antibodies can bind simultaneously to two adjacent AChRs, through the α-subunits that are present in duplicate in each receptor, to form AChR-antibody complexes that are internalized and degraded by the muscle fiber, thereby leading to loss of AChRs. Third, most of the antibodies are immunoglobulin G1 (IgG1) subclass, a subclass that binds and activates complement. As a result, the membrane attack complex is activated, leading to destruction of the postsynaptic membrane and probably causing the morphologic damage that is frequently seen. All these effects are strictly limited to the neuromuscular junction; the remainder of the muscle fiber is essentially normal.

The AChR antibodies are IgG, have high affinity, and are highly specific for the native human AChR. Although the antibodies are the effector mechanism for the loss of AChRs, their characteristics indicate that specific antibody production requires helper T cells that can recognize AChR epitopes. The

thymus gland, which is often abnormal in myasthenia, is at least one site where the immune response occurs. In early-onset myasthenia gravis, the thymus is often "hyperplastic," with numerous T- and B-cell lymphocytic infiltrates in the medulla. These infiltrates are very similar to the germinal centers found in lymph nodes, and some contain B cells that express surface immunoglobulin specific for AChRs. Plasma cells are also present and synthesize AChR antibodies. In the thymic medulla, muscle-like "myoid" cells have AChRs on their surface in both normal and myasthenic individuals; these cells probably provide the antigenic stimulus responsible for the germinal center formation and AChR antibody production in myasthenia gravis.

In late-onset myasthenia gravis, the thymus is mostly normal for age. In patients without AChR antibodies, the thymus gland is more likely to appear normal for age, particularly in patients with muscle-specific kinase antibodies. However, in patients without either AChR or muscle-specific kinase antibodies, a typical thymic hyperplasia is often present.

Thymoma

Thymoma occurs in about 10% of myasthenic patients, reaching a peak in middle age. Thymomas are epithelial cell tumors and correspond mainly to the World Health Organization types B1 and B2. The epithelial cells attract large numbers of T lymphocytes, which may be sensitized to the AChR in the tumor and then exported to the periphery. Rarely, myasthenia gravis arises after removal of a thymoma.

CLINICAL MANIFESTATIONS

Myasthenia gravis presents clinically with painless muscle weakness that increases with muscle use and improves after rest. In many patients, the weakness starts in the eye muscles, where it results in double vision and ptosis (drooping eyelids). In others, it may first affect bulbar muscles or limb muscles (Fig. 430-3). Virtually any skeletal muscle may be involved as the illness progresses. Typically, the weakness varies in distribution and severity from day to day or from week to week, and it is often worse in the evening. It may first appear following an infection. Established weakness can increase with anxiety, with infection, or with the menstrual period and tends to improve with rest.

Ptosis, which is often asymmetrical, and diplopia initially can be transient and first noticed while driving, for example. Severity can range from mild unilateral ptosis or minimal diplopia to profound bilateral ptosis, which obscures vision, combined with almost complete ophthalmoplegia. Bulbar symptoms include weakness of facial muscles with difficulties in closing eyes and a "snarling" smile, difficulty in chewing, nasal or slurred speech that can noticeably deteriorate as speech continues, impaired swallowing sometimes associated with nasal regurgitation of fluids, reduced tongue movements, and head droop related to neck weakness.

Limb muscle involvement is common, and proximal muscles are usually more involved than distal. Proximal weakness of the legs can lead to collapse when walking and can be misinterpreted as a functional (psychogenic) disorder. Weakness of elbow extension and of finger abduction may be prominent. By contrast, ankle dorsiflexion is rarely affected except in severe disease.

Respiratory muscle involvement is less common but can be life threatening, especially if associated with dysphagia. Selective involvement of the diaphragm can cause severe breathlessness in the supine posture. Wasting is uncommon but can affect the facial muscles and tongue, for example, in long-standing disease. Tendon reflexes are typically brisk. Bladder disturbances are rare, and sensory symptoms do not occur.

Subtypes of Myasthenia Gravis

Several subgroups can be distinguished on the basis of clinical and pathologic criteria and can help to inform treatment.

FIGURE 430-3. Marked ocular and facial muscle weakness in a young female with myasthenia gravis.

Ocular Myasthenia Gravis

Ocular myasthenia gravis is confined to extraocular muscles; if it remains localized for at least 2 years, subsequent generalized weakness is unlikely. AChR antibody levels are generally low and are undetectable in about 50% of patients. This subgroup rarely is associated with a thymoma. The neuromuscular junction of ocular muscles shows structural and physiologic differences from typical limb muscles. Ocular weakness is often the presenting symptom not only in myasthenia gravis but also in neurotoxin poisoning, for example, botulism (Chapter 304). Thus, physiologic factors or accessibility of the neuromuscular junctions of ocular muscles to circulating factors may make them particularly vulnerable to antibodies in myasthenia gravis.

Generalized Myasthenia Gravis with Acetylcholine Receptor Antibodies

Among patients with generalized disease and AChR antibodies, there are three clinical subgroups. Early-onset myasthenia gravis is more frequent in females and associates strongly with HLA-A1, -B8, and -DR3. The thymus is generally hyperplastic. AChR antibody titers are usually high and decline to varying degrees after successful treatments, including thymectomy.

Late-onset myasthenia gravis is becoming increasingly common with the aging of the population and, when associated with bulbar weakness, may be mistaken for amyotrophic lateral sclerosis (Chapter 418) or brain stem cerebrovascular disease. Among older patients, males are more frequently affected, and the thymus is usually normal for age.

Thymoma-associated myasthenia gravis is an important distinction because thymectomy or other specific tumor therapy is required. Most patients with thymomas and myasthenia gravis present between the ages of 30 and 60 years.

Generalized Myasthenia Gravis with Muscle-Specific Kinase Antibodies

About 15% of myasthenic patients with generalized symptoms do not have detectable AChR antibodies. A variable proportion of these patients have antibodies to another neuromuscular junction protein, the muscle-specific kinase. Muscle-specific kinase antibodies are mainly IgG4 and are absent or very infrequent in patients with AChR antibody–positive myasthenia gravis, patients with persistent ocular myasthenia gravis, and patients with thymoma. Muscle-specific kinase antibodies are found more often in younger females, including children, with marked ocular, bulbar, neck, or respiratory muscle weakness but are seen less frequently in older patients. It is not yet clear how these antibodies cause the neuromuscular junction defect.

Generalized Myasthenia Gravis with Neither Acetylcholine Receptor nor Muscle-Specific Kinase Antibodies

Some patients with generalized myasthenia gravis have neither AChR nor muscle-specific kinase antibodies. These patients can develop severe disease but usually respond well to treatment and may have low-affinity antibodies to AChR.

DIAGNOSIS

Diagnosis is based on the clinical features, serologic testing for specific antibodies, clinical electrophysiology, and, if doubt still remains or specialized facilities are not available, the clinical response to anticholinesterase medication (Table 430-2). Mediastinal imaging is needed to exclude a thymoma in patients with AChR antibodies.

AChR antibodies are present in about 85% of patients with generalized symptoms but in only 50% of patients with purely ocular involvement. In the absence of AChR antibodies, especially in subjects with generalized symptoms, testing for muscle-specific kinase antibodies is recommended. Both AChR and muscle-specific kinase antibodies are very specific, and their detection in symptomatic patients confirms the diagnosis.

The electrophysiologic abnormality is an abnormally large decrement (>10%) in the amplitude of the compound muscle action potential on low-rate (3-Hz) stimulation with increased jitter or blocking on single-fiber electromyogram (EMG). In patients with muscle-specific kinase antibodies, EMG abnormalities may be detectable only in facial muscles. These EMG changes are not specific for myasthenia gravis but can occur in any disorder that interferes with neuromuscular transmission.

Intravenous administration of edrophonium (Tensilon), a short-acting cholinesterase inhibitor, transiently improves myasthenic weakness but requires an appropriate medical setting, including resuscitative facilities and

TABLE 430-2 DIAGNOSTIC EVALUATION (EXCLUDES NEUROMYOTONIA)

	AChR MG	MuSK MG	SERONEG MG	NEONATAL MG	LEMS	CMS	BoTx	MM
Onset birth, recovery of muscle strength within 2 mo	–	–	–	+	–	AChR γ-subunit mutations, variable severity	–	–
Onset birth plus arthrogryposis	–	–	–	+	–	Rapsyn or AChR δ-subunit mutations	–	–
Onset at <1 yr and persistent	–	–	–	–	–	Any CMS Dok-7, rapsyn deficiency, and SCS may present later	+	+/–
Infantile apneas	–	–	–	+/–	–	Fast channel syndrome, rapsyn, or ChAT mutation		
AChR Ab positive	+	–	–	+/–	–	–	–	–
MuSK Ab positive	–	+	–	+/–	–	–	–	–
VGCC Ab positive	–	–	–	–	+	–	–	–
EMG decrement >10%	+/–	+/–	+/–	+/–	+/–	+/–	+/–	–
EMG jitter increased	+	+ Especially face muscles	+	+	+	+	+	+/–
Post-tetanic potentiation	–	–	–	–	+	–	+	–
AChE inhibitor response	+	Often weak	+	+	Often weak	Except *SCS, COLQ,* or *DOK7* mutations	+/–	–
Thymoma	+/–	–	–	–	–	–	–	–

AChE = acetylcholinesterase; AChR = acetylcholine receptor; BoTx = botulism; ChAT = choline acetyltransferase; CMS = congenital myasthenic syndromes; Dok-7 = downstream of kinase 7; LEMS = Lambert-Eaton myasthenic syndrome; MG = myasthenia gravis; MM = mitochondrial myopathy; MuSK = muscle-specific kinase; SCS = slow channel syndrome; seroneg = seronegative for AChR and MuSK antibodies.

the availability of atropine, because of the risk for adverse events and severe cholinergic reactions, including syncope. A test dose of 2 mg is given intravenously, followed 30 seconds later by 6 to 8 mg if no adverse event has occurred. The equivalent doses in children are a 20 μg/kg test dose followed by 60 to 80 μg/kg. Some patients improve sufficiently with the test dose that it is not necessary to give the full dose. An alternative pharmacologic test in adults is a single dose of subcutaneous or intramuscular neostigmine (1 to 2.5 mg) or of oral pyridostigmine (60 mg).

Differential Diagnosis

Congenital AChR deficiency syndromes (see later) should be considered in patients who have clinical and EMG evidence of myasthenia but are seronegative for AChR and muscle-specific kinase antibodies. Lambert-Eaton myasthenic syndrome almost always begins with difficulty in walking; ocular symptoms are rare, and specific laboratory tests are available (see later). The ocular muscle involvement that characterizes Miller-Fisher syndrome is more rapid in onset than is usual in myasthenia gravis and is associated with GQ1b antibodies. Mitochondrial myopathy may show signs that are similar to those of myasthenia gravis (e.g., asymmetrical ptosis and limitation of eye movements), and there may be increased jitter on single-fiber EMG, but this condition and oculopharyngeal dystrophy can be distinguished from myasthenia gravis by the nonfluctuating weakness and by muscle biopsy. In neurasthenia and chronic fatigue syndrome (Chapter 282), the laboratory tests for myasthenia gravis are negative.

TREATMENT   Rx

Most patients with AChR antibodies respond to oral pyridostigmine, 30 to 60 mg four or five times daily; in patients with mild disease, this dose may adequately control symptoms. Doses in excess of 90 mg are likely to cause gastrointestinal side effects, abdominal cramps and diarrhea, which can be controlled with oral propantheline bromide, 15 mg, or loperamide, 2 mg. Patients with muscle-specific kinase antibodies generally show an unsatisfactory response to pyridostigmine. In some of these patients, pyridostigmine, even at a low doses, can increase weakness and cause nicotinic side effects (muscle cramps and diffuse fasciculations).

Neonatal Myasthenia Gravis

Pyridostigmine, 3 to 5 mg, can be given every 4 hours to about an hour before a feeding. Close monitoring and respiratory support in a special unit may be required.

Ocular Myasthenia

Diplopia can sometimes be helped by the use of prisms. Ocular symptoms that respond incompletely to pyridostigmine are often improved or completely corrected by low-dose prednisone therapy (e.g., 5 mg every other day) increasing by 5 mg at weekly intervals either until symptoms are completely controlled or until a ceiling dose (e.g., 1 mg/kg) is reached. When remission is established, the dose can be slowly reduced (e.g., by 5 mg at 2-weekly intervals) until symptoms recur and then adjusted upward to define the effective minimal dose. Full withdrawal of prednisone is usually followed by a symptomatic relapse. Most centers do not recommend thymectomy for nonthymomatous ocular myasthenia gravis. In patients who fail to respond adequately to prednisone or who are intolerant of the medication, the addition of azathioprine (2 to 2.5 mg/kg body weight) or ocular muscle surgery is an option. However, the diagnosis should be reviewed in patients who show no improvement with high-dose prednisone treatment.

Thymoma

Thymoma usually represents an absolute indication for surgery, but removal of the tumor typically does not result in improvement in muscle weakness. If the tumor is found to be locally invasive, postoperative radiotherapy is indicated. If tumor spread is more extensive, chemotherapy is performed, mainly with cisplatin-containing regimens.

Generalized Nonthymomatous Myasthenia Gravis

When generalized symptoms are inadequately controlled by pyridostigmine, thymectomy is often recommended empirically even for patients without a thymoma, especially patients younger than 45 years. Despite the absence of trials and no clear consensus from observational data, thymectomy in early-onset patients with anti-AChR antibodies appears to be associated with an increased rate of remission. By comparison, thymectomy does not appear to influence the course of the disease in patients who have anti-MuSK antibodies and in whom the thymus is generally devoid of hyperplastic changes. Most patients respond to alternate-day prednisone, started at a low dose (e.g., 10 mg every other day) and increasing by 5 to 10 mg per dose to 1.0 to 1.5 mg/kg.■ Because starting prednisone can temporarily exacerbate the disease, patients are usually best managed in the hospital, especially if they have bulbar or respiratory muscle involvement. When remission is established, the dose can be reduced by 5 to 10 mg every 2 weeks (or more slowly) until symptoms recur, when it can then be adjusted upward, aiming to define the effective minimal dose. Prophylactic treatment for steroid-induced bone disease should be considered in all patients (Chapter 251).

For chronic treatment, immunosuppressive medication is required in patients who do not respond satisfactorily to prednisone or need high maintenance doses. Because these agents have a long latency of effect, they are generally combined with prednisone (see earlier) during the early phases of treatment and then used as monotherapy if steroids can be withdrawn or are contraindicated. Azathioprine (2.5 mg/kg/day) is the preferred treatment;

compared with prednisone alone, combination treatment is better tolerated and associated with fewer relapses.[2] Cyclosporine (3 to 5 mg/kg daily) is effective as monotherapy or combined with steroids[3] and is frequently used as the second-choice immunosuppressant. Although the efficacy of mycophenolate mofetil in association with prednisone is questioned,[4] this agent at the standard dose of 2000 mg/day is used in patients who are unresponsive to or intolerant of azathioprine. Tacrolimus is also used when the other agents fail or cannot be tolerated. Methotrexate (5 to 15 mg weekly) is an option for those intolerant of azathioprine, but long-term randomized studies are not yet available. When remission has been achieved, doses can be reduced slowly and cautiously; full withdrawal is likely to be followed by relapse.

Immunoglobulin infusion[5] and plasmapheresis are equally efficacious[6] for providing short-term improvement, typically persisting 4 to 6 weeks, and can be used to prepare patients for thymectomy, to cover the initiation of prednisone therapy, or to control an exacerbation of myasthenic weakness. An immunoglobulin infusion of 1 g/kg given on day 1 only is as effective as 1 g/kg given on day 1 and again on day 2.[7] Because of the short-lived benefits of these therapies, they must be accompanied by additional immunosuppressive therapy, as noted previously.

Inhibition of the production of acetylcholinesterase using a short antisense oligonucleotide was both effective and safe in a phase Ib study on patients with anti-AChR positive MG. Rituximab, a monoclonal anti-CD20 antibody that markedly reduces circulating B cells, has been used successfully in patients with refractory disease.

PROGNOSIS

The increasing use of immunologic therapies, coupled with advances in critical care, has improved the prognosis in nonthymomatous myasthenia gravis. Many patients can expect substantial improvement or remission with a normal life expectancy. The prognosis is less good, however, in those with invasive thymoma.

Lambert-Eaton Myasthenic Syndrome

DEFINITION AND EPIDEMIOLOGY

The Lambert-Eaton myasthenic syndrome, which is a rare disorder that can occur in paraneoplastic (Chapter 187) and nonparaneoplastic forms, affects all races. The incidence of the paraneoplastic form is much higher, but its shorter survival results in a similar prevalence of the two types. The paraneoplastic form affects about 2% of patients with small cell lung cancer (Chapter 197) and can also occur with lymphoma (Chapter 191). The nonparaneoplastic form associates with HLA-A1, -B8, and -DR3, as in myasthenia gravis.

PATHOBIOLOGY

Lambert-Eaton myasthenic syndrome is an antibody-mediated presynaptic disorder characterized by a reduced number of acetylcholine quanta (vesicles) released by each nerve impulse. End plate potentials recorded from intercostal muscle biopsies are consequently much reduced in amplitude. During repetitive high-frequency nerve stimulation, the end plate potential amplitude increases, probably because build-up of calcium in the motor nerve terminal leads to increased release of acetylcholine. Freeze-fracture electron microscopic studies of motor nerve terminals show that the "active zone" particles, which represent voltage-gated calcium channels, are reduced in number and disorganized. IgG binds to the presynaptic nerve terminal at the sites of acetylcholine release. The antibodies in Lambert-Eaton myasthenic syndrome appear to act principally by cross-linking the voltage-gated calcium channels on the surface of the presynaptic motor nerve membrane, thereby leading to their clustering and internalization. The antibodies also interfere with transmitter release from postganglionic parasympathetic and sympathetic neurons in injected mice, providing an explanation for the autonomic dysfunction observed in many patients.

CLINICAL MANIFESTATIONS

Almost all patients present with difficulty in walking, which exhibits a rolling characteristic. Weakness in ocular, bulbar, and respiratory muscles is less common than in myasthenia gravis. Weakness predominantly affects proximal muscles, which may show augmentation of strength during the first few seconds of a maximal contraction. Reflexes are absent or depressed but can increase after 10 seconds of maximal contraction of the muscle (post-tetanic potentiation). Autonomic symptoms such as dry mouth, constipation, and erectile dysfunction are present in most patients. Cerebellar ataxia occasionally may be present. Patients with nonparaneoplastic Lambert-Eaton myasthenic syndrome may have other autoimmune diseases, notably vitiligo.

DIAGNOSIS

Diagnosis is based on the clinical features, on a positive serum voltage-gated calcium-channel antibody test, and on the characteristic EMG findings (see Table 430-2). Antibodies specific for the α1A (P/Q) subtype of voltage-gated calcium channels are found in 90% of patients, both with and without small cell lung cancer. Patients may not respond convincingly to intravenous edrophonium. On EMG, the amplitude of the resting compound muscle action potential is reduced, but it increases by more than 100% after 10 seconds of voluntary contraction of the muscle or during high-frequency (40-Hz) nerve stimulation. Chest imaging is required in those at risk for tumor.

Differential Diagnosis

Botulinum poisoning (Chapter 304) causes blockade of presynaptic transmitter release at the neuromuscular junction as well as EMG changes similar to those in the Lambert-Eaton myasthenic syndrome. Botulism is detected by finding the toxin in serum or the *Clostridium botulinum* bacteria in the wound or feces. Myopathies (Chapters 277 and 429) can mimic Lambert-Eaton myasthenic syndrome clinically, but autonomic changes do not occur, EMG findings are different, and muscle biopsy is abnormal.

TREATMENT

Plasma exchange leads to clinical improvement within a few days in acutely ill patients, and most patients respond to immunosuppressive drugs or intravenous immunoglobulin therapy. Intravenous immunoglobulin therapy (1 g/kg for 2 days) improves strength, with an associated decline in specific antibody.[8] Specific tumor treatments (resection, local radiotherapy, chemotherapy) often lead to improvement of the neurologic disorder. Most patients respond to 3,4-diaminopyridine (10 to 20 mg four times daily).[9] This drug is available in Europe and many other countries; it has yet been approved by the U.S. Food and Drug Administration but can be obtained through some referral centers. Long-term immunosuppressive treatment with prednisone, azathioprine, or cyclosporine may be required in those with severe weakness, using doses similar to those described previously for myasthenia gravis.

PROGNOSIS

Prognosis mainly depends on the association with malignancy. Patients with paraneoplastic Lambert-Eaton myasthenic syndrome tend to have a progressive disease and a less satisfactory response to treatment. The nonparaneoplastic disease responds generally well to therapy as described previously.

● ACQUIRED NEUROMYOTONIA

DEFINITION AND EPIDEMIOLOGY

Neuromyotonia, or Isaacs' syndrome, is a rare disorder primarily characterized by myokymia (spontaneous undulating muscle contractions) that can be intermittent or continuous and may be present during sleep or general anesthesia. It results from the hyperexcitability of motor nerves. A milder variant, the cramp-fasciculation syndrome, is more common.

PATHOBIOLOGY

Neuromyotonia may be associated with other autoimmune diseases or other autoantibodies, and cerebrospinal fluid analysis may show oligoclonal bands. In about 15% of patients, it is paraneoplastic, usually associated with thymoma and occasionally with lung cancer. Occasionally, neuromyotonia appears to be triggered by infection or allergic reactions, and it may improve spontaneously within weeks to months in these cases.

CLINICAL MANIFESTATIONS

The clinical presentation is heterogeneous with a combination of muscle stiffness, cramps, myokymia (visible undulation of the muscle), pseudomyotonia (e.g., failure to relax after fist clenching), and weakness. Increased sweating is common. Myokymia persists during sleep. Cramp-fasciculation syndrome shares some features with neuromyotonia. Some patients have sensory symptoms, including paresthesias, dysesthesia, and numbness, and a few have autonomic such as constipation or cardiac irregularities and central nervous system features of an encephalopathy, including insomnia, hallucinations, delusions, and mood change (Morvan's syndrome).

DIAGNOSIS

EMG shows spontaneous motor unit discharges that occur as distinctive doublet, triplet, or multiplet bursts with high intraburst frequency (40 to 300 per second), longer continuous bursts, and postactivation contraction. The abnormal muscle activity may be generated at different sites throughout the length of the nerve, but in most cases it is principally distal. Antibodies to voltage-gated potassium channels are found in 40% of patients. The differential diagnosis includes neuromyotonia caused by acquired and inherited neuropathies and by voltage-gated potassium-channel gene mutations (Kv1.1) that can associate with neuromyotonia and episodic ataxia.

TREATMENT AND PROGNOSIS   Rx

Neuromyotonia can be improved by anticonvulsant drugs, such as carbamazepine (up to 800 to 1000 mg daily), phenytoin (up to 300 mg daily), or lamotrigine (up to 100 mg daily), that downregulate sodium channel function, thereby reducing the hyperexcitability of nerves. Plasma exchange and intravenous immunoglobulins, using the same regimen as for myasthenia gravis, may be followed by short-term improvement. Immunosuppressive medications, again using the same drugs as for myasthenia gravis, are effective in some patients. Neuromyotonia is often a monophasic disease that can be successfully managed with symptomatic and immunodulating treatment. Because it is commonly associated with myasthenia gravis, the administration of pyridostigmine can increase symptoms of motor nerve hyperexcitability. Prognosis is less favorable in cases with central nervous system involvement.

GENETIC MYASTHENIC SYNDROMES

Congenital myasthenic syndromes (see Table 430-1) are inherited disorders that result from mutations in genes encoding key proteins at the neuromuscular junction. In the United Kingdom, their prevalence is at least 6 per 1 million population.

PATHOBIOLOGY

The genetic mutations can be presynaptic, synaptic, or postsynaptic and can involve many of the genes specific for neuromuscular junction proteins. The most common is the AChR ε-subunit gene, in which the single nucleotide missense substitutions or frameshift mutations usually result in complete loss of function of the AChR ε-subunit. Because this subunit replaces the AChR γ-subunit around the time of birth, the babies are normal in development but show weakness during late pregnancy and in the neonatal period. Survival probably depends on the continued expression of the γ-subunit. AChR deficiency can also result from defects in the gene for rapsyn, a cytoplasmic protein required for the clustering of the AChRs at the neuromuscular junction. Single nucleotide changes in genes for any of the AChR subunits can affect acetylcholine-induced receptor channel openings, leading to kinetic defects. In the fast channel syndrome (recessive), the result is reduced function of AChR, whereas in the slow channel syndrome (dominant), the channel opens for prolonged periods, thereby resulting in subsynaptic accumulation of ions and degenerative changes.

Mutations in the *COLQ* gene, which gives rise to the collagen tail that anchors acetylcholinesterase in the synaptic cleft, are less common. The resulting continuous exposure of the postsynaptic membrane to acetylcholine leads to degenerative changes and progressive muscle weakness. Mutations in choline acetyltransferase, the enzyme responsible for the synthesis of acetylcholine, do not always lead to dysfunction at rest; during repetitive activity, however, the amount of acetylcholine in each packet decreases, with consequent failure of neuromuscular transmission. Mutations in *DOK7* cause a "synaptopathy" with small, simplified neuromuscular junctions. Dok-7 binds muscle-specific kinase, and the mutations are thought to impair the signaling that maintains the synaptic structure. Other gene mutations are rarely identified.

CLINICAL MANIFESTATIONS

Clinical manifestations may vary from death in utero in severe cases to mild symptoms that present in adulthood. Although most cases present in infancy with ptosis, hypotonia, and difficulties with feeding and breathing, the slightly different patterns of muscle weakness provide clues that point to which gene is involved. Arthrogryposis multiplex congenita, indicative of fetal akinesia, often associates with rapsyn mutations. Life-threatening episodic apneas can occur with mutations in choline acetyltransferase or rapsyn

or in fast-channel syndromes. Severe ophthalmoplegia occurs in endplate acetylcholinesterase deficiency, AChR deficiency due to AChR subunit mutations, and fast channel syndromes, but is rarely seen in the other genetic syndromes. Motor symptoms with *DOK7* mutations usually appear at about 2 years of age after the child first learns to walk and are characterized by a limb-girdle proximal pattern of muscle weakness.

DIAGNOSIS

The EMG findings in the AChR deficiencies and fast channel syndromes are similar to those in typical myasthenia gravis. In the slow channel syndrome and acetylcholinesterase deficiency syndrome, there may be a double response to a single nerve stimulus (see Table 430-2). Most patients show a response to cholinesterase inhibitors (edrophonium or neostigmine), with the exception of the slow channel syndrome, acetylcholinesterase deficiency, and Dok-7 congenital myasthenic syndromes. DNA screening is essential. Genetic analysis can confirm the diagnosis and help in treatment, prognosis, and counseling, although the faulty gene has not been identified in many families.

The principal differential diagnoses are spinal muscular atrophy, infant botulism, hereditary neuropathies, and congenital myopathies or muscular dystrophies. Onset in early childhood, adolescence, or adulthood, as can occasionally occur, may mean that the genetic nature of the disorder is not recognized or initially leads to the incorrect diagnosis of seronegative myasthenia gravis.

TREATMENT AND PROGNOSIS   Rx

Many of the congenital myasthenic syndromes respond to acetylcholinesterase inhibitors, as used for myasthenia gravis, and to 3,4-diaminopyridine (1 mg/kg/day in four divided doses). For the slow channel syndrome, some patients have responded to fluoxetine (60 to 100 mg/day in adults), but the use of fluoxetine in children or adolescents requires psychiatric supervision. For syndromes in which the neuromuscular junction is destabilized or there are degenerative changes, such as for Dok-7 or end plate acetylcholinesterase deficiency, treatment with ephedrine (75 to 100 mg/day in adults, 3 mg/kg/day in children) or salbutamol (0.5 to 2 mg, three times a day when ephedrine is not available) can be remarkably effective. The beneficial effects of this treatment are not seen immediately but build up over a period of 6 months or more.

Although these congenital disorders can be fatal during infancy, usually because of apneic episodes during infections, most tend to be nonprogressive and stable or even may improve during adolescence or adult life. The exceptions are the slow channel syndrome and acetylcholinesterase deficiency, which, owing to the excess AChR activations that they cause, can be associated with progressive degenerative changes at the neuromuscular junction, although this risk is largely mitigated with treatment.

Grade **A**

1. Schneider-Gold C, Gajdos P, Toyka KV, et al. Corticosteroids for myasthenia gravis. *Cochrane Database Syst Rev.* 2005;2:CD002828.
2. Palace J, Newsom-Davis J, Lecky B, et al. A randomized double-blind trial of prednisolone alone or with azathioprine in myasthenia gravis. Myasthenia Gravis Study Group. *Neurology.* 1998;50:1778-1783.
3. Hart IK, Sathasivam S, Sharshar T. Immunosuppressive agents for myasthenia gravis. *Cochrane Database Syst Rev.* 2007;4:CD005224.
4. Sanders DB, McDermott M, Thornton C, et al, for the Muscle Study Group. A trial of mycophenolate mofetil with prednisone as initial immunotherapy in myasthenia gravis. *Neurology.* 2008; 71:394-399.
5. Zinman L, Ng E, Bril V. IV immunoglobulin in patients with myasthenia gravis: a randomized controlled trial. *Neurology.* 2007;68:837-841.
6. Gajdos P, Chevret S, Clair B, et al. Clinical trial of plasma exchange and high-dose intravenous immunoglobulin in myasthenia gravis. Myasthenia Gravis Clinical Study Group. *Ann Neurol.* 1997;41:789-796.
7. Gajdos P, Tranchant C, Clair B, et al. Treatment of myasthenia gravis exacerbation with intravenous immunoglobulin: a randomized double-blind clinical trial. *Arch Neurol.* 2005;62:1689-1693.
8. Bain PG, Motomura M, Newsom-Davis J, et al. Effects of intravenous immunoglobulin on muscle weakness and calcium-channel autoantibodies in the Lambert-Eaton myasthenic syndrome. *Neurology.* 1996;47:678-683.
9. Oh SJ, Claussen GG, Hatanaka Y, et al. 3,4-Diaminopyridine is more effective than placebo in a randomized, double-blind, cross-over drug study in LEMS. *Muscle Nerve.* 2009;40:795-800.

SUGGESTED READINGS

Argov Z. Current approach to seronegative myasthenia. *J Neurol.* 2011;258:14-18. *Seronegative patients may have low-affinity antibodies or late onset of congenital myasthenia.*
Mao ZF, Mo XA, Qin C, et al. Course of prognosis of myasthenia gravis: a systematic review. *Eur J Neurol.* 2010;17:913-921. *Review.*
Skeie GO, Apostolski S, Evoli A, et al. Guidelines for treatment of autoimmune neuromuscular transmission disorders. *Eur J Neurol.* 2010;17:893-902. *Consensus guidelines.*

XXVI

EYE, EAR, NOSE, AND THROAT DISEASES

431

DISEASES OF THE VISUAL SYSTEM

MYRON YANOFF AND DOUGLAS CAMERON

The eye is a compact, complicated structure (Fig. 431-1) that is remarkably stable throughout life. Once the growth of the eye is complete, at about the age of 3 years, the structure of the eye changes very little for the next 60 to 80 years.

The eyelids physically protect the eye. The visual axis contains blood vessel–free structures, including the tear film, cornea, intraocular aqueous, crystalline lens, vitreous, and retina that, except for the crystalline lens, remain essentially transparent throughout life. Delicate intraocular structures are protected by a tough collagenous "eye wall" composed of the cornea and sclera. The optic nerve is formed from retinal ganglion cell axons and the continuation of the brain dura, arachnoid, and pia maters. The optic nerve is long enough to allow free excursions of the eye through a 100-degree arc under the influence of six coordinated and critically placed rectus muscles. All these functional components are housed in a bony cavity, the orbit, which protects the eye from external injury.

The eyelid skin, only loosely connected to underlying structures, is among the thinnest of the body. The eyelid is unique because it contains the highest density of sebaceous glands in the body. These meibomian glands produce a sebaceous (lipid) material that is the principal evaporation retardant for the tear film. Malorientation of the eyelid margin or malorientation of the cilia (trichiasis) may cause extensive scarring to the anterior surface of the cornea, even to the point of blindness. The eyelid is opened under the influence of the levator muscle. The tendon of the levator tends to degenerate over time to produce mechanical ptosis. The soft tissue of the eyelid is separated from the soft tissue of the orbit by the orbital septum, a major collagenous barrier to protect orbital soft tissue from extension of eyelid inflammation. Extension of inflammation from preseptal cellulitis or ethmoiditis may cause septic optic neuropathy. Involution of elastic tissue supporting the skin of the anterior eyelid is reduced over time, causing dermatochalasis ("baggy eyelids"). The redundant tissue may be sufficient in quantity to restrict visual field, particularly superiorly.

The conjunctiva is a mucous membrane covered by stratified, nonkeratinizing squamous epithelium containing goblet cells. The epithelium is supported by delicate fibrovascular tissue that contains lymphatic channels. Squamous cell carcinoma or malignant melanoma originating in the conjunctiva may extend through these channels to regional lymph nodes or beyond. The conjunctival epithelium contains melanocytes. Immune processing cells are present in the epithelium (Langhans cells) and in the stroma in the forms of collections of non-nodal B and T lymphocytes. Non-nodal primary lymphomas, which tend to have an indolent course in this location, may arise from this tissue. The aqueous portion of tears is formed constantly by accessory lacrimal glands in the conjunctiva and lid soft tissue and by reflex action from the lacrimal gland. Symptoms of itching and burning, as well as periodic disturbance of vision, may result from decreased tearing.

Tears drain through puncta at the nasal eyelid margin to the nasolacrimal duct that exits inferior to the inferior turbinate of the nasal cavity. The epithelium of the nasolacrimal duct also contains melanocytes and is supported by a resting lymphocyte population. Neoplasms including lymphoma, concretions (dacryoliths), and tissue injury from trauma may occlude the puncta in adults.

The cornea is avascular and lined both anteriorly and posteriorly by surface cells. Lack of an adequate tear film, called dry eye syndrome, may seriously alter the ability of the cornea to transmit light, thereby affecting visual acuity. The posterior cellular lining of the cornea is a single layer of highly modified corneal endothelial cells. Lack of effective pumping by the endothelial cells will allow excess hydration of the corneal stroma, seen clinically as corneal edema. The corneal stroma is particularly sensitive to proteolysis from collagenases found with certain inflammatory diseases such as herpes simplex keratitis. The result is progressive corneal thinning and possible perforation of the cornea with multiple recurrent episodes of herpes simplex keratitis.

The intraocular pressure is measured by indentation tomography. The amount of pressure necessary to flatten the central cornea is proportional to the intraocular pressure.

The anterior chamber is bounded by the posterior surface of the cornea, the anterior surface of the iris, and the anterior crystalline lens within the pupillary space. Aqueous material normally flows from the posterior chamber into the anterior chamber through the pupil and exits into the general circulation through the trabecular meshwork. Most causes of pathologically increased intraocular pressure and optic nerve damage, that is, glaucoma, are due to abnormalities of filtration through the trabecular meshwork. The posterior chamber is bounded by the posterior surface of the iris, the ciliary body circumferentially, and the anterior surface of the vitreous. The crystalline lens is located entirely in the posterior chamber.

The anterior segment is composed of the cornea and the anterior and posterior chambers. Most of the anterior segment is derived from the skin. The posterior segment is the remainder of the eye. Most of the posterior segment structures are derived from the central nervous system.

When first formed, the crystalline lens is a totally cellular structure bounded by a true basement membrane. Throughout life, the new cells that are continuously added from the outer layer epithelial cells compress the central cells, thereby resulting in cell degeneration in the central core (nucleus). The lens doubles in volume from birth to age 70 years at the cost of both pliability (presbyopia) and clarity (cataract). The lens is suspended in the posterior chamber by fibers (zonules) attached to the ciliary body.

The ciliary body is the posterior extent of the iris. Its surface cells produce aqueous, and its muscles function in accommodation.

The vitreous is composed mostly of water and type II collagen. The vitreous makes up the majority of the volume and weight of the eye. It functions as a biochemical sink as well as to maintain neural retinal attachment. With time, the vitreous shrinks and separates from the retina (posterior vitreous detachment). Condensed and displaced vitreous casts a shadow on the retina, which is perceived by the patient as "floaters."

The retina is the site of photochemical conversion of light to electrical energy. Ganglion cells and their axons in the internal retina aggregate at the optic disc to form the optic nerve. Only the inner half of the retina is supplied by the retinal circulation. The outer half of the retina is supplied by a large-caliber capillary lake in the choroid (the choriocapillaris). Only a 500-μm area of the posterior retina, the central macula (about 3 to 5% of the total retina), has the ability to resolve images to 20/20. The remainder of the retina has much less sensitive image resolution. Extensive biochemical support and control of stray light are performed by the retinal pigment epithelium located between the choriocapillaris and the photoreceptor outer segments. The blood-retinal barrier, which protects the biochemical integrity of the retina, is composed of anatomic attachments between neighboring retinal pigment epithelial cells, as well as attachments between vascular endothelial cells of the retinal circulation. The retina is held in place by physiologic forces that may be compromised by holes forming in the retina (rhegmatogenous retinal detachment) or by fluid accumulating in the subretinal space (serous retinal detachment).

The optic nerve is composed of approximately 1 million axons from retinal ganglion cells. Axons are separated into bundles by pial septa, which are in turn enclosed in an arachnoid layer. The dura is contiguous with the posterior sclera and the periosteum of the optic canal. The optic nerve is supplied by delicate vessels extending from the dura across the arachnoid to the pial septa. The central retinal artery is present in the axial layer of the optic nerve near the eye but does not supply blood to the optic nerve itself. The optic nerve travels through a collagenous sieve in the plane of the posterior sclera, the lamina cribrosa. The choroid is that portion of the uveal tract posterior to the retina. This layer is composed of various calibers of blood vessels that ultimately supply blood for the choriocapillaris. There are no lymphatic channels in the choroid.

The sclera is composed of dense, relatively disorganized collagen. It is opaque because of the nonhomogeneous structure of the collagen and the degree of hydration relative to the cornea. There are multiple scleral ostia for arteries, veins, and nerves, both posteriorly and anteriorly.

The orbit is composed of bones of the facial skeleton. Sutures between major bones exist in the superior nasal and superior temporal quadrants. Multiple vessels and nerves extend through the thin ethmoid bone from nasal sinus tissue medially. The orbital floor is poorly supported over the maxillary sinus and may rupture with increased intraorbital pressure. The nasolacrimal duct travels through a portion of the lacrimal bone. The optic nerve is protected by portions of the sphenoid bone. Major cranial nerves travel through the adjacent superior orbital fissure, also a portion of the sphenoid bone. There is no normal lymphoid tissue in the orbit outside of the lacrimal gland. The rectus muscle may be enlarged by inflammation in thyroid eye

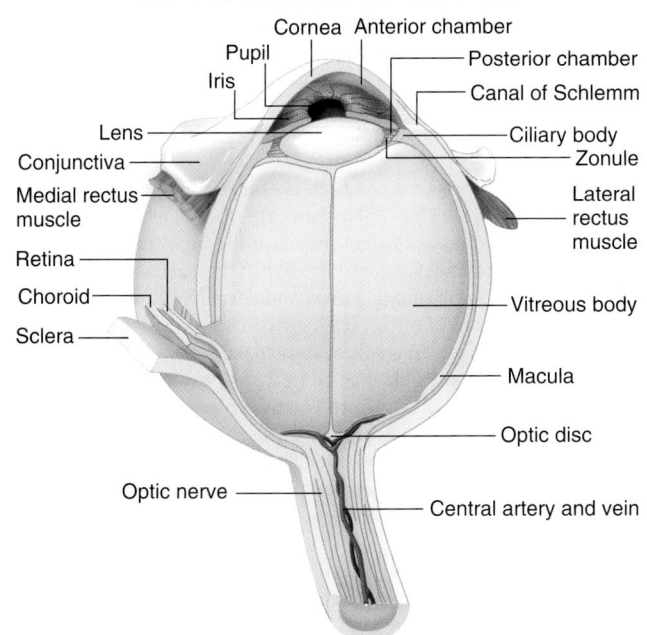

FIGURE 431-1. Anatomy of the eye.

TABLE 431-1	VISUAL ACUITIES REQUIRED FOR COMMON DAILY TASKS
20/20	Physiologic vision
20/30-20/100	Driver's license, varies by state
20/50	Newspaper print
20/70	Large-print *Reader's Digest*
20/100	Write a check
20/200	Legally blind
20/400	Paper currency

disease, but the tendinous insertion into the sclera is not inflamed early in the course of the disease.

CLINICAL MANIFESTATIONS AND DIAGNOSIS

Patients may present with complaints of diminished vision, eye pain, red eyes, or pain around the eye. The causes may be primarily ophthalmic (e.g., cataract) or systemic (e.g., diabetic retinopathy). A comprehensive ophthalmologic examination also should evaluate for possible asymptomatic local (e.g., choroidal melanoma) or systemic (e.g., hypertensive retinopathy) abnormalities in patients with normal acuity and no subjective complaints.

Functional Evaluation

The most objective and common measure of ocular function is line letter acuity, with normal vision (Table 431-1) defined as the ability to see at 20 feet what a normal person sees at 20 feet (Fig. 431-2). Less than 20/20 vision can be caused by an abnormality anywhere from the tear film to the visual cortex of the occipital lobe (see Fig. 431-1). However, normal vision also includes other functions, such as the perception of color, motion, contrast, brightness, field, and depth, for which there is greater variation among individuals and no universally adopted, standardized scales. Normal visual acuity is potentially achievable in essentially all individuals, either naturally or with visual correction.

Correction of vision is based on the refraction of light (Fig. 431-3). The diopter (D) is the unit of measurement of the ability of an optical system to refract (bend) light. The normal human eye has the refractive capacity of approximately 60 D. If the eye is too short, light will be focused behind the eye (hyperopia). If the eye is too long, light will be focused in the vitreous in front the retina (myopia). Normally, a person can voluntarily control the crystalline lens, alternating between near and distant tasks. At approximately age 45 years, the lens becomes stiff, and the eye becomes set for distance (presbyopia). Refraction is the method of determining the amount of optical correction (strength of glasses) needed to establish 20/20 (6/6) vision.

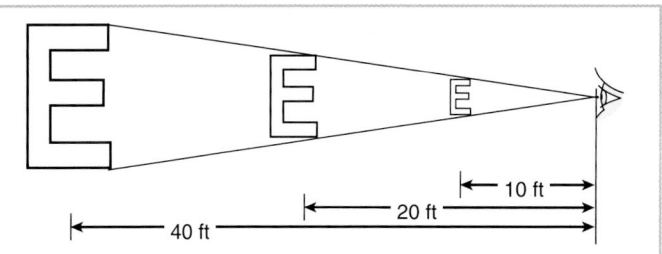

FIGURE 431-2. Snellen visual acuity. The most common test for visual acuity describes the eye's ability to resolve linear images at a test distance of 20 feet, approximating infinity (parallel rays of light). A 20/20 E subtends 5 minutes of arc at a distance of 20 feet, with each segment of the E subtending 1 minute of arc. The larger letters (e.g., 20/30, 20/40) are determined by the distance at which they subtend an angle of 5 minutes. Thus, an E that subtends 5 minutes at 40 feet, if viewed clearly at 20 feet, indicates 20/40 visual acuity.

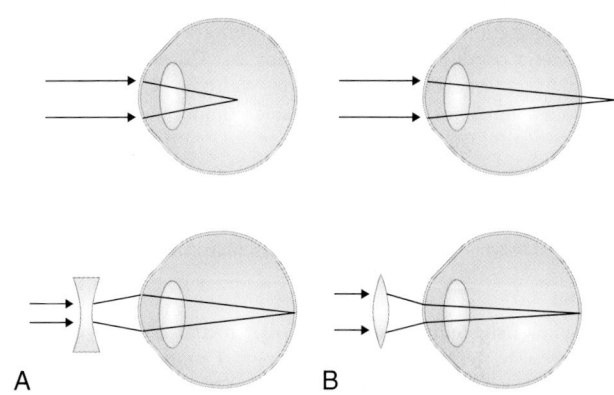

FIGURE 431-3. Myopia/hyperopia. **A,** In the myopic eye, parallel rays of light are focused anterior to the retina. A divergent lens can be used to compensate for the mismatch between refracting power and axial length. **B,** The hyperopic eye requires the additional power of a convergent lens to bring images into focus on the retina.

Examination of pupillary response assesses whether neural function is intact (see Figs. 432-2 and 432-4 in Chapter 432). Confrontational visual field testing (see Fig. 432-1 in Chapter 432) should be performed in each eye to detect gross quadrantic defects. Extraocular motility should be assessed to exclude nerve or muscle abnormalities (see Table 432-4 in Chapter 432). Color vision testing plates are a sensitive indicator of optic nerve function.

Diagnostic testing during a routine eye examination also includes external examination of the lids and adnexa, applanation tonometry to determine intraocular pressure, biomicroscopy (slit lamp examination) of the anterior segment, and ophthalmoscopic examination of the ocular fundus. Other office tests when indicated include exophthalmometry (measurement of proptosis), visual field and electrophysiologic testing, and vascular imaging (fluorescein angiography, mainly in diabetic patients; ocular computed tomography [OCT] to investigate retinal macular disease; and corneal topography).

The conjunctiva, cornea, lens, and anterior chamber are evaluated using a slit lamp. The slit lamp is composed of a binocular microscope with variable magnification (40× and 80×) in conjunction with adjustable light sources. An increased concentration of protein can be detected in the anterior chamber because of the Tyndall (flare) effect, indicating vascular incompetence associated with either inflammation or ischemia. Even individual inflammatory cells can be resolved with the slit lamp. A cobalt blue filter can be used to detect fluorescein dye that accumulates in regions of abnormal epithelium (dendrite of herpes simplex keratitis or a corneal abrasion). The slit beam is used to examine the crystalline lens to determine the degree of opacification from a cataract. By using a green filter with the 90 D lens, the retinal vessels and retinal vascular abnormalities such as microaneurysm can be seen at relatively high magnification.

COMMON CLINICAL CONDITIONS
Chronic Abnormal Vision
MYOPIA

Nearsightedness (myopia; see Fig. 431-3) is usually discovered during childhood when children cannot perform distant tasks during school (reading the blackboard) or during school screening. Myopia usually progresses until the eye is fully developed, typically by age 20 to 25 years. Rapidly progressing myopia during childhood or at any time after age 25 years requires evaluation for juvenile glaucoma, diabetes mellitus (reversible metabolic changes in the crystalline lens), trauma (development of a cataract), or use of corticosteroids (development of a cataract). Myopia is usually fully correctable with glasses. Laser in situ keratomileusis (LASIK) is a surgical procedure that may be used in adults to correct myopia and other refractive errors, with 95% of patients achieving visual acuity of 20/40 or better. Complications of LASIK include glare symptoms, dry eye, and undercorrection or overcorrection. Rare but serious complications include epithelial ingrowth, diffuse keratitis, and flap dislocation.

Pathologic myopia is a heritable condition causing progressive weakening of the posterior sclera and resulting increases in the axial length of the eye. The posterior radius of curvature of the eye increases (posterior staphyloma). The refractive error is usually above −8.00 D and may be as high as −20.00 D in severe cases. Abnormal physical forces in pathologic myopia may lead to retinal hole formation, retinal detachment, or intraocular hemorrhage. Associated systemic conditions include trisomy 21, Cornelia de Lange's syndrome, Stickler's syndrome, and Marfan syndrome. Clinical surveillance must be maintained to watch for treatable complications such as retinal detachment. Pathologic myopia is usually treated with spectacles or contact lenses. Refractive procedures are less successful in pathologic myopia because of the severity of the refractive errors and the presence of posterior segment abnormalities. Surgical and laser procedures may be required to treat retinal and choroidal lesions (e.g., subretinal neovascularization).

HYPEROPIA

In hyperopia (farsightedness; see Fig. 431-3), in contrast to myopia, the eye tends to have a shorter than average axial length. Compensatory mechanisms of the crystalline lens may functionally correct small degrees of hyperopia until age 40 years, when the crystalline lens loses its pliability. The 40-year-old hyperopic changes from latent to manifest hyperopia simultaneously. The initial pair of glasses may have to correct for both distance and near tasks (bifocals). LASIK can correct up to 5 D of hyperopia.

ASTIGMATISM

Astigmatism usually is the result of irregularities in the radius of curvature of the cornea. Astigmatism is not a pathologic state, but rather a variation in anatomy; most people have some degree of astigmatism. Trauma to the cornea can cause alteration of structure, leading to irregular astigmatism. Symptoms are predominantly blurry vision and difficulty seeing fine detail. Regular astigmatism can be corrected with spectacle lenses or with rigid contact lenses, whereas irregular astigmatism requires rigid contact lenses. Some forms of astigmatism can also be corrected with laser ablation of the cornea.

KERATOCONUS

Keratoconus is an acquired irregularity of corneal curvature, possibly caused when inappropriate activation of matrix metalloproteinase weakens the structure of the cornea, particularly in the inferior nasal quadrant. Onset generally is during adolescence, and the process often evolves over 5 years or so. The prevalence in the United States appears to be about 55 cases per 100,000 people but is probably greater when subclinical cases diagnosed by computerized videokeratography are considered.

Patients typically have astigmatism, which may be severe. The condition is usually bilateral but not symmetrical. Mild degrees of keratoconus can be corrected with glasses or contact lenses. For severe cases, corneal transplantation (graft) often is very successful.

STRABISMUS

The control of simultaneous orientation of the two eyes to ensure that the visual axes of both eyes are aligned is not complete until several years following birth. Misalignments of the two eyes (strabismus) may be the result of abnormalities in the central nuclei of the brain, malfunction of one or several peripheral nerves, or intrinsic abnormalities of the rectus or oblique muscles (see Fig. 432-6 in Chapter 432). If the eyes are not simultaneously stimulated with the images of the same degree of clarity or complexity, only one eye will develop normally. The image processing ability of the blurred eye will not develop (amblyopia). Generally, amblyopia can be corrected until about age 7 to 8 years of age, after which an amblyopic eye is not likely to develop normal (20/20) vision. In most cases, only the central vision is affected. The peripheral vision in both eyes is likely to be equal and normal.

Amblyopia also may be caused by a marked difference in refractive error between the two eyes (anisometropic amblyopia) or eyelid ptosis (deprivational amblyopia). Ptosis may be neurogenic or mechanical (e.g., congenital eyelid hemangioma). To avoid amblyopia, it is extremely important to refer a child with strabismus to an ophthalmologist as soon as the strabismus is noted.

Esotropia is deviation of one or both eyes inward. Esotropia may not be clinically evident until the child is 3 to 4 months of age. Delay in facial maturation (underdeveloped nasal bridge) may give the appearance of esotropia, even though the visual axes are correctly aligned. In true strabismus, the light reflex will be in the center of one cornea and decentered in the other.

Exotropia is deviation of one or both eyes outward. Exotropia tends to be intermittent and less likely to result in amblyopia.

Both esotropia and exotropia may be treated by using appropriate corrections of refractive error with glasses (occasionally bifocals). Occasionally extraocular muscle surgery is necessary to correct alignment. To allow the second eye to develop to its full potential, amblyopia is corrected by occluding the stronger eye with a patch or by pharmacologically occluding (blurring) the better eye with atropine. Success is directly related to compliance.

DIPLOPIA (DOUBLE VISION)

Acute onset of diplopia is an ominous sign suggestive of a third nerve palsy (Chapter 432). Diplopia of any kind is an intolerable symptom, but vertical diplopia is less tolerated than horizontal diplopia.

COLOR VISION CHANGE

Most cases of congenital color blindness go undetected for many years. Acquired color deficiency at any age may be caused by a cataract or optic nerve disease.

CHANGE IN VISION

If only one eye has a change in vision, the problem, such as a cataract or retinal detachment, is most likely in that eye. If both eyes have a change in vision, the problem generally is outside of the eye, such as homonymous hemianopia (Chapter 432). Improvement of near vision in middle age may be a sign of cataract ("second sight") or hyperglycemia. Transient complete unilateral or bilateral loss of vision may be caused by vascular abnormalities inside or outside of the eye (Table 431-2).

Acute Eye Abnormalities

PAIN

The most severe eye pain (Table 431-3), typically associated with a red eye, is caused by acute angle-closure glaucoma. Sharp, intermittent pain is usually caused by ocular surface abnormalities (e.g., corneal foreign body). Burning pain that clears with blinking generally relates to tear-film abnormalities (dry eyes). Deep boring pain most often is associated with an ocular abnormality (e.g., uveitis).

RED EYE

A red or inflamed eye can be caused by conjunctivitis, iritis (anterior uveitis), acute glaucoma, corneal trauma, or infection (Table 431-4). Of these causes, all are typically painful, with the occasional exception of conjunctivitis.

TABLE 431-2	DIFFERENTIAL DIAGNOSIS OF SUDDEN VISUAL LOSS	
UNILATERAL		**BILATERAL**
Amaurosis fugax (carotid artery stenosis)		Eclampsia
Central retinal artery occlusion		Vertebrobasilar infarct
Occipital lobe infarct		Trauma
Temporal arteritis		
Nonarteritic anterior ischemic optic neuropathy		
Hemorrhage		
Preretinal (high altitude, Valsalva)		
Vitreous		
Aqueous (hyphema)		
Trauma		

DISTORTED VISION

Distorted vision (metamorphopsia), which is the perception that straight lines are distorted or bowed, results from macular dysfunction. Causes include fluid under the retina, exudative macular degeneration, which tends to elevate the retina, and an epiretinal membrane, which tends to contract the retina.

NIGHT BLINDNESS

Retinitis pigmentosa, vitamin A deficiency, and systemic medications such as phenothiazines can cause true night blindness, in which patients have difficulty seeing any stars in the sky on a clear night and may be unable to ambulate without assistance in a dark environment. Patients with cataracts may have difficulty driving at night because of excessive glare and visual distortion.

SENSATION OF FLASHING LIGHTS

The sudden onset of flashes in the peripheral visual field suggests a posterior vitreous detachment with resulting traction of the vitreous on the peripheral retina, sometimes with a resulting retinal tear. The flashes, which may be more pronounced in the dark and with rapid eye movement, may be associated with the sudden onset of floaters, which can indicate debris or blood in the vitreous cavity. Because a tear in the retina can lead to a retinal detachment, urgent consultation with an ophthalmologist is required.

Flashing light with a migraine (Chapter 405) is described as scintillations or zigzagging lights that march across the visual field for a few minutes or as long as 30 minutes, sometimes associated with transient visual field loss. Headache is not universal.

FLOATERS

Floaters, which are caused by small aggregates in the vitreous cavity, result from the normal aging of the vitreous. The acute onset of vitreous floaters may be associated with uveitis or with the sudden onset of bleeding in the vitreous cavity owing to diabetes or sickle cell anemia. Acute floaters, however, particularly if associated with flashing lights, may indicate a poste-rior vitreous detachment or a retinal tear with an impending retinal detachment. Urgent ophthalmic referral is essential.

PHOTOPHOBIA

Photophobia, particularly if associated with eye pain, redness, and decreased vision, is a symptom of uveitis or traumatic iritis. Photophobia is also typical of acute migraine and meningeal irritation. Prompt ophthalmologic referral is prudent.

HALOS AROUND LIGHTS

Patients with cataracts commonly see halos around lights, particularly when driving at night. Episodic decreased vision, redness, and halos around lights may be symptoms of impending angle-closure glaucoma. Halos also can occur as a complication of LASIK eye surgery.

FOREIGN BODY SENSATION

A foreign body sensation is commonly caused by dry eyes. An entropion (Fig. 431-4) or misdirected lashes (trichiasis) also can cause a foreign body sensation. Most corneal abrasions cause severe pain, but minor corneal abrasions may be associated with a foreign body sensation rather than the severe pain that usually accompanies a more severe abrasion. An arc welder burn causes a punctate corneal keratopathy, and foreign body sensation may be a prominent symptom. A true conjunctival or corneal foreign body also may be present.

EXCESSIVE TEARING

Impairment of tear drainage can occur with an ectropion or any obstructions of the nasolacrimal drainage system. An entropion or abnormal lashes rubbing on the cornea (trichiasis) stimulate tear production.

EYELID TWITCHING

Any irritation of the conjunctiva or cornea can cause the eyelids to twitch. Occasional twitching of the lids usually is associated with stress or adrenergic stimulation. Benign essential blepharospasm is severe spasm of the lids leading to functional impairment. Multiple sclerosis (Chapter 419) also can cause lid spasm.

CONJUNCTIVITIS

Any ocular inflammation, including corneal ulcers, angle-closure glaucoma, endophthalmitis, and uveitis can be associated with secondary conjunctivitis. Conjunctivitis usually involves the entire conjunctiva, is associated with a discharge, and usually is not associated with pain (see Table 431-4).

PTOSIS (DROOPY EYELID)

Ptosis (Fig. 431-5) can be caused by a third nerve palsy, which usually is associated with diplopia and a reduction in elevation, depression, and medial movement of the pupil. Horner's syndrome (see Fig. 432-5 in Chapter 432) is associated with a small pupil. With myasthenia gravis (Chapter 430), other typical features of muscle weakness are usually present or can be elicited. Some patients have mild senile ptosis, especially after eye surgery.

TABLE 431-3	CAUSES OF EYE PAIN
Blepharitis	Glaucoma
Blocked tear duct	Hordeolum (stye)
Chalazion	Iritis
Conjunctivitis	Keratoconus
Corneal abrasion	Optic neuritis
Dry eyes	Scleritis
Ectropion	Trauma
Entropion	Uveitis
Foreign object	

TABLE 431-4	DIFFERENTIAL DIAGNOSIS OF COMMON CAUSES OF INFLAMED EYE*			
FEATURE	**ACUTE CONJUNCTIVITIS**	**ACUTE IRITIS**[†]	**ACUTE GLAUCOMA**[‡]	**CORNEAL TRAUMA OR INFECTION**
Incidence	Extremely common	Common	Uncommon	Common
Discharge	Moderate to copious	None	None	Watery or purulent
Vision	No effect on vision	Slightly blurred	Markedly blurred	Usually blurred
Pain	None	Moderate	Severe	Moderate to severe
Conjunctival injection	Diffuse: more toward fornices	Mainly circumcorneal	Mainly circumcorneal	Mainly circumcorneal
Cornea	Clear	Usually clear	Steamy	Change in clarity related to cause
Pupil size	Normal	Small	Moderately dilated and fixed	Normal or small
Pupillary light response	Normal	Poor	None	Normal
Intraocular pressure	Normal	Normal	Elevated	Normal
Smear	Causative organisms	No organisms	No organisms	Organisms found only in corneal ulcers related to infection

*Other less common causes of red eyes include endophthalmitis, foreign body, episcleritis, and scleritis.
†Acute anterior uveitis.
‡Angle-closure glaucoma.

FIGURE 431-4. Involutional entropion. (From Palay DA, Krachmer JH. *Primary Care Ophthalmology,* 2nd ed. Philadelphia: Elsevier Mosby; 2005.)

FIGURE 431-5. Ptosis of the right upper lid. (From Palay DA, Krachmer JH. *Primary Care Ophthalmology,* 2nd ed. Philadelphia: Elsevier Mosby; 2005.)

FIGURE 431-6. Graves' ophthalmopathy with characteristic exophthalmos and eyelid retraction.

FIGURE 431-7. Involutional ectropion. (From Palay DA, Krachmer JH. *Primary Care Ophthalmology,* 2nd ed. Elsevier Mosby, Philadelphia, 2005.)

PROPTOSIS (EXOPHTHALMOS)

Proptosis, or a prominent globe, can be a manifestation of thyroid abnormalities, especially Graves' disease (Chapter 233), in which proptosis is subacute and bilateral but sometimes asymmetrical (Fig. 431-6). An orbital pseudotumor can cause acute, usually unilateral proptosis, with severe pain, particularly with eye movement, and often with decreased vision. An optic nerve tumor causes chronic, unilateral proptosis associated with a slow onset of visual field loss. Acute cellulitis can be associated with unilateral proptosis, severe redness, and moderate to severe pain, commonly with sinusitis and an elevated white blood cell count.

SMALL PUPIL

A unilateral small pupil is best detected in dark conditions. Causes include Horner's syndrome, associated with ptosis on the same side; the bilaterally small, poorly reacting pupils of tertiary syphilis (Argyll Robertson pupils), which accommodate with normal constriction to a near object; miotic drops (e.g., pilocarpine); traumatic iritis; uveitis; and recent eye surgery.

LARGE PUPIL

Any α-adrenergic or anticholinergic agent placed into the eye can cause a large pupil. With eye trauma, the iris sphincter muscle can be damaged, and an abnormally large pupil can result. Tears in the iris sphincter can sometimes be appreciated on slit lamp examination. Third nerve palsy may cause a dilated pupil associated with ptosis and decreased elevation, depression, and medial eye movement. Adie's pupil (see Fig. 432-3 in Chapter 432) is an idiopathic, unilateral large pupil that is hypersensitive to weak cholinergic stimulation. Recent eye surgery, uveitis, closed-angle glaucoma, and traumatic iritis can cause a large pupil.

LEUKOKORIA

Leukokoria (white pupil) in a child is often a sign of retinoblastoma. However, any condition that changes transmission of ambient light to reflection of ambient light through the pupil may cause this sign. Some of the more common nonretinoblastoma conditions presenting with leukokoria (Table

TABLE 431-5	DIFFERENTIAL DIAGNOSIS OF LEUKOKORIA
Retinoblastoma
Cataract
Persistent hyperplastic primary vitreous
Retinopathy of prematurity (retrolental fibroplasia)
Coats' disease (retinal telangiectasia)
Retinal detachment
Toxocariasis
Familial exudative vitreoretinopathy (FEVR)

431-5) include cataracts, retinal detachment, persistent hyperplastic primary vitreous (a developmental anomaly of the vitreous resulting in intraocular fibrosis and retinal detachment), Coats' disease (a developmental vascular malformation of the retina leading to retinal detachment), and ocular toxocariasis (a parasitic intraocular nematode infection, which leads to intraocular scarring and retinal detachment).

Eyelid Abnormalities
ECTROPION AND ENTROPION

An ectropion is an out-turning of the lower lid (Fig. 431-7), typically with the inner part of the lower end visible between the eye globe and the lid. Causes include aging, scarring, a mass on the lower lid, and seventh nerve palsy. Common symptoms include burning, itching, tearing, and the sense of a foreign body. Treatment is symptomatic, unless the underlying cause can be surgically corrected.

FIGURE 431-8. Bilateral chalazion in the upper eyelids.

FIGURE 431-9. A lower lid stye *(1)*. (From Palay DA, Krachmer JH. *Primary Care Ophthalmology,* 2nd ed. Philadelphia: Elsevier Mosby; 2005.)

FIGURE 431-10. Staphylococcal blepharitis. The lid margins are very red and under high magnification demonstrate tiny ulcerations. (From Palay DA, Krachmer JH. *Primary Care Ophthalmology,* 2nd ed. Philadelphia: Elsevier Mosby; 2005.)

An entropion, which is an in-turning of the lower lid (see Fig. 431-4), is usually age-related and associated with irritation, burning, and a foreign body sensation. If it leads to trichiasis, in which the eyelashes rub or abrade the cornea, the lashes can be removed with forceps or surgery.

CHALAZION
A chalazion (Fig. 431-8) is a localized lipogranulomatous inflammation that results when the eyelid reacts to the contents of a ruptured sebaceous (meibomian) gland. The retained, lipid-rich sebaceous material acts as a foreign material that stimulates a lipogranulomatous foreign body inflammatory reaction. A painless or slightly tender, poorly demarcated, nonmobile nodule forms under the eyelid skin. Most lesions resolve over days to weeks with warm compresses or without specific treatment. Occasionally, an ophthalmologist may inject steroids to reduce inflammation or debulk the foreign material by incision and drainage through the tarsal conjunctiva. Some individuals may have recurrent chalazion.

HORDEOLUM (STYE)
A hordeolum (stye) (Fig. 431-9) is an extremely painful abscess in a hair or eyelash follicle or in a sebaceous gland. Styes are usually self-limited infections that respond to warm compresses and topical antibiotics (e.g., bacitracin or erythromycin ointment or moxifloxacin or gatifloxacin drops). Incision and drainage may be performed by an ophthalmologist if symptoms do not improve within 48 hours.

BLEPHARITIS
Blepharitis (Fig. 431-10), which is a nonspecific inflammation of the eyelid skin, is common, particularly in men. The condition is usually bilateral and symmetrical. Rosacea (Chapter 447) is the most common associated cutaneous condition, and *Staphylococcus aureus* is the most common infectious agent. If untreated, blepharitis becomes chronic and may lead to corneal and conjunctival inflammation (blepharoconjunctivitis). Ophthalmic antibiotic ointment (e.g., bacitracin or erythromycin) is more efficacious than eye drops, but systemic antibiotics (e.g., minocycline, 50 to 100 mg, or doxycycline, 100 mg, once daily; tetracycline, 250 mg twice daily; or erythromycin, 250 mg three times daily) are recommended if there is any evidence of inflammation of the cornea or conjunctiva.

In seborrheic blepharitis, exfoliated keratinous debris accumulates along the eyelid margin, particularly at the follicles of the eyelashes, and irritates the conjunctiva. Treatment of this chronic condition is directed at mechanically removing the keratinous debris by scrubbing the eyelid and eyelashes daily with a mild detergent ("baby shampoo") in warm water applied with a soft cloth.

BENIGN EYELID NEOPLASMS
Skin tags, also known as squamous papillomas, are the most common benign skin lesions. Other skin lesions include seborrheic keratitis, actinic keratitis, inverted follicular keratitis, and benign lesions of the eccrine and apocrine systems. Most of these benign lesions are cured by simple excision.

SEBACEOUS GLAND CARCINOMA
Sebaceous gland carcinoma originates from sebaceous glands either in the tarsal plate (meibomian gland) or associated with eyelashes (glands of Zeis) and is capable of producing widespread metastasis resulting in death. Muir-Torre syndrome is sebaceous tumors associated with visceral malignancy. Except for chronic, unilateral blepharitis, owing to the peculiar manner of spread of this tumor in the plane of the skin epithelium (pagetoid spread) without causing the formation of nodules, few symptoms occur early in the course of the disease. The tumor may progress to involve the tarsal conjunctiva, the bulbar conjunctiva, and even the corneal epithelium. A characteristic sign is regional loss of eyelashes. When the mass thickens, it may have the appearance of a chalazion, and a history of multiple chalazia in the same region of the eyelid is suggestive of sebaceous gland carcinoma.

Treatment is surgical removal. Surgical margins are difficult to estimate because of the intraepithelial extension of the tumor. In advanced cases, removal of the eyelids, eye, and orbital contents (exenteration) may be necessary.

BASAL CELL CARCINOMA
Basal cell carcinoma (Fig. 431-11), which originates from the basal cell layer of the epithelium, is a common cutaneous malignancy (Chapter 210). The lesion, which usually is asymptomatic, is often a well-demarcated, elevated nodule that may have a central region of ulceration and fine cutaneous vascular channels (telangiectasias). A common benign cutaneous lesion, sometimes confused clinically with basal cell carcinoma, is seborrheic keratosis (Chapter 448), which tends to be soft and appear hyperpigmented; the most common site is the lower eyelid, especially in the nasal quadrant. Basal cell carcinoma, particularly near the medial canthus, may extend posteriorly into the soft tissues of the orbit. Imaging before surgical excision for medial canthal lesions may be necessary to determine the true extent of the tumor. Basal cell carcinoma is treated by surgical excision, using Mohs' technique with intraoperative histologic evaluation to determine adequate margins of excision, if possible.

Metastasis is extremely rare. Generally with early detection and adequate excision of the local lesion, the prognosis is excellent.

EYELID SQUAMOUS CELL CARCINOMA

Eyelid squamous cell carcinoma, which is much less common than basal cell carcinoma, arises from the surface squamous epithelium. Ultraviolet light exposure is the major risk factor. In contrast to basal cell carcinoma, squamous cell carcinoma can metastasize, most often to regional lymph nodes. Treatment is surgical excision. Except in rare circumstances, such as in immunosuppressed patients or patients with xeroderma pigmentosa, the prognosis is excellent.

Ocular Surface Abnormalities

DRY EYES

Even minor disturbances in the tear film can cause itching, burning, pulling, and transient changes in vision. Some patients are particularly disturbed by dry eyes that cause conjunctival hyperemia without purulent discharge. Paradoxically, decreased tearing can result in irritation and secondary increased (reflux) tearing.

Most daily tear production is not by the lacrimal gland but by small collections of lacrimal glands, mucous producing glands, and sebaceous glands located throughout the conjunctiva, eyelid, and anterior orbital soft tissue. Over time, particularly in women, production of tear film diminishes. Because tear film production is lower during sleep, patients often note symptoms on awakening followed by slow resolution over minutes or hours. Wind and low humidity environments, such as in commercial airliners, can exacerbate symptoms. The reduction in aqueous components of tears is often associated with a compensatory increase in mucous production, which tends to blur vision until the patient blinks or uses supplemental tears. These symptoms are particularly prominent in persons who have rheumatoid arthritis (Chapter 272), Sjögren's syndrome (Chapter 276), Stevens-Johnson syndrome (Chapter 448), and ocular cicatricial pemphigoid (Fig. 431-12).

Treatment is not definitive and is rarely satisfactory. No medication increases the production of tears. Low-viscosity artificial tears (e.g., polyethylene glycol 400 0.4%), which do not tend to blur vision but have a short duration of action, are best used during visually important tasks. High-viscosity tears (e.g., carboxymethylcellulose sodium) have a longer duration of action but tend to blur vision; they are best used at bedtime to maintain lubrication of the ocular surface during sleep. When artificial tears do not control symptoms, occlusion of the nasolacrimal duct with synthetic plugs or permanent surgical occlusion tends to retain the tears that are produced. Anti-inflammatory drugs (e.g., cyclosporine 0.05% drops, every 12 hours indefinitely) can preserve glandular tissue that may be affected by local inflammation. For patients with systemic disease associated with dry eyes, effective treatment of the systemic disease sometimes improves the eye abnormalities.

PINGUECULA AND PTERYGIUM

A pinguecula (Fig. 431-13) consists of a limbal (at junction of cornea and sclera) and bulbar conjunctival degenerative process caused by ultraviolet light damage to the subepithelial tissue. It is very common and rarely causes symptoms. If the supportive tissue degeneration extends into the cornea, it becomes a pterygium (Fig. 431-14), which may cause visual changes and require surgical excision.

RECURRENT EROSION

Recurrent erosion of the cornea usually is a delayed reaction to minor traumatic corneal abrasion. The abrasion heals abnormally, resulting in a weakness of the epithelial attachment to underlying tissue. Weeks to months to years later, the patient is awakened in the middle of the night with extreme

FIGURE 431-11. A typical nodular basal cell carcinoma. (From Palay DA, Krachmer JH. *Primary Care Ophthalmology,* 2nd ed. Philadelphia: Elsevier Mosby; 2005.)

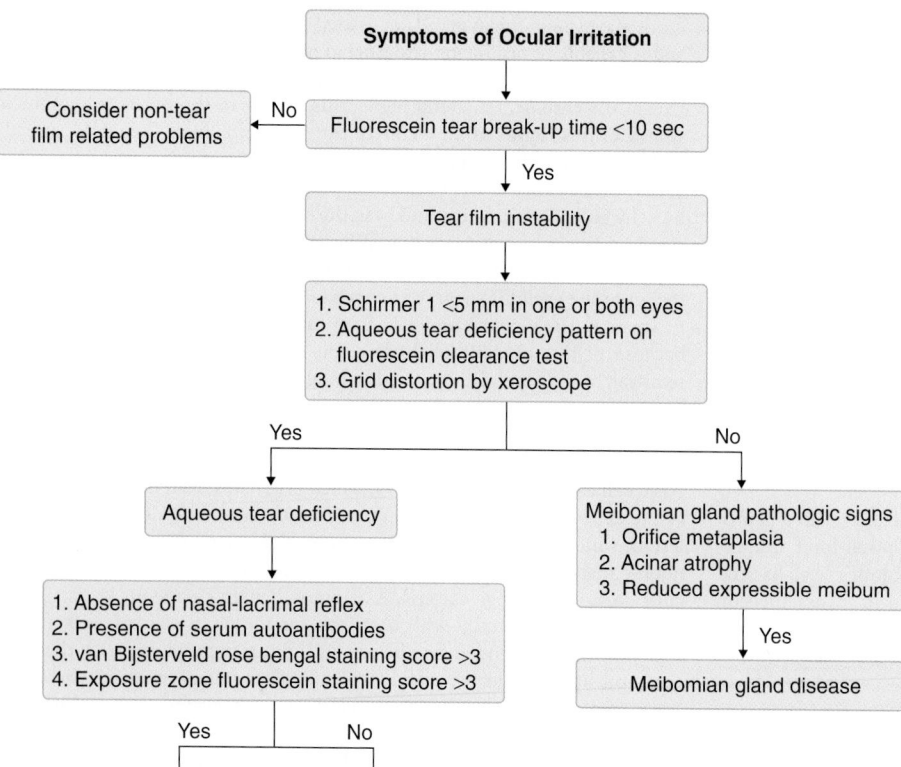

FIGURE 431-12. Diagnostic algorithm for ocular irritation. (Modified from Pflugfelder SC, Tseng SC, Sanabria O, et al. Evaluation of subjective assessments and objective diagnostic tests for diagnosing tear-film disorders known to cause ocular irritation. *Cornea.* 1998;17:38-56.)

FIGURE 431-13. **Pinguecula.** These lesions are found at the 3-o'clock and 9-o'clock positions and are extremely common, especially in older patients. (From Palay DA, Krachmer JH. *Primary Care Ophthalmology,* 2nd ed. Philadelphia: Elsevier Mosby; 2005.)

FIGURE 431-14. **Pterygium.** These lesions are found in the horizontal meridian, most common nasally. (From Palay DA, Krachmer JH. *Primary Care Ophthalmology,* 2nd ed. Philadelphia: Elsevier Mosby; 2005.)

ocular pain on opening the eyelids. The epithelium has become "stuck" to the overlying upper lid and is mechanically abraded. The condition is treated with hyperosmotic drops and ointment. There is a tendency to recurrence.

ACCIDENTAL TRAUMA
With ocular trauma, many tissues of the eye can be easily disrupted, and the effects of trauma may not be manifest for months or even years after the episode of trauma. If the traumatic episode disrupts the eye wall (cornea and sclera), surgical repair is necessary, usually urgently. If the eye wall is intact, surgical treatment is often not necessary, at least initially.

CORNEAL ABRASION
Corneal abrasion, one of the most common forms of ocular injury, may be caused by shearing trauma or hypoxia associated with overwearing of contact lenses. Symptoms are often intense and intolerable. Healing (i.e., re-epithelialization) of the cornea occurs within 24 to 48 hours. Rust from metallic fragments is toxic to the epithelium and should be removed. Fungal keratitis may complicate injuries from fingernails or vegetable matter, such as tree branches. Treatment usually consists of a topical antibiotic (e.g., erythromycin ointment, four times daily for 10 days) to prevent bacterial keratitis. Subsequent scarring usually does not occur unless deeper structures, such as Bowman's membrane, are affected. Topical anesthetics never should be prescribed to control pain because they increase the risk for microbial keratitis and scarring and may delay healing.

MAJOR OCULAR TRAUMA
Hyphema (Fig. 431-15) is hemorrhage into the anterior chamber caused by blunt trauma. If the patient is in an intensive care unit and supine, the blood will distribute uniformly over the iris to cause the appearance of increased pigmentation of the iris (heterochromia iridis). If the patient has been sitting,

FIGURE 431-15. Hyphema following cataract surgery. (Courtesy of Dr. Myron Yanoff.)

the blood may settle by gravity to form an aqueous-blood interface with the blood in the dependent portion of the anterior chamber. Hyphema, which is a sign of serious ocular damage, may lead to secondary glaucoma and blood staining of the cornea. It requires prompt evaluation by an ophthalmologist.

The most common site of rupture of a globe is at the limbus (junction of cornea and sclera), where a pigmented mass may be noted. The mass may be either a blood clot or an anteriorly displaced uveal tract (usually iris). Any manipulation of the globe may force the remaining intraocular tissue through the wound and may make the injury irreparable. Surgical repair is usually indicated.

Cataract and retinal detachment are not common except in severe accidental trauma. A unilateral cataract or unilateral glaucoma may occur decades after the injury, even when an injury is too minor to be recalled. Traumatic cataract and traumatic glaucoma are treated in the same manner as other forms of these conditions.

● INFLAMMATORY EYE DISORDERS
Uveitis
Inflammation of any part or parts of the uveal tract (iris, ciliary body, and choroid) may be called anterior or posterior uveitis, iritis, iridocyclitis, or choroiditis. Symptoms include a red eye (see Table 431-4), decreased vision, and photophobia. The inflammation is chronic, and a cause is rarely found. However, uveitis accompanies many autoimmune diseases, often without correlation with the activity of the systemic inflammation. Anterior uveitis or conjunctivitis is nearly universal in patients with reactive arthritis (Chapter 273). About 25% of patients with ankylosing spondylitis (Chapter 273) develop acute, recurrent anterior uveitis. Two to 12% of patients with inflammatory bowel disease (Chapter 143) develop anterior uveitis, which is also common with psoriatic arthritis but not with psoriasis alone (Chapters 273 and 446). Treatment with topical corticosteroids (e.g., prednisolone acetate 1%, one drop in the affected eye or eyes every 1 to 6 hours while awake) is usually sufficient to control the ocular disease.

Endophthalmitis
Endophthalmitis is extensive inflammation within the eye from any cause. Most cases of endophthalmitis involve a breach in the eye wall (cornea and sclera), associated with either accidental trauma (incidence of approximately 5%) or surgical procedures (incidence of approximately <0.1%). The initial symptom is usually decreased vision followed by dull ocular pain. The initial sign is often evidence of inflammatory cells either within the aqueous (anterior uveitis) or within the vitreous (vitreitis). The cells can be seen only by slit lamp biomicroscopy. Common microbial organisms include toxin-producing gram-positive species and gram-negative species that are often associated with rapidly destructive course. Other organism of relatively low virulence, *Propionibacterium acnes* and *Staphylococcus epidermidis,* follow a more indolent course with less potential destruction. Metastatic endophthalmitis infection from a primary source outside of the eye is an unusual cause.

Diagnosis is established by sampling anterior chamber fluid or preferably vitreous fluid (vitreous tap) and evaluation of that fluid by Gram stain and culture. Treatment often requires outpatient intravitreal injection of antibiotics. In severe cases, the microbial and inflammatory debris burden is reduced by performing a vitrectomy through a pars plana incision. Under certain

TABLE 431-6 OPHTHALMIC DISORDERS ASSOCIATED WITH CONJUNCTIVITIS

DISORDER	ACUTE OR CHRONIC	UNILATERAL OR BILATERAL	KEY SYMPTOMS	DEGREE OF INJECTION	DISCHARGE TYPE	OTHER FEATURES
Viral conjunctivitis	Acute	Bilateral, possibly asymmetrical	Itching, burning, soreness	4+	Watery	Preauricular lymphadenopathy
Bacterial conjunctivitis	Acute	Unilateral or bilateral	Burning	3+	Heavy, mucopurulent	Lids possibly adherent
Chlamydial conjunctivitis	Subacute, chronic	Usually unilateral	Burning, irritation	2+	Scant, mucopurulent	Usual occurrence in young, sexually active adults
Herpes simplex conjunctivitis	Acute	Unilateral	Photophobia, irritation	1-2+	None	Dendritic ulcer on the cornea or vesicles on the lid possible
Allergic conjunctivitis	Chronic	Bilateral	Itching	2+	Stringy, mucoid	Usual occurrence in atopic persons, possible seasonal symptoms
Blepharitis	Chronic	Bilateral	Itching, burning, foreign body sensation	1-2+	Usually none	Inflammation and crusting of lid margins
Dry eye	Chronic	Bilateral	Foreign body sensation	1+	Mucoid in severe cases	Punctate fluorescein staining of the cornea

Adapted from Palay DA, Krachmer JH. *Primary Care Ophthalmology,* 2nd ed. Philadelphia: Elsevier Mosby; 2005.

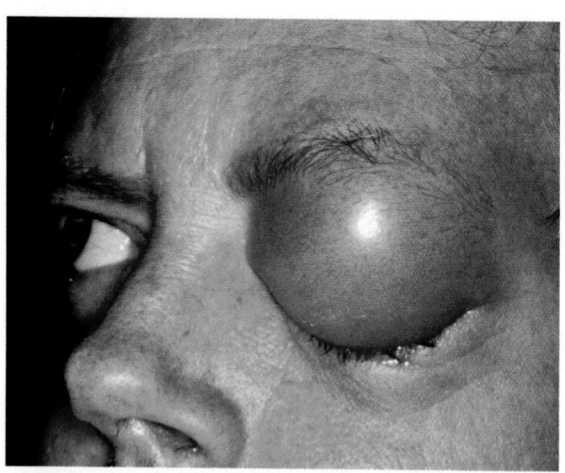

FIGURE 431-16. Eyelid abscess. Preseptal cellulitis, commonly resulting from minor penetrating trauma, may evolve into an abscess. Treatment requires incision and drainage followed by systemic antibiotics.

FIGURE 431-17. Diffuse injection of the conjunctiva with a watery discharge is evident in this case of viral conjunctivitis. (From Palay DA, Krachmer JH. *Primary Care Ophthalmology,* 2nd ed. Philadelphia: Elsevier Mosby; 2005.)

circumstances, corticosteroids and antibiotics are injected simultaneously to minimize the irreversible destructive effects of inflammation to the retina.

Allergic Conjunctivitis

Allergic conjunctivitis (Table 431-6) is commonly associated with atopy, hay fever, and allergic rhinitis (Chapter 259). Itching, a foreign body sensation, and a watery discharge are common. Treatment includes cool compresses and topical vasoconstrictors or antihistamines (e.g., naphazoline drops, four times daily during the allergic season, or levocabastine drops, four times daily). Long-term treatment with mast cell stabilizers (e.g., pemirolast drops, four times daily during the allergic season) or the combination of an antihistamine plus a mast cell stabilizer (e.g., olopatadine drops, two times daily during the allergic season) can be extremely effective in treating chronic symptoms.

● INFECTIOUS EYE DISORDERS
Cellulitis

Preseptal cellulitis (Fig. 431-16) is soft tissue inflammation of the eyelid anterior to the orbital septum. The orbital septum divides the soft tissues of the eyelid from the soft tissues of the orbit. Orbital tissue is more susceptible to damage by the inflammation than is the preseptal tissue.

The clinical signs of preseptal cellulitis include soft tissue swelling, hyperemia, and conjunctival chemosis (edema). Movement of the eye is not restricted. Extension of inflammation posterior to the orbital septum is indicated by proptosis of the globe and ophthalmoplegia (restricted motion). Treatment of preseptal cellulitis includes oral antibiotics (e.g.,

amoxicillin-clavulanate, 500 mg orally every 8 hours for 10 days). Treatment of orbital cellulitis, which can lead to septic optic neuritis, intracranial spread, and cavernous sinus thrombosis, may require intravenous antibiotics and surgical drainage of a paraorbital abscess.

Adenoviral Conjunctivitis

Viral conjunctivitis (Fig. 431-17) is common (see Table 431-6), and adenoviral conjunctivitis (especially subtypes 7, 11, and 18) is the most common type. The condition is highly contagious through direct contact or inhalation of respiratory particles. After an incubation period of 5 to 15 days, the patient presents with very red eyes (see Table 431-4), itching, burning, a foreign body sensation, and often a discharge and ocular discomfort (see Table 431-3), which persist for 5 to 15 days. Preauricular lymphadenopathy may be present, and a history of upper respiratory tract infection is common. The disease is self-limited, and treatment is aimed at patients' comfort. Cool compresses are often soothing. Patients are advised to wash their hands frequently. Topical antibiotics are not required, and topical corticosteroids are contraindicated.

Bacterial Conjunctivitis

Fewer than 5% of cases of conjunctivitis are caused by bacteria, mostly *Staphylococcus, Haemophilus,* or *Streptococcus* species. Patients have a mucoid or purulent discharge (Fig. 431-18), often with crusting and edema of the conjunctiva (chemosis) and lids. Bacterial conjunctivitis responds to broad-spectrum antibiotic solutions or ointments (e.g., topical erythromycin ointment three times daily for 2 weeks) (Table 431-7).

Chlamydial Conjunctivitis

Adult inclusion conjunctivitis is a chronic conjunctivitis caused by sexual transmission of *Chlamydia trachomatis* (Chapter 326). Patients often have preauricular lymphadenopathy. Oral erythromycin (500 mg orally, four times daily for 7 days) or azithromycin (1 g orally twice daily for 7 days) is required. Trachoma, which is a chronic cicatricial conjunctivitis after repeated chlamydial infection (Chapter 326), is the world's leading cause of corneal blindness. It causes an entropion, inversion of the eyelashes (trichiasis), corneal vascularization, and opacification. Topical erythromycin or tetracycline, twice daily for 3 to 4 weeks, can be effective, but surgical epilation or eyelid reconstruction may be required.

FIGURE 431-18. Bacterial conjunctivitis. Purulent discharge and conjunctival hyperemia suggest bacterial conjunctivitis. Viral conjunctivitis produces watery discharge, foreign body sensation, preauricular lymphadenopathy, and conjunctival follicles seen on slit lamp examination. (Reproduced with permission from the American Academy of Ophthalmology.)

FIGURE 431-19. Herpes simplex corneal epithelial keratitis in diffuse light and in light passed through a cobalt blue filter after fluorescein staining (*inset*). Note the dendritic staining pattern characteristic of herpes simplex.

TABLE 431-7 TOPICAL ANTIBIOTICS FOR EYE INFECTIONS

DRUG	TYPE	CONCENTRATION	DOSE
Moxifloxacin	Drops	0.5%	1 drop 4 times daily
Gatifloxacin	Drops	0.5%	1 drop 4 times daily
Ciprofloxacin	Drops	0.3%	1 drop 4 times daily
Gentamicin	Drops	0.3%	1 drop 4 times daily
Ofloxacin	Drops	0.3%	1 drop 4 times daily
Bacitracin	Ointment	500 U/g	Put in eye 4 times daily
Tobramycin	Ointment	0.3%	Put in eye 4 times daily
Erythromycin	Ointment	0.5%	Put in eye 4 times daily

Herpes Simplex Keratitis

Herpes simplex keratitis is the most common cause of central corneal ulcer (Fig. 431-19). Herpes simplex virus also can cause vesicular eyelid dermatitis. Initially, the main signs of primary herpes simplex keratitis are a red eye and a corneal epithelial dendritic ulcer. With appropriate antiviral therapy (e.g., trifluridine drops every 2 hours for 1 to 2 weeks), the keratitis usually heals without scarring. Recurrent herpes simplex keratitis may be precipitated by fever, menses, sunlight, irradiation, or stress. With recurrence, the disease may extend into the corneal stroma and cause a red eye, ocular discomfort, blurred vision, and corneal scarring. The treatment of stromal involvement is multifactorial and may not be successful. Corneal transplantation may be needed.

Herpes Zoster Ophthalmicus

Herpes zoster ophthalmicus (shingles, Chapter 383) has a propensity to involve one or more branches of the trigeminal nerve. The virus also can affect the uveal tract and, in immunosuppressed patients, the retina (i.e., acute retinal necrosis). When the trigeminal nerve is involved, spread to the inside of the eye (uveitis) is most likely if vesicles are present in the inner corner of the eyelids or on the nose, especially the tip of the nose. If the uvea is not involved, the skin lesions heal with some scarring but no long-term effects. In patients with moderate to severe skin involvement, treatment can be started with oral acyclovir (800 mg orally five times per day for 7 to 10 days). If uveitis develops, the treatment (e.g., prednisolone acetate drops 1% four times daily and scopolamine drops 0.25% three times daily) can be extended and difficult.

Pseudomonal and Gonococcal Keratitis

Keratitis, which is inflammation of the corneal stroma, can be caused by spread of pathogens internally from a corneal ulcer. *Pseudomonas aeruginosa* (Chapter 314), which causes a particularly virulent keratitis, is the most common gram-negative pathogen and is especially common in wearers of contact lenses. To avoid internal spread, urgent treatment is necessary (e.g., fortified tobramycin or gentamicin, 1.5 mg/mL every hour, alternating with fortified cefazolin, 50 mg/mL every hour, so a treatment is given each one-half hour around the clock). The dosage and duration of the treatment depend on the response.

Another gram-negative cause of a virulent keratitis is *Neisseria gonorrhoeae* (Chapter 306). Corneal infection is accompanied by copious weeping and a characteristic hyperpurulent discharge. Prompt treatment is essential in preventing corneal perforation.

Cytomegalovirus Retinitis

Cytomegalovirus retinitis (Chapter 384) is unusual except in immunosuppressed patients, especially patients with human immunodeficiency virus infection. Clinically, a central retinochoroiditis is seen. The presumptive diagnosis is made on the characteristic intense, retinal, wedge-shaped reaction, with considerable exudates and hemorrhages, giving the terms "pizza pie retinitis" and "hemorrhagic cottage cheese retinitis" to the entity. Treatment is antiviral drugs: ganciclovir (5 mg/kg intravenously twice daily, two to three times per week), foscarnet (90 mg/kg intravenously twice daily, twice per week), or cidofovir (5 mg/kg intravenously, weekly for 3 weeks) with follow-up maintenance.

Acanthamoeba Keratitis

Acanthamoeba species (Chapter 360) can cause a severe, blinding keratitis. Contact lens wearing is a major risk factor. A characteristic stromal ring infiltrate develops, and uveitis may occur. Using a confocal microscope, the acanthamebic parasite can be observed clinically as a pear-shaped cyst (11 to 15 μm). Numerous treatment protocols exist (e.g., polyhexamethyl biguanide 0.02% drops every hour). The duration and dose depend on the response, but the ideal treatment is not yet in hand.

Toxoplasmic Retinitis

Toxoplasma gondii (Chapter 357) causes both a congenital and acquired retinochoroiditis, which is more common in immunosuppressed patients. The lesions begin as an acute retinitis that atrophies centrally and pigments peripherally as it heals. The protozoa are found both in free and encysted forms within the retina. The condition may be self-limited and diagnosed as a healed incidental finding that does not need treatment. When active lesions are in the macula or a severe vitreitis causes at least a two-line decrease in vision, 4 to 6 weeks of quadruple therapy (pyrimethamine, 200 mg oral loading dose then 25 mg orally daily; folinic acid, 10 mg orally every other day; sulfadiazine, 2 g oral loading dose then 1 g four times daily; and oral corticosteroids, e.g., prednisone, 20 to 60 mg orally daily beginning at least 24 hours after antibiotic therapy is started and tapered 10 days before stopping antibiotics) usually produces good results. Alternative regimens may include clindamycin (150 to 450 mg orally three to four times daily) or atovaquone (1 g oral loading dose then 500 mg daily).

Fungal Endophthalmitis

Endophthalmitis is a potentially disastrous infection of the inside of the eye, often leading to blindness. The main fungal causes are *Candida, Coccidioides,* and *Aspergillus* species, which can gain access inside the eye either by traumatic introduction or through hematogenous spread. The patient presents with a red eye, ocular pain, and decreased vision. Multiple vitreous abscesses tend to be caused by fungi, whereas a solitary abscess is more likely caused by bacteria. Usually a vitreous "tap" (biopsy) is performed for culture and to guide to therapy.

Tuberculosis

About 1% of patients with pulmonary tuberculosis (Chapter 332) have uveal involvement, usually as iridocyclitis or diffuse choroiditis. Painless progressive visual loss is the most common symptom. Small yellow choroidal lesions may be seen, and retinal periphlebitis may occur secondarily. Treatment is as for the primary disease.

Syphilis

About 5% of patients with secondary syphilis (Chapter 327) develop anterior uveitis or neuroretinitis. In tertiary syphilis, the miotic Argyll Robertson pupil reacts poorly to light but briskly to accommodation. Treatment is as for the systemic disease.

● STRUCTURAL AND AGE-RELATED DISORDERS
Cataract

A cataract is an opacification of the crystalline lens. The lens doubles in volume between birth and age 70 years as new lens "fiber cells" are laid down on the external aspect of the lens cortex, beneath the lens capsule. The older fibers in the center of the lens cannot be desquamated into the surrounding aqueous and thus are compressed into the center of the lens. At birth, the lens is pliable and totally transparent. By age 45 years, the lens loses its pliability, which compromises near vision. As the process progresses, the lens loses its transparency, beginning at the center of the lens (nuclear sclerosis). The concurrent change in density of the lens nucleus may alter the optical characteristics of the eye to cause acquired nearsightedness ("second sight"). Ultimately, the cataract may become so dense that cataract surgery is necessary to restore vision.

Symptoms are typically loss of vision, especially at night, and glare. Cataract surgery, performed as an outpatient, is elective and depends on how much the decreased vision interferes with the normal lifestyle of the patient. A synthetic intraocular lens implant is inserted into the eye during surgery. Prognosis for restoration of vision is excellent, depending on the function of the retina. In general, cataracts develop asymmetrically. The worst eye (vision-wise) should have surgery first. As the second eye's cataract worsens, decreasing vision and monocularity are indications for cataract surgery in the second eye.

Glaucoma

Glaucoma results from an imbalance between the production of aqueous fluid and the drainage of aqueous fluid. The aqueous is produced by the nonpigmented ciliary epithelium of the pars plicata of the ciliary body. Aqueous fluid leaves the eye through the trabecular meshwork into the venous circulation. If the drainage function does not match the production potential, the intraocular pressure increases. If the elevated intraocular pressure is high enough or is present long enough, ganglion cells in the retina are damaged, causing loss of their axons. Loss of axons can best be appreciated clinically at their normal exit from the eye, the optic disc. Bulk loss of axons will lead to enlargement of the optic cup, which is recorded as increase in the cup-to-disc ratio.

In open-angle glaucoma, there is apparent free anatomic access to the trabecular meshwork. In closed-angle glaucoma, there is a relative or absolute anatomic barrier to the flow of aqueous.

CHRONIC OPEN-ANGLE GLAUCOMA

The most common type of glaucoma in elderly people is chronic open-angle glaucoma. The first symptom is loss of peripheral visual fields with retention of central visual function. The visual field may be reduced considerably before the patient notes loss of function. Most cases of chronic open-angle glaucoma are identified during routine eye examinations, either by discovery of abnormally high intraocular pressure or by the presence of a high cup-to-disc ratio (Fig. 431-20). Normal intraocular pressure is generally at or below 21 mm Hg, but exceptions exist depending on corneal thickness (influencing artifacts of measurement) and genetic disposition. The diagnosis of glaucoma is confirmed by characteristic visual field loss as determined by automated perimetry.

The treatment goal is to reduce intraocular pressure, initially with pharmacologic agents: β-blockers (e.g., betaxolol drops 0.5% twice daily), carbonic anhydrase inhibitors (e.g., dorzolamide drops twice daily), α-agonists (e.g., apraclonidine drops twice daily), and antiprostaglandins (e.g., latanoprost drops twice daily). Generally, the drops are taken for a lifetime. Applying energy to the structures of the trabecular meshwork with a laser (laser trabeculoplasty) often results in years of control of intraocular pressure. In resistant cases, mechanical filtration is accomplished surgically by bypassing the trabecular meshwork either by creating a fistula (trabeculectomy) between the anterior chamber and the episcleral tissue or by implanting a synthetic filtration device (a tube-shunt) from the anterior chamber through the sclera

FIGURE 431-20. Cup-to-disc ratios. **A,** Normal cup-to-disc (C/D) ratio of 0.1. **B,** Likely normal C/D ratio of 0.5. **C,** C/D ratio of 0.8 vertically with inferior notching (1) of the nerve (glaucomatous change). **D,** C/D ratio of 0.90 vertically (glaucomatous change). C = cup; D = disc. (From Palay DA, Krachmer JH. *Primary Care Ophthalmology,* 2nd ed. Philadelphia: Elsevier Mosby; 2005.)

FIGURE 431-21. Acute angle closure glaucoma. The left eye is normal. The red right eye has a nonreactive pupil. (Courtesy of Dr. Myron Yanoff.)

FIGURE 431-22. Dry age-related macular degeneration. Drusen are present in the posterior pole around a large area of geographic atrophy of the retinal pigment epithelium.

into a collection reservoir located at the equator of the eye in the soft tissues of the orbit.

PSEUDOEXFOLIATIVE GLAUCOMA

Pseudoexfoliative glaucoma syndrome is a genetically determined biochemical abnormality of the basement membrane protein, fibrillin. The syndrome occurs among people throughout the world but is especially prominent in Scandinavians and Saudi Arabians. Affected individuals are identified by accumulation of abnormal fibrillin (exfoliative material) on the surface of the crystalline lens, most easily seen in the pupillary space. Pseudoexfoliative glaucoma increases the risk of developing open-angle glaucoma five-fold, to a lifetime risk of about 10%. Treatment is as for open-angle glaucoma.

ANGLE-CLOSURE GLAUCOMA

Angle-closure glaucoma (Fig. 431-21) may occur over a short period of time and cause extreme debilitating symptoms. Alternatively, symptoms may develop over a long period of time with few specific symptoms.

The risk factors for angle-closure glaucoma closure are based on the anatomic configuration of the components of anterior chamber. Persons who are farsighted (hyperopia) have a shortened anterior-to-posterior axis of the eye, indicated clinically by a shallow anterior chamber. As the crystalline lens increases in volume with time, the iris is displaced anteriorly. At some point, the posterior surface of the iris may come in relatively tight contact with the anterior surface of the lens. Aqueous flow is restricted, and fluid accumulates in the posterior chamber, where it displaces the diaphanous peripheral iris anteriorly. When the peripheral iris comes in contact with the posterior cornea, the anterior chamber angle is suddenly occluded. Angle closure may be precipitated by pharmacologic dilation of the pupil. Patients who are farsighted (hyperopia) or have cataracts should be dilated with caution. The intraocular pressure may increase from 21 mm Hg to 50 to 70 mm Hg (nearly equaling diastolic arterial pressure). The symptoms of acute angle closure may include extreme pain, which may be poorly localized to the eye, nausea, and vomiting. Persistent vomiting may cause abdominal pain, simulating an acute abdomen.

Initial treatment is with topical (e.g., timolol 0.5% in one dose) and systemic pressure-lowering agents (e.g., carbonic acetazolamide, 250 to 500 mg intravenously or two 250-mg tablets orally in one dose if intravenous access or drug is not available), followed by creation of a fistula in the peripheral iris with a laser (YAG laser iridectomy) between the posterior chamber and the anterior chamber to bypass the obstruction. Most patients require a laser iridectomy prophylactically in the second eye to prevent angle-closure glaucoma.

Secondary glaucoma may also occur after intraocular hemorrhage, intraocular trauma, and intraocular inflammation. Some developmentally related secondary glaucomas, such as the iridocorneal endothelial syndrome, may not become evident until adulthood.

Retinal Detachment

A retinal detachment is a separation of the neural (sensory) retina from the retinal pigment epithelium. The two main types are rhegmatogenous, caused by a retinal hole, as may occur with a posterior vitreous detachment, and nonrhegmatogenous, caused by traction, such as in proliferative diabetic retinopathy or by fluid accumulation under neural retina in conditions such as malignant hypertension or eclampsia of pregnancy.

The classic symptoms are a sensation of flashes of light, floaters in the field of the involved eye owing to the causative vitreous detachment, and a shadow. Urgent treatment usually is needed. Some small peripheral rhegmatogenous

detachments may be treated by laser, but larger ones and traction retinal detachments are treated by more extensive surgery (scleral buckle surgery or vitreous surgery). In serous retinal detachment, the underlying condition should be treated.

Age-Related Macular Degeneration

Age-related macular degeneration is a neurodegenerative disease that affects the junction between the neural retina and the retinal pigment epithelium, mainly in the sixth to ninth decades of life. About 8.5% of the world's blindness is caused by age-related macular degeneration, mainly in industrialized countries. In the United States, age-related macular degeneration affects more than 1.75 million persons, and its prevalence increases with each decade after the age of 55 years. The genetic influence of age-related macular degeneration has not yet been determined, but abnormalities of complement factor H may play a role. Environmental factors such as smoking are known to accelerate this degenerative process.

Two types predominate: the "dry" or geographic type, and the "wet" or neovascular type. The wet type causes the most profound vision loss but is less common than the dry type.

The first sign of age-related macular degeneration is variation of the character and density of the retinal pigment epithelial pigment (pigment dropout) in the posterior region of the retina, the macula. The pathologic process causes abnormal protein (lipofuscin) to accumulate between the retinal pigment epithelial cells and its basement membrane complex (Bruch's membrane), designated as drusen. The drusen of macular degeneration (soft drusen) are small (30 µm), hypopigmented, poorly defined areas in the deep retina. This stage, called dry age-related macular degeneration, may antedate subjective alteration in vision by several decades. The anticipated rate of progression is difficult to determine in individual cases.

The first symptom of age-related macular degeneration is loss of vision. Loss of vision corresponds with loss of photoreceptor outer segments. The effect is in the exact center of the most sensitive portion of the retina, the fovea. The peripheral retina is not involved. As the process progresses, individuals with advanced disease will be able to walk down a street without apparent difficulty (a peripheral retinal function) but will not be able to recognize facial features of people whom they meet (a macular retinal function). Visual aids and other devices, such as special glasses and television aids, may allow patients to continue with daily functions and to continue to live independently. This phase of the process, the "dry phase," advances at a slow rate (months to decades), during which patients develop retinal features of well-defined pigment loss (geographic retinal atrophy; Fig. 431-22). No current treatment exists for the dry phase of the disease, except for a possible positive influence of dietary supplements (antioxidants). Vitamin supplementation with vitamins C and E, β-carotene, zinc, and copper may retard the progression of moderate age-related macular degeneration to severe age-related macular degeneration. ∎ β-Carotene (a vitamin A precursor) of this quantity is not recommended for cigarette smokers because of an increased risk for lung cancer. Cessation of smoking, control of blood sugar, control of blood lipid levels, and control of systemic blood pressure are particularly important behavioral modifications.

In the "wet phase" of age-related macular degeneration (Fig. 431-23), frail, neovascular channels originating from the established vascular system of the choroid may extend through a breach in Bruch's membrane into the

FIGURE 431-23. Wet age-related macular degeneration. A "dirty gray" neovascular membrane is present under the central macular area.

FIGURE 431-24. Background diabetic retinopathy. Exudates, microaneurysms, and small hemorrhages are seen in the posterior pole (right eye).

FIGURE 431-25. Severe proliferative diabetic retinopathy with cotton-wool spots, intraretinal microvascular abnormalities, and venous bleeding. (From Yanoff M, Duker JS, eds. *Ophthalmology*. Philadelphia: Mosby Elsevier; 2009.)

FIGURE 431-26. Hypertension retinopathy with narrowed arterioles whose sclerosed walls create the appearance of "nicking" when the arterioles cross venules. (From Yanoff M, Duker JS, eds. *Ophthalmology*. Philadelphia: Mosby Elsevier; 2009.)

subretinal space (subretinal neovascularization). Spontaneous hemorrhage of the vessels adds to photoreceptor loss. Hemorrhage is accompanied by acute, and usually permanent, loss of central visual acuity (i.e., the wet phase of age-related macular degeneration). Both eyes are usually affected to a similar degree. Neovascularization can be identified by fluorescein angiography and OCT. Intraocular injections of antivascular endothelial growth factors (e.g., ranibizumab) reduce the risk for visual loss in patients with neovascular age-related macular degeneration and can result in gains in vision.**2** Other treatments include argon laser photocoagulation or, in advanced cases, vitrectomy to remove subretinal neovascular membranes.

SYSTEMIC DISEASES WITH OCULAR SYMPTOMS DURING ADULTHOOD

Diabetes Mellitus

Diabetic retinopathy is one of the leading causes of blindness in the United States. More than 75% of the blind are women. Background diabetic retinopathy, with microaneurysms, hemorrhages, exudates (Fig. 431-24), and macular edema, accounts for most cases of decreased vision, but rarely causes profound vision loss. Most diabetic patients never develop the more severe proliferative diabetic retinopathy (Fig. 431-25), which generally occurs only after 15 years or more of diabetes and causes a profound loss of vision.

Diabetic retinopathy is closely correlated with the duration of diabetes mellitus (Chapter 236). The prevalence of diabetic retinopathy is about 27% among patients who have had type 1 diabetes for 5 to 10 years, 70 to 90% among patients who have had diabetes for more than 10 years, and 95% among patients who have had diabetes for 20 to 30 years. In patients with type 2 diabetes (Chapter 237), the prevalence of diabetic retinopathy is about 23% after 12 years and 60% after 16 years. Tight control of blood

glucose greatly reduced the risk for the development of diabetic retinopathy.

The treatment of diabetic retinopathy includes control of the diabetes and any hyperlipidemia,**3** laser therapy for background diabetic retinopathy,**4** and laser or surgical therapy to treat proliferative diabetic retinopathy.**4** Timely laser therapy of macular edema can reduce severe vision loss by 95%, and intravitreal steroid injection is also beneficial.**5** The benefit of antiangiogenic therapy is less clear.**6** With acute hyperglycemia, accumulation of sorbitol may lead to lenticular swelling; secondary refractive errors may persist for 6 to 8 weeks.

Hypertension

In chronic hypertension (Chapter 67), the characteristic retinal vascular findings can assess the severity of hypertension. As the severity increases, patients develop arterial narrowing, arteriovenous nicking (Fig. 431-26), nerve fiber layer infarcts, and intraretinal hemorrhages. Moderately sclerosed arterioles have a "copper wiring" appearance, whereas severely sclerosed vessels demonstrate "silver wiring." Acute hypertension may cause optic nerve edema ("papilledema"; Fig. 431-27) and serous retinal detachments that usually resolve without significant sequelae if blood pressure is controlled.

Other Systemic Diseases

In bacterial endocarditis (Chapter 76), emboli may cause conjunctival hemorrhages or the characteristic Roth's spot (Fig. 431-28). Accumulation of copper in the posterior cornea may aid in the diagnosis of Wilson's disease (Chapter 218), although its clinical diagnosis usually precedes the characteristic Kayser-Fleischer ring (see Fig. 218-1 in Chapter 218), which fades after treatment. Tay-Sachs and Niemann-Pick diseases (Chapter 215) are associated with a foveal cherry-red spot owing to the accumulation of gangliosides within perifoveal ganglion cells. Pseudoxanthoma elasticum (Chapter 268) is often associated with characteristic angioid streaks of the retina.

VASCULAR ABNORMALITIES OF THE EYE

The major vessels of the retina enter the eye at a point of relative constriction in the tissues of the lamina cribrosa of the optic disc. In persons who have

FIGURE 431-27. Papilledema. (Courtesy of Dr. Kathleen Digre.)

FIGURE 431-28. Roth's spots. Multiple white-centered hemorrhages in a man with recurrent subacute bacterial endocarditis. White-centered hemorrhages are also seen with leukemia and diabetes. The small white scars are probably the residua of previous episodes.

FIGURE 431-29. Central retinal artery occlusion. Fundus photograph shows diffuse retinal edema. The heavily pigmented fovea with its uniquely thin inner retina produces a cherry-red spot against the dusky macula. In this case, a small area of retina adjacent to the optic disc is spared, owing to the presence of a cilioretinal artery.

generalized vascular disease, particularly systemic hypertension, occlusion of either the artery or vein may lead to a sudden loss of vision. Partial occlusion of either the artery or vein is associated with less visual loss but still increases the risk of developing neovascular glaucoma.

Arterial occlusion of the central retinal artery (Fig. 431-29) presents as painless acute loss of vision. The ischemic posterior retina generally has a pale

FIGURE 431-30. Central retinal vein occlusion with diffuse intraretinal hemorrhages in all four quadrants.

gray appearance except at the fovea, where the normal color is preserved (cherry-red spot). The clinical appearance of edema resolves over time, but vision generally does not recover.

Venous occlusion of the central retinal vein (Fig. 431-30) presents as painless loss of vision. The retina, however, is characterized by extreme, generalized hemorrhages, which resolve very slowly and are often associated with opaque areas of focal retinal ischemia (cotton-wool spots). This process destroys the full-thickness of the retina. Usually, no vision returns. Central vein occlusion is associated with a major risk of developing secondary neovascular glaucoma.

Giant cell arteritis (temporal arteritis [Chapter 279]) is occlusion of the blood supply of the optic disc by inflammation of the short posterior ciliary arteries. Occlusion causes acute, painless loss of vision. Presenting symptoms before visual loss often include a vague sensation of fatigue, scalp tenderness, or jaw claudication. Diagnosis is suspected by classic characteristics and by an elevated erythrocyte sedimentation rate or elevated C-reactive protein level. Histologic confirmation is provided by a biopsy showing granulomatous inflammation in the region of the internal elastic lamina of the temporal artery. Emergent treatment, often protracted, with systemic steroids (Chapter 279) can prevent vascular occlusion and visual loss, but lost vision is not usually restored by treatment. There is a significant risk of the process developing in the second eye.

Nonarteritic optic neuropathy is caused by occlusion of the posterior ciliary arteries and infarction of the optic disc, resulting in acute, usually unilateral, painless loss of vision. There often are no antecedent symptoms except those systemic signs and symptoms associated with systemic nonarteritic vascular disease such as systemic hypertension. Occlusion is thought to be due to atherosclerosis or some other lumen-compromising mechanism. No treatment restores vision. There is a risk for the same process affecting the second eye.

IDIOPATHIC INFLAMMATORY AND AUTOIMMUNE DISORDERS

Ocular or periocular tissues may be the primary focus of isolated idiopathic or autoimmune inflammation. Pain is common, and changes in vision may occur.

Keratoconjunctivitis Sicca

Keratoconjunctivitis sicca, or the dry eye syndrome, results from deficiency of any of the tear film layers. Symptoms include gritty, foreign body sensations, burning, photophobia, and decreased visual acuity. Idiopathic inflammation in keratoconjunctivitis sicca and xerostomia represents Sjögren's syndrome (Chapter 276). Recurrent corneal erosion, keratitis, and corneal opacification can occur. Many medications can also cause dry eyes (Table 431-8).

Artificial tears, up to four times daily, and lubricating ointments are helpful. Corticosteroids (e.g., loteprednol 0.5% eyedrops four times a day) are also effective as an initial treatment. Cyclosporine eyedrops (0.05%, one drop in each eye every 12 hours) are useful when other measures fail.

TABLE 431-8 PARTIAL LIST OF SYSTEMIC MEDICATIONS CAUSING DRY EYE

MEDICATION	CLASS
Ibuprofen	Nonsteroidal anti-inflammatory
Diphenhydramine	Antihistamine
Triprolidine	Antihistamine
Chlorpheniramine	Antihistamine
Atenolol	β-Blocker
Metoprolol	β-Blocker
Propranolol	β-Blocker
Clonidine	α-Agonist
Scopolamine	Anticholinergic
Amiodarone	Antiarrhythmic
Thiabendazole	Antinematode
Isotretinoin*	Retinoid

*Severe, long-term dry eye with onset up to several years after treatment. All others tend to abate with cessation.

From Goldman L, Ausiello DA, eds. *Cecil Textbook of Medicine*, 23rd ed. Philadelphia: Saunders Elsevier; 2008:2852.

Scleritis

Episcleritis, which is an inflammation immediately underlying the conjunctiva, is distinguished from conjunctivitis because its radially oriented vessels do not move with the conjunctiva. Mild pain may be present. Episcleritis is self-limited. Instillation of 2.5% phenylephrine is helpful in making the diagnosis because it causes blanching in episcleritis but not in scleritis. Oral or topical nonsteroidal anti-inflammatory medications such as flurbiprofen or diclofenac may hasten resolution.

Scleritis, which presents as severe pain and redness, is associated with infectious or autoimmune connective tissue disease in about 50% of cases. Vision may be reduced if the posterior sclera is involved. Diffuse or sectoral hyperemia is nonmobile and does not blanch with instillation of phenylephrine. Secondary uveitis and keratitis may occur. Diagnostic evaluation includes ultrasonography or magnetic resonance imaging and laboratory tests to identify potential underlying conditions. Treatment may require topical or oral nonsteroidal anti-inflammatory medications or corticosteroids.

Mooren's Ulcer

Mooren's ulcer is idiopathic, progressive, peripheral corneal thinning, likely autoimmune. It can be unilateral or bilateral, and pain is common. Topical corticosteroids, mucolytics, and cytotoxic agents have been used. Bandage contact lenses and conjunctival recession or advancement have also been used with variable success.

Orbital Pseudotumor

Nonspecific, idiopathic orbital inflammation involving the lacrimal gland (dacryoadenitis), extraocular muscles (myositis), orbital fat, sclera, or optic nerve sheath (optic perineuritis) can be caused by orbital pseudotumor. Pain is frequent. Patients may present with proptosis, limited ocular movements, or decreased acuity. OCT or magnetic resonance imaging excludes a mass lesion. Patients respond dramatically to systemic corticosteroids within 24 hours, but the steroids must be tapered slowly over months to prevent recurrence.

Iritis

Iritis presents with pain, photophobia, and blurred vision, with about 50% of cases related to systemic disease. Slit lamp examination shows inflammatory cells and protein exudate in the anterior chamber. Symptomatic treatment is with prednisolone acetate 1% suspension four times a day and cycloplegic drugs (cyclopentolate 1 or 2% twice daily) is usually effective, but repeated episodes require evaluation for autoimmune and infectious causes.

Rheumatoid Arthritis

Juvenile rheumatoid arthritis (Chapter 272) is the most common specific childhood entity associated with uveitis. In adults, the ocular manifestations of rheumatoid arthritis mainly affect the anterior part of the eye, cornea, and

sclera. Nearly 50% of patients who have peripheral ulcerative keratitis of the cornea have an associated systemic disease, mainly collagen vascular disease, and especially rheumatoid arthritis. Similarly, almost half of patients who have scleritis have an associated systemic disease, and about 15% of these are connective tissue diseases. Scleromalacia perforans, which is aseptic necrosis of the sclera, is associated with rheumatoid arthritis about 46% of the time.

Systemic Lupus Erythematosus

Systemic lupus erythematosus (Chapter 274) causes eye manifestations from both the primary disease and its treatment with derivatives of chloroquine. The retina may show a retinal vasculitis, and the optic nerve an optic neuritis, ischemic or nonischemic. Chloroquine therapy can cause a toxic retinal degeneration, but this complication is rare if the daily dose of chloroquine does not exceed 250 mg (and 6.5 mg/kg of body weight for hydroxychloroquine).

Sarcoidosis

About 25% of patients with sarcoidosis (Chapter 95) develop chronic uveitis. Sarcoid also can involve the lids, conjunctiva, optic nerve, cranial nerves, and lacrimal glands. Anterior uveitis is treated topically with prednisolone acetate in decreasing doses, depending on degree of inflammation, and with daily cycloplegics (cyclopentolate 2%, atropine 1%). Posterior uveitis, dacryoadenitis, and neurologic manifestations require systemic corticosteroids, but the doses have not been standardized.

Sympathetic Ophthalmia

Sympathetic ophthalmia is an autoimmune disease characterized by bilateral, granulomatous uveitis following trauma to one eye. The condition is very rare, occurring in less than 1 per 10,000 cases of ocular surgical procedures and 1 per 1000 cases of accidental trauma.

The identified antigen within the eye is thought to be located in the outer retina. The disease is recognized clinically by signs of inflammation in the uninjured eye, about 2 weeks after the injury. Generally, removal of the injured eye within these 2 weeks will protect against the development of sympathetic ophthalmia in the uninjured eye, but once the uninjured eye is involved, removal of the originally injured eye will not influence the process. Left untreated, inflammation may destroy the function of both eyes. Once sympathetic ophthalmia is established, the patient will require anti-inflammation treatment (e.g., prednisolone, 1.0 to 1.5 mg/kg orally per day), most likely for an extended period.

⬤ GENETICALLY DETERMINED DISEASES THAT MAY BECOME SYMPTOMATIC DURING ADULTHOOD

Corneal Stromal Dystrophy

Most corneal dystrophies are autosomal dominant and bilateral, progress slowly, and primarily affect one layer of an otherwise normal cornea. Common types of dystrophies are anterior basement membrane, macular, granular, lattice, and Fuchs' endothelial. Some result from mutations within the same gene. For example, the *BIGH3* on 5q31 is associated with granular and lattice dystrophy and corneal dystrophy of Bowman. The main symptom, caused by opaque corneal deposits, is blurred vision. If the decreased vision interferes with activities of normal living, a corneal transplantation can be performed.

Choroidal Dystrophy

Choroidal dystrophies are progressive, inherited disorders characterized by atrophy of the retinal pigment epithelium and choroid. The main entities are central areolar choroidal sclerosis (autosomal dominant or recessive), gyrate atrophy (deficiency of the mitochondrial matrix enzyme ornithine-δ-aminotransferase), and choroideremia (deficiency of component A of Rab geranylgeranyl transferase). No treatment exists for central areolar choroidal sclerosis or choroideremia. An arginine-restricted diet may be helpful in treating gyrate atrophy.

Retinitis Pigmentosa

Retinitis pigmentosa (Fig. 431-31) is bilateral and symmetrical, starts in early adult life, and is progressive. Retinitis pigmentosa can be an autosomal dominant or recessive disease, X-linked, digenic, mitochondrial, or sporadic. The primary defect, apoptotic in nature, appears to be in the neural retinal receptors. The main findings consist of the tetrad of bone-corpuscular retinal pigmentation; a pale, waxy optic nerve; attenuation of retinal arterioles; and a

FIGURE 431-31. Retinitis pigmentosa. Fundus photograph shows "bone spicule" pigmentation of the midperipheral fundus, waxy pallor of the optic disc, and attenuated retinal vessels, the most consistent finding in retinitis pigmentosa. (Courtesy of Dr. John I. Loewenstein.)

posterior subcapsular cataract. Night blindness is the primary symptom. The electroretinogram usually shows no electrical evidence of retinal function. Vitamin A palmitate supplementation (15,000 IU daily) may slow the rate of progression. Gene therapy is under investigation.

COMMON PEDIATRIC OR ADOLESCENT DISEASES THAT MAY PERSIST INTO ADULTHOOD

Retinopathy of Prematurity
The peripheral retina, particularly the temporal retina, is not vascularized in premature infants (36 weeks or younger). In the premature infant, vessels of the immature retina may leave the plane of the retina and grow into the adjacent vitreous body, where tractional forces can cause total, irreversible retinal detachment. The detached retina forms a mass of fibrovascular tissue posterior to the crystalline lens, explaining the original name of this condition, retrolental fibroplasia. The primary risk factor for retinopathy of prematurity is the degree of prematurity of the infant and the use of supplemental oxygen. Early recognition and treatment of retinal neovascularization aid in reestablishing normal retinal vascular development.

Hemangioma of the Eyelid
Hemangioma of the eyelid is a hamartomatous (tissue normally found in the area) malformation of vessels in the soft tissues of the eyelid. The abnormal vascular channel, which may not be clinically evident until several weeks after birth, can expand to enlarge the eyelid and cause mechanical ptosis. Eyelid hemangioma may involute over time, usually in 4 to 7 years, but in the interval there is risk of developing amblyopia. Treatment includes intralesional steroid injection, laser photocoagulation, and, rarely, surgical debulking.

Congenital Cataract
Opacification of the crystalline lens occurs in many developmental and biochemical abnormalities. In congenital rubella (Chapter 376), the opacity is relatively limited to the fetal nucleus and has a pearl-like density. Cataract extraction is essential for dense cataracts of any type if amblyopia is to be prevented, but liberation of live rubella virus into the eye during cataract surgery may lead to necrotizing endophthalmitis and loss of the eye.

The cataract of galactosemia (Chapter 212) is potentially reversible with dietary restriction of galactose. Most other congenital cataracts do not progress. The degree of vision, which may be surprisingly adequate, cannot be accurately predicted by the clinical appearance of a lens opacity.

TUMORS OF THE EYE

Retinoblastoma
Retinoblastoma, the most common intraocular malignant tumor of childhood, results from uncontrolled proliferation of retinoblasts, which are pluripotential neuroectodermal cells that will differentiate into the various components of mature retina. A genetic deletion of the RB (retinoblastoma) gene occurs in the chromosomal region 13q14. The tumor initially proliferates in the plane of the retina but is capable of involving all structures within

the eye. Retinoblastoma may spread to the central nervous system through the optic nerve and through blood vessels to tissues at distant sites.

Approximately 40% of cases of retinoblastoma are heritable and generally diagnosed before age 12 months, much earlier than the nonheritable form. In 80% of heritable retinoblastomas, retinal tumors are multiple in each eye and are bilateral. These patients have a significant risk of developing a secondary primary malignant tumor (e.g., osteogenic sarcoma).

The nonheritable, sporadic form arises spontaneously and represents about 60% of cases. The average age at presentation is 24 months. Generally only a single tumor occurs in one eye, unlike the heritable form, in which multiple tumors in one eye and bilateral tumors are common. No detectable chromosomal abnormality is present, so the risk for retinoblastoma in succeeding generations is low. These children have the same risk for second primary tumors as the general population.

Retinoblastoma is often discovered by parents or relatives who notice a light reflex in one eye relative to the other either (white or "cat's eye" reflex; leukokoria). Children with retinoblastoma also may present with strabismus, iris neovascularization, dilated fixed pupil, secondary glaucoma, or tumor accumulation in the anterior chamber (neoplastic hypopyon). More advanced cases may present with signs of intraocular inflammation or ruptured globe with orbital extension. In some of cases of regressed retinoblastoma, the sole clinical sign may be a small, calcified tumor in the plane of the retina with surrounding retinal pigment epithelial scarring.

Most children are treated with chemotherapy, sometimes also with intraocular laser therapy or radiation, or both. Enucleation is used for advanced cases with no visual potential.

Malignant Melanoma
Malignant melanoma (Chapter 210) of the conjunctiva is rare. The individuals at risk are middle aged and lightly pigmented. Melanoma of the conjunctiva may arise from a preexisting nevus or de novo, but most arise from unilateral, acquired, variably pigmented regional, flat, or slightly elevated lesions in which the degree and distribution of pigmentation tend to vary over time. The regions of greatest risk are the conjunctiva at the limbus (junction of cornea and sclera), in the conjunctival fornix (deep peripheral recesses of the conjunctiva), and in the caruncle (elevated nodule between the nasal lid margins). Extensions onto the corneal surface or formation of a nodule or loss of pigmentation are indications for biopsy. Proliferation and hyperpigmentation of melanocytes without nuclear or cellular atypia is not associated with progression to melanoma, whereas associated nuclear or cellular atypia, particularly coupled with mitotic activity, is highly linked with progression to melanoma. Frank melanoma with a thickness of more than 0.8 mm is a risk factor for metastatic melanoma. Treatment is surgical excision, often supplemented with cryoablation. The long-term outcome is less favorable than for cutaneous melanoma because the tumor may metastasize early when the primary tumor is very small (e.g., 2 mm).

Malignant melanoma of the uveal tract is the most common primary intraocular malignancy of adults, but its incidence is only 2 to 6 per 1 million per year in high-risk populations (blue-eyed white people). The tumor, which arises from preexisting nevi or dendritic melanocytes anywhere in the uveal tract, is almost always unilateral, unicentric, and nodular and is usually diagnosed at an asymptomatic phase during routine screening examination of the dilated fundus. Symptomatic tumors arise near sensitive portions of the retina (e.g., the macula) or cause retinal detachment or cystoid macular edema. Iris tumors (Fig. 431-32) are generally pigmented and elevated above the surrounding contour, where they are recognized early in their course. Posterior tumors may be completely amelanotic and occasionally may have a bilobed appearance. Accuracy in diagnosing melanoma of the uveal tract by clinical means alone is greater than 98%. Treatment is controversial; options include enucleation of the eye, external beam and plaque (iodine-125) radiation, and en bloc resection. The overall survival rate is approximately 50% at 15 years. Risk factors for metastasis, most commonly to the liver, include tumor size, cell type, angiogenic mimicry, and the presence of monosomy 3 in the tumor cells.

Orbital Tumors
Primary tumors in the orbit of adults include cavernous hemangioma, schwannomas, and various proliferations of fibrous tissue (solitary fibrous tumor). Rhabdomyosarcoma may arise from ectopic rests of mesenchyme rather than from mature rectus muscle. Orbital tumors usually are diagnosed by imaging techniques. The treatment is orbital exploration and surgical removal.

FIGURE 431-32. Iris melanoma that has prominent intrinsic blood vessels. Note peaking of the pupil toward the tumor. (From Yanoff M, Duker JS, eds. *Ophthalmology*. Philadelphia: Mosby Elsevier; 2009.)

TABLE 431-9	SYSTEMIC MEDICATIONS WITH OCULAR EFFECTS
AGENT	**EFFECT**
Chloroquine	Dyschromatopsia, visual field defects
Hydroxychloroquine	Dyschromatopsia, visual field defects
Thioridazine	Blurred vision
Chlorpromazine	Blurred vision
Digoxin	Yellow vision
Ethambutol	Optic neuritis
Amiodarone	Corneal whorls, pigmentary retinopathy
Corticosteroids	Glaucoma, cataract
Plaquenil	Pigmentary maculopathy
Tamoxifen	Retinopathy
Neuroleptics	Nystagmus
Compazine	Oculogyric crisis
Vitamin A	Pseudotumor cerebri
5-Fluorouracil	Canalicular stenosis (tearing)
Isotretinoin	Severe dry eye (long-term effect)

From Goldman L, Ausiello DA, eds. *Cecil Textbook of Medicine*, 23rd ed. Philadelphia: Saunders Elsevier; 2008:2852.

Lymphoma

Orbital and conjunctival lymphomas are usually small B-cell mucosa-associated lymphoid tissue tumors (Chapter 191). Approximately 50% of cases ultimately include systemic disease that may, however, be delayed by decades. External beam radiation is used to treat isolated periocular disease, whereas systemic chemotherapy is required for systemic involvement.

Large-cell B-cell lymphoma (Chapter 191) may present in the eye as a form of vitreitis (cells suspended in the vitreous) or a subretinal or intraretinal infiltrate before it is discovered in the central nervous system. The diagnosis may be verified by cytologic examination of vitrectomy specimens. Treatment is generally systemic, but the outcome is usually poor.

The eye may infrequently be involved in multiple myeloma (Chapter 193). Retinal hemorrhages and vitreous opacification may occur. Periorbital osteolytic lesions of bone may be present.

Lacrimal Gland Tumors

Epithelial lacrimal gland neoplasms may arise in the lacrimal gland. The lacrimal gland contains a resting population of non-nodal lymphocytes and is a second common site for lymphomas. Malignant epithelial tumors (adenoid cystic carcinoma) may metastasize at an early stage through perineural spaces of large peripheral nerves to adjacent bone. Most epithelial gland tumors are treated with total surgical removal of the lacrimal gland because of the risk for recurrence and malignant transformation of residual tumor.

Ocular Metastasis

Metastasis to the orbit in adults is very uncommon because of its relatively small vascular volume. Metastasis to the rectus muscles present with adult-onset strabismus. Metastasis to the orbit is more common in childhood than adult leukemia.

Metastasis to the uveal tract is common, especially from primary breast and lung tumors. Metastatic lesions often grow rapidly and disturb visual function; serous retinal detachment is common.

● OCULAR EFFECTS OF SYSTEMIC MEDICATIONS

Innumerable medications may cause ocular side effects (Table 431-9). Therefore, patients taking systemic medications often require periodic surveillance to identify ocular toxicity.

Chloroquine and *hydroxychloroquine* may cause decreased color vision and visual field defects at high doses. Chloroquine toxicity is thought to occur after a cumulative dose of 300 g, whereas hydroxychloroquine may cause symptoms after long-term maintenance of 750 mg/day. The macular portion of the fundus develops a typical bull's-eye pattern. Corneal whorls may be seen. Symptoms are not reversible and tend to progress after drug cessation. Annual fundus examination with color testing, macular function tests, and automated visual field test may be indicated.

Pigmentary maculopathy may arise as blurred vision in patients taking *thioridazine* or *chlorpromazine*. Approximately 800 mg/day of the former or 1200 mg/day of the latter is believed sufficient to cause toxicity. Patients should be examined every 6 months.

Any of the commonly used antituberculous medications may cause optic neuropathy, although *ethambutol* carries the greatest risk. Pupillary response, color vision, acuity, and visual fields are the clinical parameters used to assess optic nerve function.

Cornea verticillata may be seen in patients taking *amiodarone* because of lysosomal accumulations within the epithelial basement membrane. *Fabry's disease* produces similar changes, as can other medications. Corneal whorls are usually reversible when caused by drug toxicity, and they rarely interfere with vision.

1. Evans J. Antioxidant supplements to prevent or slow down the progression of AMD: a systematic review and meta-analysis. *Eye (London)*. 2008;22:751-760.
2. Colquitt JL, Jones J, Tan SC, et al. Ranibizumab and pegaptanib for the treatment of age-related macular degeneration: a systematic review and economic evaluation. *Health Technol Assess.* 2008;12:1-222.
3. Chew EY, Ambrosius WT, Davis MD, et al, for the ACCORD Eye Study Group. Effects of medical therapies on retinopathy progression in type 2 diabetes. *N Engl J Med.* 2010;363:233-244.
4. Hoerle S, Kroll P. Evidence-based therapy of diabetic retinopathy. *Ophthalmologica.* 2007; 221:132-141.
5. Grover D, Li TJ, Chong CC. Intravitreal steroids for macular edema in diabetes. *Cochrane Database Syst Rev.* 2008;1:CD005656.
6. Parravano M, Menchini F, Virgili G. Antiangiogenic therapy with anti-vascular endothelial growth factor modalities for diabetic macular oedema. *Cochrane Database Syst Rev.* 2009;4:CD007419.

SUGGESTED READINGS

Cheung N, Mitchell P, Wong TY. Diabetic retinopathy. *Lancet.* 2010;376:124-136. *Review.*
Cochener B, Lafuma A, Khoshnood B, et al. Comparison of outcomes with multifocal intraocular lenses: a meta-analysis. *Clin Ophthalmol.* 2011;5:45-56. *Multifocal lenses provided better uncorrected near visual acuity and reduced the need for spectacles by about 50%.*
Dhital A, Pey T, Stanford MR. Visual loss and falls: a review. *Eye (London).* 2010;24:1437-1446. *Emphasizes the role of vision in normal ambulation.*
Friedman DI, Gordon LK, Quiros PA. Headache attributable to disorders of the eye. *Curr Pain Headache Rep.* 2010;14:62-72. *Review.*
Salim S, Shields MB. Glaucoma and systemic disease. *Surv Ophthalmol.* 2010;55:64-77. *Review.*

432

NEURO-OPHTHALMOLOGY

ROBERT W. BALOH AND JOANNA JEN

A mechanistic understanding of vision impairment along with disturbances in pupillary and oculomotor control lies close to the heart of diagnosing neurologic disorders.

VISION

One of the most difficult diagnostic problems is vision loss that cannot be explained by obvious abnormalities of the eye. To evaluate such a patient properly, the examining physician must be familiar with the anatomy and physiology of the afferent visual system. The afferent visual pathways cross the major ascending sensory and descending motor systems of the cerebral hemispheres and in their anterior portion are intimately related to the vascular and bony structures at the base of the brain. Not surprisingly, localization of lesions within the afferent visual pathways has great value in neurologic diagnosis.

Anatomy of the Visual Pathways

Light entering the eye falls on the retinal rods and cones, which transduce the stimulus into neural impulses to be transmitted to the brain. The distribution of visual function across the retina takes a pattern of concentric zones increasing in sensitivity toward the center, the fovea. The fovea consists of a "rod-free" central grouping of approximately 100,000 slender cones. The ganglion cells subserving these cones send their axons directly to the temporal aspect of the optic disc, where they form the papillomacular bundle. Axons originating from ganglion cells in the temporal retina curve above and below the papillomacular bundle and form dense arcuate bands.

The arteries supplying the optic nerve and retina derive from branches of the ophthalmic artery. The central retinal artery approaches the eye along each optic nerve and pierces the inferior aspect of the dural sheath about 1 cm behind the globe to enter the center of the nerve. The artery emerges in the fundus at the center of the nerve head, from which it nourishes the inner two thirds of the retina by superior and inferior branches. Anastomotic branches derived from the choroidal and posterior ciliary arteries, the ciliary system, supply the choroid, optic nerve head, and outer retinal layers, including the photoreceptors. In about 10% of the population, the macula is supplied by a retinociliary artery, a branch of the ciliary system. Venous drainage from the retina and nerve head flows primarily through the central retinal vein, whose course of exit from the eye parallels that of entry of the artery.

What each eye "sees" is termed its *visual field* (Fig. 432-1). The nasal side of the left retina and the temporal side of the right see the left side of the world, and the upper half of each retina sees the lower half of the world. Behind the eyes, the optic nerves pass through the optic canal to form the optic chiasm. In the chiasm, nerves from the nasal half of each retina decussate and join the fibers from the temporal half of the contralateral retina. From the chiasm, the optic tracts pass around the cerebral peduncles to reach the lateral geniculate ganglia. The orientation of the visual field is rotated 90 degrees in the lateral geniculate such that images from the inferior visual field project to the medial half, whereas images from the superior visual field project to the lateral half. The geniculocalcarine radiation initially fans out into superolateral and inferolateral projections, the latter passing around the lateral ventricle and for a short distance into the temporal lobe (Meyer's loop) before turning posteriorly to reach the striate cortex of the occipital lobe. In the occipital lobe, the striate cortex (area 17) lies along the superior and inferior bands of the calcarine fissure, with macular fibers projecting most posteriorly to the occipital pole and more peripheral retinal projections lying more anteriorly.

Localization of Lesions within Visual Pathways

Monocular vision loss is due to a lesion in one eye or optic nerve. Binocular visual loss, on the other hand, can result from disease located anywhere in the visual pathways from the corneas to the occipital poles. Lesions involving the optic chiasm produce nonhomonymous visual abnormalities (e.g., the bitemporal hemianopia illustrated by lesion 3 in Fig. 432-1). Optic tract

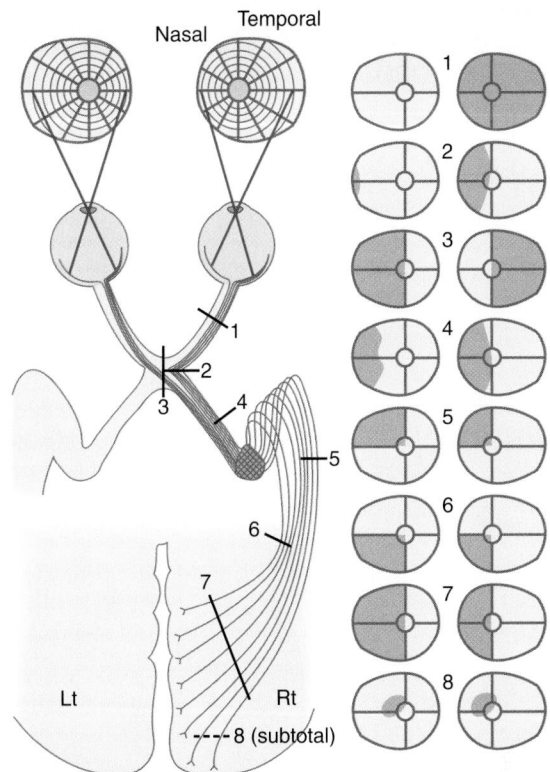

FIGURE 432-1. Visual fields that accompany damage to the visual pathways. *1,* Optic nerve: unilateral amaurosis. *2,* Lateral optic chiasm: grossly incongruous, incomplete (contralateral) homonymous hemianopia. *3,* Central optic chiasm: bitemporal hemianopia. *4,* Optic tract: incongruous, incomplete homonymous hemianopia. *5,* Temporal (Meyer's) loop of the optic radiation: congruous partial or complete (contralateral) homonymous superior quadrantanopia. *6,* Parietal (superior) projection of the optic radiation: congruous partial or complete homonymous inferior quadrantanopia. *7,* Complete parieto-occipital interruption of the optic radiation: complete congruous homonymous hemianopia with psychophysical shift of the foveal point, often sparing central vision and resulting in "macular sparing." *8,* Incomplete damage to the visual cortex: congruous homonymous scotomas, usually encroaching at least acutely on central vision.

abnormalities are comparatively rare but produce characteristic visual changes. The fibers serving identical points in the homonymous half fields do not fully commingle in the optic tract, so lesions damaging this structure produce incongruous homonymous hemianopia. Lesions of the geniculate nuclei, optic radiations, or visual cortex produce congruent hemianopic field defects that may go unrecognized unless the hemianopia intrudes on macular vision. Postgeniculate visual loss can be differentiated from pregeniculate visual loss by (1) a normal funduscopic appearance, (2) intact pupillary light reactions, and (3) appropriate lesions on brain imaging.

Examination of the Afferent Visual System

Visual function is most commonly assessed by "best-corrected visual acuity" (Chapter 431). If visual acuity is not normal, it must be determined whether acuity can be improved with lenses or at least with the use of a pinhole. The normal reference is recognition of letters at an idealized 20 feet, and acuity charts are designed with even larger letters that are normally recognized at proportionally greater distances. Thus, if one reads letters at 20 feet no better than those normally perceived at 40 feet, vision is recorded as 20/40. Small visual charts that are easily carried in the physician's case permit quick and fairly accurate bedside appraisal of acuity.

Visual fields can be tested at the bedside by confrontation, and rough estimates of their integrity can be made even in patients with reduced alertness. The fields should be tested individually for each eye because the pattern of visual field defects can provide important localizing information. A quick screen of the visual fields can be made by having the patient fixate on the examiner's nose and identify the number of fingers flashed in each of the four visual field quadrants. With practice and a cooperative subject, accurate confrontation fields can be obtained that outline even scotomas. Ophthalmoscopic examination permits direct visualization of the retina and optic disc. Corneal, lenticular, or vitreous opacities severe enough to produce visual symptoms can almost always be detected with the ophthalmoscope.

TABLE 432-1 COMMON CAUSES OF TRANSIENT MONOCULAR VISION LOSS

CATEGORY (TYPICAL DURATION)	CAUSES	DIFFERENTIAL FEATURES
Thromboembolism (1-5 min)	Atherosclerosis	Other atherosclerotic vascular disease, associated crossed hemiparesis, angiography (carotid atheroma)
	Cardiac	Valvular disease, mural thrombi, atrial fibrillation, recent myocardial infarction
	Blood dyscrasia	Blood tests positive for sickle cell anemia, macroglobulinemia, multiple myeloma, polycythemia, other
Vasospasm (5-30 min)	Migraine	Ipsilateral headache, other classic aura, family history
Vascular compression (few seconds)	Increased intracranial pressure	Precipitated by position change, Valsalva maneuver, or pressure waves
	Tumor	Associated slowly progressive monocular visual loss
Vasculitis (1-5 min)	Temporal arteritis	Associated headache, polymyalgia rheumatica, palpable temporal artery, elevated sedimentation rate

TABLE 432-2 DIFFERENTIATION OF OPTIC NEURITIS FROM PAPILLEDEMA

	OPTIC NEURITIS	PAPILLEDEMA
Central-cecocentral vision loss	Present	Absent
Distribution	Usually unilateral	Usually bilateral
Ocular pain on movement	Present	Absent
Direct light reflex	±Reduced	Intact
CT and MRI of head	White matter plaques	Tumor, venous occlusion, etc.
Visual evoked responses	Abnormal	Normal
Lumbar puncture pressure	Normal	Elevated

CT = computed tomography; MRI = magnetic resonance imaging.

Common Causes of Visual Loss

Eye

The cause of monocular vision loss secondary to ocular and retinal lesions can often be detected by ophthalmoscopic examination or by measurement of intraocular pressure (Chapter 431). *Glaucoma* caused by impaired absorption of aqueous humor results in a high intraocular pressure that usually produces gradual loss of peripheral vision, "halos" seen around lights, and occasionally, pain and redness in the affected eye. The diagnosis is made by tonometric measurement of high intraocular pressure and may be suspected by palpating an abnormally firm globe and observing a deep, pale optic cup and attenuated blood vessels. *Retinal tears* and *detachments* give rise to unilateral distortions of the visual image seen as sudden angulations or curves of objects containing straight lines (metamorphopsia). *Hemorrhages* into the vitreous humor or *infections* or *inflammatory lesions* of the retina can produce scotomas that resemble those resulting from primary disease of the central visual pathway.

Binocular vision loss secondary to retinal disease in younger subjects is often due to *heredodegenerative conditions*. Vascular diseases, diabetes (Chapter 236), and age-related macular degeneration are causes in older patients. In most cases of *pigmentary retinal degeneration*, visual loss begins peripherally and slowly proceeds centrally. By contrast, *macular degeneration* (see Figs. 431-22 and 431-23 in Chapter 431) impairs central vision early in its course. A common variant in the complement factor H (*CFH*) gene is associated with a markedly increased risk for the development of age-related macular degeneration.

Optic Nerve

Acute or subacute monocular vision loss (Table 432-1) as a result of optic nerve disease is most commonly produced by demyelinating disorders, vascular obstruction, neoplasm, or hereditary optic neuropathy. Demyelinating disease of the nerve head (*optic neuritis* or *papillitis*) produces disc edema along with loss of central vision in the affected eye only; subjectively unrecognized scotomas may sometimes be found in the other eye. Demyelination of the optic nerve behind the point where the retinal vein emerges (*retrobulbar neuritis*) initially leaves a normal-looking disc but a central or paracentral scotoma. With chronic demyelinating disorders, the optic disc becomes pale and atrophic. The clinical course and therapeutic response of optic neuritis depend on the underlying inflammatory mechanism. In more than 50% of patients initially seen with optic neuritis, typical symptoms and signs of multiple sclerosis eventually develop (Chapter 419). Optic neuritis with an associated transverse myelitis is the clinical hallmark of neuromyelitis optica,

which is a severe demyelinating disease often mistaken for multiple sclerosis but now recognized to be caused by anti–aquaporin 4 autoantibodies. Intraocular arterial occlusion may produce either central visual loss or an altitudinal field defect (*ischemic optic neuropathy*). *Tumors* (Chapter 195) invading the optic nerve or space-occupying lesions compressing it anywhere between the orbit and chiasm cause gradually decreasing central vision or a sector defect of the peripheral visual field. With such chronic lesions, the affected optic nerve becomes visibly atrophic.

Acute binocular vision loss resulting from bilateral optic nerve disease is most often caused by demyelinating disease or by toxic or nutritional factors (Chapter 425). In younger persons and those lacking a clear history of toxic exposure, demyelinating lesions overwhelmingly predominate. Symptoms are of abrupt or subacute onset with visual blurring, which may progress rapidly to blindness within hours or days. There may be pain about the eyes, particularly with movement. *Leber's optic neuropathy*, caused by a mutation in mitochondrial DNA, typically begins painlessly and centrally in one eye, with the second eye affected weeks to months later.

Papilledema is disc edema secondary to increased intracranial pressure (Table 432-2). Vision is normal except under one of two circumstances: (1) acute transient episodes of amaurosis lasting a few seconds and attributable to acute increases in intracranial pressure (plateau waves) and (2) progressive loss of peripheral vision with long-standing, severe papilledema caused by compression of the optic nerve head. Subacute or chronic binocular vision loss secondary to optic nerve disease can result from *toxic* and *nutritional* causes or from *inherited optic atrophy*. The latter sometimes accompanies spinocerebellar degeneration but may selectively affect the optic nerve. With either cause, visual loss is painless and primarily affects central vision; ophthalmoscopy shows optic atrophy.

Chiasm and Optic Tract

Patients with lesions of the optic chiasm or optic tract are often unaware of visual impairment until the deficit encroaches on central vision in one or both eyes. Intrinsic or extrinsic neoplasms and parachiasmal arterial aneurysms are the most common lesions in this location. Gliomas that arise within the chiasm or optic tract are rare in adulthood. Extrinsic lesions compressing the chiasm or tract include *pituitary adenomas* (Chapter 231), *dysgerminomas*, *craniopharyngiomas*, *meningiomas* (Chapter 195), and large *aneurysms* of the carotid or basilar artery (Chapter 415). The diagnosis rests on finding the characteristic visual field abnormalities (bitemporal hemianopia for chiasm and incongruous homonymous hemianopia for optic tract lesions) and identifying the lesion with computed tomography or magnetic resonance imaging. Pituitary apoplexy secondary to acute hemorrhage into the gland (Chapter 231) can result in sudden vision loss; prompt neurosurgical intervention under steroid coverage is required for most patients.

Visual Radiations and Occipital Cortex

Lesions involving the postgeniculate visual pathways most often result from *vascular damage, traumatic injuries, neoplasms*, or rarely, *inflammatory* or *degenerative disorders* involving the cerebral white matter. Their localization can be deduced by the resulting visual field defects. Vascular disease of the occipital lobes is the most common cause of homonymous visual field defects in the middle-aged and elderly population. *Anton's syndrome* refers to cerebral visual loss with denial of a visual defect. Affected patients not only deny that they are blind but also confabulate details of their visual environment from memory. Anton's syndrome results from bilateral lesions involving the

Pupillary Response

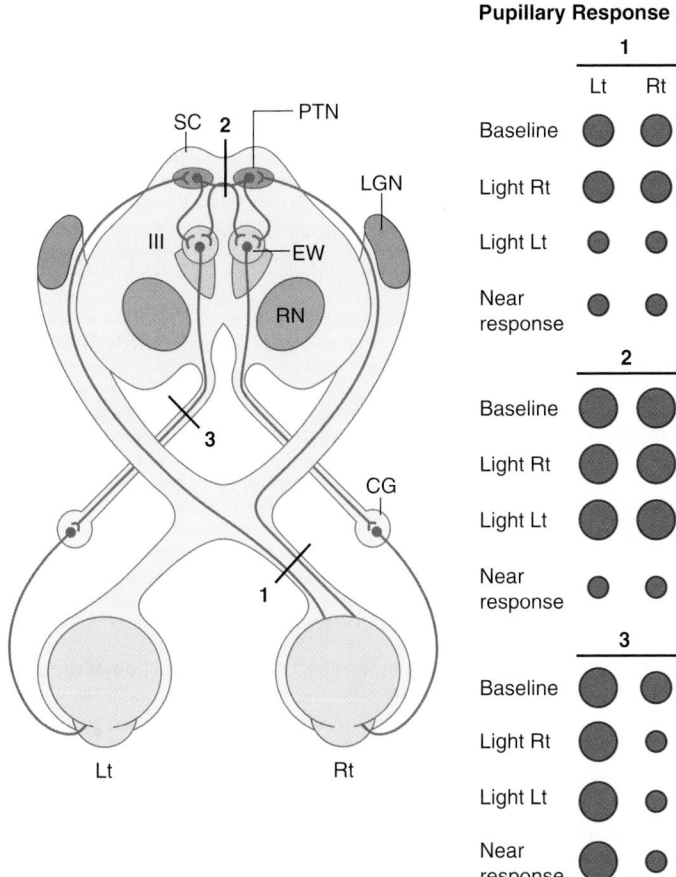

FIGURE 432-2. Pupillary responses associated with lesions of the *(1)* optic nerve, *(2)* pretectum, and *(3)* oculomotor nerve. Baseline is obtained with fixation on a distant target and the near response with a target in front of the nose. CG = ciliary ganglion; EW = Edinger-Westphal nucleus; LGN = lateral geniculate nucleus; PTN = pretectal nucleus; RN = red nucleus; SC = superior colliculus.

FIGURE 432-3. Adie's tonic pupil in the right eye of a young woman. The affected pupil is "tonic"; that is, it responds slowly to light and accommodation but on rapid testing appears unresponsive. The site of the lesion is usually obscure, but the condition is benign. There may be associated areflexia. (From Forbes CD, Jackson WF. *Color Atlas and Text of Clinical Medicine,* 3rd ed. London: Mosby; 2003.)

parieto-occipital lobes or in the setting of metabolic encephalopathy. The reversible *posterior leukoencephalopathy syndrome,* which is characterized by headache, seizures, confusion, and cortical visual loss, is associated with an abrupt increase in blood pressure, such as may be seen with eclampsia and with immunosuppressive therapy after transplantation.

⬤ PUPILLARY CONTROL

The neuromechanisms that control pupil size and reactivity are complex, yet they can be evaluated by simple clinical procedures. The diameter of the pupil is determined by the antagonistic actions of the iris sphincter and dilator muscles, with the latter playing a minor role. If the sphincter muscle is severed or ruptured, it does not retract toward one quadrant but rather continues to function, except in the altered segment. Therefore, pupillary response can be evaluated even in the presence of significant damage to the iris.

Anatomy and Localization of Lesions within Pupillary Pathways

The size of the pupil is governed by tonic balance between sympathetic and parasympathetic innervation of the muscles of the iris. Sympathetic stimulation dilates the pupil, whereas parasympathetic stimulation constricts it. In the normal resting state, light entering the eye provides the major stimulus governing the size of the pupil (Fig. 432-2). Light activates the retinal rods and cones, with maximal sensitivity in the macular area. The optic nerve fibers follow the crossed and uncrossed visual pathways to the pregeniculate portion of the optic tracts, where the receptor fibers for light diverge to the pretectal nucleus located at the midbrain-diencephalic junction. Interneurons project from this nucleus to the Edinger-Westphal nuclei atop the midbrain third nerve nuclear complex of either side. From that point, paired parasympathetic efferents leave the midbrain in the third nerves, travel in the interpeduncular space across the petroclinoid ligament and edge of the tentorium, traverse the cavernous sinus, and then enter the orbit through the superior orbital fissure. In the orbit, the parasympathetic efferents synapse in the ciliary ganglion, from which ciliary nerves enter the eye to reach the pupillary muscles.

The principal sympathetic control of the pupil originates in the ventral lateral hypothalamus (first-order neuron), from which fibers descend ipsilaterally through the brain stem tegmentum and thence to the cervical cord, where they synapse with preganglionic neurons in the intermedial lateral column of the upper three thoracic segments. Preganglionic fibers (second-order neurons) emerge with the ventral roots of C8, T1, and T2 and ascend in the neck to synapse in the superior cervical ganglion adjacent to the base of the skull. Postganglionic (third-order neurons) pupillary fibers accompany the internal carotid artery through the skull and then leave it to follow the ophthalmic branch of the trigeminal nerve to reach the pupillodilator muscle of the eye.

Examination of the Pupil

The pupillary response to light should be examined in a dimly lighted room, where the pupils are naturally dilated. First, the size and symmetry of the pupils are assessed by shining a dim light onto the face from below so that both pupils are seen simultaneously in the indirect illumination. To test light reactivity, gaze is directed at a distant object (so that constriction secondary to convergence is minimal), and first one and then the other pupil is illuminated with a bright light source. If a pupil reacts poorly to direct light, it is observed as the opposite eye is illuminated (consensual response). Pupils that react poorly to light should be tested for reactivity to the near reflex by first having the patient gaze at a distant object and then quickly fixate on an object just in front of his or her nose. *Light-near dissociation* refers to a pupil that does *not* react to light but does accommodate by constricting to a near target.

Common Causes of Pupillary Abnormalities

With so-called benign pupillary dilation or *physiologic anisocoria,* there is a long-standing difference in the size of the two pupils with normal reflex reactions; the disparity remains constant during constriction and dilation. Lesions compressing or damaging the pretectal region interrupt the afferent light reflex bilaterally to produce dilated and light-fixed pupils (e.g., lesion 2; see Fig. 432-2). Pupillary constriction to the near response is preserved until late stages. Tumors of the pineal gland (e.g., dysgerminomas) and *localized infarctions* are the most common lesions in this location. *Adie's tonic pupil* (Fig. 432-3) is a medium to large (3 to 6 mm) pupil that constricts little or not at all to light and very slowly to accommodation but constricts with the instillation of dilute (0.125%) pilocarpine (Fig. 432-4). The condition usually affects one eye (occasionally both), is more common in women 25 to 45 years of age, and carries no serious implications. It most likely results from postviral denervation of the pupillary muscles. Unexplained unilateral or bilateral dilated pupils as an isolated finding can result from *accidental or intentional instillation of mydriatic drugs.* Transdermal scopolamine is a common cause. Failure of the pupil to constrict promptly with pilocarpine (1%) gives the diagnosis if the history is unclear. Interruption of the emerging third nerve in the ventral midbrain or along the proximal part of its course produces a dilated pupil 6 to 7 mm in diameter. Important causes of compression of the third nerve in this region are *aneurysms* (Chapter 415), *neoplasia* (Chapter 195), and *brain herniation* (Chapter 195) as a result of increased intracranial pressure. In nearly all cases, the pupillary involvement is associated with other signs of third nerve involvement (see later text).

Sympathetic paralysis of the eye with ptosis, anhidrosis, and miosis (Horner's syndrome; Fig. 432-5) can result from lesions anywhere along the pathway of the sympathetic innervation to the eye (Table 432-3). The diagnosis can sometimes be made by identifying associated signs in the brain

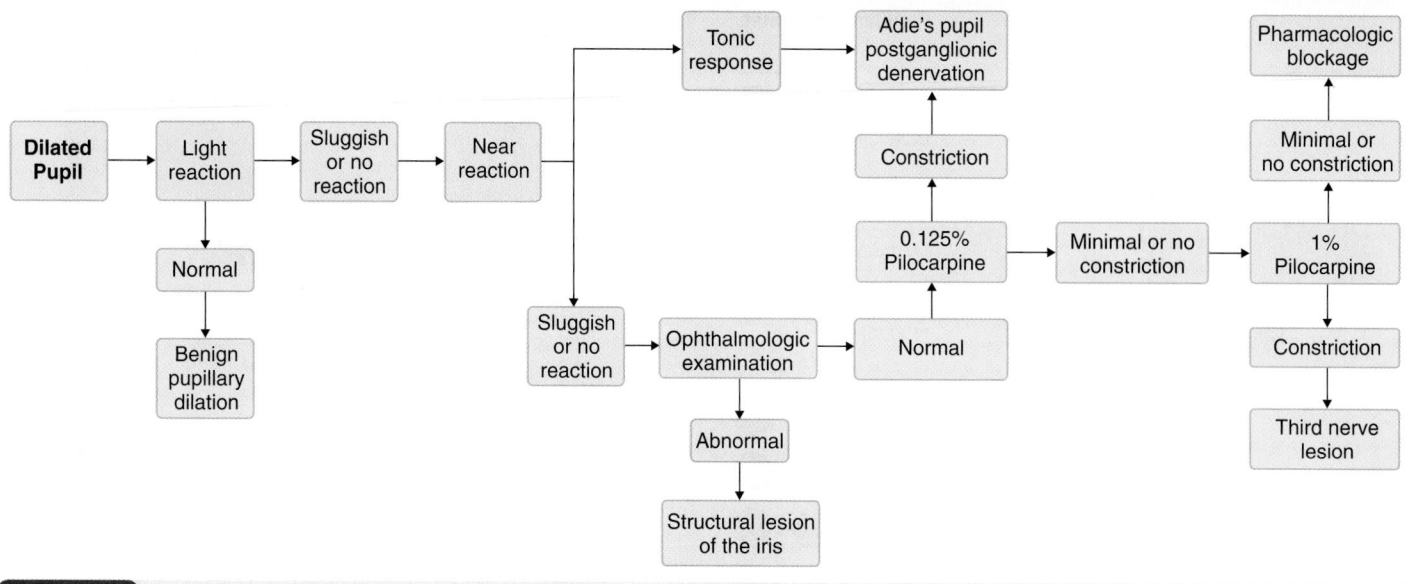

FIGURE 432-4. Use of pilocarpine to help differentiate between different causes of a dilated pupil.

FIGURE 432-5. Horner's syndrome. Note the characteristic ptosis of the left eye associated with constriction of the pupil (miosis). This patient had syringomyelia, but Horner's syndrome has many possible causes. (From Forbes CD, Jackson WF. *Color Atlas and Text of Clinical Medicine*, 3rd ed. London: Mosby; 2003.)

TABLE 432-3   HORNER'S SYNDROME RESULTS FROM LESIONS IN MULTIPLE LOCATIONS

LOCATION OF LESION	NEURON INVOLVED	TYPE OF LESION	ASSOCIATED SYMPTOMS AND SIGNS
Lateral brain stem	1st order	Infarction, glioma	Vertigo, nystagmus, imbalance, numbness, weakness
Apex of lung	2nd order	Lung cancer, trauma	Often none
Neck	3rd order	Carotid dissection or inflammation	Pain, monocular visual loss, hemiparesis

stem or neck or along the carotid artery. *Argyll Robertson pupils* are small (1 to 2 mm), unequal, irregular, and fixed to light; they constrict minimally to accommodation. Their principal cause is tertiary neurosyphilis (Chapter 327).

OCULOMOTOR CONTROL

Abnormal eye movements can result from disturbances at several levels. Disconjugate eye movements result from lesions in the individual ocular muscles, the myoneural junctions, the oculomotor nerves and their three paired nuclei in the brain stem, and the internuclear medial longitudinal fasciculus (MLF), which yokes the eyes in horizontal movements. Supranuclear lesions typically produce disorders of conjugate gaze (gaze palsies).

Anatomy and Localization of Lesions within the Oculomotor Pathways
Nuclear and Internuclear Pathways

The abducens (sixth) nerve supplies the lateral rectus muscle. Selective involvement of the abducens nerve anywhere along its pathway leads to isolated weakness of abduction of the affected eye. Destruction of the abducens nucleus in the brain stem results in a conjugate gaze paralysis (ipsilateral) because, in addition to oculomotor neurons, the nucleus contains interneurons destined for the contralateral medial rectus nucleus. The trochlear (fourth) nerve supplies the contralateral superior oblique muscle, which turns in and depresses the eye. Patients with superior oblique weakness note an increase in diplopia with head tilt toward the side of weakness and often tilt their head in the opposite direction. At rest, there is slight upward deviation of the involved eye, and downward movement is impaired when the affected eye is turned in. Patients typically complain of diplopia when reading or going down stairs. The third (oculomotor) cranial nerve supplies the remaining ocular muscles. Involvement of the third nerve nucleus in the midbrain always produces at least some bilateral oculomotor weakness; the superior rectus division of the nucleus supplies the contralateral superior rectus muscle (all other divisions supply ipsilateral muscles). Peripheral third nerve paralysis can result from lesions damaging the structure anywhere from its course within the ventral midbrain to where it enters the orbit through the superior orbital fissure. When complete, third nerve palsy produces a widely dilated pupil, severe ptosis, and an externally deviated eye held in position by unopposed contraction of the lateral rectus muscle. In such conditions, the continued trochlear action reveals itself by intorsion of the eye when the subject attempts to look down.

The MLF interconnects the abducens nucleus in the pons with the contralateral oculomotor nuclear complex in the midbrain. It terminates cephalad in the interstitial nucleus in the rostral midbrain and can be traced as far caudad as the thoracocervical region of the spinal cord (coordinating nuchal-ocular control). Lesions involving the MLF characteristically produce internuclear ophthalmoplegia (INO), in which the eyes are conjugate in the primary position but disconjugate on lateral gaze. With fully developed INO on lateral gaze away from the side of the lesion, the contralateral eye abducts and shows nystagmus, whereas the ipsilateral adducting eye does not move nasally because of failure of ascending impulses to reach the medial rectus division of the third nerve nucleus. Adduction for convergence is usually relatively maintained.

Supranuclear Pathways

Pathways descending from the frontal eye fields in the frontal lobe through the superior colliculi to the contralateral brain stem regulate rapid voluntary eye movements (*saccades*) (Table 432-4). Pathways descending from the parieto-occipital and frontal regions to the ipsilateral brain stem subserve slow visual tracking (smooth pursuit—foveal target; optokinetic—full-field target). For the vestibulo-ocular reflex, primary afferent neurons in the inner ear synapse with neurons in the vestibular nuclei, which in turn synapse with appropriate oculomotor neurons to produce compensatory eye movements. The *convergence* center is located in the rostral-dorsal midbrain near the vertical gaze center.

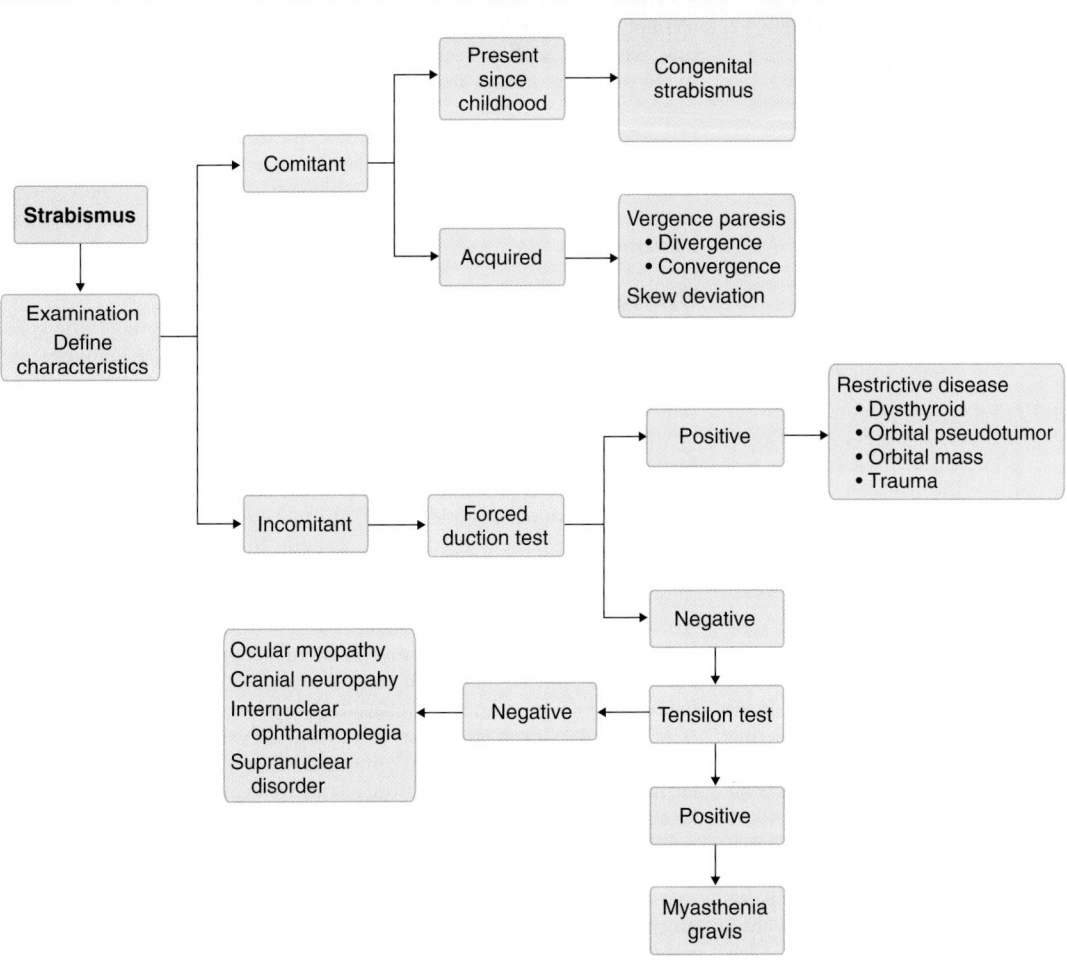

FIGURE 432-6. Diagnostic tests that help differentiate among common causes of strabismus.

TABLE 432-4	SUPRANUCLEAR OCULOMOTOR CONTROL SYSTEMS		
SYSTEM	**DESCRIPTION**	**FUNCTION**	**KEY ANATOMIC STRUCTURES**
Saccade	Fast conjugate voluntary movements	Move the fovea to a new target of interest	Frontal eye field, superior colliculus, pretectum—vertical, pontine—horizontal cerebellar dentate nucleus
Smooth pursuit/ optokinetic	Slow conjugate tracking	Match eye velocity to target velocity	Occipital, parietal, pons, cerebellar flocculus
Vestibulo-ocular	Slow conjugate compensatory eye movements	Keep eyes stable when head moves	Pontomedullary region
Vergence	Slow disconjugate tracking	Focus on near and far targets	Pretectum, tectum

TABLE 432-5	KEY DISTINGUISHING FEATURES OF PERIPHERAL AND CENTRAL TYPES OF SPONTANEOUS AND POSITIONAL NYSTAGMUS	
TYPE OF NYSTAGMUS	**PERIPHERAL (END ORGAN AND NERVE)**	**CENTRAL (BRAIN STEM AND CEREBELLUM)**
Spontaneous	Unidirectional, fast phase away from the lesion, combined horizontal torsional, inhibited with fixation	Bidirectional or unidirectional; often pure horizontal, vertical, or torsional; *not* inhibited with fixation
Static positional	Fixed or changing direction, inhibited with fixation	Fixed or changing direction, *not* inhibited with fixation
Paroxysmal positional	Vertical-torsional, occasionally horizontal-torsional, vertigo prominent, fatigability, latency	Often pure vertical, vertigo less prominent, no latency, nonfatigable

Examination of Eye Movements

Fixation and gaze holding are tested by having the patient look center, right, left, up, and down. Each position should be held steady and unwavering with the observer carefully documenting abnormal movements or ocular disconjugacies. Each supranuclear oculomotor control system is examined separately. *Saccades* are tested by having the patient alternately fixate on two targets such as the examiner's finger and nose; the speed and accuracy are noted. *Smooth pursuit* is tested by slowly moving a target back and forth and up and down and observing the patient's ability to produce smooth tracking movements. If the target velocity is low, normal subjects should be able to pursue without requiring catch-up saccades. The *vestibulo-ocular reflex* is evaluated with the head-thrust test (Chapter 436). *Convergence* is tested by having the patient follow a target moving from far to near. The degree of convergence depends to some extent on the cooperation of the patient. A clear sign that the patient is attempting to converge is simultaneous pupillary constriction.

Common Causes of Abnormal Oculomotor Control
Strabismus (Ocular Misalignment)

A comitant (same in all directions of gaze) strabismus present since childhood is usually a benign *congenital disorder*. Latent congenital strabismus can become manifested in adulthood in association with a systemic illness. An acquired skew deviation (vertical displacement of the ocular axes) indicates a lesion within the otolith-ocular pathways (generally the brain stem). Incomitant strabismus can result from restrictive disease of the orbit or from abnormal muscle or oculomotor nerve function. The presence of mechanical restriction is confirmed by the use of forced duction testing (Fig. 432-6) (After a topical anesthetic is applied to the eye, the ophthalmologist grasps

FIGURE 432-7. Internuclear ophthalmoplegia may be an initial feature of brain stem involvement in multiple sclerosis. On lateral gaze to the right, adduction of the left eye is incomplete. On convergence, eye movement was normal. The lesion is in the left medial longitudinal bundle, between the nucleus in the pons and the third nerve nucleus on the opposite side. (From Forbes CD, Jackson WF. *Color Atlas and Text of Clinical Medicine*, 3rd ed. London: Mosby; 2003.)

the muscle insertion with large blunt-toothed forceps. Failure of the eye to deviate fully in the pulled direction implies restriction.) Common causes of *orbital restrictive disease* include dysthyroid ophthalmopathy (Chapter 233), orbital pseudotumor, trauma, and orbital mass lesions (Chapter 431). Variable strabismus that increases with fatigue suggests *myasthenia gravis* (Chapter 430). A Tensilon test can usually confirm the diagnosis (see Fig. 432-6). If both restrictive disease and myasthenia gravis (Chapter 430) have been excluded, most patients with incomitant strabismus have processes affecting the oculomotor nuclei, their fascicles, or the cranial nerves themselves. Common causes of an *isolated third nerve palsy* in an adult include aneurysm (Chapter 413), small-vessel occlusive disease (including diabetes mellitus (Chapter 236), trauma (Chapter 406), and neoplasm. Typically, third nerve lesions secondary to vascular disease spare the pupil. Vascular disease and trauma are by far the most common causes of *isolated trochlear nerve palsy*. The abducens nerve is particularly vulnerable to isolated traumatic involvement because of its long pathway outside the brain stem. Lesions that produce increased intracranial pressure (Chapter 195) can lead to abducens nerve dysfunction regardless of the location and produce a "false localizing sign." Other common causes of *isolated sixth nerve palsy* are vascular disease (Chapter 414), trauma (Chapter 406), and neoplasm. About one fourth of cases of cranial nerve palsy (third, fourth, or sixth nerves) remain undiagnosed.

Internuclear Ophthalmoplegia

INO (Fig. 432-7) may be unilateral or bilateral, partial or complete, depending on the location of the lesion and the degree of damage to the MLF. *Demyelinating* and small *vascular lesions* are the most common causes of unilateral INO unaccompanied by other ocular palsies or brain stem signs. Larger brain stem lesions that damage one or more oculomotor nuclei plus the MLF often produce combinations of disconjugate eye movements coupled with nuclear oculomotor palsies. Myasthenia gravis (Chapter 430) can produce an ophthalmoparesis resembling INO as a result of greater involvement of the medial rectus than the lateral rectus. Demyelinating diseases (Chapter 419) are the most common causes of bilateral INO involvement.

Disorders of Conjugate Gaze

Acute lesions involving a frontal eye field (e.g., hemorrhage or infarction [Chapters 414 and 415]) result in a transient inability to direct the eyes contralaterally. Vertical eye movements are not affected by unilateral lesions. Bilateral damage to the frontal eye fields or their descending pathways may produce an inability to move the eyes voluntarily (horizontal or vertical) despite preserved reflex eye movements, a condition called *oculomotor apraxia*. Lesions involving the horizontal gaze center in the pons produce an ipsilateral paralysis of conjugate gaze and tonic deviation of the eyes to the contralateral side (Chapter 431). Lesions of the pretectum selectively impair vertical gaze, with the vertical upgaze center being slightly rostral and dorsal to the vertical downgaze center. Patients with the *dorsal midbrain syndrome* (Parinaud's syndrome) have a conjugate upgaze paresis. When they

attempt to make upward saccades, convergence retraction nystagmus develops. As noted earlier, impaired convergence and light-near dissociation of the pupillary reflexes are also part of the syndrome. The most common causes of the dorsal midbrain syndrome include tumors of the pineal gland (Chapter 230) (dysgerminomas), hydrocephalus (Chapter 195), and localized infarction. With the so-called locked-in syndrome (secondary to basilar artery thrombosis [Chapter 411]), voluntary horizontal eye movements are absent; the patient's only remaining motor functions are vertical eye and lid movements.

Nystagmus

Spontaneous nystagmus can be congenital or acquired. *Congenital nystagmus* typically has a high frequency and variable waveform (usually pendular) and is highly fixation dependent. It generally remains horizontal in all positions of gaze. The lifelong history and lack of symptoms confirm the diagnosis. Spontaneous nystagmus resulting from a *peripheral vestibular* lesion (i.e., in the labyrinth or vestibular nerve) usually has combined horizontal and torsional components (Table 432-5). The nystagmus resolves within a few days of the acute lesion. Acquired persistent spontaneous nystagmus indicates a lesion in the brain stem or cerebellum, or both. The latter is often purely vertical, horizontal, or torsional. Spontaneous *downbeat nystagmus* is commonly seen with lesions of the cerebellum or cervicomedullary junction (e.g., Arnold-Chiari malformation [Chapter 426]).

Gaze-evoked nystagmus is always in the direction of gaze and is usually present with and without fixation. It is most commonly produced by the ingestion of *drugs* such as phenobarbital, phenytoin, alcohol, and diazepam (Chapter 110). It can also occur in patients with such varied conditions as myasthenia gravis (Chapter 430), multiple sclerosis (Chapter 419), and cerebellar atrophy. Asymmetrical horizontal gaze-evoked nystagmus is caused by a structural brain stem or cerebellar lesion (particularly at the cerebellopontine angle), with the lesion generally being on the side of the larger-amplitude nystagmus (Bruns' nystagmus). *Rebound nystagmus* is a type of gaze-evoked nystagmus that either disappears or reverses direction as the eccentric gaze position is held. When the eyes are returned to the primary position, nystagmus occurs in the direction of the return saccade. Rebound nystagmus occurs in patients with cerebellar atrophy and focal structural lesions of the cerebellum; it is the only variety of nystagmus thought to be specific for cerebellar involvement. *Disconjugate gaze–evoked nystagmus* most commonly results from lesions of the MLF (see earlier discussion), but it can also occur with other lesions of the brain stem involving the oculomotor nuclei. Positional nystagmus is discussed in Chapter 436.

Other Ocular Oscillations

Ocular bobbing consists of a fast conjugate downward eye movement followed by a slow return to the primary position. The phenomenon accompanies severe displacement or destruction of the pons or, less often, metabolic central nervous system depression. *Ocular myoclonus* consists of continuous rhythmic pendular oscillations, most often vertical, at a rate of 1 to 3 beats per second; it often accompanies palatal myoclonus and has a similar pathogenesis. *Square-wave jerks* and *ocular flutter* consist of brief, intermittent, horizontal oscillations (back to back saccades) arising from the primary gaze position. These types of ocular oscillation are most commonly seen with cerebellar disease but can also accompany more diffuse central nervous system disorders. *Opsoclonus* consists of rapid, chaotic, conjugate, repetitive saccadic eye movements (dancing eyes). Opsoclonus accompanies the cerebellar dysfunction, with the most chaotic varieties associated with brain stem encephalitis or the remote effects of systemic neoplasm, especially neuroblastoma in children. *Ocular dysmetria* refers to overshooting and undershooting of saccadic eye movements, often followed by multiple attempts at refixation. It reflects cerebellar dysfunction.

SUGGESTED READINGS

Pula JH, Reder AT. Multiple sclerosis. Part I: neuro-ophthalmic manifestations. *Curr Opin Ophthalmol.* 2009;20:467-475. *Common visual and oculomotor finding with multiple sclerosis.*

Rucker JC. Neuro-ophthalmology of systemic disease. *Semin Neurol.* 2009;29:111-123. *Neuro-ophthalmological findings associated with common systemic disorders.*

Wilhelm H. The pupil. *Curr Opin Neurol.* 2008;21:36-42. *Review of papillary control and common clinical findings.*

433

DISEASES OF THE MOUTH AND SALIVARY GLANDS

TROY E. DANIELS

More than 200 primary lesions or diseases occur in the oral mucosa, gingiva, teeth, jaws, and minor or major salivary glands. In addition, secondary abnormalities of the oral mucosa or salivary glands can be caused by systemic diseases or drugs. The most common or important of these diseases may be observed during physical examination and are often part of a systemic process.

● ORAL MUCOSAL DISEASES
Acute Ulcerations

Painful short-term ulcerations are caused by mechanical trauma, immunologic mechanisms, or bacterial or viral infections (Table 433-1). Soon after formation, oral mucosal ulcers become covered by a white to gray pseudomembrane, analogous to scabs on dry epidermis. Pseudomembrane-covered ulcers are distinguished from white hyperkeratotic lesions by their clinical features of pain, a flat surface, and an erythematous periphery. Traumatic ulcers are characteristically located on the tongue or inside the cheeks or lips, are close to the chewing surfaces of the teeth, and have irregular borders.

APHTHOUS STOMATITIS ("CANKER SORES")

These idiopathic recurrent ulcers, which afflict up to 20% of the population, are found on all areas of the oral mucosa except the hard palate, gingiva, and vermilion, which are keratinized (Fig. 433-1). They form well-defined circular lesions that may be single or multiple. There are three clinical forms: (1) minor, which are flat and less than 1 cm in diameter and last 5 to 10 days; (2) major, which have raised borders, are greater than 1 cm, and often last for weeks or months; and (3) herpetiform, which are usually clusters of very small ulcers that resemble recurrent herpetic lesions but are not preceded by vesicles and do not occur on keratinized mucosa. A viral pathogenesis has not been established for any of these forms. Lesions clinically identical to minor aphthae occur in Behçet's syndrome (Chapter 278). Aphthae are occasionally associated with anemias or gluten-sensitive enteropathy and may become more frequent and severe in association with human immunodeficiency virus (HIV) infection (Table 433-2).

Minor or herpetiform aphthous ulcers may not require treatment unless they occur frequently.■ Topical steroids, such as fluocinonide gel or ointment, can reduce the severity and duration of the lesions only if applied with prodromal symptoms or earliest signs. Major aphthae usually require treatment with prednisone (e.g., 40 mg daily for 3 days); failure to respond significantly should prompt incisional biopsy to exclude neoplasia.

VIRAL ULCERS

Several types of virus (most commonly herpes simplex type 1; Chapter 382) cause multiple oral mucosal vesicles that last only a few hours or days and then become irregular shallow ulcers. In the initial infection by herpes simplex virus, usually in children, numerous vesicles may appear on any oral mucosal site (primary herpetic gingivostomatitis), accompanied by malaise, headache, fever, and cervical lymphadenopathy. Patients previously exposed to this virus may develop recurrent (secondary) lesions as clusters of small vesicles, most commonly on the lips (herpes labialis) and less commonly on the keratinized mucosa of the gingiva or hard palate (Fig. 433-2). Such lesions contain live virus and tend to recur at the same site but less frequently with increasing age.

Similar mucosal vesicles may also accompany the initial infection by the varicella-zoster virus in children with chickenpox (Chapter 383), and unilateral lesions may occur if herpes zoster (Chapter 383) affects branches of the trigeminal nerve. Uncommonly, oral mucosal ulcers may be caused by

TABLE 433-1	ORAL MUCOSAL ULCERS
TYPE/DISEASE	**CLINICAL FEATURES**
Insidious Onset, Chronic	
Multiple or bilateral	Shallow ulcers on mucosa, skin, or both
Pemphigus vulgaris	Begin as short-duration blisters
Mucous membrane pemphigoid	Begin as short-duration blisters
Lichen planus	Bilaterally symmetrical lesions (associated with hyperkeratosis and/or erythema)
Lupus erythematosus	Asymmetrical lesions, with or without systemic lupus (associated with hyperkeratoses and/or erythema)
Drug reaction	Variable lesions; appropriate history of drug use (e.g., penicillamine, gold)
Epidermolysis bullosa	Begin as blisters; lifelong history
Solitary	Indurated or cratered ulcers
Squamous cell carcinoma	Most common on tongue, oropharynx, lip, mouth floor
Adenocarcinomas, various	Most commonly on palate, cheeks, mouth floor
Tuberculosis	Usually painful
Actinomycosis	Often associated with draining sinus
Deep mycoses (particularly histoplasmosis, coccidioidomycosis)	Associated with systemic infection
Midline granuloma	Associated with necrosis, may perforate palate
Underlying osteonecrosis	Associated with prior cancer radiation therapy or bisphosphonate use
Acute Onset, Often Self-Limiting	
Clusters	Usually small and shallow ulcers; history of blisters
Primary herpes simplex	Any oral mucosal site, associated with fever, malaise
Recurrent herpes simplex	Only on gingiva, hard palate, or lip (keratinized mucosa)
Varicella-zoster	Unilateral lesions along neural distribution
Herpangina	Usually on oropharynx
Measles (rubeola)	Precede skin rash; associated with fever, malaise
Solitary or multiple (without clustering)	Variable, usually without history of blisters
Traumatic ulcers	Usually solitary; history of trauma
Aphthous stomatitis (canker sores)	Circular, often multiple, only on nonkeratinized mucosa
Behçet's syndrome	Oral lesions similar to recurrent aphthae
Erythema multiforme	Multiple lesions, often involve lower labial mucosa; can be recurrent or chronic
Drug reaction	Appropriate history of drug use
Necrotizing sialometaplasia	Deep ulcers, usually on palate
Primary syphilis	Solitary, indurated, painless, any site
Gonorrhea	Painful, surrounded by erythema, any site

different types of coxsackievirus (Chapter 387), appearing on any oral site in hand-foot-and-mouth disease or on the soft palate or pharynx in herpangina. After infection by the measles (rubeola) virus, small ulcers (Koplik's spots) may form on the inside of the cheeks 1 to 2 days before development of the skin rash (Chapter 375).

ERYTHEMA MULTIFORME

In this potentially recurrent disease, painful oral mucosal ulcerations develop rapidly, with or without target-like skin lesions. It may be associated with a previous viral infection or hypersensitivity to a food or drug. The affected patients, usually young adults with minimal or no systemic symptoms, have irregularly shaped ulcers that can be small and few or involve large areas of the mucosa; the most common sites are the lower labial mucosa and vermilion. These lesions can be distinguished from those of primary herpes by the absence of oral vesicles and systemic symptoms or by the presence of characteristic skin lesions (Chapter 447). A major variant of this disease is Stevens-Johnson syndrome, in which ocular, genital, and other lesions may accompany the oral lesions.

FIGURE 433-1. Aphthous ulcers. *Left,* A cluster of minor aphthae on the soft palate and buccal mucosa, present about 1 week. *Right,* A major aphthous ulcer on the labial mucosa, present about 3 weeks.

FIGURE 433-2. Clusters of recurrent herpes simplex vesicles. *Left,* on the lip; *right,* on the hard palate, both present 2 to 3 days, in different patients.

TABLE 433-2   ORAL LESIONS ASSOCIATED WITH HUMAN IMMUNODEFICIENCY VIRUS INFECTION

Kaposi's sarcoma (human herpesvirus type 8)

Candidiasis
    Pseudomembranous lesions
    Hyperplastic lesions
    Erythematous lesions

Other opportunistic fungal infections (e.g., histoplasmosis or coccidioidomycosis)

Aphthous ulcers (increased frequency, duration, or size)

Virus-associated epithelial hyperplasias
    Hairy leukoplakia (Epstein-Barr virus)
    Oral wart (human papillomavirus type 11 and other types)
    Focal epithelial hyperplasia (Heck's disease) (human papillomavirus types 13 and 32)
    Condyloma acuminatum (human papillomavirus types 6 and 11)

Herpes zoster (varicella-zoster virus)

Exaggerated forms of gingivitis and inflammatory periodontal disease

Decreased salivary gland function

Parotid gland enlargement (lymphoepithelial lesion)

Non-Hodgkin's lymphoma

VENEREAL INFECTIONS

Primary syphilis may arise as a solitary, indurated, painless ulcer on the oral mucosa that resolves spontaneously in 4 to 6 weeks (Chapter 327). Uncommonly, *Neisseria gonorrhoeae* may cause oral ulcers, usually in the pharynx, which may be confused with oral ulcers of other causes.

Oral Squamous Cell Carcinoma

About 4% of all cancers occur in the mouth, commonly as squamous cell carcinomas of the mucosal epithelium (Chapter 196). Oral carcinoma

FIGURE 433-3. Squamous cell carcinoma. Biopsy of this area of erythroplakia with slight induration in the anterior mouth floor exhibited squamous cell carcinoma.

TABLE 433-3   WHITE AND RED/BLUE ORAL MUCOSAL LESIONS

WHITE LESIONS (PLAQUES)

Squamous cell carcinoma (early)
Frictional keratosis (buccal mucosa at dental occlusal line)
Leukoplakia (with or without dysplasia)
Smokeless tobacco–associated lesions
Nicotine stomatitis (palate)
Lichen planus (reticular and plaque types)
Pseudomembranous candidiasis (thrush)
Hyperplastic candidiasis (candidal leukoplakia)
Hairy leukoplakia (HIV associated; usually on lateral tongue)
Geographic tongue
Mucous patch or condyloma latum of secondary syphilis
Pseudomembrane-covered ulcers (see Table 433-1)

RED OR BLUE LESIONS (MACULAR, MACULOPAPULAR)

Squamous cell carcinoma (early)
Erythroplakia (epithelial dysplasia)
Erythematous (atrophic) candidiasis
Median rhomboid glossitis
Mucocutaneous diseases (see Table 433-1)
Angular cheilitis
Telangiectasias and purpuras (red to blue)
Kaposi's sarcoma (blue to purple)

HIV = human immunodeficiency virus.

occurs usually in the fifth decade or beyond, in men twice as frequently as in women, and is associated with long-term use of tobacco in more than 80% of cases.

Oral carcinoma usually arises as a chronic, indurated, cratered ulcer, but white (leukoplakia) and especially red (erythroplakia) macular lesions (Table 433-3; Fig. 433-3) frequently exhibit premalignant dysplasia or early carcinoma. Oral carcinomas spread to cervical lymph nodes. The overall 5-year survival rate is about 50%, but early treatment of small, localized lesions can lead to survival rates as high as 90%.

Other Chronic Ulcerations

Prescription drugs that can be responsible for chronic oral mucosal ulcerations include barbiturates, β-blockers, nonsteroidal anti-inflammatory drugs, and many others (see *http://emedicine.medscape.com/article/1080772-overview*). Several mucocutaneous diseases can cause chronic multifocal oral mucosal lesions composed of ill-defined areas of erythema and ulceration. They are among the most difficult oral lesions to diagnose and are discussed later with the red lesions (see Table 433-3). Several microbial infections or underlying osteonecrosis (e.g., associated with bisphosphonate use) can lead to indurated, chronic oral mucosal ulcerations with moderate symptoms (see Table 433-1).

White Lesions

White plaques are commonly found in the mouth but, like ulcerations, have a wide variety of causes and outcomes (see Table 433-3). The term *leukoplakia* applies to a white plaque that does not rub off and whose appearance does not indicate another disease. Leukoplakia can occur in any area of the mouth and usually exhibits benign hyperkeratosis on biopsy (see Fig. 196-1

FIGURE 433-4. Lichen planus. A similar-appearing lesion is also present on the right buccal mucosa. Note central pseudomembrane-covered ulceration.

FIGURE 433-5. Hairy leukoplakia. These white plaques were the first visible sign of human immunodeficiency virus infection.

in Chapter 196). On long-term follow-up, 2 to 6% of these lesions undergo malignant transformation into squamous cell carcinoma. Areas of leukoplakia with a corrugated surface or mixed with areas of erythema are often found in the lower labial or buccal vestibule of patients who use smokeless tobacco.

Frictional keratoses are often found posterior to the lower molar teeth as irregular white plaques and on the buccal mucosa as white lines adjacent to the dental occlusion. Unlike leukoplakia, these lesions rarely become malignant.

LICHEN PLANUS

Oral lesions of lichen planus (Chapter 446) occur in about 1% of the population, usually as multiple, bilaterally symmetrical reticular white plaques, with or without adjacent areas of erythema (atrophy or erosion) or irregular ulcers (Fig. 433-4). The presence of mucosal atrophy, erosion, or ulceration usually causes pain and sensitivity to certain foods. Most lesions can be adequately controlled by topical application of fluocinonide or clobetasol gel or ointment (0.05%, three times a day) for periods of several weeks to several months, although recurrence is common.

ORAL CANDIDIASIS

This common fungal disease (Chapter 346) has three clinical forms: pseudomembranous (thrush), erythematous (atrophic), and hyperplastic (candidal leukoplakia). Pseudomembranous candidiasis, usually of relatively short duration, occurs on any site and consists of white fungal plaques that can be rubbed off, leaving a red or bleeding base. Lesions of hyperplastic candidiasis are white, have fungal hyphae within the surface layers of hyperkeratotic epithelium, do not rub off, and are most often found on the anterior buccal mucosa or on the tongue. Erythematous candidiasis is discussed under Red Lesions. All forms of oral candidiasis represent overgrowth or superficial infection by *Candida* species from the oral flora, induced by a variety of causes, including suppression of bacterial flora by systemic antibiotics, chronic salivary dysfunction, uncontrolled diabetes mellitus or anemia, and immunosuppression (especially in HIV-infected patients).

HAIRY LEUKOPLAKIA

The lesion of hairy leukoplakia, which is caused by Epstein-Barr virus, is a white plaque occurring most frequently on the lateral surfaces of the tongue bilaterally in immunosuppressed persons, usually HIV infected (Fig. 433-5). *Candida* may be present in the surface layers, but the lesion is not eliminated by effective antifungal therapy. The diagnosis of hairy leukoplakia by biopsy should raise suspicion of HIV infection or other forms of immunodeficiency.

GEOGRAPHIC TONGUE

Also called *benign migratory glossitis,* this benign idiopathic condition affects the dorsal tongue of about 2% of the population. It is characterized by well-defined areas of atrophied filiform papillae bordered by arcs of normal or hyperplastic filiform papillae and by gradual changes in the location of these lesions over time (Fig. 433-6). Treatment is usually not necessary.

FIGURE 433-6. Geographic tongue. The distribution of these changes on the dorsal tongue may change over time, but they are asymptomatic and diagnosed by their characteristic appearance.

SECONDARY SYPHILIS

Secondary syphilis may manifest as a well-defined white plaque on the labial or palatal mucosa, called *condyloma latum* (or "split papule," because of its lobulated periphery), or as a mucous patch.

Red Lesions

Solitary red macules or plaques (*erythroplakia*) are less common in the mouth than white lesions but should be viewed with concern because they may exhibit premalignant dysplasia, carcinoma in situ, or carcinoma (see Table 433-3 and Fig. 433-3). One exception is a red macule occurring in the midline of the posterior dorsal tongue, classified as *median rhomboid glossitis,* which is an idiopathic but uniformly benign condition that is often associated with localized overgrowth of *Candida* species.

ERYTHEMATOUS (ATROPHIC) ORAL CANDIDIASIS

This chronic condition is characterized by erythema and atrophy of the filiform papillae on the dorsal tongue or by patchy, ill-defined erythema on the palate, tongue, or buccal mucosa (Fig. 433-7). It is usually accompanied by symptoms of oral mucosal burning and sensitivity to spicy foods. It occurs most commonly in patients with chronic salivary hypofunction (e.g., Sjögren's syndrome or anticholinergic drug effects), but it also occurs in patients who wear removable dentures, in whom mucosal erythema is confined to the denture-bearing area.

Systemic or topical antifungal drugs are necessary to resolve these lesions. In patients who have clinically apparent salivary production, fluconazole (200 mg on the first day, then 100 mg every day for 2 to 4 weeks) is the drug of choice. However, systemic antifungal drugs may not be effective in patients who have severe salivary hypofunction and insufficient saliva to convey the drug from the bloodstream to oral mucosa. In such patients, with remaining natural teeth, *oral* antifungal preparations (troches or pastilles), all of which contain cariogenic amounts of sucrose or glucose, *must not be used* to avoid

FIGURE 433-7. Erythematous oral candidiasis. *Left,* Erythematous candidiasis in a 26-year-old woman with primary Sjögren's syndrome, exhibiting symptomatic angular cheilitis, atrophic mucositis, and lingual papillary atrophy. *Right,* Asymptomatic and normal-appearing mucosa after treatment with appropriate topical antifungal drugs (see text).

TABLE 433-4	PIGMENTATIONS OF THE ORAL MUCOSA (BROWN OR GRAY-BLACK IN COLOR)

INCREASED MELANIN PRODUCTION (FLAT LESIONS)

Oral melanotic macule
Ephelis (vermilion border)
Systemic diseases: Addison's disease, von Recklinghausen's disease of skin, Albright's syndrome, Peutz-Jeghers syndrome

PROLIFERATION OF MELANIN-PRODUCING CELLS (FLAT OR RAISED LESIONS)

Pigmented cellular nevi (benign and premalignant types)
Atypical melanocytic hyperplasia, melanoma in situ, radial growth phase of melanoma
Malignant melanoma

NONMELANIN PIGMENTATION

Amalgam tattoo
Focal deposition of systemically distributed metal (lead, bismuth, mercury, others) usually at sites of chronic inflammation
Systemically administered drugs (chloroquine, minocycline, ketoconazole, cyclophosphamide)

enhancing dental caries. Instead, slow oral dissolution (15 to 20 minutes for 2 weeks to 2 months) of vaginal nystatin tablets (twice daily) or miconazole tablets (50 mg daily), which contain little or no caries-supporting carbohydrates, is safe and effective; patients usually need frequent sips of water to aid in dissolving the tablets. Effective topical or systemic treatment significantly improves oral symptoms. Treatment of denture-associated candidiasis requires concurrent treatment of the denture.

The treatment end point is reached when mucosal burning symptoms cease, the patient can again tolerate acidic or spicy foods, and filiform papillae on the dorsal tongue have returned to normal; this recovery takes 2 to 12 weeks, depending on patients' salivary production and treatment compliance. Recurrence is common in patients with chronic salivary hypofunction or immunosuppression, which necessitates recurring or long-term treatment using a noncariogenic topical antifungal drug that provides a sufficient duration of oral mucosal contact (e.g., nystatin or miconazole tablets).

ANGULAR CHEILITIS

Erythema or crusting of the labial angles is usually caused by *Candida* species (see Fig. 433-7) and is usually associated with intraoral candidiasis. In such cases, topical treatment of the angular cheilitis with clotrimazole (1% cream) must be accompanied by intraoral or systemic antifungal treatment, as described previously.

MUCOCUTANEOUS DISEASES

The mucocutaneous diseases of pemphigus vulgaris, mucous membrane pemphigoid, atrophic or erosive lichen planus, and lupus erythematosus can cause similar-appearing oral lesions. Their diagnosis requires examination of a biopsy specimen by routine histopathology and direct immunofluorescence to identify characteristic deposits of various inflammatory proteins.

The first lesions of pemphigus vulgaris are usually oral mucosal vesicles that rapidly rupture, leaving painful erosions or ulcerations. These are followed by development of skin lesions. Rarely, the lesions remain confined to the mouth (Chapter 447).

Lesions of mucous membrane (cicatricial) pemphigoid are usually confined to the oral mucosa or conjunctivae and occur in patients older than 50 years. They begin as vesicles that quickly rupture, leaving ulcers that are chronic but only moderately symptomatic. Use of topical fluocinonide or clobetasol (0.05% gel or ointment, three times a day, 4 to 12 weeks) for several months, as described for lichen planus, is sometimes sufficient to treat the oral lesions, but some patients also need systemic treatment (Chapter 447).

Oral mucosal lesions of lupus may occur in patients who have systemic lupus erythematosus (SLE), in patients who do not have SLE but later develop that disease, or in patients who do not develop SLE (Chapter 274). In this latter group, the lesions of mucosal lupus may be analogous to the skin lesions of chronic discoid lupus. They take the form of reticular hyperkeratotic figures associated with erythema, often resembling lichen planus, but unlike lichen planus are usually solitary or bilaterally asymmetrical. They can be controlled by topical fluocinonide (0.05%, three times a day, 2 to 4 weeks)

or intralesional triamcinolone suspension (5 mg/mL), or respond to systemic treatment of SLE.

Pigmentations

Brown or gray-black macules on the oral mucosa are relatively common and range from benign to highly malignant. They may be caused by localized increase in melanin production, proliferation of melanin-producing cells, or deposition of local or systemically distributed pigmented substances (Table 433-4). Mucosal pigmentation may occur after long-term administration of hydroxychloroquine, minocycline, ketoconazole, methyldopa, or cyclophosphamide. Malignant melanomas can occur at any oral mucosal site, but about 85% develop on the hard palatal mucosa or gingiva, or both. Diagnosis of any of these conditions is usually established by biopsy and knowledge of relevant underlying conditions.

Lesions of Kaposi's sarcoma associated with HIV infection often appear first on the oral mucosa, especially the palate. They begin as macules with a blue or purple color, at which time they must be distinguished from purpura. Later, they spread radially and expand vertically (Chapter 400).

● ORAL SOFT TISSUE TUMORS

In addition to squamous carcinoma, a variety of oral benign soft tissue tumors are usually treated by excisional biopsy.

Connective Tissue Hyperplasias

The most common oral soft tissue tumors are small, pedunculated masses of hyperplastic fibrous connective tissue covered by normal-appearing mucosa (Table 433-5). Solitary lesions are usually found on the inside of the cheeks or lips. Similar lesions may be present at the border of an ill-fitting denture or may occur in clusters on the hard palate under an ill-fitting denture (palatal papillomatosis).

Generalized or multifocal enlargement of the gingiva (gingival hyperplasia) may be caused by chronic administration of phenytoin, cyclosporine, and many of the calcium-channel blocking drugs (e.g., diltiazem, verapamil, or nifedipine; Fig. 433-8). It can also be associated with a hereditary defect or be caused by an infiltration of atypical white blood cells in some types of leukemia (particularly acute monocytic leukemia; Chapter 189) or by uncontrolled diabetes mellitus (Chapter 236).

Reactive Hyperplasias

Small masses with surfaces that are ulcerated or only partially covered by normal-appearing mucosa usually represent reactive lesions in the form of pyogenic granulomas (whose frequency increases during pregnancy), peripheral giant cell granulomas, or lymphoid hyperplasia of the lingual or other tonsillar tissue. The granulomas are most often located on the gingiva. Rarely, such lesions may represent a metastatic neoplasm.

Epithelial Tumors

Small, white, wartlike epithelial masses are common and can occur in any area of the oral mucosa (Fig. 433-9). They are occasionally classified as

FIGURE 433-8. Drug-induced gingival hyperplasia. Similar clinical lesions may occur with prolonged use of various drugs or as a hereditary condition (see text).

FIGURE 433-9. Papillary epithelial tumors. *Left,* A solitary squamous papilloma. *Right,* multiple gingival papillomas, occurring in all quadrants, from condyloma acuminatum, associated with papilloma virus subtype 6 or 11.

TABLE 433-5 ORAL SOFT TISSUE TUMORS

CONNECTIVE TISSUE HYPERPLASIA (NORMAL-APPEARING OVERLYING MUCOSA)

Irritation fibroma
Denture-associated hyperplasia
Palatal papillomatosis
Generalized gingival hyperplasia
Drug-induced (phenytoin, nifedipine, cyclosporine)
Hereditary

REACTIVE HYPERPLASIA (ERYTHEMATOUS OVERLYING MUCOSA)

Pyogenic granuloma/pregnancy tumor
Peripheral giant cell granuloma
Inflammatory gingival hyperplasia
Hyperplastic lingual tonsil

EPITHELIAL MASSES (USUALLY IRREGULAR WHITE SURFACE)

Papilloma/oral wart
Squamous cell carcinoma
Verrucous carcinoma
Focal epithelial hyperplasia (Heck's disease)
Condyloma acuminatum (venereal wart)
Keratoacanthoma (on lips)

SALIVARY DUCT OBSTRUCTION (MINOR SALIVARY GLANDS)

Mucocele/ranula (usually fluctuant)
Salivary stone (sialolith)

SUBEPITHELIAL NEOPLASMS

Primary connective tissue or salivary gland tumors
Metastatic lesions (especially in the mandible)
Lymphoma (especially in the palate or posterior mandible)
Focal or generalized leukemic infiltrates in the gingiva (especially with acute monocytic leukemia)

TABLE 433-6 CAUSES OF SALIVARY GLAND ENLARGEMENT

USUALLY UNILATERAL

Benign or malignant salivary gland neoplasms (more than 20 different histopathologic types)
Bacterial infection
Chronic sialadenitis (single gland)

USUALLY BILATERAL AND ASSOCIATED WITH SALIVARY HYPOFUNCTION

Viral infection (mumps, cytomegalovirus, influenza, Coxsackie A)
Sjögren's syndrome (benign lymphoepithelial lesion)
Chronic granulomatous diseases (sarcoidosis, tuberculosis, leprosy)
Recurrent parotitis of childhood
Human immunodeficiency virus infection/acquired immunodeficiency syndrome

BILATERALLY SYMMETRICAL, SOFT, NONTENDER, PAROTID ONLY

Sialadenosis (asymptomatic parotid enlargement), idiopathic or associated with:
    Diabetes mellitus
    Hyperlipoproteinemia
    Hepatic cirrhosis
    Anorexia/bulimia
    Chronic pancreatitis
    Acromegaly
    Gonadal hypofunction
    Phenylbutazone use

epithelial neoplasms, but most do not continue to grow. Human papillomavirus types 2, 6, 11, 13, 32, and 57 have been identified in these wartlike lesions, which are usually classified generically as papillomas. A large wartlike lesion on the oral mucosa should raise the suspicion of verrucous carcinoma.

Mucus Retention Lesions (Mucoceles)

Mucoceles are small, chronic, or recurring vesicles or bullae that occur commonly on the inside of the cheeks and lips, the posterior palate, and the mouth floor. They are caused by injury to one of the many submucosal minor salivary glands, resulting in extravasation of mucus, which causes granulomatous inflammation or blockage of the excretory duct, leading to cyst formation. Both types of lesions require conservative surgical excision because simple incision and drainage are usually followed by recurrence.

⬤ SALIVARY GLAND DISEASES
Primary Diseases of Salivary Glands

More than 20 types of benign or malignant neoplasms appear as firm and nontender unilateral or bilateral enlargement of a major gland or as a firm submucosal nodule on the palate or the labial or buccal mucosa (Table 433-6). Their causes are unknown, except for Warthin's tumor (adenolymphoma), which has a strong association with cigarette smoking. Uncommonly, unilateral major gland enlargement may be reactive—for example, chronic sialadenitis from duct obstruction or inadequately treated bacterial sialadenitis. Detection of any of these lesions should be followed by appropriate imaging and biopsy. Both benign and malignant tumors are generally treated by surgery.

Unilateral major salivary gland enlargement that is markedly painful or tender to palpation and has a purulent exudate or nothing expressible from the duct suggests bacterial sialadenitis. Any exudate should be cultured, and initial treatment should be with an oral penicillinase-resistant antibiotic, such as cloxacillin or dicloxacillin, 500 mg, every 6 hours.

Secondary Diseases of Salivary Glands
BILATERAL SALIVARY GLAND ENLARGEMENT AND DECREASED SALIVARY SECRETION ASSOCIATED WITH SYSTEMIC DISEASES

The best-known cause of bilateral salivary gland enlargement is infection by the mumps virus (Chapter 377) in children. However, the prevalence of mumps decreased in the United States by more than 98% after the introduction of an effective vaccine in 1967, and now there are only a few hundred to a few thousand cases per year. Uncommonly, a less acute, mumpslike illness may occur in adults in association with cytomegalovirus (Chapter 384), influenza (Chapter 372), or Coxsackie A (Chapter 387) virus infection.

TABLE 433-7 CAUSES OF DECREASED SALIVARY SECRETION

TEMPORARY

Effects of short-term drug use (e.g., antihistamines)
Virus infections (e.g., mumps)
Dehydration
Psychogenic conditions (e.g., anxiety)

CHRONIC

Effects of chronically administered drugs (particularly antidepressants, monoamine oxidase inhibitors, neuroleptics, parasympatholytics, some combinations of drugs for treating hypertension)
Chronic diseases:
  Sjögren's syndrome
  Sarcoidosis
  Human immunodeficiency virus or hepatitis C infection
  Depression
  Diabetes mellitus (uncontrolled)
  Amyloidosis (primary or secondary)
  Central nervous system diseases
Other effects of treatment
  Therapeutic radiation to the head and neck
  Graft-versus-host disease
Absent or malformed glands (rare)

About 25% of patients with Sjögren's syndrome (Chapter 276) gradually develop chronic bilateral enlargement of major salivary glands, which feel firm and nontender or only slightly tender to palpation. Histologically, the tumors begin as a benign lymphoepithelial lesion (myoepithelial sialadenitis), but after years of chronicity, some transform into an indolent extranodal marginal zone lymphoma or aggressive B-cell lymphoma.

In most patients with Sjögren's syndrome, gradually progressive salivary hypofunction can impair speech and swallowing and cause a characteristic pattern of progressive dental caries that leads to excessive tooth loss if not actively prevented. In severe cases, the oral mucosa becomes dry and sticky, saliva is not expressible from the major ducts, and about one third of patients have signs and symptoms of chronic erythematous candidiasis (see earlier discussion and Fig. 433-7).

The salivary component of Sjögren's syndrome is diagnosed from a labial salivary gland biopsy specimen that contains three to five minor glands and exhibits focal lymphocytic sialadenitis in the absence of nonspecific chronic sialadenitis or another disease, such as noncaseating granuloma. A patient's symptoms of oral dryness (xerostomia) can be caused by a wide variety of conditions (Table 433-7).

Several chronic granulomatous diseases, such as sarcoidosis (Chapter 95), tuberculosis (Chapter 332), and leprosy (Chapter 334), can cause bilateral enlargement and decreased function of salivary glands. The clinical and serologic features of sarcoidosis may occasionally closely mimic those of Sjögren's syndrome, and the distinction is best made by minor salivary gland biopsy.

A few adult patients with HIV infection and most children who are infected in utero develop major salivary gland enlargement and reduced salivary secretion that are caused by lymphocytic infiltration. Parotid gland enlargement usually represents a solid or cystic lymphoepithelial lesion (see Table 433-2).

Recurrent parotitis of childhood includes episodes of unilateral or bilateral parotid enlargement. During flares of this illness, salivary secretion may be reduced, but usually without prominent secondary symptoms or signs. This condition, of unknown cause, usually subsides after puberty.

ASYMPTOMATIC PAROTID ENLARGEMENT (SIALADENOSIS)

Parotid glands can develop bilateral, symmetrical enlargement that is soft and nontender to palpation and associated with normal salivary function (see Table 433-6). Diagnosis is established by this clinical presentation and the presence of one of the systemic diseases known to be associated with it: diabetes mellitus (Chapter 236), hyperlipoproteinemia (Chapter 213), hepatic cirrhosis (Chapter 156), anorexia or bulimia (Chapter 226), chronic pancreatitis (Chapter 146), acromegaly (Chapter 231), and gonadal hypofunction. It can also result from use of phenylbutazone or be a reaction to iodine-containing contrast media. Biopsy of the affected glands is not indicated for diagnosis.

Impaired Salivary Secretion without Gland Enlargement

The common symptom of dry mouth (xerostomia) is most often a side effect of chronically administered drugs. Many classes of drugs reduce unstimulated salivary secretion through anticholinergic or other mechanisms (see Table 433-7). Patients experience these symptoms soon after beginning to use the drug but produce enough saliva during a meal for normal chewing and swallowing. However, the symptoms and associated dental caries are dose dependent and gradually increase with prolonged use of the drug. The classes of drugs producing the most profound effects are most tricyclic antidepressants, most neuroleptics, monoamine oxidase inhibitors, and all anticholinergics. A combination of drugs for treatment of hypertension may also cause symptoms of dry mouth.

Several systemic diseases affect salivary secretion. As noted earlier, most patients with Sjögren's syndrome, some with sarcoidosis, and a few patients with HIV infection experience symptoms of dry mouth to various degrees, with or without salivary gland enlargement. In addition, patients who have primary or secondary *amyloidosis* with salivary gland amyloid deposits may develop impaired secretion. The symptom of xerostomia is more prevalent in individuals who exhibit symptoms of depression but are not taking drugs for its treatment. Studies done before the availability of antidepressant drugs showed that symptoms of depression were associated with decreased salivary secretion.

Irradiation of the head and neck region to treat a malignant tumor usually produces profound dry mouth during therapy. Secretory capacity recovers only slightly in the months following treatment for patients with solid tumors, but recovers significantly for those with multifocal tumors (e.g., Hodgkin's disease).

TREATMENT

Significant chronic salivary hypofunction from any cause produces a risk for dental caries (decay) in approximate proportion to the secretory impairment, but caries can largely be prevented if appropriate measures are taken as soon as the hypofunction begins. Remaining teeth should be protected by a comprehensive dental caries prevention program, monitored by a dentist and including frequent application of appropriate topical fluorides, removal of dental plaque, counseling on control of cariogenic dietary carbohydrates, and placement of appropriate dental restorations as necessary.

Symptomatic treatment of mild to moderately severe salivary hypofunction can include sialagogues such as sugar-free hard candies or chewing gum, regular sips of water, and use of saliva substitutes at night. Symptoms of severe hypofunction can be improved by prescribing cevimeline (30 mg three times a day), **2 3** or pilocarpine (5 mg four times a day), if not contraindicated, but such treatment alone will not prevent dental caries.

Chronic erythematous oral candidiasis is a frequent sequela of chronic salivary hypofunction, and its treatment and retreatment, as noted earlier, substantially improve the patient's oral symptoms.

1. Femiano F, Buonaiuto C, Bombos F, et al. Pilot study on recurrent aphthous stomatitis (RAS): a randomized placebo-controlled trial for the comparative therapeutic effects of systemic prednisone and systemic montelukast in subjects unresponsive to topical therapy. *Oral Surg Oral Med Oral Pathol Oral Radiol Endod.* 2010;109:402-407.
2. Fife RS, Chase WF, Dore RK, et al. Cevimeline for the treatment of xerostomia in patients with Sjögren syndrome: a randomized trial. *Arch Intern Med.* 2002;162:1293-1300.
3. Chambers MS, Posner M, Jones CU, et al. Cevimeline for the treatment of postirradiation xerostomia in patients with head and neck cancer. *Int J Radiat Oncol Biol Phys.* 2007;68:1102-1109.

SUGGESTED READINGS

Adelstein DJ, Rodriguez CP. What is new in the management of salivary gland cancers? *Curr Opin Oncol.* 2011;23:249-253. *Review emphasizing use of PET or PET/CT for diagnosis and to guide newer treatment regimens.*
Carlson DL. Necrotizing sialometaplasia: A practical approach to the diagnosis. *Arch Pathol Lab Med.* 2009;133:692-698. *Summary of clinical and histopathologic features.*
Colella G, Cannavale R, Flamminio F, et al. Fine-needle aspiration cytology of salivary gland lesions: a systematic review. *J Oral Maxillofac Surg.* 2010;68:2146-2153. *The technique has an 80% sensitivity with a 96% specificity for diagnosing tumor.*
Feinstein TM, Lai SY, Lenzner D, et al. Prognostic factors in patients with high-risk locally advanced salivary gland cancers treated with surgery and postoperative radiotherapy. *Head Neck.* 2011;33:318-323. *Review showing overall 5-year survival of 55%, with advanced stage as the only significant predictor.*
Kalmar J. Oral manifestations of drug reactions. http://emedicine.medscape.com/article/1080772-overview. *Review of the many drugs associated with various oral mucosal lesions.*
Messadi DV, Younai F. Aphthous ulcers. *Dermatol Ther.* 2010;23:281-290. *Review.*

434

APPROACH TO THE PATIENT WITH NOSE, SINUS, AND EAR DISORDERS

ANDREW H. MURR

TABLE 434-1	MAJOR AND MINOR SINUSITIS FACTORS	
MAJOR FACTORS	**MINOR FACTORS**
Facial pain or pressure (in conjunction with other nasal symptoms)	Headache
	Halitosis
Facial fullness	Fatigue
Nasal obstruction	Dental pain
Nasal discharge or purulence	Fever (in nonacute rhinosinusitis)
Fever (in acute rhinosinusitis)	Cough
	Ear pressure or fullness

Patients with nose, sinus, and ear disorders may have a variety of chief complaints. Nasal symptoms most commonly relate to rhinorrhea or congestion, both of which may be due to allergic, infectious, inflammatory, or structural causes. Sinus disorders, which commonly arise as a feeling of stuffiness or congestion but are sometimes also manifested as pain or even headache (Chapter 405), have a similar set of causes. Common ear complaints include pain, loss of hearing (Chapter 436), and vestibular symptoms (Chapter 436), commonly described by the patient as dizziness but recognized by the physician as vertigo that is different from the lightheadedness that characterizes presyncope and syncope (Chapters 50 and 62). Epistaxis, which is bleeding from the nose, is usually easy to distinguish from hemoptysis from the bronchial tree (Chapter 83) or hematemesis from the gastrointestinal tract (Chapter 137).

Loss of hearing (Chapter 436) and vestibular symptoms (Chapter 436) are discussed elsewhere, as are smell, the related sensation of taste (Chapter 435), and the details of head and neck tumors (Chapter 196). This chapter focuses on the approach to patients with other common nose, sinus, and ear complaints.

NASAL AND SINUS COMPLAINTS
Rhinitis and Sinusitis

DEFINITION

Rhinitis is generally defined as any inflammatory process in the nose, with the common result being a sensation of excess mucous or nasal congestion. The patient may have a sensation of fluid dripping from the nose, either coming from the nose anteriorly or coming from the nose posteriorly. Anterior nasal drainage may be perceived by the patient as being accompanied by an activity such as eating (gustatory rhinitis) and may be visible to an observer. Posterior nasal drainage is more nebulous and subjective, but it is very common and is referred to as postnasal drip.

In general, acute rhinitis and sinusitis describe inflammatory conditions of the nose and sinuses that last less than 4 weeks. Chronic rhinitis and sinusitis persist for more than 3 months despite treatment. Recurrent acute rhinitis and sinusitis are defined by exacerbations that occur four or more times per year and last 7 to 10 days per episode. Subacute rhinitis and sinusitis define symptoms that persist between 4 and 12 weeks and resolve completely with treatment.

EPIDEMIOLOGY

The most common reason for a patient to seek the advice of a physician in the United States concerns problems relating to rhinitis and sinusitis. More than 20 million visits by patients per year are devoted to this complaint, and billions of dollars are spent on medications that are expected to improve the condition.

PATHOBIOLOGY

Humans normally produce about 2 L of mucus per day from their nasal lining. The nose functions primarily as a humidification and filtration system, with a clean and refreshed nasal mucous blanket serving to trap particulate matter and organisms. The nasal and sinus lining consists of ciliated respiratory epithelium; the cilia function in a highly organized and orderly fashion under normal circumstances to transport particulate matter trapped in the mucous blanket in a consistent fashion so that the mucus can be swallowed, thereby avoiding deposition in the bronchi. The nose also serves as the organ of olfaction (Chapter 435) to allow patients to discern tastes and avoid spoiled foods that could cause illness.

The parasympathetic nervous system controls both vascular tone and mucus production in the nose. Inflammatory conditions, such as the common cold, can cause the nasal and sinus lining to swell, thus highlighting the nasal cycle governed by parasympathetic neural control. In a normal state, one side of the nose is relatively decongested and one side is relatively congested because of vascular engorgement. This vascular dilation allows humidification and warming of inspired air and can also affect the ability to discern odors in the process of olfaction. During rhinitis, the inflammation exaggerates the normal relative comparison between the decongested and congested sides of the nose and can be perceived as an uncomfortable nasal stuffiness that shifts from side to side over a period of several hours.

Sinusitis differs from rhinitis in that the term implies an infectious cause rather than physiologic dysfunction. Nevertheless, many different mechanisms of inflammation besides infection may give rise to what is currently generally termed sinusitis.

CLINICAL MANIFESTATIONS

When normal nasal mucosal function is lost, patients often complain of nasal crusting or obstruction, hypersecretion or postnasal drip, coughing, facial pressure, and fatigue. Nasal obstruction that shifts from side to side during the day is common in many types of rhinitis and may be considered an exaggeration of normal physiology.

Major symptoms of sinusitis (Table 434-1) include facial pressure, facial congestion or fullness, nasal obstruction, nasal discharge, and anosmia. Minor symptoms include headache, halitosis, fatigue, dental pain, cough, and ear pressure. Major signs include purulence in the nose noted on examination and, with acute sinusitis, fever. Pain is a frequent complaint with acute sinusitis but infrequent with chronic sinusitis. Patients with chronic sinusitis often note a dull facial pressure that seems to worsen with dependency. Patients with acute sinusitis may have discrete facial pain or dental pain but also have obvious purulent nasal discharge, often with a frank fever. It is important to note that facial pain is not a symptom of chronic sinusitis in the absence of other nasal signs and symptoms. Generally, sinusitis is thought to be present on the basis of at least two major factors, one major factor and two minor factors, or purulence on nasal examination.

DIAGNOSIS

History

A thorough history should probe whether patients have tried over-the-counter or prescription medications, including antihistamines, decongestants, mucolytics, analgesics, mast cell stabilizers, and even steroids, and whether they have helped improve the condition. In addition, other prescription medications have side effects that affect nasal physiology, including birth control pills, antihypertensive medications that cause systemic vasodilation, aspirin, steroids, and antibiotics. Specific questions regarding allergies are important, including seasonality or environmental triggers, the presence or absence of pets, food sensitivities, recent changes in environment, and living conditions, with a focus on old or new carpets, mattresses, furnace filters, or freshly painted interior walls. A patient should be questioned about past allergy skin testing or other testing.

A recent history of other family members or coworkers being ill suggests an infectious process. An astute physician often suspects an infectious process by noting the similarity and time course of symptoms in other patients; this information can be related to patients so that they know what to expect in terms of time course and recovery. A careful past medical history should allow one to determine whether relevant conditions such as previous nasal surgery or trauma, granulomatous diseases, cystic fibrosis (Chapter 89), rheumatologic conditions, immune deficiencies (Chapter 258), or other problems may be contributing factors. Unilateral nasal congestion raises concern for either an anatomic abnormality, such as septal deviation, perhaps related to previous trauma, a polyp or other neoplastic mass, or perhaps even a foreign body.

Physical Examination

The nose should be inspected with a nasal speculum to assess nasal septal anatomy (Fig. 434-1), the most caudal aspect of the inferior turbinates (Fig. 434-2), and the possibility of large nasal polyps (Fig. 434-3) or other masses. In patients with allergic rhinitis, the physical examination may reveal pale and swollen inferior turbinates, whereas copious nasal secretions are more apparent with viral infections. By spraying the nose with a topical decongestant such as phenylephrine (Neo-Synephrine) or oxymetazoline, the middle meatus, which is the air space between the middle turbinate and lateral nasal wall, can often be visualized to assess for nasal polyps or purulent discharge. Examination of the mouth and oropharynx, including the posterior pharyngeal wall, with a tongue blade if necessary, can sometimes identify a stream of postnasal discharge or pus. Sinus palpation and transillumination, though part of the art of medicine, are not sufficiently reliable for diagnosis. The patient's ability to open the mouth without limitation helps exclude trismus, which can sometimes be caused by a deep neck infection.

A complete examination of the head and neck should be performed to look for signs of recent or old trauma such as ecchymosis under the eyelids, swelling of the soft tissue of the face, or deviation of the nasal dorsum. The neck should be palpated for adenopathy (Chapter 171) or other masses.

A basic eye examination should be performed to assess pupillary function, extraocular movements, and possible nystagmus (Chapter 432). An ear examination should be conducted to assess the tympanic membranes bilaterally. In patients with an abnormality of the tympanic membrane or concomitant complaints of hearing loss or disequilibrium (Chapter 436), pneumatoscopy using an air bulb attached to the otoscope can be used to insufflate the ear canal and assess for mobility of the tympanic membrane; decreased mobility suggests a middle ear effusion. Weber and Rinne testing using a 512-Hz tuning fork screens for conductive hearing loss, especially unilateral loss.

Endoscopic examination of the nose, almost always performed by a specialist, is the "gold standard" for evaluating rhinitis and sinusitis. A flexible or rigid fiberoptic scope can allow fine inspection of the septum, turbinates, middle meatus, and sphenoethmoid recess, as well as direct inspection of the nasopharynx, orifice of the eustachian tube, and fossa of Rosenmüller, which is just rostral to the eustachian tube in the nasopharynx and is often the site of origin of nasopharyngeal carcinoma (Chapter 196). Flexible endoscopy can be used to further inspect the oropharynx, larynx, and most of the hypopharynx (Chapter 437).

Laboratory Findings
Cultures

Cultures of the nostril or lower nasal cavity are not typically useful and are not recommended. An endoscopically guided culture of the middle meatus by a specialist may help guide treatment for acutely ill immunocompromised patients, patients with refractory chronic rhinosinusitis, or those whose sinusitis is suspected of causing secondary meningitis, epidural or subdural abscess, brain abscess, orbital involvement, or cavernous sinus thrombosis.

Other Tests

A nasal smear can reveal eosinophils, which is consistent with allergic rhinitis (Chapter 259). Likewise, skin testing or radioallergosorbent testing can help pinpoint allergic triggers (Chapter 257). In patients with acute sinusitis, a white blood cell count with differential may be useful. In patients with chronic sinusitis, serum immunoglobulin levels can be helpful: highly elevated immunoglobulin E (IgE) levels can raise suspicion for allergic fungal sinusitis, whereas low levels of IgG and other subclasses suggest immunodeficiency (Chapter 258). If the patient has chronic nasal crusting as a primary complaint, screening serologic tests for sarcoid (Chapter 95), Wegener's granulomatosis (Chapter 278), T-cell lymphomas (Chapter 191), syphilis (Chapter 327), tuberculosis (Chapter 332), Sjögren's syndrome (Chapter 276), and other chronic inflammatory diseases can be considered. Relatively rare infections such as rhinoscleroma may also be present, so biopsy and cultures may be indicated to help reveal a diagnosis. Use of illicit substances should be considered because cocaine and other illicit drugs may cause nasal crusting. In a patient with a lifelong history of sinusitis since childhood, cystic fibrosis should also be considered (Chapter 89).

FIGURE 434-1. Purulent drainage from the middle meatus seen on anterior rhinoscopy.

FIGURE 434-3. Bilateral nasal polyps in the nasal vestibules. A polyp can easily be confused with a normal inferior turbinate. (From Dhillon RS, East CA, eds. *Ear, Nose and Throat and Head and Neck Surgery,* 2nd ed. Edinburgh: Churchill Livingstone; 1994:36.)

A   B

FIGURE 434-2. Edematous inferior turbinates narrowing the nasal airway in a patient with hay fever. **A,** Physical examination. **B,** Computed tomography. (From Dhillon RS, East CA, eds. *Ear, Nose and Throat and Head and Neck Surgery,* 2nd ed. Edinburgh: Churchill Livingstone; 1994:34.)

FIGURE 434-4. Coronal computed tomography showing bilateral acute pansinusitis. There is a fluid level in the left maxillary sinus, which if aspirated, can be sent for microbiology. (From Dhillon RS, East CA, eds. *Ear, Nose and Throat and Head and Neck Surgery,* 2nd ed. Edinburgh: Churchill Livingstone; 1994:50.)

Imaging

Non–contrast-enhanced computed tomography (CT) is indicated for patients with known or suspected rhinitis and sinusitis. CT is generally performed to document the presence of disease or the effects of treatment to improve the disease. CT is also used to evaluate complications of sinusitis or to investigate sinusitis in immunocompromised patients. Finally, CT is critical before any surgical treatment of the sinuses because of the anatomic information that it provides the surgeon. Opacification or other findings on CT (Fig. 434-4) can often differentiate among the various causes of sinusitis. Plain films have little utility and are not generally recommended. Magnetic resonance imaging (MRI) is occasionally helpful, especially when evaluating tumors or processes that erode bone and are proximate to the brain or eye.

Differential Diagnosis

A rapid onset of symptoms present for a short time suggests a viral upper respiratory infection, especially if the patient also has typical systemic symptoms, such as arthralgia, myalgia, fever, chills, gastrointestinal symptoms, and cough in addition to nasal congestion, postnasal drip, and headache. By comparison, acute bacterial rhinosinusitis causes facial pressure and purulent postnasal discharge. Frequently, viral disease can progress to a secondary bacterial infection, which can become chronic. An acute onset of inhalant allergy is often seasonal or can be traced to a particular precipitant (Chapter 259). Allergic rhinitis typically responds to an empirical trial of antihistamines, whereas viral or bacterial rhinitis does not.

Chronic sinusitis must be differentiated from rhinitis, which is not accompanied by the same degree of incessant inflammation. Types of rhinitis include gustatory rhinitis associated with eating, rhinitis of pregnancy, rhinitis related to abuse of topical vasoconstrictors, rhinitis associated with illicit drug use (e.g., cocaine or methamphetamine), rhinitis of aging, vasomotor rhinitis presumably related to a hypersecretory state mediated by the parasympathetic nervous system, and perennial allergic rhinitis, whose hallmark is a lack of seasonality.

Chronic sinusitis may be caused by chronic viral infection, chronic bacterial infection, chronic fungal infection, and chronic allergy. It is often difficult to pinpoint a specific cause, but the common underlying factor is often inflammatory in nature. Although maxillary antral punctures were used for diagnosis and treatment in the pre-CT era, endoscopically guided culture techniques combined with CT are now the standard of care, except for acute bacterial maxillary sinusitis, for which surgical decompression is desirable, or for some cases of refractory sinusitis in immunocompromised patients or patients in the intensive care unit, where direct culture can guide antibiotic therapy.

Nasal polyps may be caused by Samter's triad (asthma, aspirin sensitivity, and nasal polyposis related to upregulation of leukotrienes caused by prostaglandin blockade). Human papillomavirus (Chapter 381) may cause an inverted papilloma, which responds to surgical excision but can transform to frank malignancy. Polyps are also seen in patients with cystic fibrosis (Chapter 89) and allergic fungal sinusitis, which is manifested by an elevated IgE level, positive fungal cultures (usually for aspergillosis), Charcot-Leyden crystals

on histopathology, characteristic densities on CT, and nasal polyposis that is often, but not always unilateral. Antral choanal polyps may extend into the nasal cavity or nasopharynx and cause obstruction.

CT can reveal mucoceles, which are blocked individual sinuses that continue to secrete mucus and can slowly erode bone, expand to involve the eye and brain, or become acutely infected. A mycetoma, which is an isolated "fungus ball" in a sinus, has a characteristic hyperdensity within a sinus opacification. Mycetomas (Chapter 350) are noninvasive but may erode bone via pressure necrosis over a long period. Unilateral nasal polyposis is suggestive of antral choanal polyps, malignancy, inverted papilloma, or allergic fungal sinusitis; early biopsy is recommended. Mucus retention cysts, often present in the maxillary sinus, are manifested as a spherical opacification; an estimated 10% of the population has a mucus retention cyst, which is often asymptomatic.

TREATMENT ⟨Rx⟩

Medical Therapy

Viral rhinitis is treated with supportive care, including fluid replacement and treatment of the febrile component of the syndrome with acetaminophen or nonsteroidal anti-inflammatory medications. Steam has a mild decongestant effect, and vitamin C and good nutrition may help hasten the resolution of symptoms. Oral decongestants (such as pseudoephedrine, 120 mg every 12 hours for several days), mucolytics (such as guaifenesin, 200 to 400 mg every 4 to 6 hours for several days), and ipratropium bromide (0.03 or 0.06%, two sprays on each side of the nose every 12 hours for several days) are of potential benefit.

For clinically diagnosed rhinosinusitis, antibiotics are of little benefit, except perhaps in patients with a purulent discharge, in whom a diagnosis of bacterial rhinosinusitis based on the history and physical examination is quite inaccurate.**[1]** Because any benefits of antibiotics are small and the potential side effects are not trivial, they should be reserved for patients with a high probability of bacterial infection.**[2]** For acute nonrecurrent maxillary sinusitis diagnosed on purely clinical grounds in a primary care setting without fiberoptic nasal endoscopy, neither antibiotics nor topical nasal steroids are beneficial.**[3]** By comparison, topical nasal steroids are of proven benefit when acute rhinosinusitis is confirmed by either radiography or nasal endoscopy.**[4]**

Allergic rhinitis (Chapter 259) responds to various antihistamines, such as diphenhydramine hydrochloride (25 to 50 mg every 4 to 6 hours), loratadine (5 mg twice a day or 10 mg a day), cetirizine hydrochloride (10 mg a day), fexofenadine hydrochloride (60 mg twice a day or 120 mg/day), and topical nasal steroids, including triamcinolone acetonide (two sprays [55 μg] to each side of the nose every day), mometasone furoate (two sprays [50 μg] to each naris every day), fluticasone propionate (two sprays [50 μg] to each naris every day), and budesonide (two sprays [32 μg] to each naris every day). Oral steroids such as prednisone and methylprednisolone in various doses are sometimes useful as well. Allergic desensitization is sometimes recommended when a discrete allergen elicits a strong reaction in a patient. Allergic desensitization may specifically be beneficial for some inflammatory disorders, such as allergic fungal sinusitis.**[5]**

Nasal polyps frequently respond to oral steroids, either in a tapered burst dose or, in rare cases, in small amounts of titrated daily oral steroids such as prednisone or methylprednisolone. Topical steroids may also be efficacious for treating nasal polyps.

Bacterial sinusitis should be treated with antibiotics directed toward *Haemophilus influenzae, Moraxella catarrhalis, Streptococcus pneumoniae,* and *Staphylococcus aureus.* Antibiotics such as amoxicillin, 500 mg three times a day, or erythromycin, 500 mg twice a day for 2 to 3 weeks, with subsequent follow-up examination to document resolution are reasonable first-line coverage. β-Lactamase–stable antibiotics are used as a second-line treatment, as are antibiotics that have good anaerobic coverage: amoxicillin with clavulanic acid at 875 mg twice a day for β-lactamase stability or clindamycin at 300 mg three times a day for anaerobic coverage. The use of antifungals, including itraconazole in an oral or aerosolized form and amphotericin B in an aerosolized form, remains controversial in the treatment of chronic sinusitis.

Surgical Therapy

Surgery is recommended in patients with mucoceles, inverted papilloma, antral choanal polyps, juvenile nasopharyngeal angiofibroma, and malignancies. Surgery can correct septal deviations and anatomically related nasal obstruction. Surgery on the inferior turbinates may be beneficial for refractory rhinitis. Surgery for benign nasal polyposis can improve symptomatic control and reduce the need for oral steroids. Functional endoscopic surgery, which is designed to preserve mucociliary function and is performed with endoscopes through the nostril without large incisions, can be useful for recurrent acute sinusitis and chronic rhinosinusitis.

FIGURE 434-5. Dilated nasal vessels and crusting typical of a patient with epistaxis.

- Pars flaccida
- Short process of malleus
- Malleus long process
- Light reflex
- Pars tensa

FIGURE 434-6. A normal tympanic membrane. (From Dhillon RS, East CA, eds. *Ear, Nose and Throat and Head and Neck Surgery,* 2nd ed. Edinburgh: Churchill Livingstone; 1994:2.)

TABLE 434-2 CAUSES OF OTALGIA

CAUSES OF OTALGIA	EXTERNAL EAR	MIDDLE EAR	UPPER AERODIGESTIVE TRACT
Likely	Otitis externa Herpes zoster oticus Chondritis Foreign body	Acute otitis media Acute eardrum perforation Barotrauma Chronic otitis media with impending complication	Tonsillitis Tonsil abscess Deep neck abscess Tumor (especially base of the tongue, tonsil, hypopharynx, larynx, nasopharynx)
Unlikely	Malignant otitis externa Tumor	Tumor	

Epistaxis

For a patient with epistaxis, it is first critical to determine the severity of the blood loss. Persistent bleeding may result from warfarin, antiplatelet agents, or any underlying platelet (Chapter 176) or clotting deficiency (Chapter 177). Physical examination should focus on inspection of the anterior septum, which is the most frequent point of origin for epistaxis (see Fig. 434-1). Frequently, dilated blood vessels on the caudal septum can be seen with anterior rhinoscopy (Fig. 434-5). The combination of unilateral otitis media, epistaxis, nasal congestion, and a neck mass would be concerning for nasopharyngeal carcinoma. Rare tumors that can arise with bleeding include juvenile nasopharyngeal angiofibromas in male patients.

Epistaxis can be treated by local pressure, packing (using nasal sponges, balloons, or ½ by 72-inch gauze impregnated with petroleum jelly), humidification, and hydration. Hospitalization and transfusion are rarely required. Offending medications should be reduced in dose or discontinued temporarily if possible. Topical vasoconstrictive medication such as oxymetazoline spray, two sprays on each side of the nose every 12 hours for 3 days, can help prevent persistent epistaxis. Occasionally, lasers or other types of cautery are used to improve the problem. At times, arterial clipping or interventional arterial occlusion can address a specific bleeding area.

● EAR PAIN

◗ DEFINITION

Ear pain (Table 434-2) is discomfort perceived by a patient in the area of the temporal bone. Although the discomfort can often be localized by the patient, at times the cause of the discomfort may in fact be distant from the site where the pain is felt. This referred pain can be due to problems in the oral cavity, oropharynx, hypopharynx, or larynx.

◗ PATHOBIOLOGY

The ear is well supplied with sensory nerves and is positioned on the side of the skull. The ear is divided into the outer ear, or pinna, and the ear canal; the middle ear, which encompasses the tympanic membrane and ossicles (Fig. 434-6); and the inner ear, which consists of the cochlea and the vestibular canals, including the utricle and saccule. In general, otalgia is due to

problems in the outer or middle ear. The trigeminal nerve innervates the anterior superior quadrant of the pinna, whereas the C2 and C3 cervical cutaneous nerves innervate the rest of the majority of the outer ear. However, there are contributions by the 9th and 10th nerves in the ear canal and even a small patch of sensory innervation by the 7th nerve in the posterior superior ear canal. It is the overlap in distribution of the 9th and 10th cranial nerves that establishes the anatomic basis for referred otalgia in diseases of the oral cavity, oropharynx, and larynx. Therefore, ear pain may be due to inflammatory conditions of the skin of the outer ear, the ear canal, or the middle ear, or it may be due to disease processes unrelated to the ear itself.

◗ CLINICAL MANIFESTATIONS

Patients with ear pain often have complaints referable directly to the ear itself. In cases of otitis externa, frankly obvious erythema and swelling of the skin of the ear canal may be present. Even minute physical manipulation of the ear may be excruciating. In chondritis of the pinna, which may be related to rheumatologic disorders, infection, or trauma, the entire pinna may be swollen and painful. Hearing loss accompanying otalgia may indicate middle ear disease, especially otitis media. Patients sometimes complain of pain in the ear after air travel or driving from a mountainous region. Quick changes in pressure, such as encountered in scuba diving, may indicate barotrauma (Chapter 94), in which the eustachian tube is unable to compensate rapidly enough for the changes in pressure that are encountered. Pain may also be a post-traumatic symptom from relatively minor percussion injury, more severe head trauma, or percussion injury related to a blast. Pain related to noise exposure may also indicate damage to the middle ear or even the inner ear. Deep-seated boring pain over the temporal area accompanied by retro-orbital pain can be due to petrous apex disease, including petrous apicitis.

◗ DIAGNOSIS

History

A patient with ear pain should be asked to reveal the location of the discomfort, the duration of the symptoms, and any activities related to onset of the condition. As an example, recent swimming would make otitis externa ("swimmer's ear") more likely, whereas a recent upper respiratory infection with hearing loss would suggest otitis media. Questions should address possible hearing loss, vertigo, otorrhea, hoarseness, voice change, dysphagia, odynophagia, dyspnea, hemoptysis, hematemesis, and weight loss. A social history with specific concentration on tobacco and alcohol use should be obtained. A possible family history of upper aerodigestive tract and nasopharyngeal carcinoma should be sought. A past surgical history can reveal distant ear or throat surgery.

Physical Examination

A complete head and neck examination, including general assessment for trauma and a basic eye examination, is required. The outer ear and pinna should be examined first. The ear canal should first be palpated and then inspected. An otoscope with a pneumatic bulb attachment is critical to establish the presence or absence of a middle ear effusion. Inspection of the tympanic membrane should be accomplished with notations made about patency and perforation, translucency of the eardrum, position and definition of the malleus, and the eardrum's mobility with the ear canal sealed and a puff of air delivered by the pneumatic bulb. Abnormalities may be caused by infection (Fig. 434-7) or barotrauma (Fig. 434-8). Examination with a 512-Hz tuning fork should be performed to determine lateralization of the sound (Weber test) and whether air conduction is superior to bone conduction (Rinne test). Facial nerve function should be assessed (Chapter 403) by determining

FIGURE 434-7. Otoscopic appearance in otitis media with effusion. The handle and short process of the malleus are brought into relief by retraction of the eardrum. There is a slightly yellow appearance of the eardrum related to the middle ear effusion. (From Dhillon RS, East CA, eds. *Ear, Nose and Throat and Head and Neck Surgery,* 2nd ed. Edinburgh: Churchill Livingstone; 1994:7.)

FIGURE 434-8. Blood in the middle ear (hemotympanum). Causes include otitic baro-trauma, secretory otitis media, and a high jugular bulb. (From Dhillon RS, East CA, eds. *Ear, Nose and Throat and Head and Neck Surgery,* 2nd ed. Edinburgh: Churchill Livingstone; 1994:26.)

whether the patient can close the eyes. The presence or absence of nystagmus should be recorded. Inspection of the nose, oral cavity, oropharynx, and neck should be accompanied by cranial nerve examination (Chapter 403). Palpation of the tongue and tonsils is especially important if the ear pain is intense and persistent. A careful neck examination should be performed to look for masses. Oral cavity infections (Chapter 433), such as a peritonsillar abscess or severe tonsillitis, may arise as ear pain, and the physical examination should reveal trismus, erythema, mass effect, and other common signs of pharyngitis.

Laboratory

An audiogram can assess hearing loss (Chapter 436). A tympanogram measures compliance of the middle ear system and is an accurate method for diagnosis of otitis media. Cultures are rarely performed because they require tympanocentesis, and cultures of the external ear can reveal a vast variety of organisms that are often treated empirically with antibiotics. If a fever and middle ear effusion are present and neck stiffness is found on physical examination, lumbar puncture may rarely be recommended.

Imaging

In general, imaging is indicated if complications of acute or chronic otitis media are suspected or to look for occult causes of otalgia in the upper aerodigestive tract. If a patient is suspected of having meningitis, epidural or subdural abscess, brain abscess, or sagittal sinus thrombosis, imaging is mandatory. Imaging is also useful for operative planning in patients with chronic

otitis media or (rarely) to evaluate for the presence of tumors in the middle or external ear.

Differential Diagnosis

Otitis externa, which is an infection of the skin of the ear canal, is often due to manipulating the ear after swimming or trying to scratch an ear canal that itches because of skin irritation. Patients exhibit erythema of the canal skin and extreme pain on manipulation of the ear canal. In the presence of concomitant cranial neuropathies, especially in diabetic or otherwise immunocompromised patients, malignant otitis externa with osteomyelitis should be suspected. Inspection of the tympanic membrane may reveal fluid (see Fig. 434-7) consistent with otitis media; the tuning fork examination should support the presence of conductive hearing loss. Vesicles on the conchal portion of the pinna, especially when accompanied by facial nerve paralysis, strongly suggest herpes zoster oticus with Ramsay Hunt syndrome (Chapter 383). Perforation of the eardrum suggests either acute or chronic otitis media, traumatic perforation, or possibly cholesteatoma (Chapter 436) if the perforation is in the posterior superior quadrant. Chronic draining otorrhea of long standing with a deep boring pain and perforation of the tympanic membrane suggests a complication of otitis media.

If findings on ear and cranial nerve examination are negative but the patient's complaints of otalgia are persistent, special effort needs to be made to visualize the upper aerodigestive tract, including the nasopharynx, oral cavity, oropharynx, larynx, and hypopharynx, to be sure that infection or tumor is not present in these hard-to-examine areas. MRI can be very useful in these cases.

TREATMENT Rx

Otitis externa is often treated with office suctioning of debris under a microscope and the application of antibiotic drops (ciprofloxacin, tobramycin, neomycin, polymyxin B), with or without hydrocortisone in various combinations. Frequently, a small wick or sponge is placed in the ear canal to help maintain patency of the canal and allow facile application of the medications. For otitis media, oral antibiotic treatment is directed at eradicating *H. influenzae, M. catarrhalis, S. pneumoniae,* and *S. aureus* with amoxicillin or erythromycin as for sinusitis (see earlier). The benefit is notable for children 2 years or younger with bilateral otitis and for older children with otitis plus otorrhea, whereas other patients can be observed without antibiotics. In general, antibiotics provide somewhat better short-term outcomes but at the expense of significantly more diarrhea and rashes.[6] Interestingly, the natural history of acute otitis media is acute perforation of the eardrum, which often results in otorrhea and relief of pain. Most middle ear effusions clear spontaneously within 3 months regardless of whether they are treated. Most perforations of an eardrum caused by trauma heal without surgical intervention, but if an eardrum perforation persists for more than about 3 months, surgical closure and the use of tympanoplasty with or without mastoidectomy can be contemplated. Chronic draining perforations, especially if located in the posterior superior quadrant of the tympanic membrane, may require tympanomastoid surgery.

In patients in whom herpes zoster is suspected, acyclovir can be started at 800 mg by mouth five times per day for 7 days, with or without prednisone (Chapter 383). Intracranial complications of otitis media often need to be addressed surgically.

 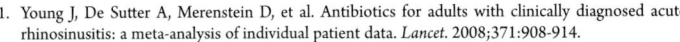

1. Young J, De Sutter A, Merenstein D, et al. Antibiotics for adults with clinically diagnosed acute rhinosinusitis: a meta-analysis of individual patient data. *Lancet.* 2008;371:908-914.

2. Falagas ME, Giannopoulou KP, Vardakas KZ, et al. Comparison of antibiotics with placebo for treatment of acute sinusitis: a meta-analysis of randomised controlled trials. *Lancet Infect Dis.* 2008;8:543-552.

3. Williamson IG, Rumsby K, Benge S, et al. Antibiotics and topical nasal steroid for treatment of acute maxillary sinusitis: a randomized controlled trial. *JAMA.* 2007;298:2487-2496.

4. Zalmanovici A, Yaphe J. Intranasal steroids for acute sinusitis. *Cochrane Database Syst Rev.* 2009; 4:CD005149.

5. Calderon M, Alves B, Jacobson M, et al. Allergen injection immunotherapy for seasonal allergic rhinitis. *Cochrane Database Syst Rev.* 2007;24:CD001936.

6. Tähtinen PA, Laine MK, Huovinen P, et al. A placebo-controlled trial of antimicrobial treatment for acute otitis media. *N Engl J Med.* 2011;364:116-126.

SUGGESTED READINGS

Coker TR, Chan LS, Newberry SJ, et al. Diagnosis, microbial epidemiology, and antibiotic treatment of acute otitis media in children: a systematic review. *JAMA.* 2010;304:2161-2169. *Review noting about a 13% improvement in short-term outcomes with antibiotics, offset by about a 5% increased risk of diarrhea or rash.*

Comstock RH 3rd, Lam K, Mikula S. Topical antibiotic therapy of chronic rhinosinusitis. *Curr Infect Dis Rep.* 2010;12:88-95. *Review suggesting topical antibiotics are preferable to the oral and intravenous routes.*

Mösges R, Bachert C, Rudack C, et al. Efficacy and safety of mometasone furoate nasal spray in the treatment of chronic rhinosinusitis. *Adv Ther.* 2011;28:238-249. *At 200 μg twice daily for 16 weeks, this steroid spray offers an effective and safe treatment for chronic rhinosinusitis.*

435

SMELL AND TASTE

ROBERT W. BALOH AND JOANNA JEN

Millions of people suffer from disorders of taste and smell, but these disorders are often neglected because they are not fatal and, unlike abnormalities of vision and hearing, are not considered serious handicaps. Chemosensory disorders, however, often reduce the enjoyment and quality of life and are important to patients who suffer from them.

DEFINITION

The sensory receptor for taste, the taste bud, is made up of 50 to 150 cells arranged to form a pear-shaped organ. The lifespan of these cells is 10 to 14 days, and they are constantly being renewed from dividing epithelial cells surrounding the bud. Taste buds are located on the tongue, soft palate, pharynx, larynx, epiglottis, uvula, and upper third of the esophagus. The taste buds located on the anterior two thirds of the tongue and on the palate are innervated by the chorda tympani branch of the seventh cranial nerve. The ninth cranial nerve innervates the posterior third of the tongue. The 9th and 10th nerves innervate taste buds in the pharynx and larynx. Afferent signals from the taste buds project to the nucleus of the solitary tract in the medulla and then via a series of relays to the thalamus and postcentral somatosensory cerebral cortex (primary ipsilateral). Free nerve endings of the fifth cranial nerve are found on the tongue and in the oral cavity, and lesions involving these pathways can also alter taste perception.

Olfactory receptors lie in a roughly dime-sized area of specialized pigmented epithelium that arches along the superior aspect of each side of the nasal mucosa. Specialized bipolar sensory cells in this region thrust short receptor hairs into the overlying mucosa to detect aromatic molecules as they dissolve. As with taste buds, the specialized receptor portion of the bipolar neuron undergoes continuous renewal, with turnover occurring approximately every 30 days. Thin axons of the bipolar neurons course through small holes in the cribriform plate of the ethmoid bone to form connections in the overlying olfactory bulb on the ventral surface of the frontal lobe. From there, second- and third-order neurons project directly and indirectly to the prepiriform cortex and parts of the amygdaloid complex of both sides of the brain, which represents the primary olfactory cortex.

PATHOBIOLOGY
Pathology

Disorders of taste interfere with digestion because taste stimulants alter salivary and pancreatic flow, gastric contractions, and intestinal motility. Smell also contributes to the anticipation and ingestion of food because much of what is tasted is derived from olfactory stimulation during ingestion and chewing. An inability to detect noxious tastes and odors can result in food or gas poisoning, particularly in elderly subjects. In the extreme, chemosensory disorders can lead to overwhelming stress, anorexia, and depression. Genes that encode for chemoreceptor proteins belong to the G protein–coupled receptor superfamily, which accounts for up to 1% of mammalian genomes. Sequence diversity in these genes encodes unique structural motifs that bind to different ligands signaling different odors and tastes. Distinct and dedicated taste receptor cells express unique receptors to detect each of the five basic tastes: sweet (sensed by the heterodimers T1R1 and T1R3), umami (detected by the heterodimers T1R2 and T1R3), bitter (sensed by an estimated 30 T2Rs), sour (sensed by PKD2L1, with membrane-tethered carbonic anhydrase IV sensing carbonation), and salty. The identity of salt receptors remains unknown. The taste receptor cells transform and transmit information to primary afferents through multiple cranial nerves (VII, IX, and X) via the solitary tract nucleus in the brain stem, with relay in the thalamus, and then onward to the primary cortex (Fig. 435-1).

Pathophysiology

Disorders of taste and smell can be divided into local, systemic, and neurologic categories (Table 435-1). The taste buds and the specialized receptor portion of the bipolar olfactory cells are constantly being renewed, and the

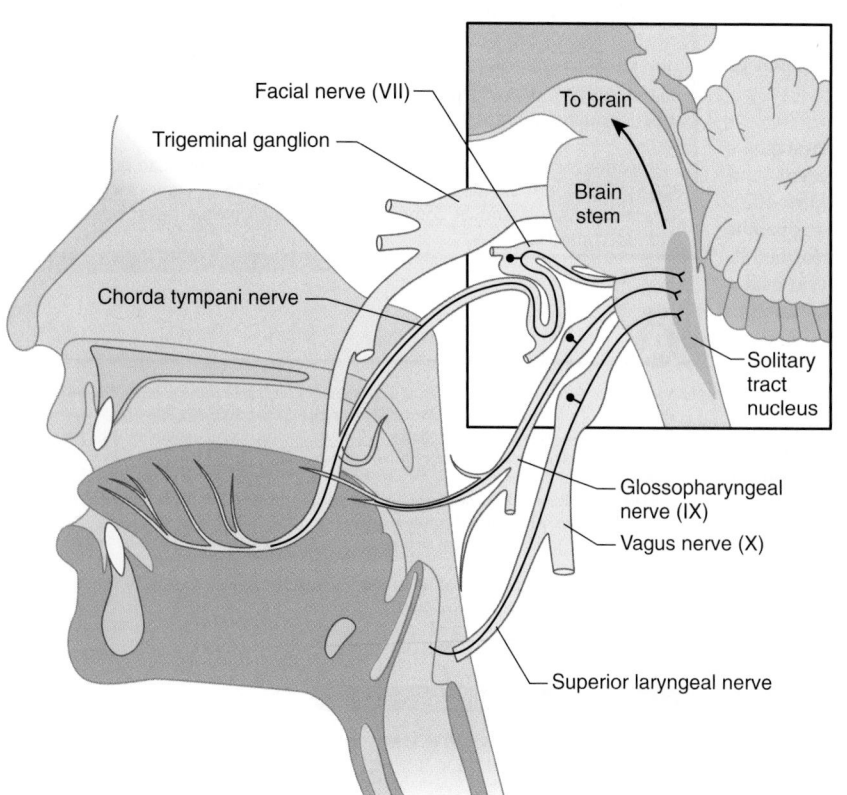

Facial nerve (VII)
Trigeminal ganglion
To brain
Brain stem
Chorda tympani nerve
Solitary tract nucleus
Glossopharyngeal nerve (IX)
Vagus nerve (X)
Superior laryngeal nerve

FIGURE 435-1. Anatomy of peripheral taste pathways. Taste information is transmitted from the mouth and the pharynx through multiple cranial nerves that project to the solitary tract nucleus in the brain stem, with relay in the thalamus before reaching the cortex. (Copyright 1999-2000 David Klemm. Reproduced from Bromley SM. Smell and taste disorders: a primary care approach. *Am Fam Physician.* 2000;61:427-436, 438.)

TABLE 435-1	COMMON CAUSES OF LOSS OF TASTE AND SMELL	
	TASTE	**SMELL**
Local	Radiation therapy, oral infections, dentures, dental procedures	Allergic rhinitis, sinusitis, nasal polyposis, upper respiratory infection
Systemic	Cancer, renal failure, hepatic failure, nutritional deficiency (vitamin B_3, zinc), Cushing's syndrome, hypothyroidism, diabetes mellitus, infection (viral), drugs (antirheumatic and antiproliferative, e.g., corticosteroids, cisplatin, carboplatin, cyclophosphamide, doxorubicin, and methotrexate)	Renal failure, hepatic failure, nutritional deficiency (vitamin B_{12}), Cushing's syndrome, hypothyroidism, diabetes mellitus, infection (viral hepatitis, influenza), drugs (nasal sprays, antihistamines, decongestants, antibiotics, and antirheumatic and antiproliferative drugs that affect taste)
Neurologic	Bell's palsy, familial dysautonomia, multiple sclerosis	Head trauma, multiple sclerosis, Parkinson's disease, Alzheimer's disease, frontal tumor

on cards. The anterior two thirds and posterior third of the tongue should be tested separately.

SUGGESTED READINGS

Doty RL. The olfactory system and its disorders. *Semin Neurol.* 2009;29:74-81. *Reviews common disorders of smell.*

Green E, Jacobson A, Haase L, et al. Reduced nucleus accumbens and caudate nucleus activation to a pleasant taste is associated with obesity in older adults. *Brain Res.* 2011;1386:109-117. *A reduced response to pleasant taste stimuli may contribute to overeating and obesity.*

Hong JH, Omur-Ozbek P, Stanek BT, et al. Taste and odor abnormalities in cancer patients. *J Support Oncol.* 2009;7:58-65. *Reviews taste and smell abnormalities seen in cancer patients.*

Schubert CR, Cruickshanks KJ, Klein BE, et al. Olfactory impairment in older adults: five-year incidence and risk factors. *Laryngoscope.* 2011;121:873-878. *The 5-year incidence of olfactory impairment was 12.5%, with a 1.8-fold increased risk for every additional 5 years of age.*

process of renewal can be affected by nutritional, metabolic, and hormonal states, as well as by therapeutic radiation, drugs, and age. For example, with interruption of mitosis by antiproliferative agents, return of normal taste function takes a minimum of 10 days, whereas return to normal olfactory function takes more than 30 days. Diuretics can block apical ion channels on a taste bud, and antifungal drugs inhibit cytochrome P-450–dependent enzymes at the level of the receptors. Numerous local conditions such as colds and allergies, chronic sinusitis, and nasal polyposis can influence the sense of smell by restricting airway patency. Accidental blows to the head can shear the fine axons of the bipolar olfactory neurons and result in loss of smell. Lesions of the fifth, seventh (*chorda tympani*), and ninth nerves can lead to disordered taste sensation. Olfactory and gustatory disturbances can serve as important diagnostic signs for focal neurologic lesions (e.g., frontal lobe tumors). Hallucinations of smell and taste occur in persons with epileptogenic lesions affecting the mesial temporal lobe and insular region, respectively. Finally, olfactory disturbances and hallucinations occur with a number of psychiatric illnesses (particularly depressive illness and schizophrenia).

CLINICAL MANIFESTATIONS

The most frequently encountered causes of loss of smell are local obstructive disease, viral infections, head injuries (Chapter 406), and normal aging (Chapter 24). Patients can lose their sense of smell not only from chronic allergies and sinusitis (Chapter 434) but also from the nasal sprays and drops that they use to treat these conditions. The most common causes of loss of the sense of taste are viral infections and drug ingestion, particularly antirheumatic and antiproliferative drugs (see Table 435-1). Many of the systemic disorders listed in Table 435-1 probably produce their effect by decreasing the rate of turnover of sensory receptors on the tongue and olfactory epithelia. Disturbances of smell and taste in malnourished patients may be due to specific deficiencies in vitamins and minerals, such as zinc. Viral illnesses such as influenza (Chapter 372) and viral hepatitis (Chapter 150) produce disorders in both taste and smell. Multifocal neurologic disorders such as multiple sclerosis (Chapter 419) can affect the central olfactory and gustatory pathways at multiple levels; as a result, abnormalities in taste and smell are common in such patients. Loss of smell is increasingly being recognized in the early stages of many neurodegenerative disorders, including Parkinson's disease, Alzheimer's dementia, motor neuron disease, and Huntington's disease.

DIAGNOSIS

Olfaction can be tested grossly at the bedside with a few easily recognized odors such as coffee, chocolate, and the roselike aroma of the compound phenylethyl alcohol. Nasal irritants should be avoided. Each nostril is tested separately to determine whether the problem is unilateral or bilateral. Gustatory sensation is typically tested with weak solutions of sugar, salt, and acetic acid, or vinegar. The patient must keep the tongue protruded and respond to questions by nodding the head or by pointing to names of the tastes written

436

HEARING AND EQUILIBRIUM

ROBERT W. BALOH AND JOANNA JEN

DEFINITION

The neural pathways subserving hearing and those most important for equilibrium and spatial orientation are anatomically proximate in much of their course from their end organs in the inner ear to their termination in the superior portion of the temporal lobe. Because of the close anatomic linkage, disorders that affect hearing often affect equilibrium, and vice versa. For this reason, they are considered together here.

PATHOBIOLOGY

Despite their anatomic propinquity, however, substantial pathophysiologic differences make clinical examination of the two systems quite different. The auditory system is physiologically relatively isolated, so that its function and dysfunction can be tested independently of other neural systems. The vestibular system, in contrast, has many close physiologic links with other neural systems (particularly the visual-oculomotor, somatosensory, and autonomic systems) and can be difficult to test in isolation of these other systems.

DIAGNOSIS

Abnormalities of the auditory system lead to only a few well-defined and unique symptoms (i.e., hearing loss or tinnitus). Abnormalities of the vestibular system can cause symptoms that mimic disorders of other neural structures. Such symptoms include dizziness, visual distortion (oscillopsia), imbalance, nausea, vomiting, and even syncope.

DISORDERS OF THE AUDITORY SYSTEM

DEFINITION
Anatomy and Physiology of Hearing

In normal hearing, sound waves are transmitted from the tympanic membrane through the three ossicles of the air-filled middle ear (air conduction) to the oval window and the basilar membrane of the fluid-sealed cochlea. The ossicles increase the gain from the tympanum to oval window about 18-fold, compensating for the loss that sound waves moving from air to fluid would otherwise suffer. In the absence of this system, sound may reach the cochlea by vibration of the temporal bone (bone conduction) but with much less efficiency (approximately 60-dB loss). Hair cells, tonotopically organized along the cochlear basilar membrane, detect the vibratory movement of that membrane and transduce vibration into nerve impulses. The nerve impulses are relayed by nerve cells that synapse at the base of hair cells and have their bodies in the spiral ganglion to the cochlear nucleus of the ipsilateral pontine tegmentum. The spiral cochlea mechanically analyzes the frequency content of sound. For high-frequency tones, only sensory cells in the basilar region are activated, whereas for low-frequency tones, all or nearly all sensory cells are activated. Therefore, with lesions of the cochlea and its afferent nerve, the hearing levels for different frequencies are usually unequal, typically resulting in better hearing sensitivity for low-frequency than for high-frequency tones. Within the brain stem, auditory signals ascend from the ventral and dorsal cochlear nuclei to reach the superior olivary nuclei of both sides. Thus, nervous system lesions central to the cochlear nucleus do not cause monaural hearing loss and, conversely, unilateral central lesions do not cause deafness. From these structures, the pathway projects by way of the lateral lemnisci to the inferior colliculi. Each inferior colliculus transmits to the other and to its ipsilateral medial geniculate body, which in turn sends the final projection to the transverse auditory gyrus lying in the superior portion of the ipsilateral temporal lobe.

The normal ear can detect sound frequencies ranging between 20 and 20,000 Hz; the upper range drops off fairly rapidly with advancing age. The ear is most sensitive between 500 and 4000 Hz, which roughly corresponds to the frequency range most important for understanding speech. The hearing level in this range has several practical implications in terms of the degree of handicap and the potential for useful correction with amplification. A 30- to 40-dB hearing level in the speech range would impair normal conversation, whereas an 80-dB hearing level would make everyday auditory communication almost impossible (the social definition of deafness).

PATHOBIOLOGY
Localization of Lesions within the Auditory Pathways

Conductive hearing loss results from lesions involving the external or middle ear. It is typically characterized by an approximately equal loss of hearing at all frequencies and by well-preserved speech discrimination once the threshold for hearing is exceeded. Patients with conductive hearing loss can hear speech in a noisy background better than in a quiet background because they can understand loud speech as well as anyone.

Sensorineural hearing loss results from lesions of the cochlea or auditory division, or both, of the eighth cranial nerve. With sensorineural hearing loss, the hearing levels for different frequencies are usually unequal, typically resulting in better hearing for low- than for high-frequency tones. Patients with sensorineural hearing loss often have difficulty hearing speech that is mixed with background noise and may be annoyed by loud speech. Three important manifestations of sensorineural lesions are diplacusis, recruitment, and tone decay. Diplacusis and recruitment are common with cochlear lesions; tone decay usually accompanies eighth nerve involvement.

Central hearing disorders result from lesions of the central auditory pathways. As a rule, patients with central lesions do not have impaired hearing for pure tones, and they can understand speech as long as it is clearly spoken in a quiet environment. If the listener's task is made more difficult with the introduction of background noise or competing messages, performance deteriorates more markedly in patients with central lesions than in normal subjects.

DIAGNOSIS
Evaluation
Bedside Test

A quick test for hearing loss in the speech range is to observe the response to spoken commands at different intensities (whisper, conversation, shouting). Tuning fork tests permit a rough assessment of the hearing level for pure tones of known frequency. The clinician can use his or her own hearing level as a reference standard. In the Rinne test, nerve conduction is compared with bone conduction by holding a tuning fork (preferably 512 Hz) against the mastoid process until the sound can no longer be heard. It is then placed 1 inch from the ear and, in normal subjects, can be heard about twice as long by air as by bone. If bone conduction is better than air conduction, the

hearing loss is conductive, but care must be taken to ensure that the bone conduction is not heard in the normal ear. In the Weber test, the tuning fork is placed on the patient's forehead or upper teeth. Normally, this sound is referred to the center of the head. If it is referred to the side of unilateral hearing loss, the hearing loss is conductive; if it is referred away from the side of unilateral hearing loss, the loss is sensorineural.

Audiometry

Pure tone testing is the cornerstone of most auditory examinations. Pure tones at selected frequencies are presented through either earphones (air conduction) or a vibrator pressed against the mastoid portion of the temporal bone (bone conduction), and the minimal level that the subject can hear (threshold) is determined for each frequency. Two speech tests are routinely used. The *speech reception threshold* (SRT) is the intensity at which the patient can correctly repeat 50% of the words presented. The SRT is a test of hearing sensitivity for speech and should reflect the hearing level for pure tones in the speech range. The *speech discrimination test* is a measure of the patient's ability to understand speech when it is presented at a level that is easily heard. In patients with eighth nerve lesions, speech discrimination scores can be severely reduced, even when pure tone thresholds are normal or nearly normal; by comparison, in patients with cochlear lesions, discrimination tends to be proportional to the magnitude of hearing loss.

Brain stem auditory evoked responses can be recorded from scalp electrodes at 0 to 10 msec (early), 10 to 50 msec (middle), and 50 to 500 msec (late) following a click (a high-frequency stimulus). The early potentials reflect electrical activity at the cochlea, eighth cranial nerve, and brain stem; the later potentials reflect cortical activity. Computer averaging of the responses to 1000 to 2000 clicks separates the evoked potential from background noise. Early evoked responses may be used to estimate the magnitude of hearing loss and to differentiate among cochlea, eighth nerve, and brain stem lesions.

Hearing Loss

PATHOBIOLOGY
Conductive Hearing Loss

The history, examination, and audiometry usually provide the key differential features for identifying common causes of hearing loss (Fig. 436-1). The most common cause of conductive hearing loss is *impacted cerumen* in the external canal. This benign condition is usually first noticed after bathing or swimming when a droplet of water closes the remaining tiny passageway. The most common serious cause of conductive hearing loss is inflammation of the middle ear, *otitis media*, either infective (suppurative; see Fig. 434-7 in Chapter 434) or noninfective (serous). Fluid accumulates in the middle ear, impairing the conduction of airborne sound to the cochlea. Because the air cavity of the middle ear is in direct connection with the mastoid air cells, infection can spread through the mastoid bone and, occasionally, into the intracranial cavity. Chronic otitis media with perforation of the tympanic membrane can result in an invasion of the middle ear and other pneumatized areas of the temporal bone by keratinizing squamous epithelium (*cholesteatoma*). Cholesteatomas can produce erosion of the ossicles and bony labyrinth, resulting in a mixed conductive sensorineural hearing loss. Barotrauma to the middle ear arises with otalgia and hearing loss and can be associated with serous effusion or hematotympanum (see Fig. 434-8 in Chapter 434). *Otosclerosis* commonly produces progressive conductive hearing loss by immobilizing the stapes with new bone growth in front of and below the oval window. The hearing loss is typically conductive, although in some persons the cochlea may be invaded by foci of otosclerotic bone, producing an additional sensorineural hearing loss. Otosclerosis usually stabilizes when the hearing level reaches 50 to 60 dB and rarely progresses to deafness. Other common causes of conductive hearing loss include trauma, congenital malformations of the external and middle ear, and glomus body tumors.

Sensorineural Hearing Loss
Hereditary Deafness

Genetically determined deafness, usually from hair cell aplasia or deterioration, may be present at birth or may develop in adulthood. The diagnosis of *hereditary deafness* rests on the finding of a positive family history. Mutations in connexin 26, a key component of gap junctions in the inner ear, account for most cases of recessively inherited deafness. *Intrauterine factors* resulting in congenital hearing loss include infection (especially rubella); toxic, metabolic, and endocrine disorders; and anoxia associated with Rh incompatibility and difficult deliveries.

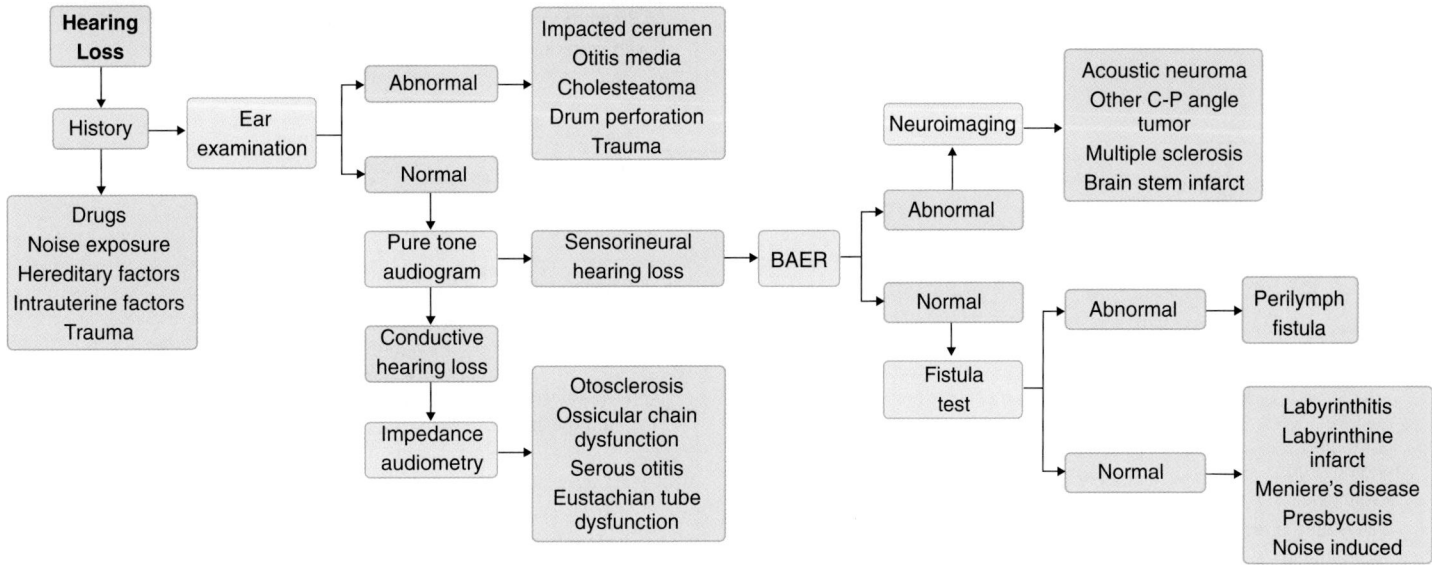

FIGURE 436-1. Evaluation of hearing loss. BAER = brain stem auditory evoked response; C-P = cerebellopontine.

Cochlear Damage

Acute unilateral deafness usually has a cochlear basis. *Bacterial or viral infections* of the labyrinth, *head trauma* with fracture or hemorrhage into the cochlea, or *vascular occlusion* of a terminal branch of the anterior inferior cerebellar artery can extensively damage the cochlea and its hair cells. An acute idiopathic, often reversible, unilateral hearing loss strikes young adults and is presumed to reflect an isolated viral infection of the cochlea and auditory nerve terminals.

Sudden unilateral hearing loss often associated with vertigo and tinnitus can result from a *perilymphatic fistula.* Such fistulas may be congenital or may follow stapes surgery or head trauma.

Drugs

Drugs cause acute and subacute bilateral hearing impairment. Salicylates, furosemide, and ethacrynic acid have the potential to produce transient deafness when taken in high doses. More toxic to the cochlea are aminoglycoside antibiotics (gentamicin, tobramycin, amikacin, kanamycin, streptomycin, and neomycin). These agents can destroy cochlear hair cells in direct relation to their serum concentrations. Some antineoplastic chemotherapeutic agents, particularly cisplatin, cause severe ototoxicity.

Meniere's Disease

Subacute relapsing cochlear deafness occurs with *Meniere's disease,* a condition associated with fluctuating hearing loss and tinnitus, recurrent episodes of abrupt and often severe vertigo, and a sensation of fullness or pressure in the ear. Recurrent endolymphatic hypertension (hydrops) is believed to cause the episodes. Pathologically, the endolymphatic sac is dilated, and the hair cells become atrophic. The resulting deafness is subtle and reversible in the early stages but subsequently becomes permanent and is characterized by diplacusis and loudness recruitment. The disorder is usually unilateral, but in about 20 to 40% of patients, bilateral involvement occurs.

Presbycusis

The gradual, progressive, bilateral hearing loss commonly associated with advancing age is called *presbycusis.* Presbycusis is not a distinct disease entity but rather represents multiple effects of aging on the auditory system. It may include conductive and central dysfunction, although the most consistent effect of aging is on the sensory cells and neurons of the cochlea. The typical audiogram of presbycusis is a symmetrical high-frequency hearing loss gradually sloping downward with increasing frequency. The most consistent pathology associated with presbycusis is degeneration of sensory cells and nerve fibers at the base of the cochlea.

Noise

The recurrent trauma of *noise-induced hearing loss* affects approximately the same region at the base of the cochlea and is also common, particularly among those with exposure to loud explosive or industrial noises. Loud, blaring, modern music has become a recent offender. The loss almost always begins at 4000 Hz and does not affect speech discrimination until late in the disease process. With only brief exposure to loud noise (hours to days), there may be only a temporary threshold shift, but with continued exposure, permanent injury begins. The duration and intensity of exposure determine the degree of permanent injury.

Acoustic Neuroma

Progressive unilateral hearing loss, which arises insidiously, initially in the high frequencies, and worsens by almost imperceptible degrees, is characteristic of benign neoplasms of the cerebellopontine angle, most commonly *acoustic neuromas.* In about 10% of cases, the hearing loss can be acute, apparently owing to either hemorrhage into the tumor or compression of the labyrinthine vasculature. Magnetic resonance imaging (MRI) with contrast reliably identifies small acoustic neuromas.

Central Hearing Loss

Central hearing loss is unilateral only if it results from damage to the pontine cochlear nuclei on one side of the brain stem from conditions such as *ischemic infarction* of the lateral brain stem (e.g., occlusion of the anterior inferior cerebellar artery [Chapter 414]), a plaque of *multiple sclerosis* (Chapter 419), or, rarely, invasion or compression of the lateral pons by a *neoplasm* or *hematoma* (Chapters 195 and 406). Bilateral *degeneration* of the cochlear nuclei accompanies some of the rare recessive inherited disorders of childhood. As noted, clinically important unilateral hearing loss never results from neurologic disease arising rostral to the cochlear nucleus. Although bilateral hearing loss could, in theory, result from bilateral destruction of central hearing pathways, in practice this is rare because involvement of neighboring structures in the brain stem or hemisphere would usually produce overwhelming neurologic disability.

TREATMENT   Rx

If an underlying disorder has not yet destroyed the auditory system and can be ameliorated medically or surgically, hearing may be improved or preserved. Most patients with otosclerosis respond to stapedectomy. Closure of a perilymph fistula may improve hearing. Antibiotic and decongestive treatment of otitis media (Chapter 434) should prevent permanent hearing loss. A brief course of high-dose steroids followed by rapid taper is commonly used for patients with idiopathic sudden unilateral sensorineural deafness, but the evidence to support this approach is limited. **1** A low-salt diet and diuretics are effective in selected cases of Meniere's disease. Folic acid supplementation appears to reduce the rate of hearing loss in the elderly. **2** Hearing aids amplify sound, usually with the goal of making speech intelligible. Patients with conductive hearing loss require simple amplification, but those with sensorineural hearing loss often need frequency-selective amplification to make hearing aids useful. Advances in acoustic technology have markedly improved the outlook for the latter. Serial audiograms in patients with noise or ototoxic drug exposure are critical for prevention of permanent hearing loss.

Evaluation of tinnitus flowchart

Tinnitus → History → Ear examination

Common offending drugs:
Quinidine
Salicylates
Indomethacin
Carbamazepine
Propranolol
Levodopa
Aminophylline
Caffeine

Ear examination →
- Audible sounds
  - Synchronous with respiration → Patent eustachian tube
  - Synchronous with pulse → Aneurysm / Vascular malformation / Vascular tumor / Venous hum
  - Continuous → Venous hum / Acoustic emissions
- No audible sounds → Neurologic examination → Normal → Audiogram
  - Conductive hearing loss → Impacted cerumen / Chronic otitis / Otosclerosis
  - Sensorineural hearing loss → BAER
    - Abnormal (neural) → Acoustic neuroma / Other C-P angle tumors / Vascular compression
    - Normal (cochlear) → Noise damage / Ototoxic drugs / Labyrinthitis / Meniere's disease / Perilymph fistula / Presbycusis
  - Normal → Idiopathic tinnitus

Neurologic examination → Brain stem signs → Multiple sclerosis / Tumor / Ischemic infarction

FIGURE 436-2. Evaluation of tinnitus. BAER = brain stem auditory evoked response; C-P = cerebellopontine.

Tinnitus

DIAGNOSIS

The evaluation of common causes of tinnitus (Fig. 436-2) begins with a careful history to identify common offending drugs.

Objective Tinnitus

With *objective tinnitus,* the patient hears a sound arising external to the auditory system, a sound that can usually be heard by the examiner with a stethoscope. Objective tinnitus usually has benign causes such as noise from temporomandibular joints, opening of eustachian tubes, or repetitive muscle contractions. Sometimes, in a quiet room, the patient can hear the pulsatile flow in the carotid artery or a continuous hum of normal venous outflow through the jugular vein. The latter can be obliterated by compression of the jugular vein or extreme lateral rotation of the neck. Pathologic objective tinnitus occurs when patients hear turbulent flow in vascular anomalies or tumors (e.g., glomus jugulare tumor). Objective tinnitus may also be an early sign of increased intracranial pressure. Such tinnitus, which probably arises from turbulent flow through compressed venous structures at the base of the brain, is usually overshadowed by other neurologic abnormalities.

Subjective Tinnitus

Subjective tinnitus can arise from sites anywhere in the auditory system. The sounds most frequently reported are metallic ringing, buzzing, blowing, roaring, or, less often, bizarre clanging, popping, or nonrhythmic beating. Tinnitus heard as a faint, moderately high pitched, metallic ring can be observed by almost anyone who concentrates attention on auditory events in a quiet room. Sustained louder tinnitus accompanied by audiometric evidence of deafness occurs in association with both conductive and sensorineural hearing loss. Tinnitus observed with otosclerosis tends to have a roaring or hissing quality, and that associated with Meniere's disease often produces sounds that vary widely in intensity with time and quality, sometimes including roaring or clanging. Tinnitus with auditory nerve lesions tends to be higher pitched and ringing in quality. Audiometric and brain stem evoked response testing can help distinguish between lesions involving the conducting apparatus, the cochlea, and the auditory nerve. Tinnitus without observable deafness appears sporadically and for variable lengths of time in many persons without other evidence of an ongoing pathologic process.

TREATMENT

Most patients with tinnitus can be helped by a careful evaluation to exclude serious underlying conditions and by subsequent reassurance when appropriate. Often, exacerbating factors such as chronic anxiety and depression can be treated. In patients with hearing loss and tinnitus, a hearing aid may improve tinnitus because the amplification of ambient sound may effectively mask the tinnitus. This mechanism probably explains the frequent observation that removal of cerumen from the external auditory canal to improve ambient hearing also improves tinnitus. Also, when cerumen is attached to the tympanic membrane, tinnitus may result from local mechanical effects on the conductive system. For patients who find their tinnitus most obtrusive when trying to sleep, a bedside frequency modulation (FM) clock radio tuned between stations can provide an effective masking sound; some such radios can be programmed to switch off after the patient falls asleep. A careful drug history should be taken (see Fig. 436-2), and a drug-free trial period should be considered when possible. Benzodiazepines (e.g., diazepam, 2 to 5 mg every 8 hours) or tricyclic amines (e.g., amitriptyline, 25 to 75 mg at bedtime) may provide temporary symptomatic relief of tinnitus, but cognitive behavioral therapy is a more effective long-term approach. **3**

Equilibrium-Vestibular System

PATHOBIOLOGY

Anatomy and Physiology of the Vestibular System

The paired vestibular end organs lie within the temporal bones next to the cochlea. Each organ consists of three semicircular canals that detect angular acceleration and two otolith structures, the utricle and saccule, that detect linear acceleration (including gravitational). Like the cochlea, these organs possess hair cells that act as force transducers, converting the forces associated with head acceleration into afferent nerve impulses. The hair cells of the three semicircular canals, each of which is oriented at right angles to the others, are located in the crista, where their cilia are embedded in a gelatinous mass called the *cupula.* Movement of the head causes the endolymph to flow either toward or away from the cupula, bending the cilia and, depending on the direction of endolymphatic movements, either exciting or inhibiting the afferent nerves at the base of the hair cells. Because the afferent nerves are tonically active, the baseline activity can be increased or decreased

FIGURE 436-3. Evaluation of vertigo. BAER = brain stem auditory evoked response; C-P = cerebellopontine; ENG = electronystagmography.

depending on the direction of hair cell bending. Furthermore, the two sets of semicircular canals are approximately mirror images of each other, so that rotational movement of the head that excites one canal inhibits the analogous canal on the opposite side. The hair cells of the utricle and saccule are located in an area called the *macule*. The macule of the utricle lies approximately in the plane of the horizontal canal, and the macule of the saccule is approximately in the plane of the anterior canal. The hair cell cilia are embedded in a membrane that contains calcium carbonate crystals or otoliths; the density of otoliths is considerably greater than that of the endolymph. Linear accelerations of the head combine with the linear acceleration of gravity to distort the otolith membrane, thereby bending the cilia of the hair cells and modulating the activity of the afferent nerve terminals at the base of the hair cells.

The afferent vestibular nerves have their cell bodies in Scarpa's ganglion. The nerve fibers travel in the vestibular portion of the eighth cranial nerve contiguous to the acoustic portion. Fibers from different receptor organs terminate in different vestibular nuclei at the pontomedullary junction. There are also direct connections with many portions of the cerebellum, the greatest representation being in the flocculonodular lobe, the so-called vestibular cerebellum. Efferent fibers from the brain stem travel through the vestibular nerve to reach hair cells of the semicircular canals and macules, where they modulate afferent activities. From the vestibular nuclei, second-order neurons make important connections to the vestibular nuclei of the other side, to the cerebellum, to motor neurons of the spinal cord, to autonomic nuclei in the brain stem, and, most important for the examining clinician, to the nuclei of the oculomotor system. Fibers from the vestibular nuclei also ascend through the brain stem and thalamus to reach the cerebral cortex bilaterally.

DIAGNOSIS

Evaluation

History

Most vestibular problems presented to the physician are episodic, and often there are neither symptoms nor signs when the physician examines the patient. The history, therefore, can become paramount for identifying vestibular dysfunction. The history should attempt to distinguish vertigo (the illusion of movement in space) from lightheadedness (presyncope), ataxia (disequilibrium of the body without true movement in space), and psychogenic symptoms (the feeling of dissociation or, sometimes, disequilibrium).

Vertigo can be caused by either the peripheral or central vestibular apparatus. In general, peripheral vertigo is more severe, is more likely to be associated with hearing loss and tinnitus, and often leads to nausea and vomiting. Nystagmus associated with peripheral vertigo is usually inhibited by visual fixation. Central vertigo is generally less severe than peripheral vertigo and is often associated with other signs of central nervous system disease. The nystagmus of central vertigo is not inhibited by visual fixation and frequently is prominent when vertigo is mild or absent.

Common Causes of Vertigo

Physiologic Vertigo

Physiologic vertigo includes common disorders that occur in healthy people such as *motion sickness, space sickness,* and *height vertigo* (Fig. 436-3). In these conditions, vertigo (defined as an illusion of movement) is minimal while autonomic symptoms predominate. With height vertigo, patients may experience acute anxiety and panic reaction. Individuals with motion sickness and space sickness typically develop perspiration, nausea, vomiting, increased salivation, yawning, and generalized malaise. Gastric motility is reduced and digestion impaired. Even the sight or smell of food is distressing. Hyperventilation is a common sign, and the resulting hypocapnia leads to changes in blood volume, with pooling in the lower parts of the body predisposing to postural hypotension and syncope. An unusual variant of motion-induced dizziness occurs when the subject returns to stationary conditions after prolonged exposure to motion (*mal de debarquement syndrome*). Typically, affected patients report that they feel the persistent rocking sensation of a boat long after returning to solid ground. Rarely, the syndrome can last for months to years after exposure to motion and can even be incapacitating. The cause is unknown.

Physiologic vertigo can often be suppressed by supplying sensory cues that help to match the signals originating from different sensory systems. Thus, motion sickness, which is caused by a mismatch of visual and vestibular signals, is exacerbated by sitting in a closed space or reading (giving the visual system the miscue that the environment is stationary). It may be improved by looking out at the horizon. Height vertigo, caused by a mismatch between sensation of normal body sway and lack of its visual detection, can often be relieved either by sitting or by visually fixating a nearby stationary object.

Benign Positional Vertigo (Canalithiasis)

Benign positional vertigo is by far the most common cause of vertigo. Patients with this condition develop brief episodes of vertigo (less than 1 minute) with position change, typically when turning over in bed, getting in and out of bed, bending over and straightening up, or extending the neck to look up (so-called top-shelf vertigo). Benign positional vertigo results when otolith debris inadvertently enters one of the semicircular canals. It can occur after head trauma or inner ear infection but most commonly occurs spontaneously in older people. The diagnosis rests on finding characteristic positional nystagmus in the plane of the affected canal (see later). It is important to recognize this syndrome because, in most patients, it can be cured by simple bedside maneuvers (Fig. 436-4). If the history or findings are atypical, the condition must be distinguished from other causes of positional vertigo that may occur with tumors or infarcts of the posterior fossa.

Acute Peripheral Vestibulopathy (Vestibular Neuritis)

One of the most common clinical neurologic syndromes at any age is the acute onset of vertigo, nausea, and vomiting lasting for several days and not associated with auditory or neurologic symptoms. A viral origin is suspected,

FIGURE 436-4. Modified Epley's (A) and Semont's (B) maneuvers for benign positional vertigo affecting the right posterior semicircular canal (PSC). The procedure is reversed for treating the left PSC. The entire sequence should be repeated until no nystagmus is elicited. (From Fife TD, Iverson DJ, Lempert T, et al. Practice parameter: therapies for benign paroxysmal positional vertigo [an evidence-based review]: report of the Quality Standards Subcommittee of the American Academy of Neurology. *Neurology.* 2008;70:2067-2074.)

but attempts to isolate an agent have been unsuccessful, except for occasional findings of a herpes zoster infection. Pathologic studies showing atrophy of one or more vestibular nerve trunks, with or without atrophy of their associ-ated sense organs, are evidence of a vestibular nerve site and, probably, viral cause for many patients with this syndrome. Many patients report an upper respiratory tract illness 1 to 2 weeks before the onset of vertigo. This syn-drome occasionally occurs in epidemics (epidemic vertigo), may affect several members of the same family, and more often erupts in the spring and early summer. Most affected patients gradually improve over 1 to 2 weeks, but residual dizziness and imbalance can persist for months.

Meniere's Disease

Meniere's disease (see earlier) accounts for about 10% of all patients with vertigo. The diagnosis is based on documenting episodic severe attacks accompanied by fluctuating hearing levels on audiometric testing beginning in the low frequencies.

Migraine

Vertigo is a common symptom with migraine (Chapter 405). It can occur with headaches or in separate isolated episodes, and it can predate the onset of headache. So-called benign paroxysmal vertigo of childhood is often the first symptom of migraine. The mechanism of vertigo with migraine is not clear, but damage to the inner ear occurs in about one fourth of patients. A few develop typical features of Meniere's disease.

Post-traumatic Vertigo

Vertigo, hearing loss, and tinnitus often follow a blow to the head (Chapter 406) that does not result in temporal bone fracture, termed *labyrinthine concussion.* Although they are protected by a bone capsule, the delicate laby-rinthine membranes are susceptible to blunt trauma. Blows to the occipital or mastoid region are particularly likely to produce labyrinthine damage. *Transverse fractures* of the temporal bone typically pass through the vestibule of the inner ear, tearing the membranous labyrinth and lacerating the ves-tibular and cochlear nerves. Complete loss of vestibular and cochlear func-tion is the usual sequela, and the facial nerve is interrupted in approximately 50% of cases. Examination of the ear often reveals hemotympanum (see Fig. 434-8 in Chapter 434), but bleeding from the ear seldom occurs because the tympanic membrane usually remains intact. As noted earlier, *benign positional vertigo* is also a common sequela of head trauma. *Fistulas* of the oval and round windows can result from impact noise, deep-water diving, severe physical exertion, or blunt head injury without skull fracture. The mechanism of the rupture is a sudden negative or positive pressure change in the middle ear or a sudden increase in cerebrospinal fluid pressure transmitted to the inner ear through the cochlear aqueduct and internal auditory canal. Clinically, the rupture leads to the sudden onset of vertigo or hearing loss, or both. Surgical exploration of the middle ear is warranted when there is a clear relationship between the onset of vertigo or hearing loss, or both, and the onset of severe exertion, barometric change, head injury, or impact noise.

Postconcussion Syndrome

The so-called postconcussion syndrome refers to a vague dizziness (rarely vertigo) associated with anxiety, difficulty in concentrating, headache, and photophobia induced by a head injury resulting in concussion (Chapter 406). Occasionally, similar but less pronounced symptoms are associated with mild head injury judged to be trivial at the time. The cause is unknown, but animal studies indicate that small multifocal brain lesions (petechiae) commonly occur after concussive brain injury.

Other Peripheral Causes of Vertigo

Vertigo can be associated with *chronic bacterial otomastoiditis,* either from direct invasion of the inner ear by the bacteria or by erosion of the labyrinth by a cholesteatoma. Radiographic studies of the temporal bone readily identify these disorders. *Autoimmune inner ear disease* typically arises with episodic vertigo and fluctuating hearing levels similar to Meniere's disease, but it is more fulminant with early bilateral involvement. It can occur in isolation or with other systemic features of autoimmune disease. About two thirds of patients have antibodies directed against heat shock protein 70. The aminoglycosides streptomycin and gentamicin are remarkably selective for vestibular ototoxicity. The patient may suffer acute vertigo if the toxic effect is asymmetrical. More often, there is a progressive symmetrical loss of vestibular function leading to imbalance but not vertigo. Unfortunately, many patients being treated with ototoxic drugs are initially bedridden and unaware of the vestibular impairment until they recover from their acute illness and try to walk. They then discover that they are unsteady on their feet and that the environment tends to jiggle in front of their eyes (*oscillopsia*). The diagnosis can be made at the bedside with a head-thrust test (bilateral corrective saccades; see later). Caloric and rotational testing can document the degree of vestibular loss. The best treatment is prevention. If the drug is discontinued early during the course of symptoms, the disorder may stabilize or improve.

Vascular Insufficiency

Vertebrobasilar insufficiency is a common cause of vertigo in elderly persons. Whether the vertigo originates from ischemia of the labyrinth, brain stem, or both structures is not always clear because the blood supplies to the labyrinth, eighth cranial nerve, and vestibular nuclei originate from the same source, the basilar vertebral circulation (Chapter 413). Vertigo with *vertebrobasilar insufficiency* is abrupt in onset, usually lasting several minutes, and is frequently associated with nausea and vomiting. Associated symptoms resulting from ischemia in the remaining territory supplied by the posterior circulation include visual illusions and hallucinations, drop attacks and weakness, visceral sensations, visual field defects, diplopia, and headache. These symptoms occur in episodes either in combination with the vertigo or alone. Vertigo may be an isolated initial symptom of vertebrobasilar ischemia, but repeated episodes of vertigo without other symptoms should suggest another diagnosis. Vertebrobasilar insufficiency is usually caused by atherosclerosis of the subclavian, vertebral, and basilar arteries. Occasionally, episodes of vertebrobasilar insufficiency are precipitated by postural hypotension, Stokes-Adams attacks, or mechanical compression from cervical spondylosis. MRI of the brain is usually normal because the vascular insufficiency is transient and function returns to normal between episodes. MR angiography can identify occlusive vascular disease most commonly involving the vertebral-basilar junction.

Vertigo is a common symptom with *infarction of the lateral brain stem or cerebellum* (Chapter 414), or both. The diagnosis is usually clear, based on the characteristic acute history and pattern of associated symptoms and neurologic findings. Occasionally, cerebellar infarction or hemorrhage arises with severe vertigo, vomiting, and ataxia without associated brain stem symptoms and signs that might suggest the erroneous diagnosis of an acute peripheral vestibular disorder. The key differential is the finding of clear cerebellar signs (extremity and gait ataxia) and of direction-changing, gaze-evoked nystagmus. Such patients must be watched carefully for several days because they may develop progressive brain stem dysfunction owing to compression by a swollen cerebellum.

Cerebellopontine Angle Tumors

Most tumors growing in the cerebellopontine angle (e.g., *acoustic neuroma, meningioma, epidermal cyst*) grow slowly, allowing the vestibular system to accommodate so that they produce only a vague sensation of disequilibrium rather than acute vertigo (Chapter 195). Occasionally, however, episodic vertigo or positional vertigo heralds the presence of a cerebellopontine angle tumor. In virtually all patients, retrocochlear hearing loss is present, best identified by audiometric testing. MRI with contrast is the most sensitive diagnostic study for identifying a cerebellopontine angle tumor.

Other Central Causes of Vertigo

Acute vertigo may be the first symptom of *multiple sclerosis* (Chapter 419), although only a small percentage of young patients with acute vertigo eventually develop multiple sclerosis. Vertigo in multiple sclerosis is usually transient and often associated with other neurologic signs of brain stem disease, in particular, internuclear ophthalmoplegia or cerebellar dysfunction. Vertigo may also be a symptom of *parainfectious encephalomyelitis* or, rarely, *parainfectious cranial polyneuritis.* In this instance, the accompanying neurologic signs establish the diagnosis. The *Ramsay Hunt syndrome* (geniculate ganglion herpes) is characterized by vertigo and hearing loss associated with facial paralysis and, sometimes, pain in the ear. The typical lesions of herpes zoster (Chapter 383), which may follow the appearance of neurologic signs, are found in the external auditory canal and over the palate in some patients. Rarely is herpes zoster responsible for vertigo in the absence of the full-blown syndrome. *Granulomatous meningitis* (Chapter 420) or *leptomeningeal metastasis* and cerebral or systemic *vasculitis* (Chapter 278) may involve the eighth nerve, producing vertigo as an early symptom. In these disorders, cerebrospinal fluid analysis usually suggests the diagnosis (Chapter 403). Patients suffering from *temporal lobe epilepsy* (Chapter 410) occasionally experience vertigo as the aura. Vertigo in the absence of other neurologic signs or symptoms is never caused by epilepsy or other diseases of the cerebral hemispheres.

Bedside Tests
Hyperventilation

If the history is not clear, bedside provocative tests to mimic the symptom may assist in making a pathophysiologic diagnosis. Hyperventilation, which lowers the arterial partial pressure of carbon dioxide ($Paco_2$) and decreases cerebral blood flow, causes a lightheaded sensation associated with syncope. Patients with compressive lesions of the vestibular nerve, such as with an acoustic neuroma or cholesteatoma, or with demyelination of the vestibular nerve root entry zone may develop vertigo and nystagmus after hyperventilation. Presumably, metabolic changes associated with hyperventilation trigger the partially damaged nerve to fire inappropriately.

Vestibulospinal Function

Bedside tests of vestibulospinal function are often insensitive because most patients can use vision and proprioceptive signals to compensate for any vestibular loss. Patients with acute unilateral peripheral vestibular lesions may past-point or fall toward the side of the lesion, but within a few days, balance returns to normal. Patients with bilateral peripheral vestibular loss have more difficulty compensating and usually show some imbalance on the Romberg and tandem walking tests (Chapter 403), particularly with eyes closed.

Doll's-Eye and Head-Thrust Tests

The vestibulo-ocular reflex can be tested at the bedside using the doll's-eye and head-thrust tests. In an alert human, rotating the head back and forth in the horizontal plane induces compensatory horizontal eye movements that are dependent on both the visual and vestibular systems. The doll's-eye test is a test of vestibular function in a comatose patient (Chapter 411) because such patients cannot generate pursuit or corrective fast components. In this setting, conjugate compensatory eye movements indicate normally functioning vestibulo-ocular pathways. Because the vestibulo-ocular reflex has a much higher frequency range than the smooth pursuit system, a qualitative bedside test of vestibular function can be made with the *head-thrust test.* It is performed by grasping the patient's head and applying brief, small-amplitude, high-acceleration head thrusts first to one side and then the other. The patient fixates on the examiner's nose and the examiner watches for corrective saccades, which are a sign of an inappropriate compensatory slow phase.

Caloric Test

The caloric test induces endolymphatic flow in the horizontal semicircular canal and horizontal nystagmus by creating a temperature gradient from one side of the canal to the other. With a cold caloric stimulus, the column of endolymph nearest the middle ear falls because of its increased density. This

TABLE 436-1 DESCRIPTION, MECHANISM, AND FOCUS OF DIAGNOSTIC WORK-UP FOR COMMON TYPES OF DIZZINESS

TYPE OF DIZZINESS	DESCRIPTION	MECHANISM	FOCUS OF DIAGNOSTIC EVALUATION
Vertigo	Spinning (environment moves), tilt, drunkenness	Imbalance in tonic vestibular activity	Auditory and vestibular systems
Near faint	Lightheaded, swimming	Decreased blood flow to entire brain	Cardiovascular system
Psychophysiologic	Dissociated from body, spinning inside (environment still)	Impaired central integration of sensory signals	Psychiatric assessment
Disequilibrium	Off balance, unsteady on feet	Loss of vestibulospinal, proprioceptive, cerebellar, or motor function	Neurologic assessment

causes the cupula to deviate away from the utricle (ampullofugal flow) and produces horizontal nystagmus with the fast phase directed away from the stimulated ear. A warm stimulus produces the opposite effect, causing ampullopetal endolymph flow and nystagmus directed toward the stimulated ear (a mnemonic is COWS, meaning cold opposite, warm same). Because of its ready availability, ice water (approximately 0° C) can be used for bedside caloric testing. To bring the horizontal canal into the vertical plane, the patient lies in the supine position with head tilted 30 degrees forward. Infusion of 1 to 3 mL of ice water induces a burst of nystagmus usually lasting about a minute. Greater than a 20% asymmetry in nystagmus duration suggests a lesion on the side of the decreased response. The ice water caloric test is a useful way to test the integrity of the oculomotor pathways in a comatose patient. In this case, ice water induces only a slow tonic deviation toward the side of stimulation.

Positional Tests

Examination for pathologic vestibular nystagmus should include a search for spontaneous and positional nystagmus (see Table 432-5 in Chapter 432). Because vestibular nystagmus secondary to peripheral vestibular lesions is inhibited with fixation, the yield is increased by impairing fixation with +30 lenses (Frenzel glasses) or infrared video recordings. Two types of positional testing are typically performed: moving the patient from the sitting to head-hanging-right and head-hanging-left positions (Dix-Hallpike test) and turning the head to the right and left while the patient lies supine. Induced positional nystagmus may be paroxysmal or persistent, and it may be in the same direction in all positions or change directions in different positions. The most common cause of positional nystagmus is otolith debris in the semicircular canals, either free floating (paroxysmal) or attached to the cupula (persistent). This type of nystagmus always occurs in the plane of the affected canal—vertical torsional for the vertical canals and horizontal torsional for the horizontal canal. By contrast, central positional nystagmus is often pure vertical or horizontal and cannot be explained by stimulating a single semicircular canal.

Nystagmography

Nystagmography tests oculomotor control by inducing and recording eye movements. A standard test battery includes (1) tests of visual ocular control (saccades, smooth pursuit, and optokinetic nystagmus), (2) a careful search for pathologic nystagmus with fixation and with eyes open in darkness, and (3) measurement of induced vestibular nystagmus (caloric and rotational). Nystagmography can be helpful in identifying a vestibular lesion and localizing it within the peripheral and central pathways.

Evaluating the "Dizzy" Patient

The history is key because it determines the type of dizziness (vertigo, near-faint, psychophysiologic disequilibrium), associated symptoms (neurologic, audiologic, cardiac, psychiatric), precipitating factors (position change, trauma, stress, drug ingestion), and predisposing illness (systemic viral infection, cardiac disease, cerebrovascular disease; Table 436-1). The history provides direction for both the examination and the diagnostic evaluation. When focal neurologic signs are found, neuroimaging usually leads to a specific diagnosis. When vertigo is present without focal neurologic symptoms or signs, head-thrust and positional testing are key to localizing the lesion to the labyrinth or eighth nerve. Audiometry and nystagmography are useful if the cause of vertigo is not clear after the history and examination. Patients with psychophysiologic dizziness should be identified early so that needless tests are not obtained. A detailed cardiac evaluation (including loop monitoring) often identifies the cause of episodic near fainting (Chapters 50 and 62).

TABLE 436-2 TREATMENT OF COMMON VERTIGO SYNDROMES

SYNDROME	TREATMENT
Benign positional vertigo	
Posterior canal variant	Epley's maneuver (see Fig. 436-4)
Horizontal canal variant	Barbecue roll toward normal side (side with less nystagmus), sleep with normal ear down
Vestibular neuritis	Methylprednisolone, 100 mg × 3 days, gradual taper over 22 days (must start within 3 days of onset)
Meniere's disease	
Medical	Low salt (1-2 g Na$^+$/day) *and* either hydrochlorothiazide 25-50 mg/day *or* hydrochlorothiazide 25 mg/day plus triamterene 50 mg/day
Surgical	Intratympanic gentamicin, vestibular nerve section

TREATMENT

Treatment of vertigo can be divided into three general categories: specific, symptomatic, and rehabilitative. When possible, treatment should be directed at the underlying disorder. Specific therapies include particle repositioning maneuvers (the Epley and Semont maneuvers; see Fig. 436-4) for benign positional vertigo.[4] For vestibular neuritis, steroids (e.g., methylprednisolone, 1 mg/kg/day for 5 days then tapered over the next 15 days) are effective.[5] For Meniere's disease, a low-salt diet and diuretics (e.g., 25 mg hydrochlorothiazide and 50 mg triamterene daily) (Table 436-2) are effective. Intratympanic gentamicin can significantly reduce vertigo in patients with unilateral Meniere's disease who do not respond to medical treatment.[6]

In many cases, however, symptomatic treatment either is combined with specific therapy or is the only treatment available. Many different classes of drugs have been found to have antivertiginous properties, and in most instances, the exact mechanism of action is uncertain. All these agents produce potentially unpleasant side effects, and the decision concerning which drug or combination to use is based on their known complications and on the severity and duration of the vertigo. An episode of prolonged, severe vertigo is one of the most distressing symptoms that a patient can experience. Affected patients prefer to lie still with eyes closed in a quiet, dark room. Antivertiginous drugs with sedation such as promethazine HCl (25 mg) or diazepam (5 mg) may be helpful. Prochlorperazine suppositories (25 mg) may stop vomiting.

In more chronic vertiginous disorders, when the patient is trying to carry on normal activity, less sedating antivertiginous medications such as meclizine (25 mg) or transdermal scopolamine (0.5 mg every 3 days) may provide relief. Chronic use of these drugs should be avoided.

Vestibular rehabilitation exercises are designed to help the patient compensate for permanent loss of vestibular function.[7] As the acute stage of nausea and vomiting subsides, the patient should attempt to focus the eyes and to move and hold them in the direction that provokes the most dizziness. A useful exercise involves staring at a visual target while oscillating the head from side to side or up and down, slow at first and then fast. The patient should try to stand and walk, at first in contact with a wall or with an assistant, and make slow supported turns. As improvement occurs, head movements should be added while standing and walking.

1. Conlin AE, Parnes LS. Treatment of sudden sensorineural hearing loss. II. A meta-analysis. *Arch Otolaryngol Head Neck Surg.* 2007;133:582-586.
2. Durga J, Verhoef P, Anteunis LJ, et al. Effects of folic acid supplementation on hearing in older adults: A randomized, controlled trial. *Lancet.* 2007;369:208-216.

3. Martinez Devesa P, Waddell A, Perera R, et al. Cognitive behavioural therapy for tinnitus. *Cochrane Database Syst Rev.* 2007;24:1.
4. Hilton M, Pinder D. The Epley (canalith repositioning) manoeuvre for benign paroxysmal positional vertigo. *Cochrane Database Syst Rev.* 2004:CD003162.
5. Strupp M, Zingler VC, Arbusow V, et al. Methylprednisolone, valacyclovir, or the combination for vestibular neuritis. *N Engl J Med.* 2004;351:354-361.
6. Postema RJ, Kingma CM, Wit HP, et al. Intratympanic gentamicin therapy for control of vertigo in unilateral Meniere's disease: a prospective, double-blind, randomized, placebo-controlled trial. *Acta Otolaryngol.* 2008;128:876-880.
7. Yardley L, Donovan-Hall M, Smith H, et al. Effectiveness of primary care-based vestibular rehabilitation for chronic dizziness. *Ann Intern Med.* 2004;141:598-605.

SUGGESTED READINGS

Baloh RW. Neurotology. *Semin Neurol.* 2009;29:471-547. *Diagnosis and treatment of the common causes of vertigo.*
Chou R, Dana T, Bougatsos C, et al. Screening adults aged 50 years or older for hearing loss: a review of the evidence for the U.S. Preventive Services Task Force. *Ann Intern Med.* 2011;154:347-355. *Consensus guidelines supporting screening.*
Martin González C, González FM, Trinidad A, et al. Medical management of Ménière's disease: a 10-year case series and review of literature. *Eur Arch Otorhinolaryngol.* 2010;267:1371-1376. *At 5 years, 94% of patients reported symptomatic improvement.*
Schreiber BE, Agrup C, Haskard DO, et al. Sudden sensorineural hearing loss. *Lancet.* 2010;375:1203-1211. *Review.*

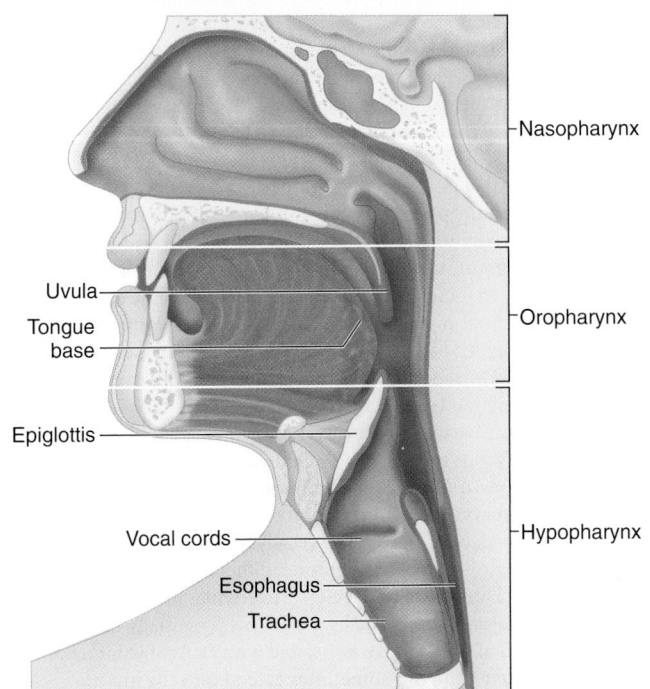

FIGURE 437-1. The pharynx (throat) is typically divided into three distinct anatomic regions (nasopharynx, oropharynx, and hypopharynx).

437

THROAT DISORDERS

THOMAS A. TAMI

The functions of deglutition, respiration, voice, and alimentation are influenced by disorders of the throat. Because the anatomy in this area is characterized by indistinct boundaries, symptoms are often difficult to ascribe to a specific anatomic area without a careful physical examination.

PATHOBIOLOGY

The pharynx is usually divided into three regions (Fig. 437-1). The *nasopharynx,* which is the region of the pharynx located above the soft palate and uvula, is usually very difficult to visualize directly unless the examiner is adept at using small nasopharyngeal mirrors or is able to use a fiberoptic endoscope introduced through the nose. Anatomic structures in the nasopharynx include the adenoids, the openings of the eustachian tubes, and the posterior tips of the inferior turbinates of the nasal cavity.

The *oropharynx* is anatomically defined as the region beginning at the level of the soft palate and extending inferiorly to the tip of the epiglottis. This anatomic area includes the faucial tonsils, the base of the tongue, the lingual tonsils, the soft palate, the uvula, and part of the posterior pharyngeal wall.

The *hypopharynx* is the lower part of pharynx extending from the tip of the epiglottis above to the introitus of the esophagus (the cricopharyngeus muscle) below. This region includes the entire larynx (epiglottis, arytenoids, glottis or true vocal cords), the pyriform sinuses (pharyngeal folds lateral to the larynx), and the posterior pharyngeal wall. Although the tip of the epiglottis can occasionally be visualized by using a routine flashlight and tongue blade during a routine oral examination, this region can usually be clearly visualized only by using a laryngeal mirror or, more commonly, a fiberoptic nasopharyngoscope.

DISEASE OF THE PHARYNX

Nasopharynx

CLINICAL MANIFESTATIONS

Typically, diseases occurring in the nasopharynx produce few symptoms until the process is well advanced and produces nasal obstruction (Chapter 434), epistaxis (Chapter 434), ear pain (Chapter 434), headache (Chapter 405), or cranial nerve abnormalities owing to extension to the skull base. Symptoms of postnasal drainage, including cough and sore throat, can be

caused by acute or chronic sinusitis or by allergic or nonallergic rhinitis. Treatment is for the underlying cause (Chapter 434). Examination using fiberoptic technology can often easily establish the appropriate diagnosis, but magnetic resonance imaging (MRI) or computed tomography (CT) can also be helpful (Chapter 434), especially when extension outside the nasopharynx is suspected.

Nasopharyngeal carcinoma (Chapter 196), which is uncommon in Western populations but more common in Asian populations, particularly southern Chinese, is related to Epstein-Barr virus infection. Common presenting symptoms include nasal obstruction, unilateral or bilateral serous otitis media, epistaxis, cervical lymph node enlargement, or cranial nerve neuropathy that often arises as diplopia.

Oropharynx

PHARYNGITIS

In the oropharynx, sore throat (pharyngitis) is the most common presenting symptom (Fig. 437-2), and tonsillitis is the most important cause. Although the faucial tonsils are occasionally the only site of infection, the lingual tonsils and the adenoids are also usually involved. The clinical evaluation must differentiate among viral pharyngitis, bacterial causes (usually streptococcus (Chapter 298), tonsillitis, peritonsillar abscess, and (rarely) acute epiglottitis (Table 437-1).

Antibiotic treatment is recommended in patients at reasonable risk for bacterial infection (Chapter 298). Penicillin (penicillin VK, 250 mg three times a day or 500 mg twice a day for 5 to 10 days) is usually chosen to treat acute bacterial pharyngitis,**1** but cefuroxime axetil (250 mg twice a day for 5 to 10 days) is even more effective for primary treatment and can be very effective for persistent infection. **2** For patients who are allergic to penicillin, azithromycin (500 mg/day for 3 days**3** or a single dose of 2 g**4**) is an alternative. Any of these regimens is reasonable for patients with a positive throat culture or rapid antigen test for group A streptococci (Chapter 298). However, azithromycin is not effective against *Fusobacterium necrophorum*, which can cause severe Lemierre's syndrome (see later). For very symptomatic sore throat, short-term corticosteroid therapy (e.g., one dose of 8 mg dexamethasone intramuscularly, or prednisone, 60 mg orally for 1 or 2 days) can reduce pain without the risk for infectious complications.**5**

Infectious mononucleosis (Chapter 385) often produces disabling tonsillitis with impressive exudative tonsillar hypertrophy (Fig. 437-3). Corticosteroids (see earlier) are very effective during the acute phase of infectious mononucleosis, particularly for patients with potential airway obstruction related to tonsillar hypertrophy. Because this systemic viral disease can also produce other medical problems, such as hepatitis and thrombocytopenia, these possibilities should be considered during the clinical evaluation.

Peritonsillar abscess can usually be diagnosed by physical examination (Fig. 437-4). A peritonsillar abscess can usually be managed in an outpatient setting using surgical or needle drainage by an ear, nose, and throat specialist and oral antibiotics, such as amoxicillin plus metronidazole or clindamycin or amoxicillin clavulanate.

By comparison, a deep neck abscess is a more serious condition because of its anatomic access to the fascial planes of the neck and chest. These patients usually present in a more toxic condition and often have swelling of the external neck, trismus, or torticollis and, occasionally, a compromised airway. These infections must be recognized immediately, often using imaging techniques, and managed aggressively, usually by external incision and drainage as well as with intravenous broad-spectrum antibiotic coverage of aerobic and anaerobic bacteria (e.g., clindamycin, 600 mg intravenously every 8 hours; ampicillin-sulbactam, 3 g every 6 hours; or penicillin G, 2 million units every 4 hours plus metronidazole 500 mg every 6 hours).

An uncommon yet quite serious complication that can result from severe infections of the pharynx is septic thrombophlebitis of the internal jugular vein (Lemierre's syndrome). Patients typically have an underlying peritonsillar abscess and present with persistent fever, difficulty swallowing, neck pain, and a neck mass. Patients may develop bacteremia and septic pulmonary emboli. The diagnosis is best made by a CT. This potentially life-threatening condition, which is almost always associated with anaerobic infection, especially with *F. necrophorum*, can sometimes extend into the intrathoracic vasculature. Treatment usually consists of antimicrobial therapy including anaerobic therapy (with either clindamycin 600 mg every 8 hours or metronidazole 500 mg every 6 hours), anticoagulation, and occasionally surgery, especially when it is associated with vascular extension or pulmonary embolization. Mortality rates can be as high as 5%.

TONSILS

Patients who have deep crypts and crevices in the tonsils can accumulate debris, such as food or sloughed mucosa, within these crypts, which provide an ideal environment for the growth of bacteria, especially anaerobes. These patients typically complain of whitish or yellow pieces of semisolid debris emanating from their tonsils. These tonsilloliths often have a foul odor and taste, and they sometimes can be associated with halitosis. Occasionally, these patients also complain of chronic sore throat owing to chronic secondary infections. Treatment usually consists of maintaining good tonsillar hygiene with frequent throat gargling and occasionally manually expressing this debris from the tonsil. If patients have symptomatic chronic, recurrent tonsillitis, adenotonsillectomy can modestly reduce the recurrence rate.[6]

APHTHOUS STOMATITIS

Aphthous stomatitis, typically encountered in the oral cavity (Chapter 433), can also occur in the oropharynx. The spectrum of causes and their treatment is similar to that for oral stomatitis.

THRUSH

Oral and pharyngeal candidiasis (thrush) is usually easily recognized by its typical "cottage cheese" exudative appearance. However, in the atrophic form of thrush, the inflammatory mucositis can be present without typical exudates. Treatment with either topical (clotrimazole or nystatin) or systemic (fluconazole) agents usually results in immediate and dramatic symptomatic improvement (Chapter 346). Underlying medical conditions commonly associated with thrush include diabetes, immune deficiency, malignancies, prolonged use of antibiotics, and xerostomia (dry mouth).

TUMORS

The most common benign tumor of the oropharynx is the squamous papilloma, which is associated with human papillomavirus (Chapter 381) infection. These small, benign, usually pedunculated tumors often have a predilection for the soft palate and uvula (Fig. 437-5). In some circumstances, these can become widely disseminated within the mouth and pharynx. Although they are rarely symptomatic, removal is recommended when these produce undue concern on the part of the patient or the physician.

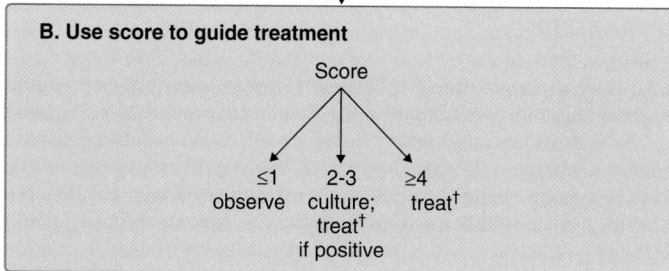

A. Calculate risk score*

	Points
• Temperature > 38° C	1
• Absence of cough	1
• Swollen, tender anterior cervical nodes	1
• Tonsillar swelling or exudate	1
• Age 3-14 yr	1
15-44 yr	0
≥45 yr	−1

B. Use score to guide treatment

Score

≤1 observe   2-3 culture; treat† if positive   ≥4 treat†

FIGURE 437-2. Approach to diagnosis and treatment of the patient with a sore throat. (*Data from McIsaac WJ, Kellner JD, Aufricht P, et al. Empirical validation of guidelines for the management of pharyngitis in children and adults. *JAMA.* 2004;291:1587-1595. †Treat for streptococcal infection; see text.)

FIGURE 437-3. Mononucleosis can produce impressive symmetrical exudative tonsillitis as shown in this patient.

TABLE 437-1 CLINICAL DIFFERENTIATION OF COMMON CONDITIONS ARISING AS SORE THROAT

FEATURE	VIRAL PHARYNGITIS	BACTERIAL TONSILLITIS	PERITONSILLAR ABSCESS	EPIGLOTTITIS
Tonsillar enlargement	Usual	Rare	None	None
Tonsillar exudates	Occasional (mononucleosis)	Usual	Often	None
Tonsillar asymmetry	None	None	Usual	None
Trismus (inability to open jaw)	None	None	Usual	None
Cervical adenopathy	Occasional	Usual (tender)	Usual (tender)	None
Tender larynx	Rare	None	None	Usual

FIGURE 437-4. If the tonsils are inflamed and appear asymmetrical with unilateral palatal swelling and uvular deviation, a peritonsillar abscess should be suspected.

FIGURE 437-5. Benign squamous papilloma. A benign squamous papilloma usually arises as a solitary lesion of the oropharynx, usually on the palate or uvula, but occasionally, especially in immunocompromised patients, the papillomatosis can become widespread on the oral and oropharyngeal mucosal surfaces.

Hypopharynx

The hypopharynx is difficult to examine and assess. Nevertheless, when the presenting symptoms cannot be easily explained on the basis of the standard oral and oropharyngeal examination, conditions in the hypopharynx and larynx should be considered.

EPIGLOTTITIS

Epiglottitis (supraglottitis) is an uncommon problem but now is more common in adults than in children because of vaccination against *Haemophilus influenzae* in children (Chapter 308). The typical adult presenting with epiglottitis has a severe sore throat and odynophagia, often with fever and occasionally with a compromised airway, despite few or no findings on the oral or oropharyngeal examination. An examination of the larynx, preferably using a nasal fiberoptic endoscope, typically reveals swelling, erythema, and occasionally exudates of the epiglottis and other supraglottic structures. During the examination, palpation or manual movement of the larynx by external palpation produces significant pain. Patients with a confirmed diagnosis of epiglottitis require intravenous antibiotics (e.g., cefotaxime, 2 g every 6 hours, or ceftriaxone, 1 to 2 g/day, intravenously) and close observation because of the risk of developing a compromised airway. Low-dose corticosteroids (e.g., prednisone, 1 mg/kg, or dexamethasone, 0.15 mg/kg, given once) appear to be as beneficial as higher doses (e.g., dexamethasone, 0.6 mg/kg given once) for croup in children. **7 8**

HOARSENESS

The symptom of hoarseness invariably points to the larynx as the site of pathology. Benign lesions are most common, including vocal nodules (screamer's nodules), vocal cord cysts, vocal cord granulomas (usually resulting from intubation trauma or laryngopharyngeal reflux), and vocal cord papillomas. Malignancies must be suspected (Chapter 196), especially in patients with a strong smoking history.

Of the malignant tumors that can occur in the hypopharynx and larynx, squamous cell carcinoma is the most common and is usually associated with tobacco and ethanol use. Squamous cell carcinoma (Chapter 196) can occur on essentially any mucosal surface in the head and neck. Symptoms can range from mild sore throat to hoarseness, severe dysphagia, and odynophagia. Pain is often referred to the jaw or ear. Associated cervical lymph node enlargement is also common in advanced disease. Successful management depends on early detection by a careful examination of the entire upper aerodigestive tract, biopsy with histopathologic examination, and aggressive treatment based on the clinical stage and site of the lesion. Symptoms of hoarseness or of odynophagia (Chapter 140), hemoptysis (Chapter 83), aspiration (Chapter 94), enlarging neck nodes (Chapters 171 and 196), and otherwise unexplained ear pain (Chapter 434), especially when present for more than 4 to 6 weeks, should be investigated carefully with a thorough head and neck examination, which must include either indirect or a direct laryngoscopy.

Neurologic conditions affecting the larynx include unilateral vocal cord paralysis, which produces a "breathy" voice because the vocal cords cannot meet in the midline. The mobile cord often compensates over several months by moving across the midline to meet the paralyzed cord, thereby improving the voice. However, when compensation is inadequate or when aspiration occurs, vocal cord medialization procedures can be considered.

Bilateral vocal cord paralysis, either iatrogenic owing to thyroid surgery or thoracic surgery or, on occasion, owing to the Arnold-Chiari malformation (Chapter 426), may not produce severe impairment of voice because the cords are often positioned very close to one another in the midline; however, airway obstruction, especially with exertion, can be severe. In spasmodic dysphonia (Chapter 415), central nervous system–mediated dystonia of the vocal cord musculature causes a strained and tight-sounding voice that worsens with continued use. Severely affected patients are often unable to maintain a voice beyond one or two words. Botulinum toxin injected directly into the vocalis muscle of the vocal cord can provide substantial symptomatic relief for up to 6 months.

DYSPHAGIA AND ESOPHAGEAL REFLUX

Dysphagia (Chapter 140) can have its origins in the hypopharynx, and the possibility of a mass lesion producing swallowing dysfunction must always be considered early in the diagnostic evaluation (see Hoarseness).

Symptoms of gastroesophageal reflux disease (GERD) may include intermittent hoarseness, chronic cough, postnasal drip, "globus" sensation, reactive airway disease, halitosis, and a brackish or acid taste in the back of the mouth and throat. Laryngoscopy typically reveals posterior laryngitis, with swollen and erythematous arytenoid cartilages, thickening of the vocal folds, interarytenoid edema, and thickening of the mucosa. When treatment aimed at nasal disorders (topical steroids, antihistamines, mucolytics, decongestants) fails to provide symptomatic relief, reflux disease should be suspected. Treatment is a therapeutic trial of a proton pump inhibitor (Chapter 140) for up to 3 months.

Spasm or thickening of the cricopharyngeus muscle, also known as the upper esophageal sphincter (Chapter 140), can cause poor pharyngeal emptying and occasionally cause spillage and penetration of secretions into the larynx with aspiration. This finding is common in patients with GERD and also seems to increase with age. Chronic cricopharyngeal spasm can result in the development of a diverticulum of the hypopharynx (Zenker's diverticulum; see Fig. 140-9 in Chapter 140). These diverticula, which can slowly enlarge, can also serve as a reservoir for lodged food, medication, or other ingested materials for hours. The hallmark of Zenker's diverticulum is regurgitation of undigested food up to 4 hours after a meal; when large or symptomatic, these diverticula can usually be managed surgically.

Progressive neurologic conditions such as multiple sclerosis (Chapter 419) or amyotrophic lateral sclerosis (Chapter 418) can arise as slowly progressive dysphagia owing to loss of coordination of the swallowing musculature. An acute stroke (Chapter 414) also can lead to impaired swallowing. Although these underlying neurologic conditions are not curable, attention to adequate alimentation and protection of the airway from aspiration are paramount. A careful evaluation by a swallowing therapist can provide invaluable management recommendations, including alterations of swallowing techniques, changes in food consistency, and timing of other interventions, such as gastrostomy tube feedings or even tracheostomy for airway management.

1. Del Mar CB, Glasziou PP, Spinks AB. Antibiotics for sore throat. *Cochrane Database Syst Rev.* 2006;4:CD000023.

2. Casey JR, Pichichero ME. Meta-analysis of cephalosporins versus penicillin for treatment of group A streptococcal tonsillopharyngitis in adults. *Clin Infect Dis.* 2004;38:1526-1534.

3. Altamimi S, Khalil A, Khalaiwi KA, et al. Short versus standard duration antibiotic therapy for acute streptococcal pharyngitis in children. *Cochrane Database Syst Rev.* 2009;1:CD004872.

4. Jorgensen DM. Single-dose extended-release oral azithromycin vs. 3-day azithromycin for the treatment of group A beta-haemolytic streptococcal pharyngitis/tonsillitis in adults and adolescents: a double-blind, double-dummy study. *Clin Microbiol Infect.* 2009;15:1103-1110.

5. Hayward G, Thompson M, Heneghan C, et al. Corticosteroids for pain relief in sore throat: systematic review and meta-analysis. *BMJ.* 2009;339:b2976.

6. Burton MJ, Glasziou PP. Tonsillectomy or adeno-tonsillectomy versus non-surgical treatment for chronic/recurrent acute tonsillitis. *Cochrane Database Syst Rev.* 2009;1:CD001802.

7. Bjornson CL, Klassen TP, Williamson J, et al. A randomized trial of a single dose of oral dexamethasone for mild croup. *N Engl J Med.* 2004;351:1306-1313.

8. Fifoot AA, Ting JY. Comparison between single-dose oral prednisolone and oral dexamethasone in the treatment of croup: a randomized, double-blinded clinical trial. *Emerg Med Australas.* 2007;19:51-58.

SUGGESTED READINGS

Cook IJ. Oropharyngeal dysphagia. *Gastroenterol Clin North Am.* 2009;38:411-431. *Review.*

Karkos PD, Asrani S, Karkos CD, et al. Lemierre's syndrome: a systematic review. *Laryngoscope.* 2009;119:1552-1559. *Review of 84 studies.*

Schwartz SR, Cohen SM, Dailey SH, et al. Clinical practice guideline: hoarseness (dysphonia). *Otolaryngol Head Neck Surg.* 2009;141:S1-S31. *Practical recommendations.*

Wald EL. Croup: common syndromes and therapy. *Pediatr Ann.* 2010;39:15-21. *Review.*

Wessels MR. Clinical practice: streptococcal pharyngitis. *N Engl J Med.* 2011;364:648-655. *Review.*

XXVII

MEDICAL CONSULTATION

PRINCIPLES OF MEDICAL CONSULTATION

GERALD W. SMETANA

APPROACH TO MEDICAL CONSULTATION

A general medical or subspecialty medical physician may receive a request to perform a consultation for a variety of purposes. In some settings a single consultative encounter will be requested, or the consultant will determine that only one visit, either in the inpatient or in the outpatient setting, is necessary. More commonly, the approach will include one or more follow-up visits to meet the goals of the consultation from the perspectives of the requesting physician, patient, and consultant. The consultant generally assumes one of four roles: cognitive consultant, procedural consultant, comanager with shared care, or comanager with principal care. The consultant as a comanager continues to care for a component of the patient's needs in an ongoing fashion while being careful to coordinate this comanagement with the continuing role of the requesting physician. Finally, in some situations it may be most appropriate for the physician who initially requested the consultation no longer to play an active role in the care of the patient but rather to transfer ongoing care exclusively to the consultant.

From a practical perspective, consulting medical physicians, whether they are generalists or subspecialists, enter into the consultative mode in a relatively limited number of ways. Surgeons may request a preoperative medical consultation to assess operative risk and obtain recommendations regarding perioperative care (Chapter 439) or, after surgery, to seek help in managing specific postoperative complications or assisting in the patient's long-term management. Both general medical physicians and medical subspecialists appropriately seek help from a subspecialist with particular knowledge in problems outside their own area of expertise to reduce uncertainty. Sometimes these requests are for specific medical procedures, but requests often seek cognitive guidance as well. Finally, noninternists may seek medical consultation for reasons other than perioperative care. For example, a psychiatrist may request a consultation to help determine whether the somatic symptoms of a particular patient represent important medical conditions (Chapter 442). In the peripartum setting, specific complications of pregnancy may require sophisticated medical consultation (Chapter 247).

Each of these settings raises different challenges for the medical consultant. In all settings, however, a number of general principles apply and can improve the effectiveness of consultations.

SETTING-SPECIFIC CONSULTATIVE ISSUES

An effective consultant must recognize the setting in which the consultation is requested and possess the required content knowledge. Distressingly, a number of studies have demonstrated that the requesting physician and the consultant often have different views on the reasons why a consultation was requested, and this initial disconnection, if present, will doom any medical consultation.

Preoperative Surgical Consultation

In the preoperative setting, the medical consultant should not "clear" a patient for surgery and must avoid the temptation to do so even if asked. Clearance may incorrectly imply that the procedure has no risk or that the medical consultant will take responsibility for having misled the patient and surgeon. Instead, the medical consultant should help determine the inherent risk associated with the proposed procedure for the particular patient, whether the patient is in the best possible condition for surgery, and whether any generic or patient-specific interventions would reduce the risk (Chapter 439). Effective consultation also requires a specialized knowledge base, whether the consultation is focusing on a particular organ system or on overall perioperative risk (Chapter 439).

Postoperative Surgical Consultation

Surgeons typically request a postoperative medical consultation when a complication has developed that is beyond their area of expertise. These problems are commonly urgent, so the goal is expeditious consultation and prompt intervention. Management of these problems does not usually differ from that used for medical patients in nonoperative settings. Another reason for a postoperative consultation is to obtain assistance in post-hospitalization care or to facilitate seamless discharge planning. Consultants should aid in the transition to the outpatient or long-term care setting by taking primary or consultative roles as appropriate.

Medical-Medical Consultations

Cross-consultations between medical subspecialists or between a subspecialist and a generalist, in either direction, are quintessential examples of collaboration. For subspecialty consultations, the key is to provide the requested expertise without overstepping into the domain of the expertise of the requesting physician. A growing example of medical-medical consultation is the situation in which a hospitalist assumes principal responsibility for an inpatient admission and then returns the patient to the primary care physician after discharge from the hospital. In this consultative interaction, close communication is critical because primary responsibility for the patient's care has shifted from the outpatient medical physician to the inpatient physician. This transfer of responsibility is not dissimilar to that occurring when a patient is submitted to the care of a subspecialist for a procedure such as cardiac catheterization or gastrointestinal endoscopy. Similar issues also arise when a critically ill patient with a condition such as a complicated myocardial infarction (Chapter 73) or shock (Chapters 106, 107, and 108) is managed principally by an inpatient-oriented medical specialist and is then expected to return to the care of the primary physician after hospital discharge. However, a key difference is that the inpatient hospitalist physician, unlike the consulting subspecialist, will not typically have any ongoing comanagement role. Because of the higher risk for discontinuity, effective communication at the time of hospitalization, whenever key issues arise during hospitalization, and at the time of discharge is even more important in the inpatient hospitalist model than in the other settings in which subspecialists may take on more of a comanagement role. Effective and comprehensive "handoffs" at the time of hospital discharge improve continuity and reduce the potential for errors and medicolegal liability.

Rapid Response Teams

A recent quality improvement initiative has been the development of rapid response teams. In this model, a prespecified consultative team urgently sees sick, hospitalized patients when a "trigger" abnormality indicates potential impending serious complications. The activation triggers for rapid response teams have varied somewhat among institutions, but there is substantial agreement on what constitutes an appropriate trigger (Table 438-1). Although implementation of these teams has not consistently reduced hospital mortality, most trials have shown a reduction in unplanned intensive care unit (ICU) transfers and in hospital length of stay. For example, in a trial of 5391 patients at a single academic medical center, patients randomly assigned to a rapid response team had a shorter length of stay, fewer unplanned ICU transfers, and lower mortality in patients with unplanned ICU transfers. **1** Other studies have shown a greater impact on unplanned ICU transfers and a reduction in hospital cardiac arrest rates.

This novel consultative strategy crosses specialties and may include general internal medicine, hospital medicine, and critical care physicians, as well as respiratory therapists and ICU nurses. When an emergency consultation is generated by a trigger event, the consultant's relationship is primarily with the patient rather than with the referring physician.

Consultations for Special Populations

When consulting for psychiatrists or in the peripartum period, the consultant requires special expertise to understand the different expressions of signs and symptoms in specific populations, as well as how and when to modify typical medical recommendations because of special circumstances (Chapters 247 and 442). Although these consultations occasionally result in long-term comanagement, more commonly they revolve around the resolution of an isolated problem. In addition, the medical consultant should not make assumptions about the requesting physician's knowledge base regarding the specific medical issues that generate the consultation. The written report and verbal communications should be comprehensive and commonly include more basic medical content and specific recommendations than may be typical of a consultation for a medical subspecialist.

Subspecialty consultations requested by primary care physicians may be for advice, a technical procedure, or ongoing comanagement (Table 438-2).

TRIGGERS: CRITERIA FOR MOBILIZING AN IN-HOSPITAL RAPID RESPONSE SERVICE

VITAL SIGNS

Heart rate
- heart rate <40/min, especially if symptoms
- heart rate >140/min

Blood pressure
- systolic blood pressure <90 mm Hg or >30-40 mm Hg below patient's usual stable blood pressure
- systolic blood pressure >200 mm Hg for >30 min
- diastolic blood pressure >110 mm Hg with symptoms

Respiratory rate
- respiratory rate <8/min or >35/min
- new onset of marked dyspnea, compromised airway, cyanosis

Oxygenation
- O_2 saturation <85% for >5 min (except patients with chronic severe hypoxemia)
- need for 100% supplemental O_2 or a non-rebreathing O_2 mask

Temperature
- fever >39°C or associated with acute decompensation

NEUROLOGIC STATUS
- acute change in mental status
- new focal findings
- prolonged or repeated seizures
- ≥2 point decline in Glasgow coma scale score

GENERAL STATUS
- uncontrollable bleeding
- decreased urine output to <50 mL over 4 hours

Based on criteria of the Joint Commission on Accreditation of Healthcare Organizations and on other sources.

TABLE 438-2 REASONS TO CONSIDER A SUBSPECIALTY CONSULTATION

To provide ongoing co-management: become a partner in in-patient care
- for an acute, unstable problem
- for a chronic condition

To perform a procedure (or advise on whether to perform it)
- diagnostic
- therapeutic

To provide one-time or periodic advice
- diagnostic guidance
- therapeutic guidance
- reassurance
- medico-legal issues

Consultations for general practitioners or family physicians generally follow the same guidelines as those for general internists. However, because both the training and ongoing practices of such physicians may or may not include the same spectrum and complexity of disease encountered by typical general internists, the subspecialty consultant must use judgment regarding both the initial consultation and the advisability of ongoing comanagement.

STRATEGIES FOR EFFECTIVE CONSULTATION

It is critical that requesting and consulting physicians agree about the reason for the consultative request. For example, the nature of a preoperative medical consultant's evaluation would differ substantially if the request were (1) routine, (2) for advice on perioperative insulin management in a patient with type 1 diabetes, or (3) to assist in determining the risks and benefits of proceeding to vascular surgery in a high-risk patient with coronary artery disease and a previous stroke. Effective communication at the time of the request will improve the value of the consultation and clarify the question. When there is doubt regarding the reason for the consultation, the consultant should speak directly to the referring physician before completing the evaluation of the patient.

Common reasons for medical consultation include assessment of perioperative risk; interpretation of a laboratory abnormality; help in performing a

procedure, in obtaining advice, or in selecting therapy; and aid in providing long-term care. Prophylactic strategies (venous thromboembolism, endocarditis, and surgical site infection) infrequently generate requests for medical consultation because they are commonly standardized to conform to practice guidelines at individual institutions.

Determining the question will also help narrow the scope of the consultant's advice and minimize the number of recommendations. This focus is especially important inasmuch as evidence indicates that adherence by the requesting physician to any of the recommendations made by the consultant is higher for consultations with fewer recommendations. Another strategy to minimize the number of recommendations is to restrict advice to pertinent issues at the time, preferably in order of their importance. For example, a consultant who is asked to aid in the care of a critically ill pregnant patient with HELLP syndrome (hemolysis, elevated liver enzymes, and low platelet count) (Chapters 163 and 247) should not also make recommendations regarding the value of cigarette cessation (Chapter 31), even though this issue will be pertinent after the mother and child have survived the acute event.

Requesting physicians are also more likely to adhere to recommendations when the patient is sicker, when the consultation is performed promptly, when advice is given to institute specific therapy rather than perform more diagnostic testing, when the consultant writes frequent follow-up notes, and when computerized order entry support systems are used to convey recommendations. When giving advice about medications, consultants should indicate specific doses and duration of treatment. If a recommendation is likely to be controversial (e.g., postpone surgery), it is always preferable to speak directly to the requesting physician before writing a consultation note in the hope that direct conversation will provide an opportunity to develop a consensus that may then be reflected in the formal consultation note. In one study of 323 physicians, the three elements of greatest perceived importance for a high-quality consultation request were to frame the question, to indicate clearly whom to call with the response, and to establish urgency.

Consultants should be careful to restrict their advice to their particular area of expertise. For example, unless a particular antipsychotic medication is contraindicated because of a medical issue (Chapter 442), it is wisest to defer decision making regarding psychiatric management to the psychiatrist. A strongly worded consultation note that advises against a particular strategy will put another physician in a difficult medicolegal position if it differs from the physician's usual or recommended practice.

Salerno and colleagues have proposed modifications of Goldman's original "Ten Commandments" for effective consultations (Table 438-3). These recommendations serve as a helpful guide for consultants to improve adherence to their advice and, as a result, improve patient outcomes.

SPECIAL CONSULTATIVE SITUATIONS

Curbside Consultation

Informal consultations are commonly termed "curbside" consultations. In the current era, ready access to online medical references may potentially reduce curbside requests. Consultants in "cognitive" specialties such as infectious diseases, rheumatology, and endocrinology provide a disproportionate amount of informal (as compared with formal) consultations. Informal consultations may occur by telephone, by e-mail, or in person. Curbside consultation is ingrained into the fabric of medical care.

Both generalists and specialists participate in an average of three to four curbside consultations per week. These consultations commonly involve questions about diagnostic tests, treatment plans, and the potential value of a formal consultation (which follows approximately a third of curbside consultations) in the future. To be effective, curbside consultations should be brief, involve a single question, and require no direct examination of the patient or medical records.

An important limitation of curbside consultations is that the consultant must rely on limited, secondhand information from the requesting physician rather than primary data from direct evaluation of the patient. Consultants report that such indirect information is often inaccurate on subsequent formal consultation. This reality, along with lack of financial compensation, leads to a greater degree of dissatisfaction with the curbside process by consultants than by requesting physicians. Salaried consultants may view a request for a curbside consultation more favorably than might those whose livelihood depends on a fee-for-service model of care.

Although requesting physicians may perceive reduced medicolegal risk when they obtain and even document a curbside consultation, consultants may fear the risk of malpractice liability themselves when offering such advice.

However, courts have consistently found that curbside consultants have no liability because no direct physician-patient relationship exists. Rather, the relationship is only between the requesting and consulting physicians.

Mandatory Consultations

In some situations, mandatory consultations may help enforce a standard of care. For example, mandatory inpatient infectious disease consultations, as part of an antimicrobial stewardship program, can improve the rational use of antimicrobial agents in the hospital and after discharge. Similarly, instituting routine consultation for patients with certain sentinel conditions, such as diabetes, may improve outcomes.

Comanagement

A consultation that begins with an initial encounter or a limited number of follow-up visits may evolve into ongoing comanagement. In such an arrangement, the physician initially serving in a consultative role becomes at least coequal to the requesting physician in the provision of ongoing care. In some situations, the consultant may actually become the primary physician. This arrangement is obvious in situations in which the consultation was requested specifically for the provision of ongoing care. Other examples include situations in which an oncologist assumes principal care of a patient with a malignancy or a nephrologist assumes principal care of a patient with end-stage renal disease who is being maintained on dialysis. In some of these situations, a general internist who initially requested the consultation may now become the consultant and provide advice on preventive care and occasional help with intercurrent medical problems.

Comanagement is also increasingly common in the hospital setting. Medical consultants may become comanagers of postoperative surgical patients, with a potential for improving outcomes. In one randomized trial of perioperative patients, formal comanagement, in which a medical physician took responsibility for managing medical problems rather than acting in a consultative role, reduced postoperative complications; in addition, both nurses and surgeons preferred this model.[2] Similar benefit has been demonstrated in a study of comanagement for elderly patients with hip fractures. In some institutions, comanagement for orthopedic or other surgical patients has become routine and does not require a specific request for consultation.

In some settings the outpatient primary care physician may retain a comanagement role even as a cardiologist cares for a patient with acute myocardial infarction, a pulmonologist cares for a patient in the ICU, a hospitalist cares for a patient in the general medical setting, or a noninternist addresses a specific problem.

RESPONSIBILITIES OF THE CONSULTANT

The consultant is responsible to two parties: the patient and the referring physician. A paternalistic approach is not desirable. The consultant should not limit communication to just the referring physician and must not withhold discussion and recommendations from the patient. However, the consultant should not usurp the role of the referring physician, who remains responsible for assembling information and advice from varied sources, as well as for developing an integrated plan with the patient. For example, in the preoperative setting, the consultant should not express a final opinion regarding the suitability of proceeding to surgery without first discussing all relevant considerations with the referring surgeon. In the trilateral deliberative model, the patient, referring physician, and consultant each have responsibilities and constraints inherent in their relationships (Fig. 438-1). Above all, the role of the consultant is to improve patient care and outcomes.

IMPACT OF CONSULTATIONS ON PATIENT OUTCOME

Few studies have investigated the impact of medical consultations on outcomes. In one study, investigators randomly assigned 355 patients whose surgeons had requested a preoperative consultation to either an outpatient medical consultation or usual care (inpatient consultation at the discretion

TABLE 438-3	GUIDELINES TO HELP MAKE CONSULTATIONS EFFECTIVE

Determine whether the goal is to obtain advice (and, if so, specifically for what) or to aid in ongoing co-management (see Table 438-2).

Understand the urgency of the consultation, so the consultation will be performed on a timely basis that meets the needs of the requesting physician and patient.

Perform a focused but careful history and physical examination—do not rely on information gathered by others.

Do not re-hash information in an overly detailed note—emphasize the key issue(s) your evaluation reinforced or discovered.

Be sure your recommendations are clearly listed and appropriately detailed—for example, indicate specific drugs, doses, and durations.

Limit the number of total number of recommendations in order to improve adherence.

Indicate how to monitor the effectiveness of your recommendations, as well as how to contact you urgently if problems arise.

Adjust your involvement (advice vs. co-management) as appropriate, in concert with the requesting physician.

Serve as a peer—teach as appropriate, but also seek to learn.

Remember that personal contact with the requesting physician, even if very brief, may be far more helpful than the best of written notes.

Do not disappear—follow the patient as frequently as appropriate, in coordination with the requesting physician.

For a more complete discussion of this topic, see Goldman L, Lee T, Rudd P. Ten commandments for effective consultations. *Arch Intern Med.* 1983;143:1753-1755 and Salerno SM, Hurst FP, Halvorson S, et al. Principles of effective consultation: an update for the 21st-century consultant. *Arch Intern Med.* 2007;167:271-275.

Relationships in Consultative Medicine

Consultant
- Listen to the patient
- Maintain confidence desired by patient
- Interpret test results
- Avoid insignificant contradictions with the primary MD
- Provide information, but remember that the primary MD is the principal source of information and advice

- Provide advice and guidance
- Interpret options for care
- Maintain role as advisor unless requested otherwise
- Defer to primary MD's judgment except when truly important

- Friend and teacher
- Provide information
- Orchestrate care
- Explain and reconcile conflicting opinions
- Ultimate responsibility for final decision making

Patient   **Primary MD**

FIGURE 438-1. Consultative relationships. The consultant must execute his or her duty to the patient while acknowledging and hopefully conforming to the collegial professional model of advising the primary physician. If, however, the patient's safety or welfare is at stake, the consultant's duty is to be sure that the patient's needs always take precedence. (Based on Emanuel LL, Richter J. The consultant and the patient-physician relationship. A trilateral deliberative model. *Arch Intern Med.* 1994;154:1785-1790, and other sources.)

of the surgeon). Length of stay did not differ between the two groups, but there were fewer unnecessary admissions (those that did not result in surgery) in the outpatient consultation group. Other reports indicate that anywhere from 5 to 50% of preoperative medical consultations result in changes in patient management.

1. Rothschild JM, Woolf W, Finn KM. et al. A controlled trial of a rapid response system in an academic medical center. *Jt Comm J Qual Patient Saf*. 2008;34:417-425.
2. Huddleston JM, Long KL, Naessens JL, et al. Medical and surgical comanagement after elective hip and knee arthroplasty. A randomized, controlled trial. *Ann Intern Med*. 2004;141:28-38.

SUGGESTED READINGS

Boulware DR, Dekarske AS, Filice GA. Physician preferences for elements of effective consultation. *J Gen Intern Med*. 2010;111:515-519. *Emphasizes how to improve the process by addressing the needs of both parties.*
Cherry K, Martinek J, Esleck S, et al. Rapid response systems: the stories. Developing and evaluating a trigger response system. *Jt Comm J Qual Patient Saf*. 2009;35:331-338. *Recommendations on developing a rapid response system and how to evaluate its efficacy.*
Foy R, Hempel S, Rubenstein L, et al. Meta-analysis: effect of interactive communication between collaborating primary care physicians and specialists. *Ann Intern Med*. 2010;152:247-258. *Interventions that enhance the quality of the exchange of information have larger effects than those that do not.*
O'Malley AS, Reschovsky JD. Referral and consultation communication between primary care and specialist physicians: finding common ground. *Arch Intern Med*. 2011;171:56-65. *Better communication can improve care.*

439

PREOPERATIVE EVALUATION

STEVEN L. COHN

PREOPERATIVE EVALUATION

Each year in the United States, more than 25 million inpatient surgical procedures and an additional 25 million outpatient procedures are performed. Although more than one third of these surgical patients are older than 65 years, overall morbidity and mortality are relatively low, in part because of modern anesthetic and surgical techniques. A crucial aspect of safety is careful preoperative evaluation of the patient, not only by the surgeon and anesthesiologist but also, in many instances, by a general medical consultant or medical subspecialist.

Operative Risk Assessment

The components of perioperative risk include those related to the patient, procedure, provider, and anesthesia. Anesthetic risk is low, with mortality less than 0.03% in a normal healthy patient—American Society of Anesthesiology (ASA) class 1—but increasing to 0.2% in ASA class 2 (mild systemic disease), 1.2% in class 3 (severe systemic disease), 8% in class 4 (severe systemic disease that is a constant threat to life), and 34% in class 5 (a moribund patient not expected to survive for 24 hours without surgery). Meta-analysis suggests that when feasible, neuraxial (spinal or epidural) anesthesia may reduce postoperative complications compared with general anesthesia (Chapter 440), but decisions regarding the anesthetic technique should be the responsibility of the anesthesiologist and not be part of the preoperative medical consultation. With respect to the provider, data support a "learning curve," with better outcomes when procedures are performed by more experienced, higher-volume surgeons.

General Risk Assessment
History and Physical Examination

The medical history and physical examination are the most important components in assessing a patient's risk for surgery. The consultation should focus on pertinent medical problems, particularly cardiopulmonary symptoms and diseases that are associated with risk and are likely to influence perioperative management (Chapter 438). The importance of the past surgical history is to determine whether the patient was able to undergo major surgery in the recent

past or had any perioperative medical or anesthetic-related complications that could occur again. The social history should assess and quantify the amount, duration, and last use of tobacco, alcohol, or illicit substances. It is important to document allergies to medications, foods, and latex as well as to obtain an accurate list of the patient's current prescription and over-the-counter medications, including doses and adherence. The family history is relevant primarily for any genetically associated complications such as malignant hyperthermia. The review of systems should include the presence or absence of chest pain and dyspnea and the patient's exercise capacity. The physical examination must include the vital signs, assessment of the airway and respiratory status, cardiovascular examination, and documentation of any neurologic deficit.

Preoperative Tests

Screening preoperative test results in otherwise healthy individuals are usually normal and, even when abnormal, rarely affect management (generally <1%) (Table 439-1). Most significant abnormalities can be predicted from the clinical information obtained, which then guides selective testing based on the history, the physical findings, and the planned type of surgery and anesthesia. Most patients undergoing low-risk surgery with local anesthesia require no preoperative testing. Repeat testing should be avoided if recent (within 3 months) results were normal, unless the patient's condition or medications have changed.

Perioperative Medications

Decisions regarding whether to continue a medication perioperatively should consider the drug's pharmacokinetics (Chapter 28) as well as its effects on the primary disease and perioperative risk, including potential interactions with anesthetic agents. Some medications are essential to continue (e.g., cardiac medications and corticosteroids), whereas others must be discontinued (e.g., oral hypoglycemic agents) or have their dose altered (e.g., insulin and anticoagulants). Still other medications should be started prophylactically to minimize perioperative risk (e.g., anticoagulants for prophylaxis against venous thromboembolism [Chapter 81] and antibiotic prophylaxis for surgical site infection or endocarditis [Chapter 76]). Data are often lacking or conflicting. Table 439-2 briefly summarizes "consensus" perioperative recommendations for the major classes of drugs.

Cardiac Risk Assessment

A significant proportion of patients who undergo surgery have either known coronary artery disease or risk factors for it, and postoperative cardiac complications are second only to direct surgical complications as a cause of perioperative mortality. The goal is to risk-stratify patients clinically and to determine whether additional testing, new medications, or cardiac interventions will be beneficial.

History and Physical Examination

Important information includes any history of previous cardiac disease (myocardial infarction [MI], angina, heart failure, arrhythmias, valvular disease), cardiac interventions (coronary artery bypass grafting, percutaneous coronary intervention), cardiac evaluation (noninvasive testing, angiography), risk factors (hypertension, diabetes mellitus, dyslipidemia, cigarette smoking), and associated diseases (peripheral arterial disease, stroke, chronic kidney disease, and chronic obstructive pulmonary disease [COPD]). Current status regarding chest pain or dyspnea, functional capacity, and medications should be assessed. The physical examination serves to confirm findings in the history as well as to assess severity and control of the disease (e.g., heart failure, hypertension, valvar disease). The preoperative electrocardiogram rarely changes management unless it demonstrates evidence of a recent or silent MI, but it is often useful as a baseline against which to compare postoperative tracings.

Cardiac Risk Indices

Over the years, a number of risk indices have been proposed to assist in preoperative cardiac evaluation. The most current of these, the revised cardiac risk index (RCRI; Table 439-3), was developed during the evaluation of several thousand patients, was validated in thousands more, and has been incorporated into the consensus guidelines developed by the American College of Cardiology and the American Heart Association. These guidelines, which are updated periodically, use a stepwise strategy based on clinical risk factors, surgery-specific risk, and exercise capacity, combined with a systematic approach to perioperative testing and treatment in patients with known or suspected cardiac disease (Fig. 439-1). Preoperative levels of brain

TABLE 439-1 RECOMMENDATIONS FOR PREOPERATIVE LABORATORY TESTING

TEST	% ABNORMAL	% INFLUENCING MANAGEMENT	INDICATIONS
Hemoglobin	1.8	0.1	Expected major blood loss, symptoms of anemia, chronic kidney disease
White blood count	0.7	0.0	Suspected infection, myeloproliferative disorder, myelotoxic medications
Platelet count	0.9	0.02	Bleeding diathesis, myeloproliferative disorder, myelotoxic medications
Prothrombin time	0.3	0.0	Bleeding diathesis, liver disease, malnutrition, antibiotic use, anticoagulants
Partial thromboplastin time	6.5	0.1	Bleeding diathesis, anticoagulant use
Electrolytes	12.7	1.8	Renal disease, medications affecting electrolytes (e.g., diuretics, digoxin, ACE inhibitor, ARBs)
Glucose	9.3	0.5	Known DM, steroids, morbid obesity
Renal function	8.2	2.6	Renal disease, DM, HTN, major surgery, older age, medications affecting renal function
Liver function tests	0.4	0.1	Known liver disease, albumin level if at risk for needing postoperative parenteral nutrition
Urinalysis	19.1	1.4	No indication unless GU symptoms or instrumentation planned
Electrocardiogram (<50 years old)	29.6 (19.7)	2.6	Age >40 yr in men or >50 yr in women or symptoms/signs of or previous known diagnosis of cardiac disease, DM, or HTN
Chest radiograph (<50 years old)	21.2 (4.9)	3.0	Age >50 yr undergoing major upper abdominal or thoracic surgery or symptoms/signs or previous known diagnosis of cardiac or pulmonary disease

ACE = angiotensin-converting enzyme; ARB = angiotensin receptor blocker; DM = diabetes mellitus; GU = genitourinary; HTN = hypertension.
Modified from Smetana GW, Macpherson DS. The case against routine preoperative laboratory testing. *Med Clin North Am.* 2003;87:7-40.

TABLE 439-2 PERIOPERATIVE MANAGEMENT OF MEDICATIONS

MEDICATION CLASS	RECOMMENDATION
Anticoagulants (heparins, warfarin)*	Continue for minor surgery Discontinue at an appropriate interval before major surgery Consider bridging anticoagulation for patients at high risk for interim thrombosis (see Chapter 37)
Antiplatelet drugs	Continue for minor surgery Discontinue clopidogrel at least 5 days before surgery and prasugrel at least 7 days before surgery If discontinuing aspirin, do so at least 5-7 days before surgery
Cardiovascular medications	Continue most agents Consider starting β-blockers in patients at high risk for perioperative cardiac morbidity (vascular or high-risk surgery) Withhold diuretics on the morning of surgery, especially if signs of volume depletion are present Stop tamsulosin before cataract surgery (floppy iris syndrome)
Lipid-lowering agents	Continue "statins" Discontinue other agents
Pulmonary agents	Continue
Gastrointestinal agents	Continue
Diabetic agents (see text)	Withhold oral hypoglycemic agents on the morning of surgery; restart when the patient resumes eating For type 1 diabetes, continue some form of insulin (long acting or intravenous) at all times For type 2 diabetes, decrease the dose of morning intermediate insulin
Thyroid agents (hypothyroidism and hyperthyroidism) (see text)	Continue thyroid replacement Continue antithyroid medication and postpone surgery until the hyperthyroidism is controlled
Oral contraceptives, hormone replacement, and SERMs	May discontinue 3 weeks before surgery only in patients at high risk for perioperative venous thromboembolism; otherwise continue
Corticosteroids (see text)	Continue chronic corticosteroids; increase the dosage to account for surgical stress
Psychotropic agents	Continue SSRIs but consider withholding them several weeks before CNS surgery Continue tricyclic antidepressants, benzodiazepines, lithium, and antipsychotics Usually discontinue MAOIs 10-14 days before surgery
Chronic opioids	Continue; substitute equianalgesic or higher doses for surgical pain
Rheumatologic agents	Continue methotrexate Discontinue other DMARDs and anticytokines Continue hypouricemic agents
Neurologic agents	Continue antiseizure medications Consider withholding antiparkinsonian agents briefly Continue agents for myasthenia gravis
Herbal agents	Discontinue all agents

*See also Table 439-8 for more detail.
CNS = central nervous system; DMARD = disease-modifying antirheumatic drug; MAOI = monoamine oxidase inhibitor; SERM = selective estrogen receptor modulator; SSRI = selective serotonin reuptake inhibitor.
Adapted from Cohn SL, Macpherson DS. Perioperative medication management. In: Cohn SL, Smetana GW, Weed HG, eds. *Perioperative Medicine: Just the Facts.* New York: McGraw-Hill, 2006.

natriuretic peptide (BNP) are independent predictors of postoperative cardiac complications, although the definition of an abnormal value has varied among studies. The emphasis of the new guideline is to minimize cardiac testing unless the results are likely to alter management.

Noninvasive Tests

A resting echocardiogram (Chapter 55) is indicated to evaluate valvular heart disease in patients with clinically suspicious murmurs and to evaluate left ventricular function in patients with heart failure. Other than for the assessment of aortic stenosis (see later), resting echocardiography is not a reliable predictor of perioperative cardiac events.

Exercise testing (with or without imaging) is preferred to pharmacologic stress testing because it assesses functional capacity (see Table 50-3 in Chapter 50), but its use is often limited by a patient's inability to achieve the target heart rate. Furthermore, patients with adequate exercise capacity by history rarely require preoperative stress testing.

Pharmacologic Stress Testing

Pharmacologic stress testing (either dipyridamole or adenosine with nuclear imaging [Chapters 56 and 71] or dobutamine echocardiography [Chapters 55 and 71]) is indicated when a patient cannot perform adequate exercise (see Table 71-6 and Fig. 71-3 in Chapter 71). Both tests have equivalent sensitivity for predicting perioperative ischemic complications, whereas stress echocardiography has fewer false-positive results. Dipyridamole and adenosine can cause bronchospasm and are best avoided in patients with symptomatic or severe asthma or obstructive lung disease, but they are preferred in patients with left bundle branch block, in whom exercise or stress echocardiography is more likely to give false-positive results. Quantitatively, the number and extent of reperfusion defects or wall motion abnormalities correlate with the severity of disease, likelihood of complications, and need for further evaluation by angiography.

Patients whose clinical condition would warrant stress testing independent of planned surgery should have such testing before elective operations. Otherwise, stress testing is recommended only in patients who are undergoing high-risk surgery (Table 439-4) and have three or more clinical risk factors (Table 439-5; see Table 439-3). Evidence for stress testing in other situations is weak, but it may be considered on an individual basis in patients with one or two risk factors if the results are likely to change management.

TABLE 439-3 CLINICAL FACTORS IMPORTANT IN ASSESSING PERIOPERATIVE CARDIAC RISK

Revised cardiac risk index criteria*
Patients are at risk and may be candidates for perioperative β-blockers if they have
Ischemic heart disease or at least two of the following:
Heart failure[†] defined as S₃ or bilateral rales on physical examination or pulmonary edema on chest radiograph
Cerebrovascular disease defined as history of transient ischemic attack or history of cerebrovascular accident
Insulin-dependent diabetes mellitus
Chronic renal insufficiency defined as baseline creatinine of 2.0 mg/dL or greater
High-risk surgery defined as intrathoracic, intra-abdominal, or suprainguinal vascular surgery

*Lee TH, Marcantonio ER, Mangione CM, et al. Derivation and prospective validation of a simple index for prediction of cardiac risk of major noncardiac surgery. *Circulation.* 1999;100:1043-1049.
†Use of β-blockers must be individualized and used with caution in patients with heart failure. From Auerbach AD, Goldman L. Assessing and reducing the cardiac risk of non-cardiac surgery. *Circulation.* 2006;113:1361-1376.

FIGURE 439-1. Cardiac evaluation and care algorithm for noncardiac surgery based on active clinical conditions, known cardiovascular disease, or cardiac risk for patients 50 years or older. *Active cardiac conditions include unstable coronary syndromes (unstable or severe angina, or recent myocardial infarction within the past 30 days), decompensated heart failure, significant arrhythmias, and severe valvular disease. †See Table 439-4. ‡Self-reported exercise capacity is considered adequate if the patient can perform 4 or more metabolic equivalents of activity (see Table 50-5 in Chapter 50). **See Table 439-3 (include all risk factors other than type of surgery, which is considered elsewhere in this algorithm). ††See Table 439-5. ‡‡See Table 439-6. HR = heart rate; METS = metabolic equivalents. (Adapted from a report of the American College of Cardiology Foundation/American Heart Association Task Force on Practice Guidelines. Developed in collaboration with the American Society of Echocardiography, American Society of Nuclear Cardiology, Heart Rhythm Society, Society of Cardiovascular Anesthesiologists, Society for Cardiovascular Angiography and Interventions, Society for Vascular Medicine, Society for Vascular Surgery. Fleishmann KE, Beckman JA, Buller CE, et al. 2009 ACCF/AHA focused update on perioperative beta blockade incorporated into the ACC/AHA 2007 guidelines on perioperative cardiovascular evaluation and care for noncardiac surgery. *J Am Coll Cardiol.* 2009;54:e13-e118.)

TABLE 439-4 RISKS OF VARIOUS SURGICAL PROCEDURES

HIGH RISK (CARDIAC RISK >5%)

Major vascular surgery
Emergent major operations
Prolonged procedures with large fluid shifts or significant blood loss

INTERMEDIATE RISK (CARDIAC RISK 1-5%)

Intraperitoneal or intrathoracic procedures
Carotid endarterectomy
Endovascular aortic aneurysm repair
Head and neck surgery
Orthopedic procedures
Prostate surgery

LOW RISK (CARDIAC RISK <1%)

Superficial operations
Cataract surgery
Breast surgery
Ambulatory surgery

TABLE 439-5 RECOMMENDATIONS FOR STRESS TESTING BEFORE NONCARDIAC SURGERY

RECOMMENDATIONS	CLASS*	LEVEL[†]
Stress testing is recommended in high-risk surgery[‡] patients with ≥3 clinical factors.	I	C
Stress testing may be considered in high-risk surgery patients with ≤2 clinical factors.[§]	IIb	B
Stress testing may be considered in intermediate-risk surgery patients.	IIb	C
Stress testing is not recommended in low-risk surgery patients.	III	C

*Class of recommendation: I = evidence and/or general agreement that a given treatment or procedure is beneficial, useful, and effective; II = conflicting evidence and/or a divergence of opinion about the usefulness/efficacy of the given treatment or procedure; IIa = weight of evidence/opinion is in favor of usefulness/efficacy; IIb = usefulness/efficacy is less well established by evidence/opinion; III = evidence or general agreement that the given treatment or procedure is not useful or effective, and in some cases may be harmful.
[†]Level of evidence: A = data derived from multiple randomized clinical trials or meta-analyses; B = data derived from a single randomized clinical trial or large nonrandomized studies; C = consensus of opinion of the experts and/or small studies, retrospective studies, registries.
[‡]See Table 439-4.
[§]See Table 439-3.
Adapted from Poldermans D, Bax JJ, Boersma E, et al. Guidelines for pre-operative cardiac risk assessment and perioperative cardiac management in non-cardiac surgery. The Task Force for Preoperative Cardiac Risk Assessment and Perioperative Cardiac Management in Non-cardiac Surgery of the European Society of Cardiology (ESC) and endorsed by the European Society of Anaesthesiology (ESA). Eur Heart J. 2009;30:2769-2812.

Risk Reduction Strategies for Ischemic Heart Disease
Medical Therapy

Prophylactic β-blockers (e.g., atenolol or bisoprolol) decreased major postoperative cardiac events in small early studies of higher-risk patients, but a number of subsequent studies failed to show a significant benefit. In by far the largest trial of prophylactic perioperative β-blockers, a high dose of extended-release metoprolol, started hours before surgery, reduced perioperative MI, but at the expense of increasing strokes and overall mortality, in part owing to more hypotension and bradycardia.[1] A meta-analysis confirmed the benefit of β-blockers in reducing perioperative MI and the side effect of increasing stroke, but found no statistically significant difference in overall mortality,[2] and a review of trials in which bisoprolol was started well before surgery found no relationship with postoperative stroke.[3] Until more evidence is available, it seems prudent to avoid starting β-blockers immediately before surgery and to avoid them in the settings of emergency surgery, prior cerebrovascular disease, or sepsis (Table 439-6). β-Blockers may benefit patients at high risk for MI but not for stroke and are more likely to be beneficial when started at a lower dose well in advance of surgery and titrated to a heart rate of 55 to 70 beats per minute.[4] Various recommended regimens are listed in Table 439-7.

If a patient has contraindications to β-blockers (bronchospasm, bradyarrhythmia, acute heart failure, advanced heart block), an α_2-adrenergic agonist

(i.e., a transdermal clonidine extended-release TTS-2 patch the night before, and 0.2 mg orally the night before and morning of surgery) may be an alternative choice based on limited data that such medications also reduce ischemia and possibly perioperative MI and death, especially in patients undergoing major vascular surgery.[5] Limited data on prophylactic calcium antagonists or nitrates have not shown major benefits in preventing complications after noncardiac surgery.

Statins (Chapter 213) reduce endovascular inflammation and stabilize endothelial plaque. Although the manufacturers' package inserts have recommend discontinuing statins before surgery, current data suggest not only that they should be continued perioperatively but also that they should be started prophylactically before surgery in patients who meet criteria for their ongoing use (Chapter 213).[6]

Invasive Therapies

Prophylactic coronary revascularization in patients who have stable cardiac symptoms and no aortic stenosis and do not meet standard criteria for the procedure (Chapter 71) does not appear to reduce perioperative myocardial infarction, death within 30 days, or long-term mortality at an average of 2.7 years in patients who receive appropriate medical therapy.[7] Preoperative coronary revascularization is indicated only if the patient meets the criteria for coronary angiography or revascularization independent of the need for surgery, but even then coronary revascularization based on the results of preoperative noninvasive testing has not been shown to improve perioperative outcomes.[8]

For bare metal stents, data suggest that surgery should be delayed for 4 to 6 weeks after stenting because of the risk for in-stent thrombosis when dual antiplatelet therapy with aspirin and clopidogrel is discontinued early or because of the alternative risk for bleeding if surgery is performed in patients receiving such antiplatelet therapy (Chapter 74). Similar concerns apply with drug-eluting stents, for which the guidelines currently recommend continuing uninterrupted dual antiplatelet therapy for a minimum of 12 months because of the risk for late stent thrombosis. For balloon angioplasty without stenting, a delay of 2 weeks is generally recommended. If antiplatelet therapy has to be discontinued, clopidogrel is usually discontinued 5 to 7 days before (and prasugrel is stopped 7 days before) the noncardiac procedure, and aspirin is continued, if possible. If aspirin also needs to be discontinued, it is usually stopped approximately 1 week before surgery.

Other Cardiovascular Diseases
Heart Failure

Heart failure, which is a major risk factor for surgery, requires treatment and optimization before surgery (Chapter 59). Routine use of *pulmonary artery catheters* does not reduce morbidity or mortality in patients undergoing elective noncardiac surgery.[9] At present, there is no evidence that treatment to lower the BNP level or use of β-blockers will reduce postoperative complications in patients with heart failure.

Aortic Stenosis

Patients with *symptomatic aortic stenosis* who meet the criteria for valve replacement (Chapter 75) independent of their need for surgery should undergo the valve surgery before the noncardiac surgery. However, patients usually survive surgery with intensified care if they refuse valve replacement or time does not permit it. Balloon aortic valvuloplasty may be an option in severe cases. An asymptomatic aortic valve gradient higher than 25 to 30 mm Hg also carries an increased risk for perioperative complications but is an indication for more careful monitoring rather than valve surgery. Endocarditis prophylaxis is appropriate for patients with mechanical heart valves, previous endocarditis, or complex congenital heart disease undergoing invasive dental or upper respiratory procedures (Chapter 76).

Hypertension

Hypertension with blood pressure lower than 110 mm Hg diastolic or 180 mm Hg systolic without significant target organ damage does not increase the risk for major perioperative cardiac complications. Even when the preoperative diastolic blood pressure is higher, limited data suggest that surgery is safe after additional antihypertensive therapy.

Arrhythmias

Although patients with arrhythmias have increased perioperative risk, the risk is increased because the arrhythmias are usually markers of more serious

TABLE 439-6 RECOMMENDATIONS FOR PERIOPERATIVE β-BLOCKER THERAPY*

2009 RECOMMENDATIONS OF AMERICAN HEART ASSOCIATION/AMERICAN COLLEGE OF CARDIOLOGY (ACCF/AHA)	RECOMMENDATIONS OF EUROPEAN SOCIETY OF CARDIOLOGY
CLASS I	
1. β-Blockers should be continued in patients undergoing surgery who are receiving β-blockers for treatment of conditions with ACCF/AHA class I guideline indications for the drugs (level of evidence: C).	1. β-Blockers are recommended in patients who have known ischemic heart disease or myocardial ischemia according to preoperative stress testing (level of evidence: B). 2. β-Blockers are recommended in patients scheduled for high-risk surgery (level of evidence: B). 3. Continuation of β-blockers is recommended in patients previously treated with β-blockers because of ischemic heart disease, arrhythmias, or hypertension (level of evidence: C).
CLASS IIA	
1. β-Blockers titrated to heart rate and blood pressure are probably recommended for patients undergoing vascular surgery who are at high cardiac risk owing to coronary artery disease or the finding of cardiac ischemia on preoperative testing (level of evidence: B). 2. β-Blockers titrated to heart rate and blood pressure are reasonable for patients in whom preoperative assessment for vascular surgery identifies high cardiac risk, as defined by the presence of more than 1 clinical risk factor† (level of evidence: C). 3. β-Blockers titrated to heart rate and blood pressure are reasonable for patients in whom preoperative assessment identifies coronary artery disease or high cardiac risk, as defined by the presence of more than 1 clinical risk factor,† who are undergoing intermediate-risk surgery‡ (level of evidence: B).	1. β-Blockers should be considered for patients scheduled for intermediate-risk surgery (level of evidence: B). 2. Continuation in patients previously treated with β-blockers because of chronic heart failure with systolic dysfunction should be considered (level of evidence: C).
CLASS IIB	
1. The usefulness of β-blockers is uncertain for patients who are undergoing either intermediate-risk procedures or vascular surgery in whom preoperative assessment identifies a single clinical risk factor in the absence of coronary artery disease† (level of evidence: C). 2. The usefulness of β-blockers is uncertain in patients undergoing vascular surgery with no clinical risk factors† who are not currently taking β-blockers (level of evidence: B).	1. β-Blockers may be considered in patients scheduled for low-risk surgery with risk factor(s) (level of evidence: B).
CLASS III	
1. β-Blockers should not be given to patients undergoing surgery who have absolute contraindications to β-blockade (level of evidence: C). 2. Routine administration of high-dose β-blockers in the absence of dose titration is not useful and may be harmful in patients not currently taking β-blockers who are undergoing noncardiac surgery (level of evidence: B).	1. Perioperative high-dose β-blockers without titration are not recommended (level of evidence: A). 2. β-Blockers are not recommended in patients scheduled for low-risk surgery without risk factors (level of evidence: B).

*See Table 439-5 for definitions of class of recommendation and level of evidence.
†See Table 439-3.
‡See Table 439-4.
Reproduced from Poldermans D, Bax JJ, Boersma E, et al. Guidelines for pre-operative cardiac risk assessment and perioperative cardiac management in non-cardiac surgery. The Task Force for Preoperative Cardiac Risk Assessment and Perioperative Cardiac Management in Non-cardiac Surgery of the European Society of Cardiology (ESC) and endorsed by the European Society of Anaesthesiology (ESA). *Eur Heart J.* 2009;30:2769-2812.

heart disease or cause hemodynamic problems. Patients with tachyar-rhythmias and bradyarrhythmias should generally be treated as in the non-operative setting (Chapters 64 and 65), except for the special circumstance of anticoagulation in the perioperative setting (Chapter 37).

Pulmonary Risk Assessment
Postoperative pulmonary complications are as common as cardiac complications and are associated with significant morbidity and mortality. Major complications include respiratory failure (e.g., reintubation, prolonged mechanical ventilation), pneumonia, atelectasis requiring bronchoscopy, and to a lesser degree, bronchospasm or an exacerbation of COPD requiring treatment and prolonged length of stay. Many postoperative pulmonary complications are due to exaggerations of the usual postoperative changes in pulmonary function: decreased lung volumes, diaphragmatic dysfunction, ventilation-perfusion mismatches and shunting, hypoventilation, hypoxemia, and impaired defense mechanisms. Pulmonary risk factors can be divided into patient-related and procedure-related factors, the latter of which includes the type of surgery, anesthesia, and related factors.

Patient-Related Factors
COPD (Chapter 88) increases the risk for postoperative pulmonary complications approximately twofold, depending on its severity, whereas well-controlled *asthma* (Chapter 87) does not increase risk. Active cigarette smokers are at increased risk, mainly related to the number of pack years smoked; smoking cessation at least 4 to 8 weeks before surgery may reduce the risk. *Obstructive sleep apnea* (Chapter 100), typically associated with obesity, confers an increased risk for hypercapnia and hypoxemia, and obese patients are at increased risk for atelectasis. Advanced age, poor functional

status, an altered mental state, and suppressed immune status from chronic steroid use, alcohol use, or diabetes may also increase the risk for postoperative pulmonary complications.

Procedure-Related Factors
The most important predictor of postoperative pulmonary complications is the type of surgery and proximity of the surgical incision to the diaphragm. Pulmonary function decreases by approximately 50% after intrathoracic surgery, upper abdominal procedures, and abdominal aortic aneurysm repair and does not fully return to normal for several weeks. Lower abdominal surgery is associated with a 25% decrease in pulmonary function. Laparoscopic procedures are usually associated with lower rates of postoperative pulmonary complications and shorter hospital stays than open procedures. Neuraxial anesthesia (epidural or spinal) may be associated with decreased risk when compared with general anesthesia, but the decision about which type of anesthesia to use is best left to the anesthesiologist. Emergency surgery, prolonged duration of anesthesia or surgery (>2 to 6 hours), and routine postoperative nasogastric tube use increase the risk for postoperative pulmonary complications.

Pulmonary Function Tests
In general, pulmonary function tests (Chapter 85) are no more predictive of pulmonary complications than is clinical risk assessment alone. Such testing may be more helpful in assessing risk for lung resection surgery when it can predict the function of the remaining lung mass. However, even a postoperative predicted forced expiratory volume in 1 second (FEV_1) of less than 800 mL for lung resection, which is thought to portend a very high risk for death or prolonged mechanical ventilation, is not an absolute

TABLE 439-7 PROTOCOLS FOR PROPHYLACTIC PERIOPERATIVE β-BLOCKERS*

GENERAL PRINCIPLES

Start β-blocker at least 1 week before surgery (if possible).

Titrate the dose to an ideal target heart rate of 55-70 beats/min.

Use half the dose if the heart rate is <65 beats/min, if systolic blood pressure is <120 mm Hg, or in a small elderly or frail patient.

Hold the dose if the heart rate is <55 beats/min or systolic blood pressure is <100 mm Hg.

Continue β-blocker postoperatively for at least 1-4 wk (or indefinitely if independent criteria such as known coronary artery disease, peripheral arterial disease, or hypertension are present). Taper the dose if discontinuing.

Before increasing the dose for postoperative tachycardia, evaluate the patient for other potential causes, including pain, bleeding, and sepsis (where β-blockers may be detrimental).

SPECIFIC DRUGS: ATENOLOL, BISOPROLOL, OR METOPROLOL

Preoperatively (recommended starting dose, then titrate to the target heart rate):
  Atenolol: start at 25 mg orally daily
  Bisoprolol: start at 5 mg orally daily at least 7 days before surgery
  Metoprolol: start at 25-50 mg orally twice daily up to 30 days preoperatively

Day of surgery—continue the usual dose or increase the oral dose to control the heart rate or give additional intravenous (IV) doses (atenolol or metoprolol, 5-10 mg) as needed if unable to take orally. Esmolol can also be used (500-μg/kg IV loading dose over a 1-min period; then infuse at 50-200 μg/kg/min and titrate to the target heart rate)

Postoperatively—continue the usual preoperative dose:
  Atenolol: 25-100 mg orally daily for at least 7 days
  Bisoprolol: 2.5-5 mg orally daily for at least 30 days
  Metoprolol: 25-100 mg orally twice daily for at least 14 days
  Substitute IV atenolol or metoprolol (5-mg doses) as needed if unable to take medication orally

*See Table 439-6 for indications.

---

contraindication to surgery. Preoperative arterial blood gas evaluation is also of little benefit in predicting postoperative pulmonary complications.

Risk Reduction Strategies

Unfortunately, many of the risk factors for postoperative pulmonary complications cannot be modified. Inhaled bronchodilators (β-agonists and anticholinergics) and steroids can optimize the respiratory status of patients with COPD and asthma. Broad-spectrum antibiotics should be used to treat exacerbations caused by bacterial infection. Chest physiotherapy may be helpful. Smoking should be stopped at least 8 weeks before surgery, if possible.

Lung expansion maneuvers (either incentive spirometry or deep-breathing exercises) can significantly improve pulmonary function, minimize atelectasis, and reduce risk, especially for thoracic and upper abdominal surgery. Pain control (Chapter 29) improves pulmonary function by allowing deeper breathing. Epidural analgesia and patient-controlled intravenous analgesia reduce postoperative pulmonary complications and, when possible, are preferable to parenteral narcotics.

Endocrine Conditions

Diabetes Mellitus

The major risks associated with surgery in diabetic patients are cardiac complications and wound infections. Complications are probably related more to associated diseases and end-organ involvement (coronary artery disease, chronic kidney disease, and autonomic neuropathy) than to the glucose level itself. Significantly, elevated glucose levels may impair wound healing and interfere with leukocyte defense mechanisms. However, current recommendations suggest a glucose target level of 140 to 180 mg/dL rather than tight perioperative control.

Patients whose diabetes is controlled by diet require only perioperative glucose monitoring (fingersticks) with short-acting insulin coverage on an as-needed basis. Patients taking oral hypoglycemic agents (Chapter 237) should not take them on the morning of surgery (chlorpropamide should be stopped 2 to 3 days before and metformin preferably 1 day before) and should be monitored with sliding-scale insulin coverage as needed. Patients taking insulin are most often given half to two thirds of their usual

intermediate-acting insulin on the morning of surgery and are then given short-acting insulin on a sliding scale and correction dose based on fingerstick monitoring (Chapter 236). Continuous intravenous insulin, which provides tighter glucose control but is associated with more episodes of hypoglycemia and requires a monitored setting, is typically used in patients undergoing cardiac surgery and in critically ill patients. There are no validated guidelines regarding the management of patients taking long-acting basal insulin (glargine). In general, it should be continued, but its dose may be reduced for ambulatory surgery or in patients with tight control. Regardless of the mode of treatment, frequent monitoring of the glucose level is critical.

Exogenous Corticosteroids and Adrenal Insufficiency

The stress of surgery activates the hypothalamic-pituitary-adrenal (HPA) axis, which in turn stimulates release of adrenocorticotropic hormone (ACTH) and subsequent secretion of cortisol (Chapter 234), but a patient who is taking exogenous corticosteroids may have suppression of the HPA axis and not be able to respond to this stress adequately. As a result, hypotension and shock may occur.

In general, a daily dose equivalent to 5 mg or less of prednisone (Chapter 234), alternate-day short-acting therapy, or corticosteroids given for less than 3 weeks do not cause clinically significant HPA suppression, so no supplemental therapy is indicated. Conversely, doses greater than 20 mg/day of prednisone for longer than 3 weeks usually suppress the HPA axis and warrant perioperative supplemental corticosteroids. In patients who are taking intermediate dosing regimens or who took large doses in the past year but are not taking corticosteroids or are taking lower doses now, the options are to perform an ACTH (cosyntropin) stimulation test, if time permits, and treat only patients with an inadequate response (Chapter 234) or to prescribe supplemental corticosteroids empirically.

When supplemental corticosteroids are appropriate, short-term therapy tailored to the level of expected stress can provide protection without adverse effects on wound healing and with only short-term problems with glucose intolerance and fluid retention. For minor procedures or local anesthesia, the recommended approach is to give the patient's usual dose before surgery without further supplementation. For moderate surgical stress (e.g., open cholecystectomy, lower extremity vascular surgery), a reasonable approach is 50 mg of hydrocortisone intravenously before surgery, followed by 25 mg every 8 hours for 1 to 2 days, and then the patient's usual dose. For major surgical stress, patients are typically given 75 to 100 mg of hydrocortisone intravenously before induction of anesthesia, followed by 50 mg every 8 hours for 1 to 3 days until the stressful period resolves, and then their usual dose.

Thyroid Disease

An inadequately treated or undiagnosed hyperthyroid patient is potentially at risk for thyroid storm postoperatively. Elective surgery should be postponed in patients who are symptomatic or have resting tachycardia until they are euthyroid. Treatment of a thyrotoxic patient undergoing urgent or emergency surgery includes a combination of β-blockers, antithyroid agents, and iodine to control the resting heart rate to less than 90 beats per minute, as well as prophylactic corticosteroid supplementation, as used for thyroid storm (Chapter 233).

Conversely, patients with mild to moderate hypothyroidism tolerate surgery reasonably well. Patients with markedly symptomatic hypothyroidism should be treated with oral levothyroxine (T₄) for several weeks before elective surgery. For emergency surgery, intravenous liothyronine (T₃) or T₄ (200 to 300 μg intravenously, then 50 to 100 μg/day) and supplemental corticosteroids (hydrocortisone, 100 mg intravenously, then 25 to 50 mg every 6 hours; also correct fluid and electrolyte abnormalities) should be given. Myxedema coma is a rare complication of surgery.

Liver Disease

Routine preoperative testing of liver function is not recommended, but elective surgery should be avoided in patients with acute viral or alcoholic hepatitis. Patients with stable mild chronic hepatitis tolerate surgery well.

Patients with alcoholic liver disease or cirrhosis are at risk for postoperative complications, including bleeding, infection, poor wound healing, and delirium. The severity of disease as assessed by Child-Turcotte-Pugh criteria and the MELD (Model for End-Stage Liver Disease) score (Chapter 157) can be used to estimate risk; the MELD score is thought to be more predictive of outcome. Aggressive treatment of coagulopathy, ascites, and encephalopathy is indicated before surgery.

TABLE 439-8	APPROACH TO ANTICOAGULATION IN THE PERIOPERATIVE PATIENT

Low thromboembolic risk/low bleeding risk
- Continue anticoagulant therapy with INR in therapeutic range.

Low thromboembolic risk/high bleeding risk
- Discontinue anticoagulant therapy 5 days before the procedure.
- Start LMWH prophylaxis once daily or UFH IV 1 day after acenocoumarol interruption and 2 days after warfarin interruption. Administer the last dose of LMWH at least 12 hr before the procedure or give UFH IV up to 4 hr before surgery.
- Resume LMWH or UFH at the preprocedural dose 1-2 days (at least 12 hr) before the procedure according to haemostatic status. Resume anticoagulant therapy 1 to 2 days after surgery at the preprocedural dose + 50% boost dose for 2 consecutive days according to the hemostatic status.
- LMWH or UFH is continued until the INR has returned to therapeutic levels.

High thromboembolic risk
- Discontinue anticoagulant therapy 5 days before the procedure.
- Start therapeutic LMWH twice daily or UFH IV 1 day after acenocoumarol interruption and 2 days after warfarin interruption. Administer the last dose of LMWH at least 12 hr before the procedure or give UFH IV up to 4 hr before surgery.
- Resume LMWH or UFH at the preprocedural dose 1-2 days (at least 12 hr) after the procedure according to hemostatic status. Resume anticoagulant therapy 1-2 days after surgery at the preprocedural dose + 50% boost dose for 2 consecutive days according to haemostatic status.
- LMWH or UFH is continued until the INR has returned to therapeutic levels.

LMWH = low-molecular-weight heparin; INR = international normalized ratio; IV = intravenous; UFH = unfractionated heparin.
Reproduced from Poldermans D, Bax JJ, Boersma E, et al. Guidelines for pre-operative cardiac risk assessment and perioperative cardiac management in non-cardiac surgery. The Task Force for Preoperative Cardiac Risk Assessment and Perioperative Cardiac Management in Non-cardiac Surgery of the European Society of Cardiology (ESC) and endorsed by the European Society of Anaesthesiology (ESA). Eur Heart J. 2009;30:2769-2812.

Hematologic Problems

Anemia is associated with an increased risk for postoperative complications, but operative patients generally tolerate hemoglobin levels as low as 7 g/dL. Preoperative transfusion should not be triggered solely by the hemoglobin level but should also consider the expected blood loss from the surgical procedure and the patient's comorbid conditions. For patients with cardiopulmonary disease, however, a goal of 10 g/dL is typically recommended for major surgery.

Patients without a personal or family history of abnormal bleeding require no preoperative testing of coagulative function, but those with such a history should be evaluated. Ideally, the prothrombin time should be within 3 seconds of control (international normalized ratio <1.5), the partial thromboplastin time within 10 seconds of control, and the platelet count above a minimum of 50,000, depending on the type of surgery.

The approach to perioperative anticoagulation, both in terms of prevention of venous thromboembolism and for the management of a patient taking warfarin, aspirin, or other antithrombotic medications, is described elsewhere (Chapter 37). For patients already on anticoagulants, perioperative recommendations depend on the short-term risks for thromboembolism and bleeding (Table 439-8).

Renal Disorders

Chronic kidney disease is an independent risk factor for postoperative cardiovascular events and death. Patients with chronic kidney disease typically have other comorbid diseases and may also have fluid and electrolyte abnormalities, anemia, and bleeding diatheses, which should be treated and optimized before surgery. Patients maintained on dialysis should ideally undergo dialysis the day before surgery to optimize their volume status, prevent hyperkalemia, and minimize acute shifts in acid-base balance.

Neurologic Problems

The risk for a postoperative stroke in unselected patients after general surgery is less than 0.5%, but patients with a history of stroke, older patients, and those undergoing vascular surgery, especially carotid surgery, have higher risk. Patients with symptomatic carotid bruits require further investigation and possible intervention before elective surgery (Chapter 414). Patients who newly receive perioperative β-blockers are at increased risk for stroke,[2] and the risk must be balanced against the protective effect of

β-blockers for perioperative MI. However, there is no evidence that continuation of chronic β-blockade increases risk for postoperative stroke. There is no evidence to support preoperative intervention in patients with asymptomatic bruits before noncardiac surgery. The general recommendation is to delay elective surgery for at least 2 to 4 weeks after a stroke.

1. Devereaux PJ, Yang H, Yusuf S, et al. Effects of extended-release metoprolol succinate in patients undergoing non-cardiac surgery (POISE trial): a randomised controlled trial. Lancet. 2008; 371:1839-1847.
2. Bangalore S, Wetterslev J, Pranesh S, et al. Perioperative beta blockers in patients having non-cardiac surgery: a meta-analysis. Lancet. 2008;372:1962-1976.
3. van Lier F, Schouten O, Hoeks SE, et al. Impact of prophylactic beta-blocker therapy to prevent stroke after noncardiac surgery. Am J Cardiol. 2010;105:43-47.
4. Dunkelgrun M, Boersma E, Schouten O, et al. Bisoprolol and fluvastatin for the reduction of perioperative cardiac mortality and myocardial infarction in intermediate-risk patients undergoing noncardiovascular surgery: a randomized controlled trial (DECREASE-IV). Ann Surg. 2009;249: 921-926.
5. Wijeysundera DN, Bender JS, Beattie WS. Alpha-2 adrenergic agonists for the prevention of cardiac complications among patients undergoing surgery. Cochrane Database Syst Rev. 2009;4: CD004126.
6. Schouten O, Boersma E, Hoeks SE, et al, for the Dutch Echocardiographic Cardiac Risk Evaluation Applying Stress Echocardiography Study Group. Fluvastatin and perioperative events in patients undergoing vascular surgery. N Engl J Med. 2009;361:980-989.
7. McFalls EO, Ward HB, Moritz TE, et al. Coronary-artery revascularization before elective major vascular surgery. N Engl J Med. 2004;351:2795-2804.
8. Poldermans D, Schouten O, Vidakovic R, et al. A clinical randomized trial to evaluate the safety of a noninvasive approach in high-risk patients undergoing major vascular surgery: the DECREASE-V Pilot Study. J Am Coll Cardiol. 2007;49:1763-1769.
9. Sandham JD, Hull RD, Brant RF, et al. A randomized, controlled trial of the use of pulmonary-artery catheters in high-risk surgical patients. N Engl J Med. 2003;348:5-14.

SUGGESTED READINGS

Bradley KA, Rubinsky AD, Sun H, et al. Alcohol screening and risk of postoperative complications in male VA patients undergoing major non-cardiac surgery. J Gen Intern Med. 2011;26:162-169. Postoperative complications were more likely with AUDIT-C scores of 5 or more within a year of surgery.
Brienza N, Giglio MT, Marucci M. Preventing acute kidney injury after noncardiac surgery. Curr Opin Crit Care. 2010;16:353-358. Review.
Fleisher LA, Beckman JA, Brown KA, et al. 2009 ACCF/AHA Focused Update on Perioperative Beta Blockade. A Report of the American College of Cardiology Foundation/American Heart Association Task Force on Practice Guidelines. Developed in Collaboration with the American Society of Echocardiography, American Society of Nuclear Cardiology, Heart Rhythm Society, Society of Cardiovascular Anesthesiologists, Society for Cardiovascular Angiography and Interventions, Society for Vascular Medicine, and Society for Vascular Surgery. J Am Coll Cardiol. 2009;54:2102-2128. Consensus guidelines.
Lobo SM, Rezende E, Knibel MF, et al. Early determinants of death due to multiple organ failure after noncardiac surgery in high-risk patients. Anesth Analg. 2011;112:877-883. Multiorgan failure is the leading cause of death in high-risk noncardiac surgery; risk factors include peritonitis, diabetes, unplanned surgery, high central venous pressure, tachycardia, abnormal pH, and elevated serum lactate levels.
Poldermans D, Bax JJ, Boersma E, et al. Guidelines for pre-operative cardiac risk assessment and perioperative cardiac management in non-cardiac surgery. The Task Force for Preoperative Cardiac Risk Assessment and Perioperative Cardiac Management in Non-cardiac surgery of the European Society of Cardiology (ESC) and endorsed by the European Society of Anaesthesiology (ESA). Eur Heart J. 2009;30:2769-2812. Consensus guidelines.

440

OVERVIEW OF ANESTHESIA

JEANINE P. WIENER-KRONISH AND LEE FLEISHER

In the United States, more than 40 million procedures, including outpatient procedures, that require an anesthetic are performed annually. With modern techniques, anesthesia causes or contributes to mortality in about 1 per 20,000 healthy patients. Perioperative mortality now more often relates to the patient's underlying diseases (Chapter 439).

PREOPERATIVE ASSESSMENT

Important aspects of preoperative risk assessment include the type of surgery to be performed, the patient's underlying medical condition, and the particular demands for anesthesia (Chapter 439). In addition, a number of other issues are relevant to management and anesthetic evaluation.

Airway Assessment

Assessment of the airway is always necessary even if regional anesthesia or monitored anesthesia care (local anesthesia with sedation) is planned because unexpected complications or compromise of airway reflexes may lead to an emergency need for ventilatory support. The laryngeal mask airway device allows many patients to be ventilated easily, but it is important to assess the ability to intubate the patient, as well as the ability to ventilate. Reasons for difficulty include airway pathology (e.g., tumors, previous surgery) or an abnormal anatomic relationship between the larynx and trachea. In many such patients, endotracheal intubation can be accomplished by placing the endotracheal tube via a fiberoptic bronchoscope through either the nose or mouth. If this approach is not successful, a surgical airway should be considered. The prevalence of difficult elective intubation in the operating room is about 6% in nonobese patients.

Malignant Hyperthermia

Malignant hyperthermia (Chapter 442) is characterized by acute hyperpyrexia developing during or immediately after general anesthesia. The channels that regulate the duration and amplitude of calcium efflux from the sarcoplasmic reticulum are the ryanodine receptors, which exist in three isoforms. Gain-of-function mutations affecting RyR1, the receptor expressed primarily in skeletal muscle, are present in 1 per 15,000 to 50,000 people and are associated with enhanced sensitivity to halothane and caffeine and with malignant hyperthermia and central core disease. More than 80 distinct mutations have been detected, and mutation of the adult skeletal muscle sodium channel SCN4A may also cause the syndrome. Patients with mutations predisposing to malignant hyperthermia function normally at resting conditions, but exposure to volatile anesthetics, including halothane, isoflurane, enflurane, desflurane, and sevoflurane, or exposure to a depolarizing muscle relaxant, succinylcholine, can precipitate life-threatening muscle contractures, increases in heart rate and body temperature, rhabdomyolysis, myoglobinuria, and metabolic acidosis. The mortality rate is 80% in untreated patients but about 5% with current treatment. Note that succinylcholine causes release of myoglobin from muscle in small amounts even in normal patients. Patients with malignant hyperthermia do not predictably respond to triggering agents, and some patients with malignant hyperthermia have had milder symptoms of malignant hyperthermia after the administration of nontriggering agents. Malignant hyperthermia now often presents differently, probably because of the decreased use of succinylcholine by anesthesiologists, diagnostic awareness of malignant hyperthermia by anesthesiologists, routine use of carbon dioxide monitors so that increases in end-expiratory carbon dioxide are detected quickly, and the availability of dantrolene. If malignant hyperthermia is suspected from a family history of adverse events with the administration of anesthetics or when a patient has a reaction suspicious for malignant hyperthermia, a muscle biopsy is usually performed for in vitro contracture testing, which evaluates the muscle contracture responses to caffeine or halothane. Genetic investigations are also recommended, but malignant hyperthermia cannot be excluded on the basis of genetic testing alone because of the diversity of mutations and genes that can be involved in this syndrome. The Malignant Hyperthermia Association of the United States (*www.mhaus.org*) is available for information to the public, and all medical personnel can get information 24 hours every day on the malignant hyperthermia hotline 1-800-MHHYPER (1-800-644-9737).

Dantrolene is the drug of choice to prevent and reverse the symptoms of malignant hyperthermia. Dantrolene decreases muscle sensitivity to caffeine, reduces calcium release from the sarcoplasmic reticulum, and produces some muscle weakness. Dantrolene comes in 20-mg bottles and must be dissolved in sterile water; the doses recommended are 2 mg/kg every 5 minutes intravenously until cardiac and respiratory symptoms stabilize, up to a total dose of 10 mg/kg; however, doses of 29 mg/kg have been reported. Side effects of dantrolene include weakness that may require mechanical ventilation. Other treatments of malignant hyperthermia include stopping use of the volatile anesthetics, hyperventilating the patient and administering 100% oxygen, administering bicarbonate for severe acidosis, controlling fevers, and maintaining temperature below 39° C without causing hypothermia by using iced fluids, surface cooling, and cooling of body cavities if necessary. Monitoring of temperature and vital signs, urinary output, muscle enzymes, glucose, coagulation studies, acid-base status, and gas exchange is recommended.

Two other diseases associated with mutations in RyR1 include central core disease and multiminicore disease, rare congenital myopathies. Central core disease causes infantile hypotonia; muscle biopsy is needed for definitive diagnosis. Multiminicore disease is a nonprogressive congenital myopathy in which infants exhibit hypotonia, ophthalmoplegia, and arthrogryposis. Scoliosis develops in these children and they may eventually require chronic ventilation. Avoidance of triggering agents is advised for these syndromes and for patients with other myopathies. Both malignant hyperthermia and central core disease are thought to be inherited as autosomal dominant diseases, but extensive genetic analysis has revealed overlapping phenotypes.

Monamine Oxidase Inhibitors, Opioid Analgesics, and Serotonin Toxicity

Anesthesiologists routinely ask whether patients are taking monoamine oxidase (MAO) inhibitors because of their many drug interactions, particularly with analgesics. In addition, serotonin toxicity has features similar to malignant hyperthermia and must be distinguished from it. Serotonin toxicity, characterized by the triad of neuromuscular hyperactivity (tremor, clonus, myoclonus, hyperreflexia, and pyramidal rigidity), autonomic hyperactivity (diaphoresis, fever, tachycardia, and tachypnea), and altered mental status (agitation, excitement, and confusion), can be precipitated by the coadministration of MAO inhibitors and serotonin re-uptake inhibitors. Rigidity, increasing arterial carbon dioxide levels, and fever with a temperature higher than 38.5°C are associated with life-threatening toxicity. Ecstasy, or 3,4-methylenedioxymethamphetamine (MDMA), combined with MAO inhibitors, including moclobemide, can lead to fatalities because they act as serotonin releasers. Tramadol, used for pain relief, and venlafaxine, an antidepressant, act as serotonin releasers and have been involved in the development of toxicity with the concurrent administration of MAO inhibitors.

● ANAPHYLAXIS IN THE PERIOPERATIVE PERIOD

The incidence of life-threatening hypersensitivity reactions during anesthesia is 1 in 4000 to 25,000. Anaphylaxis is caused by immunoglobulin E (IgE)-mediated reactions (Chapter 261), whereas anaphylactoid reactions produce the same clinical picture but are not mediated by IgE. Anaphylaxis during anesthesia can be manifested as cardiovascular collapse, airway obstruction, and flushing or edema of the skin, singly or in combination, so knowledge of any previous allergic reactions to medications and the nature of the reaction is critical information to communicate to the anesthesiologist and other members of the perioperative team. Neuromuscular blocking agents, such as succinylcholine, and opioid analgesics can cause nonimmunologic release of histamine from mast cells and produce a similar clinical syndrome. Antibiotics, protamine, and blood transfusions, all given routinely during operations (Chapter 180), can also elicit a variety of systemic reactions. About 75% of perioperative hypersensitivity reactions appear to be due to muscle relaxants, especially rocuronium and vecuronium, with a mortality of 3 to 6%. Skin tests, or prick tests to all the substances to which the patient was exposed, and IgE levels are usually performed to determine whether the patient has an allergic reaction and whether it is mediated by IgE.

Latex Allergies

For sensitized patients (Chapter 261), exposure to even low amounts of latex-containing particles is sufficient to induce a severe anaphylactic reaction. A latex-free operating environment, in which no latex gloves or accessories are used, is key in patients with known allergy. Skin prick tests with latex extracts should be considered in patients at high risk for latex allergy. Early aggressive treatment with epinephrine is critical if severe anaphylaxis occurs.

● INTRAOPERATIVE MANAGEMENT

Choice of Intraoperative Anesthesia

There are three general classes of anesthesia: general, regional, and monitored anesthesia care. General anesthesia can be achieved with a balanced drug regimen that induces loss of consciousness, which can range from deep sedation requiring only airway support to states requiring full ventilatory support because of weakness and loss of respiratory drive. Both intravenous and inhaled drugs can be used to induce and maintain general anesthesia. In contrast, monitored anesthesia care denotes a state in which patients can still control their airway, do not require ventilatory support, but are sleepy, have less pain, and may be amnestic. The same drugs are often used for general anesthesia and monitored anesthesia care; achievement of the two different conditions requires knowledge of the pharmacokinetics of the drugs (Table 440-1).

Propofol

Propofol, an alkylphenol, is perhaps the most frequently used intravenous anesthetic for induction of anesthesia and is often used for maintenance of

TABLE 440-1 COMMON ANESTHETIC APPROACHES FOR VARIOUS TYPES OF SURGERY

SURGERY ON INTRA-ABDOMINAL OR INTRATHORACIC ORGANS

Examples: cardiac surgery, lung resections, gastric bypass
General anesthesia usually administered because mechanical ventilation is often required
Drugs include premedication for anxiety with midazolam, general anesthesia with volatile anesthetics (desflurane, sevoflurane, nitrous oxide), neuromuscular blockade, and opioid analgesics*
Epidural anesthesia and analgesia also used; examples include ropivacaine, lidocaine, with fentanyl

SURGERY ON LIMBS

Examples: hip replacement, knee replacement, foot or arm surgery
Can perform with epidural or spinal anesthesia, depending on the limb. Examples of medications would include tetracaine, lidocaine, ropivacaine, and fentanyl or morphine
Can perform axillary or scalene block; examples include lidocaine and ropivacaine
For postoperative pain control: can perform regional blocks that leave the catheter in place, including femoral nerve block, axillary nerve blocks

CATARACT SURGERY—LOCAL ANESTHESIA ON EYE WITH OR WITHOUT SEDATION

Examples of drugs used for sedation include midazolam and fentanyl

*Includes the use of opioids given intraoperatively and whose effects extend into the postanesthesia care unit (PACU) or postoperative period, opioids given in the PACU, or opioids given or intended to be given after discharge from the PACU.

anesthesia during short procedures or to achieve deep sedation during monitored anesthesia care. It is lipid soluble and cleared quickly from the central compartment, so it is eliminated rapidly even after long periods of continuous infusion. However, clearance of propofol is changed by gender (men have lower clearance rates than women do), size (children require higher doses), age (elderly patients have decreased clearance rates and experience increased effects with the drug), and narcotics, which decrease its clearance. Because of its predilection for causing apnea, propofol should be administered only by someone with expertise in airway management. Propofol also decreases arterial blood pressure, causes pain with injection, and can precipitate myoclonus. Large quantities of propofol can cause propofol infusion syndrome, which is associated with cardiomyopathy, metabolic acidosis, skeletal myopathy, hyperkalemia, hepatomegaly, and lipemia. Despite these issues, propofol is frequently being used because recovery from propofol is complete within minutes, even after it is given as a prolonged continuous infusion, in contrast to the longer duration of drug effects seen after the administration of other intravenous sedatives.

Propofol is the preferred agent for healthy outpatients undergoing colonoscopy because it leads to earlier discharge and higher patient satisfaction than do other agents.**1**

When used in higher-risk populations or administered by nonanesthesiologists, however, narcotic/benzodiazepine sedation appears to be safer than propofol for such procedures.**2** At a minimum, the use of propofol requires the presence of a provider who can rescue an airway and manage decreased respiration, oxygen saturation, and hypotension.

Midazolam

Midazolam, a benzodiazepine that produces muscle relaxation through a central mechanism, is hypnotic, sedative, anxiolytic, amnesic, and anticonvulsant. Its amnesic and anticonvulsant effects are mediated through α_1 and γ-aminobutyric acid A (GABA$_A$) receptors, and the anxiolytic and muscle relaxation are mediated through α_2 and GABA$_A$ receptors. Only 20% receptor occupancy is needed to produce anxiolysis, whereas unconsciousness requires 60%. Long-term administration of benzodiazepines produces tolerance, which appears to decrease receptor binding and function. Benzodiazepines cause dose-related depression of the respiratory system, with a peak effect achieved at 3 minutes and significant depression persisting for 60 to 120 minutes. The rate of administration of the drug affects the onset of depression: the faster the drug is given, the quicker the respiratory depression occurs. Benzodiazepines and opioids appear to produce additive respiratory depression, including apnea. Unlike propofol, benzodiazepines used alone decrease blood pressure only modestly. Other drugs, particularly those that

affect the cytochrome P-450 3A4 enzyme (including azole antifungals, human immunodeficiency virus [HIV] protease inhibitors, and calcium-channel blockers), affect the clearance of midazolam and prolong its half-life *significantly*. There are several reports of prolonged amnesia in HIV-infected patients who received midazolam for conscious sedation. Midazolam also has an active metabolite and is often associated with delirium in the elderly (Chapter 27), perhaps because it impairs both implicit and relational memory.

Opioids

Opioids are classified as naturally occurring (morphine, codeine), semisynthetic (heroin), and synthetic (methadone, fentanyl, remifentanil). They can be administered both intravenously and in the neuraxial space (epidural or spinal). There are four opiate receptors (μ, κ, δ, and nociceptin receptors), which are G protein–coupled receptors. Chronic exposure to agonists leads to cellular adaptation mechanisms that are probably involved in tolerance, dependence, and withdrawal. Clinically, μ-agonists are used almost exclusively; μ-agonists include morphine, fentanyl, and meperidine. Opioid analgesics are administered because they relieve pain, but they have other important adverse effects, including respiratory depression, decreased gastric emptying, nausea and vomiting, sedation, constipation, pruritus, dependence, and tolerance, when given repeatedly. When opioids are given with propofol or benzodiazepines (or with both), there is a synergistic depressive effect on respiration, hence the rationale for monitoring patients who receive medications for conscious sedation.

Ketamine

Ketamine is unique among the intravenous agents because it has analgesic properties and decreases tolerance to opiates. Ketamine produces dose-related analgesia, which may be profound even when patients can keep their eyes open, breathe spontaneously, and protect their own airway with conserved swallowing and cough reflex. Side effects include increased lacrimation, salivation, and muscle tone. Ketamine increases cerebral blood flow, can increase seizure activity, and can produce undesirable psychological reactions; these side effects are dose related and may be minimized by the concomitant use of benzodiazepines. Ketamine is also a bronchial smooth muscle relaxant and can prevent experimentally induced bronchospasm. Ketamine is usually associated with an increase in blood pressure, heart rate, and cardiac output. These features make ketamine a useful drug for sedating patients with hemodynamic instability.

Dexmedetomidine

Dexmedetomidine is a highly selective α_2-agonist that is associated with less respiratory depression and more cooperative behavior than propofol is. Dexmedetomidine also causes hypnosis, analgesia, sympatholysis, and inhibition of insulin secretion. It induces sedation that has a respiratory pattern and electroencephalographic changes similar to those of natural sleep. Even high concentrations of dexmedetomidine are associated with preservation of spontaneous respiration; however, when dexmedetomidine is administered in combination with sympatholytic or cholinergic agents, there is a high risk for extreme bradycardia and sinus arrest. Dexmedetomidine is associated with less amnesia than the benzodiazepines are. Although propofol and benzodiazepines have commonly been used in critically ill patients to achieve sedation for procedures or for maintenance of mechanical ventilation, dexmedetomidine appears to have significant advantages over benzodiazepines because it appears to cause less delirium and appears to decrease the time that critical care patients spend on ventilators.**3**

Volatile Anesthetics

Volatile (inhalational) anesthetics include desflurane, sevoflurane, isoflurane, halothane, and nitrous oxide. Inhaled anesthetics are absorbed through the respiratory epithelium and mucous membranes of the respiratory tract, and they are excreted mainly by exhalation. Access to the circulation is almost instantaneous because of the large pulmonary surface area. The pharmacologic effects of inhaled anesthetics depend primarily on alveolar ventilation, the ventilation-perfusion ratio, coadministered gases, gas flow, and the physicochemical properties of the anesthetic gas rather than on the quantity of drug administered, the extent and rate of absorption, protein binding, excretion, secretion, or metabolism. Based on the available evidence, no inhalational agent appears to be superior to any other.

All inhalational agents, with the exception of nitrous oxide, cause dose-dependent cardiovascular depression. Severe hepatotoxicity, which resulted in discontinuation of the use of chloroform, carbon tetrachloride, and trichloroethylene anesthetics, leads to fatal hepatic necrosis in 1 in 10,000 patients anesthetized with halothane. This problem appears to occur much less frequently after isoflurane and desflurane exposure. Mild halothane hepatoxicity is self-limited and can occur with a single exposure, whereas fulminant halothane hepatitis occurs only after multiple exposures to the drug, has a high mortality rate (50%), and is associated with antibodies to halothane-altered antigens.

Nitrous oxide, which is the only nonhalogenated agent still being used, is not metabolized in human tissues. It irreversibly oxidizes the cobalt atom of vitamin B_{12}, thereby inhibiting the activity of the cobalamin-dependent enzyme methionine synthase. Individuals with vitamin B_{12} deficiency or with mutations in methionine synthase may be at risk for neurologic injury from nitrous oxide, which should not be used in patients at risk. Exposure to concentrations higher than 10**3** ppm may be associated with an increased incidence of abortions and decreased fertility, so exposure should be avoided in patients and personnel at risk. General anesthesia can be achieved only by giving combinations of drugs along with nitrous oxide to achieve the desired effects. Based on the available evidence, one anesthetic does not appear to be superior to any other.

Neuromuscular Blockers

Neuromuscular blockers are used to paralyze muscles to facilitate endotracheal intubation and mechanical ventilation, to decrease shivering during induced hypothermia, or to improve conditions for optimal surgery. Succinylcholine causes prolonged depolarization of the neuromuscular junction, which results in failure to generate an action potential. Within 9 to 13 minutes after the administration of 1 mg/kg of succinylcholine, 90% of muscle strength is restored. The very rapid onset and rapid return of muscle function make succinylcholine a most useful drug for difficult intubations. Side effects of succinylcholine include hyperkalemia, myalgia, masseter spasm, sinus bradycardia and nodal rhythms, and increased intraocular pressure.

Most of the other neuromuscular drugs used by anesthesiologists are nondepolarizing in that they compete with acetylcholine for the neuromuscular junction and can be reversed by increasing the quantity of acetylcholine. Categorization of these drugs is according to their chemical makeup; there are steroidal compounds, benzylisoquinolinium compounds, and other chemical compounds. Clinically, a drug is often chosen for its duration of action, with intermediate agents being used most frequently. These drugs act for 20 to 50 minutes and include vecuronium, rocuronium, atracurium, and cisatracurium. They have different routes of metabolism, so the choice of agent depends in part on the presence of coexisting disease.

Chronic administration of neuromuscular blocking agents is associated with prolonged paralysis, particularly in patients taking steroids concomitantly. Other notable interactions with nondepolarizing agents include the following: antibiotics can increase neuromuscular blockade; magnesium sulfate potentiates neuromuscular blockade; lithium can potentiate neuromuscular blockade with succinylcholine and with pipecuronium; antiepileptic drugs cause resistance to nondepolarizing muscle blockade, so larger doses have to be administered for paralysis; and patients receiving anticonvulsants have accelerated recovery from neuromuscular blockade.

Regional Anesthesia

Regional anesthesia involves the deposition of local anesthetics near nerves, including deposition in the epidural space and into cerebrospinal fluid (CSF). Local anesthetics, which are aminoesters or aminoamides, affect cardiac function, as well as central nervous system function when administered systemically.

Binding of the local anesthetic to sodium channels in the axoplasm prevents opening of the channels and conduction of nerve impulses. The rates of onset and recovery from nerve blockade are controlled by diffusion of the local anesthetic into and out of the whole nerve.

Examples of regional anesthesia include neuraxial techniques, deposition of local anesthetics near the brachial plexus to anesthetize the arms (axillary or interscalene blocks), deposition near the femoral or sciatic nerves to anesthetize the legs, deposition near the ulnar or radial nerves for lower arm blocks, deposition near the pudendal nerves for groin procedures, and deposition of local anesthetics into the caudal space for groin surgery. Dentists use this technique frequently when they inject local anesthetics near various nerves in the oral cavity. Many surgeries, including carotid surgery and placement of fistulas for dialysis, can be performed with regional anesthesia.

Regional anesthetics may also require supplementation with sedation or general anesthesia.

The dangers associated with regional anesthesia include injection of local anesthetic into the systemic circulation. Systemic toxicity is manifested as convulsions and respiratory depression, which can require assisted ventilation. Tinnitus, visual and auditory disturbances, and dizziness are signs of milder central nervous toxicity. Cardiac toxicity can be manifested by decreases in heart rate, prolonged conduction times, and negative inotropic effects. Bupivacaine toxicity is associated with ventricular fibrillation. Twenty percent Intralipid at various doses (1 mL/kg for three doses and then infusion at 0.25 mL/kg/min or 1.2 mL/kg as a single dose followed by infusion at 0.5 mL/kg/min) has been reported in case reports and animal studies to reverse these toxic effects, although optimal dosing has yet to be determined. Furthermore, the prolonged duration of many of the local anesthetics may require the institution of cardiopulmonary bypass until the drugs are metabolized.

Neuraxial (Spinal and Epidural) Anesthesia and Analgesia

Spinal anesthesia is achieved by instilling local anesthetics into the CSF. Epidural anesthesia is the instillation of larger volumes of local anesthetics into the epidural space, or the potential space between the dura mater and the walls of the vertebral canal. Spinal anesthesia is associated with an increased incidence of headache in younger patients, so epidural anesthesia is often used in younger patients. Complications of epidural and spinal anesthesia and analgesia include failed blocks, post–dural puncture headaches, and toxicity from the local anesthetics. Another major concern with neuraxial anesthesia is that epidural hematoma may develop in patients taking antiplatelet agents, although it remains a rare event that occurs in fewer than 1 in 150,000 operations, even in the presence of potent antiplatelet agents. Other rarer complications of epidural and spinal anesthesia, in addition to the effects of local anesthesia outlined earlier, include intracranial subdural hematoma, transverse myelitis, hypotension, and cardiac arrest.

Postoperative epidural analgesia, in which either local anesthetics or local anesthetics and narcotics are instilled into the epidural space for postoperative pain control, is associated with superior pain control, lower doses of opioids, improved bowel mobility, slightly decreased length of stay in the intensive cause unit, and a slight decrease in the requirement for mechanical ventilation.**4 5**

⬤ GENERAL VERSUS REGIONAL ANESTHESIA

The decision regarding which type of anesthesia to administer often depends on the requirements of the surgery. For example, laparoscopic surgery requires general anesthesia because insufflation of gases impairs the ability to breathe adequately. General anesthesia is also required for surgeries on the airway or thorax because mechanical ventilation is needed to sustain adequate respiration. Procedures that do not allow any movement (e.g., precise procedures in the brain) often require general anesthesia and paralysis.

Side effects of general anesthesia depend on the drugs used to achieve anesthesia, whether neuromuscular blockade is administered, and whether mechanical ventilation is needed. Complications of endotracheal intubation include local pain, airway trauma, swelling, vocal cord paralysis, increased bronchospasm, and death from improper placement. Volatile anesthetics are associated with postoperative atelectasis (Chapter 90), whereas regional anesthesia helps preserve respiratory dynamics. Postoperative cognitive dysfunction (Chapter 27) does not seem to depend on the type of anesthesia used.

⬤ NAUSEA AND VOMITING

Postoperative nausea and vomiting are more likely with volatile anesthetics but are also common when perioperative opioids are administered. Prophylactic ondansetron, dexamethasone, and droperidol each reduce postoperative nausea and vomiting independently by about 26%, with the main predictor for efficacy being the patient's risk for nausea and vomiting.**6** It should be noted that droperidol has received a "black box" warning from the Food and Drug Administration, so is not used very often in the United States. Total intravenous anesthesia with propofol reduces postoperative nausea and vomiting by only about a fifth, often because narcotics are still administered. The use of spinal or epidural anesthesia (or both) may decrease the incidence of nausea and vomiting. In addition to general anesthesia, risk factors for postoperative nausea and vomiting include female gender, a previous history of nausea and vomiting, a history of motion sickness, nonsmoking, and intended administration of opioids for postoperative analgesia. If three or more risk factors are present, it is generally recommended that patients receive at least two prophylactic pharmacologic antiemetic agents of different classes (e.g., selected among ondansetron or another 5-HT$_3$ antagonist, droperidol, dexamethasone, scopolamine, or phenothiazides) preoperatively for the prevention of nausea and vomiting.

1. Singh H, Poluha W, Cheung M, et al. Propofol for sedation during colonoscopy. *Cochrane Database Syst Rev.* 2008;4:CD006268.
2. Schilling D, Rosenbaum A, Schweitzer S, et al. Sedation with propofol for interventional endoscopy by trained nurses in high-risk octogenarians: a prospective, randomized controlled study. *Endoscopy.* 2009;41:295-298.
3. Riker RR, Shehabi Y, Bokesch PM, et al. Dexmedetomidine vs midazolam for sedation of critically ill patients. *JAMA.* 2009;301:489-499.
4. Park WY, Thompson JS, Lee KK. Effect of epidural anesthesia and analgesia on perioperative outcome: a randomized, controlled Veterans Affairs cooperative study. *Ann Surg.* 2001;234:560-569.
5. Ballantyne JC, Kupelnick B, McPeek B, et al. Does the evidence support the use of spinal and epidural anesthesia for surgery? *J Clin Anesth.* 2005;17:382-391.
6. Apfel CC, Korttila K, Abdalla M, et al. A factorial trial of six interventions for the prevention of postoperative nausea and vomiting. *N Engl J Med.* 2004;350:2441-2451.

SUGGESTED READINGS

Benca J, Hogan K. Malignant hyperthermia, coexisting disorders, and enzymopathies: risks and management options. *Anesth Analg.* 2009;109:1049-1053. *Suggestions for management when risks are uncertain.*

Brandom BW, Larach MG, Chen MS, et al. Complications associated with the administration of dantrolene 1987-2006: a report from the North American Malignant Hyperthermia Registry of the Malignant Hyperthermia Association of the United States. *Anesth Analg.* 2011;112:1115-1123. *Documents complications seen with dantrolene treatment for malignant hyperthermia.*

Brown EN, Lydic R, Schiff ND. General anesthesia, sleep, and coma. *N Engl J Med.* 2010;363:2638-2650. *Review.*

Merchant R, Bosenberg C, Brown K, et al. Guidelines to the practice of anesthesia: revised edition 2011. *Can J Anaesth.* 2011;58:74-107. *Comprehensive practice guidelines.*

Panzer O, Moitra V, Sladen RN. Pharmacology of sedative-analgesic agents: dexmedetomidine, remifentanil, ketamine, volatile anesthetics, and the role of peripheral mu antagonists. *Crit Care Clin.* 2009;25:451-469. *A comprehensive review.*

Practice guidelines for preoperative fasting and the use of pharmacologic agents to reduce the risk of pulmonary aspiration: application to healthy patients undergoing elective procedures: an updated report by the American Society of Anesthesiologists Committee on Standards and Practice Parameters. *Anesthesiology.* 2011;114:495-511. *Consensus guidelines.*

441

POSTOPERATIVE CARE AND COMPLICATIONS

DONALD A. REDELMEIER

POSTOPERATIVE CARE

Overview

Postoperative medical complications are common, sometimes serious, and vary substantially across different settings. Large national studies, for example, show about a two-fold difference in risk for mortality between high- and low-ranked hospitals. However, analyses disagree about how much these differences reflect a greater incidence of each complication (failure of prevention around the time of surgery) or a heightened lethality of each complication (failure to rescue in the aftermath of the operation). Regardless of the explanation, the purpose of medical consultation is to relieve human suffering by the prevention, detection, and correction of postoperative complications. The main constraint is that the consultant often has little ongoing direct contact with the patient before or after the perioperative interval.

Team Psychology

The medical consultant in the postoperative setting must have both knowledge of medicine and an appreciation of team psychology (Chapter 438). In contrast to other settings, the internist is not the team leader, often does not maintain an ongoing relationship with the patient, and does not have the authority of the most responsible physician. Moreover, patients may be dispersed across diverse surgical services, each with their own orientation and culture. The challenges of coordination and communication are enormous, particularly given the multiple other health care professionals involved in complex surgical cases. Considerable tact is often needed to avoid antagonizing the surgeon, disrupting the team's dynamics, or inducing a cascade of cumbersome inopportune testing.

Focusing on Recovery

Facilitating the patient's recovery from surgery differs somewhat from managing patients with acute exacerbations of chronic disease. In the postoperative setting, many therapies need to be discontinued at some point because the patient has recovered, such as discontinuing a urinary catheter because the patient can now void spontaneously or discontinuing a major tranquilizer because the patient is now orientated and coherent. Discontinuation of many other interventions requires substantial judgment, such as the decision when to discontinue intravenous access, supplemental oxygen, and intermittent laxatives. Much depends on experience and reconsideration of an individual patient's situation on a regular basis.

Reading Anesthesia Records

A focused review of the anesthesia record is essential because the consultant is rarely present during the operation. Perhaps the most basic information to identify is the date of surgery because the time elapsed helps in interpreting the patient's current state of recovery. Moreover, sometimes the date is not immediately evident if more than one surgery has been performed, a planned operation was canceled, or misquotations arise. Data about the duration of surgery, type of anesthesia (e.g., regional, spinal, or general [Chapter 440]), and major intraoperative events help establish reasonable expectations about the future course, as well as the possibility of specific complications (e.g., epidural hematoma after spinal anesthesia). Sharing some of the basic data with the patient is often helpful because a surprising number either benefit from repetition or are not otherwise informed.

Patterns of Mistakes

Medical errors (Chapter 11) that arise in postoperative care often seem mundane in retrospect yet can be lethal if undetected. Some patterns of mistakes have the feature of "double trouble," such as when a patient has both a potassium level of 2.0 mEq/L and an international normalized ratio of 2.0 but care focuses on only one of these abnormalities. Other mistakes occur because a single problem arises at an awkward moment, such as a patient in whom acute dyspnea develops when another patient is having a seizure. Still other mistakes relate to the fallibility of human memory and attention, such as when a normal blood sugar value in the morning leads clinicians to assume that the level is still normal at night. These errors can result in substantial harm, failure of clinicians to learn from past mistakes, and unprofessional reactions related to embarrassment. None of these patterns are unique to postoperative care, yet the fast and unfamiliar terrain of surgical settings can make even simple mistakes difficult to avoid.

Checking Orders

The first method for reducing errors after surgery is to check the postoperative orders already written for the patient. Such double checking is a tedious task, and clinicians often direct insufficient attention to this review in the mistaken belief that most of the work is already done. Ironically, checking orders written by another clinician sometimes requires more than customary attention because of the challenges of following someone else's legibility, sequencing, and preferences. The set of orders may need to be read twice: once for errors of commission (e.g., a calcium-channel blocker ordered at the wrong dose) and once for errors of omission (e.g., a β-blocker inadvertently not reordered after surgery). A classic mistake on postoperative orders is failure to follow through on interventions initiated immediately before surgery (e.g., endocarditis prophylaxis). A particularly vexing issue is the need for repeated rechecking on subsequent days (e.g., new orders for sedative drugs).

Recommended Prophylaxis

Some complications are sufficiently frequent and serious that routine prophylaxis is merited in the postoperative setting. For example, antibiotics are indicated for patients at high risk for endocarditis (Chapter 76). Systemic anticoagulation with heparin is indicated for patients at high risk for postoperative deep vein thrombosis (Chapters 37 and 81). Gastric acid suppression

(Chapter 141) is justified for patients at high risk for postoperative gastric bleeding. Parenteral antibiotics are indicated for patients undergoing prosthetic joint replacement. The optimal method for gauging whether a patient is at high risk for each complication is contentious and thereby leads to variation in practice patterns across different settings.

Future Prevention

A postoperative consultant who maintains communication, facilitates the patient's recovery, and avoids postoperative mistakes also has the chance to initiate unrelated medical interventions for general medical care. Such opportunities for prevention might include influenza vaccination, colon cancer screening, or cholesterol reduction. The main advantage of such comprehensive care is that it conforms to the ideal of providing all services possible to the individual. The main disadvantage of such comprehensive care is the potential for creating unintended chaos, confusion, or misquotation (Chapter 438). Such unintended consequences distract the surgical team from the primary goal and also carry some risk for complications from the comprehensive care at a time when the patient is trying to recover from surgery. Many effective postoperative consultants will defer such opportunities for prevention to the physicians who assume long-term responsibility for the patient's care.

⬤ COMPLICATIONS

Symptoms

Chest Pain

Chest pain is a common problem after surgery and has an extensive differential diagnosis (Chapter 50). In the postoperative setting, the immediate consideration is an acute ischemic myocardial event. The diagnosis of postoperative myocardial infarction (MI) differs somewhat from community-acquired MI (Table 441-1). Interpretation of a patient's symptoms, examination, and electrocardiogram is often problematic because of changes related to surgery and anesthesia. Instead, diagnosis is heavily dependent on biomarkers such as an elevated troponin level, especially since many postoperative MIs are painless. Management priorities include supplemental oxygen, heart rate control, and correction of hemoglobin. Thrombolysis is often contraindicated, but percutaneous coronary intervention may be considered. In the absence of data from randomized trials, other therapies such as aspirin, statins, and angiotensin-converting enzyme inhibitors should be used on a case-by-case basis (Chapter 73).

Dyspnea

Shortness of breath (Chapter 83) after surgery has an extensive differential diagnosis (Table 441-2). The three key considerations are fluid overload/ heart failure (Chapter 58), pulmonary embolism (Chapter 98), and air space disease (a continuum encompassing atelectasis [Chapter 90], bronchitis [Chapter 96], aspiration [Chapter 94], mucous plugging, and pneumonia). Distinguishing among these three considerations requires focusing on the speed of onset, the timing relative to surgery, vital signs, findings on oximetry, and the physical examination (Chapter 83). Fluid overload is most commonly seen soon after the cessation of positive-pressure ventilation or vasodilating neuraxial anesthesia or analgesia. It is also common 3 to 5 days postoperatively when fluid that has been "third-spaced" is mobilized into the intravascular compartment. Interventions that are safe in most situations include administration of oxygen and withholding sedation. The use of continuous positive airway pressure can reduce the rate of reintubation in hypoxemic postoperative patients.[1] Other interventions that will be helpful or harmful, depending on the specific situation, include diuretics, elaborate medical imaging, and vigorous physiotherapy.

Anorexia

Loss of appetite after surgery has an extensive differential diagnosis (Chapter 134) that can be narrowed substantially if the patient was eating properly before surgery. The immediate priority is to search for and correct underlying contributors. Oral, enteral, or parenteral support is not the priority initially, although such support may become necessary. Drug toxicity is a particularly common, easily detected when considered, and rapidly reversible contributor to postoperative anorexia. Anatomic abnormalities are usually evident by medical imaging studies. Other common metabolic contributors include abnormalities in electrolytes, calcium, phosphorus, and magnesium. Acalculous cholecystitis (Chapter 158) is an important postoperative complication that must be considered in a patient with right upper quadrant tenderness. Multiple antinausea medications are available for symptomatic relief (e.g., ondansetron, dexamethasone, droperidol) and act in an additive manner when used in combination.[2]

Vomiting

Vomiting is the extreme form of nausea in the postoperative setting, and the two symptoms share the same differential diagnosis. In most patients, vomiting is rare and unexpected and merits immediate care. Initial management is to ensure that the patient's airway is protected, discontinue oral medications (and find parenteral substitutes if necessary), and consider insertion of a nasogastric tube. In patients after gastrointestinal surgery, the priorities are to consider the possibility of an anastomotic leak, peritoneal abscess, or other anatomic abnormality. In patients after operations on more remote parts of the body, the priorities are emetogenic medications (such as postoperative chemotherapy), gastroparesis associated with autonomic neuropathy, and fecal impaction. If no reversible contributor is identified, the default diagnosis is prolonged idiopathic ileus, and a therapeutic trial of intravenous neostigmine can be considered.

Diarrhea

Diarrhea (Chapter 142) is relatively rare after surgery and involves a limited number of possibilities if the patient's bowel movements were normal before surgery. In such cases the situation represents an acute-onset diarrhea that is usually secretory in nature. The immediate priority is to exclude toxic megacolon, which is caused by overgrowth of toxigenic *Clostridium difficile* and is a potential emergency. Clinical evaluation for toxic megacolon requires assessment for tachycardia, hypotension, delirium, and other signs of sepsis rather than waiting on initial stool studies for confirmation of infection with *C. difficile*. Risk factors for antibiotic-associated diarrhea include advanced age, use of broad-spectrum antibiotics (e.g., third-generation cephalosporins), and unknown host susceptibility factors (e.g., past episodes of pseudomembranous colitis). Frequently, a definitive diagnosis is never established and treatment focuses on feeding the patient a lactose-free diet while avoiding intestinal paralytics. Complete resolution is typical, provided that adequate fluid and electrolyte levels are maintained.

Weakness

Generalized weakness after surgery is almost inevitable, but focal weakness may reflect nerve damage caused by intraoperative positioning (e.g., damage to the facial nerve after carotid endarterectomy) and rarely indicates a spontaneous new intracranial event (e.g., intracerebral bleeding [Chapter 415] secondary to anticoagulation). Such deficits are often overlooked during the initial postoperative interval and may become apparent only after the patient has regained strength elsewhere in the body. Conversely, new deficits that are

---

TABLE 441-1　CRITERIA FOR DIAGNOSING POSTOPERATIVE MYOCARDIAL INFARCTION

The diagnosis of perioperative MI requires any one of the following criteria:

Criterion 1: A typical rise in the troponin level or a typical fall in an elevated troponin level detected at its peak after surgery in a patient without a documented alternative explanation for an elevated troponin level (e.g., pulmonary embolism) or a rapid rise and fall in CK-MB only if troponin measurement is unavailable.*
This criterion requires that one of the following criteria be met:
  Ischemic signs or symptoms (e.g., chest, arm, or jaw discomfort; shortness of breath; pulmonary edema)
  Development of pathologic Q waves on an ECG
  Changes on an ECG indicative of ischemia
  Coronary artery intervention
  New or presumed new cardiac wall motion abnormality on echocardiography or new or presumed new fixed defect on radionuclide imaging

Criterion 2: Pathologic findings of acute or healing MI

Criterion 3: Development of new pathologic Q waves on an ECG if troponin levels were not obtained or were obtained at times that could have missed the clinical event

*Because CK-MB is both less sensitive and less specific than troponin levels in the perioperative setting than in other settings, it should be used for diagnostic purposes only when troponin levels are not obtainable.
CK-MB = creatine kinase MB isoenzyme; ECG = electrocardiogram; MI = myocardial infarction.
Reproduced with permission from Devereaux PJ, Goldman L, Yusuf S, et al. Surveillance and prevention of major perioperative ischemic cardiac events in patients undergoing noncardiac surgery: a review. *CMAJ.* 2005;173:779-788.

TABLE 441-2 DISTINGUISHING AMONG COMMON CAUSES OF ACUTE POSTOPERATIVE DYSPNEA

	PULMONARY AIR SPACE	FLUID OVERLOAD/HEART FAILURE	PULMONARY THROMBOEMBOLISM
CHARACTERISTICS OF TIMING			
Days since surgery	1-7 days	0-5 days	5-28 days
Speed of onset	1-3 days	1-24 hours	1-5 minutes
PREVIOUS HISTORY			
Previous lung disease	++		
Previous heart failure		++	
Previous venous thrombosis			++
ABNORMAL VITAL SIGNS			
Temperature			
Heart rate	+	+	+
Blood pressure	+	+	++
Respiratory rate	+	++	+
Oximetry	++	+	+
PHYSICAL EXAMINATION			
Jugular venous distention		+	+
Pulmonary rales	+	++	
S_3 gallop		++	
RESPONSE TO TREATMENT			
Oxygen	+	+	+
Anticholinergic bronchodilators	+	+	+
Withdrawal of sedatives	+	+	+
Aggressive physiotherapy	++		
Diuretics/afterload reduction		++	

evident early after surgery and resolve rapidly thereafter may reflect an old stroke that is fully compensated during less stressful circumstances. Medical imaging of the brain is worthwhile if no explanation is apparent on initial assessment. Nonfocal weakness commonly responds to physical therapy.

Delirium

Changes in mental status after surgery are common, especially in elderly patients (Chapter 27), and can be remarkably difficult to diagnose and correct. The immediate priority is to determine whether the impairment is acute or chronic and to detect easily reversible contributors (such as infection, hypoglycemia, alkalosis). A complete assessment is often unnecessary if the patient had normal mental status before surgery because many dementia syndromes are thereby excluded (such as vitamin B_{12} deficiency, tertiary syphilis, Alzheimer's disease). Immediate treatment usually focuses on discontinuing medications, especially anticholinergics, narcotics, and tranquilizers. The patient may also benefit from the continuous presence of friends and family members, who can provide frequent orientation and constant attention. A sense of patience is necessary because delirium rarely resolves instantly. The benefit of low-dose neuroleptics (e.g., risperidone, 0.5 mg twice daily) remains uncertain.

Seizures

The development of uncontrolled seizures (Chapter 410) after surgery is rare. The immediate priority is to exclude status epilepticus, uncover any past history of a chronic seizure disorder, and identify provocative factors. Neurosurgical patients typically undergo a standardized treatment protocol, including steroids and imaging. Other conditions that can cause abnormal movement, such as septic rigors, delirium tremens, Parkinson's disease, major psychopathology, hypothermic shivering, and hypercapnic asterixis, must be excluded. Additional considerations include detecting and correcting any underlying metabolic abnormalities such as hypocalcemia, hypoxemia, hyponatremia, hypophosphatemia, and drug toxicity. Treatment focuses primarily on reversing the underlying precipitating cause and providing nonspecific care with benzodiazepines, phenytoin, and ongoing monitoring.

Signs
Hypertension

Hypertension may reflect a variety of disorders and must be treated in a manner that neither overreacts nor underreacts to the situation. Hypertension is particularly common after neurosurgical procedures or carotid endarterectomy. The initial assessment focuses on whether the patient has chronic hypertension based on the past history, current electrocardiogram, or findings on funduscopy. Special attention should also be directed toward excluding undertreated pain, agitated delirium, fluid overload, alcohol withdrawal, and inadvertent discontinuation of chronic antihypertensive medications. In uncertain cases, systemic analgesia is often helpful, along with nitrates (e.g., nitroglycerin, 0.4 mg/hr transdermally) and β-blockers (e.g., metoprolol, 5 mg intravenously). The major complication of treatment is the potential for overcorrection and inadvertent hypotension—such errors are particularly common in patients with no evidence of past hypertension.

Hypotension

Hypotension (Chapter 7) after surgery is generally an emergency, and the immediate concern is often internal bleeding, especially after intra-abdominal operations or when anticoagulation is used to prevent venous thrombosis. The initial stages of hypotension are frequently unrecognized because of biologic stress responses by patients, psychological denial by clinicians, and misattribution to the concurrent use of analgesia. Early hypotension is particularly easy to miss if the patient has coexisting chronic hypertension and the apparently "normal" blood pressure is dismissed as unremarkable. Treatment usually entails volume supplementation, serial assessment, vasopressors as needed (Chapters 107 and 108), and a search for underlying causes, especially possible sepsis. Sometimes an extensive differential diagnosis needs to be considered if no anatomic cause related to surgery is evident (Chapter 106). Routine use of pulmonary artery catheters for diagnosis or to guide therapy is not helpful.**3**

Tachycardia

Tachycardia after surgery can be caused by a myriad of arrhythmias (Chapters 64 and 65) and may contribute to postoperative cardiac ischemia.

Distinguishing between newly identified and newly incident tachycardia can sometimes be accomplished by determining whether the patient does or does not complain of palpitations. The initial assessment almost always requires review of the electrocardiogram to distinguish atrial fibrillation from other disorders. The goal of treatment is to identify and correct precipitating factors such as pain, blood loss, hypoxia, electrolyte abnormalities, fluid overload, hypotension, pulmonary embolism, and drug withdrawal. Most arrhythmias respond to correction of the underlying abnormality. Specific antiarrhythmic treatment, when needed, is generally similar to that used in the nonoperative setting (Chapters 64 and 65). For atrial fibrillation, anticoagulation is sometimes contraindicated; in such situations, cardioversion within 48 hours merits consideration.

Fever

Fever (Chapter 288) after surgery is common, frequently perplexing, and often multifactorial. Worrisome possibilities include transfusion reactions (Chapter 180), hospital-acquired pneumonia (Chapter 97), urinary tract infection (Chapter 292), line sepsis (Chapter 290), and wound infection. In many cases no definitive cause is found, the patient recovers spontaneously, and the default diagnosis is atelectasis. Detailed evaluation, when necessary, requires culture of blood, urine, and the wound to identify specific microbiologic organisms. Selection of empirical antibiotics is usually based on local practice patterns and hospital ecology, with the main disadvantage being the breeding of resistant organisms. Hydration, nutrition, and general supportive care are important, yet frequently neglected needs of patients with prolonged elevations in body temperature.

Edema

Peripheral edema (Chapter 50), which is often first noticed by nursing staff after surgery, is rarely life-threatening unless treated with excessive diuretics. The cause is frequently multifactorial and includes both increased hydrostatic pressure (including heart failure and gravity from intraoperative positioning), decreased oncotic pressure (related to hypoalbuminemia from decreased liver production or increased losses), and capillary leak (potentially caused by medications or tissue reactions). Treatment focuses on correction of any underlying abnormalities, maintenance of nutrition, judicious use of diuretics, monitoring of renal function, provision of systemic anticoagulation against deep vein thrombosis, and efforts toward mobilization of the patient. Selected use of echocardiography, a low-salt diet, afterload reduction, and spironolactone may be helpful in patients in whom heart failure (Chapter 59) is the dominant mechanism.

Laboratory
Leukocytosis

An elevated white blood cell count (Chapter 170) can have many causes, but the immediate priority is to exclude a life-threatening septic process (Chapters 106 and 108). Direct microscopic examination of the peripheral blood smear (Chapter 160) can be helpful to check for toxic granulations (see Fig. 160-18), Döhle's bodies (Fig. 160-19), and a shift toward primitive band cells. Many cases are caused by noninfectious causes, including infarcted tissue (brain, heart, intestinal tract), inflammatory conditions (renal insufficiency, diabetic ketoacidosis, lupus erythematosus), or demargination stress reactions (dehydration, systemic corticosteroids, inotropic medications). In the absence of direct evidence, some clinicians may initiate antibiotics empirically, whereas others may elect waiting. Substantial controversy remains about the proper duration of an empirical trial of antibiotics when no cause is discovered and the patient is otherwise recovering.

Anemia

Anemia (Chapter 161) is common and sometimes underappreciated because coexisting volume depletion causes the blood hemoglobin concentration to underestimate the degree of blood loss. The initial priority is to differentiate bleeding at the surgical site from other causes. In many cases the exact cause is unclear and substantial uncertainty may arise over the need to initiate gastric acid suppression therapy or sacrifice systemic anticoagulation originally directed against venous thrombosis. Guidelines for transfusion therapy depend on the patient's cardiac reserve, as well as the available blood bank supply at the particular medical center. A reasonable goal is to maintain a hemoglobin level of 7 mg/dL or higher, except in patients with cardiovascular disease, in whom a hemoglobin goal of 10 mg/dL is reasonable. The immediate postoperative interval is not usually the appropriate time to initiate erythropoietin, oral iron replacement, or detailed evaluations for other hematologic abnormalities.

Abnormalities in Platelet Count

Patients often have abnormal platelet counts after surgery yet rarely require further evaluation or treatment. In most cases the thrombocytopenia is mild, does not require transfusion therapy, resolves in a few weeks, and is not a sign of an ominous disorder (e.g., sepsis or heparin-induced thrombocytopenia). Platelet transfusions are indicated if the decrease in platelet count is extreme, accompanied by evidence of major blood loss, or related to recent surgery on the central nervous system (including the eye). Thrombocytosis is also common about a month after surgery and is occasionally extreme. However, even postoperative thrombocytosis exceeding 1,000,000/mL rarely necessitates treatment, does not predispose patients to unwanted clotting disorders, and typically resolves spontaneously after a few weeks.

Abnormal Sodium

Both hyponatremia and hypernatremia (Chapter 118) are frequent complications in the postoperative setting. The immediate priority is to assess the patient's intravascular volume status and correct possible volume depletion. The cause of hyponatremia is often multifactorial, including excessive use of diuretics, excess intrinsic antidiuretic hormone (as a result of factors such as drugs, pain, or mechanical ventilation), and unmeasured osmoles (e.g., intravenous contrast agents). This risk for postoperative hyponatremia may be more effectively reduced by the administration of isotonic saline rather than by water restriction.■ Once hyponatremia develops, vasopressin antagonists (Chapter 118) are effective for both hypervolemic and euvolemic hyponatremia.■ Hypernatremia is always due to free water deficiency, which may indicate severe cognitive impairment or other factors interfering with the ability to express thirst or ingest water. Correction is similar to that in the nonoperative setting. Abnormalities in sodium concentration require careful follow-up, can develop or recur at any point after an operation, yet are rarely the root cause of a patient's inability to recover from surgery.

Abnormal Serum Potassium

Hyperkalemia and hypokalemia (Chapter 119) are also frequent postoperative complications. The immediate priority is to assess and stabilize the patient's electrocardiographic findings. Hyperkalemia is usually due to cellular shifts, renal failure, and tissue destruction (including hemolysis). Hyperkalemia will generally correct with treatments that shift potassium into cells (e.g., intravenous glucose with or without insulin or β-agonists) and enhance excretion (e.g., gastrointestinal binding agents). Hypokalemia is usually due to inadequate intake, excessive loss, or cellular shifts. Hypokalemia will generally correct with replacement therapy and rarely requires aldosterone antagonism. Both abnormalities can usually be treated as in the nonoperative setting (Chapter 119). The prognosis is favorable if the patient's electrocardiogram shows no major abnormalities and renal function is preserved.

Alkalosis

Systemic alkalosis (Chapter 120) typically requires volume supplementation because the cause is generally intravascular volume depletion. Blood gas determinations may be necessary in some cases to exclude the possibility of concurrent carbon dioxide retention with compensatory metabolic alkalosis. Untreated, alkalosis can result in altered mentation, cardiac arrhythmias, and delayed mobilization. Most patients with postoperative alkalosis do not require carbonic anhydrase inhibitors or intravenous acid. The prognosis is usually favorable, with gradual correction over a period of several days. Rapid correction of alkalosis, unlike rapid correction of hyponatremia, is not known to cause neurologic injury.

Azotemia

The initial assessment of an elevated serum creatinine concentration (Chapter 116) focuses on reviewing previous values (to distinguish acute from chronic renal insufficiency) and identifying contributing factors (such as prerenal volume depletion, intrarenal nephrotoxins, or postrenal urethral obstruction). A trial of intravenous fluids may be useful on both a diagnostic and therapeutic basis. Treatment is the same as in the nonoperative setting. Subsequent monitoring is always necessary, with serum creatinine measurements obtained on a daily basis. Serial measurements of urinary volume and body weight and urine cultures are occasionally helpful in selected cases. The prognosis is dependent on the underlying factors and is less favorable after cardiac surgery.

Hyperbilirubinemia

Elevations in serum bilirubin (Chapter 149) are rare after surgery, even though abnormalities in liver enzyme levels occur frequently with general anesthesia. The most benign explanation is Gilbert's syndrome, but the immediate priority is to assess for possible hepatic failure (especially in patients who have received halothane). As in the nonoperative setting, treatment involves withdrawing potential hepatotoxins, supporting the patient, and allowing time for liver function to recover (Chapter 157). Treatment of hepatic encephalopathy is particularly important because of the constipation and generalized catabolic state that follow major surgery. Monitoring should include serial measurement of liver function on a daily basis because each component (e.g., bilirubin, albumen, prothrombin time) can be altered in postoperative patients by factors unrelated to the liver. The prognosis is unfavorable if the patient's liver function fails to recover quickly.

Hypoalbuminemia

Reductions in serum albumin are common after surgery and are an ominous prognostic finding. The cause is rarely decreased production if the loss of albumin occurs rapidly. Possible explanations include nephrotic syndrome, capillary leak into extravascular spaces, and occult catabolism in unrecognized sites. Treatment with albumin infusions does not usually normalize the biochemical abnormality and does not seem to improve patient mortality rates significantly. The main priorities are to continue nutritional support, preserve skin integrity, minimize the use of systemic diuretics, correct any contributing factors, and consider correlated serum protein deficiencies (such as reduced levels of immunoglobulins or antithrombin III). Hypoalbuminemia can also cause indirect harm by the loss of carrier proteins, which predisposes patients to unwanted episodes of drug toxicity. The long-term prognosis is favorable for survivors because the serum albumin level will eventually fully return to normal.

Blood Glucose Abnormalities

In patients with diabetes mellitus (Chapter 236), serum blood sugar concentrations often become erratic after surgery because of altered dietary intake, decreased physical activity, and release of counter-regulatory hormones. The priorities are to avoid hypoglycemia, severe hyperglycemia, diabetic ketoacidosis, cerebral damage, and repeated events. Intensive control of the blood glucose level increases the risk for severe hypoglycemia and death, so a target glucose level of about 140 to 200 mg/dL is recommended.[6] Rapid reversal of sepsis or focal infection can lead to a precipitous decrease in insulin requirements; in such cases, vigilance is required because unsuspected hypoglycemia may cause permanent damage or be fatal in a patient who may seem to be sleeping. Patients need to be forewarned that temporary doses of subcutaneous insulin may be required but do not commit the patient to chronic insulin therapy. Monitoring involves serial measurement of blood sugar until the patient is eating in a reliable manner.

Special Situations
Multiplicity

Some postoperative complications are difficult to classify because no single dominant problem is apparent by symptoms, signs, or laboratory testing. Instead, the patient has two or more problems that need to be addressed simultaneously. The immediate goal is to set priorities and avoid the temptation to try to eliminate every possibility on the first day. The corollary is to continue to check progress over the many days that may be required for complete diagnosis and successful therapy. Because so many concerns require attention in the postoperative interval, the risk is that clinicians will lose track of a secondary issue and make an error that seems obvious in retrospect.

Redundancy

Postoperative complications sometimes generate multiple consultations with physicians who have overlapping abilities. An example might be a patient with a postoperative fever that prompts consultations from pulmonology, nephrology, dermatology, general medicine, and infectious diseases. In theory, gathering a critical mass of medical experts together should increase the likelihood of accurate diagnosis, timely treatment, and foolproof follow-up. In reality, however, coordination and communication are never perfect.

Personal rivalries, diffusion of responsibility, and many other psychological factors may impede interactions among consultants. Opportunities for miscommunication may be further accentuated if the patient has an exotic diagnosis that is a special draw on the consultant's attention (e.g., pheochromocytoma). Arguing in front of the patient, in view of other professionals, or in the medical record can be demoralizing. The priority is to communicate effectively with the surgical team responsible for the patient and encourage that team to make the final decision.

Ambiguity

Another vexation occurs when an urgent request is not connected to a clear rationale (Chapter 438). Diplomacy is needed to establish whether the motivation reflects medicolegal concerns rather than a biologic change in the patient. Sometimes the stimulus that drives the consultation can best be addressed by providing reassurance and confirmation. Sometimes the stimulus is an obscure preexisting disorder (e.g., moyamoya disease), and the surgical team has neither the experience nor the time to investigate how this unrelated medical condition can influence recovery from surgery. Sometimes the stimulus is an unspoken political wish to transfer the care of a burdensome patient from one physician to another. A consultant should develop an understanding of how to interact with other clinicians under such ambiguous circumstances.

Setting Priorities

Requests for consultation often arrive outside conventional working hours, are usually tinged with a sense of urgency, and sometimes cluster to encompass more than one patient. Developing an effective method for prioritizing patients is a crucial clinical skill. One communication strategy is to provide an objective estimated time of arrival for the initial request from the surgical team. An oftentimes helpful treatment strategy is to make some safe suggestions at the time of the initial request so that clear-cut recommendations can be instituted during the interval before the patient is seen and used later to help evaluate the patient's status and course.

Ending

In many postoperative cases, the original reason for consultation may resolve and no major issues remain. The situation now provides an opportunity to review the patient, particularly for the appropriate use of unrelated medications. The consultant may often detect excessive medications that were appropriate early in the hospital course but have ceased to be necessary, thereby justifying discontinuation (e.g., diuretics, antibiotics, bronchodilators). Discontinuing medications that have become superfluous requires initiative and wisdom, and the common mistake is to propagate unnecessary medications in stable patients under the rationale of "don't mess with success." The ability to watch the patient for several hours or for a day or two often presents an ideal opportunity for the safe withdrawal of medications. Ironically, discontinuing a treatment sometimes requires more skill, time, and initiative than starting it.

1. Squadrone V, Coha M, Cerutti E, et al. Continuous positive airway pressure for treatment of postoperative hypoxemia: a randomized controlled trial. *JAMA.* 2005;293:589-595.
2. Apfel CC, Korttila K, Abdalla M, et al. A factorial trial of six interventions for the prevention of postoperative nausea and vomiting. *N Engl J Med.* 2004;350:2441-2451.
3. Sandham JD, Jull RD, Brant RF, et al. A randomized, controlled trial of the use of pulmonary-artery catheters in high-risk surgical patients. *N Engl J Med.* 2003;348:5-14.
4. Neville KA, Sandeman DJ, Rubinstein A, et al. Prevention of hyponatremia during maintenance intravenous fluid administration: a prospective randomized study of fluid type versus fluid rate. *J Pediatr.* 2010;156:313-319.
5. Rozen-Svi B, Yahav D, Gheorghiade M, et al. Vasopressin receptor antagonists for the treatment of hyponatremia: systematic review and meta-analysis. *Am J Kidney Dis.* 2010;56:325-337.
6. Kansagara D, Fu R, Freeman M, Wolf F, et al. Intensive insulin therapy in hospitalized patients: a systematic review. *Ann Intern Med.* 2011;154:268-282.

SUGGESTED READINGS

Duggan M, Kavanagh BP. Perioperative modifications of respiratory function. *Best Pract Res Clin Anaesthesiol.* 2010;24:145-155. *Strategies to include smoking cessation, inspiratory muscle training, and optimizing nutritional status.*

Frenzel JC, Kee SS, Ensor JE, et al. Ongoing provision of individual clinician performance data improves practice behavior. *Anesth Analg.* 2010;111:515-519. *Ongoing personal performance feedback was the most effective approach to improve surgical practices.*

Neily J, Mills PD, Young-Xu Y, et al. Association between implementation of a medical team training program and surgical mortality. *JAMA.* 2010;304:1693-1700. *A team training program was associated with a 18% reduction in surgical mortality.*

Redelmeier DA, McAlister FA, Kandel CE, et al. Postoperative pneumonia in elderly patients receiving acid suppressants. *BMJ.* 2010;340:c2608. *No increase in the risk of postoperative pneumonia.*

442

MEDICAL CONSULTATION IN PSYCHIATRY

PETER MANU

HEALTH STATUS IN PSYCHIATRIC PATIENTS

The physical health of psychiatric patients is poor, with a higher risk for death at an early age than in the mentally sane. The magnitude of the problem is greatest in patients with schizophrenia, who have a significantly shorter lifespan compared with the general population. Poverty, social neglect, standard medical care, unhealthy life habits, and complications of psychiatric treatments are major contributors to the increased morbidity and mortality of patients with chronic psychiatric disorders, who have a 22.5-year average decline in life expectancy.

MEDICAL EVALUATION IN PSYCHIATRIC SETTINGS

Requirements for medical training in psychiatry vary. In the United States, psychiatric residents have up to 4 months of inpatient medical training. Data suggest that psychiatrists have limited skills in assessing nonpsychiatric problems in terms of history taking, a reluctance to perform physical examinations, and a tendency toward premature diagnostic closure. As a result, medical consultations are often requested for basic medical issues. For example, in one study, 1001 consecutively admitted psychiatric patients generated 2120 initial consultations and 1800 follow-up visits. The highest rate of medical utilization was for patients with dementia, schizophrenia, substance abuse disorders, and mental retardation. Because medical issues may precipitate psychiatric decompensation or be obscured by it, about 10% of psychiatric inpatients seen by a medical consultant required transfer to a medical or surgical unit.

Medical consultation in psychiatry is not more difficult than in other clinical settings but must be informed by knowledge about the serious complications of psychiatric treatments (Table 442-1). This chapter provides details about some of the most important entities specific to the psychiatric setting.

EVALUATION OF CHIEF COMPLAINTS

Medical consultation for psychiatric patients creates unique challenges in evaluation of the chief complaint. Many patients with outpatient psychiatric disorders have somatic symptoms such as fatigue, weakness, dizziness, headache, insomnia, widespread pain, and constipation. In most of these patients, the underlying mental illnesses are mood disorders (unipolar depression and dysthymia), anxiety disorders (panic disorder and generalized anxiety disorder), somatoform disorders, substance use disorders (most often alcohol, opiates, cocaine, and benzodiazepine), and borderline personality disorder. As a group, these patients have many physical complaints and resist a psychological explanation for their symptoms even when the medical evaluation fails to identify objective abnormalities.

In contrast, patients admitted for inpatient psychiatric treatment often have psychotic disorders, developmental abnormalities, or dementia with behavioral disturbance; they are frequently vague or silent about physical suffering and only rarely voice somatic delusions. Such patients may deny pain even after bowel perforation or myocardial infarction.

A rigorous diagnostic evaluation is therefore required to avoid the errors of omission created by the weak correlation between complaints and

TABLE 442-1	MAJOR MEDICAL COMPLICATIONS OF PSYCHOTROPIC DRUGS
CARDIOVASCULAR	
Cardiomyopathy	Clozapine
Hypertension	MAO inhibitors, venlafaxine
Myocarditis	Clozapine
Orthostatic hypotension	Tricyclics, trazodone, antipsychotics
QTc prolongation	Antipsychotics, tricyclics
Venous thromboembolism	Clozapine, risperidone, phenothiazines
RESPIRATORY	
Choking	Antipsychotics, tricyclics
Laryngospasm	Antipsychotics
Respiratory depression	Benzodiazepines, barbiturates, methadone, antidepressants, atypical antipsychotics
GASTROINTESTINAL	
Bowel obstruction	Tricyclics, antipsychotics
Dysphagia	Tricyclics, antipsychotics
Hepatic impairment	Carbamazepine, valproic acid, phenothiazines, mirtazapine, nefazodone, quetiapine, olanzapine, clozapine, MAO inhibitors, naltrexone
Pancreatitis	Carbamazepine, valproic acid, clozapine, olanzapine
KIDNEY AND URINARY TRACT	
Renal insufficiency	Lithium, clozapine
Urinary retention	Antipsychotics, tricyclics
ENDOCRINE	
Hyperprolactinemia	First-generation antipsychotics, risperidone
Hypothyroidism	Lithium, quetiapine
Inappropriate ADH secretion	Serotonin reuptake inhibitors, methadone, tricyclics
Metabolic syndrome	Clozapine, olanzapine, risperidone, quetiapine
HEMATOLOGIC	
Leukocytosis	Lithium
Neutropenia	Clozapine, olanzapine, risperidone, carbamazepine, valproate, mirtazapine
Thrombocytopenia	Carbamazepine, valproate
MUSCULOSKELETAL	
Rhabdomyolysis*	Antipsychotics, serotonin reuptake inhibitors, MAO inhibitors
SKIN	
Stevens-Johnson syndrome	Lamotrigine, carbamazepine, barbiturates
OTHER	
Fever*	Antipsychotics, serotonin reuptake inhibitors, MAO inhibitors
Seizure	Bupropion, MAO inhibitors, tricyclics, phenothiazines

*Includes neuroleptic malignant syndrome and serotonin syndrome.
ADH = antidiuretic hormone; MAO = monoamine oxidase.

pathology. This evaluation should include consideration of physical disorders, drug effects (adverse reaction, toxicity, or withdrawal), cognitive impairment (delirium), sensory impairment (loss of vision, hearing, speech, or postural balance), and situational maladjustment (isolation, overload, or loss of privacy). Attribution of symptoms to the patient's psychiatric condition should remain a diagnosis of exclusion.

MEDICAL COMPLICATIONS OF PSYCHIATRIC TREATMENTS

Antipsychotic-Induced Metabolic Syndrome

Metabolic syndrome is more prevalent (range, 29 to 63%) in schizophrenic and other psychiatric patients treated with atypical antipsychotic drugs such as clozapine, olanzapine, risperidone, and quetiapine than in the general population. Clozapine, olanzapine, and quetiapine are the worst offenders because they induce substantial weight gain, thereby leading to insulin resistance (with or without fasting hyperglycemia) and atherogenic dyslipidemia. This gain in weight may be related to affinity for the histamine-1 (H_1) receptor and to neurobiologic mechanisms that regulate appetite and metabolism via the production and activity of serotonin, leptin, and tumor necrosis factor-α. Within 18 months, 30% of patients treated with olanzapine will increase their body weight by more than 7%, with an average increase of 43 mg/dL in triglycerides, 15 mg/dL in blood glucose, and 0.41% in glycosylated hemoglobin. Not surprisingly, these changes result in about a two-fold increased risk for diabetes and coronary heart disease events. Nonetheless, controlled trials have identified olanzapine and clozapine as effective drugs for patients with schizophrenia and other psychotic disorders.

Because the glucose intolerance often seen in patients treated with antipsychotic agents is due to insulin resistance (Chapter 237), it is best treated by aggressive weight reduction, (Chapter 220), increasing physical activity (Chapter 15), and metformin (Chapter 237), or a combination of these. For example, in randomized trials, metformin, 850 mg twice daily, reduced the weight gain associated with the initiation of second-generation antipsychotic drugs,**1** and a single daily dose of 750 mg may prevent weight gain if initiated at the onset of olanzapine treatment.**2** In treating hypertension, β-adrenergic blockers should be used cautiously in patients receiving neuroleptics because they increase the potential for orthostatic hypotension, syncope, and falls. Smoking cessation programs combining transdermal or transmucosal nicotine replacement, bupropion, and cognitive-behavioral therapy should be strongly recommended despite the dismally high failure rates that have been reported in patients with chronic schizophrenia (Chapter 31).

Antipsychotic-Induced Myocarditis and Cardiomyopathy

Antipsychotic-induced myocarditis and cardiomyopathy (Chapter 60) are most common in patients treated with clozapine (0.9%) and fluphenazine (0.4%). In contrast, the risk for these complications is only 0.1% in patients receiving haloperidol, thioridazine, and risperidone.

The accepted pathophysiologic explanation for myocarditis is an immunoglobulin E (IgE)-mediated acute hypersensitivity reaction, similar to the allergic myocarditis produced by penicillins, sulfonamides, and methyldopa. In a small number of patients, a competing hypothesis proposes that clozapine induces hypereosinophilic myocarditis, colitis, hepatitis, pancreatitis, alveolitis, and interstitial nephritis. A direct cardiotoxic effect of drug metabolites cannot be excluded.

In patients in whom myocarditis develops, the mortality rate is as high as 50%, with almost half the deaths occurring suddenly and unexpectedly. The average duration of exposure to clozapine before diagnosis or death is 21 days, and the dosage range is 50 to 725 mg/day. Common symptoms are fever (48%), dyspnea (35%), flulike illness (30%), chest pain (22%), and fatigue (17%). Laboratory features include left ventricular hypokinesia or reduced ejection fraction (48%) or pericardial effusion (17%) on echocardiography, nonspecific repolarization abnormalities on electrocardiography (35%), peripheral eosinophilia (35%), elevated creatine kinase and troponin levels (22%), and radiographic evidence of heart failure (13%). The diagnosis can be confirmed by endomyocardial biopsy showing fraying of myocytes and perivascular infiltrates with degranulated eosinophils. Among survivors, symptoms resolve or substantially improve after discontinuation of clozapine and treatment with high-dose corticosteroids (e.g., prednisone, 1 mg/kg/day for 4 days, tapered to 0.33 mg/kg/day for the following 4 days).

Clozapine-induced dilated cardiomyopathy may be caused by an evolving myocarditis or by chronic injury mediated by free radicals, similar to the myocarditis produced by doxorubicin (Chapter 60). The demographic features are similar to those of myocarditis, but the mean duration of treatment before diagnosis is much longer (9 months vs. 3 weeks), and the mortality rate is lower (22 vs. 51%). Patients have clinical or echocardiographic evidence of left ventricular dysfunction without eosinophilia or enzymatic evidence of myocardial necrosis.

Prolonged QTc Interval and Sudden Death

Significant prolongation of the QTc interval (Chapter 65) leading to ventricular tachyarrhythmias and sudden cardiac death (Chapter 63) can occur after antipsychotic treatment with the usual doses of thioridazine, haloperidol, and sertindole. Abnormal myocardial repolarization has been observed during treatment with most antipsychotic medications and after intentional or accidental overdoses of tricyclic antidepressants, lithium, and methadone (Chapter 110). All antipsychotics affect the cardiac potassium channel by blocking the rapidly activating component of the rectifier potassium current (Chapter 61). This effect translates into a dose-dependent increase in the duration of phase 3 of the action potential. The drug concentration that produces 50% inhibition of rapid potassium outflow varies for each drug (e.g., 1 nmol/L for haloperidol and 6 nmol/L for olanzapine). Compared with nonusers of antipsychotic drugs, the risk for sudden death is twice as high for current users of conventional (first-generation) antipsychotics and is 2.25

times higher for current users of atypical (second-generation) antipsychotics. All patients about to start antipsychotic drugs should be asked about a personal history of syncope and a family history of long QT syndrome or sudden death at a young age. A baseline electrocardiogram and serum electrolytes should be obtained before starting antipsychotic drug therapy, tricyclic antidepressants, and methadone. Interval electrocardiograms should be obtained after each increase in medication in older patients, patients with known heart disease, and those starting other drugs known to produce QTc prolongation or hypokalemia (Chapter 65). A QTc interval of 500 msec or greater requires the discontinuation of all drugs that affect membrane repolarization. QTc intervals greater than 450 msec in males and 470 msec in females, QTc dispersion (difference between the longest and shortest QTc on a 12-lead electrocardiogram) greater than 100 msec, and an increase in QTc duration of more than 60 msec in comparison to the baseline measurement should prompt reevaluation of the risks and benefits associated with the drugs in question.

Choking and Laryngeal Dystonia

Asphyxia deaths from choking occur at a rate of 0.8% per 1000 psychiatric patients each year, a frequency that is more than 100 times greater than in the general population. In addition, videofluoroscopy demonstrates silent aspiration in 38% of psychiatric patients who survive a choking incident. Choking and silent aspiration are manifestations of dysphagia (Chapter 140), which is common in the mentally ill. Half the psychiatric patients with dysphagia have a fast-eating syndrome seen in association with restlessness, poor chewing skills, food pocketing in the cheeks, and attention deficits that characterize psychotic disorders and mental retardation. Bradykinetic dysphagia, which is seen in 25% of psychiatric patients with choking episodes, is due to the antidopaminergic and anticholinergic effects of psychotropic medications. This condition, which features reduced lingual range of motion, increased oral transit time, decreased pharyngeal peristalsis, and delayed initiation of the swallowing reflex, is seen in patients with neurologic features of drug-induced parkinsonism (Chapter 416). Dyskinetic dysphagia (7% of choking cases), which generally occurs in patients maintained on long-term antipsychotic medication, is part of the clinical spectrum of tardive dyskinesia (Chapter 417). The examination reveals involuntary contractions of the tongue and perioral musculature, clumsiness of voluntary movements of the tongue, and discontinuous bolus propulsion in the oral stage. In the remaining patients, the dysphagia is due to cerebrovascular disease (11%) or to pharyngeal or esophageal pathology (7%).

Laryngeal dystonia, which is a life-threatening complication of antipsychotic drug therapy, primarily with haloperidol and phenothiazines, is produced by acute spasmodic contraction of the adductor laryngeal muscles. Symptoms include respiratory distress, dysphonia, and stridor. Neuroleptic-induced bronchospasm may precede the onset of stridor. Patients typically indicate extreme subjective distress by clutching their anterior cervical area. Most patients also have other dystonias involving the head and neck, including torticollis, retrocollis, trismus, tongue protrusion, and deviation of the eyes up, down, or sideward. In general, the symptoms and signs develop in the first week after starting or rapidly increasing the dose of neuroleptic medications. Similar dystonic phenomena have been described after treatment with the antiemetics promethazine, prochlorperazine, and metoclopramide. A reduction in the dose of anticholinergic or antiparkinsonian medication used to prevent or treat extrapyramidal symptoms can also precipitate laryngeal dystonia. The condition is more common in young males and must be distinguished from epiglottitis, allergic or anaphylactic laryngeal edema or laryngospasm, mechanical obstruction, and psychogenic stridor. Intravenous administration of diphenhydramine (initial dose, 25 mg; may repeat after 5 minutes if symptoms persist) is the treatment of choice, and endotracheal intubation is seldom required.

Drug-Induced Neutropenia and Agranulocytosis

Drug-induced neutropenia with absolute neutrophil counts of less than 1500/μL has been observed during treatment with most second-generation antipsychotics (clozapine, olanzapine, risperidone, and quetiapine) and mood stabilizers (carbamazepine, valproic acid, and lamotrigine) as well as some antidepressant drugs (tricyclic antidepressants and mirtazapine). Clozapine-induced neutropenia occurs in 4 to 5% of patients within 6 months after starting treatment and progresses to agranulocytosis in 10% or more of neutropenic patients if the drug is continued. In vitro, clozapine toxicity requires peroxide and peroxidase, and the defect in oxidation is related to abnormalities in the *NQO2* (quinone oxidoreductase) gene involved in drug

TABLE 442-2 DIFFERENTIAL DIAGNOSIS OF NEUROLEPTIC MALIGNANT SYNDROME
Infection of the central nervous system
Infection in patients with drug-induced parkinsonism
Drug overdose (psychostimulants, antidepressants, lithium, anticholinergics)
Alcohol or drug withdrawal (benzodiazepines, barbiturates, antiparkinsonian drugs)
Side effects of nonpsychotropic dopamine-depleting drugs (reserpine, metoclopramide, prochlorperazine, promethazine)
Cholinergic rebound
Serotonin syndrome
Thyrotoxicosis
Malignant hyperthermia

TABLE 442-3 CLASSES OF MEDICATIONS THAT PRODUCE SEROTONIN SYNDROME IN PSYCHIATRIC PATIENTS
Selective serotonin reuptake inhibitors
Monoamine oxidase inhibitors
Atypical antipsychotics
Heterocyclic antidepressants
Trazodone
Dual-uptake inhibitors
Psychostimulants
Buspirone
Mood stabilizers
Analgesics
Antiemetics
Cough suppressants
Dietary supplements

detoxification. Treatment with clozapine should be started only if the baseline absolute neutrophil count is greater than 1500/μL. The concomitant use of carbamazepine, angiotensin-converting enzyme inhibitors, sulfonamides, and propylthiouracil, and mirtazapine should be avoided because they can produce neutropenia and increase the risk for agranulocytosis. Clozapine should be stopped and the patient evaluated immediately for fever, oral ulcerations, and symptoms or signs of infection. Complete blood counts should be obtained once a week for the first 26 weeks and every other week thereafter, and clozapine should be stopped and all medications reassessed if the absolute neutrophil count drops below 1500/μL. Clozapine-related agranulocytosis has been treated successfully with colony-stimulating factors (either granulocyte or granulocyte-macrophage colony-stimulating factor).

Neutropenia has also been associated with olanzapine, risperidone, and quetiapine in patients who have never received clozapine. Treatment with anticonvulsant mood stabilizers, particularly carbamazepine, is associated with a dose-dependent neutropenia and thrombocytopenia in approximately 10% of patients in the first 6 months of treatment and should be monitored with complete blood counts twice each month during this period.

Neuroleptic Malignant Syndrome

Neuroleptic malignant syndrome, which occurs in approximately 0.2% of patients receiving neuroleptics, must be part of the differential diagnosis of fever and rhabdomyolysis (Chapter 115) in a psychiatric patient (Table 442-2). The frequency is greater in young males and patients who are malnourished or dehydrated, have Parkinson's disease, or are treated parenterally with large doses of neuroleptics over short periods. The main diagnostic criteria are elevated temperature (higher than 104° F [40° C] in 40% of patients) and diffuse muscle rigidity (ranging from mild hypertonicity to severe "lead pipe" stiffness). In addition, two or more of the following are required for a definitive diagnosis: (1) autonomic instability (tachycardia, elevated or labile blood pressure, postural hypotension, diaphoresis, sialorrhea, and urinary incontinence), (2) changes in mental status (ranging from confusion to mutism or coma), (3) leukocytosis (up to 20,000/mL), and (4) elevated creatine kinase (up to 100,000 IU/L). Other clinical manifestations include bradykinesia, chorea, dystonias, dysphagia, dysarthria or aphonia, seizures, and tremor. The severity of rhabdomyolysis correlates with the creatine kinase level and with the presence of myoglobinemia, myoglobinuria, metabolic acidosis, and azotemia. The electroencephalogram shows nonspecific slowing in slightly more than half of patients.

The time lag from starting the drug to the onset of neuroleptic malignant syndrome is generally short, with 30% of cases developing within 48 hours and 96% within the first month of treatment. The exception appears to be clozapine-associated neuroleptic malignant syndrome, which has an average time lag of 50 days. Neuroleptic syndrome is sometimes confused with severe catatonia (Chapter 404), but the catatonic signs in neuroleptic malignant syndrome are usually restricted to mutism and akinesia. Furthermore, hyperthermia, rigidity, tremor, and rhabdomyolysis are not present in patients with catatonia. Nonetheless, close medical follow-up of severely catatonic patients is warranted because they are at very high risk (22%) for neuroleptic malignant syndrome.

Untreated, neuroleptic malignant syndrome has a mortality rate of 10% as a result of acute renal failure, aspiration pneumonia, adult respiratory distress syndrome, disseminated intravascular coagulation, and cerebellar neuronal degeneration. Most fatalities are avoidable if the diagnosis is made early, the neuroleptic agent is discontinued rapidly, and the patient is immediately transferred to an intensive care setting for supportive and specific therapy. Bromocriptine (2.5 mg three times daily orally or through a nasogastric tube; may increase by 2.5 mg three times daily to a maximal daily dose of 40 mg) or amantadine (100 mg orally or through a nasogastric tube twice daily; may increase to 300 mg/day in divided doses) should be used in moderately severe cases and continued until the muscle rigidity and metabolic abnormalities have significantly improved. The skeletal muscle relaxant dantrolene (starting with a dose of 1 mg/kg intravenously and titrated to a maximal dose of 10 mg/kg/day divided into three intravenous or oral doses) should be added to bromocriptine or amantadine in patients with fulminant hypermetabolic features and those with persistent muscle rigidity despite treatment with dopamine agonists. Refractory neuroleptic malignant syndrome improves after electroconvulsive therapy (ECT).

Serotonin Syndrome

Serotonin syndrome (Chapter 440) is an adverse drug reaction primarily produced by excess serotonergic agonism of central nervous system and peripheral serotonin receptors by selected drugs (Table 442-3). In postmarketing surveillance studies of the newer antidepressants, the syndrome has an incidence of 4 cases per 10,000 patient months in patients who start taking nefazodone, a drug that inhibits neuronal uptake of serotonin and norepinephrine and also acts as a 5-HT2 receptor antagonist. The syndrome also occurs in 15% of patients with intentional overdose of selective serotonin reuptake inhibitors (SSRIs). The serotonin syndrome is caused by overstimulation of 5-HT1A and possibly also 5-HT2 receptors through excess of serotonin precursors or agonists, increased serotonin release, reduced serotonin uptake, and decreased serotonin metabolism. Severe cases of the syndrome have been more frequently reported in patients treated with monoamine oxidase inhibitors who took over-the-counter dextromethorphan or the illegal methylenedioxymethamphetamine (Ecstasy) or who started treatment with serotonin reuptake inhibitors, meperidine, or atypical antipsychotics such as aripiprazole.

Potentially life-threatening, the syndrome is characterized by changes in mental status (ranging from agitation to confusion and coma), autonomic instability (tachycardia, labile or high blood pressure, diaphoresis, and diarrhea), neuromuscular abnormalities (myoclonus, mydriasis, ocular clonus, rigidity, hyperreflexia, tremors, and shivering), and hyperthermia. The symptoms occur within the first 24 hours and sometimes within minutes after the initial use of medication, a change in dose, addition of a new drug, or overdose attempt. Death may occur as a consequence of rhabdomyolysis with renal failure, hyperkalemia, disseminated intravascular coagulation, and acute respiratory distress syndrome. The differential diagnosis includes neuroleptic malignant syndrome, viral or bacterial meningitis or encephalitis, heat stroke (Chapter 109), anticholinergic toxidrome (Chapter 110), and drug (Chapter 33) or alcohol withdrawal (Chapter 32).

General management includes immediate discontinuation of serotonergic drugs, comprehensive supportive therapy, and benzodiazepines for control of agitation and myoclonus. Specific therapy relies on the use of cyproheptadine (an H_1-receptor antagonist with antiserotonergic and anticholinergic properties) and chlorpromazine (a 5-HT1A and 5-HT2 receptor antagonist). Cyproheptadine should be started at a dose of 12 mg administered orally or through a nasogastric tube, with additional 2-mg doses given every 2 hours until symptoms improve or the maximal dose of 32 mg has been reached. The usual maintenance dose of cyproheptadine is 8 mg three times daily. Chlorpromazine (50 mg intramuscularly; may repeat three or four times daily and increase gradually to 400 mg/day in divided doses) is indicated in patients with severe symptoms who must be treated parenterally. Rapid improvement has also been observed after single doses of olanzapine (10 mg administered sublingually). Chlorpromazine and olanzapine should be used only after the possibility of neuroleptic malignant syndrome has been excluded.

Antipsychotic-Induced Hyperprolactinemia

Drug-induced hyperprolactinemia is produced by first-generation antipsychotic medications and by risperidone, but it is quite rare with other atypical antipsychotics such as aripiprazole, olanzapine, and ziprasidone. In patients treated with prolactin-raising antipsychotic medications, hormone levels are above the normal limit in 60% of females and 40% of males. Symptomatic hyperprolactinemia (Chapter 231) occurs in about one third of these patients and is generally associated with a 10-fold increase above baseline levels. Excess prolactin leads to dysfunction of target tissues (galactorrhea, oligomenorrhea and amenorrhea, infertility, sexual impairment, and gynecomastia) as well as an increased risk for breast cancer, osteoporosis, and cardiovascular disease. The mechanism of antipsychotic-related hyperprolactinemia is suppression of dopamine inhibition of lactotroph cells in the hypothalamus. Brain imaging is required in symptomatic patients and those with significant elevated prolactin levels to exclude tumors of the pituitary and hypothalamus.

Psychogenic Polydipsia and Drug-Induced Hyponatremia

Hyponatremia is common in psychiatric patients and can lead to severe complications, including seizure, coma, brain stem herniation, and death (Chapter 118). The diagnosis is often delayed because traditional manifestations of hyponatremia, such as lethargy, restlessness, weakness, and disorientation, overlap with features of psychiatric disorders. The differential diagnosis in psychiatric settings must emphasize psychogenic polydipsia and the drug-induced syndrome of inappropriate secretion of antidiuretic hormone (SIADH) (Chapter 118).

Patients with psychogenic polydipsia typically have serum hypoosmolality and a maximally dilute urine (urine osmolality <100 mOsm/L). The incidence of polydipsia is 20% and the incidence of water intoxication is 5% in inpatient psychiatric facilities. Urinary incontinence and nocturnal enuresis may be part of the clinical manifestation. The mechanism of increased thirst is poorly understood but may involve incomplete suppression of antidiuretic hormone (ADH) by the hypothalamus as well as response to the mouth dryness produced by the anticholinergic effect of many psychotropic drugs. The differential diagnosis includes diuretic effect, renal insufficiency, glucocorticoid deficiency, and hypothyroidism. Stringent measures to restrict fluid intake are generally effective in patients with moderate hyponatremia, and clozapine limits polydipsia and improves water intoxication in refractory cases.

Drug-induced SIADH is predominantly related to SSRIs, and animal experiments have suggested that the excess serotonin stimulates release of ADH and will lead to hyponatremia, provided that water intake is sufficient. Other drugs that are commonly used by psychiatric patients and that may produce SIADH include tricyclic antidepressants, monoamine oxidase inhibitors, carbamazepine, conventional and second-generation antipsychotics, benzodiazepines, methadone, and nicotine. Elderly patients, patients with a lower body mass index, and those with a baseline plasma sodium level of less than 138 mEq/L are at higher risk. The median time to diagnosis after starting SSRIs is 9 days. Urinary excretion of sodium usually is greater than 20 mEq/L, and urine osmolality is higher than 300 mOsm/L. In patients with mild asymptomatic hyponatremia, SSRIs can be continued with careful monitoring while the patient is placed on supervised fluid restriction. For patients who cannot tolerate fluid restriction or have symptomatic hyponatremia with serum sodium levels of less than 125 mEq/L, the use of tolvaptan (initially 15 mg, titratable to 30 or 60 mg), a vasopressin V2-receptor antagonist, is effective. **3**

Risk Assessment before Electroconvulsive Therapy

ECT is highly effective for the treatment of drug-refractory major depression and other psychiatric disorders. The procedure requires a brief period of

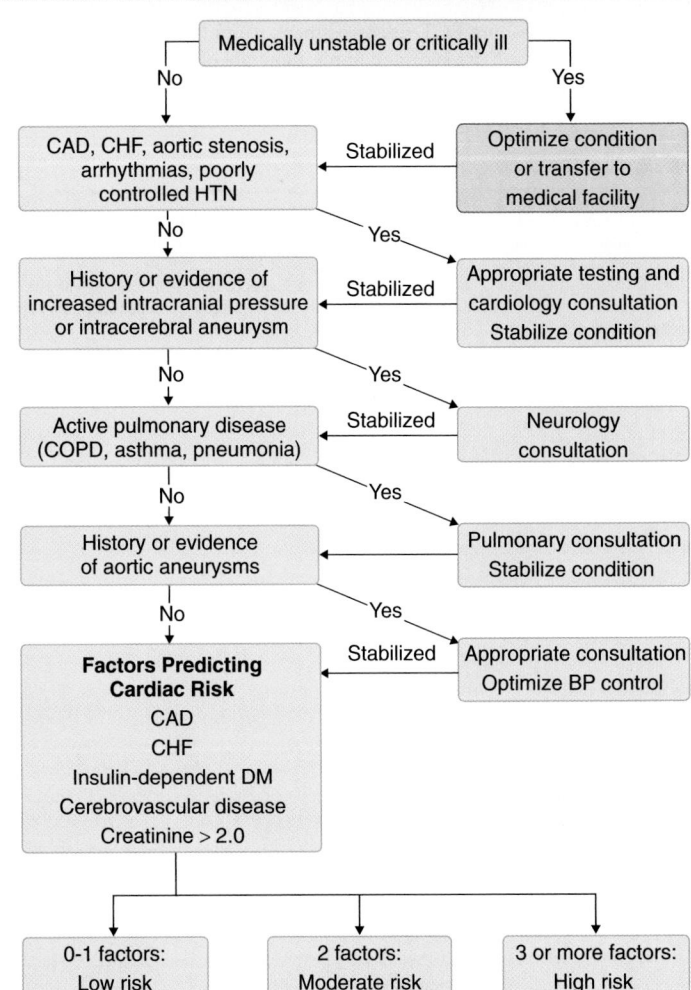

FIGURE 442-1. Risk assessment before electroconvulsive therapy. BP = blood pressure; CAD = coronary artery disease; CHF = congestive heart failure; COPD = chronic obstructive pulmonary disease; DM = diabetes mellitus; HTN = hypertension. (Modified from Frederickson A, Manu P. Risk assessment prior to electroconvulsive therapy. In Manu P, Suarez RE, Barnett BJ, eds. *Handbook of Medicine in Psychiatry*. Washington, DC: American Psychiatric Publishing; 2006:687-700.)

general anesthesia with sodium pentothal, etomidate, or propofol, as well as muscle paralysis with succinylcholine, during which the patient receives bag-valve-mask ventilation with supplemental oxygen and is monitored with continuous electrocardiography and pulse oximetry. Bronchospasm may follow induction of anesthesia, particularly in patients already at risk for respiratory compromise. During electrical stimulation of the brain, parasympathetic activation can lead to bradycardia or several seconds of asystole, which can be avoided by premedicating the patient with intravenous glycopyrrolate. The parasympathetic effect lasts until onset of the akinetic seizure, when sympathetic tone increases and produces tachycardia, an elevation in blood pressure, and increased myocardial demand for oxygen. These changes can be corrected with intravenous esmolol. At the same time, because of the enhanced neuronal metabolic rate, augmented blood flow to the brain increases intracranial pressure. This elevated sympathetic tone causes ECT-related myocardial ischemia, tachyarrhythmias, and potential rupture of aortic or intracranial aneurysms. The elevated intracranial pressure may lead to brain herniation in patients with a space-occupying lesion. Older patients have a high rate of prolonged confusion, arrhythmias, and falls after ECT. A structured medical evaluation before ECT can address risks and the potential for complications (Fig. 442-1). All effort must be made to optimize the patient's active medical conditions before ECT. For high-risk patients, one must require that ECT be performed in a setting that allows immediate access to an intensive care unit rather than in the ECT suite of a self-standing psychiatric hospital. Essential medications should be administered with a small amount of fluid 6 hours before ECT. Drugs that can increase or decrease the seizure threshold, such as lidocaine, theophylline, phenothiazine, tricyclic antidepressants, and benzodiazepines, must be discontinued before ECT. Optimal pre-ECT risk assessment, careful anesthesia, and post-ECT monitoring result in a serious complication rate of only 0.9% and essentially no fatalities.

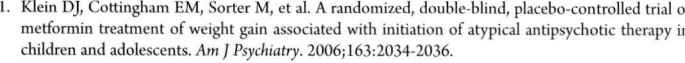

1. Klein DJ, Cottingham EM, Sorter M, et al. A randomized, double-blind, placebo-controlled trial of metformin treatment of weight gain associated with initiation of atypical antipsychotic therapy in children and adolescents. *Am J Psychiatry.* 2006;163:2034-2036.
2. Wu RR, Zhao JP, Guo XF, et al. Metformin addition attenuates olanzapine-induced weight gain in drug-naïve first-episode schizophrenia patients: a double-blind, placebo-controlled study. *Am J Psychiatry.* 2008;165:352-358.
3. Josiassen RC, Goldman M, Jessani M, et al. Double-blind, placebo-controlled, multicenter trial of a vasopressin V2-antagonist in patients with schizophrenia and hyponatremia. *Biol Psychiatry.* 2008;54:1097-1100.

SUGGESTED READINGS

Lipscombe LL, Levesque L, Gruneir A, et al. Antipsychotic drugs and hyperglycemia in older patients with diabetes. *Arch Intern Med.* 2009;169:1282-1289. *The risk for hospitalization owing to hypoglycemia was substantially increased by current use of antipsychotic drugs.*

Ray WA, Chung CP, Murray KT, et al. Atypical antipsychotic drugs and the risk of sudden cardiac death. *N Engl J Med.* 2009;360:225-235. *Both typical and atypical antipsychotic drugs increased the risk for sudden death about two-fold.*

Taylor D, Meader N, Bird V, et al. Pharmacological interventions for people with depression and chronic physical health problems: systematic review and meta-analyses of safety and efficacy. *Br J Psychiatry.* 2011;198:179-188. *Comprehensive review including medication side effects.*

XXVIII

SKIN DISEASES

443

STRUCTURE AND FUNCTION OF THE SKIN

DAVID A. NORRIS

KEY FUNCTIONS OF THE SKIN

The skin, which is the largest organ in the body, is a tough, resilient barrier that covers the body and shields the muscle compartment and internal structures. The structure of the skin varies considerably from one area of the body to another, including changes in the thickness of its components and in its specialized structures of epithelial origin (e.g., hair, nails, sweat glands, and sebaceous glands). The skin is commonly affected in diseases, and it is often damaged by external stimuli such as radiation, sunlight, toxins, irritants, allergens, and infectious agents.

The skin serves critical functions:

- *Protection.* Melanin pigment and antioxidant enzymes are positioned in the epidermis to protect the skin against radiation. The thick reticular dermis is a barrier to injury and trauma as well as a cushion for underlying structures. The epidermis resists friction and tangential stress. The stratum corneum, which is an impenetrable barrier to external substances, is thickened on the palms and soles to provide padding and protection.
- *Thermoregulation.* Evaporation from eccrine sweat glands is critical for thermoregulation. Vascular dilation and constriction help regulate the exchange of heat in the skin to preserve heat in cold climates and eliminate heat after exercise.
- *Immunologic response.* The skin is the outermost arm of the immune response and is designed to defend against infection, transformed cells, and toxins by means of highly developed innate and acquired local immune responses.
- *Barrier to water loss.* The stratum corneum is the critical component of normal skin that prevents transepidermal water loss.
- *Secretion of wastes.* Eccrine and apocrine sweat glands transport wastes and also provide excretion of odiferous substances.
- *Sensation.* The skin is the largest sensory organ. The skin and mucous membranes are the principal sites of pleasurable sensation and also sites of unpleasant sensations.

STRUCTURE OF THE SKIN

The skin consists of two distinct layers: the *epidermis* and the *dermis* (Fig. 443-1). The skin is derived from two germinal cell lineages: the ectoderm, which gives rise to the epidermis; and the mesenchyme, which produces the dermis. These two layers are joined at a basement membrane zone termed the *basal lamina*.

The epidermis, which is a stratified squamous epithelial layer, contains several different levels of structure and function. It is held together by distinctive adhesion structures termed *desmosomes* (Fig. 443-2). The *stratum corneum*, which is the product of the dying epidermis, resists the penetration of external organisms and toxins and prevents water loss. The *basal lamina* is a very complex structure of epidermal- and dermal-derived proteins that attach the epidermis to the dermis and resist shear stress.

The *papillary dermis* is a collagenous matrix containing the blood vessels that feed the epidermis. The *reticular dermis* is a tougher cushion protecting underlying tissue and containing the epidermal adnexal structures. The blood vessels and nerves are separated into a superficial plexus in the papillary dermis and a deeper plexus that serves the adnexal structures. The dermis is separated from the fascia and underlying muscle by a layer of subcutaneous adipose tissue that allows the skin to move freely relative to deeper internal structures.

The epidermally derived adnexal structures (eccrine sweat glands, apocrine sweat glands, sebaceous glands, and hair follicles) are anchored in the dermis but penetrate the epidermis and the barrier of the stratum corneum (see Fig. 443-1). The hair follicle is a cycling structure containing specialized populations of epithelial cells, pigment cells, and mesenchymal cells that control the hair cycle. Eccrine sweat glands discharge sweat directly through the stratum corneum. Apocrine sweat glands discharge their products into hair follicles. Sebaceous glands drain into sebaceous hair follicles on the scalp, face, chest, back, axilla, and groin. An extensive network of blood vessels and nerves serves the skin. The superficial vascular plexus feeds the epidermis through an extensive complex of capillary loops in the papillary dermis. The deep vascular and nerve plexus serve the adnexal structures in the dermis. The hair follicles, with their apocrine and sebaceous glands, and the eccrine sweat glands are potential avenues for transepidermal absorption of drugs because they penetrate the stratum corneum.

Cells of the Epidermis and Epidermal Differentiation

The epidermis is a stratified squamous epithelium composed mostly of keratinocytes, with other resident cells in distinct locations (melanocytes, Langerhans cells, and Merkel cells). In response to various stimuli, migrating cells such as lymphocytes, dermal macrophages, neutrophils, and eosinophils enter the epidermis. Keratinocytes are attached firmly to each other through desmosomes (see Fig. 443-2), which connect to the rigid keratin intermediate filament network and give the epidermis strength. The basal layer of the rigid epidermis connects to the basement membrane zone by means of hemidesmosomes, which are highly organized adhesion structures linked to the basal keratin network. Adherens junctions link surrounding keratinocytes and connect them to the actin microfilament network. These junctions provide more plastic adhesions that are also involved in actin-mediated movement, and the dendritic structure of melanocytes and Langerhans cells depend on attachment of these cells to keratinocytes through E-cadherin-containing adherens junctions.

Keratinocytes and Epidermal Differentiation
Epidermal Differentiation

Epidermal differentiation is a genetically programmed process by which keratinocytes differentiate from proliferating cells in the germinative layer to form tightly attached "prickle" cells in the malpighian layer, dying cells in the granular layer, and corneocytes in the stratum. During this process, keratinocytes undergo tremendous changes reflecting their different functional characteristics. Keratinocytes are named for the intermediate filament protein keratin, which forms insoluble stiff filaments that give the epidermis its strength. The keratins are made of tetramers composed of two basic and two acidic keratins (K5/14 in the basal layer, K1/10 in the spinous layer, K6/16 in the hyperproliferative epidermis, K9/19 in the palms and soles). Keratin has versatile properties and is the major component of hair and nails in humans and of beaks, hooves, and feathers in other animals.

The attachments within the epidermis are formed by desmosomes and adherens junctions. The adherens junctions that form between keratinocytes are characterized by homophilic binding of cell surface cadherins and by binding of the adhesion structure to actin microfilaments within the cell by catenins (Fig. 443-3A). Desmosomes are composed of molecules called desmogleins and desmocollins, which are homologous to cadherins and form adhesion structures with keratins through numerous associated proteins such as plakoglobin and plakophilin (see Fig. 443-3B). The basal keratinocytes are attached to the basal lamina at the hemidesmosome, a specialized adhesion structure linked to the basal cell keratin filament network (see Fig. 443-3C). The progressive differentiation of the epidermis is associated with specific changes in protein expression and function.

Functions of the Epidermal Layers

The *germinative (basal) layer* of the epidermis is responsible for cell proliferation. This layer is resistant to apoptosis because of defenses maintained by receptors for growth factors and matrix molecules. The germinative layer can become a migrating epithelial tongue to aid in wound healing.

The *spinous layer* produces a dense keratin filament network (keratins 1/10) that interacts with desmosomes, and it synthesizes involucrin (which is involved in protein cross-linking with the plasma membrane in the granular layer), a protective antioxidant network (glutathione reductase, peroxidases, catalases), cytokines, chemokines, lamellar bodies, and keratohyaline granules.

Cells in the *granular layer* undergo programmed cell death (apoptosis). Keratohyaline granule profilaggrin is activated into filaggrin, thereby inducing keratin cross-linking. Lamellar body contents are secreted into the extracellular space by fusion of the lamellar body to the cell membrane. Cross-linking of involucrin and cornifin to the cell membrane by transglutaminase produces a thickened, cornified envelope. Protein synthesis ceases as

FIGURE 443-1. **The skin and adnexal structures.** The relationship of the epidermis and its adnexal structures (sebaceous and sweat glands and hair follicles) to the dermis and subcutaneous adipose tissue is shown. Note how these structures are associated with breaks in the barrier of the stratum corneum.

Adherens junction ○ Desmosome 🛢 Hemidesmosome ⌒

FIGURE 443-2. **Cell attachment in the epidermis.** The epidermal keratinocytes, melanocytes, and Langerhans cells form a network of attachments crucial to normal epidermal function.

FIGURE 443-3. Molecular aspects of key epidermal adhesion structures and connection of the epidermis to the dermis. A-C, These structures are crucial to the normal integrity of the skin. Mutations or autoimmune damage to these structures has devastating effects on skin function. HSP = heat shock protein.

cells die to form intact corneocytes, which contain cross-linked keratin filaments and a thick cornified envelope.

Flat corneocytes surrounded by phospholipid lamellae form the impervious *stratum corneum*. Although the cornified layer provides a thin, flexible barrier to protect sensitive cells from the external environment, some molecules can diffuse through the cornified layer. Indeed, this transepidermal route is the major route of penetration of topical medications (Chapter 445). After a defined period, desquamation of superficial corneocytes occurs by enzymatic degradation of extracellular material.

Melanocytes

Melanocytes, which are dendritic cells that synthesize and secrete the pigment melanin, are derived from neural crest cells and typically migrate to the epidermal-dermal junction during embryonic development, although a few can be found in the dermis. Melanocytes are localized in the basal layer of the epidermis, with the ratio of melanocytes to keratinocytes ranging from about 1:4 to about 1:10 at different locations in the skin. The relative number of melanocytes is roughly the same for both genders and for all races, approximately 1500 melanocytes per square millimeter of skin surface. A totally separate population of melanocytes resides in hair follicles that produce pigmented hairs. Differences in the coloration of skin are therefore determined by the relative activity of these cells, not their numbers. Epidermal melanocytes are attached to the basal lamina by integrin receptors, and they are attached to surrounding keratinocytes by E-cadherin–mediated attachments. Melanin pigment is synthesized in melanocyte-specific organelles termed *melanosomes*. Melanosome transfer is achieved when

keratinocytes actively engulf the melanosome-containing cytoplasmic tips of the dendritic processes of the melanocytes. Exposure to ultraviolet (UV) light increases the rate of formation of melanosomes and enhances their rate of delivery to keratinocytes.

Melanin is a complex heteropolymer that absorbs light across the entire UV and visible spectrum; it provides the most effective protection of the skin against solar radiation. Melanization is a complex biochemical process controlled largely by three genes: tyrosinase (rate-limiting step), which oxidizes tyrosine to 3,4-dihydroxyphenylalanine (dopa); tyrosinase-related protein 1 (TyRP-1); and tyrosinase-related protein 2 (TyRP-2). Control of melanization is a complex genetic and environmental process involving more than 150 genes. One important level of control is binding of melanocyte-stimulating hormone to the melanocortin-1 receptor (MC-1R) on melanocytes. The enzymes that control melanization are transported into the melanosome, where the biochemical processes occur in a protected organelle-bound environment. The whole organelle is then transported to keratinocytes, where it resides in a "helmet" location above the nucleus. Polymorphisms in MC-1R control the relative amounts of the three key enzymes. Decreases in TyRP-1 and TyRP-2 lead to the production of pheomelanin, a brown-red pigment with inferior photoprotective properties. This type of pigment is seen in red-haired individuals and is associated with decreased sun protection, increased photoaging, and a higher rate of melanoma and nonmelanoma skin cancer. UV light can transform melanocytes into malignant melanoma, the most deadly form of skin cancer (Chapter 210).

Melanocytes are terminally differentiated cells with no stem cell population to repopulate interfollicular melanocytes. A melanocyte precursor population in the outer root sheath of the hair follicle can be mobilized to repopulate lost interfollicular melanocytes—an approach to repigmentation that is used to treat human vitiligo. However, melanocyte stem cell populations are believed to exist in the hair follicle, where they replenish the melanocytes of the hair bulb during each cycle of hair regeneration in the transition from telogen to anagen (see Hair).

Langerhans Cells

Dendritic Langerhans cells are an important subset of antigen-presenting cells located in the midportion of the epidermis. These cells become more abundant at sites of inflammatory skin disorders, including allergic reactions such as contact dermatitis (Chapter 446). Langerhans cells are migratory, and they contain characteristic striated, rodlike structures known as Birbeck granules. They also bear several important immunologic cell surface receptors (DC1, major histocompatibility complex [MHC] class II, immunoglobulin G [IgG] receptor, C3 receptor). In contact sensitization (contact dermatitis), Langerhans cells internalize and process antigen, migrate to regional lymph nodes, and present the antigen to naïve lymphocytes. When the antigen is reapplied to skin (challenge), the Langerhans cells again process and present the antigen to sensitized lymphocytes in the skin or in lymph nodes.

Merkel Cells

Merkel cells are scattered among the basal keratinocytes and are often found near or in contact with very fine, unmyelinated nerves, with which they form synapses. Merkel cells are present singly or in clusters called tactile corpuscles. They are attached to adjacent epidermal cells by numerous desmosome connections, but their tonofilaments, unlike those of keratinocytes, are not grouped into bundles. In the cytoplasm of Merkel cells are numerous membrane-bound dense granules that contain catecholamines. It is believed that Merkel cells serve as adapting mechanoreceptors. Merkel cell tumors are uncommon but are among the most deadly of skin cancers.

Dermal-Epidermal Junction

The dermal-epidermal junction is a transitional zone in which the basal layer of the epithelium is connected to penetrating deep collagenous anchors that originate in the papillary dermis. The connection is composed of collagenous rods, globular domains, and cruciate protein complexes that form a firm attachment that resists friction and tangential stress. This junction, which is the weakest structure point in the skin, is the site of blistering induced by cold, heat, and immunologically and genetically mediated blistering disorders.

Downgrowths of the epidermis form tiny ridges, called rete pegs, that add bonding surface area between the dermis and epidermis. The sandwiched basal lamina follows the ridges, which are more pronounced in areas of high abrasion. The lamina has three zones: the lamina lucida, the lamina densa, and the fibroreticular lamina. Keratin filaments in the basal cells anchor in the hemidesmosomes, which connect to anchoring filaments of the lamina lucida and then to the dense collagen and heparan sulfate proteoglycan matrix of the lamina densa. Anchoring fibrils of type VII collagen form the fibroreticular lamina and end in the anchoring plaques that intercalate with type III and VI collagen in the papillary dermis.

Dermis

The thickness of the dermis varies considerably in different parts of the body. For descriptive purposes, the dermis is divided into the papillary layer, which is the thinner layer next to the epidermis, and the reticular layer, which is composed of denser connective tissue and constitutes the bulk of the dermis. The papillary layer, which forms the dermal papillary ridges, is composed of collagen and reticular and elastic fibers that are woven into a loose network. The dermis contains many different cell types, including fibroblasts, fibrocytes, macrophages, leukocytes, and plasma cells. The vascular supply to the skin is confined to the dermis, where small arteries enter from the subcutaneous tissue and form deep and superficial sheetlike plexus. Capillary loops ascend into the dermal papillae and return through the venous plexus. The postcapillary venule portion of the vascular network, which is where leukocytes enter the tissue, is an important target of damage in allergic vasculitis. The nerve supply to the skin is very extensive and consists of both myelinated and nonmyelinated fibers. Specialized sensory structures such as pacinian and Meissner's corpuscles are located prominently in the hands and feet. Because up to 4 to 5% of the total blood volume can be stored in the dermis, it plays an important role in thermal regulation; sympathetic nerve fibers control blood flow to and from the skin.

Epidermal Appendages of the Skin

Sebaceous Glands

Sebaceous glands, or oil glands, are found throughout the dermis except for the palms of the hands and the soles of the feet. Most of these glands, which are greatly activated at the onset of puberty, discharge their contents through a single duct into the lumen of hair follicles. Where these glands occur independently of hairs (e.g., the glans penis, lips, labia minora, and eyelids), they open directly onto the surface of the skin. Sebaceous secretions contain triglycerides, waxy esters, squalene, cholesterol, and fatty acids.

Eccrine Sweat Glands

Eccrine sweat glands are positioned over the entire skin but are concentrated most densely in the palms, the soles, and the head. Eccrine sweat glands, which number about 3 million, are innervated by postganglionic, cholinergic sympathetic nerves. Excess heat causes sweating to begin on the forehead and to spread elsewhere over the body. Eccrine sweat glands secrete a watery solution that is high in sodium chloride but also contains urea, uric acid, potassium, and immunoglobulins.

Apocrine Sweat Glands

Apocrine glands are scent glands whose secretion is increased by fear, sexual excitement, and other forms of heightened tension. Apocrine glands are present in the axilla, the external genitalia, the areolar skin around nipples, and the perianal area, and they develop following the onset of puberty. Specialized apocrine glands include Moll's glands on the eyelid and ceruminous (wax) glands in the auditory canal.

Nails

The nail is composed of a proximal germinative epithelium that is called the nail matrix, a keratinized product that is called the nail plate or body, an underlying specialized epithelium that is called the nail bed and is attached to the undersurface of the nail, and a protective loop of skin that is called the proximal nail fold. Underlying the proximal part of the body of the nail is a collection of germinal cells that form an opaque spot on the nail, the lunula. The lunula is the site of the proliferating nail matrix that is responsible for growth of the nail.

Hair

There are three types of hair follicles: vellus hair follicles located over most of the body; terminal hair follicles located on the scalp, beard area, axilla, groin, and other hairy areas; and sebaceous hair follicles located on the scalp, face, beard, chest, back, axilla, and groin. Sebaceous hair follicles have a minimal hair shaft but hypertrophied sebaceous glands. Terminal hairs form the long hairs of the scalp and beard. The hair follicles of the eyelashes and eyebrows also have specialized characteristics determined by local mesenchymal factors.

Hairs are dead shafts composed of fused plates of keratin that project from the surface of the epidermis. Hair does not grow continuously but rather passes through a cycle (Fig. 443-4). Anagen is the growth phase. Then comes a short catagen stage in which portions of the hair follicle involute and growth ceases. Next is the telogen, or resting, phase. After a telogen phase of 3 to 4 months, a new anagen hair develops from the follicular stem cells, and the existing hair falls out or is easily pulled out. The hair cycle depends on synchronized cooperation among four major components of the hair follicle: the dermal papilla, the hair matrix, the outer root sheaths, and the stem cells in the bulge region. During the actively growing anagen phase of the hair cycle, signals from the dermal papilla maintain the proliferating hair matrix. When these signals terminate, the follicle enters the catagen phase in which the matrix and root sheaths of the lower follicle die by apoptosis. The follicle then enters a resting telogen phase. When the follicle re-enters the anagen phase, signals from the dermal papilla stimulate stem cells in the bulge region of the follicle, and these cells migrate to form the new matrix, initiate a new hair shaft, and cause the old hair to fall out. In normal follicles in young healthy adults, the anagen phase is almost 3 years, and the telogen phase is about 3 months. At any time, 10 to 15% of the hairs are in telogen on a healthy young scalp.

In telogen effluvium, the shift to telogen is abrupt, and hairs fall from the scalp precipitously in 3 months when new anagen hairs are formed in the follicles. This pattern is commonly seen 3 to 4 months after a severe systemic illness or at the termination of pregnancy. A gradual shift to the telogen phase occurs with age and is even greater in androgenetic alopecia.

SPECIALIZED ASPECTS OF SKIN STRUCTURE AND FUNCTION

Skin-Associated Immune System

The skin is the most external component of the immune response, with well-developed elements of both the innate and acquired immune systems (Chapter 44). The barrier of the stratum corneum is broken by adnexal structures such as hair and sweat glands, and infections in these sites are suppressed by a network of innate immune responses and defenses. The skin is also a principal site for invasion by bacteria, parasites, and viruses, and it is an important site of tumor induction; all these processes are influenced by a well-developed acquired immune response. The skin contains several populations of antigen-presenting cells, including the epidermal Langerhans cells. Trafficking of T cells to the skin occurs through skin-specific homing receptors such as the cutaneous lymphocyte antigen.

The skin's innate immune system includes macrophages, dendritic cells, and neutrophils as well as a very extensive epidermal network of cytokines (e.g., interleukin-1 [IL-1] and tumor necrosis factor-α [TNF-α]) and chemokines. The skin has a number of receptors for foreign organisms (CD14, toll-like receptors, mannose receptors), defensins and other antimicrobial peptides, and networks that augment and inhibit complement in the papillary dermis.

The skin's acquired immune system includes an epidermal network of specialized dendritic cells (Langerhans cells) plus dermal dendritic cells. The cutaneous lymphocyte antigen stimulates the trafficking of lymphocytes to the skin. Both T_H1 and T_H2 responses are well developed in skin, but most inflammatory skin diseases have a T_H1 response. Hair follicles may be immunologically privileged sites because they lack MHC class I.

Control of Apoptosis in the Skin

Apoptosis is a normal part of the cycle of epidermal differentiation. In the granular cell layer, transglutaminase-mediated cross-linking of involucrin initiates formation of the cornified envelope, which is a specialized apoptotic envelope. Unlike other apoptotic cells, the corneocyte is not phagocytized or fragmented. Epidermal stem cells, melanocytes, and proliferating transit-amplified cells of the basal and suprabasal epidermis are resistant to apoptosis, owing to defenses against apoptosis mediated by integrin and growth factor receptor ligation. Integrin and growth factor expression are lost in the differentiating epidermal compartment, and these cells are susceptible to apoptosis induced by chemotherapy, activation of death receptors such as Fas, and UV radiation (Fig. 443-5). In the granular cell layer, apoptosis initiates terminal changes in keratinocytes, thereby producing the dead corneocytes that are the "bricks" of the stratum corneum.

Endothelial cells are also resistant to apoptosis by virtue of their attachment to basement membrane proteins through integrin receptors and because of antiapoptotic proteins that are induced during inflammation to protect these cells. Conversely, during vessel remodeling, the antiapoptotic defenses decrease, and endothelial cells die.

Activated lymphocytes, Langerhans cells, and granulocytes that enter the skin are all sensitive to apoptosis. Most phototherapy protocols to treat inflammatory skin diseases rely on UV light–induced apoptosis to destroy Langerhans cells and lymphocytes, whereas the relative resistance of keratinocytes and melanocytes to UV light protects the normal underlying skin cells.

Ultraviolet Radiation and the Skin

The skin is uniquely susceptible to damage induced by exposure to radiation from the sun. Visible and UV light penetrates into the skin and produces important biologic effects. Some effects, such as photoactivation of vitamin D, are beneficial, but most are damaging.

The skin has a number of natural defenses against UV light. First, melanin, a heteropolymer that is transferred from melanocytes to keratinocytes, protects the basal keratinocytes against UV radiation. Second, antioxidant enzymes (e.g., catalase, peroxidase, thioredoxin, and superoxide dismutase) protect skin cells against oxidant damage. Macrophages are induced by UV radiation to enter the epidermis to remove damaged cells. UV radiation also induces Langerhans cells to exit the epidermis and present antigens to T cells

FIGURE 443-4. Hair follicle cycle. Communications among the dermal papilla, the matrix, the follicle sheath, and the stem cells control the hair cycle through its anagen, catagen, and telogen phases.

FIGURE 443-5. Epidermal differentiation. Differentiation of the epidermis, controlled by growth factor receptors and integrin receptors, also modulates the susceptibility of the epidermis to apoptosis induced by external and internal triggers. BM = basal membrane; EGF = epidermal growth factor; EGFR = EGF receptor; FGF = fibroblast growth factor; FGFR = FGF receptor; GF = growth factor; GFR = GF receptor; IGF = insulin-like growth factor.

TABLE 443-1 CLINICAL ASSOCIATIONS WITH PRURITUS

SKIN DISEASES

Dermatitis, including contact dermatitis
Bullous disorders, especially dermatitis herpetiformis and bullous pemphigoid
Drug effects (opiates, aspirin, quinidine)
Urticaria and angioedema
Lichen planus
Sunburn
Seborrheic dermatitis
Infestations (e.g., scabies, pediculosis)
Xerosis (dry skin)
Irritant particles (e.g., fiberglass, "itching powder")

SYSTEMIC DISEASES

Uremia
Obstructive biliary disease (primary biliary cirrhosis, cholestatic hepatitis, cholestasis of pregnancy, extrahepatic biliary obstruction)
Hematologic and myeloproliferative disorders (lymphoma, polycythemia vera, iron deficiency anemia)
Endocrine disorders (thyrotoxicosis, hypothyroidism, diabetes, carcinoid)
Carcinomas (breast, stomach, or lung)
Psychiatric disorders (e.g., delusional states, stress, psychosis)
Neurologic disorders (e.g., multiple sclerosis, notalgia paresthetica, neuropathy)
Mastocytosis (urticaria pigmentosum, telangiectasia macularis eruptiva perstans)

TABLE 443-2 TOPICAL TREATMENTS FOR PRURITUS

MEDICATION	DOSE	COMMENTS
Topical corticosteroids	Variable	Not directly antipruritic, may be useful in pruritus due to inflammatory skin dermatoses
Topical calcineurin inhibitors	Tacrolimus 0.03 and 0.1% ointment Pimecrolimus 1% cream	Particularly useful in anogenital pruritus; may cause transient burning and stinging
Doxepin	5% cream	20-25% risk for sedation
Menthol	1-3% cream or lotion	Useful in patients who report cooling as an alleviating factor
Capsaicin	0.025-0.1% cream	Particularly useful in neuropathic itch, may cause transient burning
Salicylic acid	2-6%	Useful in lichen simplex chronicus, avoid in acute inflammatory dermatoses
Local anesthetics	Pramoxine 1.0-2.5%	Useful on face and for chronic kidney disease
Cannabinoids	Creams containing N-palmitoylethanolamine	Useful in atopic dermatitis and chronic kidney disease

Adapted from Patel T, Yosipovitch G. Therapy of pruritus. *Expert Opin Pharmacother.* 2010;11:1673-1682.

in regional lymph nodes. Finally, keratinocytes release large amounts of IL-1 and TNF-α in response to UV radiation, and a complex system of antagonists and decoy receptors buffer the epidermis from cytokine-induced damage.

Despite these defenses, UV radiation damages keratinocytes and induces malignancy. UV radiation damage also induces both local and systemic immunosuppression, and it can induce autoimmunity when apoptotic keratinocyte autoantigens are presented to lymphocytes in patients with diseases such as lupus erythematosus.

Itching

The sensations of both itch and pain are transmitted by unmyelinated C fibers. It is assumed that the receptors are the free nerve endings in the dermis and epidermis. Multiple compounds induce pruritus: amines (histamine and serotonin), proteases (papain, kallikrein, trypsin), neuropeptides (substance P, vasoactive intestinal peptide, calcitonin gene–related peptide), eicosanoids, opioids, cytokine growth factors, and products of eosinophils and platelets. Many of these compounds act through their effects as mast cell degranulators. Histamine is the major itch-inducing product of mast cells, but other mediators are also involved. Pruritus is a frequent component of many skin and systemic diseases (Table 443-1).

Pruritus is a common clinical problem whose treatment is often unsatisfactory. Treatment of any underlying skin or systemic disease is necessary for long-term success. Drugs that inhibit the effects of mast cell products (H_1- or H_2-blocking antihistamines, antileukotrienes) or that inhibit mast cell degranulation (phosphodiesterase inhibitors, β-agonists) are effective as oral agents. Common options include topical therapies (Table 443-2) and systemic therapies (Table 443-3). Neuropeptide-mediated itching can be inhibited by desensitization with capsaicin. Opiate antagonists block the central opiate receptors that induce the pruritus associated with opiate use. UV radiation treatment can effectively treat the intractable pruritus that occurs in patients with renal failure.

Wound Healing

The skin is the major target of wounding in most people and is the preeminent model used to study wound healing in animals and humans. Wound healing is a complex process with three sequential phases: inflammation, proliferation and tissue formation, and tissue remodeling. The phase of tissue remodeling extends for weeks and months after the closure of wounds, and the fibroblast is the cornerstone of remodeling of the dermis, vessels, and basement membrane.

Vascular abnormalities (arterial insufficiency, venous stasis, and microangiopathy) are commonly associated with poor wound healing. Poor wound healing is also a serious problem in patients with chronic infections or malnutrition. Patients with extensive skin disease, especially mechanobullous or immunobullous disorders such as epidermolysis bullosa or pemphigus, likewise demonstrate defects in wound healing. Efforts to promote wound healing in these situations focus on repair and reversal of vascular disease,

TABLE 443-3 SYSTEMIC TREATMENTS FOR PRURITUS

MEDICATION	DOSE	COMMENTS
Antihistamines	Chlorpheniramine 4 mg Loratadine 10 mg Fexofenadine 60 to 180 mg	Sedating, but no direct effect on pruritus, except in urticaria
Antidepressants SNRIs	Mirtazapine 7.5-15 mg orally at bedtime	Nocturnal pruritus; may increase appetite and weight
SSRIs	Paroxetine 10-40 mg orally per day Fluvoxamine 25-150 mg orally per day Sertraline 75-100 mg orally per day	Psychiatric patients and paraneoplastic pruritus Psychiatric patients and paraneoplastic pruritus Cholestatic pruritus
μ-Opioid receptor antagonists	Naltrexone 25-50 mg orally per day	Pruritus associated with cholestatic or chronic kidney disease; can cause nausea, vomiting, and drowsiness
Neuroleptics	Gabapentin 100-3600 mg orally per day Pregabalin 150-300 mg orally per day	Neuropathic pruritus; can cause drowsiness and weight gain
Substance P antagonist	Aprepitant 80 mg orally per day	Sézary's syndrome
Immunosuppressants	Cyclosporine 2.5-5 mg/ kg orally per day	Short-term use for refractory atopic dermatitis; monitor blood pressure and renal function
	Azathioprine 1.0 to 2.5 mg/ kg orally per day	Refractory atopic dermatitis; monitor for myelosuppression

SNRI = serotonin-norepinephrine reuptake inhibitor; SSRI = selective serotonin reuptake inhibitor.
Adapted from Patel T, Yosipovitch G. Therapy of pruritus. *Expert Opin Pharmacother.* 2010;11:1673-1682.

reversal of tissue edema, application of growth factors to stimulate angiogenesis and keratinocyte migration, and the use of antibiotics to decrease local infection.

SUGGESTED READINGS

Buddenkotte J, Steinhoff M. Pathophysiology and therapy of pruritus in allergic and atopic disease. *Allergy.* 2010;65:805-821. *Review.*

Patel T, Yosipovitch G. Therapy of pruritus. *Expert Opin Pharmacother.* 2010;11:1673-1682. *Review.*

444

EXAMINATION OF THE SKIN AND APPROACH TO DIAGNOSING SKIN DISEASES

CHERYL A. ARMSTRONG

● EXAMINATION OF THE SKIN

The examination of the skin is a critical component of the comprehensive medical approach to the patient. By learning how to examine the skin and approach the diagnosis of skin diseases, the physician can focus on the lesions that warrant therapy or provide important information about the systemic health of the patient. Other lesions may be of cosmetic concern to the patient even though they have little or no medical significance.

As the organ system that is an interface with the environment, the skin has an extensive array of mechanical, biochemical, immunologic, and neurologic properties that both inform and protect each individual. The skin also has a vast ability to alter its cellular and acellular components in response to internal or external insults, a process that leads to changes that are subsequently defined as disorders or diseases. The physical examination of the skin can provide information about both cutaneous and systemic diseases, and the examination can sometimes diagnose serious medical conditions at an otherwise asymptomatic stage.

Skin disorders can usually be visualized directly by both the patient and the physician. For example, the patient not only feels the itch and discomfort of an allergic contact dermatitis reaction to poison ivy but also sees the vesicular and crusted skin lesions. The appearance of new lesions or a sudden change in existing lesions can elicit emotional reactions in patients or their family members. The physician must learn to see the same eruptions using a careful and systematic approach that leads to a specific and treatable diagnosis.

History and Physical Examination

Most dermatologists conduct the dermatologic history and examination simultaneously. The physician can best focus the history and full skin examination by first visualizing the lesion or lesions that constitute the patient's primary skin complaint. Because there are hundreds of described dermatoses, the systematic approach is based on pattern recognition.

Physical Examination
Setting

A skin examination can be conducted in virtually any medical setting. It is most effectively performed in an office equipped with an examination table, adequate natural or artificial fluorescent lighting, examination gowns for patients to wear, and a sink for thorough handwashing before and after each examination. If natural light through a window is used, it is critical to ensure the patient's privacy inside the examination room. A movable focused artificial light beam and a lighted magnifying glass can be used to shine obliquely on the skin to assess the elevation of skin lesions. Many dermatologists prefer to examine all lesions at a 1:1 ratio without magnification, but others prefer magnifying certain types of lesions to ascertain morphologic features. For example, the follicular plugging of the lesions of discoid lupus erythematosus (Chapter 274) or the telangiectasias associated with a basal cell carcinoma (Chapters 210 and 448) may be better appreciated with magnification. Gowns that can be positioned to uncover parts of the skin surface while leaving other parts covered help ensure the patient's comfort during the examination.

Precautions

Universal precautions against infectious diseases should be practiced during every skin examination or cutaneous procedure. Handwashing with soap and warm water or the use of hand sanitizing gels or foams ensures that the physician is taking appropriate steps to avoid spreading organisms from a previous patient. As patients become more aware of the spread of infections by health care providers, it can be useful for the physician to cleanse his or her hands in the presence of the patient, rather than outside the examination room. When examining intact skin, it is not necessary to wear gloves. For the protection of both the patient and physician, gloves should be worn when the physician touches nonintact skin surfaces. Because of the increasing incidence of allergies to latex in the health care setting, the use of nonlatex gloves should be considered for all patients. Gloves should be discarded after the examination is complete or after touching the mouth or the genital area.

Total Body Examination

A total body skin examination is usually recommended for each new patient to assess existing pigmented lesions and determine whether any are serious, although there are no data to document the yield of such an approach (Chapter 14). With the steady increase in squamous cell carcinoma, basal cell carcinoma, and cutaneous melanomas over the past several decades, the total body skin examination is an opportunity to diagnose lesions in an early treatable stage as well as to educate patients about their own risk factors for developing skin cancer. Subsequently, total body skin examinations can be scheduled at 3- to 12-month intervals for patients at high risk for developing new or recurrent malignant lesions (Chapter 210), whereas patients at low risk should be examined at less frequent intervals, such as every 1 to 3 years.

Many dermatologists approach this examination by using the following sequence: face (forehead, eyelids, lips, ears, nose, cheeks, chin), neck, scalp and hair, back, chest, abdomen, arms, hands (including palms and fingernails), legs, and feet (including soles and toenails). Having the patient change into a comfortable gown with undergarments removed facilitates the ease of the examination. Some dermatologists perform part of the examination with the patient in a sitting position and part of the examination with the patient lying back on the examination table. The goal is to ensure that the skin can be well visualized and that the patient is comfortable with the amount of skin being exposed at one time.

Assessing Skin Features

Basic skin features such as skin pigmentation, skin turgor, abnormal skin color (jaundice, pallor), and the degree of photodamage to sun-exposed skin surfaces should be assessed, and these findings guide the medical history and subsequent, detailed examination. For example, patients with lightly pigmented skin and evident photodamage to the hands and face warrant a careful history to inquire about prior skin cancers in themselves and their immediate family members as well as a full body skin examination to look for precancerous or potentially malignant lesions of which the patient may be unaware. Patients with abnormal skin color, such as a yellow hue (jaundice; Chapter 149) should be questioned about known medical conditions, examined for any other cutaneous signs associated with disease of that organ, and assessed with the appropriate laboratory studies.

It is often helpful to touch the lesion and the skin surrounding the lesion. Features such as firmness, movability from the underlying skin, fluctuance, and depressibility are helpful in characterizing the lesion. Darier's sign, which is the appearance of an urticarial wheal and flare reaction after rubbing a skin lesion, is observed in lesions that contain large numbers of mast cells (e.g., urticaria pigmentosa) and is the result of the mechanical degranulation of the mast cells and the resulting release of histamine. Nikolsky's sign is dislodgement of the epidermis with the appearance of a moist, glistening defect after pushing, rubbing, or rotating normal skin near bullous lesions; this sign is typical of disorders in which epidermal cells are not well adhered together (e.g., pemphigus and toxic epidermal necrolysis).

Obtaining the History

After seeing and palpating the lesion, the physician can obtain a more detailed history and continue with a more comprehensive examination of the skin as indicated. Pertinent questions should assess duration of the lesion or eruption, what the lesion looked like when it first began, how the lesion feels (e.g., itch, sting, tenderness, pain), and how the condition has changed since it was first noticed. It is also helpful to inquire about a history of prior similar lesions and how they progressed. A medication history is important because both systemic and topical medications can cause or exacerbate a number of skin conditions. It is also important to inquire specifically about how the patient may have tried to treat the lesion because many treatments can change the natural appearance of the lesion.

The past medical history should be targeted to obtain information about major illnesses, especially those that would lead to immunodeficiency states, as well as prior dermatologic diseases. The presence of known heritable dermatologic conditions in the family should be determined. In particular, patients should be specifically questioned about a personal or family history of atopic dermatitis, hay fever, or asthma (atopy). All patients should be asked about a personal or family history of malignant melanoma and nonmelanoma skin cancers. The social and work history can also provide critical clues to the diagnosis of a particular skin condition because many are related to occupational or recreational activities. A travel history to determine whether patients have encountered environmental stresses such as sun, heat, or cold or have been exposed to parasitic infestations can also be useful. Because psychological stress can exacerbate many dermatoses, it is useful to inquire about overall levels of anxiety and stress or recent stressful situations.

After visualizing the lesion of concern, it is often helpful to look systematically at all the skin again. It is also important to watch the patient's behavior in the examination room. Many patients think that they should not scratch lesions and they tell the physician that the lesions itch but that they do not scratch. However, direct observation shows the patient rubbing, tapping, scratching, or picking the lesion while engaged in conversation with the physician. These behaviors can change a primary lesion to a secondary lesion.

Melanoma

Patients at high risk for the development of melanoma require the most comprehensive skin examinations, commonly by a dermatologist. Photography (conventional or digital) and detailed "maps" of the nevi may be used over time to assess changes in lesions or the presence of new lesions that warrant removal. A hair dryer at the low setting can be used to blow aside the hair to allow visualization of the entire scalp. The skin of the external and internal labia is examined for pigmented lesions in women. The comprehensive skin examination is also an ideal opportunity to educate the patient about performing self-examinations that include exposed and unexposed skin including the buttocks, posterior thighs, and calves.

● DIAGNOSING SKIN DISEASES

Categorization of Skin Lesions

Four major features of skin lesions or eruptions allow the skin disease to be placed in diagnostic categories that facilitate specific diagnosis: (1) the morphologic appearance of the individual lesions, (2) the distribution of lesions over the body surface, (3) the arrangement of the lesions, and (4) the number of lesions present. This information also enables the physician to determine whether the lesions are primary or secondary in nature. Primary lesions are defined as those that represent the initial pathologic change; secondary lesions result from external forces such as scratching, picking, or infection of primary lesions. An experienced dermatologist can often make the diagnosis from this descriptive information before even seeing the patient.

Morphology of Lesions

The morphology of individual lesions can be described in the following ways (Table 444-1): (1) whether they are flat, raised above the surface of the skin, or depressed; (2) the range of their size; (3) whether they are solid or contain fluid; and (4) how their color compares with the patient's normal skin. Morphologic terms have been developed to assess alterations in the stratum corneum and dermal or subcutaneous tissue. For example, the stratum corneum in psoriatic plaques can be silvery in color with densely adherent layers so that it looks like the mineral mica; this pattern is called a *micaceous scale*. Another usual morphologic feature is whether the individual lesions are monomorphic or polymorphic: all monomorphic lesions are the same shape, size, color, and consistency. Certain diseases, such as eruptive xanthoma, almost always have monomorphic papules, whereas other diseases, such as

TABLE 444-1	TERMINOLOGY TO DESCRIBE THE MORPHOLOGY OF INDIVIDUAL SKIN LESIONS	
TERM	**DEFINITION**	**EXAMPLE**
PRIMARY SKIN LESIONS: INITIAL PATHOLOGIC CHANGE		
Macule	Circumscribed change in skin color that is flush with the surrounding skin. Lesion is <1 cm in diameter.	Solar lentigo Traumatic purpura
Patch	Circumscribed change in skin color that is flush with the surrounding skin. Lesion is ≥1 cm in diameter	Cafe au lait spot Vitiligo
Papule	A solid or cystic elevation <1 cm in diameter	Acne Eruptive xanthoma
Nodule	A solid or cystic elevation >1 cm but <2 cm in diameter	Dermatofibroma
Tumor	A solid or cystic elevation >2 cm in diameter	Follicular cyst
Plaque	An elevated lesion that is >1 cm in diameter	Psoriasis
Scale	Desiccated, thin plates of cornified epidermal cells that form flakes on the skin surface	Ichthyosis
Wheal	Circumscribed, flat-topped, firm elevation of skin with a well-demarcated and palpable margin	Urticaria
Vesicle	Circumscribed, elevated lesion containing clear serous or hemorrhagic fluid that is <1 cm in diameter	Contact dermatitis Herpes simplex
Bulla	Circumscribed, elevated lesion containing clear serous or hemorrhagic fluid that is >2 cm in diameter	Bullous pemphigoid
Pustule	A vesicle containing purulent exudate	Folliculitis
Atrophy	A depression from the surface of the skin with underlying loss of epidermal or dermal substance	Lichen sclerosis et atrophicus
Erosion	A depression from the surface of the skin with a loss of all or part of the epidermis Can be a secondary lesion	Burn Ruptured bulla
Ulceration	A depression from the surface of the skin with a loss of the entire epidermis and at least some of the dermis Can be a secondary lesion	Ecthyma Excoriation of acne papule
SECONDARY SKIN LESIONS: RESULT FROM EXTERNAL FORCES SUCH AS SCRATCHING, PICKING, INFECTION, OR HEALING OF PRIMARY LESIONS		
Lichenification	Dry, leathery thickening of the skin with exaggerated skin markings	Chronic eczema
Scar	An elevated or depressed area of fibrosis of the dermis or subcutaneous tissue resulting from an antecedent destructive process	Healing wound
Fissure	A deep linear split in the skin extending through the epidermis	Traumatized eczema
Crust	Dried exudates of serum, blood, sebum, or purulent material on the surface of the skin	Acute and/or secondarily infected eczema

acne, are more likely to have polymorphic lesions that may represent either changes over time or a basic variability.

Distribution of Lesions

Many skin diseases commonly affect particular parts of the body surface (Table 444-2). In certain cases, the pattern of distribution is consistent with our understanding of the pathogenesis of a disease. For example, acne lesions are found on the parts of the skin that contain the highest concentration of sebaceous glands, which are known to be involved in the development of acne. Other skin diseases are precipitated or caused by sun exposure, and their lesions are present only in sun-exposed areas of the body (e.g., lupus erythematosus or phototoxic drug eruptions). Dermatologic disorders that are the direct result of the patient's manipulation of the skin are found only where the patient can reach (e.g., the posterior shoulders but not the middle of the back).

The pattern of distribution, although poorly understood from a pathogenetic perspective, is extremely helpful for diagnosis (Fig. 444-1). For example, psoriasis often symmetrically affects the scalp, extensor arms and legs (elbows, knees, and shins), umbilicus, intragluteal cleft, and fingernails (Fig. 444-2; Chapter 446). Psoriatic lesions can involve the entire body surface, but an awareness of their common distribution guides the physical examination and aids accurate diagnosis. Conversely, atopic dermatitis (Chapter 446) typically involves the flexural arms and legs (antecubital fossae and popliteal fossae), wrists, nipples, and eyelids.

It is important to examine the mucous membranes of the mouth and the genital areas. Lichen planus (Chapter 446), a papulosquamous skin disease, often involves the volar wrists, shins, buccal mucosa, and shaft of the penis.

In lichen planus, the oral and genital lesions may be asymptomatic, and the medical history cannot substitute for a careful physical examination.

Arrangement of Lesions

The arrangement of several lesions in relation to each other can provide valuable diagnostic information. Terms that are commonly used to describe the relationship of lesions to each other include *clustered, grouped, linear, zosteriform, annular,* and *coalescing* (Table 444-3). *Clustered* lesions are arranged within a few millimeters of each other. When vesicular lesions are clustered on an erythematous base, the word *herpetiform* is used to describe their arrangement because this is the classic appearance of herpes simplex (Fig. 444-3; Chapters 382 and 447). *Grouped* lesions are arranged in the same body site, such as over a shoulder or elbow. A *linear* arrangement of lesions looks like a geometric line over any part of the body surface. One type of linear arrangement is called *koebnerization* (or the Koebner phenomenon), which occurs in particular skin diseases, such as psoriasis, in which new lesions evolve after traumatic injury. Linear lesions are frequently seen in allergic contact dermatitis if the offending antigen brushed against the skin to create a linear pattern of dermatitis. This pattern often results when a plant such as poison oak brushes against the skin (Fig. 444-4). A *zosteriform* arrangement refers to usually unilateral lesions in the cutaneous distribution of a spinal nerve dermatome; herpes zoster (Chapters 383 and 447) is the classic zosteriform dermatosis, but other lesions can arise in this arrangement. *Annular* lesions, which are round to oval with an area of central clearing, often consist

TABLE 444-2 PREFERENTIAL DISTRIBUTION OF SELECTED SKIN DISEASES

DISTRIBUTION ON THE SKIN	SKIN DISEASE
Skin chronically exposed to sunlight (face, neck, hands, arms)	Actinic keratosis, basal cell carcinoma, squamous cell carcinoma
Central chest, shoulders, and earlobes	Keloids
Extensor arms and legs, intragluteal cleft, umbilicus	Psoriasis
Antecubital fossa, popliteal fossa	Atopic dermatitis
Anterior surface of lower legs	Palpable purpura, pretibial myxedema, necrobiosis lipoidica diabeticorum, erythema nodosum
Axilla and inguinal areas	Hidradenitis suppurativa
Posterior neck and back	Folliculitis
Web spaces of toes and sides of feet	Tinea pedis
Web spaces of fingers and wrists	Scabies
Palms and soles	Secondary syphilis, erythema multiforme

FIGURE 444-2. The distribution of psoriatic lesions is often symmetrical over the extensor surfaces of the skin.

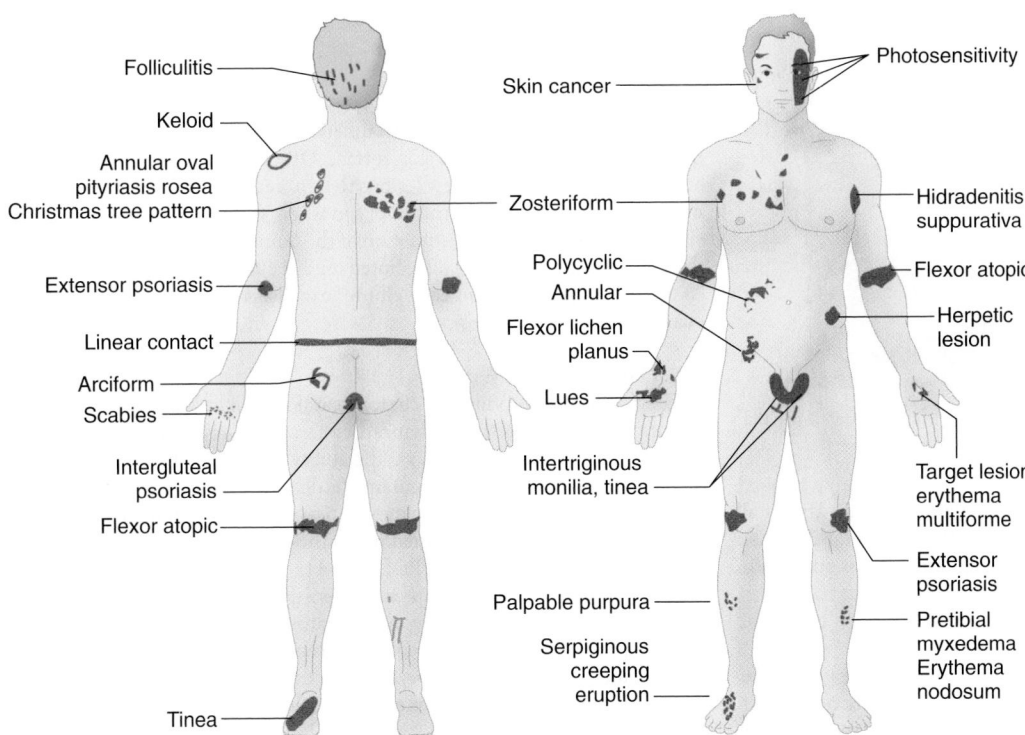

FIGURE 444-1. Configurational and regional diagnostic aids for the diagnosis of primary and secondary skin lesions.

TABLE 444-3 ARRANGEMENT OF SKIN LESIONS

TYPE OF ARRANGEMENT	EXAMPLE OF SKIN DISEASE
Clustered	Herpes simplex
Grouped	Lichen planus Granuloma annulare Dermatitis herpetiformis
Linear	Allergic contact dermatitis Epidermal nevus Morphea Koebnerized psoriasis
Zosteriform	Herpes zoster Metastatic breast carcinoma Hemangiomas of Sturge-Weber syndrome
Annular without scale	Secondary syphilis Lupus erythematosus Urticaria Hansen's disease (leprosy)
Annular with scale	Dermatophytosis Pityriasis rosea Erythema annulare centrifugum
Coalescing	Psoriasis Drug hypersensitivity eruption Viral exanthema Urticaria

FIGURE 444-3. This arrangement of vesicular lesions clustered on an erythematous base, seen here in a patient with herpes simplex, is termed *herpetiform*.

FIGURE 444-4. Allergic contact dermatitis occurring in a linear arrangement when the offending antigen, such as poison oak, is brushed against the skin in this way.

of an arrangement of smaller lesions in this configuration. Finally, almost all types of lesions can coalesce, meaning that individual lesions merge into each other. *Coalescing* lesions often assume annular or figurate patterns on the skin (Chapter 446).

Number of Lesions

At the most extreme, an eruption can cover nearly 100% of the skin surface. At the other end of the spectrum, only one or two lesions may be present. Certain diseases are characterized by an overall typical number of lesions on

TABLE 444-4 MORPHOLOGY-BASED CLASSIFICATION OF MAJOR SKIN DISORDERS

GROUP	CLINICAL MORPHOLOGY	EXAMPLES OF DISEASES IN THE GROUP
Eczematous dermatitis	Erythematous macules, papules, vesicles, lichenification, fine scaling, excoriations, crusting	Contact dermatitis, atopic dermatitis, stasis dermatitis, photodermatitis, exfoliative dermatitis
Maculopapular eruptions	Macules, erythema, papules	Viral exanthems, drug hypersensitivity reactions, Kawasaki disease, vasculitic, purpuric eruptions
Papulosquamous dermatoses	Papules, plaques, and erythema with scales	Psoriasis, reactive arthritis, pityriasis rosea, lichen planus, seborrheic dermatitis, ichthyosis, secondary syphilis, mycosis fungoides
Vesiculobullous diseases	Vesicles, bullae, erythema	Herpes simplex and zoster, hand-foot-and-mouth disease, insect bites, bullous impetigo, scalded skin syndrome, pemphigus, bullous pemphigoid, dermatitis herpetiformis, porphyria cutanea tarda, erythema multiforme
Pustular diseases	Pustules, cysts, erythema	Acne vulgaris rosacea, pustular psoriasis, folliculitis
Urticaria and cellulitis	Wheals and figured, raised erythema, scaling	Urticaria, erythema annulare centrifugum, and erysipelas
Nodular lesions	Nodules and tumors, some associated with erosions and ulceration	Benign and malignant tumors—basal cell cancer, squamous cell cancer, rheumatoid nodules, xanthomas
Telangiectasia, atrophic, scarring, ulcerative diseases	Atrophic, sclerotic telangiectasia, ulcerative changes	Connective tissue diseases, radiation dermatitis, lichen sclerosus et atrophicus, vascular insufficiency (arterial and venous), pyoderma gangrenosum
Hypermelanosis and hypomelanosis	Increased and decreased melanin deposition in skin	Acanthosis nigricans, cafe au lait spots, vitiligo, tuberous sclerosis, xeroderma pigmentosum, melasma, freckles

the skin. For example, patients with tuberculoid leprosy generally have fewer than five lesions on the entire skin surface. Other diseases, such as granuloma annulare, can range from a few lesions to hundreds of lesions. Sometimes the number of lesions is an indication of the severity of the disorder, as in widespread psoriasis. A general estimation of the number of lesions such as "more than 50 flat-topped papules distributed on the shins and wrists bilaterally" or "8 to 10 orange papules on each elbow" can also assist in guiding the physician to the correct diagnosis.

Major Classifications

After carefully identifying the clinical features of skin lesions or eruptions, the physician can use the recognized patterns to classify the disease into a general category of skin disorders. The ability to identify the clinical features of a lesion's morphology allows cutaneous disorders to be placed in categories that narrow the differential diagnosis to a reasonable number of choices, which can then be further refined by considering the distribution, arrangement, and number of lesions (Table 444-4).

Eczematous dermatitis (Chapter 446) is a common superficial skin inflammation that is characterized by erythematous macules and papules in the early and mild stages. These changes can progress to vesiculation, oozing, fine scaling, and crusting. Because eczematous dermatitis is associated with pruritus (itching), the patient often excoriates the involved skin. In the chronic setting, lichenification caused by repeated rubbing is a typical secondary

FIGURE 444-5. Allergic contact dermatitis on the arm at the site of application of a topical antibacterial ointment to treat a burn wound. This cutaneous allergic response manifests as erythematous macules, papules, and vesicles where the allergen comes in contact with the skin.

FIGURE 444-7. Psoriasis is characterized by erythematous, scaling papules and plaques.

FIGURE 444-6. Palpable purpura (nonblanching red macules and papules) on the lower legs is typical of many types of cutaneous vasculitis.

FIGURE 444-8. Arthropod bite reactions on the skin of the back appear as multiple papulovesicles with surrounding erythema from assault by sand fleas while the patient was sleeping on the beach.

clinical feature of eczematous dermatitis. The localized distribution of an eczematous eruption at the site of allergen exposure helps distinguish allergic contact dermatitis (Fig. 444-5) from other types of eczematous dermatoses, such as atopic dermatitis and stasis dermatitis, that tend to be bilaterally symmetrical and involve particular areas of the skin.

Maculopapular eruptions (Chapter 447) are characterized by erythema, macules, and papules. Many of these cutaneous eruptions, such as viral exanthems and drug eruptions, are often symmetrical, bilateral, and widespread. Cutaneous vasculitis shows clinical features of erythematous macules and papules that are commonly most prominent on the lower legs or other dependent portions of the skin. When the red macules and papules in vasculitic processes do not blanch with pressure, they are termed *palpable purpura* (Fig. 444-6).

Papulosquamous lesions (Chapter 446) are defined as papules with scaling. Psoriasis is a chronic proliferative epidermal disease that typifies the papulosquamous skin disorders. This inflammatory disease, which may have a genetic component, often begins with red macules that progress to scaly papules and plaques (Fig. 444-7). Psoriatic plaques have a propensity to develop on the elbows, knees, and scalp but can involve any part of the skin. If the psoriatic process becomes widespread, the entire skin surface can be involved, and the syndrome is then termed *erythroderma*.

In vesiculobullous diseases (Chapter 447), cleavage at particular levels in the epidermis or dermis results in the clinical appearance of vesicles or bullae, often with surrounding erythema. This broad morphologic group comprises genetic and acquired diseases with a variety of etiologies. For example, insect (arthropod) bite reactions are a common cause of vesiculobullous lesions with surrounding erythema, distributed in patterns that relate to the site of interaction with the particular offending insect (Fig. 444-8).

The hallmark of pustular skin diseases (Chapter 447) is the presence of small, circumscribed, elevated lesions containing purulent exudates, often with associated erythema. Cystic lesions are pustular lesions larger than

FIGURE 444-9. Monomorphous follicularly oriented pustules on the chest are seen in folliculitis.

1 cm. Pustules may be sterile, as in pustular psoriasis, or may contain microbial organisms, as in acne (Chapter 447). Folliculitis is a pustular skin infection located within hair follicles and often surrounded by erythema (Fig. 444-9).

Skin disorders arising as urticaria (Chapter 448) or cellulitis (Chapter 449) share clinical features of wheals, figured raised erythema, and occasionally scaling. Urticaria is an inflammatory mast cell–mediated process that may have an allergic or nonallergic cause and is characterized by clinical lesions called wheals, which are evanescent, erythematous, rounded or flat-topped, elevated (edematous) lesions (Fig. 444-10). Although the borders of a wheal are sharply demarcated, they tend to be transient and may appear and disappear in a matter of hours. Wheals may be round, oval, serpiginous, or annular in appearance and can range in size from several millimeters to more than 10 cm. Itching is often intense in the affected skin but resolves as the wheal

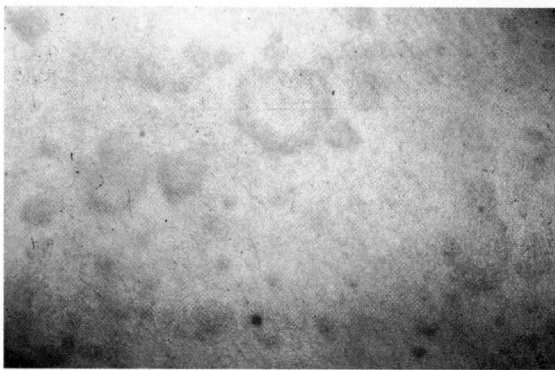

FIGURE 444-10. This eruption consisting of evanescent, annular wheals is termed *urticaria*.

FIGURE 444-11. This nodule represents a neglected basal cell carcinoma. The lesion is well defined and sharply demarcated from normal skin. The rolled smooth border with telangiectasias surrounds several crusted ulcerations.

FIGURE 444-12. This single plaque of morphea manifests as localized induration of the skin with central atrophy and hypopigmentation with a peripheral rim of erythema.

FIGURE 444-13. Widespread hypopigmented and hyperpigmented macules on sun-exposed skin are a clinical feature of xeroderma pigmentosum after exposure to normal amounts of sunlight over time.

FIGURE 444-14. *Candida albicans.* Potassium hydroxide examination of candidal skin lesion shows short, stubby hyphae and budding yeast elements.

fades. In contrast to urticaria, the erythematous, raised lesions seen in cellulitis have an infectious cause and tend to expand in a centrifugal pattern until appropriate antibiotic treatment is initiated.

Nodular lesions (Chapter 448) may be single or multiple nodules and may have associated erosions or ulcerations. Basal cell carcinoma (Chapter 210), a common malignant tumor of the skin, is linked to decades of cutaneous sun exposure (Fig. 444-11). In addition, a large variety of inflammatory and infectious diseases of the skin are associated with nodular lesions.

Skin diseases sharing the morphologic features of telangiectasia, atrophy, scarring, and ulceration can be classified together, although there is a wide range of causes, including connective tissue diseases, such as localized or systemic scleroderma. A localized type of cutaneous scleroderma, termed *morphea* (Chapter 275), is characterized by single or multiple discrete patches or plaques of indurated skin, often accompanied by cutaneous atrophy and pigmentary changes (Fig. 444-12).

Hypermelanosis and hypomelanosis (Chapter 449) occur in a wide range of cutaneous disorders in which there is increased or decreased melanin deposition in the skin. These skin lesions may appear dark (hyperpigmented), as seen with cafe au lait spots, or pale (hypopigmented), as seen with vitiligo. Xeroderma pigmentosum is a rare, genetic disease in which patients cannot repair DNA damage induced by ultraviolet irradiation and develop early freckling that progresses to widespread hypopigmented and hyperpigmented macules over time (Fig. 444-13). Most important, without meticulous protection from ultraviolet irradiation of the skin, these patients suffer from cutaneous neoplasms, including malignant melanoma (Chapter 210), in the early decades of life.

Diagnostic Tests

After a reasonable differential diagnosis has been created, diagnostic tests can narrow the differential or confirm the correct diagnosis. Several diagnostic tests can be performed in the physician's office after collecting material from the surface of the skin. The potassium hydroxide preparation of scale and pustules is used to look for microscopic hyphae or pseudohyphae that indicate the presence of a dermatophyte infection or yeast infection (Fig. 444-14; Chapter 446). The Gram stain of pustules or bullae is used to determine whether bacteria are present or whether the lesion is sterile (Chapter 447). The Tzanck preparation of the base of a vesicle is used to look for rounded, multinucleated keratinocytes that indicate a herpesvirus infection (Fig. 444-15; Chapter 447). The oil mount of skin scrapings from the base of a burrow or pruritic papule is used to look for the mites or eggs that indicate a scabies infestation (Fig. 444-16; Chapter 367). When an infection is suspected, it is often necessary to obtain specimens for culture by swabbing

FIGURE 444-15. Tzanck smear of herpes simplex. Positive Tzanck smear is seen as multinucleated giant cell.

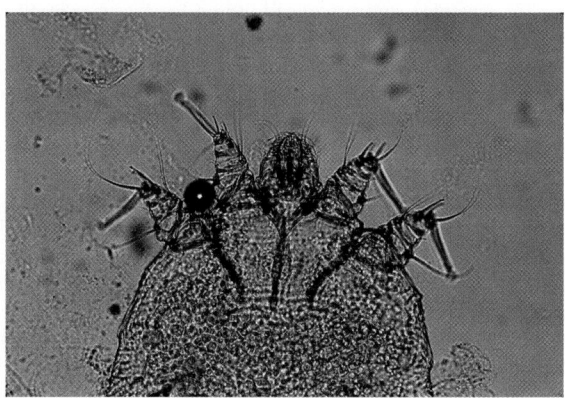

FIGURE 444-16. A scabies mite is seen on this microscopic examination of an oil mount of a scraping taken from the end of a small burrow on the wrist.

pustules, bullae, or abscesses. Any overlying crust should be removed before obtaining the culture specimen. Scale from the surface of the skin can also be sent for fungal culture to increase the detection of dermatophyte infections, especially those involving the nails.

Skin Biopsy

Skin biopsies are performed to aid in the diagnosis of cutaneous infections and in the histologic diagnosis of inflammatory and neoplastic skin disorders. If bacterial cellulitis is suspected, tissue from the dermis can be obtained by performing a punch biopsy of the affected skin and submitting the core of tissue for bacterial culture. To diagnose deep fungal or mycobacterial infections, tissue usually must be obtained by this type of biopsy and sent for culture under appropriate temperature conditions.

Skin biopsies of cutaneous growths or inflammatory eruptions are an essential tool when the diagnosis is not certain (Fig. 444-17). The term *biopsy* may also be applied to the surgical removal of benign skin lesions such as warts and skin tags. Many dermatologists follow the general practice of sending all excised skin tissue for histologic assessment.

Biopsy of Possible Malignancy

Any lesions that have features of basal cell carcinoma or squamous cell carcinoma should undergo biopsy (Chapters 210 and 448). Clinical indications for biopsy of lesions suspected to be malignant include lesions that fail to heal, increase in size, bleed easily, or ulcerate spontaneously. Actinic keratoses, which are considered to be precancerous lesions, are usually treated without preceding biopsy. The usual biopsy approach to nonmelanotic lesions that protrude from the surface of the skin is to perform either a snip biopsy (with scissors) or a shave biopsy (with a blade). If the entire lesion is removed, it can be considered an excisional biopsy.

 Excisional Biopsy	Complete lesion removed with margin of normal skin down to adipose tissue. Useful if suspect melanoma, skin cancer, small bulla	
 Incisional Biopsy	Cross-section wedge of tissue through center of lesion. Useful when lesion is too big to excise and diagnosis is unsure (e.g., keratoacanthoma vs. squamous cell carcinoma)	
 Shave Biopsy	Horizontal shave of the skin lesion with only superficial portion of dermis. Use only to remove benign lesions, as may not get entire depth of lesion. Leaves largest scar. Never use if suspect melanoma	
 Punch Biopsy	For sampling possible cancers, tumors, and inflammatory skin conditions. Multiple biopsies can be done to obtain more extensive sampling	

FIGURE 444-17. Methods of skin biopsy.

Punch Biopsy

For inflammatory skin lesions, it is usually necessary to obtain tissue down to subcutaneous fat for an accurate assessment of the inflammatory process. A punch biopsy using an instrument 3 to 8 mm in diameter to "core out" a piece of skin tissue is the preferred approach. If multiple lesions are present, it is prudent to select a lesion that is not in a cosmetically important area because a scar will occur at the punch biopsy site but to be sure to select a representative lesion that has not been altered by scratching, infection, or lichenification. The punch biopsy wound heals best when closed with one to two sutures, but it can be left to heal by granulation. Some inflammatory skin disorders, especially bullous disorders, have characteristic autoantibody deposition that can be assessed by direct immunofluorescence of biopsy tissue. This test is performed in specialized dermatopathology laboratories.

The approach to biopsy of lesions that have clinical features of malignant melanoma is critical. First, there is only one opportunity to obtain tissue correctly to maximize the chance of accurate diagnosis. Second, an improperly obtained biopsy specimen can make it impossible to assess the patient's risk for metastatic disease. When malignant melanoma is suspected, the lesion should be removed entirely with an elliptical excisional biopsy; margins of normal skin are not included in the excised tissue. A shave biopsy should be avoided because it does not allow the full depth of the lesions to be determined histologically. The thickness of the lesion remains the most accurate way to predict metastatic disease and is critical for planning adjuvant therapy (Chapters 210 and 448). A punch biopsy should be avoided because it does not provide the dermatopathologist with the full histologic architecture of the lesion. When clinical features of a pigmented lesion of the skin are highly suggestive of malignant melanoma, the patient should usually be referred to a dermatologist before performing the biopsy to ensure that the most accurate histologic information is obtained to guide clinical treatment.

SUGGESTED READINGS

Garg A, Haley H-L, Hatem D. Modern moulage—evaluating the use of 3-dimensional prosthetic mimics in a dermatology teaching program for second-year medical students. *Arch Dermatol.* 2010;146:143-146. *Teaching sessions using three-dimensional prosthetic skin lesions improved both short-term and long-term lesion recognition by medical students.*

Kantor J, Kantor DE. Routine dermatologist-performed full-body skin examination and early melanoma detection. *Arch Dermatol.* 2009;145:873-876. *Full examination of the skin by dermatologists increases diagnosis of early melanomas over skin examinations focused on lesions of concern to the patient.*

Wolff T, Tai E, Miller T. Screening for skin cancer: an update of the evidence for the U.S. preventive services task force. *Ann Intern Med.* 2009;150:194-198. *Due to a lack of controlled studies, there is no accurate estimation of the benefits of screening for skin cancer in the general primary care population.*

PRINCIPLES OF THERAPY OF SKIN DISEASES

VICTORIA P. WERTH

The goal of therapy is to improve a skin condition with the least toxic and most specific approach. Because many treatments or medications can be applied directly to the skin, the option for topical therapy is attractive for treating many dermatologic diseases. However, many diseases require systemic therapy, particularly when patients have widespread involvement of the skin or a disease that cannot be improved with topical therapy. Therapies work by improving barrier function, removing scale, altering inflammation in the skin, altering blood flow, providing antimicrobial effects, or affecting proliferating cells. Recent advances in the understanding of cutaneous biology have not been routinely accompanied by evidence-based documentation of the benefits of many specific therapies.

PRINCIPLES OF TOPICAL THERAPY

Soaks and Dressings

Water or saline applied by soaks and wet dressings can be beneficial for many skin conditions, including ulcers, by promoting healing of the epidermis and débridement of crusts. Soaked gauze is applied to involved areas for 15 to 30 minutes several times a day, and care should be taken not to allow the gauze to dry and adhere. If adherence occurs, the gauze should be soaked before the dressing is removed. Use of strong antiseptic solutions, including hydrogen peroxide, is not recommended because of toxicity to cells. Whirlpool action can enhance débridement. When large areas of skin are involved, baths are a convenient way to treat the skin with medications that reduce itching and inflammation. The best time to apply moisturizers that help trap water in the upper layers of skin is immediately after a bath or shower.

Wet-to-dry dressings are rarely used, except when initial vigorous wound débridement is necessary. Continued use after wounds are débrided traumatizes wounds and delays healing. Moist wound healing, which is often ideal, can be accomplished with a topical antibiotic such as a combination of polymyxin B and bacitracin (Polysporin) or mupirocin (Bactroban), gauze impregnated with petrolatum (Vaseline), or an occlusive hydrocolloid dressing. Little evidence indicates that débriding enzymes are beneficial. Compression with an Unna or multilayered boot, which includes an elastic dressing such as Coban, can decrease local edema and facilitate wound healing. Polysporin/petrolatum gauze or occlusive dressings are placed underneath, an approach that is helpful for chronic venous, diabetic, and pressure ulcers, as well as for acute wounds. Closed wet dressings, in which gauze is soaked and then covered with an impervious material, can help when maceration and heat retention are needed. Biologic dressings with skin substitutes or keratinocytes can be beneficial for wounds that are resistant to healing. Skin grafts can also facilitate healing of otherwise nonhealing wounds. Platelet-derived growth factor, which is approved for use on diabetic ulcers, can modestly improve wound healing.

Topical Medications

Topical medications mix an active drug with preservatives, emulsifying agents, and an appropriate base or vehicle. Systemic absorption varies among patients, sites, and vehicles. Topically applied drugs are absorbed more readily through inflamed, thin skin. The base can be any of the following: a *powder*, which promotes dryness and is used to reduce maceration in intertriginous areas; a *lotion*, which is a suspension of oil in water; *solutions*, which include water, alcohol, and propylene glycol, but not oil; *gels*, which are solid at room temperature but melt on contact with the skin; a *cream*, which is an emulsion of oil in water that leaves a thin oil coating as the water evaporates; an *ointment*, which combines oils, such as petrolatum (Vaseline), with small amounts of water and which is more occlusive and hence increases the absorption of medication but also results in a greasier appearance; a *paste*, which is a mixture of powder and ointment; or a *spray*. Lotions, solutions, and gels provide less penetration than ointments do, but they are especially useful for the treatment of hair-bearing areas such as the scalp, where greasiness is displeasing. Creams are less greasy than ointments and are useful for the face, groin, and intertriginous areas. Ointments are often more effective for dry, scaly conditions such as eczema and psoriasis and are helpful in areas that have thick skin, such as the palms and soles, but they should be avoided in infected or intertriginous areas. The choice of base is determined by the skin condition and location. Impregnated tapes are another delivery method to provide occlusion and protect the skin from manipulation.

ANTI-INFLAMMATORY AGENTS

Glucocorticoids

Topical glucocorticoids work because of their effects on vasoconstriction, proliferation, immunosuppression, and inflammation. Assays related to the ability to vasoconstrict and clinical trials of efficacy have allowed glucocorticoids to be divided into various classes based on potency (Table 445-1). These medications are typically used twice a day. Side effects include atrophy of the skin, telangiectases, purpura, striae, local skin infections (e.g., folliculitis, tinea, and candidiasis), hypopigmentation, hypertrichosis, systemic adrenal suppression when these agents are used on as little as 20% of the skin's surface area, and glaucoma when they are used around the eye. Side effects are especially prevalent when fluorinated steroids are used on thin skin (e.g., face, groin, or scrotum), and prolonged use on the face can result in facial dermatitis, acne, and an eruption resembling acne rosacea that is often exacerbated when use of the steroid is terminated. Certain conditions are more responsive to steroids, and the potency of the steroid chosen must be based on the condition and its location (Table 445-2). The superpotent class I agents should be restricted to patients with severe dermatoses, and their use should normally not exceed 2 weeks. Patients who receive these potent agents require frequent follow-up and must be carefully evaluated for the need to continue strong topical steroids. Use of any fluorinated steroid on the face requires an exact diagnosis and should be limited in the extent of application and duration of use. Intralesional glucocorticoids can be injected into individual lesions to improve delivery of the medication, and this method is commonly used to treat patients with acne cysts, hypertrophic scars, keloids, alopecia areata, granuloma annulare, discoid and panniculitic lupus erythematosus (Chapter 274), psoriasis, and lichen simplex chronicus. Triamcinolone acetonide is most frequently used, followed by the longer-acting triamcinolone hexacetonide. It is important to use proper dilutions, such as 2.5 mg/mL on the face and 5 mg/mL elsewhere, to avoid local skin atrophy.

Systemic glucocorticoids are used for acute and chronic conditions in dermatology, but they should be avoided, if possible, or minimized because of their well-known side effects (Chapter 34). Acute conditions that commonly require systemic steroids include severe contact dermatitis such as poison ivy, photodermatitis, severe atopic dermatitis, and acute urticaria. Many skin conditions such as psoriasis and eczema become exacerbated when use of the steroids is tapered, so steroids should be avoided when possible in these conditions. The dose of steroid must be individualized to the condition and its severity. Steroid-sparing drugs, such as immunosuppressive agents, can be used to minimize the long-term use of steroids for selected conditions.

TABLE 445-1	RANKING OF SOME COMMONLY USED TOPICAL STEROIDS BY POTENCY
Super potency	Clobetasol propionate (Temovate ointment and cream), betamethasone dipropionate (Diprolene cream and ointment), diflorasone diacetate (Psorcon E ointment), halobetasol propionate (Ultravate ointment)
High potency	Amcinonide, mometasone furoate ointment, diflorasone diacetate (Florone ointment), halcinonide 0.1% cream, fluocinonide, desoximetasone, triamcinolone acetonide, diflorasone diacetate ointment and cream, betamethasone dipropionate (Diprosone), betamethasone benzoate and valerate
Medium potency	Fluticasone propionate; mometasone furoate cream; halcinonide 0.25% ointment; triamcinolone acetonide 0.1% cream and lotion; fluocinolone acetonide 0.2%, 0.25%, and 0.1% cream and 0.25% ointment and 0.5% solution; hydrocortisone valerate 0.2% ointment and cream; alclometasone dipropionate 0.5% ointment; betamethasone dipropionate 0.5% lotion; hydrocortisone butyrate 0.1% cream; betamethasone benzoate 0.25% cream; betamethasone valerate 0.1% cream and 0.5% lotion; flumethasone pivalate 0.3% cream; desonide 0.5% cream
Low potency	Hydrocortisone 1% cream

TABLE 445-2	CLINICAL APPLICATION OF TOPICAL GLUCOCORTICOIDS
Super potency and high potency	Plaque and palmoplantar psoriasis, lichen planus, dyshidrotic eczema, lichen simplex chronicus, granuloma annulare, sarcoidosis
Medium potency	Dermatitis: allergic contact, atopic, neurodermatitis
Low potency	Intertrigo, pruritus ani, seborrheic dermatitis

Nonsteroidal Anti-inflammatory Agents

Psoriasis Therapies

Tars and anthralin are used for psoriasis (Chapter 446). Tars are most commonly used in conjunction with ultraviolet B (UVB) light. Tars are also used in shampoos and bath oils to treat seborrhea and psoriasis. Anthralin is a synthetic hydroxyanthrone that inhibits keratinocyte proliferation; it stains and can be irritating, but it can be effective therapy (Chapter 446).

Calcipotriol

Calcipotriol is a vitamin D derivative that has antiproliferative and immunomodulatory effects on skin. Hypercalcemia can occur if more than 100 g/wk is used, so this agent cannot be used for widespread disease. It is applied twice daily, can be irritating on thin skin, and takes 6 to 8 weeks to be effective.

Retinoids

The retinoids are a group of compounds that include vitamin A and its derivatives. Their effects are mediated through several different classes of receptors, and the receptor-drug complex has effects on other regulatory proteins that affect growth factors, oncogenes, keratins, or transglutaminases. Retinoids affect cell growth, differentiation, and morphogenesis; inhibit tumor promotion and malignant cell growth; have immunomodulatory effects; and alter cell cohesion.

Topical retinoids include all-*trans*-retinoic acid (tretinoin), which is approved for acne (Retin-A) and photoaging (Renova 0.05% cream) and is also useful for hyperpigmentation, steroid-induced atrophy, and early stretch marks. Tretinoin is available as a cream (0.025%, 0.05%, 0.1%), a gel (0.01%, 0.025%), and a solution (0.05%). Adapalene (Differin 0.1% gel) and tazarotene (Tazorac) are used for acne (Chapter 447). Tazarotene is also used for psoriasis, often in combination with topical steroids to minimize irritation. Bexarotene (Targretin) 1% gel is used for the topical treatment of cutaneous lesions in patients who have refractory or persistent stage IA or IB cutaneous T-cell lymphoma. Topical retinoids can be irritating and frequently cause an exacerbation before improvement. However, they should be used regularly on lesion-prone skin to produce improvement. Moisturizers may be needed to minimize drying effects.

Systemic retinoids commonly used for the skin include isotretinoin, acitretin, and bexarotene (Targretin). They have many applications, but most frequently isotretinoin (Accutane) is used for cystic and conglobate acne, acitretin for severe psoriasis (especially the erythrodermic and pustular forms), and bexarotene for cutaneous T-cell lymphoma. Isotretinoin and acitretin have also been used to treat several forms of ichthyosis and lupus erythematosus and for the chemoprevention of skin cancers, particularly in immunosuppressed transplant recipients. The many side effects of systemic retinoids include teratogenicity, cheilitis, hair loss, headaches, hyperlipidemia, abnormal liver enzyme levels, vertebral hyperostosis, tendon and ligament calcification, osteoporosis, and central hypothyroidism with bexarotene. Pregnancy must be avoided, and the use of retinoids in women of childbearing age therefore requires careful monitoring. Treatment of acne is reserved for cases of cystic acne not responding to less toxic therapies; in this setting, a 4- to 5-month course of Accutane, 0.5 to 1 mg/kg/day, is curative in 85 to 90% of patients.

Antimalarial Drugs

Aminoquinolines include chloroquine, hydroxychloroquine, and quinacrine. These agents have inhibitory effects on pro-inflammatory cytokine production, DNA replication, and chemotaxis. They are useful in patients with connective tissue diseases, polymorphous light eruption, sarcoidosis (Chapter 95), porphyria cutanea tarda (Chapter 447), sclerosing conditions, and vasculitis. Side effects include diarrhea, headache, irritability, psychosis, skin dyspigmentation, and rarely, retinopathy. Retinopathy is rare if doses of chloroquine are 3.5 mg/kg/day or less and doses of hydroxychloroquine are 6.5 mg/kg/day or less. Combinations of hydroxychloroquine or chloroquine with quinacrine are frequently helpful when a solitary agent is inadequate. The combination of hydroxychloroquine and chloroquine should not be used because of the additive risk for retinopathy.

Dapsone

Dapsone is a sulfone that inhibits the response of neutrophils and possibly eosinophils to chemotactic stimuli. It is useful for dermatitis herpetiformis (Chapter 447), cutaneous vasculitis (Chapter 448), pyoderma gangrenosum (Chapter 143), bullous lupus erythematosus (Chapter 274), Behçet's disease (Chapter 278), and autoimmune bullous diseases (Chapter 447). Side effects include hemolysis, methemoglobinemia, peripheral neuropathy, agranulocytosis, and rarely, a hypersensitivity syndrome with hepatitis, fevers, and rash. The glucose-6-dehydrogenase level should be checked before starting the drug, and it is common for patients with a normal glucose-6-dehydrogenase level to experience a 2-g/dL decrease in hemoglobin after achieving therapeutic doses of 100 to 200 mg/day.

Thalidomide

Thalidomide has potent anti-inflammatory effects, probably resulting from inhibition of tumor necrosis factor-α. It also modifies adhesion molecules on circulating leukocytes. Thalidomide is a serious teratogen, and patients must comply with strict birth control and monitoring. It is effective at a dose of 50 to 100 mg/day, with improvement beginning in 2 weeks and a full clinical response seen in 2 to 3 months in patients with severe cutaneous lupus erythematosus (Chapter 274), erythema nodosum leprosum (Chapter 446), aphthae, Behçet's disease (Chapter 278), actinic prurigo, chronic graft-versus-host disease (Chapter 181), multiple myeloma (Chapter 193), and numerous other inflammatory dermatoses. Besides teratogenesis, the main side effects include peripheral neuropathy, constipation, sedation, and rarely, amenorrhea.

Gold

Intramuscular gold has been used to treat pemphigus vulgaris (Chapter 447), with success as a solitary agent. A total dose of 400 to 600 mg of gold is often required to stop the formation of blisters; after the initial test doses, gold is administered at 50 mg once a week.

Colchicine

Colchicine, usually at a dose of 0.6 mg twice a day, is used for leukocytoclastic vasculitis (Chapter 447) and Behçet's disease. The main side effect of this low oral dose is diarrhea.

● ANTIMICROBIAL AGENTS

Antibacterials

Topical antibiotics are used to treat superficial skin diseases, such as acne and folliculitis, that are associated with infectious organisms, as well as skin wounds and ulcers. They may work by decreasing neutrophil chemotaxis and other anti-inflammatory mechanisms. Topical solutions, gels, pledgets, and ointments are available, depending on the agent, and antibiotics include erythromycin, clindamycin, tetracycline, and metronidazole. Benzoyl peroxide also has antibacterial properties and is quite effective for mild to moderate acne (Chapter 447). Bacitracin and Polysporin ointments are typically used for wounds, but they can cause contact hypersensitivity; neomycin should be avoided because of the high incidence of allergic reactions. Mupirocin is particularly effective against *Staphylococcus* and *Streptococcus* species, and it can be used in the nose for carriers of staphylococci. Systemic antibiotics such as penicillins, cephalosporins, and erythromycin are used in patients with soft tissue infections such as impetigo, folliculitis, furuncles, carbuncles, cellulitis, ecthyma, erysipelas, postoperative wound infections, and necrotizing fasciitis. Tetracycline, doxycycline, and minocycline are used for acne, rosacea, and perioral dermatitis. Fluoroquinolones such as ciprofloxacin are useful for the treatment of gram-negative soft tissue infections.

Antifungals

Topical antifungal agents are used in patients with limited superficial fungal infections of the skin (Chapter 446). The numerous topical antifungal drugs available include the azoles (clotrimazole, econazole, ketoconazole, oxiconazole, and miconazole), which are available as creams and lotions applied once or twice daily. The creams tend to be more effective. Topical agents used for dermatophytes, but not *Candida*, are haloprogin and tolnaftate. The newer allylamine antifungals naftifine and terbinafine have fungicidal effects. Ciclopirox 8% topical solution was recently approved for use in treating and preventing relapses of onychomycosis. Nystatin creams, oral suspensions, and vaginal tablets are effective for the treatment of *Candida* infections. The combination of antifungals with potent topical steroids such as betamethasone dipropionate is not advised because of increased side effects from the steroid and decreased efficacy of the antifungal as a result of the concomitant steroid.

Systemic antifungal agents include griseofulvin, terbinafine (allylamine), ketoconazole (imidazole), itraconazole, and fluconazole. These agents are used for extensive or severe superficial skin fungal infections (Chapter 446) caused by dermatophytes, *Candida*, or *Malassezia furfur* or for local infections not responsive to topical drugs, such as those found in the nails and scalp. Itraconazole and terbinafine are the only oral antifungals approved in the United States for the treatment of onychomycosis, and griseofulvin is the only oral agent approved for tinea capitis. Griseofulvin is best taken with a fatty meal to improve absorption and is the only antifungal drug not requiring regular monitoring of liver enzymes. Griseofulvin shows weak affinity for keratin, and thus it must be used for 18 months for onychomycosis of the toenails and 6 months for the fingernails to achieve even relatively poor cure rates. Terbinafine is the only fungicidal drug, whereas the rest are fungistatic. The number of interactions with medications is lower with terbinafine than with the triazole antifungals and ketoconazole because terbinafine does not inhibit or induce hepatic isoenzyme CYP3A4 (Chapter 28). However, terbinafine affects CYP2D6, another hepatic isoenzyme, so it is relatively contraindicated in patients who are taking cyclosporine or rifampin. Itraconazole and fluconazole have been used in pulse-dosing regimens for the treatment of onychomycosis. Fluconazole and terbinafine are not dependent on gastric acidity for optimal gastrointestinal absorption. Overall, the side effects of the systemic antifungal agents are similar and include headache and gastrointestinal symptoms (griseofulvin, terbinafine), nausea and vomiting (itraconazole, fluconazole, ketoconazole), hepatitis, and lupus-like syndromes (terbinafine).

Antivirals

Verrucae are treated with various destructive modalities, including 50 to 80% dichloroacetic acid and trichloroacetic acid solutions, podophyllin resin, and podofilox. Topical antiviral creams such as penciclovir and acyclovir do not significantly shorten the course of herpes simplex. Systemic antiviral drugs include acyclovir, valacyclovir, famciclovir, and foscarnet, which are used to treat primary and recurrent herpes simplex (Chapter 382) and herpes zoster (Chapter 383), although only acyclovir is approved for treatment of herpes zoster. These agents specifically block the function of herpesvirus DNA polymerase. Valacyclovir and famciclovir are available only orally in the United States, but their prolonged intracellular half-life allows less frequent dosing than with acyclovir. Patients with herpes zoster require higher doses than do patients with herpes simplex. Side effects include nausea and headaches. The varicella-zoster vaccine has significantly decreased the incidence of herpes zoster in individuals older than 60 years.[1]

Antiparasitics

Topical antiparasitic medications are used to treat pediculosis capitis, pediculosis pubis, and scabies. In addition, topical metronidazole has anti-inflammatory properties and is used to treat rosacea. For pediculosis and scabies, clothing and bedding must be washed, and all family members must be treated. Effective treatment includes 1% γ-benzene hexachloride (lindane), a chlorinated hydrocarbon pesticide that should not be used on young children or on pregnant or lactating women. It is ineffective against nits and thus must be reapplied after 1 week. Permethrin 5% cream (Elimite) for scabies or 1% cream rinse is particularly effective for head lice and requires just one application; 10% crotamiton (Eurax) and 5% topical sulfur ointments are less effective. Malathion is a moderately toxic organophosphate insecticide, but it must be applied overnight to treat lice. Pyrethrins (RID, Nix) are best used twice, one week apart, to treat head lice and nits.

● ANTIPRURITIC OR ANESTHETIC AGENTS

Topical Analgesics

Capsaicin, an active ingredient of cayenne peppers and other plants of the genus *Capsicum*, is used for postherpetic neuralgia and other painful

TABLE 445-3   OVERVIEW OF ANTIHISTAMINES

ANTIHISTAMINE GROUP	GENERIC NAME	AVERAGE ORAL ADULT DOSES
FIRST-GENERATION H₁-TYPE ANTIHISTAMINES		
Alkylamine	Brompheniramine (Dimetapp)	4 mg q4-6h
	Chlorpheniramine (Chlor-Trimeton)	4 mg q4-6h (short acting); 8-12 mg q8-12h (long acting)
Amino alkyl ether (ethanolamine)	Clemastine fumarate	1.34 mg bid or 2.68 mg qd-tid
	Diphenhydramine (Benadryl)	25-50 mg q4-6h
Ethylenediamine	Pyrilamine (Triaminic)	30 mg bid
Phenothiazine	Promethazine (Phenergan)	10-12.5 mg qid
	Trimeprazine (Temaril)	2.5 mg q6h
Piperidine	Azatadine	1-2 mg q8-12h
	Cyproheptadine	4 mg q8h
	Diphenylpyraline	2 mg tid-qid
Piperazine	Hydroxyzine (Atarax)	25-100 mg tid-qid
SECOND-GENERATION H₁-TYPE ANTIHISTAMINES		
Alkylamine	Acrivastine (combined with pseudoephedrine in allergy medication)	8 mg qid
Piperidine	Astemizole (Hismanal)	10 mg qd
	Loratadine (Claritin)	10 mg qd
	Fexofenadine (Allegra)	60 mg bid or 180 mg qd
Piperazine	Cetirizine (Zyrtec)	5-10 mg/day
H₂-TYPE ANTIHISTAMINES		
	Cimetidine (Tagamet)	400 mg bid
	Ranitidine (Zantac)	150 mg bid
	Famotidine	10 mg bid
	Nizatidine	300 mg hs
H₁- AND H₂-TYPE ANTIHISTAMINES		
	Doxepin (Sinequan)	10-25 mg hs

bid = twice daily; hs = at bedtime; qd = once daily; qid = four times daily; tid = three times daily.

nerve-related conditions. It causes excitation of neural afferent C fibers and reduces substance P levels. Capsaicin causes a burning sensation and is applied four to five times daily for 5 to 6 weeks. Eutectic mixture of local anesthetic (EMLA) is a mixture of lidocaine and prilocaine that is used under occlusion to induce cutaneous anesthesia before a procedure. Lidocaine can be used as a topical anesthetic, but benzocaine should be avoided because it is a sensitizer.

Antipruritic Agents

Doxepin 5% cream is used for localized pruritus. Menthol is a cyclic terpene plant alcohol used for non–histamine-related itching. Pramoxine hydrochloride is a topical anesthetic used for mild to moderate itching. Oral antihistamines play an important role in controlling pruritus in many skin conditions (Table 445-3), especially those mediated by histamine, such as urticaria, angioedema, and urticaria pigmentosa. The sedating and anticholinergic properties of many H₁-receptor antihistamines probably account for some of their efficacy. H₁-receptor antihistamines are the cornerstones of routine therapy, and if an agent from one group of H₁-receptor antihistamines is ineffective, an agent from a different class should be administered or combined. Second-generation H₁-receptor antihistamines are less sedating and are used if patients cannot tolerate or do not improve after taking first-generation agents. The combination of two different H₁-receptor antihistamines can be used when a solitary agent does not work; in particular, use of a sedating antihistamine at night and a second-generation antihistamine during the day can be helpful. The skin contains both H₁- and H₂-receptors, and occasionally combining H₁- and H₂-receptor antagonists can be beneficial. Usually, first-generation agents (e.g., hydroxyzine, 10 to 25 mg every 6 hours) are started at low doses and increased as tolerated, and regular continuous dosing is recommended. The tricyclic antidepressant doxepin, normally started at 10 to 25 mg at bedtime, has both anti–H₁- and H₂-receptor activity, but it interacts with drugs metabolized by the cytochrome P-450 pathway. Side effects of commonly used first-generation antihistamines include sedation, dry mouth, blurred vision, constipation, and urinary retention, and lower doses may be required in elderly patients. The recommended dose for second-generation antihistamines (e.g., fexofenadine, 60 mg twice daily) should not be exceeded.

AGENTS THAT IMPROVE SURFACE FUNCTIONS (LUBRICATION, SCALE)

Moisturizers

Moisturizers improve skin by diminishing scale and increasing water content. They usually contain mixtures of water and fatty substances such as petrolatum, lanolin, lanolin derivatives, and fatty alcohols. Greasy moisturizers tend to function better, but they are less acceptable cosmetically.

Keratolytics

α-Hydroxy acids (lactic acid, glycolic acid, citric acid, glucuronic acid, pyruvic acid) are extremely effective keratolytics. They are helpful in treating disorders of keratinization and photoaging, as well as acne. Propylene glycol, used in 40 to 60% aqueous solutions, can decrease scaling. Salicylic acid, which works by decreasing keratinocyte adhesion and hydrating keratins, is used in a range of concentrations with many different bases to remove scale, to soften the stratum corneum, or as destructive therapy to remove warts and calluses. Urea is used in varying concentrations to treat scaling.

IMMUNE THERAPIES

Hormonal Therapies

Systemic therapies to modulate androgen production can be beneficial in patients with acne and hidradenitis suppurativa. Such treatments for moderate acne include spironolactone and, in women, Food and Drug Administration–approved combination oral contraceptives, e.g., Ortho Tri-Cyclen (norgestimate and ethinyl estradiol), Estrostep (norethindrone acetate and ethinyl estradiol), and Yaz (drospirenone and ethinyl estradiol), as they would be prescribed for contraception (Chapter 246).**2**

Immunosuppressive Agents

Topical cytotoxic drugs include 5-fluorouracil, mechlorethamine (nitrogen mustard), carmustine (BCNU), bleomycin, and the calcineurin inhibitors tacrolimus and pimecrolimus. Topical 5-fluorouracil interferes with pyrimidine metabolism and action and blocks DNA synthesis. It is used to treat actinic keratosis, superficial basal cell cancer, Bowen's disease, bowenoid papulosis, actinic cheilitis, and warts. Topical use does not cause systemic toxicity, but expected side effects include local irritation, erythema, and pain. Nitrogen mustard and BCNU, which have alkylating agents that inhibit DNA, RNA, and protein synthesis, are used to treat cutaneous T-cell lymphoma (Chapter 190); they can cause cutaneous reactions and myelosuppression, and nitrogen mustard commonly causes a cutaneous hypersensitivity reaction.

Intralesional bleomycin, which disrupts DNA synthesis, has been used to treat warts. Topical tacrolimus (Prograf) and pimecrolimus, immunosuppressive macrolides that act on T lymphocytes to inhibit interleukin-2 (IL-2) transcription, are used for atopic dermatitis, allergic contact dermatitis, psoriasis, and several other inflammatory skin conditions. They frequently cause a burning sensation in the skin; although systemic absorption is minimal, ongoing studies are assessing whether the risk for cancer is increased by their topical use. Systemic immunosuppressives such as methotrexate, azathioprine, thioguanine, hydroxyurea, mycophenolate (CellCept), cyclophosphamide, chlorambucil, rapamycin, and cyclosporine are used for numerous inflammatory or immunologically mediated skin conditions, particularly for widespread psoriasis (Chapter 446) and as glucocorticoid-sparing agents for autoimmune blistering diseases.

Immunomodulatory Therapies

Imiquimod, available as a 5% cream, is an imidazoquinolinamine that has antitumor and antiviral activity. It induces local production of interferon-γ and is used to treat warts and superficial skin cancers. Topical 3% diclofenac in hyaluronic acid, which blocks the induced cyclooxygenase-2 found in precancerous lesions, is approved to treat actinic keratosis. Many systemic immunomodulatory drugs are currently used in dermatology. These include interferons and tumor necrosis factor-α inhibitors such as etanercept, adalimumab, and infliximab (Remicade). In addition, anti–IL-12/23 therapy with ustekinumab is used for psoriasis.**3** Anti-CD20 antibodies have been effective in the treatment of autoimmune skin-blistering diseases. Interferon alfa-2b is used both intralesionally and subcutaneously to treat genital warts, high-risk melanoma, Kaposi's sarcoma, hemangiomas, cutaneous T-cell lymphoma, keloids, Behçet's disease, cryoglobulinemia and vasculitis from hepatitis C (Chapter 151), and perhaps basal cell and squamous cell carcinoma. Total interferon doses are generally 3 million IU or less per session, and systemic doses are usually administered 3 days per week. Side effects include flulike symptoms, leukopenia, anemia, and hepatitis. Denileukin diftitox is a fusion protein consisting of a fragment of diphtheria toxin genetically fused to IL-2. It targets IL-2 receptors on the surface of malignant cells and is approved for use in patients with resistant or recurrent cutaneous T-cell lymphoma. Alefacept, which is used to treat psoriasis, affects T cells by blockade of costimulatory signals. Intravenous immunoglobulin, which is used to treat certain autoimmune skin diseases, including pemphigus vulgaris, cicatricial pemphigoid, and dermatomyositis, probably works through Fc receptor modulation and anti-idiotype interactions. Extracorporeal photochemotherapy (photopheresis), which combines 8-methoxypsoralen and ultraviolet A (UVA) irradiation of lymphocytes, is used for Sézary's syndrome, the leukemic form of cutaneous T-cell lymphoma (Chapter 190). Plasmapheresis, used in combination with other immunosuppressive therapies, can remove autoantibodies and immune complexes in patients in whom autoimmune disease or cryoglobulinemia is resistant to other therapies.

OTHER THERAPIES

Phototherapy and Laser

Ultraviolet treatments are given with different wavelengths, depending on the condition and the response to treatment. Currently, clinicians use broadband UVB (290 to 320 nm), narrow-band 311-nm UVB, PUVA (psoralen with 320- to 400-nm UVA), and UVA1 (340 to 400 nm). Both forms of UVB and PUVA are used for psoriasis and vitiligo, but other conditions such as nummular and atopic dermatitis, pruritus resulting from uremia, and cutaneous T-cell lymphoma are treated in this way. High-dose UVA1 is used, mainly in Europe, to treat atopic dermatitis, localized scleroderma, and mastocytosis. PUVA is associated with increased risk for skin cancers, including melanoma. The risks related to long-term UVA therapy are currently unknown, but photoaging is associated with UVA, and there have been reports of an increase in melanoma associated with use of suntanning beds, in which much of the exposure is to UVA. Laser therapy is used to treat vascular lesions such as port-wine stains, tattoos, psoriasis, benign skin tumors, and photodamage, as well as to remove hair. Photodynamic therapy involves activation of a photosensitizer by illumination with visible light, which leads to photochemical tissue destruction or immunomodulation. Photodynamic therapy can be used to treat actinic keratosis, Bowen's disease, and superficial basal cell carcinoma by causing selective tissue necrosis and tumor destruction.

Dermatologic Surgery

Although approaches such as desiccation and curettage can be used for some skin tumors, others require excisional surgery or Mohs' microscopic controlled surgery to ensure complete removal of lesions. If the tumors are recurrent, of a pathologic type that increases the likelihood for recurrence, or large and requiring clearance of the tumor before repair, the Mohs approach can provide rapid documentation of full removal while sparing as much normal tissue as possible. After the margins have been cleared of tumor, flaps and grafts can be used immediately for repair of the resultant defects.

Patients with extensive actinic damage resulting in either large numbers of actinic keratoses or photodamage can be treated with various ablative approaches that use either chemical peels or laser resurfacing with the carbon dioxide laser. Chemical peels can be performed at different depths and intensities, and agents can include glycolic acid, acetic acid, or even phenol. Lasers used to remove sun-induced lentigines include Q-switched lasers such as the neodymium:yttrium-aluminum-garnet, ruby, and alexandrite lasers. Many patients seek treatment of wrinkles with soft tissue augmentation that uses human-derived collagen and hyaluronic acid or with a muscle relaxer, botulinum type A exotoxin.

Hair transplants are a surgical approach to the problem of hair loss. The process includes harvesting hair grafts from the posterior of the scalp and placing the grafts in areas of alopecia.

Sunscreen

Transparent sunscreens absorb photons of light. They are rated by the sun protection factor (SPF), which is determined by the ratio of ultraviolet exposure needed to cause erythema in protected versus unprotected skin. Most sunscreens work in the UVB range or shorter UVA wavelengths. Examples of UVB-absorptive compounds include aminobenzoates, cinnamates, salicylates, and benzophenones. Short-wavelength UVA-absorptive compounds include benzophenones and anthranilates. The best UVA blocking agent in the United States is avobenzone (Parsol 1789), which can be combined with UVB screens. Some sunscreens are water resistant or waterproof, as determined by the substantivity of the sunscreen, and these agents provide continued protection after sweating or swimming. Sunscreens can cause irritation and, rarely, contact allergic reactions. Physical sunscreens, such as zinc oxide and titanium dioxide, reflect light from the skin and include newer micronized reflecting powders that provide broad-spectrum (UVB and UVA) protection. Sunscreens decrease skin cancers and photodamage. UVB is partially reflected by clothing, and sun-protective clothing can provide substantial protection (Solumbra, SPF of 30).

Cosmetics: Camouflage, Bleaching, and Hair Loss

Patients with numerous skin conditions benefit from camouflage cosmetics, which can also cause contact hypersensitivity. Products such as Dermablend can be blended to match skin colors, are thicker, can cover disfiguring lesions, and can be fixed with powder. Hydroquinones, topical retinoic acid, and azelaic acid (inhibits tyrosinase) are used to treat hyperpigmented conditions such as melasma and lentigines; these agents can be irritating and cause dyspigmentation. Topical minoxidil, 2% (available over the counter) and 5% solutions, are used for androgenic alopecia and alopecia areata. Finasteride, a 5α-reductase inhibitor, is effective in men with androgenic alopecia.

1. Kimberlin DW, Whitley RJ. Varicella-zoster vaccine for the prevention of herpes zoster. *N Engl J Med.* 2007;356:1338-1343.
2. Arowojolu AO, Gallo MF, Lopez LM, et al. Combined oral contraceptive pills for treatment of acne. *Cochrane Database Syst Rev.* 2009;8:CD004425.
3. Papp KA, Langley RG, Lebwohl M, et al. PHOENIX 2 study investigators. Efficacy and safety of ustekinumab, a human interleukin-12/23 monoclonal antibody, in patients with psoriasis: 52-week results from a randomised, double-blind, placebo-controlled trial (PHOENIX 2). *Lancet.* 2008;371:1675-1684.

SUGGESTED READINGS

Chang KH, Finn DT, Lee D, et al. Novel 16-minute technique for evaluating melanoma resection margins during Mohs surgery. *J Am Acad Dermatol.* 2011;64:107-112. *An expedited approach with equally good results.*

Grossberg AL, Gaspari AA. Topical antineoplastic agents in the treatment of mucocutaneous diseases. *Curr Probl Dermatol.* 2011;40:71-82. *Review of agents, including their indications and side effects.*

Jessop S, Whitelaw DA, Delamere FM. Drugs for discoid lupus erythematosus. *Cochrane Database Syst Rev.* 2009;4:CD002954. *Reviews current therapy.*

446

ECZEMAS, PHOTODERMATOSES, PAPULOSQUAMOUS (INCLUDING FUNGAL) DISEASES, AND FIGURATE ERYTHEMAS

HENRY W. LIM

● ECZEMA

The more commonly encountered eczemas (Table 446-1) share similar histologic characteristics. However, they have varying degrees of edema within the epidermis (spongiosis) and of infiltration with lymphocytes and macrophages in the superficial dermis.

FIGURE 446-1. Coin-shaped erythematous patches in a patient with nummular dermatitis.

TABLE 446-1 ECZEMAS
Nummular dermatitis
Dyshidrosis
Atopic dermatitis
Seborrheic dermatitis
Allergic contact dermatitis
Irritant contact dermatitis

Nummular Dermatitis

Nummular dermatitis occurs most frequently in patients who are in their 50s to 60s and is usually associated with significant dryness of the skin (xerosis). Both sexes are affected; in temperate climates, this condition is most frequently seen in the winter. The condition appears to be more frequent among Asians. The origin of nummular dermatitis is unclear, although xerosis plays a significant role in its pathogenesis.

Patients usually present with pruritic, coin-shaped, erythematous patches with some scales and occasionally with pinhead-sized vesicles (Fig. 446-1). Lesions may be excoriated and lichenified (i.e., thickened skin with accentuation of skin markings). Legs and arms are commonly affected, and lesions can also occur on the trunk, but facial involvement is uncommon. All patients should be educated about the care of dry skin, such as the use of emollients and moisturizing soaps and avoidance of long, hot showers. Topical corticosteroid ointments (e.g., triamcinolone ointment, 0.1% twice daily for 1 to 2 weeks) are helpful for active lesions, and oral antihistamines (e.g., fexofenadine, 180 mg every morning, and hydroxyzine, 25 to 50 mg at bedtime, as needed) are useful for pruritus. In severe cases, narrow-band ultraviolet B (NB-UVB) phototherapy, a short course of oral corticosteroids (prednisone, 0.5 to 1 mg/kg/day, with a maximal dose of 60 mg/day, for 1 to 2 weeks, then taper in 10 to 14 days) or day hospitalization for intensive topical and ultraviolet (UV) therapy is beneficial.

Dyshidrosis

Dyshidrosis appears as deep-seated, pinhead-sized vesicles, most commonly along the sides of the fingers (Fig. 446-2). Occasionally, the palms and soles may also be involved. Lesions are usually pruritic, associated with xerosis of the surrounding skin. Fissuring of the tip and the side of the fingers frequently occurs. Dyshidrosis is seen in individuals who wash their hands frequently, such as health care and restaurant workers and mothers of young infants. Treatment follows a sequential order: (1) minimizing of hand washing, (2) liberal use of emollients, (3) topical corticosteroid ointments (e.g., fluocinonide ointment, 0.05% twice daily for 2 weeks), and (4) oral antihistamines (e.g., fexofenadine, 180 mg every morning, and hydroxyzine, 25 to 50 mg at bedtime, as needed).

Atopic Dermatitis

Atopic dermatitis is most commonly seen among young children, but severe cases persist into adulthood. In 90% of the patients, the disease starts before the age of 5 years. The prevalence has been estimated at between 15 and 23%. Patients usually present with xerosis, erythematous scaly patches, small

FIGURE 446-2. Dyshidrosis. Deep-seated vesicles and scaliness on fingers.

FIGURE 446-4. Hypopigmentation with fine scales on the forehead and scalp of a patient with seborrheic dermatitis.

FIGURE 446-3. Atopic dermatitis. Note the erythema, excoriation, and lichenification.

vesicles, excoriations, crusting, and, not infrequently, impetiginization (Fig. 446-3). With chronic scratching and rubbing, hyperpigmentation and lichenification occur. Commonly affected sites include the periorbital area and flexor areas such as the neck, antecubital fossa, and popliteal fossa. In severe cases, the entire skin surface may be involved. Diagnosis is made by the typical morphologic features, by the distribution of the lesions, and by a family and personal history of atopy. The therapeutic ladder consists of the following: (1) emollients; (2) topical corticosteroid ointments (e.g., triamcinolone ointment, 0.1% twice daily for 1 to 2 weeks), or topical calcineurin inhibitors (tacrolimus ointment, 0.1% for 3 to 4 weeks, or pimecrolimus cream, 1% for 3 to 4 weeks)◨; (3) oral antihistamines (e.g., fexofenadine, 180 mg every morning, and hydroxyzine, 25 to 50 mg at bedtime, as needed); (4) NB-UVB phototherapy; and (5) psoralen and UVA (PUVA). It should be noted that tacrolimus and pimecrolimus have "black box" warnings from the U.S. Food and Drug Administration for their potential association with the development of malignant disease. Although some feel such data are inconclusive, continuous prolonged use (i.e., >2 to 3 months) should be minimized. In patients with recalcitrant cases, day hospitalization, oral prednisone (0.5 to 1 mg/kg/day), cyclosporine (3 to 5 mg/kg/day), and mycophenolate mofetil (1 to 2 g/day) have been successful.

Seborrheic Dermatitis

Seborrheic dermatitis is a common condition that occurs as erythematous patches with fine, greasy-appearing scales, most commonly on the malar area, midforehead, midchest, and scalp (Fig. 446-4). It is common in patients with

human immunodeficiency virus (HIV) infection (Chapter 399). The pathogenesis is unknown, although *Pityrosporum ovale* is believed to play a role. The diagnosis is made clinically. Topical corticosteroids (e.g., hydrocortisone cream 2.5%, twice daily for 1 to 2 weeks for facial lesion, fluocinolone acetonide 0.01% solution for scalp, twice daily for 3 to 4 weeks) can rapidly reduce the inflammation; then topical ketoconazole cream, 2% twice daily as needed (or shampoo 2% daily or every other day for the scalp), is safe for long-term treatment.

Allergic Contact Dermatitis and Irritant Contact Dermatitis

Allergic contact dermatitis and irritant contact dermatitis are induced by exogenous agents. Allergic contact dermatitis is a delayed hypersensitivity response to external allergens, whereas irritant contact dermatitis is a nonspecific toxic response to contact irritants. In both conditions, lesions occur in the exposed area, but in patients with severe cases, nonexposed areas may also have milder lesions, especially in allergic contact dermatitis. Patients with allergic contact dermatitis present with erythematous pruritic papules and vesicles. Lesions resolve with fine scales. Postinflammatory hyperpigmentation may be observed, especially in dark-skinned individuals. Histologically, epidermal edema and dermal histiocytic infiltrates are observed. Irritant contact dermatitis manifests with lesions morphologically similar to those of allergic contact dermatitis. However, irritant contact dermatitis is usually associated with a burning sensation rather than with pruritus. Postinflammatory hyperpigmentation is frequently observed. Histologic changes consist of necrotic keratinocytes, epidermal necrosis, and neutrophilic infiltrates. Management includes identification and removal of the offending agent, as well as symptomatic treatments such as topical corticosteroids and oral antihistamines.

⬤ PHOTODERMATOSES

Photodermatoses are cutaneous eruptions secondary to exposure to UV or visible radiation (Table 446-2). By convention, electromagnetic radiation in the UV region is divided into UVC (200 to 290 nm), UVB (290 to 320 nm), UVA-2 (320 to 340 nm), and UVA-1 (340 to 400 nm). Visible light extends from 400 to 760 nm. Because UVC emitted by the sun is absorbed by ozone in the stratosphere, UVC does not reach the Earth's surface. UVB, UVA, and less frequently, visible light are the relevant spectra in photodermatoses.

Polymorphic Light Eruption

Polymorphic light eruption, the most common immunologically mediated photodermatosis, occurs in 10 to 20% of the general population. It usually occurs in young adults, has a slight female predominance, and is seen worldwide. Affected individuals are less susceptible to cutaneous photoimmunosuppression and hence have an enhanced response to UV-induced neoantigens in the skin. Lesions usually occur in early spring within a few hours of exposure to sunlight. Lesions can manifest as pinhead papules, papules, papulovesicles, or, less commonly, vesicles (Fig. 446-5); they can also be pruritic. Usually, lesions persist for several days and resolve spontaneously. The condition tends to improve as the sunny season progresses, a phenomenon known as hardening.

FIGURE 446-5. Erythematous papules a few hours after exposure to the sun in a patient with polymorphic light eruption.

TABLE 446-2	SELECTED PHOTODERMATOSES

Polymorphic light eruption
Chronic actinic dermatitis
Solar urticaria
Phototoxicity and photoallergy
Porphyrias

The course is chronic; only 11% of patients have complete resolution of the disease in 16 years and 24% in 32 years. Diagnosis is based on the typical history and morphologic features of the lesion; the diagnosis can be confirmed by the induction of lesions with provocative phototesting. When lesions occur primarily on the face, a diagnosis of lupus must be excluded. Management consists of sun avoidance, the use of broad-spectrum sunscreens, topical corticosteroids, and oral antihistamines. In severe cases, desensitization treatment using NB-UVB or PUVA has been successful. Desensitization is usually performed in early spring by exposing patients to increasing doses of NB-UVB or PUVA three times weekly for 15 treatments.

Chronic Actinic Dermatitis

Chronic actinic dermatitis is a chronic photodermatosis that occurs most commonly in men in their 60s and 70s. It occurs in patients of all ethnic groups, but in the United States, it is more commonly seen in dark-skinned individuals. It is seen in 5 to 17% of patients referred for evaluation of photosensitivity. Chronic actinic dermatitis can evolve from photoallergic contact dermatitis, allergic contact dermatitis, or exposure to a known photosensitizing agent; however, it can also arise de novo. Investigators have postulated that this condition represents a delayed hypersensitivity response to an unidentified antigen.

Patients present with erythematous papules and plaques with superficial scaling and, frequently, with lichenification (Fig. 446-6). The distribution of lesions is primarily on sun-exposed areas, such as the forehead, nose, cheeks, V area of the neck, dorsum of the hands, and forearms. Typically, sun-protected areas, such as the postauricular area, the area underneath the chin, the area above the eyes, and the trunk, are spared. This chronic photosensitivity occurs in the absence of any continued exposure to known photosensitizers. Histologically, one sees a dermal lymphohistiocytic infiltrate; atypical mononuclear cells may be observed. On phototesting, patients have increased sensitivity to UVA, UVB, or visible light, or a combination. In a study of 178 cases, 10% resolved in 5 years and 50% in 15 years. An association with HIV infection (Chapter 399) has been reported.

FIGURE 446-6. Hyperpigmentation and lichenification in a patient with chronic actinic dermatitis. Note sparing of the sun-protected areas of the neck and infra-auricular area.

The diagnosis is based on the patient's history and on the morphologic features and distribution of the lesions. It is confirmed by phototesting.

Management is challenging. During the sunny season, it is critical that patients practice maximal photoprotection, consisting of staying in the shade, using broad-spectrum sunscreens with high SPF, clothing, and wearing a wide-brimmed hat. Other treatment modalities, in approximate sequential order, are topical tacrolimus ointment (0.1%), oral mycophenolate mofetil (1 to 2 g/day), oral cyclosporine (3 to 5 mg/kg/day), and azathioprine (50 to 200 mg/day). Treatment with oral corticosteroids (e.g., prednisone, 1 mg/kg/day) may be needed for acute flare. In recalcitrant cases, the following may be used: PUVA in conjunction with oral corticosteroids or a combination of mycophenolate mofetil, PUVA, and oral corticosteroids.

Solar Urticaria

Solar urticaria occurs worldwide. In photodermatology referral centers, it accounts for 4 to 18% of patients. The mean age at onset is usually in the fourth decade, with a slight female predominance. Patients develop urticaria that appears within minutes of sun exposure and persists for less than 24 hours. Lesions are most commonly induced by visible light, but they can also be induced by UVA or UVB. Similar to polymorphic light eruption, improvement may occur as the summer season progresses (hardening). The diagnosis is confirmed by induction of the lesion after controlled exposure to the appropriate light source. Management consists of photoprotection and the use of oral antihistamines (e.g., fexofenadine, 180 mg every morning, and hydroxyzine, 25 to 50 mg at bedtime). For patients with reactions in the visible light range as determined by phototesting, physical photoprotection is the only effective means because sunscreens do not protect against visible light. In severe cases, graduated exposure to UVA or PUVA is helpful.

Phototoxicity and Photoallergy

The terms *phototoxicity* and *photoallergy* refer to the development of skin lesions after combined exposure to an oral or topical photosensitizer and electromagnetic radiation. Phototoxicity is a nonspecific cutaneous toxic reaction, whereas photoallergy is a delayed hypersensitivity response. For most photosensitizers, the action spectrum for both lies in the UVA range. Most of the phototoxic agents are systemic medications, whereas the most common photoallergens are the various UV filters in sunscreen. In both conditions, patients present with erythematous papules and vesicles confined to sun-exposed areas. Vesicular eruption is distinctly more common in phototoxicity, whereas pruritic eczematous eruption is more common in photoallergy. Histologically, phototoxicity is characterized by necrotic keratinocytes and infiltrates consisting predominantly of neutrophils, whereas photoallergy is characterized by epidermal edema (spongiosis) and lymphohistiocytic dermal infiltrate. The diagnosis is based on a careful history for exposure to photosensitizers combined with the typical morphologic features. Management consists of identification and removal of photosensitizer and the use of topical corticosteroids (e.g., triamcinolone ointment, 0.1% twice daily for 2 weeks) and oral antihistamines (e.g., fexofenadine, 180 mg every morning, and hydroxyzine, 25 to 50 mg at bedtime as needed [Chapter 445]).

FIGURE 446-7. Erosion, crusting, and vesicles on the dorsum of the hand of a patient with porphyria cutanea tarda.

FIGURE 446-8. Erythematous plaques with silvery scales in a patient with psoriasis.

TABLE 446-3   PAPULOSQUAMOUS DISEASES

Psoriasis
Pityriasis rubra pilaris
Pityriasis rosea
Lichen planus
Lichen nitidus
Secondary syphilis
Pityriasis lichenoides
Parapsoriasis
Mycosis fungoides
Dermatophytosis
Tinea versicolor

Porphyrias

The most common cutaneous porphyria is porphyria cutanea tarda, in which patients present with skin fragility and blister formation on sun-exposed areas, most commonly the dorsum of the hands and the forearms (Fig. 446-7; Chapter 217). Patients usually have periorbital hypertrichosis and, less frequently, periorbital mottled hyperpigmentation and hypopigmentation. Sclerodermoid skin changes can occur in both sun-exposed and sun-protected areas. The defective enzyme is uroporphyrinogen decarboxylase. Porphyria cutanea tarda is associated with excessive alcohol intake, exposure to estrogens, hepatitis C infection (Chapter 151), HIV infection (Chapter 399), and hemochromatosis (Chapter 219). Patients invariably have an elevated level of ferritin and frequently have elevated liver enzyme values.

The diagnosis is suggested by the typical clinical appearance and is confirmed by the characteristic porphyrin profile (elevated levels of 8-, 7-, 6-, 5-, and 4-carboxyl porphyrins in the urine and isocoproporphyrin in feces; Chapter 217). Management consists of avoidance of precipitating factors (alcohol, iron-containing vitamins, estrogen-containing birth control pills) and weekly phlebotomy. In patients who are anemic (e.g., those with HIV infection), low-dose hydroxychloroquine (200 mg/week) is beneficial.

● PAPULOSQUAMOUS (INCLUDING FUNGAL) DISEASES

Common papulosquamous diseases are listed in Table 446-3.

Psoriasis

EPIDEMIOLOGY

Psoriasis is the most commonly recognized papulosquamous disease. It occurs in 2 to 3% of the general population, with considerable variation in different parts of the world. It affects male and female patients equally. Approximately one third of the patients have a positive family history. Psoriasis has a bimodal peak of onset, at age 22.5 years and again at age 55 years. The onset of psoriasis before the age of 15 years is associated with a higher prevalence of positive family history of psoriasis and with more severe disease.

PATHOBIOLOGY

Psoriasis involves the innate and adaptive immune systems, with abnormal keratinocyte proliferation. Factors playing a role in the pathogenesis include activation of antigen-presenting cells and development of T_H1 and T_H17 cells. Mediators include interleukin-12 (IL-12), IL-23, tumor necrosis factor-α (TNF-α), and interferon-γ. Investigators have postulated that, in genetically susceptible individuals, exposure to precipitating factors such as infections (e.g., streptococcal or HIV infections), stress, or physical injury results in activation of T cells and generation of cytokines, followed by influx of neutrophils and subsequent release of inflammatory mediators, which lead to the development of cutaneous lesions.

Psoriasis has a complex, polygenetic inheritance. Susceptibility genes include *PSORS1* to *PSORS9*, although *PSORS1*, mapped to chromosome 6p21.3, is now considered a major locus for susceptibility to psoriasis.

CLINICAL MANIFESTATIONS

Psoriasis can involve the skin, scalp, and nails. Skin lesions are characterized by erythematous macules, papules, or plaques that are usually covered with silvery scales (Fig. 446-8). On removal of the scales, pinpoint bleeding may be observed (the Auspitz sign), a finding reflecting the proliferation of blood vessels in the superficial dermis. Nail involvement includes pittings, yellowish macules underneath the nail plate ("oil drop" sign), and thickening of the nail (onychodystrophy) (Fig. 446-9). Minor injury to the skin can result in the development of psoriatic lesions (Koebner's phenomenon). The association of psoriasis with HIV infection (Chapter 399) has been well documented.

Several distinct forms of psoriasis are recognized. *Psoriasis vulgaris,* the most common type, appears as a persistent erythematous scaly papule and plaque most commonly on elbows, knees, and scalp. *Guttate psoriasis* usually occurs after viral or bacterial (most commonly streptococcal) infection; it appears as small, erythematous, scaly papules scattered over a large area of the body in a raindrop distribution (*guttate* means "droplike"). *Inverse psoriasis* refers to psoriasis that occurs in skinfold areas such as the groin, axilla, and inframammary folds. It appears as an erythematous, somewhat shiny patch; because of the constant friction in the involved areas, scales are usually absent. *Erythrodermic psoriasis* appears as widespread erythroderma with fine silvery scales. *Palmoplantar psoriasis* manifests as keratotic scaly patches and plaques on the palms and soles, very frequently with accompanying fissures. *Pustular psoriasis of von Zumbusch* is a rare variant of psoriasis occurring with

FIGURE 446-9. Thickening and crumbling of the nail plate (onychodystrophy) in a patient with psoriasis. Note the erythematous patches with silvery scales in the periungual area.

FIGURE 446-10. Pityriasis rubra pilaris. Note the erythematous orange plaques with islands of sparing.

generalized pustules that are 2 to 3 mm in diameter and associated with the onset of fever.

Five to 30% of patients with psoriasis may also have psoriatic arthritis, which may precede the appearance of cutaneous lesions (Chapter 273); 95% of these patients present with peripheral asymmetrical oligoarthritis involving the interphalangeal joints of the hands and feet, while 5% have exclusively axial or skeletal disease. Psoriatic arthritis has been associated with HLA-B57, although some studies have also reported HLA-Cw6 in more than 50% of all persons with this disease. Psoriasis is associated with ulcerative colitis, lymphoma, the metabolic syndrome, heart disease, depression, smoking, and alcohol consumption.

DIAGNOSIS

In most cases, the diagnosis of psoriasis can be made based on the history and physical examination alone. However, in patients with erythrodermic psoriasis, other causes of generalized erythroderma (including pityriasis rubra pilaris, drug eruption, and cutaneous T-cell lymphoma) must be excluded.

TREATMENT   Rx

Therapy includes topical medications, UV-based treatment, and systemic drugs. For mild disease, topical therapy with topical corticosteroids (e.g., triamcinolone ointment, 0.1% twice daily for 1 to 2 weeks), calcipotriene cream (0.005%, twice daily as needed), or tazarotene gel (0.05%, once or twice daily as needed), used alone or in combination, is effective. In patients who have widespread lesions, NB-UVB is the best option, whereas PUVA should be considered for patients in whom NB-UVB therapy has failed. For patients with recalcitrant disease, oral medications such as methotrexate (7.5 to 15 mg/week), acitretin (25 to 50 mg/day), cyclosporine (3 to 5 mg/kg/day), hydroxyurea (1 g/day), and mycophenolate mofetil (1 to 2 g/day) have all been used with success.

Biologic agents, because of their cost, are usually reserved for when conventional therapy has failed or is contraindicated (Table 446-4). TNF-α inhibitors include etanercept, a human TNF receptor/immunoglobulin G1 (IgG1) fusion protein; infliximab, a chimeric mouse anti-TNF-α antibody; and adalimumab, a human IgG1 anti-TNF-α antibody. A CD2 antagonist is alefacept, a protein that is fused to IgG and that contains the binding site of lymphocyte function–associated antigen-3, which binds to CD2 markers on the surface of memory T cells. Efalizumab, an anti-CD11a humanized monoclonal antibody, has been taken off the market because of increased incidence of progressive multifocal leukoencephalopathy Ustekinumab, a fully human monoclonal antibody against the p40 subunit of IL-12 and IL-23 (at 45 or 90 mg, repeated at 1 month) is efficacious and appears to be superior to etanercept for moderate-to-severe psoriasis.[2,3]

TABLE 446-4 BIOLOGIC AGENTS FOR PSORIASIS

BIOLOGIC AGENTS	DOSE/DURATION	MONITORING	SIDE EFFECTS
TNF-α INHIBITORS			
Etanercept (Enbrel)	50 mg SC twice a week for 12 wk, then 50 mg SC weekly indefinitely	PPD CBC, LFT	Injection site reaction, infection
Infliximab (Remicade)	5-10 mg/kg IV at weeks 0, 2, 6, then every 8 wk indefinitely	PPD CBC, LFT	Infusion reaction, sepsis, lupus-like syndrome, aplastic anemia (rare)
Adalimumab (Humira)	80 mg SC at week 0, 40 mg at wk 1, then 40 mg every 2 wk indefinitely	PPD CBC, LFT	Injection site reaction, infection
ANTI-CD2			
Alefacept (Amevive)	15 mg IM weekly for 12-16 wk; consider a second course after a 12-wk interval	CD4	Infection
ANTI–IL-12/23			
Ustekinumab (Stelara)	SC at weeks 0, 4, then every 12 wk <100 kg: 45 mg; >100 kg: 90 mg indefinitely	PPD	Infection

CBC = complete blood count; IM = intramuscularly; IV = intravenously; LFT = liver function test; PPD = purified protein derivative; SC = subcutaneously; TNF = tumor necrosis factor.

Pityriasis Rubra Pilaris

EPIDEMIOLOGY

Pityriasis rubra pilaris occurs equally in men and women; the incidence ranges from 1 in 5000 new dermatology patients in Great Britain to 1 in 50,000 in India. This disease most frequently occurs as the acquired form, although a familial form (autosomal dominant with variable expression) also occurs. Sixty percent of patients have adult-onset disease, with peak incidences in the first, second, and fifth to sixth decades. Abnormal vitamin A metabolism has been postulated as a possible cause.

CLINICAL MANIFESTATIONS

Clinically, patients present with erythematous to orange papules and plaques on all parts of the body (Fig. 446-10). Characteristically, skin appears normal between these lesions ("islands of sparing"). Erythema, hyperkeratosis, and fissures of the palms and soles are common; when severe, these lesions result in functional impairment. Many patients have follicular keratotic papules on the dorsa of the fingers and occasionally on the elbows as well as on the wrists. The nails are yellow and thickened, with distal splinter hemorrhages. In adult patients, the condition typically starts on the face and moves to the lower extremities; in the juvenile form, it usually starts in the lower half of the body. Ectropion may occur, and pruritus is observed in approximately

FIGURE 446-11. Large erythematous oval patch (herald patch) of pityriasis rosea accompanied by smaller erythematous patches.

FIGURE 446-12. Erythematous flat-topped papules on the wrist of a patient with lichen planus.

20% of patients. In contrast to psoriasis, arthritis is uncommon. Pityriasis rubra pilaris has been associated with HIV infection (Chapter 399).

DIAGNOSIS

Definitive diagnosis can usually be made based on the clinical presentations and by the characteristic histologic findings of alternating vertical and horizontal parakeratosis in the stratum corneum.

TREATMENT Rx

The most effective treatment is with oral retinoids (acitretin, 25 to 50 mg/day for 2 to 4 months). Methotrexate (7.5 to 15 mg/week), either as a monotherapy or in combination with oral acitretin, is also beneficial. Other options include PUVA or cyclosporine (3 to 5 mg/kg/day). For all patients, topical emollients should be used as needed, and topical keratolytic agents, such as ammonium lactate lotion 12%, twice daily as needed, are helpful as adjunctive therapy.

Pityriasis Rosea

EPIDEMIOLOGY AND PATHOBIOLOGY

The incidence of pityriasis rosea has been reported as 3 to 30 per 1000 patients. It occurs in all ethnic groups, most commonly in the third and fourth decades of life, with a slight female predominance. The cause is not known, and a possible association with human herpesvirus types 6 and 7 has been reported.

CLINICAL MANIFESTATIONS

In 50 to 90% of patients, pityriasis rosea starts with a primary lesion (herald patch), which is an erythematous, scaly, oval patch a few centimeters in diameter. This lesion is usually followed within a few days by smaller erythematous scaly patches on the trunk, less commonly on the proximal extremities (Fig. 446-11). As a rule, the palms and soles are spared. The distribution of the eruption, especially on the back, tends to follow the lines of cleavage of the skin, with a resulting "Christmas tree" distribution. Lesions are most commonly asymptomatic, although they may be mildly pruritic. The eruption is self-limited and resolves within 6 to 8 weeks. In rare instances, lesions may persist.

DIAGNOSIS

The diagnosis can usually be made clinically. The most important differential diagnosis is secondary syphilis, which, in contrast to pityriasis rosea, usually involves the palms and soles. In many instances, a rapid plasma reagin test is advisable to exclude syphilis.

TREATMENT Rx

Treatment is primarily symptomatic, including topical corticosteroids and oral antihistamines. NB-UVB phototherapy or PUVA should be reserved for patients with severe, recalcitrant cases.

Lichen Planus

EPIDEMIOLOGY

Lichen planus occurs most commonly in patients between 30 and 60 years of age. Women are affected more frequently than men and tend to be somewhat older at the onset of disease. The prevalence in the general population is about 1%.

PATHOBIOLOGY

Histologically, lichen planus is characterized by dense lymphocytic infiltrate at the dermal-epidermal junction. The infiltrates consist of predominantly T cells, a finding suggesting the pathogenic role of cell-mediated immunity. Because lichen planus or lichen planus–like eruptions can occur after exposure to drugs or chemicals (e.g., color film developer), the role of drugs and chemicals in inducing a T-cell–mediated response against the epidermis has been postulated. Lichen planus may be associated with hepatitis C infection (Chapter 151).

CLINICAL MANIFESTATIONS

Clinically, patients usually present with erythematous to violaceous flat-topped papules, often with white lacy lines (Wickham's striae) on the wrists, forearms, and genitalia (Fig. 446-12). *Oral lichen planus* occurs as white papules and plaques with a reticulated appearance, most commonly along the bite line on the buccal mucosa. Erosion may occur, and genital mucosa may also be involved. *Hypertrophic lichen planus* usually occurs on the lower extremities as lichenified, violaceous plaques, probably secondary to chronic rubbing and scratching of the lichen planus lesions. *Erosive lichen planus* occurs as erosion usually surrounded by violaceous discoloration at the periphery; this variant tends to occur more commonly on the feet. *Bullous lichen planus* occurs as vesicles or bullae arising from a preexisting lesion of lichen planus. *Lichen planopilaris* occurs as violaceous papules and plaques involving the scalp, most prominently surrounding the hair follicles; it progresses to scarring alopecia. *Lichen planus actinicus*, a variant of lichen planus occurring most commonly in the Middle East, tends to occur on the sun-exposed areas such as the forehead; it occurs as papules or plaques with minimally elevated rolled edges. *Atrophic lichen planus* resembles typical lichen planus lesions but with a central area of superficial atrophy. *Lichen planus of the nails* causes a thinning of the nail with longitudinal ridges; it may progress to complete loss of the nail plate (pterygium formation).

DIAGNOSIS

The diagnosis can be made by clinical appearance. It is confirmed by the characteristic histologic findings of infiltration by lymphocytes at the dermal-epidermal junction.

TREATMENT Rx

Several treatment options are available. Topical corticosteroids (e.g., triamcinolone ointment, 0.1% twice daily for 2 to 4 weeks) are helpful in patients with limited disease. Hypertrophic lichen planus can be treated with topical corticosteroids (fluocinonide 0.05% ointment, twice daily for 2 to 4 weeks), with occlusion at night, or with interlesional corticosteroid injections (triamcinolone suspension, 3 to 5 mg/mL). A 6- to 8-week course of oral corticosteroid is helpful in patients with widespread lichen planus. NB-UVB phototherapy

FIGURE 446-13. Scaly papules and plaques on the palm of a patient with secondary syphilis.

or PUVA is helpful for widespread conditions. Oral acitretin (25 to 50 mg/day) or systemic cyclosporine (3 to 5 mg/kg/day) has been used with good success in some patients. Oral lesions can be treated with topical corticosteroids (triamcinolone 0.1% paste, twice daily for 2 to 3 weeks), topical retinoids (tretinoin gel 0.01%, twice daily for 3 to 4 weeks), or cyclosporine solution (100 mg/mL, 1 mL, twice daily, swish and spit). Painful erosive lesions in the mouth and genital area are best treated with oral prednisone in combination with mycophenolate mofetil (1 to 2 g daily). Without treatment, cutaneous lesions resolve in approximately 1 year, whereas oral and hypertrophic lesions tend to be much more chronic, persisting for an average of 4.5 years and 8.5 years, respectively.

Lichen Nitidus

Lichen nitidus is a rather uncommon condition that usually occurs in children or young adults. The incidence has been estimated to be 3.4 cases per 10,000 population. It is more commonly observed in dark-skinned individuals. The cause is unclear, and no infectious agent has been identified.

The lesions are 1- to 2-mm, shiny, skin-colored discrete papules, sometimes with fine scales on their surface, occurring most commonly on the genitalia or forearms and occasionally on the trunk. A generalized form has rarely been reported. Lesions are usually asymptomatic. Histologically, one sees a dense lymphocytic infiltrate in the superficial dermis and at the dermal-epidermal junction. In contrast to lichen planus, in which the infiltrate tends to involve the entire section of the skin, the infiltrate in lichen nitidus tends to be much more focal and localized.

The diagnosis usually can be confirmed from the typical clinical appearance and the characteristic histologic changes. The condition tends to remit spontaneously in a few years, so therapy, with topical corticosteroids (e.g., triamcinolone ointment, 0.1% twice daily for 2 weeks) and oral antihistamines (e.g., fexofenadine, 180 mg every morning, and hydroxyzine, 25 to 50 mg at bedtime, as needed) should be reserved for symptomatic cases only.

Secondary Syphilis

Lesions of secondary syphilis typically occur 1 to 2 months after the development of a primary chancre lesion (Chapter 327). However, up to 25% of patients may not remember having a chancre. Once the eruption occurs, it lasts for 1 to 3 months.

Clinically, secondary syphilis may appear as erythematous macules ("roseola syphilitica"), erythematous to hyperpigmented oval or circular papules and plaques covered with scales, or a maculopapular eruption. Nodular eruption may also occur occasionally. The lesions tend to be widespread, and the palms and soles are very frequently involved (Fig. 446-13). The diagnosis is made based on the history, physical examination, and a positive rapid plasma reagin test. Skin biopsy shows the proliferation of endothelial cells in the dermis and a dense dermal infiltrate containing many plasma

FIGURE 446-14. Erythematous patches with fine scales in a patient with large plaque parapsoriasis.

cells. Intramuscular benzathine penicillin or procaine penicillin is the recommended treatment, with oral doxycycline or tetracycline as alternatives.

Pityriasis Lichenoides

Pityriasis lichenoides occurs as erythematous papules that may be minimally pruritic and covered with scales, scattered on all parts of the body. In the acute form (pityriasis lichenoides et varioliformis acuta [PLEVA]), the central part of the lesions develops vesicles, pustules, and hemorrhages, with eventual crusting of the lesions. The patient may have mild constitutional symptoms of fever and malaise. The chronic form (pityriasis lichenoides chronica [PLC]) occurs as asymptomatic erythematous to hyperpigmented papules and plaques covered with fine scales; the trunk and extremities are common sites. Histologically, both PLEVA and PLC are characterized by dense lymphocytic infiltrates in the dermis, with CD8 lymphocytes predominating in PLEVA and CD4 lymphocytes in PLC.

PLEVA usually resolves in a few months, although it can persist. PLC usually lasts for a few years. Both disorders affect patients of all ages, with a slight male predominance.

Treatment generally follows a sequential order: (1) topical corticosteroids (e.g., triamcinolone ointment, 0.1% twice daily for 1 to 2 weeks) and antihistamines, (2) tetracycline (1 to 2 g/day), or erythromycin (1 to 2 g/day), (3) NB-UVB phototherapy (three times weekly for 8 to 10 weeks with increasing doses of NB-UVB) or PUVA, and (4) methotrexate (7.5 to 15 mg/week).

Parapsoriasis

The two common variants of parapsoriasis are large plaque parapsoriasis and small plaque parapsoriasis. The peak incidence is in the fifth decade, although rare cases may begin in childhood. Large plaque parapsoriasis appears as oval to circular, erythematous to hyperpigmented macules and patches with fine scales and superficial atrophy (crinkling atrophy) scattered on all parts of the body (Fig. 446-14). These lesions are usually larger than 5 cm. Although lesions may be minimally pruritic, they are usually asymptomatic. Large plaque parapsoriasis is considered by some to be a less aggressive variant of mycosis fungoides (see later). Small plaque parapsoriasis appears as circular to oval erythematous to hyperpigmented patches or minimally elevated plaques, with lesions smaller than 5 cm in diameter and usually covered with fine scales. Digitate dermatosis is a distinct variant of small plaque parapsoriasis in which lesions appear along the lines of cleavage, usually on the lateral aspect of the trunk in the shape of fingerprints. Histologically, large plaque parapsoriasis is characterized by a dermal lymphocytic infiltrate, which may extend into the epidermis, whereas small plaque parapsoriasis is characterized by spongiotic dermatitis, with a mild superficial lymphocytic infiltrate in the dermis. In up to one third of patients, large plaque parapsoriasis may evolve into mycosis fungoides. As a result, treatment of large plaque parapsoriasis is similar to that of early-stage mycosis fungoides: high-potency topical corticosteroids, topical nitrogen mustard, NB-UVB phototherapy, and PUVA. By comparison, patients with small plaque parapsoriasis have a benign course, and management of small plaque parapsoriasis should be symptomatic only, with emollients, topical corticosteroids, and NB-UVB phototherapy.

Mycosis Fungoides

Mycosis fungoides is a variant of cutaneous T-cell lymphoma (Chapter 191). The four types of cutaneous manifestations are patch, plaque, tumor, and

FIGURE 446-15. Hyperpigmented patches in a patient with mycosis fungoides.

FIGURE 446-16. Hypopigmented patches of tinea versicolor.

erythrodermic. The patch stage of mycosis fungoides manifests as patches with fine "cigarette paper" wrinkling of the epidermis. The patches can be skin colored or minimally erythematous; hyperpigmented or hypopigmented lesions are frequently seen in dark-skinned patients. The patches can vary from a few millimeters to a few centimeters in diameter; they are more common on sun-protected areas such as the buttocks (Fig. 446-15). The patches are usually asymptomatic, although they occasionally may be mildly pruritic. Lesions may be present for years. As the disease progresses, some of the patches may become more indurated and may evolve into more elevated plaques. Nodular lesions may occur in patients without any patch or plaque lesions, although more commonly these lesions occur in conjunction with patches and plaques. Erythrodermic mycosis fungoides occurs as a generalized erythroderma with significant scaling and pruritus. Hyperkeratosis of the palms and soles, as well as fissuring of hands and feet, are quite common. In dark-skinned patients, mycosis fungoides may appear as hypopigmented patches.

The diagnosis is confirmed by histologic demonstration of atypical mononuclear cells both in the epidermis and in the dermis, as well as immunophenotypic markers showing predominance of CD4 cells in the infiltrate. Therapy for mycosis fungoides generally follows a sequential order: (1) topical nitrogen mustard (i.e., mechlorethamine, 10 mg in 60 mL of water, applied daily until lesions resolve, then taper), or NB-UVB, each of which can be combined with topical corticosteroids (e.g., triamcinolone ointment, 0.1% twice daily for 1 to 2 months); (2) PUVA; (3) topical retinoids (e.g., bexarotene gel, 1% once to four times daily, until lesions resolve); and (4) one of the following: oral bexarotene (300 mg/m²/day for 2 to 4 months) or interferon-α (3 to 9 million units subcutaneously 3 times weekly for 2 to 4 months). Erythrodermic disease is most effectively treated with extracorporeal photopheresis.

Dermatophytoses

Fungal infections that occur as papulosquamous eruptions include tinea corporis, tinea manuum, tinea cruris, and tinea pedis. Tinea corporis presents as a polycyclic erythematous scaly patch that has elevated borders and consists of papules and sometimes pustules. As the lesion progresses, the border advances centrifugally. The trunk is the most common site. Tinea cruris has similar morphologic features, except it is located in the inguinal folds and expands centrifugally from the folds. In men, the scrotum is usually spared. Tinea manuum presents as an erythematous scaly patch with an advancing active border, usually located on the dorsum of the hands, or it may occur as diffuse scaly patches with mild hyperkeratosis involving part or the entire surface of the palm and palmar aspect of the fingers. Tinea pedis also has two clinical manifestations: it can occur as scaly macerated lesions with erythema in the toe webs or as patchy or diffuse scaliness on the sole extending to the medial and lateral aspect of the foot (moccasin distribution). The latter presentation can be associated with diffuse scaliness of one but not both palms, a condition known as the "one-hand, two-feet syndrome." The diagnosis can be confirmed by examination of skin scrapings using 10% potassium hydroxide preparation or by fungal culture. Treatment consists of topical or oral antifungal medications (e.g., clotrimazole cream, 1%, twice daily for 2 to 4 weeks, or terbinafine, 250 mg for 2 to 12 weeks), depending on the site involved.

Tinea Versicolor

Tinea versicolor is a fungal infection of the skin caused by *Malassezia furfur*. It occurs in otherwise healthy young individuals, especially in warm and

TABLE 446-5	FIGURATE ERYTHEMAS
Erythema annulare centrifugum	
Erythema gyratum repens	
Erythema chronicum migrans	

moist environments during the summer. Clinically, it appears as macules and patches with very fine scales; the color can be hypopigmented, skin colored, minimally erythematous, or light brown (Fig. 446-16). The patches start as perifollicular macules, with the midchest and midback the most common sites. As the lesions progress, hypopigmentation of the skin may also occur. The lesion usually is asymptomatic. The diagnosis is confirmed by the characteristic appearance of the fungal elements on a 10% potassium hydroxide preparation: grapelike clusters of yeast and short, septate branching hyphae ("spaghetti and meatballs" appearance). Treatment is with 2.5% selenium sulfide shampoo (applied for 10 minutes then wash off, 5 times weekly for 4 to 6 weeks), topical antifungal preparations (e.g., clotrimazole cream, 1% twice daily for 4 weeks), or a 1- to 3-day course of oral ketoconazole (200 mg/day).

FIGURATE ERYTHEMIAS

These conditions appear as erythematous circular or polycyclic plaques with central clearing and, frequently, centrifugally migrating border (Table 446-5). Occasionally, fine scaling may also be observed. The extremities are the most common sites. The diagnosis can frequently be made by the typical history and morphologic features.

Erythema annulare centrifugum is most commonly idiopathic; however, it can also be a manifestation of a hypersensitivity response to medications. Management includes identification of a precipitating agent (if possible) and treatment with topical or systemic corticosteroids. *Erythema gyratum repens* occurs as concentric erythematous plaques with fine scales, resembling a wood-grain pattern. This unusual form of figurate erythema has been associated with malignant hematologic diseases and with carcinomas of the breast, lung, gastrointestinal tract, prostate, and cervix. Treatment of the underlying malignant disease results in the resolution of the skin lesion in a few months. *Erythema chronicum migrans*, which is a cutaneous manifestation of Lyme disease and is caused by the spirochete *Borrelia burgdorferi* (Chapter 329), appears as a concentric ring of erythema that progresses centrifugally from the site of a tick bite. Occasionally, it may appear as a circular erythematous patch. The diagnosis is made by a history of a tick bite, the characteristic cutaneous lesion, or elevated serum antibodies to *B. burgdorferi*. Management is the same as for Lyme disease.

1. Paller AS, Lebwohl M, Fleischer Jr AB, et al. for the US/Canada Tacrolimus Ointment Study Group. Tacrolimus ointment is more effective than pimecrolimus cream with a similar safety profile in the treatment of atopic dermatitis: results from 3 randomized, comparative studies. *J Am Acad Dermatol.* 2005;52:810-822.
2. Gottlieb A, Menter A, Mendelsohn A, et al. Ustekinumab, a human interleukin 12/23 monoclonal antibody, for psoriatic arthritis: randomised, double-blind, placebo-controlled, crossover trial. *Lancet.* 2009;373:633-640.
3. Griffiths CE, Strober BE, van de Kerkhof P, et al. Comparison of ustekinumab and etanercept for moderate-to-severe psoriasis. *N Engl J Med.* 2010;362:118-128.

SUGGESTED READINGS

Burnett ME, Wang SQ . Current sunscreen controversies: a critical review. *Photodermatol Photoimmunol Photomed.* 2011;27:58-67. *Review supporting their use.*

Darsow U, Wollenberg A, Simon D, et al. ETFAD/EADV eczema task force 2009 position paper on diagnosis and treatment of atopic dermatitis. *J Eur Acad Dermatol Venereol.* 2010;24:317-328. *Consensus guidelines including topical corticosteroids, calcineurin inhibitors, tacrolimus, and pimecrolimus, as well as phototherapy and systemic options for severe cases.*

Hwang ST, Janik JE, Jaffe ES, et al. Mycosis fungoides and Sézary syndrome. *Lancet.* 2008;371:945-957. *Review.*

Menter A, Korman NJ, Elmets CA, et al. Guidelines of care for the management of psoriasis and psoriatic arthritis Section 6. Guidelines of care for the treatment of psoriasis and psoriatic arthritis: case-based presentations and evidence-based conclusions. *J Am Acad Dermatol.* 2011. [Epub ahead of print.] *Consensus guidelines.*

Trautinger F. Phototherapy of mycosis fungoides. *Photodermatol Photoimmunol Photomed.* 2011;27:68-74. *Review of phototherapy as well as combined therapies for more advanced disease.*

447

MACULAR, PAPULAR, VESICULOBULLOUS, AND PUSTULAR DISEASES

NEIL J. KORMAN

MACULAR AND PAPULAR EXANTHEMS

An exanthem is an acute generalized eruption of the skin, and there are two major types: scarlatiniform eruptions and morbilliform eruptions. Scarlatiniform eruptions consist of confluent blanching erythema; their name was derived from their similarity to the eruption of scarlet fever (Table 447-1). Morbilliform eruptions consist of erythematous macules and papules; they are named for their resemblance to the measles eruption. Morbilliform eruptions can be caused by exposure to medications (Chapter 448) or viral infections.

Scarlatiniform Eruptions

SCARLET FEVER

Scarlet fever is caused by infection of the ears, nose, throat, and skin with toxin-producing β-hemolytic streptococci (Chapter 298). It most commonly occurs in children after streptococcal wound infections, burns, and upper respiratory tract infections. Occasional cases of scarlet fever can also be caused by *Staphylococcus aureus* (Chapter 296), *Haemophilus influenzae* (Chapter 308), and *Clostridium* species (Chapter 304). The rash is due to a circulating toxin that induces local production of inflammatory mediators and alteration of cutaneous cytokines. Patients may have an abrupt onset of fever, headache, vomiting, malaise, chills, and sore throat. The mucous membranes are usually erythematous with petechiae, and the tongue commonly has a white membrane. Red, exudative tonsils are present with pharyngeal infections. The skin eruption appears after the fever and is characterized by fine erythematous papules, first on the upper part of the trunk and then in a more general distribution. The face is flushed, and circumoral pallor is seen. This eruption lasts 4 to 5 days, followed by fine desquamation, the extent and duration of which are related to the severity of the eruption. Treatment is 1.2 million units of benzathine penicillin G given intramuscularly or oral penicillin VK, 1000 mg twice daily for 10 days. Most patients recover after 4 to 5 days, and the rash usually resolves completely over a period of several weeks.

TOXIC SHOCK SYNDROME

DEFINITION

Toxic shock syndrome is an acute febrile illness caused by toxin-producing strains of *S. aureus* (Chapter 296) or, less commonly, *Streptococcus* species (toxic shock–like syndrome [Chapter 298]).

PATHOBIOLOGY

Most cases of staphylococcal toxic shock syndrome or streptococcal toxic shock–like syndrome occur in young healthy persons aged 20 to 50 years.

TABLE 447-1   MACULAR AND PAPULAR ERUPTIONS

SCARLATINIFORM ERUPTIONS

Scarlet fever
Toxic shock syndrome
Kawasaki disease

MORBILLIFORM ERUPTIONS

Measles
Rubella
Erythema infectiosum
Roseola

PAPULAR ERUPTIONS

Molluscum contagiosum
Warts

These toxins cause massive release of tumor necrosis factor-α and interleukin-1, cytokines that mediate fever, rash, hypotension, tissue injury, and shock.

CLINICAL MANIFESTATIONS

The hallmarks of the disease are fever, rash, hypotension, and involvement of multiple organs, including the lungs, kidneys, liver, and gastrointestinal tract. Desquamation of the palms and soles follows onset of the illness by 1 to 2 weeks. There is diffuse macular erythema with flexural accentuation, mucous membrane erythema, and severe conjunctival involvement. Blood cultures are positive in 5 to 15% of patients with staphylococcal toxic shock syndrome and approximately 50% of those with streptococcal toxic shock-like syndrome.

TREATMENT

Treatment is supportive and includes hydration, vasopressors, appropriate antibiotics, and drainage of infected sites. Patients with staphylococcal toxic shock should be treated with intravenous vancomycin to cover methicillin-resistant staphylococci, 1 g every 12 hours for 10 to 15 days, with dose adjustment based on creatinine clearance. Patients with streptococcal toxic shock should be treated with both intravenous penicillin G, 3 to 4 million units every 4 hours, and intravenous clindamycin, 600 to 900 mg every 8 hours for 10 to 15 days, followed by oral therapy. Double antibiotic coverage is the standard of care for streptococcal toxic shock syndrome because this infection is characterized by extremely large numbers of stationary bacteria and penicillin alone is not effective in this scenario inasmuch as penicillin-binding proteins are not expressed during the stationary group phase of streptococci. Silver sulfadiazine cream may lead to increased toxin production; therefore, mupirocin ointment should be used for infected sites.

PROGNOSIS

The mortality rate in patients with staphylococcal toxic shock syndrome is 5 to 15%, whereas that for streptococcal toxic shock–like syndrome may be five times higher.

KAWASAKI DISEASE

EPIDEMIOLOGY

Kawasaki disease, a systemic vasculitis of unknown etiology, occurs in children of all races but is up to 20 times more common in North East Asians than in whites. Although primarily an illness of children younger than 5 years, Kawasaki disease also occurs in adults. Its epidemiologic and clinical manifestations imply that an infection is the cause, but bacterial, viral, and serologic studies have yet to confirm such an etiology.

CLINICAL MANIFESTATIONS

The clinical hallmarks are fever lasting up to 2 weeks, with spikes to 40° C (104° F), and a toxic-appearing patient. During the acute phase, the polymorphic eruption may be scarlatiniform, urticarial, morbilliform, or targetoid. Desquamation occurs in the perianal area 2 days after the onset of fever and on the extremities 2 to 3 weeks later. Patients often have hemorrhagic, dry fissured lips, conjunctival injection, a "strawberry tongue," and cervical lymphadenitis. Myocarditis and coronary artery aneurysms may develop in untreated patients, so prompt diagnosis is critical. Other findings include arthralgias and arthritis, urethritis, aseptic meningitis, pneumonitis, and diarrhea.

DIAGNOSIS

Despite the lack of specific diagnostic tests for this syndrome, the typical skin eruption accompanied by myocarditis is characteristic.

TREATMENT Rx

Recommended therapy in the acute phase of Kawasaki disease is a single infusion of 2 g/kg of intravenous gamma globulin. When this therapy is given within 5 to 10 days after the onset of fever, 85 to 90% of patients will become afebrile within 36 hours, and the risk of developing coronary artery aneurysms is significantly reduced.[1] During the subacute and convalescent phase, acetylsalicylic acid is usually given at 3 to 8 mg/kg for 6 to 8 weeks. The optimal salicylate regimen for Kawasaki disease remains uncertain, and there are no controlled trials to prove that aspirin reduces coronary artery aneurysms.

FIGURE 447-1. Reticulate macular erythema on the thigh of a patient with erythema infectiosum.

Morbilliform Eruptions

MEASLES

Measles is caused by a paramyxovirus (Chapter 375) that infects respiratory epithelium and is highly transmissible. The incubation period is 7 to 14 days. The prodrome consists of cough, coryza, and conjunctivitis. The enanthem, or Koplik's spots, predates the exanthem by 1 to 2 days and lasts 2 to 4 days. These blue-white spots surrounded by a red halo appear on the buccal mucosa and are pathognomonic for measles. The exanthem begins on the fourth or fifth day as papules on the face and behind the ears; it then spreads to the trunk and extremities. Measles is diagnosed on clinical grounds. Active immunization with live attenuated virus has dramatically reduced the incidence of measles infection (Chapter 17) and is the most important preventive measure. Treatment consists of supportive care, with attention to maintaining good hydration.

RUBELLA

Rubella is an RNA virus of the Togaviridae family (Chapter 376). Infection with this virus leads to an illness involving the skin, lymph nodes, and occasionally the joints, primarily in young children. The disease is spread by nasal droplet infection and has an incubation period of 14 to 21 days. Patients are most contagious when the rash is erupting. In children there may be no prodrome; in adults, however, fever, sore throat, and rhinitis may be present. The exanthem begins as pink macules and papules on the face that spread to the trunk and extremities; it lasts 1 to 3 days. Generalized tender lymphadenopathy, especially the suboccipital, postauricular, and cervical nodes, is the hallmark of rubella. In normal children and adolescents, the diagnosis is made clinically, and laboratory work is unnecessary. If the diagnosis is questioned, a rising immunoglobulin M (IgM) antibody titer over a 2-week period indicates recent infection. No treatment exists, and the disease is usually self-limited. Rest and fluids are appropriate. The best protection is vaccination given with measles and mumps vaccine (i.e., MMR) at 12 to 15 months and again at 4 to 6 years (Chapter 17).

ERYTHEMA INFECTIOSUM

Erythema infectiosum is an exanthem caused by human parvovirus B19 (Chapter 379). It has a 4- to 14-day incubation period and is spread by aerosolized respiratory droplets. Acute infection leads to the production of IgM antibodies and the formation of immune complexes, which are deposited in the skin and joints. Bright red erythema appears abruptly over the cheeks. Within 1 to 4 days, an erythematous morbilliform eruption occurs on the extremities; it fades within several days to a reticulate pattern (Fig. 447-1). There may also be malar erythema or a reticulate eruption on the extremities. Exposure of adults to parvovirus B19 leads to an acute polyarthropathy of the hands, wrists, knees, and ankles. Parvovirus B19 can interfere with erythropoiesis (Chapter 168) and can cause aplastic crisis in patients with sickle cell disease (Chapter 166). The diagnosis is clinical, and further testing is not generally necessary. Erythema infectiosum is usually a benign, self-limited disease.

ROSEOLA

Roseola (exanthem subitum) is caused by human herpesvirus 6 (Chapter 382). Virus replication occurs in leukocytes and salivary glands. Early invasion of the central nervous system (CNS) may lead to seizures. The classic patient is a healthy 9- to 12-month-old with an abrupt onset of high fever (40° C [104° F]) lasting 3 days. Febrile seizures occur in 15% of cases. Its rapid defervescence is striking, with the onset of a generalized pink morbilliform exanthem. The eruption lasts 2 days and consists of pink papules or blanchable macular erythema. The lack of symptoms during the febrile phase and appearance of the exanthem as the fever subsides help with the diagnosis, but rubella and measles must also be considered. In an immunocompromised child or adult, there is usually an abrupt onset of fever, malaise, and sometimes CNS involvement. Virus isolation, seroconversion (IgM), or detection of viral DNA sequences in peripheral blood mononuclear cells can confirm the diagnosis. No antiviral therapy is available for roseola, and treatment is supportive. Practically all immunocompetent patients recover from roseola without sequelae, but chronic infection with multisystem complications may develop in immunocompromised patients.

Papular Eruptions

MOLLUSCUM CONTAGIOSUM

Molluscum contagiosum is a cutaneous infection caused by a large DNA poxvirus (Chapter 380) that affects both children and adults. Firm, smooth, umbilicated papules, usually 2 to 6 mm in diameter, are present in groups or widely disseminated on the skin and mucosal surfaces. Patients infected with human immunodeficiency virus (HIV) may have hundreds of lesions, and some lesions can be larger than 15 mm (Chapter 399). The diagnosis is made on clinical grounds. Molluscum contagiosum is self-limited, with the goal of treatment being destruction of the lesions. Commonly used treatments are all topical and include cryotherapy with liquid nitrogen, curettage, cantharidin, podophyllin, and tretinoin.

WARTS

Warts are benign proliferations of skin and mucosa caused by human papillomaviruses (HPVs) (Chapter 381). More than 150 types of HPV have been identified. Certain types of HPV occur at particular anatomic sites; however, warts of any HPV type may be found at any site. Variants include common warts, genital warts, flat warts, and deep palmoplantar warts. Common warts, known as verruca vulgaris, are hard papules that range in size from 1 mm to more than 1 cm with a rough scaly surface (Fig. 447-2) and can occur anywhere on the body. Warts are transmitted by direct contact, and disruption of the epithelial barrier is a predisposing factor. HPV subtypes 6, 11, 16, 18, 31, and 35 may be associated with malignancies (Chapter 381). Malignant transformation, although uncommon, can occur in patients with genital warts or in immunocompromised patients. Infection is confined to

FIGURE 447-2. Hand of a patient with verruca vulgaris revealing many verrucous papules.

FIGURE 447-3. Purpura fulminans. Purpura and hemorrhagic blisters are seen on the arm of this patient.

TABLE 447-2 PURPURIC ERUPTIONS

NONPALPABLE PURPURA

Cutaneous Disorders

Solar purpura
Steroid purpura
Pigmented purpuric dermatosis

Systemic Disorders

Idiopathic thrombocytopenic purpura
Abnormal platelet function in renal or hepatic disease
Thrombocytosis in myeloproliferative neoplasms
Clotting factor abnormalities
Ehlers-Danlos syndrome
Scurvy
Amyloidosis
Disseminated intravascular coagulation
Thrombotic thrombocytopenic purpura
Monoclonal cryoglobulinemia
Warfarin necrosis
Emboli
    Cholesterol emboli
    Fat emboli
    Tumor emboli from atrial myxomas
    Emboli from endocarditis

PALPABLE PURPURA

Vasculitis

Leukocytoclastic vasculitis
Henoch-Schönlein purpura
Urticarial vasculitis
Polyarteritis nodosa

Infectious Emboli

Meningococcemia
Gonococcemia
Rocky Mountain spotted fever
Ecthyma gangrenosum

the epithelium and does not result in systemic viral dissemination. The diagnosis is made on clinical grounds. Viral DNA identification by Southern blot hybridization is used to identify specific HPV subtypes. All therapies are methods of physical destruction of the skin where the virus is located because there are no specific anti-HPV medications. Common topical therapies include in-office treatment with liquid nitrogen, cantharidin, or podophyllin, as well as prescription-strength tretinoin or imiquimod. Over-the-counter liquid nitrogen is neither as cold nor as effective as in-office treatment.

Purpuric Eruptions

Purpura occurs when red blood cell extravasation leads to visible hemorrhage in the skin (Table 447-2). Petechiae (<3 mm) and purpura (>3 mm) may be nonpalpable or palpable. When the condition is severe, petechiae and purpuric lesions may become confluent and form ecchymoses larger than 1 cm.

NONPALPABLE PURPURA

Dermal Causes

Frequent causes of nonpalpable purpura include solar purpura, steroid purpura, and Schamberg's disease. Solar purpura, caused by chronic sun exposure and aging, is usually found on the forearms. Steroid purpura, which is due to prolonged use of topical or systemic steroids, can occur in any location (Chapter 34). Both conditions are caused by changes in the dermal connective tissue surrounding blood vessels. Schamberg's disease, or pigmented purpuric dermatosis, is a capillaritis with yellow-brown macules and petechiae on the lower part of the legs. This capillaritis occurs as a result of red blood cell extravasation secondary to perivascular lymphocyte inflammation.

Systemic Causes

Systemic causes of nonpalpable purpura include idiopathic thrombocytopenic purpura (Chapter 175), abnormal platelet function as a result of renal or hepatic insufficiency (Chapters 132 and 157) or thrombocytosis as seen in myeloproliferative diseases (Chapter 169), and clotting factor abnormalities (Chapter 177). Fragility of the blood vessels, especially the capillaries, is found in Ehlers-Danlos syndrome (Chapter 268), scurvy (Chapter 220), and systemic amyloidosis (Chapter 194).

Thrombi

Thrombus formation within skin blood vessels also leads to purpura in patients with disseminated intravascular coagulation (Chapter 178), thrombotic thrombocytopenic purpura (Chapter 175), monoclonal cryoglobulinemia (Chapter 193), and drug reactions to warfarin (Chapter 37). Disseminated intravascular coagulation may be caused by infectious agents (bacterial, particularly meningococcemia, viral, or rickettsial) and by malignancies such as leukemia (Chapter 178). Purpura fulminans is a type of disseminated intravascular coagulation associated with fever and hypotension; it is usually found in children after a bacterial or viral infection. Widespread purpura and hemorrhagic bullae can be seen in disseminated intravascular coagulation and purpura fulminans (Fig. 447-3). Thrombotic thrombocytopenic purpura (Chapter 175) is manifested as fever, purpura, renal failure, microangiopathic hemolytic anemia, and neurologic disease. Monoclonal cryoglobulinemia may be associated with leukemia, lymphoma, multiple myeloma, and Waldenström's macroglobulinemia. Mixed cryoglobulinemia is frequently associated with hepatitis C infection (Chapter 151). Widespread purpura, along with ulcerations limited to the lower extremities or fingers and toes, can occur. Skin biopsy specimens may reveal intracapillary deposits of precipitated cryoglobulins. Disease can be worsened by exposure to cold. The vessels of the lungs, brain, and kidneys may be involved. Warfarin necrosis of the skin (Chapter 37) is an uncommon reaction that occurs between the third and tenth day of therapy and is characterized by painful erythematous to purpuric plaques in which hemorrhagic bullae develop. The most common sites include the breasts, thighs, and buttocks. The onset of disease is unrelated to the dose of warfarin, and continued warfarin therapy does not alter the course of the disease.

Emboli

Cholesterol emboli are found in the lower extremities of patients with severe atherosclerosis as a result of occlusion of small- and medium-caliber arteries

FIGURE 447-4. Palpable purpura. Leukocytoclastic vasculitis commonly causes raised purpuric and ulcerated lesions on the legs.

FIGURE 447-5. Leukocytoclastic vasculitis. Histologic evaluation reveals a smudged blood vessel in the dermis with neutrophils, neutrophilic dust, and red blood cells.

by cholesterol crystals (Chapters 80 and 127). Cholesterol emboli are triggered by vascular procedures or thrombolytic therapy, but they can also occur spontaneously. Other sources of emboli that may cause petechiae or purpura include fat emboli occurring after major injury (Chapters 98 and 112), tumor emboli from atrial myxomas (Chapter 60), emboli from infective endocarditis (Chapter 76), or nonbacterial thrombotic endocarditis (Chapters 60 and 187).

PALPABLE PURPURA

Vasculitis

Palpable purpura results from inflammatory damage to cutaneous blood vessels. Leukocytoclastic vasculitis, which is manifested as palpable purpura (Fig. 447-4), may be idiopathic or associated with sepsis, drug reactions, connective tissue diseases, cryoglobulinemia, hepatitis B or C infection, or underlying malignancies. Appropriate evaluation of patients with palpable purpura should always include histopathologic evaluation to confirm the diagnosis. Skin biopsy specimens from patients with leukocytoclastic vasculitis reveal angiocentric inflammation with endothelial cell swelling, fibrinoid necrosis of blood vessel walls, a neutrophilic cellular infiltrate with fragmentation of nuclei (karyorrhexis or leukocytoclasia) around and within blood vessel walls, and extravasated red blood cells (Fig. 447-5). Fresh skin biopsy specimens processed for direct immunofluorescence reveal deposits of immunoglobulins and complement in blood vessel walls. Once the diagnosis is confirmed, routine blood tests (including testing of renal and liver function) and urinalysis should be performed in all patients, whereas specialized tests should be targeted to specific patients with suggestive findings. If an etiologic agent can be identified and treated, the vasculitis will often resolve. Patients with idiopathic leukocytoclastic vasculitis can be treated with oral colchicine (0.6 mg twice daily), oral dapsone (up to 200 mg once daily), or in the most severe cases, immunosuppressive agents such as mycophenolate mofetil (up to 45 mg/kg for as long as the disease is active), azathioprine (up to 2.5 mg/kg for as long as the disease is active, as guided by the thiopurine

methyltransferase level), or cyclophosphamide (up to 2.5 mg/kg for as long as the disease is active).

Henoch-Schönlein purpura is a leukocytoclastic vasculitis that affects children and young adults; it is often preceded by an upper respiratory infection with associated fever, arthralgias, abdominal pain, and renal vasculitis (Chapter 123). Direct immunofluorescence reveals IgA deposits in dermal blood vessels.

Urticarial or hypocomplementemic vasculitis (Chapter 278) is characterized by urticarial lesions that last longer than 24 hours; arthritis, facial, and laryngeal edema; and low serum complement levels. In some patients, systemic lupus erythematosus (Chapter 274) may develop. In polyarteritis nodosa (Chapter 278), vasculitis of the arterial blood vessels leads to ischemia of the skin. Skin lesions usually include ulcerated nodules and ecchymoses.

Cutaneous Emboli

In addition to vasculitis, cutaneous emboli can also lead to the development of palpable purpura. Infectious emboli (Chapter 76) can be caused by gram-negative cocci, gram-negative rods, *Rickettsia* species, and in immuno-compromised patients, *Candida* species and opportunistic fungi. Acute meningococcemia (Chapter 306) occurs after an upper respiratory tract infection and is associated with headache, fever, meningitis, hypotension, and disseminated intravascular coagulation. The embolic lesions, which are found on the trunk and lower extremities, can range from 1 mm up to several centimeters. Disseminated gonococcal infection (Chapter 307) is accompanied by fever, arthralgias, tenosynovitis, and a small number of vesiculopustules with purpura or hemorrhagic necrosis over the distal ends of the extremities. Rocky Mountain spotted fever (Chapter 335) is a tick-borne disease characterized by headache, fever, chills, photophobia, and myalgias. The cutaneous eruption starts acrally and spreads centripetally as small, erythematous, blanchable macules that evolve into petechiae, palpable purpura, and ecchymoses. Ecthyma gangrenosum is manifested as erythematous papules and plaques in which central purpura and hemorrhagic necrosis develop; *Pseudomonas aeruginosa* (Chapter 314) is the most common organism, but *Klebsiella* species (Chapter 314), *Escherichia coli* (Chapter 312), and *Serratia* species (Chapter 315) have also been implicated. In immunocompromised patients, ecthyma gangrenosum may develop as a result of infection with *Candida* species or opportunistic fungi.

● VESICULOBULLOUS DISEASES

Vesicles are clear, fluid-filled lesions measuring less than 5 mm; bullae or blisters are clear, fluid-filled lesions larger than 5 mm. Vesiculobullous lesions in the skin may be caused by immunologically mediated mechanisms, hypersensitivity reactions, metabolic disorders, inherited genetic defects, and infections (Table 447-3).

Immunologically Mediated Blistering Diseases
BULLOUS PEMPHIGOID

DEFINITION

Bullous pemphigoid is an autoimmune blistering disease that occurs in elderly people. Tense blisters and urticarial plaques occur on the flexor surfaces of the arms and legs, axilla, groin, and abdomen (Fig. 447-6).

PATHOBIOLOGY

IgG autoantibodies bind to the epidermal basement membrane and activate complement, which attracts inflammatory cells. These inflammatory cells release proteases that degrade basement membrane proteins and lead to blister formation. Histology reveals a subepidermal blister with an eosinophilic infiltrate. Direct immunofluorescence shows linear deposits of IgG and C3 at the basement membrane. Indirect immunofluorescence studies using salt-split skin demonstrate circulating IgG antibodies that bind to the epidermal side.

TREATMENT ℞

Treatment is dictated by the degree of involvement and the rate of progression of the disease. The ultrapotent topical steroid clobetasol (10 to 30 g per day), applied to the skin of patients with bullous pemphigoid until 15 days after disease control is obtained and then tapered over 4 months, is effective, is superior to oral corticosteroid treatment, and is associated with fewer side effects than higher dose clobetasol in patients with both moderate and severe

FIGURE 447-6. Bullous pemphigoid. Tense subepidermal bullae are seen on an erythematous base.

FIGURE 447-7. Herpes gestationis. Multiple tense blisters and erosions on an erythematous base are present.

TABLE 447-3   VESICULOBULLOUS DISEASES

IMMUNOLOGICALLY MEDIATED DISEASES

Bullous pemphigoid
Herpes gestationis
Mucous membrane pemphigoid
Epidermolysis bullosa acquisita
Dermatitis herpetiformis
Linear immunoglobulin A bullous dermatosis
Pemphigus
    Vulgaris
    Foliaceus
    Paraneoplastic

HYPERSENSITIVITY DISEASES

Erythema multiforme minor
Erythema multiforme major (Stevens-Johnson syndrome)
Toxic epidermal necrolysis

METABOLIC DISEASES

Porphyria cutanea tarda
Pseudoporphyria
Diabetic blisters

INHERITED GENETIC DISORDERS

Epidermolysis bullosa
    Simplex
    Junctional
    Dystrophic

INFECTIOUS DISEASES

Impetigo
Staphylococcal scalded skin syndrome
Herpes simplex
Varicella
Herpes zoster

disease.[2] Nevertheless, the practicality of such potent topical steroids is controversial, and many experts use oral prednisone, 1 mg/kg in an early morning daily dose, as a foundation of therapy for patients with generalized bullous pemphigoid. Other treatments include tetracycline (500 mg four times daily), dapsone (up to 150 mg daily), azathioprine (up to 2.5 mg/kg as guided by the thiopurine methyltransferase level), methotrexate (up to 15 mg weekly), mycophenolate mofetil (35 to 45 mg/kg divided into two daily doses), and cyclophosphamide (up to about 2.5 mg/kg). The duration of therapy with all of these medications varies, depending on the activity of the disease. Left untreated, bullous pemphigoid generally persists for months to years. Spontaneous remissions and exacerbations occur. The mortality rate is relatively low, even without treatment.

Herpes Gestationis

Herpes gestationis is a rare autoimmune dermatosis of pregnancy. Despite the name, herpes gestationis has no relationship to herpesvirus infection. Most patients have intense pruritus. Periumbilical urticarial plaques progress to vesicles and blisters. The eruption spreads peripherally (Fig. 447-7), typically sparing the face, palms, soles, and mucous membranes. IgG autoantibodies are produced against bullous pemphigoid antigen II, which is critical in epidermal-dermal adhesion. Antibody binding triggers an immune response leading to blister formation. Histology reveals a subepidermal blister, and direct immunofluorescence shows linear C3 deposits at the basement membrane.

Corticosteroids are the mainstay of therapy. Patients with mild disease are treated with moderate- to high-potency topical corticosteroids, such as 0.05% fluocinonide ointment applied twice daily to affected areas, whereas patients with extensive disease usually require systemic corticosteroids, such as prednisone, 1 mg/kg given once daily as an early morning dose. Disease clears within 1 to 2 weeks after initiation of treatment. There is an increased risk for premature delivery and birth of infants who are small for gestational age, suggesting that these women should be managed by obstetricians experienced in high-risk pregnancies.

Mucous Membrane Pemphigoid

DEFINITION

Mucous membrane pemphigoid, previously called cicatricial pemphigoid, is a group of subepithelial blistering diseases that involve the mucosal surfaces. Patients have blisters of the oral, ocular, nasopharyngeal, laryngeal, anogenital, and esophageal mucosa that heal with scarring, which causes the major morbidity associated with the disease.

PATHOBIOLOGY

There are several subgroups of mucous membrane pemphigoid. Some patients have circulating IgG autoantibodies that bind to the dermal side of salt-split skin and recognize laminin 5. A second subgroup includes patients who have pure ocular disease and IgG antibodies directed against β_4 integrin. A third subgroup has mucosal disease and skin lesions. The fourth variant includes patients with oral disease but without skin disease. Histology reveals a subepidermal blister with an inflammatory cell infiltrate. Direct immunofluorescence shows linear IgG, IgA, and C3 deposits at the basement membrane. Indirect immunofluorescence reveals circulating IgG or IgA antibodies, or both.

TREATMENT   Rx

Treatment is dictated by the extent, severity, and location of disease; it ranges from topical corticosteroids, such as 0.05% fluocinonide ointment applied twice daily to affected areas under occlusion in patients with only oral disease, to prednisone, 1 mg/kg given once daily as an early morning dose, and cyclophosphamide, up to 2.5 mg/kg given as an early morning dose for up to 2 years, for severe ocular disease. Management teams should include ophthalmologists, otolaryngologists, dermatologists, and internists for patients with severe disease. Patients with both circulating IgG and IgA antibodies tend to have more severe disease.

FIGURE 447-8. **Dermatitis herpetiformis.** The elbow of a patient has eroded erythematous papules and papulovesicles.

FIGURE 447-9. **Pemphigus vulgaris.** The lower lip of a patient has confluent erosions with scattered crusting.

PROGNOSIS

Mucous membrane pemphigoid is a chronic disease. Untreated ocular disease can result in blindness.

EPIDERMOLYSIS BULLOSA ACQUISITA

Epidermolysis bullosa acquisita is an acquired autoimmune blistering disease that generally occurs in middle age. There are two types of skin lesions: non-inflammatory acral blisters that heal with scarring and milia formation and widespread inflammatory vesiculobullous disease.

PATHOBIOLOGY

Epidermolysis bullosa acquisita is characterized by IgG autoantibodies that target collagen VII, the major protein of anchoring fibrils. These autoantibodies alter dermal-epidermal adhesion and lead to blister formation. Histology reveals a subepidermal blister containing few inflammatory cells when mechanobullous lesions are sampled or a neutrophil-rich infiltrate when inflammatory blisters are sampled. Direct immunofluorescence reveals linear IgG deposits at the basement membrane. Indirect immunofluorescence shows circulating IgG autoantibodies that bind the dermal side of salt-split skin.

TREATMENT — Rx

Epidermolysis bullosa acquisita is a chronic disease that is very difficult to treat. Dapsone (at doses up to 150 mg daily), colchicine (0.6 mg twice daily), azathioprine (up to 2.5 mg/kg as guided by the thiopurine methyltransferase level), or cyclophosphamide (2.5 mg/kg given as an early morning dosage) alone or along with prednisone (60 mg given once daily as an early morning dose) is only occasionally successful. Cyclosporine at doses of up to 5 mg/kg, extracorporeal photopheresis, and intravenous immunoglobulin (at doses of 2 gm/kg given monthly) have been used successfully in patients with severe disease. Because of nephrotoxicity, cyclosporine should be reserved for crisis management of patients who have severe disease and are experiencing a major flare.

DERMATITIS HERPETIFORMIS

Dermatitis herpetiformis is an immune-mediated vesicular disease that usually occurs in young to middle-aged patients. Skin lesions are extremely pruritic, grouped vesicles and erosions located on the scalp, posterior of the neck, and extensor surfaces of the elbows, knees, and buttocks (Fig. 447-8). Most patients have a subclinical gluten-sensitive enteropathy (Chapter 142) that is reversible with a gluten-free diet. Diet alone can sometimes control the skin disease, with clearance of the cutaneous granular IgA deposits at the basement membrane. Biopsy specimens of skin lesions reveal dermal papillary neutrophilic microabscesses. Direct immunofluorescence shows dermal papillary granular IgA deposits in all patients. Most patients with dermatitis herpetiformis have circulating IgA antibodies directed against tissue transglutaminase. Dermatitis herpetiformis can be treated with dapsone, up to 200 mg daily given chronically. Dermatitis herpetiformis is a lifelong disease.

LINEAR IMMUNOGLOBULIN A BULLOUS DERMATOSIS

Linear IgA bullous dermatosis is an acquired autoimmune blistering disease of the skin. The primary lesions are papulovesicles, and involvement of the oral mucous membranes is common. The disease occurs throughout adulthood. Deposition of IgA antibody specific for a portion of bullous pemphigoid antigen II leads to complement activation and neutrophil chemotaxis. Proteolytic enzymes are released, destroy the dermal-epidermal junction, and cause blister formation. Histology reveals a subepidermal vesicle or cleft with neutrophil predominance. Direct immunofluorescence shows linear deposits of IgA at the basement membrane. Indirect immunofluorescence demonstrates circulating IgA antibodies. Most patients respond to dapsone, up to 200 mg daily, given chronically. Patients whose disease is not controlled with dapsone may benefit from the addition of oral prednisone, 1 mg/kg once daily as an early morning dose. The disease tends to be chronic in adults, but the childhood version (called chronic bullous disease of childhood) may run a several-year course and then remit.

PEMPHIGUS

DEFINITION

Pemphigus refers to a group of autoimmune blistering intraepidermal diseases of the skin and mucous membranes that are most common in middle age.

CLINICAL MANIFESTATIONS

Patients with pemphigus vulgaris have flaccid blisters and erosions in the oropharynx (Fig. 447-9), trunk, head, neck, and intertriginous areas. Pemphigus foliaceus is accompanied by erythema, scaling, and crusting of the face, scalp, and upper part of the trunk. Patients with paraneoplastic pemphigus have ocular and oral blisters and erosions along with skin lesions resembling erythema multiforme and an associated underlying malignancy that is generally lymphoreticular in origin (Chapter 187).

PATHOBIOLOGY

Autoantibodies in pemphigus vulgaris target desmoglein III, and autoantibodies in pemphigus foliaceus target desmoglein I. Circulating antibodies in paraneoplastic pemphigus recognize a complex of proteins, including desmoplakin I and II, bullous pemphigoid antigen I, envoplakin, periplakin, and desmoglein I and III.

DIAGNOSIS

Skin biopsy specimens from patients with pemphigus vulgaris reveal suprabasilar acantholysis, whereas pemphigus foliaceus biopsy specimens demonstrate subcorneal acantholysis. Biopsy specimens of paraneoplastic pemphigus show suprabasilar acantholysis and dyskeratotic keratinocytes with basal cell vacuolization.

Direct immunofluorescence demonstrates cell surface deposits of IgG in patients with pemphigus vulgaris and foliaceus, whereas indirect immunofluorescence reveals circulating IgG antibodies that recognize molecules on the epidermal cell surface. Patients with paraneoplastic pemphigus have circulating and tissue-bound IgG antibodies that are indistinguishable from those in pemphigus vulgaris and that also recognize the cell surface of simple epithelia, including the liver and heart.

TREATMENT   Rx

Treatment regimens depend on the patient's age, the degree of involvement, the rate of disease progression, and the subtype of pemphigus. Systemic corticosteroids (e.g., oral prednisone, 1 mg/kg once daily as an early morning dose) are required for the treatment of patients with pemphigus vulgaris, whereas topical corticosteroids (e.g., 0.05% fluocinonide ointment applied twice daily to affected areas) may occasionally control pemphigus foliaceus. One course of intravenous immunoglobulin (400 mg/kg/day for 5 days) appears to be a safe and effective treatment for patients whose disease is resistant to steroids.**3** Other agents include dapsone (up to 200 mg daily), hydroxychloroquine (administered at less than 6 mg/kg of lean body mass divided into two daily doses), mycophenolate mofetil (35 to 45 mg/kg/day divided into two daily doses), azathioprine (up to 2.5 mg/kg as guided by the thiopurine methyltransferase level), cyclophosphamide (up to 2.5 mg/kg given as an early morning dose), and rituximab (four weekly doses of 375 mg/m^2). The duration of therapy with each of these medications varies according to the level of disease activity. Although the use of steroid-sparing agents is supported by clinical experience, few controlled studies have demonstrated their benefit. For paraneoplastic pemphigus caused by benign tumors such as Castleman's disease (Chapter 191), tumor removal is often curative. Patients with associated malignant tumors have recalcitrant disease, although there are occasional successes with pulse corticosteroids (methylprednisolone, 1000 mg given daily for 3 consecutive days), pulse cyclophosphamide (500 to 1000 mg given monthly for 6 months to 1 year, often along with varying doses of prednisone), immuno-apheresis, immunoablative high-dose cyclophosphamide (50 mg/kg/day for 4 days), and rituximab (four weekly doses of 375 mg/m^2).

FIGURE 447-10. Erythema multiforme. Target or "bull's-eye" annular lesions with central vesicles and bullae are characteristic of erythema multiforme.

PROGNOSIS

Before the availability of corticosteroids, 60 to 90% of patients with pemphigus vulgaris died, whereas the mortality rate has now decreased to the 5 to 10% range. The prognosis of patients with paraneoplastic pemphigus is related to the type of associated neoplasm. Patients with benign tumors usually experience clearance of their lesions after tumor resection, whereas those with malignant tumors generally have a poor prognosis.

Hypersensitivity Reactions That Cause Blisters
ERYTHEMA MULTIFORME

DEFINITION

Erythema multiforme is an acute blistering eruption that occurs in all age groups. Erythema multiforme minor is localized, with minimal or no mucosal involvement. Erythema multiforme major, also known as Stevens-Johnson syndrome, is a more severe mucosal and skin disease characterized by signs and symptoms reminiscent of serum sickness (Chapter 46).

CLINICAL MANIFESTATIONS

Toxic epidermal necrolysis is at the most severe end of the erythema multiforme spectrum. The primary lesions of erythema multiforme minor are erythematous macules and edematous papules with vesicular centers that become dusky violet. Target or iris lesions are found on extensor surfaces of the extremities and spread centripetally (Fig. 447-10). The skin lesions of Stevens-Johnson syndrome resemble those of erythema multiforme minor but are likely to be generalized and show confluent erythema with urticarial and purpuric lesions. Erosions of two or more mucosal surfaces occur in Stevens-Johnson syndrome and may include hemorrhagic crusting of the lips, ulceration of the ocular mucosa, and genital involvement. Patients with erythema multiforme major have a 1- to 14-day prodrome that includes fever, cough, sore throat, vomiting, and diarrhea. Patients with toxic epidermal necrolysis may have a similar prodrome, rapidly followed by generalized macular erythema that progresses to confluent erythema with skin tenderness. Large blisters follow soon afterward, and then skin sloughing occurs as the large blisters break and leave denuded skin.

PATHOBIOLOGY

Common etiologic associations of erythema multiforme include infections such as herpes simplex (Chapter 382) (especially recurrent erythema multiforme minor), *Mycoplasma pneumoniae* (Chapter 325), and drug reactions (Chapter 262). Sulfonamides, penicillins, barbiturates, carbamazepine, phenytoin, allopurinol, and nonsteroidal anti-inflammatory drugs (NSAIDs) are the most common drugs implicated in Stevens-Johnson syndrome and toxic epidermal necrolysis.

DIAGNOSIS

The diagnosis of erythema multiforme is clinical.

TREATMENT   Rx

Chronic antiviral treatment with acyclovir (400 mg twice daily for 6 months) decreases outbreaks in a subset of patients with recurrent erythema multiforme minor. Treatment of erythema multiforme major is otherwise nonspecific, with attention to fluid and electrolyte balance and eye disease being critical. If a drug is suspected, it must be withdrawn. Systemic corticosteroid treatment is contraindicated in Stevens-Johnson syndrome. Treatment of toxic epidermal necrolysis is very difficult, but uncontrolled studies suggest that intravenous immune globulin (2 to 3 g/kg over a period of 2 to 5 days) may improve the prognosis.

PROGNOSIS

Erythema multiforme minor usually subsides within 2 to 3 weeks. Erythema multiforme major takes 3 to 6 weeks to clear and has less than a 5% mortality rate. Toxic epidermal necrolysis has a mortality rate approaching 30%, and patients are best managed in an intensive care or burn unit.

Metabolic Disorders That Cause Blisters
PORPHYRIA CUTANEA TARDA

Porphyria cutanea tarda is caused by deficient activity of the heme synthetic enzyme uroporphyrinogen decarboxylase (Chapter 217). The fragility of sun-exposed skin leads to erosions and bullae, which are worst on the dorsal surface of the hands (Fig. 447-11), forearms, and face. Healing of crusted erosions and blisters leaves scars, milia, and hyperpigmented and hypopigmented atrophic patches. Hypertrichosis is common and most florid over the temporal and malar areas. Urinary porphyrin levels are abnormally high. Histology reveals a subepidermal blister with minimal dermal infiltrate, and direct immunofluorescence demonstrates immunoglobulin and complement deposition in dermal capillaries and at the basement membrane. Phlebotomy is the standard treatment, and the goal is to reduce serum ferritin to the lower limit of the normal range. Another treatment option is oral hydroxychloroquine at a dose (200 mg twice weekly until the disease is under control) that is much lower than that used for photoprotective indications. Alcohol and estrogen use should be discontinued because they can cause the disease to flare.

PSEUDOPORPHYRIA

Pseudoporphyria is a bullous eruption that mimics porphyria cutanea tarda clinically and histologically without porphyrin abnormalities. Many medications can cause pseudoporphyria, including propionic acid–derivative NSAIDs (e.g., naproxen, diflunisal, ketoprofen, nabumetone, oxaprozin, and mefenamic acid), furosemide, tetracycline, fluoroquinolones, amiodarone, cyclosporine, dapsone, etretinate, and flutamide. The prognosis is good for patients with pseudoporphyria after the offending agent has been discontinued. However, resolution of the disease may take several months. In patients with chronic renal failure treated by hemodialysis, true porphyria cutanea tarda or pseudoporphyria may develop and is very difficult to treat.

FIGURE 447-11. Porphyria cutanea tarda. A blister and erosions are present on the dorsal surface of the hand.

FIGURE 447-13. Bullous impetigo. Multiple blisters are present on the trunk of this patient.

FIGURE 447-12. Epidermolysis bullosa simplex. Tense blisters and erosions are present on the trunk and extremities of a newborn.

FIGURE 447-14. Staphylococcal scalded skin syndrome. Confluent erythema with exfoliation of skin is seen on the trunk.

DIABETES MELLITUS

Distal extremity blisters may occasionally develop in patients with diabetes mellitus (Chapter 236). There is no correlation between the development of blisters and the severity, duration, or complications of diabetes. The mechanism of blister formation is not understood.

Inherited Genetic Disorders That Cause Blisters

Epidermolysis bullosa is a group of inherited bullous disorders characterized by blister formation in response to mechanical trauma. Subtypes include epidermolysis bullosa simplex (intraepidermal skin separation) (Fig. 447-12), junctional epidermolysis bullosa (skin separation in the lamina lucida), and dystrophic epidermolysis bullosa (sublamina densa separation). Infancy is an especially difficult time, and epidermolysis bullosa may be accompanied by blistering that is complicated by infection and sepsis. Many patients with junctional epidermolysis bullosa have severe disease that can lead to death, usually secondary to infection, and metastatic squamous cell carcinoma may develop in some patients with recessive dystrophic epidermolysis bullosa and can also lead to death. In contrast, epidermolysis bullosa simplex, milder forms of junctional epidermolysis bullosa, and dominant dystrophic epidermolysis bullosa do not usually affect life expectancy. Epidermolysis bullosa simplex is caused by mutations of the genes coding for keratins 5 and 14. Junctional epidermolysis bullosa has a variable molecular etiology, and mutations in genes coding for laminin 5 subunits, bullous pemphigoid antigen I, α_6 integrin, and β_4 integrin have been demonstrated. Dystrophic epidermolysis bullosa is caused by mutations of the type VII collagen gene. Epidermolysis bullosa is a lifelong disease. Some subtypes, especially the milder forms, improve with age. No medications are known to correct the underlying molecular defects, but gene therapy is being actively pursued.

Infectious Diseases That Cause Blisters
IMPETIGO

Impetigo is a bacterial infection of the superficial layers of the epidermis. Bullous impetigo is caused by *S. aureus* (Chapter 296), and nonbullous impetigo is caused by group A β-hemolytic streptococci (Chapter 298). Bullous impetigo is manifested as vesicles and bulla (Fig. 447-13). Lesions are common on the face but may appear anywhere. Nonbullous impetigo is characterized by fragile vesicles or pustules that rupture and leave honey-colored crusted papules or plaques, especially near the nose and mouth and on the extremities. Lesions develop on normal or traumatized skin or are superimposed on preexisting conditions, including scabies, varicella, or atopic dermatitis. The causative agent of bullous impetigo is coagulase-positive *S. aureus*, which produces exfoliatins A and B. The toxins cause cleavage within or below the stratum granulosum. Impetigo is diagnosed clinically. Culture and sensitivity studies are recommended if topical or oral treatment is ineffective. Oral antibiotics, including dicloxacillin (500 mg four times daily for 7 days) or cephalexin (500 mg three times daily for 7 days), are used for extensive disease or in patients refractory to topical mupirocin. Gentle débridement of crusts is recommended. Lesions resolve after 7 to 10 days of treatment. Acute glomerulonephritis (Chapter 123) develops in 2 to 5% of young children with nonbullous impetigo, usually within 10 days after the skin lesions appear.

STAPHYLOCOCCAL SCALDED SKIN SYNDROME

Staphylococcal scalded skin syndrome is a blistering disease caused by an exotoxin produced by *S. aureus* (Chapter 296). It is most common in young children but may occur in adults who have renal insufficiency or are immunocompromised. The site of the staphylococcal infection is usually extracutaneous. Staphylococcal scalded skin syndrome is manifested as a sudden onset of fever and tender, blanchable erythema. It starts on the central part of the face, neck, and intertriginous areas and rapidly generalizes. The palms, soles, and mucous membranes are spared. Flaccid blisters occur within 1 to 2 days and soon exfoliate in large sheets, with superficially denuded skin remaining (Fig. 447-14). The disease must be distinguished from toxic epidermal necrolysis by skin biopsy. In staphylococcal scalded skin syndrome, there is an upper epidermal blister, whereas toxic epidermal necrolysis causes a dermal-epidermal blister. Patients with the most severe staphylococcal scalded skin syndrome should be treated with intravenous nafcillin or oxacillin, 2 g every 4 to 6 hours for 10 to 14 days. If the patient is found to have methicillin-resistant staphylococci, vancomycin, 1 g every 12 hours (with dose adjustment based on creatinine clearance), should be given for 10 to 14 days. Patients with mild disease may be treated with oral dicloxacillin, 500 mg four times daily for 10 to 14 days, unless the staphylococcal isolate is methicillin resistant, in which case the choice of antibiotics should be guided by the results of sensitivity testing.

HERPES SIMPLEX VIRUS INFECTION

PATHOBIOLOGY

Herpes simplex virus (HSV) infection (Chapter 382) may be caused by type 1 or type 2 HSV. The hallmark of HSV infection is its ability to establish latent infection. Disease commonly occurs as a recurrent vesicular eruption of the oral, perioral (typically HSV-1), or genital (typically HSV-2) regions, although primary gingivostomatitis (typically in children and young adults and caused by HSV-1) and primary genital herpes (typically HSV-2) are less common.

CLINICAL MANIFESTATIONS

Patients with primary gingivostomatitis have high fever, regional lymphadenopathy, and malaise. Patients with primary genital herpes have fever, flulike symptoms, tender inguinal adenopathy, and aseptic meningitis. These infections all reveal grouped vesicles on an erythematous base. Recurrent eruptions can be triggered by skin trauma, cold or heat, concurrent infection, and menstruation. Chronic erosive ulcers of the face and anogenital areas may develop in immunocompromised patients.

DIAGNOSIS

Tzanck smear of fluid from the roof of a vesicle can be helpful in confirming the diagnosis (see Fig. 444-15 in Chapter 444), but viral culture is the diagnostic "gold standard." The direct fluorescent antibody test is an antigen-based technique that not only yields same-day results but can also distinguish HSV from varicella-zoster virus (VZV) and is becoming widely used.

TREATMENT   Rx

In healthy individuals, HSV infection is self-limited. The goal of treatment is to shorten the current attack and prevent recurrences. Acyclovir is effective in the treatment of HSV infections; valacyclovir and famciclovir are closely related, effective medications with improved oral bioavailability. The doses and duration of therapy vary depending on whether the infection is limited to the oral or genital mucous membranes or is disseminated and on whether it is primary or recurrent disease (Chapter 382).

CHICKENPOX

Chickenpox is caused by VZV (Chapter 383). It is usually a childhood disease, but affected adults have more morbidity. Skin lesions occur 10 to 21 days after exposure to VZV. Erythematous macules appear on the scalp, face, trunk, and proximal ends of the limbs, with rapid progression to papules, vesicles, pustules, and crusting (Fig. 447-15). Adults may experience a more widespread eruption, prolonged fever, and pneumonia. The diagnosis is usually made clinically, but direct fluorescent antibody or culture confirmation is sometimes needed. Treatment of healthy children is unnecessary because the disease is self-limited. Adults should be treated with oral acyclovir, 800 mg five times a day for 7 days. The varicella vaccine given once to healthy children 12 to 18 months of age and twice, in a 4- to 8-week interval, to susceptible persons older than 13 years (Chapter 17) is highly effective.

HERPES ZOSTER

PATHOBIOLOGY

Herpes zoster is caused by reactivation of VZV from a previous chickenpox infection. The disease is more common in older or immunocompromised patients.

CLINICAL MANIFESTATIONS

The typical manifestation is painful grouped herpetiform vesicles on an erythematous base confined to cutaneous surfaces innervated by one sensory nerve and preceded by radicular pain (Fig. 447-16). The major morbidity, which is pain within the affected dermatome, can be severe and persist after

FIGURE 447-15. Erythematous macules and vesicles with crusted erosions on the chest of a patient with varicella.

FIGURE 447-16. Herpes zoster. Necrotic blisters and erosions in a dermatomal pattern are seen on the trunk of this patient.

the skin lesions have resolved (postherpetic neuralgia). Immunocompromised patients have an increased risk for cutaneous dissemination and visceral involvement of the bladder, lungs, and CNS.

TREATMENT   Rx

Acyclovir (800 mg orally five times daily for 7 days) and its derivatives valacyclovir (500 mg orally three times daily for 7 days) and famciclovir (500 mg orally three times daily for 7 days) are safe and effective in the treatment of active disease and prevention of postherpetic neuralgia. In an immunocompromised patient, acyclovir should be given intravenously (10 mg/kg every 8 hours for 7 to 10 days). The earlier antiviral medications are started, the more effective they are in shortening the duration of herpes zoster and in preventing or decreasing the severity of postherpetic neuralgia. Oral steroids are not effective in reducing the incidence of acute pain or postherpetic neuralgia. Patients with postherpetic neuralgia of more than 3 months' duration benefit from the use of gabapentin, 1600 or 2400 mg daily, with a significant reduction in pain.[4] VZV vaccine markedly reduces both the morbidity from herpes zoster and postherpetic neuralgia in healthy adults older than 60 years.[5]

● PUSTULAR ERUPTIONS
Acne Vulgaris

DEFINITION

Acne vulgaris is the most common pustular skin condition. Teenagers are usually affected, but the disease may persist into adulthood. The comedo, which is the primary lesion, can be either closed (whitehead) or open (blackhead).

PATHOBIOLOGY

Androgen production after puberty stimulates the release of sebum by sebaceous glands. Sebum flow is impeded because of abnormal keratinization within the pilosebaceous canal, a process that leads to the formation of

FIGURE 447-17. Sebaceous gland hyperplasia. A large red bulbous nose known as rhinophyma is characteristic of late-stage rosacea.

FIGURE 447-18. Perioral dermatitis. Erythematous papules and pinpoint pustules are evident around the mouth.

comedones. Bacterial (*Propionibacterium acnes*) proliferation within the comedo predisposes to rupture of the pilosebaceous unit with extravasation into the surrounding dermis, which results in papules, pustules, and cysts.

TREATMENT Rx

Patients with mild disease are treated topically with benzoyl peroxide, tretinoin, adapalene, or tazarotene, which normalize follicular keratinization. In patients with mild to moderate disease, treatment with benzoyl peroxide is the most cost-effective therapy.[6] The addition of topical antibiotics helps control inflammatory papules and pustules. More significant disease is often treated with oral tetracycline (250 to 1000 mg/day), doxycycline (200 mg/day), or minocycline (200 mg/day). Dapsone gel (5%) is safe and effective.[7] Another approach is oral contraceptives containing either ethinyl estradiol and norgestimate or ethinyl estradiol and drospirenone, both of which are superior to placebo in the treatment of acne in women.[8] Isotretinoin (1 mg/kg given for 5 months), which decreases sebaceous gland size and sebum production, is reserved for severe cystic disease because of its teratogenicity, possible associated risk for depression, and other significant side effects. Acne may be exacerbated by the use of oil-based cosmetics or hair preparations. Androgenic hormones, systemic corticosteroids, lithium, phenytoin, phenobarbital, isoniazid, and endocrinologic conditions such as polycystic ovary disease and adrenal or ovarian tumors may produce acneiform eruptions or aggravate preexisting acne.

ROSACEA

Rosacea, which is a chronic inflammatory disease of the face, affects the pilosebaceous units and blood vessels and generally occurs in middle age. Erythema, telangiectases, erythematous papules, and pustules occur on the central part of the face. Ocular rosacea can lead to keratitis, iritis, blepharitis, and recurrent chalazion; it should be managed by an ophthalmologist. In its most severe form, rosacea can cause sebaceous gland hyperplasia leading to a large red bulbous nose known as rhinophyma (Fig. 447-17). Rosacea is more likely to develop in patients with a tendency toward facial flushing. Flushing can be due to heat, spicy foods, hot drinks, alcohol, or emotional stimuli. With time, the flushing reaction lasts longer and longer until it persists. Topical antibiotics, including 0.75 to 1% metronidazole, are helpful in mild disease, and the combination of a sub-antimicrobial dose (20 mg twice daily) of doxycycline plus topical 0.75% metronidazole is more efficacious than topical metronidazole alone.[9] Patients with more severe disease require oral tetracycline, 500 mg twice daily for 3 to 4 months and then slowly decreased as tolerated. Azelaic acid gel (15%) can significantly improve papulopustular rosacea.

PERIORAL DERMATITIS

Perioral dermatitis is characterized by erythematous papules and pustules as well as scaling patches around the mouth and eyes (Fig. 447-18). Most

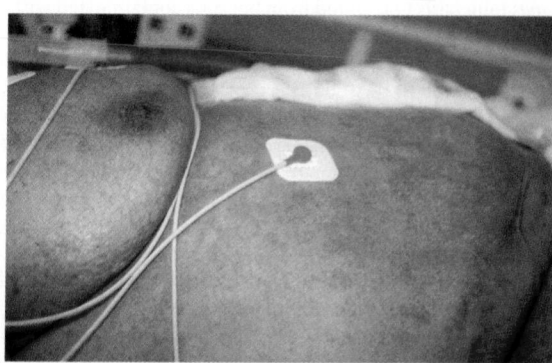

FIGURE 447-19. Acute generalized exanthematous pustulosis. Erythematous macules and numerous superficial pustules are present on the trunk of this patient.

patients have used potent topical corticosteroids inappropriately for long periods. The eruption generally clears after stopping the corticosteroid and using tetracycline, 250 mg orally twice daily for 6 weeks.

ACUTE GENERALIZED EXANTHEMATOUS PUSTULOSIS

Acute exanthematous pustulosis is a generalized pustular eruption that is associated with fever and frequently caused by antibiotics. Pustules develop within 2 days of drug administration, start on the face or in flexural areas, and rapidly disseminate (Fig. 447-19). Spontaneous resolution occurs in less than 2 weeks.

PUSTULAR PSORIASIS

Pustular psoriasis is a variant of psoriasis (Chapter 446) that localizes to the palms and soles or generalizes over the entire body. Patients with generalized disease have fever and leukocytosis and require systemic therapy. Pustules can also be seen in patients with septic emboli of bacterial or fungal origin, including gonococcemia and systemic candidiasis (see Purpuric Eruptions).

FOLLICULITIS

Folliculitis is inflammation of the hair follicles caused by infection with staphylococci. It is due to obstruction of individual hair follicles and associated pilosebaceous units. Folliculitis is more common in patients with diabetes mellitus, obesity, or immunocompromised states. The primary lesion is a pustule with a central hair. Typical affected sites are the scalp, thighs, trunk, axilla, and inguinal area. Sometimes the infection can extend deeper into the dermis and form larger erythematous nodules from one (furuncle) or more (carbuncle) follicles. Treatment with oral antibiotics such as cephalexin, 500 mg twice daily for 14 days, clears extensive infections, whereas topical

FIGURE 447-20. *Pseudomonas* **species folliculitis.** The trunk of this patient has numerous pustules on an erythematous base.

antibiotics (e.g., clindamycin solution applied twice daily for 2 weeks or longer) and antibacterial soaps (e.g., Dial or Lever 2000) help in milder disease.

Pseudomonas Folliculitis

Pseudomonas folliculitis is acquired from hot tubs contaminated with *P. aeruginosa* (Chapter 314). The typical finding is papules and pustules in areas of skin occluded by a bathing suit (Fig. 447-20). Treatment with ciprofloxacin, 500 mg twice daily for 10 to 14 days, is usually curative.

Pityrosporum folliculitis is a pruritic, acne-like eruption that occurs on the upper part of the back and the chest, arms, and face and is caused by *Pityrosporum ovale.* Treatment is with oral itraconazole, 200 mg/day for 1 week, and 2% ketoconazole shampoo applied to the affected area daily for 1 month.

Eosinophilic Pustular Folliculitis

Eosinophilic pustular folliculitis is a sterile, intensely pruritic folliculitis usually found on the face, chest, and back of patients who are positive for HIV (Chapter 399). Skin biopsy is needed to confirm the diagnosis. Treatment is difficult, but options include potent topical corticosteroids, such as 0.1% triamcinolone ointment applied twice daily for several months (although this class 4 topical corticosteroid should not be used on the face); tacrolimus ointment 0.1% is another topical option that is safe for facial use. Systemic options include antihistamines, such as hydroxyzine, 25 mg every 8 hours as needed, and ultraviolet light therapy.

1. Oates-Whitehead RM, Baumer JH, Haines L, et al. Intravenous immunoglobulin for the treatment of Kawasaki disease in children. *Cochrane Database Syst Rev.* 2003;4:CD004000.
2. Joly P, Roujeau, JC, Benichou J, et al. A comparison of two regimens of topical corticosteroids in the treatment of patients with bullous pemphigoid: A multi-center randomized study. *J Invest Dermatol.* 2009;129:1681-1687.
3. Amagai M, Ikeda S, Shimizu H, et al, for the Pemphigus Study Group. A randomized double-blind trial of intravenous immunoglobulin for pemphigus. *J Acad Dermatol.* 2009;60:595-603.
4. Rice AS, Maton S, for the Postherpetic Neuralgia Study Group. Gabapentin in post herpetic neuralgia: a randomized, double blind, placebo-controlled study. *Pain.* 2001;94:215-224.
5. Oxman MN, Levin MJ, Johnson GR, et al. A vaccine to prevent herpes zoster and postherpetic neuralgia in older adults. *N Engl J Med.* 2005;352:2271-2284.
6. Ozolins M, Eady EA, Avery AJ, et al. Comparison of five antimicrobial regimens for the treatment of mild to moderate inflammatory facial acne vulgaris in the community: randomized controlled trial. *Lancet.* 2004;364;2188-2195.
7. Draelos ZD, Carter E, Maloney JM, et al. Two randomized studies demonstrate the efficacy and safety of dapsone gel 5% for the treatment of acne vulgaris. *J Am Acad Dermatol.* 2007;56:439.
8. Koltun W, Lucky AW, Thiboutot D, et al. Efficacy and safety of 3 mg drospirenone/20 mcg ethinyl-estradiol oral contraceptive administered in 24/4 regimen in the treatment of acne vulgaris: a randomized double-blind, placebo-controlled trial. *Contraception.* 2008;77:249-256.
9. Sanchez J, Somolinos AL, Almodovar PI, et al. A randomized, double-blind, placebo-controlled trial of the combined effect of doxycycline hyclate 20-mg tablets and metronidazole 0.75% topical lotion in the treatment of rosacea. *J Am Acad Dermatol.* 2005;53:791-797.

SUGGESTED READINGS

Chayavichitsilp P, Buckwalter JV, Krakowski AC, et al. Herpes simplex. *Pediatr Rev.* 2009;30:119-129. *A comprehensive review.*

Daniel BS, Murrell DF. The actual management of pemphigus. *G Ital Dermatol Venereol.* 2010;145:689-702. *Review including systemic prednisone and adjuvant immunosuppression.*

Fuertes I, Mascaró JM, Bombí JA, et al. A retrospective study of clinical, histological, and immunological characteristics in patients with dermatitis herpetiformis. The experience of Hospital Clinic de Barcelona, Spain between 1995 and 2010 and a review of the literature. *Actas Dermosifiliogr.* 2011. [Epub ahead of print.] *Review including the finding that more than 80% of patients had celiac disease.*

Harnden A, Takahashi M, Burgner D. Kawasaki disease. *BMJ.* 2009;338:1133-1138. *A comprehensive review.*

Ingram JR, Grindlay DJ, Williams HC. Management of acne vulgaris: an evidence-based update. *Clin Exp Dermatol.* 2010;35:351-354. *Review.*

Kim JH, Kim YH, Kim SC. Epidermolysis bullosa acquisita: a retrospective clinical analysis of 30 cases. *Acta Derm Venereol.* 2011;91:307-312. *Review suggesting benefit of high-dose (>8 mg) methylprednisolone.*

Wetter DA, Camilleri MJ. Clinical, etiologic, and histopathologic features of Stevens-Johnson syndrome during an 8-year period at Mayo Clinic. *Mayo Clin Proc.* 2010;85:131-138. *Review.*

448

URTICARIA, DRUG HYPERSENSITIVITY RASHES, NODULES AND TUMORS, AND ATROPHIC DISEASES

MADELEINE DUVIC

URTICARIA

DEFINITION AND EPIDEMIOLOGY

Urticaria, also known as hives, is one of the most common cutaneous reaction patterns (Fig. 448-1). It is triggered by a wide variety of antigens or by physical stimuli, including cold, pressure, and sunlight (Table 448-1). The term *urticaria* refers to a disease spectrum ranging from simple wheals to angioedema. Clinical distinction between acute and chronic urticaria is important for diagnosis and treatment. Chronic urticaria, defined as urticaria that recurs over a period of 6 weeks or more, is often of unknown cause.

Urticaria is common worldwide in persons of all ages, although certain types of urticaria have a predilection for certain age groups. For example, acute urticaria is often seen in children with atopic dermatitis, whereas chronic urticaria peaks in the fourth decade.

PATHOBIOLOGY

Urticaria can be due to immunologic (autoimmune, immunoglobulin E [IgE]-dependent, immune complex–mediated, complement-kinin dependent) or nonimmunologic (direct mast cell–releasing agents, vasoactive stimuli, drugs) reactions. Local degranulation of mast cells with the release of histamine and other factors, such as slow-reacting substance of anaphylaxis, precipitates urticaria. Functional IgG autoantibodies, which release histamine from mast cells and basophils, are commonly found in the blood of patients with chronic urticaria. Additionally, basophils are recruited into

FIGURE 448-1. Urticaria. (From www.dermnetnz.org/reactions/urticaria.html.)

TABLE 448-1 COMMON CAUSES OF URTICARIA

URTICARIA MAY BE ACCOMPANIED BY ANGIOEDEMA AND ANAPHYLAXIS

Blood products: red cells, platelets, gamma globulin
Drugs
    Antibiotics: penicillins, cephalosporins, sulfonamides, isoniazid
    Aspirin: salicylates, benzoates, phenylbutazone
    Anticonvulsants: hydantoin
    Chemotherapy: doxorubicin, daunorubicin, L-asparaginase, chlorambucil, cyclophosphamide, melphalan, methotrexate, nitrogen mustard, procarbazine
    Dextran
    Nonsteroidal anti-inflammatory drugs
    Opiates
    Quinidine
    Radiocontrast dyes, iodine
Environmental: animal dander or proteins, formaldehyde, pollen, mold, plants, latex, plastic tubing, exercise, heat, cold, sunlight
Foods: berries, eggs, milk, nuts, tomatoes, shellfish, soy
Food additives: sodium benzoate, tartrazine (yellow dye #5)
Hormones
Infections: streptococcal, staphylococcal, sinusitis or abscesses, viral hepatitis, Epstein-Barr virus mononucleosis, *Candida* species
Insect bites or venom: Hymenoptera, mosquitoes, mites, scabies
Mechanical stimuli (dermographism, vibratory angioedema, delayed-pressure urticaria)
Vaccines

URTICARIA-LIKE ERUPTIONS AND REACTIVE ERYTHEMAS

Erythema multiforme: herpes simplex, DNA viruses, *Mycoplasma pneumoniae*, drugs
Erythema marginatum: streptococcal rheumatic fever
Juvenile rheumatoid arthritis
Erythema chronicum migrans: *Borrelia* species infections
Erythema annulare centrifugum: tinea, drugs
Figurate erythemas: erythema repens (often with underlying carcinoma)
Urticaria pigmentosa (mastocytosis)

FIGURE 448-2. Erythema marginatum. (From www.medscape.com/content/1998/00/41/73/417394/art-m5649.fig2.jpg.)

the wheals, where they sustain the response by releasing histamine. Eosinophils also contribute through leukotriene C_4 (LTC_4), leukotriene D_4 (LTD_4), leukotriene E_4 (LTE_4), and major basic protein. Urticaria is typically transient and self-limited, without leakage of blood cells into the skin or damage to the blood vessels. Leakage of plasma into the dermis from capillaries and small postcapillary venules correlates clinically with development of a demarcated, pink, raised lesion (hive).

CLINICAL MANIFESTATIONS

Urticarial lesions are pink to light red, blanch with pressure, and are raised above the surface of the skin. The center of the lesions may be paler than the leading edge. By definition, individual wheals come and go within 24 hours. A mosquito bite (Chapter 261) is the archetypal urticarial lesion. Individual hives can coalesce into giant plaques or annular rings called giant urticaria as is seen in serum sickness, in which they are accompanied by arthralgias and fever. Confluent urticaria may also be accompanied by swelling of the underlying soft tissue or the mucous membranes (angioedema) as well as by anaphylaxis with laryngeal edema, a life-threatening emergency. In otherwise normal individuals, pressure or writing on the skin will cause spontaneous local release of histamine, which induces a wheal-and-flare reaction known as dermatographism. Deep swelling develops at the site of sustained pressure and may remain for days in a condition known as delayed pressure urticaria. Affected individuals may develop lesions from tight-fitting clothing, shoes, socks, or sexual intercourse.

Other physical stimuli such as cold, heat, sun, or exercise may induce urticaria. Cold urticaria may be precipitated by putting an ice cube on the skin; the interval until hives develop and the duration of the hives correlate with the severity of the condition, which can be life-threatening if the patient is suddenly immersed in cold water. Heat, exercise, or exertion may be accompanied by small, 2- to 3-mm urticarial lesions in a condition called cholinergic urticaria. Exercise-induced anaphylaxis may be hereditary, but the defect is unknown. Patients with vibratory angioedema develop swelling and erythema within a few minutes of exposure to a vibratory stimulus. Lesions persist for about 30 minutes. Other forms of physically induced urticaria include solar urticaria and aquagenic urticaria (urticarial lesions caused by exposure to sun and water, respectively).

Food-and-exercise-induced anaphylaxis is a syndrome in which a few minutes of exercise following ingestion of certain specific foods results in angioedema or anaphylaxis. The cause of this syndrome is unknown.

DIAGNOSIS

A detailed history (duration, occupation, medications, frequency of episodes, associated illness) is critical. Urticaria typically results from exposure to antigen only minutes to a few hours before onset of the lesions. In many cases, pruritus may precede onset of the rash. The most common triggers of IgE-mediated allergic urticarial reactions are drugs (especially penicillin, sulfa drugs, antibiotics, and contrast dye), foods (shellfish, salicylates in berries, tomatoes, yeast, and penicillin in blue cheese), food additives (sodium benzoate), nuts (especially peanuts), or insect bites. Nonimmunologic mediators of urticaria include aspirin and opiates as well as physical agents that work through the prostaglandin pathway or degranulate mast cells.

Acute urticaria can also be triggered by skin contact with an antigen, such as latex, and can progress to anaphylaxis. In addition, urticaria can be a sign or prodrome of a latent infection, especially streptococcal pharyngitis in children or viral hepatitis in adults. The migratory urticarial rash accompanying rheumatic fever, erythema marginatum (Fig. 448-2), is characterized by evanescent, scalloped lesions that change location over the course of hours.

When urticarial lesions are present for more than 24 hours, underlying urticarial vasculitis should be suspected. A skin biopsy is required to distinguish urticarial vasculitis from urticaria in which no damage to the blood vessels is evident. When vascular damage is present, the lesion is termed *leukocytoclastic vasculitis,* the most severe expression of hypersensitivity reactions involving cutaneous blood vessels.

Chronic urticaria can be caused by occult infections (sinusitis, gallbladder disease, *Helicobacter pylori,* yeast infections, tooth abscesses, or silent hepatitis) as well as by collagen vascular diseases and tumors, especially Hodgkin's lymphoma. Deficiency of the C1 esterase inhibitor can be manifested as chronic urticaria with angioedema. Allergy testing is recommended if the history is unrevealing. If lesions persist for more than 24 hours, skin biopsy is indicated to determine whether vasculitis or mastocytosis is present. If infection, collagen vascular disease, or a tumor is suspected, a full serologic evaluation should be undertaken. Although a thorough medical evaluation may aid in diagnosis, the cause of chronic urticaria may remain uncertain. In the absence of a known antigen, stress is often invoked as the underlying cause of chronic recurrent idiopathic urticaria.

Systemic mastocytosis (Chapter 263) may be accompanied by urticarial lesions and gastrointestinal symptoms. In the form of mastocytosis known as *urticaria pigmentosa,* stroking the lesions produces urticaria, known as *Darier's sign.* A skin biopsy shows an increased number of dermal mast cells. Serum tryptase and histamine levels may be elevated during an attack.

TREATMENT   Rx

Management of urticaria depends on its severity and the duration of the problem (Chapter 260). For mild urticaria limited to the skin, traditional antihistamines (diphenhydramine) or the newer nonsedating agents (terfenadine, cetirizine, loratadine)■ can be administered by mouth intermittently as needed (Table 448-2). Acute urticaria is often treated with diphenhydramine orally. If the urticaria is severe, short-term corticosteroids, up to 1 mg/kg, can be used. For urticaria associated with wheezing or anaphylaxis, subcutaneous epinephrine, intravenous corticosteroids, and oxygen should be administered immediately. For chronic urticaria despite antihistamines, cyclosporine at doses of 3 mg/kg or higher for 8 to 16 weeks may be helpful.[2] Finding the cause and removing the antigen of chronic recurrent urticaria is highly preferable to chronic administration of corticosteroids or antihistamines. The patient should avoid aspirin compounds and other drugs that could be the cause.

DRUG RASHES

DEFINITION

Drugs have been associated with every type of cutaneous reaction pattern ranging from mild and self-limited to severe and life-threatening. Urticaria and exanthematous eruptions are common manifestations of cutaneous drug reactions. Less commonly seen are fixed drug, lichenoid, pustular, phototoxic, bullous, or vasculitic reactions, as well as Stevens-Johnson syndrome and toxic epidermal necrolysis.

PATHOBIOLOGY

Drug rashes, which result from drug toxicity, overdose, drug-drug interactions, or products of metabolism, may be caused by immunologic or nonimmunologic mechanisms. Drugs or their metabolites can act as haptens and induce cell-mediated or humoral responses. Mechanisms include IgE-dependent anaphylaxis and urticaria, cytotoxic reactions resulting in thrombocytopenia and resultant petechiae, immune complex–mediated serum sickness, and delayed-type hypersensitivity resulting in exanthematous or fixed drug eruptions or Stevens-Johnson syndrome.

CLINICAL MANIFESTATIONS AND DIAGNOSIS

Most drug rashes are either immediate (urticaria) or delayed hypersensitivity reactions (exanthems). Immediate reactions such as pruritus, hives, angioedema, and anaphylaxis occur within minutes to a few hours after the drug is taken. The most common drug-related rash (Table 448-3) is a T-cell–mediated hypersensitivity reaction manifested as a macular, bright pink to salmon-colored exanthem that appears as early as 7 to 10 days and as late as 14 days after a drug is first administered. Delayed hypersensitivity reactions can be macular or papular exanthems (or both), morbilliform eruptions, annular erythema, or confluent erythema (Fig. 448-3). Once sensitization to a particular drug has occurred, readministration of the same drug may trigger an eruption within 24 to 72 hours. Drug hypersensitivity reactions are typically symmetrical. They characteristically begin on the face and upper trunk and progress to the lower extremities, where they may become purpuric. Exanthems secondary to drugs most often become confluent erythematous patches after several days.

Pruritus is the most common symptom. The differential diagnosis for drug rashes includes viral exanthems (Chapter 447), graft-versus-host disease or the leukocyte recovery rash after allogeneic bone marrow transplantation, erythematous exanthems that accompany streptococcal [scarlet fever (Chapter 298)] or staphylococcal [toxic shock syndrome (Chapter 296)] infections, and the acute manifestation of collagen vascular diseases. A similar exanthem occurs when ampicillin is administered to patients who have infectious mononucleosis. A careful drug history is critical in diagnosis and treatment.

TREATMENT AND PROGNOSIS

After the offending drug is discontinued, delayed hypersensitivity reactions resolve in about a week. Therapy is mostly supportive. Corticosteroids, such as 0.01% triamcinolone cream applied several times per day to the affected area, and antihistamines given orally three to four times daily are helpful in reducing the itching and shortening the course.

Specific Syndromes
DRUG RASH WITH EOSINOPHILIA AND SYSTEMIC SYMPTOMS

An especially severe hypersensitivity *drug rash with eosinophilia and systemic symptoms* (DRESS) is most frequently seen with sulfonamides and anticonvulsants (Fig. 448-4). This condition is thought to be due to an alteration in drug metabolism. Activated T lymphocytes release interleukin-5 (IL-5),

---

TABLE 448-2 TREATMENT OF URTICARIA

1. Avoid the inciting agent!

2. Medications based on severity
   A. Mild to moderate, acute urticaria
      Oral antihistamines, e.g., diphenhydramine (Benadryl), 10-50 mg PO q12h, or hydroxyzine, 10-25 mg PO q8h; nonsedating alternatives include cetirizine (Zyrtec), 5-10 mg, or loratadine (Claritin), 10 mg/day

   B. Severe urticaria with or without angioedema
      Antihistamines, e.g., diphenhydramine (Benadryl), 25-50 mg PO q6-8h or 10-50 mg IV q2-4h, not to exceed 400 mg/24 hr
      Corticosteroids, e.g., prednisone, 10-60 mg PO every morning with tapering over a 2-wk period, triamcinolone (Kenalog), 40 mg IM for one dose, or dexamethasone, 0.6-0.75 mg/m²/day IV in divided doses q6-12h, depending on severity

   C. Anaphylaxis
      A—Airway (intubation)
      B—Breathing (oxygen)
      C—Circulation: parenteral aqueous epinephrine, 1:1000 IV, saline or volume expanders
      IV corticosteroids (e.g., methylprednisolone, 125 mg)
      Histamine H₁- and H₂-antagonists (50 mg each of diphenhydramine and ranitidine)

   D. Chronic idiopathic urticaria—combination therapy
      Nonsedating antihistamine: cetirizine, 10 mg/day, or fexofenadine, 30-180 mg twice daily, alone or with montelukast, 10 mg/day, or H₁- and H₂-antagonists (50 mg each of diphenhydramine and ranitidine) and/or low-dose corticosteroids (if unavoidable)

TABLE 448-3 DELAYED HYPERSENSITIVITY DRUG RASHES BY CATEGORY

MACULOPAPULAR EXANTHEMS—ANY DRUG CAN PRODUCE A RASH 7-10 DAYS AFTER THE FIRST DOSE

Allopurinol
Antibiotics: penicillin, sulfonamides
Antiepileptics: phenytoin, phenobarbital
Antihypertensives: captopril, thiazide diuretics
Contrast dye: iodine
Gold salts
Hypoglycemic drugs
Meprobamate
Phenothiazines
Quinine

DRUG RASH WITH EOSINOPHILIA AND SYSTEMIC SYMPTOMS (DRESS)

Anticonvulsants: phenytoin, phenobarbital, valproate, lamotrigine
Antibiotics: sulfonamides, minocycline, dapsone
Allopurinol
Phenothiazines

ERYTHEMA MULTIFORME/STEVENS-JOHNSON SYNDROME

Sulfonamides, phenytoin, barbiturates, carbamazepine, allopurinol, amikacin, phenothiazines
Toxic epidermal necrolysis: same as for erythema multiforme but also acetazolamide, gold, nitrofurantoin, pentazocine, tetracycline, quinidine

ACUTE GENERALIZED EXANTHEMIC PUSTULOSIS

Antibiotics: penicillins, macrolides, cephalosporins, clindamycin, imipenem, fluoroquinolones, isoniazid, vancomycin, minocycline, doxycycline, linezolid
Antimalarials: chloroquine, hydroxychloroquine
Antifungals: terbinafine, nystatin
Anticonvulsants: carbamazepine
Calcium-channel blockers
Furosemide
Systemic corticosteroids
Protease inhibitors

COLLAGEN VASCULAR OR LUPUS-LIKE REACTIONS

Procainamide, hydralazine, phenytoin, penicillamine, trimethadione, methyldopa, carbamazepine, griseofulvin, nalidixic acid, oral contraceptives, propranolol

ERYTHEMA NODOSUM

Oral contraceptives, penicillin, sulfonamides, diuretics, gold, clonidine, propranolol, opiates
Fixed drug reactions: phenolphthalein, barbiturates, gold, sulfonamides, meprobamate, penicillin, tetracycline, analgesics

FIGURE 448-3. Delayed hypersensitivity reaction. **A,** Drug reaction. **B,** Acral erythema.

FIGURE 448-4. Hypersensitivity drug rash caused by phenytoin.

leading to characteristic eosinophilia. DRESS may be delayed in onset by 2 to 6 weeks, persists longer than classic drug-induced eruptions, and becomes generalized and severe, even when use of the agent is discontinued. It typically begins as a morbilliform eruption, which later evolves into an edematous pustular eruption with erythroderma and purpura. The rash begins on the face, upper trunk, and extremities and later becomes generalized. Continued administration of the drug can result in exfoliative erythroderma, toxic necrolysis, and systemic hypersensitivity, including hepatitis (50%), nephritis (10%), or atypical lymphocytosis and lymphadenopathy mimicking mononucleosis or T-cell lymphoma. Less commonly seen are pneumonitis, myocarditis, and pericarditis. With visceral involvement, there is a 10% mortality rate, usually from hepatic failure. This condition is thought to be due to an alteration in drug metabolism. Activated T lymphocytes release IL-5, leading to characteristic eosinophilia.

ERYTHEMA MULTIFORME, STEVENS-JOHNSON SYNDROME, AND TOXIC EPIDERMAL NECROLYSIS

Stevens-Johnson syndrome and toxic epidermal necrolysis represent a spectrum of the same disease, of which erythema multiforme (see Fig. 447-10 in Chapter 447) is the least severe. Stevens-Johnson syndrome is defined as less than 10% body surface area involvement, and toxic epidermal necrolysis is defined as greater than 30% body surface area involvement. Erythema multiforme, a hybrid of urticaria and vasculitis, consists of symmetrically distributed red macules or papules that evolve into classic target or bull's eye lesions with deep red centers and pink urticarial rims. It is commonly precipitated by herpes simplex infections, other DNA viruses, or drugs. Stevens-Johnson syndrome is characterized by severe mucosal involvement with purpuric lesions. Widespread epidermal necrosis is seen in toxic epidermal necrolysis.

Drugs are almost always implicated when Stevens-Johnson syndrome or toxic epidermal necrolysis develops in adults (Fig. 448-5). Commonly implicated medications include nonsteroidal anti-inflammatory drugs (NSAIDs), allopurinol, phenytoin, and sulfa drugs. Alterations in drug metabolism (i.e., slow acetylators of sulfonamides) are often implicated. Extensive keratinocyte necrosis leads to separation at the dermal-epidermal junction. Symptoms include fever, severe pain, or sometimes asthenia. The condition can progress rapidly, so it is critical to determine and discontinue the causative agent immediately. Superinfection and fluid and electrolyte imbalances can lead to death in 5% of cases of Stevens-Johnson syndrome and 30% of cases of toxic epidermal necrolysis.

LEUKOCYTOCLASTIC VASCULITIS

Severe drug reactions can also be manifested as vasculitis, neutrophilic eruptions, and ulcerations. Vasculitis is further categorized by the size of the involved vessel and the nature of the cellular reaction and immune complexes. Leukocytoclastic vasculitis, which is the most common form of vasculitis induced by drugs, is manifested as palpable purpura, usually on the extremities (see Figs. 447-4 and 447-5 in Chapter 447).

NEUTROPHILIC DRUG REACTIONS

Neutrophilic drug reactions include iododermas, bromodermas, and Sweet's syndrome (acute febrile neutrophilic dermatosis. Acute generalized exanthematous pustulosis is characterized by numerous (>100), small (<5 mm), nonfollicular subcorneal pustules that arise on erythematous skin, often beginning in skin creases or on the face. High fever and peripheral neutrophilia may precede or accompany the eruption. The pustules are sterile, present for 5 to 10 days, and followed by desquamation. They usually appear less than 2 days after the administration of the causative drug. Ninety percent of cases are due to drugs, most commonly β-lactam antibiotics, macrolides, and calcium-channel blockers. This syndrome has also been called pustular drug rash, pustular psoriasis after corticosteroid withdrawal, and toxic pustuloderma. When severe, it may be confused with toxic epidermal necrolysis, but the mortality rate is only 1 to 2%. Skin patch testing is frequently positive.

FIXED DRUG ERUPTIONS

A fixed drug reaction appears at the same location 1 to 2 weeks after first drug exposure and within 24 hours of repeat exposure. The lips, hands, face, feet, and genitalia are most commonly involved. The lesion may begin as erythema and then become gray, brown, or violaceous. Trimethoprim-sulfamethoxazole, NSAIDs, tetracyclines, and pseudoephedrine are common causes. Epidermal growth factor receptor inhibitors and protein kinase inhibitors cause an acneiform eruption on the face and chest that is associated with drug response (Fig. 448-6).

PHOTOSENSITIVITY AND WITHDRAWAL REACTIONS

Light combined with drugs (Table 448-4) can produce photosensitivity reactions that can be quite severe and mimic sunburn. Ultraviolet radiation interacts with a drug or its metabolite to generate reactive oxygen species, leading to cellular damage. Tetracyclines, sulfa drugs, NSAIDs, and fluoroquinolones are often implicated in photosensitivity reactions. Photosensitizing drugs may exacerbate lupus erythematosus (Chapter 274) or porphyria cutanea tarda (Chapter 217).

FIGURE 448-5. Toxic epidermal necrolysis. **A,** Clinical appearance. **B,** Close-up appearance of epidermal sheets.

FIGURE 448-6. Epidermal growth factor receptor inhibitor–associated rash.

TABLE 448-4 DRUGS ASSOCIATED WITH SUN SENSITIVITY

PHOTOTOXIC

Chlorpromazine
Hydralazine
Levaquin
Procainamide
Psoralens
Porphyrins
Sulfonamides
Tetracyclines
Thiazide diuretics

PHOTOALLERGIC

Chlorothiazide
Griseofulvin
Hypoglycemic drugs
Promethazine

CONTACT DERMATITIS

Allergic contact dermatitis is a T-cell–mediated delayed hypersensitivity reaction following topical drug application or exposure to poison ivy, oak, or sumac. It is manifested by erythema and microvesiculation and may spread beyond the area of application (id reaction). Common contact sensitizers include Neosporin (polymyxin B/neomycin/bacitracin), bacitracin, diphenhydramine, doxepin, lidocaine, lanolin, mercury, and p-aminobenzoic acid.

⬤ BENIGN PAPULES, NODULES, AND TUMORS

The skin is heterogeneous, composed of epidermis, dermis, subcutaneous compartments, and blood vessels. The skin hosts a number of migrating cells (Chapter 443), all of which can give rise to benign or malignant tumors. Lesions that arise from epidermal keratinocytes are usually papules (warts,

TABLE 448-5 TUMORS AND NODULES OF THE SKIN

Benign, nonpigmented tumors and nodules
   Epidermal: warts, acrochordons, tricholemmomas, sebaceous hyperplasia
   Adnexal: epidermal cysts, syringomas, follicular cysts, pilomatricoma, apocrine or eccrine adenomas
   Dermal and subcutaneous: lipomas, angiolipomas, neurofibromas, leiomyomas

Benign, pigmented tumors and nodules
   Epidermal: seborrheic keratoses
   Melanocytic compound nevi (junctional nevi are flat)
   Spitz nevus
   Blue nevus
   Dermatofibromas

Malignant, nonpigmented tumors and nodules
   Basal cell carcinoma (nodular, superficial, morpheaform, pigmented)
   Squamous cell carcinoma (actinic keratoses, Bowen's disease, keratoacanthomas)
   Cutaneous T- and B-cell lymphomas
   Amelanotic melanomas
   Merkel cell carcinomas
   Adnexal carcinomas of the sebaceous and apocrine glands

Malignant, pigmented tumors and nodules
   Pigmented basal cell carcinoma
   Malignant melanoma: in situ, superficial spreading, nodular, acral lentiginous
   Dermatofibrosarcoma protuberans

Inflammatory nodules over joints
   Gottron's papules (dermatomyositis)
   Gouty tophi
   Heberden's nodes (osteoarthritis)
   Multicentric reticulohistiocytosis (paraneoplastic syndrome)
   Rheumatoid nodules
   Granuloma annulare

Inflammatory nodules of the lower extremities
   Panniculitis
   Vasculitis: periarteritis nodosa

Metabolic nodules of the skin
   Amyloidosis
   Gouty tophi
   Xanthomas, necrobiotic xanthogranuloma
   Xanthelasma

Vascular lesions
   Benign: nevus flammeus, angiokeratomas, spider hemangiomas, capillary hemangiomas, cavernous hemangiomas, blue rubber bleb nevi, pyogenic granulomas
   Malignant: Kaposi's sarcoma, angiosarcoma

sebaceous hyperplasia) or plaques (psoriasis, Bowen's disease). Nodules are deeper lesions that may be tender or asymptomatic, single or multiple, and break down to form ulcers. Nodules are classified as inflammatory (granulomas, vasculitis, or panniculitis), infectious, vascular, or metabolic; they can be benign or malignant tumors that arise from skin cells or migrant cells (Table 448-5). Nodules that are smaller and symmetrical are more likely to

FIGURE 448-7. Actinic keratoses.

FIGURE 448-8. Seborrheic keratoses.

FIGURE 448-9. Molluscum contagiosum in an immunocompromised patient.

be benign than lesions that grow rapidly, are larger, or invade surrounding tissue. Any rapidly changing skin nodule should be investigated with an excisional biopsy to the level of fat and sent for histology as well as for bacterial, fungal, and acid-fast cultures.

Benign Epidermal Tumors

The top layer of skin is the avascular epidermis composed of keratinocytes that undergo apoptosis to form the stratum corneum. Melanocytes, Langerhans cells, and inflammatory cells may enter the epidermis. Epidermal stem cells form adnexal organs such as hair follicles and sebaceous, eccrine, and apocrine glands that can give rise to tumors.

ACTINIC KERATOSES

Actinic keratoses are pink, scaly macules composed of sun-damaged keratinocytes and are precursors of in situ squamous cell carcinoma (Bowen's disease) or invasive squamous carcinomas (Chapter 210). Actinic keratoses are 0.1 to 1.0 cm and are found on sun-exposed areas such as the forearms, hands, face, and scalp (Fig. 448-7). Lesions with induration, thick crusts, ulceration, or pain are excised for biopsy to exclude invasive squamous cell carcinoma. Actinic keratoses are treated with cryotherapy and topical fluorouracil, retinoids, or imiquimod. To treat and prevent actinic keratoses, sun-exposed areas may be treated topically with 5-fluorouracil cream (5%) applied daily for 2 weeks or twice weekly for 8 weeks.

SEBORRHEIC KERATOSES

Seborrheic keratoses are common verrucous or stuck-on epidermal papules of various colors (Fig. 448-8). They are commonly seen with advancing age

but may arise suddenly (sign of Leser-Trélat) in association with internal malignancy. Seborrheic keratoses are composed from a single clone of keratinocytes and inherited as an autosomal dominant trait. Their surface may be friable, and lesions can be scraped off. Seborrheic keratoses spare the palms, soles, and mucosal surfaces. Although benign, seborrheic keratoses must be differentiated from melanocytic nevi, melanomas, and pigmented basal cell carcinoma, usually by the presence of white to yellow horn cysts on their surface, best appreciated with dermoscopy.

WARTY LESIONS

Epidermal papules include common warts (see Fig. 447-2 in Chapter 447) caused by human papillomavirus (HPV). HPV can also be detected in squamous carcinomas arising on the digits and in keratoacanthomas, which are low-grade, well-demarcated, dome-shaped papules or nodules that grow rapidly and spontaneously involute in 6 to 8 weeks. Acrodermatitis verruciformis is characterized by multiple warts with the appearance of seborrheic keratoses on the dorsal extremities and gives rise to squamous cell carcinomas. Molluscum contagiosum (Chapter 447) (Fig. 448-9), caused by a DNA virus, are small, shiny, domed-shaped, 1- to 5-mm papules with a central dell. They are common in children and immunocompromised patients.

Cowden's syndrome (Chapter 199), caused by mutations in *PTEN* gene, is associated with warty papules (tricholemmomas; Fig. 448-10), cobblestone papules on the gums and tongue, fibrous papules, and multiple hamartomas involving the breast, thyroid, intestines, ovary, and cerebellum.

ADNEXAL TUMORS

Adnexal tumors arise from hair follicles or glands and are commonly found on the face or scalp. Trichoepitheliomas resemble basal cell carcinomas. Sebaceous hyperplasia consists of small yellow papules with a central depression. Adnexal tumors of sebaceous origin, including sebaceous adenomas and sebaceous carcinomas, also found on the face, can be markers for the Muir-Torre syndrome of familial breast and colon cancer. Epidermal or sebaceous cysts, which are found in acne or as single firm nodules with a central pore, are filled with sebum or keratin. Epidermoid tumors of the scalp and a family history of colon cancer raises question of a diagnosis of Gardner's syndrome (Chapter 199).

DERMATOFIBROMAS AND COLLAGENOMAS

Fibroblasts, the resident cells of the dermis, produce collagen, elastin, and mucopolysaccharides. Accumulation of these products results in sclerosis, papules, or nodules. Fibroblasts in small dense clusters form firm brown or tan papules known as dermatofibromas. Dermatofibromas are commonly found on the extremities and may form after insect bites or trauma. They are firm and well-demarcated papules, and the skin puckers when lateral pressure is applied. Dermatofibromas can be treated, but increased scarring may occur. The malignant counterpart is dermatofibroma sarcoma protuberans, which is a poorly defined, rapidly expanding, dermal, malignant tumor. Overlying erythema or hyperpigmentation is often present.

Collagenomas and elastic tumors with the appearance of small white to yellow papules are found in the skin and bone of patients with Buschke-Ollendorff syndrome. *Pseudoxanthoma elasticum* (Chapter 268), an autosomal recessive disorder, is typically manifested as cutaneous yellow plaques on the neck or antecubital fossa from damaged elastin tissue. Mucin cysts are gray, shiny, well-demarcated, round nodules that generally arise on the

FIGURE 448-10. Cowden's syndrome: cobblestone gums *(left)* and tricholemmoma *(right)*.

FIGURE 448-11. Neurofibromatosis with cafe au lait spots and neurofibromas.

FIGURE 448-12. Schwannoma.

mucosa or on the digits, where they may have an underlying connection to the joint space.

NEURAL CREST CELL TUMORS

Benign tumors in the dermis arising from neural crest cells include neurofibromas (soft, flesh-colored papules; Fig. 448-11), schwannomas (larger subcutaneous soft tumors or plaques; Fig. 448-12), and melanocytic lesions. Although solitary neurofibromas may occur, multiple lesions with cafe au lait spots (tan macules) or axillary freckling (Crowe's sign) are diagnostic of neurofibromatosis type I, an autosomal dominant disorder caused by mutations in neurofibromin (Chapter 426). Schwannomas can become malignant and be manifested as dermal nodules. Merkel cell carcinoma, which is a neuroendocrine carcinoma of the skin, is a particularly aggressive small cell tumor arising from the cutaneous nerve endings or Meissner's corpuscles. Merkel cell polyomavirus is associated with development of Merkel cell carcinoma. Merkel cell carcinoma may present as a solitary pink to purple dome-shaped papule on the head or neck (Fig. 448-13). Treatment requires full excision, radiation therapy, and often chemotherapy because the cancer tends to recur and metastasize.

Melanocytic Lesions

Benign melanocytic moles or nevi (new) are discrete nests of melanocytes acquired during childhood and young adulthood, stimulated by sun exposure. Nevi are benign and composed of melanocytes (Chapter 210). They regress with age and change in color during pregnancy. Benign melanocytic nevi are formed by nests of melanocytes at the epidermal junction (junctional nevi), in the dermis (intradermal nevi), or in both compartments (compound nevi). Their appearance depends on type and age of the lesion. Junctional nevi (Fig. 448-14) are small, flat, and light to dark brown.

FIGURE 448-13. Merkel cell tumor.

Intradermal nevi are soft, flesh-colored to pink papules with smooth regular borders and surface. Compound nevi are papules with pigmentation. Blue nevi (Fig. 448-15) are flat, grayish blue, and regular. Small congenital nevi are dark brown, whereas dysplastic nevi (Fig. 448-16) have variegated colors and may transform into melanoma. More than 10 large, atypical moles with irregular borders and colors confer higher risk of developing melanoma, especially with a positive family history. Other recognized risk factors for melanoma include having more than 50 small nevi, red or blonde hair, or fair skin that burns and a history of blistering sunburns as a child. Patients with higher risk for melanoma should have surveillance and regular skin examinations.

Langerhans Cell Histiocytosis

Skin surveillance is mediated by antigen-presenting cells: Langerhans cells, dermal dendritic cells, and skin-homing T lymphocytes. Proliferation of

FIGURE 448-14. Junctional nevus.

FIGURE 448-15. Benign blue nevus.

FIGURE 448-16. Dysplastic nevus syndrome.

FIGURE 448-17. Histiocytosis X.

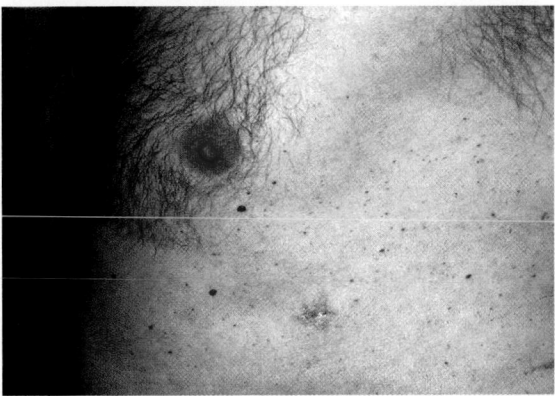

FIGURE 448-18. Benign capillary hemangioma.

Langerhans cells is called histiocytosis. Childhood histiocytosis X is manifested as severe seborrheic dermatitis of the scalp and gluteal areas with underlying purpura and may result in the hemophagocytic syndrome. In adults, lesions appear in the intertriginous areas (Fig. 448-17). Patients with the non–Langerhans cell histiocytosis have lytic bone involvement (eosinophilic granulomas) or diabetes insipidus (Hand-Schüller-Christian syndrome).

Vascular Lesions

HEMANGIOMAS

Benign capillary, or cherry, hemangiomas are bright cherry-red to purple papules, generally less than 5 mm in diameter. They appear on the trunk with aging and may be numerous (Fig. 448-18). Pyogenic granulomas can resemble hemangiomas but contain polymorphonuclear leukocytes, are friable, and bleed easily. Multiple pyogenic granulomas are seen in infectious bacillary angiomatosis in immunocompromised hosts (Chapter 323). Cavernous or strawberry hemangiomas can also appear in the neonatal period as rapidly growing vascular tumors; they may obstruct the eye or the pharynx before regressing. Corticosteroids, interferon, or antiangiogenic factors can be used to treat these lesions successfully. Cavernous hemangiomas are deeper and less likely to resolve than smaller lesions. When associated with platelet consumption, the Kasabach-Merritt syndrome is present (Chapter 174).

KAPOSI'S SARCOMA

Kaposi's sarcoma (Chapter 399) is a disseminated angiomatosis that arises from viral IL-8 production by herpesvirus 8. Lesions are symmetrical purple, red, gray, or brown patches, papules, nodules, or ulcers (Fig. 448-19). Mucosal involvement is more common in advanced disease. Kaposi's sarcoma in young African adults and Kaposi's sarcoma associated with human immunodeficiency virus (HIV) infection often have a more aggressive course than Kaposi's sarcoma in elderly men of Mediterranean background, whose disease is indolent and often confined to the lower extremities. Treatment of HIV disease with highly active antiretroviral therapy has been associated with a marked decreased incidence and severity of HIV-associated Kaposi's sarcoma. Angiosarcomas are malignant purple to red vascular tumor nodules that are more common in elderly individuals or on the extremities of patients with chronic lymphedema.

Inflammatory and Hematopoietic Papules and Tumors

Inflammatory diseases of the skin involve the superficial or dermal vessels or subcutaneous tissue. Inflammatory infiltrates can be mixed or restricted in

FIGURE 448-19. Kaposi's sarcoma. **A,** Involvement of the lower extremity (Mediterranean Kaposi's sarcoma). **B,** Histology.

FIGURE 448-20. Cutaneous sarcoidosis.

FIGURE 448-21. Leonine facies associated with lepromatous leprosy.

nature. Lymphocytes, polymorphonuclear leukocytes, histocytes, eosinophils, and plasma cells are the most common inflammatory reactions. Hematologic malignancies can present with secondary skin lesions, including patches, nodules, papules, or vasculitic lesions. Skin-homing CD4+ T cells give rise to cutaneous T-cell lymphomas. Mycosis fungoides (Chapter 191) lesions are pleomorphic pink, white, or brown patches or plaques, alopecia, or diffuse erythroderma with blood involvement (Sézary's syndrome). Early patch or plaque mycosis fungoides is indistinguishable from chronic eczematous or psoriasiform dermatitis. Tumors occur late in mycosis fungoides and can transform to a large cell lymphoma phenotype, with or without expression of CD30. Peripheral cutaneous T-cell lymphomas may also be found in subcutaneous tissue as panniculitic lesions. Lymphomatoid papulosis is characterized by crops of red to pink self-regressing papules with a histology similar to anaplastic large cell lymphoma, including expression of CD30 antigen. Lymphomatoid papulosis, CD3+ anaplastic T-cell lymphoma, and transformed CD30+ mycosis fungoides should be distinguished for treatment. Natural killer T-cell lymphomas, immunoblastic lymphomas, and plasmacytoid dendritic cell tumors appear as brown to purple dermal nodules.

Cutaneous B-cell lymphomas present as pink, infiltrated, dome-shaped shiny papules or tumors. Follicular B-cell lymphoma is commonly located on the face, scalp, or upper part of the back, whereas mucosa-associated B-cell tumors are more common on the trunk. With the exception of large cell lymphoma, many B-cell lymphomas of the skin are indolent, and some are stimulated by *Borrelia* species infection (Chapter 329) or chronic inflammation. Plasmacytomas can arise in the skin, in bone, with multiple myeloma (Chapter 193), or independently. Extramedullary hematopoiesis or endometriosis can be associated with red or brown nodules in the dermis.

Granulomatous Diseases

Sarcoidosis is an inflammatory granulomatous process manifested as ichthyosis, papules, plaques, or tumors with an apple-jelly color (Fig. 448-20).

Patients with lepromatous leprosy also can have histiocytic plaques or tumors (Fig. 448-21); treatment of leprosy may induce an inflammatory reaction called erythema nodosum leprosum. Granulomatous inflammation within the dermis can result in damage to collagen, as seen in granuloma annulare (ringlike pink to red infiltrated lesions, often on the hands or elbows), rheumatoid nodules that occur on the extensor surface of the arms, and necrobiosis lipoidica on the shins of diabetic patients. All three lesions typically include fibrin deposits within dermal blood vessels. Multicentric reticulohistiocytosis is a rare paraneoplastic syndrome in which histiocytic nodules form over joints with associated arthritis.

Inflammatory Skin Nodules

Inflammatory skin nodules arise from inflamed blood vessels (vasculitis) or adipose tissue (panniculitis). Either can arise in response to underlying infection or antigen stimulation with influx of inflammatory cells. Vasculitis is categorized by vessel size and circulating immune complexes. Damage to blood vessels results in leakage of red blood cells with the development of purpura (nonblanching red to purple lesions; Chapter 278). Erythema elevatum diutinum is manifested as multiple, infiltrated pink, yellow, red, or violaceous nodules or papules that may be painful or asymptomatic. The lesions can coalesce to form gyrate lesions on the dorsum of the hands or extensor surfaces similar to granuloma annulare. Erythema elevatum diutinum is associated with upper respiratory infections (especially *Streptococcus* species),

FIGURE 448-22. Sweet's syndrome. **A** and **B**, Sweet's syndrome in patients with leukemia.

FIGURE 448-23. Erythema nodosum. **A** and **B**, Erythema nodosum and septal panniculitis of the lower extremities.

HIV infection, and inflammatory bowel disease. The underlying histopathology is a necrotizing vasculitis with neutrophils and hyalinization of the vessels. Erythema elevatum diutinum must be distinguished from Sweet's syndrome, which is characterized by similar lesions clinically (Fig. 448-22). Sweet's syndrome is accompanied by fever, and biopsy specimens show sheets of leukocytes filling the upper dermis in the absence of infection. It occurs in patients with leukemia, inflammatory bowel disease, or rheumatoid arthritis. Sweet's syndrome, but not erythema elevatum diutinum, is highly responsive to corticosteroids, whereas dapsone can improve both conditions.

Polyarteritis Nodosa and Panniculitis

Polyarteritis nodosa (Chapter 278) arises in larger arterioles and may be associated with hepatitis C infection, mesenteric aneurysms, cryoglobulinemia, cutaneous ulceration, and livedo reticularis. Polyarteritis nodosa is distinct from small vessel leukocytoclastic vasculitis, which is characterized by smaller areas (a few millimeters) of purpura.

In the clinical setting, *panniculitis* occurs more frequently than nodular vasculitis. The diagnosis of vasculitis versus septal or lobular panniculitis requires an excisional biopsy, including fat, with appropriate cultures and stains.

Erythema nodosum (Fig. 448-23) is a septal panniculitis characterized by tender nodules that are 1 to 2 cm in diameter with warm, pink, overlying epidermis. They appear in crops on the extremities. A perivascular inflammatory infiltrate is present around small intralobular vessels without vasculitis. Erythema nodosum frequently arises in response to various infections, inflammatory bowel disease, or drug use, but often the underlying cause remains unknown (Table 448-6).

Lobular panniculitis with necrosis and purpura is called nodular vasculitis or erythema induratum. Nodular vasculitis is characterized by painful, chronic recurrent nodules on the shin or thighs that become bluish, ulcerate,

TABLE 448-6	TRIGGER FACTORS ASSOCIATED WITH ERYTHEMA NODOSUM

Infections
  Bacterial: *Streptococcus,* tuberculosis, leprosy, *Mycoplasma, Yersinia, Salmonella,* leptospirosis, tularemia
  Fungal: coccidioidomycosis, blastomycosis, histoplasmosis, dermatophytosis
  Viruses and *Chlamydia:* paravaccinia, Epstein-Barr virus, lymphogranuloma venereum, cat-scratch disease, psittacosis, hepatitis B

Drugs: sulfonamides, bromides, oral contraceptives

Malignancies: lymphoma, leukemia, carcinoma, after tumor radiation

Inflammatory: ulcerative colitis, Crohn's disease, Whipple's disease, Behçet's syndrome, Sweet's syndrome, collagen vascular diseases

Pregnancy

and heal with scarring. Erythema induratum (Fig. 448-24) is exacerbated by cold exposure and is sometimes associated with *Mycobacterium tuberculosis* (Chapter 333). True lobular panniculitis, with or without fat necrosis, is more frequent in males with underlying pancreatitis (Chapter 146) and may precede pancreatic cancer (Chapter 200). The lesions have a predilection for the anterior aspect of the shins and may be fluctuant as a result of fat necrosis. *Lupus panniculitis,* or lupus profundus, which involves the fat, is diagnosed by overlying granular immune complex deposition of IgM along the dermal-epidermal junction and must be distinguished from subcutaneous T-cell lymphomas. Lupus panniculitis of the breast, which can be mistaken for adenocarcinoma, is treated with antimalarials or corticosteroids. Lobular panniculitis with calcification of the small arterioles, which occurs in the setting of renal failure with hyperparathyroidism, is called calciphylaxis (Chapter 132).

FIGURE 448-24. Erythema induratum.

FIGURE 448-25. Atrophic skin in Ehlers-Danlos syndrome type 2.

Fungal Infections

In immunocompromised patients, necrotic or granulomatous lobular pan-niculitis can be caused by disseminated fungal infections with *Candida, Sporothrix schenckii, Cryptococcus, Histoplasma, Nocardia, Rhizopus, Aspergillus, Fusarium,* or chromomycosis. Fungal mycelia invade vessel walls, where they produce purpuric and painful lesions that may ulcerate. Osler's nodes, which are tender nodular vasculitic lesions on the extremities, occur in the setting of bacterial endocarditis (Chapter 76). Staphylococcal or streptococcal sepsis may be manifested as pustules, papules, or panniculitic lesions. *Klebsiella* and *Pseudomonas* species are associated with hemorrhagic necrosis of vessels or ecthyma gangrenosa. Granulomatous lobular panniculitis may also arise in the setting of syphilis, atypical mycobacterial infection, tuberculosis, or leprosy.

● ATROPHIC AND SCLEROTIC LESIONS
Atrophic Lesions

Atrophic lesions result from thinning or loss of the epidermal and dermal layers (Table 448-7). Examples are photoaging due to loss of epidermal thickness and collagen, discoid lupus, and genetic disorders of collagen production (e.g., Ehlers-Danlos syndrome; Fig. 448-25). Epidermal wrinkling can result in a cigarette paper appearance with prominence of the underlying blood vessels. High-potency topical corticosteroids cause loss of collagen resulting in atrophy. In Cushing's syndrome (Chapter 234), striae appear as red or purple streaks because the underlying dermis can be seen through the epidermis.

Aging skin is most pronounced in sun-exposed areas, but intrinsic aging beginning as early as 30 years of age is characterized by abnormalities in the formation of elastin fibers. Aging of the skin is accompanied by decreased rete ridges and diminished circulation. Sunlight ages the skin by inducing proteolytic enzymes that digest the underlying collagen and elastin (wrinkles). These changes can be partially prevented or restored with the use of topical vitamin A creams on a regular basis and with use of sun protection, including sunscreen. In addition, sun exposure induces pigment incontinence (freckling), increased junctional nevi, and proliferation of benign keratinocyte growths (seborrheic keratoses).

Atrophy can also result from ongoing inflammatory processes that cause scarring, such as collagen vascular disease or mycosis fungoides. The cutaneous and discoid forms of lupus erythematosus (Chapter 274) are manifested as scaly plaques with atrophy or alopecia on sun-exposed areas; the systemic form is characterized by malar rash, urticaria, or vasculitic lesions. Dermatomyositis (Chapter 277) can be associated with collagen vascular disease or malignancy; periorbital suffusion, telangiectasia of the nail beds, and Gottron's papules or scaly lesions over the joints are the skin manifestations. Anetodermas are localized sclerotic lesions (Fig. 448-26) with distinctive clinical features, from underlying inflammation.

Eosinophilic fasciitis is accompanied by nodules or sclerosis of the lower extremities, myopathy, pulmonary disease, and eosinophilia. This syndrome, which follows the ingestion of L-tryptophan or its contaminants, resembles the panniculitis seen in systemic sclerosis, in which fat lobules are replaced by new collagen formation. Eosinophilic cellulitis, or Wells' syndrome, is

TABLE 448-7	ATROPHIC SKIN CONDITIONS WITH SCARRING, ULCERATIONS, AND/OR TELANGIECTASES

ATROPHY

Epidermal: chronic corticosteroid use, photoaging, mycosis fungoides
Dermal elastin: anetoderma, cutis laxa, intrinsic aging
Dermal collagen: Ehlers-Danlos syndrome, aging
Subcutaneous: granulomatous slack skin (a mycosis fungoides variant)
Lipodystrophy (loss of fat)

SCARRING OR ATROPHY WITH TELANGIECTASIAS

Discoid and subacute cutaneous lupus erythematosus
Dermatomyositis
Keloid formation
Large plaque parapsoriasis (poikiloderma vasculare atrophicans variant of mycosis fungoides)
Photoaging
Necrobiosis lipoidica diabeticorum
Radiation dermatitis
Porphyrias
Thermal burns (erythema ab igne)

SCLEROSIS OR INFILTRATIVE PROCESSES

Amyloidosis
Systemic sclerosis, scleroderma
Localized sclerosis, morphea
Lichen sclerosis et atrophicus
Lichen myxedematosus/papular mucinosis (mucopolysaccharide deposition with paraproteinemia)
Myxedema (mucin deposits with anti–thyroid-stimulating hormone receptor antibodies)

ULCERATIONS

Secondary breakdown of any blister or nodule: infectious, inflammatory, tumor, vasculitis
Decubitus or pressure ulcers
Genital ulcers: syphilis, herpes simplex, chancroid, lymphogranuloma venereum, Behçet's syndrome
Pyoderma gangrenosum, Sweet's syndrome

manifested as nodules, papules, or ulcerative lesions, as well as red plaques where eosinophils infiltrate the area between collagen fibers.

Sclerotic Lesions

Sclerotic lesions are accompanied by more collagen production, which results in skin with a glossy appearance. Sclerosis may also result from the accumulation of mucopolysaccharides in scleromyxedema (lichen myxedematosus) or from amyloid deposits. An entity associated with renal failure and gadolinium exposure, nephrogenic fibrosing dermopathy (Fig. 448-27) is also characterized by acral fibrosis and deposition of hyaluronate in the skin. In scleroderma (Chapter 275), increased collagen deposition may be associated with Raynaud's syndrome, calcinosis, and telangiectasia. A localized form of scleroderma, termed *morphea,* may occur down the center of the face (coup de

FIGURE 448-26. Anetoderma.

FIGURE 448-28. Linear morphea.

FIGURE 448-27. Nephrogenic fibrosing dermopathy.

sabre), or as plaques on the extremities (Fig. 448-28), after radiation exposure, or with *Borrelia* species infection. Lichen sclerosis et atrophicus is a superficial inflammatory morphea characterized by white atrophic patches, especially in the genital region. Widespread systemic sclerosis may also follow bone marrow transplantation in the setting of chronic graft-versus-host disease.

Telangiectasia

Telangiectasia is prominence of skin blood vessels that frequently accompanies atrophic as well as sclerotic processes and is common in photoaged skin and following radiation therapy. Telangiectasia of the mucous membranes is found in Osler-Weber-Rendu syndrome, and vascular spiders are found both in α_1-antitrypsin deficiency and alcoholic liver disease. The presence of telangiectasia, hyperpigmentation, and hypopigmentation (poikiloderma) in sun-shielded areas of the body should alert the clinician to the diagnosis of early mycosis fungoides.

Ulcers

Ulcers are secondary skin lesions that may arise from trauma, loss of proper blood supply, aging, vasculitis, blister formation, infection, or underlying neoplasia. Ulcers may be shallow erosions (loss of the epidermis) or may be deeper and involve the dermis and underlying subcutaneous structures. Ulcers most commonly appear on the lower extremities, where they result from stasis dermatitis and venous insufficiency, arteriolar insufficiency, diabetic neuropathy, or vasculitis. *Pyoderma gangrenosum* is a trauma-induced

ulcer that is part of the spectrum of Sweet's syndrome, accompanies other conditions, and may require immunosuppressive therapy. In contrast, decubitus ulcers require débridement, elimination of local pressure, and attention to nutrition. Diagnosis requires skin biopsy, cultures, and serologic testing for other associated diseases.

After an inflammatory or ulcerated skin wound heals, scarring is common. Epidermal stem cells that reside in the bulge region of the hair follicle are capable of regenerating a normal epidermis. When a wound is deeper than the bulge region, scarring and loss of hair are likely to occur. Scarring alopecia (lichen planopilaris, discoid lupus, scarring folliculitis) results in permanent baldness and must be distinguished from the less severe, nonscarring conditions such as telogen effluvium or alopecia areata. Scarring also accompanies the most severe epidermolysis bullosa disorders caused by sub-basement membrane defects in proteins. Scarring accompanies third-degree burns, deep cryotherapy, or other trauma to the dermis. Scarring may also follow severe inflammation (discoid lupus) or infection (syphilis, leprosy).

Keloids

Some individuals have more pronounced and hypertrophic scar formation known as keloids, with an autosomal dominant inheritance pattern. Keloids are tumor-like in appearance and result from an overproduction of collagen. They are especially common on the anterior of the chest, neck, and earlobes and may require antineoplastic treatment after surgical removal.

1. Weinstein ME, Wolff AH, Bielory L. Efficacy and tolerability of second- and third-generation antihistamines in the treatment of acquired cold urticaria: a meta-analysis. *Ann Allergy Immunol.* 2010;104:518-522.
2. Vena GA, Cassano N, Colombo D, et al. Cyclosporine in chronic idiopathic urticaria: a double-blind, randomized, placebo-controlled trial. *J Am Acad Dermatol.* 2006;55:705-709.

SUGGESTED READINGS

Fine DM, Perazella MA. Nephrogenic systemic fibrosis: what the hospitalist needs to know. *J Hosp Med.* 2010;5:46-50. *Review.*

Fonacier L, Aquino M, Kim B. Clinical evaluation and treatment of chronic urticaria. *Postgrad Med.* 2010;122:148-156. *Review.*

Friedman PS, Ardern-Jones M. Patch testing in drug allergy. *Curr Opin Allergy Clin Immunol.* 2010;10:291-296. *Review emphasizing its limitations.*

449

INFECTIONS, HYPER- AND HYPOPIGMENTATION, REGIONAL DERMATOLOGY, AND DISTINCTIVE LESIONS IN BLACK SKIN

JEAN BOLOGNIA

⬤ INFECTIONS, INCLUDING CELLULITIS

Cutaneous infections can be divided into four major categories: bacterial, fungal (Chapter 446), viral, and parasitic (Table 449-1).

Bacterial Infections

Of the bacterial infections, impetigo, folliculitis, furuncles, and cellulitis are most commonly encountered.

IMPETIGO

Impetigo, which is caused by *Staphylococcus aureus* or group A β-hemolytic streptococci, is usually seen as honey-colored crusts (Fig. 449-1); less often, subcorneal (superficial) bullae are present. This infection is most commonly found on the face in children, but it can develop at any site where the cutaneous barrier has been disrupted (e.g., areas of dermatitis, sites of trauma, or arthropod bites). A deeper, but less common, bacterial infection of the skin is *ecthyma*, which is most frequently streptococcal in origin; it is characterized

by thick hemorrhagic crusts overlying erosions or ulcerations, usually 0.5 to 1.5 cm in diameter. These lesions favor the extremities, especially in the setting of lymphedema. Ecthyma should not be confused with ecthyma gangrenosum, which represents an embolic phenomenon most often caused by bacteremia with gram-negative bacilli. Although mild cases of impetigo usually respond to topical mupirocin, oral antibiotics that cover *S. aureus* (e.g., dicloxacillin, 250 mg orally four times a day, or cephalexin, 250 mg orally four times a day) are needed to treat more severe impetigo and ecthyma. Compared with furuncles and abscesses, impetigo is less often due to methicillin-resistant *S. aureus*.

FOLLICULITIS

The initial lesions of folliculitis are perifollicular pustules that are often surrounded by a rim of erythema (Chapter 447). *Pseudomonas* folliculitis, which favors the trunk, is usually associated with the use of hot tubs or whirlpools because their higher temperatures (vs. swimming pools) make eradication of *Pseudomonas* more difficult (see Fig. 447-20 in Chapter 447).

FURUNCLES

Furuncles, also called boils, represent *S. aureus* cutaneous infections that are localized primarily within the dermis. In contrast to folliculitis, the lesions are larger and manifest as tender erythematous nodules (Fig. 449-2). A central follicular structure may be noted, as may a central pustule ("pointing"). Because a furuncle is an abscess, the preferred treatment is incision and drainage◼ followed by oral antistaphylococcal antibiotics (e.g., dicloxacillin, 250 mg orally four times a day, or cephalexin, 250 mg orally four times a day);

TABLE 449-1 SKIN INFECTIONS
BACTERIAL DISEASES

Impetigo
Ecthyma
Folliculitis
Furuncle/carbuncle
Abscess
Erysipelas
Cellulitis
Necrotizing fasciitis
Ecthyma gangrenosum
Other
    Gram-negative cocci: meningococcemia, gonococcemia
    Gram-positive bacilli: erythrasma, anaerobic cellulitis
    Spirochetes: Lyme disease, syphilis, endemic treponematoses
    Mycobacteria

VIRAL DISEASES
Herpes simplex virus: oral, genital Human papillomavirus: common warts, condyloma acuminata Poxvirus: molluscum contagiosum Varicella-zoster virus Viral exanthems (e.g., enteroviruses, rubeola, rubella, parvovirus, Epstein-Barr virus, adenovirus, human immunodeficiency virus)
FUNGAL DISEASES
Candidiasis Tinea (dermatophytoses): pedis, corporis, cruris, manuum, capitis Pityriasis (tinea) versicolor Emboli (e.g., *Aspergillus, Mucor* species)
ECTOPARASITES/PARASITES
Scabies Lice: scalp, pubic, body Leishmaniasis Schistosomiasis, human and animal Onchocerciasis Strongyloidiasis Amebiasis Trypanosomiasis Hookworm infections, human and animal Filariasis Acanthamoebiasis

FIGURE 449-1. Impetigo in an infant and marked involvement of the face with honey-colored crusts and superficial erosions. (Courtesy of Yale Dermatology Residents' Slide Collection.)

FIGURE 449-2. Furuncle with surrounding cellulitis. (Courtesy of Yale Dermatology Residents' Slide Collection.)

FIGURE 449-3. Bullous and hemorrhagic cellulitis of the shin. (Courtesy of University of Southern California Dermatology Residents' Slide Collection.)

FIGURE 449-4. Erysipelas of the face with well-demarcated erythematous plaques. (Courtesy of Yale Dermatology Residents' Slide Collection.)

if methicillin-resistant *S. aureus* is likely (e.g., use of health care facilities such as dialysis units, participation in skin-to-skin contact sports, an elevated prevalence of methicillin-resistant isolates in the local community), the antibiotic should be changed to clindamycin (300 to 450 mg orally four times daily), doxycycline (100 mg orally twice daily), minocycline (100 mg orally twice daily), trimethoprim-sulfamethoxazole (160 mg/800 mg orally twice daily), or linezolid (600 mg orally every 12 hours). The duration of therapy is usually 10 to 14 days. *Carbuncles* are larger, more complex, and more extensive versions of furuncles; they may be accompanied by systemic symptoms such as fever and may require a more prolonged course of therapy.

CELLULITIS

Cellulitis is a fairly common cutaneous infection that occurs most often on the lower extremities. Locally, it manifests as erythema, edema, warmth, and tenderness; systemic findings can include fever, malaise, and leukocytosis. Most cases are bacterial in origin, but some are caused by fungal infections (e.g., *Cryptococcus* species) or chemical reactions (e.g., extravasated oxacillin or calcium salts). Bacterial cellulitis is most commonly caused by group A β-hemolytic streptococci and *S. aureus*, with the former being associated with the more severe, necrotizing variant. In patients who have diabetes or who are immunocompromised, cellulitis can be caused by gram-negative bacilli or atypical mycobacteria. Risk factors include a preceding break in the skin barrier, edema secondary to venous hypertension, lymphedema, and previous bouts of cellulitis.

Although the diagnosis of cellulitis is usually fairly straightforward (Fig. 449-3), it can sometimes be difficult in patients with chronic lower extremity edema, especially those who are afebrile. One complication of chronic lower extremity edema is lipodermatosclerosis (i.e., inflammation followed by fibrosis of subcutaneous fat), which is seen acutely as erythema, warmth, and tenderness and is easily confused with cellulitis. The skin above the medial malleolus is often the initial site of involvement with lipodermatosclerosis, but the inflammation can extend onto the shin and calf. The chronic phase of lipodermatosclerosis is characterized by induration, a permanent brown-red to violet discoloration of the skin, and an "inverted wine bottle" appearance of the distal end of the lower extremity. It is important for the clinician to realize that in patients with chronic lipodermatosclerosis and superimposed cellulitis, the skin will never return to its normal color, even after adequate antibiotic therapy.

Unless there is an associated bacteremia, the diagnosis of cellulitis is primarily clinical. In immunocompromised hosts, a saline injection followed by aspiration and culture can be helpful. Histologically, cellulitis is characterized by an infiltrate of neutrophils within the dermis. Skin biopsy can exclude disorders that may be confused with cellulitis, such as contact dermatitis, erythema migrans, inflammatory carcinoma, toxic erythema of chemotherapy, and Wells' syndrome (an idiopathic disorder in which eosinophils infiltrate the dermis). Treatment of cellulitis varies from oral cephalexin to intravenous vancomycin plus intravenous ceftazidime, depending on the suspected pathogens, the host, and the severity of systemic toxicity.

Cellulitis resides in the middle of a spectrum of soft tissue infections that includes *erysipelas* (more superficial and more sharply demarcated; Fig. 449-4) at one end and *necrotizing fasciitis* (deeper, more necrotic, and undermining) at the other. In healthy adults, erysipelas can be treated with oral penicillin (200,000 units four times daily) or, if methicillin-sensitive *S. aureus* is of concern, oral dicloxacillin (500 mg four times daily) for a 10-day course.

Necrotizing fasciitis is usually caused by multiple organisms, including anaerobic streptococci; its diagnosis requires a high index of suspicion, and it must be considered when there are areas of violaceous induration or a foul-smelling discharge. Prompt surgical débridement and broad-spectrum systemic antibiotics (e.g., a β-lactam/β-lactamase inhibitor such as intravenous piperacillin-tazobactam, 4.5 g every 6 hours for a total of 18 g/day [16 g piperacillin/2 g tazobactam]), with or without ciprofloxacin (500 mg orally or 400 mg intravenously every 12 hours), for at least 2 weeks are mandatory. Unless only a single organism is seen on Gram stain and isolated on culture, broad-spectrum antibiotic coverage should be continued because of the polymicrobial nature of necrotizing fasciitis and the difficulty of culturing anaerobes.

Although *Clostridium perfringens* can cause anaerobic cellulitis and gas gangrene, the most common cutaneous infection by gram-positive bacilli is *erythrasma*, which is manifested as interdigital toe web maceration with fissures, as well as shiny or scaly brown-red patches in the axillae and groin. The latter is often confused with tinea cruris (Chapter 446). A diagnostic finding is the presence of coral (orange-pink) fluorescence on Wood's lamp illumination (ultraviolet A). The responsible organism is *Corynebacterium minutissimum*. Treatment options include topical and oral erythromycin (e.g., 333 mg three times a day for 7 to 14 days).

TOXIC ERYTHEMAS

Eruptions caused by the release of toxins (e.g., exfoliative toxins ET-A and ET-B) produced by *S. aureus* and streptococci include *staphylococcal scalded skin syndrome* (Chapters 296 and 447), *scarlet fever* (Chapter 298), and *toxic shock syndrome* (Chapter 447). Staphylococcal scalded skin syndrome (see Fig. 447-14 in Chapter 447) is characterized by large areas of tender erythema in which superficial desquamation (peeling) develops, often with scaling and crusting in a radial array around the mouth. The areas of erythema are sterile; the conjunctivae, nasopharynx, or a distant site on the skin is the usual site of the primary staphylococcal infection. A clue to the diagnosis of scarlet fever is the presence of a strawberry tongue with prominent red papillae. Management involves treatment of the systemic infection (Chapters 296 and 447).

NEISSERIA INFECTIONS

Both *gonococcemia* (Chapter 307) and *meningococcemia* (Chapter 306) can present with cutaneous lesions. The former gives rise to a small number of vesicopustules on an erythematous base, generally acral in location (Fig. 449-5); these lesions represent septic emboli and are accompanied by fever, arthritis, and tendinitis. The earliest lesions of *acute meningococcemia* may be subtle (macular areas of erythema), but central hemorrhage (petechiae and purpura) and necrosis (gun-metal gray color) soon follow (Fig. 449-6). The lesions may become quite extensive; when accompanied by disseminated intravascular coagulation, severe peripheral ischemia may result. Cutaneous involvement in *chronic meningococcemia* is a reflection of lymphocytic or leukocytoclastic vasculitis rather than septic emboli. Management is systemic treatment (Chapters 306 and 307).

PSEUDOMONAS INFECTIONS

Pseudomonas infections of the skin vary from "hot tub" folliculitis (Chapter 447) to soft tissue infections of the external ear. Interdigital toe web infections that begin as simple tinea pedis can be complicated by superimposed

FIGURE 449-5. Disseminated gonococcal infection with an acral pustule on a red-violet base. (Courtesy of Yale Dermatology Residents' Slide Collection.)

FIGURE 449-6. Purpuric and necrotic embolic lesions of meningococcemia. (Courtesy of Yale Dermatology Residents' Slide Collection.)

FIGURE 449-7. Scabies with involvement of the penis. (From Bolognia J, Jurizzo J, Rapini R, et al. *Dermatology,* 2nd ed. Edinburgh: Mosby; 2007.)

Pseudomonas infection and result in erythema, swelling, tenderness, and drainage. Depending on its severity, treatment varies from topical antiseptics to oral or intravenous fluoroquinolones (e.g., ciprofloxacin, 500 mg orally every 12 hours for 7 to 14 days). In immunocompromised hosts, *Pseudomonas* and other gram-negative bacilli can produce cellulitis as well as secondary septic emboli in the skin. The latter begin as purpura or purpuric bullae in which central necrosis then develops. These lesions, which arise as a result of ischemic infarction of the skin, are termed *ecthyma gangrenosum*. Management is treatment of the systemic pseudomonal disease (Chapter 314).

SPIROCHETES

Spirochetal infections have a wide range of skin findings, from erythema migrans secondary to *Borrelia burgdorferi* (Chapter 329), to endemic treponematoses such as *yaws* and *pinta* (Chapter 328), to the cutaneous manifestations of the three stages of *syphilis* (Chapter 327). Syphilitic lesions include a firm, generally nontender ulceration (chancre) in primary syphilis; a generalized papulosquamous eruption (Chapter 446) plus alopecia, oral ulcers, and condylomata lata in secondary syphilis; and thick plaques and ulcers in tertiary disease. Management involves treatment of the systemic disease.

MYCOBACTERIA INFECTIONS

Infections with *Mycobacterium tuberculosis* and mycobacteria other than *M. tuberculosis* (atypical mycobacteria) are associated with skin lesions, including verrucous or crusted papules, scarring granulomatous plaques, and draining ulcers. In immunocompetent hosts in developed countries, *Mycobacterium marinum* (Chapter 333) is most commonly associated with skin disease, which is usually manifested in a lymphocutaneous (i.e., sporotrichoid) pattern. Treatment of cutaneous mycobacterial disease (Chapters 332 and 333), including leprosy (Chapter 334), is the same as for systemic disease.

Viral Infections

The most common viral infections of the skin are verrucae (warts; see Fig. 447-2 in Chapter 447), recurrent oral and genital herpes simplex (Chapters 382 and 447), molluscum contagiosum (see Fig. 448-9 in Chapter 448), and exanthems (Chapter 447). Varicella and herpes zoster are seen less frequently (Chapter 383).

Fungal Infections

A variety of fungal infections involve the skin and nails and are most commonly due to dermatophytes (tinea), *Candida* species, and *Malassezia* species (pityriasis versicolor) (Chapter 446; also see Table 449-1). Although both dermatophyte infections and pityriasis versicolor are associated with scaling, cutaneous candidiasis is characterized by erythema, a more erosive quality, and satellite pustules. Treatment is described in Chapter 446.

Septic emboli caused by *Candida* or other opportunistic fungi such as *Aspergillus* (Chapter 347) or *Fusarium* often have a clinical appearance similar to that of ecthyma gangrenosum secondary to gram-negative rods such as *Pseudomonas*. The responsible organisms can be detected histologically in biopsy specimens or by bedside examination of dermal scrapings; culture confirms the specific organism. Cutaneous plaques secondary to *Pneumocystis jirovecii* favor the internal ear. Treatment is for the underlying fungal infection.

Ectoparasites and Parasites
ECTOPARASITES: SCABIES AND LICE

The most common ectoparasitic cutaneous infestations are (1) scabies from the human variant of the *Sarcoptes* mite and (2) lice, of which there are three subtypes: head, body, and pubic. *Scabies* is characterized by pruritus in association with papules, papulovesicles, and linear burrows, as well as signs of scratching, such as excoriations and areas of dermatitis. Sites of predilection include the wrists, ankles, fingers, toes (including the web spaces), areolae, and genitalia (especially the penis) (Fig. 449-7). The number of mites living within the stratum corneum is limited in immunocompetent hosts; when scraped and examined microscopically, linear burrows provide the highest yield of mites and eggs. In elderly and immunosuppressed patients, a form of scabies known as crusted or Norwegian scabies presents as multiple areas of scaling and crusting that are teeming with mites.

Infestations with scalp *lice* are seen most commonly in children, who may be asymptomatic or have marked pruritus. In addition to the lice, multiple egg casings ("nits") are attached to the proximal portions of scalp hairs. In developed countries, body lice are seen primarily in homeless individuals; patients typically have multiple erythematous papules at the sites of "bites," as well as signs of scratching. The lice and their eggs are found in the patient's clothing. Pubic lice are sometimes called "crabs" because their bodies are shorter and broader than those of scalp or body lice and thus resemble the shape of a crab. As a result of their leg span, these lice reside primarily on pubic hairs and less often on axillary hairs or eyelashes.

The most effective U.S. Food and Drug Administration–approved treatments of head lice, pubic lice, and routine scabies are topical 0.5% malathion, 5% permethrin cream, **2** and 5% permethrin cream, respectively; each of these topical medications is applied for 8 to 12 hours on days 1 and 8. For crusted scabies, oral ivermectin (250 to 400 µg/kg; off-label use) is often required to eradicate the infestation. **3** Treatment of body lice involves discarding egg- and lice-infested clothing; for head lice, potential sources of reinfection, such as hairbrushes, should be discarded. Sexual and household contacts of patients with pubic lice and scabies, respectively, must be treated similarly to the symptomatic patient.

OTHER PARASITES

Cutaneous lesions are seen in leishmaniasis (Chapter 356), amebiasis (Chapter 360), schistosomiasis (Chapter 363), onchocerciasis (Chapter 366), strongyloidiasis (Chapter 365), and hookworm infections (Chapter 365). Exposure to water infested with the cercariae of animal schistosomes results in multiple erythematous papules, which occur most commonly on the feet and are termed *swimmer's itch*. Dog and cat hookworm infections lead to *cutaneous larva migrans*, with serpiginous erythematous tracks that correspond to the path of migration of the hookworm larvae. Both these infections are self-limited because the parasite's life cycle cannot be completed in humans. In immunocompromised hosts, cutaneous plaques can occasionally develop from free-living amebae such as *Acanthamoeba*.

⬤ DISORDERS OF HYPOPIGMENTATION AND HYPERPIGMENTATION

Disorders of pigmentation can be divided into four major categories: diffuse, linear, circumscribed, and either reticulated (in the case of hyperpigmentation) or guttate (in the case of hypopigmentation) (Table 449-2).

Hypopigmentation
ALBINISM

The primary disorder of diffuse hypopigmentation is *oculocutaneous albinism*, an autosomal recessive disorder in which there is a pigmentary dilution of melanin-containing structures (i.e., the eyes, hair, and skin). The phenotype varies from total absence of melanin pigment to a subtle decrease whose recognition requires comparison with first-degree relatives; the density of melanocytes in skin is normal, but their ability to produce pigment is absent or decreased. Ninety percent of patients with oculocutaneous albinism have mutations in the genes that encode either tyrosinase (type I) or P protein (type II). Complications of oculocutaneous albinism include decreased visual acuity, nystagmus, photophobia, and an increase in cutaneous carcinomas, especially squamous cell carcinoma. These signs and symptoms are most severe in those who produce the least pigment. The differential diagnosis includes total vitiligo (absence of melanocytes histologically) and a few inborn errors of metabolism (e.g., phenylketonuria). Treatment consists of longitudinal ophthalmologic care and minimizing sun exposure.

LINEAR HYPOPIGMENTATION

Disorders of *linear hypopigmentation* consist primarily of nevoid conditions (e.g., nevoid linear hypopigmentation, hypomelanosis of Ito, segmental or systematized nevus depigmentosus) in which streaks of hypomelanosis follow Blaschko's lines (an embryonic development pattern that involves all layers of the skin and becomes clinically apparent in the setting of mosaicism). A minority of patients have associated central nervous system and musculoskeletal abnormalities.

CIRCUMSCRIBED (PATCHY) HYPOPIGMENTATION
Vitiligo

Vitiligo (Fig. 449-8) is usually slowly progressive and occurs principally in periorificial areas (around the eyes, nose, lips, genitalia) and the hands, feet, flexor surface of the wrists, ankles, elbows, knees, and major body folds. Vitiligo, which is caused by a loss of melanocytes within the skin, is also associated with autoimmune endocrinopathies (Chapter 239) and alopecia areata (see later). T cells that recognize antigens on the surface of melanocytes (and melanoma cells) are found within the skin and in peripheral blood. Treatment includes topical corticosteroids, topical immunomodulators (e.g.,

TABLE 449-2 DISORDERS OF PIGMENTATION
HYPOPIGMENTATION
Diffuse (Pigmentary Dilution)
Oculocutaneous albinism
Hermansky-Pudlak syndrome
Chédiak-Higashi syndrome
Generalized (total) vitiligo
Inborn errors of metabolism (e.g., phenylketonuria)
Circumscribed
Decrease in pigment
Acquired: postinflammatory hypopigmentation (e.g., atopic dermatitis, sarcoidosis, systemic lupus erythematosus, mycosis fungoides), pityriasis (tinea) versicolor secondary to *Malassezia* spp infection
Congenital: nevus depigmentosus, ash-leaf spots of tuberous sclerosis
Absence of pigment
Acquired: vitiligo, chemical leukoderma, leukoderma of scleroderma, leukoderma of melanoma
Congenital: piebaldism
Linear
Nevoid linear hypopigmentation (previously referred to as hypomelanosis of Ito)
Guttate
Idiopathic guttate hypomelanosis
Confetti macules of tuberous sclerosis
HYPERPIGMENTATION
Diffuse
Drug reactions (e.g., cyclophosphamide, busulfan)
Addison's disease
Ectopic adrenocorticotropic hormone production (e.g., small cell lung cancer)
Hemochromatosis
Scleroderma
Primary biliary cirrhosis
Hyperthyroidism
Vitamin B_{12} or folate deficiency
Porphyria cutanea tarda
Melanosis secondary to metastatic melanoma
Argyria (gray hue)
Circumscribed
Postinflammatory hyperpigmentation (e.g., acne vulgaris, arthropod bites, dermatitis, lichen planus)
Melasma
Pityriasis (tinea) versicolor
Mastocytosis
Fixed drug reactions
Deposits of drugs and their metabolites
Linear
Exposure to psoralen-containing plants (e.g., limes) plus ultraviolet A light
Drug reactions (e.g., bleomycin)
Nevoid linear hyperpigmentation
Genodermatoses (e.g., incontinentia pigmenti)
Reticulated
Erythema ab igne
Genodermatoses

tacrolimus), and phototherapy. **4** The differential diagnosis is primarily chemical leukoderma secondary to compounds that are cytotoxic to melanocytes (e.g., catechols, phenols), the leukoderma of melanoma (a good prognostic sign if seen in association with immunotherapy but an indication to exclude metastases if occurs spontaneously), and the leukoderma of scleroderma with retention of perifollicular pigmentation.

Guttate Hypopigmentation

Idiopathic guttate hypomelanosis, in which well-demarcated hypopigmented macules measure only 2 to 4 mm in diameter, is the most common cause of guttate ("raindrop") leukoderma (Fig. 449-9). The favored sites for this common age-related disorder, which may be related to chronic sun exposure, are the shins and the extensor surface of the forearms.

Other Acquired Causes

Circumscribed hypomelanosis is seen in patients with pityriasis (tinea) versicolor (see Fig. 446-16) and *postinflammatory hypopigmentation*. Although

FIGURE 449-8. Striking leukoderma of the hand in a patient with vitiligo.

FIGURE 449-10. Postinflammatory hyperpigmentation secondary to arthropod bites. (Courtesy of Yale Dermatology Residents' Slide Collection.)

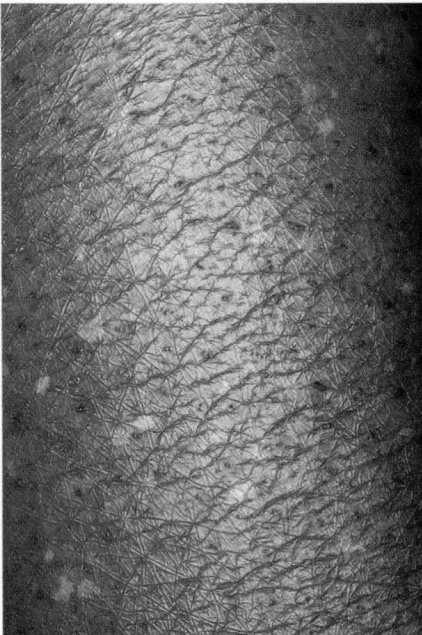

FIGURE 449-9. Idiopathic guttate hypomelanosis with small, well-demarcated hypopigmented macules on the shin.

FIGURE 449-11. Hyperpigmented patches on the cheek in a patient with melasma.

postinflammatory hypopigmentation is most often associated with atopic dermatitis, it can also occur with sarcoidosis (Chapter 95), lupus erythematosus (Chapter 274), and mycosis fungoides (Chapter 191).

Congenital Causes

Congenital circumscribed areas of hypomelanosis include *nevus depigmentosus*, a common tan "birthmark" seen in 1 in 50 infants in which there is a partial decrease in pigment; *piebaldism*, an unusual autosomal dominant disorder with areas of complete absence of pigment caused by mutations in the *KIT* gene; *nevus anemicus*, a localized area of vasoconstriction; and the *ash-leaf spots* of tuberous sclerosis (Chapter 426), with a partial decrease in pigment.

Hyperpigmentation
DIFFUSE HYPERPIGMENTATION

Diffuse hyperpigmentation is most commonly due to drugs (e.g., cyclophosphamide, zidovudine) and endocrinopathies associated with increased circulating levels of adrenocorticotropic hormone (ACTH) (e.g., Addison's disease [Chapter 234], ectopic ACTH production by tumors such as small cell lung carcinoma [Chapter 197]). ACTH, as well as melanocyte-stimulating hormone, can bind and activate the melanocortin-1 receptors on melanocytes, thereby leading to increased melanin production. Additional causes include hemochromatosis (Chapter 219), scleroderma (Chapter 275), primary biliary cirrhosis (Chapter 158), and hyperthyroidism (Chapter 233). Systemic exposure to silver (argyria; Chapter 21) can lead to a slate-gray color.

LINEAR AND RETICULATED HYPERPIGMENTATION

Linear streaks of hyperpigmentation can be due to nevoid (i.e., hamartomatous) conditions that reflect cutaneous mosaicism, as in linear hypopigmentation (see earlier) and genodermatoses (inherited disorders with cutaneous manifestations, e.g., incontinentia pigmenti secondary to mutations in the gene *NEMO*), as well as due to exposure to either plant-derived psoralens (e.g., from limes) plus ultraviolet A irradiation or systemic bleomycin (flagellate pigmentation). Reticulated hypermelanosis is also seen in several genodermatoses (e.g., dyskeratosis congenita) and after chronic exposure to heat (erythema ab igne). The latter corresponds to the cutaneous venous plexus and is seen most commonly in the lumbosacral region where heating pads have been applied or on the anterior thighs from laptop computers.

CIRCUMSCRIBED (PATCHY) HYPERPIGMENTATION

The most common causes of circumscribed hypermelanosis are tinea versicolor (which can present as both hypopigmentation and hyperpigmentation, hence its name), postinflammatory hyperpigmentation, and melasma. *Postinflammatory hyperpigmentation* (Fig. 449-10) is observed more frequently in darkly pigmented individuals and often follows acne vulgaris, arthropod bites, chronic dermatitis, and lichen planus. Additional causes of circumscribed darkening of the skin are cutaneous mastocytosis (urticaria pigmentosa; Chapter 263), deposits of drugs such as antimalarials and minocycline (blue-gray discoloration), and medications that produce fixed drug reactions, most frequently trimethoprim-sulfamethoxazole and nonsteroidal anti-inflammatory drugs. In *melasma* (Fig. 449-11), symmetrical hyperpigmented patches are seen on the lateral aspect of the forehead, upper part of the cheek, and mandibular area. At least 90% of patients with melasma are women. The lesions are exacerbated by ultraviolet light and estrogen (oral contraceptives, pregnancy). Melasma is treated with daily broad-spectrum sunscreens and lightening agents such as hydroquinone (4% cream) and retinoic acid (0.025 to 0.10% cream) for 3 to 4 months; the creams are applied daily, but should be reduced to alternate days if irritation develops.

DISTINCTIVE LESIONS IN BLACK SKIN

Although some diseases are more common in patients of African ancestry (e.g., tinea capitis, pseudofolliculitis barbae, dissecting cellulitis), others are simply more noticeable (e.g., vitiligo and postinflammatory hypopigmentation) (Table 449-3). The explanation for the increased incidence is speculative in most instances, with the exception of curled hairs leading to pseudofolliculitis barbae. Tightly curled hairs, when shaved, are usually cut at an oblique angle, which results in a sharp tip at the distal end of the hair shaft that allows penetration of the skin adjacent to the hair follicle and subsequent inflammation. Some cutaneous disorders are seen less commonly in black skin (e.g., acne rosacea and scabies).

Another entity seen more commonly in individuals of African descent is keloids (Fig. 449-12). Keloids generally appear at sites of trauma (e.g., ear piercing) but can occasionally develop spontaneously, especially on the trunk. In the former situation, they are thought to represent an exaggerated response to wound healing, with increased formation of collagen not only at the site of the trauma (as in hypertrophic scars) but also in adjacent, previously uninvolved skin. Treatment options include intralesional corticosteroids, intralesional interferon, pulsed dye laser, or excision followed by radiation therapy.

REGIONAL DERMATOSES

Some common dermatoses have a predilection for particular anatomic sites (Fig. 449-13 and Table 449-4). These locations can help narrow the differential and guide further diagnostic testing and therapy in many patients.

TABLE 449-3	DISORDERS SEEN MORE COMMONLY IN PATIENTS OF AFRICAN ANCESTRY

HEAD AND NECK

Folliculitis decalvans/dissecting cellulitis
Tinea capitis
Traction alopecia
Central centrifugal cicatricial alopecia*
Acne keloidalis nuchae
Pseudofolliculitis barbae
Pomade acne
Dermatosis papulosa nigra
Inherited patterned lentiginosis
Melasma
Discoid lupus erythematosus

PALMAR

Keratosis punctata of the palmar creases

LOWER EXTREMITIES

Ulcers secondary to sickle cell anemia

GENERALIZED

Keloids
Cutaneous sarcoidosis
Papular eczema and follicular-based inflammation

*Also termed *follicular degeneration syndrome* or *hot comb alopecia*.

FIGURE 449-12. Acne keloidalis in an African American man. (Courtesy of Kalman Watsky, MD.)

TABLE 449-4	REGIONAL DERMATOLOGY	
REGION OF SKIN	**TYPE OF SKIN LESION**	**DISEASE PROCESS**
Scalp	Papulosquamous and eczematous	Seborrheic dermatitis, psoriasis, tinea capitis, eczema (atopic, contact)
	Pustular	Folliculitis, kerion
	Papulonodular	Melanocytic nevi, seborrheic keratoses, pilar cysts, verrucae
Face	Pustular	Acne, rosacea, folliculitis (beard), tinea
	Papulosquamous and eczematous	Seborrheic dermatitis, psoriasis (hairline), contact dermatitis (e.g., cosmetics), atopic dermatitis, impetigo, systemic lupus erythematosus, photodermatitis
	Vesicular	Herpes simplex, herpes zoster, bullous impetigo
	Papulonodular	Melanocytic nevi, actinic keratoses, seborrheic keratoses, basal cell carcinomas, squamous cell carcinomas, melanomas
	Atrophic and telangiectatic	Discoid lupus erythematosus
Trunk	Papulosquamous and eczematous	Psoriasis, atopic dermatitis, contact dermatitis, tinea versicolor, pityriasis rosea, scabies, secondary syphilis, subacute cutaneous lupus (upper trunk)
	Vesiculobullous	Bullous pemphigoid, pemphigus, erythema multiforme/Stevens-Johnson syndrome, herpes zoster
	Maculopapular	Morbilliform drug reactions, viral exanthems
	Papulonodular	Melanocytic nevi, seborrheic keratoses, angiomas, lipomas, epidermoid inclusion cysts, basal and squamous cell carcinomas, keloids, neurofibromas, melanoma
	Pustular	Acne, folliculitis
	Urticarial	Hives, drug reactions, early herpes zoster
Arms and forearms	Eczematous and papulosquamous	Contact dermatitis (e.g., plants), atopic dermatitis, psoriasis, lichen planus, photodermatitis (drugs, contactants, dermatomyositis, subacute cutaneous lupus)
	Papulonodular	Melanocytic nevi, verrucae, seborrheic keratoses, actinic keratoses, squamous cell carcinomas, polymorphic light eruption
	Purpuric	Actinic (solar) purpura
	Annular	Granuloma annulare, subacute cutaneous lupus

TABLE 449-4 REGIONAL DERMATOLOGY—cont'd

REGION OF SKIN	TYPE OF SKIN LESION	DISEASE PROCESS
Legs	Eczematous and papulosquamous	Stasis dermatitis, eczema craquelé (xerotic eczema), contact dermatitis, atopic dermatitis, psoriasis, lichen planus
	Papulonodular	Melanocytic nevi, dermatofibromas, erythema nodosum, melanoma, Kaposi's sarcoma
	Purpuric	Schamberg's disease (capillaritis), vasculitis
	Ulcerative	Stasis ulcers, arterial insufficiency, pyoderma gangrenosum, trauma, spider bite, livedoid vasculopathy, squamous cell carcinoma, diffuse dermal angiomatosis
Genitalia and groin	Eczematous and papulosquamous	Seborrheic dermatitis, tinea, psoriasis, contact dermatitis, scabies, reactive arthritis (Reiter's syndrome), erythrasma, candidiasis, lichen planus, lichen simplex chronicus
	Vesiculobullous	Herpes simplex, Stevens-Johnson syndrome
	Ulcerative	Herpes simplex, syphilis, chancroid, Behçet's disease, squamous cell carcinoma, trauma
	Papulonodular	Condyloma acuminata, molluscum contagiosum, epidermoid inclusion cyst, hidradenitis suppurativa, squamous cell carcinoma
	Pustular	Folliculitis, candidiasis, hidradenitis suppurativa
Hands	Eczematous and papulosquamous	Irritant and allergic contact dermatitis, atopic dermatitis, tinea, scabies, secondary syphilis
	Vesiculobullous, pustular	Erythema multiforme, hand-foot-and-mouth disease (palmar), porphyria cutanea tarda (dorsal), epidermolysis bullosa acquisita, herpetic whitlow, blistering dactylitis, psoriasis
	Papulonodular	Warts, actinic keratoses (dorsal), squamous cell carcinomas (dorsal), pyogenic granuloma, granuloma annulare, digital mucous cysts (dorsal)
	Depigmentation	Vitiligo, chemical leukoderma
	Periungual telangiectases	Scleroderma, dermatomyositis, systemic lupus erythematosus, Osler-Weber-Rendu disease
Feet	Eczematous and papulosquamous	Tinea, psoriasis, contact dermatitis, atopic dermatitis, syphilis
	Vesiculobullous	Tinea, arthropod bites, epidermolysis bullosa (inherited and acquired), erythema multiforme, hand-foot-and mouth disease, epidermolysis bullosa acquisita
	Papules	Verrucae, corns
	Ulcerative	Neuropathic ulcers (plantar)

Psoriasis

Scalp, ears, scalpline
Palms, soles
Dorsal hands, feet
Elbows, knees/shins
Presacrum
Intergluteal fold
Nails

Inverse Psoriasis

Submammary
Inguinal fold
Umbilicus

Seborrheic Dermatitis

Scalp, ears, postauricular
Eyebrows
Nasolabial folds
Central chest
Intergluteal fold
Submammary
Inguinal fold

Atopic Dermatitis (adults)

Eyelids
Antecubital fossa
Popliteal fossa
Posterior neck
Ankles
Hands

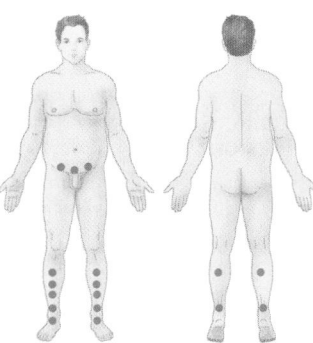

Stasis Dermatitis (adults)

Legs, below knees, but greater on shins than calves
Lower pannus

Vitiligo

Loss of color:
Around eyes
Around nose
Around mouth
Axillae, groin
Wrists (flexor)
Poliosis (streak of white hairs)
Elbows, knees, ankles
Backs of hands/feet (includes digits)
Perianal

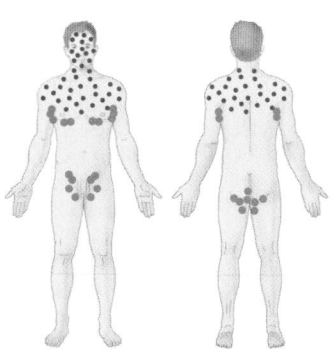

Acne Vulgaris/ Hidradenitis Suppurativa

∴ = papulopustules, blackheads or whiteheads Face/neck/upper trunk/shoulders

● = nodules of hidradenitis suppurativa

FIGURE 449-13. Regional involvement of specific skin diseases.

1. Rajendran PM, Young D, Maurer T, et al. Randomized, double-blind, placebo-controlled trial of cephalexin for treatment of uncomplicated skin abscesses in a population at risk for community-acquired methicillin-resistant *Staphylococcus aureus* infection. *Antimicrob Agents Chemother.* 2007;51:4044-4048.
2. Currie BJ, McCarthy JS. Permethrin and ivermectin for scabies. *N Engl J Med.* 2010;362:717-725.
3. Chosidow O, Giraudeau B, Cottrell J, et al. Oral ivermectin versus malathion lotion for difficult-to-treat head lice. *N Engl J Med.* 2010;362:896-905.
4. Whitton ME, Pinart M, Batchelor J, et al. Interventions for vitiligo. *Cochrane Database Syst Rev* 2010;1:CD003263.

SUGGESTED READINGS

Boissy RE, Nordlund JJ. Vitiligo: current medical and scientific understanding. *G Ital Dermatol Venereol.* 2011;146:69-75. *Review of pathogenesis, treatment, and prognosis.*
Stevens DL, Eron LL. Cellulitis and soft-tissue infections. *Ann Intern Med.* 2009;150:ITC11. *Practical approach with helpful tables.*

450

DISEASES OF HAIR AND NAILS

ANTONELLA TOSTI

HAIR DISORDERS
Normal Hair

The hair shaft is a fully keratinized structure that is produced by the hair follicle. The entire skin, with the exception of the palms and the soles, contains hair follicles. Hair follicles are of two types: terminal follicles and vellus follicles. Terminal follicles, which reach the hypodermis, produce terminal hairs, which are long, thick (60 to 80 μm), and pigmented. Terminal hairs are present since birth on the scalp, eyebrows, and eyelashes and later develop after puberty on the axillae, pubis, and beard region in males. Vellus follicles are small and localized to the superficial and mid-dermis, where they produce vellus hairs, which are thin (<30 μm), short (<2 cm), and not pigmented and cover all the glabrous skin.

The hair follicle is formed by an upper permanent portion and by a lower dynamic transient portion that migrates during the hair cycle. The transient portion includes the hair bulb, which is surrounded by the dermal papilla and contains the hair matrix that produces the hair shaft and its sheaths. The anatomic division between the permanent and the transient portion is just below the bulge region, which corresponds to the insertion of the erector pili muscle. The bulge region contains the epithelial stem cells that regenerate the follicle in each hair growth cycle; its damage results in stem cell destruction and cicatricial alopecia.

Hair Cycle

Hair follicles have a cyclic activity, characterized by alternating periods of hair shaft production and periods of resting (anagen, catagen, telogen). During the anagen phase, the follicles produce the hair shaft. Duration of anagen, which in the scalp ranges from 2 to 7 years, determines hair shaft length. Maximal length and growth rate of terminal hair varies in the different body regions. Scalp hair grows about 0.4 mm/day and may reach a length of more than 1 meter. Maximal hair length decreases with age. Catagen is a transitional phase, which lasts for 2 to 3 weeks and precedes the resting telogen phase. During telogen, hair production is absent, even if the shaft remains within the follicle to be shed only when, after 3 months, the follicle reenters the anagen phase.

The hair cycle of adjacent scalp follicles is not synchronized. In normal conditions, about 85 to 90% of follicles are in anagen and 10 to 15% in telogen.

Hair Loss and Alopecias

Hair loss distresses most patients, independently from its severity and pattern. In some cases, the decrement in quality of life attributable to hair loss is comparable with that caused by major chronic diseases.

The first diagnostic step is to assess family history, drug intake, systemic illness, and severity and duration of hair loss (Table 450-1). The second step

TABLE 450-1 CAUSES OF HAIR LOSS

DIFFUSE ALOPECIA

Telogen effluvium (e.g., after illness or stress)
Anagen effluvium (e.g., after chemotherapy or radiation therapy)
Medications (see Table 450-2)
Nutritional deficiency
Hair treatments
Androgenetic alopecia (in women)
Hormonal changes (e.g., menopause, discontinuation of oral contraceptives, hypothyroidism)

PATCHY ALOPECIA

Alopecia areata (probably autoimmune)
Cicatricial (scarring) alopecia (e.g., lichen planopilaris, discoid lupus erythematosus, folliculitis decalvans)
Traction alopecia (e.g., excessive hair straightening or braiding)
Trichotillomania (hair pulling)
Scalp infection (e.g., ringworm)

is to establish whether the hair density is normal or decreased. The severity of hair shedding should be evaluated, and if possible, the shed hairs should be examined.

Acute and severe hair loss is typical of diseases that acutely interrupt mitotic activity of anagen follicles (drugs, alopecia areata). A normal hair density suggests a diagnosis of telogen effluvium, which may be acute or chronic. A reduced hair density may involve the whole scalp (diffuse alopecia), may be limited to specific scalp regions (patterned alopecia), or may present with bald patches (patchy alopecia). In patchy alopecias, the scalp may show patches of alopecia that are completely devoid of hairs (alopecia areata, cicatricial alopecia) or have short broken hairs (trichotillomania, hair shaft disorders).

TELOGEN EFFLUVIUM
Acute Telogen Effluvium

Acute telogen effluvium results from noxious events that precipitate the entry of a large number of follicles into their resting phase (telogen). Possible causes include systemic diseases, drugs (Table 450-2), fever, stress, weight loss, delivery, iron deficiency, and inflammatory scalp disorders. For drugs, the severity of hair loss depends on the drug, its dosage, and the patient's susceptibility.

Hair loss starts approximately 3 months after the causative event, a time frame that corresponds with the duration of the telogen phase. Telogen hairs are retained within the follicle during telogen, to be shed when the follicle produces a new anagen hair. Hair loss is severe when shedding is 100 to 200 hairs. The patient usually remembers quite precisely when the increased hair shedding started. Acute telogen effluvium does not usually produce visible alopecia because about 50% of hairs need to be lost before reduction of hair density is evident.

TREATMENT AND PROGNOSIS **Rx**

Acute telogen effluvium subsides spontaneously in a few months after removal of the cause. It may, however, increase the likelihood or severity of subsequent androgenetic alopecia.

Chronic Telogen Effluvium

Chronic telogen effluvium, which is characterized by increased hair shedding lasting for more than 6 months, mostly affects middle-aged women and frequently remains unexplained. The daily shedding is mild (usually less than 100 hairs daily), but patients can be distressed and complain of progressive temporal thinning and decreased hair mass. Scalp pain (trichodynia) is frequently reported. Patients who have a high hair density may even bring in envelopes of shed hairs to prove the amount of hair loss. There is no effective treatment. Chronic telogen effluvium has a chronic course with periodic exacerbations.

DIFFUSE ALOPECIA
Anagen Effluvium

Acute hair shedding leading to diffuse alopecia is a typical side effect of cancer chemotherapy and scalp radiation. Hair shedding is caused by acute damage to the growing hair; the result is hair breaking. Hair loss is acute and severe and may produce loss of most of the scalp hair, eyebrows, and eyelashes;

TABLE 450-2   DRUGS REPORTED TO INDUCE HAIR LOSS

ACE inhibitors (captopril, enalapril, moexipril, ramipril)	Haloperidol
	Immunoglobulins
Allopurinol	Indanediones
Amiodarone	Indinavir*
Amphetamines*†	Interferons*†
Analgesics, anti-inflammatories (ibuprofen, indomethacin, naproxen)	Isonicotinic acid hydrazide§
	Leflunomide*
Androgens*¶	Levodopa
Anticoagulants (coumarin, dextran, heparin/heparinoids)*†	Lithium*
	Maprotiline
Antiepileptics (carbamazepine, hydantoins, lamotrigine, troxidone, valproic acid, vigabatrin)*†	Mesalazine
	Methyldopa
	Methysergide
Antipsychotics (flupenthixol decanoate, fluphenazine decanoate)	Metyrapone
	Minoxidil‖
Antithyroid drugs (carbimazole, iodine, thiouracil)*	Nicotinic acid
	Nitrofurantoin
Appetite suppressants	Octreotide
Aromatase inhibitors (fadrozole, 4-OHA, vorozole)*¶	Olanzapine
	Pentosan polysulfate
Benzimidazoles (albendazole, mebendazole)	Phenindione
	Piroxicam
β-Blockers (levobunolol, metoprolol, nadolol, propranolol, timolol)*	Potassium thiocyanate
	Pyridostigmine
Bromocriptine	Radiation (<700 Gy)*§
Buspirone	Retinol (vitamin A)*
Butyrophenones	Retinoids (acitretin, etretinate, isotretinoin)*†
Cantharidin	
Cholestyramine	Risperidone
Chloramphenicol	Salicylates
Cidofovir	Serotonin reuptake inhibitors (fluoxetine, fluvoxamine, paroxetine, sertraline)*
Cimetidine	
Clonazepam	Sorafenib
Clotrimazole	Strontium ranelate*†
Colchicine	Sulfasalazine
Contraceptives (oral)‖	Tamoxifen
Danazol	Terbinafine
Diclofenac	Terfenadine
Dixyrazine	Thiamphenicol
Diazoxide	Thyroxine
Ethambutol	Tocopherol (vitamin E)
Ethionamide	Trazodone
Fibrates (clofibrate, fenofibrate)	Triazoles (fluconazole, itraconazole)
Gentamicin	Tricyclic antidepressants (amitriptyline, desipramine, doxepin, imipramine, maprotiline)
Gefitinib†	
Glatiramer acetate	
Glibenclamide	Trimethadione
Gold salts	Triparanol
G-CSF (granulocyte-colony stimulating factor)	Vasopressin
	Spironolactone

*Established by multiple reports or proved by rechallenge.
†Hair loss usually severe.
‡May produce permanent alopecia.
§May produce anagen effluvium.
‖May produce telogen effluvium 3 months after discontinuation.
¶May produce androgenetic alopecia.

density at the occipital region. Severe female pattern alopecia also often involves parietal and occipital regions with diffuse thinning. In premenopausal women, androgenetic alopecia can be a sign of hyperandrogenism, together with hirsutism and acne. In most women, however, androgenetic alopecia occurs in the absence of biochemical and clinical evidence of androgen excess and may be due to excessive follicular sensitivity to androgens.

Androgenetic alopecia is a progressive disease that tends to worsen with time. Medical treatments of androgenetic alopecia include 2% topical minoxidil in women and 5% topical minoxidil **2** or oral finasteride, 1 mg daily, in men.**3** Clinical improvement is mostly due to thickening of the preexisting hair.

Treatments for androgenetic alopecia should be continued for at least 6 months before assessing their efficacy, and regular drug use is mandatory for maintaining results. Interruption of minoxidil produces an acute telogen effluvium, which becomes evident 3 to 4 months often interruption and cannot be prevented by concomitant finasteride treatment. Interruption of finasteride is followed by gradual hair loss with return to the pretreatment status after 1 year. Hair transplantation is a good option for men with severe androgenetic alopecia, and treatment with finasteride, 1 mg daily, improves the long-term results of surgery. Hair transplantation in women is more complicated because the hair thinning is often diffuse in the parietal and occipital regions, so there is not a good hair donor area. In addition, surgery may induce an effluvium of the preexisting hair in the recipient area, which, in women, produces significant temporary worsening of the hair thinning.

⬤ PATCHY ALOPECIA

Alopecia Areata

Alopecia areata is a common form of nonscarring, usually patchy hair loss affecting up to 2% of the population. The etiology is unknown, but evidence is consistent with an autoimmune disease, to which both a genetic predisposition and environmental factors contribute. In genetically predisposed individuals, various triggering factors cause a predominantly CD8-driven, T_H1-type T-cell autoimmune reaction against the hair follicles, thereby resulting in acute hair loss.

The disease occurs in all ethnic groups and in both sexes. It can start at any age, but severe forms often start during childhood and are more frequent in males. Clinical examination reveals one or multiple well-circumscribed smooth patches of nonscarring absence of hair that enlarge in a centrifugal way (Fig. 450-1). The margins of the patches often are composed of hair 3 mm in length with a broken pigmented tip (exclamation mark hairs), which indicates that the disease is progressing.

Alopecia areata may affect all hairy body areas. Severe forms involve the entire scalp (alopecia areata totalis) or all body hair (alopecia areata universalis). Involvement of the scalp margins (ophiasis) is associated with a poor prognosis. Alopecia areata may be associated with other autoimmune diseases, most commonly thyroid diseases (Chapter 233). Other possible associations include celiac disease (Chapter 142), vitiligo (Chapter 449), and atopy (Chapter 446). Nail abnormalities are common, especially in children.

The natural history of alopecia areata is unpredictable. Studies indicate that 34 to 50% of patients will recover within 1 year and 15 to 25% will progress to total loss of scalp hair or loss of hair from the entire scalp and body, a condition for which full recovery is only about 10%. To date, there is no cure for alopecia areata, and available treatments may induce temporary hair regrowth but do not change the long-term prognosis.**4**

Relapses often occur in a high percentage of patients, even during therapy. High-dose pulse corticosteroid therapy is effective in about 60% of patients with acute alopecia areata but is not useful in ophiasis or long-standing alopecia totalis or alopecia universalis. Intralesional steroids can be used in localized forms of alopecia, including alopecia areata of the eyebrows. High-potency topical steroids (clobetasol propionate cream 0.05%) under occlusion induce regrowth in about 25% of patients with long-standing alopecia totalis or alopecia universalis, but relapses are common. Clobetasol propionate 0.05% in foam can be used in patchy alopecia areata. Topical immunotherapy with diphenylcyclopropenone (DPCP) or squaric acid dibutylester (SADBE), which is used in Europe but is not approved by the U.S. Food and Drug Administration, induces hair regrowth in about 20% of patients with severe alopecia totalis or alopecia universalis. Medium- and low-potency topical steroids and topical minoxidil are probably only placebo treatments for alopecia areata.

Trichotillomania

Trichotillomania is a compulsive disorder that is more common in children. Repetitive hair pulling and plucking produces patches of irregular alopecia. The scalp is not completely bald, but rather shows broken hairs of various

other body hairs are less commonly involved. Hair shedding usually starts 4 to 6 weeks after drug intake and may be very severe, with up to 1000 hairs shed daily. Regrowth of hair is usually fast after discontinuation of therapy, but hair shape and color may be different. Permanent alopecia may occur with high dose radiation and certain drug regimens, such as busulphan. Scalp hypothermia may prevent or reduce hair loss during chemotherapy.**1** Topical minoxidil accelerates hair regrowth but does not prevent hair loss.

Patterned Alopecia (Androgenetic Alopecia)

Androgenetic alopecia, which is the most common form of hair loss, affects up to 80% of men and 50% of women in the course of their life. Androgenetic alopecia is caused by a progressive reduction in the diameter, length, and pigmentation of the hair. Hair thinning is not diffuse, but rather is limited to the frontal, temporal, and vertex areas, where hair follicles are sensitive to the effects of the testosterone metabolite, dehydrotestosterone (DHT). This sensitivity to DHT, which requires the 5-α-reductase enzymes, is genetically determined. In male pattern hair loss, androgenetic alopecia involves the frontotemporal areas and the vertex, following a pattern that corresponds to the Hamilton-Norwood scale. In female pattern alopecia, androgenetic alopecia produces diffuse thinning of the crown region with maintenance of the frontal hairline (Ludwig pattern), a pattern that can easily be appreciated by making a central parting and comparing hair density at the top with hair

FIGURE 450-1. Alopecia areata: patchy hair loss. The alopecic area is devoid of hairs, and the scalp does not present inflammatory changes.

FIGURE 450-2. Trichotillomania: patchy hair loss. The alopecic area has an irregular shape and present hairs broken at different lengths. Also note scalp excoriations.

lengths (Fig. 450-2). The frontal, parietal, and occipital scalp are most commonly affected, but other terminal hairs can be involved, especially the upper eyelashes.

Occasionally, patients develop the habit of chewing or eating the pulled hairs. Patients with trichotillomania frequently do not admit their habit, and parents of affected children may be recalcitrant to accept the diagnosis. Psychiatric referral may be indicated, especially in adults.

Cicatricial Alopecias (Scarring Alopecia)

The hallmark of cicatricial alopecias is loss of follicular ostia. Cicatricial alopecias include diseases that primarily affect the hair follicles as well as diseases that affect the dermis and secondarily cause follicular destruction. In cicatricial alopecia, the scalp has atrophic bald areas that may slowly enlarge centrifugally. The differential diagnosis among the different diseases (e.g., lichen planopilaris, discoid lupus erythematosus, folliculitis decalvans) that cause cicatricial alopecia requires the evaluation of pathologic specimens because clinical features are usually not diagnostic. The biopsy should be taken from scalp areas that show active evidence of inflammation because biopsy of atrophic scalp will typically show only follicular or dermal fibrosis.

LICHEN PLANOPILARIS

In lichen planopilaris, which is the most common form of cicatricial alopecia, the hair follicles surrounding the alopecic patches show perifollicular erythema and follicular plugging. The patient usually complains of severe itching. A variant of lichen planopilaris is frontal fibrosing alopecia, which typically affects the frontal hairline of postmenopausal women with a bandlike scarring

FIGURE 450-3. Frontal fibrosing alopecia. Scarring alopecia of the hair margin with recession of the frontal hairline.

alopecia, often associated with marked decrease or complete loss of the eyebrows (Fig. 450-3). The pathogenesis is unknown, but lichen planopilaris may be a hair-specific autoimmune reaction, in which T lymphocytes target follicular antigens located mainly in the bulge area, with relative sparing of the interfollicular dermis. No consistently effective treatment for lichen planopilaris is available, but attempted treatments include intralesional or systemic steroids, oral tetracyclines, and systemic antimalarials.

DISCOID LUPUS ERYTHEMATOSUS

In discoid lupus erythematosus, the alopecic area shows active inflammation with erythema, edema, scaling, and follicular plugging, as well as atrophy with variable degrees of telangiectasia and dyspigmentation.

Females are more often affected, and the disease is more common in African American women. Approximately 5 to 10% of adults with discoid lupus erythematosus will develop systemic lupus erythematosus (Chapter 274), especially those with widespread discoid lesions. In localized lesions, treatment with high-potency topical steroids (see Table 445-1 in Chapter 445) is usually effective. Antimalarials are a second-line treatment. Hair regrowth may occur when treatment is promptly started. Therapeutic strategy should include photoprotection of the involved area.

FOLLICULITIS DECALVANS

In folliculitis decalvans, the scalp shows papulopustular lesions that often coalesce to form exudative crusted areas that result in cicatricial alopecia. A frequent clinical finding is tufted folliculitis, that is, tufts of 5 to 15 hairs that emerge together from the scalp. The cause is unknown, but the condition may reflect an abnormal host response to bacterial antigens. *Staphylococcus aureus* is often isolated from active lesions. Folliculitis decalvans sometimes responds to oral antibiotics (e.g., trimethoprim-sulfamethoxazole or clindamycin with or without rifampin for 8 to 10 weeks) but usually relapses after interruption of therapy. The disease tends to have a prolonged course with frequent inflammatory relapses and, sometimes, severe scarring.

● HAIR DISORDERS IN CHILDREN

Hereditary and congenital alopecias are present since birth or appear in the first years of life. Aplasia cutis congenita is the most common form of focal alopecia in newborns. Patterned hair loss in a prepubertal child does not exclude the diagnosis of androgenetic alopecia because the disease may appear at the time of pubarche in the absence of any endocrinologic abnormality.

Hereditary hair shaft abnormalities associated with increased hair fragility produce diffuse or patchy alopecia that appears during childhood. The most common hereditary hair shaft disorder is monilethrix, in which hair shaft fragility is associated with follicular hyperkeratosis. The hair is dull and fragile and breaks easily, especially in the nape and occipital areas. Diagnosis is confirmed by finding hair beading on microscopic examination of the hair shaft.

Congenital triangular alopecia is usually noticed by the age of 6 years as an irregularly triangular patch of alopecia on the frontotemporal region. The presence of vellus hairs in the area is diagnostic and suggests a possible nevoid origin of the alopecia.

The loose anagen hair syndrome is characterized by a defective anchorage of the hair to the follicle, thereby resulting in hairs that are easily and painlessly pulled out from the scalp. The condition is typical of children and may manifest with patchy hair loss due to hair pulling while playing.

RACIAL DIFFERENCES

The frequency and clinical aspects of hair disorders vary in different races. Androgenetic alopecia, for instance, is more frequent in whites than in blacks and Asians, whereas black and Asian hair is more susceptible to weathering and fragility.

The black hair shaft is flat in shape, highly twisted, and difficult to manage without strong chemical or hair styling procedures, which often cause considerable damage to the hair. Hair straightening and braiding are responsible for traction alopecia, which is common and typically produces cicatricial alopecia of the frontal and lateral margins.

In Asians, the hair shaft is round in shape, thick, robust, and straight. Asian hair is very difficult to style and dye, and it is often damaged by its treatment with high concentrations or long exposure to chemicals.

EXCESSIVE HAIR GROWTH

Hirsutism describes excessive terminal hair with male distribution in a female. Hirsutism should be distinguished from hypertrichosis, which is characterized by the presence of an excessive amount of hair in a non–androgen-dependent area.

Hirsutism

Hirsutism is a common condition that affects up to 10% of women. The prevalence of hirsutism is influenced by genetic and racial factors. It is more frequent in Hispanic and Mediterranean women than in Asian or African women. Hirsutism may or not be associated with hyperandrogenism or with acne and androgenetic alopecia. Idiopathic hirsutism accounts for about 15% of cases.

Hypertrichosis

Hypertrichosis results from the presence of terminal hairs in anatomic areas that are normally characterized by vellus hair. Hypertrichoses can be congenital or acquired, localized or generalized. Acquired hypertrichoses are most commonly iatrogenic, metabolic (e.g., Cushing's syndrome, porphyria, hyperthyroidism), nutritional (e.g., anorexia nervosa), or paraneoplastic (Chapter 187).

NAIL DISORDERS

Normal Nail

The nail plate is a keratinized hard structure produced by the nail matrix, which is a specialized epithelium located above the distal phalanx of the finger. In longitudinal sections, the matrix consists of a dorsal, an apical, and a ventral portion. The proximal matrix (dorsal portion and apex) produces the dorsal nail plate (two thirds upper plate), and the distal matrix (ventral portion) produces the ventral plate (one third lower plate). The nail plate is produced continuously throughout life. Nails grow slowly, and the nail plate can reflect illnesses that occurred several months before nail abnormality is evident. Complete replacement takes about 6 months for a fingernail and 12 to 18 months for a toenail. Many medications (e.g., anticonvulsants, neuroleptics, antifungals), drugs (e.g., amphetamine, cocaine, doping substances), and poisons (e.g., mercury, arsenic) are retained in the nails, whose fragments (nail clippings) can be used to monitor previous exposure.

NAIL DISORDERS

Nail abnormalities can be congenital or acquired and may caused by developmental, traumatic, inflammatory, infective, and neoplastic disorders or by medications. The diagnosis of nail dystrophies usually relies on a careful clinical examination and an accurate history, but radiographic or magnetic resonance imaging investigation of the digit and pathology may be required.

Koilonychia (Spoon Nails)

In koilonychia (Fig. 450-4), which is also called spooning of the nails, the nail plate is thin and has a concave appearance. Koilonychia is physiologic in children. In adults, it can be occupational or, more rarely, a sign of iron deficiency (Chapter 162).

Clubbing

Clubbing (Fig. 450-5) develops when enlargement of the soft tissue of the distal digit causes a bulbous digit with an enlarged and overcurved nail plate. The angle between the proximal nail fold and the nail plate (Lovibond's angle) is greater than 180 degrees. Clubbing may be congenital (i.e., in congenital heart disease; Chapter 69) or acquired. Other causes of acquired clubbing include intrathoracic and gastrointestinal neoplasms (Chapter 187), chronic intrathoracic suppurative disease (Chapter 90), inflammatory bowel disease (Chapter 143), and liver disorders.

FIGURE 450-4. Spooning. (Available at McGraw-Hill's Access Medicine: http://www.accessmedicine.com/search/searchAMResultImg.aspx?rootterm=koilonychia&rootID=41210&searchType=1.)

FIGURE 450-5. Clubbing. (Available at The Dermatologists' Image Resource: http://www.dermnet.com/image.cfm?passedArrayIndex=3&moduleID=13&moduleGroupID=183. Accessed May 24, 2006.)

Beau's Lines and Onychomadesis

Beau's lines (Fig. 450-6) and onychomadesis are due to a temporary reduction or arrest of the mitotic activity of the proximal matrix. Beau's lines appear as transverse grooves of various depth; onychomadesis as a full-thickness transverse groove of the proximal nail plate. Causes (Table 450-3) include trauma, skin diseases involving the proximal nail fold and the matrix, and systemic diseases. In the latter case, Beau's lines or onychomadesis involve all the nails and are localized at the same level.

Pitting

Pitting (Fig. 450-7) appears as punctate depressions of the dorsal nail plate, with variable breadth and depth. Pitting is caused by inflammatory skin disorders such as psoriasis (Chapter 446), alopecia areata, and eczema (Chapter 446).

Longitudinal Grooves and Striations

Normal nails often show superficial thin longitudinal ridges that increase in number with aging. Deep longitudinal fissures, which indicate damage to the proximal matrix, can be caused by nail lichen planus, vascular insufficiency, trauma, and tumors involving or compressing the matrix.

Leukonychia

Leukonychia describes a whitish discoloration of the nail, which may be due to persistence of nuclei in the cells of the ventral nail plate (true leukonychia), or to a pallor of the nail bed (apparent leukonychia). True leukonychia does not fade with pressure and moves distally with nail growth; it is most commonly caused by trauma. Apparent leukonychia, which does not follow nail

FIGURE 450-6. Beau's lines after a severe infection. The lines affect all the nails at the same level.

TABLE 450-3	CAUSES OF BEAU'S LINES AND ONYCHOMADESIS

SYSTEMIC

Acrodermatitis enteropathica
Severe metabolic stress
High fever
Viral infections (Kawasaki disease, measles, hand-foot-and-mouth syndrome)
Typhus
Stevens-Johnson syndrome
Drugs
Bullous disorders (pemphigus, pemphigoids)
Deep saturation, high altitude
Hemodialysis
Myocardial infarction

LOCAL

Trauma (including manicure)
Paronychia
Congenital malalignment (big toenails)

growth and fades with pressure, may be a sign of systemic diseases such as liver cirrhosis (Terry's nails; Chapter 148), chronic renal diseases (half-and-half nails, characterized by apparent leukonychia of the proximal half of the nail; Chapter 132), hypoalbuminemia (Chapter 123), and systemic chemotherapy (Muehrcke's lines; Fig. 450-8).

Yellow Nail Syndrome

The yellow nail syndrome is a chronic nail disorder characterized by an arrest or a reduction of nail growth, resulting in nail thickening, hardening, and yellow discoloration. Fingernails and toenails are excessively curved from side to side, and cuticles are absent (Fig. 450-9). Yellow nail syndrome may occasionally be paraneoplastic (Chapter 187). The pathogenesis of yellow nail syndrome is unknown, but a congenital abnormality of the lymphatic vessels may be involved. Typical cases have associated lymphedema or respiratory disturbances. The nail abnormalities improve with treatment of the associated respiratory disorders. Oral Vitamin E (1200 mg/day for several months) is useful in some cases.

Splinter Hemorrhages

Splinter hemorrhages (see Fig. 50-11 in Chapter 50) appear as longitudinal thin red-brown lines of variable length. Splinter hemorrhages are usually localized in the distal nail and are commonly seen in inflammatory diseases, including eczema (Chapter 446), psoriasis (Chapter 446), and onychomycosis. Multiple splinter hemorrhages localized in the proximal nail plate can be a sign of systemic diseases, including infectious or marantic endocarditis (Chapter 76), trichinosis (Chapter 365), and the antiphospholipid syndrome.

Onycholysis

Onycholysis (Fig. 450-10) describes detachment of the nail plate from the bed. The detachment usually occurs at the free lateral margins of the nail. The

FIGURE 450-7. Pitting and onycholysis in nail psoriasis.

FIGURE 450-8. Muehrcke's lines. (From Wikipedia Commons.)

FIGURE 450-9. Yellow nail syndrome. The nails are yellow, overcurved, and thickened and do not grow.

onycholytic area is white owing to the presence of air, but it may acquire a green-brown color if the space if colonized by bacteria, such as *Pseudomonas aeruginosa.*

Onycholysis of the fingernails is a common sign of nail psoriasis (Chapter 446). It may also be due to prolonged and frequent contact with water, detergents, or irritants (idiopathic onycholysis). Toenail onycholysis is almost exclusively caused by trauma or onychomycosis. When onycholysis is limited to one digit, the possibility of a nail tumor should always be considered.

Paronychia

Paronychia, which describes the acute or chronic inflammation of the proximal and lateral nail folds, is common in the fingernails at any age. In acute paronychia, the affected digit is painful, with erythema, swelling, and pus discharge localized to one corner of the proximal nail fold. Acute paronychia usually follows a trauma to the nail fold, as in children who pick or bite the cuticles or in women after a manicure. Treatment with mild-potency topical steroids (see Table 445-1 in Chapter 445) and antibiotics (e.g., amoxicillin and clavulanic acid, 1 mg per day for 5 days in adults) promptly induces regression of the condition.

FIGURE 450-10. Onycholysis. Note the detachment of the distal nail from the nail bed. (From Dartmouth University and Dermnet Weekly Clinic, July 30, 2001.)

In chronic paronychia, prolonged mechanical or environmental trauma (such as contact with water and irritants) damages the cuticle, allowing penetration of dirt, bacteria, and other particles under the proximal nail fold. The result is an inflammatory reaction of the proximal nail fold and nail matrix, with edema and redness of the fold, absence of the cuticles, Beau's lines, and abnormalities of the nail plate surface. Treatment includes protective measures, such as use of cotton and rubber gloves to avoid contact with irritants, as well as topical steroids and topical antimicrobials.

Onychomycosis

Fungal nail infections most commonly affect the toenails of adults. Dermatophytes (particularly *Trichophyton rubrum*) are responsible for most infections. The clinical presentation varies depending on the modality of the nail invasion. In distal subungual onychomycosis, which is the most common form, fungi spread from plantar skin and invade the nail bed. The affected nail shows subungual hyperkeratosis, onycholysis, and yellow streaks. In white superficial onychomycosis, which only affects toenails, fungi colonize the surface of the nail plate, where they cause multiple white friable patches. Proximal subungual onychomycosis produces a true leukonychia, owing to the presence of fungal hyphae in the deep layers of the plate. Proximal subungual onychomycosis caused by *T. rubrum* is typical in immunosuppressed patients. Treatment of onychomycosis depends on the clinical type, the number of affected nails, and severity of nail involvement. A systemic treatment is always required for proximal subungual onychomycosis and for distal subungual onychomycosis involving the proximal nail. Terbinafine (250 mg per day) for 2 (fingernails) or 3 (toenails) months is the most effective treatment for dermatophyte infections.**5**

Ingrowing Toenails

Ingrown toenails are a common condition, especially in young patients. Nail ingrowing most commonly affects one or both the big toes and is related to genetic factors, hyperhidrosis, and poorly fitting shoes. Ingrowing is usually precipitated by incorrect nail trimming, with formation of a sharp edge (spicule) of the lateral nail plate that penetrates and injures the soft tissues of the lateral nail fold. Depending on severity, treatment varies from simple disembedding of the spicule to chemical destruction of the lateral nail matrix by phenolization.**6**

Nail Pigmentation

Nail pigmentation is usually caused by staining from external agents, such as nicotine or hair dyes. It may rarely be due to drugs deposition in the nail plate or into the nail bed (i.e., antimalarials) or systemic diseases (argyria). In these cases, the proximal margin of the pigmentation follows the shape of the lunula.

Melanonychia

Melanonychia is defined by the presence of melanin within the nail plate. It appears more often as a longitudinal brown-black band starting from the matrix and extending to the free edge of the nail plate. Less often, the pigmentation can involve the whole nail plate or present as a transverse band.

Melanonychia results from production of melanin by melanocytes of the nail matrix, where melanocytes are usually quiescent but may become active and start melanin synthesis. Melanonychia has three main causes: simple melanocytic activation, benign melanocyte proliferations (lentigo, nevus), and malignant melanocyte proliferation (melanoma; Chapter 210).

Common causes of longitudinal melanonychia due to melanocytic activation include inflammatory and traumatic nail disorders, drugs

FIGURE 450-11. Melanonychia and apparent leukonychia (Muehrcke's lines) in a patient undergoing systemic chemotherapy with cisplatin.

FIGURE 450-12. Nail melanoma. Melanonychia and periungual pigmentation (Hutchinson's sign).

(chemotherapy, azidothymidine, antimalarials, PUVA therapy) (Fig. 450-11), and systemic diseases (acquired immunodeficiency syndrome [Chapter 399]; Addison's disease [Chapter 234]).

Nail melanoma is rare and most frequently involves the thumb of middle-aged individuals. Diagnosis is often delayed, and the 5-year survival is only 15%. Hutchinson's sign, extension of the pigmentation to the proximal or lateral nail folds, is an important indicator of nail melanoma (Fig. 450-12).

1. Macduff C, Mackenzie T, Hutcheon A, et al. The effectiveness of scalp cooling in preventing alopecia for patients receiving epirubicin and docetaxel. *Eur J Cancer Care*. 2003;12:154-161.
2. Olsen EA, Whiting D, Bergfeld W, et al. A randomized clinical trial of 5% topical minoxidil versus 2% topical minoxidil and placebo in the treatment of androgenetic alopecia in men. *J Am Acad Dermatol*. 2002;47:377-385.
3. Acra E, Açikgöz G, Taştan HB, et al. An open, randomized, comparative study of oral finasteride and 5% topical minoxidil in male androgenetic alopecia. *Dermatology*. 2004;209:117-125.
4. Delamere FM, Sladden MM, Dobbins HM, et al. Interventions for alopecia areata. *Cochrane Database Syst Rev*. 2008;2:CD004413.
5. Sigurgeirsson B, Olafsson JH, Steinsson JB, et al. Long-term effectiveness of treatment with terbinafine vs itraconazole in onychomycosis: a 5-year blinded prospective follow-up study. *Arch Dermatol*. 2002;13:353-357.
6. Bos AM, van Tilburg MW, van Sorge AA, et al. Randomized clinical trial of surgical technique and local antibiotics for ingrowing toenail. *Br J Surg*. 2007;94:292-296.

SUGGESTED READINGS

Baran R. The nail in the elderly. *Clin Dermatol*. 2011;29:54-60. *Review*.
Camacho-Martinez FM. Hair loss in women. *Semin Cutan Med Surg*. 2009;28:19-32. *Review emphasizing the potential role for finasteride or dutasteride in postmenopausal women.*
Rathnayake D, Sinclair R. Male androgenetic alopecia. *Expert Opin Pharmacother*. 2010;11:1295-1304. *Review*.

Appendix

LABORATORY REFERENCE INTERVALS AND VALUES

REFERENCE INTERVALS AND LABORATORY VALUES*

RONALD J. ELIN

Reference intervals are valuable guidelines for the clinician to assess health and disease, but they should not be used as absolute indicators of health and disease. For essentially every test, significant overlap exists between healthy and diseased populations. Many factors may influence the determination of the reference interval. The method and mode of standardization are variables for the reference interval, particularly for immunologic and enzymatic tests. The selection of the "normal" population is also important because factors such as age, gender, race, diet, personal habits (e.g., alcohol consumption, smoking), and exercise may influence the reference interval for a given analyte. Finally, the statistics chosen to define the reference interval are also a factor. These multiple variables for determining the reference interval indicate why differences exist among institutions for the same analyte.

The values in this chapter are primarily for adults in the fasting state. Values for other groups, when included, are clearly identified. Prefixes and abbreviations are listed in Table Appendix-1. For convenience, this chapter is divided into the following three sections: clinical chemistry, toxicology, and serology (Table Appendix-2); hematology and coagulation (Table Appendix-3); and drugs; therapeutic and toxic (Table Appendix-4). The list includes reference intervals for the most common tests used in the practice of internal medicine.

All laboratory values are given in conventional and international units. If the value and units for a reference interval are the same for conventional and international units, the interval is listed only in the column for international units. The temperature for all enzyme assays listed in the chapter is 37° C. The pertinent prefixes denoting the decimal factors and abbreviations are listed in Table Appendix-1.

*The material in this chapter was partially extracted from Tietz NW, ed. *Clinical Guide to Laboratory Tests*. Philadelphia: WB Saunders; 1995. The material for the section on therapeutic drug concentrations was partially extracted from Burtis CA, Ashwood ER, eds. *Tietz Textbook of Clinical Chemistry*. Philadelphia: WB Saunders; 1994. The main contributors to this section of the book are P. C. Painter, J. Y. Cope, and J. L. Smith.

TABLE APPENDIX-1 PREFIXES AND ABBREVIATIONS

Prefixes Denoting Decimal Factors

PREFIX	SYMBOL	FACTOR
mega	M	10^6
kilo	k	10^3
hecto	h	10^2
deca	da	10^1
deci	d	10^{-1}
centi	c	10^{-2}
milli	m	10^{-3}
micro	μ	10^{-6}
nano	n	10^{-9}
pico	p	10^{-12}
femto	f	10^{-15}

ABBREVIATIONS

AU	Arbitrary units
CSF	Cerebrospinal fluid
EDTA	Ethylenediaminetetraacetic acid
EU	Ehrlich unit
GD	General diagnostics
Hb	Hemoglobin
hpf	High-power field
IFA	Immunofluorescence assay
IU	International unit (of hormone activity)
Kat	Katal
Pa	Pascal
RBC	Red blood cell
RIA	Radioimmunoassay
RID	Radial immunodiffusion
S	Substrate
U	International unit (of enzyme activity)
WBC	White blood cell

TABLE APPENDIX-2 CLINICAL CHEMISTRY, TOXICOLOGY, AND SEROLOGY

TEST	SPECIMEN	REFERENCE INTERVAL (CONVENTIONAL UNITS)	REFERENCE INTERVAL (INTERNATIONAL UNITS)
Acetoacetate Semiquantitative	Serum or plasma (fluoride/oxalate)	Negative (<1 mg/dL)	Negative (<0.1 mmol/L)
Acetone Semiquantitative	Urine Serum or plasma (fluoride or oxalate)	Negative Negative (<1 mg/dL)	Negative Negative (0.17 mmol/L)
Adrenocorticotropic hormone (ACTH)	Plasma (heparin)	0800 hr: <120 pg/mL 1600-2000 hr: <85 pg/mL	<26 pmol/L <19 pmol/L
Alanine aminotransferase (ALT, SGPT)	Serum	M: 10-40 U/L F: 7-35 U/L	0.17-0.68 μKat/L 0.12-0.60 μKat/L
Albumin Nephelometric, colorimetric Turbidimetric	Serum CSF Urine	3.4-4.8 g/dL <45 mg/dL <80 mg/day at rest <150 mg/day ambulatory	34-48 g/L <450 mg/L <80 mg/day <150 mg/day
Aldolase	Serum	1.0-7.5 U/L	0.2-0.13 μKat/L
Aldosterone	Plasma (heparin EDTA) or serum	Adult, average sodium diet Supine: 3-16 ng/dL Upright: 7-30 ng/dL	0.8-0.44 nmol/L 0.19-0.83 nmol/L
Alkaline phosphatase (S:4-NPP)	Serum	Adult (>20 yr) 25-100 U/L	0.43-1.70 μKat/L
Aluminum	Serum	<5.41 μg/L	<0.2 μmol/L

TABLE APPENDIX-2 CLINICAL CHEMISTRY, TOXICOLOGY, SEROLOGY—cont'd

TEST	SPECIMEN	REFERENCE INTERVAL (CONVENTIONAL UNITS)	REFERENCE INTERVAL (INTERNATIONAL UNITS)
δ-Aminolevulinic acid (δ-ALA)	Serum	15-23 µg/dL	1.1-8 µmol/L
	Urine	1.5-7.5 mg/day	11.4-57.2 µmol/day
Ammonia nitrogen Resin or enzymatic	Serum or plasma (Na-heparin) Urine, 24-hr	Adult 15-45 µg N/dL 140-1500 mg/day	11-32 µmol/L 10-107 mmol/day
Amylase (S:Beckman, defined substrate)	Serum Urine, timed specimen	27-131 U/L	0.46-2.23 µKat/L 1-17 U/hr
Angiotensin I	Peripheral venous plasma (EDTA)	<25 pg/mL	<25 ng/L
Angiotensin II	Plasma (EDTA) Arterial blood	10-60 pg/mL	10-60 ng/L
α₁-Antitrypsin (nephelometry)	Serum	78-200 mg/dL	0.78-2 g/L
Anion gap $[Na^+-(Cl^- + HCO_3^-)]$	Serum or plasma (heparin)	7-16 mEq/L	7-16 mmol/L
Arsenic	Whole blood (heparin)	0.2-2.3 µg/dL Chronic poisoning: 10-50 µg/dL Acute poisoning: 60-93 µg/dL	0.3-0.31 µmol/L 1.33-6.65 µmol/L 7.98-12.37 µmol/L
Ascorbic acid (see Vitamin C)			
Aspartate aminotransferase (AST, SGOT)	Serum	10-30 U/L	0.17-0.51 µKat/L
Base excess	Whole blood (heparin)	−2 to 3 mEq/L	−2 to 3 mmol/L
Bicarbonate	Serum	22-29 mEq/L	22-29 mmol/L
Bile acids, total	Serum, fasting Serum, 1-hr postprandial Feces	0.3-2.3 µg/mL 1.8-3.2 µg/mL 120-225 mg/day	0.74-5.64 µmol/L 4.41-7.84 µmol/L 294-551 µmol/day
Bilirubin, conjugated (direct)	Serum	0-0.2 mg/dL	0-3.4 µmol/L
Bilirubin, total	Serum Urine	0.3-1.2 mg/dL	5-21 µmol/L Negative
B-type natriuretic peptide (BNP)	Whole blood or plasma (EDTA)	<100 pg/mL	<28.8 pmol/L
Calcium, ionized (iCa)	Serum	4.65-5.28 mg/dL	1.16-1.32 mmol/L
Calcium, total	Serum Urine, 24-hr CSF	8.6-10.0 mg/dL 100-300 mg/day 4.2-5.4 mg/dL	2.15-2.50 mmol/L 2.5-7.5 mmol/day 1.5-1.35 mmol/L
Cancer antigen 125 (CA 125)	Serum	<35 U/mL	<35 kU/L
Cancer antigen 15-3 (CA 15-3)	Serum	<30 U/mL	<30 kU/L
Carbohydrate antigen 19-9 (CA 19-9)	Serum	<37 U/mL	<37 kU/L
Carbon dioxide, partial pressure (P_{CO_2})	Whole blood, arterial (heparin)	M: 35-48 mm Hg F: 32-45 mm Hg	4.66-6.38 kPa 4.26-5.99 kPa
Carbon dioxide, total (T_{CO_2})	Serum or plasma (heparin)	23-29 mEq/L	23-29 mmol/L
Carcinoembryonic antigen (CEA)	Serum	Nonsmokers: <2.5 ng/mL	<2.5 µg/L
β-Carotene	Serum	10-85 µg/dL	0.19-1.58 µmol/L
Catecholamines, total	Urine, 24-hr	<100 µg/day	<5.91 nmol/day
Ceruloplasmin	Serum	18-45 mg/dL	180-450 mg/L
Chloride	Serum or plasma (heparin) CSF Urine, 24-hr	98-106 mEq/L 118-132 mEq/L 110-250 mEq/day	98-106 mmol/L 118-132 mmol/L 110-250 mmol/day
Cholesterol, total	Serum or plasma (EDTA)	Recommended: <200 mg/dL Moderate risk: 200-239 mg/dL High risk: ≥240 mg/dL	<5.18 mmol/L 5.18-6.19 mmol/L 6.22 mmol/L
Chorionic gonadotropin, β-subunit (β-HCG)	Serum or plasma (EDTA)	M and nonpregnant F: <5.0 mIU/mL	<5.0 IU/L
Complement, total hemolytic	Serum	26-58 U/mL	26-58 kU/L
Copper	Serum Erythrocyte (heparin) Urine, 24-hr	M: 70-140 µg/dL F: 80-155 µg/dL 90-150 µg/dL 3-35 µg/day	10.99-21.98 µmol/L 12.56-24.34 µmol/L 14.13-23.55 µmol/L 0.47-0.55 µmol/day
Coproporphyrin	Urine, 24-hr Feces, 24-hr	34-234 µg/day <30 µg/g dry wt 400-1200 µg/day	51-351 nmol/day <45 nmol/g dry wt 600-1800 nmol/day
Corticosterone	Serum	0800 hr: 130-820 ng/dL 1600 hr: 60-220 ng/dL	4-24 nmol/L 2-6 nmol/L

TABLE APPENDIX-2 CLINICAL CHEMISTRY, TOXICOLOGY, SEROLOGY—cont'd

TEST	SPECIMEN	REFERENCE INTERVAL (CONVENTIONAL UNITS)	REFERENCE INTERVAL (INTERNATIONAL UNITS)
Cortisol	Serum or plasma (heparin)	0800 hr: 5-23 μg/dL 1600 hr: 3-15 μg/dL 2000 hr: ≤50% of 0800 hr	138-635 nmol/L 82-413 nmol/L Fraction of 0800 hr: ≤0.50
Cortisol, free	Urine, 24-hr	20-90 μg/day	55-248 nmol/day
C-peptide	Serum	0.78-1.89 ng/mL	0.26-0.62 nmol/L
C-reactive protein	Serum	68-8200 ng/mL	68-8200 μg/L
Creatine kinase (CK)	Serum		M: 38-174 U/L F: 26-140 U/L
Isoenzymes, fraction 2 (MB)	Serum	<4-6% of total (method-dependent)	Fraction of total: <0.4-0.6
Creatinine Jaffe, kinetic or enzymatic	Serum or plasma Urine, 24-hr	M: 0.7-1.3 mg/dL F: 0.6-1.1 mg/dL M: 14-26 mg/kg/day F: 11-20 mg/kg/day	62-115 μmol/L 53-97 μmol/L 124-230 μmol/kg/day 97-177 μmol/kg/day
Creatinine clearance (endogenous)	Serum or plasma, and urine	M: 90-139 mL/min/1.73 m² F: 80-125 mL/min/1.73 m²	0.87-1.34 mL/sec/m² 0.77-1.20 mL/sec/m²
Dehydroepiandrosterone (DHEA)	Serum	M: 1.8-12.5 ng/mL F: 1.3-9.8 ng/mL	6.2-43.3 nmol/L 4.5-34 nmol/L
11-Deoxycortisol (compound S)	Serum	12-158 ng/dL	0.3-4.6 nmol/L
Erythropoietin	Serum		5-36 U/L
Estrogens, total	Serum Urine, 24-hr	M: 20-80 pg/mL F, cycle: Postmenopausal: ≤130 pg/mL Follicular phase: 60-200 pg/mL Luteal phase: 160-400 pg/mL	20-80 ng/L ≤130 ng/L 60-200 ng/L 160-400 ng/L M: 15-40 μg/day F: Preovulation: 4-25 μg/day Ovulation: 28-100 μg/day Luteal peak: 22-80 μg/day Pregnancy, term: <45,000 μg/day Postmenopausal: <20 μg/day
Fat, fecal	Feces, 72-hr		<7 g/day Fat-free diet: <4 g/day
Fatty acids, nonesterified (free)	Serum or plasma (heparin)	8-25 mg/dL	0.28-0.89 mmol/L
Ferritin	Serum	M: 20-250 ng/mL F: 10-120 ng/mL	20-250 μg/L 10-120 μg/L
α₁-Fetoprotein	Serum	<10 ng/mL	<10 μg/L
Fibrinogen (see Table Appendix-3)			
Folate	Serum Erythrocytes (EDTA)	3-16 ng/mL 140-628 ng/mL packed cells	7-36 nmol/L 317-1422 nmol/L packed cells
Follitropin (FSH)	Serum or plasma (heparin) Urine, 24-hr	M: 4-25 mIU/mL F: Follicular phase: 1-9 mIU/L Ovulatory peak: 6-26 mIU/mL Luteal phase: 1-9 mIU/mL Postmenopausal: 30-118 mIU/mL	4-25 IU/L 1-9 IU/L 6-26 IU/L 1-9 IU/L 30-118 IU/L M: 3-11 IU/day F: 2-15 IU/day
Gastrin	Serum	25-90 pg/mL	25-90 ng/L
Glucose Quantitative, enzymatic Qualitative	Serum Whole blood (heparin) CSF Urine Urine	Adult: 74-106 mg/dL >60 yr: 80-115 mg/dL 65-95 mg/dL 40-70 mg/dL <0.5 g/day	4.1-5.9 mmol/L 4.4-6.4 mmol/L 3.6-5.3 mmol/L 2.2-3.9 mmol/L <2.8 mmol/day Negative
Glucose, 2-hr postprandial	Serum	<126 mg/dL	<7.0 mmol/L

TEST	SPECIMEN		mg/dL			mmol/L	
Glucose, tolerance test (GTT), oral	Serum		Normal	Diabetic		Normal	Diabetic
		Fasting:	70-105	>140		3.9-5.8	>7.8
		60 min:	120-170	≥200		6.7-9.4	≥11
		90 min:	100-140	≥200		5.6-7.8	≥11
		120 min:	70-120	≥140		3.9-6.7	≥7.8

TEST	SPECIMEN	REFERENCE INTERVAL (CONVENTIONAL UNITS)	REFERENCE INTERVAL (INTERNATIONAL UNITS)
γ-Glutamyltransferase (GGT) (Szasz method)	Serum	M: 2-30 U/L F: 1-24 U/L	0.03-0.51 μKat/L 0.02-0.41 μKat/L

TABLE APPENDIX-2 CLINICAL CHEMISTRY, TOXICOLOGY, SEROLOGY—cont'd

TEST	SPECIMEN	REFERENCE INTERVAL (CONVENTIONAL UNITS)	REFERENCE INTERVAL (INTERNATIONAL UNITS)
Growth hormone (hGH, somatotropin)	Serum	Adult, M: 0-4 ng/mL	0-4 µg/L
		F: 0-18 ng/mL	0-18 µg/L
		>60 yr, M: 1-9 ng/mL	1-9 µg/L
		F: 1-16 ng/mL	1-16 µg/L
Haptoglobin (see Table Appendix-3)			
HDL cholesterol (HDLC) (5th percentile from Lipid Research Clinics)	Serum or plasma (EDTA)	M: >29 mg/dL	>0.75 mmol/L
		F: >35 mg/dL	>0.91 mmol/L
Hemoglobin A$_{1c}$ (electrophoresis)	Whole blood (heparin, EDTA, or oxalate)	4.0-6.0% of total Hb	Fraction of Hb: 0.040-0.060
Homovanillic acid (HVA)	Urine, 24-hr	1.4-8.8 mg/day	8-48 µmol/day
17-Hydroxycorticosteroids (17-OHCS)	Urine, 24-hr	M: 3.0-10.0 mg/day	8.3-27.6 µmol/day
		F: 2.0-8.0 mg/day	5.5-22.1 µmol/day
5-Hydroxyindole acetic acid (5-HIAA)			
Qualitative	Urine, fresh random		Negative
Quantitative	Urine, 24-hr	2-6 mg/day	10.4-31.2 µmol/day
17-Hydroxyprogesterone (17-OHP)	Serum	M: 0.5-2.5 ng/mL	1.5-7.5 nmol/L
		F: Follicular: 0.2-1.0 ng/mL	0.6-3.0 nmol/L
		Luteal: 1.-5.0 ng/mL	3.0-15.5 nmol/L
		Postmenopausal: ≤0.7 ng/mL	≤2.1 nmol/L
Immunoglobulin A (IgA)	Serum	40-350 mg/dL	400-3500 mg/L
Immunoglobulin D (IgD)	Serum	0-8 mg/dL	0-80 mg/L
Immunoglobulin E (IgE)	Serum	0-380 IU/mL	0-380 kIU/L
Immunoglobulin G (IgG)	Serum	650-1600 mg/dL	6.5-16 g/L
	CSF	0.5-5 mg/dL	5-50 mg/L
Immunoglobulin M (IgM)	Serum	55-300 mg/dL	550-3000 mg/L
Insulin (12-hr fasting), immunoreactive	Serum	0.7-9.0 µIU/mL	5-63 pmol/L
Intrinsic factor (see Vitamin B$_{12}$)			
Iron	Serum	M: 65-175 µg/dL	11.6-31.3 µmol/L
		F: 50-170 µg/dL	9.0-30.4 µmol/L
Iron-binding capacity, total (TIBC)	Serum	250-450 µg/dL	44.8-80.6 µmol/L
Iron saturation	Serum		Fraction of iron saturation:
		M: 20-50	0.20-0.5
		F: 15-50	0.15-0.5
17-Ketogenic steroids (17-KGS)	Urine, 24-hr	M: 5-23 mg/day	17-80 µmol/day
		F: 3-15 mg/day	10-52 µmol/day
Ketone bodies	Serum	Negative (0.5-3.0 mg/dL)	Negative (5-30 mg/L)
Qualitative	Urine, random		Negative
17-Ketosteroids, total (17-KS)	Urine, 24-hr	M: 10-25 mg/day	37-87 µmol/day
		F: 6-15 mg/day	21-52 µmol/day
L-Lactate	Whole blood (heparin)	Venous: 8.1-15.3 mg/dL	0.9-1.7 mmol/L
		Arterial: <11.3 mg/dL	<1.3 mmol/L
Lactate dehydrogenase (LDH)	Serum		208-378 U/L
Lead	Whole blood (heparin)	<25 µg/dL	<1.21 µmol/L
		Toxic: ≥100 µg/dL	≥4.83 µmol/L
	Urine	<80 µg/dL	<0.39 µmol/L
Light chains, free	Serum		
Kappa		0.33-1.94 mg/dL	3.3-19.4 mg/L
Lambda		0.571-2.63 mg/dL	5.71-26.3 mg/L
K/L ratio			0.26-1.65
Lipase	Serum	31-186 U/L	0.5-3.2 µKat/L
Low-density-lipoprotein cholesterol (LDLC)	Serum or plasma (EDTA)	Recommended: <130 mg/dL	<3.37 mmol/L
		Moderate risk: 130-159 mg/dL	3.37-4.12 mmol/L
		High risk: ≥160 mg/dL	≥4.14 mmol/L
Lutropin (LH)	Serum or plasma (heparin)	M: 1-8 mU/mL	1-8 U/L
		F: Follicular phase: 1-2 mU/mL	1-12 U/L
		Midcycle: 16-104 mU/mL	16-104 U/L
		Luteal: 1-12 mU/mL	1-12 U/L
		Postmenopausal: 16-66 mU/mL	16-66 U/L
	Urine		M: 9-23 U/day
			F: non-midcycle, 4-30 U/day

TABLE APPENDIX-2 CLINICAL CHEMISTRY, TOXICOLOGY, SEROLOGY—cont'd

TEST	SPECIMEN	REFERENCE INTERVAL (CONVENTIONAL UNITS)	REFERENCE INTERVAL (INTERNATIONAL UNITS)
Lysozyme	Serum, plasma	0.4-1.3 mg/dL	4-13 mg/L
Magnesium	Serum	1.3-2.1 mEq/L	0.65-1.05 mmol/L
	Urine, 24-hr	6.0-10.0 mEq/day	3.00-5.00 mmol/day
Mercury	Whole blood (EDTA)	<5.0 µg/dL	<0.25 µmol/L
	Urine, 24-hr	<20 µg/L	<0.1 µmol/L
		Toxic: >150 µg/L	<0.75 µmol/L
Metanephrine, total	Urine, 24-hr	0.05-1.20 µg/mg creatinine	0.03-0.69 mmol/mol creatinine
Myelin basic protein	CSF		<2.5 µg/L
Myoglobin	Serum		M: 19-92 µg/L
			F: 12-76 µg/L
	Urine, random		Negative
Osmolality	Serum		275-295 mOsmol/kg
	Urine, random		50-1200 mOsmol/kg, depending on fluid intake
			After 12-hr fluid restriction:
			>850 mOsmol/kg
	Urine, 24-hr		~390-900 mOsmol/kg
Oxalate	Serum	1-2.4 µg/mL	11-27 µmol/L
		Ethylene glycol poisoning: >20 µg/mL	Ethylene glycol poisoning: >228 µmol/L
Oxygen (Po₂)	Whole blood, arterial (heparin)	83-108 mm Hg	11-14.4 kPa
Oxygen saturation	Whole blood, arterial (heparin)	95-98%	Fraction saturated: 0.95-0.98
Parathyroid hormone	Serum	Varies with laboratory	
		N-terminal 8-24 pg/mL	8-24 ng/L
		C-terminal 50-330 pg/mL	50-330 ng/L
		Intact 10-65 pg/mL	10-65 ng/L
pH (37° C)	Whole blood, arterial (heparin)		7.35-7.45
Phosphorus, inorganic	Serum	2.7-4.5 mg/dL	0.87-1.45 nmol/L
		>60 yr, M: 2.3-3.7 mg/dL	0.74-1.2 nmol/L
		F: 2.8-4.1 mg/dL	0.90-1.3 nmol/L
	Urine, 24-hr	0.4-1.3 g/day	13-42 mmol/d
Porphobilinogen (PBG)			
Quantitative	Urine, 24-hr	0-2.0 mg/day	0-8.8 µmol/d
Qualitative	Urine, fresh random		Negative
Potassium	Serum	3.5-5.1 mEq/L	3.5-5.1 mmol/L
	Plasma (heparin)	3.5-4.5 mEq/L	3.5-4.5 mmol/L
	Urine, 24-hr	25-125 mEq/day	25-125 mmol/day
Pregnanediol	Urine, 24-hr	M: 0-1.9 mg/day	0-5.9 µmol/day
		F: Follicular: <2.6 mg/day	<8 µmol/day
		Luteal: 2.6-10.6 mg/day	8-33 µmol/day
		Postmenopausal: 0.2-1.0 mg/day	0.6-3.1 µmol/day
Progesterone	Serum	M: 0.13-0.97 ng/mL	0.4-3.1 nmol/L
		F: Follicular: 0.15-0.70 ng/mL	0.5-2.2 nmol/L
		Luteal: 2.0-25 ng/mL	6.4-79.5 nmol/L
Prolactin (hPRL)	Serum	M: 3.0-14.7 ng/mL	3.0-14.7 µg/L
		F: 3.8-23.2 ng/mL	3.8-23.2 µg/L
Prostate-specific antigen (PSA)	Serum, freeze	M: <4 ng/mL	<4 µg/L
Protein			
Total	Serum	6.4-8.3 g/dL	64.0-83.0 g/L
Electrophoresis (cellulose acetate)	Serum	Albumin: 3.5-5.0 g/dL	35-50 g/L
		α₁-Globulin: 0.1-0.3 g/dL	1-3 g/L
		α₂-Globulin: 0.6-1.0 g/dL	6-10 g/L
		β-Globulin: 0.7-1.1 g/dL	7-11 g/L
		γ-Globulin: 0.8-1.6 g/dL	8-16 g/L
Total	Urine, 24-hr	♪	50-80 mg/day at rest
Total	CSF	Lumbar: 15-45 mg/dL	150-450 mg/L
Pyruvic acid	Whole blood (heparin)	0.3-0.9 mg/dL	0.03-0.10 mmol/L
Renin (normal diet)	Plasma (EDTA)	Supine: 0.2-1.6 ng/mL/hr	0.2-1.6 µg/L/hr
		Standing: 0.7-3.3 ng/mL/hr	0.7-3.3 µg/L/hr
Riboflavin (see Vitamin B₂)			
Sediment	Urine, fresh, random		Hyaline: occasional (0-1) casts/hpf
Casts			RBC: not seen
			WBC: not seen
			Tubular epithelial: not seen
			Transitional and squamous epithelial: not seen

Note: The "Protein inorganic" phosphorus international units appear as nmol/L in source (likely mmol/L).

TABLE APPENDIX-2 CLINICAL CHEMISTRY, TOXICOLOGY, SEROLOGY—cont'd

TEST	SPECIMEN	REFERENCE INTERVAL (CONVENTIONAL UNITS)	REFERENCE INTERVAL (INTERNATIONAL UNITS)
Sediment Cells			RBC: 0-2/hpf WBC: M: 0-3/hpf F: 0-5/hpf Epithelial: few Bacteria: Unspun: no organisms/oil immersion field Spun: <20 organisms/hpf
Sodium	Serum or plasma (heparin) Urine, 24-hr	136-146 mEq/L 40-220 mEq/day	136-146 mmol/L 40-220 mmol/day
Specific gravity	Urine, random Urine, 24-hr		1.002-1.030 1.015-1.025
Testosterone, free	Serum	M: 50-210 pg/mL F: 1.0-8.5 pg/mL	174-729 pmol/L 3.5-29.5 pmol/L
Testosterone, total	Serum Urine	M: 280-1100 ng/dL F: 15-70 ng/dL 20-50 yr, M: 50-135 µg/day F: 2-12 µg/day >50 yr, M: 40-60 µg/day F: 2-8 µg/day	9.7-38.2 nmol/L 0.5-2.4 nmol/L 173-470 nmol/day 7-42 nmol/day 139-210 nmol/day 7-28 nmol/day
Thiamine (see Vitamin B_1)	Serum	0.10-0.54 µg/dL	2.9-16.1 nmol/L
Thyroglobulin (Tg)	Serum	3-42 ng/mL	3-42 µg/L
Thyroglobulin antibodies	Serum		<1 : 10
Thyroid microsomal antibodies	Serum		Nondetectable (hemagglutination) or <1 : 10 (IFA)
Thyrotropin (hTSH)	Serum or plasma	0.4-4.2 µU/mL	0.4-4.2 mU/L
Thyrotropin-releasing hormone	Plasma	5-60 pg/mL	5-60 ng/L
Thyroxine, free (FT_4)	Serum	0.8-2.4 ng/dL	10-31 pmol/L
Thyroxine (T_4), total	Serum	M: 4.6-10.5 µg/dL F: 5.5-11.0 µg/dL	59-135 nmol/L 71-142 nmol/L
Thyroxine-binding globulin (TBG)	Serum	15.0-34.0 µg/mL	15.0-34.0 mg/L
Thyroxine index, free	Serum		4.2-13.0
Transcortin	Serum	M: 18.8-25.2 mg/L F: 14.9-22.9 mg/L	323-433 nmol/L 256-393 nmol/L
Transferrin	Serum	200-400 mg/dL >60 yr: 180-380 mg/dL	2.0-4.0 g/L 1.80-3.80 g/L
Transthyretin (prealbumin)	Serum	10-40 mg/dL	100-400 mg/L
Triglycerides (TG)	Serum, after ≥12-hr fast	Recommended: <250 mg/dL	2.83 mmol/L
Tri-iodothyronine, free	Serum	260-480 pg/dL	4.0-7.4 pmol/L
Tri-iodothyronine, total (T_3)	Serum	100-200 ng/dL	1.54-3.08 mmol/L
Tri-iodothyronine resin uptake test (T_3RU)	Serum	24-34%	24-34 AU (arbitrary units)
Troponin-I (cTnI)	Serum	Method dependent	<0.8 µg/L
Troponin-T (cTnT)	Serum	Method dependent	<0.01 µg/L
Urea nitrogen	Serum or plasma Urine	6-20 mg/dL 12-20 g/day	2.1-7.1 mmol/L 0.43-0.71 mol/day
Urea nitrogen/creatinine ratio	Serum		12 : 1-20 : 1
Uric acid (uricase)	Serum Urine, 24-hr	M: 3.5-7.2 mg/dL F: 2.6-6.0 mg/dL 250-750 mg/day	0.21-0.42 mmol/L 0.15-0.35 mmol/L 1.48-4.43 mmol/day
Urinary sediment (see Sediment)			
Urobilinogen	Urine, 2-hr Urine, 24-hr Feces	0.1-0.8 EU 0.5-4.0 EU 75-275 EU/100 g 75-400 EU/day 40-280 mg/day	0.1-0.8 U 0.5-4.0 U 750-2750 U/kg 75-400 U/day 67-473 µmol/day
Uroporphyrin	Urine, 24-hr Feces, 24-hr specimen Erythrocytes (heparin or EDTA)	<50 µg/day 10-40 µg/day	<60 nmol/day 12-48 nmol/day Negative
Vanillylmandelic acid (VMA)	Urine, 24-hr	2-7 mg/day	10.1-35.4 µmol/day
Viscosity	Serum		1.10-1.22 centipoise

TABLE APPENDIX-2 CLINICAL CHEMISTRY, TOXICOLOGY, SEROLOGY—cont'd

TEST	SPECIMEN	REFERENCE INTERVAL (CONVENTIONAL UNITS)	REFERENCE INTERVAL (INTERNATIONAL UNITS)
Vitamin A	Serum	30-80 µg/dL	1.05-2.8 µmol/L
Vitamin B$_1$ (Thiamine)	Serum	0-2 µg/dL	0-75 nmol/L
Vitamin B$_2$ (Riboflavin)	Serum	4-24 µg/dL	106-638 nmol/L
Vitamin B$_6$	Plasma (EDTA)	5-30 ng/mL	20-121 nmol/L
Vitamin B$_{12}$	Serum	200-835 pg/mL	148-616 pmol/L
Vitamin C	Plasma (oxalate, heparin, or EDTA)	0.5-1.5 mg/dL	28-85 µmol/L
	Urine, 24-hr	5-50 µg/day	0.67-0.665 µmol/day
Vitamin D$_3$, 1,25-dihydroxy	Serum	16-65 pg/mL	42-169 pmol/L
Vitamin D$_3$, 25-hydroxy	Serum or plasma (heparin)	Summer: 15-80 ng/mL	37.4-200 nmol/L
		Winter: 14-42 ng/mL	34.9-105 nmol/L
Vitamin E	Serum	5.0-18.0 µg/mL	12-42 µmol/L
Zinc	Serum	70-150 µg/dL	10.7-22.9 µmol/L

TABLE APPENDIX-3 HEMATOLOGY AND COAGULATION

TEST	SPECIMEN	REFERENCE INTERVAL (CONVENTIONAL UNITS)	REFERENCE INTERVAL (INTERNATIONAL UNITS)
Activated partial thromboplastin time (APTT)	Plasma (Na citrate)		25-35 sec
Antithrombin III	Plasma (Na citrate)	85-115% of normal human plasma	0.85-1.15
Bleeding time (BT)	Blood from skin		Normal: 2-7 min
Ivy			Borderline: 7-11 min
Simplate (G-D)			2.75-8 min
Blood volume	Whole blood (heparin)		M: 52-83 mL/kg
			F: 50-75 mL/kg
Bone marrow	Bone marrow aspirate	% (mean)	Number fraction (mean)
Differential count			
Myeloblasts		0.3-5.0 (2.0)	0.003-0.05 (0.02)
Promyelocytes		1.0-8.0 (5.0)	0.01-0.08 (0.05)
Myelocytes:			
Neutrophilic		5.0-19.0 (12.0)	0.05-0.19 (0.12)
Eosinophilic		0.5-3.0 (1.5)	0.005-0.03 (0.015)
Basophilic		0.0-0.5 (0.3)	0.00-0.005 (0.003)
Metamyelocytes		13.0-32.0 (22.0)	0.13-0.32 (0.22)
Polymorphonuclear neutrophils		0.7-3.0 (2.0)	0.007-0.03 (0.02)
Polymorphonuclear eosinophils		0.5-4.0 (2.0)	0.005-0.04 (0.02)
Polymorphonuclear basophils		0.0-0.7 (0.2)	0.0-0.007 (0.002)
Lymphocytes		3.0-17.0 (10.0)	0.03-0.17 (0.10)
Plasma cells		0.0-2.0 (0.4)	0.00-0.02 (0.004)
Monocytes		0.5-5.0 (2.0)	0.005-0.05 (0.02)
Reticulum cells		0.1-2.0 (0.2)	0.001-0.02 (0.002)
Megakaryocytes		0.3-3.0 (1.0)	0.003-0.03 (0.01)
Pronormoblasts		1.0-8.0 (4.0)	0.01-0.08 (0.04)
Normoblasts		7.0-32.0 (18.0)	0.07-0.32 (0.18)
Clot lysis, 37° C	Whole clotted blood		47-72 hr
Clot retraction screen	Whole blood (no anticoagulant)		Retraction begins at 1 hr maximum at 24 hr
Clotting time, Lee-White, 37° C	Whole blood (no anticoagulant)		5-8 min
Differential count (see Bone marrow, Differential count or Leukocyte, Differential count)			
Eosinophil count	Whole blood (EDTA); capillary blood	50-400 cells/µL (mm^3)	50-400 × 10^6 cells/L
Erythrocyte count (RBC count)	Whole blood (EDTA)	×10^6 cells/µL	×10^{12} cells/L
		M: 4.3-5.7	4.3-5.7
		F: 3.8-5.1	3.8-5.1
Erythrocyte sedimentation rate (ESR), Wintrobe			M: 0-15 mm/hr
			F: 0-20 mm/hr
Ferritin (see Table Appendix-2)			
Fibrin degradation products (agglutination, Thrombo-Wellco test)	Whole blood: special tube containing thrombin and proteolytic inhibitor	<10 µg/mL	<10 mg/L
	Urine: 2 mL in special tube (see above)	<0.25 µg/mL	<0.25 mg/L
Fibrinogen	Plasma (Na citrate)	200-400 mg/dL	2.00-4.00 g/L
Glucose-6-phosphate dehydrogenase (G6PD) in erythrocytes	Whole blood (ACD, EDTA, or heparin)	12.1 ± 2.09 U/g Hb (1 SD)	0.78 ± 0.13 MU/mol Hb (1 SD)

TABLE APPENDIX-3 HEMATOLOGY AND COAGULATION—cont'd

TEST	SPECIMEN	REFERENCE INTERVAL (CONVENTIONAL UNITS)		REFERENCE INTERVAL (INTERNATIONAL UNITS)	
Haptoglobin (Hp)	Serum; avoid hemolysis	26-85 mg/dL		260-1850 mg/L	
Hematocrit (HCT, Hct) Calculated from MCV and RBC (electronic displacement or laser)	Whole blood (EDTA)	M: 39-49% F: 35-45%		0.39-0.49 volume fraction 0.35-0.45 volume fraction	
Hemoglobin (Hb)	Whole blood (EDTA)	M: 13.5-17.5 g/dL F: 12.0-16.0 g/dL		2.09-2.71 mmol/L 1.86-2.48 mmol/L	
	Plasma (heparin, ACD) Urine, fresh, random	<3 mg/dL		<0.47 μmol/L Negative	
Hemoglobin electrophoresis	Whole blood (EDTA, citrate, or heparin)	HbA > 95% HbA_2 = 1.5-3.5% HbF < 2%		HbA > 0.95 HbA_2 = 0.015-0.035 HbF < 0.02	
International Normalized Ratio (INR) (see Prothrombin time)					
Leukocyte count (WBC count)	Whole blood (EDTA) CSF	$4.5-11.0 \times 10^3$ cells/μL (mm³) 0.5 mononuclear cells/μL		$4.5-11.0 \times 10^9$ cells/L 0.5×10^6 cells/L	
Leukocyte	Whole blood (EDTA)	% Cells/μL (mm³)		Number fraction cells $\times 10^6$/L	
Differential count					
Myelocytes		0	0	0	0
Neutrophils-bands		3-5	150-400	0.03-0.05	150-400
Neutrophils-segmented		54-62	3000-5800	0.54-0.62	3000-5800
Lymphocytes		23-33	1500-3000	0.23-0.33	1500-3000
Monocytes		3-7	285-500	0.03-0.07	285-500
Eosinophils		1-3	50-250	0.01-0.03	50-250
Basophils		0-0.75	15-50	0-0.0075	15-50
Leukocyte	CSF	%		Number fraction	
Differential count					
Lymphocytes		62 ± 34		0.62 ± 0.34	
Monocytes (includes pia-arachnoid mesothelial cells)		36 ± 20		0.36 ± 0.20	
Neutrophils		2 ± 5		0.02 ± 0.05	
Histocytes				Rare	
Ependymal cells				Rare	
Eosinophils				Rare	
Mean corpuscular hemoglobin (MCH)	Whole blood (EDTA)	26-34 pg/cell		0.40-0.53 fmol/cell	
Mean corpuscular hemoglobin centration (MCHC)	Whole blood (EDTA)	31-37% Hb/cell or gHb/dL RBC		4.81-5.74 mmol Hb/L RBC	
Mean corpuscular volume (MCV)	Whole blood (EDTA)			80-100 fL	
Methemoglobin (MetHb)	Whole blood (EDTA, heparin, or ACD)	0.06-0.24 g/dL		9.3-37.2 μmol/L	
Plasma volume	Plasma (heparin)	M: 25-43 mL/kg F: 28-45 mL/kg		0.025-0.043 L/kg 0.028-0.045 L/kg	
Platelet count (thrombocyte count)	Whole blood (EDTA)	$150-450 \times 10^3$/μL (mm³)		$150-450 \times 10^9$/L	
Prothrombin consumption	Whole blood (no anticoagulant)			>30 sec	
Prothrombin time, one-stage International Normalized Ratio (INR) for prothrombin time (PT)	Plasma (Na citrate)	Reference values will vary with the type of thromboplastin Relevant only for patients on warfarin $INR = \left[\dfrac{\text{Patient PT}}{\text{Normal mean PT}} \right]^{ISI\dagger}$ $\dagger$ISI = International Sensitivity Index of thromboplastin Therapeutic INR > 2.0		In general: 11-15 sec	
RBC count (see Erythrocyte count)					
Red cell volume	Whole blood (heparin)	M: 20-36 mL/kg F: 19-31 mL/kg		M: 0.020-0.036 L/kg F: 0.019-0.031 L/kg	
Reticulocyte count	Whole blood (EDTA, heparin, or oxalate)	0.5-1.5% of erythrocytes		0.005-0.015 (number fraction)	
Sulfhemoglobin	Whole blood (EDTA, heparin, or EDTA)	≤1.0% of total Hb		<0.010 of total Hb (mass fraction)	
Thrombin time	Plasma (citrate)			Variable depending on reagent—instrument used, 17-23 sec	
Thromboplastin time, activated (see Activated partial thromboplastin time [APTT])					

TABLE APPENDIX-4 DRUGS: THERAPEUTIC AND TOXIC

DRUG	SPECIMEN	REFERENCE INTERVAL (CONVENTIONAL UNITS)		REFERENCE INTERVAL (INTERNATIONAL UNITS)
Acetaminophen	Serum or plasma (hep or EDTA)	Therapeutic:	10-30 μg/mL	66-199 μmol/L
		Toxic:	>200 μg/mL	>1324 μmol/L
Amikacin	Serum or plasma (EDTA)	Therapeutic:		
		Peak	25-35 μg/mL	43-60 μmol/L
		Trough (severe infection)	4-8 μg/mL	6.8-13.7 μmol/L
		Toxic:		
		Peak	>35 μg/mL	>60 μmol/L
		Trough	>10 μg/mL	>17 μmol/L
ε-Aminocaproic acid	Serum or plasma (hep or EDTA); trough	Therapeutic:	100-400 μg/mL	0.76-3.05 mmol/L
Amitriptyline	Serum or plasma (hep or EDTA); trough (>12 hr after dose)	Therapeutic:	120-250 ng/mL	433-903 nmol/L
		Toxic:	>500 ng/mL	>1805 nmol/L
Amobarbital	Serum	Therapeutic:	1-5 μg/mL	4-22 μmol/L
		Toxic:	>10 μg/mL	>44 μmol/L
Amphetamine	Serum or plasma (hep or EDTA)	Therapeutic:	20-30 ng/mL	148-222 nmol/L
		Toxic:	>200 ng/mL	>1480 nmol/L
Bromide	Serum	Toxic:	>1250 μg/mL	>15.6 mmol/L
Caffeine	Serum or plasma (hep or EDTA)	Therapeutic:	3-15 μg/mL	15-77 μmol/L
		Toxic:	>50 μg/mL	>258 μmol/L
Carbamazepine	Serum or plasma (hep or EDTA); trough	Therapeutic:	4-12 μg/mL	17-51 μmol/L
		Toxic:	>15 μg/mL	>63 μmol/L
Carbenicillin	Serum or plasma	Therapeutic:	Dependent on minimum inhibitory concentration of specific organism	Same
		Toxic:	>250 μg/mL	>660 μmol/L
Chloramphenicol	Serum or plasma (hep or EDTA); trough	Therapeutic:	10-25 μg/L	31-77 μmol/L
		Toxic:	>25 μg/L	>77 μmol/L
Chlordiazepoxide	Serum or plasma (hep or EDTA); trough	Therapeutic:	400-3000 ng/mL	1.3-10 μmol/L
		Toxic:	>3500 ng/mL	>11.7 μmol/L
Chlorpromazine	Serum or plasma (hep or EDTA); trough	Therapeutic:	50-300 ng/mL	157-942 nmol/L
		Toxic:	>1000 ng/mL	>3140 nmol/L
Cimetidine	Serum or plasma (hep or EDTA); trough	Therapeutic:	0.78-3.9 μg/mL	3.1-15.5 μmol/L
Clonazepam	Serum or plasma (hep or EDTA); trough	Therapeutic:	20-80 ng/mL	63-254 nmol/L
		Toxic:	>80 ng/mL	>254 nmol/L
Clonidine	Serum or plasma (hep or EDTA)	Therapeutic:	1.0-2.0 ng/mL	4.4-8.7 nmol/L
Clorazepate	Serum or plasma (hep or EDTA)	As desmethyldiazepam:		
		Therapeutic:	0.12-1.0 μg/mL	0.36-3.01 μmol/L
Cocaine	Serum or plasma (hep or EDTA) on ice	Therapeutic:	100-500 ng/mL	330-1650 nmol/L
		Toxic:	>1000 ng/mL	>3300 nmol/L
Codeine	Serum	Therapeutic:	10-100 ng/mL	33-334 nmol/L
		Toxic:	>200 ng/mL	>668 nmol/L
Cyclosporine	Serum (12 hr after dose)	Therapeutic:	100-400 ng/mL	83-333 nmol/L
		Toxic:	>400 ng/mL	>333 nmol/L
Desipramine	Serum or plasma (hep or EDTA); trough (≥12 hr after dose)	Therapeutic:	75-300 ng/mL	281-1125 nmol/L
		Toxic:	>400 ng/mL	>1500 nmol/L
Diazepam	Serum or plasma (hep or EDTA); trough	Therapeutic:	200-1500 ng/mL	0.70-5.27 μmol/L
		Toxic:	>3000 ng/mL	>10.53 μmol/L
Digitoxin	Serum or plasma (hep or EDTA) ≥6 hr after dose	Therapeutic:	10-30 ng/mL	13-39 nmol/L
		Toxic:	>45 ng/mL	>59 nmol/L
Digoxin	Serum or plasma (hep or EDTA) trough (≥12 hr after dose)	Therapeutic:	0.8-1.5 mg/mL	1.0-1.9 nmol/L
		CHF Arrhythmias:	1.5-2.0. ng/mL	1.9-2.6 nmol/L
		Toxic:	>2.5 ng/mL	>3.2 nmol/L
Diphenylhydantoin (see Phenytoin)				
Disopyramide	Serum or plasma (hep or EDTA); trough	Therapeutic: Arrhythmias:		
		Atrial	2.8-3.2 μg/mL	8.3-9.4 μmol/L
		Ventricular	3.3-7.5 μg/mL	9.7-22 μmol/L
		Toxic:	>7 μg/mL	>20.7 μmol/L
Doxepin	Serum or plasma (hep or EDTA); trough (≥12 hr after dose)	Therapeutic:	30-150 ng/mL	107-537 nmol/L
		Toxic:	>500 ng/mL	>1790 nmol/L

TABLE APPENDIX-4 DRUGS: THERAPEUTIC AND TOXIC—cont'd

DRUG	SPECIMEN	REFERENCE INTERVAL (CONVENTIONAL UNITS)		REFERENCE INTERVAL (INTERNATIONAL UNITS)
Ephedrine	Serum	Therapeutic:	0.05-0.10 µg/mL	0.30-0.61 µmol/L
		Toxic:	>2 µg/mL	>12.1 µmol/L
Ethchlorvynol	Serum or plasma (hep or EDTA)	Therapeutic:	2-8 µg/mL	14-55 µmol/L
		Toxic:	>20 µg/mL	>138 µmol/L
Ethosuximide	Serum or plasma (hep or EDTA); trough	Therapeutic:	40-100 µg/mL	283-708 µmol/L
		Toxic:	>150 µg/mL	>1062 µmol/L
Fenoprofen	Plasma (EDTA)	Therapeutic:	20-65 µg/mL	82-268 µmol/L
Fentanyl	Serum, plasma	Therapeutic:	1-3 ng/mL	3-9.2 nmol/L
		Toxic:	>3 ng/mL	>9.2 nmol/L
Flecainide	Serum or plasma (hep or EDTA); trough	Therapeutic:	0.2-1.0 µg/mL	0.5-2.4 µmol/L
		Toxic:	>1.0 µg/mL	>2.4 µmol/L
Flurazepam	Serum or plasma (EDTA)	Therapeutic:	0.02-0.1 µg/mL	0.05-0.26 µmol/L
		Toxic:	>0.2 µg/mL	
Furosemide	Serum (30 min after dose)	Therapeutic:	1-2 µg/mL	3-6 µmol/L
Gentamicin	Serum or plasma (EDTA)	Therapeutic:		
		Peak (severe infection)	8-10 µg/mL	16.7-20.9 µmol/L
		Trough (severe infection)	<2-4 µg/mL	<4.2-8.4 µmol/L
		Toxic:		
		Peak	>10 µg/mL	>21 µmol/L
		Trough	>4 µg/mL	>8.4 µmol/L
Glutethimide	Serum	Therapeutic:	0.2-5 µg/mL	0.92-23 µmol/L
		Toxic:	>10 µg/mL	>46 µmol/L
Haloperidol	Serum or plasma (hep or EDTA)	Therapeutic:	5-15 ng/mL	13.3-39.9 nmol/L
		Toxic:	>50 ng/mL	>133 nmol/L
Ibuprofen	Serum or plasma (hep or EDTA)	Therapeutic:	10-50 µg/mL	49-243 µmol/L
		Toxic:	100-700 µg/mL	485-3395 µmol/L
Imipramine	Serum or plasma (hep or EDTA); trough (≥12 hr after dose)	Therapeutic:	125-250 ng/mL	446-893 nmol/L
		Toxic:	>500 ng/mL	>1784 nmol/L
Isoniazid	Serum or plasma (hep or EDTA)	Therapeutic:	1-7 µg/mL	7-51 µmol/L
		Toxic:	>20 µg/mL	>146 µmol/L
Kanamycin	Serum or plasma (EDTA)	Therapeutic:		
		Peak	25-35 µg/mL	52-72 µmol/L
		Trough (severe infection)	4-8 µg/mL	8-16 µmol/L
		Toxic:		
		Peak	>35 µg/mL	>72 µmol/L
		Trough	>10 µg/mL	>21 µmol/L
Lidocaine	Serum or plasma (hep or EDTA); ≥45 min following bolus dose	Therapeutic:	1.5-6.0 µg/mL	6.4-26 µmol/L
		Toxic:		
		CNS or cardiovascular depression	6-8 µg/mL	26-34.2 µmol/L
		Seizures, obtundation, decreased cardiac output	>8 µg/mL	>34.2 µmol/L
Lithium	Serum or plasma (hep or EDTA); (>12 hr after last dose)	Therapeutic:	0.6-1.2 mEq/L	0.6-1.2 nmol/L
		Toxic:	>1.5 mEq/L	>1.5 mmol/L
Lorazepam	Serum or plasma (hep or EDTA)	Therapeutic:	50-240 ng/mL	156-746 nmol/L
Meperidine	Serum or plasma (hep or EDTA)	Therapeutic:	70-500 ng/mL	283-2020 nmol/L
		Toxic:	>1 µg/mL	>4043 nmol/L
Meprobamate	Serum	Therapeutic:	5-10 µg/mL	23-46 µmol/L
		Toxic:	>10 µg/mL	>46 µmol/L
Methadone	Serum or plasma (hep or EDTA)	Therapeutic:	100-400 ng/mL	0.32-1.29 µmol/L
		Toxic:	>2000 ng/mL	>6.46 µmol/L
Methamphetamine	Serum	Therapeutic:	0.01-0.05 µg/mL	0.07-0.34 µmol/L
		Toxic:	>0.5 µg/mL	>3.35 µmol/L
Methaqualone	Serum or plasma (hep or EDTA)	Therapeutic:	1-3 µg/mL	4-12 µmol/L
		Toxic:	>3-5 µg/mL	>12-20 µmol/L
Methotrexate	Serum or plasma (hep or EDTA)	Therapeutic:	variable	variable
		Toxic:		
		Low-dose therapy (1-2 wk)	>9.1 ng/mL	>20 nmol/L
		High-dose therapy (48 hr)	>227 ng/mL	>0.5 µmol/L
Methsuximide (N-desmethyl methsuximide)	Serum	Therapeutic:	10-40 µg/mL	53-212 µmol/L
		Toxic:	>40 µg/mL	>212 µmol/L

TABLE APPENDIX-4 DRUGS: THERAPEUTIC AND TOXIC—cont'd

DRUG	SPECIMEN	REFERENCE INTERVAL (CONVENTIONAL UNITS)		REFERENCE INTERVAL (INTERNATIONAL UNITS)
Methyldopa	Plasma (EDTA)	Therapeutic: Toxic:	1-5 µg/mL >7 µg/mL	4.7-23.7 µmol/L >33 µmol/L
Methyprylon	Serum	Therapeutic: Toxic:	8-10 µg/mL >50 µg/mL	43-55 µmol/L >273 µmol/L
Morphine	Serum or plasma (hep or EDTA)	Therapeutic: Toxic:	10-80 ng/mL >200 ng/mL	35-280 nmol/L >700 nmol/L
N-Acetylprocainamide	Serum or plasma (hep or EDTA); trough	Therapeutic: Toxic:	5-30 µg/mL >40 µg/mL	18-108 µmol/L >144 µmol/L
Netilmicin	Serum or plasma (EDTA)	Therapeutic: Peak (severe infection) Trough (severe infection) Toxic: Peak Trough	 8-10 µg/mL <4 µg/mL >12 µg/mL >4 µg/mL	 17-21 µmol/L <8 µmol/L >25 µmol/L >8 µmol/L
Nortriptyline	Serum or plasma (hep or EDTA); trough (≥12 hr after dose)	Therapeutic: Toxic:	50-150 ng/mL >500 ng/mL	190-570 nmol/L >1900 nmol/L
Oxazepam	Serum or plasma (hep or EDTA)	Therapeutic:	0.2-1.4 µg/mL	0.70-4.9 µmol/L
Oxycodone	Serum	Therapeutic: Toxic:	10-100 ng/mL >200 ng/mL	32-317 nmol/L >634 nmol/L
Pentazocine	Serum or plasma (EDTA) Urine	Therapeutic: Toxic: Toxic:	0.05-0.2 µg/mL >1 µg/mL >3 µg/mL	0.2-0.7 µmol/L >3.5 µmol/L >10.5 µmol/L
Pentobarbital	Serum or plasma (hep or EDTA); trough	Therapeutic, hypnotic: Therapeutic coma: Toxic:	1-5 µg/mL 20-50 µg/mL >10 µg/mL	4-22 µmol/L 88-221 µmol/L >44 µmol/L
Phenacetin	Plasma (EDTA)	Therapeutic: Toxic:	5-20 µg/mL >50 µg/mL	28-112 µmol/L >279 µmol/L
Phenobarbital	Serum or plasma (hep or EDTA); trough	Therapeutic: Toxic: Slowness, ataxia, nystagmus Coma with reflexes Coma without reflexes	15-40 µg/mL 35-80 µg/mL 65-117 µg/mL >100 µg/mL	65-170 µmol/L 151-345 µmol/L 280-504 µmol/L >430 µmol/L
Phensuximide (both parent and N-desmethyl metabolites)	Serum or plasma (hep or EDTA)	Therapeutic:	40-60 µg/mL	228-324 µmol/L
Phenylbutazone	Plasma (EDTA)	Therapeutic: not well defined Toxic:	50-100 µg/mL >100 µg/mL	162-324 µmol/L >324 µmol/mL
Phenytoin	Serum or plasma (hep or EDTA); trough	Therapeutic: Toxic:	10-20 µg/mL >20 µg/mL	40-79 µmol/L >79 µmol/L
Primidone	Serum or plasma (hep or EDTA) trough	Therapeutic: Toxic:	5-12 µg/mL >15 µg/mL	23-55 µmol/L >69 µmol/L
Procainamide	Serum or plasma (hep or EDTA); trough	Therapeutic: Toxic: Also consider effect of metabolite, N-acetylprocainamide	4-10 µg/mL >10-12 µg/mL	17-42 µmol/L >42-51 µmol/L
Propoxyphene	Plasma (EDTA)	Therapeutic: Toxic:	0.1-0.4 µg/mL >0.5 µg/mL	0.3-1.2 µmol/L >1.5 µmol/L
Propranolol	Serum or plasma (hep or EDTA); trough	Therapeutic:	50-100 ng/mL	193-386 nmol/L
Protriptyline	Serum or plasma (hep or EDTA); trough (≥12 hr after dose)	Therapeutic: Toxic:	70-250 ng/mL >500 ng/mL	266-950 nmol/L >1900 nmol/L
Quinidine	Serum or plasma (hep or EDTA); trough	Therapeutic: Toxic:	2-5 µg/mL >6 µg/mL	6-15 µmol/L >18 µmol/L
Ranitidine	Serum, plasma (hep or EDTA)	Therapeutic:	34-94 ng/mL	114-299 nmol/L
Salicylates	Serum or plasma (hep or EDTA); trough	Therapeutic: Toxic:	150-300 µg/mL >300 µg/mL	1086-2172 µmol/L >2172 µmol/L
Secobarbital	Serum	Therapeutic: Toxic:	1.5-5.0 µg/mL >7 µg/mL	6.3-21.0 µmol/L >29.4 µmol/L
Theophylline	Serum or plasma (hep or EDTA)	Therapeutic: Toxic:	8-20 µg/mL >20 µg/mL	44-111 µmol/L >110 µmol/L

TABLE APPENDIX-4 DRUGS: THERAPEUTIC AND TOXIC—cont'd

DRUG	SPECIMEN	REFERENCE INTERVAL (CONVENTIONAL UNITS)		REFERENCE INTERVAL (INTERNATIONAL UNITS)
Thiocyanate	Serum or plasma (EDTA)	Nonsmoker:	1-4 µg/mL	17-69 µmol/L
		Smoker:	3-12 µg/mL	52-206 µmol/L
		Therapeutic, after nitroprusside infusion:	6-29 µg/mL	103-499 µmol/L
	Urine	Nonsmoker:	1-4 mg/day	17-69 µmol/L
		Smoker:	7-17 mg/day	120-292 µmol/L
Thiopental	Serum or plasma (hep or EDTA); trough	Hypnotic:	1-5 µg/mL	4.1-20.7 µmol/L
		Coma:	30-100 µg/mL	124-413 µmol/L
		Anesthesia:	7-130 µg/mL	29-536 µmol/L
		Toxic conc:	>10 µg/mL	>41 µmol/L
Thioridazine	Serum or plasma (hep or EDTA)	Therapeutic:	0.1-2 µg/mL	0.27-5.4 µmol/L
		Toxic:	>2.5 µg/mL	>6.75 µmol/L
Tobramycin	Serum or plasma (hep or EDTA)	Therapeutic:		
		Peak (severe infection)	8-10 µg/mL	17-21 µmol/L
		Trough (severe infection)	<4 µg/mL	<9 µmol/L
		Toxic:		
		Peak	>10 µg/mL	>21 µmol/L
		Trough	>4 µg/mL	>9 µmol/L
Tocainide	Serum or plasma (hep or EDTA)	Therapeutic:	4-10 µg/mL	21-52 µmol/L
Tolbutamide	Serum	Therapeutic:	50-100 µg/mL	185-370 µmol/L
		Toxic:	>400 µg/mL	>1480 µmol/L
Valproic acid	Serum or plasma (hep or EDTA); trough	Therapeutic:	50-100 µg/mL	347-693 µmol/L
		Toxic:	>100 µg/mL	>693 µmol/L
Vancomycin	Serum or plasma (hep or EDTA); trough	Therapeutic:	5-10 µg/mL	3-7 µmol/L
		Toxic: not well established	>80-100 µg/mL	>55-69 µmol/L
Verapamil	Serum or plasma (hep or EDTA)	Therapeutic:	100-500 ng/mL	220-1100 nmol/L
Warfarin	Serum or plasma (hep or EDTA)	Therapeutic:	1-10 µg/mL	3-32 µmol/L

INDEX

Page numbers followed by "f" indicate figures, "t" indicate tables, and "b" indicate boxes. **Boldface** numbers refer to main discussions; **boldface** terms indicate supplemental online material.

A

Abatacept, 167
ABCA1 (ATP binding cassette A1), 1347t, 1348
Abciximab, 176
  in acute coronary syndrome, 430t
Abdomen. *See also* Abdominal pain
  Actinomyces infection of, 1969
  auscultation of, 833-837
  caput medusae of, 954, 954f
  distention of, 838-839
  examination of, 25
    in abdominal pain, 833-837, 834t-837t
    in cardiovascular disease, 252
    in cirrhosis, 1003
    in gastrointestinal disease, 829
    in heart failure, 301
    in liver disease, 954-955, 954f-955f, 956t
    in nutritional assessment, 1386t
    in pelvic inflammatory disease, 1858
    in trauma, 690-691, 690f
  fluid in. *See* Ascites
  pain in. *See* Abdominal pain
  palpation of, 25
    in abdominal pain, 833-837
    in gastrointestinal disease, 829
  percussion of, 833-837
Abdominal guarding, 833-837
Abdominal pain, **832**
  acute, 832, 834t-836t
    clinical manifestations of, 832-844, 834t-836t
    diagnosis of, 828, 831t-832t, 834t-836t, 836f, 837, 838f
    differential diagnosis of, 834t-836t, 836f
    in extra-abdominal conditions, 833
    in hospitalized patient, 837
    imaging in, 837
    patient history in, 832-833
    physical examination in, 833-837, 837t
    in special populations, 837
  in appendicitis, 921
  chronic, 837
    clinical manifestations of, 834t-836t
    diagnosis of, 831t-832t, 834t-836t, 837, 839f
    in chronic pancreatitis, 941, 943t
    duration of, 832
    in female, 833
    in liver disease, 952, 956t
    location of, 836f
    pathobiology of, 832
    postprandial, 1723
Abetalipoproteinemia, 905, 1344t, 1348
Abnormal uterine bleeding, **1537**
ABO blood group
  in blood transfusion, 1155
  in transplantation, 236
  Vibrio cholerae infection and, 1866
Abortion, infection with, 1842-1844, 1849
Abscess
  abdominal, 834t-836t
    in Crohn's disease, 919
  brain. *See* Brain abscess
  cutaneous, 1816, **2544**, 2544f
  epidural, **2373**, 2373t, 2374f
  glomerulonephritis with, 767
  hepatic, 988t
    amebic, 988t, 990-996, 2045, 2046f
    pyogenic, 988, 988t

Abscess (*Continued*)
  neck, 2470
  perianal, **945**
  peritonsillar, 2470, 2470t, 2471f
  retropharyngeal, 514t
  tubo-ovarian, 1969
Absence seizures, 2286t, 2288, 2290-2291, 2292t
Absolute risk reduction, 31
Abstinence, in infection prevention, 1799, 2182
Abulia, 2274
Abuse
  alcohol. *See* Alcohol use/abuse
  drug. *See* Drug abuse
  physical, 1413, 2229
Acamprosate, in alcohol dependence treatment, 152-153, 152t
Acanthamoeba spp. infection, 2047, 2047t
  corneal, 2435
Acanthosis nigricans, **1195**, 1196t, 1197f, 1276, 1420
Acarbose, 1496t
Accelerated aerobic glycolysis, 646
Accelerated idioventricular rhythm, 444
Accessory pathway tachycardia, 353-355, 354f
Accidents. *See* Burn injury; Trauma; Traumatic brain injury
Acebutolol
  in hypertension, 382t
  in stable myocardial ischemia, 423t
Acetaminophen, 135
  metabolism of
    occult ingestion of, 673
    sodium in, 384-385
    toxicity of, 132, 674t-677t, 679t-683t, 981-982, 981t
Acetazolamide
  in high-altitude syndromes, 575-576, 576b
  potassium effects of, 739
Acetylcholine
  in asthma, 531
  in neuromuscular transmission, 2417-2418, 2418f
Acetylcholine challenge, in Prinzmetal's angina, 424
Acetylcholine receptor, 2417-2418, 2418f
  antibodies against, 2418-2420, 2419f
  deficiency of, 2419t, **2423**
  in neuromuscular transmission, 2417-2418, 2418f
Acetylcholinesterase deficiency, 2419t, **2423**
N-Acetylcysteine
  in acetaminophen toxicity, 679t-683t
  in contrast-related injury prevention, 760
Acetylhydrolase, in anaphylaxis, 1636
Acetylsalicylic acid. *See* Aspirin
Achalasia, **881**, 881f, 1273
Achilles tendon
  inflammation of, 1681
  rupture of, 1681
Achondroplasia, **1610**
Acid(s)
  gastric, 891
  nonvolatile, 742
  urinary, 743
  volatile, 741

Acid-base balance, 741-744
  disorders of, **741-753**. *See also* Acidosis; Alkalosis
    clinical manifestations of, 743
    compensatory changes in, 744-745, 745t
    definition of, 741
    diagnosis of, 743, 744f, 744t
    epidemiology of, 741
    hypovolemia and, 724
    pathobiology of, 741-743
    kidneys in, 742-743, 742f
    lungs in, 741-742
Acid peptic disease. *See* Dyspepsia, functional (nonulcer); Gastroesophageal reflux disease (GERD); Peptic ulcer disease
Acidosis
  metabolic, 744f, **745**
    alcohol intoxication and, 746t, 747-752
    anion gap, 744f, 745, 746t
      in acute poisoning, 673
      potassium level in, 737
    clinical manifestations of, 745
    compensatory changes in, 744-745, 745t
    diabetic, 746t
    diagnosis of, 744t
    epidemiology of, 745
    ethanol intoxication and, 747-752
    ethylene glycol and, 746t, 747-748
    hyperchloremic, 744t, 748
      of nonrenal origin, 748
      of renal origin, 748-752, 749t, 750f
    isopropyl alcohol and, 748
    lactic, **746-752**, 746t, 1343t
    methanol and, 746t, 748
    pathobiology of, 745
    potassium level in, 737
    propylene glycol and, 748
    salicylate intoxication and, 746t, 747
    treatment of, 749b
    uremic, 745
  renal tubular. *See* Renal tubular acidosis (RTA)
  respiratory, 742, 744f, 744t, **752**
    compensatory changes in, 744-745, 745t
  in shock, 646, 648
Aciduria, 1343t
  orotic, 1345-1346
Acinetobacter baumannii infection, 1782t, 1882, 1882f
Acinetobacter spp. infection, **1881-1884**
  bloodstream, 1882
  bone, 1882
  burn injury, 1882
  clinical manifestations of, 1882
  CNS, 1882, 2364
  cutaneous, 1882, 1882f
  definition of
  respiratory tract, 1882
  soft tissue, 1882
  treatment of, 1883b
  urinary tract, 1882
  wound, 1882
Acitretin, 2511
Acne, 1420
  pyogenic arthritis with, **1671-1672**
  in women of reproductive potential, 1550t
Acne keloidalis, 2549, 2549f
Acne vulgaris, **2530-2532**, 2550f
Acoustic neuroma, 1250, 2463

Acquired immunodeficiency syndrome (AIDS). *See* Human immunodeficiency virus (HIV) infection
Acrivastine, 2512t
Acrocyanosis, 497
Acrodermatitis chronica atrophicans, 1933
Acrodermatitis enteropathica, 1403t-1404t
Acrodermatitis verruciformis, 2537
Acromegaly, **1436-1437**
  clinical manifestations of, 1436-1437, 1436f
  diagnosis of, 1437, 1437t
  GRFoma and, 1296
  osteoarthritis in, 1749
  pathobiology of, 1436
  treatment of, 1438b
ACTH. *See* Adrenocorticotropic hormone (ACTH)
ACTH stimulation test, 1434t, 1440, 1468-1469
ACTHoma, 1293t
Actigraphy, 2300-2301
Actin, 320t, 1113, 1114f
Actinic keratoses, **2537**
Actinomycosis, **1847-1851**, 1847t, **1967-1969**
  abdominal, 1969
  cervicofacial, 1968, 1968f
  clinical manifestations of, 1849t, 1968
  CNS, 1969
  definition of, 1967-1969
  diagnosis of, 1850t, 1969
  epidemiology of, 1967
  vs. mycetoma, 2006-2007
  pathobiology of, 1967-1968
  pelvic, 1969
  prognosis for, 1969
  thoracic, 1968-1969, 1968f
  treatment of, 1849b-1850b, 1850t, 1969b
Action potential, cardiac, 260, 261f, 334-335, 334f-335f
Activated charcoal, in acute poisoning, 679t-684t
Activated protein C
  recombinant
    in DIC, 1146b-1147b
    in septic shock, 664-665
    resistance to, 1149
    in viral hemorrhagic fevers, 2154
Activated protein C resistance, 1149
Activin, 1426, 1442
Activities of daily living (ADLs), in geriatric assessment, 101, 115
Acupuncture, 179
Acute chest syndrome, in sickle cell disease, 1070-1071, 1073, 1073t
Acute coronary syndrome, 29, **425-434**. *See also* Angina pectoris; Myocardial infarction (MI)
  biomarkers in, 427
  definition of, 425
  diagnosis of, 426-427, 427t
  differential diagnosis of, 428-429
  electrocardiography in, 427
  epidemiology of, 425
  noninvasive testing in, 427
  primary, 425
  risk assessment in, 428, 428t, 429f
  secondary, 425
  substance abuse and, 427
  treatment of, 429b-432b
Acute disseminated encephalomyelitis, **2354**

	CHAPTER	SPECIFIC TABLES OR FIGURES
SYMPTOMS		
Constitutional		
Fever	288	Tables 288-1 to 288-8
Fatigue	282	Table 282-3
Poor appetite	134	Table 134-1
Weight loss	134, 226	Figure 134-4; Tables 134-4, 226-1, 226-2
Obesity	227	Figure 227-1
Snoring, sleep disturbances	100, 412	Tables 412-2, 412-4
Head, Eyes, Ears, Nose, Throat		
Headache	405	Tables 405-1, 405-2
Visual loss, transient	431, 432	Tables 431-1, 432-2
Ear pain	434	Table 434-2
Hearing loss	436	Figure 436-1
Ringing in ears (tinnitus)	436	Figure 436-2
Vertigo	436	Figure 436-3
Nasal congestion, rhinitis or sneezing	259, 434	Figure 259-1, Table 259-2
Loss of smell or taste	435	Table 435-1
Dry mouth	433	Table 433-7
Sore throat	437	Figure 437-2; Table 437-1
Hoarseness	437	
Cardiopulmonary		
Chest pain	50	Tables 50-2, 139-5, 139-6
Bronchitis	90	Table 90-1
Shortness of breath	50	Figures 50-1, 83-3
Palpitations	50, 62	Figure 62-1; Tables 50-4, 62-2, 62-3
Dizziness	50, 62	Figure 62-1
Syncope	62	Figure 62-1; Tables 62-1, 62-2, 62-3
Cardiac arrest	63	Figures 63-2, 63-3
Cough	83	Figure 83-1; Tables 83-1, 83-2
Hemoptysis	83	Tables 83-4, 83-5
Gastrointestinal		
Nausea and vomiting	134	Figure 134-5; Table 134-5
Dysphagia, odynophagia	134, 140	Table 134-1
Hematemesis	137, 156	Figure 137-3; Table 137-1
Heartburn/dyspepsia	134, 139, 140, 141	Figures 134-6, 139-3, 140-2; Table 141-1
Abdominal pain:		
Acute	134, 144	Figure 134-1; Tables 134-2, 134-3, 144-1
Chronic	134, 139	Figure 134-2; Tables 134-2, 139-1
Diarrhea	139, 142	Figures 139-1, 142-2, 142-3, 142-4, 142-8
Melena, blood in stool	137	Figures 137-3, 137-4, 137-6; Table 137-4
Constipation	138, 139	Figures 138-3, 138-5, 139-1; Table 138-2
Fecal incontinence	147	Figure 147-3
Anal pain	147	
Genitourinary		
Dysuria	292, 293	Tables 292-4, 292-8, 293-2
Frequency	292	Tables 292-4
Incontinence	25	Tables 25-1 to 25-3
Urinary obstruction	125	Tables 125-1 to 125-3
Renal colic	128	Figure 128-3
Vaginal discharge	293	
Menstrual irregularities	244	Figure 244-3; Tables 244-3, 244-4
Female infertility	244	Table 244-5
Hot flushes	248	Table 248-1
Erectile dysfunction	242	
Male infertility	242	Figures 242-8, 242-9; Table 242-7
Scrotal mass	206	Figure 206-1

	CHAPTER	SPECIFIC TABLES OR FIGURES
Genital ulcers or warts	293	
Musculoskeletal		
Neck or back pain	407	Figures 407-4, 407-5; Tables 407-3 to 407-6
Painful joints	264	Table 264-2
Extremities		
Swollen feet, ankles, or legs		
Bilateral	50	Figure 50-8
Unilateral	81	Figure 81-2; Table 81-2
Claudication	79	Table 79-2
Acute limb ischemia	79	Figure 79-5; Table 79-3
Neurologic		
Weakness	403, 428, 429, 430	Tables 403-1, 428-2, 429-2, 429-4
Sensory loss	403, 428	Figure 428-1; Tables 428-1, 428-4 to 428-7
Memory loss	409	Figures 409-1, 409-2; Tables 409-1 to 409-6
Abnormal gait	403	Table 403-2
Seizures	410	Tables 410-1 to 410-6
Integumentary		
Abnormal bleeding	174	Table 174-1
Rash	444, 449	Figure 444-1; Tables 444-1 to 444-4, 449-4
Hives	261, 448	Figure 261-1; Tables 261-1, 448-1
Abnormal pigmentation	449	Table 449-2
Hirsutism and alopecia	450	Tables 261-1, 450-1, 450-2
Nail disorders	450	Table 450-3
SIGNS		
Vital Signs		
Fever	288, 289	Figure 289-1; Tables 288-1 to 288-8, 289-2
Hypothermia	7, 109	Table 109-4
Tachycardia/bradycardia	7, 62, 64, 65	Figures 62-2, 62-3; Tables 64-4, 65-2
Hypertension	67	Table 67-4
Hypotension/shock	7, 106	Figures 106-3, 108-3; Tables 106-1, 107-1, 107-2
Altered respiration	7, 86, 104	Tables 86-1, 86-2, 104-2
Head, Eyes, Ears, Nose, Throat		
Eye pain	431	Table 431-3
Red eye	431	Tables 431-4, 431-6
Dilated pupil	432	Figure 432-4
Nystagmus	432	Table 432-5
Papilledema	432	Table 432-2
Strabismus	432	Figure 432-6
Jaundice	149	Figure 149-3; Tables 149-1 to 149-3
Otitis	434	Table 434-2
Sinusitis	259, 434	Tables 259-3, 434-1
Oral ulcer	433	Tables 433-1 to 433-4
Salivary gland enlargement	433	Table 433-6
Neck		
Neck mass	196	Figure 196-3
Lymphadenopathy	171	Tables 171-1 to 171-6
Thyroid nodule	233	Figure 233-4
Thyromegaly/goiter	233	Figures 233-1, 233-3
Breast		
Breast mass	204	
Lungs		
Wheezes	83	Table 83-3
Cardiac		
Heart murmur or extra sounds	50	Figure 50-6; Tables 50-7, 50-8
Jugular venous distention	50	Table 50-6
Carotid pulse abnormalities	50	Figure 50-5